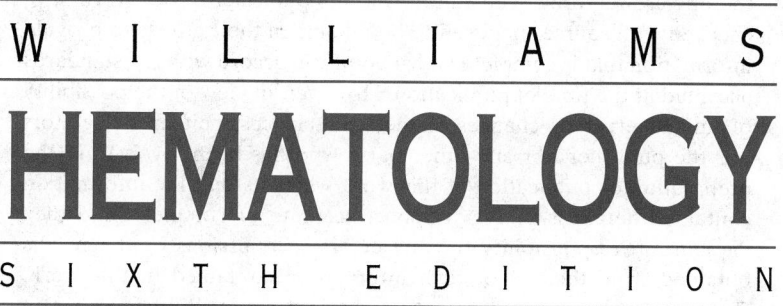

WILLIAMS
HEMATOLOGY
SIXTH EDITION

NOTICE

Medicine is an ever-changing science. As new research and clinical experience broaden our knowledge, changes in treatment and drug therapy are required. The editors and the publisher of this work have checked with sources believed to be reliable in their efforts to provide information that is complete and generally in accord with the standards accepted at the time of publication. However, in view of the possibility of human error or changes in medical sciences, neither the editors nor the publisher nor any other party who has been involved in the preparation or publication of this work warrants that the information contained herein is in every respect accurate or complete, and they disclaim all responsibility for any errors or omissions or the results obtained from the use of such information contained in this work. Readers are encouraged to confirm the information contained herein with other sources. For example and in particular, readers are advised to check the product information sheet included in the package of each drug they plan to administer to be certain that the information contained in this work is accurate and that changes have not been made in the recommended dose or in the contraindications for administration. This recommendation is of particular importance in connection with new or infrequently used drugs.

WILLIAMS

HEMATOLOGY

SIXTH EDITION

EDITORS

ERNEST BEUTLER, M.D., Ph.D. (HON)

Professor and Chairman
Department of Molecular and Experimental Medicine
The Scripps Research Institute
Clinical Professor of Medicine
University of California, San Diego
La Jolla, California

BARRY S. COLLER, M.D.

Murray M. Rosenberg Professor and Chairman
Department of Medicine
Mount Sinai School of Medicine
Director and Chief of Medicine
Mount Sinai Hospital
New York, New York

MARSHALL A. LICHTMAN, M.D.

Professor of Medicine and of Biochemistry and
Biophysics
University of Rochester School of Medicine and
Dentistry
Rochester, New York

THOMAS J. KIPPS, M.D., Ph.D.

Professor and Head
Division of Hematology/Oncology
Deputy Director, UCSD Cancer Center
University of California at San Diego
La Jolla, California

URI SELIGSOHN, M.D.

Chairman
Department of Hematology and
Director of the Institute of Thrombosis and Hemostasis
The Chaim Sheba Medical Center
Tel-Hashomer
Professor of Hematology
Sackler Faculty of Medicine
Tel-Aviv University
Tel-Aviv, Israel

McGRAW-HILL
MEDICAL PUBLISHING DIVISION

New York / St. Louis / San Francisco / Auckland / Bogota / Caracas / Lisbon / London / Madrid
Mexico City / Milan / Montreal / New Delhi / San Juan / Singapore / Sydney / Tokyo / Toronto

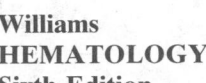

McGraw-Hill

A Division of The McGraw·Hill Companies

Williams
HEMATOLOGY
Sixth Edition

1234567890   DOW   DOW   09876543210

ISBN 0-07-070397-3 (domestic)

This book was set in Times Roman by York Graphic Services. The editors were Martin Wonsiewicz and Karen G. Edmonson. The index was prepared by Irving Tullar; the production supervisor was Robert Laffler. The text and cover designer was Marsha Cohen/Parallelogram Graphics. Donnelly-Willard was the printer and binder.

This book is printed on acid-free paper

Library of Congress Cataloging-in-Publication Data

Williams hematology/authors, Ernest Beutler . . . [et al.].—6th ed.
    p. cm.
Includes bibliographic references and index.
ISBN 0-07-070397-3
   1. Blood—Diseases.   2. Hematology. I. Beutler, Ernest, 1928– II. Williams, William J. (William Joseph), 1926–
   [DNLM: 1. Hematologic Diseases. WH 100 W721 2001]
RC633.H43 2001
616.1'5—dc21

                                               00-058746

ISBN: 0-07-116293-3 (international)

Exclusive rights by The McGraw-Hill Companies, Inc., for manufacture and export. This book cannot be re-exported from the country to which it is consigned by McGraw-Hill. The International Edition is not available in North America.

C O N T E N T S

P A R T I
CLINICAL EVALUATION OF THE PATIENT

P A R T I I
GENERAL HEMATOLOGY

P A R T V

THE ERYTHROCYTE

PART VI

NEUTROPHILS, EOSINOPHILS, BASOPHILS AND MAST CELLS

PART VII

MONOCYTES AND MACROPHAGES

PART VIII

LYMPHOCYTES AND PLASMA CELLS

PART IX

MALIGNANT DISEASES

PART X

HEMOSTASIS AND THROMBOSIS

COLOR PLATES I–XXV (BETWEEN PAGES 1676 AND 1677)

PART XI

TRANSFUSION MEDICINE

CAMILLE N. ABBOUD M.D., F.A.C.P. [4]
Professor of Medicine
Hematology/Oncology Unit
University of Rochester Medical Center
Rochester, New York

CHARLES S. ABRAMS, M.D. [120]
Assistant Professor of Medicine
Division of Hematology-Oncology
University of Pennsylvania School of
    Medicine
University of Pennsylvania Hospital
Philadelphia, Pennsylvania

ALICE ALEXANDER, PH.D. [109]
Research Scientist
Department of Medicine
New York Harbor Health Care Center
New York, New York

BERNARD M. BABIOR, M.D., PH.D. [25, 37, 66]
Professor and Head
Division of Biochemistry
Department of Molecular & Experimental
    Medicine
The Scripps Research Institute
La Jolla, California
Adjunct Professor of Medicine
UCSD School of Medicine
San Diego, California

FEDOR BACHMANN, M.D., [136]
Emeritus Professor in Medicine
Department of Medicine
University of Lausanne Medical School
Lausanne, Switzerland

DOROTHY F. BAINTON, M.D. [64]
Professor of Pathology
Vice Chancellor, Academic Affairs
University of California, San Francisco
San Francisco, California

STEPHEN M. BAIRD, M.D. [80, 104]
Professor of Clinical Pathology
University of California, San Diego
Chief, Pathology and Laboratory Medicine
VA Medical Center
San Diego, California

NICHOLAS A. BANDARENKO, M.D. [141]
Assistant Professor of Pathology and
    Laboratory Medicine
Associate Director
Transfusion Medicine Service
Director of Apheresis
University of North Carolina Hospitals
Chapel Hill, North Carolina

PETER M. BANKS, M.D. [101]
Clinical Professor of Pathology
University of North Carolina–Chapel Hill
Chapel Hill, North Carolina
Director of Hematopathology
Department of Pathology
Carolinas Medical Center
Charlotte, North Carolina

BART BARLOGIE, M.D., PH.D. [106]
Director
Arkansas Cancer Research Center
University of Arkansas
Little Rock, Arkansas

JOEL S. BENNETT, M.D. [120]
Professor of Medicine & Pharmacology
Department of Medicine
University of Pennsylvania
Philadelphia, Pennsylvania

FRED E. BERTRAND, M.D. [82]
Research Associate
University of Minnesota Cancer Center
Minneapolis, Minnesota

ROBERT F. BETTS, M.D. [90]
Professor of Medicine
University of Rochester School of
    Medicine & Dentistry
Department of Medicine and Infectious
    Diseases Unit
Rochester, New York

STEVEN M. BEUTLER, M.D. [17]
Assistant Clinical Professor of Medicine
University of California at Irvine
Irvine, California
Associate Director
Division of Infectious Diseases
Arrowhead Regional Medical Center
Colton, California

ERNEST BEUTLER, M.D. [1, 9, 23, 26, 29, 35, 36, 39, 45, 47,
    48, 49, 53, 54, 61, 63, 65; 79]
Professor and Chairman
Department of Molecular and Experimental
    Medicine
The Scripps Research Institute
Clinical Professor of Medicine
University of California, San Diego
La Jolla, California

KARL G. BLUME, M.D. [18]
Professor of Medicine
Departments of Medicine and Bone Marrow
    Transplantation
Stanford University
Stanford Hospital and Clinics
Stanford, California

LAURENCE A. BOXER, M.D. [67, 72]
Professor of Pediatrics
University of Michigan
Director of Pediatric Hematology/
    Oncology
Womens Hospital
Ann Arbor, Michigan

DAVID J. BRANDHAGEN, M.D. [42]
Assistant Professor of Medicine
Division of Gastroenterology and
    Hepatology
Mayo Clinic
Rochester, Minnesota

MARK E. BRECHER, M.D. [141]
Professor, Department of Pathology &
    Laboratory Medicine
University of North Carolina
Director, Transplantation & Transfusion
    Services
University of North Carolina Hospitals
Chapel Hill, North Carolina

JAMES K. BRENNAN, M.D. [92]
Associate Professor of Medicine
Hematology Oncology Unit
University of Rochester Medical
    Center
Rochester, New York

BRIAN S. BULL, M.D. [22]
Professor and Chair
Department of Pathology and Human
    Anatomy
Vice President & Dean
Loma Linda University
School of Medicine
Loma Linda, California

JOEL N. BUXBAUM, M.D. [107, 109]
Professor
Department of Molecular and Experimental
    Medicine
The Scripps Research Institute
La Jolla, California

LONI CALHOUN, M.T. (A.S.C.P.), S.B.B. [137]
Senior Technical Specialist
Department of Transfusion
    Medicine
UCLA Medical Center
Los Angeles, California

JAIME CARO, M.D. [33]
Professor of Medicine
Jefferson Medical College of Thomas
    Jefferson University
Cardeza Foundation for Hematologic
    Research
Philadelphia, Pennsylvania

DENNIS A. CARSON, M.D. [12]
Professor of Medicine
Department of Medicine
University of California, San Diego
Director of the Sam and Rose Stein Institute
    for Research on Aging
La Jolla, California

BRUCE A. CHABNER, M.D. [16]
Professor of Medicine
Harvard Medical School
Clinical Director
Massachusetts General Hospital Cancer
    Center
Chief, Hematology and Oncology
Massachusetts General Hospital
Boston, Massachusetts

EDWARD A. CLARK, PH.D. [15]
Professor of Microbiology & Immunology
University of Washington Medical Center
Seattle, Washington

BARRY S. COLLER, M.D. [1, 111, 115, 119]
Murray M. Rosenberg Professor and
　Chairman
Department of Medicine
Mount Sinai School of Medicine
Director and Chief of Medicine
Mount Sinai Hospital
New York, New York

GERALD A. COLVIN, D.O. [14]
Assistant Professor of Medicine
University of Massachusetts Medical
　School
Worcester, Massachusetts

TIMOTHY COOLEY, M.D. [89]
Boston Medical Center
Boston University School of Medicine
Boston, Massachusetts

DAVID C. DALE, M.D. [71]
Professor of Medicine
Department of Medicine
University of Washington Medical Center
Seattle, Washington

STEVEN D. DOUGLAS, M.D. [73]
Professor of Pediatrics
Associate Chair, Academic Affairs
Chief, Section of Immunology
Director
Clinical Immunology Laboratories
The Children's Hospital of Philadelphia
Philadelphia, Pennsylvania

ANN DVORAK, M.D. [69]
Professor of Pathology
Harvard Medical School
Senior Pathologist
Department of Pathology
Beth Israel Deaconess Medical Center
Boston, Massachusetts

NEIL M. ELLISON, M.D. [21]
Clinical Professor of Medicine
Jefferson University College of Medicine
Professor of Clinical Medicine
Penn State College of Medicine
Philadelphia, Pennsylvania
Director of Palliative Medicine Program
Geisinger Health System
Danville, Pennsylvania

JOSHUA EPSTEIN, D.SC. [106]
Professor of Medicine
University of Arkansas for Medical Sciences
Director of Laboratory Affairs
Myeloma and Transplantation Research
　Center
Little Rock, Arkansas

ALLAN J. ERSLEV, M.D. [32, 33, 34, 40, 41, 50, 52, 60]
Distinguished Professor of Medicine
Jefferson Medical College of Thomas
　Jefferson University
Cardeza Foundation for Hematologic
　Research
Philadelphia, Pennsylvania

NAOMI L. ESMON, PH.D. [114]
OMRF Associate Professor
Department of Pathology
University of Oklahoma Health Sciences
　Center
Associate Member
Cardiovascular Biology Research Program
Oklahoma Medical Research Foundation
Oklahoma City, Oklahoma

VIRGIL F. FAIRBANKS, M.D. [24, 38, 42]
Professor Emeritus
Department of Laboratory Medicine and
　Pathology
Department of Internal Medicine
Mayo Clinic and Mayo Medical School
Rochester, Minnesota

RICHARD I. FISHER, M.D. [103]
Dorothy W. & J.D. Stetson Coleman
　Professor of Oncology
Professor of Medicine
Loyola University Medical Center
Director, Cardinal Bernardin Cancer Center
Director, Division of Hematology/Oncology
Maywood, Illinois

KENNETH A. FOON, M.D. [103]
Professor of Medicine
University of Cincinnati
Director of The Barrett Cancer Center
Cincinnati, Ohio

BERNARD G. FORGET, M.D. [27]
Professor and Chief
Section of Hematology
Department of Internal Medicine
Yale University School of Medicine
Attending Physician
Department of Internal Medicine
Yale-New Haven Hospital
New Haven, Connecticut

ALISON G. FREIFELD, M.D. [20]
Associate Professor of Medicine
University of Nebraska Medical Center
Omaha, Nebraska

DEBORAH L. FRENCH, M.D. [119]
Assistant Professor
Department of Medicine
Mount Sinai School of Medicine
New York, New York

KENNETH D. FRIEDMAN, M.D. [143]
Associate Professor
Medical College of Wisconsin
Associate Medical Director
Director of Hemostasis Laboratory
The Blood Center of Southeastern
　Wisconsin
Milwaukee, Wisconsin

PATRICK G. GALLAGHER, M.D. [43, 44]
Associate Professor
Department of Pediatrics
Yale University School of Medicine
Attending Physician
Department of Pediatrics
Yale-New Haven Hospital
New Haven, Connecticut

STEPHEN J. GALLI, M.D. [69]
Mary Hewitt Loveless Professor
Professor of Pathology, Microbiology and
　Immunology
Chair, Department of Pathology
Stanford University School of Medicine
Stanford University Medical Center
Stanford, California

TOMAS GANZ, M.D., PH.D. [74, 75]
Professor of Medicine & Pathology
Department of Medicine
UCLA School of Medicine
Los Angeles, California

JAMES N. GEORGE, M.D. [117]
Professor of Medicine
Hematology-Oncology Section
The University of Oklahoma Health Sciences
　Center
Oklahoma City, Oklahoma

DAVID GINSBURG, M.D. [135]
Professor, Departments of Internal
　Medicine & Human Genetics
University of Michigan
Investigator
Howard Hughes Medical Institute
Ann Arbor, Michigan

DAVID W. GOLDE, M.D. [66]
Professor of Medicine
Cornell University
Physician-in-Chief
Memorial Sloan-Kettering Cancer Center
New York, New York

SCOTT H. GOODNIGHT, M.D. [127]
Professor of Medicine & Pathology
Department of Hematology & Medical
　Oncology
Oregon Health Sciences University
Portland, Oregon

ROBERTA A. GOTTLIEB, M.D. [11]
Associate Professor
Department of Molecular & Experimental
　Medicine
The Scripps Research Institute
La Jolla, California

JOHN H. GRIFFIN, PH.D. [113, 127]
Professor
Department of Molecular & Experimental
　Medicine
The Scripps Research Institute
La Jolla, California

KATHERINE A. HAJJAR, M.D. [114, 116]
Stavros S. Naircons Professor of Pediatrics
Weill Medical College of Cornell University
Attending Pediatrician
New York Presbyterian Hospital
New York, New York

CHAIM HERSHKO, M.D. [59]
Professor of Medicine
Hebrew University School of Medicine
Head, Department of Medicine
Shaare Zedek Medical Center
Jerusalem, Israel

ROBERT S. HILLMAN, M.D. [59]
Professor of Medicine
Chairman Emeritus
Department of Medicine
Maine Medical Center
Portland, Maine

WEN-ZHE HO, M.D. [73]
Associate Professor of Pediatrics
Division of Immunology
The Children's Hospital of Philadelphia
Philadelphia, Pennsylvania

MAUREANE R. HOFFMAN, M.D. [112, 123]
Associate Professor of Pathology
Assistant Professor of Immunology
Duke University
Director, Hematology and Blood Bank
Durham VA Medical Center
Durham, North Carolina

MCDONALD K. HORNE, III, M.D. [20]
Senior Clinical Investigator
Hematology Service
Clinical Pathology Department
Warren G. Magnuson Clinical Center
National Institute of Health
Bethesda, Maryland

SANDRA J. HORNING, M.D. [102]
Professor of Medicine
Stanford University
Palo Alto, California

KUO-LIANG HUANG, M.D. [90]
Assistant Clinical Professor
Department of Medicine
University of California—Irvine Medical
    Center
Orange, California
Director, Section of Infectious Diseases
Department of Internal Medicine
Arrowhead Regional Medical Center
Colton, California

RUSSELL D. HULL, M.D. [129, 133]
Professor
Department of Medicine
University of Calgary
Active Staff
Department of General Internal Medicine
Foothills Hospital
Calgary, Canada

DANIEL R. JACOBSON, M.D. [107]
Associate Professor
Department of Medicine
New York University
Attending Physician
Research Service
New York Harbor Health Care Center
New York, New York

MARSHALL E. KADIN, M.D. [100]
Professor of Pathology
Harvard Medical School
Director of Hematopathology
Beth Israel Deaconess Medical Center
Boston, Massachusetts

A. BARRY KAY, M.D., PH.D. [68]
Professor and Head
Department of Allergy and Clinical
    Immunology
National Heart and Lung Institute
London, United Kingdom

THOMAS J. KIPPS, M.D., PH.D. [1, 5, 13, 81, 83, 84, 86, 87,
    96, 98, 108]
Professor and Head
Division of Hematology/Oncology
Deputy Director, UCSD Cancer Center
University of California at San Diego
La Jolla, California

DAVID J. KUTER, M.D., D. PHIL. [110]
Associate Professor
Department of Medicine
Harvard Medical School
Chief, Clinical Hematology
Massachusetts General Hospital
Harvard Medical School
Boston, Massachusetts

LEWIS L. LANIER, M.D. [85]
Professor
Department of Microbiology & Immunology
University of California–San Francisco
San Francisco, California

MICHELLE M. LEBEAU, PH.D. [10]
Professor of Medicine
Section of Hematology/Oncology
University of Chicago
Chicago, Illinois

TUCKER W. LEBIEN, PH.D. [82]
Professor of Laboratory Medicine/Pathology
University of Minnesota
Deputy Director, University of Minnesota
    Cancer Center
Minneapolis, Minnesota

ROBERT I. LEHRER, M.D. [74, 75]
Professor of Medicine
Department of Medicine
UCLA Center for the Health Sciences
Los Angeles, California

ALEXANDRA M. LEVINE, M.D. [89]
Professor of Medicine
Chief, Division of Hematology
University of Southern California
Keck School of Medicine
Medical Director
USC/Norris Cancer Hospital
Los Angeles, California

MARSHALL A. LICHTMAN, M.D. [1, 4, 8, 70, 76, 77, 78, 91, 92,
    93, 95, 105]
Professor of Medicine and of Biochemistry
    and Biophysics
University of Rochester School of Medicine
    and Dentistry
Rochester, New York

HOWARD LIEBMAN, M.D. [89]
Associate Professor of Medicine and
    Pathology
University of Southern California
Los Angeles, California

JANE L. LIESVELD, M.D. [93, 94]
Associate Professor of Medicine
Director, Samuel E. Durand Blood and
    Marrow Transplantation Unit
University of Rochester Medical Center
Rochester, New York

JOHNSON M. LIU, M.D. [19]
Investigator
Hematology Branch
National Heart, Lung, and Blood Institute
Bethesda, Maryland

JOSEPH LOSCALZO, M.D., PH.D. [134]
Wade Professor and Chairman
Department of Medicine
Boston University School of Medicine
Director, Whitaker Cardiovascular
    Institute
Boston, Massachusetts

THOMAS P. LOUGHRAN, JR., M.D. [100]
Professor of Internal Medicine
University of South Florida
Program Leader, Hematologic Malignancies
H. Lee Moffitt Cancer Center & Research
    Institute
Tampa, Florida

NAOMI L. C. LUBAN, M.D. [58]
Professor of Pediatrics & Pathology
George Washington University School of
    Medicine
Director of Transfusion Medicine
Children's Hospital Medical Center
Washington, District of Columbia

EBERHARD F. MAMMEN, M.D. [125]
Professor Emeritus
Department of Obstetrics and Gynecology
C.S. Mott Center
Wayne State University
Detroit, Michigan

AARON J. MARCUS, M.D. [114]
Professor of Medicine and Pathology
Weill Medical College of Cornell
    University
Chief, Hematology-Oncology
VA New York Harbor Health Care
    System
New York, New York

JOSE MARTINEZ, M.D. [51]
Professor of Medicine
Professor of Biochemistry & Molecular
    Pharmacology
Jefferson Medical College of Thomas
    Jefferson University
Associate Director
Cardeza Foundation for Hematologic
    Research
Philadelphia, Pennsylvania

DONNA JO MAYO, R.N., M.A. [20]
Research Nurse Specialist
National Institute of Health
Bethesda, Maryland

JEFFREY MCCULLOUGH, M.D. [139]
Professor
Department of Laboratory Medicine &
Pathology
Director, Division of Laboratory Medicine &
Section of Transfusion Medicine
University of Minnesota Medical School
Minneapolis, Minnesota

BRUCE C. MCLEOD, M.D. [144]
Professor of Medicine & Pathology
Rush Medical College
Director, Blood Center
Rush-Presbyterian—St. Luke's Medical
Center
Chicago, Illinois

JAY E. MENITOVE, M.D. [143]
Clinical Professor of Medicine
University of Missouri-Kansas City School of
Medicine
Executive Director and Medical Director
Community Blood Center of Greater Kansas
City
Kansas City, Missouri

DEAN D. METCALFE, M.D. [69]
Chief, Laboratory of Allergic Diseases
NIAID/National Institute of Health
Bethesda, Maryland

DOUGALD M. MONROE, III, PH.D. [112]
Associate Professor of Medicine
Division of Hematology-Oncology
University of North Carolina School of
Medicine
Chapel Hill, North Carolina

MICHAEL W. MOSESSON, M.D. [124]
Professor
Department of Medicine
University of Wisconsin Medical School
Madison, Wisconsin
Senior Investigator
The Blood Research Institute
The Blood Center of Southeastern Wisconsin
Milwaukee, Wisconsin

WILLIAM MULLER, M.D., PH.D. [114]
Associate Professor
Department of Pathology
Weill Medical College of Cornell
University
New York, New York

NIKHIL MUNSHI. M.D. [106]
Professor of Medicine
Department of Myeloma and Transplantation
Research Center
University of Arkansas for Medical Sciences
Little Rock, Arkansas

SCOTT MURPHY, M.D. [142]
Adjunct Professor of Medicine
University of Pennsylvania
Chief Medical Officer
American Red Cross, Penn-Jersey
Region
Philadelphia, Pennsylvania

ROBERT S. NEGRIN, M.D. [18]
Associate Professor of Medicine
Departments of Medicine and Bone Marrow
Transplantation
Stanford University
Stanford Hospital and Clinics
Stanford, California

ARTHUR W. NIENHUIS, M.D. [19]
St. Jude Professor of Medicine &
Pediatrics
University of Tennessee, Memphis
Director, St. Jude Children's Research
Hospital
Memphis, Tennessee

CHARLES H. PACKMAN, M.D. [55, 56, 57]
Clinical Professor of Medicine
University of North Carolina School of
Medicine
Chapel Hill, North Carolina
Chief, Section of Hematology/Oncology
Department of Internal Medicine
Carolinas Medical Center
Charlotte, North Carolina

JAMES PALIS, M.D. [7]
Associate Professor of Pediatrics in
Oncology
University of Rochester Medical Center
Rochester, New York

LESLIE V. PARISE, PH.D. [111]
Professor
Department of Pharmacology
University of North Carolina at Chapel Hill
Chapel Hill, North Carolina

RICHARD B. PATT, M.D. [21]
Associate Professor of Anesthesiology
Baylor School of Medicine
President & Chief Medical Officer
The Patt Center for Cancer Pain &
Wellness
Houston, Texas

LAWRENCE D. PETZ, M.D. [137]
Professor of Pathology & Laboratory
Medicine
UCLA Medical Center
Los Angeles, California

GRAHAM F. PINEO, M.D. [129, 133]
Professor of Medicine
Department of Medicine and Oncology
University of Calgary
Department of Medicine
Foothills Hospital
Calgary, Alberta, Canada

CHING-HON PUI, M.D. [97]
Professor of Pediatrics
University of Tennessee, Memphis—College
of Medicine
Director, Leukemia/Lymphoma Division
Vice Chairman, Department of Hematology/
Oncology
St. Jude Children's Research Hospital
Memphis, Tennessee

PETER J. QUESENBERRY, M.D. [14]
Professor of Medicine
University of Massachusetts School of
Medicine
Cancer Center, University of Massachusetts
Medical Center
Worcester, Massachusetts

JAYASHREE RAMASETHU, M.B.B.S., M.D. [58]
Assistant Clinical Professor of Pediatrics
Georgetown University School of Medicine
Assistant Professor of Pediatrics
Division of Neonatology
Georgetown University Hospital
Washington, District of Columbia

JACOB H. RAND, M.D. [128]
Professor of Medicine
Hematology Division
Director, Coagulation Laboratory
Mount Sinai-NYU Medical Center and
Health System
New York, New York

HELEN M. RANNEY, M.D. [28]
Professor of Medicine, Emeritus
University of California, San Diego
San Diego, California

GARY E. RASKOB, PH.D. [129, 133]
Samuel Roberts Noble Presidential Professor
Departments of Medicine, Biostatistics and
Epidemiology
University of Oklahoma Health Sciences
Center
Associate Vice President for Clinical
Research
Oklahoma City, Oklahoma

MUJAHID A. RIZVI, M.D., M.P.H. [117]
Resident
Department of Medicine
University of Florida Health Science Center
Gainesville, Florida

HAROLD R. ROBERTS, M.D. [112, 123]
Sarah Graham Kenan Distinguished
Professor of Medicine & Pathology
University of North Carolina at Chapel Hill
Attending Physician
University of North Carolina Hospitals
Chapel Hill, North Carolina

FRED S. ROSEN, M.D. [88]
James L. Gamble Professor of Pediatrics
Harvard Medical School
Boston, Massachusetts

DANIEL H. RYAN, M.D. [2, 3]
Professor of Pathology & Laboratory
Medicine
Director of Clinical Laboratories
University of Rochester Medical Center
Rochester, New York

SHIGERU SASSA, M.D., PH.D. [62]
Associate Professor & Physician
Emeritus & Head of Laboratory for
Biochemical Hematology
The Rockefeller University
New York, New York

ALAN SAVEN, M.D. [99]
Adjunct Professor
Department of Molecular and Experimental
    Medicine
The Scripps Research Institute
Head, Division of Hematology/Oncology
Director, Ida M. and Cecil H. Green Cancer
    Center
The Scripps Clinic
La Jolla, California

ANDREW I. SCHAFER, M.D. [118]
The Bob and Vivian Smith Professor of
    Medicine
Chairman, Department of Medicine
Baylor College of Medicine
Houston, Texas

MATHIAS SCHMID, M.D. [12]
University of Ulm
Internal Medicine III
Hematology, Oncology, Rheumatology &
    Infectious Diseases
Ulm, Germany

PAUL I. SCHNEIDERMAN, M.D. [121]
Associate Clinical Professor
Department of Dermatology
Columbia University College of Physicians &
    Surgeons
New York, New York

SAM SCHULMAN, M.D. [132]
Assistant Professor
Coagulation Unit
Department of Hematology
Karolinska Hospital
Stockholm, Sweden

GEORGE B. SEGEL, M.D. [7]
Professor of Pediatrics, Medicine, Genetics &
    Oncology
Chief, Pediatric Hematology/Oncology &
    Genetics
University of Rochester Medical Center
Rochester, New York

URI SELIGSOHN, M.D. [1, 115, 122, 126]
Chairman
Department of Hematology and
Director of the Institute of Thrombosis and
    Hemostasis
The Chaim Sheba Medical Center
Tel-Hashomer
Professor of Hematology
Sackler Faculty of Medicine
Tel-Aviv University
Israel

RICHARD KINGSLEY SHADDUCK, M.D. [31]
Clinical Professor of Medicine
University of Pittsburgh School of Medicine
Director, The Western Pennsylvania Cancer
    Institute
Pittsburgh, Pennsylvania

JEAN A. SHAFER, B.S., M.A.
Assistant Professor of Medicine and
    Pathology
University of Rochester Medical Center
Rochester, New York

VIJAY S. SHARMA, M.D. [28]
Professor of Medicine
Department of Medicine
University of California at San Diego
La Jolla, California

SANFORD J. SHATTIL, M.D. [120]
Professor, Department of Vascular
    Biology
The Scripps Research Institute
La Jolla, California
Adjunct Professor of Medicine
University of California, San Diego
San Diego, California

JOHN SHAUGHNESSY JR., PH.D. [106]
Assistant Professor
University of Arkansas Medical School
Director
Lambert Laboratory for Myeloma Genetics
Little Rock, Arkansas

JAMES E. SMOLEN, PH.D. [67]
Associate Professor
Department of Pediatrics, Section of
    Leukocyte Biology
Baylor College of Medicine
Houston, Texas

SUSAN S. SMYTH, M.D., PH.D. [111]
Clinical Instructor
Department of Medicine
Division of Hematology
SUNY at Stony Brook
Stony Brook, New York

KAREN A. SULLIVAN, PH.D. [138]
Research Professor of Medicine
Director, Histocompatibility &
    Immunogenetics Laboratory
Tulane University Health Sciences
    Center–School of Medicine
New Orleans, Louisiana

JEFFREY SUPKO, M.D. [16]
Assistant Professor of Medicine
Harvard Medical School
Director, Clinical Pharmacology
    Laboratory
Massachusetts General Hospital Cancer
    Center
Boston, Massachusetts

MARK B. TAUBMAN, M.D. [130]
Irene and Dr. Arthur Fishberg Professor of
    Medicine (Cardiology)
Department of Medicine
Mount Sinai School of Medicine
New York, New York

GIORGIO TRINCHIERI, M.D. [85]
Professor
Immunology Program
The Wistar Institute
Philadelphia, Pennsylvania

CHRISTOPHER E. WALSH, M.D. [19]
Assistant Professor of Internal Medicine
University of North Carolina Gene Therapy
    Center
Chapel Hill, North Carolina

PETER A. WARD, MD [6]
Godfrey D. Stobbe Professor of
    Pathology
Chairman
Department of Pathology
University of Michigan Medical
    School
Ann Arbor, Michigan

A.J. WARDLAW, M.D., PH.D. [68]
Professor of Respiratory Medicine
Department of Respiratory Medicine
Glenfield Hospital
Leicester, United Kingdom

JEFFREY S. WARREN, M.D. [6]
Warthin-Weller Endowed Professor
Director, Division of Clinical
    Pathology
University of Michigan Medical
    School
Ann Arbor, Michigan

SIR DAVID J. WEATHERALL, M.D. [46]
Regius Professor of Medicine
University of Oxford
Honorary Director, Institute of Molecular
    Medicine
John Radcliffe Hospital
Headington Oxford, United Kingdom

HARVEY J. WEISS, M.D. [131]
Professor Emeritus of Medicine
Columbia University College of Physicians &
    Surgeons
Division of Hematology/Oncology
St. Luke's–Roosevelt Hospital Center
New York, New York

GILBERT C. WHITE, II, M.D. [122]
John C. Parker Distinguished Professor of
    Medicine and Pharmacology
Division of Hematology-Oncology
Director, Center for Thrombosis and
    Hemostasis
University of North Carolina School of
    Medicine
Chapel Hill, North Carolina

WILLIAM J. WILLIAMS, M.D. [1, 8]
Edward C. Reifenstein Professor of
    Medicine
Department of Medicine
Upstate Medical University
State University of New York
Syracuse, New York

WYNDHAM WILSON, M.D. [16]
Senior Investigator
Medicine Branch
National Cancer Institute
National Institute of Health
Bethesda, Maryland

THEODORE J. YUN, M.D. [15]
Department of Microbiology
University of Washington
Seattle, Washington

In the five years that have passed since the appearance of the 5th Edition of Williams Hematology, there has been enormous progress in many areas in hematology including the mechanisms of hematopoiesis, the role of cytokines, the regulation of genes and of cell growth, the functioning of the immune system, and the understanding of hemostasis and thrombosis.

As we prepared the sixth edition of this text, we were very fortunate to be able to add to the group of editors, Dr. Uri Seligsohn, whose broad knowledge of hematology and special expertise in the field of hemostasis and thrombosis have been a great resource. All of the contributors are acknowledged experts in their fields. Nonetheless, as in the previous editions, the editors have carefully reviewed each chapter and whenever necessary, extensively revised or even rewritten the contributed material to maintain uniformity and to make certain that the chapter will be useful to the reader.

Attempting to encompass adequately the new knowledge that has accrued in the past five years and at the same time produce a readable, single-volume work has been a great challenge to the editors. To accomplish this goal we decided to eliminate the section of the book pertaining to laboratory techniques. This part of the book had been a valuable feature since the First Edition and seemed to fill an important need. More than most medical specialties, hematology is laboratory-based, and having ready access to the required techniques is essential. When we published our first edition it was quite possible for a clinical trainee to take the book to the laboratory and to perform many of the studies that were needed to establish a diagnosis, sometimes, perhaps, with the aid of an experienced "special hematology" technician. The automation of laboratory procedures has dramatically diminished the role of trainees in performing assays, and while this trend has undoubtedly improved the reliability of the results, it has made it less important for trainees to have detailed information about the specifics of the assays. It does not, however, diminish our belief that trainees should know how the studies are performed and critically interpreted; therefore, we have included discussion of important elements of tests and their interpretation in the text of relevant chapters. In addition, we encourage trainees to consult other standard references or the manuals supplied by the instrument and assay manufacturers for details that we may not have been able to include in this text.

When we reviewed the allocation of space in the 5th edition we realized that in the previous editions nearly as much space had been devoted to the red blood cell as to the entire area of hemostasis. The immune system as represented in Part VIII "Lymphocytes and Plasma Cells" was only allocated about one-half that space. Red cells are, of course, of great importance to the hematologist and, indeed, to the general physician. After all, anemias are some of the most common manifestations of disease. Yet, the dynamic nature of science has required us to reallocate space. In part it has been possible to accomplish this by removing some of the comprehensive compilations of the genetic variants of hemoglobin, glucose-6-phosphate dehydrogenase, and various plasma proteins. At one time our text was the most readily available resource in which such complete listings could be found; now this information is increasingly available in continually updated form at various web sites. We have established a web site at *williamshematology.com* that provides either links to such information or the information itself. A few new features designed to aid the user of the text have been added. A brief summary has been added to the beginning of each chapter. To save the reader the task of searching for a definition, those few acronyms or abbreviations that the editors have allowed contributors to use are now defined at the beginning of each chapter.

The production of this text has required the cooperation of our many contributors. We are grateful to them for providing us with the chapters that have made possible this comprehensive work. In this edition we have revised and expanded the color plates. Most of the blood and marrow photomicrographs were provided by Jean A. Shafer, B.S., M.A., Assistant Professor of Medicine (Hematology) and Pathology at the University of Rochester School of Medicine and Dentistry. Joshua Z. Sickel, M.D. at El Camino Hospital, Mountain View, California, formerly in the Department of Pathology and Laboratory Medicine at the University of Rochester School of Medicine and Dentistry provided the photomicrographs of the lymph node sections in Plate XIV-6 and XXII-4 to XXII-10. Michelle Le Beau, Ph.D. provided the photomicrographs for Plate XXIV. Paul Schneiderman, M.D. provided the photographs for Plate XXV-1 through 42. Virgil Fairbanks, M.D. provided the photograph for Plate XXV-43. Karl Blume, M.D. provided the photographs for Plate XXV-44 and 45.

Several colleagues were helpful to us in reviewing and criticizing parts of the text. We thank Daniel Salomon, M.D. of the Scripps Research Institute and George B. Segal, M.D. of the University of Rochester for their contributions in this regard. Organizing and tracking the production of the many chapters of this text and troubleshooting whenever necessary was an awesome task, and we are grateful to Mrs. Jane Verenini for having performed this task and for having coordinated the production of *Williams Hematology* in La Jolla. We also thank Ms. Alice Nahum, Ruth Aped, Suzanne Rivera, and Susan M. Daley for their attention to detail and their assistance in bibliographic searches, record-keeping, typing, proofreading, and communications with the publisher, editors, and authors. Last but not least, it is the families of the editors and their infinite patience that made this edition possible.

SI UNIT CONVERSION TABLE

Constituent[a]	Traditional units	Multiplication factor[b]	SI units[c]
δ-Aminoleuvulinic acid (U)	mg per day	7.63	μmol per day
Bilirubin			
Direct (S)	mg per dl	17.1	μmol per liter
Total (S)	mg per dl	17.1	μmol per liter
Calcium (S)	mg per dl	0.25	mmol per liter
Coproporphyrin (U)	μg per dl	1.5	nmol per day
Erythrocyte count	number per μl	10^6	number per liter
Fibrinogen[d] (Factor I) (P)	mg per dl	0.01	g per liter
	mg per dl	0.029	μmol per liter
Folic acid (S)	ng per dl	1.0	μg per liter
	ng per dl	2.27	nmol per liter
Haptoglobin (S)	mg per dl	0.01	g per liter
Hematocrit (B)	%	0.01	ratio
Hemoglobin[l] (B)	g per dl	1.0	g per dl
Iron (S)	μg per dl	0.179	μmol per liter
Iron-binding capacity (S)	μg per dl	0.179	μmol per liter
Leukocyte count (B)	number per μl	10^6	number per liter
Mean corpuscular hemoglobin	pg	1.0	pg
Mean corpuscular hemoglobin concentration	%	1.0	g per dl
Mean corpuscular volume	μm^3	1.0	fl
Packed cell volume	%	0.01	ratio
Phosphorus (S)	mg per dl	0.323	mmol per liter
Platelet count (B)	number per μl	10^6	number per liter
Porphobilinogen (U)	mg per day	4.42	μmol per day
Protoporphyrin (erythrocyte)	μg per dl	0.018	μmol per liter
Reticulocyte count (B)	%	0.01	ratio
	number per μl	10^6	number per liter
Transferrin (S)	mg per dl	0.01	g per liter
Urea nitrogen (B)	mg per dl	0.36	mmol per liter
Uric acid	mg per dl	0.36	mmol per liter
Uroporphyrin (U)	μg per dl	1.2	nmol per day
Vitamin B$_{12}$(S)	pg per ml	1.0	ng per liter

[a]The following abbreviations are used: B = blood; S = serum; P = plasma; U = urine.

[b]Conventional units multiplied by this factor will yield SI units.

[c]The following units are used:

fl = femtoliter (10^{-15} liter)	fmol = femtomole	fg = femtogram
pl = picoliter (10^{-12} liter)	pmol = picomole	pg = picogram
nl = nanoliter (10^{-9} liter)	nmol = nanomole	ng = nanogram
μl = microliter (10^{-6} liter)	μmol = micromole	μg = microgram
ml = milliliter (10^{-3} liter)	mmol = millimole	mg = milligram
dl = deciliter (10^{-1} liter)		

[d]The molar concentration is calculated assuming a molecular weight of 340,000.

[e]Hemoglobin is not usually expressed in molar terms because of the uncertainty regarding the polymeric state of the molecule. If the unit molecular weight is assumed to be 16,000, the multiplication factor is 0.62 to convert g per dl to mmol per liter [2]. If the molecular weight of 64,500 is assumed, the conversion factor is 0.1555 [3]

Sources

1. Baron DN, Broughton PMG, Cohen M, Lansley TS, Lewis SM, Shinton NK: The use of SI units in reporting results obtained in hospital laboratories. *J Clin Pathol* 27:590, 1974.

2. Young DS: "Normal laboratory values" (case records of the Massachusetts General Hospital) in SI units. *N Engl J Med* 292:795, 1975.

3. Lehmann HP: Metrication of clinical laboratory data in SI units. *Am J Clin Pathol* 65:2, 1976.

PART I

CLINICAL EVALUATION OF THE PATIENT

APPROACH TO THE PATIENT

ERNEST BEUTLER
MARSHALL A. LICHTMAN
BARRY S. COLLER
THOMAS J. KIPPS
URI SELIGSOHN
WILLIAM J. WILLIAMS

Ideally, the physician's goal is to prevent illness, and many opportunities exist for hematologists to prevent the development of hematologic disorders. These opportunities include identification of individual genetic risk factors and either avoidance of situations that may make a latent disorder manifest or actual prophylactic therapy, as for example in avoiding venous stasis in patients heterozygous for protein C deficiency or administering prophylactic subcutaneous heparin after major surgery in such patients. Hematologists may also prevent disease by participating in public health and community medicine efforts, such as eliminating sources of environmental lead that may result in childhood anemia. Prenatal diagnosis of hematologic disorders can provide information to families in which a fetus is affected with a hematologic disorder.

When preventive opportunities are not available or fail, the care of a patient begins with a systematic attempt to determine the nature of the illness by eliciting an in-depth medical history and performing a physical examination. The physician should identify the important symptoms and obtain as much relevant information as possible about their origin and evolution and about the general health of the patient by appropriate questions designed to explore the patient's recent and remote experience. Reviewing previous records may add important data for understanding the onset or progression of illness. Hereditary and environmental factors should be carefully sought and evaluated. The physician follows the medical history with a physical examination to obtain data on the patient's general health and to permit a careful search for signs of the illnesses suggested by the history. Additional history is obtained during the physical examination, as findings suggest an additional or alternative diagnosis. Thus, the history and physical examination should be considered as a unit, providing the basic information with which further diagnostic information is integrated.

Primary hematologic diseases are uncommon, while hematologic manifestations secondary to other diseases occur frequently. For example, the signs and symptoms of anemia and the presence of enlarged lymph nodes are common clinical findings that may be related to hematologic disease but occur even more frequently as secondary manifestations of disorders not considered primarily hematologic. A wide variety of diseases may produce signs or symptoms of hematologic illness. Thus, in patients with metastatic carcinoma, all the signs and symptoms of anemia may be elicited and lymphadenopathy may be pronounced, but additional findings are usually present that indicate primary involvement of some system besides the blood and lymph nodes. In this discussion, therefore, emphasis is placed on the clinical findings resulting from either primary hematologic disease or the complications of hematologic disorders in order to avoid presenting an extensive catalog of signs and symptoms encountered in general clinical medicine.

In each discussion of specific diseases in subsequent chapters, the signs and symptoms that accompany the particular disorder are presented, and the clinical findings are covered in detail. In this chapter a more general systematic approach is taken.

HISTORY[1-4]

DRUGS AND CHEMICALS

DRUGS

Drug therapy, either self-prescribed or ordered by a physician, is extremely common in our society. Drugs often induce or aggravate hematologic disease, and it is therefore essential that a careful history of drug ingestion, including beneficial and adverse reactions, be obtained from all patients. Drugs taken regularly often become a part of the patient's way of life and are often forgotten or are not recognized as "drugs." Agents such as aspirin, laxatives, tranquilizers, medicinal iron, vitamins, other nutritional supplements, and sedatives belong to this category. Further, drugs may be ingested in unrecognized form, such as antibiotics in food or quinine in tonic water. Specific, persistent questioning, often on several occasions, may be necessary before a complete history of drug use is obtained. It is very important to obtain detailed information on alcohol consumption from every patient. The four "CAGE" questions—about *c*utting down, being *a*nnoyed by criticism, having *g*uilt feelings, and needing an *e*ye-opener—provide an effective approach to the history of alcohol use. Patients should also be asked about the use of recreational drugs. The use of "alternative medicines" and herbal medicines are common, and many patients will not consider these medications or may actively withhold information about their use. Nonjudgmental questioning may be successful in identifying agents in this category that the patient is taking.

CHEMICALS

In addition to drugs, most people are exposed regularly to a variety of chemicals in the environment, some of which may be potentially harmful agents in hematologic disease. Similarly, occupational exposure to chemicals must be considered. When a toxin is suspected, the patient's daily activities and environment must be carefully reviewed, since significant exposure to toxic chemicals may occur incidentally.

VACCINATION

Vaccinations can be potent triggers of exacerbations of immune thrombocytopenia.

NUTRITION

Nutrition information can be useful in deducing the possible role of dietary deficiency in anemia. The avoidance of certain food groups, as might be the case with vegans, or the ingestion of uncooked fish or meat can be clues to the pathogenesis of anemia.

Acronyms and abbreviations that appear in this chapter include: PS, performance status.

GENERAL SYMPTOMS

Performance status (PS) is a useful concept in establishing the seriousness of the patient's disability at the outset and in evaluating the effects of therapy.[2] A well-founded set of criteria for evaluating performance status is presented in Table 1-1.

Weight loss is a frequent accompaniment of many serious diseases, including primary hematologic entities, but it is not a prominent accompaniment of most hematologic disease. Many "wasting" diseases, such as disseminated carcinoma or tuberculosis, cause anemia, and pronounced emaciation should suggest one of these diseases rather than anemia as the primary disorder.

Fever is a common manifestation of the lymphomas or leukemias, usually because of secondary infection but sometimes as a result of the disease itself. In patients with "fever of unknown origin," leukemia or lymphoma, and particularly Hodgkin's disease, should be considered. Myelofibrosis and chronic lymphocytic leukemia may also cause fever. In rare patients with severe pernicious anemia or hemolytic anemia, fever may be pronounced. *Chills* may accompany severe hemolytic processes and the bacteremia that may complicate the immunocompromised or neutropenic patient. *Night sweats* suggest the presence of low-grade fever and may occur in patients with lymphoma or leukemia.

Fatigue, malaise, and *lassitude* are such common accompaniments of both physical and emotional disorders that their evaluation is complex and often difficult. In patients with serious disease, these symptoms may be readily explained by fever, muscle wasting, or other associated findings. Patients with anemia frequently complain of fatigue, malaise, or lassitude, and these symptoms may accompany the hematologic malignancies. Fatigue or lassitude may occur also with iron deficiency even in the absence of sufficient anemia to account for the symptom. In slowly developing chronic anemias, the patient may not recognize reduced exercise tolerance, etc., except in retrospect, after a remission has been induced by appropriate therapy. Anemia may be responsible for more symptoms than has been traditionally recognized, as suggested by the remarkable improvement in quality of life of most uremic patients treated with erythropoietin.[3]

Weakness may accompany anemia or the wasting of malignant processes, in which cases it is manifest as a general loss of strength or reduced capacity for exercise. The weakness may be localized as a result of neurologic complications of hematologic disease. In pernicious anemia there may be weakness of the lower extremities, accompanied by numbness, tingling, and unsteadiness of gait. Peripheral neuropathy also occurs with dysproteinemias. Weakness of one or more extremities in patients with leukemia, myeloma, or lymphoma may signify central or peripheral nervous system invasion or compression. Myopathy secondary to malignancy occurs with the hematologic malignancies and is usually manifest as weakness of proximal muscle groups. Foot drop or wrist drop may occur in lead poisoning, amyloidosis, systemic autoimmune diseases, or as a complication of vincristine therapy. Paralysis may occur in acute intermittent porphyria.

SPECIFIC SYMPTOMS

NERVOUS SYSTEM

Headache may be due to a number of causes related to hematologic diseases. Anemia or polycythemia may cause mild to severe headache. Invasion or compression of the brain by leukemia or lymphoma, or infection of the central nervous system by *Cryptococcus* or tuberculosis, may also cause headache in patients with hematologic malignancies. Hemorrhage into the brain or subarachnoid space in patients with thrombocytopenia or other bleeding disorders may cause sudden, severe headache.

Paresthesias may occur because of peripheral neuropathy in pernicious anemia or secondary to hematologic malignancy or amyloidosis. They may also result from therapy with vincristine.

Confusion may accompany malignant or infectious processes involving the brain, sometimes as a result of the accompanying fever. Confusion may also occur with severe anemia, hypercalcemia, or glucocorticoid therapy. Confusion or apparent senility may be a manifestation of pernicious anemia. Frank psychosis may develop in acute intermittent porphyria or with glucocorticoid therapy.

Impairment of consciousness may be due to increased intracranial pressure secondary to hemorrhage or tumor in the central nervous system. It may also accompany severe anemia or polycythemia, or it may be due to hyperviscosity secondary to a paraprotein in the plasma.

EYES

Visual disturbances may be manifestations of anemia, polycythemia, leukemia, or macroglobulinemia. Occasionally blindness may result from retinal hemorrhages secondary to anemia and thrombocytopenia or severe hyperviscosity. Diplopia or disturbances of ocular movement may occur with orbital tumors or paralysis of the third, fourth, or sixth cranial nerves because of compression by tumor.

EARS

Vertigo, tinnitus, and "roaring" in the ears may occur with marked anemia, polycythemia, or macroglobulinemia-induced hyperviscosity.

NASOPHARYNX AND MOUTH

Epistaxis may occur with any bleeding disorder. *Anosmia* or *olfactory hallucinations* occur in pernicious anemia. The nasopharynx may be invaded by a malignant tumor, with the symptoms dependent on the structures invaded. *Sore tongue* occurs in pernicious anemia and may accompany iron deficiency or vitamin deficiencies. *Macroglossia* occurs in amyloidosis. *Bleeding gums* may occur with bleeding disorders. Infiltration of the gingiva with leukemic cells occurs in acute monocytic leukemia. *Ulceration* of the tongue or oral mucosa may be severe in the leukemias or in patients with neutropenia. *Dryness of the mouth* may be due to hypercalcemia, secondary, for example, to plasma cell myeloma. *Dysphagia* may be seen in patients with severe mucous membrane atrophy associated with chronic iron-deficiency anemia.

TABLE 1-1   CRITERIA OF PERFORMANCE STATUS

Able to carry on normal activity; no special care is needed.	
100%	Normal; no complaints, no evidence of disease.
90%	Able to carry on normal activity; minor signs or symptoms of disease.
80%	Normal activity with effort; some signs or symptoms of disease.
Unable to work; able to live at home, care for most personal needs; a varying amount of assistance is needed.	
70%	Cares for self; unable to carry on normal activity or to do active work.
60%	Requires occasional assistance but is able to care for most personal needs.
50%	Requires considerable assistance and frequent medical care.
Unable to care for self; requires equivalent of institutional or hospital care; disease may be progressing rapidly.	
40%	Disabled; requires special care and assistance.
30%	Severely disabled; hospitalization is indicated though death not imminent.
20%	Very sick; hospitalization necessary; active supportive treatment necessary.
10%	Moribund; fatal processes progressing rapidly.
0%	Dead.

SOURCE: *Cancer* 1:634, 1948.

NECK

Painless swelling in the neck is characteristic of lymphoma but may be due to a number of other diseases as well. Occasionally, the enlarged lymph nodes of lymphomas may be tender or painful because of secondary infection or rapid growth. *Diffuse swelling* of the neck and face may occur with obstruction of the superior vena cava due to lymphoma.

CHEST AND HEART

Both *dyspnea* and *palpitations*, usually on effort but occasionally at rest, may occur because of anemia. *Congestive heart failure* may supervene, and *angina pectoris* may become manifest in anemic patients. The impact of anemia on the circulatory system depends in part on the rapidity with which it develops, and chronic anemia may become severe without producing major symptoms; with acute blood loss, the patient may develop shock with a nearly normal hemoglobin level. *Cough* may result from enlarged mediastinal nodes. *Chest pain* may arise from involvement of the ribs or sternum with lymphoma or multiple myeloma, nerve-root invasion or compression, or herpes zoster; the pain of herpes zoster usually precedes the skin lesions by several days. *Tenderness of the sternum* may be quite pronounced in chronic myelogenous or acute leukemia, in myelofibrosis, or if the sternal marrow is invaded by lymphoma or myeloma.

GASTROINTESTINAL SYSTEM

Dysphagia has already been mentioned under ''Nasopharynx.'' *Anorexia* frequently occurs but usually has no specific diagnostic significance. Hypercalcemia and azotemia cause anorexia, nausea, and vomiting. A variety of ill-defined gastrointestinal complaints grouped under the heading ''indigestion'' may occur with hematologic diseases. *Abdominal fullness, premature satiety, belching,* or *discomfort* may occur because of a greatly enlarged spleen, but such splenomegaly may also be entirely asymptomatic. *Abdominal pain* may arise from intestinal obstruction by lymphoma, retroperitoneal bleeding, lead poisoning, ileus secondary to therapy with the *Vinca* alkaloids, acute hemolysis, allergic purpura, the abdominal crises of sickle cell disease, or acute intermittent porphyria. *Diarrhea* may occur in pernicious anemia. It also may be prominent in the various forms of intestinal malabsorption, although significant malabsorption may occur without diarrhea. Malabsorption may be a manifestation of small-bowel lymphoma. *Gastrointestinal bleeding* related to thrombocytopenia or other bleeding disorder may be entirely occult but often is manifest as *hematemesis* or *melena*. *Constipation* may occur in the patient with hypercalcemia or in one receiving treatment with the *Vinca* alkaloids.

GENITOURINARY AND REPRODUCTIVE SYSTEMS

Impotence or *bladder dysfunction* may occur with spinal cord or peripheral nerve damage due to one of the hematologic malignancies or with pernicious anemia. Priapism may occur in leukemia or sickle cell disease. *Hematuria* may be a manifestation of any of the bleeding disorders. *Red urine* may also occur with intravascular hemolysis (hemoglobinuria), myoglobinuria, or porphyrinuria. Injection of anthracycline drugs or ingestion of drugs such as pyridium regularly causes the urine to turn red. Beeturia also occurs as a benign genetic trait. *Amenorrhea* may accompany any serious disease. It may also be induced by certain drugs, such as antimetabolites or alkylating agents. *Menorrhagia* is a common cause of iron deficiency, and care must be taken to obtain an accurate history of the extent of menstrual blood loss. Semiquantification can be obtained from estimates of the number of days of heavy bleeding (usually 1 to 2), the number of days of any bleeding (usually 5 to 7), number of tampons or pads used, degree of blood soaking, and clots formed. Menorrhagia may occur in patients with bleeding disorders.

BACK AND EXTREMITIES

Back pain may accompany acute hemolytic reactions or be due to involvement of bone or the nervous system in malignant disease. It is one of the commonest manifestations of myeloma.

Arthritis or *arthralgia* may occur with gout secondary to increased uric acid production in patients with hematologic malignancies, myelofibrosis, or hemolytic anemia. They also occur in the plasma cell dyscrasias, acute leukemias, and sickle cell disease without evidence of gout, and in allergic purpura. Arthritis may accompany hemochromatosis. Hemarthroses in patients with severe bleeding disorders cause marked joint pain. Autoimmune diseases may present as anemia and/or thrombocytopenia, and arthritis appears as a later manifestation. *Shoulder pain* on the left may be due to infarction of the spleen and on the right from gall bladder disease associated with chronic hemolytic anemia such as hereditary spherocytosis. *Bone pain* may occur with bone involvement by the hematologic malignancies or metastatic tumor; it is common in the congenital hemolytic anemias, such as sickle cell anemia, and may occur in myelofibrosis. In patients with Hodgkin's disease, ingestion of alcohol may induce pain at the site of any lesion, including those in bone. *Edema* of the lower extremities, sometimes unilateral, may occur because of obstruction to veins or lymphatics by enlarged lymph nodes. *Leg ulcers* are a common complaint in sickle cell anemia and occur rarely in other hereditary anemias.

SKIN

Skin manifestations of hematologic disease may be of great importance; they include changes in texture or color, itching, and the presence of specific or nonspecific lesions. The skin in iron-deficient patients may become dry, the hair dry and fine, and the nails brittle. In hypothyroidism, which may cause anemia, the skin is dry, coarse, and scaly. *Jaundice* may be apparent with pernicious anemia or congenital or acquired hemolytic anemia. The skin of patients with pernicious anemia is said to be ''lemon yellow'' because of the simultaneous appearance of jaundice and pallor. Jaundice may also occur in patients with hematologic diseases as a result of liver involvement or biliary tract obstruction. *Pallor* is a common accompaniment of anemia, although some severely anemic patients may not appear pale. Widespread *erythroderma* occurs in cutaneous T-cell lymphoma and in some cases of chronic lymphocytic leukemia or lymphocytic lymphoma. The skin is often involved, sometimes severely, in graft-versus-host disease following marrow transplantation. Patients with hemachromatosis may have bronze or grayish pigmentation of the skin. *Cyanosis* occurs with methemoglobinemia, either hereditary or acquired; sulfhemoglobinemia; abnormal hemoglobins with low oxygen affinity; and primary and secondary polycythemia. Cyanosis of the ears or the fingertips may occur after exposure to cold in individuals with cryoglobulins or cold agglutinins.

Itching may occur in the absence of any visible skin lesions in Hodgkin's disease and may be extreme. Mycosis fungoides or other lymphomas with skin involvement may also present as itching. A significant number of patients with polycythemia vera will complain of itching after bathing.

Petechiae and *ecchymoses* are most often seen in the extremities in patients with thrombocytopenia, nonthrombocytopenic purpura, or nonthrombocytopenic bleeding disorders. Unless secondary to trauma, these lesions usually are painless, although the lesions of psychogenic purpura and erythema nodosum are painful. *Easy bruising* is a common complaint, especially among women, and when no other hemorrhagic symptoms are present, usually no abnormalities are found after detailed study. This symptom may, however, indicate a mild hereditary bleeding disorder, such as von Willebrand's disease or one of the platelet disorders.

Infiltrative lesions may occur in the leukemias and lymphomas and are sometimes the presenting complaint. *Necrotic lesions* may occur with intravascular coagulation, purpura fulminans, warfarin-induced skin necrosis, or rarely with exposure to cold in patients with circulating cryoproteins or cold agglutinins.

FAMILY HISTORY

A carefully obtained family history may be of great importance in the study of patients with hematologic disease. In the case of hemolytic disorders, questions should be asked regarding jaundice, anemia, and gallstones in relatives. In patients with disorders of hemostasis or venous thrombosis, particular attention must be given to bleeding manifestations, and clots in family members. In the case of autosomal recessive disorders such as pyruvate kinase deficiency the parents are usually not affected, but a similar clinical syndrome may have occurred in siblings. It is particularly important to inquire about siblings who may have died in infancy, since these may be forgotten, especially by older patients. When sex-linked inheritance is suspected, it is necessary to inquire about symptoms in the maternal grandfather, maternal uncles, male siblings, and nephews. In patients with disorders with dominant inheritance, such as hereditary spherocytosis, one may expect to find that one of the parents and possibly siblings and children of the patient have stigmata of the disease. Ethnic background may be important in the consideration of certain diseases such as thalassemia, sickle cell anemia, glucose-6-phosphate dehydrogenase deficiency, or other inherited disorders that are concentrated in geographic areas.

SEXUAL HISTORY

Because of the epidemic of infections with the human immunodeficiency viruses, it is important to ascertain the sexual preferences and risk factors of patients.

PHYSICAL EXAMINATION

A detailed physical examination should be performed on every patient, with sufficient attention paid to all systems to obtain a full evaluation of the general health of the individual. Certain body areas are especially pertinent to hematologic disease and therefore deserve special attention. These are the skin, eyes, tongue, lymph nodes, skeleton, spleen and liver, and nervous system.

SKIN

PALLOR AND FLUSHING

The color of the skin is due to the pigment contained therein and to the blood flowing through the skin capillaries. The component of skin color related to the blood may be a useful guide to anemia or polycythemia, since pallor may result when the hemoglobin level is reduced and redness when the hemoglobin level is increased. The amount of pigment in the skin will modify skin color and may mislead the clinician, as in individuals with pallor due to decreased pigment, or make skin color useless as a guide because of the intense pigmentation present.

Alterations in blood flow and in hemoglobin content may change skin color; this too may mislead the clinician. Thus emotion may cause either pallor or blushing. Exposure of the skin to cold or heat may similarly cause pallor or blushing. Chronic exposure to wind or sun may lead to permanent redness of the skin, and chronic ingestion of alcohol to a flushed face. The degree of erythema of the skin can be evaluated by pressing the thumb firmly against the skin, as on the forehead, so that the capillaries are emptied, and then comparing the color of the compressed spot with the surrounding skin immediately after the thumb is removed.

The mucous membranes and nail beds are usually more reliable guides to anemia or polycythemia than the skin. The conjunctivae and gums may be inflamed, however, and therefore not reflect the hemoglobin level, or the gums may appear pale because of pressure from the lips. The gums and the nail beds may also be pigmented and the capillaries correspondingly obscured. In some individuals, the color of the capillaries does not become fully visible through the nails unless pressure is applied to the fingertip, either laterally or on the end of the nail.

The palmar creases are useful guides to the hemoglobin level and appear pink in the fully opened hand unless the hemoglobin is 7 g/dl or less. Liver disease may induce flushing of the thenar and hypothenar eminences of the palm, even in patients with anemia.

CYANOSIS

The detection of cyanosis, like the detection of pallor, may be made difficult by skin pigmentation. Cyanosis is a function of the total amount of reduced hemoglobin, methemoglobin, or sulfhemoglobin present. The minimum amounts of these pigments that cause detectable cyanosis are about 5 g of reduced hemoglobin, 1.5 to 2.0 g of methemoglobin, and 0.5 g of sulfhemoglobin per deciliter of blood.

JAUNDICE

Jaundice may be observed in the skin of individuals who are not otherwise deeply pigmented or in the conjunctivae or the mucous membranes. The patient should be examined in daylight rather than under incandescent or fluorescent light, because the yellow color of the latter masks the yellow color of the patient. Jaundice is due to actual staining of the skin by bile pigment, and bilirubin glucuronide (direct-reacting or conjugated bilirubin) stains the skin more readily than the unconjugated form. Jaundice of the skin may not be visible if the bilirubin level is below 2 to 3 mg/dl. Yellow pigmentation of the skin may also occur with carotenemia, especially in young children.

PETECHIAE AND ECCHYMOSES

Petechiae are small (1 to 3 mm), round, red or brown lesions resulting from hemorrhage into the skin and are present primarily in areas with high venous pressure, such as the lower legs. These lesions do not blanch on pressure, and this can be demonstrated most readily by compressing the skin with a glass microscope slide or magnifying lens. Petechiae may occasionally be elevated slightly, i.e., palpable; this finding suggests vasculitis. Ecchymoses may be of various sizes and shapes and may be red, purple, blue, or yellowish green, depending on the intensity of the skin hemorrhage and its age. They may be flat or elevated; some are painful and tender. The lesions of hereditary hemorrhagic telangiectasia are small, flat, nonpulsatile, and violaceous. They blanch with pressure.

EXCORIATION

Itching may be intense in some hematologic disorders such as Hodgkin's disease, even in the absence of skin lesions. Excoriation of the skin from scratching is the only physical manifestation of this severe symptom.

LEG ULCERS

Open ulcers or scars from healed ulcers are often found in the region of the internal or external malleoli in patients with sickle cell anemia and, rarely, in other hereditary anemias.

NAILS

Detection of pallor or rubor by examining the nails was discussed earlier. The fingernails in chronic, severe iron-deficiency anemia may be ridged longitudinally and flattened or concave rather than convex. The latter change is referred to as *koilonychia* and is uncommon in present practice.

EYES

Jaundice, pallor, or *plethora* may be detected from examination of the eyes. Jaundice is usually more readily detected in the sclerae than in the skin. Ophthalmoscopic examination is also essential in patients with hematologic disease. *Retinal hemorrhages* and *exudates* occur in patients with severe anemia and thrombocytopenia. These hemorrhages are usually the typical "flame-shaped" hemorrhages, but they may be quite large and elevate the retina so that they may appear as a darkly colored tumor. Round hemorrhages with white centers are also often seen. *Dilatation of the veins* may be seen in polycythemia; in patients with macroglobulinemia, the veins are engorged and segmented, resembling link sausages.

MOUTH

Pallor of the mucosa has already been discussed. *Ulceration* of the oral mucosa occurs commonly in neutropenic patients. In leukemia there may also be infiltration of the gums with swelling, redness, and bleeding. *Bleeding* from the mucosa may occur with a hemorrhagic disease. A dark line of lead sulfide may be deposited in the gums at the base of the teeth in lead poisoning. The *tongue* may be completely smooth in pernicious anemia and iron-deficiency anemia. Patients with an upper dental prosthesis may also have papillary atrophy, presumably on a mechanical basis. The tongue may be smooth and red in patients with nutritional deficiencies. This may be accompanied by fissuring at the corners of the mouth, but fissuring may also be due to ill-fitting dentures.

LYMPH NODES

Lymph nodes are widely distributed in the body, and in disease any node or group of nodes may be involved. The major concern on physical examination is the detection of enlarged or tender nodes in the cervical, supraclavicular, axillary, epitrochlear, inguinal, or femoral regions. Under normal conditions in adults, the only readily palpable lymph nodes are in the inguinal region, where several firm nodes 0.5 to 2.0 cm long are normally attached to the dense fascia below the inguinal ligament and in the femoral triangle. In children, multiple small (0.5 to 1.0 cm) nodes may be palpated in the cervical region as well. Supraclavicular nodes may sometimes be palpable only when the patient performs the Valsalva maneuver.

Enlarged lymph nodes are ordinarily detected in the superficial areas by palpation, although they are sometimes large enough to be seen. Palpation should be gentle and is best performed with a circular motion of the fingertips, using slowly increasing pressure.

Nodes too deep to palpate may be detected by radiologic examination, including computerized tomography, magnetic resonance imaging, radiographic lymphangiography, isotopic lymphangiography, or by ultrasound.

CHEST

Increased rib or sternal tenderness is an important physical sign often ignored. Increased bone pain may be generalized, as in leukemia, or spotty, as in plasma cell myeloma or in metastatic tumors. The superficial surfaces of all bones should be examined thoroughly by applying intermittent firm pressure with the fingertips to locate potential areas of disease.

SPLEEN[5–8]

The normal adult spleen is usually not palpable on physical examination but occasionally may be felt. Palpability of the normal spleen

may be related to body habitus, but there is disagreement on this point. Enlarged spleens may be detected by percussion, palpation, or a combination of these two methods. Some enlarged spleens may be visible through the abdominal wall.

The normal spleen weighs about 150 g and lies in the peritoneal cavity against the diaphragm and the posterolateral abdominal wall at the level of the lower three ribs. As it enlarges it remains close to the abdominal wall, while the lower pole moves downward, anteriorly, and to the right. Spleens enlarged only 40 percent above normal may be palpable, but significant splenic enlargement may occur and the organ still not be felt on physical examination. A good but imperfect correlation has been reported between spleen size estimated from radioisotope scanning or ultrasonography and spleen weight determined after splenectomy or at autopsy. Although it is common to fail to palpate an enlarged spleen on physical examination, palpation of a normal-sized spleen is unusual, and therefore a palpable spleen is usually a significant physical finding.

In examining for an enlarged spleen, it should be remembered that the organ lies just beneath the abdominal wall and that it is identified by its movement during respiration. The splenic notch may be evident if the organ is moderately enlarged. During the examination the patient lies in a relaxed, supine position. The examiner, standing on the patient's right, gently palpates the left upper abdomen with the right hand while exerting pressure forward with the palm of the left hand placed over the lower ribs posterolaterally. If nothing is felt, the palpation should be performed repeatedly, moving the examining hand about 2 cm toward the inguinal ligament each time. It is often advantageous to carry out the examination initially with the patient lying on the right side with left knee flexed and to repeat it with the patient supine.

It is not always possible to be sure that a left upper quadrant mass is spleen; masses in the stomach, colon, kidney, or pancreas may mimic splenomegaly on physical examination. When there is uncertainty regarding the nature of a mass in the left upper quadrant, imaging procedures will usually permit accurate diagnosis.

LIVER[7–11]

Palpation of the edge of the liver in the right upper quadrant of the abdomen is commonly used to detect hepatic enlargement, although the inaccuracies of this method have been demonstrated. It is necessary to determine both the upper and lower borders of the liver by percussion in order to properly assess liver size. The normal liver may be palpable as much as 4 to 5 cm below the right costal margin but is usually not palpable in the epigastrium. The height of liver dullness is best measured in a specific line 8, 10, or 12 cm to the right of the midline. Techniques should be standardized so that serial measurements can be made. The vertical span of the normal liver determined in this manner will range about 10 cm in an average-size man and about 2 cm smaller in women. Because of variations introduced by technique, each physician should determine the normal area of liver dullness by his or her own procedure. Correlation of radioisotope imaging data with results from routine physical examinations indicates that often a liver of normal size is considered enlarged on physical examination and an enlarged liver is considered normal. Imaging procedures are useful in demonstrating localized infiltrative lesions.

NERVOUS SYSTEM

A thorough evaluation of neurologic function is necessary in many patients with hematologic disease. Vitamin B_{12} deficiency impairs cerebral, olfactory, spinal cord, and peripheral nerve function, and severe chronic deficiency may lead to irreversible neurologic degeneration. Leukemic meningitis is often manifested by headache, visual impairment, or cranial nerve dysfunction. Tumor growth in the brain or spinal cord compression may be due to malignant lymphoma or plasma cell myeloma. A variety of neurologic abnormalities may develop in patients with various leukemias and lymphomas as a consequence of infiltration, bleeding, or infection.

JOINTS

Deformities of the knees, elbows, ankles, shoulders, wrists, or hips may be the result of repeated hemorrhage in patients with hemophilia A, hemophilia B, or severe factor VII deficiency. Often, a target joint is prominently affected.

REFERENCES

1. Bates B: *A Guide to Physical Examination and History Taking,* 6th ed. Lippincott, Philadelphia, 1995.
2. Mor V, Laliberte L, Morris JN, Wiemann M: The Karnovsky Performance Status Scale: an examination of its reliability and validity in a research setting. *Cancer* 53:2002, 1984.
3. Sackett DL: A primer on the precision and accuracy of the clinical examination. *JAMA* 267:2638, 1992.
4. Enelow AJ, Forde DL, Brummel-Smith K: *Interviewing and Patient Care,* 4th ed. Oxford University Press, Oxford, 1996.
5. Arkles LB, Gill GD, Nolan MP: A palpable spleen is not necessarily enlarged or pathological. *Med J Aust* 145:15, 1986.
6. Barkun AN, Camus M, Green L, et al: The bedside assessment of splenic enlargement. *Am J Med* 91:512, 1991.
7. Halpern S, Coel M, Ashburn W, et al: Correlation of liver and spleen size: determinations by nuclear medicine studies and physical examination. *Arch Intern Med* 134:123, 1974.
8. Downey MT: Estimation of splenic weight from ultrasonographic measurements. *Can Assn Rad J* 43:273, 1992.
9. Castell DO, O'Brien KD, Muench H, Chalmers TC: Estimation of liver size by percussion in normal individuals. *Ann Intern Med* 70:1183, 1969.
10. Bennett WF, Dova JG: Review of hepatic imaging and a problem-oriented approach to liver masses. *Hepatology* 12:761, 1990.
11. Barloon TJ, Brown BP, Abu-Yousef MM, et al: Teaching physical examination of the adult liver with the use of real-time sonography. *Acad Radiol* 5:101, 1998.

EXAMINATION OF THE BLOOD

DANIEL H. RYAN

Examination of the blood is central to the diagnosis and management of hematologic diseases. In few other disciplines can the physician make a specific diagnosis and monitor therapy with easily accessible tissue samples and readily available methodologies, many of which can be performed in a physician's office. Assessment of the prevalence of red cells, of the several types of leukocytes, and of platelets, usually from automated particle counters, and examination of the blood film for qualitative changes in the appearance of red cells, leukocytes, and platelets, and the presence of marrow precursors, malignant cells, and intracellular parasites can be used to diagnose specific diseases, gain insight into pathophysiology, and measure the response to treatment.

The blood is examined in order to answer two principal questions: Is the marrow producing sufficient numbers of mature cells in the hematopoietic lineages? Is the development of each hematopoietic lineage qualitatively normal? Quantitative measures routinely available from automated cell counters are generally reliable and provide a rapid and cost-effective way to screen for major disturbances of hematopoiesis. Morphologic observation of the blood film is essential to confirm certain quantitative results and to investigate qualitatively abnormal differentiation of the hematopoeitic lineages. Based on examination of the blood, the physician is directed toward a more focused assessment of the marrow or to systemic disorders which secondarily involve the hematopoietic system. Table 2-1 lists blood cell values in a normal population.

The complete blood count is a necessary part of the diagnostic workup in a broad variety of clinical conditions. Similarly, the leukocyte differential count and examination of the blood film, in spite of limitations as a screening test for occult disease,[1] is important in sorting out the differential diagnosis in most ill patients. Quantitative and morphologic examination of the formed elements of the peripheral blood are for convenience considered separately in this chapter, but it should be understood that the distinction between these two is not absolute, and measures once strictly confined to the "qualitative" realm can become quantifiable and routinely measurable as technology advances.

QUANTITATIVE MEASURES OF HEMATOPOIETIC ELEMENTS IN THE BLOOD

In a typical automated blood cell counter, the aspirated blood sample is separated into two portions, one of which is lysed and diluted to permit measurement of hemoglobin concentration and leukocyte enumeration, and the other which is diluted without lysis to enable counting and sizing of red cells and platelets. Some recently developed instruments offer automated reticulocyte counting as well.

RED CELLS

Most automated blood cell counters measure the red cell count, MCV (mean corpuscular volume), and hemoglobin concentration directly. All other red cell parameters, including the hematocrit, are derived from these primary values. The red cell count is most commonly measured by passing a well-mixed sample of blood diluted in an electrolyte solution through a small orifice through which the electrical impedance can be measured.[2] Each cell causes a jump in impedance as it passes through the opening, since it cannot readily conduct an electrical signal through its lipid membrane. Red cells are distinguished from platelets by the magnitude of the impedance signal, which is proportional to cell size. Alternatively, red cells and other hematopoietic elements can be counted and sized by measuring the intensity and angle at which laser light is scattered as the cells pass by.

MEASUREMENT OF THE RED CELL COUNT AND HEMATOCRIT

In electronic instruments the hematocrit (proportion of blood volume occupied by erythrocytes) is calculated from direct measurements of the erythrocyte count and the mean corpuscular volume: (Hct $(\mu l/100\ \mu l)$ = [RBC in millions per $\mu l \times$ MCV in fl] ÷ 10). Falsely elevated MCV and decreased red cell counts can be observed when red cell autoantibodies are present and retain binding capability at room temperature, particularly cold agglutinins and in some cases of autoimmune hemolytic anemia.[3] This causes red cells to clump and, by affecting the accuracy of both RBC count and MCV, also affects the derived hematocrit.

The hematocrit may also be determined by subjecting the blood to sufficient centrifugal force to pack the cells into as small a volume as possible.[4] Before standardized methods for hemoglobin quantitation were available, the hematocrit was the best method of determining adequacy of red cell production. However, the "spun" hematocrit is a manual procedure not well adapted to routine processing in a high-volume clinical laboratory. The microhematocrit includes plasma trapped between red cells in the packed cell volume,[5] which is a source of systematic bias between the "spun" and automated hematocrit. The amount of plasma remaining in the packed cells is typically about 2 to 3 percent.[6,7] Microhematocrits from blood containing abnormal erythrocytes (sickle cell anemia, thalassemia, iron deficiency, spherocytosis, macrocytosis) are relatively increased because of enhanced plasma trapping that generally is due to increased red cell rigidity.[6,7] Fully oxygenated blood also has about a 2 percent lower hematocrit than deoxygenated blood.[8] In polycythemic samples (Hct > 55), plasma trapping is commonly increased. Therefore, although automated hematocrit values are adjusted to be equivalent to spun hematocrit for normal samples, in abnormal samples, the spun hematocrit may be artifactually elevated (up to 6% in microcytosis[9]). In general, the automated hematocrit is more accurate and easier to routinely obtain than the spun hematocrit, although the hemoglobin determination is preferred to either, as it is directly measured.

MEASUREMENT OF HEMOGLOBIN

Hemoglobin is intensely colored, and this property has been utilized in methods for estimating its concentration in blood. Erythrocytes contain a mixture of hemoglobin, oxyhemoglobin, carboxyhemoglobin, methemoglobin, and minor amounts of other forms of hemoglobin. To determine hemoglobin concentration in the peripheral blood, red cells are lysed and hemoglobin variants are converted to the stable compound cyanmethemoglobin for quantitation by absorption at 540 nm.[10] All forms of hemoglobin are readily converted to cyanmethemo-

TABLE 2-1   BLOOD CELL VALUES IN A NORMAL POPULATION*

	MEN	WOMEN
White cell count, 10^3/ml blood	7.8 (4.4–11.3)	
Red cell count, 10^6/ml blood	5.21 (4.52–5.90)	4.60 (4.10–5.10)
Hemoglobin, g/dl blood	15.7 (14.0–17.5)	13.8 (12.3–15.3)
Hematocrit (%)	46 (42–50)	40 (36–45)
Mean corpuscular volume, fl/red cell	88.0 (80.0–96.1)	
Mean corpuscular hemoglobin, pg/red cell	30.4 (27.5–33.2)	
Mean corpuscular hemoglobin concentration, g/dl RBC	34.4 (33.4–35.5)	
Red cell distribution width, CV (%)	13.1 (11.5–14.5)	
Platelet count, 10^3/ml blood	311 (172–450)	

*The mean and reference intervals (normal range) are given. Because the distribution curves may be nongaussian, the reference interval is the nonparametric central 95 percent confidence interval. Results are based on 426 normal adult men and 212 normal adult women, with studies performed on the Coulter Model S-Plus IV. This table is provided as a guide. Normal ranges should be validated by the clinical laboratory for the specific methods in use.

globin except sulfhemoglobin, which is rarely present in significant amounts. In automated blood cell counters, hemoglobin is accurately and directly measured, and hence this determination is preferable to the hematocrit for the diagnosis of anemia. In practice, the major interference with this measurement is chylomicronemia.[11] Methodological improvements in recent instrumentation may minimize this interference.[12]

The hemoglobin level varies with age (see Table 2-2). Changes in hemoglobin in the neonatal period are discussed in Chap. 7. After the first week or two of extrauterine life, the hemoglobin falls from levels of about 17 g/dl to levels of about 12 g/dl by 2 months of age. Thereafter the levels remain relatively constant throughout the first year of life. Any child with a hemoglobin level below 11 g/dl should be considered to be anemic.[13,14] Changes in hemoglobin levels in the elderly are discussed in Chap. 8.

DETERMINATION OF SIZE AND HEMOGLOBIN CONTENT OF ERYTHROCYTES (RED CELL INDICES)

The size and hemoglobin content of erythrocytes (red cell indices) have traditionally been used to assist in the differential diagnosis of anemia.[15] In current practice, the most useful parameter is the MCV.[16,17]

Automated blood counters measure the MCV directly using the Coulter principle,[2] in which the cross-sectional area of a nonconducting particle (i.e., any cell) in an electrolyte solution is proportional to the increase in electrical impedance as the particle passes through a narrow orifice.[18] The MCV has been used to guide the diagnostic workup in patients with anemia, for example, testing patients with microcytic

anemia for iron deficiency or thalassemia,[17] and those with macrocytic anemia for folate or B_{12} deficiency.[19] This assumption has practical value, but its limitations should be recognized,[20] for instance, in elderly patients with megaloblastic anemia, who may have an MCV in the normal range.[21] In about one-third of elderly patients, the cause of an elevated MCV is not evident.[22] Numerous mathematical manipulations of the red cell indices, particularly the MCV and red cell count, have been devised to assist in the differential diagnosis of iron deficiency anemia and thalassemia,[23] but their utility has been questioned[24] due to significant overlap and the availability of more definitive tests for these conditions.

The other red cell indices are less useful in clinical decision-making. The MCH (mean corpuscular hemoglobin, or the amount of hemoglobin per red cell) is calculated by the formula MCH (pg/cell) = [hemoglobin in g/dl ÷ red cell count in millions/μl] × 10. Changes in MCH accompany similar alterations in the MCV and generally provide little additional diagnostic information. The MCHC (mean corpuscular hemoglobin concentration, or the concentration of hemoglobin in the red cell volume) is calculated by the formula MCHC (g/dl) = [hemoglobin in g/dl ÷ hematocrit in μl/100 μl] × 100. An MCHC greater than 35 has been associated with hereditary spherocytosis,[25] and low MCHC is typical of iron deficiency,[26] but its diagnostic usefulness is limited.[27] The dynamic range of the MCHC measurement in most automated instruments is limited by technical considerations,[28] but technical improvements in newer instruments may improve the usefulness of this parameter.[12] In the clinical laboratory, the MCHC is useful as a warning of potential interferences with the measurement of MCV or RBC count. For instance, an abnormally low MCHC suggests the possibility of artifactually high MCV due to osmotic shifts that occur when red cells from patients with severe hyperglycemia are diluted in saline prior to analysis.[29]

The MCV, MCH, and MCHC are average quantities and therefore may not detect abnormalities in blood with mixed-cell populations. For example, patients with sideroblastic anemia usually have a dimorphic blood picture, with both hypochromic and normochromic cells. The indices may be in the normal range, and the important finding of the mixed-cell population would not be detected. It is possible to identify mixed populations by direct examination of a histogram of MCV (or

TABLE 2-2   NORMAL LEUKOCYTE COUNT, DIFFERENTIAL COUNT, AND HEMOGLOBIN CONCENTRATION AT VARIOUS AGES*

AGE	LEUKOCYTES (× 10^3/μl)	NEUTROPHILS			EOSINOPHILS	BASOPHILS	LYMPHOCYTES	MONOCYTES	HEMOGLOBIN g/dl BLOOD
		TOTAL	BAND	SEGMENTED					
12 mo	11.4(6.0–17.5)	3.5(1.5–8.5) *31*	0.35 *3.1*	3.2(1.0–8.5) *28*	0.30(0.05–0.70) *2.6*	0.05(0–0.20) *0.4*	7.0(4.0–10.5) *61*	0.55(0.05–1.1) *4.8*	12.6(11.1–14.1)
4 yr	9.1(5.5–15.5)	3.8(1.5–8.5) *42*	0.27(0–1.0) *3.0*	3.5(1.5–7.5) *39*	0.25(0.02–0.65) *2.8*	0.05(0–0.2) *0.6*	4.5(2.0–8.0) *50*	0.45(0–0.8) *5.0*	12.7(11.2–14.3)
6 yr	8.5(5.0–14.5)	4.3(1.5–8.0) *51*	0.25(0–1.0) *3.0*	4.0(1.5–7.0) *48*	0.23(0–0.65) *2.7*	0.05(0–0.2) *0.6*	3.5(1.5–7.0) *42*	0.40(0–0.8) *4.7*	13.0(11.4–14.5)
10 yr	8.1(4.5–13.5)	4.4(1.8–8.0) *54*	0.24(0–1.0) *3.0*	4.2(1.8–7.0) *51*	0.20(0–0.60) *2.4*	0.04(0–0.2) *0.5*	3.1(1.5–6.5) *38*	0.35(0–0.8) *4.3*	13.4(11.8–15.0)
21 yr	7.4(4.5–11.0)	4.4(1.8–7.7) *59*	0.22(0–0.7) *3.0*	4.2(1.8–7.0) *56*	0.20(0–0.45) *2.7*	0.04(0–0.2) *0.5*	2.5(1.0–4.8) *34*	0.30(0–0.8) *4.0*	M 15.5(13.5–17.5) F 13.8(12.0–15.6)

*For leukocyte and differential count, see PL Altman and DS Dittmer (eds), *Blood and Other Body Fluids*. Federation of American Societies for Experimental Biology, Washington, DC, 1961. By permission. For hemoglobin concentration, see AM Rudolph and JI Hoffman (eds), in *Pediatrics*, 18th ed, pp 1011, 1012. Appleton and Lange, Norwalk, CT, 1987. The numbers in italic type are mean percentages. This table is provided as a guide. Normal ranges should be validated by the clinical laboratory for the specific methods in use.

red cell hemoglobin concentration, in instruments that measure this parameter on individual cells[30]) values for individual cells that is printed out by the instrument but typically not included in the laboratory report. Another index, the red cell distribution width (RDW), is specifically designed to reflect the variability of red cell size. It is based on the width of the red blood cell volume distribution curve, with larger values indicating greater variability. An elevated RDW may be an early sign of iron deficiency anemia,[31,32] and, although proposed as an aid in distinguishing iron deficiency from other causes of microcytic anemia,[33] the RDW is not sufficiently diagnostic to obviate the need for more specific tests.[34] The RDW can be used in the laboratory as a flag to select which samples submitted for automated blood count should have manual review of the blood film for red cell morphology.

As with any laboratory test, the clinical use of these red cell parameters depends on the prevalence of disease and the clinical setting. For instance, the Centers for Disease Control recommends routine hemoglobin screening and a 1-month therapeutic trial of oral iron for those with anemia in populations at particularly high risk of iron-deficiency anemia (9- to 18-month-old infants, pregnant women). In the absence of clinical evidence for other causes of anemia, a further workup beyond hemoglobin measurement is recommended only if the hemoglobin is not increased by at least 1 g/dl during the therapeutic trial.[35] In contrast, for other populations, anemia detected during routine medical examinations should be fully evaluated for its cause.[35]

LEUKOCYTES

LEUKOCYTE COUNT

Leukocyte counts are performed by automated blood counters on blood samples appropriately diluted with a solution that lyses the erythrocytes (e.g., acid or a detergent) but preserves leukocyte integrity. Manual counting of leukocytes is used only when the instrument reports a potential interference or the count is beyond instrument linearity limits. Manual counts are subject to much greater technical variation than automated counts due to technical and statistical factors. Leukocyte counts may be falsely elevated due to cryoglobulins or cryofibrinogen,[36] clumped platelets or fibrin from an inadequately anticoagulated or mixed sample,[37] EDTA-induced platelet aggregation,[38] nucleated red blood cells (RBCs),[37] or nonlysed RBCs. These interferences cause a population of small-sized particles to appear in the leukocyte volume histogram and trigger a flag for manual review.[39]

LEUKOCYTE DIFFERENTIAL

Leukocytes in the peripheral blood serve different functions and arise from different hematopoietic lineages, so it is important to separately evaluate each of the major leukocyte types. The size differences among lymphocytes, monocytes, and neutrophils were initially used to produce a "three-part" leukocyte differential. Modern automated instruments use additional parameters (typically light scatter at different angles or electrical conductivity) to identify and enumerate the five major morphologic leukocyte types in peripheral blood. Complex algorithms flag samples likely to contain abnormal cells (or variants such as immature granulocytes and reactive lymphocytes) for manual review.[40] "Band neutrophils" cannot be specifically identified by any current automated cell counter but usually trigger a manual review flag if present in increased numbers. Current instruments can perform an accurate automated "five-part" differential without need for manual review in about 50 to 80 percent of samples from medical center patient populations.[40,41] It should be recognized, however, that small numbers of abnormal cells can escape detection by either automated or manual methods. The false negative rate for detection of abnormal cells varies from 1 to 20 percent, depending on the instrument and

the detection limit desired (1–5% abnormal cells).[42–44] Lymphoma cells and reactive lymphocytes are the most problematic[41] for both automated instruments and the human observer. If one needs to search for infrequent abnormal cells or evaluate leukocyte morphology, there is still no substitute for examination of a properly stained blood film by a trained observer. In spite of instrumentation that permits automated analysis of a majority of clinical samples, the test is still quite labor-intensive relative to other high-volume laboratory tests, and its value as a case-finding tool in screening of asymptomatic patients has been questioned.[1,45]

The normal differential leukocyte count varies with age (see Table 2-2). As described in Chap. 7, in the first few days after birth polymorphonuclear neutrophils are predominant, but thereafter lymphocytes account for the majority of leukocytes. This persists up to about 4 to 5 years of age, when the polymorphonuclear leukocyte again becomes the predominant cell and remains so throughout the rest of childhood and adult life. Changes in the leukocyte count in the elderly are discussed in Chap. 8. The leukocyte count may decrease slightly in older subjects because of a fall in the lymphocyte count. The reference range for neutrophil counts is lower in African Americans, Africans, and some Middle Eastern populations than caucasians (Table 2-3).[46–49]

PLATELETS

Platelets are usually counted electronically by enumerating particles in the unlysed sample within a specified volume window (e.g., 2–20 fl). The platelet count was more difficult to automate than the red cell count, because of the small size, tendency to aggregate, and potential overlap of platelets with more numerous red cells. Current instruments typically construct a platelet volume histogram based on measured platelet size within the platelet volume window and mathematically extrapolate this histogram to account for platelets whose size overlaps with debris or small red cells. The normal platelet count is lower in individuals of African ethnic origin[49] (Table 2-3).

Since platelet volumes in health or disease follow a log-normal distribution,[50] volume histograms not consistent with such a distribution are flagged for manual review. Automated platelet counting by current instrumentation is accurate and reliable, even in the thrombocytopenic range,[51] and far more precise than manual methods.[51] Platelet counts by either manual or automated methods may be falsely decreased if the sample is incompletely anticoagulated (often indicated by small clots in the specimen or fibrin strands on the stained film). Infrequently, it may be necessary to confirm automated results by a manual (phase contrast) platelet count or platelet estimate from the blood film when potential interferences are present. These include severe microcytosis and leukocyte fragmentation (falsely elevated count) or platelet clumping/"satellitism" (falsely decreased count). Current instruments are able to identify and flag samples when these interferences are present. Some newer automated cell counters incorporate novel approaches, such as staining with antiglycoprotein IIIa antibody or volume/refractive index two-parameter measurement, to minimize the need for manual review of the platelet count.[12] Platelet clumping, or platelet satellitism (adherence of platelets to neutrophils), may occur due to platelet reactive antibodies,[52] which cause no clinical symptoms. Paradoxically, these antibodies recognize epitopes on adhesion molecules which are exposed in the absence of divalent cations, and so become activated in EDTA- or citrate-anticoagulated blood specimens.[52] This condition occurs in about 0.1 percent of hospitalized patients, and the origin of the thrombocytopenia in such cases can be suspected by the appearance of small particles (representing the platelet clumps) on the leukocyte volume histogram.[39] Platelet counting under these conditions is difficult but can be minimized by collecting blood in

TABLE 2-3   ETHNIC DIFFERENCES IN NORMAL BLOOD CELL VALUES

	Men			Women		
	CAUCASIAN n = 100	AFROCARRIBEAN n = 51	AFRICAN n = 65	CAUCASIAN n = 100	AFROCARRIBEAN n = 51	AFRICAN n = 50
White cell count*	5.7 (3.6–9.2)	5.2 (2.8–9.5)	4.5 (2.8–7.2)	6.2 (3.5–10.8)	5.7 (3.3–9.9)	5.0 (3.2–7.8)
Neutrophil count	3.2 (1.7–6.1)	2.5 (1.0–5.8)	2.0 (0.9–4.2)	3.6 (1.7–7.5)	3.0 (1.4–6.5)	2.4 (1.3–4.2)
Lymphocyte count	1.7 (1.0–2.9)	1.9 (1.0–3.6)	1.8 (1.0–3.2)	1.8 (1.0–3.5)	2.0 (1.2–3.4)	2.0 (1.1–3.6)
Monocyte count	0.34 (0.18–0.62)	0.33 (0.18–0.52)	0.29 (0.15–0.58)	0.30 (0.14–0.61)	0.31 (0.16–0.59)	0.28 (0.15–0.39)
Eosinophil count	0.12 (0.03–0.48)	0.13 (0.03–0.58)	0.12 (0.02–0.79)	0.13 (0.04–0.44)	0.10 (0.03–0.33)	0.10 (0.02–0.41)
Platelet count	218 (143–332)	196 (122–313)	183 (115–290)	246 (169–358)	236 (149–374)	207 (125–342)

*Adapted from Bain et al.[49] All counts expressed ×10³/μl; geometric mean and 95% reference range, with studies performed on the Bayer-Technicon H.2 counter. This table is provided as a guide. Normal ranges should be validated by the clinical laboratory for the specific methods in use.

citrate[39] or estimating platelet count from a freshly prepared fingerstick blood smear.

Platelet volume is measured in the same fashion as red cell size, and the mean platelet volume (MPV) has been proposed as a clinically useful tool in the differential diagnosis of thrombocytopenias[53] and as a risk factor for thrombotic disease.[54,55] Increased MPV may be related in a complex way to thrombopoietic stimulus[56] and not platelet age per se.[57] However, in spite of the known association of increased platelet size on blood films with consumptive thrombocytopenias, platelet size is a difficult parameter to accurately quantitate and use diagnostically, because of a wide physiologic variation of the MPV in normal subjects (i.e., Mediterranean macrothrombocytopenia[58,59]) and susceptibility of anticoagulated platelets to time-dependent swelling in vitro.[60] A platelet volume distribution width (PDW) can be calculated just as the RDW and is correlated with platelet count and MPV.[61] This measurement has yet to find an established clinical use, although a higher-than-expected PDW has been observed in thrombocytoses due to myeloproliferative disease.[61]

MORPHOLOGIC EXAMINATION OF THE BLOOD

Microscopic examination of the blood spread on a glass slide or coverslip yields useful information regarding all the formed elements of the blood. The process of preparing a thin blood film causes mechanical trauma to the cells. Also, the cells flatten on the glass during drying, and the fixation and staining involve exposure to methanol and water. Some artifacts are inevitably introduced, but these can be minimized by good technique. The optimal part of the stained blood film to use for morphologic examination of the formed blood elements should be sufficiently thin that only a few erythrocytes in a 100× field touch each other but not so thin that no red cells are touching. Selection of a portion of the blood film for analysis that is too thick or too thin for proper morphologic evaluation is by far the most common error in blood film interpretation. For example, leukemic blasts may appear dense and rounded and lose their characteristic features when viewed in the thick part of the film. For specific purposes, the thick portion or side and "feathered" edges of the film are of interest (for instance, to detect microfilariae and malarial parasites or to search for large abnormal cells and platelet clumps). It is sometimes advantageous to examine fresh blood diluted in saline under the microscope to avoid artifacts of fixation or staining which may mimic spherocytosis or acanthocytosis.

The blood film is first scanned at medium power (×20) to confirm reasonably even distribution of leukocytes and check for abnormally large or immature cells in the side and feathered edges of the film. The feathered edge is examined for platelet clumps. Abnormal cells, red cell aggregation or rouleaux, background bluish staining consistent with paraproteinemia, and parasites are all findings that can be sug-

gested by medium-power examination. The optimal portion of the film is then examined at high power (50–100×, oil immersion) to systematically assess the size, shape, and morphology of the major hematopoietic lineages.

RED CELL MORPHOLOGY

Erythrocytes should be examined for size, shape, hemoglobin concentration and distribution, staining properties, distribution on the film, and inclusions (see Plates I–IV).

Normal erythrocytes on dried films are nearly uniform in size, with a normal distribution about a mean of 7.2 to 7.9 μm. Erythrocyte diameter can be evaluated by the use of a micrometer disc inserted into the microscope, although experienced morphologists usually evaluate erythrocyte size without this aid. It is helpful to compare erythrocyte size with the similar diameter of small lymphocyte nuclei. Note that the MCV is a more sensitive measure of red cell volume than the red cell diameter. However, an experienced observer should be able to recognize abnormalities in average red cell size when the MCV is markedly elevated or decreased. *Anisocytosis* is used to describe variation in erythrocyte size and is the morphologic correlate of the RDW. *Macrocytes* may be seen in a number of disease states. Cells are considered to be macrocytes if they are well hemoglobinized and their diameters exceed 9 μm. Early ("shift") *reticulocytes* (i.e., those with the most residual RNA) appear in stained films as large, bluish cells, often referred to as *polychromatophilic* cells. *Microcyte* is the term used to describe a cell less than 6 μm in diameter.

The normal erythrocyte on a dried film is round with central pallor. *Poikilocytosis* is a term used to describe variations in the shape of erythrocytes. The predominant appearance of a specific abnormality in red cell shape can be an important diagnostic clue in patients with anemia. These are described in detail in Chap. 22 and Plates I–IV. Erythrocytes with evenly spaced spikes (crenated cells) can be an artifact caused by prolonged storage or may reflect metabolic erythrocyte abnormalities.

The normal erythrocyte appears as a disc with a rim of hemoglobin and a clear central area. The central pallor normally occupies less than one-half the diameter of the cells. Increased central pallor (*hypochromia*) is associated with disorders characterized by diminished hemoglobin synthesis. Evaluation of red cell hemoglobinization as well as red cell size is completely dependent on examining the proper part of the blood film. Cells at the far feathered edge will always be large and lack central pallor, while cells in the thick part of the film will look small and rounded and will also lack central pallor. A sharp refractile border demarcating the central area of pallor is an artifact secondary to inadequate drying of the film before staining (due to high humidity, and more common in anemic samples). *Spherocytes* are more densely stained and appear smaller because of their rounded shape and will show decreased or absent central pallor. Some automated blood counters produce a histogram of red cell hemoglobin concentration that identifies hypochromic, normochromic, and hyperchromic populations.[62] The hemoglobin may appear to be abnormally distributed in erythrocytes, particularly in a form of cell in which there is a spot or disc of hemoglobin in the center surrounded by a clear area which is in turn surrounded by a rim of hemoglobin at the outer edge of the cell, giving the appearance of a target—a *target cell*. This is in reality a cup-shaped cell which is distorted as it is flattened on the glass slide. These cells are typically found in disorders of hemoglobin synthesis (e.g., thalassemia, iron deficiency), where the cell surface to cell volume ratio is high.

Erythrocytes are usually distributed evenly throughout the film. In some films the cells become aligned in aggregates (rouleaux) resembling stacks of coins. Such rouleaux formation is normal in the thicker part of the film; when found in the optimal viewing portion of the film, it may be due to the presence of a paraprotein and suggests the diagnosis of plasma cell myeloma or macroglobulinemia.

Inclusions that may be observed in erythrocytes on films stained with Wright stain are described in Chap. 22.

PLATELET MORPHOLOGY

Platelets appear in normal stained blood as small blue or colorless bodies with red or purple granules (see Plates XII and XIII). Normal platelets average about 1 to 2 μm in diameter but show wide variation in shape, from round to elongated, cigar-shaped forms. A rough estimate of the platelet count can be made by observation of the stained blood film. If the platelet count is normal, approximately 8 to 15 platelets (individually or in small clumps) should be visible in each $100\times$ oil-immersion field. There should be one platelet present for every 10 to 30 erythrocytes. This is a valuable check when the automated platelet count is in question or an unexpected result is obtained.

In improperly prepared films, platelets may form large aggregates in some areas and appear to be diminished or absent in others. The occurrence of giant platelets or platelet masses may indicate a myeloproliferative disorder (see Chap. 118) or improper collection of the blood specimen. The latter circumstance can occur when venipuncture technique is faulty and platelets become activated before the blood sample is thoroughly mixed with anticoagulant. These platelet masses are readily recognized (typically in the feathered edge of the film), but this maldistribution may create a mistaken impression of thrombocytopenia if the aggregates are not detected. Platelet clumping throughout the blood film, or platelet satellitism (adherence of platelets to neutrophils), may be due to platelet agglutinins as previously discussed (see Plates XII and XIII).

A platelet will occasionally overlie an erythrocyte, where it may be mistaken for an inclusion body or a parasite. The differentiation depends on the observation of a halo around the platelet, determination that it lies above the plane of the erythrocyte, and observation of the characteristics of a normal platelet in the ''inclusion.''

LEUKOCYTE MORPHOLOGY

The distribution of leukocytes on glass slides is not uniform, and the larger cells, such as monocytes and polymorphonuclear leukocytes, tend to be concentrated on the side and feathered edges of the film. The cells that are normally found in blood are polymorphonuclear leukocytes of the neutrophilic, eosinophilic, and basophilic types; lymphocytes; and monocytes (see Plates VII and VIII). These cell types are described below, and normal values for the differential count are presented in Table 2-2.

Neutrophils are round cells ranging from 10 to 14 μm in diameter (see Plate VII). The nucleus is lobulated, with two to five lobes connected by a thin chromatin thread. The defining feature of the mature neutrophil is the round lobes with condensed chromatin, since the chromatin thread may overlie the nucleus and not be visible. The chromatin stains purple and is coarse and arranged in clumps. The nucleus of 1 to 16 percent of the neutrophils from females may have an appendage that is shaped like a drumstick and is attached to one lobe by a strand of chromatin (see Plate VII). Nuclear spicules or appendages attached by a broad base occur in normal individuals but may be increased in number in chronic illnesses or after cytotoxic or radiation therapy.[63] The cytoplasm is clear and contains many small tan to pink granules distributed evenly throughout the cell, although they may not be apparent when they lie over the nucleus.

Bands are identical to mature polymorphonuclear leukocytes except that the nucleus is U-shaped or has rudimentary lobes connected by a band containing chromatin rather than by a thin thread (see Plate VII). The nuclear chromatin is slightly less condensed than the mature neutrophil.

Eosinophils are on the average slightly larger than neutrophils. The nucleus usually has only two lobes. The chromatin pattern is the same as that in the neutrophil, but the nucleus tends to be more lightly stained. The differentiating characteristic of these cells is the presence of many refractile, orange-red granules that are distributed evenly throughout the cell and may be visible overlying the nucleus (see Plate VII). These granules are larger than those in the neutrophil and are more uniform in size. Occasionally some of the granules in eosinophils stain light blue rather than orange-red.

Basophils are similar to the other polymorphonuclear cells and are slightly smaller than neutrophils. The nucleus may stain more faintly and usually is less segmented and has less distinct chromatin condensation than is the case in neutrophils. The large deeply basophilic granules are fewer in number and less regular in size and shape than in the eosinophil. The granules are visible overlying the nucleus and, in some cells, almost completely obscure the lightly stained nuclear chromatin. Because the granular constituents are water-soluble, some granules may stain only faintly or not at all (see Plate V).

Lymphocytes on blood films are usually small, about 10 μm in diameter, but larger forms up to 20 μm in diameter are seen. The small lymphocyte, the predominant type in normal blood, is round and contains a relatively large, round, densely stained nucleus in which the chromatin is distributed in coarse masses (see Plate V). The cytoplasm is scanty and stains pale to dark blue. In the large lymphocytes the nuclear/cytoplasmic ratio is lower and the chromatin is less condensed than in the small lymphocytes. The nucleus is usually round but may be oval or indented. The cytoplasm is abundant and may contain a few azurophilic granules. Large lymphocytes containing azurophilic granules and relatively abundant cytoplasm are designated *large granular lymphocytes* and often represent cytotoxic T cells or NK cells. *Reactive lymphocytes*, as seen in viral infections caused by EBV, CMV, adenovirus, or other organisms, are large with indented nuclei and abundant blue cytoplasm. Nuclear chromatin condensation is variable, and nucleoli may be evident. A low nuclear/cytoplasmic ratio distinguishes these reactive T lymphocytes from neoplastic cells.

Monocytes are the largest normal cells in the blood, usually measuring from 15 to 22 μm in diameter. The nucleus is of various shapes—round, kidney-shaped, oval, or lobulated—and frequently appears to be folded (see Plate VII). The chromatin is arranged in fine strands with sharply defined margins. The cytoplasm is light blue or gray, contains numerous fine lilac or purple granules, and is frequently vacuolated, especially in films made from blood anticoagulated with EDTA. The gray (as opposed to blue) color of monocyte cytoplasm is due to fine granules (staining pink) seen on the back-

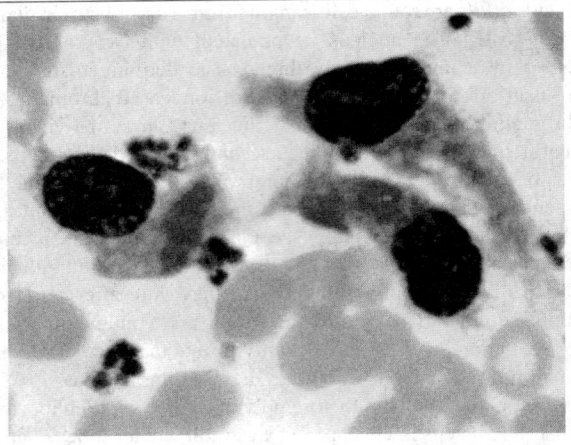

FIGURE 2-1   Endothelial cells in blood film. (Courtesy of Dr. HA Wurzel.)

ground of RNA-containing cytoplasm (staining blue) and helps to distinguish between monocytes and reactive lymphocytes. The monocyte nuclear chromatin contains a fine stringlike structure as opposed to the coarser clumps of the lymphoid chromatin. Nuclear shape and cytoplasmic vacuolation are less reliable distinguishing features between monocytic and lymphoid cells.

LEUKOCYTE INCLUSIONS

Leukocytes may contain abnormal inclusions as a result of genetic or acquired disorders.

ABNORMAL GRANULES

In patients with conditions associated with a systemic inflammatory reaction, neutrophil granules may appear larger than normal and stain more darkly, often assuming a dark blue-black color. This has been called *toxic granulation*. These granules can be confused with the larger granules of basophils. In *mucopolysaccharidoses*, coarse, dark granules may be found in the neutrophils (the Alder-Reilly anomaly), and large azurophilic granules are often found in some lymphocytes (Gasser cells) and monocytes. Huge misshapen granules are found in the polymorphonuclear leukocytes, and giant azurophilic granules are present in the lymphocytes of patients exhibiting the *Chédiak-Higashi* anomaly (see Chap. 72).[64] *Auer rods* are sharply outlined, red-staining rods found in the cytoplasm in blast cells, and occasionally in more

mature leukemic cells, in the blood of some patients with acute myelogenous leukemia (see Plate XVI).

ABNORMAL RNA AGGREGATIONS

Light blue round or oval bodies about 1 to 2 μm in diameter may be seen in the cytoplasm of neutrophils of patients with infections, burns, and other inflammatory states. These have been named *Döhle bodies*. The blue staining is due to RNA, since it is blocked by treating the slide with ribonuclease prior to staining. Ultrastructurally, Döhle bodies contain rough-surfaced endoplasmic reticulum. Similar blue inclusions are seen in patients with the *May-Hegglin* anomaly. The staining of May-Hegglin inclusions is also attributable to RNA, but ultrastructurally they differ from Döhle bodies, suggesting alterations in the RNA.[65]

LEUKOCYTE ARTIFACTS

CRUSHED ("SMUDGE," "BASKET") CELLS

During the process of preparing the film, leukocytes may be damaged, with consequent alteration in their appearance and staining. In some damaged leukocytes the nucleus appears enlarged, with alteration of the chromatin so that the strands appear more homogeneous, stain with a distinct reddish hue, and are more widely separated; the cytoplasm may or may not appear intact. Such cells may appear to have a large blue nucleolus. There is no specific association with disease other than chronic lymphocytic leukemia, where the neoplastic lymphocytes are fragile and smudge cells are frequent.

RADIAL NUCLEAR SEGMENTATION

This refers to abnormal segmentation of the nuclei of leukocytes on the blood film, in which the lobes appear to radiate from a single point, giving a cloverleaf or cartwheel picture. This change is common in cytocentrifuged preparations (i.e., from a body fluid), EDTA anticoagulated blood after excessive storage, or samples collected in oxalate.

VACUOLATION

Vacuoles may develop in the nucleus and cytoplasm of leukocytes, especially monocytes and neutrophils, with prolonged storage in EDTA anticoagulated blood. Vacuoles may be associated with swelling of the nuclei and loss of granules from the cytoplasm. In blood films prepared without anticoagulation, vacuoles in neutrophils suggest sepsis.

ENDOTHELIAL CELLS

If the blood film is prepared from the first drop of blood issuing from the microsampling wound, endothelial cells may be present singly or in clumps. Such cells are illustrated in Fig. 2-1. These cells appear quite immature and may be misinterpreted as blasts or metastatic tumor cells.

THE NEED FOR EXAMINATION OF THE BLOOD FILM

The quantitative determinations discussed earlier in this chapter—hemoglobin level, hematocrit, and erythrocyte, platelet, and leukocyte counts—describe the blood in sufficient detail that the physician will often recognize the need for further laboratory and clinical study. Quantitative analysis of the peripheral blood may suggest diseases involving erythrocytes, leukocytes, and/or platelets that can then be con-

TABLE 2-4   CONDITIONS IN WHICH THE BLOOD COUNT MAY BE RELATIVELY UNREMARKABLE BUT EXAMINATION OF THE BLOOD FILM WILL SUGGEST OR CONFIRM THE DISORDER

DISEASE	FINDINGS ON BLOOD FILM
Compensated acquired hemolytic anemia	Spherocytosis, polychromatophilia Erythrocyte agglutination if immune-mediated
Hereditary spherocytosis	Spherocytosis, polychromatophilia
Hemoglobin C disease	Target cells
Elliptocytosis	Elliptocytes
Lead poisoning	Basophilic stippling (not a sensitive indicator)
Multiple myeloma, macroglobulinemia	Rouleaux formation
Malaria, babesiosis	Parasites in the erythrocytes
Consumptive coagulopathy	Schizocytes (not a sensitive indicator)
Mechanical hemolysis	Schizocytes
Severe infection	Neutrophilia with immature granulocytes; Döhle bodies, neutrophil vacuoles
Infectious mononucleosis	Atypical lymphocytes
Acute leukemia (early relapse)	Blast cells

firmed by examination of a stained blood film. A number of diseases in which the blood counts may be relatively unremarkable but in which examination of the blood film will suggest the disorder are listed in Table 2-4. Based on the quantitative and morphologic examination of the peripheral blood, the physician can assess the need for direct examination of the marrow, as described in Chap. 3.

REFERENCES

1. Shapiro MF, Hatch RL, Greenfield S: Cost containment and labor-intensive tests. The case of the leukocyte differential count. *JAMA* 252:231, 1984.
2. Coulter WH: High speed automatic blood cell counter and cell size analyzer. *Proc Natl Elect Conf* 12:1034, 1956.
3. Bessman JD, Banks D: Spurious macrocytosis, a common clue to erythrocyte cold agglutinins. *Am J Clin Pathol* 74:797, 1980.
4. Wintrobe MM: Macroscopic examination of the blood. *Am J Med Sci* 185:58, 1933.
5. England JM, Walford DM, Waters DA: Re-assessment of the reliability of the haematocrit. *Br J Haematol* 23:247, 1972.
6. Pearson TC, Guthrie DL: Trapped plasma in the microhematocrit. *Am J Clin Pathol* 78:770, 1982.
7. Fairbanks VF: Nonequivalence of automated and manual hematocrit and erythrocyte indices. *Am J Clin Pathol* 73:55, 1980.
8. Dacie JV, Lewis SL: *Practical Hematology.* Churchill Livingstone, Edinburgh, 1991.
9. England JM: *Blood Cell Sizing.* Churchill Livingstone, New York, 1991.
10. International Committee for Standardization in Haematology; Expert Panel on Haemoglobinometry: Recommendations for reference method for haemoglobinometry in human blood (ICSH standard 1986) and specifications for international haemoglobincyanide reference preparation (3rd edition). *Clin Lab Haematol* 9:73, 1987.
11. Gagne C, Auger PL, Moorjani S, et al: Effect of hyperchylomicronemia on the measurement of hemoglobin. *Am J Clin Pathol* 68:584, 1977.
12. Kickler TS: Clinical analyzers. Advances in automated cell counting. *Anal Chem* 71:363R, 1999.
13. Dallman PR, Bart GD, Allen CM, et al: Hemoglobin concentration in white, black and Oriental children: Is there a need for separate criteria in screening for anemia? *Am J Clin Nutr* 31:377, 1978.
14. Dallman PR, Siimes MA: Percentile curves for hemoglobin and red cell volume in infancy and childhood. *J Pediatr* 94:26, 1979.
15. Wintrobe MM: Anemia: Classification and treatment on the basis of differences in the average volume and hemoglobin content of the red corpuscles. *Arch Intern Med* 54:256, 1934.
16. Hillman RS: After sixty years: the MCV is still alive and well. *J Gen Intern Med* 5:264, 1990.
17. Rund D, Filon D, Strauss N et al: Mean corpuscular volume of heterozygotes for beta-thalassemia correlates with the severity of mutations. *Blood* 79:238, 1992.
18. Segel GB, Cokelet GR, Lichtman MA: The measurement of lymphocyte volume: Importance of reference particle deformability and counting solution tonicity. *Blood* 57:894, 1981.
19. Griner PF, Oranburg PR: Predictive values of erythrocyte indices for tests of iron, folic acid, and vitamin B$_{12}$ deficiency. *Am J Clin Pathol* 70:748, 1978.
20. Seward SJ, Safran C, Marton KI, Robinson SH: Does the mean corpuscular volume help physicians evaluate hospitalized patients with anemia? *J Gen Intern Med* 5:187, 1990.
21. Carmel R: Pernicious anemia. The expected findings of very low serum cobalamin levels, anemia, and macrocytosis are often lacking. *Arch Intern Med* 148:1712, 1988.
22. Mahmoud MY, Lugon M, Anderson CC: Unexplained macrocytosis in elderly patients. *Age Ageing* 25:10, 1996.
23. Eldibany MM, Totonchi KF, Joseph NJ, Rhone D: Usefulness of certain red blood cell indices in diagnosing and differentiating thalassemia trait from iron-deficiency anemia. *Am J Clin Pathol* 111:676, 1999.
24. Lafferty JD, Crowther MA, Ali MA, Levine M: The evaluation of various mathematical RBC indices and their efficacy in discriminating between thalassemic and non-thalassemic microcytosis. *Am J Clin Pathol* 106:201, 1996.
25. Michaels LA, Cohen AR, Zhao H, Raphael RI, Manno CS: Screening for hereditary spherocytosis by use of automated erythrocyte indexes. *J Pediatr* 130:957, 1997.
26. Bentley SA, Ayscue LH, Watson JM, Ross DW: The clinical utility of discriminant functions for the differential diagnosis of microcytic anemias. *Blood Cells* 15:575, 1989.
27. Mahu JL, Leclercq C, Suquet JP: Usefulness of red cell distribution width in association with biological parameters in an epidemiological survey of iron deficiency in children. *Int J Epidemiol* 19:646, 1990.
28. Rose MS: Epitaph for the M.C.H.C. *Br Med J* 4:169, 1971.
29. Holt JT, DeWandler MJ, Arvan DA: Spurious elevation of the electronically determined mean corpuscular volume and hematocrit caused by hyperglycemia. *Am J Clin Pathol* 77:561, 1982.
30. Liu TC, Seong PS, Lin TK: The erythrocyte cell hemoglobin distribution width segregates thalassemia traits from other nonthalassemic conditions with microcytosis. *Am J Clin Pathol* 107:601, 1997.
31. McClure S, Custer E, Bessman JD: Improved detection of early iron deficiency in nonanemic subjects. *JAMA* 253:1021, 1985.
32. Patton WN, Cave RJ, Harris RI: A study of changes in red cell volume and haemoglobin concentration during phlebotomy induced iron deficiency and iron repletion using the Technicon H1. *Clin Lab Haematol* 13:153, 1991.
33. Bessman JD, Gilmer PR Jr, Gardner FH: Improved classification of anemias by MCV and RDW. *Am J Clin Pathol* 80:322, 1983.
34. Flynn MM, Reppun TS, Bhagavan NV: Limitations of red blood cell distribution width (RDW) in evaluation of microcytosis. *Am J Clin Pathol* 85:445, 1986.
35. Anonymous: Recommendations to prevent and control iron deficiency in the United States. Centers for Disease Control and Prevention. *MMWR* 47:1, 1998.
36. Gulati GL, Hyun BH, Gagaldon H: Falsely elevated automated leukocyte count on cryoglobulinemic and/or cryofibrinogenic blood samples. *Lab Med* 8:14, 1977.
37. Williams LJ: Cell histograms: New trends in data interpretation and classification. *J Med Technol* 1:189, 1984.
38. Lombarts AJ, deKieviet W: Recognition and prevention of pseudothrombocytopenia and consomitant pseudoleukocytosis. *Am J Clin Pathol* 89:534, 1988.
39. Bartels PC, Schoorl M, Lombarts AJ: Screening for EDTA-dependent deviations in platelet counts and abnormalities in platelet distribution histograms in pseudothrombocytopenia. *Scand J Clin Lab Invest* 57:629, 1997.
40. Ferrero-Vacher C, Sudaka I, Jambou D, et al: Evaluation of the ABX Cobas Vega automated hematology analyzer and comparison with the Coulter STKS. *Hematol Cell Ther* 39:149, 1997.
41. Cornbleet PJ, Myrick D, Levy R: Evaluation of the Coulter STKS five-part differential. *Am J Clin Pathol* 99:72, 1993.
42. Thalhammer-Scherrer R, Knobl P, Korninger L, Schwarzinger I: Automated five-part white blood cell differential counts. Efficiency of software-generated white blood cell suspect flags of the hematology analyzers Sysmex SE-9000, Sysmex NE-8000, and Coulter STKS. *Arch Pathol Lab Med* 121:573, 1997.
43. Warner BA, Reardon DM, Marshall DP: Automated haematology analysers: a four-way comparison. *Med Lab Sci* 47:285, 1990.
44. Zaccaria A, Celso B, Raspadori D, et al: Comparative evaluation of differential leukocyte counts by Coulter VCS cytometer and direct microscopic observation. *Haematologica* 75:412, 1990.
45. Atwater S, Corash L: Advances in leukocyte differential and peripheral blood stem cell enumeration. *Cur Opin Hematol* 3:71, 1996.
46. Reed WW, Diehl F: Leukopenia, neutropenia, and reduced hemoglobin levels in healthy American blacks. *Arch Intern Med* 151:501, 1991.
47. Haddy TB, Rana SR, Castro O: Benign ethnic neutropenia: what is a normal absolute neutrophil count? *J Lab Clin Med* 133:15, 1999.
48. Caramihai E, Karayalcin G, Aballi AJ, et al: Leukocyte count differences in healthy white and black children 1 to 5 years of age. *J Pediatr* 86:252, 1975.
49. Bain BJ: Ethnic and sex differences in the total and differential white cell count and platelet count. *J Clin Pathol* 49:664, 1996.
50. Paulus JM: Platelet size in man. *Blood* 46:321, 1975.
51. Lawrence JB, Yomtovian RA, Dillman C, et al: Reliability of automated platelet counts: comparison with manual method and utility for prediction of clinical bleeding. *Am J Hematol* 48:244, 1995.

52. Fiorin F, Steffan A, Pradella P, et al: IgG platelet antibodies in EDTA-dependent pseudothrombocytopenia bind to platelet membrane glyco-protein IIb. *Am J Clin Pathol* 110:178, 1998.

53. Levin J, Bessman JD: The inverse relation between platelet volume and platelet number. Abnormalities in hematologic disease and evidence that platelet size does not correlate with platelet age. *J Lab Clin Med* 101:295, 1983.

54. Bath PM, Butterworth RJ: Platelet size: measurement, physiology and vascular disease. *Blood Coagul Fibronol* 7:157, 1996.

55. van der Loo B, Martin JF: A role for changes in platelet production in the cause of acute coronary syndromes. *Arterioscler Thromb Vasc Biol* 19:672, 1999.

56. Bessman JD: The relation of megakaryocyte ploidy to platelet volume. *Am J Hematol* 16:161, 1984.

57. Thompson CB, Love DG, Quinn PG, Valeri CR: Platelet size does not correlate with platelet age. *Blood* 62:487, 1983.

58. Behrens WE: Mediterranean macrothrombocytopenia. *Blood* 46:199, 1975.

59. Altes A, Pujol-Moix N, Muniz-Diaz E, et al: Hereditary macrothrom-bocytopenia and pregnancy. *Thrombosis and Haemostasis* 76:29, 1996.

60. O'Malley T, Ludlam CA, Fox KA, Elton RA: Measurement of platelet volume using a variety of different anticoagulant and antiplatelet mix-tures. *Blood Coagul Fibronol* 7:431, 1996.

61. Osselaer JC, Jamart J, Scheiff JM: Platelet distribution width for differen-tial diagnosis of thrombocytosis. *Clin Chem* 43:1072, 1997.

62. Ross DW, Bentley SA: Evaluation of an automated hematology system (Technicon H*1). *Arch Pathol Lab Med* 10:803, 1986.

63. Bessis M: *Living Blood Cells and Their Ultrastructure,* Springer-Verlag, New York, 1973.

64. Brunning RD: Morphologic alterations in nucleated blood and marrow cells in genetic disorders. *Hum Pathol* 1:99, 1970.

65. Jenis EH, Takeuchi A, Dillon DE, et al: The May-Hegglin anomaly: Ultrastructure of the granulocytic inclusion. *Am J Clin Pathol* 55:187, 1971.

EXAMINATION OF THE MARROW

DANIEL H. RYAN

The examination of the marrow in concert with the prior examination of the blood remains the dyad required for the diagnosis of many hematologic diseases. The marrow examination provides a semi-quantitative and qualitative assessment of the state of hematopoiesis and the normalcy of the blood cell precursors of all lineages. It can provide the diagnosis of several hereditary and acquired benign and malignant diseases. The marrow is a source of cells for clonal hematopoietic cell assays, cells for histocytologic, immunocytologic, cytogenetic, and molecular analysis. It is an easy, safe, and inexpensive means to arrive at the diagnosis of important abnormalities of the hematopoietic system. It is an important test to assess the response to treatment of the leukemias and some lymphomas. It can be useful in assessing the state of iron stores and of metabolic diseases that affect macrophages, such as Gaucher disease. It represents the cornerstone of hematologic diagnosis, even as hematology moves to a more molecularly- and genetically-based discipline.

Marrow progenitors give rise to all hematopoietic lineages in the adult. Therefore, direct visual examination of the marrow has long been a mainstay of hematologic diagnosis. Even with the advent of specialized biochemical and molecular assays that capitalize on advances in understanding of the biology of hematopoiesis, the primary diagnosis of hematologic malignancies and many nonneoplastic hematologic disorders relies on visual examination of the marrow. Marrow may be obtained without significant risk and with only minor discomfort and is quickly and easily processed for examination.

At birth all bones contain hematopoietic marrow. Fat cells begin to replace hematopoietic marrow in the extremities in the fifth to seventh year, and by adulthood the hematopoietic marrow is limited to the axial skeleton and the proximal portions of the extremities.[1,2] The structure and function of the marrow and the distribution of marrow in the skeleton are discussed in Chap. 4. Fatty marrow appears yellow, while hematopoietic marrow is red. Red marrow does contain fat, however, and fat droplets are visible grossly in aspirated marrow specimens. Histologically, yellow marrow consists almost entirely of fat cells and supporting connective tissue, while red marrow contains an abundance of hematopoietic cells along with fat cells and connective tissue. The marrow fills the spaces between the trabeculae of bone in the marrow cavity. It is soft and friable and can be readily aspirated or biopsied with a needle.

INDICATIONS FOR MARROW ASPIRATE OR BIOPSY

The marrow should be examined when the clinical history, laboratory test results, or blood film suggests the possibility of a primary or secondary hematologic disorder for which morphologic analysis or special studies of the marrow would aid in the diagnosis. Although marrow aspiration and biopsy techniques are safe, they should be performed with a clear idea as to how the results will aid in distinguishing the differential diagnoses under consideration or provide assessment of treatment. In some hematologic disorders, such as most cases of iron deficiency anemia, thalassemia, pernicious anemia, and Gaucher disease, examination of the blood and specialized laboratory tests may be sufficient to make the diagnosis without the need for a marrow examination.

When examination of the marrow is indicated, it should be decided whether an aspirate only or aspirate plus biopsy is desired. The aspirate is always performed, because of the superior morphology offered by examination of the marrow aspirate film. However, a marrow biopsy is superior to the aspirate in quantitating marrow cellularity and diagnosing infiltrative diseases of the marrow and should be performed when these conditions are part of the differential diagnosis.[3–7] In low-grade lymphoma the marrow is frequently involved at the time of diagnosis, and this involvement is most sensitively detected by marrow biopsy.[8] Marrow biopsy is also useful in diagnosing and following the course of disorders that are commonly associated with fibrosis, such as megakaryoblastic leukemia, hairy-cell leukemia, and the chronic myeloproliferative disorders.[9,10] In myelodysplastic syndromes, marrow biopsy is useful in evaluating the abnormal localization of immature precursor cells (ALIP) as well as evaluating abnormal megakaryocytes.[9] Marrow necrosis and gelatinous transformation are more readily detected in marrow sections than in aspirate films. In some clinical settings where the diagnostic question is very targeted, such as diagnosis of childhood ITP or surveillance follow-up of leukemia patients, marrow aspirate alone may be appropriate. It is important to anticipate whether additional sample volume is required for cytogenetic or molecular studies.

MARROW ASPIRATION TECHNIQUE

The posterior iliac crest (Fig. 3-1) is the preferred site for both marrow aspiration and biopsy. In adults, the sternum and the anterior iliac crest can also be utilized (Fig. 3-2). The sternum should be used for aspiration only, and the anterior iliac crest is less preferred than the posterior crest in adults due to its thick cortical bone. The anteromedial surface of the tibia is an option for infants less than 1 year old (particularly newborns), but the posterior iliac crest is still the preferred site. The spinous processes of the vertebrae, the ribs, or other marrow-containing bones are rarely used. The hazards of marrow aspiration include hemorrhage, infection, and reactions to anesthetic agents, but these are very rare when the procedure is carefully performed. Penetration of the bone with damage to the underlying structures is possible with all marrow aspirations, but the hazard is greatest in sternal aspirations, since the sternum at the second interspace is only about 1 cm thick in the adult.

For either marrow biopsy or aspirate, conscious sedation minimizes anxiety and pain,[11] particularly in children, but must be performed with proper patient monitoring to minimize risk. Marrow biopsies and aspirates performed for staging purposes can often be done while a patient is under anesthesia for other reasons (insertion of central line). Several different types of needles, most of which are satisfactory, are available for marrow aspiration. For adults an 18-gauge needle is sufficiently large to permit aspiration of adequate specimens; larger needles are unnecessary. The patient is prone or in the left or right lateral decubitus position. Sterile precautions must be observed. The skin over the puncture site is shaved if necessary and cleansed with a disinfectant solution, and the skin, subcutaneous tissues, and periosteum are infiltrated with a local anesthetic solution such as 1% lidocaine. Adequate infiltration of the anesthetic at the periosteal surface is important, but no more than 20 ml of 1% lidocaine

Acronyms and abbreviations that appear in this chapter include: ALIP, abnormal localization of immature precursor cells; M/E, myeloid/erythroid.

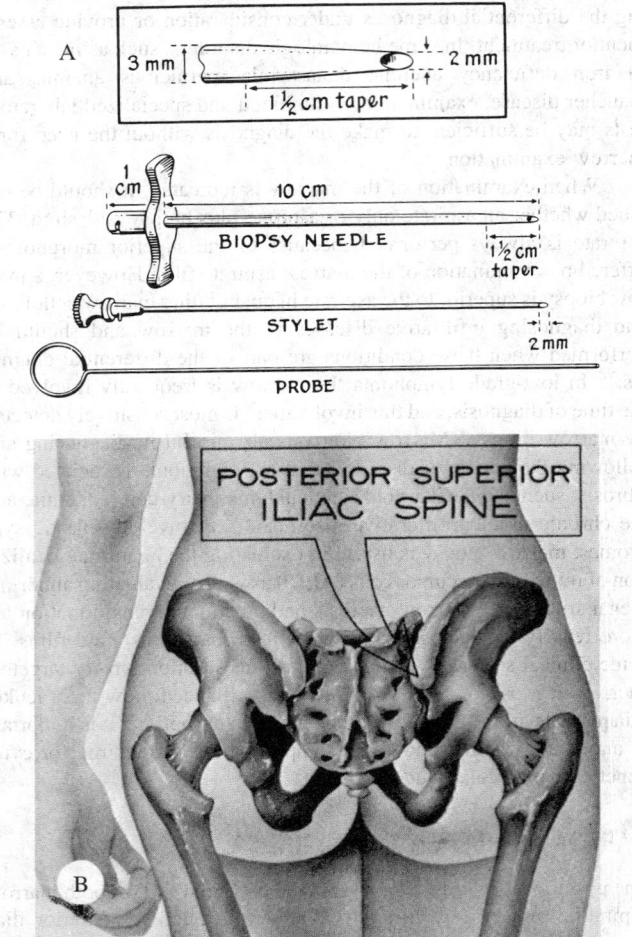

FIGURE 3-1 (a) Jamshidi biopsy instrument. (b) Site of marrow biopsy. [(a) *From Jamshidi and Swaim*[13] *by permission;* (b) *from Ellis, Jensen, and Westerman*[3] *by permission.*]

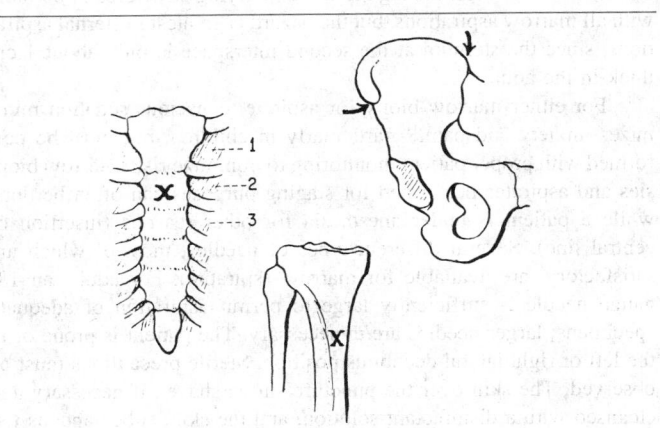

FIGURE 3-2 Sites used for marrow aspiration. (*Modified from SO Schwartz, WH Hartz Jr, and JH Robbins,* Hematology in Practice, *part 1, p 36. McGraw-Hill, New York, 1961.*)

should be used in an adult.[12] An air gun may be used to anesthetize the skin surface prior to application of anesthetic to the periosteal surface by injection. After the anesthesia has taken effect, the marrow needle is inserted through the skin, subcutaneous tissue, and cortex of the bone with a slight twisting motion. In obese patients, the length of the needle must be sufficient to reach the iliac crest. The stylet should be locked into place on the hub of the needle to prevent plugging of the needle with tissue prior to entry into the marrow cavity. Penetration of the cortex can be sensed by a slight, rapid forward movement accompanied by a sudden increase in the ease of advancing the needle. The stylet of the needle is removed promptly, the hub is attached to a 10- or 20-ml syringe, and about 0.2 to 0.5 ml of fluid is aspirated. The actual aspiration of the marrow causes a transient painful sensation for most patients. If additional specimen volume is required, another syringe is fitted on the marrow needle and marrow is aspirated. The stylet may be reinserted and the marrow needle slightly repositioned between aspirations. When aspiration is complete, the stylet is reinserted and the needle removed from the bone immediately. Pressure is applied to the skin over the aspiration site for at least 5 min to minimize bruising at the site. In a thrombocytopenic patient, firm pressure should be applied for at least 10 to 15 min.

The bloody fluid that is aspirated contains light-colored particles of marrow from 0.5 to 1 mm in diameter. They are often readily visible in the syringe but may not be detected until the syringe contents are discharged on a glass slide to prepare films.

Occasionally nothing enters the syringe when aspiration is performed. This may mean that the needle has not been properly placed in the marrow cavity. It may be cautiously advanced 1 to 2 mm after reinsertion of the stylet and aspiration may be attempted again, or it may be more desirable to remove the needle from the bone and reinsert it in a nearby site in the anesthetized area. The thickness of the bone must be kept in mind when one is attempting to adjust the needle in the bone. Occasionally the needle must be rotated on its longitudinal axis, or in a larger orbit, in order to loosen the marrow mechanically before it can be aspirated. If a small amount of blood has been aspirated, it is wise to use a new needle because of the probability of clotting of the aspirate when it is finally obtained. Aspiration with a 50-ml syringe may succeed when failure has been encountered with a smaller syringe. Leukemic marrow may be so densely packed in the bone as to resist all attempts at aspiration, in which case biopsy is necessary. The marrow in myelofibrosis also may be impossible to aspirate. The commonest cause of failure to obtain marrow is faulty positioning of the needle, and a second attempt at aspiration will usually succeed.

NEEDLE BIOPSY TECHNIQUE

Needle biopsy is usually performed with the Jamshidi needle,[13] using the same preparation as described above. The Jamshidi instrument (Fig. 3-1) consists of a cylindrical needle of constant bore except for a concentrically tapered distal portion ending in a sharp, beveled cutting tip. The stylet fits precisely inside the opening at the tapered tip, interlocks at the hub of the needle, and extends 1 to 2 mm beyond the end of the needle. An 11-gauge needle is most commonly used in the United States. After one has anesthetized the skin and the periosteum of the biopsy site, a 3-mm incision is made in the skin, and the needle, with obturator in place, is inserted into the skin incision and through the subcutaneous tissue to the cortex of the bone. The needle is directed toward the posterior iliac spine and advanced with a twisting motion. Penetration of the cortex is sensed by a decreased resistance to forward movement of the needle. The obturator is then removed, and the needle is slowly advanced with reciprocal clockwise-counterclockwise twisting motions around the long axis. After sufficient penetration of the bone (up to about 3 cm), the needle is rotated several times on its axis and withdrawn about 2 to 3 mm. The needle is then reinserted to the original depth at a slightly different angle, with care taken not to bend the needle, and rotated several times in order to free the specimen from attachments in the marrow cavity. Next the needle is slowly withdrawn, using the same twisting motion employed during insertion. The core of marrow inside the needle is removed by inserting the probe through the cutting tip and extruding the specimen through the hub of the needle. The smaller size of the cutting aperture relative to the bore of the shaft of the Jamshidi instrument yields a specimen which fits loosely inside the needle and is therefore less subject to compression, distortion, or fragmentation. This technique reliably produces biopsy specimens of good quality. Marrow biopsy should be performed before marrow aspiration is attempted (or in a slightly different site on the iliac crest) to avoid hemorrhage and distorted marrow architecture in the biopsy core.

With the availability of the biopsy needles described above, open (surgical) biopsies are rarely necessary but may be performed, for example, for the diagnosis of deeply situated bone lesions.

PREPARATION OF MARROW SPECIMENS FOR STUDY

Several types of preparations can be made from the marrow aspirate to make maximal use of the diagnostic material. Most important is the direct film, which is made immediately from the unmanipulated aspirate. This is the best preparation for evaluation of cellular morphology and differential counts of the marrow. The particle film is best for estimation of marrow cellularity and megakaryocyte abundance, but morphology is obscured in the thicker parts of the film. A concentrate film, prepared from a buffy coat of the marrow, is useful to detect low abundance cells, such as megakaryoctyes and metastatic tumor, or when the marrow is hypocellular. However, the relative proportions of cell lineages are not reliably maintained in this preparation (often erythroid precursors are relatively enriched). This preparation is also subject to anticoagulant-induced changes in nuclear morphology or cytoplasmic vacuolation. The touch imprint from the biopsy is essential to evaluate cellular morphology in case of a "dry tap"[14] and provides cytologic detail of cells that may not appear in the aspirate specimen.[15]

FILMS

After aspiration, about 0.5 ml of marrow is placed on a glass slide, and the rest mixed into an EDTA-anticoagulated tube. The marrow specimen is examined to be sure that "spicules" or particles of marrow containing bony or fatty pieces are present, indicating successful aspiration of the marrow cavity. Direct marrow films are immediately prepared by transferring drops of the unanticoagulated marrow pool to fresh slides and making push films with coverslips. Sufficient slides should be made for special stains. Heparinization of the aspirate is not necessary if the operator works rapidly and should be avoided as it may introduce artifacts.

It is useful to prepare a film enriched in marrow particles ("particle film") by picking up with a pipette several spicules from the pool of marrow, discharging a drop or two on a slide, covering the particles with a second slide, pressing these gently together to express most of the blood into a gauze sponge, and then pulling the slides apart longitudinally. Such preparations may contain an increased number of broken cells if too much pressure is applied, but they provide a large number of particles from which cellularity of the marrow may be estimated and which are useful for estimation of the amount of hemosiderin present.

An aliquot of the EDTA-anticoagulated sample is centrifuged (1500 g for 10 min) in a Wintrobe tube to concentrate the cellular elements of the marrow. After centrifugation, the fatty layer and plasma are removed, and the "buffy coat" is mixed with an equal amount of plasma; then multiple films are made of this preparation ("bone marrow concentrate"). These slides should be air dried, labeled, and retained as unstained preparations in case special stains are required.

TOUCH PREPARATIONS

After one has obtained a biopsy with a Jamshidi needle, the biopsy specimen should be extruded through the hub of the needle and then gently rolled across a glass slide (using forceps to move the specimen) before it is placed in fixative, taking care to avoid crushing. The touch preparations are allowed to dry and are stained in the same manner as films.

SPECIAL STUDIES

One of the reasons that it is essential to formulate the diagnostic question before performing a marrow aspiration is to be sure that adequate sample is obtained for all the special studies that may be needed to make the correct diagnosis. A sterile anticoagulated sample containing viable unfixed cells in single-cell suspension is the best substrate for nearly all special studies that are likely to be required on a marrow sample. Specifically, flow cytometry is best performed on an EDTA- or heparin-anticoagulated aspirate specimen, which is stable for at least 24 h at room temperature. For cytogenetic or cell culture analysis, anticoagulated marrow should be added to tissue culture medium and analyzed as soon as possible to maintain optimal cell viability. Cytogenetic samples are generally not adversely affected by overnight incubation.[16]

For molecular analysis of genomic DNA, sample preparation and storage as described for cell marker studies is adequate, since DNA is relatively stable. DNA can be extracted and analyzed even from paraffin-embedded tissue sections. However, RT-PCR assays, involving amplification of cDNA prepared from cellular messenger RNA, are often needed for molecular diagnosis of translocations associated with leukemia and lymphoma. Messenger RNA has a variable half-life in an intact cell and is degraded rapidly (on the order of seconds to minutes) in a cell lysate by ubiquitous RNAses. For maximal mRNA recovery, cell suspensions (typically buffy coat or mononuclear cell preparations) should be lysed in an appropriate RNAse-inhibitor containing buffer as soon as possible after sampling. Air-dried films may retain varying amounts of detectable mRNA.[17] EDTA is the preferred anticoagulant, as heparin can interfere with some molecular assays.

Archival storage of marrow specimens is of increasing interest in light of advances in molecular diagnosis that may necessitate validation studies using samples of known origin or testing of diagnostic material from a patient now in remission. Isolated DNA or RNA can be stored for long periods at $-70°C$ ($-158°F$), while viable, intact cells are most reliably preserved by controlled rate freezing in DMSO and storage in liquid nitrogen.

HISTOLOGIC SECTIONS

A variety of techniques have been advocated for preparing aspirated material for histologic study. All are designed to collect a sufficient number of marrow particles in a small volume so that adequate sections may be prepared. This may be accomplished by discharging the marrow aspirate onto a glass slide, allowing the particles to settle for a few seconds, and then gently tilting the slide so that the excess blood runs off. The particles are then pushed together with an applicator stick, and the remaining blood is allowed to clot. The clot is then promptly fixed in Zenker solution, B5, or buffered formalin[18] for tissue processing and sectioning. An alternative method employing filtration of anticoagulated aspirate specimen has been described.[19]

The core marrow biopsy specimen is processed for histologic examination by fixation in Zenker solution, B5 fixative, or neutral buffered formalin, followed by decalcification and embedding in paraffin. Sections of high quality cut at 4 μm and stained with hematoxylin and eosin or Giemsa stain are eminently satisfactory for routine work. Refinements in fixation and embedding techniques have made it possible to use most immunologic markers in decalcified paraffin-embedded marrow biopsy specimens.[19] Fixation in neutral buffered formalin and embedding in plastic has the advantage of superior morphology[20] and suitability for most immunochemical procedures,[21] but is technically more demanding and expensive.[22]

MORPHOLOGIC INTERPRETATION OF MARROW PREPARATIONS

OVERVIEW

The Wright-Giemsa-stained direct marrow aspirate film should be examined as quickly as possible to provide a preliminary assessment of the marrow morphology and allow specialized testing based on this preliminary evaluation to be set up while the sample is still fresh. The final interpretation of the marrow biopsy and aspirate should be integrated with results from the blood film, cell counts, laboratory data, clinical history, cell marker studies, and molecular or cytogenetic data. There is no other histologic specimen in which a state-of-the-art interpretation is dependent on such an array of supportive data. This is a result of the wealth of basic biologic information gained from in vitro studies of blood cells which has been translated into useful diagnostic tests. The challenge for the hematopathologist and hematologist is to understand the advantages and limitations of each diagnostic approach, so that apparently conflicting results can be reconciled and put into perspective.

ADEQUACY OF THE MARROW SAMPLE

The first question in interpreting the marrow is whether the sample is adequate for diagnosis. The best indicator at the time of the procedure that the needle entered the medullary cavity and marrow was successfully withdrawn is the presence of marrow particles in the aspirate. Marrow particles are bony with a glistening appearance caused by fat in the particles. A biopsy specimen should minimally contain at least a 0.5-cm length of marrow cavity. Correlation of biopsy specimen length with positivity rate for metastatic neoplasia suggests that a length of at least 1.2 cm is preferred for this purpose.[23] Specimens containing cortical bone, muscle, or other tissue with little or no medullary bone are inadequate for marrow interpretation (although they may provide other information). Also inadequate are samples with extensive crush artifact or hemorrhage, underscoring the importance of proper technique in obtaining a readable sample.

The marrow cavity was entered if the aspirate contains marrow particles or hematopoietic precursors (e.g., megakaryocytes, nucleated red cells) not found in the blood film. This does not ensure, however, that the specimen is adequate for diagnosis, since the amount of marrow actually aspirated can vary significantly in disease states, as discussed below.[24] Also, some cell types, notably fibroblasts and metastatic tumor cells, are not as readily removed from the marrow space by aspiration as are normal precursors. Lack of particles or precursor cells does not prove that the marrow cavity was not entered, as marrow packed with leukemic cells or infiltrated with fibroblasts may yield a "dry tap."[14] Marrow aspirations resulting in a dry tap are usually due to significant

pathology (only 7 percent show normal histology on biopsy[14]), indicating the necessity of examining a biopsy specimen in these cases.

An unspoken assumption is that the piece of marrow provided for diagnostic evaluation is representative of the marrow as a whole. This is generally a reasonable assumption, but studies employing bilateral biopsies,[25] comparison with radiologic studies,[26] or immunologic markers[27] indicate that the focal nature of tumor deposits contributes to false-negative results of marrow biopsy staging.

BONE MARROW CELLULARITY

The "gold standard" for overall marrow cellularity is examination of an adequate marrow biopsy specimen.[28,29] The normal cellularity (percent of the nonbony marrow space occupied by hematopoietic cells as opposed to fatty and nonhematopoietic tissue) of iliac crest marrow decreases from a mean of 80 percent in early childhood to 50 percent by age 30, with further decreases after age 70.[30] Marrow cellularity should therefore be evaluated with reference to normal individuals of the same age as the patient.[31] The normal range of iliac crest marrow cellularity is broader than one might expect.[30] In evaluating cellularity, it must be remembered that marrow spaces directly adjacent to cortical bone are frequently fatty in the elderly and are not representative of the cellularity of the deeper marrow spaces.[32]

Cellularity assessment by examination of the direct marrow aspirate film is more difficult because of loss of histologic structure and mixture with blood. The aspirate may suggest that the marrow is more hypocellular than indicated by the biopsy.[29] Marrow particles (seen in the direct film or a particle preparation) are the best indicators of cellularity. These particles are like "minibiopsies" and contain sufficient hematopoietic and fatty elements to give some idea of the cellularity of the marrow. Cellularity estimates from careful examination of particles in the aspirate preparation agree well with cellularity estimated from the marrow biopsy.[31]

The degree of dilution of marrow aspirate specimens with blood during the aspiration is quite variable and may affect interpretation of marrow cellularity. Adult marrows with over 30 percent lymphocytes plus monocytes are likely to be substantially admixed with blood, as shown by cytokinetic studies of paired marrow aspirate and biopsy preparations.[33] Radiolabeled erythrocytes and serum albumin have been used to estimate the admixture of nucleated cells from blood with those from marrow in sternal marrow aspirates.[24] In patients with hematologic disease, from 6 to 93 percent of the nucleated cells were derived from the blood.[24] The greatest admixture occurred in patients with leukemia. Substantial dilution with blood may occur in difficult aspirates or when multiple draws are taken from the same puncture site. Based on cell markers and progenitor assays, the first 1.0 ml of marrow aspirated from healthy donors was found to be only 8 percent contaminated with peripheral blood nucleated cells, while subsequent aspirates performed for marrow harvesting were 20 percent contaminated with nucleated blood cells.[34] The bulk volume of the "marrow" aspirate (i.e., plasma, red cells) is almost completely derived from blood, even if the nucleated cells are mostly marrow derived.[34] Assessment of marrow cellularity by measuring the buffy coat observed after centrifugation of the aspirate specimen is unreliable.[29]

Cellularity of individual lineages is also best assessed by examination of the biopsy. Erythroid cells are typically arranged in clusters, while megakaryocytes are scattered throughout the biopsy. Erythroid and megakaryoctic cellularity is best appreciated at low power. In the aspirate, a myeloid/erythroid (M/E) ratio is frequently calculated to give some impression of the relative cellularity of these two major lineages. The rule of thumb is that this value should normally lie between 2:1 and 4:1 (for normal ranges in men and women, see Table 3-1). The relative proportions of cell types should be assessed only

TABLE 3-1   NORMAL VALUES FOR MARROW DIFFERENTIAL CELL COUNT AT DIFFERENT AGES (PERCENT OF CELLS)**

	Rosse et al[50] Infants Tibial Marrow			Glaser et al[55] Subjects Aged 1-20 Sternal Marrow, 1 ml Aspirated	Bain[35] Subjects Aged 21-56 Years Iliac Marrow 0.1-0.2 ml Aspirated	
Type of Cell	<1 Month (n = 57)	1 Month (n = 7)	18 Months (n = 19)		Men (n = 30)	Women (n = 20)
Myeloblast	—	—	—	1.2 (0–3)	1.4 (0–3.0)	
Promyelocyte	0.79±0.91	0.76±0.65	0.64±0.59	1.8 (0–4)	7.8 (3.2–12.4)	
Myelocyte	3.95±2.93	2.50±1.48	2.49±1.39	16.5 (8–25)		
Neutrophilic					7.6 (3.7–10.0)	
Eosinophilic					1.3 (0–2.8)	
Basophilic						
Metamyelocyte	19.37±4.84	11.34±3.59	12.42±4.15	23 (14–34)	4.1 (2.3–5.9)	
Band	28.89±7.56	14.10±4.63	14.20±5.63	—	†	
Segmented						
Neutrophil	7.37±4.64	3.64±2.97	6.31±3.91	12.9 (4.5–29)	32.1 (21.9–42.3)	37.4 (28.8–45.9)
Eosinophil	2.70±1.27	2.61±1.40	2.70±2.16	—	2.2 (0.3–4.2)	
Basophil	0.12±0.20	0.07±0.16	0.10±0.12	—	0.1 (0–0.4)	
Lymphocyte	14.42±5.54	47.05±9.24	43.55±8.56	16 (5–36)	13.1 (6.0–20.0)	
Monocyte	0.88±0.85	1.01±0.89	2.12±1.59	—	1.3 (0–2.6)	
Plasma cell	0.00±0.02	0.02±0.06	0.06±0.08	—	0.6 (0–1.2)	
Proerythroblast	0.02±0.06	0.10±0.14	0.08±0.13	0.5 (0–1.5)		
Erythroblast					28.1 (16.2–40.1)‡	22.5 (13.0–32.0)‡
Basophilic	0.24±0.25	0.34±0.33	0.50±0.34	1.7 (0–5)		
Polychromatophilic	13.06±6.78	6.90±4.45	6.97±3.56	18 (5–34)		
Orthochromatic	0.09±0.73	0.54±1.88	0.44±0.49	2.7 (0–8)		
Megakaryocyte	0.06±0.15	0.05±0.09	0.07±0.12	—	31 (6–77) §	
Macrophage					0.4 (0–1.3)	
Others					¶	
Transitional cells*	1.18±1.13	1.95±0.94	1.99±1.00	—		
Broken cell	5.79±2.78	5.50±2.46	5.05±2.15	—		
M/E ratio	4.4	4.4	4.8	2.9 (1–5)	2.1 (1.1–4.1)	2.8 (1.6–5.2)

*Immature lymphoid cells.
†Bands included in segmented neutrophil count.
‡All erythroblast forms (basophilic, polychromatophilic, orthochromatic) grouped together.
§Number of megakaryocytes near the advancing edge of the smear (mean, range).
¶Osteoclasts noted in 8/50 subjects, osteoblasts in 5/50, no mast cells observed.
**Data expressed as percent of cells counted.

on the direct marrow film or particle preparation, not a concentrate film, which has been manipulated by centrifugation. A decreased M/E ratio could be interpreted as either myeloid hypocellularity or erythroid hyperplasia, depending on the overall marrow cellularity. Megakaryoctye numbers can be assessed in the direct marrow aspirate film, where there should be at least 5 megakaryocytes in the optimal portion of the smear. In the particle preparation, most large particles should contain one or more megakaryocytes. Megakaryocyte number varies markedly in direct marrow aspirate films of normal subjects[35] (Table 3-1) and is dependent on the degree of admixture of the specimen with blood. Megakaryocytes are variably enriched in the feathered edge of concentrate films.

INFILTRATIVE DISEASES OF THE MARROW

METASTATIC TUMOR

Metastatic nonhematopoietic tumor in the marrow biopsy is characterized by disruption of the marrow architecture with groups of cytologically abnormal cells. Assessment of the tissue of origin is primarily based on morphology, clinical history, and immunocytochemical staining. The tendency of carcinoma cells to form tightly adherent clusters is frequently helpful in recognizing these neoplasms. Such clumps can also appear on the marrow aspirate, but the aspirate is less sensitive than the biopsy for detection of metastatic tumor. Tumor clumps may be infrequent in the aspirate, often appearing only on side or feathered edges of the film or only in the concentrate preparation. These tumor

clumps must be distinguished from clumps of damaged hematopoietic cells which commonly appear in aspirate preparations, especially the concentrate. This is best accomplished by examining cells at the periphery of the clumps to determine if they show the morphology of hematopoietic precursors or cytologically atypical cells. Isolated nonhematopoietic tumor cells are infrequent in aspirate preparations, even when tumor is obvious in the biopsy, due to the adherent nature of most nonhematopoietic tumors. Examination of multiple films may be necessary to find isolated tumor cell clumps.[36]

Myeloma[37] and lymphomas[8] are also more reliably detected in the biopsy preparation. Lymphoma cells frequently form abnormal lymphoid aggregates which must, however, be distinguished from lymphoid aggregates found in reactive conditions or in older patients.[38] Neoplastic aggregates are more likely to show cytologic atypia, monomorphous cellular population, and are often adjacent to bony trabeculae, but the distinction can be difficult in some cases. The cellular morphology can often be appreciated better on the marrow aspirate, but the key histologic features are lost. Lymphoma cells do not form the tight clusters seen in nonhematopoietic tumors on the marrow aspirate smear. In hairy cell leukemia, however, the hematopoietic cells are sufficiently adherent to each other and the marrow matrix that aspirate specimens are often "dry," while the biopsy shows extensive infiltration with tumor. Special studies such as in situ hybridization for kappa versus lambda light-chain mRNA[39] or immunohistochemistry/flow cytometry to determine cell lineage and demonstrate surface light-chain restriction may be necessary to distinguish a reactive process from malignant lymphoma. Flow cytometry and morphologic examination of the bone marrow are complementary and can improve detection of lymphomatous involvement when used together.[56]

FIBROSIS

Bone marrow fibrosis is typically recognizable only on a marrow biopsy specimen, with the aspirate merely showing reduced or absent recovery of hematopoietic cells. Early stages of fibrosis are characterized by increased stainable marrow reticulin fibers. Fibrosis may accompany either primary hematopoietic disorders (e.g., myelofibrosis) or infiltrative diseases such as metastatic tumor.

STORAGE DISEASES

Storage disorders, such as Gaucher and Niemann-Pick diseases (described in Chap. 79), are characterized by abnormal macrophages containing stored material in various forms. These cells can be appreciated on both the biopsy and aspirate. In the latter preparation, they are typically more common in the feathered edge of the films. Reactive cells, such as the histiocytes with ''sea-blue'' inclusion granules or pseudo-Gaucher cells,[40] which are seen in chronic myelogenous leukemia can resemble those seen in storage disorders.

INFECTIONS

Infectious organisms with an intracellular location, such as *Leishmania*,[41] *Histoplasma*,[45] and *Toxoplasma*,[42] can be visualized in monocytic cells by morphologic examination of the marrow. Identification of mycobacterial organisms in the marrow by acid-fast staining lacks sensitivity but allows early diagnosis in one-third of cases of HIV-related *Mycobacterium avium* complex infection.[43] Morphologic examination and culture of the marrow is the most sensitive diagnostic test for disseminated leishmaniasis, a troublesome problem in HIV-infected patients who are exposed to this organism.[44] Marrow morphology is also a sensitive diagnostic tool for detection of disseminated histoplasmosis in patients with AIDS.[45] The presence of marrow granulomas, recognizable only on biopsy specimens, necessitates examination by special stains for fungal and mycobacterial organisms, but the differential diagnosis is extensive.[46]

NECROSIS AND GELATINOUS TRANSFORMATION

Marrow necrosis may occur in a variety of disorders, particularly sickle cell disease and neoplastic processes involving the marrow.[47] Aspirates of necrotic marrow stained with polychrome stains contain cells with indistinct margins and smudged basophilic nuclei surrounded by acidophilic material. In advanced necrosis all nuclei become acidophilic, with blurred outlines. Sections of marrow stained with hematoxylin and eosin or with polychrome stains show loss of normal marrow architecture, indistinct cellular margins, and a background of amorphous eosinophilic material. Patients with severe weight loss may develop gelatinous transformation of the marrow, characterized by amorphous extracellular material (proteoglycans), fat atrophy, and marrow hypoplasia.[48] The findings of gelatinous transformation are reversible.[49]

DIFFERENTIATION OF THE HEMATOPOIETIC LINEAGES

OVERVIEW

The marrow aspirate films should be examined under low-power magnification to assess the relative amounts of fat and hematopoietic cells in particles and the number of megakaryocytes, plasma cells, and mast cells present. Low-power examination will also permit detection of osteoclasts or osteoblasts, groups of malignant cells, Gaucher cells, lymphoid follicles, and granulomas. The entire film should be examined, including the particles, and higher magnification should be employed to study any abnormalities discovered. Similarly, biopsy sections are examined at low power to assess adequacy, cellularity, presence of infiltrative disease, and cellularity of the major hematopoietic lineages.

After the low-power survey, the films should be examined under oil-immersion magnification to determine the various hematopoietic cell types present and assess adequacy of differentiation in each hematopoietic lineage. For most diagnostic questions, a careful and systematic visual examination of the marrow is sufficient to assess differentiation, but a marrow differential count can be performed to quantify the status of hematopoietic differentiation, particularly in the granulocytic lineages. Because a large variety of cell types are normally present in the marrow and their distribution is irregular, an accurate marrow differential count requires examination of 300 to 500 nucleated cells. Normal values for these determinations are presented in Table 3-1, including data for infants from birth to 18 months of age.[50] Between birth and age 1 month there is an increase in lymphocytes and a decrease in erythroid and granulocytic precursors. After 1 month the marrow differential count varies little to age 18 months, the duration of the study.[50] The proportion of polymorphonuclear neutrophils is increased with large volumes of aspirate, probably because of dilution of marrow cells by mature granulocytes in the blood.[51] The range of normal for all cell types is broad, and differential counts and M/E ratios are to be considered rough guides to the character of the marrow as a whole.

Morphologically recognizable cells in the normal marrow include mature granulocytes and their precursors, erythroid precursors, lymphocytes in varying stages of development, plasma cells, monocytes, macrophages (histiocytes), stromal cells, megakaryocytes, osteoblasts, osteoclasts, and mast cells. It should be recognized that typically only the later stages of differentiation, in which progenitors become fully committed to a given lineage, are morphologically recognizable. The earliest committed progenitors of all lineages are typically rather unremarkable cells without distinctive morphologic attributes.

The morphologic characteristics of each cell type are briefly described below. Detailed descriptions of the normal development and differentiation in the major hematopoietic lineages are found in the specific chapters related to the erythroid (Chaps. 22 and 29), granulocytic (Chaps. 64, 65, 68, and 69), monocytic (Chaps. 73 and 75), megakaryocytic (Chap. 110), and lymphoid (Chap. 80) series.

GRANULOCYTES

The term *granulocytes* is used to refer to the precursors and mature forms of leukocytes characterized by neutrophilic, eosinophilic, or basophilic granules in their cytoplasm in the more mature stages of development. This series is sometimes referred to as the *myeloid series*. The overall trend is a gradual decrease in nuclear size and enhanced clumping of nuclear chromatin as cells lose proliferative capacity, while granules of varying types progressively appear in the cytoplasm.

The *myeloblast* (Plate X-1) is round and large, about 14 to 18 μm in diameter on a dried film. The nucleus occupies most of the cell. The nuclear chromatin is very fine, and two to five nucleoli are present. The cytoplasm is basophilic but less so than that of the erythroid series. No granules are present.

The *promyelocyte* (progranulocyte) (Plate X-2) is larger than the myeloblast. The chromatin pattern is coarser than that of the myeloblast, but nucleoli are usually present. The cytoplasm is basophilic with a clear Golgi area and is characterized by a small number of prominent, large red granules. These are called *primary, nonspecific*, or *azurophilic* granules, and in the marrow they usually mark the cell as a granulocyte precursor, although similar-appearing granules (with different enzymatic composition, however) may occur in large lympho-cytes.

The *myelocyte* (Plate X-7) is slightly smaller than the promyelo-cyte. This is the most mature dividing cell in the granulocytic lineage. Its nucleus is round or oval and is often located eccentrically. The chromatin pattern is coarser than that of the promyelocyte, and nucleoli are usually not visible. The defining feature is the presence of specific (secondary) granules in the cytoplasm, which identify the cell lineage. These may be neutrophilic (fine, variable size, lilac color), eosinophilic (larger, round, orange-red), or basophilic (larger still, irregular in size, deep blue). Based on the type of specific granules present, myelocytes, metamyelocytes, and bands are described as being either neutrophilic, eosinophilic, or basophilic. These granules first appear in the perinu-clear area. The cytoplasm is only slightly basophilic.

The *metamyelocyte* (Plate X-8) is about the same size as the myelocyte and resembles it closely, except that the nucleus is indented, the chromatin is more coarse, and the cytoplasm is less basophilic.

The *band* cell (Plate X-6) is characterized by a nucleus which is horseshoe-shaped or lobulated but not segmented in that the rudimen-tary lobes are connected by a thick band of chromatin rather than the thin thread or filament which characterizes the mature polymorphonu-clear leukocyte. The cytoplasm is yellowish pink or nearly colorless. Fine neutrophilic granules are abundant in the cytoplasm. Nuclear chromatin is dense, but less so than the segmented granulocyte.

Polymorphonuclear (segmented) granulocytes (Plate X-6) differ from the band cell by the multilobed character of the nucleus. At least two separate lobes are defined by a complete rounded shape, whether or not the thin filament joining them is seen. Nuclear chromatin is very dense. The mature eosinophil typically has only two lobes, while the neutrophil averages three to four lobes. Basophil nuclei are often obscured by the abundant basophilic granules.

MONOCYTES
Monocytes in normal marrow are identical morphologically to those in the blood (Plate VII). Promonocytes have more delicate chromatin, visible nucleoli, often a few fine granules, and somewhat more baso-philic cytoplasm.

MACROPHAGES (HISTIOCYTES)
These cells are derived from monocytes but are larger, reaching 20 to 30 μm in the longest dimension. The nucleus is oval with delicate reticular chromatin and one or two small nucleoli. The cytoplasm ranges from blue-gray to pale and colorless and often contains phago-cytosed cells, degenerating cell debris, and vacuoles. Normally, intact red cells are rarely visible inside marrow histiocytes. However, uncon-trolled activation of histiocytic cells leads to a "hemophagocytic syn-drome," which is associated with a variety of neoplastic, viral, and reactive conditions.[52]

ERYTHROID CELLS
During erythroid differentiation, the nucleus progressively becomes smaller and nuclear chromatin more condensed, as the cell's prolifera-tive capacity decreases, while cytoplasm gradually loses the bluish color imparted by mRNA, replacing it with the pink-staining hemoglo-bin. Cells in the erythroid series are termed "erythroblasts" or "nor-moblasts." The latter term was used to distinguish the normal sequence from that observed in megaloblastic anemia, in which the erythroid precursors are called "megaloblasts" because of their large size. It should be recognized that these stages are arbitrary divisions within a continuum of differentiation.

The *proerythroblast* (Plate V-1) is a large round cell measuring from 15 to 20 μm in diameter. The nucleus occupies most of the cell. The chromatin is present in a fine reticular or stippled pattern, but is

more densely stained than the chromatin of the myeloblast. Nucleoli are present and are often bluish. The cytoplasm is typically more basophilic than the myeloblast.

The *basophilic erythroblast* (Plate V-2) is smaller than the pro-erythroblast, and the nucleus occupies less of the cell. The chromatin pattern is stippled, and the small, condensed masses of chromatin are sharply defined and separated by pale parachromatin. The cytoplasm is deeply basophilic.

The *polychromatophilic erythroblast* (Plate V-3) is smaller than the basophilic erythroblast. The nucleus occupies even less of the cell, and the chromatin pattern is more condensed, with larger masses of chromatin sharply defined by pale parachromatin. The cytoplasm is gray or grayish-pink due to the increasing amounts of hemoglobin.

The *orthochromatic erythroblast* (Plate V-4) is only slightly larger than the mature erythrocyte. The nucleus is small and pyknotic. The cytoplasm is red, like that of the mature erythrocyte.

The *erythrocyte* (Plate I-1) is the mature anucleate red cell. *Polychromatophilic erythrocytes* are mature anucleate red cells that are just released from the marrow and still have sufficient residual mRNA to impart a slight grayish tinge to the cytoplasm. The gray color of the cytoplasm is due to a combination of cytoplasmic RNA and hemoglobin.

MEGAKARYOCYTES
Megakaryocytes are large cells (30 to 150 μm) with darkly stained, irregularly lobed nuclei (Plate XI). The cytoplasm is blue cotton-candy-textured, and the more mature cells contain many purple-red granules. About half the megakaryocytes should have platelets adjacent to their periphery.

LYMPHOCYTES
In normal marrow lymphocytes similar to those found in the blood occur in variable numbers dependent on the degree of peripheral blood contamination of the marrow. Immature lymphoid cells with very high nuclear/cytoplasmic ratio and moderately dense but finely distributed chromatin are often seen in pediatric marrow aspirates and may cause diagnostic difficulty in some clinical settings, such as the "rebound" lymphocytosis that occurs after cessation of maintenance chemother-apy for acute lymphoblastic leukemia.[53] These mostly represent vary-ing stages of B-cell precursor development.[54] Mature lymphocytes and smaller numbers of immature lymphoid forms are prominent in infant marrows but diminish in number with age.

PLASMA CELLS
Normal plasma cells vary somewhat in size but are usually 12 to 16 μm in diameter. They are round or oval. The nucleus is small, round, eccentrically placed, and stained densely purple. The chromatin is coarse and clumped. Nucleoli are not visible. The cytoplasm is deep blue, often with a paranuclear clear zone. Binucleate forms may be found in normal marrow (Plate XVI-1, -2, and -3).

OTHER CELL TYPES
Mast cells are readily recognized by their content of dark-blue granules, which usually completely fill the cytoplasm and may obscure the nucleus. The cells are round or spindle-shaped and are often located deep in the particles, frequently lying along blood vessels. The nucleus is often not visible, but, when seen, it is round or oval with a vesicular chromatin pattern (Plate VII-5).

Osteoclasts and *osteoblasts* are uncommon and are seen more frequently in marrow obtained from children and from adults with hyperparathyroidism or osteoblastic reactions to tumors (Plate XV). Osteoclasts are large cells and may be more than 100 μm in diameter. They superficially resemble megakaryocytes but contain multiple separated nuclei which have a moderately fine chromatin pattern with nucleoli. The cytoplasm varies from slightly basophilic to intensely eosinophilic due to the content of eosinophilic granules. Osteoclasts may contain coarse basophilic debris.

Osteoblasts are usually oval cells up to 30 μm in the longest diameter. They often occur in groups. The nucleus is usually eccentric and is relatively small. The chromatin pattern is uniform, and there are one to three nucleoli. The cytoplasm is light blue and may contain a few red granules. Osteoblasts may be mistaken for plasma cells. In osteoblasts the pale centrosomal region of the cytoplasm is separated from the nucleus, in contrast to that of the plasma cell, in which it abuts the nucleus directly.

EVALUATION OF IRON STORES

Marrow examination should include evaluation of the iron stores, especially if the patient is anemic. This is accomplished by staining a marrow film or section by the Prussian blue technique. Marrow macrophages are evaluated for storage iron, and erythroblasts are examined for the presence of iron granules in the cytoplasm (sideroblasts). In order to sensitively detect presence of iron stores in macrophages, a film containing marrow particles should be examined. Late erythroblasts are readily identified by their small size and the size, shape, and chromatin pattern of the nucleus. The proportion of late erythroblasts in normal subjects which contain one or more Prussian blue granules is extremely variable (3 to 69 percent).[35] Abnormal sideroblasts are characterized by increased number (>5) or size of iron granules, particularly if these are arranged in a ring around the nucleus, reflecting accumulation of iron in mitochondria.

REFERENCES

1. Piney A: Anatomy of bone marrow. *Br Med* 2:792, 1922.
2. Custer RP, Ahlfeldt FE: Studies on the structure and function of bone marrow: II. Variations in cellularity in various bones with advancing years of life and their relative response to stimuli. *J Lab Clin Med* 17:960, 1932.
3. Ellis LD, Jensen WN, Westerman MP: Needle biopsy of bone marrow: an experience with 1,445 biopsies. *Arch Intern Med* 114:213, 1964.
4. Sabharwal BD, Malhotra V, Aruna S, Grewal R: Comparative evaluation of bone marrow aspirate particle smears, imprints and biopsy sections. *J Postgrad Med* 36:194, 1990.
5. Bearden JD, Ratkin GA, Coltman CA: Comparison of the diagnostic value of bone marrow biopsy and bone marrow aspiration in neoplastic disease. *J Clin Pathol* 27:738, 1974.
6. Pasquale D, Chikkappa G: Comparative evaluation of bone marrow aspirate particle smears, biopsy imprints, and biopsy sections. *Am J Hematol* 22:381, 1986.
7. Kidd PG, Saminathan T, Drachtman RA, Ettinger LJ: Comparison of the cellularity and presence of residual leukemia in bone marrow aspirate and biopsy specimens in pediatric patients with acute lymphoblastic leukemia (ALL) at day 7–14 of chemotherapy. *Med Pediatr Oncol* 29:541, 1997.
8. Montserrat E, Villamor N, Reverter JC, et al: Bone marrow assessment in B-cell chronic lymphocytic leukaemia: aspirate or biopsy? A comparative study in 258 patients. *Br J Haematol* 93:111, 1996.
9. Winfield DA, Polacarz SU: Bone marrow histology 3: value of bone marrow core biopsies in acute leulemia, myelodysplastic syndromes, and chronic myeloid leukemia. *J Clin Pathol* 45:855, 1992.
10. Bartl R, Frisch B, Wilmanns W: Potential of bone marrow biopsy in chronic myeloproliferative disorders (MPD). *Eur J Haematol* 50:41, 1993.
11. Dunlop TJ, Deen C, Lind S, et al: Use of combined oral narcotic and benzodiazepine for control of pain associated with bone marrow examination. *South Med J* 92:477, 1999.
12. Cannell H: Evidence for safety margins of lignocaine local anaesthetics for peri-oral use. *Br Den J* 181:243, 1996.
13. Jamshidi K, Swaim WR: Bone marrow biopsy with unaltered architecture: a new biopsy device. *J Lab Clin Med* 77:335, 1971.
14. Humphries J: Dry tap bone marrow aspiration: clinical significance. *Am J Hematol* 247, 1990.
15. James L, Stass S, Schumacher H: Value of imprint preparation of bone marrow biopsies in hematologic diagnosis. *Cancer* 46:173, 1980.
16. Dewald G, Allen JE, Strutzenberg DK: A cytogenetic method for mailed in bone marrow specimens for the study of hematologic disorders. *Lab Med* 13:225, 1982.
17. Akoury DA, Seo JJ, James CD, Zaki SR: RT-PCR detection of mRNA recovered from archival glass slide smears. *Mod Pathol* 6:195, 1993.
18. Lillie RD, Fullmer HM: *Histopathologic Technique and Practical Histochemistry*. McGraw-Hill, New York, 1976.
19. Hyun BH, Stevenson AJ, Hanau CA: Fundamentals of bone marrow examination. *Hematol Oncol Clin North Am* 8:651, 1994.
20. Moosavi H, Lichtman MA, Donnelly JA, Churukian CJ: Plastic-embedded human marrow biopsy specimens: improved histochemical methods. *Arch Pathol Lab Med* 105:269, 1981.
21. Blythe D, Hand NM, Jackson P, et al: Use of methyl methacrylate resin for embedding bone marrow trephine biopsy specimens. *J Clin Pathol* 50:45, 1997.
22. Brown DC, Gatter KC: The bone marrow trephine biopsy. A review of normal histology. *Histopathology* 22:411, 1992.
23. Bishop PW, McNally K, Harris M: Audit of bone marrow trephines. *J Clin Pathol* 45:1105, 1992.
24. Holdrinet RSG, Egmond J, Wessels JMC, Haanen C: A method for quantification of peripheral blood admixture in bone marrow aspirates. *Exp Hematol* 8:103, 1980.
25. Juneja SK, Wolf MM, Cooper IA: Value of bilateral bone marrow biopsy specimens in non-Hodgkin's lymphoma. *J Clin Pathol* 43:630, 1990.
26. Perrin-Resche I, Bizais Y, Buhe T, Fiche M: How does iliac crest bone marrow biopsy compare with imaging in the detection of bone metastases in small cell lung cancer? *EurJ Nucl Med* 20:420, 1993.
27. Cheung NK, Heller G, Kushner BH, et al: Detection of metastatic neuroblastoma in bone marrow: when is routine marrow histology insensitive? *J Clin Oncol* 15:2807, 1997.
28. Ozkaynak MF, Scribano P, Gomperts E, et al: Comparative evaluation of the bone marrow by the volumetric method, particle smears, and biopsies in pediatric disorders. *Am J Hematol* 29:144, 1988.
29. Gruppo RA, Lampkin BC, Granger S: Bone marrow cellularity determination: comparison of the biopsy, aspirate, and buffy coat. *Blood* 49:29, 1977.
30. Hartsock RJ, Smith EB, Petty CS: Normal variations with aging of the amount of hemopoietic tissue in bone marrow from the anterior iliac crest. *Am J Clin Path* 43:326, 1965.
31. Tuzuner N, Cox C, Rowe JM, Bennett JM: Bone marrow cellularity in myeloid stem cell disorders: impact of age correction. *Leuk Res* 18:559, 1994.
32. Wilkins BS: Histology of normal haemopoiesis: bone marrow histology I. *J Clin Pathol* 45:645, 1992.
33. Abrahamsen JF, Lund-Johansen F, Laerum OD, et al: Flow cytometric assessment of peripheral blood contamination and proliferative activity of human bone marrow cell populations. *Cytometry* 19:77, 1995.
34. Batinic D, Marusic M, Pavletic Z, et al: Relationship between differing volumes of bone marrow aspirates and their cellular composition. *Bone Marrow Transplant* 6:103, 1990.
35. Bain BJ: The bone marrow aspirate of healthy subjects. *Br J Haematol* 94:206, 1996.
36. Atac B, Lawrence C, Goldberg S: Metastatic tumor: the complementary role of the marrow aspirate and biopsy. *Am J Med Sci* 302:211, 1991.
37. Terpstra W, Lokhorst H, Blomjous F: Comparison of plasma cell infiltration in bone marrow biopsies and aspirates in patients with multiple myeloma. *Br J Haematol* 82:46, 1992.
38. Navone R, Valpreda M, Pich A: Lymphoid nodules and nodular lymphoid hyperplasia in bone marrow biopsies. *Acta Haematol* 74:19, 1985.
39. Erber WN, Asbahr HD, Phelps PN: In situ hybridization of immunoglobulin light chain mRNA on bone marrow trephines using biotinylated probes and the APAAP method. *Pathology* 25:63, 1993.
40. Anastasi J, Musvee T, Roulston D, et al: Pseudo-Gaucher histiocytes identified up to 1 year after transplantation for CML are BCR/ABL-positive. *Leukemia* 12:233, 1998.
41. Magill AJ, Grogl M, Gasser RA Jr, et al: Visceral infection caused by

Leishmania tropica in veterans of Operation Desert Storm. *N Engl J Med* 328:1383, 1993.

42. Brouland JP, Audouin J, Hofman P, et al: Bone marrow involvement by disseminated toxoplasmosis in acquired immunodeficiency syndrome: the value of bone marrow trephine biopsy and immunohistochemistry for the diagnosis. *Hum Pathol* 27:302, 1996.

43. Hussong J, Peterson LR, Warren JR, Peterson LC: Detecting disseminated *Mycobacterium avium* complex infections in HIV- positive patients. The usefulness of bone marrow trephine biopsy specimens, aspirate cultures, and blood cultures. *Am J Clin Pathol* 110:806, 1998.

44. Agostoni C, Dorigoni N, Malfitano A, et al: Mediterranean leishmaniasis in HIV-infected patients: epidemiological, clinical, and diagnostic features of 22 cases. *Infection* 26:93, 1998.

45. Neubauer MA, Bodensteiner DC: Disseminated histoplasmosis in patients with AIDS. *South Med J* 85:1166, 1992.

46. Eid A, Carion W, Nystrom JS: Differential diagnoses of bone marrow granuloma. *West J Med* 164:510, 1996.

47. Norgard MJ, Carpenter JTJ, Conrad ME: Bone marrow necrosis and degeneration. *Arch Intern Med* 139:905, 1979.

48. Seaman JP, Kjeldsberg CR, Linker A: Gelatinous transformation of the bone marrow. *Hum Pathol* 9:685, 1978.

49. Tavassoli M, Eastlund DT, Yam LT, et al: Gelatinous transformation of bone marrow in prolonged self-induced starvation. *Scand J Haematol* 16:311, 1976.

50. Rosse C, Krauner MJ, Dillon TL, et al: Bone marrow cell populations of normal infants: the predominance of lymphocytes. *J Lab Clin Med* 89:1225, 1977.

51. Dresch C, Faille A, Poirier O, Kadouche J: The cellular composition of the granulocyte series in the normal human bone marrow according to the volume of the sample. *J Clin Pathol* 27:106, 1974.

52. Janka G, Imashuku S, Elinder G, et al: Infection- and malignancy-associated hemophagocytic syndromes. Secondary hemophagocytic lymphohistiocytosis. *Hematol Oncol Clin North Am* 12:435, 1998.

53. Pritchard-Jones K, Toogood IR, Rice MS: The significance of an M2 bone marrow at cessation of chemotherapy in childhood acute lymphoblastic leukemia. *Am J Pediatr Hematol Oncol* 10:292, 1988.

54. Longacre TA, Foucar K, Crago S, et al: Hematogones: a multiparameter analysis of bone marrow precursor cells. *Blood* 73:543, 1989.

55. Glaser K, Limarzi LR, Poncher HG: Cellular composition of the bone marrow in normal infants and children. *Pediatrics* 6:789, 1950.

56. Duggan PR, Easton D, Linder J, Auer IA: Bone marrow staging of patients with non-Hodgkin lymphoma by flow cytometry: correlation with morphology. *Cancer* 88:894, 2000.

PART II

GENERAL
HEMATOLOGY

CHAPTER 4

STRUCTURE OF THE MARROW AND THE HEMATOPOIETIC MICROENVIRONMENT

CAMILLE N. ABBOUD

MARSHALL A. LICHTMAN

The marrow, located in the medullary cavity of bone, is the sole site of effective hematopoiesis in human beings. It produces about 6 billion cells per kilogram of body weight per day. Hematopoietically active (red) marrow regresses after birth until late adolescence, after which time it is focused in the lower skull, vertebrae, shoulder and pelvic girdles, ribs, and sternum. Fat cells replace hematopoietic cells in the bones of the hands, feet, legs, and arms (yellow marrow). Fat comes to occupy about 50 percent of the space of red marrow in the adult, and further fatty metamorphosis continues slowly with aging. In very old individuals, a gelatinous transformation of fat to a mucoid material may occur (white marrow). Yellow marrow can revert to hematopoietically active marrow if prolonged demand is present, such as hemolytic anemia. Thus, hematopoiesis can be expanded by increasing the volume of red marrow and decreasing the development (transit) time from progenitor to mature cell.

The marrow stroma consists principally of a network of sinuses that originate at the endosteum from cortical capillaries and terminate in collecting vessels that enter the systemic venous circulation. The trilaminar sinus wall is composed of endothelial cells; an underdeveloped, thin basement membrane; and adventitial reticular cells that are fibroblasts capable of transforming into adipocytes. The endothelium and reticular cells are sources of hematopoietic cytokines. Hematopoiesis takes place in the intersinus spaces and is controlled by a complex array of stimulatory and inhibitory cytokines, cell-to-cell contacts, and the effects of extracellular matrix components on proximate cells. In this unique environment, lymphohematopoietic stem cells differentiate into all the blood cell lineages. Mature cells are produced and released to maintain steady-state blood cell levels. The system can also go into overdrive to meet increased demands for additional cells as a result of blood loss, hemolysis, inflammation, immune cytopenias, and other causes. Stem cells can leave and reenter marrow as part of their normal circulation. Their extramedullary circulation can be increased by exogenous cytokines and chemokines.

The evolutionary pressures that led to hematopoiesis being confined to the medullary cavity of bone is unclear, but advances in knowledge of the chemical links between the two tissues may provide the answers.

The marrow, one of the largest organs in the human body, is the principal site for blood cell formation. In the normal adult its daily production amounts to about 2.5 billion red cells, 2.5 billion platelets, and 1.0 billion granulocytes per kilogram of body weight. The rate of production is adjusted to actual needs and can be varied from nearly zero to many times normal.[1] Until the late nineteenth century, blood cell formation was thought to be the prerogative of the lymph nodes or the liver and spleen. In 1868 Neuman[2] and Bizzozero[3] independently observed nucleated blood cells in material squeezed from the ribs of human cadavers and proposed that the marrow is the major source of blood cells.[4] The first in vivo marrow biopsy was probably done in 1876 by Mosler,[5] who used a regular wood drill to obtain marrow particles from a patient with leukemia. Fifty years passed before Arinkin's studies in 1929 established marrow aspiration as a safe, easy, and useful technique.[6]

Kinetic studies of marrow cells, using radioisotopes and in vitro cultures, have shown that cell lines consist of mature end cells with a finite functional life span, capable of limited proliferation before their full maturation but without the capacity for self-renewal. Sustained cellular production, on the other hand, depends on the presence of pools of primordial cells capable both of differentiation and of self-replication.[7] The most primitive pool consists of pluripotential stem cells with the capacity for continuous self-renewal. The more mature pools consist of differentiated unipotential progenitor cells with their maturation restricted to single cell lines and with no capacity for self-renewal. The proliferative activity of these pools involves humoral feedback from peripheral target tissues[8] as well as cell-to-cell interactions within the microenvironment of the marrow.[9,10] The marrow stroma has evolved to provide a unique structural and chemical environment to support the survival, differentiation, and proliferation of pluripotential (lymphohematopoietic) stem cells. These stem cells can be identified and isolated using a unique array of surface antigen-receptor expression, especially CD34 and Thy-1, but lacking CD38 and CD33.[11–14] Isolated cell populations enriched in stem cells can be quantified using in vitro progenitor assays[15–18] and surrogate in vivo long-term repopulating assays in severely immunodeficient mice and xenogeneic animal models[19–22] (see Chap. 14).

HEMATOPOIETIC LOCATION

EMBRYOGENESIS AND EARLY STEM CELL DEVELOPMENT

The yolk sac and later the fetal liver are sites of early erythropoiesis and contain cells with multilineage differentiation capabilities beginning at day 8 of gestation (yolk sac).[23] Non-yolk-sac regions such as the paraaortic splanchnopleura give rise to B-cell progenitors when transplanted into mice with severe combined immunodeficiency.[24] The aorta-gonad-mesonephros region (AGM) contains pluripotential stem cells during embryogenesis.[25] Stem cells in the AGM region appear

Acronyms and abbreviations that appear in this chapter include: AGM, aorta-gonad-mesonephros; b-FGF, basic fibroblast growth factor; BMP, bone morphogenetic protein; ECMs, extracellular matrix proteins; ELAM-1, endothelial leukocyte adhesion molecule 1; GAGs, glycosaminoglycans; G-CSF, granulocyte colony stimulating factor; GCSFR, G-CSF receptor; GM-CSF, granulocyte-macrophage colony stimulating factor; HCA, hematopoietic cell antigen; HCAM, homing cell adhesion molecule; IAP, integrin-associated protein; ICAM-1, intercellular adhesion molecule 1; LIF, leukemia inhibitory factor; M-CSF, macrophage colony stimulating factor; MIP-1, macrophage inflammatory protein 1; MMP-9, matrix metalloproteinase 9; NK, natural killer; ODF, osteoclast differentiation and activation factor; OPG, osteoprotegrin; PCLP1, podocalyxin-1; PDGF, platelet-derived growth factor; PRR2, poliovirus receptor-related 2 protein; PSGL-1, P-selectin glycoprotein ligand; SDF-1, stroma-derived factor 1; SHP-1, Src homology 2 domain-bearing protein tyrosine phosphatase 1; TGF-β, transforming growth factor beta; TSP, thrombospondin; IIICS, type III connecting segment; VAP-1 vascular adhesion protein 1; VCAM-1, vascular cell adhesion molecule 1; VEGF, vascular endothelial growth factor; VLA-4, very late antigen 4.

before the fetal liver, indicating the importance of this mesodermal region of the embryo in stem cell migration. Early lymphoid precursors have been identified in the day 8 yolk sac[26] and the body of embryos beginning at the 10- to 12-somite stage.[27] The earliest repopulating lymphohematopoietic stem cells in the day 9 yolk sac have been detected in vivo, using primary conditioned newborn mice,[28] and in vitro.[29]

The early inductive microenvironment for pluripotential stem cells elaborates KIT ligand, encoded by the Sl locus; a later transition from early independent to the late KIT-ligand-dependent fetal hematopoiesis in the embryo occurs.[30] Similarly, KIT-negative stem cells have been shown to give rise to KIT-positive cells with pluripotential stem cell activity.[31] Murine embryonic stem cells require multiple growth factors such as leukemia inhibitory factor (LIF), KIT ligand, and basic fibroblast growth factor (b-FGF) acting in concert.[32,33] Direct interactions and soluble growth factors from AGM stromal[34] or endothelial cells[35] and marrow-derived stromal cells improve the survival of primitive hematopoiesis.[34–36] This action is exerted via intimate cell-cell interactions of CD34-positive stem cells, which are HLA-DR-negative and uncommitted, with adventitial reticular cells.[36]

Locally expressed cytokines may lead to differences in the functions of the stromal cells of early blood islands[27,32] and those of marrow or spleen.[37] Morphologic studies of marrow recovering from aplasia show that early hematopoiesis is localized to the endosteum and vascular endothelium.[38] The intimate relationship of angiogenesis and early hematopoiesis is validated by the demonstration that AGM-derived single cells at day 10.5 postcoitum express the receptor tyrosine kinase, TEK, and give rise to hematopoietic cells in the presence of IL-3 and endothelial cells when exposed to angiopoietin-1, defining them as hemangioblasts.[39] Podocalyxin-1 (PCLP1), a highly glycosylated protein with similarity to CD34, a high-endothelial venule ligand for L-selectin, has been found on AGM-derived hemangioblasts.[40] These PCLP1-positive, CD45-negative cells give rise to hematopoietic cells and endothelial cells when cultured over stromal cells.[40] Expression of the alpha₄-integrin, in CD45-negative vascular E (VE)-cadherin-positive or -negative cells, defines the earliest precursor of hematopoietic cell lineage diverged from endothelial cells.[41] Primitive stem cells obtained from human fetal liver or marrow reconstitute all lymphohematopoietic-derived cells and part of the stromal microenvironment in in vivo repopulation assays.[42] These observations are consistent with the early derivation of hematopoietic, vascular, and stromal cells from a CD34-negative, vascular-endothelial cell growth factor 2 receptor (known as *KDR*) -positive, multipotential mesenchymal stem cell.[43–47] These findings are also underscored by the identification of AC133-positive, CD34-negative, CD7-negative hematopoietic stem cells[685] and by the presence of endothelial precursors in AC133-positive progenitor cells.[686] The presence of long-term reconstituting hematopoietic stem cells in murine skeletal tissue,[48] and in brain-derived neural cells,[49] emphasizes the plasticity of these totipotential cells. (See Chap. 14.)

HISTOGENESIS

Cavities within bone occur in the human being at about the fifth fetal month and soon become the exclusive site for granulocytic and megakaryocytic proliferation. Erythropoietic activity at the time is confined to the liver, and it is not until the end of the last trimester that the microenvironment in the marrow becomes supportive of erythroblasts (Fig. 4-1). At birth, the bone cavities are the only sites of significant hematopoietic activity and are completely engorged with hematopoietic cells.[50,51] The sequential appearance and disappearance of hematopoietic activity is governed by signaling via chemokine receptors (CXCR4) for stroma-derived factor 1 (SDF-1)[52,53] and cellular

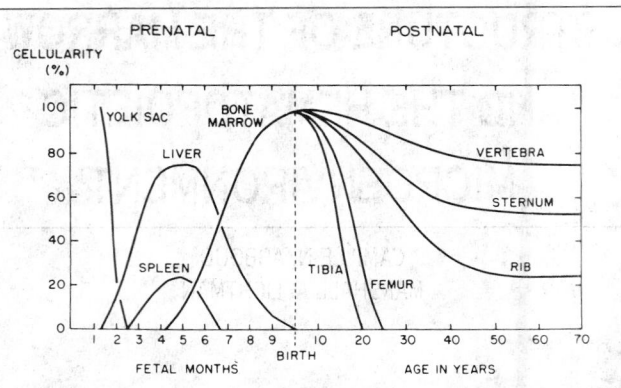

FIGURE 4-1   Expansion and recession of hematopoietic activity in extramedullary and medullary sites.

adhesion molecule-ligand pair interactions, such as, alpha₄-integrin with vascular cell adhesion molecule 1 (VCAM-1) or alpha₄-integrin with fibronectin.[54,55]

By the fourth year of life, a significant number of fat cells have appeared in the diaphysis of the human long bones.[56] These cells slowly replace hematopoietic elements and expand centripetally until, at about the age of 18 years, hematopoietic marrow is found only in the vertebrae, ribs, skull, pelvis, and proximal epiphyses of the femora and humeri. Direct measurements of the volume of bone cavities reveal that the bone cavity volume increases from 1.4 percent of body weight at birth to 4.8 percent in the adult,[50,57] while the blood volume decreases from 8 percent of body weight in the newborn to about 7 percent in the adult.[58] The expansion of marrow space continues throughout life, resulting in a further gradual increase in the amount of fatty tissue in all bone cavities, especially in the long bones.[59,60] The preference of hematopoietic tissue for centrally located bones has been ascribed to higher central tissue temperature with greater vascularity.[61] However, since complete reactivation of fatty marrow can occur in experimental animals in which hematopoietic expansion is induced, other factors must be involved.[62,63]

MARROW STRUCTURE

VASCULATURE

The blood supply comes from two major sources.[64] The nutrient artery, the principal source, penetrates the cortex through the nutrient canal. In the marrow cavity, it bifurcates into ascending and descending medullary arteries from which radial branches travel to the inner face of the cortex. After repenetrating the endosteum, the radial vessels diminish in caliber to structures of capillary size that course within the canalicular system of the cortex. Here arterial blood from the nutrient artery mixes with blood that enters the cortical capillary system from the periosteal capillaries derived from muscular arteries. After reentering the marrow cavity, the cortical capillaries form a sinusoidal network. Hematopoietic cells are located in the intersinusoidal tissue spaces (Fig. 4-2). Some arteries have specialized, thin-walled segments that arise abruptly as continuations of arteries with walls of normal thickness.[65] These vessels give off nearly perpendicular branches analogous to the arterial branching observed in the spleen and kidney, permitting volume compensation for changes in intramedullary pressure. In the marrow cavity, blood flows through a highly branching network of medullary sinuses. These sinuses collect into a large central sinus from which the blood enters the systemic venous circulation through emissary veins.

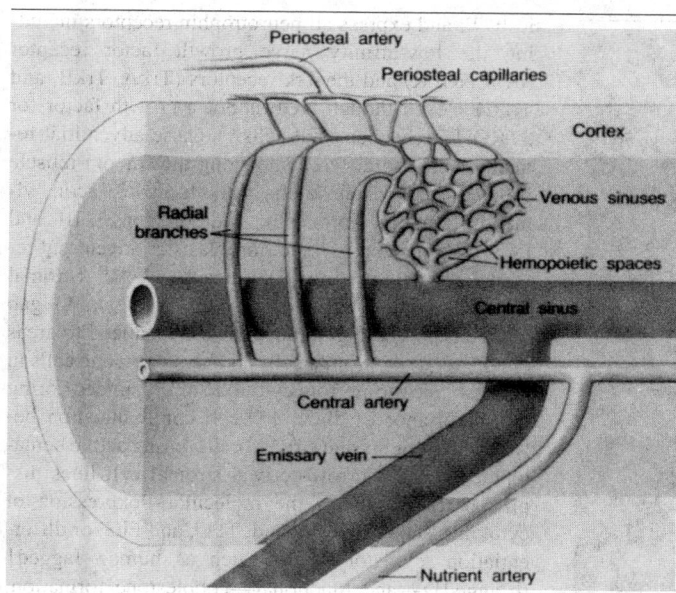

FIGURE 4-2 Schematic diagram of the circulation of the marrow. See text for further explanation.

Vascular networks consisting of cells expressing CD31, CD34, and CD105 (endoglin) but lacking intercellular adhesion molecule 1 (ICAM-1), ICAM-2, ICAM-3, or endothelial leukocyte adhesion molecule 1 (ELAM-1, E-selectin) can form also within the stroma of long-term marrow cultures, underscoring the intimate relationship of blood vessels to hematopoietic activity.[66] A study of early hematopoiesis of human marrow from long bones (ages 6 to 28 weeks) has shown an absence of CD34-positive hematopoietic progenitors before onset of hematopoiesis, a predominance of CD68-positive cells mediating chondrolysis, and CD34-positive endothelial cells developing into specific vascular structures organized by endothelial cells and myoid cells.[67] The vascular endothelial growth factor (VEGF) receptors found on CD34-positive cells[46] and AGM primitive stem cells underscore that common ontogeny.[68,69] Subsets of CD34-positive cells expressing the AC133 antigen and the human vascular endothelial receptor-2 define the functional endothelial precursor phenotype.[687]

INNERVATION

Myelinated and nonmyelinated nerve fibers are present in periarterial sheaths in marrow,[70] where they are thought to regulate arterial vessel tone. Nerve terminals are distributed between layers of periarterial adventitial cells or localize next to arterial smooth muscle cells.[71] Nonmyelinated fibers terminate in the hematopoietic spaces, implying that neurohumors elaborated from free-nerve terminals may affect hematopoiesis. Intimate cell-cell communication between sympathetic nerve cells and structural elements within the marrow sinuses occurs at less than 5 percent of nerve terminals that terminate within the hematopoietic parenchyma or on sinus walls. This anatomic unit, termed a *neuroreticular complex*, consists of efferent (autonomic) nerves and marrow stromal cells connected by gap junctions.[71]

Nerve growth factor receptor antibody reacts with adventitial reticular cells.[72] Tachykinins have demonstrated stimulatory and inhibitory hematopoietic activities within the marrow microenvironment,[73,74] and substance P stimulates CD34-positive cell proliferation by modulating stromal cell release of cytokines such as IL-3, IL-6, granulocyte colony stimulating factor, granulocyte-macrophage colony stimulating

factor (GM-CSF), and KIT ligand.[75,76] Interactions between neurokinins and cytokines such as platelet-derived growth factor and IL-1 result in fibroblast proliferation.[77] Neurokinin 1 receptors for substance P are present on marrow vascular endothelium,[78] and both noradrenergic and peptidergic innervation have been demonstrated in mouse marrow with dense fibers seen predominantly around blood vessels but also ramifying among marrow cells.[79] Thus, adrenergic responses to stress may regulate marrow blood flow and cellular release directly[80-83] or by altering endogenous nitric oxide levels within the marrow.[84] Exposure of marrow mononuclear cells to hypoxia increases the expression of neurokin-2 receptor and alters the proliferation of myeloid and erythroid progenitors.[85] Furthermore, the positive regulation of hematopoiesis by adrenergic agents after syngeneic marrow transplantation[86] supports the concept of neural influences. This issue remains controversial. In one study, no neuronal regulation of marrow function was elicited after neonatal sympathectomy or hind limb denervation in mice.[87]

SINUS ARCHITECTURE AND CELLULAR ORGANIZATION

In mammals, hematopoiesis takes place in the extravascular spaces between marrow sinuses. The sinus wall is composed of a luminal layer of endothelial cells and an abluminal coat of adventitial reticular cells, which forms an incomplete outer lining (Fig. 4-3). A thin, interrupted basement lamina is present between these cell layers.

ENDOTHELIAL CELLS

Endothelial cells are broad flat cells that completely cover the inner surface of the sinus.[88-90] They form the major barrier and control the system for chemicals and particles entering and leaving the hematopoietic spaces, with overlapping or interdigitating unions permitting volume expansion.[89] The endothelium of marrow sinusoids is actively endocytic and contains clathrin-coated pits, clathrin-coated vesicles, lysosomes, phagosomes, transfer tubules, and diaphragmed fenestrae.[91,92] Particles are endocytosed by endothelial cells primarily through clathrin-coated pits.[93]

Such endocytic features are in keeping with studies demonstrating colony-stimulating factor receptors on endothelial cells[94] and their shared antigenic determinants with macrophages.[95,96] Marrow endothelial cells express von Willebrand factor antigen,[97] type IV collagen, and laminin[98]; they also constitutively express two adhesion molecules: VCAM-1 and E-selectin.[99] The distribution of sialic acid and other carbohydrates on the luminal surface of marrow sinus endothelium is discontinued at diaphragmed fenestrae and coated pits, suggesting that such sugars play a role in endothelial membrane function.[93,100] Marrow microvascular endothelium can be isolated using the *Ulex europeaus* lectin, as well as CD34 monoclonal antibodies.[101-105] Marked attenuation of endothelial cell cytoplasm, short of discontinuity, can occur such that a short length of cytoplasm thins to approach a double plasma membrane in thickness (fenestra with a diaphragm).[106]

There is reciprocal regulation of CD34 expression and adhesion molecules by vascular endothelial cells exposed to inflammatory stimuli such as IL-1, interferon-γ, and tumor necrosis factor-α.[107] Receptors for the complement component C1q are upregulated on marrow microvascular endothelium by inflammatory cytokines.[108] Other receptors that may mediate marrow cellular trafficking include fractalkine, a novel endothelial membrane-bound chemokine with a mucin stalk, also upregulated by cytokines.[109] Marrow sinusoidal endothelium specifically expresses sialylated CD22 ligands, which are homing receptors for recirculating B lymphocytes.[110]

ADVENTITIAL RETICULAR CELLS

The abluminal or adventitial surface of the vascular sinus is composed of reticular cells.[88,111,112] The reticular cell bodies are contiguous with

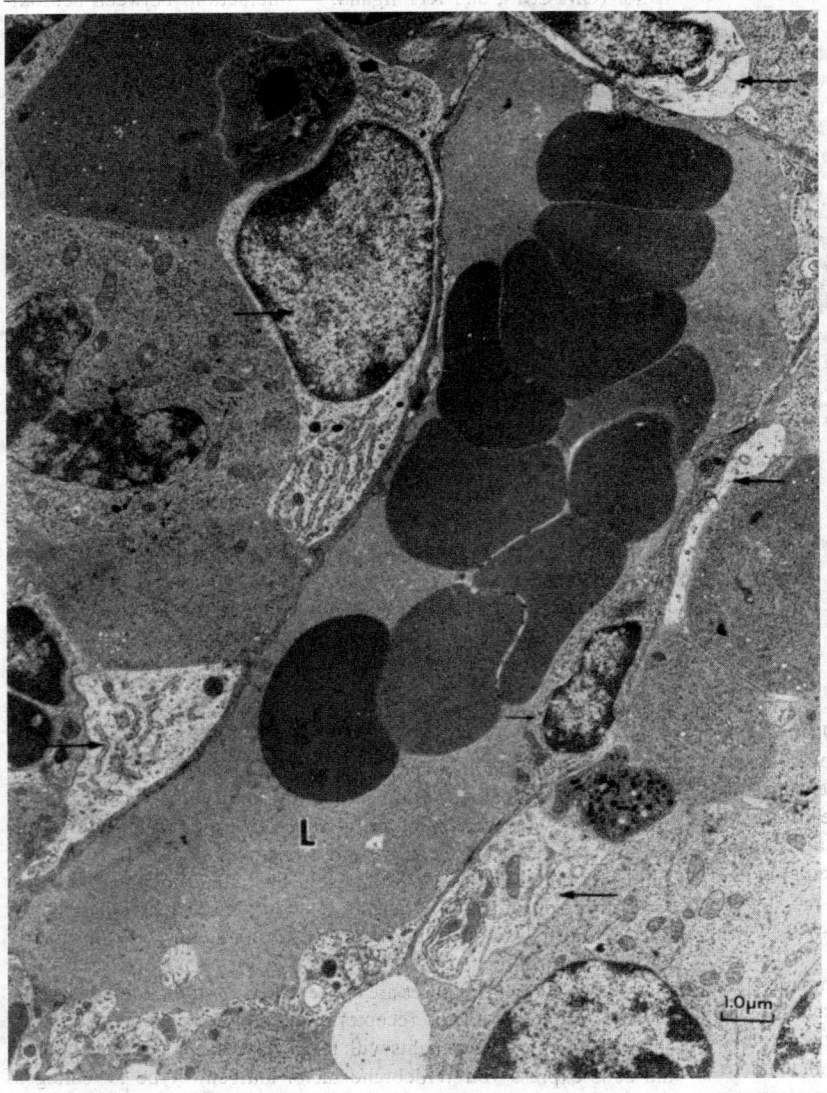

FIGURE 4-3 Transmission electron micrograph (TEM) of a mouse marrow sinus. The small arrow in the sinus lumen (L) indicates the perikaryon of an endothelial cell. Several endothelial cell junctions are present along the circumference of the sinus endothelial wall. Thus, the wall is composed of the cytoplasm of endothelial cells that overlap or interdigitate. Two adventitial reticular cells are identified by arrows at the top and upper left of the sinus. The cytoplasm of the adventitial reticular cells is discontinuous as it is followed around the sinus. Four cytoplasmic processes of adventitial reticular cells are indicated by arrows. Other, smaller processes of reticular cell cytoplasm can be found on close inspection of the sinus periphery and the hematopoietic spaces. The scattered rough endoplasmic reticulum and dense bodies are characteristic of the reticular cell cytoplasm. (Reprinted from Lichtman,[70] with permission.)

the sinus, forming part of its adventitial coat (Fig. 4-4). Their extensive branching cytoplasmic processes envelop the outer wall of the sinus to form an adventitial sheath. This sheath is interrupted and has been estimated to cover about two-thirds of the abluminal surface area of sinuses. The reticular cells synthesize reticular (argentophilic) fibers that, along with their cytoplasmic processes, extend into the hematopoietic compartments and form a meshwork on which hematopoietic cells rest. The cell bodies, their broad processes, and their fibers constitute the reticulum of the marrow.

Adventitial reticular cells have a high concentration of alkaline phosphatase in their membranes; express CD10, CD13, and class I HLA antigens[88]; react with the 6/19 and STRO-1 monoclonal antibod-

ies[114,115]; and express all neurotrophin receptors including the low-affinity nerve growth factor receptor (p75LNGFR) and the Trk receptors (TrkA, TrkB, and TrkC)[116] even though NGF is not a growth factor for STRO-1-derived stromal cells.[117] These adventitial reticular cells can differentiate along the smooth-muscle pathway and contain alpha smooth-muscle actin, vimentin, laminin, fibronectin, and collagens I, III, and IV.[118,119] Unlike embryonic fibroblasts,[120] adventitial reticular cells are usually CD34-negative.[89,119,121] Stromal cells display cell-cell contacts via connexin-43 gap junctions.[122] These gap junctions are localized to areas of adherence of stromal cells and hematopoietic cells in marrow recovering from cytotoxic injury, underscoring the importance of direct cell-cell communication between progenitors and stromal cells during active hematopoiesis.[123,124] Marrow-derived stromal cell lines display heterogeneity at the molecular—expression of cytokines such as KIT ligand, TPO, and Flt3, or differentiation regulatory genes such as human Jagged1 (hJagged1)—and functional—cobblestone formation, CD34+ cell proliferation—levels, with variable expression of ICAM-1, VCAM-1, and collagens I, III, and IV.[125]

More specialized contractile reticular "barrier cells" have been described in both spleen and marrow in mice after hematopoietic stress, such as malarial infection or administration of IL-1.[126,127] Barrier cells increase in number and seem to enclose developing hematopoietic progenitors in these animals. These cells may regulate the release of precursors into the circulation.[127] Human counterparts of barrier cells are alpha smooth-muscle-positive cells that appear in culture after 2 weeks and are represented by myoid cells lining sinuses at the abluminal side of endothelial cells in marrow biopsies.[119] These cells also have been described in fetal marrow and are increased in areas of active marrow proliferation after inflammation.[127]

ADIPOCYTES

Adipocytes in marrow develop by lipogenesis in fibroblast-like cells, most likely the adventitial reticular cells (Fig. 4-5). Reticular cells in mouse marrow and human marrow can undergo transformation to fat cells in vitro and can transform into fibroblasts in culture by a process of lipolysis.[88,129] Marrow fat cells are relatively resistant to lipolysis during starvation. Their proportion of saturated fatty acids is lower than in other fat deposits, but their composition depends to a certain extent on whether they are located in red, hematopoietically active, or yellow, hematopoietically inactive, marrow.[129] Adipocytes express leptin, osteocalcin, and increased prolactin receptors during their differentiation, thereby promoting hematopoiesis and influencing osteogenesis.[130-133] Adipocyte maturation in vitro is inhibited by stromal-derived cytokines such as IL-1 and IL-11.[134,135] Marrow adipocyte leptin may modulate adjacent hematopoietic progenitor growth.[129] Adipocyte differentiation by marrow stromal cells is inhibited by bone morphogenetic proteins[136] and leptin,[137] supporting the reciprocal regulation of osteogenesis and adipogenesis in the marrow microenvironment.

STROMAL CELLS

Stromal cells are obtained from animal or human marrow and studied in cultures. They presumably are derived from fibroblasts. They have

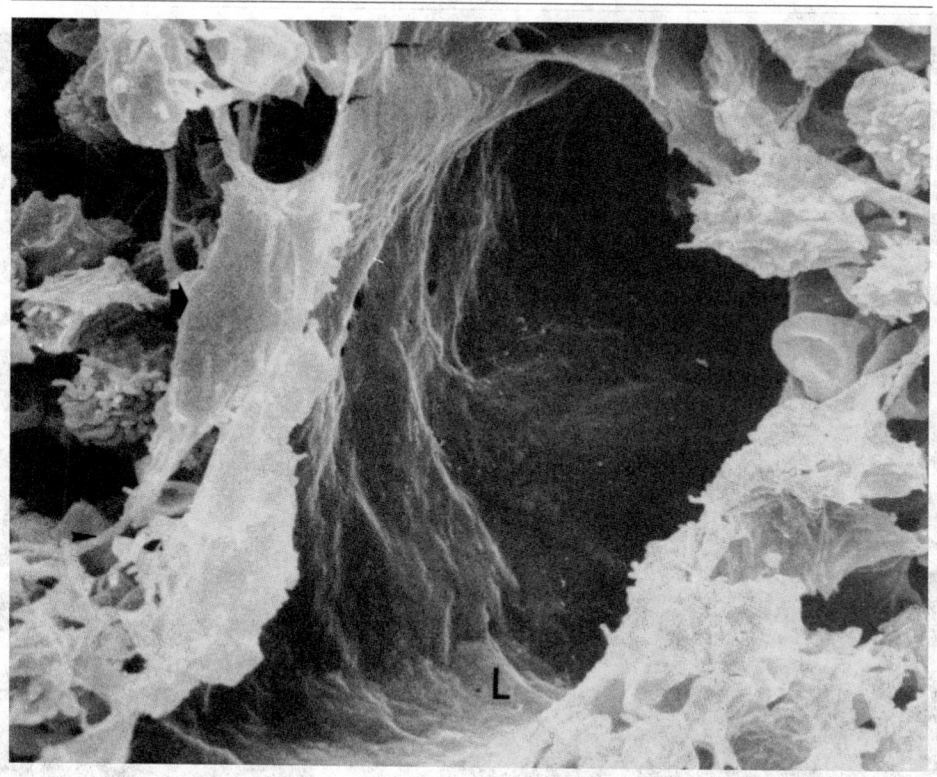

FIGURE 4-4   Scanning electron micrograph (SEM) of rat marrow sinus. The floor of the lumen is labeled *L*. The arrow on the left indicates the cell body of an adventitial reticular cell, which is just beneath the endothelial cell layer. Reticular cell processes can be seen coursing between the sinus wall and the hematopoietic compartment. Several of these are indicated by small arrows. (Reprinted from Lichtman,[70] with permission.)

unique phenotypic and functional characteristics that allow them to nurture hematopoietic development in highly specialized microenvironmental niches.[125] These cells express nerve growth factor receptor, VCAM-1, tenascin, endoglin, and collagens IV and VI but do not express intercellular adhesion molecules[138]; unlike marrow fibroblasts, marrow stromal cells fail to upregulate collagenase when exposed to IL-1.[139] Stromal cells and cell lines differ in their capacities to support the growth of myeloid,[140–142] pro-B,[143,144] and T-cell precursors.[145] This nurturing function is mediated by different combinations of early acting growth factors such as Flt3-ligand,[146] KIT ligand,[147] thrombopoietin,[148–151] LIF,[152] and IL-6,[153] all released by stromal cells. Other interactions that regulate hematopoietic cell survival and differentiation are mediated by cell-cell contact via negative regulators of hematopoiesis such as transforming growth factor beta (TGF-β), which downregulates *c-KIT* expression[147,154]; the Notch/Jagged pathway, which inhibits myeloid differentiation[155]; and specific receptors (e.g., WNT protein family[156] or angiogenins such as neuropilin-1[157]) and adhesion molecules (MUC18, CD164, and HCA) on stromal cells and hematopoietic CD34-positive cells.[158–160]

BONE CELLS

Osteoblasts, osteoclasts, and elongated flat cells with a spindle-shaped nucleus form the marrow endosteal lining.[161] Resting endosteal cells express vimentin, tenascin, alpha smooth-muscle actin, osteocalcin, CD51, and CD56 and do not react with CD3, CD15, CD20, CD34, CD45, CD68, or CD117.[162] Enriched CD56-positive, CD45-negative, CD34-negative endosteal cells grown in the presence of cytokines

[insulin growth factor 1, basic fibroblast growth factor (b-FGF), KIT ligand, IL-3, and GM-CSF] do not give rise to hematopoietic cells, suggesting that they are not totipotent mesenchymal stem cells in these culture conditions.[162] Cultured human bone cells have high levels of α_1/β_1, α_3/β_1, α_5/β_1, α_v/β_5 integrins.[163] Endosteal cells are a rich source of stem cells (using the in vivo CFU-S assay, see Chap. 14)[164] and provide a homing niche for newly transplanted hematopoietic stem cells.[165] Mesenchymal stem cells positive for the STRO-1 antibody can differentiate into adipocyte, chondrocytic, and osteogenic cells,[166–169] and similar osteogenic potential is found in STRO-1-positive vascular pericytes.[170] This process of mesenchymal stem cell to osteogenic differentiation is associated with the loss of the activated leukocyte adhesion molecule (CD166).[171]

OSTEOBLAST

Bone-forming osteoblast progenitor cells, like stromal precursors, reside in the CD34-negative, STRO-1-positive nonadherent marrow cell population.[172–174] Bone morphogenetic protein 2, b-FGF, and TGF-β promote the growth and differentiation of these cells.[172,175] Osteoblasts expand early hematopoietic progenitor survival in long-term cultures and secrete hematopoietic growth factors such as macrophage colony stimulating factor (M-CSF), granulocyte colony stimulating factor (G-CSF), GM-CSF, IL-1, and IL-6.[176,177] Osteoblasts also produce hematopoietic cell-cycle inhibitory factors such as TGF-β, which may contribute to their intimate role in stem cell regulation within the marrow microenvironment.[178] These cells can be transplanted in nonablated mouse[179] and facilitate the engraftment of purified allogeneic hematopoietic stem cells, in keeping with their ability to support hematopoie-

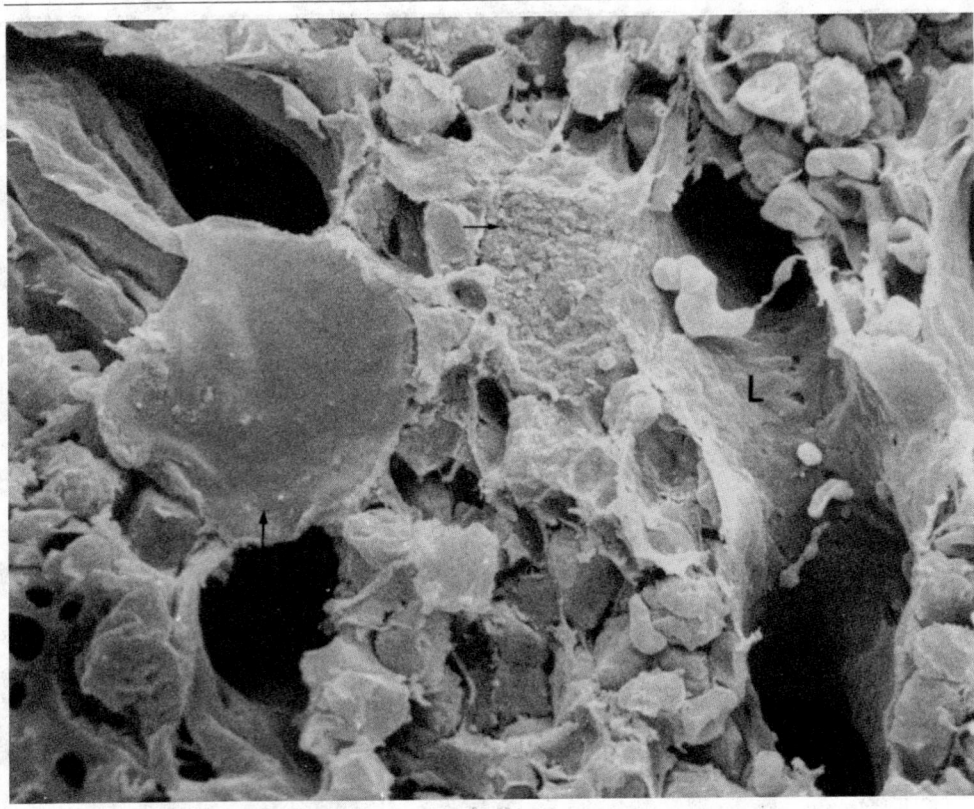

FIGURE 4-5   **SEM** of rat marrow. Several sinuses are evident. The exposed lumen of one branching sinus is labeled *L*. The short horizontal arrow points to the cytoplasm of a transected megakaryocyte. The longer, vertical arrow points to the remnant of a fat cell. The rat femoral marrow contains a modest number of fat cells. (Reprinted from Lichtman,[70] with permission.)

sis.[180] Subcapsular renal explants of bone are able to form a suitable hematopoietic microenvironment for early stem cells, underscoring the potential for osteoblasts to nurture hematopoiesis.[181] Direct cell-cell communication has been shown in marrow[123] as well as in osteoblastic cell networks,[182] indicating a potential regulatory role for these anatomic gap junctions in hematopoiesis.[122]

OSTEOCLAST

Bone-resorbing osteoclasts are derived from hematopoietic progenitors (CD34-positive, STRO-1-negative) and branches from the monocyte-macrophage lineage early during differentiation.[183,184] The essential role of M-CSF in osteoclastogenesis is demonstrated by the op/op mouse, which has osteopetrosis and congenital deficiency of M-CSF[185] and which improves after M-CSF treatment.[186] KIT ligand and M-CSF act synergistically on osteoclast maturation,[187] and M-CSF is essential for the proliferation and maturation of osteoclast progenitors.[188] The major form of secreted M-CSF is a proteoglycan.[189] It binds to bone-derived collagens and can be extracted from the bone matrix,[190] implying a local role for this factor in bone development and remodeling. Targeted disruption of oncogenes such as *C-FOS*[191] and pp60 *C-SRC*[192] prevents osteoclast differentiation leading to osteopetrosis. Osteoprotegrin (OPG), or osteoclastogenesis inhibitory factor, is a cytokine of the tumor necrosis factor receptor superfamily, which inhibits osteoclast differentiation.[193] Osteoclast maturation requires osteoprotegrin ligand (TRANCE/RANKL), an osteoclast differentiation and activation factor (ODF) elaborated by stromal cells and osteoblasts.[194] ODF together with M-CSF induces osteoclast formation without requiring stromal cells.[195–197] Cross-linking antibodies to the adhesion receptor CD44 inhibit osteoclast formation in primary marrow cultures treated with 1 alpha 25-dihydroxyvitamin D_3.[198] Similarly, blocking the expression of cadherin-6 interferes with heterotypic interactions between osteoclasts and stromal cells, impairing their ability to support osteoclast formation.[199] CD9, a tetraspan transmembrane adhesion protein on stromal cells, is known to influence myelopoiesis in long-term marrow cultures.[200] Inhibition of stromal cell CD9-mediated signaling by a blocking antibody reduces ODF transcription, leading to reduced osteoclastogenesis.[201] Such cell-cell cross-talk underscores the functional heterogeneity of hematopoietic inductive signals within the marrow microenvironment.

MACROPHAGES AND LYMPHOCYTES

Macrophages and lymphocytes form part of the marrow microenvironment through growth factor production (IL-3, MIP-1α) and cell-cell interactions with developing progenitors.[70,88,202–206] Macrophages[207] and lymphocytes[140,208] are an integral part of the adherent monolayer found in long-term lymphohematopoietic cultures. Mature T and B lymphocytes and plasma cells are found near foci of granulopoiesis in the adherent layers of long-term cultures in humans.[209] Marrow stroma can support thymocyte differentiation,[210] and an early T-cell progenitor maturation pathway occurs in the marrow.[211] Marrow stroma regulates B lymphopoiesis by different stromal cell niches and homing receptors (VCAM-1) and the production of cytokines such as Flt3 ligand, KIT ligand, IL-7, and TGF-β.[212–214] Stromal cells facilitate the maturation of natural killer cells,[215] an effect likely mediated by stromal-derived Flt3 ligand and IL-15.[216]

Stromal cells elaborate and respond to peptide growth factors such as platelet-derived growth factor (PDGF).[217] PDGF upregulates M-CSF secretion by stromal cells, establishing a paracrine stimulatory loop between these two cell types.[218] The addition of PDGF to macrophages expressing PDGF receptors upregulates interleukin-1 secretion and thereby activates primitive hematopoietic cells.[219] Macrophages also modulate the structure and composition of the extracellular matrix and its fibronectin content.[220] Marrow macrophage phenotype[221] is regulated by adjoining stromal cell–accessory cell–derived colony-stimulating factors and cytokines,[222] such as M-CSF upregulation of $\alpha_4\beta_1$ and $\alpha_5\beta_1$ integrin expression[223] and Flt3 ligand-promoting macrophage outgrowth with B-cell-associated antigens.[224] Macrophages express sialic-acid-binding receptors[225] and play an integral role in erythropoiesis.[226]

EXTRACELLULAR MATRIX

Mesenchymal cells forming the cellular stroma in marrow are active in laying down a rich carpet of extracellular matrix proteins (ECMs)[227] such as proteoglycans or glycosaminoglycans (GAGs),[227,228] fibronectin,[227,229] tenascin,[227,230] collagen,[227,230] laminin,[98,230] hemonectin,[231] and thrombospondin.[227,232] Localizing signals are provided by stromal, ECM hematopoietic cell adhesive interactions,[233,234] in concert with chemoattractant small molecules, the chemokines[235] and cytokines, bound to heparin-like structures in the GAGs.[236] These interactions form specialized niches that may facilitate lymphocytic (B and T) or lineage-specific development along the erythroid, myeloid, or megakaryocytic pathways.[237,238] Other functions of these niches include stem cell survival[239] and quiescence.[237,240] Cytokines that are presented on the surface of stromal cells and matrix-binding chemokines and cytokines are shown in Table 4-1.[236,241–253] Sl/Sl[d] mice that have a deficient hematopoietic microenvironment as a result of a deficiency in KIT ligand[147,254] processing or membrane presentation are anemic and have alterations in their extracellular matrix composition.[255] The addition of hemonectin improves stem cell adhesion to a stromal line derived from Sl/Sl[d] mice.[256]

TABLE 4-1 CELL MEMBRANE PRESENTATION AND MATRIX ASSOCIATION OF CYTOKINES AND CHEMOKINES

Cell Membrane	Matrix Association
Chemokine	*Chemokine*
Fractalkine	RANTES, PF-4, IP-10, IL-8
	Macrophage inflammatory proteins (MIP-1 α/β)
	Stromal cell derived growth factor 1 (SDF-1 α/β)
	Monocyte chemoattractant protein 1 (MCP-1)
Cytokine	*Cytokine*
c-KIT ligand	Granulocyte-macrophage colony-stimulating factor
Tumor necrosis factor alpha (TNF-α)	Interferon gamma (IFN-γ)
Interleukin-1 (IL-1)	Leukemia inhibitory factor (LIF)
Macrophage colony-stimulating factor (M-CSF)	Interleukins (IL-1α, β, IL-2, IL-3, IL-4, IL-5, IL-6, IL-7, IL-12)
	Basic fibroblast growth factor (b-FGF)
Transforming growth factor alpha (TGF-α)	Hepatocyte growth factor (HGF)
	Transforming growth factor beta (TGF-β) (binding to endoglin and heparan sulfate)

RANTES, *Regulated upon Activation Normal T cell Expressed* presumed *Secreted*; PF-4, platelet factor 4; IP-10, interferon inducible protein 10; IL-8, interleukin 8.

In long-term marrow cultures, collagen, fibronectin, and laminin are secreted early, and extracellular deposition of these proteins coincides with active hematopoiesis.[255] GM-CSF is found to prominently stain adipocyte membranes.[257] Cultures actively generating granulocyte-macrophage precursors produce M-CSF and GM-CSF and, to a lesser extent, KIT ligand and G-CSF within the adherent layer.[258] GM-CSF, G-CSF, and b-FGF are detected on the surface of endothelial cells and fibroblasts, and GM-CSF localizes to the extracellular matrix as shown by double-labeling of heparan sulfate proteoglycans and GM-CSF.[259] Negative regulators like TGF-β exert their effects early on long-term marrow cultures by limiting megakaryocyte progenitor and stem cell expansion.[260]

PROTEOGLYCANS

Proteoglycans are polyanionic macromolecules (heparan sulfate, dermatan, chondroitin sulfate, and hyaluronic acid) that are distributed on the surface of adventitial reticular cells as well as within the extracellular matrix.[227,261] Heparan sulfate is the main cell-surface glycosaminoglycan in long-term marrow cultures, and chondroitin sulfate is the major secreted species.[255,262] D-xylosides, which stimulate artificial sulfated glycosaminoglycan synthesis, cause an increase in chondroitin sulfate synthesis and hematopoietic cell production.[262] Hyaluronic acid and chondroitin sulfate-containing proteoglycans are prominent in the adherent and nonadherent compartments of long-term marrow cultures.[261] Heparin-containing and heparan-sulfate-containing proteoglycans interact with laminin and type IV collagen[263] and may play a role in cell-cell interactions, cytokine presentation, and cell differentiation.[264–267] They also mediate progenitor binding to stroma, along with other extracellular matrix molecules such as fibronectin.[268–272]

Another important lymphocyte-progenitor cell-associated proteoglycan, CD44, uses hyaluronate as a ligand and promotes stromal adhesive interactions.[208,273] A binding site for lymphocyte CD44 on the carboxy-terminal heparin-binding domain of fibronectin is present,[274] and neutralizing antibodies to CD44 inhibit hematopoiesis in long-term marrow cultures.[275] Cytokines (GM-CSF, IL-3, and KIT ligand) rapidly induce CD44 expression and increase CD44-mediated adhesion of CD34-positive hematopoietic progenitors to hyaluronan.[276] Chondroitin sulfates A and B mediate monocyte and B-cell activation via a CD44-dependent pathway,[277] while hyaluronate, the CD44 ligand, enhances hematopoiesis by releasing IL-1 (CD44-dependent) and IL-6 (CD44-independent pathway), supporting the important role of this proteoglycan receptor in hematopoiesis.[278] Heparan sulfate mediates IL-7-dependent lymphopoiesis[249] and modulates hematopoiesis and stromal cell-matrix remodeling[282] by anchoring both hepatocyte growth factor[250,279] and b-FGF.[280–282] Marrow stromal cell surface heparan-sulfate-containing proteoglycans consist mainly of syndecan-3 and -4 and glypican-1, while the major extracellular matrix-associated form is perlecan.[283] Syndecan-3 is expressed in marrow stromal cells as a variant form with a core protein of 50 to 55 kDa, suggesting it may play a role in hematopoiesis.[283] Perlecan promotes b-FGF receptor binding and mitogenesis and is able to bind GM-CSF.[277,284] Heparan sulfate expression is also induced in early erythroid differentiation of multipotential hematopoietic stem cells.[285] Glypican-4, another member of this family, has been found on marrow stromal cells and progenitor cells.[286] Syndecan-1 expression in B lymphoid cells is reduced by IL-6, which may imply similar regulatory pathways in other cell types.[287] Biglycan, a matrix glycoprotein *sc1* with homology to osteonectin, and the molecule SIM selectively increase IL-7-dependent proliferation of B cells.[288] Interactions of B cells with other components of the immune system are mediated by syndecan-4, which facilitates the formation of dendritic processes[289] and regulates focal adhesion, stress fiber formation, and cell migration.[290] Taken together, these observations underscore the major contribution of proteoglycans in the formation of specialized microenvironmental niches to promote lineage-specific hematopoiesis.

FIBRONECTIN

Fibronectin localizes at sites of attachment of hematopoietic cells and marrow stromal cells in vitro,[229,291] at sites of interaction between these cells and developing granulocytes or monocytes.[292] Early erythroid progenitors attach to the cell-binding domain of fibronectin,[293,294] and this association can be inhibited by blocking antibodies to the fibronectin integrin receptors $\alpha_5\beta_1$ and $\alpha_4\beta A_1$.[295] Adhesion of hematopoietic progenitor cells to stroma is mediated in part by fibronectin,[268,296] and this binding can be enhanced by protein kinase C activators such as phorbol esters, suggesting the involvement of integrin receptors in this process.[297–299] The alternatively spliced form of fibronectin (type III connecting segment, IIICS) is expressed uniquely within the marrow microenvironment[122,299] and associates with the $\alpha_4\beta_1$ integrin receptor on hematopoietic stem cells.[300] Additional IIICS fibronectin variants have been detected in marrow stroma, providing for a fine control using mRNA splicing of progenitor–stem cell interactions.[301] Fibronectin adhesion to peptide domains, such as the CS1 domain (which activates alpha₄ integrins) or stromal cells, has dual effects of stimulation as well as inhibition of hematopoietic progenitor growth.[302–305]

The integrins very late antigen 4 (VLA-4) and VLA-5, as well as CD44, cooperate to promote these fibronectin adhesive interactions.[302,306–308] Cytokines such as IL-3, KIT ligand, and thrombopoietin augment the magnitude of the fibronectin-mediated hematopoietic progenitor cell adhesion and migration.[309–312] Fibronectin facilitates the maturation of CD34-positive progenitor-derived dendritic cells[313] and is involved in the adhesion of mature cells like megakaryocytes,[314,315] mast cells,[316] chemokine-activated T lymphocytes,[317] eosinophils,[318] and neutrophils.[319] Fibronectin is required for the expression of gelatinase in macrophages[320] and regulates the cytokine release by M-CSF-activated macrophages[321] and chondrocytes.[322] These interactions of fibronectin and its integrin counterreceptors on hematopoietic cells are associated with activation of the sodium-hydrogen exchanger and result in improved cell survival or stimulation.[323]

TENASCIN

Tenascin is an extracellular matrix glycoprotein family consisting of three members: tenascin-C, tenascin-R (restrictin), and tenascin-X.[230,324] Tenascin-C is expressed on the surface of stromal cells in the marrow and, like fibronectin and collagen III, is found in the microenvironment surrounding maturing hematopoietic cells.[227,325] In a long-term marrow culture system (Whitlock-Witte), the thiol 2-mercaptoethanol induced the expression of tenascin-C and improved lymphoid-lineage differentiation.[326] Glucocorticoids, on the other hand, promote myeloid differentiation in long-term marrow cultures and downregulate tenascin expression.[327] Tenascin-C has distinct functional domains that promote hematopoietic cell adhesion to stroma or extracellular matrix proteins, or mediate a strong mitogenic signal to marrow mononuclear cells.[328] In tenascin-C-deficient mutant mice, the colony-forming capacity of marrow is markedly decreased.[329] Long-term marrow cultures from these tenascin-deficient animals result in a decreased progenitor cell output.[329] Addition of tenascin-C to these cultures restores hematopoietic cell production.[329] Mutant tenascin-C-deficient animals also display decreased fibronectin in their marrow, suggesting a possible mechanistic interaction between tenascin-C and fibronectin in the marrow microenvironment.[330] These studies underscore the important role of extracellular matrix proteins such as fibronectin and tenascin-C in hematopoiesis.

COLLAGEN

Collagen type I and type III are associated with microvascular walls, whereas type IV collagen is confined to basal lamina beneath endothelial cells.[96,255,331] Marrow-derived capillary networks grow in collagen gel cultures,[332] and inhibition of collagen synthesis reduces hematopoiesis in vitro,[333] underscoring the importance of the underlying matrix in reconstituting an intact hematopoietic microenvironment.[262,334] Erythroid and granulocytic progenitors adhere to collagen type I in vitro,[335] and a low-molecular-weight collagen has been described in lithium-stimulated marrow cultures,[336] emphasizing the effects of cytokines on matrix composition and stromal support of hematopoiesis.[220,337] Marrow-derived fibroblasts and stromal cells synthesize collagens I, III, IV, V, and VI.[338] Collagen VI is a strong cytoadhesive component of the marrow microenvironment. It binds von Willebrand factor.[339] Collagen type XIV, another fibril-associated collagen, promotes hematopoietic cell adhesion of myeloid and lymphoid cell lines.[340] Collagen-induced, intracellular calcium-mediated signaling events occur in megakaryocytes.[341] In situ immunolocalization of ECMs in murine marrow showed that collagen types I, IV, and fibronectin localize to the endosteum.[342] The distinct spatial distribution of these matrix proteins underscores their role in the preferential homing of engrafted hematopoietic stem cells to marrow.[165]

LAMININ

A multidomain glycoprotein with mitogenic and adhesive sites, laminin is a major component of the extracellular matrix and basement membranes.[227,343] Laminin interacts with collagen type IV and basement membrane components such as proteoglycans and entactin[344] and thus can regulate leukocyte chemotaxis.[345,346] Similarly, CD34-positive granulocytic progenitors,[347] mature monocytes,[348] and neutrophils[349] adhere to laminin. Its role within the cytomatrix may be to strengthen adhesive interactions with integrin receptors, $\alpha_5\beta_1$ (VLA-5) and $\alpha_6\beta_1$ (VLA-6), on hematopoietic cells.[350,351] VLA-6 mediates mast cell adhesion to laminin,[352] while the Lutheran blood group glycoproteins serve as laminin receptors on erythroid cells.[353] A 67-kDa laminin receptor has been identified on acute myeloid leukemia cells displaying monocytic differentiation. Laminins are heterodimers composed of alpha, beta, and gamma polypeptides. Laminin-1 ($\alpha_1\beta_1\gamma_1$) is not expressed in marrow, which expresses laminin-2 ($\alpha_2,\beta_1,\gamma_1$), laminin-8 ($\alpha_4\beta_1\gamma_1$), and laminin-10 ($\alpha_5\beta_1\gamma_1$).[355] Laminins containing the α_5 chain bind to multipotential hematopoietic cells (FDCP-mix cells), in contrast to laminin-1 heterodimers.[355] Stromal cells in cultures as well as cytokine-expanded CD34-positive cells also express laminin β_2, which is found in the pericellular space in marrow and intracellularly in megakaryocytes.[354,356] Laminin promotes the M-CSF-dependent proliferation of marrow-derived macrophages and macrophage cell lines. This effect is partially mediated via an α_6 integrin subunit.[357]

HEMONECTIN

Hemonectin, a 60-kDa glycoprotein, mediates the attachment of granulocytes to marrow.[231] This protein is expressed in hematopoietic tissues as they develop in murine embryos.[358] Hemonectin is related to the plasma glycoprotein fetuin.[359] Granulocytic adhesion to marrow-derived hemonectin is mediated by galactose and mannose.[360] The exact nature of this molecule and its receptor has yet to be identified, hence the role of hemonectin in the marrow hematopoietic microenvironment remains unclear.

THROMBOSPONDIN

Thrombospondin (TSP) is a 450-kDa multifunctional extracellular matrix protein, initially identified in platelet α granules. TSP has domains that interact with collagen and fibronectin and may participate in stem cell lodgement.[361] Receptors on hematopoietic and nonhematopoietic cells can interact with thrombospondin, including CD36[362–364] and a protein, CLA-1, of the CD36/LIMP II gene family.[365] Perlecan mediates the binding of thrombospondin to endothelial cells.[366] The

TSP receptor CD36 is expressed during erythroid (CFU-E stage) and megakaryocytic maturation.[367] TSP has a dual range of activities from suppression of megakaryopoiesis,[368] to an early stimulatory effect on early hematopoietic stem cells,[271] erythropoiesis,[369] and natural killer cells.[370] The inhibition of megakaryocytopoiesis is partially reversed by a low-molecular-weight heparin, suggesting a role for the N-terminal heparin-binding domain in this interaction.[368] Other modulatory effects like the natural killer cell expansion, are a consequence of TSP's ability to activate latent TGF-β.[370,371] All-*trans* retinoic acid-induced granulocytic differentiation of HL-60 cells is associated with an increase in TSP secretion. This process is delayed by a blocking anti-TSP antibody.[372] TSP decreases the proliferation and promotes the differentiation of HL-60 cells; these effects are not mediated by latent TGF-β activation.[372] A 140-kDa fragment of TSP binds b-FGF and has antiangiogenic properties.[373] Endothelial cell TSP expression is inhibited by proangiogenic inflammatory cytokines such as IL-1 and TNF-α.[374] TSP stimulates matrix metalloproteinase-9 activity in endothelial cells[375] and is chemotactic to monocytes and neutrophils.[376] These multiple cellular and microenvironmental interactions underscore TSP's importance in hematopoietic stem cells homing and differentiation.

VITRONECTIN

Vitronectin, also known as *serum spreading factor*, is a 75-kDa protein present in plasma, platelets, and connective tissue.[230] Vitronectin, a major cytoadhesive glycoprotein, binds to specific integrin receptors ($\alpha_V\beta_3$) on fibroblasts, endothelial cells, and mature hematopoietic cells,[378] namely, megakaryocytes,[379] mast cells,[380] bone cells[381] such as osteoblasts and osteoclasts,[382,383] monocyte-macrophages,[384,385] neutrophils, and platelets.[386] Transendothelial migration of monocytes and neutrophils is mediated through the $\alpha_V\beta_3$ vitronectin receptor.[385,386] Metargidin (ADAM-15) is a type I transmembrane glycoprotein (ADAM, a disintegrin and metalloprotease domain) that binds the $\alpha_V\beta_3$ receptor on a monocytic cell line.[387] It uses a different integrin receptor ($\alpha_5\beta_1$) to mediate adhesion of a lymphoid cell line, underscoring the complexity of cell adhesive interactions in different hematopoietic cells. The $\alpha_V\beta_3$ vitronectin receptor cooperates with TSP and CD36 in the recognition and phagocytosis of apoptotic cells.[388–390] Vitronectin and a platelet-derived GAG, serglycin, augment megakaryocyte proplatelet formation.[391–393] Soluble vitronectin inhibits b-FGF-mediated endothelial cell adhesion by interfering with its interaction with the $\alpha_V\beta_3$ receptor.[394] Cytotoxic T lymphocytes,[395] γ/δ lymphocytes[396] and natural killer cells,[397] utilize the $\alpha_V\beta_3$ vitronectin receptor as a costimulatory molecule mediating activation signals and cell proliferation. The TSP receptor integrin-associated protein CD47, together with the $\alpha_V\beta_3$ vitronectin receptor, mediate monocyte activation and cytokine release after interacting with soluble CD23.[398] Hence, vitronectin appears to contribute mainly to terminal megakaryocyte maturation and platelet formation, while exerting a major role in apoptotic cell clearance, cellular activation, and trafficking to areas of inflammation, bone remodeling, and angiogenesis.

HEMATOPOIETIC CELLS

The hematopoietic cells lie in cords or wedges between the vascular sinuses. Erythroblasts are arranged against the outside surface of the vascular sinuses in distinctive clusters, erythroblastic islands,[399] which consist of one or more concentric circles of erythroblasts closely surrounding a macrophage. The inner erythroblastic cells are less mature than the peripheral ones. The central macrophage sends out extensive slender membranous processes that envelop each erythroblast and may phagocytize defective erythroblasts and extruded nuclei.[400] The optimal microenvironmental niche for the terminal ery-

throid maturation into erythroblasts and erythrocytes consists of closely associated fibroblasts, macrophages, and endothelial cells.[401] Erythropoiesis is stimulated by stromal cell-derived activin A,[402,403] a member of the TGF-β family, while mesodermal erythroid islands are induced by stromal cell-derived growth factors acting in concert, BMP-4 plus activin A or b-FGF.[404] The additional ability of b-FGF and HGF to enhance erythropoiesis[405,406] underscores the complex cell-cell interactions required for steady-state erythropoiesis in vivo.

Megakaryocytes also lie directly outside the vascular wall[407] in normal and myeloproliferative diseases,[408] while granulocytes mature deeper in the hematopoietic cords, away from the vascular sinuses. Such discrete spatial structural distribution may be determined by specific adhesive interactions and the provision of specific growth factors for a given cell lineage.[88,231,409] The intimate relation of megakaryocyte to sinus endothelium is explained by their expression of CXCR4, the receptor for the marrow endothelial cell-derived chemokine (SDF-1).[410] SDF-1 increases transendothelial migration of megakaryocytes and, unlike thrombopoietin, enhances platelet formation.[411,412] Thrombopoiesis is also regulated by locally produced synergistic cytokines such as IL-11,[413] KIT ligand,[414] IL-6,[153,415] LIF,[152,416] thrombopoietin,[148,417] and extracellular matrix proteins.[315,391] Stem cells and granulocytic progenitor cells are concentrated in the subcortical regions of the hematopoietic cords.[418]

Lymphocytes and macrophages concentrate around arterial vessels, near the center of the hematopoietic cords. Computer-assisted three-dimensional reconstruction analysis of human marrow confirms the megakaryocyte apposition against the sinus wall and the position of granulocytic cells along the wall of the central arteriole.[419] Erythropoietic cells located mainly around the sinus wall form a continuous network or cord instead of separate ''islands.'' On this basis, the unitary structure of marrow has been defined as a hematopoietic cord with a central arteriole and surrounded by sinuses.[419] A similar structure termed a *hematon* serves as a multicellular functional unit of marrow and contains adipocytes, stromal elements, macrophages, and hematopoietic stem cells in a compact spheroid.[420]

Macrophages are a source of stem cell stimulators, such as IL-1, and inhibitors, such as macrophage inflammatory protein (MIP) 1 alpha and tumor necrosis factor α, and play an important role in local control of hematopoiesis.[421–423] Stromal cells and accessory cells are needed for optimum hematopoietic cell development.[424] Signals regulating the pluripotential hematopoietic stem cells are not entirely defined but require intimate cell-cell contact for signaling through cytokine-chemokine receptors, integrin receptors, alone or together with heparan sulfate or chondroitin-sulfate-containing glycoproteins.

This regulatory paradigm is underscored by several studies: (1) a neutralizing antibody to KIT, while able to abrogate myelopoiesis in stromal–stem cell cocultures, did not affect stem cell survival[425]; (2) stromal-cell-derived BMPs (BMP-2, -4, -7) regulate the proliferation and differentiation of CD34-positive, CD38-negative, lineage-negative cells, with high amounts of BMP-2 and -7 inhibiting proliferation and maintaining repopulating capacity, while BMP-4 at higher concentrations extends the survival of these repopulating cells ex vivo[426]; (3) several adhesion receptors of the sialomucin family mediate inhibitory signals to limit stem cell expansion or differentiation[427]; (4) direct contact of enriched CD34-positive, lineage-negative cells and stroma induces a soluble factor that increases primitive hematopoietic cell production.[428]

CELL ADHESION AND HOMING

Hematopoietic stem-progenitor cells (mostly expressing the CD34 antigen[12]) have multiple adhesion receptors, allowing them to attach to cellular and matrix components within the marrow sinusoidal

TABLE 4-2　HEMATOPOIETIC AND MICROENVIRONMENT ADHESION RECEPTORS AND THEIR LIGANDS

RECEPTOR SUBGROUPS	RECEPTOR	CELLULAR DISTRIBUTION	LIGAND
Integrins			
β_1 subgroup (CD29)	CD49d, $\alpha_4\beta_1$ (VLA-4)	CD34+ cells, (erythroid, and lymphomyeloid progenitors)	VCAM-1 (CD106), FN, thrombospondin (TSP)
	CD49e, $\alpha_5\beta_1$ (VLA-5)	CD34+ cells, bone cells	Fibronectin (FN), laminin
	CD49f, $\alpha_6\beta_1$ (VLA-6)	Rare CD34+ cells, monocytes	Collagen, laminin
β_2 subgroup (CD18)	CD11a/CD18, $\alpha L\beta_2$ (LFA-1)	CD34+ cell subsets, not on repopulating stem cells	ICAM-1, -2, -3, DYNAM-1
	CD11b/CD18, Mβ_2 (Mac-1)	CD34+ subsets, monocytes	ICAM-1, -2, iC3b, Fibrinogen
β_3 subgroup	Vβ_3 (VNR)	Megakaryocytes, osteoclast	Fibrinogen, TSP, CD31
β_7 subgroup	$\alpha_4\beta_7$, (LPAM-1)	Lymphoid progenitor cells, mature myeloid cells	MAdCAM-1, VCAM-1, FN
Immunoglobulins			
	CD31 (PECAM-1)	Endothelial cells (ECs), CD34+ cells, monocytes	CD31 homophilic adhesion, $\alpha V\beta_3$ (VNR), CD38
	CD50 (ICAM-3, -R)	CD34+ cells, monocytes	$\alpha L\beta_2$ (LFA-1), CD11d/CD18 ($\alpha D\beta_2$)
	CD54 (ICAM-1)	CD34+ cells, stroma, activated ECs	$\alpha L\beta_2$ (LFA-1), $\alpha M\beta_2$ (Mac-1)
	CD58 (LFA-3)	CD34+ progenitors, stroma, ECs	CD2
	CD102 (ICAM-2)	Endothelial cells, monocytes	$\alpha L\beta_2$, (LFA-1)
	CD106 (VCAM-1)	Stroma, activated ECs	$\alpha_4\beta_1$ (VLA-4), $\alpha_4\beta_7$ (LPAM-1)
	CD117 (*c-KIT*)	CD34+ progenitors	Membrane KIT ligand
	PRR2 (related to CD155, the poliovirus receptor)	CD34+, CD33+, CD41+, myelomonocytic, megakaryocytic, ECs	PRR2 homophilic adhesion
Lectins			
	CD62L (L-selectin)	Stroma, CD34+ cells	GlyCAM-1, MAdCAM-1, CD162, CD34, s-Lex, PCLP1
	CD62E (E-selectin)	Activated ECs, (marrow ECs express CD62E constitutively)	CD15, s-Lea, CD162, CLA, s-Lex
	CD62P (P-selectin)	Activated ECs	CD162, s-Lex, CD24 (HSA)
Sialomucins			
	CD34	CD34+ cells, endothelial cells	Selectins, other ligands?
	CD43	CD34+, monocytes, NK cells	CD54 (ICAM-1)
	CD162 (PSGL-1)	CD34+ cells, endothelial cells	CD62L, CD62E, CD62P
	CD164 (MGC-24v)	CD34+ cells, stroma, monocytes	Unknown
	CD166 (HCA, ALCAM)	CD34+ cells, stromal cells, ECs	CD6, CD166
Hyaladherin			
	CD44	CD34+ cells, broad distribution	Hyaluronan, b-FGF, HGF
Other			
	CD38	CD34+ subsets, early T and B cells, plasma cells, thymocytes	CD31, hyaluronan
	CD144 (VE-cadherin)	CFU-E, stromal cells, Ecs	E-cadherin
	CD157 (BST-1)	Stroma, T and B, myeloid cells	Unknown

ALCAM, activated leukocyte adhesion molecule; b-FGF, basic fibroblast growth factor; CD, cluster designation; CFU-E, colony-forming unit–erythroid; CLA, cutaneous lymphocyte antigen; EC, endothelial cell; FN, fibronectin; GlyCAM, glycosylation-dependent cell adhesion molecule; HCA, hematopoietic cell antigen; HGF, hepatocyte growth factor; HSA, heat-stable antigen; ICAM, intercellular adhesion molecule; iC3b, inactive complement 3b complex; LFA, lymphocyte function antigen; LPAM, lymphocyte Peyer's patch specific adhesion molecule; MAdCAM, mucosal addressin cell adhesion molecule; MGC-24, multi-glycosylated core of 24 kDa; PCLP: podocalyxin-like protein; PECAM, platelet/endothelial cell adhesion molecule; PRR2; poliovirus receptor-related protein 2; PSGL, P-selectin glycoprotein ligand; s-Le, sialyl Lewis; TSP thrombospondin; VLA, very late antigen; VCAM, vascular cell adhesion molecule; VNR vitronectin receptor.

spaces,[295–300] thereby facilitating their homing and lodgement in the marrow, and providing the close cell-cell contacts required for cell survival and regulated steady-state proliferation.[427,429] Adhesive receptors and their ligands, present on hematopoietic stem-progenitor cells, and components of the hematopoietic microenvironment, are shown in Table 4-2. Six subgroups of receptors, the integrins,[299,430] immunoglobulins,[427,431] lectins (selectins),[432,433] sialomucins,[434,435] hyaladherin (CD44, H-CAM),[436,437] and other receptors such as CD38 (ADP-ribosyl cyclase),[438] CD144 [439,440] (cadherin), and CD157 (BST-1),[441] are shown, listing mostly interactions involving CD34-positive cells and progenitors.[429,442] Thus receptor-ligand interactions that regulate the trafficking of mature leukocytes are not included exhaustively.[443]

INTEGRINS

Members of this family are divalent cation-requiring heterodimeric proteins (17 α and 8 β subunits), and they mediate important cellular functions including embryonic development, cell differentiation, and adhesive interactions between hematopoietic cells and inflammatory cells and surrounding vascular and stromal microenvironment.[299,444] They are subdivided based on the β-chain composition, and as shown in Table 4-2, α chains can associate with more than one β-chain subunit. The principal integrin receptors of the β_1 subgroup involved in hematopoietic stem cells endothelial and stromal interactions are $\alpha_4\beta_1$ (VLA-4), $\alpha_5\beta_1$ (VLA-5), and $\alpha_L\beta_2$ (LFA-1) of the β_2 subgroup. $\alpha_4\beta_1$-based stromal adhesion events in vitro,[445] or in vivo,[446] alone or in conjunction with the integrin-associated protein (IAP, CD47)[447] regulate erythropoiesis. This receptor also mediates selective granulopoiesis over established marrow stromal cells in cooperation with PECAM-1 (CD31), an immunoglobulin superfamily member,[448] and is essential for pre-B cell growth and differentiation over stromal cells expressing IL-7, KIT ligand, and Flt3 ligand.[449–452] An acquired defect in stromal function, characterized by a deficiency in VCAM-1 and IL-7 expression,[453–457] accounts for the delayed B lymphoid reconstitution seen after marrow transplantation.

Integrins also are signaling molecules,[458,459] and after engaging their ligands, or subsequent to activation by monoclonal antibodies, multiple events (tyrosine phosphorylation of focal adhesion kinase, paxillin, and ERK-2) are triggered (inside-out signaling), culminating with *RAS* activation.[460-464] Integrin receptor cross-talk[465] with other adhesive receptor members, such as the immunoglobulin superfamily [natural killer cell-T cell ($\alpha_1\beta_2$/DYNAM-1), CD34-positive-endothelial cell PECAM-1,[466-469] or selectins[470]], results also from outside-in signaling events that regulate receptor-binding affinity[451,471] and mediates inhibitory signals for erythroid, myeloid, and lymphoid progenitor growth.[472-476] Also, integrin-binding to their counterreceptors, such as $\alpha_4\beta_1$/VCAM-1[477] or $\alpha_4\beta_1$/FN,[312] in early CD34-positive progenitors, is associated with a decreased rate of apoptosis. Unchecked tyrosine kinase activation, as is the case in chronic myeloid leukemia cells,[478] alters integrin affinity and allows the cells to egress from the marrow.[479] Inhibition of the *Abl* kinase activity directly,[480] or indirectly, using alpha interferon,[481] restores the adhesive properties of these progenitors.

IMMUNOGLOBULIN SUPERFAMILY

The immunoglobulin superfamily[233] designates a group of molecules containing one or more amino acid repeats also found in immunoglobulins and consists of PECAM-1 (CD31), ICAM-3/R (CD50) and ICAM-1 (CD54), LFA-3 (CD58), ICAM-2 (CD102), VCAM-1 (CD106), *KIT* (CD117),[482-503] and PRR2, a molecule related to CD155, which serves as a poliovirus receptor.[503] (See Table 4-2.) VCAM-1 is upregulated by inflammatory cytokines (IL-4, IL-13).[500,501] Immunoglobulin-like adhesion molecules also include NCAM, a neural adhesion molecule that binds lymphocytes but not hematopoietic progenitors; Thy-1, a stem cell antigen MHC classes I and II; and CD2, CD4, and CD8.[233] (See Table 4-2.)

LECTINS (SELECTINS)

Homing of stem cells requires lectin receptors with galactosyl and mannosyl specificities.[504,505] The selectins are a family of adhesion molecules, each containing type C lectin structures. The leukocyte selectin (L-selectin, CD62L) is expressed on hematopoietic stem-progenitors[506] and mediates adhesive interactions with other receptors (addressins), such as the CD34 sialomucin present on specialized endothelium, using sialylated fucosyl-glucoconjugates. (See Table 4-2.) The CD34 receptor on stem cells, however, does not bind L-selectin,[506] as a putative L-selectin ligand yet to be defined exists on these cells. The selectin family also contains CD62E, which is an E-selectin constitutively expressed on marrow sinusoidal endothelium, and regulates the transmigration of leukocytes as well as CD34-positive stem cell homing. The third member of this family is P-selectin, which is found on platelets and is able to bind hematopoietic stem cells, using a mucin receptor, the P-selectin glycoprotein ligand (PSGL-1), which binds to all three selectins. (See Table 4-2.) These proteins are responsible for leukocyte rolling over endothelial surfaces and tethering, thereby allowing integrin-mediated firm adhesion to the endothelium to form, and mediating cellular homing events using specialized high endothelial venule lymphocyte homing sites.[507-516]

SIALOMUCINS

The mucin family includes the CD34 stem cell antigen,[517,518] not an L-selectin ligand on these cells,[519] and CD43, an antiadhesion large glycoprotein (leukosialin)[520] able to regulate hematopoietic progenitor survival.[521] Both CD34 and CD43 signal via tyrosine kinases when capping their surface receptors[517,522,523] and, in the case of CD43, clustering of cytoskeleton with CD44 and ICAM-2.[522] CD162 (PSGL-1) is important in cell trafficking and stem cell homing,[524-530] CD164 (MGC-24v), another sialomucin receptor,[531] transmits inhibitory signals to

stem-progenitor cells like CD162 and CD34.[233] Lastly, CD166, the hematopoietic cell antigen (HCA, ALCAM), forms homodimers (CD166) and heterodimers with CD6.[532]

HYALADHERIN

The fifth subgroup shown in Table 4-2 is the cartilage-related proteoglycan, CD44, also known as the *lymphocyte homing cell adhesion molecule* (HCAM). This adhesion receptor is expressed on hematopoietic stem-progenitor cells and facilitates their homing and adhesion to marrow in concert with VLA-4 and ICAM-1, -3. CD44 has several isoforms expressed in normal and tumor tissues. The CD44 variant v10 has been shown to regulate hematopoietic progenitor mobilization, underscoring its importance in mediating cellular matrix-stromal cell adhesion.[533-536]

OTHER ADHESION MOLECULES

CD38 is a newly recognized adhesion receptor that binds the CD31 receptor and matrix hyaluronan. It is expressed on early T and B cells and subsets of CD34-positive hematopoietic progenitors.[537,538] Cadherins are large molecules involved in cell-cell junctions and vascular integrity. CD144, E-cadherin, is expressed on CD34-positive progenitors as well as marrow stroma and endothelial cells, thereby providing another pathway for stem cell lodgement.[539] The stromal adhesion receptor BST-1, CD157, is an ADP-ribosyl cyclase, with similarity to CD38. CD157 is expressed on marrow stroma, T and B cells, and myeloid cells and promotes pre-B cell adhesion and growth.[540-543]

CELLULAR HOMING

The control of lymphocyte and leukocyte cellular trafficking[544,545] is a multistep process that involves: (1) selectin-mediated tethering and rolling over vascular endothelial cells expressing in a tissue-specific distribution selectin-binding sialomucins like GlyCAM-1 on lymphatic tissue high endothelial venules,[546] MAdCAM-1 on Peyer's patch endothelium,[547] the peripheral lymph node addressin PNAd,[548] and the vascular adhesion protein 1 (VAP-1)[549] molecule (both mediating CD8 T-lymphocyte migration)[547]; (2) a triggering step, at sites of inflammation, by short-acting signals such as platelet activating factor,[550] cytokine[551,552] or chemokine-activating[553,554]; integrins; (3) tight adhesion and spreading of cells over endothelial surfaces mediated by the immunoglobulin receptors (ICAM-1, -2, VCAM-1)[555-557]; (4) CD31-mediated diapedesis,[558] in concert with selectin-mediated tethering at vascular endothelial cell junctions.[559] Other molecules can promote rolling of cells, such as tenascin,[560] and cooperation between different adhesion receptors is frequently seen during the transmigration process.[561]

Chemokines bind heparan sulfate proteoglycans and thereby play a central role in directing cellular trafficking at sites of inflammation[244,245,562] and, in the case of SDF-1,[247] regulate cellular trafficking under steady-state conditions. Fractalkine, an endothelial transmembrane mucin-chemokine hybrid molecule, is strategically placed on the surface of activated endothelium and mediates the rapid capture, firm adhesion, and activation under physiologic flow of circulating monocytes, resting or IL-2-activated CD8 lymphocytes, and natural killer (NK) cells.[563] The cytokines, TNF-α, and IL-1 upregulate fractalkine, in keeping with the need to recruit effector cells rapidly at sites of inflammation.[564] Tissue-restricted chemokines modulate hematopoietic cell adhesive interactions by providing local activation signals, thereby enhancing the specificity of cellular trafficking.[235]

Unlike lymph nodes, no specific marrow sinusoidal addressins have been defined. A study comparing the adhesive capacity of human marrow or umbilical-cord-derived endothelial cell lines[565] did not show any major differences in CD34-positive progenitor adhesion. This interaction is blocked to varying degree by combinations of monoclonal antibodies against $\alpha_4\beta_1$, CD18, and/or E-selectin.[565] These findings support the concept of a complex stem cell homing and lodgement process that relies on several short-range signals—adhesive interactions between homing CD34-positive cells and marrow sinusoidal endothelial cells.[566,567]

Thus, stem cell homing and lodgement to the marrow appears to rely on the distinct characteristics of marrow endothelium and stroma and intrinsic properties of hematopoietic stem and progenitor cells. First, the marrow sinusoidal endothelial cells express constitutively E-selectin, and upon activation both E-selectin and P-selectin are upregulated[568]; they also express VCAM-1,[569,570] while the homing CD34-positive progenitors express PSGL-1 (CD162), a highly glycosylated sialomucin that binds all selectins,[524,525] as well as the integrin receptor $\alpha_4\beta_1$, which engages VCAM-1.[451] Secondly, L-selectin on CD34-positive progenitors[571] may influence the engraftment process by providing a carbohydrate interaction with sinus cavity E-selectin[510] and with underlying stroma; L-selectin may also improve progenitor survival as shown by its ability to improve the clonogenic potential of CD34-positive cells.[572,573] While the sinusoidal endothelial cells rarely express PSGL-1 (CD162), they display other L-selectin ligands such as chondroitin sulfate[574] and heparan sulfate proteoglycans,[575] in addition to VEGF-driven E-selectin.[576] Thirdly, stromal cells and endothelial cells elaborate SDF-1, a potent chemokine known to enhance integrin activation,[576] mediate endothelial CD34-positive cell arrest under flow,[577] and enhance CD34-positive cell transmigration.[570,576] The fourth element in this complex homing process is based upon the constitutive stromal cell expression of VCAM-1,[573] leading to $\alpha_4\beta_1$ integrin-mediated firm adhesion to marrow stroma,[573] of $\alpha_4\beta_1$-positive early reconstituting hematopoietic stem cells[41] and CD34-positive progenitor cells.[54,55]

Additional homing signals could result from $\alpha_5\beta_1$ integrin binding to fibronectin,[297,311] CD44 binding to cytomatrix hyaluronan,[276] ubiquitin binding sites on stroma cells interacting with progenitors,[578] and L-selectin interacting with PCLP1.[40,516] This heterotypic adhesion occurs because both CD34-positive stem cells and endothelial cells express this receptor/ligand pair. Other immunoglobulin superfamily receptors, PECAM-1 (CD31), ICAM-1, -2 (CD54, CD102), and CD117, also participate in the stem cell lodgement process.[427] CD117 (KIT) can interact with membrane-bound KIT ligand to promote adhesion as well as cross-activate other integrin receptors.[427]

Another homotypic adhesion receptor in this family is the human poliovirus receptor-related 2 protein (PRR2), which is expressed on endothelial cells at the intercellular junctions and on the majority of CD34-positive cells, as well as precursors differentiating along the myelomonocytic and megakaryocytic lineages (CD33- and CD41-positive).[503] PRR2 isoforms can homodimerize or heterodimerize, on the cell surface of endothelial cells, in a fashion similar to PECAM-1 (CD31)-mediated aggregation. The latter PECAM-1-signaling events involve phosphorylation of tyrosine on the receptor's intracytoplasmic tail and by recruitment and activation of Src homology 2 domain-bearing protein tyrosine phosphatase 1 (SHP-1) and SHP-2.[579]

This cellular trafficking model is supported by experiments in mutant mice deficient in E and P selectins,[573] showing decreased marrow progenitor homing in vivo. Similar results are obtained after the administration of blocking antibodies to VLA-4-VCAM-1[566,567] or to SDF-1-CXCR4.[579] These events result in decreased stromal–stem cell adhesion[451] and in diminished CD34-positive cell–endothelial cell transmigration,[53,570] leading to impaired homing of transplanted stem cells.[580]

TABLE 4-3   NORMAL PRECURSOR CELL KINETICS

CELL TYPE	MARROW		
	NUMBER, CELLS/kg	TRANSIT TIME, DAYS	PRODUCTION RATE, CELLS/kg PER DAY
I. Red cells			
Erythroblasts	5.3×10^9	~5.0	3.0×10^9
Reticulocytes	8.2×10^9	2.8	3.0×10^9
II. Megakaryocytes	15.0×10^6	~7.0	2.0×10^6
III. Granulocytes			
Proliferation pool	2.1×10^9	~5.0	0.85×10^9
Postmitotic pool	5.6×10^9	6.6	0.85×10^9

SOURCE: Finch, Harker, and Cook,[595] with permission.

CELL PROLIFERATION AND MATURATION

The earliest stem cells are pluripotential and capable of differentiation to either lymphopoietic or hematopoietic multipotential stem cells (Chap. 14). These pluripotential stem cells and progenitor cells are in a dormant state[12] and are able to withstand the normal hypoxic milieu within the marrow sinusoidal spaces.[581] Hematopoietic stem-progenitor cells are prevented from unchecked proliferation by matrix-associated negative regulators such as BMPs[426] and TGF-β,[582–584] alone or with locally induced inhibitory chemokines like MIP-1α[585] and MCP-1.[586,587] Direct inhibitory signals are also triggered by stromal-hematopoietic progenitor binding using sialomucins such as CD34,[427] CD162,[512] and CD164.[159]

Later unipotential progenitor cells respond to lineage-specific cytokines and mature into precursor cells that may undergo four or five cell divisions before terminating in functional blood cells (Chap. 14). Hematopoietic growth factors and cytokines are produced locally by stromal cells and other cellular elements of marrow. Such factors as KIT ligand are expressed in a membrane-bound form,[147] bind to proteoglycans and heparan sulfate moieties within the cytomatrix, and mediate hematopoietic cell attachment, where they are presented in an active form to receptor-bearing hematopoietic progenitors.[284,588] (See "Extracellular Matrix" and Table 4-1.) Cellular attachment to the marrow cytomatrix is an active process leading to signaling and activation of focal adhesion kinases within regions of integrin receptor clustering.[589] These properties explain the ability of stromal cells to promote the self-renewal of stem cells[590] and inhibit apoptosis of hematopoietic cells.[591–594]

After maturation of committed progenitor cells, the erythroid and granulocytic blast cells undergo four to five mitotic divisions, while the megakaryocytic blast cells divide perhaps once and then undergo five or six endomitotic (nuclear) divisions. The number of precursor cells in the marrow of humans has been calculated primarily through the study of marrow films and sections relating differential counts of marrow samples to their content of injected radioactive iron. A number of assumptions and approximations need to be made,[595] but the summary data given in Table 4-3 agree well with many other observations on the cellular content and kinetics of normal marrows.

CELLULAR RELEASE

Cell migration occurs between adventitial cells but through endothelial cell channels that develop at the time of cell transit. Migrating cells make the hole that develops in the endothelial cell cytoplasm. A number of releasing factors have been implicated in the initiation of marrow egress. The best characterized are those for granulocytes, which include G-CSF,[596,597] GM-CSF,[598] the C3$_e$ component of complement,[599] zymosan-activated plasma-containing complement fragments,[600] glucocorticoid hormones,[601] androgenic steroids,[602] and endotoxin.[603] Cellular migration is under the complex control of a family of small cytokines termed *chemokines* with overlapping tissue and target cell specificity, allowing them to regulate effector cell trafficking throughout the body. The chemokine superfamily has several branches based on the cysteine motifs: the "C-X-C" family (platelet factor 4, IL-8, melanocyte growth-stimulating activity/groα, neutrophil activating protein 2, and granulocyte chemotactic protein 2), all mediating neutrophil migration and activation, and the "C-C" family (MIP-1α and β, RANTES, and MCP-1, -2, -3, -4, -5) mediating mostly monocyte and in some cases lymphocyte chemotaxis.[235,564] Neutrophils residing in the marrow venous sinusoids are rapidly released into the circulation by IL-8.[604] Eosinophil and eosinophil progenitors are recruited from marrow selectively in allergic states, after exposure to IL-5,[605] by the chemokines eotaxin[606] or RANTES.[607] In both systems, migration is inhibited by blocking the β_2 integrin CD18, underscoring the importance of integrin activation as well as surface proteolytic activation in mediating transendothelial migration.[607,608] Similarly, SDF-1 and KIT ligand cooperate to enhance hematopoietic progenitor chemotaxis.[609] Table 4-4 has a detailed listing of chemokine receptors as well as cellular targets and ligands interacting with each receptor subgroup.[610–614] Chemokines-receptors active on CD34-positive cells are shown in bold font.

Releasing factors for reticulocytes and platelets have been more difficult to identify and may also be of less biological significance, since early release of these cells has little impact on the large pool of circulating cells. Erythropoietin therapy in uremic patients accelerates the egress of reticulocytes.[615] Adventitial reticular cell cytoplasm is a barrier to the reticulocytes on the abluminal surface of the endothelium.[616] Phlebotomy, phenylhydrazine-induced hemolytic anemia, and erythropoietin result in marked reduction of the adventitial cell cover of the sinus, a process that is thought to facilitate cell egress through the endothelium.[617]

To leave the marrow, the reticulocyte depends on a pressure gradient across the membrane to drive it through the pore[616,617] (see Fig. 4-6). The pressures within the marrow sinuses are pulsatile, and pressures sufficient to cause egress may be transient.[618] Anemia and the administration of erythropoietin markedly increase blood flow to marrow and bone,[83,619] while G-CSF increases blood flow to marrow only.[620] This effect is not blocked by denervation[83] and may explain the egress of cells after G-CSF administration.[620]

Electron micrographs of leukocytes partially translocated across endothelium indicate that marked deformation of these cells occurs as they penetrate the cytoplasm of the endothelial cell to enter the sinus lumen.[621] As with reticulocytes, egress occurs adjacent to junctions of endothelial cells.[400] The nucleus of the granulocyte, usually segmented,

TABLE 4-4   CHEMOKINE RECEPTORS, INTERACTING CHEMOKINE LIGANDS, AND CELLULAR SPECIFICITY

RECEPTORS	RECEPTOR EXPRESSION	CHEMOKINE LIGANDS
CXCR1	Neutrophils (Neu)	CXCL8 (IL-8), CXCL6 (GCP-2)
CXCR2	Neutrophils, IL-5 primed eosinophils (Eos)	CXCL8, CXCL1,2,3 (GROα/β/γ), CXCL5 (ENA78), CXCL6, CXCL7 (NAP-2)
CXCR3	Activated memory and naive T cells, natural killer cells; T (preferentially Th1) cells	CXCL9 (MIG), CXCL10 (IP-10), CXCL11 (I-TAC)
CXCR4	Neutrophils, monocytes, megakaryocytes, CD34+ and pre-B cell precursors, resting and activated T cells	CXCL12 (SDF-1α,β, stromal cell-derived factor)
CXCR5	B lymphocytes	CXCL13 (BCA-1/BLC)
CX3CR1	Monocytes, dendritic cells, CD34+ cells, natural killer cells (NK); in nodal tissues activated T helper lymphocytes, activated B cells, and follicular dendritic cells (DC)	CXCL1 (Fractalkine/neurotactin)
XCR1	Resting T cells, natural killer cells	XCL1 (lymphotactin/SCM-1α/ATAC) XCL2 (SCM-1β)
CCR1	Monocytes, Eos, basophils, activated Neu, and T cells, CD34+ cells, and immature DCs	CCL5 (RANTES), CCL3 (MIP-1α), MIP-5, CCL7 (MCP-3), CCL8 (MCP-2), CCL14 (MCP-4), CCL23 (CK-β8/-β8-1/MPIF-1)
	Monocytes, T cells (not Neu, Eos, or B cells)	CKCCL14 (HCC-1), CCL16 (HCC-4/LEC) CCL15 (HCC-2/MIP-1δ)
CCR2	Monocytes, basophils, dendritic cells, T cells, activated memory CD4 T cells, and NK cells	CCL2 (MCP-1), CCL7 (MCP-3), CCL8 (MCP-2), CCL13 (MCP-4), CCL12 (MCP-5), CCL5 (RANTES), CCL11 (Eotaxin-1), CCL24 (Eotaxin-2/MPIF-2)
CCR3	Eosinophils, thymocytes, basophils, dendritic cells, activated memory CD4 T cells	CCL11, CCL24, CCL26 (Eotaxin-3), CCL5, MCP-2, -3, -4, MIP-5, vMIP-II
CCR4	Activated T cells, immature dendritic cells	CCL17 (TARC),
	Monocyte-derived DCs, activated NK cells	CCL22 (MDC)
	Thymocytes (CD3+, CD4+, CD8^{low})	CCL22 (MDC)
CCR5	Monocytes, activated memory CD4 T cells	CCL5 (RANTES), MCP-2, -3, -4
	Immature DCs, CD34+ cells, and NK cells	CCL3 (MIP-1α), CCL4 (MIP-1β)
	Human thymocytes	CCL4 (MIP-1β)
CCR6	T cells, CD34+ -derived dendritic cells	CCL20 (MIP-3α/LARC/exodus-1)
CCR7	Activated T (naïve and memory T cells) > B lymphocytes, NK cells subsets, CD34+ macrophage progenitors, and mature DCs	CCL19 (MIP-3β/ELC/CK-β11/exodus-3), CCL21 (SLC/exodus-2/TCA4/6Ckine) (6Ckine inactive on B cells)
CCR8	Monocytes, T (TH2) cells	CCL1 (I309), CCL17 (TARC), vMIP-1, vMIP-II
CCR9	Thymocytes (CD4+/CD8+, CD4+/CD8−), activated macrophages	CCL25 (TECK)
CCR10	Skin-homing memory T cells, CD4/CD8 cells	CCL27 (CTACK/ILC/ESkine)
CCR1 and CCR3	Neutrophils, monocytes and lymphocytes	CCL15 (Leukotactin-1/HCC-2/MIP-1δ)
Not known	Resting T cells	CCL18 (DC-CK1/PARC)

BLC, B-cell homing chemokine that activates Burkitt's lymphoma receptor 1 (BLR1); CTACK, cutaneous T-cell-attracting chemokine; DC-CK-1, dendritic cell chemokine 1; ELC, EBI1-ligand chemokine; HCC, human, hemofiltrate C-C-chemokine; IL-8 is also chemotactic for a specific subset of (CD3+, CD8+, CD56+, CD26-) T cells; I-TAC, interferon inducible T-cell alpha chemoattractant; LARC, liver and activation-regulated chemokine; leukotactin-1 (Lkn-1), a beta chemokine, is identical to CK-β8, CK-β8-1 is alternatively spliced, Ck-β8 is 17 amino acids shorter. MDC, macrophage-derived chemokine; MCP-3 binding does not transduce a signal and is a natural antagonist of the CCR5 receptor. MDC is chemotactic to eosinophils, in a CCR3 and CCR4 independent manner; vMIP-II is a human herpes virus 8–encoded chemokine antagonist of CC, CXC, and CXCR1 receptors. MPIF-1, -2, myeloid progenitor inhibitory factor 1, 2; MPIF-1 is identical to CKβ-8 and MIP-3, MPIF-2 is also known as CKβ-6 or eotaxin-2; PARC, pulmonary and activation-regulated chemokine; SLC, secondary lymphoid-tissue chemokine, also known as exodus-2 and 6Ckine; TARC, thymus and activation-regulated chemokine; TECK, thymus-expressed chemokine.

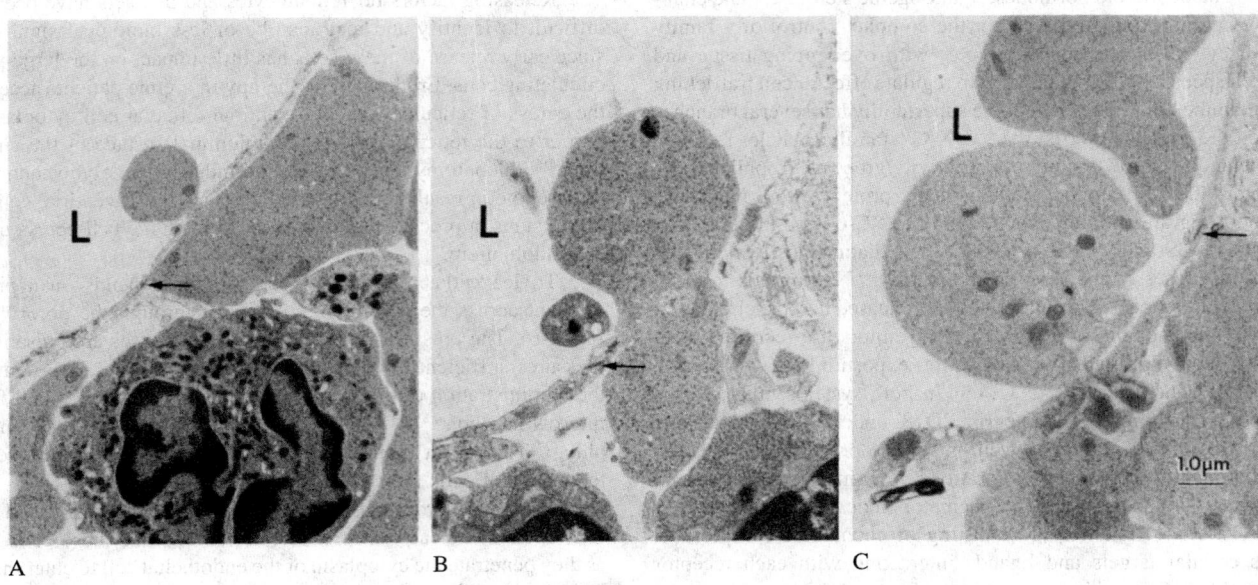

FIGURE 4-6   Composite TEM of reticulocytes in egress. (A) Small protrusion of marrow reticulocyte into sinus lumen (L). (B) A reticulocyte in egress with about half the cell in the sinus lumen. (C) A reticulocyte virtually completely in the sinus. Egress occurs through a migration pore which is parajunctional in position (arrows point to endothelial cell junctions). (Reprinted from Lichtman and Waugh,[400] with permission.)

does not require as marked a deformation to traverse the migration pore as do the nuclei of monocytes and lymphocytes.[621] The immature granulocytes in marrow are anchored to adventitial reticular cells through lectinlike adhesion molecules. Gradual loss of these molecules (e.g., shedding of L-selectin) during maturation or after activation, could permit movement toward the sinus wall.[622] Transient changes in surface glycoproteins (upregulation of α-2,6 sialylation of CD11b and CD18) of maturing marrow myeloid cells lead to decreased stromal and fibronectin adhesion and may favor contact with endothelium and cell egress.[623] Activated neutrophils can adhere under flow using the VLA-4 integrin pathway.[624] Neutrophil egress occurs mostly at the endothelial cell borders and is entirely P selectin mediated.[625] C5a and G-CSF administration recruit neutrophils by altering integrins (low CD11a with G-CSF) and decreased L-selectin expression (with both agents).[626,627] Similar findings obtained in mice lacking two or all three selectins underscore the essential role selectins play in neutrophil recruitment.[628]

The release of platelets is initiated by megakaryocytes that invaginate the abluminal surface of the marrow sinus endothelial cell until a pore is made. Cytoplasm flows through this pore into the marrow sinus and is eventually separated from the body of the megakaryocyte, resulting in a multiplatelet fragment or proplatelet.[407,629] The proplatelets often are stringbean-shaped structures and are found in the marrow sinus lumen. Eventually they fragment into single platelets.[391–393] Megakaryocyte nuclei are left in marrow after platelet release and are degraded and phagocytized there.[630] The entry of either nuclear remnants or entire megakaryocytes with residual cytoplasm has been observed in both normal individuals[631] and patients with marrow disorders.[632] The latter regulatory events are mediated by the chemokine SDF-1[411] and by c-Mpl ligand.[412]

Occasional immature granulocytes and megakaryocyte nuclei or whole megakaryocytes are present in cell concentrates of normal blood.[631] Nucleated red cells rarely escape from the marrow under normal conditions. The absence of circulating erythroblasts may also relate to the capacity of the spleen to sequester and enucleate circulating erythroblasts. The late myelocytes and metamyelocytes have the capacity to move, respond to chemoattractants, and deform, albeit less well

than the mature neutrophils, and thus may occasionally exit marrow by normal mechanisms. The invasion of marrow by neoplastic cells or the replacement of marrow by fibrous tissue is associated with an increased prevalence of immature cells in the circulation. Damage to the architecture of marrow with a breakdown of the integrity of sinus walls may allow cells to enter the circulation less discriminately. Tumor cells elaborate chemoattractive cytokines (chemokines), and this explains their ability to facilitate cell egress from marrow.[633]

The intramedullary expression of SDF-1 and KIT ligand may allow stem cells to localize to that space.[634] KIT ligand upregulates CXCR4 expression on CD34-positive cells, enhancing their chemotactic response, while mobilized blood CD34-positive progenitors have a defective response to SDF-1.[635] CXCR4 is expressed on early lymphohematopoietic progenitors,[636] providing a model in which mobilized CD34-positive cells have alterations in their adhesion repertoire and chemotactic capacities, allowing them to leave their sinusoidal niches to the peripheral circulation.[637] Enhanced hematopoietic progenitor mobilization is also seen when the chemokine MIP-2 is combined with G-CSF.[638]

The homing and egress processes require the interaction between separate adhesion pathways on hematopoietic stem and progenitor cells and marrow endothelium and stroma, as seen in a mouse model using blocking antibodies to $\alpha_4\beta_1$ and CD44.[639] Marrow stem cell homing depends on the $\alpha_4\beta_1$/VCAM-1 adhesion pathway, while CD44 affects homing to marrow and spleen. Inhibition of CD44 and/or $\alpha_4\beta_1$ adhesion rapidly mobilized stem cells.[639] The CS1 domain FN fragment did not mobilize progenitors, and antibody to $\alpha_5\beta_1$ did not alter homing.[640] G-CSF augments the mobilizing action of $\alpha_4\beta_1$/VCAM-1 integrin-blocking antibodies in primates,[641] while c-KIT signaling cooperates with this integrin-based mobilization process,[642] confirming the complexity of the stem cell egress process.[643]

STEM CELL CIRCULATION

Stem cells circulate in the blood and can reenter marrow and reestablish hematopoiesis in the marrow cords. Whole-body irradiation of an animal with shielding of a single bone results in the repopulation of the irradiated marrow, strongly implying transfer of stem cells from shielded marrow into irradiated marrow.[644] Also, marrow or blood cells from a syngeneic or histocompatible allogeneic donor can reenter marrow and reconstitute hematopoiesis of an animal or human recipient.[645] The expression of L-selectin,[646] and CD44,[647] in blood CD34-positive progenitors seems to correlate with faster engraftment and platelet recovery. Umbilical cord blood CD34-positive cells express L-selectin on their surface in higher amounts than steady-state adult blood progenitors, thereby displaying a preferential homing capacity to the marrow.[648] High proliferative potential colony-forming cells in the CD34-positive, CD38-negative subgroup are detectable in the circulation, very early after allogeneic transplantation, coinciding with rapid recovery of blood counts and implying a role for in vivo stem cell recirculation leading to a sustained engraftment process.[649]

The entry of stem cells into the marrow is mediated by a lectin-sugar interaction[650,651] and may be facilitated by alterations in the sinus endothelium induced by the conditioning therapy.[652,653] However, c-KIT-positive primitive hematopoietic stem cells, when infused in a nonirradiated host model, home more efficiently to areas of marrow, spleen, lung, and thymus than after sublethal irradiation.[654] Unpurified marrow cells labeled with the membrane dye PKH-2 appear to be governed by a nonspecific seeding process rather then by a selective homing signal,[655] suggesting that stem cells display adhesive and chemotactic properties that allow them to preferentially seek marrow endothelial sinusoidal spaces. Indeed, marrow endothelial cells under the influence of VEGF constitutively express E-selectin and VCAM-1 and elaborate chemotactic signals such as SDF-1 to attract CD34-positive cells.[656,657] Similar findings have been seen when the in vivo homing of long-term repopulating stem cells is analyzed in a serial marrow transplantation model.[658]

Blood stem cell mobilization for marrow transplantation has been facilitated by improvements in CD34 cell collection and processing[659] and the growing availability of recombinant cytokines[660] such as G-CSF, GM-CSF, Flt3 ligand, KIT ligand, IL-3, interleukin-7, and thrombopoietin, all of which enhance the release of stem cells into the circulation.[661–667] The KIT ligand receptors are downregulated in certain hematopoietic cell lines exposed to growth factors.[668] This explains the propensity of KIT ligand to mobilize stem cells, since it can alter receptor affinity and/or density and thus decrease the anchorage of stem cells to the membrane-bound KIT ligand on marrow stromal cells.[147,637]

As discussed earlier, both CD44-mediated adhesion and $\alpha_4\beta_1$/VCAM-1 interactions affect hematopoietic stem cell egress and homing.[539,643] Antibodies directed to the CD44v10 isoform release hematopoietic progenitors into the circulation.[536] Moreover, intracellular pools of hyaluronate receptor (RHAMM) and CD44 have been identified in early stem cells (CD34-positive, CD45-low/medium). Steady-state marrow CD34-positive progenitors have larger intracellular CD44 and intracellular RHAMM pools then do cells obtained from G-CSF mobilized blood collections which show a depleted intracellular RHAMM compartment.[669] Progenitor adhesion is blocked by anti-CD44 and anti-β_1 integrin antibodies, whereas motility is inhibited by antibodies to β_1 integrin and RHAMM, suggesting a reciprocal role between these two molecules during stem cell trafficking.

A working model of stem cell egress can be divided into five events shown in Table 4-5. This complex process does not rely on any one feature of stem cells and the marrow microenvironment; rather, the process assumes a continuous series of interactions affecting blood flow,[620] adventitial reticular cell-microvascular endothelial cell contraction,[670] altered integrin, selectin, cytokine and cytoskeletal receptor expression,[669] or functional activation. Chemokines such as IL-8 can efficiently mobilize hematopoietic stem cells.[671] IL-8, a potent activator of neutrophil integrin function, causes shedding of L-selectin and degranulation, exposing nearby matrix components to proteolytic enzymes such as elastase and gelatinase B, known also as *matrix*

TABLE 4-5   FACTORS REGULATING MARROW STEM CELL EGRESS

1. Increased marrow blood flow[620]
2. Adventitial reticular cell/microvascular endothelial cell contraction[670]
3. Altered adhesive interactions of CD34 cells and underlying cytomatrix:
   a) Integrin receptor ($\alpha_4\beta_1$) affinity[551] and expression (blocking antibody)[638,640]
   b) Decreased L-selectin affinity and expression[571]
   c) *C-KIT*- KIT ligand interactions[588,637,641]
   d) β_1-mediated integrin-cytoskeletal interactions[553]
   e) Alteration in intracellular RHAMM and CD44 pools[669]
   f) CD44v10 blocking antibody, progenitor egress with CD44v10 receptor globulin[536,639]
4. Increased enzyme production by:
   a) CD34 cells [gelatinase A (MMP-2) and gelatinase B (MMP-9)][684]
   b) Neutrophils activated by cytomatrix adherence, IL-8, and/or G-CSF (elastase and gelatinase B)[683]
5. Chemokine gradient(s) across sinusoidal barrier:
   a) Heparan sulfate containing matrix proteins binding to chemokines[241–249]
   b) Decreased CXCR4 receptor expression and SDF-1 expression by stromal cell or microvascular endothelial cell[147,570]

MMP, matrix metalloproteinase; RHAMM, hyaluronan receptor.

metalloproteinase 9 (MMP-9).[235,433,610] Antibodies against gelatinase B inhibit stem cell mobilization in this model.[672] Also, G-CSF administration in vivo is accompanied by a surge in IL-8 that may potentiate stem cell release.[673] This action is an indirect one, since long-term repopulating stem cells mobilized by IL-8 do not express $\alpha_L\beta_1$,[674] while anti-$\alpha_L\beta_1$ antibody administration blocks IL-8-induced stem cell egress.[675]

Another example of cooperation between cytokines and chemoattractants is provided by the study of G-CSF receptor (GCSFR)-deficient neutrophils, showing that a functional GCSFR is needed for β integrin activation.[676] In that GCFR knockout model, Flt3 ligand mobilizes progenitors, whereas IL-8 fails to do so.[677] Indeed, a functional GCFR is needed to activate β_2 integrins and mediate the IL-8 activation process, with subsequent gelatinase B release.[678] The inhibitory effects of anti-$\alpha_L\beta_1$ antibodies and the requirement for a functional G-CSF receptor imply that this mobilization process involves intramedullary activation of neutrophils, leading to enhanced stem cell egress.[675] This localized proteolysis (elastase, gelatinase B) is necessary for active cell migration[679] and is enhanced by cooperating signals from IL-8-, G-CSF-activated neutrophils adhering to matrix heparan sulfates.[680–683] In addition, CD34-positive progenitor cells elaborate gelatinase A and B, a process also augmented by cytokines.[684]

Hence, stem cell egress is affected by gelatinase expression coupled with altered integrin-, hyuloronan-based anchorage-migration ($\alpha_4\beta_1$-VCAM-1, CD44), by cytokine enhanced blood flow, and by E-selectin-chemokine driven transendothelial migration. This model (see Table 4-5) also takes into account the ability of antibody to gelatinase B, and to β_2 integrin, to block the IL-8 mobilization cascade. Integrin signaling and cross-talk with CD44, and the localized production of cytokines (such as KIT ligand, Flt3 ligand, G-CSF, thrombopoietin), create a complex matrix of interactions resulting in upmodulation (or downregulation) of CD34 active chemokine-chemokine receptors (SDF-1/CXCR4, IL-8/CXCR2, RANTES/CCR1, MIP-1α/CCR1, and SLC/CCR7), thereby setting the stage for multiple stem cell mobilization strategies.

REFERENCES

1. Testa NG, Molineux G: *Haemopoiesis: a Practical Approach.* IRL Press/Oxford University Press, New York, 1993.
2. Neuman E: Ueber die Bedeutung des Knochenmarks für die Blutbildung. *Cbl Med Wiss* 6:689, 1868.
3. Bizzozero G: Sulla fungione ematopoietica del midolo delle ossa. *Gazz Med Ital-Lomb,* vol 46, 1868.

4. Neuman E: Du Role de la möelle des os dans la formation du sang. *CR Acad Sci (Paris)*, 68:1112, 1869.

5. Mosler F: Klinische Symptome und Therapie der medullalären Leukemi. *Berl Klin Wochenschr* 13:233, 1876.

6. Arinkin MJ: Die intravitale Untersuchungsmetodik des Knochenmarks. *Folia Haematol (Leipz)* 38:233, 1929.

7. Lajtha LG: The common ancestral cell, in *Blood Pure and Eloquent*, edited by MM Wintrobe, p 81. McGraw-Hill, New York, 1980.

8. Erslev AJ: Feedback circuits in the control of stem cell differentiation. *Am J Pathol* 65:629, 1971.

9. Trentin JJ: Determination of bone marrow stem cell differentiation by stroma hemopoietic inductive microenvironment (HIM). *Am J Pathol* 65:621, 1971.

10. Zipori D: The renewal and differentiation of hemopoietic stem cells. *FASEB J* 6:2691, 1992.

11. Simmons DL, Satterthwaite AB, Tenen DG, Seed B: Molecular cloning of a cDNA encoding CD34, a sialomucin of human hematopoietic stem cells. *J Immunol* 148:267, 1992.

12. Ogawa M: Differentiation and proliferation of hematopoietic stem cells. *Blood* 81:2844, 1993.

13. Craig W, Kay R, Cutler RL, Lansdorp PM: Expression of Thy-1 on human hematopoietic progenitor cells. *J Exp Med* 177:1331, 1993.

14. Goodell MA, Rosenzweig M, Kim H, et al: Dye efflux studies suggest the existence of CD34-negative/low hematopoietic stem cells in multiple species. *Nat Med* 3:1337, 1997.

15. Bertoncello I, Bradford GB: Surrogate assays for hematopoietic stem cell activity, in *Colony-Stimulating Factors: Molecular and Cellular Biology*, edited by JM Garland, PJ Quesenberry, DJ Hilton, pp 35–47. Marcel Dekker, New York, 1997.

16. Sato T, Laver JH, Ogawa M: Reversible expression of CD34 by murine hematopoietic stem cells. *Blood* 94:2548, 1999.

17. Fujisaki T, Berger MG, Rose-John S, Eaves CJ: Rapid differentiation of a rare subset of adult human Lin- CD34- CD38- cells stimulated by multiple growth factors in vitro. *Blood* 94:1926, 1999.

18. Punzel M, Wissink SD, Miller JS, et al: The myeloid-lymphoid initiating cell (ML-IC) assay assesses the fate of multipotent human progenitors in vitro. *Blood* 93:3750, 1999.

19. Bahtia M, Bonnet D, Murdoch B, et al: A newly discovered class of human hematopoietic cells with SCID- repopulating activity. *Nat Med* 4:1038, 1998.

20. Kim DK, Fujiki Y, Fukushima T, et al: Comparison of hematopoietic activities of human bone marrow and umbilical cord blood CD34 positive and negative cells. *Stem Cells* 17:286, 1999.

21. Novelli EM, Ramirez M, Civin CI: Human hematopoietic stem/progenitor cells generate CD5+ B lymphoid cells in NOD/SCID mice. *Stem Cells* 17:242, 1999.

22. Zanjani ED, Almeida-Porada G, Flake AW: The human/sheep xenograft model: a large animal model of human hematopoiesis. *Int J Hematol* 63:179, 1996.

23. Moore MAS: Embryologic and phylogenetic development of the haemopoietic system. *Adv Biosci* 16:87, 1975.

24. Godin IE, Garcia-Porrero JA, Coutinho A, et al: Para-aortic splanchnopleura from early mouse embryos contains B1a cell progenitors. *Nature* 364:67, 1993.

25. Medvinski A, Dzierzak EA: Definitive hematopoiesis is autonomously initiated by the AGM region. *Cell* 86:897, 1996.

26. Yoder MC, Hiatt K, Dutt P, et al: Characterization of definitive lymphohematopoietic stem cells in the day 9 murine yolk sac. *Immunity* 7:335, 1997.

27. Cumano A, Furlonger C, Paige CJ: Differentiation and characterization of B-cell precursors detected in the yolk sac and embryo body of embryos beginning at the 10- to 12-somite stage. *Proc Natl Acad Sci USA* 90:6429, 1993.

28. Yoder MC, Hiatt K, Mukherjee P: In vivo repopulating hematopoietic stem cells are present in the murine yolk sac at day 9.0 postcoitus. *Proc Natl Acad Sci USA* 94:6776, 1997.

29. Palis J, Starr M, Koniski A, Yoder MC: Temporal and spatial emergence of high proliferative potential colony forming cells (HPP-CFC) during mammalian embryogenesis. *Blood* 94(suppl 1):32a, 1999.

30. Ogawa M, Nishikawa S, Yoshinaga K, et al: Expression and function of c-Kit in fetal hemopoietic progenitor cells: transition from the early c-Kit-independent to the late c-Kit-dependent wave of hematopoiesis in the murine embryo. *Development* 117:1089, 1993.

31. Ortiz M, Wine JW, Lohrey N, et al: Functional characterization of a novel hematopoietic stem cell and its place in the c-Kit maturation pathway in bone marrow cell development. *Immunity* 10:173, 1999.

32. Matsui Y, Zsebo K, Hogan BL: Derivation of pluripotential embryonic stem cells from murine primordial germ cells in culture. *Cell* 70:841, 1992.

33. Conquet F, Brulet P: Developmental expression of myeloid leukemia inhibitory factor gene in preimplantation blastocysts and in extraembryonic tissue of mouse embryos. *Mol Cell Biol* 10:3801, 1990.

34. Xu MJ, Tsuji K, Ueda T, et al: Stimulation of mouse and human primitive hematopoiesis by murine embryonic aorta-gonad-mesonephros-derived stromal cell lines. *Blood* 92:2032, 1998.

35. Ohneda O, Fennie C, Zheng Z, et al: Hematopoietic stem cell maintenance and differentiation are supported by embryonic aorta-gonad-mesonephros region-derived endothelium. *Blood* 92:908, 1998.

36. Verfaille CM: Soluble factor(s) produced by human bone marrow stroma increase cytokine-induced proliferation and maturation of primitive hematopoietic progenitors while preventing their terminal differentiation. *Blood* 82:2045, 1993.

37. Fukushima N, Nishina H, Koishihara Y, Ohkawa H: Enhanced hematopoiesis in vivo and in vitro by splenic stromal cells derived from the mouse with recombinant granulocyte colony-stimulating factor. *Blood* 80:1914, 1992.

38. Islam A, Glomski C, Henderson ES: Endothelial cells and hematopoiesis: a light microscopic study of fetal, normal, and pathologic human bone marrow in plastic-embedded sections. *Anat Rec* 233:440, 1992.

39. Hamaguchi I, Huang X-L, Takakura N, et al: In vitro hematopoietic and endothelial cell development from cells expressing TEK receptor in murine aorta-gonad-mesonephros region. *Blood* 93:1549, 1999.

40. Hara T, Nakano Y-K, Tanaka M, et al: Identification of podocalyxin-like protein 1 as a novel cell surface marker for hemangioblasts in the murine aorta-gonad-mesonephros region. *Immunity* 11:567, 1999.

41. Ogawa M, Kizumoto M, Nishikawa S, et al: Expression of α4-integrin defines the earliest precursor of hematopoietic cell lineage diverged from endothelial cells. *Blood* 93:1168, 1999.

42. Almeida-Porada GD, Hoffman R, Manalo P, et al: Detection of human cells in human/sheep chimeric lambs with in vitro human stroma-forming potential. *Exp Hematol* 24:482, 1996.

43. Osawa M, Hanada K-I, Hamada H, et al: Long-term lymphohematopoietic reconstitution by a single CD34-low/negative hematopoietic stem cell. *Science* 273:242, 1996.

44. Zanjani ED, Almeida-Porada G, Livingston AG, et al: Human bone marrow CD34- cells engraft in vivo and undergo multilineage expression that includes giving rise to CD34+ cells. *Exp Hematol* 26:353, 1998.

45. Dieterlen-Lievre F: Hematopoiesis: progenitors and their genetic program. *Curr Biol* 8:R727, 1998.

46. Ziegler BL, Valtieri M, Almeida-Porada G, et al: KDR receptor: a key marker defining hematopoietic stem cells. *Science* 285:1553, 1999.

47. Nakamura Y, Ando K, Chargui J, et al: Ex vivo generation of CD34+ cells from CD34- hematopoietic cells. *Blood* 94:4053, 1999.

48. Jackson KA, Mi T, Goodell MA: Hematopoietic potential of stem cells isolated from murine skeletal muscle. *Proc Natl Acad Sci USA* 96:14482, 1999.

49. Bjornson CR, Rietze RL, Reynolds BA, et al: Turning brain into blood: a hematopoietic fate adopted by adult neural stem cells in vivo. *Science* 283:534, 1999.

50. Hudson G: Bone marrow volume in the human foetus and newborn. *Br J Haematol* 11:446, 1965.

51. Rosse C, Kraemer MJ, Dillon TL, et al: Bone marrow cell populations of normal infants: the predominance of lymphocytes. *J Lab Clin Med* 89:1225, 1977.

52. Nagasawa T, Hirota S, Tachibana K, et al: Defects of B-cell lymphopoiesis and bone marrow myelopoiesis in mice lacking the CXC chemokine PBSF/SDF-1. *Nature* 382:635, 1996.

53. Imai K, Kobayashi M, Wang J, et al: Selective transendothelial migration of hematopoietic progenitor cells: a role in homing of progenitor cells. *Blood* 93:149, 1999.

54. Arroyo AG, Yang JT, Rayburn H, et al: α4 integrins regulate the proliferation/differentiation balance of multilineage hematopoietic progenitors in vivo. *Immunity* 11:555, 1999.

55. Roy V, Verfaille CM: Expression and function of cell adhesion molecules on fetal liver, cord blood and bone marrow hematopoietic progenitors: implications for anatomical localization and developmental stage specific regulation of hematopoiesis. *Exp Hematol* 27:302, 1999.

56. Custer RP, Ahlfeldt FE: Studies on the structure and function of the bone marrow. *J Lab Clin Med* 17:960, 1932.

57. Mechanik N: Untersuchange über das Gewicht des Knochenmarks des Menschen. *Z Ges Anat* 79:58, 1926 (summarized by RE Ellis, *Phys Med Biol* 5:255, 1961).

58. Gregersen MI, Rawson RA: Blood volume. *Physiol Rev* 39:307, 1969.

59. Christy M: Active marrow distribution as a function of age in humans. *Phys Med Biol* 26:389, 1981.

60. Babyn PS, Ranson M, McCarvelle ME: Normal bone marrow signal characteristics and fatty conversion. *Med Clin North Am* 6:473, 1998.

61. Huggins C, Blocksom BH Jr: Changes in outlying bone marrow accompanying a local increase in temperature within physiologic limits. *J Exp Med* 64:253, 1936.

62. Maniatis A, Tavassoli M, Crosby WH: Factors affecting the conversion of yellow to red marrow. *Blood* 37:581, 1971.

63. Crosby WH: Experience with injured and implanted bone marrow: relation of function to structure, in *Hemopoietic Cellular Proliferation,* edited by F Stohlman Jr, p 87. Grune & Stratton, New York, 1970.

64. Brookes M: *The Blood Supply of Bone.* Butterworth, London, 1971.

65. Tavassoli M: Arterial structure of the bone marrow in rabbits with special reference to thin walled arteries. *Acta Anat (Basel)* 90:608, 1974.

66. Wilkins BS, Jones DB: Vascular networks within the stroma of human long-term bone marrow cultures. *J Pathol* 177:295, 1995.

67. Charbord P, Tavian M, Humeau L, Peault B: Early ontogeny of the human marrow from long bones: an immunohistochemical study of hematopoiesis and its microenvironment. *Blood* 87:4109, 1996.

68. Eichman A, Corbel C, Nataf V, et al: Ligand-dependent development of the endothelial and hematopoietic lineages from embryonic mesodermal cells expressing vascular endothelial growth factor receptor 2. *Proc Natl Acad Sci USA* 94:141, 1997.

69. Marshall CJ, Moore RL, Thorogood P, et al: Detailed characterization of the human aorta-gonad-mesonephros region reveals morphological polarity resembling a hematopoietic stromal layer. *Dev Dyn* 215:139, 1999.

70. Lichtman MA: The ultrastructure of the hemopoietic environment of the marrow: a review. *Exp Hematol* 9:391, 1981.

71. Yamazaki K, Allen TD: Ultrastructural morphometric study of efferent nerve terminals on murine bone marrow stromal cells, and the recognition of a novel anatomical unit: the "neuro-reticular complex." *Am J Anat* 187:261, 1990.

72. Cattoretti G, Schiro R, Orazi A, et al: Bone marrow stroma in humans: anti-nerve growth factor receptor antibodies selectively stain reticular cells in vivo and in vitro. *Blood* 81:1726, 1993.

73. Rameshwar P, Gascon P: Induction of negative hematopoietic regulators by neurokinin-A in bone marrow stroma. *Blood* 88:98, 1996.

74. Rameshwar P, Gascon P: Substance P (SP) mediates production of stem cell factor and interleukin-1 in bone marrow stroma: potential autoregulatory role for these cytokines in SP receptor expression and induction. *Blood* 86:482, 1995.

75. Rameshwar P, Gascon P: Hematopoietic modulation by the tachykinins. *Acta Haematol* 98:59, 1997.

76. Hiramoto M, Aizawa S, Iwase O, et al: Stimulatory effects of substance P on CD34 positive cell proliferation and differentiation in vitro are mediated by the modulation of stromal cell function. *Int J Mol Med* 1:347, 1998.

77. Rameshwar P, Poddar A, Zhu G, Gascon P: Receptor induction regulates the synergistic effects of substance P with IL-1 and platelet-derived growth factor on the proliferation of bone marrow fibroblasts. *J Immunol* 158:3417, 1997.

78. Greeno EW, Mantyh P, Vercellotti GM, Moldow CF: Functional neurokin 1 receptors for substance P are expressed by human vascular endothelium. *J Exp Med* 177:1269, 1993.

79. Tabarowski Z, Gibson-Berry K, Felten SY: Noradrenergic and peptidergic innervation of mouse femur bone marrow. *Acta Histochem* 98:453, 1996.

80. Afran AM, Broome CS, Nicholls SE, et al: Bone marrow innervation regulates cellular retention in the murine haematopoietic system. *Br J Haematol* 98:569, 1997.

81. Iversen PO, Stokland A, Rolstad B, Benestad HB: Adrenaline-induced leucocytosis: recruitment of blood cells from rat spleen, bone marrow and lymphatics. *Eur J Appl Physiol* 68:219, 1994.

82. Tang Y, Shankar R, Gamelli R, Jones S: Dynamic norepinephrine alterations in bone marrow: evidence of functional innervation. *J Neuroimmunol* 96:182, 1999.

83. Iversen PO: Blood flow to the haemopoietic bone marrow. *Acta Physiol Scand* 159:269, 1997.

84. Iversen PO, Nicolaysen G, Benestad HB: Endogenous nitric oxide causes vasodilatation in rat bone marrow, bone, and spleen during accelerated hematopoiesis. *Exp Hematol* 22:1297, 1994.

85. Quinlan DP Jr, Rameshwar P, Qian J, et al: Effect of hypoxia on the hematopoietic and immune modulator preprotachykinin-I. *Arch Surg* 133:1328, 1998.

86. Maestroni GJM, Conti A, Pedrinis E: Effect of adrenergic agents on hematopoiesis after syngeneic bone marrow transplantation in mice. *Blood* 80:1178, 1992.

87. Benestad HB, Strom-Gundersen I, Iversen PO, et al: No neuronal regulation of murine bone marrow function. *Blood* 91:280, 1998.

88. Abboud CN, Liesveld JL, Lichtman MA: The architecture of marrow and its role in hematopoietic cell lodgement, in *The Hematopoietic Microenvironment,* edited by MW Long, MS Wicha, pp 2–20. Johns Hopkins University Press, Baltimore and London, 1993.

89. Tavassoli M, Shaklai M: Absence of tight junctions in endothelium of marrow sinuses: possible significance for marrow cell egress. *Br J Haematol* 41:303, 1979.

90. Abboud CN: Human bone marrow microvascular endothelial cells: elusive cells with unique structural and functional properties. *Exp Hematol* 23:1, 1995.

91. Bankston PW, DeBruyn PPH: The permeability to carbon of the sinusoidal lining cells of the embryonic rat liver and rat bone marrow. *Am J Anat* 141:281, 1974.

92. Lichtman MA, Packman CH, Constine LS: Molecular and cellular traffic across the marrow sinus wall, in *Blood Cell Formation: The Role of Hemopoietic Microenvironment,* edited by M. Tavassoli, pp 87–140. Humana Press, Clifton, NJ, 1989.

93. Kataoka M, Tavassoli M: Identification of lectin-like substances recognizing galactosyl residues of glycoconjugates on the plasma membrane of marrow sinus endothelium. *Blood* 65:1163, 1985.

94. Bussolino F, Colotta F, Bocchietto E, et al: Recent developments in the cell biology of granulocyte-macrophage colony-stimulating factor and granulocyte colony-stimulating factor: Activities on endothelial cells. *Int J Clin Lab Res* 23:8, 1993.

95. Koch AE, Burrows JC, Domer PH, et al: Monoclonal antibodies defining shared human macrophage-endothelial antigens. *Pathobiology* 60:59, 1992.

96. Penn PE, Jiang D-Z, Fei R-G, et al. Dissecting the hematopoietic microenvironment: IX. Further characterization of murine bone marrow stromal cells. *Blood* 81:1205, 1993.

97. Hasthorpe S, Bogdanovski M, Rogerson J, Radley JM: Characterization of endothelial cells in murine long-term marrow culture: Implication for hemopoietic regulation. *Exp Hematol* 20:386, 1992.

98. Perkins S, Fleischman RA: Stromal cell progeny of murine bone marrow fibroblast colony-forming units are clonal endothelial-like cells that express collagen IV and laminin. *Blood* 75:620, 1990.

99. Schweitzer KM, Drager AM, van der Valk P, et al: Constitutive expression of E-selectin and vascular cell adhesion molecule-1 on endothelial cells of hematopoietic tissues. *Am J Pathol* 148:165, 1996.

100. DeBruyn PPH, Michelson S: Changes in the random distribution of sialic acid at the surface of the myeloid sinus endothelium resulting from the presence of diaphragmed fenestrae. *J Cell Biol* 82:708, 1979.

101. Masek LC, Sweetenham JW, Whitehouse JMA, Schumacher U: Immuno-, lectin-, and enzyme-histochemical characterization of human bone marrow endothelium. *Exp Hematol* 22:1203, 1994.

102. Kuemmel TA, Thiele J, Hafenrichter EG, et al: Distribution of lectin binding sites in human bone marrow. Identification by use of ultrastructural postembedding technique. *J Submicrosc Cytol Pathol* 28:537, 1996.

103. Garlanda C, Berthier R, Garin J, et al: Characterization of MEC 14.7, a new monoclonal antibody recognizing mouse CD34: a useful reagent for identifying and characterizing blood vessels and hematopoietic precursors. *Eur J Cell Biol* 73:368, 1997.

104. Rafii S, Shapiro F, Rimarachin J, et al: Isolation and characterization

of human bone marrow microvascular endothelial cells: hematopoietic progenitor adhesion. *Blood* 84:10, 1994.

105. Bazzoni G, Dejana E, Lampugnani MG: Endothelial adhesion molecules in the development of the vascular tree: the garden of forking paths. *Curr Opin Cell Biol* 11:573, 1999.

106. DeBruyn PPH, Michelson S, Becker RP: Endocytosis, transfer tubules and lysosomal activity in myeloid sinusoidal endothelium. *J Ultrastruct Res* 53:133, 1975.

107. Delia D, Lampugnani MG, Resnati M, et al: CD34 expression is regulated reciprocally with adhesion molecules in vascular cells in vitro. *Blood* 81:1001, 1993.

108. Guo WX, Ghebrehiwet B, Weksler B, et al: Up-regulation of endothelial cell binding proteins/receptors for complement component C1q by inflammatory cytokines. *J Lab Clin Med* 133:541, 1999.

109. Imai T, Hieshima K, Haskell C, et al: Identification and molecular characterization of fractalkine receptor CX3CR1, which mediates both leukocyte migration and adhesion. *Cell* 91:521, 1997.

110. Nitschke L, Floyd H, Ferguson DJ, Crocker PR: Identification of CD22 ligands on bone marrow sinusoidal endothelium implicated in CD22-dependent homing of recirculating B cells. *J Exp Med* 189:1513, 1999.

111. Weiss L, Chen L-T: The organization of hemopoietic cords and vascular sinuses in bone marrow. *Blood Cells* 1:617, 1975.

112. Leblond PF, Chamberlain JK, Weed RI: Scanning electron microscopy of erythropoietin-stimulated bone marrow. *Blood Cells* 1:639, 1975.

113. Lichtman MA: The relationship of stromal cells to hemopoietic cells in marrow, in *Long-Term Bone Marrow Culture,* edited by DG Wright, JS Greenberger, pp 3–26. Liss, New York, 1984.

114. Abboud CN, Duerst RE, Frantz CN, et al: Lysis of human fibroblast colony-forming cells and endothelial cells by monoclonal antibody (6-19) and complement. *Blood* 68:1196, 1986.

115. Simmons PJ, Torok-Storb B: Identification of stromal cell precursors in human bone marrow by a novel monoclonal antibody, STRO-1. *Blood* 78:55, 1991.

116. Labouyrie E, Dubus P, Groppi A, et al: Expression of neurotrophins and their receptors in human bone marrow. *Am J Pathol* 154:405, 1999.

117. Gronthos S, Simmons PJ: The growth factor requirements of STRO-1-positive human bone marrow stromal precursors under serum-deprived conditions in vitro. *Blood* 85:929, 1995.

118. Charbord P, Lerat H, Newton I, et al: The cytoskeleton of stromal cells from human bone marrow cultures resembles that of cultured smooth muscle cells. *Exp Hematol* 18:276, 1990.

119. Galmiche MC, Koteliansky VE, Briere J, et al: Stromal cells from human long-term marrow cultures are mesenchymal cells that differentiate following a vascular smooth muscle differentiation pathway. *Blood* 82:66, 1993.

120. Brown J, Greaves MF, Molgaard HV: The gene encoding the stem cell antigen, CD34, is conserved in mouse and expressed in haemopoietic progenitor cell lines, brain, and embryonic fibroblasts. *Int Immunol* 3:175, 1991.

121. Simmons PJ, Torok-Storb B: CD34 expression by stromal precursors in normal adult bone marrow. *Blood* 78:2848, 1991.

122. Dorshkind K, Green L, Godwin A, Fletcher WH: Connexin-43-type gap junctions mediate communication between bone marrow stromal cells. *Blood* 82:38, 1993.

123. Rosendaal M, Green CR, Rahman A, Morgan D: Up-regulation of the connexin43+ gap junction network in haemopoietic tissue before the growth of stem cells. *J Cell Sci* 107:29, 1994.

124. Krenacs T, Rosendaal M: Connexin43 gap junctions in normal, regenerating, and cultured mouse bone marrow and in human leukemias: their possible involvement in blood formation. *Am J Pathol* 152:993, 1998.

125. Torok-Storb B, Iwata M, Graf L, et al: Dissecting the marrow microenvironment. *Ann NY Acad Sci* 872:164, 1999.

126. Weiss L: Barrier cells in the spleen. *Immunol Today* 12:24, 1991.

127. Weiss L, Geduldig U: Barrier cells: stromal regulation of hematopoiesis and blood cell release in normal and stressed murine bone marrow. *Blood* 78:975, 1991.

128. Schmitt-Gräff A, Skalli O, Gabbiani G: Alpha-smooth muscle actin is expressed in a subset of bone marrow stromal cells in normal and pathological conditions. *Virchows Archiv [B]* 57:291, 1989.

129. Tavassoli M: Fatty evolution of marrow and the role of adipose tissue in hematopoiesis, in *Handbook of the Hemopoietic Microenvironment,* edited by M Tavassoli, pp 157–187. Humana Press, Clifton, NJ, 1989.

130. Laharrague P, Larrouy D, Fontanilles AM, et al: High expression of leptin by human bone marrow adipocytes in primary cultures. *FASEB J* 12:747, 1998.

131. Benayahu D, Shamay A, Wientroub S: Osteocalcin (BGP), gene expression, and protein production by marrow stromal adipocytes. *Biochem Biophys Res Commun* 13:442, 1997.

132. McAveny KM, Gimble JM, Yu-Lee L: Prolactin receptor expression during adipocyte differentiation of bone marrow stroma. *Endocrinology* 137:5723, 1996.

133. Gimble JM, Robinson CE, Wu X, Kelly KA: The function of adipocytes in the bone marrow stroma: an update. *Bone* 19:421, 1996.

134. Delikat S, Harris RJ, Galvani DW: IL-1 beta inhibits adipocyte formation in human long-term bone marrow culture. *Exp Hematol* 21:31, 1993.

135. Keller DC, Du XX, Srour EF, et al: Interleukin-11 inhibits adipogenesis and stimulates myelopoiesis in human long-term marrow cultures. *Blood* 82:1428, 1993.

136. Gimble JM, Morgan C, Kelly K, et al: Bone morphogenetic proteins inhibit adipocyte differentiation by bone marrow stromal cells. *J Cell Biochem* 58:393, 1995.

137. Thomas T, Gori F, Khosla S, et al: Leptin acts on human marrow stromal cells to enhance differentiation to osteoblasts and to inhibit differentiation to adipocytes. *Endocrinology* 140:1630, 1999.

138. Wilkins BS, Jones DB: Immunophenotypic characterization of stromal cells in aspirated human bone marrow samples. *Exp Hematol* 26:1061, 1998.

139. Takahashi GW, Moran D, Andrews DF III, Singer JW: Differential expression of collagenase by human fibroblasts and bone marrow stromal cells. *Leukemia* 8:305, 1994.

140. Liesveld JL, Abboud CN, Duerst RE, et al: Characterization of human marrow stromal cells: role in progenitor cell binding and granulopoiesis. *Blood* 73:1794, 1989.

141. Aiuti A, Friedrich C, Sieff CA, Gutierrez-Ramos J-C: Identification of distinct elements of the stromal microenvironment that control human hematopoietic stem/progenitor cell growth and differentiation. *Exp Hematol* 26:143, 1998.

142. Li J, Sensebe L, Herve P, Charbord P: Nontransformed colony-derived stromal cell lines from normal human marrows: III. The maintenance of hematopoiesis from CD34+ cell populations. *Exp Hematol* 25:582, 1997.

143. Osmond DG, Kim N, Manoukina R, et al: Dynamics and localization of early B-lymphocyte precursor cells (pro-B cells) in the bone marrow of scid mice. *Blood* 79:1695, 1992.

144. Moreau I, Duvert V, Caux C, et al: Myofibroblastic stromal cells isolated from human bone marrow induce the proliferation of both early myeloid and B lymphoid cells. *Blood* 82:2396, 1993.

145. Tamir M, Eren R, Globerson A, et al: Selective accumulation of lymphocyte precursor cells mediated by stromal cells of hemopoietic origin. *Exp Hematol* 18:332, 1990.

146. Lisovsky M, Braun SE, Ge Y, et al: Flt3-ligand production by human bone marrow stromal cells. *Leukemia* 10:1012, 1996.

147. Besmer P: Kit-ligand-stem cell factor, in *Colony-Stimulating Factors: Molecular and Cellular Biology,* edited by JM Garland, PJ Quesenberry, DJ Hilton, pp 369–404. Marcel Dekker, New York, 1997.

148. Kaushansky K: Thrombopoietin and the hematopoietic stem cell. *Blood* 92:1, 1998.

149. Solar GP, Kerr WG, Zeigler FC, et al: Role of c-mpl in early hematopoiesis. *Blood* 92:4, 1998.

150. Guerriero A, Worford L, Holland HK, et al: Thrombopoietin is synthesized by bone marrow stromal cells. *Blood* 90:3444, 1997.

151. Matsunaga T, Kato K, Miyazaki H, Ogawa M: Thrombopoietin promotes the survival of murine hematopoietic long-term reconstituting cells: comparison with the effects of FLT3/FLK-2 ligand and interleukin-6. *Blood* 92:452, 1998.

152. Waring PM: Leukemia inhibitory factor, in *Colony-Stimulating Factors: Molecular and Cellular Biology,* edited by JM Garland, PJ Quesenberry, DJ Hilton, pp 467–513. Marcel Dekker, New York, 1997.

153. Sui X, Tsuji K, Ebihara Y, et al: Soluble interleukin-6 (IL-6) receptor with IL-6 stimulates megakaryopoiesis from human CD34+ cells through glycoprotein (gp)130 signaling. *Blood* 93: 2525, 1999.

154. Heberlein C, Friel J, Laker C, et al: Downregulation of c-kit (stem cell factor receptor) in transformed hematopoietic precursor cells by stroma cells. *Blood* 93:554, 1999.

155. Walker L, Lynch M, Silverman S, et al: The Notch/Jagged pathway

inhibits proliferation of human hematopoietic progenitors in vitro. *Stem Cells* 17:162, 1999.

156. Van Den Berg DJ, Sharma AK, Bruno E, Hoffman R: Role of members of the Wnt gene family in human hematopoiesis. *Blood* 92:89, 1998.

157. Tordjman R, Ortega N, Coulombel L, et al: Neuropilin-1 is expressed on bone marrow stromal cells: a novel interaction with hematopoietic cells? *Blood* 94:2301, 1999.

158. Filshie RJ, Zannettino AC, Makrynikola V, et al: MUC18, a member of the immunoglobulin superfamily, is expressed on bone marrow fibroblasts and a subset of hematological malignancies. *Leukemia* 12:414, 1998.

159. Zannettino ACW, Buhring H-J, Niutta S, et al: The sialomucin CD164 (MCG-24v) is an adhesive glycoprotein expressed by human hematopoietic progenitors and bone marrow stromal cells that serves as a potent negative regulator of hematopoiesis. *Blood* 92:2613, 1998.

160. Cortes F, Deschaseaux F, Uchida N, et al: HCA, an immunoglobulin-like adhesion molecule present on the earliest human hematopoietic precursor cells, is also expressed by stromal cells in blood-forming tissues. *Blood* 93:826, 1999.

161. Deldar A, Lewis H, Weiss L: Bone lining cells and hematopoiesis: an electron microscopic study of canine bone marrow. *Anat Rec* 213:187, 1985.

162. Sillaber C, Walchshofer S, Mosberger I, et al: Immunophenotypic characterization of human bone marrow endosteal cells. *Tissue Antigens* 53:559, 1999.

163. Saito T, Albelda SM, Brighton CT: Identification of integrin receptors on cultured human bone cells. *J Orthop Res* 12:384, 1994.

164. Gong J: Endosteal marrow: a rich source of hematopoietic stem cells. *Science* 199:1443, 1978.

165. Nilsson SK, Dooner MS, Tiarks CY, et al: Potential and distribution of transplanted hematopoietic stem cells in a nonablated mouse model. *Blood* 89:4013, 1997.

166. Park SR, Oreffo RO, Triffitt JT: Interconversion potential of cloned human marrow adipocytes in vitro. *Bone* 24:549, 1999.

167. Dennis JE, Merriam A, Awadallah, A et al: A quadripotential mesenchymal progenitor cell isolated from the marrow of an adult mouse. *J Bone Miner Res* 14:700, 1999.

168. Pittenger MF, Mackay AM, Beck SC, et al: Multilineage potential of adult human mesenchymal stem cells. *Science* 284:143, 1999.

169. Oyajobi BO, Lomri A, Hott M, Marie PJ: Isolation and characterization of human clonogenic osteoblast progenitors immunoselected from fetal bone marrow stroma using STRO-1 monoclonal antibody. *J Bone Miner Res* 14:351, 1999.

170. Doherty MJ, Ashton BA, Walsh S, et al: Vascular pericytes express osteogenic potential in vitro and in vivo. *J Bone Miner Res* 13:828, 1999.

171. Bruder SP, Ricalton NS, Boynton RE et al: Mesenchymal stem cell surface antigen SB-10 corresponds to activated leukocyte cell adhesion molecule and is involved in osteogenic differentiation. *J Bone Miner Res* 13:655, 1998.

172. Long MW, Robinson JA, Ashcraft EA, Mann KG: Regulation of human bone marrow-derived osteoprogenitor cells by osteogenic growth factors. *J Clin Invest* 95:881, 1995.

173. Gronthos S, Zannettino AC, Graves SE, et al: Differential cell surface expression of the STRO-1 and alkaline phosphatase antigens on discrete developmental stages in primary cultures of human bone cells. *J Bone Miner Res* 14:47, 1999.

174. Stewart K, Walsh S, Screen J, et al: Further characterization of cells expressing STRO-1 in cultures of adult human bone marrow stromal cells. *J Bone Miner Res* 14:1345, 1999.

175. Hanada K, Dennis JE, Caplan AI: Stimulatory effects of basic fibroblast growth factor and bone morphogenetic protein-2 on osteogenic differentiation of rat bone marrow-derived mesenchymal stem cells. *J Bone Miner Res* 12:1606, 1997.

176. Taichman RS, Emerson SG: The role of osteoblasts in the hematopoietic microenvironment. *Stem Cells* 16:7, 1998.

177. Ahmed N, Khokher MA, Hassan HT: Cytokine-induced expansion of human CD34+ stem/progenitor and CD34+CD41+ early megakaryocytic marrow cells cultured on normal osteoblasts. *Stem Cells* 17:92, 1999.

178. Gehron Robey P, Young MF, Flanders KC, et al: Osteoblasts synthesize and respond to transforming growth factor-type β (TGF-beta) in vitro. *J Cell Biol* 105:457, 1987.

179. Nilsson SK, Dooner MS, Weier HU, et al: Cells capable of bone produc-

180. El-Badri NS, Wang B-Y, Cherry, Good RA: Osteoblasts promote engraftment of allogeneic hematopoietic stem cells. *Exp Hematol* 26:110, 1998.

181. Gurevitch O, Fabian I: Ability of the hemopoietic microenvironment in the induced bone to maintain the proliferative potential of early hemopoietic precursors. *Stem Cells* 11:56, 1993.

182. Civitelli R, Beyer EC, Warlow PM, et al: Connexin43 mediates direct intercellular communication in human osteoblastic cell networks. *J Clin Invest* 91:1888, 1993.

183. Matayoshi A, Brown C, DiPersio JF, et al: Human blood-mobilized hematopoietic precursors differentiate into osteoclasts in the absence of stromal cells. *Proc Natl Acad Sci USA* 93:10785, 1996.

184. Roodman GD: Cell biology of the osteoclast. *Exp Hematol* 27:1229, 1999.

185. Yoshida H, Hayashi S-I, Kunisada T, et al: The murine mutation osteopetrosis is in the coding region of the macrophage colony-stimulating factor gene. *Nature* 345:442, 1990.

186. Wiktor-Jedrzejczak W, Urbanowska E, Aukerman SL, et al: Correction by CSF-1 of defects in the osteopetrotic op/op mouse suggests local, developmental, and humoral requirements for this growth factor. *Exp Hematol* 19:1049, 1991.

187. Demulder A, Suggs SV, Zsebo KM, et al: Effects of stem cell factor on osteoclast-like cell formation in long-term human marrow cultures. *J Bone Min Res* 7:1337, 1992.

188. Tanaka S, Takahashi N, Udagawa N, et al: Macrophage colony-stimulating factor is indispensable for both proliferation and differentiation of osteoclast progenitors. *J Clin Invest* 91:257, 1993.

189. Price LK, Choi HU, Rosenberg L, Stanley ER: The predominant form of secreted colony-stimulating factor-1 is a proteoglycan. *J Biol Chem* 267:2190, 1992.

190. Ohtsuki T, Suzu S, Hatake K, et al: A proteoglycan form of macrophage colony-stimulating factor that binds to bone-derived collagens and can be extracted from bone matrix. *Biochem Biophys Res Commun* 190:215, 1993.

191. Grigoriadis AE, Wang ZQ, Ceccini MG, et al: c-Fos a key regulator of osteoclast-macrophage lineage determination and bone remodeling. *Science* 266:443, 1994.

192. Soriano P, Montgomery C, Geske R, Bradley A: Targeted disruption of the c-src proto-oncogene leads to osteopetrosis in mice. *Cell* 64:693, 1991.

193. Shalhoub V, Faust J, Boyle WJ, et al: Osteoprotegrin and osteoprotegrin ligand effects on osteoclast formation from human peripheral blood mononuclear cell precursors. *J Cell Biochem* 72:251, 1999.

194. Takahashi N, Udagawa N, Suda T: A new member of tumor necrosis factor ligand family, ODF/OPGL/TRANCE/RANKL, regulates osteoclast differentiation and function. *Biochem Biophys Res Commun* 256:449, 1999.

195. Yasuda H, Shima N, Nakagawa N, et al: A novel molecular mechanism modulating osteoclast differentiation and function. *Bone* 25:109, 1999.

196. Burgess TL, Qian Y, Kaufman S, et al: The ligand for osteoprotegrin (OPGL) directly activates mature osteoclasts. *J Cell Biol* 145:527, 1999.

197. Hsu H, Lacey DL, Dunstan CR, et al: Tumor necrosis factor receptor family member RANK mediates osteoclast differentiation and activation induced by osteoprotegrin ligand. *Proc Natl Acad Sci USA* 96:3540, 1999.

198. Kania JR, Kehat-Stadler T, Kupfer SR: CD44 antibodies inhibit osteoclast formation. *J Bone Miner Res* 12:1155, 1997.

199. Mbalaviele G, Nishimura R, Myoi A, et al: Cadherin-6 mediates the heterotypic interactions between the hemopoietic osteoclast cell lineage and stromal cells in a murine model of osteoclast differentiation. *J Cell Biol* 141:1467, 1998.

200. Oritani K, Wu X, Medina K, et al: Antibody ligation of CD9 modifies production of myeloid cells in long-term cultures. *Blood* 87:2252, 1996.

201. Tanio Y, Yamazaki H, Kunisada T, et al: CD9 molecule expressed on stromal cells is involved in osteoclastogenesis. *Exp Hematol* 27:853, 1999.

202. Quesenberry PJ, Crittenden RB, Lowry P, et al: In vitro and in vivo studies of stromal niches. *Blood Cells* 20:97, 1994.

203. Gibson FM, Scopes J, Daly S, et al: IL-3 is produced by normal stroma in long-term bone marrow cultures. *Br J Haematol* 90:518, 1995.

tion engraft from whole bone marrow transplants in nonablated mice. *J Exp Med* 189:729, 1999.

204. Verfaillie CM, Catanzarro PM, Li WN: Macrophage inflammatory protein 1 alpha, interleukin-3 and diffusible marrow stromal factors maintain human hematopoietic stem cells for at least eight weeks in vitro. *J Exp Med* 179:643, 1994.

205. Garland JM, Rudin CE: Introduction to the hematopoietic system, in *Colony-Stimulating Factors: Molecular and Cellular Biology,* edited by JM Garland, PJ Quesenberry, DJ Hilton, pp 1-33. Marcel Dekker, New York, 1997.

206. Crocker PR, Morris L, Gordon S: Novel cell surface adhesion receptors involved in interactions between stromal macrophages and haematopoietic cells. *J Cell Sci* 9(suppl):185, 1988.

207. Wang QR, Wolf NS: Dissecting the hematopoietic microenvironment: VIII. Clonal isolation and identification of cell types in murine CFU-F colonies by limiting dilution. *Exp Hematol* 18:355, 1990.

208. Kincade PW: Cell interaction molecules and cytokines which participate in B lymphopoiesis. *Baillieres Clin Haematol* 5:575, 1992.

209. Berneman ZN, Chen ZZ, van Bockstaele D, et al: The nature of the adherent hemopoietic cells in human long-term bone marrow cultures (HLTBMCs): presence of lymphocytes and plasma cells next to the myelomonocytic population. *Leukemia* 9:648, 1989.

210. Tong J, Kishi H, Matsuda T, Muraguchi A: A bone marrow-derived stroma line, ST2, can support the differentiation of fetal thymocytes from CD4+ CD8+ double negative to the CD4+ CD8+ double positive differentiation stage in vitro. *Immunology* 97:672, 1999.

211. Dejbakhsh-Jones S, Strober S: Identification of an early T cell progenitor for a pathway of T cell maturation in the bone marrow. *Proc Natl Acad Sci USA* 96:14493, 1999.

212. Kurosaka D, LeBien TW, Priby JAR: Comparative studies of different stromal cell microenvironments in support of human B-cell development. *Exp Hematol* 27:1271, 1999.

213. Funk PE, Stephan RP, Witte PL: Vascular adhesion molecule-1-positive reticular cells express interleukin-7 and stem cell factor in the bone marrow. *Blood* 86:2661, 1995.

214. Tang J, Nuccie BL, Ritterman I, et al: TGF-beta down-regulates stromal IL-7 secretion and inhibits proliferation of human B cell precursors. *J Immunol* 159:117, 1997.

215. Tsuji JM, Pollack SB: Maturation of murine natural killer precursor cells in the absence of exogenous cytokines requires contact with bone marrow stroma. *Nat Immun* 14:44, 1995.

216. Yu H, Fehniger TA, Fuschsuber P, Thiel KS, et al: Flt3 ligand promotes the generation of a distinct CD34(+) human natural killer cell progenitor that responds to interleukin-15. *Blood* 92:3647, 1998.

217. Abboud SL: A bone marrow stromal cell line is a source and target for platelet-derived growth factor. *Blood* 81:2547, 1993.

218. Abboud SL, Pinzani M: Peptide growth factors stimulate macrophage colony-stimulating factor in murine stromal cells. *Blood* 78:103, 1991.

219. Yan XQ, Brady G, Iscove NN: Platelet-derived growth factor (PDGF) activates primitive hematopoietic precursors (pre-CFCmulti) by upregulating IL-1 in PDGF receptor-expressing macrophages. *J Immunol* 150:2440, 1993.

220. Lerat H, Lissitzky JC, Singer JW, et al: Role of stromal cells and macrophages in fibronectin biosynthesis and matrix assembly in human long-term marrow cultures. *Blood* 82:1480, 1993.

221. Baldus SE, Wickenhauser C, Stefanovic A, et al: Enrichment of human bone marrow mononuclear phagocytes and characterization of macrophage subpopulations by immunoenzymatic double staining. *Histochem J* 30:285, 1998.

222. Wijffels JF, de Rover Z, Kraal G, Beelen RH: Macrophage phenotype regulation by colony-stimulating factors at bone marrow level. *J Leukoc Biol* 53:249, 1993.

223. Shima M, Teitelbaum SL, Holers VM, et al: Macrophage-colony-stimulating factor regulates expression of the integrins alpha 4 beta 1 and alpha 5 beta 1 by murine marrow macrophages. *Proc Natl Acad Sci USA* 92:5179, 1995.

224. Dannaeus K, Johannisson A, Nilsson K, Jonsson JI: Flt3 ligand induces the outgrowth of Mac-1+ B22+ mouse bone marrow progenitor cells restricted to macrophage differentiation that coexpress early B cell-associated genes. *Exp Hematol* 27:1646, 1999.

225. Munday J, Floyd H, Criker PR: Sialic acid binding receptors (siglecs) expressed by macrophages. *J Leukoc Biol* 66:705, 1999.

226. Sadahira Y, Mori M: Role of the macrophage in erythropoiesis. *Pathol Int* 49:841, 1999.

227. Klein G: The extracellular matrix of the hematopoietic microenvironment. *Experimentia* 51:914, 1995.

228. Singer JW, Keating A, Wright TN: The human haemopoietic microenvironment, in *Recent Advances in Haematology,* edited by AV Hoffbrand, pp 1-24. Churchill Livingstone, London, 1985.

229. Bentley SA, Tralka TS: Fibronectin-mediated attachment of hematopoietic cells to stromal elements in continuous bone marrow culture. *Exp Hematol* 11:129, 1983.

230. Postlethwaite A, Kang AH: Fibroblasts and matrix proteins, in *Inflammation Basic Principles and Clinical Correlates,* 3rd ed, edited by JI Gallin, R Snyderman, pp 227-263. Lippincott Williams and Wilkins, Philadelphia, 1999.

231. Campbell AD, Long MW, Wicha MS: Haemonectin: a bone marrow adhesion protein specific for cells of granulocytic lineage. *Nature* 329:445, 1987.

232. Lawler J: The structural and functional properties of thrombospondin. *Blood* 67: 1197, 1986.

233. Simmons PJ, Levesque JP, Zannettino AC: Adhesion molecules in haemopoiesis. *Baillieres Clin Haematol* 10:485, 1997.

234. Verfaille CM: Adhesion receptors as regulators of the hematopoietic process. *Blood* 92:2609, 1998.

235. Broxmeyer HE, Kim CH: Regulation of hematopoiesis in a sea of chemokine family members with a plethora of redundant activities. *Exp Hematol* 27:1113, 1999.

236. Gordon MY: Extracellular matrix- and membrane-bound cytokines, in *Colony-Stimulating Factors: Molecular and Cellular Biology,* edited by JM Garland, PJ Quesenberry, DJ Hilton, pp 133-144. Marcel Dekker, New York, 1997.

237. Long MW: Hematopoietic microenvironments, in *Colony-Stimulating Factors: Molecular and Cellular Biology,* edited by JM Garland, PJ Quesenberry, DJ Hilton, pp 117-132. Marcel Dekker, New York, 1997.

238. Oritani K, Kanakura Y, Aoyama K, et al: Matrix glycoprotein SC1/ECM2 augments B lymphopoiesis. *Blood* 90:3404, 1997.

239. Koller MR, Oxender M, Jensen TC, et al: Direct contact between CD34+ lin- cells and stroma induces a soluble activity that specifically increases primitive hematopoietic cell production. *Exp Hematol* 27:734, 1999.

240. Varnum-Finney B, Purton LE, Yu M, et al: The Notch ligand, Jagged-1, influences the development of primitive hematopoietic precursor cells. *Blood* 91:4084, 1998.

241. Hoogewerf AJ, Kuschert GS, Proudfoot AE, et al: Glycosaminoglycans mediate cell surface oligomerization of chemokines. *Biochemistry* 36:13570, 1997.

242. Luster AD, Greenberg SM, Leder P: The IP-10 chemokine binds to a specific cell surface heparan sulfate site shared with platelet factor 4 and inhibits endothelial cell proliferation. *J Exp Med* 182: 219, 1995.

243. Tanaka T, Adams DH, Hubscher S, et al: T-cell adhesion induced by proteoglycan immobilized cytokine MIP-1β. *Nature* 361:78, 1993.

244. Chakravarty L, Rogers L, Quach T, et al: Lysine 58 and histidine 66 at the C-terminal alpha-helix of monocyte chemoattractant protein-1 are essential for glycosaminoglycan binding. *J Biol Chem* 273:29641, 1998.

245. Spillman D, Witt D, Lindahl U: Defining the interleukin-8-binding domain of heparan sulfate. *J Biol Chem* 273:15487, 1998.

246. Koopman W, Ediriwickrema C, Krangel MS: Structure and function of the glycosaminoglycan binding site of chemokine macrophage-inflammatory protein-1 beta. *J Immunol* 163:2120, 1999.

247. Amara A, Lorthioir O, Valenzuela A, et al: Stromal cell derived factor-1 alpha associates with heparan sulfates through the first beta-strand of the chemokine. *J Cell Biol Chem* 274:23916, 1999.

248. Wolff EA, Greenfield B, Taub DD, et al: Generation of artificial proteoglycans containing glycosaminoglycan-modified CD44. Demonstration of the interaction between rantes and chondroitin sulfate. *J Biol Chem* 274:2518, 1999.

249. Lipscombe RJ, Nakhoul AM, Sanderson CJ, Coombe DR: Interleukin-5 binds to heparin/heparan sulfate. A model for an interaction with extracellular matrix. *J Leukoc Biol* 63:342, 1998.

250. Borghesi LA, Yamashita Y, Kincade PW: Heparan sulfate proteoglycans mediate interleukin-7-dependent B lymphopoiesis. *Blood* 93:140, 1999.

251. Lyon M, Deakin JA, Nakamura T, Gallagher JT: Interaction of hepatocyte growth factor with heparan sulfate. Elucidation of major heparan sulfate structural determinants. *J Biol Chem* 269:11216, 1994.

252. Kiefer MC, Stephans JC, Crawford K, et al: Ligand-affinity cloning

and structure of a cell surface heparan sulfate proteoglycan that binds basic fibroblast growth factor. *Proc Natl Acad Sci USA* 87:6985, 1990.

253. Robledo MM, Ursa MA, Sanchez-Madrid F, Teixido J: Associations between TGF-beta1 receptors in human bone marrow stromal cells. *Br J Haematol* 102:804, 1998.

254. Kapur R, Cooper R, Xiao X, et al: The presence of novel amino acids in the cytoplasmic domain of stem cell factor results in hematopoietic defects in the *Steel*[17H] mice. *Blood* 94:1915, 1999

255. Gay RE, Prince CW, Zuckerman KS, Gay S: The collagenous hemopoietic microenvironment, in *Handbook of the Hemopoietic Microenvironment,* edited by M Tavassoli, pp 369–398. Humana Press, Clifton, NJ, 1989.

256. Anklesaria P, Greenberger JS, Fitzgerald TJ, et al: Hemonectin mediates adhesion of engrafted murine progenitors to a clonal bone marrow stromal cell line from *Sl/Sl*[d] mice. *Blood* 77:1691, 1991.

257. De Wynter E, Allen T, Coutinho L, et al: Localization of granulocytic macrophage colony-stimulating factor in human long-term bone marrow cultures. Biological and immunocytochemical characterization. *J Cell Sci* 106:761, 1993.

258. Deschaseaux ML, Herve P, Charbord P: The detection of colony-stimulating factors and steel factor in adherent layers of human long-term marrow cultures using reverse-transcriptase polymerase chain reaction. *Leukemia* 8:513, 1994.

259. Liu J, de Wynter E, Testa NG, et al: Immunoelectron microscopic localization of growth factors and other markers of human long-term bone marrow cultures. *Chin Med Sci J* 11:129, 1996.

260. Waegell WO, Higley HR, Kincade PW, Dasch JR: Growth acceleration and stem cell expansion in Dexter-type cultures by neutralization of TGF-beta. *Exp Hematol* 22:1051, 1994.

261. Wight TN, Kinsella MG, Keating A, Singer JW: Proteoglycans in human long-term bone marrow cultures: Biochemical and ultrastructural analyses. *Blood* 67:1333, 1986.

262. Allen TD, Dexter TM, Simmons PJ: Marrow biology and stem cells, in *Colony Stimulating Factors, Molecular and Cellular Biology*, edited by TM Dexter, JM Garland, NG Testa, Immunology Series, vol 49, pp 1–38. Marcel Dekker, New York, 1990.

263. Yurchenco PD, Schittny JC: Molecular architecture of basement membranes. *FASEB J* 4:1577, 1990.

264. Keating A, Gordon MY: Hierarchical organization of hematopoietic microenvironments: role of proteoglycans. *Leukemia* 2:766, 1988.

265. Gordon MY, Riley GP, Clarke D: Heparan sulfate is necessary for adhesive interactions between human early hemopoietic progenitor cells and the extracellular matrix of the marrow microenvironment. *Leukemia* 2:804, 1988.

266. Uhlman DL, Luikart SD: The role of proteoglycans in the adhesion and differentiation of hematopoietic cells, in *The Hematopoietic Microenvironment,* edited by MW Long, MS Wicha, pp 232–245. Johns Hopkins University Press, Baltimore and London, 1993.

267. Bruno E, Luikart SD, Long MW, Hoffman R: Marrow-derived heparan sulfate proteoglycan mediates the adhesion of hematopoietic progenitor cells to cytokines. *Exp Hematol* 23:1212, 1995.

268. Minguell JJ, Hardy C, Tavassoli M: Membrane-associated chondroitin sulfate proteoglycan and fibronectin mediate the binding of hemopoietic progenitor cells to stromal cells. *Exp Cell Res* 201:200, 1992.

269. Han ZC, Bellucci S, Shen ZX, et al: Glycosaminoglycans enhance megakaryopoiesis by modifying the activities of hematopoietic growth regulators. *J Cell Physiol* 168:97, 1996.

270. Gordon MY, Lewis Jl, Marley SB, et al: Stromal cells negatively regulate primitive haematopoietic progenitor cell activation via a phosphatidyl-inositol-anchored cell adhesion/signalling mechanism. *Br J Haematol* 96:647, 1997.

271. Gupta P, Oegema TR Jr, Brazil JJ, et al: Structurally specific heparan sulfates support primitive human hematopoiesis by formation of a multi-molecular stem cell niche. *Blood* 92:4641, 1998.

272. De Prato, Valentini P, Testi R , et al: Differential activity of glycosaminoglycans on colony-forming cells from cord blood. Preliminary results. *Leuk Res* 23:1015, 1999.

273. Lewinsohn DM, Nagler A, Ginzton N, et al: Hematopoietic progenitor cell expression of the H-CAM (CD44) homing-associated adhesion molecule. *Blood* 75:589, 1990.

274. Jalkanen S, Jalkanen M: Lymphocyte CD44 binds the COOH-terminal heparin-binding domain of fibronectin. *J Cell Biol* 116:817, 1992.

275. Miyake K, Medina KL, Mayashi S-I, et al: Monoclonal antibodies to Pgp-1/CD44 block lympho-hemopoiesis in long-term bone marrow cultures. *J Exp Med* 171:477, 1990.

276. Legras S, Levesque JP, Charrad R, et al: CD44-mediated adhesiveness of human hematopoietic progenitors to hyaluronan is modulated by cytokines. *Blood* 89:1905, 1997.

277. Rachmilewitz J, Tykocinski ML: Differential effects of chondroitin sulfates A and B on monocyte and B cell activation: evidence for B-cell activation via a CD44-dependent pathway. *Blood* 92:223, 1998.

278. Khaldoyanidi S, Moll J, Karakhanova S, et al: Hyaluronate-enhanced hematopoiesis: two different receptors trigger the release of interleukin-1β and interleukin-6 from bone marrow macrophages. *Blood* 94:940, 1999.

279. Weimar IS, Miranda N, Muller EJ, et al: Hepatocyte growth factor/scatter factor (HGF/SF) is produced by bone marrow stromal cells and promotes proliferation, adhesion and survival of human hematopoietic progenitor cells (CD34+). *Exp Hematol* 26:885, 1998.

280. Pivak-Kroizman T, Lemmon MA, Dikic I, et al: Heparin-induced oligomerization of FGF molecules is responsible for FGF receptor dimerization, activation, and cell proliferation. *Cell* 79:1015, 1994.

281. Ratajczak MZ, Ratajczak J, Slorska M, et al: Effect of basic (FGF-2) and acidic (FGF-1) fibroblast growth factors on early haematopoietic cell development. *Br J Haematol* 93:772, 1996.

282. Sternberg D, Peled A, Shezen E, et al: Control of stroma-dependent hematopoiesis by basic fibroblast growth factor: stromal phenotypic plasticity and modified myelopoietic functions. *Cytokines Mol Ther* 2:29, 1996.

283. Schofield KP, Gallagher JT, David G: Expression of proteoglycan core proteins in human bone marrow stroma. *Biochem J* 343:663, 1999.

284. Klein G, Conzelmann S, Beck S, et al: Perlecan in human bone marrow: a growth-factor-presenting, but anti-adhesive, extracellular matrix component for hematopoietic cells. *Matrix Biol* 14:457, 1995.

285. Drzeniek Z, Stoocker G, Siebertz B, et al: Heparan sulfate proteoglycan expression is induced during early erythroid differentiation of multipotential hematopoietic stem cells. *Blood* 93:2884, 1999.

286. Siebertz B, Stocker G, Drzeniek Z, et al: Expression of glypican-4 in haematopoietic-progenitor and bone-marrow-stromal cells. *Biochem J* 344:937, 1999.

287. Sneed TB, Stanley DJ, Young LA, Sanderson RD: Interleukin-6 regulates expression of the syndecan-1 proteoglycan on B lymphoid cells. *Cell Immunol* 153:456, 1994.

288. Oritani K, Kincade PW: Identification of stromal cell products that interact with pre-B cells. *J Cell Biol* 134:771, 1996.

289. Yamashita Y, Oritani K, Miyoshi EK, et al: Syndecan-4 is expressed by B lineage lymphocytes and can transmit a signal for formation of dendritic processes. *J Immunol* 162:5940, 1999.

290. Longley RL, Woods A, Fleetwood A, et al: Control of morphology, cytoskeleton and migration by syndecan-4. *J Cell Sci* 112:3421, 1999.

291. Zukerman KS, Wicha MS: Extracellular matrix production by the adherent cells of long-term murine bone marrow cultures. *Blood* 61:540, 1983.

292. Sorrel JM: Ultrastructural localization of fibronectin in bone marrow of the embryonic chick and its relationship to granulopoiesis. *Cell Tissue Res* 252:565, 1988.

293. Tsai S, Patel V, Beaumont E, et al: Differential binding of erythroid and myeloid progenitors to fibroblasts and fibronectin. *Blood* 69:1587, 1987.

294. Vuillet-Gaugler MH, Breton-Gorius J, Vainchenker W, et al: Loss of attachment to fibronectin with terminal human erythroid differentiation. *Blood* 75:865, 1990.

295. Rosemblatt M, Vuillet-Gaugler MH, Leroy C, Coulombel L: Coexpression of two fibronectin receptors, VLA-4 and VLA-5, by immature human erythroblastic precursor cells. *J Clin Invest* 87:6, 1991.

296. Liesveld JL, Winslow J, Kempski MC, et al: Adhesive interactions of normal and leukemic human CD34+ myeloid progenitors: Role of marrow stroma, fibroblasts and cytomatrix components. *Exp Hematol* 19:63, 1991.

297. Kerst JM, Sanders JB, Slaper Cortenbach IC, et al: Alpha 4 beta 1 and alpha 5 beta 1 are differentially expressed during myelopoiesis and mediate the adherence of human CD34+ cells to fibronectin in an activation-dependent way. *Blood* 81:344, 1993.

298. Ryan DH, Nuccie BL, Abboud CN, Winslow JM: Vascular cell adhesion molecule-1 and the integrin VLA-4 mediate adhesion of human B cell

precursors to cultured bone marrow adherent cells. *J Clin Invest* 88:995, 1991.

299. Hynes RO: Integrins: versatility, modulation, and signaling in cell adhesion. *Cell* 69:11, 1992.

300. Williams DA, Rios M, Stephens C, Patel VP: Fibronectin and VLA-4 in haematopoietic stem cell-microenvironment interactions. *Nature* 352:438, 1991.

301. Schofield KP, Humphries MJ: Identification of fibronectin IIICS variants in human bone marrow stroma. *Blood* 93:410, 1999.

302. Verfaillie CM, Benis A, Iida J, et al: Adhesion of committed human hematopoietic progenitors to synthetic peptides from the C-terminal heparin-binding domain of fibronectin: cooperation between the integrin alpha 4 beta 1 and the CD44 adhesion receptor. *Blood* 84:1802, 1994.

303. Hassan HT, Sadovinkova E Yu, Drize NJ, et al: Fibronectin increases both non-adherent cells and CFU-GM while collagen increases adherent cells in human normal long-term bone marrow cultures. *Haematologica (Budapest)* 28:77, 1997.

304. Yokota T, Oritani K, Mitsui H, et al: Growth-supporting activities of fibronectin on hematopoietic stem/progenitor cells in vitro and in vivo: structural requirements for fibronectin activities of CS1 and cell-binding domains. *Blood* 91:3263, 1998.

305. Hurley RW, McCarthy JB, Verfaillie CM: Direct adhesion to bone marrow stroma via fibronectin receptors inhibits hematopoietic progenitor proliferation. *J Clin Invest* 96:511, 1995.

306. Goltry KL, Patel VP: Specific domains of fibronectin mediate adhesion and migration of early murine erythroid progenitors. *Blood* 90:138, 1997.

307. Van der Loo JC, Xiao X, McMillin D, et al: VLA-5 is expressed by mouse and human long-term repopulating hematopoietic cells and mediates adhesion to extracellular matrix protein fibronectin. *J Clin Invest* 102:1051, 1998.

308. Robledo MM, Sanz-Rodrigues F, Hidalgo A, Teixido J: Differential use of very late antigen-4 and -5 integrins by hematopoietic precursors and myeloma cells to adhere to transforming growth factor-beta-1-treated bone marrow stroma. *J Biol Chem* 273:12056, 1998.

309. Schofield KP, Rushton G, Humphries MJ, et al: Influence of interleukin-3 and other growth factors on alpha$_4$beta$_1$ integrin-mediated adhesion and migration of human hematopoietic progenitor cells. *Blood* 90:1858, 1997.

310. Levesque JP, Haylock DN, Simmons PJ: Cytokine regulation of proliferation and cell adhesion are correlated events in human CD34+ hemopoietic progenitors. *Blood* 88:1168, 1996.

311. Cui L, Ramsfjell V, Borge OJ, et al: Thrombopoietin promotes adhesion of primitive human hemopoietic cells to fibronectin and vascular cell adhesion molecule-1: role of activation of very late antigen (VLA)-4 and VLA-5. *J Immunol* 159:1961, 1997.

312. Schofield KP, Humphries MJ, de Wynter E, et al: The effect of $\alpha 4\beta 1$-integrin binding sequences of fibronectin on growth of cells from human hematopoietic progenitors. *Blood* 91:3230, 1998.

313. Staquet MJ, Jacquet C, Dezutter-Dambuyant C, Schmitt D: Fibronectin upregulates in vitro generation of dendritic Langerhans cells from human cord blood CD34+ progenitors. *J Invest Dermatol* 109:738, 1997.

314. Berthier R, Jacquier-Sarlin M, Schweitzer A, et al: Adhesion of mature polypoid megakaryocytes to fibronectin is mediated by beta 1 integrins and leads to cell damage. *Exp Cell Res* 242:315, 1998.

315. Schick PK, Wojenski CM, He X, et al: Integrins involved in the adhesion of megakaryocytes to fibronectin and fibrinogen. *Blood* 92:2650, 1998.

316. Krugger-Krasagakes S, Grutzkau A, Krasagakis K, et al: Adhesion of human mast cells to extracellular matrix provides a co-stimulatory signal for cytokine production. *Immunology* 98:253,1999.

317. Lloyd AR, Oppenheim JJ, Kelvin DJ, Taub DD: Chemokines regulate T cell adherence to recombinant adhesion molecules and extracellular matrix proteins. *J Immunol* 156:932, 1996.

318. Higashimoto I, Chihara J, Kawabata M, et al: Adhesion to fibronectin regulates expression of intercellular adhesion molecule-1 on eosinophilic cells. *Int Arch Allergy Immunol* 120(suppl 1):34, 1999.

319. Xu X, Hakansson L: Simultaneous analysis of eosinophil and neutrophil adhesion to plasma and tissue fibronectin, fibrinogen, and albumin. *J Immunol Methods* 226:93, 1999.

320. Xie B, Laouar A, Huberman E: Fibronectin-mediated cell adhesion is required for induction of 92-kDa type IV collagenase/gelatinase (MMP-9) gene expression during macrophage differentiation. The signaling role of protein kinase C-beta. *J Biol Chem* 273:11576, 1998.

321. Kremlev SG, Chapoval AI, Evans R: Cytokine release by macrophages after interacting with CSF-1 and extracellular matrix proteins: characteristics of a mouse model of inflammatory responses in vitro. *Cell Immunol* 185:59, 1998.

322. Yonezawa I, Kato K, Yagita H, et al: VLA-5-mediated interactions with fibronectin induces cytokine production by human chondrocytes. *Biochem Biophys Res Commun* 219:261, 1996.

323. Rich IN, Brackmann I, Worthington-White D, Dewey MJ: Activation of sodium/hydrogen exchanger via the fibronectin-integrin pathway results in hematopoietic stimulation. *J Cell Physiol* 177:109, 1998.

324. Klein G, Beck S, Muller CA: Tenascin is a cytoadhesive extracellular matrix component of the human hematopoietic microenvironment. *J Cell Biol* 123:1027, 1993.

325. Chiquet-Ehrismann R, Matsuoka Y, Hofer U, et al: Tenascin variants: differential binding to fibronectin and distinct distribution in cell cultures and tissues. *Cell Regul* 2:927, 1991.

326. Sakai T, Ohta M, Kawakatsu H, et al: Tenascin-C induction in Whitlock-Witte culture: a relevant role of the thiol moiety in lymphoid-lineage differentiation. *Exp Cell Res* 217:395, 1995.

327. Ekblom M, Fassler R, Tomasini-Johansson B, et al: Downregulation of tenascin expression by glucocorticoids in bone marrow stromal cells and in fibroblasts. *J Cell Biol* 123:1037, 1993.

328. Seiffert M, Beck SC, Schermutzki F, et al: Mitogenic and adhesive effects of tenascin-C on human hematopoietic cells are mediated by various functional domains. *Matrix Biol* 17:47, 1998.

329. Ohta M, Sakai T, Saga Y, et al: Suppression of hematopoietic activity in tenascin-C-deficient mice. *Blood* 91:4074, 1998.

330. Mackie EJ, Tucker RP: The tenascin-C knockout revisited. *J Cell Sci* 112:3847, 1999.

331. Bentley SA: Collagen synthesis by bone marrow stromal cells: a quantitative study. *Br J Haematol* 50:491, 1982.

332. Mori M, Sadahira Y, Kawasaki S, et al: Formation of capillary networks from bone marrow cultured in collagen gel. *Cell Struct Funct* 14:393, 1989.

333. Zukerman KS, Rhodes RK, Goodrum DD, et al: Inhibition of collagen deposition in the extracellular matrix prevents the establishment of a stroma supportive of hematopoiesis in long-term murine bone marrow cultures. *J Clin Invest* 75:970, 1985.

334. Zukerman KS, Prince CW, Gay S: The hemopoietic extracellular matrix, in *Handbook of the Hemopoietic Microenvironment,* edited by M Tavassoli, pp 399–432. Humana Press, Clifton, NJ, 1989.

335. Koenigsmann M, Griffin JD, DiCarlo J, Cannistra SA: Myeloid and erythroid progenitor cells from normal bone marrow adhere to collagen type I. *Blood* 79:657, 1992.

336. Waterhouse EJ, Quesenberry PJ, Balian G: Collagen synthesis by murine bone marrow cell culture. *J Cell Physiol* 127:397, 1987.

337. Charbord P, Tamayo E, Saeland S, et al: Granulocyte-macrophage colony-stimulating factor (GM-CSF) in human long-term bone marrow cultures: Endogenous production in the adherent layer and effect on exogenous GM-CSF on granulomonopoiesis. *Blood* 78:1230, 1991.

338. Chichester CO, Fernández M, Minguel JJ: Extracellular matrix gene expression by human bone marrow stroma and by marrow fibroblasts. *Cell Adhesion Commun* 1:93, 1993.

339. Klein G, Muller CA, Tillet E, et al: Collagen type VI in the human bone marrow microenvironment: a strong cytoadhesive component. *Blood* 86:1740, 1995.

340. Klein G, Kibler C, Schermutzki F, et al: Cell binding properties of collagen type XIV for human hematopoietic cells. *Matrix Biol* 16:307, 1998.

341. Briddon SJ, Melford SK, Turner M, et al: Collagen mediates changes in intracellular calcium in primary mouse megakaryocytes through syk-dependent and -independent pathways. *Blood* 93: 3847, 1999.

342. Nilsson SK, Debatis ME, Dooner MS, et al: Imunofluorescence characterization of key extracellular matrix proteins in murine bone marrow in situ. *J Histochem Cytochem* 46:371, 1998.

343. Kleinman HK, Weeks BS: Laminin: structure, function and receptors. *Curr Opin Cell Biol* 1:964, 1989.

344. Senior RM, Gresham HD, Griffin GL, et al: Entactin stimulates neutrophil adhesion and chemotaxis through interactions between its Arg-Gly-Asp (RGD) domain and the leukocyte response integrin. *J Clin Invest* 90:2251, 1992.

345. Bryant G, Rao CN, Brentani M, et al: A role for the laminin receptor in leukocyte chemotaxis. *J Leukocyte Biol* 41:220, 1987.

346. Lundgren-Akerlund E, Olofsson AM, Berger E, Arfors KE: CD11b/CD18-dependent polymorphonuclear leucocyte interaction with matrix proteins in adhesion and migration. *Scand J Immunol* 37:569, 1993.

347. Liesveld JL, Ryan DH, Kempski MC, et al: Quantitation of the binding of human CD34 positive myeloid progenitors to marrow stroma fibroblasts, and components of the extracellular matrix, in *Hematopoiesis*, edited by SC Clark, DW Golde, *UCLA Symposia on Molecular and Cellular Biology New Series*, pp 157–169. Wiley-Liss, New York, 1990.

348. Tobias JW, Bern MM, Netland PA, Zetter BR: Monocyte adhesion to subendothelial components. *Blood* 69:1265, 1987.

349. Bohnsack JF, Akiyama SK, Damsky CH, et al: Human neutrophil adherence to laminin in vitro: evidence for a distinct neutrophil integrin receptor for laminin. *J Exp Med* 171:1221, 1990.

350. Bohnsack JF: CD11/CD18-independent neutrophil adherence to laminin is mediated by the integrin VLA-6. *Blood* 79:1545, 1992.

351. Thompson HL, Matsushima K: Human polymorphonuclear leucocytes stimulated by tumour necrosis factor-alpha show increased adherence to extracellular matrix proteins which is mediated via the CD11b/18 complex. *Clin Exp Immunol* 90:280, 1992.

352. Fehlner-Gardiner C, Uniyal S, von Ballestrem C, et al: Integrin VLA-6 (alpha 6 beta 1) mediates adhesion of mouse bone marrow-derived mast cells to laminin. *Allergy* 51:650, 1996.

353. El-Nemer W, Gane P, Colin Y, et al: The Lutheran blood group glycoproteins, the erythroid receptors for laminin, are adhesion molecules. *J Biol Chem* 273:16686, 1998.

354. Monturi N, Selleri C, Risitano AM, et al: Expression of the 67-kDa laminin receptor in acute myeloid leukemia cells mediates adhesion to laminin and is frequently associated with monocytic differentiation. *Clin Cancer Res* 5:1465, 1999.

355. Gu Y, Sorokin L, Durbeej M, et al: Characterization of bone marrow laminins and identification of α5-containing laminins as adhesive proteins for multipotent hematopoietic FDCP-mix cells. *Blood* 93:2533, 1999.

356. Vogel W, Kanz L, Brugger W, et al: Expression of laminin β2 chain in normal human bone marrow. *Blood* 94:1143, 1999.

357. Ohki K, Kohashi O: Laminin promotes proliferation of bone marrow-derived macrophages and macrophage cell lines. *Cell Struct Funct* 19:63, 1994.

358. Peters C, OShea KS, Campbell AD, et al: Fetal expression of hemonectin: An extracellular matrix hematopoietic cytoadhesion molecule. *Blood* 75:357, 1990.

359. White H, Totty N, Panayotou G: Haemonectin, a granulocytic-cell-binding protein, is related to the plasma glycoprotein fetuin. *Eur J Biochem* 213:523, 1993.

360. Sullenbarger BA, Petitt MS, Chong P, et al: Murine granulocytic cell adhesion to bone marrow hemonectin is mediated by mannose and galactose. *Blood* 86:135, 1995.

361. Long MW, Dixit VM: Thrombospondin functions as a cytoadhesion molecule for human hematopoietic progenitor cells. *Blood* 75:2311, 1990.

362. Stomski FC, Gani JS, Bates RC, Burns GF: Adhesion to thrombospondin by human embryonic fibroblasts is mediated by multiple receptors and includes a role for glycoprotein 88 (CD36). *Exp Cell Res* 198:85, 1992.

363. Li WX, Howard RJ, Leung LL: Identification of SVTCG in thrombospondin as the conformation-dependent, high affinity binding site for its receptor, CD36. *J Biol Chem* 268:16179, 1993.

364. Suchard SJ, Burton MJ, Dixit VM, Boxer LA: Human neutrophil adherence to thrombospondin occurs through a CD11/CD18-independent mechanism. *J Immunol* 146:3945, 1991.

365. Calvo D, Vega MA: Identification, primary structure, and distribution of CLA-1, a novel member of the CD36/LIMPII gene family. *J Biol Chem* 268:18929, 1993.

366. Vischer P, Feitsma K, Schon P, Volker W: Perlecan is responsible for thrombospondin 1 binding on the surface of cultured porcine endothelial cells. *Eur J Cell Biol* 73:332, 1997.

367. Nakahata T, Okumura N: Cell surface antigen expression in human erythroid progenitors: erythroid and megakaryocytic markers. *Leuk Lymphoma* 13:401, 1994.

368. Chen YZ, Incardona F, Legrand C, et al: Thrombospondin, a negative modulator of megakaryopoiesis. *J Lab Clin Med* 129:231, 1997.

369. Dallalio G, van Laer A, Means RT: Effects of thrombospondin and CD36 on erythroid colony formation in vitro. *Blood* 94(suppl 1, part 2):163b, 1999.

370. Pierson BA, Gupta K, Hu WS, Miller JS: Human natural killer cell expansion is regulated by thrombospondin-mediated activation of transforming growth factor-beta 1 and independent accessory cell-derived contact and soluble factors. *Blood* 87:180, 1996.

371. Crawford SE, Stellmach V, Murphy-Ullrich JE, et al: Thrombospondin-1 is a major activator of TGF-beta 1 in vivo. *Cell* 93:1159, 1998.

372. Touhami M, Fauvel-Lafeve F, Da Silva N, et al: Induction of thrombospondin-1 by all-*trans* retinoic acid modulates growth and differentiation of HL-60 myeloid leukemia cells. *Leukemia* 11:2137, 1997.

373. Taraboletti G, Belotti D, Borsotti P, et al: The 140-kilodalton antiangiogenic fragment of thrombospondin-1 binds to basic fibroblast growth factor. *Cell Growth Differ* 8:471, 1997.

374. Loganadane LD, Berge N, Legrand C, Fauvel-Lafeve F: Endothelial cell proliferation regulated by cytokines modulates thrombospondin-1 secretion into the subendothelium. *Cytokine* 9:740, 1997.

375. Qian X, Wang TN, Rothman VL, et al: Thrombospondin-1 modulates angiogenesis in vitro by up-regulation of matrix metalloproteinase-9 in endothelial cells. *Exp Cell Res* 235:403, 1997.

376. Mansfield PJ, Suchard SJ: Thrombospondin promotes both chemotaxis and haptotaxis of human peripheral blood monocytes. *J Immunol* 153:4219, 1994.

377. Mansfield PJ, Suchard SJ: Thrombospondin promotes both chemotaxis and haptotaxis in neutrophil-like HL-60 cells. *J Immunol* 150:1959, 1993.

378. Horton MA: The alpha,beta$_3$ integrin "vitronectin receptor." *Int J Biochem Cell Biol* 29:721, 1997.

379. Molla A, Mossuz P, Berthier R: Extracellular matrix receptors and the differentiation of human megakaryocytes in vitro. *Leuk Lymphoma* 33:15, 1999.

380. Shimizu Y, Irani AM, Brown EJ, et al: Human mast cells derived from fetal liver cells cultured with stem cell factor express a functional CD51/CD61 (alpha,beta$_3$) integrin. *Blood* 86:930, 1995.

381. Hughes DE, Salter DM, Dedhar S, Simpson R: Integrin expression in human bone. *J Bone Miner Res* 8:527, 1993.

382. Mbalaviele G, Jaiswal N, Meng A, et al: Human mesenchymal stem cells promote human osteoclast differentiation from CD34+ bone marrow hematopoietic progenitors. *Endocrinology* 140:3736, 1999.

383. Boissy P, Machuca I, Pfaff M, et al: Aggregation of mononucleated precursors triggers cell surface expression of alpha,beta$_3$ integrin, essential to formation of osteoclast-like multinucleated cells. *J Cell Sci* 111:2563, 1998.

384. Murphy JF, Bordet JC, Wyler B, et al: The vitronectin receptor (alpha,beta$_3$) is implicated, in cooperation with P-selectin and platelet-activating factor, in the adhesion of monocytes to activated endothelial cells. *Biochem J* 304:537, 1994.

385. Weerasinghe D, McHugh KP, Ross FP, et al: A role for the alpha,beta$_3$ integrin in the transmigration of monocytes. *J Cell Biol* 142:595, 1998.

386. Rainger GE, Buckley CD, Simmons DL, Nash GB: Neutrophils sense flow-generated stress and direct their migration through alpha$_v$beta$_3$-integrin. *Am J Physiol* 276:H858, 1999.

387. Nath D, Slocombe PM, Stephens PE, et al: Interactions of metargidin (ADAM-15) with alpha,beta$_3$ and alpha$_5$beta$_1$ integrins on different haemopoietic cells. *J Cell Sci* 112:579, 1999.

388. Savill J, Hogg N, Ren Y, Haslett C: Thrombospondin cooperates with CD36 and the vitronectin receptor in macrophage recognition of neutrophils undergoing apoptosis. *J Clin Invest* 90:1513, 1992.

389. Fadok VA, Warner ML, Bratton DL, Henson PM: CD36 is required for phagocytosis of apoptotic cells by human macrophages that use either a phosphatidylserine receptor or the vitronectin receptor (alpha,beta$_3$). *J Immunol* 161:6250, 1998.

390. Rubartelli A, Poggi A, Zocchi MR: The selective engulfment of apoptotic bodies by dendritic cells is mediated by the alpha$_{(v)}$beta$_3$ integrin and requires intracellular calcium and extracellular calcium. *Eur J Immunol* 27:1893, 1997.

391. Leven RM, Tablin F: Extracellular matrix stimulation of guinea pig megakaryocyte proplatelet formation in vitro is mediated through the vitronectin receptor. *Exp Hematol* 20:1316, 1992.

392. Hunt P, Hokom MM, Hornkohl A, et al: The effect of platelet-derived

glycosaminoglycan serglycin on in vitro proplatelet-like process formation. *Exp Hematol* 21:1295, 1993.

393. Leven RM: Differential regulation of integrin-mediated proplatelet formation and megakaryocyte spreading. *J Cell Physiol* 163:597, 1995.

394. Rusnati M, Tanghetti E, Dell'Era P, et al: Alpha,beta₃ integrin mediates the cell-adhesive capacity and biological activity of basic fibroblast growth factor (FGF-2) in cultured endothelial cells. *Mol Cell Biol* 8:2449, 1997.

395. Ybarrondo B, O'Rouke AM, McCarthy JB, Mescher MF: Cytotoxic T-lymphocyte interaction with fibronectin and vitronectin: activated adhesion and cosignalling. *Immunology* 91:186, 1997.

396. Roberts K, Yokoyama WM, Kehn PJ, Shevach EM: The vitronectin receptor serves as an accessory molecule for the activation of a subset of gamma/delta T cells. *J Exp Med* 173:231, 1991.

397. Rabinowich H, Lin WC, Amoscato A, et al: Expression of vitronectin receptor on human NK cells and its role in protein phosphorylation, cytokine production, and cell proliferation. *J Immunol* 154:1124, 1995.

398. Hermann P, Armant M, Brown E, et al: The vitronectin receptor and its associated CD47 molecule mediates proinflammatory cytokine synthesis in human monocytes by interactions with soluble CD23. *J Cell Biol* 144:767, 1999.

399. Bessis M: L'ilot èrythroblastique, unitè fonctionelle de le moelle osseuse. *Rev Hematol* 13:8, 1958.

400. Lichtman MA, Waugh RE: Red cell egress from the marrow: Ultrastructural and biophysical aspects, in *Regulation of Erythropoiesis,* edited by ED Zanjani, M Tavassoli, J Ascencao, pp 15–35. PMA, Great Neck, NY, 1989.

401. Zuhrie SR, Wickramasinghe SN: Stromal cell-dependent terminal maturation of K562 erythroleukemia cells. *Leuk Res* 975, 1991.

402. Yu AW, Shao LE, Frigon NL Jr, Yu J: Detection of functional and dimeric activin A in human marrow microenvironment. Implications for the modulation of erythropoiesis. *Ann N Y Acad Sci* 718:285, 1994.

403. Mizugushi T, Kosaka M, Saito S: Activin A suppresses proliferation of interleukin-3-responsive granulocyte-macrophage colony-forming progenitors and stimulates proliferation and differentiation of interleukin-3-responsive erythroid burst-forming progenitors in peripheral blood. *Blood* 81:2891, 1993.

404. Huber TL, Zhou Y, Mead PE, Zon LI: Cooperative effects of growth factors involved in the induction of hematopoietic mesoderm. *Blood* 92:4128, 1998.

405. Koristschoner NP, Bartunek P, Knespel S, et al: The fibroblast growth factor receptor FGFR-4 acts as a ligand dependent modulator of erythroid cell proliferation. *Oncogene* 18:5904, 1999.

406. Iguchi T, Sogo S, Hisha H, et al: HGF activates signal transduction from EPO receptor on human cord blood CD34+/CD45+ cells. *Stem Cells* 17:82, 1999.

407. Lichtman MA, Chamberlain JK, Simon W, et al: Parasinusoidal location of megakaryocytes in marrow: a determinant of platelet release. *Am J Hematol* 4:303, 1978.

408. Thiele J, Galle R, Sander C, Fischer R: Interactions between megakaryocytes and sinus wall: an ultrastructural study of bone marrow tissue in primary (essential) thrombocythemia. *J Submicrosc Cytol Pathol* 23:595, 1991.

409. Avraham H, Cowley S, Chi SY, et al: Characterization of adhesive interactions between human endothelial cells and megakaryocytes. *J Clin Invest* 91:2378, 1993.

410. Riviere C, Subra F, Cohen-Solal K, et al: Phenotypic and functional evidence for the expression of CXCR4 receptor during megakaryopoiesis. *Blood* 93:1511, 1999.

411. Hamada T, Mohle R, Hesselgesser J, et al: Transendothelial migration of megakaryocytes in response to stromal cell-derived factor 1 (SDF-1) enhances platelet formation. *J Exp Med* 188:539, 1998.

412. Ito T, Ishida Y, Kashiwagi R, Kuriya S: Recombinant human c-Mpl ligand is not a direct stimulator of proplatelet formation in mature human megakaryocytes. *Br J Haematol* 94:387, 1996.

413. Bruno E, Briddell RA, Cooper RJ, Hoffman R: Effects of recombinant interleukin 11 on human megakaryocyte progenitor cells. *Exp Hematol* 19:378, 1991.

414. Gordon MS, Hoffman R: Growth factors affecting human thrombopoiesis: potential agents for the treatment of thrombocythemia. *Blood* 80:302, 1992.

415. Ishibashi T, Kimura H, Shikama Y, et al: Interleukin-6 is a potent thrombopoietic factor in vivo in mice. *Blood* 74:1241, 1989.

416. Metcalf D, Hilton D, Nicola NA: Leukemia inhibitory factor can potentiate murine megakaryocyte production in vitro. *Blood* 77:2150, 1991.

417. Kaushansky K: Thrombopoietin. *N Engl J Med* 339:746, 1998.

418. Lambertsen RH, Weiss L: A model of intramedullary hemopoietic microenvironments based on stereologic study of the distribution of endoclonal colonies. *Blood* 63:287, 1984.

419. Naito K, Tamahashi N, Chiba T, et al: The microvasculature of the human bone marrow correlated with the distribution of hematopoietic cells: a computer-assisted three-dimensional reconstruction study. *Tohoku J Exp Med* 166:439, 1992.

420. Blazsek I, Misset JL, Benavides M, et al: Hematon, a multicellular functional unit in normal human bone marrow: structural organization, hemopoietic activity, and its relationship to myelodysplasia and myeloid leukemias. *Exp Hematol* 18:259, 1990.

421. Wright EC, Pragnell IB: Stem cell proliferation inhibitors. *Baillieres Clin Hematol* 5:723, 1992.

422. Jacobsen SEW, Ruscetti FW, Dubois CM, Keller JR: Tumor necrosis factor α directly and indirectly regulates hematopoietic progenitor cell proliferation: role of colony-stimulating factor receptor modulation. *J Exp Med* 175:1759, 1992.

423. Rogers JA, Berman JW: A tumor necrosis factor-responsive long-term-culture-initiating cell is associated with the stromal layer of mouse long-term bone marrow cultures. *Proc Natl Acad Sci USA* 90:5777, 1993.

424. Knospe WH, Husseini SG, Zipori D, Fried W: Hematopoiesis on cellulose ester membranes: XIII. A combination of cloned stromal cells is needed to establish a hematopoietic microenvironment supportive of trilineal hematopoiesis. *Exp Hematol* 21:257, 1993.

425. Winerman JP, Nishikawa S, Muller-Sieburg CE: Maintenance of high levels of pluripotent hematopoietic stem cells in vitro: Effect of stromal cells and c-kit. *Blood* 81:365, 1993.

426. Bhatia M, Bonnet D, Wu D, et al: Bone morphogenetic proteins regulate the developmental program of human hematopoietic stem cells. *J Exp Med* 189:1139, 1999.

427. Simmons PJ, Zannettino A, Gronthos S, Leavesley D: Potential adhesion mechanisms for localization of haemopoietic progenitors to bone marrow stroma. *Leuk Lymphoma* 12:353, 1994.

428. Koller MR, Oxender M, Jensen TC, et al: Direct contact between CD34+ lin- cells and stroma induces a soluble activity that specifically increases primitive hematopoietic cell production. *Exp Hematol* 27:734, 1999.

429. Simmons PJ, Haylock DN, Levesque J-P: Influence of cytokines and adhesion molecules on hematopoietic stem cell development, in *Ex Vivo Cell Therapy,* edited by K Schindhelm, R Nordon, pp 51–83. Academic Press, San Diego, 1999.

430. Coulombel L, Auffray I, Gaugler MH, Rosemblatt M: Expression and function of integrins on hematopoietic progenitor cells. *Acta Haematol* 97:13, 1997.

431. Wang J, Springer TA: Structural specializations of immunoglobulin superfamily members for adhesion to integrins and viruses. *Immunol Rev* 163:197, 1998.

432. Kansas GS: Selectins and their ligands: current concepts and controversies. *Blood* 88:3259, 1996.

433. Robinson LA, Steeber DA, Tedder TA: The selectins in inflammation, in *Inflammation Basic Principles and Clinical Correlates,* 3rd ed, edited by JI Gallin, R Snyderman, pp 571–583. Lippincott Williams and Wilkins, Philadelphia, 1999.

434. Lasky LA: Sialomucin ligands for selectins: a new family of cell adhesion molecules. *Princess Takamatsu Symp* 24:81, 1994.

435. Butcher EC, Picker LJ: Lymphocyte homing and homeostasis *Science* 272:60, 1996.

436. Lesley J, Hyman R, Kincade PW: CD44 and its interaction with extracellular matrix. *Adv Immunol* 54:271, 1993.

437. Borland G, Ross JA, Guy K: Forms and functions of CD44. *Immunology* 93:139, 1998.

438. Deaglio S, Morra M, Mallone R, et al: Human CD38 (ADP-ribosyl cyclase) is a counter-receptor of CD31, an Ig superfamily member. *J Immunol* 160:395, 1998.

439. Hynes RO: Specificity of cell adhesion in development: the cadherin superfamily. *Curr Opin Genet Dev* 2:621, 1992.

440. Steinberg MS, McNutt PM: Cadherins and their connections: adhesion junctions have broader functions. *Curr Opin Cell Biol* 11:554, 1999.

441. Okuyama Y, Ishihara K, Kimura N, et al: Human BST-1 expressed on myeloid cells functions as a receptor molecule. *Biochem Biophys Res Commun* 228:838, 1996.

442. Liesveld JL, DiPersio JF, Abboud CN: Integrins and adhesive receptors in normal and leukemic CD34+ progenitor cells: potential regulatory checkpoints for cellular traffic. *Leuk Lymphoma* 14:19, 1994.

443. Kishimoto TK, Baldwin ET, Anderson DC: The role of β_2 integrins in inflammation, in *Inflammation Basic Principles and Clinical Correlates*, 3rd ed, edited by JI Gallin, R Snyderman, pp 537–569. Lippincott Williams and Wilkins, Philadelphia, 1999.

444. Ruoslahti E: Integrins. *J Clin Invest* 87:1, 1991.

445. Yanai N, Sekine C, Yagita H, Obinata M: Roles for integrin very late activation antigen-4 in stroma-dependent erythropoiesis. *Blood* 83:2844, 1994.

446. Hamamura K, Matsuda H, Takeuchi Y, et al: A critical role of VLA-4 in erythropoiesis in vivo. *Blood* 87:2513, 1996.

447. Furasawa T, Yanai N, Hara T, et al: Integrin-associated protein (IAP, also termed CD47) is involved in stroma-supported erythropoiesis. *J Biochem (Tokyo)* 123:101, 1998.

448. Iguchi A, Okuyama R, Koguma M, et al: Selective stimulation of granulopoiesis in vitro by established bone marrow stromal cells. *Cell Struct Funct* 22:357, 1997.

449. Dittel BN, McCarthy JB, Wayner EA, LeBien TW: Regulation of human B-cell precursor adhesion to bone marrow stromal cells by cytokines that exert opposing effects on the expression of vascular cell adhesion molecule-1 (VCAM-1). *Blood* 81:2272, 1993.

450. Ryan DH, Nuccie BL, Ritterman I, et al: Cytokine regulation of early human lymphopoiesis. *J Immunol* 152:5250, 1994.

451. Oostendorp RA, Dormer P: VLA-4-mediated interactions between normal human hematopoietic progenitors and stromal cells. *Leuk Lymphoma* 24:423, 1997.

452. Ryan DH, Nuccie BL, Ritterman I, et al: Expression of interleukin-7 receptor by lineage-negative human bone marrow progenitors with enhanced lymphoid proliferative potential and B-lineage differentiation capacity. *Blood* 89:929, 1997.

453. Dittel BN, LeBien TW: Reduced expression of vascular cell adhesion molecule-1 on bone marrow stromal cells isolated from marrow transplant recipients correlates with a reduced capacity to support human B lymphopoiesis in vitro. *Blood* 86:2833, 1995.

454. Novitzky N, Mohamed R: Alterations in both the hematopoietic microenvironment and the progenitor cell population follow the recovery from myeloablative therapy and bone marrow transplantation. *Exp Hematol* 23:1661, 1995.

455. Funk PE, Stephan RP, Witte PL: Vascular cell adhesion molecule 1-positive reticular cells express interleukin-7 and stem cell factor in the bone marrow. *Blood* 86:2661, 1995.

456. Funk PE, Kincade PW, Witte PL: Native associations of early hematopoietic stem cells and stromal cells isolated in bone marrow cell aggregates. *Blood* 83:361, 1994.

457. Galotto M, Berisso G, Delfino L, et al: Stromal damage as a consequence of high-dose chemo/radiotherapy in bone marrow transplant recipients. *Exp Hematol* 27:1460, 1999.

458. Dedhar S: Integrins and signal transduction. *Curr Opinion Hematol* 6:37, 1999.

459. Lowell CA, Berton G: Integrin signal transduction in myeloid leukocytes. *J Leukoc Biol* 65:313, 1999.

460. Aplin AE, Howe A, Alahari SK, Juliano RL: Signal transduction and signal modulation by cell adhesion receptors: the role of integrins, cadherins, immunoglobulin-cell adhesion molecules and selectins. *Pharmacol Rev* 50:197, 1998.

461. Jarvis LJ, Maguire JE, LeBien TW: Contact between human bone marrow stromal cells and B lymphocytes enhances very late antigen-4/vascular cell adhesion molecule-1-independent tyrosine phosphorylation of focal adhesion kinase, paxillin, and ERK-2 in stromal cells. *Blood* 90:1626, 1997.

462. Shibayama H, Anzai N, Braun SE, et al: H-Ras is involved in the inside-out signaling pathway of interleukin-3-induced integrin activation. *Blood* 93:1540, 1999.

463. Levesque J-P, Simmons PJ: Cytoskeleton and integrin-mediated adhesion signaling in human CD34+ hemopoietic progenitor cells. *Exp Hematol* 27:579, 1999.

464. Arai A, Nosaka Y, Kohsaka H, et al: CrkL activates integrin-mediated hematopoietic cell adhesion through the guanine nucleotide exchange factor C3G. *Blood* 93:3713, 1999.

465. Porter JC, Hogg N: Integrin cross talk: activation of lymphocyte function-associated antigen-1 on human T cells alters alpha$_4$beta$_1$- and alpha$_5$.beta$_1$-mediated function. *J Cell Biol* 138:1437, 1997.

466. Shibuya A, Campbell D, Hannum C, et al: DYNAM-1, a novel adhesion molecule involved involved in the cytolytic function of T lymphocytes. *Immunity* 4:573, 1996.

467. Shibuya K, Lanier LL, Phillips JH, et al: Physical and functional association of LFA-1 with DYNAM-1 adhesion molecule. *Immunity* 11:615, 1999.

468. Rodriguez-Fernandez JL, Gomez M, Luque A, et al: The interaction of activated integrin lymphocyte function-associated antigen 1 with ligand intercellular adhesion molecule 1 induces activation and redistribution of focal adhesion kinase and proline-rich tyrosine kinase 2 in T lymphocytes. *Mol Biol Cell* 10:1891, 1999.

469. Leavesley DI, Oliver JM, Swart BW, et al: Signals from platelet/endothelial cell adhesion molecule enhance the adhesive activity of the very late antigen-4 integrin of human CD34+ hematopoietic progenitor cells. *J Immunol* 153:4673, 1994.

470. Vestweber D, Blanks JE: Mechanisms that regulate the function of the selectins and their ligands. *Physiol Rev* 79:181, 1999.

471. Gotoh A, Ritchie A, Takahira H, Broxmeyer HE: Thrombopoietin and erythropoietin activate inside-out signaling of integrin and enhance adhesion to immobilized fibronectin in human growth-factor-dependent hematopoietic cells. *Ann Hematol* 75:207, 1997.

472. Liesveld JL, Winslow JM, Frediani KE, et al: Expression of integrins and examination of their adhesive function in normal and leukemic hematopoietic cells. *Blood* 81:112, 1993.

473. Ryan DH, Nuccie BL, Abboud CN: Inhibition of human bone marrow lymphoid progenitor colonies by antibodies to VLA integrins. *J Immunol* 149:3759, 1992.

474. Sugahara H, Kanakura Y, Furitsu T, et al: Induction of programmed cell death in human hematopoietic cell lines by fibronectin via its interaction with very late antigen 5. *J Exp Med* 179:1757, 1994.

475. Hurley RW, McCarthy JB, Wayner EA, Verfaillie CM: Monoclonal antibody crosslinking of the alpha 4 beta 1 integrin inhibits committed clonogenic hematopoietic progenitor proliferation. *Exp Hematol* 25:321, 1997.

476. Oostendorp RA, Spitzer E, Reisbach G, Dormer P: Antibodies to the beta 1-integrin chain, CD44, or ICAM-3 stimulate adhesion of blast colony-forming cells and may inhibit their growth. *Exp Hematol* 25:345, 1997.

477. Wang MW, Consoli U, Lane CM, et al: Rescue from apoptosis in early (CD34-selected) versus late (non-CD34-selected) human hematopoietic cells by very late antigen 4- and vascular cell adhesion molecule (VCAM) 1-dependent adhesion to bone marrow stromal cells. *Cell Growth Differ* 9:105, 1998.

478. Bhatia R, Munthe HA, Verfaillie CM: Role of abnormal integrin-cytoskeletal interactions in impaired $\beta 1$ integrin function in chronic myelogenous leukemia hematopoietic progenitors. *Exp Hematol* 27:1384, 1999.

479. Verfaillie CM, Hurley R, Zhao RC, et al: Pathophysiology of CML: do defects in integrin function contribute to the premature circulation and massive expansion of the BCR/ABL positive clone? *J Lab Clin Med* 129:584,1997.

480. Bahtia R, Munthe HA, Verfaillie CM: Tyrphostin AG957, a tyrosine kinase inhibitor with anti-BCR/ABL tyrosine kinase activity restores beta$_1$ integrin-mediated adhesion and inhibitory signaling in chronic myelogenous leukemia hematopoietic progenitors. *Leukemia* 12:1708,1998.

481. Bahtia R, Verfaillie CM: The effect of interferon-alpha on beta-1 integrin mediated adhesion and growth regulation in chronic myelogenous leukemia. *Leuk Lymphoma* 28:241, 1998.

482. Sun QH, Paddock C, Visentin GP, et al: Cell surface glycosaminoglycans do not serve as ligands for PECAM-1. PECAM-1 is not a heparin-binding protein. *J Biol Chem* 273:11483, 1998.

483. Muller WA, Randolph GJ: Migration of leukocytes across endothelium and beyond: molecules involved in the transmigration and fate of monocytes. *J Leukoc Biol* 66:698, 1999.

484. Chiba R, Nakagawa N, Kurasawa K, et al: Ligation of CD31 (PECAM-1) on endothelial cells increases adhesive function of $\alpha_v\beta_3$

integrin and enhances β_1 integrin-mediated adhesion of eosinophils to endothelial cells. *Blood* 94:1319, 1999.

485. Duncan GS, Andrew DP, Takimoto H, et al: Genetic evidence for functional redundancy of platelet/endothelial cell adhesion molecule-1 (PECAM-1): CD31-deficient mice reveal PECAM-1-dependent and PECAM-1-independent functions. *J Immunol* 162:3022, 1999.

486. Nakada MT, Amin K, Christofidou-Solomidou M, et al: Antibodies against the first Ig-like domain of human platelet endothelial cell adhesion molecule-1 (PECAM-1) that inhibit PECAM-1-dependent homophilic adhesion block in vivo neutrophil recruitment. *J Immunol* 164:452, 2000.

487. Arkin S, Naprstek B, Guarini L, et al: Expression of intercellular adhesion molecule-1 (CD54) on hematopoietic progenitors. *Blood* 77:948, 1991.

488. Gunji Y, Nakamura M, Hagiwara T, et al: Expression and function of adhesion molecules on human hematopoietic stem cells: CD34+ LFA-1(neg) cells are more primitive than CD34+ LFA-1+ cells. *Blood* 80:429, 1992.

489. Makgoba MW, Sanders ME, Ginther Luce GE, et al: ICAM-1, a ligand for LFA-1-dependent adhesion of B, T and myeloid cells. *Nature* 331:86, 1988.

490. Rao SG, Chitnis VS, Deora A, et al: An ICAM-1-like cell adhesion molecule is responsible for CD34-positive haemopoietic stem cells adhesion to bone-marrow stroma. *Cell Biol Int* 20:255, 1996.

491. Staunton DE, Dustin ML, Springer TA: Functional cloning of ICAM-2, a cell adhesion ligand for LFA-1 homologous to ICAM-1. *Nature* 339:61, 1989.

492. Fawcett J, Holness CLL, Needham LA, et al: Molecular cloning of ICAM-3, a third ligand for LFA-1, constitutively expressed on resting leukocytes. *Nature* 360:481, 1992.

493. Campanero MR, Sanchez-Mateos P, del Pozo MA, Sanchez-Madrid F: ICAM-3 regulates lymphocyte morphology and integrin-mediated T cell interactions with endothelial cell and extracellular matrix ligands. *J Cell Biol* 127:867, 1994.

494. Wang JH, Smolyar A, Tan K, et al: Structure of a heterophilic adhesion complex between the human CD2 and CD58 (LFA-3) counterreceptors. *Cell* 97:791, 1999.

495. Nielsen M, Gerwien J, Geisler C, et al: MHC class II ligation induces CD58 (LFA-3)-mediated adhesion in human T cells. *Exp Clin Immunogenet* 15:61, 1998.

496. LeGuiner S, Le Drean E, Labarriere N, et al: LFA-3 co-stimulates cytokine secretion by cytotoxic T lymphocytes by providing a TCR-independent activation signal. *Eur J Immunol* 28:1322, 1998.

497. Itzhaky D, Raz N, Hollander N: The glycosylphosphatidylinositol-anchored form and the transmembrane form of CD58 associate with protein kinases. *J Immunol* 60:4361, 1998.

498. Kirby AC, Cahen P, Porter SR, Olsen I: LFA-3 (CD58) mediates T-lymphocyte adhesion in chronic inflammatory infiltrates. *Scand J Immunol* 50:469, 1999.

499. DE Waele M, Renmans W, Jochmans K, et al: Different expression of adhesion molecules on CD34+ cells in AML and B lineage ALL and their normal bone marrow counterparts. *Eur J Haematol* 63:192, 1999.

500. McCarty JM, Yee EK, Deisher TA, et al: Interleukin-4 induces endothelial vascular cell adhesion molecule-1 (VCAM-1) by an NF-kappa b-independent mechanism. *FEBS Lett* 372:194, 1995.

501. Bochner BS, Klunk DA, Sterbinsky SA, et al: IL-13 selectively induces vascular cell adhesion molecule-1 expression in human endothelial cells. *J Immunol* 154:799, 1995.

502. Kinashi T, Springer TA: Regulation of cell-matrix adhesion by receptor tyrosine kinases. *Leuk Lymphoma* 18:203, 1995.

503. Lopez M, Aoubala M, Jordier F, et al: The human poliovirus receptor related 2 protein is a new hematopoietic/endothelial homophilic adhesion molecule. *Blood* 92:4602, 1998.

504. Aizawa S, Tavassoli M: In vitro homing of hemopoietic stem cells mediated by a recognition system with galactosyl and mannosyl specificities. *Proc Natl Acad Sci USA* 84:4485, 1987.

505. Tavassoli M, Hardy CL: Molecular basis of homing of intravenously transplanted stem cells. *Blood* 76:1059, 1990.

506. Sackstein R: Expression of an L-selectin ligand on hematopoietic progenitor cells. *Acta Haematol* 97:22, 1997.

507. Karakantza M, Gibson FM, Cavenagh JD, et al: Sle(x) expression of normal CD34 positive bone marrow haemopoietic progenitor cells. *Brit J Haematol* 86:883, 1994.

508. Tu L, Murphy PG, Li X, Tedder TF: L-selectin ligands expressed by human leukocytes are HECA-452 antibody-defined carbohydrate epitopes preferentially displayed by P-selectin glycoprotein ligand-1. *J Immunol* 161:1140, 1998.

509. Mazo IB, Gutierrez-Ramos JC, Frenette PS, et al: Hematopoietic progenitor cell rolling in bone marrow microvessels: parallel contributions by endothelial selectins and vascular cell adhesion molecule 1. *J Exp Med* 188:465, 1998.

510. Zollner O, Lenter MC, Blanks JE, et al: L-selectin from human, but not mouse, neutrophils binds directly to E-selectin. *J Cell Biol* 136:707, 1997.

511. Von Andrian UH, M-Rini C: In situ analysis of lymphocyte migration to lymph nodes. *Cell Adhes Commun* 6:85, 1998.

512. Levesque J-P, Zannettino ACW, Pudney M, et al: PSGL-1-mediated adhesion of human hematopoietic progenitors to P-selectin results in suppression of hematopoiesis. *Immunity* 11:369, 1999.

513. Van der Merwe PA: Leukocyte adhesion: High-speed cells with ABS. *Curr Biol* 9:R419, 1999.

514. Vest weber D, Blanks JE: Mechanisms that regulate the function of the selectins and their ligands. *Physiol Rev* 79:181, 1999.

515. Puri KD, Finger EB, Gaudernack G, Springer TA: Sialomucin CD34 is the major L-selectin ligand in human tonsil high endothelial venules. *J Cell Biol* 131:261, 1995.

516. Sassetti C, Tangemann K, Singer MS, et al: Identification of podocalyxin-like protein as a high endothelial venule ligand for L-selectin: parallels to CD34. *J Exp Med* 187:1965, 1998.

517. Tada J, Omine M, Suda T, Yamaguchi N: A common signaling pathway via *Syk* and *Lyn* tyrosine kinases generated from capping of the sialomucins CD34 and CD43 in immature hematopoietic cells. *Blood* 93:3723, 1999.

518. Young PE, Baumhueter S, Lasky LA: The sialomucin CD34 is expressed on hematopoietic cells and blood vessels during murine development. *Blood* 85:96, 1995.

519. Oxley SM, Sackstein R: Detection of an L-selectin ligand on a hematopoietic progenitor cell line. *Blood* 84:3299, 1994.

520. Stockton BM, Cheng G, Manjunath N, et al: Negative regulation of T cell homing by CD43. *Immunity* 8:373, 1998.

521. Bazil V, Brandt J, Chen S, et al: A monoclonal antibody recognizing CD43 (leukosialin) initiates apoptosis of human hematopoietic progenitor cells but not stem cells. *Blood* 87:1272, 1996.

522. Yonemura S, Hirao M, Doi Y, et al: Ezrin/radixin/moesin (ERM) proteins bind to a positively charged amino acid cluster in the juxta-membrane cytoplasmic domain of CD44, CD43, and ICAM-2. *J Cell Biol* 140:885, 1998.

523. Anzai N, Gotoh A, Shibayama H, Broxmeyer HE: Modulation of integrin function in hematopoietic progenitor cells by CD43 engagement: possible involvement of protein tyrosine kinase and phospholipase C-γ. *Blood* 93:3317, 1999.

524. Spertini O, Cordey AS, Monai N, et al: P-selectin glycoprotein ligand 1 is a ligand for L-selectin on neutrophils, monocytes, and CD34+ hematopoietic progenitor cells. *J Cell Biol* 135:523, 1996.

525. Tracey JB, Rinder HM: Characterization of the P-selectin ligand on human hematopoietic progenitors. *Exp Hematol* 24:1494, 1996.

526. Zannettino AC, Berndt MC, Butcher C, et al: Primitive human hematopoietic progenitors adhere to P-selectin (CD62P). *Blood* 85:3466, 1995.

527. Blanks JE, Moll T, Eytner R, Vestweber D: Stimulation of P-selectin glycoprotein ligand-1 on mouse neutrophils activates beta 2-integrin mediated cell attachment to ICAM-1. *Eur J Immunol* 28:433, 1998.

528. Yang J, Hirata T, Croce K, et al: Targeted gene disruption demonstrates that P-selectin glycoprotein ligand 1 (PSGL-1) is required for P-selectin-mediated but not E-selectin-mediated neutrophil rolling and migration. *J Exp Med* 190:1769, 1999.

529. Fuhbridge RC, Kieffer JD, Armerding D, Kupper TS: Cutaneous lymphocyte antigen is a specialized form of PSGL-1 expressed on skin-homing T cells. *Nature* 389:978, 1997.

530. Aigner S, Sthoeger ZM, Fogel M, et al: CD24, a mucin-type glycoprotein, is a ligand for P-selectin on human tumor cells. *Blood* 89:3385, 1997.

531. Watt SM, Buhring HJ, Rappold I, et al: CD164, a novel sialomucin on CD34(+) and erythroid subsets, is located on human chromosome 6q21. *Blood* 92:849, 1998.

532. Bowen MA, Aruffo A: Adhesion molecules, their receptors, and their

regulation: analysis of CD6-activated leukocyte cell-adhesion molecule (ALCAM/CD166) interactions. *Transplant Proc* 31:795, 1999.

533. Stamenkovin I, Aruffo A, Amiot M, Seed B: The hematopoietic and epithelial forms of CD44 are distinct polypeptides with different adhesion potentials for hyaluronate-bearing cells. *EMBO J* 10:343, 1991.

534. Dougherty GJ, Lansdorp PM, Cooper DL, Humphries RK: Molecular cloning of CD44R1 and CD44R2, two novel isoforms of the human CD44 lymphocyte "homing" receptor expressed by hemopoietic cells. *J Exp Med* 174:1, 1991.

535. Herrlich P, Zöller M, Pals ST, Ponta H: CD44 splice variants: Metastases meet lymphocytes. *Immunol Today* 14:395, 1993.

536. Rosel M, Khaldoyanidi S, Zawadski V, Zoller M: Involvement of CD44 variant isoform v10 in progenitor cell adhesion and maturation. *Exp Hematol* 27:698, 1999.

537. Funaro A, Malavasi F: Human CD38, a surface receptor, an enzyme, an adhesion molecule and not a simple marker. *J Biol Regul Homeost Agents* 13:54, 1999.

538. Hoenstein AL, Stokinger H, Imhof BA, Malavasi F: CD38 binding to human myeloid cells is mediated by mouse and human CD31. *Biochem J* 330:1129, 1998.

539. Turel KR, Rao SG: Expression of the cell adhesion molecule E-cadherin by the human bone marrow stromal cells and its probable role in CD34(+) stem cell adhesion. *Cell Biol Int* 22:641, 1998.

540. Kaisho T, Ishikawa J, Oritani K, et al: BST-1, a surface molecule of bone marrow stromal cell lines that facilitates pre-B-cell growth. *Proc Natl Acad Sci USA* 91:5325, 1994.

541. Hirata Y, Kimura N, Sato K, et al: ADP ribosyl cyclase activity of a novel bone marrow stromal cell surface molecule, BST-1. *FEBS Lett* 356:244, 1994.

542. Vicari AP, Bean AG, Zlotnik A: A role for BP-3/BST-1 antigen in early T cell development. *Int Immunol* 8:183, 1996.

543. Okuyama Y, Ishihara K, Kimura N, et al: Human BST-1 expressed on myeloid cells functions as a receptor molecule. *Biochem Biophys Res Commun* 228:838, 1996.

544. Springer TA: Traffic signals for lymphocyte recirculation and leukocyte emigration: the multistep paradigm. *Cell* 76:301, 1994.

545. Steeber DA, Tedder TF: Molecular basis of lymphocyte migration, in *Inflammation Basic Principles and Clinical Correlates*, 3rd ed, edited by JI Gallin, R Snyderman, pp 593–605. Lippincott Williams and Wilkins, Philadelphia, 1999.

546. Imai Y, Lasky LA, Rosen SD: Sulphation requirement for GlyCAM-1, an endothelial ligand for L-selectin. *Nature* 361:555, 1993.

547. Berg EL, McEvoy LM, Berlin C, et al: L-selectin-mediated lymphocyte rolling on MAdCAM-1. *Nature* 366:695, 1993.

548. Lawrence MB, Berg EL, Butcher EC, Springer TA: Rolling of lymphocytes and neutrophils on peripheral node addressin and subsequent arrest on ICAM-1 in shear flow. *Eur J Immunol* 25:1025, 1995.

549. Salmi M, Hellman J, Jalkanen S: The role of two distinct endothelial molecules, vascular adhesion protein-1 and peripheral lymph node addressin, in the binding of lymphocyte subsets to human lymph nodes. *J Immunol* 160:5629, 1998.

550. Weber C, Springer TA: Neutrophil accumulation on activated, surface-adherent platelets in flow is mediated by interaction of Mac-1 with fibrinogen bound to alphaIIbbeta3 and stimulated by platelet-activating factor. *J Clin Invest* 100:2085, 1997.

551. Kovach NL, Lin N, Yednock T, et al: Stem cell factor modulates avidity of alpha 4 beta 1 and alpha 5 beta 1 integrins expressed on hematopoietic cell lines. *Blood* 85:159, 1995.

552. Levesque JP, Leavesley DI, Niutta S, et al: Cytokines increase human hemopoietic cell adhesiveness by activation of very late antigen (VLA)-4 and VLA-5 integrins. *J Exp Med* 181: 1805, 1995.

553. Weber C, Alon R, Moser B, Springer TA: Sequential regulation of alpha 4 beta 1 and alpha 5 beta 1 integrin avidity by CC chemokines in monocytes: implications for transendothelial chemotaxis. *J Cell Biol* 134: 1063, 1996.

554. Suehiro Y, Muta K, Umemura T, et al: Macrophage inflammatory protein 1alpha enhances in a different manner adhesion of hematopoietic progenitor cells from bone marrow, cord blood, and mobilized peripheral blood. *Exp Hematol* 27:1637,1999.

555. Issekutz AC, Rowter D, Springer TA: Role of ICAM-1 and ICAM-2 and alternate CD11/CD18 ligands in neutrophil transendothelial migration. *J Leukoc Biol* 65:117, 1999.

556. Meerschaert J, Furie MB: The adhesion molecules used by monocytes for migration across endothelium include CD11a/CD18, CD11b/CD18, and VLA-4 on monocytes and ICAM-1, VCAM-1, and other ligands on endothelium. *J Immunol* 154:4099, 1995.

557. Weber C, Springer TA: Interaction of very late antigen-4 with VCAM-1 supports transendothelial chemotaxis of monocytes by facilitating lateral migration. *J Immunol* 161:6825, 1998.

558. Yong KL, Watts M, Shaun TN, et al: Transmigration of CD34+ cells across specialized and non-specialized endothelium requires prior activation by growth factors and is mediated by PECAM-1 (CD31). *Blood* 91:1196, 1998.

559. Muller WA: The role of PECAM-1 (CD31) in leukocyte emigration: studies in vitro and in vivo. *J Leukoc Biol* 57:523, 1995.

560. Clark RA, Erickson HP, Springer TA: Tenascin supports lymphocyte rolling. *J Cell Biol* 137:755, 1997.

561. Imhof BA, Weerasinghe D, Brown EJ, et al: Cross talk between alpha(v)beta3 and alpha4beta1 integrins regulates lymphocyte migration on vascular cell adhesion molecule 1. *Eur J Immunol* 27: 3242, 1997.

562. Muller WA: Leukocyte-endothelial cell adhesion molecules in transendothelial migration, in *Inflammation Basic Principles and Clinical Correlates*, 3rd ed, edited by JI Gallin, R Snyderman, pp 585–592. Lippincott Williams and Wilkins, Philadelphia, 1999.

563. Fong AM, Robinson LA, Steeber DA, et al: Fractalkine and CX3CR1 mediate a novel mechanism of leukocyte capture, firm adhesion, and activation under physiologic flow. *J Exp Med* 188:1413, 1998.

564. Bacon KB, Greaves DR, Dairaghi DJ, Schall TJ: The expanding universe of C, CX3C and CC chemokines, in *The Cytokine Handbook*, 3rd ed, edited by AW Thompson, pp 753–775. Academic Press, San Diego, 1998.

565. Rood PML, Gerristen WR, Kramer D, et al: Adhesion of hematopoietic progenitor cell to human bone marrow or umbilical vein derived endothelial cell lines: a comparison. *Exp Hematol* 27:1306, 1999.

566. Papayannopoulou T, Craddock C, Nakamoto B, et al: The VLA4/VCAM-1 adhesion pathway defines contrasting mechanisms of lodgement of transplanted murine hemopoietic progenitors between bone marrow and spleen. *Proc Natl Acad Sci USA* 92:9647, 1995.

567. Papayannopoulou T, Craddock C: Homing and trafficking of hematopoietic progenitor cells. *Acta Hematol* 97:97, 1997.

568. Mazo IB, von Andrian UH: Adhesion and homing of blood-borne cells in bone marrow microvessels. *J Leukoc Biol* 66:25, 1999.

569. Schweitzer KM, Vicart P, Delouis C, et al: Characterization of a newly established human bone marrow endothelial cell line: distinct adhesive properties for hematopoietic progenitors compared with human umbilical vein endothelial cells. *Lab Invest* 76:25, 1997.

570. Mohle R, Bautz F, Rafii S, et al: The chemokine receptor CXCR-4 is expressed on CD34+ hematopoietic progenitors and leukemic cells and mediates transendothelial migration induced by stromal cell-derived factor-1. *Blood* 91:4523, 1998.

571. Mohle R, Murea S, Kirsch M, Haas R: Differential expression of L-selectin, VLA-4, from LFA-1 on CD34+ progenitor cells from bone marrow and peripheral blood during G-CSF-enhanced recovery. *Exp Hematol* 23:1535, 1995.

572. Koenig JM, Baron S, Luo D, et al: L-selectin expression enhances clonogenesis of CD34+ cord blood progenitors. *Pediatr Res* 45:867, 1999.

573. Frenette PS, Subbarao S, Mazo IB, et al: Endothelial selectins and vascular cell adhesion molecule-1 promote hematopoietic progenitor homing to bone marrow. *Proc Natl Acad Sci USA* 95:14423, 1998.

574. Derry CJ, Faveeuw C, Mordsley KR, Ager A: Novel chondroitin sulfate-modified ligands for L-selectin on lymph node high endothelial venules. *Eur J Immunol* 29:419, 1999.

575. Norgard-Sumnicht K, Varki A: Endothelial heparan sulfate proteoglycans that bind to L-selectin have glucosamine residues with unsubstituted amino groups. *J Biol Chem* 270:12012, 1995.

576. Naiyer AJ, Jo DY, Ahn J, et al: Stromal derived factor-1-induced chemokinesis of cord blood CD34(+) cells (long-term culture-initiating cells) through endothelial cells is mediated by E-selectin. *Blood* 94:4011, 1999.

577. Peled A, Grabovsky V, Habler L, et al: The chemokine SDF-1 stimulates integrin-mediated arrest of CD34(+) cells on vascular endothelium under shear flow. *J Clin Invest* 104:1199, 1999.

578. Parakh KA, Kannan K: Demonstration of a ubiquitin binding site on

murine haemopoietic progenitor cells: implications of ubiquitin in homing and adhesion. *Br J Haematol* 84:212, 1993.

579. Hua CT, Gamble JR, Vadas MA, Jackson DE: Recruitment and activation of SHP-1 protein-tyrosine kinase phosphatase by human platelet endothelial cell adhesion molecule-1 (PECAM-1). Identification of immunoreceptor tyrosine-based inhibitory motif-like binding motifs and substrates. *J Biol Chem* 273:28332, 1998.

580. Peled A, Petit I, Kollet O, et al: Dependence of human stem cell engraftment and repopulation of NOD/SCID mice on CXCR4. *Science* 283:845, 1999.

581. Cipolleschi MG, Dello Sbarba P, Olivotto M: The role of hypoxia in the maintenance of hematopoietic stem cells. *Blood* 82:2031, 1993.

582. Jacobsen SE, Ruscetti FW, Ortiz M, et al: The growth response of Lin-Thy1+ hematopoietic progenitors to cytokines is determined by the balance between synergy of multiple stimulators and negative cooperation of multiple inhibitors. *Exp Hematol* 22:985, 1994.

583. Tang J, Nuccie BL, Ritterman I, et al: TGF-beta down-regulates stromal IL-7 secretion and inhibits proliferation of human B cell precursors. *J Immunol* 159:117, 1997.

584. Sakamaki S, Hirayama Y, Matsunaga T, et al: Transforming growth factor-β1 (TGF-β1) induces thrombopoietin from bone marrow stromal cells which stimulates the expression of TGF-β receptor on megakaryocytes and, in turn, renders them susceptible to suppression by TGF-β itself with high specificity. *Blood* 94:1961, 1999.

585. Cashman JD, Clark-Lewis I, Eaves AC, Eaves CJ: Differentiation stage-specific regulation of primitive human hematopoietic progenitor cycling by exogenous and endogenous inhibitors in an in vivo model. *Blood* 94:3722, 1999.

586. Gautam SC, Noth CJ, Janakiraman N, et al: Induction of chemokine mRNA in bone marrow stromal cells: modulation by TGF-beta 1 and IL-4. *Exp Hematol* 23:482, 1995.

587. Cashman JD, Eaves CJ, Sarris AH, Eaves AC: MCP-1, not MIP-1alpha, is the endogenous chemokine that cooperates with TGF-beta to inhibit the cycling of primitive normal but not leukemic (CML) progenitors in long-term human marrow cultures. *Blood* 92:2338, 1998.

588. Kinashi T, Springer TA: Steel factor and c-kit regulate cell matrix adhesion. *Blood* 83:1033, 1994.

589. Juliano RL, Haskill S: Signal transduction from the extracellular matrix. *J Cell Biol* 120:577, 1993.

590. Issaad C, Croisille L, Katz A, et al: A murine stromal cell line allows the proliferation of very primitive human CD34++/CD38- progenitor cells in long-term cultures and semisolid assays. *Blood* 81:2916, 1993.

591. Sachs L, Lotem J: Control of programmed cell death in normal and leukemic cells: new implications for therapy. *Blood* 82:15, 1993.

592. Gibson LF, Piktel D, Narayanan R, et al: Stromal cells regulate bcl-2 and bax expression in pro-B cells. *Exp Hematol* 24:628, 1996.

593. Liesveld JL, Harbol AW, Abboud CN: Stem cell factor and stromal cell co-culture prevent apoptosis in a subculture of the megakaryoblastic cell line, UT-7. *Leuk Res* 20:591, 1996.

594. Borge OJ, Ramsfjell V, Cui L, Jacobsen SE: Ability of early acting cytokines to directly promote survival and suppress apoptosis of human primitive CD34+CD38- bone marrow cells with multilineage potential at the single-cell level: key role of thrombopoietin. *Blood* 90:2282, 1997.

595. Finch CA, Harker LA, Cook JD: Kinetics of the formed elements of human blood. *Blood* 50:699, 1977.

596. Yong KL: Granulocyte colony-stimulating factor (G-CSF) increases neutrophil migration across vascular endothelium independent of an effect on adhesion: comparison with granulocyte-macrophage colony-stimulating factor (GM-CSF). *Br J Haematol* 94:40, 1996.

597. Ulich TR, del Castillo J, Souza L: Kinetics and mechanisms of recombinant human granulocyte-colony stimulating factor-induced neutrophilia. *Am J Pathol* 133:630, 1988.

598. DiPersio JF, Abboud CN: Activation of neutrophils by granulocyte-macrophage colony-stimulating factor, in *Granulocyte Responses to Cytokines: Basic and Clinical Research,* edited by RG Coffey, pp 457–484. Immunology Series, vol 57, Marcel Dekker, New York, 1992.

599. Ghebrehiwet B, Muller-Eberhard HJ: C3e: an acidic fragment of human C3 with leukocytosis-inducing activity. *J Immunol* 123:616, 1979.

600. Kubo H, Graham L, Doyle NA, et al: Complement fragment-induced release of neutrophils from bone marrow and sequestration within pulmonary capillaries in rabbits. *Blood* 92:283, 1998.

601. Deinard AS, Page AR: A study of steroid-induced granulocytosis. *Br J Haematol* 28:333, 1974.

602. Vogel MJ, Yankee RA, Kimball HR, et al: The effect of etiocholanolone on granulocyte kinetics. *Blood* 30:474, 1967.

603. Cybulsky MI, McCoumb DJ, Movat HZ: Neutrophil leukocyte emigration induced by endotoxin: Mediator roles of interleukin-1 and tumor necrosis factor alpha. *J Immunol* 140:3144, 1988.

604. Terashima T, English D, Hogg JC, van Eeden SF: Release of polymorphonuclear leukocytes from the bone marrow by interleukin-8. *Blood* 92:1062, 1998.

605. Wang JM, Rambaldi A, Biondi A, et al: Recombinant human interleukin 5 is a selective eosinophil chemoattractant. *Eur J Immunol* 19:701, 1989.

606. Palframan RT, Collins PD, Williams TJ, Rankin SM: Eotaxin induces a rapid release of eosinophils and their progenitors from the bone marrow. *Blood* 91:2240, 1998.

607. Ebisawa M, Yamada T, Bickel C, et al: Eosinophil transendothelial migration induced by cytokines: III. Effect of the chemokine RANTES. *J Immunol* 153:2153, 1994.

608. Lundahl J, Moshfegh A, Gronneberg R, Hallden G: Eotaxin increases the expression of CD11b/CD18 and adhesion properties in IL-5, but not fMLP-prestimulated human peripheral blood eosinophils. *Inflammation* 22:123, 1998.

609. Dutt P, Wang JF, Groopman JE: Stromal cell-derived factor-1 alpha and stem cell factor/kit ligand share signaling pathways in hemopoietic progenitors: a potential mechanism for cooperative induction of chemotaxis. *J Immunol* 161:3652, 1998.

610. Hedrick JA, Helms A, Vicari A, Zlotnik A: Characterization of a novel chemokine, HCC-4, whose expression is increased by interleukin-10. *Blood* 91:4242, 1998.

611. Kim CH, Broxmeyer HE: Chemokines: signal lamps for trafficking of T and B cells for development and effector function. *J Leukoc Biol* 65:6, 1999.

612. Kim CH, Broxmeyer HE: SLC/exodus2/6Ckine/TCA4 induces chemotaxis of hematopoietic progenitor cells: differential activity of ligands of CCR7, CXCR3, or CXCR4 in chemotaxis vs. suppression of progenitor proliferation. *J Leukoc Biol* 66:455, 1999.

613. Morales J, Homey B, Vicari AP, et al: CTACK, a skin-associated chemokine that preferentially attracts skin-homing memory T cells. *Proc Natl Acad Sci USA* 96:14470, 1999.

614. Zlotnik A, Yoshie O: Chemokines: a new classification system and their role in immunity. *Immunity* 12:121, 2000.

615. Tanaka H, Tatsumi N, Kan E, et al: EPO test in hemodialysis patients. *Biomater Artif Cells Immobil Biotechnol* 21:221, 1993.

616. Chamberlain JK, Weiss L, Weed RI: Bone marrow sinus cell packing: a determinant of cell release. *Blood* 46:91, 1975.

617. Waugh RE, Sassi M: An in vitro model of erythroid egress in bone marrow. *Blood* 68:250, 1986.

618. Dabrowski A, Szygula Z, Miszta H: Do changes in bone marrow pressure contribute to the egress of cells from the bone marrow? *Acta Physiol Pol* 32:729, 1981.

619. Iversen PO, Nicolaysen G, Benestad HB: Blood flow to bone marrow during development of anemia or polycythemia in the rat. *Blood* 79:594, 1992.

620. Iversen PO, Nicolaysen G, Benestad HB: The leukopoietic cytokine granulocyte colony-stimulating factor increases blood flow to rat bone marrow. *Exp Hematol* 21:231, 1993.

621. Lichtman MA, Chamberlain JK, Santillo PA: Factors thought to contribute to the regulation of egress of cells from marrow, in *The Year in Hematology 1978,* edited by R Silber, J LoBue, A Gordon, pp 243–279. Plenum, New York, 1978.

622. Van Eeden SF, Miyagashima R, Haley L, Hogg JC: A possible role for L-selectin in the release of polymorphonuclear leukocytes from bone marrow. *Am J Physiol* 272:H1717, 1997.

623. LeMarer N, Skacel PO: Up-regulation of alpha2,6 sialylation during myeloid maturation: a potential role in myeloid cell release from the bone marrow. *J Cell Physiol* 179:315, 1999.

624. Reinhardt PH, Elliott JF, Kubes P: Neutrophils can adhere via alpha$_2$beta$_1$-integrin under flow conditions. *Blood* 89:3837, 1997.

625. Burns AR, Bowden RA, Abe Y, et al: P-selectin mediates neutrophil adhesion to endothelial cell borders. *J Leukoc Biol* 65:299, 1999

626. Jagels MA, Chambers JD, Arfors KE, Hugli TE: C5a- and tumor necrosis factor-alpha-induced leukocytosis occurs independently of beta 2 inte-

grins and L-selectin: differential effects on neutrophil adhesion molecule expression in vivo. *Blood* 85:2900, 1995.

627. Stroncek DF, Kaszcz W, Herr GP, et al: Expression of neutrophil antigens after 10 days of granulocyte-colony-stimulating factor. *Transfusion* 38:663, 1998.

628. Jung U, Ley K: Mice lacking two or all three selectins demonstrate overlapping and distinct functions for each selectin. *J Immunol* 162:6755, 1999.

629. Scurfield G, Radley JM: Aspects of platelet formation and release. *Am J Hematol* 10:285, 1981.

630. Radley JM, Haller CJ: Fate of senescent megakaryocytes in bone marrow. *Br J Haematol* 53:277, 1983.

631. Efrati P, Rozenszajn L: The morphology of buffy coats in normal human adults. *Blood* 16:1012, 1960.

632. Tinggaard-Pedersen N, Laursen B: Megakaryocytes in cubital venous blood in patients with chronic myeloproliferative diseases. *Scand J Haematol* 30:50, 1983.

633. Mantovani A, Vecchi A, Sozzani S, et al: Tumors as a paradigm for the in vivo role of chemokines in leukocyte recruitment, in *Chemokines and Cancer, Contemporary Cancer Research,* edited by BJ Rollins, pp 35–49. Humana Press Inc, NJ, 1999.

634. Kim CH, Broxmeyer HE: In vitro behavior of hematopoietic progenitor cells under the influence of chemoattractants: stromal cell-derived factor-1, steel factor, and the bone marrow environment. *Blood* 91:100, 1998.

635. Aiuti A, Webb IJ, Bleul C, et al: The chemokine SDF-1 is a chemoattractant for human hematopoietic progenitor cells and provides a new mechanism to explain the mobilization of CD34+ progenitors to peripheral blood. *J Exp Med* 185:111, 1997.

636. Aiuti A, Tavian M, Cipponi A, et al: Expression of CXCR4, the receptor for stromal cell-derived factor-1 on fetal and adult human lympho-hematopoietic progenitors. *Eur J Immunol* 29:1823, 1999.

637. Roberts MM, Swart BW, Simmons PJ, et al: Prolonged release and c-kit expression of haemopoietic precursor cells mobilized by stem cell factor and granulocyte colony stimulating factor. *Br J Haematol* 104:778, 1999.

638. Wang JB, Mukaida N, Zhang Y, et al: Enhanced mobilization of hematopoietic progenitor cells by mouse MIP-2 and granulocyte colony-stimulating factor. *J Leuk Biol* 62:503, 1997.

639. Vermeulen M, Le Pesteur F, Gagnerault MC, et al: Role of adhesion molecules in the homing and mobilization of murine hematopoietic stem and progenitor cells. *Blood* 92:894, 1998.

640. Craddock CF, Nakamoto B, Elices M, Papayannopoulou TH: The role of CS1 moiety of fibronectin in VLA mediated haemopoietic progenitor trafficking. *Br J Haematol* 98:828, 1997.

641. Craddock CF, Nakamoto B, Andrews RG, et al: Antibodies to VLA4 integrin mobilize long-term repopulating cells and augment cytokine-induced mobilization in primates and mice. *Blood* 90:4779, 1997.

642. Papayannopoulou T, Priestley GV, Nakamoto B: Anti-VLA4/VCAM-1-induced mobilization requires cooperative signaling through the kit/mkit ligand pathway. *Blood* 91:2231, 1998.

643. Papayannopoulou T: Hematopoietic stem/progenitor cell mobilization. A continuing quest for etiologic mechanisms. *Ann NY Acad Sci* 872:187, 1999.

644. Maloney MA, Patt HM: Migration of cells from shielded to irradiated marrow. *Blood* 39:804, 1972.

645. Link H, Arseniev L, Bahre O, et al: Combined transplantation of allogeneic bone marrow and CD34+ blood cells. *Blood* 86:2500, 1995.

646. Dercksen MW, Gerristen WR, Rodenhuis S, et al: Expression of adhesion molecules on CD34+ cells: CD34+ L-selectin+ cells predict a rapid platelet recovery after blood stem cell transplantation. *Blood* 85:3313, 1995.

647. Watanabe T, Dave B, Heiman DG, et al: Cell adhesion molecule expression on CD34+ cells in grafts and time to myeloid and platelet recovery after autologous stem cell transplantation. *Exp Hematol* 26:10, 1998.

648. Timeus F, Crescenzio N, Marranca D, et al: Cell adhesion molecules in cord blood hematopoietic progenitors. *Bone Marrow Transplant* 22(suppl 1):S61, 1998.

649. Katayama Y, Mahmut N, Takimoto H, et al: Hematopoietic progenitor cells from allogeneic bone marrow transplant donors circulate in the very early post-transplant period. *Bone Marrow Transplant* 23:659, 1999.

650. Hardy CL: The homing of hematopoietic stem cells to the bone marrow. *Am J Med Sci* 309:260, 1995.

651. Pipia GG, Long MW: Human hematopoietic progenitor cell isolation based on galactose-specific cell surface binding. *Nat Biotechnol* 15:1007, 1997.

652. Shirota T, Tavassoli M: Alterations of bone marrow sinus endothelium induced by ionizing irradiation: implications in homing of intravenously transplanted marrow cells. *Blood Cells* 18:197, 1992.

653. Yamazaki K, Allen TD: The structure and function of the blood-marrow barrier: early ultrastructural changes in irradiated bone marrow sinus endothelial cells detected by vascular perfusion fixation (comment). *Blood Cells* 18:215, 1992.

654. Bolante-Cervantes R, Li S, Sahota A, et al: Pattern of localization of primitive hematopoietic cells in vivo using a novel mouse model. *Exp Hematol* 27:1346, 1999.

655. Cui J, Wahl RL, Shen T, et al: Bone marrow cell trafficking following intravenous administration. *Br J Haematol* 107:895, 1999.

656. Imai K, Kobayashi M, Wang J, et al: Selective secretion of chemoattractants for haemopoietic progenitor cells by bone marrow endothelial cells: a possible role in homing of haemopoietic progenitor cells to bone marrow. *Br J Haematol* 106:905, 1999.

657. Jo DY, Rafii S, Hamada T, Moore MA: Chemotaxis of primitive hematopoietic cells is in response to stromal cell-derived factor-1. *J Clin Invest* 105:101, 2000.

658. Lanzkron SM, Collector MI, Sharkis SJ: Hematopoietic stem cell trafficking in vivo: a comparison of short-term and long-term repopulating cells. *Blood* 93:1916, 1999.

659. Kessinger A: Collection of autologous peripheral blood stem cells in steady state, in *Peripheral Stem Cells in Bone Marrow Transplantation,* edited by NC Gorin, pp 19–26, *Baillieres Best Practice and Research Clinical Haematology,* vol 12, #1/2, 1999.

660. Shpall EJ: The utilization of cytokines in stem cell mobilization strategies. *Bone Marrow Transplant* 23(suppl 2):S13, 1999.

661. Facon T, Harousseau JL, Maloisel F, et al: Stem cell factor in combination with filgastrim after chemotherapy improves peripheral blood progenitor cell yield and reduces apheresis requirements in multiple myeloma patients: a randomized, controlled trial. *Blood* 94:1218, 1999.

662. Lyman SD: Biologic effects and potential clinical applications of Flt3 ligand. *Curr Opin Hematol* 5:192, 1998.

663. Fischmeister G, Kurz M, Haas OA, et al: G-CSF versus GM-CSF for stimulation of peripheral blood progenitor cells (PBPC) and leukocytes in healthy volunteers: comparison of efficacy and tolerability. *Ann Hematol* 78:117, 1999.

664. Chao NJ, Schriber JR, Grimes K, et al: Granulocyte colony-stimulating factor "mobilized" peripheral blood progenitor cells accelerate granulocyte and platelet recovery after high-dose chemotherapy. *Blood* 81:2031, 1993.

665. Damia G, Komschlies KL, Faltynek CR, et al: Administration of recombinant human interleukin-7 alters the frequency and number of myeloid progenitor cells in the bone marrow and spleen of mice. *Blood* 79:1121, 1992.

666. Somlo G, Sniecinski I, ter Veer A, et al: Recombinant human thrombopoietin in combination with granulocyte colony-stimulating factor enhances mobilization of peripheral blood progenitor cells, increases peripheral blood platelet concentration, and accelerates hematopoietic recovery following high-dose chemotherapy. *Blood* 93:2798, 1999.

667. MacVittie TJ, Farese AM, Davis TA, et al: Myelopoietin, a chimeric agonist of human interleukin 3 and granulocyte colony-stimulating factor receptors, mobilizes CD34+ cells that rapidly engraft lethally x-irradiated nonhuman primates. *Exp Hematol* 27:1557, 1999.

668. Welham MJ, Schrader JW: Modulation of c-*kit* mRNA and protein by hemopoietic growth factors. *Mol Cell Biol* 11:2901, 1991.

669. Pilarski LM, Pruski E, Wizniak J, et al: Potential role for hyaluronan and the hyaluronan receptor RHAMM in mobilization and trafficking of hematopoietic progenitor cells. *Blood* 93:2918, 1999.

670. Chamberlain JK, Leblond PF, Weed RI: Reduction of adventitial cell cover: an early direct effect of erythropoietin on bone marrow ultrastructure. *Blood Cells* 1:655, 1975.

671. Pruijt JF, Williamze R, Fibbe WE: Mechanisms underlying hematopoietic stem cell mobilization induced by the CXC chemokine interleukin-8. *Curr Opin Hematol* 6:152, 1999.

672. Pruijt JF, Fibbe WE, Laterveer L, et al: Prevention of interleukin-8-induced mobilization of hematopoietic progenitor cells in rhesus monkeys by inhibitory antibodies against the metalloproteinase gelatinase B (MMP-9). *Proc Natl Acad Sci USA* 96:10863, 1999.

673. Watanabe T, Kawano Y, Kanamaru S, et al: Endogenous interleukin-8 (IL-8) surge in granulocyte colony-stimulating factor-induced peripheral blood stem cell mobilization. *Blood* 93:1157, 1999.

674. Pruijt JF, van Kooyk Y, Figdor CG, et al: Murine hematopoietic progenitor cells with colony-forming or radioprotective capacity lack expression of the beta 2-integrin LFA-1. *Blood* 93:107, 1999.

675. Pruijt JF, van Kooyk Y, Figdor CG, et al: Anti-LFA-1 blocking antibodies prevent mobilization of hematopoietic progenitor cells induced by interleukin-8. *Blood* 91:4099, 1998.

676. Semerad, CL, Poursine-Laurent J, Liu F, et al: A role for G-CSF receptor signaling in the regulation of hematopoietic cell function but not lineage commitment or differentiation. *Immunity* 11:153, 1999.

677. Liu F, Poursine-Laurent J, Link D: The granulocyte colony-stimulating factor receptor is required for the mobilization of murine hematopoietic progenitors into peripheral blood by cyclophosphamide or interleukin-8 but not Flt-3 ligand. *Blood* 90:2522, 1997.

678. Betsuyaku T, Liu F, Senior RM, et al: A functional granulocyte-macrophage colony-stimulating factor receptor is required for normal chemoattractant-induced neutrophil activation. *J Clin Invest* 103:825, 1999.

679. Murphy G, Gavrilovic J: Proteolysis and cell migration: creating a path? *Curr Opin Cell Biol* 11:614, 1999.

680. Webb LM, Ehrengruber MU, Clark-Lewis I, et al: Binding of heparan sulfate or heparin enhances neutrophil responses to interleukin-8. *Proc Natl Acad Sci USA* 90:7158, 1993.

681. Dias Baruffi M, Pereira-da-Silva G, Jamur MC, Roque-Barreira MC: Heparin potentiates in vivo neutrophil migration induced by IL-8. *Glyconj J* 15:523, 1998.

682. Rainger GE, Rowley AF, Nash GB: Adhesion-dependent release of elastase from human neutrophils in a novel, flow-based model: specificity of different chemotactic agents. *Blood* 92:4819, 1998.

683. Wize J, Sopata I, Smerdel A, Maslinski S: Ligation of selectin L and integrin CD11b/CD18 (Mac-1) induces release of gelatinase B (MMP-9) from human neutrophils. *Inflamm Res* 47:325, 1998.

684. Janowska-Wieczorek A, Marquez LA, Nabholtz J-M, et al: Growth factors and cytokines upregulate gelatinase expression in bone marrow CD34+ cells and their transmigration through reconstituted basement membrane. *Blood* 93:3379, 1999.

685. Gallacher L, Murdoch B, Wu DM, Karanu FN, et al: Isolation and characterization of human CD34(−)Lin(−) and CD34(+)Lin(−) hematopoietic stem cells using cell surface markers AC133 and CD7. *Blood* 95:2813, 2000.

686. Gehling UM, Ergun S, Schumacher U, Wagener C, et al: In vitro differentiation of endothelial cells from AC133-positive progenitor cells. *Blood* 95:3106, 2000.

687. Peichev M, Naiyer AJ, Pereira D, Zhu Z, et al: Expression of VEGFR-2 and AC133 by circulating human CD34(+) cells identifies a population of functional endothelial precursors. *Blood* 95:952, 2000.

THE LYMPHOID TISSUES

THOMAS J. KIPPS

The lymphoid tissues can be divided into primary and secondary lymphoid organs. Primary lymphoid tissues are sites where lymphocytes develop from progenitor cells into functional and mature lymphocytes. The major primary lymphoid tissue is the marrow, the site where all lymphocyte progenitor cells reside and initially differentiate. This organ is discussed in Chap. 4. The other primary lymphoid tissue is the thymus, the site where progenitor cells from the marrow differentiate into mature thymus-derived (T) cells. Secondary lymphoid tissues are sites where lymphocytes interact with each other and nonlymphoid cells to generate immune responses to antigens. These include the spleen, lymph nodes, and mucosa-associated lymphoid tissues (MALT). The structure of these tissues provides insight into how the immune system discriminates between self-antigens and foreign antigens and develops the capacity to orchestrate a variety of specific and nonspecific defenses against invading pathogens.

THE THYMUS

The thymus is the site for development of thymic-dependent lymphocytes, or T cells. It is a primary lymphoid organ in that it is a major site of lymphopoiesis (lymphocyte development). In this organ, developing T cells, called thymocytes, differentiate from lymphoid stem cells derived from the marrow into functional, mature T cells. It is here that T cells acquire their repertoire of specific antigen receptors to cope with the antigenic challenges received throughout one's life span. Once they have completed their maturation, the T cells leave the thymus and circulate in the blood and through secondary lymphoid tissues.

THYMIC ANATOMY

The thymus is located in the superior mediastinum, overlying, in order, the left brachiocephalic (or innominate) vein, the innominate artery, the left common carotid artery, and the trachea. It overlaps the upper limit of the pericardial sac below and extends into the neck beneath the upper anterior ribs. It receives its blood supply from the internal thoracic arteries. Venous blood from the thymus drains into the brachiocephalic and internal thoracic veins, which communicate above with the inferior thyroid veins.

Arising from the third and fourth brachial pouches as an epithelial organ populated by lymphoid cells, the thymus develops at about the eighth week of gestation. The thymus increases in size through fetal and postnatal life and remains ample into puberty,[1] when it weighs

Acronyms and abbreviations that appear in this chapter include: CT, computed tomography; MALT, mucosa-associated lymphoid tissues; MHC, major histocompatibility complex; PALS, periarteriolar lymphoid sheath; T, thymus-derived; TCR, T-cell receptor.

about 40 g. Thereafter, the size progressively decreases with aging as a consequence of thymic involution.[2,3]

The volume of the thymus can be estimated by sonography. In one study of 149 healthy term infants within 1 week of birth, there was a significant correlation between the estimated thymic volume and the weight of the infant.[4] However, no correlation was apparent between the estimated thymic volume and the infant's sex, length, or gestational age. Also, there was no apparent correlation between estimated volume and the proportions of CD4+ T cells or CD8+ T cells found in the blood. The estimated thymic volume of healthy infants increases from birth to 4 and 8 months of age and then decreases.[1] Most of the individual variation at 4 and 10 months of age appears to correlate with breast-feeding status, body size, and, to a lesser extent, illness. Breast-fed infants at 4 months of age have significantly larger estimated thymic volumes than do age-matched formula-fed infants with similar thymic volumes at birth.[5]

THYMIC STRUCTURE

A longitudinal fissure divides the thymus into two asymmetrical lobes, a larger right and a smaller left, that are derived from the right and left brachial pouches, respectively. These two developmentally separate parts of the thymus are easily separated from each other by blunt dissection.

Each lobe of the thymus is divided into multiple lobules by fibrous septa. Each lobule consists of an outer cortex and an inner medulla. The cortex contains dense collections of thymocytes that appear as lymphocytes of slightly variable size with scattered, rare mitoses. The lighter-staining medulla is more sparsely populated with cells. It contains loosely arranged mature thymocytes and characteristic tightly packed whorls of squamous-appearing epithelial cells, called Hassall's corpuscles. These appear to be remnants of degenerating cells and are rich in high-molecular-weight cytokeratins.

The thymus contains several other important cell types in addition to thymocytes. There are three types of specialized epithelial cells within the thymus: the medullary epithelial cells, which are organized into clusters; the cortical epithelial cells, which form an epithelial network; and the epithelial cells of the outer cortex.[6] The epithelial cells in the cortex and medulla often have a stellate shape, display desmosomal connections to one another, and may function as nurse cells to developing thymocytes. In addition, the thymus contains marrow-derived antigen-presenting cells, primarily interdigitating dendritic cells and macrophages, particularly at the corticomedullary junction.

After puberty, thymic involution begins within the cortex. This region may disappear completely with aging, while medullary remnants persist throughout life. Corticosteroids also may induce atrophy of the cortex secondary to glucocorticoid-induced apoptosis of cortical thymocytes.[7] This also may be seen in conditions that are associated with increases in circulating steroids, for example, pregnancy or stress.[8,9]

THYMIC IMMUNE FUNCTION

Prothymocytes originate in the marrow and migrate to the thymus, where they mature into T cells (see Chaps. 82 and 84). Maturation of T cells is accompanied by the sequential acquisition by thymocytes of the various T-cell markers (Fig. 5-1). Terminal deoxynucleotidyl transferase is found in prothymocytes and immature thymocytes but is absent in mature T cells.

Pre–T cells enter the cortex via small blood vessels and are double negative for CD4 and CD8 antigens. One of the earliest identifiable

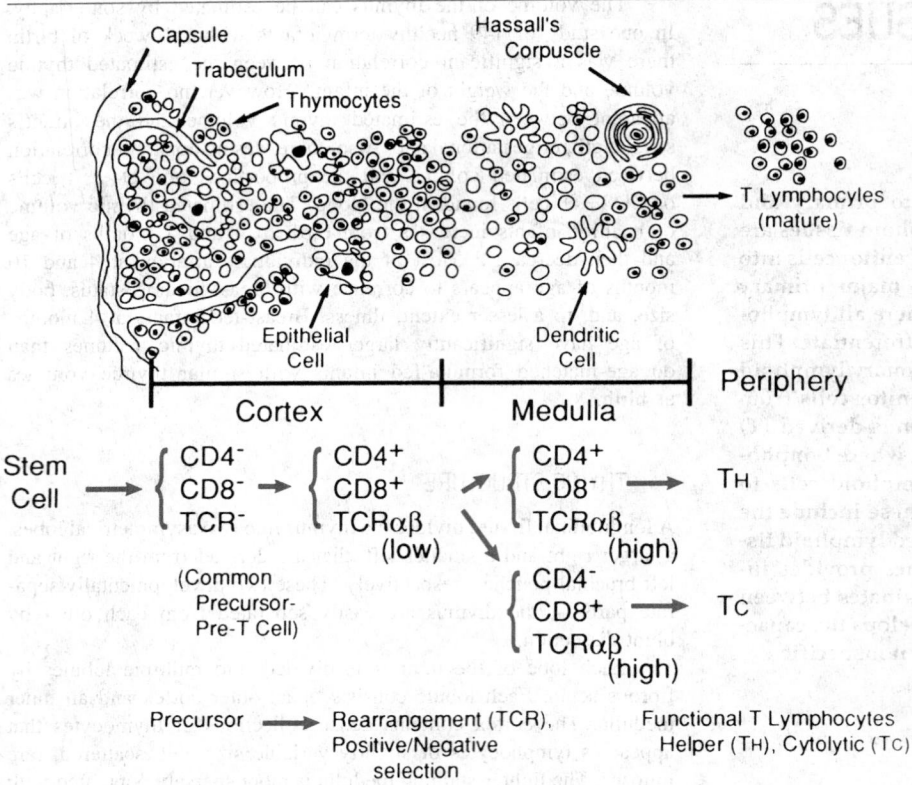

FIGURE 5-1 Structure of the thymus. The top half of the figure provides a cross section of a thymic lobule, indicating the outer cortex *(left)*, inner medulla *(center)*, and periphery *(far right)*. The marked arrows indicate various structures and cell types. As thymocytes mature, they migrate from the cortex toward the medullary region and acquire phenotypic features that are outlined at the bottom of the figure, as described in the text (see Chap. 82).

T-cell membrane antigens is CD2. As the thymocytes proliferate and differentiate in the cortex, they acquire CD4 and CD8 antigens. They subsequently acquire the CD3 antigen and the T-cell receptor for antigen as they migrate toward the medulla.

Positive and negative selection of maturing T cells takes place in the thymus. "Double-positive" (CD4+ and CD8+) thymocytes undergo an initial positive selection step that is mediated exclusively by thymic cortical epithelium.[10] Thymocytes that have T-cell receptors (TCR) capable of interacting with the major histocompatibility complex (MHC) molecules expressed by thymic cortical epithelial cells will undergo expansion, while thymocytes with defective TCR will undergo apoptosis.[11,12] As these positively selected cells migrate toward the medulla, they experience negative selection. Those thymocytes that have TCR that react too vigorously with the MHC molecules of the medullary epithelium and marrow-derived cells will undergo apoptosis.[12-14] Most of the developing thymocytes are destroyed. In this way, only those T cells that have the right level of low affinity for self-MHC molecules will reach the final maturation stages and be allowed to exit the thymus.

The selected thymocytes enter the thymic medulla, where they further mature and differentiate to become "single positive" for either CD4 or CD8 and acquire the capacity for future helper and cytolytic functions, respectively. Here they also may interact with scattered B cells during their final stages of thymic education (see Chaps. 15, 82, and 84). A small percentage of the lymphocytes produced in the thymus finally exit the medulla via efferent lymphatics as mature, naive T cells.

THE SPLEEN

The spleen is a secondary lymphoid organ. Secondary lymphoid tissues provide an environment in which the cells of the immune system can interact with antigen and with one another to develop an immune response to antigen. The spleen is a major site of immune response to blood-borne antigens. In addition, the splenic red pulp contains macrophages that are responsible for clearing the blood of unwanted foreign substances and senescent erythrocytes, even in the absence of specific immunity. Thus, it acts as a filter for the blood.

SPLENIC ANATOMY

The spleen is located within the peritoneum in the left upper quadrant of the abdomen between the fundus of the stomach and the diaphragm. It receives its blood supply from the systemic circulation via the splenic artery, which branches off the celiac trunk, and the left gastroepiploic artery.[15] The blood returning from the spleen drains into the portal circulation via the splenic vein. Therefore, the spleen can become congested with blood and increase in size when there is portal hypertension.

About 10 percent of individuals have one or more accessory spleens. Accessory spleens are usually 1 cm in diameter and resemble lymph nodes. However, they usually are covered with peritoneum, as is the spleen itself. Accessory spleens typically lie along the course of the splenic artery or its gastroepiploic branch, but they may be elsewhere.[16] The commonest location is near the hilus of the spleen, but approximately one in six accessory spleens can be found embedded in the tail of the pancreas, where they may be occasionally mistaken for a pancreatic mass lesion.[17-21]

The average weight of the spleen in the adult human is 135 g, ranging from 100 to 250 g. However, when emptied of blood it weighs only about 80 g. On autopsy of 539 subjects with normal spleens, there was a positive correlation between the spleen weight and both the degree of acute splenic congestion and the subject's height and weight but not with the subject's sex or age.[22]

The splenic volume can be estimated by computed tomography (CT) of the abdomen.[23,24] In one study, the splenic volume was calculated from the linear and the maximal cross-sectional area measurements of the spleen, using the following formula: splenic volume = 30 cm^3 + 0.58 × the product of the measured width, length, and thickness of the spleen.[23] Using this formula, the mean value of the calculated splenic volume for 47 normal subjects was 214.6 cm^3, with a range from 107.2 to 314.5 cm^3. The calculated splenic volume did not appear to vary significantly with the subject's age, gender, height, weight, body mass index, or the diameter of the first lumbar vertebra, the latter being considered representative of body habitus on CT.

The splenic volume also can be estimated by sonography. In one study of 32 normal spleens from adult corpses, the ultrasound measurements of maximal height, width, and breadth of the spleen were compared with the actual volume displaced by the excised organ.[25] The mean actual splenic volume was approximately 148 cm^3 (± 81 cm^3 SD), whereas mean splenic volume estimated from ultrasound was

$284\ cm^3$ ($\pm\ 168\ cm^3$ SD). Despite the differences between the actual and estimated volumes, these investigators did find a roughly linear correlation between actual splenic volume and the estimated splenic volume measured by ultrasound. However, there may be operator-to-operator variation in measurement of the estimated splenic volume, making the use of sonography in longitudinal studies technically demanding.

SPLENIC STRUCTURE

The spleen has an "open" circulation, which lacks endothelial continuity from artery to vein.[26] When isolated spleens are perfused in washout studies, erythrocytes that appear in the splenic vein appear to be flushed out from three compartments. The red cells that are flushed out first come from a compartment that presumably is formed by the splenic vessels. The erythrocytes that are flushed out next come from a second compartment, where they presumably are loosely held within the filtration beds. The erythrocytes that are flushed out last presumably were adherent to cells of the filtration beds. Although 90 percent of the blood flow passes through the splenic vessels, only about 10 percent of the total splenic red cells are found within this first compartment. The second compartment is perfused by 9 percent of the total inflow yet contains 70 percent of the splenic red cells. The last compartment is perfused by only 1 percent of the inflow but contains 20 percent of the splenic red cells.

These compartments reflect the anatomy of the spleen and its stroma. The stroma is composed of branched, fibroblast-like cells called reticular cells. These cells produce slender collagen fibers, the reticular fibers, which are rich in type IV collagen. The reticular cells and fibers form a meshwork, or reticulum, which filters the blood. Three major types of filtration beds can be distinguished by their structure and content: the white pulp, the marginal zone, and the red pulp.

WHITE PULP

The white pulp contains the lymphocytes and other mononuclear cells that surround the arterioles branching off the splenic artery. After the splenic artery pierces the splenic capsule at the hilum, it divides into progressively smaller branches. Each branch is called a central artery because it runs through the central longitudinal axis of a distinctive filtration bed that surrounds each central artery (Fig. 5-2). This is composed of a cuff of lymphocytes called the periarteriolar lymphoid sheath (or PALS). The PALS is contained within a protective and supporting fibrous trabecula and is composed mostly of T lymphocytes, about two-thirds of which are CD4+ T cells. Attached to the PALS are lymphoid follicles, some of which contain pale kernels of activated lymphocytes interspersed with large, pale macrophages and dendritic cells called germinal centers.[27] On gross inspection of the surface of a freshly cut spleen, these appear as white dots referred to as Malpighian corpuscles. These corpuscles predominantly contain a germinal center and have the same anatomic features and functions as secondary follicles in the lymph node (Fig. 5-3).

Branches coming off the central artery deliver disproportionate amounts of plasma and lymphocytes to the rims of the PALS. These branches tend to run at acute angles, leading to a selective loss of plasma from the blood, a phenomenon referred to as skimming. After

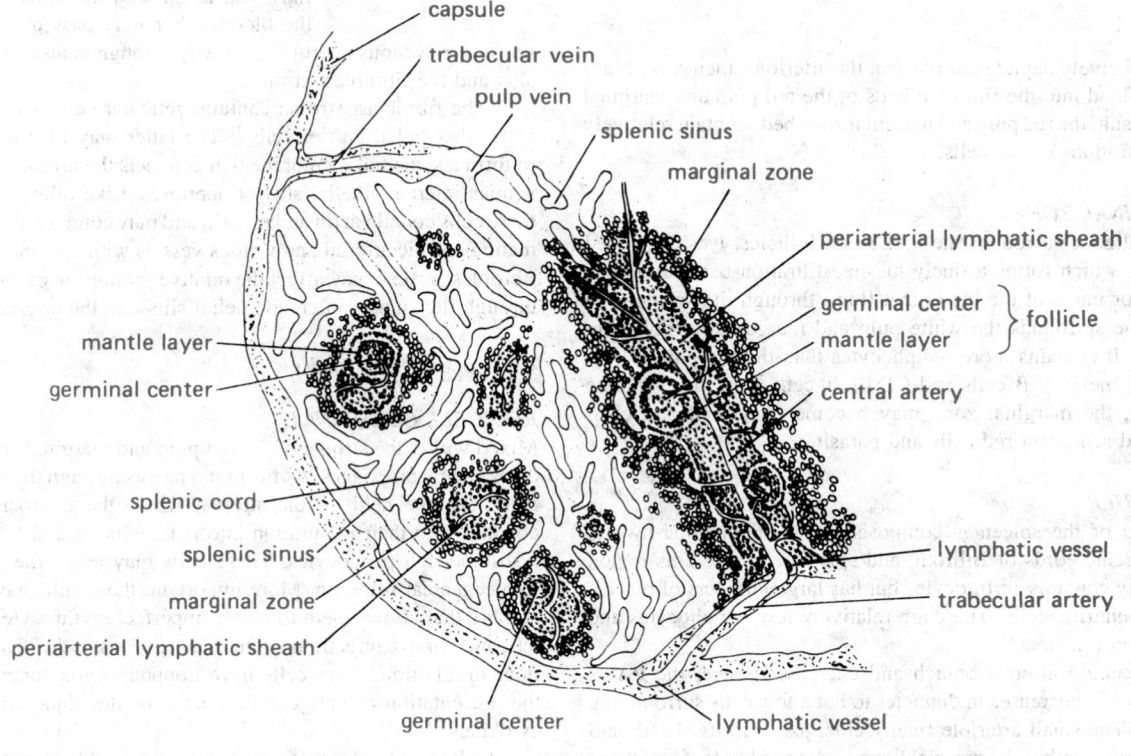

FIGURE 5-2   Structure of the spleen. A branch of the splenic artery enters the pulp and becomes a central artery. Surrounding the central artery is a PALS. At the circumference of the PALS is the marginal zone, which generally separates the white pulp of the PALS from the red pulp. Follicles of B cells with occasional germinal centers (Malpighian corpuscles) are located at the outer margins of the PALS for the depicted central artery and the PALS of central arteries that are in a different plane from that of the figure.

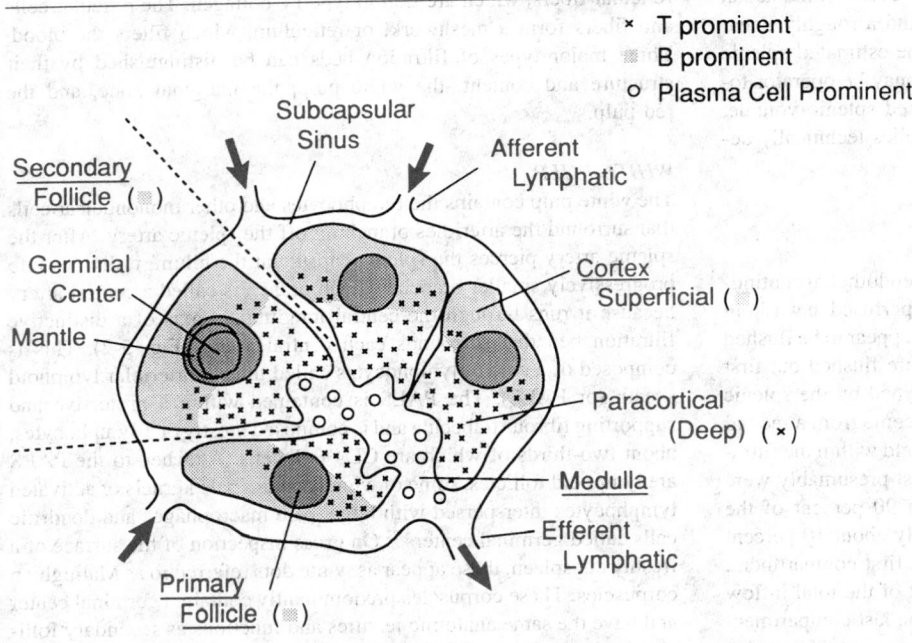

× T prominent
▦ B prominent
○ Plasma Cell Prominent

FIGURE 5-3   Structure of the lymph node. The lymph enters via afferent lymphatic channels and exits via the efferent lymphatic channel. The large arrows indicate the direction of the lymphatic flow into and out of the lymph node. The legend shows the symbols used for the T-cell zone *(x)* and the B-cell zone *(shaded)* of each follicle. The follicle in the lower left part of the node contains a primary follicle lacking a germinal center. The follicle immediately above this follicle contains a germinal center. Thus, the entire follicle delineated by the dashed lines is a secondary follicle. The cortex, paracortical area, and medulla are also shown.

becoming relatively depleted of plasma, the arterioles then carry high-hematocrit blood into the filtration beds of the red pulp and marginal zone. As a result, the red pulp and marginal zone beds contain relatively high concentrations of red cells.

THE MARGINAL ZONE

The marginal zone surrounds the PALS and follicles. It is composed of reticulum, which forms a finely meshed filtration bed, serving as a vestibule for much of the blood that flows through the spleen. The marginal zone surrounds the white pulp and merges insensibly into the red pulp. It contains more lymphocytes than the red pulp. These are primarily memory B cells and CD4+ T cells.[28-30] However, like the red pulp, the marginal zone may become congested and clear imperfect and senescent red cells and parasites.

THE RED PULP

The red pulp of the spleen is composed of a reticular meshwork, called the splenic cords of Billroth, and splenic sinuses. This region predominantly contains erythrocytes but has large numbers of macrophages and dendritic cells. There are relatively few lymphocytes and plasma cells in this area.

As the central arteries branch and decrease in size, the PALS also branches and decreases in diameter to but a few cells surrounding the arteriole. The small arteriole finally emerges from its sheath and then terminates in either the marginal zone or the red pulp. Here these vessels are suspended and anchored by adventitial reticular cells in the periarterial beds. They often terminate abruptly as arteriolar capillaries or as vessels with a trumpetlike flare with widened slits called interendothelial slits. The blood flows through these slits into filtration beds composed of large-meshed loculi that open to one another.

The blood in the red pulp and marginal zone drains into venous sinuses that form anastomosing, blind-ending vessels. These venous sinuses actually are specialized postcapillary venules. The endothelial cells are shaped as tapered rods that are stiffened by basal, longitudinal, intermediate cytoskeletal filaments and contractile filaments of actin and myosin. These intracellular contractile filaments can shorten the vein, causing the endothelium to buckle and form interendothelial gaps, favoring transmural passage.

The endothelial cells are attached to a basement membrane. While this appears to be fashioned of fibers, the basement membrane actually is an extracellular membranous wall with large, regular defects that expose considerable basal endothelial surface. This includes the interendothelial slits, through which blood may flow from the filtration bed and into the vein. Ordinarily the interendothelial slits are narrow or even closed unless forced apart by cells in transmural transit or by endothelial contraction.

Splenic arterioles terminate at varied distances from the walls of venous vessels. Blood flowing from arterioles that terminate at the venous vessel wall may flow directly into the splenic vein. However, blood flowing from arterioles that terminate at a distance from a vein must traffic through the spleen. In so doing, the blood either may pass quickly through a nonsinusal venous aperture or slowly through sinusal interendothelial slits and the fibroblast stroma.

The fibroblast stroma contains reticular cells and myofibroblast cells, also called barrier cells.[31] The latter may fuse with each other to form a syncytial membrane that connects the arterial terminals with venous interendothelial slits or apertures. Like other myofibroblasts, these cells contain actin and myosin and may contract, thereby approximating splenic arterial and venous vessels with one another. Thus, the fibroblast stroma may affect the relative proportion of blood that flows through the sinusal interendothelial slits and the stroma itself.

SPLENIC FUNCTION

RED CELL CLEARANCE

Mixed within the stroma of the red pulp and marginal zone are monocytes and macrophages. As the blood passes through the stroma, monocytes may be held on the stroma, where the microenvironment is conducive to their maturation into macrophages and large, dendritic, lysosome-rich phagocytes. These cells may assist the reticular cells in mechanical filtration. More important, these cells have phagocytic activity that allows them to ingest imperfect erythrocytes, store platelets, and remove infectious agents, such as *Plasmodia*, from the circulation. In addition, these cells have nonphagocytic functions, such as the presentation of antigens to T cells or the elaboration of certain cytokines.

Collectively, the anatomy of the spleen allows the marginal zone and red pulp to cull defective erythrocytes. As the blood passes slowly through the sinusal interendothelial slits and the fibroblast stroma, the erythrocytes must undergo alterations in shape to squeeze through the mechanical barrier generated by this filtration compartment. Normal red cells that are supple may pass through readily because the interendothelial slits can open to about 0.5 μm. However, blood cells containing large, rigid inclusions, such as plasmodium-containing erythrocytes, are delayed or sequestered. Moreover, splenic macrophages residing within these filtration beds can sequester erythrocytes that are coated with antibody.

When these filtration beds sequester imperfect red cells, the blood pools inside the spleen, causing stasis and congestion. This stimulates sphincterlike contraction of the distal vein, resulting in proximal plasma transudation that produces a viscous luminal mass of high-hematocrit blood. During episodes of enhanced red cell sequestration, as occur during malarial crises or hemolytic episodes in sickle cell disease, the splenic volume and weight may increase ten- to twenty-fold.[32,33] Although the white pulp may enlarge, particularly in germinal centers, the marginal zones and red pulp become greatly widened with pooled erythrocytes and macrophages in this setting.

SPLENIC IMMUNE FUNCTION

The spleen and its responses to antigens are similar to those of lymph nodes, the major difference being that the spleen is the major site of immune responses to blood-borne antigens, while lymph nodes are involved in responses to antigens in the lymph. Antigens and lymphocytes enter the spleen through the vascular sinusoids, since the spleen lacks high endothelial venules. Upon entry, the lymphocytes home to the white pulp. T cells migrate to the PALS and B cells to the lymphoid nodules. T cells and B cells migrate within these compartments for about 5 and 7 h, respectively. In the absence of an immune response, these cells migrate through a reticulum arranged around the circumference of the central artery.

Upon immune activation in response to antigen, the lymphocytes may remain in the spleen to sustain a primary or secondary immune response. Activation of B cells is initiated in the marginal zones that are adjacent to CD4+ T cells in the PALS. Activated B cells then migrate into germinal centers or into the red pulp.[34] Lymphoid nodules appear and expand by recruiting lymphocytes from the blood and the peripheral zone of the follicles, termed the mantle zone. These cells then proliferate and differentiate in the center of a lymphoid nodule, forming a germinal center.[35] In their path from the marginal zone to the follicles, B cells pass the PALS, where they remain in contact with T lymphocytes for a few hours, allowing ample time for T-B cell interaction in response to antigens. If they are not recruited in an immune response to antigen, both T and B lymphocytes exit the spleen via deep efferent lymphatics, not the splenic veins.

These efferent lymphatics are not distinguished as separate structures within the PALS, being quite thin-walled and often packed with efferent lymphocytes. However, they are important in moving nonreactive lymphocytes out of the spleen and in producing high-hematocrit pulp blood. After leaving the spleen, the efferent lymphocytes become the afferent lymphatics of the perisplenic mesenteric lymph nodes or empty into the thoracic duct. This duct empties into the left subclavian vein, thus returning the lymphocytes to the venous circulation.

LYMPH NODES

The lymphoid nodes are secondary lymphoid tissues. They form part of a network that filters antigens from the interstitial tissue fluid and lymph during its passage from the periphery to the thoracic duct. Thus, the lymph nodes are the primary sites of immune response to tissue antigens.

LYMPH NODE ANATOMY

The lymph nodes are round or kidney-shaped clusters of mononuclear cells that normally are less than 1 cm in diameter. A collagenous capsule surrounds a typical lymph node and has an indentation called the hilus where blood vessels enter and leave.

Lymph nodes typically are present at the branches of the lymphatic vessels and form part of the extensive network of lymphatic channels that extends throughout the body. Several afferent lymphatic channels that drain lymph from regional tissues into the lymph node perforate the capsule of each lymph node. The lymph draining from the node leaves through one efferent lymphatic vessel at the hilus. The lymph from the node, in turn, empties into efferent lymphatic vessels that eventually drain into larger lymphatic channels leading eventually to the thoracic duct. The thoracic duct in turns drains into the left subclavian vein, thus returning lymph into the systemic circulation.

Clusters of lymph nodes are placed strategically in areas that drain various superficial and deep regions of the body, such as the neck, axillae, groin, mediastinum, and abdominal cavity. The lymph nodes that receive lymph that drains from the skin, termed somatic nodes, are superficial. The lymph nodes that receive their lymph from the mucosal surface of the respiratory, digestive, or genitourinary tract, termed visceral nodes, are usually deep within body cavities.

LYMPH NODE STRUCTURE

Beneath the collagenous capsule is the subcapsular sinus, into which the afferent lymphatic channels drain (see Fig. 5-3). This sinus is lined with phagocytic cells. Fibrous trabeculae radiate from the medulla adjacent to the hilus of the node to the subcapsular sinus, thus breaking the node into several follicles, called cortical follicles. These trabeculae, together with the capsule and a network of reticulin fibers, support the various cellular components of the node and serve as the scaffolding for lymphatic spaces, namely, the subcapsular and cortical sinuses. These lymphatic spaces are continuous with medullary sinuses and the solitary efferent lymphatic channel exiting the hilus.

Each cortical follicle contains dense collections of small, mature, recirculating lymphocytes. These consist of a B-cell area (cortex), a T-cell area (paracortex), and a central medulla with cellular cords that contain T cells, B cells, plasma cells, and macrophages. Some follicles contain lightly staining areas of 1- to 2-mm in diameter, called germinal centers. Germinal centers are the specialized sites for the generation of memory B cells and antibody affinity maturation via the process of immunoglobulin variable-region somatic hypermutation.[36,37] Follicles without germinal centers are called primary follicles, and those with germinal centers are called secondary follicles. Primary lymphoid follicles contain nodules that consist predominantly of small, mature, recirculating B lymphocytes.

Within 1 week after antigenic stimulation, secondary follicles develop a germinal center, which contains proliferating B cells and macrophages.[27,38] The small, nonreactive B cells are apparently forced to the periphery of the follicle, where they form a dense follicular mantle. The B cells within the germinal center, on the other hand, are highly activated, typically forming blasts that have abundant cytoplasm and round, cleaved, or convoluted shapes. Follicular dendritic cells also are found within the germinal centers. These cells can trap and retain antigens for months, possibly in the form of immune complexes.[39] The germinal centers of the secondary follicle may gradually regress after the antigenic stimulus is eliminated.

Surrounding the lymphoid follicles of the superficial cortex are sheets of lymphocytes that extend to the deep cortex, the so-called paracortex, that blend into medullary cords of cells. The paracortical zones are formed mostly of T cells. The ratio of T cells to B cells in these zones is about 3:1. The medulla, however, contains scattered B cells, dendritic cells, macrophages, and, during an immune response, plasma cells. The superficial cortex and medulla of the lymph nodes are the thymic-independent areas, while the deep cortex is particularly enriched with T cells, forming an area that sometimes is referred to as the thymic-dependent area. The major T-cell population found within the lymph node consists of CD4+ T cells. The scattering of CD4+ T cells in the follicles, and in more prominent numbers in the interfollicular zones, reveals the proximity of CD4+ T and B cells important for T-B cooperation during proliferation and maturation of antigen-stimulated B cells.[40]

Lymphocytes primarily enter lymphatic tissues from the blood by migrating across the tall, active endothelium of specialized post-capillary venules called high endothelial venules.[41] Cellular adhesion molecules and various chemokines are responsible for the pattern of lymphocyte trafficking and determine the microanatomy of the lymphoid tissues.[42]

LYMPH NODE FUNCTION

The lymph node is the site where different types of lymphocytes, macrophages, and dendritic cells can interact with one another to generate an immune response to antigens carried within the lymph. As the lymph passes across the nodes from afferent to efferent lymphatic vessels, particulate antigens are removed by the phagocytic cells and transported into the lymphoid tissue of the lymph node. Abnormal cells within the lymph, such as neoplastic cells, also can be trapped within the lymph node.

Within the lymph node, antigen is presented to T cells as processed peptides by MHC molecules of antigen-presenting cells (see Chap. 84). Various T-cell subsets comprise a network of interactive cells. CD4+ and CD8+ cell-mediated contacts, as well as T cell–derived soluble factors, induce and regulate the immune response (see Chap. 15). T-cell recognition is mediated by the TCR for antigen (see Chap. 84). Which T cells are activated is determined by the specificity of the TCRs (see Chap. 86), the structure of MHC molecules, and the nature of antigen-presenting cells, including the dendritic reticular cells, macrophages, and B cells.

However, along with TCR recognition of processed antigen presented in the MHC of the antigen-presenting cell, adequate T-cell activation requires second signals, or costimulation, delivered through accessory molecules, such as CD28 on T cells (see Chap. 84).[43] Without these second signals, the T cells may become anergic, or specifically nonresponsive to antigen stimulation. This specific suppression is thought to play an important regulatory role in the maintenance of self-tolerance.[44,45]

T-cell recognition of specific antigen may induce release of soluble factors, such as the interleukins, that can activate T cells, B cells, and/or monocytes.[46–49] Also, the activated T cells express surface molecules, such as CD40 ligand, that also can activate B cells, dendritic cells, or macrophages.[50,51]

The T-dependent immune response includes the formation of early germinal centers within days after antigen exposure. There is a mixture of B cells and activated CD4+ T cells in the lymphoid follicles. T-B cooperation involves the accessory B-cell antigen CD40 and the CD40 ligand expressed on activated T cells (see Chap. 15). Activated B cells become blasts and comprise the largest numbers of cells in the early germinal center.[27] Subsequently, B-cell blasts give rise to smaller B cells, the centrocytes. B cells undergo affinity maturation within the germinal center. During this process, the genes encoding the surface immunoglobulin of B cells undergo high rates of mutation, called somatic hypermutation.[35,52] B cells, including the centrocytes, that express immunoglobulin with little or no affinity for antigen undergo apoptosis.[53] The resulting cellular debris is tingible, or capable of being stained, and is found prominently within macrophages specifically designated tingible body macrophages. On the other hand, B cells expressing surface immunoglobulin with high affinity for antigen

are selected to proliferate and differentiate to memory B cells or plasma cells.[38] As well as promoting activation of B cells, CD4+ T cells, and CD8+ T cells, the T-cell limb of the primary immune response may generate circulating CD4+ and CD8+ memory T cells.[54,55]

Following release of specific antibody, antigen-antibody complexes may form and become sequestered on the surface of follicular dendritic cells within the germinal centers. These antigen-antibody complexes produce a coating of small, beadlike, immune complex–coated bodies called iccosomes. Iccosomes may be presented to CD4+ T cells by B cells and dendritic cells. Iccosomes also appear to assist in anamnestic recall of high levels of antibody following reentry of antigen in the host.[56] T-cell and B-cell memory functions and self-tolerance depend upon persistence of antigen.[54,57–59]

PERIPHERAL LYMPHOID TISSUES

MUCOSA-ASSOCIATED LYMPHOID TISSUES

The MALT are diffusely organized aggregates of lymphocytes that protect the respiratory and gastrointestinal epithelium. The lymphoid aggregates associated with the respiratory epithelium are sometimes referred to as the bronchial-associated lymphoid tissue. The lymphoid aggregates associated with the intestinal epithelium are sometimes referred to as the gut-associated lymphoid tissue.[60] These tissues include the tonsils, adenoids, appendix, and specialized structures called Peyer's patches found in the ileum, and they collect antigen from the epithelial surfaces of the gastrointestinal tract.

Solitary lymph nodules with follicular and germinal center structures occur in the mucosa and submucosa of the respiratory tract, the gastrointestinal tract (particularly within the ileum), the urinary tract, and the vagina. During states of chronic inflammation, lymphoid nodules may form as a localized center of lymphocytes with marked follicular activity. Waldeyer's ring of pharyngeal lymphoid tissues and Peyer's patches in the ileum contain prominent aggregated nodular lymphoid tissue. No capsule or efferent or afferent lymphatic vessels are present in these accessory lymphoid tissues.

These MALT are rich in plasma cells and eosinophils. The plasma cells are a source of secretory immunoglobulin that is transferred into the lumina of the bronchi and gastrointestinal tract. The majority of plasma cells in the mucosa of the bronchi and gut contain IgA. IgA is released from the plasma cell and then combines with a secretory piece synthesized within the mucosal epithelium to become secretory IgA (see Chap. 83). Secretory IgA then is secreted across the microvilli of mucosal epithelium into the lumen, where it may prevent colonization of mucosal membranes by pathogens. Lymphoid nodules along mucosa-lined tracts serve as precursors of IgA-producing cells. These nodules form a barrier against many microorganisms and antigens. Microfolds overlying specialized epithelial cells in the gut transport antigenic material by pinocytosis, with subsequent immunization and IgA secretion.

PEYER'S PATCHES

Peyer's patches are the most important and highly organized of the gut-associated lymphoid tissues. They are found in the lamina propria of the small intestine (beneath the mucosa near the ileocolonic junction) and consist of up to 50 or more lymphoid nodules covered by a single layer of columnar epithelium. They are well developed in youth and regress with age. Antigens from the intestinal epithelium are collected by specialized epithelial cells called M cells, allowing for generation of specific immune responses against intestinal pathogens.[61] Peyer's patches are the sites at which B cells differentiate, in response to these antigens, into the plasma cells found within the intestine.[62]

TONSILS

The tonsils are the major component of Waldeyer's ring of pharyngeal lymphoid tissues. They are covered by variable epithelial surfaces that have deep, branching depressions called crypts. Fused lymphatic nodules lie adjacent to the crypts, and germinal centers are prominent. A pseudocapsule of condensed connective tissue surrounds the tonsils, and septae within the structures form lobulations. Together with the other lymphoid tissues of Waldeyer's ring, the tonsils provide the initial barrier to pathogens entering the oral pharynx.

REFERENCES

1. Hasselbalch H, Jeppesen DL, Ersbøll AK, Engelmann MD, Nielsen MB: Thymus size evaluated by sonography: A longitudinal study on infants during the first year of life. *Acta Radiol* 38:222, 1997.

2. Pawelec G, Adibzadeh M, Solana R, Beckman I: The T cell in the ageing individual. *Mech Ageing Dev* 93:35, 1997.

3. Haynes BF, Hale LP: The human thymus: A chimeric organ comprised of central and peripheral lymphoid components *Immunol Res* 18:175, 1998.

4. Hasselbalch H, Jeppesen DL, Ersbøll AK, Lisse IM, Nielsen MB: Sonographic measurement of thymic size in healthy neonates: Relation to clinical variables. *Acta Radiol* 38:95, 1997.

5. Hasselbalch H, Jeppesen DL, Engelmann MD, Michaelsen KF, Nielsen MB: Decreased thymus size in formula-fed infants compared with breastfed infants. *Acta Paediatr* 85:1029, 1996.

6. Röpke C: Thymic epithelial cell culture. *Microsc Res Tech* 38:276, 1997.

7. Cifone MG, Migliorati G, Parroni R, et al: Dexamethasone-induced thymocyte apoptosis: Apoptotic signal involves the sequential activation of phosphoinositide-specific phospholipase C, acidic sphingomyelinase, and capsases. *Blood* 93:2282, 1999.

8. Rijhsinghani AG, Thompson K, Bhatia SK, Waldschmidt TJ: Estrogen blocks early T cell development in the thymus. *Am J Reprod Immunol* 36:269, 1996.

9. Ayala A, Herdon CD, Lehman DL, Ayala CA, Chaudry IH: Differential induction of apoptosis in lymphoid tissues during sepsis: Variation in onset, frequency, and the nature of the mediators. *Blood* 87:4261, 1996.

10. Laufer TM, Glimcher LH, Lo D: Using thymus anatomy to dissect T cell repertoire selection. *Semin Immunol* 11:65, 1999.

11. Blackman M, Kappler J, Marrack P: The role of the T cell receptor in positive and negative selection of developing T cells. *Science* 248:1335, 1990.

12. Müller-Hermelink HK, Wilisch A, Schultz A, Marx A: Characterization of the human thymic microenvironment: Lymphoepithelial interaction in normal thymus and thymoma. *Arch Histol Cytol* 60:9, 1997.

13. Takahama Y, Shores EW, Singer A: Negative selection of precursor thymocytes before their differentiation into CD4+CD8+ cells. *Science* 258:653, 1992.

14. Oukka M, Colucci-Guyon E, Tran PL, et al: CD4 T cell tolerance to nuclear proteins induced by medullary thymic epithelium. *Immunity* 4:545, 1996.

15. Romero-Torres R: The true splenic blood supply and its surgical applications. *Hepato-Gastroenterology* 45:885, 1998.

16. Paul R, Bielmeier J, Breul J, Nathrath WBJ, Hartung R: Accessory spleen of the spermatic cord. *Urol Ausg A* 36:262, 1997.

17. Takayama T, Shimada K, Inoue K, Wakao F, Yamamoto J, Kosuge T: Intrapancreatic accessory spleen. *Lancet* 344:957, 1994.

18. Harris GN, Kase DJ, Bradnock H, McKinley MJ: Accessory spleen causing a mass in the tail of the pancreas: MR imaging findings. *Am J Roentgenol* 163:1120, 1994.

19. Ota T, Tei M, Yoshioka A, et al: Intrapancreatic accessory spleen diagnosed by technetium-99m heat-damaged red blood cell SPECT. *J Nucl Med* 38:494, 1997.

20. Churei H, Inoue H, Nakajo M: Intrapancreatic accessory spleen: Case report. *Abdom Imaging* 23:191, 1998.

21. Lauffer JM, Baer HU, Maurer CA, Wagner M, Zimmermann A, Buchler MW: Intrapancreatic accessory spleen: A rare cause of a pancreatic mass. *Int J Pancreatol* 25:65, 1999.

22. Sprogøe-Jakobsen S, Sprogøe-Jakobsen U: The weight of the normal spleen. *Forensic Sci Int* 88:215, 1997.

23. Prassopoulos P, Daskalogiannaki M, Raissaki M, Hatjidakis A, Gourtsoyiannis N: Determination of normal splenic volume on computed tomography in relation to age, gender, and body habitus. *Eur Radiol* 7:246, 1997.

24. Watanabe Y, Todani T, Noda T, Yamamoto S: Standard splenic volume in children and young adults measured from CT images. *Surg Today* 27:726, 1997.

25. Rodrigues Júnior AJ, Rodrigues CJ, Germano MA, Rasera Júnior I, Cerri GG: Sonographic assessment of normal spleen volume. *Clin Anat* 8:252, 1995.

26. Weiss L: The cell: The blood and hematopoietic tissues, in *Histology: Cell and Tissue Biology,* 6th ed, p 3. Urban & Schwarzenburg, Baltimore, 1988.

27. Tarlinton D: Germinal centers: Form and function. *Curr Opin Immunol* 10:245, 1998.

28. Dunn-Walters DK, Isaacson PG, Spencer J: Analysis of mutations in immunoglobulin heavy chain variable region genes of microdissected marginal zone (MgZ) B cells suggests that the MgZ of human spleen is a reservoir of memory B cells. *J Exp Med* 182:559, 1995.

29. Spencer J, Perry ME, Dunn-Walters DK: Human marginal-zone B cells. *Immunol Today* 19:421, 1998.

30. Tierens A, Delabie J, Michiels L, Vandenberghe P, De Wolf-Peeters C: Marginal-zone B cells in the human lymph node and spleen show somatic hypermutations and display clonal expansion. *Blood* 93:226, 1999.

31. Weiss L: Barrier cells in the spleen. *Immunol Today* 12:24, 1991.

32. Weiss L, Geduldig U, Weidanz W: Mechanisms of splenic control of murine malaria: Reticular cell activation and the development of a blood-spleen barrier. *Am J Anat* 176:251, 1986.

33. Smith NC, Fell A, Good MF: The immune response to asexual blood stages of malaria parasites. *Chem Immunol* 70:144, 1998.

34. Rizzo LV, Secord EA, Tsiagbe VK, et al: Components essential for the generation of germinal centers. *Dev Immunol* 6:325, 1998.

35. Hollowood K, Goodlad JR: Germinal centre cell kinetics. *J Pathol* 185:229, 1998.

36. Varade WS, Insel RA: Isolation of germinal center-like events from human spleen RNA: Somatic hypermutation of a clonally related V_H6DJ_H rearrangement expressed with IgM, IgG, and IgA. *J Clin Invest* 91:1838, 1993.

37. Han S, Zheng B, Takahashi Y, Kelsoe G: Distinctive characteristics of germinal center B cells. *Semin Immunol* 9:255, 1997.

38. Przylepa J, Himes C, Kelsoe G: Lymphocyte development and selection in germinal centers. *Curr Top Microbiol Immunol* 229:85, 1998.

39. Burton GF, Masuda A, Heath SL, Smith BA, Tew JG, Szakal AK: Follicular dendritic cells (FDC) in retroviral infection: Host/pathogen perspectives. *Immunol Rev* 156:185, 1997.

40. Gulbranson-Judge A, Casamayor-Palleja M, MacLennan IC: Mutually dependent T and B cell responses in germinal centers. *Ann NY Acad Sci* 815:199, 1997.

41. Butcher EC, Williams M, Youngman K, Rott L, Briskin M: Lymphocyte trafficking and regional immunity. *Adv Immunol* 72:209, 1999.

42. Warnock RA, Askari S, Butcher EC, von Andrian UH: Molecular mechanisms of lymphocyte homing to peripheral lymph nodes. *J Exp Med* 187:205, 1998.

43. Greenfield EA, Nguyen KA, Kuchroo VK: CD28/B7 costimulation: A review. *Crit Rev Immunol* 18:389, 1998.

44. Van Parijs L, Abbas AK: Homeostasis and self-tolerance in the immune system: Turning lymphocytes off. *Science* 280:243, 1998.

45. Malvey EN, Telander DG, Vanasek TL, Mueller DL: The role of clonal anergy in the avoidance of autoimmunity: Inactivation of autocrine growth without loss of effector function. *Immunol Rev* 165:301, 1998.

46. Mosmann TR, Li L, Hengartner H, Kagi D, Fu W, Sad S: Differentiation and functions of T cell subsets. *Ciba Found Symp* 204:148, 1997.

47. Mosmann TR, Li L, Sad S: Functions of CD8 T-cell subsets secreting different cytokine patterns. *Semin Immunol* 9:87, 1997.

48. Takatsu K: Cytokines involved in B-cell differentiation and their sites of action. *Proc Soc Exp Biol Med* 215:121, 1997.

49. Seder RA, Gazzinelli RT: Cytokines are critical in linking the innate and adaptive immune responses to bacterial, fungal, and parasitic infection. *Adv Intern Med* 44:353, 1999.

50. Grewal IS, Flavell RA: CD40 and CD154 in cell-mediated immunity. *Annu Rev Immunol* 16:111, 1998.

51. van Kooten C, Banchereau J: Functions of CD40 on B cells, dendritic cells and other cells. *Curr Opin Immunol* 9:330, 1997.

52. Vora KA, Ravetch JV, Manser T: Insights into the mechanisms of antibody-affinity maturation and the generation of the memory B-cell compartment using genetically altered mice. *Dev Immunol* 6:305, 1998.

53. Liu YJ, de Bouteiller O, Fugier-Vivier I: Mechanisms of selection and differentiation in germinal centers. *Curr Opin Immunol* 9:256, 1997.

54. Doherty PC, Topham DJ, Tripp RA: Establishment and persistence of virus-specific CD4+ and CD8+ T cell memory. *Immunol Rev* 150:23, 1996.

55. Callan MF, Annels N, Steven N, et al: T cell selection during the evolution of CD8+ T cell memory in vivo. *Eur J Immunol* 28:4382, 1998.

56. Liu YJ, Grouard G, de Bouteiller O, Banchereau J: Follicular dendritic cells and germinal centers. *Int Rev Cytol* 166:139, 1996.

57. Choe J, Kim HS, Armitage RJ, Choi YS: The functional role of B cell antigen receptor stimulation and IL-4 in the generation of human memory B cells from germinal center B cells. *J Immunol* 159:3757, 1997.

58. Freitas AA, Rocha B: Peripheral T cell survival. *Curr Opin Immunol* 11:152, 1999.

59. Slifka MK, Ahmed R: Long-lived plasma cells: A mechanism for maintaining persistent antibody production. *Curr Opin Immunol* 10:252, 1998.

60. Isaacson PG, Spencer J: Low-grade B-cell lymphoma of gut-associated lymphoid tissue (GALT): A model of the structure and migration pathways of the B-cell component of normal human GALT. *Digestion* 46:274, 1990.

61. Porta C, James PS, Phillips AD, Savidge TC, Smith MW, Cremaschi D: Confocal analysis of fluorescent bead uptake by mouse Peyer patch follicle-associated M-cells. *Exp Physiol* 77:929, 1992.

62. Dunn-Walters DK, Isaacson PG, Spencer J: Sequence analysis of human IgV(H) genes indicates that ileal lamina propria plasma cells are derived from Peyer's patches. *Eur J Immunol* 27:463, 1997.

THE INFLAMMATORY RESPONSE

JEFFREY S. WARREN

PETER A. WARD

The inflammatory response is characterized by a series of events that encompass a rapid and relatively short-lived increase in local blood flow, an increase in microvascular permeability, and the sequential recruitment of different types of leukocytes. Superimposed upon the inflammatory response is a series of reparative processes (e.g., parenchymal regeneration, angiogenesis, production of extracellular matrix material, and scar formation). Early hemodynamic changes at a site of an inflammation establish conditions that enable marginated leukocytes to engage in low-affinity selectin-mediated rolling interactions with endothelial cells. In response to locally produced soluble and cell surface mediators, endothelial cells and rolling leukocytes become activated and sequentially express several sets of complementary adhesion molecules which include β_2 integrins, members of the selectin family, and members of the immunoglobulin superfamily. Leukocyte and endothelial cell adhesion molecules mediate the high-affinity adhesive interactions necessary for leukocyte emigration from the vascular space and across specific chemotactic gradients. Analogous, temporally regulated soluble mediators and cellular adhesion molecules also orchestrate the monocyte- and lymphocyte-rich chronic inflammatory response. This basic paradigm is modulated by a large number of surface-active and soluble inflammatory mediators which include vasoactive amines and lipids, reactive oxygen and nitrogen intermediates, cytokines, chemokines, and many plasma proteins (e.g., complement system, kinins, and coagulation cascade).

HISTORY

The sentinel clinical features of acute inflammation, rubor, calor, tumor, and dolor, have been recognized for at least five thousand years. Dr. John Hunter, the renowned late eighteenth century Scottish surgeon, observed that the inflammatory response is not a disease *per se* but rather a nonspecific and salutary response to a variety of insults. Through his microscopic examinations of transparent vital membrane preparations, Julius Cohnheim concluded that the inflammatory response is fundamentally a vascular phenomenon. Leukocytic phagocytosis was discovered late in the nineteenth century by Eli Metchnikoff and his colleagues. Morphologic studies, using both live animals and fixed histologic preparations, transformed our understanding of inflammation and led to the currently held concepts of inflammation-associated hemodynamic alterations, "acute" inflammation, and "chronic" inflammation.[1] It has been during the past thirty to forty years that the modern techniques of biochemistry (e.g., protein and lipid purification and the measurements of reactive oxygen and nitrogen species), tissue culture, monoclonal antibody production, recombinant DNA technology, and the genetic manipulation of isolated cells and whole animals, have enabled a more detailed understanding of the cellular and molecular mechanisms which characterize the inflammatory response. These studies, in concert with "experiments of nature" such as chronic granulomatous disease (see Chaps. 67 and 72) and the leukocyte adhesion deficiency disorders (see Chap. 72), have provided for the formulation of complex, yet elegant, models of acute and chronic inflammation and the development of incisive therapeutic approaches that promise to exploit this knowledge. A vast array of human diseases is marked by either defects in the development of the inflammatory response or the deleterious effects of the inflammatory response itself.

GENERAL CHARACTERISTICS OF INFLAMMATION

While necessarily contrived, it remains useful to consider inflammation as an acute or chronic process. "Acute" inflammation lasts from minutes to several days and is characterized by local hemodynamic and microvascular changes and leukocyte accumulation.[2] The acute inflammatory response is consistently marked by microvascular leakage and the accumulation of neutrophils. The four cardinal signs of inflammation, alluded to above, can be accounted for within the physiologic terms of acute inflammation.

In contrast, the chronic inflammatory response lasts much longer and is more varied in its effects.[2] Cellular infiltrates are composed primarily of lymphocytes and monocytes but there are many variations in the cellular composition, anatomic distribution, and tempo of development of chronic inflammatory lesions. The chronic inflammatory response is also marked by the proliferation of resident fibroblasts and the growth of new capillaries. Chronic inflammatory processes are classified according to these variations. For example, granulomatous inflammation is a chronic process marked by nodular aggregates of mononuclear phagocytes that have become "transformed" into so-called epithelioid histiocytes because of their similar appearance to epithelial cells. In many cases there are accompanying multinucleate giant cells. Granulomas may be distributed along blood vessels (e.g., angiocentric), along airways (e.g., bronchocentric), or randomly throughout the interstitium or parenchyma of an organ. Some chronic inflammatory processes are marked by the appearance of plasma cells or eosinophils.

Superimposed upon the acute and chronic inflammatory response is repair.[2] Repair may entail the regeneration of parenchymal cells damaged as the result of an insult *per se* or damaged secondary to the inflammatory response to the insult. Repair is characterized by the growth of new capillaries (angiogenesis) and the activation of fibroblasts which produce extracellular matrix molecules (e.g., scar tissue). In some circumstances an acute inflammatory response is self-contained and nonprogressive. In other situations the response progresses to a chronic process which can persist for years (e.g., tuberculous granulomas).

Acronyms and abbreviations that appear in this chapter include: cGMP, cyclic guanosine 3,5-monophosphate; EDRF, endothelium-derived relaxing factor; ELAM-1, endothelial cell leukocyte adhesion molecule-1; GMP-140, granule membrane protein-140; 5-HPETE, 5-hydroperoxyeicosatetraenoic acid; ICAM-1, intercellular adhesion molecule-1; ICAM-2, intercellular adhesion molecule-2; ICAM-3, intercellular adhesion molecule-3; IFN-γ, interferon-γ; IL-1, interleukin-1; IL-6, interleukin-6; IL-8, interleukin-8; IL-β, interleukin-β; γ-IP-10, γ-interferon-inducible protein; LAM-1, leukocyte adhesion molecule-1; LTB$_4$, leukotriene B$_4$; LTC$_4$, leukotriene C$_4$; LTD$_4$, leukotriene D$_4$; LDE$_4$, leukotriene E$_4$; LFA-1, lymphocyte function-associated antigen-1; MCP-1, monocyte chemoattractant protein-1; MGSA (or GROα), melanocyte growth-stimulatory activity; MIP-1α, macrophage inflammatory protein-1α; MIP-1β, macrophage inflammatory protein-1β; NADPH, reduced nicotinamide adenine dinucleotide phosphate; NOS, nitric oxide synthase; PAF, platelet-activating factor; PECAM-1, platelet endothelial cell adhesion molecule; PF4, platelet factor 4; RANTES, regulated upon activation, normal T cell expressed and presumably secreted; RGD; TNF-α, tumor necrosis factor-α; VCAM-1, vascular cell adhesion molecule-1; VLA-4, very late antigen 4.

This chapter will first address acute inflammation, which encompasses localized changes in blood flow, alterations in microvascular permeability, and neutrophil exudation. There has been a rapid advance in understanding of the processes of endothelial cell activation, leukocyte-endothelial cell rolling and adhesive interactions, leukocyte emigration, and leukocyte activation. The second section of this chapter will introduce the vast array of soluble and surface-active mediators that orchestrate both acute and chronic inflammatory responses. These mediators include substances that range from short-lived reactive oxygen and nitrogen intermediates to entire regulatory systems (e.g., complement system and coagulation cascade). Finally, a brief overview of chronic inflammation and tissue repair will be provided. The goal of this chapter is to provide a framework for understanding the basic processes of inflammation while gaining an appreciation for the highly complex and integrated nature of the regulated inflammatory response.

ACUTE INFLAMMATION

HEMODYNAMIC CHANGES

The hemodynamic changes that occur early in the acute phase of inflammation include arteriolar vasodilatation and localized increases in microvascular permeability. In many but not all circumstances arteriolar vasodilatation follows a rapidly developing (within seconds) and brief (seconds) period of vasoconstriction.[3] Arteriolar vasodilation results in increased blood flow, thus explaining the familiar redness and warmth which characterize a site of acute inflammation. The increase in blood flow, coupled with increases in microvascular permeability, results in hemoconcentration and increased local viscosity. These localized hemodynamic changes are critical to subsequent leukocyte emigration because selectin-mediated low-affinity rolling leukocyte-endothelial adhesive interactions can efficiently occur only under such conditions of low shear force (see below). Experimental studies using in vitro flow chambers and live animals indicate that selectin-mediated leukocyte-endothelial rolling adhesive interactions cannot occur in the face of the shear forces exerted by normal blood flow. Increased microvascular permeability leads to the exudation of protein-rich plasma which is a fundamental characteristic of acute inflammation. Microvascular leakage occurs through a variety of mechanisms that include venular endothelial cell contraction, which is accompanied by widening of intercellular junctions; so-called endothelial cell retraction, which is not well understood but involves cytoskeletal changes; leukocyte-mediated endothelial cell injury; direct endothelial injury; and leakage via new capillaries which do not yet possess fully "closed" intercellular junctions.[4,5] Increases in rate of transcytosis in which plasma constituents cross endothelial cells in vesicles or vacuoles have a role in neoplastic blood vessels and may play a role in inflammation.[6] Alterations in local blood flow occur at the level of arterioles which are regulated largely by the autonomic nervous system, vasoactive peptides, and eicosanoids. A variety of soluble mediators [e.g., histamine, leukotrienes, complement components C3a and C5a, interleukin-1, tumor necrosis factor-α (TNF-α), and interferon-γ (IFN-γ)] can induce increases in microvascular permeability through several of the above-mentioned mechanisms.

LEUKOCYTE RECRUITMENT

The orchestrated recruitment of leukocytes into a site of inflammation is a fundamental characteristic of the inflammatory response.[6] The importance of white blood cells in host defense is highlighted in patients with genetic defects in white blood cell function [e.g., absence respiratory burst in patients with chronic granulomatous disease (Chap. 67) and diminished leukocyte emigration in patients with leukocyte

adhesion deficiency (Chap. 72)]. Leukocytes are critical because of their central role in the phagocytosis and containment or killing of microbes and in the digestion of necrotic tissue debris. Leukocyte-derived products such as proteolytic enzymes and reactive oxygen intermediates contribute to tissue injury.

Leukocyte Adhesion and Transmigration

When vascular stasis occurs as the result of the hemodynamic changes of early acute inflammation, leukocytes are pushed from the central axial column of blood cells to a position along the endothelial surface. This process, called margination, occurs under conditions of slow blood flow.[2] Individual leukocytes adhere transiently and weakly to the endothelial surface. Studies using vital membrane preparations and flow chamber studies using endothelial cell monolayers and suspensions of purified leukocytes have revealed that cells roll along the endothelial surface.[6-13] Rolling neutrophil-endothelial adhesive interactions occur early (minutes) after the initiation of an acute inflammatory response and can, depending upon the time within the evolution of an inflammatory response, involve neutrophils, lymphocytes, monocytes, basophils, or eosinophils. The leukocyte-endothelial cell rolling adhesive interaction is a specific and necessary step that precedes tight adhesion and emigration.[10] Studies indicate that early rolling adhesive interactions are mediated largely by selectins.[11] In turn, the cell surface expression of selectins (and other intercellular adhesion molecules, see below) is regulated by a number of locally produced proinflammatory mediators.[6-13]

Selectins contain a C-terminal cytoplasmic tail, a lipophilic transmembrane domain, a series of complement regulatory domains, an epidermal growth factor–like domain, and an extracellular N-terminal carbohydrate-binding region which is homologous to mammalian lectins (Table 6-1).[9-13] P-selectin (previously known as GMP-140) is expressed by endothelial cells and platelets, E-selectin (formerly ELAM-1) by endothelial cells, and L-selectin (also known as LAM-1) by most white blood cells. P-selectin is stored in endothelial intracytoplasmic granules called Weibel-Palade bodies.[14,15] When endothelial cells are exposed to histamine, thrombin, or platelet-activating factor, P-selectin is rapidly (minutes) translocated to the endothelial surface where it engages marginated leukocytes via carbohydrate moieties that contain sialic acid residues (e.g., sialyl Lewis^X glycoprotein).[9-13] This transient, low-affinity binding interaction which can withstand only the low-flow shear force conditions found in stasis, accounts in part for the early rolling leukocyte-endothelial cell adhesive interactions (Fig. 6-1). Exposure of endothelial cells to TNF-α or IL-β results in protein synthesis–dependent expression of E-selectin, a response that occurs within 1–2 hours and peaks at 4–6 hours.[16,17] As in the case of P-selectin–mediated leukocyte adhesion, E-selectin–mediated adhesion occurs via a series of sialylated and fucosylated carbohydrate moieties related to the sialyl Lewis^X (SLe^X) and sialyl Lewis^A (SLe^A) blood group antigens on leukocytes (Table 6-1).[13,18] L-selectin is constitutively expressed by leukocytes, participates in white blood cell-endothelial cell adhesive interactions via mucin-like glycoproteins (e.g., CD34, GlyCAM), and is shed when the leukocyte is activated (Table 6-1).[9,19] It is believed that L-selectin shedding facilitates leukocyte emigration by allowing the white blood cell to detach from the endothelium. Low-affinity rolling adhesive interactions set the stage for β-integrin and immunoglobulin superfamily-mediated high-affinity adhesive interactions and leukocyte transmigration.[10]

Relatively weak selectin-mediated and high-affinity adhesive interactions are not temporally or mechanistically discrete. For example, TNF-α and IL-β induce both E-selectin, which is not expressed by quiescent cells, and increases in endothelial expression of ICAM-1 and VCAM-1, which are constitutively expressed in low concentrations and are involved in the recruitment of all types of leukocytes in the

TABLE 6-1   ADHESION MOLECULES IN INFLAMMATION

FAMILY	STRUCTURE	MEMBERS	TISSUE DISTRIBUTION	COUNTERRECEPTOR
Selectin	N-terminal lectin domain, epidermal growth factor domain, multiple complement regulatory repeats, transmembrane, and short cytoplasmic tail	P-selectin E-selectin L-selectin	Endothelium, platelets Endothelium Leukocytes	Sle^X glycoprotein, others? Sle^X glycoprotein, others? Mucin-like: GlyCAM-1, CD34
Immunoglobulin superfamily	Multiple immunoglobulin domains, transmembrane region and cytoplasmic tail	ICAM-1 ICAM-2 ICAM-3	Endothelium	CD11a/CD18 CD11b/CD18
		VCAM-1	Endothelium	VLA-4
Integrins	Heterodimers: distinct α subunits with common β subunits	CD11a/CD18 (LFA-1)	Neutrophils, monocytes, macrophages, and lymphocytes	ICAM-1 ICAM-2 ICAM-3
		CD11b/CD18 (Mac-1)	Neutrophils, monocytes, and macrophages	ICAM-1, iC3b, LPS, and fibronectin
		VLA-4	Monocytes, lymphocytes	VCAM-1 and fibronectin

case of ICAM-1, and chronic inflammatory leukocytes (lymphocytes, monocytes, eosinophils, and basophils) in the case of VCAM-1.[6–12,20] Intercellular adhesion molecule-1 binds to β_2 (leukocyte) integrins (e.g., CD11a/CD18, CD11b/CD18) and VCAM-1 binds to β_1 integrins (e.g., VLA-4/$\alpha 4\beta 1$) (Table 6-1).[21] It is believed that activated endothelial cells secrete such mediators as platelet-activating factor and IL-8 which in turn activate overlying leukocytes.[6] Leukocyte CD11a/CD18 (LFA-1) undergoes a conformational change by which there is an increase in its binding affinity for endothelial ICAM-1. The β_2 integrins are heterodimeric structures which contain varied alpha chains (CD11a, CD11b, CD11c) and a common beta chain (CD18).[21] The role of CD11c/CD18 is less clearcut than those of CD11a/CD18 and CD11b/CD18. Intercellular adhesion molecules (ICAM-1, ICAM-2, ICAM-3) are found on a variety of cell types aside from endothelial cells.[22–24] CD11a/CD18 interacts with both ICAM-1 and ICAM-2 while CD11b/CD18 binds to ICAM-2 and the complement activation product, iC3b (see below). The role of ICAM-3 in leukocyte-endothelial adhesion is less well established. β_1 integrins, notably VLA-4, are found primarily on chronic inflammatory leukocytes (e.g., lymphocytes, monocytes, basophils, and eosinophils) and mediate leukocyte binding via VCAM-1.[25–27] β_1-integrin–mediated adhesive interactions occur via RGD amino acid sequences within VCAM-1 as well as other molecules (e.g., fibronectin). β_2 integrin-ICAM and β_1-VCAM-1–mediated adhesive interactions occur later (hours-days) in the inflammatory response than do selectin-mediated interactions. Studies indicate that additional adhesive interactions are also involved in leukocyte transmigration [e.g., CD31 or PECAM-1 (platelet endothelial cell adhesion molecule)].[28] The functional importance of the various complementary leukocyte-endothelial adhesive interactions has been clarified by in vitro leukocyte-endothelial binding studies and in vivo studies that have employed neutralizing antibodies directed against adhesion molecules, pharmacologic antagonists of adhesion molecules, and knockout mice.[29–31] The functional importance of leukocyte integrins (CD11a/CD18, CD11b/CD18, CD11c/CD18) has also been highlighted by clinical and experimental observations in patients with leukocyte adhesion deficiencies (see Chap. 72).[32]

LEUKOCYTE CHEMOTAXIS AND ACTIVATION

Leukocytes that are tightly bound to endothelium emigrate from the vascular space into the interstitium by extending pseudopods between intercellular junctions (Fig. 6-1). Secreted specific granule proteases play a role in the passage or ''invasion'' of leukocytes through subendothelial extracellular matrix material (e.g., basement membrane). Leukocyte emigration and movement through the interstitium is facilitated by binding interactions between leukocyte integrins and complementary sites on extracellular matrix molecules (e.g., fibronectin).[33] A wide variety of soluble mediators can provide the motive force (chemotaxis) for this process.[34] Chemotactic factors for neutrophils include peptides derived from bacteria (e.g., N-formyl-methionyl peptides), complement-derived peptides (e.g., C5a, see below), chemotactic lipids [e.g., leukotriene B4 (LTB$_4$) and others, see below], and locally produced cytokines (e.g., TNF-α and IL-1β) and chemokines (e.g., IL-8, see below). Chemotactic factors vary with respect to their specificity for different types of leukocytes. For example, C5a and N-formyl peptides both induce neutrophil and monocyte chemotaxis, IL-8 induces neutrophil chemotaxis, and monocyte chemoattractant protein-1 (MCP-1) induces chemotactic responses in monocytes and a specific subset of memory T lymphocytes. Each of these chemotactic factors activates ''target'' cells by engaging specific, cell surface receptors which in turn are linked to the contractile cell motility apparatus (e.g., microfilament proteins such as myosin and actin, and actin-regulating proteins such as gelsolin, filamen, profilin, and calmodulin) via complex signal-transduction pathways.[33,34] In addition to chemotaxis, soluble and cell surface mediators induce leukocyte activation which is manifested by a wide array of changes in cellular function (e.g., adhesion molecule upregulation and increased adhesion molecule binding avidity (e.g., CD11a/CD18), selectin shedding (e.g., L-selectin), lysosome degranulation, and initiation of the respiratory burst). There have been great advances in understanding of the biochemical pathways involved in chemotaxis and cell activation. While there are many nuances in the signal-transduction pathways involved

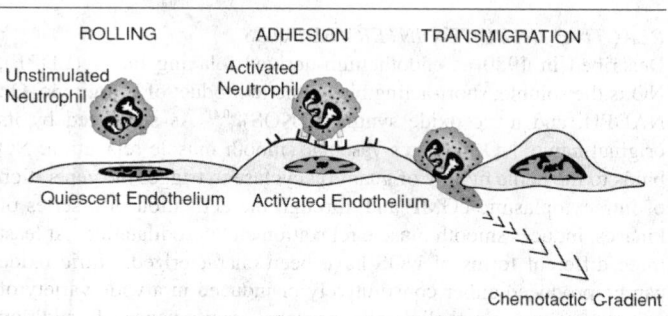

ROLLING   ADHESION   TRANSMIGRATION

Unstimulated Neutrophil

Activated Neutrophil

Quiescent Endothelium   Activated Endothelium

Chemotactic Gradient

FIGURE 6-1   Leukocyte-endothelial adhesive interactions. Early in the acute inflammatory response, marginated leukocytes engage in transient, low-affinity, selectin-mediated adhesive interactions with endothelial cells. As the response evolves, activated leukocytes and endothelial cells engage in high-affinity β_2-integrin and immunoglobulin superfamily-mediated adhesive interactions. A variety of chemotactic factors can provide the motive force for leukocyte emigration. [Modified and redrawn from multiple references (7-11)].

in these processes, several themes have emerged. Cell surface receptors are activated by specific ligands (e.g., C5a, LTB_4, IL-8, etc.) and receptor activation is transduced via specific G proteins and membrane-associated phospholipases which in turn leads to mobilization of intracellular calcium, influx of extracellular calcium, and protein phosphorylation. Genetic defects in the regulation of many of these processes have been described and are detailed elsewhere throughout this text.

The principal result of neutrophil and monocyte recruitment are to provide 1) high concentrations of activated leukocytes that can release lytic substances and reactive oxygen and nitrogen intermediates needed to destroy foreign invaders, and 2) a vehicle to contain foreign particulates through phagocytosis. The products and functions of activated inflammatory cells are at once salutary because they contain and destroy invaders and deleterious because they cause tissue damage.

Leukocyte activation, especially that of neutrophils and mononuclear phagocytes, induced either by soluble mediators or by the process of phagocytosis, results in the secretion of many lysosomal substances (e.g., myeloperoxidase by neutrophils), the generation of reactive oxygen and nitrogen intermediates (e.g., O_2^-, H_2O_2, NO), the generation of arachidonate metabolites (e.g., leukotrienes and prostaglandins), and the production of other mediators (see below).[35,36] In some circumstances these materials are released into phagolysosomes where they contribute to the destruction of engulfed microbes while in other circumstances they are secreted into the extracellular milieu where they may amplify the inflammatory response and cause tissue damage.

Phagocytosis involves three distinct steps: recognition and attachment, engulfment, and degradation (killing) of the ingested material.[37,38] Phagocytosis is enhanced greatly when particles (e.g., bacteria) are coated with opsonins which in turn function as ligands for leukocyte surface receptors. The major opsonins include the Fc domain of IgG and IgM immunoglobulins and the complement-derived fragments, C3b and iC3b, which covalently link to the surfaces of particles and large molecules. There are a variety of Fc receptors (FcγRI, FcγRII, FcγRIII, etc.) and complement receptors (e.g., CR1, CR2, CR3) which specifically engage their respective opsonins when the latter coat foreign particulates. As noted in Table 6-1, some enhanced phagocytic reactions occur independently of opsonins (e.g., CR3, the β_2 integrin Mac-1, binds lipopolysaccharide directly). Engulfment is triggered as the result of engagement of FcγR and is enhanced by the concurrent engagement of complement receptors. In some circumstances, engulfment is enhanced by the simultaneous binding of the leukocyte to specific extracellular matrix molecules (e.g., fibronectin) or soluble cytokines. Engulfment results in the formation of phagosomes which fuse with lysosomes to form phagolysosomes in which the foreign particle is degraded. Numerous mechanisms for killing and/or degradation of microbes have been elucidated (Table 6-2). Although these mechanisms are classified as either oxygen-dependent or oxygen-independent, both types of processes may be involved in

TABLE 6-2　KILLING AND DEGRADATION OF MICROORGANISMS IN PHAGOCYTES

Oxygen-Dependent		Oxygen-Independent
Superoxide anion	(O_2^-)	Arachidonate metabolites (prostaglandins, leukotrienes)
Hydrogen peroxide	(H_2O_2)	Platelet-activating factor
Hydroxyl radical	$(HO \cdot)$	Lysosomal proteases
Singlet oxygen	$(^1O_2)$	Lactoferrin
N-chloramines	$(R-NHC1, R-NCl_2)$	Lysozyme
Hypohalous acids	$(HO-X)$	Cationic proteins (e.g., major basic protein, defensins)

the destruction of a given microorganism, and a given microorganism may vary greatly in its susceptibility to various mechanisms of destruction.[35,39]

REGULATION OF THE INFLAMMATORY RESPONSE

The foregoing sections provide a conceptual framework for the inflammatory response, specifically, the hemodynamic alterations, mechanisms of specific leukocyte-endothelial adhesive interactions, chemotaxis, and leukocyte activation and phagocytosis. The many steps that constitute this paradigm are regulated by a variety of soluble mediators that are produced by endothelial cells and leukocytes at a site of inflammation, by other resident cells (e.g., tissue macrophages, fibroblasts, mast cells), and as by-products of blood-borne proteins (e.g., complement system, coagulation cascade). These inflammatory mediator systems are summarized in Table 6-3.

REACTIVE OXYGEN INTERMEDIATES

Since the early 1970s it has been recognized that activated phagocytes exhibit a transient but marked increase in oxygen consumption and the generation of reduced oxygen metabolites.[35] Although small quantities of reactive oxygen intermediates are produced as by-products of a variety of biochemical pathways, the chief source is the leukocyte membrane-associated NADPH oxidase, an enzyme complex that is defective in patients with chronic granulomatous disease (see Chap. 67). Reactive oxygen intermediates include superoxide anion (O_2^-), hydrogen peroxide (H_2O_2), hydroxyl radical (HO ·), and singlet oxygen ($^1O_2$). These reduced oxygen products play a major role in intraphagolysosomal killing of microorganisms and when released extracellularly are directly or indirectly responsible for a variety of inflammatory processes including endothelial cell lysis, extracellular matrix degradation, activation of latent proteolytic enzymes (collagenase, gelatinase), inactivation of antiproteases, interaction with toxic metabolites of L-arginine, and generation of chemotactic factors from arachidonic acid and the complement component, C5. In addition to their role in endothelial cytotoxicity, reactive oxygen intermediates have been shown to be cytotoxic for fibroblasts, erythrocytes, tumor cells, and various parenchymal cells. The biochemical mechanisms implicated include lipid peroxidation, the formation of carbonyl moieties and nitrosylation products, intracellular enzyme inactivation, protein oxidation, and oxidant-mediated DNA damage. Studies indicate that reactive oxygen intermediates (e.g., O_2^-) can also undergo reactions with reactive nitrogen intermediates (e.g., NO, see below) to generate toxic NO derivatives.

REACTIVE NITROGEN INTERMEDIATES

Described in 1980 as endothelium-derived relaxing factor (EDRF), NO is the soluble, short-acting biosynthetic product of L-arginine, O_2, NADPH, and nitric oxide synthase (NOS).[40,41] As suggested by its original name, NO mediates vascular smooth muscle relaxation. NO binds to the heme moiety of guanylyl cyclase to trigger the generation of intracytoplasmic cGMP and, through the activation of a series of kinases, induces smooth muscle relaxation and vasodilatation. At least three different forms of NOS have been characterized. Nitric oxide can be produced either constitutively or induced in a wide variety of cell types (e.g., endothelial cells, neurons, macrophages). In addition to its activity as a vasodilator, NO plays important roles in the inhibition of smooth muscle proliferation and in inflammation. For instance, NO can react with reactive oxygen intermediates to form both reactive oxygen and nitrogen species (e.g., $NO + O_2^- \rightarrow NO_2^- + HO \cdot$), it can inhibit DNA synthesis, it can directly kill microbes and tumor cells, and it can inactivate cytosolic glutathione and a number of sulfhydryl enzymes. In vivo studies have confirmed that inhibition of NO synthe-

TABLE 6-3   INFLAMMATORY MEDIATOR SYSTEMS

MEDIATOR SYSTEM	SOURCE	MAJOR ACTIONS
Reactive oxygen intermediates (O_2^-, H_2O_2, HOX, HO·)	Leukocytes, endothelial cells	Tissue damage through cytolysis, matrix degradation, activation of complement, and generation of chemotactic lipids
Reactive nitrogen intermediates (NO·, $ONOO^-$, NO_2^-, NO_3^-)	Monocytes, macrophages, lymphocytes, endothelial cells	Cytostasis of cells, inhibition of DNA synthesis, inhibition of mitochondrial respiration, and formation of OH·
Lysosomal granule constituents (proteases, lysozyme, lactoferrin, cationic proteins)	Neutrophils, monocytes	Tissue damage through proteolysis, matrix degradation, and catalysis of oxidant-generating reactions
Cytokines and chemokines (TNF, IL-1, IL-8, MCP-1, etc.)	Monocytes, macrophages, and endothelial cells	Cell activation, induction of adhesion, chemotaxis, fever, and acute-phase response
Platelet-activating factor	Leukocytes, endothelial cells	Vascular permeability and cell activation
Arachidonic acid metabolites (prostaglandins, 5-HPETE, leukotrienes)	Cell membranes (endothelial cells, platelets, leukocytes)	Coagulation, vasodilatation, vascular permeability, cell activation, and chemotaxis
Kinins (bradykinin, kallikrein)	Plasma	Pain, vascular permeability, and vasodilatation
Vasoactive amines (serotonin, histamine)	Platelets, mast cells, and basophils	Vascular permeability, induction of adhesion
Complement	Plasma, macrophages	Chemotaxis, vascular permeability, and cell activation
Coagulation	Plasma	Chemotaxis, vascular permeability, and complement activation

sis with antagonistic L-arginine analogs can reduce tissue injury in models of inflammation.[42,43]

LYSOSOMAL GRANULE CONSTITUENTS
The activation of neutrophils, monocytes, and macrophages results in the release, either through exocytosis or as the result of cell death, of a wide variety of proinflammatory mediators that have important roles in the inflammatory response.[44] Neutrophils contain two major types of granules (see Chaps. 64, 65, and 67). Large, primary (azurophilic) granules contain lysozyme, a variety of cationic proteins, myeloperoxidase, defensins, phospholipase, acid hydrolases, and neutral proteases (e.g., proteinase 3, collagenases, elastase). Smaller, secondary (specific) granules contain lysozyme, lactoferrin, type IV collagenase, alkaline phosphatase, membrane-associated NADPH oxidase, and the β_2 integrins. Acid proteases function most efficiently within phagolysosomes where the pH is low, while neutral proteases can function efficiently within extracellular inflammatory exudates. Lysosomal granule constituents contribute to the inflammatory response and tissue injury through a wide array of mechanisms (e.g., degradation of extracellular matrix, proteolytic generation of chemotactic peptide, catalysis of reactive oxygen metabolite generation).

CYTOKINES AND CHEMOKINES
Cytokines are relatively small (5–20kD) proteins that modulate the function of other cell types. A large number of cytokines and chemokines have been identified and characterized in recent years.[45–47] In addition to their important roles in regulating various aspects of the immune response, many cytokines participate in inflammatory processes. Among the most thoroughly characterized cytokines are IL-1 and TNF-α. Interleukin 1 and TNF-α are structurally dissimilar but share many biologic activities and function as autocrine, paracrine, and endocrine mediators (Table 6-4).

IL-1 is a 17 kD protein that exhibits a wide variety of biological activities. Initially termed "endogenous pyrogen" due to its ability to induce temperature elevation and the acute-phase response, IL-1 is now known to be relevant to acute inflammation because of its ability to induce cytokine production in monocytes, macrophages, fibroblasts, and endothelial cells (TNF-α, IL-1, and IL-6). Interleukin-1 can also induce NOS. As noted in the section that describes endothelial-leukocyte adhesive interactions, IL-1 can activate endothelial cells, resulting in the expression of adhesion molecules.

Tumor necrosis factor-α (TNF-α), or cachectin, is also a 17 kD protein. Like IL-1, TNF-α can induce cytokine production in a variety of cells. TNF-α can induce neutrophil activation and the expression of adhesion molecules on endothelial cells. In contrast to IL-1, TNF-α possesses potent cytotoxic activities for certain types of cells. Both IL-1 and TNF-α are produced in response to endotoxemia and both can initiate a systemic shock-like response.

Chemokines, or "intercrines," are cytokines which exhibit prominent chemotactic activities.[48–51] The two major subfamilies include the alpha, or "C-X-C-," chemokines and the beta, or "C-C," chemokines. "C-X-C" chemokines are so-designated because the first two N-terminal cystine residues are separated by a single amino acid. Alpha chemokines, of which IL-8 is the prototype, consistently exhibit neutrophil chemotactic activity, while the beta, or "C-C," chemokines, of which monocyte chemoattractant protein-1 (MCP-1) is the prototype, exhibit monocyte chemotactic activity (Table 6-5). Chemokines activate leukocytes through membrane receptors (serpentines) which contain seven transmembrane domains and are linked to cytosolic surface G proteins.[52]

INFLAMMATORY LIPIDS
Arachidonic acid is a 20-carbon polyunsaturated fatty acid (5, 8, 11, 14-eicosatetraenoic acid) derived either from dietary sources or by conversion from linoleic acid. Arachidonic acid is maintained in cell

TABLE 6-4   INTERLEUKIN-1 AND TUMOR NECROSIS FACTOR IN INFLAMMATION

Acute Phase Response
  Fever
  Shock
  Neutrophilia
  Somnolence
  Anorexia
  Acute phase proteins
Endothelial Activation
  Induction of IL-1, IL-6, IL-8
  Procoagulant phenotype
  Leukocyte adherence
Fibroblast Activation
  Proliferation
  Collagen synthesis
  Collagenase and protease induction

TABLE 6-5   CHEMOKINES

FAMILY	MEMBERS	ABBREVIATIONS	PRIMARY TARGET CELLS
α-Chemokines (C-X-C)	Interleukin-8	IL-8	Neutrophils
	Platelet factor 4	PF4	Neutrophils
	Melanocyte growth-stimulatory activity	MGSA or GROα	Neutrophils
	Neutrophil-activating peptide-2	NAP-2	Neutrophils
	γ-Interferon-inducible protein	γ-IP-10	Neutrophils
β-Chemokines (C-C)	Monocyte chemoattractant protein-1	MCP-1/MCAF or JE	Monocytes, basophils
	Regulated upon activation, normal T cell expressed and presumably secreted	RANTES	Monocytes, eosinophils, basophils
	Macrophage inflammatory protein-1α	MIP-1α	Monocytes, eosinophils
	Macrophage inflammatory protein-1β	MIP-1β	Monocytes

membranes as an esterified phospholipid. The two families of inflammatory mediators derived from arachidonic acid are generated via the cyclooxygenase and lipoxygenase pathways (resulting in the appearance of prostaglandins and leukotrienes, respectively).[53] Cell activation or mechanical stress can result in the release of arachidonic acid. Activation of the cyclooxygenase family of phospholipases results in prostaglandins synthesis. Members of this group of mediators exhibit several proinflammatory activities which include vasodilatation, vasoconstriction, increases in permeability, and platelet activation (aggregation). Activation of the lipoxygenase pathway results in the synthesis of 5-hydroperoxyeicosatetraenoic acid (5-HPETE), which is a potent chemoattractant of neutrophils and is further modified to yield a series of leukotrienes. Leukotriene B_4 (LTB$_4$) induces neutrophil chemotaxis, aggregation, degranulation, and adherence, while LTC$_4$, LTD$_4$, and LTE$_4$ trigger smooth muscle constriction and increases in vascular permeability. Members of both of these families of lipid-derived mediators have been detected in inflammatory exudates. Nonsteroidal antiinflammatory agents and aspirin, which inhibit cyclooxygenase, emphasize the importance of these mediators in the development of an acute inflammatory response.

Platelet-activating factor (PAF) is a potent proinflammatory lipid produced by a variety of cell types including neutrophils, monocytes, endothelial cells, and IgE-sensitized basophils.[54] Derived from the cell membrane constituent, choline phosphoglyceride, PAF is an acetyl glycerol ether phosphocholine which is synthesized following the activation of phospholipase A_2. PAF triggers platelet aggregation and degranulation, increases vascular permeability, and promotes leukocyte accumulation and activation. In vivo studies using specific PAF antagonists have suggested a role for PAF in ischemia-reperfusion of the heart and gut and in immune complex–mediated injury in the skin, lung, and kidney.[54] In addition, a PAF-like lipid has been measured in the blood of patients with angioedema and cold urticaria.

KININS

The kinin system is activated by contact activation of clotting factor XII (Hageman factor) (see Chap. 112).[55] Activation of the kinin system results in the generation of the vasoactive nine amino acid peptide, bradykinin. Bradykinin possesses several activities, including the capacity to increase vascular permeability, to induce smooth muscle contraction, to trigger vasodilation, and to cause pain.[55] Activated Hageman factor (factor XIIa), also known as the prekallikrein activator, converts plasma prekallikrein to kallikrein. Kallikrein cleaves high-molecular-weight kininogen to produce bradykinin. Models of septic shock have revealed decreases in plasma kininogen that parallel decreases in peripheral arterial resistance.[55] The presence of plasma kininases precludes the routine measurement of bradykinin by functional or immunochemical approaches.

VASOACTIVE AMINES

Histamine and serotonin (5-hydroxytryptamine) are low molecular weight vasoactive amines. Histamine is contained in mast cell and basophil granules while platelets are the chief source of serotonin.[56] Localized release of histamine results in wheal formation due to increases in vascular permeability. Histamine induces the formation of reversible openings in endothelial tight junctions, triggers the formation of prostacyclin in endothelium, and induces NO release from the endothelium. In addition, histamine, like thrombin, can induce the rapid upregulation of endothelial P-selectin.[57] Serotonin, which acts through receptors on vascular smooth muscle cells, is responsible for vasoconstriction, whereas interaction with endothelial receptors results in vasodilation (via release of NO) and increased permeability. Release of histamine and serotonin from mast cells and platelets can be triggered by IgE-mediated type I hypersensitivity reactions, directly by C3a or C5a, and directly by neutrophil granule-derived cationic proteins.

COMPLEMENT

The complement system, including its soluble and cell membrane–associated regulators, consists of nearly two dozen plasma proteins that give rise to mediators of chemotaxis, increased vascular permeability, opsonic activity, phagocytic activation, and cytolysis.[58] In a manner analogous to coagulation, the complement system is activated through a cascade of proteolytic cleavage reactions. There are two convergent pathways (Figure 6-2). The first of these, the classical pathway, is initiated by complement-fixing immune complexes (IgG and IgM), while the second, the alternative pathway, is triggered by a variety of substances that include IgA aggregates, endotoxin, cobra venom factor, and the polysaccharide components of some bacterial and fungal cell walls. The classical pathway is initiated by the fixation of C1 (C1qr$_2$s$_2$) by the Fc portion of surface-bound IgG or IgM immunoglobulins. Activated C1 (C1qr$_2$s$_2$) cleaves C2 and C4 which leads to the formation of "classical pathway" C3 convertase, C4b2a. Activation of the alternative pathway results in the formation of an "alternative pathway" C3 convertase following direct cleavage of C3 and subsequent interactions of C3b with factors B and D in the presence of Mg^{2+}. The resulting complex, C3bBb is stabilized by properdin, leading to a stable C3 convertase, C3bBbP. C3 convertases generated via either pathway can cleave C3 to form C3a and C3b. C3b can bind to either the classical or alternative pathway C3 convertase to form a C5 convertase, which cleaves C5 into C5a and C5b. C5a is released into the fluid phase, like C3a, whereas C5b combines first with C6 and then C7 to form C5b-7 which in turn binds with C8 and multiple C9 molecules to form C5b-9, the membrane attack complex. In addition to the cell-activating and cytolytic activities of C5b-9, individual complement cleavage products and complexes have a wide variety of specific and

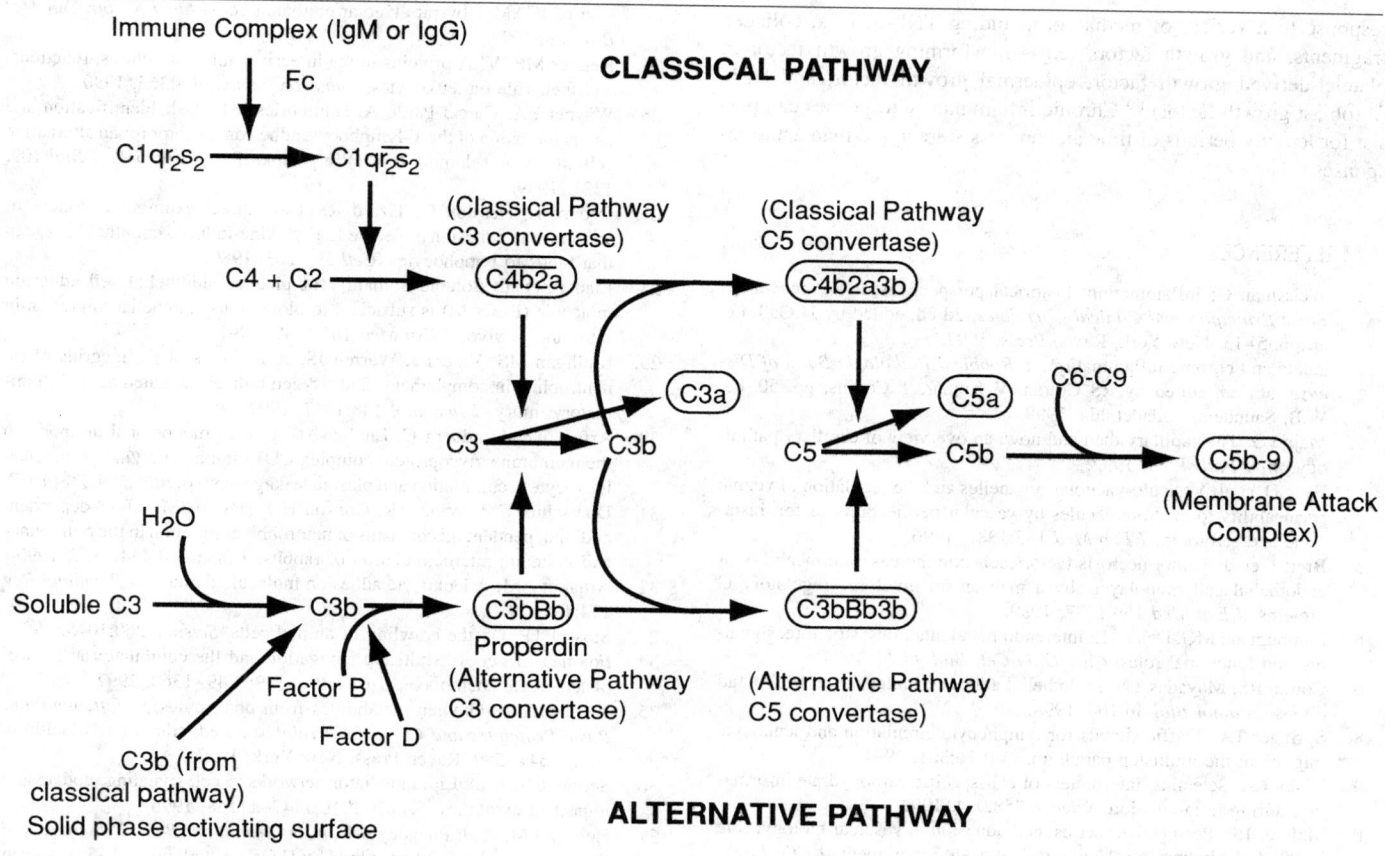

FIGURE 6-2   The complement system. The complement system consists of a series of soluble and surface-associated mediators which are functionally organized into the classical and alternative pathways. The classical and alternative pathways of complement converge and lead to the production of the pore-forming membrane attack complex. The classical pathway is most often activated by IgG- and IgM-containing immune complexes while the alternative pathway can be activated by a variety of particulates. In both cases, complex multicomponent enzyme complexes called C3 and C5 convertases are formed. A variety of proinflammatory peptide fragments (e.g., C3a, C5a) are generated as a result of complement activation.

potent proinflammatory activities.[58] These various functions, combined with the rapid amplification in numbers of complement-derived mediators, emphasize the vital role of complement in acute inflammation. The most important activation products of complement appear to be the major chemotactic factor, C5a, and the anaphylatoxins (C3a, C4a, C5a), of which C3a is the most abundant. C5b-9 appears to be a major cytotoxic product, provided that this complex is assembled on the surface of a susceptible cell (e.g., bacterium). A series of soluble and cell membrane–associated complement proteins play important roles in the regulation of the complement cascade.[58]

COAGULATION SYSTEM

The coagulation system, its disorders, and the clinical management of its disorders, are reviewed in detail in Chaps. 112 through 134. Activation of the clotting cascade results in the generation of fibrinopeptides which increase vascular permeability and are chemotactic for leukocytes. Thrombin has been shown to induce endothelial expression of P-selectin, resulting in increased neutrophil adhesion.[59] In addition, plasmin is responsible for the activation of Hageman factor, which then can activate the kinin system, and can cleave C3 into its active components; it can also generate fibrin-split products. The induction of procoagulant activity in endothelial cells exposed to TNF-α and IL-1 further links the coagulation system to the inflammatory response.[60]

CHRONIC INFLAMMATION AND REPAIR

The chronic inflammatory response and repair processes are, like the acute inflammatory response, highly regulated. Chronic inflammation is characterized by the recruitment of lymphocytes, monocytes, and plasma cells as well as by the proliferation of new capillaries (angiogenesis) and increases in the deposition of extracellular matrix molecules.[1-3] The recruitment of this wide variety of cell types is achieved by a complex interaction among cytokines, chemokines, and indigenous cells. Great advances in understanding of angiogenesis and extracellular matrix molecule metabolism have been made in recent years. The characteristics of individual chronic inflammatory responses are dependent upon the location of the injury and the type of injurious agent. For instance, lymphocyte- and monocyte-binding interactions with endothelial cells are mediated by selectins, β_1 and β_2 integrins, and both ICAM and VCAM-1. Bacterium-derived chemotactic peptides play a role in monocyte recruitment, and members of the β chemokine subfamily induce monocyte and lymphocyte recruitment. These several factors have been observed to play a key role in the development of some models of chronic inflammation (Table 6-5).

The proliferation of fibroblasts and the induction of angiogenesis that accompany chronic inflammation are mediated by a variety of cytokines and growth factors derived from platelets, macrophages, and lymphocytes. For instance, fibroblast chemotaxis has been observed in response to a variety of mediators including TNF-α, C5a, collagen fragments, and growth factors (e.g., transforming growth factor-β, platelet-derived growth factor, epidermal growth factor, and basic fibroblast growth factor).[1-3] Chronic inflammatory responses can persist for lengthy periods of time and are less stereotypic than acute responses.

REFERENCES

1. Weissman G: Inflammation: historical perspectives, in *Inflammation: Basic Principles and Clinical Correlates*, 2d ed, edited by JJ Gallin et al, pp. 5–13. New York, Raven Press, 1992.
2. Acute and chronic inflammation, in *Robbins' Pathologic Basis of Disease*, 6th ed, edited by RS Cotran, V Kumar, T Collins, pp. 50–88. W.B. Saunders, Philadelphia, 1999.
3. Majno G: The capillary then and now: an overview of capillary pathology. *Mod Pathol* 5:9, 1992.
4. Feng D, et al: Vesiculo-vacuolar organelles and the regulation of venule permeability to macromolecules by vascular permeability factor, histamine and serotonin. *J Exp Med* 183:1981, 1996.
5. Brett J, et al: Tumor necrosis factor/cachectin increases permeability of endothelial cell monolayers by a mechanism involving regulatory G proteins. *J Exp Med* 169:1977, 1989.
6. Lampugnani MG, Dejana E: Interendothelial junctions: structure, signaling and functional roles. *Curr Opin Cell Biol* 9:674, 1997.
6. Cotran RS, Mayadas TN: Endothelial adhesion molecules in health and disease. *Pathol Biol* 46:164, 1998.
8. Springer TA: Traffic signals for lymphocyte circulation and leukocyte migration: the multistep paradigm. *Cell* 76:301, 1994.
9. Lasky LA: Selectins: interpreters of cell-specific carbohydrate information during inflammation. *Science* 258:964, 1992.
10. McEver RP: Perspectives series: cell adhesion in vascular biology: role in PSGL-1 binding to selectins in leukocyte recruitment. *J Clin Invest* 100:485, 1997.
11. Bevilacqua MP, Nelson RM: Selectins. *J Clin Invest* 91:379, 1993.
12. Ley K, Gaehtgens P, Fennie C, et al: Lectin-like cell adhesion molecule 1 mediates leukocyte rolling in mesenteric venules in vivo. *Blood* 77:2553, 1991.
13. Polley MJ, Phillips ML, Wayner E, et al: CD62 and endothelial cell-leukocyte adhesion molecule-1 (ELAM-1) recognizes the same carbohydrate ligand, sialyl Lewis^X. *Proc Natl Acad Sci USA* 88:6224, 1991.
14. Lorant DE, et al: Inflammatory roles of P-selectin. *J Clin Invest* 92:559, 1993.
15. Geng JG, Bevilacqua MP, Moore KL, et al: Rapid neutrophil adhesion to activated endothelium mediated by GMP-140. *Nature* 343:757, 1990.
16. Bevilacqua MP, Stengelin S, Gimbrone MAJ, Seed B: Endothelial leukocyte adhesion molecule 1: an inducible receptor for neutrophils related to complement regulatory proteins and lectins. *Science* 243:1160, 1989.
17. Cotran RS, Briscoe DM: Endothelial cells in inflammation, in *Textbook of Rheumatology*, 5th ed, edited by W. Kelley et al, pp. 183–198. WB Saunders, Philadelphia, 1997.
18. Lowe JB, Stoolman LM, Nair RP, et al: ELAM-1 dependent cell adhesion to vascular endothelium determined by a transfected human fucosyltransferase cDNA. *Cell* 63:475, 1990.
19. Picker LJ, Warnock RA, Burns AR, et al: The neutrophil selectin LECAM-1 presents carbohydrate ligands to the vascular selectins ELAM-1 and GMP-140. *Cell* 66:921, 1991.
20. Smith CW, Marlin SD, Rothlein R, et al: Role of ICAM-1 in the adherence of human neutrophils to human endothelial cells *in vitro*, in *Structure and Function of Molecules Involved in Leukocyte Adhesion*, edited by TA Springer, DC Anderson, R Rothlein, AS Rosenthal, p 170. Springer-Verlag, New York, 1989.
21. Arnout MA: Structure and function of the leukocyte integrins (CD18/CD11). *Blood* 75:1037, 1990.
22. Bevilacqua MP, Pober JS, Mendrick DL, et al: Identification of an inducible endothelial leukocyte adhesion molecule. *Proc Natl Acad Sci USA* 84:9238, 1987.
23. Larson RS, Springer TA: Structure and function of leukocyte integrins. *Immunol Rev* 114:181, 1990.
24. Christensen PJ, Kim S, Simon RH, et al: Differentiation-related expression of ICAM-1 by rat alveolar epithelial cells. *Am J Respir Cell Mol Biol* 8:9, 1993.
25. Hemler ME: VLA proteins in the integrin family: structures, functions, and their role on leukocytes. *Annu Rev Immunol* 8:365, 1990.
26. Wayner EA, Garcia-Pardo A, Humphries MJ, et al: Identification and characterization of the T-lymphocyte adhesion receptor for an alternative cell attachment domain (CS-1) in plasma fibronectin. *J Cell Biol* 109:1321, 1989.
27. Osborn L, Hession C, Tizard R, et al: Direct expression cloning of vascular cell adhesion molecule 1, a cytokine-induced endothelial protein that binds to lymphocytes. *Cell* 59:1203, 1989.
28. Liao F, et al: Soluble domain 1 of platelet-endothelial cell adhesion molecule (PECAM) is sufficient to block transendothelial migration in vitro and in vivo. *J Exp Med* 185:1349, 1997.
29. Mulligan MS, Varani J, Warren JS, et al: Roles of β_2 integrins of rat neutrophils in complement- and oxygen radical-mediated acute inflammatory injury. *J Immunol* 148:1847, 1992.
30. Arfors KE, Lundberg C, Lindom L, et al: A monoclonal antibody to the membrane glycoprotein complex CD18 inhibits polymorphonuclear leukocyte accumulation and plasma leakage in vivo. *Blood* 69:338, 1987.
31. Doerschuk CM, Winn RK, Coxson HO, Harlan JM: CD18-dependent and -independent mechanisms of neutrophil emigration in the pulmonary and systemic microcirculation of rabbits. *J Immunol* 144:2327, 1990.
32. Arnaout AM: A leukocyte adhesion molecule deficiency. *Immunol Rev* 114:145, 1990.
33. Stossel TP: On the crawling of animal cells. *Science* 260:1045, 1993.
34. Foxman EF, et al: Multistep navigation and the combinatorial control of leukocyte chemotaxis. *J Cell Biol* 139:1349–1360, 1997.
35. Klebanoff SJ: Oxygen metabolites from phagocytes, in *Inflammation: Basic Principles and Clinical Correlates*, 2d ed, edited by JJ Gallin et al, pp. 541–589. Raven Press, New York, 1992.
36. Serhan CN, et al: Lipid mediator networks in cell signaling: update and impact of cytokines. *FASEB J* 10:1147–11158, 1996.
37. Henson PM, et al: Phagocytosis, in *Inflammation: Basic Principles and Clinical Correlates*, 2d ed, edited by JJ Gallin et al, pp. 511–541. Raven Press, New York, 1992.
38. Gallin JJ (eds.): Disorders of phagocytic cells, in *Inflammation: Basic Principles and Clinical Correlates*, 2d ed, edited by JJ Gallin et al, pp. 859–875. Raven Press, New York, 1992.
39. Martin E, Gantz T, Lehrer RI: Defensins and other endogenous peptide antibiotics of vertebrates. *J Leukoc Biol* 58:128–136, 1995.
40. Furchgott RF and Zawadzki JV: The obligatory role of endothelial cells in the relaxation of arterial smooth muscle by acetylcholine. *Nature* 288:373, 1980.
41. MacMicking JD, et al: Nitric oxide and macrophage function. *Annu Rev Immunol* 15:323, 1997.
42. Mulligan MS, Warren JS, Smith CW, et al: Lung injury after deposition of IgA immune complexes: requirements for CD18 and L-arginine. *J Immunol* 148:3086, 1992.
43. Mulligan MS, Moncada S, Ward PA: Protective effects of inhibitors of nitric oxide synthase in immune complex-induced vasculitis. *Br J Pharmacol* 107:1159, 1992.
44. Venge P, et al: Neutrophils and eosinophils, in *Textbook of Rheumatology*, 5th ed, edited by W. Kelley et al, pp. 146–160. Philadelphia, WB Saunders, 1997.
45. Gauldie J, Baumann H: Cytokines and acute-phase protein expression, in *Cytokines in Inflammation*, edited by ES Kimball, pp. 275–298. CRC Press, Boca Raton, FL, 1992.
46. Beutler B: TNF, immunity and inflammatory disease: lessons of the past decade. *J Invest Med* 43:227–235, 1995.
47. Dinarello CA: Biologic basis for interleukin-1 in disease. *Blood* 87:2095–2147, 1996.
48. Taub DD, Oppenheim JJ: Review of the chemokines. The Third International Meeting of Chemotactic Cytokines. *Cytokine* 5:175, 1993.
49. Adams DH, Lloyd AR: Chemokines: leukocyte recruitment and activation cytokines. *Lancet* 349:490–495, 1997.
50. Schall TJ: Biology of RANTES/SIS cytokine family. *Cytokine* 3:165, 1991.
51. Wolpe SD, Cerami A: Macrophage inflammatory proteins 1 and 2: members of a novel superfamily of cytokines. *FASEB J* 3:2565, 1989.

52. Kelvin DJ, et al: Chemokines and serpentines. *J Leukocyte Biol* 54: 605, 1993.

53. Zurier RB: Prostaglandins, leukotrienes, and related compounds. In Kelley WN, et al (eds.): *Textbook of Rheumatology*, 4th ed. pp. 201–212. W. B. Saunders Co., Philadelphia, 1992.

54. Zimmerman G, et al: A fluid phase and cell-associated mediator of inflammation. In Gallin JJ, et al (eds.): *Inflammation: Basic Principles and Clinical Correlates*, 2nd ed. pp. 149–176. Raven Press, New York, 1992.

55. Carmeliet P, Collen D: Molecular genetics of the fibrinolytic and coagulation systems in haemostasis, thrombogenesis, restenosis and atherosclerosis. *Curr Opin Lipidol* 8:118–125, 1997.

56. Busse W: Histamine mediator and modulator in inflammation, in *Chemical Messengers of the Inflammatory Process*, edited by JC Houck, p 1. Elsevier, Amsterdam, 1979.

57. Bonfanti R, Furie BC, Furie B, Wagner DD: PADGEM (GMP-140) is a component of Weibel-Palade bodies of human endothelial cells. *Blood* 73:1109, 1989.

58. Asghar SS, Pasch MC: Complement as a promiscuous signal transduction device. *Lab Invest* 78:1203, 1998.

59. McEver RP, Beckstead JH, Moore KL, et al: GMP-140, a platelet alpha-granule membrane protein, is also synthesized by vascular endothelial cells and is localized in Weibel-Palade bodies. *J Clin Invest* 84:92, 1989.

60. Argiles JM, et al: Journey from cachexia to obesity by TNF. *FASEB J* 11:743–751, 1997.

CHAPTER 7

HEMATOLOGY OF THE NEWBORN

GEORGE B. SEGEL

JAMES PALIS

A newborn represents the culmination of developmental events from conception and implantation through organogenesis. The embryo requires red cells for the transport of maternal oxygen to permit this growth and development. Birth brings dramatic changes in circulation and oxygenation, which affect hematopoiesis, as the newborn makes the transition to a separate biological existence. This chapter discusses the ontogeny of hematopoiesis and focuses on hematopoiesis of the normal newborn.

FETAL HEMATOPOIESIS

PRODUCTION OF EMBRYONIC AND FETAL HEMATOPOIETIC CELLS

During embryogenesis, hematopoiesis occurs in spatially and temporally distinct sites, including the extraembryonic yolk sac, the fetal liver, and the preterm bone marrow. Erythropoiesis is established soon after implantation of the blastocyst, with primitive erythroid cells appearing in yolk sac blood islands by day 18 of gestation.[1,2] The origin of hematopoietic cells in mammals is tied closely to gastrulation and the formation of mesoderm. Inducers of mesoderm, including transforming growth factor β (TGF-β), fibroblast growth factor, and bone morphogenetic protein-4 (BMP-4), likely are important molecules regulating the onset of hematopoiesis.[3] Yolk sac erythroblasts arise in close association with the first embryonic blood vessels, suggesting that endothelial cells and blood cells arise from a common hemangioblast precursor.

YOLK SAC HEMATOPOIESIS

The development of primitive erythroblasts in the yolk sac is critical for embryonic survival. In the mouse, targeted disruption of the murine transcription factors SCL (TAL1), LMO2 (RBTN2), and GATA-1 each abrogates primitive erythropoiesis in the yolk sac and leads to early embryonic death.[4-6] Yolk sac erythroblasts have several characteristics distinguishing them from their later definitive counterparts. Primitive erythroblasts differentiate within the vascular network rather than in the extravascular space and remain nucleated as they circulate. Primitive erythroblasts are characterized by more rapid maturation, increased sensitivity to erythropoietin, and a shortened life span compared to fetal and adult erythroblasts.[7] Yolk sac erythroblasts are extremely large red cells (megaloblasts) with an estimated mean cell volume (MCV) of >450 fl/cell.

Acronyms and abbreviations that appear in this chapter include: AGM, aorta-gonad-mesonephros; BFU-E, burst forming unit–erythroid; BMP, bone morphogenetic protein; BPG, bisphosphoglycerate; CFU-E, colony forming unit–erythroid; CFU-GEMM, colony forming unit–granulocyte-erythroid-monocyte-macrophage; CFU-GM, colony forming unit–granulocyte-monocyte; G-CSF, granulocyte colony stimulating factor; GM-CSF, granulocyte-monocyte colony stimulating factor; IL, interleukin; MCV, mean cell volume; NBT, nitroblue tetrazolium; SIDS, sudden infant death syndrome; TNF, tumor necrosis factor

The erythroid progenitors, burst-forming units-erythroid (BFU-E), and the later erythroid progenitors, colony-forming units-erythroid (CFU-E), are present in the yolk sac at 4 weeks gestation.[8] Primitive erythroblasts and erythroid progenitors then enter the embryo proper through the circulation. BFU-E appear in the fetal liver as early as 5 weeks of gestation, and CFU-E are evident soon thereafter.[8] Erythroid and nonerythroid progenitors are evident also in the nonliver regions of the embryo proper.[9] After 7 weeks gestation, hematopoietic progenitors are no longer detected in the yolk sac.[10] Yolk sac derived primitive erythroblasts continue to circulate until approximately 12 weeks of gestation.

HEPATIC HEMATOPOIESIS

The liver serves as the primary source of red cells from the 9th to the 24th weeks of gestation. Between 7 and 15 weeks gestation, 60 percent of the liver cells are hematopoietic.[11] Erythroid cells differentiate in close association with macrophages and extrude their nuclei prior to entering the blood stream. These fetal liver-derived definitive "macrocytes" are smaller than yolk sac megaloblasts and contain one-third the amount of hemoglobin. Differentiation of erythroid cells in the fetal liver is dependent on erythropoietin signaling through its receptor and the JAK2 kinase.[12,13] Fetal liver-derived erythroid progenitors will differentiate in vitro with erythropoietin alone, in contrast to adult bone marrow-derived BFU-E that require erythropoietin plus interleukin-3 (IL-3).[14,15] Erythropoietin transcripts are present during the first trimester in the liver.[9] The liver remains the primary site of erythropoietin transcription throughout fetal life.[16] Erythropoietin transcripts also are present in the developing human kidney as early as 17 weeks of gestation and increase after 30 weeks.[16] Erythropoietin is expressed both in the fetal liver and in the postnatal kidney.[16] Like primitive erythropoiesis in the yolk sac, definitive erythropoiesis in the fetal liver is necessary for continued survival of the embryo. Targeted disruption of the c-myb and EKLF transcription factors in the mouse each blocks fetal liver erythropoiesis and leads to fetal death.[17,18] These mutations do not effect yolk sac erythropoiesis, indicating fundamental differences in the transcriptional regulation of these distinct forms of erythropoiesis.

In contrast to the yolk sac, where hematopoiesis is restricted to erythroid and macrophage cells, hematopoiesis in the fetal liver also includes other myeloid as well as lymphoid lineages. Megakaryocytes are present in the liver by 6 weeks of gestation. Platelets are first evident in the circulation at 8–9 weeks gestation.[11] Small numbers of circulating leukocytes are present at the 11th week of gestation.[2] Granulopoiesis is present in the liver parenchyma and in some areas of connective tissue as early as 7 weeks gestation. Despite the low number and immature appearance of hepatic neutrophils, the fetal liver contains abundant hematopoietic progenitor cells, including colony-forming unit–granulocyte-erythroid-monocyte-macrophage (CFU-GEMM) and colony-forming unit–granulocyte-monocyte (CFU-GM).[19,20] CFU-GM growth depends upon several cytokines, including granulocyte colony stimulating factor (G-CSF), granulocyte-monocyte colony stimulating factor (GM-CSF), and interleukins.[21] When compared to adult bone marrow-derived myeloid progenitors, these fetal liver derived myeloid progenitors have a similar dose response in vitro to G-CSF.[22] G-CSF is expressed by hepatocytes at 14 weeks gestation.[23]

MARROW HEMATOPOIESIS

Hematopoietic cells are first seen in the marrow of the 10- to 11-week embryo,[1,2] and they remain confined to the diaphyseal regions of long bones until 15 weeks gestation.[24] Initially there are approximately equal numbers of myeloid and erythroid cells in the fetal marrow. However, myeloid cells predominate by 12 weeks gestation, and the myeloid to erythroid ratio approaches the adult level of 3 to 1 by 21 weeks gestation.[11] Macrophage cells in the fetal marrow, but not in the fetal liver, express the lipopolysaccharide receptor CD14.[23] The marrow becomes the major site of hematopoiesis after the 24th week of gestation.

LYMPHOPOIESIS

Lymphopoiesis is present in the lymph plexuses and the thymus beginning at 9 weeks gestation.[11] B cells with surface IgM are present in the liver, and circulating lymphocytes also are seen at 9 weeks gestation.[2] Lymphocyte subpopulations are detected by 13 weeks gestation in fetal liver.[25] Absolute numbers of major lymphoid subsets in 20–26-week-old fetuses, as defined by the antigens CD2, CD3, CD4, CD8, CD19, CD20 and CD16 (see Chapter 14 for functional significance of these phenotypes), are similar to those in newborns (see "Neonatal Lymphopoiesis").[26,27]

ONTOGENY OF HEMATOPOIETIC STEM CELLS

The reconstitution of hematopoiesis by transplantation with cord blood indicates that hematopoietic stem cells are present at birth.[28] However, the developmental origin of hematopoietic stem cells has not yet been defined. It was first postulated that hematopoietic stem cells originate independently in each hematopoietic site (yolk sac, liver, and bone marrow) of the embryo.[29] However, experiments in the mammalian embryo indicate that the liver rudiment is seeded by exogenous hematopoietic cells.[30,31] The marrow also is seeded by exogenously derived blood cells. Fetal liver provides a source of stem cells for myeloid and lymphoid reconstitution of fetal sheep and monkey transplant recipients.[32] The immunological reconstitution of an immunodeficient human fetus with fetal liver-derived cells also indicates that hematopoietic stem cells exist in the fetal liver.[13]

Yolk sac stem cells were first thought to seed the liver and eventually the bone marrow.[33] However, later experiments in avian and amphibian embryos indicated that the hematopoietic stem cells that seed the marrow arise within the body of the embryo proper rather than from the yolk sac.[34,35] Investigations in the mouse embryo also suggest that prior to the fetal liver, the aorta-gonad-mesonephros (AGM) region of the embryo proper contains stem cells capable of engrafting myeloablated adult recipients.[36] This correlates anatomically with the transient appearance of CD34-positive blood cells closely associated with the ventral wall of the aorta in several mammalian species, including the 5-week gestation human embryo.[37,38] These studies suggest that the AGM-region-derived stem cells seed the liver and the marrow to provide lifelong hematopoiesis. The underlying relationship of primitive hematopoiesis in the yolk sac to definitive hematopoiesis in the fetal liver and the marrow is unclear.

SYNTHESIS OF FETAL HEMOGLOBINS

Human hemoglobin is a tetramer composed of two α-type and two β-type globin chains (Table 7-1). The α-globin gene cluster is located on chromosome 16 and contains the ζ gene 5′ to the pair of α-globin genes. The β-globin gene cluster is located on chromosome 11 and contains five globin genes oriented 5′ to 3′ as ε-γ^A-γ^G-δ-β.[39] During embryogenesis the genes on both chromosomes are activated sequentially from the 5′ to the 3′ end. This globin "switching" is related not only to the relative positions of the globin genes within their respective chromosomal clusters, but also to interacting upstream "locus control regions."[40]

Hb Gower 1 ($\zeta_2\varepsilon_2$), is the major hemoglobin in embryos less than 5 weeks of gestation (see Table 7-1).[41] Hb Gower 2 ($\alpha_2\varepsilon_2$) has been found in embryos with a gestational age as young as 4 weeks and is absent in embryos older than 13 weeks.[42] Hb Portland ($\zeta_2\gamma_2$) is found in young embryos but persists in infants with homozygous α thalassemia.[11] Synthesis of the ζ and ε chains decreases as that of α and γ chains increases (Figure 7-1). The ζ to α globin switch precedes the ε to γ globin switch as the liver replaces the yolk sac as the main site of erythropoiesis.[43,44]

Hb F ($\alpha_2\gamma_2$) is the major hemoglobin of fetal life[45] (see Figure 7-1). Synthesis of Hb A can be demonstrated in fetuses as young as 9 weeks of gestation.[46,47] In fetuses of 9 to 21 weeks of gestation, the amount of Hb A ($\alpha_2\beta_2$) rises from 4 to 13 percent of the total hemoglobin.[47] These levels of Hb A have enabled the antenatal diagnosis of β thalassemia using globin chain synthesis. After 34 to 36 weeks of gestation the percentage of Hb A rises, while that of Hb F decreases (see Figure 7-1). The mean synthesis of Hb F in term infants was 59.0 ± 10 percent (1 SD) of total hemoglobin synthesis as assessed by ^{14}C-leucine uptake.[48] The amount of Hb F in blood varies in term infants from 53 to 95 percent of total hemoglobin.[49,50]

The fetal hemoglobin concentration in blood decreases after birth by approximately 3 percent per week and is generally less than 2 to 3 percent of the total hemoglobin by 6 months of age. This rate of decrease in Hb F production is closely related to the gestational age of the infant and is not affected by the changes in environment and oxygen tension that occur at the time of birth.[51] Hb A₂ ($\alpha_2\delta_2$) has not been detected in fetuses. Normal adult levels of Hb A₂ are achieved by four months of age.[52] Increased proportions of Hb F at birth have been reported in infants who are small for gestational age, who have experienced chronic intrauterine hypoxia, or who have trisomy 13.[53–56] Decreased levels of Hb F at birth are found in trisomy 21.[57] Persistence of the embryonic Hb Gower-1, Hb Gower-2, and Hb Portland has been described in some infants with developmental abnormalities, while persistently elevated levels of fetal hemoglobin have been observed in infants dying from the sudden infant death syndrome (SIDS).[58]

FETAL BLOOD

The fetal blood composition changes markedly during the second and third trimesters. The mean hemoglobin in fetuses progressively increases from 9.0 ± 2.8 g/dl at age 10 weeks to 16.5 ± 4.0 g/dl at 39 weeks.[59] There is a concomitant decrease in the MCV of fetal red cells from a mean of 134 fl/cell at 18 weeks to 118 fl/cell at 30 weeks gestation.[60] The total white blood cell count during the middle trimester is between 4 and 4.5 × 10⁹/liter, with an 80 to 85 percent preponderance of lymphocytes and 5 to 10 percent neutrophils.[60] The percentage of circulating nucleated red cells decreases from a mean of 12 percent at 18 weeks to 4 percent at 30 weeks.[60] The platelet count remains greater than 150,000/μl from 15 weeks gestation to term.[60,61]

Large numbers of committed hematopoietic progenitors circulate in the fetal blood. Blood samples obtained by fetoscopy at 12 to 19 weeks of gestation reveal a mean of 20,450 BFU-E/ml and 12,490 CFU-GM/ml.[62] This is in striking contrast to adult peripheral blood, which contains essentially no erythroid progenitors and 30 to 250 CFU-GM/ml.[63] The cycling rate of 26 to 28 week gestation fetal

TABLE 7-1 EMBRYONIC HEMOGLOBINS

HEMOGLOBIN	CHAIN COMPOSITION	PRIMARY SITE	APPEARANCE
Gower 1	$\zeta_2\varepsilon_2$	Yolk sac	<5–6 weeks
Gower 2	$\alpha_2\varepsilon_2$	Yolk sac	4–13 weeks
Portland	$\zeta_2\gamma_2$	Yolk sac	4–13 weeks
Fetal, F	$\alpha_2\gamma_2$	Liver	Early, 53–95% at term
Adult, A	$\alpha_2\beta_2$	Marrow	9 weeks, 5–45% at term

hematopoietic progenitors is nearly maximal (70–80%) compared to the relative quiescence (0–5%) of adult marrow-derived progenitors.[63]

NEONATAL HEMATOPOIESIS

RED CELLS

NEONATAL ERYTHROPOIESIS

Hemoglobin, Hematocrit, and Indices   The mean hemoglobin level in cord blood at term is 16.8 g/dl, with 95 percent of the values falling between 13.7 and 20.1 g/dl.[64] This variation reflects perinatal events, particularly asphyxia,[65] and also the amount of blood transferred from the placenta to the infant after delivery. Delay of cord clamping may increase the blood volume and red cell mass of the infant by as much as 55 percent.[66,67] The mean total blood volume after birth is 86.3 ml/kg for the term infant and 89.4 ml/kg for the premature infant.[68] The blood volume per kilogram decreases over the ensuing weeks, reaching a mean value of about 65 ml/kg by 3 to 4 months of age.

Normally the hemoglobin and hematocrit values rise in the first several hours after birth because of the movement of plasma from the intravascular to the extravascular space.[69] A venous hemoglobin concentration of less than 14 g/dl in a term infant and/or a fall in hemoglobin or hematocrit level in the first day of life are abnormal. Normal red cell values from capillary blood samples are shown in Table 7-2 for term infants in the first 12 weeks of life.[70] Capillary hematocrit values in newborns are higher than those in simultaneous venous samples, particularly during the first days of life, and the capillary/venous ratio is approximately 1.1 : 1.[71] This difference reflects circulatory factors and is greater in preterm and sick infants.

The red cells of the newborn are macrocytic, with a mean cell volume (MCV) in excess of 110 fl/cell. The MCV begins to fall after the first week, reaching adult values by the ninth week (see Table 7-2).[70,72] The blood film from a newborn infant shows macrocytic normochromic cells, polychromasia, and a few nucleated red blood cells. Even in healthy infants there may be mild anisocytosis and poikilocytosis.[73] Three to 5 percent of the red cells may be fragments, target cells, or distorted. By 3 to 5 days after birth, nucleated red blood cells are not found normally in the blood of term or premature infants, but they may be present in markedly elevated numbers in the presence of hemolysis or hypoxic stress.

There are significant numbers of circulating progenitor cells in cord blood.[74–77] Cord blood BFU-E and CFU-E differentiate more rapidly than their adult counterparts.[78] Furthermore, the proportion of cord blood hematopoietic progenitors in the mitotic cycle is approximately 50 percent, intermediate between the proportions found in fetal and adult progenitor cells.[76]

In several,[79,80] but not all, studies[81] premature infants at birth had lower hemoglobin levels, higher reticulocyte counts, and higher nucleated red cell counts than the term infants. The reticulocyte counts of premature infants are inversely proportional to their gestational age, with a mean of 8 percent reticulocytes evident at 32 weeks gestation and 4 to 5 percent at term.[82] Infants who are small for their gestational ages have higher red cell counts, hematocrit levels, and hemoglobin concentrations compared to infants whose size is appropriate for their gestational age.[80,83]

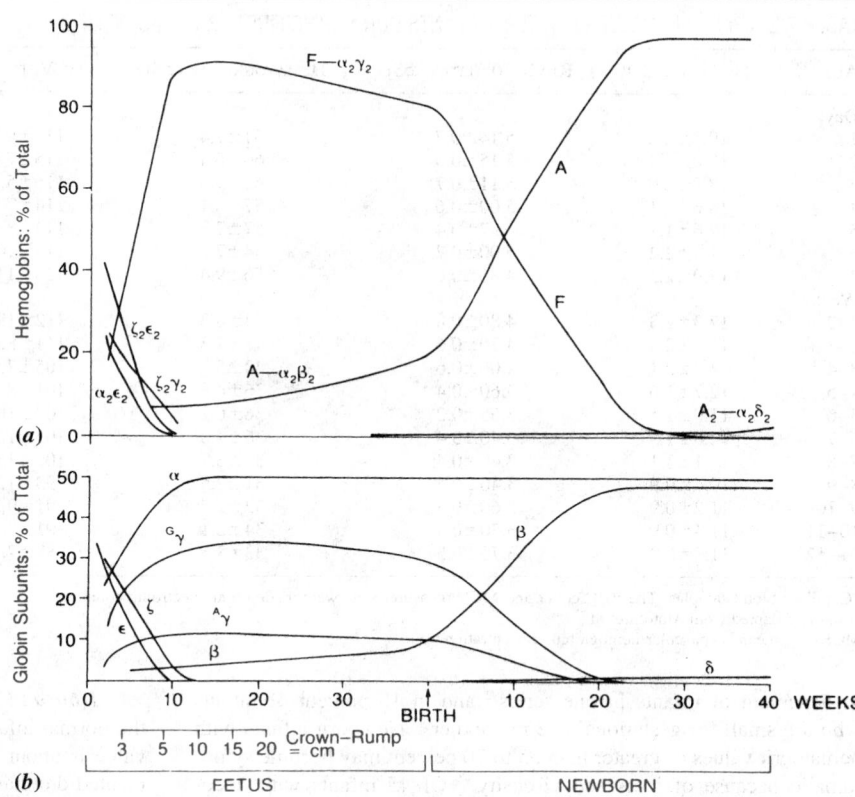

FIGURE 7-1   Changes in hemoglobin tetramers (a) and in globin subunits (b) during human development from embryo to early infancy. (Reproduced from HF Bunn and BG Forget, *Hemoglobin: Molecular, Genetic and Clinical Aspects*, Saunders, Philadelphia, 1986, with permission.)

Erythropoietin and Physiologic Anemia of the Newborn   Erythropoietin is the primary regulator of erythropoiesis. While erythropoietin is present in cord blood, it falls to undetectable levels after birth in healthy infants.[84] Subsequently, the reticulocyte count falls to less than one percent by the sixth day of life.[85] The red cell, hemoglobin, and hematocrit values decrease only slightly during the first week but decline more rapidly in the following 5 to 8 weeks (see Table 7-2),[70] producing the physiologic anemia of the newborn.[86] The lowest hemoglobin values in the term infant occur at about 2 months of age.[72] When the hemoglobin concentration falls below 11 g/dl, erythropoietic activity begins to increase. Erythropoietin can be measured after the 60th day of life,[87] corresponding to the recovery from physiologic anemia. If there is sufficient stimulus, such as hemolytic anemia or cyanotic heart disease, the newborn infant is able to produce erythropoietin during the first several months of life.[84]

In the premature infant the fall in hemoglobin level is more pronounced. In one study of premature infants the mean hemoglobin level at 2 months was 9.4 g/dl, with a 95 percent range of 7.2 to 11.7 g/dl.[88] In healthy premature infants erythropoietin becomes detectable when the hemoglobin level falls to about 12 g/dl. In infants with a lower percentage of Hb F (as from transfusion) and consequently better oxygen delivery, erythropoietin does not rise until the hemoglobin falls to about 9.5 g/dl.[89] The mean values for iron-sufficient premature infants reached those of term infants by 4 months for red cell count, 5 months for hemoglobin level, and 6 months for mean corpuscular volume and mean corpuscular hemoglobin.[88]

Blood Viscosity   The viscosity of blood increases logarithmically in relation to the hematocrit.[90,91] Hyperviscosity has been found

TABLE 7-2   RED CELL VALUES FOR TERM INFANTS DURING THE FIRST 12 WEEKS OF LIFE*

AGE	HB, G/DL ±SD	RBC×10¹²/LITER ±SD	HEMATOCRIT, % ±SD	MCV, FL ±SD	MCHC, G/DL ±SD	RETICULOCYTES, % ±SD
Days						
1	19.3±2.2	5.14±0.7	61±7.4	119±9.4	31.6±1.9	3.2±1.4
2	19.0±1.9	5.15±0.8	60±6.4	115±7.0	31.6±1.4	3.2±1.3
3	18.8±2.0	5.11±0.7	62±9.3	116±5.3	31.1±2.8	2.8±1.7
4	18.6±2.1	5.00±0.6	57±8.1	114±7.5	32.6±1.5	1.8±1.1
5	17.6±1.1	4.97±0.4	57±7.3	114±8.9	30.9±2.2	1.2±0.2
6	17.4±2.2	5.00±0.7	54±7.2	113±10.0	32.2±1.6	0.6±0.2
7	17.9±2.5	4.86±0.6	56±9.4	118±11.2	32.0±1.6	0.5±0.4
Weeks						
1–2	17.3±2.3	4.80±0.8	54±8.3	112±19.0	32.1±2.9	0.5±0.3
2–3	15.6±2.6	4.20±0.6	46±7.3	111±8.2	33.9±1.9	0.8±0.6
3–4	14.2±2.1	4.00±0.6	43±5.7	105±7.5	33.5±1.6	0.6±0.3
4–5	12.7±1.6	3.60±0.4	36±4.8	101±8.1	34.9±1.6	0.9±0.8
5–6	11.9±1.5	3.55±0.2	36±6.2	102±10.2	34.1±2.9	1.0±0.7
6–7	12.0±1.5	3.40±0.4	36±4.8	105±12.0	33.8±2.3	1.2±0.7
7–8	11.1±1.1	3.40±0.4	33±3.7	100±13.0	33.7±2.6	1.5±0.7
8–9	10.7±0.9	3.40±0.5	31±2.5	93±12.0	34.1±2.2	1.8±1.0
9–10	11.2±0.9	3.60±0.3	32±2.7	91±9.3	34.3±2.9	1.2±0.6
10–11	11.4±0.9	3.70±0.4	34±2.1	91±7.7	33.2±2.4	1.2±0.7
11–12	11.3±0.9	3.70±0.3	33±3.3	88±7.9	34.8±2.2	0.7±0.3

*Capillary blood samples. The RBC count and MCV measurements were made on an electronic counter.
SOURCE: Adapted from Matoth et al.[70]
MCHC = mean corpuscular hemoglobin concentration.

in 5 percent of infants in one series[92] and in 18 percent of infants who are small for gestational age in another.[93] Newborn infants with hematocrit values of greater than 65 to 70 percent may become symptomatic because of increased viscosity.[94] Of 45 infants with documented hyperviscosity and a mean hematocrit greater than 65 percent, 17 (38%) had symptoms of irritability, hypotonia, tremors, or poor suck reflex.[95] Partial plasma exchange transfusion reduced blood viscosity, improved cerebral blood flow, and relieved the symptoms. However, cerebral blood flow was normal in the asymptomatic infants with hyperviscosity, and there consequently was no benefit from exchange transfusion.[95]

Red Cell Antigens   The blood group antigens on neonatal red cells differ from those of the older child and adult. The i antigen is expressed strongly while the I antigen and the A and B antigens are expressed only weakly on neonatal red cells. The i antigen is a straight-chain carbohydrate which is replaced by the branched-chain derivative, I antigen, as a result of the developmental acquisition of a glycosyl-transferase.[96] By one year of age the i antigen has become undetectable, and the ABH antigens increase to adult levels by age 3. The ABH, Kell, Duffy and Vel antigens can be detected on the cells of the fetus in the first trimester and are present at birth.[97] The Lu^a and Lu^b antigens also are detectable on fetal red cells and are more weakly expressed at birth, increasing to adult levels by age 15.[97] The Xg antigen is variably expressed in the fetus and is weaker on newborn than adult red cells. Moreover, particularly poor expression of Xg has been noted in newborns with trisomy 13, 18, and 21.[97] The Lewis group (Le^a/Le^b) antigens are adsorbed on the red cell membrane and become detectable within 1 to 2 weeks after birth as the receptor sites develop. Anti-A and anti-B as isohemagglutinins develop during the first 6 months of life, reaching adult levels by 2 years of age.

Red Cell Life Span   The life span of the red cells in the newborn infant is shorter than that of red cells in the adult. The average of several studies of mean half-life of newborn red cells labeled with chromium was 23.3 days in term infants and 16.6 days in premature infants. When corrected for the elution rate of chromium from newborn cells, the estimate of mean red cell survival in the newborn is 60 to 80 days.[98] The reasons for this shortened survival are unclear, but the known susceptibility to oxidant injury of newborn red cells may be a contributing factor.

Iron and Transferrin   The serum iron level in cord blood of the normal infant is elevated compared to maternal levels. The mean value is about 150 ± 40 μg/dl (1 SD).[99] Infants on an iron-supplemented diet have a median serum iron level of 125 μg/dl at 1 month of age and of about 75 μg/dl at 6 months of age. The total iron-binding capacity rises throughout the first year of life. The median transferrin saturation falls from almost 65 percent at 0.5 months to 25 percent at 1 year, and saturations as low as 10 percent may be observed in the absence of iron deficiency.[100] The mean serum ferritin levels in iron-sufficient infants are high at birth, 160 μg/l, rise further during the first month, and then fall to a mean of 30 μg/l by 1 year of age.[101] The amount of stainable iron in the marrow at birth is small but increases in both term and premature infants during the first weeks of life. Stainable marrow iron begins to decrease after 2 months and is gone by 4 to 6 months in term infants and earlier in premature infants.[102]

RED CELL FUNCTIONS

Oxygen Delivery   The oxygen affinity of cord blood is greater than that of maternal blood, since the affinity of Hb F for 2,3-bisphos-phoglycerate (2,3-BPG) is less than that of Hb A.[103] Levels of 2,3-BPG are lower in newborn red cells than in adult cells and even more decreased in the red cells of premature infants,[104] and this low 2,3-BPG level further heightens the oxygen affinity of newborn red cells. Thus, the red cell oxygen equilibrium curve of the newborn is shifted to the left of that of the adult (Figure 7-2). The mean partial pressure of oxygen at which hemoglobin is 50 percent saturated with oxygen at 1 day of age in term infants is 19.4 ± 1.8 torr, as compared with the normal adult value of 27.0 ± 1.1 torr.[105] This results in a decrease in the oxygen released at the tissue level, as shown in Figure 7-2. As the P_{O_2} falls from 90 torr in arterial to 40 torr in the venous blood, 3.0 ml/dl of oxygen are released from newborn blood, while 4.5 ml/dl are released from adult, Hb A-containing blood. The shift to the left of the oxygen equilibrium curve is even more pronounced in the premature infant, requiring a larger fall in P_{O_2} to release an equivalent amount of oxygen. After birth the oxygen equilibrium curve shifts gradually to the right, reaching the position of the adult curve by 6 months of age. The position of the curve in the premature infant correlates with gestational age rather than with postnatal age,[105] and its shift to the adult position is more gradual.

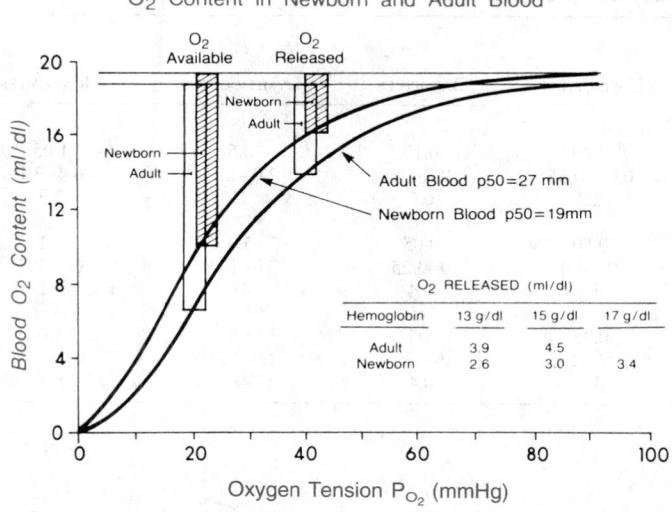

O₂ Content in Newborn and Adult Blood

FIGURE 7-2 The oxygen equilibrium curves are based on the assumption that the Hb concentration is 15 g/dl and that there is full O_2 saturation of Hb at a Pa_{O_2} of 100 torr. The O_2 released is the difference in O_2 content between a Pa_{O_2} of 90 torr and the mixed venous P_{O_2} of 40 torr. The O_2 available is the difference in O_2 content between a Pa_{O_2} of 90 torr and a mixed venous Pa_{O_2} of 20 torr. This is the maximum O_2 available without evoking compensatory mechanisms such as increased cardiac output.

Metabolism Many differences have been found between the metabolism of the red cells of newborn infants and that of adults.[106,107] Some of the differences may be explained by the younger mean cell age in the newborn, but others seem to be properties of the fetal cell. The glucose consumption in newborn cells is lower than that in adult cells.[108] Elevated levels of glucose phosphate isomerase, glyceraldehyde-3-phosphate dehydrogenase, phosphoglycerate kinase, and enolase beyond those explainable by the young cell age have been found in neonatal cells.[104,109] The level of phosphofructokinase is low in red cells of term and premature infants.[104,109,110] The pentose phosphate shunt is active in red cells of term and premature infants,[111] but there is glutathione instability and a heightened susceptibility to oxidant injury. Furthermore, there is relative instability of the 2,3-BPG concentration. Lower-than-adult activities have been found for several other red cell enzymes, including NADP-dependent methemoglobin reductase[112] and glutathione peroxidase.[113] The levels of ATP and ADP are higher in the red cells of term and preterm infants[110] but may merely reflect the younger age of the erythrocyte population.[114]

Membrane The membrane of the newborn red cell also is different from that of the adult red cell. Ouabain-sensitive ATPase is decreased,[115] and active potassium influx is significantly less in neonatal red cells.[116] Newborn cells are more sensitive to osmotic hemolysis and to oxidant injury than are adult cells. Newborn red cell membranes have higher total lipid, phospholipid, and cholesterol per cell than adult red cells.[117,118] The patterns of phospholipid and phospholipid fatty acid composition also differ from those in adult red cells. Red cells of newborns have the same pattern of membrane proteins on polyacrylamide gel electrophoresis[119] and the same rate of mobility in an electric field[120] as do red cells from adults. After trypsin treatment of newborn and adult cells, however, there is a difference in electrophoretic mobility, indicating that the surface trypsin-resistant proteins are different.[120] The relationship of the metabolic and membrane alterations in neonatal red cells to their shorter life span is not clear.

WHITE CELLS

NEONATAL GRANULOPOIESIS

Colony-Stimulating Factors and Granulo-monopoiesis The absolute number of neutrophils in the blood of term and premature infants is usually greater than that found in older children (Table 7-3).[121] The neutrophil count tends to be lower in the premature than in the term infant, and the proportion of myelocytes and band neutrophils is higher.[122] Serum and urinary colony-stimulating activity are elevated during the period of neutrophilia.[123,124] When granulopoiesis was studied in cord blood, blood, and marrow of infants, the macrophage colony-forming unit was predominant in spite of the clinical neutrophilia, and this pattern was not altered by different sources of colony-stimulating factors.[125,126] The endogenous cytokines produced by mononuclear cells from cord or systemic venous blood support the growth of neutrophil colonies in assays using marrow from adults.[125] However, there is diminished GM-CSF, G-CSF, and IL-3 production and diminished mRNA expression in stimulated newborn compared to adult mononuclear cells,[127–129] which may limit the response to bacterial infection in the newborn. Smaller numbers of CFU-GM colonies were observed in the blood of sick infants, who have diminished endogenous production of CSF in culture.[126] Dysregulation of neonatal granulopoiesis may impair the neonatal response to infection.[130] The administration of stem cell factor with G-CSF to newborn rats reduces the mortality of experimental group B streptococcal infection, and this approach may be useful in human disease.[131]

White Cell and Differential Counts The values for the white cell and differential counts during the first 2 weeks of life are given in Table 7-3. The absolute number of segmented neutrophils rises in both term and premature infants in the first 24 h of life.[132] In term infants the mean value increases from 8×10^9/liter (8000/μl) to a peak of 13×10^9/liter (13,000/μl) and then falls to 4×10^9/μl) by 72 h of age, remaining at this level through the following 7 days. In the premature infant the mean values for neutrophils are 5×10^9/liter (5000/μl) at birth, 8×10^9/liter (8000/μl) at 12 h, and 4×10^9/liter (4000/μl) at 72 h. The mean count then falls gradually to 2.5×10^9/liter (2500/μl) by the 28th day of life. The level after the first 72 h is very stable for an individual infant, whether term or premature. Immature forms, including an occasional promyelocyte and blast cell, may be seen in the blood of healthy infants in the first few days of life and are more frequent in premature infants than in term infants.[132] Segmented granulocytes are the predominant cells in the first few days of life. As their number decreases, the lymphocyte becomes the most numerous cell and remains so during the first 4 years of life. An absolute eosinophil count of greater than 0.7×10^9/liter (700/μl) was found in 76 percent of premature infants at 2 to 3 weeks of age. The onset of the eosinophilia coincided with the establishment of steady weight gain in the infants.[133] It is increased by the use of total parenteral nutrition, endotracheal intubation, and blood transfusions.

PHAGOCYTE FUNCTIONS

Bacterial infections are a major cause of morbidity and mortality in the newborn period.[134] The infections are frequently due to organisms of low virulence in normal children and adults, including *Staphylococcus*, Lancefield group B β-hemolytic streptococci, *Pseudomonas*, and other gram-negative bacilli. Cellular defense mechanisms and humoral immunity of the newborn differ from those found later in life, and these undoubtedly contribute to the unusual susceptibility to infection noted in the neonatal period.[134]

Opsonins and Complement Engulfment and destruction of bacteria by neutrophils depend on opsonic activity of the plasma and on chemotaxis, phagocytosis, and the bacteriocidal capacity of the

TABLE 7-3　THE WHITE CELL COUNT AND THE DIFFERENTIAL COUNT DURING THE FIRST 2 WEEKS OF LIFE*

| Age | Leukocytes | Neutrophils | | | Eosinophils | Basophils | Lymphocytes | Monocytes |
		Total	Seg.	Band				
Birth								
Mean	18.0	11.0	9.4	1.6	0.40	0.10	0.5	1.05
Range	9.0–30.0	6.0–26.0	—	—	0.02–0.85	0–0.64	2.0–11.0	0.4–3.1
Mean %	—	61	52	9	2.2	0.6	31	5.8
7 days								
Mean	12.2	5.5	4.7	0.83	0.50	0.05	5.0	1.1
Range	5.0–21.0	1.5–10.0	—	—	.07–1.1	0–0.25	2.0–17.0	0.3–2.7
Mean %	—	45	39	6	4.1	0.4	41	9.1
14 days								
Mean	11.4	4.5	3.9	0.63	0.35	.05	5.5	1.0
Range	5.0–20.0	1.0–9.5	—	—	0.07–1.0	0–0.23	2.0–17.0	0.2–2.4
Mean %	—	40	34	5.5	3.1	0.4	48	8.8

*All white cell counts are expressed as cells $\times$ 10^9/liter.
SOURCE: From Altman and Dittmer,[121] with permission.

leukocyte. The serum factors necessary for optimal phagocytosis (opsonins) include the immunoglobulins and complement components. In term infants, opsonic activity is normal for *Staphylococcus aureus*,[135,136] but it is low for yeast[137] and *Escherichia coli*.[136] Diminished opsonic antibody has been associated with group B streptococcal infection and represents one risk factor for neonatal infection.[138]

In premature infants, opsonic activity is low for *Staphylococcus aureus* and *Serratia marcescens*[135] but is normal for *Pseudomonas aeruginosa*.[139] When serum concentrations of fibronectin and IgG subclasses C3 and C4 were measured at birth, 1 month, 3 months, and 6 months, early gestational age was correlated with lower initial levels.[140] The decreased opsonic activity for some organisms in premature infants has been attributed to diminished IgG levels, since additional IgG will correct the opsonic defect both in vivo and in vitro.[135] The added IgG improves bacterial opsonization by serum of premature infants in part because complement consumption and deposition of C3 on the bacterial surface is augmented.[141,142]

Complement components appear in fetal blood before 20 weeks of gestation and increase markedly during the third trimester. However, in many newborns both the classical and alternative complement pathways are decreased in activity and in levels of individual components.[143] The mean level of C3, the first common component of the two pathways of complement activation, is about 65 percent of that in normal adults.[144–146] There is no transplacental transfer of this protein, and levels in infants are lower than those in their mothers.[144] Total hemolytic complement (CH50) and alternative pathway activity (PH50) in newborns are lower than in adults, as are mean levels of C1q, C2–C9, properdin, and factors B, I and H.[145–147] In general, the mean levels in full-term infants are greater than 50 percent of those in normal adult controls and may be somewhat less in premature infants. There is considerable overlap, however, between levels in infants and in controls. A functional deficiency in the alternative pathway has been detected in infants.[148]

Fibronectin mediates more efficient interactions between phagocytes and infectious agents. Fibronectin, a 450 kD glycoprotein found in plasma and in the intercellular matrix, promotes the attachment of staphylococci to neutrophils[149] and enhances opsonic activity of antibodies against group B streptococci.[150] Since both these bacteria are common pathogens for neonates, the deficiency in fibronectin observed in neonates[151] may further compromise opsonic capacity and hence bactericidal activity in the neonate.

The administration of intravenous IgG may be useful in the treatment or prophylaxis of infection in preterm infants based on the reduced placental transfer of maternal antibody and the restricted endogenous synthesis of IgG.[152] IgG administered to septic neonates appears to enhance serum opsonic capacity as well as to increase the quantity of circulating neutrophils.[153] Added IgG heightens phagocytosis of granulocytes from premature neonates,[154] and intravenous IgG has been reported to effectively treat infected premature neonates, but these reports involved small numbers of subjects.[155,156] The clinical efficacy of IgG prophylaxis against neonatal pathogens is not firmly established.[157,158] New IgG preparations with consistent, adequate levels of antibodies directed against neonatal pathogens can be achieved by selection of sera with high levels of functional antibodies,[159] or potentially by the addition of monoclonal antibodies, and these may prove more clearly effective.

Chemotaxis　Chemotactic function of leukocytes is low in neonates, while random motility is normal.[160–162] Neonatal serum does not generate as much chemotactic factor as does adult serum, even after the addition of purified C3. The defect in chemotaxis may be related to decreased granulocyte deformability and impaired capping of cell surface receptors.[163] The role of observed cAMP and membrane potential alterations in the defective chemotaxis is not clear.[163]

The densities of the C3bi receptor (CD11b/CD18) and of the low-affinity receptor for immunoglobulin, FcRIII (CD16), are decreased on neutrophils of premature infants, whereas term infants' cells show a lesser impairment.[164–167] The deficient up-regulation of C3bi has been correlated with decreased adherence and chemotaxis by neonatal neutrophils.[168] Low FcRIII was associated with impaired chemotaxis of neonatal neutrophils,[169] although decreased FcRIII might also be responsible for subtle defects in adherence and subsequent phagocytosis of opsonized[159] and unopsonized[170] organisms by neutrophils.

Phagocytic and Bactericidal Activity　Phagocytosis of bacteria and latex granules by neutrophils from premature and term infants is normal.[135–139,172,173] Bactericidal activity varies according to the conditions of testing and the clinical status of the neonates. The intracellular killing of *Staphylococcus aureus* and *Serratia marcescens* in cells from most term and low-birth-weight infants is normal,[135,174] as is that of *Escherichia coli* in term infants.[136] Similar studies have shown defective bactericidal activity against *S. aureus* in some infants in the first 12 h of life,[172] *P. aeruginosa* in cells from premature infants,[139] and *Candida albicans* in granulocytes from term and premature infants.[175] With bacteria/neutrophil ratios of 1 : 1, newborn cells kill *S. aureus* and *E. coli* as effectively as controls; however, at the higher ratio of 100 : 1 killing and oxidative response as measured by chemiluminescence are markedly depressed, although phagocytosis is normal.[173] Depressed activity also has been found in cells from newborns who have had clinical stress, either from infection or other disorders, shown both as decreased chemiluminescence and impaired bactericidal activity against *S. aureus*, *E. coli*, and group B streptococci.[176–178] The decreased granulocyte function shown in these studies also is found in liquid culture, where neutrophils from newborns do not survive as long as those from adults, perhaps because of decreased resistance to autoxidation.[179] Although superoxide dismutase levels are normal and superoxide production is normal or increased in neutrophils from newborns, glutathione peroxidase and catalase levels are decreased.[180,181] The relationship of these in vitro cellular defects to bacterial infections in the newborn is still not clear.

Monocytes from newborn infants have normal nitroblue tetrazolium (NBT) reduction,[182] normal antibody-dependent cellular cytotoxicity,[183] and normal in vitro killing of *S. aureus* and *E. coli*.[184] However, they are slower than monocytes from adults in phagocytosis of polystyrene spheres,[185] and they have reduced ATP production.[186] Furthermore, chemotaxis to serum-derived factors is decreased, as is monocyte appearance in skin windows.[187] These functional aspects may contribute to the observed susceptibility of newborns to a variety of infectious agents.

Cytokine Effects on Neonatal Phagocytic Function   There is a complex interaction between cytokines produced by lymphocytes and macrophages, and the activation status of neutrophils during infection. There is decreased production of γ-interferon by neonatal leukocytes.[188–190] γ-interferon causes the up-regulation of the C3bi receptor and induces the surface expression of the high-affinity immunoglobulin receptor FcRI (CD64)[191] on neutrophils. C3bi is required for adherence and efficient chemotaxis by neutrophils. Complement-mediated phagocytosis and oxidative metabolism also are impaired by low levels of this receptor. FcRI mediates oxidative responses as well, and appears on neutrophils of adults during infection. The diminished production of G-CSF and GM-CSF by neonatal mononuclear cells[127–129] may not only limit progenitor colony growth but also impair neonatal neutrophil functions, including chemotaxis, superoxide production, and C3bi expression, which are enhanced by these factors.[192,193] Tumor necrosis factor alpha (TNF-α) and interleukin 4 (IL-4), cytokines which modulate neutrophil functions, also may be produced at lower levels in neonates.[194] Interleukin 8 (IL-8), a cytokine that enhances neutrophil functions, has not been adequately studied in neonates.

PLATELETS

NEONATAL THROMBOPOIESIS

The platelet counts in term and preterm infants are between 150 and 400×10^9/liter (150,000 to 400,000/μl), comparable to adult values.[195–196] Thrombocytopenia of less than 100×10^9/liter (100,000/μl) may occur in high-risk infants with respiratory distress or sepsis,[197] small-for-date infants,[198] and newborns with trisomy syndromes.[199] Even normal newborns are unable to regulate thrombopoiesis and myelopoiesis in a totally effective manner.[200] Although committed megakaryocyte progenitors (CFU-Meg) are increased in the marrow and cord blood of newborns, they are less able to produce adequate numbers of platelets when severely stressed. Thrombopoiesis-stimulating activity appears lower in cord serum than in adult serum,[201] and reduced levels of G-CSF, GM-CSF, IL-3, and IL-11 may play a role in the impaired response.[202] IL-11 and IL-3 act synergistically to enhance mouse CFU-Meg, and the role of these growth factors and others, such as TPO, IL-6, and Steel factor are currently being explored.

PLATELET FUNCTIONS

Bleeding Time   The expected inverse relationship between the platelet count and bleeding time has been described in term and preterm newborns.[203] However, the bleeding time often is longer than would be predicted by the platelet count because of sepsis or respiratory distress resulting in impaired platelet function, aggravating the effects of thrombocytopenia.

The bleeding time reflects platelet function and capillary integrity as well as the platelet count and traditionally has been used to assess these parameters. However, there are technical difficulties in applying a technique for measuring bleeding time to neonates or preterm infants because of the need for venous occlusion of the forearm, where the test normally is performed, and for a minimal incision to avoid scarring of the skin. Bleeding times were measured using an automatic device to minimize trauma in normal neonates, with venous occlusion of 20 torr for infants less than 1000 g, 25 torr for those 1000 to 2000 g, and 30 torr for those over 2000 g. In 82 observations, 97 percent of the measurements were below 3.5 min, which was suggested as the upper limit for normal in these infants.[204] A similar upper limit (200 s) for the bleeding time of normal infants has been obtained using an automated device and vertical incisions.[205] Generally, newborn infants have shorter bleeding times than those of children and adults, and this may reflect their higher hematocrit, increased concentration of von Willebrand factor, and higher proportion of high molecular weight multimers of von Willebrand factor.[206] Children have longer bleeding times than either adults or newborns,[207] and the upper limit measured with an automated pediatric device may be as high as 13 min before age 10, compared to an upper limit of 7 min in adults measured with the same device.[207]

The bleeding times in newborns may be prolonged for a variety of reasons, including neonatal infection and respiratory distress syndrome, which do not necessarily result in thrombocytopenia.[208] The use of indomethacin for treatment of patent ductus arteriosus in preterm infants has been questioned because this agent interferes with prostaglandin metabolism and the production of thromboxane A_2, an important initiator of platelet aggregation. Although bleeding times are prolonged from a normal of 3.5 min to approximately 9 min in indomethacin-treated patients,[209] indomethacin did not result in an increase in periventricular or intraventricular hemorrhage in preterm infants treated for patent ductus arteriosus.

Platelet Aggregation and Metabolism   A variety of differences have been described in the platelet function of neonates. These include decreased ADP release, platelet factor 3 activity, platelet adhesiveness, and platelet aggregation in response to ADP, epinephrine, collagen, or thrombin.[210,211] These defects result from intrinsic differences in neonatal compared to adult platelets.[212] Paradoxically, these insufficiencies have little effect on the bleeding time of neonates. The in vitro findings do not appear related to a significant defect in prostaglandin synthesis or to storage pool deficiency of adenine nucleotides.[210] Further, electron micrographs of neonatal platelets do not differ from those of platelets from normal adults.[213] This leaves unexplained the in vitro observations in neonatal platelets, which may be related to platelet membrane immaturity. These in vitro abnormalities may aggravate the impairment in platelet function and the predisposition to bleeding which results from neonatal diseases, particularly respiratory distress syndrome and sepsis.

Aspirin ingestion by mothers also results in abnormalities in platelet aggregation in response to collagen.[214,215] However, aspirin has been studied extensively in patients with preeclampsia, and there is no significant bleeding in the fetus or newborn.[216,217]

Newborn infants commonly have petechiae, particularly on the head, neck, and shoulders after vertex deliveries. They are presumably due to trauma associated with passage through the birth canal and disappear within a few days. Petechiae usually are not present in infants delivered by cesarean section.

Platelet Antigens and Glycoproteins   The glycoprotein complex GPIIb/IIIa represents about 15 percent of platelet surface protein and exhibits two allelic forms, Pl[A1] and Pl[A2].[218] The Pl[A1] antigen can be

TABLE 7-4　LYMPHOCYTE SUBSETS IN NEONATAL (CORD) BLOOD

	MEAN (25–75 PERCENTILE RANGE)		
LYMPHOCYTE SUBSET	INFANTS (2 DAYS–11 MONTHS)	CHILDREN* (1–6 YEARS)	ADULTS (18–70 YEARS)
Lymphocytes, total	47% (39–59) 4.1×10^9/liter (2.7–5.4)	46 (38–53) 3.6 (2.9–5.1)	32 (28–39) 2.1 (1.6–2.4)
CD3	64% (58–67) 2.5×10^9/liter (1.7–3.6)	64 (62–69) 2.5 (1.8–3.0)	72 (67–76) 1.4 (1.1–1.7)
CD4	41% (38–50) 2.2×10^9/liter (1.7–2.8)	37 (30–40) 1.6 (1.0–1.8)	42 (38–46) 0.8 (0.7–1.1)
CD8	21% (18–25) 0.9×10^9/liter (0.8–1.2)	29 (25–32) 0.9 (0.8–1.5)	35 (31–40) 0.7 (0.5–0.9)
CD4/CD8 ratio	1.9 (1.5–2.9)	1.3 (1.0–1.6)	1.2 (1.0–1.5)
NK (CD3−/CD16 or CD56+)	11% (8.0–17) 0.5×10^9/liter (0.3–0.7)	11 (8.0–15) 0.4 (0.2–0.6)	14 (10–19) 0.3 (0.2–0.4)
CD20	23% (19–31) 0.9×10^9/liter (0.5–1.5)	16 (12–22) 0.4 (0.3–0.5)	13 (11–16) 0.3 (0.2–0.4)

*Age 7–17 years, similar to adults.
SOURCE: Based on Erkeller-Yuksel, et al.[223]

identified on fetal platelets by 16 weeks gestation.[210] PI^{A1} antigen is observed in a higher percentage of fetuses between 18 and 26 weeks than in adults. Approximately 2 percent of the population in the United States of European descent is homozygous for PI^{A2} and hence PI^{A1} negative. The complete expression of the PI^{A1} antigen during early gestation likely permits early sensitization in women who are PI^{A1} negative even during their first pregnancy.[219] The membrane glycoprotein GPIb, as well as the GPIIb/IIIa complex, is expressed by 18 weeks of gestation.[219] The gene for GPIIb/IIIa has been cloned, and the difference between PI^{A1} and PI^{A2} is a leucine 33/ proline 33 amino acid polymorphism in glycoprotein IIIA.[218] Prenatal diagnosis of the glycoprotein genotype using DNA from amniocytes and the polymerase chain reaction can establish the potential for neonatal alloimmune thrombocytopenia[220] as well as the diagnosis of Glanzmann's thrombasthenia. Rarely, other fetal platelet antigens such as PI^{E2}, DUZO^a, Ko^a and Bak^a have caused maternal sensitization and neonatal alloimmune thrombocytopenia.[221] The gestational ages for expression of these antigens have not been defined but are sufficiently early to permit sensitization.

NEONATAL LYMPHOPOIESIS

T-LYMPHOCYTE FUNCTIONS—CELLULAR IMMUNITY

The absolute number of lymphocytes in the newborn is equivalent to that in older children (Table 7-4), with lower values in premature infants at birth. Thymus-derived cells (T cells) develop early in gestation.[222] The various lymphocyte subsets in newborns are shown in Table 7-4.[223] The absolute number of CD3+ and CD4+ (helper/ inducer phenotype) T-cell subsets in blood of newborns is significantly higher than in adults.[13,224] This is due to an increased total lymphocyte count in neonates (and older children) compared to adults.[225] The percentages of major lymphoid subsets (CD2, CD3, CD4, CD8, CD19, CD16) are not markedly different in neonates, children, and adults when measured by flow cytometry methods.[226] There is a trend to increased CD4 and decreased CD8 lymphocytes in newborns and children, resulting in an increased CD4/CD8 ratio.[227,228] In spite of this, T-cell suppressor activity may be increased in newborns.[229] Most responses of the cellular immunity system, such as antigen recognition and binding, antibody-dependent cytotoxicity and graft-versus-host reactivity are present in the newborn,[229] although some are decreased in comparison with

adults.[230] The in vitro response to phytohemagglutinin of cord blood lymphocytes is increased,[231,232] but the response of the newborn to 2,4-dinitrofluorobenzene, a potent inducer of delayed hypersensitivity, is not as consistent as that seen in older children.[233] Impaired T-cell production of γ interferon and other lymphokines may be related to immature macrophage rather than T-lymphocyte function, since intercellular cooperation is a requisite for these processes.[234] Further, cord blood T-lymphocytes form a functional IL-2 receptor complex and have normal IL-2 receptors, but they do not up-regulate γ interferon in response to IL2.[235]

B-LYMPHOCYTE FUNCTIONS— HUMORAL IMMUNITY

Humoral (B-cell) immunity also develops early in gestation,[222] but it is not fully active until after birth. In the newborn, about 15 percent of lymphocytes have immunoglobulin on their surface, with all Ig isotypes represented.[236] A percentage of these cells are CD5+ B cells (B-1 cells), which produce polyreactive autoantibodies whose function is yet unclear.[237] The proportion of CD5+ B cells is markedly higher in the fetus compared to adults. The percentages of B cells expressing specific immunoglobulin isotypes are not related to the plasma levels of those isotypes. Variation in antibody response to specific antigens relates to the interaction of macrophages, T cells, and B cells; B lymphocytes are well represented in newborns.[238]

Fetal lymphocytes synthesize little immunoglobulin, presumably because of the sheltered environment in utero. Animals kept germ-free after birth have few plasma cells and markedly decreased production of immunoglobulins.[239] IgG levels of term infants are similar to maternal levels because of transplacental transfer.[240] IgM, IgD, and IgE do not cross the placenta,[240,241] and the levels of these immunoglobulins and of IgA are low or not detectable at birth. Breast feeding provides some transfer of antibodies, particularly secretory IgA, lysozyme, and lactoferrin. Large numbers of lymphocytes and monocytes (10^6 cells/ ml) are found in colostrum and milk during the first two months postpartum.[242] These may provide local gastrointestinal protection against infection,[243] and there is some evidence for absorption of immunoglobulin and transfer of tuberculin sensitivity to the infant.

Although the newborn infant can produce specific IgG antibody,[244] only small amounts of IgG are usually produced by the fetus. IgG levels in premature infants are reduced in relation to gestational age because of the low placental transport early in pregnancy.[245–247] The ability of the fetus to produce IgM and IgA with appropriate stimuli is indicated by the presence of these antibodies in many newborn infants who have had prenatal infections[248] and by the presence of IgM isohemagglutinins in more than one-half of term newborn infants.[249] In human newborns and in fetal animals the IgM response is predominant, and the appearance of IgG after exposure to specific antigens is delayed. These differences from the adult may relate to functional immaturity of B and T lymphocytes,[250–252] to increased activity of suppressor T cells[239,250] and perhaps to altered macrophage function.[253]

Newborns also may have relative splenic hypofunction, suggested by the large number of "pocked" red cells seen in the blood films of neonates, particularly premature infants. These "pocks" represent residual intraerythrocyte inclusions, which remain because of monocyte and macrophage hypofunction.[254,255]

TABLE 7-5   REFERENCE VALUES FOR COAGULATION TESTS IN PRETERM AND FULL-TERM INFANTS*

Coagulation Test	Preterm 28–31 Week Infants Day 1	Preterm 30–36 Week Infants			Full-Term Infants			Adults
		Day 1	Day 30	Day 180	Day 1	Day 30	Day 180	
PT (s)	15.4 (14.6–16.9)	13.0 (10.6–16.2)	11.8 (10.0–13.6)	12.5 (10.0–15.0)	13.0 (10.1–15.9)	11.8 (10.0–14.3)	12.3 (10.7–13.9)	12.4 (10.8–13.9)
INR	1.0 (0.61–1.70)	1.0 (0.61–1.70)	0.79 (0.53–1.11)	0.91 (0.53–1.48)	1.00 (0.53–1.62)	0.79 (0.53–1.26)	0.88 (0.61–1.17)	0.89 (0.64–1.17)
APTT (s)	108 (80.0–168)	53.6 (27.5–79.4)	44.7 (26.9–62.5)	37.5 (27.2–53.5)	42.9 (31.3–54.5)	40.4 (32.0–55.2)	35.5 (28.1–42.9)	33.5 (26.6–40.3)
TCT (s)		24.8 (19.2–30.4)	24.4 (18.8–29.9)	25.2 (18.9–31.5)	23.5 (19.0–28.3)	24.3 (19.4–29.2)	25.5 (19.8–31.2)	25.0 (19.7–30.3)
Fibrinogen (g/L)	2.56 (1.60–5.50)	2.43 (1.50–3.73)	2.54 (1.50–4.14)	2.28 (1.50–3.60)	2.83 (1.67–3.99)	2.70 (1.62–3.78)	2.51 (1.50–3.87)	2.78 (1.56–4.00)
II (U/mL)	0.31 (0.19–0.54)	0.45 (0.20–0.77)	0.57 (0.36–0.95)	0.87 (0.51–1.23)	0.48 (0.26–0.70)	0.68 (0.34–1.02)	0.88 (0.60–1.16)	1.08 (0.70–1.46)
V (U/mL)	0.65 (0.43–0.80)	0.88 (0.41–1.44)	1.02 (0.48–1.56)	1.02 (0.58–1.46)	0.72 (0.34–1.08)	0.98 (0.62–1.34)	0.91 (0.55–1.27)	1.06 (0.62–1.50)
VII (U/mL)	0.37 (0.24–0.76)	0.67 (0.21–1.13)	0.83 (0.21–1.45)	0.99 (0.47–1.51)	0.66 (0.28–1.04)	0.90 (0.42–1.38)	0.87 (0.47–1.27)	1.05 (0.67–1.43)
VIII (U/mL)	0.79 (0.37–1.26)	1.11 (0.50–2.13)	1.11 (0.50–1.99)	0.99 (0.50–1.87)	1.00 (0.50–1.78)	0.91 (0.50–1.57)	0.73 (0.50–1.09)	0.99 (0.50–1.49)
vWF (U/mL)	1.41 (0.83–2.23)	1.36 (0.78–2.10)	1.36 (0.66–2.16)	0.98 (0.54–1.58)	1.53 (0.50–2.87)	1.28 (0.50–2.46)	1.07 (0.50–1.97)	0.92 (0.50–1.58)
IX (U/mL)	0.18 (0.17–0.20)	0.35 (0.19–0.65)	0.44 (0.13–0.80)	0.81 (0.50–1.20)	0.53 (0.15–0.91)	0.51 (0.21–0.81)	0.86 (0.36–1.36)	1.09 (0.55–1.63)
X (U/mL)	0.36 (0.25–0.64)	0.41 (0.11–0.71)	0.56 (0.20–0.92)	0.77 (0.35–1.19)	0.40 (0.12–0.68)	0.59 (0.31–0.87)	0.78 (0.38–1.18)	1.06 (0.70–1.52)
XI (U/mL)	0.23 (0.11–0.33)	0.30 (0.08–0.52)	0.43 (0.15–0.71)	0.78 (0.46–1.10)	0.38 (0.10–0.66)	0.53 (0.27–0.79)	0.86 (0.49–1.34)	0.97 (0.67–1.27)
XII (U/mL)	0.25 (0.05–0.35)	0.38 (0.10–0.66)	0.43 (0.11–0.75)	0.82 (0.22–1.42)	0.53 (0.13–0.93)	0.49 (0.17–0.81)	0.77 (0.39–1.15)	1.08 (0.52–1.64)
PK (U/mL)	0.26 (0.15–0.32)	0.33 (0.09–0.57)	0.59 (0.31–0.87)	0.78 (0.40–1.16)	0.37 (0.18–0.69)	0.57 (0.23–0.91)	0.86 (0.56–1.16)	1.12 (0.62–1.62)
HK (U/mL)	0.32 (0.19–0.52)	0.49 (0.09–0.89)	0.64 (0.16–1.12)	0.83 (0.41–1.25)	0.54 (0.06–1.02)	0.77 (0.33–1.21)	0.82 (0.36–1.28)	0.92 (0.50–1.36)
XIII$_a$ (U/mL)		0.70 (0.32–1.08)	0.99 (0.51–1.47)	1.13 (0.65–1.61)	0.79 (0.27–1.31)	0.93 (0.39–1.47)	1.04 (0.46–1.62)	1.05 (0.55–1.55)
XIII$_b$ (U/mL)		0.81 (0.35–1.27)	1.07 (0.57–1.57)	1.15 (0.67–1.63)	0.76 (0.30–1.22)	1.11 (0.39–1.73)	1.10 (0.50–1.70)	0.97 (0.57–1.37)

*All factors except fibrinogen are expressed as units per milliliter (U/mL), where pooled plasma contains 1.0 U/mL. All values are expressed as the mean of 40 to 77 samples for each population. The range of values encompassing 95% of the population is shown in brackets.

ABBREVIATIONS: PT, prothrombin time; APTT, activated partial thromboplastin time; TCT, thrombin clotting time; vWF, von Willebrand factor; PK, prekallikrein; HK, high molecular weight kininogen; INR, international normalized ratio.

SOURCE: Modified from Andrew M[259,262] with permission.

COAGULATION IN THE NEONATE

PLASMA COAGULATION FACTORS

When the term newborn is compared to older children and adults, several differences in the coagulation and fibrinolytic systems have been described.[256-261] A comprehensive evaluation of the developmental changes in the levels of clotting factors and coagulation tests in preterm and term infants has been published.[262,263] The term newborn has reduced mean plasma levels (<60% of adult levels) of factors II, IX, X, XI, XII, prekallikrein, and high molecular weight kininogen (Table 7-5). In contrast, the plasma concentration of factor VIII is similar and von Willebrand factor is increased compared to older children and adults. In spite of the lower levels of factors, the functional tests (prothrombin and partial thromboplastin times) are only slightly prolonged compared to adult normal values (see Table 7-5). Although different coagulation factors show different postnatal patterns of maturation, near-adult values are achieved for most components by 6 months of life.[259]

Factor II (prothrombin), VII, IX, and X require vitamin K for the final gamma glutamyl carboxylation step in their synthesis.[264] These factors decrease during the first 3 to 4 days after birth. This fall may be lessened by administration of vitamin K,[265] effectively preventing classical, early-occurring (first few days of life) hemorrhagic disease of the newborn. Inactive prothrombin molecules have been found in the plasma of some newborns, but they disappear after administration of vitamin K.[266] Early-occurring hemorrhagic disease is most often associated with maternal administration of medications such as phenytoin (Dilantin)[267] and warfarin[268] which reduce the vitamin K-dependent factors. In rare cases no contributing factor is found.

A hemorrhagic diathesis also may occur later, 2 to 12 weeks after birth, due to lack of vitamin K and is called late hemorrhagic disease of the newborn, or acquired prothrombin complex deficiency.[269,270] The etiology of the vitamin K lack is unclear but may result from poor dietary intake, particularly related to breast feeding, alterations in liver function with cholestasis and decreased vitamin K absorption, or a toxic or infectious impairment of hepatic utilization.[269] Unfortunately, intracranial hemorrhage frequently is the presenting event in this condition. This problem can be prevented by parenteral or oral vitamin K, but the preferred route of administration remains controversial.[271] The parenteral route may result rarely in neuromuscular complications,[272] and an association of intramuscular vitamin K prophylaxis and cancer in infancy was suggested but not substantiated. Oral administration, however, may be less reliable and require repeated doses.[269] The most current recommendation of the Scientific and Standardization Subcommittee on Perinatal Haemostasis suggests that present practice should not be changed at this time.[270] Many institutions in the United States administer 1 mg vitamin K_1 intramuscularly at birth with effective prophylaxis. A new mixed micellar vitamin K_1 preparation is particularly well absorbed[273] and may permit prophylaxis with a single oral dose.

The values for coagulation factors in healthy 30- to 36-week-gestation premature infants are shown in Table 7-5. More prominent decreases in factors IX, XI, and XII are noted, which tend to prolong the partial thromboplastin time. The values for coagulation factors in 28- to 31-week-gestation infants also are shown in Table 7-5. All of the coagulation factors are lower at earlier gestational ages.

There are no significant differences in mean prothrombin time determinations between 30- to 36-week-premature and full-term infants who have not received vitamin K.[274] Premature infants given vitamin K have a longer mean prothrombin time than term infants similarly treated. In some small infants there is no improvement in prothrombin time or levels of prothrombin and factors VII and X after the intramuscular administration of vitamin K.[265,275] These results suggest a greater degree of "immaturity" of the liver in the small infants.

BLEEDING AND THROMBOSIS

Significant bleeding occurs more often in low-birth-weight infants than in term newborn infants. Increased capillary fragility is frequently found in premature infants in the first 2 days after birth and is not associated with thrombocytopenia.[265] Bleeding under the scalp or in other superficial areas may be due to trauma coupled with increased capillary fragility. The more serious disorders of periventricular-intraventricular hemorrhage and pulmonary hemorrhage probably are not primarily due to coagulation disorders, although such disorders may increase the bleeding.[276] Hypoxia seems to affect the clotting status of low birth weight infants.[277] Many infants with markedly abnormal prothrombin times have had hypoxia during delivery or shortly thereafter.[274] Cardiovascular collapse seen with episodes of cardiac arrest or with profound shock may cause disseminated intravascular coagulation and generalized bleeding. In many sick premature infants, a combination of shock, sepsis, liver immaturity, hypoxia, and other factors may contribute to the pathogenesis of coagulation abnormalities.

Arterial and venous thromboses are relatively frequent in newborns compared to other age groups, but greater than 90 percent of arterial and greater than 80 percent of venous clots are related to catheters. Spontaneous thromboses are much less common, and most involve the renal veins or rarely the pulmonary vasculature.[278] Relative hypercoagulability in the newborn could result from a difference in the vascular endothelium, activation of the coagulation cascade, diminished coagulation inhibitor activity, or a defect in fibrinolysis. Inhibi-

TABLE 7-6   REFERENCE VALUES FOR INHIBITORS OF COAGULATION IN PRETERM AND FULL-TERM INFANTS*

INHIBITOR LEVELS	PRETERM 30–36 WEEK INFANTS			FULL-TERM INFANTS			ADULT
	DAY 1	DAY 30	DAY 180	DAY 1	DAY 30	DAY 180	
AT (U/mL)	0.38 (0.14–0.62)	0.59 (0.37–0.81)	0.90 (0.52–1.28)	0.63 (0.39–0.87)	0.78 (0.48–1.08)	1.04 (0.84–1.24)	1.05 (0.7901.31)
α_2M (U/mL)	1.10 (0.56–1.82)	1.38 (0.72–2.04)	2.09 (1.10–3.21)	1.39 (0.95–1.83)	1.50 (1.06–1.94)	1.91 (1.49–2.33)	0.86 (0.52–1.20)
C_1E-INH (U/mL)	0.65 (0.31–0.99)	0.74 (0.40–1.24)	1.40 (0.96–2.04)	0.72 (0.36–1.08)	0.89 (0.47–1.31)	1.41 (0.89–1.93)	1.01 (0.71–1.31)
α_1AT (U/mL)	0.90 (0.36–1.44)	0.76 (0.38–1.12)	0.82 (0.48–1.16)	0.93 (0.49–1.37)	0.62 (0.36–0.88)	0.77 (0.47–1.07)	0.93 (0.55–1.31)
HCll (U/mL)	0.32 (0.10–0.60)	0.43 (0.15–0.71)	0.89 (0.45–1.40)	0.43 (0.10–0.93)	0.47 (0.10–0.87)	1.20 (0.50–1.90)	0.96 (0.66–1.26)
Protein C (U/mL)	0.28 (0.12–0.44)	0.37 (0.15–0.59)	0.57 (0.31–0.83)	0.35 (0.17–0.53)	0.43 (0.21–0.65)	0.59 (0.37–0.81)	0.96 (0.64–1.28)
Protein S (U/mL)	0.26 (0.14–0.38)	0.56 (0.22–0.90)	0.82 (0.44–1.20)	0.36 (0.12–0.60)	0.63 (0.33–0.93)	0.87 (0.55–1.19)	0.92 (0.60–1.24)

*All values are expressed in units per milliliter (U/mL) where pooled plasma contains 1.0 U/mL. All values are expressed as the mean of 40 to 75 samples for each population. The range of values encompassing 95% of the population is shown in brackets.

ABBREVIATIONS: AT, antithrombin; α_2M, α_2-macroglobulin; C_1E-INH, c_1 esterase inhibitor; α_1AT, α_1-antitrypsin; HCll, heparin cofactor II.

SOURCE: Modified from Andrew M[259,262] with permission.

TABLE 7-7   HEMATOLOGIC EFFECTS OF MATERNAL DRUGS ON THE FETUS AND NEWBORN

Drug	Effect	Certainty*	Mechanism	Reference
Aspirin	Bleeding	Known	Interference with platelet function	210, 214, 215
	Kernicterus	Potential	Displacement of bilirubin from albumin	293
Coumadin	Bleeding		Known depletion of vitamin K–dependent coagulation factors by blocking carboxylation	267, 268
Diazoxide	Bleeding	Questionable	Thrombocytopenia	283
Dilantin/phenobarbitol	Bleeding	Suspected	Depletion of vitamin K–dependent coagulation factors by hepatic enzyme induction and factor degradation	267
		Questionable	Thrombocytopenia	287
Nalidixic acid	Hyperbilirubinemia	Potential	Oxidant damage to hemoglobin	291
Nitrofurantoin	Hyperbilirubinemia	Potential	Oxidant damage to hemoglobin	290, 292
Rifampin/isoniazid	Bleeding	Suspected	Depletion of vitamin K–dependent coagulation factors	289
Sulfonamides	Kernicterus	Known	Displacement of bilirubin from albumin	293
Thiazides	Bleeding	Suspected	Thrombocytopenia	284, 285

*Certainty reflects the level of confidence in the data, assigned in increasing order from potential through questionable, suspected, and known.
SOURCE: Based on Miller, et al.[283]

tors of coagulation include antithrombin, heparin cofactor II, protein C, and protein S.[263,279] The levels of proteins C and S, which are vitamin K-dependent, as well as antithrombin and heparin cofactor II, are low in the newborn; they are in a range associated with thrombotic episodes in adults with inherited deficiencies.[279] In addition, the presence of factor V Leiden may occur in as many as 6 percent of newborns.[280] This produces resistance to the action of protein C and may heighten the susceptibility to thrombosis. Further, hyperprothrombinemia secondary to the 20210A allele prothrombin gene may affect 1 percent of the population[281] and has been associated with heightened venous thrombosis.[282] The combined deficiency of these anticoagulant proteins may further intensify the thrombotic risk. However, the precise role of these inhibitors of coagulation in newborn hypercoagulability is uncertain, since a proportionate decrease in vitamin K dependent procoagulant factors (II, VII, IX, X) also is present, and an additional inhibitor, α_2-macroglobulin, is increased. The values for plasma inhibitors of coagulation in premature and term infants are shown in Table 7-6.

HEMATOLOGIC EFFECTS OF MATERNAL DRUGS ON THE FETUS AND NEWBORN

HEMOSTATIC EFFECTS

A number of maternally administered pharmacologic agents have been implicated in hematologic abnormalities of the fetus or newborn (Table 7-7). Maternal aspirin ingestion results in impaired platelet aggregation but does not foster neonatal bleeding. Other agents taken by the mother, including diazoxide and thiazides, may be associated with neonatal thrombocytopenia.[283–285]

The newborn's plasma coagulation factors may be depressed by maternal warfarin ingestion.[268] This drug is best avoided during pregnancy, as it is teratogenic (first trimester) and may cause growth retardation of the fetus as well as bleeding.[268] In contrast, heparin does not cross the placenta, and maternal treatment with heparin appears to be safe for the fetus.[286]

Dilantin and/or phenobarbital also may reduce the newborn's vitamin-K dependent factors, possibly by microsomal enzyme induction, which enhances their degradation.[267] Furthermore, phenytoin (Dilantin) may depress the platelet count as a result of prenatal exposure[287] and cause teratogenic effects, e.g., the fetal hydantoin syndrome.[288] The decision to use this agent during pregnancy should reflect an assessment of the need for this specific drug, and also the risk of maternal seizures to the fetus and mother versus the potential side effects of treatment. Newborns of mothers taking rifampin and isoniazid also may have depressed vitamin K-dependent factors.[289]

BILIRUBIN/KERNICTERUS

Nitrofurantoin and nalidixic acid may cause oxidant injury to the red cell membrane and hemoglobin.[290,291] If there is glucose-6-phosphate dehydrogenase deficiency or if reduced glutathione is diminished, as in newborn red cells, these drugs have the potential to induce hemolysis and heighten neonatal hyperbilirubinemia. Although this problem has not been documented by transplacental transfer of nitrofurantoin or nalidixic acid, hemolysis has occurred in glucose-6-phosphate dehydrogenase–deficient infants who acquired the drugs from breast milk.[291,292] Alternatively, sulfonamides may cause displacement of bilirubin bound to albumin and heighten the risk of kernicterus.[293] Salicylates, phenylbutazone, and naproxen may have a similar effect at very high plasma concentrations.[293]

Ideally, all these medications should be avoided during pregnancy unless their indication outweighs the potential risk to the fetus and newborn.

REFERENCES

1. Bloom W, Bartelmez GW: Hematopoiesis in young human embryos. *Am J Anat* 67:21, 1940.
2. Gilmour JR: Normal hemopoiesis in intrauterine and neonatal life. *J Pathol* 52:25, 1942.
3. Zon L: Developmental biology of hematopoiesis. *Blood* 86:2876, 1995.
4. Shivdasani RA, Mayer EL, Orkin SH: Absence of blood formation in mice lacking T-cell leukemia oncoprotein tal-1/SCL. *Nature* 373:432, 1995.
5. Warren AJ, Colledge WH, Carlton MBL, Evans M, Smith AJH, Rabbitts TH: The oncogenic cysteine-rich LIM domain protein is essential for erythroid development. *Cell* 78:45, 1994.
6. Fujiwara Y, Browne CP, Cuniff K, Goff SC, Orkin SH: Arrested development of embryonic red cell precursors in mouse embryos lacking transcription factor GATA-1. *Proc Natl Acad Sci* 93:12355, 1996.
7. Peschle C, Migliaccio AR, Migliaccio G, Ptrini M, Calandrini M, Russo G, et al: Embryonic to fetal Hb switch in humans: studies on erythroid bursts generated by embryonic progenitors from yolk sac and liver. *Proc Natl Acad Sci USA* 81:2416, 1984.
8. Migliaccio G, Migliaccio AR, Petti S, et al: Human embryonic hemopoiesis. Kinetics of progenitors and precursors underlying the yolk sac—liver transition. *J Clin Invest* 78:51, 1986.
9. Huyhn A, Dommergues M, Izac B, Croisille L, Katz A, Vainchenker W, Coulombel L: Characterization of hematopoietic progenitors from human yolk sacs and embryos. *Blood* 86:4474, 1995.
10. Dommergues M, Aubeny E, Dumez Y, Durandy A, Coulombel L: Hematopoiesis in the human yolk sac: quantitation of erythroid and granulopoietic progenitors between 3.5 and 8 weeks of development. *Bone Marrow Transplant* 9:23, 1992.
11. Keleman E, Calvo W, Fliedner TM: *Atlas of Human Hemopoietic Development*, Springer-Verlag, Berlin, 1979.

12. Lin C-S, Lim S-K, D'Agati V, Constantini F: Differential effects of an erythropoietin receptor gene disruption on primitive and definitive erythropoiesis. *Genes Dev* 10:154, 1996.

13. Neubauer H, Cumano A, Muller M, Wu H, Huffstadt U, Pfeffer K: Jak2 deficiency defines an essential developmental checkpoint in definitive hematopoiesis. *Cell* 93:397, 1998.

14. Valtieri M, Gabbianelli M, Pelosi E, Bassano E, Petti S, Russo G, et al: Erythropoietin alone induces erythroid burst formation by human embryonic but not adult BFU-E in unicellular serum-free culture. *Blood* 74:460, 1989.

15. Emerson SG, Shanti T, Ferrara JL, Greenstein JL: Developmental regulation of erythropoiesis by hematopoietic growth factors: analysis on populations of BFU-E from bone marrow, peripheral blood, and fetal liver. *Blood* 74:49, 1989.

16. Dame C, Fahnenstich H, Feitag P, Hofmann D, Abdul-Nour T, Bartmann P, Fandrey J: Erythropoietin mRNA expression in human fetal and neonatal tissue. *Blood* 92:3218, 1998.

17. Mucenski ML, McLain K, Kier AB, Swerdlow SH, Schreiner MC, Miller TA, et al: A functional c-myb gene is required for normal murine fetal hepatic hematopoiesis. *Cell* 65:677, 1991.

18. Nuez B, Michalovich D, Bygrave A, Ploemacher R, Grosveld F: Defective haematopoiesis in fetal liver resulting from inactivation of the EKLF gene. *Nature* 375:316, 1995.

19. Hann IM, Bodger MP, Hoffbrand AV: Development of pluripotent hematopoietic progenitor cells in the human fetus. *Blood* 62:118, 1983.

20. Porcellini A, Manna A, Manna M, et al. Ontogeny of granulocyte-macrophage progenitor cells in the human fetus. *Int J Cell Clon* 1:92, 1983.

21. Nicola NA, Metcalf D: Specificity of action of colony-stimulating factors in the differentiation of granulocytes and macrophages. *CIBA Found Symp* 118:7, 1986.

22. Ohls RK, Li Y, Abdel-Mageed A, Buchanan G Jr., Mandell L, Christensen RD. Neutrophil pool sizes and granulocyte colony-stimulating factor production in human mid-trimester fetuses. *Pediatric Res* 37(6):806, 1995.

23. Slayton WB, Juul SE, Calhoun DA, Li Y, Braylan RC, Christensen RD: Hematopoiesis in the liver and marrow of human fetuses at 5 to 16 weeks postconception: quantitative assessment of macrophage and neutrophil populations. *Pediatric Res* 43:774, 1998.

24. Charbord P, Tavian M., Humeau L, Peault B: Early ontogeny of the human marrow from long bones: an immunohistochemical study of hematopoiesis and its microenvironment. *Blood* 87:4109, 1996.

25. Gupta S, Pahwa R, O'Reilly R, et al: Ontogeny of lymphocyte subpopulation in human fetal liver. *Proc Natl Acad Sci USA* 73:919, 1976.

26. Rainaut M, Pagniez M, Hercend T, Daffos F, Forestier F: Characterization of mononuclear cell subpopulations in normal fetal peripheral blood. *Hum Immunol* 18:331, 1987.

27. Hann IM, Gibson BES, Letsky EA: *Fetal and Neonatal Haematology*, Baillaire Tindale, Philadelphia, 1991.

28. Cairo MS, Wagner JE: Placental and/or umbilical cord blood: an alternative source of hematopoietic stem cells for transplantation. *J Am Soc Hematol* 90:4665, 1997.

29. Maximow AA: Relation of blood cells to connective tissues and endothelium. *Physiol Rev* IV(4):532, 1924.

30. Houssaint E: Differentiation of the mouse hepatic primordium. II. Extrinsic origin of the haemopoietic cell line. *Cell Differ* 10:243, 1981.

31. Cudennec CA, Johnson GR: Presence of multipotential hemopoietic cells in teratocarcinoma cultures. *J Embryol Exp Morphol* 61:51, 1981.

32. Gupta S, Pahwa R, O'Reilly R, et al: Ontogeny of lymphocyte subpopulation in human fetal liver. *Proc Natl Acad Sci USA* 73:919, 1976.

33. Moore MAS, Owen JJT: Stem-cell migration in developing myeloid and lymphoid systems. *Lancet* i:658, 1967.

34. Dieterlen-Lievre F: On the origin of hematopoietic stem cells in the avian embryo: an experimental approach. *J Embryol Exp Morphol* 33:607, 1975.

35. Carpenter KL, Turpen JB: Experimental studies on hemopoiesis in the pronephros of *Rana pipiens*. *Differentiation* 14:167, 1979.

36. Muller AM, Medvinsky A, Strouboulis J, Grosveld F, Dzierzak E: Development of hematopoietic stem cell activity in the mouse embryo. *Immunity* 1:291, 1994.

37. Smith RA, Glomski CA: "Hemogenic endothelium" of the embryonic aorta: does it exist? *Dev Comp Immunol* 6:359, 1982.

38. Tavian M, Coulombel L, Luton D, San Clemente H, Dieterlen-Lievre F, Peault B: Aorta-associated CD-34+ hematopoietic cells in the early human embryo. *Blood* 87:67, 1996.

39. Proudfoot NJ, Shander MH, Manley JL, Gefter ML, Maniatis T: Structure and in vitro transcription of human globin genes. *Science* 209:1329, 1980.

40. Grosveld F, van Assendelft GB, Greaves DR, Kolias B: Position independent, high-level expression of the human β globin gene in transgenic mice. *Cell* 51:975, 1987.

41. Hecht F, Motulsky AG, Lemire RJ, et al: Predominance of hemoglobin Gower 1 in early human embryonic development. *Science* 152:91, 1966.

42. Huehns ER, Dance N, Beaven GH, et al: Human embryonic hemoglobins. *Cold Spring Harbor Symp Quant Biol* 29:327, 1964.

43. Gale RE, Clegg JB, Huehns ER: Human embryonic haemoglobins Gower 1 and Gower 2. *Nature* 280:162, 1979.

44. Peschle C, Mavilio F, Care A, Migliaccio G, Migliaccio AR, Salvo G, et al: Haemoglobin switching in human embryos: asynchrony of the ζ to α and ε to γ globin switches in primitive and definitive erythropoietic lineage. *Nature* 313:235, 1985.

45. Pataryas HA, Stomatoyannopoulos G: Hemoglobins in human fetuses: evidence of adult hemoglobin production after the 11th gestational week. *Blood* 39:688, 1972.

46. Thomas ED, Lochte HL Jr, Greenough WB III, et al: In vitro synthesis of foetal and adult haemoglobin by foetal haematopoietic tissues. *Nature* 185:396, 1960.

47. Kazazian HH, Woodhead AP: Hemoglobin A synthesis in the developing fetus. *N Engl J Med* 289:58, 1973.

48. Bard H: The effect of placental insufficiency on fetal and adult hemoglobin synthesis. *Am J Obstet Gynecol* 120:67, 1974.

49. Kirschbaum T: Fetal hemoglobin content of cord blood determined by column chromatography. *Am J Obstet Gynecol* 84:1375, 1962.

50. Armstrong D, Schroeder WA, Fenninger W: A comparison of the percentage of fetal hemoglobin in human umbilical cord blood as determined by chromatography and by alkali denaturation. *Blood* 22:554, 1963.

51. Bard H: Postnatal fetal and adult hemoglobin synthesis in early preterm newborn infants. *J Clin Invest* 52:1789, 1973.

52. Metaxotou-Mavromati AD, Antonopoulou HK, Laskari SA, Tsiarta HK, Ladis VA, Kattamis CA: Developmental changes in hemoglobin F levels during the first two years of life in normal and heterozygous β-thalassemia infants. *Pediatrics* 69:734, 1982.

53. Bard H, Makowski EL, Meschia G, et al: The relative rates of synthesis of hemoglobins A and F in red cells of newborn infants. *Pediatrics* 45:766, 1970.

54. Bromberg YN, Abrahamov A, Salzberger M: The effect of maternal anoxemia on the foetal haemoglobin of the newborn. *J Obstet Gynaecol Br Commonw* 63:875, 1956.

55. Huehns ER, Hecht F, Keil JV, et al: Developmental hemoglobin anomalies in a chromosomal triplication. *Proc Natl Acad Sci USA* 51:89, 1964.

56. Lee CSN, Boyer SH, Bowen P, et al: The D1 trisomy syndrome: three subjects with unequally advancing development. *Johns Hopkins Med J* 118:374, 1966.

57. Wilson MG, Schroeder WA, Graves DA: Postnatal change of hemoglobins F and A_2 in infants with Down's syndrome (G trisomy). *Pediatrics* 42:349, 1968.

58. Giulian GG, Gilbert EF, Moss RL: Elevated fetal hemoglobin levels in sudden infant death syndrome. *N Engl J Med* 316:1122, 1987.

59. Brown MS: Fetal and neonatal erythropoieses, in *Developmental and Neonatal Hematology*, edited by JA Stockman, III and C Pochedly, pp 39. Raven Press, New York, 1988.

60. Forestier F, Daffos F, Galacteros F, et al: Haematological values of 163 normal fetuses between 18 and 30 weeks of gestation. *Paediat Res* 20:342, 1986.

61. Millar DS, Davis LR, et al. Normal blood cell values in the early mid-trimester fetus. *Prenat Diagn*, 5:367, 1985.

62. Linch DC, Knott LJ, et al. Studies of circulating hemopoietic progenitor cells in human fetal blood. *Blood* 59:976, 1982.

63. Christensen RD. Hematopoiesis in the fetus and neonate. *Pediatr Res* 26:531, 1989.

64. Marks J, Gairdner D, Roscoe JD: Blood formation in infancy. III. Cord blood. *Arch Dis Child* 30:117, 1955.

65. Linderkamp O, Versmold HT, Messow-Zahn K, et al: The effect of intrapartum and intra-uterine asphyxia on placental transfusion in premature and full-term infants. *Eur J Pediatr* 127:91, 1978.

66. Yao AC, Hirvensalo M, Lind J: Placental transfusion rate and uterine contraction. *Lancet* 1:380, 1968.

67. Usher R, Shepard M, et al: The blood volume of the newborn and placental transfusion. *Acta Paediatr* 52:497, 1963.

68. Bratteby LE: Studies on erythro-kinetics in infancy. XI. The change in circulating red cell volume during the first five months of life. *Acta Paediatr Scand* 57:215, 1968.

69. McCue CM, Garner FB, Hurt WG, et al: Placental transfusion. *J Pediatr* 72:15, 1968.

70. Matoth Y, Zaizor R, Varsano I: Postnatal changes in some red cell parameters. *Acta Paediatr Scand* 60:317, 1971.

71. Linderkamp O, Versmold HT, Strohhacker I, et al: Capillary-venous hematocrit differences in newborn infants. *Eur J Pediatr* 127:9, 1977.

72. Saarinen UM, Simmes MA: Developmental changes in red blood cell counts and indices of infants after exclusion of iron deficiency by laboratory criteria and continuous iron supplementation. *J Pediatr* 92:412, 1978.

73. Zipursky A, Brown E, Palko J, et al: The erythrocyte differential count in newborn infants. *Am J Pediatr Hematol Oncol* 5:45, 1983.

74. Shannon KM, Naylor GS, Torkildson JC, et al: Circulating erythroid progenitors in the anemia of prematurity. *N Engl J Med* 317:728, 1987.

75. Linch DC, Knott LJ, Rodeck CH, Huehns ER: Studies of circulating hemopoietic progenitor cells in human fetal blood. *Blood* 59:976, 1983.

76. Christensen RD: Circulating pluripotent hematopoietic progenitor cells in neonates. *J Pediatr* 11:622, 1987.

77. Clapp DW, Baley JE, Gerson SL: Gestational age dependent changes in circulating hematopoietic stem cells in newborn infants. *J Lab Clin Med* 113:422, 1989.

78. Holbrook SR, Christensen RD, Rothstein G: Erythroid colonies derived from fetal blood display different growth patterns from those derived from adult marrow. *Pediatr Res* 24:605, 1988.

79. Burman D, Morris AF: Cord hemoglobin in low birth weight infants. *Arch Dis Child* 49:382, 1974.

80. Meberg A: Haemoglobin concentrations and erythropoietin levels in appropriate and small for gestational age infants. *Scand J Haematol* 24:162, 1980.

81. Zaizov R, Matoth Y: Red cell values on the first postnatal day during the last 16 weeks of gestation. *Am J Hematol* 1:275, 1976.

82. Lockridge S, Pass R, Cassidy G: Reticulocyte counts in intrauterine growth retardation. *Pediatrics* 47:919, 1971.

83. Humbert JR, Abelson H, Hathaway WE, et al: Polycythemia in small for gestational age infants. *J Pediatr* 75:1812, 1969.

84. Halvorsen S, Finne PH: Erythropoietin production in the human fetus and newborn. *Ann NY Acad Sci* 149:576, 1968.

85. Seip M: The reticulocyte level and the erythrocyte production judged from reticulocyte studies in newborn infants during the first week of life. *Acta Paediatr Scand* 44:355, 1955.

86. Stockman JA III, Oski FA: Physiological anaemia of infancy and the anaemia of prematurity. *Clin Haematol* 7:3, 1978.

87. Mann DL, Sites ML, Donati RM, et al: Erythropoietic stimulating activity during the first ninety days of life. *Proc Soc Exp Biol Med* 118:212, 1965.

88. Lundstrom U, Simmes MA: Red blood cell values in low-birth-weight infants: Ages at which values become equivalent to those of term infants. *J Pediatr* 96:1040, 1980.

89. Stockman JA III, Garcia JF, Oski FA: The anemia of prematurity: factors governing the erythropoietin response. *N Engl J Med* 296:647, 1977.

90. MackIntosh TF, Walker CHM: Blood viscosity in the newborn. *Arch Dis Child* 48:547, 1973.

91. Bergqvist G: Viscosity of the blood in the newborn infant. *Acta Paediatr Scand* 63:858, 1974.

92. Wirth FH, Goldberg WR, Lubchenco L: Neonatal hyperviscosity. I. Incidence. *Pediatrics* 63:833, 1979.

93. Hakanson DO, Oh W: Hyperviscosity in the small-for-gestational age infant. *Biol Neonate* 37:190, 1980.

94. Ramamurthy RS, Berlanga M: Postnatal alteration in hematocrit and viscosity in normal and polycythemic infants. *J Pediatr* 110:929, 1987.

95. Bada HS, Korones SB, Pourcyrous M, et al: Asymptomatic syndrome of polycythemic hyperviscosity: Effect of partial plasma exchange transfusion. *J Pediatr* 120:579, 1992.

96. Bierhuizen MFA, Mattei MG, Fukuda M: Expression of the developmental I antigen by a cloned human cDNA encoding a member of a b-1,6-N-acetylglucosaminyltransferase gene family. *Gene Dev* 7:468, 1993.

97. Race RR, Sanger R: *Blood Groups in Man,* 6th ed. Blackwell Scientific Publications, London, 1975.

98. Pearson HA: Life-span of the fetal red blood cell. *J Pediatr* 70:166, 1967.

99. Weipple G, Pantlitschko M, Bauer P, et al: Normal values and distribution of serum iron in cord blood. *Clin Chim Acta* 44:147, 1973.

100. Saarinen UM, Siimes MA: Developmental changes in serum iron, total iron-binding capacity, and transferrin saturation in infancy. *J Pediatr* 91:875, 1977.

101. Saarinen UM, Siimes MA: Serum ferritin in assessment of iron nutrition in healthy infants. *Acta Paediatr Scand* 67:745, 1978.

102. Seip M, Halvorsen S: Erythrocyte production and iron stores in premature infants during the first months of life. The anemia of prematurity—etiology, pathogenesis, iron requirement. *Acta Paediatr Scand* 45:600, 1956.

103. Bauer C, Ludwig I, Ludwig M: Different effects of 2,3-diphosphoglycerate and adenosine triphosphate on oxygen affinity of adult and fetal hemoglobin. *Life Sci* 7:1339, 1968.

104. Oski FA: Red cell metabolism in the newborn infant. V. Glycolytic intermediates and glycolytic enzymes. *Pediatrics* 44:84, 1969.

105. Oski FA, Delivoria-Papadopoulos M: The red cell, 2, 3-diphosphoglycerate, and tissue oxygen release. *J Pediatr* 77:941, 1970.

106. Zipursky A: The erythrocytes of the newborn infant. *Semin Hematol* 2:167, 1965.

107. Oski FA, Komazawa M: Metabolism of the erythrocytes of the newborn infant. *Semin Hematol* 12:209, 1975.

108. Oski FA, Smith CA: Red cell metabolism in the premature infant. III. Apparent inappropriate glucose consumption for cell age. *Pediatrics* 41:473, 1968.

109. Konrad PN, Valentine WN, Paglia DE: Enzymatic activities and glutathione content of erythrocytes in the newborn: comparison with red cells of older normal subjects and those with comparable reticulocytosis. *Acta Haematol* 48:193, 1972.

110. Gross RT, Schroeder EAR, Brounstein SA: Energy metabolism in the erythrocytes of premature infants compared to full term newborn infants and adults. *Blood* 21:755, 1963.

111. Oski FA: Red cell metabolism in the premature infant. II. The pentose phosphate pathway. *Pediatrics* 39:689, 1967.

112. Ross JD: Deficient activity of DPNH-dependent methemoglobin diaphorase in cord blood erythrocytes. *Blood* 21:51, 1963.

113. Gross RT, Bracci R, Rudolph N, et al: Hydrogen peroxide toxicity and detoxification in erythrocytes of newborn infants. *Blood* 29:481, 1967.

114. Travis SF, Kumar SP, Delivoria-Papadopoulos M: Red cell metabolic alterations in postnatal life in term infants: glycolytic intermediates and adenosine triphosphate. *Pediatr Res* 15:34, 1981.

115. Whaun JM, Oski FA: Red cell stromal adenosine triphosphatase (ATPase) of newborn infants. *Pediatr Res* 3:105, 1969.

116. Blum SF, Oski FA: Red cell metabolism in the newborn infant. IV. Transmembrane potassium flux. *Pediatrics* 43:396, 1969.

117. Crowley J, Ways P, Jones JW: Human fetal erythrocyte and plasma lipids. *J Clin Invest* 44:989, 1965.

118. Neerhout RC: Erythrocyte lipids in the neonate. *Pediatr Res* 2:172, 1968.

119. Shapiro DL, Pasqualini P: Erythrocyte membrane proteins of premature and full-term infants. *Pediatr Res* 12:176, 1978.

120. Kosztolanyi G, Jobst K: Electrokinetic analysis of the fetal erythrocyte membrane after trypsin digestion. *Pediatr Res* 14:138, 1980.

121. Altman PL, Dittmer, DS: *Blood and Other Body Fluids.* Federation of American Societies for Experimental Biology, Washington, DC, 1961.

122. Coulombel L, Dehan M, Tchernia G, Hill C, et al: The number of polymorphonuclear leukocytes in relation to gestational age in the newborn. *Acta Paediatr Scand* 68:709, 1979.

123. Barak Y, Blachar Y, Levin S: Neonatal neutrophilia: Possible role of a humoral granulopoietic factor. *Pediatr Res* 14:1026, 1980.

124. Laver J, Duncan E, Abboud M, et al: High levels of granulocyte and granulocyte-macrophage colony-stimulating factors in cord blood of normal full-term neonates. *Pediatr Res* 116:627, 1990.

125. Ijima H, Suda T, Miura Y: Predominance of macrophage-colony formation in human cord blood. *Exp Hematol* 10:234, 1982.

126. Prindull G, Ben-Ishay Z, Gabriel M, et al: A comparison of spontaneous and CSF added CFU-MG colony formation in healthy, sick and hypotrophic pre-term infants. *Blut* 45:167, 1982.

127. Cairo MS, Suen Y, Knoppel E, Van De Ven C, Nguyen A, Sender L: Decreased stimulated GM-CSF production and GM-CSF gene expression but normal numbers of GM-CSF receptors in human term newborns compared with adults. *Pediatr Res* 30:362, 1991.

128. English BK, Hammond WP, Lewis DB, Brown CB, Wilson CB: Decreased granulocyte-macrophage colony-stimulating factor production by human neonatal blood mononuclear cells and T cells. *Pediatr Res* 31:211, 1992.

129. Cairo MS, Suen Y, Knoppel E, et al: Decreased G-CSF and IL-3 production and gene expression from mononuclear cells of newborn infants. *Pediatr Res* 31:574, 1992.

130. Rosenthal J, Cairo MS: The role of cytokines in modulating neonatal myelopoiesis and host defense. *Cytokin Mol Ther* 1:165, 1995.

131. Cairo MS, Plunkett JM, Nguyen A, Van De Ven C: Effect of stem cell factor with and without granulocyte colony-stimulating factor on neonatal hematopoiesis: in vivo induction of newborn myelopoiesis and reduction of mortality during experimental group B streptococcal sepsis. *Blood* 80:96, 1992.

132. Xanthou M: Leucocyte blood picture in healthy full-term and premature babies during neonatal period. *Arch Dis Child* 45:242, 1970.

133. Gibson EL, Vaucher Y, Corrigan JJ Jr: Eosinophilia in premature infants. Relationship to weight gain. *J Pediatr* 95:99, 1979.

134. Siegel JD, McCracken GH Jr: Sepsis neonatorum. *N Engl J Med* 304:642, 1981.

135. Forman ML, Stiehm ER: Impaired opsonic activity but normal phagocytosis in low-birth-weight infants. *N Engl J Med* 281:926, 1969.

136. Dossett JH, Williams RC Jr, Quie PG: Studies on interaction of bacteria, serum factors and polymorphonuclear leukocytes in mothers and newborns. *Pediatrics* 44:49, 1969.

137. Miller ME: Phagocytosis in the newborn infant: humoral and cellular factors. *J Pediatr* 74:255, 1969.

138. Hill HR, Shigeoka AO, Pincus S, Christensen RD: Intravenous IgG in combination with other modalities in the treatment of neonatal infection. *Pediatr Inf Dis* 5:180, 1986.

139. Cocchi P, Marianelli L: Phagocytosis and intracellular killing of *Pseudomonas aeruginosa* in premature infants. *Helv Paediatr Acta* 22:110, 1967.

140. Drossou V, Kanakoudi F, Diamanti E, et al: Concentrations of main serum opsonins in early infancy. *Arch Dis of Childhood* (Fetal and Neonatal Edition) 72:F172, 1995.

141. Yang KD, Bathras JM, Shigeoka AO, James J, Pincus SH, Hill HR: Mechanisms of bacterial opsonization by immune globulin intravenous correlation of complement consumption with opsonic activity and protective efficacy. *J Infect Dis* 159:701, 1989.

142. Shaio MF, Yang KD, Bohnsack JF, Hill HR: Effect of immune globulin intravenous on opsonization of bacteria by classic and alternative complement pathways in premature serum. *Pediatr Res* 25:634, 1989.

143. Hill H: Host defenses in the neonate: prospects for enhancement. *Semin Perinatol* 9:2, 1985.

144. Propp RP, Alper CA: C3 synthesis in the human fetus and lack of transplacental passage. *Science* 162:672, 1968.

145. Johnston RB Jr, Altenburger KM, Atkinson AW Jr, et al: Complement in the newborn infant. *Pediatrics* 64:781, 1979.

146. Strunk RC, Fenton LJ, Gaines JA: Alternative pathway of complement activation in full term and premature infants. *Pediatr Res* 13:641, 1979.

147. Davis CA, Vallota EH, Forristal J: Serum complement levels in infancy: age related changes. *Pediatr Res* 13:1043, 1979.

148. Mills EL, Bjorksten B, Quie PG: Deficient alternative complement pathway activity in newborn sera. *Pediatr Res* 13:1341, 1979.

149. Proctor RA, Prendergast E, Mosher DF: Fibronectin mediates attachment of *Staphylococcus aureus* to human neutrophils. *Blood* 59:681, 1982.

150. Hill HR, Shigeoka AO, Augustine NH, Pritchard D, Lundblad JL, Schwartz RS: Fibronectin enhances the opsonic and protective activity of monoclonal and polyclonal antibody against group B streptococci. *J Exp Med* 159:1618, 1984.

151. Harris MC, Levitt J, Douglas SD, Gerdes JS, Polin RA: Effect of fibronectin on adherence of neutrophils from newborn infants. *J Clin Microbiol* 21:243, 1985.

152. Hill HR, Shigeoka AO, Gonzales LA, Christensen RD: Intravenous immune globulin use in newborns. *J Allergy Clin Immunol* 84:617, 1989.

153. Christensen RD, Brown MS, Hall DC, Lassiter HA, Hill HR: Effect on neutrophil kinetics and serum opsonic capacity of intravenous administration of immune globulin to neonates with clinical signs of early-onset sepsis. *J Pediatr* 118:606, 1991.

154. Fujiwara T, Taniuchi S, Hattori K, Kobayashi T, Kinoshita Y, Kobayashi Y: Effect of immunoglobulin therapy on phagocytosis by polymorphonuclear leucocytes in whole blood of neonates. *Clin Exp Immunol* 107:435, 1997.

155. Weisman LE, Stoll BJ, Kueser TJ, et al: Intravenous immune globulin therapy for early-onset sepsis in premature neonates. *J Pediatr* 121:434, 1992.

156. Schreiber JR, Berger M: Intravenous immune globulin therapy for sepsis in premature neonates. *J Pediatr* 121:401, 1992.

157. Baker CJ, Melish ME, Hall RT, et al: Intravenous immune globulin for the prevention of nosocomial infection in low-birth-weight infants. *N Engl J Med* 327:213, 1992.

158. Fanaroff A, Wright E, Korones S, Wright L: A controlled trial of prophylactic intravenous immunoglobulin to reduce nosocomial infections in VLBW infants. *Pediatr Res* 31:202A, 1992.

159. Fischer GW, Weisman LE, Hemming VG: Directed immune globulin for the prevention or treatment of neonatal group B streptococcal infections: A review. *Clin Immunol Immunopathol* 62:S92, 1992.

160. Miller ME: Chemotactic function in the neonate. Humoral and cellular aspects. *Pediatr Res* 5:487, 1971.

161. Klei RB, Fischer TJ, Gard SE, et al: Decreased mononuclear and polymorphonuclear chemotaxis in human newborns, infants, and young children. *Pediatrics* 60:467, 1977.

162. Tono-oka T, Nakayama M, Uehara H, et al: Characteristics of impaired chemotactic function in cord blood leukocytes. *Pediatr Res* 13:148, 1979.

163. Hill HR, Augustine NH, Newton JA, Shigeoka AO, Morris E, Sacchi F: Correction of a developmental defect in neutrophil activation and movement. *Am J Pathol* 128:307, 1987.

164. Bruce MC, Baley JE, Medvik KA, Berger M: Impaired surface membrane expression of C3bi but not C3b receptors on neonatal neutrophils. *Pediatr Res* 21:306, 1987.

165. Anderson DC, Freeman KLB, Heerdt B, Hughes BJ, Jack RM, Smith CW: Abnormal stimulated adherence of neonatal granulocytes: impaired induction of surface MAC-1 by chemotactic factors or secretagogues. *Blood* 70:740, 1987.

166. Smith JB, Campbell DE, Ludomirsky A, et al: Expression of the complement receptors CR1 and CR3 and the type III Pc-gamma receptor on neutrophils from newborn infants and from fetuses with Rh disease. *Pediatr Res* 28:120, 1990.

167. Carr R, Davies JM: Abnormal PcRIII expression by neutrophils from very preterm neonates. *Blood* 76:607, 1990.

168. Anderson DC, Rothlein R, Marlin SD, Krater SS, Smith CW: Impaired transendothelial migration by neonatal neutrophils: abnormalities of Mac-1(CD11b/CD18)-dependent adherence reactions. *Blood* 76:2613, 1990.

169. Masuda K, Kinoshita Y, Kobayashi Y: Heterogeneity of Fc expression in chemotaxis and adherence of neonatal neutrophils. *Pediatr Res* 25:6, 1989.

170. Tosi MF, Berger M: Functional differences between the 40 kDa and 50 kDa IgG Fc receptors on human neutrophils revealed by elastase treatment and antireceptor antibodies. *J Immunol* 141:2097, 1988.

171. Salmon JE, Kapur S, Kimberly RP: Opsonin-independent ligation of Fc-gamma receptors. *J Exp Med* 166:1798, 1987.

172. Coen R, Grush O, Kander E: Studies of bactericidal activity and metabolism of the leukocyte in full-term neonates. *J Pediatr* 78:400, 1969.

173. Mills EL, Thompson T, Bjorksten B, et al: The chemiluminescence response and bactericidal activity of polymorphonuclear neutrophils from newborns and their mothers. *Pediatrics* 63:429, 1979.

174. Park BH, Holmes B, Good RA: Metabolic activities in leukocytes of newborn infants. *J Pediatr* 76:237, 1970.

175. Xanthou M, Valassi-Adam E, Kintronidou E, et al: Phagocytosis and killing ability of *Candida albicans* by blood leucocytes of healthy term and preterm babies. *Arch Dis Child* 50:72, 1975.

176. Wright WC Jr, Ank BJ, Herbert J, et al: Decreased bactericidal activity of leukocytes of stressed newborn infants. *Pediatrics* 56:569, 1975.

177. Shigeoka AO, Santos JI, Hill HR: Functional analysis of neutrophil granulocytes from healthy, infected, and stressed neonates. *J Pediatr* 95:454, 1979.

178. Shigeoka AO, Charette RP, Wyman ML, et al: Defective oxidative metabolic responses of neutrophils from stressed neonates. *J Pediatr* 98:392, 1981.

179. Strauss RG, Snyder EL: Neutrophils from human infants exhibit decreased viability. *Pediatr Res* 15:794, 1981.

180. Strauss RG, Snyder EL, Wallace PO, et al: Oxygen-detoxifying enzymes in neutrophils of infants and their mothers. *J Lab Clin Med* 95:897, 1980.

181. Yamazaki M, Matsuoka T, Yasui K, Komiyama A, Akabane T: Increased production of superoxide anion by neonatal polymorphonuclear leukocytes stimulated with a chemotactic peptide. *Amer J Hematol* 27:169, 1988.

182. Kretschmer RR, Papierniak CK, Stewardson-Krieger P, et al: Quantitative nitrobluetetrazolium reduction by normal newborn monocytes. *J Pediatr* 91:306, 1977.

183. Milgrom H, Shore SL: Assessment of monocyte function in the normal newborn infant by antibody-dependent cellular cytotoxicity. *J Pediatr* 91:612, 1977.

184. Orlowski JP, Sieger L, Anthony BF: Bactericidal capacity of monocytes of newborn infants. *J Pediatr* 89:797, 1976.

185. Schuit KE, Powell DA: Phagocytic dysfunction in monocytes of normal newborn infants. *Pediatrics* 65:501, 1980.

186. Das M, Henderson T, Feig SA: Neonatal mononuclear cell metabolism: Further evidence for diminished monocyte function in the neonate. *Pediatr Res* 13:632, 1979.

187. Mills EL: Mononuclear phagocytes in the newborn: their relation to the state of relative immunodeficiency. *Am J Pediatr Hematol* 5:189, 1983.

188. Bryson YJ, Winter HS, Gard SE, Fisher TJ, Stiehm ERL: Deficiency of immune interferon production by leukocytes of normal newborns. *Cell Immunol* 55:191, 1987.

189. Frenkel L, Bryson YJ: Ontogeny of phytohemagglutinin-induced gamma interferon by leukocytes of healthy infants and children: evidence for decreased production in infants younger than 2 months of age. *J Pediatr* 111:97, 1987.

190. Wilson CB, Westall J, Johnston L, Lewis DB, Dower SK, Alper AR: Decreased production of interferon-gamma by human neonatal cells. *J Clin Invest* 77:860, 1986.

191. Perussia B, Dayton ET, Lazarus R, Fenning V, Trinchieri G: Immune interferon induces the receptor for monomeric IgG on human monocytic and myeloid cells. *J Exp Med* 158:1092, 1983.

192. Cairo MS: Review of G-CSF and GM-CSF effects on neonatal neutrophil kinetics. *Am J Pediatr Hematol Oncol* 11:238, 1989.

193. Cairo MS, VandeVen C, Toy C, Suen Y, Mauss D, Sender L: GM-CSF primes and modulates neonatal PMN motility: up-regulation of C3bi (Mol) expression with alteration in PMN adherence and aggregation. *Am J Pediatr Hematol Oncol* 13:249, 1991.

194. Sautois B, Fillet G and Beguin Y. Comparative cytokine production by in vitro stimulated mononucleated cells from cord blood and adult blood. *Exp Hematol* 25:103, 1997.

195. Fogel BJ, Arais D, Kung F: Platelet counts in healthy premature infants. *J Pediatr* 73:108, 1968.

196. Sell EJ, Corrigan JJ: Platelet counts, fibrinogen concentrations and factor V and factor VIII levels in healthy infants according to gestational age. *J Pediatr* 82:1028, 1973.

197. Mehta P, Vasa R, Neumann L, Karpatkin M: Thrombocytopenia in the high-risk infant. *J Pediatr* 97:791, 1980.

198. Meberg A, Halvorsen S, Orstavik I: Transitory thrombocytopenia in small-for-dates infants, possibly related to maternal smoking. *Lancet* 2:303, 1977.

199. Thuring W, Tonz O: Neonatale Thrombozytenwere be: Kindern mit Down-Syndrom und anderen autosomalen Trisomien. *Helv Paediatr Acta* 34:545, 1979.

200. Cairo, MS: The regulation of hematopoietic growth factor production from cord mononuclear cells and its effect on newborn rat hematopoiesis. *J Hematother* 2:217, 1993.

201. Sirota L, Bessler H, Weissman Z, Dulitzky F, Djaldetti M: Thrombopoietic activity in preterm newborns and infants. *Arch Dis Childhood* 61:585, 1986.

202. Suen Y, Chang M, Lee SM, Buzby JS, Cairo MS: Regulation of interleukin-11 protein and mRNA expression in neonatal and adult fibroblasts and endothelial cells. *Blood* 84:4125, 1994.

203. Feusner JH: Normal and abnormal bleeding times in neonates and young children utilizing a fully standardized template technic. *Am Soc Clin Pathol* 74:73, 1980.

204. Rennie JM, Gibson T, Cooke RWI: Micromethod for bleeding time in the newborn. *Arch Dis Child* 60:51, 1985.

205. Andrew M, Paes B, Bowker J, Vegh P: Evaluation of an automated bleeding time device in the newborn. *Am J Hematol* 35:275, 1990.

206. Weinstein MJ, Blanchard R, Moake JL, Vosburgh E, Moise K: Fetal and neonatal von Willebrand factor (vWF) is unusually large and similar to the vWF in patients with thrombotic thrombocytopenic purpura. *Br J Haematol* 72:68, 1989.

207. Andrew M, Vegh P, Johnston M, Bowker J, Ofosu F, Mitchell L: Maturation of the hemostatic system during childhood. *Blood* 80:1998, 1992.

208. Andrew M, Castle V, Saigal S, et al: Clinical impact of neonatal thrombocytopenia. *J Pediatr* 110:457, 1987.

209. Corazza MS, Davis RF, Merritt TA, et al: Prolonged bleeding time in preterm infants receiving indomethacin for patent ductus arteriosus. *J Pediatr* 105:292, 1984.

210. Stuart MJ: Platelet function in the neonate. *Am J Pediatr Hematol Oncol* 1:227, 1979.

211. Israels SJ, Daniels M, McMillan EM: Deficient collagen-induced activation in the newborn platelet. *Pediatr Res* 27:337, 1990.

212. Rajasekhar D, Kestin AS, Bednarek FJ, Ellis PA, Barnard MR, Michelson AD: Neonatal platelets are less reactive than adult platelets to physiological agonists in whole blood. *Thromb Haemost* 72:957, 1994.

213. Ts'ao C, Green D, Schultz K: Function and ultrastructure of platelets of neonates; enhanced ristocetin aggregation of neonatal platelets. *Br J Haematol* 32:225, 1976.

214. Blieyer WA, Breckenridge RT: Studies on the detection of adverse drug reactions in the newborn. II. The effects of prenatal aspirin on newborn hemostasis. *JAMA* 213:2049, 1970.

215. Corby DG, Schulman I: The effects of antenatal drug administration on aggregation of platelets of newborn infants. *J Pediatr* 79:307, 1971.

216. Hauth JC, Goldenberg RL, Parker CR Jr, Cutter GR, Cliver SP: Low-dose aspirin: lack of association with an increase in abruptio placentae or perinatal mortality. *Obstet Gynecol* 85:1055, 1995.

217. Sibai BM, Caritis SN, Thom E, Shaw K, McNellis D: Low-dose aspirin in nulliparous women: safety of continuous epidural block and correlation between bleeding time and maternal-neonatal bleeding complications. National Institute of Child Health and Human Developmental Maternal-Fetal Medicine Network. *Am J Obstet Gynecol* 172:1553, 1995.

218. Newman PJ, Derbes RS, Aster RH: The human platelet alloantigens, PIA1 and PIA2, are associated with a leucine 33/proline 33 amino acid polymorphism in membrane glycoprotein IIIa, and are distinguishable by DNA typing. *J Clin Invest* 83:1778, 1989.

219. Gruel Y, Boizard B, Daffos F, Forestier F, Caen J, Wautier JL: Determination of platelet antigens and glycoproteins in the human fetus. *Blood* 68:488, 1986.

220. McFarland JG, Aster RH, Bussel JB, Gianopoulos JG, Derbes RS, Newman PJ: Prenatal diagnosis of neonatal alloimmune thrombocytopenia using allele-specific oligonucleotide probes. *Blood* 78:2276, 1991.

221. Shulman NR, Jordan JV Jr: Platelet immunology, in *Hemostasis and Thrombosis: Basic Principles and Clinical Practice*, 2nd ed, edited by RW Colman, J Hirsh, VJ Marder, EW Salzman, pp 476–483. JB Lippincott, Philadelphia, 1987.

222. Pabst HF: Ontogeny of the immune response as a basis of childhood diseases. *J Pediatr* 97:519, 1980.

223. Erkeller-Yuksel FM, Deneys V, Yuksel B, et al: Age related changes in human blood lymphocyte subpopulations. *J Pediatr* 120:216, 1992.

224. De Waele M, Foulon W, Renmans W, et al: Hematologic values and lymphocyte subsets in fetal blood. *Am J Clin Pathol* 89:742, 1988.

225. Hicks MJ, Jones JF, Minnich LL, Weigle KA, Thies AC, Layton JM: Age-related changes in T- and B-lymphocyte subpopulations in the peripheral blood. *Arch Pathol Lab Med* 107:518, 1983.

226. Kotylo PA, Baenziger JC, Yoder MC, Engle WA, Bolinger CD: Rapid analysis of lymphocyte subsets in cord blood. *Am J Clin Pathol* 93:263, 1990.

227. Slukvin II, Chernishov VP: Two-color flow cytometric analysis of natural killer and cytotoxic T-lymphocyte subsets in peripheral blood of normal human neonates. *Biol Neonate* 61(3):156–61, 1992.

228. Neubert R, Delgado I, Abraham K, Schuster C, Helge H: Evaluation of the age-dependent development of lymphocyte surface receptors in children. *Life Sci* 62:1099, 1998.

229. Miller ME: Immune-inflammatory response in the human neonate. *Am J Pediatr Hematol* 3:199, 1981.

230. Stiehm ER, Winter HS, Bryson YF: Cellular (T cell) immunity in the human newborn. *Pediatrics* 64:814, 1979.

231. Carr MC, Stites DP, Fudenberg HH: Cellular immune aspects of the human fetal-maternal relationship. I. In vitro response of cord blood lymphocytes to phytohemagglutinin. *Cell Immunol* 5:21, 1972.

232. Papiernick M: Comparison of human foetal with child blood lymphocytic kinetics. *Biol Neonate* 19:163, 1971.

233. Uhr JW, Dancis J, Newmann CG: Delayed-type hypersensitivity in premature neonatal humans. *Nature* 187:1130, 1960.

234. Blaese RM, Poplack DG, Muchmore AV: The mononuclear phagocyte system: Role in expression of immunocompetence in neonatal and adult life. *Pediatrics* 64(suppl):829, 1979.

235. Von Freeden U, Zessack N, Van Valen F, Burdach S: Defective interferon gamma production in neonatal T cells is independent of interleukin-2 receptor binding. *Pediatr Res* 30:270, 1991.

236. Sterm CMM: Changes in lymphocytes subpopulations in the blood of healthy and sick newborn infants. *Pediatr Res* 13:792, 1979.

237. Raveche ES: Possible immunoregulatory role for CD5+ B cells. *Clin Immuno Immunopath* 56:135, 1990.

238. Lawton AR, Cooper MD: B cell ontogeny: immunoglobulin genes and their expression. *Pediatrics* 64:750, 1979.

239. Gustafsson BE, Laurell CB: Gamma globulin production in germ free rats after bacterial contamination. *J Exp Med* 110:675, 1959.

240. Gitlin D: The differentiation and maturation of specific immune mechanisms. *Acta Pediatr Scand* 172(suppl):60, 1967.

241. Stiehm ER: Fetal defense mechanisms. *Am J Dis Child* 129:438, 1975.

242. Goldman AS, Garza C, Nichols BL, Goldblum RM: Immunological factors in human milk during the first year of lactation. *J Pediatr* 100:563, 1982.

243. Goldman AS, Ham Pong AJ, Goldblum RM: Host defenses: development and maternal contributions. *Adv Pediatr* 32:71, 1985.

244. Rothberg RM: Immunoglobulin and specific antibody synthesis during the first weeks of life of premature infants. *J Pediatr* 75:391, 1969.

245. Harworth JC, Norris M, Dilling L: A study of the immunoglobulins in premature infants. *Arch Dis Child* 40:243, 1965.

246. Thom H, McKay E, Gray DWG: Protein concentrations in the umbilical cord plasma of premature and mature infants. *Clin Sci* 33:433, 1967.

247. Yeung CY, Hoffs JR: Serum g-G-globulin levels in normal, premature, postmature, and "small-for-dates" newborn babies. *Lancet* 1:1167, 1968.

248. Sever JH: Immunological responses to perinatal responses to perinatal infections. *J Pediatr* 75:1111, 1969.

249. Thomaidis T, Agathopoulos A, Matsaniotis N: Natural isohemagglutinin production by the fetus. *J Pediatr* 74:39, 1969.

250. Morito T, Bankhurst AD, Williams RC Jr: Studies of human cord blood and adult lymphocyte interactions with in vitro immunoglobulin production. *J Clin Invest* 64:990, 1979.

251. Miyagawa Y, Sugita K, Komiyama A, et al: Delayed in vitro immunoglobulin production by cord lymphocytes. *Pediatrics* 65:497, 1980.

252. Ferguson AC, Cheung SC: Modulation of immunoglobulin M and G synthesis by monocytes and T lymphocytes in the newborn infant. *J Pediatr* 98:385, 1981.

253. Blaese RM, Poplack DG, Muchmore AV: The mononuclear phagocyte system: role in expression of immunocompetence in neonatal and adult life. *Pediatrics* 64:829, 1977.

254. Holroyde CP, Oski FA, Gardner FH: The "pocked" erythrocyte. *N Engl J Med* 281:516, 1969.

255. Freedman RM, Johnston D, Mahoney MJ, et al: Development of splenic reticuloendothelial function in neonates. *J Pediatr* 96:466, 1980.

256. Gross SJ, Stuart MJ: Hemostasis in the premature infant. *Clin Perinatol* 4:259, 1977.

257. Barnard DR, Hathaway WE: Neonatal thrombosis. *Am J Pediatr Hematol Oncol* 1:235, 1979.

258. Bleyer WA, Hakami N, Shepard TH: The development of hemostasis in the human fetus and newborn infant. *J Pediatr* 79:838, 1971.

259. Andrew M, Paes B, Milner B, et al: Development of the human coagulation system in the full-term infant. *Blood* 70:165, 1987.

260. Andrew M, Paes B, Milner R, et al: Development of the human coagulation system in the healthy premature infant. *Blood* 72:1651, 1988.

261. Corrigan JJ Jr: Neonatal thrombosis and the thrombolytic system: pathophysiology and therapy. *Am J Pediatr Hematol Oncol* 10:83, 1988.

262. Andrew M, Paes B, Johnston M: Development of the hemostatic system in the neonate and young infant. *Am J Pediatr Hematol Oncol* 12:95, 1990.

263. Andrew M: The relevance of developmental hemostasis to hemorrhagic disorders of newborns. *Semin Perinatol* 21:70, 1997.

264. Furie B, Furie BC: Molecular basis of gamma-carboxylation. Role of the propeptide in the vitamin K-dependent proteins. *Ann NY Acad Sci* 614:1, 1991.

265. Aballi AJ, deLamerens S: Coagulation changes in the neonatal period and in early infancy. *Pediatr Clin North Am* 9:785, 1962.

266. Muntean W, Petek W, Rosanelli K, et al: Immunologic studies of prothrombin in newborns. *Pediatr Res* 13:1262, 1979.

267. Lane PA, Hathaway WE: Vitamin K in infancy. *J Pediatr* 106:351, 1985.

268. Stevenson RE, Burton OM,, Ferlauto GJ, et al: Hazards of oral anticoagulants during pregnancy. *JAMA* 243:1549, 1980.

269. Shearer MJ: Annotation: Vitamin K and vitamin K-dependent proteins. *Br J Haematol* 75:156, 1990.

270. von Kries R, Hanawa Y: Neonatal vitamin K prophylaxis. Report of Scientific and Standardization Subcommittee on Perinatal Haemostasis. *Thromb Haemost* 69:293, 1993.

271. Sutor AH, Gobel U, Kries RV, Kunzer W, Landbeck G: Vitamin K prophylaxis in the newborn. *Blut* 60:275, 1990.

272. Hathaway WE, Isarangkura PB, Mahasandana C, et al: Comparison of oral and parenteral vitamin K prophylaxis for prevention of late hemorrhagic disease of the newborn. *J Pediatr* 119:461, 1991.

273. Amadee-Manesme O, Labert WE, Alagille D, De Leenheer AP: Pharmacokinetics and safety of a new solution of vitamin K₁ (20) in children with cholestasis. *J Pediatr Gastroenterol Nutr* 14:160, 1996.

274. Aballi AJ: The action of vitamin K in the neonatal period. *South Med J* 58:48, 1965.

275. Gray OP, Ackerman A, Fraser AJ: Intracranial haemorrhage and clotting in low birth weight infants. *Lancet* 1:543, 1968.

276. Volpe JJ: Neonatal intraventricular hemorrhage. *N Engl J Med* 304:886, 1981.

277. Appleyard WJ, Cottom DG: Effect of asphyxia on thrombotest values in low birthweight infants. *Arch Dis Child* 45:705, 1970.

278. Schmidt B, Zipursky A: Thrombotic disease in newborn infants. *Clin Perinatol* 2:461, 1984.

279. Rodgers GM, Shuman MA: Congenital thrombotic disorders. *Am J Hematol* 21:419, 1986.

280. Sifontes MT, Nuss R, Hunger SP, Jacobson LJ, Waters J, Manco-Johnson MJ: Correlation between the functional assay for activated protein C resistance and factor V Leiden in the neonate. *Pediatr Res* 42:776, 1997.

281. Leroyer C, et al: Prevalence of 20210 A allele of the prothrombin gene in venous thromboembolism patients. *Thromb Haemost* 80:49, 1998.

282. Poort SR, Rosendaal FR, Reitsma PH, Bertina RM: A common genetic variation in the 3'-untranslated region of the prothrombin gene is associated with elevated plasma prothrombin levels and an increase in venous thrombosis. *Blood* 88:3698, 1996.

283. Miller RK, Kellogg CR, Saltzman RA: Reproductive and perinatal toxicology, in *Handbook of Toxicology*, edited by TJ Haley, WO Berndt, pp 209–309. Hemisphere Publishing, Washington, DC, 1987.

284. Gray MJ: Use and abuse of thiazides in pregnancy. *Clin Obstet Gynecol* 11:568, 1968.

285. Leikin SL: Thiazide and neonatal thrombocytopenia. *N Engl J Med* 271:161, 1964.

286. Ginsberg JS, Kowalchuk G, Hirsh J, Brill-Edwards P, Burrows R: Heparin therapy during pregnancy. *Arch Intern Med* 149:2233, 1989.

287. Page TE, Hoyme HE, Markarian M, et al: Neonatal hemorrhage secondary to thrombocytopenia: an occasional effect of prenatal hydantoin exposure. *Birth Defects* 18:47, 1982.

288. Hanson JW, Buehler BA: Fetal hydantoin syndrome: current status. *J Pediatr* 101:816, 1982.

289. Eggermont E, Logghe N, van de Casseye W, et al: Haemorrhagic disease of the newborn in the offspring of rifampin and isoniazid treated mothers. *Acta Pediatr Belg* 29:87, 1976.

290. Powell RD, DeGowin RL, Alving AS, et al: Nitrofurantoin-induced hemolysis. *J Lab Clin Med* 62:1002, 1963.

291. Belton EM, Jones RV: Haemolytic anaemia due to nalidixic acid. *Lancet* 2:691, 1965.

292. Varsano I, Fischl J, Tikvah P, et al: The excretion of orally ingested nitrofurantoin in human milk. *J Pediatr* 82:886, 1973.

293. Brodersen R: Prevention of kernicterus, based on recent progress in bilirubin chemistry. *Acta Paediatr* 66:625, 1977.

HEMATOLOGY IN THE AGED

MARSHALL A. LICHTMAN

WILLIAM J. WILLIAMS

The hematopoietic system is modestly affected by aging, and these effects become particularly notable after age 65. There is a continuous decrease in the volume of the hematopoietic marrow with age, which does not cause significant alterations in either granulocyte, monocyte, or platelet counts, although a slight ($\leq$1.0 g/dl) decrease in population mean hemoglobin concentration in men occurs. The recruitment of neutrophils in response to exogenous stimuli is slightly decreased, but the response to infection does not appear impaired. Neutrophil function is not significantly decreased with age of the subject. Although the population mean vitamin B_{12} and folate levels decrease with age, these changes do not result in decreased hematopoiesis as judged by blood counts, except in individual patients with significant deficiencies. Anemia in older individuals should be evaluated in the same manner as anemia in younger individuals. Certain coagulation proteins are altered significantly with aging, and a propensity to accelerated coagulation and compensatory fibrinolysis is present, leading to a new steady state. Decreased immune cell function is the most consistent change in older persons and perhaps the most important functionally. Although there is a tendency to decreased lymphocyte counts in the blood, the major effects are mediated by dysregulation of T lymphocyte function, perhaps as a result of the prolonged period since thymic atrophy in older subjects. This change affects both cellular immune functions and antibody responses to antigens because of the T helper cell function required. Many studies of aging have to be interpreted in the light of inadequate population samples for study, the difficulty and therefore the rarity of using longitudinal as contrasted with cross-sectional analyses, the small sample sizes after stratification for gender and decade of age, and the need to study smaller age intervals in the 8th through 10th decades of life because of more dramatic changes over short intervals at these ages.

In 1998, individuals 65 years of age or older accounted for 12.7 percent of the population of the United States; this group is expected to grow to 23.0 percent of the population by the year 2040. Currently, there are 4.0 million people in the United States who are 85 years old or older.[1] Data from 1985 through 1989 indicate that life expectancy at age 65 is 14 years for males and 18 years for females in most developed countries.[2] As a result, physicians are increasingly caring for older patients and are being called upon to interpret hematologic data in

Acronyms and abbreviations that appear in this chapter include: BPG, bisphosphoglycerate; EPO, erythropoietin; G-CSF, granulocyte colony stimulating factor; GM-CSF, granulocyte-monocyte colony stimulating factor; IL, interleukin; MCHC, mean corpuscular hemoglobin concentration; MCV, mean corpuscular volume; SEER, National Cancer Institute Surveillance Epidemiology End Results.

the context of the age of the patient. Age-related effects on cellular DNA results in a dramatic increase in the incidence of clonal hematopoietic diseases, especially leukemia, lymphoma, myeloma, and closely related diseases in the decades after age 50. In addition, the decrease in immune function has an impact on vaccine use and resistance to infection in older individuals.

AGING AND HEMATOPOIESIS

Throughout embryogenesis and early infancy nearly all cells of the body have mitotic capacity. Subsequently, certain cells of the body lose their ability to divide (e.g., nervous tissue, muscles).[3] Others continue to divide until full growth has been achieved. Thereafter, cells usually do not divide at a significant rate except under conditions of stress, when they become capable of rapid cell division. These cells are said to be "potentially mitotic" or "discontinuous replicators," as exemplified by hepatic cells and renal tubular cells.[3] Cells of organs that require continuous self-renewal, such as the marrow, the scalp hair follicles, and the gastrointestinal mucosa, are continuously mitotic throughout life.[3]

Studies of diploid human cells maintained in continuous culture have led to the assertion that there is a limit to the number of divisions a cell may undergo,[4–6] a state of replication senescence, which may be related in part to telomere shortening.[7] However, there is no evidence of exhaustion of marrow stem cells with extreme aging. The proliferative capacity of marrow cells from older animals and humans has been studied by a variety of techniques, both in vivo and in vitro.[8–41] Most studies indicate that marrow can sustain normal blood cell counts in older animals,[27–30,32,35,42] but the reserve capacity may be limited during periods of exaggerated demand.[11,14,15,19,22–24,29,199] The hematopoietic limitations observed in older animals could be intrinsic to marrow stem cells or to cells of the hematopoietic stroma and/or their cytokine production.[17,28,32,33,35] The short-term hematopoietic responses to the growth factors granulocyte-monocyte colony-stimulating factor (GM-CSF), interleukin-3 (IL-3), and erythropoietin (EPO) are well maintained in older subjects,[39,40] although the response of multipotential (CD34+) cells to granulocyte colony-stimulating factor (G-CSF) in culture in older patients is decreased, and the mobilization of neutrophils by G-CSF in vivo is diminished.[40,41] There is no evidence, however, that the effects of aging on marrow proliferative capacity, or, ultimately on steady-state blood cell levels, are clinically significant within existing life-spans.[12,14–16]

MARROW CELLULARITY

The cellularity of the marrow decreases with aging, as estimated from studies of histologic sections.[43–45] Magnetic resonance imaging confirms an age-related reduction in marrow cellularity.[46] Studies of marrow from the anterior iliac crest demonstrate a progressive decrease in cellularity from 80–100 percent to about 50 percent over the first 30 years of life.[47] Cellularity of about 40 percent has been found in sternal marrow from normal adults.[48] In iliac crest marrow there is a plateau of about 50 percent cellularity to age 65, after which a decrease in cellularity to about 30 percent occurs over the succeeding decade.[44] This latter decline may be due to an increase in fat related to osteoporosis, with reduction of the volume of cancellous bone, rather than to a decrease in hematopoietic cells.[49] These changes may account for the more pronounced marrow hypocellularity in the subcortical zone.

CHROMOSOME STUDIES

Three principal cytogenetic changes in hematopoietic cells have been identified in relationship to human aging: loss of chromosomes, increased micronucleus formation, and telomere shortening. There is an exponential increase during aging in the proportion of adult women whose phytohemagglutinin-stimulated blood lymphocytes display X chromosome aneuploidy as a result of X chromosome loss. Thus, the proportion of women with X chromosome aneuploidy increases from about 1 percent of women under age 25 years to about 15 percent of women over 45 years of age.[50,51] This alteration is not evident, however, in marrow erythroid or granulocytic cells. Loss of the Y chromosome also increases with age and is a feature of marrow hematopoietic cells. Y chromosome loss is very unusual under age 50 years but occurs in about 10 percent of men beyond age 50 years, with a continuously increasing frequency each decade between 50 and 90 years of age.[52] Loss of the Y chromosome in men with clonal hemopathies occurs at a rate expected in unaffected males of the same age and thus is an aging rather than a neoplastic phenomenon. Autosome loss increases in frequency with age. Smaller chromosomes are lost more frequently than larger chromosomes.[51] An increase in stable aberrations of chromosomes, including insertions, translocations, and dicentric and acentric chromosome fragments, are evident with aging.[53,54] An increase in somatic mutations occurs with age when studied in blood lymphocytes, but this may reflect an accumulation with time rather than an age-dependent increase in mutation rate.[55]

An increase in micronuclei is evident in the blood lymphocytes of older as compared with younger individuals.[54] In women this phenomenon is directly correlated with X chromosome aneuploidy, since fluorescence in situ hybridization demonstrates lost portions of the X chromosome within micronuclei.[51,56]

The termini of chromosomes contain telomeres consisting of specific proteins and tandemly repeated sequences of DNA that have the base structure TTAGGG. Telomeres shorten during ''aging'' of cells in culture and in the cells of humans (and other species) as they age. Aging of hematopoietic tissues is complex because of the potential lengthy dormancy and the self-renewal capability of stem cells, whereas their derivative cells die and are replaced in relatively short periods of time. Telomere length has been examined in blood leukocytes. A shortening of telomere length with age of the host occurs but does so in a complex, not linear, fashion, which may have to do with the relative proliferative rate at the time of study.[57–59]

ERYTHROCYTES

HEMOGLOBIN LEVEL

Many population studies of hematologic variables in aging subjects suffer from several limitations: sampling is often done by convenience rather than random selection of a free-living, defined population; cross-sectional rather than cohort studies are conducted; and small sample sizes, especially after stratification for gender and decade of age, permit undue influence by a few deviant values. Most studies have shown that the mean hemoglobin level or hematocrit[60–64] for a population of men falls slightly after middle age. Although statistically significant in some cases, mean hemoglobin levels decrease by less than 1.0 g/dl in the sixth through eighth decades.[60–66] In a group of men age 96 to 106 years the mean hemoglobin level was 12.4 g/dl,[67] but a later report of centenarians did not find a decrease in mean hemoglobin as compared with other men.[68] In a group of men aged 84 to 98 years the mean hemoglobin level was 14.8 g/dl, only 0.8 g/dl less than that of a younger comparison group.[62] The lowest levels, however, are found in the oldest patients.[63,64,69] The hemoglobin levels in women may increase slightly with age[60,65,70] or remain unchanged.[71] Small mean decreases in hemoglobin levels in older women have been reported.[61,63,64,66,67] In studies that have identified a decrease in hemoglobin level of both men and women, the decrease is less in women than in men. The narrowing of the difference in hemoglobin level between

older men and woman may be the result of decreased androgen levels in older men and decreased estrogen levels in older women.

Iron deficiency and the anemia of chronic disease have usually been responsible for low hemoglobin levels in the majority of asymptomatic elderly people.[61,69,73,74] Iron absorption is not impaired in the elderly, but utilization of orally administered iron for hemoglobin production is reduced.[75] Since hemoglobin concentration does not decrease significantly with age, elderly patients with anemia should be evaluated for a cause (e.g., iron, folate, or vitamin B_{12} deficiency or underlying malignancy or renal disease, etc.) before ascribing it to age.[76–78]

Unexplained anemia is also frequently observed in studies of elderly people.[61,69,74] One set of studies found that the red cells of older individuals separated in vitro had a greater proportion of dense cells in each density fraction, a greater proportion of reticulocytes, and an increase in autologous IgG antibodies per cell. In vitro erythrophagocytosis by macrophages was increased when red cells from older individuals were the target particles.[79,80] The inference drawn was that shortened red cell survival may play a role in the unexplained mild decrease in hemoglobin concentration in some older individuals.

ERYTHROCYTE 2,3-BISPHOSPHOGLYCERATE CONCENTRATION (2,3-BPG)

The erythrocyte 2,3-bisphosphoglycerate (2,3-BPG) level has been reported to fall with age from a mean value of 14.9 μmol/g hemoglobin at ages 18 to 24 to 13.9 μmol/g hemoglobin at ages 75 to 84.[81,82] This decrease is statistically significant. It could account for a slight increase in oxygen affinity of hemoglobin, but is of doubtful physiologic significance.

OSMOTIC FRAGILITY

Erythrocyte osmotic fragility is increased in older individuals in comparison with younger subjects.[83,84] This phenomenon is associated with an increased mean corpuscular volume (MCV) and decreased mean corpuscular hemoglobin concentration (MCHC) of the red cells of older people.[84]

SERUM IRON, IRON-BINDING CAPACITY, AND FERRITIN LEVELS

In individuals of both sexes with normal hemoglobin levels, and presumably with normal iron stores, the serum iron level falls after the ages of 20 to 30.[70,85] In one study the values fell from a mean of about 130 μg/dl (28 μmol/liter) in males and 116 μg/dl (21 μmol/liter) for females to a mean at age 71 to 80 of about 75 μg/dl (13 μmol/liter) in men and 66 μg/dl (12 μmol/liter) in women.[85] Levels of 50 μg/dl (9 μmol/liter) or less were found in 40 percent of men and women above the age of 50.[86] The iron-binding capacity also falls in the elderly.[70,87,88]

Serum ferritin levels rise from a median of 25 μg/liter to 94 μg/liter in males in the third decade and then to a median of 124 μg/liter above age 45.[89] Ferritin levels in females remain low until middle age and then increase from a median of 25 μg/liter to 89 μg/liter in women after menopause.[89] Serum ferritin levels appear to reflect iron stores in elderly people.[73,90]

SERUM ERYTHROPOIETIN CONCENTRATION

Serum erythropoietin levels in nonanemic elderly individuals appear to be the same as those found in younger people,[91–93] although elevated levels were found in one study[94] and lower levels in another.[95] Serum erythropoietin levels are generally inversely related to hemoglobin levels,[91–93] suggesting that the erythropoietin response in the elderly is similar to that in younger individuals. The peak and trough of the diurnal variation in erythropoietin levels is the same in younger and older individuals.[90]

SERUM VITAMIN B12 AND FOLATE LEVELS

Low serum vitamin B_{12} levels are found in a significant number of older individuals who do not have clinical findings of vitamin B_{12} deficiency (i.e., anemia or a neurologic disorder).[47,96–102] They are very nonspecific screening measurements. The absorption of pure vitamin B_{12} ("Schilling test") is normal in older individuals,[88] but absorption of protein-bound vitamin B_{12} may be reduced[103] in such patients and also in apparently healthy adults over 55 years of age.[104] Reexamination of this question, however, showed normal absorption of free and protein-bound cobalamin in older subjects.[105] On the other hand, untreated patients with pernicious anemia may have only a moderate reduction in the serum vitamin B_{12} level and not have anemia or macrocytosis.[106] These data require that reductions in the serum vitamin B_{12} level be evaluated carefully.[106–108] Some individuals with low serum vitamin B_{12} levels have been followed for a 4-year period without developing anemia or other signs of vitamin B_{12} deficiency.[109] Serum and urine methylmalonic acid and serum homocysteine assays may be helpful in assessing such patients. Patients with metabolically significant decreases in plasma vitamin B_{12} concentration will usually have elevated levels of methylmalonic acid and homocysteine, and their levels decrease to normal after vitamin B_{12} replacement (see Chap. 25).

Both serum[66,101,107] and red cell[66] folate levels were below the usual lower limit of normal (3 μg/liter) in a small proportion (3–7%) of both males and females over age 65. Low median values compared to those in young subjects were found for the plasma folate levels of a group of individuals in the eighth decade.[108] Similarly low levels were also found, however, in young people who were clinically well and apparently on a normal diet,[110,112] creating uncertainty regarding the "normal" level of serum folate and making the interpretation of these results difficult. None of the patients with low serum folate levels were anemic, and the significance of these findings is uncertain.

The MCV increases slightly but significantly with age.[62,70–73,113–115] Cigarette smoking may also cause an increase in the MCV,[114,115] and it has been reported that older persons who smoke may have a MCV of 100 fl or more in the absence of any demonstrable cause of macrocytosis.[115]

LEUKOCYTES

TOTAL AND DIFFERENTIAL LEUKOCYTE COUNT

There is no consistent, significant variation in the total leukocyte count in older subjects. Normal leukocyte and neutrophil counts were found in nonagenarian[67] and centenarian populations.[68] Some investigators have found that above age 65 the total leukocyte count tends to be lower in both sexes,[69] due primarily to a decrease in the lymphocyte count.[116–121] Others have reported a decrease in the leukocyte count due to a fall in the lymphocyte and the neutrophil count in women, but not in men, over age 50.[22,123] The absolute lymphocyte count has also been reported to be unchanged in the aged.[124–126]

LEUKOCYTE RESPONSE TO INFECTION

Medical lore has it that the leukocyte count does not rise as high in response to infection in elderly individuals as in young people and that often the principal manifestation of a leukocyte response is an increase in the number of band forms in an otherwise normal leukocyte count.[127,128] However, in two series of cases of acute appendicitis and one of pneumonia, the leukocytosis of patients over age 60 was the same as that found in younger patients.[129,130] The leukocyte count and

the proportion of neutrophils rise much less in response to bacterial pyrogen in individuals over age 70 than in young adults.[131] Similarly, the neutrophilic leukocytosis that occurs 5 h after the oral administration of 40 mg prednisolone is diminished in patients over 55 years of age.[132] These observations suggest a diminished marrow granulocyte reserve in the elderly and/or a decrease in hematopoietic growth factor release.[133] The decreased responsiveness of older individuals to granulocyte colony-stimulating factor-induced release of neutrophils from the marrow supports these suppositions.[40,41] Leukocyte function and serum opsonic capacity is well preserved in elderly individuals,[134,135] but defects in phagocytic ability[136,137] and diminished responses to chemotactic peptides[138,139] and to oxidative stress[140] have been documented. Defects in neutrophil function in elderly subjects may be due to inhibitory substances detected in plasma.[141] Splenic function in elderly subjects may be impaired, as evidenced by an increase in the percentage of pitted erythrocytes in the blood.[142]

IMMUNE RESPONSES

There is compelling experimental evidence that a decrease in immune function mediated by lymphocytes is the most significant change with aging.[200] Thymus involution occurs after puberty, and total thymic atrophy occurs by late middle age. With these changes, thymic-mediated T lymphocyte development disappears, and older individuals are dependent on their existing T lymphocyte pool to mediate T cell–dependent immune responses.[124–126,143,144]

T cells in older subjects have impaired responsiveness to mitogens and antigens,[145,146] in part due to a decrease in expression of CD28 costimulator on the cell surface.[146] The clonal expansion of T cells in culture is decreased, suggesting an inadequate response to antigen stimulation. Clones do not reach full development because of fewer doublings when T cells are obtained from older individuals.[147,148] In the absence of thymic function, the number of naive T cells decreases in older individuals and memory T cells are the predominant type.[149] Spontaneous T cell clonal expansion is a feature of older individuals and may occur among CD4+[150,151] and CD8+ cell subsets.[151] Although likened to benign monoclonal gammopathy, the T cell clones may be stable and less prone to malignant progression.[151]

B lymphocyte function is dependent on T cell accessory roles, and the decreased ability to generate antibody responses, especially to primary antigens,[126,152,153] may be the result of T cell inadequacies rather than an intrinsic fault of B lymphocytes. The response to T cell–dependent antigens is characterized by the formation of low-affinity antibodies and anti-idiotypic autoantibodies.[153] Although variable from study to study, total B lymphocyte,[68,154] T lymphocyte,[68,154] and T lymphocyte subset[68,155,156] concentrations in the blood have been found to be decreased in older individuals. Natural killer cells are increased in number, but their function is disturbed.[68,154,157,201] Not unexpectedly, delayed hypersensitivity reactions are reduced in the elderly.[158–161] These immunologic deficits are correlated with overall mortality in individuals over age 60.[162]

Serum immunoglobulin M and G concentrations do not change significantly in older subjects. Serum IgA levels increase with age.[163] An increased prevalence of autoantibodies (e.g., anti-IgG rheumatoid factor) occurs in older people.[118,152,163] Monoclonal plasma immunoglobulins (essential monoclonal gammopathy) are found with increasing frequency with age, reaching three percent in people over age 70 and nearly six percent in those from 80 to 89[164,165] (see Chap 105).

PLATELETS

The platelet count does not change with age.[68,69] Increased plasma levels of two platelet α-granule constituents, β-thromboglobulin and

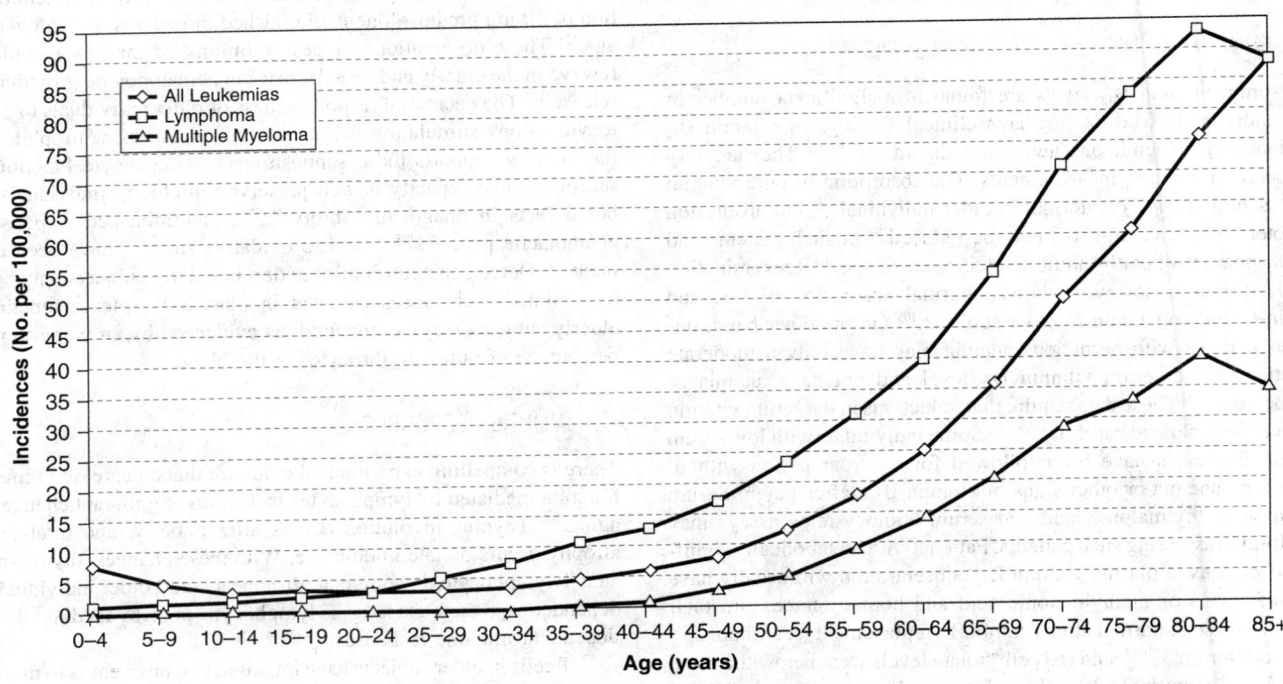

Age-Specific Incidence Rates 1988-1992

FIGURE 8-1   The abscissa depicts age in intervals of 5 years. The ordinate represents the incidence per 100,000 Americans of myeloma, lymphoma, and leukemia. The rates for each of the four major leukemias and the various subtypes of lymphoma are aggregated. The increment at 0 to 4 years among the leukemias reflects a mode in acute lymphocytic leukemia at that age. These data were obtained from the National Cancer Institute Surveillance Epidemiology End Results (SEER) Program.

platelet factor 4, have been found in individuals over 65 years of age in comparison with younger individuals.[166,167] Enhanced in vitro reactivity to platelet-aggregating agents has been observed.[168-173] Decreased platelet membrane protein kinase C activity and translocation to the cytosol after platelet activation was noted in platelets from older subjects.[174]

PLASMA COAGULATION FACTORS

Several studies have emphasized the changes in the level of proteins involved in the formation or dissolution of fibrin.[175-177] Plasma concentrations of factor VII coagulant activity and antigen,[175-179] and factor VIIIC,[175,176,180] as well as von Willebrand factor,[175,180] fibrinogen,[175,176,178,181] fibrinopeptide A,[175,176,182] and tissue plasminogen activator antigen[175,183] are increased with age. Fibrinogen level has been found to be a risk factor for thrombotic vascular disease.[181] In healthy centenarians, levels of activated factor VII, activation peptides of prothrombin, factors IX and X, and thrombin-antithrombin complex concentration were increased, signs of higher-than-expected coagulation enzyme activity.[176] Higher D-dimer and plasmin-antiplasmin complexes indicate an accompanying increase in fibrinolytic activity.[176] Thus, coagulant and fibrinolytic activities appear to be increased in the older subjects by both in vitro,[176,184-187] and in vivo studies.[182,188] Older patients may show an exaggerated anticoagulant response to warfarin.[189]

ERYTHROCYTE SEDIMENTATION RATE AND C REACTIVE PROTEIN

The erythrocyte sedimentation rate increases significantly with age.[62,190-193] Mean values of 14 mm/h (Westergren) and individual values as high as 69 mm/h were found in apparently well women age 70 to 89 years who were followed for 3 to 11 years.[193] The erythrocyte sedimentation rate is of limited value in detecting disease in elderly patients. Estimation of levels of acute-phase proteins appears to offer no advantage over the erythrocyte sedimentation rate.[195,196] The C-reactive protein content of serum also is mildly elevated in older individuals without an apparent inflammatory process.[197,198]

THE INCIDENCE OF CLONAL HEMOPATHIES

Several hematologic diseases are increased in frequency with age; for example, pernicious anemia. The notable increase in clonal (neoplastic) diseases of hematopoiesis is shown in Figure 8-1, which depicts the rate of occurrence of the leukemias (the aggregate of the four major types), lymphoma, and myeloma at 5-year intervals. The inclusion of acute lymphocytic leukemia, which has a mode at about 3.5 years and then increases in frequency again after middle age, does not dampen the dramatic age-dependent incidence rate. The curves do not provide insight into the cause of the relationship, which could reflect the accumulated injury resulting from external factors, the accumulated effects of spontaneous somatic mutations, or some combination of these events.

REFERENCES

1. WWW.census.gov/population/estimates/nation/intfile2-1.txt
2. Kinsella KG: Changes in life expectancy 1900–1990. *Am J Clin Nutr* 55:1196S, 1992.
3. Landsdorp PM: Self-renewal of stem cells. *Biol Blood Marrow Transplantation* 3:171, 1997.

4. Hayflick L: Mortality and immortality at the cellular level. A review. *Biochemistry* 62:1180, 1997.

5. Perillo NL, Walford RL, Newman MA, Effros RB: Human T lymphocytes possess a limited in vitro life span. *Exp Gerontol* 24:177, 1989.

6. Kirkland JL: The biochemistry of mammalian senescence. *Clin Biochem* 25:61, 1992.

7. Rubin H: Cell aging in vivo and vitro. *Mech Ageing Dev* 100:209, 1998.

8. Cudkowicz G, Upton AC, Shearer GM, Hughes WL: Lymphocyte content and proliferative capacity of serially transplanted mouse bone marrow. *Nature* 201:165, 1964.

9. Siminovitch L, Till JE, McCulloch EA: Decline in colony-forming ability of marrow cells subjected to serial transplantation into irradiated mice. *J Cell Comp Physiol* 64:23, 1964.

10. Yuhas JM, Storer JB: The effect of age on two modes of radiation death and on hematopoietic cell survival in the mouse. *Radiat Res* 32:596, 1967.

11. Davis ML, Upton AC, Satterfield LC: Growth and senescence of the bone marrow stem cell pool in RFM/Un mice. *Proc Soc Exp Biol Med* 137:1452, 1971.

12. Lajtha LB, Schofield R: Regulation of stem cell renewal and differentiation of possible significance in aging. *Adv Gerontol Res* 3:131, 1971.

13. Vos O, Dolans MJAS: Self-renewal of colony forming units (CFU) in serial bone marrow transplantation experiments. *Cell Tissue Kinet* 5:371, 1972.

14. Harrison DE: Normal production of erythrocytes by mouse marrow continuous for 73 months. *Proc Natl Acad Sci USA* 70:3184, 1973.

15. Relucke U, Burlington H, Cronkite EP, Laissue J: Hayflick's hypothesis: an approach to in vivo testing. *Fed Proc* 34:71, 1975.

16. Harrison DE: Normal function of transplanted marrow cell lines from aged mice. *J Gerontol* 30:279, 1975.

17. Harrison DE: Defective erythropoietic responses of aged mice not improved by young marrow. *J Gerontol* 30:286, 1975.

18. Mauch P, Botnick LE, Hannon EC, et al: Decline in bone marrow proliferative capacity as a function of age. *Blood* 60:245, 1982.

19. Inoui T, Cronkite EP: The influence of in vivo incubation of aged murine spleen colony-forming units on their proliferative capacity. *Mech Ageing Dev* 23:177, 1983.

20. Boggs DR, Saxe DF, Boggs SS: Aging and hematopoiesis. II. The ability of bone marrow cells from young aged mice to cure and maintain cure in W/W. *Transplantation* 37:300k, 1984.

21. Lipschitz DA, Udupa KB, Milton KY, Thompson CO: Effect of age on hematopoiesis in man. *Blood* 63:502, 1984.

22. Udupa KB, Lipschitz DA: Erythropoiesis in the aged mouse. II. Response to stimulation in vitro. *J Lab Clin Med* 103:581, 1984.

23. Boggs DR, Patrene KD: Hematopoiesis and aging. III. Anemia and a blunted erythropoietic response to hemorrhage in aged mice. *Am J Hematol* 19:327, 1985.

24. Williams LH, Udupa KB, Lipschitz DA: Evaluation of the effect of age on hematopoiesis in the C57BL/6 mouse. *Exp Hematol* 14:827, 1986.

25. Stead NW: Defective mononuclear cell support of erythropoiesis in the elderly. *Am J Med Sci* 293:85, 1987.

26. Hirota Y, Okamura S, Kimura N, et al: Haematopoiesis in the aged as studied by in vitro colony assay. *Eur J Haematol* 40:83, 1988.

27. Schofield R, Dexter TM, Lord BI, Tasta NG: Comparison of haemopoiesis in young and old mice. *Mech Ageing Dev* 34:1, 1986.

28. Boggs D, Patrene K, Steinberg H: Aging and hematopoiesis. VI. Neutrophilia and other leukocyte changes in aged mice. *Exp Hematol* 14:372, 1986.

29. Williams LH, Udupa KB, Lipschitz DA: Evaluation of the effect of age on hematopoiesis in the C57BL/6 mouse. *Exp Hematol* 14:827, 1986.

30. Maggio-Price L, Wolf NS, Priestley GV, et al: Evaluation of stem cell reserve using serial bone marrow transplantation and competitive repopulation in a murine model of chronic hemolytic anemia. *Exp Hematol* 16:653, 1988.

31. Baldwin JG: Hematopoietic function in the elderly. *Arch Intern Med* 148:2544, 1988.

32. Harrison DE, Astle CM, Stone M: Numbers and functions of transplantable primitive immunohematopoietic stem cells: effects of age. *J Immunol* 142:3833, 1989.

33. Lee MA, Segal GM, Bagby GC: The hematopoietic microenvironment in the elderly: defects in IL-1-induced CSF expression in vitro. *Exp Hematol* 17:952, 1989.

34. Tejero C, Testa NG, Hendry JH: Decline in cycling of granulocyte-macrophage colony-forming cells with increasing age in mice. *Exp Hematol* 17:66, 1989.

35. Sharp A, Zipori D, Toledo J, et al: Age related changes in hemopoietic capacity of bone marrow cells. *Mech Ageing Dev* 48:91, 1989.

36. Morrison SJ, Wandycz AM, Akashi K, et al: The aging of hematopoietic stem cells. *Nat Med* 2:1011, 1996.

37. Boggs SA, Patrene KD, Austin CA, et al: Latent deficiency of the hematopoietic microenvironment of aged mice as revealed in W/W^v mice given +1/+ cells. *Exp Hematol* 19:683, 1991.

38. Keating A: The hematopoietic stem cell in elderly patients with leukemia. *Leukemia* 10(suppl 1):530, 1996.

39. Shank WA Jr, Balducci L: Recombinant hemopoietic growth factors: comparative hemopoietic response in younger and older subjects. *J Am Geriatr Soc* 40:151, 1992.

40. Chatta GS, Andrews RG, Rodger E, et al: Hematopoietic progenitors and aging: alterations in granulocyte precursors and responsiveness to recombinant human G-CSF, GM-CSF, and IL-3. *J Gerontol* 48:M207, 1993.

41. Chatta GS, Price TH, Dale DC, et al: The effects of in vivo rhG-CSF on the neutrophil response in healthy young and elderly volunteers. *Blood* 84:2923, 1994.

42. Egusa Y, Fujiwara Y, Syahrrudin E, et al: Effect of age on human peripheral blood stem cells. *Oncol Rep* 5:398, 1998.

43. Custer RP, Ahlfeldt FE: Studies on the structure and function of the bone marrow. *J Lab Clin Med* 17:960, 1932.

44. Hartsock RJ, Smith EB, Petty CS: Normal variations with aging on the amount of hematopoietic tissue in bone marrow from the anterior iliac crest. *Am J Clin Pathol* 43:326, 1965.

45. Kricun ME: Red-yellow marrow conversion: its effect on location of some solitary bone lesions. *Skeletal Radiol* 14:10, 1985.

46. Ricci C, Cova M, Kang YS, et al: Normal age-related patterns of cellular and fatty bone marrow distribution in the axial skeleton: MR imaging study. *Radiology* 177:83, 1990.

47. Callander ST, Spray GH: Latent pernicious anemia. *Br J Haematol* 8:230, 1962.

48. Beutler E, Drennan W, Block M: The bone marrow and liver in iron-deficiency anemia: a histopathologic study of sections with special reference to the stainable iron content. *J Lab Clin Med* 43:427, 1954.

49. Mangolas SC, Jilka RL: Bone marrow, cytokines, and bone remodelling. *N Engl J Med* 332:305, 1995.

50. Nowinski GP, Van Dyke DL, Tilley BC, et al: The frequency of aneuploidy in cultured lymphocytes is correlated with age and gender but not with reproductive history. *Am J Hum Genet* 46:1101, 1990.

51. Stone JF, Sandberg AA: Sex chromosome aneuploidy and aging. *Mutat Res* 338:107, 1995.

52. United Kingdom Cancer Cytogenetics Group: Loss of Y chromosome from normal and neoplastic bone marrow. *Genes, Chromosomes, Cancer* 5:83, 1992.

53. Ramsey MJ, Moore DH II, Briner JF, et al: The effects of age and lifestyle factors on the accumulation of cytogenetic damage as measured by chromosome painting. *Mutat Res* 338:95, 1995.

54. Bolognesi C, Abbondandolo A, Barale R, et al: Age-related increase of baseline frequencies of sister chromatid exchanges, chromosome aberrations, and micronuclei in human lymphocytes. *Cancer Epidemiol Biomark Prevent* 6:249, 1997.

55. Grist SA, McCarron M, Kutlaca A, et al: In vivo human somatic mutation: frequency and spectrum with age. *Mutat Res* 266:189, 1992.

56. Catalan J, Autio K, Wessman M, et al: Age-associated micronuclei containing centromeres and the X chromosome in lymphocytes of women. *Cytogen Cell Genet* 68:11, 1995.

57. Frenck RW Jr, Blackburn EH, Shannon KM: The rate of telomere sequence loss in human leukocyte varies with age. *Proc Natl Acad Sci USA* 95:5607, 1998.

58. Notario R, Cimmino A, Tabarini D, et al. In vivo telomere dynamics of human hematopoietic stem cells. *Proc Natl Acad Sci USA* 94:13782, 1997.

59. Batliwalla F, Monteiro J, Serrano D, Gregorson PK: Oligoclonality of CD8+ T cells in health and disease: aging, infection, or immune regulation. *Hum Immunol* 48:68, 1996.

60. McDonough JR, Hames CG, Garrison GE, et al: The relationship of

hematocrit to cardiovascular states of health in the negro and white population of Evans County, Georgia. *J Chron Dis* 18:243, 1965.

61. McLennan WJ, Andrews GR, Macleod C, Caird FI: Anaemia in the elderly. *Q J Med* 42:1, 1973.

62. Zauber NP, Zauber AG: Hematologic data of healthy very old people. *JAMA* 257:2181, 1987.

63. Nilsson-Ehle H, Jagenburg R, Landahl S, et al: Decline of blood haemoglobin in the aged: a longitudinal study of an urban Swedish population from age 70 to 81. *Br J Haematol* 71:437, 1989.

64. Salive ME, Cornoni-Huntley J, Guralnik JM, et al: Anemia and hemoglobin level in older persons: relationship with age, gender, and health status. *J Am Geriat Soc* 40:489, 1992.

65. Cruickshank JM: Some variations in the normal haemoglobin concentration. *Br J Haematol* 18:523, 1970.

66. Elwood PC, Shinton NK, Wilson CD, et al: Haemoglobin, vitamin B_{12} and folate levels in the elderly. *Br J Haematol* 21:557, 1971.

67. Zaino EC: Blood counts in the nonagenarian. *NY State J Med* 81:1199, 1981.

68. Sansoni P, Cossarizza A, Brianti V, et al: Lymphocyte subsets and natural killer cell activity in healthy old people and centenarians. *Blood* 82:2767, 1993.

69. Nilsson-Ehle H, Jagenburg R, Landahl S, et al: Haematological abnormalities and reference intervals in the elderly: a cross-sectional comparative study of three Swedish population samples aged 70, 75 and 81 years. *Acta Med Scand* 224:595, 1988.

70. Yip R, Johnson C, Dallman PR: Age-related changes in laboratory values used in the diagnosis of anemia and iron deficiency. *Am J Clin Nutr* 39:427, 1984.

71. Jernigan JA, Gudat JC, Blake JL, et al: Reference values for blood findings in relatively fit elderly persons. *J Am Geriatr Soc* 28:308, 1980.

72. Kelly A, Munan L: Haematologic profile of natural populations: red cell parameters. *Br J Haematol* 35:153, 1977.

73. Htoo MSH, Kofkoff RL, Freedman ML: Erythrocyte parameters in the elderly: an argument against new geriatric normal values. *J Am Geriatr Soc* 27:547, 1979.

74. Lipschitz DA, Mitchell CO, Thompson C: The anemia of senescence. *Am J Hematol* 11:47, 1981.

75. Marx JJM: Normal iron absorption and decreased red cell iron uptake in the aged. *Blood* 53:204, 1979.

76. Garry PJ, Goodwin JS, Hunt WC: Iron status and anemia in the elderly: new findings and a review of previous studies. *J Am Geriatr Soc* 31:389, 1983.

77. Timiras ML, Brownstein H: Prevalence of anemia and correlation of hemoglobin with age in a geriatric screening clinic population. *J Am Geriatr Soc* 35:639, 1987.

78. Baldwin JG: Hematopoietic function in the elderly. *Arch Intern Med* 148:2544, 1988.

79. Glass GA, Gershon D, Gershon H: Some characteristics of the human erythrocyte as a function of donor and cell age. *Exp Hematol* 13:1122, 1978.

80. Sheibon E, Gershon H: Recognition and sequestration of young and old erythrocytes from young and elderly human donors: in vitro studies. *J Lab Clin Med* 121:493, 1993.

81. Purcell Y, Brozovic B: Red cell 2,3-diphosphoglycerate concentration in man decreases with age. *Nature* 241:511, 1974.

82. Kalofoutis A, Paterakis S, Koutselenis A, Spanos V: Relationship between erythrocyte 2,3-diphosphoglycerate and age in a normal population. *Clin Chem* 22:1918, 1976.

83. Detraglia M, Cook FB, Stasiw DM, Cerny LC: Erythrocyte fragility in aging. *Biochim Biophys Acta* 345:213, 1974.

84. Araki K, Rifkind JM: Age dependent changes in osmotic hemolysis of human erythrocyte. *J Gerontol* 35:499, 1980.

85. Pirrie R: The influence of age upon serum iron in normal subjects. *J Clin Path* 5:10, 1952.

86. Powell DEB, Thomas JH, Mills P: Serum iron in elderly hospital patients. *Gerontol Clin (Basel)* 10:21, 1968.

87. Rechenberger J: über die Eisenbildungskapazität des Blutserums in den verscheidenen Lebensaltern. *Z Alternsforsch* 9:98, 1955.

88. Powell DEB, Thomas JH: The iron-binding capacity of serum in elderly hospital patients. *Gerontol Clin (Basel)* 11:36, 1969.

89. Cook JD, Finch CA, Smith NJ: Evaluation of the iron status of a population. *Blood* 48:449, 1976.

90. Guyatt GH, Patterson C, Ali M, et al: Diagnosis of iron deficiency anemia in the elderly. *Am J Med* 88:205, 1990.

91. Mori M, Murai Y, Hirai M, et al: Serum erythropoietin titers in the aged. *Mech Ageing Dev* 46:105, 1988.

92. Powers JS, Lichtenstein MJ, Collins JC, et al: Serum erythropoietin in healthy older persons. *J Am Geriatr Soc* 37:388, 1989.

93. Powers JS, Krantz SB, Collins JC, et al: Erythropoietin response to anemia as a function of age. *J Am Geriatr Soc* 39:30, 1991.

94. Kario K, Matsuo T, Nakao K: Serum erythropoietin levels in the elderly. *Gerontology* 37:345, 1991.

95. Pasqualetti P, Casale R: No influence of aging on the circadian rhythm of erythropoietin in healthy subjects. *Gerontology* 43: 206, 1997.

96. Henderson JG, Strachen RW, Swanson Beck J, et al: The antigastrin-antibody test as a screening procedure for vitamin B_{12} deficiency in psychiatric practice. *Lancet* 2:809, 1966.

97. Schilling RF, Fairbanks VF, Miller R, et al: ''Improved'' vitamin B_{12} assays: a report on two commercial kits. *Clin Chem* 29:582, 1983.

98. Cooper BA, Fehedy V, Blanshay P: Recognition of deficiency of vitamin B_{12} using measurement of serum concentration. *J Lab Clin Med* 107:447, 1986.

99. Thompson WG, Babitz L, Cassino C, et al: Evaluation of current criteria used to measure vitamin B_{12} levels. *Am J Med* 82:291, 1987.

100. Nilsson-Ehle H, Landahl S, Lindstedt G, et al: Low serum cobalamin levels in a population study of 70- and 75-year-old subjects: gastrointestinal causes and hematologic effects. *Dig Dis Sci* 34:716, 1989.

101. Lindenbaum J, Rosenberg IH, Wilson PWF, et al: Prevalence of cobalamin deficiency in the Framingham elderly population. *Am J Clin Nutr* 60:2, 1994.

102. Carmel R: Cobalamin, the stomach and aging. *Am J Clin Nutr* 66: 750, 1997.

103. Carmel R, Sinow RM, Siegel ME, Samloff IM: Food cobalamin malabsorption occurs frequently in patients with unexplained low serum cobalamin levels. *Arch Intern Med* 148:1715, 1988.

104. Scarlett JD, Read H, O'Dea K: Protein-bound cobalamin absorption declines in the elderly. *Am J Hematol* 39:79, 1992.

105. van Asselt DZ, van den Broek MJ, Lamers CB, et al: Free and protein-bound cobalamin absorption in healthy middle-aged and older subjects. *J Amer Geriatr Soc* 44:949, 1996.

106. Carmel R: Pernicious anemia. The expected findings of very low serum cobalamin levels, anemia, and macrocytosis are often lacking. *Arch Intern Med* 148:1712, 1988.

107. Herbert V: Don't ignore low serum cobalamin (vitamin B_{12}) levels. *Arch Intern Med* 148:1705, 1988.

108. Carmel R, Sinow RM, Karnaze DS: Atypical cobalamin deficiency: subtle biochemical evidence of deficiency is commonly demonstrable in patients with megaloblastic anemia and is often associated with protein-bound cobalamin malabsorption. *J Lab Clin Med* 109:454, 1987.

109. Pathy MS, Newcombe RG: Temporal variation of serum levels of vitamin B_{12}, folate, iron, and total iron-binding capacity. *Gerontology* 26: 34, 1980.

110. Girdwood RH, Thompson AD, Williamson J: Folate status in the elderly. *Br Med J* 2:670, 1967.

111. Osterlind PO, Alafuzoff I, Lofgren A-C, et al: Blood components in an elderly population. *Gerontology* 30:247, 1984.

112. Hall CA, Bardwell SA, Allen ES, Rappazzo ME: Variation in plasma folate levels among groups of healthy persons. *Am J Clin Nutr* 28:854, 1975.

113. Okuno T: Red cell size as measured by the Coulter model S. *J Clin Pathol* 25:599, 1972.

114. Okuno T: Smoking and blood changes. *JAMA* 225:1387, 1973.

115. Helman N, Rubenstein LS: The effects of age, sex, and smoking on erythrocytes and leukocytes. *Am J Clin Pathol* 63:35, 1975.

116. Caird FI, Andrews GR, Gallie TB: The leukocyte count in old age. *Age and Ageing* 1:239, 1972.

117. Conrad RA, Demoise CF, Scott WA, Makar M: Immunohematological studies of Marshall Islanders sixteen years after fallout radiation exposure. *J Gerontol* 26:28, 1971.

118. Diaz-Jouanen E, Strickland RG, Williams RC Jr: Studies of human lymphocytes in the newborn and the aged. *Am J Med* 58:620, 1975.

119. MacKinney AA Jr: Effect of aging on the peripheral blood lymphocyte count. *J Gerontol* 33:213, 1978.

120. Jamil NAK, Millard RE: Studies of T, B, and "null" blood lymphocytes in normal persons of different age groups. *Gerontology* 27:79, 1981.

121. Polednak AP: Age changes in differential leukocyte count among female adults. *Hum Biol* 50:30, 1978.

122. Allan RN, Alexander MK: A sex difference in the leukocyte count. *J Clin Pathol* 21:691, 1968.

123. Cruickshank JM, Alexander MK: The effect of age, sex, parity, haemoglobin level, and oral contraceptive preparations on the normal leukocyte count. *Br J Haematol* 18:541, 1970.

124. Globerson A: T lymphocytes and aging. *Int Arch Allergy Immunol* 107:491, 1995.

125. Miller RA: The aging immune system. *Science* 273:70, 1996.

126. Wick G, Grubeck-Lobenstein B: The aging immune system: primary and secondary alterations of immune reactivity in elderly. *Exp Gerontol* 32:401,1997.

127. Thomas JH, Powell DEB: *Blood Disorders in the Elderly,* p 18. John Wright and Sons, Bristol, UK, 1971.

128. Thorbjarharson B, Loehr WJ: Acute appendicitis in patients over the age of sixty. *Surg Gynecol Obstet* 125:1277, 1967.

129. Peitokallio P, Jauhiainen K: Acute appendicitis in the aged patients: study of 300 cases after the age of 60. *Arch Surg* 100:140, 1970.

130. Sasso RD, Hanna EA, Moore DL: Leukocyte and neutrophil counts in acute appendicitis. *Am J Surg* 120:563, 1970.

131. Fedullo AJ, Swinburne AJ: Relationship of patient age to clinical features and outcome for in-hospital treatment of pneumonia. *J Gerontol* 40:29, 1985.

132. Timaffy M: A comparative study of bone marrow function in young and old individuals. *Gerontol Clin (Basel)* 4:13, 1962.

133. Cream JJ: Prednisolone-induced granulocytosis. *Br J Haematol* 15:259, 1968.

134. Buchanan JP, Peters CA, Rasmussen CJ, Rothstein G: Impaired expression of haematopoietic growth factors: a candidate mechanism for the hematopoietic defect of aging. *Exp Gerontol* 31:135, 1996.

135. Corberand JX, Laharrague PF, Fillola G: Neutrophils of healthy aged humans are normal. *Mech Ageing Dev* 36:57, 1986.

136. Nagel JE, Han K, Coon PJ, et al: Age differences in phagocytosis by polymorphonuclear leukocytes measured by flow cytometry. *J Leukoc Biol* 39:399, 1986.

137. Emanuelli G, Lanzio M, Anfossi T, et al: Influence of age on polymorphonuclear leukocytes in vitro: phagocytic activity in healthy human subjects. *Gerontology* 32:308, 1986.

138. Lipschitz DA, Udupa KB, Boxer LA: The role of calcium in the age-related decline of neutrophil function. *Blood* 71:659, 1988.

139. Rao KMK, Currie MS, Padmanabhan J, Cohen HJ: Age-related alterations in actin cytoskeleton and receptor expression in human leukocytes. *J Gerontol* 47:B37, 1992.

140. Niwa Y, Ishimoto K, Kanoh T: Induction of superoxide dismutase in leukocytes by paraquat: correlation with age and possible predictor of longevity. *Blood* 76:835, 1990.

141. Dantew B, Spagnuolo PJ, Goldsmith GGH, Marino JA: Neutrophil adhesion in the elderly: inhibitory effects of plasma from elderly patients. *Clin Immunol Immunopathol* 54:247, 1990.

142. Markus HS, Toghill PJ: Impaired splenic function in elderly people. *Age and Ageing* 20:287, 1991.

143. Grubeck-Lobenstein: Changes in the aging immune system. *Biologicals* 25:205, 1997.

144. Yoshikawa TT: Perspective: aging and infectious diseases: past, present and future. *J Infect Dis* 176:1053, 1997.

145. Song L, Kim YH, Chopra RK, et al: Age-related effects in T cell activation and proliferation. *Exp Gerontol* 28:313, 1993.

146. Effros RB, Boucher N, Porter V, et al: Decline in CD2 T cells in centenarians and in long-term T cell cultures: a possible cause for both in vivo and in vitro immunosenescence. *Exp Gerontol* 29:60, 1994.

147. Grubeck-Lobenstein B, Lechner H, Trieb K: Long-term in vitro growth of human T cell clones: can postmitotic senescent cell population be defined? *Int Arch Allergy Immunol* 110:278, 1996.

148. Lechner H, Amort M, Steger MM, et al: Regulation of CD 95 (APO-1) expression and the induction of apoptosis in human T cells: changes in old age. *Int Arch Allergy Immunol* 110:238, 1996.

149. Cossarizza A, Ortolani C, Paganelli R, et al: CD4 isoform expression on CD4+ and CD8+ T cells throughout life, from newborn to centenarians. Implication for T cell memory. *Mech Aging Dev* 86:173, 1996.

150. Posnett DN, Sinka R, Kabak S, Russo C: Clonal populations of T cells in normal elderly humans: the T cell equivalent to "benign monoclonal gammopathy." *J Exp Med* 179:609, 1994.

151. Schwab R, Szabo P, Manavalan JS, et al: Expanded CD4+ and CD8+ T cell clones in elderly humans. *J Immunol* 158:4493, 1997.

152. Schulze DH, Goidl EA: Age-associated changes in antibody-forming cells (B cells). *Proc Soc Exp Biol Med* 196:253, 1991.

153. Powers DC: Immunological principles and emerging strategies of vaccination for the elderly. *J Am Geriatr Soc* 40:81, 1992.

154. McArthur WP, Bloom K, Taylor M, et al: Peripheral blood leukocyte populations in the elderly with and without periodontal disease. *J Clin Periodontol* 23:846, 1996.

155. Miyaji C, Watanabe H, Minagawa M, et al: Numerical and functional characteristics of lymphocyte subsets in centenarians. *J Clin Immunol* 17:420, 1997.

156. Ruiz M, Esparza B, Perez C, et al: CD8+ T cell subsets in aging. *Immunol Invest* 24:891, 1995.

157. McNerlan SE, Rea IM, Alexander HD, Morris TCM: Changes in natural killer cells, the CD57CD8 subset, and related cytokines in health aging. *J Clin Immunol* 18:31, 1998.

158. Moesgaard F, Nielsen ML, Larsen N, et al: Cell-mediated immunity assessed by skin testing (Multitest®). I. Normal values in healthy Danish adults. *Allergy* 42:591, 1987.

159. Stead WW, To T: Significance of the tuberculin skin test in elderly patients. *Ann Intern Med* 107:837, 1987.

160. Marrie TJ, Johnson S, Durant H: Cell-mediated immunity of healthy adult Nova Scotians in various age groups compared with nursing home and hospitalized senior citizens. *J Allergy Clin Immunol* 81:836, 1988.

161. Castle SC, Norman DC, Perls TT, et al: Analysis of cutaneous delayed-type hypersensitivity reaction and T cell proliferative response in elderly nursing home patients: an approach to identifying immunodeficient patients. *Gerontology* 36:217, 1990.

162. Wayne SJ, Rhyne RL, Garry PJ, Goodwin JS: Cell-mediated immunity as a predictor of morbidity and mortality in subjects over 60. *J Gerontol* 45:M45, 1990.

163. Lichtman MA, Vaughn JH, Hames CG: The distribution of serum immunoglobulins, anti-gamma G globulins ("rheumatoid factors"), and antinuclear antibodies in Evans County, Georgia. *Arthr Rheum* 10:204, 1967.

164. Axelsson U, Bachmann R, Hällén J: Frequency of pathological proteins (M-components) in 6995 sera from an adult population. *Acta Med Scand* 179:235, 1966.

165. Hällén J: frequency of "abnormal" serum globulins (M-components) in the aged. *Acta Med Scand* 173:737, 1963.

166. Van Rensburg EJ, Heyns A du P: The effect of age, arteriosclerosis and hypercholesterolemia on platelet function tests, in *Thrombotic and Haemorrhagic Disorders,* Springer-Verlag, 1990.

167. Zahavi J, Jones NRG, Leyton J, et al: Enhanced in vivo platelet "release reaction" in old healthy individuals. *Thromb Res* 17:329, 1980.

168. Fetkovska N, Amstein R, Ferraein F, et al: 5HT-kinetics and sensitivity of human blood platelets: variations with age, gender and platelet number. *Thromb Haemost* 60:486, 1988.

169. Kasjanovova D, Balaz V: Age-related changes in human platelet function in vitro. *Mech Ageing Dev* 37:175, 1986.

170. Winther K, Naesh O: Aging and platelet β-adrenoceptor function. *Eur J Pharmacol* 136:219, 1987.

171. Vericel E, Croset M, Sedivy P, et al: Platelets and aging. I. Aggregation, arachidonate metabolism and antioxidant status. *Thromb Res* 49:331, 1988.

172. Winther K, Naesh O: Platelet alpha-adrenoreceptor function and aging. *Thromb Res* 46:677, 1987.

173. Bastyr EJ, Kadrofske MM, Vinik AI: Platelet activity and phosphoinositide turnover increase with advancing age. *Am J Med* 88:601, 1990.

174. Wang H-Y, Bashore TR, Friedman E: Exercise reduces age-dependent decrease in platelet protein kinase C activity and translocation. *J Gerontol* 50A:M12, 1995.

175. Kario K, Matsuo T, Kobayashi H, et al: Close relationship between hemostatic factors and acute-phase reaction as normal aging process. *J Am Geriatr Soc* 44:614, 1996.

176. Mari D, Mannucci PM, Coppola R, et al: Hypercoagulability in centenarians: the paradox of successful aging. *Blood* 85:3144, 1995.

177. Haverkate F, Thompson SG, Duckert F: Haemostasis factors in angina

pectoris: relation to gender, age and acute phase reaction: results from the ECAT Angina Pectoris Study Group. *Thromb Haemost* 73:561, 1995.

178. Balleisen L, Bailey J, Epping P-H, et al: Epidemiological study on factor VII, factor VIII and fibrinogen in an industrial population. I. Baseline data on the relation to age, gender, body weight, smoking, alcohol, pill-using, and menopause. *Thromb Haemost* 54:475, 1985.

179. Scarabin PY, Van Dreden P, Bonithon-Kop C, et al: Age-related changes in factor VII activation in healthy women. *Clin Sci* 75:341, 1988.

180. Conlan MG, Folsom AR, Finch A, et al: Associations of Factor VIII and von Willebrand factor with age, race, sex, and risk factors for atherosclerosis. *Thromb Haemost* 70:380, 1993.

181. Ernst E, Rosch KL: Fibrinogen as a cardiovascular risk factor: a meta-analysis and review of the literature. *Ann Intern Med* 118:956, 1993.

182. Bauer KA, Weiss LM, Sparrow D, et al: Aging associated changes in indices of thrombin generation and protein C activation in humans: normative aging study. *J Clin Invest* 80:1527, 1987.

183. Sundell B, Nilsson TK, Rainby M, et al: Fibrinolytic variables are related to age, sex, blood pressure, and body build measurements: a cross-sectional study in Norsjo, Sweden. *J Clin Epidemiol* 42:719, 1989.

184. Eliasson M, Evrin PE, Lundblad D, et al: Influence of gender, age, sampling time on fibrinolytic variables and fibrinogen. A population study. *Fibrinolysis* 7:316, 1993.

185. Siegert G, Bergmann S, Jaross W: Influence of age, gender and lipoprotein metabolism parameters on the activity of plasminogen activator inhibitor and the fibrinogen concentration. *Fibrinolysis* 6 (suppl 3): 47, 1992.

186. Cawkwell RC: Patient's age and the activated partial thromboplastin time test. *Thromb Haemost* 39:780, 1978.

187. Ibbotson SH, Tate GM, Davies JA: Thrombin activity by intrinsic activation of plasma in-vitro accelerates with increasing age of the donor. *Thromb Haemost* 67:377, 1992.

188. Kario K, Matsuo T, Kobayashi H: Which factors affect high D-dimer levels in the elderly? *Thromb Res* 62:501, 1991.

189. Gurwitz JH, Avorn J, Ross-Oegnan D, et al: Aging and the anticoagulant response to warfarin therapy. *Ann Intern Med* 116:901, 1992.

190. Boyd RV, Hoffbrand BI: Erythrocyte sedimentation rate in elderly hospital in-patients. *Br Med J* 1:901, 1966.

191. Böttiger LE, Svedberg CA: Normal erythrocyte sedimentation rate and age. *Br Med J* 2:85, 1967.

192. Sharland DE: Erythrocyte sedimentation rate: the normal range in the elderly. *J Am Geriatr Soc* 28:346, 1980.

193. Sparrow D, Rowe JW, Silbert JE: Cross-sectional and longitudinal changes in the erythrocyte sedimentation rate in man. *J Gerontol* 36:180, 1981.

194. Shearn MA, Kang IY: Effect of age and sex on the erythrocyte sedimentation rate. *J Rheumatol* 13:297, 1986.

195. Katz PR, Gutman SJ, Richman G, et al: Erythrocyte sedimentation rate and C-reactive protein compared in the elderly. *Clin Chem* 35:466, 1989.

196. Katz PR, Karuza J, Gutman SI, et al: A comparison between erythrocyte sedimentation rate (ESR) and selected acute-phase proteins in the elderly. *Am J Clin Pathol* 94:637, 1990.

197. Ballou SP, Lozanski GP, Hadder S, et al: Quantitative and qualitative alterations of acute phase proteins in healthy elderly persons. *Age and Ageing* 25:224, 1996.

198. Caswell M, Pike LA, Bull BS: Effect of patients' age on tests of the acute-phase response. *Arch Pathol Lab Med* 117:906, 1993.

199. Globerson A: Hematopoietic stem cells and aging. *Exp Gerontol* 34:137, 1999.

200. Pawelec G, Solana R, Remarque E, Mariani E: Impact of aging on innate immunity. *J Leuk Biol* 64:703, 1998.

201. Solana R, Alonso MC, Pena J: Natural killer cells in healthy aging. *Exp Gerontol* 34:435, 1999.

PART III

MOLECULAR AND CELLULAR HEMATOLOGY

C H A P T E R   9

GENETIC PRINCIPLES AND MOLECULAR BIOLOGY

ERNEST BEUTLER

The understanding of hematology is more than ever dependent upon an appreciation of genetic principles and the tools that can be used to study genetic variation. All of the genetic information that makes up an organism is encoded in the DNA. This information is *transcribed* into RNA, and then the triplet code of the RNA is *translated* into protein. Mutations that change the DNA code, either present in the germline or acquired after birth, can cause a variety of hematologic disorders. A variety of changes in DNA occur, including single base changes, deletions, and insertions. The detection of defined mutations that cause a variety of diseases is now possible and has become a routine method for the diagnosis of some disorders, particularly prenatally. Inheritance patterns depend upon the characteristics of the disorder and the chromosomal location of the mutation. Common autosomal recessive hematologic diseases include sickle cell disease, the thalassemias, and Gaucher disease. Hereditary spherocytosis, thrombophilia due to factor V Leiden, most forms of von Willebrand disease, and acute intermittent porphyria are characterized by autosomal dominant inheritance. Mutations that cause glucose-6-phosphate dehydrogenase deficiency, hemophilia A and B, and the most common form of chronic granulomatous disease are all carried on the X-chromosome and therefore manifest sex-linked inheritance, with transmission of the disease state from mother to son. Understanding of the genetics of a disorder is necessary for accurate genetic counselling.

Many of the hematologic diseases described in this text have a genetic basis. Often the disease is caused by a mutation in a single gene. Some of these disorders, such as sickle cell disease (Chap. 47), thalassemia (Chap. 46), glucose-6-phosphate dehydrogenase deficiency (Chap. 45), and factor V Leiden (Chap. 127) are extremely common. Others, such as congenital dyserythropoietic anemia type I (Chap. 35), chronic granulomatous disease (Chap. 72), or afibrinogenemia (Chap. 124) are rare, but all are due to mutations in a gene that results in the formation of a defective protein or an insufficient amount of a normal protein. The principal focus of this chapter is such genetic disorders. However, a number of acquired hematologic diseases, including lymphomas, leukemias, and paroxysmal nocturnal hemoglobinuria, are now understood to result from damage to the genetic apparatus that is not inherited but rather occurs in a cell at some time during

the lifetime of the patient. Understanding these diseases requires an appreciation of how the genetic apparatus functions.

All of the information required for the development of a complete adult organism is encoded in the DNA of a single cell, the zygote. This information, designated the *genome,* includes the data needed for the synthesis of all enzymes; of all the plasma proteins, including clotting factors, complement components, and transport proteins; of all the membrane proteins, including receptors; and of all of the cytoskeletal proteins. The units of information into which the genome is organized are the *genes.* Some of these genes direct the formation of ribosomal RNA and of proteins that regulate the function of genes. The remainder encode the proteins involved in the structure and function of the body. Genetic diseases are the result of changes, or *mutations,* in these genes.

THE PATTERN OF INHERITANCE

The inheritance of each genetic disease follows a distinctive pattern. The concept of dominant and recessive inheritance is one of the most deeply ingrained in our genetic thinking. It has long played a primary role in the introduction of every high school student of biology to genetics and is used extensively in the classification of genetic disease. A dominant disease is one that is expressed when the patient has only a single copy of the mutant gene, i.e., in the heterozygous state. A recessive disease, on the other hand, is expressed only when both copies of the gene are abnormal. If the mutations on both alleles are the same, as is the case with some very common diseases, and with some less common diseases when the parents are related, then the patient is said to be *homozygous.* If two different abnormal alleles have been inherited, then the patient is designated as being a *compound heterozygote* (or less accurately, a *mixed heterozygote* or *double heterozygote*). It is often implied that genes are dominant or recessive. This is incorrect. It is disease states, or phenotypes, that are dominant or recessive. The gene for sickle cell hemoglobin is expressed in the heterozygous state, so that the carrier of this gene has sickle cell trait. Sickle cell trait is therefore dominant, but sickle cell disease, which occurs in the homozygote, is recessive. By definition, the heterozygous phenotype of a recessive disease does not differ from the homozygous normal state, but it can usually be identified by biochemical means.

X LINKAGE AND X INACTIVATION

The principles of dominant and recessive disease can be readily applied to mutations occurring on the *autosomes* (chromosomes other than the X chromosome), but the situation is somewhat different in the case of genes on the X chromosome. Although the X chromosome is involved, at least indirectly, in the sex determination process, most of the genes on the X chromosome have nothing whatsoever to do with sex determination. Hematologically, some of the more important of these ''sex-linked'' genes include those which code for G-6-PD, phosphoglycerate kinase, factor VIII, factor IX, Bruton-type agammaglobulinemia, and one form of chronic granulomatous disease.

The chromosomal complement of males differs from that of females in that males have one X chromosome and one Y chromosome, while females have two X chromosomes. However, early in embryonic development one of the two X chromosomes of somatic cells of female mammals becomes genetically inactive: in some cells the paternally derived chromosome is inactivated; in others, the maternally derived chromosome is inactivated.[1,2] Inactivation remains fixed, so that all the progeny of the cell in which the maternally derived X chromosome is inactive show only the gene products from the paternal X. Female heterozygotes for sex-linked genes such as G-6-PD deficiency, phosphoglycerate kinase deficiency, factor VIII deficiency, or factor IX deficiency are therefore a mosaic of cells, some of which manifest

Acronyms and abbreviations that appear in this chapter include: BAC, bacterial artificial chromosome; G-6-PD, glucose-6-phosphate dehydrogenase; PAC, P1-derived artificial chromosome; PCR, polymerase chain reaction; poly(A), polyriboadenylic acid; RFLP, restriction fragment length polymorphism; RT, reverse transcription; YAC, yeast artificial chromosome.

the full-blown deficiency, as it is found in affected males, and some of which are normal. The final proportion of cells with one or the other X chromosome active depends upon random factors, i.e., the binomial probability distribution, and on selection between cell populations, which may occur following the inactivation process.[3,4] The process of X inactivation is not only useful in understanding the expression of X-linked diseases in women but has been valuable in studying the possible clonal origin of a variety of disorders. As shown in Fig. 9-1, the progeny of a single cell of a female heterozygous for an X-linked gene will manifest only the phenotype of the original cell. Examination of electrophoretically distinguishable variants of G-6-PD has made it possible to demonstrate in this way that the red cells are a clone in chronic myelogenous leukemia,[5] in paroxysmal nocturnal hemoglobinuria,[6] and probably in acute myelogenous leukemia.[7,8] This indicates that each of these disorders arises through transformation of a single cell and that in the case of the leukemias erythroid cells as well as leukocytes are part of the malignant clone.

With the development of DNA-based technology it has been possible to use X-linked genes as a clonal marker even when there is not a different protein product from the two alleles. A different pattern of methylation of cytidines distinguishes the active from the inactive X-chromosome.[9] This fact, together with the existence of restriction endonucleases that distinguish methylated from unmethylated cytidine, has made it possible to utilize restriction fragment length polymorphisms to determine the clonal origin of neoplasms,[10,11] even when no polymorphism involving an X-linked enzyme is available. The existence of polymorphisms involving the coding region of genes also makes possible the detection of clones by reverse transcription and amplification of mRNA.[12,13]

The pattern of genetic transmission of sex-linked genes is characteristic: a father cannot transmit a sex-linked gene to his son, since the offspring is a boy by virtue of the fact that he inherited the father's Y chromosome, not his X chromosome. Conversely, it is a truism that males always inherit sex-linked genes from their mother and that the mother must therefore be either heterozygous or homozygous for the gene. Because X inactivation is random, however, the degree of

expression of X-linked genes in females is highly variable. This is why, even with the most sophisticated methodology, it is not always possible to detect the heterozygous state in the mother of an affected individual. It also explains why even identical twin carriers of diseases such as factor VIII deficiency can have very different levels of the clotting factor.

MITOCHONDRIAL INHERITANCE

The vast majority of the genetic material in cells is encoded in the chromosomal DNA. However, mitochondria have their own replicating DNA. Apparently having arisen from symbiotic bacteria over a billion years ago, the DNA of mitochondrial DNA (mtDNA) exists as a closed circular molecule of 16,569 nucleotides. This DNA encodes 13 polypeptides, all of which are subunits of the mitochondrial energy-producing pathway; a small and a large ribosomal RNA; and 22 transfer RNAs.[14] Some proteins found in mitochondria are, however, encoded in nuclear DNA. Mitochondria are transmitted through the egg; thus, inheritance is entirely maternal.[15,16] Cells contain several hundred mitochondria, each with its own circle of mtDNA. To become clinically significant, mitochondrial mutations must confer some selective advantage upon the mitochondrion with the mutation; mutations that affect only a few of the hundreds of mitochondria in each cell are unlikely to produce a phenotype. Mitochondrial mutations, often consisting of deletions, are responsible for a number of neurologic diseases.[15] Some of the childhood myelodysplastic syndromes,[17,18] particularly Pearson marrow-pancreas syndrome,[19] are hematologic manifestations of mitochondrial mutations.

THE FAMILY HISTORY

A carefully taken family history can give a physician considerable insight into the nature of a hematologic disorder. One should ascertain whether another member of the family has had a similar disease. In the case of patients with anemia, this is often difficult, since so many women have a history of anemia, usually due to iron deficiency. To estimate the severity of anemia it is particularly germane to inquire whether transfusion was required. A history of gallstones, particularly at an early age, may indicate that a hemolytic disorder was present. Similarly, episodes of jaundice in family members may be the only clue to the existence of familial hemolytic anemia.

Presence of the disease in one of the parents strongly suggests a dominant mode of transmission. If neither parent is affected, but several siblings have the disease, an autosomal recessive transmission is more likely. Consanguinity of the patient's parents makes it highly probable that a disease is an autosomal recessive disorder. Occurrence primarily in male siblings and maternal uncles, with mild or absent manifestations of the disease in the mother, suggests a sex-linked mode of inheritance. Father-to-son transmission rules out sex linkage.

Lack of any family history does not rule out the genetic basis of a disease. In some instances the disease may be so mild in other family members that it is not recognized. Whenever possible, the physician should examine the family members, rather than relying solely on history. In some instances, of course, the gene mutation causing the disorder may have arisen in the generation in which the disease presents.

Once the mode of genetic transmission is clear, the diagnostic alternatives have been narrowed considerably. For example, methemoglobinemia transmitted as an autosomal dominant disorder is due to hemoglobin M, while methemoglobinemia transmitted as an autosomal recessive disorder is due to NADH diaphorase deficiency. Hemolytic anemia with autosomal dominant transmission is likely to be due to hereditary spherocytosis, but sex-linked transmission of the hemolytic

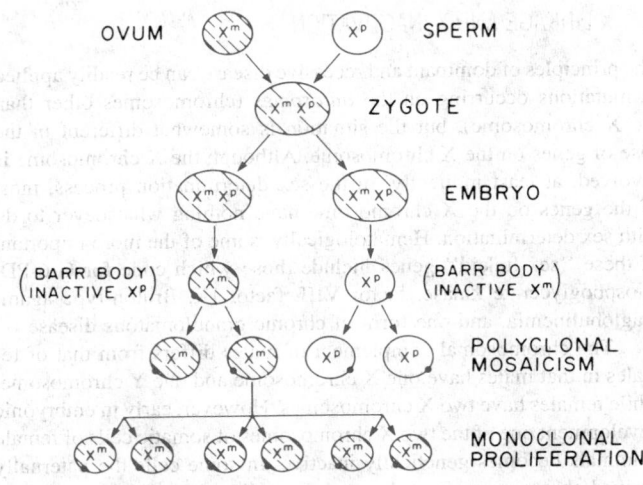

FIGURE 9-1   At fertilization, the female zygote inherits one maternal chromosome (X^m) and one paternal X chromosome (X^p). At some time early in embryogenesis, one X in each cell is inactivated at random and condenses to form the Barr body. The active X remains active not only for the lifetime of that cell but for the lifetime of all of its progeny. A tumor with a clonal origin will consist entirely of cells in all of which either X^m or X^p are active. A tumor with a multicentric origin may contain both X^m and X^p cells.

state suggests a deficiency of G-6-DP or, more rarely, phosphoglycerate kinase. A bleeding disorder that is transmitted in a sex-linked fashion may be due to a deficiency of factor VIII or factor IX, but autosomal recessive inheritance should suggest to the physician a deficiency of other clotting factors, such as X, XI, or V. Careful analysis of the family history not only will make possible more appropriate genetic counseling to the patient and family but also will shorten the road to a correct diagnosis.

LINKAGE

In human somatic cells chromosomes are present in pairs—one pair of sex chromosomes (two X chromosomes in females and an X and a Y in males) and 22 pairs of autosomes. One chromosome of each pair is distributed into the gametes, so that eggs and sperm of humans each contain 23 chromosomes.

If two genes are located on different chromosomes or are far apart on the same chromosome they are said to be unlinked: the offspring of a carrier of these two genes has one chance in two of inheriting either of the genes, and the probability of inheriting one or the other, both, or neither is governed by the laws of chance. For example, if a woman is a carrier of pyruvate kinase deficiency and of sickle cell trait, two genes that are on different autosomes, the probabilities of inheritance of pyruvate kinase deficiency, on the one hand, and sickle cell trait, on the other, are entirely independent. One-fourth the offspring will inherit both pyruvate kinase deficiency and sickle cell trait, one-fourth the offspring will inherit neither, one-fourth will inherit only sickle cell trait, and one-fourth will inherit only pyruvate kinase deficiency.

If the two genes in question are close together on the same chromosome, however, the situation may be quite different. For example, the genes for hemophilia A and for G-6-PD deficiency are both sex-linked. If a woman carries both these genes on one of her X chromosomes, the probability of her child's inheriting either both of the abnormal genes or neither of the abnormal genes is much greater than the probability of its inheriting one or the other. Yet the inheritance of only one of these two genes is not an impossibility, because of the phenomenon of crossing-over during meiosis. In the course of the formation of germ cells, homologous pairs of chromosomes come into side-by-side apposition and regularly exchange chromosomal material. Thus, two genes that were originally on the same X chromosome may find themselves on separate chromosomes after germ cell formation (Fig. 9-2). The probability of their being separated during meiosis is a function of their distance from one another on the chromosome, and this distance is expressed in terms of map units, or morgans. One-hundredth of a morgan, a centimorgan, represents the genetic distance

that gives a one percent probability per generation of a crossover between the two genes. A rule of thumb is that this corresponds to a physical distance of 1,000,000 base pairs, but the actual physical distance represented by a centimorgan varies a great deal from one location in the genome to another; the tendency to cross over varies greatly from place to place. It is not unusual for genes on the same chromosome to be so far apart that the probability of finding them in separate germ cells is just as great as though they had been on separate chromosomes. For this reason, genes on the same chromosome may be linked but may also be unlinked; in the latter case they are referred to as syntenic. G-6-PD and hemophilia A are both on the X chromosome, with a map distance estimated at approximately 0.04 morgans, or 4 centimorgans.[20] Therefore, if two mutant genes at this locus are on the same X chromosome in a female, there is a four percent chance of the genes being in separate gametes. The genes for both G-6-PD and the Xg blood group are also on the X chromosome, but are apparently unlinked.[21]

DNA AND THE GENETIC CODE

Understanding how the massive amount of information required to allow a complex organism to grow and survive is coded has been one of the major advances of modern biology. The information is all contained in polynucleotides, deoxyribonucleic acid (DNA). DNA contains only four different bases—adenine (A), guanine (G), thymine (T), and cytosine (C). DNA exists as a double helix in which A is always paired with T, and G is always paired with C.

The two ends of a strand of DNA are not the same. The nucleosides that make up each strand are linked to each other through a molecule of phosphoric acid attached to the 3' carbon of the deoxyribose of one nucleoside and to the 5' carbon of the next one. A linear strand of DNA thus has one end in which the hydroxyl group attached to the 5' carbon is free; at the other end it is the hydroxyl group attached to the 3' carbon that is not involved in a link. These ends are designated the 5' and 3' ends respectively, and by convention the 5' end is drawn at the left and is called the "upstream" end. The 3' end, then, is designated as "downstream". In the pairing of two complementary strands of DNA the polarity of the two strands is opposite, i.e., the 5' end of each strand is paired with the 3' end of the other. By convention, the strand shown at the top is the coding, or "sense" strand, but the strand at the bottom is the one that actually serves as a template for RNA synthesis. Thus, the sequence of the mRNA is that of the top strand, and the triplet code may be read from this strand.

It is the faithful pairing of A with T and C with G in double-stranded DNA that makes possible the accurate replication of the genetic code. When cells divide, the two DNA strands separate. As this occurs the bases of the separate strands pair with the complementary purine or pyrimidine nucleotide, which become linked to each other, forming a complementary strand of nucleotides. In this way the cell forms two double strands that are identical with the original double strand.

The sequence of base pairs in the DNA strand specifies the sequence of amino acids in proteins. Each base cannot represent a single amino acid, since only four bases are found in DNA and there are 20 commonly occurring amino acids in proteins. Similarly, pairs of bases are not sufficient; they could code for only 16 amino acids. A triplet code is therefore the minimum number of bases that is required to code for 20 amino acids. The genetic code has been found in fact to consist of triplets: each amino acid is specified by one or more sequences of three bases. Long stretches of the triplet code are colinear with the amino acid sequence of the protein the synthesis of which the gene specifies, but these stretches are separated by interven-

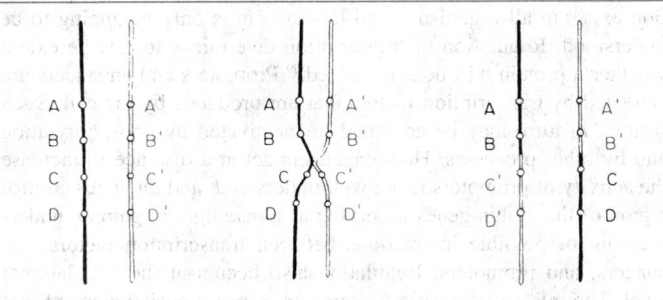

FIGURE 9-2   Schematic representation of equal crossing-over during meiosis. There has been an exchange of chromosomal material between the maternally derived and paternally derived chromosome, but all genes are represented on the products of the crossover.

ing sequences, or introns, that do not code for the amino acid sequence of the protein (see Fig. 47-2). Moreover, DNA does not directly assemble amino acids into protein. This is achieved through a mechanism that involves another polynucleotide, ribonucleic acid (RNA). There are two differences between DNA and RNA. First of all, the nucleotide units contain ribose instead of deoxyribose. Secondly, in RNA uridine (U) is used instead of the thymidine (T) component of DNA. Messenger ribonucleic acid (mRNA) is synthesized with a base sequence determined by the nuclear DNA, which serves as a template in a copying process that is designated as *transcription*.

GENE EXPRESSION

TRANSCRIPTION

The transcription of DNA into mRNA is the first step in gene expression. In order for a gene to be transcribed a promoter must be located "upstream" (i.e., in the 5′ direction) from the DNA. Typical promoters have certain sequences in common. These include a "CAT box," the cytosine- and guanine-rich CCAAT sequence, and a "TAATA box," an adenine- and thymine-rich sequence. Mutations in these regions impair transcription of a gene; such lesions have been identified as causes of the thalassemias and are discussed in greater detail in Chap. 46. The effectiveness of a promoter may be increased by more distant DNA sequences, known as enhancers, which may be either upstream or downstream from the gene. The identification of sequences that enhance expression of the globin genes has been of particular importance in designing vectors for gene transfer to remedy the hemoglobinopathies[22,23] (see Chap. 19).

RNA PROCESSING

The mRNA that is formed on the DNA template by RNA polymerase is not ready to be translated to a polypeptide. First it must be processed, by adding a cap to the 5′ end and a poly-A tail to the 3′ end and by removing introns. Capping consists of formation of an atypical 5′ to 5′ triphosphate bond between the 5′ terminus of the mRNA and a molecule of 7-methylguanosine. The addition of a poly-A tail serves to stabilize the mRNA. Recognition of a sequence (AAUAAA) serves as a signal that a poly-A tail should be added at a point that is approximately 15 bases downstream from the signal when another consensus sequence, YGUGUUYY (where Y stands for a pyrimidine, i.e. uridine or cytidine), is present further downstream. Sometimes more than one adenylation signal is present, and then additional species of mRNA with 3′ portions differing in length are formed.

Excision of introns is particularly important, since they interrupt the coding sequence. The first 5′ bases of the intron are always GpU and the last 3′ bases always ApG (the p represents the phosphate bond between the nucleotides). But there are many such couplets in the RNA, and additional information is required for an actual splice site to exist. The nature of this information has not been clearly defined, but a "consensus" sequence has been defined that most splice sites resemble closely. Removal of the intron is a complex enzymatic process involving the prior formation of a "lariat" structure.[24] Splicing of a given normal mRNA does not always occur in the same manner. Sometimes "alternative splicing" occurs, so that after mRNA is processed some of the molecules contain an exon that is missing from other messenger molecules. This is a powerful mechanism that allows a single gene to direct the synthesis of more than one polypeptide. Potentially the type of polypeptide made can be modulated according to need, and different tissues and different developmental stages may utilize different splice sites to make tissue-specific polypeptides. Alternative splicing has been important, for example, in producing different

forms of erythrocyte membrane band 4.1[25] and different forms of pyruvate kinase for the liver and for the erythrocyte.[26]

TRANSLATION

Processed mRNA contains the code for the synthesis of proteins, and an elaborate mechanism has evolved for the *translation* of the triplet code in the mRNA into protein. A ribosomal complex, consisting of ribosomal RNA (rRNA) subunits and protein components, attaches to the 5′ end of the mRNA. The transport of the needed amino acids to the ribosomal complex is achieved by clover-shaped RNA molecules designated transfer RNA (tRNA). tRNA molecules contain a recognition site which binds to a triplet on mRNA and a site that carries the amino acid appropriate for that triplet to the mRNA, where the ribosomal complex creates the peptide bond between it and the amino acid that is immediately 5′ to it. The initiation of protein synthesis is always at a AUG codon, usually one quite near the 5′ end of the messenger RNA. A consensus sequence[27] around this codon marks it for the starting point of protein synthesis. The ribosome moves down the mRNA, adding amino acids to the nascent protein chain as it goes, until it reaches a termination codon, which serves as the signal to stop protein synthesis. The ribosome is then released and can begin the synthesis of another protein molecule. This complex process requires the presence of initiation factors (IF-1 through IF-6) and elongation factors (EF-1 through EF-3), as well as a releasing factor (RF). Both ATP and GTP are required.[28] The cycle through which the peptide is formed on the ribosome is illustrated schematically in Fig. 9-3.

Since the initiation codon AUG codes for methionine, the amino terminus of the primary translated protein is always a methionine, but this is usually cleaved from the protein during *processing*. Modification of the protein may include changes such as the removal of a leader sequence that directs the protein to a membrane, the addition of sugars to glycoproteins, the addition of fatty acids, and the formation of internal sulfhydryl bonds.

REGULATION OF GENE EXPRESSION

NORMAL REGULATORY PROCESSES

Many genes are highly specialized in their function. Hemoglobin is made only by erythrocyte precursors, crystallin only by the lens, and immunoglobulins only by lymphoid cells. Such genes must be silenced in other types of cells. On the other hand, so-called *housekeeping genes* produce their products in all cells. The latter include the enzymes of the basic metabolic processes that provide energy to all cells, such as hexokinase, phosphoglycerate kinase, and G-6-PD, or that provide basic structural proteins.

Clearly, an elaborate system for the regulation of protein production exists in all organisms, and this system is only beginning to be understood. Regulation of transcription determines to a large extent whether a protein will be synthesized.[29] Promoters and enhancers are activated by transcription factors that are produced by the cell. Such factors, in turn, may be activated or inactivated by phosphorylation and by other processes. How enhancers act at a distance to increase the activity of promoters is not well understood, and the locus control region of the globin genes is serving as a paradigm in gaining understanding of possible interactions between transcription factors, enhancers, and promoters. Regulation also occurs at the translational level. The mRNA of ferritin contains an iron-responsive element that binds to a 87-kDa regulatory protein in the absence of iron, effectively shutting off translation.[30] The same type of binding site in the 3′ untranslated region of the transferrin receptor mRNA serves to stabilize the message by allowing the protein to bind in the absence of iron.[30]

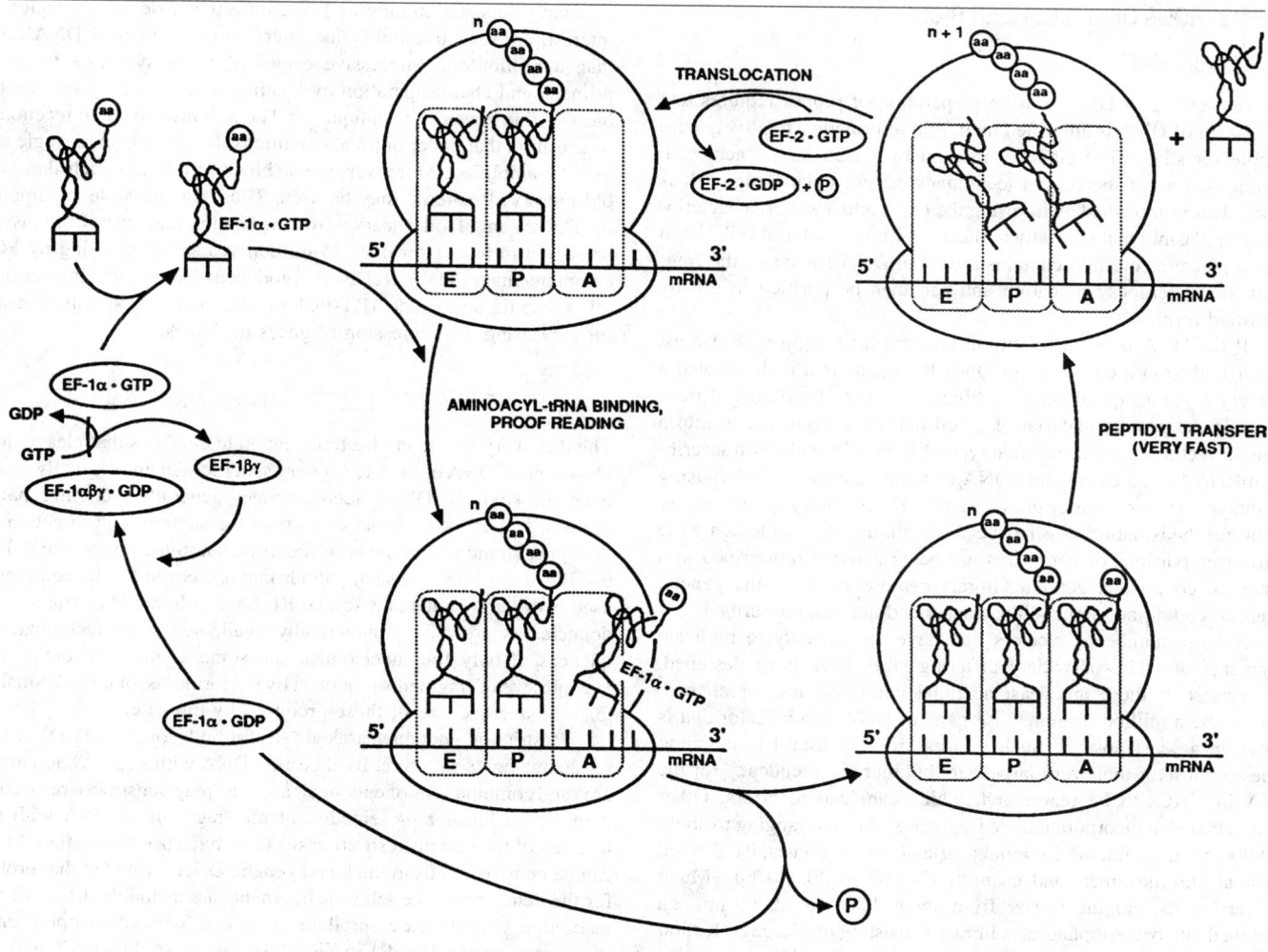

FIGURE 9-3   The elongation of a polypeptide as the ribosome moves down the mRNA. Each amino acid (aa) is added to the preceding one by the coordinated activity of elongation factors (EF). From Merrick,[28] by permission.

Similarly, a UA-rich portion in the 3′ untranslated portion of the tumor necrosis factor gene serves to inhibit translation of that mRNA.[31] It is also likely that the stability of the mRNA itself is regulated by nucleases.[32,33]

EXPERIMENTAL INTERFERENCE WITH GENE EXPRESSION

It is possible to interdict the expression of a gene at several different levels. Genes can be interrupted in murine embryonic stem cells by the process of *targeted disruption*, destroying their function.[34,35] The resulting ''knockout mice'' (a subset of transgenic mice, see ''Transgenic Animals,'' below) can provide valuable insights into the function of genes and serve as animal models of human disease (see Chap. 10).

The translation of mRNA can be inhibited and the RNA degraded by placing *antisense* RNA or DNA into cells. These molecules have a sequence complementary to the mRNA that is to be inactivated. When such oligonucleotides are present they inhibit gene expression through a variety of mechanisms. For example, they form a double strand with the RNA, just as two complementary strands of DNA will hybridize to form the normal double-stranded form of DNA. Because the double-stranded form cannot be translated and is probably degraded rapidly, the production of its protein product is inhibited specifically.

Since antisense RNA can be produced in vivo by transcribing the complementary strand of a gene, it may represent a natural regulatory mechanism.[36–38] In experimental systems, antisense DNA or stable DNA analogs such as the methyl phosphonates[39] can be transfected directly into cells, or the RNA can be made by a plasmid with the appropriate DNA template and a promotor. Some of the uses of this approach include the suppression of lymphoma growth with DNA oligonucleotides antisense to introns of the oncogene *c-myc*,[40] the suppression of the growth of marrow cells from patients with chronic myelogenous leukemia by antisense DNA directed at the BCR-ABL junction,[41] the down-regulation of growth of BCL-2-positive lymphoma cells in culture by BCL-2 antisense,[42] and the inhibition of Friend murine erythroleukemia cell growth by transfection with a plasmid that produces antisense to *c-jun*.[43]

The discovery of the enzymatic activity of certain forms of RNA represents a major advance in our understanding of how life may have originated on earth. Cleaving RNA at defined sequences, much as restriction endonucleases cleave DNA, is one of the known enzymatic functions of RNA, and this function provides a means by which the expression of a gene can be interdicted in experimental systems. This *ribozyme* approach has been used, for example, in preventing replication of the HIV-1 virus[44,45] and for cleaving BCR-ABL with a view to developing a treatment for chronic myelogenous leukemia.[46]

THE METHODS OF MOLECULAR BIOLOGY

CLONING DNA

The sequencing of DNA and the preparation of probes requires that a fragment of DNA is amplified manyfold to provide a relatively pure sample for study. The classical method by which this is achieved, cloning, is one of the central techniques of molecular biology. It is generally accomplished by inserting the DNA into a vector, a bacteriophage or plasmid that normally replicates within a bacterial cell. When such a phage or plasmid contains a foreign DNA fragment, the fragment too undergoes replication and can then be purified in greatly amplified form.

If the DNA is not available in pure form to begin with it must be purified from a collection of DNA fragments that is designated a "library". An adequate genomic library consists of millions of fragments of the genetic material of a cell that have been ligated into a suitable vector. Another valuable type of library is made by transcribing mRNA from a tissue into cDNA ("complementary" DNA) using the enzyme reverse transcriptase. Such a cDNA library is particularly useful for the isolation of genes because in it are represented only the intron-free portions of genes that are being actively transcribed in a tissue. In contrast, a genomic library represents all of the genetic material, coding and noncoding, transcribed and nontranscribed.

A large number of vectors that have the capacity to replicate fragments of DNA of widely differing sizes have been designed. The largest of these are yeast artificial chromosomes, which may incorporate a million or more base pairs of DNA into a vector that is grown in a yeast host.[47,48] Such vectors are very useful in mapping genes because of their very large size, but there is a tendency for the DNA in YACs to be rearranged, which can lead to errors. Other vectors that also incorporate large fragments of DNA, ranging to about 100,000 bp in length, are bacterial artificial chromosomes, P1-derived artificial chromosomes, and cosmids (20,000 to 30,000 bp). Much smaller inserts, ranging in size from about 3,000 to 12,000 bp, can be cloned into bacteriophages. A library consisting of a large collection of the vector containing many different inserts is plated on a confluent layer ("lawn") of micro-organisms; bacteria transfected with a plasmid library are plated on a semisolid culture medium. It is then necessary to detect the amplified wanted DNA fragment. If the exact sequence of at least 17 nucleotides is known, a probe consisting of a radioactively labeled synthetic complementary sequence can be used to detect the clone that is wanted. The precise base sequence cannot be deduced from the amino acid sequence, because there is more than one codon for most amino acids. However, if an appropriate portion of the amino acid sequence is selected, several different complementary sequences, encompassing all of the possibilities, may be used as probes.

Antibodies against the gene product may also serve as probes by using an "expression vector" in which a promotor is present upstream from the cloned DNA. When the fragment is in the correct orientation and when it is "in frame" so that the triplets are read correctly, sufficient gene product may be formed to allow immunologic detection. Colonies (or, in the case of phage vectors, plaques) that react with the probe are picked and subcultured at lower density until a single reactive colony or plaque is isolated.

THE POLYMERASE CHAIN REACTION

Amplification of the desired part of the genome may be achieved when some of the sequence is already known by using the polymerase chain reaction, a technique that is much simpler than cloning. For example, one may wish to determine the sequence of a portion of a gene for diagnostic purposes, but cloning the gene(s) of interest is too time-consuming and labor intensive to be practical. Two primers, matching opposite strands of DNA on either side of the region of interest, are used to amplify the intervening segment of DNA more than a millionfold. Successive cycles of DNA synthesis from the primers, and chain separation by heating between the cycles, are the basis of this powerful technique.[49,50] The polymerase chain reaction is so sensitive that under optimal conditions the DNA from a single cell may be amplified. Moreover, the stability of DNA is such that very old preserved material may be used. Thus, it is possible to amplify the DNA from blood smears,[51] from mummies, and even from insects preserved in amber for over 25 million years.[52] Amplifying by PCR complementary DNA (cDNA) produced by reverse-transcribing mRNA in tissue extracts (RT-PCR) provides a very sensitive means for measuring the expression of genes in tissues.

CUTTING DNA WITH RESTRICTION ENDONUCLEASES

The discovery that many bacteria elaborate enzymes that cleave double-stranded DNA at the sites of very specific sequences greatly facilitated the study of DNA. Such enzymes generally recognize palindromes, i.e., DNA sequences that read the same in one direction on the upper strand and in the opposite direction in the lower strand. Fig. 9-4 illustrates how one such palindrome is cleaved by the commonly used restriction endonuclease Eco RI. Several hundred restriction endonucleases are now commercially available. Some recognize sequences of only four nucleotides and some as many as eight. The average size of fragments produced by the former is, of course, smaller than the average size of those produced by the latter.

Restriction endonucleases are useful both for cloning DNA and for analyzing its structure. By digesting DNA with various endonucleases and combinations of endonucleases one may construct a restriction map, i.e., a linear representation of the fragment of DNA with the location of the various restriction sites that have been identified. Maps can be constructed from uncloned genetic DNA, provided that probes for the detection of the relevant fragments are available. Many of the restriction endonucleases produce fragments with overlapping ends (see, for example, Eco RI in Fig. 9-4). Such "sticky ends" may be used for the ligation (i.e., splicing) of DNA fragments into a vector by using a vector with complementary sticky ends. The seal is made permanent with the enzyme DNA ligase.

The size of restriction fragments produced after digesting whole genomic DNA with restriction endonucleases may be appreciated using the technique of Southern blotting, a useful procedure named after the investigator who developed it.[53] The DNA is digested with one or more restriction endonucleases and then subjected to electrophoresis in a gel that separates fragments by size. It is then transferred to a membrane that binds DNA, and the appropriate DNA fragments are detected using labeled probes. Alternatively, the segment of DNA that is of interest may be amplified using the PCR technique and digested by a restriction endonuclease to determine whether or not target sites are present.

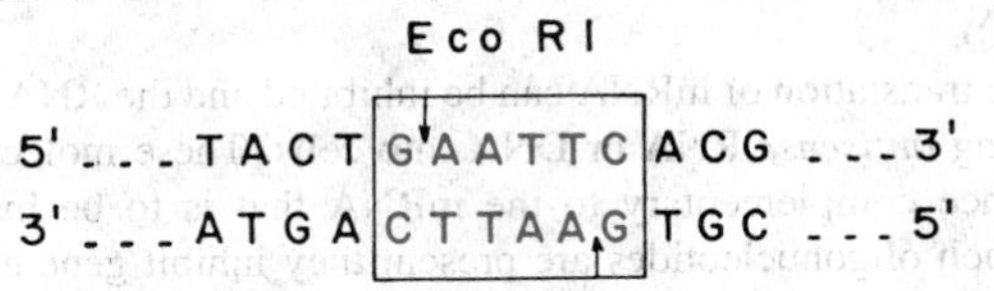

Eco RI

5' ...TACT G A A T T C ACG ...3'
3' ...ATGA C T T A A G TGC ...5'

FIGURE 9-4   A schematic representation of ECO R1 cleaving its recognition sequence, which is outlined by the rectangle. Whenever this restriction endonuclease encounters the palindromic sequence GAATTC, it cleaves DNA at the position shown by the arrows.

One of the most powerful uses of restriction endonucleases is in the detection of genetic variability. Changes in nucleotides may create or abolish restriction sites. Thus, they change the size of fragments that are formed when the DNA is digested. Such areas of variability represent restriction fragment length polymorphisms (RFLP). In some cases the changes in nucleotide sequence may be the ones that cause the disease itself. For example, the sickle cell mutation causes disappearance of a restriction site recognized by the enzyme *Mst* II,[54] and the G-6-PD A− mutation causes formation of a restriction site recognized by *Nla* III; such changes have proved valuable in diagnosis (see Chaps. 45 and 47).

Deletions of chromosomal material, as occur in α-thalassemia, also produce changes in fragment sizes. Larger fragments may appear if the deleted fragment contains a restriction site, or smaller fragments if it does not. If the area covered by the probe is deleted in its entirety, as occurs in hydrops fetalis, no band will be seen at all. Even when the lesion that causes the disease does not directly affect a restriction site, RLFPs may be valuable in disease detection by virtue of close linkage of the restriction site to a disease-causing gene. Multiple restriction sites near the gene of interest produce haplotypes that may unequivocally identify a chromosome. Such haplotypes have been particularly useful in the prenatal diagnosis of the thalassemias (see Chap. 46).

SEQUENCING

The chain termination technique[55] is most commonly used to determine the sequence of DNA. It depends upon synthesizing a labeled strand of DNA, with the DNA to be sequenced serving as the template. The mixture of nucleotides used contains, in addition to the native deoxynucleotides, a nucleotide analog that results in chain termination when incorporated. The normal nucleotides are present in excess, and therefore chain termination occurs only sporadically, but always when the analog is incorporated. Four different incubation mixtures are used, each with an analog of one of the four nucleotides. Gel electrophoresis of the labeled products produces "ladders" of polynucleotides. The size of each fragment depends on the point at which there exists a nucleotide corresponding to the chain-terminating analog in the mixture (Fig. 9-5). Sequencing can now be carried out rapidly and accurately by automated methods.[56]

While DNA sequencing formerly required cloning of the fragment to be studied, amplification by PCR serves as a simpler alternative when the surrounding sequences are known.[57,58]

DETECTING MUTATIONS IN INDIVIDUAL PATIENTS

The cloning and sequencing of DNA is too time-consuming to permit application for diagnostic purposes to individual patients. Fortunately, there are shortcuts that can be used when the nature of the lesion is known and a yes-or-no answer is sought with regards to the existence of a certain substitution. The value of restriction sites in this regard has been discussed above, but since many substitutions neither abolish nor create restriction sites the use of restriction endonucleases is not feasible in every case. However, a mismatch in one of the amplifying primers used in amplifying DNA by PCR, selected so as to create a restriction site where none existed before, is a technique that has been used successfully to detect mutations.[59] Using amplifying primers that fit one genotype but not the other has been used in "color PCR"[60] and in the amplification refractory mutation system (ARMS).[61] The failure of fragments of DNA to ligate when aligned on a template in which there is a misfit of the terminal nucleotide also has been used to detect mutations.[62–64] The hybridization of labeled oligonucleotide probes with a defined sequence to an amplified DNA target, but not

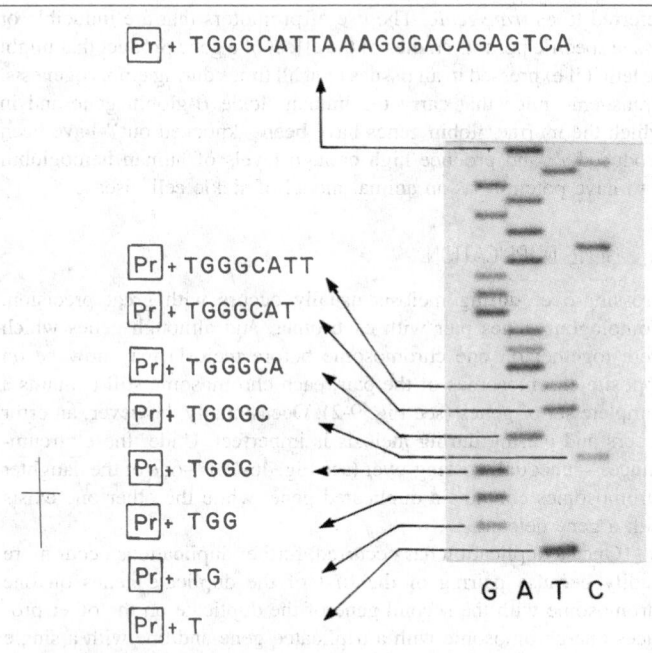

FIGURE 9-5   Radioautograph of a gel being used to determine the sequence of the glucocerebrosidase gene by the chain termination method. Four reaction mixtures are used. Each mixture contains a polynucleotide primer (Pr) that has a sequence complementary to the beginning of the strand to be sequenced, and all four normal deoxynucleoside triphosphates labeled with ^{32}P. The "G" mixture also contains dideoxyguanosine triphosphate to act as a chain terminator when a guanine is reached. The "A" mixture contains the adenine chain terminator, and so on. Each mixture is placed in a slot: the "G" mixture in G, and so on. Upon electrophoresis the gel separates polynucleotides by size. Thus, the positions to which polynucleotides move in the gel correspond to the positions at which the indicated nucleotides are added to the end of the DNA strand as it is being synthesized. The sequence of the DNA can then be deduced. The apparent sequence of some of the bands are shown at the left.

to a DNA target harboring even a single nucleotide change, a method designated allele-specific oligonucleotide hybridization (ASOH), is also very useful.[65,66] Probes containing approximately 17 nucleotides fitting either the normal or the mutant sequence are hybridized to PCR-amplified DNA. A single mismatch in an oligonucleotide of this size produces a sufficient change in melting temperature (i.e., the temperature at which the strands of DNA separate) that the two sequences can be distinguished from one another.

When the mutation is not known, other techniques may prove useful. Single-stranded conformation polymorphism (SSCP) analysis takes advantage of the fact that a single base substitution will usually change the conformation of single-stranded DNA and change its migration in a gel when it is subjected to electrophoresis. This technique has been found to be particularly powerful, revealing most mutations in segments of DNA between 200 and 400 bases in length.[67,68] Alternatively single base mismatches may be detected by hybridizing mRNA with a known sequence to the DNA and cleaving the duplexes with ribonuclease,[69] or by measuring the denaturation of mismatched double-stranded DNA (heteroduplexes) in a gradient.[70]

TRANSGENIC ANIMALS

The mechanical insertion of DNA fragments into the nucleus of a fertilized ovum provides a means for altering the genetic constitution of animals. Animals that have been engineered in this manner are referred to as *transgenic*. The use of promotors that are inducible or tissue specific permits studies of the effect of a gene product that might be lethal if expressed in all tissues or at all times during embryogenesis. Transgenic mice that carry the human sickle β-globin gene and in which the murine globin genes have been "knocked out" have been produced[71,72] and produce high enough levels of human hemoglobin S to have potential as an animal model of sickle cell disease.

GENE DUPLICATION

Crossing-over during meiosis usually occurs with great precision. Homologous genes pair with each other, and although genes which were together on one chromosome before meiosis may now be on opposite chromosomes of the pair, each chromosome still contains a complete set of genes (see Fig. 9-2). Occasionally, however, an error occurs and pairing during meiosis is imperfect. Under these circumstances—unequal crossing-over (see Fig. 46-10)—one of the daughter chromosomes contains a duplicated gene, while the other one exists with a gene deleted.

Once a duplication has occurred, further duplications occur more readily because pairing of the first of the duplicate genes on one chromosome with the second gene of the duplicate on the other produces one chromosome with a triplicated gene and one with a single gene. Duplication has probably played a very important role in the course of evolution[73] because the presence of two genes with the same function allows experiments of nature, mutations, to occur on one of the genes without totally losing the original function, which is still carried out by the duplicate. Examples of the results of gene duplication abound in hematology, particularly with respect to the hemoglobin loci. The α-chain loci are duplicated, and there are also two nearly identical copies of the γ-chain locus (see Chap. 46). Furthermore, the close similarity of their amino acid sequence and the fact that they are tightly linked indicate that the β, γ, and δ loci represent the result of duplication of a single ancestral gene. The process of unequal crossing-over takes place not only between genes, but also within genes. When this occurs, one would anticipate that a portion of the amino acid sequence of a protein is represented twice on one chromosome and is missing on the other. The Lepore hemoglobins, leading to a thalassemic clinical state, are an example of this type of unequal crossing-over (see Fig. 46-6). These abnormal hemoglobins have the amino acid sequence of the δ chain at the amino end, and the sequence of the β chain at the carboxyl end. The complement to this kind of abnormality, the "anti-Lepore" hemoglobin, also has been found (see Chap. 46). Similarly, a mutation of the glucocerebrosidase gene causing Gaucher disease has been found to be the result of a crossover between the active gene and the pseudogene.[74]

PSEUDOGENES

Pseudogenes are DNA sequences that resemble the corresponding functional genes, but do not result in the production of a gene product. Pseudogenes exist, for example, for the β-globin chain, von Willebrand factor, ferritin, and glucocerebrosidase. These pseudogenes apparently arose by gene duplication and simulate the true gene even in having introns. They have apparently lost their ability to function, through mutations either in the coding region or in their promoter. Some pseudogenes are devoid of introns. They may well have arisen in evolution as a result of the reverse transcription of a processed mRNA by retroviral reverse transcriptase. Unlike genes that arose by tandem duplication as a result of unequal crossover, such pseudogenes can be found anywhere in the genome. For example, a functional glutathione-S-transferase gene is on chromosome 11 and a pseudogene is located on chromosome 12.[75]

TYPES OF MUTATIONS

Mutations can occur in structural genes (the part of the DNA that specifies the amino acid sequence of protein), in the poorly understood regulatory apparatus that determines whether or not a gene will be available for transcription, in introns, or in portions of the DNA between genes that have no known function. As shown in Table 9-1, hematologic diseases provide examples of every known mechanism for causing mutations.

A change of one nucleotide to another without a change in the number of nucleotides in the sequence is called a point mutation. Other types of mutations are deletions and insertions (e.g., duplication of stretches of DNA in a gene). Mutations do not occur at random. Changes in the dinucleotide CpG to TpG are particularly common because invertebrate DNA cytidines followed by guanine are readily methylated and the methylcytosine formed is susceptible to oxidation to thymine. Thus, in both hemophilia A[76] and G-6-PD deficiency[77] an unusually high proportion of point mutations are found in CpG dinucleotides. Deletions or duplications of portions of genes tend to occur in areas in which the same sequence is repeated more than once. Thus, there are "hot spots" in the genome in which, for one reason or another, mutations are particularly likely to occur.

Another mechanism by which mutation appears to occur is that of *gene conversion*. This poorly understood phenomenon results in the sequence of one gene being transferred en bloc to another. This phenomenon is thought to account for the maintenance of identical sequence between duplicated genes.[78,79]

Many mutations affect the amount of processed mRNA that is formed. For example, mutations that cause abnormal splicing may produce a messenger that cannot be translated. Regulatory mutations that impair the rate at which a gene is transcribed into mRNA can be the consequence of mutations in promoter or enhancer elements. Mutations that cause thalassemia by impairing transcription of the

TABLE 9-1   EXAMPLES OF GENETIC MECHANISMS IN HEMATOLOGIC DISEASE

Diseases Due to Inherited Mitochondrial Mutations	Mechanism*	Where Discussed
myelodysplastic syndromes	del	Chap. 92
Diseases Due to Inherited X-linked Mutations		
G-6-PD deficiency	del, spl, pm	Chap. 45
chronic granulomatous disease	pm, del, spl, ins	Chap. 72
Bruton agammaglobulinemia	pm, del, spl, ins	Chap. 88
hemophilia	pm, del, spl, ins, tr	Chap. 123
Diseases Due to Inherited Autosomal Dominant Mutations		
hereditary spherocytosis	pm, del, spl, ins	Chap. 43
pyruvate kinase deficiency	pm, del, spl, ins	Chap. 45
thalassemia major	pm, del, spl, ins	Chap. 46
sickle cell disease	pm	Chap. 47
unstable hemoglobinopathies	pm, del	Chap. 48
acute intermittent porphyria	pm, del, spl, ins	Chap. 62
Gaucher disease	pm, del, spl, ins, tr	Chap. 79
inherited autosomal recessive dysfibrinogenemia	pm	Chap. 124
von Willebrand disease	pm, del, ins	Chap. 135
factor V Leiden	pm	Chap. 127
Diseases Due to Acquired X-linked Mutations		
paroxysmal nocturnal hemoglobinuria	pm, del, spl, ins	Chap. 36
Diseases Due to Acquired Autosomal Dominant Mutations		
chronic granulocytic leukemia	tr	Chap. 94

*del = deletion; ins = insertion; spl = splicing mutation; pm = point mutation; tr = chromosomal translocation.

hemoglobin β locus are the best characterized of these (see Chap. 46). However, most mutations causing hematologic disease seem to be structural mutations, those in which the sequence of the coding region of the gene is altered.

Errors in the base sequence of the structural gene result in failure to form any protein, in the formation of a very unstable protein that may never appear in the fully assembled form, or in the formation of an abnormal protein. The latter circumstance appears to be the most common. The abnormal protein may maintain all, some, or none of the functional properties of the normal protein. Even when it has lost the functional properties of the original protein it may retain the antigenic properties, and it is then designated cross-reacting material (CRM). Its stability may be normal or reduced. Mutations that result in the formation of stable proteins with normal functional properties are not clinically significant, but they may be very valuable from the point of view of population and family studies, or as genetic markers for various types of biologic investigations. Some "deficiencies" of enzymes are also clinically harmless. For example, genetic absence of the glycosyl transferases that convert the H antigen to the A or B antigen (see Chap. 137) results in the appearance of blood group O, surely a clinical state that cannot be considered a disease. Genetic variants that reach a frequency of more than one percent in a population are known as polymorphisms. Sometimes genetic variants such as the sickle cell gene or the G-6-PD deficiency gene reach polymorphic levels because the deleterious effects that they may have are counterbalanced by beneficial effects on survival, such as increased resistance to malaria. They are known as balanced polymorphisms.

All cells receive the same complement of genes. Nonetheless some mutations are tissue-specific. Several circumstances can account for this. Some enzymes that appear to perform the same function are encoded by different genes in different tissues. For example, the pyruvate kinase of leukocytes and that of erythrocytes are under separate genetic control (see Chap. 45). In other cases, alternative splicing of the primary mRNA can produce different polypeptides.[80,81] Differences in posttranslational processing, including proteolysis and glycosylation of the same polypeptide by different enzymes in different tissues, can lead to different final products. However, in most instances a mutation that affects an enzyme in one type of blood cell will also affect the same enzyme in other blood cells, in liver, in brain, and in other tissues.

The types of enzyme deficiencies encountered clinically are limited by the ability of the affected individual to survive. Thus, complete absence of a key glycolytic enzyme from all tissues is incompatible with the basic process of energy metabolism and would almost surely be lethal long before birth. In contrast, the inheritance of enzyme deficiencies that are manifested only in erythrocytes is apparently quite compatible with survival, and thus many of the enzyme defects that are observed in humans are ones that only affect the red blood cell.

MUTATION NOMENCLATURE

Historically, mutations were first detected by sequencing the protein, usually hemoglobin. Indeed, the mutation in sickle cell disease was described before the genetic code had been deciphered. Thus, mutations were designated by indicating the amino acid change. Amino acid-based nomenclature does not unambiguously define the mutation, since the same amino acid substitution can be caused by different nucleotide substitutions. Further ambiguity is introduced by the fact that three different starting points for the numbering of amino acids in protein are commonly employed: (1) the methionine start codon; (2) the amino acid after the methionine start codon; and (3) the amino terminal amino acid of the processed protein. Finally, there are many mutations, such as those that change splice sites or promoters, that

cannot be designated by an amino acid substitution. Nonetheless, designations based on amino acid mutation have been so widely used that they serve as useful "nicknames" for mutations; the nucleotide-based designation would simply not be recognized by workers in the field. Moreover, knowing the amino acid change sometimes provides valuable information regarding the effect of the mutation at the protein level. Therefore, while the more robust nucleotide-based mutation is preferred in this text, the amino acid–based notation is used when it is the one that is generally recognized by workers in the field. Standards have been established for the different notations that are in use.[82–85]

GENOTYPE-PHENOTYPE CORRELATIONS

Even before detection of mutations at the DNA level was feasible, clinicians could deduce that the same genotype did not always produce the same clinical disease picture (phenotype). Sibs inheriting autosomal recessive disorders from their parents often have been observed to have discordant clinical presentations—one severely affected, one mildly so—even though the same pair of disease-producing genes was inherited. With the development of the ability to define genotypes directly, the great degree of genotype-phenotype dissociation has become even more evident. Thus, persons inheriting the same sickle cell, G-6-PD, factor VIII, or glucocerebrosidase mutations may have mild or severe sickle cell disease, hemolytic anemia, hemophilia A, or Gaucher disease respectively. The factors that modify disease expression are usually not understood. In the case of G-6-PD deficiency, a second mutation, one in the UDP-glucuronosyltransferase-1 gene, has been shown to determine whether severe jaundice will be present.[86,87]

REFERENCES

1. Beutler E, Yeh M, Fairbanks VF: The normal human female as a mosaic of X-chromosome activity: Studies using the gene for G-6-PD deficiency as a marker. *Proc Natl Acad Sci USA* 48:9, 1962.
2. Lyon MF: Sex chromatin and gene action in the mammalian X-chromosome. *Am J Hum Genet* 14:135, 1962.
3. Gartler SM, Linder D: Developmental and evolutionary implications of the mosaic nature of the G-6-PD system. *Cold Spring Harb Symp Quant Biol* 29:253, 1964.
4. Beutler E: The distribution of gene products among populations of cells in heterozygous humans. *Cold Spring Harb Symp Quant Biol* 29:261, 1964.
5. Fialkow PJ, Gartler SM, Yoshida A: Clonal origin of chronic myelocytic leukemia in man. *Proc Natl Acad Sci USA* 58:1468, 1967.
6. Oni SB, Osunkoya BO, Luzzatto L: Paroxysmal nocturnal hemoglobinuria: Evidence for monoclonal origin of abnormal red cells. *Blood* 36:145, 1970.
7. Beutler E, West C, Johnson C: Involvement of the erythroid series in acute myeloid leukemia. *Blood* 53:1203, 1979.
8. Fialkow PJ, Singer JW, Raskind WH, et al: Clonal development, stem-cell differentiation, and clinical remissions in acute nonlymphocytic leukemia. *N Engl J Med* 317:468, 1987.
9. Lindsay S, Monk M, Holliday R, et al: Differences in methylation on the active and inactive human X chromosomes. *Ann Hum Genet* 49:115, 1985.
10. Gilliland DG, Blanchard KL, Bunn HF: Clonality in acquired hematologic disorders. *Annu Rev Med* 42:491, 1991.
11. Gilliland DG, Blanchard KL, Levy J, Perrin S, Bunn HF: Clonality in myeloproliferative disorders: analysis by means of the polymerase chain reaction. *Proc Natl Acad Sci USA* 88:6848, 1991.
12. Curnutte JT, Hopkins PJ, Kuhl W, Beutler E: Studying X-inactivation. *Lancet* 339:749, 1992.
13. Prchal JT, Guan YL, Prchal JF, Barany F: Transcriptional analysis of the active X-chromosome in normal and clonal hematopoiesis. *Blood* 81:269, 1993.
14. Wallace DC: Mitochondrial DNA sequence variation in human evolution and disease. *Proc Natl Acad Sci USA* 91:8739, 1994.

15. Graeber MB, Muller U: Recent developments in the molecular genetics of mitochondrial disorders. *J Neurol Sci* 153:251, 1998.

16. Ohno S: The one ancestor per generation rule and three other rules of mitochondrial inheritance. *Proc Natl Acad Sci USA* 94:8033, 1997.

17. Bader-Meunier B, Rotig A, Mielot F, et al: Refractory anaemia and mitochondrial cytopathy in childhood. *Br J Haematol* 87:381, 1994.

18. Superti-Furga A, Schoenle E, Tuchschmid P, et al: Pearson bone marrow-pancreas syndrome with insulin-dependent diabetes, progressive renal tubulopathy, organic aciduria and elevated fetal haemoglobin caused by deletion and duplication of mitochondrial DNA. *Eur J Pediatr* 152:44, 1993.

19. Cormier V, Rötig A, Quartino AR, et al: Widespread multi-tissue deletions of the mitochondrial genome in the Pearson marrow-pancreas syndrome. *J Pediatr* 117:599, 1990.

20. Boyer SH, Graham JB: Linkage between the X chromosome loci for glucose-6-phosphate dehydrogenase electrophoretic variation and hemophilia A. *Am J Hum Genet* 17:320, 1965.

21. Siniscalco M, Filippi G, Latte B, et al: Failure to detect linkage between Xg and other X-borne loci in Sardinians. *Ann Hum Genet* 29:231, 1966.

22. Jarman AP, Wood WG, Sharpe JA, et al: Characterization of the major regulatory element upstream of the human alpha-globin gene cluster. *Mol Cell Biol* 11:4679, 1991.

23. Orkin SH: Globin gene regulation and switching: circa 1990. *Cell* 63:665, 1990.

24. Keller W: The RNA lariat: A new ring to the splicing of mRNA precursors. *Cell* 39:423, 1984.

25. Conboy JG, Chan J, Mohandas N, Kan YW: Multiple protein 4.1 isoforms produced by alternative splicing in human erythroid cells. *Proc Natl Acad Sci USA* 85:9062, 1988.

26. Noguchi T, Yamada K, Inoue H, Matsuda T, Tanaka T: The L- and R-type isozymes of rat pyruvate kinase are produced from a single gene by use of different promoters. *J Biol Chem* 262:14366, 1987.

27. Kozak M: Compilation and analysis of sequences upstream from the translational start site in eukaryotic mRNAs. *Nucl Acids Res* 12:857, 1984.

28. Merrick WC: Mechanism and regulation of eukaryotic protein synthesis. *Microbiol Rev* 56:291, 1992.

29. Maniatis T, Goodbourn S, Fischer JA: Regulation of inducible and tissue-specific gene expression. *Science* 236:1237, 1987.

30. Rouault T, Klausner R: Regulation of iron metabolism in eukaryotes. *Curr Top Cell Regul* 35:1–19, 1997.

31. Han J, Brown T, Beutler B: Endotoxin-responsive sequences control cachectin/tumor necrosis factor biosynthesis at the translational level. *J Exp Med* 171:465, 1990.

32. Han J, Beutler B, Huez G: Complex regulation of tumor necrosis factor mRNA turnover in lipopolysaccharide-activated macrophages. *Biochim Biophys Acta* 1090:22, 1991.

33. Beutler E, Gelbart T, Han J, Koziol JA, Beutler B: Evolution of the genome and the genetic code: Selection at the dinucleotide level by methylation and polyribonucleotide cleavage. *Proc Natl Acad Sci USA* 86:192, 1989.

34. Gridley T: Insertional versus targeted mutagenesis in mice. *New Biol* 3:1025, 1991.

35. Waldman AS: Targeted homologous recombination in mammalian cells. *Crit Rev Oncol Hematol* 12:49, 1992.

36. Weintraub HM: Antisense RNA and DNA. *Sci Am* 262:40, 1990.

37. Simons RW: Naturally occurring antisense RNA control—a brief review. *Gene* 72:35, 1988.

38. Weintraub LR, Goral A, Grasso J, et al: Pathogenesis of hepatic fibrosis in experimental iron overload. *Br J Haematol* 59:321, 1985.

39. Smith CC, Aurelian L, Reddy MP, Miller PS, Ts'o POP: Antiviral effect of an oligo(nucleoside methylphosphonate) complementary to the splice junction of herpes simplex virus type 1 immediate early pre-mRNAs 4 and 5. *Proc Natl Acad Sci USA* 83:2787, 1986.

40. McManaway ME, Neckers LM, Loke SL, et al: Tumour-specific inhibition of lymphoma growth by an antisense oligodeoxynucleotide. *Lancet* 335:808, 1990.

41. Szczylik C, Skorski T, Nicolaides NC, et al: Selective inhibition of leukemia cell proliferation by BCR-ABL antisense oligodeoxynucleotides. *Science* 253:562, 1991.

42. Cotter FE, Johnson P, Hall P, et al: Antisense oligonucleotides suppress

43. Smith MJ, Prochownik EV: Inhibition of c-jun causes reversible proliferative arrest and withdrawal from the cell cycle. *Blood* 79:2107, 1992.

44. Chen CJ, Banerjea AC, Harmison GG, Haglund K, Schubert M: Multitarget-ribozyme directed to cleave at up to nine highly conserved HIV-1 env RNA regions inhibits HIV-1 replication—potential effectiveness against most presently sequenced HIV-1 isolates. *Nucl Acids Res* 20:4581, 1992.

45. Heidenreich O, Eckstein F: Hammerhead ribozyme-mediated cleavage of the long terminal repeat RNA of human immunodeficiency virus type 1. *J Biol Chem* 267:1904, 1992.

46. Kuwabara T, Warashina M, Tanabe T, et al: Comparison of the specificities and catalytic activities of hammerhead ribozymes and DNA enzymes with respect to the cleavage of BCR-ABL chimeric L6 (b2a2) mRNA. *Nucl Acids Res* 25:3074, 1997.

47. Burt MJ, Smit DJ, Pyper WR, Powell LW, Jazwinska EC: A 4.5-megabase YAC contig and physical map over the hemochromatosis gene region. *Genomics* 33:153, 1996.

48. Schuler GD, Boguski MS, Stewart EA, et al: A gene map of the human genome. *Science* 274:540, 1996.

49. Amplification of nucleic acid sequences: The choices multiply. *J NIH Res* 3:81, 1991.

50. Innis MA, Gelfand DH, Sninsky JJ, White TJ (eds): *PCR Protocols: A Guide to Methods and Applications*. Academic Press, San Diego, 1990.

51. De Melo MB, Sales TSI, Lorand-Metze I, Costa FF: Rapid method for isolation of DNA from glass slide smears for PCR. *Acta Haematol (Basel)* 87:214, 1992.

52. DeSalle R, Gatesy J, Wheeler W, Grimaldi D: DNA sequences from a fossil termite in Oligo-Miocene amber and their phylogenetic implications. *Science* 257:1933, 1992.

53. Southern E: Gel electrophoresis of restriction fragments. *Methods Enzymol* 68:152, 1979.

54. Chang JC, Kan YW: Antenatal diagnosis of sickle cell anaemia by direct analysis of the sickle mutation. *Lancet* 2:1127, 1981.

55. Sanger F, Nicklen S, Coulson AR: DNA sequencing with chain-terminating inhibitors. *Proc Natl Acad Sci USA* 74:5463, 1977.

56. Rosenthal N: Molecular medicine. Recognizing DNA. *N Engl J Med* 333:925, 1995.

57. Winship PR: An improved method for directly sequencing PCR amplified material using dimethyl sulphoxide. *Nucl Acids Res* 17:1266, 1989.

58. Beutler E, Kuhl W, Gelbart T, Forman L: DNA sequence abnormalities of human glucose-6-phosphate dehydrogenase variants. *J Biol Chem* 266:4145, 1991.

59. Kumar R, Dunn LL: Designed diagnostic restriction fragment length polymorphisms for the detection of point mutations in ras oncogenes. *Oncogene Res* 4:235, 1989.

60. Chehab FF, Kan YW: Detection of specific DNA sequences by fluorescence amplification: A color complementation assay. *Proc Natl Acad Sci USA* 86:9178, 1989.

61. Mistry PK, Smith SJ, Ali M, et al: Genetic diagnosis of Gaucher's disease. *Lancet* 339:889, 1992.

62. Landegren U, Kaiser R, Sanders J, Hood L: A ligase-mediated gene detection technique. *Science* 241:1077, 1988.

63. Barany F: Genetic disease detection and DNA amplification using cloned thermostable ligase. *Proc Natl Acad Sci USA* 88:189, 1991.

64. Kalin I, Shephard S, Candrian U: Evaluation of the ligase chain reaction (LCR) for the detection of point mutations. *Mutat Res* 283:119, 1992.

65. Beutler E, Gelbart T, West C, et al: Mutation analysis in hereditary hemochromatosis. *Blood Cells Mol Dis* 22:187, 1996.

66. Cai SP, Zhang JZ, Huang DH, Wang ZX, Kan YW: A simple approach to prenatal diagnosis of beta-thalassemia in a geographic area where multiple mutations occur. *Blood* 71:1357, 1988.

67. Mashiyama S, Murakami Y, Yoshimoto T, Sekiya T, Hayashi K: Detection of p53 gene mutations in human brain tumors by single-strand conformation polymorphism analysis of polymerase chain reaction products. *Oncogene* 6:1313, 1991.

68. Orita M, Iwahana H, Kanazawa H, Hayashi K, Sekiya T: Detection of polymorphisms of human DNA by gel electrophoresis as single-strand conformation polymorphisms. *Proc Natl Acad Sci USA* 86:2766, 1989.

69. Myers RM, Larin Z, Maniatis T: Detection of single base substitutions

by ribonuclease cleavage at mismatches in RNA:DNA duplexes. *Science* 230:1242, 1985.

70. Abrams ES, Murdaugh SE, Lerman LS: Comprehensive detection of single base changes in human genomic DNA using denaturing gradient gel electrophoresis and a GC clamp. *Genomics* 7:463, 1990.

71. Ryan TM, Ciavatta DJ, Townes TM: Knockout-transgenic mouse model of sickle cell disease. *Science* 278:873, 1997.

72. Paszty C, Brion CM, Manci E, et al: Transgenic knockout mice with exclusively human sickle hemoglobin and sickle cell disease. *Science* 278:876, 1997.

73. Ohno S: *Evolution by Gene Duplication*. Springer Verlag, Berlin, 1970.

74. Zimran A, Sorge J, Gross E, et al: A glucocerebrosidase fusion gene in Gaucher disease. Implications for the molecular anatomy, pathogenesis and diagnosis of this disorder. *J Clin Invest* 85:219, 1990.

75. Board PG, Coggan M, Woodcock DM: The human Pi class glutathione transferase sequence at 12q13-q14 is a reverse-transcribed pseudogene. *Genomics* 14:470, 1992.

76. Youssoufian H, Kazazian HH Jr, Phillips DG, et al: Recurrent mutations in haemophilia A give evidence for CpG mutation hotspots. *Nature* 324:380, 1986.

77. Vulliamy TJ, D'Urso M, Battistuzzi G, et al: Diverse point mutations in the human glucose 6-phosphate dehydrogenase gene cause enzyme deficiency and mild or severe hemolytic anemia. *Proc Natl Acad Sci USA* 85:5171, 1988.

78. Baltimore D: Gene conversion: Some implications for immunoglobulin genes. *Cell* 24:592, 1981.

79. Hess JF, Schmid CW, Shen CK: A gradient of sequence divergence in the human adult alpha-globin duplication units. *Science* 226:67, 1984.

80. Amara SG, Jonas V, Rosenfeld MG, Ong ES, Evans RM: Alternative RNA processing in calcitonin gene expression generates mRNAs encoding different polypeptide products. *Nature* 298:240, 1982.

81. Pihlajaniemi T, Myllyla R, Seyer J, Kurkinen M, Prockop DJ: Partial characterization of a low molecular weight human collagen that undergoes alternative splicing. *Proc Natl Acad Sci USA* 84:940, 1987.

82. Ad Hoc Committee on Mutation Nomenclature: Update on nomenclature for human gene mutations. *Hum Mutat* 8:197, 1996.

83. Antonarakis SE: Recommendations for a nomenclature system for human gene mutations. Nomenclature Working Group. *Hum Mutat* 11:1, 1998.

84. Beaudet AL, Tsui LC: A suggested nomenclature for designating mutations. *Hum Mutat* 4:245, 1993.

85. Beutler E, McKusick VA, Motulsky AG, Scriver CR, Hutchinson F: Mutation nomenclature: Nicknames, systematic names, and unique identifiers. *Hum Mutat* 8:203, 1996.

86. Kaplan M, Renbaum P, Levy-Lahad E, et al: Gilbert syndrome and glucose-6-phosphate dehydrogenase deficiency: A dose-dependent genetic interaction crucial to neonatal hyperbilirubinemia. *Proc Natl Acad Sci USA* 94:12128, 1997.

87. Sampietro M, Lupica L, Perrero L, et al: The expression of uridine diphosphate glucuronosyltransferase gene is a major determinant of bilirubin level in heterozygous beta-thalassaemia and in glucose-6-phosphate dehydrogenase deficiency. *Br J Haematol* 99:437, 1997.

CYTOGENETICS AND GENE REARRANGEMENT

MICHELLE M. LE BEAU

Cytogenetic analysis provides pathologists and clinicians with a powerful tool for the diagnosis and classification of hematologic malignant diseases. The detection of an acquired, somatic mutation establishes the diagnosis of a neoplastic disorder and rules out a reactive hyperplasia or morphological changes due to toxic injury or vitamin deficiency. Specific cytogenetic abnormalities identify homogeneous subsets of various malignant diseases and enable clinicians to predict their clinical course and their likelihood of responding to particular treatments. In many cases, the prognostic information derived from cytogenetic analysis is independent of that provided by other clinical features. Patients with favorable prognostic features benefit from standard therapies with well-known spectra of toxicities, whereas those with less favorable clinical or cytogenetic characteristics may be better treated with more intensive or investigational therapies. The disappearance of a chromosomal abnormality present at diagnosis is an important indicator of complete remission following treatment, and its reappearance invariably heralds relapse of the disease. Pretreatment cytogenetic analysis can be useful in choosing among postremission therapies that differ widely in cost, acute and chronic morbidity, and effectiveness.

The malignant cells in many patients who have leukemia or lymphoma have acquired clonal chromosomal abnormalities. A number of specific cytogenetic abnormalities have been recognized that are very closely, and sometimes uniquely, associated with morphologically and clinically distinct subsets of leukemia or lymphoma.[1-4] The detection of one of these recurring abnormalities can be helpful in establishing the correct diagnosis, influencing selection of therapy, and providing prognostic information. The appearance of new abnormalities in the karyotype of a patient under observation often signals a change in the pace of the disease, usually to a more aggressive disorder. Further

detailed information regarding recurring chromosomal rearrangements is contained in reviews.[1-5]

GENETIC CONSEQUENCES OF CHROMOSOMAL REARRANGEMENTS

The genes that are located at the breakpoints of a number of the recurring chromosomal translocations have been identified (Table 10-1). Alterations in the expression of the genes or in the properties of the encoded proteins resulting from the rearrangement play an integral role in the process of malignant transformation.[5,6] The altered genes fall into several functional classes, including those that encode for tyrosine or serine protein kinases, cell surface receptors, and growth factors (see Table 10-1). However, the largest class are those that encode transcriptional regulating factors; these proteins are involved in the initiation of gene transcription, often functioning in a tissue-specific fashion to regulate growth and differentiation.

There are two general mechanisms by which chromosomal translocations result in altered gene function. The first is deregulation of gene expression. This mechanism is characteristic of the translocations in lymphoid neoplasms that involve the immunoglobulin genes in B lineage tumors and the T cell–receptor genes in T lineage tumors. These rearrangements result in inappropriate expression of an oncogene with no alteration in its protein structure. The second mechanism is the expression of a novel fusion protein, resulting from the juxtaposition of coding sequences from two genes that are normally located on different chromosomes. Such chimeric proteins are "tumor-specific" in that the fusion gene does not exist in nonmalignant cells; thus, the detection of such a fusion gene or its protein product can be important in diagnosis, or in the detection of residual disease or early relapse. Moreover, they may also be appropriate targets for tumor-specific therapies. An example is the chimeric BCR/ABL protein resulting from the t(9;22) in chronic myelogenous leukemia. All of the translocations cloned to date in the myeloid leukemias result in a fusion protein.

Chromosomal translocations result in the activation of genes in a dominant fashion. A number of human tumors are believed to result from homozygous, recessive mutations.[7] These mutations lead to the *absence* of a functional protein product, suggesting that these genes function as "suppressor" genes whose normal role is to limit cellular proliferation. The hallmark of tumor suppressor genes is the loss of genetic material in malignant cells, resulting from chromosomal loss or deletion, as well as by other genetic mechanisms.

METHODS

Cytogenetic analysis of malignant diseases is based upon the study of the tumor cells themselves. In leukemia, the specimen is usually obtained by marrow aspiration and is either processed immediately (direct preparation) or cultured for 24–72 hours. When a marrow aspirate cannot be obtained, a marrow biopsy (bone core specimen) or a blood sample, for patients who have circulating immature myeloid or lymphoid cells, can often be studied successfully. An involved lymph node or tumor mass may be sampled. The use of amethopterin to synchronize dividing cells in culture, combined with brief exposures to mitotic inhibitors such as colchicine or to DNA binding agents (ethidium bromide) are used by some laboratories to obtain elongated chromosomes that have an increased number of bands.

For specimen collection, 1 to 5 ml of marrow are aspirated aseptically into a syringe coated with preservative-free sodium heparin (preservatives in heparin can suppress cell growth) and transferred to a sterile 15-ml centrifuge tube containing 5 ml of culture medium (RPMI 1640, 100 units sodium heparin). If a marrow aspirate cannot be obtained, a bone marrow biopsy may be taken and placed into the collection tube. For blood specimens, 10 ml are drawn aseptically by

TABLE 10-1　EXAMPLES OF TRANSFORMING GENES FOUND AT TRANSLOCATION JUNCTIONS: FUNCTIONAL CLASSIFICATION

GENE	LOCATION	TRANSLOCATION	CONSEQUENCE	DISEASE
SRC Family (TYRProtein Kinases)				
ABL	9q34	t(9;22)	fusion protein	CML/ALL
Serine Protein Kinase				
BCR*	22q11	t(9;22)	fusion protein	CML/ALL
Cell Surface Receptor				
TAN1*	9q34	t(7;9)	deregulated expression	T-ALL
Growth Factor				
IL3	5q31	t(5;14)	deregulated expression	Pre B-ALL
Bcl-2 Family (Antiapoptotic) Protein				
BCL2*	18q21	t(14;18)	deregulated expression	NHL
Transcriptional Regulating Factors†				
BCL3*	19q13	t(14;19)	deregulated expression	B CLL
PBX1*	1q23	t(1;19)	fusion protein	Pre-B ALL
E2A	19p13	t(1;19)	fusion protein	Pre-B ALL
HOX11*	10q24	t(10;14)/t(7;10)	deregulated expression	T ALL
LYL1*	19p13	t(7;19)	deregulated expression	T ALL
MYC	8q24	t(8;14)	deregulated expression	B ALL
PML*	15q22	t(15;17)	fusion protein	APL
RARA	17q11.2	t(15;17)	fusion protein	APL
AML1*	21q22	t(8;21)/t(3;21)	fusion protein	AML
		t(12;21)	fusion protein	ALL
TEL*	12p12	t(12;21)	fusion protein	ALL
TAL1(SCL)*	1p32	t(1;14)	deregulated expression	T ALL
RBTN1(TTG1)*	11p15	t(11;14)	deregulated expression	T ALL
RBTN2*	11p13	t(11;14)	deregulated expression	T ALL

*Gene first identified by cloning breakpoints
†Partial list of transcription factors

venipuncture into a syringe coated with preservative-free heparin. Specimens should be maintained at room temperature and transported in culture medium. To avoid loss of cell viability, it is critical that the specimen be transported to the cytogenetics laboratory without delay. Overnight shipment of specimens frequently results in loss of cell viability, and most laboratories experience a high proportion (25–50%) of inadequate analyses using such specimens. For specimens handled optimally, 95 to 98 percent of all cases should be adequate for cytogenetic analysis. Those cases that are inadequate generally represent samples from patients with hypocellular bone marrows. Overall, approximately 75 percent of bone core biopsies will yield adequate numbers of metaphase cells for complete analysis.

To prepare metaphase cells, the sample is exposed sequentially to mitotic inhibitors to accumulate cells in mitosis, hypotonic KCl (0.075 M) to swell the cells, and fixative (absolute methanol:glacial acetic acid, 3:1). Slides are prepared by dropping the cell suspension onto precleaned glass microscope slides, and the slides are air dried. The most popular chromosomal banding techniques is trypsin-Giemsa banding. Using this technique, a consistent chromosome banding pattern is induced by exposing cells to a dilute trypsin solution (0.1–0.25 percent), followed by staining in phosphate-buffered Giemsa stain.

Cytogenetic analysis of human tumors is often technically difficult, due to the presence of multiple abnormalities and multiple cell lines, and requires highly skilled personnel. These factors have led investigators to seek alternative methods for identifying chromosomal abnormalities, such as Southern blot analysis of DNA, RT-PCR analysis of RNA from tumor cells, or FISH.[8]

The technique of FISH is based upon the same principle as Southern blot analysis, namely, the ability of single-stranded DNA to anneal to complementary DNA. In the case of FISH, the target DNA is the nuclear DNA of interphase cells, or the DNA of metaphase chromosomes that are affixed to a glass microscope slide (FISH can also be accomplished with bone marrow or blood films or with fixed and sectioned tissue). The test probe is labeled with biotin- or digoxigenin-labeled nucleotides and detected with fluorescein isothiocyanate (FITC)- or CY3-conjugated avidin or

with rhodamine-labeled antidigoxigenin antibodies. Probes that are directly labeled with fluorochrome are also available for hybridization, thereby simplifying the technique by eliminating the probe detection steps. With the development of dual- and triple-pass filters, most laboratories now have the capacity to hybridize and detect 2 to 3 probes simultaneously.

Several types of probes can be used to detect chromosomal abnormalities by FISH. Hybridization of centromere-specific probes has been used to detect monosomy, trisomy, and other aneuploidies in both leukemias and solid tumors (Plate XXIV-A). Chromosome-specific libraries, which paint the chromosomes, are particularly useful in identifying marker chromosomes (rearranged chromosomes of unidentified origin), or structural rearrangements such as translocations (Plate XXIV-B). Translocations and deletions can also be identified in interphase or metaphase cells by using genomic probes that are derived from the breakpoints of recurring translocations or within the deleted segment (Plate XXIV-C). The newest innovation in FISH technology is spectral karyotyping, or multiplex FISH.[9] Using this approach 24 differentially labeled painting probes representing each chromosome are cohybridized; Fourier spectroscopy is used to distinguish each spectrally overlapping probe and imaging software assigns a unique color to each chromosome (Plate XXIV-D). Often referred to as "color karyotyping," this method is applicable to the identification of numerical abnormalities as well as many structural abnormalities.

FISH techniques have a number of applications (Table 10-2). In some cases, FISH analysis provides more sensitivity, in that cytogenetic abnormalities have been identified by FISH in samples that appeared to be normal by morphological and conventional cytogenetic analyses. FISH is most powerful when the analysis is targeted towards those abnormalities that are known to be associated with a particular tumor or disease. An example of how FISH could be used in a clinical setting is as follows: Cytogenetic analysis could be performed at the time of diagnosis to identify the chromosomal abnormalities in an individual patient's malignant cells. Thereafter, FISH with the appropriate probes could be used to detect residual disease or early relapse and to assess the efficacy of therapeutic regimens. For example, the

TABLE 10-2 APPLICATIONS AND ADVANTAGES OF FISH

Applications

Detection of numerical and structural chromosomal abnormalities

Identification of marker chromosomes (rearranged chromosomes of uncertain origin)

Monitoring the effects of therapy and detection of minimal residual disease or early relapse

Identification of the origin of bone marrow cells following bone marrow transplantation

Identification of the lineage of neoplastic cells

Examination of the karyotypic pattern of nondividing or interphase cells

Detection of gene amplification

Advantages

Rapid technique: large numbers of cells can be analyzed in a short time.

The efficiency of hybridization and detection is high.

The sensitivity and specificity is very high.

Cytogenetic data can be obtained from nondividing or terminally differentiated cells, from tumors with a low mitotic index (e.g., CLL), or from posttreatment samples that contain too few cells for routine cytogenetic studies.

Permits the direct correlation of cytogenetic and cytologic/morphologic features, which enables pathologists to differentiate malignant from benign conditions in equivocal cases.

Automated systems for analysis of hybridized slides are available.

use of FISH to detect the t(9;22) in CML patients following transplantation or interferon therapy and for the sex chromosome composition of cells in the recipient after a sex-mismatched transplant has become frequent.

CHROMOSOME TERMINOLOGY

Chromosomal abnormalities are described according to the International System for Human Cytogenetic Nomenclature (Table 10-3).[10] To describe the chromosomal complement, the total chromosome number is listed first, followed by the sex chromosomes, then by numerical and structural abnormalities in ascending order. The observation of at least two cells with the same structural rearrangement, e.g., a translocation, deletion, inversion, or gain of the same chromosome, or of three cells showing loss of the same chromosome, is considered evidence for the presence of an abnormal clone. However, one cell with a normal karyotype is considered evidence for the presence of a normal cell line. Patients whose cells show no alteration or nonclonal (single cell) abnormalities are considered to be normal. An exception to this is a single cell characterized by a recurring structural abnormality. In such instances it is likely that this represents the karyotype of the malignant cells in that particular patient.

SPECIFIC DISORDERS

CHRONIC MYELOGENOUS LEUKEMIA

The first consistent chromosome abnormality in any malignant disease was identified in CML. The Philadelphia, or Ph chromosome, was initially thought to be a deletion of chromosome 22 but was later shown to be a translocation involving chromosomes 9 and 22 [t(9;22)(q34;q11.2)], Fig. 10-1). The t(9;22) occurs in a pluripotent stem cell that gives rise to both lymphoid and myeloid lineage cells. The standard t(9;22) is identified in about 92 percent of CML patients; another 6 percent have variant translocations that involve a third chromosome in addition to numbers 9 and 22. The genetic consequences of the t(9;22) or the complex translocations is to move a portion of the Abelson (ABL) proto-oncogene on chromosome 9 adjacent to a portion of the BCR gene on 22. Analyses of leukemia cells from rare patients with typical CML who lack the t(9;22) has revealed a rearrangement involving ABL and BCR that is detectable only at the molecular level (1–2% of cases).[12]

TABLE 10-3 GLOSSARY OF CYTOGENETIC TERMINOLOGY

Aneuploidy An abnormal chromosome number due to either gain or loss of chromosomes.

Banded chromosomes Chromosomes with alternating dark and light segments due to special stains or pretreatment of metaphase cells with enzymes before staining. Each chromosome pair has a unique pattern of bands.

Breakpoint A specific site on a chromosome containing a DNA break that is involved in a structural rearrangement such as a translocation or deletion.

Centromere The constriction along the length of the chromosome that is the site of the spindle fiber attachment. The position of the centromere determines whether chromosomes are metacentric (X-shaped, e.g., chromosomes 1–3, 6–12, X, 16, 19, 20) or acrocentric (inverted V-shaped, e.g., chromosomes 13–15, 21, 22, Y). During mitosis, the two exact copies of the DNA in each chromosome are separated by shortening of the spindle fibers attached to opposite sides of the dividing cell.

Clone In the cytogenetic sense, this is defined as two cells with the same additional or structurally rearranged chromosome or three cells with loss of the same chromosome.

Deletion A segment of a chromosome is missing as the result of two breaks and loss of the intervening piece (interstitial deletion). Molecular studies of many recurring chromosomal deletions have shown that in each case the deletions were interstitial rather than terminal (single break with loss of the terminal segment).

Diploid Having the normal chromosome number and composition of chromosomes.

Haploid Having only one-half the normal complement, i.e., 23 chromosomes in human cells.

Hyperdiploid Having additional chromosomes and therefore, in human cells, a modal number of 47 or greater.

Hypodiploid Having a loss of chromosomes and therefore, in human cells, a modal number of 45 or less.

Inversion Two breaks occurring in the same chromosome, with rotation of the intervening segment. If both the breaks were on the same side of the centromere, it is called a paracentric inversion. If they were on opposite sides, it is called a pericentric inversion.

Isochromosome A chromosome that consists of identical copies of one chromosome arm with loss of the other arm. Thus, an isochromosome for the long arm of chromosome 17 [i(17q)] contains two copies of the long arm (separated by the centromere), with loss of the short arm of the chromosome.

Karyotype Arrangement of chromosomes from a particular cell according to a well-established system such that the largest chromosomes are first and the smallest ones are last. A normal female karyotype is described as 46,XX, and a normal male karyotype is 46,XY. An *idiogram* is an idealized representation (diagram) of the chromosomes.

Ploidy The particular multiple of the haploid set of chromosomes. Diploid, triploid, tetraploid, etc. are the terms used for the respective multiple of the haploid number. In human cells, these are respectively 46, 69, 92 chromosomes, etc. *Polyploidy* indicates three or more haploid sets.

Pseudodiploid Having a diploid number of chromosomes accompanied by structural chromosomal abnormalities.

Recurring abnormality A numerical or structural abnormality noted in multiple patients who have a similar neoplasm. Such abnormalities are characteristic or diagnostic of distinct subtypes of leukemia and lymphoma that have unique morphologic and/or immunophenotypic features. Recurring abnormalities represent genetic mutations that are involved in the pathogenesis of the corresponding diseases; many recurring abnormalities have prognostic significance.

Translocation A break in at least two chromosomes with exchange of material. In a reciprocal translocation, there is no obvious loss of chromosomal material. Translocations are indicated by t; the chromosomes involved are noted in the first set of brackets and the breakpoints in the second set of brackets. The Ph translocation is t(9;22)(q34;q11.2).

Nomenclature symbols:

p Short arm

q Long arm

+ If before the chromosome, indicates a gain of a whole chromosome (e.g., +8).

− If before the chromosome, indicates a loss of a whole chromosome (e.g., −7); if after the chromosome, indicates loss of part of the chromosome (e.g., 5q−, loss of part of the long arm of chromosome 5)

? Indicates uncertainty about the identity of the chromosome or band listed just after the ?.

t translocation

del deletion

inv inversion

i isochromosome

mar marker chromosome

r ring chromosome

SOURCE: Modified from Rowley JD: Chromosome abnormalities in human cancer, in *Practice and Principles of Oncology*, 3rd ed., edited by VT De Vita, S Hellman, S Rosenberg. JP Lippincott, Philadelphia, 1991.

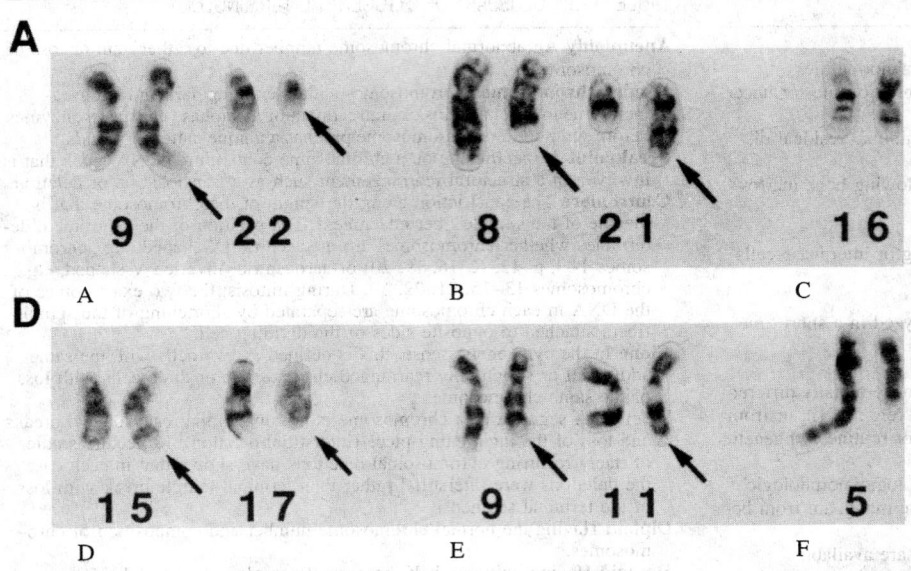

A

9   2 2   8   21   1 6

A   B   C

D

1 5   1 7   9   1 1   5

D   E   F

FIGURE 10-1   Partial karyotypes from trypsin-Giemsa-banded metaphase cells depicting recurring chromosomal rearrangements observed in myeloid leukemias. (a) t(9;22)(q34;q11), CML. (b) t(8;21)(q22;q22), AML-M2. (c) inv(16)(p13q22), AMMoL-M4Eo. (d) t(15;17)(q22;q11–12), APL. (e) t(9;11) (p22;q23), AMoL-M5. (f) del(5)(q13q33), t-AML. The rearranged chromosomes are identified with arrows.

Marrow cells from rare "CML" patients lack both a Ph chromosome and the *BCR/ABL* fusion but often have a normal karyotype or trisomy 8.[13] These patients have a substantially shorter survival than do those whose cells have the t(9;22). Most of these patients have a myelodysplastic syndrome (MDS), most commonly chronic myelomonocytic leukemia or refractory anemia with excess blasts, or the poorly understood disorder of "atypical CML." Thus, the t(9;22) and resultant *BCR/ABL* fusion is the *sine qua non* of CML.[13]

The BCR/ABL protein is located on the cytoplasmic surface of the cell membrane and acquires a novel function in transmitting growth-regulatory signals from cell surface receptors to the nucleus via the RAS signal transduction pathway.[13,14] The *BCR/ABL* fusion gene can be detected with standard Southern blot analysis of DNA or with RT-PCR analysis of mRNA for diagnosis and detection of residual disease. FISH can also be used to detect the Ph chromosome in both metaphase and interphase cells (Plate XXIV-C).

As they enter the terminal acute phase, most CML patients (80%) show karyotypic evolution, with the appearance of new chromosomal abnormalities in very distinct patterns in addition to the Ph chromosome.[11] A change in the karyotype is considered to be a grave prognostic sign.[11] With the exception of an isochromosome of the long arm of chromosome 17, i(17)(q10), which is usually associated with myeloid blast transformation, there is no association of a particular karyotype with lymphoid or myeloid blast transformation. The additional abnormalities are not correlated with the response to therapy during the acute phase.[11] The most common changes, a gain of chromosomes 8 or 19, or a second Ph (by gain of the first), or an i(17q), frequently occur in combination to produce modal chromosome numbers of 47 to 50.[11]

OTHER MYELOPROLIFERATIVE DISORDERS

POLYCYTHEMIA VERA

A cytogenetically abnormal clone is present in 14 percent of untreated polycythemia vera patients compared with 39 percent of treated pa-

tients.[2,11] When the disease transforms to acute myeloid leukemia (AML), 85 percent have an abnormal clone. The presence of a chromosome abnormality at diagnosis does not necessarily predict a short survival or the development of leukemia. A change in the karyotype may be an ominous sign. Marrow cells frequently contain additional chromosomes (+8 or +9); these abnormalities also occur together, which is otherwise rare.[11] Structural rearrangements most often involve a deletion of the long arm of chromosome 20, noted in 30 percent of patients, or a duplication of the long arm of chromosome 1, in 20 percent of patients. Loss of chromosome 7 (20 percent of patients) and del(5q) (40 percent of patients) are often observed in the leukemic phase. These changes may be related to the prior cytotoxic treatment received by these patients.

IDIOPATHIC MYELOFIBROSIS

Cytogenetic analysis of myeloid metaplasia with myelofibrosis has revealed clonal abnormalities in 35 percent of patients.[2] These abnormalities are similar to those noted in other myeloid disorders; the most common anomalies are +8, −7, del(7q), del(11q), del(13q), and del(20q).[1,2] A change in the karyotype may signal evolution to acute leukemia.

THROMBOCYTHEMIA

Fewer than 5 percent of patients with essential thrombocytosis have an abnormal clone. No consistent abnormalities have been identified.

MYELODYSPLASTIC SYNDROMES

The myelodysplastic syndromes (MDS) are a heterogeneous group of clonal hemopathies including chronic myelomonocytic leukemia (CMMoL), refractory anemia (RA), refractory anemia with ringed sideroblasts (RARS), refractory anemia with excess blasts (RAEB), and RAEB in transformation (RAEB-T). Clonal chromosome abnormalities can be detected in marrow cells of 40 to 70 percent of patients with MDS at diagnosis (RA, 30%; RARS, 27%; RAEB, 70%; RAEB-T, 70%; CMMoL, 30%).[2,15,16] The proportion varies with the risk that a subtype will transform to AML, which is highest for RAEB and RAEB-T. The common chromosome changes, +8, −5/del(5q), −7/del(7q), and del(20q), are similar to those seen in AML. The recurring abnormalities that are closely associated with the distinct morphologic subsets of AML de novo are almost never seen in MDS. With the exception of the 5q− syndrome, the chromosome changes show no close association with the specific subtypes of MDS. The 5q− syndrome occurs in a subset of older patients, frequently women, with RA, generally low blast counts, and normal or elevated platelet counts.[17] These patients have an interstitial deletion of 5q, typically as the sole abnormality. The deletions vary in size but are similar to those noted in AML. These patients can have a relatively benign course which extends over several years.[17]

Cytogenetic abnormalities in MDS are predictive of survival and progression to AML.[15,16] Patients with a "good outcome" have normal karyotypes, −Y alone, del(5q) alone, or del(20q) alone; those with an "intermediate outcome" have other abnormalities; and those with a "poor outcome" have complex karyotypes (≥3 abnormalities, typically with abnormalities of chromosome 5 and/or 7) or chromosome 7 abnormalities.[16]

ACUTE MYELOID LEUKEMIA DE NOVO

THE 8;21 TRANSLOCATION

With initial banding analyses, clonal abnormalities were detected in 50 percent of patients with AML. This percentage has increased with improved banding and culture techniques; many laboratories are currently finding that at least 80 percent of patients have an abnormal karyotype.[2,4] The most frequent abnormalities are a gain of chromosome 8 and a loss of chromosome 7, which are seen in most subtypes of AML.[2,4] Specific rearrangements are closely associated with particular subtypes of AML as defined by the FAB classification (Table 10-4).[2,4,18,19] The 8;21 translocation [t(8;21)(q22;q22)] was described in 1973 and was the first translocation identified in AML (see Fig. 10-1). The t(8;21) is common and is observed in 18 percent of all AML cases with an abnormal karyotype and in 30 percent of those patients with AML with maturation (AML-M2).[21] This translocation is the most frequent abnormality in children with AML, and occurs in 15 to 20 percent of karyotypically abnormal cases. Loss of a sex chromosome (−Y in males, −X in females) accompanies the t(8;21) in 75 percent of cases. Most cases with the t(8;21) are classified as AML with maturation, but some cases have been diagnosed as acute myelomonocytic leukemia. Although AML-M2 is heterogeneous, the presence of the t(8;21) identifies a morphologically and clinically distinct subset. AML-2 with the t(8;21) has a favorable prognosis in adults, but the outcome in children is poor.[19]

At the molecular level, the t(8;21) involves the *AML1* gene, which encodes a transcription factor that is critical in hematopoiesis.[20,21] The *AML1* gene on chromosome 21 is fused to the *ETO* gene on chromosome 8 and results in an AML1/ETO chimeric protein.[20,21] Transformation by AML1/ETO likely results from altered transcriptional regulation of normal AML1 target genes, combined with the activation of new target genes that prevent programmed cell death or cause aberrant proliferation.

THE 15;17 TRANSLOCATION

The t(15;17)(q22;q11.2–12) (see Fig. 12) is highly specific for acute promyelocytic leukemia (APL) and has not been found in any other disease. Although the t(15;17) was believed to be present in all cases of APL initially, it is now recognized that there are rare variant translocations, which occur in less than two percent of cases. These include the t(11;17)(q23;q11.2–12) and t(5;17)(q34;q11.2–12).[22] Establishing the diagnosis of APL with the typical t(15;17) is important, because this disease is sensitive to therapy with all-*trans*-retinoic acid and arsenic trioxide, whereas other cases of AML and the APL-like disorders associated with the variant translocations do not respond to retinoic acid. The t(15;17) results in a fusion retinoic-acid-receptor-alpha protein (PML/RARA), which is thought to interfere with the retinoic acid receptor pathway that regulates terminal differentiation of myeloid precursors.[22]

ABNORMALITIES OF CHROMOSOME 16

Another clinical-cytogenetic association involves acute myelomonocytic leukemia with abnormal eosinophils (AMMoL-M4Eo), including large and irregular basophilic granules and positive reactions with periodic-acid-Schiff and chloroacetate esterase. Most patients have

TABLE 10-4   RECURRING CHROMOSOME ABNORMALITIES IN MALIGNANT MYELOID DISEASES

Disease*	Chromosome Abnormality	Frequency†	Involved Genes‡	
CML	t(9;22)(q34;q11.2)	~98% (100%)§	*ABL*	*BCR*
CML Blast Phase	t(9;22) with +8, +Ph, +19, or i(17q)	~70%	*ABL*	*BCR*
AML-M2	t(8;21)(q22;q22)	18% (30%)	*ETO*	*AML1*
AML-M3, M3V	t(15;17)(q22;q11–12)	14% (98%)	*PML*	*RARA*
AMMoL-M4Eo	inv(16)(p13q22) or t(16;16)(p13;q22)	8% (~100%)	*MYH11*	*CBFB*
AMMoL-M4,	t(9;11)(p22;q23)	11% (30%) for	*AF9*	*MLL*
AMoL-M5	t(10;11)(p11–p15;q23)	all t(11q23)	*AF10*	*MLL*
	t(11;17)(q23;q25)		*MLL*	*AF17*
	t(11;19)(q23;p13.3)		*MLL*	*ENL*
	t(11;19)(q23;p13.1)		*MLL*	*ELL*
	t(6;11)(q27;q23)		*AF6*	*MLL*
	Other t(11q23)		*MLL*	
	del(11)(q23)			
AML	+8	10%		
	+11	1–2%	*MLL*	
	−7 or del(7q)	10%		
	−5 or del (5q)	10%		
	t(6;9)(p23;q34)	1%	*DEK*	*CAN*
	t(3;3)(q21;q26) or inv (3)(q21q26)	2%	*EVI1*	
	del(20q)	5%		
	t(12p) or del(12p)	2%		
Therapy-related AML	−7 or del(7q) and/or	75%		
	−5 or del(5q)			
	der(1;7)(q10;p10)	2%	*MLL*	
	t(9;11)(p22;q23)/t(11)(q23)	3%	*AML1*	
	t(21q22)	2%		
CMMoL	t(5;12)(q33;p12)	2–5%	*PDGFRB*	*TEL*

*AML-M2, acute myeloblastic leukemia with maturation; AMMoL, acute myelomonocytic leukemia; AMMoL-M4Eo, acute myelomonocytic leukemia with abnormal eosinophils; AMoL, acute monoblastic leukemia; AML, acute myeloid leukemia; APL-M3, M3V, hypergranular (M3) and microgranular (M3V) acute promyelocytic leukemia; CML, chronic myelogenous leukemia; CMMoL, chronic myelomonocytic leukemia.
†The percentage refers to the frequency within the disease overall. The numbers in the parentheses refers to the frequency within the morphological or immunological subtype of the disease (Ref. 2).
‡Genes are listed in order of citation in the karyotype, e.g., for CML, *ABL* is at 9q34 and *BCR* at 22q11.
§Some patients with CML have an insertion of *ABL* adjacent to *BCR* in a normal-appearing chromosome 22.

an inversion of chromosome 16, inv(16)(pl3q22) (see Fig. 10-1), but some have a t(16;16)(pl3;q22); these aberrations are relatively common, occurring in 25 percent of AMMoL patients.[2,4,19] They have a good response to intensive chemotherapy, with a complete remission rate of approximately 90 percent and an overall 5-year survival of 75 percent.[19] The breakpoint at 16q22 occurs within the *CBFB* gene, which encodes one subunit of the AML1/CBFB transcription factor. Thus, like the t(8;21), the inv(16) disrupts the AML1 pathway regulating hematopoiesis.[20,21]

ABNORMALITIES OF CHROMOSOME 11

Recurring translocations involving 11q23 are seen in approximately 35 percent of AML-M5 patients, and are of interest for at least three reasons.[2,23] First, there are over 30 different recurring rearrangements that involve 11q23, and thus, along with 14q32, 11q23 is one of the bands most frequently involved in rearrangements in human tumor cells.[2,3,23] The breakpoints in the translocation partners include 1p32, 4q21, and 19p13.3 in acute lymphoblastic leukemia (ALL), and 1q21, 2q21, 6q27, 9p22, 10p11, 17q25, 19p13.3, and 19p13.1 in AML. Second, these translocations occur in both lymphoid and myeloid leukemias. One common translocation in infants, t(4;11)(q21;q23), has a lymphoblastic phenotype, whereas other translocations, such as the t(9;11) (q22;q23) (see Fig. 12) and t(11;19)(q23;p13.1), are common in monoblastic leukemias. Translocations involving 11q23 have a very unusual age distribution; they comprise about three-quarters of the chromosome abnormalities in leukemia cells of children under one year of age.[23] With the exception of the t(9;11) which may have an intermediate outcome, translocations of 11q23 are associated with a poor outcome.[19] Translocations of 11q23 involve *MLL*, a very large gene (>100 Kb) with multiple transcripts of 12 to 15 Kb.[20] All breakpoints fall within an 8.3-Kb breakpoint cluster region encompassing exons 5–11; thus, *MLL* translocations can be detected by Southern blot analysis of DNA using a small cDNA probe containing these exons.[23] The MLL protein is likely to be a transcription factor but may also function in chromatin remodeling; the translocations result in fusion proteins.

Trisomy 11 is a rare abnormality, noted as a sole aberration in one to two percent of all AML or MDS cases,[2,20] and has an unfavorable outcome. Trisomy 11 is notable in that duplications of the *MLL* gene are detected in 90 percent of AMLs with +11 as the sole abnormality, and in 10 percent of AML cases with an apparently normal karyotype.[20] The rearrangement is the result of a partial tandem duplication of *MLL* exons 2–6 or 2–8, mediated by recombination between *Alu* repetitive elements, and may produce a partially duplicated protein.

OTHER CHROMOSOME ABNORMALITIES

Each of the other recurring rearrangements in AML occurs in less than three percent of patients.[3] A unique feature of abnormalities involving the long arm of chromosome 3, inv(3)(q2l;q26) or t(3;3) (q2l;q26) is the presence of platelet counts above 100,000/μl, sometimes over $10^6/\mu$l, and an increase in bone marrow megakaryocytes, especially micromegakaryocytes.[4] It is noteworthy that most of the structural rearrangements described above occur in younger patients with a median age in the thirties, whereas some of the other abnormalities, such as −5/del(5q) or −7/del(7q) occur in patients with a median age over 50. Moreover, many of the latter patients have occupational exposure to mutagenic agents such as chemicals, including solvents, petroleum, and pesticides.[18]

ACUTE MYELOID LEUKEMIA AND MYELODYSPLASTIC SYNDROMES ASSOCIATED WITH PRIOR CYTOTOXIC TREATMENT (T-MDS AND T-AML)

Therapy-related MDS and AML (t-MDS/t-AML) has been recognized as a late complication of cytotoxic therapy used in the treatment of

both malignant and nonmalignant diseases.[24] In patients who received alkylating agents the characteristic recurring chromosome abnormalities observed are loss of part or all of chromosomes 5 and/or 7 (−5/del[5q] or −7/del[7q]) (see Fig. 12). In our experience, 93 percent of t-MDS/t-AML patients had an abnormal karyotype and 75 percent had an abnormality of chromosome 5, chromosome 7, or both (Refs. 4 and 24 and unpublished data); this has been confirmed in other series. In contrast, only about 16 percent of patients with AML de novo have a similar abnormality of chromosomes 5 or 7 or both.[2,18]

By cytogenetic analysis of 177 patients with malignant myeloid diseases and a del(5q) we identified a small segment of 5q, consisting of band 5q31, that was deleted in each patient.[25] This segment has been termed the *commonly deleted segment*. By molecular analyses we have narrowed the commonly deleted segment to a region of approximately 1 Mb containing the *EGR1* tumor suppressor gene and the *CDC25C* G2 checkpoint gene.[25] Five hematopoietic growth factor genes mapped to 5q31 (GM-CSF, IL3, IL4, IL5, and IL9) are excluded from this region. We have detected no mutations of the remaining *EGR1* or *CDC25C* alleles, suggesting that a novel tumor suppressor gene in 5q31 is involved in the pathogenesis of t-AML.[25]

A second subtype of t-AML has been identified that is distinctly different from the more common leukemia that follows alkylating agents or irradiation. This type of t-AML is seen in patients receiving drugs known to inhibit topoisomerase II, e.g., etoposide, teniposide, and doxorubicin.[24,26] Clinically, these patients have a shorter latency period (1–2 years); present with overt leukemia, usually with monocytic features rarely present with MDS; and have a more favorable response to intensive remission induction therapy. Balanced translocations involving the *MLL* gene at 11q23 or the *AML1* gene at 21q22 are common in this subgroup.[26]

MALIGNANT LYMPHOPROLIFERATIVE DISORDERS

ACUTE LYMPHOBLASTIC LEUKEMIA

The most useful prognostic indicators in acute lymphoblastic leukemia (ALL)—the most frequent leukemia in children—are age, white cell count, immunophenotype, karyotype (including ploidy), and CNS status.[2,27,28] Children who are between 2 and 10 years old, with a white cell count of less than 10,000/μl, and whose leukemia cells express the common ALL antigen (CALLA, CD10) have the best prognosis. A number of recurring cytogenetic abnormalities are associated with distinct immunologic phenotypes of ALL (Table 10-5) with distinct outcomes.[2-4]

The 9;22 Translocation   The incidence of the t(9;22) in ALL is 30 percent in adults and 5 percent in children. Thus, the Ph chromosome is the most frequent rearrangement in adult ALL. About one-half of the patients show additional abnormalities, a frequency that is substantially higher than that observed in CML. Monosomy 7 is a common secondary abnormality in Ph+ ALL and is associated with a poorer outcome.[27] A chromosomally normal cell line is frequently noted in the bone marrow of Ph+ ALL patients (70 percent), but is rare in untreated CML. Most cases have a precursor B phenotype; however, some cases have had both B cell and myeloid markers.[29] The disease in both adults and children is characterized by high WBC counts, a high percentage of circulating blasts, and a poor prognosis. As in CML, the t(9;22) in ALL results in a *BCR/ABL* fusion gene; however, in over half of the patients the break in *BCR* is more proximal, resulting in a smaller fusion protein.[29]

Abnormalities of Chromosome 11   Translocations involving the *MLL* gene at 11q23 are observed in 5 to 7 percent of ALL patients.[2,4,23] Of these, the most common is the t(4;11)(q21;q23) (see Fig. 10-2). The t(11;19)(q23;p13.3) is second in frequency; however, this rearrangement is not limited to ALL, in that approximately 50 percent of these cases have AML, usually AML-M5. Of note is the high

TABLE 10-5   CYTOGENETIC-IMMUNOPHENOTYPIC CORRELATIONS IN MALIGNANT LYMPHOID DISEASES

PHENOTYPE	CHROMOSOME ABNORMALITY	FREQUENCY*	INVOLVED GENES†	
Acute lymphoblastic leukemia				
Precursor B	t(12;21)(p12;q22)	25%	TEL	AML1
	t(9;22)(q34;q11)	10%‡	ABL	BCR
	t(4;11)(q21;q23)	5%	AF4	MLL
	t(17;19)(q21-22;p13)	1%	HLF	E2A
	t(11;19)(q23;p13.3)	1%	MLL	ENL
Pre-B	t(1;19)(q23;p13)	6% (30%)	PBX1	TCF3 (E2A)
B(SIg+)	t(8;14)(q24;q32)	5% (95%)	MYC	IGH
	t(2;8)(p12;q24)	<1% (1%)	IGK	MYC
	t(8;22)(q24;q11)	<1% (4%)	MYC	IGL
Other	Hyperdiploidy (50–60)	10%		
	del(12p),t(12p)	10%		
T	t(11;14)(p15;q11)	1%	RBTN1	TCRA
	t(11;14)(p13;q11)	3%	RBTN2	TCRA
	t(8;14)(q24;q11)	<1%	MYC	TCRA
	inv(14)(q11q32)	<1%	TCRA	TCL1
	t(10;14)(q24;q11)	3%	HOX11	TCRA
	t(1;14)(p32;q11)	1%	TAL1	TCRD
	t(7;9)(q34–35;q32)		TCRB	TAL2
	t(7;9)(q34–35;q34)	2%	TCRB	
	t(7;19)(q34–35;p13)	<1%		
	del(9p),t(9p)	<1% (10%)	CDKN2A	
Lymphoma				
B cell lymphoma				
Burkitt	t(8;14)(q24;q32)	95%	MYC	IGH
	t(2;8)(p12;q24)	1%	IGK	MYC
	t(8;22)(q24;q11)	4%	MYC	IGL
Follicular	t(14;18)(q32;q21)	80%	IGH	BCL2
DLCL	t(14;18)(q32;q21)	20%		
DLCL	t(3;22)(q27;q11)	45% for all	BCL6	IGL
	t(3;14)(q27;q32)	t(3q27)	BCL6	IGH
MCL	t(11;14)(q13;q32)		CCND1	IGH
LPL	t(9;14)(p13;q32)		PAX5	IGH
SLL	t(14;19)(q32;q13.3)		IGH	BCL3
MALT	t(11;18)(q21;q21)			
T cell lymphoma				
(Ki-1+) lymphoma ALCL	t(2;5)(p23;q35)	75%	ALK	NPM
Chronic lymphocytic leukemia				
B	t(11;14)(q13;q32)	10%	CCND1	IGH
	t(14;19)(q32;q13)	10%	IGH	BCL3
	t(2;14)(p13;q32)	5%		IGH
	t(14q32)	20%		
	del(13q)	30%		
	+12	30%		
T	t(8;14)(q24;q11)	5%	MYC	TCRA
	inv(14)(q11q32)	5%	TCRA/D	IGH
	inv(14)(q11q32)	5%	TCRA/D	TCL1
Multiple myeloma				
B	t(11;14)(q13;q32)	10%	CCND1	IGH
	t(14q32)			
Adult T cell	t(14;14)(q11;q32)		TCRA	IGH
leukemia/lymphoma	inv(14)(q11q32)		TCRA/D	IGH
	+3			

*The percentage refers to the frequency within the disease overall. The number in the parentheses refers to the frequency within the morphological or immunological subtype of the disease.
†Genes are listed in order of citation in karyotype; e.g. for precursor B ALL, TEL is at 12p12 and AML1 at 21q22.
‡By cytogenetic analysis, the frequency in children is about 5% and in adults about 25%; using molecular probes this frequency is 30% in adults.

frequency of translocations involving 11q23 in infant ALL (60–80%). A recent study using RT-PCR detected the t(4;11) in 80 percent of infant ALL cases.[27,29] Patients with the t(4;11) have high leukocyte counts (median WBC 183,000/μl), L1 or L2 morphology, an immature precursor B phenotype (CD10−, CD19+), with coexpression of monocytic or, less commonly, T cell markers.[27,28] Clinically, they have aggressive features with hyperleukocytosis, extramedullary disease, and a poor response to conventional chemotherapy. Adults with the t(4;11) have a CR rate of 75 percent, but a median event-free survival (EFS) of only 7 months.[28] Children with the t(4;11) have a similar poor outcome.[27] Rearrangements affecting MLL represent a major

class of mutations in acute leukemia and identify patients with a poor outcome.

The 12;21 Translocation   A translocation, t(12;21)(p12;q22), has been identified in a high proportion (~25 percent) of childhood precursor B leukemia.[27,30] The translocation is not easily detected by cytogenetic analysis due to the similarity in size and banding pattern of 12p and 21q. However, the rearrangement can be detected reliably using RT-PCR or FISH analysis. The t(12;21) defines a distinct subgroup of patients characterized by an age between 1 and 10 years, B lineage immunophenotype (CD10+, CD19+), and a favorable outcome.[27,30] It is not seen in T cell ALL and is uncommon in adults

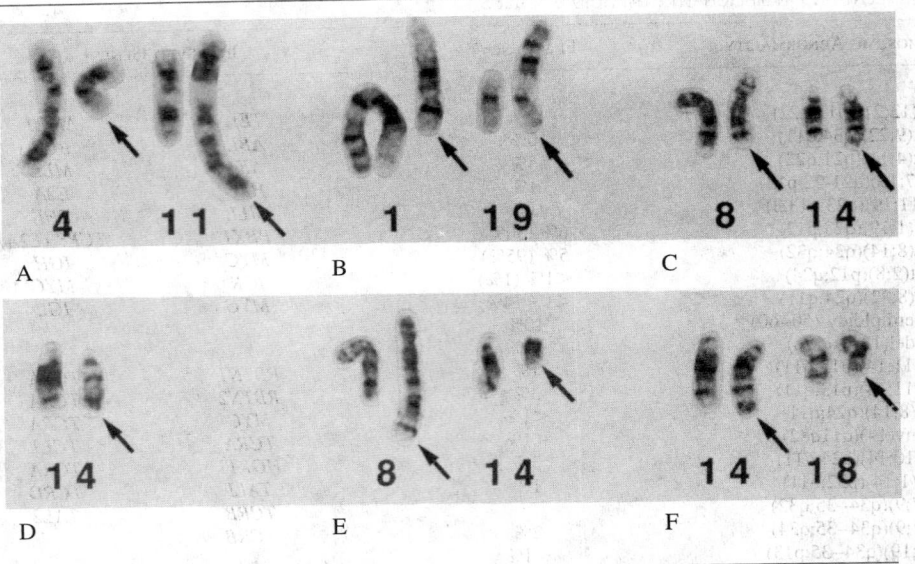

FIGURE 10-2 (A–D) Photomicrographs of metaphase and interphase cells following FISH. In panels A–C, the cells are counterstained with 4,6-diamidino-2-phenylindole-dihydrochloride (DAPI). (A) Hybridization of a directly labeled centromere-specific probe for chromosome 8 (CEP8™ Spectrum Green, Vysis Inc.) to metaphase and interphase cells from an AML with trisomy 8. Centromere-specific probes hybridize to the repetitive DNA sequences that are present at the centromeres of human chromosomes. The chromosome 8 homologs are identified with arrows. (B) Hybridization of a directly labeled chromosome 8-specific painting probe (WCP8™ Spectrum Green, Vysis Inc.) to a metaphase cell with trisomy 8 from an AML. (C) Hybridization of a locus-specific probe for the detection of a recurring translocation, the t(9;22)(q34;q11.2) in CML. The probe is a mixture of digoxigenin-labeled DNA probes (detected with rhodamine-labeled antibodies) for the major breakpoint cluster region of the *BCR* gene at 22q11.2, and biotin-labeled probes (detected with FITC-avidin) for the *ABL* gene at 9q34 (M-bcr/abl probe, Oncor). In cells with the t(9;22), only one green signal (arrowhead) and one red signal (short arrow) is observed on the normal 9 and 22 homologs, and a yellow fusion signal (long arrow) is observed on the Ph chromosome as a result of the juxtaposition of the *ABL* and *BCR* sequences. (D) Spectral karyotyping analysis of a metaphase cell from an AML-M7. Twenty-four differentially labeled probes, each representing one human chromosome, are cohybridized, and imaging analysis software assigns a unique color to each. A complex karyotype was identified by conventional cytogenetic analysis, including a derivative chromosome 1 with additional material of unknown origin on 1p, a deletion of 8p, a derivative chromosome 11 resulting from an unbalanced translocation involving 1 and 11, and a derivative chromosome 12, consisting of 11q and 12q. The results of spectral karyotyping confirmed the identity of the rearranged chromosome 12 (arrowhead) and clarified the other abnormalities. The additional material on 1p was derived from chromosome 8 (long arrow, blue signal), and the der(11) actually consisted of material from chromosomes 1, 11, and 12 (short arrow, 11p white signal; chromosome 12 brown signal; 1p blue-pink signal).

(approximately four percent of ALL cases). In a recent series, patients with the t(12;21) had a 5-year EFS of 91 percent, as compared with 65 percent for patients without this rearrangement. One-half of these patients would have fallen into a high-risk group using standard risk factors; thus, the t(12;21) may identify a subset of patients within the high-risk group who would benefit from well-tolerated, less toxic antimetabolite therapy.

Hyperdiploidy The leukemia cells of some patients with ALL are characterized by a gain of many chromosomes. Two distinct subgroups are recognized: a group with one to four extra chromosomes (47–50), and the more common group with >50 chromosomes. Chromosome numbers usually range from 51 to 60, and a few patients may have up to 65 chromosomes. Hyperdiploidy (>50 chromosomes) is common in children (~30%) but is rarely observed in adults (<5%). Certain additional chromosomes are common (X chromosome and chromosomes 4, 6, 10, 14, 17, 18, and 21). Chromosome 21 is gained most frequently (100 percent of cases).[2,4] Patients who have hyperdiploidy with >50 chromosomes have all of the previously recognized clinical factors that indicate a good prognosis, including age between

one and nine years, low WBC count (median 6,700/μl), and favorable immunophenotype (early pre-B or pre-B).[27,28] In a recent analysis of 186 children with hyperdiploidy ALL, it was observed that ALL defined by 51 to 55 chromosomes and ALL defined by 56 to 65 chromosomes may be distinct clinical entities.[31] The 105 patients in the first group (51 to 55 chromosomes) had an EFS at 5 years of 72 percent, compared with 86 percent ($P = 0.04$) for those patients with >56 chromosomes (63 patients).

The 1;19 and 8;14 Translocations The t(1;19)(q23;p3) has been identified in about 25 percent of patients with a pre-B phenotype; that is, the leukemia cells have cytoplasmic immunoglobulin and are CD10+ (Fig. 10-2).[27,30] A reciprocal translocation involving the long arms of chromosomes 8 and 14 [t(8;14)(q24;q32)] is observed in B cell ALL (L3) (see Fig. 10-2).[2] These patients have a high incidence of CNS involvement and/or abdominal nodal involvement at diagnosis. Although the outcome for both children and adults with a t(8;14) has been poor, the use of high intensity chemotherapy has markedly improved the outcome (EFS of 80 percent in children).[27]

T CELL ACUTE LYMPHOBLASTIC LEUKEMIA

A distinct pattern of recurring karyotypic abnormalities in T cell neoplasms has emerged.[2,29] Rearrangements involving 14q11 (see Fig. 10-2) and two regions of chromosome 7 (7q34–35 and 7p15) are particularly frequent in T cell malignancies (see Table 10-5). The most common are the t(11;14) (p13;q11) (~3%), t(10;11)(q24;q11) (~3%), and t(7;9)(q34–35;q34) (~2%).[1,3,29] In addition to their occurrence in T cell leukemia, these abnormalities have also been observed in lymphomas of T cell origin. The genes that are located at the breakpoints of a number of these abnormalities have been identified (see also Table 10-5). Patients with T cell ALL are most often young males and often have a mediastinal tumor mass, high WBC count, and leukemia cells in the cerebrospinal fluid. These same clinical characteristics are associated with lymphoblastic lymphoma, another T cell malignancy.

CHRONIC LYMPHOCYTIC LEUKEMIA

Unfortunately, only half of CLL patients have an adequate number of metaphase cells in unstimulated cultures for thorough evaluation. Trisomy 12 is the most common cytogenetic abnormality reported in patients with B cell CLL; it is found in 20 to 60 percent of those with a cytogenetic abnormality.[32] Abnormalities involving band 14q32 are also common, e.g., t(14;19)(q32;q13) (see Table 10-5). FISH is a sensitive alternative method for detecting abnormalities in interphase CLL cells. Using FISH, 30 percent of patients are found to have trisomy 12, and this abnormality is associated with a poorer survival.[32] Similarly, a del(13q) can be detected in 30 percent of CLL cases using FISH. T cell CLL and large granular lymphocytic leukemia are uncommon disorders in which the malignant mature lymphocytes have a T cell immunophenotype. Rearrangements involving band 14q11, with or without an accompanying break in 14q32, have been reported in T-CLL as well as in T cell lymphomas (Table 10-5).[1-3] The most common of these rearrangements is an inv(14)(q11q32) (see Fig. 10-2).

LYMPHOMA

Cytogenetic analyses of lymphoma have been reported in a number of large series.[2,4,33-35] These investigations have demonstrated that over 90 percent of cases are characterized by clonal chromosomal abnormalities and, more importantly, many of the recurring abnormalities correlate with histology and immunophenotype (see Table 10-5). For example, the t(14;18) is observed in a high proportion of follicular small cleaved cell lymphomas (70–90%), most patients with a t(3;22)(q27;q11) or t(3;14)(q27;q32) have diffuse large cell lymphomas (B cell), and patients with a t(8;14)(q24;q32) have either small noncleaved cell or diffuse large cell lymphomas (DLCL). Band 14q32, the location of the Ig heavy chain gene (IGH) is frequently involved in translocations in B cell neoplasms (~70%). In contrast, a large proportion of T cell neoplasms are characterized by rearrangements that involve 14q11, 7q34–35, or 7p15, the locations of the T cell receptor genes.

In 1972 a consistent abnormality (14q+) was identified in the cells of fresh Burkitt lymphomas (BL) and in cultured cell lines. Several years later the rearrangement was shown to be a reciprocal translocation involving chromosomes 8 and 14, t(8;14)(q24;q32) (see Fig. 10-2). The t(8;14) is characteristic of both endemic and nonendemic Burkitt tumors, as well as Epstein-Barr virus (EBV) negative and EBV-positive tumors. The t(8;14) has also been observed in other lymphomas, particularly small noncleaved cell (non-Burkitt) and large-cell immunoblastic lymphomas, AIDS-associated BL (100%), and AIDS-related DLCL (30%).[33-35] As additional Burkitt tumors were examined, it became apparent that at least two other related translocations occur, t(2;8)(p12;q24) and t(8;22)(q24;q11). All three translocations involve chromosome band 8q24. As discussed earlier, these same translocations have been seen in some patients with B cell ALL. The t(8;14) involves a break within the IGH locus on chromosome 14 and a break either 5' or within MYC on chromosome 8, and it relocates the MYC coding exons to chromosome 14.[5,33] MYC is a transcription factor that plays a role in a number of cellular processes including proliferation and apoptosis, and its oncogenic properties are due to its constitutive expression.

Between 70 and 90 percent of follicular lymphomas and 20 percent of diffuse B cell lymphomas have the t(14;18) (see Fig. 10-2), in which the BCL2 gene at 18q21 is juxtaposed to the IGH J segment, leading to the deregulated expression of BCL2.[33,34] Other malignancies which overexpress BCL2 but do not harbor the t(14;18) include hairy cell leukemia and CLL. The BCL2 gene encodes a 26 kDa membrane protein that functions to increase cell survival (antiapoptosis). Thus, this class of oncogene contributes to the development of a neoplastic state by preventing programmed cell death, rather than by promoting proliferation.

The t(11;14) (q13;q32) is observed in a relatively new pathologic entity known as mantle cell lymphoma.[36] In most series, the percentages of cases having the t(11;14) by molecular analysis have varied between 30 and 55 percent of cases, but these may be underestimates, as only the major breakpoint cluster regions have been looked for. Besides mantle cell lymphomas, the t(11;14) has also been reported in 3 percent of multiple myeloma and up to 20 percent of prolymphocytic leukemias.[36] Mantle cell lymphomas are currently regarded as a poor prognostic group, with a median survival from diagnosis of three years. This translocation results in the activation of the cyclin D1 (CCND1)

gene by the IGH gene.[33] Interestingly, the CCND1 gene is located 100 to 130 Kb away from the breakpoint on 11q13. The D-type cyclins act as growth factor sensors, causing cells to go through the restriction start point of the cell cycle at G_1 and committing them to divide.

The BCL6 gene was cloned from the recurring breakpoint at 3q27 in cells characterized by a t(3;22)(q27;q11), t(3;14)(q27;q32), or rarely t(2;3)(p12;q27).[33] BCL6 rearrangements occur in 40 percent of DLCL and, in some series, up to 10 percent of follicular lymphomas. The translocations lead to the truncation of the BCL6 gene within the first exon or the first intron, substitution of its promoter sequences with an IG promoter, and deregulated expression. The BCL6 gene product is a 96 kDa nuclear protein that acts as a potent transcriptional repressor. It is predominantly expressed in the B cell lineage, particularly in mature B cells, but not in immature bone marrow precursors or the more mature plasma cell.

A number of recurring chromosomal abnormalities have been recognized in T cell leukemias and lymphomas (see Table 10-5). Similar to B cell neoplasms, in which rearrangements frequently involve the chromosomal bands containing the immunoglobulin gene loci, T cell neoplasms often have rearrangements involving band q11 of chromosome 14, the site of the T cell receptor α-chain and δ-chain genes (TCRA, TCRD) or, less often, one of two regions of chromosome 7 (7q34–35 or 7p15) to which the T cell receptor β-chain (TCRB) and γ-chain (TCRG) genes have been localized respectively.[1,3] These translocations result from aberrant recombination events during V-D-J recombination. With few exceptions, the involved gene on the partner chromosome encodes a transcription factor, whose expression is deregulated or activated as a result of the rearrangement (see Table 10-5).[3,4] A chromosomal rearrangement which brings an oncogene under the controlling influence of promoters or enhancers active for immunoglobulin synthesis in B cells or T cell–receptor synthesis in T cells may, as a consequence, impart a proliferative advantage to the affected cell and result in malignant clonal expansion.

A distinctive subtype of lymphoma, namely, Ki-1(CD30)-positive anaplastic large cell lymphoma (Ki-1+ ALCL) has been characterized during the past few years. Patients with Ki-1+ ALCL tend to be young, and they present with skin and/or lymph node infiltration by large, often bizarre lymphoma cells, which preferentially involve the paracortical areas and lymph node sinuses. The majority of such tumors express one or more T cell antigens, a minority express B cell antigens, and some express both T and B cell antigens (the null phenotype). A reciprocal translocation, t(2;5)(p23;q35), appears to be restricted to ALCL of either T cell or null phenotype and is present in a high percentage of these cases.[33] This translocation has also been found in CD30+ primary cutaneous lymphomas.

REFERENCES

1. Mitelman F: *Catalog of Chromosome Aberrations in Cancer*, 5th ed. Wiley-Liss, New York, 1994.
2. Heim S, Mitelman F: *Cancer Cytogenetics*, 2d ed. New York, Wiley-Liss, 1995.
3. Mitelman F, Mertens F, Johansson B: A breakpoint map of recurrent chromosomal rearrangements in human neoplasia. *Nat Genet* 15: 417, 1997.
4. Le Beau MM, Larson RA: Cytogenetics and neoplasia, in *Hematology: Basic Principles and Practices*, 3d ed, edited by R Hoffman, EJ Benz, SJ Shattil, B Furie, HJ Cohen, LE Silbersein, P McGlave. Churchill Livingstone, New York, 1998.
5. Rabbitts T: Chromosomal translocations in human cancer. *Nature* 372:143, 1994.
6. Look AT: Oncogenic transcription factors in the human acute leukemias. *Science* 278:1059, 1997.
7. Brown MA: Tumor suppressor genes and human cancer. *Adv Hum Genet* 36:45, 1997.

8. Le Beau MM: Fluorescence *in situ* hybridization in cancer diagnosis, in *Important Advances in Oncology*, edited by VT De Vita, S Hellman, SA Rosenberg. Lippincott, Philadelphia, 1993:29.

9. Le Beau MM: One FISH, two FISH, red FISH, blue FISH. *Nat Genet* 12:341, 1996.

10. ISCN: *An International System for Human Cytogenetic Nomenclature*, edited by F Mitelman. Karger, Basel, 1995.

11. Rowley JD, Testa JR: Chromosome abnormalities in malignant hematologic diseases. *Adv Cancer Res* 36:103, 1982.

12. Ganesan TS, Rassool F, Guo A-P, et al: Rearrangement of the *bcr* gene in Philadelphia chromosome-negative chronic myeloid leukemia. *Blood* 68:957, 1986.

13. Gordon MY, Goldman JM: Cellular and molecular mechanisms in chronic myeloid leukemia. *Br J Haematol* 95:10, 1996.

14. Witte ON: Role of the BCR/ABL oncogene in human leukemia. *Cancer Res* 53:485, 1993.

15. Morel P, Hebbar M, Lai JL, et al: Cytogenetic analysis has strong prognostic value in de novo myelodysplastic syndromes and can be incorporated in a new scoring system: a report on 408 cases. *Leukemia* 7:1315, 1993.

16. Greenberg P, Cox C, Le Beau MM, et al: International scoring system for evaluating prognosis in myelodysplastic syndromes. *Blood* 89:2079, 1997.

17. Boultwood J, Lewis S, Wainscoat JS: The 5q− syndrome. *Blood* 84:3253, 1994.

18. Fourth International Workshop on Chromosomes in Leukemia. *Cancer Genet Cytogenet* 71:249, 1984.

19. Mrozek K, Heinonen K, de la Chapelle A, et al: Clinical significance of cytogenetics in acute myeloid leukemia. *Sem Oncol* 24:17, 1997.

20. Caligiuri MA, Strout MP, Gilliland DG: Molecular biology of acute myeloid leukemia. *Semin Oncol* 24:32, 1997.

21. Nucifora G, Rowley JD: *AML1* and the 8;21 and 3;21 translocations in acute and chronic myeloid leukemia. *Blood* 86:1, 1995.

22. Pandolfi PP: *PML, PLZF*, and *NPM* genes in the molecular pathogenesis of acute promyelocytic leukemia. *Haematologica* 81:472, 1996.

23. Rowley JD: Rearrangements involving chromosome band 11q23 in acute leukemia. *Semin Cancer Biol* 4:377, 1993.

24. Thirman M, Larson RA: Therapy-related myeloid leukemia. *Hematol Oncol Clin North Am* 10:293, 1996.

25. Zhao N, Stoffel A, Wang PW, et al: Molecular delineation of the smallest commonly deleted region of chromosome 5 in malignant myeloid diseases to 1–1.5 Mb and preparation of a PAC-based physical map. *Proc Natl Acad Sci USA* 94:6948, 1997.

26. Pedersen-Bjergaard, Rowley JD: The balanced and the unbalanced chromosome aberrations of acute myeloid leukemia may develop in different ways and may contribute differently to malignant transformation. *Blood* 83:2780, 1994.

27. Camitta BM, Pullen J, Murphy S: Biology and treatment of acute lymphoblastic leukemia in children. *Semin Oncol* 24:83, 1997.

28. Bloomfield CD, Goldman AI, Alimena G, et al: Chromosomal abnormalities identify high-risk and low-risk patients with acute lymphoblastic leukemia. *Blood* 67:415, 1986.

29. Thandla S, Aplan PD: Molecular biology of acute lymphocytic leukemia. *Sem Oncol* 24:45, 1997.

30. Rubnitz JE, Downing JR, Pui C-H, et al: *TEL* gene rearrangement in acute lymphoblastic leukemia: a new genetic marker with prognostic significance. *J Clin Oncol* 15:1150, 1997.

31. Raimondi SC, Pui C-H, Hancock ML, et al: Heterogeneity of hyperdiploid (51–67) childhood acute lymphoblastic leukemia. *Leukemia* 10:213, 1996.

32. Döhner H, Stilgenbauer S, Fischer K, et al: Cytogenetic and molecular cytogenetic analysis of B cell chronic lymphocytic leukemia: specific chromosome aberrations identify prognostic subgroups of patients and point to loci of candidate genes. *Leukemia* 11:S19, 1997.

33. Ong ST, Le Beau MM: Chromosomal abnormalities and molecular genetics of non-Hodgkin's lymphoma. *Sem Oncol* 25:447, 1998.

34. Fifth International Workshop on Chromosomes in Leukemia-Lymphoma: Correlation of chromosome abnormalities in non-Hodgkin's lymphoma and adult T-cell leukemia lymphoma. *Blood* 70:1554, 1987.

35. Offit K, Wong G, Filippa DA, et al: Cytogenetic analysis of 434 consecutively ascertained specimens of non-Hodgkin's lymphoma: Clinical correlations. *Blood* 77:1508, 1991.

36. Raffeld M, Jaffe ES: *bcl-1*, t(11;14), and mantle cell-derived lymphomas. *Blood* 78:259, 1991.

APOPTOSIS

ROBERTA A. GOTTLIEB

Apoptosis is a physiologic form of cell death that has evolved in multicellular organisms as a mechanism of eliminating unwanted cells. Apoptosis is a cell-autonomous process that may be triggered through a receptor or through the detection of cellular damage. It involves a coordinated series of enzymatic steps orchestrated by activation of a special class of proteases (caspases) and is controlled by inhibitors at each step, conferring tight control over this lethal process. The cell destruction process is accompanied by alterations in most organelles—particularly mitochondria—as well as changes to the cytoskeleton, plasma membrane, and ion transport systems, and culminates in the degradation of nuclear DNA through the action of endonucleases.

Apoptosis is a term originally coined by Kerr, Wyllie, and Currie[1] to describe a form of cell death characterized by cell shrinkage and nuclear condensation, and is derived from the Greek term for the shedding of leaves or petals. This physiologic, tightly regulated process is initiated by eukaryotic cells in response to internal or external cues. Apoptosis occurs in all multicellular organisms as the means to balance cell proliferation in continuously renewing tissues in order to maintain a constant organ size.

In the hematopoietic system, cell production is delicately balanced against cell death and removal through the monocyte-macrophage system.

A panoply of cytokines and growth factors regulate cell survival, proliferation, and apoptosis.[2] Stem cell factor, Flt ligand, thrombopoietin, and IL-3 suppress apoptosis, while IL-6 and IL-11 stimulate proliferation of early progenitors. Granulocyte-macrophage colony-stimulating factor (GM-CSF) can both suppress apoptosis and trigger proliferation. Tumor necrosis factor α (TNF-α), Fas ligand, TNF-related apoptosis-inducing ligand (TRAIL), and interferon-gamma promote apoptosis of cells expressing the appropriate receptors.

Apoptosis occurs at defined times and locations during development, thus earning it the name *programmed cell death*. It is a critical process during embryogenesis, where remodeling requires highly regulated cell death. Programmed cell death is the process by which tadpoles lose their tails, and its occurrence has been studied in detail in the nematode *Caenorhabditis elegans*. Three of the most important genes that control apoptosis have been identified through studies of development in *C. elegans*. Two of them—designated *ced-3* and *ced-4* (*C. elegans* death gene)—were shown to be essential for programmed cell death to occur, and one gene, *ced-9*, was shown to be essential for opposing cell death.[3,4] These genes are conserved throughout evolution and are represented by large families of mammalian homologs. Ced-3 is a cysteine protease with the unusual characteristic of cleaving

peptides after aspartic acid residues. The first mammalian homolog of Ced-3 to be identified was interleukin-1β–converting enzyme (ICE). Subsequently, a family of more than 10 related cysteine proteases (''death proteases'') has been identified; they have been designated caspases, for cysteine aspartases.[5,6] The nematode death gene, *ced-4*, encodes a protein that controls the activation of the caspase, Ced-3. Ced-4 is in turn regulated through interaction with Ced-9. Apaf-1 has been shown to be the mammalian homolog of Ced-4. Bcl-2 is the mammalian homolog of the anti-apoptosis gene, *ced-9*, and was first identified as an oncogene created by a chromosomal 8;14 translocation in B-cell lymphoma.[7] Studies of the mammalian homologs of the *C. elegans* death genes have led to an understanding of the critical elements of the ''death machinery'' of apoptosis.

FEATURES OF PROGRAMMED CELL DEATH

Mitochondrial alterations, caspase activation, and chromatin fragmentation are among the key events that characterize apoptosis and are discussed in greater detail below. Upon initiation of the death program, cells undergo dramatic volume loss, membrane blebbing, cytoplasmic acidification, rearrangement of the cytoskeleton, and loss of contact with adjacent cells and extracellular matrix. Cells exhibit disordered ion homeostasis characterized by diminished proton elimination (and/or increased proton production), and volume loss accomplished largely through potassium and chloride efflux, which is accompanied by water loss. Calcium homeostasis is also disturbed, since mitochondrial sequestration of calcium is impaired. Membrane blebbing and phosphatidylserine externalization have been attributed to proteolytic cleavage of the membrane cytoskeletal protein fodrin (a spectrin homolog) and to activation of the phospholipid scramblase, which is activated by low pH and elevated calcium levels. Cytoskeletal alterations are due in part to proteolytic cleavage of actin, as well as to changes in the activity of kinases and G proteins that regulate the state of assembly of cytoskeletal components. A variety of signaling pathways that participate in survival signaling are proteolytically inactivated.[8]

The cell is marked for ingestion by neighboring cells or professional phagocytes through the upregulation of certain adhesion markers and through the externalization of phosphatidylserine. In the intact organism, apoptotic cells are removed before membrane integrity is lost, thereby preventing spillage of cellular contents. The magnitude of this clearance process is demonstrated by the clearance of inflammatory cells during the resolution of pneumonia.[9]

MITOCHONDRIAL ALTERATIONS

The mitochondria are complex organelles consisting of an outer membrane, an inner membrane, an intermembrane space, and the matrix, which is enclosed by the inner membrane. The outer membrane is permeable to small molecules, while the inner membrane is highly impermeable and able to maintain a proton gradient equivalent to 1 pH unit. The electron transport system is embedded in the inner membrane and oxidizes substrates in order to move protons across the inner membrane. This proton gradient is the driving force for ATP synthesis. The inner membrane, which has extensive infoldings (cristae) to increase the available sites for ATP synthesis on the matrix face of the inner membrane, has a much greater surface area than does the outer membrane. Cytochrome c, which serves as an electron carrier, is located in the intermembrane space and is electrostatically associated with the inner membrane.

In addition to their role in ATP production, the mitochondria play a key role in the regulation of apoptosis. Sequestered in the space between the inner and outer mitochondrial membranes are cytochrome c, which is a cofactor for caspase activation; some caspases; and

Acronyms and abbreviations that appear in this chapter include: AIF, apoptosis-inducing factor; CAD, caspase-activated DNase; FADD, Fas-associated death domain; GM-CSF, granulocyte-macrophage colony-stimulating factor; ICAD, CAD inhibitor; MTP, mitochondrial permeability transition pore (MPT); TNF-α, tumor necrosis factor α; TRAIL, TNF-related apoptosis-inducing ligand.

apoptosis-inducing factor (AIF), which promotes DNA fragmentation and chromatin condensation.

Two major mitochondrial alterations occur in apoptosis: loss of cytochrome c and depolarization of the inner membrane. The earliest event is the dissociation of cytochrome c from the electron transport chain, followed somewhat later by its release from the mitochondria to the cytosol, where it may participate in caspase activation. Loss of cytochrome c from its normal association with the electron transport chain prevents delivery of electrons to complex IV and thence to oxygen. However, it may be possible for electrons to "bleed off" at the upstream site of ubiquinone, leading to superoxide production. This may explain the production of free radicals frequently observed in apoptosis. Effective mitochondrial respiration is shut down, and dissipation of the proton gradient may result in loss of membrane potential across the inner membrane. In some cases, the F_0F_1 ATPase may run in reverse, hydrolyzing any available ATP so as to maintain mitochondrial inner membrane potential through proton pumping. The mitochondria also become engaged in futile calcium cycling (uptake and release); the combination of the two processes may lead to a crisis state for the mitochondria, at which point the inner mitochondrial membrane becomes freely permeable to solutes, resulting in loss of mitochondrial membrane potential. This is often referred to as opening of the mitochondrial permeability transition (MPT) pore, although the event may be less specific than the term *pore* implies. Loss of ion homeostasis across the inner mitochondrial membrane may lead to swelling of the mitochondrial matrix compartment and eventual rupture of the outer mitochondrial membrane, leading to release of cytochrome c, caspases, and AIF.

The participation of the mitochondria in these apoptotic events is regulated by members of the Bcl-2 family, some of which oppose apoptosis while others promote apoptosis. Bcl-2, some of which opposes apoptosis, is able to prevent the release of cytochrome c from mitochondria, while the proapoptotic Bax promotes cytochrome c release.[10,11] Proteolytic processing of Bid, or dephosphorylation of Bad, results in their translocation to the mitochondria, where they cause cytochrome c release. Bax has also been reported to translocate from cytosol to mitochondria during apoptosis. Since these molecules bear structural similarity to the pore-forming colicins, much attention has been directed toward their potential role as pore formers in the outer mitochondrial membrane. They may interact with the voltage-dependent anion channel, a large-conductance porin in the outer mitochondrial membrane, as well as with the adenine nucleotide transporter, an inner-membrane protein believed to be a component of the MTP pore in addition to its primary role in ATP-ADP exchange.[12] Bcl-2 family members are extremely important in the regulation of cell death. Bcl-2 family members and their function (pro- or antiapoptotic) are shown in Fig. 11-1 and reviewed in ref. 13.

CASPASE ACTIVATION

The caspases can now be grouped into three functional categories. The first group includes ICE (also designated caspase-1) and two related caspases: caspase-4 and caspase-5. Although ICE primarily participates in cytokine processing, the function of the other members of this group is not clear. The second group consists of the effector caspases, such as caspase-3, which possess a short prodomain (<3 kDa). The effector caspases are responsible for cleaving many of the important intracellular protein substrates that are degraded during apoptosis.[14] The third, and perhaps most interesting, group includes the signaling caspases, which possess a large prodomain. Most cells express multiple caspases, probably related to the observed redundancy in pathways that initiate cell death; it also appears that the caspases may work in a cascade fashion, perhaps analogous to the amplification

seen in the clotting system. The caspase family is diagrammed in Fig. 11-2.

Caspases are synthesized as proenzymes with an amino-terminal prodomain that is removed by proteolytic processing. The enzyme is further processed into large ($\approx$20 kDa) and small ($\approx$10 kDa) fragments, which form a heterodimer. Two heterodimers assemble to form the active tetrameric protease (Fig. 11-3). Caspases are capable of autoprocessing under certain circumstances. Recently it has been suggested that effector caspases are dependent on proteolytic activation, while the signaling caspases, such as caspase-9, depend on interaction with a cofactor, such as Apaf-1.[15,16]

Activation of caspases may be accomplished through multiple pathways, two of which have been worked out in detail (Fig. 11-4). The receptor-mediated pathway involves a cell surface receptor, such as Fas or the receptor for TNF-α. Occupancy of the receptor with its ligand causes recruitment of a cytosolic adapter molecule containing a protein-protein interaction region termed the death domain. The adapter molecule [e.g., Fas-associated death domain (FADD) or TNFR–associated death domain (TRADD)] then recruits a signaling procaspase such as caspase-8 or caspase-10, which docks with the adapter molecule and undergoes proximity-induced processing. Caspase-8 or caspase-10 may directly activate caspase-3 and related effector caspases.[17]

An alternative pathway exists involving activation of caspase-9 through interaction of Apaf-1, which must bind cytochrome c and dATP or ATP (Fig. 11-5).[18] Apaf-1, which has homology to Ced-4, is present in the cytosol and inactive until cytochrome c is available for interaction. It possesses a caspase activation and recruitment domain (CARD) that is essential for its function. Additional Apaf-1-like molecules are now being identified that presumably will be activated through different pathways.

Cytotoxic T lymphocytes inject granzyme B into cells to trigger apoptosis. Granzyme B is a serine protease that cleaves caspases after Asp residues to generate active caspases. The introduction of granzyme B into the cytosol of target cells results in the rapid activation of caspase-3 and subsequent cell death.

It is generally believed that activation of proteases constitutes an irreversible event and that the caspases are the ultimate effectors of apoptotic cell destruction. There are exceptions however. For example, caspase-3 is activated in a subset of T cells and participates in processing of IL16 without leading to apoptosis. Conversely, inhibition of caspases may not always prevent cell death. Since multiple enzymatic pathways are activated in apoptosis, it is reasonable to think that completion of any subset of processes will result in the death of the cell or, at the very least, in loss of its ability to divide.

NUCLEAR ALTERATIONS

The classic histologic manifestations of apoptosis are the condensation of nuclear chromatin and fragmentation of the nucleus. DNA condensation and classic apoptotic body formation depend on proteolysis of lamin by one or more caspases.[19] DNA digestion is accomplished by several distinct endonucleases, eventually resulting in fragments representing multiples of the approximately 200 base pair nucleosome (the so-called nucleosomal ladder). The search for the responsible endonucleases has yielded several candidates, including DNase I and DNase II. DNA fragmentation factor (DFF) consists of a 40-kDa caspase-activated DNase (CAD) bound to its 45-kDa inhibitor (ICAD). Cleavage of CAD releases it from ICAD, thereby enabling it to function as an endonuclease.[20] Although DNA fragmentation is commonly observed in apoptosis, it is not an essential feature.

In addition to the characteristic morphologic changes in the nucleus, it is possible to detect DNA fragmentation using a histologic

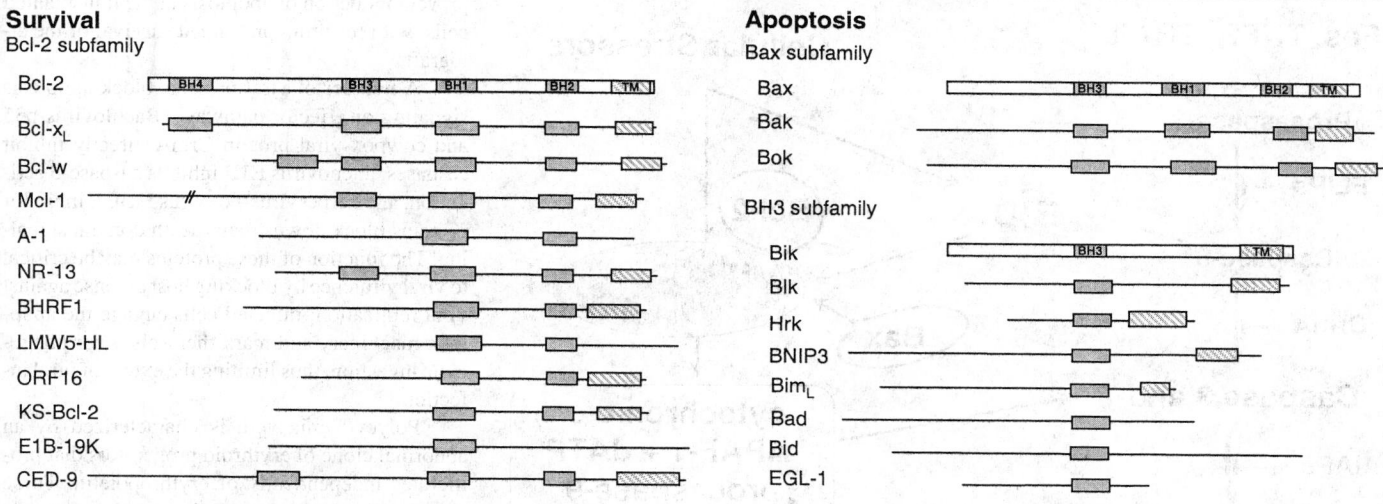

FIGURE 11-1 Bcl-2 family members and their role in apoptosis regulation. Bcl-2 homology (BH) domains represent conserved sequences among family members. TM designates the transmembrane domain. The Bcl-2 subfamily promotes cell survival. Proapoptotic members are grouped into the Bax subfamily and the BH3 subfamily, which has high sequence divergence outside the BH3 domain. (Adapted from JM Adams,[29] with permission.)

method known as terminal deoxynucleotidyl transferase dUTP nick end labeling (TUNEL), in which labeled deoxynucleotides are incorporated into nuclear DNA at sites of nicking. The incorporated nucleotides are then detected using conventional histochemical staining or fluorescence detection. This method has become widely utilized to detect DNA fragmentation in tissue sections and in cell suspensions evaluated by flow cytometry.

ENDOGENOUS PREVENTION OF APOPTOSIS

Cells have evolved a variety of safeguards to prevent inappropriate apoptosis. Viruses have also exploited these safeguards to prevent the cell from undergoing apoptosis in response to the presence of the virus. Bcl-2, which opposes apoptosis, has corresponding viral homologs, including E1B-19K. The cell also has inhibitors of apoptosis (IAPs), which bind to caspases and inhibit their activity. The cowpox response modifier protein, CrmA, is a viral gene product that performs the same

function. Transcriptional regulation of antiapoptotic genes is mediated in part through NFκB, which is mimicked by the viral transcription factor v-Rel.

APOPTOSIS IN HUMAN DISEASE

The occurrence of apoptosis in pathophysiologic settings or its absence in physiologic settings result in human disease. More simply, diseases can be grouped according to whether there is too much apoptosis or too little.

INSUFFICIENT APOPTOSIS

Since apoptosis must occur at defined times during development, a failure of apoptosis to occur in the appropriate settings would be expected to give rise to developmental defects. However, genetically

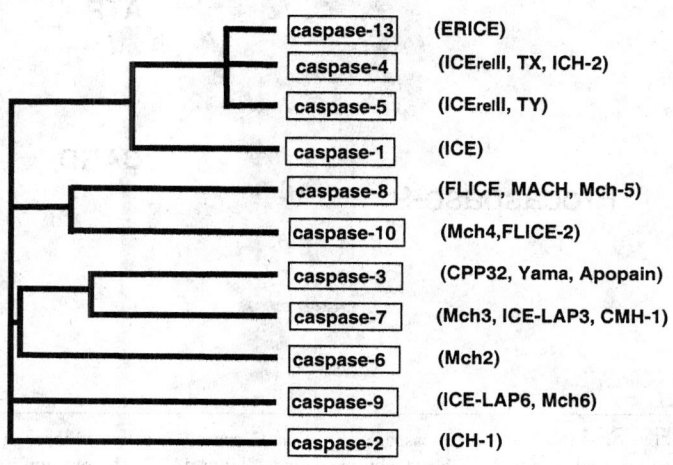

FIGURE 11-2 Phylogenetic tree for the caspase family. Caspase designations and their aliases are shown. (Adapted from ES Alnemri et al[5] and EW Humke et al,[30] with permission.)

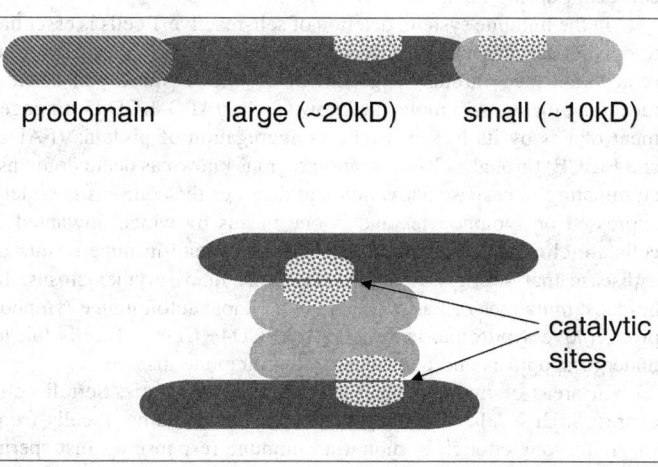

FIGURE 11-3 Diagram of caspase processing and assembly. Members of the cysteine aspartate protease (caspase) family are characterized by an amino-terminal prodomain and a catalytic domain, which is processed by cleavage after Asp residues to release large ($\approx$20 kDa) and small ($\approx$10 kDa) subunits. The two fragments assemble into a heterodimer. Two heterodimers form a tetramer in the active form of the caspase.

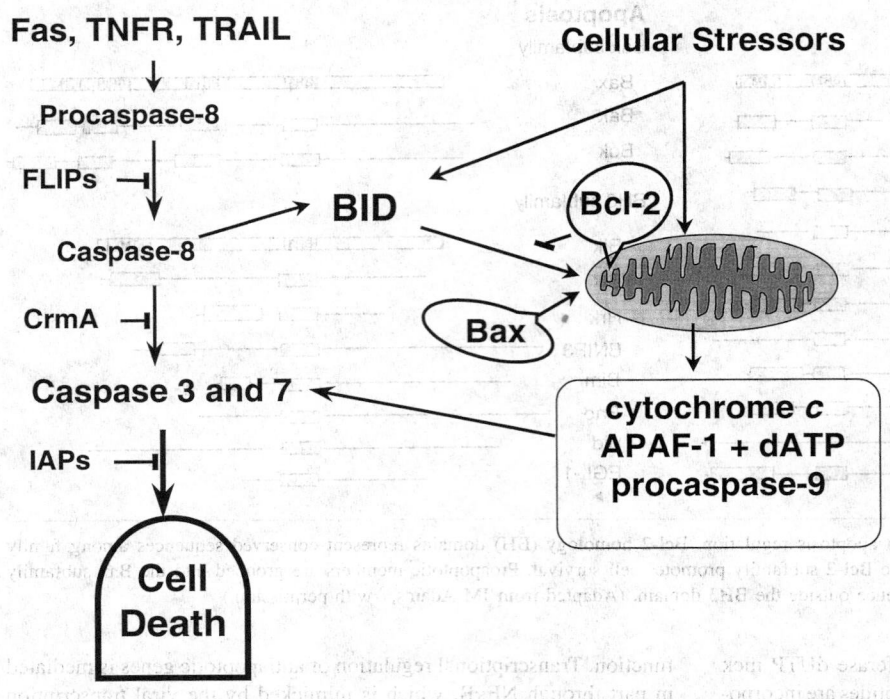

FIGURE 11-4   Two main signaling cascades lead to caspase activation. Extracellular signaling from the death receptors TNFR, Fas, and TRAIL lead to activation of caspase-8 and/or caspase-10, which leads to activation of caspase-3 and other end effectors of apoptosis. Caspase-8 and caspase-10 are inhibited by CrmA. Cell stressors and related signals lead to mitochondrial alterations resulting in caspase-3 activation through the interaction of Apaf-1, cytochrome c, and caspase-9. Bcl-2 opposes the pathway that involves mitochondria.

prevent induction of apoptosis in the transplanted cells, with resulting prolonged survival of the allograft.

A number of viral proteins block apoptosis signaling or effector pathways. Baculovirus p35 and cowpox viral protein CrmA directly inhibit caspases; adenovirus E1B inhibits caspase-3 activation, and herpesvirus-poxvirus FLICE inhibitor proteins block downstream death domain signaling. The function of these proteins may be critical to viral virulence by blocking host defense against viral replication; infected cells engage the apoptotic machinery and mark themselves for phagocytic ingestion, thus limiting the extent of viral infection.

Polycythemia vera is characterized by an abnormal clone of erythroid progenitors that proliferates independently of erythropoietin. These clonal cells overexpress Bcl-x_L, which prevents apoptosis and may contribute to the survival of erythroid progenitors in the absence of erythropoietin.[23]

Tumor growth rate is determined by the imbalance between apoptosis and mitosis. For example, the function of the Bcl-2 gene product was discovered because its overexpression prevents the normal death of B cells, leading to a lymphoma associated with a normal rate of proliferation but reduced apoptosis.[24] A malignant cell may arise when a cell fails to undergo apoptosis when it should have. Loss of a neces-

defined abnormalities in known elements of the process of apoptosis have not been identified in human developmental disorders. Some insights have been derived from gene knockout studies in mice. Deletion of the gene encoding caspase-3, arguably the most important death protease, results in mice that die in utero or soon after birth with an excess of brain tissue, owing to a failure of normal programmed cell death during neuronal development.

In the immune system, deletion of self-reactive T cells is essential to prevent autoimmune disorders.[21] Signaling for lymphocyte deletion is accomplished through engagement of one or more cell surface receptors, including a molecule known as Fas/APO-1/CD95. Engagement of Fas by its ligand results in aggregation of proteins (FADD and FLICE) through self-association regions known as death domains, culminating in caspase activation and death of the cell. Fas is widely expressed on lymphocytes and is one means by which unwanted T cells are eliminated. Mutation of Fas or its ligand in mice results in a disease that strongly resembles systemic lupus erythematosus. In humans, mutations of Fas occur in the heritable autoimmune lymphoproliferative syndrome, in which CD3+CD4−CD8− T cells fail to undergo apoptosis and contribute to autoimmune disease.[22]

In areas of immune sanctuary, such as the testis, Sertoli cells express high levels of Fas ligand to prevent invading T cells from surviving long enough to mount an immune response against sperm cells (which are recognized as foreign by the body). A similar mechanism of protection is involved in limiting inflammatory responses in viral infections in sensitive organs such as the eye. Immune-mediated rejection of transplanted organs rests in part on the induction of apoptosis in the foreign cells. This mechanism has been exploited by genetic manipulation to express Fas ligand on pancreatic islet cells to

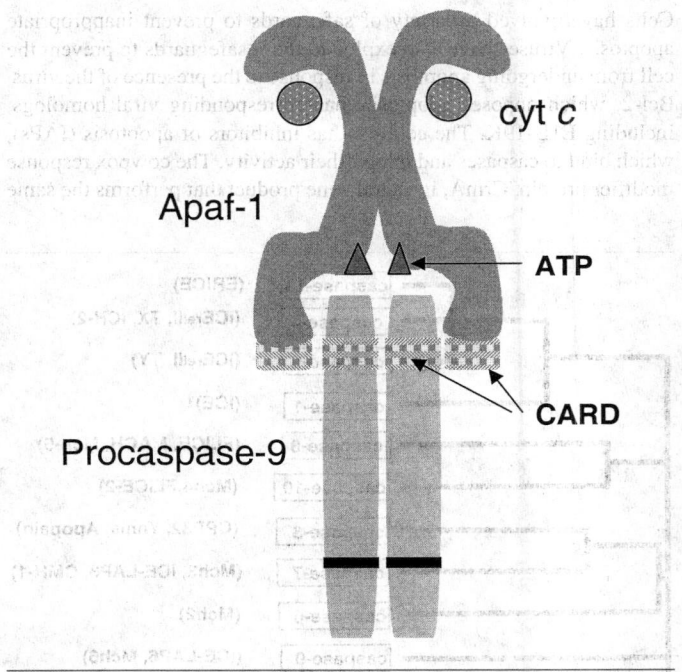

FIGURE 11-5   Model for caspase activation. Caspase-9 is activated through an interaction with Apaf-1, cytochrome c, and ATP or dATP. The reaction is normally held in check by sequestration of cytochrome c within the mitochondria. However, in response to apoptotic stimuli, cytochrome c becomes accessible to the other components. Activated caspase-9 cleaves the downstream effector caspase-3, resulting in widespread cleavage of cellular proteins.

sary growth factor or removal from the normal extracellular matrix should trigger a cell to commit suicide. If, however, the cell fails to die, it may survive and proliferate sufficiently for its progeny to acquire other mutations, including loss of p53 and activation of other oncogenes. The p53 gene product is a transcription factor activated by DNA damage to induce a family of p53-dependent genes that regulate the cell cycle and induce apoptosis.[25] Mutations of p53 have been found in many malignant tumors and in some families with hereditary cancer syndromes. Thus, the first step in oncogenesis may be a failure of apoptosis. Chronic myelogenous leukemia represents another example of the blockage of normal apoptosis due to the effects of the BCR-ABL oncogene. Modulation of apoptosis is widely considered a key target for cancer therapy.[26] Although malignant cells are generally considered more resistant to the induction of apoptosis, they still possess the necessary cellular machinery and, when exposed to appropriate chemotherapeutic agents (or radiation), usually die by apoptosis, not necrosis.[27] Efforts to decrease their resistance to apoptosis are directed at targets such as Bcl-2. Evaluation of apoptosis in response to chemotherapeutic agents may correlate with prognosis and might eventually direct the selection of agents on an individualized basis.

One hypothesis about mechanisms of aging is that too little apoptosis occurs, permitting the survival of cells that have sustained DNA damage. Such damaged cells would function inefficiently at best, owing to the accumulation of mutations in essential genes, and could undergo malignant transformation. Eventually, such marginally functioning and precancerous cells would predominate, with more generalized cellular dysfunction as time went on.

EXCESSIVE APOPTOSIS

Excessive cell death is of particular concern in organs that are populated by terminally differentiated, nondividing cells. Any cells lost, whether by apoptosis or necrosis, are irreplaceable. In settings where cell death is inevitable, inhibiting the enzymatic processes of apoptosis may not salvage the cell but may merely convert its demise to a necrotic form. However, if a cell is damaged beyond repair, a tidy, noninflammatory apoptotic death may still be preferable, avoiding collateral damage from inflammation.

Excessive apoptosis is now being recognized in a variety of hematopoietic disorders. In some cases, this may be due to unavailability of a necessary growth factor, an inability to respond to the growth factor, or alterations in the balance of proapoptotic and antiapoptotic Bcl-2 family members. The myelodysplastic syndrome, which is characterized by peripheral cytopenias and (at least in the early stages) marrow hyperplasia, is now recognized to be associated with excessive apoptosis in the later stages of myeloid differentiation, resulting in ineffective myelopoiesis. Eventually, apoptosis-resistant clones often emerge, with concomitant progression to acute myelogenous leukemia. Fanconi's anemia is accompanied by increased susceptibility to apoptosis mediated by Fas and TNF-α. It seems likely that abnormalities in apoptosis will be recognized as features of additional myeloid disorders.[28]

REFERENCES

1. Wyllie AH, Kerr JFR, Currie AR: Cell death: the significance of apoptosis. *Int Rev Cytol* 68:251, 1980.
2. Wickremasinghe RG, Hoffbrand AV: Biochemical and genetic control of apoptosis: relevance to normal hematopoiesis and hematological malignancies. *Blood* 93:3587, 1999.
3. Ellis HM, Horvitz HR: Genetic control of programmed cell death in the nematode *C. elegans*. *Cell* 44:817, 1986.
4. Metzstein MM, Stanfield GM, Horvitz HR: Genetics of programmed cell death in *C. elegans*: past, present and future. *Trends Genet* 14:410, 1998.
5. Alnemri ES, Livingston DJ, Nicholson DW, et al: Human ICE/CED-3 protease nomenclature [letter to the editor]. *Cell* 87:171, 1996.
6. Li H, Yuan J: Deciphering the pathways of life and death. *Curr Opin Cell Biol* 11:261, 1999.
7. Korsmeyer SJ: Chromosomal translocations in lymphoid malignancies reveal novel proto-oncogenes. *Annu Rev Immunol* 10:785, 1992.
8. Wolf BB, Green DR: Suicidal tendencies: Apoptotic cell death by caspase family proteinases. *J Biol Chem* 274:20049, 1999.
9. Savill J, Haslett C: Granulocyte clearance by apoptosis in the resolution of inflammation. *Semin Cell Biol* 6:385, 1995.
10. Kluck RM, Bossy-Wetzel E, Green DR, Newmeyer DD: The release of cytochrome c from mitochondria: a primary site for Bcl-2 regulation of apoptosis. *Science* 275:1132, 1997.
11. Yang J, Liu X, Bhalla K, et al: Prevention of apoptosis by Bcl-2: release of cytochrome c from mitochondria blocked. *Science* 275:1129, 1997.
12. Tsujimoto Y: Role of Bcl-2 family proteins in apoptosis: apoptosomes or mitochondria? *Genes Cells* 3:697, 1998.
13. Reed JC: Bcl-2 family proteins. *Oncogene* 17:3225, 1998.
14. Tewari M, Quan LT, O'Rourke K, et al: Yama/CPP32, a mammalian homolog of CED-3, is a Crm-A-inhibitable protease that cleaves the death substrate poly(ADP-ribose) polymerase. *Cell* 81:801, 1995.
15. Salvesen GS, Dixit VM: Caspases: intracellular signaling by proteolysis. *Cell* 91:443, 1997.
16. Salvesen GS: Programmed cell death and the caspases. *APMIS* 107:73, 1999.
17. Ashkenazi A, Dixit VM: Death receptors: signaling and modulation. *Science* 281:1305, 1998.
18. Li P, Nijhawan D, Budihardjo I, et al: Cytochrome c and dATP-dependent formation of Apaf-1/caspase-9 complex initiates an apoptotic protease cascade. *Cell* 91:479, 1997.
19. Lazebnik YA, Takahashi A, Moir RD, et al: Studies of the lamin proteinase reveal multiple parallel biochemical pathways during apoptotic execution. *Proc Natl Acad Sci USA* 92:9042, 1995.
20. Sakahira H, Enari M, Nagata S: Cleavage of CAD inhibitor in CAD activation and DNA degradation during apoptosis. *Nature* 391:96, 1998.
21. Los M, Wesselborg S, Schulze-Osthoff K: The role of caspases in development, immunity, and apoptotic signal transduction: lessons from knockout mice. *Immunity* 10:629, 1999.
22. Straus SE, Sneller M, Lenardo MJ, Puck JM, Strober W: An inherited disorder of lymphocyte apoptosis: the autoimmune lymphoproliferative syndrome. *Ann Intern Med* 130:591, 1999.
23. Fernandez-Luna JL: Apoptosis and polycythemia vera. *Curr Opin Hematol* 6:94, 1999.
24. Hockenberry DG, Nunez C, Milliman RB, Schreiber RD, Korsmeyer SJ: Bcl-2 is an inner mitochondrial membrane protein that blocks programmed cell death. *Nature* 348:334, 1990.
25. el-Deiry WS: Regulation of p53 downstream genes. *Semin Cancer Biol* 8:345, 1998.
26. Hannun YA: Apoptosis and the dilemma of cancer chemotherapy. *Blood* 89:1845, 1997.
27. Brown JM, Wouters BG: Apoptosis, p53, and tumor cell sensitivity to anticancer agents. *Cancer Res* 59:1391, 1999.
28. Haurie C, Dale DC, Mackey MC: Cyclical neutropenia and other periodic hematological disorders: a review of mechanisms and mathematical models. *Blood* 92:2629, 1998.
29. Adams JM, Cory S: The Bcl-2 protein family: arbiters of cell survival. *Science* 281:1322, 1998.
30. Humke EW, Ni J, Dixit VM: ERICE, a novel FLICE-activatable caspase. *J Biol Chem* 273:15702, 1998.

CELL CYCLE REGULATION AND HEMATOLOGICAL DISORDERS

MATHIAS SCHMID
DENNIS A. CARSON

Complex feedback pathways regulate the passage of cells through the G_1, S, G_2, and M phases of the growth cycle. Two key checkpoints control the commitment of cells to replicate DNA synthesis and to mitosis. Many oncogenes and tumor suppressor genes promote malignant change by stimulating cell cycle entry, or disrupting the checkpoint response to DNA damage. This chapter presents the pathways that regulate cell replication and tabulates the various oncogenes that have been shown to be involved in hematologic and some other malignancies.

INTRODUCTION

Cell mitosis is the final step of a defined program—the cell cycle—which can be separated into four phases: the G_1-, S-, G_2-, and M phases (Fig. 12-1). A number of surveillance systems (checkpoints) control the cell cycle and interrupt its progression when DNA damage occurs or when the cells have failed to complete a necessary event.[1] These checkpoints have been given an empirical definition: When the occurrence of an event B is dependent on the completion of a prior event A, the dependence is due to a checkpoint if a loss-of-function mutation can be found that relieves the dependence.[1] Three major cell cycle checkpoints have been discovered: the DNA damage checkpoint, the spindle checkpoint, and the spindle pole body duplication checkpoint.[2-4]

The functional consequence of cell cycle checkpoint failure is usually death by apoptosis. However, small numbers of genetically altered cells may survive. Cells with defective checkpoints have an advantage when selection favors multiple genetic changes. Cancer cells are often missing one or more checkpoints, which facilitates a greater rate of genomic evolution.[5]

Most of the basic principles of cell cycle regulation were worked out in yeast, but the underlying principles are equally applicable to the mammalian cell cycle. One must understand basic cell cycle regulation in order to understand the mechanisms that lead to hematological malignancies and the importance of tumor suppressor genes and oncogenes.

CYCLINS AND CYCLIN-DEPENDENT KINASES (TABLE 12-1)

Early experiments on the control of mitosis in human cells provided evidence for the existence of factors called *M-phase* and *S-phase*

promoting factors (MPF, SPF).[6] The key element of SPF was thought to be cdc2. Experiments performed in Xenopus eggs showed that cdc2 is an M-phase-specific histone H1 kinase[7] but is just one subunit of a regulatory complex. A second component is cyclin B, which is synthesized in interphase and degraded in mitosis. At least eight members of the mammalian cyclin family have been cloned to date (cyclins A-H). These cyclins all interact with a group of cdc2-related kinases called *cyclin-dependent kinases* (cdk).[8,9] The cyclin/cdk complex is the mammalian counterpart of the cdc2/cdc13 complex in yeast. Phosphorylation of tyrosine 15 is the key event in regulating human cdc2 activity. Threonine 14 also is phosphorylated in G_2 phase. Both phosphorylation sites are required for mitotic initiation. Cdc2 interacts with cyclin B in mitosis, whereas the cdc2/cyclin A complex is formed before mitosis and probably is required for progression through late G_2 phase[10] Thus, cyclins A and B are also called the *mitotic* cyclins, since they are upregulated in late G_2 or G_2/M and undergo proteolysis in M phase.

The exit from mitosis is characterized by the abrupt ubiquitination and subsequent degradation of cyclin B. Cells with a defective cyclin B degradation mechanism or without mitotic cyclin B easily become aneuploid. The exact role of the other mitotic cyclin, cyclin A, is still unclear. There is evidence that it both acts at the G_2/M transition and binds cdk2 in S phase. Overexpression of cyclin A in G_1 phase leads to an accelerated entry into S phase.[11] Since cdc2 is able to interact with mitotic and G_1 cyclins, it seems likely that one protein kinase potentially can fulfill several different functions in the cell cycle at various checkpoints. The redundancy of cyclin functions makes it difficult to ascertain the exact function of each protein in all cell types.

There are several cdc2-related protein kinases in humans that interact with the corresponding cyclins. Originally, three cdc2-related proteins were isolated which were able to replace deficient cdc28 function in budding yeast: cdk1, cdk2, and cdk3.[12-15] Another group of cdks that bind to cyclin D (a G_1 cyclin) have been named cdk4,[16] cdk5,[17] and cdk6.[18] Cdk4 has been in the focus of tumor suppressor gene research for the last several years, since it complexes with cyclin D1. This complex is an important element in the *p16^{INK4A}*-retinoblastoma (rb) gene pathway, which is commonly disrupted in cancer (see below). Three other cyclin-dependent kinases have been partially characterized: cdk7 (*p40^{MO15}*) interacts with cyclin H and is responsible for phosphorylating pcdc2 on threonine 161.[19-21] Cdk8 interacts with cyclin C and is associated with RNA polymerase II.[22-24] Cdk9 binds cyclin T1 and displays a tissue-specific expression pattern.[25-27] The fact that cdk9/cyclin T1 specifically interacts with the tat element of the human immunodeficiency virus 1 (HIV-1) links this cyclin-dependent kinase directly to the replication pathway of HIV, and circumstantially to HIV-1 related malignancies (e.g., Kaposi sarcoma).[28-30]

All cyclins share an approximately 150 amino acid region, called the *cyclin box*, which interacts with the cdks.[31] The G_1 cyclins (C, D, and E) and the mitotic cyclins (A and B)[32] form distinct categories, although cyclin H and the type T cyclins (T_1, T_2a, and T_2b) fall outside these two major groups.

Cyclin A binds and activates cdk2 mainly in S phase. However, microinjection of anticyclin A antibodies into cells causes cell cycle arrest just before S phase.[10] The integration of the hepatitis B virus into the cellular genome is accompanied by the formation of a chimeric cyclin A, lacking the cyclin destruction box, and with a prolonged half-life.[33] This observation, together with the finding that overexpression of cyclin A leads to accelerated S-phase entry, suggests that cyclin A is involved in transformation.[11] The other cyclin that interacts with cdk2, cyclin E, may control the progression from G_1 to S phase, but the exact timepoint when cdk2 "switches" from cyclin E to cyclin A binding is unknown. Cdk2/cyclin E activity peaks during late G_1 phase, and declines in early S phase.[34] Cells overexpressing cyclin E progress

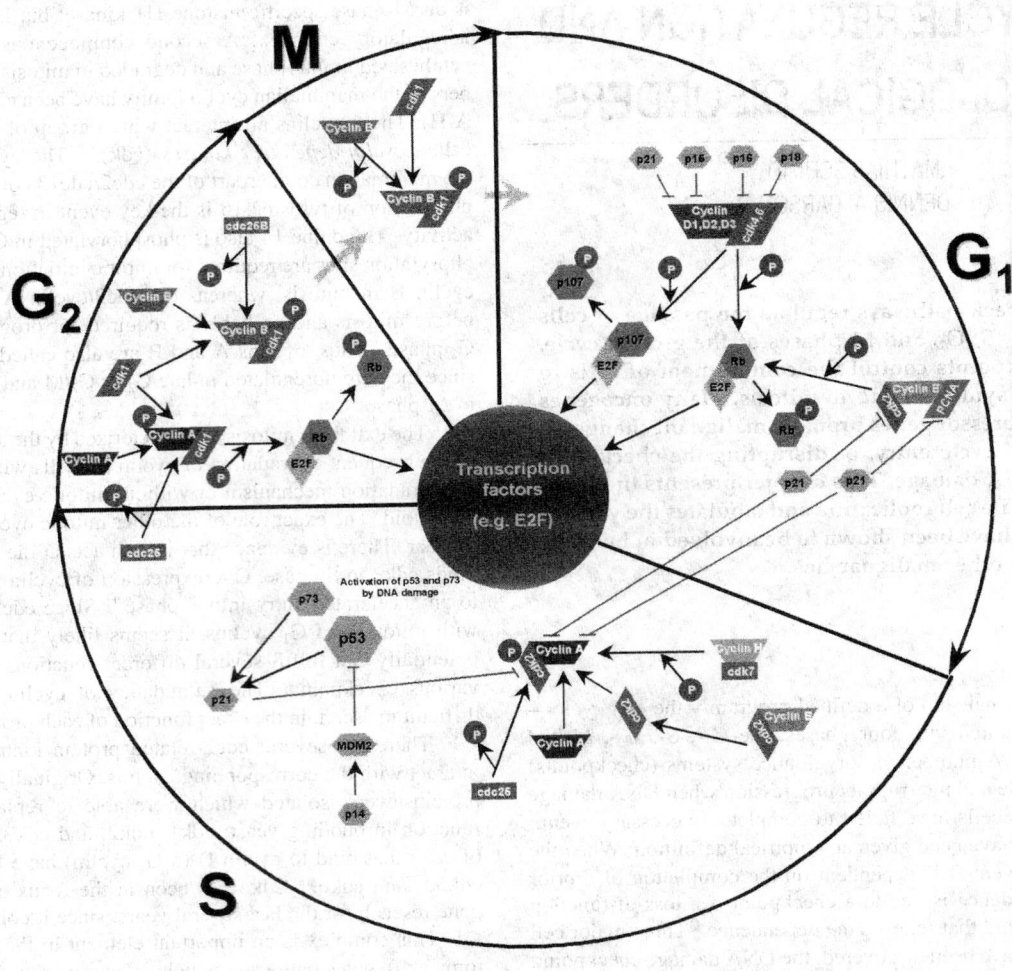

FIGURE 12-1   Cell cycle regulation in mammalian cells.

much faster through G_1 into S phase, but the time required for DNA synthesis remains normal.[35] Cyclin E levels also are regulated by environmental factors, including TGF-β and irradiation. These effects are, in part, mediated by small proteins, the cyclin-dependent kinase inhibitors (CDI). In addition to its role at the G_1/S boundary, cyclin A acts in late G_2 phase, where it complexes with cdk1. It has been suggested that this interaction might be necessary for the reorganization of the cytoskeleton prior to mitosis.[36]

The B-type cyclins associate with cdk1 and cdk2 to form the

classical mitotic cyclin/cdk complexes.[37] Cyclin B is synthesized in S phase and accumulates together with cdk2. Ubiquitin mediates the degradation of cyclin B, allowing the cell to exit from mitosis. The cyclin B/cdk2 checkpoint is very often defective in malignant cells, leading to uncontrolled M-phase entry and aneuploidy. The cellular localization of the cdk1-cyclin B complexes also is strictly cell-cycle–dependent. Although the complexes accumulate in the cytoplasm during G_2 and S phase, they move to the nucleus in mitosis and bind to the mitotic spindle.[38–41]

The three different cyclin D molecules (D_1, D_2, and D_3) function mainly in late G_1 phase, where they bind cdk4 and cdk6. These complexes phosphorylate rb, restraining its inhibitory effects on E2F, and related transcription factors. Cyclin D_1 is the major D cyclin in most cell types. All three cyclin D molecules act in late G phase, just before entry into S phase. Forced overexpression of cyclin D_1 shortens the G_1 phase. Many tumors have high cyclin D_1 levels without amplification or mutation of the cyclin D_1 structural gene. Instead, cycle D levels may be regulated by a feedback loop dependent on rb. Alterations of the retinoblastoma gene in cancer may secondarily cause upregulation of cyclin D transcription.

The most recently identified member of the cdk-family, cdk9, partners with cyclin T, an 87-kDa cyclin C type protein with three subunits.[25] The cdk9/cyclin T complex is an essential component of the P-TEFb human transcription elongation factor.[26] P-TEFb can hyperphosphorylate the C-terminal domain of RNA polymerase II, simi-

TABLE 12-1   CDKs, ASSOCIATED CYCLINS, AND THE STAGE OF THE CELL CYCLE WHERE THEY ACT

Cdk	Associated Cyclin	Cell Cycle Stage
CdK1	Cyclin A, B	G_2/M
Cdk2	Cyclin A, D, E; cyclin H?	G_1/S; S; G_2/M?
Cdk3	?	?
Cdk4	Cyclin D	G_1/S; S
Cdk5	Cyclin D	G_1/S
Cdk6	Cyclin D	G_1/S; S
Cdk7	Cyclin H	G_1/S; transcriptional regulation
Cdk8	Cyclin C	G_1/S; G_2/M, transcriptional regulation
Cdk9	Cyclin T1, T2	Acts on differentiation, interaction with tat, the transcriptional regulator of the HIV virus

lar to the cyclin H/cdk7/MAT1 complex.[28] In addition, P-TEFb forms a complex with the HIV tat protein that binds the transactivation response element (TAR). The modification of RNA polymerase II by cdk9/cyclin T facilitates the efficient multiplication of the viral genome.[42,43] The fact that the cyclin T1/cdk9 complex is upregulated during T-cell activation enables the HIV to utilize this complex for replication.[44] Another binding partner of cdk9 is a tumor necrosis factor signal transducer molecule, TRAF2.[45]

SUBSTRATES AND INHIBITORS OF CYCLIN-DEPENDENT KINASES

Many cyclin-cdk substrates have been identified by immunoprecipitation or two-hybrid assays, but only a few of them are thought to exert a direct function in cell cycle control. In G_1 phase, the most important substrate of the cdk4-cyclin D and cdk6-cyclin D complexes is rb (Fig. 12-2). In its hypophosphorylated state, rb binds to and inhibits a class of transcription factors, of which the best characterized is the E2F transcription factor. Hyperphosphorylation causes rb to detach from its binding site, permitting transcriptional activation of genes necessary for DNA synthesis and cell division. This phosphorylation of rb is regulated in a cell-cycle–dependent manner.[46–48] Interference with rb function impairs G_1 checkpoint regulation, fosters unrestrained cell growth, and is a nearly universal characteristic of malignancy. Causes of reduced rb activity include changes in the structural gene, the sequestration and inactivation of the protein by viral oncogene products, and hyperphosphorylation of rb due to increased cdk4 and cyclin D activity or to deletion of the gene for the $p16^{INK4A}$ inhibitor of cdk4. Deletions, mutations, and translocations of rb are common in various malignancies, while homozygous deletions of the $p16^{INK4A}$ gene are even more frequent. Many different transforming viruses, such as papilloma virus and simian virus 40, produce proteins that interact with rb. Both cyclin D_1/cdk4 and cyclin $D_1(D_2, D_3)$/cdk6 complexes are able to phosphorylate the rb.[49,50] The timepoint

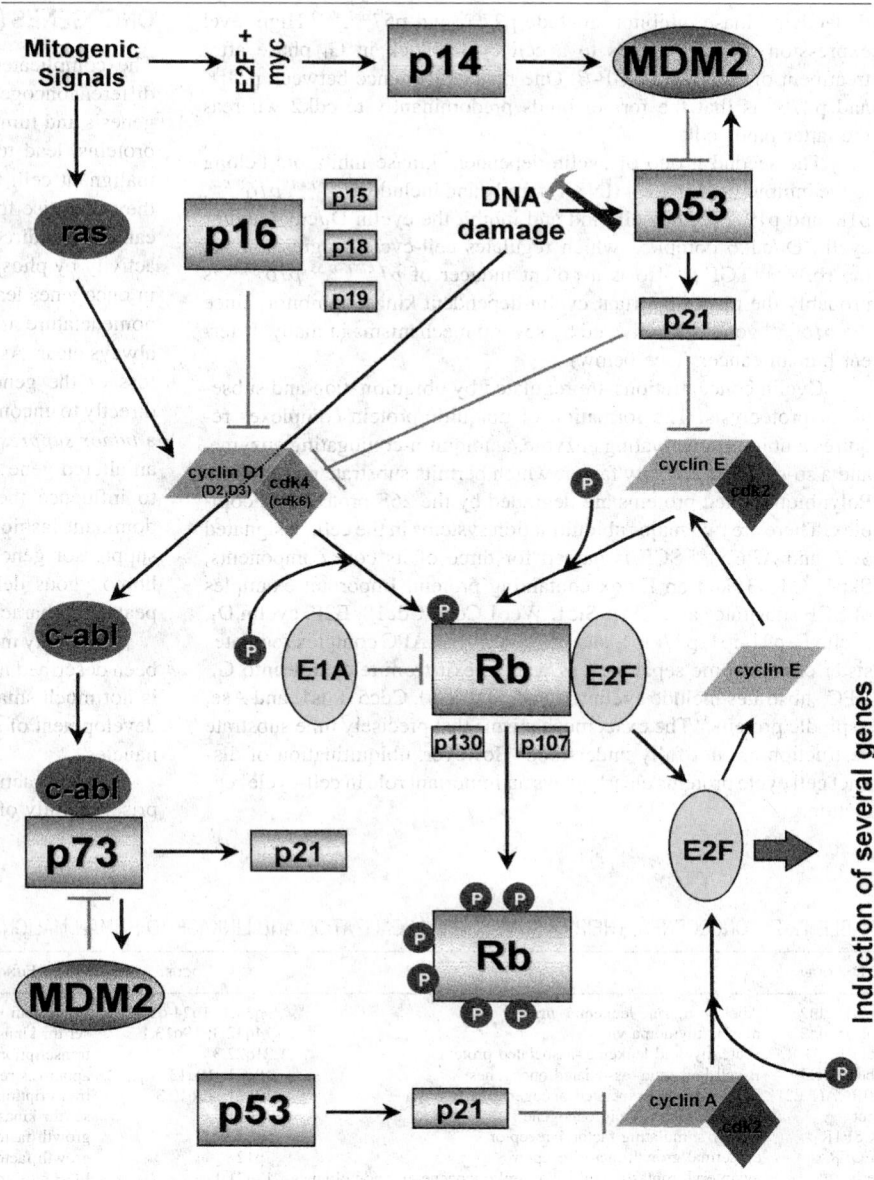

FIGURE 12-2   Interactions between cyclin-dependent kinase inhibitors (p16, p14, p21), p53, and the retinoblastoma protein (rb).

of rb-phosphorylation correlates strongly with the appearance of the cyclin D_1/cdk4 complex. The link between rb and cyclin D is supported by the observation that loss of rb function leads to a decrease in the cellular cyclin D level.[51,52] However, cyclin D may not be the only cyclin that is involved in the rb regulatory pathway.[53,54] Ectopic expression of both cyclin A and cyclin E restores rb hyperphosphorylation and causes cell cycle arrest in cancer cell lines. Perhaps the cdk2-cyclin A complex contributes to additional phosphorylation of rb, whereas cdk2/cyclin E prolongs the phosphorylation time.[53]

Two rb-related proteins, p107 and p130, also form complexes with the transcription factor E2F,[52,55,56] bind to the region of the adenovirus E1A protein required for transformation, and are able to induce G_1 arrest when they are overexpressed in human malignant cell lines.[57–59] Unlike the rb, the p107 and p130 proteins contain a so-called spacer region that interacts with cdk2/cyclin A and cdk2/cyclin E,[60,61] although it seems to be unlikely that these two complexes regulate the activity of p107 and p130.[53] Instead, p107 may bind and inactivate the cyclin

A and cyclin E complexes. Thus, p107 may regulate the cell cycle by several different mechanisms. Since both p107 and p130 are regulated through phosphorylation, efficient cell cycle entry is accompanied by phosphorylation of all the rb-related proteins.

The cyclin-dependent kinases themselves are also controlled by several different mechanisms. Besides their regulation by phosphorylation, specific protein inhibitors of enzyme activity have been identified.[62,63] The cyclin-dependent kinase inhibitors cause cells to arrest in G_1 phase, followed by differentiation and/or senescence. The first cyclin-dependent kinase inhibitor identified was p21^{cip1}.[64] It binds to several cyclin/cdk complexes including cyclin A/cdk2, cyclin D/cdk4, and cyclin E/cdk2 (Fig. 12-2).[46–48,65–67] Several different cell cycle regulatory pathways involve p21^{cip1}. This molecule has a p53 binding site in its promoter, and an increase in p53 levels results in transcriptional activation of p21^{cip1}, slowing down cell-cycle progression. The p21^{cip1} cyclin-dependent kinase inhibitor also plays a role in cellular differentiation in myoblasts.[68] Other members of the p21^{cip1} family of cyclin-dependent kinase inhibitors include p27^{kip1} and p57^{kip2}.[49,50] High-level expression of p27^{kip2} leads to a cell cycle block in G$_1$ phase after treatment of cells with TGF-β. One major difference between p21^{cip1} and p27^{kip1} is that the former binds predominantly to cdk2 whereas the latter binds cdk4.

The second group of cyclin-dependent kinase inhibitors belong to the inhibitor of kinase 4 (INK4) family and include *p15^{INK4B}*, *p16^{INK4A}*, p18, and p19.[51-56] They all bind and inhibit the cyclin D$_1$/cdk4 and/or cyclin D$_1$/cdk6 complex, which regulates cell-cycle progression via the rb.[51,54,55] TGF-β also is a potent inducer of *p15^{INK4B}*.[55] *p16^{INK4A}* is probably the most important cyclin-dependent kinase inhibitor, since the *p16^{INK4A}* gene is inactivated by several mechanisms in many different human cancers (see below).

Cyclin concentrations are regulated by ubiquitination and subsequent proteolysis. The formation of ubiquitin/protein complexes requires a ubiquitin-activating enzyme, a ubiquitin-conjugating enzyme, and a so-called specificity factor, which permits substrate recognition. Polyubiquitinated proteins are degraded by the 26S proteasome complex. There are two major ubiquitination systems in the cell, designated *SCF* and *APC*.[57-60] SCF is named for three of its core components, Skp1, Cdc53, and an F-box containing protein. Important examples of SCF substrates are: Cln1, Sic1, Wee1 Cdc6/Cdc18, E2F, cyclin D$_1$, cyclin E, p21cip1, p27kip1, and p57kip2.[61] The APC complex regulates sister chromosome separation as well as exit from telophase into G$_1$. APC substrates include cyclins A and B, Cdc20, Cdc5, Pds1, and Ase, a spindle protein.[69] The exact mechanisms that precisely time substrate destruction are not fully understood. However, ubiquitination of distinct cell cycle proteins clearly plays an important role in cell-cycle regulation.

ONCOGENES (TABLE 12-2)

The complicated cell-cycle network has its parallel in the several different oncogenes and tumor suppressor genes that influence carcinogenesis and tumor progression. The products of oncogenes, the oncoproteins, lead to or faciltitate the transformation of a normal into a malignant cell. Oncogenes can be carried into the cell by viruses or they can arise from mutations in normal cellular genes. Oncoproteins can interact directly with cell-cycle regulatory proteins or control their activity by phosphorylation and dephosphorylation. Not all mutations in oncogenes lead to an altered function of the resulting product. The nomenclature in the oncogene tumor suppressor gene field is not always clear. As a general guideline, if a mutation causes a functional loss of the gene product, and the recessive loss of function leads directly to uncontrolled cell division, the underlying gene can be named a *tumor suppressor gene*. On the other hand, if the mutation leads to an altered gene product that interacts abnormally with other proteins to influence the cell cycle, this gene is an *oncogene*, acting in a dominant fashion. Mutations are found in both oncogenes and tumor suppressor genes. Translocations are typical of oncogenes, whereas homozygous deletions and hypermethylation of CpG-nucleotide repeats are characteristic features of tumor suppressor genes.

Probably more than 100 oncogenes and oncogene candidates have been described in the literature. The number of tumor suppressor genes is not much smaller. They are both involved in the pathogenesis and development of all kinds of tumors, especially the hematologic malignancies.

Mutant-activated receptor protein-tyrosine kinases (rPTK) comprise a family of very well characterized oncogenes. The constitutive

TABLE 12-2   ONCOGENES, THEIR CHROMOSOMAL LOCALIZATION AND LINKAGE TO HUMAN MALIGNANCIES

ONCOGENE	DESCRIPTION	LOCUS	FUNCTION	POTENTIAL ASSOCIATED MALIGNANCIES
abl1; abl2	Abelson murine leukemia virus	9q34.1; 1q24-q25	tyr protein kinase	lymphoid and myeloid neoplasms
akt1; akt2	murine thymoma virus	14q32.3; 19q13.1	ser/thr kinase	breast cancer, thymoma
aml1	acute myeloid leukema–associated protein	21q22.3	transcription factor	acute myeloid leukemia
bcl2, bcl3	B-cell leukemia–associated oncogenes	18q21; 19q13.1-q13.2	apoptosis regulation	B-cell leukemias, lymphomas
BRCA(1+2)	breast cancer–associated oncogene, early onset	17q21; 13q12.3	transcription factor	breast cancer
cot	cancer Osaka thyroid oncogene	10p11.2	ser/thr kinase	breast and thyroid cancer
CSF1R	colony stimulating factor 1 receptor	5q33-q35	growth factor receptor	lung cancer
EGFR	epidermal growth factor receptor	7p12	growth factor receptor	several human neoplasms
erb	avian erythroblastic leukemia viral oncogene and homologues	17q21.1	EGF receptor	brain tumors, breast cancer, several others
erg	v-ets avian erythroblastosis virus E26 oncogene homologues	21q22.3	transcription factor	acute myeloid leukemia
eto	involved in the t(8;21) in acute myeloid leukemia	8q22	transcription factor?	acute myeloid leukemia
ews	involved in t(11;22)(q24;q12)	22q12	RNA binding protein	Ewing sarcoma
fgr	Gardner-Rasheed feline sarcoma virus	1p36.2-p36.1	tyr kinase	myeloid leukemias
fli1	friend leukemia virus integration 1	11q24.1-q24.3	transcription factor	Ewing sarcoma
fos	murine osteosarcoma virus	14q24.3	transcription factor	several human neoplasms
fyn	oncogene related to src, fgr yes	6q21	tyr kinase	several human neoplasms
gli	glioma-associated oncogene	12q13.2-q13.3	transcription factor	glioma, soft tissue sarcomas, skin tumors
jun	avian sarcoma virus 17	1p32-p31	transcription factor	ovarian, breast, colon, lung, leukemia, several others
kit	Hardy-Zuckerman 4 feline sarcoma virus	4p11-p12	receptor tyr kinase	acute myeloid leukemia
lyn	Yamaguchi sarcoma virus related	8q13	tyr kinase	lymphoid and myeloid neoplasms
myb	avian myeloblastosis virus	6q22-q23	transcription factor	hematological disorders, several human neoplasms
myc	MC29 myelocytoma virus	8q24.12-q24.13	transcription factor	myeloid, lymphatic neoplasms, renal cancer
npm1	nucleophosmin (nuclear phosphoprotein)	5q35	tyr kinase	childhood acute myeloid leukemia
pim1	murine leukemia virus	6p21.2	ser/thr kinase	T-cell lymphoma
pml	involved in t(15;17) in promyelocytic leukemia	15q22	transcription factor	promyelocytic leukemia
raf	murine leukemia virus	3p25	ser/thr kinase	several human neoplasms
rar	retinoic acid receptor	17q12	transcription factor	(pro-)myelocytic leukemia
ras	Harvey sarcoma viral oncogene, several related proteins exist	Several	G-protein	myeloid neoplasms, several human neoplasms
ret	involved in the MEN II syndrome	10q11.2	receptor tyrosine kinase	MEN II, medullary thyroid carcinoma
ros	avian UR2 sarcoma virus	6q21-q22	tyr kinase	brain tumors
ski	avian sarcoma virus	1q22-q24	transcription factor?	rhabdomyosarcoma?
spi	spleen focus forming virus	11p12-p11.22	transcription factor	myeloid leukemias, lymphomas?
src	Rous sarcoma virus	20q11.2-q12	tyr kinase	lymphomas
tax1	human T-cell leukemia virus binding protein (2 forms)	chr7 and chr16	binding protein	acute T-cell leukemia
tel	t(5;12) involved oncogene	12p13	transcription factor	myeloid leukemia
tml1	TCL1/ MTCP1-like protein	14q32.1	?	T-cell leukemia and lymphoma
yes	Yamaguchi sarcoma virus	18p11.31-p11.21	tyr kinase	Colon, breast, melanoma cancer

activation of rPTK usually is achieved by mutations that lead to the dimerization and activation of their cytoplasmic cytalytic domains.[70] Prominent examples include Neu/ERbB and CSF-1 oncogenes. NeuERbB2 is frequently mutated in breast cancer as well as in brain tumors.[71-73] Another possible cause of rPTK dimerization is chromosomal translocations that create chimeric proteins. In the t(2;5) translocation, found in several anaplastic large cell lymphomas, N-terminal nucleophosmin sequences on the long arm of chromosome 5 are fused to the cytoplasmic domain of the Alk protein on chromosome 2.[74,75] The characteristic translocation of chronic myelomonocytic leukemia (CMML), t(5;12), fuses sequences from the transcription factor Tel to the cytoplasmic domain of the platelet-derived growth factor-β receptor (PDGF-α rPTK), resulting in the formation of a Tel/PDGFβR fusion protein and the constitutive activation of the PTK.[76] The chromosomal area surrounding the Tel gene is a fragile site, since the Tel gene is involved in several other translocations in human acute leukemias [e.g., t(12;9)]. The t(9;21) translocation, also called the *Philadelphia chromosome*, is a characteristic feature of chronic myelogenous leukemia (CML) and, less frequently, of other chronic myeloproliferative syndromes. It fuses the c-abl and bcl-2 oncogenes. Amplification of the fusion sequence is frequently used to detect minimal residual disease in patients under therapy with interferon-α and after bone marrow- or stem cell transplantation.[77-79] Other oncogenes that belong to this family are Ret (mutations in Ret cause multiple endocrine neoplasia type 2A and type 2B)[80], and c-Cbl, the homolog of the *C. elegans* gene *Sli1*.[81]

For several years, oncogene research focused on growth factor receptors because of the possibilities for therapeutic intervention. For example, the murine myeloproliferative leukemia virus protein (v-Mpl) is actually a mutant form of the human thrombopoietin receptor (c-Mpl). V-Mpl has part of the viral Env protein fused to the C-terminal end of c-Mpl and is activated through dimerization. This blocks normal differentiation and leads to uncontrolled cell growth. It has been suggested that one of the TGF-β receptors also is involved in oncogenesis, since mutations have been found frequently in colon cancer. TGF-β receptor signalling acts through the Smad family of transcription factors.

Two very important oncogene families encode the ras and rho family proteins. Ras itself is a G-protein, and activating mutations in H-Ras, K-Ras, and N-Ras have been found in nearly all kinds of human cancers. Several different Ras mutations are able to transform normal cells in tissue culture.[82-85] Mutations in many different Ras family members have been identified in cancer (e.g., Raf1, p110 PI3 kinase, Rin1, Mekk1), but the exact downstream signalling effects of each mutation are still unclear. The Ras and the Rho family of oncoproteins are linked by a small G-protein called *Rac*, which is required for transformation by Ras.[86-88] The Rho family of small G-proteins also regulates actin stress fiber formation.[89] The regular formation of actin filaments is required for G_1/S-phase entry. Thus, alterations in the Rho pathway may lead to premature entry into S phase by interference with cytoskeletal organization. The NF2 tumor suppressor gene also encodes a cytoskeletal protein.[90] The two oncogenes BRCA1 and BRCA2 are frequently mutated in affected families with breast cancer.[91-93] Their oncogenic activity might be associated with the transactivating property of the C-terminal ends of the genes, since mutations in this area inactivate this activity.[94]

Mitogen-activated protease kinases are potential downstream effectors of the Ras pathway.[95,96] The three different MAP kinase cascades are the ERK-, JNK/SAPK-, and the p38 pathways. The MAP kinase pathways consist of three types of kinases in a series, MAPK, MAPKK, and MAPKKK. The MAP kinase cascades all transmit responses from several different surface receptors to the nucleus.[97] Acti-

vation of the Ras-ERK pathway causes cyclin D overexpression and therefore promotes G_1-phase progression.[98]

Several oncogene proteins are localized in the nucleus and include transcription factors and chromatin regulatory proteins. A characteristic feature of acute promyelocytic leukemia (APL) is a t(15;17) translocation that fuses the Pml protein to the retinoic acid receptor-α (RAR-α). The chimeric protein disrupts a nuclear structure called *PODS* in a retinoic acid reversible fashion.[99,100] The detection and molecular characterization of the t(15;17) translocation, together with the development of retinoic acid therapy, was a direct result of oncogene research.[101-103] A variant of this chromosomal translocation results in a fusion protein between RAR-α and the promyelocytic leukemia Kruppel-like zink finger (PLZF) protein, which is observed in a subset of patients with APL.[104]

Recent experiments on oncoproteins have focused on apoptosis, the lethal response of a cell to either DNA damage or to signaling through cell surface "death" receptors. Key regulators of apoptosis induced by DNA damage are the multiple members of the bcl family of proteins, which include bcl, bcl-X_L, bax, and bad. Bcl-2 is involved in the t(14;18) chromosomal translocation, which is found in many leukemias and lymphomas of B-cell origin.[105-107] The disruption of these loci increases expression of bcl, and results in the uncontrolled accumulation of malignant B cells, due to an impaired balance between growth and apoptosis.[108-110] Apoptosis also is controlled by certain tumor suppressor genes, such as p53, that influence the cellular response to DNA damage. The nuclear histone deacetylase complex, which regulates the structural conformation of DNA and therefore the activation of several genes, is targeted by Eto, the fusion partner of the acute myelogenous leukemia AML1 gene. The t(8;21) translocation that occurs in acute myelogenous leukemia allows the formation of a stable complex between the histone deacetylase complex and Eto, with resultant leukemogenesis.[111-113] Other ongogenes that target the histone deacetylase complex are PLZF, PLZF-RAR-α, and BCL-6.[114-116] This implies that specific histone deacetylase inhibitors might be useful drugs in the treatment of myeloid leukemias. Recent reports provide evidence for this hypothesis (see below) and underline the important role of epigenetic phenomena in hematologic malignancies.

TUMOR SUPPRESSOR GENES (TABLE 12-3)

Almost every cancer harbors one or more abnormalities of tumor suppressor genes. These include mutations, translocations, and deletions. In addition, at least two epigenetic mechanisms, the hypermethylation of CpG islands in the promoter and the abberant acetylation of histones (especially histone H4), can silence tumor suppressor genes in a variety of human cancer cell lines and primary tumors.

It is remarkable that the products of the three most important tumor suppressor genes (rb, p53, and *p16^{INK4A}*) are interconnected biochemically. The retinoblastoma gene maps to chromosome 13q14 and has several downstream effectors, among which the transcription factor E2F is the best characterized.[117] The retinoblastoma gene family consists of three closely related proteins, rb, p107, and p130. All three proteins are able to interact with several E2F family members. Transcriptional activation and repression are mediated via complexes consisting of rb family members, E2F family members, and so-called DP proteins.[118] Besides its role in cell cycle control, rb can modulate RNA polymerase activity, thus linking cell-cycle progression to transcriptional regulation. More than 30 separate cellular proteins have been identified that bind to rb. These proteins can be divided into different groups, including transcription factors, growth factors, protein kinases, protein phosphatases and nuclear matrix proteins. Mutations of rb are frequent in leukemias, soft tissue sarcomas, breast,

TABLE 12-3 CHARACTERIZATION OF HUMAN TUMOR SUPPRESSOR GENES

TSG	CHROM. LOCUS	DISEASES	MAJOR MECHANISM(S) OF INACTIVATION
Cadherin 1 (E-cadherin)	16q22.1	malignomas of the gastrointestinal tract	hypermethylation of CpG islands, mutation
CDKN1A (p21, Cip1)	6p21.2	several human malignant and non-malignant diseases	homozygous deletion?
CDKN1C (p57, Kip2)	11p15.5	breast cancer?, Wilms tumor	Hypermethylation of CpG islands, mutations?
CDKN2A (p16)	9p21	several human cancers	homozygous deletion, hypermethylation of CpG-islands, mutations
CDKN2B (p15)	9p21	several human cancers	homozygous deletion, hypermethylation of CpG islands
p14^{ARF}	9p21	several human cancers	homozygous deletion, hypermethylation of CpG-islands, mutations
p53	17p13.1	several human cancers	mutations
WT1	11p13	Wilms tumor, nephroblastoma	Homozygous deletion, mutation
DMBT1	10q25.3-26.1	malignant brain tumors	Homozygous deletion
PTEN	10q23	glioblastoma, breast cancer	mutation
p73	1p36	leukemia, lymphoma	hypemethylation of CpG islands, mutation?
VHL	3p	von-Hippel-Lindau disease	hypermethylation of CpG islands
H19	11p15.5	hepatoblastoma, Wilms-Tu.	hypermethylation of CpG islands
HIC1	17p13	AML, HCC, breast cancer	hypermethylation of CpG islands
Rb	13q14.2	several human cancers	mutation
nm23	17q21.3-22	neuroblastoma, breast-, prostate cancer, melanoma	mutation, hypermethylation of CpG-islands?
H-cadherin	16q24	lung cancer	hypermethylation of CpG islands
N33	?	glioblastoma multiforme	hypermethylation of CpG-islands, mutation
S100A2	?	breast cancer	hypermethylation of CpG-islands, mutation
APC	5q21-q22	adenomatosis polyposis coli	homozygous deletion, hypermethylation of CpG-islands, mutation
NF-1, NF-2	17q11.2, 22q12.2	neurofibromatosis, bilateral acoustic neuroma	mutation

esophagus, prostate, and renal carcinomas.[119] Several viral or oncoproteins can bind to and inactivate rb.[120]

The p53 gene has been called a "guardian" of the genome because it transmits signals arising from various forms of DNA damage, leading to cell cycle arrest or apoptosis. The major regulator of p53 expression is MDM2. The MDM2 protein inhibits p53 transcription and stimulates p53 degradation.[121,122] The MDM2 binding region includes several phosphorylation sites, although the exact mechanism by which MDM2 regulates p53 degradation is still not clear.[121-124] The recently discovered p14^{ARF} tumor suppressor gene, which is encoded within the p16^{INK4A} locus by alternate splicing, controls MDM2 activity.[125,126] The p14^{ARF} gene shares exons 2 and 3 with p16^{INK4A} but has a distinct exon 1. The discovery that two important tumor suppressor genes are encoded by the same chromosomal locus and share several exons was unexpected and is unique in human biology. The p16^{INK4A} gene function depends on p53, since overexpression of p16^{INK4A} causes cell cycle arrest in p53-wild type cells but not in p53-dependent cells.[127] The transcription of p16^{INK4A} is regulated by E2F, which is under the control of rb.[128] This indicates the existence of yet another feedback loop, which links the rb pathway to p53.[129] The Ras protein is another recently identified p16^{INK4A} factor involved in MDM2-p53-p21-rb regulation.[130-132]

Abnormalities of p53 are found in slightly more than 50 percent of all human tumors and, surprisingly, even in some normal cells. It is unclear if these "normal" cells represent a pool of premalignant cells in an otherwise healthy body or if p53 changes are just one step in multistage tumorigenesis. Recently, a human p53 homologue, p73, has been described, which has DNA binding, transactivation, and oligomerization domains similar to p53. The p73 gene has been localized to chromosome 1p36, a common region of cytogenetic changes in cancer. If p73 is overexpressed, the pzl cyclin-dependent kinase inhibitor, a downstream element in the p53 pathway, is also upregulated.[133] The p73 protein also can bind p53, inhibiting its transcriptional regulatory activity.[134] Although p53 mutations are found in many cancers, p73 mutations apparently are much more rare. However, the p73 gene is inactivated by hypermethylation of CpG-islands in its promoter region in both leukemias and lymphomas.[135] This finding supports the hypothesis that p73 is a tumor suppressor gene on chromosome 1p.

Homozygous deletions of the p16^{INK4A}/p14^{ARF} gene locus on human chromosome 9p21 have been detected in gliomas,[56,136,137] primary cancers of the lung,[56,138,139] bladder,[140-142] head and neck,[143-145] as well as in acute T-cell leukemias[146-148] and mesotheliomas.[149] Since inherited mutations of p16^{INK4A} exon 2 may interfere with its expression and/or function, without causing an amino acid change in p14^{ARF}, it is clear that p16^{INK4A} inactivation alone is an important step in the evolution of malignant disease. However, in established tumor cell lines, nearly all chromosome 9p21 deletions disable the entire p16^{INK4A}/p14^{ARF} locus. The p15^{INK4B} gene, also located on chromosome 9p21, about 20 kDa centromeric of p16^{INK4A}, is deleted somewhat less frequently. Analyses of primary tumors, however, have shown that not all 9p21 deletions encompass these three tumor suppressor genes. One mechanism for disruption of the p15^{INK4B}/p14^{ARF}/p16^{INKA} region in T-cell leukemias may be the action of an illegitimate V(D)J recombinase.[150]

Hypermethylation of CpG islands in the promoter areas of both p16^{INK4A} and p15^{INK4B} are frequently found in hematological malignancies.[151-155] The availability of demethylating agents such as 5-aza-2'-deoxycytidine (decitabine) makes this phenomenon interesting for chemotherapy.[156,157] Decitabine has been used to treat patients suffering from different hematological malignancies and was reported to have activity in advanced myelodysplastic syndrome, accompanied by demethylation of the p16^{INK4A} promoter.[158-161] Transcriptional regulation by methylation is mediated by a multiprotein complex consisting of a MeCP2, a methylcytosine-binding protein with a transcriptional repressor domain that binds the corepressor mSin3A, which is itself one element of a multiprotein complex that includes histone deacetylase HDAC1 and HDAC2.[162,163] Therefore, reexpression of silenced genes can be achieved by demethylating DNA or by destabilizing histone deacetylases. A mammalian protein with specific demethylase activity for methylated CpG islands has been detected recently[164] indicating that gene silencing by epigenetic mechanisms is highly regulated in vertebrate organisms. Histone deacetylase inhibitors and demethylating agents act synergistically to induce genes silenced in cancer by hypermethylation.[165] Based on these findings, the MeCP2/SIN3A/HDAC1/2 complex may represent a new target for antineoplastic therapy.

In addition to the three major tumor suppressor gene pathways described above, several others have been identified. It is noteworthy that many different tumor suppressors can be inactivated by hypermethylation.

REFERENCES

1. Hartwell LH, Weinert TA: Checkpoints: controls that ensure the order of cell cycle events. *Science* 246:629, 1989.

2. Elledge SJ: Cell cycle checkpoints: preventing an identity crisis. *Science* 274:1664, 1996.

3. Russell P: Checkpoints on the road to mitosis. *Trends Biochem Sci* 23:399, 1998.

4. Murray AW: The genetics of cell cycle checkpoints. *Curr Opin Genet Dev* 5:5, 1995.

5. Hartwell LH, Kastan MB: Cell cycle control and cancer. *Science* 266:1821, 1994.

6. Rao PN, Johnson RT: Mammalian cell fusion: studies on the regulation of DNA synthesis and mitosis. *Nature* 225:159, 1970.

7. Lohka MJ, Hayes MK, Maller JL: Purification of maturation-promoting factor, an intracellular regulator of early mitotic events. *Proc Natl Acad Sci U S A* 85:3009, 1988.

8. Sherr CJ: Mammalian G1 cyclins. *Cell* 73:1059, 1993.

9. Pines J: Cyclins and cyclin-dependent kinases: take your partners. *Trends Biochem Sci* 18:195, 1993.

10. Pagano M, Pepperkok R, Verde F, Ansorge W, Draetta G: Cyclin A is required at two points in the human cell cycle. *Embo J* 11:961, 1992.

11. Resnitzky D, Hengst L, Reed SI: Cyclin A-associated kinase activity is rate limiting for entrance into S phase and is negatively regulated in G1 by p27Kip1. *Mol Cell Biol* 15:4347, 1995.

12. Meyerson M, Enders GH, Wu CL, Su LK, Gorka C, Nelson C, Harlow E, Tsai LH: A family of human cdc2-related protein kinases. *Embo J* 11:2909, 1992.

13. Ninomiya-Tsuji J, Nomoto S, Yasuda H, Reed SI, Matsumoto K: Cloning of a human cDNA encoding a CDC2-related kinase by complementation of a budding yeast cdc28 mutation. *Proc Natl Acad Sci U S A* 88:9006, 1991.

14. Solomon MJ: Activation of the various cyclin/cdc2 protein kinases. *Curr Opin Cell Biol* 5:180, 1993.

15. Lew J, Wang JH: Neuronal cdc2-like kinase. *Trends Biochem Sci* 20:33, 1995.

16. Matsushime H, Ewen ME, Strom DK, Kato JY, Hanks SK, Roussel MF, Sherr CJ: Identification and properties of an atypical catalytic subunit (p34PSK- J3/cdk4) for mammalian D type G1 cyclins. *Cell* 71:323, 1992.

17. Xiong Y, Zhang H, Beach D: D type cyclins associate with multiple protein kinases and the DNA replication and repair factor PCNA. *Cell* 71:505, 1992.

18. Meyerson M, Harlow E: Identification of G1 kinase activity for cdk6, a novel cyclin D partner. *Mol Cell Biol* 14:2077, 1994.

19. Fesquet D, Labbe JC, Derancourt J, et al: The MO15 gene encodes the catalytic subunit of a protein kinase that activates cdc2 and other cyclin-dependent kinases (CDKs) through phosphorylation of Thr161 and its homologues. *Embo J* 12:3111, 1993.

20. Fisher RP, Morgan DO: A novel cyclin associates with MO15/CDK7 to form the CDK-activating kinase. *Cell* 78:713, 1994.

21. Makela TP, Tassan JP, Nigg EA, Frutiger S, Hughes GJ, Weinberg RA: A cyclin associated with the CDK-activating kinase MO15. *Nature* 371:254, 1994.

22. Tassan JP, Jaquenoud M, Leopold P, Schultz SJ, Nigg EA: Identification of human cyclin-dependent kinase 8, a putative protein kinase partner for cyclin C. *Proc Natl Acad Sci U S A* 92:8871, 1995.

23. Leclerc V, Tassan JP, O'Farrell PH, Nigg EA, Leopold P: Drosophila Cdk8, a kinase partner of cyclin C that interacts with the large subunit of RNA polymerase II. *Mol Biol Cell* 7:505, 1996.

24. Rickert P, Seghezzi W, Shanahan F, Cho H, Lees E: Cyclin C/CDK8 is a novel CTD kinase associated with RNA polymerase II. *Oncogene* 12:2631, 1996.

25. Wei P, Garber ME, Fang SM, Fischer WH, Jones KA: A novel CDK9-associated C-type cyclin interacts directly with HIV-1 Tat and mediates its high-affinity, loop-specific binding to TAR RNA. *Cell* 92:451, 1998.

26. Peng J, Zhu Y, Milton JT, Price DH: Identification of multiple cyclin subunits of human P-TEFb. *Genes Dev* 12:755, 1998.

27. Bagella L, MacLachlan TK, Buono RJ, Pisano MM, Giordano A, De Luca A: Cloning of murine CDK9/PITALRE and its tissue-specific expression in development. *J Cell Physiol* 177:206, 1998.

28. Zhou Q, Chen D, Pierstorff E, Luo K: Transcription elongation factor P-TEFb mediates Tat activation of HIV-1 transcription at multiple stages. *Embo J* 17:3681, 1998.

29. Chen D, Fong Y, Zhou Q: Specific interaction of Tat with the human but not rodent P-TEFb complex mediates the species-specific Tat activation of HIV-1 transcription. *Proc Natl Acad Sci U S A* 96:2728, 1999.

30. Napolitano G, Licciardo P, Gallo P, Majello B, Giordano A, Lania L: The CDK9-associated cyclins T1 and T2 exert opposite effects on HIV-1 Tat activity. *AIDS* 13:1453, 1999.

31. Hunt T: Cyclins and their partners: from a simple idea to complicated reality. *Semin Cell Biol* 2:213, 1991.

32. Lees EM, Harlow E: Sequences within the conserved cyclin box of human cyclin A are sufficient for binding to and activation of cdc2 kinase. *Mol Cell Biol* 13:1194, 1993.

33. Wang J, Zindy F, Chenivesse X, Lamas E, Henglein B, Brechot C: Modification of cyclin A expression by hepatitis B virus DNA integration in a hepatocellular carcinoma. *Oncogene* 7:1653, 1992.

34. Dulic V, Lees E, Reed SI: Association of human cyclin E with a periodic G1-S phase protein kinase. *Science* 257:1958, 1992.

35. Ohtsubo M, Roberts JM: Cyclin-dependent regulation of G1 in mammalian fibroblasts. *Science* 259:1908, 1993.

36. Verde F, Dogterom M, Stelzer E, Karsenti E, Leibler S: Control of microtubule dynamics and length by cyclin A- and cyclin B- dependent kinases in Xenopus egg extracts. *J Cell Biol* 118:1097, 1992.

37. McGowan CH, Russell P, Reed SI: Periodic biosynthesis of the human M-phase promoting factor catalytic subunit p34 during the cell cycle. *Mol Cell Biol* 10:3847, 1990.

38. Buendia B, Draetta G, Karsenti E: Regulation of the microtubule nucleating activity of centrosomes in Xenopus egg extracts: role of cyclin A-associated protein kinase. *J Cell Biol* 116:1431, 1992.

39. Maldonado-Codina G, Glover DM: Cyclins A and B associate with chromatin and the polar regions of spindles, respectively, and do not undergo complete degradation at anaphase in syncytial Drosophila embryos. *J Cell Biol* 116:967, 1992.

40. Gallant P, Nigg EA: Cyclin B2 undergoes cell cycle-dependent nuclear translocation and, when expressed as a non-destructible mutant, causes mitotic arrest in HeLa cells. *J Cell Biol* 117:213, 1992.

41. Ookata K, Hisanaga S, Okano T, Tachibana K, Kishimoto T: Relocation and distinct subcellular localization of p34cdc2-cyclin B complex at meiosis reinitiation in starfish oocytes. *Embo J* 11:1763, 1992.

42. Fujinaga K, Cujec TP, Peng J, et al: The ability of positive transcription elongation factor B to transactivate human immunodeficiency virus transcription depends on a functional kinase domain, cyclin T1, and Tat. *J Virol* 72:7154, 1998.

43. Isel C, Karn J: Direct evidence that HIV-1 Tat stimulates RNA polymerase II carboxyl-terminal domain hyperphosphorylation during transcriptional elongation. *J Mol Biol* 290:929, 1999.

44. Garriga J, Peng J, Parreno M, Price DH, Henderson EE, Grana X: Upregulation of cyclin T1/CDK9 complexes during T cell activation. *Oncogene* 17:3093, 1998.

45. MacLachlan TK, Sang N, De Luca A, Puri PL, Levrero M, Giordano A: Binding of CDK9 to TRAF2. *J Cell Biochem* 71:467, 1998.

46. Gu Y, Turck CW, Morgan DO: Inhibition of CDK2 activity in vivo by an associated 20K regulatory subunit. *Nature* 366:707, 1993.

47. Harper JW, Adami GR, Wei N, Keyomarsi K, Elledge SJ: The p21 Cdk-interacting protein Cip1 is a potent inhibitor of G1 cyclin-dependent kinases. *Cell* 75:805, 1993.

48. Xiong Y, Hannon GJ, Zhang H, Casso D, Kobayashi R, Beach D: p21 is a universal inhibitor of cyclin kinases [see comments]. *Nature* 366:701, 1993.

49. Nourse J, Firpo E, Flanagan WM, et al: Interleukin-2-mediated elimination of the p27Kip1 cyclin-dependent kinase inhibitor prevented by rapamycin. *Nature* 372:570, 1994.

50. Kato JY, Matsuoka M, Polyak K, Massague J, Sherr CJ: Cyclic AMP-induced G1 phase arrest mediated by an inhibitor (p27Kip1) of cyclin-dependent kinase 4 activation. *Cell* 79:487, 1994.

51. Serrano M, Hannon GJ, Beach D: A new regulatory motif in cell-cycle control causing specific inhibition of cyclin D/CDK4 [see comments]. *Nature* 366:704, 1993.

52. Guan KL, Jenkins CW, Li Y, et al: Growth suppression by p18, a p16^{INK4A}INK4/MTS1- and p14^{INK4B}/MTS2-related CDK6 inhibitor, correlates with wild-type prb function. *Genes Dev* 8:2939, 1994.

53. Chan FK, Zhang J, Cheng L, Shapiro DN, Winoto A: Identification of human and mouse p19, a novel CDK4 and CDK6 inhibitor with homology to p16^{INK4A}ink4. *Mol Cell Biol* 15:2682, 1995.

54. Hirai H, Roussel MF, Kato JY, Ashmun RA, Sherr CJ: Novel INK4 proteins, p19 and p18, are specific inhibitors of the cyclin D-dependent kinases CDK4 and CDK6. *Mol Cell Biol* 15:2672, 1995.

55. Hannon GJ, Beach D: p15^{INK4BINK4B} is a potential effector of Tgf-beta-induced cell cycle arrest [see comments]. *Nature* 371:257, 1994.

56. Nobori T, Miura K, Wu DJ, Lois A, Takabayashi K, Carson DA: Deletions of the cyclin-dependent kinase-4 inhibitor gene in multiple human cancers. *Nature* 368:753, 1994.

57. Schwob E, Bohm T, Mendenhall MD, Nasmyth K: The B-type cyclin kinase inhibitor p40SIC1 controls the G1 to S transition in *S. cerevisiae* [published erratum appears in *Cell* 1996 Jan 12;84(1):following 174]. *Cell* 79:233, 1994.

58. Bai C, Sen P, Hofmann K, et al: SKP1 connects cell cycle regulators to the ubiquitin proteolysis machinery through a novel motif, the F-box. *Cell* 86:263, 1996.

59. Feldman RM, Correll CC, Kaplan KB, Deshaies RJ: A complex of Cdc4p, Skp1p, and Cdc53p/cullin catalyzes ubiquitination of the phosphorylated CDK inhibitor Sic1p [see comments]. *Cell* 91:221, 1997.

60. Skowyra D, Koepp DM, Kamura T, et al: Reconstitution of G1 cyclin ubiquitination with complexes containing SCFGrr1 and Rbx1 [see comments]. *Science* 284:662, 1999.

61. Koepp DM, Harper JW, Elledge SJ: How the cyclin became a cyclin: regulated proteolysis in the cell cycle. *Cell* 97:431, 1999.

62. Hunter T, Pines J: Cyclins and cancer. II: Cyclin D and CDK inhibitors come of age [see comments]. *Cell* 79:573, 1994.

63. Sherr CJ, Roberts JM: Inhibitors of mammalian G1 cyclin-dependent kinases. *Genes Dev* 9:1149, 1995.

64. Zhang H, Xiong Y, Beach D: Proliferating cell nuclear antigen and p21 are components of multiple cell cycle kinase complexes. *Mol Biol Cell* 4:897, 1993.

65. El-Deiry WS, Harper JW, O'Connor PM, et al: WAF1/CIP1 is induced in p53-mediated G1 arrest and apoptosis. *Cancer Res* 54:1169, 1994.

66. Noda A, Ning Y, Venable SF, Pereira-Smith OM, Smith JR: Cloning of senescent cell-derived inhibitors of DNA synthesis using an expression screen. *Exp Cell Res* 211:90, 1994.

67. Li Y, Jenkins CW, Nichols MA, Xiong Y: Cell cycle expression and p53 regulation of the cyclin-dependent kinase inhibitor p21. *Oncogene* 9:2261, 1994.

68. Deng C, Zhang P, Harper JW, Elledge SJ, Leder P: Mice lacking p21CIP1/WAF1 undergo normal development, but are defective in G1 checkpoint control. *Cell* 82:675, 1995.

69. Dirick L, Nasmyth K: Positive feedback in the activation of G1 cyclins in yeast. *Nature* 351:754, 1991.

70. Rodrigues GA, Park M: Dimerization mediated through a leucine zipper activates the oncogenic potential of the met receptor tyrosine kinase. *Mol Cell Biol* 13:6711, 1993.

71. Mezzelani A, Alasio L, Bartoli C, et al: c-eRbB2/neu gene and chromosome 17 analysis in breast cancer by Fish on archival cytological fine-needle aspirates. *Br J Cancer* 80:519, 1999.

72. Haapasalo H, Hyytinen E, Sallinen P, Helin H, Kallioniemi OP, Isola J: c-eRbB-2 in astrocytomas: infrequent overexpression by immunohistochemistry and absence of gene amplification by fluorescence in situ hybridization. *Br J Cancer* 73:620, 1996.

73. Engelhard HH, Wolters M, Criswell PS: Analysis of c-eRbB2 protein content of human glioma cells and tumor tissue. *J Neurooncol* 23:31, 1995.

74. Morris SW, Kirstein MN, Valentine MB, Dittmer KG, Shapiro DN, Saltman DL, Look AT: Fusion of a kinase gene, ALK, to a nucleolar protein gene, NPM, in non-Hodgkin's lymphoma [published erratum appears in *Science* 1995 Jan 20;267(5196):316-7]. *Science* 263:1281, 1994.

75. Fujimoto J, Shiota M, Iwahara T, et al: Characterization of the transforming activity of p80, a hyperphosphorylated protein in a Ki-1 lymphoma cell line with chromosomal translocation t(2;5). *Proc Natl Acad Sci U S A* 93:4181, 1996.

76. Golub TR, Barker GF, Lovett M, Gilliland DG: Fusion of PDGF receptor beta to a novel ets-like gene, tel, in chronic myelomonocytic leukemia with t(5;12) chromosomal translocation. *Cell* 77:307, 1994.

77. Mittebauer G, Nemeth P, Wacha S, et al: Quantification of minimal residual disease in patients with BCR-ABL- positive acute lymphoblastic leukaemia using quantitative competitive polymerase chain reaction. *Br J Haematol* 106:634, 1999.

78. Elmaagacli AH, Beelen DW, Opalka B, Seeber S, Schaefer UW: The risk of residual molecular and cytogenetic disease in patients with Philadelphia-chromosome positive first chronic phase chronic myelogenous leukemia is reduced after transplantation of allogeneic peripheral blood stem cells compared with bone marrow [see comments]. *Blood* 94:384, 1999.

79. Bose S, Deininger M, Gora-Tybor J, Goldman JM, Melo JV: The presence of typical and atypical BCR-ABL fusion genes in leukocytes of normal individuals: biologic significance and implications for the assessment of minimal residual disease. *Blood* 92:3362, 1998.

80. Hoppener JW, Lips CJ: RET receptor tyrosine kinase gene mutations: molecular biological, physiological and clinical aspects. *Eur J Clin Invest* 26:613, 1996.

81. Galisteo ML, Dikic I, Batzer AG, Langdon WY, Schlessinger J: Tyrosine phosphorylation of the c-cbl proto-oncogene protein product and association with epidermal growth factor (EGF) receptor upon EGF stimulation. *J Biol Chem* 270:20242, 1995.

82. Graham SM, Cox AD, Drivas G, et al: Aberrant function of the Ras-related protein TC21/R-Ras2 triggers malignant transformation. *Mol Cell Biol* 14:4108, 1994.

83. Graham SM, Oldham SM, Martin CB, et al: TC21 and Ras share indistinguishable transforming and differentiating activities. *Oncogene* 18:2107, 1999.

84. Cox AD, Brtva TR, Lowe DG, Der CJ: R-Ras induces malignant, but not morphologic, transformation of NIH3T3 cells. *Oncogene* 9:3281, 1994.

85. Saez R, Chan AM, Miki T, Aaronson SA: Oncogenic activation of human R-ras by point mutations analogous to those of prototype H-ras oncogenes. *Oncogene* 9:2977, 1994.

86. Khosravi-Far R, Solski PA, Clark GJ, Kinch MS, Der CJ: Activation of Rac1, RhoA, and mitogen-activated protein kinases is required for Ras transformation. *Mol Cell Biol* 15:6443, 1995.

87. Qiu RG, Chen J, Kirn D, McCormick F, Symons M: An essential role for Rac in Ras transformation. *Nature* 374:457, 1995.

88. Qiu RG, Chen J, McCormick F, Symons M: A role for Rho in Ras transformation. *Proc Natl Acad Sci U S A* 92:11781, 1995.

89. Nobes CD. Hall A: Rho, rac, and cdc42 GTPases regulate the assembly of multimolecular focal complexes associated with actin stress fibers, lamellipodia, and filopodia. *Cell* 81:53, 1995.

90. Belliveau MJ, Lutchman M, Claudio JO, Marineau C, Rouleau GA: Schwannomin: new insights into this member of the band 4.1 superfamily. *Biochem Cell Biol* 73:733, 1995.

91. Turner BC, Harrold E, Matloff E, et al: BRCA1/BRCA2 germline mutations in locally recurrent breast cancer patients after lumpectomy and radiation therapy: implications for breast-conserving management in patients with BRCA1/BRCA2 mutations. *J Clin Oncol* 17:301724, 1999.

92. Neuhausen SL, Ostrander EA: Mutation testing of early-onset breast cancer genes BRCA1 and BRCA2. *Genet Test* 1:75, 1997.

93. Yang X, Lippman ME: BRCA1 and BRCA2 in breast cancer. *Breast Cancer Res Treat* 54:1, 1999.

94. Chapman MS, Verma IM: Transcriptional activation by BRCA1 [letter; comment]. *Nature* 382:678, 1996.

95. Coso OA, Chiariello M, Yu JC, et al: The small GTP-binding proteins Rac1 and Cdc42 regulate the activity of the JNK/SAPK signaling pathway. *Cell* 81:1137, 1995.

96. Minden A, Lin A, Claret FX, Abo A, Karin M: Selective activation of the JNK signaling cascade and c-Jun transcriptional activity by the small GTPases Rac and Cdc42Hs. *Cell* 81:1147, 1995.

97. Johnson NL, Gardner AM, Diener KM, et al: Signal transduction pathways regulated by mitogen-activated/extracellular response kinase kinase induce cell death. *J Biol Chem* 271:3229, 1996.

98. Lavoie JN, Rivard N, L'Allemain G, Pouyssegur, J: A temporal and biochemical link between growth factor-activated MAP kinases, cyclin D1 induction and cell cycle entry. *Prog Cell Cycle Res* 2:49, 1996.

99. Dyck JA, Maul GG, Miller WH Jr, Chen JD, Kakizuka A, Evans RM: A novel macromolecular structure is a target of the promyelocyte-retinoic acid receptor oncoprotein. *Cell* 76:333, 1994.

100. Koken MH, Puvion-Dutilleul F, Guillemin MC, et al: The t(15;17) translocation alters a nuclear body in a retinoic acid-reversible fashion. *Embo J* 13:1073, 1994.

101. Martinelli G, Ottaviani E, Visani G, Testoni N, Montefusco V, Tura S: Long-term disease-free acute promyelocytic leukemia patients really can be cured at molecular level [letter]. *Haematologica* 83:860, 1998.

102. Fenaux P, Chomienne C, Degos L: Acute promyelocytic leukemia: biology and treatment. *Semin Oncol* 24:92, 1997.

103. Hussey CE, Lyon E, Millson A, Lay MJ, Wittwer CT, Segal GH: A rapid practical RT-PCR-based approach for the detection of the PML/RAR alpha fusion transcript in acute promyelocytic leukemia. *Am J Clin Pathol* 112:256, 1999.

104. Chen Z, Brand NJ, Chen A, et al: Fusion between a novel Kruppel-like zinc finger gene and the retinoic acid receptor-alpha locus due to a variant t(11;17) translocation associated with acute promyelocytic leukaemia. *Embo J* 12:1161, 1993.

105. Monni O, Franssila K, Joensuu H, Knuutila S: BCL2 overexpression in diffuse large B-cell lymphoma. *Leuk Lymphoma* 34:45, 1999.

106. Kramer MH, Hermans J, Wijburg E, et al: Clinical relevance of BCL2, BCL6, and MYC rearrangements in diffuse large B-cell lymphoma. *Blood* 92:3152, 1998.

107. Kojima K, Taniwaki M, Yoshino T, et al: Trisomy 12 and t(14;18) in B-cell chronic lymphocytic leukemia. *Int J Hematol* 67:199, 1998.

108. Bonnotte B, Favre N, Moutet M, et al: Bcl-2-mediated inhibition of apoptosis prevents immunogenicity and restores tumorigenicity of spontaneously regressive tumors. *J Immunol* 161:1433, 1998.

109. Yin DX, Schimke RT: Inhibition of apoptosis by overexpressing Bcl-2 enhances gene amplification by a mechanism independent of aphidicolin pretreatment. *Proc Natl Acad Sci U S A* 93:3394, 1996.

110. Marin MC, Jost CA, Irwin MS, DeCaprio JA, Caput D, Kaelin WG Jr: Viral oncoproteins discriminate between p53 and the p53 homolog p73. *Mol Cell Biol* 18:6316, 1998.

111. Gelmetti V, Zhang J, Fanelli M, Minucci S, Pelicci PG, Lazar MA: Aberrant recruitment of the nuclear receptor corepressor-histone deacetylase complex by the acute myeloid leukemia fusion partner ETO. *Mol Cell Biol* 18:7185, 1998.

112. Lutterbach B, Westendorf JJ, Linggi B, et al: ETO, a target of t(8;21) in acute leukemia, interacts with the N-CoR and mSin3 corepressors. *Mol Cell Biol* 18:7176, 1998.

113. Wang J, Hoshino T, Redner RL, Kajigaya S, Liu JM: ETO, fusion partner in t(8;21) acute myeloid leukemia, represses transcription by interaction with the human N-CoR/mSin3/HDAC1 complex. *Proc Natl Acad Sci U S A* 95:10860, 1998.

114. Wong CW, Privalsky ML: Components of the SMRT corepressor complex exhibit distinctive interactions with the POZ domain oncoproteins PLZF, PLZF-RARα, and BCL-6. *J Biol Chem* 273:27695, 1998.

115. David G, Alland L, Hong SH, Wong CW, DePinho RA, Dejean A: Histone deacetylase associated with mSin3A mediates repression by the acute promyelocytic leukemia-associated PLZF protein. *Oncogene* 16:2549, 1998.

116. Dhordain P, Lin RJ, Quief S, et al: The LAZ3(BCL-6) oncoprotein recruits a SMRT/mSIN3A/histone deacetylase containing complex to mediate transcriptional repression. *Nucleic Acids Res* 26:4645, 1998.

117. Yunis JJ, Ramsay N: Retinoblastoma and subband deletion of chromosome 13. *Am J Dis Child* 132:161, 1978.

118. Grana X, Garriga J, Mayol X: Role of the retinoblastoma protein family, pRB, p107 and p130 in the negative control of cell growth. *Oncogene* 17:3365, 1998.

119. Bookstein R, Lee WH: Molecular genetics of the retinoblastoma suppressor gene. *Crit Rev Oncog* 2:211, 1991.

120. Chellappan S, Kraus VB, Kroger B, et al: Adenovirus E1A, simian virus 40 tumor antigen, and human papillomavirus E7 protein share the capacity to disrupt the interaction between transcription factor E2F and the retinoblastoma gene product. *Proc Natl Acad Sci U S A* 89:4549, 1992.

121. Haupt Y, Maya R, Kazaz A, Oren M: Mdm2 promotes the rapid degradation of p53. *Nature* 387:296, 1997.

122. Kubbutat MH, Jones SN, Vousden KH: Regulation of p53 stability by Mdm2. *Nature* 387:299, 1997.

123. Honda R, Tanaka H, Yasuda H: Oncoprotein MDM2 is a ubiquitin ligase E3 for tumor suppressor p53. *FEBS Lett* 420:25, 1997.

124. Roth J, Dobbelstein M, Freedman DA, Shenk T, Levine AJ: Nucleocytoplasmic shuttling of the hdm2 oncoprotein regulates the levels of the p53 protein via a pathway used by the human immunodeficiency virus rev protein. *Embo J* 17:554, 1998.

125. Quelle DE, Zindy F, Ashmun RA, Sherr CJ: Alternative reading frames of the^{INK4A} tumor suppressor gene encode two unrelated proteins capable of inducing cell cycle arrest. *Cell* 83:993, 1995.

126. Chin L, Pomerantz J, DePinho RA: The^{INK4A}/ARF tumor suppressor: one gene—two products—two pathways. *Trends Biochem Sci* 23:291, 1998.

127. Kamijo T, Zindy F, Roussel MF, et al: Tumor suppression at the mouse^{INK4A} locus mediated by the alternative reading frame product p19ARF. *Cell* 91:649, 1997.

128. Bates S, Phillips AC, Clark PA, et al: p14arf links the tumour suppressors Rb and p53 [letter]. *Nature* 395:124, 1998.

129. Palmero I, Pantoja C, Serrano M: p19arf links the tumour suppressor p53 to Ras [letter]. *Nature* 395:125, 1998.

130. Prives C: Signaling to p53: breaking the MDM2-p53 circuit. *Cell* 95:5, 1998.

131. Sherr CJ: Tumor surveillance via the ARF-p53 pathway. *Genes Dev* 12:2984, 1998.

132. Prives C, Hall PA: The p53 pathway. *J Pathol* 187:112, 1999.

133. Jost CA, Marin MC, Kaelin WGJr: p73 is a simian [correction of human] p53-related protein that can induce apoptosis [see comments] [published erratum appears in *Nature* 1999 Jun 24;399(6738):817]. *Nature* 389:191, 1997.

134. Di Como CJ, Gaiddon C, Prives C: p73 function is inhibited by tumor-derived p53 mutants in mammalian cells. *Mol Cell Biol* 19:1438, 1999.

135. Kawano S, Miller CW, Gombart AF, et al: Loss of p73 gene expression in leukemias/lymphomas due to hypermethylation. *Blood* 94:1113, 1999.

136. Nishikawa R, Furnari FB, Lin H, et al: Loss of P16^{INK4A}INK4 expression is frequent in high grade gliomas. *Cancer Res* 55:1941, 1995.

137. Olopade OI, Jenkins RB, Ransom DT, et al: Molecular analysis of deletions of the short arm of chromosome 9 in human gliomas. *Cancer Res* 52:2523, 1992.

138. Okami K, Cairns P, Westra WH, et al: Detailed deletion mapping at chromosome 9p21 in non-small cell lung cancer by microsatellite analysis and fluorescence in situ hybridization. *Int J Cancer* 74:588, 1997.

139. Schmid M, Malicki D, Nobori T, et al: Homozygous deletions of methylthioadenosine phosphorylase (MTAP) are more frequent than p16^{INK4AINK4A} (CDKN2) homozygous deletions in primary non-small cell lung cancers (NSCLC). *Oncogene* 17:2669, 1998.

140. Stadler WM, Olopade OI: The 9p21 region in bladder cancer cell lines: large homozygous deletion inactivate the CDKN2, CDKN2B and MTAP genes. *Urol Res* 24:239, 1996.

141. Balazs M, Carroll P, Kerschmann R, Sauter G, Waldman FM: Frequent homozygous deletion of cyclin-dependent kinase inhibitor 2 (MTS1, p16^{INK4A}) in superficial bladder cancer detected by fluorescence in situ hybridization. *Genes Chromosomes Cancer* 19:84, 1997.

142. Orlow I, Lacombe L, Hannon GJ, et al: Deletion of the p16^{INK4A} and p15^{INK4B} genes in human bladder tumors [see comments]. *J Natl Cancer Inst* 87:1524, 1995.

143. Gonzalez MV, Pello MF, Lopez-Larrea C, Suarez C, Menendez MJ, Coto E: Deletion and methylation of the tumour suppressor gene p16^{INK4A}/CDKN2 in primary head and neck squamous cell carcinoma. *J Clin Pathol* 50:509, 1997.

144. Matsuura K, Shiga K, Yokoyama J, Saijo S, Miyagi T, Takasaka T: Loss of heterozygosity of chromosome 9p21 and 7q31 is correlated with high incidence of recurrent tumor in head and neck squamous cell carcinoma. *Anticancer Res* 18:453, 1998.

145. Waber P, Dlugosz S, Cheng QC, Truelson J, Nisen PD: Genetic alterations of chromosome band 9p21 in head and neck cancer are not restricted to p16^{INK4AINK4A}. *Oncogene* 15:1699, 1997.

146. Yamada Y, Hatta Y, Murata K, et al: Deletions of p15^{INK4B} and/or p16^{INK4A} genes as a poor-prognosis factor in adult T-cell leukemia. *J Clin Oncol* 15:1778, 1997.

147. Hatta Y, Hirama T, Miller CW, Yamada Y, Tomonaga M, Koeffler HP: Homozygous deletions of the p15^{INK4B} (MTS2) and p16^{INK4A} (CDKN2/MTS1) genes in adult T-cell leukemia. *Blood* 85:2699, 1995.

148. Hori Y, Hori H, Yamada Y, et al: The methylthioadenosine phosphorylase gene is frequently co-deleted with the p16^{INK4AINK4A} gene in acute type adult T-cell leukemia. *Int J Cancer* 75:51, 1998.

149. Kratzke RA, Otterson GA, Lincoln CE, et al: Immunohistochemical analysis of the p16^{INK4A}INK4 cyclin-dependent kinase inhibitor in malignant mesothelioma. *J Natl Cancer Inst* 87:1870, 1995.

150. Cayuela JM, Gardie B, Sigaux F: Disruption of the multiple tumor

suppressor gene MTS1/p16$^{INK4A(INK4A)}$/CDKN2 by illegitimate V(D)J recombinase activity in T-cell acute lymphoblastic leukemias. *Blood* 90:3720, 1997.

151. Jaffrain-Rea ML, Ferretti E, Toniato E, Cannita K, Santoro A, Di Stefano, Ricevuto E, Maroder M, Tamburrano G, Cantore G, Gulino A, Martinotti S: p16 (INK4a, MTS-1) gene polymorphism and methylation status in human pituitary tumours. *Clin Endocrinol (Oxf)* 51(3):317, 1999.

152. Melki JR, Vincent PC, Clark SJ: Concurrent DNA hypermethylation of multiple genes in acute myeloid leukemia. *Cancer Res* 59:3730, 1999.

153. Nakamura M, Sugita K, Inukai T, et al: p16^{INK4A}/Mts1/^{INK4A} gene is frequently inactivated by hypermethylation in childhood acute lymphoblastic leukemia with 11q23 translocation. *Leukemia* 13:884, 1999.

154. Baylin SB, Herman JG, Graff JR, Vertino PM, Issa JP: Alterations in DNA methylation: a fundamental aspect of neoplasia. *Adv Cancer Res* 72:141, 1998.

155. Drexler HG: Review of alterations of the cyclin-dependent kinase inhibitor INK4 family genes p15^{INK4B}, p16^{INK4A}, p18 and p19 in human leukemia-lymphoma cells. *Leukemia* 12:845, 1998.

156. Timmermann S, Hinds PW, Munger K: Re-expression of endogenous p16^{INK4AINK4A} in oral squamous cell carcinoma lines by 5-aza-2'-deoxycytidine treatment induces a senescence-like state. *Oncogene* 17:3445, 1998.

157. Bender CM, Pao MM, Jones PA: Inhibition of DNA methylation by 5-aza-2'-deoxycytidine suppresses the growth of human tumor cell lines. *Cancer Res* 58:95, 1998.

158. Kantarjian HM, O'Brien SM, Keating M, et al: Results of decitabine therapy in the accelerated and blastic phases of chronic myelogenous leukemia. *Leukemia* 11:1617, 1997.

159. Zagonel V, Lo Re G, Marotta G, et al: 5-Aza-2'-deoxycytidine (Decitabine) induces trilineage response in unfavourable myelodysplastic syndromes. *Leukemia* 7(suppl 1):30, 1993.

160. Petti MC, Mandelli F, Zagonel V, et al: Pilot study of 5-aza-2'-deoxycytidine (Decitabine) in the treatment of poor prognosis acute myelogenous leukemia patients: preliminary results. *Leukemia* 7(suppl 1):36, 1993.

161. Quesnel B, Guillerm G, Vereecque R, et al: Methylation of the p15$^{INK4B(INK4B)}$ gene in myelodysplastic syndromes is frequent and acquired during disease progression. *Blood* 91:2985, 1998.

162. Razin A: CpG methylation, chromatin structure and gene silencing—a three-way connection. *Embo J* 17:4905, 1998.

163. Jones PL, Veenstra GJ, Wade PA, et al: Methylated DNA and MeCP2 recruit histone deacetylase to repress transcription. *Nat Genet* 19:187, 1998.

164. Bhattacharya SK, Ramchandani S, Cervoni N, Szyf M: A mammalian protein with specific demethylase activity for mCpG DNA [see comments]. *Nature* 397:579, 1999.

165. Cameron EE, Bachman KE, Myohanen S, Herman JG, Baylin SB: Synergy of demethylation and histone deacetylase inhibition in the re-expression of genes silenced in cancer. *Nat Genet* 21:103, 1999.

THE CLUSTER OF DIFFERENTIATION ANTIGENS

THOMAS J. KIPPS

DEFINITION AND HISTORY

The advent of monoclonal antibody technology revolutionized the classification of cell surface antigens. The availability of virtually unlimited quantities of monospecific typing reagents permitted the identification and study of previously unrecognized lymphoid and myeloid-specific surface proteins. However, as the number of monoclonal antibodies (mAbs) detecting cell surface differentiation antigens grew, it became apparent that international standardization was required.

Accordingly, six international workshops have been held to exchange monoclonal antibodies to compare their ability to react with human cells and/or human cell proteins. Monoclonal antibodies that have similar patterns of reactivity with various tissues or cell types are assigned to a cluster group. An antigen that is recognized by a cluster of antibodies can be assigned a cluster of differentiation number, or CD number. If only one monoclonal antibody defines a cluster, or if all monoclonal antibodies defining a cluster originate from the same laboratory, a suffix w is added to the CD designation. The last conference, held in Kobe, Japan, November 1996, compiled the data obtained from testing hundreds of different monoclonal antibodies.[1] This conference culminated in the classification of over three dozen new CD antigens.

All CD antigens defined at this and previous workshops are presented in Table 13-1, along with any common names used before a CD number was assigned in the column marked *Other Names*. Table 13-1 summarizes what is known about each CD antigen's: molecular size, orientation or attachment to the plasma membrane (O), tissue distribution, and known or suspected physiology. Table 13-1 also indicates the chromosomal location of the gene encoding each CD antigen and the GenBank accession number of the reference cDNA encoding the antigen in the column marked *Genetics*. Finally, in the column labeled *Selected References*, Table 13-1 cites a few key primary papers and review articles for each CD antigen.

Additional information regarding the CD antigens can be found on the Internet. The accession numbers provided in the column labeled *Genetics* can be used to obtain the primary nucleic acid and protein sequences of each CD antigen using the GenBank website on the Internet (see http://www.ncbi.nlm.nih.gov or http://www3.ncbi.nm.nih.gov/Entrez/) or by email at: retrieve@ncbi.nlm.nih.gov. Other useful websites for analyzing protein or genomic structure are the websites for the European Bioinformatics Institute (see http://www.ebi.ad.uk), the SWISSPROT protein structure database (see http://www.expasy.ch/), the central repository for genomic mapping data from the Human Genome Initiative (see http://gdbwww.gdb.org/), or the archive of three-dimensional structures from the Brookhaven Na-tional Laboratory (see http://pdbpdb.bnl.gov/). A comprehensive list of other useful servers is provided by SWISSPROT on the Internet, at http://www.expasy.ch/alinks.htm.

GENERAL STRUCTURE OF MEMBRANE ANTIGENS

Membrane antigens are classified into different groups, depending on how they orient or anchor themselves to the plasma membrane (Fig. 13-1).

TYPE I TRANSMEMBRANE PROTEINS (I)

Type I transmembrane molecules have their COOH-termini in the cytoplasm and their NH_2-termini outside the cell. Each of these molecules generally has a signal sequence at the NH_2-terminus that is cleaved off after the molecule passes into the endoplasmic reticulum. Afterwards it may be glycosylated in the Golgi apparatus (if it contains glycosylation sites) and then expressed on the cell surface. These proteins commonly serve as cell surface receptors and/or ligands. Many belong to the immunoglobulin superfamily (see Chap. 83, Functions of B lymphocytes and Plasma Cells, and Chap. 84, Functions of T Lymphocytes).

Each type I protein generally has a transmembrane domain of approximately 25 hydrophobic amino acid residues followed by a cluster of basic amino acids that bind the protein to phospholipid head groups inside the surface membrane bilayer. The transmembrane domain does not contain any charged amino acid residues, such as Arg, Asn, Asp, Glu, Gln, His, or Lys, except when it associates with the transmembrane domain of another cell surface protein to form a multimeric complex. An example of this is the multimeric complex formed by the CD3 proteins and the two chains of the T-cell receptor for antigen (see Chap. 84, Functions of T Lymphocytes).

TYPE II TRANSMEMBRANE PROTEINS (II)

Type II transmembrane proteins have an opposite orientation to that of type I transmembrane proteins. The NH_2-terminus is located inside the cell, and the COOH-terminus is extracellular. These proteins often have uncleaved signal sequences for transmembrane domains, allowing for their cleavage and release from the cell surface. As such, these proteins may double as cell surface antigens and plasma proteins, each often having a physiologic effect on cells bearing the respective ligand.

TYPE III TRANSMEMBRANE PROTEINS (III)

Type III transmembrane proteins cross the plasma membrane more than once. Some pass through the bilayer as many as 12 times, such as the multidrug resistance transporter protein, MDR1. Because they cross the membrane multiple times, these molecules can form channels that often are used to transport ions or small molecules through the lipid bilayer. An important subgroup of type III transmembrane proteins that commonly are found on leukocytes is the tetra-span family. These proteins each pass through the surface bilayer 4 times and have both their COOH-termini and NH_2-termini inside the cell. Most of the type III transmembrane proteins listed in Table 13-1 belong to this family. An example is CD20, a molecule that is postulated to form a calcium channel for B lymphocytes that is required for B-cell activation.

TYPE IV TRANSMEMBRANE PROTEINS (IV)

Type IV proteins can be distinguished from type III proteins by the presence of a water-filled transmembrane channel. None of the current CD antigens have such a membrane organization.

Acronyms and abbreviations that appear in this chapter include: CD, cluster of differentiation; GPI, glycosyl-phosphatidylinositol; mAbs, monoclonal antibodies; MDR1, multidrug resistance transporter protein; PI-PLC, phosphatidylinositol phospholipase C; PNH, paroxysmal nocturnal hemoglobinuria; sIg, surface immunoglobulin.

TABLE 13-1　CLUSTER OF DIFFERENTIATION ANTIGENS DEFINED AS OF THE SIXTH INTERNATIONAL WORKSHOP ON LEUKOCYTE TYPING

ANTIGEN	OTHER NAMES	SIZE	O	GENETICS	DISTRIBUTION	PHYSIOLOGY	SELECTED REFERENCES
CD1a–e	T6	43–49	I	1q22-23 X04450..1a M28826..1b M28827..1c J04142..1d X14975..1e	cortical thymocytes, DC, Langerhans cells (CD1a), brain astrocytes, dermal cells, some B cells (CD1c, d)	There exist six different isoforms with functional domains of each encoded by separate exons. Each is involved in "nonclassical" presentation of antigens, including lipids, that is involved in the delivery of signals for lymphocyte activation.	Curr Opin Immunol 11:100, 1999 Curr Opin Microbiol 2:89, 1999 Immunol Today 19:362, 1998
CD2	Sheep red blood cell-Rc; Leukocyte function antigen-2 (LFA-2); Leu-5; T11; Tp50	45–58	I	1p13 M16445	thymocytes, T cells, NK cells	Serves as a ligand for CD48 and CD58 (LFA-3) that enhances adhesion between T cells and APC that also may have role in signal transduction.	Immunol Rev 163:217, 1998 Immunol Today 17:177, 1996 Nature 384:134, 1996
CD3	CD3γ	25–28	I	11q23 X04145	pan T cell	A family of proteins that form the signal transduction complex for T cell Rc for antigen (see Chap. 84).	Adv Immunol 72:103, 1999 Seminars in Hematology 35:310, 1998
	CD3δ	20	I	11q23 X03934			Curr Opin Immunol 8:282, 1996 Science 274:209, 1996
	CD3ε	20	I	11q23 X03884			Nature 384:134, 1996 Curr Opin Immunol 8:93, 1996
	CD3ζ	16	I	1q22 J04132			
CD4	T4; Leu-3	55	I	12pter-p12 M12807	thymocytes, helper/inducer T cells, monocytes, MØ, DC	Serves as a Rc for class II MHC to facilitate recognition of peptide antigens and also may have role in signal transduction. CD4 also is a co-Rc for HIV gp120.	Transplant Proc 31:820, 1999 Int J Biochem Cell Bio 29:871, 1997 Curr Top Microbiol Immunol 205, 1996
CD5	Tp67, Leu-1	67	I	11q13 M15177	T cells and some B cells	Scavenger Rc previously thought to serve as ligand for CD72 that may modulate signals transduced by the Rc for antigen.	Cur Opin Hematol 6:30, 1999 Immunol Today 19:106, 1998 Science 269:535, 1995
CD6	T12, Tp120	120	I	11 X60992	blood T cells, medullary thymocytes, some cortical thymocytes, brain	Scavenger Rc that serves as ligand for CD166 that plays role in T cell development.	Transplant Proc 31:795, 1999 J Exp Med 181:2213, 1995
CD7	gp40, Tp41	40	I	17 X06180	thymocytes, some T cells, monocytes, NK cells, hematopoietic stem cells	Associates with PI 3 kinase via YXXM motif upon cross-linking, implying that it may be involved in cell activation.	J Clin Immunol 17:265, 1997 J Immunol 155:2407, 1995
CD8	T8; Leu-2 α chain	68 (32–34)	I	2p12 M27161	cytotoxic/suppressor-T cells, some NK cells, most thymocytes	Forms a heterodimer with CD8β to form Rc for class I MHC to facilitate recognition of peptide antigens presented in the context of MHC class I antigens.	Sem Immunol 9:87, 1997 J Immunol 157:4287, 1996
CD8B	β chain of CD8 heterodimer	68(32–34)	I	2 X13444	see CD8	Forms a heterodimer with CD8α to act as Rc for class I MHC (see above).	Immunity 1:243, 1994
CD9	p24	24	III Tet.	12p13 M38690	plts, monocytes, pre-B and act. T cells, eos, basophils	Plays role in signal transduction leading to cell activation, adhesion, and/or aggregation.	Immunol Today 15:588, 1994 Mol Biol Cell 7:193, 1996
CD10	CALLA, Neutral endopeptidase; Metalloendopeptidase	95–100	II	3q21-27 Y00811	pre-B and pre-T cells, germinal center B cells, some PMN, epithelial cells	A zinc-binding metalloprotease that cleaves peptides on the amino side of hydrophobic amino acids, thereby reducing the local concentration of peptide hormones.	J Exp Med 181:2271, 1995 Blood 82:1052, 1993
CD11a	αL chain of β₂ integrins; Leukocyte function antigen-1 (LFA-1)	180	I	16p13.1-11 Y00796	lymphocytes, PMN, monocytes, MØ	Associates with CD18 to form Rc for CD54 (ICAM-1) and CD102 (ICAM-2), thereby facilitating homotypic or heterotypic adhesion and cell activation.	Curr Opin Cell Biol 9:643, 1997 Immunol Rev 146:82, 1995 Immunol Today 16:479, 1995
CD11b	Complement Rc 3 (CR3), C3biR, Mac-1, Mo-1; αM chain of β₂ integrins	155	I	16p13.1-11 J03925	monocytes, MØ, PMN, DC, some B and NK cells	Assembles with CD18 to form a Rc for C3bi, clotting factor X, and fibrinogen that facilitates adhesion to endothelium and plts, homotypic adhesion, phagocytosis, and/or chemotaxis.	Structure 3:1333, 1995 Cell 80:631, 1995 Immunol Today 14:145, 1996
CD11c	gp150/95; αX chain of β₂ integrins; Leu M5	150	I	16p13.1-11 M81695	monocytes, PMN, some B cells	Assembles with CD18 to form an adhesion Rc for fibrinogen and Rc for C3bi. Binding of ligand to heterodimer induces cellular activation and helps trigger neutrophil respiratory burst.	Immunol Today 5:209, 1996 Immunity 5:653, 1996 J Immunol 156:3780, 1996
CD11d	Integrin αD subunit	150	I	16p13.1-11 U37028	red pulp MØ (strong), blood WBC (moderate)	Forms a heterodimer with CD18 to make a Rc that binds CD50 (ICAM-3), but not CD54 or CD106.	Immunity 3:683, 1995
CDw12		90–120	–		monocytes, PMN, NK cells (weak)	Unknown.	Leucocyte Typing VI, Garland Pub, NY, p961, 1998
CD13	Aminopeptidase N (EC 3.4.11.2); gp150	150–170	II	15q25-26 X13276	myeloid cells	A zinc-binding metalloprotease that catalyzes removal of NH₂-terminal amino acids from peptides, thereby reducing local concentration of peptide hormones.	J Exp Med 184:183, 1996 J Exp Med 194:1183, 1996 Transplantation 61:600, 1996
CD14	gp55; GPI-linked glycoprotein	53–55	GPI	5q31 X06882	monocytes, DC	Rc for lipopolysaccharide (LPS) that can transduce signal(s), leading to oxidative burst and/or synthesis of tumor necrosis factor alpha.	Infect. Dis. Clinics of N. Am. 13:341, 1999 Curr Opin Immunol 11:19, 1999 Biochem Soc Trans 26:644, 1998
CD15	Lewisˣ (LeX); 3-fucosyl-N-acetyl-lactosamine (3-FAL)	185–260		none	PMN, eos, monocytes	A carbohydrate determinant that is found on several glycoproteins (e.g. CD11/CD18, CD66) and is dependent on the activity of alpha 3-fucosyltransferase (FucT-IV).	Histo Histopathol 11:1007, 1996 Histochem J 24:811, 1992 Biochem J 268:275, 1990
CD15s	sialyl Lewisˣ (sLeX)	185–260		none	PMN, basophils, monocytes, myeloid cells, some T cells (weak)	The sialyated form of CD15, the major ligand for CD62E (ELAM-1), and is dependent upon fucosyl transferase VII (FucT-VII).	Am J Pathol 143:1220, 1993 J Leukoc Biol 53:541, 1993

TABLE 13-1   CLUSTER OF DIFFERENTIATION ANTIGENS DEFINED AS OF THE SIXTH INTERNATIONAL WORKSHOP ON LEUKOCYTE TYPING (*CONTINUED*)

ANTIGEN	OTHER NAMES	SIZE	O	GENETICS	DISTRIBUTION	PHYSIOLOGY	SELECTED REFERENCES
CD16(A)	Transmembrane form of FcγRIIIA (low-affinity FcRc)	50–65	I	1q23 X52645	NK cells, MØ, mast cells	Low-affinity Rc for aggregated IgG that also may be involved in lysis of cells independent of IgG. CD16 (A) associates with the FcεRIγ, CD3ζ, or FcεRI β chain (mast cells) for signal transduction.	*J Immunol 162:735, 1999* *Proc Natl Acad Sci USA 96:5640, 1999* *J Clin Invest 100:1059, 1997*
CD16(B)	GPI anchored form of FcγRIII (low-affinity FcRc); FcγRIIIB	48–60	GPI	1q23 X16863	PMN	This is the GPI isoform of CD16 that is deficient in patients with PNH. Cross-linking CD16B may transduce a different signal than that of CD16A.	*J Leuk Biol 65:875, 1999* *Transfusion 39:593, 1999* *J Biol Chem 271:3659, 1996*
CDw17	Lactosylceramide (LacCer)				PMN, basophils, plts, monocytes, some B cells	A glycosphingolipid that may play role in granule content packaging, exocytosis, and signaling.	*J Biol Chem 273:34349, 1998* *Circ Res 82:540, 1998*
CD18	Beta chain of the β2 integrins	95	I	21q22.3 M15395	same as CD11a–d combined	Assembles into a heterodimer with one of several α chains (CD11a->d) and appears responsible for signal transduction via the heterodimer.	*Int J Biochem Cell Biol 30:179, 1998* *Curr Opin Cell Biol 9:643, 1997* *Eur J Biochem 245:215, 1997*
CD19	B4	95	I	16p11.2 M28170	all B cells and B cell precursors, some FDC	Forms a noncovalent complex with CD21, CD81, Leu 13 that modulates signal transduction by the B cell receptor for antigen.	*Curr Opin Immunol 8:378, 1996* *Sem Immunol 10:267, 1998* *Curr Opin Immunol 9:324, 1997*
CD20	B1, Bp35	95 (33, 35, 37)	III Tet.	11q13 X12530	B cells but not plasma cells	May act as a Ca²⁺ channel involved in regulating cell cycle progression that can be targeted by mAb for therapy of B cell lymphomas.	*Biochem Soc Trans 25:705, 1997* *Curr Opin Hematol 5:237, 1998*
CD21	CR2, EBV-Rc, C3d-Rc	145	I	1q32 M26004	B cells, FDC, pharyngeal and cervical epithelial cells, some T cells, astrocytes	Rc for C3d and Epstein-Barr virus. Binding of C3d to CD21 enhances B cell antigen receptor signal transduction. Also, in concert with CD23, it may regulate production of IgE.	*Adv Exp Med Biol 452:181, 1998* *Sem Immunol 10:279, 1998* *Immunol Lett 54:201, 1996* *Immunol Today 14:56, 1993*
CD22	Bgp 135, B lymphocyte cell adhesion molecule (BL-CAM), Leu-14, Lyb-8	110–130	I	19p13.1 X52785-a X59350-b	mature B cells but not plasma cells	Binds sialoglycoconjugates (NeuAcα2->6Galβ1->4G1cNAc) on some CD45 isoforms and glycoproteins to modulate B cell signal transduction. The 2 isoforms (α/β) are formed by alternative splicing.	*Adv Exp Med Biol 452:181, 1998* *Curr Opin Immunol 8:378, 1996* *Ann Rev Immunol 15:481, 1997* *Immunity 6:509, 1997*
CD23	FcεRII, BLAST-2; (alternatively spliced forms are called FcεRIIa and FcεRIIb)	45–50	II	19p13.3 M15059	sIgM⁺/sIgD⁺ B cells, monocytes, some T cells, FDC, eos, NK cells, plts	A Ca²⁺-dependent (C-type) lectin with low affinity for IgE, CD21, CD11a, and CD11b that plays a role in the regulation of IgE synthesis and in cell-cell adhesion. Secreted form of CD23 may act as growth factor.	*Int Rev Immunol 16:113, 1997* *Biochem Soc Trans 25:393, 1997* *Curr Opin Immunol 7:355, 1995* *Immunol Today 19:313, 1998*
CD24	Heat-stable antigen (HSA)	35–45	GPI	6q21 M58664 L33930	B cells, pre-B cells, PMN, epithelium, ≤ 2% of thymocytes	May play a role in regulation of B cell proliferation and/or differentiation and serve as a ligand for CD62P.	*Blood 89:3385, 1997* *Int Immunol 7:155, 1995*
CD25	IL-2 Rc, TAC-antigen; α-chain of the IL-2 Rc	55	I	10p14-15 X01057	act. T and act. B cells, some thymocytes, early myeloid cells	A low-affinity Rc for IL-2 that can associate with CD122 and CD132 to form a heterotrimeric Rc with high affinity for IL-2.	*Adv Immunol 59:225, 1995* *Cell 75:5, 1995* *J Biol Chem 266:2681, 1991*
CD26	Dipeptylpeptidase IV, gp120	110	II	2q24.3 X60708	intestinal epithelial cells, renal proximal tubule, bile duct, prostate, memory or act. T cells, medullary thymocytes	A serine-type exopeptidase that cleaves dipeptides from the amino-termini of proteins with a penultimate proline residue. With an intracellular domain that associates with adenosine deaminase, it also can function as a T cell co-stimulatory molecule. Also binds collagen.	*Immunol Rev 161:43, 1998* *Curr Med Chem 6:311, 1999* *Adv Exp Med Biol 421:109, 1997* *Immunol Today 15:180, 1994*
CD27		110(55)	I	12p13 M63928	some T, B, and NK cells, medullary thymocytes	A ligand for CD70 and a member of the nerve-growth-factor-receptor superfamily.	*Sem Immunol 10:491, 1998* *Immunol Today 15:307, 1994*
CD28	Tp44 antigen	80(44)	I	2q33 J02988	95% of CD4 T cells, 50% of CD8 T cells, most plasma cells	Interacts with CD80 and CD86. Cross-linking CD28 serves as co-stimulatory signal and enhances the transcription and stability of IL-2 mRNA.	*Immunol Rev 165:287, 1998* *Crit Rev Immunol 18:389, 1998* *Adv Immunol 62:131, 1996*
CD29	VLA β chain, platelet GPIIa; Integrin β1 subunit	110–130	I	10p11.2 X07979	plts and all leukocytes with higher levels on memory T cells	Assembles into a heterodimer with one of several α chains (CD49a–f or α1–α6) to form Rc involved in cell-cell or cell-matrix adhesion. Highly conserved cytoplasmic domain can interact with cytoskeleton.	*Int J Biochem Cell Biol 30:179, 1998* *Artif Organs 20:828, 1996* *Annu Rev Cell Dev Biol 11:549, 1995* *J Cell Biol 132:211, 1996*
CD30	Ki-1 antigen; Ber-H2	120(105)	I	1p36 M83554	Act. T and B cells, Reed-Sternberg cells, embryonal CA	Member of the nerve-growth-factor-receptor superfamily that may play a role in cell activation and/or differentiation.	*Sem Immunol 10:457, 1998* *Apmis 106:169, 1998*
CD31	platelet endothelial cell adhesion molecule-1 (PECAM-1)	130–140	I	17q23-ter M28526 M37780	monocytes, myeloid cells, plts: cell-cell junctions of endothelium, some T cells	Interacts with itself and with integrin αVβ3 and glycosaminoglycans. Ligation of CD31 activates leukocyte integrins.	*J Exp Med 184:229, 1996* *N Eng J Med 334:286, 1996* *J Cell Sci 109:16037, 1996*
CD32	FcγRII, gp40; Isoforms (A, B1->3, and C) arise through alternative splicing.	40	I	1q23 M31932...A M31935.B1 M31934.B2 M31933.B3 X17652...C	monocytes, MØ, plts; B cells express only the B isoforms whereas PMN express isoforms A and C.	Rc for aggregated IgG that can trigger IgG-mediated phagocytosis and oxidative burst. It transduces an inhibitory signal on B cells and its expression on placental epithelia suggests a role in transport of IgG.	*Biomembranes 3:269, 1996* *Adv Immunol 57:1, 1994* *Immunol Today 14:215, 1993*
CD33	gp67	67	I	19q13.3 M23197	cells of myelomonocytic lineage but not stem cells	Binds to sialoglycoconjugates NeuAcα2->3Galβ1->3(4)G1cNAc and NeuAcα2->3Galβ1->3GalNAc and may mediate cell-cell adhesion.	*Blood 85:2005, 1995* *Biochem Soc Trans 24:150, 1996*

TABLE 13-1   CLUSTER OF DIFFERENTIATION ANTIGENS DEFINED AS OF THE SIXTH INTERNATIONAL WORKSHOP ON LEUKOCYTE TYPING (*Continued*)

ANTIGEN	OTHER NAMES	SIZE	O	GENETICS	DISTRIBUTION	PHYSIOLOGY	SELECTED REFERENCES
CD34	My10; Spg90	105–120	I	1q32 M81104	1–4% of marrow cells including hematopoietic stem cell, endothelium	May play a role in signal transduction or leukocyte-endothelial interactions through its ability to interact with CD62L, CD62P, and CD62E.	*Blood* 87:3550, 1996 *Blood* 87:479, 1996 *Acta Haematol* 97:22, 1997
CD35	Complement Receptor type 1 (CR1), C3b/C4b Rc	160–285	I	1q32 Y00816 X05309	monocytes, PMN, DC, rbc, B cells, some T cells, some astrocytes, glomerular podocytes	Facilitates phagocytosis and/or binding to immune complexes or cells coated with C3b or C4b. CD35 is one of the few CD antigens with allotypic polymorphism resulting in varied molecular sizes.	*J Immunol* 157:1242, 1996 *J Hematother* 4:357, 1995 *Proc Natl Acad Sci USA* 93:3357, 1996
CD36	Platelet GPIV; GPIIIb; OKM5; PAS IV	78–90	VI	7q11.2 M24795	plts, monocytes, MØ, adipocytes, some epithelial, endothelial cells	Signal transducing Rc for thrombospondin, collagen, oxidized low-density lipoprotein, fatty acids, anionic phospholipids, and *Plasmodium falciparum*–infected rbc.	*J Biol Chem* 271:22315, 1996 *Platelets* 7:117, 1996 *Annu Rev Biochem* 63:601, 1994
CD37	gp52-40	40–52	III Tet.	19p13-q13.4 X14046	mature B cells, some T cells/monocytes (weak)	Associates with MHC class II, CD19, CD21, CD53, CD81, and CD82 in B cell membrane, suggesting a role in signal transduction.	*Immunol Today* 15:588, 1994 *Mol Immunol* 33:867, 1996
CD38	T10	46	II	4p15 M34461	plasma cells, early or act. B and T cells, thymocytes, NK cells, brain, myeloid progenitors	Can synthesize cyclic ADP-ribose (ADPR) from nicotinamide adenine dinucleotide and hydrolyze cADPR to ADP-ribose. May play a role in cell activation, proliferation, or survival.	*Immunol Today* 16:469, 1995 *FASEB J* 10:1408, 1996 *J Immunol* 15:741, 1997
CD39		78		10q23.1-24.1 S73813	endothelial cells, MØ, DC, act. cells of the NK-, B-, or T-cell lineage (not on resting cells or germinal center B cells)	Facilitates B cell homotypic adhesion and has ectoapyrase activity that may inhibit platelet adhesion and aggregation by digesting ADP and protect activated cells through hydrolysis of extracellular ATP.	*J Biol Chem* 271:9898, 1996 *J Immunol* 153:3574, 1994 *Biochem Biophys Res Comm* 218:916, 1996
CD40	Bp50	48	I	20q12-13.2 X60592	mature B cells, monocytes, DC, some epithelial cells	Member of the nerve-growth-factor-receptor superfamily that induces cell activation and/or differentiation upon binding its ligand, CD154.	*Adv Immunol* 61:1, 1996 *Int J Mol Med* 3:343, 1999 *Immunol Today* 19:502, 1998
CD41	GPIIb of the GPIIb/GPIIIa complex; αIIβ integrin	13 (120, 23)	I	17q21.32 J02764	plts and megakaryocytes	Associates with CD61 to form Rc for fibrinogen, fibronectin, vitronectin, vWF, and thrombospondin to facilitate platelet adhesion and aggregation.	*N Engl J Med* 332:1553, 1995 *J Biol Chem* 271:6017, 1996 *J Biol Chem* 271:18610, 1996
CD42a	GPIX	22	I	17pter-p12 X52997	plts and megakaryocytes	GPIbα, GPIbβ, GPIX, and GPV form a complex with 2:2:2:1 stoichiometry to form the GP1b complex that binds to subendothelial vWF, allowing for platelet adhesion to damaged blood vessels.	*Blood* 87:1377, 1996 *Blood* 81:2339, 1993 *Proc Natl Acad Sci USA* 86:6773, 1989
CD42b	CD42bα, GPIbα	160–170	I	17pter-p12 J02940	plts and megakaryocytes	Serves as binding site of the GP1b complex for vWF by forming disulfide-linked heterodimer with CD42c that noncovalently associates with CD42a and CD42d.	*J Biol Chem* 269:23716, 1996 *Immunol Today* 13:100, 1992 *Proc Natl Acad Sci USA* 84:5615, 1987
CD42c	CD42bβ, GPIbβ	22	I	17pter-p12 JO3259	plts and megakaryocytes	Forms disulfide-linked heterodimer with CD42b that associates with CD42a and CD42d.	*Proc Natl Acad Sci USA* 85:2135, 1988
CD42d	GPV	82	I	22 Z23091	plts and megakaryocytes	Associates with CD42a, CD42b, and CD42c to form Rc for vWF.	*Biochemistry* 35:906, 1996 *Proc Natl Acad Sci USA* 90:8327, 1993
CD43	Leukosialin, sialophorin	95–135	I	16p11.2 J04168	thymocytes, T cells, PMN, MØ, monocytes, NK cells, plts, brain, act. B cells (weak), plasma cells, hematopoietic stem cells	Sialoglycoprotein that may interact with CD54 or albumin and function as an anti-adhesion molecule, inhibiting T cell interactions, including T cell killing. It may play a costimulatory role on T cells. A soluble form is present in human serum.	*Immunol Today* 19:546, 1998 *Nature* 377:535, 1995 *J Exp Med* 182:139, 1995 *Proc Natl Acad Sci USA* 89:663, 1992
CD44	Phagocytic glycoprotein-1 (Pgp-1); Hermes antigen; Extracellular matrix Rc type III (ECMRIII); Hutch-1	80–90	I	11pter-p13 M59040	most cell types except plts, hepatocytes, cardiac muscle, renal tubular epithelium, testis	A Rc for hyaluronate that facilitates lymphocyte binding to high endothelial venules (HEV). Variants of CD44 have attached chondroitin sulfate and are able to bind fibronectin, laminin, and collagen. Also is Rc for chemotactic cytokine osteopontin.	*Exp Hematol* 27:978, 1999 *Immunology* 93:139, 1998 *Int J Biochem Cell Biol* 30:299, 1998 *Mol Pathol* 51:191, 1998 *Science* 271:509, 1996
CD44R	CD44R1, Restricted (exon 9 of CD44); CD44	85–95	I	11pter-p13 X56794	epithelial cells, rbc, monocytes, act. leukocytes	Serves as the protein backbone of rbc Lutheran antigen and, like CD44, may be involved in leukocyte attachment and rolling on endothelium for homing to lymphoid tissue and sites of inflammation.	*Immunol Today* 14:395, 1993 *J Cell Biol* 132:1199, 1996 *J Immunol* 156:1557, 1996
CD45	T200; Leukocyte common antigen (LCA)	180–240	I	1q31-32 Y00638	all hematopoietic cells except rbc	A tyrosine phosphatase that modulates signal transduction by surface antigen Rc. Changes in the extracellular domain do not affect the intracellular phosphatase activity of the cytoplasmic domain.	*Immunol Res* 16:101, 1997 *Adv Immunol* 66:1, 1997 *Immunol Cell Biol* 75:430, 1997
CD45RA	B220	240	I	1q31-31 Y00638	B cells, subset of naïve CD4 T cells, monocytes	Formed by joining the 8–amino acid NH2-terminal sequence to that encoded by exons A, B, and C, this is the largest of the CD45 isoforms.	*Immunology* 2:246, 1999 *Eur J Immunol* 29:2098, 1999 *Int Immunol* 10:1837, 1998
CD45RB	T200	205, 220	I	1q31-32 Y00638	memory T-cell subset, monocytes, PMN (weak)	Formed by joining the 8–amino acid NH2-terminal sequence to that encoded by exons B and C.	*Eur J Immunol* 28:3435, 1998 *Cell Immunol* 167:56, 1996
CD45RC		190, 205, 220	I	1q31-32 Y00638	some T cells	Formed by joining the 8–amino acid NH2-terminal sequence to that encoded by exon C.	*Immunol Rev* 146:82, 1995

TABLE 13-1   CLUSTER OF DIFFERENTIATION ANTIGENS DEFINED AS OF THE SIXTH INTERNATIONAL WORKSHOP ON LEUKOCYTE TYPING (*CONTINUED*)

ANTIGEN	OTHER NAMES	SIZE	O	GENETICS	DISTRIBUTION	PHYSIOLOGY	SELECTED REFERENCES
CD45RO	Restricted T200;	180	I	1q31-32 *Y00638*	thymocytes act., some memory T-cells	Formed by joining the 8–amino acid NH_2-terminal sequence to the CD45 backbone without A, B, or C, and thus is the smallest of the CD45 iso-forms.	*Leuk Lymph 28:583, 1998* *Eur J Immunol 29:2098, 1999*
CD46	Membrane cofactor protein (MCP); HuLy-m5; Trophoblast leukocyte-common antigen (TLX)	46–63 (51–68)	I	1q32 *M58050*	endothelial cells, epithelial cells, fibroblasts, placenta, sperm, all blood cells except rbc	Acts as a cofactor that binds to CD3b or CD4b, thereby permitting factor I, a serine protease, to convert them into inactive complement fragments. CD46 also may be the Rc used by measles virus.	*Int J Mol Med 1:809, 1998* *Virus Res 48:1, 1997* *Int J Hematol 64:1996*
CD47	Integrin associated protein (IAP); Ovarian CA antigen (OV-3); Rh-related antigen	47–52	III Tet.	3q13.1-2 *Z25521*	all hematopoietic cells	Associates with CD61 integrins to form Rc for thrombospondin, suggesting a role in chemotaxis and cell-cell adhesion. It forms part of the Rh complex on rbc and is not expressed on Rh_{null} rbc.	*Science 274:795, 1996* *J Cell Biol 123:485, 1993* *J Biol Chem 271:21, 1996*
CD48	HuLy-m3; Blast-1; BCM1; MEM-102	40–47	GPI	1q21-23 *M37766*	all hematopoietic cells except PMN, plts, rbc	Low affinity ligand for CD2 that may play role in signal transduction. On T cells, the cytoplasmic domain associates with the lck and fyn tyrosine kinases.	*Immunol Today 17:177, 1996* *Immunogenetics 42:59, 1995* *Eur J Immunol 171:2115, 1993*
CD49a	very late antigen (VLA)-1 α subunit; Integrin α_1 subunit	200 (210)	I	5 *X68742*	monocytes, endothelium, smooth muscle, act. T and B cells	Assembles into a heterodimer with CD29 to form a Rc for collagen and laminin.	*Annu Rev Immunol 8:365, 1990* *J Biol Chem 268:2989, 1993*
CD49b	very late antigen (VLA)-2 α subunit; Integrin α_2 subunit; Ia subunit of platelet glycoprotein Ia-IIa; ECMRI; Collagen Rc	160	I	5q23-31 *X17033*	monocytes, plts, T, B, and NK cells, thymocytes, fibroblasts, endothelium, osteoclasts, epithelium	Assembles with CD29 to form a Rc for laminin and collagen types I, II, III, and IV that is responsible for Mg^{2+}-dependent adhesion of platelets to collagen.	*Annu Rev Immunol 114:365, 1990* *Eur J Immunol 22:1109, 1992* *J Cell Biol 109:397, 1989*
CD49c	very late antigen (VLA)-3 α subunit; Integrin α_3 subunit	150 (25/130)	I	17q *M59911*	monocytes, T and B cells, kidney glomerulus, thyroid, some basement membranes	Assembles with CD29 to form a Rc for laminin and epilgrin (kalinin) that also binds weakly to collagen and fibronectin, suggesting a role in cell-cell adhesion.	*J Biol Chem 268:8651, 1993* *Cell 65:599, 1991* *Mol Biol Cell 7:194, 1996*
CD49d	very late antigen (VLA)-4 α subunit; Integrin α_4 subunit	180 (150)	I	2q31-32 *X16983*	T, B, and NK cells, eos, monocytes, erythroblasts, thymocytes, mast cells, DC, basophils, myeloblasts	Assembles with CD29 or β_7 integrin to form VLA-4 or $\alpha_4\beta_7$, respectively. These integrins bind VCAM-I (CD106) and some forms of fibronectin. $\alpha_4\beta_7$ also binds mucosal addressin MAdCAM-1. These integrins help mediate cell *arrest and adhesion to endothelium*.	*J Clin Invest 94:1722, 1994* *J Immunol 156:3727, 1996* *Cell 80:413, 1995* *J Cell Biol 128:1243, 1995*
CD49e	very late antigen (VLA)-5 α subunit; Integrin α_5 subunit; Ic subunit to GPIc-IIa	155 (135/25)	I	12q11-13 *X06256*	thymocytes, T cells, monocytes, plts, act. or very early B cells	Assembles with CD29 to form a Rc for fibronectin and invasin via binding to RGD. Upon binding, it activates the Na^+/H^+ antiporter and may act as accessory molecule for T cell activation.	*Annu Rev Immunol 114:365, 1990* *Cell 69:11, 1992* *J Immunol 145:59, 1990*
CD49f	very late antigen (VLA)-6 α subunit; Integrin α_6 subunit; subunit of laminin Rc, platelet GPIc	140 (120/30)	I	2 *X53586*	plts, MØ, monocytes, thymocytes, T cells, adherent epithelia	Assembles with CD29 or the β_4 integrin chain (CD104) to form a Rc for laminin on basement membranes of vessels.	*Proc Natl Acad Sci USA 88:10183, 1991* *Trends Cell Biol 5:419, 1995* *Annu Rev Immunol 114:365, 1990*
CD50	Intercellular adhesion molecule-3 (ICAM-3)	120–160	I	19p13.3-2 *X69711*	thymocytes, T and B cells, monocytes, PMN	Serves as a ligand for LFA-1 (CD11a/CD18).	*Biochem Soc Trans 26:644, 1998*
CD51	Vitronectin Rc α chain; α_v subunit of $\alpha_v\beta_3$ integrin (CD51/CD61)	150 (125/24)	I	2q31-32 *M14648*	endothelial cells, monocytes, MØ, plts (weak), some B cells (weak)	Assembles with CD61(β_3) to form a Rc for vitronectin, vWF, thrombospondin, fibrinogen, and collagen. These Rc facilitate plt aggregation and/or endothelial cell adhesion and may play a role in monocyte migration through subendothelium. CD51 also can associate with the β_5 integrin to form an alternate vitronectin Rc.	*Curr Opin Cell Bio 5:864, 1993* *Int J Exp Pathol 71:741, 1990* *Annu Rev Cell Biol 6:329, 1990* *Thromb Haemost 70:87, 1993*
CD52	CAMPATH-1	21–28	GPI	1p36 *X62466*	lymphocytes, monocytes, few PMN (weak), seminal vesicles, epididymis, spermatozoa	Some anti-CD52 mAbs are strongly mitogenic, suggesting that CDw52 plays a role in signal transduction.	*Biochim Biophys Acta 1446:334, 1999* *Eur J Immunol 21:1677, 1991* *Transplantation 54:97, 1992*
CD53	OX-44	35–42	III Tet.	1p12-13.3 *M37033*	leukocytes, plts, osteoblasts, osteoclasts	Can transduce signals in B cells, monocytes, and PMN, leading to cell activation.	*Immunol Today 15:588, 1994* *J Immunol 157:2039, 1996*
CD54	Intercellular adhesion molecule-1 (ICAM-1)	90	I	19p13.3-2 *X06990*	leukocytes, endothelial and epithelial cells, expression increased with activation	Functions as a ligand for LFA-1 (CD11a/CD18), Mac-1 (CD11b/CD18), and CD11c/CD18 (p150,95). CD54 also is Rc for rhinovirus, can bind CD43, and can bind to *Plasmodium falciparum*–infected rbc.	*J Exp Med 182:1231, 1995* *Eur J Immunol 154:6080, 1995* *Eur J Immunol 25:1008, 1995*
CD55	Decay accelerating factor (DAF)	70	GPI	1q32 *M35156*	all cells in contact with serum, CNS, epithelial cells	Neutralizes complement activation on autologous tissue by preventing the assembly of C3 convertase or accelerating disassembly of preformed convertase.	*Pharmacol Rev 50:59, 1998* *Adv Immunol 61:201, 1996*
CD56	Neural cell adhesion molecule (NCAM); Leu 19, NKH1	120–220	I or GPI	11q23.1 *X16841*	NK cells, embryonic cells, muscle, neural cells, epithelium, some act. T cells.	Facilitates homotypic adhesion and may play a role in contact-dependent growth inhibition and NK cell cytotoxicity.	*Ann Hematol 74:51, 1997* *Proc Natl Acad Sci USA 93:6421, 1996* *Neuron 17:413, 1996*
CD57	Human Natural Killer-1 (HNK-1); Leu 7	110			NK cells, some T, few B, some Schwann cells	Unknown.	*Trends Neurosci 18:183, 1995* *Prog Brain Res 105:183, 1995*

TABLE 13-1   CLUSTER OF DIFFERENTIATION ANTIGENS DEFINED AS OF THE SIXTH INTERNATIONAL WORKSHOP ON LEUKOCYTE TYPING (*CONTINUED*)

ANTIGEN	OTHER NAMES	SIZE	O	GENETICS	DISTRIBUTION	PHYSIOLOGY	SELECTED REFERENCES
CD58	Leukocyte function associated-3 (LFA-3)	45–70	I or GPI	1p13.1 Y00636	most hematopoietic cells, fibroblasts; endothelium	Binds CD2 and enhances T cell Ag recognition. The CD58 homologue on sheep rbc allows these cells to form rosettes with human T cells.	*Cell* 97:791, 1999 *Proc Natl Acad Sci USA* 96:4289, 1999
CD59	Complement protectin, MIRL, H19, MACIF, HRF20, P-18	19	GPI	11p13 X16447	leukocytes, rbc, endothelial and epithelial cells, placenta, spermatozoa, body fluids	Inhibits complement membrane attack by binding to activated C8 and C9. It also is a minor ligand for CD2 and may be involved in T cell signal transduction.	*Int J Oncol* 13:305, 1998 *Adv Immunol* 61:201, 1996
CD60	NeuAc-NeuAc-Gal; UM4D4				T cell subset; plts, some monocytes, melanocytes	May play a role in signal transduction leading to cell activation. Minimal antigenic epitope consists of NeuAc2-[>8NeuAc2->3Galβ_1->4.	*Cell Immunol* 187:117, 1998 *J Exp Med* 179:1385, 1994
CD61	GPIIIa, integrin β_3 subunit, vitronectin Rc β chain	90 (105)		17q21.3 J02703	plts, megakaryocytes, monocytes, MØ, endothelial cells	Associates with CD41 to form the GPIIb-IIIa heterodimer that facilitates plt aggregation, or with CD51 to form a Rc for vitronectin.	*Blood* 88:1666, 1996 *Thromb Haemost* 2:492, 1994
CD62E	E-Selectin; Endothelial leukocyte adhesion molecule-1 (ELAM-1); LECAM-2	115	I	1q23-25 M30640	endothelium	Facilitates adhesion of PMN, monocytes, and some T cells to vascular endothelium by binding sialyl Lewis^x, sialyl Lewis^a, and related fucosylated *N*-acetyl-lactosamines of leukocyte glycolipids and glycoproteins.	*Cell* 84:563, 1996 *Nature* 367:532, 1994 *FASEB J* 9:866, 1995
CD62L	L-Selectin; TQ1; gp90^{MEL-14}; Leukocyte adhesion molecule-1 (LAM-1); LECAM-1, Leu-8	75–80	I	1q23-25 M25280	B cells, T cells, PMN, thymocytes monocytes, eos, basophils, erythroid and myeloid progenitor cells, NK cells.	Functions as a peripheral lymph node homing Rc. Facilitates binding to endothelium at inflammatory sites or at high endothelial venules (HEV) of peripheral lymph nodes by binding to endothelial heparin-like chains and the vascular sialomucin, CD34. It is involved in leukocyte rolling in mesenteric venules.	*Annu Rev Biochem* 64:113, 1995 *J Clin Invest* 98:1081, 1996 *Science* 272:60, 1996 *Nature* 380:720, 1996 *J Exp Med* 184:1343, 1996
CD62P	P-Selectin; GMP-140; LECAM-3; PADGEM; CD62	130–150	I	1q21-24 M25322	plts, endothelial cells, megakaryocytes	Facilitates adhesion of monocytes and neutrophils to activated platelets and endothelial cells by binding sialylated, fucosylated lactosaminoglycans, including sialyl Lewis^x, on neutrophils.	*Curr Biol* 6:261, 1996 *J Biol Chem* 270:11025, 1995 *Science* 273:252, 1996 *Cell* 84:563, 1996
CD63	Platelet 53-kDa activation antigen; ME491; MLA1; PTLGP40; granulophysin	53	III Tet.	12q12-13 X07982	act. plts, monocytes, MØ, secretory granules of vascular endothelial cells, platelet dense granules	Facilitates adhesion to activated endothelium.	*Biochem Biophys Res Comm* 246:841, 1998 *Immunol Today* 15:588, 1994 *J Immunol* 157:2039, 1996
CD64	FcγRI	75	I	1q21.1 X14356...A M91645...B M91647...C	monocytes (B and C forms), MØ, act. PMN	There exist at least 3 isoforms (A, B, and C) that each act as a high affinity Rc for IgG and that mediate release of cytokines, including IL-1, IL-6, and TNF-α.	*Mol Immunol* 35:989, 1998 *J Immunol* 157:541, 1996 *Immunol Today* 14:215, 1994
CD65	Ceramide-dodecasaccharide 4c; VIM-2				myeloid cells, some monocytic cells	CDw65 is a carbohydrate determinant with a minimal epitope consisting of NeuAcα2->3Galβ1->4GlcNAcβ1->3Galβ1->4GlcNAc(Fucα1->3)β1->3Galβ. Associated glycoprotein is involved in signal transduction leading to formation of the respiratory burst.	*J Biochem* 119:456, 1996 *J Biol Chem* 263:10186, 1988
CD66a	Phosphorylated glycoprotein; Biliary glycoprotein-1 (BGP-1); nonspecific cross-reacting antigen-160 (NCA-160)	160–180 (113, 96, 74)	I	19q13.1-2 X16354	PMN, histiocytes, some myeloid progenitor cells, brush border of colonic epithelial cells	A biliary glycoprotein member of the carcinoembryonic antigen family of adhesion molecules that facilitate Ca^{2+}-independent homotypic and heterotypic adhesion and neutrophil activation. CD66 possesses Lewis^x and sialyl Lewis^x determinants.	*Eur J Immunol* 28:3664, 1998 *Am J Pathol* 152:1401, 1998 *J Histochem Cytochem* 45:957, 1997 *J Histochem Cytochem* 44:35, 1996
CD66b	Formerly CD67; CGM6; p100; nonspecific cross-reacting antigen-95 (NCA-95)	95–100	GPI	19q13.1-2 X52378	PMN	CD66b is one GPI isoform of CD66. Cross-linking of CD66b induces aggregation and activation, possibly via binding to CD62E.	*Blood* 91:663, 1998 *J Leukoc Biol* 60:106, 1996
CD66c	nonspecific cross-reacting antigen-90 (NCA-90)	90	GPI	19q13.1-2 M29541	myeloid restricted, pre-B ALL	CD66c is another GPI isoform of CD66. Cross-linking of CD66c induces aggregation and activation possibly via binding to CD62E.	*Leukemia* 13:779, 1999 *Tissue Antigens* 52:1, 1998
CD66d	CGM1	30	I	19q13.1-2 L00692	PMN	Member of carcinoembryonic antigen family of adhesion molecules that facilitates homotypic adhesion and neutrophil activation.	*J Leukoc Biol* 60:106, 1996
CD66e	Carcinoembryonic antigen (CEA)	180–200	GPI	19q13.1-2 M17303	tissues derived from all three germ layers during embryogenesis; adult colon epithelial cells (very weak)	May facilitate Ca^{2+}-independent homotypic and heterotypic adhesion during embryogenesis. CD66e binds weakly to other nonspecific cross-reacting antigens CD66a–c.	*Semin Cancer Biol* 9:67, 1999 *Cancer Res* 55:3873, 1995 *Cancer Res* 56:4805, 1996
CD66f	PSG (Pregnancy-specific glycoprotein), Sp-1	54–72	GPI	19q13.1-2 U18469	tissues derived from all three germ layers during embryogenesis; adult colon epithelial cells (very weak)	Its function is unknown, but appears necessary for successful pregnancy and may be involved in protection of the fetus from maternal immune recognition.	*Semin Cancer Biol* 9:67, 1999 *Cancer Res* 55:3873, 1995 *Cancer Res* 56:4805, 1996
CD68	gp110, macrosialin (mouse)	110	I	17p13 S57235	monocytes/MØ, osteoclasts, mast cells, cytoplasmic granules, large lymphocytes	A sialomucin belonging to a family of highly glycosylated, acidic lysosomal glycoproteins (LGPs) that include LAMP-1 (CD107a) and LAMP-2 (CD107b). It may protect the lysosomal membranes from attack by hydrolases.	*Proc Natl Acad Sci USA* 93:14833, 1996 *Genomics* 54:165, 1998 *Proc Natl Acad Sci USA* 92:9580, 1995 *Am J Clin Pathol* 103:425, 1995

TABLE 13-1 CLUSTER OF DIFFERENTIATION ANTIGENS DEFINED AS OF THE SIXTH INTERNATIONAL WORKSHOP ON LEUKOCYTE TYPING (CONTINUED)

ANTIGEN	OTHER NAMES	SIZE	O	GENETICS	DISTRIBUTION	PHYSIOLOGY	SELECTED REFERENCES
CD69	Activation inducer molecule (AIM); early activation antigen (EA 1); MLR-3; Leu-23	60 (28/33)	II	12p12.3-13.2 L07555	plts, act. lymphocytes, CD4$^+$ or CD8$^+$ thymocytes	Member of the Ca^{2+}-dependent (C-type) lectin superfamily of type II transmembrane proteins. Forms a homodimer that may function as signal transducer enhancing cell activation and/or platelet aggregation.	J Immunol 162:3978, 1999 Clin Exp Immunol 114:66, 1998 Scand J Immunol 48:196, 1998
CD70	Ki-24 antigen; CD27-ligand	29	II	19p13.3 L08096	act. B and some act. T cells	Member of the TNF family that binds CD27 and may provide costimulatory signal for T cell activation.	Semin Immunol 10:491, 1998
CD71	Transferrin Rc, T9	180 (95/95)	II	3q26.2-qter X01060	act. or proliferating cells	Binds 2 molecules of the serum iron-transport protein transferrin, facilitating cellular iron uptake.	Proc Natl Acad Sci USA 93:8175, 1996 Crit Rev Oncog 4:241, 1993
CD72	Lyb-2, Ly-32.2	86 (39/43)	II	9p M54992	all B cells (except plasma cells), MØ (weak)	May be involved in B cell activation. The binding of CD72 by CD5 remains controversial.	Eur J Immunol 28:3003, 1998 J Immunol 160:4662, 1998
CD73	Ecto-5'-nucleotidase	69	GPI	6q14-21 X55740	some B cells, some T cells, thymocytes (weak), some epithelial and endothelial cells, DC	Catalyzes 5' dephosphorylation of pyrimidine and purine ribo- and deoxyribonucleoside monophosphates to nucleosides.	Immunol Rev 161:95, 1998 Blood 82:1052, 1993
CD74	Class II-associated invariant chain; Ii; Iγ	33/35/41	II	5q32 X03339 X03340	B cells, monocytes (weak), DC, act. T cells	Associates with the α and β chains of MHC class II proteins in the endoplasmic reticulum to prevent binding of endogenous peptides. It is released from the MHC protein in the acidic lysosomal compartment.	Hum Immunol 54:159, 1997 Immunology 79:331, 1993
CDw75		53 and 87	II	3q21-28 (SiaT-1)	mature B cells but not plasma cells	Requires β-galactoside α2,6-sialyltransferase (SiaT-1) activity in the Golgi, indicating it is a sialylated protein of unknown function.	Blood 87:5113, 1996 J Cell Biol 116:423, 1992
CDw76					mature B cells (strong, particularly on mantle zone B cells), some T cells (weak), melanocytes, endothelial cells, hepatocytes, kidney tubules	Neuraminidase-sensitive carbohydrate determinant (NeuAcα2-6Galβ1-4G1cNAcβ1-3Galβ1-4G1c-β1-1'Cer) that is dependent on β-galactoside α2,6-sialyltransferase activity in the Golgi.	Blood 87:5113, 1996 Eur J Immunol 22:2777, 1992
CD77	Globotriaosylceramide (Gβ3), P^k blood group, Burkitt lymphoma associated antigen (BLA), ceramide trihexoside				germinal center B cells, FDC, endothelium, some epithelial cells	May serve as Rc for vero toxin of E. coli and the Shiga toxin of Shigella dysenteriae. Ligation may induce apoptosis.	Eur J Immunol 21:1131, 1991 J Exp Med 180:191, 1994
CDw78					B cells (increased after activation), tissue MØ	May be involved in signal transduction.	Leucocyte Typing VI, Oxford Univ. Press. p. 178, 1998
CD79a	MB-1 (Igα)	82–95 (32–33)	I	19q13.2 L32754	B cells	An accessory molecule that mediates sIg expression and signal transduction (see Chap. 83).	Curr Opin Cell Biol 7:163, 1995
CD79b	B29(Igβ)	82–95 (37–39)	I	17q23 L27587	B cells	An accessory molecule that mediates sIg expression and signal transduction (see Chap. 83).	Immunity 4:145, 1996
CD80	B7; B7-1; BB1	60	I	3q21 M27533	act. B cells, monocytes, FDC	Interacts with CD28 or CD152 (CTLA-4) for costimulation or inhibition of T cells, respectively.	Annu Rev Immunol 14:233, 1996 Curr Opin Immunol 9:858, 1997
CD81	Target of anti-proliferative antibody-I (TAPA-1)	22	III Tet.	11p15.5 M33680	many cell types including lymphocytes	Involved in signal transduction and cell adhesion. Also, CD81 can serve as the Rc for hepatitis C.	Annu Rev Immunol 16:89, 1998 Science 282:938, 1998
CD82	R2; IA4; 4F9; KAI1	50–53	III Tet.	11p11.2	epithelia, endothelium, monocytes, PMN, plt, act. lymphocytes	Involved in signal transduction.	Immunol Today 15:588, 1994 Biochem Biophys Acta 1287:67, 1996
CD83	HB15	45	I	6p23-21.3 Z11697	DC (not FDC), Langerhans cells, B cells (weak), interdigitating reticular cells	May play a role in antigen presentation or the cellular interactions that follow lymphocyte activation. Currently one of the best markers for mature DC.	J Immunol 154:3821, 1995 J Immunol 156:541, 1996
CDw84		72–86			monocytes, plts, germinal center B cells (strong), mantle zone B cells (weak)	Unknown.	Leucocyte Typing VI, Garland Pub., NY, p. 193, 1998
CD85		110 (83)			plasma cells (strong), NK, B cells, monocytes, HCL	Unknown.	Leucocyte Typing VI, Garland Pub., NY, p. 196, 1998
CD86	B7-2, B70	80	I	3q13-23 U404343	monocytes, act. B and T cells, and DC	Interacts with CD28 to provide a costimulatory signal or with CD152 (CTLA-4) to provide an inhibitory signal for T cell activation.	Annu Rev Immunol 14:233, 1996 J Biol Chem 271:26762,1996
CD87	urokinase plasminogen activator Rc (uPAR), Mo3	50–65	GPI	19q13 M83246	monocytes, PMN, act. NK and LGL cells	The Rc for uPA that can retain and concentrate uPA at the plasma membrane, allowing for local conversion of plasminogen to plasmin.	J Immunol 156:297, 1996 J Immunol 152:505, 1994 J Immunol 148:3636, 1992
CD88	Rc for C5a (C5aR)	40	III	19q13.3-13.4 X57250	PMN, MØ, eos, mast cells, hepatocytes, smooth muscle, endothelium	A G protein–coupled Rc that triggers chemotaxis, activation, respiratory burst, and degranulation upon binding to C5a.	Nature 383:86, 1996 Annu Rev Immunol 12:758, 1994 Nature 349:614, 1991
CD89	FcRc for IgA; FcαR	55–75	I	19q13.4 X54150	PMN, monocytes, MØ, mucosa, some T and B cells	Binds Fc of IgA$_1$ or IgA$_2$ with high affinity to trigger granulocyte respiratory burst. As such, it amplifies the protective effects of IgA.	J Exp Med 172:1665, 1990 J Immunol 156:4442, 1996 Immunogenetics 43:246, 1996
CD90	Thy-1, theta	18	GPI	11q23.3 M11749	pro-thymocytes, brain, other non-lymphoid tissues	May contribute to formation of neuron memory and to growth regulation of hematopoietic stem cells.	Nature 379:826, 1996 Science 216:696, 1982
CD91	Rc for α$_2$ macroglobulin; low density lipoprotein (LDL) Rc-associated protein	600 (515/85)	I	12q13.1-13.3 X13916	monocytic and macrophage phagocytes, astrocytes, fibroblasts, epithelial cells	Member of the low density lipoprotein receptor family that binds to α$_2$ macroglobulin, is involved in lipoprotein metabolism, and may facilitate endocytosis of coated pits.	Ann NY Acad Sci 737:1, 1994

TABLE 13-1　CLUSTER OF DIFFERENTIATION ANTIGENS DEFINED AS OF THE SIXTH INTERNATIONAL WORKSHOP ON LEUKOCYTE TYPING (*CONTINUED*)

ANTIGEN	OTHER NAMES	SIZE	O	GENETICS	DISTRIBUTION	PHYSIOLOGY	SELECTED REFERENCES
CDw92		70			PMN, monocytes, and weak on lymphocytes, endothelium	Unknown.	*Leucocyte Typing VI, Garland Pub., NY, p. 1031, 1998*
CDw93		110–120			PMN, monocytes, endothelial cells	An *O*-sialoglycoprotein of unknown function.	*Leucocyte Typing VI, Garland Pub., NY, p. 1032, 1998*
CD94	Kp43	70 (30,43)	II	12P12.3-13.1 *U30610*	NK (increased upon activation), a few T cells	Plays a role in NK recognition of MHC class I molecules. Ligation on NK cells can inhibit target cell killing.	*Immunity 5:163, 1996* *J Immunol 157:4741, 1996*
CD95	Apo-1; FAS	42	I	10q 24.1 *M67454*	act. lymphocytes, fibroblasts, monocytes, PMN, liver	Cross-linking CD95 can induce apoptosis.	*Curr Opin Immunol 8:355, 1996* *Cell 85:781, 1996*
CD96	Tactile T cell ACTivation Increased Late Expression (TACTILE)	240/180/160 (160)	I	— *M88282*	T and NK cells (increased upon activation)	Expressed primarily upon activation, suggesting that it may have binding activity for some unknown ligand.	*J Immunol 148:2600, 1992*
CD97		74,80,89	III	19p13.12-2 *X84700*	PMN, monocytes, act. T and B cells	Has 7 potential membrane-spanning domains and 3 extracellular EGF domains with 1 RGD sequence.	*J Exp Med 184:1185, 1996* *J Immunol 155:1942, 1995*
CD98	4F2; FRP-1	120 (40/80)	II	11q *J02939*	strong on monocytes, myocardial, act. T cells, but weak on T, B, and NK cells	May play a role in cell growth and death. CD98 mAbs can inhibit lectin-induced T cell mitogenesis and/or induce cell fusion, homotypic aggregation, and/or tyrosine phosphorylation.	*Blood 87:3676, 1996* *J Immunol 155:3585, 1995*
CD99	MIC 2; E2; 12E7; HuLy-m6; FMC29	32	I	Xp22.32-pter and Yp11.2-pter *X16996*	all WBC, especially thymocytes, CD99 is found on surface of Xg(a+) rbc and in cytoplasm of Xg(a-) rbc.	Involved in rosette formation with sheep rbc. The gene encoding CD99 is pseudoautosomal. MIC2Y or MIC2X is expressed by males or females, respectively. MIC2X does not undergo X inactivation.	*Immunol Invest 24:173, 1995* *J Immunol 154:26, 1995*
CD100		300 (150)	I	— *U60800*	B, T, and NK cells, most myeloid cells—expression increases upon activation	Member of Semaphorin (sema) family that plays a role in lymphocyte activation by modifying the signaling of other Rc, such as CD40 or CD45.	*Immunol Invest 24:173, 1995* *Nature Genet 8:285, 1994* *Cell and Mol Life Sci 54:1265, 1998*
CD101	V7, p126	200 (126)	I	1p13 *Z33642*	PMN, monocytes, some mucosal T cells, act. T	May play a costimulatory role in T cell activation.	*J Immunol 157:3366, 1996*
CD102	ICAM-2 (Intercellular adhesion molecule-2)	54–68	I	17q23-25 *X15606*	endothelial cells (strong), plts (strong), subset of lymphocytes, monocytes, DC, splenic sinusoids	Acts as a ligand for LFA-1 (CD11a/CD18), but unlike CD54, it does not bind to Mac-1 (CD11b/CD18) or undergo upregulation upon cellular activation. It may facilitate recirculation of memory T cells.	*Nature 339:61, 1989* *J Biol Chem 268:21474, 1993*
CD103	Integrin αE subunit; human mucosal lymphocyte-1 integrin (HML-1)	175 (150,25)	I	— *L25851*	intraepithelial, 1–2% of blood lymphocytes, testis, prostate, ovary, pancreas	Associates with the β_7 integrin to form a Rc that binds E-cadherin to facilitate adhesion to epithelia.	*J Immunol 150:3459, 1993* *J Biol Chem 269:6016, 1994* *Semin Immunol 7:335, 1995*
CD104	Integrin β_4 subunit of laminin Rc	210 (220)	I	17q11-qter *X51841*	epithelia, thymocytes, few neuronal cells, basement membranes, Schwann cells	Associates with α_6 (CD49f) to form a Rc for laminin (and possibly epiligrin), facilitating adhesion of cells to the extracellular matrix.	*J Cell Biol 134:559, 1996* *Nature Genet 10:229, 1995*
CD105	Endoglin; Rc for transforming growth factor-beta (TGF-β) types I and III	170 (95)	II	9q34.1 *X72012*	endothelium, act. monocytes, MØ, pro-erythroblasts, FDC	Has binding activity for TGF-β_1 and TGF-β_3 in association with TGF-β Rc I and Rc II and is involved in regulation of cell differentiation and migration.	*Nature Genet 8:345, 1994* *J Cell Biol 133:1109, 1996* *J Immunol 154:4456, 1995*
CD106	Vascular cell adhesion molecule-1 (VCAM-1); INCAM-110	100–110	I	1p31–32 *M73255*	act. endothelial cells, MØ, FDC, marrow stroma, myoblasts, some MØ, myotubes	Serves as a ligand for VLA-4 ($\alpha_4\beta_1$ integrin or CD49d/CD29) and, to a lesser degree, $\alpha_4\beta_7$ integrin. CD106 facilitates recruitment of leukocytes to sites of inflammation, and is involved in lymphocyte-dendritic cell interactions and in myogenesis.	*Nature 373:539, 1995* *J Immunol 156:2851, 1996* *Blood 84:2068, 1994*
CD107a	Lysosome-associated membrane protein-1 (LAMP-1)	120	I	13q34 *J04182*	act. plts, PMN, T cells, MØ, DC, endothelial cells, tonsillar epithelium	Serves as ligand for galaptin, an S-type lectin (galectin) in the extracellular matrix. Contains sialylated Lewis^x (sLe^x) structures that can bind CD62E.	*J Biol Chem 266:21327, 1991* *Biochem Biophys Res Commun 215:757, 1995*
CD107b	Lysosome-associated membrane protein-2 (LAMP-2)	120	I	Xq24 *J04183*	act. plts, PMN, act. endothelial cells, tonsillar epithelium, melanoma	Same as CD107a above.	*J Biol Chem 266:21327, 1991* *Biochem Biophys Res Commun 215:757, 1995*
CDw108	JMH erythrocyte blood group antigen	75 (80)	GPI	—	weakly expressed on some lymphocytes, myeloid, stromal cells	Unknown.	*Transfusion 35:566, 1995*
CD109	Gov$^{a/b}$ alloantigen	175	GPI	—	endothelium, plt, act.T cell	Unknown.	*Blood 86:2807, 1995*
CD114	Granulocyte-colony stimulating factor Rc	150	I	1p35-34.3 *X55721*	monocytes, MØ, PMN, and their precursors	Class I cytokine receptor for G-CSF that plays a role in the regulation of myeloid proliferation and differentiation.	*Blood 88:761, 1996*
CD115	Colony-stimulating factor (CSF)-1 Rc, c-fms proto-oncogene	150	I	5q33.2-33.3 *X03663*	placenta, MØ, monocytes, and their precursors	Class III cytokine Rc for macrophage-CSF. M-CSF induces tyrosine phosphorylation of CD115, leading to the proliferation and differentiation of monocytes and their progenitors.	*Blood 75:1, 1990* *Cell 61:203, 1990*
CDw116	Rc for granulocyte-macrophage colony-stimulating factor (GM-CSFR); CSF-1 R; HGM-CSFR	70–85	I	Xp22.32; Yp11.3; pseudoautosomal *X17648*	monocytes, PMN, endothelial cells, DC, fibroblasts	CDw116 is the Rc for GM-CSF. The low affinity of the α subunit for GM-CSF is increased when it forms a heterodimer with a 120–140 kDa β subunit common to the IL3-Rc (CD123) and the IL5-Rc (CD125). Binding of CDw116 to GM-CSF stimulates cell proliferation and differentiation.	*Annu Rev Biochem 59:783, 1990* *Cell 67:1, 1991*

TABLE 13-1　CLUSTER OF DIFFERENTIATION ANTIGENS DEFINED AS OF THE SIXTH INTERNATIONAL WORKSHOP ON LEUKOCYTE TYPING (*CONTINUED*)

ANTIGEN	OTHER NAMES	SIZE	O	GENETICS	DISTRIBUTION	PHYSIOLOGY	SELECTED REFERENCES
CD117	Rc for stem cell factor (SCFR); c-kit; steel factor Rc (SCR)	145	I	4 cen->q21	hematopoietic progenitors, mast cells, melanocytes, spermatogonia, oocytes, some NK cells	Class III cytokine Rc for "steel factor" that induces its tyrosine kinase activity, leading to cellular proliferation and/or differentiation.	*Oncogene 7:1259, 1992* *J Exp Med 178:1079, 1993*
CD119	Rc for Interferon (IFNγ-R)	90–100	I	6q23-q24 *J03143*	MØ, monocytes, T, B, and NK cells, PMN, epithelial cells, endothelium, fibroblasts	Class II cytokine Rc for IFN-γ that is responsible for binding IFN-γ, but cannot transduce a signal in transfected cell lines without IFN-γ accessory factor-1 (AF-1).	*Annu Rev Immunol 11:571, 1993* *Cell 76:793, 1994*
CD120a	55-kDa Rc for tumor necrosis factor alpha (TNF-α); TNFRI	55	I	12p13.2 *M33294*	many cell types—highest levels on epithelial cells, germinal center dendritic reticulum cells	Functions as a high affinity Rc for tumor necrosis factor alpha (TNF-α) and tumor necrosis factor beta (TNF-β).	*Biol Chem 266:18324, 1991* *Int Rev Exp Pathol 34 Pt B:149, 1993*
CD120b	75-kDa Rc for tumor necrosis factor alpha (TNF-α); TNFRII	75	I	1p36.3-p36.2 *M35857*	many cell types—highest levels on epithelial cells, germinal center dendritic reticulum cells	Functions as a high affinity Rc for tumor necrosis factor alpha (TNF-α) and tumor necrosis factor beta (TNF-β) or lymphotoxin alpha.	*J Exp Med 176:1015, 1992* *Int Rev Exp Pathol 34 Pt B:149, 1993*
CDw121a	Rc for IL-1 (type I); IL-1R	80	I	2q12 *M27492*	T cells, thymocytes, chondrocytes, synovial cells, endothelial cells, fibroblasts, keratinocytes, hepatocytes	Rc for interleukin-1 alpha (IL-1α) and interleukin-1 beta (IL-1β) that induces cellular proliferation and/or activation upon binding IL-1.	*Proc Natl Acad Sci USA 90:6155, 1993*
CDw121b	Rc for IL-1 (type II); IL-1R	68	I	2q12 *M59770*	B cells, monocytes, PMN, MØ	Nonsignal transducing Rc for IL-1α and IL-1β that may inhibit IL-1 effects by competing with CD120a for IL-1 binding.	*Science 261:472, 1993*
CD122	β chain of the IL-2 Rc; p75, IL-2R-beta	75	I	22q11.2-q13 *M26062*	act. T cells, B cells, monocytes, NK cells	Associates with CD25 and CD132 to form a heterotrimeric Rc with high affinity for IL-2.	*Annu Rev Immunol 11:245, 1993* *Cell 73:147, 1993*
CDw123	IL-3 Rc alpha chain	70	I	Xp22.3, Yp13.3 *M74782*	pluripotent stem cells and committed hematopoietic progenitor cells	A low affinity Rc for IL-3 that associates with CDw131 to form a high affinity Rc for IL-3 that, upon binding to IL-3, stimulates proliferation and/or differentiation.	*Biochem Biophys Res Commun 208:360, 1995* *J Biol Chem 270:22422, 1995*
CD124	HIL-4R; IL-4 Rc alpha chain	140	I	16p11.2-p12.1 *X52425*	mature B cells, T cells, epithelium, endothelium, hematopoietic precursors, fibroblasts	A Rc for IL-4 that forms a heterodimer with CD132 to induce cellular differentiation and/or activation upon binding IL-4.	*Annu Rev Biochem 59:783, 1990* *J Exp Med 171:861, 1990*
CDw125	IL-5 Rc alpha chain	55–60	I	3p26 *X61176-8* *X62156*	eos, basophils, act. B cells	Associates with CDw131 to form the IL-5 Rc that stimulates proliferation and/or differentiation upon binding IL-5.	*EMBO J 14:3395, 1995* *Immunity 4:483, 1996*
CD126	IL-6 Rc alpha chain	80	I	1q21 *X12830*	plasma cells (high), act. B (high), WBC (weak), epithelial cells, fibroblasts, neural cells, hepatocytes	Associates with CD130 to form IL-6 Rc that stimulates cell growth and/or differentiation upon binding IL-6.	*Annu Rev Immunol 15:797, 1997* *Science 241:825, 1988* *Cell 63:1149, 1990* *Annu Rev Immunol 8:253, 1990*
CD127	HIL-7R; IL-7 Rc alpha chain; p90 IL-7R	75	I	5p13 *M29696*	B cell precursors, thymocytes, mature T cells, monocytes	Specific Rc for IL-7. Forms functional high-affinity complex in association with γc chain (CD132). Critical role for IL-7/IL-7R system in lymphoid development.	*Leucocyte Typing VI, Garland Pub., NY, p. 838, 1998* *J Leuk Biol 58:623, 1995* *Annu Rev Biochem 59:783, 1990* *Cell 60:941, 1990*
CDw128	IL-8 Rc type A (type I), CXCR1; IL-8 Rc type B (type II), CXCR2	58–67	III	2q35 *M68932*	PMN, basophils, monocytes, keratinocytes, some T cells	G-protein-coupled Rc for IL-8 that induces chemotaxis and/or cell activation upon binding IL-8.	*Seminars in Immunology 11:95, 1999* *Crit Rev Immunol 19:1, 1999* *Leucocyte Typing VI, Garland Pub., NY, p. 840, 1998*
CD129	IL-9 Rc	64	I	Xq28, Yq12 *M84747*	act. T cells, B cells, myeloid and erythroid precursors, mast cells	Associates with CD132 to form an IL-9 Rc that stimulates cell growth and/or differentiation with IL-9.	*J Biol Chem 273:9255, 1998* *Proc Natl Acad Sci USA 89:5690, 1992* *Adv Immunol 54:79, 1993*
CD130	gp130; subunit of Rc for IL-6, Oncostatin-M, Leukemia inhibitory factor, IL-11, or ciliary neurotrophic factor	130–140	I	5q11 *M57230*	most WBC, epithelial cells, fibroblasts, hepatocytes, neural cells	A low affinity Rc for oncostatin-M. Together with each respective specific alpha chain, forms high-affinity Rc for IL-6, oncostatin-M, leukemia inhibitory factor, IL-11, or cardiotrophin I.	*Annu Rev Immunol 15:797, 1997* *Science 260:1808, 1993* *Science 260:1805, 1993*
CDw131	IL-3 Rc common beta chain	140	I	22q12.2–13.1 *M59941*	myeloid, blood, and progenitor cells, neutrophils, some B cells	Common beta subunit of IL-3, IL-5, and GM-CSF Rc.	*Blood 82:1960, 1993* *Leukemia Suppl 3:418, 1997* *Cell 66:1165, 1991*
CD132	IL-2 Rc common gamma chain	64	I	Xq13 *D11086*	thymocytes, most WBC, increased with activation	Common gamma subunit for IL-2, IL-4, IL-7, IL-9, IL-15 Rc.	*Immunol Today 20:71, 1999* *Crit Rev Immunol 18:503, 1998*
CD134	MRC OX40, Rc for OX40-ligand	50	I	1p36 *X7562*	medullary thymocytes, act. CD4 T cells	Member of TNF-Rc family that is the Rc for OX40-ligand. Costimulatory molecule for B cell activation.	*J Immunol 163:3007, 1999* *J Exp Med 183:979, 1996* *Adv Immunol 61:1, 1996*
CD135	STK-1, FLT3, flk-2	130 (160)	I	13q12 *U02687*	hematopoietic stem cell	Type III Rc tyrosine kinase that is the Rc for FLT3-ligand.	*Proc Natl Acad Sci USA 91:459, 1994* *Nature 368, 648, 1994*
CDw136	*Récepteur d'Origine Nantaise* (RON)	180 (150/40)	I	3p21.1-22	monocytes, epithelial cells	Heterodimeric Rc tyrosine kinase that provides signal transduction, leading to cell growth and differentiation.	*Oncogene 8:1195, 1993* *Oncogene 13:2167, 1996*
CDw137	4-1BB, ILA (induced by lymphocyte act.)	85 (39)	I	1p36 *U03397*	act. T cells, thymocytes, some non-lymphoid cells	Member of TNF-Rc family that is the Rc for 4-1BBL that serves as costimulatory signal for T cell growth.	*Eur J Immunol 24:2219, 1994* *Blood 85:1043, 1995*
CD138	Syndecan-1, heparan sulfate proteoglycan	80–250	I	2p23 *J05392*	pre-B, immature B, plasma cells, epithelial, mesenchymal cells	Extracellular matrix Rc that can serve as co-Rc for fibroblast growth factor 2, fibronectin, collagen, thrombospondin, and antithrombin III.	*J Cell Biochem 61:578, 1996* *J Biol Chem 265:6884, 1990* *Annu Rev Cell Biol 8:365, 1992*
CD139		209 (228)			B cells, monocytes, FDC, endothelial cells	Unknown.	*Leucocyte Typing VI, Garland Pub., NY, p. 255, 1998*
CD140a	alpha chain of the Rc for platelet-derived growth factor	160, 175	I	4q11–12 *Y10208*	mesenchymal cells, plts, various cancers	Split-tyrosine kinase that serves as Rc for PDGF that is involved in signal transduction induced by PDGF binding.	*Arterioscler Thromb Vasc Biol 19:900, 1999* *Proc Natl Acad Sci USA 93:2884, 1996*

TABLE 13-1 CLUSTER OF DIFFERENTIATION ANTIGENS DEFINED AS OF THE SIXTH INTERNATIONAL WORKSHOP ON LEUKOCYTE TYPING (*CONTINUED*)

Antigen	Other Names	Size	O	Genetics	Distribution	Physiology	Selected References
CD140b	beta chain of the Rc for platelet-derived growth factor	160, 180	I	5q23-31	mesenchymal cells, monocytes, PMN, various cancers	Same as CD140a.	*Biochim Biophys Acta 1305:63, 1996* *J Biol Chem 269:32023, 1994*
CD141	thrombomodulin, feto-modulin	75	I		endothelial cells, PMN, keratino-cytes, smooth muscle, megakar-yocytes, monocytes, synovial lin-ing	C-type lectin that is critical for activa-tion of protein C.	*Hematol Rev 9:251, 1996* *J Biol Chem 271:16603, 1996* *Blood 89:652, 1997*
CD142	tissue factor, thrombo-plastin, coagulation factor III	45–47	I		keratinocyte, epithelia, adventitia, stromal cells, act. monocytes and endothelial cells, some PMN	Serine protease cofactor that acts as major initiator of clotting in normal hemostasis and thrombotic diseases.	*FASEB J 9:883, 1995* *Blood Coag Fibrinol 4:281, 1993*
CD143	peptidyl dipeptidase A, ACE (angiotensin-converting enzyme), kininase II	170	I	17q23 *P12821*	endothelial cells, proximal renal tu-bules, neuronal cells, mesenchy-mal tissues, some T cells	Acts as a peptidyl dipeptide hydrolase to metabolize angiotensin II, bradyki-nin, substance P, LH-RH, and other dipeptides.	*J Hypertension 13:S3, 1995* *J Biol Chem 269:26806, 1994*
CD144	VE-cadherin, cadherin-5	135	I	Unknown *P33151*	endothelium	Involved in homotypic binding.	*Blood 87:630, 1996* *J Clin Invest 98:886, 1996*
CDw145		110, 90, 25			endothelium, stromal cells	Unknown.	*Leucocyte Typing VI, Garland Pub., NY, p. 754, 1998*
CD146	MCAM, Muc 18, S-ENDO Mel-CAM, A32	118 (130)	I		endothelium, sm. muscle, subset act. T cells, FDC	Potential adhesion molecule, esp. of neu-ral crest cells during development.	*Curr Topics Micobiol Immunol 213:95, 1996*
CD147	M6, EMMPRIN (extra-cellular matrix metal-loproteinase inducer)	54 (65)	I	19p13.3 X64364	act. lymphocytes, monocytes, rest-ing WBC (weak)	Binds an unknown ligand on fibroblasts to induce production of collagenase and extracellular MMP.	*Cancer Res 55:434, 1995* *Biochem Biophys Res Commun 224:33, 1996*
CD148	HTPT-η, DEP-1 (high cell density-enhanced phosphotyrosine phosphatase-1), p260	220–250	I	11p11.2 D37781	PMN, monocytes, plts, fibroblasts, DC, nerve cells	Phosphotyrosine phosphatase that in-creases on contact between cells and may be involved in contact inhibi-tion, lymphocyte signal transduction, and T cell activation.	*J Immunol 161:3249, 1998* *Blood 91:2800, 1998* *Cancer Res 56:4236, 1996*
CDw149	MEM-133	120		Not cloned	blood lymphocytes, weakly on plt, PMN, monocytes	Unknown.	*Leucocyte Typing VI, Garland Pub., NY, p. 581, 1998*
CDw150	SLAM, IPO-3	70	I	Unknown U33017	thymocytes, some memory T, some B, act. lymphocytes	IgSF that associates with protein kinases and CD45 that may function as co-stimulatory molecule that also modu-lates the sensitivity to apoptosis.	*J Immunol 162:5719, 1999* *Nature 376:260, 1995* *Immunol Today 17:177, 1996*
CD151	PETA-3, SFA-1	27	III Tet.	Unknown U14650	plt, megakaryocytes, monocytes, ep-ithelial and endothelial cells	May play a role in platelet activation, in-tegrin Rc signaling, as well as tumor cell migration and metastasis.	*Cancer Research 59:3812, 1999* *J Cell Biol 146:477, 1999* *Blood 86:1348, 1995* *Immunol Today 15:588, 1994*
CD152	CTLA-4	50 (33)	I	2q33 M74363	act. T cells	Ligand for CD80 and CD86 that nega-tively regulates T cell activation.	*Science 271:1734, 1996* *J Exp Med 185:393, 1997*
CD153	CD30-ligand	40	II	9q33 L09753	act. T cells, act. MØ, neutrophils, B cells	TNF family member that serves as li-gand for CD30.	*Blood 85:3378, 1995*
CD154	CD40-ligand; gp39	39	II	Xq26.3-27.1 Z15017	act. CD4+ T cells, few act. CD8+ T cells	Ligand for CD40 that induces activa-tion, proliferation, and/or differentia-tion of CD40-expressing cells.	*Adv Immunol 61:1, 1996* *Annu Rev Immunol 14:591, 1996*
CD155	poliovirus Rc	80–90	I	19q13 P15151	monocytes	Can serve as Rc for poliovirus possibly in association with CD44.	*Virology 195:798, 1993*
CD156	ADAM 8, MS2	69	I	10q26.3 P78325	monocytes, PMN	A *d*isintegrin and *m*etalloprotease (ADAM) that possibly is involved in leukocyte extravasation.	*Leucocyte Typing VI, Garland Pub., NY, p. 1083, 1998*
CD157	Mo5, BST-1, BP-3	42–45	GPI	4p15 Q10588	monocytes, PMN, marrow stroma, FDC, synovial cells, endothelial cells	ADP-ribosyl cyclase and cADP-ribose hydrolase.	*Int Immunol 8:1395, 1996* *Int Immunol 8:183, 1996*
CD158a	Killer cell inhibitory re-ceptor (KIR)-cl.42, NKAT1, p58.1, EB6-reactive	58/50	I	19q13.4 L41267	subset of NK cells, some T cells	Ligand for HLA-Cw2, 3, 4, 5, and 6 that regulates NK-mediated cytotoxic-ity (p58 is inhibitory and p50 is acti-vating).	*Annu Rev Immunol 14:619, 1996* *Immunol Today 17:86, 1996* *Science 268:405, 1995*
CD158b	Killer cell inhibitory re-ceptor (KIR)-cl.6, NKAT2, p58.2, p50.2, GL183-reac-tive	58/50	I	19q13.4 L41268	subset of NK cells, some T cells	Ligand for HLA-Cw1, 3, 7, and 8 that regulates NK-mediated cytotoxicity (p58 is inhibitory and p50 is activat-ing).	*Annu Rev Immunol 14:619, 1996* *Immunological Reviews, Vol. 155, 1997*
CD161	NKR-P1A	80–85 (40–44)	II	12p12.3-p13.1 U11276	NK cells, weakly on some T cells, monocytes	May function as a specific Rc for cer-tain NK cell targets.	*Annu Rev Immunol 11:613, 1993*
CD162	P-selectin glycoprotein ligand 1	220 (120)	I	12q24 U02297	PMN, monocytes, most lympho-cytes	Binds to CD62P, CD62E, and CD62L, and helps mediate cell migration.	*J Biol Chem 271:6342, 1996* *Curr Biol 6:261, 1996*
CD163	M130 Antigen, GHI/61, Ber-Mac3, Ki-M8, SM4	110 (130)		Unknown Z22971	monocytes, MØ	Scavenger Rc Group B family member may play a role in the regulation of the immune response in inflamma-tory processes.	*Biochem Biophys Res Comm 260:466, 1996* *J Immunol 161:1883, 1998* *Eur J Immunol 23:2320, 1993*
CD164	MUC-24, Multi-glyco-sylated core protein 24 (MGC-24)	160 (80)	I	6q21 Q04900	epithelial cells, monocytes, marrow stroma	Mucin-like molecule that may mediate adhesion between marrow stroma and hematopoietic progenitors and may also be involved in negatively regulating CD34+ hematopoietic pro-genitor cell growth.	*Blood 92:849, 1998* *Blood 92:2613, 1998* *J Biochem Tokyo 112:609, 1992*
CD165	AD2, gp37	37 (42)			plts, thymocytes, T, B, and NK cells, few monocytes	May play a role in intercellular adhe-sion between thymocytes and thymic epithelial cells.	*J Immunol 154:2012, 1995*
CD166	ALCAM, CD6L, BEN, SC-1, DM-GRASP, neurolin, Kg-CAM	105	I	3q13.1–2 L38608	thymic epithelial cells, act. T cells, CD34+ marrow cells, endothe-lial cells	May interact with CD6 and play a role in T cell development.	*Blood 93:826, 1999* *J Exp Med 181:2213, 1995*

The CD designation is listed in the far-left column labeled *Antigen*. Common names of an antigen before it was given CD status are listed in the column marked *Other Names*. The molecular size of the nonreduced CD antigen is provided in the column marked *Size*. If the molecular size of the reduced CD antigen is different, then this is provided in parentheses. The orientation or anchorage to the plasma membrane of each protein is indicated in the column labeled *O*. The chromosomal location of the gene encoding a surface antigen and the GenBank accession number of the cDNA encoding the molecule are indicated in the column labeled *Genetics*. Tissue and cell types that are known to express a particular CD are provided in the column marked *Distribution*. The preposed or known physiology of a CD antigen is given in the column marked *Physiology*. A few key references and/or reviews concerning each CD antigen is provided in the column marked *Selected References*.

ABBREVIATIONS: act, activated; ALL, acute lymphocytic leukemia; DC, dendritic cells; eos, eosinophils; esp., especially; FDC, follicular dendritic cells; GPI, glycosyl-phosphatidylinositol; HCL, hairy cell leukemia; HEV, high endothelial venules; ICAM, intercellular adhesion molecule; IFN, interferon; IgSF, member of the immunoglobulin supergene family; IL, interleukin; LFA, leukocyte function antigen; LGL, large granular lymphocyte; MHC, major histocompatibility complex; MØ, macrophages; NK, natural killer cells; O, orientation/anchorage of the antigen in the plasma membrane; PDGF, platelet-derived growth factor; PHN, paroxysmal nocturnal hemoglobinuria; plts, platelets; PMN, polymorphonuclear neutrophils; rbc, red blood cells; Rc, receptor; RGD, amino acid sequence, arginine-glycine-aspartic acid; TGF, transforming growth factor; TNF, tumor necrosis factor; vWF, von Willebrand factor; WBC, white blood cells.

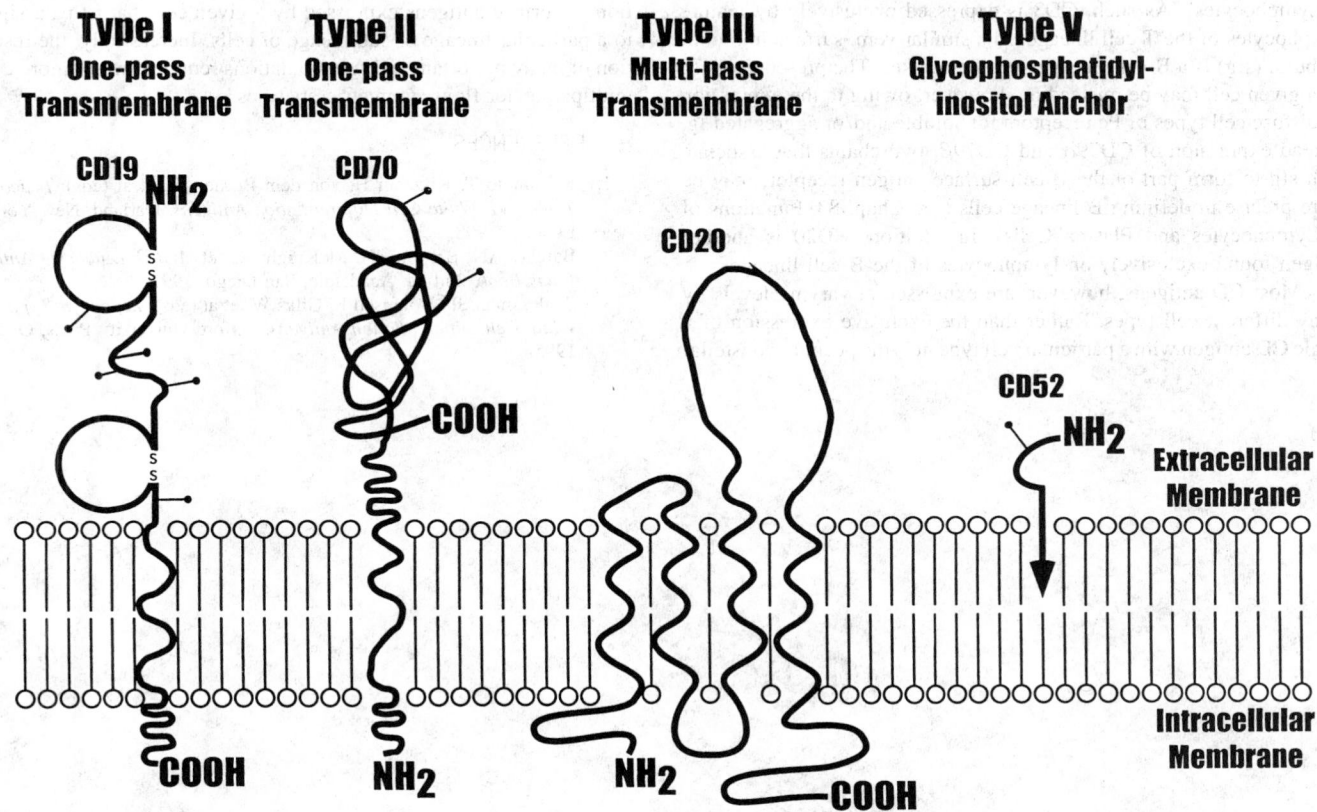

FIGURE 13-1   This figure depicts the major different types of surface proteins with respect to how they integrate into the membrane bilayer. The types of membrane protein are indicated at the top of the figure. The straight lines attached to the open circles represent the lipid bilayer. The dark black lines represent the polypeptide backbones, and the thin black pegs extending from the polypeptide backbone represent carbohydrates. At the far left is CD19, a type I transmembrane protein that passes through the membrane once and has the C-terminus (COOH) in the cytoplasm and N-terminus (NH$_2$) outside the cell. To the immediate right is CD70, a type II single-pass transmembrane protein with the N-terminus inside the cell. To the right of this is CD20, a type III multispan protein that also is a tetraspan molecule in that it traverses the lipid bilayer four times. The tetraspan proteins have both the N-terminus and C-terminus in the cytoplasm. To the far right is CD52, a glycosyl-phosphatidylinositol (GPI)-anchored protein. The labels at the far right indicate the extracellular and intracellular membranes.

TYPE V GLYCOSYL-PHOSPHATIDYLINOSITOL-ANCHORED PROTEINS

Type V proteins use lipid to attach themselves to the plasma membrane. The most common attachment for extracellular proteins in this category is the glycosyl-phosphatidylinositol (GPI) anchor. The GPI anchor can be cleaved by the bacterial enzyme, phosphatidylinositol phospho-lipase C (PI-PLC). Release of an antigen from the cell surface by treatment with PI-PLC often is used to verify that the surface protein has a GPI anchor. However, this criterion is not absolute, as some GPI-anchored proteins may be resistant to PI-PLC.

Newly synthesized proteins destined to receive a GPI anchor each contain a secretion signal sequence at the NH$_2$-terminus and another signal sequence at the COOH-terminus. The latter directs cleavage and subsequent appendage of a GPI anchor soon after the molecule's biosynthesis and extrusion into the endoplasmic reticulum. This biosynthetic pathway is defective in paroxysmal nocturnal hemoglobinuria (PNH) (see Chap. 36, Paroxysmal Nocturnal Hemoglobinuria).

The site of attachment for the GPI generally precedes a hydrophobic domain of 7 to 20 amino acids that sometimes may double as an actual transmembrane domain. In this case, the molecule may exist as either of two isoforms, one attached to the membrane via a GPI anchor and another as a type I transmembrane protein. Because GPI-anchored proteins associate specifically with sphingomyelin lipids, follow a different path of transport to the cell surface than type I transmembrane proteins, are excluded from coated pits, and are not able to associate directly with intracellular proteins, a GPI isoform of a given surface protein usually has a physiology that is distinct from that of its respective type I transmembrane isoform.

TISSUE DISTRIBUTION OF MEMBRANE ANTIGENS

The tissue distribution for each CD antigen listed in Table 13-1 summarizes the work of many laboratories. For most CD antigens, however, a comprehensive analysis of the full gamut of different tissues has not been performed. Therefore, failure to list a cell type in this table for a particular CD antigen does not necessarily mean that cell type does not express that antigen. A complete review of the tissue distributions of the CD antigens is reviewed in the summary books published after each workshop.[1-3] References to these books are implied, but not necessarily cited, for each CD antigen listed.

Some of surface antigens are useful for delineating the cell lineage of leukocytes. Unique assignment of a surface antigen to a particular lineage is best when the antigen is related to a unique functional property of a given cell type. The CD3 surface antigens form part of the T-cell receptor complex for antigen (see Chap. 84, Functions of

T Lymphocytes). As such, CD3 is expressed exclusively by mature lymphocytes of the T cell lineage. In a similar vein, surface immunoglobulin (sIg) is a B-cell lineage specific marker. The presence of sIg on a given cell may be misleading, however, owing to the expression on diffuse cell types of Fc receptors for soluble and/or aggregated Ig. Instead expression of CD79α and CD79β, two chains that associate with sIg to form part of the B-cell surface antigen receptor, may be more precise in defining B-lineage cells (see Chap. 83, Functions of B Lymphocytes and Plasma Cells). In addition, CD20 is another antigen found exclusively on lymphocytes of the B-cell lineage.

Most CD antigens, however, are expressed at varying levels by many different cell types. Rather than the exclusive expression of a single CD antigen with a particular cell type, it is the peculiar constella-

tion of surface antigens expressed by a given cell that helps assign it to a particular lineage or sublineage of cells. Increasingly, the resolution of many important cell subpopulations requires two or more color multiparameter flow cytometric analyses.

REFERENCES

1. Kishimoto T, Kikutani H, von dem Borne AE, et al (eds): *Leucocyte Typing VI, White Cell Differentiation Antigens.* Garland, New York & London, 1998.
2. Barclay AN, Brown MH, McKnight AJ, et al: *The Leucocyte Antigen Facts Book,* 2nd ed. Academic, San Diego, 1997.
3. Schlossman SF, Boumsell L, Gilks W, et al (eds): *Leucocyte Typing V. White Cell Differentiation Antigens.* Oxford University Press, Oxford, 1995.

HEMATOPOIETIC STEM CELLS, PROGENITOR CELLS, AND CYTOKINES

PETER J. QUESENBERRY

GERALD A. COLVIN

HEMATOPOIESIS

GENERAL CONSIDERATIONS

The blood in mammalian species includes a number of different cell types essential for survival. Erythrocytes transport oxygen; platelets mediate blood clotting and support tissue integrity; neutrophil, eosinophil, and basophil granulocytes and monocytes are essential to host defense against bacteria, fungi, parasites, and viruses; T lymphocytes, natural killer cells, and dendritic cells all function as antigen-presenting cells and in cell-mediated immunity; and B lymphocytes are the source of antibodies. The level of these cell types is controlled by multiple humoral and cellular factors and adjusts rapidly to meet need. Infection by a variety of microorganisms results in almost immediate release of mature neutrophils from the marrow storage pool, followed by an increase in production of granulocytes, and usually also monocytes, until the infectious agents are cleared. Hemorrhage or acute hemolysis results in a rapid release of marrow reticulocytes, followed by a sustained increase in red cell production until the red cell numbers return to normal. Platelet production and release responds to several stimuli, including decreases in platelet number, acute anemia, and tissue destruction or inflammation. The modulation of T- and B-cell production is complex and occurs in response to immune stimuli (e.g., foreign antigens), and the modulation of increased production may occur within different subsets of these cells (see Chaps. 83 and 84).

Mature cell types derive ultimately from marrow stem cells, which differentiate into progenitor cells that are controlled by circulating or membrane-bound cytokines or various adhesion proteins. A very small proportion of circulating cells are progenitor cells and stem cells, which can be isolated from the blood by special techniques.

STEM CELLS

A hematolymphopoietic stem cell is defined as a cell with extensive self-renewal and proliferative potential, coupled with the capacity to differentiate into the progenitors of all the blood cell lineages, that is,

---

Acronyms and abbreviations that appear in this chapter include: AGM, aortogonadal mesonephros; BFU-E, burst-forming unit-erythroid; BRDU, bromodeoxyuridine; CFU-E, colony-forming unit-erythroid; CFU-GM, granulocyte-macrophage colony-forming unit; CFU-S, colony-forming unit spleen; CSF-1, colony-stimulating factor-1; FOG, friend of GATA-1; G-CSF, granulocyte colony-stimulating factor; GM-CSF, granulocyte-macrophage colony-stimulating factor; IL, interleukin; LIF, leukemia inhibitory factor; LTC-IC, long-term culture-initiating cell; MCAP, monocyte chemotactic and activating factor; M-CSF, macrophage colony-stimulating factor; MIP, macrophage inflammatory protein; MPLV, myeloproliferative leukemia virus; NK, natural killer; PDGF, platelet-derived growth factor; PTB, phosphotyrosine binding; SHZ, Src-homology; VLA, very late antigen.

---

erythrocytes, neutrophil, eosinophil, and basophil granulocytes, mast cells, monocytes and macrophages, platelets, B lymphocytes, T lymphocytes, natural killer cells, and dendritic cells. *Self-renewal* refers to the potential to produce daughter cells with identical characteristics. Self-renewal resulting in production of identical stem cells without any new differentiated characteristics has not been established experimentally, but renewal on a cell population basis clearly occurs. The sequential development of progenitor cells and mature cells from stem cells is presented in Fig. 14-1.

Studies of both murine and human hematopoietic cells indicate that two daughter cells from a primitive undifferentiated cell can have totally different lineages, for example, one cell giving rise to neutrophils and monocytes, while the daughter cell may give rise to erythrocytes, megakaryocytes, and mast cells.[1-7] These observations suggest a less-ordered or stochastic system in which the commitment decision to produce different lineages is made within one cell cycle transit, although concordance of daughter cells is still the rule, indicating a model in which there is ordered and progressive lineage restriction with differentiation. In general, as differentiated characteristics are attained, self-renewal potential declines precipitously.

The "gold standard" for the definition of a stem cell is the ability of that single cell to repopulate long-term hematopoiesis in the whole animal. The majority of stem cell studies have been carried out in mice, although one can infer the existence of long-term repopulating cells in humans based on the repopulation in patients given marrow ablative treatment and allogeneic marrow transplant. Studies in mice using unique radiation-induced chromosome abnormalities or retroviral markers have established the capacity of a very few cells (approaching one cell) to totally repopulate the lymphohematopoietic system.[8-11] When relatively small numbers of marked stem cells, obtained by limiting dilution of sorted marrow cells, are transplanted, lymphohematopoiesis may be clonal or oligoclonal initially. Normal polyclonal lymphohematopoiesis derives from a relatively large number of clones. Studies of competitive marrow repopulation and mathematical modeling support the model of polyclonal hematopoiesis.[12]

COLONY-FORMING UNIT SPLEEN

Studies on the potential of single lymphohematopoietic cells to give rise to clones of progeny cells in vivo or in vitro provided the model systems for the detailed definition of lymphohematopoietic stem progenitor cells. The observation of "bumps" on the spleen after marrow infusion into lethally irradiated mice resulted in the first clonal hematopoietic stem cell assay.[13-27] These splenic nodules were clones of hematopoietic cells containing erythroid, granulocytic, and megakaryocytic lineages, and the cells giving rise to the clones were termed *colony-forming unit spleen* (CFU-S). This assay is rarely carried out today, but characteristics of this cell illustrate the nature of stem/progenitor cells. This cell (the CFU-S) gave rise to variable, but large, numbers of differentiated cells, was influenced by the splenic microenvironment, was in a relatively quiescent (G_0/G_1) state, and reproduced itself. The CFU-S assay monitors cells with varying engraftment and growth potential but did not appear to be an assay for the most primitive long-term repopulating stem cell.

Perhaps the major breakthrough in the hematopoiesis field was the description of marrow cells with the capacity to form colonies of granulocytes and macrophages in vitro in the obligate presence of stimulatory factors present in conditioned media or serum (Fig. 14-2).[28,29]

The characterization of the granulocyte-macrophage colony-forming cell (CFU-GM) and the molecules, which stimulated or inhibited its growth, was followed by the description of a number of different progenitors with different growth and lineage potential in in vitro clonal culture. These included clones with a single lineage such as

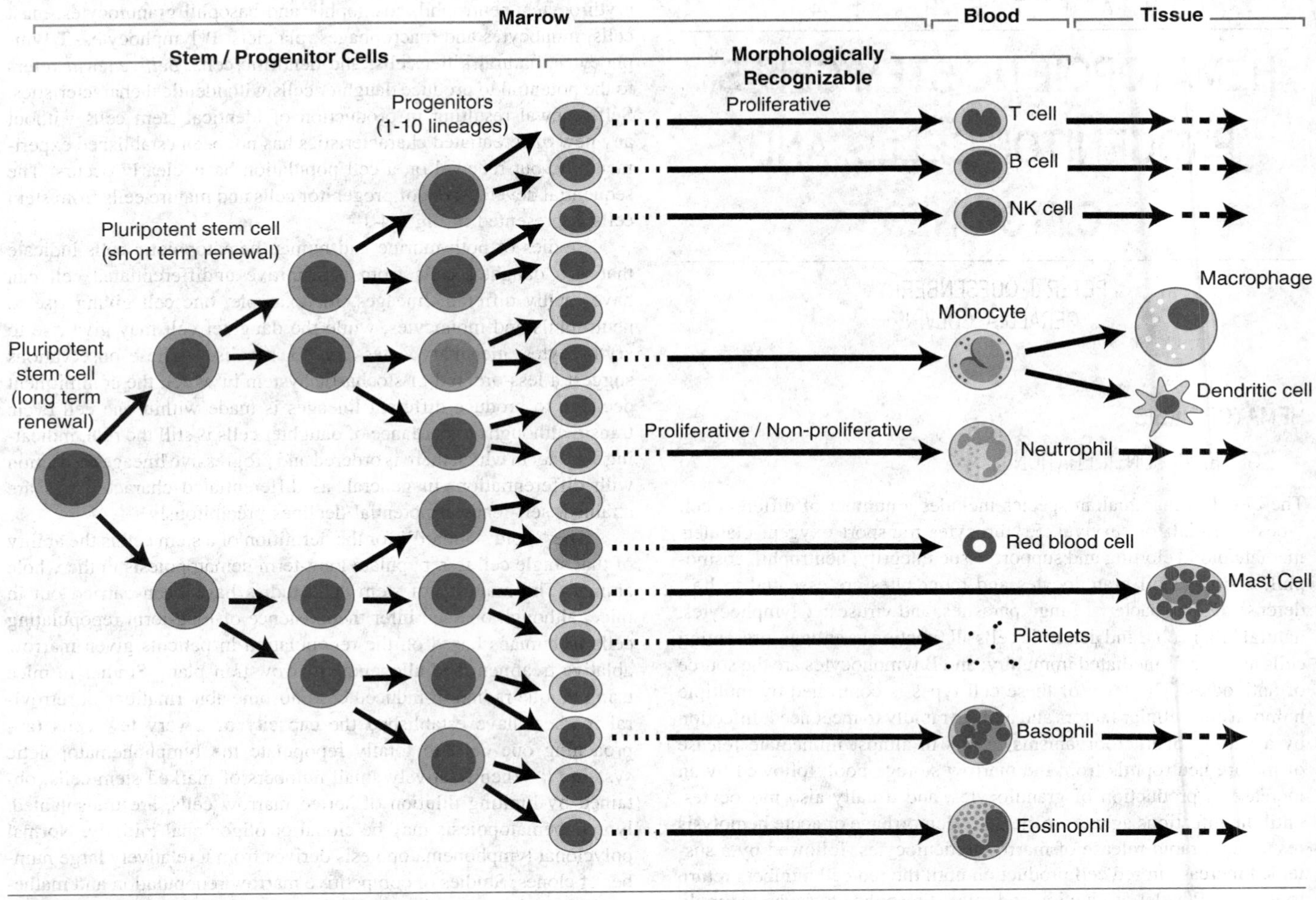

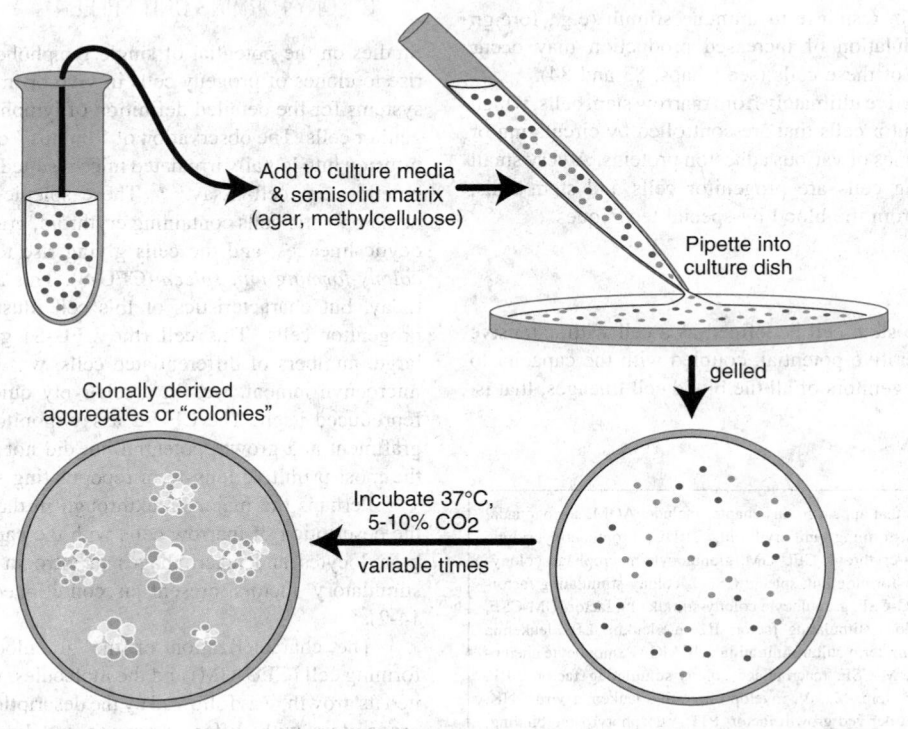

Marrow

Stem / Progenitor Cells

Blood

Tissue

Progenitors
(1-10 lineages)

Morphologically Recognizable

Proliferative

Pluripotent stem cell
(short term renewal)

Pluripotent
stem cell
(long term
renewal)

T cell

B cell

NK cell

Macrophage

Monocyte

Dendritic cell

Proliferative / Non-proliferative

Neutrophil

Red blood cell

Mast Cell

Platelets

Basophil

Eosinophil

FIGURE 14-1 Hierarchical model of lymphohematopoiesis.

Add to culture media
& semisolid matrix
(agar, methylcellulose)

Pipette into
culture dish

gelled

Clonally derived
aggregates or "colonies"

Incubate 37°C,
5-10% CO_2

variable times

FIGURE 14-2 Clonal assay for granulocyte-macrophage progenitor cells.

TABLE 14-1   HEMATOPOIETIC STEM/PROGENITOR CELLS ASSAYED IN VITRO

Cell Type (assay)	Lineage	Primary Cytokine
Granulocyte-macrophage colony-forming cell (CFU-GM)	Neutrophil-macrophage	GM-CSF
Macrophage-colony-forming cell (CFU-M)	Macrophage	CSF-1
Granulocyte colony-forming cell (CFU-G)	Neutrophil	G-CSF
Eosinophil colony-forming cell (CFU-EOS)	Eosinophil	IL-5 IL-3 GM-CSF
Burst-forming unit erythroid (BFU-e) (primitive progenitor)	Erythroid	Erythropoietin and "primitive" cytokines (IL-3, KIT ligand, GM-CSF, IL-4, others)
Colony-forming unit erythroid (CFU-E) (more mature progenitor)	Erythroid	Erythropoietin
Burst-forming unit megakaryocyte (BFU-meg) (primitive progenitor)	Megakaryocyte	IL-3, GM-CSF, phorbol ester, cholera toxin, C-mpl ligand
Colony-forming unit megakaryocyte (CFU-meg) (more mature progenitor)	Megakaryocyte	IL-3, GM-CSF, c-mpl ligand, IL-11, IL-6, leukemia-inhibitory factor (LIF), G-CSF, KIT ligand, IL-4
Mast cell colony-forming unit	Basophil; mast cell	IL-3, KIT ligand, GM-CSF
Macrophage-B-cell colony-forming unit (fetal liver)	Macrophage; B-lymphocyte	IL-7; other unknown factors
Colony-forming unit granulocyte/erythroid/macrophage & megakaryocyte (CFU-GEMM)	Neutrophil, erythroid, IL-3, macrophage possible T-cell	GM-CSF, erythropoietin
Long-term culture-initiating cell (LTC-IC), LTC-IC extended and cobblestone-forming cell, - stromal based	Not clear, probably assays both more or less primitive progenitor/stem cells—usefulness not yet established	Stromal-cell–derived cytokines
High proliferative potential colony-forming cell (HPP-CFC)	Dependent on numbers of cytokines. Two cytokines yield macrophage colonies. Three or more end in neutrophil, macrophage, megakaryocyte, and other cell types	CSF-1, IL-3, IL-1α, KIT ligand, G-CSF, GM-CSF, IL-6, others
Colony-forming unit blast (CFU-B1)	Early multiple lineage progenitor cell	Defined by cytokine stimulators

granulocytic or erythroid or clones with multiple lineages including lymphocytes. In parallel with the description of these clonal entities, a growing number of cytokine regulators was described, purified, and then molecularly cloned. The different stem/progenitor clones are outlined in Table 14-1. General characteristics of lymphohematopoietic stem cells are presented in Table 14-2. Progenitor cells in general have a higher proliferative rate, i.e., are progressing through cell cycle, have less total proliferative potential, and show a restricted number of differentiated cell types. They are also responsive to a smaller number of cytokines; in essence they are defined by a limited number of cytokine receptors.

The erythroid progenitors and their primary regulator, erythropoietin, were the first to be extensively studied. The presence of reticulocytes and iron incorporation to mark newly produced red blood cells and the capacity of induced polycythemia to shut off in vivo erythropoiesis provided an in vivo model for the study of erythroid regulation.[30-34] A mouse was made polycythemic inhibiting its own erythropoiesis, a

putative erythroid regulator was administered, and then red blood cell production was monitored by reticulocyte number or iron incorporation. These cumbersome in vivo models allowed for the initial definition of erythropoietin, but it took in vitro culture systems and the application of biochemical and molecular genetic techniques to provide biochemical characterization and molecular cloning of erythropoietin.

The studies with in vitro clonal culture system showed erythroid progenitors with different proliferative and differentiative potential.[35-37] The more primitive erythroid progenitors termed *burst-forming unit-erythroid* (BFU-E) were defined by a high proliferative response to multiple cytokines, while the more differentiated colony-forming unit-erythroid (CFU-E) was responsive to erythropoietin and had limited proliferative potential (Fig. 14-3).

Erythropoietin was found to be active in vivo and in vitro[30,31,35-37] and acted via a cell membrane receptor to induce erythroid differentiation[38,39] and to suppress apoptosis or programmed cell death.[40,41] It is one of the most specific of the lymphohematopoietic cytokines acting

TABLE 14-2   PLURIPOTENTIAL HEMATOPOIETIC STEM AND PROGENITOR CELLS

Characteristic	Stem Cell	Progenitor Cell
Proliferative potential	Large	More limited
Renewal	On a population basis	Probably none
Potential for differentiation	All lymphohematopoietic lineages	Restricted
Differentiated characteristics	Minimal—lineage negative	Progressively increases to lineage specific cell
Cycle status	Dormant	Cycling
Cytokine responsiveness	Large number of cytokines needed for expression of phenotype	Restricted
Cell of origin	Unknown	Stem cell
Staining with rhodamine & Hoechst dyes (partial measure of p170 activity)	Stains dimly (p170 very active)	Rhodamine "bright" (p170 less active)
Producing long-term hemopoiesis after in vivo transplant	Defines these cells	Limited to none
Adheres to marrow stroma	Yes	Limited to none

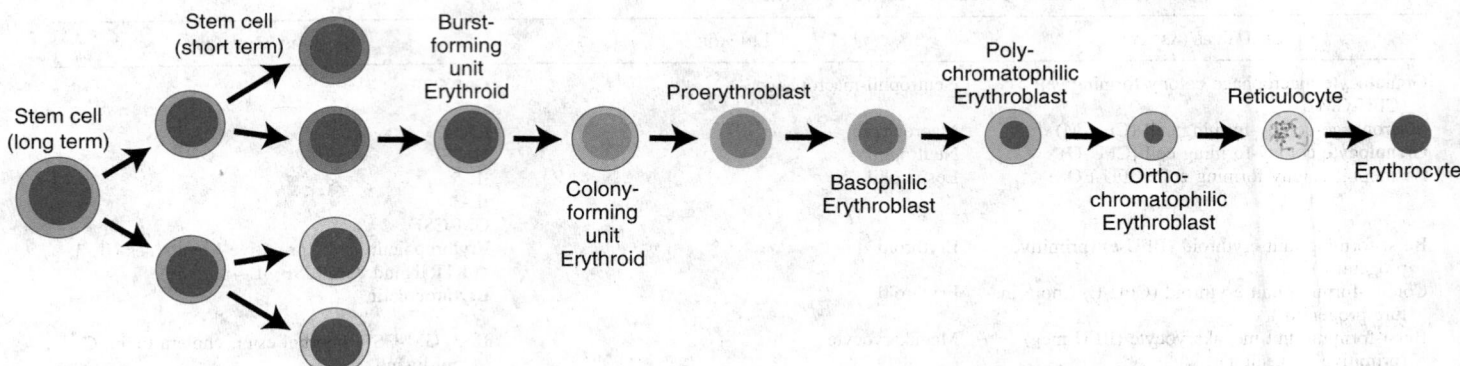

FIGURE 14-3   The erythroid differentiation pathway.

on erythroid cells, while many other cytokines show action on multiple lineages. The explicit actions of erythropoietin are described in Chap. 29, and its use in the treatment of anemia associated with a relative erythropoietin deficiency state (i.e., renal failure) is described in Chap. 33.

The CFU-GM, CFU-G, and CFU-M are progenitors in the granulocyte macrophage pathway regulated by a number of cytokines, but primarily granulocyte colony-stimulating factor (G-CSF), granulocyte-macrophage CSF (GM-CSF), and macrophage CSF (M-CSF) or CSF-1 (Figure 14-4). These cytokines are active in vivo and G-CSF and GM-CSF are in use clinically for neutropenic states.

The GM and G progenitors are also in cycle, have restricted lineages, and respond to a relatively small number of cytokines. As with erythropoietin, CSF-1 and to a lesser extent G-CSF are relatively lineage-specific, stimulating predominantly the production of monocyte-macrophages and granulocytes, respectively. These cytokines stimulate proliferation and differentiation and inhibit apoptosis through cell-surface–based receptors which send second messenger signals activating nuclear transcriptional mechanisms which then turn on or off various genetic programs.

There are a very large number of cytokines regulating hematopoiesis, certainly exceeding 60 to 70 in numbers. These cytokines and their most prominent hematopoietic activity are presented in Tables 14-3, 14-4, and 14-5. There are an intimidating number of cytokines with a wide range of effects on lymphohematopoietic cells. These agents, however, have certain common features. The cytokines are

glycoproteins acting at very low concentrations on receptor molecules to signal the cell to live, die, proliferate, differentiate, or function; many cytokines act on primitive stem cells and their functioning terminally differentiated progeny. These actions, particularly at the more primitive stem cell levels, may be on survival, proliferation, or differentiation or, alternatively, especially in mature cells, on function. Cytokines usually act on multiple lineages and multiple cell types and frequently act synergistically (or additively) to stimulate or inhibit. In many ways the progenitors are defined by their cytokine receptors.

SPECIFIC CYTOKINES

The broad-based actions of cytokines on hematopoietic cells are complex and evolving. Most cytokines have many actions on different lineages and stages of differentiation. Descriptions of the biologic, biochemical, and molecular genetic characteristics of these cytokines follows.

ERYTHROPOIETIN

Erythropoietin was first defined in in vivo assays. The initial definition was provided in the 1950s.[30,31] The hormone was later purified, its sequence determined, and the gene encoding its production cloned.[117-119] The clonal culture systems for BFU-E, CFU-E, and intermediate erythroid progenitor cells facilitated investigation of the biology of erythropoietin (Fig. 14-3). Erythropoietin is produced in the

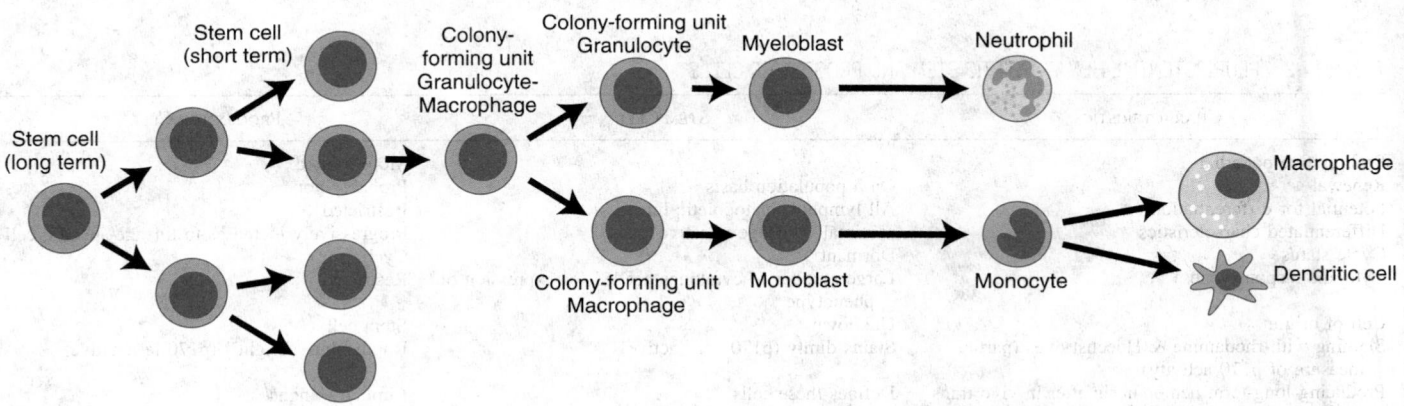

FIGURE 14-4   The granulocyte-monocyte-macrophage differentiation pathway.

TABLE 14-3   CYTOKINES ACTIVE ON LYMPHOHEMATOPOIESIS STEM AND PROGENITOR CELLS

CYTOKINE	PRINCIPAL ACTIVITY
IL-1	Induces production of other cytokines from many cells, co-stimulates early stem cells with other cytokines, immune response modulator.[42,43]
IL-2	T-cell growth factor. Inhibits myelopoiesis and erythropoiesis.[44–46]
IL-3	Multilineage stimulator of neutrophilic, erythroid, lymphoid, and megakaryocytic cells. In vivo increases blood monocytes, neutrophils, eosinophils, and platelets.[47–50]
IL-4	Stimulates B cells and modulates immune response—co-stimulates CFU-GM and CFU-E.[51,52]
IL-5	Simulates B cells and eosinophils.[53–55]
IL-6	Stimulates megakaryopoiesis and synergizes with IL-1, 2, 3, 4, GM-CSF, and CSF. Enhances plasma cell proliferation. Role in Castleman's disease and atrial myxoma.[56,57]
IL-7	Pre-B cell (with KIT ligand) and early stem cells.[58,59]
IL-8	Stimulates production and function of neutrophils and acts as proinflammatory factor. Marrow progenitor and stem cell mobilizer.[60–64]
IL-9	Co-stimulates CFU-GM and CFU-mixed. Stimulates BFU-E with erythropoietin. Enhances T-cell production and, with IL-3, mast cell production.[65]
IL-10	Inhibits cytokine production, modulates immune cells and stimulates mast cells.[66]
IL-11	Shares most of the activities of IL-6. Increases neutrophil and platelets in blood in primate model.[67–69]
IL-12	Increases generation of immunocompetent cells.[70]
IL-13	Enhances KIT ligand induced proliferation of lineage negative, stem cell, and antigen-positive murine marrow stem cells. Inhibits cytokine production by monocytes. Stimulates B cells and activates T cells.[71]
IL-14	B-cell growth factor.[72]
IL-15	Modulates T-cell activity.[73]
IL-16	Acts as immunomodulator and lymphocyte chemoattractant ligand for CD-4.[74]
IL-17	Induces production of other cytokines such as IL-6, IL-8, and G-CSF and enhances expression of adhesion molecules.[75,76]
IL-18	Induces GM-CSF and interferon gamma production. Inhibits IL-10 production.[77,78]

renal peritubular interstitial cells[121,122] or renal tubular cells.[123] There are also measurable erythropoietin levels in anephric animals and humans presumably of hepatic origin.[124–127] Hepatocytes and Kupffer cells have been implicated as the cell of origin for hepatic erythropoietin.[128] Marrow macrophages may also be a source of erythropoietin.[129] The tissue oxygen-sensing mechanisms that are linked to erythropoietin elaboration may involve a heme protein.[130] Further details of the structure, function, and regulation of erythropoietin are presented in Chap. 29.

The response of BFU-E and CFU-E to erythropoietin correlates directly with the presence of erythropoietin receptors. Two classes of erythropoietin receptor, high and low affinity, have been identified on erythroblasts obtained from the spleens of mice infected with the

TABLE 14-4   CYTOKINES ACTIVE ON LYMPHOHEMATOPOIETIC STEM OR PROGENITOR CELLS (GROWTH FACTORS)

CYTOKINE	PRINCIPAL OR HIGHLIGHTED ACTIVITY
CSF-1 (M-CSF)	Enhances production and function of monocytes.[79,80]
G-CSF	Stimulates granulocyte production and function. Co-stimulates early progenitors in synergy with several other cytokines. Stimulates pre-B cells. In vivo stimulates granulocyte production.[81,82]
GM-CSF	Stimulates CFU GM and production of monocytes, neutrophils, eosinophils, and basophils. Synergizes with IL-4 to produce dendritic cells. Co-stimulates many types of progenitors, including early multipotent stem cells.[83–87]
Erythropoietin	Stimulates erythrocyte production in vitro and in vivo. Co-stimulates BFU-E and CFU-meg and stimulates CFU-E.[30,31,88,89]
FLT-3 ligand	Co-stimulates multipotential stem cells, especially with thrombopoietin and KIT ligand. Stimulates generation of dendritic cells. Induces tumor regression in vivo.[90–94]
KIT ligand	Stimulates survival and growth of primitive stem cells in synergism with many factors. Enhances generation of mast cells.[91,95–97]
Thrombopoietin	Major regulator of proliferation and differentiation of megakaryocytes. Co-stimulates multipotential stem cells in combination with KIT ligand and IL-11. Promotes erythropoiesis in synergy with erythropoietin.[98,99]

anemia strain of Friend virus.[39] The receptor has been cloned[38] and belongs to the hemopoietic family of receptor proteins. The cell cycle behavior of BFU-E[131] in vivo is not influenced by hypoxia (increased erythropoietin) or hypertransfusion (decreased erythropoiesis), and BFU-E can proliferate in vitro in the absence of exogenous erythropoietin when in the presence of other cytokines.[132] Actinomycin given to mice blocks the action of erythropoietin on CFU-E and more mature erythroid cells, virtually eliminating them in vivo, but has no effect on the numbers of marrow and splenic BFU-E.[133] Monoclonal antibody purified blood BFU-E do not require erythropoietin until after 72 h of culture. Initially only 20 percent of BFU-E have erythropoietin receptors, but with maturation in vitro over 4 days 100 percent of the cells bind ^{125}I erythropoietin. The peak receptor number occurs at the CFU-E stage, the main target cell for the action of erythropoietin. CFU-E does not have the proliferative potential of BFU-E but requires erythropoietin for limited proliferation, survival, and terminal maturation.[88] CFU-E is responsive to low concentrations of erythropoietin.[89] Adding erythropoietin to CFU-E in vitro leads to rapid expression of mRNA for alpha and beta globins, and hemoglobin synthesis commences soon thereafter.[134] Erythropoietin also stimulates the proliferation of proerythroblasts and basophilic erythroblasts,[135] but with maturation beyond the basophilic erythroblast stage, the erythroid cells no longer appear to require erythropoietin for maturation or function[136]; many erythroid cells, including late-stage erythroid progenitors, undergo programmed cell death or apoptosis, and this is prevented by erythropoietin. The action of erythropoietin on second messenger and transcriptional factors is outlined below.

EARLY-ACTING ERYTHROID CYTOKINES

A critical observation was that erythropoietin does not act on BFU-E or other early progenitors alone, but rather in concert with other cytokines. These include IL-3,[137,138] GM-CSF,[139] IL-9,[140] steel factor,[137] interleukin 4,[141] and insulin-like growth factor.[1] This list will grow with increased purity of the progenitors or omissions of serum from the cultures.

There are strong similarities between erythropoietin growth control and the action of other lymphohematopoietic cytokines. These include (1) an action on proliferation and maturation; (2) an effect on

TABLE 14-5   CYTOKINES ACTIVE ON LYMPHOHEMATOPOIETIC STEM CELLS: CYTOKINE INHIBITORY FACTORS AND OTHERS

CYTOKINE	PRINCIPAL OR HIGHLIGHTED ACTIVITY
MIP-1 alpha	Inhibits early multipotent colony formation, but stimulates committed precursor colonies.[100,101]
Transforming growth factor beta	Suppresses early multipotent progenitors, but stimulates later progenitors.[102,103]
MCAF, platelet factor 4, H-subunit ferritin	Similar to TGF beta.[102]
Tumor necrosis factor	Similar to TGF beta but a more pronounced effect on BFU-E and CFU-E.[104]
Activin	Enhances IL-3 and erythropoietin stimulated BFU-E and CFU-E. Inhibits IL-3 stimulated CFU-GM.[105]
Inhibin	Inhibits CFU-MIX, CFU-GM, & BFU-E.[102,105]
Interferon—alpha, beta, and gamma	Coinhibits CFU-MIX, CFU-GM, & BFU-E. Inhibits or stimulates production of cytokines. Immune modulators.[102]
Prostaglandin E and 2	Suppresses CFU-M with less or no activity on CFU-GM, CFU-G. Enhances BFU-E indirectly through CD8+ lymphocytes.[102]
Glu-Glu-Asp-Asp-Lys (pentapeptide)	Inhibits CFU-S proliferation and CFU-GM.[106]
N-acetyl-Ser-As-Lys-Pro (tetrapeptide)	Inhibits CFU-S and other progenitors entry into cell cycle.[107]
Leukemia inhibitory factor	Inhibits GM- & G-CSF stimulated CFU-GM and CFU-G, respectively.[108,109]
Insulin-like growth factor II	Stimulates erythroid and granulocyte progenitors.[110,111]
Hepatocyte growth factor	Synergistic activity on progenitors.[112]
Basic fibroblast growth factor	Acts in concert with other cytokines on early multipotential and megakaryocyte progenitors.[113-115]
Platelet-derived growth factor	Stimulates erythroid and granulocyte progenitors.[116]

cell survival inhibiting apoptosis; (3) an action mediated through cell surface receptors; and (4) synergistic interactions with a number of other cytokines.

COLONY-STIMULATING FACTORS

These were first defined by the stimulation of granulocyte-macrophage colonies in soft agar culture. The four colony-stimulating factors are CSF-1 or M-CSF, GM-CSF, G-CSF, and IL-3 (multi-CSF).

GRANULOCYTE-MACROPHAGE COLONY-STIMULATING FACTOR

GM-CSF was first defined by its ability to stimulate colonies of neutrophils and macrophages in soft-agar culture, but it acts on many cell types, including relatively early multipotential stem cells, megakaryocyte, eosinophil erythroid, dendritic progenitors, and mature neutrophils and macrophages.[83-87] GM-CSF was first isolated from murine lungs[142] and later from a human T-cell leukemia line.[143] Human GM-CSF is a glycoprotein with a M_r of 22,000, and murine GM-CSF is a glycoprotein with a M_r of 23,000.

The murine gene was cloned from a murine lung cDNA library[144] while the human cDNA was isolated from a human leukemia cell line.[145,146] The human GM-CSF contains 127 amino acids with an M_r of 14,000, and the human gene was isolated on chromosome 5 [147,148] with a control region 5 prime of the gene.[149] GM-CSF stimulates proliferation and maturation of bipotential neutrophil and macrophage progenitors and has multiple actions on mature cells including stimulation of synthesis of membrane and nucleoproteins in murine granulocytes,[87] increased adhesion protein expression in neutrophils,[150] inhibition of neutrophil migration,[143] and stimulation of cytotoxic and phagocyte activity against bacteria, yeast, parasites, and antibody-coated tumor cells,[151-154] enhanced survival and cytotoxicity of human neutrophils and eosinophils in vitro,[155] and increased basophil histamine release. GM-CSF also increases neutrophil superoxide production in response to bacterial chemoattractants and increases neutrophil arachidonic acid release and leukotriene B4 synthesis in response to calcium ionophore and chemoattractants.[156,157] GM-CSF also induces changes in neutrophil calcium flux and pH after treatment with a chemotactic agent.

GM-CSF mediates its effects by binding to a specific cell receptor (see below).[158,160] GM-CSF controls the proliferation of GM-CSF–dependent cells during the GI phase of cell cycle.[161]

The availability of recombinant growth factor has permitted studies of bioactivity of GM-CSF in vivo. Administration of GM-CSF

to murine species and to primates causes increases in granulocytes, monocytes, eosinophils, and, to a lesser extent, other white cell types in both normal animals or animals subjected to cytotoxic or irradiation-induced marrow suppression.[162-168] GM-CSF may also raise the platelet count and possibly the reticulocyte level,[162,164,166] although in some patients the platelet count is lowered.

Administration of GM-CSF to humans with AIDS results in a dose-dependent increase in neutrophils, eosinophils, and monocytes.[169] The administration of GM-CSF during chemotherapy lessens the fall in the neutrophil count.[170,171] GM-CSF stimulates proliferation of about one-third of human cancer cell lines, including small-cell lung carcinoma, ovary, breast, colon, and melanoma. Other effects of GM-CSF include lowering of serum cholesterol, mobilization of blood progenitors, induction of inflammatory recall, and a capillary leak syndrome. GM-CSF is licensed for therapeutic use.

GRANULOCYTE COLONY-STIMULATING FACTOR

G-CSF was first defined as a factor that had the capacity both to stimulate normal granulocyte colonies and to induce maturation of leukemic cell lines.[81,82] It has been purified to homogeneity from mouse lung ($M_r = 25,000$).[172] Human G-CSF has a similar molecular size and cross-reacts with both human and murine cells. cDNAs for both murine and human G-CSFs have been cloned.[172,173] The human cDNA encodes a polypeptide with a 30 amino acid signal sequence followed by mature G-CSF sequence of 177 amino acids. The molecular mass is 19 KD. These proteins stimulate predominantly neutrophil colony formation. The gene for human G-CSF has been localized on chromosome 17.[174] G-CSF can initiate the proliferation of some granulocyte-macrophage progenitors but does not sustain this beyond several days. G-CSF interacts with a number of cytokines to stimulate blast colony and high proliferative potential colony-forming cell development in vitro, induces terminal maturation in WEHI-3B myelomonocytic leukemic cells,[85] and stimulates pre-B cells in vitro.[175] G-CSF also affects mature progeny; priming human neutrophils to undergo oxidative metabolism in response to formyl-methionlleucylphenylanine, as well as increasing antibody-dependent cell-mediated cytotoxicity of human neutrophils. G-CSF primes human neutrophils for enhanced arachidonic acid release, and receptors for G-CSF have been identified on both human neutrophils and leukemic cell lines.[176] G-CSF also stimulates proliferation and variable degrees of maturation in acute myelogenous leukemia blast cells[177,178] and stimulates proliferation of a variety of human solid tumor cell lines. G-CSF is active in vivo in mice, hamsters, primates, and humans, stimulating impressive neutrophil increases with lesser increases of monocytes, lymphocytes, and possibly platelets.[179-188]

G-CSF has been licensed for therapeutic use.

COLONY-STIMULATING FACTOR 1 (MACROPHAGE COLONY-STIMULATING FACTOR)

CSF-1 (M-CSF) stimulates a population of progenitor cells with a high predilection for macrophage maturation, although early in the culture period there may be some granulocyte production. CSF-1 binds rapidly to mature macrophages and is internalized and degraded. Low levels of CSF-1 support survival of murine marrow macrophages while decreasing their level of protein catabolism. Higher levels of CSF-1 stimulate protein synthesis, cell division,[189,190] and various macrophage functions, including antitumor activity,[191] secretion of products of oxygen reduction,[192] and plasminogen activator.[193-195] CSF-1 also induces production of IL-1 from macrophages.[196] The product of the FMS gene is the receptor for CSF-1.[197-199] The receptor is a tyrosine kinase, which autophosphorylates. The number of monocyte receptors increases with maturation and may be induced by other growth factors, including IL-3 and IL-1, explaining the synergistic effects of the combinations either of CSF-1 or IL-3 and IL-1 on in vitro macrophage colony formation.[79,200,201] CSF-1 induces macrophage cell lines to progress through cell cycle by modulating levels of specific cyclins.[202] CSF-1 can increase neutrophil levels and lower cholesterol in vivo.

CSF-1 has been purified to homogeneity[79,80,203-205] from both murine and human sources. Human urinary CSF-1 is a heavily glycosylated homodimer of 45 kD,[206] whereas the material purified from L-cell-conditioned medium is a glycoprotein of 70 kD.[79,80,203] Its basic structure is that of a homodimeric protein of 28 kD consisting of two 14-kD peptide chains. Varying degrees of glycosylation explain, in part, different estimates of molecular size. Genes for both human and murine CSF-1 have been cloned and expressed in vitro.[207,208] The human CSF-1 gene is a single gene encoding several differentially spliced mRNA transcripts ranging from 1.5 to 4.5 kb. Several different sizes of human CSF-1 have also been purified from natural sources; the smaller variety possibly being a proteolytic degradation product of a larger 70- to 90-kD glycoprotein. Higher-molecular-weight forms bound to proteoglycans have been reported.[209]

INTERLEUKIN-3 (MULTI-COLONY-STIMULATING FACTOR)

A fourth murine T-cell-derived regulator, interleukin-3 (IL-3) or multi-CSF, has been characterized,[49] purified,[210-214] and genetically cloned.[215-219] It stimulates growth of granulocytes and monocytes, but also has megakaryocyte, erythroid, mast cell, and possibly T-cell growth stimulatory activity. Il-3 was cloned from a gibbon T-cell line.[50] Il-3 was initially believed to be T-cell specific[49,220] but has now been established as a major multilineage stimulator with direct megakaryocyte-, mast cell-, basophil-, B-cell-, and eosinophil-stimulating ability. It also interacts with erythropoietin to stimulate primitive erythroid stem cells,[221] with CSF-1, GM-CSF, and IL-1α to stimulate the growth of high proliferative potential colony-forming cells[222] and supports the formation of early multilineage blast cells in vitro.[223] It is identical to the "stem cell activating factor" that induced CFU-S to proliferate. Recombinant IL-3 is an activating factor for basophils, mast cells, and eosinophils but not neutrophils. In vivo administration to mice induces 10-fold increases in blood eosinophils and 3-fold increases in granulocytes and monocytes. Splenic hematopoiesis is increased with prominent effects on mast cells, and many tissues show an increase in macrophages or mast cells.[47] Single injections of IL-3 induce most types of murine marrow progenitors into cell cycle. In murine species, IL-3, GM-CSF, and CSF-1 in low doses, act synergistically to induce progenitor cell cycling,[48,224] and sequential treatment of primates with recombinant human IL-3 followed by low-dose re-combinant human GM-CSF synergistically increases blood neutrophil, monocyte, lymphocyte, and eosinophil levels. IL-3 alone augments reticulocyte and platelet levels in nonhuman primates.[225] Administration of IL-3 to normal or myelosuppressed humans stimulates increases in a similar range of cell types, but its ability to raise platelet levels has been marginal.[226,227] This, along with a relatively high incidence of toxic side effects, has lessened the enthusiasm for the use of IL-3 as a single agent in therapy.

THE OTHER INTERLEUKINS

Cytokines with pleiotropic actions are referred to as *interleukins*. Their principal actions on lymphohematopoiesis are presented in Table 14-3.

INTERLEUKIN-1

IL-1, identical with the previously described endogenous pyrogen- and lymphocyte-activating factor, was initially defined as a macrophage product that induces IL-2 receptor expression on T lymphocytes.[42,43] It is produced by many different cell types in response to inflammatory stimuli and has two molecular forms, IL-1-α and IL-1-β, which have a low level of homology but similar activities and share a common receptor. The activity of IL-1 is further modulated by the IL-1 receptor antagonist.[228] IL-1 shares many properties with IL-6 (and probably also IL-11) and is involved in the regulation of the immune system, induction of fever, acute phase protein production, tissue repair, and cytotoxicity.[42,43,229] IL-1 has apparent direct effects on early hemopoietic stem cells and acts synergistically with many other factors to augment proliferation of high proliferative potential colony-forming cells, CFU-blast, and myelogenous leukemia blasts.[230-234] IL-1 is also an inducer of other growth factors such as G-CSF, GM-CSF, and IL-3 from different cell types including fibroblasts, endothelial cells, monocytes, keratinocytes, and thymic nonlymphoid cells.[235-240] Studies in vivo in mice and humans indicate that IL-1 augments hemopoietic recovery probably by an action on early stem cells.[241,242] In addition, it interacts synergistically in vivo with other cytokines to accomplish the same end. Its use as a sole agent clinically may be limited by toxic manifestations including hypotension, hypoglycemia, fever, rigors, and headache.

INTERLEUKIN-2

IL-2 is T-cell growth factor[44] (see Chap. 84). It augments production of other lymphokines such as gamma interferon and is produced by T cells and stimulates and activates B cells and natural killer cells, modulating the expression of histocompatibility antigens.[243] IL-2 may inhibit both granulocyte-macrophage colony formation and erythropoiesis.[45,46] The immune modulatory functions of IL-2 have been applied to the treatment of cancers. IL-2 alone, or in combination with other cytokines and cell populations, has some effects against melanoma and renal cell carcinoma.

INTERLEUKIN-4

IL-4, also known as B-cell stimulating factor 1, B-cell differentiation factor, and IgG induction factor,[51,52,244,245] stimulates B-cell maturation, immunoglobulin synthesis, and generation of cytotoxic and helper T lymphocytes (see Chaps. 83 and 84). It interacts with a variety of other growth factors to stimulate granulocyte-macrophage, mast cell, erythroid, and megakaryocyte proliferation in murine systems.[246,247] It also interacts with IL-11 to stimulate the proliferation of dormant hemopoietic progenitors cells[247] and conversely may exert inhibitory influences on IL-3-dependent erythroid colony formation.[248] It also stimulates proliferation and differentiation of dendritic cells.

INTERLEUKIN-5

IL-5, also known as T-cell replacing factor,[249] B-cell growth factor-2,[250] and eosinophil differentiation factor,[53] supports the proliferation, maturation, and function of eosinophils (see Chap. 68). IL-5 also can stimulate both proliferation and differentiation of different leukemic blasts from different subsets of patients with acute myelocytic leukemia. IL-5 has a variety of effects on promoting maturation of proliferation of B cells and like CSF-1 is a homodimer.

INTERLEUKIN-6

IL-6, also previously called *interferon B-2, hybridoma growth factor, B-cell stimulating factor 2, B-cell differentiation factor,* and *hybridoma plasmacytoma growth factor,* is produced by a variety of different cell types and was originally cloned from a T-lymphocyte cDNA library as a molecule inducing immunoglobulin production by B lymphocytes.[56,57,251–253] IL-6 also has direct proliferative effects on hemopoietic cells and interacts synergistically with other growth factors to stimulate myeloid proliferation.[57,254–256] It is a potent mitogen for B cells and also induces T-cell growth and maturation. It has activity on hematopoietic blast colony-forming cells and is a major factor in the immune response and inflammation. IL-6 augments colony formation induced by other growth factors and stimulates granulocyte-macrophage and megakaryocyte colony formation. IL-6 also has in vivo activity stimulating platelet production in normal and myelosuppressed mice, primates, and humans.[257–259] Neutrophil elevations are also seen. IL-6 stimulates blasts from patient with acute myelocytic leukemia[260] and has been implicated as an autocrine or paracrine factor in multiple myeloma (see Chap. 106).[261] Other diseases in which IL-6 may play a role, and be responsible for the systemic manifestations, include atrial myxoma, Castleman's disease, and rheumatoid arthritis.[262]

INTERLEUKIN-7

IL-7, also known as *lymphopoietin-1,* is a B-cell activating factor that appears to have effects on T-cell stimulation and on immature blood granulocyte and splenic megakaryocyte regeneration in irradiated mice.[58,59,263] IL-7 shows potent interactions with KIT ligand in inducing pre-B cells in culture[264] (see Chap. 94).

INTERLEUKIN-8

IL-8 is a chemotactic factor for granulocytes that has been termed *neutrophil-activating peptide.*[60–62] It induces immediate inflammatory responses on intracutaneous injection and a granulocytosis after intravenous injection, apparently by redistributing blood and/or splenic granulocytes.[63,64] It is part of the family of proinflammatory molecules linked by amino acid homology, chromosome location of their genes, and a position-invariant cysteine motif.[64] These include, under the chemokine β classification, Gro-α, macrophage inflammatory protein-2-β (MIP-2-β), platelet factor 4 (PF4), IL-8, neutrophil activating protein-2 (NAP-2) and interferon-inducible protein-10 (IP-10).[64,265–267] The following all inhibit in progenitor assays: MIP-1α, MIP-2α, PF4, IL-8, IP-10, and monocyte chemotactic and activating factor (MCAF); they also show synergistic inhibition when tested in combination.[267] These molecules tend to inhibit more primitive progenitors and may stimulate growth of more mature progenitors. They are potent mobilizers of stem and progenitor cells.

INTERLEUKIN-9

IL-9, or *mouse T-cell growth factor,* P40, supports the development of erythroid bursts (BFU-E) in cultures supplemented with erythropoietin.[268,269] Recombinant murine and human IL-9 were cloned from T-cell lines, and the sequence of recombinant human IL-9 bears homology with mouse T-cell growth factor, P40.[269,270] IL-9 also has mast cell growth-promoting activity and stimulates maturation of multilineage and myeloid colony-forming cells from fetal cells.[65,271]

INTERLEUKIN-10

IL-10 was initially characterized as cytokine synthesis inhibitory factor and is able to inhibit interferon-γ production by activated T-cell clones.[272] IL-10 also appears to have direct effects on mature T cells, increasing the frequency of cytotoxic T-cell precursors and increasing cytotoxic effect or function.[273] It also synergistically stimulates mast cell growth and induces MHC class II antigen expression on and increased viability of B cells.[66,274]

INTERLEUKIN-11

IL-11 has many of the biologic effects produced by IL-6.[67–69,275–277] IL-11 stimulates B-cell, megakaryocyte, and mast cell lineages, along with early multipotential progenitor cells (e.g., CFU-blast).[68,69,275–277] IL-11 stimulates platelet production in mice and primates[278,279] but also stimulates increased neutrophil levels.

INTERLEUKIN-12

IL-12 is a natural killer cell stimulatory factor or cytotoxic lymphocyte maturation factor.[70,280–284] IL-12, in synergy with IL-2, increases generation of cytotoxic T cells and of lymphokine-activated killer cells, increases cytotoxic activity of natural killer cells, promotes proliferation of activated T cells and natural killer cells, and induces interferon-γ production by resting or activated natural killer cells and T cells.

INTERLEUKIN-13

IL-13, a T-cell–derived cytokine, was cloned and shown to share many biologic activities with IL-4.[71,285] Both IL-4 and IL-13 inhibit cytokine production by blood monocytes, affect the proliferation and maturation of B cells to antibody-producing cells,[285] and cause a switch to IgG4- and IgE-producing cells by naive human B cells. IL-13, in contrast to IL-4, induces the production of interferon-γ by large granular lymphocytes and, in contrast to IL-4, has growth stimulatory effects on activated T cells.

INTERLEUKIN-14

IL-14, also known as *high-molecular-weight B-cell growth factor,* induces B-cell proliferation, inhibits immunoglobulin synthesis/secretion, and acts as a B-cell growth stimulant for certain subpopulations.[286,287] IL-14 is produced by T cells and some B-cell malignancies such as B-cell precursor acute lymphocytic leukemia, chronic lymphocytic leukemia, and B-cell lymphoma.[287–289] Exogenous IL-14 has been shown to have putative proliferative activity on B-lymphoma cells in vitro when other B-cell stimulatory cytokines such as IL-2, IL-4, IL-6, or tumor necrosis factor do not have increased activity, suggesting a paracrine effect. IL-14 also has been shown to have an autocrine growth factor effect for intermediate to high-grade B-lymphoma cells. In fact, in vitro studies suggest that many of the B-cell malignancies could be immunomodulated to inhibit proliferation by an antisense oligonucleotide to IL-14.[288]

INTERLEUKIN-15

IL-15 shares biologic activity with IL-2 as well as components of the IL-2 receptor. IL-15 is a cytokine, having multiple levels of receptor and signaling pathways and expression control. Expression occurs at many tissue beds throughout the body, stimulating the proliferation of activated CD4+, CD8+, $\gamma\delta$ subset of T cells, natural killer (NK) cells, and mast cells. Il-15 acts as a potent T-cell chemoattractant and acts as a costimulator with IL-12 to facilitate production of IFNγ and TNFα. IL-15 may act as an anabolic agent that increases muscle mass and help with the differentiation and maturation of the immune system.

Unlike IL-2, IL-15 is not expressed by T cells, but it does stimulate mast cells and is believed to be responsible for inducing the pathological propagation of mast cells that leads to mastocytosis.[290–294]

INTERLEUKIN-16

IL-16 is an immunomodulatory and proinflammatory cytokine that acts as a CD4+ T-lymphocyte chemoattractant and growth factor stimulant.[295,296] IL-16 is synthesized as an 80-kDa peptide precursor molecule that gets processed to a biologically active 14- to 17-kDa protein. Functional bioactivity is dependent on autoaggregation of the pepide to homotetramers (56 kDa).[296] The gene is located on chromosome 15 (q26.1).[297] The gene location and IL-16 structure are unique, without significant homology to other interleukins or chemokines. IL-16 synthesis is produced by stimulated CD4 and CD8 T cells, eosinophils, mast cells, and epithelial lung cells stimulated by chronic inflammation of asthma.[295–297] Prominent immunomodulatory effects are seen with this cytokine with repression of HIV/SIV transcription and replication.[295–298] IL-16 activity has been associated with granulomatous disease states (sarcoidosis, tuberculosis), asthmatic inflammation,[299] primary IgA nephropathy,[300] rheumatoid synovitis (possible anti-inflammatory effects),[301] systemic lupus erythematosus,[320] and allergic contact dermatitis.[303]

INTERLEUKIN-17

IL-17, also referred to as *cytotoxic T-lymphocyte–associated antigen 8* or *murine CTLA-8* is a 155 amino acid glycoprotein homodimer, which stimulates adherent cells such as macrophage, epithelial, endothelial, keratinocyte, or fibroblast to secrete a variety of cytokines including IL-6, IL-8, G-CSF, LIF, TNF-alpha, IL-1 beta, IL-10, IL-12, and IL-1R antagonist. It induces ICAM-1 surface expression, proliferation of T cells, growth and differentiation of CD34+ human progenitors into neutrophils when cocultured with irradiated fibroblasts, and osteoclast progenitor differentiation to osteoclasts.[304–317] It also inhibits IFN-gamma- and TNF-alpha-induced production of Rantes. It stimulates granulopoiesis in vivo, and it is produced by CD4+ and CD8+ T cells and alpha-beta TCR + CD4 − CD8- T cells.[308,318,319]

INTERLEUKIN-18

Interleukin-18 is also known as *interferon-γ–inducing factor* or *interleukin-1 γ*. Functional properties are similar to IL-12. Produced by a wide variety of cells, it augments cell-mediated immunity, modulates T, B, and NK function, induces interferon gamma in type 1 helper T and NK cells, initiating immune and antitumor effects, augmenting GM-CSF, and decreasing IL-10 production. Pretreatment or early treatment with IL-18 in mice confers resistance or protection in many types of tumors.[320–334]

KIT LIGAND (STEEL FACTOR)

The SI/SI^d and W/W^v mice exhibit macrocytic anemia, pigmentation, and germ cell defects.[335–343] These mice have a macrocytic anemia and other more subtle defects in multilineage hematopoiesis. They also have germ cell (sterility) and melanocyte (coat color) defects. The W/W^v mouse has a CFU-S stem cell deficiency, whereas the S1/S1^d mouse has a stromal cell (microenvironmental) defect, since stromal (irradiated spleen) cells from W/W^v will cure the anemia of S1/S1^d mice, while marrow stem cells from S1/S1^d will cure the anemia of W/W^v mice. The defect in W/W^v mice was found to be due to abnormalities in the tyrosine kinase KIT receptor,[344–351] while subsequently the defect in S1/S1^d has found to be due to a deficiency of the ligand for the KIT receptor.[352–355] This protein exists in both membrane and soluble forms and may serve both to bind and stimulate stem cells. This protein KIT ligand is the same as hemolymphopoietic

growth factor-1[175] and synergizes with a large number of cytokines to stimulate early high proliferative potential colony form cells, possibly acting as a survival factor. It exerts action on all myeloid pathways and in the presence of IL-7 stimulates pre-B cell generation in vitro. It also stimulates the functional activation of mast cells. KIT-ligand has multilineage effects in mice, primates, and humans, but its mast cell activation and associated allergic toxicities may limit its clinical use, at least as a single agent.

THROMBOPOIETIN

A number of investigators strived to define the humoral regulator of megakaryocytopoiesis and platelet production.[356–358] Critical insights were generated studying the transforming oncogene (v-mpl) of MPLV, an acute transforming murine retrovirus,[359,360] which induces a pan-myeloid disorder.[361] Thrombopoietin was cloned in 1994[362–365] and was found to be the ligand for c-Mpl, the normal cellular receptor and counterpart to v-Mpl. Thrombopoietin appears to be the major regulator of megakaryocyte proliferation, differentiation, and platelet production. It also induces platelet-specific proteins and ultrastructural features and increased endomitosis.[366] It also has action on multiple other hematopoietic lineages and is a major regulator of primitive multilineage stem cells. Administration of thrombopoietin to normal or myelo-suppressed mice increased progenitor cells of all hematopoietic lineages and hastened hematopoietic recovery.[367,368] Other studies have indicated that thrombopoietin exerts potent effects on early multipotent hematopoietic stem cells inducing entry into cell cycle[369] maintaining or expanding LTC-IC in vitro.[370] Furthermore, hematopoietic repopulating cells appear to be localized to the mpl + population[371] and disruption of the mpl gene reduces murine stem cells as assayed in a competitive repopulation assay.[372]

OTHER CYTOKINES THAT AFFECT HEMATOPOIETIC STEM CELLS

There are a daunting number of other regulators that impact on the lymphohemopoietic pathways either as stimulators or inhibitors, some showing both effects dependent on the stage of maturation of the lineage under consideration. Leukemia inhibitory factor (LIF), which supports proliferation of the IL-3-dependent cell line DA-1,[108] also sustains the proliferation of embryonic stem cells, inhibits adipogenesis, induces renal cell differentiation, neuronal development and differentiation, and bone remodeling. It stimulates proliferation of megakaryocyte progenitors and possibly CFU-S.[109]

Basic fibroblast growth factor also is a pleiotropic growth factor that stimulates primitive marrow stem cells, megakaryocyte progenitors, and marrow stromal cells.[113–115] Insulin-like growth factors I and II stimulate erythroid and myeloid progenitors,[110,111] and hepatocyte growth factor synergizes with other factors at the progenitor's cell level.[112] Platelet-derived growth factor acts on erythroid and granulopoietic progenitors and indirectly on early multilineage stem cells.[116]

Flt-3 ligand acts on relatively primitive progenitor stem cells showing synergies with G-CSF, GM-CSF, M-CSF, IL-3, and SCF and stimulates dendritic cell formation[90–93]; Flt-3 ligand can also induce tumor regression in vivo.[94]

INHIBITORS OF HEMATOPOIESIS

Inhibitors of hematopoiesis have been difficult to study due to questions of the specificity and physiologic relevance of their effects. However, with the progressive definition of cytokines, coupled with advances in cell purification and the use of serum-free culture systems, a number of molecules have been established as having specific inhibitory effects on different stem or progenitor cells. Some of these molecules may exert inhibitory effects on early, more primitive stem cells, while stimulating their latter, more differentiated progeny. A number of inhibitors with varying action are presented in Table 14-5.

Transforming growth factor beta has received the most attention for its ability to inhibit early stem cells, while stimulating more mature cells,[103,104] possibly through modulating surface cytokine receptor expression.[373]

The chemokine family of inhibitors and the small peptides are presented in Table 14-5. The chemokine family was outlined in the description of IL-8. The beta subfamily contains a position invariant cysteine-x-cysteine motif, and its genes are on human chromosome 17, while the alpha subfamily contains position invariant cysteine-x-cysteine motif, and its genes are on human chromosome 4. These inhibitor molecules are potential marrow cell protectors, since they can block entry of stem cell into S phase of the cell cycle (tetrapeptide),[107] remove cells from S phase (pentapeptide),[106] or do both (MIP-1α and related family members) in a rapid and reversible manner.

CYTOKINE RECEPTORS

Cytokines influence cell behavior by binding to cell-surface-receptor proteins and then sending messages for various cell responses. There are a number of receptor families that have been described.

The hematopoietic receptor family includes IL-2, IL-3, IL-4, IL-5, IL-6, IL-7, IL-9, G-CSF, GM-CSF, and erythropoietin.[374-377] The extracellular binding domains of these receptors contain four conserved cysteine residues and a WS-X-WS motif (X is a variable nonconserved amino acid). Some also have immunoglobulin-like structures. GM-CSF, IL-3, and IL-5 receptors contain specific low-affinity alpha chains and a high-affinity beta chain shared by each receptor.[377] The common beta chain plays a role in the competitive binding of these ligands.

The tyrosine kinase receptor family includes receptors for FLT-3 ligand, c-KIT, PDGF, CSF-1, and thrombopoietin.[90,197-199,349-351] These receptors have an immunoglobulin-like structure and conserved cysteines in the extracellular domain with tyrosine kinase activity in the cytoplasmic domain.

Typical steps for the action of a cytokine on a hematopoietic cell (or any other cell) include receptor oligomerization with activation of tyrosine kinase activity, phosphorylation of the receptor, and recruitment of Src-homology (SHZ) and phosphotyrosine binding (PTB) domain proteins to the receptor. What follows varies between different cytokines but in essence represents a series of enzymatic phosphorylation-dephosphorylation steps with final evolution of a protein or protein complex that binds to DNA to initiate genetic programs. Signaling through the GM-CSF, IL-3, and IL-5 receptors, which share a common beta chain, illustrates some specifics of these complex and evolving second messenger systems. The beta chain without kinase activity induces tyrosine phosphorylation of itself along with an increasing number of cytoplasmic proteins including kinases such as PI-3 kinase,[378] adapters illustrated by Grb2,[379] the insulin receptor substrate-2,[380] Cbl,[381,382] and SHC[383,384]; guainine nucleotide exchange factors such as Vav[382,383,385]; phosphatases such as SH-2–domain protein tyrosine phosphatase-2[378,379,383,386] and SH2 containing inositol phosphatase[387] and transcription factors such as STAT 5.[386-388] Receptor phosphorylation is mediated by receptor-associated kinases such as JAK2[389] and Src-family kinases.[390] These sequential interactions lead to proteins, usually in complexes that bind to regions of DNA and in turn prompt initiation of transcription, guiding different genetic programs which modify or effect cell death, proliferation, differentiation, or function.[391]

These transcription factors have been characterized in adult mammals and perhaps most extensively in a variety of developmental studies utilizing mouse, xenopus, drosophila, *c. elegans,* and zebra fish and employing transgenic techniques for knock-outs, knock-ins, and overexpression. This is also an evolving field, but certain transcription factors appear to be responsible for certain differentiation pathways. Factors acting at the earliest stem cell levels include C-myb, p45-NF-E2, GATA-2, AML-1, and tal-1/SCL, while IKaros and PU-1 may act at the earliest lymphoid level. In the myeloid pathways, PU-1 appears to influence granulocyte and monocyte differentiation; PAX-5 B-lymphoid development; GATA-1 erythroid, mast cell, and megakaryocyte lineages; and P45-NF-EC the megakaryocyte lineage. FOG (friend of GATA-1) acts in concert with GATA-1.[392]

These transcription factors appear to act in complexes, binding to DNA regions. An example is the recently described complex of SCL, LMO-2, GATA-1, E47, and Lbdl/NLI.[393] Further definition of these systems promises to define the genetic bases for lymphohematopoietic regulation.

FEATURES OF STEM CELLS

LOCATION OF LYMPHOHEMATOPOIETIC STEM CELLS

Current theories of hematopoietic stem cell sites of origin and the hematopoietic potential of marrow cells have been reexamined as a result of unexpected findings. Convincing evidence has been found that cloned neural (brain) stem cells can repopulate an irradiated host giving rise to multilineage hematopoiesis.[394] Further studies have indicated that isolated muscle satellite cells can also give rise to hematopoiesis.[395] These data indicate that cells in other tissues when exposed to the hematopoietic microenvironment may have lymphohematopoietic potential. Moreover, marrow contains mesenchymal stem cells capable of giving rise to muscle cells, adipocytes, chondrocytes, and osteocytes[396] and cells that give rise to hepatocytes.[397] The relationship of these mesenchymal stem cells to lymphohematopoietic stem cells is yet to be elucidated.

EMBRYONIC ORIGIN OF LYMPHOHEMATOPOIETIC STEM CELLS

Controversy exists over the embryonic origin of lymphohematopoietic stem cells, either from the yolk sac or from the aortogonadal mesonephros (AGM) mesenchymal region. One line of study indicates that hematopoietic stem cells originate in murine yolk and from there migrate to fetal liver and then to marrow. Alternatively, a mesenchymal region has been proposed as the source for stem cells for both avian and murine species.[399-405] It now appears that during development, there are two temporally separate phases of hematopoiesis, the first in the yolk sac giving rise to primitive hematopoiesis restricted to nucleated embryonic erythrocytes, while definitive hematopoiesis arises later in the aortagonadal mesonephric area, giving rise to all hematopoietic lineages and cells that can repopulate lethally irradiated recipients. A cell bipotential for vascular and hematopoietic lineages, the hemangioblast may give rise to the hematopoietic lineages.[406] The yolk sac region may also be a source of some definitive hematopoiesis[407] (see Chaps. 4 and 7).

STEM CELL LOCATION AND MODULATION

Hematopoietic stem cells in the adult reside most prominently in the marrow and less so in the spleen. Stem cells are also present in blood, and the number in blood may be dramatically increased by a number of hematopoietic stresses (anemia, endotoxin, infection), by cytotoxic therapy (e.g., cyclophosphamide) or by the administration of a variety of cytokines (most prominently G-CSF, KIT ligand, FLT-3, IL-8, GM-CSF, or thrombopoietin).

STEM CELL PHENOTYPE

The hematopoietic stem cell in both murine and human species has been characterized as to surface protein, physical, metabolic, and cell cycle characteristics and these characteristics used to purify stem cells. Early stem cells express a relatively large number of cytokine receptors at low levels, with a restricted number of receptors expressed at higher levels after differentiation.[408] Certain other proteins have been found to be present on relatively primitive classes of stem cells: in the mouse, Ly6, c-Kit, c-mpl, CD34, Thy-1, and Flk-2/Flk-3,[371,409-412] and in the human, CD34, c-Kit, Thy-1, Flk-2/Flt-3, and AC133.[412-415] Other features of primitive stem cells include lack of expression of HLA-DR, CD38, and differentiated lineage markers.[416,417] Human and mouse CD34 negative cells may have significant stem cell potential and give rise to CD34+ cells[418,419] or, alternatively, that CD34 expression may vary, depending on the activation state of the stem cell.[420] The most primitive stem cells appear to be dormant in G_0 or a prolonged G_1. The stem cell membrane has a strong p170 membrane pump activity. This pump is the MDR-1 which extrudes certain chemotherapeutic agents and the supravital dyes, rhodamine and Hoechst, from cells.[421] Thus the most primitive stem cells are characterized by an absence of lineage markers and low staining with rhodamine and Hoechst.[422-425] These properties have been used to purify or selectively enrich stem cells for study and clinical application.

PLURIPOTENTIAL LYMPHOHEMATOPOIETIC (MARROW-REPOPULATING) STEM CELL

This cell is ultimately defined by in vivo repopulation and renewal; as noted above, under the appropriate circumstances a single stem cell may renew and restore hematopoiesis in a mouse.[9-11] Thus the cell has tremendous renewal, proliferation, and differentiation potential. These cells have been characterized most definitively in murine species, where in vivo repopulation or population can be assessed in detail. In humans, of necessity, this cell has been defined by surrogate assays of questionable validity. This cell appears to be quiescent (G_0 or prolonged G_1). BRDU studies suggesting a constant cycling state for these cells[426] may be monitoring DNA damage and repair rather than cell cycling.[427] However, the stem cell is easily stimulated to enter active cell cycle transit by in vitro exposure to cytokines[428] or by in vivo engraftment.[429] This cell also appears to have a high level of baseline motility and is rapidly stimulated to demonstrate directed movement by exposure to a variety of cytokines, perhaps most prominently, stromal-derived factor-1 (SDF-1) and KIT ligand.[430] It rapidly binds in vitro to stromal populations,[431] expresses a variety of adherence proteins (vide infra), and migrates toward stromal cells. The murine lineage negative, rhodamide low, Hoechst low cells appear to respond to SFD-1 and KIT ligand in the presence of stroma with extension of lamellipodia in up to 10 to 15 percent of cells.[430] These cells may also differ from differentiated cells in their adhesion receptor profile.

The stem cell appears capable of renewal and expansion under certain experimental conditions such as MDR-1 transfection,[432] or certain serial transfer experiments, but most attempts to expand the engraftable stem cells in vitro, usually in the presence of stroma and/or cytokines, have been unsuccessful.[413] There has been intense interest in such approaches for their potential for retroviral vector-based gene therapy or stem cell transplantation.

A critical feature of this cell is its plasticity, especially with cell cycle transit. The engraftment phenotype of this cell varies dramatically and reversibly when stimulated by cytokines (IL-11, IL-3, IL-6, steel factor) to transit the cell cycle.[433-435] During the first cell cycle transit, long-term engraftment appears to be lost in late S-early G2 and regained in G1.[435] Multiple other phenotypic features of this cell change

with cytokine-induced cell cycle transit, including cytokine and adhesion receptor, transcription factor, and cell cycle factor expression.[436-439] The critical observation is that the phenotype of this cell can go from high to low to high engraftment. These observations suggest a cell cycle model of hematopoiesis.

ADHESION PROTEINS AND RECEPTORS

Adhesion receptors and their ligands mediate cell-to-matrix and cell-to-cell interaction and include the selectins, the integrins, the immunoglobulin family, and miscellaneous others. First defined in studies on lymphoid homing, these proteins now have been found to play a role in anchoring of hematopoietic cells in marrow or in the promotion of differentiation.[440,441] The integrin class of adhesion receptors are heterodimers of the noncovalently associated α and β chains. There are at least 18 different α and β chains. The β chain associates with α_1 through α_6 to form the very late antigen (VLA) group. $\alpha_5\beta_1$ is the classical fibrinogen receptor, and $\alpha_6\beta_1$ is a laminin receptor. L-selectin, PECAM-1, CD44, β_1, and α_4 through α_6 are all expressed on primitive human or murine stem cells, and their modulation appears to correlate with engraftment efficiency. Immature blasts, erythroid progenitors, monocytes, and CD34+ cells show α_4 and α_5, and these decrease with maturation. There also appears to be differential binding of hematopoietic cells to different extracellular matrix components: erythroid cells to fibronectin[442,443] and CFU-GM and BFU-E to collagen.[444] Several groups have implicated VLA-4 and VCAM-1 or CD44 in marrow homing and engraftment. VLA-4 binding to the CS-1 peptide of alternatively spliced fibronectin mediates binding of murine CFU-S[445] or human long-term marrow culture initiating cells,[446] and an antibody to VLA-4 caused mobilization of hematopoietic progenitors in normal or cytokine-treated primates or mice.[447,448] c-KIT receptor was also found to be important for optimal mobilization by anti-VLA-4 or VCAM-1 in W/W^v or $S1/S1^d$ mice.[449]

The non-integrin adhesion receptors also play a role in engraftment. These include CD44,[450] PECAM,[451] and a receptor for a ligand bearing galactosyl and mannosyl residues from stroma.[452] Both PECAM and L-selectin are affected by cytokines, and hematopoietic progenitors can bind to thrombospondin,[453,454] interleukin-3, and KIT ligand,[448] and these cytokines bind to heparin sulfate proteoglycans. Studies with E- and P- selectin knockout mice,[455] also employing VCAM-1 blocking antibodies, has implicated the selectins and VLA-4 as receptors that are critical for stem cell homing. Adhesion receptor expression on hematopoietic progenitor or stem cells is summarized in Table 14-6.

STEM CELL HOMING AND THE MICROENVIRONMENT

A critical aspect of hematopoiesis is the milieu in which hematopoietic stem cells reside: the microenvironment. The latter consists of stromal cells and the extracellular matrix. Stem cells home to stromal cells

TABLE 14-6   HEMATOPOIETIC STEM AND PROGENITOR CELL ADHESION RECEPTORS AND LIGANDS

Ligand	Receptor
VCAM-, alternatively spliced fibronectin	VLA-4
Fibronectin (RGD)	VLA-5
Laminin	VLA-6
Sulfated glycosaminoglycans	PECAM
Sialyl Lewis x_1	L-selectin
Sialyl Lewis a_1	
CD34, Gly CAM-1	
Hyaluronic acid, collagen, mucosal addressin	CD44

during development, in the steady state, or after transplantation, and these same cells function to regulate hematopoiesis.[456-460] Early studies showed the dramatic influence of microenvironment in the spleen on lineage expression in spleen colonies,[26-28] and the introduction of the Dexter long-term stromal-based culture system provided an in vitro model of stromal supported hematopoiesis.[461,462] In this latter system adherent stromal cells, consisting of hematopoietically derived macrophages, preadipocytic fibroblasts, and other cells (variable with the system) could support virtually all engraftable stem cells, CFUs, and a variety of different progenitor cells.[463-466] The marrow stromal cells in this system produce a variety of cytokines and express a number of adhesion molecules, both playing important roles in regulation of lymphohematopoiesis.[467-471] Adhesion proteins are critical for stem cell binding to stromal cells in vitro and homing to marrow in vivo when stem cells are infused subsequently and move to the endosteal surface of marrow (Chap. 4).[472]

MOBILIZATION OF STEM OR PROGENITOR CELLS

Long-term repopulating stem cells and their progenitors are mobilized into the blood by a number of cytokines including GM-CSF, CSF-1, IL-1, KIT ligand, FLT-3, IL-11, IL-12, IL-3, IL-8, IL-7, MIP-1α, and epo.[473-480] In addition, previous exposure to cyclophosphamide or other cytoxic agents also mobilizes stem cell, presumptively as a result of cytokine effects. Mobilization has been utilized to collect stem and progenitor cells for transplantation. Pretreatment with cyclophosphamide followed by treatment with KIT ligand and G-CSF may be the most potent mobilization regimen. In general, mobilized progenitor and stem cells appear to restore hematopoiesis more rapidly than unstimulated marrow, although marrow "primed" with in vivo cytokines may be equivalent to mobilized blood cells for rapid engraftment. Whether these mobilized stem cells will have the same long-term repopulation capacity as marrow cells remains to be established (Chaps. 4 and 141).

REFERENCES

1. Nakahata T, Ogawa M: Clonal origin of murine hemopoietic colonies with apparent restriction to granulocyte-macrophage-megakaryocyte (GMM) differentiation. *J Cell Physiol* 111:239, 1982.
2. Ogawa M, Pharr PN, Suda T: Stochastic nature of stem cell functions in culture. Progress in Clinical & Biological Research, in *Hematopoietic Stem Cell Physiology*, edited by E Cronkite, N Dainiak, R McCaffrey, J Palek, P Quesenberry, pp 11–19. Alan Liss, New York, 1985.
3. Suda J, Suda T, Ogawa M: Analysis of differentiation of mouse hemopoietic stem cells in culture by sequential replating of paired progenitors. *Blood* 64:393, 1984.
4. Nakahata T, Ogawa M: Hemopoietic colony-forming cells in umbilical cord blood with extensive capability to generate mono- and multipotential hemopoietic progenitors. *J Clin Invest* 70:1324, 1982.
5. Nakahata T, Ogawa M: Identification in culture of a class of hemopoietic colony-forming units with extensive capability to self-renew and generate multipotential hemopoietic colonies. *Proc Natl Acad Sci USA* 79:3843, 1982.
6. Suda T, Suda J, Ogawa M: Single-cell origin of mouse hemopoietic colonies expressing multiple lineages in variable combinations. *Proc Natl Acad Sci USA* 80:6689, 1983.
7. Suda T, Suda J, Ogawa M: Disparate differentiation in mouse hemopoietic colonies derived from paired progenitors. *Proc Natl Acad Sci USA* 81:2520, 1963.
8. Becker AF, McCulloch EA, Till JE: Cytological demonstration of the clonal nature of spleen colonies derived from transplanted mouse marrow cells. *Nature* 197:452, 1963.
9. Wu AM, Till JE, Siminovitch L, McCulloch EA: A cytological study of the capacity for differentiation of normal hemopoietic colony-forming cells. *J Cell Physiol* 69:177, 1967.
10. Abramson S, Miller RG, Phillips RA: The identification in adult bone marrow of pluripotent and restricted stem cells of the myeloid and lymphoid systems. *J Exp Med* 145:1567, 1977.
11. Lemischka IR, Raulet DH, Mulligan RC: Developmental potential and dynamic behavior of hematopoietic stem cells. *Cell* 45:917, 1986.
12. Harrison DE, Lerner C, Hoppe PC, Carlson GA, Alling D: Large numbers of primitive stem cells are active simultaneously in aggregated embryo chimeric mice. *Blood* 69:773, 1987.
13. Till JE, McCulloch EA: A direct measurement of the radiation sensitivity of normal mouse bone marrow cells. *Radiat Res* 14:213, 1961.
14. Siminovitch L, McCulloch EA, Till JE: The distribution of colony forming cells among spleen colonies. *J Cell Comp Physiol* 62:327, 1963.
15. Lewis JP, Trobaugh FE Jr: Hematopoietic stem cells. *Nature* 204:589, 1964.
16. Juraskova V, Tkadlecek L: Character of primary and secondary colonies of hematopoiesis in the spleen of irradiated mice. *Nature* 206:951, 1965.
17. Quesenberry PJ, Stanley K: A statistical analysis of murine stem cell suicide techniques. *Blood* 56:1000, 1980.
18. Moffatt DJ, Rosse C, Yoffey JM: Identity of the hemopoietic stem cell. *Lancet* 2:547, 1967.
19. Van Bekkum DW, van Noord MJ, Maat B, Dicke KA: Attempts at identification of hemopoietic stem cell in mouse. *Blood* 38:547, 1971.
20. Rubinstein AS, Trobaugh FE Jr: Ultrastructure of presumptive hematopoietic stem cells. *Blood* 42:61, 1973.
21. Magli MC, Iscove NN, Odartchenko N: Transient nature of early hematopoietic spleen colonies. *Nature* 295:527, 1982.
22. Curry JL, Trentin JJ: Hemopoietic spleen colony studies. I. Growth and differentiation. *Dev Biol* 15:395, 1967.
23. Siminovitch LF, Till JE, McCulloch EA: Radiation responses of hemopoietic colony forming cells derived from different sources. *Radiat Res* 24:482, 1965.
24. Barnes DW, Loutit JF: Hematopoietic stem cells in the peripheral blood. *Lancet* 2:1138, 1967.
25. Wu AM, Till JE, Siminovitch L, McCulloch EA: Cytological evidence for a relationship between normal hematopoietic colony forming cells and cells of the lymphoid system. *J Exp Med* 127:455, 1968.
26. Curry JL, Trentin JJ: Hemopoietic spleen colony studies. IV. Phytohemagglutinin and hemopoietic regeneration. *J Exp Med* 126:819, 1967.
27. Fowler JH, Wu AM, Till JE, et al: The cellular composition of hemopoietic spleen colonies. *J Cell Physiol* 69:65, 1967.
28. Pluznik DH, Sachs L: The cloning of normal "mast" cells in tissue culture. *J Cell Physiol* 66:319, 1965.
29. Bradley TR, Metcalf D: The growth of mouse bone marrow cells in vitro. *Aust J Exp Biol Med Sci* 44:287, 1966.
30. Reissman KR: Studies on the mechanisms of rats during hypoxia. *Blood* 5:372, 1950.
31. Erslev AJ: Humoral regulation of red cell production. *Blood* 8:349, 1953.
32. Cotes PM, Bangham DR: Bioassay of erythropoietin in mice made polycythemic by exposure to air at a reduced pressure. *Nature* 191:1065, 1961.
33. Jacobson LO, Goldwasser E, Plzak L, et al: Studies on erythropoiesis. IV. Reticulocyte response of hypophysectomized and polycythemic rodents to erythropoietin. *Proc Soc Exp Biol* 94:243, 1957.
34. Plzak LF, Fried W, Jacobson LO, et al: Demonstration of stimulation of erythropoiesis by plasma from anemic rats using Fe[59]. *J Lab Clin Med* 46:671, 1955.
35. Axelrad AA, McLeod DL, Shreeve MM, Health DS: Properties of cells that produce erythrocytic colonies *in vitro*, in *Hemopoiesis in Culture: Second International Workshop*, edited by WA Robinson, p 226. HEW Publication, NIH Government Printing Office, Washington, 1973.
36. McLeod DL, Shreeve MM, Axelrad AA: Improved plasma culture system for production of erythrocytic colonies in vitro: quantitative assay method for CFU-E. *Blood* 44:517, 1974.
37. Iscove NN, Sieber F: Erythroid progenitors in mouse bone marrow detected by macroscopic colony formation in culture. *Exp Hematol* 3:32, 1975.
38. D'Andrea AD, Lodish HF, Wong GG: Expression cloning of the murine erythropoietin receptor. *Cell* 57:277, 1989.
39. Sawyer ST, Krantz SB, Goldwasser E: Binding and receptor-mediated endocytosis of erythropoietin in Friend virus-infected erythroid cells. *J Biol Chem* 262:5554, 1987.
40. Koury MJ, Bondurant MC: Maintenance by erythropoietin of viability

and maturation of murine erythroid precursor cells. *J Cell Physiol* 137:65, 1988.

41. Koury MJ, Bondurant MC: A survival model of erythropoietin action. *Blood* 74(suppl 1):48a, 1989.

42. Dinarello CA: Interleukin-1. *Rev Infect Dis* 6:51, 1984.

43. Dinarello CA: Biology of interleukin-1. *FASEB J* 2:108, 1988.

44. Smith KA: Interleukin-2, inception, impact and implications. *Science* 240:1169, 1988.

45. Naldini A, Fleischmann WR, Ballas ZK, et al: Interleukin-2 inhibits *in vitro* granulocyte macrophage colony formation. *J Immunol* 139:1880, 1987.

46. Burdach SE, Levitt LJ: Receptor specific inhibition of bone marrow erythropoiesis by recombinant DNA-derived interleukin-2. *Blood* 69:1368, 1987.

47. Metcalf D, Bagby GC, Johnson GR, et al: Effects of purified bacterially synthesized murine multi-colony stimulating factor (interleukin-3) on hematopoiesis in normal adult mice. *Blood* 68:46, 1986.

48. Broxmeyer HE, Williams DE, Cooper S, et al: Comparative effects *in vivo* of recombinant murine interleukin-3, natural murine colony stimulating factor-1 and recombinant murine granulocyte-macrophage colony stimulating factor on myelopoiesis in mice. *J Clin Invest* 79:721, 1987.

49. Ihle JN: Biochemical and biological properties of interleukin-3: a lymphokine mediating the differentiation of a lineage of cells which includes prothymocytes and mast-like cells. *J Immunol* 131:282, 1983.

50. Clark SC, Kamen R: The human hematopoietic colony-stimulating factors. *Science* 236:1229, 1987.

51. Howard M, Farrar J, Hilfiker M, et al: Identification of a T cell derived B cell growth factor distinct from interleukin-2. *J Exp Med* 155:914, 1982.

52. Vitetta ES, Brooks K, Chen YW, et al: T cell derived lymphokines that induce IgM and IgG secretion in activated murine B cells. *Immunol Rev* 78:137, 1984.

53. Campbell HD, Tucker WQJ, Hort Y, et al: Molecular cloning and expression of the gene encoding human eosionophil differentiation factor (interleukin-5). *Proc Natl Acad Sci USA* 84:6629, 1987.

54. Van Damme J, DeLey M, Van Snick J, et al: The role of interferon-B1 and the 26-kDa protein (interferon-B2) as mediators of the antiviral effect of interleukin-1 and tumor necrosis factor. *J Immunol* 139:1867, 1987.

55. Hirano T, Taga T, Yasukawa K, et al: Human B cell differentiation factor defined by an anti-peptide antibody and its possible role in autoantibody production. *Proc Natl Acad Sci USA* 84:228, 1987.

56. Yasukawa K, Hirano T, Watanabe Y, et al: Structure and expression of human B cell stimulatory factor 2 (BSF-2) gene. *EMBO J* 6:2939, 1987.

57. Wong GG, Witek-Giannotti JS, Temple PA, et al: Stimulation of murine hemopoietic colony formation by human IL-6. *J Immunol* 40:3040, 1988.

58. Namen AE, Lupton S, Hjerrild K, et al: Stimulation of B cell progenitors by cloned murine interleukin-7. *Nature* 333:571, 1988.

59. Namen AE, Schmierer AE, March CJ, et al: B cell precursor growth-promoting activity: Purification and characterization of a growth factor active on lymphocyte precursors. *J Exp Med* 167:988, 1988.

60. Yoshimura T, Matsushima K, Tanaka S, et al: Purification of a human monocyte-derived neutrophil chemotactic factor that has peptide sequence similarity to other host defense cytokines. *Proc Natl Acad Sci USA* 84:9233, 1987.

61. Shroder JM, Mrowietz U, Morita E, Christophers E: Purification and partial biochemical characterization of a human monocyte-derived neutrophil-activating peptide that lacks interleukin-1 activity. *J Immunol* 139:3474, 1987.

62. Lindley I, Aschauer H, Seifert J-M, et al: Synthesis and expression in *Escherichia coli* of the gene encoding monocyte-derived neutrophil-activating factor: biological equivalence between natural and recombinant neutrophil-activating factor. *Proc Natl Acad Sci USA* 85:9199, 1988.

63. Kimberly JVZ, Fischer E, Hawes AS, et al: Effects of intravenous IL-8 administration in nonhuman primates. *J Immunol* 148:1746, 1992.

64. Oppenheim JJ, Zachariae COC, Mukaida N, Matsushima K: Properties of the novel pro-inflammatory super gene "intercrine" cytokine family. *Ann Rev Immunol* 9:617, 1991.

65. Holbrook ST, Ohls RK, Schibler KR, et al: Effect of interleukin-9 on clonogenic maturation and cell cycle status of fetal and adult hematopoietic progenitors. *Blood* 77:2129, 1991.

66. Thompson-Sniper LA, Dhar V, Bond M, et al: Interleukin-10: a novel stimulatory factor for mast cells and their progenitors. *J Exp Med* 173:507, 1991.

67. Paul SR, Yang Y-C, Donahue RE, et al: Stromal cell-associated hematopoiesis: Immortalization and characterization of a primate bone marrow-derived cell line. *Blood* 77:1723, 1991.

68. Paul SR, Bennett F, Calbretti JA, et al: Molecular cloning of a cDNA encoding interleukin-11, a stromal lymphopoietic and hematopoietic cytokine. *Proc Natl Acad Sci USA* 87:7512, 1990.

69. Musashi M, Yang Y-C, Paul SR: Direct and synergistic effects of interleukin-11 on murine hemopoiesis in culture. *Proc Natl Acad Sci USA* 88:765, 1991.

70. Gubler U, Chua AO, Schoenhaut DS, et al: Coexpression of two distinct genes is required to generate secreted bioactive cytotoxic lymphocyte maturation factor. *Proc Natl Acad Sci USA* 88:4143, 1991.

71. Minty A, Chalon P, Derocq JM, et al: Interleukin-13 is a new human lymphokine regulating inflammatory and immune responses. *Nature* 362:248, 1993.

72. Ambrus JL, Pippin J, Joseph A, et al: Identification of a cDNA for a human high-molecular-weight B cell growth factor. *Proc Natl Acad Sci USA* 90:6330, 1993.

73. Agostini C, Trentin L, Sancetta R, et al: Interleukin-15 triggers activation and growth of the CD-8 T cell pool in extravascular tissues of patients with acquired immunodeficiency syndrome. *Blood* 90: 1115, 1997.

74. Baier M, Bannert N, Werner A, Lang K, Kurth R: Molecular cloning, sequence, expression, and processing of the interleukin-16 precursor. *Proc Natl Acad Sci USA* 94:5273, 1997.

75. Fossiez F, Djossou O, Chomarat P, et al: T cell IL-17 induces stromal cells to produce proinflammatory and hematopoietic cytokines. *J Exp Med* 183: 2593, 1996.

76. Yao Z, Painter SL, Fanslow WC, et al: Human IL-17: a novel cytokine derived from T cells. *J Immunol* 155: 5483, 1995.

77. Micallef MJ, Ohtsuki T, Kohno K, et al: Interferon-gamma-inducing factor enhances T helper 1 cytokine production by stimulated human T cells: synergism with interleukin-12 for interferon-gamma production. *Eur J Immunol* 26: 1647, 1996.

78. Okamura H, Tsutsi H, Komatsu T, et al: Cloning of a new cytokine that induces INF-gamma production by T cells. *Nature* 378: 88, 1995.

79. Waheed A, Shadduck R: Purification and properties of L cell-derived colony-stimulating factor. *J Lab Clin Med* 94:180, 1979.

80. Stanley ER, Guilbert LF: Methods of purification, assay, characterization and target cell binding of a colony-stimulating factor (CSF-1). *J Immunol Meth* 42:253, 1981.

81. Nicola NA, Metcalf D, Matsumoto M, et al: Purification of a factor inducing differentiation in murine myelomonocytic leukemia cells. Identification as granulocyte colony stimulating factor. *J Biol Chem* 258:9017, 1983.

82. Nicola NA, Begley CG, Metcalf D: Identification of the human analogue of a regulator that induces differentiation in murine leukemia cells. *Nature* 314:625, 1985.

83. Sieff CA, Emerson SF, Donahue RE, Nathan DG: Human recombinant granulocyte-macrophage colony stimulating factor: a multilineage hematopoietic. *Science* 230:1171, 1985.

84. Metcalf D, Burgess AW, Johnson GR, et al: *In vitro* actions on hemopoietic cells of recombinant murine GM-CSF purified after production in *Escherichia coli*. Comparison with purified native GM-CSF. *J Cell Physiol* 128:421, 1986.

85. Robinson BE, McGrath HE, Quesenberry PJ: Recombinant murine granulocyte-macrophage colony stimulating factor has megakaryocyte colony stimulating activity and augments megakaryocyte colony stimulation by interleukin-3. *J Clin Invest* 79:1648, 1987.

86. Quesenberry PJ, Ihle JN, McGrath HE: The effect of interleukin-3 and GM-CSA-2 on megakaryocyte and myeloid clonal colony formation. *Blood* 65:214, 1985.

87. Stanley IJ, Burgess AW: Granulocyte-macrophage colony stimulating factor stimulates the synthesis of membrane and nuclear proteins in murine neutrophils. *J Cell Biochem* 23:241, 1983.

88. Eaves AC, Eaves CJ: Erythropoiesis in culture. *Clin Haematol* 13:371, 1984.

89. Gregory CJ, Eaves AC: Three stages of erythropoietic progenitor cell differentiation distinguished by a number of physical and biological properties. *Blood* 51:527, 1978.

90. Lyman DJ, James L, Vanden BT, et al: Molecular cloning of ligand for fH3/flk-2 tyrosine kinase receptor: a proliferative factor. *Cell* 75:1157, 1993.

91. Lyman S, Jacobson S: C-kit ligand and FLT-3 ligand: stem progenitor cell factors with overlapping yet distinct activities. *Blood* 91:1101, 1998.

92. Strobl H, Bello-Fernandez C, Riedl E, et al: FLT-3 ligand in cooperation with transforming growth factor-61 potentiates in vitro development of Langerhans-type dendritic cells and allows single-cell dendritic cell cluster formation under serum-free conditions. *Blood* 90:1425, 1997.

93. Maraskovsky E, Brasel K, Teepe M, et al: Dramatic increase in the numbers of functionally mature dendritic cells in FT-3 ligand-treated mice: multiple dendritic cell subpopulations identified. *J Exp Med* 184:1993, 1996.

94. Lynch DH, Andersen A, Maraskovsky E, Whitmore J, Miller RE, Schuh JCL: FLT-3 ligand induces tumors regression and antitumor immune responses in vivo. *Nat Med* 3:625, 1997.

95. Toksoz D, Zsebo KM, Smith KA, et al: Support of human hematopoiesis in long-term bone marrow cultures by murine stromal cells selectively expressing the membrane-bound and secreted forms of the human hematology of the steel gene product, stem cell factor. *Proc Natl Acad Sci USA* 89:7350, 1992.

96. Lowry PA, Zsebo KM, Deacon DH, Eichman CE, Quesenberry PJ: Effects of rrSCF on multiple cytokine responsive HPP-CFC generated from SCA+Lin- murine hematopoietic progenitors. *Exp Hematol* 19:994, 1991.

97. Lowry PA, Deacon DH, Witefield P, McGrath HE, Quesenberry PH: SCF induction of in vitro murine hematopoietic colony formation by "subliminal" cytokine combinations: the role of "anchor factors." *Blood* 80:663-669, 1992.

98. De Savvage FJ, Carver-Moore K, Luoh S, et al: Physiological regulation of early and late stages of megakaryocyteopoiesis by thrombopoietin. *J Exp Med* 183:651, 1996.

99. Kaushanksy K, Lin N, Grossman A, Homen J, Sprugel KH, Brouchy VC: Thrombopoietin expands erythroid granulocyte and macrophage and megakarocyte progenitor cells in normal and myelosuppressed mice. *Exp Hematol* 23:265, 1996.

100. Plumb M, Graham GJ. Grove M, Reid A, Pragnell IB: Molecular aspects of a negative regulator of haemopoiesis. *Br J Cancer* 64:990, 1991.

101. Broxmeyer HE, Sherry B, Lu L, Cooper S, Oh K-O, Tekamp-Olson P, Kwon BS, Corami A: Enhancing and suppressing effects of recombinant murine macrophage inflammatory proteins on colony formation in vitro by bone marrow myeloid progenitor cells. *Blood* 76:1110, 1998.

102. Broxmeyer HE: Suppressor cytokines and regulation of myelopoiesis. *Am J Ped Hematol/Oncol* 14:22, 1992.

103. Keller JR, McNeice IK, Sill KT, et al: Transforming growth factor-beta directly regulates primitive murine hematopoietic cell proliferation. *Blood* 75:596, 1990.

104. Jacobsen SEW, Veiby OP, Myklebust J, Okkenhaug C, Lyman SD: Ability of FLT-3 ligand to stimulate the in vitro growth of primitive murine hematopoietic progenitor is potentially and directly inhibited by transforming growth factors-β and tumor increases factor-α. *Blood* 87:5010, 1996.

105. Broxmeyer HE, Lu L, Cooper S, Schwa RH, Mason AJ, Nikolias K: Selective and indirect modulation of human multi-potential and erythroid hematopoietic progenitor cell proliferation by recombinant human activin and inhibin. *Proc Natl Acad Sci USA* 85:9052, 1998.

106. Laerum OD, Paukovits WR: Inhibitory effects of a synthetic pentapeptide on hemopoietic stem cells *in vitro* and *in vivo*. *Exp Hematol* 12:7, 1984.

107. Bonnet D, Cesaire R, Lamoine F, et al: The tetrapeptide AcSDKP an inhibitor of the cell cycle status for normal human hematopoietic progenitors, has no effect on leukemia cells. *Exp Hematol* 20:251, 1992.

108. Moreau JF, Donaldson DD, Bennet F, et al: Leukemia inhibitory factor is identical to the myeloid growth factor human interleukin for DA cells. *Nature* 336:690, 1988.

109. Fletcher FA, Williams DE, Maliszewski C, et al: Murine leukemia inhibitory factor enhances retroviral-vector infection efficiency of hematopoietic progenitors. *Blood* 76:1098, 1990.

110. Kurtz A, Jelkman W, Bauer C: A new candidate for the regulation of erythropoiesis-insulin-like growth factor-1. *FEBS Lett* 149:105, 1982.

111. Merchav S, Tatarsky I, Hochberg Z: Enhancement of human granulopoiesis *in vitro* by biosynthetic insulin-like growth factor-I/Somatomedin C and human growth hormone. *J Clin Invest* 81:791, 1988.

112. Kmiecik TE, Keller JR, Rosen E, Vandewoude GF: Hepatocyte growth factor is a synergistic factor for growth of hematopoietic progenitor cells. *Blood* 80:2454, 1992.

113. Wilson EL, Rifkin DB, Kelly T, et al: Basic fibroblast growth factor stimulates myelopoiesis in long-term human bone marrow cultures. *Blood* 77:954, 1991.

114. Gabbianelli M, Sargiacomo M, Pelesi E, et al: "Pure" human hematopoietic progenitors: permissive action of basic fibroblast growth factor. *Science* 249:1561, 1990.

115. Bruno E, Cooper RJ, Wilson EL, et al: Basic fibroblast growth factor promotes the proliferation of human megakaryocyte progenitor cells. *Blood* 82:430, 1993.

116. Xia-Qiang Y, Brady G, Iscove NN: Platelet-derived growth factor (PDGF) activates primitive hematopoietic precursors (pre-CFC multi) by upregulating IL-1 in PDGF receptor expressing macrophages. *J Immunol* 150:2440, 1993.

117. Miyake T, Kung CKH Goldwasser E: Purification of human erythropoietin. *J Biol Chem* 252:5558, 1977.

118. Jacobs K, Shoemaker C, Rudersdorf R, et al: Isolation and characterization of genomic and cDNA clones of human erythropoietin. *Nature* 313:806, 1985.

119. Lai PH, Everett R, Wang FF, et al: Structural characterization of human erythropoietin. *J Biol Chem* 261:3116, 1986.

120. Jacobson LO, Goldwasser E, Fried W, et al: Role of the kidney in erythropoiesis. *Nature* 179:633, 1957.

121. Koury ST, Bondurant MC, Koury MK: Localization of erythropoietin synthesizing cells in murine kidneys by in situ hybridization. *Blood* 71:524, 1988.

122. Lacombe C, DaSilva JL, Bruneval P: Peritubular cells are the site of erythropoietin synthesis in the murine hypoxic kidney. *J Clin Invest* 81:620, 1988.

123. Maxwell AP, Lappin TRJ, Johnson CF, et al: Erythropoietin production in kidney tubular cells. *Br J Haematol* 74:535, 1990.

124. Jacobson LO, Marks EK, Gaston EO, et al: Studies on erythropoiesis. XI. Reticulocyte response of transfusion induced polycythemic mice to anemic plasma from nephrectonized mice and to plasma from nephrectonized rate exposed to low oxygen. *Blood* 14:635, 1959.

125. Fried W: The liver as a source of extrarenal erythropoietin. *Blood* 40:671, 1972.

126. Mirand EA, Murphy GP, Steeves RA, et al: Extrarenal production of erythropoietin in man. *Acta Haematol* 39:359, 1968.

127. Naets JP, Witteck M: Presence of erythropoietin in the plasma of one anephric patient. *Blood* 31:249, 1968.

128. Fried W, Baronc-Varelas J, Morley C: Factors that regulate extrarenal erythropoietin production. *Blood Cells* 10:287, 1984.

129. Rich IN, Hart W, Kubanek B: Extrarenal erythropoietin production by macrophages. *Blood* 60:1007, 1982.

130. Goldberg MA, Dunning SP, Bunn HF: Regulation of the erythropoietin gene: evidence that the oxygen sensor is a heme protein. *Science* 242:1412, 1988.

131. Iscove NN: The role of erythropoietin in regulation of population size and cell cycling of early and late erythroid precursors in mouse bone marrow. *Cell Tissue Kinet* 10:323, 1977.

132. Iscove NN: Erythropoietin-independent stimulation of early erythropoiesis in adult marrow cultures by conditioned medium from lectin-stimulated mouse spleen cells, in *ICN-UCLA Symposium on Hematopoietic Cell Differentiation*, edited by DW Golde, MJ Cline, D Metcalf, et al. Academic Press, New York, 1978.

133. Zuckerman K, Sullivan R, Quesenberry PJ: Effects of actinomycin-D *in vivo* on murine erythroid stem cells. *Blood* 51:957, 1978.

134. Nihof W, Wierenga PK, Sahr K, et al: Induction of globin mRNA transcription by erythropoietin in differentiating erythroid precursor cells. *Exp Hematol* 15:779, 1987.

135. Glass J, Lavidor LM, Robinson SH: Use of cell separation and short term culture techniques to study erythroid cell development. *Blood* 46:705, 1975.

136. Landschulz KT, Noyes AN, Rogers O, et al: Erythropoietin receptors on murine erythroid colony forming units: natural history. *Blood* 137:65, 1988.

137. Migliaccio G, Migliaccio AR, Visser JW: Synergism between erythropoietin and interleukin-3 in the induction of hematopoietic stem cell proliferation and erythroid burst colony formation. *Blood* 72:944, 1988.

138. Umemura T, Papayannopoulou T, Stamatoyannopoulos G: The mechanism of expansion of late erythroid progenitors during erythroid regeneration: Target cells and effect of erythropoietin and interleukin-3. *Blood* 73:1993, 1989.

139. Sonoda Y, Yang YC, Wong GG, et al: Erythroid burst-promoting activity of purified recombinant human GM-CSF and interleukin-3: studies with anti-GM-CSF and anti-IL-3 sera and studies in serum free culture. *Blood* 72:1381, 1988.

140. Donahue RE, Yang YC, Clark SC: Human P40 T cell growth factor (interleukin-9) supports erythroid colony formation. *Blood* 72:2271, 1990.

141. Peschel C, Paul WE, Ohara J, Green I: Effects of B-cell stimulatory factor-1/interleukin 4 on hematopoietic progenitor cells. *Blood* 70:254-263, 1987.

142. Burgess AW, Camarakis J, Metcalf D: Purification and properties of colony stimulating factor from mouse lung-conditioned medium. *J Biol Chem* 252:1998, 1977.

143. Gasson JC, Weisbart RH, Kaufman SE, et al: Purified human granulocyte-macrophage colony stimulating factor: direct action on neutrophils. *Science* 226:1339, 1984.

144. Gough NM, Gough J, Metcalf D, et al: Molecular cloning of cDNA encoding a murine hematopoietic growth regulator, granulocyte-macrophage colony stimulating factor. *Nature* 309:763, 1984.

145. Lee F, Yokota T, Otsuka T, et al: Isolation of cDNA for a human granulocyte-macrophage colony stimulating factor by functional expression in mammalian cells. *Proc Natl Acad Sci USA* 82:4360, 1985.

146. Wong GG, Witek JS, Temple PA, et al: Human GM-CSF: molecular cloning of complementary DNA and purification of the natural and recombinant proteins. *Science* 228:810, 1985.

147. Huebner K, Iscobe M, Croce CM, et al: The human gene encoding GM-CSF is a 5121-q32, the chromosome region deleted in the 5q-anomaly. *Science* 230:1282, 1985.

148. LeBeau MM, Westbrook CA, Diaz MO, et al: Evidence for the involvement of GM-CSF and fms in the deletion (5q) in myeloid disorders. *Science* 231:984, 1986.

149. Chan JY, Slaman DF, Nimer SD, et al: Regulation of expression of human granulocyte/macrophage colony stimulating factor. *Proc Natl Acad Sci USA* 83:8669, 1986.

150. Arnaout MA, Wang EA, Clark SC, et al: Human recombinant granulocyte-macrophage colony stimulating factor increases cell to cell adhesion and surface expression of adhesion-promoting surface glycoproteins on mature granulocytes. *J Clin Invest* 78:597, 1986.

151. Fleischman J, Golde DW, Weisbart RH, Gasson JC: Granulocyte-macrophage colony stimulating factor enhances phagocytosis of bacteria by human neutrophils. *Blood* 68:708, 1986.

152. Metcalf D, Begley CG, Johnson GR: Biologic properties in vitro of a recombinant human granulocyte-macrophage colony stimulating factor. *Blood* 67:37, 1986.

153. Vadas MA, Nicola NA, Metcalf D: Activation of antibody dependent cell mediated cytotoxicity of the human neutrophils and eosinophils by separate colony stimulating factors. *J Immunol* 130:795, 1983.

154. Handman E, Burgess AW: Stimulation by granulocyte-macrophage colony stimulating factor of *Leishmania tropica* killing by macrophages. *J Immunol* 122:1134, 1979.

155. Begley CG, Lopez AF, Nicola NA, et al: Purified colony stimulating factors enhance the survival of human neurophils and eosinophils in vitro: a rapid and sensitive microassay for colony-stimulating factors. *Blood* 68:162, 1986.

156. Weisbart RH, Golde DW, Clark SC, et al: Human granulocyte-macrophage colony stimulating factor is a neutrophil activator. *Nature* 314:361, 1985.

157. Dispersio J, Billing P, Kaufman S, et al: The human GM-CSF receptor: Mechanisms of tranmembrane signaling and neutrophil priming. *Blood* 70:170a, 1987.

158. Walker F, Nicola NA, Metcalf D, et al: Hierarchical down-modulation of hemopoietic growth factor receptors. *Cell* 43:269, 1985.

159. Walker F, Burgess AW: Specific binding of radio-iodinated granulocyte-macrophage colony stimulating factor to hemopoietic cells. *EMBO J* 4:933, 1985.

160. Park LS, Friend D, Gillis S, Urdal DL: Characterization of the cell surface receptor for human granulocyte/macrophage colony stimulating factor. *J Exp Med* 164:251, 1986.

161. Pluznik DH, Cunningham RE, Noguchi PD: Colony stimulating factor (CSF) controls proliferation of CSF-dependent cells by acting during G1 phase of cell cycle. *Proc Natl Acad Sci USA* 81:7451, 1984.

162. Donahue R, Wang E, Stone D, et al: Stimulation of haematopoiesis in primates by continuous infusion of recombinant human GM-CSF. *Nature* 321:872, 1986.

163. Metcalf D, Bagby CG, Williamson DF, et al: Hemopoietic responses in mice injected with purified recombinant murine granulocyte-macrophage colony stimulating factor. *Exp Hematol* 15:1, 1987.

164. Monroe RL, Skelly RR, Taylor P, et al: Recovery from severe hematopoietic suppression using recombinant human graulocyte-macrophage colony-stimulating factor. *Exp Hematol* 16:344, 1988.

165. Nienhaus AW, Donahue RE, Karlsson S, Clark SC, et al: Recombinant human granulocyte-macrophage colony-stimulating factor (GM-CSF) shortens the period of neutropenia after autologous bone marrow transplantation in a primate model. *J Clin Invest* 80:573, 1987.

166. Monray RL, Skelly RR, MacVittie TJ, et al: The effect of recombinant GM-CSF on the recovery of monkeys transplanted with autologous bone marrow. *Blood* 70:1696, 1987.

167. Mayer P, Lam C, Obenhaus H, et al: Recombinant human GM-CSF induces leukocytosis and activates peripheral blood polymorphonuclear neutrophils in nonhuman primates. *Blood* 70:206, 1987.

168. Welte K, Bonilla MA, Gillo AP, et al: Recombinant human granulocyte colony-stimulating factor. Effects on hematopoiesis in normal cyclophosphamide-treated primates. *J Exp Med* 165:941, 1987.

169. Groopman JE, Mitsuasu RT, Deleo MJ, et al: Effect of recombinant human granulocyte-macrophage colony stimulating factor on myelopoiesis in the acquired immunodeficiency syndrome. *N Engl J Med* 317:593, 1987.

170. Antman K, Griffin J, Elias A, et al: Effect of recombinant human granulocyte-macrophage colony-stimulating factor on chemotherapy-induced myelosuppression. *N Engl J Med* 319:593, 1988.

171. Grosh WW, Quesenberry PJ: Recombinant human hematopoietic growth factors in the treatment of cytopenias. *Clin Immunol Immunopathol* 62:S25, 1992.

172. Tsuchiya M, Asano S, Kaziro Y, Nagata S: Isolation and characterization of the cDNA for murine granulocyte colony stimulating factor. *Proc Natl Acad Sci USA* 83:7633, 1986.

173. Nagata S, Tsuchiym, Asano S, et al: The chromosomal gene structure and two mRNAs for human granulocyte colony stimulating factor. *Embo J* 5:575, 1989.

174. Simmers RN, Webber LM, Shannon MF, et al: Localization of the G-CSF gene on chromosome 17 proximal to the breakpoint in the t(15;17) in acute promyelocytic leukemia. *Blood* 70:330, 1987.

175. Woodward TA, McNeice IK, Witte PL, et al: Further studies on growth factor production by the TC-1 stromal cell line: pre-B stimulating activity. *Blood* 75:2130, 1990.

176. Avalos BR, Hedzat C, Baldwin GC, et al: Biological activities of human G-CSF and characterization of the human G-CSF receptor. *Blood* 70:165a, 1987.

177. Vallenga E, Young DC, Wagner K, et al: The effects of GM-CSF and G-CSF in promoting growth of clonogenic cell in acute myeloblastic leukemia. *Blood* 69:1771, 1987.

178. Miyauchi J, Kelleher CA, Yang Y, et al: The effects of three recombinant growth factors IL-3, GM-CSF and G-CSF on the blast cells of acute myeloblastic leukemia maintained in short term suspension culture. *Blood* 70:657, 1987.

179. Okabe T, Takaku F: In vivo granulocytopoietic activities of human recombinant granulocyte colony stimulating factor. *Exp Hematol* 14:475, 1986.

180. Moore MAS, Welte K, Gabrilove JL, et al: In vivo action of recombinant human G-CSF in chemotherapy or radiation myelosuppressed mice. *Blood* 69:173a, 1986.

181. Cohen AM, Zsebo K, Hines D, et al: In vivo activity of recombinant human granulocyte colony stimulating factor. *Exp Hematol* 14:489, 1986.

182. Welte K, Bonilla MA, Gillio AP, et al: *In vivo* effects of combined recombinant human G-CSF and GM-CSF on hematopoiesis in primates. *Blood* 68:183a, 1986.

183. Monroe RL, Skelly RR, MacVittie TJ, et al: The effect of recombinant GM-CSF on the recovery of monkeys transplanted with autologous bone marrow. *Blood* 70:1696, 1987.

184. Welte K, Bonilla MA, Gabrilove JL, et al: Recombinant human granulo-cyte-colony stimulating factor: in vitro and in vivo effects on myelopoiesis. *Blood Cells* 13:17, 1987.

185. Tamura M, Hattori K, Nomura H, et al: Induction of neutrophilic granulo-cytosis in mice by administration of purified human granulocyte colony stimulating factor (G-CSF). *Biochem Biophys Res Comm* 142:454, 1987.

186. Shimamura M, Kobayashi Y, You A, et al: Effect of human recombinant granulocyte colony stimulating factor on hematopoietic injury in mice induced by 5-fluorouracil. *Blood* 69:353, 1987.

187. Gabrilove J, Jakubowski A, Fain K, et al: A Phase I/II study or rhG-CSF in cancer patients at risk for chemotherapy induced neutropenia. *Blood* 70:135a, 1987.

188. Bronchud MH, Scarffe JH, Thatcher N, et al: Phase I/II study of recombi-nant human granulocyte colony stimulating factor in patients receiving intensive chemotherapy for small cell lung cancer. *Br J Cancer* 56:809, 1987.

189. Tushinski RJ, Stanley ER: The regulation of mononuclear phagocyte entry into S phase by the colony stimulating factor, CSF-1. *J Cell Physiol* 122:221, 1985.

190. Tushinski RJ, Stanley ER: The regulation of macrophage protein turn-over by a colony stimulating factor (CSF-1). *J Cell Physiol* 116:67, 1983.

191. Wing EJ, Waheed A, Shadduck R, et al: Effect of colony stimulating factor on murine macrophages. *J Clin Invest* 69:270, 1982.

192. Wing EF, Ampel NM, Waheed A, et al: Macrophage CSF (M-CSF) enhances the capacity of murine macrophages to secrete oxygen reduc-tion products. *J Immunol* 135:2052, 1985.

193. Lin HS, Gordon S: Secretion of plasminogen activator by bone marrow derived mononuclear phagocytes and its enhancement by colony stimu-lating factor. *J Exp Med* 150:231, 1979.

194. Hamilton JA, Stanley ER, Burgess AW, et al: Stimulation of macrophage plasminogen activator activity by colony stimulating factors. *J Cell Physiol* 103:435, 1980.

195. Chen BD-M, Lin HS: Colony stimulating factor (CSF-1): Its enhance-ment of plasminogen activator production and inhibition of cell growth in a mouse macrophage cell line. *J Immunol* 132:2955, 1984.

196. Moore RN, Oppenheim JJ, Farrar JJ, et al: Production of lymphocytes-activating factor (interleukin-1) by macrophages activated with colony stimulating factors. *J Immunol* 125:1302, 1980.

197. Sherr CF, Rettenmier CW, Sacca R, et al: The c-fms proto-oncogene product is related to the receptor for the mononuclear phagocyte growth factor, CSF-1. *Cell* 41:665, 1985.

198. Sacca R, Stanley ER, Sherr CJ, et al: Specific binding of the mononuclear phagocyte colony stimulating factor CSF-1 to the product of the c-fms oncogene. *Proc Natl Acad Sci USA* 8:3331, 1986.

199. Rettenmier CW, Sacca R, Furman WL, et al: Expression of the human c-fms proto-oncogene product (colony stimulating factor-1) receptor on peripheral blood mononuclear cells and choriocarcinoma cell lines. *J Clin Invest* 77:1740, 1986.

200. Jubinsky PT, Stanley ER: Purification of hemopoietin 1: A multilineage hemopoietic growth factor. *Proc Natl Acad Sci USA* 82:2764, 1985.

201. Mochizuki DY, Eisenman JR, Conlon PJ, et al: Interleukin-1 regulates hematopoietic activity, a role previously ascribed to hemopoietin 1. *Proc Natl Acad Sci USA* 84:5267, 1987.

202. Matsushima H, Roussel MF, Ashman RA, Scherr CJ: Colony-stimulating factor-1 regulates novel cyclins during the G1 phase of the cell cycle. *Cell* 65:701, 1991.

203. Stanley ER, Heard PM: Factors regulating macrophage production and growth. Purification and some properties of the colony stimulating factor from medium. *J Biol Chem* 252:4305, 1977.

204. Waheed A, Shadduck R: Purification of colony-stimulating factor by affinity chromatography. *Blood* 60:238, 1982.

205. Das Sk, Stanley ER, Guilbert LF, Forman LW: Human colony stimulat-ing factor (CSF-1) radioimmunoassay: resolution of three subclasses of human colony stimulating factors. *Blood* 58:630, 1981.

206. Das SK, Stanley ER: Structure-function studies of a colony stimulating factor (CSF-1). *J Biol Chem* 257:13679, 1982.

207. Kawaski ES, Lander MB, Wang AM, et al: Molecular cloning of a complementary DNA encoding human macrophage-specific colony stimulating actor (CSF-1). *Science* 230:291, 1985.

208. DeLamarter JF, Hession C, Semon D, et al: Nucleotide sequence of a cDNA encoding murine CSF-1 (macrophage-CSF). *Nucleic Acid Res* 15:2389, 1987.

209. Price LKH, Choi HU, Kosenberg L, Stanley ER: The predominant form of secreted colony stimulating factor-1 is a proteoglycan. *J Biol Chem* 267:2190, 1992.

210. Ihle JN, Keller J, Henderson L, et al: Procedures for the purification of IL-3 to homogeneity. *J Immunol* 129:2431, 1982.

211. Clark Lewis I, Kent SBH, Schrader JW: Purification to apparent homoge-neity of a factor stimulating the growth of multiple lineages of hemopoi-etic cells. *J Biol Chem* 259:7488, 1984.

212. Prestidge RL, Watson JD, Urdal DL, et al: Biochemical comparison of murine colony stimulating factors secreted by a T cell lymphoma and a myelomonocytic leukemia. *J Immunol* 133:293, 1984.

213. Cutler RL, Metcalf D, Nicola NA, et al: Purification of a multipotential colony stimulating factor from pokeweed mitogen-stimulated mouse spleen cell conditioned medium. *J Biol Chem* 260:6579, 1985.

214. Watson JD, Crosier PS, March CF, et al: Purification to homogeneity of a human hematopoietic growth factor that stimulates the growth of a murine IL-3-dependent cell line. *J Immunol* 137:854, 1986.

215. Fung MC, Hapel AJ, Ymer S, et al: Molecular cloning of cDNA for murine interleukin-3. *Nature* 307:233, 1984.

216. Yokota T, Lee F, Rennick D, et al: Isolation and characterization of a mouse cDNA clone that expresses mast cell growth factor activity in monkey cells. *Proc Natl Acad Sci USA* 81:1070, 1984.

217. Miyatake S, Yokota T, Lee F, Arai K: Structure of the chromosomal gene for murine interleukin-3. *Proc Natl Acad Sci USA* 82:316, 1985.

218. Campbell HD, Ymer S, Fung M-C, Young IG: Cloning and nucleotide sequence of the murine interleukin-3 gene. *Eur J Biochem* 150:297, 1985.

219. Todokoro K, Yamamoto A, Amanuma H, Ikawa Y: Isolation and charac-terization of a genomic DDD mouse interleukin-3 gene. *Gene* 39:103, 1985.

220. Hapel AJ, Osborne JM, Fung MC, et al: Expression of 20-hydroxysteroid dehydrogenase in mouse macrophages, hemopoietic cells and cell lines and its induction by colony stimulating factors. *J Immunol* 134:2492, 1985.

221. Prystowsky MB, Ihle JN, Rich I, et al: Two biologically distinct colony stimulating factors are secreted by a T lymphocyte clone. *J Cell Biochem* 6:37, 1983.

222. McNiece IK, Bertoncello I, Kriegler AB, Quesenberry PJ: Colony form-ing cells with high proliferative potential (HPP-CFC). *Int J Cell Cloning* 8:146, 1990.

223. Koike K, Ihle JN, Ogawa M: Declining sensitivity to interleukin 3 of murine multipotential hemopoietic progenitors during their develop-ment. Application to a culture system that favors blast cell colony formation. *J Clin Inv* 77:894, 1986.

224. Broxmyer HE, Williams DE, Hangoc G, et al: Synergistic myelopoietic actions *in vivo* after administration to mice of combinations of purified natural murine colony stimulating facotr-1, recombinant murine interleu-kin-3 and recombinant murine granulocyte/macrophage colony stimulat-ing factor. *Proc Natl Acad Sci USA* 84:3871, 1987.

225. Donahue RE, Seehra J, Metzger M, et al: Human IL-3 and GM-CSF act synergistically in stimulating hematopoiesis in primates. *Science* 241:1820, 1988.

226. Ganser A, Lindemann A, Seipelt G, et al: Effects of recombinant human interleukin-3 in a plastic anemia. *Blood* 76:1287, 1990.

227. Kuzrock R, Talpaz M, Estrov Z, et al: Phase I study of recombinant human interleukin-3 in patients with bone marrow failure. *J Clin Oncol* 9:1241, 1991.

228. Arend WP, Welgus HG, Thompson RC, Eisenbery SP: Biologic proper-ties of recombinant human monocyte-derived interleukin-1 receptor an-tagonist. *J Clin Invest* 85:1694, 1990.

229. Dinarello CA: Interleukin-1 and the pathogenesis of the acute phase response. *N Engl J Med* 311:1413, 1984.

230. Ikebuchi K, Ihle JN, Hirai Y: Synergistic factors for stem cell proliferation: further studies of the target stem cells and the mechanism of stimulation by interleukin-1, interleukin-6 and granulocyte colony stimulating factor. *Blood* 72:2007, 1988.

231. Hoang T, Haman A, Goncalves O, et al: Interleukin-1 enhances growth factor-dependent proliferation of the clonogenic cells in acute myeloblas-tic leukemia and of normal human primitive hemopoietic precursors. *J Exp Med* 168:463, 1988.

232. Zhou Y-Q, Stanley ER, Clark SC, et al: Interleukin-3 and interleukin-1-alpha allow earlier bone marrow progenitors to respond to human colony stimulating factor-1. *Blood* 72:1870, 1988.

233. Zsebo KM, Wypych J, Yuschenkoff VN, et al: Effects of hematopoietin-1 and interleukin-1 activities on early hematopoietic cells of the bone marrow. *Blood* 71:962, 1988.

234. Warren DJ, Moore MAS: Synergism amon interleukin-1, interleukin-3 and interleukin-5 in the production of eosinophils from primitive hemopoietic stem cells. *J Immunol* 140:94, 1989.

235. Kupper TS, Lee F, Birchall N, et al: Interleukin-1 binds to specific receptors on human keratinocytes and induces granulocyte-macrophage colony stimulating factor mRNA and protein. *J Clin Invest* 82:1787, 1988.

236. Seelentag WK, Mermod J-J, Montesano R, Vassalli P: Additive effects of interleukin-1 and tumor necrosis factor-alpha on the accumulation of the three granulocytes and macrophage colony stimulating factor mRNAs in human endothelial cells. *EMBO J* 6:2261, 1987.

237. Hermann F, Oster W, Meuer SC, et al: Interleukin-1 stimulates T lymphocytes to produce granulocyte-monocyte colony stimulating factor. *J Clin Invest* 81:1415, 1988.

238. Fibbe WE, Van Damme J, Billiou A, et al: Interleukin-1 stimulates T lymphocytes to produce granulocyte-monocyte colony stimulating factor. *J Clin Invest* 81:1415, 1988.

239. Zucali JR, Dinarello CA, Oblon DF, et al: Interleukin-1 stimulates fibroblasts to produce granulocyte-macrophage colony stimulating activity and prostaglandin E2. *J Clin Invest* 77:1857, 1986.

240. Rennick D, Yang G, Gemmell L, Lee F: Control of hemopoiesis by a bone marrow stromal cell clone: lipopolysaccharide and interleukin-1 inducible production of colony stimulating factors. *Blood* 69:682, 1987.

241. Kimura H, Ishibashi T, Shikama Y, et al: Interleukin-1β (IL-1β) induces thrombocytosis in mice: possible implication of IL-6. *Blood* 76:2493, 1990.

242. Crown J, Jakubowski A, Kemeny N, et al: A phase I trial of recombinant human interleukin-1β alone and in combination with myelosuppressive doses of 5-fluorouracil in patients with gastrointestinal cancer. *Blood* 78:1420, 1991.

243. Waldman TA, Goldman CK, Robb RJ, et al: Expression of interleukin-2 receptors on activated human B cell. *J Exp Med* 160:1450, 1984.

244. Noma Y, Sideras P, Naito T, et al: Cloning of cDNA encoding the murine IgG1 induction factor by a novel strategy using SP6 promoter. *Nature* 319:640, 1986.

245. Coffman RL, Ohara J, Bond MW, et al: B cell stimulatory factor-1 enhances the IgE response of lipoplysacchardie-activated B cells. *J Immunol* 136:4538, 1986.

246. Broxmeyer HE, Lu L, Cooper S, et al: Synergistic effects of purified recombinant human and murine B cell growth factor-1/interleukin-4 on colony formation *in vitro* by hematopoietic progenitor cells. *J Immunol* 141:3852, 1988.

247. Musashi M, Clark SC, Sudo T, et al: Synergistic interactions between interleukin-11 and interleukin-4 in support of proliferation of primitive hematopoietic progenitors of mice. *Blood* 78:1448, 1991.

248. DeWolf JTM, Beentijes JAM, Esselink MT, et al: Interleukin-4 suppresses the interleukin-3 dependent erythroid colony formation form normal human bone marrow cells. *Br J Haematol* 74:246, 1990.

249. Takatsu K, Tominaga A, Mamaoka T: Antigen induced T cell replacing factor (TRF). I. Functional characterization of TRF-producing helper T cell subset and genetic studies on TRF production. *J Immunol* 124:2414, 1980.

250. Swain SL, Dutton RW: Production of a B cell growth-promoting activity, (DL) BCGF, from a cloned T cell line and its assay on the BCL1 B cell tumor. *J Exp Med* 156:1821, 1982.

251. Tanabe O, Akira S, Kamiya T, et al: Genomic structure of the murine IL-6 gene. *J Immunol* 141:3875, 1988.

252. Sehgal PB, May LT, Tamm I, Vilcek J: Human B2 interferon and B cell differentiation factor BSF-2 are identical. *Science* 235:731, 1987.

253. Gauldie J, Richards C, Harnish D, et al: Interferon beta 2/B-cell stimulatory factor type 2 shares identity with monocyte-derived hepatocyte-stimulating factor and regulates the major acute phase protein response in liver cells. *Proc Natl Acad Sci USA* 84:7251, 1987.

254. Ikebuchi K, Wong GG, Clark SC, et al: Interleukin-6 enhancement of interleukin-3-dependent proliferation of multipotential hemopoietic progenitors. *Proc Natl Acad Sci USA* 84:9035, 1987.

255. Chiu CP, Moulds C. Coffman RL, et al: Multiple biological activities are expressed by a mouse interleukin-6 cDNA clone isolated from bone marrow stromal cells. *Proc Natl Acad Sci USA* 85:7009, 1988.

256. Quesenberry PJ, McGrath HE, Williams ME, et al: Multifactor stimulation of megakaryocytopoiesis: effects of IL-6. *Exp Hematol* 19:35, 1991.

257. Ishibashi T, Kimura H, Shikama Y, et al: Inteleukin-6 is a potent throbopoietic factor *in vivo* in mice. *Blood* 74:1241, 1989.

258. Herodin F, Mestries J-C, Janodet D, et al: Recombinant glycosylated human interleukin-6 accelerates peripheral blood platelet count recovery in radiation-induced bone marrow depression in baboons. *Blood* 80:688, 1992.

259. Cooper RJ, Gordon MS, Weber J, Hoffman R: The *in vivo* administration of recombinant human interleukin-6 (IL-6) to patients with advanced malignancies has a profound effect on thrombopoiesis. *Exp Hematol* 21:1117, 1993.

260. Hoang T, Haman A, Goncalves O, et al: Interleukin-6 enhances growth factor-dependent proliferation of the blast cells of acute myeloblastic leukemia. *Blood* 72:823, 1988.

261. Klein B, Zhang X-G, Jourdan M, et al: Paracrine rather than autocrine regulation of myeloma-cell growth and differentiation by interleukin-6. *Blood* 73:517, 1989.

262. Yoshizaki K, Matsuda T, Nishimoto N, et al: Pathogenic significance of interleukin-6 (IL-6/BSF-2) in Castleman's disease. *Blood* 74:1360, 1989.

263. Faltynek CR, Wang S, Miller D, et al: Administration of human recombinant IL-7 to normal and irradiated mice increases the number of lymphocytes and some immature cells of myeloid lineage. *J Immunol* 149:1276, 1992.

264. McNiece IK, Langley KE, Zsebo KM: The role of recombinant stem cell factor in early B cell development. *J Immunol* 146:378, 1991.

265. Schall TJ, Bacon K, Camp RDR, et al: Human macrophage inflammatory protein-1α (MIP-1α) and MIP 1β chemokines attract distinct populations of lymphocytes. *J Exp Med* 177:1821, 1993.

266. Volpe SD, Cerami A: Macrophage inflammatory protein 1 and 2: members of a novel super family of cytokines. *FASEB J* 3:2565, 1989.

267. Broxmeyer HE, Benninger L, Hague N, et al: Suppressive effects of the chemokine (macrophage inflammatory protein) family of cytokines on proliferation of normal and leukemia myeloid cell proliferation, in *The Negative Regulation of Hematopoiesis: From Fundamental Aspects to Clinical Applications*, edited by M Guigon. Inserum Eurotext Libbey, Paris, 1993.

268. Donahue RE, Yang Y-C, Clark SC: Human P40 T cell growth factor (interleukin-9) supports erythroid colony formation. *Blood* 75:2271, 1990.

269. VanSnick J, Goethals A, Renauld JC, et al: Cloning and characterization of a cDNA for a new mouse T cell growth factor (P40). *J Exp Med* 169:363, 1989.

270. Yang Y-C, Ricciardi S, Ciarletta A, et al: Expression cloning of a cDNA encoding a novel human hematopoietic growth factor human homologue of murine T cell growth factor P40. *Blood* 74:1880, 1989.

271. Hueltner L, Moeller J, Schmitt E, et al: Thiol-sensitive mast cell lines derived from mouse bone marrow respond to a mast cell growth-enhancing activity different from both IL-3 and IL-4. *J Immunol* 142:3440, 1989.

272. Suda T, O'Garra A, MacNeil I, et al: Identification of a novel thymocyte growth-promoting factor derived from B cell lymphomas. *Cell Immunol* 147:528, 1991.

273. Chen W-F, Zlotnick A: IL-10: a novel cytotoxic T cell differentiation factor. *J Immunol* 147:528, 1991.

274. Go NF, Castle BE, Barrett R, et al: Interleukin-10, a novel B cell stimulatory factor: unresponsiveness of x chromosome-linked immunodeficiency B cells. *J Exp Med* 172:1625, 1990.

275. Yin T, Schendel P, Yu-Chung Y: Enhancement of in vitro and in vivo antigen-specific antibody responses by interleukin-11. *J Exp Med* 175:211, 1992.

276. Bruno E, Briddell RA, Cooper RJ, Hoffman R: Effects of recombinant interleukin-11 on human megakaryocyte progenitor cells. *Exp Hematol* 19:378, 1991.

277. Musashi M, Clark SC, Sudo T, et al: Synergistic interactions between interleukin-11 and interleukin-4 in support of proliferation of primitive hematopoietic progenitors of mice. *Blood* 78:1448, 1991.

278. Goldman S, Loebelenz J, McCarthy K, et al: Recombinant human in-

terleukin-11 stimulates megakaryoctyic maturation and increase in peripheral platelet number *in vivo. Blood* 78:1329, 1991 (abstract).

279. Du XX, Neben T, Goldman S, Williams DA: Effects of recombinant humaninterleukin-11 on hematopoietic reconstitution in transplant mice: acceleration of recovery of peripheral blood neutrophils and platelets. *Blood* 81:27, 1993.

280. Wolf SF, Temple PA, Kobayashi M, et al: Cloning of cDNA for natural killer cells stimulatory factor, a heterodimeric cytokine with multiple biologic effects on T and natural killer cells. *J Immunol* 146:3074, 1991.

281. Kobayashi M, Fitz L, Ryan M, et al: Identification and purification of natural killer cell stimulatory factor (NKSF), a cytokine with multiple biologic effects on human lymphocytes. *J Exp Med* 170:827, 1989.

282. Gately MK, Desai BB, Wolitzky AG, et al: Regulation of human lymphocyte proliferation by a heterodimeric cytokine, IL-12 (cytotoxic lymphocyte maturation factor). *J Immunol* 147:874, 1991.

283. Chan SH, Perussia B, Gupta JW, et al: Induction of interferon γ production by natural killer cell stimulatory factor: characterization of the responder cells and synergy with other inducers. *J Exp Med* 173:869, 1991.

284. Kiniwa M, Gately M, Gubler U, et al: Recombinant interleukin-12 suppresses the synthesis of immunoglobulin E by interleukin-4-stimulated human lymphocytes. *J Clin Invest* 90:262, 1992.

285. McKenize ANJ, Culpepper JA, de Waal Malefyt R, et al: Interleukin-13, a novel T-cell-derived cytokine that regulates human monocyte and B cell function. *Proc Natl Acad Sci USA* 90:3735, 1993.

286. Ambrus JL Jr., Chesky L, Stephany D, McFarland P, Mostowski H, Fauci AS: Functional studies examining the subpopulation of human B lymphocytes responding to high molecular weight B cell growth factor. *J Immunol* 145:3949, 1990.

287. Ambrus JL Jr., Pippin J. Joseph A. et al: Identification of a cDNA for a human high-molecular-weight B-cell growth factor [published erratum appears in *Proc Natl Acad Sci USA* 1996 Jul 23;93(15):8154]. *Proc Natl Acad Sci USA* 90:6330, 1993.

288. Ford R, Tamayo A, Martin B, Niu K, Claypool K, Cabanillas F, Ambrus J Jr: Identification of B-cell growth factors (interleukin-14; high molecular weight B-cell growth factors) in effusion fluids from patients with aggressive B-cell lymphomas. *Blood* 86:283, 1995.

289. Uckun FM, Fauci AS, Chandan-Langlie M, Myers DE, Ambrus JL: Detection and characterization of human high molecular weight B cell growth factor receptors on leukemic B cells in chronic lymphocytic leukemia. *J Clin Invest* 84:1595, 1989.

290. Bamford RN, Battiata AP, Waldmann TA: IL-15: the role of translational regulation in their expression. *J Leuk Biol* 59:476, 1996.

291. Giri J, Anderson DM, Kumaki S, et al: IL-15, a novel T cell growth factor that shares activities and receptor components with IL-2, *J Leuk Biol* 57:763, 1995.

292. Kennedy MK, Park LS: Characterization of interleukin-15 (IL-15) and the IL-15 receptor complex. *J Clin Immunol* 16:134, 1996.

293. Tagaya Y, Bamford RN, DeFilippis AP, Waldman TA: IL-15: a pleoriophic cytokine with diverse receptor/signaling pathways whose expression is controlled at multiple levels. *Immunity* 4:329, 1996.

294. Kirman I, Vainer B, Nielsen OH: Interleukin-15 and its role in chronic inflammatory diseases. *Inflam Res* 47:285, 1998.

295. Center DM, Kornfeld H, Cruikshank WW: Interleukin-16. *Int J Biochem Cell Biol* 29:1231, 1997.

296. Center DM, Kornfeld H, Cruikshank WW: Interleukin-16 and its function as a CD4 ligand. *Immunol Today* 17:476, 1996.

297. Cruikshank WW, Kronfeld H, Center DM: Signaling and functional properties of interleukin-16. *Int Rev Immunol* 16:523, 1998.

298. Amiel C, Darcissac E, Truong MJ, et al: Interleukin-16 (IL-16) inhibits human immunodeficiency virus replication in cells from infected subjects, and serum IL-16 levels drop with disease progression. *J Infect Dis* 179:83, 1999.

299. Mashikian MV, Tarpy RE, Saukkonen JJ, et al: Identification of IL-16 as the lymphocyte chemotactic activity in the bronchoalveolar lavage fluid of histamine-challenged asthmatic patients. *J Allergy Clin Immunol* 101:786, 1998.

300. Antonaci S, Serlenga E, Garofalo AR, et al: Imbalance of T cell immunoregulatory subsets in primary IgA nephropathy. *Cytobios* 59:95, 1989.

301. Klimiuk PA, Goronzy JJ, Weyand CM: IL-16 as an anti-inflammatory cytokine in rheumatoid synovitis. *J Immunol* 162:4293, 1999.

302. Lee S, Kaneko H, Sekigawa I, et al: Circulating interleukin-16 in systemic lupus erythematosus. *Br J Rheum* 37:1334, 1998.

303. Laberge S, Ghaffar O, Boguniewicz M, et al: Association of increased CD4+ T-cell infiltration with increased IL-16 gene expression in atopic dermatitis. *J Allergy Clin Immunol* 102:645, 1998.

304. Spriggs, MK: Interleukin-17 and its receptor. *J Clin Immunol* 17:366, 1997.

305. Fossiez F, Banchereau J, Murray R, et al: Interleukin-17. *Inter Rev Immunol* 16:541, 1998.

306. Yao Z, Spriggs MK, Derry JM, et al: Molecular characterization of the human interleukin (IL)-17 receptor. *Cytokine* 9:794, 1997.

307. Aarvak T, Chabaud M, Miossec P, Natvig JB: IL-17 is produced by some proinflammatory Th1/Th0 cells but not by Th2 cells. *J Immunol* 162:1246, 1999.

308. Shin HC, Benbernou N, Fekkar H, et al: Regulation of IL-17, IFN-gamma and IL-10 in human CD8(+) T cells by cyclic AMP-dependent signal transduction pathway. *Cytokine* 10:841, 1998.

309. Chabaud M, Durand JM, Buchs N, et al: Human interleukin-17: a T cell-derived proinflammatory cytokine produced by the rheumatoid synovium. *Arthritis Rheum* 42:963, 1999.

310. Awane M, Andres PG, Li DJ, Reinecker HC: NF-kappa B-inducing kinase is a common mediator of IL-17-, TNF-alpha-, and IL-1 beta-induced chemokine promoter activation in intestinal epithelial cells. *J Immunol* 162:5337, 1999.

311. VanKooten C, Boonstra JG, Paape ME, et al: Interleukin-17 activates human renal epithelial cells in vitro and is expressed during renal allograft rejection. *J Am Soc Nephrol* 9:1526, 1998.

312. Cai XY, Gommoll CP Jr, Justice L, et al: Regulation of granulocyte colony-stimulating factor gene expression by interleukin-17. *Immunol Letters* 62:51, 1998.

313. Jovanvic DV, Di Battista JA, Martel-Pelletier J, et al: IL-17 stimulates the production and expression of proinflammatory cytokines, IL-beta and TNF-alpha, by human macrophages. *J Immunol* 160:3513, 1998.

314. Shalom-Barak T, Quach J, Lotz M: Interleukin-17-induced gene expression in articular chondrocytes is associated with activation of mitogen-activated protein kinases and NF-kappaB. *J Biol Chem* 273:27467, 1998.

315. Teunissen MB, Koomen CW, de Waal Malefyt R, et al: Interleukin-17 and interferon-gamma synergize in the enhancement of proinflammatory cytokine production by human keratinocytes. *J Invest Derm* 111:645, 1998.

316. Albanesi C, Cavani A, Girolomoni G: IL-17 is produced by nickel-specific T lymphocytes and regulates ICAM-1 expression and chemokine production in human keratinocytes: synergistic or antagonist effects with IFN-gamma and TNF-alpha. *J Immunol* 162:494, 1999.

317. Hoshino H, Lotvall J, Skoogh BE, Linden A: Neutrophil recruitment by interleukin-17 into rat airways in vivo. Role of tachykinins. *Am J Resp Crit Care Med* 159:1423, 1999.

318. Hoshino H. Lotvall J. Skoogh BE. Linden A. Neutrophil recruitment by interleukin-17 into rat airways in vivo. Role of tachykinins. *Am J Resp Crit Care Med* 159:1423, 1999.

319. Schwarzenberger P, La Russa V, Miller A, et al: IL-17 stimulates granulopoiesis in mice: use of an alternate, novel gene therapy-derived method for in vivo evaluation of cytokines. *J Immunol* 161:6383, 1998.

320. Gillespie MT. Horwood NJ: Interleukin-18: perspectives on the newest interleukin. *Cytokine Growth Factor Rev* 9:109, 1998.

321. Dinarello CA, Novick D, Puren AJ, et al: Overview of interleukin-18: more than an interferon-gamma inducing factor. *J Leuk Biol* 63:658, 1998.

322. Okamura H, Kashiwamura S, Tsutsui H, et al: Regulation of interferon-gamma production by IL-12 and IL-18. *Curr Opin Immunol* 10:259, 1998.

323. Brummer E: Human defenses against *Cryptococcus neoformans:* an update. *Mycopathologia* 143:12, 1998–99.

324. Fantuzzi G, Dinarello CA: Interleukin-18 and interleukin-1 beta: two cytokine substrates for ICE (caspase-1). *J Clin Immunol* 19:1, 1999.

325. Corsini E, Galli CL: Cytokines and irritant contact dermatitis. *Toxicol Lett* 102-103:277, 1998.

326. Dinarello CA: Interleukin-1 beta, interleukin-18, and the interleukin-1 beta converting enzyme. *Ann N Y Acad Sci* 856:1, 1998.

327. Dinarello CA: IL-18: A TH1-inducing, proinflammatory cytokine and new member of the IL-1 family. *J Allergy Clin Immunol* 103:11, 1999.

328. Okamura H, Tsutsui H, Kashiwamura S, et al: Interleukin-18: a novel

cytokine that augments both innate and acquired immunity. *Adv Immunol* 70:281, 1998.

329. Martin TJ, Romas E, Gillespie MT: Interleukins in the control of osteoclast differentiation. *Crit Rev Eukaryotic Gene Expression*. 8:107, 1998.

330. Dinarello CA: Interleukin-1, interleukin-1 receptors and interleukin-1 receptor antagonist. *Int Rev Immunol* 16:457, 1998.

331. Rothe H. Kolb H: The APC1 concept of type I diabetes. *Autoimmunity* 27:179, 1998.

332. Murphy KM: Lymphocyte differentiation in the periphery. *Curr Opin Immunol* 10:226, 1998.

333. Revoltella RP: Natural and therapeutically-induced antibodies to cytokines. *Biotherapy*. 10:321, 1998.

334. Fukumoto H, Nishio M, Nishio K, et al: Interferon-gamma-inducing factor gene transfection into Lewis lung carcinoma cells reduces tumorigenicity in vivo. *Jap J Cancer Res* 88:501, 1997.

335. Russell ES, Smith LJ, Lawson FA: Implantation of normal blood-forming tissue in radiated genetically anemic hosts. *Science* 124:1076, 1956.

336. Russell ES, Bernstein SE: Proof of whole-cell implant in therapy of W-series anemia. *Arch Biochem Biophys* 125:594, 1968.

337. Russell ES: Hereditary anemias of the mouse: a review of geneticists. *Adv Genet* 20:357, 1979.

338. Mintz B, Russell ES: Gene-induced embryological modifications of primordial germ cells in the mouse. *J Exp Zool* 134:207, 1957.

339. Bernstein SE, Russell ES, Keighley G: Two hereditary mouse anemias (S1/S1^d and W/W^v) deficient in response to erythropoietin. *Ann N Y Acad Sci* 149:475, 1968.

340. Fried W, Camberlin W, Knospe WH, et al: Studies on the defective hematopoietic microenvironment of S1/S1^d mice. *Br J Haematol* 24:643, 1973.

341. McCulloch EA, Siminovitch L, Till JE, et al: The cellular basis of the genetically determined hemopoietic defect in anemic mice of genotype S1/S1^d. *Blood* 26:399, 1965.

342. Mayer TC, Green MC: An experimental analysis of the pigment defect caused by mutations at the W and S1 loci in mice. *Dev Biol* 18:62, 1968.

343. Mayer TC: A comparison of pigment cell development in albino, stell and dominant-spotting mutant mouse embryos. *Dev Biol* 23:297, 1970.

344. Chabot B, Stephenson DA, Chapman VM, et al: The proto-oncogene c-Kit encoding a transmembrane tyrosin kinase receptor maps to the mouse W locus. *Nature* 335:88, 1988.

345. Geissler EN, Ryan MA, Housman DE: The dominant-whitespotting (W) locus of the mouse encodes the c-Kit proto-oncogene. *Cell* 55:185, 1988.

346. Yarden Y, Kuang W-J, Yang-Feng T, Coussens L, et al: Human protooncogene c-Kit: a new cell surface receptor tyrosine kinase for an unidentified ligand. *EMBO J* 6:3341, 1987.

347. Tan JC, Nocka K, Ray P, et al: The dominant W^{42} spotting phenotype results from a missense mutation in the c-Kit receptor kinase. *Science* 247:209, 1990.

348. Nocka K, Majumder S, Chabot B, et al: Expression of c-Kit gene products in known cellular targets of W mutations in normal and W mutant mice—evidence for an impaired c-Kit kinase in mutant mice. *Genes Dev* 3:816, 1989.

349. Nocka, K, Tan JC, Chiu E, et al: Molecular basis of dominant negative and loss of function mutations at the murine c-Kit receptor. *Genes Dev* 4:390, 1990.

350. Reith AD, Rottapel R, Giddens E, et al: W mutant mice with mild or severe developmental defects contain distinct point mutations in the kinase domain of the c-Kit receptor. *Genes Dev* 4:390, 1990.

351. Majumder S, Brown K, Qiu F-H, Besmer P: c-Kit protein, a transmembrane kinase: identification in tissues and characterization. *Mol Cell Biol* 8:4896, 1988.

352. Nocka K, Buck J, Levi E, Besmer P: Candidate ligand for the c-Kit transmembrane kinase receptor: KL, a fibroblast derived growth factor stimulates most cells and erythroid progenitors. *Embo J* 9:3287-94, 1990.

353. Zsebo KM, Wypych J, McNiece IK, et al: Identification, purification, and biological characterization of hematopoietic stem cell factor from buffalo rat liver conditioned media. *Cell* 63:195-201, 1990.

354. Copeland NG, Gilbert DJ, Cho BC, et al: Most cell growth factor maps near the steel locus on mouse chromosome 10 and is deleted in a number of steel alleles. *Cell* 63:175, 1990.

355. Wehrle-Haller B, Weston JA: Soluble and cell-bound forms of steel factor activity play distinct roles in melanocyte precursor dispersal and

survival on the lateral neural crest migration pathway. *Development* 121:731, 1995.

356. McDonald TP: Thrombopoietin: its biology, purification and characterization. *Exp Hematol* 16:201, 1988.

357. Hill RJ, Levin J: Regulators of thrombopoiesis: their biochemistry and physiology. *Blood Cells* 15:141, 1989.

358. Ebbe S: Forward, in *Thrombopoiesis and Thrombopoietins: Molecular, Cellular, Preclinical, and Clinical Biology*, edited by DJ Kuter, P Hunt, W Sheridan, D Zucker-Franklin, pp V-XI. Human Press, Totowa, NJ, 1997.

359. Vigon I, Mornon JP, Cocault L, et al: Molecular cloning and characterization of MPL, the human hemolog of the v-mpl oncogene: identification of a member of the hematopoietic growth factor receptor superfamily. *Proc Natl Acad Sci USA* 89:5640, 1992.

360. Souyri M, Vigon I, Penciolelli J-F et al: A putative truncated cytokine receptor gene transduced by the myeloproliferative leukemia virus immortalization hematopoietic progenitors. *Cell* 63:1137, 1990.

361. Wendling F, Varlet P, Charon M, et al: A retrovirus complex inducting an acute myeloproliferative leukemia disorder in mice. *Virology* 149:242, 1986.

362. DeSauvage FJ, Hass PE, Spencer SD, et al: Stimulation of megakaryocytopoiesis and thrombopoiesis by the c-Mpl ligand. *Nature* 369:533, 1994.

363. Lok S, Kaushansky K, Holly RD, et al: Cloning and expression of murine thrombopoietin eDNA and stimulation of platelet production in vivo. *Nature* 369:565, 1994.

364. Bartley TD, Bogenberger J, Hunt P, et al: Identification and cloning of a megakaryocyte growth and development factor that is a ligand for the cytokine receptor Mpl. *Cell* 77:1117, 1994.

365. Sohma Y, Akahori H, Seki N, et al: Molecular cloning and chromosomal localization of the human thrombopoietin gene. *FEBS Lett* 353:57, 1994.

366. Kaushansky K: Thrombopoietin: the primary regulator of platelet production. *Blood* 86:419, 1995.

367. Kaushansky K, Lin N, Grossman A, et al: Thrombopoietin expands erythroid, granulocyte-macrophage and megakaryocyte progenitor cells in normal and myelosuppressed mice. *Exp Hematol* 23:265, 1996.

368. Forese AM, Hunt P, Grab LB, Mac Vittre: Combined administration of recombinant human megakaryocyte growth and development factor and granulocyte colony-stimulating factor enhances multi-lineage hematopoietic reconstitution in non-human primates after irradiation induced marrow aplasia. *J Clin Invest* 97:2145, 1996.

369. Ku H, Yonemura Y, Kaushonsky K, Ogawa M: Thrombopoietin, the ligand for the Mpl receptor, synergizes with steel factor and other early-acting cytokines in supporting proliferation of primitive hematopoietic progenitors of mice. *Blood* 87:4544, 1991.

370. Petzor AL, Sandstra PW, Piret JM, Eaves CJ: Differential cytokine effects on primitive (CD34+ CD38-) human hematopoietic cells: novel responses to Flt-3 ligand and thrombopoietin. *J Exp Med* 183:2551, 1996.

371. Solar GP, Kerr WG, Zeigler FC, et al: Role of c-Mpl in early hematopoiesis. *Blood* 92:4, 1998.

372. Kimura S, Roberts AW, Metcalf D, Alexander WS: Hematopoietic stem cell deficiencies in mice lacking c-Mpl, the receptor for thrombopoietin. *Proc Natl Acad Sci USA* 95:1195, 1998.

373. Jacobsen SEM, Ruscetti FW, Dubois CM, et al: Transforming growth factor beta transmodulates the expression of colony stimulating factor receptors on murine hematopoietic progenitor cell lines. *Blood* 77:1706, 1991.

374. Cosman D, Lyman SD, Idzerda RL, et al: A new cytokine receptor superfamily. *Trends Biochem Sci* 15:265, 1990.

375. D'Andrea AD, Fasman GD, Lodish HF: A new hematopoietic growth factor receptors superfamily: structural features and implications for signal transduction. *Curr Opin Cell Biol* 2:648, 1990.

376. Bazan JF: Structural design and molecular evolution of a cytokine receptor superfamily. *Proc Natl Acad Sci USA* 87:6934, 1990.

377. Miyajima A, Hayashida K, Itoh N, et al: Molecular structure of the receptors for GM-CSF, IL-3 and IL-5, in *Molecular Biology of Hematopoiesis*, edited by NG Abraham et al vol 2, p 119. Intercept, Ltd, 1992.

378. Welham MJ, Dechert U, Leslie KB, et al: Interleukin (IL)-3 and granulocyte/macrophage colony-stimulating factor, but not IL-4, induce tyrosine phosphorylation, activation, and association of SHPTP2 and Grb2 and phosphatidylinsoitol 3'-kinase. *J Biol Chem* 269:23764, 1994.

379. Okuda K, Smith L, Griffin JD, et al: Signaling functions of the tyrosine

residues in the Bc chain of the glanulocyte-macrophage colony-stimulating factor receptor. *Blood* 90:4759, 1997.

380. Welham MJ, Bone H, Levings M, et al: Insulin receptor substrate-2 is the major 170-kDa protein phoespharylaed on tyrosine in response to cytokines in murine lymphohematopoietic. *J Biol Chem* 272:1377, 1997.

381. Odai H, Sasaki K, Iwamatsu A, et al: The proto-oncogene product c-Cbl becomes tyrosine phosphorylated by stimulation with GM-CSF or Epo and constitutively binds to the SH3 domain of Grb2/Ash in human hematopoietic cells. *J Biol Chem* 270:10800, 1995.

382. Hanazono Y, Odai H, Sasaki K, et al: Proto-oncogene products Vav and c-Cb1 are involved in the signal transduction through Grb2/Ash in hematopoietic cells. *Acta Hematol* 95:236, 1996.

383. Inhorn RC, Carlesso N, Durstin M, et al: Identification of a viability domain in the granulocyte/macrophage colony-stimulating factor receptor beta-chain involving tyrosine-750. *Proc Natl Acad Sci USA* 92:8665, 1995.

384. Sato N, Sakamaki K, Teroda N, et al: Signal transduction by the high affinity GM-CSF receptor: two distinct cytoplasmic regions of the common B subunit responsible for different signaling. *Embo J* 12:4181, 1993.

385. Matsuguchi T, Inhorn RC, Carlesso N, et al: Tyrosine phosphorylation of p95 Vav in myeloid cells is regulated by GM-CSF, IL-3 and steel factor and is constitutively increased by p210 BCR/ABL, *Embo J* 14:257, 1995.

386. Itoh T, Liu R, Yokota T, et al: Definition of the role of tyrosine residues of the common beta subunit regulating multiple signaling pathways of granulocyte macrophage colony-stimulating factor receptor. *Mol Cell Biol* 18:742, 1998.

387. Odai H, Sasaki K, Iwamatsu A, et al: Purification and molecular cloning of SH2 and SH3-containing inosital polyphosphate-5-phosphatase, which is involved in the signaling pathway of granulocyte-macrophage colony-stimulating factor, erythropoietin, and Bcr-Abl. *Blood* 89:2745, 1997.

388. Mui A-IF, Wakao H., O'Farrell A-M, et al: Interleukin-3, granulocyte-macrophage colony stimulating factor and interleukin-5 transduce signals through two STAT5 homologs. *Embo J* 14:1166, 1995.

389. Quelle FW, Sato N, Wilthuhn BA, et al: JAK2 associates with the Bc chain of the receptor for granulocyte-macrophage colony-stimulating factor, and its activation requires the membrane proximal region. *Mol Cell Biol* 14:4335, 1994.

390. Chaturvedi P, Reddy MV, Reddy EP: Src kinases and not JAK's activate STATS during IL-3 induced myeloid cell proliferation. *Oncogene* 16:1749, 1998.

391. Guthridge MA, Stomski FC, Thomas D, et al: Mechanism of activation of the GM-CSF, IL-3, and IL-5 family of receptors. *Stem Cells* 16:301, 1998.

392. Weissman SM, Perkins AS: Stem cell transcription, in *Stem Cell Biology and Gene Therapy*, edited by PJ Quesenberry, GS Stein, B Forget, S Weissman, pp 81–131. Wiley-Liss, New York.

393. Wadman IA, Osacla H, Grutz GG, et al: The LIM - only protein Lmo2 is a bridging molecule resembling an erythroid, DNA-binding complex which includes the TALI, E47, GAT-1 and Ldbl/NLI proteins. *Embo J* 16:3145, 1997.

394. Bjornson CRR, Rietze RL, Reynolds BA, Magli MC, Vescovi AL. Turning brain into blood: a hematopoietic fate adopted by adult neural stem cells in vivo. *Science* 283:534, 1999.

395. Jackson KA, Ticjugn MI, Goudell MA: Hematopoietic stem cells in adult skeletal muscle. Presented at Inter Soc Exp Hematol meeting, Monte Carlo, July 12, 1999.

396. Bruder SP, Kurth AA, Shea M, Hayes WC, Jaiswal N, Kadiyala S: Bone regeneration by implantation of purified culture-expanded human mesenchymal stem cells. *J Orthop Res* 16:155, 1998.

397. Petersen BE, Bowen WC, Patrene KD, et al: Bone marrow as a potential source of hepatic oval cells. *Science* 284:1168, 1999.

398. Moore MA, Metcalf D: Ontogenesis of the haemopoietic system: yolk sac origin of in vivo and in vitro colony forming cells in the developing mouse embryo. *Br J Haematol* 18:279, 1970.

399. Dieterlen-Lievre F: On the origin of haemopoietic stem cells in the avian embryo: an experimental approach. *J Embryol Exp Morphol* 33:607, 1975.

400. Cumaro A, Furlonger C, Paige CJ: Differentiation and characterization of B-cell precursors detected in the yolk sac and embryo body of embryos

beginning at the 10- to 12-somite stage. *Proc Natl Acad Sci USA* 90:6429, 1993.

401. Cumaro A, Dieter-lenLievre F, Godin I: Lymphoid potential, probed before circulation in mouse, is restricted to caudal intraembryonic splanchnopleura. *Cell* 86:907, 1996.

402. Godin I, Garcia-Porrono JA, Coutin HO, et al: Para-aortic splanchnopleura from early mouse embryos contains B1a cell progenitors. *Nature* 364:67, 1993.

403. Meduinsky A, Dzierzak E: Definitive hematopoiesis is autonomously initiated by the A6M region. *Cell* 86:897, 1996.

404. Meduinsky AL, Samoylina NL, Muller AM, Dzierzak EA: An early pre-liver intra-embryonic source of CFU-s in the developing mouse. *Nature* 364:64 1993.

405. Muller AM, Meduinsky A, Strouboulis J, et al: Development of hematopoietic stem cells activity in the mouse embryo. *Immunity* 1:291, 1994.

406. Choi H, Kennedy M, Kazarov A, et al: A common precursor for hematopoietic and endothelial cells. *Development* 125:725, 1998.

407. Liao EC, Zon LI: Conservation of themes in vertebrate blood development, in *Cell Lineage and Fate Determination*, edited by SA Moody, pp 569–578. Academic Press, New York, 1999.

408. Quesenberry PJ: Unpublished observation, 1999.

409. Sprangrude GJ, Heimfeld S, Weissman IL: Purification and characterization of mouse hematopoietic stem cells. *Science* 241:58, 1988.

410. Ogawa M, Matsuzaki Y, Nichikawa S, et al: Expression and function of c-kit in hematopoietic progenitor cells. *J Exp Med* 174:67, 1991.

411. Zeigler FC, Bennett BD, Jordan CT, et al: Cellular and molecular characterization of the role of the FLK-2/FLT-3 receptor tyrosine kinase in heamatopoietic stem cells. *Blood* 84:2422, 1994.

412. Krause DS, Fackler MJ, Civin CL, May WS: CD34: Structure, biology and clinical utility. *Blood* 87:1, 1996.

413. Pettergell R, Moore MAS: Hematopoietic stem cells: proliferation, purification and clinical application, in *Stem Cell Biology and Gene Therapy*, edited by PJ Quesenberry, GS Stein, B Forget, S Weissman, pp 133–159. Wiley-Liss, New York.

414. Watt SM, Visser JW: Recent advances in the growth and isolation of primitive haemopoietic progenitor cells. *Cell Prolif* 25:263, 1992.

415. Miraglia S, Godrey W, Yin AH, et al: A novel five-transmembrane hematopoietic stem cell antigen: isolation, characterization and molecular cloning. *Blood* 90:5013, 1997.

416. Craig W, Kay R, Cutler RL, Landsdorp PM: Expression of Thy-1 on human hematopoietic progenitor cells. *J Exp Med* 177:1331, 1993.

417. Landsdorp PM, Dragowska W, Mayan H: Ontogene-related changes in proliferative potential of human hematopoietic cells. *J Exp Med* 178:787, 1993.

418. Osawa M, Hanada K, Homeda H, Nakauch H: Long-term lympho hematopoietic reconstitution by a single D34-low/negative hematopoietic stem cell. *Science* 273:242, 1996.

419. Zanjani ED, Almeida-Porada G, Livingston AG, Flae AW, Ogowa M: Human bone marrow CD34- cells engraft in vivo and undergo multilineage expression that includes giving rise to CD34+ cells. *Exp Hematol* 26:353, 1998.

420. Sato T, Laver JH, Ogawa M: Reversible expression of CD34 by murine hematopoietic stem cells. *Blood* 94:2548, 1999.

421. Chaudry PM, Roninson IB: Expression and activity of P-glycoprotein: a multidrug efflux pump in human hematopoietic stem cells. *Cell* 66:85, 1991.

422. Bertoncello I, Hodgson GS, Bradley TR: Multiparameter analysis of transplantable hemopoietic stem cells. The separation and enrichment of stem cells homing to marrow and spleen on the basis or rhodamine-124 fluorescence. *Exp Hematol* 13:99, 1985.

423. Mulder AH, Visser JWM: Separation and functional analysis of bone marrow cells separated by rhodamine-123 fluorescence. *Exp Hematol* 15:99, 1987.

424. Ploemacher RE, Brons NHC: Cells with marrow and spleen repopulating ability and forming spleen colonies on days 16, 12 and 8 are sequentially ordered on the basis of increasing rhodamine-123 retention. *J Cell Physiol* 136:531, 1988.

425. Sitnicka E, Bartelmez SH, Wolf NS: Separation of distinct subpopulations of primitive hematopoietic stem cells: in vivo and in-vitro characteristics. *Exp Hematol* 21:378, 1993.

426. Bradford GB, Williams B, Rossi R, Bertoncello I: Quiescence, cycling

and turnovers in the primitive hemapoietic stem cell compartment. *Exp Hematol* 25:445, 1997.

427. Pang L, Reddy PV, Quesenberry PJ: Are bone marrow stem cells quiescent? *Exp Hematol* 27(suppl 1):106, 1999.

428. Reddy GPV, Tiarks CY, Pang L, Quesenberry PJ: Synchronization and cell cycle analysis of pluripotent hematopoietic progenitor stem cells. *Blood* 90:2293, 1997.

429. Nilsson SK, Dooner MS, Quesenberry PJ: Synchronized cell-cycle induction of engrafting long-term repopulating stem cells. *Blood* 90:4646, 1997.

430. Frimberger AE, McAuliffe CI, Tuft RA, Quesenberry PJ: Studies of hematopoietic stem cell movement and membrane protrusions. Submitted *International Society for Experimental Hematology*, 1999.

431. Frimberger AE, Stering AI, Tuft RA, et al: An in vitro model of hematopoietic stem cell homing. *Blood* 92:585a, 1998.

432. Bunting KD, Galipeau J, Topham D, et al: Effects of retro-viral-mediated MDRI expression on hematopoietic stem cell self-renewal and differentiation in culture, in *Hematopoietic Stem Cells Biology and Transplantation*, edited by D Orlic, TA Bock, L Kanz, pp 125–141. New York Academy of Science, New York, 1999.

433. Peters SO, Kittler EL, Ramshaw HS, Quesenberry PJ: Murine marrow cells expanded in culture with IL-3, IL-6, IL-11, and SCF acquire an engraftment defect in normal hosts. *Exp Hematol* 23:461, 1995.

434. Peters SO, Kittler ELW, Ramshaw HS, Quesenberry PJ: Ex vivo expansion of murine marrow cells with interleukin-3, interleukin-6, interleukin-11, and stem cell factor leads to impaired engraftment in irradiated hosts. *Blood* 87:30, 1996.

435. Hababian HK, Peters SO, Hsieh CC, et al: The fluctuating phenotype of the lympho-hematopoietic stem cell with cell cycle transit. *J Exp Med* 188:393, 1998.

436. Cooper CL, Brady G, Bilia F, et al: Expression of the Id family helix-loop-helix regulators during growth and development in the hematopoietic system. *Blood* 89:3135, 1997.

437. Shakoori R, van Wijnen AJ, Cooper C, et al: Cytokine-induciton of proliferation and expression of CDC2 and cyclin A in FDC- P1 myeloid hematopoietic progenitor cells: regulation of ubiquitous and cell cycle dependent histone gene transcription factors. *J Cell Biochem* 58:1, 1995.

438. Pearson-White S, Deacon D, Crittenden R, et al: The ski/sno proto-oncogene family in hematopoietic development. *Blood* 86:2146, 1995.

439. Becker PS, Nilsson SK, Zhifang L, et al: Adhesion receptor expression by hematopoietic cell lines and murine progenitors: modulation by cytokines and cell cycle status. *Exp Hematol* 27:533, 1999.

440. Carlos TM, Harlan JM: Leukocyte-endothelial adhesion molecules. *Blood* 84:2068, 1994.

441. Long MW: Blood cell cytoadhesion molecules. *Exp Hematol* 20:288, 1992.

442. Giancotti FG, Comoglio PM, Tarone G: Fibronectin plasma membrane interaction in the adhesion of hemopoietic cells. *J Cell Biol* 103:429, 1986.

443. Tsai S, Patel V, Beaumont E, Lodish HF: Differential binding of erythroid and myeloid progenitors to fibroblasts and fibronectin. *Blood* 69:1587, 1987.

444. Koenigsmann M, Griffin JD, DiCarlo J, Cannistra SA: Myeloid and erythroid progenitor cells from normal bone marrow adhere to collagen type I. *Blood* 79:657, 1992.

445. Williams DA, Rios M, Stephens C, Patel VP: Fibronectin and VLA-4 in hematopoietic stem cell-microenvironment interactions. *Nature (London)* 352:438, 1991.

446. Verfaillie CM, Mcarthy JB, McGlave PB: Differentiation of primitive human multipotent hematopoietic progenitors into single lineage clonogenic progenitors is accompanied by alterations in their interaction with fibronectin. *J Exp Med* 174:693, 1991.

447. Papayannopoulou T, Nakamoto B: Peripheralization of hemopoietic progenitors in primates treated with anti-VLA4 integrin. *Proc Natl Acad Sci USA* 90:9374, 1993.

448. Papayannopoulou T, Craddock C, Nakamoto B, et al: The VLA4/VCAM-1 adhesion pathway defines contrasting mechanisms of lodgement of transplanted murine hemopoietic progenitors between bone marrow and spleen. *Proc Natl Acad Sci USA* 92:9647, 1995.

449. Papayannopoulou T, Priestley GV, Nakamoto B: Anti-VLA4/CAM-1-induced mobilization requires cooperative signaling through the kit/mkit ligand pathway. *Blood* 91:2231, 1998.

450. Lewinsohn DM, Nagler A, Ginzton N, et al: Hematopoietic progenitor cell expression of the H-CAM (CD44) homing-associated adhesion molecule. *Blood* 75:589, 1990.

451. Yong KL, Watts M, Thomas NS, et al: Transmigration of CD34+ cells across specialized and non-specialized endothelium requires prior activation by growth factors and is mediated by PECAM-1 (CD31). *Blood* 91:1196, 1998.

452. Aizawa S, Tavassoli M: In vitro homing of hematopoietic stem cells is mediated by a recognition system with galactosyl and mannosyl specificities. *Proc Natl Acad Sci USA* 84:4485, 1987.

453. Long MW, Briddell R, Walter AW, et al: Human hematopoietic stem cell adherence to cytokines and matrix molecules. *J Clin Invest* 90:251, 1992.

454. Bruno E, Luikart SD, Long MW, Hoffman R: Marrow-derived heparan sulfate proteoglycan mediates the adhesion of hematopoietic progenitor cells to cytokines. *Exp Hematol* 23:1212, 1995.

455. Frenette PS, Subbarao S, Mazo IB, et al: Endothelial selectins and vascular cell adhesion molecule-1 promote hematopoietic progenitor homing to bone marrow. *Proc Natl Acad Sci* 95:14423, 1998.

456. Wolf NS, Trentin JJ: Hemopoietic colony studies. V. Effect of hemopoietic organ stroma on differentiation of pluripotent stem cells. *J Exp Med* 127:205, 1968.

457. Curry JL, Trentin JJ, Wolf N: Hemopoietic spleen colony studies. II. Erythropoiesis. *J Exp Med* 125:703, 1967.

458. Bernstein SE: Tissue transplantation as an analytic and therapeutic tool in hereditary anemias. *Am J Surg* 119:448, 1970.

459. Bessis M, Mize C, Prenant M: Erythropoiesis: comparison of in vivo and in vitro amplification. *Blood Cells* 4:155, 1978.

460. Lichtman MA: The ultrastructure of the hemopoietic environment of the marrow: a review. *Exp Hematology* 9:391, 1981.

461. Quesenberry PJ: Stromal cells in long-term bone marrow cultures, in *Handbook of the Hemopoietic Microenvironment*, edited by M Tavassoli, pp 253–285. Humana Press, New Jersey, 1989.

462. Quesenberry PJ: Stroma-dependent hematolymphopoietic stem cells, in *Current Topics in Microbiology and Immunology*, edited by C Muller-Sieburg, vol 177, *Hematopoietic Stem Cells*, pp 151–166. Springer-Verlag, Berlin-Heidelberg, 1992.

463. Levitt L, Quesenberry PJ: The effect of lithium on murine hematopoiesis in a liquid culture system. *N Engl J Med* 302:713, 1980.

464. Quesenberry PJ, Coppola MA, Gualtieri RJ, et al: Lithium stimulation of murine hematopoiesis in a liquid culture system: an effect mediated by radioresistant stromal cells. *Blood* 63:121, 1984.

465. Song ZX, Quesenberry PJ: Radioresistant murine marrow stromal cells: a morphologic and functional characterization. *Exp Hematol* 12:523, 1984.

466. Doukas M, Niskanen E, Quesenberry PJ: The effect of lithium on stem cell and stromal cell proliferation in vitro. *Exp Hematol* 14:215, 1986.

467. Gualtieri RJ, Shadduck RF, Baker DG, Quesenberry PJ: Hematopoietic regulatory factors produced in long-term bone marrow cultures and the effect of in vitro irradiation. *Blood* 64:516, 1984.

468. Song ZX, Shadduck RK, Innes DJ Jr, et al: Hematopoietic factor production by a cell line (TC-1) derived from adherent murine marrow cells. *Blood* 66:273, 1985.

469. Quesenberry PJ, Song Z, McGrath HE, et al: Multilineage synergistic activity produced by a murine adherent marrow cell line. *Blood* 69:827, 1987.

470. Alberico T, Ihle JN, McGrath HE, et al: Stromal growth factor production in irradiated lectin exposed long-term murine bone marrow cultures. *Blood* 69:1120, 1987.

471. McGrath HE, Liang C, Alberico T, Quesenberry PJ: The effect of lithium on growth factor production in long-term bone marrow cultures. *Blood* 70:1136, 1987.

472. Nilsson S, Dooner M, Tiarks C, et al: Potential and distribution of transplanted hematopoietic stem cells in a nonablated mouse model. *Blood* 89:4013, 1997.

473. Fibbe WE, Pruijt JFM, Welders GA, et al: Biology of IL-8 induced stem cell mobilization. *Ann N Y Acad Sci* 872:71, 1999.

474. Sheridan WP, Begley CG, Juttner CA, et al: Effect of peripheral blood progenitor cell mobilized by filarastim (G-CSF) on platelet recovery after high doses of chemotheraphy. *Lancet* 339:640, 1992.

475. Gianni AM, Siena S, Bregni M., et al: Granulocyte-macrophage colony-stimulating factor to harvest circulating hematopoietic stem cells for auto transplantation. *Lancet* 21:580, 1989.

476. Papayannopoulou T: Hematopoietic stem/progenitor cell mobilization a continuing quest for etcolegic mechanisms, in *Hematopoietic Stem Cells—Biology and Transplantation*, edited by D Orlic, TA Bock, Kanz L, pp 187–197. New York Academy of Sciences, New York, 1999.

477. Sheridan W: Cytokine-only approaches to mobilization of progentior cells, in *Cell Therapy*, edited by G Morstyn, W Sheridan, pp 146–198. Cambridge University, New York, 1996.

478. Gately MK, Gubler E, Brunde MJ, et al: Interleukin 12: a cytokine with therapeutic potential in oncology and infectious diseases. *Ther Immunol* 1:187, 1994.

479. Korbling M: In vivo expansion of the circulating stem cell pool, in *Characteristics and Potentials of Blood Stem Cells*, edited by TM Fleidner, D Hoelzer D, pp 131–138. Univ. Alpha Med. Press, 1998.

480. Mauch P, Lamont C, Neben TY, et al: Hematopoietic stem cells in the blood after stem cell factor and interleukin-11 administration: evidence for different mechanisms of mobilization. *Blood* 86:4673, 1995.

IMMUNE ACCESSORY MOLECULES AND SIGNAL TRANSDUCTION

THEODORE J. YUN
EDWARD A. CLARK

This chapter describes the accessory molecules and signal transduction pathways that are important in lymphocyte function and turnover. In addition, this chapter provides a description of immune deficiency disorders that result from defects in the expression of signaling of immune accessory molecules.

The development, migration, activation, and maturation of lymphocytes are dependent on cell-cell interactions that are regulated and coordinated by cell surface accessory molecules and antigen receptors.[1-5] During their development, lymphoid cells migrate to a number of sites in the body. Lymphocyte progenitors interact with accessory cells, such as epithelial cells in the thymus or stromal cells in the marrow. These cells nurture and instruct lymphoid precursor cells to express antigen-receptor genes, to proliferate, and to differentiate into mature cells. The newly formed lymphocytes then enter the blood and home to peripheral lymphoid tissues via cell-cell interactions with specialized endothelial cells in highly endothelial venules. Once in the spleen or lymph node, a naive B lymphocyte may encounter antigens and yet another set of cells, including T cells, dendritic cells, and, as germinal centers (GCs) are formed, follicular dendritic cells and activated T cells. In the presence of these cells and a T-cell-dependent antigen, the B lymphocyte is induced to become a memory B cell or a plasma cell.

Several families of surface molecules are involved in cell-cell interactions.[6,7] These families include: (1) the integrin family, (2) the selectin family, (3) the type II C-lectin family, (4) the immunoglobulin (Ig) superfamily, (5) the tumor necrosis factor (TNF) family, (6) the TNF receptor (TNFR) family, (7) the complement control protein family, (8) the scavenger receptor family, and (9) the tetraspan, or transmembrane 4 pass, family.

T-CELL-DEPENDENT B-CELL MATURATION

After entering a lymph node, the B cells that have surface immunoglobulin receptors specific for foreign antigen trapped within the lymphoid

Acronyms and abbreviations that appear in this chapter include: BCR, B-cell receptor; DAG, diacylglycerol; DD, death domain; DED, death effector domain; EBV, Epstein-Barr virus; GAS, gamma-activated site; GCs, germinal centers; IFN, interferon; Ig, immunoglobulin; IL-2, interleukin-2; IL-2R, IL-2 receptor; IREs, interferon response elements; ITAM, immunoreceptor tyrosine-based activation motif; JAK, Janus kinase; MAP, mitogen-activated protein; MAPK, MAP kinases; MAPKK, MAP kinase kinases; MAPKKK, MAP kinase kinase kinases; PH, Pleckstrin homology; PI3K, phosphatidylinositol-3 kinase; PLC-γc, phospholipase C-γc; PTK, protein tyrosine kinase; PY, phosphotyrosine; SAP, SLAM-associated protein; SH, src-homology; STATs, signal transducers and activators of transcription; TCR, T-cell receptor; TNF, tumor necrosis factor; TNFR, TNF receptor; V, Ig variable; XLP, X-linked chromosome lymphoproliferative disease.

tissue migrate into T-cell-rich paracortical regions of secondary lymphoid tissues (see Chap. 5). Here they may capture and process soluble antigen. Some T cells in this region already may have recognized antigenic peptides processed and presented in association with MHC class II molecules of potent antigen-presenting cells, such as extrafollicular dendritic cells (see Chap. 84). The activated T cells, and perhaps dendritic cells, then signal a few antigen-specific B cells to migrate to follicles and interact with folicular dendritic cells. The latter cells are large, spiny, nonhematopoietic cells that retain antigen-antibody immune complexes and induce B-cell proliferation and the formation of germinal centers. Somatic mutation of Ig variable (V) region genes occurs soon after antigenic stimulation during germinal center development (see Chap. 83).[8] After somatic mutation occurs, B cells with high-affinity receptors for antigen are selected, and switching from IgM to another immunoglobulin class ("Ig class switching") occurs. Four key cell types are required for this process: activated B cells, CD4+ T cells, GC dendritic cells, and follicular dendritic cells. Eventually germinal center B cells mature into memory B cells or plasmablasts.

Several cell-cell interaction receptor-ligand pairs are involved in T-cell-dependent B-cell maturation.[8-10] In the paracortical regions, CD4+ T cells are activated by recognizing MHC class II molecules plus peptide on dendritic cells. Interdigitating dendritic cells are especially effective antigen-presenting cells because they express not only high levels of MHC class II and CD40 but also other key accessory molecules, such as CD54, CD58, CD80, and CD86. Since the affinity of the TCR for MHC class II + peptide is low, the binding of CD4 and CD2 ligands on T cells to their ligands, MHC class II and CD58 on antigen-presenting cells facilitates cell-cell interactions leading to T-cell activation. Cross-linking of the T cell receptor (TCR) and its coreceptors in turn leads to the rapid activation of an avid CD11a/18 complex,[11] which then can bind to its ligand CD54. The fact that tissue dendritic cells, unlike resting B cells, express key accessory molecules, such as CD54, CD58, CD80, and CD86, may explain why naive T cells are activated by dendritic cells but not by resting B cells. Once B cells are activated initially by T cells and later by follicular dendritic cells, they express an array of surface accessory molecules that enable them to become efficient antigen-presenting cells.

ACCESSORY MOLECULES INVOLVED IN IMMUNE ACTIVATION

Two surface molecules of antigen-presenting cells, CD40 and CD80/CD86, have ligands found on activated or resting T cells. These receptor-ligand pairs are engaged during a cognate T-B dialogue, allowing T cells and B cells to sense each other's state of activation and then respond appropriately.[4]

CD40, a member of the TNFR family, is expressed on antigen-presenting cells, such as B cells, dendritic cells, and activated macrophages. The ligand for CD40 is a TNF family member, CD154 (CD40L). It is expressed primarily on activated CD4+ T cells but not on resting T cells.[10,12] When the CD154-CD40 interaction is blocked in vitro, B cells cannot proliferate or produce IgG in the presence of T cells.[13] Patients with an X-linked chromosome defect in CD154 expression or function do not form germinal centers in response to antigen, and their B cells do not switch Ig classes in vivo.[14] Thus, T cells and CD154-CD40 interactions are required for both germinal-center formation and Ig class switching.

While the CD154-CD40 interaction enables the B cell to respond to an activated T cell, a second critical receptor-ligand interaction through CD80 and CD28 allows peripheral T cells to respond to an activated B-cell partner, to divide, and to produce the cytokines required for T-cell differentiation. CD80 is expressed on activated B cells, macrophages, and some dendritic cells. It has two known ligands:

CD28, found on both resting and activated T cells, and CD152 (CTLA-4), found on activated T cells. The binding of CD80 to CD28 on T cells, which previously were stimulated via the cross-linking of their TCRs, enhances interleukin-2 (IL-2) production and T-cell proliferation.[15] Interference with the CD80 signal to T cells blocks T-cell proliferation and T-cell-dependent B-cell maturation. In contrast, weakly immunogenic tumors can be made immunogenic, i.e., able to induce a protective T-cell response, by transfecting them with the CD80 cDNA,[16] demonstrating that the immunogenicity of a cellular antigen(s) is dependent on the coexpression of CD80.

Another ligand for CD28 and CD152 related to CD80 that has been identified on antigen-presenting cells is designated *CD86*.[17,18] Monoclonal antibodies to CD86 inhibit CD28-dependent T-cell activation.[17] Unlike CD80, CD86 is expressed on natural killer cells and is upregulated rapidly on antigen-presenting cells after activation.[17,18] The fact that CD86, unlike CD80, is constitutively expressed on resting B cells suggests that it may provide one of the first costimulatory signals to T cells.

Once CD80/CD86 is expressed on an antigen-presenting cell, it in turn can signal the T cell via CD28 (see Chap. 84).[10] There is an additional level of reciprocity in this T-B dialogue: cross-linking CD28 on activated T cells increases the expression of CD154,[19] while cross-linking CD40 on B cells increases the expression of both CD80 and CD86.[17,20] This "reciprocal dialogue" may occur in peripheral lymphoid T-cell zones and perhaps in the basal light zones of germinal centers, where T cells expressing CD154 have been identified.

Initiation of this sequential reciprocal dialogue must be carefully regulated to prevent the activation of autoreactive or bystander T cells or B cells. The presence of just CD40 and class II on resting B cells and the TCR/CD3 complex and CD28 on resting T cells is not sufficient for mutual T-B cell activation to commence, since resting B cells do not activate resting T cells. Rather, antigen-specific resting B cells induce tolerance in T cells to protein antigens.[9] Similarly, activated T cells can provide contact-dependent helper activity for B cells, but resting T cells cannot.[9] However, a reciprocal dialogue may ensue if *either* the T cell *or* the B cell has been activated. If the activated T cell expresses CD154, it is able to induce resting B cells to express CD80.[20] Similarly, activated cells expressing CD80/CD86 are able to induce T cells to express CD154. In other words, the presence of either CD154 or CD80/CD86 enables both the T cell and the B cell to be activated in the presence of antigen. Theoretically, a number of agents that can stimulate the expression of CD80 on B cells, such as cross-linking of antigen receptors or class II, might promote a production dialogue. However, the antigen specificity of the T-B dialogue is maintained overall, since signaling through either CD40 on B cells, or CD28 on T cells, is most efficient after B or T cells have been stimulated through their antigen receptors.[15]

The CD40 signal to B cells and the CD28 signal to T cells have a number of similar and potentially reciprocal properties. Just as antibodies to CD28 promote the proliferation of T cells after TCR/CD3 cross-linking, antibodies to CD40 can promote the proliferation of B cells stimulated by immunoglobulin receptor cross-linking.[10] Signaling T cells through their specific TCR alone without the CD28 signal from CD80 may lead to induction of T-cell tolerance or anergy. Cross-linking of CD28 not only can prevent anergy but also can prevent T cells from undergoing programmed cell death, or apoptosis.[15] Similarly, apoptosis occurring in germinal center B cells, or induced by cross-linking surface IgM on immature B cells, can be blocked by cross-linking CD40. Thus, the presence or absence of T-cell help through CD40, or an antigen-presenting-cell signal through CD28, may determine whether antigen-stimulated B cells or T cells are activated or induced to die.

The reciprocal T-B cell signaling involving CD154-CD40 and CD28/CD152-CD80 is not the only means by which T cells and B cells interact. Other signaling pairs are involved in regulating reciprocal signaling. For example, the CD11a/18-CD54 integrin pair in particular is important in T-B cell cognate interactions. Furthermore, cross-linking CD40 on B cells promotes T-cell proliferation via CD11a/18-CD54-dependent interactions. Signaling through CD150 and a recently described member of the CD28/CD152 family, ICOS, can also promote T cell activation.

In addition, the binding affinities of the accessory molecules involved in cognate cell-cell interactions can be influenced by the activation states of the interacting cells. For example, cross-linking the TCR increases the affinity of the T cell's CD11a/18 and CD2 surface molecules for their respective ligands, CD54 and CD58, on antigen-presenting cells.[11,21,22] Furthermore, T-cell activation also induces increased expression of CD49d/29 (VLA-4), an integrin with binding activity for CD106 (VCAM-1) and fibronectin. The affinity of CD8 for its respective ligand, namely MHC class I proteins, also is increased after T-cell antigen recognition.[23] The consequences of these increased affinities depend on the receptor-ligand pairs. For example, activated CD8, after avidly binding to MHC class I molecules, initiates hydrolysis of phosphatidylinositol, but adhesion of CD49d or CD49e to fibronectin does not[23]; the avid binding to fibronectin instead may amplify this signaling pathway. Cyclic AMP induces increased CD2 avidity to CD58[22] but decreases avidity of CD11a/18 to CD54.[11] This may be because activation induces the CD2 molecule to associate with tubulin in the cytoskeleton but induces CD11a/18 to interact with talin, and thus presumably with the actin cytoskeleton.

SIGNAL TRANSDUCTION THROUGH EXTRACELLULAR RECEPTORS

Although the key pathway for activating resting B and T lymphocytes is through their specific antigen receptors, certain other signals via accessory receptors or cytokine receptors may modulate or provide additional signals. The fate of antigen-receptor signaling depends on the context in which the interactions occur. In T-cell activation, signals that CD28 generates upon ligation by CD80/CD86 enhance the activation process. Likewise, signals through CD40 are important in B-cell activation. Throughout T- or B-cell maturation, signals generated from costimulatory receptors or cytokine receptors influence the signal from the antigen receptor. The combination of all extracellular stimuli determines the fate of an individual cell. For example, antigen-receptor cross-linking may induce immature T cells or B cells to undergo apoptosis, affect stimulation of mature T cells, or rescue germinal center B cells from undergoing apoptosis.[24–26]

Understanding how a cell can integrate various extracellular stimuli and transmit these to the nucleus is an area of active research. Although a comprehensive description of all possible transduction pathways that a lymphocyte uses is beyond the scope of this chapter, we will focus on major pathways by which signals are transmitted from the membrane, through the cytosol and to the nucleus. Activation of other transcription factors, such as NF-κB and NF-AT follow similar principles.

ANTIGEN RECEPTOR SIGNALING

TCR or B cell receptor (BCR) complexes not only contain receptors for specific antigens but also have associated molecules that inform the cell interior that antigen has been recognized. Although Fig. 15-1 shows only a model for how the BCR may be activated, the BCR and TCR complexes have a number of similar features[26,27] and thus likely have similar signaling mechanisms.[3,28–30]

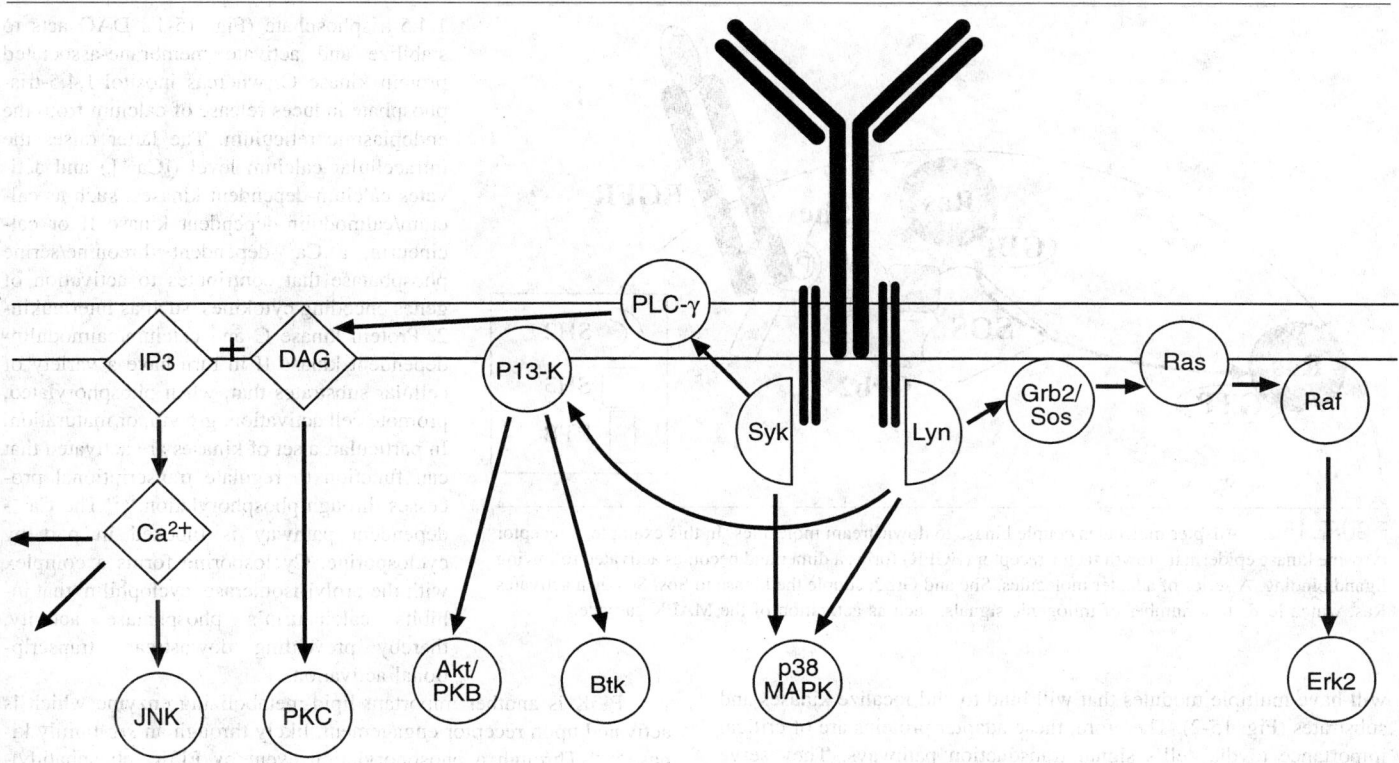

FIGURE 15-1   Proximal signaling events after surface Ig stimulation in B cells. A simple model on the early kinases involved that initiate a cascade of effector molecules that exert a broad range of biological effects. In particular, tyrosine kinases such as Syk and Lyn can independently or cooperatively activate multiple substrates. Lipid-modifying enzymes, such as PLC-γ and PI3-K, are activated by Syk or Lyn and can produce a variety of lipid products that activate the cell, such as DAG, IP3, and PIP3. The MAPK pathways can also be activated by these proximal events. This scheme generalizes the activation process, and in vivo this process is much more complex and mysterious. Other molecules, such as costimulatory molecules and cytokine receptors, are likely to be involved in modifying the signals transduced to the nucleus.

The TCR and BCR differ from the classic protein tyrosine kinase (PTK) receptors, such as the epidermal growth factor receptor or platelet-derived growth factor receptor, in that they do not themselves have protein tyrosine kinase activity. However, they are associated with potentially potent PTKs at the cell membrane, such as the *src* or Syk/ZAP-70 family kinases. These PTKs are inactive during the resting state, perhaps because they have been phosphorylated and are folded up upon themselves.[31]

After antigen-receptor cross-linking, a cell surface protein tyrosine phosphatase, CD45, apparently dephosphorylates inactive PTKs, freeing them to become active and to begin the signaling cascade.[3,32] One initial event is the phosphorylation of TCR- or BCR-associated surface molecules on certain tyrosine residues. The phosphotyrosine residues are flanked by a characteristic set of amino acids making a phosphotyrosine motif, termed *immunoreceptor tyrosine-based activation motif* (ITAM). Phosphorylated ITAMs can be recognized by proteins containing one or more *src*-homology (SH) region 2 domains, called *SH2 domains* (see below).[33,34] The SH2 domains in signaling components, such as phospholipase C-γ (PLC-γ) or phosphatidylinositol-3 kinase (PI3K), bind with high affinity to certain phosphotyrosine (PY) motifs and thereby assemble to form a cytosolic signaling apparatus beneath the cell surface membrane. The tyrosine residues of the *src*-family kinases also are phosphorylated and contain an SH2 motif. As such, they may bind to each other or to other PY-containing proteins following activation (Fig. 15-1).

In T cells, *src*-family PTKs, probably Fyn and Lck, initiates phosphorylation on the TCR complex. Then, ZAP-70, in mature T cells, is recruited into the receptor complex by binding to tyrosine phosphorylated molecules. This adds an additional kinase specificity to the signaling pathway that, through tyrosine phosphorylation of substrates, can form additional distinctive signaling apparati. Together these apparati transmit distinct messages to the cell interior.

In B cells, the initial activation events are likely different from those in T cells (Fig. 15-1). Both Lyn, an *src*-family PTK, and Syk are excellent candidates for participation in the early events in receptor activation. Contrasting the sequential model of T-cell activation, BCR engagement can activate Syk and Lyn simultaneously, leading to parallel activation of both signaling pathways. This model is supported by the fact that the BCR can transmit signals in either Lyn- or Syk-deficient B cells.

ADAPTER MOLECULES

One perplexing problem of signal transduction is the multiple substrate specificity of a given kinase. Also, multiple kinases can phosphorylate a single substrate. How does a cell achieve specificity by activating certain transduction pathways through a single receptor? A solution to this problem may be found in the emerging members of adapter proteins.

Adapter proteins are functionally defined as molecules that have no intrinsic kinase activity; however, these proteins contain "modules" that can specifically couple with other molecules, such as kinases.[35,36] These modules, such as SH2, SH3, or PH domains, can recognize peptide motifs or phospholipids. Typically, adapter proteins

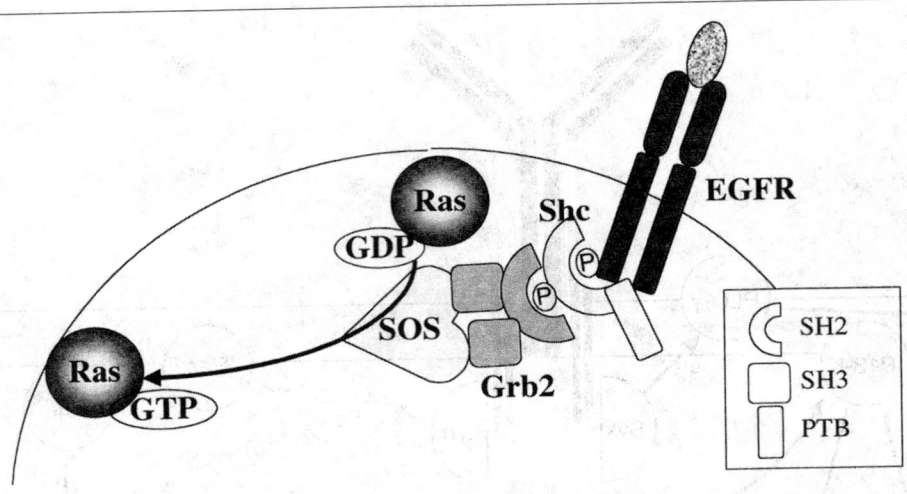

FIGURE 15-2   Adapter molecules couple kinase to downstream molecules. In this example, a receptor tyrosine kinase epidermal growth factor receptor (EGFR) forms a dimer and becomes activated following ligand binding. A series of adapter molecules, Shc and Grb2, couple the kinase to Sos. Sos then activates Ras, which leads to a number of mitogenic signals, such as activation of the MAPK cascade.

will have multiple modules that will bind to and localize kinases and substrates (Fig. 15-2). Therefore, these adapter proteins are of critical importance to the cell's signal transduction pathways. They serve to localize and organize specific pathways to certain receptors or subcellular sites.

Several different types of modules have been described. A module is typically 30 to 100 residues with a characteristic motif. The variable residues in the motif are thought to direct specificity with binding sites on target proteins. There are two types of SH domains that are commonly found in adapter proteins.[34] SH2 domains often direct interaction with phosphotyrosine located in a specific motif. Some SH2 domains are also able to bind to certain phospholipids. Many receptor and nonreceptor tyrosine kinases become phosphorylated themselves. This may allow binding of SH2-containing adapter proteins to the kinases, which will functionally serve to couple the kinase with target molecules that are also bound to the adapter protein. SH3 domains have been described to interact with proline rich sequences in proteins, often containing the motif PXXP.

Pleckstrin homology (PH) domains can also be found in many signaling proteins.[37] These modules can direct both protein-protein interactions and protein-phospholipid interactions. The interaction with phospholipid is especially important as these PH domains containing adapter proteins can cause recruitment of bound molecules to discrete regions of the cell membrane. Through protein-binding modules, adapter proteins can recruit and organize kinases and their targets. This can be a daunting task, especially in complex signaling apparatus such as lymphocyte antigen receptors, where multiple costimulatory and downregulatory molecules are within proximity to the antigen receptors, which themselves are associated with a number of kinases.[38] The number of characterized adapter molecules is increasing, and soon it may be possible to delineate molecules that are involved in a particular transduction cascade initiating from the membrane and ending at the nucleus.

LIPID METABOLITES

One result of cross-linking antigen receptors is that the enzymes PLC-γ1 or PLC-γ2 are activated to metabolize phosphatidylinositol bisphosphate into two second messengers, diacylglycerol (DAG) and inositol-

1,4,5-trisphosphate (Fig. 15-1). DAG acts to stabilize and activate membrane-associated protein kinase C, whereas inositol-1,4,5-trisphosphate induces release of calcium from the endoplasmic reticulum. The latter raises the intracellular calcium level ($[Ca^{2+}]_i$) and activates calcium-dependent kinases, such as calcium/calmodulin-dependent kinase II or calcineurin, a Ca^{2+}-dependent threonine/serine phosphatase that contributes to activation of genes encoding cytokines, such as interleukin-2. Protein kinase C and calcium/calmodulin-dependent kinase II in turn have a variety of cellular substrates that, when phosphorylated, promote cell activation, growth, or maturation. In particular, a set of kinases are activated that can function to regulate transcriptional processes through phosphorylation.[39,40] The Ca^{2+}-dependent pathway is blocked in part by cyclosporine. Cyclosporine forms a complex with the prolyl-isomerase, cyclophilin, that inhibits calcineurin's phosphatase activity, thereby preventing downstream transcriptional activation.

PI3K is another important lipid-metabolizing enzyme which is activated upon receptor engagement, likely through an *src*-family kinase.[41-44] Through a phosphorylation event by PI3K, phosphatidylinositol and its derivatives can form potent second messengers, PtdIns(3)P, PtdIns(3,4)P2, and PtdIns(3,4,5)P. Inhibition of PI3K enzymatic activity generally results in suppression of many cellular responses, such as cell survival or proliferation.[45]

Via SH2 or PH domains, certain proteins can specifically bind to distinct lipid products. These domains regulate protein-phospholipid and protein-phosphoprotein interactions. Through these domains, multiple kinases can be brought in proximity at the membrane. A number of examples exist. The SH2 domain of *src* has been demonstrated to bind to PtdIns(3,4,5)P3. Akt/PKB, a Ser/Thr kinase that has been implicated in cell survival, is downstream of PI3K.[46] The PH domain of Akt/PKB has been shown to bind to PtdIns(3,4)P2, so Akt/PKB could be recruited to the membrane. In B-cell signaling, Btk may also be recruited to the membrane through its PH domain binding to PI3K lipid products. Btk is a critical regulator of B-lymphocyte signaling, since genetically Btk-deficient humans or mice lack functional B cells. In summary, following cellular stimulation, PI3K generates lipid products that mediate recruitment of upstream signaling molecules (Fig. 15-1).

MITOGEN-ACTIVATED PROTEIN KINASE PATHWAY

Mitogen-activated protein (MAP) kinase signaling cascades are a major means by which signals are transduced from the membrane to the nucleus. The cascade is composed of three analogous pathways (Fig. 15-3). At the core of each pathway there are three kinases that are categorized as MAP kinase kinase kinases (MAPKKK), MAP kinase kinases (MAPKK), or MAP kinases (MAPK). A straightforward model proposes that there is sequential activation of these kinases, i.e., one MAPKKK activates a MAPKK, which in turn activates a MAPK. These proteins are Ser/Thr kinases that are activated through mitogenic or stress-induced stimuli. The importance of this cascade is underscored by the fact that homologous pathways exist in diverse species such as yeast to human. The final outcome of activating the MAPK pathways can lead to a variety of biological effects, including cell proliferation, cell differentiation, and stress response induction. Currently, the ability of the kinases to cross-talk between other members of the parallel MAPK pathways is not known.

Receptor activation is linked to activating the ERK MAPK by Ras. Ras is a guanine nucleotide binding protein that is involved in a variety of mitogenic signals. Although several mechanisms are known to exist that couple receptor activation to Ras activation, a general model can be proposed where receptor dimerization results in autophosphorylation and recruitment of SH2-containing adapter molecules, such as Grb2. Grb2 is able to recruit Sos, a guanine nucleotide exchange factor, which activates Ras by guanine nucleotide exchange (Fig. 15-2). Bound to GTP, Ras becomes a potent activator of signal transduction. The first ''tier'' of MAPKKK proteins in this cascade then become activated.[47] Raf, the MAPKKK in the ERK2 pathway, is activated following membrane translocation and dimerization.

The activated MAPKKK phosphorylates MAPKKs on serine residues. Once activated, the MAPKK can then activate its respective MAPK family substrates (Fig. 15-3). The MAP kinases include ERK, JNK/SAPK (jun-N terminal or stress-activated protein kinase), and p38 MAPK/Hog. Finally, these three kinases can activate distinct but overlapping sets of transcription: ERK can activate Elk, Ets-1 and -2, and c-fos; JNK can activate Elk, c-jun, and ATF; and p38 can activate ATF2, Elk, CHOP, MEF2c, and Max (Fig. 15-3).[48,49]

CYTOKINE RECEPTORS

Within the past decade, tremendous advances in understanding cytokine signaling have been made. In some ways, delineating the pathways of their signals has been as daunting as understanding antigen receptor signaling. Like antigen receptors, many cytokine receptors also lack intrinsic kinase activity. Furthermore, a cell can express multiple cytokine receptors, which are often multimeric complexes. Also, some cytokine receptor complexes share individual components. How can a cell integrate multiple signals originating from very similar receptors? Some cytokine receptors, such as the IL-2 receptor (IL-2R) complex,[50] resemble the TCR, insofar as they may associate with *src*-family kinases such as p56[lck]. Different regions within the cytoplasmic tails of the IL-2Rβ chain and IL-2Rγ chain appear to link to distinct signaling pathways.[50,51] Activation through the *src*-family protein tyrosine kinases requires a distal region of IL-2Rβ chain's cytoplasmic tail and the SH2 region in the tail of IL-2Rγ chain. This protein tyrosine kinase group may be required for activation of the MAPK cascade, leading to expression of the *c-fos* and *c-jun* genes.

A region of IL-2Rγ chain more proximal to the plasma cell membrane is required for activation of another protein tyrosine kinase that possibly is a member of the Janus kinase (JAK) family of protein kinases. Discovery of the JAK-STAT transduction pathway has begun to explain some of the mysteries regarding cytokine transduction.[52] Janus kinases are a family of nonreceptor tyrosine kinases that can associate with some cytokine receptors. JAK activation can lead to recruitment of another family of molecules, signal transducers and activators of transcription (STATs), which, upon activation, translocate to the nucleus and bind a consensus motif called *gamma-activated site* (GAS) (Fig. 15-4).[52] Much remains to be elucidated about this family, in terms of structure-function, regulation, and possible characterization of other family members. Homologous JAK-STAT pathways

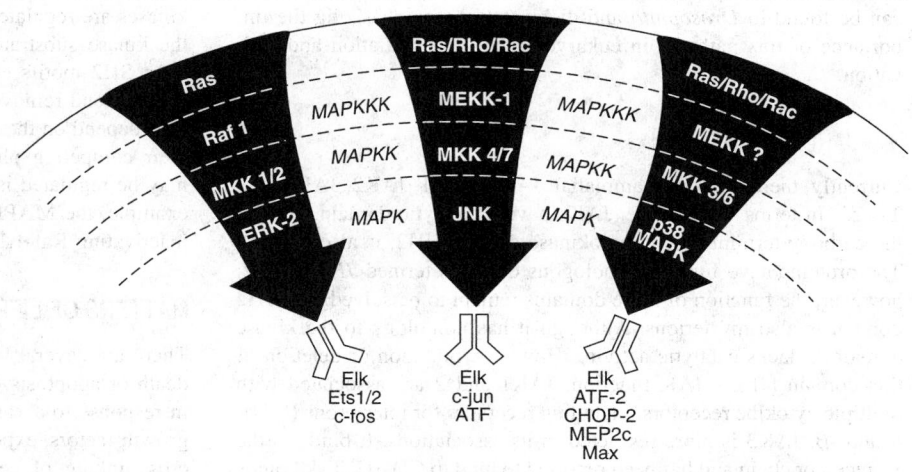

FIGURE 15-3 Depiction of the multiple, parallel pathways of the MAPK cascade. The MAPK cascade transduces signals from cell-surface-associated kinases to the nucleus via a series of Ser/Thr kinases. In each pathway, the MAPKKK family member activates its respective MAPKK, which then activates the MAPK. Activated MAPKs can then phosphorylate and activate a set of transcription factors that mediate a wide variety of biological effects.

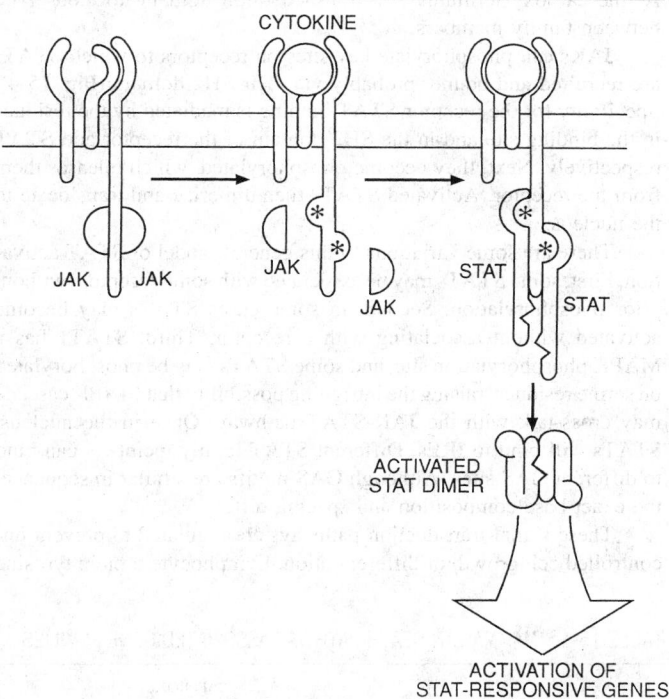

FIGURE 15-4 Diagram showing a general model of JAK-STAT activation. This figure illustrates a general model where cytokine binding to its appropriate receptor leads to cell activation or differentiation. Prior to cytokine binding, JAKs are associated with a chain of a cytokine receptor. Upon ligand binding, JAKs become activated, dissociate from the receptor, and phosphorylate the receptor chain. STATs then bind to the phosphorylated sites on the receptor. Next, bound STATs become phosphorylated, dissociated from the receptor, dimerize, and then translocate to the nucleus, where they bind to GAS sequences and activate transcription.

can be found in *Drosophila* and dichtostelium, emphasizing the importance of this pathway in eukaryotic cell differentiation and activation.

JANUS KINASES

Currently, there are four mammalian JAKs: JAK1, JAK2, JAK3, and Tyk2.[52] In terms of structure, JAKs have a catalytic domain, JH1, at the carboxy terminus. A pseudokinase domain, JH2, is also present. The proteins have further homologous domains termed *JH3* to *JH7*; however, the function of these domains remain to be solved. The JH2 domain is also mysterious. Although it has homology to the kinase domain, it lacks catalytic activity. However, mutation or deletion of this domain affects JAK function. JAK1 and 2 are associated with multiple cytokine receptors, including receptors for interferons (IFN)-α and -β. JAK3 is more restricted in its associations. It binds to the γc receptor chain and has been reported to bind to CD40.[53] Tyk2 binds to gp130 chain that is shared among several cytokine receptor complexes.

SIGNAL TRANSDUCERS AND ACTIVATORS OF TRANSCRIPTION

Additional specificity in cytokine signaling is achieved via the STAT family of transcription factors. STATs are cytoplasmic proteins which, when activated, translocate to the nucleus where they bind to GAS motif in interferon (IFN) response elements (IREs). Structurally, they have a DNA-binding domain, as well as SH2 and SH3 domains.[52] The latter two domains most likely mediate protein-protein interactions. At the carboxy terminus is a transactivation domain not conserved between family members.

JAKs can phosphorylate key sites on receptors to which STATs are recruited and bound, probably via their SH2 domain (Fig. 15-4). Specificity for the receptor-STAT binding is mediated by the residues in the binding site and in the SH2 domain of the receptor and STAT respectively. Next, they become phosphorylated, which releases them from the receptor. Activated STATs then dimerize and translocate to the nucleus.

There are some variations to this general model of STAT activation. First, some STATs may be associated with some receptors without prior phosphorylation. Second, in some cases STATs may become activated without associating with a receptor. Third, STAT1 has a MAPK phosphorylation site, and some STATs may be phosphorylated on serine residues, raising the intriguing possibility that MAPK cascade may cross-talk with the JAK-STAT pathway. Once in the nucleus, STATs will bind to IREs. Different STAT family members can bind to different GAS sites. Although GAS motifs are similar in sequence, the exact base composition and spacing differs.

These signal-transduction pathways are regulated to prevent uncontrolled cell growth or differentiation. Lymphocyte protein tyrosine kinases are regulated by protein tyrosine phosphatases that inactivate the kinase substrates or the kinase itself. Some phosphatases even have SH2 motifs enabling them to bind to tyrosine-phosphorylated proteins and remove phosphates. Whether a cellular response ensues may depend on the balance of activities between tyrosine kinases and their competing phosphatases.[54] Another way a signaling pathway may be regulated is via contact with another signaling pathway. For example, the MAPK cascade may be inhibited by protein kinase A, inactivating Raf-1.[55]

MATTERS OF LIFE AND DEATH

There are several ways to induce cells to undergo programmed cell death or apoptosis (see Chap. 12a).[56,57] Cells may undergo apoptosis in response to a variety of stimuli, including withdrawal of essential growth factors, exposure to radiation or glucocorticoids, or following cross-linking of certain surface membrane receptors, such as Fas (CD95). Unlike necrosis, apoptosis requires new gene expression. Studies using homozygous null gene "knockout" mice have shown that expression of certain proteins is essential for inducing apoptosis or for preventing it from occurring.[56,57] On the other hand, the c-myc protein is required for TCR-mediated apoptosis of some T cells. However, this or other proteins in other contexts can have the opposite or no effect. For example, the tumor suppressor p53 is required for irradiation-induced apoptosis of lymphocytes but does not play an apparent role in steroid-induced apoptosis of thymocytes. How different stimuli, such as those provided by TCR cross-linking, irradiation, or glucocorticoids, induce apoptosis is not yet defined.

Recent excitement has focused on defining molecules which are involved in cell survival or death.[58] There appear to be two active pathways present in a cell that responds to extracellular signals which induce the apoptotic program, or an intrinsic signal when the cell "senses" to undergo cell death.[59] An example of the former situation is signaling through the CD95/Fas receptor, a prototype TNFR family member generally associated with signaling cell death. Response to growth factor withdrawal exemplifies the latter case. These two pathways probably converge.

A tremendous advance in our understanding of apoptotic mechanisms comes from genetically defining three genes in *Caenorhabditis elegans,* a nematode. These genes, *CED-3, CED-4,* and *CED-9,* are involved in the development of *C. elegans* where 131 of 1030 somatic cells must undergo cell death in order for proper progression in development. Mammalian orthologs have been described for these three genes, and *CED-3* encodes for a protease. In higher vertebrates, a family of *CED-3*-related molecules exist, called *caspases,* and form a proteolytic cascade. *APAF* is a gene that resembles *CED-4;* it functions as a scaffolding molecule that bridges *CED-3* to *CED-9.* The mammalian homologs of *CED-9,* the bcl-2-related proteins, are a growing family of molecules that can either protect or activate apoptosis. Bcl-2 is a mitochondria protein with structural similarity to an ion channel; however, how this protein functions in mitochondria physiology and how this overall affects cell survival are still unanswered questions. Mice without the *BCL*-2 protooncogene display normal embryonic development and hematopoiesis. However, soon after birth these *BCL*-2-null mice undergo massive apoptotic involution in the thymus and spleen, demonstrating that *BCL*-2 plays a key role in preventing lymphocyte apoptosis.[60]

Although many TNFR family receptors can transduce an apoptotic signal, we will use

TABLE 15-1   MAMMALIAN DEATH PATHWAY-ASSOCIATED GENE FAMILIES

DEATH GENE FAMILY	EXAMPLES	APPROX. NO.	SPECIAL FEATURES
Death Domain	FADD, TRADD, DAP kinase, RIP	7	Cytosolic proteins binding each other or DD receptor subgroup
Death Effector Domain (DED)	FADD, FLIP, Caspase 8, 10	4	Links receptor complexes to caspase specialized regulator (FLIP/MRIT/Caspar)
Caspases	Caspase 1, 3	12	Protease initiators/effectors of death
TRAFs	TRAF1, 2, 3	6	Anti-apoptotic via activation of NF-kB
Bcl-2 family	Bcl-2, Bax, Bcl-x, Bad	15	Anti-apoptotic or pro-apoptotic; associated with mitochondria

CD95/Fas as the prototype example. Similar features of this cascade can be found in apoptotic cascades transduced by other receptors.

In the case of CD95, adapter molecules associate with the cytoplasmic tail via modules defined as *death domains* (DDs). Molecules containing DD motifs can potentially dimerize via these sequences (see Table 15-1). Although the homology among different DDs is low, the unique sequences mediate specificity of interactions. FADD is an adapter that associates with CD95.[61–63] FADD contains a C-terminal DD and an N-terminal motif called a *death effector domain* (DED).[63,64] Analogous to DDs, DEDs can associate, effectively bringing together molecules forming a death-inducing signaling complex.[65] One critical DED-containing molecule in the CD95 apoptotic cascade is caspase-8.[66] The entire molecule is actually an holoenzyme, and when activated, the procaspase-8 is cleaved into active p18 and p10 subunits. This initiates the apoptotic-signaling cascade that includes cleavage and activation of other proteases such as caspase-1, -3, -6 and -7, and kinases, such as Mst-1.

IMMUNODEFICIENCIES DUE TO DEFECTS IN SIGNAL TRANSDUCTION

Several X-linked chromosome immunodeficiency disorders are due to mutations in genes required for lymphocyte activation (see Chap. 88). Patients with the hyper-IgM syndrome have mutations in the *CD40L* gene (Xq25) such that their T cells either do not express CD154 or express a defective CD154 that is unable to bind CD40. Because of this, the T cells of these patients are unable to induce B cells to proliferate or switch immunoglobulin classes.[14] As a result, these patients produce IgM only in response to antigens and do not form germinal centers. Patients with X-linked chromosome hypogammaglobulinemia (XLA) have a defective *XLA* gene (Xq22) encoding the B-cell tyrosine kinase critical for the development of B lymphocytes.[67,68] Also, a group of patients with X-linked chromosome severe combined immunodeficiency have nonsense mutations in the gene encoding the γ chain of the IL-2 receptor, *IL-2RG* (Xq13).[69] These patients have reduced or absent levels of immature and mature T cells, demonstrating that IL-2Rγ is essential for T-cell development. However, since the IL-2Rγ chain also can associate with the receptors for IL-4 and IL-7 to form higher-affinity receptors for their respective cytokine, it is not clear whether the immunodeficiency of such patients is due solely to a defect in the IL-2R signaling. Another X-linked immunodeficiency results from mutations in an adapter molecule called *SLAM-associated protein* (SAP).[70] This molecule associates with CD150, which is a costimulatory molecule that can modulate signals in T cells and B cells. Patients with mutation in SAP are susceptible to X-linked chromosome lymphoproliferative disease (XLP) after infection by Epstein-Barr virus (EBV). These patients have an uncontrolled proliferation of T and B cells that results in fatality in 51 percent of patients.[71]

On the other hand, defects that interfere with the regulation of lymphocyte cell growth or activation can lead to lymphoproliferative or autoimmune disease. The *lpr* mutation in mice interferes with expression of the Fas (CD95) antigen.[72] The lymphocytes of mice that are homozygous for this mutation do not express Fas and, consequently, have prolonged and inappropriate life spans, resulting in lymphocyte accumulation and eventual lymphoproliferative disease. Homozygous motheaten mice (*me/me*) have a defect in a protein tyrosine phosphatase, designated the SHP-1 phosphatase.[73] This defect impairs T-cell development and results in an autoimmune disease syndrome.

REFERENCES

1. Miyajima A, Kitamura T, Harada N, et al: Cytokine receptors and signal transduction. *Annu Rev Immunol* 10:295, 1992.
2. Perlmutter R, Levin SD, Appleby MW, et al: Regulation of lymphocyte function by protein phosphorylation. *Annu Rev Immunol* 11:451, 1993.
3. Weiss A: T cell antigen receptor signal transduction: a tale of tails and cytoplasmic protein-tyrosine kinases. *Cell* 73:209, 1993.
4. Moller GB (editor): Accessory molecules in the immune response. *Immunol Rev* 153:1, 1996.
5. Parham P (editor): The anatomy of antigen-specific immune responses. *Immunol Rev* 156:1, 1997.
6. Barclay A, Birkeland ML, Brown MH, et al: *The Leukocyte Antigen Fact Book*. Academic, London, 1993.
7. Schlossman S, Boumsell L, Gilks W, et al (editors): *Leukocyte Typing V: White Cell Differentiation Antigens*. Oxford University Press, Oxford, 1994.
8. Liu Y-J, Arpin C: Germinal center development. *Immunol Rev* 156:111, 1997.
9. Parker D: T cell-dependent B cell activation. *Annu Rev Immunol* 11:331, 1993.
10. Clark E, Ledbetter JA: How T cells talk to B cells. *Nature* 367:425, 1994.
11. Dustin M, Springer TA: Role of lymphocyte adhesion receptors in transient interactions and cell locomotion. *Annu Rev Immunol* 9:27, 1991.
12. Armitage R, Fanslow WC, Strockbine L, et al: Molecular and biological characterization of a murine ligand for CD *Nature* 357:80, 1992.
13. Armitage R, Maliszewski CR, Alderson MR, et al: CD40-L: A multi-functional ligand. *Semin Immunol* 5:401, 1993.
14. Hill A, Chapel H: The fruits of cooperation. *Nature* 361:494, 1993.
15. Linsley P, Ledbetter JA: The role of the CD28 receptor during T cell responses to antigen. *Annu Rev Immunol* 11:191, 1993.
16. Chen L, Ashe S, Brady WA, et al: Costimulation of antitumor immunity by the B7 counterreceptor for the T lymphocyte molecules CD28 and CTLA-4. *Cell* 71:1093, 1992.
17. Azuma M, Ito D, Yagita H, et al: B70 Antigen is a second ligand for CTLA-4 and CD28. *Nature* 366:76, 1993.
18. Freeman G, Gribben JG, Boussiotis VA, et al: Cloning of B7-2: a CTLA-4 counter-receptor that costimulates human T cell proliferation. *Science* 262:909, 1993.
19. Klaus S, Pinchuk L, Fanslow WC, et al: Costimulation through CD28 receptors enhances T-cell-dependent B cell activation via a CD40′ CD40-L interaction. *J Immunol* 152:5643, 1994.
20. Ranheim E, Kipps TJ: Activated T cells induce expression of B7/BB1 on normal or leukemic B cells through a CD40-dependent signal. *J Exp Med* 177:925, 1993.
21. Mobley J, Reynolds PJ, Shimizu Y: Regulatory mechanisms underlying T cell-integrin receptor function. *Semin Immunol* 5:227, 1993.
22. Bierer B, Hahn WC: T cell adhesion, avidity regulation and signaling: a molecular analysis of CD2. *Semin Immunol* 5:249, 1993.
23. O'Rourke A, Mescher MF: Cytotoxic T-lymphocyte activation involves a cascade of signaling and adhesion events. *Nature* 358:253, 1992.
24. Schwartz L, Osborne BA: Programmed cell death, apoptosis and killer genes. *Immunol Today* 14:582, 1993.
25. MacLennan I, Gulbranson-Judge A, Toellner K-M, et al: The changing preference of T and B cells for partners as T-dependent antibody responses develop. *Immunol Rev* 156:53, 1997.
26. Craxton A, Otipoby KL, Jiang A, et al: Signal transduction pathways that regulate the fate of B lymphocytes. *Adv Immunol* 73:79, 1999.
27. Cambier J: Signal transduction by T- and B-cell antigen receptors: converging structures and concepts. *Curr Opin Immunol* 4:257, 1992.
28. Alberola-Ila J, Takaki S, Kerner JD, Perlmutter RM: Differential signaling by lymphocyte antigen receptors. *Annu Rev Immunol* 15:125, 1997.
29. DeFranco A: The complexity of signaling pathways activated by the BCR. *Curr Opin Immunol* 9:296, 1997.
30. Kurosaki T: Molecular mechanisms in B cell antigen receptor signaling. *Curr Opin Immunol* 9:309, 1997.
31. Cooper J, Howell B: The when and how of Src regulation. *Cell* 73:1051, 1993.
32. Law C, Craxton A, Otipoby KL: Regulation of signaling through B lymphocyte antigen receptors by cell-cell interaction molecules. *Immunol Rev* 153:123, 1996.

33. Mayer B, Baltimore D: Signaling through SH3 and SH2 domains. *Trends Cell Biol* 3:8, 1993.

34. Mayer B, Gupta R: Functions of SH2 and SH3 domains. *Curr Top Microbiol Immunol* 228:1, 1998.

35. Rudd C: Adaptors and molecular scaffolds in immune cell signaling. *Cell* 96:5, 1999.

36. Pawson T: Signaling through scaffold, anchoring, and adaptor proteins. *Science* 278:2075, 1997.

37. Lemmon M, Ferguson KM: Pleckstrin homology domains. *Curr Top Microbiol Immunol* 228:39, 1998.

38. Koretzky G: The role of Grb2-associated proteins in T-cell activation. *Immunol Today* 18:401, 1997.

39. Hunter T, Karin M: The regulation of transcription by phosphorylation. *Cell* 70:375, 1993.

40. Glimcher L, Singh H: Transcription factors in lymphocyte development—T and B cells get together. *Cell* 96:13, 1999.

41. Yamanashi Y, Fukui Y, Wongsasant B, et al: Activation of Src-like protein-tyrosine kinase Lyn and its association with phosphatidylinositol 3-kinase upon B-cell antigen receptor-mediated signaling. *Proc Natl Acad Sci USA* 89:1118, 1992.

42. Pleiman C, Hertz WM, Cambier JC: Activation of phosphatidylinositol-3' kinase by Src-family kinase SH3 binding to the p85 subunit. *Science* 263:1609, 1994.

43. Downward J: Lipid-regulated kinases: some common themes at last. *Science* 279:673, 1998.

44. Toker A, Cantley LC: Signalling through the lipid products of phospho-inositide-3-OH kinase. *Nature* 387:673, 1997.

45. Franke T, Kaplan DR, Cantley LC, Toker A: Direct regulation of the Akt proto-oncogene product by phosphatidylinositol-3,4-bisphosphate. *Science* 275:665, 1997.

46. Burgering B, Coffer, PJ: Protein kinase B (c-Akt) in phosphatidylinositol-3-OH kinase signal transduction. *Nature* 376:599, 1995.

47. Reif K, Cantrell DA: Networking Rho family GRPases in lymphocytes. *Immunity* 8:395, 1998.

48. Su B, Karin M: Mitogen-activated protein kinase cascades and regulation of gene expression. *Curr Opin Immunol* 8:402, 1996.

49. Treisman R: Regulation of transcription by MAP kinase cascades. *Curr Opin Cell Biol* 8:205, 1996.

50. Taniguchi T, Minami Y: The IL-2/IL-2 receptor system: a current overview. *Cell* 73:5, 1993.

51. Mills GB (editor): Transmembrane signaling. *Semin Immunol* 5:297, 1993.

52. O'Shea JJ: Jaks, STATs, cytokine signal transduction, and immunoregulation: are we there yet? *Immunity* 7:1, 1997.

53. Hanissian S, Geha RS: Jak3 is associated with CD40 and is critical for CD40 induction of gene expression in B cells. *Immunity* 6:379, 1997.

54. Tan Y: Yin and Yang of phosphorylation in cytokine signaling. *Science* 262:376, 1993.

55. Marx J: Two major signal pathways linked. *Science* 262:998, 1993.

56. Williams G, Smith CA: Molecular regulation of apoptosis: genetic controls on cell death. *Cell* 74:777, 1993.

57. Cohen J, Duke RC, Fadok VA, Sellins KS: Apoptosis and programmed cell death in immunity. *Annu Rev Immunol* 10:267, 1992.

58. Winoto A: Cell death in the regulation of immune responses. *Curr Opin Immunol* 9:365, 1997.

59. Gruss H-J, Dower SK: Tumor necrosis factor ligand superfamily: involvement in the pathology of malignant lymphomas. *Blood* 85:3378, 1995.

60. Veis D, Sorenson CM, Shuttler JR, Korsmeyer SJ: Bcl-2 deficient mice demonstrate fulminant lymphoid apoptosis, polycystic kidneys, and hypopigmented hair. *Cell* 75:229, 1993.

61. Boldin M, Goncharov TM, Goltsev YV, Wallach D: Involvement of MACH, a novel MORT1/FADD-interacting protease, in Fas/APO-1- and TNF receptor-induced cell death. *Cell* 85:803, 1996.

62. Chinnaiyan A, O'Rourke K, Tewari M, Dixit VM: FADD, a novel death domain-containing protein, interacts with the death domain of Fas and initiates apoptosis. *Cell* 81:505, 1996.

63. Chinnaiyan A, Dixit VM: The cell-death machine. *Curr Biol* 6:555, 1996.

64. Fernandes-Alnemri T, Armstrong RC, Krebs J, et al: In vitro activation of CPP32 and Mch3 by Mch4, a novel human apoptotic cysteine protease containing two FADD-like domains. *Proc Natl Acad Sci USA* 93:7464, 1996.

65. Kischkel F, Hellbardt S, Behrmann I, et al: Cytotoxicity-dependent APO-1 (Fas/CD95)-associated proteins form a death-inducing signaling complex (DISC) with the receptor. *EMBO J* 14:5579, 1995.

66. Muzio M, Chinnaiyan AM, Kischkel FC, et al: FLICE, a novel FADD-homologous ICE/CED-3-like protease, is recruited to the CD95 (Fas/APO-1) death-inducing signaling complex. *Cell* 85:817, 1996.

67. Vetrie D, Vorechovsky I, Sideras P, et al: The gene involved in X-linked agammaglobulinemia is a member of the src-family of protein-tyrosine kinases. *Nature* 361:226, 1993.

68. Tsukada S, Saffran DC, Rawlings DJ, et al: Deficient expression of a B cell cytoplasmic tyrosine kinase in human X-linked agammaglobulinemia. *Cell* 72:279, 1993.

69. Noguchi M, Yi H, Rosenblatt HM, et al: Interleukin-2 receptor g chain mutation results in X-linked severe combined immunodeficiency in humans. *Cell* 73:147, 1993.

70. Sayos J, Wu C, Morra M, et al: The X-linked lymphoproliferative-disease gene product SAP regulates signals induced through the co-receptor SLAM. *Nature* 395:462, 1998.

71. Klein G, Klein E: Sinking surveillance's flagship. *Nature* 395:441, 1998.

72. Watenabe-Fukunaga R, Brannan CI, Copeland NG, et al: Lymphoproliferation disorder in mice explained by defects in Fas antigen that mediates apoptosis. *Nature* 356:314, 1992.

73. Schultz LD, Schweitzer PA, Rajan T, et al: Mutation at the murine moth-eaten locus are within the hemopoietic cell protein tyrosine phosphatase (Hcph) gene. *Cell* 73:1445, 1993.

THERAPEUTIC PRINCIPLES

PHARMACOLOGY AND TOXICITY OF ANTINEOPLASTIC DRUGS

BRUCE A. CHABNER

WYNDHAM WILSON

JEFFREY SUPKO

The safe and effective use of anticancer drugs in the treatment of hematological malignancies requires an in-depth knowledge of the pharmacology of these agents. In no other field of medicine is the margin of safety more narrow or the potential for serious if not fatal toxicity more real. At the same time, anticancer drugs are capable of curing many of these otherwise aggressive malignancies, and their discovery and development have provided a paradigm for approaches to the improved treatment of the more common solid tumors.

The intelligent use of these drugs begins with an understanding of their mechanism of action. Most anticancer drugs inhibit the synthesis of DNA or directly attack the integrity of DNA through the formation of DNA adducts or enzyme-mediated breaks. These DNA-directed actions are recognized by repair processes and by the checkpoints that monitor DNA integrity, including most prominently p53. If DNA damage can not be repaired, and if the DNA damage reaches thresholds for activating programmed cell death, then DNA damage is translated into tumor regression. Resistance to drug action can arise from alterations in any one of the critical steps required for drug activity; these steps include drug transport in the blood stream or across the blood-brain barrier, transport across the cell membrane, transformation of the parent drug to its active form within the tumor cell or in the liver, interaction of the drug with its target protein or nucleic acid, enzymatic or chemical inactivation of the agent and its transport out of the cell, and elimination of the agent from the body through the kidneys or bile. The underlying mutability of tumors leads to the generation of cells with alterations in one or more of these critical steps in drug action, leading to the selection and outgrowth of drug-resistant tumor. Combination chemotherapy logically evades resistance that carries specificity for single agents, but increasingly, research has revealed mutations that lead to multidrug resistance (MDR), including overexpression of transporters such as the multidrug resistance (*MDR*) gene, as well as loss of the apoptotic response.

In addition to the molecular determinants of drug action, pharmacokinetics (the disposition of drugs in humans) play a critical role in determining drug effectiveness and toxicity. Because of the potential of these agents for toxicity, it is critical for oncologists to understand the pathways of drug clearance and to adjust dose in the presence of compromised organ function. Drugs such as methotrexate, hydroxyurea, and the newer purine antagonists (fludarabine and cladribine) are eliminated primarily by renal excretion and should not be used in full doses in patients with renal dysfunction. Similarly, hepatic dysfunction with elevated serum bilirubin concentrations should alert clinicians to decrease doses of the taxanes, vinca alkaloids, and (with less certainty) the anthracyclines. In addition, clinicians must be alert to the potential for drug interactions, particularly the ability of drugs that induce CYP 3A4 and CYP 2B6 to accelerate the metabolism of paclitaxel and of allopurinol to inhibit the metabolic breakdown of orally administered 6-mercaptopurine.

Clinicians must be alert to the potential for genetically determined differences in drug toxicity and response. The most important of these familial syndromes affecting treatment of leukemia is the deficiency of thiopurine methyltransferase, which slows the elimination of 6-mercaptopurine and leads to unanticipated toxicity during maintenance chemotherapy for acute lymphocytic leukemia. Pharmacokinetic monitoring has a standard role in the use of certain therapies, particularly high-dose methotrexate, and in the evaluation of new drugs or new drug combinations. Major cancer centers must have the capability of performing pharmacokinetic studies in conjunction with their clinical research programs.

To assure appropriate dose reduction, regimen choice, and management of toxicity, there is no substitute for therapy based on standard protocols and peer reviewed clinical trials. Adherence to protocols assures that the pharmacologic and pharmacogenetic variables affecting cancer chemotherapy can be recognized early in the course of treatment and that serious untoward events can be avoided while maintaining effective therapy.

The leukemias and lymphomas have been the proving ground for chemotherapy. The first evidence for antitumor activity of a chemical agent came from experiments with nitrogen mustard in a patient with Hodgkin disease in 1942.[1] The even more startling discovery of remission induction by antifolates in acute lymphocytic leukemia 6 years later ushered in the era of chemotherapy in cancer treatment.[2] Subsequent clinical experiments in these diseases established the basic principles of cyclic combination therapy and dose intensification, developed effective strategies for marrow transplantation, and demonstrated the importance of specific mechanisms of drug resistance. These principles have led to curative regimens for acute leukemias and lymphomas, effective therapies for chronic leukemias and multiple myeloma, and they have provided the conceptual basis for the current practice of medical oncology.

BASIC PRINCIPLES OF CANCER CHEMOTHERAPY

The safe and effective use of chemotherapy in clinical practice requires a thorough understanding of the basic aspects of drug action as well

Portions of this chapter are based on Chapter 28, by Joseph Bertino, in the fourth edition of this book.

Acronyms and abbreviations that appear in this chapter include: ABVD, Adriamycin (doxorubicin), bleomycin, vinblastine, and dacarbazine; APL, acute promyelocytic leukemia; ADH, antidiuretic hormone; ALL, acute lymphocytic leukemia; AML, acute myelogenous leukemia; ara-C, cytosine arabinoside; ara-U, uracil arabinoside; BCNU, bischloroethylnitrosourea; CDA, chlorodeoxyadenosine; CLL, chronic lymphocytic leukemia; CML, chronic myelogenous leukemia; CYP, cytochrome P450; DCF, deoxycoformycin; DHFR, dihydrofolate reductase; HPRT, hypoxanthine-guanine phosphoribosyl transferase; IL, interleukin; MDR, multidrug resistance; MP, mercaptopurine; MRP, multidrug resistance–associated protein; MTD, maximum tolerated dose; RAR-α, retinoic acid-α receptor; TG, thioguanine; TGB, transforming growth factor; tRA, all-*trans*-retinoic acid.

as knowledge of the important clinical toxicities, pharmacokinetics, and drug interactions. Antineoplastic chemotherapy is often complex, and there is the potential for serious or fatal side effects. Patients are best served, usually, if their treatment is derived from the recommendations made from clinical trials. The modification of doses and schedules of drug administration should be made, where possible, on the recommendations derived from clinical trials. The choice of a specific protocol of treatment should depend not only on the stage and histology of the tumor but on an assessment of individual patient tolerance and susceptibility to specific potential toxicities. Thus, bleomycin would not usually be an appropriate choice for a patient with serious underlying lung disease, nor would doxorubicin be an appropriate drug for use in a patient with a history of congestive heart failure.

With the development of techniques for marrow or blood stem cell storage and reinfusion, previously fatal doses of chemotherapy can be administered in an attempt to cure malignancies refractory to standard chemotherapy. In general, these regimens produce a spectrum of organ toxicities not seen at conventional doses—including pulmonary dysfunction, cardiac failure, and hepatic and renal insufficiency—and are ordinarily reserved for patients of younger age and with normal baseline organ function[3] (see Chap. 18).

Since the malignant process is characterized by uncontrolled proliferation, it is logical that chemotherapy should target DNA replication. Most effective cancer drugs either interfere with the synthesis of DNA or produce chemical lesions in DNA. The mechanism by which most drugs cause cell death is unclear. In some cells apoptosis, or programmed cell death, follows exposure to cytotoxic agents, whereas other cells may proceed through mitosis before dying. The greater susceptibility of malignant cells to drug toxicity, while evident in the course of remission induction, cannot be explained at present but may result from the existence of normal stem cells in a nonreplicating phase of the cell cycle, where they are less susceptible to damage by DNA-directed agents. In addition, there is growing evidence that cancer cells lack the normal checkpoints in the cell cycle that would otherwise block the entry of damaged cells into DNA synthesis and mitosis and would thus allow repair of DNA strand breaks, base deletions, or other lesions induced by chemotherapy.[4] These factors allow normal cells to escape with less intrinsic damage and favor their recovery from chemotherapy-induced injury. While most antimetabolites and alkylating agents target DNA, other drugs attack the mitotic spindle (vinca alkaloids), inhibit protein synthesis (L-asparaginase), or induce cell differentiation (all-*trans*-retinoic acid). Cancer drug discovery efforts have evolved and now target a number of specific processes fundamental to tumor initiation or progression, including receptor signaling, intracellular signal transduction, angiogenesis, and metastasis.[5]

COMBINATION CHEMOTHERAPY

While most leukemias and lymphomas are highly drug sensitive, with the exception of Burkitt lymphoma treated with cyclophosphamide, these tumors are rarely cured with single-agent chemotherapy. Combination chemotherapy has proven to be much more effective in forestalling the emergence of drug-resistant cells and thus has curative potential in settings where individual agents are ineffective. Certain empirical principles have resulted from the clinical experience of the past four decades of combination therapy. Drugs selected for combination therapy should, with few exceptions (such as the rescue agent leucovorin), have demonstrable antineoplastic activity of their own against the tumor in question. The individual agents should have different mechanisms of action and should not share a common mechanism of resistance such as MDR. The dose-limiting toxicities of the agents chosen should not overlap; otherwise, they could not be used together at or near full doses. Finally, the clinical use of specific combinations should be designed on preclinical evidence of synergistic interaction. Favorable drug interactions may be very dependent on specific sequences and schedules of administration. For these reasons, clinical protocols should attempt to duplicate the most favorable preclinical regimens.

Another important consideration in designing clinical protocols is dose intensity, the dose administered per unit time, which should be maintained throughout a treatment regimen. Achieving this objective may require the use of hematopoietic growth factors to hasten marrow recovery, prevent repeated episodes of febrile neutropenia, and allow on-time administration of the next treatment cycle. Interdigitation of chemotherapy with surgery and irradiation makes it possible to take advantage of favorable cytokinetic or radiosensitizing effects of chemotherapy, while avoiding enhancement of toxicity. Thus, 5-fluorouracil and cisplatin are used with radiation therapy to enhance local tumor control in malignancies of the head and neck,[6] esophagus,[7] and anus.[8] Surgical reduction of tumor bulk increases the response rate of ovarian tumors to chemotherapy, perhaps by eliminating poorly perfused tumor masses.[9] In the treatment of lymphomas, the toxicity of radiation therapy to sensitive organs such as skin, lung, heart, and brain may be significantly increased by concurrent administration of anthracyclines, a consideration that has prompted the use of radiation therapy either separated from or sandwiched between cycles of chemotherapy that include doxorubicin.

CELL KINETICS AND CANCER CHEMOTHERAPY

The cell-killing characteristics of cancer chemotherapeutic agents vary according to their mechanism of action. Many of the most effective agents in antileukemic therapy belong to the antimetabolite class, including cytosine arabinoside, 6-thioguanine, and methotrexate. These drugs kill cells most effectively during the DNA-synthetic phase (S phase) of the cell cycle. They have greatly diminished toxicity for nondividing cells. For these agents, a prolonged period of tumor exposure to drug is essential in order to maximize the number of cells exposed during the vulnerable period of the cell cycle. As would be predicted, the antimetabolite drugs are primarily active against rapidly dividing tumors such as acute leukemias and intermediate and high-grade lymphomas. High-dose regimens achieve a number of worthwhile objectives for these agents, including an enhancement of cross-membrane transport, saturation of anabolic pathways inside the cell, and prolongation of the period of effective drug concentration. However, achieving these objectives is realized at the cost of increased toxicity to normal proliferating marrow precursor cells and may produce significant and unexpected damage to normal organs, such as hepatic veno-occlusive disease (alkylating agents), cerebellar toxicity (cytosine arabinoside), or pulmonary toxicity (nitrosoureas and alkylating agents). Because hematopoietic stem cells can be harvested, stored, and reinfused, dose-limiting toxicities of high-dose chemotherapy are generally those affecting nonhematologic organs.

A number of other anticancer drugs do not require cells to be exposed during a specific phase of the cell cycle, although like the antimetabolites, these drugs are generally more effective against actively proliferating cells as compared to resting cells. These agents include the anthracyclines, the epipodophyllotoxins, and certain alkylating agents such as cyclophosphamide. Still others, most notably the nitrosoureas and busulfan, are equally toxic to dividing and nondividing cells and deplete marrow stem cells. In general, the duration of exposure to alkylating agents such as the nitrosoureas and cyclophosphamide is less important than the total dose of drug, while for the cell cycle–specific drugs (such as methotrexate and cytosine arabinoside), both drug concentration and duration of exposure determine cytocidal effect. For these agents, cytotoxicity is best related to the area under

TABLE 16-1   DOSE MODIFICATION IN PATIENTS WITH RENAL OR HEPATIC
DYSFUNCTION

RENAL DYSFUNCTION (creatinine clearance<60 mL/min)
• Reduce dose in proportion to reduction in creatinine clearance.

Drugs

1. Methotrexate
2. Cisplatin
3. Carboplatin
4. Bleomycin
5. Etoposide

6. Hydroxyurea
7. Deoxycoformycin
8. Fludarabine phosphate
9. 2-Chlorodeoxyadenosine
10. Topotecan

HEPATIC DYSFUNCTION
• For bilirubin>1.5 mg/dL reduce initial dose by 50%.
• For bilirubin>3.0 mg/dL reduce initial dose by 75%.

Drugs

1. Amsacrine
2. Doxorubicin
3. Daunorubicin
4. Vincristine

5. Vinblastine
6. Paclitaxel
7. Mitoxantrone

the plasma concentration-time curve of the drug. However, for drugs that act through alternate mechanisms, such as the taxanes, myelosuppression correlates best with the duration of exposure above a threshold plasma concentration, which is approximately 50 to 100 nM for paclitaxel and 200 nM for docetaxel.[10]

The choice of an appropriate dose and schedule of drug administration depends on a number of factors: (1) the drug's cell cycle dependence, (2) its pattern of toxicity to marrow and other organs as a function of dose and schedule, (3) pharmacokinetic behavior, (4) potential interactions with other drugs, and (5) patient tolerance. The last factor will vary among individuals and will depend on physiologic parameters such as renal and hepatic functions (Table 16-1), which determine the patient's ability to eliminate drug, and on the patient's prior treatment experience, performance status, and age. Protocols for cancer chemotherapy must contain provisions for adjusting the dose or duration of drug infusion to accommodate these variables and should be followed diligently when employing those drugs.

DRUG RESISTANCE

Inadequate treatment of a sensitive tumor tends to select for the outgrowth of drug-resistant clones of the original tumor. It has been proposed that the basis for drug resistance is the spontaneous generation of resistant mutants, with subsequent selection of the drug-resistant mutant under the pressure of chemotherapeutic drugs.[11] While formal proof of the clonal selection hypothesis is lacking, experimental models of drug resistance fit the hypothesis quite well, with the additional caveat that cancer drugs and irradiation are mutagenic themselves and increase significantly the rate at which drug-resistant mutants are generated. The hypothesis implies that the use of multiple drugs that do not share a common mechanism of resistance should be more effective than single agents; the hypothesis further suggests that multiple agents should be used simultaneously, since the likelihood of there being a doubly or triply resistant cell is the product of the probabilities of the independent drug-resistant mutations occurring at the same time in a single cell. The probability of a cell division resulting in mutation at any given genetic locus is approximately 10^{-6} for somatic cells; thus the probability of multiple independent mutations arising in the same cell will be 10^{-12} or lower. However, mutation rates may be distinctly higher in tumor cells and may be further increased by exposure to alkylating agents and irradiation.

In choosing drugs for combination therapy, one must bear in mind potential mechanisms of resistance. Classical MDR due to increased

expression of drug efflux pumps such as the P-glycoprotein or the MRP proteins[12–14] confers resistance to a broad spectrum of agents derived from natural products, including taxanes, anthracyclines, vinca alkaloids, and epipodophyllotoxins. Other mechanisms, such as dihydrofolate reductase amplification,[15] are highly specific for a single drug, methotrexate. The common mechanisms are listed in Table 16-2. While none of these biochemical changes are routinely measured either prior to or following therapy, these mechanisms should be considered in developing new protocols and in choosing new therapy for patients who relapse from primary treatment.

In addition to drug-specific mechanisms of resistance, it is now recognized that mutations affecting recognition of DNA damage, such as the mismatch repair genes,[16] lead to cisplatin, thiopurine, or alkylating agent resistance, while other mutations that block the induction of apoptosis, such as loss of p53,[17] or overexpression of the antiapoptotic factors such as BCL-2[18] may render tumor cells insensitive to a broad array of drugs and modalities, including ionizing irradiation, alkylating agents, antimetabolites, and anthracyclines. Although the specific contribution of these factors to clinical resistance is still uncertain, emerging evidence suggests that mutations involving genes that control cell cycle and apoptosis, such as loss of p53 function, are strongly associated with clinically resistant and aggressive tumors[17] and may be more relevant causes of drug resistance in the clinic than are the classical drug-specific mechanisms.

CELL CYCLE-ACTIVE AGENTS

METHOTREXATE

The folate antagonist aminopterin was shown by Farber and his associates to induce a complete remission in children with ALL.[2] Unfortunately, these remissions were short-lived, and the leukemia invariably became resistant within months to further treatment. Subsequently, methotrexate supplanted aminopterin because it had a better therapeutic index. Methotrexate continues to be a key drug in maintenance therapy of ALL and in combination therapy of intermediate- and high-grade lymphomas. It is also used for treatment and prophylaxis of meningeal leukemia.

MECHANISMS OF ACTION

Methotrexate enters cells through an active uptake process mediated in most tumor cells by the reduced folate transporter,[19] although a second transporter, the membrane folate binding protein,[20] may contribute to the cellular uptake of other antifolates. Methotrexate inhibits the enzyme DHFR, which recycles oxidized folates to their active reduced state. Inhibition of DHFR leads to rapid depletion of intracellular folate coenzymes. Since folate coenzymes are required for thymidylate and purine biosynthesis, DNA synthesis is blocked and cell replication stops. Methotrexate is retained in certain cells for long periods of time as a consequence of an enzymatic process that adds up to five additional glutamate moieties to the γ-carboxyl group of the drug (see Chap. 25). Polyglutamation may be an important determinant of methotrexate selectivity, since cells that effect this conversion efficiently, such as leukemic myeloblasts and lymphoblasts, are more susceptible to the drug than are normal myeloid precursors, which have limited capability for polyglutamation.[21] Hyperdiploid lymphoblasts are particularly efficient in producing polyglutamated species and have a high cure rate with chemotherapy.[22] Acquired resistance to methotrexate in patients with leukemia is due to increased levels of dihydrofolate reductase as a consequence of gene amplification,[15] defective polyglutamation,[23] and impaired drug uptake.[19] Alterations of the DHFR enzyme leading to decreased binding of methotrexate have also been observed.[24]

TABLE 16-2 MECHANISMS OF RESISTANCE TO ANTICANCER DRUGS

MECHANISMS	DRUGS AFFECTED	EVIDENCE FOR CLINICAL ROLE
1. Decreased drug uptake		
Reduced folate transporter	Methotrexate	ALL
Nucleoside transporter	Cytosine arabinoside	AML
2. Increased drug efflux		
mdr transporter (P-glycoprotein)	Anthracyclines, vincas, taxanes, etoposide	Multiple myeloma, ANLL, non-Hodgkin lymphoma
mrp transporter	Anthracyclines, vincas, taxanes, etoposide	Uncertain
3. Decreased drug activation in tumor		
Deoxycytidine kinase deletion	Cytosine arabinoside (likely fludarabine and cladribine as well)	AML
Hypoxanthine phosphoribosyl transferase deletion	6-Mercaptopurine	Uncertain
Folyl polyglutamation	Methotrexate	Acute leukemias
4. Increased drug inactivation		
Thiopurine methyl transferase	6-Mercaptopurine	ALL
Bleomycin hydrolase	Bleomycin	Uncertain
Glutathione transferase	Alkylating agents	Uncertain
5. Decreased target enzyme		
Topoisomerase I	Camptothecins	Uncertain
Topoisomerase II	Anthracyclines, etoposide	Uncertain
6. Increased target enzyme		
Dihydrofolate reductase	Methotrexate	Acute leukemia
Thymidylate synthase	5-fluorouracil	Solid tumors
Adenosine deaminase	Deoxycoformycin	Uncertain
7. Altered intracellular target		
Dihydrofolate reductase	Methotrexate	Uncertain
Tubulin	Vincas, taxanes	Uncertain
Topoisomerase I	Camptothecins	Uncertain
Topoisomerase II	Anthracyclines, etoposide	Uncertain
8. Increase DNA repair		
Guanine-0–6 methyl transferase	Procarbazine, nitrosoureas	Brain tumors
Nucleotide excision repair	Platinating drugs	Ovarian cancer
9. Decreased DNA damage recognition		
p53 mutation	Many cancer drugs, radiation	Leukemias, lymphomas
Mismatch DNA repair mutations	Platinating agents, thiopurines	Colon cancer

ABBREVIATIONS: ANLL, acute non-lymphocytic leukemia; ALL, acute lymphocytic leukemia; mdr, multidrug resistance gene; mrp, multidrug resistance protein.
REFERENCES: See text for references and explanation.

CLINICAL PHARMACOLOGY

Methotrexate is well absorbed when administered orally at low doses (5–10 mg/m²), but when doses exceed 30 mg/m² absorption is progressively decreased and more variable. Therefore, doses greater than 25 mg/m² should be administered parenterally. Poor absorption resulting in low blood levels of the drug (i.e., <16 μM) is associated with an increased risk of relapse in children with ALL receiving maintenance therapy with methotrexate.[25]

The concentration of methotrexate in plasma declines in a polyexponential manner. There is a very rapid initial disposition phase that persists for only a few minutes after intravenous administration. The intermediate disposition phase has a 2- to 3-h half-life and persists for 12 to 24 h after dosing. The terminal phase of drug decay is considerably slower, with an 8- to 10-h half-life. Methotrexate is primarily excreted unchanged by the kidney, although with large doses a minor fraction of the drug (7–30%) is inactivated by hepatic enzyme–mediated hydroxylation at the 7 position. Thus, patients with renal impairment should not be treated with methotrexate, since the prolonged exposure to high blood levels may result in life-threatening hematologic and gastrointestinal toxicity. When renal toxicity occurs following methotrexate treatment, large (100 mg/m²) and frequent (every 6 h) doses of leucovorin should be administered until the concentration of methotrexate in the blood decreases to nontoxic levels.[26] High-dose methotrexate (>0.5 g/m²) together with leucovorin rescue is used to treat patients with high-grade lymphoma or ALL. This is usually accomplished by administering six to eight doses of 10 to 15 mg/m² leucovorin at 6-h intervals, starting 6 to 24 h after the injection of methotrexate, and continuing until plasma concentrations of the drug fall below 1 μM. In patients receiving high-dose methotrexate, drug levels are routinely assayed 24 to 48 h after dosing to determine the rate of drug elimination and the safety for discontinuing leucovorin administration. In patients receiving such therapy, renal toxicity is generally the cause of decreased drug clearance, which may result from intrarenal precipitation of the parent drug or its 7-OH metabolite. Renal dysfunction can be prevented by alkalinizing the urine to pH 7.0 with intravenous sodium bicarbonate prior to and during therapy, or alternately, by intensive hydration. Both methotrexate and its hydroxylated metabolite are organic acids, which, like uric acid, are much more soluble in weakly alkaline urine. If drug concentrations in plasma exceed 1 μM during routine monitoring, leucovorin should be continued at doses of 50 to 100 mg/m² every 6 h until methotrexate concentrations fall below 0.1 μM. In cases of extreme renal failure, with stable drug levels in the 10 μM range, leucovorin will not be effective and dialysis will not provide a sustained reduction in drug levels. The only effective measure in this circumstance is the administration of carboxypeptidase G, a bacterial enzyme that degrades antifolates.[27] The enzyme can be obtained from the Cancer Therapy Evaluation Program of the National Cancer Institute and may be life saving.

ADVERSE EFFECTS

The dose-limiting toxicities of methotrexate are myelosuppression and gastrointestinal toxicity. Toxic doses of methotrexate can induce thrombocytopenia and/or leukopenia, although leukopenia is more common. An early indication of methotrexate toxicity to the gastrointestinal tract is oral mucositis, while more severe toxicity may be manifested by diarrhea and gastrointestinal bleeding. Less common toxic effects of methotrexate are skin rash (10%), pneumonitis, and chemical hepatitis. The latter is reversible in most patients, but low-dose chronic administration may lead to fibrosis and cirrhosis of the liver in a small percentage of patients.

Methotrexate given intrathecally in doses of 12 mg every 4 days is used to treat meningeal leukemia and lymphoma. Toxicities due to this route of administration include acute arachnoiditis with nuchal rigidity and headache, as well as more chronic CNS toxicities, including dementia, motor deficits, seizures, and coma.[28] Rarely these neurotoxicities develop hours after intrathecal drug administration, but more commonly they occur in the days or weeks after initiation of intrathecal treatment. Leucovorin is ineffective in reversing or preventing these toxicities. Patients exhibiting such signs should undergo evaluation to rule out progressive CNS leukemia or lymphoma, and if neither of these is present intrathecal cytosine arabinoside should be given instead of methotrexate.

CYTOSINE ARABINOSIDE (CYTARABINE)

Ara-C is an antimetabolite analog of cytidine differing in the configuration at the C_2' position of the sugar, with the C_2'-hydroxyl group being *cis*-oriented relative to the C_1'-N glycosyl bond, as opposed to the *trans* configuration of the ribose nucleoside. Ara-C is a mainstay in the induction of remission in patients with AML. When used with an anthracycline, remissions may be achieved in 60 to 80 percent of patients with this disease.

High doses (1–3 g/m^2) of ara-C given at 12-h intervals for 6 to 12 doses are more effective alone or in a combination with anthracyclines than conventional doses (100–150 mg/m^2 q 12 h) in consolidation therapy of AML, and they confer particular benefit in patients with cytogenetic abnormalities t(8:21), inv [16], t(9:16), and del (16) related to the core binding factor that regulates hematopoiesis.[29] Ara-C has also been used to treat ALL, lymphoma, and both the chronic and the blast phases of CML, but its exact role in the treatment of these malignancies is less well defined.

MECHANISM OF ACTION

Ara-C is converted to the nucleoside triphosphate (ara-CTP) intracellularly. Ara-CTP is an inhibitor of DNA polymerase and is also incorporated into DNA, where it terminates strand elongation.[30] Ara-C and its mononucleotide are inactivated by two intracellular enzymes, cytidine deaminase and deoxycytidylate deaminase respectively. The ara-U formed as a consequence of ara-C deamination is more slowly cleared from plasma than is ara-C and may inhibit subsequent inactivation of ara-C in high-dose regimens.

Acquired ara-C resistance in experimental leukemias consistently results from the loss of deoxycytidine kinase, the initial activating enzyme in the ara-C pathway.[31] Other changes implicated in experimental tumors include decreased drug uptake, increased deamination, increased pool size of competitive deoxycytidine triphosphate, and inhibition of the apoptotic pathway. Some of these changes have been reported in studies of human leukemia, but these results have not been confirmed in definitive trials.[18,31,32]

CLINICAL PHARMACOLOGY

Ara-C is administered intravenously either as a bolus injection or continuous infusion. It is not orally bioavailable due to degradation by cytidine deaminase present in the gastrointestinal epithelium and liver. Ara-C distributes rapidly throughout total body water and is eliminated from plasma with a biological half-life of 7 to 20 min. Most of the dose is excreted as ara-U, an inactive metabolite, which

is formed in plasma, the liver, granulocytes, and other tissues. Product inhibition of ara-C deamination by ara-U is believed to be responsible for the prolongation of the biological half-life of the drug as larger doses are administered.[33] Single bolus injections and short infusions (0.5- to 1-h duration) at doses as high as 5 g/m^2 produce little myelotoxicity because of the drug's rapid clearance, whereas continuous intravenous infusion of only 1g/m^2 over 48 h produces severe marrow toxicity. Unlike most drugs, a relatively high concentration of ara-C is achieved in the cerebrospinal fluid after intravenous administration, which may approach 50 percent of the corresponding concentration in plasma.

Ara-C is also used intrathecally to treat meningeal leukemia. Doses of 70 mg in adults are usually employed and afford cerebrospinal fluid levels of the drug near 1.0 mM, which decline with a half-life of 2 h. Ara-C has been impregnated into a gel matrix for sustained release into the cerebrospinal fluid, thus avoiding the need for repeated spinal taps. Initial clinical results in spinal lymphomatous meningitis resistant to methotrexate is promising.[34]

ADVERSE EFFECTS

The dose-limiting toxicity for conventional dosing regimens of ara-C, 100 to 150 mg/m^2 per day for 5 to 10 days, is myelosuppression. Some nausea and vomiting also occur at these doses, the severity of which increases markedly when higher doses are employed, although repeated administration of the drug results in some tolerance. The nadir of the white count and platelet count occurs at about day 7 to 10 after the last dose of drug. Neurologic, gastrointestinal, and liver toxicity have also been observed when high-dose regimens are used. Hepatotoxicity ranges from abnormalities in serum transaminase levels to frank jaundice. The severity of these effects increases as the duration of therapy is prolonged; however, toxic effects rapidly subside upon discontinuation of treatment. Pulmonary infiltrates due to noncardiogenic pulmonary edema are frequently observed in leukemic patients receiving ara-C, as are gastrointestinal ulcerations with bleeding and infrequently perforation. Ara-C treatment is also reported to predispose to *Streptococcus viridans* pneumonia.[35]

In patients over 50 years of age, high-dose ara-C (3 g/m^2 q12 h) causes cerebellar toxicity, manifested as ataxia and slurred speech.[36] Confusion and dementia may supervene, leading to a fatal outcome. Cerebellar toxicity is more frequent in patients with abnormal renal function, despite the fact that the drug is primarily eliminated by metabolism, not by renal excretion, and is thought to result from slowed elimination of ara-U, with consequent inhibition of ara-C deamination. Intrathecal ara-C is usually well tolerated, but neurologic side effects have been reported (seizures, alterations in mental status).

5-AZACYTIDINE

The only riboside nucleoside to attract clinical interest, 5-azacytidine, exhibits cytotoxic activity and also induces differentiation of malignant cells at low doses. The latter action is believed to result from an inhibition of methylation of cytosine bases in DNA, leading to enhanced transcription of otherwise silent genes. The differentiating effects of 5-azacytidine are the basis for its experimental use in the induction of fetal hemoglobin synthesis in patients with sickle cell anemia and thalassemia[37] and in low-dose therapy of myelodysplastic syndromes. The usual doses administered are 150 to 200 mg/m^2 per day for 5 days.

5-Azacytidine is rapidly deaminated, affording a chemically unstable metabolite which immediately degrades into inactive products.[38] Pharmacologic activity results from phosphorylation of the parent compound by cytidine kinase, with subsequent conversion to a triphosphate nucleotide that becomes incorporated into RNA and DNA. The precise mechanism of cytotoxicity has not been defined. The primary clinical toxicities include reversible myelosuppression, rather severe nausea and vomiting, hepatic dysfunction, myalgias, and fever and rash.

PURINE ANALOGS

Purine analogs have won an important role in remission induction and maintenance for ALL, and in the past decade new analogs have shown remarkable activity in chronic leukemias and small cell lymphomas. With methotrexate, 6-mercaptopurine (6-MP) is a critical component in the maintenance phase of curative therapy of childhood ALL. Other clinically useful purine analogs include azathioprine, a 6-MP precursor and potent immunosuppressive agent; allopurinol, an inhibitor of xanthine oxidase, useful in the prevention of uric acid nephropathy; 2-chlorodeoxyadenosine, effective in the treatment of hairy cell leukemia and other lymphoid malignancies; 6-thioguanine (6-TG), an antileukemic agent; fludarabine-phosphate (2-fluoro-ara-adenosine monophosphate), an effective agent for chronic lymphocytic leukemia; and antiviral compounds such as ara-A (vidarabine). Deoxycoformycin, a potent inhibitor of adenosine deaminase, is effective in the treatment of T-cell malignancies and hairy cell leukemia.

MECHANISM OF ACTION OF 6-THIOPURINES

Both 6-MP and 6-TG have a thiol group substituted for the 6-oxo or 6-hydroxy group of hypoxanthine or guanine, respectively. Both compounds are converted to nucleotides by the enzyme HPRT. The exact mechanism whereby these analogs exert their cytotoxic effects is not known.[39] De novo purine synthesis is blocked by the 6-TG nucleotide, as is the conversion of inosine monophosphate to adenosine and guanosine monophosphates.[40] The nucleotides of both 6-MP and 6-TG are incorporated into DNA. Thiopurines incorporated into DNA are recognized by the mismatch repair system, triggering apoptosis.[16] Cell death correlates with the extent of their incorporation into DNA.

In experimental tumor cells, resistance is most commonly due to decreased activity of HPRT.[41] In human ALL, resistance has also been ascribed to an increase in activity of membrane alkaline phosphatase capable of degrading the nucleotides.[42] Absence of HPRT activity is an uncommon cause of resistance in human AML; an alteration of this enzyme leading to decreased thiopurine binding is present in the blast cells of some patients. Resistance may also be mediated by methylation of the thiol group by 5-thiopurine methyl transferase.[40,43] Low levels of red blood cell thiopurine nucleotides correlate with a high risk of clinical relapse in patients with ALL.[44]

Methotrexate and 6-MP are highly synergistic, possibly because methotrexate blocks the de novo synthesis of purines and enhances the utilization of preformed purines and purine analogs such as 6-MP.

CLINICAL PHARMACOLOGY OF 6-THIOPURINES

Both 6-TG and 6-MP are given orally at doses of 50 to 100 mg/m² per day. Oral absorption of 6-MP is erratic, as only 16 to 50 percent of an oral dose is systemically available.[45] Food and antibiotics may decrease absorption. 6-MP is inactivated by metabolism to 6-thiouric acid, a reaction catalyzed by xanthine oxidase. Allopurinol inhibits the metabolism of 6-MP but not of 6-TG. Therefore, it is generally recommended that dosages of 6-MP must be reduced by 75 percent in patients receiving allopurinol. 6-TG is inactivated primarily by S-methylation, followed by oxidation and desulfuration. Dose reduction is not necessary when 6-TG and allopurinol are administered together.

ADVERSE EFFECTS OF 6-THIOPURINES

The two drugs, 6-TG and 6-MP, are equally myelotoxic, with marrow toxicity following the pattern typical of cytotoxic drugs, producing nadirs of white blood cells and platelets at 7 to 10 days after treat

ment. Moderate nausea and vomiting may also be observed. Mild but rapidly reversible hepatotoxicity may be experienced by patients after treatment with either compound. Cirrhosis has occurred in some children with leukemia receiving long-term therapy with 6-MP. Thiopurine methyl transferase, which inactivates 6-thiopurines, occurs in several polymorphic forms that fail to metabolize the analogs. About 10 percent of the Caucasian population are heterozygous for ineffective polymorphic forms of the enzyme and have increased sensitivity to thiopurines, while 1 in 300 patients is homozygous for the inactive forms and at risk for overwhelming toxicity. Thiopurine nucleotide levels in lymphoblasts and in red cells are inversely related to enzyme activity.[46]

FLUDARABINE PHOSPHATE

Originally synthesized as a deamination-resistant analog of adenosine, fludarabine phosphate has outstanding activity in CLL.[47] It is strongly immunosuppressive, like the other purine analogs, and has potential use in nonmyeloablative allogeneic bone marrow transplantation[48] and in the treatment of collagen vascular diseases.

The pharmacology of fludarabine requires dephosphorylation to allow cellular uptake, and then intracellular phosphorylation. Fludarabine phosphate undergoes rapid dephosphorylation in plasma to the nucleoside fludarabine, which readily enters cells, and is restored intracellularly to the monophosphate level by deoxycytidine kinase. The triphosphate inhibits DNA polymerase and becomes incorporated into DNA and into RNA.[49] Its mechanism of cytotoxicity is believed to result from DNA chain termination and induction of apoptosis.[50,51]

The drug is available in the United States as an intravenous preparation, although in Europe it can be given orally. It has 60 to 80 percent bioavailability. Because it is resistant to adenosine deaminase, fludarabine is eliminated primarily by renal excretion, although specific guidelines for dose reduction in patients with compromised renal function have not been established. In CLL, the recommended doses are 20 to 30 mg/m² per day for 5 days given as 2-h infusions and repeated every 4 weeks. When administered at these doses, fludarabine causes only moderate myelosuppression. In CLL patients its antileukemic effect will lead to a progressive but relatively slow improvement in marrow function over a period of 2 to 3 cycles of treatment, with a median time to disease progression of 31 months.[47] However, the drug also exerts cytotoxic effects against both B and T lymphocytes, lowering CD4 T-cell counts to 150 to 200 cells per mm³ and predisposing patients to opportunistic infection. In patients with a large tumor burden, rapid tumor lysis may rarely lead to hyperuricemia, renal failure, and hypocalcemia (tumor lysis syndrome).[52] Thus, patients should be well hydrated and their urine alkalinized prior to beginning therapy. Peripheral sensory and motor neuropathy may occur during standard-dose therapy; and rare episodes of hemolytic anemia with both warm and cold antibodies have been reported.[53] At higher doses (125 mg/m² per day for 5 days) altered mental status, seizures, coma, and optic neuritis have been reported.

2-CHLORODEOXYADENOSINE (CLADRIBINE)

The extreme sensitivity of normal and malignant lymphocytes to deamination-resistant purine analogs is further exemplified by the potent activity of 2-CdA in hairy cell leukemia, chronic lymphocytic leukemia, and low-grade lymphomas.[54,55] A single course of 2-CdA, typically 0.09 mg/kg per day for 7 days by continuous intravenous infusion, induces complete response in 80 percent of patients with hairy cell leukemia, with partial responses in the remainder. Administration by subcutaneous injection or by 2-h intravenous infusions for 5 days to the same total dose achieves similar results. The drug has much the same intracellular fate as fludarabine, undergoing phosphorylation by deoxycytidine kinase and further conversion to a triphosphate that becomes incorporated into DNA. The triphosphate of 2-CdA has a very long intracellular half-life of 9.7 h in CLL cells isolated from patients treated with the drug.[56] The triphosphate also accumulates in mitochondria, disrupting oxidative phosphorylation, and inhibits ribonucleotide reductase and depletes NAD levels in tumor cells. All of these actions might help explain the drug's toxicity to slowly dividing lymphoid malignancies such as hairy cell leukemia and CLL. The actual mechanisms by which 2-CdA induces DNA strand breaks are not completely understood. However, similar to fludarabine, it inhibits DNA chain extension and daughter strand synthesis.[57] Furthermore, the drug induces apoptosis (programmed cell death) in some cell lines.[58]

2-CdA is eliminated primarily by renal excretion, with a terminal plasma half-life of 21 h. 2-CdA retains effectiveness in at least a fraction of hairy cell leukemia patients resistant to deoxycoformycin or fludarabine, although clinical experience with sequential use of these drugs is limited. Toxicities of 2-CdA include transient myelosuppression, fever, and occasional infections possibly related to immunosuppression. The development of cumulative thrombocytopenia during treatment with repeated courses of the drug may limit its use.

2-DEOXYCOFORMYCIN (PENTOSTATIN)

DCF contains a unique 7-carbon primary ring system that closely resembles the transition-state intermediate of the adenosine deaminase reaction. As such, DCF is a potent inhibitor of the enzyme, leading to accumulation of intracellular adenosine and deoxyadenosine nucleotides.[59] In addition, the triphosphate of DCF is incorporated into DNA. The imbalance in purine nucleotide pools produced by DCF probably accounts for its cytotoxicity.

Although initial trials of DCF demonstrated striking renal and neurologic toxicities at doses of 10 mg/m^2 per day or greater, lower doses (4 mg/m^2 biweekly) have proven to be extremely effective in inducing pathologically confirmed complete responses in hairy cell leukemia. At this lower dose, severe depletion of normal T cells occurs and may predispose to opportunistic infection.[60] The optimal dose may be lower than 4 mg/m^2 biweekly. The drug is eliminated entirely by renal excretion, necessitating proportional dose reduction in patients with reduced creatinine clearance.

HYDROXYUREA

Hydroxyurea inhibits ribonucleotide reductase, the enzyme that converts ribonucleotide diphosphates to deoxyribonucleotides. Hydroxyurea is most commonly used in the treatment of polycythemia vera and the chronic phase of CML and to lower the leukocyte count rapidly during blast crisis of CML. Resistance to hydroxyurea occurs in experimental tumors as a consequence of an increase in ribonucleotide reductase activity, or through mutations that produce an enzyme that binds the drug with decreased affinity.

CLINICAL PHARMACOLOGY
Hydroxyurea is usually administered orally and is well absorbed, even when large doses such as 50 to 75 mg/kg are given. Peak plasma levels following oral administration are achieved at about 1 h and decline rapidly thereafter. Renal excretion is the major route of drug elimination.

ADVERSE EFFECTS
The major toxicities of hydroxyurea are leukopenia and the induction of megaloblastic changes. Except for nausea, little other toxicity has been observed with this drug, even when large doses are administered.

Hydroxyurea, like cytosine arabinoside, is an S phase–specific agent. Accordingly, single large doses effect little toxicity other than myelosuppression. The nadir of the leukocyte count occurs 6 to 7 days after a single dose of drug, and the leukocyte count recovers rapidly. When hydroxyurea is used as therapy for essential thrombocythemia, there may be an increase in the incidence of acute myelogenous leukemia.[134] The agent is also used in nonmalignant disorders, notably sickle cell anemia (see Chap. 47).

THE VINCA ALKALOIDS

Among the three vinca alkaloids that have been extensively evaluated during the past three decades—vinblastine, vincristine, and vindesine—only the first two are now available commercially in the United States. Both of these drugs are used widely in the treatment of hematologic neoplasms; vinblastine because of its excellent activity in the treatment of Hodgkin disease and testicular cancer, and vincristine in lymphomas, breast cancer and childhood leukemia, and other solid tumors. Another drug belonging to this class of compounds, Navelbine, is used primarily for the treatment of breast and lung cancers.

MECHANISM OF ACTION
The vinca alkaloids exert their cytotoxic action by binding to tubulin, a protein found in the cytoplasm of cells. Microtubules, assembled through polymerization of tubulin dimers, form the spindle along which the chromosomes migrate during mitosis and maintain cell structure. Binding of the vinca alkaloids to tubulin leads to inhibition of the process of assembly of the mitotic spindle,[61] arresting cells in metaphase and inducing apoptosis. Resistance to the vinca alkaloids may be acquired through the development of the MDR phenotype,[12] which causes increased efflux of the drugs from the resistant cells. Alternatively, resistant cells may contain mutant tubulin with decreased avidity of vinca binding.[62] The clinical significance of these resistance mechanisms, however, is still unproven.

CLINICAL PHARMACOLOGY
Vincristine and vinblastine are both administered by the intravenous route. The average single dose of vincristine is 1.4 mg/m^2 and that of vinblastine 8 to 9 mg/m^2. Sequential doses of the drugs are usually given at 2- to 4-week intervals. These doses provide peak plasma drug concentrations of approximately 1 μM. The plasma concentration–time profile of vincristine is characterized by a very rapid initial disposition phase followed by two slower phases of decay, with half-lives of 3 h and 23 to 85 h. In comparison, the intermediate and terminal disposition phases of vinblastine have half-lives of 1 h and 20 h respectively. Almost 70 percent of a dose of vincristine is metabolized by the liver and excreted in the feces. Metabolism is also the major route of inactivation of vinblastine, but details are lacking with respect to the site of metabolism and the identity of metabolic products. Accordingly, the dose of vincristine or vinblastine should be reduced in patients with hepatic impairment. While specific guidelines for dose reduction have not been completely developed, a 50 percent decrease in dose is recommended for patients presenting with a bilirubin greater than 3 mg/dL. Dose reduction is not necessary for patients with impaired renal function, as very little intact drug is excreted in urine.

ADVERSE EFFECTS
The dose-limiting side effect of vincristine is neurotoxicity, which usually occurs when the total dose received exceeds 6 mg/m^2. The initial signs of neurotoxicity are paresthesia of the fingers and lower extremities and loss of deep-tendon reflexes. Continued administration may lead to profound loss of motor strength, such as weakness of dorsiflexion of the foot and extension of the wrists. Elderly patients

are particularly susceptible to such toxicities. Occasionally cranial nerve palsies may lead to vocal chord paralysis or diplopia, and severe jaw pain may result from vincristine administration. At high doses of vincristine (>3 mg total single dose), autonomic neuropathy may cause obstipation and paralytic ileus. Sensory changes and reflex abnormalities slowly improve when the drug is discontinued; however, motor impairment improves less rapidly and may be irreversible. Inappropriate ADH release, resulting in symptomatic dilutional hyponatremia is sometimes observed.

While marrow suppression is not common with vincristine administration, some marrow toxicity may be noted in patients with impaired marrow function as a consequence of prior treatment with other drugs. The primary toxicity of vinblastine is leukopenia. The white count reaches a nadir at day 7 and reverses rapidly thereafter. Mucositis may result from higher doses (>8 mg/m²) of vinblastine or when it is used in combination with other cytotoxic drugs. Neurotoxicity is rare, but ileus may occur at high doses.

Both drugs cause severe pain and local toxicity if extravasated. Neither drug should be given intrathecally, since deaths have been reported from vincristine administered inadvertently into the cerebrospinal fluid.

TAXANES

The newest of the antimitotic drugs are the taxanes, paclitaxel (Taxol) and docetaxel (Taxotere). Paclitaxel was purified from an extract of the bark of *Taxus brevifolia,* while docetaxel is a closely related semisynthetic derivative. Neither drug has won an important role in the treatment of hematological malignancies, although paclitaxel has modest activity in the lymphomas.[63] Taxanes are highly active in a number of solid tumors, including breast, ovarian, and lung cancers. They bind to the β-tubulin subunit of microtubules and promote the polymerization of microtubules, leading to disordered mitotic spindle formation and a block in the progression through mitosis.[64] Both drugs induce apoptosis in tumor cells irrespective of p53 status of the cells and kill cells at 1 to 10 nM concentrations in cell culture in a time-dependent manner.[65,66] The taxanes are subject to MDR mediated by the *mdr* and *mrp* genes, and also β-tubulin mutations. Because they are highly insoluble in aqueous solution, both drugs are formulated in lipid-based solvents that cause occasional hypersensitivity reactions. Thus, paclitaxel is given after pretreatment with antihistamines (cimetidine and Benadryl) and Decadron. Both drugs are cleared primarily by hepatic CYP metabolism, with terminal plasma half-lives of 10 to 13 h. Their metabolism is stimulated by Dilantin and other CYP-inducing drugs and inhibited by CYP substrates such as ketoconazole. Their major toxicities, aside from hypersensitivity, are a sharp but brief leukopenia, milder thrombocytopenia, and mucositis. High-dose or repeated cycles of the taxanes cause a sensory and motor peripheral neuropathy that is reversible with drug discontinuation. Occasional patients have experienced atrial conduction block or atrial or ventricular arrhythmias after paclitaxel administration, and the combination of paclitaxel with doxorubicin may produce a greater incidence of congestive heart failure than seen with doxorubicin alone.[67] A syndrome of progressive fluid retention and peripheral edema occurs in patients receiving multiple cycles of docetaxel and can be at least partially prevented by pretreatment with corticosteroids.[68]

CAMPTOTHECINS

This group of compounds includes synthetic derivatives of 20 (*S*)-camptothecin, a naturally occurring compound initially isolated from the *Camptotheca accuminata* bush. The campothecins interact with a unique target, topoisomerase I, stabilizing the enzyme's complex with

DNA and preventing the resealing of DNA single-strand breaks induced by the enzyme. Resistance arises through mutation, deletion, or decreased expression of the topoisomerase I gene. The primary agents in clinical use are irinotecan, which is approved for treatment of colon cancer, and topotecan, approved for use against ovarian cancer and small cell lung cancer. Irinotecan, most commonly administered intravenously at a dose of 125 mg/m², once each week for 4 weeks every 42 days, has shown promise against lymphomas in phase II trials, but has received limited evaluation in the United States for this indication.[69] In contrast, topotecan has impressive remission-inducing activity in patients with myelodysplasia and chronic myelomonocytic leukemia, both as a single agent (1.5 mg/m²/day for 5 days) and in combination with ara-C.[70] The two drugs differ substantially in their profile of toxicities and pharmacokinetic behavior. Irinotecan is a water-soluble prodrug which affords the active species, SN-38, by carboxyl esterase–mediated cleavage of the basic promoiety. SN-38 and its parent drug are eliminated by biliary excretion, either directly as in the case of the parent drug or upon glucuronidation of the active metabolite SN-38. Therefore, irinotecan must be used with caution and at lower doses in patients with Gilbert disease or hepatic dysfunction.[71] Approximately two-thirds of the dose of topotecan is eliminated by renal excretion, with the remainder being cleared by biliary excretion. Dose adjustment proportional to creatinine clearance is indicated in patients with renal failure.[72] Topotecan toxicity consists mainly of myelosuppression, and to a lesser degree mucositis, while irinotecan causes a profound diarrhea that is responsive to loperamide, and a more modest myelosuppression.

ANTHRACYCLINE ANTIBIOTICS

The anthracyclines in general clinical use are doxorubicin, daunorubicin, and idarubicin, and in Europe, epirubicin. Mitoxantrone (Novantrone), a closely related anthracenedione, has very similar pharmacologic properties. The anthracyclines are produced by a *Streptomyces* species, while mitoxantrone is a synthetic compound not containing a sugar moiety. Doxorubicin (Adriamycin) has a broad spectrum of activity against neoplastic disease; it is an important drug in the treatment of hematological malignancies, especially Hodgkin disease and the other lymphomas. Daunorubicin (daunomycin) and idarubicin are used almost exclusively in combination with ara-C for the treatment of AML. Mitoxantrone is employed for the treatment of AML and breast cancer.

MECHANISM OF ACTION

These drugs exert their effects by forming a complex with DNA and topoisomerase II, leading to double-stranded DNA strand breaks. The various anthracycline analogs differ in their specificity for binding to DNA base sequences.[73] To varying degrees they also generate free radicals through oxidation-reduction cycling of their quinone groups, an action that may contribute to their cardiac toxicity. The anthracyclines enter cells through a passive transport process and are pumped out by both the MRP protein and the P-glycoprotein transport system.[12] Other mechanisms for anthracycline resistance include decreased or altered topoisomerase II activity.

CLINICAL PHARMACOLOGY

Doxorubicin and daunorubicin are converted to active hydroxyl metabolites, and thereafter to a spectrum of inactive products in the liver. Only a minor fraction of the dose is excreted in the urine as the parent drug or active metabolite. The pharmacokinetics of the clinically useful anthracyclines are predominantly influenced by their terminal disposition phases, which exceed 10 h. While prolongation of the half-life of doxorubicin has been reported in studies of patients with compromised liver function, no clear correlations with toxicity have been established. Idarubicin is the only anthracycline that exhibits reasonable oral bioavailability, being 20 percent for the parent drug and 40 percent for parent plus idarubicinol, the primary active metabolite.[74] Idarubicinol has a very prolonged biological half-life, ranging from 50 to 60 h, and is likely responsible for the antitumor activity of this drug. In contrast to doxorubicin and daunorubicin, it is eliminated significantly by renal excretion. Mitoxantrone has a brief initial plasma half-life of 1.1 h and a considerably longer terminal half-life of 23 to 42 h. Only a minor fraction of unchanged drug is excreted in the urine ($<10\%$) or stool ($<20\%$). The majority of the drug is probably metabolized or bound to tissues. Patients with impaired hepatic function may have a more prolonged elimination of mitoxantrone.

The usual dose of doxorubicin when administered as a single agent by bolus intravenous injection is 60 to 75 mg/m^2 every 3 to 4 weeks. Less cardiac toxicity may result from schedules that avoid high peak plasma concentrations, such as weekly doses (15–25 mg/m^2) or continuous intravenous infusion over 48 to 96 h. When given in combination with other myelotoxic agents such as cyclophosphamide, the dose of doxorubicin is usually decreased by one-third to one-half. Although daunorubicin has been used as the anthracycline of choice in the treatment of AML, usually in combination with ara-C, doxorubicin and mitoxantrone and idarubicin may be equally effective.

ADVERSE EFFECTS

Myelosuppression is the primary toxicity of this class of drugs, with a nadir occurring 7 to 10 days after single-dose administration and recovery by 2 weeks. Mitoxantrone produces less nausea and vomiting than does daunorubicin or doxorubicin. Doxorubicin may cause mucositis, especially when used in maximally tolerated divided doses given over 2 to 3 days or when used in combination with other drugs that cause mucositis. These drugs may also cause a reaction in previously irradiated tissues, especially when the drug is administered just prior to or in the weeks following irradiation. Alopecia often occurs. Extravasation of these drugs results in tissue necrosis.

Cardiac toxicity is a major toxic effect of doxorubicin and daunorubicin.[75] Cardiac toxicity appears to be mediated by free radical formation catalyzed by the quinone function of the anthracycline nucleus and can be averted by free radical–scavenging agents (sulfhydryl compounds) or by iron chelators such as dexrazoxane (ICRF-187).[76] It is not known whether these modulators affect antitumor activity. Both acute effects, manifested by arrhythmias and conduction abnormalities and a "pericarditis-myocarditis syndrome," and chronic congestive heart failure may occur. Ejection fraction measurements have been helpful as a noninvasive technique to demonstrate a decline in myocardial function and a rising risk of myocardial failure with increasing doses. Anthracycline therapy should be discontinued when the ejection fraction falls below 40 percent. Most patients will tolerate total doses of 450 to 550 mg/m^2 doxorubicin or daunorubicin before the risk of cardiac damage exceeds 5 percent.[77] There is a high risk of cardiac damage at lower cumulative doses in patients receiving mantle irradiation. Once clinically overt cardiac toxicity occurs, usually manifested by congestive heart failure, the mortality rate is high. Congestive heart failure usually occurs during therapy or less than 1 month following cessation of treatment; rarely, heart failure may occur many months later or may be elicited by a second drug, such as mitoxantrone or mitomycin C. Children treated with anthracyclines may show abnormal cardiac development and late congestive heart failure in their teenage years.[78] Those who receive greater than 300 mg/m^2 demonstrate decreased myocardial contractility and increased ventricular dimension when tested years later,[79] thus leading to the recommendation that total anthracycline dose be limited to no more than 300 mg/m^2 in children. Low-dose schedules cause less cardiac

toxicity. Treatment with idarubicin or mitoxantrone is associated with a lower risk of cardiac toxicity, but the data are less complete for these newer agents.

EPIPODOPHYLLOTOXINS

Two semisynthetic derivatives of podophyllotoxin, VP-16 (etoposide) and VM-26 (teniposide), have significant clinical activity in hematologic malignancies. Etoposide has been incorporated into combination therapy regimens for Hodgkin disease, diffuse aggressive lymphomas, and leukemias and is frequently used as a component of high-dose chemotherapy regimens. Teniposide has been used investigationally to treat various forms of childhood acute leukemia and appears to be synergistic with ara-C.[80]

These compounds induce double-stranded breaks in DNA through their sequence-specific binding to DNA in complex with topoisomerase II, a DNA repair enzyme.[81] One mechanism of resistance is increased expression of the MDR phenotype (12). A second mechanism results from decreased topoisomerase II activity or mutation of the enzyme, resulting in decreased drug binding.[82,83]

CLINICAL PHARMACOLOGY

Etoposide has excellent oral bioavailability and may be administered either orally or intravenously. The usual intravenous dose schedule used for etoposide is 100 to 120 mg/m^2 per day for 3 days, either consecutively or every other day. When administered orally, the dose should be increased twofold over the intravenous dose, since 50 to 67 percent of the dose is absorbed. Approximately 30 to 40 percent of an intravenous dose of etoposide is excreted intact in the urine; thus, doses of etoposide require modification for patients with compromised renal function but not hepatic dysfunction.[84] The biological half-life of etoposide is 15 h. The clinical activity of etoposide is highly schedule dependent. Single conventional doses are essentially without antitumor effect as compared to consecutive daily doses for 3 to 5 days. The oral administration of 50 mg per day for 2 to 3 weeks is a commonly used regimen that takes advantage of that schedule dependency.

The pharmacokinetics of teniposide are very similar to those of etoposide, with a terminal plasma half-life of 20 to 48 h. However, little parent drug appears intact in the urine, and dose modification for patients with renal dysfunction is unnecessary.

ADVERSE EFFECTS

When administered intravenously, both etoposide and teniposide should be infused over a 30-min period to avoid hypotensive episodes. The major toxicity of both drugs is leukopenia, which is rapidly reversible. Thrombocytopenia is less common. Nausea and vomiting often follow etoposide administration. Alopecia may occur with both drugs. Other toxicities, such as fever, mild elevation of liver function tests, or peripheral neuropathy, are relatively uncommon. Because the major toxicity of etoposide is limited to the marrow, this drug is under intensive investigation as a component of high-dose regimens followed by marrow transplantation. In high-dose etoposide protocols (3 to 4 g/m^2 given over 3 to 5 days) oropharyngeal mucositis becomes a prominent toxicity. Less frequent high-dose toxicities include hepatocellular damage and rarely anaphylactic-like symptoms, probably related to the Cremophor-based vehicle. Reports of secondary acute myeloid leukemia following etoposide treatment in children with ALL[85] and in adults with testicular cancer have alerted clinicians to this potential complication.[86]

BLEOMYCIN

Bleomycin is a mixture of peptides produced by the fungus *Streptomyces verticillis*.[87] Because it has antitumor effects with little or no marrow toxicity, it is commonly used as part of combination regimens (ABVD) to treat Hodgkin disease, the aggressive lymphomas, and germ cell tumors. Bleomycin acts by causing both single- and double-strand breaks in DNA. These breaks form as a consequence of a bleomycin:Fe(II) complex with DNA leading to proton abstraction from the deoxyribose and cleavage at the 4'-carbon.[88–90] In experimental tumors, resistance to bleomycin has been attributed to increased concentrations of an aminohydrolase that cleaves and inactivates the drug.[91] Some resistant cell lines exhibit enhanced capacity to repair strand breaks, and in others resistance results from decreased drug accumulation. Additional factors, such as increased free radical detoxification may also influence toxicity. The tumor specificity of this drug and the lack of toxicity of bleomycin to marrow and the gastrointestinal tract may be due to different levels of a bleomycin-inactivating enzyme in these tissues. The aminohydrolase is found in low concentrations in the lung and skin, a possible explanation for the susceptibility of these two normal organs to damage by this drug. Cell killing occurs throughout the cell cycle.

CLINICAL PHARMACOLOGY

Bleomycin may be administered intravenously or intramuscularly for systemic therapy, as well as intrapleurally or intraperitoneally for control of malignant effusions. The half-life of drug elimination from plasma has been estimated to be 2 to 3 h. After a single intravenous injection, over half the dose is excreted in the urine during 24 h.[92] Bleomycin elimination may be markedly impaired in patients with poor renal function; such patients are at risk of overwhelming skin and lung toxicity. Dose reduction proportional to creatinine clearance should be considered in these patients.

ADVERSE EFFECTS

Bleomycin has few or no effects on normal marrow; however, in patients given other myelosuppressive drugs or recovering from marrow toxicity from these agents, additional mild myelosuppression may be observed. The primary toxicities that result from bleomycin are pulmonary fibrosis and skin changes. In experimental settings, the drug induces the secretion of numerous cytokines, including IL-6 and TGB-β, by alveolar macrophages, leading to collagen deposition.[93] The risk of pulmonary toxicity is related to the cumulative dose administered, increasing to 10 percent in patients given more than 450 mg.[94] Risk is also greater in patients over the age of 70, in patients with underlying lung disease, in patients receiving bleomycin who are given high oxygen concentrations, or in patients who have had previous radiotherapy to the lungs. Single doses of 25 mg/m^2 or more are more likely to predispose to this toxic effect. Symptoms of pulmonary toxicity include cough and dyspnea. Chest x-rays show nonspecific infiltrates, especially in the lower lobes. Open lung biopsy may be required to distinguish bleomycin pulmonary toxicity from infection or malignant disease. Findings of bleomycin toxicity include an inflammatory alveolar infiltrate with edema, pulmonary hyaline formation, and squamous metaplasia of the alveolar lining cells. These changes progress to intraalveolar and interstitial fibrosis over a period of months. Patients with bleomycin lung toxicity have a defect in carbon monoxide diffusing capacity, a test of possible value in predicting potential pulmonary toxicity.[95] Since there is no specific therapy for patients with bleomycin lung toxicity, close attention should be paid to early pulmonary symptoms and radiographic changes. In patients with bleomycin pulmonary toxicity, some improvement may be seen on discontinuation of the drug, but the pulmonary fibrosis is usually not reversible. Glucocorticoids are of no proven benefit once fibrosis has occurred.

The dermatological toxicity of bleomycin is also dose related. Erythema, hyperpigmentation, hyperkeratosis, and even ulceration may occur when the drug is given in conventional daily doses for longer than 2 to 3 weeks. Areas of skin pressure, especially of the hands, fingers, and joints, are initially affected. Nail changes and alopecia may also occur with continued use of the drug. In combination regimens (e.g., ABVD) where bleomycin is used intermittently, skin toxicity usually does not occur.

Fever and malaise are common symptoms and may be alleviated with the use of acetaminophen. Hypersensitivity reactions have also been observed. Idiosyncratic cardiovascular collapse has been rarely noted. A 1-mg or 2-mg test dose administered to such susceptible patients may result in hypotension, tachycardia, pulmonary insufficiency, or anaphylactoid reactions within 30 to 60 min. Their occurrence precludes further treatment with bleomycin.

ASPARAGINASE

The enzyme L-asparaginase is used clinically in the treatment of lymphoid malignancies, in particular in poor-risk B-cell ALL, T-cell ALL, and the lymphomas.

MECHANISM OF ACTION

The cells causing these lymphoid malignancies require exogenous L-asparagine for growth, and they obtain this amino acid from the circulating pool of amino acids generated primarily by the liver. The enzyme L-asparaginase, which catalyzes the hydrolysis of asparagine to aspartic acid and ammonia, is capable of rapidly depleting the serum level of L-asparagine. This induces an asparagine deficiency in lymphoid malignant cells. Resistant tumors are able to respond by rapid induction of asparagine synthetase.[96] Resistance can be detected by in vitro incubation of leukemic cells with asparaginase.[97]

Three preparations of L-asparaginase are available for clinical use in the United States. The product purified from *Escherichia coli* is employed as a first-line agent, while a second preparation (pegaspargase), derived by attachment of polyethylene glycol to the *E. coli* enzyme, is primarily reserved for patients with hypersensitivity to the unmodified enzyme and has a longer half-life. A third preparation, purified from *Erwinia chrysanthemi*, can be obtained from the National Cancer Institute of the United States for patients hypersensitive to the *E. coli* enzyme. The enzyme from *E. coli* is primarily used in the clinical treatment of ALL and high-grade lymphomas. The various preparations differ in their pharmacokinetics and recommended doses.[98,99]

CLINICAL PHARMACOLOGY

L-Asparaginase is administered either intravenously or intramuscularly. Dose schedules commonly used are 6000 IU/m^2, or in European trials, 5000 to 10,000 IU/m^2 every third day for 3 to 4 weeks for the unmodified enzyme and 2500 IU every 2 weeks for the pegaspargase.[99,100] Blood levels of L-asparaginase are detectable for at least three days after a single dose is administered intravenously or intramuscularly. Blood and cerebrospinal fluid concentrations of L-asparagine fall below 1 μM within minutes after enzyme injection and begin to be measurable again 7 to 10 days after a single dose. The half-life of the unmodified *E. coli* enzyme in plasma is 14 to 24 h, while that of pegaspargase is fivefold to tenfold longer.

ADVERSE EFFECTS

Reactions to the first dose are uncommon, but after two or more doses of the drug, hypersensitivity may develop, varying from urticarial reactions to hypotension, laryngospasm, and cardiac arrest. Skin testing to predict allergic reactions is helpful in some but not all cases and should be performed to confirm a clinical suspicion of hypersensitivity. Hypersensitive patients may have antibodies to L-asparaginase in their plasma. However, more than half the patients with such circulating antibodies will not display an overt allergic reaction to the drug,[100] but they may have more rapid disappearance of drug from plasma and an inadequate clearance of asparagine from plasma and cells. Patients who are treated with L-asparaginase should be observed carefully for several hours after dosing, and epinephrine should be available in case anaphylactic reactions occur. Anaphylaxis is less likely when L-asparaginase is given intramuscularly than when it is administered by the intravenous route.

The other major toxic effects of L-asparaginase are due to the ability of this drug to inhibit protein synthesis in normal tissues.[101] Inhibition of protein synthesis in the liver will result in hypoalbuminemia, a decrease in clotting factors, a decrease in serum lipoproteins, and a marked increase in plasma triglycerides. Inhibition of insulin production may lead to hypoglycemia. The clotting abnormalities that are regularly observed as a consequence of L-asparaginase treatment include initial decreases in the anticoagulant factors antithrombin III, protein C, and protein S, leading to either arterial or venous thrombosis in occasional patients. With more prolonged therapy, bleeding sequelae may result from inhibition of the synthesis of procoagulant proteins such as fibrinogen and factors II, VII, IX, and X. Monitoring coagulation factors is therefore recommended. High doses of L-asparaginase may cause cerebral dysfunction manifested as confusion, stupor, and coma, and cortical sinus thrombosis has been documented by MRI scan in such patients.[102] Acute nonhemorrhagic pancreatitis occurs as a complication of L-asparaginase treatment, especially in patients who have extreme elevations of plasma triglycerides (>2 g/dL).[103]

USE IN COMBINATION CHEMOTHERAPY

Inasmuch as L-asparaginase manifests little toxicity in marrow or gastrointestinal mucosa, this drug has been used in combination with other drugs that do have such toxicities. It rescues normal marrow cells from methotrexate toxicity, perhaps through its inhibition of protein synthesis, and can be used to prevent myelosuppression if administered following high-dose methotrexate.[104] This combination has produced clinical responses in patients with acute leukemia refractory to conventional methotrexate doses.

AGENTS ACTIVE THROUGHOUT THE CELL CYCLE

THE ALKYLATING DRUGS

These drugs are important in the treatment of hematopoietic malignancies either as single agents or as components of combination regimens. Their role as treatment for both acute and chronic hematologic malignancies results from their lack of cell cycle specificity. In combination with cell cycle–specific agents they may eradicate noncycling cells that escape cycle-active components of the treatment. While these agents share the common property of forming covalent bonds with electron-rich sites on DNA (oxygen and nitrogen substituents), they exhibit important differences in their intrinsic reactivity, route of cellular uptake, favored sites of alkylation on DNA bases, and the specific mechanism of DNA repair that determines cell survival. These differences are borne out in experimental settings, where cross-resistance to alkylating agents is not complete. Thus, protocols employing multiple alkylators, particularly in high-dose regimens, have a rational basis.[105] Alkylating agents differ as well in their patterns of toxicity. The majority of these drugs cause myelosuppression and mucositis as their primary acute toxicities, as well as delayed pulmonary fibrosis and late secondary leukemias. They also cause vascular endothelial damage in occasional patients when used in high doses. However, cyclophosphamide and BCNU cause less mucositis in high-dose regimens, although cyclophosphamide rarely produces a hemorrhagic myocarditis.

4-Hydroperoxycyclophosphamide, an activated analog of cyclophosphamide, appears to spare marrow stem cells relative to tumor cells and is used for in vitro purging of marrow in autologous transplantation.[106]

MECHANISM OF ACTION

All alkylating agents have in common the generation of highly reactive carbonium intermediates that attack electron-rich sites on DNA, such as the N-7, O-2, and O-6 positions of guanine and the N-1, N-3, and N-7 positions of adenine. For many of these agents, the alkylating group must undergo a preliminary activation reaction mediated either by chemical rearrangement of the molecule, as in the case of nitrogen mustard and the nitrosoureas, or by metabolic activation followed by chemical rearrangement, as for cyclophosphamide, ifosfamide, and procarbazine. In some alkylating agents the reactive intermediate contains two reactive centers, usually chloroethyl groups, and therefore may cross-link opposing strands of DNA. Methylating agents produce only single-strand alkylation but may be highly carcinogenic, as, for example, procarbazine and dacarbazine. In general, the most commonly used drugs of this class, including cyclophosphamide, ifosfamide, melphalan, and chlorambucil, produce the same spectrum of myelosuppressive, carcinogenic, and genotoxic actions.

Mechanisms of resistance to alkylating agents that are unique to these compounds have been elucidated in experimental systems.[107] Some mechanisms are specific for certain alkylating agents (e.g., impaired uptake of nitrogen mustard as a consequence of an alteration in the membrane carrier for choline, or deletion of the amino acid carrier used by melphalan), while others appear to be less specific (e.g., drug inactivation associated with an increase in intracellular sulfhydryl compounds, and enhanced nucleotide excision-repair of DNA cross-links). The primary resistance mechanisms for various alkylating drugs, as documented in experimental tumors, include: increased degradation by aldehyde dehydrogenase (cyclophosphamide)[108]; increased conjugation of the reactive intermediates with glutathione or glutathione transferase (all chloroethylating agents and platinum analogs); increased repair of the O-6 guanine alkyl lesions by a specific alkyl transferase (nitrosoureas, procarbazine, dacarbazine)[109]; increased nucleotide excision repair (all platinum derivatives and chloroethylating agents, except nitrosoureas); decreased uptake (melphalan, nitrogen mustard); and decreased ability to recognize DNA damage (alkylating agents and platinum derivatives). The clinical basis of alkylating agent resistance is incompletely understood.

CLINICAL PHARMACOLOGY

In general, the alkylating agents and their reactive intermediates have short residence times in the systemic circulation and within cells. They are eliminated predominantly by hydrolysis, chemical or biochemical conjugation to the sulfhydryl groups of glutathione or proteins, or by oxidative metabolism; therefore, dose reduction is not required in patients with diminished renal function. Cyclophosphamide and ifosfamide are closely related molecules that undergo hepatic activation. Their active metabolites generate a highly toxic metabolite, acrolein, that is excreted in the urine.[110] In order to counteract toxicity to kidneys and bladder, mercaptoethane sulfonate (MESNA) is administered simultaneously in equivalent doses to patients receiving ifosfamide or high-dose cyclophosphamide. Nitrogen mustard is a highly reactive compound that may be administered topically, intravenously, or intrapleurally. It is a potent vesicant, and care must be taken in the mixing and administration of the drug. Extravasation may lead to severe tissue injury. The second-generation alkylating agents, which include cyclophosphamide, melphalan, busulfan, and chlorambucil, are more chemically stable and absorbed reasonably well when given orally.

TABLE 16-3 DOSE-LIMITING EXTRAMEDULLARY TOXICITIES OF SINGLE-AGENT CHEMOTHERAPY

DRUG	MAXIMUM TOLERATED DOSE, MG/M^2*	INCREASE OVER STANDARD DOSE†	MAJOR TOXICITIES‡
Cyclophosphamide	7000	7.0	Cardiac
Ifosfamide	16,000	2.7	Renal, CNS
Thiotepa§	1005	18.0	GI, CNS
Melphalan§	180	5.6	GI
Busulfan§	640	9.0	GI, hepatic
BCNU§	1050	5.3	Lung, hepatic
Cisplatin	200	2.0	Renal, neuropathy
Carboplatin§	2000	5.0	Hepatic, renal
Etoposide	3000	6.0	GI
Cytosine arabinoside	6000	10–30	Neurologic, mucositis

*Independent of hematopoietic toxicity.[112–118,133]
†This is an approximation because standard doses may vary.
‡All drugs listed in this table cause vascular endothelial damage and venoocclusive disease, as well as late secondary leukemias.
§With stem cell support.
NOTE: GI, gastrointestinal; CNS, central nervous system; PN, peripheral neuropathy; BCNU, bischloroethylnitrosourea.

ADVERSE EFFECTS

Marrow toxicity, which is cumulative and a function of total dose, is the most important toxic effect of these compounds. Other toxicities, including lung, cardiac, and endothelial damage, have been described above. Since alkylating agents all react with DNA, mutations and secondary leukemias are major long-term effects of these agents. This hazard appears to be related to the total dose administered. The monofunctional methylating agents (e.g., procarbazine) are especially potent in this regard and may have a major role in the increased incidence of secondary malignancies noted in patients who have been treated with chemotherapy. The dose-limiting toxicity of one of these drugs, dacarbazine, is nausea and vomiting rather than marrow suppression.

Nitrosoureas produce a characteristic delayed myelosuppression that reaches a nadir 4 to 6 weeks after administration. Busulfan, like the nitrosoureas, depletes stem cells and can cause profound marrow hypoplasia or permanent aplasia when administered over prolonged periods of time and must be used with caution. All alkylating agents, but particularly busulfan and the nitrosoureas, may produce pulmonary fibrosis. The nitrosoureas also cause nephrotoxicity, particularly after total doses of 1200 mg/m^2 BCNU or methylcyclohexylchloroethylnitrosourea.[111]

HIGH-DOSE ALKYLATING AGENT THERAPY

The development of marrow stem cell rescue techniques has made it clinically possible to administer doses of chemotherapy that would otherwise produce life-threatening aplasia. In order to be of benefit, however, high-dose therapy must employ agents that have a relatively steep dose–response relationship and must not have lethal extramedullary toxicity at high doses. Among the classes of cytotoxics, alkylators have a particularly favorable linear relationship between dose and cytotoxicity in experimental systems. Their hematopoietic toxicity is generally limiting within standard dose ranges, but other organ toxicities are infrequent until doses are increased manyfold, making them ideal candidates for high-dose regimens. When agents are administered with stem cell rescue, marrow toxicity ceases to be dose limiting and extramedullary toxic effects are seen. Depending on the agent and the toxicity profile, doses may only be escalated by as little as 2-fold, as seen with cisplatin because of renal toxicity, or to as high as 18-fold in the case of thiotepa (Table 16-3).[112–118] However, when agents are combined into a high-dose regimen, overlapping extramedullary toxicities of the agents must be considered in order to avoid serious new additive and/or synergistic toxicities (Table 16-4). Overlapping extramedullary toxicities (particularly the risk of pulmonary or hepatic

dysfunction or secondary leukemia) cannot be completely avoided, but rational drug selection can minimize the dose reductions of the individual agents, compared to their single-agent maximum tolerated dose, that are required to make a combination regimen safe. This is illustrated in Table 16-4, which shows the fraction of the single agent MTD that can be administered in combination with other drugs. As might be expected, this fraction is quite variable depending on the drug combinations, with the average fractional MTD used in combination ranging from 0.5 to 1. Depending on the regimen, significant gastrointestinal, pulmonary, hepatic, and/or renal toxicities are encountered and become dose limiting. For these reasons, high-dose regimens are safest in patients who are younger (<70 years) and who have had minimal prior chemotherapy and radiation therapy.

DIFFERENTIATING AGENTS

A variety of chemical agents have the ability to cause differentiation of malignant cells.[119] The most prominent of these are members of the vitamin A family (carotenes and retinoids), vitamin D and its analogs, phenylacetic acid, cytotoxic agents used in low concentrations (such as cytosine arabinoside and 5-azacytidine), and a broad chemical class known as polar-planar differentiation agents, of which hexamethylene bisacetamide (HMBA) is the most extensively studied.[120] In addition, biological agents such as the interferons and interleukins induce differentiation of both malignant and normal cells, but the role of differentiation in the anticancer action of these drugs in humans is uncertain, as they have multiple biological effects. Among the differentiating agents, the retinoids are the only drugs that have clearly identified therapeutic value in the treatment and prevention of cancer, although HMBA has produced interesting early results.

RETINOIDS

Two retinoids, 13-*cis*-retinoic acid (cRA) and all-*trans*-retinoic acid (tRA), are used clinically. cRA prevents the development of second malignancy in patients with head and neck cancer[121] and when used with interferon induces a 50 percent response rate in squamous carcinomas of the skin[122] and cervix,[123] while tRA induces complete responses in a high percentage of patients with APL.[124] This discussion will be confined to tRA, although other retinoids may find clinical utility in the treatment of hematologic disease in the future.

tRA acts through binding to a nuclear receptor formed by the heterodimerization of the RAR-α receptor and the retinoid X receptor. In APL, an abnormal fusion protein, composed of portions of the RAR-α receptor and a unique transcription factor (the *PML* gene product) results from the characteristic 15;17 chromosomal translocation found in this disease.[125] The basis for the transforming properties of this mutant protein and the reasons for the sensitivity of APL cells to the differentiating activity of retinoids undoubtedly relate to the disordered retinoid receptor status but are not understood. It is not known whether the fusion protein has physiologic activity, although a functional RAR-α receptor seems essential to the expression of the differentiating effects of tRA in leukemic cells. In experimental settings, resistance to tRA differentiating activity results from mutation in the *PML-RAR-α* fusion gene, indicating that the fusion gene product

TABLE 16-4   TOXICITIES AND DOSES OF HIGH-DOSE REGIMENS ADMINISTERED WITH STEM CELL SUPPORT

REGIMEN	DOSE, MG/M^2	FRACTION OF MTD* (AVERAGE)	MAJOR TOXICITIES	TUMOR TARGETS	REFERENCES
Cyclophosphamide	6000	0.86	GI, cardiac	Breast	134
Thiotepa	500	0.5			
Carboplatin	800	0.4			
		(0.59)			
Cyclophosphamide	6000	0.86	Lung, GI	Lymphomas	135
BCNU	300	0.29			
Etoposide	750	0.25			
		(0.47)			
Busulfan	640	1.0	Lung, GI, hepatic	Leukemia	136
Cyclophosphamide	8000	1.0		Lymphomas	
		(1.0)			
Ifosfamide	16,000	1.0	Renal, hepatic, GI	Lymphomas	137
Carboplatin	1800	0.9		Breast	
Etoposide	1500	0.5		Testicular	
		(0.8)			
Cyclophosphamide	5625	0.8	Cardiac, hepatic, renal	Breast	105
BCNU	600	0.57			
Cisplatin	164	0.82			
		(0.73)			
Cyclophosphamide	5250	0.75	GI, renal	Breast	138
Etoposide	1200	0.4			
Cisplatin	180	0.9			
		(0.68)			

*This is the fraction of the single-agent MTD (Table 16-3, Col. 2). Calculation based on Eder et al.[134]
ABBREVIATIONS: MTD, maximum tolerated dose; GI, gastrointestinal; BCNU, bischloroethylnitrosourea.

plays a role in retinoid responsiveness, and sensitivity can be restored by transfection of a functional *RAR-α* gene.[126]

tRA is administered to APL patients in doses of 45 mg/m^2 per day until complete remission is achieved and reaches peak serum levels of 300 ng/mL 1 to 2 h after administration.[127] It disappears from serum with a half-life of less than 1 h during the initial course of treatment, but its rate of clearance greatly accelerates with continued treatment, a factor that may contribute to resistance to tRA therapy. Induction of CYP-mediated metabolism is suspected to underlie this accelerated clearance.[128] The primary toxicities of tRA resemble those of other retinoids and vitamin A, specifically dry skin, cheilitis, mild and reversible hepatic dysfunction, bone tenderness and hyperostosis on x-ray, and occasional cases of pseudotumor cerebri; in addition, about 15 percent of patients with APL, particularly those with an initial white blood cell count greater than 5000 per mm^3, develop a syndrome of hyperleukocytosis, fever, and respiratory failure (the "retinoic acid syndrome").[129] Hyperleukocytosis results from a rapid increase in the number of mature leukemic cells in the blood and from the increased expression of integrins on the leukemic cell surface in response to tRA. In patients with white blood cell counts above 20 × 10^3 cells per μL (20 × 10^9 cells/liter), pleural and pericardial effusions and peripheral edema develop rapidly, and respiratory distress, cardiac failure, and renal insufficiency may lead to death. Anecdotal reports indicate that high-dose glucocorticoids may reverse these findings, which is mediated by leukocyte adhesion and clogging of small vessels and/or by cytokine release.[129] The early introduction of cytotoxic chemotherapy during remission induction, or the use of Decadron (10 mg twice daily for 3 or more days), may lower the incidence of the syndrome.[130]

ARSENIC TRIOXIDE

Arsenic had been used in the treatment of chronic myelogenous leukemia and other malignancies in the 1930s with little effect. It has reappeared as an effective therapy for promyelocytic leukemia when used in the form of arsenic trioxide (As_2O_3), which induces differentiation and apoptosis in APL cells[131] and produces remissions in most patients refractory to tRA and conventional chemotherapy. Remissions appeared in 2 to 3 months after beginning doses of 0.15 mg/kg/day for 25 days every 3 to 6 weeks, with evidence of leukemic cell differentiation and a progressive peripheral blood leukocytosis after 2 weeks of therapy.[132,133] No consistent side effects have been observed, although occasional patients complain of fatigue, dysesthesias, and lightheadedness. A maximum plasma concentration of 5.5 to 7.3 μM was achieved in the initial studies from China, and small amounts of drug are eliminated in the urine, the rest residing in tissues.[133]

REFERENCES

1. Goodman LS, Wintrobe MM, Dameshek W, et al: Nitrogen mustard therapy: Use of methylbis (B-chlorethyl) amino hydrochloride for Hodgkin's disease, lymphosarcoma, leukemia and certain allied and miscellaneous disorders. *JAMA* 132:126, 1946.
2. Farber S, Diamond LK, Mercer RD, et al: Temporary remissions in acute leukemia in children produced by folic acid antagonist, 4-aminopteroylglutamic acid (aminopterin). *N Engl J Med* 238:787, 1948.
3. Doney K, Fisher LD, Appelbaum FR, et al: Treatment of adult acute lymphoblastic leukemia with allogeneic bone marrow transplantation. Multivariate analysis of factors affecting acute graft-versus-host disease, relapse and relapse-free survival. *Bone Marrow Transplant* 7:453, 1991.
4. Hartwell L: Defects in a cell cycle checkpoint may be responsible for the genomic instability of cancer cells. *Cell* 71:543, 1992.
5. Boral A, Dessain S, Chabner B: Clinical evaluation of biologically targeted drugs: obstacles and opportunities. *Cancer Chemother Pharmacol* 42(suppl):S3, 1998.
6. Vokes EE, Schilsky RL, Weichselbaum RR, et al: Induction chemotherapy with cisplatin, fluorouracil, and high-dose leucovorin for locally advanced head and neck cancer: A clinical and pharmacologic analysis. *J Clin Oncol* 8:241, 1990.
7. Seitz JF, Giovanni M, Padaut-Cesana J, Fuentes C: Inoperable nonmetastatic squamous cell carcinoma of the esophagus managed by concomitant chemotherapy (5-fluorouracil and cisplatin) and radiation therapy. *Cancer* 66:214, 1990.
8. Leichman L, Nigro N, Vaitkevicius VK, et al: Cancer of the anal canal: Model for preoperative adjuvant combined modality therapy. *Am J Med* 78:211, 1985.
9. Omura GA, Bundy BN, Berek JS, et al: Randomized trial of cyclophos-

phamide plus cisplatin with or without doxorubicin in ovarian carcinoma: A Gynecologic Oncology Group study. *J Clin Oncol* 7:457, 1989.

10. Bruno R, Hille D, Riva A, et al: Population pharmacokinetics/pharmacodynamics of docetaxel in Phase II studies in patients with cancer. *J Clin Oncol* 16:187, 1998.

11. Goldie JH, Coldman AJ: A mathematical model for relating the drug sensitivity of tumors to their spontaneous mutation rate. *Cancer Treat Rep* 63:1727, 1979.

12. Endicott JA, Ling V: The biochemistry of p-glycoprotein-mediated multidrug resistance. *Annu Rev Biochem* 58:137, 1989.

13. Van der Kolk, de Vries E, Loning J, et al: Activity and expression of the multidrug resistance proteins MRP1 and MRP2 in acute myeloid leukemia cells, tumor cell lines, and normal hematopoietic CD34+ peripheral blood cells. *Clin Cancer Res* 4:1727, 1998.

14. Dalton WS, Grogan TM: Does P-glycoprotein predict response to chemotherapy, and if so, is there a reliable way to detect it? *J Natl Cancer Inst* 83:80, 1991.

15. Göker E, Waltham M, Kheradpour A, et al: Amplification of the dihydrofolate reductase gene is a mechanism of acquired resistance to methotrexate in patients with acute lymphoblastic leukemia and is correlated with p53 gene mutations. *Blood* 86:677, 1995.

16. Fink D, Aebi S, Howell S: The role of DNA mismatch repair in drug resistance. *Clin Cancer Res* 4:1, 1998.

17. Kirsch D, Kastan M: Tumor-suppressor p53: implications for tumor development and prognosis. *J Clin Oncol* 16:3158, 1998.

18. Hannun Y: Apoptosis and the dilemma of cancer chemotherapy. *Blood* 89(6):1845, 1997.

19. Moscow JA, Connolly T, Myers TG, et al: Reduced folate carrier gene (RFC1) expression and anti-folate resistance in transfected and non-selected cell lines. *Int J Cancer* 72:184, 1997.

20. Ross JF, Chaudhuri PK, Ratnam M: Differential regulation of folate receptor isoforms in normal and malignant tissues in vivo and in established cell lines. Physiologic and clinical implications. *Cancer* 73:2432, 1994.

21. Galpin A, Schuetz J, Mason E, et al: Differences in folylpolyglutamate synthetase and dihydrofolate reductase expression in human B-lineage versus T-lineage leukemic lymphoblasts: mechanisms for lineage differences in methotrexate polyglutamylation and cytoxicity. *Mol Pharmacol* 52:155, 1997.

22. Synold TW, Relling MV, Boyett JM, et al: Blast cell methotrexate-polyglutamate accumulation in vivo differs by lineage, ploidy, and methotrexate dose in acute lymphoblastic leukemia. *J Clin Invest*, 94:1996, 1994.

23. Longo GS, Gorlick R, Tong WP, et al: Gamma-glutamyl hydrolase and folylploglutamate synthetase activities predict polyglutamylation of methotrexate in acute leukemia. *Oncol Res* 9:259, 1997.

24. Dicker AP, Volkenandt M, Schweitzer BI, et al: Identification and characterization of a mutation in the dihydrofolate reductase gene from the methotrexate-resistant Chinese hamster ovary cell line Pro-3 MTX^RIII. *J Biol Chem* 265:8317, 1990.

25. Evans W, Crom W, Abromowitch M, et al: Clinical pharmacodynamics of high-dose methotrexate in acute lymphocytic leukemia: identification of a relation between concentration and effect. *N Engl J Med* 314:471, 1986.

26. Stoller RG, Hande KR, Jacobs SA, et al: Use of plasma pharmacokinetics to predict and prevent methotrexate toxicity. *N Engl J Med* 297:630, 1977.

27. Widemann BC, Balis FM, Murphy RF, et al: Carboxypeptidase-G2, thymidine, and leucovorin rescue in cancer patients with methotrexate-induced renal dysfunction. *J Clin Oncol* 15:2125, 1997.

28. Shapiro WR, Allen JC, Horten BC: Chronic methotrexate toxicity to the central nervous system. *Clin Bull Memorial-Sloan Kettering* 10:49, 1980.

29. Bloomfield CD, Lawrence D, Byrd JC, et al: Frequency of prolonged remission duration after high-dose cytarabine intensification in acute myeloid leukemia varies by cytogenetic subtype. *Cancer Res* 58:4173, 1998.

30. Kufe DW, Munroe D, Herrick D, et al: Effects of 1-β-D-arabinofuranosylcytosine incorporation on eukaryotic DNA template function. *Mol Pharmacol* 26:128, 1984.

31. Owens JK, Shewach DS, Ullman B, Mitchell RS: Resistance to 1-β-D-arabinofuranosylcytosine in human T-lymphoblasts mediated by mutations within the deoxycytidine kinase gene. *Cancer Res* 52:2389, 1992.

32. Flasshove M, Strumberg D, Ayscue L, et al: Structural analysis of the deoxycytidine kinase gene in patients with the acute myeloid leukemia and resistance to cytosine arabinoside. *Leukemia* 8:780, 1993.

33. Capizzi RL, Powell BL: Sequential high-dose ara-C and asparaginase versus high-dose ara-C alone in the treatment of patients with relapsed and refractory acute leukemias. *Semin Oncol* 14(suppl 1):40, 1987.

34. Glantz MJ, Jaeckle KA, Chamberlain MC, et al: A Randomized controlled trial comparing intrathecal sustained-release cytarabine (Depo-Cyt) to intrathecal methotrexate in patients with neoplastic meningitis from solid tumors. *Clin Cancer Res* 5:3394, 1999.

35. Kern W, Kurrle E, Schmeiser T: Streptococcal bacteremia in adult patients with leukemia undergoing aggressive chemotherapy. A review of 55 cases. *Infection* 18:138, 1990.

36. Herzig RH, Hines JD, Herzig GP, et al: Cerebellar toxicity with high-dose cytosine arabinoside. *J Clin Oncol* 5:927, 1987.

37. Ley TJ, DeSimone J, Anagnon NP, et al: 5-Azacytidine selectively increases gamma chain synthesis in a patient with β-thalassemia. *N Engl J Med* 307:1469, 1982.

38. Drake JC, Stoller RG, Chabner BA: Characteristics of the enzyme uridine-cytidine kinase isolated from a cultured human cell line. *Biochem Pharmacol* 26:64, 1977.

39. Christie NT, Drake S, Meyn RE, et al: 6-Thiopurine-induced DNA damage as a determinant of cytotoxicity in cultured Chinese hamster ovary cells. *Cancer Res* 44:3665, 1984.

40. Lilleyman J, Lennard L: Mercaptopurine metabolism and risk of relapse in childhood lymphoblastic leukaemia. *Lancet* 343:1188, 1994.

41. Van Diggelen OP, Donahue TF, Shin SI: Basis for differential cellular sensitivity to 8-azaguanine and 6-thioguanine. *J Cell Physiol* 98:59, 1979.

42. Scholar EM, Calabresi P: Increased activity of alkaline phosphatases in leukemic cells from patients resistant to thiopurines. *Biochem Pharmacol* 28:445, 1979.

43. Lennard L, Lillyman JS: Are children with lymphoblastic leukaemia given enough 6-mercaptopurine? *Lancet* 2:785, 1987.

44. Lennard L, Lilleyman JS, Van Loon J, Weinshilboum RM: Genetic variation in response to 6-mercaptopurine for childhood acute lymphoblastic leukaemia. *Lancet* 336:225, 1990.

45. Zimm S, Collins JM, Riccardi R, et al: Variable bioavailability of oral 6-mercaptopurine: Is maintenance chemotherapy in acute lymphoblastic leukemia being optimally delivered? *N Engl J Med* 308:1005, 1983.

46. Lennard L, Davies HA, Lilleyman JS: Is 6-thioguanine more appropriate than 6-mercaptopurine for children with acute lymphoblastic leukaemia. *Br J Canc* 68:186, 1993.

47. Keating MJ, O'Brien S, Lerner S, et al: Long-term follow-up of patients with chronic lymphocytic leukemia (CLL) receiving fludarabine regimens as initial therapy. *Blood* 92(4):1165, 1998.

48. Slavin S, Nagler A, Naparstek E, et al: Nonmyeloablative stem cell transplantation and cell therapy as an alternative to conventional bone marrow transplantation with lethal cytoreduction for the treatment of malignant and nonmalignant hematologic diseases. *Blood* 91(3):756, 1998.

49. Brockman RW, Cheng Y-C, Schabel FM Jr, et al: Metabolism and chemotherapeutic activity of 9-β-D-arabinofuranosyl-2-fluoroadenine against murine leukemia L1210 and evidence for its phosphorylation by deoxycytidine kinase. *Cancer Res* 40:3610, 1980.

50. Plunkett W, Gandhi V: Pharmacology of purine nucleoside analogues. *Hematol Cell Ther* 38(suppl 2):67, 1996.

51. Fan S, el-Deiry WS, Bae I, et al: p53 Gene mutations are associated with decreased sensitivity of human lymphoma cells to DNA damaging agents. *Cancer Res* 54:5824, 1994.

52. Cheson B, Frame J, Vena D, et al: Tumor lysis syndrome: an uncommon complication of fludarabine therapy of chronic lymphocytic leukemia. *J Clin Oncol* 16:2313, 1998.

53. Cheson BD: Immunologic and immunosuppressive complications of purine analogue therapy. *J Clin Oncol* 13:2431, 1995.

54. Estey EH, Kurzrock R, Kantarjin HM, et al: Treatment of hairy cell leukemia with 2-chlorodeoxyadenosine (2-CdA). *Blood* 79:882, 1992.

55. Kay AC, Saven A, Carrera CJ, et al: 2-Chlorodeoxyadenosine treatment of low-grade lymphomas. *J Clin Oncol* 10:371, 1992.

56. Albertoni F, Lindemalm S, Reichelova V, et al: Pharmacokinetics of cladribine in plasma and its 5-monophosphate and 5-triphosphate in

leukemic cells of patients with chronic lymphocytic leukemia 1. *Clin Cancer Res* 4:653, 1998.

57. Beutler E: Cladribine (2-chlorodeoxyadenosine). *Lancet* 340:952, 1992.

58. Saven A, Piro L: 2-chlorodeoxyadenosine: A newer purine analogue active in the treatment of indolent lymphoid malignancies. *Ann Intern Med* 120:784, 1994.

59. Mitchell BS, Edwards NL, Koller CA: Deoxyribonucleoside triphosphate accumulation by leukemic cells. *Blood* 62:419, 1983.

60. Steis R, Urba WJ, Kopp WC, et al: Kinetics of recovery of CD4+ cells in peripheral blood of deoxycoformycin-treated patients. *J Natl Cancer Inst* 83:1678, 1992.

61. Madoc-Jones H, Mauro F: Interphase action of vinblastine and vincristine: Differences in their lethal action through the mitotic cycle of cultured mammalian cells. *J Cell Physiol* 72:185, 1968.

62. Cabral FR, Brady RC, Schiber MJ: A mechanism of cellular resistance to drugs that interfere with microtubule assembly. *Ann NY Acad Sci* 46:748, 1986.

63. Wilson WH, Chabner BA, Bryant G, et al: A phase II study of paclitaxel (Taxol) in relapsed non-Hodgkin's lymphomas. *J Clin Oncol* 13:381, 1995.

64. Rowinsky EK, Donehower RC: Paclitaxel (Taxol). *N Engl J Med* 332:1004, 1995.

65. Consolini R, Ching-Hon P, Behn FG: In vitro cytoxicity of docetaxel in childhood acute leukemias. *J Clin Oncol* 16(3):907, 1998.

66. Lopes NM, Adams EG, Pitts TW, et al: Cell kill kinetics and cell cycle effects of Taxol on human hamster ovarian cell lines. *Cancer Chemother Pharmacol* 32:235, 1993.

67. Gianni L, Vigano L, Locatelli A, et al: Human pharmacokinetic characterization and in vitro study of the interaction between doxorubicin and paclitaxel in patients with breast cancer. *J Clin Oncol* 15:1906, 1997.

68. Semb K, Aamdal S, Oian P: Capillary protein leak syndrome appears to explain fluid retention in cancer patients who receive docetaxel treatment. *J Clin Oncol* 16(10):3426, 1998.

69. Ohno R, Okada K, Masaoka T, et al: An early phase II study of CPT-11: A new derivative of camptothecin, for the treatment of leukemia and lymphoma. *J Clin Oncol* 8:1907, 1990.

70. Beran M, Kantarjian H, Obrien S, et al: Topotecan, a topoisomerase I inhibitor, is active in the treatment of myelodysplastic syndrome and chronic myelomonocytic leukemia. *Blood* 88:2473, 1996.

71. Iyer L, King C, Whitington P, et al: Genetic predisposition to the metabolism of irinotecan (CPT-11). Role of uridine glucuronosyltransferase isoform 1A1 in the glucuronidation of its active metabolite (SN-38) in human liver microsomes. *J Clin Invest* 101:847, 1998.

72. Grochow LB, Rowinski EK, Johnson R, et al: Pharmacokinetics and pharmacodynamics of topotecan in patients with advanced cancer. *Drug Metab Dispos* 20:706, 1992.

73. Capranico G, Butelli E, Zunnino F: Change of the sequence specificity of daunorubicin-stimulated topoisomerase II DNA cleavage by epimerization of the amino group of the sugar moiety. *Cancer Res* 55:312, 1995.

74. Reid JM, Pendergrass TW, Krailo MD, et al: Plasma pharmacokinetics and cerebrospinal fluid concentrations of idarubicin and idarubicinol in pediatric leukemia patients: A Children's Cancer Study Group report. *Cancer Res* 50:6525, 1990.

75. Moreb JS, Oblon DJ: Outcome of clinical congestive heart failure induced by anthracycline chemotherapy. *Cancer* 70:2637, 1992.

76. Speyer JL, Green MD, Kramer E, et al: Protective effect of the bispiperazinedione, ICRF-187, against doxorubicin-induced cardiac toxicity in women with advanced breast cancer. *N Engl J Med* 319:745, 1988.

77. Billingham ME, Bristow MR, Glatstein E, et al: Adriamycin cardiotoxicity: Endomyocardial biopsy evidence of enhancement by irradiation. *Am J Surg Pathol* 1:17, 1977.

78. Lipschultz SE, Colan SD, Gelber RD, et al: Late cardiac effects of doxorubicin in therapy for acute lymphoblastic leukemia in childhood. *N Engl J Med* 324:808, 1991.

79. Nysom K, Holm K, Lipsita S: Relationship between cumulative anthracycline dose and late cardiotoxicity in childhood acute lymphoblastic leukemia. *J Clin Oncol* 16(2):545, 1998.

80. Odom LF, Gordon EM: Acute monoblastic leukemia in infancy and early childhood: Successful treatment with an epipodophyllotoxin. *Blood* 64:875, 1984.

81. Capranico G, Zunino F: Antitumor inhibitors of DNA topoisomerases. *Curr Pharm Des* 1:1, 1995.

82. Zwelling LA, Hinds M, Chan D, et al: Characterization of an amsacrine-resistant line of human leukemia cells. Evidence for a drug resistant form of topoisomerase II. *J Biol Chem* 264:16411, 1989.

83. Buggs BY, Danks MK, Beck WT, Suttle DP: Expression of a mutant topoisomerase II in CCRF-CEM human leukemia cells selected for resistance to teniposide. *Proc Natl Acad Sci USA* 88:7654, 1991.

84. Stewart CF, Arbuck SG, Fleming RA, et al: Changes in the clearance of total and unbound etoposide in patients with liver dysfunction. *J Clin Oncol* 8:1874, 1990.

85. Winick N, McKenna R, Shuster JJ, et al: Secondary acute myeloid leukemia in children with B-lineage acute lymphoblastic leukemia treated with an epipodophyllotoxin. *J Clin Oncol* 11:209,1993.

86. Ratain MJ, Kaminer LS, Bitran JD, et al: Acute nonlymphocytic leukemia following etoposide and cisplatin combination chemotherapy for advanced non-small-cell carcinoma of the lung. *Blood* 70:1412, 1987.

87. Umezawa H, Maeda K, Takeuchi T, et al: New antibiotics, bleomycin A and B. *J Antibiot Ser A* 19:200, 1966.

88. Petering DH, Byrnes RW, Antholine WE: The role of redox-active metals in the mechanism of action of bleomycin. *Chem Biol Interact* 73:133, 1990.

89. Burger RM, Drlica K, Birdsall B: The DNA cleavage pathway of iron BLM strand scission precedes deoxyribose 3-phosphate bond cleavage. *J Biol Chem,* 269:25978, 1994.

90. Burger R: Cleavage of nucleic acids by bleomycin. *Chem Rev* 98:1153, 1998.

91. Sebti SM, Jani JP, Mistry JS, et al: Metabolic inactivation: A mechanism of human tumor resistance to bleomycin. *Cancer Res* 51:227, 1991.

92. Alberts DS, Chen HSG, Liu R, et al: Bleomycin pharmacokinetics in man: I. Intravenous administration. *Cancer Chemother Pharmacol* 1:177, 1978.

93. Karmiol S, Remick DG, Kunkel SL, Phan SL: Regulation of rat pulmonary endothelial cell interleukin-6 production by bleomycin: Effects of cellular fatty acid composition. *Am J Respir Cell Mol Biol,* 9:628, 1993.

94. Blum RH, Carter SK, Agre K: A clinical review of bleomycin—a new antineoplastic agent. *Cancer* 31:903, 1973.

95. Comis RL: Detecting bleomycin pulmonary toxicity: A continued conundrum. *J Clin Oncol* 8:765, 1990.

96. Hutson RG, Kitoh T, Moraga Amador DA: Amino acid control of asparagine synthetase: relation to asparaginase resistance in human leukemia cells. *Am J Physiol* 272:1691, 1997.

97. Kaspers GJ, Veerman AJ, Pieters R, et al: In vitro cellular drug resistance and prognosis in newly diagnosed childhood acute lymphoblastic leukemia. *Blood* 90:2723, 1997.

98. Asselin BL, Whitin JC, Coppola DJ, et al: Comparative pharmacokinetic studies of three asparaginase preparations, *J Clin Oncol.* 11:1780, 1993.

99. Holle LM: Pegaspargase: An alternative? *Ann Pharmacother* 31:616, 1997.

100. Killander D, Dohlwitz S, Engstedt L, et al: Hypersensitive reactions and antibody formation during L-asparaginase treatment of children and adults with acute leukemia. *Cancer* 37:220, 1976.

101. Semeraro N, Montemurro P, Giordano P, et al: Unbalanced coagulation fibrinolysis potential during L-asparaginase therapy in children with acute lymphoblastic leukaemia. *Thromb Haemost* 64:38, 1990.

102. Bushara KO, Rust RS: Reversible MRI lesions due to pegaspargase treatment of non-Hodgkin's lymphoma. *Pediatr Neurol* 17:185, 1997.

103. Parsons SK, Skapek SX, Neufeld EJ, et al: Asparaginase-associated lipid abnormalities in children with acute lymphoblastic leukemia. *Blood* 89:1886, 1997.

104. Capizzi R: Improvement in the therapeutic index of L-asparaginase by methotrexate. *Cancer Chemother Rep* 6(3):37, 1975.

105. Peters WP, Shpall EJ, Jones RB, et al: High-dose combination alkylating agents with bone marrow support as initial treatment for metastatic breast cancer. *J Clin Oncol* 6:1368, 1988.

106. Yeager AM, Kaizer H, Santos GW, et al: Autologous bone marrow transplantation in patients with acute nonlymphocytic leukemia using ex vivo marrow treatment with 4-hydroperoxycyclophosphamide. *N Engl J Med* 315:141, 1986.

107. Tew KD, Colvin M, Chabner BA: Alkylating agents, in *Cancer Chemotherapy and Biotherapy: Principles and Practice,* 2nd ed, edited by BA Chabner, DL Longo, pp 297–332. Lippincott, Philadelphia, PA, 1996.

108. Hilton J: Role of aldehyde dehydrogenase in cyclophosphamide-resistant L1210 leukemia. *Cancer Res* 44:5156, 1984.

109. Erickson L: The role of *O*-6 methylguanine DNA methyltransferase (MGMT) in drug resistance and strategies for its inhibition. *Sem Cancer Biol* 2:257, 1991.

110. Droller MJ, Saral R, Santos G: Prevention of cyclophosphamide-induced hemorrhagic cystitis. *Urology* 20:256, 1982.

111. Schacht RG, Baldwin DS: Chronic interstitial nephritis and renal failure due to nitrosourea (NU) therapy. *Kidney Int* 14:661, 1978.

112. Gianni AM, Bregni M, Siena S, et al: Recombinant human granulocyte-macrophage colony stimulating factor reduces hematologic toxicity and widens clinical applicability of high-dose cyclophosphamide treatment in breast cancer and non-Hodgkin's lymphoma. *J Clin Oncol* 8:768, 1990.

113. Elias AD, Eder JP, Shea T, et al: High-dose ifosfamide with mesna uroprotection: A phase I study. *J Clin Oncol* 8:170, 1990.

114. Lazarus HM, Reed MD, Spitzer TR, et al: High-dose IV thiotepa and cryopreserved autologous bone marrow transplantation for therapy of refractory cancer. *Cancer Treat Rep* 71:689, 1987.

115. Peters WP, Henner WD, Grochow LB, et al: Clinical and pharmacologic effects of high dose single agent busulfan with autologous bone marrow support in the treatment of solid tumors. *Cancer Res* 47:6402, 1987.

116. Phillips GL, Wolff SN, Fay JW, et al: Intensive 1,3-bis(2-chloroethyl)-1-nitrosourea (BCNU) monochemotherapy and autologous marrow transplantation for malignant glioma. *J Clin Oncol* 4:639, 1986.

117. Ozols RF, Corden BJ, Jacob J, et al: High dose cisplatin in hypertonic saline. *Ann Intern Med* 100:19, 1984.

118. Shea TC, Flaherty M, Elias A, et al: A phase I clinical and pharmacokinetic study of carboplatin and autologous bone marrow support. *J Clin Oncol* 7:651, 1989.

119. Parkinson DR, Smith MA: Retinoid therapy for acute promyelocytic leukemia: A coming of age for the differentiation therapy of malignancy (Editorial). *Ann Intern Med* 117:338, 1992.

120. Andreeff M, Stone R, Michaeli J, et al: Hexamethylene bisacetamide in myelodysplastic syndrome and acute myelogenous leukemia: A phase II clinical trial with a differentiation-inducing agent. *Blood* 80:2504, 1992.

121. Hong WK, Lippman SM, Itri LM, et al: Prevention of second primary tumors with isotretinoin in squamous-cell carcinoma of the head and neck. *N Engl J Med* 323:795, 1990.

122. Lippman SM, Parkinson DR, Weber RS, et al: Isotretinoin plus alpha interferon: Effective therapy of advanced squamous cell carcinoma (scc) of the skin. *Proc Am Soc Clin Oncol* 10:A650, 1991.

123. Lippman SM, Kavanagh JJ, Paredes-Espinoza J, et al: 13-*cis*-Retinoic acid plus interferon alpha-2a: Highly active systemic therapy for squamous cell carcinoma of the cervix. *J Natl Cancer Inst* 84:241, 1992.

124. Warrell RP Jr, Frankel SR, Miller WH Jr, et al: Differentiation therapy of acute promyelocytic leukemia with tretinoin (all-*trans* retinoic acid). *N Engl J Med* 324:1385, 1991.

125. Kazizuka A, Miller WH Jr, Umesono K, et al: Chromosomal translocation t(15;17) in human acute promyelocytic leukemia fuses RARα with a novel putative transcription factor, PML. *Cell* 66:663, 1991.

126. Robertson KA, Emami B, Collins SJ: Retinoic acid-resistant HL-60R cells harbor a point mutation in the retinoic acid receptor ligand binding domain that confers dominant negative activity. *Blood* 80:1885, 1992.

127. Muindi JRF, Frankel SR, Huselton C, et al: Clinical pharmacology of oral all-*trans* retinoic acid in patients with acute promyelocytic leukemia. *Cancer Res* 52:2138, 1992.

128. Muindi J, Frankel SR, Miller WH Jr, et al: Continuous treatment with all-*trans* retinoic acid causes a progressive reduction in plasma drug concentrations: Implications for relapse and retinoid "resistance" in patients with acute promyelocytic leukemia. *Blood* 79:299, 1992.

129. Frankel SR, Eardley A, Lauwers G, et al: The "retinoic acid syndrome" in acute promyelocytic leukemia. *Ann Intern Med* 117:292, 1992.

130. De Botton S, Dombret H, Sanz M, et al: Incidence, clinical features, and outcome of all *trans*-retinoic acid syndrome in 413 cases of newly diagnosed acute promyelocytic leukemia. *Blood* 92(8):2712.

131. Soignet SL, Maslak P, Wang Z-G, et al: Complete remission after treatment of acute promyelocytic leukemia with arsenic trioxide. *N Engl J Med* 339(19):1341, 1998.

132. Chen G-Q, Shi X-G, Tang W, et al: Use of arsenic trioxide (As_2O_3) in the treatment of acute promyelocytic leukemia (APL): I. As_2O_3 exerts dose-dependent dual effects on APL cells. *Blood* 89:3345, 1997.

133. Shen Z-X, Chen G-Q, Ni J-H, et al: Use of arsenic trioxide (As_2O_3) in the treatment of acute promyelocytic leukemia (APL): II. Clinical efficacy and pharmacokinetics in relapsed patients. *Blood* 89(9):3354, 1997.

134. Eder JP, Elias A, Shea TC, et al: A phase I–II study of cyclophosphamide, thiotepa, and carboplatin with autologous bone marrow transplantation in solid tumor patients. *J Clin Oncol* 8:1239, 1990.

135. Kessinger A, Armitage JO, Smith DM, et al: High-dose therapy and autologous peripheral blood stem cell transplantation for patients with lymphoma. *Blood* 74:1260, 1989.

136. Jones RJ, Piantadosi S, Mann RB, et al: High-dose cytotoxic therapy and bone marrow transplantation for relapsed Hodgkin's disease. *J Clin Oncol* 8:527, 1990.

137. Wilson WH, Jain V, Bryant G, et al: Phase I and II study of high-dose ifosfamide, carboplatin, and etoposide with autologous bone marrow rescue in lymphomas and solid tumors. *J Clin Oncol* 10:1712, 1992.

138. Dunphy FR, Spitzer G, Buzdar AU, et al: Treatment of estrogen receptor-negative or hormonally refractory breast cancer with double high-dose chemotherapy intensification and bone marrow support. *J Clin Oncol* 8:1207, 1990.

139. Sterkers Y, Preudhomme C, Lai J-L, et al: Acute myeloid leukemia and myelodysplastic syndromes following essential thrombocythemia treated with hydroxyurea: high proportion of cases with 17p deletion. *Blood* 91:616, 1998.

TREATMENT OF INFECTIONS IN THE IMMUNOCOMPROMISED HOST

STEVEN M. BEUTLER

Infection is a major cause of morbidity and mortality in patients receiving chemotherapy for treatment of hematologic neoplasms. Bacterial infections may result in rapid clinical deterioration and, if not treated appropriately, death. Fungal, viral, and parasitic infections may also result in potentially lethal complications during and after chemotherapy. Recognition and treatment of such infections in the context of different clinical situations is addressed. The introduction of home antibiotic therapy is noted and may be appropriate for certain patients. Since prevention of infection during periods of neutropenia should reduce morbidity and improve outcome, attention is also focused on various means of prophylaxis of bacterial, parasitic, viral, and fungal infections.

The profound pancytopenia that results from cytoreductive chemotherapy is a common and dramatic manifestation of stem cell failure. During the periods of neutropenia that follow such chemotherapy, infection will develop in most patients. Patients with neoplasms of the lymphoid system commonly manifest altered humoral and cellular immunity, resulting in an increased incidence of nonbacterial infection.

RISK FACTORS AND INFECTING ORGANISMS

Bacterial, fungal, viral, and parasitic organisms may cause infection in neutropenic patients. Bacterial infections are the most frequent and usually the most serious. The risk for bacterial infection increases somewhat when the neutrophil count falls below $500/\mu l$ (0.5×10^9/liter) and becomes especially pronounced at neutrophil counts below 100 ml (0.1×10^9/liter; see Fig. 17-1).[1] The duration of the neutropenia and rate of decline of the granulocyte count are also important in determining the risk of bacterial infection. Disruption of integumental barriers further favors the development of infection by providing portals of entry.

Historically, gram-negative bacilli have been the most commonly isolated pathogens. These organisms include *Pseudomonas, Klebsiella, Escherichia coli,* and *Proteus* and are responsible for a broad variety of infections, including pneumonia, soft tissue infections, perirectal infections, and primary bacteremia. Urinary tract infections are surprisingly infrequent unless a urinary catheter is present or urinary tract obstruction has developed. Meningitis is also uncommon.

During the past two decades, the incidence of gram-positive infection has increased.[2] Staphylococcal species, enterococcus, and *Corynebacterium* are now the pathogens most frequently isolated from neutropenic patients. This may be due, in part, to the popularity of semipermanent venous catheters. Several recent reports document the increasing frequency of *Streptococcus viridans* as a major pathogen in neutropenic patients,[3] especially in those receiving marrow transplant, perhaps because these patients have a higher incidence of mucositis. Septic shock may occur in these patients.[4] Anaerobic infections are less common unless there is coexisting dental or gastrointestinal pathology.

Patients with Hodgkin's disease, other lymphomas, or chronic lymphocytic leukemia primarily suffer from impaired cell-mediated immunity and diminished antibody production.[5] Consequently, the spectrum of infections in these patients differs from that found in the neutropenic patient. Bacterial infections, when they occur, tend to be due to encapsulated organisms such as *Pneumococcus* or *Haemophilus*. *Listeria* and *Nocardia* infections are also seen more frequently in this group of patients.

Fungal infections are also common during periods of prolonged neutropenia as well as in patients with lymphomas or chronic lymphocytic leukemia. *Candida* species are most frequently isolated, but *Aspergillus* and *Phycomycetes* are also found. The gastrointestinal tract serves as a reservoir for *Candida*; thrush and erosive esophagitis may develop. *Candida* may also enter the bloodstream via indwelling catheters. *Aspergillus* and *Phycomycetes* tend to colonize and infect the sinuses and bronchopulmonary tree. Since cell-mediated immunity is required for defense against fungal infections, it is not surprising that infections with *Cryptococcus, Aspergillus, Coccidioides, Histoplasma,* and *Candida* are more common in patients with leukemia or lymphoma who have required glucocorticoid treatment.

Viral infections are especially frequent in patients with impaired cell-mediated immunity. Among viruses that cause infections in immunocompromised hosts, herpes simplex, varicella zoster, CMV, and adenoviruses are the most important. Cutaneous lesions and mucositis are often caused by herpes simplex. Herpes zoster infections may be especially severe and have a propensity for dissemination. Primary varicella infections are associated with a high mortality rate if not treated. CMV may cause febrile illnesses associated with pneumonia, hepatitis, and/or gastrointestinal tract ulcerations. This virus may be isolated by culture or demonstrated by the presence of viral antigens or viral DNA in clinical specimens.[6] Respiratory infections caused by RSV have been documented in about 18 percent of marrow transplant recipients with pulmonary symptoms during the winter months.[7] Influenza, picorna viruses, and others have also been isolated.

Pneumocystis carinii, a ubiquitous, endogenous parasite, may cause pneumonia in neutropenic patients as well as in those with defective cell-mediated immunity. It often becomes clinically evident after glucocorticoids have been tapered or discontinued. *Toxoplasma gondii,* another protozoan parasite, may be responsible for brain abscesses in patients with lymphoma or chronic lymphocytic leukemia, especially those treated with glucocorticoids. Glucocorticoid-treated patients are also at risk for *Strongyloides* hyperinfection.

The association between lymphoid malignancies and tuberculosis has been recognized for over a century. With the resurgence of tuberculosis and the increased prevalence of drug-resistant strains, this threatens to become a more frequent, serious problem.[8] Atypical mycobacterial infections, while very common in HIV-positive patients, are fairly rare in patients receiving chemotherapy.

RECOGNITION AND DIAGNOSIS OF INFECTION

The development of an infection in a neutropenic patient may be accompanied by dramatic clinical manifestations or by none at all. Fever, if it develops, is very suggestive of infection. However, hypothermia, declining mental status, myalgias, or lethargy may indicate

Acronyms and abbreviations that appear in this chapter include: CMV, cytomegalovirus; G-CSF, granulocyte colony-stimulating factor; GM-CSF, granulocyte-macrophage colony-stimulating factor; PCR, polymerase chain reaction; RSV, respiratory syncytial virus.

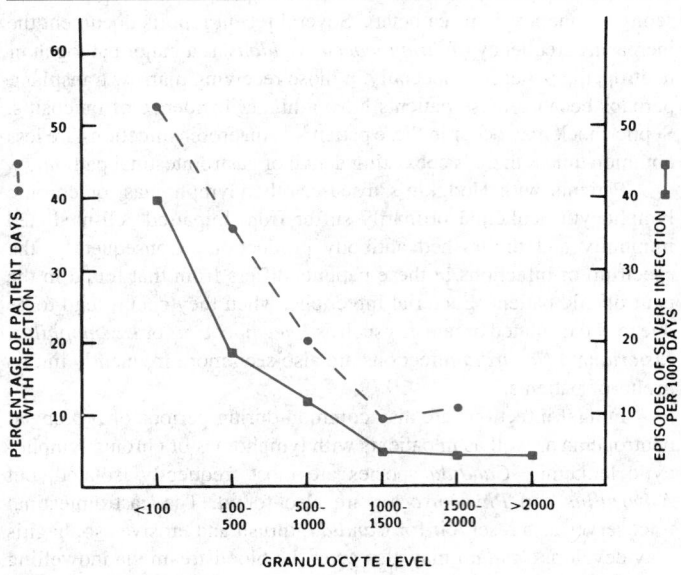

FIGURE 17-1   Relationship between the granulocyte count and the percentage of patient days with infection (●---●) and the episodes of severe infections per 1000 days (■---■). (Based on the data of Bodey et al.[1])

infection in these patients. The usual local signs of infection may be absent or delayed because these are mediated by neutrophils.[9]

A careful physical examination should be performed when such a change in condition is observed. Special attention should be paid to the mouth and teeth for evidence of thrush or periodontal disease. The skin should be examined in detail. Innocuous-appearing skin lesions may actually be septic emboli, and trivial injuries inflicted by venipuncture or intravenous catheters may become infected and result in septicemia. There is an increased incidence of perianal and perirectal infection in the neutropenic patient[10]; examination of the rectum may provide a clue to the source of fever in patients without other clinical findings. While such examinations should not be performed unnecessarily on an immunocompromised patient, rectal or pelvic examination should not be deferred when searching for a cause of fever.

Chest x-rays should be obtained initially and may need to be repeated, although this practice has been questioned in patients without respiratory complaints.[11] Chest computed tomography may reveal lesions not detected on routine radiograms.[12] Sinus x-rays may be helpful if symptoms are present.

Blood cultures should be collected prior to the institution of antibiotic therapy and periodically thereafter if fever persists. If an indwelling venous catheter is present, some of the cultures should be obtained from the catheter. There does not seem to be a physiologic or experimental basis for the common practice of separating blood cultures by 10 to 15 min. However, obtaining two to three cultures improves the likelihood of recovering fastidious organisms. To improve the likelihood of isolating fungal pathogens, the specimens should be retained by the laboratory for at least 10 days. Urine cultures and sputum cultures may be helpful. Results of the latter, however, must be interpreted with caution, since they may reflect the flora colonizing the oropharynx rather than the pathogens infecting the lung. Skin lesions of a suspicious nature should be biopsied and cultured. Stools should be examined for *Clostridium difficile* toxin in patients with diarrhea. Potentially infected intravenous lines should be cultured upon removal. Nasal cultures may be useful in predicting pulmonary aspergillosis.[13] Fungal infections, which may be difficult to document

using conventional culture techniques, may be diagnosed by PCR and by antigen detection.[14,15] However, there are currently only limited data available validating these assays, and they are not routinely available at the present time.

Open lung biopsies were once advocated for further evaluation of the neutropenic patient with pulmonary infiltrates.[16] However, since this procedure rarely establishes a treatable diagnosis, it should not be routinely performed in immunocompromised patients with pneumonia. It may be useful under certain limited circumstances, for example, when further empiric therapy would be unacceptably toxic in a patient whose clinical condition is deteriorating.

Transbronchial lung biopsies are generally considered to be unsafe in patients with thrombocytopenia because the risk of uncontrolled bleeding is high. Obtaining material via bronchial brushing or lavage carries a lower risk and may yield useful information.[17]

TREATMENT

INITIAL TREATMENT

BACTERIAL INFECTIONS

The need for prompt, effective therapy is dramatized by the finding that mortality rates approach 100 percent in bacteremic neutropenic patients treated with regimens lacking activity against the organisms subsequently isolated.[18] In contrast, patients receiving appropriate therapy have mortality rates that are much lower.[19] Therefore, it is critical to select potent, broad-spectrum agents when initiating empiric antimicrobial therapy in the neutropenic patient. It is particularly important that therapy effective against gram-negative organisms be given; gram-positive organisms tend to be less virulent, and brief delays in treating these organisms may not be attended by increased mortality,[20] at least in institutions where methicillin-resistant *Staphylococcus aureus* or fulminant gram-positive infections are uncommon.[21]

In general, antibiotics should be given at the maximum recommended doses (see Table 17-1). Aminoglycoside and vancomycin levels should be measured to establish proper doses. High peak levels of aminoglycosides are desirable. The increasingly common practice of administering aminoglycosides as a single, daily dose seems to be effective in neutropenic patients.[22,23] Aminoglycoside selection will depend on institutional sensitivity patterns. In the case of β-lactam drugs, frequent or continuous administration following a loading dose ensures constant therapeutic levels[24] and may be advantageous.

Many different regimens have been evaluated and found to be acceptable for empiric therapy in neutropenic patients.[21] Several are listed in Table 17-2. Generally, combinations of two or three drugs have been favored for initial empiric therapy, but single-drug therapy may also be efficacious. Imipenem,[25] meropenem,[26,27] cefipime,[25,28] and ceftazidime[27] have each been studied as single agents. These drugs are active against most of the virulent pathogens infecting neutropenic patients, and subsequent modification of therapy can serve to optimize treatment. Antibiotic toxicity is reduced by omitting the aminoglycoside from the regimen. However, development of resistant organisms during single-drug therapy is of concern. Aminoglycosides may provide synergy against gram-negative bacilli and further broaden the spectrum of antimicrobial activity. It is also important to note that none of these agents is active against methicillin-resistant staphylococcus or against *Corynebacterium*. Cefipime and ceftazidime lack activity against enterococcus.

Therapy with two β-lactam drugs has been advocated by some, but development of resistant organisms has been a problem, and the second β-lactam drug may increase the frequency of toxicity without improving efficacy. Quinolones, usually in conjunction with another

TABLE 17-1   MAXIMUM RECOMMENDED DOSES OF ANTIBIOTICS

Drug Category	Drug	Brand Name	Dose	Adjustment for Renal Insufficiency	Activity	Toxicity
Antipseudomonal penicillins	Ticarcillin-clavulanic acid	Timentin	3.1 g q 4 h	++	Methicillin-sensitive *Staphylococcus* (ticarcillin-clavulanic acid, piperacillin-tazobactam), *Streptococcus*, anaerobes, *Pseudomonas aeruginosa*	Hypokalemia, antiplatelet effect
	Piperacillin	Pipracil	4 g q 4 h	+		
	Piperacillin-tazobactam	Zosyn	4.5 g q 4 h	+		
Antipseudomonal cephalosporins	Ceftazidime	Fortaz	2 g q 8 h	+++	*Pseudomonas aeruginosa*, enteric gram-negative rods, methicillin-sensitive *Staphylococcus*	
		Tazicef	2g q 8 h	++		
	Cefipime	Maxipime	2g q 12 h			
Aminoglycosides	Amikacin	Amikin	15 (mg/kg)/d*	+++	Enteric gram-negative rods and *Pseudomonas aeruginosa*	Nephrotoxicity, ototoxicity
	Tobramycin	Nebcin	4–5 (mg/kg)/d*			
	Gentamicin	Garamycin	4–5 (mg/kg)/d*			
Glycopeptide	Vancomycin	Vancocin	30 (mg/kg)/d in 2 doses*	+++	*Staphylococcus* (including MRSA), *Streptococcus*, *Corynebacterium*	Ototoxicity, red-man syndrome with rapid infusion
Carbopenem	Imipenem	Primaxin	0.5–1 g q 6 h [30–60 (mg/kg)/d]	++–++++	Gram-negative rods, *Pseudomonas aeruginosa*, *Staphylococcus*, enterococcus, anaerobes	Nausea, seizures (Primaxin)
	Meropenem	Merrem	1 g q 8 h	+(?)		
Monobactam	Aztreonam	Azactam	2 g q 6 h	+	Gram-negative rods, *Pseudomonas aeruginosa*	
Sulfonamides	Trimethoprim-sulfamethoxazole	Bactrim Septra	10–20 (mg/kg)/d (based on trimethoprim) in 2–4 doses/d	++	*Pneumocystis carinii*, gram-negative rods, *Haemophilus*, *Staphylococcus*	Sulfa allergy, increased creatinine, nausea, rash
Fluoroquinolones	Ciprofloxacin	Cipro	500–750 mg q 12 h or 200–400 mg IV q 12 h	+	Gram-negative rods, *Pseudomonas aeruginosa* (Cipro)	Nausea. Not for use in children
	Levofloxacin	Levaquin	500 mg PO or IV q 24 h	+++		
Nucleosides	Acyclovir	Zovirax	15 (mg/kg)/d IV [30 (mg/kg)/d IV for encephalitis or for herpes zoster] in 3 divided doses; comparable oral dose approximately twice as high	+–++	Herpes simplex and zoster	Crystalluria
	Valacyclovir	Valtrex	1000 mg b.i.d. (t.i.d. in herpes zoster) PO	++	Herpes simplex and zoster	
	Famciclovir	Famvir	250–500 mg t.i.d. PO	+++	CMV, herpes simplex	
	Ganciclovir	Cytovene	10 (mg/kg)/d in 2 divided doses	++		Neutropenia
Phosphonoformate	Foscarnet	Foscavir	180 (mg/kg)/d in 3 doses	++	CMV	Renal failure, electrolyte abnormalities
Polyene antifungals	Amphotericin B	Fungizone	0.7–1.0 (mg/kg)/d in a single daily dose over 2–6 h	0	*Candida, Aspergillus, Torulopsis*, other fungus	Nausea, vomiting, chills, fever, renal failure, hypokalemia, hypomagnesemia
	Ampho B lipid complex	Abelcet	5 (mg/kg)/d		*Candida, Aspergillus, Torulopsis*, other fungus	Fever, chills, nausea, vomiting, increased creatinine
	Ampho B cholest complex	Amphotec	4 (mg/kg)/d		*Candida, Aspergillus, Torulopsis*, other fungus	Fever, chills, nausea, vomiting, increased creatinine
	Ampho B liposomal ampho	Ambisome	5 (mg/kg)/d		*Candida, Aspergillus, Torulopsis*, other fungus	Fever, chills, nausea, vomiting, increased creatinine
	Ampho B coll dispersion	Amphocil	6 (mg/kg)/d		*Candida, Aspergillus, Torulopsis*, other fungus	Fever, chills, nausea, vomiting, increased creatinine
Azole	Fluconazole	Diflucan	400 mg/d PO/IV	++	*Candida albicans, Cryptococcus, Coccidiodes immitis*, histoplasmosis, *Aspergillus*	Nausea, LFT abnormality
	Itraconazole	Sporanox	400 mg/d in 2 doses PO	0		Nausea
Diamidine	Pentamidine	Pentam	4 mg/kg q 24 h IV	++(?)	*Pneumocystis carinii*	Renal failure, hypotension, hypoglycemia

*Adjust dose based on levels.

NOTE: 0, no adjustment required; +, small adjustment for creatinine clearance less than 20; ++, moderate adjustment required; +++, nearly complete renal excretion; dose to be reduced proportionately to renal function.

ABBREVIATIONS: b.i.d, twice a day; CMV, cytomegalovirus; IV, intravenous; LFT, liver function tests; MRSA, methicillin-resistant *Staphylococcus aureus*; t.i.d., three times a day.

TABLE 17-2   REGIMENS FOR EMPIRIC THERAPY IN NEUTROPENIC
            PATIENTS

Ceftazidime + aminoglycoside ± vancomycin
Imipenem (or meropenem) + aminoglycoside ± vancomycin
Piperacillin + aminoglycoside ± vancomycin
Cefipime + aminoglycoside ± vancomycin
Ciprofloxacin + aminoglycoside
Ciprofloxacin + ceftazidime
"Monotherapy" (imipenem, meropenem, ceftazidime, or cefipime)

antibiotic, are effective in patients who have not received quinolone prophylaxis.[29]

The use of single-drug therapy cannot be recommended for all patients with stem cell failure. Single-drug therapy may be appropriate for patients with less profound neutropenia, those who are not frankly septic, and those who may have problems tolerating aminoglycosides. Differences in institutional sensitivity patterns will also influence antibiotic selection.

Vancomycin-resistant enterococcus is being isolated with increasing frequency and presents a major challenge.[30] Several regimens have been employed, including chloramphenicol as a single agent or combination therapy with penicillin, vancomycin, and one or two other agents (rifampin and/or a quinolone.) None of these strategies has met with consistent success. Synercid (quinupristin/dalfopristin), is active against about 86 percent of vancomycin-resistant enterococci.[31] There is limited clinical experience with this drug in neutropenic patients.

Therapeutic use of granulocytes is rarely necessary (see Chap. 141), may result in the transmission of CMV disease, and may cause severe reactions.

FUNGAL INFECTIONS

Amphotericin B is the drug of choice for the majority of fungal infections that develop in the neutropenic host. The dose should be advanced rapidly so that the full therapeutic dose is given by the first or second day. Serum creatinine, potassium, and magnesium levels should be monitored. Fever and chills associated with administration of this drug may be treated or prevented with meperidine (Demerol) or diphenhydramine hydrochloride (Benadryl) and acetaminophen. This will not be necessary in all patients, and systemic reactions tend to decrease after several doses. Twenty-five to 100 mg hydrocortisone added to the infusion may attenuate the reactions. Infusions should be given over 2 to 6 h. More rapid infusions have been studied but are not recommended for routine use.[32]

Flucytosine provides synergy against *Cryptococcus neoformans* and some strains of *Candida* but not against *Aspergillus*. This drug is myelotoxic and may cause hepatitis and colitis; therefore, it should not be used routinely in the treatment of fungal infections in this group of patients.

Several preparations of liposomal amphotericin B have recently become available.[33] They are more likely than nonliposomal amphotericin B to cause infusion-related symptoms[34] but are less nephrotoxic.[35,36] Higher doses are required to achieve a clinical response, and the cost is considerably higher than that of amphotericin B. Therefore, those formulations should be reserved for patients who have underlying renal insufficiency or who have experienced nephrotoxicity with amphotericin B.[33]

Fluconazole, an azole drug that may be administered orally or intravenously, is approved for treatment of *Candida albicans, Cryptococcus neoformans,* and *Coccidioides immitis.* It is less active against non-*albicans Candida* species and is completely inactive against *Candida krusei.* It can be used to treat patients with sensitive strains of fungus who are unable to tolerate amphotericin B or who fail

treatment with it. It has been used as first-line therapy in hepatosplenic candidiasis (see below) and may be appropriate for patients with nonsystemic fungal infections.

Itraconazole is not approved for the treatment of candidiasis. It can be used in the treatment of *Aspergillus* infection, although amphotericin is more potent and reliable. Currently it is only available orally; an intravenous preparation is expected to be released in the near future. Ketoconazole and miconazole have no role in the treatment of seriously ill patients with fungal infections.

VIRAL INFECTIONS

There are a limited number of options for the treatment of viral infections. Acyclovir is active against herpes simplex and, at higher doses, against varicella zoster. It is not useful against CMV or Epstein-Barr virus. Newer agents (e.g., famciclovir and valacyclovir) may be administered less frequently but are not available for intravenous administration. Valacyclovir has been shown to be efficacious in the prevention of CMV in renal transplant patients,[37] but otherwise these agents have not been well studied in immunosuppressed patients.

Ganciclovir and foscarnet have documented efficacy in the treatment of CMV disease and are also active against herpes simplex. They are most effective when used early in the course of the infection. Hence, frequent screening for antigenemia in high-risk (e.g., marrow transplant) patients may allow for improved outcomes.[38] Both agents have been used successfully in conjunction with CMV immunoglobulin to treat CMV pneumonia in marrow transplant patients.[39] Ganciclovir results in neutropenia in a significant percentage of patients who receive it. Foscarnet therapy may be complicated by azotemia and electrolyte abnormalities. Ribavirin can be used to treat RSV. Rimantadine should be used if influenza A is suspected.

PARASITIC INFECTIONS

Pneumocystis carinii may be treated with trimethoprim-sulfamethoxazole or with pentamidine. Doses are listed in Table 17-1. A number of other regimens, including dapsone-trimethoprim, primaquine-clindamycin, and atovaquone, have proven efficacious in patients with AIDS but are largely untested in patients with chemotherapy-related immunosuppression.

ADJUSTING THERAPY

For several reasons, it may prove necessary to adjust or modify the initial antimicrobial regimen. Results of cultures may suggest that another regimen would be more active or less toxic. All cultures may remain negative while the patient fails to respond to the regimen employed. Fever may recur following an initial response to therapy, raising the possibility of a superinfection.

Adjusting therapy based on a culture report is usually straightforward, but the other two situations may pose dilemmas. In these circumstances, resistant organisms or noninfectious causes of fever need to be considered. Repeat cultures and careful clinical reappraisal may prove to be helpful. Empiric modification of the antibiotic regimen to enhance the effect on gram-positive or fungal pathogens may be successful. Vancomycin is active against gram-positive organisms; antifungal therapy should be strongly considered if a combination of antibacterial agents proves ineffective after 5 to 7 days of treatment.[21] Addition of a nonsteroidal anti-inflammatory agent may eliminate fever caused by tumor or tumor lysis.

DURATION OF THERAPY

Antibiotics should usually be discontinued when the neutropenia has resolved if there is no clinical evidence of infection. Often, however, the fever may resolve, while neutropenia is expected to continue for a prolonged period of time. Antibiotic therapy is commonly continued until the granulocyte count reaches 500 μl (0.5×10^9/liter). While this reduces the number of relapsing infections, it is likely to increase the risk of superinfection and the risk of antibiotic toxicity. Marrow recovery may be delayed by cephalosporins and sulfa drugs. Therefore, it is reasonable to discontinue antibiotics after an appropriate course in patients who have responded promptly and completely to therapy.[21,40,41] If antibiotics are discontinued, close observation is required and therapy should be reinstituted at any suggestion of recurrent infection.

The duration of antifungal therapy will vary considerably. Parasitic infection with *Pneumocystis* requires 2 to 3 weeks of therapy. Herpetic infections are generally treated for 7 days.

FEVER FOLLOWING RECOVERY FROM CHEMOTHERAPY

Occasionally fevers will persist after the granulocyte count has returned to normal levels. Drug fever is a consideration in this setting, but more commonly a deep-seated infection is present.[42] Pulmonary and hepatic[43] fungal infections must be considered. Elevations of serum alkaline phosphatase levels and a characteristic image on computed tomography are common with hepatic involvement.[44] Hepatic ultrasound[45] and magnetic resonance imaging[46] have also been reported to be diagnostically useful, but biopsy may be required to establish this diagnosis. Hepatosplenic candidiasis requires prolonged therapy. Several regimens have been proposed, including fluconazole[47] and liposomal amphotericin B.[48] Cure is difficult to achieve regardless of the regimen employed.

Indwelling catheter infection should also be considered when fevers continue after marrow recovery.

CATHETER-RELATED INFECTIONS

Minor exit site infections generally respond promptly to therapy. Infection of indwelling catheters with *Staphylococcus epidermidis* and other avirulent pathogens can often be cured with a prolonged course (at least 2 weeks) of an appropriate antibiotic. If a tunnel infection is present, successful therapy is less likely. Gram-negative infections or fungal infections[49] of the catheter usually necessitate its removal. This may be followed, if necessary, by insertion of a new catheter at a different site. Catheters impregnated with antibiotics may resist infection but have not been widely studied in neutropenic patients or with tunneled catheters. Chlorhexidine and silver-impregnated central venous catheters do not appear to prevent bloodstream infections in neutropenic patients.[50] Catheter infections and their management are considered in greater detail in Chap. 21 and have been reviewed elsewhere.[51]

OUTPATIENT THERAPY

Ten years ago, treatment of the febrile neutropenic patient outside of the hospital would have been unthinkable. More recently, economic pressures, coupled with the widespread availability of home intravenous antibiotic services and more potent oral antibiotics, have made outpatient therapy an option for some of these patients.[52,53] Outcomes seem to be comparable to those observed in hospitalized patients, provided that the patients are selected properly and that appropriate monitoring can be ensured. Suitable candidates for home intravenous therapy include those patients who are expected to have a short duration of neutropenia. Individuals who remain febrile, who require multiple antibiotics, or who are unreliable are not candidates for home intravenous therapy. Nurses must be experienced in the evaluation of chemo-

therapy patients and familiar with catheter care and maintenance. Rigorous family education is a crucial ingredient for a successful outcome.

PREVENTION OF INFECTIONS

PREVENTION OF BACTERIAL INFECTIONS

In view of the high mortality rate associated with infections in neutropenic patients, preventive measures remain a priority. Instrumentation should be avoided whenever possible. Intravenous access sites should be carefully maintained. The earliest strategies included administration of nonabsorbable oral antibiotics usually consisting of gentamicin, vancomycin, and nystatin.[54] Unfortunately, this combination is poorly tolerated. Therefore, this practice has been abandoned in favor of systemic antibiotics. Trimethoprim-sulfamethoxazole has been especially well studied and is of benefit in some patients, particularly those with severe neutropenia expected to last over 2 weeks.[21] It has the advantage of also preventing *Pneumocystis*, but it will cause a rash in 5 to 10 percent of individuals. Its use may be associated with infections with resistant organisms, and it may result in a delay of marrow recovery.[55]

The fluorinated quinolones have received considerable attention for their ability to prevent gram-negative infections in neutropenic patients.[56–58] Unfortunately, indiscriminate use of these agents in the community have diminished their value as resistant bacteria have developed. Infection with gram-positive organisms is more common in patients receiving quinolones prophylactically.[59,60] Prophylactic use would also eliminate these agents for therapeutic use in the same patient.

Prophylactic antibiotics are of benefit in some patients with acute leukemia receiving induction chemotherapy. The best regimen remains to be determined and may vary from institution to institution. Perhaps equally important for preventing infection is careful attention to sterile technique and personal hygiene.[61] Isoniazid hydrazide therapy is recommended for all tuberculin-positive patients who require chemotherapy unless they have previously been treated.

The ability of GM-CSF and G-CSF to raise the granulocyte count in neutropenic patients may serve as another means of preventing bacterial infections in this group of patients (see Chap. 15). While some series show a small reduction in the infection rate in patients receiving these agents,[62] others do not.[63–65] Although it is likely that a subset of patients will benefit from this therapy, definitive data are lacking.

Immunotherapy of various forms has been reviewed.[66] Intravenous immunoglobulin has been advocated for prevention of bacterial infection in some patients with chronic severe hypogammaglobulinemia, such as may occur in chronic lymphocytic leukemia and multiple myeloma, but its value has not been proven. The value of special diets and reverse isolation has not been established. Granulocyte transfusions have no role in the prevention of infection.

PREVENTION OF PARASITIC INFECTIONS

Pneumocystis carinii pneumonia can be prevented with trimethoprim-sulfamethoxazole. Pentamidine administered monthly in aerosolized form also appears to be effective.[67] Although *P. carinii* is a ubiquitous organism, it appears that there is institutional variability in the incidence of infection. Therefore, the need for prophylaxis will vary.

PREVENTION OF VIRAL INFECTIONS

Acyclovir has proven useful for the prevention of recurrent herpes simplex infections in patients receiving chemotherapy and marrow transplantation.[68,69] Such prophylaxis is probably unnecessary in patients who lack antibodies to herpes simplex virus. Varicella zoster immunoglobulin given to susceptible individuals reduces the incidence of varicella following exposure.

The incidence of CMV infection can be reduced by the avoidance of blood products from CMV-seropositive individuals.[70] Passive immunization has provided benefit in some studies. Acyclovir, while ineffective in treating CMV infections, may reduce their incidence.[71] Ganciclovir[72] and foscarnet[73] have been used successfully to prevent CMV infections in marrow recipients, but these strategies have not been applied to patients receiving conventional chemotherapy.

Active immunizations with killed vaccines (e.g., influenza) are of some benefit. Attenuated vaccines (e.g., measles) should be avoided.

PREVENTION OF FUNGAL INFECTIONS

Studies on prevention of fungal infections in neutropenic patients are difficult to evaluate. Results of the various studies have been conflicting, partly because different definitions have been applied and different doses of antifungal agents have been administered and partly because of the small numbers of patients.

Nystatin,[74] amphotericin B,[75] clotrimazole,[76] and ketoconazole[77] have been studied. Each has been effective in reducing colonization and mucositis, but none has been consistently effective in preventing systemic fungal infections and improving survival.

Several studies have documented a statistically significant reduction in superficial and invasive fungal infections when fluconazole is used prophylactically.[78,79] However, many failures have also been reported, including breakthrough fungemia.[80] Not all studies have documented a benefit of using fluconazole prophylactically.[81,82] Superinfection with *Aspergillus*, *Torulopsis glabrata*, and *Candida krusei* have been seen when fluconazole has been used prophylactically.[83] Itraconazole may be effective in preventing infection with *Aspergillus*.[84]

Thus, while antifungal prophylaxis appears to diminish the incidence of mucositis, close observation and early treatment of mucositis would also be a reasonable approach to this problem. The ability of antifungal agents to prevent systemic infection is not consistent. Prophylactic use of these agents may prove to select more resistant strains of fungus and may not reduce mortality. Therefore, pending the results of additional studies, earlier and more aggressive empiric antifungal therapy may be preferable to prophylaxis. Exceptions to this approach would include patients undergoing marrow transplantation and patients in facilities where there is a high incidence of invasive infections with *C. albicans*.

INFECTIONS IN MARROW TRANSPLANTATION RECIPIENTS

Patients receiving marrow transplants are at risk for the same infections occurring in patients rendered neutropenic by chemotherapy. Graft-versus-host disease and the immunosuppressive agents used to treat it result in a particularly high incidence of infection in this group of patients. Viral infections, especially CMV and varicella zoster virus, are especially troublesome. Infection in marrow transplant patients has been reviewed[85,86] and is discussed in Chap. 18.

REFERENCES

1. Bodey GP, Buckley M, Sathe YS, Freireich EJ: Quantitative relationships between circulating leukocytes and infection in patients with acute leukemia. *Ann Intern Med* 64:328, 1966.
2. Oppenheim BA: The changing pattern of infection in neutropenic patients. *J Antimicrob Chemother* 41(suppl D):7, 1998.
3. Spanik S: *Viridans* streptococcal bacteraemia due to penicillin-resistant and penicillin-sensitive streptococci: Analysis of risk factors and outcome in 60 patients from a single cancer centre before and after penicillin is used for prophylaxis. *Scand J Infect Dis* 29:245, 1997.
4. Martino R, Manteiga R, Sanchez I, et al: *Viridans* streptococcal shock syndrome during bone marrow transplantation. *Acta Haematol* 94:69, 1995.
5. Morrison VA: The infectious complications of chronic lymphocytic leukemia. *Semin Oncol* 25:98, 1998.
6. Matsunaga T, Sakamaki S, Ishigaki S, et al: Use of PCR serum in diagnosing and monitoring cytomegalovirus reactivation in bone marrow transplant recipients. *Int J Hematol* 69:105, 1999.
7. Whimbey E, Champlin RE, Couch RB, et al: Community respiratory virus infections among hospitalized adult bone marrow transplant recipients. *Clin Infect Dis* 5:778, 1966.
8. Libshitz HI, Pannu HK, Elting LS, Cooksley CD: Tuberculosis in cancer patients: An update. *J Thorac Imaging* 12:41, 1997.
9. Sickles EA, Greene EA, Wiernik PH: Clinical presentation of infection in granulocytopenic patients. *Arch Intern Med* 135:715, 1975.
10. Cohen JS, Paz BI, O'Donnell MR: Treatment of perianal infection following bone marrow transplantation. *Dis Colon Rectum* 39:981, 1996.
11. Korones DN, Hussong MR, Gullace MA: Routine chest radiography of children with cancer hospitalized for fever and neutropenia. *Cancer* 80:1160, 1997.
12. Heussel CP, Kauczor HU, Heussel G, Fischer B, Mildenberger P, Thelen M: Early detection of pneumonia in febrile neutropenic patients: Use of thin-section CT. *Am J Roentgenol* 169:1347, 1997.
13. Aisner J, Murillo J, Schimpff SC, Steere AC: Invasive aspergillosis in acute leukemia: Correlation with nose cultures and antibiotic use. *Ann Intern Med* 90:4, 1979.
14. Einsele H, Hebart H, Roller C, et al: Detection and identification of fungal pathogens in blood by using molecular probe. *J Clin Microbiol* 35:1353, 1997.
15. Richardson MD, Kokki MH: Diagnosis and prevention of fungal infection in the immunocompromised patient. *Blood Rev* 12:24, 1998.
16. Toledo-Pereyra LH, DeMeester TR, Kinealey A, et al: The benefits of open lung biopsy in patients with previous nondiagnostic transbronchial lung biopsy. *Chest* 77:647, 1980.
17. Pagano L, Pagliari G, Busso A, et al: The role of bronchoalveolar lavage in the microbiological diagnosis of pneumonia in patients with haematological malignancies. *Ann Med* 29:535, 1997.
18. Love LJ, Schimpff SC, Schiffer CA, Wiernik PH: Improved prognosis for granulocytopenic patients with gram-negative bacteremia. *Am J Med* 68:643, 1980.
19. Elting LS: Outcomes of bacteremia in patients with cancer and neutropenia: Observations from two decades of epidemiological clinical trials. *Clin J Infect Dis* 25:247, 1997.
20. Dompeling EC, Donnelly JP, Deresinski SC, Feld R, Lane-Allman EF, De Pauw BE: Early identification of neutropenic patients at risk of gram-positive bacteraemia and the impact of empirical administration of vancomycin. *Eur J Cancer* 32:1332, 1996.
21. Hughes WT, Armstrong O, Bodey GP, et al: Guidelines for the use of antimicrobial agents in neutropenic patients with unexplained fever. Infectious Diseases Society of America. *Clin Infect Dis* 25:551, 1997.
22. Gerberding JL: Aminoglycoside dosing: Timing is of the essence. *Am J Med* 105:256, 1998.
23. Hatala R, Dinh TT, Cook DJ: Single daily dosing of aminoglycosides in immunocompromised adults: A systematic review. *Clin Infect Dis* 24:810, 1997.
24. Daenen S, Erjavec Z, Uges DRA, De Vries-Hospers HG, De Jonge P, Halie MR: Continuous infusion of ceftazidime in febrile neutropenic patients with acute myeloid leukemia. *Eur J Clin Microbiol Infect Dis* 14:188, 1995.
25. Biron P, Fuhrmann C, Cure H, et al: Cefepime versus imipenem-cilastatin as empirical monotherapy in 400 febrile patients with short duration neutropenia (CEMIC): Study Group of Infectious Diseases in Cancer. *J Antimicrob Chemother* 42:511, 1998.
26. Behre G, Link H, Maschmeyer G, et al: Meropenem monotherapy versus combination therapy with ceftazidime and amikacin for empirical treatment of febrile neutropenic patients. *Ann Hematol* 76:73, 1998.
27. Lindblad R, Rodjer S, Adriansson M, et al: Empiric monotherapy for febrile neutropenia: A randomized study comparing meropenem with ceftazidime. *Scand J Infect Dis* 30:237, 1998.

28. Yamamura D, Gucaip R, Carlisle P, Cimino M, Roberts J, Rostein C: Open randomized study of cefepime versus piperacillin-gentamicin for treatment of febrile neutropenic cancer patients. *Antimicrob Agents Chemother* 41:1704, 1997.

29. Ghazal HH, Ghazal CD, Tabbara IA: Ceftazidime and ciprofloxacin as empiric therapy in febrile neutropenic patients undergoing hematopoietic stem cell transplantation. *Clin Ther* 19:520, 1997.

30. Moellering RO: Vancomycin-resistant enterococci. *Clin Infect Dis* 26:1196, 1998.

31. Eliopoulos GM, Wennersten GB, Gold HS, et al: Characterization of vancomycin-resistant *Enterococcus faecium* isolates from the United States and their susceptibility in vitro to dalfopristin-quinupristin. *Antimicrob Agents Chemother* 42:1088, 1998.

32. Cruz JM, Peacock JE Jr, Loomer L, et al: Rapid intravenous infusion of amphotericin B: A pilot study. *Am J Med* 93:123, 1992.

33. Wong-Beringer A, Jacobs RA, Guglielmo BJ: Lipid formulations of amphotericin B: Clinical efficacy and toxicities. *Clin Infect Dis* 27:603, 1998.

34. White MH, Bowden RA, Sandier ES, et al: Randomized, double-blind clinical trial of amphotericin B colloidal dispersion vs. amphotericin B in the empirical treatment of fever and neutropenia. *Clin Infect Dis* 27:296, 1998.

35. Lube RG, Boyle JA: Renal effects of amphotericin B lipid complex. *Am J Kidney Dis* 31:780, 1998.

36. Prentice HG, Hann IM, Herbrecht R, et al: A randomized comparison of liposomal versus conventional amphotericin B for the treatment of pyrexia of unknown origin in neutropenic patients. *Br J Haematol* 98:711, 1997.

37. Lowance D, Neumayer HH, Legendre CM, et al: Valacyclovir for the prevention of cytomegalovirus disease after renal transplantation: International Valacyclovir Cytomegalovirus Prophylaxis Transplantation Study Group. *N Engl J Med* 340:1462, 1999.

38. Stocchi R, Ward KN, Fanin R, Baccarani M, Apperley JF: Management of human cytomegalovirus infection and disease after allogeneic bone marrow transplantation. *Haematologica* 84:71, 1999.

39. Ljungman P: Cytomegalovirus pneumonia: Presentation, diagnosis, and treatment. *Semin Respir Infect* 10:209 1995.

40. Dinubile MJ: Stopping antibiotic therapy in neutropenic patients. *Ann Intern Med* 108:289,1988.

41. Cornelissen JJ, Rozenberg-Arska M, Dekker AW: Discontinuation of intravenous antibiotic therapy during persistent neutropenia patients receiving prophylaxis with oral ciprofloxacin. *Clin Infect Dis* 21:1300, 1995.

42. Barton TD, Schuster MG: The cause of fever following resolution of neutropenia in patients with acute leukemia. *Clin J Infect Dis* 22:1064, 1996.

43. Sallah S: Hepatosplenic candidiasis in patients with acute leukemia: Increasingly encountered complications. *Anticancer Res* 19:757, 1999.

44. Thaler M, Pastakia B, Shawker TH, et al: Hepatic candidiasis in cancer patients: The evolving picture of the syndrome. *Ann Intern Med* 108:88, 1988.

45. Karthaus M, Huebner G, Elser C, Geissler RG, Heil G, Ganser A: Early detection of chronic disseminated candida infection in leukemia patients with febrile neutropenia: Value of computer-assisted serial ultrasound documentation. *Ann Hematol* 77:41, 1998.

46. Sallah S, Semelka R, Kelekis N, Worawattanakul S, Sallah W: Diagnosis and monitoring response to treatment of hepatosplenic candidiasis in patients with acute leukemia using magnetic resonance imaging. *Acta Haematol* 100:77, 1998.

47. Torres-Valdivieso MJ, Lopes J, Melero O, et al: Hepatosplenic candidosis in an immunosuppressed patient responding to fluconazole. *Mycoses* 37:443, 1994.

48. Walsh TJ, Whitcomb P, Piscitelli S, et al: Safety, tolerance, and pharmacokinetics of amphotericin B lipid complex in children with hepatosplenic candidiasis. *Antimicrob Agents Chemother* 41:1944, 1997.

49. Klein NC, Gill MV, Cunha BA: Unusual organisms causing intravenous line infections in compromised hosts: II. Fungal infections. *Infect Dis Clin Pract* 5:303, 1996.

50. Logghe C, Van Ossel C, D'Hoore W, Ezzedine H, Wauters G, Haxhe JJ: Evaluation of chlorhexidine and silver-sulfadiazine impregnated central venous catheters for the prevention of bloodstream infection in leukaemic patients: A randomized controlled trial. *J Hosp Infect* 37:145, 1997.

51. Mayhall CG: Diagnosis and management of infections of implantable devices used for prolonged venous access, in *Current Clinical Topics in Infectious Diseases,* edited by JS Remington, MN Swartz, vol 12, p 83. Blackwell, Cambridge, MA, 1992.

52. Escalante CP, Rubenstein KB, Roiston KV: Outpatient antibiotic therapy for febrile episodes in low-risk neutropenic patients with cancer. *Cancer Invest* 15:237, 1997.

53. Tice AD: Outpatient parenteral antibiotic therapy for fever and neutropenia. *Infect Dis Clin North Am,* 12:963, 1998.

54. Schimpff SC, Greene WH, Young VM, et al: Infection prevention in acute nonlymphocytic leukemia. *Ann Intern Med* 82:351, 1975.

55. Kovatch AL, Wald ER, Albo VD, et al: Oral trimethoprim-sulfamethoxazole for prevention of bacterial infection during the induction phase of cancer chemotherapy in children. *Pediatrics* 76:754, 1985.

56. Engels BA, Lau J, Barza M: Efficacy of quinolone prophylaxis in neutropenic cancer patients: A meta-analysis. *J Clin Oncol* 16:1179, 1998.

57. Cruciani M, Rampazo R, Malena M, et al: Prophylaxis with fluoroquinolones for bacterial infections in neutropenic patients: A meta-analysis. *Clin Infect Dis* 23:795, 1996.

58. Bow EJ, Loewen R, Vaughan D: Reduced requirement for antibiotic therapy targeting gram-negative organisms in febrile, neutropenic patients with cancer who are receiving antibacterial chemoprophylaxis with oral quinolones. *Clin Infect Dis* 20:907, 1995.

59. Bochud PY, Calandra T, Francioli P: Bacteremia due to *viridans* streptococci in neutropenic patients: A review. *Am J Med* 97:256, 1994.

60. Patrick CC: Use of fluoroquinolones as prophylactic agents in patients with neutropenia. *Pediatr Infect Dis J* 12:135, 1997.

61. Schimpff SC: Infection prevention during granulocytopenia, in *Current Clinical Topics in Infectious Disease,* edited by JS Remington, MN Swartz, vol 1, p 85. McGraw-Hill, New York, 1980.

62. Mitchell PLR, Morland B, Stevens MOG, Dick G, et al: Granulocyte colony-stimulating factor in established febrile neutropenia: A randomized study of pediatric patients. *J Clin Oncol* 15:1163, 1997.

63. Pui OH, Boyett JM, Hughes WI, et al: Human granulocyte colony-stimulating factor after induction chemotherapy in children with acute lymphoblastic leukemia. *N Engl J Med* 336:1781, 1997.

64. Ohno R, Miyawaki S, Hatake K, et al: Human urinary macrophage colony-stimulating factor reduces the incidence and duration of febrile neutropenia and shortens the period required to finish three courses of intensive consolidation therapy in acute myeloid leukemia: A double-blind controlled study. *J Clin Oncol* 15:2954, 1997.

65. Hartmann LC, Tschetter LK, Habermann TM, et al: Granulocyte colony-stimulating factor in severe chemotherapy-induced afebrile neutropenia. *N Engl J Med* 336:1776, 1997.

66. Siber GR, Snydman DR: Use of immune globulins in the prevention and treatment of infections. *Curr Clin Top Infect Dis* 12:208, 1992.

67. Weinthal J, Frost JD, Briones G, Cairo MS: Successful *Pneumocystis carinii* pneumonia prophylaxis using aerosolized pentamidine in children with acute leukemia. *J Clin Oncol* 12:136, 1994.

68. Saral R, Ambinder RF, Burns WH, et al: Acyclovir prophylaxis against herpes simplex virus infection in patients with leukemia: A randomized, double-blind placebo-controlled study. *Ann Intern Med* 99:773, 1983.

69. Wade JO, Newton B, Fluornoy N, Meyers JD: Oral acyclovir for prevention of herpes simplex virus reactivation after marrow transplantation. *Ann Intern Med* 100:823, 1984.

70. Bowden ERA, Sages M, Gleaves CA, Banaji M, Newton B, Meyers JD: Cytomegalovirus. Seronegative blood components for the prevention of primary cytomegalovirus infection after marrow transplant. Considerations for blood banks. *Transfusion* 27:478, 1987.

71. Prentice HG, Gluckman E, Powles RL, et al: Long-term survival in allogeneic bone marrow transplant recipients following acyclovir prophylaxis for CMV infections: The European Acyclovir for CMV Prophylaxis Study Group. *Bone Marrow Transplant* 19:129, 1997.

72. Verdonck LF, Dekker AW, Rozenberg-Arska M, van den Hoek MR: A risk-adapted approach with a short course of ganciclovir to prevent cytomegalovirus (CMV) pneumonia in CMV-seropositive recipients of allogeneic bone marrow transplants. *Clin Infect Dis* 24:901, 1997.

73. Reusser P, Gambertoglio JG, Lilleby K, Meyers JD: Phase I-II trial of foscarnet for prevention of cytomegalovirus infection in autologous and allogeneic marrow transplant recipients. *J Infect Dis* 166:473, 1992.

74. Pizzuto J, Conte G, Aviles A, Ambriz R, Morales M: Nystatin prophylaxis in leukemia and lymphoma (letter). *N Engl J Med* 299:661, 1978.

75. Perfect JR, Klotman ME, Gilbert CC, et al: Prophylactic intravenous amphotericin B in neutropenic autologous bone marrow transplant recipients. *J Infect Dis* 156:891, 1992.

76. Cuttner J, Troy KM, Funaro L, et al: Clotrimazole treatment for prevention of oral candidiasis in patients with acute leukemia undergoing chemotherapy. *Am J Med* 61:771, 1986.

77. Hansen RM, Einerio N, Sohnle PG, et al: Ketoconazole in the prevention of candidiasis in patients with cancer: A prospective randomized, controlled, double-blind study. *Arch Intern Med* 147:710, 1987.

78. Goodman JL, Winston DJ, Green RA, et al: A controlled trial of fluconazole to prevent fungal infections in patients undergoing bone marrow transplantation. *N Engl J Med* 362:845, 1992.

79. Rotstein C, Bow EJ, Laverdiere M, Ioannou S, Carr D, Moghaddam N: Randomized placebo-controlled trial of fluconazole prophylaxis for neutropenic cancer patients: benefit based on purpose and intensity of cytotoxic therapy. The Canadian Fluconazole Prophylaxis Study Group. *Clin Infect Dis* 28:331, 1999.

80. Girmenia C, Martino P: Breakthrough candidemia during antifungal treatment with fluconazole in patients with hematologic malignancies. *Blood* 87:838, 1996.

81. Kern W, Behre G, Rudolf T, Kerkhoff A: Failure of fluconazole prophylaxis to reduce mortality or the requirement of systemic amphotericin B therapy during treatment for refractory acute myeloid leukemia: Results of a prospective randomized phase III study. German AML Cooperative Group. *Cancer* 83:291, 1998.

82. Schaffner A, Schaffner M: Effect of prophylactic fluconazole on the frequency of fungal infections, amphotericin B use, and health care costs in patients undergoing intensive chemotherapy for hematologic neoplasias. *J Infect Dis* 172:1035, 1995.

83. Wingard JR, Merz WG, Rinaldi MG, Johnson TR, Karp JE, Saral R: Increase in *Candida krusei* infection among patients with bone marrow transplantation and neutropenia treated prophylactically with fluconazole. *N Engl J Med* 325:1274, 1991.

84. Lamy T, Bernard M, Courtois A, et al: Prophylactic use of itraconazole for the prevention of invasive pulmonary aspergillosis in high-risk neutropenic patients. *Leuk Lymphoma* 30:63, 1998.

85. Winston DJ: Prophylaxis and treatment of infections in the bone marrow transplant recipient. *Curr Clin Top Inf Dis* 113:293, 1993.

86. Thomas ED, Blume KG, Forman SJ (eds): *Hematopoietic Cell Transplantation*, 2d ed. Blackwell Science, Boston, 1999.

ALLOGENEIC AND AUTOLOGOUS HEMATOPOIETIC CELL TRANSPLANTATION

ROBERT S. NEGRIN

KARL G. BLUME

Hematopoietic cell transplantation has developed from a treatment of "last resort" to an effective therapy for patients with a variety of hematologic diseases. Developments in this field have dramatically reduced the morbidity and mortality of transplantation. Most notable has been the introduction of peripheral blood progenitor cells as a source of hematopoietic stem cells. Here we emphasize the theoretical framework for curative therapy as the biological basis of transplantation. Important developments in the field include the sources of hematopoietic stem cells, novel approaches to preparative regimens, uses of monoclonal antibodies and nonmyeloablative preparative regimens. Advances in engraftment and supportive care including the utilization of hematopoietic growth factors and other supportive care measures have greatly reduced the morbidity associated with transplantation. In this chapter, the biological basis, as well as clinical results, of both autologous and allogeneic hematopoietic cell transplantation will be discussed. Emphasis will be placed on the biological mechanisms underlying and facilitating transplantation. Results of transplantation in the hematologic diseases are stressed, in particular, acute myelogenous leukemia, acute lymphocytic leukemia, and chronic myelogenous leukemia. Additional information can be found in the individual chapters that focus on specific disease entities (see Chaps. 46, 47, 92–94, 97, and 103). Novel indications for transplantation are also reviewed with particular reference to the biological basis for these interventions. The major challenges facing patients undergoing transplantation, including complications such as graft-versus-host disease, veno-occlusive disease, infection, and relapse of the underlying disease, remain formidable. Major advances that are likely to have a dramatic impact on the treatment outcome and that will further enhance the field of hematopoietic cell transplantation in years to come continue to be made in the fields of cell biology, hematology, and immunology.

Acronyms and abbreviations that appear in this chapter include: ALL, acute lympho-blastic leukemia; AML, acute myelogenous leukemia; ATG, antithymocyte globulin; AT-III, antithrombin-III; BEAM, carmustine (BCNU), etoposide, cytosine arabino-side, and melphalan; BMT, bone marrow transplantation; CI, confidence interval; CLL, chronic lymphocytic leukemia; CML, chronic myelogenous leukemia; CMV, cytomegalovirus; CR, complete remission; CSF, colony-stimulating factors; CTL, cytotoxic T lymphocytes; EPO, erythropoietin; FACS, fluorescent activated cell sort-ing; G-CSF, granulocyte colony-stimulating factors; GM-CSF, granulocyte-macro-phage colony-stimulating factor; 4HC, 4-hydroperoxycyclophosphamide; HLA, hu-man leukocyte antigen; IL, interleukin; MACOP-B, Methotrexate, Adiramycin, Cyclophosphamide, Vincristine, Prednisone, Bleomycin; MDS, myelodysplastic syn-dromes; MHC, major histocompatibility complex; MoAb, monoclonal antibody; NK, natural killer; PCR, polymerase chain reaction; PUVA, psoralen plus ultraviolet radia-tion; SCF, stem-cell factor; SCID, severe combined immunodeficiency disorder; TNF, tumor necrosis factor; tPA, tissue-type plasminogen activator; TPN, total parenteral nutrition; TPO, thrombopoietin; WBC, white blood count.

HISTORY

The transplantation of marrow to rescue patients from lethal radiation or chemotherapy or to replace abnormal marrow has evolved over the past three decades from an act of desperation administered only to patients with end-stage disease to an acceptable and, in some instances, "first-line" form of therapy employed early in the course of a variety of malignant and nonmalignant disorders. Advances in transplantation biology and supportive care have made that evolution possible and have helped to usher in the modern era of marrow transplantation.

The first documented human marrow transplant was attempted in 1939, when a woman with gold-induced aplasia was given marrow intravenously from a brother with identical blood group antigens. The transplant was not successful, and the patient died five days later.[1] In the early 1950s, laboratory experiments demonstrated that splenic shielding or intravenous administration of marrow cells protected animals from lethal radiation.[2,3] Subsequently, patients with end-stage hematologic malignancies were treated with myeloablative doses of radiation and chemotherapy followed by marrow infusion. These initial attempts at human marrow transplantation were generally unsuccessful but demonstrated at least transient engraftment in some patients and provided a framework for future studies.[4] Sustained engraftment was first documented in 1965 in a patient with acute lymphoblastic leuke-mia who received irradiation and chemotherapy followed by intrave-nous infusion of marrow from six different related donors.[5] En-graftment from one of the donors was demonstrated by erythrocyte phenotype, acceptance of a skin graft from that donor, and development of graft-versus-host disease. The patient died of recurrent leukemia 20 months after marrow infusion.

Studies in dogs demonstrated the importance of immunological matching for a successful outcome.[6] Discovery of the human leukocyte antigen (HLA) system and development of histocompatibility typing methods in the 1960s led to a new phase of marrow transplantation. The first successful marrow transplants were in children with severe combined immunodeficiency performed in 1968,[7,8] as was a successful transplant in a patient with Wiskott-Aldrich syndrome.[9] The latter report also demonstrated the need for immunosuppressive therapy prior to marrow infusion in order to ensure engraftment in immuno-competent patients. Between 1969 and 1975, increasing numbers of patients with acute leukemia who had failed conventional therapy and patients with advanced aplastic anemia underwent marrow transplanta-tion from identical twin donors[10] and histocompatible siblings.[11,12] For the first time, a significant percentage of patients became long-term, disease-free survivors.[13]

Since 1975, patients have been considered suitable candidates for marrow transplantation earlier in the clinical course of their disease. The number of marrow transplant centers continues to increase throughout the world. During the past 15 years, autologous marrow grafting (use of the patient's own marrow) has also become a viable treatment modality for selected candidates to the extent that autologous marrow transplantation is now more frequently performed than alloge-neic marrow transplantation. More recently, the introduction of periph-eral blood progenitor cells has reduced the morbidity and mortality associated with transplantation.

THEORETICAL CONCEPTS FOR CURATIVE THERAPY IN HEMATOPOIETIC CELL TRANSPLANTATION

The beneficial effects of hematopoietic cell transplantation are due to both the high-dose chemotherapy that allows for enhanced tumor-cell killing and the ability to overcome drug resistance, as well as the immunological effects referred to as the graft-versus-tumor effect. Dose escalation of chemotherapy and radiation therapy is possible if the dose-limiting effects of hematopoietic toxicity are circumvented with the infusion of the stem-cell graft. This is the underlying concept in autologous hematopoietic cell transplantation, where there are no immunological effects due to the infused stem cells. The dramatic dose escalation of chemotherapy and radiation therapy that can be achieved with autologous transplantation allows for the possibility of curative therapy in malignancies where dose escalation results in significantly greater tumor-cell killing.

In the allogeneic setting, the importance of graft-versus-tumor effects has been central to the success of the transplant procedure. This has been demonstrated in a number of ways. Comparison of results following allogeneic transplantation to those of syngeneic transplantation, where the donor and recipient are genetically identical, have been particularly informative. Here it has been well documented that the relapse rate is significantly higher for patients who undergo syngeneic transplantation than for patients who undergo an allogeneic transplant procedure.[14] It is interesting to note that this phenomenon appears to be disease dependent, since those patients with chronic myelogenous leukemia (CML) and acute myelogenous leukemia (AML) exhibit a much more demonstrable graft-versus-tumor effect than do patients with acute lymphoblastic leukemia (ALL). The cells responsible for the graft-versus-tumor effect include T cells, since depletion of T cells from the allograft results in control of graft-versus-host disease; however, it markedly increases the risk of relapse of the underlying malignancy.[15] In addition, a variety of clinical studies have demonstrated that those patients who develop some degree of graft-versus-host-disease, especially chronic graft-versus-host disease, have a reduction in the risk of relapse.[16,17] All of these studies are consistent with the concept that immunological effector cells within the donor inoculum are capable of immunological control of the minimal disease that remains following the transplant. Further support of this concept comes from the utilization of donor leukocyte infusions in patients who suffer a relapse following an allogeneic transplant procedure, after which a significant percentage of patients reenter a complete remission (CR).[18-20]

STEM-CELL MODELS OF HEMATOPOIESIS

The role of hematopoietic stem cells is central to the biological basis of transplantation. A variety of early in vitro and in vivo assay systems have been developed to identify the biological activity of hematopoietic stem cells. Through these assay systems, it has become clear that immature populations of cells capable of giving rise to all of the hematolymphoid cells are present in the marrow. Various accessory and antigen-presenting cells found in the liver, gastrointestinal tract, lung, and brain are also derived from hematopoietic stem cells. Hematopoietic stem cells are biologically defined as those cells that are capable of rescuing lethally irradiated animals, a definition that is conceptually clear but difficult to apply to humans.

In murine systems, monoclonal antibodies have been developed that recognize proteins on the surface of both immature hematopoietic stem cells and mature progenitor cells. Using fluorescence-activated cell sorting, populations of highly purified murine marrow cells have been identified that are capable of rescuing lethally irradiated animals.[21] In murine systems, the phenotype of cells with this biological activity is positive for stem-cell antigen 1 and Thy-1 yet does not express the various markers found on committed cells (lineage negative).[21] These cells also have been found capable of excreting the vital dye rhodamine. Cells with this phenotype are present in the murine marrow with the frequency of approximately $1:10^3$ and $1:10^4$. Morphologically, they appear to be similar to normal lymphocytes. These hematopoietic stem

cells are capable of self-renewal and multilineage differentiation into progenitor cells that in turn mature into the various committed cells that are released from the marrow. As few as 25 purified hematopoietic stem cells are capable of rescuing more than half of lethally irradiated animals, and 100 stem cells are capable of rescuing virtually all of the animals.[21]

Using a similar approach of monoclonal antibody staining and fluorescence-activated cell sorting, it has been possible to isolate and characterize a population of human putative hematopoietic stem cells capable of multilineage growth in in vitro and surrogate in vivo assays. Human hematopoietic stem cells express the antigen CD34 and also are lineage negative. They also have been found to express low amounts of Thy-1,[22,23] lack DR expression,[24] and excrete the dye rhodamine 123.[25] More recently, a population of hematopoietic stem cells that do not express CD34 and that are functionally capable of excreting the vital DNA-binding dye Hoechst 33342 has also been described.[26] However, in clinical transplantation, the CD34+ cells infused correlated closely with the functional capability of the hematopoietic graft.[27] Despite the fact that the most useful marker in clinical marrow transplantation to define cells capable of multilineage hematopoietic reconstitution has been CD34, it is recognized that only a fraction of CD34+ cells are true hematopoietic stem cells. Subset separation of CD34+ cells has been successful on a clinical scale, and preliminary trials using highly purified hematopoietic stem cells demonstrate that this population of cells, despite its relatively rare frequency, is capable of reconstituting multilineage hematopoiesis in a timely fashion.[28]

SOURCES OF HEMATOPOIETIC STEM CELLS

A variety of sources have been utilized for the collection of hematopoietic stem cells for transplantation procedures. These include marrow; peripheral blood, especially following mobilization; and umbilical cord blood obtained at the time of delivery.

MARROW

Marrow has served as the traditional source of hematopoietic stem cells for both allogeneic and autologous transplantation. The technique of marrow harvesting has become relatively routine.[29] Marrow is aspirated from the posterior iliac crests under either regional or general anesthesia. The cell dose required for stable long-term engraftment has not been defined with certainty; however, typical collections contain more than 2×10^8 nuclear cells per kilogram of recipient body weight. This generally requires between 700 and 1500 ml of marrow for an adult recipient. Current guidelines indicate that collection of up to 15 ml/kg is generally considered safe.

Complications of marrow harvesting are rare and generally involve complications of anesthesia. In one report of 1270 allogeneic marrow harvests from normal donors, there were six (0.5%) life-threatening complications.[30] This is similar to the rate described in individuals undergoing autologous collection.[31] The National Marrow Donor Program has reviewed the experience of volunteer donors in the first 493 harvests. In this cohort of donors, there was only one serious event (apnea), and three patients (0.6%) required a blood transfusion that was from nonautologous sources. However, the marrow collection procedure was not without significant morbidity, since it took up to 16 days for patients to fully recover, and 10 percent of the donors still had not completely recovered at the end of the first month following harvest.[32]

PERIPHERAL BLOOD

Hematopoietic stem cells circulate in the peripheral blood at extremely low levels. Following the administration of colony-stimulating factors

(CSF) and/or chemotherapy, a time-dependent increase in hematopoietic stem cells and progenitor cells—termed mobilization—is observed. The products obtained after stimulation have been termed peripheral-blood progenitor cells. A number of CSF have been found to be effective mobilizing agents, including G-CSF, GM-CSF, IL-3, and thrombopoietin (TPO).[33,34] The most common mobilization regimen involves the administration of G-CSF at 10 μg/kg/day, followed by apheresis on the fourth and fifth days.[35-37] A variety of other doses and schedules have been utilized with both CSF alone or in combination with chemotherapy. An earlier-acting cytokine termed stem-cell factor (SCF) or c-kit ligand has been found to synergize with G-CSF in mobilization of CD34+ cells.[38] Another novel cytokine, Flt-3 ligand, has been shown to enhance the mobilization of peripheral-blood progenitor cells, as well as dendritic cells, in a time-dependent fashion in synergy with G-CSF.[39] Administration of mobilized peripheral-blood progenitor cells has resulted in more rapid hematopoietic reconstitution than has been observed following a marrow transplant.[40] This advantage significantly reduced the morbidity and mortality of the transplant procedure, and the use of mobilized peripheral-blood progenitor cells has gained wide acceptance in the autologous setting.

The optimal methodology for mobilizing peripheral-blood progenitor cells has yet to be defined; however, the absolute number of CD34+ cells/kg recipient weight has proven to be a reliable and practical method for determining the adequacy of the stem-cell product. Most laboratories measure CD34+ cell content by FACS. A major effort has been made to standardize and validate this process. The optimal cell dose is controversial. However, most transplant centers have observed that stem-cell products containing more than 2×10^6 CD34+ cells/kg result in rapid hematopoietic recovery. Higher stem-cell doses may lead to more rapid platelet recovery.[41] The minimum cell dose required for hematopoietic engraftment has not been defined with certainty; however, cell doses below 1×10^6 CD34+ cells/kg are felt to be inadequate. A significant problem has been that approximately 10 to 40 percent of patients do not mobilize progenitor cells adequately using G-CSF alone or chemotherapy plus G-CSF. In addition, it has been difficult to identify prospectively those patients who are poor mobilizers. To achieve improved CD34+ cell mobilization, higher doses of G-CSF, between 20 and 40 μg/kg, have been utilized to improve the CD34+ cell yield and reduce the number of days of apheresis required to reach the collection goal.[42] Compared to G-CSF alone, combinations of cytokines using both G-CSF and SCF have resulted in improved CD34+ cell yields in a randomized study of breast cancer patients undergoing autologous transplantation.[43] However, SCF also activates mast cells, which may produce serious unwanted side effects.

The clinical significance of tumor cells in mobilized peripheral-blood progenitor-cell collections has generated considerable debate. There is no doubt that tumor-cell contamination of peripheral-blood progenitor cells does occur, especially when sensitive assays, such as the polymerase chain reaction (PCR) or immunofluorescence techniques, are utilized.[44,45] In one comparative study, the difference in tumor burden between the marrow and peripheral blood was measured at less than 1 log.[46] Since the absolute number of cells infused with an unmanipulated peripheral-blood progenitor cell graft is on the order of ten- to fifteenfold higher than with marrow, the total number of tumor cells infused could conceivably be greater with peripheral-blood progenitor cells. Therefore, methodologies designed to purge the stem-cell product of possible malignant-cell contamination have been developed, as discussed below.

Mobilized peripheral-blood progenitor cells have been largely utilized in the autologous setting; however, this approach has also been explored in the allogeneic setting in an effort to enhance hematopoietic recovery. The concern with the use of mobilized peripheral-blood progenitor cells in the allogeneic setting is that the large numbers of T cells in the inoculum may increase the risk of graft-versus-host disease. However, despite the large number of T cells in the inoculum, initial studies did not show an increase in the incidence of acute graft-versus-host disease,[40,47,48] but the incidence of chronic graft-versus-host disease may be higher.[49] The reason for this phenomenon is unclear. However, it may be related to the increased production of cytokines of the TH$_2$ type, such as IL-4 and IL-10, which may decrease the risk of graft-versus-host disease.[50] The relative merits of marrow versus G-CSF–mobilized peripheral-blood progenitor cells in allogeneic transplantation are currently being evaluated in randomized prospective clinical trials.

UMBILICAL CORD BLOOD

Umbilical cord blood obtained from the umbilical blood vessels and placenta following delivery has been found to be a rich source of hematopoietic stem cells. The relative immaturity of the cord blood cells may allow for engraftment across immunological barriers more easily than when other stem-cell sources are used.[51] Registries that allow for the collection, cryopreservation, typing, and quality control of cord blood products have been established. These can then be accessed following a search of the database. This approach may be particularly useful for securing donors for patients of minority groups that are relatively underrepresented in the donor registries. In addition, since the cord blood samples are collected and cryopreserved, there is less delay once a potential donor has been identified.

HISTOCOMPATIBILITY SYSTEM AND TYPES OF HEMATOPOIETIC STEM-CELL DONORS

The antigens of the HLA system are a series of cell-surface molecules critical for immune function. They are encoded by genes on chromosome 6. Gene clusters have been recognized that have been designated class I, class II, and class III. Class I and class II genes have been shown to be important for the success of organ grafts. The genes of class I and class II HLA molecules are similar and contain a peptide binding groove that is critical for proper cellular immune recognition. A large number of class I genes and pseudogenes have been identified. Those encoding for HLA-A, -B, and -C antigens are the most important. More than 15 different class II genes also have been identified, the most important of which are the HLA-D region genes, which include DR, DQ, DO, DN, and DP, with DR being the most relevant for marrow transplantation.

Typing for the HLA class I and II molecules is routinely performed by serologic assays. More recently, the use of DNA-based genotyping has had a significant impact in establishing identity between donors and recipients, especially when unrelated donors are utilized. Most centers utilize serologic typing for sibling matches; if the identified genes are serologically identical, they are most likely genotypically identical, since the donor and recipient are related. However, in the unrelated setting, there is no such assurance, and multiple different alleles have been identified for a given HLA antigen. Cytotoxic T lymphocyte analysis has also identified minor histocompatibility antigens that have an important additional function following transplantation.[52]

The importance of HLA matching has been well documented following allogeneic marrow transplantation. With greater HLA incompatibility, the risk of graft-versus-host disease and graft failure increases. For example, in one study, the rate of graft failure using marrows from donors who were only haplotype matched was 12.3 percent. In contrast, the rate of graft failure is only approximately 2 percent in recipients of stem cells from HLA-matched donors.[53] Among sibling donors, the degree of incompatibility has been correlated with the severity of graft-versus-host disease. More than one antigen mismatch results in an unacceptable incidence of graft-versus-host disease using conventional unmanipulated marrow transplant techniques. A single antigen mismatch resulted in increased incidence and severeity of graft-versus-host disease; however, overall survival was not impacted.[53] Mismatches at HLA-B appear to be tolerated best, followed by those at HLA-A, with mismatches at HLA-DR being the least well tolerated. However, since only approximately 30 percent of potential marrow transplant recipients have an HLA-matched or single antigen–mismatched donor, other sources of marrow cells are required. One approach has been to utilize the large numbers of volunteer donors, either through the National Marrow Donor Program or related registries. To date, more than 3 million altruistic individuals have enrolled in the National Marrow Donor Program and have volunteered to serve as marrow donors.

Such registries have provided large lists of potential donors that can be searched to identify appropriate donors throughout the world. Registry donors are especially useful for Caucasian recipients; minority donors are less represented, although this discrepancy is improving with time. Initial results of transplant procedures performed from unrelated donors demonstrated that this form of transplantation was feasible and successful, although initial results were inferior to those achieved with matched related donors.[54] Multiple reasons were associated with these poorer outcomes, including patient candidacy, increased risk of opportunistic infection, increased risk of graft failure, and graft-versus-host disease. With the development of molecular typing, especially at the class II region, results have improved substantially. Molecular donor-recipient identity at the HLA/DR1 and DQB1 alleles has reduced the risk of acute lethal graft-versus-host disease and has improved survival following unrelated donor marrow transplantation.[55,56] The use of molecular typing for the class II region has become part of routine practice for identifying appropriate donors for unrelated donor transplantation.

Molecular typing has also been developed for HLA class I alleles. This technology has revealed considerable heterogeneity. Some of the incompatibilities that have been identified by molecular typing and were not recognized by standard serologic typing have been associated with immunological reactions as assessed by cytotoxic T-lymphocyte (CTL) reactivity. In one study, 128 patients and 484 potential unrelated donors were evaluated by both serologic typing and molecular typing. Of the 187 individuals who were identified serologically as being matched, only 52.9 percent were found to be fully matched following DNA typing.[57] A higher level of disparity was noted for HLA-B than for HLA-A alleles. It is unclear as to which of these HLA disparities are clinically most important. The effect of matching of class I HLA alleles has been correlated with outcome in one study from Japan. In this study of 440 recipients of unrelated donor transplantation who were serologically identical with respect to recipients for HLA, -A, -B, and -DR antigens, the degree of HLA-A and HLA-C molecular incompatibility was found to be an independent risk factor for severe acute graft-versus-host disease. In addition, mismatching for HLA-A, but not HLA-C, alleles was an independent risk factor for higher mortality, and mismatching of HLA-C alleles was a significant risk factor for relapse of underlying leukemia.[58] These data require confirmation in a larger patient population. These clinical studies underline the importance of high resolution typing for identifying donors; however, it is clear that with increasing the requirement for molecular matching, an ever smaller donor pool will be available for each individual patient. Identifying which disparities are clinically relevant is a significant task that must be completed in order to fully evaluate these data.

Another alternative for patients, especially children, who do not have an appropriate HLA-matched sibling donor is the use of placental cord blood obtained from unrelated sources. Following cord blood transplantation, engraftment has been achieved; however, it is considerably delayed compared to engraftment following marrow transplantation. In one study of 562 recipients of placental cord blood transplants from unrelated donors, durable engraftment was achieved in 81 percent of recipients by day 42 for neutrophils and 85 percent by day 180 for platelets. The speed of hematopoietic engraftment was related to the leukocyte content of the graft, whereas transplantation-related mortality was associated with the degree of HLA disparity, the patient's underlying disease, and the experience of the transplantation center. Severe grade II to IV acute graft-versus-host disease occurred in 23 percent of patients, and chronic graft-versus-host disease occurred in 25 percent.[59] The relatively small number of cells collected on routine umbilical cord blood processing has made this type of transplantation primarily useful for children and small adults, although some clinical investigators are attempting to expand umbilical cord blood stem cells in vitro to transplant adult patients.

The use of three-antigen–mismatched or haplotype-matched donors has been mostly unsuccessful due to the high risk of graft-versus-host disease and graft failure. Higher stem-cell doses may overcome the problem of graft rejection in this donor-recipient setting. This has been accomplished with the use of G-CSF mobilized peripheral blood progenitor cells. Using this stem-cell source and highly immunosuppressive preparative regimens that include total body irradiation, high-dose chemotherapy, and antithymocyte globulin, extensively T-cell–depleted haplotype-matched grafts have been successfully engrafted without graft-versus-host disease.[60,61] The successful use of haplotype-matched related donors would greatly increase the availability of donors, since virtually all patients have a haplotype-matched donor. Impressive results have been obtained in patients with advanced leukemias; however, prolonged immunosuppression, with resultant risk of infection, remains a significant obstacle.[61]

The choice between these various sources of hematopoietic stem cells depends largely upon the underlying disease and remission status, as well as the approach chosen by the given transplant center.

PREPARATIVE REGIMENS

The purpose of the preparative regimen is twofold, namely, to eradicate the underlying disease and to provide sufficient immunosuppression to allow for the administration of the graft without subsequent rejection. The transplanted graft provides an immunologic reaction, the graft-versus-tumor effect. The relative contribution of these diverse mechanisms to successful transplantation is not known with certainty. However, it has become increasingly apparent that the graft-versus-tumor effect makes a major contribution. In the autologous setting, the sole purpose of the preparatory regimen is to provide substantial dose escalation in an attempt to overcome drug resistance, with subsequent rescue using hematopoietic cells.

RADIATION-BASED REGIMENS

Total-body irradiation has been utilized in preparatory regimens since the inception of transplantation. Initial approaches used radiation delivered in a single fraction; however, this technique was associated with significant multiple-organ toxicity that occasionally proved life threatening. The advent of fractionated radiation administered over several days has resulted in decreased toxicity in both immediate and long-term complications with respect to nausea, vomiting, and cataract formation.[62] The total dose of fractionated total-body irradiation administered ranges from 1200 to 1575 cGy. The major dose-limiting toxicities of fractionated total-body irradiation include mucositis, lung toxicity, and infertility. The maximally tolerated dose of total-body irradiation is approximately 1500 cGy. In randomized studies of two different doses of total-body irradiation (1220 versus 1575 cGy), a decreased relapse rate was noted with the higher radiation dose. However, this advantage was not associated with improved survival due to the increased incidence of regimen-related mortality.[63,64] Therefore, most groups have utilized fractionated total-body irradiation in the dose range noted above (1200–1320 cGy). The most commonly utilized regimen includes fractionated total-body irradiation with cyclophosphamide at a total dose of 120 mg/m^2.[65] Others have used fractionated total-body irradiation with etoposide and have found the maximally tolerated dose of etoposide to be 60 mg/kg.[66] In addition, excellent results have been reported combining fractionated total-body irradiation with etoposide and cyclophosphamide in both the autologous and allogeneic settings.[67–69] The major dose-limiting toxicity of fractionated total-body irradiation includes mucositis, lung toxicity, and infertility.

NON-RADIATION-BASED REGIMENS

A variety of regimens that do not include radiation have been developed and utilized in both the autologous and the allogeneic setting. The most widely utilized of these regimens combines the effects of oral busulfan at the dose of 16 mg/kg given over 4 days with cyclophosphamide at 120 mg/kg administered over 2 days.[70] A randomized comparison between fractionated total-body irradiation and cyclophosphamide and busulfan and cyclophosphamide did not show significant differences in long-term survival in patients with chronic myelogenous leukemia.[71] Because of the overall ease of administration of the busulfan-cyclophosphamide regimen, this continuation may be the preferred approach in some settings.[72] Total-body irradiation plus etoposide has been compared to busulfan and cyclophosphamide for patients with advanced leukemias. In this study, both regimens were well tolerated, and no significant differences were noted with respect to toxicity, incidence of acute graft-versus-host disease, overall survival, or disease-free survival. In those patients with good-risk disease, estimated disease-free survival was 55 percent ($\pm$11%) for those patients receiving fractionated total-body irradiation and etoposide. In contrast, 34 percent ($\pm$10%) of those patients who received busulfan and cyclophosphamide experienced disease-free survival.[73] Other regimens utilizing etoposide in combination with busulfan have also had excellent results in autologous marrow transplantation of patients with acute nonlymphocytic leukemia.[74–76]

A variety of other regimens that contain carmustine in the range of 300 to 500 mg/m^2 in addition to cyclophosphamide and etoposide have been utilized in the autologous setting.[77,78] In addition, the BEAM regimen, which contains carmustine (BCNU), etoposide, cytosine arabinoside, and melphalan, has been widely utilized in patients with lymphomas following autologous transplantation.[77] Other regimens, including the use of cisplatin and carboplatin, have been explored in patients with breast cancer and ovarian cancer.[78–80]

MULTIPLE CYCLES OF HIGH-DOSE CHEMOTHERAPY FOLLOWED BY PERIPHERAL-BLOOD PROGENITOR-CELL SUPPORT

With the introduction of mobilized peripheral-blood progenitor cells, it has become clear that sufficient numbers of stem cells could be collected to allow for multiple transplant procedures. Pilot studies using this general approach have been reported from a number of different institutions.[81–83] These studies have demonstrated feasibility but have been associated with significant toxicity. A variety of diseases have been treated in this fashion, including metastatic breast cancer, Hodgkin's disease, and lymphoma, with good response rates. However,

long-term studies have not demonstrated improved disease-free survival. In addition, a randomized comparative study between single and double transplants in patients with multiple myeloma did not demonstrate any benefit with the double-transplant approach.[84]

RADIOLABELED MONOCLONAL ANTIBODIES

Although higher doses of radiation may be associated with better disease-free control of the underlying disease, they have been associated with increased mortality due to toxicity. The fact that higher doses of radiation show an advantage in controlling the malignancy has led to the concept of using targeted radiotherapy to augment the preparative regimen. Several different monoclonal antibodies and radiation isotopes have been utilized, with the goal of delivering increased doses of radiation to the sites of disease, for example, the marrow. In one study, anti-CD33 antibodies conjugated to ^{131}I were utilized in nine patients. In four of these patients, biodistribution studies demonstrated that the marrow and spleen received more radiation than any normal nonhematopoietic organ. Therefore, those patients were treated with between 110 and 130 mCi of ^{131}I conjugated to anti-CD33 followed by the standard transplant regimen of cyclophosphamide plus total-body irradiation. This regimen was relatively well tolerated, with expected toxicities.[85] ^{131}I-labeled anti-CD45 monoclonal antibodies have also been utilized in combination with cyclophosphamide and total-body irradiation. In one study, 20 patients were treated with a dose of ^{131}I and estimated doses of 3.5 cGy and 7 cGy to the liver, and 4 to 30 cGy to the marrow, followed by 120 mg/kg of cyclophosphamide and 12 cGy of total-body irradiation. The toxicity observed was not thought to be greater than that of cyclophosphamide and total-body irradiation alone. Nine of 13 patients with acute myelogenous leukemia (AML) or refractory anemia with excess blasts and 2 of 7 patients with acute lymphoblastic leukemia were alive and disease-free from 8 to 41 months (median 17 months) after bone marrow transplantation (BMT).[86] These innovative studies demonstrate that radiolabeled monoclonal antibodies can be combined with standard preparative regimens and higher doses of radiation can be successfully delivered. Demonstration of improved disease-free survival using radiolabeled antibodies is currently being evaluated.

NONMYELOABLATIVE PREPARATIVE REGIMENS

The demonstration of the beneficial effects of immune-mediated mechanisms in controlling minimal residual disease has challenged the concept of using the relatively toxic myeloablative preparative regimens. Regimens with reduced toxicity may be particularly useful in older patients who may not be able to tolerate the aggressive preparative regimens that are currently in use for allogeneic transplantation and for those patients with relatively indolent disease. Less toxic regimens could also be extremely useful in patients with genetic disorders or autoimmune conditions.

The goal in this therapeutic approach is to use the minimum amount of immunosuppressive therapy required to achieve engraftment and to develop mixed chimerism. Once mixed chimerism is established, additional donor leukocytes could be utilized if required to treat the underlying malignancy by immunological mechanisms. In one study, conditioning included six daily infusions of fludarabine at 30 mg/m^2, busulfan at 4 mg/kg/day for 2 consecutive days, and anti-T-lymphocyte globulin at 10 mg/kg/day for 4 consecutive days. Patients then received G-CSF–mobilized peripheral-blood progenitor cells from an HLA-matched sibling donor. This resulted in acceptable, although significant, toxicity in patients who underwent this procedure. Hematopoietic toxicity was minimal, and these patients received only cyclosporine, since graft-versus-host disease prophylaxis resulted in either stable partial or complete chimerism. Using this approach, those patients who achieved some degree of chimerism were eligible for donor leukocyte infusions in an effort to control the underlying disease.[87]

Another approach has been utilized in 15 patients with chronic lymphocytic leukemia (CLL) who were treated with fludarabine at doses between 90 and 150 mg/m^2 and cyclophosphamide at doses between 900 and 2000 mg/m^2, followed by an allogeneic hematopoietic cell infusion from an HLA-matched sibling donor. Those patients who developed mixed chimerism then received an additional donor leukocyte infusion if no graft-versus-host disease was present. In this initial study, 11 patients had prompt engraftment of donor cells, and the remaining 4 patients recovered autologous hematopoiesis. Eight of the 11 patients achieved CR, indicating the feasibility and potential clinical efficacy of this approach.[88] However, remissions in some patients were not long-lasting, and the procedure was associated with a high morbidity and mortality.

An alternative approach based upon careful experimentation in the canine model has utilized low-dose radiation of 200 cGy followed by immunosuppression with mycophenolate mofetil and cyclosporine in an attempt to suppress the recipient T cells from rejecting the graft. Studies have been initiated in patients with a variety of malignancies, resulting in striking hematopoietic engraftment with chimerism achieved in all lineages.[89] These novel concepts require validation in larger numbers of patients with demonstration of long-term control of disease. However, the finding that either stable partial or complete chimerism can be achieved with minimal immunosuppression and low doses of chemotherapy or radiation is a striking finding. It will likely find utility in the future treatment of a variety of malignant conditions that are relatively indolent, as well as the treatment of patients with genetic disorders or autoimmune diseases.

STEM-CELL PROCUREMENT AND GRAFTING PROCEDURES

Details of stem-cell collection and processing are discussed in Chap. 141. Transplant donors must be in generally good health. The donor must have a performance status that will permit the safe collection of the cells, either from the marrow or blood. Thus, the donor must be able to tolerate anesthesia (either general or regional) and have adequate cardiac, pulmonary, hepatic, and renal functions. Pediatric donors are only used for autologous collection or donation to siblings. Donors with ongoing malignancies or a history of a malignant condition other than minor skin cancers (e.g., basal cell carcinomas) are generally excluded from further consideration.

In the unusual situation in which there is more than one sibling donor, cytomegalovirus (CMV) status is usually used to decide which donor to select, especially if the recipient is CMV seronegative. A CMV-seronegative donor is preferred, since the risk of subsequent infection with CMV will be greatly reduced, assuming that the patient receives CMV-seronegative blood products. There is some evidence that transplant procedures from parous female donors have a slightly increased risk of graft-versus-host disease, although this has not been observed in all studies.[16]

ABO INCOMPATIBILITY

HLA identity does not ensure red blood cell ABO compatibility. Major ABO compatibilities can result in serious hemolytic reactions upon infusion of the graft as a result of infusion of incompatible erythrocytes. Accordingly, the red blood cells must be removed.[90] Red cell depletion can be accomplished by a variety of methods, including hydroxyethyl starch sedimentation and cell separation techniques.[91] Minor ABO incompatibilities occasionally can lead to hemolytic complications from donor-derived isoagglutinins[92]; however, generally these types of ABO disparities do not require treatment.

The infusion of marrow and peripheral-blood progenitor cells is generally associated with minimal to minor toxicities of cough, flushing, and low-grade fever. Severe complications are rare but can occur and may occasionally even be life threatening.[93] Selection of CD34+ cells has been associated with decreased infusional toxicities.[43] However, it is not clear that this reason alone justifies the utilization of this methodology.

TUMOR-CELL PURGING

Tumor cells may be present in the stem-cell products utilized in autologous transplantation. The relative contributions of tumor-cell contamination of the stem-cell product and of residual disease in the patient are difficult, if not impossible, to evaluate. However, it seems reasonable to assume that both sources of tumor cells are capable of contributing to eventual relapse. In addition, as patient selection and treatment are optimized, tumor-cell contamination of the graft is likely to be even more important to address.

A number of retrospective studies have suggested that the infusion of products containing tumor cells is associated with higher rates of relapse. Among patients with acute leukemia, ex vivo treatment with the activated form of cyclophosphamide (4-hydroperoxycyclophosphamide) or the related drug mafosfamide has been associated with a lower relapse rate than seen in historical control patients who received unmanipulated marrow.[94,95] Moreover, further analysis of 4-hydroperoxycyclophosphamide–treated marrow grafts revealed that patients who had fewer than 1 percent of pretreatment CFU-GM following the purging procedure had a lower relapse rate and improved leukemia-free survival of 36 percent versus 12 percent, (p = 0.006) in patients with more than 1 percent CFU-GM. These data suggest that the intensity of marrow purging had an impact on relapse rate.[96]

These studies utilized either historical control subjects or surrogate assays to evaluate the effects of chemical treatment of the marrow. 4-Hydroperoxycyclophosphamide treatment does result in delayed hematopoietic engraftment, however. Other approaches have been utilized to purge the marrow, including monoclonal antibody-mediated methods and positive selection of stem cells. Generally a cocktail of monoclonal antibodies is used for B-cell lymphoma. Sensitive PCR-based methods have been utilized to evaluate the efficacy of tumor-cell removal.[45,97]

In one study, 114 patients with lymphoma who had the t(14;18) chromosomal translocation underwent marrow purging with monoclonal antibodies and complement. In a retrospective analysis, 57 patients were successfully purged to PCR-negativity and had a dramatically reduced rate of subsequent relapse.[98]

Direct demonstration that tumor cells contained within the graft can contribute to relapse comes from gene-marking studies in which marrow products were transduced by a retrovirus, allowing for detection of the viral genome PCR following infusion. In some patients who were transplanted with neuroblastoma, acute leukemia, or chronic myelogenous leukemia, tumor cells transduced by the retrovirus were detected following relapse.[99,100] Positive selection of CD34+ cells also has been performed using several different column-based techniques. In these studies, it could be demonstrated that tumor-cell contamination can be reduced by 2 to 4 logs.[101] Despite these suggestive data, as yet there have been no prospective randomized clinical trials assessing the role of purging in autologous marrow transplantation.

With the emergence of peripheral-blood progenitor cells as the preferred source of stem cells for autologous transplantation, several approaches have been employed to deplete tumor cells from the products. Column-based approaches have been employed to positively select for CD34+ progenitor cells and deplete tumor cells passively.[102] An alternative methodology uses an enrichment step for CD34+ cells followed by tumor-cell depletion with monoclonal antibodies and complement,[103] column-based techniques,[104] or immunomagnetic beads.[105] Further purification of human stem cells has also been pursued by selecting for CD34+ cells that coexpress Thy-1. This has resulted in significant depletion of myeloma and other malignant cells.[106] These methods are effective in significantly reducing the tumor-cell burden in many different clinical settings; however, further studies are required to demonstrate that a reduction in tumor-cell burden translates into superior disease-free survival.

ENGRAFTMENT AND SUPPORTIVE CARE

Progress in the supportive care of patients has been critically important in improving overall treatment results. Advances in hematopoietic support, antibiotics, antifungal agents, and antiviral drugs, as well as better medications to control such side effects of treatment as nausea, vomiting, diarrhea, and pain, have all had a major beneficial impact on the clinical course of the transplant patient.

Probably the single most important advance in reducing the morbidity and mortality of autologous transplantation has been the introduction of mobilized peripheral-blood progenitor cells as the source of stem cells. The more rapid hematologic recovery observed with the peripheral-blood progenitor cells has significantly reduced the duration of antibiotic therapy, the degree of mucositis, the length of hospitalization, and the risk of the transplant procedure itself. Other developments are discussed below.

HEMATOPOIETIC SUPPORT

Cloned hematopoietic growth factors, including G-CSF, GM-CSF, erythropoietin (EPO), TPO, and megakaryocyte growth and development factor, have been explored in the treatment of the transplant patient. The use of hematopoietic growth factors have been explored in two clinical settings, namely, following transplantation to accelerate hematopoietic recovery and in the mobilization process.

G-CSF AND GM-CSF
G-CSF and GM-CSF have resulted in clear clinical benefits in the transplant setting. The initial studies were performed following autologous BMT. In the phase I and II studies, a reduced number of days required for neutrophil engraftment was observed in all studies, with an associated reduction in the days of antibiotic therapy and length of hospitalization in some studies. Subsequent randomized clinical phase III trials confirmed these benefits derived from both GM-CSF and G-CSF.[107–111] These results led to the U.S. Food and Drug Administration (FDA) approval of both drugs for the treatment of patients following an autologous BMT to enhance neutrophil recovery. However, the positive results in these trials were limited to neutrophil engraftment and neutropenia-related complications. Red blood cell and platelet engraftment was not enhanced and patient-survival was not demonstrably improved.

MOBILIZATION
As discussed above, the observation that hematopoietic growth factor administration produces a time-limited enhancement in stem-cell mobilization has had a major impact on autologous transplantation with ongoing evaluation in the allogeneic setting. Upon reinfusion of mobilized peripheral-blood progenitor cells, hematopoietic engraftment of all lineages is accelerated significantly.[112]

A prospective randomized clinical trial comparing the use of G-CSF–mobilized autologous peripheral-blood progenitor cells to that of autologous marrow in 58 patients with relapsed Hodgkin's disease and lymphoma was performed. The patients who received mobilized peripheral-blood progenitor cells had a shorter time to platelet recovery above 20,000/μl (16 versus 23 days), a shorter time to neutrophil recovery, reduced hospital stays, and lower costs compared to control patients.[113,114] Early posttransplant morbidity, mortality, and overall survival (median follow-up 311 days) were similar in both groups.

Accelerated hematopoietic engraftment has also been noted in the allogeneic setting with the use of G-CSF mobilization.[47,48,115] However, the overall long-term benefit remains to be determined due to the potential risk of graft-versus-host disease, especially chronic graft-versus-host disease.[49] Randomized clinical trials are currently under way in North America and Europe.

The role of CSF following peripheral-blood progenitor-cell transplantation is less well defined. The addition of G-CSF may modestly accelerate neutrophil engraftment. Many centers employ G-CSF following infusion of the peripheral-blood progenitor cell autograft.[116,117] The dose of G-CSF used varies between 5 and 10 μg/kg per day. This is generally continued until stable neutrophil engraftment is established.

ERYTHROPOIETIN
Erythropoietin has been used in an effort to accelerate the recovery of red blood cells following transplantation. The rationale for this developed in part from the observation that EPO levels were lower than predicted for the degree of anemia following transplantation.[118]

In the autologous setting, small randomized studies have not shown reductions in transfusional requirements.[119,120] Modest increases in recovery of reticulocytes was observed in one study where patients were treated with both G-CSF and EPO.[120] Following allogeneic transplantation, mixed results have been observed. Initial small trials suggested that EPO administration produced more rapid recovery of red blood cells and reduced transfusional requirements.[121,122] Larger randomized trials have also been performed. One such trial randomized 215 patients undergoing allogeneic BMT to placebo or EPO therapy (150 U/kg per day as a continuous infusion) from marrow infusion until stable hemoglobin levels were achieved for 7 days. The median time to transfusion independence was reduced from 27 to 19 days, but total transfusion requirements for the two groups were similar. Another trial from Australia evaluated 91 patients who underwent allogeneic hematopoietic cell transplantation followed by randomization to placebo or EPO (300 U/kg three times weekly). Erythropoietin therapy was associated with increases in the reticulocyte count, hemoglobin concentration, and marrow erythropoiesis on day 14; however, red blood cell transfusional requirements were not different in the two groups.[123]

MUCOSITIS AND NUTRITIONAL SUPPORT

The majority of patients who undergo hematopoietic cell transplantation, especially those who receive fractionated total-body irradiation as part of the preparative regimen, develop significant mucositis and have difficulty maintaining an adequate caloric intake. These patients are generally treated with total parenteral nutrition (TPN) until they are able to maintain adequate oral nutritional intake.[124]

In a randomized trial of prophylactic TPN therapy in 137 patients, patients who received TPN had improved overall survival compared to hydration with 5% dextrose.[125] A second randomized trial administered in the outpatient setting reported different results. In this double-blinded study, 258 patients were randomized to either TPN or hydration. The patients who received TPN had a delay in the resumption of more than 85 percent of their caloric requirement, suggesting that the administration of TPN may suppress normal appetite recovery.[126] In this study, there was no effect of TPN on hospital readmission, relapse, or survival. In other studies, supplementation of TPN with glutamine was reported to reduce infection (13% versus 43% in one trial) and microbial colonization following BMT.[127] However, a second randomized study did not confirm these results.[128]

Mucositis remains an important clinical complication and is often regarded as the most difficult problem from the patient's perspective. Current management approaches include the use of topical and intravenous pain medications, acyclovir, and good oral hygiene. Many patients who undergo hematopoietic cell transplantation require narcotic pain medication. The length of time in which intravenous narcotics are needed is one of the best indicators of the degree of mucositis. New approaches are greatly needed, since the severity of mucositis and the requirement for pain medications is one of the principal reasons that patients undergoing transplantation require hospitalization.

Novel strategies include the use of recombinant growth factors, such as keratinocyte growth factor, which is now entering clinical trials. This agent reduces the degree of mucositis and improves survival in animal models in which the degree of mucositis and associated risk of infection are associated with measurable mortality.[129,130]

INFECTION

Patients who undergo transplantation, especially allogeneic transplantation, are at risk for bacterial, fungal, and viral infections (see Chap. 17).[131] Bacterial infections are frequent during the period of severe neutropenia and are most commonly due to gram-positive organisms, although gram-negative infections also occur. The early administration of broad-spectrum antibiotics in febrile, neutropenic patients is critically important.[132] Indwelling catheters and tissue damage from the preparative regimen or graft-versus-host disease, especially to the mouth, skin, and gut, are frequent mechanisms by which organisms enter the circulation. Infections caused by *Streptococcus mitis* can be particularly virulent following transplantation.[133]

A variety of measures are instituted at different transplant centers in an effort to reduce the risk for infection. These include protective isolation, handwashing, masking, gowning, and low-microbial diets. Decontamination of the gastrointestinal tract with oral antibiotics, such as ciprofloxacin or nonabsorbable broad-spectrum antibiotics, is utilized in many transplant centers. Immunoglobulin infusions also have been utilized to reduce the incidence of infectious complications following allogeneic BMT. In one trial, 383 transplant recipients were randomized to receive intravenous immunoglobulin (500 mg/kg weekly to day 90, then monthly to day 360) or no intravenous immunoglobulin. Patients treated with intravenous immunoglobulin had a significantly lower incidence of interstitial pneumonia among patients seropositive for CMV (13% versus 22%), a reduced risk of gram-negative septicemia (relative risk 0.38), and, in patients more than 20 years of age, a lower incidence of acute graft-versus-host disease (34% versus 51%) compared to control patients.[134] Neither survival nor the risk of relapse was altered by intravenous immunoglobulin. A subsequent randomized trial of 250 patients conducted by the same group of investigators evaluated the effects of intravenous immunoglobulin (500 mg/kg per month) given between days 90 and 360. In this study, no beneficial effects on the incidence of bacteremia, septicemia, localized infection, or obliterative bronchiolitis or on the incidence or mortality of chronic graft-versus-host disease were observed.[135] Therefore, many transplant centers utilize biweekly infusions of intravenous immunoglobulin (500 mg/kg) only until day 100 following the transplant.

Fungal infections are particularly worrisome in BMT recipients and are a frequent cause of transplant-related mortality. A variety of different fungal organisms have been observed, with the most common infections caused by *Candida* and *Aspergillus* species. However, other fungal infections can occur, such as coccidioidomycosis.[136] Treatment of established fungal infections is difficult, and prevention is clearly preferred.

Studies of prophylaxis against severe fungal infections are difficult to perform due to the relatively low incidence of such infections and the challenge in clearly documenting an invasive fungal infection. As a result, other trial endpoints, such as surveillance cultures or colonization, have been utilized. However, they may not be truly predictive. Retrospective analyses from two transplant centers have suggested that low-dose amphotericin B may lower the risk of fungal infections.[137,138] Newer agents, such as the liposomal amphotericin products, have been utilized mainly for treatment of established disease and have not been widely used for prophylaxis, due to their high cost.[139]

Prophylaxis with fluconazole has been explored in a randomized trial of 356 patients. In this study, fluconazole (400 mg/day) or placebo was administered prophylactically from the start of the conditioning regimen until the neutrophil count recovered to more than $1000/\mu l$. By the end of the treatment period, patients treated with fluconazole had a lower incidence of positive fungal cultures from any site (30% versus 67%) and of systemic fungal infections (3% versus 16%).[140]

VIRAL INFECTIONS

Viral infections are common following transplantation and are an important source of morbidity. Fortunately, major advances in this field have occurred with the introduction of effective drugs.

Cytomegalovirus Infection The most serious viral infection is due to CMV, a complication that typically occurs between 35 to 100 days following transplantation. The incidence of CMV infection following autologous transplantation is not significantly different from that observed following allogeneic transplantation; however, the incidence of CMV disease is clearly higher among patients receiving allogeneic transplants.[141] Cytomegalovirus infection can arise from viral activation within the patient or from infusion of CMV-positive blood products. Transfusing exclusively seronegative blood products effectively eliminates the risk of CMV disease in patients who are CMV negative and who have CMV-negative donors.[142] The introduction of ganciclovir has ushered in a new era in the prevention and treatment of this previously lethal infection. The early introduction of ganciclovir to patients who are at risk for CMV infection decreases the incidence of clinically significant infection dramatically and is associated with an improved overall outcome.[143-145] In addition, expansion of cytotoxic T lymphocytes directed against CMV have also been effective in preventing CMV disease.[146]

Despite these successes, a number of issues remain, since ganciclovir prophylaxis is expensive and associated with significant toxicity to the marrow, kidney, and central nervous system. The best method of detecting patients at risk for CMV infection, the optimal dose and timing of ganciclovir therapy, the required duration of treatment, and the benefits of combined therapy with other agents remain the focus of ongoing clinical studies. In addition, some patients develop recurrent CMV disease, which can present challenging clinical problems.

Herpetic Infections Mucocutaneous herpetic infections caused by herpes simplex viruses I and II are extremely common following BMT and result in significant pain and difficulty in alimentation. Intravenous acyclovir (5 mg/kg every 8 h if renal function is normal) is an effective agent against herpes simplex viruses I and II and is typically used prophylactically for patients who are seropositive during the period of neutropenia.[147,148]

Varicella zoster virus causes another common viral infection (occurring in 30 to 40% of patients) following transplantation.[149] Although varicella zoster virus infection is rarely life threatening, it can be a cause of significant pain and disability. Varicella zoster virus infections are usually dermatomal but occasionally disseminate. Infections typically occur within the first 12 months following hematopoietic cell transplantation. Other viral infections, such as respiratory syncytial virus infections, can occur in BMT patients and can result in fatalities.[150–152] Outbreaks of respiratory syncytial virus infections within a medical center have been reported, suggesting a nosocomial spread.[153] Respiratory syncytial virus infections can be effectively treated with combination therapy with aerosolized ribavirin and intravenous immunoglobulin.[154] The use of intravenous immunoglobulin or antibodies with high titers of antibodies against respiratory syncytial virus may improve upon these results. Human herpes virus 6 has been isolated from patients undergoing transplantation and has been associated with fatalities.[155,156] Infection with the BK strain of adenovirus has been associated with hemorrhagic cystitis.[157,158]

LATE INFECTIONS

Due to prolonged immunosuppression, patients undergoing allogeneic transplantation are at greater risk of infection following neutrophil recovery than are autologous transplant patients. Infections occurring beyond day +50 have been noted to be more frequent following unrelated donor transplantation (84.7%) than following related donor transplantation (68.2%; p = 0.009).[159]

BLOOD PRODUCT SUPPORT

Virtually all patients undergoing hematopoietic cell transplantation require blood product support in the form of red blood cell and platelet transfusions until the transplanted stem cells engraft. In the allogeneic setting, transfusion requirements are generally greater due to the immunosuppressive effects of drugs such as cyclosporin, methotrexate, and ganciclovir, as well as to complications such as graft-versus-host disease. Following allogeneic hematopoietic cell transplantation, all CMV-negative patients who receive cells from a CMV-negative donor should receive seronegative blood products. In addition, all transplant centers utilize either irradiated or filtered blood products to avoid the risk of transfusion-associated graft-versus-host disease.

The indications for transfusion of red blood cells vary. However, most centers utilize a threshold hematocrit of approximately 30 percent. The need for red cell transfusions may be influenced by a number of factors, including the number of days from hematopoietic cell transplantation, the clinical condition of the patient, evidence of engraftment of other cell types, and the reticulocyte count. Patients with graft-versus-host disease or those being treated with immunosuppressive drugs such as cyclosporin may have continued blood product requirements from bleeding and/or microangiopathic hemolysis.

Patients who are thrombocytopenic and bleeding require platelet transfusions. Such support is required by most transplanted patients. In comparison, the role of prophylactic platelet transfusions remains controversial. Many transplant centers have relied upon threshold values of platelet counts to determine the timing of platelet transfusions. This practice has been questioned due to the risk of alloimmunization, the relatively short life span of transfused platelets, and the expense of transfusion. Seven hundred ninety-eight patients transplanted at 18 centers in the United States and Canada were evaluated for the pace of platelet recovery and incidence of bleeding complications. A number of variables were identified that were associated with accelerated platelet recovery, including a higher CD34+ cell count of the infused stem-cell product, a higher platelet count at the start of myeloablative therapy, and a graft from an HLA-identical sibling donor.[160] Platelet

recovery was more rapid in patients who received progenitor cells from the peripheral blood than in those who received them from the marrow. Patients who had received prior radiation therapy, who had posttransplant fever, who had hepatic veno-occlusive disease, or who required posttransplant growth factors recovered platelet counts more slowly. In this retrospective study, 11 percent of all patients had a significant bleeding event during the first 60 days following the transplant, contributing to death in 2 percent; however, these deaths were strikingly independent of the platelet count.[160] Similar results were observed in studies of patients who become thrombocytopenic after chemotherapy for acute leukemia. Reducing the platelet transfusion threshold from 20,000/μl to 10,000/μl led to decreased utilization of platelet transfusions without any significant effect on morbidity and only a small adverse effect on bleeding.[161–163]

A significant concern among patients and their family members is the risk of transfusion-transmitted viral diseases. Fortunately, with improved and systematic testing of blood products, the risks per unit of blood are low and in the range of 1 in 493,000 units for HIV, 1 in 103,000 units for hepatitis C virus, and 1 in 63,000 units for hepatitis B virus (see Chap. 140).[164] Ongoing improvements in screening may reduce these risks even further.

CLINICAL RESULTS OF MARROW TRANSPLANTATION

ACUTE MYELOGENOUS LEUKEMIA

Bone marrow transplantation has been extensively studied in patients with AML as postremission therapy. Allogeneic BMT was initially utilized for patients with refractory disease, in whom it was observed that 10 to 20 percent of patients with advanced disease enjoyed long-term disease-free survival, some of whom are now alive for more than 20 years.[65] Many other studies have confirmed these early results and demonstrated that the outcome following BMT is highly dependent upon the remission status of the patient. Advances in tissue typing, graft-versus-host disease prophylaxis, and supportive care have made it feasible to consider BMT for patients with more favorable disease. Subsequently, the use of allogeneic BMT early in the course of disease, for example, following remission induction, was studied. Five-year disease-free survival rates range from 45 to 65 percent, with relapse rates varying between 10 and 25 percent.[165–173] In these studies, it was observed that the primary cause of treatment failure was related to complications from hematopoietic cell transplantation and not due to relapse of the underlying disease. This observation is in marked contrast to findings in patients who are treated with chemotherapy or an autologous BMT, where the predominant cause of treatment failure is relapse of AML.

To further document the potential efficacy of allogeneic BMT in AML patients in first CR, randomized studies have been performed. These studies employed a biological randomization whereby those patients with an HLA-matched sibling donor received the transplant and those without received chemotherapy. Some of these studies further randomized patients who did not have an HLA-matched sibling donor between autologous BMT and chemotherapy, which is discussed below. In these studies, it was assumed that having an HLA-matched sibling donor or not was a random event. Many randomized studies comparing allogeneic BMT to chemotherapy have been reported that have demonstrated a consistent, although not always statistical, benefit in disease-free survival for patients who underwent allogeneic BMT (Table 18-1). In six of these trials, a statistically significant difference in disease-free survival was reported.[174–179] In the other studies, a trend toward improved overall survival was evident, with a reduction in the risk of relapse. The primary causes of treatment failure in transplanted patients are graft-versus-host disease, interstitial pneumonitis, and infection.

TABLE 18-1   ALLOGENEIC MARROW TRANSPLANTATION VERSUS AUTOLOGOUS MARROW TRANSPLANTATION VERSUS CHEMOTHERAPY FOR AML IN FIRST REMISSION

	TREATMENT	# OF PTS	DISEASE-FREE SURVIVAL	P VALUE	OVERALL SURVIVAL	P VALUE	RELAPSE	P VALUE
Royal Marsden (1982)[174]	AlloBMT	53	54%	p < 0.005				
	ChemoRx	51	21%					
Seattle (1984, 1988)[176,177]	AlloBMT	33	48%	p < 0.05				
	ChemoRx	43	21%					
	AlloBMT	43	40%	p = 0.07				
	ChemoRx	43	21%					
†UCLA (1985)[564]	AlloBMT	23			40%	p = NS	40%	p < 0.01
	ChemoRx	44			27%		71%	
Genova (1985)[175]	AlloBMT	19	64%	p < 0.05	70%	p = NR		
	ChemoRx	18	13%		21%			
M.D. Anderson (1988)[565]	AlloBMT	11			36%	p = NS	9%	p < 0.01
	ChemoRx	27			15%		85%	
Spain (1988)[566]	AlloBMT	14	70%	p = NS			10%	p < 0.005
	ChemoRx	25	10%				88%	
France (1989)[178]	AlloBMT	20	66%				18%	
	ABMT	12	41%	p < 0.004			50%	p < 0.0002
	ChemoRx	20	16%				83%	
Netherlands (1990)[187]	AlloBMT	23	51%	p = NS	66%	p = 0.05	34%	p = 0.03
	ABMT	32	35%		37%		60%	
UCLA (1992)[567]	AlloBMT	42	45%	p = NS	45%	p = NS	32%	p = 0.05
	ChemoRx	28	38%		53%		60%	
†ECOG (1992)[568]	AlloBMT	54	42%	p = NS	43%	p = NS		
	ChemoRx	29	30%		42%			
†France (1994)[569]	AlloBMT	27	41%	p = NS	41%	p = NS	43%	p = 0.1
	ChemoRx	31	27%		46%		67%	
†Boston (1995)[191]	AlloBMT	23	62%	p = NS			0%	p = SGNFCT
	ABMT	27	62%				38%	
	AlloBMT	31	56%	p = NS			20%	p = 0.04
	ABMT	53	45%				50%	
Southwestern Oncology Group (1995)[570]	AlloBMT	34	38%	p = NS				
	ChemoRx	110	28%					
†EORTC/GIMEMA (1995)[570]	AlloBMT	168	55%		59%		27%	
	ABMT	128	48%	p = SGNFCT*	56%	p = NR	41%	p = NR
	ChemoRx	126	30%		46%		57%	
GOELAM (1997)[194]	AlloBMT	67	45%				38%	
	ABMT	67	47%	p = NS			44%	p = NS
	ChemoRx	61	53%				43%	
†U.S. Intergroup (1998)[192]	AlloBMT	113	43%		46%	p = 0.04	29%	
	ABMT	116	34%	p = NS	43%	p = 0.05	48%	
	ChemoRx	117	34%		52%		62%	
	AlloBMT	92	47%	p = NR	45%	p = NR		
	ABMT	63	48%		55%			

ABBREVIATIONS: AML, acute myeloid leukemia; AlloBMT, allogeneic marrow transplantation; ABMT, autologous marrow transplantation; ChemoRx, chemotherapy; SGNFCT, significant; NS, not significant; NR, not reported.
†Patients assigned to transplantation based on availability of matched siblings or to chemotherapy and analyzed according to intent-to-treat.

More recently, it has become apparent that patients with AML have a variable prognosis and can be placed into risk categories based upon cytogenetic features at diagnosis. Patients with low-risk disease are characterized by the chromosomal abnormalities t(15;17), t(8;21), and (inv16). Due to this relatively favorable prognosis, some centers have elected not to consider transplantation for these patients until first relapse or during second CR. In contrast, patients with a myelodysplastic syndrome; cytogenetic abnormalities involving chromosomes 5, 7, and 8; or complex cytogenetic abnormalities fare poorly with chemotherapy and should be transplanted early in the course of their disease. Patients with intermediate prognosis, which includes the large group of individuals with normal cytogenetics, may be offered allogeneic BMT in first CR. One potential algorithm for the treatment of adults with AML is presented in Fig. 18-1.

Acute myeloblastic anemia patients who do not enter CR with one or two courses of chemotherapy are also considered candidates for allogeneic BMT. In one report, 16 such patients with induction failures underwent allogeneic BMT utilizing HLA-matched sibling donors. With follow-up ranging from 18 months to 11 years, 8 of these patients were alive and free of disease.[180] Similar results were reported to the International Bone Marrow Transplant Registry, where 21 percent (CI 14–31%) of patients with induction failures were alive and disease free at 3 years of follow-up.[181]

The role of autologous transplantation in patients with AML is considerably more complex. Only a few patients with advanced disease (beyond first CR) can be salvaged with autologous BMT.[182] One early study demonstrated a disease-free survival rate of 43 percent in a group of patients with AML in second or third remission who underwent transplantation with 4HC-purged marrow.[94] A follow-up of this study reported continued disease-free survival for 28 percent of those patients, with minimum follow-up of 4 years.[183] Other investigators have reported similar rates of disease-free survival in AML patients who had suffered a relapse.[74,184]

The role of purging in autologous transplantation has been controversial. In vitro data discussed above have suggested that the intensity of purging with 4HC, as assessed by normal CFU-GM survival, has had an impact on relapse rate and disease-free survival.[187] In addition, retrospective analyses also have revealed a benefit for those patients

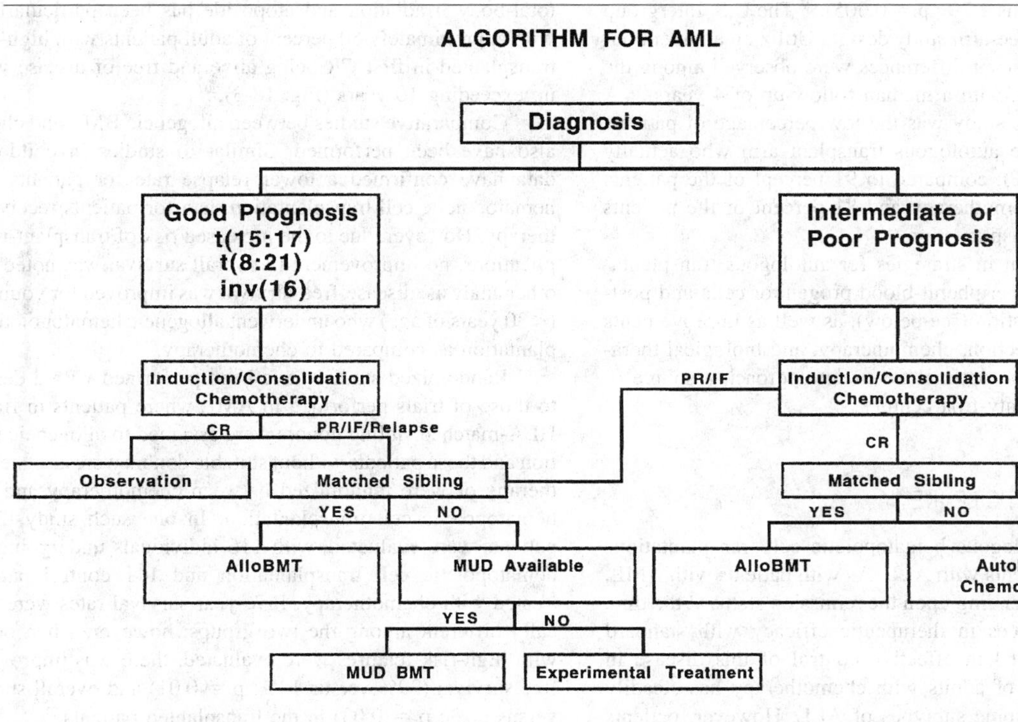

ALGORITHM FOR AML

```
                              ┌─────────────┐
                              │  Diagnosis  │
                              └─────────────┘
              ┌────────────────────────┴────────────────────────┐
    ┌───────────────────┐                          ┌───────────────────┐
    │  Good Prognosis   │                          │  Intermediate or  │
    │     t(15:17)      │                          │   Poor Prognosis  │
    │      t(8:21)      │                          └───────────────────┘
    │     inv(16)       │
    └───────────────────┘
    ┌───────────────────┐                          ┌───────────────────┐
    │Induction/Consolidation│      PR/IF           │Induction/Consolidation│
    │    Chemotherapy   │──────────────────────────│    Chemotherapy   │
    └───────────────────┘                          └───────────────────┘
      CR        PR/IF/Relapse                               CR
   ┌──────────┐ ┌────────────────┐            ┌──────────────────┐
   │Observation│ │ Matched Sibling│────────────│  Matched Sibling │
   └──────────┘ └────────────────┘            └──────────────────┘
                YES        NO                    YES        NO
            ┌────────┐ ┌──────────────┐      ┌────────┐ ┌──────────────┐
            │AlloBMT │ │ MUD Available│      │AlloBMT │ │  AutoBMT or  │
            └────────┘ └──────────────┘      └────────┘ │ Chemotherapy │
                        YES        NO                   └──────────────┘
                     ┌─────────┐ ┌────────────────────┐
                     │ MUD BMT │ │Experimental Treatment│
                     └─────────┘ └────────────────────┘
```

FIGURE 18-1   Algorithm for the treatment of acute myelogenous leukemia. (From KE Stockerl-Goldstein, KG Blume,[563] with permission.)

who underwent autologous BMT with mafosfamide-purged marrow, especially early after remission induction.[95] Despite the considerable suggestive evidence that purging may have a role in reducing relapse rates following autologous BMT for AML patients, there has not been a randomized trial directly demonstrating the benefit of such graft manipulation. Because of this and the myelotoxicity, 4HC has not yet been approved by the FDA. An alternative approach to purging has been the use of high-dose chemotherapy and transplantation of peripheral-blood progenitor cells early following recovery, a procedure termed in vivo purging.[186]

The role of autologous transplantation in first CR has been controversial. A number of phase II studies have reported a broad range in disease-free survival from 35 to 76 percent, with relapse rates ranging from 22 to 60 percent.[74–76,95,187–189] Where allogeneic BMT has been compared directly to autologous hematopoietic cell transplantation in first CR, there is either a better outcome following the allogeneic transplant[187,190] or no difference between the two groups.[179,191,192] Comparisons between autologous hematopoietic cell transplantation and chemotherapy for first CR AML patients have yielded conflicting results. The Medical Research Council 10 trial of 1966 patients from 163 institutions assigned patients to allogeneic transplantation if they had an HLA-matched sibling donor and randomized the remaining patients to autologous BMT or to four courses of intensive chemotherapy. In this study, 381 patients were randomized, and of the 190 patients who were assigned to the autologous BMT arm, 126 (66%) actually underwent the procedure. Using an intention-to-treat analysis, those patients who underwent autologous BMT had a lower relapse rate (37% versus 58%; p = 0.0007) and superior disease-free survival at 7 years of follow-up (53% versus 40%; p = 0.040) as compared to patients who received intensive chemotherapy (Fig. 18-2).[193] In another large study of 623 patients, a similar study design was employed. Here again the relapse rate was lower for patients who underwent autologous BMT than for those who received chemotherapy

(41% versus 57%). Disease-free survival was superior in the autologous BMT the group as compared to the group treated with chemotherapy (48% versus 30%). However, overall survival was not different due to the use of salvage therapy with hematopoietic cell transplantation for those patients who relapsed following chemotherapy.[179]

Other randomized clinical trials have not supported the conclusion that autologous transplantation results in a superior outcome than that using chemotherapy alone.[192,194,195] In a study of 232 children with AML in first CR who were randomized between autologous BMT and chemotherapy, there were no differences in event-free survival (36% versus 38%). A lower relapse rate was observed following autologous transplantation (31% versus 58%; p < 0.001), but this again was offset by higher treatment-related mortality in the trans-

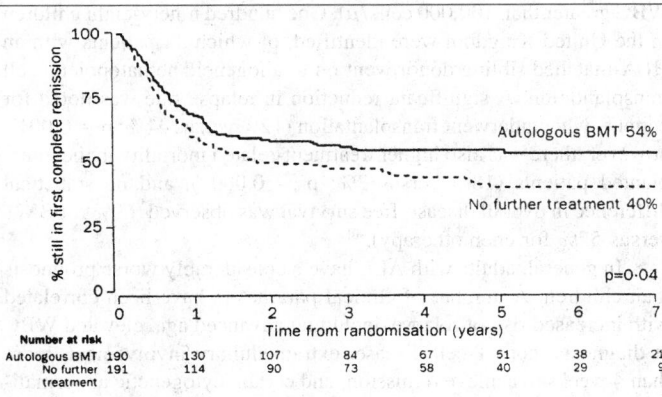

FIGURE 18-2   Randomized comparison of autologous transplantation versus conventional chemotherapy for acute myelogenous leukemia. (From AK Burnett et al,[193] with permission.)

planted patients (15% versus 2.7%; p = 0.005).[195] The U.S. Intergroup Trial also had a similar three-arm study design. Utilizing an intention-to-treat analysis, no significant differences were observed among the different treatment groups, with a median follow-up of 4 years.[192] A significant problem in this study was the low percentage of patients who were assigned to the autologous transplant arm who actually received the therapy (54%), compared to 91 percent of the patients who were assigned to chemotherapy and 81 percent of the patients assigned to allogeneic transplantation.

Ongoing improvement in strategies for autologous transplantation, including the use of peripheral-blood progenitor cells and post-transplant immune modulation (see below), as well as improvements in results with patient selection, chemotherapy, and biological therapies, are likely to make the optimal treatment approach a source of ongoing debate in the twenty-first century.

ACUTE LYMPHOBLASTIC LEUKEMIA

Both allogeneic and autologous hematopoietic cell transplantations have been utilized for patients with ALL. As with patients with AML, results vary markedly, depending upon the remission status at the time of transplantation. Advances in therapeutic efficacy with standard chemotherapy have resulted in effective control of this disease in most children. Treatment of adults with chemotherapy has steadily improved, especially for some subtypes of ALL. However, patients with high risk of recurrence can be defined at diagnosis or once a first remission has been attained. Therefore, hematopoietic cell transplantation studies have focused on patients with relapsed disease or adults with high-risk disease in first CR.

A number of clinical trials indicate that children with ALL who suffer a relapse can be salvaged with allogeneic BMT, with 40 to 64 percent of patients enjoying long-term survival.[196–199] Comparative analyses of results expected with chemotherapy have been performed based upon registry data. In one such study, results for allogeneic hematopoietic cell transplantation in 376 children in second CR reported to the International Bone Marrow Transplant Registry were compared to 540 children treated with chemotherapy on Pediatric Oncology Group trials. At a mean of 5 years of follow-up, the relapse rate was significantly lower for the patients undergoing hematopoietic cell transplantation (45% versus 80%; p < 0.001) and the probability of leukemia-free survival higher in the transplanted patients (40% versus 17%; p < 0.001).[200]

Allogeneic BMT has been compared to chemotherapy for children with high-risk disease, defined as those patients presenting with a WBC greater than 100,000 cells/μl. One hundred ninety-eight children in the United Kingdom were identified, of which 34 patients with an HLA-matched sibling donor went on to allogeneic hematopoietic cell transplantation. A significant reduction in relapse rate was noted for patients who underwent transplantation (12% versus 41%; p = 0.001); however, there was also higher treatment-related mortality in the transplanted patients (18% versus 3%; p = 0.0007), and no statistical difference in overall disease-free survival was observed (69% for BMT versus 52% for chemotherapy).[201]

In general, adults with ALL have a considerably worse prognosis than children. A number of clinical parameters have been correlated with increased risk of relapse, including advanced age, elevated WBC at diagnosis, non–T-cell disease, extramedullary involvement, more than 4 weeks to achieve remission, and certain cytogenetic abnormalities, especially the Philadelphia (Ph) chromosome. Allogeneic BMT has been utilized to treat adult patients beyond first CR or patients in first CR with high-risk features. Approximately 42 to 71 percent of patients achieve long-term remissions.[202–206] The use of fractionated

total-body irradiation and etoposide has been particularly effective, with approximately 60 percent of adult patients with high-risk disease transplanted in first CR being alive and free of disease with follow-up exceeding 10 years (Fig. 18-3).[207]

Comparative studies between allogeneic BMT and chemotherapy also have been performed. Similar to studies in children, registry data have confirmed a lower relapse rate for patients undergoing hematopoietic cell transplantation than for patients receiving chemotherapy. However, due to the increased risk of transplant-related complications, no improvement in overall survival was noted.[208,209] In another analysis, disease-free survival was improved for younger patients (<30 years of age) who underwent allogeneic hematopoietic cell transplantation as compared to chemotherapy.[210]

Randomized studies have been performed with a design similar to those of trials performed in AML where patients in first CR with HLA-matched sibling donors were assigned to allogeneic transplantation and those patients without suitable donors were assigned to chemotherapy or were randomized between chemotherapy and autologous hematopoietic cell transplantation. In one such study, 257 eligible patients were evaluated, with 116 individuals undergoing allogeneic hematopoietic cell transplantation and 141 control patients being treated with chemotherapy. Five-year survival rates were not statistically different among the two groups; however, when only patients with high-risk features were evaluated, there was improved disease-free survival (39% versus 14%; p = 0.01) and overall survival (44% versus 20%; p = 0.03) in the transplanted patients.[211]

Patients with ALL who have the Ph chromosome have an extremely poor prognosis following chemotherapy treatment, with the vast majority of them ultimately suffering a relapse.[212,213] In one study of 23 Ph-positive ALL patients prepared with fractionated total-body irradiation and etoposide who underwent transplantation with HLA-matched sibling marrow while in first CR, disease-free survival at 3 years of follow-up was 65 percent.[214] Hematopoietic cell transplantation from matched unrelated donors has also been successfully employed for 18 patients with Ph-positive ALL in first CR with a 2-year probability of disease-free survival of 49 percent.[215] Patients with remission-induction failure are also a very poor risk group for whom allogeneic hematopoietic cell transplantation has been attempted as salvage therapy. In one study of 21 patients, 16 of whom had AML and 5 of whom had ALL, the probability of disease-free survival at 10 years was 43 percent.[180] However, only 1 of the 5 ALL patients was alive and free of disease.

Autologous hematopoietic cell transplantation for patients with ALL has resulted in variable outcomes. In patients with advanced disease (beyond first CR), such treatment has achieved only modest success, with 18 to 46 percent of patients enjoying long-term survival.[216–222] In addition, only a subset of relapsed patients (in one study approximately 50%) actually underwent hematopoietic cell transplantation.[223] Patients with long first remissions of at least 24 months fared better, with an event-free survival of 53 percent among 51 children who underwent transplantation with purged marrow in second CR.[224] Better results have been achieved in first CR patients, varying from 30 to 65 percent.[205,217,225,226]

The role of purging in autologous transplants for ALL has been controversial, although it is widely utilized. Monoclonal antibody (MoAb)-based techniques, immunotoxins, and chemotherapy in the form of 4-hydroperoxycyclophosphamide have been utilized.[218,227,228] In some of these studies, PCR-based methods have been used to document the efficacy of the purging procedure.[229] There are no direct comparisons between purged and unpurged stem-cell grafts.

In ALL, unique chromosomal rearrangements, such as the bcr/abl translocation, or immunoglobulin and T-cell receptor genes can be amplified by PCR. Molecular features serve as extremely sensitive markers for disease. Bcr/abl transcripts have been detected following transplantation and found to be a sensitive predictor of relapse, especially for patients with the p190 bcr/abl splice variant.[230,231] Rearrangements of immunoglobulin heavy-chain variable loci have also been utilized to detect minimal residual disease and have been found to be useful and sensitive markers for relapse following transplantation.[232] Utilizing a semiquantitative PCR technique, children and adolescent patients were grouped as having high-level disease, low-level disease, or no detectable disease using PCR amplification of immuno-globulin or T-cell receptor gene loci prior to allogeneic hematopoietic cell transplantation performed in either first or second CR. Two-year event-free survival for these groups of patients was 0 percent for high level, 36 pecent for low level, and 72 percent for those patients without PCR detectable disease prior to hemato-poietic cell transplantation, respectively (p < 0.001).[233] In the future, it may be possible to use sensitive minimal residual disease assays for the identification of patients who are at high risk of relapse, in whom innovative new approaches should be considered; of patients likely to benefit from hematopoietic cell transplantation; and of other patients who may already be cured of their disease, in whom the risk of transplantation could be avoided.

CHRONIC MYELOGENOUS LEUKEMIA

Allogeneic hematopoietic cell transplantation for CML has been widely studied and has been established as the primary therapy for this disorder. As discussed in Chap. 94, CML progresses from a relatively indolent disorder readily controllable with oral chemother-apy in chronic phase to a more aggressive disorder in accelerated phase to a frankly acute leukemic condition in blastic phase, which is often refractory to therapy. Many studies have documented that the results obtained with allogeneic hematopoietic cell transplantation are directly related to the phase of disease at the time of the transplant.[234–237] Early trials demonstrated that CML could be effectively treated with myeloablative chemoradiotherapy followed by syngeneic[10] or alloge-neic marrow[234] grafting. The finding that relapse rates are higher fol-lowing syngeneic than following allogeneic transplantation serves as one of the primary observations leading to the concept of a graft-versus-leukemia effect.[14,238]

The most important prognostic factor for survival following allo-geneic hematopoietic cell transplantation for CML is disease phase.[235,239,240] Fifty to 75 percent of CML patients transplanted in the first or second chronic phase of their disease achieve long-term remissions.[235,237,239–243] Disease-free survival falls to 30 to 40 percent of patients with accelerated phase,[237,244] and only 5 to 15 percent of patients in blastic phase obtain long-term disease-free survival with allogeneic hematopoietic cell transplantation.

Younger age may also influence survival,[239,240] while splenomeg-aly or splenectomy appears to have no impact on outcome following BMT.[240] A number of studies have documented that early hematopoi-etic cell transplantation during the first year after diagnosis is a favor-able prognostic factor in part related to the negative impact of prior exposure to chemotherapy, especially busulfan.[237,240] In the subgroup of CML patients under the age of 50 who undergo allogeneic trans-plantation from an HLA-matched sibling donor BMT during the first

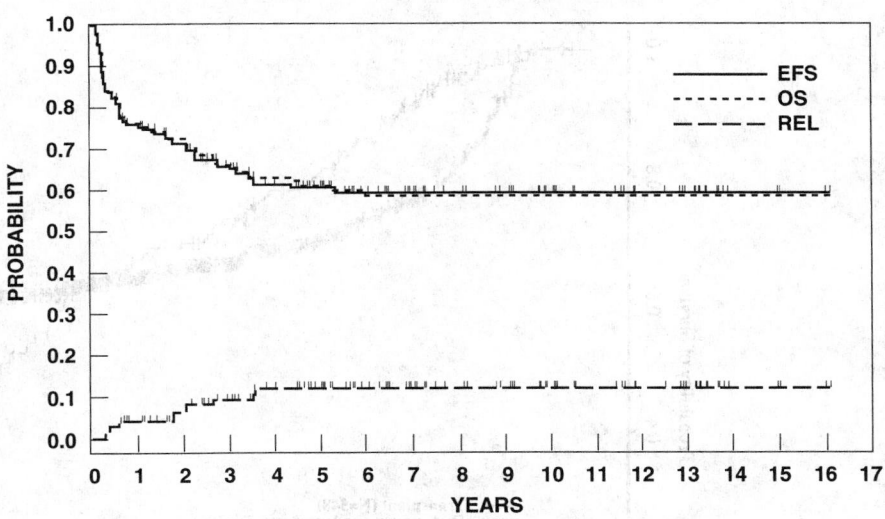

FIGURE 18-3 Long-term follow-up of allogeneic marrow transplantation for patients with high-risk features of acute lymphocytic leukemia. All patients received the preparatory regimen of fractionated total-body irradiation and high-dose etoposide followed by marrow from HLA-matched siblings EFS, event free survival; OS, overall survival; REL, relapse. (From NJ Chao et al,[207] reprinted and updated with permission.)

year of diagnosis, nearly 80 percent will be alive and free of disease 5 years later. This makes BMT the treatment of choice for younger patients with CML.

Randomized clinical trials exploring the use of non-radiation-containing preparative regimens such as busulfan/cyclophosphamide have been compared to fractionated total-body irradiation with cyclo-phosphamide. In these studies, there were no differences in disease-free survival.[71,245] However, a decreased risk of relapse in busulfan/cyclophosphamide–treated patients was reported in one study.[245] Plasma busulfan levels below the median of 917 ng/ml were associated with a higher relapse rate in one small study of 45 patients transplanted with the busulfan/cyclophosphamide regimen.[246]

Alternative therapies for CML have emerged, such as interferon-α, with documented improvements in long-term disease-free survival for a certain subset of patients (see Chap. 94). However, there have been no prospective trials comparing the role of allogeneic BMT to interferon-α. An analysis of historical data has been performed comparing results obtained for allogeneic BMT submitted to the Inter-national Bone Marrow Transplantation Registry (n = 548) to results obtained from the randomized trial of the German CML study group, which had accrued patients to therapy with hydroxyurea (n = 121) or interferon-α (interferon-α, n = 75).[237] In this analysis, as expected, there was a higher mortality risk in the transplant group for the first 18 months. Approximately 3.5 years after diagnosis, the survival curves crossed, indicating that there was significant improvement in overall survival for the transplanted patients at 4.7 years. At 7 years, the overall survival of the group treated by transplantation was 58 percent, while only 21 percent of those treated with hydroxyurea or interferon-α survived (Fig. 18-4).[248] Similar results were obtained for all risk categories. However, those patients with intermediate-, or high-risk disease manifested improved survival at an even earlier timepoint.

For patients without HLA-matched sibling donors, matched unre-lated donor transplantation has been explored. Due to the relatively indolent nature of CML, there is usually adequate time to perform a search. The outcome for matched unrelated donor transplantation for patients with CML in chronic phase was initially reported to be in the range of 35 to 40 percent, with patients with more advanced disease

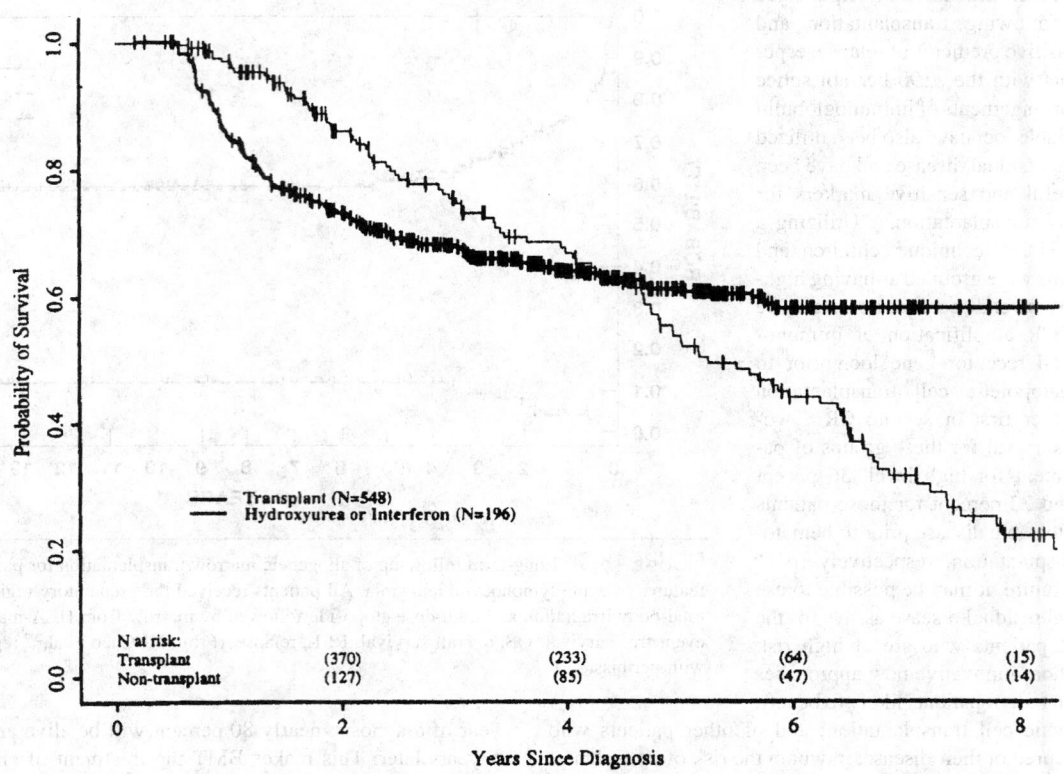

FIGURE 18-4   Historical comparison of allogeneic transplantation versus hydroxyurea or interferon-α for patients with chronic myelogenous leukemia. (From RP Gale et al,[248] with permission.)

faring worse.[54,249] Advances in donor-recipient typing, supportive care, graft-versus-host disease prophylaxis, and infectious disease prevention have resulted in significant improvements in results after matched unrelated donor transplantation. Five-year estimates of survival for patients who are 50 years of age or younger and undergo a transplant procedure within 1 year of diagnosis from an HLA-matched unrelated donor were reported to be 74 percent. This favorable outcome approximates what can be achieved with HLA-matched sibling donors (Fig. 18-5).[56]

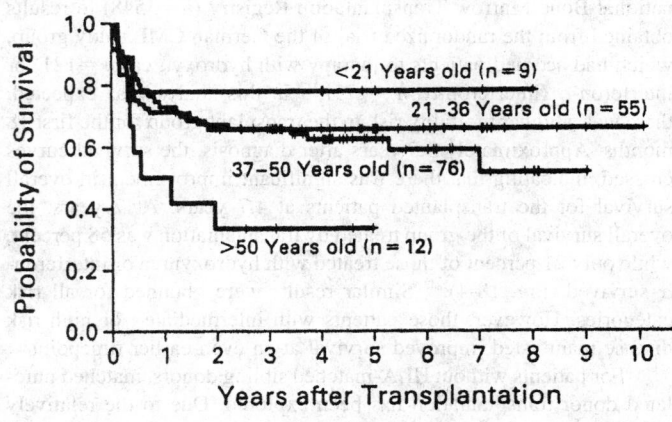

FIGURE 18-5   Results of matched unrelated donor transplantation for patients with chronic myelogenous leukemia in chronic phase stratified by recipient age. (From JA Hansen et al,[56] with permission.)

The decision to proceed to unrelated donor transplantation versus the use of interferon-α is often difficult for patients who lack an HLA-matched sibling donor. Decision analysis has been applied to this question. It was concluded that, for younger patients with newly diagnosed CML, transplantation within the first year of diagnosis provided the greatest quality-adjusted expected survival[250] and that this modality had an acceptable cost-effectiveness ratio.[251] Umbilical cord blood transplantation has also been utilized in small numbers of patients with CML.[252,253]

An alternative approach to the use of immunosuppressive drugs for the prevention of graft-versus-host disease has been T-cell depletion. This has resulted in less graft-versus-host disease, but a higher risk of leukemic relapse.[254] Donor leukocyte infusion has been utilized for those patients who suffer a relapse following the transplant. Comparable results have been obtained using unrelated donors.[255,256] Currently, a multi-institutional prospective randomized clinical trial comparing T-cell depletion to conventional marrow transplantation with matched unrelated donors is ongoing.

There has been considerable debate as to whether pretreatment of patients with interferon-α affects outcome following BMT. The argument is complicated by the fact that those patients who delay transplantation have a worse outcome independent of interferon-α usage. Nonetheless, a number of retrospective analyses have addressed this question. In one study, prolonged use of interferon-α was associated with a worse outcome, mainly due to an increased risk of infection and graft failure.[257] Another study in the matched unrelated donor setting supported the concept that prolonged interferon-α treatment of more than 6 months was associated with a worse outcome following transplantation.[258] Other studies have, however, found no impact of interferon-α use on the outcome of subsequent transplantation.[259,260]

Autologous hematopoietic cell transplantation has also been explored for a limited number of patients with CML. Registry data and single-institution studies have suggested that patients who undergo autologous hematopoietic cell transplantation while in chronic phase may attain a prolonged chronic phase of their disease and possibly enjoy improved survival.[261–263] These beneficial effects do not appear to extend to patients in accelerated phase or blastic phase.[261] A variety of strategies have been employed in an effort to enrich for normal unaffected stem cells in the graft, including in vitro culture,[200] cell selection by FACS,[264] and collection of cells upon recovery from chemotherapy.[263,265,267] Autologous transplantation may serve as a platform for subsequent immunotherapeutic strategies, such as with IL-2, autologous NK cells,[267] or CD3+CD56+ effector cells.[268]

An occasional problem in the management of CML patients is that of massive splenomegaly. This can complicate the posttransplant course by causing refractory cytopenias. Both splenectomy and splenic irradiation have been utilized without an adverse effect on the outcomes.[269] One randomized study of splenic irradiation to a total dose of 10 Gy performed in 239 patients with CML did not indicate a significant benefit.[270] However, in another study, 37 patients who received splenic radiation (2.5–5 Gy) within 10 days of hematopoietic cell transplantation had an overall survival of 82 percent.[271]

MYELODYSPLASTIC SYNDROMES

Hematopoietic cell transplantation has been used to treat patients with myelodysplastic syndromes (MDS) but is limited by donor availability and the advanced age of most patients with these conditions. With improvements in supportive care and prevention of graft-versus-host disease, a number of groups have extended the upper age limit for allogeneic BMT to 60 years. However, many MDS patients are older than 60 years of age. Therefore, this treatment modality can only be offered to a subset of individuals with this disease.

In one study, 93 patients were treated with transplantation, all of whom had severe neutropenia, thrombocytopenia, or more than 5 percent marrow blasts. The patients were prepared with either total-body irradiation and cyclophosphamide (total-body irradiation/cyclophosphamide; 88 patients) or busulfan/cyclophosphamide (busulfan/cyclophosphamide; 5 patients). Sixty-five patients received grafts from HLA-matched sibling donors, and 28 patients received either marrow grafts from other family members or unrelated donors. With a follow-up of 4 years, 41 percent of patients were alive and free of disease. Twenty-eight percent of patients relapsed, and 43 percent died of transplant-related complications. Those patients who had the best overall result were younger (<40 years) or had less than 5 percent marrow blasts at the time of hematopoietic cell transplantation.[272]

Similar results have been reported employing regimens using total-body irradiation-based regimens primarily combined with cyclophosphamide.[273–275] Regimens not employing radiation have the potential advantage of less toxicity and have also been used to prepare patients for allogeneic hematopoietic cell transplantation. Thirty-eight patients were prepared with busulfan/cyclophosphamide. The overall survival rate at 2 years was 45 percent, with a 24 percent probability of relapse.[276] The busulfan/cyclophosphamide regimen has been also used in 27 younger patients, where results using grafts from sibling donors were significantly better, with a projected 78 percent of patients alive and free of disease.[277]

In a retrospective analysis of 131 patients with MDS who underwent allogeneic BMT using HLA-matched sibling donors, the 5-year disease-free survival was 34 percent, and overall survival was 41 percent.[278] The same variables reported previously[272] were predictive of improved outcome, including younger age, shorter disease duration, and absence of excess marrow blasts.

The results of matched unrelated donor transplantation for patients with MDS were disappointing in early reports. However, with better matching techniques and supportive care, the results have continued to improve. In one series of 52 patients with MDS or MDS-related AML who underwent matched unrelated donor transplantation, a 2-year disease-free survival of 38 percent was reported.[279] Transplant-related mortality was 58 percent for a cohort of 118 patients with MDS, including 12 patients with CML. Overall survival at 2 years was 28 percent. Again, patients with low-risk disease had a lower relapse rate.[280]

Allogeneic hematopoietic cell transplantation carries significant risks, especially in an elderly patient population. In addition, MDS is a highly variable disease. Therefore, predicting which patients are likely to benefit from hematopoietic cell transplantation is important. In one study of 60 patients, those patients with poor risk cytogenetics, as defined by the International MDS Workshop categorization,[281] had a much worse outcome (event-free survival 6% versus 40–51% for the intermediate and good risk groups) and significantly higher relapse rate (82% versus 12–19%, p = 0.002).[282]

T-cell–depleted grafts have also been explored for the treatment of patients with MDS. The advantage of this approach may be the relatively lower transplant-related mortality due to a decrease in the incidence of graft-versus-host disease. In one study of 35 patients, 24 percent were alive and free of disease with 3 years of follow-up.[283]

Rarely, children develop MDS, and a limited number of pediatric patients have undergone allogeneic hematopoietic cell transplantation. This effort has resulted in long-term survival for a significant percentage.[284,285]

One question that often arises in patients with MDS, especially in those with advanced disease, is whether leukemic induction therapy should be pursued prior to hematopoietic cell transplantation. Due to the extremely poor outcome and difficulty in successfully inducing patients with MDS into remission, most transplant centers prefer to proceed directly to transplantation without prior chemotherapy.[286] Treatment of MDS patients with chemotherapy increases the risk of further complications such as infection and tissue damage. Patients with MDS are chronically immunosuppressed and are at increased risk for a variety of occult infections, including fungal infections. For patients who relapse, small numbers have undergone donor leukocyte infusions (see "Treatment and Prevention of Relapse"), with occasional responses.[19,287,288]

These studies indicate that a subset of MDS patients can be cured following allogeneic hematopoietic cell transplantation. This observation is in contrast to all other treatment modalities that have been evaluated for this difficult disease. However, because of the advanced age of the majority of MDS patients, only a small percentage of patients are candidates for transplantation. The development of less toxic preparative regimens capable of inducing a state of mixed chimerism may allow for the treatment of older patients with this disorder, especially those patients with relatively indolent disease. However, this novel concept requires further evaluation.

Autologous hematopoietic cell transplantation has been attempted in some patients with MDS. However, it has been evaluated in only limited numbers of patients due to the low CR rates obtained with induction chemotherapy. Therefore, any positive results are tempered by the fact that these patients are highly selected. Nevertheless, efforts have been made to develop strategies to collect normal stem cells in these patients. The use of in vivo mobilization and purging, similar to the strategy used in CML, has been attempted in small numbers of patients with defined karyotypic abnormalities. Karyotypically normal leukapheresis products were collected from six of nine patients following recovery from intensive chemotherapy.[265] Results of autologous transplantation for 79 patients with MDS or secondary AML who were successfully induced into CR revealed a disease-free survival of 39 percent at 2 years.[289] Therefore, autologous transplantation may be considered for those unusual patients who are successfully induced into CR and who do not have an HLA-matched donor.

MYELOPROLIFERATIVE DISORDERS

Patients with myeloproliferative disorders other than CML are occasionally considered for BMT. The variability of these disorders, as well as the small number of patients who have undergone hematopoietic cell transplantation, make it difficult to come to firm conclusions. Due to the relatively favorable prognosis of patients with polycythemia vera, there has been no role for BMT except for those patients who progress to acute leukemia. Occasionally, patients with myelofibrosis are suitable candidates for hematopoietic cell transplantation, although the decision of when to consider transplantation is often difficult. The presence of marrow fibrosis has been associated with delayed engraftment.[290] Nevertheless, occasionally patients demonstrated that long-term remission can be achieved in this disorder. It is interesting to note that, following the transplant, the marrow fibrosis resolves over a period of several months.[291]

The reported experience with 12 patients with agnogenic myeloid metaplasia further supports the view that allogeneic hematopoietic cell transplantation can be effective in patients with this disease.[292] With a median follow-up of 25 months, the 4-year overall survival was 71 percent and event-free survival was 59 percent, despite the fact that these patients were heavily pretreated. Other reports also have documented the potential utility of allogeneic hematopoietic cell transplantation for the treatment of myeloproliferative disorders other than CML.

SEVERE APLASTIC ANEMIA

Allogeneic hematopoietic cell transplantation has been extensively evaluated in patients with severe aplastic anemia. The largest single-center experience in this disease comes from Seattle, where a number of reports have highlighted the progressive increase in survival achieved by utilizing improved regimens for prophylaxis for graft-versus-host disease and the addition of antithymocyte globulin (ATG) to the preparative regimen. Using cyclophosphamide and ATG in the preparative regimen has resulted in approximately 90 percent disease-free survival for patients with severe aplastic anemia who underwent hematopoietic cell transplantation with marrow derived from an HLA-matched sibling donor.[294] A recent update demonstrates that those patients continue to enjoy excellent long-term disease-free survival, with an actuarial estimate of survival of 92 percent at 8 years posttransplantation.[295] Excellent long-term results have also been observed from other groups of investigators using similar approaches.[296]

A report from the International Bone Marrow Transplantation Registry has highlighted continued improvements in the treatment of severe aplastic anemia patients using hematopoietic cell transplantation. In this study of 1305 patients who had undergone allogeneic hematopoietic cell transplantation between 1976 and 1992 and were reported to the registry, survival was compared in three different intervals between the years 1976 and 1980, 1981 and 1987, and 1988 and 1992. Five-year survival increased from 48 percent for the earliest cohort of patients to 66 percent for those patients transplanted between 1988 and 1992.[297] The improvements in disease-free survival were due mainly to reductions in mortality in the first 3 months following hematopoietic cell transplantation, with the introduction of cyclosporine being the most important factor.

Improvements have also occurred in the therapy of severe aplastic anemia with immunosuppressive agents without hematopoietic cell

transplantation. There are no prospective randomized trials comparing immunosuppressive therapy with hematopoietic cell transplantation. However, several studies have attempted to compare historical results achieved with hematopoietic cell transplantation to immunosuppressive therapy with ATG or more recently ATG, cyclosporine, and prednisone. The advantage of the immunosuppressive approach is that it can be applied to all patients and does not carry the risk of graft-versus-host disease. The difficulties with this analysis are the long follow-up required; the variability of the patients treated with the two approaches, with the more severely affected patients generally being referred for BMT; and the overall improvements ongoing with both treatments. Nevertheless, a number of retrospective analyses have been performed. Of 155 patients who were treated with ATG, 71 percent of patients with moderate aplastic anemia were alive at 6 years, compared to 48 percent of patients with severe aplastic anemia and 38 percent of patients with very severe aplastic anemia.[298] When the outcomes of BMT for patients with severe and very severe aplastic anemia were compared, no significant differences were noted. However, it was clear from the analysis that patients who were transplanted in the more recent era, 1984 to 1989, had an overall survival of 72 percent, compared to 43 percent for those patients transplanted prior to 1984. A similar result was found in children. Estimated survival rates for pediatric patients who underwent transplantation were 75.6 percent, compared to 73.8 percent for those patients who underwent immunosuppressive therapy.[299]

In a retrospective study of 395 patients with severe aplastic anemia, actuarial survival at 15 years was 69 percent for the patients who underwent BMT, compared to 38 percent for patients who received immunosuppressive therapy (Fig. 18-6).[300] The quality of life of patients who underwent hematopoietic cell transplantation was recently reviewed with up to 26 years of follow-up. Two hundred twelve patients who survived for more than 2 years were studied in greater detail. Survival at 20 years was 69 percent for those patients who developed chronic graft-versus-host disease, compared to 89 percent for those patients who did not.[301] It is interesting to note that at least half of the patients preserved or regained the ability to become pregnant or father a child. This fact is in marked contrast to other patients who undergo hematopoietic cell transplantation with more aggressive regimens for malignant diseases.

A significant long-term problem that has been identified following successful treatment for severe aplastic anemia has been the development of new malignancies. The 10-year cumulative risk of developing new cancers following therapy was 18.8 percent after immunosuppressive therapy and 3.1 percent after BMT.[302] Another series of 700 patients transplanted for severe aplastic anemia or Fanconi anemia was subsequently reported. In this cohort of patients, 23 developed a new malignancy at a median of 91 months following hematopoietic cell transplantation. The actuarial estimate at 20 years was found to be 14 percent.[303] In the patients who were transplanted and did not have Fanconi anemia, the major risk factors were the use of azithioprine for prevention or therapy of graft-versus-host disease and total-body irradiation in the preparative regimen. Since neither of these approaches is any longer routinely utilized in the treatment of severe aplastic anemia with hematopoietic cell transplantation, it is reasonable to expect the risk of new malignancies to drop with subsequent cohorts of patients.

CHRONIC LYMPHOCYTIC LEUKEMIA

Patients with CLL are generally elderly and, due to the relatively benign course of the disease, until recently generally have not been considered candidates for transplantation. With improvements in long-term survival of patients with other diseases of B-cell origin, such as

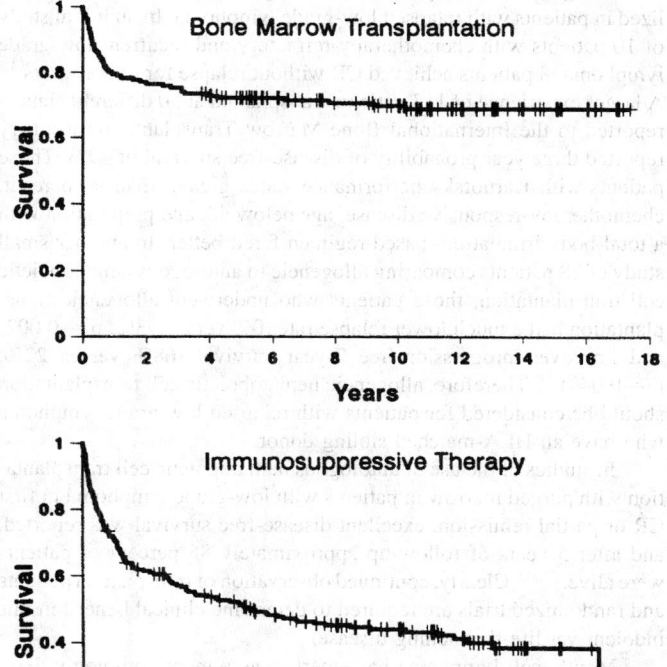

FIGURE 18-6   Historical comparison of long-term results of allogeneic marrow transplantation and immunosuppressive therapy for patients with severe aplastic anemia. (From K Doney et al,[300] with permission.)

lymphoma and multiple myeloma, and with the reduction in procedure-related morbidity and mortality, especially with autologous hematopoietic cell transplantation, an increasing number of patients are being considered for transplantation for CLL. Both allogeneic and autologous hematopoietic cell transplantations have been explored. In CLL, patient selection is of primary importance. This limits the interpretation of results with transplantation.

One of the first reports was a study of 17 patients with a median age of 40 years who underwent allogeneic hematopoietic cell transplantation. The preparative regimen consisted of fractionated total-body irradiation and cyclophosphamide, with additional chemotherapy given to some patients. With follow-up of 2 years, nine patients were alive and in continued remission.[304] An additional eight patients were prepared with fractionated total-body irradiation and cyclophosphamide and underwent transplantation with HLA-matched sibling donor marrow. Seven of these patients entered CR, and six of them were alive and free of disease at the time of the report; however, follow-up was only approximately 1 year.[305] Similar results were reported elsewhere.[306] These studies demonstrate the feasibility of performing allogeneic hematopoietic cell transplantation in patients with CLL and underscore the important finding that the majority of patients enter CR following the treatment, something that is rarely observed with conventional chemotherapy. However, patient selection, the limited number of patients treated, and the short follow-up limit the interpretation of these findings. Larger studies that utilize uniform criteria for patient selection are in progress.

Autologous hematopoietic cell transplantation has also been explored in patients with CLL. Again, the criteria used to select patients were variable and in some instances not reported, complicating the interpretation of the results. In some studies, the stem-cell grafts were treated in an effort to purge CLL cells, and the methodology used varied among centers. In one report of 12 patients who underwent autografting with marrow purged with MoAb and complement, 10 achieved CR.[305] A follow-up study evaluating minimal residual disease using PCR demonstrated that persistence of PCR positivity following either autologous or allogeneic transplantation was correlated with a high risk of subsequent relapse.[307] Clearly, much work still needs to be done in order to determine the role of hematopoietic cell transplantation in the treatment of patients with CLL.

LYMPHOMA

Hematopoietic cell transplantation for patients with lymphoma has met with considerable success. The most extensive experience has been utilizing autologous hematopoietic cell transplantation in patients with relapsed intermediate-grade lymphoma. A number of phase II studies have documented improved disease-free survival for patients with chemosensitive relapses who underwent autologous hematopoietic cell transplantation, with disease-free survival ranging from 20 to 60 percent.[67,68,308–313]

A criticism of these studies has been the lack of control groups and the possibility that the improved results were due to patient selection. To address these issues, a prospective randomized clinical trial utilizing an intention-to-treat analysis has been performed. In this study, called the PARMA trial, a total of 215 patients were enrolled, of whom 109 patients (58%) had a response to combination chemotherapy and were randomized to either an additional cycle of chemotherapy or autologous hematopoietic cell transplantation. At 5 years of follow-up, event-free survival was 46 percent in the transplant group and 12 percent in the chemotherapy group (p = 0.001). Overall survival was 53 percent for the transplant group and 32 percent for the chemotherapy group (p = 0.038), mainly due to the fact that some of the patients in the chemotherapy group could be salvaged upon relapse with stem-cell transplantation (Fig. 18-7).[314] These results have clearly documented the benefit for autologous hematopoietic cell transplantation for patients with chemosensitive relapsed lymphoma. With the introduction of peripheral-blood progenitor cells, transplant-related morbidity and mortality have decreased considerably.[315] In addition, tech-

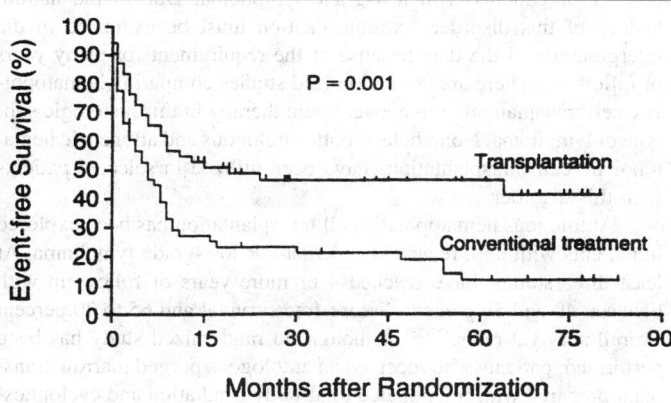

FIGURE 18-7   Results of a prospective randomized controlled trial comparing autologous transplantation with conventional chemotherapy for patients with chemotherapy-sensitive relapsed lymphoma. (From T Philip,[314] with permission.)

niques have been developed to purge peripheral-blood progenitor cells and reduce tumor burden, as discussed above. These advances are likely to result in additional improvements in results with transplantation.

A significant problem in the application of hematopoietic cell transplantation to patients with relapsed lymphoma has been the high level of drug resistance observed in this patient population. Since approximately 40 percent of patients with lymphoma enjoy long-term disease-free survival with standard chemotherapy,[316] attempts have been made to predict which patients are at high risk for relapse based upon clinical parameters of their disease at presentation. A large international effort has produced such a scoring index, based upon age, tumor stage, serum lactate dehydrogenase, performance status, and number of extranodal disease sites, which identified four risk groups.[317]

Autologous hematopoietic cell transplantation has been pursued in patients as up-front therapy, and it has been observed that patients with high-risk disease appeared to benefit from the procedure.[318,319] Randomized prospective clinical trials to formally test this hypothesis are underway.

In a randomized trial of 916 patients with lymphoma who achieved CR, the patients were assigned to either sequential chemotherapy or autologous hematopoietic cell transplantation. In the first analysis of this study, no differences were observed.[320] Subsequent analysis with additional follow-up revealed a significant 5-year disease-free survival rate for the higher-risk patients, with 57 percent of the transplanted patients and 39 percent of the patients treated with chemotherapy (p = 0.01) alive and free of disease.[321] This observation not only helps guide therapy but also demonstrates the requirement for adequate follow-up to observe differences in outcome when relapse is the major cause for treatment failure. In addition, further analysis of the PARMA trial based upon the international prognostic index demonstrated benefit primarily for patients with at least one high-risk feature.[322]

Other studies have also addressed this issue. Utilization of autologous hematopoietic cell transplantation in patients with a slow response to conventional chemotherapy did not result in improved disease-free survival.[323] Another approach utilized high doses of sequential chemotherapy followed by autologous hematopoietic cell transplantation in comparison to conventional chemotherapy with MACOP-B (see Chap. 103) for patients with aggressive lymphoma. In this study, event-free survival was 76 percent for the transplanted patients versus 49 percent for the patients who received chemotherapy (p = 0.004).[324]

Hematopoietic cell transplantation has been explored in a limited number of patients with low-grade lymphoma. Due to the natural history of this disorder, extreme caution must be exercised in the interpretation of the data because of the requirement for many years of follow-up. There are no randomized studies comparing hematopoietic cell transplantation to conventional therapy in this histologic subtype of lymphoma. Nonetheless, both autologous and allogeneic hematopoietic cell transplantations have been utilized in selected patients with this disorder.

Autologous hematopoietic cell transplantation has been explored in patients with both recurrent and first-CR low-grade lymphoma. At least three studies have reached 4 or more years of follow-up with between 40 and 50 percent disease-free survival and 65 to 70 percent overall survival rates.[325–327] Although no randomized study has been performed, patients who received an autologous purged marrow transplant prepared with fractionated total-body irradiation and cyclophosphamide have been compared to a historical cohort of patients treated with chemotherapy who were matched for disease status characteristics. There were no survival differences; however, those patients who underwent transplantation had improved freedom from progression.[325]

Allogeneic hematopoietic cell transplantation has also been utilized in patients with relapsed low-grade lymphoma. In an initial study of 10 patients with chemotherapy-refractory and recurrent low-grade lymphoma, 8 patients achieved CR without relapse for over 2 years.[328] A larger experience of 113 patients transplanted at 50 different centers reported to the International Bone Marrow Transplantation Registry reported three year probability of disease-free survival of 49%. Those patients with Karnofsky performance status greater than 90 percent, chemotherapy-responsive disease, age below 40, and preparation with a total-body irradiation–based regimen fared better. In another small study of 28 patients comparing allogeneic to autologous hematopoietic cell transplantation, those patients who underwent allogeneic transplantation had a much lower relapse rate (0% versus 93%; p = 0.002) and improved progression-free 2-year survival (68% versus 22%; p = 0.049).[330] Therefore, allogeneic hematopoietic cell transplantation should be considered for patients with relapsed low-grade lymphoma who have an HLA-matched sibling donor.

In studies of the use of autologous hematopoietic cell transplantation with purged marrow in patients with low-grade lymphoma in first CR or partial remission, excellent disease-free survival was reported, and after 5 years of follow-up approximately 85 percent of patients were alive.[331,332] Clearly, continued observation of transplanted patients and randomized trials are required to determine clinical benefit in this indolent yet life-threatening disease.

Mantle-cell lymphoma has emerged as a more commonly diagnosed subtype of lymphoma. These patients respond poorly to standard-dose chemotherapy, and many are elderly.[333] Several studies utilizing autologous hematopoietic cell transplantation have been reported, with widely variable results, depending primarily on the remission status of the patients prior to transplantation. In one study of 28 patients, 8 of whom were in first CR, the estimated 4-year disease-free survival was only 31 percent.[334] Similar results were reported in another investigation.[335] In contrast, others have reported much more optimistic results in this disorder.[322,336–338] Clearly, additional studies are required to better define the role of autologous hematopoietic cell transplantation in this disorder. However, it appears clear that, if transplantation is to be considered, it should be pursued early in the clinical course of the disease.

Burkitt's lymphoma is successfully treated with standard chemotherapy in the majority of cases; however, patients with recurrent disease can be salvaged with autologous hematopoietic cell transplantation.[318,339,340]

Patients with advanced-stage lymphoblastic lymphoma have a poor outcome with standard chemotherapy, and autologous hematopoietic cell transplantation has been successful in patients in first CR and patients with chemosensitive relapse.[341–343] Allogeneic hematopoietic cell transplantation has been applied to limited numbers of patients with lymphoma, as discussed above. Similar to other diseases, the relapse rate is generally lower following allogeneic hematopoietic cell transplantation; however, overall survival is offset by the increased risk of procedure-related complications. In patients with high-risk lymphoblastic lymphoma, results with allogeneic hematopoietic cell transplantation are similar in first CR but appear to be superior to autologous hematopoietic cell transplantation in patients with recurrent disease.[341,344]

HODGKIN'S DISEASE

Since the majority of patients with Hodgkin's disease respond well to chemotherapy, hematopoietic cell transplantation has been reserved for patients who do not enter CR (induction failures) and for patients with relapsed disease. The development of a prognostic score in Hodgkin's disease may allow for the identification of a high-risk group of patients in whom hematopoietic cell transplantation could be considered in first CR.[345] Patients with induction failures respond poorly to standard chemotherapy, and 35 to 50 percent of such patients can be salvaged with autologous hematopoietic cell transplantation.[346–350]

Patients who relapse following chemotherapy fare poorly.[351] A number of studies have addressed the issue of whether high-dose therapy with autologous hematopoietic cell transplantation can improve the outcome for these patients. Both radiation-containing and chemotherapy-only preparative regimens have been utilized. Four studies of more than 100 patients have been reported with greater than 3-year progression-free survival of 25 to 50 percent.[349,352–354] As in all phase II studies, there is the potential for patient selection that may bias results. Matched case-control analyses have been performed comparing 60 patients who underwent autologous hematopoietic cell transplantation at Stanford University with a group of patients selected with similar clinical characteristics from a database. Overall survival, event-free survival, and freedom from progression at 4 years favored the patients who underwent transplantation (overall survival 54% versus 47%, p = 0.25; event-free survival 53% versus 27%, p < 0.01; freedom from progression 62% versus 32%, p < 0.01).[355]

There has been only one prospective randomized clinical trial in which autologous hematopoietic cell transplantation was compared to salvage chemotherapy. Patients with relapsed or refractory Hodgkin's disease were randomized to receive mini-BEAM, which was the conventional dose arm, or to receive the same drugs at higher doses followed by autologous hematopoietic cell transplantation. At 3 years, event-free survival favored the patients who received the higher doses of BEAM.[356]

MULTIPLE MYELOMA

High-dose therapy and hematopoietic cell transplantation has been used in the treatment of patients with multiple myeloma. Since the majority of patients respond to standard-dose chemotherapy, the concept of using high-dose therapy to treat multiple myeloma is intellectually attractive. The use of high-dose therapy followed by autologous hematopoietic cell transplantation has been studied, and response rates of 60 to 80 percent and CR rates of 20 to 75 percent have been documented.[357–362] High-dose sequential chemotherapy similar to that used in patients with lymphoma also has been applied to patients with multiple myeloma, with a CR achieved in 10 of 13 patients (77%). Overall survival using this approach was superior to that of historical controls.[363] Tandem autologous transplants utilizing high-dose melphalan followed by fractionated total-body irradiation and melphalan has been explored. In one study of 496 newly diagnosed patients, 95 percent completed the first transplant with high-dose melphalan (200 mg/m²), and 73 percent completed the second transplant with fractionated total-body irradiation and melphalan. Complete remission was achieved in 36 percent, with 7 percent treatment-related mortality.[364] Median event-free survival and overall survival were 26 and 41 months, respectively, with low β_2-microglobulin and C-reactive protein being the most significant prognostic factors associated with prolonged event-free survival. In a subsequent analysis, 123 previously untreated patients who underwent this treatment strategy and also received interferon-α following hematopoietic cell transplantation were compared to 1123 matched patients drawn from clinical trials. The event-free survival was 49 months for the transplanted patients, compared to 22 months (p = 0.0001) for historical patients who had standard chemotherapy. Overall survival was also prolonged (62 versus 48 months; p = 0.01).[365] These results have recently been updated and confirmed.[366] In the meantime, the use of historical control patients has been challenged in another analysis. The median survival of patients with multiple myeloma who are considered candidates for hema-

topoietic cell transplantation was found to be 5 years, similar to that achieved with hematopoietic cell transplantation.[367] High-dose therapy with autologous hematopoietic cell transplantation has also been utilized in patients with late-stage multiple myeloma and found to be primarily of benefit early in the course of the disease.[368,369]

Two hundred previously untreated patients with multiple myeloma less than 65 years of age were randomized to receive either conventional chemotherapy or high-dose therapy and autologous hematopoietic cell transplantation. Analysis was performed on an intent-to-treat basis with 75 of the 100 patients randomized to undergo hematopoietic cell transplantation actually receiving the therapy. Complete remission was achieved in 22 percent of the hematopoietic cell transplantation patients and 5 percent of the patients treated with conventional chemotherapy. At 5 years, both event-free survival (28% versus 10%; p = 0.01) and overall survival (52% versus 12%; p = 0.03) was superior for patients undergoing hematopoietic cell transplantation, with similar treatment-related mortality for the two groups of patients (Fig. 18-8).[370] This seminal study has demonstrated the clinical benefit of hematopoietic cell transplantation in multiple myeloma; however, in contrast to studies in other disorders, it is not clear whether patients are in fact cured of their disease, since a plateau state has not been reached and patients continue to relapse. Therefore, additional approaches are needed to address the minimal residual disease state achieved by hematopoietic cell transplantation.

To improve upon the results obtained with hematopoietic cell transplantation in multiple myeloma, a number of approaches have been explored. Since clonal B cells are readily detected in the marrow and peripheral-blood progenitor-cell collections obtained from these patients,[371–373] a number of techniques have been explored to decrease the tumor burden in the graft. The use of monoclonal antibody– and

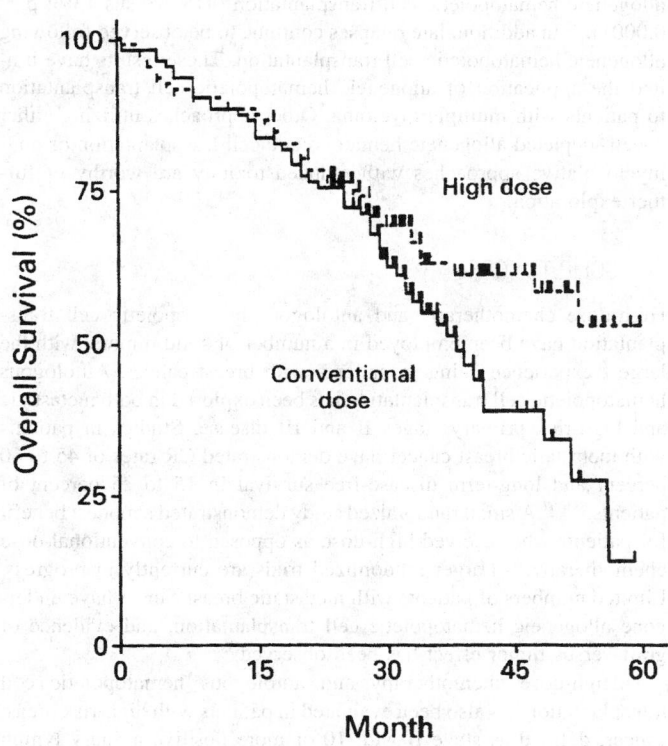

FIGURE 18-8   Prospective randomized trial of autologous transplantation compared to conventional chemotherapy for patients with newly diagnosed multiple myeloma. (From M Attal et al,[370] with permission.)

complement-based methods has demonstrated that the marrow samples can be depleted of antigen-positive cells below the limits of detection of cell sorting (approximately 1%).[374] Positive stem-cell collection has also been pursued in this disease by CD34+ cell columns or by FACS to purify the CD34+Thy1+ stem cells. A randomized trial comparing CD34+ selected versus unmanipulated grafts has been performed, with preliminary results showing equivalent engraftment, no change in infection risk, and similar event-free survival, although further follow-up is required to evaluate any impact on relapse rates and survival.[375]

In another approach, interferon-α has been used following hematopoietic cell transplantation, since this agent has shown efficacy in some studies following standard chemotherapy. In one randomized study of 85 patients, no differences in progression-free survival in the two groups were noted.[376] Vaccination is an attractive concept, since the immunoglobulin produced is monoclonal and may be recognizable by the immune system. Healthy sibling donors have been shown to have anti-idiotypic responses that could be transferred to the recipient.[377] Idiotypic vaccination has also been explored in the autologous setting by isolating the patient's idiotype protein, pulsing dendritic cells, and reinfusing the pulsed dendritic cells into the patient. Immune responses against the paraprotein have been observed in a minority of patients.[378]

Allogeneic hematopoietic cell transplantation has also been pursued in patients with multiple myeloma in an effort to exploit a graft-versus-myeloma effect.[379] Results have generally been disappointing because of significant transplant-related mortality.[380,381] A retrospective case-matched analysis comparing allogeneic versus autologous hematopoietic cell transplantation in multiple myeloma has been performed. Overall survival was superior for autologous hematopoietic cell transplantation (46 months for autologous, 30 months for allogeneic; p = 0.0003), mainly due to higher treatment-related mortality following allogeneic hematopoietic cell transplantation (41% versus 13%; p = 0.0001).[382] In addition, late relapses continue to be observed following allogeneic hematopoietic cell transplantation. These results have limited the application of allogeneic hematopoietic cell transplantation to patients with multiple myeloma. Other approaches utilizing either T-cell–depleted allogeneic hematopoietic cell transplantation or nonmyeloablative approaches with reduced toxicity are worthy of further exploration.

SOLID TUMORS

High-dose chemotherapy and autologous hematopoietic cell transplantation have been employed in a number of solid tumors, with the largest experience being in patients with breast cancer. Autologous hematopoietic cell transplantation has been explored in both metastatic and high-risk primary stages II and III disease. Studies in patients with metastatic breast cancer have demonstrated CR rates of 45 to 60 percent and long-term disease-free survival in 15 to 25 percent of patients.[383–386] A small randomized study demonstrated a modest benefit for patients who received high-dose as opposed to conventional-dose chemotherapy.[387] Larger randomized trials are currently in progress. Limited numbers of patients with metastatic breast cancer have undergone allogeneic hematopoietic cell transplantation, and evidence of graft-versus-tumor effect has been observed.[388]

High-dose chemotherapy and autologous hematopoietic cell transplantation has also been evaluated in patients with high-risk breast cancer, defined as stage II with 10 or more positive axillary lymph nodes or stage III disease. Patients undergoing autologous hematopoietic cell transplantation appear to have improved survival compared to historical control subjects.[80,386] Two large randomized trials that should help provide more definitive evidence of the potential efficacy

of autologous hematopoietic cell transplantation in this clinical setting are in progress. High-dose chemotherapy with autologous hematopoietic cell transplantation has also been explored in breast cancer patients with four to nine axillary lymph nodes, with promising results.[389] A randomized study comparing high-dose therapy with autologous hematopoietic cell transplantation to conventional, albeit high-dose, therapy without transplantation is currently being performed.

Autologous hematopoietic cell transplantation has also been utilized in patients with recurrent or refractory ovarian cancer, with disease-free survival rates of approximately 10 to 33 percent.[390,391] Ongoing studies continue to evaluate this form of therapy in patients earlier in the course of this disease. Patients with recurrent or refractory germ-cell tumors have also undergone autologous hematopoietic cell transplantation.[392] In one recent study of 21 patients, 52 percent are alive and free of disease.[393]

In pediatric patients, the use of autologous hematopoietic cell transplantation has resulted in prolonged disease-free survival in patients with advanced stage, poor-prognosis neuroblastoma who are not likely to be cured with standard therapy.[394–397] Since neuroblastoma cells can be found in the marrow and blood progenitor cells, strategies have been developed to "purge" these stem-cell products.[396,398]

FANCONI ANEMIA

Early attempts at hematopoietic cell transplantation for the treatment of Fanconi anemia with high-dose cyclophosphamide resulted in unacceptable toxicity and only modest success rates of 20 to 50 percent.[399,400] Improved outcomes have been reported utilizing much lower doses of cyclophosphamide combined with low-dose total-body irradiation[401] or without total-body irradiation.[402] All potential related marrow donors must be screened for chromosomal changes indicative of Fanconi anemia. Patients with Fanconi anemia appear to be at increased risk of developing malignancies following hematopoietic cell transplantation. In one study of 79 patients with this disorder, the actuarial risk of developing any malignancy by 20 years after hematopoietic cell transplantation was 42 percent.[303]

THALASSEMIA

Hematopoietic cell transplantation has been very successful for the treatment of selected patients with severe thalassemia who have an HLA-matched sibling donor. In one report of 222 patients who underwent allogeneic hematopoietic cell transplantation, event-free survival of 75 percent was achieved.[403] Patients with hepatomegaly and portal fibrosis had a worse outcome. Those individuals with both of these risk factors had an event-free survival of 61 percent, compared to an event-free survival of 94 percent for those patients without either of these problems.[403] Initial results of allogeneic hematopoietic cell transplantation in thalassemic patients more than 16 years of age were poor. However, refinements have resulted in improved outcomes, with event-free survival of approximately 75 percent.[404,405]

SICKLE CELL ANEMIA

The eradication of sickle cell anemia in an 8-year-old child who underwent allogeneic hematopoietic cell transplantation for AML was reported in 1984.[406] Since then, several reports have appeared detailing the use of allogeneic hematopoietic cell transplantation to treat this disorder. The major challenge has been in identifying patients with sufficiently advanced disease to warrant accepting the risks inherent in allogeneic hematopoietic cell transplantation, yet not so far advanced that they are unable to tolerate the procedure. In one study of 22 children with symptomatic sickle cell disease who were under 16 years of age and had an HLA-matched sibling donor, 20 patients were alive at a median follow-up of 2 years. Sixteen of the patients had stable engraftment of donor hematopoietic cells. Actuarial estimates of event-free survival at 4 years was 73 percent.[407,408] A larger study of 50 patients with this disorder reported similarly impressive results.[409] Further exploration in this area is clearly warranted.

IMMUNODEFICIENCY SYNDROMES AND INHERITED METABOLIC DISORDERS

A variety of other diseases have been treated with allogeneic hematopoietic cell transplantation. In fact, one of the first successful reports of a marrow transplant procedure was for the treatment of children with immunodeficiency syndromes in 1968.[7-9] Hematopoietic cell transplantation has become the treatment of choice for patients with severe combined immunodeficiency disorder (SCID), with success rates of 70 to 80 percent.[410] It is interesting to note that patients with SCID do not require conditioning prior to allogeneic hematopoietic cell transplantation but generally need some form of immunosuppression to avoid graft rejection if T-cell depletion is performed. Unrelated donor transplants have also been performed to treat SCID patients.[411,412] Long-term follow-up of 193 SCID patients who underwent allogeneic hematopoietic cell transplantation was recently reported. At 6 months following transplantation, 116 patients (60%) were alive. Normal T-cell function was achieved at a median of 8.7 months following the transplant procedure, while normal B-cell reconstitution required a median of 14.9 months.[413]

Allogeneic hematopoietic cell transplantation has also been utilized in an effort to correct a wide array of other inherited metabolic disorders. These disorders include Gaucher's disease, mucopolysaccharidosis (Hurler's syndrome), metachromatic leukodystrophy, infantile osteopetrosis, and congenital erythropoietic porphyria.[414-417]

AUTOIMMUNE DISORDERS

Considerable interest has centered around the application of hematopoietic cell transplantation to the treatment of autoimmune disorders. Studies in animal models have demonstrated the potential for this treatment modality, as have anecdotal reports of patients with concomitant autoimmune disorders who underwent hematopoietic cell transplantation for treatment of another disease and appeared to derive benefit. Other reports have appeared, however, that have shown early recurrence or no effect on the autoimmune disease.[418] Studies designed for direct evaluation of the effect of hematopoietic cell transplantation on autoimmune disorders are underway. Early reports using autologous hematopoietic cell transplantation for the treatment of multiple sclerosis and other autoimmune diseases have been encouraging.[419,420] Clearly, further evaluation is required. Major questions concerning the source of the graft (allogeneic versus autologous), preparative regimen, and the requirement for and extent of T-cell depletion in the autologous setting all need to be addressed with carefully conducted clinical trials.

COMPLICATIONS AND THEIR MANAGEMENT

GRAFT-VERSUS-HOST DISEASE

Graft-versus-host disease remains one of the most serious and challenging complications following hematopoietic cell transplantation. Graft-versus-host disease results from immunologically competent donor-derived T cells that react with recipient tissue antigens. In 1966, Billingham formulated the requirements for developing graft-versus-host disease, including (1) the graft must contain immunologically competent cells; (2) the recipient must express tissue antigens not found in the donor; and (3) the recipient must be immunologically suppressed enough that an effective response against the transplanted cells cannot be made.[421] Risk factors for developing graft-versus-host disease include HLA disparity between donor and recipient, age, gender disparity, type and status of underlying disease, and prophylaxis utilized.

By definition, acute graft-versus-host disease occurs prior to day 100, while chronic graft-versus-host disease occurs beyond day 100. Graft-versus-host disease primarily affects three organs: the skin, gastrointestinal tract, and liver. A severity system ranging between grades 0 and IV has been established that takes into account the degree of involvement of each organ system and defines an overall grade between II and IV for clinically significant disease. Graft-versus-host disease is a clinical diagnosis, although tissue biopsy results can be helpful in making a definitive diagnosis. However, severity on pathological specimens must always be tempered by an assessment of the clinical condition of the patient.

Clinically significant acute graft-versus-host disease occurs in 9 to 50 percent of patients who receive an allogeneic hematopoietic cell transplant from a histocompatible sibling donor. Patients who develop moderate (grade II) to severe (grades III–IV) acute graft-versus-host disease have a significantly enhanced risk of mortality. Established acute graft-versus-host disease is difficult to treat, and intensive efforts have been extended toward prophylaxis. Two general approaches have been utilized in an effort to prevent acute graft-versus-host disease, namely, immunosuppressive medications and T-cell depletion.

A number of different drugs have been utilized as prophylaxis against graft-versus-host disease. Methotrexate, cyclosporine, and prednisone have been the mainstays of prophylaxis, generally in combination. A series of randomized clinical trials have established cyclosporine given over at least 6 months and methotrexate administered on days 1, 3, 6, and 11 following the transplant as an effective regimen.[422,423] Subsequent updates of these studies have documented that effective prophylaxis with cyclosporine/methotrexate did not result in a significant increase in the risk of relapse, which is always a concern with any agent that prevents acute graft-versus-host disease.[424]

In an initial prospective study, cyclosporine and prednisone prophylaxis resulted in a reduced rate of grade II to IV graft-versus-host disease of 28 percent, compared to methotrexate and prednisone.[425] The regimen of cyclosporine/prednisone was compared to methotrexate/prednisone, with the methotrexate administered on days 1, 3, and 6 in a randomized trial and with all patients receiving the preparative regimen of fractionated total-body irradiation and etoposide. Patients who received the two-drug regimen had an incidence of grade II to IV graft-versus-host disease of 23 percent, compared to 9 percent for patients who received the three-drug regimen (p = 0.02).[426] No differences in the relapse rate of the risk of chronic graft-versus-host disease were observed in the two groups.[427] A trial comparing cyclosporine/methotrexate to the three-drug regimen is underway.

Tacrolimus (FK506) has also been utilized to prevent acute graft-versus-host disease. Prospective randomized clinical trials have been performed in the setting of an HLA-matched sibling and matched unrelated allogeneic hematopoietic cell transplantation. In the former study, 329 patients from 16 transplant centers were randomized to receive FK506 or cyclosporine, with both groups also receiving methotrexate. The incidence of grade II to IV acute graft-versus-host disease was significantly lower in the group of patients randomized to FK506 (31.9% versus 44.4%, respectively; p = 0.01).[428] No differences in severe (grade III–IV) acute graft-versus-host disease, chronic graft-versus-host disease, or relapse rates were noted. However, paradoxically, 2-year disease-free survival was superior in the cyclosporine arm, a result thought to be due to a larger number of patients with advanced disease randomized to receive FK506.

FK506 has also been utilized with methotrexate for the prevention of acute graft-versus-host disease in the unrelated donor setting. Phase II studies have resulted in a 42 to 50 percent incidence of grade II to IV acute graft-versus-host disease, which appears promising.[429,430] In a randomized trial, 136 patients received either FK506 or cyclosporine-based regimens. For those 69 patients who received unrelated donor transplants, the incidence of acute graft-versus-host disease was reduced from 51.4 percent in the cyclosporine group to 20.6 percent in the FK506 group (p < 0.05).[431] These results will require confirmation in a larger group of patients but are consistent with a reduction in the incidence of acute graft-versus-host disease with the use of FK506 over cyclosporine.

An alternative approach to the prevention of graft-versus-host disease has been to deplete donor T cells from the graft prior to infusion. A variety of techniques have been employed, including physical separation such as elutriation or density gradient centrifugation, MoAb-based depletion, or CD34+ cell selection. As discussed above, extensive removal of donor derived T cells has been very effective in eradicating graft-versus-host disease but has been associated with an unacceptably high risk of graft rejection and relapse.[15,254,432–435] Modifications of T-cell depletion that result in only partial removal have met with considerable success.

Thirty-nine patients with AML underwent T-cell depletion utilizing the soybean lectin agglutination and sheep red blood cell rosetting, which results in approximately a 3-log depletion of T cells. They were prepared for transplantation with fractionated total-body irradiation, thiotepa, and cyclophosphamide, with many also receiving additional immunosuppression with antithymocyte globulin. No cases of rejection or acute graft-versus-host disease were noted. Disease-free survival at a median follow-up of 4 years or more was 77 percent for patients treated in first remission and 50 percent for patients who underwent hematopoietic cell transplantation in second remission.[436]

Partial T-cell depletion with monoclonal antibodies resulted in significant reductions in graft-versus-host disease without a high incidence of graft failure or relapse.[437–439] Patients who receive T-cell–depleted hematopoietic cell transplantation are at higher risk of Epstein-Barr virus–associated lymphoproliferative disease and have delayed T-cell reconstitution, which is especially true in adults, presumably due to thymic involution.[440]

A somewhat different approach is the use of CAMPATH antibodies in which an IgM (CAMPATH-IM) is used for in vitro depletion of the graft and an IgG (CAMPATH-IG) is used for in vivo depletion of the recipient prior to graft infusion. Fifty patients treated with CAMPATH antibodies were compared to 459 patients reported to the International Bone Marrow Transplantation Registry who received nondepleted grafts and conventional graft-versus-host disease prophylaxis with cyclosporine/methotrexate. The incidence of acute graft-versus-host disease, chronic graft-versus-host disease, and transplant-related mortality were all lower in the patients who received the CAMPATH antibodies. Survival of the patients who were treated with the T-cell depletion approach was better at 6 months (92% versus 78%); however, at 5 years there was no difference (60% versus 52%).[441]

T-cell depletion has also been employed in the unrelated donor setting with encouraging results.[256,442] Clearly, the only effective way of comparing these two very different strategies for reducing the incidence of graft-versus-host disease is through a prospective randomized clinical trial. Such a trial is underway comparing T-cell depletion using the T10B9 MoAb and complement with unmanipulated marrow in the unrelated setting.

Treatment of established acute graft-versus-host disease is often a difficult clinical problem. The mainstay of treatment of established graft-versus-host disease is corticosteroids. Dosing generally ranges between 1 to 2 mg/kg of prednisone, with subsequent tapering depending upon response. Low-dose intravenous 6-methylprednisolone (2 mg/kg per day) has been compared to high-dose (10 mg/kg per day) in 95 patients with acute graft-versus-host disease. Response in the two groups was similar (68% versus 71%), with no differences noted in evolution to grade III to IV graft-versus-host disease, CMV infection, or survival.[443] A variety of other approaches have been explored in the treatment of acute graft-versus-host disease, including anti-T-cell antibodies such as ATG, OKT3 directed against CD3, BT1-322 directed against CD2 or the IL-2 receptor.[293,444] Responses have been noted in many of these studies. However, progression of graft-versus-host disease occurs following discontinuation of the antibody in most of the patients. Elevated levels of cytokines, in particular tumor necrosis factor (TNF), are thought to be central to the pathogenesis of graft-versus-host disease. In murine models, anti-TNF monoclonal antibodies prevent graft-versus-host disease. The use of anti-TNF MoAb has been explored in limited clinical trials of 19 patients with moderate to severe acute graft-versus-host disease, of whom 14 responded.[445]

A variety of newer pharmacologic agents are under investigation for the treatment of both acute and chronic graft-versus-host disease. Mycophenolate mofetil has been explored in combination with cyclosporine and prednisone. In one study of 17 patients with established acute graft-versus-host disease who were treated with 2 g of mycophenolate mofetil per day, improvements were observed in 11 patients (65%). In addition, three of six patients with chronic graft-versus-host disease also had clinical improvements.[446] Myelosuppression was the most common side effect, although discontinuation of the drug was not required by any patient.

Chronic graft-versus-host disease is another significant complication following hematopoietic cell transplantation. By definition, chronic graft-versus-host disease occurs beyond 100 days from the transplant. The clinical manifestations of chronic graft-versus-host disease are broad and resemble those of autoimmune disorders such as scleroderma and dermatomyositis.[447,448] Patients with extensive chronic graft-versus-host disease have an increased mortality rate, especially patients with platelet counts less than 100,000 platelets/μl on day +100, patients who progress from acute to chronic graft-versus-host disease, patients with lichenoid changes on skin biopsy, and patients with significant liver involvement.[449] Treatment for chronic graft-versus-host disease involves the use of immunosuppressive drugs, with cyclosporine or FK506 and prednisone being the mainstays of treatment.[450] Due to the chronic nature of the disease, long-term treatment is often required. Alternate-day dosing has been found to help reduce some of the toxicity of the immunosuppressive medications.[451]

A number of other medications have been explored for the treatment of chronic graft-versus-host disease. Thalidomide, which was initially used as a sedative but abandoned because it produced phocomelia in the offspring of pregnant women taking the drug, was found to have immunosuppressive properties and has been used to treat chronic graft-versus-host disease in both adults and children, with encouraging responses observed.[452–455] Side effects have included somnolence and constipation. It is interesting to note that thalidomide was not effective in preventing the onset of chronic graft-versus-host disease. Instead, there was a paradoxically higher incidence in patients treated with the drug in a small randomized trial.[456] Psoralen plus ultraviolet radiation (PUVA) has shown encouraging results in small numbers of patients with chronic graft-versus-host disease.[457] The use of etretinate, which is a synthetic vitamin A derivative, has recently been reported in a series of 32 patients with refractory sclerodermatous chronic graft-versus-host disease. Response was evaluated after 3 months, and positive effects were observed in 20 of 27 evaluable patients.[458] Low-dose total lymphoid irradiation (100 cGy) has also been reported to result in significant improvement in chronic graft-versus-host disease in small numbers of patients.[459]

Infection, especially by gram-positive organisms, is a common problem in patients with chronic graft-versus-host disease. Monthly intravenous immunoglobulin or rotating antibiotics is sometimes helpful in patients with recurrent infections, especially patients who are hypogammaglobulinemic as a result of chronic graft-versus-host disease. Graft-versus-host disease remains a significant and often debilitating clinical problem. New approaches to the treatment of this complication are clearly needed.

VENO-OCCLUSIVE DISEASE

Veno-occlusive disease of the liver is one of the most feared complications of allogeneic and autologous hematopoietic cell transplantations. The incidence of veno-occlusive disease varies significantly from center to center, depending upon which diagnostic criteria are used.[460,461] The typical signs and symptoms of veno-occlusive disease include unexplained weight gain, jaundice, right upper quadrant pain, and ascites. Definitive diagnostic tests are not available. However, reversal of hepatic blood flow, elevated hepatic wedge pressure, and elevated serum plasminogen activator inhibitor-1 have all been associated with patients who have or develop clinically significant veno-occlusive disease.[462] A definitive diagnosis often requires a liver biopsy, which is frequently dangerous and impractical early after hematopoietic cell transplantation in patients with liver dysfunction. Approximately 25 to 30 percent of cases are severe, and mortality in these patients is almost universal. Patients with prior hepatic B or C infection and liver function abnormalities or those with seropositive donors are at increased risk for developing veno-occlusive disease.[463,464] No single preparative regimen has been implicated as being causative in the development of veno-occlusive disease. However, a higher incidence of veno-occlusive disease appears to occur in patients who receive busulfan-containing regimens, especially if busulfan levels reach an area under the curve of greater than 1500 μmol/min per liter.[72,463,465] No therapy for veno-occlusive disease has been shown in a controlled study to be effective, and, as a result, treatment of this disorder is largely supportive.

Patients with mild to moderate veno-occlusive disease may respond spontaneously without any particular treatment. In one series, for example, survival at day +100 was 91 percent with mild veno-occlusive disease and 77 percent with moderate disease.[460] Most patients who recover from veno-occlusive disease of any severity regain normal liver function and do not develop sequelae of chronic liver disease, such as portal hypertension or esophageal varices. In contrast, the prognosis in patients with severe veno-occlusive disease, which occurs in 25 to 30 percent of cases, is typically poor. Such patients develop fulminant acute liver failure, coagulopathy, hepatic encephalopathy, hepatorenal syndrome, and multiorgan failure.

Attempts have been made to identify risk factors associated with disease progression and death in patients who develop clinical features of veno-occlusive disease. In one study, risk factors associated with the development of severe veno-occlusive disease at different time points following hematopoietic cell transplantation were ascertained in a cohort of 355 patients.[466] This model was then validated prospectively by predicting outcomes in a separate cohort of 392 patients. A logistic regression model identified the serum bilirubin and percent weight gain within 1 to 2 weeks of hematopoietic cell transplantation as the most important independent predictors of progression to severe disease.

Treatment of established veno-occlusive disease has had limited effectiveness. Several studies have evaluated the use of recombinant tissue-type plasminogen activator (tPA) and heparin based upon the hypothesis that damage to the vascular endothelium produces localized hypercoagulability and clotting. In general, a response rate of approximately 30 to 40 percent was seen in association with a significant risk of hemorrhage.[389,467,468] Based upon these findings, the authors recommended that treatment with tPA and heparin *not* be used in patients with severe veno-occlusive disease who already have developed multiorgan dysfunction. In most studies, the dose of tPA utilized has been relatively low, with a median of 60 mg total dose administered over 2 to 4 days followed by infusion of heparin.[469] Higher-dose tPA is associated with a greater risk of bleeding and does not appear to improve response.[470] Similar results have been obtained in children.[468]

Defibrotide is a polydeoxyribonucleotide derived from mammalian tissue with multiple antithrombotic and fibrinolytic activities.[471] Defibrotide has little systemic anticoagulant activity, suggesting that it might have a therapeutic advantage over tPA and heparin. Encouraging results were obtained in a retrospective study of 19 patients with severe veno-occlusive disease and multiorgan dysfunction.[472] Treatment was begun a median of 6 days after diagnosis. Defibrotide was given intravenously in doses ranging from 5 to 60 mg/kg per day for 14 days, with resolution of veno-occlusive disease in 8 patients (42%). No significant treatment-related toxicities were observed. A larger prospective study is in progress.

A number of other agents have been explored for the treatment of veno-occlusive disease. Antithrombin-III (AT-III) concentrates have been used in patients with veno-occlusive disease who have documented deficiency of this plasma protein. In one report, 10 patients with severe veno-occlusive disease and AT-III levels less than 88 percent of normal were treated with AT-III, with clinical improvement observed in all patients 1 to 10 days after beginning therapy.[473]

Surgical approaches also have been explored for the treatment of severe veno-occlusive disease. Insertion of a transjugular intrahepatic portosystemic stent-shunt has been performed in small numbers of patients with veno-occlusive disease, with some patients having regression of the hepatic and renal symptoms.[474] Orthotopic liver transplantation has been successfully performed in selected patients with severe veno-occlusive disease[475]; however, the majority of patients are not capable of undergoing such a rigorous surgical procedure.

In the absence of specific effective therapy, efforts have been made to develop nontoxic prophylactic regimens to reduce the incidence and severity of veno-occlusive disease. Protocols using ursodeoxycholic acid and heparin appear promising. A pilot study and a subsequent randomized controlled trial demonstrated that ursodeoxycholic acid used prophylactically can reduce the incidence of veno-occlusive disease.[476,477] In the controlled study, 67 patients undergoing allogeneic hematopoietic cell transplantation were randomized to receive ursodeoxycholic acid or placebo *prior* to the preparative regimen of busulfan/cyclophosphamide. The incidence of veno-occlusive disease was significantly lower in patients randomized to receive ursodeoxycholic acid (15% versus 40%; p = 0.03).

The efficacy of a low-dose continuous infusion of heparin has been evaluated in a prospective randomized clinical trial of 161 patients who underwent allogeneic or autologous hematopoietic cell transplantation. Patients were randomized to either low-dose heparin (100 units/kg total dose per day by continuous intravenous infusion) or placebo. The infusion of heparin was initiated prior to the start of the preparative regimen and continued until 30 days after hematopoietic cell transplantation. A lower incidence of veno-occlusive disease was noted in the heparin-treated group (2.5% versus 13.7%; p < 0.01); this benefit was most pronounced in those undergoing allogeneic hematopoietic cell transplantation (0 versus 18%). There was no increase in bleeding risk or other toxicities in the patients treated with heparin.[478,479]

A second study of heparin prophylaxis in children also found a statistically significant reduction in veno-occlusive disease for patients who received heparin prophylaxis compared to a historic control group.[480] Another randomized trial did not confirm the benefit of heparin therapy; however, heparin was initiated on the day of stem-cell infusion, not at the beginning of the preparative regimen.[481] Other retrospective analyses have also not found benefit for the prophylactic use of heparin.[482]

Treatment with low-molecular-weight heparin was associated with a lower incidence of veno-occlusive disease in a pilot study of 61 patients undergoing BMT who were randomized to receive low-molecular-weight heparin (enaxaparin 40 mg/day) or placebo from prior to conditioning until day +40 posttransplant.[483]

PULMONARY COMPLICATIONS

Lung toxicity is a relatively common problem following either allogeneic or autologous hematopoietic cell transplantation. The causes of lung injury or interstitial pneumonitis can be infection (bacterial or viral, e.g., CMV), chemical (BCNU, or carmustine, being the most common), bleeding, or idiopathic. Interstitial pneumonitis occurs in 10 to 15 percent of patients, the etiology of which can often be difficult to discern.[484,485] Diagnostic bronchoscopy is usually required to rule out bacterial or viral (especially CMV) infection. Risk factors for developing interstitial pneumonitis include increasing age and prior history of lung irradiation.[486] Idiopathic interstitial pneumonitis is typically treated with corticosteroids. Pulmonary toxicity has been associated with carmustine in patients with solid tumors and can be fatal if not treated promptly with corticosteroids, generally with a daily dose of prednisone of 1 mg/kg with weekly taper.[487] Pulmonary function tests with carbon monoxide diffusion capacity measurements generally are required to confirm this diagnosis.

Diffuse alveolar hemorrhage is a clinical syndrome that generally occurs within the first 40 days following hematopoietic cell transplantation and is characterized by dyspnea, hypoxia, diffuse pulmonary infiltrates on chest x-ray, and progressive blood fluid on bronchoalveolar lavage. Diffuse alveolar hemorrhage has been reported in up to 20 percent of patients undergoing autologous hematopoietic cell transplantation, but the incidence varies significantly among transplant centers.[488] Prompt treatment with high-dose corticosteroids has been successful in this disorder, which otherwise carries a high mortality risk.[489]

OTHER COMPLICATIONS

Cardiac complications, which can often be life threatening, can occur following hematopoietic cell transplantation.[490,491] In one retrospective analysis of 170 patients, fatal cardiac toxicity, which could not be predicted with routine noninvasive cardiac evaluation, occurred in 2 percent of patients.[492] Use of high doses of cyclophosphamide has been implicated in some cases of cardiac dysfunction that have occurred early in the posttransplant setting.[493]

Neurologic complications occur infrequently in patients undergoing hematopoietic cell transplantation but occasionally can be severe and even life threatening. Infection and drug toxicity are the usual causes of neurologic complications in this setting. Cyclosporine has been associated with neurologic toxicity, which can vary from tremor to significant neurologic effects.[494,495] Ganciclovir also has been associated with neurologic toxicity.

Cystitis can occur following hematopoietic cell transplantation, usually as a consequence of high-dose cyclophosphamide. The BK strain of adenovirus has been found in the urine of some patients with hemorrhagic cystitis.[158]

Endocrine toxicity is a major concern, due to the high incidence of infertility and the generally young age of many patients who undergo hematopoietic cell transplantation. Sperm banking in men is an accept-

able solution and should be offered to all prospective patients. Successful pregnancies after allogeneic hematopoietic cell transplantation using embryos collected prior to the transplant have been reported; however, this approach is obviously far from ideal.[496]

Gynecologic abnormalities, such as atrophic vaginitis and problems related to ovarian failure, are commonly observed yet can be effectively reversed with estrogen administration.[497] Growth and developmental problems can occur in pediatric patients, with total-body irradiation being implicated as the likely causative agent.[498] Hypothyroidism is also occasionally observed and is readily correctable with thyroid replacement therapy.[499]

Cataracts occur in patients who receive total-body irradiation–based preparatory regimens.[62] Fractionation of the total-body irradiation reduces but does not eliminate this problem.[500]

Transplantation-associated thrombotic thrombocytopenic purpura and hemolytic uremic syndrome have occurred following both allogeneic and autologous hematopoietic cell transplantations.[501] Cyclosporine has been implicated in this disorder. Withdrawal of the drug and plasmapheresis have been used as treatment; however, this complication is associated with a significant mortality risk.

SECONDARY MALIGNANCIES

The success of transplantation has led to the unfortunate realization that patients who are long-term survivors are at increased risk for second malignancies. This is especially true in patients with severe aplastic anemia and Fanconi anemia, as discussed above, but has also been observed following hematopoietic cell transplantation for a variety of malignancies. For example, following autologous hematopoietic cell transplantation for lymphoma or Hodgkin's disease, the estimated risk of secondary MDS and AML at 5 years is 8 to 18 percent.[502–505] Occult cytogenetic abnormalities detected in the marrow prior to stem-cell collection may help identify patients at risk for this complication.[506] The chemotherapy administered to patients prior to hematopoietic cell transplantation has been implicated as a likely cause of MDS by the observation that patients with multiple myeloma who were exposed to prolonged alkylator therapy had a much higher risk of developing MDS following transplantation.[507] Secondary malignancies also occur following allogeneic hematopoietic cell transplantation. In one retrospective analysis of 557 patients, 9 patients developed 10 secondary cancers for a cumulative actuarial risk of 12 percent at 11 years after hematopoietic cell transplantation. The age-adjusted incidence of secondary cancer was 4.2 times higher than that expected from a similar population of individuals in the general population.[508] In another large retrospective analysis of 19,229 patients who underwent allogeneic or syngeneic hematopoietic cell transplantation, the risk of developing new solid cancers was 8.3 times higher at 10 years after transplantation than that for age-adjusted individuals.[509] Despite the higher risk, the cumulative incidence at 10 years was only 2.2 percent.

TREATMENT AND PREVENTION OF RELAPSE FOLLOWING TRANSPLANTATION

Relapse of the underlying disease is an unfortunate and ominous event following hematopoietic cell transplantation. Typically, patients who suffer a relapse do so within the first 2 years following transplantation. Once a patient relapses, the likelihood of curative therapy is very low. Many patients are able to tolerate and are capable of responding to chemotherapy or radiation therapy, which may result in prolonged survival, especially for those patients who relapse several years after the transplant procedure.[510] A number of novel therapies are under consideration in an effort to treat or preferentially prevent relapses. Second transplants have rarely been successful, due to toxicity and tumor resistance.[511–514]

A major goal is to harness the immune system to prevent and/or treat patients who develop recurrent disease. The rationale for utilizing immunotherapy following hematopoietic cell transplantation is based upon the demonstration of a graft-versus-tumor effect, the minimal residual disease state that most patients enter following hematopoietic cell transplantation, and the rapid advances in our understanding of basic tumor immunology. Both CTL and natural killer (NK) cells have been implicated in the graft-versus-tumor effect. The CTL recognize target cells through the appropriate expression of specific peptides in the context of major histocompatibility complex (MHC) molecules. In order for a productive interaction to occur, costimulation through the CD28-B7 system or other costimulatory molecules must occur or anergy develops.[515] The discovery of highly efficient antigen-presenting cells, termed dendritic cells, has opened an exciting new path of investigation (see Chap. 84).[516] The NK cells, in contrast, are inhibited by the appropriate expression of certain MHC class I molecules, and the lack of expression or altered peptide presentation results in the loss of a "no-kill" signal, which triggers lysis.[517] Upon appropriate engagement, both CTL and NK cells lyse target cells through the exocytosis of cytolytic granules that contain perforin and granzymes. Perforin induces pore formation in the membrane of the target cells. This allows for the introduction of granzymes, which induce apoptosis of the target cell.[518] In addition, CTL and NK cells express fas ligand (fasL), which can induce target-cell apoptosis through engagement of the fas receptor on the target cell.[519]

These insights into tumor cell recognition have identified a number of potential mechanisms by which tumor cells may evade immunological recognition. With respect to T-cell recognition, the lack of tumor-specific antigens or the down-regulation of HLA class I molecules could result in an inability of the T cells to recognize and respond to tumor cells. The lack of costimulatory molecules on the tumor cells may result in the development of anergy. In addition, a number of tumor cells have been found to express fasL, which could theoretically inactivate fas-expressing effector cells.[520,521] In addition, functional defects in T cells, the heterogeneity of human tumor cells, and the possibility of ongoing mutations add complexity to the potential application of immunotherapy. With respect to NK-cell–mediated attack, the appropriate expression of self-MHC class I molecules could inactivate host NK cells. In addition, soluble factors have been described that are capable of inhibiting NK cells in vitro.[522]

CLINICAL APPLICATION OF IMMUNOTHERAPY FOLLOWING HEMATOPOIETIC CELL TRANSPLANTATION

Following autologous transplantation it has been observed that IL-2 production is impaired. Yet, peripheral-blood lymphocytes isolated from patients retain the ability to respond to IL-2.[523,524] Phase I and II clinical trials with IL-2 with or without in vitro activated cells suggest a clinical impact of IL-2 therapy.[205,525–528] Another approach has been to combine IL-2 with interferon-α. This combination has had considerable toxicity. However, in one study of patients who underwent hematopoietic cell transplantation for lymphoma, 80 percent of the IL-2/interferon-α-treated patients were alive and free of disease at a median follow-up of 34 months, compared to 52.5 percent of historical control subjects after a median follow-up of 23 months (p < 0.01).[529] This approach is currently under evaluation in a randomized clinical trial. IL-2 therapy was not beneficial in a modest-sized randomized clinical trial following autologous hematopoietic cell transplantation for

ALL.[530] Other cytokines, such as IL-12 and IL-15, also are in the early stages of clinical development.

An alternative approach has been to utilize cellular immunotherapy to treat malignancies. For example, patients who have suffered a relapse following allogeneic hematopoietic cell transplantation have been treated with donor leukocyte infusions. Since the initial reports in the 1980s, a number of studies have documented that reinfusion of unmanipulated leukocytes derived from the HLA-matched donor can result in significant clinical responses in relapsed patients, especially those with CML.[18,20,531–533] Responses have also been noted in other diseases such as AML or multiple myeloma, but have been less effective in patients with ALL. Two large retrospective studies have highlighted both the promise and the problems associated with donor leukocyte infusion. In an analysis of results obtained from 135 patients treated at 27 transplant centers,[19] 73 percent of patients with relapsed CML were reinduced into a CR with donor leukocyte infusion. Patients with AML did not respond as well, with only five (29%) developing a CR. None of the ALL patients responded. Remissions were durable, with many of the patients continuing in complete hematologic and molecular remission for years. Donor leukocyte infusion treatment had considerable toxicity, with 42 percent of the patients developing clinically significant graft-versus-host disease and 34 percent of the patients developing myelosuppression. Seventeen (12.6%) of the patients died of causes other than their underlying malignancy. In a second large retrospective analysis of results from donor leukocyte infusion, a similar response rate of 60 percent among CML patients was observed.[288] As expected, responses were superior either for patients with only cytogenetic relapses or for patients treated with donor leukocyte infusion while in chronic phase, compared to patients who had progressed to either accelerated phase or blastic phase. Results were not favorable for patients with AML (15.4% CR) or ALL (18.2% CR). Again, complications included graft-versus-host disease (60%) and pancytopenia (18.6%).

Overall, these results confirm the favorable clinical results of donor leukocyte infusion, especially for patients with CML that have not progressed to an advanced stage. An interesting approach will be to study those patients who develop only molecular relapses, which have been shown to be predictive of eventual relapse, especially if persistently positive and found after 6 months from the transplant.[232] The use of donor leukocyte infusion in patients with relapsed acute leukemia has been less successful, possibly due to the more rapid proliferative capacity of the malignant cells, while donor leukocyte infusion reactions often take months for full benefit. Some investigators have advocated the use of chemotherapy to first "debulk" the disease prior to donor leukocyte infusion.

As discussed above, a major complication of donor leukocyte infusion is the risk of graft-versus-host disease. This is frequently manifested as chronic graft-versus-host disease. The development of graft-versus-host disease is further complicated by the difficulty of evaluating the appropriate time to intervene with treatment, since graft-versus-host disease has been related to leukemic response in most studies, although patients have clearly been identified who develop a graft-versus-leukemia response without graft-versus-host disease. One approach to limiting the risk of graft-versus-host disease has been to explore the dose of cells infused in an effort to find a dose that has effective antileukemic properties without causing significant graft-versus-host disease. In one study of CML patients who relapsed following a T-cell–depleted transplant, a dose of 1×10^7 CD3+ T cells/kg was defined that resulted in excellent efficacy without causing significant graft-versus-host disease.[534] However, it remains unclear whether this dose level also applies to patients who relapse following transplantation of a non–T-cell-depleted graft. Attempts have been made either to deplete CD8+ cells or to enrich for CD4+ cells in an effort to reduce the risk of graft-versus-host disease while retaining a graft-versus-leukemia effect.[535] Another approach to graft-versus-host disease after donor leukocyte infusion has been to modify the donor leukocytes so that they are susceptible to certain drug treatments that allow for their eradication if graft-versus-host disease develops.[536] The major complication observed following donor leukocyte infusion has been myelosuppression and, in some instances, aplasia, which has been encountered primarily in patients who had no evidence of donor hematopoiesis at the time of donor leukocyte infusion treatment.[537]

Excellent results have also been obtained with interferon-α in patients with CML who have relapsed following allogeneic hematopoietic cell transplantation, especially when patients are treated early following a relapse at a time of only cytogenetic relapse.[538,539] Whether such patients will benefit from donor leukocyte infusion remains to be evaluated.

The specificity of CTL for tumor cells has made isolating cells with antitumor activity an attractive clinical goal. The potential clinical efficacy of CTL has been demonstrated in pilot studies directed against defined viral antigens, such as CMV and Epstein-Barr virus.[146,540–542] Whether these results can be extended to patients with malignancies where there are not clearly defined antigens remains to be determined. Tumor-specific HLA-restricted CTL have developed against metastatic breast cancer and leukemic cells.[543–545]

Another approach has been to expand T cells termed cytokine-induced killer cells, which share functional and phenotypic properties with NK cells.[546,547] Cytokine-induced killer cells have been shown to have in vivo activity in animal model systems, and clinical trials are underway.[268,548]

The successful isolation and expansion of professional antigen-presenting cells, such as dendritic cells, which express all of the molecules required for a productive immunological reaction, has generated considerable interest. The in vivo application of dendritic cells with defined experimental antigens has been explored in murine model systems with clear efficacy. Early clinical trials have been performed in which dendritic cells were pulsed with idiotype proteins in patients with follicular lymphomas and multiple myeloma.[378,549] Antitumor cellular responses have been observed in vitro, with clinical responses noted in some patients. Despite the obvious appeal of dendritic-cell–mediated immunotherapy, technical and theoretical problems need to be addressed. These include the requirement for cell culturing, individualized therapy, and HLA restriction of the peptide antigens. The optimal approach to dendritic-cell–based immunotherapy remains to be established. Issues that require optimization include the choice of dendritic cells, method of expansion and activation, source of antigen (peptide, whole protein, tumor cell extract, or genetic transfection), and the immunological competence of the recipient.[550]

Immunomodulation therapies have also been explored in the post-hematopoietic cell transplantation setting. Following withdrawal of cyclosporine, animals develop a syndrome similar to graft-versus-host disease.[551] This strategy of inducing autologous graft-versus-host disease has been extended to clinical trials, where a reduction in relapse rate and an event-free survival benefit was observed in patients with lymphoma who were treated with cyclosporine compared to historical control subjects.[552] Additional studies have been performed in patients with breast cancer treated with cyclosporine in combination with interferon-α.[553]

Monoclonal antibodies are also attractive reagents for immunotherapy due to their high degree of specificity. Humanized anti-CD20 MoAb has been used to treat patients with relapsed lymphoma.[554] Clinical trials using the anti-CD20 MoAb and anti-Her2/Neu MoAb are underway in patients with lymphoma and breast cancer, respectively. Bispecific antibodies that couple tumor-cell markers with T cells also may be useful in the clinic in the future.[555]

QUALITY OF LIFE

The success of hematopoietic cell transplantation has resulted in long-term survival of a rapidly rising number of patients, bringing issues of quality of life to the forefront. A number of studies have evaluated the quality of life of hematopoietic cell transplantation survivors. The first study examining survivors of allogeneic hematopoietic cell transplantation revealed that the majority of individuals were employed and in good health, with acceptable objective and subjective levels of functioning. However, a minority of individuals (10–15%) had evidence of psychosocial stress.[556] Another study revealed mild to moderate cognitive dysfunction among patients who received total-body irradiation as part of the preparative regimen.[557] Other reports have confirmed that the quality of life of long-term survivors of allogeneic hematopoietic cell transplantation is generally excellent, with more than 90 percent of patients having Karnofsky performance scores of 80 percent or higher.[558,559] The major limitations in quality of life were generally associated with chronic graft-versus-host disease.[560] Similar results were obtained for patients who survive for more than 5 years after allogeneic hematopoietic cell transplantation, in whom 93 percent of patients were in good health and 89 percent had returned to full-time work or school.[561] Quality of life of patients following autologous hematopoietic cell transplantation is generally excellent. In one study at 1 year after hematopoietic cell transplantation, 88 percent of patients who were surveyed reported a quality of life of above average or excellent, and 78 percent were employed.[562]

REFERENCES

1. Osgood EE, Riddle MC, Mathew TJ: Aplastic anemia treated with daily transfusions and intravenous marrow: Case report. *Ann Intern Med* 13:357, 1939.
2. Jacobson LO, Marks EK, Robson MJ, et al: Effect of spleen protection on mortality following X-irradiation. *J Lab Clin Med* 34:1538, 1949.
3. Lorenz E, Uphoff D, Reid TR, Shelton E: Modification of irradiation injury in mice and guinea pigs by bone marrow injections. *J Natl Cancer Inst* 12:157, 1951.
4. Thomas ED, Lochte HL, Lu WC, Ferrebee JW: Intravenous infusion of bone marrow in patients receiving radiation and chemotherapy. *N Engl J Med* 257:491, 1957.
5. Mathe G, Amiel JL, Schwarzenberg L, et al: Successful allogeneic bone marrow transplantation in man: Chimerism, induced specific tolerance and possible anti-leukemic effects. *Blood* 25:179, 1965.
6. Storb R, Epstein RB, Graham TC, et al: Methotrexate regimens for control of graft-versus-host disease in dogs with allogeneic marrow grafts. *Transplantation* 9:240, 1970.
7. Gatti RA, Meuwissen HJ, Allen HD, Hong R, Good RA: Immunological reconstitution of sex-linked lymphopenic immunological deficiency. *Lancet* 2:1366, 1968.
8. Hong R, Cooper MD, Allan MJ, et al: Immunological restitution in lymphopenic immunological deficiency syndrome. *Lancet* 1:503, 1968.
9. Bach FH, Albertini RJ, Joo P, Anderson JL, Bortin MM: Bone-marrow transplantation in a patient with the Wiskott-Aldrich syndrome. *Lancet* 2:1364, 1968.
10. Fefer A, Cheever MA, Greenberg PD, et al: Treatment of chronic granulocytic leukemia with chemoradiotherapy and transplantation of marrow from identical twins. *N Engl J Med* 306:63, 1982.
11. Buckner CD, Epstein RB, Rudolph RH, et al: Allogeneic marrow engraftment following whole body irradiation in a patient with leukemia. *Blood* 35:741, 1970.
12. Santos GW, Sensenbrenner LL, Burke PJ, et al: Allogeneic marrow grafts in man using cyclophosphamide. *Transplant Proc* 6:345, 1974.
13. Thomas ED, Storb R, Clift RA, et al: Bone-marrow transplantation. *N Engl J Med* 292:832, 895, 1975.
14. O'Reilly RJ: Allogenic bone marrow transplantation: Current status and future directions. *Blood* 62:941, 1983.
15. Martin PJ, Hansen JA, Buckner CD, et al: Effects of in vitro depletion of T cells in HLA-identical allogeneic marrow grafts. *Blood* 66:664, 1985.
16. Weiden PL, Flournoy N, Thomas ED, et al: Antileukemic effect of graft-

versus-host disease in human recipients of allogeneic-marrow grafts. *N Engl J Med* 300:1068, 1979.

17. Sullivan KM, Weiden PL, Storb R, et al: Influence of acute and chronic graft-versus-host disease on relapse and survival after bone marrow transplantation from HLA-identical siblings as treatment of acute and chronic leukemia. *Blood* 73:1720, 1989.

18. Kolb HJ, Mittermuller J, Clemm CH, et al: Donor leukocyte transfusions for treatment of recurrent chronic myelogenous leukemia in marrow transplant patients. *Blood* 76:2462, 1990.

19. Kolb HJ, Schattenberg A, Goldman JM, et al: Graft-versus-leukemia effect of donor lymphocyte transfusions in marrow grafted patients. *Blood* 86:2041, 1995.

20. Collins RH Jr, Pineiro LA, Nemunaitis JJ, et al: Transfusion of donor buffy coat cells in the treatment of persistent or recurrent malignancy after allogeneic bone marrow transplantation. *Transfusion* 35:891, 1995.

21. Spangrude GJ, Heimfeld S, Weissman IL: Purification and characterization of mouse hematopoietic stem cells. *Science* 241:58, 1988.

22. Baum CM, Weissman IL, Tsukamoto AS, Buckle AM, Peault B: Isolation of a candidate human hematopoietic stem-cell population. *Proc Natl Acad Sci USA* 89:2804, 1992.

23. Craig W, Kay R, Cutler RL, Lansdorp PM: Expression of thy-1 on human hematopoietic progenitor cells. *J Exp Med* 177:1331, 1993.

24. Brandt J, Baird N, Lu L, Srour E, Hoffman R: Characterization of a human hemopoietic progenitor cell capable of blast cell containing colonies in vitro. *J Clin Invest* 82:1017, 1988.

25. Uchida N, Combs J, Chen S, et al: Primitive human hematopoietic cells displaying differential efflux of the rhodamine-123 dye have distinct biological activities. *Blood* 88:1297, 1996.

26. Goodell MA, Rosenzweig M, Kim H, et al: Dye efflux studies suggest that hematopoietic stem cells expressing low or undetectable levels of CD34 antigen exist in multiple species. *Nature Med* 3:1337, 1997.

27. Berenson RJ, Andrews RG, Bensinger WI, et al: Antigen CD34+ marrow cells engraft lethally irradiated baboons. *J Clin Invest* 81:951, 1988.

28. Negrin RS, Atkinson KA, Leemhuis T, et al: Transplantation of highly purified CD34+Thy-1+ hematopoietic stem cells in patients with metastatic breast cancer. *Biol Blood Marrow Transplant* 6:262, 2000.

29. Thomas ED, Storb R: Technique for human marrow grafting. *Blood* 36:507, 1970.

30. Buckner CD, Clift RA, Sanders JE, et al: Marrow harvesting from normal donors. *Blood* 64:630, 1984.

31. Jin NR, Hill RS, Feterson FB, et al: Marrow harvesting for autologous marrow transplantation. *Exp Hematol* 13:879, 1985.

32. Stroncek DF, Holland PV, Bartch G, et al: Experiences of the first 493 unrelated marrow donors in the National Marrow Donor Program. *Blood* 81:1940, 1993.

33. Siena S, Bregni M, Brando B, et al: Circulation of CD34+ hematopoietic progenitor cells in the peripheral blood of high-dose cyclophosphamide-treated patients: Enhancement by intravenous human granulocyte-macrophage colony-stimulating factor. *Blood* 74:1905, 1989.

34. Socinski MA, Elias A, Schnipper L, et al: Granulocyte-macrophage colony stimulating factor expands the circulating haematopoietic progenitor cell compartment in man. *Lancet* 1:1194, 1988.

35. Chao NJ, Schriber JR, Grimes K, et al: Granulocyte colony-stimulating factor "mobilized" peripheral blood progenitor cells accelerate granulocyte and platelet recovery after high-dose chemotherapy. *Blood* 81:2031, 1993.

36. Bensinger WI, Longin K, Appelbaum F, et al: Peripheral blood stem cells (PBSCs) collected after recombinant granulocyte colony stimulating factor (rhG-CSF): An analysis of factors correlating with the tempo of engraftment after transplantation. *Br J Haematol* 87:825, 1994.

37. Tricot G, Jagannath S, Vesole D, et al: Peripheral blood stem cell transplants for multiple myeloma: Identification of favorable variables for rapid engraftment in 225 patients. *Blood* 85:588, 1995.

38. Glaspy JA, Shpall EJ, LeMaistre CF, et al: Peripheral blood progenitor cell mobilization using stem cell factor in combination with filgrastim in breast cancer patients. *Blood* 90:2939, 1997.

39. Lyman SD: Biologic effects and potential clinical applications of Flt3 ligand. *Current Opin Hematol* 5:192, 1998.

40. Schmitz N, Bacigalupo A, Labopin M, et al: Transplantation of peripheral blood progenitor cells from HLA-identical sibling donors: European Group for Blood and Marrow Transplantation (EBMT). *Br J Haematol* 95:715, 1996.

41. Shpall EJ, Champlin R, Glaspy JA: Effect of CD34+ peripheral blood progenitor cell dose on hematopoietic recovery. *Biol Blood Marrow Transplant* 4:84, 1998.

42. Weaver CH, Birch R, Greco FA, et al: Mobilization and harvesting of peripheral blood stem cells: Randomized evaluations of different doses of filgrastim. *Br J Haematol* 100:338, 1998.

43. Shpall EJ, LeMaistre CF, Holland K, et al: A prospective randomized trial of buffy coat versus CD34-selected autologous bone marrow support in high-risk breast cancer patients receiving high-dose chemotherapy. *Blood* 90:4313, 1997.

44. Gribben JG, Neuberg D, Barber M, et al: Detection of residual lymphoma cells by polymerase chain reaction in peripheral blood is significantly less predictive for relapse than detection in bone marrow. *Blood* 83:3800, 1994.

45. Negrin RS, Pesando J: Detection of tumor cells in purged bone marrow and peripheral blood mononuclear cells by polymerase chain reaction amplification of bcl-2 translocations. *J Clin Oncol* 12:1021, 1994.

46. Leonard BM, Hetu F, Busque L, et al: Lymphoma cell burden in progenitor cell grafts measured by competitive polymerase chain reaction: Less than one log difference between bone marrow and peripheral blood sources. *Blood* 91:331, 1998.

47. Bensinger WI, Weaver CH, Appelbaum FR, et al: Transplantation of allogeneic peripheral blood stem cells mobilized by recombinant human granulocyte colony-stimulating factor. *Blood* 85:1655, 1995.

48. Korbling M, Przepiorka D, Huh YO, et al: Allogeneic blood stem cell transplantation for refractory leukemia and lymphoma: Potential advantage of blood over marrow grafts. *Blood* 85:1659, 1995.

49. Storek J, Gooley T, Siadek M, et al: Allogeneic peripheral blood stem cell transplantation may be associated with a high risk of chronic graft-versus-host disease. *Blood* 90:4705, 1997.

50. Pan L, Delmonte J Jr, Jalonen CK, Ferrara JL: Pretreatment of donor mice with granulocyte colony-stimulating factor polarizes donor T lymphocytes toward type-2 cytokine production and reduces severity of experimental graft-versus-host disease. *Blood* 86:4422, 1995.

51. Gluckman E, Rocha V, Boyer-Chammard A, et al: Outcome of cord-blood transplantation from related and unrelated donors: Eurocord Transplant Group and the European Blood and Marrow Transplantation Group. *N Engl J Med* 337:373, 1997.

52. Goulmy E, Schipper R, Pool J, et al: Mismatches of minor histocompatibility antigens between HLA-identical donors and recipients and the development of graft-versus-host disease after bone marrow transplantation. *N Engl J Med* 334:281, 1996.

53. Anasetti C, Amos D, Beatty PG, et al: Effect of HLA compatibility on engraftment of bone marrow transplants in patients with leukemia or lymphoma. *N Engl J Med* 320:197, 1989.

54. Kernan NA, Bartsch G, Ash RC, et al: Analysis of 462 transplantations from unrelated donors facilitated by the National Marrow Donor Program. *N Engl J Med* 328:593, 1993.

55. Petersdorf EW, Longton GM, Anasetti C, et al: The significance of HLA-DRB1 matching on clinical outcome after HLA-A, B, DR identical unrelated donor marrow transplantation. *Blood* 86:1606, 1995.

56. Hansen JA, Gooley TA, Martin PJ, et al: Bone marrow transplants from unrelated donors for patients with chronic myeloid leukemia. *N Engl J Med* 338:962, 1998.

57. Prasad VK, Kernan NA, Heller G, O'Reilly RJ, Yang SY: DNA typing for HLA-A and HLA-B identifies disparities between patients and unrelated donors matched by HLA-A and HLA-B serology and HLA-DRB1. *Blood* 93:399, 1999.

58. Sasazuki T, Juji T, Morishima Y, et al: Effect of matching of class I HLA alleles on clinical outcome after transplantation of hematopoietic stem cells from an unrelated donor. Japan Marrow Donor Program. *N Engl J Med* 339:1177, 1998.

59. Rubinstein P, Carrier C, Scaradavou A, et al: Outcomes among 562 recipients of placental-blood transplants from unrelated donors. *N Engl J Med* 339:1565, 1998.

60. Henslee-Downey PJ, Abhyankar SH, Parrish RS, et al: Use of partially mismatched related donors extends access to allogeneic marrow transplant. *Blood* 89:3864, 1997.

61. Aversa F, Tabilio A, Velardi A, et al: Transplantation for high-risk acute leukemia with high doses of T-cell-depleted hematopoietic stem cells from full-haplotype incompatible donors. *N Engl J Med* 339:1186, 1998.

62. Deeg HJ, Flournoy N, Sullivan KM, et al: Cataracts after total body

irradiation and marrow transplantation: A sparing effect of dose fractionation. *Int J Radiat Oncol Biol Phys* 10:957, 1984.

63. Clift RA, Buckner CD, Appelbaum FR, et al: Allogeneic marrow transplantation in patients with acute myeloid leukemia in first remission: A randomized trial of two irradiation regimens. *Blood* 76:1867, 1990.

64. Clift RA, Buckner CD, Appelbaum FR, et al: Allogeneic marrow transplantation in patients with chronic myeloid leukemia in the chronic phase: A randomized trial of two irradiation regimens. *Blood* 77:1660, 1991.

65. Thomas ED, Buckner CD, Banaji M, et al: One hundred patients with acute leukemia treated by chemotherapy, total body irradiation, and allogeneic marrow transplantation. *Blood* 49:511, 1977.

66. Blume KG, Forman SJ, O'Donnell MR, et al: Total body irradiation and high-dose etoposide: A new preparatory regimen for bone marrow transplantation in patients with advanced hematologic malignancies. *Blood* 69:1015, 1987.

67. Horning SJ, Negrin RS, Chao NJ, et al: Fractionated total-body irradiation, etoposide, and cyclophosphamide plus autografting in Hodgkin's disease and non-Hodgkin's lymphoma. *J Clin Oncol* 12:2552, 1994.

68. Weaver CH, Petersen FB, Appelbaum FR, et al: High-dose fractionated total-body irradiation, etoposide, and cyclophosphamide followed by autologous stem-cell support in patients with malignant lymphoma. *J Clin Oncol* 12:2559, 1994.

69. Long GD, Amylon MD, Stockerl-Goldstein KE, et al: Fractionated total-body irradiation, etoposide and cyclophosphamide followed by allogeneic bone marrow transplantation for patients with high-risk or advanced-stage hematological malignancies. *Biol Blood Marrow Transplant* 3:324, 1997.

70. Tutschka PJ, Copelan EA, Klein JP: Bone marrow transplantation for leukemia following a new busulfan and cyclophosphamide regimen. *Blood* 70:1382, 1987.

71. Clift RA, Buckner CD, Thomas ED, et al: Marrow transplantation for chronic myeloid leukemia: A randomized study comparing cyclophosphamide and total body irradiation with busulfan and cyclophosphamide. *Blood* 84:2036, 1994.

72. Ringden O, Remberger M, Ruutu T, et al: Increased risk of chronic graft-versus-host disease, obstructive bronchiolitis and alopecia with busulfan versus total body irradiation: Long term results of a randomized trial in allogeneic marrow recipients with leukemia. *Blood* 93:1, 1999.

73. Blume KG, Kopecky KJ, Henslee-Downey JP, et al: A prospective randomized comparison of total body irradiation-etoposide versus busulfan-cyclophosphamide as preparatory regimens for bone marrow transplantation in patients with leukemia who were not in first remission: A Southwest Oncology Group study. *Blood* 81:2187, 1993.

74. Linker CA, Ries CA, Damon LE, et al: Autologous bone marrow transplantation for acute myeloid leukemia using bulsulfan plus etoposide as a preparative regimen. *Blood* 81:311, 1993.

75. Chao NJ, Stein AS, Long GD, et al: Busulfan/etoposide: Initial experience with a new preparatory regimen for autologous bone marrow transplantation in patients with acute nonlymphoblastic leukemia. *Blood* 81:319, 1993.

76. Linker CA, Ries CA, Damon LE, Rugo HS, Wolf JL: Autologous bone marrow transplantation for acute myeloid leukemia using 4-hydroperoxycyclophosphamide-purged bone marrow and the busulfan/etoposide preparative regimen: A follow-up report. *Bone Marrow Transplant* 22:865, 1998.

77. Reece DE, Barnett MJ, Connors JM, et al: Intensive chemotherapy with cyclophosphamide, carmustine, and etoposide followed by autologous bone marrow transplantation for relapsed Hodgkin's disease. *J Clin Oncol* 10:1871, 1991.

78. Wheeler C, Antin JH, Churchill WH, et al: Cyclophosphamide, carmustine, and etoposide with autologous bone marrow transplantation in refractory Hodgkin's disease and non-Hodgkin's lymphoma: A dose-finding study. *J Clin Oncol* 8:648, 1990.

79. Gaspard MH, Maraninchi D, Stoppa AM, et al: Intensive chemotherapy with high doses of BCNU, etoposide, cytosine arabinoside, and melphalan (BEAM) followed by autologous bone marrow transplantation: Toxicity and antitumor activity in 26 patients with poor-risk malignancies. *Cancer Chemother Pharmacol* 22:256, 1988.

80. Peters WP, Ross M, Vredenburgh JJ, et al: High-dose chemotherapy and autologous bone marrow support as consolidation after standard-

dose adjuvant therapy for high-risk primary breast cancer. *J Clin Oncol* 11:1132, 1993.

81. Shea TC, Mason JR, Storniolo AM, et al: Sequential cycles of high-dose carboplatin administered with recombinant human granulocyte-macrophage colony-stimulating factor and repeated infusions of autologous peripheral-blood progenitor cells: A novel and effective method for delivering multiple courses of dose-intensive therapy. *J Clin Oncol* 10:464, 1992.

82. Crown J, Kritz A, Vahdat L, et al: Rapid administration of multiple cycle of high-dose myelosuppressive chemotherapy in patients with metastatic breast cancer. *J Clin Oncol* 11:1144, 1993.

83. Long GD, Negrin RS, Hoyle CF, et al: Multiple cycles of high dose chemotherapy supported by hematopoietic progenitor cells as treatment for patients with advanced malignancies. *Cancer* 76:860, 1995.

84. Attal M, Harousseau JL: Standard therapy versus autologous transplantation in multiple myeloma. *Hematol Oncol Clin North Am* 11:133, 1997.

85. Appelbaum FR, Matthews DC, Eary JF, et al: The use of radiolabeled anti-CD33 antibody to augment marrow irradiation prior to marrow transplantation for acute myelogenous leukemia. *Transplantation* 54:829, 1992.

86. Matthews DC, Appelbaum FR, Eary JF, et al: Development of a marrow transplant regimen for acute leukemia using targeted hematopoietic irradiation delivered by ^{131}I-labeled anti-CD45 antibody, combined with cyclophosphamide and total body irradiation. *Blood* 85:1122, 1995.

87. Slavin S, Nagler A, Naparstek E, et al: Nonmyeloablative stem cell transplantation and cell therapy as an alternative to conventional bone marrow transplantation with lethal cytoreduction for the treatment of malignant and nonmalignant hematologic diseases. *Blood* 91:756, 1998.

88. Khouri IF, Keating M, Körbling M, et al: Transplant-lite: Induction of graft-versus-malignancy using fludarabine-based nonablative chemotherapy and allogeneic blood progenitor-cell transplantation as treatment for lymphoid malignancies. *J Clin Oncol* 16:2817, 1998.

89. McSweeney PA, Storb R: Mixed chimerism: preclinical studies and clinical applications. *Biol Blood Marrow Transplant* 5:192, 1999.

90. Sniecinski IJ, Oien L, Petz L, Blume KG: Immunohematologic consequences of major ABO-mismatched bone marrow transplantation. *Transplantation* 45:530, 1988.

91. Bensinger WI, Buckner CD, Clift RA, et al: Comparison of techniques for dealing with major ABO-incompatible marrow transplants. *Transplant Proc* 19:4605, 1987.

92. Hows J, Beddow K, Gordon-Smith E, et al: Donor-derived red blood cell antibodies and immune hemolysis after allogeneic bone marrow transplantation. *Blood* 67:177, 1986.

93. Crawford SW, Schwartz DA, Petersen FB, Clark JG: Mechanical ventilation after marrow transplantation: Risk factors and clinical outcome. *Am Rev Respir Dis* 137:682, 1988.

94. Yeager AM, Kaizer H, Santos GW, et al: Autologous bone marrow transplantation in patients with acute nonlymphocytic leukemia using ex vivo marrow treatment with 4-hydroperoxycyclophosphamide. *N Engl Med* 315:141, 1986.

95. Gorin NC, Aegerter P, Auvert B, et al: Autologous bone marrow transplantation for acute myelocytic leukemia in first remission: A European survey of the role of marrow purging. *Blood* 75:1606, 1990.

96. Rowley SD, Jones RJ, Piantadosi S, et al: Efficacy of ex vivo purging for autologous bone marrow transplantation in the treatment of acute nonlymphoblastic leukemia. *Blood* 74:501, 1989.

97. Negrin RS, Kiem HP, Schmidt-Wolf IG, Blume KG, Cleary ML: Use of the polymerase chain reaction to monitor the effectiveness of ex vivo tumor cell purging. *Blood* 77:654, 1991.

98. Gribben JG, Freedman AS, Neuberg D, et al: Immunologic purging of marrow assessed by PCR before autologous bone marrow transplanation for B-cell lymphoma. *N Engl J Med* 325:1525, 1991.

99. Brenner MK, Rill DR, Moen RC, et al: Gene-marking to trace origin of relapse after autologous bone marrow transplantation. *Lancet* 341:85, 1993.

100. Deisseroth AB, Zu Z, Claxton D, et al: Genetic marking shows that Ph+ cells present in autologous transplants of chronic myelogenous leukemia (CML) contribute to relapse after autologous bone marrow in CML. *Blood* 83:3068, 1994.

101. Shpall EJ, Bast RC Jr, Joines WT, et al: Immunomagnetic purging of breast cancer from bone marrow for autologous transplantation. *Bone Marrow Transplant* 7:145, 1991.

102. Voso MT, Hohaus S, Moos M, Haas R: Lack of t(14;18) polymerase chain reaction-positive cells in highly purified CD34+ cells and their CD19 subsets in patients with follicular lymphoma. *Blood* 89:3763, 1997.

103. Negrin RS, Kusnierz-Glaz CR, Still BJ, et al: Transplantation of enriched and purged peripheral blood progenitor cells from a single apheresis product in patients with non-Hodgkin's lymphoma. *Blood* 85:3334, 1995.

104. Bertolini F, Thomas T, Battaglia M, et al: A new "two step" procedure for 4.5 log depletion of T and B cells in allogeneic transplantation and of neoplastic cells in autologous transplantation. *Bone Marrow Transplant* 19:615, 1997.

105. Rambaldi A, Borleri G, Dotti G, et al: Innovative two-step negative selection of granulocyte colony-stimulating factor-mobilized circulating progenitor cells: Adequacy for autologous and allogeneic transplantation. *Blood* 91:2189, 1998.

106. Gazitt Y, Reading CC, Hoffman R, et al: Purified CD34+Lin-Thy+ stem cells do not contain clonal myeloma cells. *Blood* 86:381, 1995.

107. Nemunaitis J, Rabinowe SN, Singer JW, et al: Recombinant granulocyte-macrophage colony-stimulating factor after autologous bone marrow transplantation for lymphoid cancer. *N Engl J Med* 324:1773, 1988.

108. Link H, Boogaerts MA, Carella AM, et al: A controlled trial of recombinant human granulocyte-macrophage colony-stimulating factor after total body irradiation, high dose chemotherapy, and autologous bone marrow transplantation for acute lymphoblastic leukemia or malignant lymphoma. *Blood* 80:2188, 1992.

109. Advani R, Chao NJ, Horning SJ, et al: Granulocyte-macrophage colony stimulation factor (GM-CSF) as an adjunct to autologous hemopoietic stem cell transplantation for lymphoma. *Ann Intern Med* 116:183, 1992.

110. Gorin NC, Coiffier B, Hayat M, et al: Recombinant human granulocyte-macrophage colony-stimulating factor after high-dose chemotherapy and autologous bone marrow transplantation with unpurged and purged marrow in non-Hodgkin's lymphoma: A double blind placebo-controlled trial. *Blood* 80:1149, 1992.

111. Gulati SC, Bennett CL: Granulocyte-macrophage colony-stimulating factor (GM-CSF) as adjunct therapy in relapsed Hodgkin's disease. *Ann Intern Med* 116:177, 1992.

112. Sheridan WP, Begley CG, Juttner CA, et al: Effect of peripheral-blood progenitor cells mobilised by filgrastim (G-CSF) on platelet recovery after high-dose chemotherapy. *Lancet* 339:640, 1992.

113. Schmitz N, Linch DC, Dreger P, et al: Randomized trial of filgrastim-mobilised peripheral blood progenitor cell transplantation versus autologous bone-marrow transplantation in lymphoma patients. *Lancet* 347:353, 1996.

114. Smith TJ, Hillner BE, Schmitz N, et al: Economic analysis of a randomized clinical trial to compare filgrastim-mobilized peripheral-blood progenitor-cell transplantation and autologous bone marrow transplantation in patients with Hodgkin's and non-Hodgkin's lymphoma. *J Clin Oncol* 15:5, 1997.

115. Powles R, Smith C, Milan S, et al: Human recombinant GM-CSF in allogeneic bone-marrow transplantation for leukaemia: double-blind, placebo-controlled trial. *Lancet* 336:1417, 1990.

116. Spitzer G, Adkins DR, Spencer V, et al: Randomized study of growth factors post-peripheral-blood stem-cell transplant: Neutrophil recovery is improved with modest clinical benefit. *J Clin Oncol* 12:661, 1994.

117. Suzue T, Takaue Y, Watanabe A, et al: Effects of rhG-CSF (filgrastim) on the recovery of hematopoiesis after high-dose chemotherapy and autologous peripheral blood stem cell transplantation in children: A report from the Children's Cancer and Leukemia Study Group of Japan. *Exp Hematol* 22:1197, 1994.

118. Beguin Y, Clemons GK, Oris R, Fillet G: Circulating erythropoietin levels after bone marrow transplantation: Inappropriate response to anemia in allogeneic transplants. *Blood* 77:868, 1991.

119. Chao NJ, Schriber JR, Long GD, et al: A randomized study of erythropoietin and granulocyte colony-stimulating factor (G-CSF) versus placebo and G-CSF for patients with Hodgkin's and non-Hodgkin's lymphoma undergoing autologous bone marrow transplantation. *Blood* 83:2823, 1994.

120. Vannucchi AM, Bosi A, Ieri A, et al: Combination therapy with G-CSF and erythropoietin after autologous bone marrow transplantation for lymphoid malignancies: A randomized trial. *Bone Marrow Transplant* 17:527, 1996.

121. Steegmann JL, Lopez J, Otero MJ, et al: Erythropoietin treatment in allogeneic BMT accelerates erythroid reconstitution: Results of a prospective controlled randomized trial. *Bone Marrow Transplant* 10:541, 1992.

122. Klaesson S, Ringden O, Ljungman P, Lonnqvist B, Wennberg L: Reduced blood transfusion requirements after allogeneic bone marrow transplantation: Results of a randomised, double-blind study of high-dose erythropoietin. *Bone Marrow Transplant* 13:397, 1994.

123. Biggs JC, Atkinson KA, Booker V, et al: Prospective randomized double-blind trial of the in vivo use of recombinant human erythropoietin in bone marrow transplantation from HLA-sibling donors: The Australian Bone Marrow Transplant Study Group. *Bone Marrow Transplant* 15:129, 1995.

124. Schmidt GM, Blume KG, Bross KJ, et al: Parenteral nutrition in bone marrow transplant recipients. *Exp Hematol* 8:506, 1980.

125. Weisdorf SA, Lysne J, Wind D, et al: Positive effect of prophylactic total parenteral nutrition on long-term outcome of bone marrow transplantation. *Transplantation* 43:833, 1987.

126. Charuhas P, Fosberg K, Bruemmer B, et al: A double-blind randomized trial comparing outpatient parenteral nutrition with intravenous hydration: Effect on resumption of oral intake after marrow transplantation. *J Patenteral Enteral Nutr* 21:157, 1997.

127. Ziegler TR, Young LS, Benfell K, et al: Clinical and metabolic efficacy of glutamine-supplemented parenteral nutrition after bone marrow transplantation. *Ann Intern Med* 116:821, 1992.

128. Coghlin-Dickson T, Wong R, Negrin RS, et al: Effect of oral glutamine supplementation during bone marrow transplantation. *J Parenter Enteral Nutri* 24:61, 2000.

129. Playford RJ, Marchbank T, Mandir N, et al: Effects of keratinocyte growth factor (KGF) on gut growth and repair. *J Pathol* 184:316, 1998.

130. Farrell CL, Bready JV, Rex KL, et al: Keratinocyte growth factor protects mice from chemotherapy and radiation-induced gastrointestinal injury and mortality. *Cancer Res* 58:933, 1998.

131. Van der Meer JWM, Guiot HFL, van den Broek PJ, et al: Infections in bone marrow transplant recipients. *Semin Hematol* 21:123, 1984.

132. Momin F, Chandrasekar P: Antimicrobial prophylaxis in bone marrow transplantation. *Ann Intern Med* 123:205, 1995.

133. Villablanca JG, Steiner M, Kersey J, et al: The clinical spectrum of infections with *viridans* streptococci in bone marrow transplant patients. *Bone Marrow Transplant* 6:387, 1990.

134. Sullivan KM, Kopecky KJ, Jocom J, et al: Immunomodulatory and antimicrobial efficacy of intravenous immunoglobulin in bone marrow transplantion. *N Engl J Med* 323:705, 1990.

135. Sullivan KM, Storek J, Kopecky KJ, et al: A controlled trial of long-term administration of intravenous immunoglobulin to prevent late infection and chronic graft-vs.-host disease after marrow transplantation: Clinical outcome and effect on subsequent immune recovery. *Biol Blood Marrow Transplant* 2:44, 1996.

136. Riley D, Galgiani J, O'Donnell M, et al: Coccidioidomycosis in bone marrow transplant recipients. *Transplantation* 56:1531, 1993.

137. Rousey SR, Russler S, Gottlieb M, et al: Low-dose amphotericin B prophylaxis against invasive aspergillus infections in allogeneic marrow transplantation. *Am J Med* 91:484, 1991.

138. O'Donnell M, Schmidt GM, Tegtmeier BR, et al: Prediction of systemic fungal infection in allogeneic marrow recipients: Impact of amphotericin prophylaxis in high-risk patients. *J Clin Oncol* 12:827, 1994.

139. Wingard JR: Fungal infections after bone marrow transplant. *Biol Blood Marrow Transplant* 5:55, 1999.

140. Goodman JL, Winston DJ, Greenfield RA, et al: A controlled trial of fluconazole to prevent fungal infections in patients undergoing bone marrow transplantation. *N Engl J Med* 326:845, 1992.

141. Zaia JA: Epidemiology and pathogenesis of cytomegalovirus disease. *Semin Hematol* 27:5, 1990.

142. Bowden RA, Sayers M, Flournoy N, et al: Cytomegalovirus immune-globulin and seronegative blood products to prevent primary cytomegalovirus infection after marrow transplantation. *N Engl J Med* 314:1006, 1986.

143. Schmidt GM, Horak DA, Niland JC, et al: A randomized, controlled trial of prophylactic ganciclovir for cytomegalovirus pulmonary infection in recipients of allogeneic bone marrow transplants. *N Engl J Med* 324:1005, 1991.

144. Goodrich JM, Mori M, Gleaves CA, et al: Early treatment with gan-

ciclovir to prevent cytomegalovirus disease after allogeneic bone marrow transplantation. *N Engl J Med* 325:1601, 1991.

145. Winston DJ, Ho WG, Bartoni K, et al: Ganciclovir prophylaxis of cytomegalovirus infection and disease in allogeneic bone marrow transplant recipients. *Ann Intern Med* 118:179, 1993.

146. Walter EA, Greenberg PD, Gilbert MJ, et al: Reconstitution of cellular immunity against cytomegalovirus in recipients of allogeneic bone marrow by transfer of T-cell clones from the donor. *N Engl J Med* 333:1038, 1995.

147. Saral R, Burns WH, Laskin OL, et al: Acyclovir prophylaxis of herpes-simplex-virus infections. *N Engl J Med* 305:63, 1981.

148. Wade JC, Newton B, McLaren C, et al: Intravenous acyclovir to treat mucocutaneous herpes simplex virus infection after marrow transplantation: A double blind trial. *Ann Intern Med* 96:265, 1982.

149. Atkinson K, Meyers JD, Storb R, et al: Varicella-zoster infection after marrow transplantation for aplastic anemia or leukemia. *Transplantation* 29:47, 1980.

150. Englund J, Sullivan C, Jordan C, et al: Respiratory syncytial virus infection in immunocompromised adults. *Ann Intern Med* 109:203, 1988.

151. Martin M, Bock M, Phaller M, Wenzel R: Respiratory synctial virus infections in adult bone marrow transplant recipients. *Lancet* 1:1396, 1988.

152. Hertz M, Englund J, Snover D, et al: Respiratory syncytial virus-induced acute lung injury in adult patients with bone marrow transplants: A clinical approach and review of the literature. *Medicine* 68:269, 1989.

153. Harrington R, Hooton T, Hackman R, et al: An outbreak of respiratory syncytial virus in a bone marrow transplant center. *J Infect Dis* 165:987, 1992.

154. Whimbey E, Champlin R, Englund J, et al: Combination therapy with aerosolized ribavirin and intravenous immunoglobulin for respiratory syncytial virus disease in adult bone marrow transplant recipients. *Bone Marrow Transplant* 16:393, 1995.

155. Cone R, Hackman R, Huang M, et al: Human herpevirus 6 in lung tissue from patients with pneumonitis after bone marrow transplantation. *N Engl J Med* 329:156, 1993.

156. Drobyski W, Knox K, Majewski D, Carrigan D: Brief report: Fatal encephalitis due to variant B human herpesvirus-6 infection in a bone marrow transplant recipient. *N Engl J Med* 330:1356, 1994.

157. Shields AF, Hackman RC, Fife KH, Corey L, Meyers JD: Adenovirus infections in patients undergoing bone-marrow transplantation. *N Engl J Med* 312:529, 1985.

158. Arthur RR, Shah KV, Baust SJ, et al: Association of BK viruria with hemorrhagic cystitis in recipients of bone marrow transplants. *N Engl J Med* 315:230, 1986.

159. Ochs L, Shu X, Miller J, et al: Late infections after allogeneic bone marrow transplantation: comparison of incidence in related and unrelated donor transplant recipients. *Blood* 86:3979, 1995.

160. Bernstein SH, Nademanee AP, Vose JM, et al: A multicenter study of platelet recovery and utilization in patients after myeloablative therapy and hematopoietic stem cell transplantation. *Blood* 91:3509, 1998.

161. Beutler E: Platelet transfusions: The 20,000/μL trigger. *Blood* 81:1411, 1993.

162. Rebulla R, Finazzi G, Marangoni F, et al: A multicenter randomized study of the threshold for prophylactic platelet transfusions in adults with acute myeloid leukemia: Gruppo Italiano Malattie Ematologiche Maligne dell'Adulto. *N Engl J Med* 337:1870, 1997.

163. Heckman KD, Weiner GJ, Davis CS, et al: Randomized study of prophylactic platelet transfusion threshold for adult acute leukemia: 10,000/μL versus 20,000/μL. *J Clin Oncol* 15:1143, 1997.

164. Schreiber G, Busch M, Kleinman S, Korelitz J: The risk of transfusion-transmitted viral infections. *N Engl J Med* 334:1685, 1996.

165. Thomas ED, Buckner CD, Clift RA, et al: Marrow transplantation for acute nonlymphoblastic leukemia in first remission. *N Engl J Med* 301:597, 1979.

166. Blume KG, Beutler E, Bross KJ, et al: Bone-marrow ablation and allogeneic marrow transplantation in acute leukemia. *N Engl J Med* 302:1041, 1980.

167. Powles RL, Morgenstern G, Clink HM, et al: The place of bone-marrow transplantation in acute myelogenous leukaemia. *Lancet* 1:1047, 1980.

168. Bacigalupo A, Frassoni F, Van Lint MT, et al: Bone marrow transplantation (BMT) for acute nonlymphoid leukemia (ANLL) in first remission. *Acta Haematol* 74:23, 1985.

169. Clift RA, Buckner CD, Thomas ED, et al: The treatment of acute non-lymphoblastic leukemia by allogeneic marrow transplantation. *Bone Marrow Transplant* 2:243, 1987.

170. Feig SA, Nesbit ME, Buckley J, et al: Bone marrow transplantation for acute non-lymphocytic leukemia: A report from the Childrens Cancer Study Group of sixty-seven children transplanted in first remission. *Bone Marrow Transplant* 2:365, 1987.

171. McGlave PB, Haake RJ, Bostrom BC, et al: Allogeneic bone marrow transplantation for acute nonlymphocytic leukemia in first remission. *Blood* 72:1512, 1988.

172. Blaise D, Maraninchi D, Archimbaud E, et al: Allogeneic bone marrow transplantation for acute myeloid leukemia in first remission: A randomized trial of a busulfan-Cytoxan versus Cytoxan-total body irradiation as preparative regimen: A report from the Group d'Etudes de la Greffe de Moelle Osseuse . *Blood* 79:2578, 1992.

173. Snyder DS, Chao NJ, Amylon MD, et al: Fractionated total body irradiation and high-dose etoposide as a preparatory regimen for bone marrow transplantation for 99 patients with acute leukemia in first complete remission. *Blood* 82:2920, 1993.

174. Powles RL, Watson JG, Morgenstern GR, Kay HE: Bone-marrow transplantation in leukaemia remission [letter]. *Lancet* 1:336, 1982.

175. Marmot A, Bacigalupo A, Van Lint MT, Frassoni F, Carella A: Bone marrow transplantation versus chemotherapy alone for acute non-lymphoblastic leukemia. *Exp Hematol* 13(suppl 17):40, 1985.

176. Appelbaum FR, Dahlberg S, Thomas ED, et al: Bone marrow transplantation or chemotherapy after remission induction for adults with acute nonlymphoblastic leukemia: A prospective comparison. *Ann Intern Med* 101:581, 1984.

177. Appelbaum FR, Fisher LD, Thomas ED: Chemotherapy v. marrow transplantation for adults with acute nonlymphocytic leukemia: A five-year follow-up. *Blood* 72:179, 1988.

178. Reiffers J, Gaspard MH, Maraninchi D, et al: Comparison of allogeneic or autologous bone marrow transplantation and chemotherapy in patients with acute myeloid leukaemia in first remission: A prospective controlled trial. *Br J Haematol* 72:57, 1989.

179. Zittoun RA, Mandelli F, Willemze R, et al: Autologous or allogeneic bone marrow transplantation compared with intensive chemotherapy in acute myelogenous leukemia: European Organization for Research and Treatment of Cancer (EORTC) and the Gruppo Italiano Malattie Ematologiche Maligne dell'Adulto (GIMEMA) Leukemia Cooperative Groups. *N Engl J Med* 332:217, 1995.

180. Forman SJ, Schmidt GM, Nademanee AP, et al: Allogeneic bone marrow transplantation as therapy for primary induction failure for patients with acute leukemia. *J Clin Oncol* 9:1570, 1991.

181. Biggs JC, Horowitz MM, Gale RP, et al: Bone marrow transplants may cure patients with acute leukemia never achieving remission with chemotherapy. *Blood* 80:1090, 1992.

182. Gorin NC: Autologous stem cell transplantation in acute myelocytic leukemia. *Blood* 92:1073, 1998.

183. Santos GW, Yeager AM, Jones RJ: Autologous bone marrow transplantation. *Ann Rev Med* 40:99, 1989.

184. Ball ED, Mills LE, Cornwell GGd, et al: Autologous bone marrow transplantation for acute myeloid leukemia using monoclonal antibody-purged bone marrow. *Blood* 75:1199, 1990.

185. Miller CB, Zehnbauer BA, Piantadosi S, Rowley SD, Jones RJ: Correlation of occult clonogenic leukemia drug sensitivity with relapse after autologous bone marrow transplantation. *Blood* 78:1125, 1991.

186. Stein AS, O'Donnell MR, Chai A, et al: In vivo purging with high-dose cytarabine followed by high-dose chemoradiotherapy and reinfusion of unpurged bone marrow for adult acute myelogenous leukemia in first complete remission. *J Clin Oncol* 14:2206, 1996.

187. Löwenberg B, Verdonck LJ, Dekker AW, et al: Autologous bone marrow transplantation in acute myeloid leukemia in first remission: results of a Dutch prospective study. *J Clin Oncol* 8:287, 1990.

188. McMillan AK, Goldstone AH, Linch DC, et al: High-dose chemotherapy and autologous bone marrow transplantation in acute myeloid leukemia. *Blood* 76:480, 1990.

189. Cassileth PA, Andersen J, Lazarus HM, et al: Autologous bone marrow transplant in acute myeloid leukemia in first remission. *J Clin Oncol* 11:314, 1993.

190. Reiffers J, Stoppa AM, Attal M, et al: Allogeneic vs autologous stem cell transplantation vs chemotherapy in patients with acute myeloid

leukemia in first remission: The BGMT 87 study. *Leukemia* 10:1874, 1996.

191. Mitus AJ, Miller KB, Schenkein DP, et al: Improved survival for patients with acute myelogenous leukemia. *J Clin Oncol* 13:560, 1995.

192. Cassileth PA, Harrington DP, Appelbaum FR, et al: Chemotherapy compared with autologous or allogeneic bone marrow transplantation in the management of acute myeloid leukemia in first remission. *N Engl J Med* 339:1649, 1998.

193. Burnett AK, Goldstone AH, Stevens RM, et al: Randomised comparison of addition of autologous bone-marrow transplantation to intensive chemotherapy for acute myeloid leukaemia in first remission: Results of MRC AML 10 trial, UK Medical Research Council Adult and Children's Leukaemia Working Parties. *Lancet* 351:700, 1998.

194. Harousseau JL, Cahn JY, Pignon B, et al: Comparison of autologous bone marrow transplantation and intensive chemotherapy as postremission therapy in adult acute myeloid leukemia: The Groupe Ouest Est Leucémies Aiguës Myéloblastiques (GOELAM). *Blood* 90:2978, 1997.

195. Ravindranath Y, Yeager AM, Chang MN, et al: Autologous bone marrow transplantation versus intensive consolidation chemotherapy for acute myeloid leukemia in childhood: Pediatric Oncology Group. *N Engl J Med* 334:1428, 1996.

196. Brochstein JA, Kernan NA, Groshen S, et al: Allogeneic bone marrow transplantation after hyperfractionated total-body irradiation and cyclophosphamide in children with acute leukemia. *N Engl J Med* 317:1618, 1987.

197. Sanders JE, Thomas ED, Buckner CD, Doney K: Marrow transplantation for children with acute lymphoblastic leukemia in second remission. *Blood* 70:324, 1987.

198. Coccia PF, Strandjord SE, Warkentin PI, et al: High-dose cytosine arabinoside and fractionated total-body irradiation: an improved preparative regimen for bone marrow transplantation of children with acute lymphoblastic leukemia in remission. *Blood* 71:888, 1988.

199. Dopfer R, Henze G, Bender-Götze C, et al: Allogeneic bone marrow transplantation for childhood acute lymphoblastic leukemia in second remission after intensive primary and relapse therapy according to the BFM- and CoALL-protocols: results of the German Cooperative Study. *Blood* 78:2780, 1991.

200. Barnett MJ, Eaves CJ, Phillips GL, et al: Autografting with cultured marrow in chronic myeloid leukemia: Results of a pilot study. *Blood* 84:724, 1994.

201. Chessells JM, Bailey C, Wheeler K, Richards SM: Bone marrow transplantation for high-risk childhood lymphoblastic leukaemia in first remission: Experience in MRC UKALL X. *Lancet* 340:565, 1992.

202. De la Cámara R, Figuera A, Steegmann JL, et al: Allogeneic bone marrow transplantation for high risk acute lymphoblastic leukemia: Results from a single institution. *Bone Marrow Transplant* 9:433, 1992.

203. Blume KG, Forman SJ, Snyder DS, et al: Allogeneic bone marrow transplantation for acute lymphoblastic leukemia during first complete remission. *Transplantation* 43:389, 1987.

204. Vernant JP, Marit G, Maraninchi D, et al: Allogeneic bone marrow transplantation in adults with acute lymphoblastic leukemia in first complete remission. *J Clin Oncol* 6:227, 1988.

205. Blaise D, Gaspard MH, Stoppa AM, et al: Allogeneic or autologous bone marrow transplantation for acute lymphoblastic leukemia in first complete remission. *Bone Marrow Transplant* 5:7, 1990.

206. von Bueltzingsloewen A, Bélanger R, Perreault C, et al: Allogeneic bone marrow transplantation following busulfan-cyclophosphamide with or without etoposide conditioning regimen for patients with acute lymphoblastic leukaemia. *Br J Haematol* 85:706, 1993.

207. Chao NJ, Forman SJ, Schmidt GM, et al: Allogeneic bone marrow transplantation for high-risk acute lymphoblastic leukemia during first complete remission. *Blood* 78:1923, 1991.

208. Horowitz MM, Messerer D, Hoelzer D, et al: Chemotherapy compared with bone marrow transplantation for adults with acute lymphoblastic leukemia in first remission. *Ann Intern Med* 115:13, 1991.

209. Zhang MJ, Hoelzer D, Horowitz MM, et al: Long-term follow-up of adults with acute lymphoblastic leukemia in first remission treated with chemotherapy or bone marrow transplantation: The Acute Lymphoblastic Leukemia Working Committee. *Ann Intern Med* 123:428, 1995.

210. Oh H, Gale RP, Zhang MJ, et al: Chemotherapy vs HLA-identical sibling bone marrow transplants for adults with acute lymphoblastic leukemia in first remission. *Bone Marrow Transplant* 22:253, 1998.

211. Sebban C, Lepage E, Vernant JP, et al: Allogeneic bone marrow transplantation in adult acute lymphoblastic leukemia in first complete remission: A comparative study: French Group of Therapy of Adult Acute Lymphoblastic Leukemia. *J Clin Oncol* 12:2580, 1994.

212. Linker CA, Levitt LJ, O'Donnell M, Forman SJ, Ries CA: Treatment of adult acute lymphoblastic leukemia with intensive cyclical chemotherapy: A follow-up report. *Blood* 78:2814, 1991.

213. Larson RA, Dodge RK, Burns CP, et al: A five-drug remission induction regimen with intensive consolidation for adults with acute lymphoblastic leukemia: Cancer and leukemia group B study 8811. *Blood* 85:2025, 1995.

214. Snyder DM, Nademanee AP, O'Donnell MR, et al: Long-term follow-up of 23 patients with Philadelphia chromosome-positive acute lymphoblastic leukemia treated with allogeneic bone marrow transplant in first complete remission. *Leukemia* 13:2053, 1999.

215. Sierra J, Radich J, Hansen JA, et al: Marrow transplants from unrelated donors for treatment of Philadelphia chromosome-positive acute lymphoblastic leukemia. *Blood* 90:1410, 1997.

216. Schmid H, Henze G, Schwerdtfeger R, et al: Fractionated total body irradiation and high-dose VP-16 with purged autologous bone marrow rescue for children with high risk relapsed acute lymphoblastic leukemia. *Bone Marrow Transplant* 12:597, 1993.

217. Simonsson B, Burnett AK, Prentice HG, et al: Autologous bone marrow transplantation with monoclonal antibody purged marrow for high risk acute lymphoblastic leukemia. *Leukemia* 3:631, 1989.

218. Ritz J, Sallan SE, Bast RC Jr, et al: Autologous bone-marrow transplantation in CALLA-positive acute lymphoblastic leukemia after in-vitro treatment with J5 monoclonal antibody and complement. *Lancet* 2:60, 1982.

219. Sallan SE, Niemeyer CM, Billett AL, et al: Autologous bone marrow transplantation for acute lymphoblastic leukemia. *J Clin Oncol* 7:1594, 1989.

220. Uckun FM, Kersey JH, Haake R, et al: Pretransplantation burden of leukemic progenitor cells as a predictor of relapse after bone marrow transplantation for acute lymphoblastic leukemia. *N Engl J Med* 329:1296, 1993.

221. Messina C, Cesaro S, Rondelli R, et al: Autologous bone marrow transplantation for childhood acute lymphoblastic leukaemia in Italy: AIEOP/FONOP-TMO Group, Italian Association of Paediatric Haemato-Oncology. *Bone Marrow Transplant* 21:1015, 1998.

222. Maldonado MS, Diaz-Heredia C, Badell I, et al: Autologous bone marrow transplantation with monoclonal antibody purged marrow for children with acute lymphoblastic leukemia in second remission. *Bone Marrow Transplant* 22:1043, 1998.

223. Martino R, Bellido M, Brunet S, et al: Allogeneic or autologous stem cell transplantation following salvage chemotherapy for adults with refractory or relapsed acute lymphoblastic leukemia. *Bone Marrow Transplant* 21:1023, 1998.

224. Billett AL, Kornmehl E, Tarbell NJ, et al: Autologous bone marrow transplantation after a long first remission for children with recurrent acute lymphoblastic leukemia. *Blood* 81:1651, 1993.

225. Gilmore MJ, Hamon MD, Prentice HG, et al: Failure of purged autologous bone marrow transplantation in high risk acute lymphoblastic leukaemia in first complete remission. *Bone Marrow Transplant* 8:19, 1991.

226. Doney K, Buckner CD, Fisher L, et al: Autologous bone marrow transplantation for acute lymphoblastic leukemia. *Bone Marrow Transplant* 12:315, 1993.

227. Ramsay N, LeBien T, Nesbit M, et al: Autologous bone marrow transplantation for patients with acute lymphoblastic leukemia in second or subsequent remission: Results of bone marrow treated with monoclonal antibodies BA-1, BA-2, and BA-3 plus complement. *Blood* 66:508, 1985.

228. Uckun FM, Kersey JH, Vallera DA, et al: Autologous bone marrow transplantation in high-risk remission T-lineage acute lymphoblastic leukemia using immunotoxins plus 4-hydroperoxycyclophosphamide for marrow purging. *Blood* 76:1723, 1990.

229. Martin H, Atta J, Zumpe P, et al: Purging of peripheral blood stem cells yields bcr-abl-negative autografts in patients with bcr-abl-positive acute lymphoblastic leukemia. *Exp Hematol* 23:1612, 1995.

230. Miyamura K, Tanimoto M, Morishima Y, et al: Detection of Philadelphia chromosome-positive acute lymphoblastic leukemia by polymerase chain reaction: Possible eradication of minimal residual disease by marrow transplantation. *Blood* 79:1366, 1992.

231. Radich J, Gehly G, Lee A, et al: Detection of bcr-abl transcripts in Philadelphia chromosome-positive acute lymphoblastic leukemia after marrow transplantation. *Blood* 89:2602, 1997.

232. Radich JP, Gehly G, Gooley T, et al: Polymerase chain reaction of the bcr-abl fusion transcript after allogeneic marrow transplantation for chronic myeloid leukemia: Results and implications in 346 patients. *Blood* 85:2632, 1995.

233. Knechtli CJ, Goulden NJ, Hancock JP, et al: Minimal residual disease status before allogeneic bone marrow transplantation is an important determinant of successful outcome for children and adolescents with acute lymphoblastic leukemia. *Blood* 92:4072, 1998.

234. Champlin R, Ho W, Arenson E, Gale RP: Allogeneic bone marrow transplantation for chronic myelogenous leukemia in chronic or accelerated phase. *Blood* 60:1038, 1982.

235. Goldman JM, Apperley JF, Jones L, et al: Bone marrow transplantation for patients with chronic myeloid leukemia. *N Engl J Med* 314:202, 1986.

236. McGlave P: Bone marrow transplants in chronic myelogenous leukemia: An overview of determinants of survival. *Semin Hematol* 27:23, 1990.

237. Biggs JC, Szer J, Crilley P, et al: Treatment of chronic myeloid leukemia with allogeneic bone marrow transplantation after preparation with BuCy2. *Blood* 80:1352, 1992.

238. Gale RP, Horowitz MM, Ash RC, et al: Identical twin bone marrow transplants for leukemia. *Ann Intern Med* 120:646, 1994.

239. McGlave P, Arthur D, Haake R, et al: Therapy of chronic myelogenous leukemia with allogeneic bone marrow transplantation. *J Clin Oncol* 5:1033, 1987.

240. Thomas ED, Clift RA, Fefer A, et al: Marrow transplantation for the treatment of chronic myelogenous leukemia. *Ann Intern Med* 104:155, 1986.

241. Bacigalupo A, Gualandi F, Van Lint MT, et al: Multivariate analysis of risk factors for survival and relapse in chronic granulocytic leukemia following allogeneic marrow transplantation: Impact of disease related variables (Sokal score). *Bone Marrow Transplant* 12:443, 1993.

242. Snyder DS, Negrin RS, O'Donnell MR, et al: Fractionated total-body irradiation and high-dose etoposide as a preparatory regimen for bone marrow transplantation for 94 patients with chronic myelogenous leukemia. *Blood* 84:1672, 1994.

243. Gratwohl A, Hermans J, Niederwieser D, et al: Bone marrow transplantation for chronic myeloid leukemia: long-term results: Chronic Leukemia Working Party of the European Group for Bone Marrow Transplantation. *Bone Marrow Transplant* 12:509, 1993.

244. Clift RA, Buckner CD, Thomas ED, et al: Marrow transplantation for patients in accelerated phase of chronic myeloid leukemia. *Blood* 84:4368, 1994.

245. Devergie A, Blaise D, Attal M, et al: Allogeneic bone marrow transplantation for chronic myeloid leukemia in first chronic phase: A randomized trial of busulfan-cytoxan versus cytoxan-total body irradiation as preparative regimen: A report from the French Society of Bone Marrow Graft (SFGM). *Blood* 85:2263, 1995.

246. Slattery JT, Clift RA, Buckner CD, et al: Marrow transplantation for chronic myeloid leukemia: the influence of plasma busulfan levels on the outcome of transplantation. *Blood* 89:3055, 1997.

247. Hehlmann R, Heimpel H, Hasford J, et al: Randomized comparison of interferon-alpha with busulfan and hydroxyurea in chronic myelogenous leukemia: The German CML Study Group. *Blood* 84:4064, 1994.

248. Gale RP, Hehlmann R, Zhang MJ, et al: Survival with bone marrow transplantation versus hydroxyurea or interferon for chronic myelogenous leukemia: The German CML Study Group. *Blood* 91:1810, 1998.

249. McGlave P, Bartsch G, Anasetti C, et al: Unrelated donor marrow transplantation therapy for chronic myelogenous leukemia: Initial experience of the National Marrow Donor Program. *Blood* 81:543, 1993.

250. Lee SJ, Kuntz KM, Horowitz MM, et al: Unrelated donor bone marrow transplantation for chronic myelogenous leukemia: a decision analysis. *Ann Intern Med* 127:1080, 1997.

251. Lee SJ, Anasetti C, Kuntz KM, et al: The costs and cost-effectiveness of unrelated donor bone marrow transplantation for chronic phase chronic myelogenous leukemia. *Blood* 92:4047, 1998.

252. Bogdanic V, Nemet D, Kastelan A, et al: Umbilical cord blood transplantation in a patient with Philadelphia chromosome-positive chronic myeloid leukemia. *Transplantation* 56:477, 1993.

253. Laporte JP, Gorin NC, Rubinstein P, et al: Cord-blood transplantation

254. Goldman JM, Gale RP, Horowitz MM, et al: Bone marrow transplantation for chronic myelogenous leukemia in chronic phase: Increased risk for relapse associated with T-cell depletion. *Ann Intern Med* 108:806, 1988.

255. Drobyski WR, Ash RC, Casper JT, et al: Effect of T-cell depletion as graft-versus-host disease prophylaxis on engraftment, relapse, and disease-free survival in unrelated marrow transplantation for chronic myelogenous leukemia. *Blood* 83:1980, 1994.

256. Hessner MJ, Endean DJ, Casper JT, et al: Use of unrelated marrow grafts compensates for reduced graft-versus-leukemia reactivity after T-cell-depleted allogeneic marrow transplantation for chronic myelogenous leukemia. *Blood* 86:3987, 1995.

257. Beelen DW, Graeven U, Elmaagacli AH, et al: Prolonged administration of interferon-alpha in patients with chronic-phase Philadelphia chromosome-positive chronic myelogenous leukemia before allogeneic bone marrow transplantation may adversely affect transplant outcome. *Blood* 85:2981, 1995.

258. Morton AJ, Gooley T, Hansen JA, et al: Association between pretransplant interferon-alpha and outcome after unrelated donor marrow transplantation for chronic myelogenous leukemia in chronic phase. *Blood* 92:394, 1998.

259. Giralt SA, Kantarjian HM, Talpaz M, et al: Effect of prior interferon alfa therapy on the outcome of allogeneic bone marrow transplantation for chronic myelogenous leukemia. *J Clin Oncol* 11:1055, 1993.

260. Horowitz MM, Giralt S, Szydlo R, Goldman J, Veumstone J: Effect of prior interferon therapy on outcome of HLA-identical sibling bone marrow transplants for chronic myelogenous leukemia (CML) in first chronic phase. *Blood* 88:682a, 1996.

261. McGlave PB, De Fabritiis P, Deisseroth A, et al: Autologous transplants for chronic myelogenous leukaemia: Results from eight transplant groups. *Lancet* 343:1486, 1994.

262. Hoyle C, Gray R, Goldman J: Autografting for patients with CML in chronic phase: An update: Hammersmith BMT Team LRF Centre for Adult Leukaemia. *Br J Haematol* 86:76, 1994.

263. Carella A, Lerma E, Corsetti MT, et al: Autografting with Philadelphia chromosome-negative mobilized hematopoietic progenitor cells in chronic myelogenous leukemia. *Blood* 93:1534, 1999.

264. Verfaillie CM, Miller WJ, Boylan K, McGlave PB: Selection of benign primitive hematopoietic progenitors in chronic myelogenous leukemia on the basis of HLA-DR antigen expression. *Blood* 79:1003, 1992.

265. Carella AM, Chimirri F, Podestà M, et al: High-dose chemo-radiotherapy followed by autologous Philadelphia chromosome-negative blood progenitor cell transplantation in patients with chronic myelogenous leukemia. *Bone Marrow Transplant* 17:201, 1996.

266. Verfaillie CM, Bhatia R, Steinbuch M, et al: Comparative analysis of autografting in chronic myelogenous leukemia: Effects of priming regimen and marrow or blood origin of stem cells. *Blood* 92:1820, 1998.

267. Cervantes F, Pierson BA, McGlave PB, Verfaillie CM, Miller JS: Autologous activated natural killer cells suppress primitive chronic myelogenous leukemia progenitors in long-term culture. *Blood* 87:2476, 1996.

268. Hoyle C, Bangs CD, Chang P, et al: Expansion of Philadelphia chromosome-negative CD3+CD56+ cytotoxic cells from chronic myeloid leukemia patients: in vitro and in vivo efficacy in severe combined immunodeficiency disease mice. *Blood* 92:3318, 1998.

269. Kalhs P, Schwarzinger I, Anderson G, et al: A retrospective analysis of the long-term effect of splenectomy on late infections, graft-versus-host disease, relapse, and survival after allogeneic marrow transplantation for chronic myelogenous leukemia. *Blood* 86:2028, 1995.

270. Gratwohl A, Hermans J, von Biezen A, et al: No advantage for patients who receive splenic irradiation before bone marrow transplantation for chronic myeloid leukaemia: Results of a prospective randomized study. *Bone Marrow Transplant* 10:147, 1992.

271. Jabro G, Koc Y, Boyle T, et al: The role of splenic irradiation in patients with chronic myeloid leukemia undergoing allogeneic bone marrow transplantation. *Biol Blood Marrow Transplant* 5:173, 1999.

272. Anderson JE, Appelbaum FR, Fisher LD, et al: Allogeneic bone marrow transplantation for 93 patients with myelodysplastic syndrome. *Blood* 82:677, 1993.

273. O'Donnell MR, Nademanee AP, Snyder DS, et al: Bone marrow trans-

plantation for myelodysplastic and myeloproliferative syndromes. *J Clin Oncol* 5:1822, 1987.

274. Bunin NJ, Casper JT, Chitambar C, et al: Partially matched bone marrow transplantation in patients with myelodysplastic syndromes. *J Clin Oncol* 6:1851, 1988.

275. Longmore G, Guinan EC, Weinstein HJ, et al: Bone marrow transplantation for myelodysplasia and secondary acute nonlymphoblastic leukemia. *J Clin Oncol* 8:1707, 1990.

276. O'Donnell MR, Long GD, Parker PM, et al: Busulfan/cyclophosphamide as conditioning regimen for allogeneic bone marrow transplantation for myelodysplasia. *J Clin Oncol* 13:2973, 1995.

277. Ratanatharathorn V, Karanes C, Uberti J, et al: Busulfan-based regimens and allogeneic bone marrow transplantation in patients with myelodysplastic syndromes. *Blood* 81:2194, 1993.

278. Runde V, de Witte T, Arnold R, et al: Bone marrow transplantation from HLA-identical siblings as first-line treatment in patients with myelodysplastic syndromes: Early transplantation is associated with improved outcome: Chronic Leukemia Working Party of the European Group for Blood and Marrow Transplantation. *Bone Marrow Transplant* 21:255, 1998.

279. Anderson JE, Anasetti C, Appelbaum FR, et al: Unrelated donor marrow transplantation for myelodysplasia (MDS) and MDS-related acute myeloid leukaemia. *Br J Haematol* 93:59, 1996.

280. Arnold R, de Witte T, van Biezen A, et al: Unrelated bone marrow transplantation in patients with myelodysplastic syndromes and secondary acute myeloid leukemia: An EBMT survey: European Blood and Marrow Transplantation Group. *Bone Marrow Transplant* 21:1213, 1998.

281. Greenberg P, Cox L, LeBeau MM, et al: International scoring system for evaluating prognosis in myelodysplastic syndromes. *Blood* 89:2079, 1997.

282. Nevill TJ, Fung HC, Shepherd JD, et al: Cytogenetic abnormalities in primary myelodysplastic syndrome are highly predictive of outcome after allogeneic bone marrow transplantation. *Blood* 92:1910, 1998.

283. Ballen KK, Gilliland DG, Guinan EC, et al: Bone marrow transplantation for therapy-related myelodysplasia: Comparison with primary myelodysplasia. *Bone Marrow Transplant* 20:737, 1997.

284. Locatelli F, Pession A, Bonetti F, et al: Busulfan, cyclophosphamide and melphalan as conditioning regimen for bone marrow transplantation in children with myelodysplastic syndromes. *Leukemia* 8:844, 1994.

285. Rubie H, Attal M, Demur C, et al: Intensified conditioning regimen with busulfan followed by allogeneic BMT in children with myelodysplastic syndromes. *Bone Marrow Transplant* 13:759, 1994.

286. Anderson JE, Gooley TA, Schoch G, et al: Stem cell transplantation for secondary acute myeloid leukemia: Evaluation of transplantation as initial therapy or following induction chemotherapy. *Blood* 89:2578, 1997.

287. Tsuzuki M, Maruyama F, Kojima H, Ezaki K, Hirano M: Donor buffy coat infusions for a patient with myelodysplastic syndrome who relapsed following allogeneic bone marrow transplantation. *Bone Marrow Transplant* 16:487, 1995.

288. Collins RH, Shpilberg O, Drobyski WR, et al: Donor leukocyte infusions in 140 patients with relapsed malignancy after allogeneic bone marrow transplantation. *J Clin Oncol* 15:433, 1997.

289. De Witte T, Van Biezen A, Hermans J, et al: Autologous bone marrow transplantation for patients with myelodysplastic syndrome (MDS) or acute myeloid leukemia following MDS: Chronic and Acute Leukemia Working Parties of the European Group for Blood and Marrow Transplantation. *Blood* 90:3853, 1997.

290. Rajantie J, Sale GE, Deeg HJ, et al: Adverse effect of severe marrow fibrosis on hematologic recovery after chemoradiotherapy and allogeneic bone marrow transplantation. *Blood* 67:1693, 1986.

291. Wolf JL, Spruce WE, Bearman RM, et al: Reversal of acute ("malignant") myelosclerosis by allogeneic bone marrow transplantation. *Blood* 59:191, 1982.

292. Guardiola P, Esperou H, Cazals-Hatem D, et al: Allogeneic bone marrow transplantation for agnogenic myeloid metaplasia: French Society of Bone Marrow Transplantation. *Br J Haematol* 98:1004, 1997.

293. Przepiorka D, Giralt S, Khouri I, Champlin R, Bueso-Ramos C: Allogeneic marrow transplantation for myeloproliferative disorders other than chronic myelogenous leukemia: Review of forty cases. *Am J Hematol* 57:24, 1998.

294. Storb R, Etzioni R, Anasetti C, et al: Cyclophosphamide combined with antithymocyte globulin in preparation for allogeneic marrow transplants in patients with aplastic anemia. *Blood* 84:941, 1994.

295. Storb R, Leisenring W, Anasetti C, et al: Long-term follow-up of allogeneic marrow transplants in patients with aplastic anemia conditioned by cyclophosphamide combined with antithymocyte globulin. *Blood* 89:3890, 1997.

296. Reiter E, Keil F, Brugger S, et al: Excellent long-term survival after allogeneic marrow transplantation in patients with severe aplastic anemia. *Bone Marrow Transplant* 19:1191, 1997.

297. Passweg JR, Socié G, Hinterberger W, et al: Bone marrow transplantation for severe aplastic anemia: Has outcome improved? *Blood* 90:858, 1997.

298. Paquette RL, Tebyani N, Frane M, et al: Long-term outcome of aplastic anemia in adults treated with antithymocyte globulin: Comparison with bone marrow transplantation. *Blood* 85:283, 1995.

299. Gillio AP, Boulad F, Small TN, et al: Comparison of long-term outcome of children with severe aplastic anemia treated with immunosuppression versus bone marrow transplantation. *Biol Blood Marrow Transplant* 3:18, 1997.

300. Doney K, Leisenring W, Storb R, Appelbaum FR: Primary treatment of acquired aplastic anemia: Outcomes with bone marrow transplantation and immunosuppressive therapy: Seattle Bone Marrow Transplant Team. *Ann Intern Med* 126:107, 1997.

301. Deeg HJ, Leisenring W, Storb R, et al: Long-term outcome after marrow transplantation for severe aplastic anemia. *Blood* 91:3637, 1998.

302. Socié G, Henry-Amar M, Bacigalupo A, et al: Malignant tumors occurring after treatment of aplastic anemia: European Bone Marrow Transplantation–Severe Aplastic Anaemia Working Party. *N Engl J Med* 329:1152, 1993.

303. Deeg HJ, Socié G, Schoch G, et al: Malignancies after marrow transplantation for aplastic anemia and Fanconi anemia: A joint Seattle and Paris analysis of results in 700 patients. *Blood* 87:386, 1996.

304. Michallet M, Corront B, Hollard D, et al: Allogeneic bone marrow transplantation in chronic lymphocytic leukemia: 17 cases: Report from the EBMTG. *Bone Marrow Transplant* 7:275, 1991.

305. Rabinowe SN, Soiffer RJ, Gribben JG, et al: Autologous and allogeneic bone marrow transplantation for poor prognosis patients with B-cell chronic lymphocytic leukemia. *Blood* 82:1366, 1993.

306. Khouri IF, Keating MJ, Vriesendorp HM, et al: Autologous and allogeneic bone marrow transplantation for chronic lymphocytic leukemia: Preliminary results. *J Clin Oncol* 12:748, 1994.

307. Provan D, Bartlett-Pandite L, Zwicky C, et al: Eradication of polymerase chain reaction-detectable chronic lymphocytic leukemia cells is associated with improved outcome after bone marrow transplantation. *Blood* 88:2228, 1996.

308. Philip T, Armitage JO, Spitzer G, et al: High-dose therapy and autologous bone marrow transplantation after failure of conventional chemotherapy in adults with intermediate-grade or high-grade non-Hodgkin's lymphoma. *N Engl J Med* 316:1493, 1987.

309. Takvorian T, Canellos GP, Ritz J, et al: Prolonged disease-free survival after autologous bone marrow transplantation in patients with non-Hodgkin's lymphoma with a poor prognosis. *N Engl J Med* 316:1499, 1987.

310. Phillips GL, Fay JW, Herzig RH, et al: The treatment of progressive non-Hodgkin's lymphoma with intensive chemoradiotherapy and autologous marrow transplantation. *Blood* 75:831, 1990.

311. Freedman AS, Takvorian T, Anderson KC, et al: Autologous bone marrow transplantation in B-cell non-Hodgkin's lymphoma: Very low treatment-related mortality in 100 patients in sensitive relapse. *J Clin Oncol* 8:784, 1990.

312. Bosly A, Coiffier B, Gisselbrecht C, et al: Bone marrow transplantation prolongs survival after relapse in aggressive-lymphoma patients treated with the LNH-84 regimen. *J Clin Oncol* 10:1615, 1992.

313. Gulati S, Yahalom J, Acaba L, et al: Treatment of patients with relapsed and resistant non-Hodgkin's lymphoma using total body irradiation, etoposide, and cyclophosphamide and autologous bone marrow transplantation. *J Clin Oncol* 10:936, 1992.

314. Philip T, Guglielmi C, Hagenbeek A, et al: Autologous bone marrow transplantation as compared with salvage chemotherapy in relapses of chemotherapy-sensitive non-Hodgkin's lymphoma. *N Engl J Med* 333:1540, 1995.

315. Stockerl-Goldstein KE, Horning SJ, Negrin RS, et al: Influence of preparatory regimen and source of hematopoietic cells on outcome of

autotransplantation for non-Hodgkin's lymphoma. *Biol Blood Marrow Transplant* 2:76, 1996.

316. Fisher RI, Gaynor ER, Dahlberg S, et al: Comparison of a standard regimen (CHOP) with three intensive chemotherapy regimens for advanced non-Hodgkin's lymphoma. *N Engl J Med* 328:1002, 1993.

317. Shipp MA, Harrington DP, et al: A predictive model for aggressive non-Hodgkin's lymphoma: The International Non-Hodgkin's Lymphoma Prognostic Factors Project. *N Engl J Med* 329:987, 1993.

318. Nademanee A, Molina A, O'Donnell MR, et al: Results of high-dose therapy and autologous bone marrow/stem cell transplantation during remission in poor-risk intermediate- and high-grade lymphoma: International index high and high-intermediate risk group. *Blood* 90:3844, 1997.

319. Fanin R, Silvestri F, Geromin A, et al: Autologous stem cell transplantation for aggressive non-Hodgkin's lymphomas in first complete or partial remission: A retrospective analysis of the outcome of 52 patients according to the age-adjusted International Prognostic Index. *Bone Marrow Transplant* 21:263, 1998.

320. Haioun C, Lepage E, Gisselbrecht C, et al: Comparison of autologous bone marrow transplantation with sequential chemotherapy for intermediate-grade and high-grade non-Hodgkin's lymphoma in first complete remission: A study of 464 patients: Groupe d'Etude des Lymphomes de l'Adulte. *J Clin Oncol* 12:2543, 1994.

321. Haioun C, Lepage E, Gisselbrecht C, et al: Benefit of autologous bone marrow transplantation over sequential chemotherapy in poor-risk aggressive non-Hodgkin's lymphoma: Updated results of the prospective study LNH87-2: Groupe d'Etude des Lymphomes de l'Adulte. *J Clin Oncol* 15:1131, 1997.

322. Blay JY, Sebban C, Surbiguet C, et al: High-dose chemotherapy with hematopoietic stem cell transplantation in patients with mantle cell or diffuse centrocytic non-Hodgkin's lymphomas: A single center experience on 18 patients. *Bone Marrow Transplant* 21:51, 1998.

323. Verdonck LF, vanPutten WL, Hagenbeek A, et al: Comparison of CHOP chemotherapy with autologous bone marrow transplantation for slowly responding patients with aggressive non-Hodgkin's lymphoma. *N Engl J Med* 332:1045, 1995.

324. Gianni AM, Bregni M, Siena S, et al: High-dose chemotherapy and autologous bone marrow transplantation compared with MACOP-B in aggressive B-cell lymphoma. *N Engl J Med* 336:1290, 1997.

325. Rohatiner AZ, Johnson PW, Price CG, et al: Myeloablative therapy with autologous bone marrow transplantation as consolidation therapy for recurrent follicular lymphoma. *J Clin Oncol* 12:1177, 1994.

326. Bierman PJ, Vose JM, Anderson JR, et al: High-dose therapy with autologous hematopoietic rescue for follicular low-grade non-Hodgkin's lymphoma. *J Clin Oncol* 15:445, 1997.

327. Freedman AS, Neuberg D, Mauch P, et al: Long-term follow-up of autologous bone marrow transplantation in patients with relapsed follicular lymphoma. *Blood* 94:3325, 1999.

328. van Besien KW, Khouri IF, Giralt SA, et al: Allogeneic bone marrow transplantation for refractory and recurrent low-grade lymphoma: The case for aggressive management. *J Clin Oncol* 13:1096, 1995.

329. van Besien K, Sobocinski KA, Rowlings PA, et al: Allogeneic bone marrow transplantation for low-grade lymphoma. *Blood* 92:1832, 1998.

330. Verdonck LF, Dekker AW, Lokhorst HM, Petersen EJ, Nieuwenhuis HK: Allogeneic versus autologous bone marrow transplantation for refractory and recurrent low-grade non-Hodgkin's lymphoma. *Blood* 90:4201, 1997.

331. Freedman AS, Gribben JG, Neuberg D, et al: High-dose therapy and autologous bone marrow transplantation in patients with follicular lymphoma during first remission. *Blood* 88:2780, 1996.

332. Horning SJ, Negrin RS, Hoppe RT, et al: High dose therapy and autografting for follicular lymphoma in first remission. *Blood* 90(suppl 1):594a, 1997.

333. Weisenburger DD, Armitage JO: Mantle cell lymphoma: An entity comes of age. *Blood* 87:4483, 1996.

334. Freedman AS, Neuberg D, Gribben JG, et al: High-dose chemoradiotherapy and anti-B-cell monoclonal antibody-purged autologous bone marrow transplantation in mantle-cell lymphoma: No evidence for long-term remission. *J Clin Oncol* 16:13, 1998.

335. Stewart DA, Vose JM, Weisenburger DD, et al: The role of high-dose therapy and autologous hematopoietic stem cell transplantation for mantle cell lymphoma. *Ann Oncol* 6:263, 1995.

336. Haas R, Brittinger G, Meusers P, et al: Myeloablative therapy with

337. Milpied N, Gaillard F, Moreau P, et al: High-dose therapy with stem cell transplantation for mantle cell lymphoma: results and prognostic factors: A single center experience. *Bone Marrow Transplant* 22:645, 1998.

338. Kröger N, Hoffknecht M, Dreger P, et al: Long-term disease-free survival of patients with advanced mantle-cell lymphoma following high-dose chemotherapy. *Bone Marrow Transplant* 21:55, 1998.

339. Philip T, Biron P, Philip I, et al: Massive therapy and autologous bone marrow transplantation in pediatric and young adults Burkitt's lymphoma (30 courses on 28 patients): A 5-year experience. *Eur J Cancer Clin Oncol* 22:1015, 1986.

340. Sweetenham JW, Pearce R, Taghipour G, et al: Adult Burkitt's and Burkitt-like non-Hodgkin's lymphoma: Outcome for patients treated with high-dose therapy and autologous stem-cell transplantation in first remission or at relapse: Results from the European Group for Blood and Marrow Transplantation. *J Clin Oncol* 14:2465, 1996.

341. Milpied N, Ifrah N, Kuentz M, et al: Bone marrow transplantation for adult poor prognosis lymphoblastic lymphoma in first complete remission. *Br J Haematol* 73:82, 1989.

342. Baro J, Richard C, Sierra J, et al: Autologous bone marrow transplantation in 22 adult patients with lymphoblastic lymphoma responsive to conventional dose chemotherapy. *Bone Marrow Transplant* 10:33, 1992.

343. Verdonck LF, Dekker AW, de Gast GC, Lokhorst HM, Nieuwenhuis HK: Autologous bone marrow transplantation for adult poor-risk lymphoblastic lymphoma in first remission. *J Clin Oncol* 10:644, 1992.

344. Chopra R, Goldstone AH, Pearce R, et al: Autologous versus allogeneic bone marrow transplantation for non-Hodgkin's lymphoma: A case-controlled analysis of the European Bone Marrow Transplant Group Registry data. *J Clin Oncol* 10:1690, 1992.

345. Hasenclever D, Diehl V: A prognostic score for advanced Hodgkin's disease: International Prognostic Factors Project on Advanced Hodgkin's Disease. *N Eng J Med* 339:1506, 1998.

346. Jagannath S, Dicke KA, Armitage JO, et al: High-dose cyclophosphamide, carmustine, and etoposide and autologous bone marrow transplantation for relapsed Hodgkin's disease. *Ann Intern Med* 104:163, 1986.

347. Carella AM, Congiu AM, Gaozza E, et al: High-dose chemotherapy with autologous bone marrow transplantation in 50 advanced resistant Hodgkin's disease patients: An Italian study group report. *J Clin Oncol* 6:1411, 1988.

348. Lazarus HM, Crilley P, Ciobanu N, et al: High-dose carmustine, etoposide, and cisplatin and autologous bone marrow transplantation for relapsed and refractory lymphoma. *J Clin Oncol* 10:1682, 1992.

349. Chopra R, McMillan AK, Linch DC, et al: The place of high-dose BEAM therapy and autologous bone marrow transplantation in poor-risk Hodgkin's disease: A single-center eight-year study of 155 patients. *Blood* 81:1137, 1993.

350. Reece DE, Barnett MJ, Shepherd JD, et al: High-dose cyclophosphamide, carmustine (BCNU), and etoposide (VP16-213) with or without cisplatin (CBV ± P) and autologous transplantation for patients with Hodgkin's disease who fail to enter a complete remission after combination chemotherapy. *Blood* 86:451, 1995.

351. Longo DL, Duffey PL, Young RC, et al: Conventional-dose salvage combination chemotherapy in patients relapsing with Hodgkin's disease after combination chemotherapy: The low probability for cure. *J Clin Oncol* 10:210, 1992.

352. Bierman PJ, Bagin RG, Jagannath S, et al: High dose chemotherapy followed by autologous hematopoietic rescue in Hodgkin's disease: Long-term follow-up in 128 patients. *Ann Oncol* 4:767, 1993.

353. Horning SJ, Chao NJ, Negrin RS, et al: High-dose therapy and autologous hematopoietic progenitor cell transplantation for recurrent or refractory Hodgkin's disease: Analysis of the Stanford University results and prognostic indices. *Blood* 89:801, 1997.

354. Wheeler C, Eickhoff C, Elias A, et al: High-dose cyclophosphamide, carmustine, and etoposide with autologous transplantation in Hodgkin's disease: A prognostic model for treatment outcomes. *Biol Blood Marrow Transplant* 3:98, 1997.

355. Yuen AR, Rosenberg SA, Hoppe RT, Halpern JD, Horning SJ: Comparison between conventional salvage therapy and high-dose therapy with

blood stem cell transplantation is effective in mantle cell lymphoma. *Leukemia* 10:1975, 1996.

autografting for recurrent or refractory Hodgkin's disease. *Blood* 89:814, 1997.

356. Linch DC, Winfield D, Goldstone AH, et al: Dose intensification with autologous bone-marrow transplantation in relapsed and resistant Hodgkin's disease: Results of a BNLI randomised trial. *Lancet* 341:1051, 1993.

357. Attal M, Hueguet F, Rubie H, et al: Prevention of hepatic veno-occlusive disease after bone marrow transplantation by continuous infusion of low-dose heparin: A prospective, randomized trial. *Blood* 79:2834, 1992.

358. Jagannath S, Vesole DH, Glenn L, Crowley J, Barlogie B: Low-risk intensive therapy for multiple myeloma with combined autologous bone marrow and blood stem cell support. *Blood* 80:1666, 1992.

359. Cunningham D, Paz-Ares L, Milan S, et al: High-dose melphalan and autologous bone marrow transplantation as consolidation in previously untreated myeloma. *J Clin Oncol* 12:759, 1994.

360. Harousseau JL, Attal M, Divine M, et al: Autologous stem cell transplantation after first remission induction treatment in multiple myeloma: A report of the French Registry on autologous transplantation in multiple myeloma. *Blood* 85:3077, 1995.

361. Marit G, Faberes C, Pico JL, et al: Autologous peripheral-blood progenitor-cell support following high-dose chemotherapy or chemoradiotherapy in patients with high-risk multiple myeloma. *J Clin Oncol* 14:1306, 1996.

362. Long GD, Chao NJ, Hu WW, et al: High dose etoposide-based myeloablative therapy followed by autologous blood progenitor cell rescue in the treatment of multiple myeloma. *Cancer* 78:2502, 1996.

363. Gianni AM, Tarella C, Bregni M, et al: High-dose sequential chemoradiotherapy, a widely applicable regimen, confers survival benefit to patients with high-risk multiple myeloma. *J Clin Oncol* 12:503, 1994.

364. Vesole DH, Tricot G, Jagannath S, et al: Autotransplants in multiple myeloma: What have we learned? *Blood* 88:838, 1996.

365. Barlogie B, Jagannath S, Vesole DH, et al: Superiority of tandem autologous transplantation over standard therapy for previously untreated multiple myeloma. *Blood* 89:789, 1997.

366. Barlogie B, Jagannath S, Desikan KR, et al: Total therapy with tandem transplants for newly diagnosed multiple myeloma. *Blood* 93:55, 1999.

367. Bladé J, San Miguel JF, Fontanillas M, et al: Survival of multiple myeloma patients who are potential candidates for early high-dose therapy intensification/autotransplantation and who were conventionally treated. *J Clin Oncol* 14:2167, 1996.

368. Alexanian R, Dimopoulos M, Smith T, et al: Limited value of myeloablative therapy for late multiple myeloma. *Blood* 83:512, 1994.

369. Alexanian R, Dimopoulos MA, Hester J, Delasalle K, Champlin R: Early myeloablative therapy for multiple myeloma. *Blood* 84:4278, 1994.

370. Attal M, Harousseau JL, Stoppa AM, et al: A prospective, randomized trial of autologous bone marrow transplantation and chemotherapy in multiple myeloma: Intergroupe Francais du Myelome. *N Engl J Med* 335:91, 1996.

371. Billadeau D, Quam L, Thomas W, et al: Detection and quantitation of malignant cells in the peripheral blood of multiple myeloma patients. *Blood* 80:1818, 1992.

372. Witzig TE, Gertz MA, Pineda AA, Kyle RA, Greipp PR: Detection of monoclonal plasma cells in the peripheral blood stem cell harvests of patients with multiple myeloma. *Br J Haematol* 89:640, 1995.

373. Bird JM, Bloxham D, Samson D, et al: Molecular detection of clonally rearranged cells in peripheral blood progenitor cell harvests from multiple myeloma patients. *Br J Haematol* 88:110, 1994.

374. Anderson KC, Andersen J, Soiffer R, et al: Monoclonal antibody-purged bone marrow transplantation therapy for multiple myeloma. *Blood* 82:2568, 1993.

375. Vescio R, Schiller G, Stewart AK, et al: Multicenter phase III trial to evaluate CD34+ selected versus unselected autologous peripheral blood progenitor cell transplantation in multiple myeloma. *Blood* 93:1858, 1999.

376. Cunningham D, Powles R, Malpas J, et al: A randomized trial of maintenance interferon following high-dose chemotherapy in multiple myeloma: Long-term follow-up results. *Br J Haematol* 102:495, 1998.

377. Kwak LW, Taub DD, Duffey PL, et al: Transfer of myeloma idiotype-specific immunity from an actively immunised marrow donor. *Lancet* 345:1016, 1995.

378. Reichardt VL, Okada CY, Liso A, et al: Idiotype vaccination using

dendritic cells after autologous peripheral blood stem cell transplantation for multiple myeloma: A feasibility study. *Blood* 93:2411, 1999.

379. Tricot G, Vesole DH, Jagannath S, et al: Graft-versus-myeloma effect: proof of principle. *Blood* 87:1196, 1996.

380. Gahrton G, Tura S, Ljungman P, et al: Allogeneic bone marrow transplantation in multiple myeloma; European Group for Bone Marrow Transplantation. *N Engl J Med* 325:1267, 1991.

381. Bensinger WI, Buckner CD, Anasetti C, et al: Allogeneic marrow transplantation for multiple myeloma: An analysis of risk factors on outcome. *Blood* 88:2787, 1996.

382. Björkstrand BB, Ljungman P, Svensson H, et al: Allogeneic bone marrow transplantation versus autologous stem cell transplantation in multiple myeloma: A retrospective case-matched study from the European Group for Blood and Marrow Transplantation. *Blood* 88:4711, 1996.

383. Peters WP, Shpall EJ, Jones RB, et al: High-dose combination alkylating agents with bone marrow support as initial treatment for metastatic breast cancer. *J Clin Oncol* 6:1368, 1988.

384. Williams SF, Mick R, Desser R, et al: High-dose consolidation therapy with autologous stem cell rescue in stage IV breast cancer. *J Clin Oncol* 7:1824, 1989.

385. Dunphy FR, Spitzer G, Buzdar AU, et al: Treatment of estrogen receptor-negative or hormonally refractory breast cancer with double high-dose chemotherapy intensification and bone marrow support. *J Clin Oncol* 8:1207, 1990.

386. Antman KH, Rowlings PA, Vaughan WP, et al: High-dose chemotherapy with autologous hematopoietic stem-cell support for breast cancer in North America. *J Clin Oncol* 15:1870, 1997.

387. Bezwoda WR, Seymour L, Dansey RD: High-dose chemotherapy with hematopoietic rescue as primary treatment for metastatic breast cancer: A randomized trial. *J Clin Oncol* 13:2483, 1995.

388. Eibl B, Schwaighofer H, Nachbaur D, et al: Evidence for a graft-versus-tumor effect in a patient treated with marrow ablative chemotherapy and allogeneic bone marrow transplantation for breast cancer. *Blood* 88:1501, 1996.

389. Bearman SI, Overmoyer BA, Bolwell BJ, et al: High-dose chemotherapy with autologous peripheral blood progenitor cell support for primary breast cancer in patients with 4–9 involved axillary lymph nodes. *Bone Marrow Transplant* 20:931, 1997.

390. Stiff PJ, Bayer R, Kerger C, et al: High-dose chemotherapy with autologous transplantation for persistent/relapsed ovarian cancer: A multivariate analysis of survival for 100 consecutively treated patients. *J Clin Oncol* 15:1309, 1997.

391. Holmberg LA, Demirer T, Rowley S, et al: High-dose busulfan, melphalan and thiotepa followed by autologous peripheral blood stem cell (PBSC) rescue in patients with advanced stage III/IV ovarian cancer. *Bone Marrow Transplant* 22:651, 1998.

392. Broun ER, Nichols CR, Kneebone P, et al: Long-term outcome of patients with relapsed and refractory germ cell tumors treated with high-dose chemotherapy and autologous bone marrow rescue. *Ann Intern Med* 117:124, 1992.

393. Mandanas RA, Saez RA, Epstein RB, Confer DL, Selby GB: Long-term results of autologous marrow transplantation for relapsed or refractory male or female germ cell tumors. *Bone Marrow Transplant* 21:569, 1998.

394. Dini G, Lanino E, Garaventa A, et al: Myeloablative therapy and unpurged autologous bone marrow transplantation for poor-prognosis neuroblastoma: Report of 34 cases. *J Clin Oncol* 9:962, 1991.

395. Stram DO, Matthay KK, O'Leary M, et al: Consolidation chemoradiotherapy and autologous bone marrow transplantation versus continued chemotherapy for metastatic neuroblastoma: A report of two concurrent Children's Cancer Group studies. *J Clin Oncol* 14:2417, 1996.

396. Matthay KK, Seeger RC, Reynolds CP, et al: Allogeneic versus autologous purged bone marrow transplantation for neuroblastoma: A report from the Children's Cancer Group. *J Clin Oncol* 12:2382, 1994.

397. Ladenstein R, Philip T, Lasset C, et al: Multivariate analysis of risk factors in stage 4 neuroblastoma patients over the age of one year treated with megatherapy and stem-cell transplantation: A report from the European Bone Marrow Transplantation Solid Tumor Registry. *J Clin Oncol* 16:953, 1998.

398. Handgretinger R, Greil J, Schürmann U, et al: Positive selection and transplantation of peripheral CD34+ progenitor cells: Feasibility and

purging efficacy in pediatric patients with neuroblastoma. *J Hematother* 6:235, 1997.

399. Gluckman E, Berger R, Dutreix J: Bone marrow transplantation for Fanconi anemia. *Semin Hematol* 21:20, 1984.

400. Flowers ME, Doney KC, Storb R, et al: Marrow transplantation for Fanconi anemia with or without leukemic transformation: An update of the Seattle experience. *Bone Marrow Transplant* 9:167, 1992.

401. Socié G, Devergie A, Girinski T, et al: Transplantation for Fanconi's anaemia: Long-term follow-up of fifty patients transplanted from a sibling donor after low-dose cyclophosphamide and thoraco-abdominal irradiation for conditioning. *Br J Haematol* 103:249, 1998.

402. Flowers ME, Zanis J, Pasquini R, et al: Marrow transplantation for Fanconi anaemia: Conditioning with reduced doses of cyclophosphamide without radiation. *Br J Haematol* 92:699, 1996.

403. Lucarelli G, Galimberti M, Polchi P, et al: Bone marrow transplantation in patients with thalassemia. *N Engl J Med* 322:417, 1990.

404. Lucarelli G, Galimberti M, Polchi P, et al: Bone marrow transplantation in adult thalassemia. *Blood* 80:1603, 1992.

405. Lucarelli G, Clift RA, Galimberti M, et al: Bone marrow transplantation in adult thalassemic patients. *Blood* 93:1164, 1999.

406. Johnson FL, Look AT, Gockerman J, et al: Bone-marrow transplantation in a patient with sickle-cell anemia. *N Engl J Med* 311:780, 1984.

407. Walters MC, Patience M, Leisenring W, et al: Bone marrow transplantation for sickle cell disease. *N Engl J Med* 335:369, 1996.

408. Walters MC, Patience M, Leisenring W, et al: Barriers to bone marrow transplantation for sickle cell anemia. *Biol Blood Marrow Transplant* 2:100, 1996.

409. Vermylen C, Cornu G, Ferster A, et al: Haematopoietic stem cell transplantation for sickle cell anaemia: The first 50 patients transplanted in Belgium. *Bone Marrow Transplant* 22:1, 1998.

410. Lenarsky C, Parkman R: Bone marrow transplantation for the treatment of immune deficiency states. *Bone Marrow Transplant* 6:361, 1990.

411. O'Reilly RJ, Dupont B, Pahwa S, et al: Reconstitution in severe combined immunodeficiency by transplantation of marrow from an unrelated donor. *N Engl J Med* 297:1311, 1977.

412. Filipovich AH, Shapiro RS, Ramsay NK, et al: Unrelated donor bone marrow transplantation for correction of lethal congenital immunodeficiencies. *Blood* 80:270, 1992.

413. Haddad E, Landais P, Friedrich W, et al: Long-term immune reconstitution and outcome after HLA-nonidentical T-cell-depleted bone marrow transplantation for severe combined immunodeficiency: A European retrospective study of 116 patients. *Blood* 91:3646, 1998.

414. Parkman R: The application of bone marrow transplantation to the treatment of genetic diseases. *Science* 232:1373, 1986.

415. Peters C, Shapiro EG, Anderson J, et al: Hurler syndrome: II. Outcome of HLA-genotypically identical sibling and HLA-haploidentical related donor bone marrow transplantation in fifty-four children: The Storage Disease Collaborative Study Group. *Blood* 91:2601, 1998.

416. Eapen M, Davies SM, Ramsay NK, Orchard PJ: Hematopoietic stem cell transplantation for infantile osteopetrosis. *Bone Marrow Transplant* 22:941, 1998.

417. Tezcan I, Xu W, Gurgey A, et al: Congenital erythropoietic porphyria successfully treated by allogeneic bone marrow transplantation. *Blood* 92:4053, 1998.

418. Euler HH, Marmont AM, Bacigalupo A, et al: Early recurrence or persistence of autoimmune diseases after unmanipulated autologous stem cell transplantation. *Blood* 88:3621, 1996.

419. Fassas A, Anagnostopoulos A, Kazis A, et al: Peripheral blood stem cell transplantation in the treatment of progressive multiple sclerosis: first results of a pilot study. *Bone Marrow Transplant* 20:631, 1997.

420. Burt RK, Traynor AE, Pope R, et al: Treatment of autoimmune disease by intense immunosuppressive conditioning and autologous hematopoietic stem cell transplantation. *Blood* 92:3505, 1998.

421. Billingham RE: The biology of graft-versus-host reactions. *Harvey Lect* 62:21, 1966.

422. Storb R, Deeg HJ, Whitehead J, et al: Methotrexate and cyclosporine compared with cyclosporine alone for prophylaxis of acute graft versus host disease after marrow transplantation for leukemia. *N Engl J Med* 314:729, 1986.

423. Storb R, Deeg HJ, Farewell V, et al: Marrow transplantation for severe aplastic anemia: Methotrexate alone compared with a combination of

424. Storb R, Pepe M, Deeg HJ, et al: Long-term follow-up of a controlled trial comparing a combination of methotrexate plus cyclosporine with cyclosporine alone for prophylaxis of graft-versus-host disease in patients administered HLA-identical marrow grafts for leukemia [letter]. *Blood* 80:560, 1992.

425. Forman SJ, Blume KG, Krance RA, et al: A prospective randomized study of acute graft-v-host disease in 107 patients with leukemia: Methotrexate/prednisone v. cyclosporine A/prednisone. *Transplant Proc* 19:2605, 1987.

426. Chao NJ, Schmidt GM, Niland JC, et al: Cyclosporine, methotrexate, and prednisone compared with cyclosporine and prednisone for prophylaxis of acute graft-versus-host disease. *N Engl J Med* 329:1225, 1993.

427. Ross M, Forman SJ, Wong RM, et al: A prospective randomized trial comparing cyclosporine-A and prednisone (CSA/PSE) versus cyclosporine-A, methotrexate and prednisone (CSA/MTX/PSE) for the prevention of acute graft-versus-host disease: Effect on chronic graft-versus-host disease and long term survival. *Blood* 90(suppl 1):590a, 1997.

428. Ratanatharathorn V, Nash RA, Przepiorka D, et al: Phase III study comparing methotrexate and tacrolimus (prograf, FK506) with methotrexate and cyclosporine for graft-versus-host disease prophylaxis after HLA-identical sibling bone marrow transplantation. *Blood* 92:2303, 1998.

429. Nash RA, Piñeiro LA, Storb R, et al: FK506 in combination with methotrexate for the prevention of graft-versus-host disease after marrow transplantation from matched unrelated donors. *Blood* 88:3634, 1996.

430. Devine SM, Geller RB, Lin LB, et al: The outcome of unrelated donor bone marrow transplantation in patients with hematologic malignancies using tacrolimus (FK506) and low dose methotrexate for graft-versus-host disease prophylaxis. *Biol Blood Marrow Transplant* 3:25, 1997.

431. Hiroka A: Results of a phase III study on prophylactic use of FK506 for acute GVHD compared with cyclosporin in allogeneic bone marrow transplantation. *Blood* 90(suppl 1):561a, 1997.

432. Filipovich AH, Vallera DA, Youle RJ, et al: Ex-vivo treatment of donor bone marrow with anti-T-cell immunotoxins for prevention of graft-versus-host disease. *Lancet* 1:469, 1984.

433. Prentice HG, Blacklock HA, Janossy G, et al: Use of anti-T-cell monoclonal antibody OKT3 to prevent acute graft-versus-host disease in allogeneic bone-marrow transplantation for acute leukaemia. *Lancet* 1:700, 1982.

434. Kernan NA, Flomenberg N, Dupont B, O'Reilly RJ: Graft rejection in recipients of T-cell-depleted HLA-nonidentical marrow transplants for leukemia: Identification of host-derived antidonor allocytotoxic T lymphocytes. *Transplantation* 43:842, 1987.

435. Racadot E, Hervé P, Beaujean F, et al: Prevention of graft-versus-host disease in HLA-matched bone marrow transplantation for malignant diseases: A multicentric study of 62 patients using 3-pan-T monoclonal antibodies and rabbit complement. *J Clin Oncol* 5:426, 1987.

436. Papadopoulos EB, Carabasi MH, Castro-Malaspina H, et al: T-cell-depleted allogeneic bone marrow transplantation as postremission therapy for acute myelogenous leukemia: Freedom from relapse in the absence of graft-versus-host disease. *Blood* 91:1083, 1998.

437. Hervé P, Cahn JY, Flesch M, et al: Successful graft-versus-host disease prevention without graft failure in 32 HLA-identical allogeneic bone marrow transplantations with marrow depleted of T cells by monoclonal antibodies and complement. *Blood* 69:388, 1987.

438. Champlin R, Ho W, Gajewski J, et al: Selective depletion of CD8+ T lymphocytes for prevention of graft-versus-host disease after allogeneic bone marrow transplantation. *Blood* 76:418, 1990.

439. Soiffer RJ, Murray C, Mauch P, et al: Prevention of graft-versus-host disease by selective depletion of CD6-positive T lymphocytes from donor bone marrow. *J Clin Oncol* 10:1191, 1992.

440. Small TN, Avigan D, Dupont B, et al: Immune reconstitution following T-cell depleted bone marrow transplantation: Effect of age and posttransplant graft rejection prophylaxis. *Biol Blood Marrow Transplant* 3:65, 1997.

441. Hale G, Zhang MJ, Bunjes D, et al: Improving the outcome of bone marrow transplantation by using CD52 monoclonal antibodies to prevent graft-versus-host disease and graft rejection. *Blood* 92:4581, 1998.

442. Soiffer RJ, Mauch P, Fairclough D, et al: CD6+ T cell depleted alloge-

neic bone marrow transplantation from genotypically HLA nonidentical related donors. *Biol Blood Marrow Transplant* 3:11, 1997.

443. Van Lint MT, Uderzo C, Locasciulli A, et al: Early treatment of acute graft-versus-host disease with high- or low-dose 6-methylprednisolone: A multicenter randomized trial from the Italian Group for Bone Marrow Transplantation. *Blood* 92:2288, 1998.

444. Hervé P, Wijdenes J, Bergerat JP, et al: Treatment of corticosteroid resistant acute graft-versus-host disease by in vivo administration of anti-interleukin-2 receptor monoclonal antibody (B-B10). *Blood* 75:1017, 1990.

445. Hervé P, Flesch M, Tiberghien P, et al: Phase I-II trial of a monoclonal anti-tumor necrosis factor alpha antibody for the treatment of refractory severe acute graft-versus-host disease. *Blood* 79:3362, 1992.

446. Basara N, Blau WI, Römer E, et al: Mycophenolate mofetil for the treatment of acute and chronic GVHD in bone marrow transplant patients. *Bone Marrow Transplant* 22:61, 1998.

447. Shulman HM, Sale GE, Lerner KG, et al: Chronic cutaneous graft-versus-host disease in man. *Am J Pathol* 91:545, 1978.

448. Shulman HM, Sullivan KM, Weiden PL, et al: Chronic graft-versus-host syndrome in man: A long-term clinicopathologic study of 20 Seattle patients. *Am J Med* 69:204, 1980.

449. Wingard JR, Piantadosi S, Vogelsang GB, et al: Predictors of death from chronic graft-versus-host disease after bone marrow transplantation. *Blood* 74:1428, 1989.

450. Sullivan KM, Shulman HM, Storb R, et al: Chronic graft-versus-host disease in 52 patients: adverse natural course and successful treatment with combination immunosuppression. *Blood* 57:267, 1981.

451. Sullivan KM, Witherspoon RP, Storb R, et al: Alternating-day cyclosporine and prednisone for treatment of high-risk chronic graft-v-host disease. *Blood* 72:555, 1988.

452. Vogelsang GB, Farmer ER, Hess AD, et al: Thalidomide for the treatment of chronic graft-versus-host disease. *N Engl J Med* 326:1055, 1992.

453. Parker PM, Chao N, Nademanee A, et al: Thalidomide as salvage therapy for chronic graft-versus-host disease. *Blood* 86:3604, 1995.

454. Cole CH, Rogers PC, Pritchard S, Phillips G, Chan KW: Thalidomide in the management of chronic graft-versus-host disease in children following bone marrow transplantation. *Bone Marrow Transplant* 14:937, 1994.

455. Rovelli A, Arrigo C, Nesi F, et al: The role of thalidomide in the treatment of refractory chronic graft-versus-host disease following bone marrow transplantation in children. *Bone Marrow Transplant* 21:577, 1998.

456. Chao NJ, Parker PM, Niland JC, et al: Paradoxical effect of thalidomide prophylaxis on chronic graft-vs.-host disease. *Biol Blood Marrow Transplant* 2:86, 1996.

457. Kapoor N, Pelligrini AE, Copelan EA, et al: Psoralen plus ultraviolet A (PUVA) in the treatment of chronic graft versus host disease: Preliminary experience in standard treatment resistant patients. *Semin Hematol* 29:108, 1992.

458. Marcellus DC, Altomonte VL, Farmer ER, et al: Etretinate therapy for refractory sclerodermatous chronic graft-versus-host disease. *Blood* 93:66, 1999.

459. Socie G, Devergie A, Cosset JM, et al: Low-dose (one gray) total-lymphoid irradiation for extensive, drug-resistant chronic graft-versus-host disease. *Transplantation* 49:657, 1990.

460. McDonald GB, Hinds MS, Fisher LD: Veno-occlusive disease of the liver and multiorgan failure after bone marrow transplantation: A cohort study of 355 patients. *Ann Intern Med* 118:255, 1993.

461. Bearman SI: The syndrome of hepatic veno-occlusive disease after marrow transplantation. *Blood* 85:3005, 1995.

462. Salat C, Holler E, Kolb HJ, et al: Plasminogen activator inhibitor-1 confirms the diagnosis of hepatic veno-occlusive disease in patients with hyperbilirubinemia after bone marrow transplantation. *Blood* 89:2184, 1997.

463. Rozman C, Carreras E, Qian C, et al: Risk factors for hepatic veno-occlusive disease following HLA-identical sibling bone marrow transplants for leukemia. *Bone Marrow Transplant* 17:75, 1996.

464. Locasciulli A, Alberti A, Bandini G, et al: Allogeneic bone marrow transplantation from HBsAg7+ donors: A multicenter study from the Gruppo Italiano Trapianto di Midollo Osseo (GITMO). *Blood* 86:3236, 1995.

465. Dix SP, Wingard JR, Mullins RE, et al: Association of busulfan area

under the curve with veno-occlusive disease following BMT. *Bone Marrow Transplant* 17:225, 1996.

466. Bearman SI, Anderson GL, Mori M, et al: Venoocclusive disease of the liver: Development of a model for predicting fatal outcome after marrow transplantation. *J Clin Oncol* 11:1729, 1993.

467. Bearman SI, Shuhart MC, Hinds MS, et al: Recombinant human tissue plasminogen activator for the treatment of established veno-occlusive disease of the liver after bone marrow transplantation. *Blood* 80:2458, 1992.

468. Leahey AM, Bunin NJ: Recombinant human tissue plasminogen activator for the treatment of severe hepatic veno-occlusive disease in pediatric bone marrow transplant patients. *Bone Marrow Transplant* 17:1101, 1996.

469. Bearman SI, Lee JL, Baron AE, McDonald GB: Treatment of hepatic venoocclusive disease with recombinant human tissue plasminogen activator and heparin in 42 marrow transplant patients. *Blood* 89:1501, 1997.

470. Haaglund H, Ringden O, Ericzon BG, et al: Treatment of hepatic venoocclusive disease with recombinant human tissue plasminogen activator or orthotopic liver transplantation after allogeneic bone marrow transplantation. *Transplantation* 62:1076, 1996.

471. Bacher P, Kindel G, Walenga JM, Fareed J: Modulation of endothelial and platelet function by a polydeoxyribonucleotide derived drug "defibrotide": A dual mechanism in the control of vascular pathology. *Thromb Res* 70:343, 1993.

472. Richardson PG, Elias AD, Krishnan A, et al: Treatment of severe veno-occlusive disease with defibrotide: Compassionate use results in response without significant toxicity in a high-risk population. *Blood* 92:737, 1998.

473. Morris JD, Harris RE, Hashmi R, et al: Antithrombin-III for the treatment of chemotherapy-induced organ dysfunction following bone marrow transplantation. *Bone Marrow Transplant* 20:871, 1997.

474. Levy V, Azoulay D, Rio B, et al: Succesful treatment of severe hepatic veno-occlusive disease after allogeneic bone marrow transplantation by transjugular intrahepatic portosystemic stent-shunt (TIPS). *Bone Marrow Transplant* 18:443, 1996.

475. Rosen HR, Martin P, Schiller GJ, et al: Orthotopic liver transplantation for bone-marrow transplant-associated veno-occlusive disease and graft-versus-host disease of the liver. *Liver Transplant Surg* 2:225, 1996.

476. Essell JH, Thompson JM, Harman GS, et al: Pilot trial of prophylactic ursodiol to decrease the incidence of veno-occlusive disease of the liver in allogeneic bone marrow transplant patients. *Bone Marrow Transplant* 10:367, 1992.

477. Essell JH, Schroeder MT, Harman GS, et al: Ursodiol prophylaxis against hepatic complications of allogeneic bone marrow transplantation: A randomized, double-blind, placebo-controlled trial. *Ann Intern Med* 128:975, 1998.

478. Attal M, Huguet F, Schlaifer D, et al: Intensive combined therapy for previously untreated aggressive myeloma. *Blood* 79:1130, 1992.

479. Hagglund H, Remberger M, Klaesson S, et al: Norethisterone treatment, a major risk-factor for veno-occlusive disease in the liver after allogeneic bone marrow transplantation. *Blood* 92:4568, 1998.

480. Rosenthal J, Sender L, Secola R, et al: Phase II trial of heparin prophylaxis for veno-occlusive disease of the liver in children undergoing bone marrow transplantation. *Bone Marrow Transplant* 18:185, 1996.

481. Marsa-Vila L, Gorin NC, Laporte JP, et al: Prophylactic heparin does not prevent liver veno-occlusive disease following autologous bone marrow transplantation. *Eur J Haematol* 47:346, 1991.

482. Carreras E, Bertz H, Arcese W, et al: Incidence and outcome of hepatic veno-occlusive disease after blood or marrow transplantation: a prospective cohort study of the European Group for Blood and Marrow Transplantation: European Group for Blood and Marrow Transplantation Chronic Leukemia Working Party. *Blood* 92:3599, 1998.

483. Or R, Nagler A, Shpilberg O, et al: Low molecular weight heparin for the prevention of veno-occlusive disease of the liver in bone marrow transplantation patients. *Transplantation* 61:1067, 1996.

484. Bearman SI, Appelbaum FR, Buckner CD, et al: Regimen-related toxicity in patients undergoing bone marrow transplantation. *J Clin Oncol* 6:1562, 1988.

485. Wingard JR, Sostrin MB, Vriesendorp HM, et al: Interstitial pneumonitis following autologous bone marrow transplantation. *Transplantation* 46:61, 1988.

486. Pecego R, Hill R, Appelbaum FR, et al: Interstitial pneumonitis following autologous bone marrow transplantation. *Transplantation* 42:515, 1986.

487. Seiden MV, Elias A, Ayash L, et al: Pulmonary toxicity associated with high dose chemotherapy in the treatment of solid tumors with autologous marrow transplant: An analysis of four chemotherapy regimens. *Bone Marrow Transplant* 10:57, 1992.

488. Robbins RA, Linder J, Stahl MG, et al: Diffuse alveolar hemorrhage in autologous bone marrow transplant recipients. *Am J Med* 87:511, 1989.

489. Chao NJ, Duncan SR, Long GD, Horning SJ, Blume KG: Corticosteroid therapy for diffuse alveolar hemorrhage in autologous bone marrow transplant recipients. *Ann Intern Med* 114:145, 1991.

490. Cazin B, Gorin NC, Laporte JP, et al: Cardiac complications after bone marrow transplantation: A report on a series of 63 consecutive transplantations. *Cancer* 57:2061, 1986.

491. Trigg ME, Finlay JL, Bozdech M, Gilbert E: Fatal cardiac toxicity in bone marrow transplant patients receiving cytosine arabinoside, cyclophosphamide, and total body irradiation. *Cancer* 59:38, 1987.

492. Hertenstein B, Stefanic M, Schmeiser T, et al: Cardiac toxicity of bone marrow transplantation: Predictive value of cardiologic evaluation before transplant. *J Clin Oncol* 12:998, 1994.

493. Braverman AC, Antin JH, Plappert MT, Cook EF, Lee RT: Cyclophosphamide cardiotoxicity in bone marrow transplantation: A prospective evaluation of new dosing regimens. *J Clin Oncol* 9:1215, 1991.

494. Reece DE, Frei-Lahr DA, Shepard JD, et al: Neurologic complications in allogeneic bone marrow transplant patients receiving cyclosporin. *Bone Marrow Transplant* 8:393, 1991.

495. Palmer BF, Toto RD: Severe neurologic toxicity induced by cyclosporine A in three renal transplant patients. *Am J Kidney Dis* 18:116, 1991.

496. Lipton JH, Virro M, Solow H: Successful pregnancy after allogeneic bone marrow transplant with embryos isolated before transplant. *J Clin Oncol* 15:3347, 1997.

497. Schubert MA, Sullivan KM, Schubert MM, et al: Gynecological abnormalities following allogeneic bone marrow transplantation. *Bone Marrow Transplant* 5:425, 1990.

498. Sanders JE, Pritchard S, Mahoney P, et al: Growth and development following marrow transplantation for leukemia. *Blood* 68:1129, 1986.

499. Sklar CA, Kim TH, Ramsay NK: Thyroid dysfunction among long-term survivors of bone marrow transplantation. *Am J Med* 73:688, 1982.

500. Tichelli A, Gratwohl A, Egger T, et al: Cataract formation after bone marrow transplantation. *Ann Intern Med* 119:1175, 1993.

501. van der Lelie H, Baars JW, Rodenhuis S, et al: Hemolytic uremic syndrome after high dose chemotherapy with autologous stem cell support. *Cancer* 76:2338, 1995.

502. Miller JS, Arthur DC, Litz CE, et al: Myelodysplastic syndrome after autologous bone marrow transplantation: an additional late complication of curative cancer therapy. *Blood* 83:3780, 1994.

503. Stone RM, Neuberg D, Soiffer R, et al: Myelodysplastic syndrome as a late complication following autologous bone marrow transplantation for non-Hodgkin's lymphoma. *J Clin Oncol* 12:2535, 1994.

504. Bhatia S, Ramsay NK, Steinbuch M, et al: Malignant neoplasms following bone marrow transplantation. *Blood* 87:3633, 1996.

505. André M, Henry-Amar M, Blaise D, et al: Treatment-related deaths and second cancer risk after autologous stem-cell transplantation for Hodgkin's disease. *Blood* 92:1933, 1998.

506. Chao NJ, Nademanee AP, Long GD, et al: Importance of bone marrow cytogenetic evaluation before autologous bone marrow transplantation for Hodgkin's disease. *J Clin Oncol* 9:1575, 1991.

507. Govindarajan R, Jagannath S, Flick JT, et al: Preceding standard therapy is the likely cause of MDS after autotransplants for multiple myeloma. *Br J Haematol* 95:349, 1996.

508. Lowsky R, Lipton J, Fyles G, et al: Secondary malignancies after bone marrow transplantation in adults. *J Clin Oncol* 12:2187, 1994.

509. Curtis RE, Rowlings PA, Deeg HJ, et al: Solid cancers after bone marrow transplantation. *N Engl J Med* 336:897, 1997.

510. Mansi JL, Cunningham D, Viner C, et al: Repeat administration of high dose melphalan in relapsed myeloma. *Br J Cancer* 68:983, 1993.

511. Sanders JE, Buckner CD, Clift RA, et al: Second marrow transplants in patients with leukemia who relapse after allogeneic marrow transplantation. *Bone Marrow Transplant* 3:11, 1988.

512. Wagner JE, Vogelsang GB, Zehnbauer BA, et al: Relapse of leukemia after bone marrow transplantation: effect of second myeloablative therapy. *Bone Marrow Transplant* 9:205, 1992.

513. Mrsíc M, Horowitz MM, Atkinson K, et al: Second HLA-identical sibling transplants for leukemia recurrence. *Bone Marrow Transplant* 9:269, 1992.

514. Kishi K, Takahashi S, Gondo H, et al: Second allogeneic bone marrow transplantation for post-transplant leukemia relapse: results of a survey of 66 cases in 24 Japanese institutes. *Bone Marrow Transplant* 19:461, 1997.

515. Jenkins MK: The ups and downs of T cell costimulation. *Immunity* 1:443, 1994.

516. Hart DNJ: Dendritic cells: Unique leukocyte populations which control the primary immune response. *Blood* 90:3245, 1997.

517. Karre K: Express yourself or die: Peptides, MHC molecules, and NK cells. *Science* 267:978, 1995.

518. Liu CC, Walsh CM, Young JD: Perforin: Structure and function. *Immunol Today* 16:194, 1995.

519. Henkart PA: Lymphocyte-mediated cytotoxicity: Two pathways and multiple effector molecules. *Immunity* 1:343, 1994.

520. Hahne M, Rimoldi D, Schroter M, et al: Melanoma cell expression of fas (Apo-1/CD95) ligand: implications for tumor immune escape. *Science* 274:1363, 1996.

521. Walker PR, Saas P, Dietrich PY: Role of fas ligand (CD95) in immune escape: The tumor cell strikes back. *J Immunol* 158:4521, 1997.

522. Lu PH, Negrin RS: Cellular immunotherapy following autologous hematopoietic progenitor cell transplantation. *Biol Blood Marrow Transplant* 3:113, 1997.

523. Welte KG, Ciobanu N, Moore MAS, et al: Defective interleukin-2 production in patients after bone marrow transplantation and in vitro restoration of defective T lymphocyte proliferation by highly purified interleukin-2. *Blood* 64:380, 1984.

524. Cayeux S, Meuer S, Pezzutto A, et al: T-cell ontogeny after autologous bone marrow transplantation: Failure to synthesize interleukin-2 (IL-2) and lack of CD2- and CD3-mediated proliferation by both CD4- and CD8+ cells even in the presence of exogeneous IL-2. *Blood* 74:2270, 1989.

525. Higuchi CM, Thompson JA, Petersen FB, Buckner CD, Fefer A: Toxicity and immunomodulatory effects of interleukin-2 after autologous bone marrow transplantation for hematologic malignancies. *Blood* 77:2561, 1991.

526. Bosly A, Guillaume T, Brice P, et al: Effects of escalating doses of recombinant human interleukin-2 in correcting functional T-cell defects following autologous bone marrow transplantation for lymphomas and solid tumors. *Exp Hematol* 20:962, 1992.

527. Benyunes MC, Massumoto C, York A, et al: Interleukin-2 with or without lymphokine-activated killer cells as consolidative immunotherapy after autologous bone marrow transplantation for acute myelogenous leukemia. *Bone Marrow Transplant* 12:159, 1993.

528. Hamon MD, Prentice HG, Gottlieb DJ, et al: Immunotherapy with interleukin 2 after ABMT in AML. *Bone Marrow Transplant* 11:399, 1993.

529. Nagler A, Ackerstein A, Or R, Naparstek E, Slavin S: Immunotherapy with recombinant human interleukin-2 and recombinant interferon-alpha in lymphoma patients postautologous marrow or stem cell transplantation. *Blood* 89:3951, 1997.

530. Attal M, Blaise D, Marit G, et al: Consolidation treatment of adult acute lymphoblastic leukemia: A prospective, randomized trial comparing allogeneic versus autologous bone marrow transplantation and testing the impact of recombinant interleukin-2 after autologous bone marrow transplantation. *Blood* 86:1619, 1995.

531. Drobyski WR, Keever CA, Roth MS, et al: Salvage immunotherapy using donor leukocyte infusions as treatment for relapsed chronic myelogenous leukemia after allogeneic bone marrow transplantation: Efficacy and toxicity of a defined T-cell dose. *Blood* 82:2310, 1993.

532. Porter DL, Roth MS, McGarigle C, Ferrara JL, Antin JH: Induction of graft-versus-host disease as immunotherapy for relapsed chronic myeloid leukemia. *N Engl J Med* 330:100, 1994.

533. Slavin S, Naparstek E, Nagler A, et al: Allogeneic cell therapy with donor peripheral blood cells and recombinant human interleukin-2 to treat leukemia relapse after allogeneic bone marrow transplantation. *Blood* 87:2195, 1996.

534. Mackinnon S, Papdopoulos EB, Carabasi MH, et al: Adoptive immunotherapy evaluating escalating doses of donor leukocytes for relapse of

chronic myeloid leukemia after bone marrow transplantation. *Blood* 86:1261, 1995.

535. Alyea EP, Soiffer RJ, Canning C, et al: Toxicity and efficacy of defined doses of CD4+ donor lymphocytes for treatment of relapse after allogeneic bone marrow transplant. *Blood* 91:3671, 1998.

536. Bonini C, Ferrari G, Verzeletti S, et al: HSV-TK gene transfer into donor lymphocytes for control of allogeneic graft-versus-leukemia. *Science* 276:1719, 1997.

537. Keil F, Haas OA, Fritsch G, et al: Donor leukocyte infusion for leukemic relapse after allogeneic marrow transplantation: Lack of residual donor hematopoiesis predicts aplasia. *Blood* 89:3113, 1997.

538. Higano CS, Chielens D, Raskind W, et al: Use of alpha-2a-interferon to treat cytogenetic relapse of chronic myeloid leukemia after marrow transplantation. *Blood* 90:2549, 1997.

539. Elmaagacli AH, Beelen DW, Schaefer UW: A retrospective single centre study of the outcome of five different therapy approaches in 48 patients with relapse of chronic myelogenous leukemia after allogeneic bone marrow transplantation. *Bone Marrow Transplant* 20:1045, 1997.

540. Rooney CM, Smith CA, Ng CYC, et al: Use of gene-modified virus-specific T lymphocytes to control Epstein-Barr-virus related lymphoproliferation. *Lancet* 345:9, 1995.

541. Heslop HE, Ng CY, Li C, et al: Long-term restoration of immunity against Epstein-Barr virus infection by adoptive transfer of gene-modified virus-specific T lymphocytes. *Nature Med* 2:551, 1996.

542. Rooney CM, Smith CA, Ng CY, et al: Infusion of cytotoxic T cells for the prevention and treatment of Epstein-Barr virus-induced lymphoma in allogeneic transplant recipients. *Blood* 92:1549, 1998.

543. Linehan DC, Goedegebuure PS, Peoples GE, Rogers SO, Eberlein TJ: Tumor-specific and HLA-A2-restricted cytolysis by tumor-associated lymphocytes in human metastatic breast cancer. *J Immunol* 155:4486, 1995.

544. Faber LM, van Luxemburg-Heijs SAP, Willemze R, Falkenburg JHE: Generation of leukemia-reactive cytotoxic T lymphocyte clones from the HLA-identical bone marrow donor of a patient with leukemia. *J Exp Med* 176:1283, 1992.

545. Faber LM, van der Hoeven J, Goulmy E, et al: Recognition of clonogenic leukemic cells, remission bone marrow and HLA-identical bone marrow by CD8+ or CD4+ minor histocompatibility antigen-specific cytotoxic T lymphocytes. *J Clin Invest* 96:877, 1995.

546. Schmidt-Wolf IGH, Negrin RS, Kiem HP, Blume KG, Weissman IL: Use of a SCID mouse/human lymphoma model to evaluate cytokine-induced killer cells with potent antitumor cell activity. *J Exp Med* 174:139, 1991.

547. Schmidt-Wolf IG, Lefterova P, Mehta BA, et al: Phenotypic characterization and identification of effector cells involved in tumor cell recognition of cytokine-induced killer cells. *Exp Hematol* 21:1673, 1993.

548. Lu PH, Negrin RS: A novel population of expanded human CD3+CD56+ cells derived from T cells with potent in vivo antitumor activity in mice with severe combined immunodeficiency. *J Immunol* 153:1687, 1994.

549. Hsu FJ, Benike C, Fagnoni F, et al: Vaccination of patients with B-cell lymphoma using autologous antigen-pulsed dendritic cells. *Nature Med* 2:52, 1996.

550. Engleman EG: Dendritic cells in the treatment of cancer [editorial]. *Biol Blood Marrow Transplant* 2:115, 1996.

551. Geller RB, Esa AH, Beschorner WE, et al: Successful in vitro graft-versus-tumor effect against an Ia-bearing tumor using cyclosporine-induced syngeneic graft-versus-host disease in the rat. *Blood* 74:1165, 1989.

552. Jones RJ, Vogelsang GB, Ambinder RF, et al: Autologous marrow transplantation (ABMT) with cyclosporine (CsA)-induced autologous

graft-versus-host disease (GVHD) for relapsed aggressive non-Hodgkin's lymphoma (NHL). *Blood* 78:287a, 1991.

553. Kennedy MJ, Vogelsang GB, Jones RJ, et al: Phase I trial of interferon gamma to potentiate cyclosporine-induced graft-versus-host disease in women undergoing autologous bone marrow transplantation for breast cancer. *J Clin Oncol* 12:249, 1994.

554. Maloney DG, Liles TM, Czerwinski DK, et al: Phase I clinical trial using escalating single-dose infusion of chimeric anti-CD20 monoclonal antibody (IDEC-C2B8) in patients with recurrent B-cell lymphoma. *Blood* 84:2457, 1994.

555. Link BK, Weiner GJ: Production and characterization of a bispecific IgG capable of inducing T-cell-mediated lysis of malignant B cells. *Blood* 81:3343, 1993.

556. Wolcott DL, Wellisch DK, Fawzy FI, Landsverk J: Adaptation of adult bone marrow transplant recipient long-term survivors. *Transplantation* 41:478, 1986.

557. Andrykowski MA, Altmaier EM, Barnett RL, et al: Cognitive dysfunction in adult survivors of allogeneic marrow transplantation: relationship to dose of total body irradiation. *Bone Marrow Transplant* 6:269, 1990.

558. Wingard JR, Curbow B, Baker F, Piantadosi S: Health, functional status, and employment of adult survivors of bone marrow transplantation. *Ann Intern Med* 114:113, 1991.

559. Schmidt GM, Niland JC, Forman SJ, et al: Extended follow-up in 212 long-term allogeneic bone marrow transplant survivors: Issues of quality of life. *Transplantation* 55:551, 1993.

560. Syrjala KL, Chapko MK, Vitaliano PP, Cummings C, Sullivan KM: Recovery after allogeneic marrow transplantation: Prospective study of predictors of long-term physical and psychosocial functioning. *Bone Marrow Transplant* 11:319, 1993.

561. Duell T, van Lint MT, Ljungman P, et al: Health and functional status of long-term survivors of bone marrow transplantation. EBMT Working Party on Late Effects and EULEP Study Group on Late Effects: European Group for Blood and Marrow Transplantation. *Ann Intern Med* 126:184, 1997.

562. Chao NJ, Tierney DK, Bloom JR, et al: Dynamic assessment of quality of life after autologous bone marrow transplantation. *Blood* 80:825, 1992.

563. Stockerl-Goldstein KE, Blume KG: Allogeneic hematopoietic cell transplantation for adult patients with acute myeloid leukemia. *Hematopoietic Cell Transplantation*, 2nd ed, edited by ED Thomas, KG Blume, SJ Forman, p 823. Blackwell Science, Malden, MA, 1999.

564. Champlin RE, Ho WG, Gale RP, et al: Treatment of acute myelogenous leukemia: A prospective controlled trial of bone marrow transplantation versus consolidation chemotherapy. *Ann Intern Med* 102:285, 1985.

565. Zander AR, Keating M, Dicke K, et al: A comparison of marrow transplantation with chemotherapy for adults with acute leukemia of poor prognosis in first complete remission. *J Clin Oncol* 6:1548, 1988.

566. Conde E, Iriondo A, Rayon C, et al: Allogeneic bone marrow transplantation versus intensification chemotherapy for acute myelogenous leukaemia in first remission: A prospective controlled trial. *Br J Haematol* 68:219, 1988.

567. Schiller GJ, Nimer SD, Territo MC, et al: Bone marrow transplantation versus high-dose cytarabine-based consolidation chemotherapy for acute myelogenous leukemia in first remission. *J Clin Oncol* 10:41, 1992.

568. Cassileth PA, Lynch E, Hines JD, et al: Varying intensity of postremission therapy in acute myeloid leukemia. *Blood* 79:1924, 1992.

569. Archimbaud E, Thomas X, Michallet M, et al: Prospective genetically randomized comparison between intensive postinduction chemotherapy and bone marrow transplantation in adults with newly diagnosed acute myeloid leukemia. *J Clin Oncol* 12:262, 1994.

570. Hewlett J, Kopecky KJ, Head D, et al: A prospective evaluation of the roles of allogeneic marrow transplantation and low-dose monthly maintenance chemotherapy in the treatment of adult acute myelogenous leukemia (AML): A Southwest Oncology Group study. *Leukemia* 9:562, 1995.

GENE THERAPY

CHRISTOPHER E. WALSH

JOHNSON M. LIU

ARTHUR W. NIENHUIS

Understanding vector cell–host interactions will guide the field of gene transfer. These complex interactions require the understanding of virology, cell biology, host response and immunology, and the disease processes. Initial enthusiasm for genetic correction of several inherited hematopoietic disorders has now been tempered by the lack of efficient gene transfer in several clinical studies. The development and application of vectors designed to infect hematopoietic cells has led to pseudotyping, chimeric vectors, and nonviral methods for gene repair.

The development of recombinant DNA technology during the past 20 years has created the potential that genetically defined diseases, whether hereditary or acquired, can be treated by genetic therapy. Human gene therapy consists of the insertion of a functioning gene into appropriate target cells of an affected individual to correct for a defective gene or to add a new function to these cells. This chapter reviews the basic principles of gene transfer and the results of selected clinical gene transfer studies.

GENE TRANSFER: A MULTISTEP PATHWAY

Effective genetic therapy requires a safe and efficient means of gene delivery. Viral vectors attempt to capitalize on the inherent efficiency of viruses to transfer and express their genetic information in eukaryotic cells. For gene therapy applications, vectors are designed that allow entry of the recombinant virus with subsequent integration into the cellular genome or maintenance as an episome without alteration of cell metabolism or production of new virus. Retroviruses, adenoviruses, and AAV are currently being developed for use in humans. Physical methods of DNA transfer widely used in the research laboratory are also being considered for therapeutic applications. (For the definition of *vector* and other terms used in this chapter, see Table 19-1.)

Typically, viruses bind and enter host cells via receptor-mediated endocytosis (Fig. 19-1). During productive infection, the viral genome is transported to the nucleus, where it usurps host cellular machinery to direct the synthesis of viral-specific proteins and assembly of new viral particles. This complex process is shown in Fig. 19-1. Virus entry can be accomplished by binding to cell surface receptors or through nonspecific attachment. A list of cell receptors for specific viral vectors is shown in Table 19-2.

Upon binding and entry into the target cell, vector nucleic acid must be modified and transported to the nucleus. Retroviral vectors carry reverse transcriptase and convert their single-stranded RNA genomes to double-stranded DNA. The preintegration nuclear protein complex of oncoretroviruses, such as murine leukemia virus, is relatively unstable and cannot traverse the nuclear membrane. Therefore, such vectors are able to integrate their genome in dividing cells. In contrast, the preintegration complex of lentivirus, such as those based on HIV, is relatively stable and transported through the intact nuclear membrane.[1] Lentiviral vectors have a greater capacity to integrate their genome into quiescent cells. Both oncoretroviral and lentiviral vectors integrate into the host cell genome randomly. Random insertion may allow for inhibition of transgene expression due to transcriptional silencing.[2]

DNA vectors such as AAV or adenovirus behave differently. The rAAV genome is composed of single-stranded DNA molecules flanked by palindromic inverted terminal repeats. Upon entry into the nucleus, the single-stranded genome must be converted into a double-stranded form before the encoded gene can be transcribed. The double-stranded genome may remain episomal, it may form large tandem concatemers, or the genome may integrate into either single- or multicopy configuration. Persistent gene expression can be achieved in both episomal and integrated states. The double-stranded DNA genome of adenoviral vectors remains episomal, and therefore these vectors are useful for achieving transient expression in a proliferating cell population.

Host immunologic responses to viral capsid or coat proteins limit infection or readministration of virus. For example, the cell-mediated immune response directed against adenoviral coat proteins produces a significant inflammatory response.[3] Host response to the transgene protein product is dependent on the antigenicity of the expressed product. The expression of a new transgene protein may trigger cell- and humoral-mediated immune responses.

VECTORS

Retroviral Vectors

Retroviral vectors for gene transfer studies are derived from the murine leukemia virus family. Figure 19-2 outlines the integrated proviral form of the Moloney murine leukemia virus. The genome is flanked by LTRs that contain the transcriptional control elements, polyadenylation signals, and sequences required for replication and integration.[4,5] The viral genome contains coding sequences for structural proteins (GAG), reverse transcriptase (POL) and other viral enzymes, and ENV. A packaging signal, located at the 5′ end of the coding sequence ψ, facilitates incorporation of RNA into the capsid. Retroviruses capable of infecting murine cells and a few rat cell lines are described as having ecotropic specificity, which is based on interaction of the viral ENV (gp70) with a defined transmembrane protein that acts as a receptor.[6,7] Retroviruses that have a broader host range that includes human cells are termed amphotropic; the cellular receptor for amphotropic viruses has been identified as an anion transport protein. Retroviral amphotropic receptor is expressed at very low levels on murine and human stem cells.[8] Limiting amounts of virus receptor and the requirement for cell cycling explain the low transduction of human stem/progenitor cells. To enhance virus binding, amphotropic or ecotropic retroviral ENV can be substituted (pseudotyped) with ENV from other viruses, such as gibbon ape leukemia virus[9] or the rhabdovirus vesicular stomatitis virus.[10] Virus pseudotyping confers the receptor specificity of the ENV and improves the susceptibility of target cells to the new hybrid virus.[11]

Packaging cell lines have been engineered to produce retroviral vectors carrying genes of interest without the production of replication-competent virus (see Fig. 19-2). Such cell lines express a ''helper'' genome or genomes encoding the viral structural proteins, while a separate proviral genome contains the gene to be transferred and retains the *cis*-active elements required for genome encapsidation, replication, and integration.[12,13] Typically, 10^6 to 10^7 infectious vector particles per

TABLE 19-1   GLOSSARY OF TERMS

Episome: Transferred DNA remains separate from cellular DNA. Episomes, which lack elements required for replication, are eventually lost with successive cell divisions.

Gene marking: The introduction of foreign viral sequences into the chromosomal DNA of a patient's marrow to follow cell trafficking.

Integration: Process whereby exogenous genetic material becomes incorporated into the cell genome; usually refers to the latent or proviral state of certain viruses in infected cells.

Pseudotype: Engineered vector that expresses different coat proteins, allowing for improved target cell binding and entry.

Selectable marker: To optimize and enrich for transduced cells, genes encoding for bacterial antibiotic-resistance proteins (e.g., neomycin-resistance or hygromycin-resistance genes) are incorporated into the vector. Following transduction, incubation with the antibiotic allows for survival of only transduced cells.

Transduction: The transfer of genetic material into a cell. The efficiency of DNA transfer into cells depends on the particular method used, i.e., viral vs. nonviral.

Vector: Specific RNA or DNA recombinant system employed to introduce genes into cells.

---

milliliter of culture are necessary to achieve gene transfer into target hematopoietic cells. Pseudotyped retrovirus can withstand ultracentrifugation, and concentrated virus ($>10^9$ particles per milliliter) can be prepared. Retroviral gene transduction requires that target cells be actively replicating; quiescent (G_0) cells are refractory to proviral integration.[14,15] Pseudotyped lentiviral vectors offer a potential solution to the two problems of low viral receptor expression and quiescent human stem cells.

Replication-competent (wild-type or helper) virus contamination of retroviral vector stocks must also be eliminated. Studies showed that lethally irradiated rhesus monkeys developed thymic lymphomas following autologous transplantation of marrow cells that had been transduced with a vector preparation contaminated with replication-competent virus.[16] Multiple copies of a proviral genome or genomes were detected in the tumor cell DNA, implicating insertional mutagenesis as a mechanism of carcinogenesis. To prevent the production of replication-competent virus by recombination between vector and helper genomes, areas of homology between the two have been eliminated. Mutations have been introduced into residual viral coding sequences in the vector genome, and/or the structural genes required for helper function have been separated into two transcriptional units. Newer packaging lines have virtually eliminated detectable production of replication-competent virus. Similar packaging strategies employed for HIV-based vectors are paramount to avoid any possibility of wild-type HIV production.

ADENO-ASSOCIATED VIRUS VECTORS

Adeno-associated viruses are single-stranded DNA parvoviruses that require helper virus proteins (adenovirus or herpesvirus proteins) for replication and subsequent viral production in permissive cells. In the absence of helper virus, AAVs can persist in host cell genomic DNA as a multi-molecular concatenate and as an episome.[17] Some or all of these molecular species can be detected, depending on the cell or tissue type transduced. Unlike other potential viral vectors, wild-type AAV is unique with respect to its site-specific integration into a particular region on chromosome 19.[18] Viral integration has no apparent effect on cell growth or morphology. Adeno-associated virus has a broad host range through its use of heparan sulfate as an attachment molecule; virtually every mammalian cell line can be productively or latently infected. Despite its wide host range, no disease has been associated with AAVs in human or animal populations.

Recombinant AAV production relies on the cotransfection of helper and vector plasmids into a permissive cell line. Concomitant

infection with adenovirus for AAV replication provides the necessary complementing functions (Fig. 19-3). Contaminating adenovirus can be removed by gradient centrifugation or inactivated by heating; adenovirus is heat sensitive, but AAV is heat resistant. Advances in rAAV preparation have eliminated the production of adenovirus, and rapid purification can be performed using heparan-affinity chromatography. Recombinant AAV purification now yields titers of 10^{12} to 10^{14} particles. The ability to produce high-titer virus, along with its tropism for muscle, liver, and central nervous system, has broadened the appeal of this vector.[19] Recombinant AAV vectors used in a phase I clinical trial for cystic fibrosis patients indicate that they are safe[20] (Fig. 19-4).

NONVIRAL METHODS OF TRANSDUCTION

Several nonviral methods have been developed to permit target cells to take up DNA. Originally, these methods allowed for nonspecific binding and entry of DNA, either as calcium-phosphate complexes or

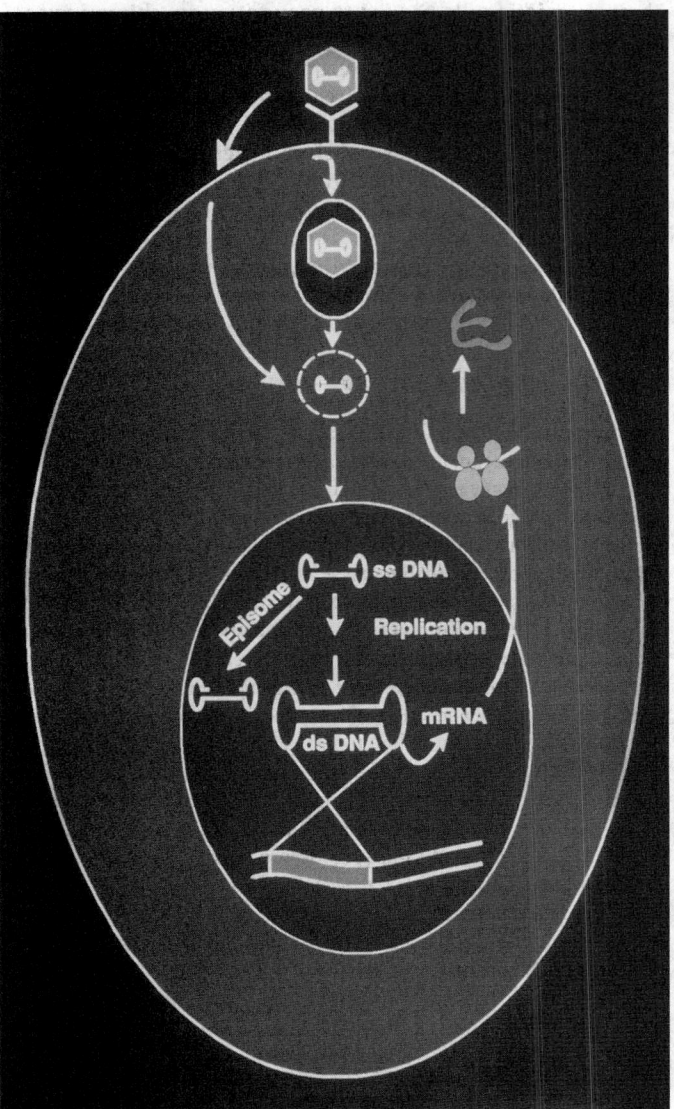

FIGURE 19-1   Vector–target cell interaction. Schematic representation of recombinant virus binding and internalizing through the cell membrane with release of the vector genome from the endosome. Following vector genome trafficking to the nucleus, episomal or integrated vector species allow for transcription of the vector transgene and translation into a functional protein.

liposomes or by direct microinjection of DNA into single cells.[21] These methods appear to be less efficient in gene transduction than are viral vectors, and gene expression is transient. Transduction of long-term repopulating stem cells using these methods has not yet been achieved.

The use of RNA or DNA oligonucleotides to repair mutations or alter RNA splicing mutations has gained interest. Hybrid DNA-RNA oligonucleotides designed to repair the single base change responsible for sickle cell disease have achieved correction of the mutation in cell lines.[22] Oligonucleotide targeting of mutant stem cells could generate permanently corrected progeny without the need for permanent transgene insertion. Oligo-based correction of aberrant RNA splicing in thalassemic cells has been described.[23]

Mammalian artificial chromosomes, suitable for large cDNAs or large genomic sequence capacity, are currently being tested. Mammalian artificial chromosomes include genetic elements that allow for their own replication. These self-replicating artificial chromosomes exist as episomes. Strategies to overcome limited mammalian artificial chromosome introduction into cells are under investigation.[24]

INHERITED GENETIC DISORDERS

HEMATOPOIETIC DISORDERS

Correction or treatment of genetic disorders affecting marrow is likely to be based on gene transfer into hematopoietic stem cells. If successfully targeted for gene transfer, stem cells would ensure the continuous production of genetically modified hematopoietic cells over the lifetime of the patient. In general, the more mature hematopoietic cells are inappropriate targets for gene transfer due to the lack of self-renewal and long-term survival. An important exception is lymphocytes, which have a long life span.

Stem cells can be highly purified based on their immunophenotype, including an absence of lineage-specific markers and the class II histocompatibility antigen HLA-DR and the presence of certain markers, such as CD34 and Thy1 (see Chap. 141). Cells having the stem cell immunophenotype that contributes to marrow repopulation are found in the blood after cytotoxic drug and/or cytokine administra-

tion. CD34+ mobilized peripheral blood, marrow, and umbilical cord blood stem cells are appropriate for therapeutic gene transfer. More primitive CD34+/CD38− cells, which maintain a greater repopulating potential, are resistant to Moloney-based retroviral transduction. The identification of CD34−[25] and fetal neuronal cells[26] capable of multilineage bone marrow reconstitution are new targets for hematopoietic gene transfer.

Efforts have been focused on enhancing the efficiency of retroviral-mediated gene transfer into hematopoietic stem cells. Cytokine-mobilized peripheral blood stem cells, cytokine combinations (e.g., stem cell factor, IL-3, IL-6, Flt3-ligand, and thrombopoietin), recombinant fibronectin support, and pseudotyping or stromal cells have been used to sustain stem cells during vector exposure in vitro and to enhance the probability of cell division required to achieve integration of the proviral genome.[27] Sixty to eighty percent of murine repopulating stem cells, and ten to twenty percent of the primate stem cells are susceptible to retroviral-mediated gene transfer under current conditions of in vitro culture during exposure to virus.[28] Alternative target cells for therapeutic gene transfer are circulating T lymphocytes. Such

TABLE 19-2   VECTORS USED IN GENE THERAPY AND THEIR RECEPTORS

Vector	Cellular Receptors
Retroviruses	
Amphotropic retrovirus	Sodium-dependent phosphate transporter (Pit 1, Pit 2)
Ecotropic retrovirus	Cationic amino acid transport protein (CAT 1)
Lentivirus (HIV-1)	CD4, CCR5, and CXCR4
Pseudotyped Retrovirus	
Vesicular stomatitis virus (VSV)	Phosphatidylserine
Gibbon ape leukemia virus (GAL-V)	Phosphate transport protein
Adenovirus	Coxsackievirus/adenovirus receptor protein integrin (CAR)
	$\alpha_v \beta_5$
AAV	Heparan sulfate
	Integrin $\alpha_v \beta_5$
	Fibroblast growth factor

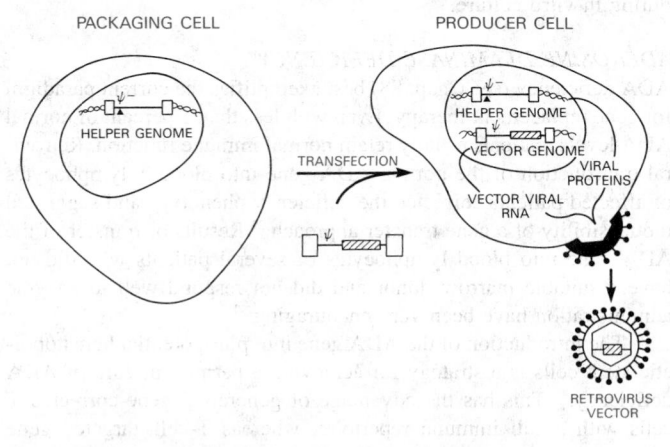

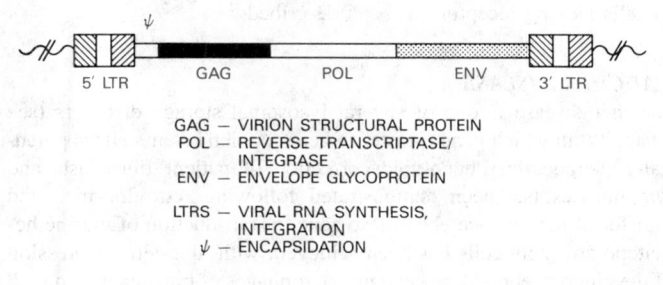

FIGURE 19-2   Schematic representation of the Moloney murine leukemia proviral form. GAG, virion structural protein; POL, reverse transcriptase/ integrase; ENV, envelope glycoprotein; LTR, viral RNA synthesis, integration; ψ, encapsidation.

FIGURE 19-3   Generation of recombinant RNA retroviral vectors. The diagram depicts the strategy to generate amphotropic recombinant virus containing a gene of interest (hatched area). Plasmid DNA containing the recombinant proviral genome of interest and the retroviral ψ (packaging) region is introduced into a packaging cell containing an integrated wild-type helper genome lacking the ψ region. Integration of the vector provirus allows for the stable production of retroviral particles. Clones identified as producing the highest concentration of vector particles are subsequently used to generate virus for gene transfer studies.

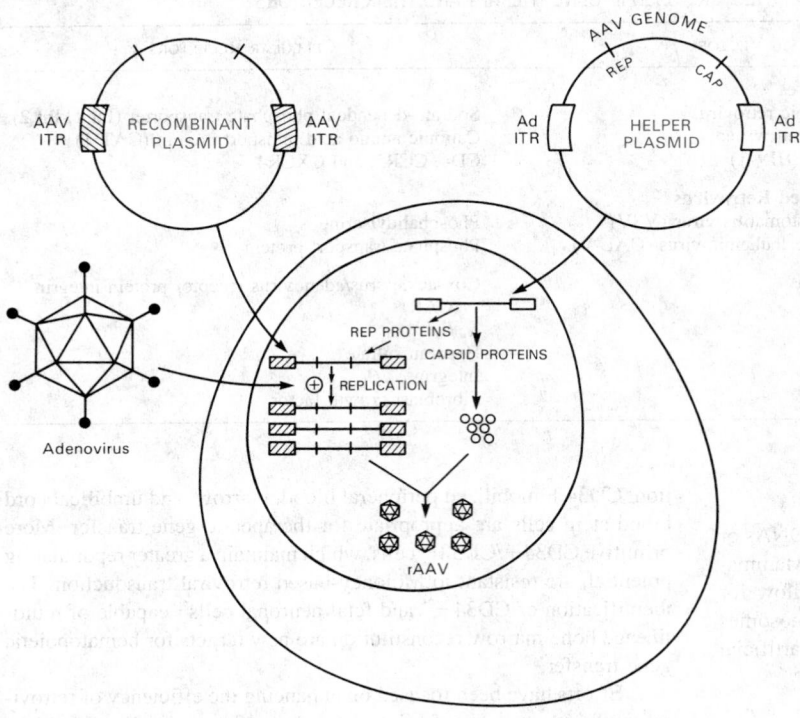

FIGURE 19-4   Recombinant DNA AAV production. A permissive cell line is cotransfected with helper and recombinant plasmids and infected with adenovirus. Both adenovirus and the helper plasmid (which produces the REP and CAP proteins) are necessary for rAAV replication and packaging. Due to the lack of homology between the two plasmids, no wild-type AAV is generated. Recombinant virion formation occurs in the cell nucleus, and both rAAV and adenovirus are released following cell lysis. Adenovirus is either inactivated by heating or removed by density centrifugation.

cells can be induced to divide many times in vitro, with a resulting several-fold amplification of the initial cell population. Interleukin-2 and an anti–T-cell-receptor antibody synergistically act as mitogens during in vitro culture.

ADENOSINE DEAMINASE DEFICIENCY

ADA deficiency (see Chap. 88) best exemplifies the current paradigm for gene replacement therapy. Even with less than 5 percent of normal ADA levels, patients usually retain normal immune function. Retroviral transduction of the normal ADA gene into blood T lymphocytes of affected patients corrected the deficiency phenotype and suggested the feasibility of a gene transfer approach.[29] Results of transfer of the ADA gene into blood lymphocytes of several patients who did not have a suitable marrow donor and did not respond well to enzyme administration have been very encouraging.[30]

The introduction of the ADA gene into pluripotential hematopoietic stem cells is a strategy for achieving a permanent cure of ADA deficiency.[31] This has the advantage of generating gene-corrected T cells with a full immune repertoire, whereas T-cell–targeted gene transfer is likely to correct cells of an already determined antigen specificity. Amplification of the gene-corrected T cell population is hypothesized to provide a selective growth advantage, despite the low efficiency of gene transfer into stem cells. This was tested using stem cells derived from umbilical cord blood harvested from ADA-affected newborns.[32] Four years after three newborns were given infusions of transduced autologous umbilical cord blood CD34+ cells, the frequency of gene-marked peripheral T lymphocytes remained at a level of 1 to 10 percent. On cessation of ADA replacement enzyme, a

decline in immune function occurred in one patient despite evidence of gene transfer.

HEMOGLOBINOPATHIES

High-level regulated globin gene expression is required for therapy of severely affected patients with sickle cell disease and β thalassemia.[33] Introduction of a normal β-globin gene into hematopoietic cells should be useful for correcting the defect in homozygous β thalassemia. In sickle cell disease, both the increased expression of a normal globin gene and a decrease in the amount of the β^S chain in mature red cells are required to be therapeutically effective. Increased fetal hemoglobin production ameliorates the severity of sickle cell disease and thalassemia. Production of γ-globin chains leading to accumulation of HbF ($\alpha_2\gamma_2$) in erythroid cells may therefore be therapeutic. This result might be achieved by introduction of genetic information that alters the pattern of globin gene expression.

Retroviral vectors have been used to transfer the β-globin gene into murine hematopoietic stem cells. The human β-globin gene was expressed in the erythroid cells of most animals for long periods but only at a level of 1 to 2 percent of normal murine β-globin levels.[34] Regulatory sequences upstream from the globin gene cluster, collectively termed the LCR, offer new hope for the design of therapeutic vectors.[35] Globin genes linked to LCR elements exhibit high-level expression in transgenic mouse models and erythroleukemia cell lines.[36] Producer clones for most vectors that have LCR elements have low titers, however, and these vectors are prone to rearrangement on insertion into target hematopoietic cells. Retroviral vectors utilizing truncated LCR elements linked to a human β-globin gene have produced levels of expression equivalent to that of endogenous genes in both erythroleukemia cell lines and murine hematopoietic cells.[37] Retroviral vectors have been modified extensively to eliminate sequences prone to produce viral rearrangement.[38] The use of α-globin LCR elements linked to β- or γ-globin genes is an alternative approach.[39]

Transfer and regulated high-level expression of a human globin gene linked to required transcriptional control elements have been achieved in erythroleukemia cells with an rAAV vector.[40] Primary hematopoietic progenitors may be transduced, but receptor levels may vary among individuals. Stable integration may not occur in all cells that initially take up and express the rAAV genome. Differences in AAV transduction of CD34+ cells are the result of variable heparan sulfate surface expression. Modification of rAAVs to facilitate binding to cells lacking receptor has been described.[41]

GAUCHER DISEASE

Gaucher disease is one of several lysosomal storage disorders (see Chap. 79) in which gene transfer to hematopoietic stem cells is potentially therapeutic. Phenotypic correction of patient fibroblasts and lymphocytes has been demonstrated following retroviral-mediated transfer of the glucocerebrosidase gene.[42] Transduction of murine hematopoietic stem cells has been achieved, with long-term expression of the glucocerebrosidase gene in macrophages of transplanted mice.[43] Expression in human hematopoietic cells has also been described after transduction of progenitors and cells capable of initiating long-term marrow cultures.[44] Two clinical trials using Moloney-based retroviral vectors targeted to CD34+ cells yield similar results with low transduction of peripheral blood cells.[45,46]

CHRONIC GRANULOMATOUS DISEASE

Phenotypic correction of phox 91 and phox 47 knockout mice was produced following bone marrow retroviral transduction.[47,48] Following treatment, knockout mice resisted bacterial and fungal infection due to a functional NADPH oxidase. These results led to clinical trials for phox-47-deficient CGD patients who received Moloney retroviral–based transduced mobilized peripheral blood.[49] Superoxide generation in blood granulocytes of patients could be detected in the peripheral blood for several weeks, suggesting that long-term stem cells were not transduced. Since mothers heterozygous for the X-linked form of the disease who have only 10 percent of normal granulocytes are clinically normal, long-term correction of only a small percentage of cells should result in therapeutic benefit.

FANCONI ANEMIA

The Fanconi anemia complementing genes A and C (*FANCA* and *FANCC*) have been genetically engineered into retroviral and rAAV viral vectors.[50,51] Phenotypic correction of Fanconi anemia lymphoblastoid cell lines was demonstrated by cell growth in the presence of clastogenic agents to which Fanconi anemia cells are typically sensitive and by reduced susceptibility to chromosomal breakage. Gene-corrected stem cells should have a selective growth advantage when transplanted into patients. These vectors were used to transduce purified hematopoietic progenitors from patients carrying defective FANCA and FANCC alleles. Retroviral-mediated gene transfer performed in four FANCC patients indicated gene marking of blood cells, improved clonogenic growth, and transient improvement in bone marrow cellularity and blood counts.

INHERITED COAGULATION DEFICIENCIES

HEMOPHILIA

Sustained therapeutic levels of factors VIII and IX would significantly affect the clinical course for the hemophilias. Transfer of factors VIII and IX into hemophilic A and B animals has been established.[52,53] Adenoviral vectors carrying the factor VIII or IX cDNAs produce high levels of circulating factor. However, due to the elimination of the virus by the host immune response, factor production lasts for only a period of weeks.

The use of rAAVs for hemophilia is promising. A single intramuscular or intravascular injection of vector produces sustained long-term factor IX expression (>1.5 years) in mice[54] and hemophilia B canines.[55,56] Targeting to either skeletal muscle or liver in hemophilic B canines produces 1 to 3 percent of normal factor IX levels. Unlike adenoviral vectors, toxicity is limited to adenoviral contamination and a modest humoral immune response to rAAV capsid.

ACQUIRED DISORDERS

ACQUIRED IMMUNODEFICIENCY SYNDROME

Gene transfer approaches to treating HIV-1 infection have emerged. Because of HIV tropism for lymphocytes, gene targeting to hematopoietic stem cells has been proposed as a mechanism for achieving a desired therapeutic effect in differentiating T cells. Current gene transfer–based strategies for therapy of HIV are targeted at (1) elimination of infected cells, (2) interruption of viral replication, or (3) inhibition of cellular infection.[57] Strategies designed to interfere with HIV receptor binding and cellular entry are currently being explored.

NEOPLASTIC DISORDERS

Graft-versus-host disease associated with the therapeutic infusion of donor lymphocytes after allogeneic bone marrow transplantation can be effectively controlled by the expression of herpes simplex virus thymidine kinase suicide gene into the allogeneic lymphocytes.[58] This was achieved by the selective elimination of transduced lymphocytes by ganciclovir infusion. This clinical trial has demonstrated the best evidence to date for effective gene transfer.

GENE-AUGMENTED IMMUNOTHERAPY

Various strategies have been proposed to enhance the immune response to neoplastic cells for therapeutic benefit.[59] TIL cells may serve as vehicles to carry tumor-inhibitory or immune-enhancing cytokines, such as tumor necrosis factor (TNF) or IL-2, into tumors after retroviral-mediated gene transfer in vitro. Another strategy attempts to augment cytotoxic T cell and/or natural killer cell response to tumor antigens by expression of cytokine or HLA genes in neoplastic cells. Explanted tumor cells are transduced in vitro and reimplanted subcutaneously into the patient from whom they were obtained. Substantial data from murine models support this approach.[60] Initial phase I clinical trials provided evidence for some resolution of tumors. Current efforts using gene-transduced tumor vaccines is directed at optimizing dendritic cell activation by cytokine genes and overexpressing relevant tumor-associated peptides.[61]

CHEMOPROTECTION

Hematopoietic toxicity associated with intensive chemotherapy is frequently dose limiting. Gene transfer into stem cells of patients undergoing autologous transplantation might be used to create marrow resistant to subsequently administered chemotherapy. This concept has been tested in oncology patients using a retroviral vector that confers multidrug resistance through expression of P glycoprotein (gp140).[62] Patients receiving chemotherapy for a variety of solid malignancies exhibited no significant hematopoietic protection.[63,64] These results highlight the low transduction efficiency of stem/progenitor cells. Overexpression of *mdr-1* produces a myelodysplastic marrow in mice, suggesting that alternative dominant selectable agents be employed.

FETAL AND NEONATAL GENE THERAPY

Advances in prenatal diagnosis and fetoscopic technique now allow for the transfer of genetic material in utero. Introduction of adenoviral vectors into the fetal airway or umbilical vein of neonatal sheep expressed marker and therapeutic genes in many organs.[65] Antiadenoviral immunologic reactions limited transgene expression in late-stage gestation. Neonatal gene transfer using rAAVs led to widespread correction of pathology in a murine model of lysosomal storage.[66] Risks of in utero gene therapy apply to the mother, the fetus, and future generations, given the potential for vector insertion into the germ line. Currently there are insufficient safety data to support a phase I trial.[67]

REFERENCES

1. Naldini L, Blomer U, Gage F, Trono D, Verma I: Efficient transfer, integration, and sustained long-term expression of the transgene in adult rat brains injected with a lentiviral vector. *Proc Natl Acad Sci USA* 93:11382, 1996.

2. Challita P, Kohn D: Lack of expression from a retroviral vector after transduction of murine hematopoietic stem cells is associated with methylation *in vivo. Proc Natl Acad Sci USA* 91:2567, 1994.

3. Kafri T, Morgan D, Krahl T, et al: Cellular immune response to adenoviral vector infected cells does not require de novo viral gene expression: Implications for gene therapy. *Proc Natl Acad Sci USA* 95:11377, 1998.

4. Shoemaker C, Goff S, Gilboa E, Paskind M, Mitra SW, Baltimore D: Structure of the cloned circular Moloney murine leukemia virus DNA molecule containing an inverted segment: Implications for retroviral integration. *Proc Natl Acad Sci USA* 77:3932, 1980.

5. Leis J, Baltimore D, Bishop JM, et al: Standardized and simplified

nomenclature for proteins common to all retroviruses. *J Virol* 62: 1808, 1988.

6. Hunter E, Swanstrom R: Retrovirus envelope glycoproteins. *Curr Top Microbiol Immunol* 171:95, 1991.

7. Levy J: Xenotropism: The elusive viral receptor finally uncovered. *Proc Natl Acad Sci USA* 96:802, 1999.

8. Orlic D, Girard L, Jordan C, et al: The level of mRNA encoding the amphotropic retrovirus receptor in mouse and human hematopoietic stem cells is low and correlates with the efficiency of retrovirus transduction. *Proc Natl Acad Sci USA* 93:11097, 1996.

9. Miller A, Garcia J, von Suhr N, et al: Construction and properties of retrovirus packaging cells based on gibbon ape leukemia virus. *J Virol* 65:2220, 1991.

10. Burns J, Friedmann, Driever W, Burrascono M, Yee J: Vesicular stomatitis virus G glycoprotein pseudotyped retroviral vectors: Concentration to very high titer and efficient gene transfer into mammalian and non-mammalian cells. *Proc Natl Acad Sci USA* 90:8033, 1993.

11. Miller A: Cell-surface receptors for retroviruses and implications for gene transfer. *Proc Natl Acad Sci USA* 93:11407, 1996.

12. Nienhuis A, Walsh C, Liu J: Viruses as therapeutic gene transfer vectors, in *Viruses and Bone Marrow: Basic Research and Clinical Practice*, p 353. Marcel Dekker, New York, 1993.

13. Miller A: Retroviral vectors. *Curr Top Microbiol Immunol* 171:95, 1991.

14. Harel J, Rassert E, Jolicoeur P: Cell cycle dependence of synthesis of unintegrated viral DNA in mouse cells newly infected with murine leukemia virus. *Virology* 110:202, 1981.

15. Miller D, Adam M, Miller A: Gene transfer by retrovirus vectors occurs only in cells that are actively replicating at the time of infection. *Mol Cell Biol* 10:4239, 1990.

16. Donahue RE, Kessler SW, Bodine D, et al: Helper virus induced T-cell lymphoma in non-human primates after retroviral mediated gene transfer. *J Exp Med* 176:1125, 1992.

17. Rabinowitz J, Samulski J: Adeno-associated virus expression systems for gene transfer. *Curr Opin Biotechnol* 9:470, 1998.

18. Samulski R: Adeno-associated virus: Integration at a specific chromosomal locus. *Curr Opin Genet Dev* 3:74, 1993.

19. Ferrari F, Xiao X, McCarty D, Samulski R: New developments in the generation of Ad-free, high-titer rAAV gene therapy vectors. *Nat Med* 3:1295, 1997.

20. Flotte T, Carter B, Conrad C, et al: A phase I study of an adeno-associated virus-CFTR gene vector in adult CF patients with mild lung disease. *Hum Gene Ther* 7:1145, 1996.

21. Mulligan R: The basic science of gene therapy. *Science* 260:926, 1993.

22. Cole-Strauss A, Yoon K, Xiang Y, et al: Correction of the mutation responsible for sickle cell anemia by an RNA-DNA oligonucleotide. *Science* 273:1386, 1996.

23. Gorman L, Suter D, Emerick V, Schumperli D, Kole R: Stable alteration of pre-mRNA splicing patterns by modified U7 small nuclear RNAs. *Proc Natl Acad Sci USA* 95:4929, 1998.

24. Vos J: Mammalian artificial chromosomes as tools for gene therapy. *Curr Opin Genet Dev* 8:351, 1998.

25. Goodell M, Brose K, Paradis G, Conner A, Mulligan R: Isolation and functional properties of murine hematopoietic stem cells that are replicating *in vivo*. *J Exp Med* 183:1797, 1996.

26. Bjornson C, Rietze R, Reynolds B, Magli M, Veccovi A: Turning brain into blood: A hematopoietic fate adopted by adult neural stem cells *in vivo*. *Science* 283:534, 1999.

27. Hanenberg H, Xiao X, Dilloo D, et al: Colocalization of retrovirus and target cells on specific fibronectin fragments increases genetic transduction of mammalian cells. *Nat Med* 2:876, 1996.

28. Kiem H, Andrews R, Morris J, et al: Improved gene transfer into baboon marrow repopulating cells using recombinant human fibronectin fragment CH-296 in combination with interleukin-6, stem cell factor, FLT-3 ligand, and megakaryocyte growth and development factor. *Blood* 92:1878, 1998.

29. Kantoff P, Kohn D, Mitsuya H, et al: Correction of adenosine deaminase deficiency in cultured human T and B cells by retrovirus-mediated gene transfer. *Proc Natl Acad Sci USA* 83:6563, 1986.

30. Blaese R: Development of gene therapy for immunodeficiency: Adenosine deaminase deficiency. *Pediatr Res* 33(suppl 1):S49, 1993.

31. Bodine D, Moritz T, Donahue R, et al: Long-term expression of a murine adenosine deaminase gene in rhesus monkey hematopoietic cells of

multiple lineages after retroviral mediated gene transfer into CD34+ bone marrow cells. *Blood* 82:1975, 1993.

32. Kohn D, Hershfield M, Carbonaro D, et al: T lymphocytes with a normal ADA gene accumulate after transplantation of transduced autologous umbilical cord blood CD34+ cells in ADA-deficient SCID neonates. *Nat Med* 4:775, 1998.

33. Walsh CE, Liu JM, Miller JL, Nienhuis AW, Samulski RJ: Gene therapy for human hemoglobinopathies. *Proc Soc Exp Biol Med* 204:289, 1993.

34. Dzierzak E, Papayannopoulou T, Mulligan R: Lineage-specific expression of a human β-globin gene in murine bone marrow transplant recipients reconstituted with retrovirus-transduced stem cells. *Nature* 331:35, 1988.

35. Grosveld F, van Assendelft B, Greaves D, Kollias G: Position independent, high level expression of the human β-globin gene in transgenic mice. *Cell* 51:975, 1987.

36. Novak U, Harris EA, Forrester W, Groudine M, Gelinas R: High-level β-globin expression after retroviral transfer of locus activation region containing human β-globin gene derivatives into murine erythroleukemia cells. *Proc Natl Acad Sci USA* 87:3386, 1990.

37. Plavec I, Papayannopoulou T, Maury C, Meyer G: A human β-globin gene fused to the human β-globin locus control region is exposed at high levels in erythroid cells of mice engrafted with retrovirus transduced hematopoietic stem cells. *Blood* 81:1384, 1993.

38. Pawliuk R, Bachelot T, Raftopoulos H, et al: Retroviral vectors aimed at the gene therapy of human beta-globin gene disorders. *Ann NY Acad Sci* 850:151, 1998.

39. Ren S, Wong B, Li J, et al: Production of genetically stable high-titer retroviral vectors that carry a human gamma-globin gene under the control of the alpha-globin locus control region. *Blood* 87:2518, 1996.

40. Walsh CE, Liu JM, Xiao X, Young NS, Nienhuis AW, Samulski RJ: Regulated high level expression of a human γ-globin gene introduced into erythroid cells by an adeno-associated virus vector. *Proc Natl Acad Sci USA* 89:7257, 1992.

41. Bartlett J, Kleinschmidt J, Boucher R, Samulski R: Targeted adeno-associated virus vector transduction of nonpermissive cells mediated by a bispecific F(ab′gamma)2 antibody. *Nat Biotechnol* 17:181, 1999.

42. Sorge J, Kuhl W, West C, Beutler E: Complete correction of the enzymatic defect of type 1 Gaucher disease fibroblasts by retroviral gene transfer. *Proc Natl Acad Sci USA* 84:906, 1987.

43. Nolta J, Sender L, Barranger J, Kohn D: Expression of human glucocerebrosidase in murine long-term bone marrow culture after retroviral vector-mediated transfer. *Blood* 75:787, 1990.

44. Correll PH, Fink JK, Brady RO, Perry LK, Karlsson S: Production of human glucocerebrosidase in mice after retroviral gene transfer into multipotential hematopoietic progenitor cells. *Proc Natl Acad Sci USA* 86:8912, 1989.

45. Barranger J, Rice E, Swaney W: Gene transfer approaches to the lysosomal storage disorders. *Neurochem Res* 24:601, 1999.

46. Dunbar C, Kohn D, Schiffmann R, et al: Retroviral transfer of the glucocerebrosidase gene into CD34+ cells from patients with Gaucher disease: *In vivo* detection of transduced cells without myeloablation. *Gene Ther* 9:2629, 1998.

47. Ding C, Kume A, Bjorgvinsdottir H, et al: High-level reconstitution of respiratory burst activity in a human X-linked chronic granulomatous disease (X-CGD) cell line and correction of murine X-CGD bone marrow cells by retroviral-mediated gene transfer of human gp91phox. *Blood* 88:1834, 1996.

48. Mardiney MR, Jackson S, Spratt S, et al: Enhanced host defense after gene transfer in the murine p47phox-deficient model of chronic granulomatous disease. *Blood* 89:2268, 1997.

49. Malech H, Maples P, Whiting-Theobald N, et al: Prolonged production of NADPH oxidase-corrected granulocytes after gene therapy of chronic granulomatous disease. *Proc Natl Acad Sci USA* 94:12133, 1997.

50. Fu K, Foe J, Joenje H, et al: Functional correction of Fanconi anemia group A hematopoietic cells by retroviral gene transfer. *Blood* 90:3296, 1997.

51. Walsh C, Nienhuis A, Samulski R, et al: Phenotypic correction of Fanconi anemia in human hematopoietic cells with a recombinant adeno-associated virus vector. *J Clin Invest* 94:1440, 1994.

52. Kay M, Rothenberg S, Landen C, et al: In vivo gene therapy of hemophilia B: Sustained partial correction of factor IX-deficient dogs. *Science* 262:117, 1993.

53. Connelly S, Andrews J, Gallo A, et al: Sustained phenotypic correction of murine hemophilia A by in vivo gene therapy. *Blood* 91:3273, 1998.

54. Herzog R, Hagstrom J, Kung S-H, et al: Stable gene transfer and expression of human coagulation factor IX after intramuscular injection of recombinant adeno-associated virus. *Proc Natl Acad Sci USA* 94:5804, 1997.

55. Monahan P, Samulski R, Tazelaar J, et al: Direct intramuscular injection with recombinant AAV vectors results in sustained expression in a dog model of hemophilia. *Gene Ther* 5:40, 1998.

56. Herzog R, Yang E, Couto L, et al: Long-term correction of canine hemophilia B by gene transfer of blood coagulation factor IX mediated by adeno-associated viral vector. *Nat Med* 5:56, 1999.

57. Morgan RA: Gene therapy for HIV infection. *Clin Exp Immunol* 107(suppl 1):41, 1997.

58. Bonini C, Ferrari G, Verzeletti S, et al: HSV-TK gene transfer into donor lymphocytes for control of allogeneic graft-versus-leukemia. *Science* 276:1719, 1997.

59. Pardoll D: Immunotherapy with cytokine gene-transduced tumor cells: The next wave in gene therapy for cancer. *Curr Opin Oncol* 4:1124, 1992.

60. Fearon ER, Pardoll DM, Itaya T, et al: Interleukin-2 production by tumor cells bypasses T helper function in the generation of an antitumor response. *Cell* 60:397, 1990.

61. Dranoff G, Soiffer R, Lynch T, et al: A phase I study of vaccination with autologous, irradiated melanoma cells engineered to secrete human granulocyte-macrophage colony stimulating factor. *Hum Gene Ther* 8:111, 1997.

62. Sorrentino B, Brandt S, Gottesman M, et al: Positive selection *in vivo* for hematopoietic cells expressing the multidrug resistance gene following retroviral mediated gene transfer. *Science* 257:99, 1992.

63. Hanania E, Giles R, Kavanagh J, et al: Results of MDR-1 vector modification trial indicate that granulocyte/macrophage colony-forming unit cells do not contribute to posttransplant hematopoietic recovery following intensive systemic therapy. *Proc Natl Acad Sci USA* 93:15346, 1996.

64. Hesdorffer C, Ayello J, Ward M, et al: Phase I trial of retroviral-mediated transfer of the human MDR1 gene as marrow chemoprotection in patients undergoing high-dose chemotherapy and autologous stem-cell transplantation. *J Clin Oncol* 16:165, 1998.

65. Yang E, Cass D, Sylvester K, Wilson J, Adzick N: BAPS Prize—1997. Fetal gene therapy: Efficacy, toxicity, and immunologic effects of early gestation recombinant adenovirus. *J Pediatr Surg* 34:235, 1999.

66. Daly T, Vogler C, Levy B, Haskins M, Sands M: Neonatal gene transfer leads to widespread correction of pathology in a murine model of lysosomal storage disease. *Proc Natl Acad Sci USA* 96:2296, 1999.

67. Moulton G: Panel finds in utero gene therapy proposal is premature. *J Natl Cancer Inst* 91:407, 1999.

THE USE OF VENOUS ACCESS DEVICES

McDonald K. Horne

Donna Jo Mayo

Alison G. Freifeld

Venous access devices are important in the management of advanced hematologic diseases. Several designs, including tunneled and nontunneled devices, are available, and the choice should be individualized to the needs of the patient. Careful maintenance of devices is required to prevent occlusion, thrombus formation, or infection. The latter may be confined to the catheter exit site or the tunnel, or it may include bacteremia or septicemia. Both thrombotic and infectious complications are common and require specific therapeutic interventions.

Central venous access is essential in the management of advanced hematologic diseases requiring intensive therapy. Repeatedly catheterizing central veins, however, is impractical and hazardous. Therefore, VADs have been developed to provide a continuous portal to the central veins for extended periods of time. These devices are silicone rubber or plastic tubes that have been engineered to maximize their longevity.

BASIC DESIGNS

Although a variety of devices are available, there are a few basic designs (Table 21-1).[1] Tunneled devices pass through the subcutaneous tissues of the anterior chest wall or neck for several centimeters before entering a central vein. Their exterior end either exits through the skin (Figure 21-1) or terminates in a reservoir (a port) that is buried beneath the skin (Figure 21-2). Because of this feature, ports can only be entered by a percutaneous puncture with a noncoring needle. Externalized devices have a fibrous cuff that anchors them in the tunnel as the insertion wound heals. Ports are secured by sutures in their subcutaneous pouches.

Nontunneled devices are inserted directly into a peripheral arm vein (PICCs) or a subclavian vein (central catheters).[2] They are secured to the skin with tape or sutures.

Catheters are manufactured with one to three lumens of differing internal diameters (0.5–2.6 mm). The number and size of the lumens determines the external diameter of the catheter, which is measured in French (one French equals 0.33 mm). The catheter tips may be continuously open (e.g., Hickman or Broviac type) or fitted with a valve that opens with positive or negative pressure (e.g., Groshong type).

SELECTION OF A VENOUS ACCESS DEVICE

In order to minimize intravenous obstruction and trauma, the external diameter of the devices should be as small as possible while still providing the needed access. The choice of lumen diameter depends on the viscosity and desired flow rates of the fluids to be administered. When the catheter is intended only for standard chemotherapy and fluids, for example, small lumens are adequate, whereas apheresis procedures require large-bore devices.

The length of time that the catheter will be needed is also important. Tunneled catheters are more likely to function well for months to years, whereas the nontunneled varieties are more appropriate for short-term use.

Patient preferences should also be considered, since external devices present cosmetic problems and may restrict activities. Furthermore, all catheters require continuous care, which may be impossible for a patient to provide for themselves.

PLACEMENT AND REMOVAL OF DEVICES

Before an attempt is made to insert a catheter, a careful history and physical examination are required to determine whether the candidate vein has been previously catheterized or is likely to be compressed by a tumor mass. These circumstances suggest the possibility of distorted venous anatomy that may preclude placement of the device.[3] A venogram may be required to assess the situation.

Tunneled devices should be placed by a surgeon or interventional radiologist in an operating suite under local anesthesia. Removal of a tunneled percutaneous catheter is complicated by the need to dissect the subcutaneous cuff, while removal of a port requires a more extensive procedure. PICCs, in contrast, can usually be inserted and removed by trained nurses in an outpatient setting, greatly reducing the cost and inconvenience of establishing central venous access.

The tip of the catheter should be placed in the superior vena cava, just outside the right atrium. If the tip resides inside the right atrium a right atrial thrombus may develop. If the tip is left in a subclavian or innominate vein there is an increased chance of catheter occlusion or venous damage from sclerosing infusates.

CATHETER MAINTENANCE

Immediately following insertion of a venous access device, surgical wound care is necessary. PICCs often cause sterile phlebitis in the upper arm or shoulder, but this usually resolves spontaneously or with the help of warm compresses.

Long-term maintenance of devices consists principally of periodic flushes to promote patency. Because of their locations nontunneled catheters are very difficult for patients to care for alone, whereas self-care is much easier for devices implanted in the chest wall. The optimal flushing program has never been established for any of the catheters. The routine programs have been rather arbitrarily developed and based largely on convenience. The lumens of open-ended devices constantly communicate with the blood. These are typically flushed daily with heparinized saline, unless they have a port buried beneath the skin. Then they are flushed monthly. The incidence of catheter occlusion is about the same whether the flushes are daily or monthly and regardless of whether they contain heparin or only saline.[4,5]

COMPLICATIONS OF VENOUS ACCESS DEVICES

CATHETER OCCLUSION

Reduced flow is a common problem.[22] If fluid can neither be infused nor withdrawn easily, the catheter is probably kinked or pinched by a suture or is defective. However, it may have become blocked with

TABLE 20-1   COMMON VENOUS ACCESS DEVICES

| | USES | | | | INSERTION | | | |
DESIGN	BLOOD DRAWING	IV FLUID	BLOOD PRODUCT	DURATION OF USE	SITE *	OPERATOR	SECURED BY	ROUTINE FLUSH
Tunneled								
Open-ended (Hickman type)	++++	++++	++++	Weeks to years	SC, IJ	Surgeon Radiologist	Fibrous cuff	Daily
Valved (Groshong type)	++++	++++	++++	Weeks to years	SC, IJ	Surgeon Radiologist	Fibrous cuff	Weekly
Ports (open or valved end)	++++	++++	++++	Months to years	SC	Surgeon	Implantation	Monthly
Nontunneled								
Peripheral (PICC, open or valved end)	+	++++	+	<3 months	AC	Nurse	Tape	Daily or weekly
Central	++++	++++	++++	<3 weeks	SC, IJ	Physician	Suture	Daily

*SC, subclavian vein; IJ, internal jugular vein; AC, antecubital vein

lipid or with precipitates of drugs or of calcium phosphate. These occlusions can sometimes be cleared with instillations of 0.1 N hydrochloric acid or 70% ethanol.

A more common type of occlusion is limited to withdrawal only. This not only interferes with blood sampling but also suggests the possibility that the catheter tip has migrated into a small vein and lodged against the vessel wall. Concentrated chemotherapeutic agents infused through such a catheter will not be quickly diluted and may damage the small vein. Therefore, withdrawal occlusion should be relieved or investigated before the catheter is used. The problem can

often be remedied by having the patient change body position or perform a Valsalva maneuver in order to move the tip of the catheter. If this does not resolve the problem, an occlusive fibrin sheath may be present.

Virtually all devices become coated with fibrin within a few days of insertion. If this coating progresses to involve the catheter tip, it may block the lumen when negative pressure is applied. One or two milliliters of urokinase (5000 units/ml) injected into the catheter and permitted to remain in the lumenal arm for up to 30 min will relieve most fibrin occlusions. If this treatment fails, the obstruction should be evaluated radiologically.

A chest x-ray may reveal that the catheter tip has migrated into a small vessel. If this is not the case a small amount of x-ray contrast material should be injected through the catheter under fluoroscopy. If an occlusive fibrin sheath is present the flow of dye will be diverted or may move retrograde along the outside of the catheter.[6] In extreme cases the sheath may extend from the catheter tip to the insertion site in the vein, where contrast material extravasates. If sclerosing medications are infused through the catheter they may follow the same path and damage extravascular tissues.

Fibrin sheaths that are refractory to urokinase instillations can often be lysed by continuous infusions of urokinase through the occluded lumen. An effective and safe regimen is to infuse 5000 units/

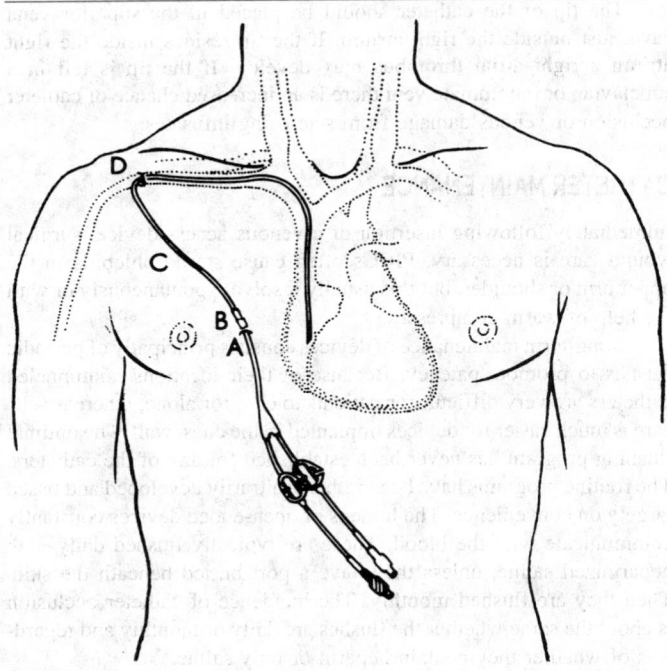

FIGURE 20-1   Schematic illustration of an external catheter in place. (*a*) Exit site and end of subcutaneous tunnel. (*b*) Dacron cuff in subcutaneous tunnel, traditional placement. (*c*) Midsubcutaneous tunnel; optimal placement for cuff to minimize accidental dislodgement. (*d*) Subclavian vein insertion site. Tip should be placed as close as possible to the superior vena cava—right atrial junction. (Used with permission from Alexander HR, Lucas A: Long-term venous access catheters and implantable ports, in *Vascular Access: The Cancer Patient.* Lippincott, Philadelphia, 1994.)

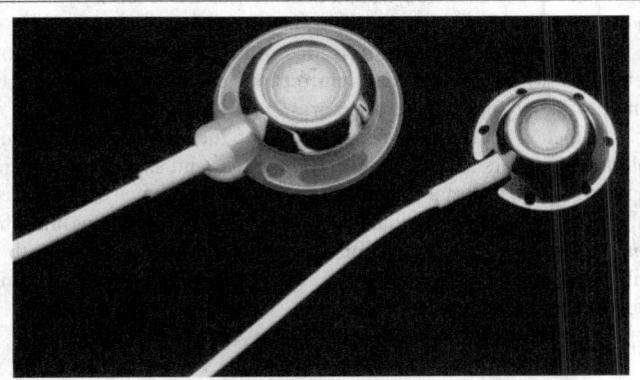

FIGURE 20-2   Photograph of standard and low-profile ports. The low-profile port is suitable for younger or aesthenic patients with little subcutaneous tissue. (Used with permission from Alexander HR, Lucas A: Long-term venous access catheters and implantable ports, in *Vascular Access: The Cancer Patient.* Lippincott, Philadelphia, 1994.)

ml of urokinase at 8 ml/h.[7]* The occlusion may be relieved within a few hours. If more than 12 h of treatment is needed, it is unlikely to be successful.

VENOUS THROMBOSIS

The reported incidence of mural thrombi associated with venous access devices varies greatly, from virtually 0 to almost 40 percent.[3,4,8] Thrombi tend to occur at the site where the catheter enters the vein or near the catheter tip, particularly if it is not properly placed in the vena cava.[3,7] Usually these thrombi are asymptomatic because they only partially obstruct flow and/or because collateral veins rapidly develop.[3] However, they may enlarge and cause pain and swelling of the ipsilateral arm or supraclavicular fossa and dilatation of the subcutaneous veins.

In the management of thrombi associated with venous access devices, several issues should be considered. If central venous access is still needed, the device should not be removed except in extreme cases. Symptomatic relief is often achieved by arm elevation. Full heparinization followed by chronic oral anticoagulation is recommended.[9] Although pulmonary emboli have been reported in up to 15 percent of patients with access-device–related thrombi, the risk appears to be much lower with newer silicone catheters.[9,10] There is also the fear that emboli will break off of a thrombus when the device is removed. Radiographically this has been shown to happen, but serious clinical events related to these emboli are unusual.[6] Therefore, there is no established role for a course of anticoagulation prior to removing a device through a thrombus.

Chronic symptoms are reported to persist in 23 percent of the cases of device-associated thrombosis.[11] However, they are usually tolerable and obscured by events related to the patient's primary disease. Another long-term concern for many patients is future venous access, since a thrombosed vein rarely recanalizes sufficiently to admit another device if needed. If restoring venous patency is a high priority, thrombolytic agents are usually necessary.

Systemically administered agents generally bypass the clot by going through collateral veins. Regional delivery of thrombolytic drugs is much safer and more effective. If the tip of the catheter is lodged in a thrombus, infusion of urokinase through the device itself will deliver the drug where it is needed. The same urokinase protocol recommended for fibrin sheaths can be used, although longer treatment may be required and heparin may be needed if local venous flow is stagnant.

If the mural thrombus is peripheral to the catheter tip, the patient must be heparinized and the thrombus injected with urokinase or tissue plasminogen activator delivered through a different catheter.* Unless the thrombus is several weeks old or the vein has become stenotic or compressed by extravascular structures, such treatment is usually both safe and successful.[12]

PROPHYLACTIC ANTICOAGULATION

Prophylactic anticoagulation to prevent catheter-related thrombosis may be warranted in high-risk patients. One milligram of warfarin/day or a daily injection of low molecular weight heparin is reported to be effective.[8,13]

INFECTIONS

Ten to 40 percent of long-term tunneled devices become infected, and the rate is generally even higher for nontunneled catheters.[14,23] In most studies, totally implanted infusion ports appear to be less prone to infection than externally tunneled catheters.[14,15]

The least serious of these complications is an exit site infection, which is an area of cellulitis within 2 cm of where the catheter penetrates the skin. Systemic symptoms are unusual. Sterile inflammation can sometimes also present in this manner and may be distinguished from infection by a semiquantitative culture of the area.[15,16]

An infection of the tunnel track or the pocket of a subcutaneously implanted catheter is more serious. It presents as cellulitis extending more than 2 cm into the catheter tunnel. Tenderness and erythema along the track of the catheter are prominent. Fever is common, and bacteremia occurs in nearly half of the cases.[15]

Catheter-related septicemia typically presents with fever, chills, and constitutional symptoms, often following an intravenous infusion or flush through the catheter. In some cases, however, intermittent fever may be the only sign that the catheter lumen is infected.

The patient's own cutaneous flora represents the major source of contamination. Accordingly, the most common pathogens in catheter-related infections are coagulase-negative staphylococci and *Staphylococcus aureus*. Coagulase-negative staphylococci are particularly adept at adhering to polymer surfaces, where they encase themselves in a polysaccharide slime that allows them to avoid host defense mechanisms.[17] *Candida* species and enterococci, including vancomycin-resistant strains, are increasingly common causes of bacteremia in patients with catheters.[15]

The management of catheter-related infections requires two decisions: which antibiotics to use and whether to remove the catheter. In most cases exit site infections can be treated with antibiotics and local care alone without catheter removal. The exceptions are exit site infections with *Pseudomonas* species and atypical mycobacteria, which do require device explantation. Tunnel and pocket infections, which are usually caused by *S. aureus*, also require catheter removal, as well as intravenous antibiotics for 10 to 14 days.[16,18]

Catheter-related septicemia, in contrast, can usually be managed without removing the device.[14,17] Coagulase-negative staphylococci, the most common etiologic agents, are rapidly cleared with vancomycin administered for 7 to 10 days through the infected catheter. Many infections with gram-negative bacilli can also be managed with antibiotics given through the catheter, provided that the patient remains hemodynamically stable and blood cultures taken through all catheter lumens are negative 48 hours after the initiation of treatment. *Pseudomonas* and *S. aureus* infections are the exceptions and usually require catheter removal in order to clear the bacteremia and avoid recurrence.[16]

Although catheter removal was once considered essential for bloodstream infections due to *Candida* species, it appears that uncomplicated catheter-related candidemia can be treated with 10 to 14 days of amphotericin B or fluconazole. High-grade or complicated candidemia or persistence of positive blood cultures after 48 hours of therapy, however, requires that the catheter be removed.[16]

Urokinase infusions have been studied as an adjunct to antibiotics for treatment of intraluminal infections with the intent to dissolve thrombi that harbor bacteria. In randomized studies, however, urokinase did not improve the outcome.[19]

Antiseptic and antibiotic impregnated cuffs reduce infections of short-term central venous catheters, but this may not be the case for long-term or tunneled devices.[20,21] Prophylactic vancomycin plus heparin flushes have also been shown to decrease rates of gram-positive infections, but this practice is discouraged because of the risk that resistant bacteria will emerge.

The most effective tactic to prevent catheter-related infections is to establish an experienced team devoted to the insertion and maintenance of all catheters within an institution.[16]

---

*Neither urokinase nor tissue plasminogen activator has been approved for this purpose by the U.S. Food and Drug Administration at the time of publication.

REFERENCES

1. Ryder M: Device selection: a critical strategy in the reduction of catheter-related complications. *Nutrition* 12:143, 1996.
2. Ng PK, Ault MJ, Ellrodt AG, Maldonado L: Peripherally inserted central catheters in general medicine. *Mayo Clin Proc* 72:225, 1997.
3. Horne MK, Mayo DJ, Alexander HR, et al.: Venographic surveillance of tunneled venous access devices in adult oncology patients. *Ann Surg Oncol* 2:174, 1995.
4. Mueller BU, Skelton J, Callender DPE, et al.: A prospective randomized trial comparing the infectious and noninfectious complications of an externalized catheter versus a subcutaneously implanted device in cancer patients. *J Clin Oncol* 10:1943, 1992.
5. Smith S, Dawson S, Hennessey R, Andrew M: Maintenance of the patency of indwelling central venous catheters: is heparin necessary? *Am J Pediatr Hem/Onc* 13:141, 1991.
6. Brismar B, Hardstedt C, Jacobson S: Diagnosis of thrombosis by catheter phlebography after prolonged central venous catheterization. *Ann Surg* 194:779, 1981.
7. Horne MK, Mayo DJ: Low-dose urokinase infusions to treat fibrinous obstruction of venous access devices in cancer patients. *J Clin Oncol* 15:2709, 1997.
8. Bern MM, Lokich JJ, Wallach SR, et al.: Very low doses of warfarin can prevent thrombosis in central venous catheters. *Ann Intern Med* 112:423, 1990.
9. Gould JR, Carloss HW, Skinner WL: Groshong catheter-associated subclavian venous thrombosis. *Am J Med* 95:419, 1993.
10. Monreal M, Raventos A, Lerma R, et al.: Pulmonary embolism in patients with upper extremity DVT associated to venous central lines—a prospective study. *Thromb Haemost* 72:548, 1994.
11. Becker DM, Philbrick JT, Walker FB: Axillary and subclavian venous thrombosis. *Arch Intern Med* 151:1934, 1991.
12. Chang R, Horne MK, Mayo DJ, Doppman JL: Pulse-spray treatment of subclavian and jugular venous thrombosis with recombinant tissue plasminogen activator. *JVIR* 7:845, 1996.
13. Monreal M, Alastrue A, Rull M, et al.: Upper extremity deep venous thrombosis in cancer patients with venous access devices—prophylaxis with a low molecular weight heparin (fragmin). *Thromb Haemost* 75:251, 1996.
14. Groeger JS, Lucas AB, Thaler HT, et al.: Infectious morbidity associated with long-term use of venous access devices in patients with cancer. *Ann Intern Med* 119:1168, 1993.
15. The Hospital Infection Control Panel Advisory Committee: Guideline for prevention of intravascular device-related infections. *Am J Infect Control* 24:262, 1996.
16. Raad II, Bodey GP: Infectious complications of indwelling vascular catheters. *Clin Infect Dis* 15:197, 1992.
17. Peters G, Locci R, Pulverer G: Adherence and growth of coagulase-negative staphylococci on surfaces of intravenous catheters. *J Infect Dis* 146:479, 1982.
18. Newman KA, Reed WP, Schimpff SC, et al.: Hickman catheters in association with intensive cancer chemotherapy. *Support Care Cancer* 1:92, 1993.
19. Atkinson JB, Chamberlin K, Boody BA: A prospective randomized trial of urokinase as an adjuvant in the treatment of proven Hickman catheter sepsis. *J Pediatr Surg* 33:714, 1998.
20. Veenstra DL, Saint S, Saha S, et al: Efficacy of antiseptic-impregnated catheters in preventing catheter-related bloodstream infection. *JAMA* 281:261, 1999.
21. Daroucche RO, Raad II, Heard SO, et al: A comparison of two antimicrobial impregnated central venous catheters. *New Engl J Med* 340:1, 1999.
22. Cobos E, Dixon S, Keung Y-K: Prevention and management of central venous catheter thrombosis. *Curr Opin Hematol* 5:355, 1998.
23. Sotir MJ, Lewis C, Bisher EW, et al: Epidemiology of device-associated infections related to long-term implantable vascular access device. *Inf Cont Hosp Epidemiol* 20:187, 1999.

PAIN MANAGEMENT

RICHARD B. PATT

NEIL M. ELLISON

Hematologic disorders comprise a wide range of disease entities, many with the capacity to produce acute and chronic pain. In addition to pain associated with procedures and complications related to hematologic diseases, such as biopsies, catheter insertions, severe infections, splenic infarctions, and their treatment, pain is a frequent and central problem in sickle cell disease, myeloma, and acquired immunodeficiency syndrome. When present, pain in patients with lymphoma is typical of the somatic and neuropathic pains that accompany the progression of solid tumors. In addition, patients with leukemia and receiving stem cell transplantation often describe persistent low-grade migratory pain that is idiopathic in nature. The guidelines described here for assessment and treatment are applicable to pain problems that coexist in patients with other underlying hematologic disorders.

MULTIDIMENSIONAL NATURE OF PAIN

Pain is defined by the International Association for the Study of Pain as an unpleasant sensory and emotional experience associated with actual or potential tissue damage.[1] Acute pain is usually associated with signs of sympathetic nervous system hyperactivity (e.g., tachycardia, hypertension, and diaphoresis) and heightened distress.[2] Chronic pain persists for weeks or months, and usually the source has been investigated and is known or suspected. Chronic pain implies that the underlying cause cannot be readily eliminated and requires some combination of palliative treatment, especially with analgesics and adjustment of lifestyle.[3]

PAIN MECHANISMS

Pain is regarded as either nociceptive or neuropathic.[13] This distinction signifies the presence or absence of an intact nervous system, and indicates that its functional status does or does not directly influence the cause of symptoms. Nociceptive pain may be somatic or visceral in origin. Somatic pain emanates from skin, bone, muscle, and other soft tissue, is characteristically localized, and is usually described with familiar adjectives (e.g., dull, aching, gnawing, or sharp). Visceral pain tends to be vague, less well localized, and is characteristically described as deep, dull, aching, dragging, squeezing, or pressure-like. Nociceptive pain of both somatic and visceral origin tends to respond to treatment with the opioids and, despite a ceiling effect, the nonsteroidal anti-inflammatory drugs (NSAIDs).[10] Bone pain of mild or moderate intensity, as well as pain that is accompanied by inflammation, tends to be especially responsive to treatment with the NSAIDs. In addition, bisphosphonates (classified as adjuvant analgesics; see Adjuvant Analgesics, below) have recently been observed to be efficacious for neoplastic bone pain.[4]

Neuropathic pain results from injury to the peripheral or central nervous system.[5] Pain is often accompanied by altered sensation, with or without objective findings of nerve injury, and is expressed in unfamiliar, sometimes bizarre terms that are distinct from prior experiences of pain. Complaints are dysesthetic in nature, and sensations are commonly described as burning, tingling, numbing, pressing, squeezing, or itching. Neuropathic pain may be constant, intermittent, or shocklike. The latter phenomenon has been likened to seizures, and may be characterized as shooting, lancinating, electrical, or jolting in nature. In contrast to nociceptive pain, neuropathic pain is less responsive to treatment with opioids and NSAIDs, but often responds favorably to adjuvant analgesics or coanalgesics, including the heterocyclic antidepressants, anticonvulsants, oral local anesthetics, and others (see below).[6] Despite the utility of the above clinical distinctions, the underlying mechanisms of pain, especially when due to progressive cancer are often mixed. The presence of mixed pain together with more obscure features that influence clinical responses idiosyncratically often call for implementing trials of analgesics on an individualized empiric basis. This is best achieved when drugs are introduced in low doses, ideally on an around-the-clock schedule, after which doses are rapidly titrated to achieve the optimal balance between therapeutic effect and toxicity.

CANCER PAIN

Pain accompanies a diagnosis of cancer in about two-thirds of cases, including about 25 percent of patients being treated with antineoplastic therapies and up to 90 percent of those with advanced disease.[7,8] About 80 percent of patients will respond with analgesia when oral and transdermal medications are used carefully to achieve a favorable balance between comfort and side effects. Most patients with moderate to severe pain who do not respond to conservative management with oral or transdermal medications can achieve comfort with parenteral opioids,[11,12] adjuvant medications,[13] or combined approaches offered by anesthesiologists or neurosurgeons.[14] It is the rare individual who will not respond to appropriate interventions. Surprisingly, despite the availability of effective treatment, unrelieved cancer pain remains an epidemic public health problem in the United States[8] and abroad.[9] Undertreatment is more closely related to cultural than medical factors. Prominent among these barriers are a failure to distinguish medical treatment from drug abuse, providers' exaggerated concerns regarding addiction and regulatory reprisal, a failure to embrace the principle of titration to effect, inadequate skills in treating side effects and using adjuvant medications, and an overall lack of accountability.[11,15] These issues are being addressed by legislation, scientific-based guidelines, and consumer-based initiatives. Pain associated with diagnostic procedures is a frequent problem in patients with hematologic disorders, especially children. Venipuncture, lumbar puncture, and bone marrow sampling are typical examples of tests that can be performed with little pain or distress with adequate planning.[16,17]

ASSESSMENT

A pain history is intended to determine the etiology of pain. Given the subjective nature of symptoms, the process includes evaluation of factors that are unique to the individual and may influence therapeutic recommendations, an endeavor that is best undertaken with a team approach that includes nursing staff. Questionnaires are available that are simple to administer and have been validated in patients with cancer pain.[18,19]

Clinicians should document pain intensity based on patient self-report and apply the same schema on return visits to guide therapy.

Acronyms and abbreviations that appear in this chapter include: AIDS, acquired immunodeficiency syndrome; CNS, central nervous system; HIV, human immunodeficiency virus; INF, interferon; NSAID, nonsteroidal anti-inflammatory drug.

Options include numerical rating scales (e.g., zero to ten, with zero an absence of pain and ten the worst pain a given patient can imagine), visual analgesic scales, or categorical scales that rate pain as absent, mild, moderate, severe, or excruciating. Easily incorporated into daily practice, these schema permit patients to guide clinicians in establishing the need to modify therapies.

TREATMENT FOR CANCER PAIN

NONSTEROIDAL ANTI-INFLAMMATORY DRUGS
When tolerated, around-the-clock administration of an NSAID may relieve pain that is mild. The NSAIDs may be combined with stronger analgesics for moderate to severe pain. The NSAIDs interfere with prostaglandin synthesis and thus are particularly effective in the management of pain of inflammatory and bony metastatic origin. The potential benefits of traditional NSAIDs should be weighed against their toxicity (gastrointestinal, renal, hematologic, and masking of fever), particularly in the presence of hematologic disorders and older age.[20] The nonacetylated salicylates (e.g., sodium salicylate and choline magnesium trisalicylate) have less effect on platelet aggregation, have less risk of gastrointestinal bleeding, and are well tolerated by asthma-

tics.[21,22] Parenteral ketorolac is equianalgesic with low doses of morphine, but is associated with the same range of potential side effects as oral NSAIDs, and treatment with oral or parenteral formulations is restricted to five days.[23] In contrast to opioids, treatment with the NSAIDs has a ceiling effect, above which dose escalations do not result in further analgesia but may result in increased toxicity. Regular, as opposed to intermittent, use promotes anti-inflammatory effects that may enhance analgesia. Although structurally distinct, NSAIDs are indistinguishable in most respects. Selection is based on the patient's prior experience, toxicity profiles, physician experience, schedule of administration, and cost. A new class of NSAIDs, referred to as COX-2 inhibitors (e.g., celecoxib and rofecoxib), has been introduced. These agents promise efficacy similar to that of less-sensitive NSAIDs with minimal toxicity and are currently being evaluated for potential chemopreventative roles, especially in colon cancer.[24,25]

OPIOIDS CONVENTIONALLY USED TO TREAT MODERATE PAIN ("WEAK" OPIOIDS)
When NSAIDs provide insufficient relief of pain, are poorly tolerated, or are contraindicated, the addition or substitution of a combination codeine-type preparation (e.g., codeine, oxycodone, hydrocodone, or dihydrocodeine combined with aspirin or acetaminophen) is an analgesic of intermediate potency. Although these agents comprise the "second step" of the World Health Organization–endorsed analgesic ladder, practitioners rely excessively on these agents, continuing their use after they are no longer effective in an attempt to avoid prescribing more potent opioids, which are also more highly regulated.[26] This practice may result in acetaminophen or aspirin toxicity, persistent pain, or side effects when symptoms would be more appropriately managed with "stronger" opioid analgesics. While continuing NSAIDs or adjuvants to exploit additive or synergistic effects to achieve an opioid-sparing effect is sometimes reasonable, this approach should be weighed against toxicities. The demonstration of equianalgesic activity for single-entity preparations of oxycodone substituted for morphine, together with the acceptance of transdermal preparations of fentanyl, which, although 100 times more potent than morphine, is prescribed in micrograms, has established that, overall, characterizing this class of drugs as "weak" is medically germane only insofar as the inclusion of acetaminophen or aspirin imposes a ceiling dose above which toxicity can be anticipated.

TABLE 21-1   COMPARISON OF POTENT OPIOID AGONISTS USED IN CANCER PAIN MANAGEMENT*

GENERIC NAME	TRADE NAME	DOSE, MG	ROUTE	DURATION, H
Morphine sulfate	Various	10	IV, SC	2–4
Morphine sulfate immediate release	MSIR, Roxanol, etc.	20–30[†]	Oral	2–4
Morphine sulfate controlled-release tablets	MS Contin, Oramorph	20–30	Oral	12–8
Morphine sulfate controlled-release capsules	Kadian	20–30	Oral	24–12
Morphine sulfate	Various	20	Rectal	3–4
Hydromorphone	Dilaudid	1.5	IV, SC	2–4
Hydromorphone	Dilaudid	7.5	Oral	2–4
Hydromorphone	Dilaudid	6	Rectal	3–4
Oxymorphone	Numorphan	1	IV	3–6
Oxymorphone	Numorphan	5–10	Rectal	4–6
Methadone	Dolophine	20	Oral	4–12*
Methadone	Dolophine	10	IV	4–12*
Levorphanol	Levodromoran	4	Oral	4–8
Levorphanol	Levodromoran	2	IV	4–8
Oxycodone immediate release	Roxycodone, Oxy-IR, etc.	20–30	Oral	2–4
Oxycodone controlled release	Oxycontin	20–30	Oral	12–8
Fentanyl	Sublimaze	0.1	IV	$\frac{1}{2}$–1
Fentanyl	Duragesic	‡	TD	
Fentanyl	Actiq	§	OTFC	
Meperidine	Demerol	75–100	IV	2–3
Meperidine	Demerol	300	Oral	2–3

Abbreviations: IV, intravenous; SC, subcutaneous; TD, transdermal; OTFC, oral transmucosal fentanyl citrate.
*Indicates conversion in acute care settings. Data from patients chronically treated with methadone suggests greater relative potency over time due to accumulation.
*Relative potencies and a guide for initiating treatment or converting from drug to drug. The correct dose is variable and should be individualized.
†Data from single-dose studies suggest that 10 mg parenteral morphine = 60 mg oral morphine is superceded in chronic pain management by extensive survey data suggesting an equivalency of 3:1 and, sometimes, 2:1.
‡Usual starting dose for relatively opioid naive individuals is 25 μg/h; if converting from moderate to high doses of a potent opioid, refer to package insert for recommended conversions and titrate to effect.
§Oral transmucosal fentanyl citrate (OTFC) is a new means of delivering fentanyl for the management of breakthrough pain in cancer patients. Drug is impregnated in a sugar-based lozenge mounted on a stick. Treatment should be commenced with the lowest available dosing unit and titrated to effect.

OPIOIDS USED TO TREAT SEVERE PAIN ("POTENT" OPIOIDS)
Individualization and Dosing Guidelines for Opioid Analgesics   Therapeutic and adverse effects of opioids vary widely based on factors such as age, previous drug history, drug metabolism and clearance, extent of disease, neuropathic pain, pain on movement, and other factors.[27,28] Effective doses may exceed guidelines recommended for acute pain in standard texts, and the correct opioid dose is the one

that relieves the pain without inducing intolerable side effects (Tables 21-1 and 21-2).[10] Because the early appearance of side effects erodes compliance, treatment is instituted in low doses that are gradually increased until either pain control is achieved or side effects occur.

Adverse Effects of Opioid Analgesics

Constipation is very frequent and should be treated prophylactically, usually with a mild stimulant and softener. Alternative laxatives (e.g., lactulose, a prokinetic agent, or enemas) can be used until regular bowel habit is reestablished.[29] When constipation is not relieved or alternates with diarrhea, fecal impaction or bowel obstruction should be excluded. When a new opioid is started or the dose is increased, tolerance to respiratory depression occurs rapidly, but transient nausea and sedation are common. With continued use, symptoms usually resolve spontaneously over a few days.[29] Unless symptoms are dramatic, patients should be encouraged to adhere to their analgesics and, if necessary, use an antiemetic (e.g., haloperidol, chlorpromazine, metoclopramide, scopolamine, glucocorticoids, odansetron, etc.), which should be gradually tapered. The possibility of severe constipation as an etiology of nausea and vomiting should be considered. Sedation that is related to opioid use may respond to an alternate opioid or treatment with a psychostimulant (methylphenidate, commencing with 10 mg on awakening and 5 mg with the noon-time meal, or dextroamphetamine).[30] Sudden cognitive changes in patients maintained on relatively stable opioid doses are unlikely to be related to the analgesic, and other causes should be considered.[31]

When side effects persist, a trial of a different opioid analgesic is warranted, since side effects are often idiosyncratic and may not be triggered by even pharmacologically similar agents.[32] The presence of intractable side effects may be an indication for invasive therapeutic modalities, such as nerve blocks or intraspinal opioids.[14]

TABLE 21-2   DOSAGE EQUIVALENCY FOR TRANSDERMAL FENTANYL*

Oral Morphine, mg/24 h†	IM Morphine, mg/24 h‡	TD Fentanyl, µg/h
45–134	8–22	25
135–224	23–37	50
225–314	38–52	75
315–404	53–67	100
405–494	68–82	125
495–584	83–97	150
585–674	98–112	175
675–764	113–127	200
765–854	128–142	225
855–944	143–157	250
945–1034	158–172	275
1035–1124	173–187	300

Abbreviations: IM, intramuscular; TD, transdermal; IV, intravenous.
*Hourly dose based on 24-h morphine equivalents.
†Conversion from oral morphine: Based on a *conservative* analgesic activity ratio of 60 mg oral morphine to 10 mg IM morphine (6:1 oral:parenteral conversion ratio rather than the widely accepted 3:1 ratio). As a result, converting from oral morphine to transdermal fentanyl using this chart, while generally quite safe, may result in underdosing of up to half of patients, who will then require rapid upward titration to achieve analgesia.
‡Conversion from IV or IM morphine: An analgesic activity ratio of 10 mg IM morphine: 100 ug IV fentanyl was used to derive the equivalence of parenteral morphine to transdermal fentanyl. *These recommendations tend to be reliable.*
SOURCE: Modified from package insert, Janssen Pharmaceutica.

TABLE 21-3   *CONTEMPORARY* DESCRIPTION OF PHENOMENA *HISTORICALLY* ASSOCIATED WITH ADDICTION

Phenomenon	Etiology	Definition	Incidence	Management
Physical dependence	Physiologic, pharmacologic	Withdrawal if opioids abruptly stopped or naloxone administered	Almost invariable	Avoid by gradual taper
Tolerance[1]	Physiologic, pharmacologic	Increased dose required to achieve analgesia†	Almost invariable	Reestablish analgesia with upward titration
Addiction (psychological dependence)	Psychological, questionable genetic influences	Nonmedical use despite harm	Rare (<1%)	Identify, multidisciplinary management
Withdrawal (abstinence syndrome)	Physiologic, pharmacologic	Characteristic signs and symptoms‡	Almost invariable	Avoid, reverse with opioids

[1]Although inevitable to some degree, this phenomenon is considerably less frequent than previously thought. It is recognized instead that dose increases in cancer patients are most likely due to disease progression.
†Tolerance develops to most adverse effects as well, especially nausea and sedation, but slowly, if at all, to constipation and miosis.
‡Characteristic signs and symptoms include lacrimation, diaphoresis, rhinorrhea, pupillary dilation, gooseflesh, muscle tremor, nausea and vomiting, abdominal cramping, diarrhea, raised heart rate, respiratory rate, and blood pressure, chills, hyperthermia, flushing, yawning, restlessness, irritability, anorexia, disturbed sleep, and generalized body aches.

Although a feared side effect of opioid therapy, addiction (Table 21-3) is an uncommon outcome of medical treatment. It has been reported in less than one of 3000 exposures for cancer-related pain[33] and in less than 3 percent of patients treated for sickle cell–related pain.[34] Addiction refers to a behavioral pattern of aberrant drug use aimed at achieving psychic, and not analgesic, effects of opioids, and implies loss of control and interference with routine activities.[40] Addiction is considered to be synonymous with psychological dependence and is unrelated to physical dependence and tolerance, pharmacologic phenomena that are, to some extent inevitable with chronic use.[35] Although common, tolerance appears to be a less dramatic phenomenon than was once thought and clinically is rarely problematic, since the dose can be raised, as tolerance also occurs to most side effects. Patients should be taught to expect that physical dependence will lead to withdrawal syndrome if treatment is abruptly stopped or an antagonist is administered and should be reassured that if pain remits, doses can be tapered without difficulties. The term *pseudoaddiction* has been used to refer to an iatrogenic syndrome of drug seeking resulting from underprescribing.[36]

FOLLOW-UP

Once a drug regimen has been established, it is the clinician's responsibility to reassess adequacy. Patients may be reluctant to ask for more potent analgesics and may not describe changes in the character of pain that signify new events, such as impending spinal cord compression or fracture. Pharmacologic tolerance is first manifested by decreased duration of analgesic effect and is best managed by an upward dose adjustment rather than decreasing the interval between administration. Increased drug requirements after a period of stable analgesia are most commonly related to disease progression or recurrence.

SCHEDULE OF USE

A time-contingent (around-the-clock) schedule for the administration of analgesics is usually preferred to symptom-contingent (prn) administration. When withheld until pain becomes severe, analgesics may be ineffective due to sympathetic arousal and established patterns of anticipation and memory of pain. Most cancer pain is relatively constant, with intermittent exacerbations (breakthrough pain), and is ideally treated with a combination of maintenance therapy with a basal, long-acting analgesic (e.g, controlled-release morphine or controlled-release oxycodone or transdermal fentanyl) and "escape doses" or "rescue doses" of a short-acting agent (e.g., immediate-release morphine, hydromorphone, oxycodone, or oral transmucosal fentanyl citrate) administered as necessary for breakthrough and incident pain.[37] The frequency with which rescue doses are utilized serves as a gauge of the efficacy of maintenance therapy. Patients are instructed to maintain records that reflect analgesic use: a need for rescue doses in excess of three to four times over a 24-h period signifies the need to raise the dose of the long-acting analgesic, whereas the absence of a need for rescue doses may permit maintenance doses to be lowered. Rescue doses are usually commenced at a dose equivalent to 5 to 15 percent of the 24-h dose of the long-acting analgesic, administered ideally at 4-h, but sometimes as often as 2-h, intervals as necessary.[10] Although the empirically derived "5 to 15 percent rule" is safe and usually effective, studies of oral transmucosal fentanyl citrate failed to reveal such a correlation,[38] presumably reflecting the heterogeneity of breakthrough pain. A common clinical oversight involves gradually raising the background dose of basal analgesic without considering altering the rescue dose. This dilemma is often best resolved by allowing reliable patients to use a range of prn dosing predicated on the breakthrough event.

Breakthrough pain that is predominantly movement-related (incident pain, as opposed to end-of-dose failure or idiopathic breakthrough pain), as in the case of an unstable fracture or decubitus ulcer, is the most clinically challenging of pain syndromes.[33-35] Rapid changes in pain intensity and in dose requirements are not readily addressed by most oral agents. The need for erratic dosing that is contingent on activity may not allow patients to tolerate side effects. Oral transmucosal fentanyl citrate (OTFC) a sweetened lozenge impregnated with fentanyl[38] and mounted on a stick may provide pain relief within 5 to 10 min after patients start to consume a unit. Available in doses ranging from 200 to 1600 μg, units usually require 15 min for complete consumption. Rapid onset relates to the proportion of drug that is rapidly absorbed across the highly vascular buccal mucosa. While this route is not subject to first-pass hepatic metabolism, the remaining drug is inevitably swallowed, providing a duration of relief ranging from 2 to 4 h.

ADJUVANT ANALGESICS

Adjuvant analgesics are drugs developed for purposes other than pain relief that have been observed to promote pain relief in specific clinical settings. Because efficacy is contingent on the underlying mechanism of pain, the adjuvants are generally reserved for specific settings, usually neuropathic pain. Other indications for adjuvant analgesics include the use of psychostimulants (e.g., methylphenidate or amphetamines) to enhance arousal and the use of glucocorticoids for bone pain and other syndromes.

Selected antidepressants relieve pain, especially when neuropathic, independent of mood, a property that has been confirmed in controlled clinical trials.[5,6] Amitriptyline and its analogs (e.g., nortriptyline and imipramine) induce pain relief in doses inadequate to combat depression (10–100 mg nightly). The tricyclics appear most likely to be effective in the presence of constant neuropathic pain that is dysesthetic (e.g., burning, numb, or tingling) in character. Pain that is predominantly intermittent, shocklike, or stabbing may be best treated first with an anticonvulsant,[39] such as carbamazepine, gabapentin phenytoin, valproic acid, and clonazepam. Specific applications for these agents include postherpetic neuralgia, diabetic neuropathy, phantom limb pain, and postmastectomy or postthoracotomy pain, chemotherapy-

mediated polyneuropathy, and tumor invasion of neural structures. Gabapentin has garnered considerable favor because, when doses are raised gradually from 100 mg tid, adverse effects are infrequent, even in doses of up to 3600 mg/day.[40] Mexiletene, an antiarrhythmic and oral local anesthetic, has been shown to be useful as a second-line agent for refractory neuropathic pain.[41] Oral glucocorticoids are effective for various cancer pain syndromes, especially when bulky tumor is present (e.g., rectal, pelvic, and esophageal cancer, and brachial and lumbosacral plexopathy), presumably due to reduction of peritumoral edema and inflammation.[42] There are few data to support a direct analgesic effect of antihistamines, antipsychotics, or anxiolytics. Since adjuvant analgesics are not as consistently effective as opioids, treatment is usually in sequential drug trials. Most require regular use for up to one week before efficacy is established, and thus these agents should not be relied on in the presence of a "pain emergency." They are typically used in conjunction with opioid therapy and must be carefully titrated to avoid adverse effects and drug interactions.

ROUTE OF DRUG ADMINISTRATION

When possible, analgesics should be administered orally or transdermally to promote independence and mobility. Parenteral administration is not more efficacious than oral administration, so treatment by these routes should be reserved for conditions that render oral administration unreliable (e.g., weakness, dry mouth, dysphagia, nausea, vomiting, malabsorption, or intestinal obstruction). Alternative routes should be considered when excessive numbers of tablets must be ingested or when rapid pain control is required. Morphine, because it is easily available in a variety of formulations, has been regarded as the initial opioid of choice for moderate to severe pain, although concerns have arisen regarding the potential for the accumulation of M-6-glucuronide, which can produce refractory nausea or sedation in a minority of patients.[43]

SPECIFIC OPIOIDS

Preferred agents for prolonged basal analgesia include controlled-release morphine (MS Contin or Oramorph[44] q 12–8 h, or Kadian capsules q 24–12 h[45]), controlled-release oxycodone (Oxycontin q 12–8 h), or transdermal fentanyl (Duragesic patches applied q 72–48 h),[46] titrated to effect. While controlled-release tablets should never be broken, crushed, or chewed, the contents of Kadian capsules can be sprinkled in food or placed through feeding tubes. All long-acting agents should be prescribed in adequate doses to avoid the need for shorter intervals between administrations. Transdermal fentanyl is especially well accepted by patients and may be associated with less constipation than other opioids. Conversion factors in Table 21-1 are conservative, thus necessitating upward titration in some patients. A small proportion of patients may need patches changed as often as q 48 h. The epidermis and a subcutaneous depot effect requires a period of time before equilibration occurs for both upward and downward titration. Thus, transdermal therapy is not useful to treat acute pain.

If controlled-release agents are poorly tolerated, short-acting opioids can be used around the clock, or inherently long-acting analgesics, such as methadone or levorphanol, can be considered. Methadone and, to a lesser extent, levorphanol have long half-lives that exceed the duration of analgesia. Patients at increased risk of respiratory depression include those who are opioid naive, patients with receding pain, older patients, and those with altered renal function.[47,48] In addition to its opioid effects, methadone binds to the newly recognized n-methyl-D-aspartate (NMDA) receptor,[49] and thus may provide better analgesia than other opioids, especially when pain has neuropathic features.

DRUGS TO AVOID: MEPERIDINE AND THE AGONIST-ANTAGONIST OPIOIDS

Chronic administration of meperidine should be avoided, particularly when renal function is impaired (see "Pain in Sickle Cell Disease"). When administered chronically, especially in high doses, all opioids have the potential to cause muscle twitching (myoclonus), usually manifest as whole body jerking, but meperidine is the only clinically relevant opioid that may produce seizures. The accumulation of normeperidine may result in naloxone-resistant grand mal seizures.[50] Predisposing factors include older age, oral use, prolonged use, and renal dysfunction.

The agonist-antagonist opioids (e.g., pentazocine, nalbuphine and butorphanol) and partial agonist opioids (e.g., buprenorphine and dezocine) are not recommended for cancer pain management[10] because of their characteristic ceiling doses, above which further analgesia does not accrue, the potential for physiologic withdrawal when combined with pure opioid agonists, unreliable reversal with naloxone, a higher incidence of dysphoria, and limited formulations.

While sedatives, antidepressants, and anxiolytics have important roles in the management of various symptoms, these agents should not be utilized as substitutes for the more reliable opioid analgesics.

OTHER PAIN THERAPIES

Whenever possible, specific therapies directed at modifying the underlying disease process should be considered for pain relief, although, when the outcome of these strategies is uncertain or is likely to be time consuming, pharmacotherapy should be instituted concomitantly.

Traditional pharmacologic therapies are inadequate in certain settings. In some patients, behavioral and physical modalities, such as relaxation training, guided imagery, hypnosis, therapeutic massage, acupuncture, and music therapy, may be useful. When pharmacologic therapy has failed, consideration should be given to more specialized interventional therapies, including neural blockade, CNS opioid therapy, neurosurgery, and electrical stimulation.[13,14]

PAIN IN SICKLE CELL DISEASE

Pain is a very frequent feature of sickle cell disease (see Chap. 47). Although the pain associated with vaso-occlusive crisis is abrupt in onset and severe in intensity, many patients experience lower-level chronic pain between episodes. Pain has been cited as a cause of death in sickle cell patients,[51,52] serves as a marker of disease severity,[53] and should be treated effectively so that patients may function more effectively.[54] Except in the presence of specific evidence, physicians should assume that the patient's report of pain is reliable and on this basis should evaluate its cause and provide symptomatic relief.[55]

As with other pain states, treatment should be individualized, and relatively large doses of analgesics often are required to control pain. When pain is chronic, it is essential to broaden therapeutic goals to maintain function and comfort. Adequate analgesia implies uninterrupted nighttime sleep, the maintenance of normal daily activities, and relative freedom from side effects such as sedation, nausea, and vomiting. Despite clinician perception,[56] the incidence of addiction in sickle cell patients is low, and drug-seeking behavior may be more intimately related to undertreatment (pseudoaddiction).[36]

PHARMACOLOGIC MANAGEMENT OF PAINFUL CRISES IN SICKLE CELL DISEASE

CHOICE OF ANALGESIC

Only one nonopioid analgesic is available in the United States in parenteral form (ketorolac), and although efficacy for the management of sickle cell pain has not been specifically demonstrated, when not contraindicated, it is a reasonable nonhabituating therapeutic option.[55,57] All opioid analgesics have been used for the management of sickle cell pain. Although meperidine (Demerol) is the most commonly used parenteral therapy, it is a poor choice for repetitive administration, in that it is the least potent of the strong opioids, it has a relatively short duration of effect (2 to 3 h), and its low oral bioavailability renders outpatient treatment ineffective and hazardous.[50,58] Normeperidine, a primary metabolite, may accumulate as a result of its half-life of 18 h. Although it is not an analgesic, its stimulant properties can produce nervousness, tremors, agitation, multifocal myoclonus, and generalized seizures, effects that are not reversible with naloxone.[50] In addition, mean peak meperidine concentrations are lower in sickle cell patients than in postoperative patients, and unexplained diurnal variations in meperidine plasma levels and efficacy have been noted in patients with painful sickle cell disease.[59] These factors taken together indicate that, despite its time-honored role, meperidine should be avoided for the management of acute or chronic pain in the sickle cell patient and should not be a first-line analgesic. Treatment of pain in patients with sickle cell disease is in most respects similar to treatment of cancer-related pain.[55]

Opioid agonist-antagonists (e.g., butorphanol, pentazocine, and nalbuphine) and partial agonists (e.g., buprenorphine and dezocine) should in general play a very limited role in the treatment of chronic sickle cell disease–related pain. The advantages of less rigorous scheduling and a ceiling effect on respiratory depression are outweighed by various other characteristics of these agents. With the exception of pentazocine, no drugs from these classes are available orally, although butorphanol has recently been introduced for intranasal administration. These agents also are associated with psychotomimetic side effects (e.g., jitteriness, hallucinations, and delirium), which are most pronounced with pentazocine. Buprenorphine may be difficult to antagonize with naloxone, and the potential of other agents to antagonize pure opioid agonists reduces flexibility and enhances the risk of undesirable drug interactions.

ROUTE OF ADMINISTRATION

Oral opioids can be used in the treatment of acute sickle cell–related pain.[60,61] Treatment with oral meperidine or morphine has resulted in significant reductions in the frequency of emergency room visits, lengths of stay, and both the frequency and dose of parenteral opioids.[60] In another emergency room–based study,[61] 88 percent of patients with uncomplicated sickle cell pain achieved relief within 30 min of starting a treatment regimen composed mostly of oral morphine sulfate elixir. After an initial dose of 60 mg oral morphine elixir, additional 15-mg doses were provided q 20 min until analgesia or sedation occurred. Once acceptable analgesia was obtained, 30- to 60-mg doses of oral morphine were administered q 2 h as needed, with aspirin or another NSAID and oral hydration (200–300 ml/h).

Although continuous intravenous infusions of morphine [0.08 mg/(kg · h)] and meperidine [0.58 mg/(kg · h)] are often used in hospitalized children with severe sickle cell pain, treatment should be provided cautiously.[62] Reports of three children with signs and symptoms of "acute chest syndrome" experienced respiratory arrest during treatment with opioids administered by a continuous intravenous infusion. A diagnosis of acute chest syndrome should be considered at least a relative contraindication to such treatment.

Patient-controlled analgesia for the management of hospitalized patients with acute sickle cell–related pain has considerable appeal. Use in postoperative and cancer pain management and preliminary experiences in sickle cell–related pain,[63,64] suggests that patients will titrate to a minimally effective analgesic concentration without over-dose, sedation, or respiratory depression.

Patient-controlled analgesia for sickle cell pain is usually safe and efficacious in children as young as 11 years of age. Although reductions in opioid use typically accompany the resolution of pain, exaggerated concerns may arise regarding the potential for addiction in adolescent populations.[59,63] In one study, 30 percent of 46 patients reported problems, which included dislike of treatment and, in one patient, respiratory insufficiency that required the administration of naloxone occurred.[63]

The application of a "cancer pain model" to sickle cell pain has met with considerable success in one inner city hospital. The short-term use of intravenous analgesics and maintenance therapy with controlled release oral morphine resulted in a 67 percent decrease in emergency department visits, a 44 percent reduction in hospital admissions, 57 percent fewer inpatient days, and a 23 percent reduction in length of stay.[55]

PREVALENCE OF ADDICTION

The management of pain in other medical illnesses, such as cancer, headache, and burns, by the chronic administration of opioids need not be complicated by a high prevalence of drug abuse or addiction.[33,65,66] Concern among practitioners regarding the risk of addiction as a consequence of treating sickle cell pain is demonstrated by a recent survey documenting that 23 percent and 53 percent of hematologists and emergency physicians, respectively, believed there was a greater than 20 percent incidence of addiction among patients with sickle cell disease.[56] While few studies have carefully investigated the risk of addiction in patients with sickle cell disease, several suggest that the perception of risk is exaggerated. One report of more than 600 patients followed in the United Kingdom failed to reveal any evidence of drug addiction, while a U.S. study of 101 patients found three patients with abuse and seven with "drug dependence." Patients with a prior history of drug abuse are at an increased risk of addiction. A report of 160 patients with sickle cell disease treated for pain found that 14 adults used emergency room facilities and hospitals excessively, tampered with infusion pumps to deliver unauthorized opioids, or engaged in trafficking in prescription drugs or cocaine.

PAIN IN MYELOMA

Bone pain occurs in about 70 percent of patients at the time of diagnosis of myeloma (see Chap. 106). Pain is characteristically severe and sudden in onset and predominantly involves the vertebrae, ribs, and long bones. As a result of osteolytic lesions and osteopenia, pathologic fractures occur in nearly two-thirds of patients. Exaggerated secretion of cytokines such as IL-1, IL-6, lymphotoxin, and INF induce osteoclastic activity, with subsequent bone resorption.[67,68] Associated pain is often severe. The resultant decreased mobility increases the likelihood of hypercalcemia. Multiple approaches can be used to alleviate pain. Successful cytotoxic therapy is the principal approach. Radiation therapy and surgery are reserved for specific localized sites requiring rapid prophylactic or palliative treatment, especially to prevent or treat fractures. Radiation therapy can relieve pain, even at modest doses, if there are no better, less cytotoxic options.

Direct inhibition of osteoclastic activity with bisphosphonates and related compounds is of significant value, when these drugs are given concurrently with antimyeloma chemotherapy, in decreasing myeloma-induced skeletal complications, including total number of pathologic fractures, delayed onset of new pathologic fractures, a reduced need for palliative radiation therapy, less overall use of analgesics, and more relief of bone pain than on patients treated with chemotherapy alone.[69,70] Side effects from recommended monthly doses of

90 mg pamidronate were relatively few, and the drug is quite well tolerated (see Chap. 106).

PAIN IN ACQUIRED IMMUNODEFICIENCY SYNDROME

Patients with the human immunodeficiency virus (HIV) infection experience a broad spectrum of pain syndromes with incidences and severities similar to those observed in cancer patients, although undertreatment is much more prevalent.[71] In addition to the impediments to pain control that have been identified in other disease states, pain may be overlooked as a consequence of the overwhelming impact of the disease, its stigma, and a history of drug abuse in some affected individuals. HIV infection is associated with a heterogeneous group of pain syndromes, of which variants of neuropathic pain are especially common. Disease-specific pain syndromes exist,[71] and, as is true for cancer, pain severity correlates with disease progression.[72] Reports of pain prevalence, intensity, and pain-related interference with function are similar among patients independent of a history of prior injection drug use, although undertreatment is much more prevalent in those with a history of drug abuse.[73]

About 50 percent of patients admitted to a hospital for care had pain, and 30 percent of hospital admissions were primarily for pain[74]; and, in a survey of outpatients, pain was identified in about 50 percent of 100 outpatients studied.[75] In some communities, pain is the second most frequent reason for hospitalizing patients,[76] and persistent or frequent pain over the most recent two-week interval was reported in 226 of 336 patients interviewed; 85 percent had inadequate analgesic therapy.[77] In the latter study, less than 8 percent of 110 patients with severe pain were given a "strong" opioid, and adjuvant analgesics were used in only 10 percent of cases.[77] Pain and discomfort are even more prevalent during the last two weeks of life. Up to 93 percent of patients developed pain for at least 48 h during this interval, and up to 38 percent experienced no relief.[78]

Although further studies investigating the relationship between AIDS and pain are needed, the application of established guidelines with a combination of opioid and adjuvant analgesics similar to that described for the management of cancer pain is recommended.[10]

REFERENCES

1. Merskey H: Classification of chronic pain. *Pain* (suppl 3):226, 1986.
2. Sternbach RA: Acute versus chronic pain, in *Textbook of Pain*, 2nd ed, edited by PD Wall, R Melzack, p 242. Churchill Livingstone, Edinburgh, 1989.
3. Sanders A: Behavioral assessment and treatment of clinical pain: appraisal and current status, in *Progress in Behavior Modification*, edited by M Hersen, RM Eisler, PM Miller, pp 249–291. *Academic*, New York, 1979.
4. Ernst DS, MacDonald RN, Paterson AH, Jensen J, Brasher P, Bruera E: A double-blind, crossover trial of intravenous clodronate in metastatic bone pain. *J Pain Symptom Manage* 7:4, 1992.
5. Bennett GJ: Neuropathic pain, in *Textbook of Pain*, 3rd ed, edited by PD Wall, R Melzack, pp 201–224. Churchill Livingstone, Edinburgh, 1994, pp 201–224.
6. Portenoy RK, Kanner RM: Nonopioid and adjuvant analgesics, in *Pain Management: Theory and Practice*, edited by RK Portenoy, RM Kanner, pp 219–247. FA Davis, Philadelphia, 1996.
7. Bonica JJ: Management of cancer pain. *Recent Results Cancer Res* 89:13, 1984.
8. Cleeland CS, Gonin R, Hatfield AK, et al: Pain and its treatment in outpatients with metastatic cancer. *N Engl J Med* 330:592, 1994.
9. World Health Organization: *Cancer Pain Relief.* World Health Organization, Geneva, 1986.
10. Jacox A, Carr DB, Payne R, et al: *Management of Cancer Pain: Clinical Practice Guideline No. 9.* Agency for Health Care Policy and Research, Rockville, MD, 1994, AHCPR Publication No. 94-0592.

11. Bruera E, Brenneis C, Macmillan K, et al: The use of the subcutaneous route for the administration of narcotics. *Cancer* 62:407, 1988.

12. Portenoy RK, Mouline DE, Rogers A, et al: IV infusion of opioids for cancer pain: clinical review and guidelines for use. *Cancer Treat Rep* 70:575, 1986.

13. Patt RB, Burton A: Pain associated with advanced malignancy, including adjuvant analgesic drugs in cancer pain management, in Aronoff (ed): *Evaluation and Treatment of Chronic Pain,* 3d ed. Baltimore, Williams & Wilkins, 1998, pp 337–376.

14. Patt RB: The current status of anesthetic approaches to cancer pain management, in Payne R, Patt RB, Hill CS Jr (eds): *Assessment and Treatment of Cancer Pain: Progress in Pain Research and Management,* vol 12. Seattle, IASP Press, 1998, pp 195–211.

15. Joranson DE, Gilson AA: Regulatory barriers to pain management. *Semin Oncol Nurs* 14:158, 1998.

16. Miser AW, Miser JS: The treatment of cancer pain in children. *Pediatr Clin North Am* 36:979, 1989.

17. Berde C, Ablin A, Glazer J, et al: American Academy of Pediatrics Report of the Subcommittee on Disease-Related Pain in Childhood Cancer. *Pediatrics* 86:818, 1990.

18. Janjan NA, Payne R, Gillis T, et al: Presenting symptoms in patients referred to a multidisciplinary clinic for bone metastases. *J Pain Symtom Manage* 16:171, 1998.

19. Philip J, Smith WB, Craft P, Lickiss A: Concurrent validity of the modified Edmonton Symptom Assessment System with the Rotterdam Symptom Checklist and the Brief Pain Inventory. *Support Care Cancer* 6:539, 1998.

20. Schlegel SI, Paulus HE: Nonsteroidal and analgesic use in the elderly. *Clin Rheum Dis* 12:245, 1996.

21. Rothwell KG: Efficacy and safety of a non-acetylated salicylate, choline magnesium trisalicylate in the treatment of rheumatoid arthritis. *J Int Med Res* 11:343, 1983.

22. Leonards JR, Levy A: Gastrointestinal blood loss from aspirin and sodium salicylate tablets in man. *Clin Pharmacol Ther* 14:62, 1973.

23. Gillis JC, Brogden RA: Ketorolac: a reappraisal of its pharmacodynamic and pharmacokinetic properties and therapeutic use in pain management. *Drugs* 53:139, 1997.

24. Vane JR, Bakhle YS, Botting RA: Cyclooxygenases 1 and 2. *Annu Rev Pharmacol Toxicol* 38:97, 1998.

25. Hawkey CJ: COX-2 inhibitors. *Lancet* 353:307, 1999.

26. Portenoy RA: Inadequate outcome of opioid therapy for cancer pain: influences on practioners and patients, in *Cancer Pain,* edited by RB Patt, pp 119–128 Lippincott, Philadelphia, 1993.

27. Kaiko RF, Wallenstein SL, Rogers AG, et al: Sources of variation in analgesic responses in cancer patients with chronic pain receiving morphine. *Pain* 15:191, 1983.

28. Bruera E, Schoeller T, Wenk R, et al: A prospective multicenter assessment of the Edmonton staging system for cancer pain. *J Pain Symptom Manage* 10:348, 1995.

29. Ellison NA: Opioid analgesics: toxicities and their treatments, in *Cancer Pain,* edited by RB Patt, pp 185–194. Lippincott, Philadelphia, 1993.

30. Bruera E, Fainsinger R, MacEachern T, Hanson J: The use of methylphenidate in patients with incident cancer pain receiving regular opiates: a preliminary report. *Pain* 50:75, 1992.

31. Bruera E, Chadwick S, Weinlick A, et al: Delirium and severe sedation in a patient with terminal cancer. *Cancer Treat Rep* 71:787, 1987.

32. de Stoutz ND, Bruera E, Suarez-Almazor A: Opioid rotation for toxicity reduction in terminal cancer patients. *J Pain Symptom Manage* 10:378, 1995.

33. Porter J, Jick A: Addiction rare in patients treated with narcotics. *N Engl J Med* 302:123, 1980.

34. Brozovic M, Davies SC, Yardumian A, et al: Pain relief in sickle cell crisis. *Lancet* 624, 1986.

35. Portenoy RA: Opioid therapy in nonmalignant pain. *J Pain Symptom Manage* 5:546, 1990.

36. Weissman DE: Understanding pseudoaddiction. *J Pain Symptom Manage* 9:74, 1994.

37. Patt RB, Ellison NA: Breakthrough pain in cancer patients: characteristics, prevalence, and treatment. *Oncology* 12:1035, 1998.

38. Christie JM, Simmonds M, Patt R, et al: Dose-titration, multicenter study of oral transmucosal fentanyl citrate for the treatment of breakthrough pain in cancer patients using transdermal fentanyl for persistent pain. *J Clin Oncol* 16:3238, 1998.

39. Rosner H, Rubin A: Gabapentin adjunctive therapy in neuropathic pain states. *Clin J Pain* 12:56, 1996.

40. Backonja M, Beydoun A, Edwards KR, et al: Gabapentin for the symptomatic treatment of painful neuropathy in patients with diabetes mellitus: a randomized controlled trial. *JAMA* 280:1831, 1998.

41. Jarvis B, Coukell AA: Mexiletine: a review of its therapeutic use in painful diabetic neuropathy. *Drugs* 56:691, 1998.

42. Bruera E, Roca E, Cedaro L, Carraro S, Chacon A: Action of oral methylprednisolone in terminal cancer patients: a prospective randomized double-blind study. *Cancer Treat Rep* 69:751, 1985.

43. Christrup LL: Morphine metabolites. *Acta Anaesthesiol Scand* 41:116, 1997.

44. Bloomfield SS, Cissell GB, Mitchell J, et al: Analgesic efficacy and potency of two oral controlled-release morphine preparations. *Clin Pharmacol Ther* 53:469, 1993.

45. Broomhead A, Kerr R, Tester W, et al: Comparison of a once-a-day sustained-release morphine formulation with standard oral morphine treatment for cancer pain. *J Pain Symptom Manage* 14:63, 1997.

46. Ahmedzai S, Brooks A: Transdermal fentanyl versus sustained-release oral morphine in cancer pain: preference, efficacy, and quality of life: the TTS-Fentanyl Comparative Trial Group. *J Pain Symptom Manage* 13:254, 1997.

47. Gourlay GK, Cherry DA, Cousins MJ: A comparative study of the efficacy and pharmacokinetics of oral methadone and morphine in the treatment of severe pain in patients with cancer. *Pain* 25:297, 1986.

48. Plummer JL, Gourlay GK, Cherry DA, Cousins MJ: Estimation of methadone clearance: application in the management of cancer pain. *Pain* 33:313, 1988.

49. Ebert B, Thorkildsen C, Andersen S, Christrup LL, Hjeds A: Opioid analgesics as noncompetitive *n*-methyl-D-aspartate (NMDA) antagonists. *Biochem Pharmacol* 56:553, 1998.

50. Kaiko RF, Foley KM, Grabinski PY, et al: Central nervous system excitatory effects of meperidine in cancer patients. *Ann Neurol* 13:180, 1983.

51. Parfrey NA, Moore GW, Hutchins GM: Is pain crises a cause of death in sickle cell disease? *Am J Clin Pathol* 84:209, 1985.

52. Thomas AN, Pattison C, Serjeant GA: Causes of death in sickle-cell disease in Jamaica. *Br Med J* 285:633, 1982.

53. Platt OG, Thornston BD, Brambilia DJ, et al: Pain in sickle cell disease: rates and risk factors. *N Engl J Med* 325:11, 1991.

54. Payne R, Foley KM (eds): Cancer pain. *Med Clin North Am* 71:153, 1987.

55. Brookoff D, Polomano A: Treating sickle cell pain like cancer pain. *Ann Intern Med* 116:364, 1992.

56. Shapiro BS, Benjamin LJ, Payne R, Heidrich G: Sickle cell-related pain: perceptions of medical practitioners. *J Pain Symptom Manage* 14:168, 1997.

57. Wright SW, Norris RL, Mitchell TR: Ketorolac for sickle cell vaso-occlusive crisis pain in the emergency department: lack of a narcotic-sparing effect. *Ann Emerg Med* 21:925, 1992.

58. Tang R, Shimomura SK, Rotblatt M: Meperidine-induced seizures in sickle cell patients. *Hosp Formul* 15:764, 1980.

59. Ritschell WA, Bykadi G, Ford DJ, et al: A pilot study on disposition and pain relief after IM administration of meperidine during the day or night. *Int J Clin Pharmacol Ther Toxicol* 21:218, 1983.

60. Friedman EW, Weber AB, Osborn HH, et al: Oral analgesia for treatment of painful crises in sickle cell anemia. *Ann Emerg Med* 15:43, 1986.

61. Powers RD: Management protocol for sickle-cell disease patients with acute pain: impact on emergency department and narcotic use. *Am J Emerg Med* 4:267, 1986.

62. Cole TB, Sprinkle RH, Smith SJ, et al: Intravenous narcotic therapy for children with severe sickle cell pain crises. *Am J Dis Child* 140:1255, 1986.

63. Schecter NL, Berrien FB, Katz SM: The use of patient-controlled analgesia in adolescents with sickle cell pain crises: a preliminary report. *J Pain Symptom Manage* 3:109, 1988.

64. Trentadue NO, Kachoyeanos MK, Lea G: Comparison of two regimens of patient-controlled analgesia for children with sickle cell disease. *J Pediatr Nurs* 13:9, 1998.

65. Perry S, Heidrich G: Management of pain during debridement: a survey of US burn units. *Pain* 13:267, 1982.

66. Medina JL, Diamond S: Drug dependency in patients with chronic headache. *Headache* 17:12, 1977.

67. Lichtenstein A, Berenson J, Norman D, et al: Production of cytokines by bone marrow cells obtained from patients with multiple myeloma. *Blood* 74:266, 1989.

68. Stashenko P, Dewhirst FE, Peros WJ, et al: Synergistic interactions between interleukin 1 tumor necrosis factor and lymphotoxin in bone resorption. *J Immunol* 138:1464, 1987.

69. Berenson J, Lichentenstein A, Porter L, et al: Efficacy of pamidronate in reducing skeletal events in patients with advanced multiple myeloma. *N Engl J Med* 334:488, 1996.

70. Berenson J, Lichtenstein A, Porter L, et al: Long term pamidronate treatment of advanced multiple myeloma patients reduces skeletal events. *J Clin Oncol* 16:593, 1998.

71. Hewitt DJ, McDonald M, Portenoy RK, Rosenfeld B, Passik S, Breitbart W: Pain syndromes and etiologies in ambulatory AIDS patients. *Pain* 70:117, 1997.

72. Singer EJ, Zorilla C, Femy-Chandon B, et al: Painful symptoms reported for ambulatory HIV-infected men in a longitudinal study. *Pain* 54:15, 1993.

73. Breitbart W, Rosenfeld B, Passik S, Kaim M, Funesti Esch J, Stein K: A comparison of pain report and adequacy of analgesic therapy in ambulatory AIDS patients with and without a history of substance abuse. *Pain* 72:235, 1997.

74. Lebovits AH, Lefkowitz M, McCarthy D, et al: The prevalence and management of pain in patients with AIDS: a review of 134 cases. *Clin J Pain* 5:245, 1989.

75. Schofferman J, Brody R: Pain in far advanced AIDS. *Adv Pain Res Ther* 16:379, 1990.

76. Lewis MS, Warfied CA: Management of pain in AIDS. *Hosp Pract* 25:51, 1990.

77. Breitbart W, Rosenfeld BD, Passik SD: The undertreatment of pain in ambulatory AIDS patients. *Pain* 65:243, 1996.

78. Kimball LR, McCormick WC: The pharmacologic management of pain and discomfort in persons with AIDS near the end of life: use of opioid analgesia in the hospital setting. *J Pain Symp Mnmt* 11:88, 1996.

PART V

THE
ERYTHROCYTE

MORPHOLOGY OF THE ERYTHRON

BRIAN S. BULL

THE ERYTHRON

Collectively the progenitor and adult red cells have been termed the *erythron* to reinforce the idea that they function as an organ. The widely dispersed cells that make up this organ arise from undifferentiated, pluripotential stem cells. Following commitment, erythroid progenitors progress through several replicative stages, becoming more functionally specialized with maturation (Table 22-1). Eventually the reticulocyte and finally the mature, circulating erythrocyte are produced.

ERYTHROID PROGENITOR AND STIMULATING FACTORS

BURST-FORMING UNIT—ERYTHROID

The earliest progenitor committed to the erythroid lineage is the BFU-E. This cell is defined by its ability to create a "burst" on semisolid media, that is, a colony consisting of several hundred cells.

COLONY-FORMING UNIT—ERYTHROID

As maturation progresses a late progenitor, CFU-E, develops. The CFU-E is very sensitive to erythropoietin (see Chap. 14 and Table 22-1).

THE ERYTHROBLASTIC ISLAND

The anatomic unit of erythropoiesis in the normal adult is the *erythroblastic island*.[46] It consists of one or two centrally located macrophages surrounded by maturing erythroid cells (Fig. 22-1). The adhesion between erythroid cells and macrophages occurs at the CFU-E stage of maturation.[47] Phase-contrast microcinematography reveals that the macrophage is far from passive or immobile. Its pseudopodium-like cytoplasmic extensions move rapidly over cell surfaces of the surrounding wreath of erythroblasts. In scanning electron micrographs the central macrophage of the erythroblastic island is spongelike, with surface invaginations in which the erythroblasts lie. As the erythroblast matures it moves along a cytoplasmic extension of the macrophage away from the main body. When sufficiently mature for nuclear expulsion, the erythroblast makes contact with an endothelial cell, passes through a pore in the cytoplasm of the endothelial cell, and enters the circulation (see Chap. 29). The nucleus is ejected prior to egress from the marrow, phagocytized and degraded by the marrow macrophages.

In addition to fibronectin[48,49] there is probably a cell-cell recognition system that undergirds the formation of the erythroblastic island. Marrow macrophages express hemagglutinin ligands, sialoadhesins (Sn), and erythroblast receptors (EbR).[50] This cell recognition system is also operative in vitro. Erythroblastic islands form in long-term marrow cultures with an adherent stromal cell layer. Likewise, erythroblasts grown from BFU-E in methylcellulose or in plasma clots will also form erythroid islands if the clots are lysed, permitting erythroblast-macrophage association.[51,52]

The erythroblastic island is, however, a fragile structure and is usually disrupted in the process of obtaining a marrow specimen by needle aspiration. Maturing erythroblasts juxtaposed to a macrophage fragment are only occasionally encountered in stained films of marrow aspirates. These cell fragments are typically rich in iron and thus more easily seen in iron-stained preparations. Only in clinical situations with accelerated erythroblastic activity, such as acute hemolytic anemia and erythroleukemia, are erythroblastic islands commonly seen in marrow films.

MARROW IRON METABOLISM

Details of iron metabolism are discussed in Chap. 24. In normal humans, the marrow macrophage plays a major role in iron conservation. Aged and damaged erythrocytes, identified and trapped within the marrow microcirculation, are phagocytosed by the macrophage. Lysosomes release their lytic enzymes into the primary phagosome of the macrophage, and within 60 min digestion of the engulfed red cell is virtually complete. The membrane is reduced to multiple myelin laminae, and erythrocyte iron is transformed into aggregates of ferritin (Fig. 22-2).

Ferritin is a 440-kDa protein consisting of 243 subunits arranged to form a hollow sphere. The central cavity may store 4500 iron atoms[53] in the form of electron-dense particles of about 6 nm (60 Å) (Fig. 22-2). Microdiffraction techniques have shown that the iron cores display a hexagonal structure.[54] Hemosiderin is the intracellular yellowish iron-containing pigment visible under light microscopy in iron-loaded tissues. Under electron microscopy it is largely composed of dense clusters of ferritin, most of which are membrane enclosed.[55] Ferritin is converted into hemosiderin upon partial degradation of its protein shell by lysosomal enzymes.[56]

The outer membrane of erythroblasts possesses transferrin receptors on clathrin-coated pits. The adherence of transferrin to these portions of the cell membrane initiates a local membrane invagination, and intracytoplasmic vesicles are formed. These rapidly shed their clathrin coats and fuse with lysosomes to form endosomes.[53,57] The acid pH in the endosome permits the transfer of iron from transferrin[53] to mobilferrin, which in turn shuttles the iron to the sites of hemoglobin formation.[58] The apotransferrin and the transferrin receptor molecules are cycled back to the cell membrane, where apotransferrin is released into the extracellular medium. Ferritin molecules are also endocytosed by coated pits on erythroblasts. This phenomenon was termed *rhopheocytosis*[59] before it became evident that this mechanism for acquiring iron was only one example of a more general cellular mechanism for recycling receptors. Immunocytochemical labeling of the transferrin receptors has shown that the same pit may contain both the transferrin receptor and ferritin molecules.[60] Calculations suggest that the coated vesicle transfers 1000 times more iron via ferritin than via transferrin.[57]

Despite the efficiency of this transfer mechanism, it is still not clear whether ferritin iron can support the biosynthesis of heme in mitochondria.[61,62] Possibly the cytosolic ferritin in early red cell precursors is utilized for hemoglobin synthesis, while the ferritin clusters in mature erythroblasts represent storage of excess iron. The H ferritin (see Chap. 24) mRNA accumulates specifically during early erythroid differentiation.[63]

Uncomplexed iron together with superoxide provides a lethal mixture containing reactive hydroxyl radicals. These radicals cause lipid peroxidation, DNA strand breakage, and degradation of other biomolecules. By retaining iron in the safe, bound ferric form, extracellular transferrin and intracellular ferritin (and membrane-encapsulated iron stored as hemosiderin) serve as effective iron detoxifiers.[64]

TABLE 22-1   ANTIGENIC DISTRIBUTION DURING ERYTHROID DIFFERENTIATION

CFU-GEMM	BFU-E	CFU-E	Proerythroblast	Erythroblast	RBC	CD	Synonym or Function	Reference
x	x					34	Multipotent Stem Cells	1, 2, 3
x	x						AC133 antigen	4
x						13	FLT3/FLK2, STK-1, tyrosine kinase receptor, growth factor receptor	5
x	x					33	Myeloid precursors	6
x	x					62	PSGL-1, P-selectin glycoprotein-ligand	7, 8, 9
x	x					62	Leu8, L-selectin, LECAM	10
x	x					11	LFA-1 Integrin alpha L-Chain (leukocyte function-associated molecule-1)	10
x	x	x				44	H-CAM, Pgp-1	10
x	x	x				49	integrin alpha4, VLA-alpha4 chain	10
x	x	x					HLA-DR	3, 6, 11–15
x	x	x				41	platelet Gp IIbIIIa	15, 16
x	x	x				41	platelet Gp IIb	15
	x	x					HTK (receptor tyrosine kinase)	17
	x	x					Undetermined (measured by moAb 7B9)	18
	x	x	x	x		11 7	c-Kit (stem cell factor receptor)	19–25
	x	x	x	x			Fibronectin receptor	26
	x	x	x	x		71	T9, transferrin receptor	15, 27, 28
	x	x	x	x	x		Glycophorin C	29
	x	x	x	x	x		Carbonic anhydrase 1 (CA1)	30, 31
							IGF-1 receptor (insulin-like growth factor-1 receptor)	32
	x	x	x	x			EpoR (erythropoietin receptor)	21, 33, 34
	x	x	x	x		36	Platelet gpIV, thrombospondin receptor	15, 35
		x	x	x	x		Blood group A antigen	15
		x	x	x			Undetermined (measured by moAb 9C4)	36
		x	x	x	x		E-cadherin, L-CAM (liver cell adhesion molecule)	36
			x	x			HLe-1	28
			x	x		43	O-glycosylated leukosialin	37
			x	x	x		Glycophorin A	15, 29, 38, 39
			x	x	x		Spectrin	38–40
			x	x	x		Ankyrin	40, 41
			x	x	x		Band 4.1	40, 41
			x	x	x		Adducin	42
			x	x	x		Band 3	40, 41, 43
				x	x		Hb alpha	15
				x	x		O-glycosylated glycophorin A (expresses M/N blood groups)	44, 45

*This table is based on serologic assessment using the antibodies specific for the CD designation indicated. However, since integrin receptors are composed of two different subunits, and neither subunit is exposed on the surface of cells without the other, the "Synonym or Function" column gives the entire integrin receptor designation. For other synonyms for the receptors, see Chap. 14.

NOTE: This table shows the pattern of the antigenic distribution during adult erythroid differentiation. CFU-GEMM is the pluripotential stem cell capable, upon appropriate stimulation in vitro, of developing into mixed colonies of granulocytes, erythroblasts, macrophages, and megakaryocytes. CD34 and the AC133 antigen, which are expressed on all progenitors, disappear by the CFU-E stage.

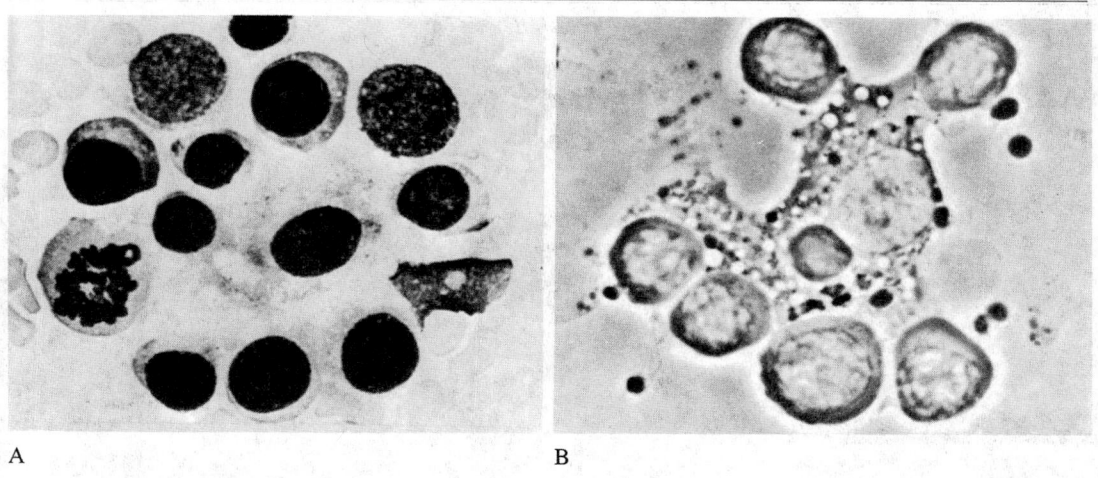

FIGURE 22-1   Erythroblastic island. (*a*) Erythroblastic island as seen in a Giemsa-stained marrow. (*b*) Erythroblastic island in the living state examined by phase-contrast microscopy. The macrophage shows dynamic movement in relation to its surrounding erythroblasts.

THE ERYTHROBLASTIC SERIES

EARLY PROGENITORS

Numerically the BFU-E and CFU-E represent only a minute proportion of human marrow. In mice CFU-E can be generated in large numbers and then enriched by centrifugal elutriation and Percoll density gradient centrifugation. Under the electron microscope these cells show large nucleoli, abundant polyribosomes, and large mitochondria.[65] Blasts from human marrow, enriched for CFU-E using a monoclonal antibody, exhibit similar ultrastructural characteristics (Fig. 22-3).[66]

PROERYTHROBLASTS

On stained films the proerythroblast (Fig. 22-4) is a large cell, 20 to 25 μm in diameter, irregularly rounded or slightly oval. The nucleus occupies approximately 80 percent of its area and contains fine chromatin delicately distributed in small clumps. One or several well-defined nucleoli are present.

Polyribosomes arranged in groups of two to six are numerous in the cytoplasm and are characteristic of the cytoplasm of proerythroblasts. It is this high concentration of polyribosomes that gives the cytoplasm of these cells its characteristic intense basophilia. At high

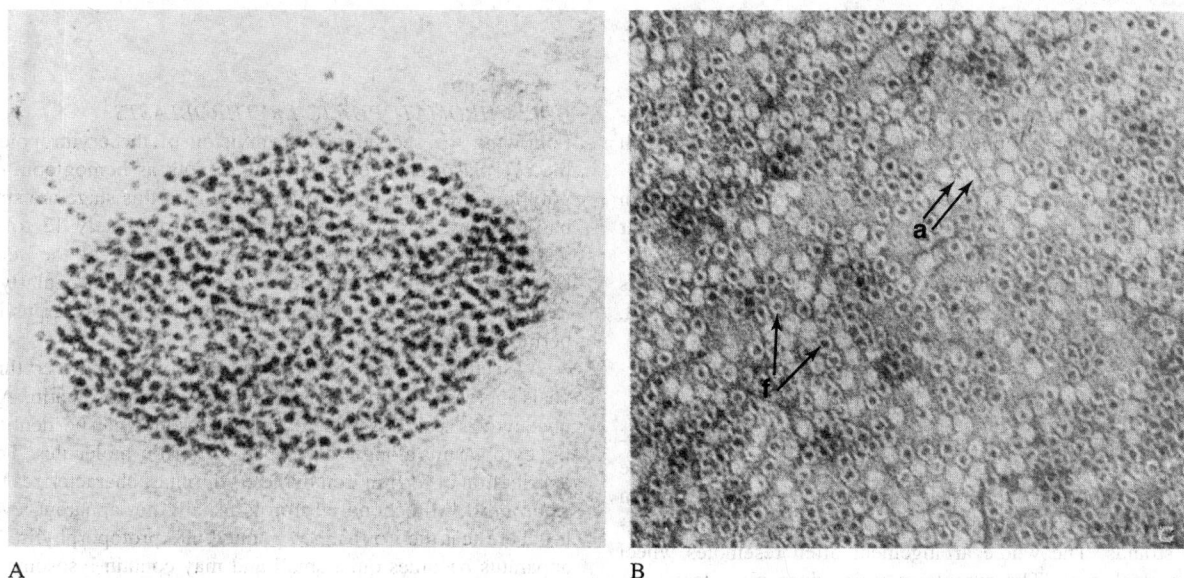

FIGURE 22-2   Ultrastructural aspects of ferritin. (*a*) Electron micrograph of a membrane-bound erythroblast siderosome, showing that it is composed of individual ferritin molecules. (*b*) Electron micrograph of negatively stained ferritin and apoferritin mixture, showing the ferritin molecule (f) with its protein coat and central dense iron core; apoferritin molecules (a) lack the central iron cores. (From Bessis and Breton-Gorius.[174])

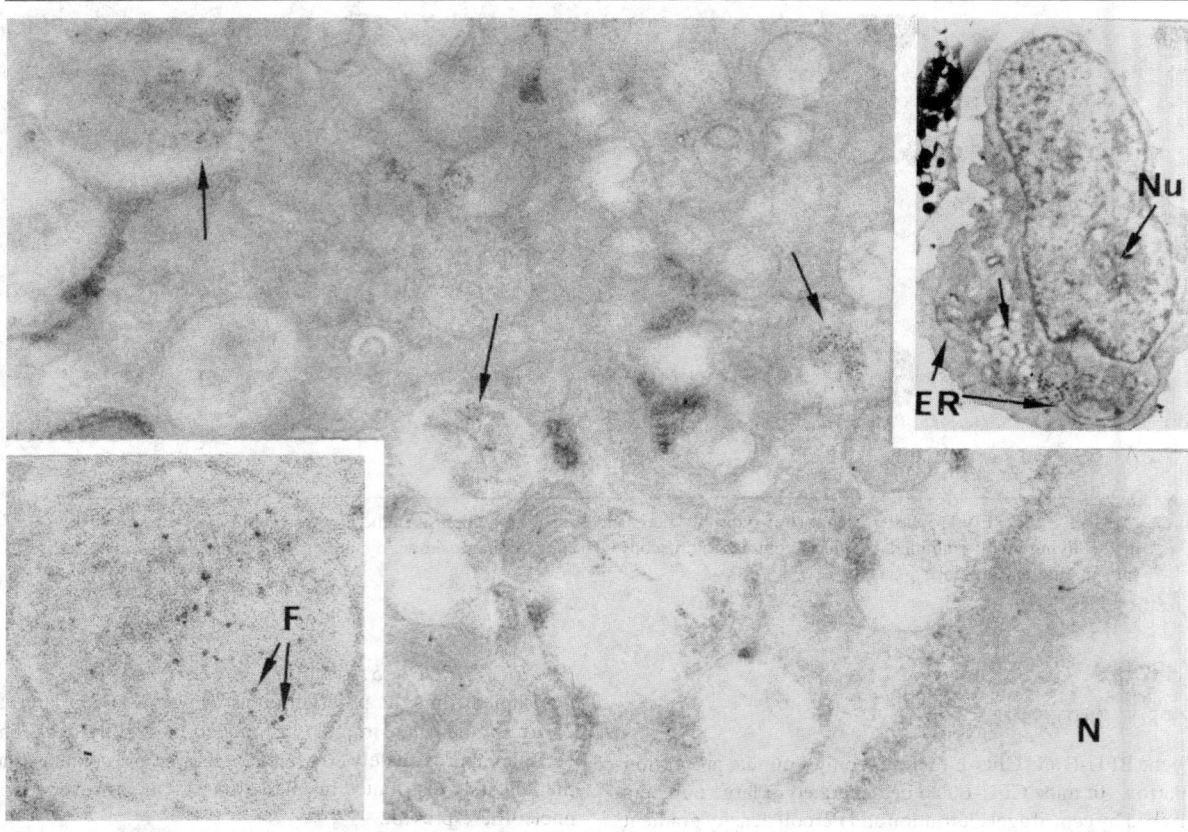

FIGURE 22-3   *Right inset:* Unstained section of a normal presumptive CFU-E which was enriched by panning from marrow, using the monoclonal antibody FA-152.[175] This blast has a large nucleolus (Nu). The incubation in diaminobenzidine medium reveals weak peroxidase activity in the endoplasmic reticulum (ER). In the Golgi zone, several granules appear as vacuoles (arrow). *Main figure:* On enlargement of the Golgi zone, a portion of the nucleus (N) can be seen surrounded by a perinuclear cistern containing weak peroxidase activity. Several granules with a pale matrix contain ferritin molecules (arrows). *Left inset:* High magnification of a granule showing ferritin molecules (F) of characteristic structure and density. (Adapted from Breton-Gorius, et al,[66] with permission.)

magnification, ferritin molecules can be seen dispersed singly throughout the cytoplasm, and rhopheocytosis is easily observed at cell margins.

Three to twelve granules present in the Golgi zone also contain ferritin molecules.[67] They stain for acid phosphatase, indicating their lysosomal nature, and differ from another class of small granules: the catalase-containing granules. Diffuse cytoplasmic density on sections stained for peroxidase indicates that hemoglobin is already present. Dispersed glycogen particles are present in the cytoplasm.[68]

BASOPHILIC ERYTHROBLASTS

The basophilic erythroblast is smaller than the proerythroblast, measuring 16 to 18 μm (Fig. 22-5). The nucleus occupies three-fourths of the cell area and is composed of characteristic dark violet heterochromatin interspersed with pink-staining clumps of euchromatin linked by irregular linear strands. The whole arrangement often resembles wheel spokes or a clock face. The cytoplasm stains deep blue, leaving a perinuclear halo enlarged to a juxtanuclear clear zone around the Golgi apparatus.

The cytoplasmic basophilia at this stage is due to the continued presence of polyribosomes. Microtubules are often seen connecting two erythroblasts in mitosis.

POLYCHROMATOPHILIC ERYTHROBLASTS

Following the second mitotic division of the erythropoietic series, the cytoplasm changes from blue to pink as hemoglobin dilutes the polyribosome content (Fig. 22-6). Cells at this stage are smaller than basophilic erythroblasts, measuring approximately 12 to 15 μm in diameter. The nucleus occupies less than half of the cell area. Its heterochromatin is in well-defined clumps spaced regularly about the nucleus, producing a checkerboard pattern. The nucleolus is lost; the perinuclear halo persists.

Electron microscopy of the polychromatophilic erythroblast reveals increased aggregation of nuclear heterochromatin. Active rhopheocytosis is always evident, and siderosomes can be identified within the cytoplasm[46] along with dispersed ferritin molecules. This normal distribution of ferritin iron in the erythroblast characterizes the *normal sideroblast*. Mitochondrial iron is usually not apparent, even though it is here that the iron is incorporated into protoporphyrin. The Golgi apparatus becomes quite small and may contain lysosomes.

ORTHOCHROMIC ERYTHROBLASTS

After the final mitotic division of the erythropoietic series, the concentration of hemoglobin increases within the erythroblast. More than any of its predecessors, this cell stains like a mature erythrocyte

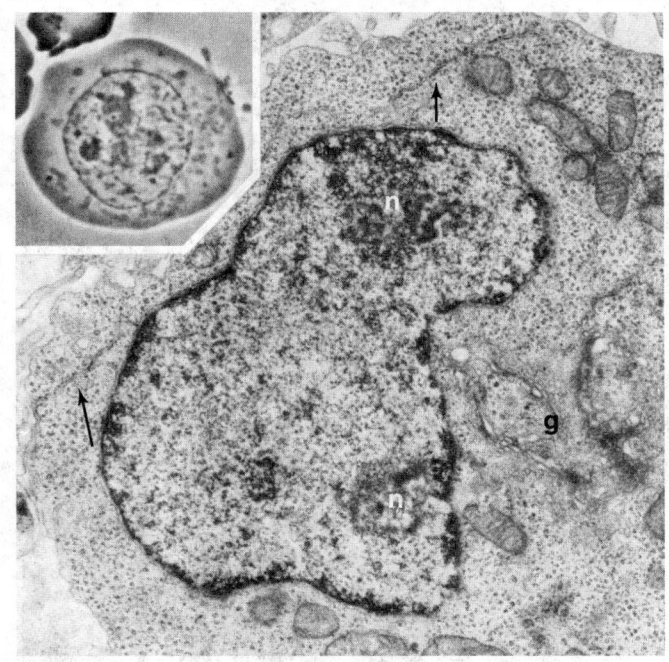

FIGURE 22-4 Proerythroblast. Phase-contrast micrograph *(inset)* of a proerythroblast, showing the immature nucleus with nucleoli and finely dispersed nuclear chromatin. The centrosome (juxtanuclear clear zone) is apparent with its dense accumulation of mitochondria. Electron microscopic section of the proerythroblast shows nucleoli (Nu) in contact with the nuclear membrane. Chromatin is finely dispersed and forms small aggregates in the fixed nuclear membrane. The perinuclear canal is narrow but well defined. Polyribosome groups, many in helical configuration, are dispersed throughout the cytoplasm. The Golgi apparatus (g) is well developed, and regions of endoplasmic reticulum (arrows) are seen.

(Fig. 22-7). However, because of the residual monoribosomes and polyribosomes it is always somewhat polychromatophilic.

Under the light microscope the nucleus appears almost completely dense and featureless; it is measurably decreased in size. This cell is the smallest of the erythroblastic series; it varies from 10 to 15 μm in diameter. The nucleus occupies approximately one-fourth of the cell area and is eccentric.

Under the phase-contrast microscope a surprising motility can be appreciated. Round projections appear suddenly in different parts of the cell periphery and are just as quickly retracted. The movements are probably in preparation for ejection of the nucleus.[46]

The ultrastructure of the cell is characterized by irregular borders, reflecting its motile state. The nucleus is eccentric; the heterochromatin forms large masses. The cytoplasmic ribosomes are further dispersed into diribosomes and monoribosomes. Mitochondria are reduced in number and size. Hemoglobin is present within the nucleus itself.[68,69]

THE RETICULOCYTE

BIRTH

Prior to enucleation, intermediate filaments and the marginal band of microtubules disappear. Vimentin decreases in quantity throughout the cytoplasm. However, tubulin and actin become concentrated at

the point where the nucleus will exit.[70] These changes, accompanied by microtubular rearrangements, play a role in nuclear expulsion.[71,72]

The expulsion of the nucleus in vitro is by no means an instantaneous phenomenon; it requires a period of minutes.[46] The process begins with several vigorous contractions around the midportion of the cell, followed by a division of the cell into unequal portions. The smaller portion consists of the expelled nucleus accompanied by a thin rim of hemoglobinized cytoplasm. It is this loss of a "corona" of hemoglobin with the nucleus that leads, in part, to an increase in the "early peak" of stercobilin when the rate of erythropoiesis is increased.[73]

In vivo, expulsion of the nucleus may take place while the erythroblast is still part of an erythroblastic island (Fig. 22-8), or the nucleus may be lost during passage through the wall of a marrow sinus. The nucleus, unable to traverse the small opening, remains in the marrow. In either case, the expelled nucleus is rapidly ingested by a macrophage.

Two proposals have been advanced to explain how the reticulocyte exits the marrow; the precise mechanism is still unknown. The reticulocyte may actively traverse the sinus epithelium[74] or more likely, since it appears incapable of directed amoeboid motion, it may be driven across by a pressure differential.[75,76]

MATURATION

As it enters the circulation the reticulocyte retains mitochondria, small numbers of ribosomes, the centriole, and remnants of the Golgi bodies. The reticulocyte contains no endoplasmic reticulum. Supravital staining with brilliant cresyl blue or new methylene blue produces aggre-

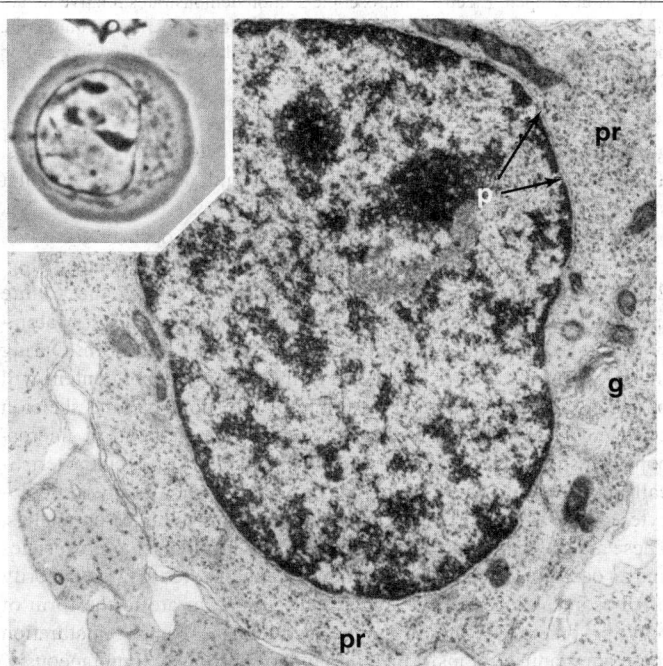

FIGURE 22-5 Basophilic erythroblast. Phase-contrast photomicrograph *(inset)* shows increased clumping of the nuclear chromatin and further rounding of the cell, with aggregation of the mitochondria and centrosome into the regions of nuclear indentation. Electron microscopic section shows clumping of the nuclear chromatin, nuclear pores (p), organization of the nucleoli, increased density of polyribosomes (pr), well-developed Golgi apparatus (g), and a decrease in smooth endoplasmic reticulum.

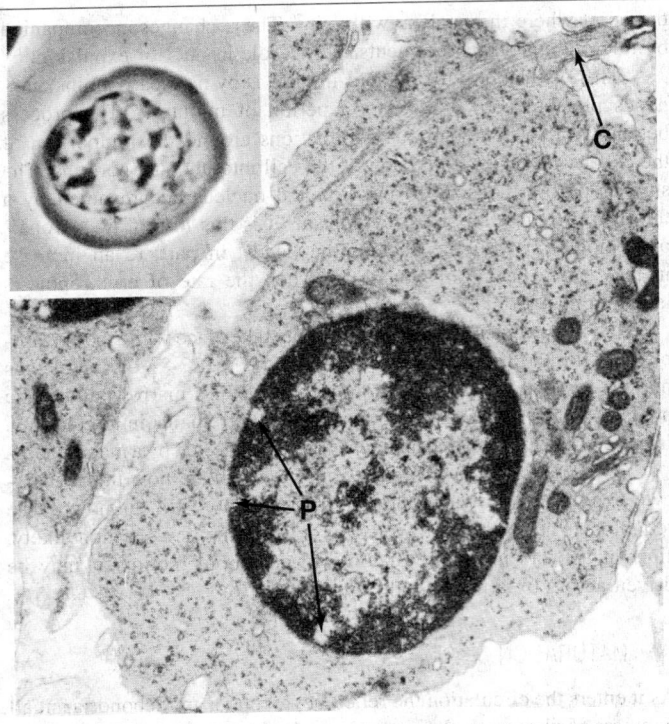

FIGURE 22-6   Polychromatophilic erythroblast. Phase-contrast micrograph *(inset)* demonstrates a diminution in the size of this cell in comparison with its precursor, with further clumping of nuclear chromatin to give the nucleus a checkerboard appearance. The centrosome is condensed, and a perinuclear halo has developed. Electron microscopic section demonstrates relative reduction of the density of polyribosomes and dilution by the moderately osmiophilic hemoglobin in the cytoplasm. Nuclear chromatin shows a marked increase in clumping, and nuclear pores (P) are enlarged.

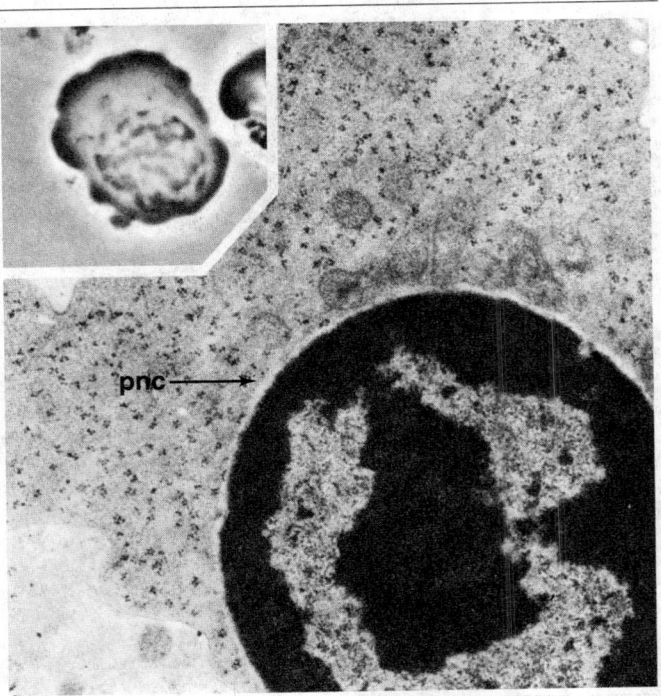

FIGURE 22-7   Orthochromic erythroblast. Phase-contrast appearance of this cell in the living state *(inset)* shows the irregular borders indicative of its characteristic motility, the eccentric nucleus making contact with the plasmalemma, further pyknosis of the nuclear chromatin, and condensation of the centrosome. Electron microscopic section shows further dilution of polyribosomes, some of which appear to be disintegrating into monoribosomes, by the increasing hemoglobin. The number of mitochondria is decreased, and some are degenerating. Nuclear chromatin is clumped into large masses, and a perinuclear canal (pnc) is seen.

gates of ribosomes, mitochondria, and other cytoplasmic organelles. These artifactual aggregates stain deep blue and, arranged in reticular strands, give the reticulocyte its name.

The in vitro maturation is very similar to that occurring in vivo. However, in a plasma clot the naked nuclei remain undamaged (Fig. 22-9). If the clot is lysed, the macrophages present in the culture immediately recognize and phagocytose the expelled nuclei. Maturation of the circulating reticulocyte requires from 24 to 48 h. During this period some 20 percent of the ultimate hemoglobin content will be synthesized and the final assembly of the submembrane skeleton completed. Living reticulocytes observed by phase-contrast microscopy are slightly motile, irregularly shaped cells with a characteristically puckered exterior. Examined by electron microscopy, reticulocytes are irregular in shape and contain many remnant organelles. These are grouped in the hilar region along with small smooth vesicles and an occasional centriole. In "young" reticulocytes the vast majority of ribosomes dispersed throughout the cytoplasm are in the form of polyribosomes. As protein synthesis diminishes during maturation these are gradually transformed into monoribosomes. Simultaneously, there is loss of transferrin receptors,[77,78] and eventually the capacity for endocytosis disappears as well.[79]

PATHOLOGIC ERYTHROBLASTS

MEGALOBLASTS AND DYSERYTHROPOIESIS

The morphologic abnormalities that characterize megaloblastic maturation and the dyserythropoietic anemias are described in Chap. 37.

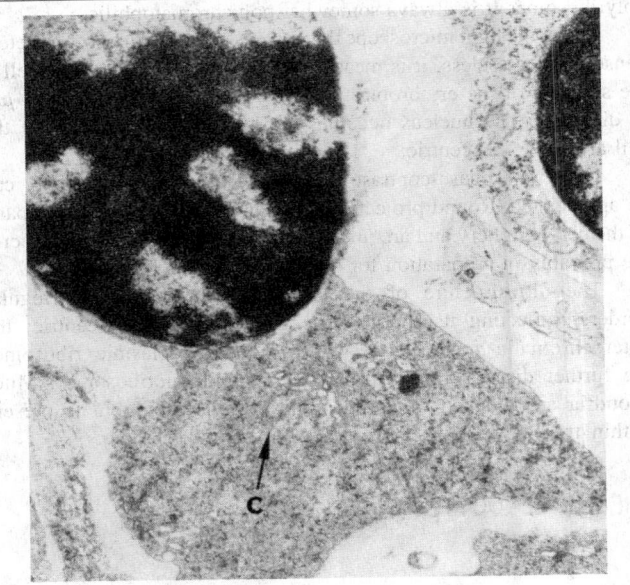

FIGURE 22-8   Orthochromatic erythroblast ejecting its nucleus. A thin rim of cytoplasm surrounds the nucleus. In the cytoplasm, a single centriole (c) is partially encircled by some Golgi saccules.

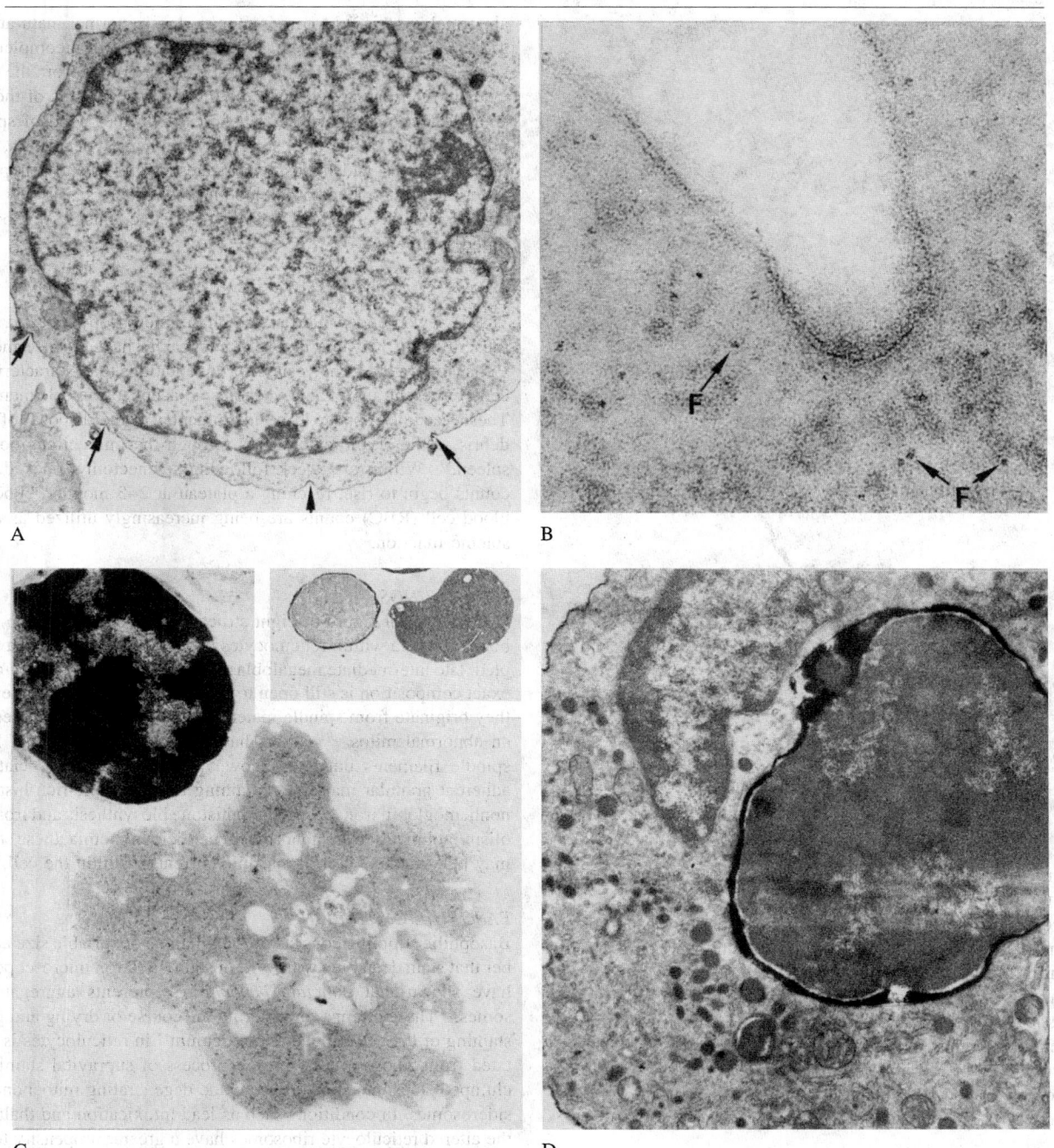

FIGURE 22-9   Erythroblast maturation in an in vitro plasma clot from BFU-E. (*a*) At day 9 of culture, a cell resembling the in vivo proerythroblast exhibits numerous rhopheocytotic invaginations (arrows). (*b*) One invagination seen at high magnification. Note the numerous ferritin molecules (F) dispersed in the cytoplasm. (*c*) At day 12 of culture, an extruded nucleus is seen close to a reticulocyte. *Insert:* When the hemoglobin is emphasized by cytochemical staining, the thin rim of cytoplasm surrounding the nucleus is clearly visible. (*d*) In the cell suspension produced by clot lysis a macrophage phagocytoses a hemoglobin-rimmed erythroblast nucleus that has been recently extruded. (Parts *c* and *d* are adapted from Breton-Gorius, et al,[52] with permission.)

PATHOLOGIC SIDEROBLASTS

A heterogeneous group of erythrocyte maturation disorders is accompanied by ineffective erythropoiesis and hyperferremia. These disorders include acquired idiopathic sideroblastic anemia, pyridoxine-responsive anemia, alcohol-induced sideroblastic anemia, lead intoxi-

cation, dyserythropoietic anemia, and certain hemoglobinopathies (see Chaps. 35, 53, 63). All these conditions are characterized by the presence of pathologic sideroblasts. When stained for iron these cells may show small iron-containing granules arranged in a ring around the nucleus. For this reason they are commonly referred to as *ringed sideroblasts*.[80] Iron stains of normal erythroid precursors demonstrate

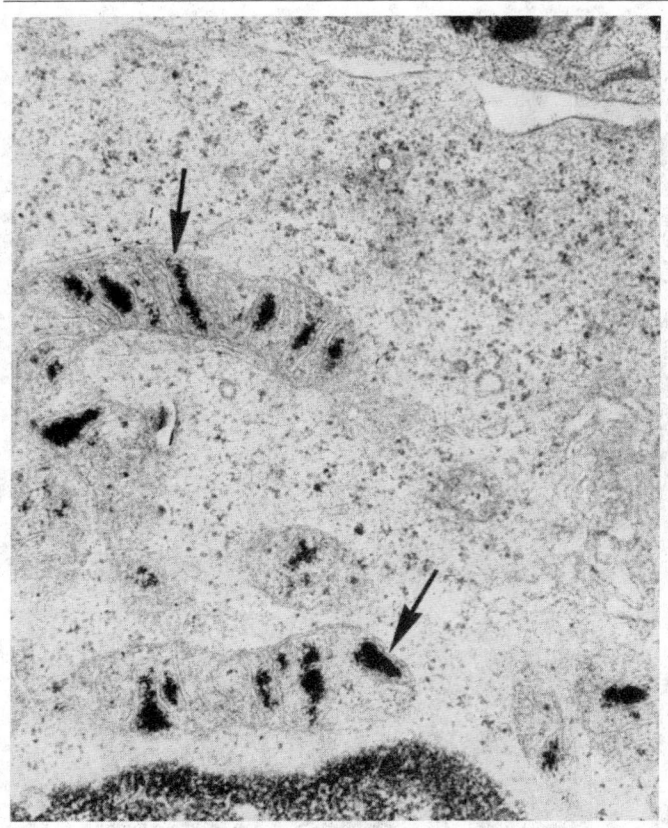

FIGURE 22-10   The pathologic sideroblast is an erythroblast characterized by the presence of mitochondrial deposits of iron-containing ferruginous micelles (arrows) between the cristae.

a few very fine granules that are difficult to see without carefully focusing up and down through the cell.

Electron microscope studies show granules in ringed sideroblasts to be iron-loaded mitochondria. Because this mitochondrial iron is distinct from ferritin antigenically, ultrastructurally, and by electron probe analysis, it has been termed *ferruginous micelles*.[46] In hereditary sideroblastic anemia these mitochondrial iron deposits occur primarily in the late, polychromatophilic erythroblasts. In acquired sideroblastic anemia the iron overload affects the early proerythroblast.[81] In cells with these iron-loaded mitochondria, many ferritin molecules are deposited between adjacent erythroblast membranes (Fig. 22-10).[82]

PATHOLOGY OF THE RETICULOCYTE AND ERYTHROCYTE

The reticulocyte may show pathologic alterations in size or staining properties. It may also contain inclusions visible by light microscopy or identifiable only on ultrastructural analysis. The majority of pathologic inclusions usually attributed to erythrocytes are actually found in reticulocytes (Table 22-2) and are nuclear or cytoplasmic remnants derived from the late-stage normoblasts.

HOWELL-JOLLY BODIES[83]
Howell-Jolly bodies are small nuclear remnants that have the color of a pyknotic nucleus on Wright-stained films and give a positive Feulgen reaction for DNA.[84] They are spherical in shape, usually no larger than 0.5 μm in diameter. Generally only one is present, but they may be numerous. In pathologic situations they appear to represent chromosomes that have been separated from the mitotic spindle during

abnormal mitosis.[85] More commonly, during normal maturation they arise from nuclear fragmentation (karyorrhexis) or incomplete expulsion of the nucleus.[86] Howell-Jolly bodies are pitted from the reticulocytes in their passage through the interendothelial slits of the splenic sinus. They are characteristically present in the blood of splenectomized persons and in those suffering from hemolytic anemia, megaloblastic anemia, and hyposplenic states. More recently, hyposplenic states and post-splenectomy blood has been more sensitively and specifically characterized by pocked red cell counts. (See Pocked [or pitted] red cells.)

POCKED (OR PITTED) RED CELLS
When viewed under interference-phase microscopy, pocked red cells (described by Koyama in 1962)[87] appear to have surface membrane "pits" or craters. The vesicles or indentations that characterize these cells represent autophagic vacuoles adjacent to the cell membrane.[88] These vacuoles appear to be instrumental in the disposal of cellular debris as the erythrocyte passes through the microcirculation of the spleen.[89] Within one week following splenectomy, pocked red cell counts begin to rise, reaching a plateau at 2–3 months.[90] Pocked red blood cell (RBC) counts are being increasingly utilized as a test of splenic function.

CABOT RINGS
The ringlike or figure-of-eight structures sometimes seen in megaloblastic anemia within reticulocytes and in an occasional, heavily stippled, late intermediate megaloblast[91] are designated *Cabot rings*. Their exact composition is still open to question. Some have suggested that they originate from spindle material that has been mishandled during an abnormal mitosis.[92] Others have found no indication of DNA or spindle filaments but have shown the rings to be associated with adherent granular material containing both arginine-rich histone and nonhemoglobin iron.[93] Since both histone biosynthesis and iron metabolism/mobilization are abnormal in pernicious anemia, these structures may be a marker of "cytoplasmic currents" within the cell.[46]

BASOPHILIC STIPPLING
Basophilic stippling consists of granulations of variable size and number that stain deep blue with Wright stain. Electron microscope studies have shown that *punctate basophilia* represents aggregated ribosomes.[94] These clumps form during the course of drying and postvital staining of the cells, much as "reticulum" in reticulocytes is precipitated from ribosomes during the process of supravital staining. The clumped ribosomes may also include degenerating mitochondria and siderosomes. In conditions such as lead intoxication and thalassemia, the altered reticulocyte ribosomes have a greater propensity to aggregate. As a result, the basophilic granulation appears larger and is referred to as *coarse basophilic stippling*.

HEINZ BODIES
Heinz bodies are composed of denatured proteins, primarily hemoglobin, that form in red cells as a result of chemical insult (see Chap. 53); in hereditary defects of the hexose monophosphate shunt (see Chap. 45); the thalassemias (see Chap. 46); unstable hemoglobin syndromes (see Chap. 48); or sickle cell disease.[95] Not seen on ordinary Wright- or Giemsa-stained blood films, Heinz bodies are readily visible in red cells that have been stained supravitally with brilliant cresyl blue or with crystal violet. They tend to adhere to the interior of the red cell membrane, protruding into the cytoplasm. Their position in dried and stained blood films is characteristically about one-third of the distance in from the edge of the disc, where membrane curvature is at a minimum, presumably because of the membrane stiffening that

TABLE 22-2   ERYTHROCYTE AND RETICULOCYTE INCLUSIONS

INCLUSIONS	COMPOSITION	CELL TYPE	APPEARANCE ON WRIGHT-STAINED FILM	COMMENTS	REFERENCE
"Reticulo-filamentous substance"	Artifactual aggregation of ribosomes	Reticulocytes	Invisible	Visible after supravital staining	46
Howell-Jolly bodies	Nuclear fragment containing aberrant chromosomes	Reticulocytes; rarely erythrocytes	Dense blue spherical granule(s)	Visible in unstained cells	83–86
Cabot rings	Spindle remnant or histone-rich and iron-rich "cytoplasmic currents"	Reticulocytes; heavily stippled late intermediate megaloblasts	Ring or figure-eight strand stained purple	Visible in some hemolytic states	46, 91–93
Basophilic stippling	Pathologic precipitation of ribosomes	Reticulocytes	Dispersed blue granulations		94
Heinz bodies	Denatured hemoglobin	Erythrocytes; occasionally reticulocytes	Rarely visible	Refractile inclusions after staining with methylene or Nile blue dyes	95, 96
Hemoglobin H inclusions	Denatured hemoglobin (induced in vitro by exposure to brilliant cresyl blue, methylene blue, new methylene blue)	Erythrocytes; reticulocytes	Invisible	Gives "golf-ball" appearance to erythrocytes after incubation with appropriate supravital stains	97–101

they cause. Membrane stiffening also results in their removal from red cells as the cells traverse the interepithelial slits of the splenic sinus.[96]

HEMOGLOBIN H INCLUSIONS

Hemoglobin H is composed of β_4 tetramers, indicating that β chains are present in excess as a result of impaired α-chain production. Exposure to redox dyes such as brilliant cresyl blue, methylene blue, or new methylene blue results in denaturization and precipitation of the abnormal hemoglobin.[97] Brilliant cresyl blue causes the formation of a large number of small membrane-bound inclusions, giving the cell a characteristic "golf-ball-like" appearance when viewed by light microscopy. Methylene blue and new methylene blue generate a smaller number of variably sized membrane-bound and floating inclusions.[98] Most frequently seen in β-thalassemia, these changes may also be found in patients with unstable hemoglobin[99] and in rare cases of erythroleukemia.[100,101]

SIDEROSOMES AND PAPPENHEIMER BODIES

Normal or pathologic cells containing siderosomes ("iron bodies") are usually reticulocytes. In the pathologic state the iron granulations are larger and more numerous, and electron microscopy has shown that many of these are mitochondria containing ferruginous micelles rather than the ferritin aggregates that characterize the normal siderocyte.[102] Siderosomes are usually found in the periphery of the cell, whereas basophilic stippling tends to be distributed homogeneously throughout the cell. Pappenheimer bodies are siderosomes that stain with Wright stain. Electron microscopy of these bodies shows that the iron is often contained within a lysosome, as confirmed by the presence of acid phosphate. Siderosomes may also contain degenerating mitochondria, ribosomes, and other cellular remnants.

MACRORETICULOCYTES

In the presence of an intense erythropoietin response to acute anemia, or experimentally in response to large doses of exogenously administered erythropoietin, "stress" reticulocytes are released into the circulation.[103] These cells may be up to twice the normal volume, with a corresponding increase in hemoglobin content. Whether this increase results from one less mitotic division during maturation or from some other process is not yet clear. In contrast, even under moderate erythro-

poietic stress some of the reticulocytes in the marrow pool are shifted to the circulating pool. These "shift" reticulocytes contain a higher RNA content than normal and can now be quantified. This is commonly done by applying a fluorescent stain to the aggregated ribosomal material and then dividing reticulocytes into high, medium, and low fluorescence categories using a fluorescence-sensitive flow cytometer. The "stress" reticulocytes of the older literature likely fall in the high and medium fluorescence categories.[103,104–106]

STRUCTURE AND SHAPE OF THE ERYTHROCYTE

The normal resting shape of the erythrocyte is a biconcave disc. Variations in the shape and dimensions of the red cell are useful in the differential diagnosis of anemias. Normal human red cells have a diameter of 7.5 to 8.7 μm, which decreases slightly with cell age. They have an average volume of 90 fl[107] and a surface area of approximately 136 μm².[108] The membrane is present in sufficient excess to allow the cell to swell to a sphere of approximately 150 fl or to enter a capillary of 2.8 μm in diameter. The normal erythrocyte stains reddish-brown in Wright-stained blood films and pink with Giemsa stain. The central one-third of the cell appears relatively pale compared with the periphery, reflecting its biconcave shape. Red cells on dried blood films are 0.6 μm thick, having lost about two-thirds of their normal thickness.[46] Many artifacts can be produced in the preparation of the blood film. They may result from contamination of the glass slide or coverslip with traces of fat, detergent, or other impurities.[109] Friction and surface tension involved in the preparation of the blood film produce fragmentation, "doughnut cells" or annulocytes, crescent-shaped cells, etc.[109] Observed in the phase-contrast or interference microscope, the red cell shows a characteristic internal scintillation known as red cell flicker.[110] This is due to thermally excited undulations of the red cell membrane. Frequency analysis of these surface undulations has provided an estimate of the curvature elastic constant and of changes in this constant due to alcohol, cholesterol loading, and exposure to cross-linking agents.[111]

RED CELL SHAPE AND SURVIVAL IN THE CIRCULATION

The red cell spends most of its circulatory life within the capillary channels of the microcirculation. During its 100- to 120-day life span it travels a distance of approximately 250 km. That it survives this long is at least partially due to the unique capacity of its membrane to "tank-tread"—rotate around the red cell contents.[112] This arrangement transmits shocks from wall contact through the membrane to the viscous hemoglobin solution in the interior rather than concentrating the energy of contact in the membrane. The physical arrangement of membrane skeletal proteins in a uniform shell[113] of highly folded hexagonal/pentagonal units[114-116] permits this unusual behavior and is also responsible for the characteristic biconcave shape of the resting cell.[117] Subtle differences in the discoid shape that resting cells assume are probably related to variations in the elastic properties of the submembrane skeleton.[108] A deficiency in the amount of spectrin or the presence of mutant spectrin in the submembrane skeleton results in the abnormal discoid cells in hereditary spherocytosis, elliptocytosis, and pyropoikilocytosis (see Chap. 43).[118] In regions of circulatory standstill or very slow flow, red cells travel in aggregates of two to a dozen cells, forming rouleaux.[119] Within large vessels, aggregation is disrupted by the increased shear forces.

NOMENCLATURE OF COMMON RED CELL SHAPES

An international terminology using uniform Greek word stems has been introduced to describe cells on the basis of their three-dimensional morphology (Table 22-3).[120]

The *discocyte* is the form that a red cell assumes when it is not subjected to external deforming stress. It is a smooth, biconcave disc. A discocyte can be reversibly and rapidly transformed by a variety of environmental agents into two other forms, the *stomatocyte*, a uniconcave cup-shaped cell, and the *echinocyte*, covered by 10 to 30 short projections evenly spaced over the cell surface. In general these changes can be superimposed on other red cell shapes, which suggests that they represent membrane energy equilibrium states.[117]

The *acanthocyte* has an irregular shape, with 2 to 10 hemispherically tipped spicules of variable length and variable diameter. The bases of the spicules on the acanthocyte are of varying girth, unlike those on echinocytes, where the spicules are of remarkably uniform dimensions.

Notwithstanding the time-honored use of the word, *spherocytes* are not truly spherical cells. Their thickness is greatly increased, so that the central concavity is significantly reduced and may be overlooked. On scanning electron microscopic examination the spherocyte frequently bears a small dimple or irregular area suggesting derivation from a stomatocyte.

Schizocyte refers to a red cell fragment that characteristically assumes a half-disc shape with two or three pointed extremities. Because it is produced by the sealing of two opposing membrane surfaces followed by physical cleavage or fragmentation of a red cell, it is smaller than the normal discocyte and may display one or more regions of stiffened and distorted membrane where the sealing and cleavage has occurred.

Drepanocyte (sickle cell) is a term that describes the sickle cell and a variety of shapes induced by the polymerization of sickle hemoglobin. Such cells vary in shape from bipolar, spiculated forms to cells with long, irregular spicules and holly-leaf configurations.

The *elliptocyte* (ovalocyte) is basically an oval biconcave disc showing varying degrees of elliptical aberration, from a slightly oval to an almost cylindrical, bipolar, elongated cell.

A relative excess of membrane in the *codocyte* (target cell) results in membrane recurvature in the center of the dimple. Hemoglobin accumulates where the upper and lower cell membranes separate when the cell is on a blood film, forming the central density, or "bulls eye," of the target.

Dacryocyte refers to cells characterized by a single elongated or pointed extremity. This cell shape has previously been referred to as a *teardrop, racket,* or *tail poikilocyte.*

The *leptocyte* is a wafer-thin cell which is generally large in diameter and displays a thin rim of hemoglobin at the periphery with a large area of central pallor. Such a cell reflects an increased surface/volume ratio.

Keratocytes are red cells with a relatively normal cell volume that have been deformed by removal of a region of apposed and sealed membranes so that they present with two or more points.

"Bite" cells are red cells that have had one or more semicircular portions removed from the cell margin when Heinz bodies are pitted out by the splenic macrophages.[121]

If necessary, any shape variation of the red cell may be described precisely by the use of compound terms such as *spherostomatocyte.* The addition of modifiers such as *micro* to denote a changed volume may add to descriptive precision, as in *microspherocyte* or *macroleptocyte.*

Variability in the size of red cells is designated *anisocytosis,* and any type of shape abnormality is designated as *poikilocytosis* (see Chap. 2).

THE NORMAL PHYSIOLOGY AND THE PATHOPHYSIOLOGY OF RED CELL SHAPE

THE BICONCAVE DISC

The means by which a healthy red blood cell maintains its normal biconcave shape are still in dispute. However, most proposals can be subsumed under two headings: (1) The red cell is a reference shape into which the membrane is cast, much as a latex rubber glove is cast in the shape of a human hand,[122] or (2) it is a dynamic equilibrium form controlled by the minimization of bending energy in the membrane.[123] Among the observations that undermine the reference-shape hypothesis is the ability of the discocyte to withstand the relocation of the biconcavities anywhere on the membrane surface without significantly changing its shape.[124] Against the minimization-of-bending-energy hypothesis are the measured values of the membrane-bending modulus. All estimates thus far are too low by one-half an order of magnitude[125] to account for the observed membrane behavior.

Proposals that the submembrane skeleton behaves as an ionic gel[126] and that the spectrin network functions as an entropic spring[127] have served notice that the mechanical properties of the red blood cell membrane are exceedingly complex and still far from being completely understood.

The Stomatocyte-Echinocyte-Discocyte Equilibrium   At physiologic pH and in the presence of normal levels of plasma proteins (particularly albumin), healthy red cells will always be smooth, biconcave discs (Fig. 22-11). As the pH is raised or the albumin concentration lowered, or in the presence of lysolecithin or anionic phenothiazine derivatives, the rim of the disc becomes bumpy. These bumps are low, are widely spaced, and involve only the membrane of the red cell rim. This form is an echinocyte I. Further environmental stress will result in transformation to echinocytes II and III. These cells bear 10 to 30 projections of surprisingly uniform dimensions, equally spaced over the entire cell surface. Should the environmental stress be sufficiently intense or of sufficient duration so that the echinocyte III becomes a spheroechinocyte I or spheroechinocyte II, the process is irreversible.

Environmental stress caused by low pH, excess albumin, or cationic phenothiazine derivatives will transform the discocyte into an intermediate form with deeper biconcavities, and then into a cup-shaped cell with only a single concavity, a stomatocyte. Thus far the changes are readily reversible, but if the single deep depression

TABLE 22-3   NOMENCLATURE OF RED CELL SHAPES AND ASSOCIATED DISEASE STATES

TERMINOLOGY (GREEK MEANING)	OLD TERMS, SYNONYMS	DESCRIPTION	MICROGRAPH	ASSOCIATED DISEASE STATES
Discocyte (disc)	Biconcave disc	Biconcave disc form of RBC		
Echinocyte (I–III) (sea urchin)	"Burr cell," crenated cell, "berry cell"	Spiculated RBC with short, equally spaced projections over entire surface; progressing from the "crenated disc" (echinocyte I) to the crenated sphere (echinocyte IV—not shown) with nearly complete loss of spicules		Uremia, liver disease Low-potassium red cells Immediately posttransfusion with aged or metabolically depleted blood Carcinoma of stomach and bleeding peptic ulcers
Acanthocyte (spike)	"Spur cell," acanthoid cell, acanthrocyte	Irregularly spiculated RBC with projections of varying length and position		Abetalipoproteinemia Alcoholic liver disease Postsplenectomy state Malabsorptive states
Stomatocyte (I–III) (mouth)	Mouth cell, cup form, mushroom cap, uniconcave disc, microspherocyte	Bowled-shaped RBC with single concavity; progressing from shallow bowl (I) to near sphere with small dimple (seen as mouth-shaped form in peripheral film)		Hereditary spherocytosis Hereditary stomatocytosis Alcoholism, cirrhosis, obstructive liver disease Erythrocyte sodium-pump defect
Spherostomatocyte (sphere)	Spherocyte, prelytic sphere, microspherocyte	Spherical RBC with dense hemoglobin content; SEM shows a persistent minimal dimple		Hereditary spherocytosis (cells actually spherostomatocytes) Immune hemolytic anemia Posttransfusion Heinz body hemolytic anemia Water-dilution hemolysis Fragmentation hemolysis
Schizocyte (cut)	Schistocyte, helmet cell, fragmented cell	Split RBC, often showing half-disc shape with two or three pointed extremities; may be small, irregular fragment		Microangiopathic hemolytic anemia (TTP, DIC, vasculitis, glomerulonephritis, renal graft rejection) Carcinomatosis Heart-valve hemolysis (prosthetic or pathologic valves) Severe burns March hemoglobinuria
Elliptocyte (oval)	Ovalocyte	Oval to elongated ellipsoid RBC (with polarization of hemoglobin)		Hereditary elliptocytosis Thalassemia Iron deficiency Myelophthisic anemias Megaloblastic anemias
Drepanocyte (sickle)	Sickle cell	RBC containing polymerized hemoglobin S; showing varying shapes from bipolar, spiculated forms to holly-leaf and irregularly spiculated forms		Sickle cell disorders (SS, S trait, SC, SD, S thalassemia, etc.) Hemoglobin C-Harlem Hemoglobin Memphis/S

TABLE 22-3   NOMENCLATURE OF RED CELL SHAPES AND ASSOCIATED DISEASE STATES (*CONTINUED*)

TERMINOLOGY (GREEK MEANING)	OLD TERMS, SYNONYMS	DESCRIPTION	MICROGRAPH	ASSOCIATED DISEASE STATES
Codocyte (bell)	Target cell	Bell-shaped RBC that assumes a target shape on dried films of blood		Obstructive liver disease Hemoglobinopathies (S, C) Thalassemia Iron deficiency Postsplenectomy state LCAT deficiency
Dacryocyte (tear)	Teardrop cell	RBC with a single elongated or pointed extremity		Myelofibrosis with myeloid metaplasia Myelophthisic anemias Thalassemia
Leptocyte (thin)	Thin cell, wafer cell	Thin, flat RBC with hemoglobin at periphery		Thalassemia Obstructive liver disease (± iron deficiency)
Keratocyte (horn)	Horn cell	RBC with spicules resulting from ruptured vacuole; cell appears half-moon shaped or spindle shaped		DIC or vascular prosthesis

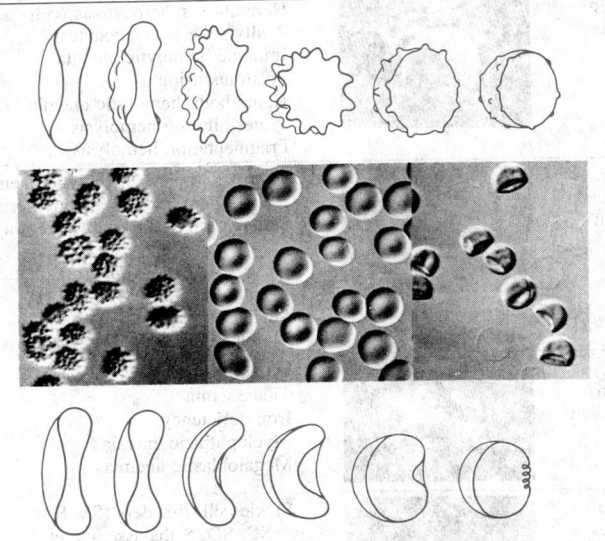

FIGURE 22-11   The discocyte-echinocyte and the discocyte-stomatocyte transformation. The upper panel schematically depicts the echinocytic transformation as induced by a rise in pH, a lack of albumin in the suspension, or exposure to an anionic phenothiazine derivative. Note particularly that the low protuberances that herald the echinocytogenic transformation appear preferentially over the rim of the biconcave disc. The lower panel schematically depicts stomatocyte formation as induced by a cationic phenothiazine derivative, a lowering of pH, or an excess of albumin in the suspending medium. Note that the intermediate form between the disc and the early cup is not a bent disc but rather a bow-tie form with very steep sides to the dimples.[176] The microscopic appearance in wet preparations of stomatocytes (*right*), discocytes (*middle*), and echinocytes (*left*) is shown in the center panel.

on the stomatocyte surface is obliterated by membrane loss, the transformation becomes irreversible and a spherostomatocyte is the result.

In addition to pH and albumin there exists a wide array of pharmacologic agents that effect stomatocytic-echinocytic changes in red cell shape. These are thought to act by preferentially expanding the outer half of the phospholipid bilayer (echinocytogenic) or the inner half (stomatocytogenic). This explanation is sometimes referred to as the *bilayer-couple hypothesis*.[128] While this hypothesis does account for the effects of these membrane-active pharmacologic agents on the red cell membrane, it is probably not a complete explanation for all stomatocytes or echinocytes. It is unlikely that pH and albumin are acting by directly expanding the inner or outer half of the phospholipid bilayer.[117]

THE AGED CELL

While there is general agreement that the reticulocyte loses membrane as it matures into a discocyte, it is less certain that membrane loss continues throughout the erythrocyte life span. The notion that erythrocyte aging is synonymous with membrane loss, increasing MCHC, and decreasing deformability is largely the result of studies on density-separated cells and the equating of dense cells with aged cells. Indeed, dense cells are dense because their MCHC is elevated, and an elevated MCHC exerts a profoundly depressant effect on red cell deformability. Thus dense cells will always be relatively nondeformable—but whether they are aged is still not settled. One thing is clear: unlike the reticulocyte, the aged red cell is not easily distinguished morphologically. Red cell aging and senescence are discussed in Chap. 29.

THE CODOCYTE

In the circulation the codocyte is a bell-shaped cell that assumes a target configuration when dried on a slide in the preparation of a blood film.[109] On a flat surface the codocyte tends to evert its concavity into a central projection into which hemoglobin redistributes. This results in a central density (target) on the blood film. The codocyte is characterized by relative membrane excess due either to increased red cell surface area or to decreased intracellular hemoglobin. In patients with obstructive liver disease there is a depression of lecithin cholesterol acetyltransferase (LCAT) activity. This increases the cholesterol/phospholipid ratio[129] and produces an absolute increase in the surface area of the red cell membrane. In contrast, the membrane excess is only relative in patients with iron-deficiency anemia and thalassemia, because of the reduced quantity of intracellular hemoglobin.

THE ACANTHOCYTE

Acanthocytes are generated from normal red blood cells under conditions that alter their membrane lipid content, possibly by loss of glycerophospholipids resulting in a relative increase in sphingomyelin.[130] Once produced, the shape is irreversible except in the rare McLeod syndrome, where incubation of the acanthocytic cells with phosphatidylserine or chlorpromazine will restore the discoid shape.[131] A markedly increased membrane cholesterol/lecithin ratio is common to acanthocytes from patients with hepatocellular disease and abetalipoproteinemia.

THE DISCOCYTE-DREPANOCYTE TRANSFORMATION

The sickle cell, or drepanocyte, displays a characteristic variation of form on stained blood films. Most commonly encountered is the fusiform cell in the shape of a crescent with two pointed extremities. Examination by phase-contrast microscopy of deoxygenated sickle cell blood reveals varied cell forms characterized by pointed extremities in holly-leaf and poikilocytic configurations, many with multiple spicules several microns in length. The spicules are quite fragile and are easily avulsed from the cell. If sickle cell formation is observed, the earliest change with deoxygenation is the loss of flicker,[132] followed by slight deformation at the border of the discocyte with displacement of the hemoglobin to one region of the cell. The cell then elongates and becomes rigid due to polymerization of hemoglobin S in rods or filaments.[133] The rods are 15 to 18 nm (150 to 180 Å) in diameter and composed of monomolecular filaments of 6 to 7 nm (60 to 70 Å) intertwined into a six-stranded helix.[134] In partially sickled cells such polymers display random orientation, but as polymerization increases the polymeric filaments undergo lateral reorientation into rods that are generally aligned with the long axis of the drepanocyte. Upon reoxygenation the drepanocyte resumes the discocyte form and in so doing loses membrane by microspherulation and fragmentation during the retraction of long spicules.[135] There is suggestive evidence that more of the typical sickle-shaped cells form under slow deoxygenation. Thus, the cell membrane will be maximally stressed, and more of it will be lost during the unsickling cycle after slow deoxygenation.[136] The unsickling process also leads to the formation of micro-Heinz bodies that adhere to the internal surface of the red cell membrane and contribute to the increased membrane rigidity and cation leak.[95] With each sickle-unsickle cycle membrane damage accumulates, until the cells become incapable of reversion to the biconcave disc shape even when fully oxygenated. They thus become *irreversibly sickled cells.*[137] These cells have an increased hemoglobin concentration and increased cation permeability, with decreased potassium and increased sodium. In addition, there is a marked decrease in membrane deformability.[137] In addition to irreversibly sickled cells, the blood of patients with sickle cell anemia contains small numbers of another rigid, membrane-damaged cell—the sequestrocyte. These cells are characterized by linear zones of membrane fusion that entrap lakes of hemoglobin. In the light microscope they appear massively vacuolated. They presumably arise from a combination of physical damage from sickle-

unsickle cycles and oxidative membrane damage that causes transcellular cross-bonding of the cell membrane.[138]

THE SCHIZOCYTE

Fibrin strands in damaged blood vessels may be arrayed so that they sieve the passing red cells. Should a passing red cell fold over or otherwise attach to the strand, the bloodstream will pull on the arrested cell and stretch and eventually fragment it.[139,140] If prior to rupture the two inner surfaces of the red cell membrane become approximated, the torn membranes will seal[141] and the schizocyte will contain hemoglobin. The more rigid schizocytes and those with a low relative surface area are rapidly removed by the spleen; the remainder may circulate for many days.

THE SPHEROCYTE

Red cells sensitized with antibodies, complement, or immune complexes undergo loss of cholesterol and thus of surface area, displaying the increased osmotic fragility of the spherocyte.[142] Heinz body formation leads to membrane depletion by fragmentation, with spherocyte formation.[143] A spherogenic mechanism common to both Heinz body hemolytic anemias and immune hemolysis is partial phagocytosis of portions of the cell containing aggregates of denatured hemoglobin[143] and portions of the sensitized membrane,[144] respectively. Stomatocytosis is a rare form of spherocytosis.[145] The anomaly is due to an abnormal ion permeability of the red cell membrane resulting in high levels of sodium and low levels of potassium in the cell interior (see Chap. 43). The cells take up water, become macrocytic and hypochromic, and show a dramatic increase in osmotic fragility. On blood films numerous spherocytic stomatocytes are present. These spherocytes, in contrast to those seen in hereditary spherocytosis, are large and hypochromic.

A spectrum of abnormal cells varying from normal discocytes to stomatocytes, spherostomatocytes, and dense microspherocytes is seen in hereditary spherocytosis.[146]

HEAT-INDUCED SHAPE CHANGES

Heating red cells to temperatures above 49°C will depolymerize spectrin. If the heating episode is brief and the inner surfaces of the biconcavities are in contact, these surfaces will fuse upon cooling.[147] More vigorous heating causes marked spherulation of the entire cell. Microspherocytes bud from the cell surface, and the entire cell becomes transformed into small spherical fragments. Such fragments may be recovered from the blood after severe burns.

ELLIPTOCYTES

In blood films of normal subjects, elliptical or oval cells usually constitute less than one percent of the erythrocytes. In various pathologic situations, with or without anemia (thalassemia trait, folate and iron deficiency, etc.), the number of elliptocytes can increase to 10 percent. Exceptionally, as in dyserythropoiesis, the proportion can be as high as 50 percent. In hereditary elliptocytosis (see Chap. 43) the number of elliptical erythrocytes varies greatly, from 0 to 98 percent.[148] Such fluctuations have forced hematologists to substitute a biochemical and functional (rheologic) definition of hereditary elliptocytosis for the original morphologic one.[148] Both qualitative and quantitative anomalies of spectrin[118,149-151] and protein 4.1,[152,153] two major proteins of the membrane skeleton, are associated with hereditary elliptocytosis. As a consequence, rheologic membrane properties are impaired.[149,154] A severe hemolytic anemia, however, is seen only in the homozygous form of the disease where schizocytes are typically present.

DACRYOCYTES

These cells are typically found in the bloodstream of patients with marrow fibrosis, often accompanied by extramedullary hemopoiesis.

How these marrow changes give rise to dacryocytes is still unknown. Aspiration of red cell membrane into a micropipette of appropriate dimensions will produce a morphologically similar shape change; however, the cell usually recovers completely within minutes. Similar deformation in a reticulocyte might be permanent since it would occur while the assembly of the submembrane skeleton was still in process. A delay during egress from the marrow would provide such an opportunity.

KERATOCYTES ("HORN CELLS" OR "HELMET CELLS")
Keratocytes are erythrocytes with one or more roughly circular bites removed from the discocyte margin. They differ from schizocytes in that their hemoglobin content is normal or only slightly lower than normal; they have not been formed by the bisection of a red cell. Rather, they appear to arise when all the hemoglobin is squeezed out of a portion near the edge of a discocytic red cell and the two opposite membrane surfaces fuse.[155] This process forms a pseudovacuole which soon ruptures, probably because of stiffening of the membrane skeleton in the fused portion. The result is a notch with bordering spicules or horns. Experimentally, membrane fusion with pseudovacuole formation can be produced by heat in excess of 49°C[147] and by mechanical stress.[141] In vitro exposure to diamide and N-ethylmaleimide[156] will produce this characteristic form.

"BITE" CELLS
"Bite" cells are formed when the Heinz bodies are pitted from the cells by splenic macrophages.[121] Emphasis on the missing portion rather than on the horns that remain has led to the term *bite cell*.[157] In vivo exposure to sulfonamide drugs such as dapsone and sulfasalazine and the urinary tract antiseptic phenazopyridine will result in "bite" cells[158] in susceptible individuals. Bite cells are obviously a form of keratocyte. It is, however, worthwhile to distinguish them from other keratocytes because their method of formation involves removal of denatured hemoglobin (and membrane), whereas keratocytes in general appear to be formed by membrane apposition and subsequent removal of the apposed membranes.

CRYSTALS OF HEMOGLOBIN C DISEASE
In splenectomized patients with homozygous hemoglobin C disease, as many as 10 percent of the circulating cells may contain tetrahedral crystals.[159] In blood films from nonsplenectomized patients crystal-containing cells are rare or absent.[160] The efficiency in splenic removal may be due to spherocyte formation from the release of osmotically active particles as the hemoglobin C crystals "melt" while undergoing deoxygenation in the spleen. "Melting" upon deoxygenation occurs readily in vitro, behavior that is opposite to that of sickle hemoglobin crystals.[161] In vitro dehydration of hemoglobin C–containing cells for a 24-h period between slide and coverslip[162] or hypertonic dehydration of red cells in 3% NaCl buffer for 4 to 12 h readily produces crystals. In homozygous hemoglobin C disease up to 75 percent of the cells may show crystals; lower percentages occur in hemoglobin SC and other hemoglobin C variants. Molecular subunits in a tetragonal or hexagonal arrangement may be identified within the hemoglobin C crystals.[163] Hemoglobin Setif, like hemoglobin C, may also precipitate as intracellular crystals when the tonicity of the suspending medium is raised.[164] This takes place in oxygenated solutions and at osmolarities achieved in the renal medulla. Even so, there have been no reported clinical symptoms among heterozygous carriers of the Setif gene.

OSMOTIC BEHAVIOR

The red cell behaves as an osmometer.[165] When placed into a hypertonic solution it shrinks, and the inner surfaces of the biconcavities touch over a progressively larger central region. When red cells in hypotonic solutions reach their critical hemolytic volume, holes greater than 10 nm (100 Å) in size appear[166] and the hemoglobin exits. Alternatively, a large tear may develop in the red cell membrane. Following hemolysis (exit of the hemoglobin), the holes or tears close and the cell resumes its original biconcave shape.

DEFORMABILITY

An important determinant of the survival of a red cell in the circulation is its deformability. The deformability of the intact cell is made up of contributions from the intrinsic deformability of the membrane itself, the internal viscosity (for practical purposes, the MCHC), and the surface/volume ratio of the cell. The deformability of the intact cell can be measured by the time it takes a red cell suspension to traverse a filter of known pore size[167]; or the cells may be suspended in a viscous medium and exposed to a shear force, and the change in shape observed microscopically, as in the rheoscope,[168] or by laser diffraction, as in the ektacytometer.[169] Additional information can be obtained from ektacytometric analysis by varying the osmolarity of the suspending medium and thus changing the surface/volume ratio as well as the internal viscosity of the cells during the analytical procedure.[170] Alternatively, the red cell may be folded over a spiderweb strand in the presence of rapidly flowing buffer. From the relationship between the flow rate of the buffer and the deformation of the red cell, the deformability of the membrane can be estimated.[171]

An increase of the MCHC by 20 percent results in an increase in the internal viscosity of about 600 percent.[172] An increase of this magnitude leaves the red cell with sufficient deformability to survive in the circulation. This is not the case for erythrocytes from patients with xerocytosis or dessicocytosis. Here the erythrocytes are always perilously close to the upper limits of internal viscosity consistent with traversing the vasculature.[173]

In the circulation the primary cause of decreased red cell deformability is likely to be insufficient membrane (spherocytosis) rather than stiffening of the membrane. The interendothelial slits of the splenic sinus stress cells with a normal surface/volume ratio, and splenic phagocytes remove those with a ratio that is lower than normal. It is self-evident that a perfectly spherical red cell will be rigid no matter how low the MCHC or how flexible the isolated membrane might be.

REFERENCES

1. Satterthwaite AB, Borson R, Tenen DG: Regulation of the gene for CD34, a human hematopoietic stem cell antigen, in KG-1 cells. *Blood* 75:2299, 1990.
2. Civin CI, Strauss LC, Fackler MJ, Trischmann TM, Wiley JM, Loken MR: Positive stem cell selection—basic science. *Prog Clin Biol Res* 333:387, 1990.
3. Lu L, Walker D, Broxmeyer HE, Hoffman R, Hu W, Walker E: Characterization of adult human marrow hematopoietic progenitors highly enriched by two-color cell sorting with My10 and major histocompatibility class II monoclonal antibodies. *J Immunol* 139:1823, 1987.
4. Yin AH, Miraglia S, Zanjani ED, et al: AC133, a novel marker for human hematopoietic stem and progenitor cells. *Blood* 90:5002, 1997.
5. Rappold I, Ziegler BL, Kohler I, et al: Functional and phenotypic characterization of cord blood and bone marrow subsets expressing FLT3 (CD135) receptor tyrosine kinase. *Blood* 90:111, 1997.
6. Wagner JE, Collins D, Fuller S, et al: Isolation of small, primitive human hematopoietic stem cells: distribution of cell surface cytokine receptors and growth in SCID-Hu mice. *Blood* 86:512, 1995.
7. Zannettino AC, Berndt MC, Butcher C, Butcher EC, Vadas MA, Simmons PJ: Primitive human hematopoietic progenitors adhere to P-selectin (CD62P). *Blood* 85:3466, 1995.

8. Tracey JB, Rinder HM: Characterization of the P-selectin ligand on human hematopoietic progenitors. *Exp Hematol* 24:1494, 1996.

9. Laszik Z, Jansen PJ, Cummings RD, Tedder TF, McEver RP, Moore KL: P-selectin glycoprotein ligand-1 is broadly expressed in cells of myeloid, lymphoid, and dendritic lineage and in some nonhematopoietic cells. *Blood* 88:3010, 1996.

10. Kobayashi M, Imamura M, Uede T, et al: Expression of adhesion molecules on human hematopoietic progenitor cells at different maturational stages. *Stem Cells (Dayt)* 12:316, 1994.

11. Harvey K, Higgins N, Akard L, et al: Lineage commitment of HLA-DR/CD38-defined progenitor cell subpopulations in bone marrow and mobilized peripheral blood assessed by four-color immunofluorescence. *J Hematother* 6:243, 1997.

12. Sieff C, Bicknell D, Caine G, Robinson J, Lam G, Greaves MF: Changes in cell surface antigen expression during hemopoietic differentiation. *Blood* 60:703, 1982.

13. Greaves M, Robinson J, Delia D, Sutherland R, Newman R, Sieff C: Mapping cell surface antigen expression of haemopoietic progenitor cells using monoclonal antibodies. *Ciba Found Symp* 84:109, 1981.

14. Brandt J, Baird N, Lu L, Srour E, Hoffman R: Characterization of a human hematopoietic progenitor cell capable of forming blast cell containing colonies in vitro. *J Clin Invest* 82:1017, 1988.

15. Nakahata T, Okumura N: Cell surface antigen expression in human erythroid progenitors: erythroid and megakaryocytic markers. *Leuk Lymphoma* 13:401, 1994.

16. Papayannopoulou T, Brice M, Farrer D, Kaushansky K: Insights into the cellular mechanisms of erythropoietin-thrombopoietin synergy. *Exp Hematol* 24:660, 1996.

17. Inada T, Iwama A, Sakano S, Ohno M, Sawada K, Suda T: Selective expression of the receptor tyrosine kinase, HTK, on human erythroid progenitor cells. *Blood* 89:2757, 1997.

18. Brashem-Stein C, Flowers DA, Smith FO, Staats SJ, Andrews RG, Bernstein ID: Ontogeny of hematopoietic stem cell development: reciprocal expression of CD33 and a novel molecule by maturing myeloid and erythroid progenitors. *Blood* 82:792, 1993.

19. Uoshima N, Ozawa M, Kimura S, et al: Changes in c-Kit expression and effects of SCF during differentiation of human erythroid progenitor cells. *Br J Haematol* 91:30, 1995.

20. Inada T, Iwama A, Sakano S, Ohno M, Sawada K, Suda T: Selective expression of the receptor tyrosine kinase, HTK, on human erythroid progenitor cells. *Blood* 89:2757, 1997.

21. deJong MO, Westerman Y, Wagemaker G, Wognum AW: Coexpression of Kit and the receptors for erythropoietin, interleukin 6 and GM-CSF on hemopoietic cells. *Stem Cells (Dayt)* 15:275, 1997.

22. Sakabe H, Kimura T, Zeng Z, et al: Haematopoietic action of flt3 ligand on cord blood-derived CD34-positive cells expressing different levels of flt3 or c-kit tyrosine kinase receptor: comparison with stem cell factor. *Eur J Haematol* 60:297, 1998.

23. Lian Z, Toki J, Yu C, et al: Intrathymically injected hemopoietic stem cells can differentiate into all lineage cells in the thymus: differences between c-kit+ cells and c-kit < low cells. *Stem Cells (Dayt)* 15:430, 1997.

24. Sogo S, Inaba M, Ogata H, et al: Induction of c-kit molecules on human CD34+/c-kit < low cells: evidence for CD34+/c-kit < low cells as primitive hematopoietic stem cells. *Stem Cells (Dayt)* 15:420, 1997.

25. McNiece IK, Briddell RA: Stem cell factor. *J Leukoc Biol* 58:14, 1995.

26. Coulombel L, Vuillet-Gaugler MH, Leroy C, Rosemblatt M, Breton-Gorius J: Adhesive properties of human erythroblastic precursor cells. *Blood Cells* 17:65, 1991.

27. Shintani N, Kohgo Y, Kato J, et al: Expression and extracellular release of transferrin receptors during peripheral erythroid progenitor cell differentiation in liquid culture. *Blood* 83:1209, 1994.

28. Loken MR, Shah VO, Dattilio KL, Civin CI: Flow cytometric analysis of human bone marrow: I. Normal erythroid development. *Blood* 69:255, 1987.

29. Villeval JL, LeVanKim C, Bettaieb A, et al: Early expression of glycophorin C during normal and leukemic human erythroid differentiation. *Cancer Res* 49:2626, 1989.

30. Villeval JL, Testa U, Vinci G, et al: Carbonic anhydrase I is an early specific marker of normal human erythroid differentiation. *Blood* 66:1162, 1985.

31. Harrison PR: Molecular analysis of erythropoiesis. A current appraisal. *Exp Cell Res* 155:321, 1984.

32. Ratajczak J, Zhang Q, Pertusini E, Wojczyk BS, Wasik MA, Ratajczak MZ: The role of insulin (INS) and insulin-like growth factor-I (IGF-I) in regulating human erythropoiesis. Studies in vitro under serum-free conditions—comparison to other cytokines and growth factors. *Leukemia* 12:371, 1998.

33. Broudy VC, Lin N, Brice M, Nakamoto B, Papayannopoulou T: Erythropoietin receptor characteristics on primary human erythroid cells. *Blood* 77:2583, 1991.

34. Wojchowski DM, He TC: Signal transduction in the erythropoietin receptor system. *Stem Cells (Dayt)* 11:381, 1993.

35. Kieffer N, Bettaieb A, Legrand C, et al: Developmentally regulated expression of a 78 kDa erythroblast membrane glycoprotein immunologically related to the platelet thrombospondin receptor. *Biochem J* 262:835, 1989.

36. Buhring HJ, Muller T, Herbst R, et al: The adhesion molecule E-cadherin and a surface antigen recognized by the antibody 9C4 are selectively expressed on erythroid cells of defined maturational stages. *Leukemia* 10:106, 1996.

37. Bettaieb A, Farace F, Mitjavila MT, et al: Use of a monoclonal antibody (GA3) to demonstrate lineage restricted O-glycosylation on leukosialin during terminal erythroid differentiation. *Blood* 71:1226, 1988.

38. Yurchenco PD, Furthmayr H: Expression of red cell membrane proteins in erythroid precursor cells. *J Supramol Struct* 13:255, 1980.

39. Ekblom M: Expression of spectrin in normal and malignant erythropoiesis. *Scand J Haematol* 33:378, 1984.

40. Wickrema A, Koury ST, Dai CH, Krantz SB: Changes in cytoskeletal proteins and their mRNAs during maturation of human erythroid progenitor cells. *J Cell Physiol* 160:417, 1994.

41. Hanspal M, Prchal JT, Palek J: Biogenesis of erythrocyte membrane skeleton in health and disease. *Stem Cells (Dayt)* 11(suppl 1):8, 1993.

42. Nehls V, Drenckhahn D, Joshi R, Bennett V: Adducin in erythrocyte precursor cells of rats and humans: expression and compartmentalization. *Blood* 78:1692, 1991.

43. Nehls V, Zeitler Zapf P, Drenckhahn D: Different sequences of expression of band 3, spectrin, and ankyrin during normal erythropoiesis and erythroleukemia. *Am J Pathol* 142:1565, 1993.

44. Loken MR, Civin CI, Bigbee WL, Langlois RG, Jensen RH: Coordinate glycosylation and cell surface expression of glycophorin A during normal human erythropoiesis. *Blood* 70:1959, 1987.

45. Ekblom M, Gahmberg CG, Andersson LC: Late expression of M and N antigens on glycophorin A during erythroid differentiation. *Blood* 66:233, 1985.

46. Bessis M: *Living Blood Cells and Their Ultrastructure*. Springer-Verlag, New York, 1973.

47. Breton-Gorius J, Vuillet-Gaugler MH, Coulombel L, et al: Association between leukemic erythroid progenitors and bone marrow macrophages. *Blood Cells* 17:127, 1991.

48. Wright SD, Meyer BC: Fibronectin receptor of human macrophages recognizes the sequence Arg-Gly-Asp-Ser. *J Exp Med* 162:762, 1985.

49. Patel VP, Lodish HF: The fibronectin receptor on mammalian erythroid precursor cells: Characterization and developmental regulation. *J Cell Biol* 102:449, 1986.

50. Fraser IP, Gordon S: Murine erythroleukemia (MEL) cells bear ligands for the sialoadhesin and erythroblast receptor macrophage hemagglutinins. *Eur J Cell Biol* 64:217, 1994.

51. Parmley RT, Ogawa M, Spicer SS: Human marrow erythropoiesis in culture: Ultrastructural and cytochemical studies of cellular interactions. *Exp Hematol* 6:78, 1978.

52. Breton-Gorius J, Guichard J, Vainchenker W: Absence of erythroblastic islands in plasma clot culture and their possible reconstitution after clot lysis. *Blood Cells* 5:461, 1979.

53. Klausner RD, Harford JB, Rao K, et al: Molecular aspects of the regulation of cellular iron metabolism, in *Proteins of Iron Storage and Transport*, edited by G Spik, J Montreuil, RR Crichton, J Mazurier, p 111. Elsevier, Amsterdam, 1985.

54. Quintana C, Bonnet N, Jeantet AY, Chemelle P: Crystallographic study of the ferritin molecule: New results obtained from natural crystals in situ (mollusk oocyte) and from isolated molecules (horse spleen). *Biol Cell* 59:247, 1987.

55. Iancu TC: Iron and neoplasia: ferritin and hemosiderin in tumor cells. *Ultrastruct Pathol* 13:573, 1989.

56. Richter GW: Studies of iron overload. Rat liver siderosome ferritin. *Lab Invest* 50:26, 1984.

57. Pearse BMF: Coated vesicles from human placenta carry ferritin, transferrin and immunoglobulin G. *Proc Natl Acad Sci USA* 79:451, 1982.

58. Conrad ME, Umbreit JN, Moore EG, Heiman D: Mobilferrin is an intermediate in iron transport between transferrin and hemoglobin in K562 cells. *J Clin Invest* 98:1449, 1996.

59. Policard A, Bessis M: Sur un mode d'incorporation des macromolecules par la cellule, visible au microscope électronique. *CR Seances Soc Biol Fil* 146:3194, 1958.

60. Parmley RT, Hajdu I, Denys FR: Ultrastructural localization of the transferrin receptor and transferrin on marrow cell surfaces. *Br J Haematol* 54:633, 1983.

61. Speyer BE, Fielding J: Ferritin as a cytosol iron transport intermediate in human reticulocytes. *Br J Haematol* 42:255, 1979.

62. Grasso JA, Hillis TJ, Mooney-Frank JA: Ferritin is not a required intermediate for iron utilization in heme synthesis. *Biochim Biophys Acta* 797:247, 1984.

63. Drysdale J, Jain SK, Boyd D: Human ferritins: Genes and proteins, in *Proteins of Iron Storage and Transport*, edited by G Spik, J Montreuil, RR Crichton, J Mazurier, p 343. Elsevier, Amsterdam, 1985.

64. Harrison PM, Arosio P: The ferritins: molecular properties, iron storage function and cellular regulation. *Biochim Biophys Acta* 1275:161, 1996.

65. Nijhof W, Wierenga PK: Isolation and characterization of the erythroid progenitor cell: CFU-E. *J Cell Biol* 96:386, 1983.

66. Breton-Gorius J, Villeval JL, Mitjavila MT, et al: Ultrastructural and cytochemical characterization of blasts from early erythroblastic leukemias. *Leukemia* 1:173, 1987.

67. Bessis M, Breton-Gorius J: Ultrastructure du proerythroblaste. *Nouv Rev Fr Hematol* 1:529, 1961.

68. Breton-Gorius J, Reyes F: Ultrastructure of human bone marrow cell maturation. *Int Rev Cytol* 46:251, 1976.

69. Dvorak AM, Dvorak HF, Karnovsky MJ: Cytochemical localization of peroxidase activity in the developing erythrocyte. *Am J Pathol* 67:303, 1972.

70. Xue SP, Zhang SF, Du Q, et al: The role of cytoskeletal elements in the two-phase denucleation process of mammalian erythroblasts in vitro observed by laser confocal scanning microscope. *Cell Mol Biol (Noisy-le- Grand)* 43:851, 1997.

71. Lazarides E: From genes to structural morphogenesis: The genesis and epigenesis of a red blood cell. *Cell* 51:345, 1987.

72. Chasis JA, Prenant M, Leung A, Mohandas N: Membrane assembly and remodeling during reticulocyte maturation. *Blood* 74:1112, 1989.

73. Bessis M, Breton-Gorius J, Thiery JP: Role possible de l'hemoglobine accompagnant le noyau des erythroblastes dans l'origine de la stercobiline élimnée précocement. *CR Acad Sci III* 252:2300, 1961.

74. Wilson JG, Tavassoli M. Microenvironmental factors involved in the establishment of erythropoiesis in bone marrow. *Ann NY Acad Sci* 718: 271, 1994.

75. Lichtman MA, Santillo P: Red cell egress from the marrow: Vis-a-tergo. *Blood Cells* 12:11, 1986.

76. Waugh RE, Hsu LL, Clark P, Clark A Jr: Analysis of cell egress in bone marrow, in *White Cell Mechanics: Basic Science and Clinical Aspects*, edited by HJ Meiselman, MA Lichtman, PL LaCelle, pp 221–236. Alan R. Liss, New York, 1984.

77. Nunez MT, Fischer S, Glass J, et al: Transferrin receptors in developing murine erythroid cells. *Br J Haematol* 36:519, 1977.

78. Pan BT, Johnstone RM: Fate of transferrin receptor during maturation of sheep reticulocytes in vitro: Selective externalization of the receptor. *Cell* 33:967, 1983.

79. Zweig S, Singer SJ: Concanavalin A induced endocytosis in rabbit reticulocytes, and its decrease with reticulocyte maturation. *J Cell Biol* 80:487, 1979.

80. Bowman WD: Abnormal (ringed) sideroblasts in various hematologic disorders. *Blood* 18:662, 1961.

81. Hines JD, Grasso JA: The sideroblastic anemias. *Semin Hematol* 7:86, 1970.

82. Flandrin G, Daniel MT, Breton-Gorius J, et al: Ilot erythroblastic abnormal du au développement de jonctions intercellulaires (synarthese erythroblastique). Un nouveau mécanisme d'anémie. Problèmes poses par le diagnostic. *Nouv Rev Fr Hematol* 14:161, 1971.

83. Jolly J: Recherches sur la formation des globules rouges des mammifères. *Arch Anat Microsc* 9:133, 1907.

84. Discombe G: L'Origine des corps de Howell-Jolly et des anneaux de Cabot. *Sangre* 29:262, 1948.

85. Rondanelli EG, Trenta A, Magliulo E, et al: Morphogenese des micronoyaux supplementaires (pseudo-corps de Jolly) dans les cellules erythropoietiques irradiées. *Acta Haematol* 35:232, 1966.

86. Koyama S: Studies on Howell-Jolly body. *Acta Haematol Jpn* 23:20, 1960.

87. Koyama S, Kihira H, Aoki S, Ohnishi H: Postsplenectomy vacuole: a new erythrocytic inclusion body. *Mie Med J* 11:425, 1962.

88. Holroyde CP, Gardner FH: Acquisition of autophagic vacuoles by human erythrocytes: physiological role of the spleen. *Blood* 36:566, 1970.

89. O'Grady JG, Harding B, Egan EL, Murphy B, O'Gorman TA, McCarthy CF: "Pitted" erythrocytes: impaired formation in splenectomized subjects with congenital spherocytosis. *Br J Haematol* 57:441, 1984.

90. Buchanan GR, Holtkamp CA, Horton JA: Formation and disappearance of pocked erythrocytes: studies in human subjects and laboratory animals. *Am J Hematol* 25:243, 1987.

91. Kass L: Origin and composition of Cabot Rings in pernicious anemia. *Am J Clin Pathol.* 64:53, 1975.

92. Van Oye E: L'Origine des anneaux de Cabot. *Rev Hematol* 9:173, 1954.

93. Kass L, Gray RH: Ultrastructural visualization of Cabot Rings in pernicious anemia. *Experientia* 32:507, 1976.

94. Jensen WN, Moreno GD, Bessis MC: An electron microscopic description of basophilic stippling in red cells. *Blood* 25:933, 1965.

95. Lessin L, Wallas CP: Biochemical basis for membrane alterations in the irreversibly sickled cell. *Blood* 42:978, 1973.

96. Heinz R: Uber Blutdegeneration und Regeneration. *Beitr Pathol* 29:299, 1901.

97. Chinprasertsuk S, Piankijagum A, Wasi P: In vivo induction of intraerythrocytic inclusion bodies in Hemoglobin H disease: an electron microscopic study. *Birth Defects Orig Artic Ser* 23:317, 1987.

98. Wickramasinghe SN, Hughes M, Fucharoen S, Wasi P. The morphology of redox-dye-treated HbH-containing red cells: differences between cells treated with brilliant cresyl blue, methylene blue and new methylene blue. *Clin Lab Haematol* 7:353, 1985.

99. Sansone G, Sciarratta GV, Ivaldi G, Chiappara G. Hb H-like inclusions in red cells of patients with unstable haemoglobin. *Haematologica* 72:481, 1987.

100. Wickramasinghe SN, Hughes M, Higgs DR, Weatherall DJ. Ultrastructure of red cells containing haemoglobin H inclusions induced by redox dyes. *Clin Lab Haematol* 3:51, 1981.

101. Beaven GH, Coleman PN, White JC: Occurrence of Haemoglobin H in leukaemia: a further case of erythroleukaemia. *Acta Haemat* 59:37, 1978.

102. Bessis M, Breton-Gorius J: Iron particles in normal erythroblasts and pathological erythrocytes. *J Biophys Biochem Cytol* 3:503, 1957.

103. Brecher G, Haley JE, Prenant M, Bessis M: Macronormoblasts, macroreticulocytes, and macrocytes. *Blood Cells* 1:547, 1975.

104. Major A, Bauer C, Breymann C, Huch A, Huch R: rh-Erythropoietin stimulates immature reticulocyte release in man. *Br J Haematol* 87:605, 1994.

105. Davis BH, DiCorato M, Bigelo NC, Langweiler MH. Proposal for standardization of flow cytometric reticulocyte maturity index (RMI) measurements. *Cytometry* 14:318, 1993.

106. Watanabe K, Kawai Y, Takeuchi K, Shimizu N, Iri H, Ikeda Y, Houwen B. Reticulocyte maturity as an indicator for estimating qualitative abnormality of erythropoiesis. *J Clin Pathol* 47:736, 1994.

107. Bull BS, Hay KL: Are red cell indices international? *Arch Pathol Lab Med* 109:604, 1985.

108. Korpman RA, Dorrough DC, Brailsford JD, Bull BS: The red cell shape as an indicator of membrane structure: Ponder's rule reexamined. *Blood Cells* 3:315, 1977.

109. Bessis M: *Blood Smears Reinterpreted*. Springer, Berlin, 1977.

110. Burton AL, Anderson WL, Andrews RV: Quantitative studies on the flicker phenomenon in the erythrocyte. *Blood* 32:819, 1968.

111. Fricke K, Wirthensohn K, Laxhuber R, Sackmann E: Flicker spectroscopy of erythrocytes: A sensitive method to study subtle changes of membrane bending stiffness. *Eur Biophys J* 14:67, 1986.

112. Schmid-Schonbein H, Wells R: Tank treading of erythrocytes. *Science* 165:288, 1969.

113. Brailsford JD, Korpman RA, Bull BS: The red cell shape from discocyte to hypotonic spherocyte—a mathematical delineation based on a uniform shell hypothesis. *J Theor Biol* 60:131, 1976.

114. Byers TJ, Branton D: Visualization of the protein associations in the erythrocyte membrane skeleton. *Proc Natl Acad Sci USA* 82:6153, 1985.

115. Shen BW, Josephs R, Steck TL: Ultrastructure of the intact skeleton of the human erythrocyte membrane. *J Cell Biol* 102:997, 1986.

116. Liu SC, Derick LH, Palek J: Visualization of the hexagonal lattice in the erythrocyte membrane skeleton. *J Cell Biol* 104:527, 1987.

117. Bull BS, Brailsford JD: Red cell shape, in *The Red Cell,* edited by J Parker, P Agre, pp 401–421. Harvard University Press, Cambridge, 1988.

118. Liu SC, Derick LH, Palek J: Alteration of the erythrocyte membrane ultrastructure in hereditary spherocytosis, hereditary elliptocytosis and pyropoikilocytosis. *Blood* 76:198, 1990.

119. Branemark PI, Bagge U: Intravascular rheology of erythrocytes in man. *Blood Cells* 3:11, 1977.

120. Bessis M, Weed R, LeBlond P (eds): *Red Cell Shape: Physiology, Pathology, Ultrastructure.* Springer-Verlag, New York, 1973.

121. Prasad AS: Acquired hemolytic anemias, in *Hematology Clinical and Laboratory Practice,* edited by Bick RL, et al, p 391. Mosby, St, Louis, 1993.

122. Evans EA, Skalak R: *Mechanics and Thermodynamics of Biomembranes.* CRC Press, Boca Raton, FL, 1980.

123. Canham PB: The minimum energy of bending as a possible explanation of the biconcave shape of the human red blood cell. *J Theor Biol* 26:61, 1970.

124. Bull B: Red cell biconcavity and deformability: A macromodel based on flow chamber observations. *Nouv Rev Fr Hematol* 12:835, 1972.

125. McMillan DE, Mitchell TP, Utterback NG: Deformational strain energy and erythrocyte shape. *J Biomechanics* 19:275, 1986.

126. Tanaka T, Fillmore D, Sun ST, et al: Phase transitions in ionic gels. *Phys Rev Lett* 45:1636, 1980.

127. Elgsaeter A, Stokke BT, Mikkelsen A, Branton D: The molecular basis of erythrocyte shape. *Science* 234:1217, 1986.

128. Sheetz MP, Painter RG, Singer SJ: Biological membranes as bilayer couples. III. Compensatory shape changes induced in membranes. *J Cell Biol* 70:193, 1976.

129. Cooper RA, Jandl JH: Bile salts and cholesterol in the pathogenesis of target cells in obstructive jaundice. *J Clin Invest* 47:809, 1968.

130. Clark MR, Aminoff MJ, Chiu DT, et al: Red cell deformability and lipid composition in two forms of acanthocytosis: Enrichment of acanthocytic populations by density gradient centrifugation. *J Lab Clin Med* 113:469, 1989.

131. Redman CM, Huima T, Robbins E, et al: Effect of phosphatidyl serine on the shape of McLeod red cell acanthocytes. *Blood* 74:1826, 1989.

132. Padilla F, Bromberg PA, Jensen WN: The sickle-unsickle cycle: A cause of cell fragmentation leading to permanently deformed cells. *Blood* 41:653, 1973.

133. Bessis M, Normarski G, Thiery JP, Breton-Gorius J: Études sur la falciformation des globules rouges au microscope polarisant et au microscope electronique. *Rev Hematol* 13:249, 1958.

134. White JG: The fine structure of sickled hemoglobin in situ. *Blood* 31:561, 1968.

135. Jensen WN, Lessin LS: Membrane alterations associated with hemoglobinopathies. *Semin Hematol* 7:409, 1970.

136. Horiuchi K, Ballas SK, Asakura T: The effect of deoxygenation rate on the formation of irreversibly sickled cells. *Blood* 71:46, 1988.

137. Bertles JF, Milner PFA: Irreversibly sickled erythrocytes: A consequence of the heterogeneous distribution of hemoglobin types in sickle-cell anemia. *J Clin Invest* 47:1731, 1968.

138. Weinstein RS, Warth JA, Near K, Marikovsky Y: Sequestrocytes: A manifestation of transcellular cross-bonding of the red cell membrane in sickle cell anemia. *J Cell Science* 94:593, 1989.

139. Bull BS, Kuhn IN: The production of schistocytes by fibrin strands (a scanning electron microscope study). *Blood* 35:104, 1970.

140. Young TW, Keeney GL, Bull BS: Red cell fragmentation in human disease (a light and scanning electron microscope study). *Blood Cells* 10:493, 1984.

141. Bull BS, Weinstein RS, Korpman RA: On the thickness of the red cell membrane skeleton: Quantitative electron microscopy of maximally narrowed isthmus regions of intact cells. *Blood Cells* 12:25, 1986.

142. Cooper RA: Loss of membrane components in the pathogenesis of antibody-induced spherocytosis. *J Clin Invest* 51:16, 1972.

143. Rifkind RA, Danon D: Heinz body anemia—an ultrastructural study. I. Heinz body formation. *Blood* 25:885, 1965.

144. Rabinovitch M: Phagocytosis: The engulfment stage. *Semin Hematol* 5:134, 1968.

145. Lock SP, Sephton Smith R, Hardisty RM: Stomatocytosis: A hereditary red cell anomaly associated with haemolytic anemia. *Br J Haematol* 7:303, 1961.

146. Leblond PF, De Boisfleury A, Bessis M: La forme des erythrocytes dans la sphèrocytose héréditaire. *Nouv Rev Fr Hematol* 13:873, 1973.

147. Bull BS: Commentary on Holey red cells: A brief note. *Blood Cells* 9:173, 1983.

148. Dhermy D, Feo C, Garbarz M, et al: Prenatal diagnosis of hereditary elliptocytosis with molecular defect of spectrin. *Prenat Diagn* 7:471, 1987.

149. Dhermy D, Garbarz M, Lecomte MC, et al: Hereditary elliptocytosis: Clinical, morphological and biochemical studies of 38 cases. *Nouv Rev Fr Hematol* 28:129, 1986.

150. Coetzer T, Palek J, Lawler J, et al: Structural and functional heterogeneity of alpha spectrin mutations involving the spectrin heterodimer self-associations site: Relationships to hematologic expression of homozygous hereditary elliptocytosis and hereditary pyropoikilocytosis. *Blood* 75:2235, 1990.

151. Marchesi SL, Knowles WJ, Morrow JS, Bologna M, Marchesi VT: Abnormal spectrin in hereditary elliptocytosis. *Blood* 67:141, 1986.

152. Agre P, Zinkham WH, Casella JF, Bennett V: Spectrin deficiency is common to all forms of hereditary spherocytosis (HS): The degree of deficiency correlates with osmotic fragility. *Blood* 62(suppl 1):42a, 1983.

153. Marchesi SL, Conboy J, Agre P, et al: Molecular analysis of insertion/ deletion mutations in protein 4.1 in elliptocytosis. *J Clin Invest* 86:516, 1990.

154. Bull BS, Feo C, Bessis M: The behavior of elliptocytes under shear stress in the rheoscope and ektacytometer. *Cytometry* 3:300, 1983.

155. Santillo PA, Lichtman MA: Holey red cells: A brief note. *Blood Cells* 9:169, 1983.

156. Fischer TM: Role of spectrin in cross bonding of the red cell membrane. *Blood Cells* 13:377, 1988.

157. Greenberg MS: Heinz body hemolytic anemia. "Bite cells"—a clue to diagnosis. *Arch Intern Med* 136:153, 1976.

158. Yoo D, Lessin L: Drug-associated "bite cell" hemolytic anemia. *Am J Med* 92:243, 1992.

159. Diggs LW, Kraus AP, Morrison DB, Rudnicki RPT: Intraerythrocytic crystals in a white patient with hemoglobin C in the absence of other types of hemoglobin. *Blood* 9:1172, 1954.

160. Fabry ME, Kaul DK, Raventos C, et al: Some aspects of the pathophysiology of homozygous HbCC erythrocytes. *J Clin Invest* 67:1248, 1981.

161. Hirsch RE, Raventos-Suarez C, Olson JA, Nagel RL: Ligand state of intraerythrocytic circulating HbC crystals in homozygote CC patients. *Blood* 66:775, 1985.

162. Charache S, Conley CL, Waugh DF, et al: Pathogenesis of hemolytic anemia in homozygous hemoglobin C disease. *J Clin Invest* 46:1795, 1967.

163. Lessin LS, Jensen WN, Ponder E: Molecular mechanism of hemolytic anemia in homozygous hemoglobin C disease. *J Exp Med* 130:443, 1969.

164. Charache S, Raik E, Holtzclaw D, Hathaway PJ: Pseudosickling of hemoglobin Setif. *Blood* 1:237, 1987.

165. Ponder E: *Hemolysis and Related Phenomena.* Grune and Stratton, New York, 1948.

166. Seeman P: Transient holes in the erythrocyte membrane during hypotonic hemolysis and stable holes in the membrane after lysis by saponin and lysolecithin. *J Cell Biol* 32:55, 1967.

167. Stuart J, Bull BS, Juhan-Vague I: Microrheological techniques for the measurement of erythrocyte deformability, in *Investigative Microtechniques in Medicine and Biology,* edited by J Chayen, L Bitensky, pp 297–325. Marcel Dekker, New York, 1984.

168. Schmid-Schonbein H, Gosen JV, Heinich L, et al: A counter-rotating "rheoscope chamber" for the study of the microrheology of blood cell aggregation by microscopic observation and microphotometry. *Microvasc Res* 6:366, 1973.

169. Bessis M, Mohandas N, Feo C: Automated ektacytometry: A new method of measuring red cell deformability and red cell indices. *Blood Cells* 6:315, 1980.

170. Mohandas N, Clark MR, Shohet SB: Analysis of factors regulating erythrocyte deformability. *J Clin Invest* 66:563, 1980.

171. Bull BS, Brailsford JD: A new method of measuring the deformability of the red cell membrane. *Blood* 45:581, 1975.

172. Williams AR, Morris DR: The internal viscosity of the human erythrocyte may determine its lifespan in vivo. *Scand J Haematol* 24:57, 1980.

173. Clark MR, Mohandas N, Caggiano V, Shohet SB: Effects of abnormal cation transport on deformability of desiccytes. *J Supramol Struct* 8:521, 1978.

174. Bessis M, Breton-Gorius J: Iron metabolism in the bone marrow seen by electron microscopy: A critical review. *Blood* 19:635, 1962.

175. Edelman P, Vinci G, Villeval JL, et al: A monoclonal antibody against an erythrocyte ontogenic antigen identifies fetal and adult erythroid progenitors. *Blood* 67:56, 1986.

176. Jay AWL: Geometry of the human erythrocyte. I. Effect of albumin on cell geometry. *Biophys J* 15:205, 1975.

COMPOSITION OF THE ERYTHROCYTE

ERNEST BEUTLER

Quantitative data have been published about many of the components of the red cell, including minerals, carbohydrates, enzymes and other proteins, vitamins and lipids. Some of these are marred by the failure to rigorously remove white cells from the red cell pellet, but this chapter provides access to some of the large amount of data that is available.

The erythrocyte is a complex cell. The membrane is composed of lipids and proteins, and the interior of the cell contains metabolic machinery designed to maintain hemoglobin function. Each component of red blood cells may be expressed as a function of red cell volume, grams of hemoglobin, or square centimeters of cell surface. These expressions are usually interchangeable, but under certain circumstances each may have specific advantages. However, because disease may produce changes in the average red cell size, hemoglobin content, or surface area, the use of any of these measurements individually may, at times, be misleading.

For convenience and uniformity, data in the accompanying tables (Tables 23-1 through 23-9) have been expressed in terms of cell constituent per milliliter of red cell and per gram of hemoglobin; in many instances this has required recalculation of published data. These recalculations assume a hematocrit value of 45 percent and 33 g per deciliter concentration of hemoglobin in red cells. To obtain concentration per g hemoglobin the concentration per ml RBC may be multiplied by 3.03. Only some of the most commonly referred to constituents of the erythrocyte are listed here. More comprehensive data may be found at www.williamshematology.com. The reference on which each value is based is the first number presented in the last column of each table. Where applicable, additional confirmatory references are shown. Additional data and references may be found elsewhere.[99,100] In some instances, only the percentage of the total of the type of constituent present is given. Data regarding activities of red cell enzymes are presented in Chap. 35. (The reader should be aware of the fact that proper care has not always been taken to remove leukocytes in isolating red cells, and in the case of constituents that are present in leukocytes at a much higher concentration than is present in erythrocytes this can produce misleading data.)

TABLE 23-1   HUMAN ERYTHROCYTE PROTEIN AND WATER CONTENT

COMPONENT	mg/ml RBC	REFERENCE
Water	721 ± 17.3	1,2
Total protein	371	2–5
Nonhemoglobin protein	9.2	2,3
Insoluble stroma protein	6.3	3
Protein from enzymes	2.9	3

TABLE 23-2   HUMAN ERYTHROCYTE LIPIDS

LIPID	mg/ml RBC	mg/g Hb	REFERENCE
Total lipid	5.10 ± 0.51	15.45 ± 1.54	6
Phospholipid	2.98 ± 0.2	9.03 ± 0.61	6
Plasmalogen	0.56	1.69	6
Total cholesterol (unesterified)	1.20 ± 0.08	3.63 ± 0.21	6,7
Fatty acids	2.00	6.06	6,8
Other	0.92 ± 0.18	2.78 ± 0.54	6
Fatty Acids as Percent of Total Fatty Acid			
Lauric (n-C_{12})		0.3	9
Myristic (n-C_{14})		0.8	9
Pentoenoic (n-C_{15})		0.3	9
Palmitoleic (16:1)		1.1	9
Palmitic (n-C_{16})		41.0	9
(C_{17}) branched		0.3	9
(n-C_{17})		0.3	9
Linoleic		15.3	9
Oleic		18.9	9
Oleic isomer		Trace	9
Stearic (n-C_{18})		7.9	9
Arachidonic (20:4)		7.9	9
C_{22} unsaturated (a)		2.5	9
C_{22} unsaturated (b)		2.0	9
Long-Chain Aldehydes as Percent of Total Aldehydes			
n-C_{14}		Trace	9
Branched C_{15}		0.8	9
n-C_{15}		0.6	9
Highly branched C_{16}		Trace	9
C_{16} monoene		0.4	9
n-C_{16}		24.2	9
Highly branched C_{17}		1.7	9
Branched C_{17}		7.5	9
n-C_{17}		1.3	9
C_{18} monoene		6.0	9
Isomeric C_{18} monoene		2.8	9
n-C_{18}		42.5	9
Unknown C_{19}		2.9	9
Unknown C_{20}		3.1	9
Unknown C_{21}		5.6	9
Fatty Acids as Percent of Total Neutral Lipids Fatty Acids			
n-C_{10}		0.0–0.6	10
n-C_{12}		1.1–2.2	10
n-C_{14}		5.9–17.3	10
16:1		3.2–6.0	10
n-C_{16}		15.2–22.6	10
18.2 and 3		11.4–21.1	10
18:1		28.8–29.1	10
n-C_{18}		5.7–10.7	10
Unsaturated C_{19}A		Trace	10
Arachidonic		7.4–8.3	10
Polyunsaturated C_{20}		Trace	10

NOTE: Some results are shown as mean±standard deviation.β.

TABLE 23-3   HUMAN ERYTHROCYTE PHOSPHOLIPIDS

LIPID	AMOUNT	REFERENCE
Total phospholipids	2.98 ± 0.20 mg/ml RBC	6
Cephalin	1.17 (0.38–1.91) mg/ml RBC	6
Ethanolamine phospho-glyceride	29% of total phospholipid	6
Mean plasmalogen content	67% of ethanolamine phospho-glyceride	6
Serine phosphoglyceride	10% of total phospholipid	6
Mean plasmalogen content	8% of serine phosphoglyceride	6
Lecithin	0.32 (0.03–0.95) mg/ml	11
Sphingomyelin	0.12–1.13 mg/ml	11
Lysolecithin	1.82% of total phospholipids	12

NOTE: Some results are shown as mean±standard deviation.

TABLE 23-4   FATTY ACID COMPOSITIONS OF ERYTHROCYTE PHOSPHOLIPIDS[6,7] (MOLE PERCENT)

SHORTHAND DESIGNATION*	MIXED PHOSPHOLIPIDS (METHANOL FRACTION)	ETHANOLAMINE	SERINE	CHOLINE
12:0	0.1	. . .	. . .	0.1
14:0	0.5	0.2	Trace	0.5
14:0	0.3	0.2	Trace	0.3
16:0	28.8	18.9	7.1	33.0
cis 16:1[9]	0.7	0.6	0.4	0.1
17:0	0.4	Trace	0.3	0.5
18:0	15.1	8.0	41.6	11.7
cis 18:1[9]	18.3	21.6	7.9	17.9
trans 18:1[9]	2.9	3.6	5.1	2.7
cis,cis 18:2[9,12]	10.6	7.0	2.8	18.2
cis,cis,cis 18:3[9,12,15]	. . .	Trace	. . .	. . .
19:0 iso or ante-iso	Trace	0.2	. . .	. . .
20:0	0.1	. . .	Trace	0.2
20:1[11]	0.2	0.3	Trace	0.2
20:2[8,11]	. . .	Trace	. . .	. . .
20:2[11,14]	0.1	0.1	. . .	0.2
20:3[5,8,11]	1.6	1.0	2.1	1.6
20:4[5,8,11,14]	10.8	21.9	19.7	5.0
20:5[5,8,11,14,17]	0.8	1.4	0.3	0.5
(22:unsat.?)	1.7	4.7	2.2	0.3
22:5	0.7	0.8	0.9	1.7
22:5	2.3	2.3	2.0	2.7
22:5[7,10,13,16,19]	1.0	. . .	. . .	1.0
22:6[4,7,10,13,16,19]	2.1	3.9	4.2	1.1
14:0	Trace	. . .	. . .	0.8
Branched 15:0	2.8	2.6	5.5	. . .
15:0 iso or ante-iso	0.1	0.4	. . .	. . .
15:0	0.2	0.3	. . .	. . .
Unknown	0.1	. . .	1.6	1.0
cis 16:1[9]	Trace	. . .	. . .	0.2
16:0	18.2	15.9	17.1	49.8
Branched 17:0 unsat.?	0.9	1.5	. . .	. . .
Branched 17:unsat.?	2.4	3.0	. . .	. . .
Branched 17:0	5.8	5.5	11.3	6.9
17:0 iso or ante-iso	1.1	0.8	0.7	2.9
cis,cis 18:2[9,12]	Trace	. . .	1.4	. . .
cis 18:1[9]	6.8	7.0	5.4	5.3
18:1 isomer	13.2	18.8	10.5	7.7
18:0	37.1	40.4	32.3	19.2
Unknown	1.3	2.1	. . .	. . .

TABLE 23-5   NUCLEOTIDES

COMPOUND	μmol/ml RBC	REFERENCE
Adenosine monophosphate	0.021 ± 0.003	13–19
Adenosine diphosphate	0.216 ± 0.036	13–18
Adenosine triphosphate	1.35 ± 0.035	15–17, 19–22
Cyclic adenosine monophosphate	0.015 ± .0024	23
Cyclic guanosine monophosphate	0.013 ± .0042	23
Guanosine diphosphate	0.018 ± 0.005	15
Guanosine triphosphate	0.052 ± 0.012	14,15
Inosine monophosphate	0.031 ± 0.005	15–19
Nicotinamide adenine dinucleotide		24,25
Reduced	0.0018 ± .001	24,25
Oxidized	0.049 ± .006	
Nicotinamide adenine dinucleotide phosphate		24,25
Reduced	0.032 ± .002	24,25
Oxidized	0.0014 ± .0011	
S-adenosylmethionine	0.005	26
Total nucleotide	1.534 ± 0.033	27
Uridine diphosphoglucose	0.031 ± 0.005	15,28
Uridine diphosphate N-acetyl glucosamine	0.018	28

NOTE: The results are given as mean±standard deviation.

TABLE 23-6   AMINO ACIDS AND OTHER NITROGEN-CONTAINING COMPOUNDS

Compound	μmol/ml RBC	Reference
Alanine	0.275 ± 0.060	29,30,31,32,33
α-Amino butyrate	0.016 ± 0.009	29,30,31
Arginine	0.040 ± 0.013	29,30,31,34,35
Asparagine	0.121 ± 0.041	29,30
Aspartate	0.306 ± 0.081*	29
Carnitine	0.23	36,37
Citrulline	0.036 ± 0.005*	29
Glutamate	0.265 ± 0.089	29,31,38
Glutamine	0.624 ± 0.136	29,31,39
Glycine	0.347 ± 0.070	29,30
Histidine	0.086 ± 0.013	29,31,35,40
Isoleucine	0.058 ± 0.013	29,30
Leucine	0.110 ± 0.009	29,30
Lysine	0.139 ± 0.032	29,31,35
Methionine	0.015 ± 0.006	29,31,35
Ornithine	0.120 ± 0.028	29,31
Phenylalanine	0.049 ± 0.006	29,30,31,35
Proline	0.137 ± 0.035	29,30,31
Serine	0.149 ± 0.032	29,30
Taurine	0.349 ± 0.057	29
Threonine	0.116 ± 0.022	29,30,31
Tyrosine	0.059 ± 0.009	29,30,31,35
Valine	0.171 ± 0.028	29,30,31,35
Creatine	0.33 ± 0.11	41
Creatinine	0.159	42
Cystine	0.016 ± 0.002	35
Ergothioneine	0.355 ± 0.112	31
Ethanolamine	0.007	31
Glutathione oxidized	0.0036 ± 0.0014	43
Glutathione reduced	2.234 ± 0.354	13
Tryptophan	0.024 ± 0.004	31,34,35,44
Uric acid	0.113	31,42
Urea	4.121 ± 0.420	31

*Measured in samples treated with sodium sulfite before analysis.
NOTE: The results are given as mean±standard deviation.

TABLE 23-7   HUMAN ERYTHROCYTE COENZYME AND VITAMINS

Compound	μmol/ml RBC	Reference
Ascorbic acid	0.0199 ± 0.0023	45,46,47
Choline (free)	Trace	48
Cocarboxylase	0.00021	49
Coenzyme A	0.0027	50
Nicotinic acid	0.105	51
Pantothenic acid	0.001 ± 0.00028	52
Pyridoxine (pyridoxal, pyridoxamine)	$1\% - 10^{-5}$	53
Riboflavin	0.00059 ± 0.00021	54
Flavin adenine dinucleotide	0.000398 ± 0.000042	55
Thiamine	0.00027	56

NOTE: The results are given as mean±standard deviation.

TABLE 23-8   HUMAN ERYTHROCYTE CARBOHYDRATES, ORGANIC ACIDS, AND METABOLITES

Compound	μmol/ml RBC	Reference
Deoxyribonucleic acid	Trace	57
Dihydroxyacetone phosphate	0.0094 ± 0.0028	13
2,3-Diphosphoglycerate	4.171 ± 0.636	13,17,21,22
Fructose 6-P	0.0093 ± 0.002	13,16,21,58
Fructose 3-P	0.013 ± .001	59,60
Fructose 2,6-bisphosphate	48 ± 13*	61
Fructose 1,6-diphosphate	0.0019 ± 0.0006	13,16,17,21,58
Glucuronic acid	Trace	62
Glucose	In equilibrium with plasma	63,64
Glucose 6-P	0.0278 ± 0.0075	13,16,21,58
Glucose 1,6-diphosphate	0.18–0.30	16,65
Glyceraldehyde 3-P	Not detectable	13
Lactic acid	0.932 ± 0.211	3,13,66
Mannose 1,6-diphosphate	0.150	65
Octulose 1,8-diphosphate	Trace	67
Pyruvate	0.0533 ± 0.0215	13
3-Phosphoglycerate	0.0449 ± 0.0051	13,21
2-Phosphoglycerate	0.0073 ± 0.0025	13,21
Phosphoenol pyruvate	0.0122 ± 0.0022	13
Ribonucleic acid	1.355 mg	68
Ribose 1,5-diphosphate	<0.02	69,70
Ribulose 5-P	Trace	71
Sedoheptulose 7-P	Trace	71
Sedoheptulose diphosphate	Trace	72
Sialic acid	0.825 ± 0.028	69
Sorbitol	31.1 ± 5.3	60,73

*Values given in pmol.
NOTE: The results are given as mean±standard deviation.

TABLE 23-9   HUMAN ERYTHROCYTE ELECTROLYTES

Electrolyte	μmol/ml RBC	Reference
Aluminum	0.0026	74
Bromide	0.1225	75,76
Calcium	0.0089 ± 0.0030	76,77,78
Chloride	78	76,79
Chromium	0.0004	80
Cobalt	0.0002	76,81
Copper	0.018	80,82,83
Fluoride	0.0131	84
Iodine, protein-bound	0.0013	85
Lead	0.0082	74,86,83,76
Magnesium	3.06	80,87,88,89
Manganese	0.0034	74,90
Nickel	0.0009	80
Phosphorus (acid soluble):		
Total P	13.2	91
Inorganic P	0.466	91
Lipid P	3.840	92
Unidentified P	0.955	91
Potassium	102.4 ± 3.9	93,94,95,87,96,97
Rubidium	0.054	76
Silicon	Trace	47
Silver	Trace	74
Sodium	6.2 ± 0.8	93,94,95
Sulfur	0.0044	98
Tin	0.0022	74
Zinc	0.153	80,99,100

NOTE: The results are given as mean.

REFERENCES

1. Nichols G, Nichols N: Electrolyte equilibria in erythrocytes during diabetic acidosis. *J Clin Invest* 32:113, 1953.
2. Ponder E: *Hemolysis and Related Phenomena.* Grune & Stratton, New York, 1948.
3. Behrendt H: *Chemistry of Erythrocytes.* Charles C Thomas, Springfield, IL, 1957.
4. Guidotti G: The protein of human erythrocyte membranes. I. Preparation, solubilization and partial characterization. *J Biol Chem* 243:1985, 1968.
5. Silverman L, Glick D: Measurement of protein concentration by quantitative electron microscopy. *J Cell Biol* 40:773, 1969.
6. Farquhar JW: Human erythrocyte phosphoglycerides. I. Quantification of plasmalogens, fatty acids and fatty aldehydes. *Biochim Biophys Acta* 60:80, 1962.
7. Myher JJ, Kuksis A, Pind S: Molecular species of glycerophospholipids and sphingomyelins of human erythrocytes: improved method of analysis. *Lipids* 24:396, 1989.
8. Doris AB, Wahle K, MacDonald A, et al: Red cell membrane fatty acids, cytosolic phospholipase-A2 and schizophrenia. *Schizophr Res* 31:185, 1998.
9. Kates M, Allison AC, James AT: Phosphatides of human blood cells and their role in spherocytosis. *Biochim Biophys Acta* 48:571, 1961.
10. James AT, Lovelock JE, Webb JPW: The lipids of whole blood. I. Lipid biosynthesis in human blood in vitro. *Biochem J* 73:106, 1959.
11. Kirk E: The concentration of lecithin, cephalin, ether-insoluble phosphatide, and cerebrosides in plasma and red blood cells of normal adults. *J Biol Chem* 123:637, 1938.
12. Phillips GB, Roome NS: Quantitative chromatographic analysis of the phospholipids of abnormal human red blood cells. *Proc Soc Exp Biol Med* 109:360, 1962.
13. Beutler E: *Red Cell Metabolism,* 3d ed. Grune & Stratton, New York, 1984.
14. Bishop C, Rankine DM, Talbott JH: The nucleotides in normal human blood. *J Biol Chem* 234:1233, 1959.
15. Mandel P, Chambon P, Karon H, et al: Nucleotides libres des globules rouges et des reticulocytes. *Folia Haematol (Leipz)* 78:525, 1961–1962.
16. Bartlett GR: Human red cell glycolytic intermediates. *J Biol Chem* 234:449, 1959.
17. Gerlach E, Fleckenstein A, Gross E: Der Intermediäre Phosphat-Stoffwechsel des Menschen-Erythrocyten. *Pfluegers Arch* 266:528, 1958.
18. Löhr GW, Waller HD: The biochemistry of erythrocyte aging. *Folia Haematol (Leipz)* 78:384, 1961.
19. Yoshikawa H, Nakao M, Miyamoto K, Tachibana M: Phosphorus metabolism in human erythrocyte. II. Separation of acid-soluble phosphorus compounds incorporating p32 by column chromatography with ion exchange resin. *J Biochem* 47:635, 1960.
20. Beutler E, Mathai CK: A comparison of normal red cell ATP levels as measured by the firefly system and the hexokinase system. *Blood* 30:311, 1967.
21. Minakami S, Suzuki C, Saito T, Yoshikawa H: Studies on erythrocyte glycolysis. I. Determination of the glycolytic intermediates in human erythrocytes. *J Biochem* 58:543, 1965.
22. Ramos JLA, Nonoyama K, Quintal VS, Barretto OCDO: Red cell enzymes and intermediates in AGA term newborns, AGA preterm newborns and SGA term newborns. *Acta Paediatr Scand* 79:32, 1990.
23. Patterson WD, Hardman JG, Sutherland EW: A comparison of cyclic nucleotide levels in plasma and cells of rat and human blood. *Endocrinology* 95:325, 1974.
24. Canepa L, Ferraris AM, Miglino M, Gaetani GF: Bound and unbound pyridine dinucleotides in normal and glucose-6-phosphate dehydrogenase—deficient erythrocytes. *Biochim Biophys Acta* 1074:101, 1991.
25. Micheli V, Simmonds HA, Bari M, Pompucci G: HPLC determination of oxidized and reduced pyridine coenzymes in human erythrocytes. *Clin Chim Acta* 220:1, 1993.
26. Lagendijk J, Ubbink JB, Vermaak WJH: Quantification of erythrocyte S-adenosyl-l-methionine levels and its application in enzyme studies. *J Chromatogr Biomed Appl* 576:95, 1992.
27. Overgard-Hansen K, Jorgensen S: Determination and concentration of adenine nucleotides in human blood. *Scand J Clin Lab Invest* 12:10, 1960.
28. Mills GC: Uridine diphosphate glucose and uridine diphosphate *N*-acetylglucosamine in erythrocytes. *Texas Rep Biol Med* 18:446, 1960.
29. Hagenfeldt L, Arvidsson A: The distribution of amino acids between plasma and erythrocytes. *Clin Chim Acta* 100:133, 1980.
30. Leighton WP, Rosenblatt S, Chanley JD: Determination of erythrocyte amino acids by gas chromatography. *J Chromatog* 164:427, 1979.
31. McMenamy RH, Lund CC, Neville GJ, Wallach DFH: Studies of unbound amino acid distributions in plasma, erythrocytes, leukocytes and urine of normal human subjects. *J Clin Invest* 39:1675, 1960.
32. Gutman GE, Alexander B: Studies of amino acid metabolism blood glycine and alanine and their relationship to the total amino acids in normal subjects. *J Biol Chem* 168:527, 1947.
33. Wiss O, Kruger R: Der Einfluss Enteral und Parenteral Verabreichter Glucose auf den Alaningehalt des Blutes. *Helv Chim Acta* 31:1774, 1948.
34. Hier SW, Bergeim O: The microbiological determination of certain free amino acids in human and dog plasma. *J Biol Chem* 163:129, 1946.
35. Johnson CA, Bergeim O: The distribution of free amino acids between erythrocytes and plasma in man. *J Biol Chem* 188:833, 1951.
36a. Borum PR, York CM, Bennett SG: Carnitine concentration of red blood cells. *Am J Clin Nutr* 41:653, 1985.
37. Reichmann HV, Lindeneiner N: Carnitine analysis in normal human red blood cells, plasma, and muscle tissue. *Eur Neurol* 34:40, 1994
38. Divino Filho JC, Hazel SJ, Furst P, Bergstrom J, Hall K: Glutamate concentration in plasma, erythrocyte and muscle in relation to plasma levels of insulin-like growth factor (IGF)-I, IGF binding protein-1 and insulin in patients on haemodialysis. *J Endocrinol* 156:519, 1998.
39. Iyer GYN: Distribution of glutamine, glutamic acid, and aspartic acid between erythrocytes and plasma. *Ind J Med Res* 44:201, 1956.
40. Von Euler H, Heller L: Free histidine in the blood serum of normal and Jensen sarcoma-bearing rats. *Arkiv Mineral Geol* 24A:23, 1947.
41. Griffiths WJ, Fitzpatrick M: The effect of age on the creatine in red cells. *Br J Haematol* 13:175, 1967.
42. Jellinek EM, Looney JM: Statistics of some biochemical variables on healthy men in the age range of twenty to forty-five years. *J Biol Chem* 128:621, 1939.
43. Srivastava SK, Beutler E: Oxidized glutathione levels in erythrocytes of glucose-6-phosphate-dehydrogenase--deficient subjects. *Lancet* 2:23, 1968.
44. Steele BF, Reynolds MS, Baumann CA: Amino acids in the blood and urine of human subjects ingesting different amounts of the same proteins. *J Nutr* 40:145, 1950.
45. Barkhan P, Howard AN: Distribution of ascorbic acid in normal and leukaemic human blood. *Biochem J* 70:163, 1958.
46. Butler AM, Cushman M: Distribution of ascorbic acid in the blood and its nutritional significance. *J Clin Invest* 19:459, 1940.
47. Sargent F: A study of the normal distribution of ascorbic acid between the red cells and plasma of human blood. *J Biol Chem* 171:471, 1947.
48. Luecke R, Pearson PB: The microbiological determination of free choline in plasma and urine. *J Biol Chem* 153:259, 1944.
49. Beerstecher E, Spangler S: In *Blood and Other Body Fluids,* edited by DS Dittmer, p 108. *Fed Am Soc Exp Biol,* Washington, DC, 1961.
50. Kaplan NO, Lipmann F: The assay of distribution of coenzyme A. *J Biol Chem* 174:37, 1948.
51. Klein JR, Perlzweig WA, Handler P: Determination of nicotinic acid in blood cells and plasma. *J Biol Chem* 145:27, 1942.
52. Pearson PB: The pantothenic acid content of the blood of mammalia. *J Biol Chem* 140:423, 1941.
53. Marsch ME, Greenberg LD, Rinehart JF: The relationship between pyridoxine ingestion and transaminase activity. *J Nutr* 56:115, 1955.
54. Burch HB, Bessey OA, Lowry OH: Fluorometric measurements of riboflavin and its natural derivatives in small quantities of blood serum and cells. *J Biol Chem* 175:457, 1948.
55. Beutler E: Glutathione reductase: stimulation in normal subjects by riboflavin supplementation. *Science* 165:613, 1969.
56. Burch HB, Bessey OA, Love RH, Lowry OH: The determination of thiamine and thiamine phosphates in small quantities of blood and blood cells. *J Biol Chem* 198:477, 1952.
57. Metais P, Mandel P: Teneur en acide desoxypentosenucleique des leucocytes chez l'homme normal et a l'etat pathologique. *CR Soc Biol (Paris)* 144:277, 1950.
58. Lionetti FJ, McLellan WL, Fortier NL, Foster JM: Phosphate esters produced from inosine in human erythrocyte ghosts. *Arch Biochem* 94:7, 1961.
59. Petersen A, Szwergold BS, Kappler F, et al: Identification of sorbitol

3-phosphate and fructose 3-phosphate in normal and diabetic human erythrocytes. *J Biol Chem* 265:17424, 1990.

60. Kawaguchi M, Fujii T, Kamiya Y, et al: Effects of fructose ingestion on sorbitol and fructose 3-phosphate contents of erythrocytes from healthy men. *Acta Diabetologica* 33:100, 1996.

61. Colomer D, Pujades A, Carballo E, Vives Corrons JL: Erythrocyte fructose 2,6-bisphosphate content in congenital hemolytic anemias. *Hemoglobin* 15:517, 1991.

62. Deichmann WB, Dierker M: The spectrophotometric estimation of hexuronates (expressed as glucuronic acid) in plasma or serum. *J Biol Chem* 163:753, 1946.

63. Jung CY: Carrier-mediated glucose transport across human red cell membranes, in *The Red Blood Cell*, edited by DM Surgenor, 2nd ed, pp 705–751. Academic, New York, 1975.

64. Lacko L, Wittke B, Geck P: The temperature dependence of the exchange transport of glucose in human erythrocytes. *J Cell Physiol* 82:213, 1973.

65. Bartlett GR: Glucose and mannose diphosphates in the red blood cell. *Biochim Biophys Acta* 156:231, 1968.

66. Johnson RE, Edward HT, Dill DB, Wilson JW: Blood as a physicochemical system. XIII. The distribution of lactate. *J Biol Chem* 157:461, 1945.

67. Bartlett GR, Bucolo G: Octulose phosphates from the human red blood cell. *Biochem Biophys Res Commun* 3:474, 1960.

68. Mandel P, Métais P: Les acides nucléiques du plasma sanguin chez l'homme. *CR Soc Biol* 142:241, 1948.

69. Aminoff D, Anderson J, Dabich L, Gathmann WD: Sialic acid content of erythrocytes in normal individuals and patients with certain hematologic disorders. *Am J Hematol* 9:381, 1980.

70. Vanderheiden BS: Ribosediphosphate in the human erythrocyte. *Biochem Biophys Res Commun* 6:117, 1961.

71. Bruns FH, Noltmann E, Vahlhaus E: Über den Stoffwechsel von Ribose-5-phosphat in Hämolysaten I. Aktivitätsmessung und Eigenschaften der Phosphoribose-isomerase. II. Der Pentose-phosphat-Cyclus in roten Blutzellen. *Biochem Z* 330:483, 1958.

72. Bucolo G, Bartlett GR: Sedoheptulose diphosphate formation by the human red blood cell. *Biochem Biophys Res Commun* 3:620, 1960.

73. Inoue S, Lin SL, Chang T, et al: Identification of free deaminated sialic acid (2-keto-3-deoxy-D-glycero-D-galacto-nononic acid) in human red blood cells and its elevated expression in fetal cord red blood cells and ovarian cancer cells. *J Biol Chem* 273:27199, 1998.

74. Kehoe RA, Cholak J, Story RV: A spectrochemical study of the normal ranges of concentration of certain trace metals in biological materials. *J Nutr* 19:579, 1940.

75. Hunter G: Micro-determination of bromide in body fluids. *Biochem J* 60:261, 1955.

76. Ojo JO, Oluwole AF, Durosinmi MA, Ogunsola OJ, Akanle OA, Spyrou NM: Baseline levels of elemental concentrations in whole blood, plasma, and erythrocytes of Nigerian subjects. *Biol Trace Elem Res* 43–45: 461–470, 1994.

77. Bernard JF, Bournier O, Boivin P: Human erythrocyte calcium concentration in hemolytic anemia. *Biomedicine* 23:431, 1975.

78. Shoji S, Komiyama A, Nakamura M, Nomoto S: Calcium content of healthy human erythrocytes. *Clin Chem* 35:1264, 1989.

79. Bernstein RE: Potassium and sodium balance in mammalian red cells. *Science* 120:459, 1954.

80. Herring WB, Leavell BS, Paixao LM, Yoe JH: Trace metals in human plasma and red blood cells: a study of magnesium, chromium, nickel, copper and zinc. I. Observations of normal subjects. *Am J Clin Nutr* 8:846, 1960.

81. Heyrovsky A: The biochemistry of cobalt. III. Amounts of cobalt in plasma, erythrocytes, urine, and feces of normal subjects. *Cas Lek Cesk* 91:680, 1952.

82. Lahey ME, Gubler CJ, Cartwright GE, Wintrobe MM: Studies on copper metabolism. VI. Blood copper in normal human subjects. *J Clin Invest* 32:322, 1953.

83. Mahalingam TR, Vijayalakshmi S, Prabhu RK, et al: Studies on some trace and minor elements in blood—a survey of the Kalpakkam (India) population. 2. Reference values for plasma and red cells, and correlation with coronary risk index. *Biol Trace Elem Res* 57:207, 1997.

84. Largent EJ, Cholak J: In *Blood and Other Body Fluids*, edited by DS Dittmer. *Fed Am Soc Exp Biol*, Washington DC, 1961.

85. McClendon JF, Foster WC: Protein-bound iodine in erythrocytes and plasma and elsewhere. *Am J Med Sci* 207:549, 1944.

86. Jensovsky L, Roth Z: Der normale Bleigehalt im menschlichen Blute. *Naturwissenschaften* 48:382, 1961.

87. McCance RA, Widdowson EM: The effect of development, anaemia, and undernutrition on the composition of the erythrocytes. *Clin Sci* 15:409, 1956.

88. Huijgen HJ, Sanders R, van Olden RW, Klous MG, Gaffar FR, Sanders GT: Intracellular and extracellular blood magnesium fractions in hemodialysis patients; is the ionized fraction a measure of magnesium excess? *Clin Chem* 44:639, 1998.

89. Martin BJ, Lyon TD, Fell GS, McKay P: Erythrocyte magnesium in elderly patients: not a reliable guide to magnesium status. *J Trace Elem Med Biol* 11:44, 1997.

90. Miller DO, Yoe JH: Spectrophotometric determination of manganese in human plasma and red cells with benzohydroxamic acid. *Anal Chim Acta* 26:224, 1962.

91. Bartlett GR, Savage E, Hughes L, Marlow AA: Carbohydrate intermediates and related cofactors in the human erythrocyte. *J Appl Physiol* 6:51, 1953--1954.

92. Ferranti F, Giannetti O: The microdetermination of phosphorus (inorganic, acid-soluble, lipoid and total) in the blood and excretions. *Diagn Tec Lab Napoli Riv Mens* 4:664, 1933.

93. Overman RR, Davis AK: The application of flame photometry to sodium and potassium determinations in biological fluids. *J Biol Chem* 168:641, 1947.

94. Fortes Mayer KD, Starkey BJ: Simpler flame photometric determination of erythrocyte sodium and potassium: the reference range for apparently healthy adults. *Clin Chem* 23(2):275, 1977.

95. Bernard JF, Bournier O, Renoux M, et al: Unclassified haemolytic anaemia with splenomegaly and erythrocyte cation abnormalities: a disease of the spleen? *Scand J Haematol* 12:231, 1976.

96. Hald PM: Notes on the determination and distribution of sodium and potassium in cells and serum of normal human blood. *J Biol Chem* 163:429, 1946.

97. Streef GM: Sodium and calcium content of erythrocytes. *J Biol Chem* 129:661, 1939.

98. Reed L, Denis W: On the distribution of the non-protein sulfur of the blood between serum and corpuscles. *J Biol Chem* 73:623, 1927.

99. Vallee BL, Gibson JG: The zinc content of normal human whole blood, plasma, leucocytes, and erythrocytes. *J Biol Chem* 176:445, 1948.

100. Zak B, Nalbandian RM, Williams LA, Cohen J: Determination of human erythrocyte zinc: hemoglobin ratios. *Clin Chim Acta* 7:634, 1962.

101. Friedeman H, Rapoport SM: Enzymes of the red cell: a critical catalogue, in *Cellular and Molecular Biology of Erythrocytes*, edited by H Yoshikawa, SM Rapoport, p 181. University Park Press, Baltimore, 1974.

102. Pennell RB: Comparison of normal human red cells, in *The Red Blood Cell*, edited by DM Surgenor, p 98. Academic, New York, 1974.

IRON METABOLISM

VIRGIL F. FAIRBANKS
ERNEST BEUTLER

Iron is a component of all living organisms. It plays an important role, particularly in electron transfer reactions. Much of the iron in the human body is in circulating red cells, which contain 1 mg of iron per 1 ml of packed cells. Iron is stored in the form of ferritin or hemosiderin. Smaller amounts of iron are present in myoglobin and in many enzymes. Because little iron is lost from the body, the iron content of the body is regulated by modulating iron absorption. Separate pathways exist for the absorption of heme and inorganic iron. The precise mechanism by which iron passes across the intestinal mucosa into the plasma has not yet been elucidated. The process appears to involve a ferrireductase, a divalent iron transporter DMT1, hephaestin, an integrin, and very likely the HFE protein. Iron absorption is increased in the presence of iron deficiency, and it decreases when there is iron overload. Once it enters the plasma, iron in the ferric form is bound by transferrin, which transports the metal into cells after being bound by the transferrin receptor. The transferrin receptor is internalized together with bound transferrin and iron, and the iron is released inside the cell into an acidified vacuole. The transferrin receptor then moves back to the cell surface.

Many of the proteins involved in iron transport are regulated by the amount of available iron through iron responsive elements (IREs), which exist as stem loop structures in RNA. IREs can serve to regulate either translation of mRNA or stability of mRNA. This regulation is achieved by IRPs (iron regulatory proteins). The major IRP is cytoplasmic aconitase, which binds to the IRE when it is not complexed with iron and does not bind when iron is present.

Iron is a key element in the metabolism of all living organisms. In plants, ferredoxins are essential for an early step of photosynthesis. DNA synthesis requires the enzyme ribonucleotide reductase to convert ribonucleotides to deoxyribonucleotides. Neither bacteria nor nucleated cells proliferate when the supply of iron is insufficient. Iron is a part of heme, which is the active site of electron transport in cytochromes and cytochrome oxygenase, essential coenzymes in the Krebs cycle. Heme is also the site of O_2 uptake by myoglobin and hemoglobin, providing the means of O_2 transport to tissues. In the root nodules of legumes hemoglobin catalyzes the fixation of atmo-

spheric N_2 by symbiotic bacteria. This is an important natural means of fertilization of soil and for synthesis of plant proteins. Heme is also the active site of peroxidases that protect cells from oxidative injury by reducing peroxides to water.

Many iron proteins are structurally related. Iron-sulfur proteins have an Fe-S cluster at the active sites. These include ferredoxins in plants, ribonucleotide reductase, aconitase, and succinic dehydrogenase. Heme proteins include hemoglobin, myoglobin, the cytochromes, cytochrome oxidase, homogentisic oxidase, peroxidases, and catalase. Iron flavoproteins include cytochrome c reductase, NADH dehydrogenase, acyl coenzyme A dehydrogenase, and xanthine oxidase. A heterogeneous group of proteins contain iron in a variety of molecular configurations.[1]

Aconitase catalyzes a critical, early step in the Krebs cycle, the interconversion of citric, isocitric, and cis-aconitic acids (Fig. 24-1). When iron is abundant within the cytosol, the cubane (cubelike) structure of the aconitase molecule contains a 4Fe-4S cluster (Fig. 24-2, left). In this form, it is an active enzyme. When iron is scarce, the cluster opens as 3Fe-4S.[2-4] Then it is not an enzyme but the iron regulatory protein IRP-1 (Fig. 24-2, right) that interacts with iron-responsive elements (discussed later) to increase the synthesis of proteins that determine the cellular uptake of iron. Nearly half the enzymes and cofactors of the Krebs tricarboxylic acid cycle either contain iron or require its presence.

IRON COMPARTMENTS IN MAN

Several iron compartments are shown in Table 24-1 and are discussed below.

HEMOGLOBIN

Approximately 2 g of body iron of men and 1.5 g in women is in hemoglobin, which is 0.34 percent iron by weight. One mL of packed erythrocytes contains approximately 1 mg of iron.

STORAGE COMPARTMENT

Iron is stored either as ferritin or as hemosiderin. The former is water-soluble; the latter is water-insoluble. Ferritin is composed of a core ferrihydrite crystal $(Fe_2O_3 \cdot 9 H_2O)_x$ within an apoferritin shell.[5]

Apoferritin is composed of 24 similar or identical subunits arranged as 12 dimers forming a dodecahedron that approximates a hollow sphere (Fig. 24-3a and b). The apoferritin monomers are of H (heavy) or L (light) type. L monomers have 15 hydrophilic residues that may bind iron, thereby promoting its retention and serving as sites for ferrihydrite crystal growth. H monomers have fewer hydrophilic residues but contribute an iron-binding histidyl to the intermonomeric pore (where iron atoms enter or exit). H monomers have ferroxidase activity, thereby enabling apoferritin to take up or release iron quite rapidly (Fig. 24-4).[6-9] Apoferritin that is rich in H monomers takes up iron more readily but retains it less avidly than does ferritin composed predominantly of L monomers.[5,10] Much of the storage iron in liver and spleen is in ferritin containing mostly L monomers.

Apoferritin synthesis is regulated in accordance with iron sufficiency or lack, as described below in the section entitled "The Intracellular Regulation of Iron Metabolism."

Ferritin occurs in virtually all cells of the body and also in tissue fluids. In blood plasma ferritin is present in minute concentration. It is largely composed of H monomers. The plasma (serum) ferritin concentration usually correlates with total-body iron stores, which makes this measurement important in the diagnosis of disorders of iron metabolism (see Chaps. 38 and 42).

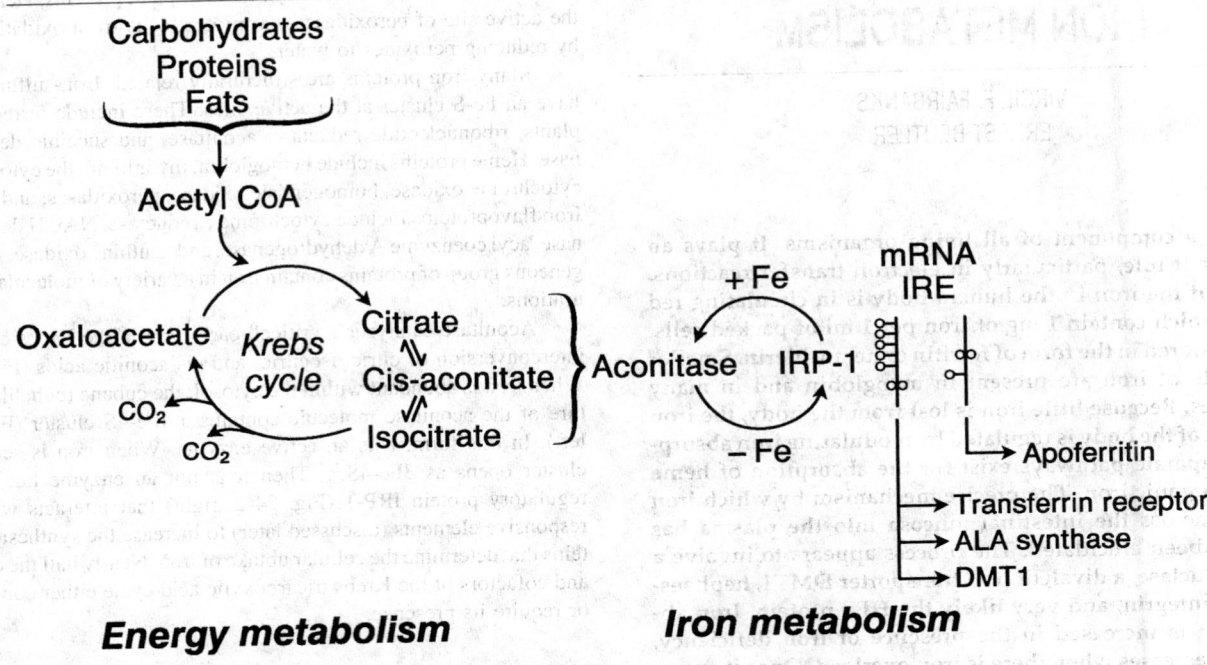

Energy metabolism   **Iron metabolism**

FIGURE 24-1   The interrelationship of iron metabolism and energy metabolism. Aconitase is critical to the regulation of both. Mitochondrial aconitase is a critical enzyme in the Krebs cycle (*left*). On the *right*, iron metabolism is regulated at the mRNA/ribosomal level by cytoplasmic aconitase, that, when iron-depleted becomes IRP-1.

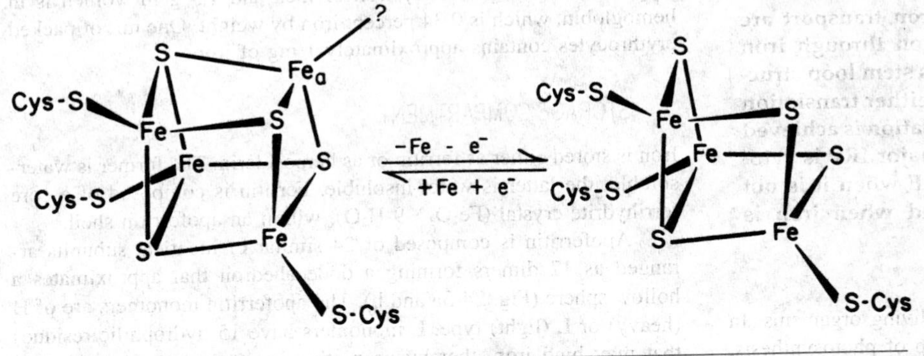

FIGURE 24-2   The iron-sulfur cluster of aconitase. *Left*: The active enzyme, with its Fe-S cluster in the cubane (cubelike) structure, catalyzes the interconversion of citric, cis-aconitic, and iso-citric acids in the Krebs cycle. *Right*: When iron is insufficient in the cytosol, the Fe-S cluster opens; it then becomes the iron regulatory protein. (*From Beinert H. and Kennedy MC,*[4] with permission of the Federation of American Societies for Experimental Biology, FASEB).

TABLE 24-1   IRON COMPARTMENTS IN NORMAL MAN*

COMPARTMENT	IRON CONTENT, MG	TOTAL BODY IRON, %
Hemoglobin iron	2000	67
Storage iron (ferritin, hemosiderin)	1000	27
Myoglobin iron	130	3.5
Labile pool	80	2.2
Other tissue iron	8	0.2
Transport iron	3	0.08

*These values represent estimates for an "average" person, that is, 70 kg, 177 cm (70 in) in height. They are derived from data in several sources.

Hemosiderin occurs predominantly in macrophages of the monocyte-macrophage system (marrow, liver, and spleen). It can be seen microscopically in unstained tissue sections or marrow films as clumps or granules of golden refractile pigment. Hemosiderin contains approximately 25 to 30 percent iron by weight. Under pathologic conditions, it may accumulate in large quantities in almost every tissue of the body. Hemosiderin consists of aggregates of ferrihydrite core crystals,[11–13] largely devoid of apoferritin.

The size of the storage compartment is quite variable. Normally in adult men it amounts to 800 to 1000 mg; in adult women it is a few hundred milligrams. Depletion of the storage iron occurs when iron loss exceeds iron absorption. The mobilization of storage iron involves the reduction of Fe^{+++} to Fe^{++}, its release from the core crystal and its diffusion out of the apoferritin shell. As it passes from cytosol to plasma, it must be reoxidized, either by hephaestin in the cell membrane or by ceruloplasmin in plasma, before it binds to transferrin.

MYOGLOBIN

Myoglobin is structurally similar to hemoglobin, but it is monomeric: Each myoglobin molecule consists of a heme group nearly surrounded by loops of a long polypeptide chain containing approximately 150 amino acid residues. Myoglobin is present in small amounts in all skeletal and cardiac muscle cells, in which it may serve as an oxygen reservoir to protect against cellular injury during periods of oxygen deprivation.

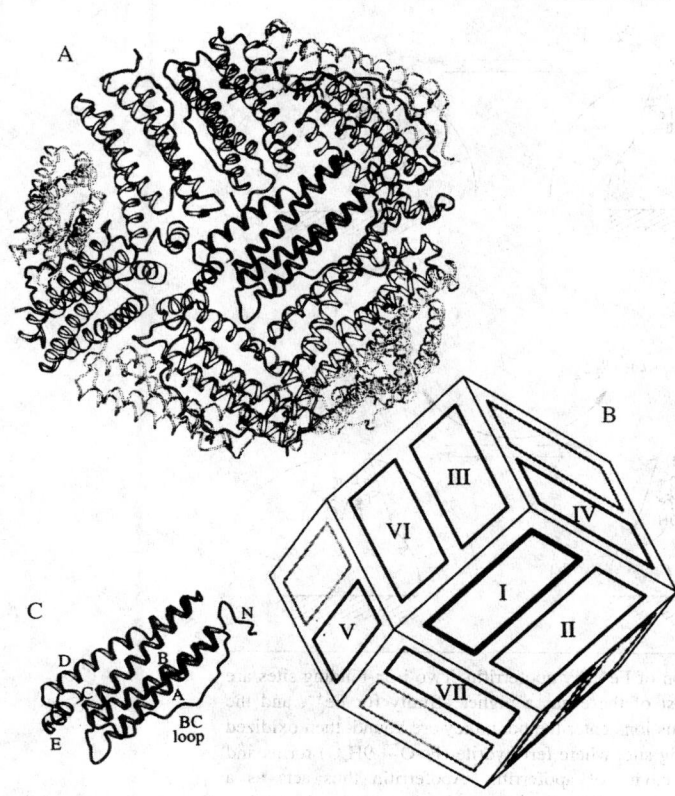

FIGURE 24-3 The quaternary structure of apoferritin. Twenty-four subunits or apoferritin monomers are joined in 12 pairs, to form a dodecahedron, or 12-sided structure, that approximates a hollow sphere. As shown in *c, lower left,* each monomer consists of 4 long helices (A–D) nearly parallel to each other, and a short E helix. In *upper left (a),* the apoferritin shell is composed of 24 monomers shown in helical configurations. In *lower right (b)* is a scheme for the pairing of monomers to form a dodecahedron. *(From Hempstead et al,*[5] *by permission of Journal of Molecular Biology).*

LABILE IRON POOL

The labile iron pool was postulated from studies of the rate of clearance of injected ^{59}Fe from plasma.[14,15] Iron leaves the plasma and enters the interstitial and intracellular fluid compartments for a brief time before it is incorporated into heme or storage compounds. Some of the iron reenters plasma, causing a biphasic curve of ^{59}Fe clearance 1 to 2 days after injection. The change in slope defines the size of the labile pool, normally 80 to 90 mg of iron.

TISSUE IRON COMPARTMENT

Tissue iron normally amounts to 6 to 8 mg. This comprises cytochromes and iron-containing enzymes. Although a small compartment, it is an extremely vital one that is sensitive to iron deficiency.[16–21]

TRANSPORT COMPARTMENT

From the standpoint of its total iron content, normally about 3 mg, the transport compartment of plasma is the smallest but the most active of the iron compartments: Its iron normally turns over at least 10 times each day. This is a common pathway for interchange of iron between compartments (Fig. 24-4).

Transferrins and lactoferrins comprise a group of glycoproteins that transport iron in plasma and in milk, respectively. They are single polypeptide chains with an M_r of approximately 80 kDA. Each molecule has two binding sites for Fe^{+++} and bicarbonate. Each is bilobed, and within each lobe the iron-binding site is in a cleft between two domains that are designated *N* and *C* (for *aminoterminal* and *carboxy-terminal*). Thus, each complete transferrin or lactoferrin molecule has two N domains and two C domains. Within each lobe, Fe^{+++} is bound to both the N and C domains, which fold over and enclose the Fe^{+++}.[22,23]

Normally, approximately one-third of the transferrin iron-binding sites are occupied by iron. About 200 mg (2.5 μmol) of transferrin, carrying about 100 μg (1.8 μmol) of iron per deciliter is normally present in human plasma.

Apotransferrin (transferrin devoid of iron) is synthesized by hepatocytes and by cells of the monocyte-macrophage system.[24,25] At least 19 genetically determined molecular variants of transferrin have been described[26,27] in humans. Their iron-binding and kinetic properties seem to be identical.

DIETARY IRON

The iron content of the diet is variable. An average American male ingests 10 to 20 mg of iron daily.[28,29] Table 24-2 shows daily requirements that are age- and sex-specific. The amount of iron absorbed by a normal adult male need only balance the small amount that is excreted, mostly in the stool, approximately 1 mg per day. A higher iron requirement exists during growth periods or when there is blood loss. In women, iron absorbed must be sufficient to replace that lost through menstruation or diverted to the fetus during pregnancy

The iron gained by food during cooking or other food processing is in the form of simple inorganic salts or iron-amino acid complexes. Heme, as from hemoglobin and myoglobin, normally comprises about one-third of dietary iron.

IRON ABSORPTION

Iron is absorbed at the brush border of epithelial cells of the intestinal villi, particularly in the duodenum and upper jejunum. It is absorbed in the form of heme, or as ferric or ferrous ions (Fig. 24-5). In humans little of the heme absorbed by mucosal cells passes directly into plasma.[30,31] In microsomes, *heme oxygenase* converts heme to biliverdin, CO, and Fe^{+++}.[32,33]

Gastric juice stabilizes dietary ferric iron, preventing its precipitation as insoluble ferric hydroxide.[34,35] This may be due in part to chelation of Fe^{+++} by small molecules in the gastric juice, such as amino acids and keto sugars.[36,37] At pH less than 3, Fe^{+++} is stable and binds loosely to mucin.[38] Within the brush border of the epithelial cell, a transmembrane ferric reductase converts Fe^{+++} to Fe^{++}.[39]

It is still uncertain how iron passes from the luminal to the abluminal (basal and lateral portions of the cell) membrane. This

TABLE 24-2 MINIMAL DAILY IRON REQUIREMENTS

	Amounts That Must Be Absorbed Daily for Hemoglobin Synthesis, mg	Minimal Amount That Should Be Ingested Daily, mg
Infants	1	10
Children	0.5	5
Young nonpregnant women	2	20
Pregnant women	3	30
Men and postmenopausal women	1	10

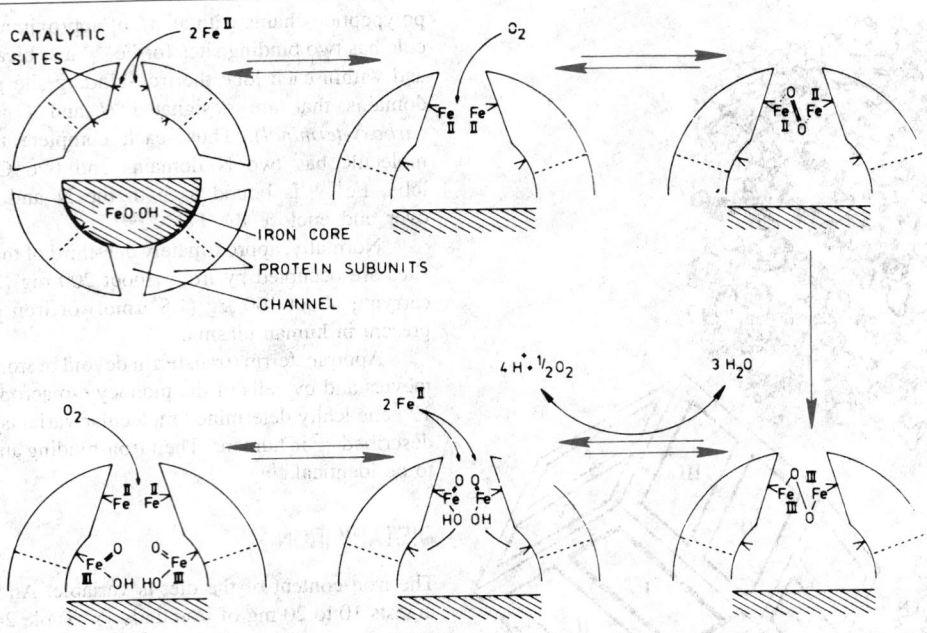

FIGURE 24-4   A scheme for the uptake and oxidation of Fe^{++} by apoferritin. Two iron-binding sites are hypothesized within each pore channel. The outermost of these has a higher affinity for Fe^{++}, and the innermost has a higher affinity for Fe^{+++}. As two ferrous ions enter the pore, they are bound, then oxidized to Fe^{+++}. The iron is then displaced to the inner binding site, where ferrihydrite ($Fe_2O_3 \cdot 9H_2O$) forms and is added to the ferrihydrite crystal in the central cavity of apoferritin. Apoferritin thus acts as a ferroxidase in the oxidation of Fe^{++} to Fe^{+++}. (*Crichton and Roman,*[8] *by permission of the* Journal of Molecular Catalysis.)

process may require a β_3-integrin, mobilferrin (calreticulin or calnexin), a flavomonooxygenase,[40] the divalent metal transporter DMT1 (also called *Nramp2* or *DCT-1* for divalent cation transporter 1), and hephaestin.

Hephaestin is a transmembrane protein of the basal membrane that is essential for the release of iron to plasma. It is structurally homologous to ceruloplasmin.[41] Both are ferroxidases. Ceruloplasmin serves as a scavenger of Fe^{++} in plasma, converting it to Fe^{+++}, which may then be taken up by monoferric transferrin. In the absence of plasma ceruloplasmin, ferrous iron atoms readily enter cells and are deposited in tissues throughout the body, with serious consequences (see aceruloplasminemia, Chap. 42).

Whereas the epithelial cells of villi of the duodenal mucosa are the principal site of iron absorption, the programming of these cells for rate of iron absorption occurs in the crypt epithelial cells.[42] In the latter cells, HFE protein and transferrin receptor (TfR) colocalize in the perinuclear endoplasmic reticulum.[43] (This localization is unique to the crypt epithelial cells of the upper small bowel. In most other cells, TfR is a membrane protein, HFE protein spans the cell membrane, and in the membrane HFE protein modulates iron uptake through its binding with TfR.) In the perinuclear endoplasmic reticulum of crypt epithelial cells, the HFE-TfR complex somehow modulates the iron-absorbing function that the cell will have as it migrates along the villus toward the lumen, becoming an absorptive cell.

Iron may also be trapped in ferritin within the epithelial cells of the gastrointestinal tract, thereby preventing its absorption when body iron stores are high.[44-47] With the passage of time the mucosal cell advances to the tip of the villus, is sloughed and lost in the feces, together with its retained iron.

The absorption of iron is modulated to meet the body's needs: The absorbed fraction is reduced when body iron stores are high. Yet this physiological mechanism is easily overcome by large oral doses of medicinal iron or by accidental ingestion of iron by a child. There is no "mucosal block" of iron absorption: For each increment in dose of an inorganic iron compound there is a corresponding increment in the amount of iron absorbed.[48-51] (Fig. 24-6).

Iron absorption is enhanced when there is chronic liver disease.[52,53] The mechanism is unknown. Pancreatic disorders appear not to influence iron absorption.[54-57] Bile may facilitate iron absorption.[58]

Oxalates, phytates, and phosphates complex with iron and retard its absorption. Many simple reducing substances increase iron absorption. Among these are hydroquinone, ascorbate, lactate, pyruvate, succinate, fructose, cysteine, and sorbitol.[59-63] There is contradictory evidence concerning the effect of ethanol on iron absorption.[64,65]

Among the factors operating outside the alimentary tract to increase iron absorption are hypoxia, anemia, depletion of iron stores, and increased erythropoiesis. Each of these factors appears to exert an independent effect, but it is not known how they "instruct" the bowel to absorb more iron. The degree of transferrin saturation, the plasma iron concentration, the rate of plasma iron clearance, and the plasma erythropoietin concentration have each been considered as humoral messengers. The fine control of the rate of iron absorption may depend on more than one humoral mechanism.

TRANSPORT OF IRON

Once an atom of iron enters the body, it is virtually in a closed system (Fig. 24-7) in which it cycles almost endlessly from the plasma to the developing erythroblast (where it is utilized in hemoglobin synthesis), thence into the circulating blood for about 4 months, and then to phagocytic macrophages. Here it is removed from hemoglobin and released back into the plasma to repeat the cycle.

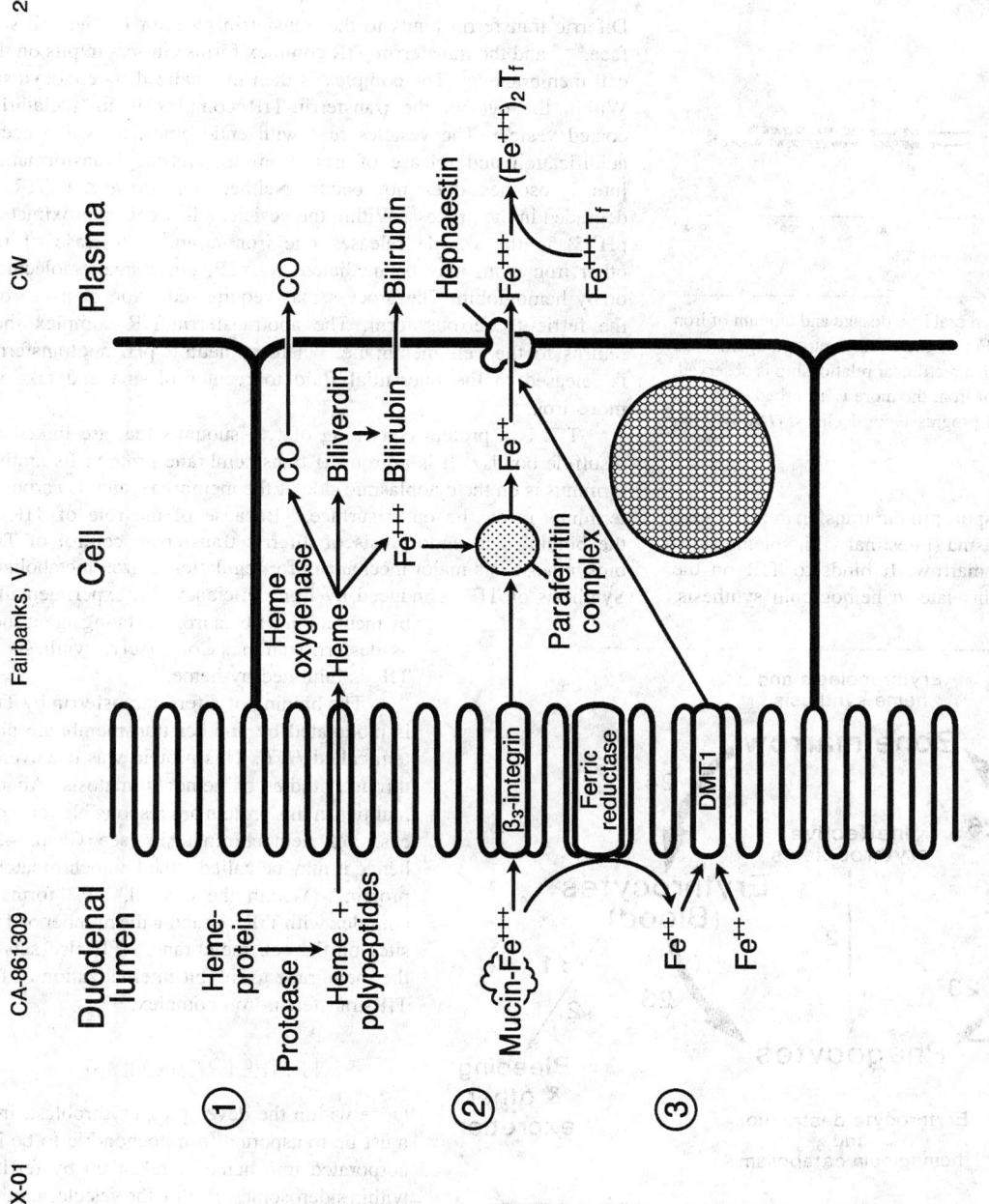

FIGURE 24-5 A scheme for the mechanism of iron uptake by epithelial cells of the duodenum and its transport across the epithelial cell to plasma of the subepithelial capillaries. At least nine proteins appear to be involved in this mechanism. They are mucin in the gastric and duodenal lumen; ferric reductase, β_3-integrin, DMT1, HFE, and hephaestin, which are cell membrane proteins; ceruloplasmin and transferrin, in plasma of the capillary network. Heme appears to enter the cell directly, by means as yet unknown. The iron is released by heme oxygenase. The uptake of Fe^{++} at the brush border may be mediated by DMT1. Fe^{++} traverses the cytosol. At the ablumenal (basal) membrane, it is bound to hephaestin, a ceruloplasmin-like membrane protein that oxidizes it to Fe^{+++}. Thus, it exits the cell, and in plasma, it is bound by monoferric-transferrin. The absorption of ferric iron is not well understood. A ferric reductase on the membrane of the brush border may reduce it to the ferrous state, enabling it to enter the cell. Fe^{++} that is complexed with mucin also appears to bind to a protein of the brush border membrane that is β_3-integrin. The iron-β_3-integrin complex may then be internalized to form, within the cytosol, a complex with calreticulin (mobilferrin). This complex has been called *paraferritin*, although it neither contains nor resembles ferritin. In this complex, Fe^{+++} is reduced to Fe^{++}. In the ferrous form, it may traverse the cell to be taken up by hephaestin, which oxidizes it to Fe^{++} and releases it to plasma.

The avidity of villus epithelial cells for iron is "programmed" when they are in the crypts, before they migrate up the villi. In the crypts, HFE protein somehow determines whether, a few days later as absorptive cells, they will absorb little iron or much iron.

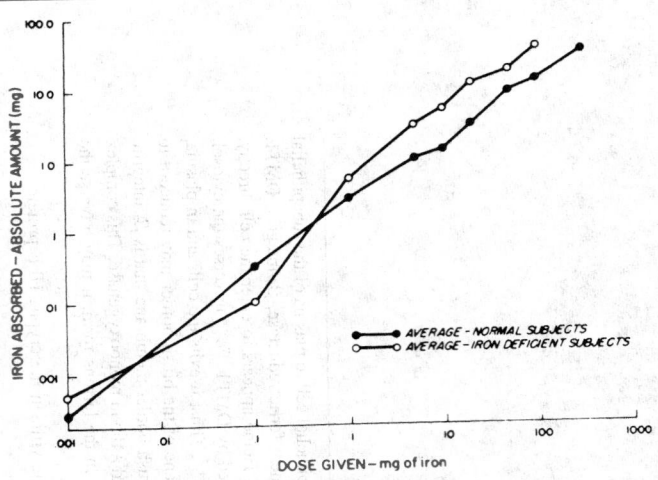

FIGURE 24-6   The relationship between oral iron dosage and amount of iron absorbed in humans. When the logarithm of the dose is plotted against the logarithm of the amount of iron absorbed, a rectilinear relationship is observed. Thus, at all levels, the greater the dose of iron, the more is absorbed, although the percent of the dose that is absorbed progressively declines. (*Drawn from data of Smith and Pannacciuli.*[48])

The major function of the transport protein transferrin is to move iron from wherever it enters the plasma (intestinal villi, splenic sinusoids) to the erythroblasts of the marrow. It binds to TfR on the erythroblast membrane.[66–68] Even this late in hemoglobin synthesis,

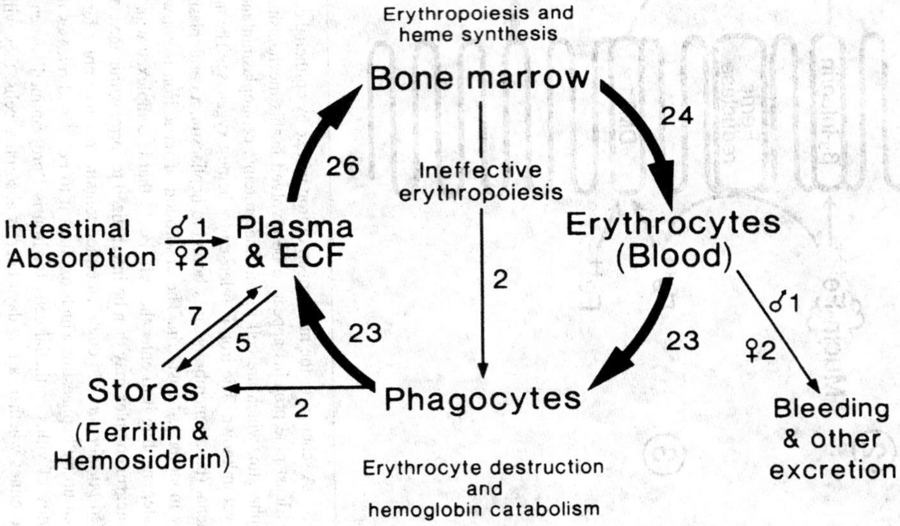

FIGURE 24-7   The iron cycle in humans. Iron is tightly conserved in a nearly closed system in which each iron atom cycles repeatedly from plasma and extracellular fluid (ECF) to the marrow, where it is incorporated into hemoglobin. Then it moves into the blood within erythrocytes and circulates for 4 months. It then travels to phagocytes of the reticuloendothelial system, where senescent erythrocytes are engulfed and destroyed, hemoglobin is digested, and iron is released to plasma, where the cycle continues. With each cycle, a small proportion of iron is transferred to storage sites, where it is incorporated into ferritin or hemosiderin, a small proportion of storage iron is released to plasma, a small proportion is lost in urine, sweat, feces, or blood, and an equivalent small amount of iron is absorbed from the intestinal tract. In addition, a small proportion (about 10%) of newly formed erythrocytes normally is destroyed within the bone marrow and its iron released, bypassing the circulating blood part of the cycle (ineffective erythropoiesis). The numbers indicate the approximate amount of iron (in mg) that enters and leaves each of these iron compartments every day in healthy adults who do not have bleeding or other blood disorders.

the membrane of a reticulocyte can still bind from 25,000 to 50,000 diferric transferrin molecules per minute.

Relatively small amounts of iron are transported to other tissues, especially in a slow exchange with the iron in ferritin and hemosiderin and to a much lesser extent with other tissue forms of iron.

ENDOCYTOSIS OF TRANSFERRIN

Diferric transferrin binds to the transferrin receptor on the cell surface,[69–72] and the transferrin-TfR complex forms clusters in pits on the cell membrane.[73,74] The complex is then internalized by endocytosis. Within the cytosol the transferrin-TfR complex is in a clathrin-coated vesicle. The vesicles fuse with endosomes, in which occur acidification and release of iron from transferrin. Transformation into lysosomes does not occur. Neither transferrin nor TfR is degraded in the process. Within the vesicle, a low pH (approximately pH 5) in the vesicle releases one iron atom.[75,76] Release of the other iron atom may be mediated by ATP, other small molecules, or by hemoglobin. The process may require reduction of iron from the ferric to ferrous form. The apotransferrin-TfR complex then returns to the cell membrane, where at neutral pH, apotransferrin is released to the interstitial fluid to reenter plasma and take up more iron.[74,75]

TfR is a protein consisting of two subunits that are linked by disulfide bonds.[77] It is a group II transmembrane protein: Its amino-terminus is on the cytoplasmic side of the membrane, and its carboxy-terminus is on the outer surface.[78] Because of the role of TfR in the binding and endocytosis of diferric transferrin, control of TfR biosynthesis is a major mechanism for regulation of iron metabolism. Synthesis of TfR is induced by iron deficiency, or, experimentally, by incubation with an iron chelating agent such as desferrioxamine. Conversely, synthesis of TfR is inhibited by heme.[79]

The binding of diferric transferrin by TfR is modulated by another transmembrane protein called *HFE*. This protein was discovered through studies of hemochromatosis: Abnormalities in this protein are responsible for most cases of hemochromatosis (see Chap. 42), hence it may be called "the hemochromatosis protein." Within the cytosol, HFE forms a complex with TfR, reducing the number of TfR sites on the cell membrane. HFE also acts at the membrane to inhibit internalization of the TfR-transferrin-iron complex.[80–82]

IRON IN THE ERYTHROBLAST

Once within the developing erythroblast, iron must be transported to mitochondria to be incorporated into heme or taken up by ferritin within siderosomes. Within the vesicle, another protein called *DMT1* (divalent metal transporter 1) effects the release of Fe^{+++} into the cytosol, where it is taken up by mitochondria for heme synthesis (Fig. 24-8).

Within mitochondria, iron is inserted into protoporphyrin by heme synthetase (ferrochelatase). When heme synthesis is impaired, as in lead poisoning or in the sideroblastic anemias (see Chap. 63), the mitochondria accumulate excessive amounts of amorphous iron aggregates.[83] The mitochondria can then be stained by the Prussian blue reaction and are seen by

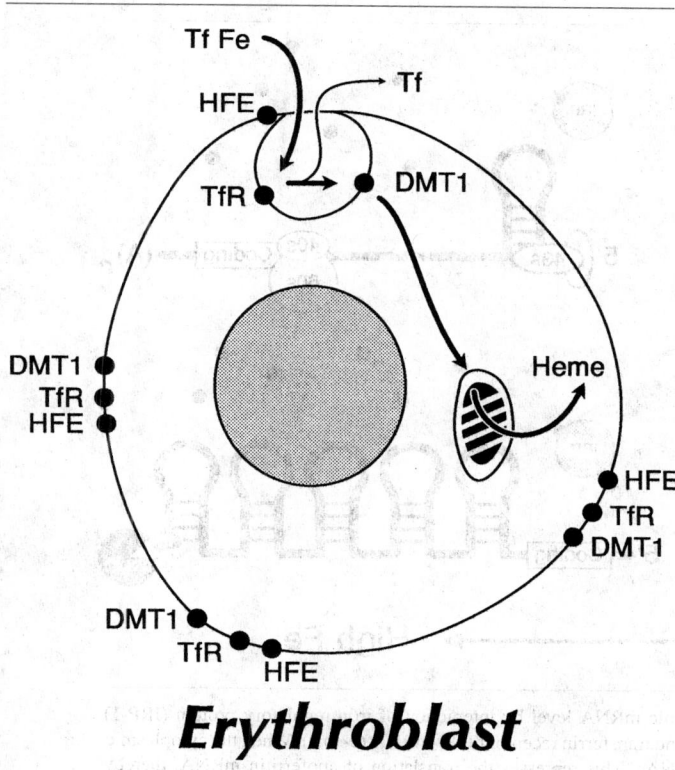

Erythroblast

FIGURE 24-8   The cellular uptake and cycling or iron, shown for an erythroblast in the bone marrow. (See text for explanation.)

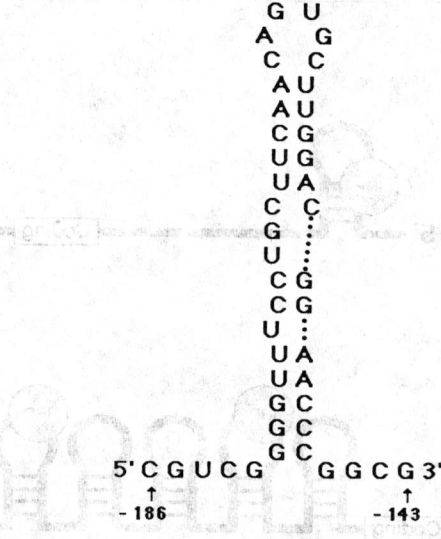

FIGURE 24-9   The stem-loop structure that is the iron-responsive element of apoferritin mRNA. (*From Hentze and coworkers,*[112] *with permission.*)

light microscopy as a ring of large blue siderotic granules encircling the erythroblast nucleus (ringed sideroblast). In normal marrow, siderotic granules are also demonstrable in erythroblast cytoplasm. However, these are very small, usually only one to three in number, and randomly distributed in the cytoplasm. These normal siderotic granules are ferritin aggregates located in lysosomal organelles designated siderosomes.[84] Erythroblasts containing these siderotic granules are called *sideroblasts* and normally represent 20 to 50 percent of the erythrocyte precursors of the marrow. In iron deficiency and in anemia that accompanies chronic disorders, sideroblasts almost disappear from the marrow. Conversely, in some states of iron overload, they may become more numerous and contain more siderotic granules than normally.

THE INTRACELLULAR REGULATION OF IRON METABOLISM

The regulation of synthesis of apoferritin, TfR, ALA synthase, apotransferrin, aconitase, DMT1, and possibly other proteins that are important in iron metabolism, is at the level of translation of mRNA by ribosomes. The mRNA for each of these proteins contains one or several IREs. Each IRE consists of a stem and loop structure, in which the loop is the nucleotide sequence CAGUGC (Fig. 24-9). The apoferritin mRNA has, as its IRE, a single stem-loop structure in the 5′ (upstream) untranslated region. In contrast to the apoferritin IRE, those for TfR consist of as many as 5 stems-loops in the 3′ (downstream) untranslated portion of TfR mRNA.[79,85-89]

IRP-1 (iron regulatory protein 1, or desferri-aconitase) binds to the apoferritin IRE to down-regulate apoferritin synthesis. The presence of iron in the cytosol causes IRP-1 to convert to the cubane form as aconitase, thereby displacing it from the IRE and reducing the inhibition of apoferritin synthesis.[87,89-96] Iron also causes translocation of preformed apoferritin messenger RNA to polyribosomes, where syn-

thesis of apoferritin occurs. The effect of binding of IRP-1 to the IREs for apotransferrin, TfR, DMT1, and ALA synthase is to *increase* synthesis of these proteins; conversely, when the iron content of cytosol is high, the displacement of IRP-1 from these IREs leads to *decreased* synthesis of these proteins. Fig. 24-10 illustrates these relationships for the regulation of synthesis of apoferritin and TfR.

There is some redundancy in iron regulatory protein: in addition to IRP-1, there is an IRP-2 that also acts on IREs. IRP-2 is structurally different; it does not contain an iron-sulfur cluster. It undergoes proteolysis when the iron concentration is low.[3,97,98]

In addition to mechanisms for regulation of iron metabolism at the mRNA level, there is regulation at the DNA level of the expression of the genes for proteins important in iron metabolism. As yet, little is known about these regulatory mechanisms that reside within the cell nucleus. However, present evidence indicates that the cellular uptake and metabolism of iron are predominantly regulated at the level of cytoplasmic mRNA, as described above, rather than at the level of DNA.

ROLE OF THE MONOCYTE-MACROPHAGE SYSTEM

Destruction of aged erythrocytes and hemoglobin degradation occur within macrophages. This proceeds at a rate sufficient to release approximately 20 percent of the hemoglobin iron within a few hours. As iron is released, it is bound to transferrin and ultimately redistributed, approximately 80 percent being rapidly reincorporated into hemoglobin. Thus, about 40 percent of the hemoglobin iron of nonviable erythrocytes reappears in circulating red cells in 12 days. The rate of reutilization is normally about 19 to 69 percent in 12 days. The remainder of the iron enters the storage pool as ferritin or hemosiderin and then turns over very slowly. In normal subjects, approximately 40 percent of this iron remains in storage after 140 days. When there is an increased iron demand for hemoglobin synthesis, however, storage iron may be mobilized more rapidly.[99] Conversely, in the presence of infection or other inflammatory process or malignancy, iron is much more slowly reutilized in hemoglobin synthesis.[99-102]

These perturbations in iron reutilization are believed to be due to changes in the rate of iron-release macrophages. Chronic inflammatory disease causes reduction in the rate of release of iron by phagocytic

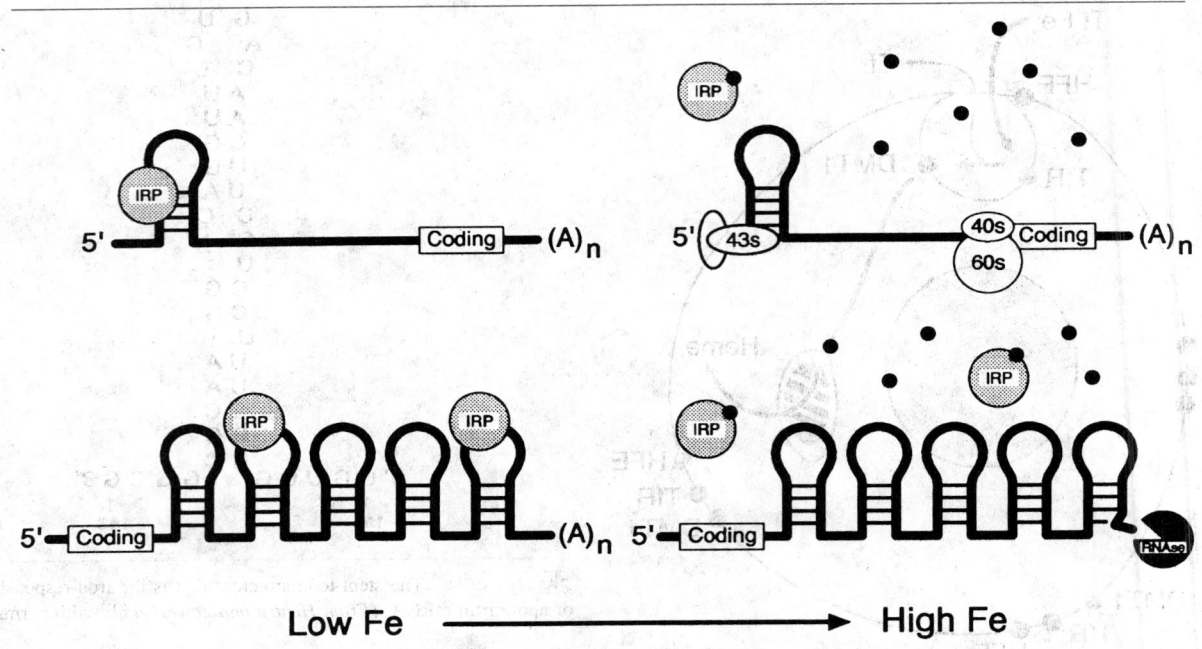

Low Fe ──────────────────────▶ **High Fe**

FIGURE 24-10   The regulation of iron metabolism at the cytoplasmic mRNA level by interaction of iron regulatory protein (IRP-1) and the iron-responsive elements (IREs) of apoferritin mRNA (*above*) and transferrin receptor (TfR) mRNA (*below*). When the cytoplasmic iron concentration is low (*left*), IRP-1 binds to the IREs of both mRNAs. This represses the translation of apoferritin mRNA, thereby reducing the amount of apoferritin formed, and stabilizes and increases the translation of TfR mRNA, thereby increasing the amount of TfR formed, which in turn increases the ability of the cell to bind diferric transferrin. Conversely, when there is an abundance of iron in the cytoplasm (*right*), IRP-1 is displaced from both species of mRNA. This results in derepression of apoferritin synthesis and destabilization and degradation of TfR mRNA. Then, apoferritin increases within the cytosol, and there is reduction in the number of TfR molecules on the cell membrane. (*Modified from: Knisely,*[113] *by permission of Mosby/Year Book.*)

cells, increased storage of iron in the monocyte-macrophage system, slowing of delivery of iron to erythropoietic cells, and slowing of erythropoiesis. Microcytic anemia is a consequence of the reduced flow of iron from the monocyte-macrophage system to the developing erythroblasts.

In addition to their role in regulating the size of iron stores, macrophages contribute to regulation of the plasma transferrin concentration through synthesis of apotransferrin and the internalization and degradation of transferrin.[103–105]

IRON EXCRETION

The body conserves iron with remarkable efficiency: less than a thousandth of it is lost each day, an amount easily replaced if dietary sources are adequate. Almost all this iron loss occurs by way of the feces, and it normally amounts to about 1 mg per day. Exfoliation of skin and dermal appendages results in a much smaller loss, as does perspiration. Even in tropical climates, the loss of iron in sweat is minimal.[106] Iron is excreted also in urine, but in very small amounts. In humans, lactation may cause excretion of about 1 mg iron daily, thus doubling the overall rate of iron excretion. Blood loss by normal menstruation contributes to negative iron balance (see Chap. 38).

While total daily iron excretion is normally about 1 mg for males and about 2 mg for menstruating women, persons with marked iron overload, as in hemochromatosis, may lose as much as 4 mg of iron daily by these mechanisms, a quantity insufficient to prevent the accumulation of storage iron.[46]

GENETIC DISORDERS RELATED TO IRON METABOLISM

During the past few years, much has been learned of genetic disorders that are related to iron metabolism. Those associated with hemochromatosis are discussed in detail in Chap. 42.

A syndrome of congenital cataracts and hyperferritinemia has been reported in several families.[107,108] This disorder has been attributed to mutation in the stem-loop structure of the apoferritin mRNA. Serum ferritin concentrations are thousands of μgm/L. The ferritin in these cases appears to contain only L monomers.

Deficiency of hephaestin is responsible for a congenital microcytic anemia in the *sla* (sex-linked anemia) inborn strain of mice.[41] Microcytic anemia (*mk*) mice are unable to absorb iron from the intestinal tract. They also fail to respond to parenterally administered iron. Thus, their red blood cell precursors are also unable to take up iron from plasma. Remarkably, the same DMT1 mis-sense mutation that was found in mk mice, G185R, causes marked reduction in iron absorption in Belgrade laboratory rats, an inbred strain with a hereditary microcytic anemia.[109,111]

REFERENCES

1. Beutler E: Iron enzymes in iron deficiency. VI. Aconitase activity and citrate metabolism. *J Clin Invest* 38:1605, 1959.
2. Paraskeva E, Hentze MW: Iron-sulphur clusters as genetic regulatory switches: the bifunctional iron regulatory protein-1. [Review] [50 refs]. *FEBS Lett* 389:40, 1996.
3. Henderson BR, Menotti E, Kuhn LC: Iron regulatory proteins 1 and 2 bind distinct sets of RNA target sequences. *J Biol Chem* 271:4900, 1996.

4. Beinert J, Kennedy MC: Aconitase, a two-faced protein: enzyme and iron regulatory factor. *FASEB J* 7:1442, 1993.

5. Hempstead PD, Yewdall SJ, Fernie AR, et al: Comparison of the three-dimensional structures of recombinant human H and horse L ferritins at high resolution. *JMB* 268:424, 1997.

6. Hoy TG, Harrison PM, Shabbir M, Macara IG: The release of iron from horse spleen ferritin to 1,10-phenanthroline. *Biochem J* 137:67, 1974.

7. Jones T, Spence R, Walsh C: Mechanism and kinetics of iron release from ferritin by dihydroflavins and dihydroflavin analogues. *Biochemistry* 17:4011, 1978.

8. Crichton RR, Roman F: A novel mechanism for ferritin iron oxidation and deposition. *J Mol Catal* 4:75, 1978.

9. Crichton RR, Roman F, Roland F, et al: Ferritin iron deposition and mobilisation. *J Mol Catal* 7:267, 1980.

10. Harrison PM, Arosio P: The ferritins: molecular properties, iron storage function and cellular regulation. [Review] [477 refs]. *Biochim Biophys Acta* 1275:161, 1996.

11. Richter GW: Electron microscopy of hemosiderin: Presence of ferritin and occurrence of crystalline lattices in hemosiderin deposits. *J Biophys Biochem Cytol* 4:55, 1958.

12. Fischbach FA, Gregory DW, Harrison PM, Hoy TG, Williams JM: On the structure of hemosiderin and its relationship to ferritin. *J Ultrastruct Res* 73:495, 1971.

13. Hoy TG, Jacobs A: Ferritin polymers and the formation of haemosiderin. *Br J Haematol* 49:593, 1981.

14. Pollycove M, Mortimer R: The quantitative determination of iron kinetics and hemoglobin synthesis in human subject. *J Clin Invest* 40:753, 1961.

15. Hosain F, Marsaglia G, Finch CA: Blood ferrokinetics in normal man. *J Clin Invest* 46:1, 1967.

16. Beutler E: Iron enzymes in iron deficiency. I. Cytochrome C. *Am J Med Sci* 234:517, 1957.

17. Beutler E, Blaisdell RK: Iron enzymes in iron deficiency. III. Catalase in rat red cells and liver with some further observations on cytochrome C. *J Lab Clin Med* 52:694, 1958.

18. Beutler E, Blaisdell RK: Iron enzymes in iron deficiency. V. Succinic dehydrogenase in rat liver, kidney and heart. *Blood* 15:30, 1960.

19. Jacobs A: Iron-containing enzymes in the buccal epithelium. *Lancet* 2:1331, 1961.

20. Dallan PR, Sunshine P, Leonard Y: Intestinal cytochrome response with repair of iron deficiency. *Pediatrics* 39:863, 1967.

21. Srivastava SK, Sanwal GG, Tewari KK: Biochemical alterations in rat tissue in iron deficiency anemia and repletion with iron. *Indian J Biochem* 2:257, 1965.

22. Bailey S, Evans RW, Garratt RC, et al: Molecular structure of serum transferrin at 3.3-A resolution. *Biochemistry* 27:5804, 1988.

23. Van Haeringen B, de Lange F, van Stokkum IHM, et al: Dynamic structure of human serum transferrin from transient electric birefringence experiments. *Proteins: Structure, Function Genet* 23:233, 1998.

24. Haurani FI, Meyer A, O'Brien R: Production of transferrin by the macrophage. *J Reticuloendothel Soc* 14:309, 1973.

25. Thorbecke GJ, Liem HH, Knight S, Cox K, Muller-Eberhard U: Sites of formation of the serum proteins transferrin and hemopexin. *J Clin Invest* 52:725, 1973.

26. Giblett ER: *Genetic Markers in Human Blood*. Philadelphia, Davis, 1969.

27. Aisen P: The transferrins, in *Iron in Biochemistry and Medicine*, edited by A Jacobs, M Worwood, p 87. Academic, New York, 1980.

28. Moore CV: Iron nutrition and requirements. *Ser Haematol* 6:1, 1965.

29. Pennington JAT, Young BE, Wilson DB, Johnson RD, Vanderveen JE: Mineral content of foods and total diets: the selected minerals in foods survey, 1982 to 1984. *J Am Diet Assoc* 86:876, 1986.

30. Turnbull A, Cleton F, Finch CA: Iron absorption. IV. The absorption of hemoglobin iron. *J Clin Invest* 41:1897, 1962.

31. Weintraub R, Weinstein MB, Huser H-J, Rafal S: Absorption of hemoglobin iron: the role of a heme-splitting substance in the intestinal mucosa. *J Clin Invest* 47:531, 1968.

32. Conrad ME, Benjamin BI, Williams HL, Foy AL: Human absorption of hemoglobin-iron. *Gastroenterology* 53:5, 1967.

33. Raffin SB, Woo CH, Roost KT, Price DC, Schmid R: Intestinal absorption of hemoglobin iron-heme cleavage by mucosal heme oxygenase. *J Clin Invest* 54:1344, 1975.

34. Beutler F, Fairbanks VF, Fahey JL: *Clinical Disorders of Iron Metabolism*. Grune & Stratton, New York, 1963.

35. Jacobs A: Gastric factor in iron absorption. *Lancet* 1:1313, 1968.

36. Van Campen D: Enhancement of iron absorption from ligated segments of rat intestine by histidine, cysteine, and lysine: Effects of removing ionizing groups and of stereoisomerism. *J Nutr* 103:139, 1973.

37. Davis PS, Deller DJ: Prediction and demonstration of iron chelating ability of sugars. *Nature* 212:405, 1966.

38. Conrad ME, Umbreit JN, Moore EG: A role for mucin the absorption of inorganic iron and other metal cations. A study in rats. *Gastroenterology* 100:129, 1991.

39. Eckmekcioglu C, Fkeyertag J, Marktl W: A ferric reductase activity is found in brush border membrane vesicles isolated from Caco-2 cells. *J Nutr* 126:2209, 1996.

40. Conrad ME, Umbreit JN, Moore EG, Heiman D: Mobilferrin is an intermediate in iron transport between transferrin and hemoglobin in K562 cells. *J Clin Invest* 98:1449, 1996.

41. Vulpe CD, Kuo YM, Murphy TL, et al: Hephaestin, a ceruloplasmin homologue implicated in intestinal iron transport, is defective in the sla mouse. *Nature Genet* 21:195, 1999.

42. Waheed A, Parkkila S, Saarnio J, et al: Association of HFE protein with transferrin receptor in crypt enterocytes of human duodenum. *Proc Natl Acad Sci USA* 96:1579, 1999.

43. Parkkila S, Waheed A, Britton RS, et al: Immunohisotchemistry of HLA-H, the protein defective in patients with hereditary hemochromatosis, reveals a unique pattern of expression in gastrointestinal tract. *Proc Natl Acad Sci USA* 94:2534, 1997.

44. Conrad ME Jr, Crosby WH: Intestinal mucosal mechanisms controlling iron absorption. *Blood* 22:406, 1963.

45. Hartman RS, Conrad ME, Jr., Hartman RE, Joy RJT, Crosby WH: Ferritin containing bodies in human small intestinal epithelium. *Blood* 22:397, 1963.

46. Crosby WH, Conrad ME Jr, Wheby MS: The rate of iron accumulation in iron storage disease. *Blood* 22:429, 1963.

47. Wheby MS, Crosby WH: The gastrointestinal tract and iron absorption. *Blood* 22:416, 1963.

48. Smith MD, Pannacciulli IM: Absorption of inorganic iron from graded doses: Its significance in relation to iron absorption tests and the 'mucosal block' theory. *Br J Haematol* 4:428, 1958.

49. Bonnet JD, Hagedorn AB, Owen CA Jr: A quantitative method for measuring gastrointestinal absorption of iron. *Blood* 15:36, 1960.

50. Brown EB Jr, Dubach R, Moore CV: Studies in iron transportation and metabolism. XI. Critical analysis of mucosal block by large doses of inorganic iron in human subjects. *J Lab Clin Med* 52:335, 1958.

51. Beutler E, Kelly BM, Beutler F: The regulation of iron absorption. II. Relationship between iron dosage and iron absorption. *Am J Clin Nutr* 11:559, 1962.

52. Murray MJ, Stein N: A gastric factor promoting iron absorption. *Lancet* 1:614, 1968.

53. Smith RS: Iron absorption in cystic fibrosis. *Br Med J* 1:608, 1964.

54. Biggs JC, Davis AE: The exocrine pancreas and iron absorption. *Aust Ann Med* 15:36, 1966.

55. Kavin H, Charlton RW, Jacobs P, Green R, Torrance JD, Bothwell TH: Effect of the exocrine pancreatic secretions on iron absorption. *Gut* 8:556, 1967.

56. Murray MJ, Stein N: Does the pancreas influence iron absorption? A critical review of information on iron absorption. *Gastroenterology* 51:694, 1966.

57. Balcerzak SP, Peternel WW, Heinle EW: Iron absorption in chronic pancreatitis. *Gastroenterology* 53:257, 1967.

58. Wheby MS, Conrad ME, Hedberg SE, Crosby WH: The role of bile in the control of iron absorption. *Gastroenterology* 42:319, 1962.

59. Herndon JF, Rice EG, Tucker RG, VanLoon EJ, Greenberg SM: Iron absorption and metabolism. III. The enhancement of iron absorption in rats by D-sorbitol. *J Nutr* 64:615, 1958.

60. Hallberg L, Sölvell L: Iron absorption studies: [1] Determination of the absorption rate of iron in man. [2] Absorption of a single dose of iron in man. [3] Iron absorption during constant intragastric infusion of iron in man. [4] Effect of iron and transferrin intravenously on iron absorption and turnover in man (Sölvell alone). *Acta Med Scand* 168(suppl 358):1, 1960.

61. Pollack S, Kaufman RM, Crosby WH: Iron absorption: effects of sugars and reducing agents. *Blood* 24:577, 1964.

62. Slatkavitz CA, Clydesdale FM: Solubility of inorganic iron as affected by proteolytic digestion. *Am J Clin Nutr* 47:487, 1988.

63. Taylor PG, Martinez-Torres C, Romano EL, Layrisse M: The effect of cysteine-containing peptides released during meat digestion on iron absorption in humans. *Am J Clin Nutr* 43:68, 1986.

64. Charlton RW, Jacobs P, Seftel H, Bothwell TH: Effect of alcohol on iron absorption. *Br Med J* 2:1427, 1964.

65. Celada A, Rudolf H, Donath A: Effect of single ingestion of alcohol on iron absorption. *Am J Hematol* 5:225, 1978.

66. Jandl JH, Inman JK, Simmons RL, Allen DW: Transfer of iron from serum iron-binding protein to human reticulocytes. *J Clin Invest* 38:161, 1959.

67. Katz JH: The delivery of iron to the immature red cell: a critical review. *Ser Haematol* 6:15, 1965.

68. Jandl JH, Katz JH: The plasma-to-cell cycle of transferrin. *J Clin Invest* 42:314, 1963.

69. Bergamaschi G, Eng MJ, Huebers HA, Finch CA: The effect of transferrin saturation on internal iron exchange. *Proc Soc Exp Biol Med* 183:66, 1986.

70. Konopka K, Mareschal JC, Crichton RR: Iron transfer from transferrin to ferritin mediated by polyphosphate compounds. *Biochim Biophys Acta* 677:417, 1981.

71. Octave JN, Schneider YJ, Crichton RR, Trouet A: Transferrin protein and iron uptake by isolated rat erythroblasts. *FEBS Lett* 137:119, 1982.

72. Morgan EH, Baker E: Role of transferrin receptors and endocytosis in iron uptake by hepatic and erythroid cells. *Ann NY Acad Sci* 526:65, 1988.

73. Cheng TPO: Redistribution of cell surface transferrin receptors prior to their concentration in coated pits as revealed by immunoferritin labels. *Cell Tissue Res* 244:613, 1986.

74. Dautry-Varsait A: Receptor-mediated endocytosis: the intracellular journey of transferrin and its receptor. *Biochemie* 68:375, 1986.

75. Dautry-Varsat A, Ciechanover A, Lodish HF: pH and the recycling of transferrin during receptor mediated endocytosis. *Proc Natl Acad Sci USA* 80:2258, 1983.

76. Chan RYY, Loh TT: Perturbation of intracellular pH by DIDS on endocytosis of transferrin and iron update in rabbit reticulocytes. *Biochem Biophys Res Commun* 150:1256, 1988.

77. Schneider C, Williams JG: Molecular dissection of the human transferrin receptor. *J Cell Sci* 3(suppl):139, 1985.

78. Zerial M, Melancon P, Schneider C, Garoff H: The transmembrane segment of the human transferrin receptor functions as a signal peptide. *EMBO J* 5:1543, 1986.

79. Rouault T, Rao K, Harford J, Mattia E, Klausner RD: Hemin chelatable iron, and the regulation of transferrin receptor biosynthesis. *J Biol Chem* 260:14862, 1985.

80. Recalcati S, Pometta R, Levi S, Conte D, Cairo G: Response of monocyte iron regulatory protein activity to inflammation: abnormal behavior in genetic hemochromatosis. *Blood* 91:2565, 1998.

81. Andrews NC, Levy JE: Iron is hot: an update on the pathophysiology of hemochromatosis. *Blood* 92:1845, 1998.

82. Salter-Cid L, Brunmark A, Li Y, et al: Transferrin receptor is negatively modulated by the hemochromatosis protein HFE: implications for cellular iron homeostasis. *Proc Natl Acad Sci USA* 96:5434, 1999.

83. Fawwaz RA, Winchell HS, Pollycove M, Sargent T: Hepatic iron deposition in humans. I. First-pass hepatic deposition of intestinally absorbed iron in patients with low plasma latent iron-binding capacity. *Blood* 30:417, 1967.

84. Cartwright GE, Deiss A: Sideroblasts, siderocytes, and sideroblastic anemia. *N Engl J Med* 292:185, 1975.

85. Casey JL, Di Jeso B, Rao KK, Rouault TA, Klausner RD, Harford JB: Deletional analysis of the promotor region of the human transferrin receptor gene. *Nucl Acids Res* 16:629, 1988.

86. Müller EW, Kühn LC: A stem-loop in the 3' untranslated region mediates iron-dependent regulation of transferrin receptor mRNA stability in the cytoplasm. *Cell* 53:815, 1988.

87. Casey JL, Hentze MW, Koeller DM, et al: Iron-responsive elements: Regulatory RNA sequences that control mRNA levels and translation. *Science* 240:924, 1988.

88. Casey JL, Di Jeso B, Rao K, Klausner RD, Harford JB: Two genetic loci participate in the regulation by iron of the gene for the human transferrin receptor. *Proc Natl Acad Sci USA* 85:1787, 1988.

89. Casey JL, Di Jeso B, Rao K, Rouault TA, Klausner RD, Harford JB: The promoter region of the human transferrin receptor gene. *Ann NY Acad Sci* 526:54, 1988.

90. Rouault TA, Hentze MW, Caughman SW, Harford JB, Klausner RD: Binding of a cytosolic protein to the iron-responsive element of human ferritin messenger RNA. *Science* 241:1207, 1988.

91. Hentze MW, Caughman SW, Casey JL, et al: A model for the structure and functions of iron-responsive elements. *Gene* 72:201, 1988.

92. Rouault TA, Hentze MW, Haile DJ, Harford JB, Klausner RD: The iron-responsive element binding protein: a method for the affinity purification of a regulatory RNA-binding protein. *Proc Natl Acad Sci USA* 86:5768, 1989.

93. Leibold EA, Guo B: Iron-dependent regulation of ferritin and transferrin receptor expression by the iron-responsive element binding protein. *Annu Rev Nutr* 12:345, 1992.

94. Tang CK, Chin J, Harford JB, Klausner RD, Rouault TA: Iron regulates the activity of the iron-responsive element binding protein without changing its rate of synthesis or degradation. *J Biol Chem* 267:24466, 1992.

95. Haile DJ, Rouault TA, Tang CK, Chin J, Harford JB, Klausner RD: Reciprocal control of RNA-binding and aconitase activity in the regulation of the iron-responsive element binding protein: role of the iron-sulfur cluster. *Proc Natl Acad Sci USA* 89:7536, 1992.

96. Kühn LC, Hentze MW: Coordination of cellular iron metabolism by post-transcriptional gene regulation. *J Inorg Biochem* 47:183, 1992.

97. Rouault T, Klausner R: Regulation of iron metabolism in eukaryotes. *Curr Top Cell Reg* 35:1, 1997.

98. Henderson BR, Kuhn LC: Differential modulation of the RNA-binding proteins IRP-1 and IRP-2 in response to iron. IRP-2 inactivation requires translation of another protein. *J Biol Chem* 270:20509, 1995.

99. Noyes WD, Bothwell TH, Finch CA: The role of the reticulo-endothelial cell in iron metabolism. *Br J Haematol* 6:43, 1960.

100. Haurani FI, Burke W, Martinez EJ: Defective reutilization of iron in the anemia of inflammation. *J Lab Clin Med* 65:560, 1965.

101. Haurani FI, Young K, Tocantins LM: Reutilization of iron in anemia complicating malignant neoplasms. *Blood* 22:73, 1963.

102. O'Shea MJ, Kershenobich D, Tavill AS: Effects of inflammation on iron and transferrin metabolism. *Br J Haematol* 25:707, 1973.

103. MacSween RNM, MacDonald RA: Iron metabolism by reticuloendothelial cells in vitro uptake of transferrin-bound iron by rat and rabbit cells. *Lab Invest* 21:230, 1969.

104. MacDonald RA, MacSween RNM, Pechet GA: Iron metabolism by reticuloendothelial cells in vitro: physical and chemical conditions, lipotrope deficiency, and acute inflammation. *Lab Invest* 21:236, 1969.

105. Hemmaplardh D, Morgan EH: Transferrin and iron uptake by human cells in culture. *Exp Cell Res* 87:207, 1974.

106. Green R, Charlton R, Seftel H, Bothwell T: Body iron excretion in man: a collaborative study. *Am J Med* 45:336, 1968.

107. Beaumont C, Leneuve P, Devaux I, et al: Mutation in the iron responsive element of the L ferritin mRNA in a family with dominant hyperferritinaemia and cataract. *Nature Genet* 11:444, 1995.

108. Girelli D, Corrocher R, Bisceglia L, et al: Hereditary hyperferritinemia-cataract syndrome caused by a 29-base pair deletion in the iron responsive element of ferritin L-subunit gene. *Blood* 90:2084, 1997.

109. Fleming MD, Trenor CC III, Su MA, et al: Microcytic anaemia mice have a mutation in Nramp2, a candidate iron transporter gene. *Nature Genet* 16:383, 1997.

110. Su MA, Trenor CC, Fleming JC, Fleming MD, Andrews NC: The G185R mutation disrupts function of the iron transporter Nramp2. *Blood* 92:2157, 1998.

111. Fleming MD, Romano MA, Su MA, Garrick LM, Garrick MD, Andrews NC: Nramp2 is mutated in the anemic Belgrade (b) rat: evidence of a role for Nramp2 in endosomal iron transport. Proceedings of the *Natl Acad Sci USA* 95:1148, 1998.

112. Hentze MW, Rouault TA, Wright-Caughman S, Dancis A, Harford JB, Klausner RD: A cis-acting element is necessary and sufficient for translational regulation of human ferritin expression in response to iron. *Proc Natl Acad Sci USA* 84:6730, 1987.

113. Knisely AS: Neonatal hemochromatosis. *Adv Pediatr* 39:383, 1992.

METABOLIC ASPECTS OF FOLIC ACID AND COBALAMIN

BERNARD M. BABIOR

Folate in its tetrahydro form is a transporter of one-carbon fragments, which it can carry at any of three oxidation levels: methanol, formaldehyde, and formic acid. The oxidation levels of the folate-bound one-carbon fragments can be altered in oxidation and reduction reactions that require NADP and NADPH, respectively. The chief source of the folate-bound one-carbon fragments is serine, which is converted to glycine as it passes its terminal carbon to folate. The one-carbon fragments are used for the biosynthesis of purines, thymidine, and methionine. During the biosynthesis of purines and methionine, free folate is released in its tetrahydro form, but, during the biosynthesis of thymidine, the tetrahydrofolate is oxidized to the dihydro form and has to be re-reduced by dihydrofolate reductase in order to continue to function in one-carbon metabolism. Methotrexate acts as an anticancer agent because it is an exceedingly powerful inhibitor of dihydrofolate reductase.

In the cell, folates are conjugated by the addition of a chain of 6 or 7 glutamic acid residues. These serve to prevent the folates from leaking out of the cell. When folates are absorbed from the intestine, a process that takes place chiefly in the duodenum and proximal jejunum, all but one of the glutamates are removed by an enzyme known as conjugase. Folates travel in the blood stream and are taken up by the cells mainly in the form of unconjugated methyltetrahydrofolate. In the cell, the newly absorbed folates are rapidly reconjugated. If reconjugation is prevented, the folates leak back out of the cell, resulting in an intracellular deficiency of folate.

Cobalamin is required for two reactions: the conversion of methylmalonyl CoA (a product of catabolism of branched-chain amino acids) to succinyl CoA, a Krebs cycle intermediate, and the conversion of homocysteine to methionine, a reaction in which the methyl group of methyltetrahydrofolate is donated to the sulfur atom of homocysteine. In cobalamin deficiency, methyltetrahydrofolate accumulates, because for practical purposes donation of the methyl group to homocysteine is the only way to generate free tetrahydrofolate from methyltetrahydrofolate. Free tetrahydrofolate is an excellent substrate for the conjugase, but methyltetrahydrofolate is a poor substrate. Consequently, much of the methyltetrahydrofolate taken up by a cobalamin-deficient cell leaks out of the cell before it can be conjugated. The megaloblastic anemia of cobalamin deficiency is actually due to an intracellular folate deficiency that arises because of the limited ability of the cell to conjugate methyltetrahydrofolate.

The absorption of cobalamin is a highly complex process. On first arriving in the stomach, cobalamin is taken up by R-binder (also called *haptocorrin* or *cobalophilin*), a glycoprotein that is found in virtually all secretions. When the cobalamin-R binder complex enters the duodenum, the R binder is digested and the cobalamin is released into the intestinal lumen, where it is taken up by intrinsic factor, a protein secreted by the gastric parietal cells. The cobalamin-intrinsic factor complex is absorbed by cells in the ileum, where the cobalamin is released and transported to the blood stream. Here the vitamin binds to transcobalamin II, which delivers its cargo of cobalamin to cells throughout the body. Folic acid (pteroylglutamic acid) and cobalamin (vitamin B_{12}) play key roles in the metabolic economy of proliferating cells.

FOLIC ACID

CHEMISTRY

Folic acid (pteroylglutamic acid) is composed of a pteridine derivative, a *p*-aminobenzoate residue, and an L-glutamic acid residue (Fig. 25-1a). The first two together are called *pteroic acid*.[1] In nature, folic acid occurs largely as conjugates in which multiple glutamic acids are linked by peptide bonds involving their γ-carboxyl groups (Fig. 25-1b). Conjugates are named according to the length of the glutamate chain (e.g., pteroylglutamate, pteroyldiglutamate, pteroylhexaglutamate). Therapeutic folic acid (abbreviated *PteGlu*, or *F*) has one glutamic acid.

To form a functional compound, folate must be reduced to tetrahydrofolate (FH_4) (see Fig. 25-1b). In this reduction, dihydrofolate (FH_2) is an intermediate. A single enzyme, *dihydrofolate reductase*, catalyzes both $F \rightarrow FH_2$ and $FH_2 \rightarrow FH_4$.

The folate family consists largely of FH_4 derivatives bearing a one-carbon substituent (symbolized as FH_4-C). The varieties of FH_4-C differ in the identity of the one-carbon unit and the site of its attachment to FH_4 (Fig. 25-2). One-carbon substituents of biochemical significance include the following:

formyl $-CH=O$
formimino $-CH=NH_2$
methenyl $-CH=$
methylene $-CH_2$
methyl $-CH_3$

These substituents are attached to FH_4 through N^5, N^{10}, or both (see Fig. 25-2). Specific enzymes interconvert these various FH_4 derivatives.

Reduced derivatives of folic acid are usually sensitive to air oxidation. An exception of clinical importance is N^5-formyl FH_4, also called *citrovorum factor*, *leucovorin*, and *folinic acid*.

NUTRITION

SOURCES

There are many sources for folic acid. The richest vegetable sources are asparagus, broccoli, endive, spinach, lettuce, and lima beans; each contains more than 1 mg of folate per 100 g dry weight. The best fruit sources are lemons, bananas, and melons. Folates are also abundant in liver, kidney, yeast, and mushrooms. An average daily U.S. diet contains 400 to 600 μg of folate.[2] Foods are readily depleted of their

---

†Acronyms and abbreviations that appear in this chapter include: AICAR, 5-amino-4-imidazole carboxamide ribotide; ATP, adenosine 5′9-triphosphate; NADP, nicotinamide adenine dinucleotide phosphate; NADPH, nicotinamide adenine dinucleotide phosphate (reduced form); TC II, transcobalamin II.

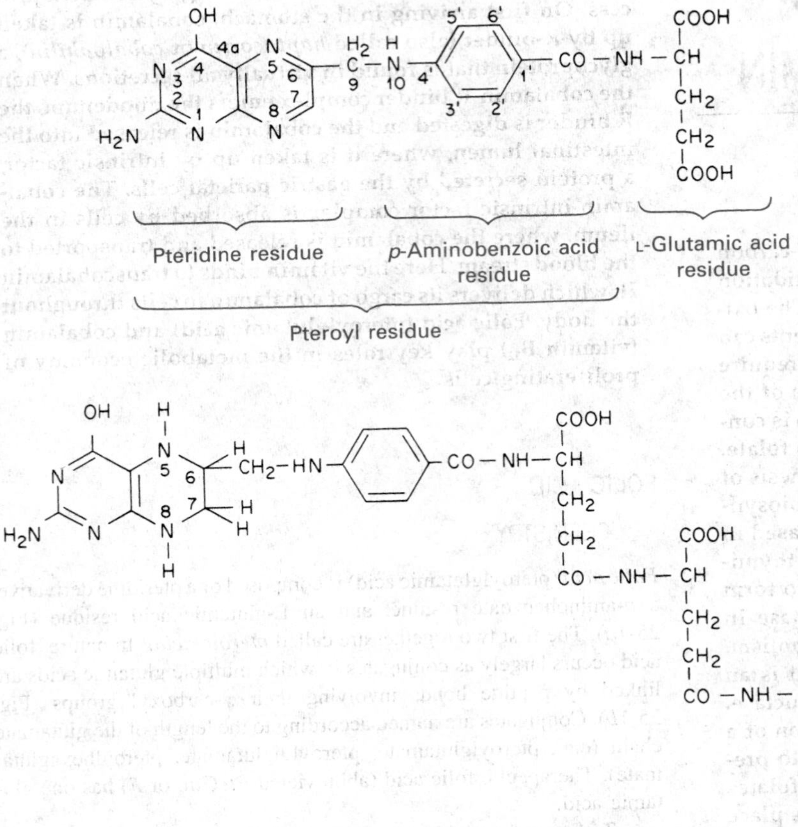

FIGURE 25-1   Folic acid. (a) Folic acid (pteroylglutamic acid) and its components. (b) Tetrahydrofolate triglutamate.

folate, however, by excessive cooking, especially with large amounts of water.

DAILY REQUIREMENTS

In the normal adult, the minimum daily requirement for folic acid is approximately 50 μg. The average diet contains many times this amount, but some may be unavailable. Accordingly, the officially recommended daily allowance of *food* folate for the adult is 0.4 mg.[3] The body is thought to contain approximately 5 mg of folate[4]; when folate intake is reduced to 5 μg/day, megaloblastic anemia develops in about 4 months.[5]

Increased requirements for folic acid occur in hemolytic anemia, leukemia, and other malignant diseases; in alcoholism[6]; during growth; and in pregnancy and lactation, which increase requirements threefold to sixfold.[7] For reasons described in Chap. 38, adequate folate supplies are particularly important in pregnant women, in whom the recommended intake is 400 μg per day.[8]

FOLATE METABOLISM

FOLATE-DEPENDENT ENZYMES

FH$_4$ is an intermediate in reactions involving the transfer of one-carbon units from a donor X—C to an acceptor Y:

$$X-C + FH_4 \rightarrow FH_4-C + X$$
$$\underline{FH_4-C + Y \rightarrow Y-C + FH_4}$$
$$\text{Sum: } X-C + Y \rightarrow Y-C + X$$

The metabolic systems of animal tissues known to require folic acid coenzymes are summarized in Table 25-1 and reviewed in references 3, 6, 25, and 26.

One-carbon units enter the folate pool principally by way of the serine hydroxymethyltransferase reaction[9]:

$$\text{Serine} + FH_4 \leftrightarrow \text{Glycine} + N^5,N^{10}\text{-methylene } FH_4 + H_2O$$

which requires pyridoxal phosphate as cofactor. In addition, the conversion of methionine to polyamines is accompanied by the production of one-carbon fragments that combine with folate at the oxidation level of formate[10,11] (Fig. 25-3). Less important sources of one-carbon units are the catabolism of histidine[12] and the ATP-dependent formation of N^5-formyl FH$_4$ (folinic acid) from formic acid and FH$_4$.[13]

Among the one-carbon transfers mediated by folic acid, the one that appears to be clinically the most important is the methylation of deoxyuridylate to thymidylate, catalyzed by the enzyme thymidylate synthase.[14] This reaction is an essential step in the synthesis of DNA (Fig. 25-4). In carrying out this reaction, N^5,N^{10}-methylene FH$_4$ simultaneously transfers and reduces a one-carbon group, itself serving as the hydrogen donor for the reduction.[15] The reaction generates FH$_2$ (Fig. 25-5), which must be reduced again to FH$_4$ by dihydrofolate reductase and NADPH before it can again be utilized as a coenzyme:

$$dUMP + N^5,N^{10}\text{-methylene } FH_4 \rightarrow FH_2 + dTMP$$
$$FH_2 + NADPH + H^+ \rightarrow FH_4 + NADP^+$$

Limitation of thymidylate synthesis in folic acid deficiency causes uracil to be incorporated into DNA instead of thymine.[16]

Deficiency of folate also diminishes purine biosynthesis by slowing (1) the folate-dependent formylation of glycinamide ribotide to N-formylglycinamide ribotide, the reaction that places the C-8 in the purine ring, and (2) the folate-dependent conversion of 5-amino-4-imidazole carboxamide ribotide (AICAR) to 5-formamido-4-imidazole carboxamide ribotide, the reaction that places the C-2 in the purine ring.[17] The decrease in purine synthesis, however, is offset by the

TABLE 25-1   METABOLIC SYSTEMS REQUIRING FOLIC ACID COENZYMES IN ANIMAL CELLS

SYSTEM	RELATED TRANSFORMATIONS OF FOLIC ACID COENZYMES
Serine ⇌ glycine	Serine + FH$_4$ ⇌ N^5,N^{10}-methylene FH$_4$ + glycine
Thymidylate synthesis	Deoxyuridylate (dUMP) + N^5,N^{10}-methylene FH$_4$ → FH$_2$ + thymidylate (dTMP)
Histidine catabolism	Formiminoglutamate + FH$_4$ → N^5-formimino FH$_4$ + glutamate
Methionine synthesis	Homocysteine + N^5-methyl FH$_4$ → FH$_4$ + methionine
Purine synthesis	Glycinamide ribotide + N^{10}-formyl FH$_4$ → FH$_4$ + formylglycinamide ribotide
Purine synthesis	5-Amino-4-imidazole carboxamide ribotide + N^{10}-formyl FH$_4$ → FH$_4$ + 5-formamido-4-imidazole carboxamide ribotide

ability of AICAR to slow purine degradation by inhibiting both adenosine deaminase and adenylate deaminase.[1] This may explain why no clinical manifestations have thus far been traced to the block in purine synthesis. Interference with the breakdown of histidine (Fig. 25-6) leads to the excretion of formininoglutamic acid (FIGlu) in the urine of folate-deficient patients.

Additional pteridine-dependent reactions of potential metabolic importance are the hydroxylation of phenylalanine to tyrosine, the oxidation of long-chain alkyl ethers of glycerol to fatty acid, the hydroxylation of tryptophan to 6-hydroxytryptophan (a precursor of serotonin), the 17-α-hydroxylation of progesterone,[1,17,18] and the production of nitric oxide (NO).[19–21] The cofactor for these reactions is biopterin, a nonfolate pteridine derivative. Tetrahydrofolic acid is weakly active in some of these systems in vitro[22,23]; whether it plays any such role in vivo is not known.

SIGNIFICANCE OF FOLYLPOLYGLUTAMATES

Intracellular folates exist primarily as polyglutamate conjugates.[24–26] About 75 percent of the folate in human erythrocytes and leukocytes is conjugated.[27,28] Plasma folate, however, consists almost exclusively of the monoglutamate N^5-methyl FH_4[29] and is transported into the cells in this form. Inside the cells, the polyglutamate chain is added by an ATP-dependent *folylpoly-γ-glutamyl synthase*.[30,31] The activity of the human synthase depends strongly on the form of the folate substrate, declining in the order N^5, N^{10}-methylene $FH_4 \rightarrow N^{10}$-formyl $FH_4 \rightarrow N^5$-methyl FH_4, toward which the enzyme is almost inert.[32] In humans, conjugated folates carry on average seven to eight glutamyl residues[33]; the length of the polyglutamate chain may be determined by the ability of the higher folate polyglutamates to inhibit folylpolyglutamyl synthase.[34] There is evidence that folylpolyglutamyl synthase is regulated within cells, its activity closely paralleling rates of DNA synthesis.[35]

Intracellular folylmonoglutamates leak out of the cells at a fairly rapid rate, while the polyglutamates do not, presumably because of the highly charged polyglutamate tail.[36] Attachment of the polyglutamate chain is therefore essential for retaining folates within cells. Moreover, folylpolyglutamates are superior to monoglutamates as substrates for folate-dependent enzyme reactions.[37,38]

PHYSIOLOGY

INTESTINAL ABSORPTION

The proximal jejunum is the principal site of folate absorption. Absorption of a dose of either unconjugated or conjugated folate begins within minutes, and peak levels are reached in 1 to 2 h. Since only folylmonoglutamate appears in plasma, all folylpolyglutamates are deconjugated during absorption across the intestine.[39,40]

Deconjugating enzymes ("conjugases") play an important but poorly understood role in the intestinal absorption of folate.[40,41] Folylpolyglutamate may be hydrolyzed within the lumen of the intestine, and the monoglutamate product may be absorbed subsequently.[42,43] Alternatively, hydrolysis may occur at the brush border of the intestinal

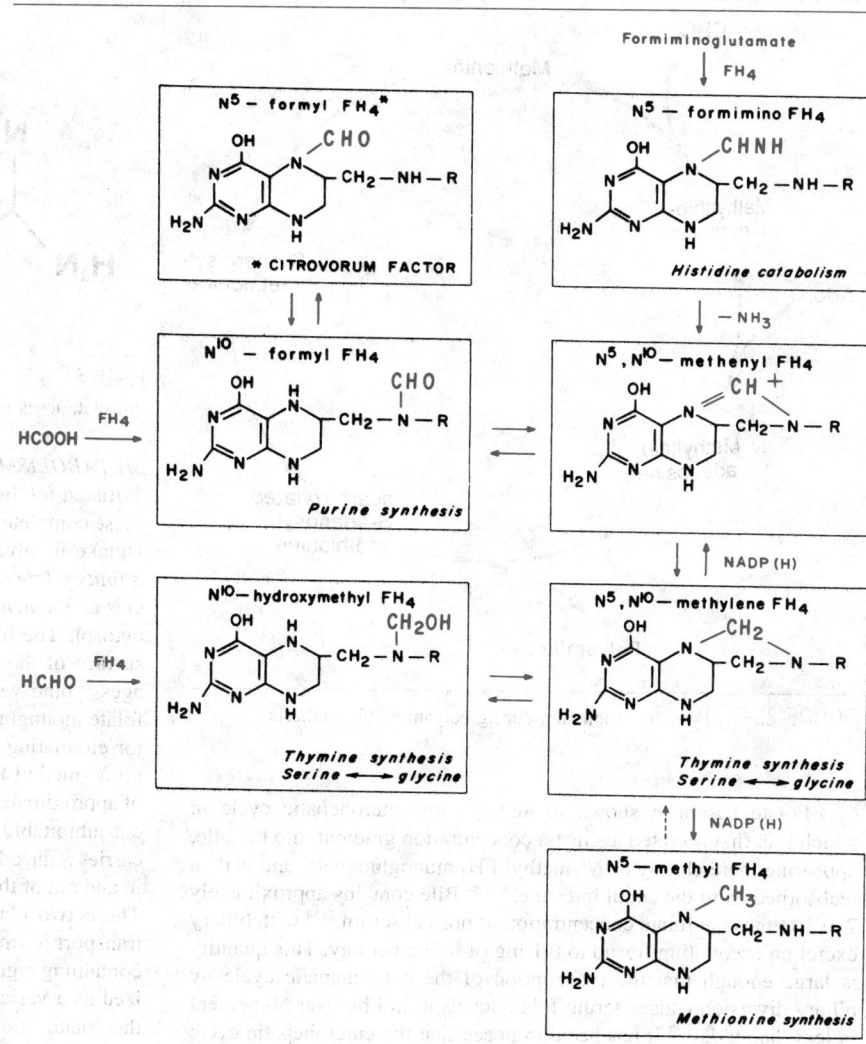

FIGURE 25-2   Derivatives of tetrahydrofolic acid (FH_4), their interconversions, and the metabolic pathways in which they participate. One-carbon substituents are shown in blue.

cell (Fig. 25-7). A brush border conjugase purified from human jejunum catalyzes the Zn^{2+}-dependent deconjugation of folate polyglutamates ranging from $PteGlu_2$ to at least $PteGlu_7$ ($K_m = 0.6$ μM for both substrates).[44] It is an exopeptidase, successively removing single glutamate residues from the end of the polyglutamate chain to yield the folylmonoglutamate.

Conjugases are not found only in the intestine. Human plasma, for example, contains sufficient conjugase to convert polyglutamates containing more than three glutamyl residues to monoglutamates.[45] Other conjugases appear to be lysosomal carboxypeptidases[31,46] that have nothing to do with the absorption of folates from the intestine.

Once deconjugated, the folates are actively transported across the intestinal epithelium[47,48] by a carrier-mediated mechanism ($K_m = 1$ to 2 μM) that is independent of Na^+, K^+, and transmembrane potential.[49] This mechanism uses the pH gradient between the jejunal lumen (pH~6) and the interior of the epithelial cell to drive folate into the cell against a concentration gradient.[50] Passive transport may also occur.[51] In the intestinal cell, the absorbed folate monoglutamates are reduced if necessary, then converted to N^5-methyl FH_4 (some N^{10}-formyl FH_4 is made as well) and transported into the bloodstream without further change.[29,52]

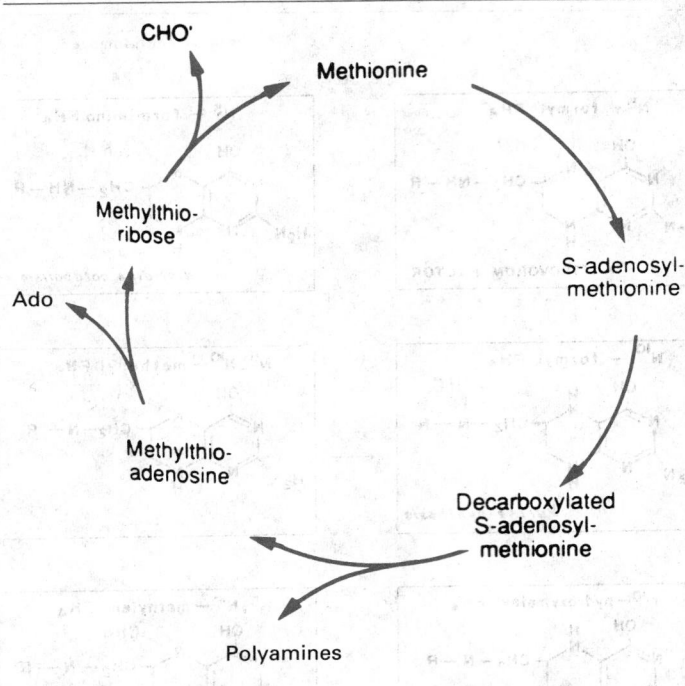

FIGURE 25-3   Formate production during polyamine biosynthesis.

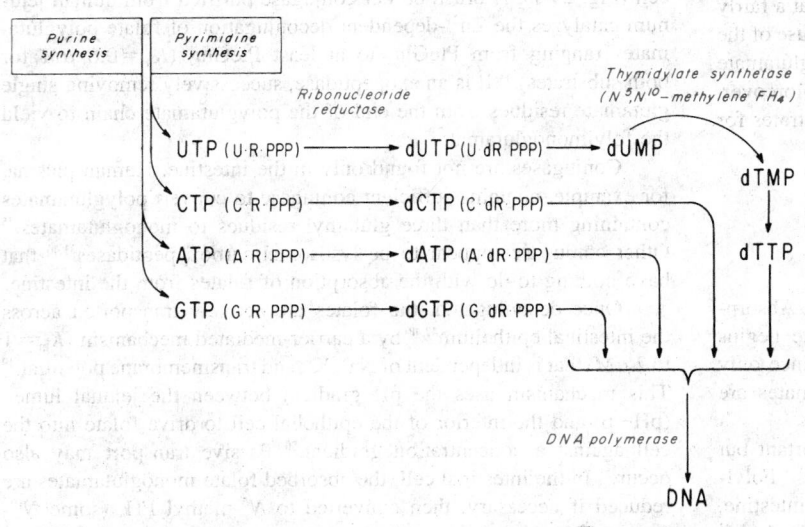

FIGURE 25-4   Pathways of deoxynucleotide and DNA synthesis.

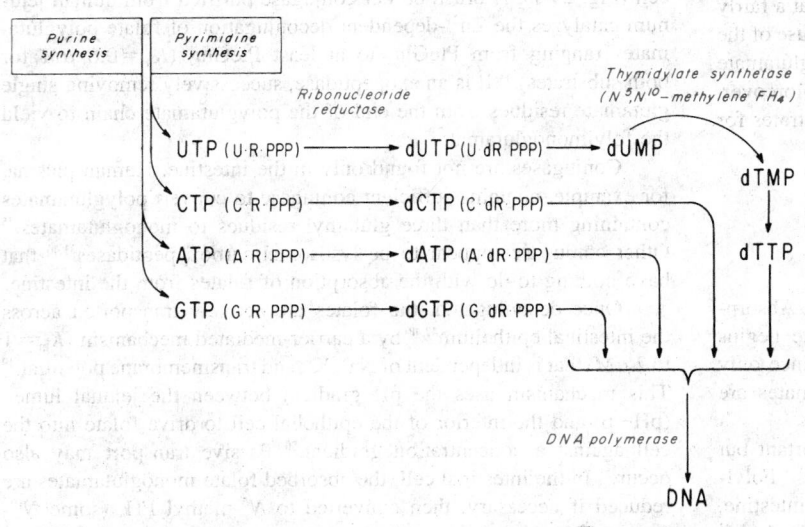

FIGURE 25-5   Dihydrofolate (FH_2). The double bond formed when tetrahydrofolate loses two hydrogens is shown in blue.

METABOLISM

Tritiated folylmonoglutamate (^{3}H-F) administered intravenously is almost completely removed from the bloodstream in a few minutes.[57] Uptake involves two classes of folate-binding proteins[56,58]: the *high-affinity folate receptors*[59–62] that concentrate folate in intracellular vesicles and a *membrane folate transporter* that transports folate into the cytosol. The high-affinity receptors, which are attached to the outer surface of the cell membrane by glycosyl-phosphatidylinositol linkages,[63] bind very tightly (K_d's in the nM range) to most physiologic folate monoglutamates,[56,58,64–66] in particular to N^5-methyl FH_4, the major circulating folate.[67] Their very high affinity enables them to take up N^5-methyl FH_4 from the plasma even at its ambient concentration of approximately 10 nM. The membrane folate transporter is a probenecid-inhibitable organic anion carrier anion that among other things carries reduced folates and methotrexate (but not oxidized folate itself) in and out of the cytoplasm.[56,58,67,68] Its K_m for folate is in the μM range. These two classes of receptors cooperate in the following way to transport N^5-methyl FH_4 into the cell[67,69,70]: (1) A region of membrane containing a group of folate-loaded high-affinity receptors is internalized as a vesicle (the *caveola*), (2) the caveola is acidified, releasing the folate into the vesicle lumen, (3) the folate is passed from the caveola to the cytoplasm by the membrane folate transporter, and, finally, (4) the caveola recycles to the cell surface, where its high-affinity receptors take on another load of N^5-methyl FH_4.

Once internalized, the folates are retained by the cells partly through polyglutamylation, as was discussed above,[71] but also through tight association with a set of intracellular folate-binding proteins.[67,72–74] Three of these proteins are enzymes involved in methyl group metabolism: sarcosine dehydrogenase and dimethylglycine dehydrogenase (mitochondrial)[75] and glycine N-methyl transferase (cytosolic).[76] It is not known why these enzymes bind folate so avidly or whether this binding affects overall methyl group metabolism, although it has been speculated that glycine N-methyl transferase regulates methyl group metabolism by controlling the tissue concentration of S-adenosylhomocysteine, one of its reaction products and a potent inhibitor of most methyltransferases.

Folates have been found in all body tissues that have been analyzed. The principal form of the vitamin in tissues as well as blood appears to be the N^5-methyl form.[75,77–79] Human liver contains 0.7 to 17 μg of folate per gram.[80]

The total folate pool turns over very slowly.[81] A portion of this turnover is accounted for by degradation; p-aminobenzoylglutamate has been identified as a breakdown product. The fate of the pteridine moiety is unknown.

Folate has been shown to undergo an enterohepatic cycle in which it is first secreted against a concentration gradient into the bile, appearing there chiefly as N^5-methyl FH_4 monoglutamate, and is then reabsorbed from the small intestine.[29,53,54] Bile contains approximately 2 to 10 times the folate concentration of normal serum,[29,54] with biliary excretion accounting for up to 0.1 mg of folate per day. This quantity is large enough that the interruption of the enterohepatic cycle by biliary diversion causes serum folate levels to fall by over 50 percent in less than a day.[53] It has been proposed that the enterohepatic cycle serves to redistribute folate between hepatic stores and peripheral tissues according to the state of the exogenous folate supplies[55]; this view, however, has been disputed.[56]

FOLATE-BINDING PROTEINS OF SERUM AND MILK

The soluble folate-binding proteins of serum and milk are high-affinity folate receptors that have been released from cell membranes by proteolysis.[56,82] These proteins can be detected in approximately 15 percent of normal individuals[83] and are found at increased levels in some pregnant women, women on oral contraceptives, folate-deficient alcoholics (but not patients with cobalamin deficiency),[84] and patients with uremia, hepatic cirrhosis, and chronic myelogenous leukemia.[85,86] In normal subjects, the proteins are about two-thirds saturated and show a total folate-binding capacity of approximately 175 pg per milliliter of serum.[87] Failure to detect the proteins in some subjects seems to be due to their prior saturation with unlabeled folate.[88] The serum protein has an M_r of 40,000 and prefers oxidized to reduced folates.[88]

Folate-binding proteins have also been found in milk and in normal granulocytes.[89,90] Folate bound to the milk folate binder is absorbed chiefly in the ileum[91] rather than the jejunum, the principal site of absorption of free folate. The milk folate binder, a glycoprotein, also promotes folate transport into the liver via the asialoglycoprotein receptor.[92] It has been speculated that the milk folate binder protects an infant's folate supply by preventing bacteria from sequestering the vitamin away from the intestinal lumen.[56] The folate-binding protein in granulocytes has been localized to the specific granules, from which it is released when the granulocytes are stimulated.[93]

EXCRETION

Folates are both resorbed and secreted by the kidney. Resorption is accomplished by means of a membrane-bound high-affinity folate receptor (K_m for N^5-methyl $FH_4 = 0.4$ nM) located in the brush borders of the proximal tubules.[94] Filtered folate is carried rapidly by this receptor into the proximal tubule cell and from there makes its way slowly into the bloodstream.[95,96] At the same time, folate is secreted into the proximal tubule by a nonspecific probenecid-sensitive organic anion carrier that is closely related or identical to the membrane folate transporter and is also responsible for the renal secretion of p-aminohippuric acid (which blocks renal folate secretion), penicillin, and uric acid.[96] The net result of these two processes is the resorption of most of but not all the filtered folate.

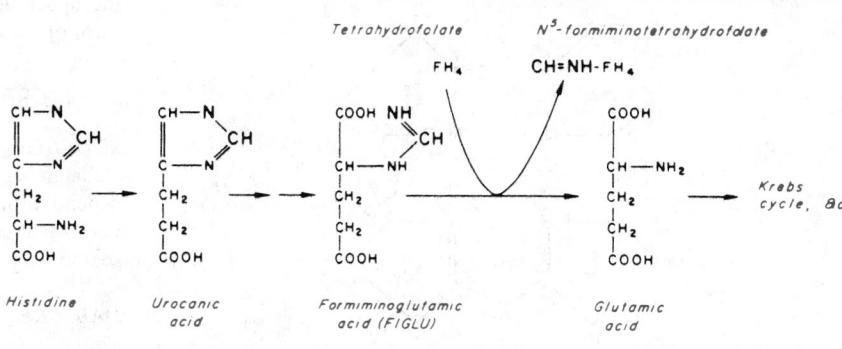

FIGURE 25-6   The catabolism of histidine.

In humans, intact folates and their cleavage products are excreted by the kidney at a rate of 2 to 5 μg/day.[97] Folates given in doses lower than 15 μg/kg are excreted in the urine in reduced forms, particularly as N^{10}-formyl FH_4.[98] With doses of folate greater than 15 μg/kg, large amounts are excreted unchanged.

A small percentage of parenterally administered ^{3}H-F is recoverable in the feces. This mainly represents overflow from the enterohepatic cycle discussed above.

ASSAY OF SERUM FOLATE

Microbiological assays for folate were in use for many years. Now, however, they have been largely supplanted by isotopic methods employing various folate binders. These isotopic folate assays are identical in principle to radioimmunoassays.

COBALAMIN

CHEMISTRY

STRUCTURE AND NOMENCLATURE

The cobalamin molecule has two major portions: a porphyrinlike near-planar macrocycle known as *corrin* and a nucleotide that lies almost perpendicular to the corrin ring (Fig. 25-8). The corrin moiety contains four reduced pyrrole rings[8,16,32,81] that bind a central cobalt atom whose two remaining coordination positions are occupied by a 5,6-dimethyl-benzimidazolyl group (below the ring) and various ligands (above the ring; in this case, —CN).

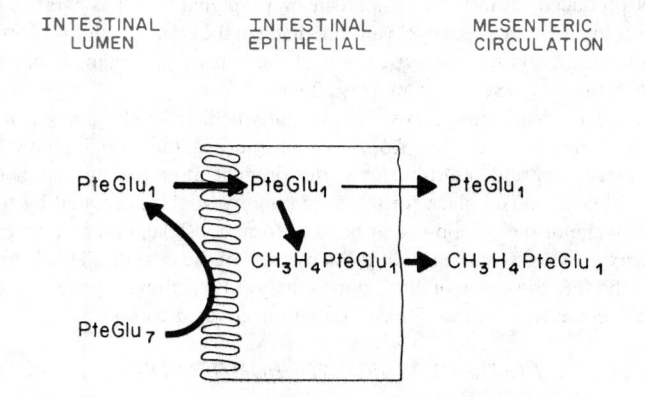

FIGURE 25-7   Digestion and absorption of folate polyglutamate by the intestine. The polyglutamate (in this case, PteGlu7) is hydrolyzed in the intestinal lumen or at the brush border. The resulting pteroylglutamate (PteGlu) is transported into the intestinal cell, where it is reduced and methylated, appearing in the circulation chiefly as N^5-methyl FH_4.

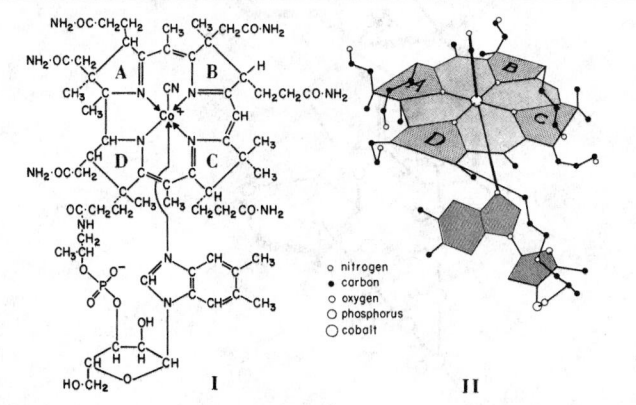

FIGURE 25-8   *I,* structure of cyanocobalamin (CNCbl; vitamin B_{12}). *II,* partial structure of CNCbl, showing the relationship between the corrin ring and the nucleotide.

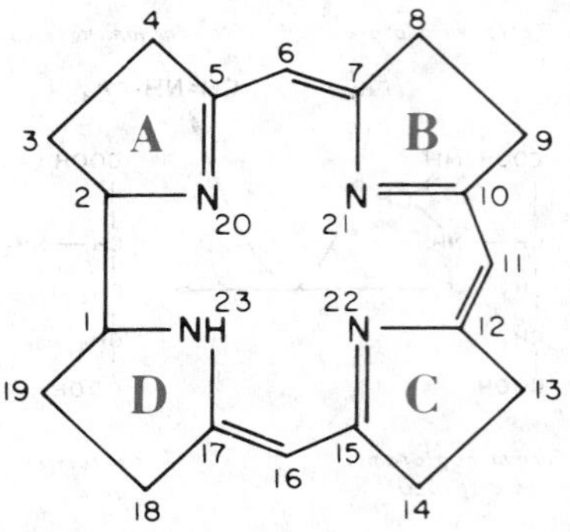

FIGURE 25-9   The corrin ring, showing ring designations and standard numbering of the atoms.

Compounds containing the corrin ring are known as *corrinoids*. The cobalamins are corrinoids whose nucleotide contains 5,6-dimethylbenzimidazole. There are two connections between the corrin and the nucleotide: (1) a bond between the nucleotide phosphate and a side chain in ring D and (2) a bond between cobalt and a nitrogen atom of benzimidazole. The numbering and ring designations of the corrin system are summarized in Fig. 25-9.

The term *vitamin B12* is sometimes employed as a generic term for the corrinoids. It is probably best reserved, however, as an alternative name for cyanocobalamin, the usual therapeutic corrinoid.

Four cobalamins are of importance in animal cell metabolism. Two are *cyanocobalamin* (CNCbl; vitamin B_{12}) and *hydroxocobalamin* (OHCbl). The other two are alkyl derivatives that are synthesized from hydroxocobalamin and serve as coenzymes. In one, *adenosylcobalamin* (AdoCbl), a 5-deoxyadenosyl replaces OH as the cobalt ligand above the ring (Fig. 25-10).[99] In the second, *methylcobalamin* (MeCbl),

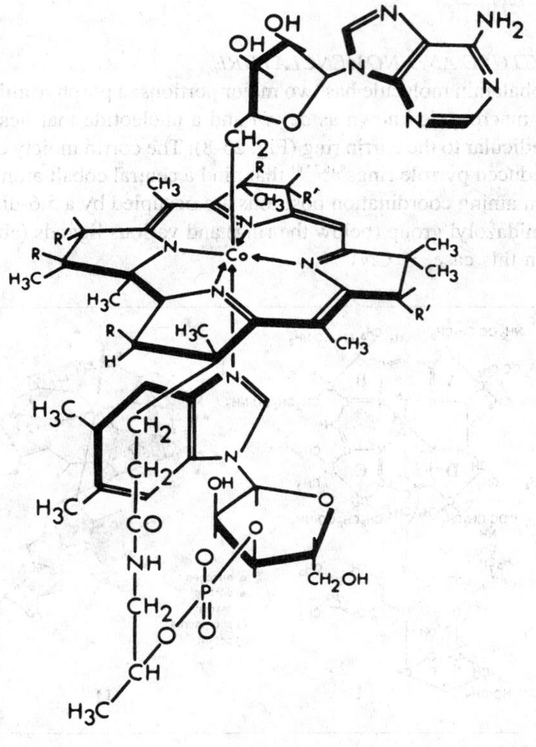

FIGURE   25-10   Adenosylcobalamin   (AdoCbl).   R=CH2CONH2; R'=CH2CH2CONH2.

the upper ligand is a methyl group. Methylcobalamin is the major form of cobalamin in human blood plasma.[100]

NUTRITION

SOURCES
Cobalamin is synthesized only by certain microorganisms, and animals depend ultimately on microbial synthesis for their cobalamin supply. Foods that contain cobalamin are those of animal origin: meat, liver, seafood, and dairy products. Cobalamin has not been found in plants.

DAILY REQUIREMENTS
The average daily diet in Western countries contains 5 to 30 μg of cobalamin. Of this, 1 to 5 μg is absorbed.[101] Less than 250 ng appears in the urine; the unabsorbed remainder appears in the feces. Total body content is 2 to 5 mg in an adult,[102] with approximately 1 mg in the liver. The kidneys are also rich in cobalamin.[103] Relative to the daily requirement, body reserves of cobalamin are much larger than those of folate.

Cobalamin has a daily rate of obligatory loss of approximately 0.1 percent of the total body pool, irrespective of the pool size. For this reason, a deficiency state will not develop for several years after the cessation of cobalamin intake. The officially recommended daily allowance for adults is 5 μg[3]; growth, hypermetabolic states, and pregnancy increase daily requirements. For infants during the first year the recommended daily allowance is 1 to 2 μg. In cobalamin-deficient subjects, a normal diet containing about 15 μg per day will replenish depleted body stores.[104]

ROLE IN METABOLISM
The only two recognized cobalamin-dependent enzymes in human cells are adenosylcobalamin-dependent *methylmalonyl CoA mutase* and methylcobalamin-dependent *methyltetrahydrofolate-homocysteine methyltransferase*. The presence in humans of a third cobalamin-dependent enzyme, leucine 2,3-aminomutase, is controversial.[104,105]

METHYLMALONYL CoA MUTASE
Methylmalonyl CoA mutase is a mitochondrial enzyme that participates in the disposal of the propionate formed during the breakdown of valine and isoleucine. The enzyme is a homodimer of a 78-kD subunit that is encoded by a gene on chromosome 6.[106,107] In the reaction catalyzed by methylmalonyl CoA mutase, methylmalonyl CoA, which is produced during the catabolism of propionate,[108] is converted to succinyl CoA, a Krebs cycle intermediate. In the course of this reaction, a hydrogen on the methyl carbon of the substrate exchanges places with the —COSCoA group (Fig. 25-11).

The coenzyme serves as an intermediate hydrogen carrier, accepting the hydrogen from the substrate in the initial phase of the reaction and returning it to the product after the migration of —COSCoA. The place for the migrating hydrogen is created by the cleavage of the carbon-cobalt bond to form cob(II)alamin and the 5'-deoxyadenos-5'-yl radical at the active site of the enzyme. This is one of the few examples of an enzyme-catalyzed reaction mediated by an active-site free radical situated on an unactivated carbon.

N^5-METHYLTETRAHYDROFOLATE:HOMOCYSTEINE METHYLTRANSFERASE
Methylcobalamin participates in the cobalamin-dependent synthesis of methionine according to the scheme shown in Fig. 25-12.[109–111] S-adenosylmethionine and methionine synthase reductase are required for methyltransferase activity, probably to reactivate enzyme molecules whose coenzyme has become inactivated by oxidation of the

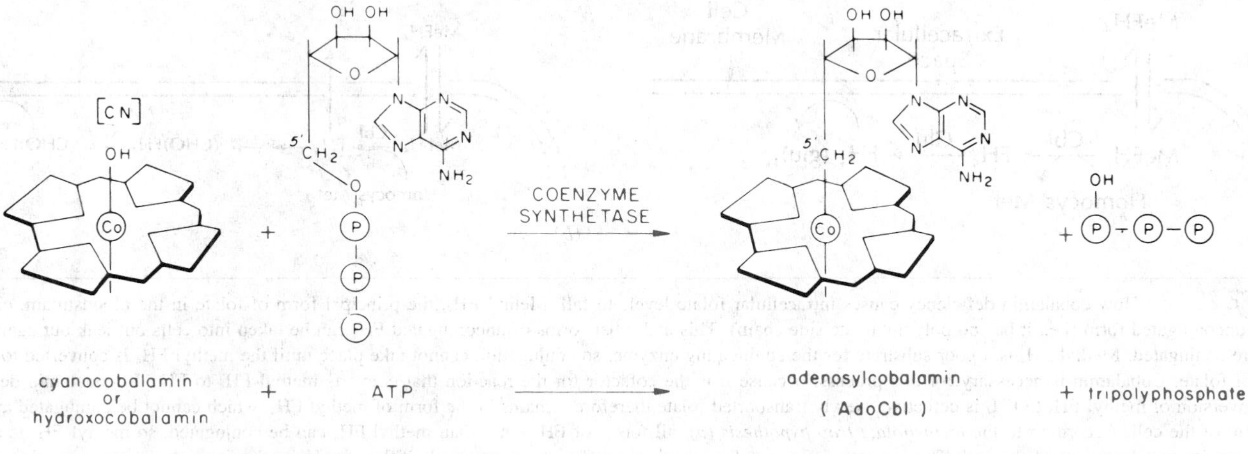

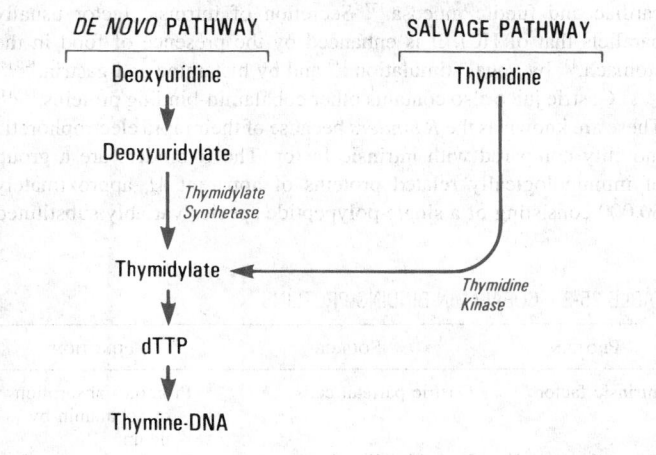

FIGURE 25-11   Biosynthesis of AdoCbl.

cobalt.[112] The reductase converts the oxidized cobalt to the readily alkylatable Co[1+], which then accepts a methyl group from S-adenosyl-methionine, a powerful biological methylating agent, thereby restoring the activity of the methyltransferase. In humans this pathway also serves as a mechanism for converting N^5-methyltetrahydrofolate to tetrahydrofolate. The demethylation of N^5-methyl FH$_4$ is a prerequisite for the attachment of the polyglutamate chain to newly acquired folate, which is largely taken up by the cell in the form of N^5-methyl FH$_4$ monoglutamate.[29] Nitrous oxide (N$_2$O) impairs the methyltransferase by oxidizing cob(I)alamin (a catalytic intermediate in the methyltransferase reaction) to cob(II)alamin.[113] This depletes MeCbl and produces a cobalamin deficiency–like state.[114]

NONENZYMATIC METABOLISM
Since cobalamin has the capacity to bind cyanide, it is possible that it participates in the metabolism of this toxin in humans. Tobacco and certain foods (fruits, beans, and nuts) contain cyanide. Although the evidence is inconclusive, it is thought that cobalamin may play a role in neutralizing cyanide taken in via these substances.[115]

THE FOLATE-COBALAMIN RELATIONSHIP
In both folate deficiency and cobalamin deficiency, the megaloblastic anemias are fully corrected by treatment with the appropriate vitamin.

FIGURE 25-12   Incorporation of thymidine into DNA via the *de novo* and salvage pathways. (Adapted from Metz.[219])

The megaloblastic anemia of cobalamin deficiency is also largely corrected by folic acid supplementation even if no cobalamin is given, while, conversely, the anemia of folate deficiency is not helped at all by cobalamin. These clinical observations indicate that in cobalamin deficiency, the megaloblastic anemia is actually a result of an abnormality in folate metabolism.[36] Further evidence that folate metabolism is deranged by cobalamin deficiency is provided by the observation that urinary excretion of FIGlu and AICAR, normally regarded as a sign of folate deficiency, is seen occasionally in pure cobalamin deficiency.[116]

Two explanations have been offered to account for the folate responsiveness of cobalamin-deficient megaloblastic anemia: the *methylfolate trap* hypothesis, which has been accepted by the majority of authorities, and the *formate starvation* hypothesis (Fig. 25-13).

The Methylfolate Trap Hypothesis   The methylfolate trap hypothesis[117,118] is based on the fact that the folate-requiring enzyme N^5-methyl FH$_4$ homocysteine methyltransferase is also dependent on cobalamin. This hypothesis states that in cobalamin deficiency, tissue folates are gradually diverted into the N^5-methyl FH$_4$ pool because of the slowing of the methyltransferase reaction,[119,120] the only route out of that pool for folate. As N^5-methyl FH$_4$ levels increase, levels of the other forms of folate decline, with a consequent fall in the rates of reactions in which those forms participate. In particular, the synthesis of dTMP is slowed, and megaloblastic anemia ensues.

In its simplest form, this hypothesis predicts that in cobalamin deficiency, tissue levels of N^5-methyl FH$_4$ should be abnormally high and those of other forms of folate should be abnormally low. Although serum N^5-methyl FH$_4$ levels are elevated in cobalamin deficiency,[118,121] tissue folate levels actually decline, while increases in the fraction of tissue folates in the form of N^5-methyl FH$_4$ may[78,120] or may not[25,122] occur. The folates whose relative levels do consistently fall as total folate levels decline are the polyglutamates.[28,122,123] Their fall appears to be related to the substrate specificity of the folate-conjugating enzyme. This enzyme works very poorly with N^5-methyl FH$_4$ and is therefore unable to carry out normal γ-glutamylation of newly internalized N^5-methyl FH$_4$ monoglutamate in cobalamin-deficient cells because the freshly acquired folate cannot be converted into a suitable substrate (i.e., free FH$_4$ or formyl FH$_4$). Thus, while sequestration of tissue folates in an expanded N^5-methyl FH$_4$ pool may account for some of the effects of the blockade in methyltransferase activity, the major problem seems to be a failure to convert newly acquired folate into a form that can be retained by the cell, the upshot being the development of a tissue folate deficiency as the unconjugated

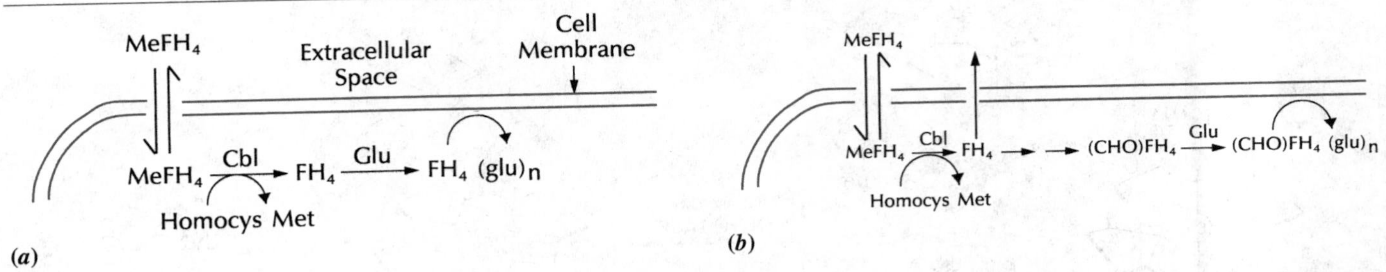

FIGURE 25-13   How cobalamin deficiency causes intracellular folate levels to fall. Methyl FH$_4$, the principal form of folate in the bloodstream, circulates in the unconjugated form (i.e., it has no polyglutamate side chain). This and other forms of unconjugated FH$_4$ can be taken into cells but leak out again unless they are conjugated. Methyl FH$_4$ is a poor substrate for the conjugating enzyme, so conjugation cannot take place until the methyl FH$_4$ is converted to another form of folate. Cobalamin is necessary for this process, because it is the cofactor for the reaction that converts methyl FH$_4$ to FH$_4$. In cobalamin deficiency the conversion of methyl FH$_4$ to FH$_4$ is defective. Newly transported folate therefore remains in the form of methyl FH$_4$, which cannot be conjugated and leaks back out of the cell. According to the *methylfolate trap hypothesis (a)*, all forms of FH$_4$ other than methyl FH$_4$ can be conjugated, so methyl FH$_4$ is the only folate species that leaks out of the cell. The *formate deficiency hypothesis (b)* differs from the methylfolate trap hypothesis solely in assuming that only the formylated folates (N^{10}-formyl FH$_4$ and/or N^5,N^{10}-methenyl FH$_4$) can be conjugated, so newly transported methyl FH$_4$, N^5,N^{10}-methylene FH$_4$, and free FH$_4$ all leak out of the cell. (CH$_2$) FH$_4$ = N^5,N^{10}-methylene FH$_4$; (CHO) FH$_4$ = N^{10}-formyl FH$_4$ or N^5,N^{10}-methenyl FH$_4$.

folate leaks out (Fig. 25-14). This whole process is aggravated by a drop in tissue levels of S-adenosylmethionine as the methionine supply is curtailed because of the diminished activity of the methyltransferase.[36,124,125] S-adenosylmethionine, which is necessary for methyltransferase activity as discussed above, is also a powerful inhibitor of N^5,N^{10}-methylene FH$_4$ reductase,[36,124] the enzyme responsible for the production of N^5-methyl FH$_4$. The relief of this inhibition as S-adenosylmethionine levels fall accelerates the flow of folates toward N^5-methyl FH$_4$, further aggravating the metabolic imbalance that results from the impairment in methyltransferase activity.

This problem could be overcome if N^5-methyl FH$_4$ could be converted into a substrate for the conjugating enzyme by another route. In theory, this could be accomplished by the reversal of the N^5,N^{10}-methylene FH$_4$ reductase reaction or by the catabolism of N^5-methyl FH$_4$ via the methylation of biogenic amines.[22,23,109] In fact, however, the N^5,N^{10}-methylene FH$_4$ reductase reaction is for practical purposes irreversible in vivo,[126] and the methylation of biogenic amines by N^5-methyl FH$_4$ is too slow to provide much relief.

The Formate Starvation Hypothesis   This hypothesis holds that formate starvation is the basis for the folate-responsive megaloblastic anemia of cobalamin deficiency.[124,127] This theory is based on the diminished capacity of cobalamin-deficient lymphoblasts to incorporate formaldehyde into purine and methionine[125] and on experiments showing that N^5-formyl FH$_4$ is more effective than FH$_4$ at correcting some of the abnormalities in folate metabolism seen in cobalamin deficiency.[124,128,129] The hypothesis states that with the fall in methionine production in cobalamin-deficient states, the generation of formate is depressed (since normally the methyl group of excess methionine is rapidly oxidized to formate[124,130,131]), leading to a decline in the production of N^5-formyl FH$_4$. If N^5-formyl FH$_4$ but not FH$_4$ is a substrate

for the conjugating enzyme,[128] then the low tissue folate levels seen in cobalamin deficiency cannot be due merely to impaired demethylation of N^5-methyl FH$_4$ by a cobalamin-deficient homocysteine methyltransferase but must reflect a decreased production of methionine, the source of the formate needed to produce the conjugable substrate, N^5-formyl FH$_4$.

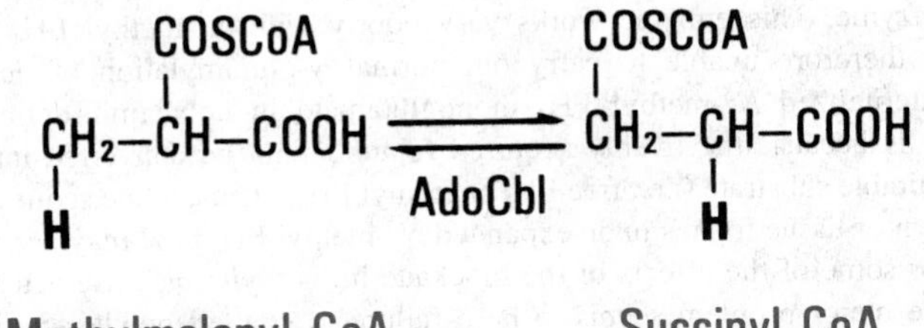

PHYSIOLOGY

INTESTINAL ABSORPTION: THE INTRINSIC FACTOR MECHANISM

Intrinsic factor is one of a number of proteins to which cobalamin is bound as it makes its way through the body (Table 25-2). Intrinsic factor is needed for the absorption of cobalamins given orally at physiologic dosage levels. Human intrinsic factor is a glycoprotein (M_r approximately 44,000) encoded by a gene on chromosome 11.[132] It has binding sites for cobalamin and for a specific ileal receptor, the former situated near the carboxy terminus and the latter near the amino terminus of the intrinsic factor molecule.[133] Binding to cobalamin is very tight.[134-136] Its properties are summarized in Table 25-3. Bound vitamin alters the conformation of intrinsic factor, producing a more compact form that is resistant to proteolytic digestion. In humans, intrinsic factor is synthesized and secreted by the parietal cells of the cardiac and fundic mucosa.[137] Secretion of intrinsic factor usually parallels that of HCl. It is enhanced by the presence of food in the stomach,[138] by vagal stimulation,[139] and by histamine and gastrin.[140,141]

Gastric juice also contains other cobalamin-binding proteins.[142,143] These are known as the *R binders* because of their rapid electrophoretic mobility compared with intrinsic factor. The R binders are a group of immunologically related proteins of apparent M_r approximately 60,000 consisting of a single polypeptide species variably substituted

FIGURE 25-14   The methylmalonyl CoA mutase reaction.

TABLE 25-2   COBALAMIN-BINDING PROTEINS

PROTEIN	SOURCE	FUNCTION
Intrinsic factor	Gastric parietal cells	Promotes absorption of cobalamin by ileum
Transcobalamin II	Probably all cells	Promotes uptake of cobalamin by cells
Cobalophilins	Exocrine glands, phagocytes	Helps dispose of cobalamin analogs (?)

TABLE 25-3   PROPERTIES OF HUMAN INTRINSIC FACTOR

PROPERTY	VALUE	REFERENCE
M_r (approximate)	44,000	105
$E_{1cm}^{1\%}$ at 279 nm	9.5	107
$S_{20,w}^0$	5.75	107
Cyanocobalamin-binding capacity, μg/mg	30.1	105
Association constant for cyanocobalamin, M^{-1}	1.5×10^{10}	105
Composition:		
Carbohydrate content, %	15.0	105
Hexoses, including fucose, %	6.9	107
Hexosamine, residues/mol	4.1	107
Sialic acid, residues/mol	1.7	107

with oligosaccharides that terminate with different quantities of sialic acid.[144,145] These proteins are found in milk, plasma, saliva, gastric juice, and numerous other body fluids. They appear to be synthesized by mucosal cells of the organs that secrete them[146] and by phagocytes.[147] Though they bind cobalamin, they lack intrinsic factor activity, i.e., they are unable to promote the intestinal absorption of the vitamin.

Cobalamins in foods are liberated in the stomach by peptic digestion.[148] They are then bound not to intrinsic factor but to R binders, because, at the acid pH of the stomach, cobalamin binds much more tightly to R binders than to intrinsic factor.[149] On entering the duodenum, cobalamin is released from the cobalamin–R binder complex by digestion with pancreatic proteases, which in normal subjects act by selectively degrading R binders and the cobalamin–R binder complex while sparing intrinsic factor.[149] It is at this point that the cobalamin finally reaches the intrinsic factor to form the intrinsic factor–cobalamin complex.

The intrinsic factor–cobalamin complex, which is very resistant to digestion,[150] then journeys down the intestine until it reaches the intrinsic factor receptor *cubulin*,[151,152] a 460-kDa peripheral membrane protein that is located in the microvillus pits of the ileal mucosa.[153] (The same receptor is found in the brush border of renal proximal tubule cells.[154–157] Its purpose there is unknown.) The ileal mucosa occupies the distal half of the small intestine, and the cubulin is found all along this portion of the intestine, its concentration rising progressively until a maximum is reached near the terminal ileum.[158] A specific site on the intrinsic factor molecule avidly attaches to the receptor in a binding reaction that requires a pH of 5.4 or greater and Ca^{2+} (or other divalent cations) but no energy.[159–161]

Following attachment of intrinsic factor–cobalamin to receptor, the vitamin is taken into the ileal mucosal cells over 30 to 60 min by endocytosis,[161–163] then over many hours is passed by the mucosal cells into the portal blood, while the receptors recycle to the surfaces of the microvilli for another load of intrinsic factor–cobalamin.[163] During its sojourn in the ileal enterocyte the vitamin first appears in the lysosomes, but by 4 h most of it is located in the cytosol.[164] During absorption the entire intrinsic factor–cobalamin complex appears to be taken into the cell, where the cobalamin is released while the intrinsic factor is degraded.[161,165–167]

It requires 3 to 4 h for the cobalamin from a small oral dose (10 to 20 μg) to start to appear in the blood and 8 to 12 h for the vitamin to reach a peak level. In the portal blood, the cobalamin is complexed with a cobalamin-transporting protein known as *transcobalamin II* (TC II).[168] The cobalamin–TC II complex is probably formed in the ileal enterocyte, one of a variety of cells that have been shown to synthesize the transcobalamin.[169–173] Large oral doses (1 mg) of cobalamin are absorbed by simple diffusion that is not mediated by intrinsic factor. In these instances, vitamin appears in blood within minutes, again as the cobalamin–TC II complex.

Like the folates, the cobalamins participate in an enterohepatic cycle. In humans, between 0.5 and 9 μg/day of cobalamins is secreted into the bile, where the cobalamins bind to an R binder and enter the intestine.[174] In the intestine, the cobalamin–R binder complexes of biliary origin are treated exactly like those delivered from the stomach: The cobalamin is released by digestion of the R binder by pancreatic proteases then is taken up by intrinsic factor and reabsorbed. It has been estimated that 65 to 75 percent of the biliary cobalamin is reabsorbed by this mechanism.[175] Because of the size of the cobalamin storage pool and the existence of this enterohepatic circulation, it takes a very long time—sometimes 20 years—to develop clinically significant cobalamin deficiency from a diet providing insufficient cobalamin (e.g., a strictly vegetarian diet). Patients who fail to absorb the vitamin, however, become clinically deficient in only 3 to 6 years, because biliary as well as dietary cobalamin is lost.[176]

COBALAMIN IN THE CELL: TRANSCOBALAMIN II[177]

The Uptake of Cobalamin by Cells   Transcobalamin II (TC II) is the plasma protein that mediates the transport of cobalamin into the tissues. A simple protein of $M_r = 43,000$,[178,179] it binds cobalamin with exceedingly high affinity ($K_a = 10^{11}/M$).[180] Unlike intrinsic factor, whose binding is relatively specific for cobalamins, TC II can also bind certain corrins that are chemically related to the cobalamins but are without function in mammalian systems and have come to be known as cobalamin "analogs."[181] TC II is synthesized by many types of cells, including enterocytes, hepatocytes, mononuclear phagocytes, fibroblasts, hematopoietic precursors in the marrow, and probably others.[161,169–173]

Although circulating TC II carries only a minor fraction of the cobalamin in the plasma, it is the protein to which newly acquired cobalamin is first bound. Cobalamin given parenterally associates almost immediately with unsaturated TC II,[182] while cobalamin absorbed through the intestine is probably carried into the portal blood as the preformed cobalamin–TC II complex. Within minutes after their appearance in the bloodstream, these cobalamin–TC II complexes are transported into the tissues.[182,183] The transport process begins with the binding of the cobalamin–TC II complex to a membrane receptor that is present on a wide variety of cells.[184,185] The receptor-bound complex is then internalized by pinocytosis and delivered to a lysosome, where the TC II is digested and the cobalamin is freed.[185–188] The cobalamin is then actively exported from the lysosome into the cytosol by a specific Mg^{2+}-dependent carrier (K_m for CNCbl = 3.5 μM) that uses a proton gradient as the energy source.[189,190]

Formation of AdoCbl and MeCbl   To be useful to the cell, CNCbl and OHCbl have to be converted to AdoCbl and MeCbl, the coenzymatically active cobalamins. This is accomplished by reduction and alkylation. CNCbl and OHCbl are first reduced to the Co^{2+} form [cob(II)alamin] by NADPH- and NADH-dependent reductases that are present in both mitochondria and microsomes.[191,192] (NADPH–cobalamin reductase activity may be identical to that of NADPH–cytochrome c reductase[193] and NADH–cobalamin reductase to the cytochrome b_5/cytochrome b_5 reductase system.)[194] The CN^- and OH^- are displaced from the metal during reduction. Some of the cob(II)alamin in the mitochondria is reduced further to the intensely nucleophilic Co^+ form [cob(I)alamin]. This is then alkylated by ATP to form AdoCbl in a reaction in which the 5′-deoxyadenosyl moiety of ATP is transferred to the cobalamin and the three phosphates of ATP are released as inorganic triphosphate.[195–197] The rest of the cobalamin binds to cytosolic N^5-methyltetrahydrofolate–homocysteine methyltransferase, where it is converted to MeCbl.[198,199] The fate of cobalamin in the cell is summarized in Fig. 25-15.

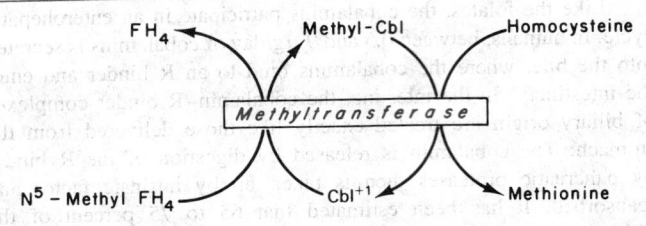

FIGURE 25-15 The N^5-methyl FH₄:homocysteine methyltransferase reaction.

THE PLASMA COBALOPHILINS: TRANSCOBALAMINS I AND III

Transcobalamin I (TC I) is the principal R binder of plasma and carries most of the circulating cobalamin. It is a glycoprotein of M_r=approximately 50,000 containing nine potential glycosylation sites[200] and is encoded by a gene on chromosome 11, the same chromosome that carries the intrinsic factor gene.[201] In contrast to TC II, its clearance from the plasma is very slow ($T_{1/2}$ 9 to 10 days).[202] The cobalamin–TC I complexes are eliminated chiefly by the hepatocytes, into which they are carried by the asialoglycoprotein receptor, there to be degraded and their load of cobalamins excreted in the bile.[202-204] TC I binds its ligands more tightly than does either intrinsic factor or TC II and is less restrictive than either with respect to ligand specificity, avidly taking up corrinoids of widely varying structure.[181,205,206] The ligand-binding properties of TC I, together with its mode of clearance by the liver, have led to the suggestion that TC I helps clear the system of nonphysiologic cobalamin analogs that may be accidentally acquired in the normal course of events.[207] As the liver metabolizes analog–TC I complexes, it will secrete the analogs into the bile. Since these analogs are bound poorly by intrinsic factor,[180,208] they will be poorly reabsorbed from the intestine and instead will be eliminated in the feces. An alternative proposal is that TC I is a storage protein for cobalamins.[209] In reality, however, the physiologic role of TC I is unknown.

A second circulating R binder is known as transcobalamin III (TC III).[210] This protein is found in the plasma as well as in granulocytes,[202,207,211] where it constitutes the cobalamin-binding protein of the specific granules and from which it is released into the serum when blood clots.[212] Structurally, TC I is richer in sialic acid than is TC III. It is likely that the plasma R binders actually consist of half a dozen or more species whose pI values range from 2.9 to 4.0, with ''TC I'' and ''TC III'' representing the arbitrary division of these R binders into a low-pI group and a high-pI group.

ASSAY OF SERUM COBALAMIN AND THE TRANSCOBALAMINS

Cobalamin As with folate, cobalamin is measured using a radioisotope assay employing a cobalamin-binding protein.[213] The misleading results formerly given by this assay were explained by the discovery in serum and tissue of a class of cobalamin analogs that are detected by the radioisotope assay when the binder is R binder but not when intrinsic factor is used as the binder.[208] Current assays use intrinsic factor as binder and give accurate values for serum cobalamin. The chemical nature and biological significance of the analogs are unknown.[214] The *transcobalamins* TC I and TC II are present in plasma in trace quantities (about 7 and 20 μg/liter, respectively), while TC III is often undetectable. In fasting plasma, 70 percent or more of the circulating cobalamin is bound to TC I.[215,216] Nevertheless, TC I has substantial unsaturated binding capacity.[217]

TC II binds only 10 to 25 percent of the total plasma cobalamin[202,218] but provides the majority (about 75 percent) of the total

TABLE 25-4 LEVELS AND BINDING CAPACITY OF COBALAMIN-BINDING PROTEINS IN DISEASE[213]

BINDER	DISEASE
Increased TC I (cobalophilin)	Myeloproliferative disorders
	Polycythemia vera
	Myelofibrosis
	Benign neutrophilia
	Chronic myelocytic leukemia
	Hepatoma (occasionally)
	Metastatic cancer
Increased TC II	Myeloproliferative disorders
	Liver disease
	Inflammatory disorders
	Gaucher disease
	Anti-TC II antibodies
Unsaturated cobalamin binders*	
Increased	Transient neutropenia
	Elevated TC I
Decreased	Liver disease
	Elevated serum cobalamin

*UBBC=unsaturated B₁₂ binding capacity.

unsaturated cobalamin-binding capacity of plasma.[217] Less than 2 percent of the TC II in plasma is saturated at any given moment.

Alterations in unsaturated cobalamin-binding capacity and in TC I and TC II levels in various disease states are listed in Table 25-4.

REFERENCES

1. Baggott JE, Vaughn WH, Hudson BB: Inhibition of 5-aminoimidazole-4-carboxamide ribotide transformylase, adenosine deaminase and 5'-adenylate deaminase by polyglutamates of methotrexate and oxidized folates and by 5-aminoimidazole-4-carboxamide riboside and ribotide. *Biochem J* 236:193, 1986.
2. Butterworth CE Jr., Santini R Jr., Frommeyer WB Jr.: The pteroylglutamate components of American diets as determined by chromatographic fractionation. *J Clin Invest* 42:1929, 1963.
3. Food and Nutrition Board: National Research Council: Recommended dietary allowances. Washington, DC, National Academy of Sciences, 1968.
4. Von der Porten AE, Gregory JF III, Toth JP, et al: In vivo folate kinetics during chronic supplementation of human subjects with deuterium-labeled folic acid. *J Nutr* 122:1293, 1992.
5. Herbert V: Minimal daily adult folate requirement. *Arch Intern Med* 110:649, 1962.
6. Halsted CH: Folate deficiency in alcoholism. *Am J Clin Nutr* 33:2736, 1980.
7. Alperin JB, Hutchinson HT, Levin WC: Studies of folic acid requirements in megaloblastic anemia of pregnancy. *Arch Intern Med* 117:681, 1966.
8. Schwarz RH, Johnston RB Jr.: Folic acid supplementation—when and how. *Obstet Gynecol* 88:886, 1996.
9. Ulevitch R, Kallen RG: Purification and characterization of pyridoxal 5'-phosphate dependent serine hydroxymethylase from lamb liver and its action upon β-phenylserines. *Biochemistry* 16:5342, 1977.
10. Trackman PC, Abeles RH: The metabolism of 1-phospho-5-methylribose. *Biochem Biophys Res Commun* 103:1238, 1981.
11. Johnson FB, Sinclair DA, Guarente L: Molecular biology of aging. *Cell* 96:291, 1999.
12. Tabor H, Wyngaarden L: The enzymatic formation of formiminotetrahydrofolic acid, 5,10-methyltetrahydrofolic acid and 10-formiminohydrofolic acid in the metabolism of formiminoglutamic acid. *J Biol Chem* 234:1830, 1959.
13. Himes RH, Harmony JA: Formyltetrahydrofolate synthetase. *CRC Crit Rev Biochem* 1:501, 1973.
14. Deacon R, Chanarin I, Perry J, Lumb M: Marrow cells from patients with untreated pernicious anaemia cannot use tetrahydrofolate normally. *Br J Haematol* 46:523, 1980.
15. Wahba AJ, Friedkin M: The enzymatic synthesis of thymidylate. I. Early

steps in the purification of thymidylate synthetase of *Escherichia coli*. *J Biol Chem* 237:3794, 1962.

16. Blount BC, Mack MM, Wehr CM, et al: Folate deficiency causes uracil misincorporation into human DNA and chromosome breakage: implications for cancer and neuronal damage. *Proc Natl Acad Sci USA* 94:3290, 1997.

17. Huennekens FM: Folic acid coenzymes in the biosynthesis of purines and pyrimidines. *Vitam Horm* 26:375, 1968.

18. Kaufman S: The phenylalanine hydroxylating system from mammalian liver. *Adv Enzymol* 35:245, 1971.

19. Tanaka K, Kaufman S, Milstein S: Tetrahydrobiopterin, the cofactor for aromatic amino acid hydroxylases, is synthesized by and regulates proliferation of erythroid cells. *Proc Natl Acad Sci USA* 86:5864, 1989.

20. Marletta MA: Nitric oxide: biosynthesis and biological significance. *Trends Biochem Sci* 14:488, 1989.

21. Kwon NS, Nathan CF, Stuehr DJ: Reduced biopterin as a cofactor in the generation of nitrogen oxides by murine macrophages. *J Biol Chem* 264:20496, 1989.

22. Pearson AGM, Turner AJ: Folate-dependent 1-carbon transfer to biogenic amines mediated by methylene-tetrahydrofolate reductase. *Nature* 258:173, 1975.

23. Banerjee SP, Snyder SH: Methyltetrahydrofolic acid mediates N- and O-methylation of biogenic amines. *Science* 182:74, 1973.

24. Leslie GI, Baugh CM: The uptake of pteroyl-^{14}C glutamic acid into rat liver and its incorporation into the natural pteroyl poly-γ-glutamates of organ. *Biochemistry* 13:4957, 1974.

25. Lavoie A, Tripp E, Parsa K, Hoffbrand AV: Polyglutamate forms of folate in resting and proliferating mammalian tissues. *Clin Sci Mol Med* 48:67, 1975.

26. Bird OD, McGlohom VM, Vaitkus JW: Naturally occurring folates in the blood and liver of rats. *Anal Biochem* 12:18, 1965.

27. Hoffbrand AV, Newcombe BFA: Leukocyte folate in vitamin B$_{12}$ folate deficiency in leukemia. *Br J Haematol* 13:954, 1967.

28. Chanarin I, Perry J, Lumb M: The biochemical lesion in vitamin B$_{12}$ deficiency in man. *Lancet* 1:1251, 1974.

29. Pratt RF, Cooper BA: Folates in plasma and bile in man after feeding folic acid-^{3}H and 5-formyltetrahydrofolate (folinic acid). *J Clin Invest* 50:455, 1971.

30. McGuire JJ, Hsieh P, Coward JK, Bertino JR: Enzymatic synthesis of folypolyglutamates: characterization of the reaction and its products. *J Biol Chem* 255:233, 1970.

31. Kisliuk RL: Pteroylpolyglutamates. *Mol Cell Biochem* 39:331, 1979.

32. Atkinson I, Garrow T, Brenner A, Shane B: Human cytosolic folypoly-gamma-glutamate synthase. *Methods Enzymol* 281:134, 1997.

33. Sussman DJ, Milman G, Shane B: Characterization of human folypolyglutamate synthetase expressed in chinese hamster ovary cells. *Somatic Cell Mol Genet* 12:531, 1986.

34. Cook JD, Cichowicz DJ, George S, et al: Mammalian folypoly-β-glutamate synthetase. IV. In vitro and in vivo metabolism of folates and analogues and regulation of folate homeostasis. *Biochemistry* 26:530, 1987.

35. Siddarth R, Beck WS: Evidence that folypolyglutamate synthetase is under regulatory control. *Clin Res* 29:552A, 1981.

36. Shane B, Stokstad EL: Vitamin B$_{12}$-folate interrelationships. *Annu Rev Nutr* 5:115, 1985.

37. Kisliuk RL, Gaumont Y, Baugh CM: Polyglutamyl derivative of folate as substrates and inhibitors of thymidylate synthetase. *J Biol Chem* 249:4100, 1974.

38. Coward JK, Chello PL, Cashmore AR, et al: 5-Methyl-5,6,7,8-tetrahydropteroyl oligo-γ-L-glutamates: synthesis and kinetic studies with methionine synthetase from bovine brain. *Biochemistry* 14:1548, 1975.

39. Godwin HA, Rosenberg IH: Comparative studies of the intestinal absorption of [^{3}H]pteroylmonoglutamate and [^{3}H]pteroylheptaglutamate in man. *Gastroenterology* 69:364, 1975.

40. Butterworth CE Jr., Baught CM, Krumdieck C: A study of folate absorption and metabolism in man utilizing carbon-14-labeled polyglutamates synthesized by the solid phase method. *J Clin Invest* 48:1131, 1969.

41. Rosenberg IH, Godwin HA: The digestion and absorption of dietary folate. *Gastroenterology* 60:445, 1971.

42. Horne DW, Krumdieck CL, Wagner C: Properties of folic acid gamma-glutamyl hydrolase (conjugase) in rat bile and plasma. *J Nutr* 111:442, 1981.

43. Kesavan V, Noronha JM: Folate malabsorption in aged rats related to low levels of pancreatic folyl conjugase. *Am J Clin Nutr* 37:262, 1983.

44. Chandler CJ, Wang TTY, Halsted CH: Pteroylpolyglutamate hydrolase from human jejunal brush borders: purification and characterization. *J Biol Chem* 261:928, 1986.

45. Wolff R, Drouet PL, Karlin R: Recherches sur la vitamin-B$_c$-conjugase: action de quelques effecteurs sur l'activité conjugasique du plasma. *Bull Soc Chim Biol* 31:1439, 1949.

46. Elsenhans B, Ahmad O, Rosenberg IH: Isolation and characterization of pteroylpolyglutamate hydrolase from rat intestinal mucosa. *J Biol Chem* 259:6364, 1984.

47. Hepner GW, Booth CC, Cowan J, et al: Absorption of crystalline folic acid in man. *Lancet* 2:302, 1962.

48. Cohen N: Differential microbiological assay in study of folic acid absorption in vitro by everted intestinal sacs. *Clin Res* 13:252, 1965.

49. Schron CM: pH Modulation of the kinetics of rabbit jejunal, brush-border folate transport. *J Membr Biol* 120:192, 1991.

50. The transmembrane pH gradient drives uphill folate transport in rabbit jejunum: direct evidence for folate/hydroxyl exchange in brush border membrane vesicles. *J Clin Invest* 76:2030, 1985.

51. Zimmerman J, Selhub J, Rosenberg IH: Role of sodium ion in transport of folic acid in the small intestine. *Am J Physiol* 251:G218, 1986.

52. Perry J, Chanarin I: Intestinal absorption of reduced folate compounds in man. *Br J Haematol* 18:329, 1970.

53. Steinberg SE, Campbell CL, Hillman RS: Kinetics of the normal folate enterohepatic cycle. *J Clin Invest* 64:83, 1979.

54. Herbert V: Excretion of folic acid in bile. *Lancet* 1:913, 1965.

55. Steinberg SE: Mechanisms of folate homeostasis. *Am J Physiol* 246:G319, 1984.

56. Henderson GB: Folate-binding proteins. *Annu Rev Nutr* 10:319, 1990.

57. Johns DG, Sperti S, Burgen ASV: The metabolism of tritiated folic acid in man. *J Clin Invest* 40:1684, 1961.

58. Antony AC: The biological chemistry of folate receptors. *Blood* 79:2807, 1992.

59. Antony AC, Utley C, Van Horne KC, Kolhouse JF: Isolation and characterization of a folate receptor from human placenta. *J Biol Chem* 256:9684, 1981.

60. Henderson GB, Grezelokowska-Sztabert B, Zevely EM, Huennekens FM: Binding properties of the 5-methyltetrahydrofolate/methotrexate transport system in L1210 cells. *Arch Biochem Biophys* 202:144, 1980.

61. McHugh M, Cheng Y-C: Demonstration of a high affinity folate binder in human cell membranes and its characterization in cultured human KB cells. *J Biol Chem* 254:11312, 1979.

62. Weitman SD, Weinberg AG, Coney LR, et al: Cellular localization of the folate receptor: potential role in drug toxicity and folate homeostasis. *Cancer Res* 52:6708, 1992.

63. Luhrs CA, Slomiany BL: A human membrane-associated folate binding protein is anchored by a glycosyl-phosphatidylinositol tail. *J Biol Chem* 264:21446, 1989.

64. Reisenauer AM, Chandler CJ, Halsted CH: Folate binding and hydrolysis by pig intestinal brush-border membranes. *Am J Physiol* 251:G481, 1986.

65. Henderson GB, Suresh MR, Vitols KS, Huennekens FM: Transport of folate compounds in L1210 cells: kinetic evidence that folate influx proceeds via the high-affinity transport system for 5-methyltetrahydrofolate and methotrexate. *Cancer Res* 46:1639, 1986.

66. Green T, Ford HC: Human placental microvilli contain high-affinity binding sites for folate. *Biochem J* 218:75, 1984.

67. Rothberg KG, Ying Y, Kolhouse JF, Kamen BA, Anderson RGW: The glycophospholipid-linked folate receptor internalizes folate without entering the clathrin-coated pit endocytic pathway. *J Cell Biol* 110:637, 1990.

68. Morshed KM, Ross DM, McMartin KE: Folate transport proteins mediate the bidirectional transport of 5-methyltetrahydrofolate in cultured human proximal tubule cells. *J Nutr* 127:1137, 1997.

69. Kamen BA, Smith AK, Anderson RGW: The folate receptor works in tandem with a probenecid-sensitive carrier in MA104 cells in vitro. *J Clin Invest* 87:1442, 1991.

70. Matsue H, Rothberg KG, Takashima A, Kamen BA, Anderson RGW, Lacey SW: Folate receptor allows cells to grow in low concentrations of 5-methyltetrahydrofolate. *Proc Natl Acad Sci USA* 89:6006, 1992.

71. Hilton JG, Cooper BA, Rosenblatt DS: Folate glutamate synthesis and turnover in cultured human fibroblasts. *J Biol Chem* 254:8498, 1979.

72. Corrocher R, DeSandre G, Pacor ML, Hoffbrand AV: Hepatic protein binding of folate. *Clin Sci Mol Med* 46:551, 1980.

73. Suzuki N, Wagner C: Purification and characterization of a folate binding protein from rat liver cytosol. *Arch Biochem Biophys* 199:236, 1980.

74. Zamierowski MM, Wagner C: High molecular weight complexes of folic acid in mammalian tissues. *Biochem Biophys Res Commun* 60:81, 1974.

75. Duch DS, Bowers SW, Nichols CA: Analysis of folate cofactor levels in tissues using high-performance liquid chromatography. *Anal Biochem* 130:385, 1983.

76. Cook RJ, Wagner C: Glycine N-methyltransferase is a folate binding protein of rat liver cytosol. *Proc Natl Acad Sci USA* 81:3631, 1984.

77. Herbert V, Larrabee AR, Buchanan JM: Studies on the identification of a folate compound of human serum. *J Clin Invest* 41:1134, 1962.

78. Wilson SD, Horne DW: Effect of nitrous oxide inactivation of vitamin B_{12} on the levels of folate coenzymes in rat bone marrow, kidney, brain, and liver. *Arch Biochem Biophys* 244:248, 1986.

79. Rosenblatt DS, Cooper BA, Lue-Shing S, et al: Folate distribution in cultured human cells: studies on 5,10-CH_2-H_4 Pte Glu reductase deficiency. *J Clin Invest* 63:1019, 1979.

80. Chanarin I, Hutchinson M, McLean A, Moule M: Hepatic folate in man. *Br Med J* 1:396, 1966.

81. Stites TE, Bailey LB, Scott KC, Toth JP, Fisher WP, Gregory JF: Kinetic modeling of folate metabolism through use of chronic administration of deuterium-labeled folic acid in men. *Am J Clin Nutr* 65:53, 1997.

82. Elwood PC, Deutsch JC, Kolhouse JF: The conversion of the human membrane-associated folate binding protein (folate receptor) to the soluble folate binding protein by a membrane-associated metalloprotease. *J Biol Chem* 266:2346, 1991.

83. Colman N, Herbert V: Total folate binding capacity of normal human plasma and variations in uremia, cirrhosis, and pregnancy. *Blood* 48:911, 1976.

84. Waxman S: Folate binding proteins. *Br J Haematol* 29:23, 1975.

85. Rothenberg B, daCosta M: Further observations on the folate binding factor in some leukemic cells. *J Clin Invest* 50:719, 1971.

86. Waxman S, Schreiber C: Measurement of serum folate binding factor in some leukemic cells. *Blood* 42:281, 1973.

87. Colman N, Herbert V: Folate-binding proteins. *Annu Rev Med* 31:433, 1980.

88. Waxman S, Schreiber C: Characteristics of folate acid-binding protein in folate deficient serum. *Blood* 42:291, 1973.

89. Ford JE, Salter DN, Scott KJ: The folate-binding protein in milk. *J Dairy Res* 36:435, 1969.

90. Rothenberg SP: A macromolecular factor in some leukemic cells which binds folic acid. *Proc Soc Exp Biol Med* 133:428, 1970.

91. Mason JB, Selhub J: Folate binding protein and the absorption of folic acid in the small intestine of the suckling rat. *Am J Clin Nutr* 48:620, 1988.

92. Rubinoff M, Abramson R, Schreiber C, Waxman S: Effect of a folate-binding protein on the plasma transport and tissue distribution of folic acid. *Acta Haematol (Basel)* 65:145, 1981.

93. Colman N, Herbert V: Studies using the calcium ionophore A23187 suggest localization of the human granulocyte folate binder in specific (secondary) granules. *Clin Res* 27:291A, 1979.

94. Selhub J, Emmanouel D, Stavropoulos T, Arnold R: Renal folate absorption and the kidney folate binding protein. I. Urinary clearance studies. *Am J Physiol* 252:F750, 1987.

95. Selhub J, Nakamura S, Carone FA: Renal folate absorption and the kidney folate binding protein. II. Microinfusion studies. *Am J Physiol* 252:F757, 1987.

96. Williams WM, Huang KC: Renal tubular transport of folic acid and methotrexate in the monkey. *Am J Physiol* 242:F484, 1982.

97. O'Brien JS: Urinary excretion of folic acid and folinic acids in normal adults. *Proc Soc Exp Biol Med* 104:354, 1960.

98. McLean A, Chanarin I: Urinary excretion of 5-methyltetrahydro-folate in man. *Blood* 27:386, 1966.

99. Lenhert PG, Hodgkin DC: Structure of the 5,6-dimethyl-benzimida-zolylcobamide coenzyme. *Nature* 192:937, 1961.

100. Stahlberg KG: Studies on methyl-B_{12} in man. *Scand J Haematol* 4(suppl 1):1, 1967.

101. Heyssel RM, Bozian RC, Darby WC, Bell MC: Vitamin B_{12} turnover in man: the assimilation of vitamin B_{12} from natural foodstuff by man and estimates of minimal daily dietary requirements. *Am J Clin Nutr* 18:176, 1966.

102. Gräsbeck R: Calculations on vitamin B_{12} turnover in man. *Scand J Clin Lab Invest* 11:250, 1959.

103. Hsu JM, Kawin B, Minor P, Mitchell JA: Vitamin B_{12} concentrations in human tissues. *Nature* 210:1264, 1966.

104. Poston JM: Cobalamin-dependent formation of leucine and β-leucine by rat and human tissue. Changes in pernicious anemia. *J Biol Chem* 255:10067, 1980.

105. Stabler SP, Lindenbaum J, Allen RH: Failure to detect beta-leucine in human blood or leucine 2,3-aminomutase in rat liver using capillary gas chromatography-mass spectrometry. *J Biol Chem* 263:5581, 1988.

106. Jansen R, Kalousek F, Fenton W, et al: Cloning of full-length methyl-malonyl-CoA mutase from a cDNA library using the polymerase chain reaction. *Genomics* 4:198, 1989.

107. Nham SU, Wilkemeyer MF, Ledley FD: Structure of the human meth-ylmalonyl-CoA mutase (MUT) locus. *Genomics* 8:710, 1990.

108. Beck WS, Flavin M, Ochoa S: Metabolism of propionic acid in animal tissues. III. Formation of succinate. *J Biol Chem* 229:997, 1957.

109. Taylor RT, Hanna ML: 5-Methyltetrahydrofolate aromatic alkylamine N-methyltransferase: an artefact of 5,10-methylene-tetrahydrofolate reductase activity. *Life Sci* 17:111, 1975.

110. Loughlin RE, Elford HL, Buchanan JM: Enzymatic synthesis of the methyl group of methionine. VII. Isolation of a cobalamin-containing transmethylase (5-methyltetrahydrofolate homocysteine) from mammalian liver. *J Biol Chem* 239:2888, 1964.

111. Peytremann R, Thorndike J, Beck WS: Studies on N^5-methyltetrahy-drofolate-homocysteine methyltransferase in normal and leukemic leukocytes. *J Clin Invest* 56:1293, 1975.

112. Taylor RT, Weissbach H: Enzymatic synthesis of methionine: formation of a radioactive cobamide enzyme with N^5-methyl-^{14}C-tetrahydrofolate. *Arch Biochem Biophys* 119:572, 1967.

113. Banks RGS, Henderson RJ, Pratt JM: Reactions of gases in solution. III. Some reactions of nitrous oxide with transition-metal complexes. *J Chem Soc* (A):2886, 1968.

114. Chanarin I: Cobalamins and nitrous oxide: a review. *J Clin Pathol* 33:909, 1980.

115. Matthews DM, Wilson J: Cobalamins and cyanide metabolism in neurological diseases, in *The Cobalamins: A Glaxo Symposium*, edited by HRV Arnstein, RJ Wrighton, p 115. Williams & Wilkins, Baltimore, 1971.

116. Knowles JP, Prankerd TA: Abnormal folic acid metabolism in vitamin B_{12} deficiency. *Clin Sci* 22:233, 1962.

117. Norohna JM, Silverman M: On folic acid, vitamin B_{12}, methionine and formiminoglutamic acid metabolism, in *Vitamin B_{12} and Intrinsic Faktor, 2d Europäisches Symposion*, edited by HC Heinrich, p 728. Enke, Stuttgart, 1962.

118. Herbert V, Zalusky R: Interrelations of vitamin B_{12} and folic acid metabolism: folic acid clearance studies. *J Clin Invest* 41:1263, 1962.

119. Kano Y, Sakamoto S, Hida K, et al: 5-Methyltetrahydrofolate related enzymes and DNA polymerase α activities in bone marrow cells from patients with vitamin B_{12} deficient megaloblastic anemia. *Blood* 59:832, 1982.

120. Lumb M, Chanarin I, Perry J, Deacon R: Turnover of the methyl moiety of 5-methyltetrahydropteroylglutamic acid in the cobalamin-inactivated rat. *Blood* 66:1171, 1985.

121. Waters AH, Mollin DL: Observations on the metabolism of folic acid in pernicious anaemia. *Br J Haematol* 9:319, 1963.

122. Smith RM, Osborne-White WS: Folic acid metabolism in vitamin B_{12}-deficient sheep: depletion of liver folates. *Biochem J* 136:279, 1973.

123. Jeejeebhoy KN, Pathare SM, Noronha JM: Observations on conjugated and unconjugated blood folate levels in megaloblastic anemia and the effects of vitamin B_{12}. *Blood* 26:354, 1965.

124. Chanarin I: The methyl-folate trap and the supply of S-adenosylmethionine. *Lancet* 2:755, 1965.

125. Boss GR: Cobalamin inactivation decreases purine and methionine synthesis in cultured lymphoblasts. *J Clin Invest* 76:213, 1985.

126. Katzen HM, Buchanan JM: Enzymatic synthesis of the methyl group of methionine. VIII. Repression-derepression, purification and properties of 5,10-methylenetetrahydrofolate reductase from *E. coli*. *J Biol Chem* 240:825, 1980.

127. Chanarin I, Deacon R, Lumb M, Perry J: Vitamin B$_{12}$ regulates folate metabolism by the supply of formate. *Lancet* 2:505, 1980.

128. Perry J, Chanarin I, Deacon R, Lumb M: The substrate for folate poly-glutamate biosynthesis in the vitamin B$_{12}$-inactivated rat. *Biochem Biophys Res Commun* 91:678, 1979.

129. Taheri MR, Wickremasinghe RG, Jackson BF, Hoffbrand AV: The effect of folate analogues and vitamin B$_{12}$ on provision of thymine nucleotides for DNA synthesis in megaloblastic anemia. *Blood* 59:634, 1982.

130. Deacon R, Bottiglieri T, Chanarin I: Methylthioadenosine serves as a single carbon source to the folate coenzyme pool in rat bone marrow cells. *Biochim Biophys Acta* 1034:342, 1990.

131. Chanarin I, Deacon R, Lumb M, et al: Cobalamin and folate: recent developments. *J Clin Pathol* 45:277, 1992.

132. Hewitt JE, Gordon MM, Taggart RT, et al: Human gastric intrinsic factor: characterization of cDNA and genomic clones and localization to human chromosome 11. *Genomics* 10:432, 1991.

133. Tang LH, Chokshi H, Hu CB, et al: The intrinsic factor (IF)-cobalamin receptor binding site is located in the amono-terminal portion of IF. *J Biol Chem* 267:22982, 1992.

134. Allen RH, Mehlman CS: Isolation of gastric vitamin B$_{12}$ binding proteins using affinity chromatography. I. Purification and properties of human intrinsic factor. *J Biol Chem* 248:3660, 1973.

135. Christensen JM, Hippe E, Olesen H: Purification of human intrinsic factor by affinity chromatography. *Biochim Biophys Acta* 310:510, 1973.

136. Visuri K, Gräsbeck R: Human intrinsic factor: isolation by improved conventional methods and properties of the preparation. *Biochim Biophys Acta* 303:319, 1973.

137. Levine JS, Nakane PK, Allen RH: Immunocytochemical localization of human intrinsic factor: the nonstimulated stomach. *Gastroenterology* 79:493, 1980.

138. Deller DJ, Germar H, Witts LJ: Effect of food on absorption of radioactive vitamin B$_{12}$. *Lancet* 1:574, 1961.

139. Meikle DD, Bull J, Callendar ST, Truelove SC: Intrinsic factor secretion after vagotomy. *Br J Surg* 96:795, 1977.

140. Irvine WJ: Effect of gastrin I and II on the secretion of intrinsic factor. *Lancet* 1:736, 1965.

141. Lawrie JH, Anderson NM: Secretion of gastric intrinsic factor. *Lancet* 1:68, 1967.

142. Marcouillis G, Gräsbeck R: Vitamin B$_{12}$-binding proteins in human gastric mucosa: general pattern and demonstration of intrinsic isoproteins typical of mucosa. *Scand J Clin Lab Invest* 35:5, 1975.

143. Stenman UH: Vitamin B$_{12}$-binding proteins of R-type cobalophilin: characterization and comparison of cobalophilin from different sources. *Scand J Haemat* 14:91, 1975.

144. Jacob E, Baker SJ, Herbert V: Vitamin B$_{12}$-binding proteins. *Physiol Rev* 60:918, 1980.

145. Burger RL, Allen RH: Characterization of vitamin B$_{12}$-binding proteins isolated from human milk and saliva by affinity chromatography. *J Biol Chem* 249:7220, 1974.

146. Hurlimann J, Zuber C: Vitamin B$_{12}$ binders in human body fluids. II. Synthesis in vitro. *Clin Exp Immunol* 4:141, 1974.

147. Simons K, Weber T: The vitamin B$_{12}$ binding protein in human leukocytes. *Biochim Biophys Acta* 117:201, 1966.

148. Cooper BA, Castle WB: Sequential mechanisms in the enhanced absorption of vitamin B$_{12}$ by intrinsic factor in the rat. *J Clin Invest* 39:199, 1966.

149. Allen RH, Seetharam B, Podell ER, Alpers DH: Effect of proteolytic enzymes on the binding of cobalamin to R protein and intrinsic factor: in vitro evidence that a failure to partially degrade R protein is responsible for cobalamin malabsorption in pancreatic insufficiency. *J Clin Invest* 61:47, 1978.

150. Abels J, Schilling RF: Protection of intrinsic factor by vitamin B$_{12}$. *J Lab Clin Med* 64:375, 1964.

151. Birn H, Verroust PJ, Nexo E, Hager H, Jacobsen C, Christensen EI, Moestrup SK: Characterization of an epithelial approximately 460-kDa protein that facilitates endocytosis of intrinsic factor-vitamin B12 and binds receptor-associated protein. *J Biol Chem* 272:26497, 1997.

152. Titenko-Holland N, Jacob RA, Shang N, Balaraman A, Smith MT: Micronuclei in lymphocytes and exfoliated buccal cells of postmenopausal women with dietary changes in folate. *Mutat Res* 417:101, 1998.

153. Levine JS, Allen RH, Alpers DH: Immunocytochemical localization of

154. the intrinsic factor-cobalamin receptor in dog ileum: distribution of intracellular receptor during cell maturation. *J Cell Biol* 98:1111, 1984.

154. Seetharam B, Levine JS, Ramasamy M, et al: Purification, properties, and immunochemical localization of a receptor for intrinsic factor-cobalamin complex in the rat kidney. *J Biol Chem* 263:4443, 1988.

155. Ramanujam KS, Seetharam S, Ramasamy M, et al: Renal brush border membrane bound intrinsic factor. *Biochim Biophys Acta* 1030:157, 1990.

156. Ramanujam KS, Seetharam S, Dahms NM, et al: Functional expression of intrinsic factor-cobalamin receptor by renal proximal tubular epithelial cells. *J Biol Chem* 266:13135, 1991.

157. Seetharam S, Ramanujam KS, Seetharam B: Synthesis and brush border expression of intrinsic factor-cobalamin receptor from rat renal cortex. *J Biol Chem* 267:7421, 1992.

158. Hagedorn CH, Alpers DH: Distribution of intrinsic factor-vitamin B$_{12}$ receptors in human intestine. *Gastroenterology* 73:1019, 1977.

159. Herbert V, Castle WB: Divalent cation and pH dependence of rat intrinsic factor action in everted sacs and mucosal hemogenates in rat small intestine. *J Clin Invest* 40:1978, 1961.

160. Mackenzie IL, Donaldson RM, Jr.: Effect of divalent cations and pH on intrinsic factor-mediated attachment of B$_{12}$ to intestinal microvillous membranes. *J Clin Invest* 51:2465, 1972.

161. Kapadia CR, Serfilippi D, Voloshin K, Donaldson RM Jr.: Intrinsic factor-mediated absorption of cobalamin by guinea pig ileal cells. *J Clin Invest* 71:440, 1983.

162. Seetharam B, Presti M, Frank C: Intestinal uptake and release of cobalamin complexed with rat intrinsic factor. *Am J Physiol* 248:G326, 1985.

163. Robertson JA, Gallagher MD: In vivo evidence that cobalamin is absorbed by receptor-mediated endocytosis in the mouse. *Gastroenterology* 88:908, 1985.

164. Horadagoda NU, Batt RM: Lysosomal localisation of cobalamin during absorption by the ileum of the dog. *Biochim Biophys Acta* 838:206, 1985.

165. Jenkins WJ, Empson R, Jewell DP, Taylor KB: Subcellular localisation of vitamin B$_{12}$ absorption. *Gut* 22:617, 1981.

166. Cooper BA: Complex of intrinsic factor and B$_{12}$ in human ileum during vitamin B$_{12}$ absorption. *Am J Physiol* 214:832, 1968.

167. Rothenberg SP, Weisberg H, Ficarra A: Evidence for the absorption of immunoreactive intrinsic factor into the intestinal epithelial cell during vitamin B$_{12}$ absorption. *J Lab Clin Med* 79:578, 1972.

168. Hall CA: Transcobalamins I and II as natural transport proteins of vitamin B$_{12}$. *J Clin Invest* 56:1125, 1975.

169. Chanarin I, Muir M, Hughes A, Hoffbrand AV: Evidence for intestinal origin of transcobalamin II during vitamin B$_{12}$ absorption. *Br Med J* 1:1453, 1978.

170. Rothenberg SP, Weiss JP, Cotter R: Formation of transcobalaminII-vitamin B$_{12}$ complex by guinea pig ileal mucosa in organ culture after in vivo incubation with intrinsic factor-vitamin B$_{12}$. *Br J Haematol* 40:401, 1978.

171. Rabinowitz R, Rachmilewitz B, Rachmilewitz M, Schlesinger M: Production of transcobalamin II by various murine and human cells in culture. *Isr J Med Sci* 18:740, 1982.

172. England JM, Clarke HGM, Down MC, Chanarin I: Studies on transcobalamins. *Br J Haematol* 25:737, 1973.

173. Savage CR, Green PD: Biosynthesis of transcobalamin II by adult rat liver parenchymal cells in culture. *Arch Biochem Biophys* 173:691, 1976.

174. Gräsbeck R, Nyberg W, Reizenstein P: Biliary and fecal vitamin B$_{12}$ excretion in man: an isotope study. *Proc Soc Exp Biol Med* 97:780, 1958.

175. Booth MA, Spray GH: Vitamin B$_{12}$ activity in the serum and liver of rats after total gastrectomy. *Br J Haematol* 6:288, 1960.

176. Dorscherholmen A, Hagen PS, Liu M: A dual mechanism of vitamin B$_{12}$ plasma absorption. *J Clin Invest* 36:1551, 1957.

177. Seetharam B, Alpers DH: Cellular uptake of cobalamin. *Nutr Rev* 43:97, 1985.

178. Platica O, Janeczko R, Quadros EV, et al: The cDNA sequence and the deduced amino acid sequence of human transcobalamin II show homology with rat intrinsic factor and human transcobalamin I. *J Biol Chem* 266:7860, 1991.

179. Seetharam S, Dahms N, Li N, Seetharam B: Functional expression of transcobalamin II cDNA in Xenopus laevis oocytes. *Biochem Biophys Res Commun* 181:1151, 1991.

180. Hippe E, Olesen H: Nature of vitamin B$_{12}$ binding. III. Thermodynamics

of binding to human intrinsic factor and transcobalamins. *Biochim Biophys Acta* 243:83, 1999.

181. Kolhouse JF, Allen RH: Absorption, plasma transport and cellular retention of cobalamin analogues in the rabbit. *J Clin Invest* 60:1381, 1977.

182. Donaldson RM, Brand M, Serfilippi D: Changes in circulating transcobalamin II after injection of cyanocobalamin. *N Engl J Med* 296:1427, 1977.

183. Schneider RJ, Burger RL, Hehlman CS, Allen RH: The role and fate of rabbit and human transcobalamin II in the plasma transport of vitamin B_{12} in the rabbit. *J Clin Invest* 57:27, 1978.

184. Seligman PA, Allen RH: Characterization of receptor for transcobalamin II isolation from human placenta. *J Biol Chem* 253:1766, 1978.

185. Youngdahl-Turner P, Rosenberg LE, Allen RH: Binding and uptake of transcobalamin II by human fibroblasts. *J Clin Invest* 61:133, 1978.

186. Youngdahl-Turner P, Mellman IS, Allen RH: Protein mediated vitamin uptake: adsorptive endocytosis of the transcobalamin II-cobalamin complex by cultured human fibroblasts. *Exp Cell Res* 118:127, 1999.

187. Newmark P, Newman GE, O'Brien JRP: Vitamin B_{12} in the rat kidney: evidence for an association with lysosomes. *Arch Biochem Biophys* 141:121, 1970.

188. Pletsch QA, Coffey JW: Properties of the proteins that bind vitamin B_{12} in subcellular fractions of rat liver. *Arch Biochem Biophys* 151:157, 1972.

189. Rosenblatt D, Hosack A, Matiaszuk NV, et al: Defect in vitamin B_{12} release from lysosomes: newly described inborn error of vitamin B_{12} metabolism. *Science* 228:1319, 1985.

190. Idriss J-M, Jonas AJ: Vitamin B_{12} transport by rat liver lysosomal membrane vesicles. *J Biol Chem* 266:9438, 1991.

191. Watanabe F, Nakano Y, Tachikake N, et al: Occurrence and subcellular location of NADH- and NADPH-linked aquacobalamin reductases in human liver. *Int J Biochem* 23:531, 1991.

192. Watanabe F, Nakano Y: Comparative biochemistry of vitamin B_{12} (cobalamin) metabolism: biochemistry diversity in the systems for intracellular cobalamin transfer and synthesis of the coenzymes. *Int J Biochem* 23:1353, 1991.

193. Watanabe F, Nakano Y, Saido H, et al: NADPH-cytochrome c (P-450) reductase has the activity of NADPH-linked aquacobalamin reductase in rat liver microsomes. *Biochim Biophys Acta* 119:175, 1992.

194. Watanabe F, Nakano Y, Saido H, Tamura Y, Yamanaka H: Cytochrome b_5/cytochrome b_5 reductase complex in rat liver microsomes has NADH-linked aquacobalamin reductase activity. *J Nutr* 122:940, 1992.

195. Shuster S, Marks J, Chanarin I: Folic acid deficiency in patients with skin disease. *Br J Dermatol* 79:398, 1967.

196. Hild D: Folate losses from the skin in exfoliative dermatitis. *Arch Intern Med* 123:51, 1969.

197. Van Scott EJ, Auerback R, Weinstein GD: Parental methotrexate in psoriasis. *Arch Dermatol* 89:550, 1964.

198. Ardeman S, Chanarin I: Steroids and Addisonian pernicious anemia. *N Engl J Med* 273:1352, 1965.

199. Boddington MM, Spriggs AI: The epithelial cells in megaloblastic anaemias. *J Clin Pathol* 12:228, 1969.

200. Johnston J, Bollekens J, Allen RH, Berliner N: Structure of the cDNA encoding transcobalamin I, a neutrophil granule protein. *J Biol Chem* 264:15754, 1989.

201. Johnston J, Yang-Feng T, Berliner N: Genomic structure and mapping of the chromosomal gene for transcobalamin I (TCN1): comparison to human intrinsic factor. *Genomics* 12:459, 1992.

202. Burger RL, Schneider RJ, Mehlman CS, Allen RH: Human plasma R-type vitamin B12-binding proteins. II. The role of transcobalamin I, transcobalamin III, and the normal granulocyte vitamin B12-binding protein in the plasma transport of vitamin B12. *J Biol Chem* 250:7707, 1975.

203. Ashwell G, Morrell AG: The role of surface carbohydrates in the hepatic recognition and transport of circulating glycoproteins. *Adv Enzymol* 41:99, 1974.

204. Gueant JL, Monin B, Boissel P, et al: Biliary excretion of cobalamin and cobalamin analogues in man. *Digestion* 30:151, 1984.

205. Allen RH, Seetharam B, Allen NC: Correction of cobalamin malabsorption in pancreatic insufficiency with a cobalamin analogue that binds with high affinity R protein but not to intrinsic factor. *J Clin Invest* 61:1628, 1978.

206. Gottlieb C, Retief FP, Herbert V: Blockage of vitamin B_{12}-binding sites in the gastric juice, serum and saliva by analogues and derivatives of vitamin B_{12} and by antibody to intrinsic factor. *Biochim Biophys Acta* 141:560, 1967.

207. Allen RH: Human vitamin B12 transport proteins. *Prog Hematol* 9:57, 1975.

208. Kolhouse JF, Kondo H, Allen NC, Podell E, Allen RH: Cobalamin analogues are present in human plasma and can mask cobalamin deficiency because current radioisotope dilution assays are not specific for true cobalamin. *N Engl J Med* 299:785, 1978.

209. Retief FP, Gottlieb CW, Herbert V: Delivery of Co57 B_{12} by human and mouse tumour cells. *Nature* 191:393, 1961.

210. Carmel R: Vitamin B_{12} binding abnormality in subjects without myeloproliferative disease. I. Elevated serum B_{12} binding capacity in patients with leucocytosis. *Br J Haematol* 22:43, 1972.

211. Stenman UH, Simons K, Gräsbeck R: Vitamin B_{12} binding proteins in normal and leukemic leukocytes and sera. *Scand J Clin Invest* 21 (suppl 101):103, 1974.

212. Carmel R, Herbert V: Vitamin B_{12}-binding protein of leukocytes as a possible major source of the third vitamin B_{12}-binding protein of serum. *Blood* 40:452, 1972.

213. Kelly A, Herbert V: Coated charcoal assay of erythrocyte vitamin B_{12}. *Blood* 29:139, 1967.

214. Kondo H, Kolhouse JF, Allen RH: Presence of cobalamin analogues in animal tissues. *Proc Natl Acad Sci USA* 77:817, 1980.

215. Fernandes-Costa F, Metz J: Vitamin B_{12} binders (transcobalamins) in serum. *CRC Crit Rev Clin Lab Sci* 18:1, 1982.

216. Hom BL: Plasma turnover of ^{57}cobalt-vitamin B_{12} bound to transcobalamin I and II. *Scand J Haemat* 4:321, 1967.

217. Hom BL, Ahluwalia BK: The vitamin B_{12} binding capacity of transcobalamin I and II on normal serum. *Scand J Haemat.* 5:64, 1967.

218. Carmel R: The distribution of endogenous cobalamin among cobalamin-binding proteins in the blood of normal and abnormal states. *Am J Clin Nutr* 41:713, 1985.

219. Metz J: The deoxyuridine suppression test. *CRC Crit Rev Clin Lab Sci* 20:205, 1984.

CHAPTER 26

ENERGY METABOLISM AND MAINTENANCE OF ERYTHROCYTES

ERNEST BEUTLER

Red cells possess an active metabolic machinery that provides energy to pump ions against electrochemical gradients and to maintain hemoglobin in the reduced form. The main source of metabolic energy comes from glucose. Glucose is metabolized through the glycolytic pathway and through the hexose monophosphate shunt. Glycolysis catabolizes glucose to pyruvate and lactate, which represent the end-products of glucose metabolism in the erythrocyte, because it lacks the mitochondria required for further oxidation of pyruvate. ADP is phosphorylated to ATP and NAD$^+$ is reduced to NADH in glycolysis. Bisphosphoglycerate, an important regulator of the oxygen affinity of hemoglobin, is generated during glycolysis. The hexose-monophosphate shunt oxidizes glucose-6-phosphate, reducing NADP$^+$ to NADPH. In addition to glucose, the red cell has the capacity to utilize some other sugars and nucleosides as a source of energy. The red cell lacks the capacity for de novo purine synthesis but has a salvage pathway which permits synthesis of purine nucleotides from purine bases. The red cell contains high concentrations of glutathione, which is maintained almost entirely in the reduced state by NADPH through the catalytic activity of glutathione reductase. Glutathione is synthesized from glycine, cysteine, and glutamic acid in a two-step process that requires ATP as a source of energy. Catalase and glutathione peroxidase serve to protect the red cell from oxidative damage. The maturation of reticulocytes into erythrocytes is associated with a rapid decrease in the activity of several enzymes. However, the decrease in enzymatic activities of enzymes occurs much more slowly or not at all with ageing.

Although the binding, transport, and delivery of oxygen do not require the expenditure of metabolic energy by the red blood cell, a source of energy is required if the red cell is to perform its function efficiently and to survive in the circulation for its full life span of approximately 120 days. This energy is needed to maintain (1) the iron of hemoglobin in the divalent form, (2) the high potassium and low calcium and sodium levels within the cell against a gradient imposed by the high

Acronyms and abbreviations that appear in this chapter include: ADA, adenosine deaminase; ADP, adenosine diphosphate; APRT, adenine phosphoribosyltransferase; ATP, adenosine triphosphate; 2,3-BPG, 2,3-bisphosphoglycerate; cAMP, cyclic adenosine 3′,5′-monophosphate; cGMP, cyclic guanosine 3′,5′-monophosphate; G-6-PD, glucose-6-phosphate dehydrogenase; GSH, reduced glutathione; GSSG, oxidized glutathione; HGPRT, hypoxanthine-guanine phosphoribosyltransferase; LDH, lactate dehydrogenase; NAD, nicotinamide adenine dinucleotide; PEP, phosphoenolpyruvate; R-1-P, ribose 1-phosphate; SCID, severe combined immunodeficiency; UDPG, uridine diphosphoglucose.

plasma calcium and sodium and low plasma potassium levels, (3) the sulfhydryl groups of red cell enzymes, hemoglobin, and membranes in the active, reduced form, and (4) the biconcave shape of the cell. If the red cell is deprived of a source of energy, it becomes sodium- and calcium-logged and potassium-depleted, and the red cell shape changes from a biconcave disc to a sphere. Such a cell is quickly removed from the circulation by the filtering action of the spleen and by a perceptive monocyte-macrophage system. Even if it survived, such an energy-deprived cell would gradually turn brown as hemoglobin is oxidized to methemoglobin by the very high concentrations of oxygen within the erythrocyte. The cell would then be unable to perform its function of transporting oxygen and carbon dioxide.

The process of extracting energy from a substrate, such as glucose, and of utilizing this energy is carried out by a large number of enzymes. Since the red cell loses its nucleus before it enters the circulation and most of its RNA within 1 or 2 days of its release into the circulation, it does not have the capacity to synthesize new enzyme molecules to replace those that may become degraded during its life span. The enzymes present in the red cells were formed largely by the nucleated marrow cell and to a lesser extent by the reticulocyte.

GLUCOSE METABOLISM

Glucose is the normal energy source of the red cell.[1] It is metabolized by the erythrocyte along two major routes, the glycolytic pathway and the hexose monophosphate shunt. The steps in these pathways are essentially the same as those found in other tissues and in other organisms, including even relatively simple ones such as *Escherichia coli* and yeast. Unlike most other cells, however, the red cell lacks a citric acid cycle. Only the reticulocytes maintain some capacity for the breakdown of pyruvate to CO_2 with the attendant highly efficient production of ATP. The mature red cell must content itself with extracting energy from glucose almost solely by anaerobic glycolysis. Before glucose can be metabolized by the red cell, it must pass through the membrane. The membrane contains a carrier[2] that can combine with glucose and other sugars at the cell surface and release them at the interior surface of the membrane. The red cell membrane contains insulin receptors,[3,4] but the transport of glucose into red cells is independent of insulin.[5]

PATHWAYS OF GLUCOSE METABOLISM

THE DIRECT GLYCOLYTIC PATHWAY

In the Embden-Meyerhof direct glycolytic pathway (Fig. 26-1), glucose is catabolized anaerobically to pyruvate or lactate. Although 2 moles of high-energy phosphate in the form of ATP are utilized in preparing glucose for its further metabolism, up to 4 moles of ADP may be phosphorylated to ATP during the metabolism of each mole of glucose, giving a net yield of 2 moles of ATP per mole of glucose metabolized. The rate of glucose utilization is limited largely by the hexokinase and phosphofructokinase reactions. Both of the enzymes catalyzing these reactions have a relatively high pH optimum; they have very little activity at pH levels lower than 7. For this reason, red cell glycolysis is very pH-sensitive, being stimulated by a rise in pH. However, at higher-than-physiologic pH levels, the stimulation of hexokinase and phosphofructokinase activity merely results in the accumulation of fructose diphosphate and triose phosphates, because the availability of NAD$^+$ for the glyceraldehyde phosphate dehydrogenase reaction becomes a limiting factor.

Branching of the metabolic stream after the formation of 1,3-bisphosphoglycerate provides the red cell with flexibility in regard to the amount of ATP formed in the metabolism of each mole of glucose. 1,3-Bisphosphoglycerate may be metabolized to 2,3-bisphosphoglycerate (2,3-BPG), also known as 2,3-diphosphoglycerate (2,3-DPG),

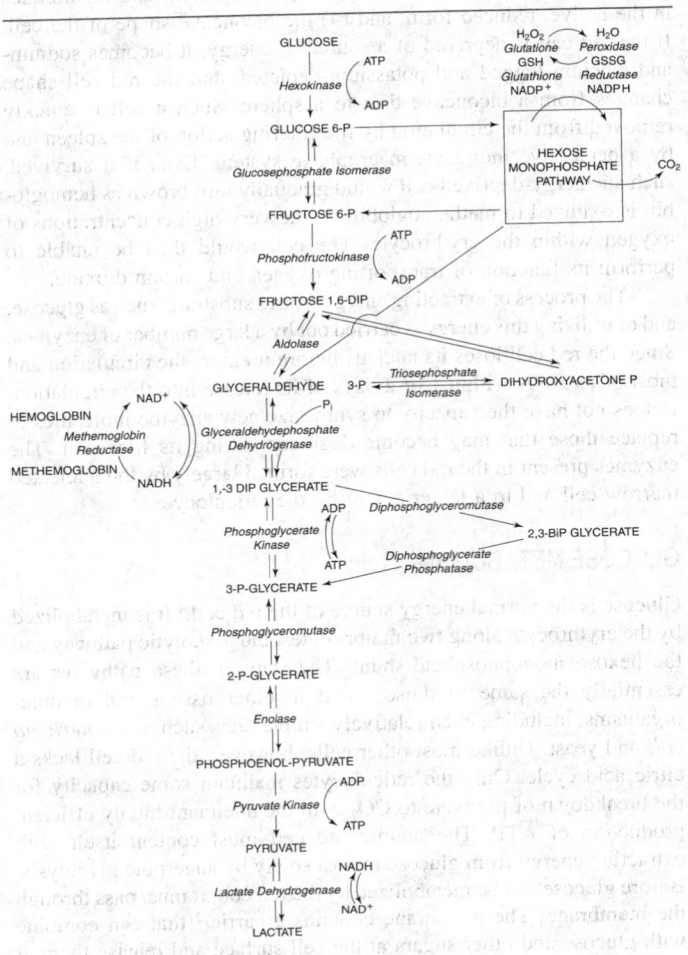

FIGURE 26-1   Glucose metabolism of the erythrocyte. The details of the hexose monophosphate pathway are shown in Fig. 26-2.

thus "wasting" the high-energy phosphate bond in position 1 of the glycerate. Removing the phosphate group at position 2 by bisphosphoglycerate phosphatase results in the formation of 3-phosphoglycerate. Alternatively, 3-phosphoglycerate may be formed directly from 1,3-bisphosphoglycerate through the phosphoglycerate kinase step, resulting in phosphorylation of a mole of ADP to ATP. While metabolism of glucose through the 2,3-BPG step occurs without any net gain of high-energy phosphate bonds in the form of ATP, metabolism through the phosphoglycerate kinase step results in the formation of two such bonds per mole of glucose metabolized. This portion of the direct glycolytic pathway has been called the "energy clutch."[6] Regulation of metabolism at this branch point determines not only the rate of ADP phosphorylation to ATP but also the concentration of 2,3-BPG, an important regulator of the oxygen affinity of hemoglobin (see Chap. 28). The concentration of 2,3-BPG depends on the balance between its rate of formation from 1,3-BPG by bisphosphoglycerate mutase and its degradation by bisphosphoglycerate phosphatase. Hydrogen ions inhibit the bisphosphoglycerate mutase reaction and stimulate the phosphatase reaction. Thus red cell 2,3-BPG levels are exquisitely sensitive to pH: A rise in pH causes a rise in 2,3-BPG levels, while acidosis results in 2,3-BPG depletion. It may be that the ratio of oxyhemoglobin to deoxyhemoglobin also influences 2,3-BPG synthesis by virtue of the fact that only deoxyhemoglobin binds this compound, thus affecting the concentration of free 2,3-BPG that is available for feedback inhibition of the enzymes that lead to its formation.

However, the available evidence suggests that the pH is the primary controlling factor.[7]

Metabolism of glucose by way of the Embden-Meyerhof pathway may also yield reducing energy in the form of NADH. The reduction of NAD^+ to NADH occurs in the glyceraldehyde phosphate dehydrogenase step. If NADH is reoxidized in reducing methemoglobin to hemoglobin, the end product of glucose metabolism is pyruvate. If NADH is not reoxidized by methemoglobin, however, pyruvate is reduced in the lactate dehydrogenase step, forming lactate as the final end product of glucose metabolism.[1] The lactate or pyruvate formed is transported from the red cell[8] and is metabolized elsewhere in the body. Thus the erythrocyte has a flexible Embden-Meyerhof pathway that can adjust the amount of ADP phosphorylated per mole of glucose according to the requirement of the cell.

The regulation of red cell glycolytic metabolism is very complex. Products of some reactions may stimulate others. For example, the pyruvate kinase reaction is exquisitely sensitive to fructose diphosphate, the product of phosphofructokinase. Conversely, other metabolic products may serve as strong enzyme inhibitors. Attempts have been made to construct computer models that simulate this network of reactions,[9–12] but the usefulness of such models has been limited by the fact that all of the interactions are not well understood.

THE HEXOSE MONOPHOSPHATE SHUNT

Not all the glucose metabolized by the red cell passes through the direct glycolytic pathway. A direct oxidative pathway of metabolism, the hexose monophosphate shunt, also functions. In this pathway glucose 6-phosphate is oxidized at position 1, yielding carbon dioxide. In the process of glucose oxidation, $NADP^+$ is reduced to NADPH. The pentose phosphate formed when glucose is decarboxylated undergoes a series of molecular rearrangements, eventuating in the formation of a triose, glyceraldehyde 3-phosphate, and a hexose, fructose 6-phosphate (Fig. 26-2). These are normal intermediates in anaerobic glycolysis and thus can rejoin that metabolic stream. Because the glucose phosphate

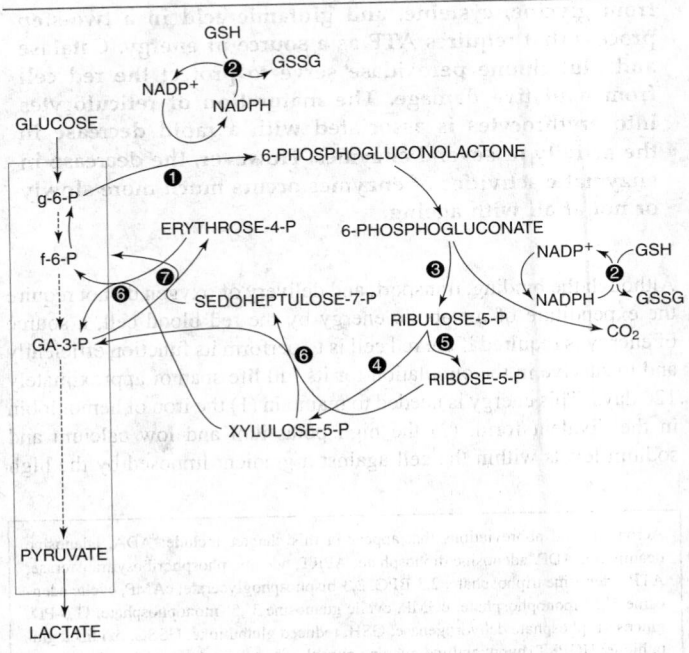

FIGURE 26-2   The hexose monophosphate pathway of the erythrocyte: (1) glucose-6-phosphate dehydrogenase, (2) glutathione reductase, (3) phosphogluconate dehydrogenase, (4) ribulosephosphate epimerase, (5) ribosephosphate isomerase, (6) transketolase, and (7) transaldolase.

isomerase reaction is freely reversible, allowing fructose 6-phosphate to be converted to glucose 6-phosphate, recycling through the hexose monophosphate pathway is also possible. Unlike the anaerobic glycolytic pathway, the hexose monophosphate pathway does not generate any high-energy phosphate bonds. Its primary function appears to be the reduction of $NADP^+$, and, indeed, the amount of glucose passing through this pathway appears to be regulated by the amount of $NADP^+$ that has been made available by the oxidation of NADPH. NADPH appears to function primarily as a substrate for the reduction of glutathione-containing disulfides in the erythrocyte through mediation of the enzyme glutathione reductase, which catalyzes the conversion of oxidized glutathione (GSSG) to reduced glutathione (GSH) and the reduction of mixed disulfides of hemoglobin and GSH.[13] $NADP^+$ also strongly binds to catalase and may effect its activity.[14,15]

As in the case of anaerobic glycolysis, efforts have been made to construct a computer model of the hexose monophosphate pathway of red cells.[16–18]

ENZYMES OF GLUCOSE METABOLISM

HEXOKINASE

Hexokinase catalyzes the phosphorylation of glucose in position 6 by ATP (Fig. 26-1). It thus serves as the first step in the utilization of glucose, whether by the anaerobic or the hexose monophosphate pathway. Mannose or fructose may also serve as a substrate for this enzyme.[19] Red cell hexokinase does not phosphorylate galactose.[20] The average normal activity of the hexokinase reaction (Table 26-1) is about 5 times the rate of glucose utilization by intact cells. Reticulocytes have much higher levels of hexokinase activity than do mature red cells.[26–28]

Hexokinase has an absolute requirement for magnesium. It is strongly inhibited by its product, glucose 6-phosphate, and is apparently released from this inhibition by the inorganic phosphate ion[29] and by high concentrations of glucose.[30] Inorganic phosphate enhances the rate of glucose utilization by red cells. It has been suggested that this effect is not exerted through hexokinase, but rather through stimulation of the phosphofructokinase reaction, resulting in a lowered glucose 6-phosphate concentration within the cell and thus releasing hexokinase from inhibition.[31] GSSG[32] and other disulfides and 2,3-BPG[33,34] inhibit hexokinase.

The human enzyme resolves into two major bands by electrophoresis.[35,36] Designated types I_A and I_F, both bands actually correspond to type I liver enzyme. Separated chromatographically, the two major fractions of red cell hexokinase have been designated HK and HK_R, the latter fraction being unique to erythrocytes and particularly to reticulocytes.[37] The hexokinase I gene has been cloned and its structure determined.[38] Evidence of an alternative red-blood-cell-specific exon 1 located upstream of the 5′ flanking region of the gene has been obtained[38] and a hexokinase cDNA that appears to be unique to erythrocytes has been isolated.[39]

Rabbit reticulocytes appear to contain hexokinase fractions that are membrane bound and free.[40,41] It has been proposed that the ubiquitin-ATP proteolytic system selectively degrades the membrane-bound form of the enzyme, but the physiologic significance of such a process is not clear.[42] A small amount of type III hexokinase is also present in erythrocytes.

Hexokinase deficiency is a rare cause of hereditary nonspherocytic hemolytic anemia[43,44] (see Chap. 44).

GLUCOSE PHOSPHATE ISOMERASE

Glucosephosphate isomerase catalyzes the interconversion of glucose 6-phosphate and fructose 6-phosphate.[1] Electrophoresis resolves the normal enzyme into three bands, all of which are products of the same

gene[45]; mutations that affect electrophoretic mobility are known.[45] The human GPI gene has been cloned and its structure and coding sequence determined.[45,47] Glucose phosphate isomerase deficiency is one of the causes of hereditary nonspherocytic hemolytic anemia (see Chap. 45).

PHOSPHOFRUCTOKINASE

Red cells contain two distinct types of phosphofructokinase. The classical (or type I) form of the enzyme catalyzes the phosphorylation of the 1-carbon of fructose 6-phosphate by ATP. The type II enzyme, fructose 6-phosphate-2-kinase, phosphorylates the second carbon of fructose 6-phosphate.[48] The product of this reaction, fructose 2,6-diphosphate, is a potent allosteric activator of type I phosphofructokinase. The type I enzyme requires magnesium for activity and is stimulated by ADP, inorganic phosphate, ammonia, and fructose 2,6-diphosphate.[49] The existence of the latter effector has been demonstrated in red cells.[48]

TABLE 26-1   THE ACTIVITIES OF SOME RED CELL ENZYMES

ENZYME	ACTIVITY AT 37°C (IU/g Hb) (MEAN ± STANDARD DEVIATION)	REFERENCES
Acetylcholinesterase	36.93 ± 3.83	1
Adenosine deaminase	1.11 ± 0.23	1
Adenylate kinase	258 ± 29.3	1
Aldolase	3.19 ± 0.86	1
ATPase (Na⁺-K⁺)*	0.121 ± .031	1
ATPase (Mg²⁺)	0.278 ± .066	21
Catalase	153,117 ± 2390	1
Bisphosphoglyceromutase	4.78 ± 0.65	1
Enolase	5.39 ± 0.83	1
Galactose-4-epimerase	0.231 ± 0.061	1
Galactokinase	0.0291 ± 0.004	1
Glucose phosphate isomerase	60.8 ± 11.0	1
Glucose-6-phosphate dehydrogenase	8.34 ± 1.59	1
γ-glutamyl cysteine synthetase	1.05 ± 0.19	22
Glutathione peroxidase*	30.82 ± 4.65	1
Glutathione reductase without FAD†	7.18 ± 1.09	1
Glutathione reductase with FAD	10.4 ± 1.50	1
Glutathione-S-transferase	6.66 ± 1.81	1
Glutathione synthetase	0.34 ± 0.06	22
Glyceraldehyde phosphate dehydrogenase	226 ± 41.9	1
GOT without pyridoxal phosphate	3.02 ± 0.67	1
GOT with pyridoxal phosphate	5.04 ± 0.90	1
Hexokinase	1.78 ± 0.38	1
Lactate dehydrogenase	200 ± 26.5	1
Monophosphoglyceromutase	37.71 ± 5.56	1
NADH-methemoglobin reductase	19.2 ± 3.85 (30°C)	1
NADPH diaphorase	2.26 ± 0.16	1
Nucleoside phosphorylase	359 ± 32	23
Phosphofructokinase	11.01 ± 2.33	1
Phosphoglucomutase	5.50 ± 0.62	1
Phosphoglycerate kinase	320 ± 36.1	1
Phosphoglycolate phosphatase	1.23 ± 0.10	1
Phosphomannose isomerase	0.054 ± 0.026	19
Pyrimidine 5′ nucleotidase	0.138 ± .018	1
Pyruvate kinase	15.0 ± 1.99	1
6-Phosphogluconolactonase	50.6 ± 5.9	24
6-Phosphogluconate dehydrogenase	8.78 ± 0.78	1
Ribosephosphate isomerase	200	1
Superoxide dismutase	2255 ± 303	1
Transaldolase	1.21 ± 0.24	25
Transketolase	0.725 ± 0.17	25
Triosephosphate isomerase	2111 ± 397	1

*For U.S.-European subjects.
†Flavin adenine dinucleotide.

Red cell type I phosphofructokinase exists as a series of tetramers comprised of muscle (M) and liver (L) subunits. A platelet (P) subunit has also been identified.[50] The M and L subunits of phosphofructokinase I and phosphofructokinase II have been cloned and sequenced.[51-53] Deficiency of type I phosphofructokinase, which may be associated with mild hemolytic anemia and with type VII glycogen storage disease, is discussed in Chap. 44.

ALDOLASE

Aldolase reversibly cleaves fructose 1,6-diphosphate into two trioses. The "upper" half of the fructose 1,6-diphosphate molecule becomes dihydroxyacetone phosphate (DHAP), and the "lower" half glyceraldehyde-3-phosphate. Red cells contain aldolase A, as is found in muscle, and no aldolase B (liver aldolase). On isoelectric focusing of hemolysates, however, five isoenzymes can be resolved, as is the case with other tissues.[54] The isoenzymes presumably represent mixed tetramers of native α polypeptide chains and chains that have undergone posttranscriptional deamidation, α' chains. Young red cells contain more of the nondeamidated isoenzymes. Aldose A has been cloned and sequenced.[55,56] Aldolase deficiency is a rare cause of hereditary nonspherocytic hemolytic anemia (see Chap. 44).

TRIOSEPHOSPHATE ISOMERASE

Triosephosphate isomerase (TPI) is the enzyme of the anaerobic glycolytic pathway that has the highest activity. Its metabolic role is to catalyze interconversion of the two trioses formed by the action of aldolase—dihydroxyacetone phosphate and glyceraldehyde-3-phosphate.[1] Although equilibrium is in favor of dihydroxyacetone phosphate, glyceraldehyde-3-phosphate undergoes continued oxidation through the action of glyceraldehyde phosphate dehydrogenase and is thus removed from the equilibrium. The gene encoding TPI has been cloned and sequenced.[57] A polymorphism in the promotor region[58] of uncertain significance has been identified.[59] A deficiency of TPI has been found in patients with hereditary nonspherocytic hemolytic anemia associated with a severe neuromuscular disorder (see Chap. 44).

GLYCERALDEHYDE PHOSPHATE DEHYDROGENASE

Glyceraldehyde phosphate dehydrogenase performs the dual functions of oxidizing and phosphorylating glyceraldehyde-3-phosphate, producing 1,3-BPG. In the process, NAD^+ is reduced to NADH. This enzyme is closely associated with the red cell membrane.[60] A two- to threefold stimulation of activity by hemoglobin could have a regulatory role.[61]

PHOSPHOGLYCERATE KINASE

Phosphoglycerate kinase effects the transfer to ADP of the high-energy phosphate from the 1-carbon of 1,3-BPG to form ATP. The reaction is readily reversible. Electrophoretically detectable mutations of the enzyme have been described,[62,63] and their transmission in families confirms that the structural gene for phosphoglycerate kinase is sex-linked. The amino acid sequence of phosphoglycerate kinase has been determined,[64] the cDNA for phosphoglycerate kinase has been cloned and sequenced,[65] and linkage relationships on the X-chromosome determined.[66] Deficiency of phosphoglycerate kinase is a cause of nonspherocytic hemolytic anemia, often associated with neuromuscular abnormalities (see Chap 54).

BISPHOSPHOGLYCEROMUTASE-BISPHOSPHOGLYCERATE PHOSPHATASE

The same protein molecule is responsible for both bisphosphoglycerate mutase and bisphosphoglycerate phosphatase activities in the erythrocyte.[67,68] This enzyme is particularly important because it regulates the concentration of 2,3-BPG of erythrocytes. In its role as a bisphosphoglyceromutase, the enzyme competes with phosphoglycerate kinase

for 1,3-bisphosphoglycerate as a substrate. It changes 1,3-bisphosphoglycerate to 2,3-bisphosphoglycerate, thereby dissipating the energy of the high-energy acylphosphate bond.[69] It is inhibited by its product, 2,3-bisphosphoglycerate, and by inorganic phosphate, and it is activated by 2-phosphoglycerate and by increased pH levels. It requires 3-phosphoglycerate for activity. Bisphospoglycerate phosphatase catalyzes the removal of the phosphate group from carbon 2 of 2,3-BPG.[69] It is inhibited by its product, 3-phosphoglycerate, and by sulfhydryl reagents. It is most active at a slightly acid pH and is strongly stimulated by bisulfite and phosphoglycolate.

A deficiency of bisphosphoglyceromutase-bisphosphoglycerate phosphatase results in a marked decrease in red cell 2,3-BPG levels. The consequent left shift of the oxygen dissociation curve leads to polycythemia (Chap. 61). The cDNA of the enzyme has been cloned and sequenced.[70,71]

Phosphoglycolate, the most potent activator of phosphatase activity, is present in erythrocytes at very low concentrations,[72,73] but the source of this substance in red cells is a mystery.[74-76] Phosphoglycolate phosphatase, the enzyme that hydrolyzes phosphoglycolate has also been identified in erythrocytes.[77,78]

MONOPHOSPHOGLYCEROMUTASE

An equilibrium is established between 3-phosphoglycerate and 2-phosphoglycerate by phosphoglyceromutase.[79,80] 2,3-Bisphosphoglycerate acts as an essential cofactor for the transformation.

ENOLASE

Enolase establishes an equilibrium between 2-phosphoglycerate and phosphoenolpyruvate (PEP).[81] Electrophoresis of red cell enolase gives three bands, supporting the suggestion that it is composed of two different subunits that associate randomly into dimers.[82]

PYRUVATE KINASE

The transfer of phosphate from PEP to ADP, forming ATP and pyruvate, is catalyzed by pyruvate kinase.[83] This is one of the energy-yielding steps of glycolysis. There are two major types of pyruvate kinase. The R type of enzyme found in erythrocytes closely resembles the L or liver enzyme; both are products of the same gene. The minor differences between the liver and red cell enzyme are due to differences in RNA processing[84] (see Chap. 8). Leukocytes contain type M or muscle enzyme. It is quite different in its kinetic properties and is the product of a different gene. Red cell pyruvate kinase is an allosteric enzyme, manifesting sigmoid kinetics with respect to PEP in the absence of fructose diphosphate. Hyperbolic kinetics are observed in the presence of even minute amounts of fructose diphosphate,[85,86] so that at low concentrations of PEP the enzyme activity is greatly increased by fructose diphosphate. Genes for both the L and M type enzymes have been cloned.[87,88] Pyruvate kinase deficiency is the most common cause of nonspherocytic hemolytic anemia (Chap. 44).

LACTATE DEHYDROGENASE

Lactate dehydrogenase (LDH) catalyzes the reversible reduction of pyruvate to lactate by NADH. The enzyme is composed of H (heart) and M (muscle) subunits. In red cells the predominant subunit is LDH-H.[89] However, hereditary absence of the H subunit seems to be a benign condition, usually without clinical manifestations,[89-92] although one case with hemolysis has been reported.[93] Absence of the M subunit has been reported as well[89] and was unaccompanied by hematologic manifestations. Judging from the origin of the reports, LDH deficiency appears to be most common in Japan, where population surveys show a gene frequency of approximately 0.05 for each deficiency,[94,95] and several frame-shift mutations have been identified.[95]

GLUCOSE-6-PHOSPHATE DEHYDROGENASE

G-6-PD is the most extensively studied erythrocyte enzyme.[94,96] It catalyzes the oxidation of glucose 6-phosphate to 6-phosphogluconolactone, which is rapidly hydrolyzed to 6-phosphogluconic acid. NADP$^+$ is reduced to NADPH in the reaction. The enzyme has been crystallized,[97] and its gene[98] and cDNA[99-101] cloned and sequenced. The structure of the *Leuconostoc mesenteroides* enzyme has been deduced from its crystal structure.[102]

Much information is available regarding substrate specificity, Michaelis constants, and pH optimum curves. The M_r of the highly purified enzyme has been reported to be 240,000 daltons,[97] but in its natural state the M_r is probably approximately 105,000 daltons.[103,104] In the absence of NADP$^+$ G-6-PD dissociates into inactive subunits. The computed subunit M_r is 59,256. The enzyme is strongly inhibited by physiologic amounts of NADPH[105] and, to a lesser extent, by physiologic concentrations of ATP.[106,107] It is much more active in reticulocytes than mature red cells.[27,28] Many electrophoretic mutations are known, as are others involving the activity, stability, and kinetic properties of the enzyme (see Chap. 44).

PHOSPHOGLUCONOLACTONASE

Although 6-phosphogluconolactone, the direct product of the oxidation of glucose-6-phosphate by glucose-6-phosphate dehydrogenase hydrolyzes spontaneously at a relatively rapid rate at a physiologic pH, enzymatic hydrolysis is much more rapid and is required for normal metabolic flow through the stimulated hexose monophosphate pathway.[108,109] Partial deficiency of the enzyme has been observed[110] and is probably benign.[111]

PHOSPHOGLUCONATE DEHYDROGENASE

Phosphogluconate dehydrogenase catalyzes the oxidation of phosphogluconate to ribulose 5-phosphate and CO_2 and the reduction of NADP$^+$ to NADPH. Variability of electrophoretic mobility of the enzyme is common in humans and in several animal species.[112] Deficiency of the enzyme has been observed only rarely and appears to be essentially innocuous.[113]

RIBOSEPHOSPHATE ISOMERASE

Ribosephosphate isomerase catalyzes the interconversion of ribulose 5-phosphate and ribose 5-phosphate.[33,114]

RIBULOSEPHOSPHATE EPIMERASE

Ribulosephosphate epimerase converts ribulose 5-phosphate to xylulose 5-phosphate.[33] The exact activity of this enzyme in human hemolysates has not been reported but seems to be less than that of ribosephosphate isomerase.

TRANSKETOLASE

Transketolase effects the transfer of two carbon atoms from xylulose 5-phosphate to ribose 5-phosphate, resulting in the formation of the 7-carbon sugar sedoheptulose 7-phosphate and the 3-carbon sugar glyceraldehyde 3-phosphate.[33,115] It can also catalyze the reaction between xylulose 5-phosphate and erythrose 4-phosphate, producing fructose 6-phosphate and glyceraldehyde 3-phosphate. Thiamine pyrophosphate is a coenzyme for transketolase, and the activity of erythrocyte transketolase has been used as an index of the adequacy of thiamine nutrition.[116,117]

TRANSALDOLASE

The conversion of seduhepulose 7-phosphate and glyceraldehyde 3-phosphate into erythrose 4-phosphate and fructose 6-phosphate is catalyzed by transaldolase.[115] This is another one in the series of molecular rearrangements that eventuate in the conversion of the 5-carbon sugar

formed in the phosphogluconate dehydrogenase step to metabolic intermediates of the Embden-Meyerhof pathway.

L-HEXONATE DEHYDROGENASE

Red cells contain L-hexonate dehydrogenase, an enzyme that has the capacity to reduce aldoses such as glucose, galactose, or glyceraldehyde to their corresponding polyol (i.e., glucose to sorbitol, galactose to dulcitol, and glyceraldehyde to glycerol). NADPH serves as a hydrogen donor for this reaction.[118] Aldose reductase,[119] another enzyme that can catalyze this reaction, may also be present in red cells.

THE UTILIZATION OF SUBSTRATES OTHER THAN GLUCOSE AS ENERGY SOURCES

The red cell has the capacity to utilize several other substrates in addition to glucose as a source of energy. Among these are adenosine, inosine, fructose, mannose, galactose, dihydroxyacetone, and lactate. Although in the circulation red cells normally rely on glucose as their energy source, the utilization of other substrates, particularly during blood storage (see Chap. 138) and in certain experimental situations, is of interest.

ADENOSINE AND INOSINE

Adenosine has been used as an experimental blood preservative, and it has been suggested that it may also be metabolized by human red cells in vivo.[120] Adenosine is deaminated to inosine by the enzyme adenosine deaminase (ADA)[121]:

$$\text{Adenosine} \xrightarrow{\text{ADA}} \text{inosine} + NH_3$$

It apparently plays a regulatory role in the concentration of purine nucleotides in the red cell. Deficiency of ADA is associated with SCID[122,123] (Chap. 86). In this disorder, large quantities of deoxyadenine nucleotides, not normally present in erythrocytes, accumulate. Hereditary increase in activity of erythrocyte ADA results in the depletion of red cell ATP and nonspherocytic hemolytic anemia.[124] For reasons that are not understood, ADA activity also increases in the red cells of AIDS patients[125,126] and of those with Diamond-Blackfan anemia.[127]

Inosine formed in the ADA reaction or added directly to red cells may enter the erythrocyte and undergo phosphorolysis to form hypoxanthine and ribose 1-phosphate (R-1-P):

$$\text{Inosine} + P_i \xrightarrow{\text{nucleoside phosphorylase}} \text{R-1-P} + \text{hypoxanthine}$$

This reaction is of particular interest because it results in the introduction of a phosphorylated sugar, R-1-P, into the erythrocyte without the utilization of ATP.[121,128] The R-1-P may then be further metabolized to yield high-energy phosphate. The nucleoside phosphorylase reaction appears to be the only practical means by which ATP may be formed in the cell without first expending ATP to prepare an unphosphorylated substrate for further metabolism. The use of inosine has therefore received much attention in the field of blood banking (see Chap. 138). A deficiency of nucleoside phosphorylase has been associated with immunodeficiency.[123]

FRUCTOSE

Fructose is readily utilized by the erythrocyte, although at a rate somewhat slower than that of glucose.[129] Fructose undergoes phosphorylation at position 6 in the hexokinase reaction:

$$\text{Fructose} + \text{ATP} \xrightarrow[Mg^{2+}]{\text{hexokinase}} \text{fructose 6-P} + \text{ADP}$$

Fructose 6-phosphate is a normal metabolic intermediate in the anaerobic glycolytic pathway. Thus, the result of fructose phosphorylation is exactly the same as the result of the phosphorylation of glucose.

Fructose may also be metabolized by another red cell enzyme, sorbitol dehydrogenase.[130,131] This enzyme reduces fructose to its corresponding polyol, sorbitol, with NADH serving as a hydrogen donor. The reaction is reversible, and a pathway therefore exists for the formation of fructose from glucose through L-hexonate dehydrogenase and sorbitol dehydrogenase. An enzyme that facilitates sorbitol permeation through the erythrocyte membrane has been described.

MANNOSE

Mannose is also phosphorylated in the hexokinase reaction[19]:

$$\text{Mannose} + \text{ATP} \xrightarrow[\text{Mg}^{2+}]{\text{hexokinase}} \text{mannose 6-P} + \text{ADP}$$

Mannose 6-phosphate must be isomerized to fructose 6-phosphate before it is further metabolized by erythrocytes. This is accomplished by phosphomannose isomerase[132,133]:

$$\text{Mannose 6-P} \xrightleftharpoons{\text{PMI}} \text{fructose 6-P}$$

Phosphomannose isomerase of red cells has very low activity, even at its pH optimum of 5.9.[19] The rate of mannose utilization is therefore limited by the activity of phosphomannose isomerase. Young red cells have enhanced phosphomannose isomerase activity and can therefore utilize mannose at a more rapid rate than can mature red cells.

GALACTOSE

The utilization of galactose by erythrocytes is more complex than that of most other substrates. At low concentrations of galactose, metabolism occurs by way of galactokinase, galactose-1-phosphate uridyl transferase, and phosphoglucomutase.[134] Unlike fructose, mannose, and glucose, galactose is phosphorylated at position 1:

$$\alpha\text{-Galactose} + \text{ATP} \xrightarrow[\text{Mg}^{2+}]{\text{galactokinase}} \alpha\text{-galactose-1-P} + \text{ADP}$$

The galactose-1-phosphate formed in the galactokinase reaction exchanges with the glucose-1-phosphate moiety of uridine diphosphoglucose (UDPG) in the galactose-1-phosphate uridyl transferase reaction:

$$\alpha\text{-Galactose-1-P} + \text{UDPG} \xrightleftharpoons{\text{transferase}} \alpha\text{-glucose 1-P} + \text{UDPgalactose}$$

The uridine diphosphogalactose (UDPgalactose) formed in this reaction is epimerized to UDPG:

$$\text{UDPgalactose} \xrightleftharpoons[\text{NAD}^+]{\text{epimerase}} \text{UDPG}$$

The α-glucose-1-phosphate in the transferase reaction is transformed to α-glucose-6-phosphate in the phosphoglucomutase (PGM) reaction[135] with glucose 1,6-diphosphate acting as coenzyme:

$$\alpha\text{-Glucose-1-P} \xrightleftharpoons[\text{glucose 1,6-diP}]{\text{PGM}} \alpha\text{-glucose-6-P}$$

The α-glucose-6-phosphate formed may join the direct metabolic stream after conversion by phosphoglucose isomerase to fructose 6-phosphate. It may also undergo anomerization to β-glucose-6-phosphate and enter the hexose monophosphate pathway, if NADP$^+$ is available. Very high concentrations of galactose appear to be metabolized by way of another pathway, as yet poorly delineated. This pathway is known not to involve galactose-1-phosphate uridyl transferase or to have the capacity to reduce NAD$^+$.[20]

DIHYDROXYACETONE AND GLYCERALDEHYDE

As indicated earlier, glyceraldehyde can be reduced in erythrocytes to glycerol in the L-hexonate dehydrogenase reaction. In addition, glyceraldehyde and dihydroxyacetone can each be phosphorylated by ATP in the presence of the enzyme triokinase.[136] Like other kinases, this enzyme has a requirement for magnesium. A remarkable feature of this enzyme is its extraordinarily low K_m for dihydroxyacetone. It is one-half saturated with this substrate at a concentration of only 0.5 μM. The products of the triokinase reaction, dihydroxyacetone phosphate or glyceraldehyde-3-phosphate, are normal metabolic intermediates and can be metabolized in the usual fashion. Because of its capacity to act as an alternative substrate for red cell energy metabolism and 2,3-BPG formation, dihydroxyacetone had been studied as an experimental additive for blood storage.[137,138]

GLYCOGEN METABOLISM

Red cells have the capacity to form and to break down glycogen. They contain the enzymes UDPG-glycogen glucosyltransferase and α-1,4-glucan: α-1,4-glucan-6-glycosyltransferase (the brancher enzyme) for the formation of glycogen from glucose 1-phosphate. Red cells also contain the enzymes phosphorylase and amylo-1,6-glucosidase (the debrancher enzyme) for the breakdown of glycogen.[139] Only very little glycogen is present in normal red cells,[140] and most of what was thought to be in red cells may actually be platelet and leukocyte glycogen.[141] The function of glycogen in red cell metabolism is not understood.

GLUTATHIONE METABOLISM OF THE ERYTHROCYTE

The red cell contains a high concentration (approximately 2 mM) of the sulfhydryl-containing tripeptide reduced glutathione.[1] Red cell GSH appears to undergo a rapid turnover, with a $T_{1/2}$ approximately 4 days.[142] Synthesis occurs in two steps:

$$\text{Glutamate} + \text{cysteine} + \text{ATP} \longrightarrow$$
$$\gamma\text{-glutamyl cysteine} + \text{ADP} + \text{P}_i$$

$$\gamma\text{-Glutamyl cysteine} + \text{glycine} + \text{ATP} \longrightarrow \text{GSH} + \text{ADP} + \text{P}_i$$

Both steps are catalyzed by red cell hemolysates.[22] The red cell requires a system for the synthesis of GSH because of the active transport of GSSG from the erythrocyte.[143] It has also been suggested that a requirement for GSH synthesis comes from the amino acid transporting function of the γ-glutamyl cycle.[144] However, this pathway is not present in red cells.[145-147]

One important function of GSH in the erythrocyte appears to be the detoxification of low levels of hydrogen peroxide that may form spontaneously or as a result of drug administration. In either event, the superoxide radical may be formed first and then be converted to H_2O_2 by the action of the copper-containing enzyme superoxide dismutase.[148] Hydrogen peroxide is reduced to water through the mediation of the enzyme glutathione peroxidase.[149,150] Glutathione peroxidase is a selenium-containing enzyme.[151] In New Zealand, dietary selenium intake is extremely low, and glutathione peroxidase activities are much lower than are observed elsewhere.[152] A polymorphism affecting the activity of the enzyme which is most common in persons of Mediterranean descent[153] has also been described. The consequent decreases in enzyme activity are without clinical effect. The genes for several glutathione peroxidases, including that of the erythrocyte, have been cloned.[154] The triplet UGA usually acts as a stop codon in this particular message and inserts selenocysteine in the proper location.[155] A unique tRNA that has complementary UCA anticodons is aminoacylated with serine. The seryl-tRNA is then converted to selenocysteyl-tRNA and is delivered to the ribosome.[156] Recognition elements within the mRNAs are essential for translation of UGA as selenocysteine rather than the usual stop codon.[156]

GSH also functions in maintaining integrity of the erythrocyte by reducing sulfhydryl groups of hemoglobin, membrane proteins, and enzymes that may become oxidized.[157] In the process of reducing peroxides or oxidized protein sulfhydryl groups, GSH is converted to GSSG or may form mixed disulfides. GSSG, like certain other disulfides, has the capacity to inhibit red cell hexokinase,[32,158] although greater-than-physiologic levels appear to be needed for this effect. It may also complex with hemoglobin A to form hemoglobin A3.[159] Glutathione reductase provides an efficient mechanism for the reduction of GSSG to GSH in the red cell. It is a flavin enzyme, and either NADPH or NADH may serve as a hydrogen donor.[160,161] In the intact cell, only the NADPH system appears to function.[162] The same enzyme system appears to have the capacity to reduce mixed disulfides of GSH and proteins.[13] Although inherited deficiencies of this enzyme exist,[163] the activity of red cell glutathione reductase is strongly influenced by the riboflavin content of the diet.[164] Red cells also contain thioltransferase that can catalyze GSH-dependent reduction of some disulfides.[165]

Oxidized glutathione is actively extruded from the erythrocyte[166,167] by a system consisting of at least two GSSG-activated ATPases that serve as an enzymatic basis for this transport process.[168] In addition to transporting GSSG, the system appears to have the capacity to transport thioether conjugates of GSH and electrophiles formed by the action of glutathione-S-transferase.[169,170] Blood cells, specifically including erythrocytes, contain a glutathione-S-transferase that is distinct from the predominant liver forms of the enzyme. This enzyme, designated type III or ρ to distinguish it from the liver enzymes catalyzes the formation of a thioether bond between GSH and a variety of xenobiotics. The role of glutathione-S-transferase in the erythrocyte has not been established. It may be that it serves to cleanse the blood of xenobiotics to which the red cell membrane is permeable. Glutathione-S-transferase could conjugate such substances to glutathione, and the detoxified product of conjugation would be transported out of the red cell for subsequent disposal. The enzyme has the capacity to reversibly bind heme, and a possible role in heme transport has been postulated.[171]

Fairly severe deficiency of this enzyme has been associated with hemolytic anemia, but a cause-and-effect relationship has not been established.[172]

METHEMOGLOBIN REDUCTION

The reduction of methemoglobin in normal red cells is achieved primarily through a NADH-linked system[173] (Chap. 48). A methemoglobin reductase (known also as *NADH diaphorase* or *cytochrome b5 reductase*) utilizes NADH generated in the glyceraldehyde-phosphate dehydrogenase reaction to reduce cytochrome b5, which in turn reduces the iron of methemoglobin from the trivalent to the divalent form. The gene for this enzyme has been cloned and sequenced.[174,175]

Red cells also contain a NADPH-linked methemoglobin-reducing system[176,177] that functions only in the presence of an artificial electron carrier, such as methylene blue. Nonenzymatic reduction of methemoglobin by GSH and ascorbic acid accounts for only a small portion of the total methemoglobin-reducing rate of red cells.

OTHER RED CELL ENZYMES

Erythrocytes contain a high concentration of carbonic anhydrase I. In catalyzing the equilibrium between carbon dioxide and carbonic acid, this enzyme aids in oxygen and carbon dioxide transport of the erythrocyte. This enzyme has been obtained from red cells in a highly purified state, and the cDNA has been cloned.[178]

The red blood cell is a rich source of catalase, the enzyme that decomposes hydrogen peroxide to water and oxygen. Hereditary lack of catalase does not seem to cause any hematologic disorder.[179,180] This enzyme functions efficiently only when relatively high concentrations of peroxide are present. Low concentrations of peroxide are detoxified by the enzyme glutathione peroxidase.[149,150] There has been an ongoing controversy regarding whether catalase or glutathione peroxidase is the more important means for the protection of the erythrocyte against free radicals[15,181-183]; however, it is difficult to understand why one would have to be more important than the other. Either system alone appears to suffice, since deficiencies of either are well tolerated. Superoxide dismutase, a copper-containing enzyme, is also present in erythrocytes.[184] It presumably plays an important role in the protection of hemoglobin and other red cell components against a highly reactive superoxide anion. It has been suggested that red cells contain thioredoxin, thioredoxin reductase,[185] and glutaredoxin,[186] but it is possible that these enzymes might have been present in contaminating leukocytes, since these were inadequately removed. If this system does exist in erythrocytes, it could serve as another defense mechanism against the oxidative damage to which erythrocytes are vulnerable because of their large load of oxygen that is continually being bound by and released by hemoglobin. Erythrocytes are a primary means for the removal not only of nitric oxide but also of nitric oxide synthase-1.[187]

The red cell membrane contains large amounts of acetylcholinesterase.[188] Although the activity of this enzyme is diminished in paroxysmal nocturnal hemoglobinuria, this does not play an etiologic role. It is merely a manifestation of the underlying defect in the phosphotidyl-inositol anchor (see Chap. 35). Hereditary lack of red cell cholinesterase activity is not associated with any clinical hematologic effects.[189] AMP-deaminase[190] seems to be particularly important because of the regulatory role that it plays in the levels of adenine nucleotides in the red cell. An entirely separate enzyme from ADA, AMP deaminase removes ammonia from the adenine moiety of AMP, converting it to inosine monophosphate. A severe deficiency of this enzyme has been reported,[191] and this resulted in elevated red cell ATP levels. However, there were no hematologic consequences.

Red cell membranes also contain protein kinase activities.[192] Several such enzymes catalyze the transfer of the terminal phosphate from ATP to various cytoskeletal protein acceptors, primarily band 2 of spectrin and "band 3" (see Chap. 26). One protein kinase is relatively insensitive to stimulation by cAMP and unaffected cGMP. It has the capacity to phosphorylate exogenous protein acceptors, such as casein and histones, as well as endogenous cytoskeletal proteins. In rabbit erythrocytes membrane-associated casein kinase was found to show striking age-dependency.[193] The role of this enzyme in the structural properties of the red cell membrane is not yet clear. Several proteolytic systems have been defined in erythrocytes. One of these, calpain, is activated by high concentrations of calcium.[194] Reticulocytes contain ubiquitin that, together with ATP and several partially defined enzyme activities, may serve as an important mechanism for the destruction of mitochondrial matrix and unneeded enzymes as the red cell matures from the reticulocytes to the erythrocyte stage.[195] The red cell membrane is also believed to contain neutral protease activities.[196] Multicatalytic proteinase[197–199] or enzymes that closely resemble it have also been found.[200]

Several distinct membrane ATPases have been characterized. Each seems to serve a transport function, and each is stimulated to hydrolyze ATP by the substance that is transported. Thus, the Na⁺-K⁺-ATPase is a membrane enzyme that functions to move sodium out of the red cell and potassium in at a fixed ratio of two potassium ions for each three sodium ions.[201] It appears to have a requirement for bound lipid[202,203] and is inhibited by ouabain. A Ca^{2+}-ATPase[204,205] serves to extrude calcium from the red cell. It binds calmodulin,[204] a regulator of calcium transport that has also been identified in red cells.[206] The function of Mg^{2+}-ATPase[207] is less clear, since all ATPases require magnesium ions for their function. Guanosine triphosphatase[208] and inosine triphosphate[209,210] activities have also been characterized in red cells. G-proteins are present.[211,212]

An aldehyde dehydrogenase of red cells makes it possible for erythrocytes to utilize aldehydes such as formaldehyde as substrates for methemoglobin reduction,[213,214] and the enzyme may play a role in drug detoxification.[215,216] The presence and usually the characteristics of amino acid-activating enzymes,[217] dipeptidases,[218] formate-activating enzyme,[219] glutamic-oxaloacetic transaminase,[1] glyoxalase,[220] pyridoxine kinase,[221,222] uroporphyrinogen 1 synthetase,[223] ribonucleases,[224] pyrroline-5-carboxylate reductase,[225] acid phosphatase,[226] prolidase,[227,228] nucleoside diphosphokinase,[229] (ADP-ribose)ₙ glycohydrolase,[230] ribonuclease,[224] ribonuclease inhibitor,[231] arylamine-N-acetyltransferase,[232] phosphatidylinositol 3-monophosphate-4-kinase,[233] phosphatidylinositol 4-kinase,[233] protein palmitoyl acyltransferase,[234] calpromotin,[216,235] D-dopachrome tautomerase,[236] thiopurine methyltransferase,[237] UMP synthetase,[238] and numerous other enzymes[239] have been reported in erythrocytes.

NUCLEOTIDE SYNTHESIS

Most cells achieve the de novo synthesis of purine nucleotides by constructing the heterocyclic purine ring in a series of enzymatic reactions that begin with the synthesis of phosphoribosyl pyrophosphate (PRPP) from ribose 5-phosphate and ATP. Methyl groups are added through the mediation of folate coenzymes, and nitrogens are supplied by glutamine, lysine, and aspartic acid. The initial product of the de novo pathway, inosine 5′-monophosphate (IMP), is then converted to AMP and to guanosine 5′-phosphate through further enzymatic transformations. Pyrimidine nucleotides are synthesized de novo through pathways beginning with the reaction of carbamyl phosphate and aspartic acid to form carbamyl aspartate. Further intermediates include dihydroorotate, orotate, and orotidine 5′-phosphate, which is finally converted to uridine 5′-phosphate.

Although all the reactions for synthesis of purine and pyrimidine nucleotides presumably occur in erythroid precursors, the mature erythrocyte depends on the so-called salvage pathway for its supply of purine nucleotides. The adenine phosphoribosyltransferase (APRT) and hypoxanthine-guanine phosphoribosyltransferase (HGPRT) reactions serve to incorporate adenine (in the case of APRT) or hypoxanthine or guanine (in the case of HGPRT) into nucleotides:

$$\text{Adenine} + \text{PRPP} \xrightarrow{\text{APRT}} \text{AMP}$$

$$\text{Guanine (or hypoxanthine)} + \text{PRPP} \xrightarrow{\text{HGPRT}} \text{GMP (or IMP)}$$

The first of these reactions is the basis for the use of adenine in blood preservatives (Chap. 138). Absence of APRT,[240] inherited as an autosomal recessive disorder, results in nephrolithiasis, deoxyadenine stones being deposited in the kidneys.[241–243] The function of HGPRT in red cells is unclear, since the role of guanine and inosine nucleotides remains undefined. Absence of this enzyme, inherited as a sex-linked disorder, results in hyperuricemia and a neurologic disorder characterized by self-mutilation, the so-called Lesch-Nyhan syndrome.[244,245] Red cells are also able to synthesize adenine nucleotides by phosphorylating adenosine. This reaction is catalyzed by adenosine kinase.[246] The bridge between ribonucleotides and deoxyribonucleotides is provided by the enzyme ribonucleotide reductase. All dividing cells require deoxyribonucleotides for DNA synthesis. Ribonucleotides are needed not only for the synthesis of RNA for protein synthesis but also to perform many other functions. For example, ATP and GTP provide the energy for many biochemical processes and serve as precursors of cyclic nucleotides, the regulators of many enzymatic reactions. Uridine nucleotides are sugar carriers that serve as intermediates in various carbohydrate transformations and in the synthesis of glycoproteins and glycolipids.

The mature erythrocyte contains small quantities of pyrimidine nucleotides. Little is known of their function in this cell. The capacity of erythrocytes to metabolize galactose reflects one function of a pyrimidine nucleotide, UDPGlucose, in the erythrocyte. However, since the red cell is a trivial site of galactose metabolism in the body, this function of the pyrimidine nucleotide can hardly be considered of much physiologic importance. The enzyme pyrimidine 5′-nucleotidase[247] specifically dephosphorylates pyrimidine mononucleotides and thus presumably plays a role in the catabolism of ribose polynucleotides in the red cell.

The nicotinic acid nucleotides NAD⁺ and NADP⁺ are also a vital component of the biochemical machinery of the cell, and pathways for their synthesis exist. NAD⁺ is synthesized from nicotinic acid as shown in Fig. 26-3. PRPP is attached to the nicotinic acid ring through the mediation of the enzyme desamido-NMN pyrophosphorylase, forming desamido nicotinic acid mononucleotide. After attachment of AMP through a pyrophosphate bond, glutamine provides an amino group for completion of the synthesis of NAD⁺.[248–250] The only known pathway for the synthesis of NADP⁺ involves phosphorylation of NAD⁺ by ATP in the presence of NAD kinase.[218,251] Large oral doses of nicotinic acid promote an increase in the concentration of red cell NAD⁺ but not of NADP⁺.[252] NAD⁺ is degraded by the enzyme NADase, which hydrolyzes the pyridine nucleotides at the nicotinamide-ribose linkage. The enzymes can catalyze the exchange of free nicotinamide with pyridine nucleotide-bound nicotinamide.[218] A deficiency of this activity, apparently without significant effect, has been documented.[253]

RETICULOCYTE METABOLISM

The energy metabolism of reticulocytes is more active than that of older erythrocytes. The activity of enzymes that are important in regulating the rate of glycolysis is increased in reticulocytes. Evidence is mounting that there is an abrupt decrease of a number of glycolytic enzymes as reticulocytes mature.[27,254–256] These observations stand in contrast to the earlier held view that a gradual decrease in activities of red cell enzymes occurred throughout their life span.[257] This concept was based on the assumption that there was a sufficiently consistent increase in density of erythrocytes during their ageing in the circulation to make possible meaningful separations of red cells into different age groups by density centrifugation. In reality, this does not seem to occur, and the apparent decrease in the activity of many enzymes

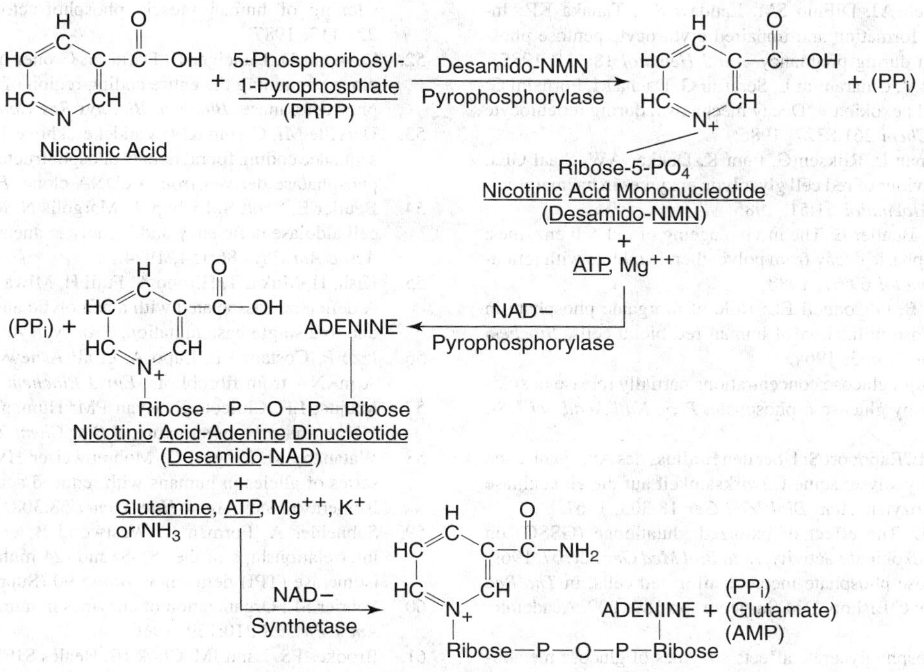

FIGURE 26-3   The nicotinic acid pathway for the biosynthesis of nicotinamide adenine dinucleotide.

based on such studies may well be due to decreasing contamination of layers of different density with reticulocytes.

In addition to their capacity to carry out glycolysis at a relatively rapid rate, reticulocytes have mitochondria with a complete complement of mitochondrial enzymes.[258] This enables them to metabolize glucose not only through the Embden-Meyerhof pathway and hexose monophosphate shunt but also through the Krebs cycle. The rate of oxygen consumption of reticulocytes is 60 times that of mature red cells; the rate of glucose consumption is 7.5 times as great.[259] This metabolic capacity provides these cells with the potential of phosphorylating ADP to ATP at a greatly accelerated rate and of providing succinate for the synthesis of heme.

REFERENCES

1. Beutler E: *Red Cell Metabolism: A Manual of Biochemical Methods.* Grune & Stratton, New York, 1984.
2. Baldwin SA, Lienhard GE: Purification and reconstitution of glucose transporter from human erythrocytes. *Methods Enzymol* 174:39, 1989.
3. Herzberg V, Boughter JM, Carlisle S, Hill DE: Evidence for two insulin receptor populations on human erythrocytes. *Nature* 286:279, 1980.
4. Robinson TJ, Archer JA, Gambhir KK, Hollis VW Jr, Carter L, Bradley C: Erythrocytes: a new cell type for the evaluation of insulin receptor defects in diabetic humans. *Science* 205:200, 1979.
5. Eadie GS, MacLeod JJR, Noble EC: Insulin and glycolysis. *Am J Physiol* 65:462, 1923.
6. Keitt AS, Bennett DC: Pyruvate kinase deficiency and related disorders of red cell glycolysis. *Am J Med* 41:762, 1966.
7. Gerlach E, Duhm J, Deuticke B: Metabolism of 2,3-diphosphoglycerate in red blood cells under various experimental conditions, in *Red Cell Metabolism and Function*, edited by E Beutler, p 155–174. Plenum, New York, 1970.
8. Poole RC, Halestrap AP: Identification and partial purification of the erythrocyte L-lactate transporter. *Biochem J* 283:855, 1992.
9. Heinrich R, Rapoport SM: The utility of mathematical models for the understanding of metabolic systems. *Biochem Soc Trans* 11:31, 1983.
10. Joshi A, Palsson BO: Metabolic dynamics in the human red cell. Part II—Interactions with the environment. *J Theor Biol* 141:529, 1989.

11. Reddy VN, Liebman MN, Mavrovouniotis ML: Qualitative analysis of biochemical reaction systems. *Comput Biol Med* 26:9, 1996.
12. Mulquiney PJ, Kuchel PW: Model of the pH-dependence of the concentrations of complexes involving metabolites, haemoglobin and magnesium ions in the human erythrocyte. *Eur J Biochem* 245:71, 1997.
13. Srivastava SK, Beutler E: Glutathione metabolism of the erythrocyte. The enzymic cleavage of glutathione-haemoglobin preparations by glutathione reductase. *Biochem J* 119:353, 1970.
14. Scott MD, Wagner TC, Chiu DTY: Decreased catalase activity is the underlying mechanism of oxidant susceptibility in glucose-6-phosphate dehydrogenase-deficient erythrocytes. *Biochim Biophys Acta* 1181:163, 1993.
15. Gaetani GF, Ferraris AM, Rolfo M, Mangerini R, Arena S, Kirkman HN: Predominant role of catalase in the disposal of hydrogen peroxide within human erythrocytes. *Blood* 87:1595, 1996.
16. Thorburn DR, Kuchel PW: Regulation of the human-erythrocytehexose-monophosphate shunt under conditions of oxidative stress. *Eur J Biochem* 150:371, 1985.
17. Ni TC, Savageau MA: Application of biochemical systems theory to metabolism in human red blood cells—signal propagation and accuracy of representation. *J Biol Chem* 271:7927, 1996.
18. Schuster R, Jacobasch G, Holzhütter HG: Mathematical modelling of metabolic pathways affected by an enzyme deficiency—energy and redox metabolism of glucose-6-phosphate-dehydrogenase-deficient erythrocytes. *Eur J Biochem* 182:605, 1989.
19. Beutler E, Teeple L: Mannose metabolism in the human erythrocyte. *J Clin Invest* 48:461, 1969.
20. Beutler E, Mathai CK: Genetic variation in red cell galactose-1-phosphate uridyl transferase, in *Hereditary Disorders of Erythrocyte Metabolism*, edited by E Beutler, p 66–86. Grune & Stratton, New York, 1968.
21. Beutler E, Kuhl W: *Unpublished* 1991.
22. Beutler E, Gelbart T: Improved assay of the enzymes of glutathione synthesis: gamma-glutamylcysteine synthetase and glutathione synthetase. *Clin Chim Acta* 158:115, 1986.
23. Oski FA, Sugerman HJ, Miller LD: Experimentally induced alterations in the affinity of Hb for oxygen: I. In vitro restoration of erythrocyte 2,3-DPG and its relationship to erythrocyte purine nucleoside phosphorylase activity in a variety of species. *Blood* 39:522, 1972.
24. Beutler E, Kuhl W, Gelbart T: Blood cell phosphogluconolactonase: assay and properties. *Br J Haematol* 62:577, 1986.

25. Lachant NA, Gottlieb AJ, DiFino SM, Landaw SA, Tanaka KR: Increased Heinz body formation and impaired erythrocyte pentose phosphate shunt function during pregnancy. *Am J Hematol* 18:131, 1985.

26. Magnani M, Stocchi V, Chiarantini L, Serafini G, Dacha M, Fornaini G: Rabbit red blood cell hexokinase. Decay mechanism during reticulocyte maturation. *J Biol Chem* 261:8327, 1986.

27. Jansen G, Koenderman L, Rijksen G, Punt K, Dekker AW, Staal GEJ: Age dependent behaviour of red cell glycolytic enzymes in haematological disorders. *Br J Haematol* 61:51, 1985.

28. Zimran A, Torem S, Beutler E: The in vivo ageing of red cell enzymes: direct evidence of biphasic decay from polycythemic rabbits with reticulocytosis. *Br J Haematol* 69:67, 1988.

29. Rose IA, Warms JVB, O'Connell EL: Role of inorganic phosphate in stimulating the glucose utilization of human red blood cells. *Biochem Biophys Res Commun* 15:33, 1964.

30. Fujii S, Beutler E: High glucose concentrations partially release hexokinase from inhibition by glucose-6-phosphate. *Proc Natl Acad Sci USA* 82:1552, 1985.

31. Gerber G, Kloppick E, Rapoport S: Über den Einfluss des Anorganischen Phosphats auf die Glykolyse; seine Unwirksamkeit auf die Hexokinase des Menschenerythrozyten. *Acta Biol Med Ger* 18:305, 1967.

32. Beutler E, Teeple L: The effect of oxidized glutathione (GSSG) on human erythrocyte hexokinase activity. *Acta Biol Med Ger* 22:707, 1969.

33. Dische Z: The pentose phosphate metabolism in red cells, in *The Red Blood Cell*, edited by C Bishop, DM Surgenor, pp 189–209. Academic, New York, 1964.

34. Beutler E: 2,3-Diphosphoglycerate affects enzymes of glucose metabolism in red blood cells. *Nature (New Biol)* 232:20, 1971.

35. Kaplan JC, Beutler E: Hexokinase isoenzymes in human erythrocytes. *Science* 159:215, 1968.

36. Altay C, Alper CA, Nathan DG: Normal and variant isoenzymes of human blood cell hexokinase and the isoenzyme patterns in hemolytic anemia. *Blood* 36:219, 1970.

37. Murakami K, Blei F, Tilton W, Seaman C, Piomelli S: An isozyme of hexokinase specific for the human red blood cell (HK$_R$). *Blood* 75:770, 1990.

38. Ruzzo A, Andreoni F, Magnani M: Structure of the human hexokinase type I gene and nucleotide sequence of the 5′ flanking region. *Biochem J* 331:607, 1998.

39. Murakami K, Piomelli S: Identification of the cDNA for human red blood cell-specific hexokinase isozyme. *Blood* 89:762, 1997.

40. Magnani M, Stocchi V, Dacha M, Fornaini G: Rabbit red blood cell hexokinase: Intracellular distribution during reticulocytes maturation. *Mol Cell Biochem* 63:59, 1984.

41. Stocchi V, Magnani M, Piccoli G, Fornaini G: Hexokinase microheterogeneity in rabbit red blood cells and its behaviour during reticulocytes maturation. *Mol Cell Biochem* 79:133, 1988.

42. Thorburn DR, Beutler E: Ubiquitin-dependent proteolysis of reticulocyte hexokinase. *Blood* 74:218A, 1989.

43. Rijksen G, Akkerman JWN, van den Wall Bake AWL, Pott Hofstede O, Staal GEJ: Generalized hexokinase deficiency in the blood cells of a patient with nonspherocytic hemolytic anemia. *Blood* 61:12, 1983.

44. Hirono A, Forman L, Beutler E: Enzymatic diagnosis in non-spherocytic hemolytic anemia. *Medicine (Baltimore)* 67:110, 1988.

45. Detter JC, Ways PO, Giblett ER, et al: Inherited variations in human phosphohexose isomerase. *Ann Hum Genet* 31:329, 1968.

46. Xu WM, Lee P, Beutler E: Human glucose phosphate isomerase: exon mapping and gene structure. *Genomics* 29:732, 1995.

47. Walker JIH, Morgan MJ, Faik P: Structure and organization of the human glucose phosphate isomerase gene (GPI). *Genomics* 29:261, 1995.

48. Fujii S, Matsuda M, Okuya S, Yoshizaki Y, Miura-Kora Y, Kaneko T: Fructose-6-phosphate, 2-kinase activity in human erythrocytes. *Blood* 70:1211, 1987.

49. Bosca L, Aragon JJ, Sols A: Modulation of muscle phosphofructokinase at physiological concentration of enzyme. *J Biol Chem* 260:2100, 1985.

50. Vora S: Isozymes of human phosphofructokinase: Biochemical and genetic aspects, in *Isozymes: Current Topics in Biological and Medical Research*, edited by MC Rattazzi, JG Scandalios, GS Whitt, pp 3–23. Liss, New York, 1983.

51. Nakajima H, Noguchi T, Yamasaki T, Kono N, Tanaka T, Tarui S: Cloning of human muscle phosphofructokinase cDNA. *FEBS Lett* 223:113, 1987.

52. Levanon D, Danciger E, Dafni N, Groner Y: Construction of a cDNA clone containing the entire coding region of the human liver-type phosphofructokinase. *Biochem Biophys Res Commun* 147:1182, 1987.

53. Darville MI, Crepin KM, Vandekerckhove J, et al: Complete nucleotide sequence coding for rat liver 6-phosphofructo-2-kinase/fructose-2,6-bisphosphatase derived from a cDNA clone. *FEBS Lett* 224:317, 1987.

54. Beutler E, Scott S, Bishop A, Margolis N, Matsumoto F, Kuhl W: Red cell aldolase deficiency and hemolytic anemia: a new syndrome. *Trans Assoc Am Phys* 86:154, 1974.

55. Kishi H, Mukai T, Hirono A, Fujii H, Miwa S, Hori K: Human aldolase A deficiency associated with a hemolytic anemia: thermolabile aldolase due to a single base mutation. *Proc Natl Acad Sci USA* 84:8623, 1987.

56. Izzo P, Costanzo P, Lupo A, et al: A new human species of aldolase A mRNA from fibroblasts. *Eur J Biochem* 164:9, 1987.

57. Maquat LE, Chilcote R, Ryan PM: Human triosephosphate isomerase cDNA and protein structure. *J Biol Chem* 260:3748, 1989.

58. Watanabe M, Zingg BC, Mohrenweiser HW: Molecular analysis of a series of alleles in humans with reduced activity at the triosephosphate isomerase locus. *Am J Hum Genet* 58:308, 1996.

59. Schneider A, Forman L, Westwood B, et al: New insights into the interrelationships of the -5, -8, and -24 mutations with triosephosphate isomerase (TPI) deficiency. *Blood* 90 (Suppl 1):273a, 1997.

60. Schrier SL: Organization of enzymes in human erythrocyte membranes. *Am J Physiol* 210:139, 1966.

61. Brookes PS, Land JM, Clark JB, Heales SJR: Stimulation of glyceraldehyde-3-phosphate dehydrogenase by oxyhemoglobin. *FEBS Lett* 416:90, 1997.

62. Chen S-H, Malcolm LA, Yoshida A, Giblett ER: Phosphoglycerate kinase: an X-linked polymorphism in man. *Am J Hum Genet* 23:87, 1971.

63. Yoshida A, Watanabe S, Chen S-H, Giblet ER, Malcolm LA: Human phosphoglycerate kinase II. Structure of a variant enzyme. *J Biol Chem* 247:446, 1972.

64. Huang IY, Rubinfien E, Yoshida A: Complete amino acid sequence of human phosphoglycerate kinase. Isolation and amino acid sequence of tryptic peptides. *J Biol Chem* 255:6408, 1980.

65. Michelson AM, Markham AF, Orkin SH: Isolation and DNA sequence of a full-length cDNA clone for human X chromosome-encoded phosphoglycerate kinase. *Proc Natl Acad Sci USA* 80:472, 1983.

66. Raskind WH, Wijsman E, Pagon RA, et al: X-linked sideroblastic anemia and ataxia: linkage to phosphoglycerate kinase at Xq13. *Am J Hum Genet* 48:335, 1991.

67. Rosa R, Gaillardon J, Rosa J: Diphosphoglycerate mutase and 2,3-diphosphoglycerate phosphatase activities of red cells: Comparative electrophoretic study. *Biochem Biophys Res Commun* 51:536, 1973.

68. Ikura K, Sasaki R, Narita H, Sugimoto E, Chiba H: Multifunctional enzyme, bisphosphoglyceromutase/2,3-bisphosphoglycerate phosphatase/phosphoglyceromutase from human erythrocytes. *Eur J Biochem* 66:515, 1976.

69. Rose ZB: The enzymology of 2,3-bisphosphoglycerate. *Adv Enzymol* 51:211, 1980.

70. Joulin V, Peduzzi J, Romeo PH, et al: Molecular cloning and sequencing of the human erythrocyte 2,3-bisphosphoglycerate mutase cDNA: revised amino acid sequence. *EMBO J* 5:2275, 1986.

71. Yanagawa S, Hitomi K, Sasaki R, Chiba H: Isolation and characterization of cDNA encoding rabbit reticulocyte 2,3-bisphosphoglycerate synthase. *Gene* 44:185, 1986.

72. Rose ZB, Salon J: The identification of glycolate-2-P as a constituent of normal red blood cells. *Biochem Biophys Res Commun* 87:869, 1979.

73. Vora S, Spear D: Demonstration and quantitation of phosphoglycolate in human red cells. *Clin Res* 34:664A, 1986.

74. Fujii S, Beutler E: Glycolate kinase activity in human red cells. *Blood* 65:480, 1985.

75. Fujii S, Beutler E: Where does phosphoglycolate come from in red cells? *Acta Haematol (Basel)* 73:26, 1985.

76. Sasaki H, Fujii S, Yoshizaki Y, Nakashima K, Kaneko T: Phosphoglycolate synthesis by human erythrocyte pyruvate kinase. *Acta Haematol (Basel)* 77:83, 1987.

77. Badwey JA: Phosphoglycolate phosphatase in human erythrocytes. *J Biol Chem* 252:2441, 1977.

78. Beutler E, West C: An improved assay and some properties of phospho-glycolate phosphatase. *Anal Biochem* 106:163, 1980.

79. Hass LF, Kappel WK, Muller KB, Engle RL: Evidence for structural homology between human red cell phosphoglycerate mutase and 2,3-bisphosphoglycerate synthase. *J Biol Chem* 253:77, 1978.

80. Chen S-H, Anderson JE, Giblett ER: Human red cell 2,3-diphosphoglyc-erate mutase and monophosphoglycerate mutase: genetic evidence for two separate loci. *Am J Hum Genet* 29:405, 1977.

81. Hoorn RKJ, Filkweert JP, Staal GEJ: Purification and properties of enolase of human erythrocytes. *Int J Biochem* 5:845, 1974.

82. Chen S-H, Giblett ER: Enolase: Human tissue distribution and evidence for three different loci. *Ann Hum Genet* 39:277, 1976.

83. Valentine WN, Tanaka KR, Paglia DE: Hemolytic anemias and erythro-cyte enzymopathies. *Ann Intern Med* 103:245, 1985.

84. Noguchi T, Yamada K, Inoue H, Matsuda T, Tanaka T: The L- and R-type isozymes of rat pyruvate kinase are produced from a single gene by use of different promoters. *J Biol Chem* 262:14366, 1987.

85. Blume KG, Hoffbauer RW, Busch D, Arnold H, Löhr GW: Purification and properties of pyruvate kinase in normal and in pyruvate kinase deficient human red blood cells. *Biochim Biophys Acta* 227:364, 1971.

86. Kahn A, Marie J, Garreau H, Sprengers ED: The genetic system of the L-type pyruvate kinase forms in man. Subunit structure, interrelation and kinetic characteristics of the pyruvate kinase enzymes from erythro-cytes and liver. *Biochim Biophys Acta* 523:59, 1978.

87. Tani K, Yoshida MC, Satoh H, et al: Human M_2-type pyruvate kinase: cDNA cloning, chromosomal assignment and expression in hepatoma. *Gene* 73:509, 1988.

88. Tani K, Fujii H, Tsutsumi H, et al: Human liver type-pyruvate kinase: cDNA cloning and chromosomal assignment. *Biochem Biophys Res Commun* 143:431, 1987.

89. Takayasu S, Fujiwara S, Waki T: Hereditary lactate dehydrogenase M-subunit deficiency: lactate dehydrogenase activity in skin lesions and in hair follicles. *J Am Acad Dermatol* 24:339, 1991.

90. Kitamura M, Iijima N, Hashimoto F, Hiratsuka A: Hereditary deficiency of subunit H of lactate dehydrogenase. *Clin Chim Acta* 34:419, 1971.

91. Miwa S, Nishina T, Kakehashi Y, Kitamura M, Hiratsuka A, Shizumo K: Studies on erythrocyte metabolism in a case with hereditary deficiency of H-subunit of lactate dehydrogenase. *Acta Haematol Jpn* 34:2, 1971.

92. Joukyuu R, Mizuno S, Amakawa T, Tsukada T, Nishina T, Kitamura M: Hereditary complete deficiency of lactate dehydrogenase H-subunit. *Clin Chem* 35:687, 1989.

93. Wakabayashi H, Tsuchiya M, Yoshino K, Kaku K, Shigei H: Hereditary deficiency of lactate dehydrogenase H-subunit. *Intern Med* 35:550, 1996.

94. Beutler E: G6PD: Population genetics and clinical manifestations. *Blood Rev* 10:45, 1996.

95. Maekawa M, Sudo K, Nagura K, Li SS, Kanno T: Population screening of lactate dehydrogenase deficiencies in Fukuoka Prefecture in Japan and molecular characterization of three independent mutations in the lactate dehydrogenase-B(H) gene. *Hum Genet* 93:74, 1994.

96. Yoshida A, Beutler E (eds): *Glucose-6-Phosphate Dehydrogenase.* Aca-demic, Orlando, FL, 1986.

97. Yoshida A, Stamatoyannopoulos G, Motulsky A: Negro variant of glu-cose-6-phosphate dehydrogenase deficiency (A-) in man. *Science* 155:97, 1967.

98. Chen EY, Cheng A, Lee A, et al: Sequence of human glucose-6-phos-phate dehydrogenase cloned in plasmids and a yeast artificial chromo-some (YAC). *Genomics* 10:792, 1991.

99. Martini G, Toniolo D, Vulliamy T, et al: Structural analysis of the X-linked gene encoding human glucose 6-phosphate dehydrogenase. *EMBO J* 5:1849, 1986.

100. Persico MG, Viglietto G, Martino G, et al: Isolation of human glucose-6-phosphate dehydrogenase (G6PD) cDNA clones: primary structure of the protein and unusual 5′ non-coding region. *Nucl Acids Res* 14:2511, 1986.

101. Takizawa T, Huang IY, Ikuta T, Yoshida A: Human glucose-6-phosphate dehydrogenase: primary structure and cDNA cloning. *Proc Natl Acad Sci USA* 83:4157, 1986.

102. Naylor CE, Rowland P, Basak AK, et al: Glucose 6-phosphate dehydro-genase mutations causing enzyme deficiency in a model of the tertiary structure of the human enzyme. *Blood* 87:2974, 1996.

103. Rattazzi MC: Glucose-6-phosphate dehydrogenase from human erythro-cytes: Molecular weight determination by gel filtration. *Biochem Biophys Res Commun* 31:16, 1968.

104. Kirkman HN, Hendrickson EM: Glucose-6-phosphate dehydrogenase from human erythrocytes. II. Subactive states of the enzyme from normal persons. *J Biol Chem* 237:2371, 1962.

105. Yoshida A: Hemolytic anemia and G-6-PD deficiency. *Science* 179:532, 1973.

106. Avigad G: Inhibition of glucose-6-phosphate dehydrogenase by adeno-sine-5-triphosphate. *Proc Natl Acad Sci USA* 56:1543, 1966.

107. Ben-Bassat I, Beutler E: Inhibition by ATP of erythrocyte glucose-6-phosphate dehydrogenase variants. *Proc Soc Exp Biol Med* 142:410, 1973.

108. Beutler E, Kuhl W: Limiting role of 6-phosphogluconolactonase in erythrocyte hexose monophosphate pathway metabolism. *J Lab Clin Med* 106:573, 1985.

109. Rakitzis ET, Papandreou P: Kinetic analysis of 6-phosphogluconolac-tone hydrolysis in hemolysates. *Biochem Mol Biol Int* 37:747, 1995.

110. Beutler E, Kuhl W, Gelbart T: 6-Phosphogluconolactonase deficiency, a hereditary erythrocyte enzyme deficiency: Possible interaction with glucose-6-phosphate dehydrogenase deficiency. *Proc Natl Acad Sci USA* 82:3876, 1985.

111. Thorburn DR, Kuchel PW: Computer simulation of the metabolic conse-quences of the combined deficiency of 6-phosphogluconolactonase and glucose-6-phosphate dehydrogenase in human erythrocytes. *J Lab Clin Med* 110:70, 1987.

112. Shih L, Justice P, Hsia DY: Purification and characterization of genetic variants of 6-phosphogluconate dehydrogenase. *Biochem Genet* 1:359, 1968.

113. Parr CW, Fitch LI: Inherited quantitative variations of human phospho-gluconate dehydrogenase. *Ann Hum Genet* 30:339, 1967.

114. Bruns FH, Noltmann E, Vahlhaus E: Über den Stoffwechsel von Ribose-5-phosphat in Hämolysaten. I. Aktivitäts-messung und Eigenschaften der Phosphoribose-isomerase. II. Der Pentosephosphate-Cyclus in roten Blutzellen. *Biochem Z* 330:483, 1958.

115. Brownstone YS, Denstedt OF: The pentose phosphate metabolic path-way in the human erythrocyte. II. The transketolase and transaldolase activity of the human erythrocyte. *Can J Biochem* 39:533, 1961.

116. Nakasaki H, Ohta M, Soeda J, et al: Clinical and biochemical aspects of thiamine treatment for metabolic acidosis during total parenteral nutrition. *Nutrition* 13:110, 1997.

117. Wolfe SJ, Brin M, Davidson CS: The effect of thiamine deficiency on human erythrocyte metabolism. *J Clin Invest* 37:1476, 1958.

118. Beutler E, Guinto E: The reduction of glyceraldehyde by human erythro-cytes. L-hexonate dehydrogenase activity. *J Clin Invest* 53:1258, 1974.

119. Das B, Srivastava SK: Purification and properties of aldose reductase and aldehyde reductase II from human erythrocyte. *Arch Biochem Biophys* 238:670, 1985.

120. Kim HD: Is adenosine a second metabolic substrate for human red blood cells? *Biochim Biophys Acta* 1036:113, 1990.

121. Gabrio BW, Finch CA, Huennekens FM: Erythrocyte preservation: a topic in molecular biochemistry. *Blood* 11:103, 1956.

122. Resta R, Thompson LF: SCID: the role of adenosine deaminase defi-ciency. *Immunol Today* 18:371, 1997.

123. Mitchell BS, Kelley WN: Purinogenic immunodeficiency diseases: clini-cal features and molecular mechanisms. *Ann Intern Med* 92:826, 1980.

124. Valentine WN, Paglia DE, Tartaglia AP, Gilsanz G: Hereditary hemo-lytic anemia with increased red cell adenosine deaminase (45- to 70-fold) and decreased adenosine triphosphate. *Science* 195:783, 1977.

125. Casoli C, Lisa A, Magnani G, et al: Prognostic value of adenosine deaminase compared to other markers for progression to acquired immu-nodeficiency syndrome among intravenous drug users. *J Med Virol* 45:203, 1995.

126. Palomba E, David O, Boltri A, Gabiano C, Tevo P-A: Increased erythro-cyte adenosine deaminase activity in children with perinatal human immunodeficiency virus infection. *Pediatr Infect Dis J* 8:862, 1989.

127. Glader BE, Backer K, Diamond LK: Elevated erythrocyte adenosine deaminase activity in congenital hypoplastic anemia. *N Engl J Med* 309:1486, 1983.

128. Accorsi A, Piacentini MP, Piatti E, Fazi A: Purine nucleoside phos-phorylase from human erythrocytes: a kinetic study of the fully separated isoenzymes. *Biochem Int* 24:23, 1991.

129. Valentine WN, Oski FA, Paglia DE, Baughan MA, Schneider AS,

Naiman NL: Erythrocyte hexokinase and hereditary hemolytic anemia, in *Hereditary Disorders of Erythrocyte Metabolism*, edited by E Beutler, p 288. Grune & Stratton, New York, 1968.

130. Morsches B, Holzmann H, Bettingen C: Zum Nachweis der Sorbit-dehydrogenase in menschlichen Erythrocyten. *Klin Wochenschr* 47:672, 1969.

131. Barretto OCO, Beutler E: The sorbitol oxidizing enzyme of red blood cells. *J Lab Clin Med* 85:645, 1975.

132. Bruns FH, Noltmann E: Phosphomannoisomerase, an SH-dependent metal-enzyme complex. *Nature* 181:1467, 1958.

133. Bruns FH, Noltmann E, Willemsen A: Phosphomannose-isomerase. I. Über die Aktivitätsmessung und die Sulfhydryl-sowie die Metallabhängigkeit der Enzymwirkung in einigen tierischen Geweben. *Biochem Z* 330:411, 1958.

134. Beutler E: Galactosemia: screening and diagnosis. *Clin Biochem* 24:293, 1991.

135. Noltmann E, Bruns FH: Über die Phosphoglucomutase der Erythrocyten und des Serums. *Hoppe-Seyler's Z Physiol Chem* 313:194, 1959.

136. Beutler E, Guinto E: Dihydroxyacetone metabolism by human erythrocytes: Demonstration of triokinase activity and its characterization. *Blood* 41:559, 1973.

137. Brake JM, Deindoerfer FH: Preservation of red blood cell 2,3-diphosphoglycerate in stored blood containing dihydroxyacetone. *Transfusion* 13:84, 1973.

138. Wood L, Beutler E: The effect of ascorbate and dihydroxyacetone on the 2,3-diphosphoglycerate and ATP levels of stored human red cells. *Transfusion* 14:272, 1974.

139. Moses SW, Chayoth R, Levin S, Lazarovitz E, Rubinstein D: Glucose and glycogen metabolism in erythrocytes from normal and glycogen storage disease type III subjects. *J Clin Invest* 47:1343, 1968.

140. Sidbury JB Jr, Cornblath M, Fisher J, House E: Glycogen in erythrocytes of patients with glycogen storage disease. *Pediatrics* 27:103, 1961.

141. Bartels H: Untersuchungen zur Frage des Glykogen-Gehaltes von Erythrocyten, in *Metabolism and Membrane Permeability of Erythrocytes and Thrombocytes*, edited by E Deutsch, E Gerlach, K Moser, p 132. Georg Thieme Verlag, Stuttgart, 1968.

142. Dimant E, Landberg E, London IM: The metabolic behavior of reduced glutathione in human and avian erythrocytes. *J Biol Chem* 213:769, 1955.

143. Lunn G, Dale GL, Beutler E: Transport accounts for glutathione turnover in human erythrocytes. *Blood* 54:238, 1979.

144. Viña JR, Palacin M, Puertes IR, Hernandez R, Viña J: Role of the gamma-glutamyl cycle in the regulation of amino acid translocation. *Am J Physiol* 257:E916, 1989.

145. Board PG, Smith JE: Erythrocyte gamma-glutamyl transpeptidase. *Blood* 49:667, 1977.

146. Srivastava SK, Awasthi YC, Miller SP, Yoshida A, Beutler E: Studies on gamma-glutamyl transpeptidase in human and rabbit erythrocytes. *Blood* 47:645, 1976.

147. Young JD, Ellory JC, Wright PC: Evidence against the participation of the gamma-glutamyltransferase-gamma-glutamylcyclotransferase pathway in amino acid transport by rabbit erythrocytes. *Biochem J* 152:713, 1975.

148. Winterbourn CC, Hawkins RE, Brian M, Carrell RW: The estimation of red cell superoxide dismutase activity. *J Lab Clin Med* 85:337, 1975.

149. Mills GC, Randall HP: Hemoglobin catabolism II. The protection of hemoglobin from oxidative breakdown in the intact erythrocyte. *J Biol Chem* 232:589, 1958.

150. Cohen G, Hochstein P: Glutathione peroxidase: the primary agent for the elimination of hydrogen peroxide in erythrocytes. *Biochemistry* 2:1420, 1963.

151. Rotruck JT, Pope AL, Ganther HE, Swanson AB, Hafeman DG, Hoekstra WG: Selenium: biochemical role as a component of glutathione peroxidase. *Science* 179:588, 1973.

152. Thomson CD, Rea HM, Doesburg VM, Robinson MF: Selenium concentrations and glutathione peroxidase activities in whole blood of New Zealand residents. *Br J Nutr* 37:457, 1977.

153. Beutler E, Matsumoto G: Ethnic variation in red cell glutathione peroxidase activity. *Blood* 46:103, 1975.

154. Burk RF: Molecular biology of selenium with implications for its metabolism. *FASEB J* 5:2274, 1991.

155. Chambers I, Harrison PR: A new puzzle in selenoprotein biosynthesis: selenocysteine seems to be encoded by the "stop" codon, UGA. *TIBS Rev* 12:255, 1987.

156. Stadtman TC: Selenocysteine. *Ann Rev Biochem* 65:83, 1996.

157. Jacob HS, Jandl JH: Effects of sulfhydryl inhibition on red blood cells. I. Mechanism of hemolysis. *J Clin Invest* 41:779, 1962.

158. Magnani M, Stocchi V, Ninfali P, Dacha M, Fornaini G: Action of oxidized and reduced glutathione on rabbit red blood cell hexokinase. *Biochim Biophys Acta* 615:113, 1980.

159. Huisman THJ, Dozy AM: Studies on the heterogeneity of hemoglobin. V. Binding of hemoglobin with oxidized glutathione. *J Lab Clin Med* 60:302, 1962.

160. Wong KK, Blanchard JS: Human erythrocyte glutathione reductase: pH dependence of kinetic parameters. *Biochemistry* 28:3586, 1989.

161. Icen A: Glutathione reductase of human erythrocytes purification and properties. *Scand J Clin Lab Invest* 96:1, 1967.

162. Beutler E, Yeh MKY: Erythrocyte glutathione reductase. *Blood* 21:573, 1963.

163. Loos H, Roos D, Weening R, Houwerzijl J: Familial deficiency of glutathione reductase in human blood cells. *Blood* 48:53, 1976.

164. Beutler E: Glutathione reductase: Stimulation in normal subjects by riboflavin supplementation. *Science* 165:613, 1969.

165. Mieyal JJ, Starke DW, Gravina SA, Hocevar BA: Thioltransferase in human red blood cells: kinetics and equilibrium. *Biochemistry* 30:8883, 1991.

166. Srivastava SK, Beutler E: The transport of oxidized glutathione from human erythrocytes. *J Biol Chem* 244:9, 1969.

167. Kondo T, Dale GL, Beutler E: Glutathione transport by inside-out vesicles from human erythrocytes. *Proc Natl Acad Sci USA* 77:6359, 1980.

168. Kondo T, Kawakami Y, Taniguchi N, Beutler E: Glutathione disulfide-stimulated Mg^{2+}-ATPase of human erythrocyte membranes. *Proc Natl Acad Sci USA* 84:7373, 1987.

169. Board PG: Transport of glutathione S-conjugate from human erythrocytes. *FEBS Lett* 124:163, 1981.

170. Kondo T, Murao M, Taniguchi N: Glutathione S-conjugate transport using inside-out vesicles from human erythrocytes. *Eur J Biochem* 125:551, 1982.

171. Harvey JW, Beutler E: Binding of heme by glutathione S-transferase: a possible role of the erythrocyte enzyme. *Blood* 60:1227, 1982.

172. Beutler E, Dunning D, Dabe IB, Forman L: Erythrocyte glutathione S-transferase deficiency and hemolytic anemia. *Blood* 72:73, 1988.

173. Prchal JT, Borgese N, Moore MR, Moreno H, Hegesh E, Hall MK: Congenital methemoglobinemia due to methemoglobin reductase deficiency in two unrelated American black families. *Am J Med* 89:516, 1990.

174. Katsube T, Sakamoto N, Kobayashi Y, et al: Exonic point mutations in NADH-cytochrome b5 reductase genes of homozygotes for hereditary methemoglobinemia, types I and III: putative mechanisms of tissue-dependent enzyme deficiency. *Am J Hum Genet* 48:799, 1991.

175. Tomatsu S, Kobayashi Y, Fukumaki Y, Yubisui T, Orii T, Sakaki Y: The organization and the complete nucleotide sequence of the human NADH-cytochrome b5 reductase gene. *Gene* 80:353, 1989.

176. Sass MD: Observations on the role of TPNH dehydrogenase in human red cells. *Clin Chim Acta* 21:101, 1968.

177. Xu F, Quandt KS, Hultquist DE: Characterization of NADPH-dependent methemoglobin reductase as a heme-binding protein present in erythrocytes and liver. *Proc Natl Acad Sci USA* 89:2130, 1992.

178. Fraser PJ, Curtis PJ: Molecular evolution of the carbonic anhydrase genes: calculation of divergence time for mouse carbonic anhydrase I and II. *J Mol Evol* 23:294, 1986.

179. Takahara S: Acatalasemia in Japan, in *Hereditary Disorders of Erythrocyte Metabolism*, edited by E Beutler, p 21. Grune & Stratton, New York, 1968.

180. Wen J-K, Osumi T, Hashimoto T, Ogata M: Molecular analysis of human acatalasemia. Identification of a splicing mutation. *J Mol Biol* 211:383, 1990.

181. Scott MD, Lubin BH, Zuo L, Kuypers FA: Erythrocyte defense against hydrogen peroxide: preeminent importance of catalase. *J Lab Clin Med* 118:7, 1991.

182. Scott MD, Zuo L, Lubin BH, Chiu DTY: NADPH, not glutathione, status modulates oxidant sensitivity in normal and glucose-6-phosphate dehydrogenase-deficient erythrocytes. *Blood* 77:2059, 1991.

183. Mueller S, Riedel HD, Stremmel W: Direct evidence for catalase as the predominant H_2O_2-removing enzyme in human erythrocytes. *Blood* 90:4973, 1997.

184. Roth EF Jr, Gilbert HS: The pyrogallol assay for superoxide dismutase: Absence of a glutathione artifact. *Anal Biochem* 137:50, 1984.

185. Cha MK, Kim IH: Thioredoxin-linked peroxidase from human red blood cell: evidence for the existence of thioredoxin and thioredoxin reductase in human red blood cell. *Biochem Biophys Res Commun* 217:900, 1995.

186. Papov VV, Gravina SA, Mieyal JJ, Biemann K: The primary structure and properties of thioltransferase (glutaredoxin) from human red blood cells. *Protein Sci* 3:428, 1994.

187. Jubelin BC, Gierman JL: Erythrocytes may synthesize their own nitric oxide. *Am J Hypertens* 9:1214, 1996.

188. Lawson AA, Barr RD: Acetylcholinesterase in red blood cells. *Am J Hematol* 26:101, 1987.

189. Johns RJ: Familial reduction in red-cell cholinesterase. *N Engl J Med* 267:1344, 1962.

190. Sasaki R, Ikura K, Katsura S, Chiba H: Regulation of human erythrocyte AMP deaminase by ATP and 2,3-biphosphoglycerate. *Agricult Biol Chem* 40:1797, 1976.

191. Ogasawara N, Goto H, Yamada Y, et al: Deficiency of AMP deaminase in erythrocytes. *Hum Genet* 75:15, 1987.

192. Tuy FPD, Henry J, Rosenfield C, Kahn A: Protein kinases in normal human blood cells. *Am J Hematol* 15:105, 1983.

193. Jindal HK, Ai Z, Gascard P, Horton C, Cohen CM: Specific loss of protein kinase activities in senescent erythrocytes. *Blood* 88:1479, 1996.

194. Michetti M, Salamino F, Tedesco I, et al: Autolysis of human erythrocyte calpain produces two active enzyme forms with different cell localization. *FEBS Lett* 392:11, 1996.

195. Raviv O, Heller H, Hershko A: Alterations in components of the ubiquitin-protein ligase system following maturation of reticulocytes to erythrocytes. *Biochem Biophys Res Commun* 145:658, 1987.

196. Vettore L, De Matteis MC, DiIorio EE, Winterhalter KH: Erythrocytic proteases: Preferential degradation of alpha hemoglobin chains. *Acta Haematol (Basel)* 70:35, 1983.

197. Kinoshita M, Hamakubo T, Fukui I, Murachi T, Toyohara H: Significant amount of multicatalytic proteinase identified on membrane from human erythrocyte. *J Biochem (Tokyo)* 107:440, 1990.

198. Sacchetta P, Battista P, Santarone S, Di Cola D: Purification of human erythrocyte proteolytic enzyme responsible for degradation of oxidant-damaged hemoglobin. Evidence for identifying as a member of the multicatalytic proteinase family. *Biochim Biophys Acta* 1037:337, 1990.

199. Ohkubo I, Gasa S, Namikawa C, Makita A, Sasaki M: Human erythrocyte multicatalytic proteinase: activation and binding to sulfated galacto- and lactosylceramides. *Biochem Biophys Res Commun* 174:1133, 1991.

200. Fagan JM, Waxman L: Purification of a protease in red blood cells that degrades oxidatively damaged haemoglobin. *Biochem J* 277:779, 1991.

201. Glynn IM, Karlish SJ: The sodium pump. *Annu Rev Physiol* 37:13, 1975.

202. Giraud F, Claret M, Bruckdorfer KR, Chailley B: The effects of membrane lipid order and cholesterol on the internal and external cationic sites of the Na^+-K^+ pump in erythrocytes. *Biochim Biophys Acta* 647:249, 1981.

203. Roelofsen B: The (non)specificity in the lipid-requirement of calcium- and (sodium plus potassium)-transporting adenosine triphosphatases. *Life Sci* 29:2335, 1981.

204. James P, Maeda M, Fischer R, et al: Identification and primary structure of a calmodulin binding domain of the Ca^{2+} pump of human erythrocytes. *J Biol Chem* 263:2905, 1988.

205. Smallwood JI, Gugi B, Rasmussen H: Regulation of erythrocyte Ca^{2+} pump activity by protein kinase C. *J Biol Chem* 263:2195, 1988.

206. Larsen FL, Katz S, Roufogalis BD: Calmodulin regulation of Ca^{2+} transport in human erythrocytes. *Biochem J* 200:185, 1981.

207. Auland ME, Morris MB, Roufogalis BD: Separation and characterization of two Mg^{2+}-ATPase activities from the human erythrocyte membrane. *Arch Biochem Biophys* 312:272, 1994.

208. Beutler E, Kuhl W: Guanosine triphosphatase activity in human erythrocyte membranes. *Biochim Biophys Acta* 601:372, 1980.

209. Vanderheiden BS: Genetic studies of human erythrocyte inosine triphosphatase. *Biochem Genet* 3:289, 1969.

210. Zachara B, Kopff M: Activity of inosine triphosphate pyrophosphohydrolase in fresh and stored human erythrocytes. *Haematologia (Budap)* 14:277, 1981.

211. Carty DJ, Iyengar R: A 43 kDa form of the GTP-binding protein G_{i3} in human erythrocytes. *FEBS Lett* 262:101, 1990.

212. Damonte G, Sdraffa A, Zocchi E, et al: Multiple small molecular weight guanine nucleotide-binding proteins in human erythrocyte membranes. *Biochem Biophys Res Commun* 166:1398, 1990.

213. Metzenthin M, Meier-Tackmann D, Agarwal DP, Zschaber R, Weh HJ: Aldehyde dehydrogenase-mediated metabolism of acetaldehyde and mafosfamide in blood of healthy subjects and patients with malignant lymphoma. *Adv Exp Med Biol* 414:147, 1997.

214. Matthies H: Untersuchungen Über eine Aldehyd-dehydrogenase in kernlosen Erythrocyten. *Biochem Z* 329:421, 1957.

215. Johnson RD, Bahnisch J, Stewart B, Shearman DJC, Edwards JB: Optimized spectrophotometric determination of aldehyde dehydrogenase activity in erythrocytes. *Clin Chem* 38:584, 1992.

216. Dockham PA, Sreerama L, Sladek NE: Relative contribution of human erythrocyte aldehyde dehydrogenase to the systemic detoxification of the oxazaphosphorines. *Drug Metab Dispos* 25:1436, 1997.

217. Izak G, Wilner T, Mager J: Amino acid activating enzymes in red blood cells of normal anemic and polycythemic subjects. *J Clin Invest* 39:1763, 1960.

218. Kaplan NO: Metabolic pathways involving niacin and its derivatives, in *Metabolic Pathways*, edited by DM Greenberg, p 627. Academic Press, New York, 1961.

219. Bertino JR, Simmons B, Donohue DM: Purification and properties of the formate-activating enzyme from erythrocytes. *J Biol Chem* 237:1314, 1962.

220. Valentine WN, Tanaka KR: The glyoxalase content of human erythrocytes and leukocytes. *Acta Haematol (Basel)* 26:303, 1961.

221. Anderson BB, Mollin DL: Red-cell metabolism of pyridoxine in sideroblastic anaemias and related anaemias. *Br J Haematol* 23:159, 1972.

222. Chern CJ, Beutler E: Pyridoxal kinase: Decreased activity in red blood cells of Afro-Americans. *Science* 187:1084, 1975.

223. Rimington C: A review of the enzymic errors in the various porphyrias. *Scand J Clin Lab Invest* 45:291, 1985.

224. Yasuda T, Mizuta K, Kishi K: Purification and characterization of two ribonucleases from human erythrocytes: immunological and enzymological comparison with ribonucleases from human urine. *Arch Biochem Biophys* 279:130, 1990.

225. Micheli V, Simmonds HA, Sestini S, Ricci C: Importance of nicotinamide as an NAD precursor in the human erythrocyte. *Arch Biochem Biophys* 283:40, 1990.

226. Dissing J, Johnsen AH, Sensabaugh GF: Human red cell acid phosphatase (ACP1). The amino acid sequence of the two isozymes Bf and Bs encoded by the ACP1*B allele. *J Biol Chem* 266:20619, 1991.

227. Endo F, Tanoue A, Nakai H, et al: Primary structure and gene localization of human prolidase. *J Biol Chem* 264:4476, 1989.

228. Holmgren A, Luthman M: Tissue distribution and subcellular localization of Bovine thioredoxin determined by radioimmunoassay. *Biochemistry* 17:4071, 1978.

229. Presecan E, Vonica A, Lascu I: Nucleoside diphosphate kinase from human erythrocytes: purification, molecular mass and subunit structure. *FEBS Lett* 250:629, 1989.

230. Tanuma S, Endo H: Purification and characterization of an (ADP-ribose)$_n$ glycohydrolase from human erythrocytes. *Eur J Biochem* 191:57, 1990.

231. Moenner M, Vosoghi M, Ryazantsev S, Glitz DG: Ribonuclease inhibitor protein of human erythrocytes: characterization, loss of activity in response to oxidative stress, and association with Heinz bodies. *Blood Cells Mol Dis* 24:149, 1998.

232. Ward A, Hickman D, Gordon JW, Sim E: Arylamine N-acetyltransferase in human red blood cells. *Biochem Pharmacol* 44:1099, 1992.

233. Graziani A, Ling LE, Endemann G, Carpenter CL, Cantley LC: Purification and characterization of human erythrocyte phosphatidylinositol 4-kinase. Phosphatidylinositol 4-kinase and phosphatidylinositol 3-monophosphate 4-kinase are distinct enzymes. *Biochem J* 284:39, 1992.

234. Das AK, Dasgupta B, et al: Purification and biochemical characterization of a protein-palmitoyl acyltransferase from human erythrocytes. *J Biol Chem* 272:11021, 1997.

235. Moore RB, Shriver SK, Jenkins LD, Mankad VN, Shah AK, Plishker GA: Calpromotin, a cytoplasmic protein, is associated with the formation of dense cells in sickle cell anemia. *Am J Hematol* 56:100, 1997.

236. Bjoerk P, Aman P, Hindemith A, et al: A new enzyme activity in human

blood cells and isolation of the responsible protein (D-dopachrome tautomerase) from erythrocytes. *Eur J Haematol* 57:254, 1996.

237. Kröplin T, Weyer N, Iven H: Determination of thiopurine methyltransferase activity in erythrocytes using 6-thioguanine as the substrate. *Adv Exp Med Biol* 431:741, 1998.

238. Micheli V, Jacomelli G, Zammarchi E, Pompucci G: Erythrocyte UMP synthetase activity—an HPLC-linked non-radiochemical assay in normal subjects and in one case of oroticaciduria. *Adv Exp Med Biol* 431:161, 1998.

239. Friedemann H, Rapoport SM: Enzymes of the red cell; a critical catalogue, in *Cellular and Molecular Biology of Erythrocytes*, edited by H Yoshikawa, SM Rapoport, p 181. University Park Press, Baltimore, 1974.

240. Hidaka Y, Palella TD, O'Toole TE, Tarle SA, Kelley WN: Human adenine phosphoribosyltransferase. Identification of allelic mutations at the nucleotide level as a cause of complete deficiency of the enzyme. *J Clin Invest* 80:1409, 1987.

241. Cartier P, Hamet M: Une nouvelle maladie metabolique: Le deficit complet en adenine-phosphoribosyltransferase avec lithiase de 2,8-dihydroxyadenine. *C R Acad Sci (Paris)* 279:883, 1974.

242. Van Acker KJ, Simmonds A, Potter C, Cameron JS: Complete deficiency of adenine phosphoribosyltransferase. Report of a family. *N Engl J Med* 297:127, 1977.

243. Kamatani N, Hakoda M, Otsuka S, Yoshikawa H, Kashiwazaki S: Only three mutations account for almost all defective alleles causing adenine phosphoribosyltransferase deficiency in Japanese patients. *J Clin Invest* 90:130, 1992.

244. Nyhan WL: The recognition of Lesch-Nyhan syndrome as an inborn error of purine metabolism. *J Inherit Metab Dis* 20:171, 1997.

245. Seegmiller JE, Rosenbloom FM, Kelley WN: Enzyme defect associated with a sex-linked human neurological disorder and excessive purine synthesis. *Science* 155:1682, 1967.

246. Kyd JM, Bagnara AS: Adenosine kinase from human erythrocytes: determination of the conditions required for assay in crude hemolysates. *Clin Chim Acta* 103:145, 1980.

247. Amici A, Emanuelli M, Ferretti E, Raffaelli N, Ruggieri S, Magni G: Homogeneous pyrimidine nucleotidase from human erythrocytes: enzymic and molecular properties. *Biochem J* 304:987, 1994.

248. Rocchigiani M, Sestini S, Micheli V, Bari M, Simmonds HA: NAD synthesis in human erythrocytes: determination of the activities of some enzymes. *Adv Exp Med Biol* 309B:337, 1991.

249. Sestini S, Ricci C, Micheli V, Pompucci G: Nicotinamide mononucleotide adenylyltransferase activity in human erythrocytes. *Arch Biochem Biophys* 302:206, 1993.

250. Preiss J, Handler P: Biosynthesis of diphosphopyridine nucleotide II. Enzymatic aspects. *J Biol Chem* 233:493, 1958.

251. Pescarmona GP, Bracone A, David O, Sartori ML, Bosia A, et al: Regulation of NAD and NADP synthesis in human red cell. *Acta Biol Med Ger* 36:759, 1977.

252. Beutler E: Red cell metabolism. A. Defects not causing hemolytic disease. B. Environmental modification. *Biochim Biophys Acta* 54:759, 1972.

253. Ng WG, Donnell GN, Bergren WR: Deficiency of erythrocyte nicotinamide adenine dinucleotide nucleosidase (NADase) activity in the negro. *Nature* 217:64, 1968.

254. Kostic MM, Rapoport SM: Maturation-dependent changes of the rabbit reticulocyte energy metabolism. *FEBS Lett* 250:40, 1989.

255. Thorburn DR, Beutler E: The loss of enzyme activity from erythroid cells during maturation, in *Red Blood Cell Aging*, edited by M Magnani, A DeFlora, p 15. Plenum, New York, 1991.

256. Zimran A, Forman L, Suzuki T, Dale GL, Beutler E: In vivo aging of red cell enzymes: study of biotinylated red blood cells in rabbits. *Am J Hematol* 33:249, 1990.

257. Seaman C, Wyss S, Piomelli S: The decline in energetic metabolism with aging of the erythrocyte and its relationship to cell death. *Am J Hematol* 3:31, 1980.

258. Rapoport S: Reifung und Alterungsvorgaenge in Erythrozyten. *Folia Haematol (Leipz)* 78:364, 1961.

259. Rapoport S, Rosenthal S, Schewe T, Schultze M, Miller N: The metabolism of the reticulocyte, in *Cellular and Molecular Biology of the Erythrocytes*, edited by H Yoshikawa, SM Rapoport, pp 93–141. University Park Press, Baltimore, 1974.

THE RED CELL MEMBRANE

PATRICK G. GALLAGHER

BERNARD G. FORGET

The easy accessibility of the red cell has allowed the human erythrocyte membrane to become the most thoroughly studied biologic membrane. It is composed of three major structural elements: a lipid bilayer primarily composed of phospholipids and cholesterol; integral proteins embedded in the lipid bilayer that span the membrane; and a membrane skeleton on the internal side of the red cell membrane. The erythrocyte membrane has many important functions. The lipid bilayer provides an impermeable barrier between the cytoplasm and the external environment and helps maintain a slippery exterior so that erythrocytes do not adhere to endothelial cells or aggregate and occlude the micro-circulation. The red cell membrane and its skeleton provide the erythrocyte with its unique deformability, durability, and tensile strength to undergo large deformations during repeated passages through narrow microcirculatory channels. The erythrocyte membrane also assembles and organizes the proteins of the lipid bilayer and the underlying skeleton. This allows the red cell to participate in a wide range of functions. These include influencing cellular metabolism by selectively and reversibly binding and inactivating glycolytic enzymes, retaining organic phosphates and other vital compounds, removing metabolic waste, and sequestering the reductants required to prevent corrosion by oxygen. During erythropoiesis, the membrane imports the iron required for the synthesis of hemoglobin. At the level of the organism, the membrane participates in the maintenance of pH homeostasis, participating in the exchange of chloride and bicarbonate. Investigation of disorders of the erythrocyte membrane such as hereditary spherocytosis, elliptocytosis, and pyropoikilocytosis has advanced our understanding of the normal structure/function relationships of the membrane as well as providing us with an understanding of the inheritance and expression of these disorders.

INTRODUCTION

The erythrocyte membrane accounts for only 1 percent of total weight of the red cell, yet it plays an integral role in the maintenance of erythrocyte integrity. The red cell membrane and its skeleton provide the erythrocyte the flexibility, durability, and tensile strength to undergo large deformations during repeated passages through narrow microcirculatory channels. The red cell membrane maintains a slippery exterior so that erythrocytes do not adhere to endothelial cells or

aggregate and occlude the microcirculation. The membrane plays an important role in metabolism by selectively and reversibly binding and inactivating glycolytic enzymes. The membrane retains organic phosphates and other vital compounds and helps remove metabolic waste. The membrane sequesters the reductants required to prevent corrosion by oxygen. During erythropoiesis, the membrane responds to erythropoietin and imports the iron required for the synthesis of hemoglobin. At the level of the organism, the membrane participates in the maintenance of pH homeostasis, participating in the exchange of chloride and bicarbonate.

The easy accessibility of the human erythrocyte membrane has allowed it to become the most thoroughly studied biologic membrane. Erythrocytes are the cells about which the most detailed information is available concerning the normal structure and function of their membrane and about the molecular pathology of disorders due primarily to abnormal membrane or cytoskeletal structure. The erythrocyte membrane remains the paradigm for ongoing studies of other cell types. Although the primary structure (Fig. 27-1) and a number of the important functions of the red cell membrane are known, its study continues to yield important insights into our understanding of membrane structure and function. Genetic investigation of disorders of the erythrocyte membrane has advanced our understanding of the normal structure/function relationships of the membrane as well as provided us with an understanding of the inheritance and expression of these disorders.

COMPOSITION OF THE ERYTHROCYTE MEMBRANE

The erythrocyte membrane is composed of three major structural elements: a lipid bilayer primarily composed of phospholipids and cholesterol that provides a permeability barrier between the external environment and the red cell cytoplasm; integral proteins embedded in the lipid bilayer that span the membrane; and a membrane skeleton on the internal side of the red cell membrane that provides structural integrity to the cell.

MEMBRANE LIPIDS

COMPOSITION

Lipids comprise 50 to 60 percent of red cell membrane mass. The principal membrane lipids are phospholipids and cholesterol, which are present in nearly equal amount.[1] Small amounts of glycolipids, primarily globoside, are also present. The primary phospholipids are phosphatidylcholine (28 percent of total phospholipids), phosphatidylethanolamine (27 percent), sphingomyelin (26 percent), phosphatidylserine (13 percent), and phosphatidylinositol.

Membrane phosphoinositides are phospholipids that contain phosphatidylinositol (PI) or its phosphorylated forms, PI-4-monophosphate and PI-4,5-biphosphate (PIP and PIP-2 respectively). In nucleated cells, phosphoinositides are precursors of important intracellular second messengers such as inositol-1,4,5-triphosphate and diacylglycerol that participate in regulation of many cellular processes. In mature erythrocytes, phosphoinositides represent 2 to 5 percent of total phospholipids, residing largely at the inner membrane surface and undergoing rapid phosphorylation and dephosphorylation. In red cells, they are involved in regulation of calcium transport and interaction of transmembrane and skeletal proteins (e.g., glycophorin C and protein 4.1), and they have been proposed to participate in the control of the discocyte-echinocyte shape transformation.[2]

In the erythrocyte, cholesterol is present in a free, unesterified form, and it is almost entirely hydrophobic. Its primary role appears to be to control membrane fluidity even under conditions that might lead to phospholipid crystallization and rigidification of the bilayer.

Acronyms and abbreviations that appear in this chapter include: AE1, anion exchanger-1; AQP1, aquaporin-1; ATP, adenosine 5'-triphosphate; HE, hereditary elliptocytosis; LCAT, lecithin-cholesterol acyltransferase; MAGUK, membrane-associated guanylate kinase; PAS, periodic acid-Schiff; PI, phosphatidylinositol; PIP, PI-4-monophosphate; PIP-2, PI-4,5-biphosphate; SDS, sodium dodecyl sulfate.

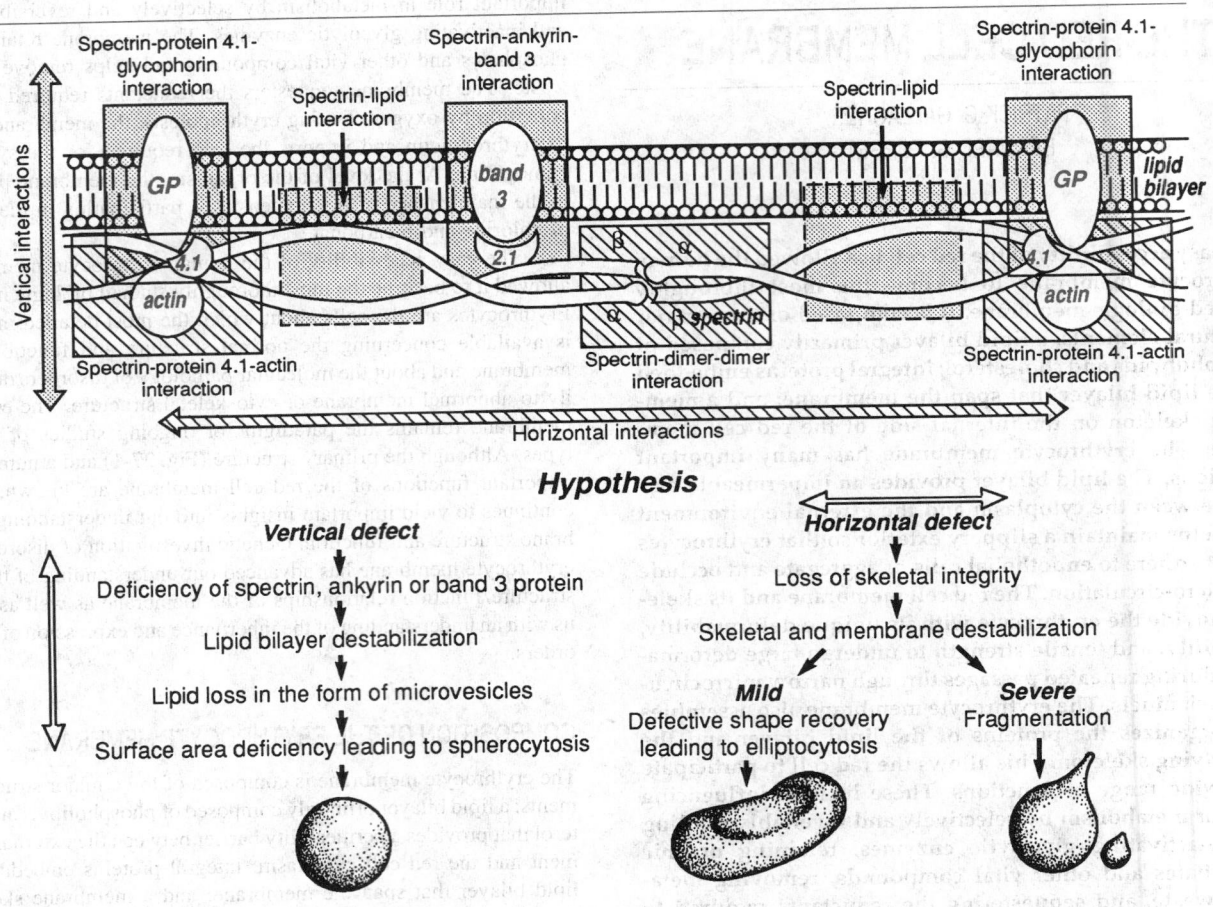

FIGURE 27-1   A schematic diagram illustrating the molecular assembly of the major erythrocyte membrane proteins and a model of the principal molecular defect in hereditary spherocytosis (HS), elliptocytosis (HE), and pyropoikilocytosis (HPP). Membrane protein-protein and protein-lipid associations can be divided into two categories: *(1) vertical interactions*, which are perpendicular to the plane of the membrane and involve spectrin-ankyrin-band 3 interaction, spectrin-protein 4.1-glycophorin C connection, and weak interactions between spectrin and the negatively charged lipids of the inner half of the membrane lipid bilayer, and *(2) horizontal interactions*, which are parallel to the plane of the membrane.

MEMBRANE LIPID DISTRIBUTION

Phospholipids are asymmetrically distributed in the red cell membrane with phosphatidylserine and phosphatidylethanolamine primarily in the inner hemileaflet, while sphingomyelin and phosphatidylcholine are outwardly oriented. This asymmetric distribution of phospholipids is a dynamic system involving a constant exchange ("flip-flop")[3] between the phospholipids of the two-bilayer leaflets. Maintenance of this asymmetry appears to be important in the regulation of hemostasis, as PS on the outer leaflet provides a site for prothrombinase binding, causing the red cell surface to become prothrombotic. Phospholipid flipping may contribute to the occurrence of thromboses in a variety of disorders including sickle cell disease (see Chap. 47) and diabetes.[4] The presence of PS on the outer surface of the red cell is one of the earliest changes in apoptosis, and it has been correlated with complement activation and red cell clearance by macrophages.

Enzymes called *flippases* actively translocate PS and PE to the inner leaflet; *floppases* catalyze translocation to the outer leaflet. Asymmetry seems to depend on the fact that flipping occurs at a higher rate than flopping. Flippase activity is mediated by a 130-kDa integral membrane protein that is a member of the Mg^{++}-dependent, P-glycoprotein ATPases.[5] Floppase activity in red cell membranes appears to be mediated by the multidrug resistance protein 1 (MRP1).[6,7]

A *scramblase* activated by elevated intracellular calcium that promotes randomization and loss of asymmetry has been isolated and cloned.[8,9] This scramblase mediates redistribution of membrane phospholipids in activated, injured, or apoptotic cells and is activated by calcium.[10,11] Derangements within the red cell often raise intracellular calcium by direct or indirect damage to ion channels and pumps. Scott's syndrome is a congenital bleeding disorder in which red cells and platelets expose subnormal amounts of PS on the outer surface in response to calcium, but it does not appear to be due to scramblase deficiency.[12,13]

Glycolipids and cholesterol are intercalated between the phospholipids in the bilayer with their long axes perpendicular to the bilayer plane. Red cell glycolipids are located entirely in the external half of the bilayer with their carbohydrate moieties extending into the aqueous phase. They carry several important red cell antigens, including A, B, H, and P, and may serve other important functions. The location of membrane cholesterol is less certain, but it appears that cholesterol is present in about equal proportions on both sides of the bilayer.

LIPID SYNTHESIS AND RENEWAL

The synthesis and assembly of red cell membrane lipids takes place during erythropoiesis. Mature erythrocytes are unable to synthesize fatty acids, phospholipids, or cholesterol de novo and depend on lipid exchange and fatty acid acylation for phospholipid repair and renewal.

These renewal pathways, although limited, permit a slow replacement of membrane lipid components.

Lipid exchange rates vary considerably. The exchange of unesterified cholesterol takes place in several hours, while the outer bilayer phospholipid phosphatidylcholine and sphingomyelin exchange with the phospholipids of plasma lipoproteins over a period of days. Because of their inaccessibility, the inner bilayer phospholipids phosphatidylserine and phosphatidylethanolamine are unable to participate in lipid exchange. Unesterified membrane cholesterol exchanges readily with the unesterified cholesterol in plasma lipoproteins where it is partially converted to esterified cholesterol by lecithin-cholesterol acyltransferase (LCAT). Because the newly formed cholesteryl ester cannot return to the red cell membrane, LCAT catalyzes a unidirectional pathway that depletes the membrane of cholesterol and decreases its surface area, and there is virtually no esterified cholesterol in the membrane. This process is reversed when this enzyme is absent or inactive, leading to a net accumulation of free cholesterol in the cells.

In addition to passive exchange, free fatty acids can be incorporated into red cell phospholipids in a two-step reaction requiring lysophospholipid, ATP, magnesium, and coenzyme A. Following the acylcoenzyme A formation, the fatty acid is incorporated into the lysophospholipid at the inner bilayer leaflet. This pathway also participates in the maintenance of phospholipid asymmetry, as evidenced by a rapid outward translocation of the newly synthesized phosphatidylcholine. Although this pathway consumes a small amount of energy, it may be important for detoxification of naturally formed lysophosphatides in the cells, as evidenced by their gradual accumulation during ATP depletion.

LIPID BILAYER FLUIDITY

Under physiologic conditions, the lipid bilayer is in a liquid state, allowing both the transmembrane proteins and the cell surface molecules (such as surface antigens) to move in the plane of the membrane. Lipid bilayer fluidity is influenced by several factors including: (1) temperature, which determines the phase transition between a liquid state and gel state; (2) free cholesterol content, as the rigid sterol ring of cholesterol decreases lipid bilayer fluidity; and (3) the length and the degree of phospholipid fatty acid saturation. Saturated fatty acids with a relatively rigid backbone resist motion, while the unsaturated fatty acids have relatively unrestricted movements, thereby increasing the fluidity of the lipid bilayer. Because of the differences in the composition of phospholipids between the two-bilayer halves, the bilayer is asymmetric in terms of the fluidity of the two hemileaflets.

MEMBRANE PROTEINS

Several general observations can be made about erythrocyte membrane proteins. Most of these proteins also are present in nonerythroid cells, where they fulfill similar functions. Many of these proteins are members of super families of proteins that are structurally related but genetically distinct. This genetic diversity explains why the clinical expression of many (but not all) red cell membrane protein mutations is confined to the erythroid lineage. Tissue- and developmental stage-specific alternative splicing or the usage of alternate initiation codons or alternate promoters creates multiple isoforms of many of these proteins. Finally, many are large, multifunctional proteins. As a result, mutations within a given region of the protein may lead to distinct differences in abnormalities of function and clinical phenotype.

Membrane proteins are classified according to the ease with which they can be removed from whole red cell membrane preparations in the laboratory. Integral proteins are firmly embedded into or through the lipid bilayer by hydrophobic domains within their amino acid sequences; only harsh reagents such as detergents can extract them. Peripheral proteins are more loosely associated; they are extractable by high- or low-salt or high-pH extraction. Peripheral proteins are attached indirectly to the lipid bilayer by means of covalent or noncovalent binding to the (usually) cytoplasmic domains of embedded or anchored proteins and typically are associated with only one face of the membrane (i.e., exterior or extracellular versus interior or cytoplasmic), whereas many integral proteins often protrude into both spaces. The affinity with which proteins associate with the membrane is not a static property. Rather, proteins can become more or less tightly bound according to their state of phosphorylation, methylation, glycosylation, or lipid modification (myristylation, palmitylation, or farnesylation).[2]

Fairbanks and colleagues assigned names to the proteins extracted from red cell membranes (Fig. 27-1 and Table 27-1).[14] These designations were based on their mobility in a sodium dodecyl sulfate (SDS)-acrylamide gel system; the slowest migrating band was band (or protein) 1, the next slowest band, band 2, etc. Subbands were designated with decimals. After further analysis, some of these proteins, such as bands 1 and 2, alpha and beta spectrin, were renamed. Other proteins, such as protein 4.1, were never renamed.

INTEGRAL MEMBRANE PROTEINS

Band 3 Band 3 (anion exchanger-1, AE1) is an abundant (10^6 copies per cell) transmembrane glycoprotein with a molecular mass of about 100 kDa. It serves as a regulator of ion content, red cell deformability, intermediary metabolism, and red cell senescence.[15,16] The NH_2-terminus of the protein encodes a 43-kDa cytoplasmic domain with COOH-terminus of the protein folded into helices and β sheets to form the membrane-spanning domain. The region between the NH_2-terminus and the first membrane-spanning segment forms an interhinge domain.

Band 3 is the major anion (chloride-bicarbonate) exchanger of the red cell. It regulates metabolic pathways by sequestering key pathway enzymes, such as the glycolytic enzymes glyceraldehyde-3-phosphate dehydrogenase, phosphoglycerate kinase, and aldolase, as well as carbonic anhydrase II. Band 3 contains important binding sites for interaction with other membrane proteins including ankyrin, protein 4.1, protein 4.2, and possibly spectrin.[17,18] Binding of the cytoplasmic domain to ankyrin is a critical mechanism for attachment of the membrane skeleton to the plasma membrane, and the interdomain hinge at this attachment point may be a crucial determinant of the flexibility or rigidity of the erythrocyte.[19]

The Glycophorins Glycophorins are the most abundant integral membrane glycoproteins in erythrocytes, and, because of their high sialic acid content, they account for more than 95 percent of the periodic acid–Schiff (PAS)-staining capacity of erythrocytes.[20] The glycophorins are 0-glycosylated and are composed of a single extracellular hydrophilic NH_2-terminal domain, a single membrane-spanning domain, and a COOH-terminal cytoplasmic tail. Characterization of cDNA and genomic clones encoding the glycophorins has revealed that they fall into two distinct subgroups.[21] Glycophorins A and B are homologous to each other and are encoded by two closely linked genes. Glycophorins C and D arise from a single locus bearing no particular homology to the genes for glycophorins A and B. Glycophorin D differs from glycophorin C by use of an alternate translation start site created by alternative splicing. Another gene linked in tandem with those for glycophorins A and B, glycophorin E, has been cloned, but no protein product has been identified.[22]

The functional roles of the glycophorins are beginning to be revealed. Because the glycophorins constitute more than 60 percent of the net negative surface charge of red cells, they may modulate red cell–red cell and red cell–endothelial cell interactions. GPC, which interacts in a complex with protein 4.1 and p55, plays a critical role in regulating the stability, deformability, and shape of the membrane. GPC deficiency leads to elliptocytic erythrocytes that are less stable

TABLE 27-1   MAJOR RED CELL MEMBRANE PROTEINS

BAND	PROTEIN	M_r (GEL)	M_r (CALC)	COPIES PER CELL ($\times 10^3$)	(%) OF TOTAL[a]	GENE SYMBOL	CHROMOSOMAL LOCALIZATION	AMINO ACIDS	GENE SIZE, KB	# OF EXONS	INVOLVEMENT IN HEMOLYTIC ANEMIAS
1	α Spectrin	240	280	240	16	SPTA1	1q22-q23	2429	80	52	HE, HS
2	β Spectrin	220	246	240	14	SPTB	14q23-q24.2	2137	>100	32	HE, HS
2.1	Ankyrin[b]	210	206	120	4.5	ANK1	8p11.2	1881	>100	40	HS
2.9	α Adducin[c]	103	81	30	2	ADDA	4p16.3	737	85	16	N
2.9	β Adducin[c]	97	80	30	2	ADDB	2p13-2p14	726	~100	17	N
3	Anion exchanger-1	90–100	102	1200	27	EPB3	17q21-qter	911	17	20	HS, SAO, HAc
4.1	Protein 4.1	80	66	200	5	EL11	1p33-p34.2	588[d]	>100	23	HE
4.2	Pallidin	72	77	200	5	EB42	15q15-q21	691	20	13	HS
4.9	Dematin[e]	48 + 52	43	40[f]	1	EPB49	8p21.1	383	—	—	N
4.9	p55[e]	55	53	80	—	MPP1	Xq28	466	—	—	N
5	β-Actin	43	42	400–500	5.5	ACTB	7pter-q22	375	>4	6	N
5	Tropomodulin	43	41	30		TMOD	9q22	359	—	—	N
6	G-3P-D[g]	35	37	500	3.5[g]	GAPD	12p13.31-p13.1	335	5	9	N
7	Stomatin	31	32	—	2.5	EPB72	9q33-q34	288	12	7	HSt
7	Tropomyosin	27 + 29	28	80	1	TPM3	1q31	239	—	—	N
PAS-1	Glycophorin A[h]	36		500–1000	85	GYPA	4q28-q31	131	>40	7	HE
PAS-2	Glycophorin C[h]	32	14	50–100	4	GYPC	2q14-q21	128	14	4	N
PAS-3	Glycophorin B[h]	20		100–300	10	GYPB	4q28-q31	72	>30	5	N
	Glycophorin D[h]	23		20	1	GYPD	2q14-q21	107	14	4	N
	Glycophorin E					GYPE	4q28-q31	59	>30	4	N

[a] Quantitation based on scanning of SDS-PAGE gels of red cell membranes prepared from healthy blood donors. For glycophorins, the values indicate the fraction of PAS-positive material.
[b] Bands 2.1, 2.2, 2.3, and 2.6 are protein isoforms of erythroid ankyrin, at least some of which are produced by alternative splicing of ankyrin mRNA.
[c] Since adducin comigrates with band 3, no numerical band designation is available.
[d] Numerous erythroid and nonerythroid isoforms of protein 4.1 produced by alternative splicing have been described. The values correspond to the major erythroid protein 4.1 isoform.
[e] Both dematin and p55 migrate within the 4.9 band.
[f] 40,000 of dematin trimers are present in one red cell.
[g] Variable amounts of band 6 are detected in red cell membranes.
[h] Detectable on PAS-stained gels only.
NOTE: HS, hereditary spherocytosis; HE, hereditary elliptocytosis; HPP, hereditary pyropoikilocytosis; SAO, Southeast Asian ovalocytosis; HAc, hereditary acanthocytosis; HSt, hereditary stomatocytosis; G-3-PD, glyceraldehyde-3-phosphate dehydrogenase; N, no hematologic abnormalities reported.

and less deformable than normal red cells. The glycophorins play important roles in clinical immunohematology, carrying a number of blood group antigens including MN, Ss, Miltenberger V, En(a-), $M^K M^k$, and Gerbich (see Chap. 137).

Other Integral Membrane Proteins The red cell membrane contains other integral membrane proteins including the Rh D protein (see Chap. 137) and various ion pumps and channels (see below).

PERIPHERAL MEMBRANE PROTEINS

The major proteins of the erythrocyte membrane skeleton are spectrin; ankyrin; actin; proteins 4.1, 4.2, and 4.9; p55; and the adducins. These proteins form an interlocking network that attaches to the inner face of the membrane primarily by binding to the cytoplasmic domains of band 3 and the glycophorins.

Spectrin Spectrin is the most abundant and largest protein of the erythrocyte membrane skeleton, constituting 75 percent of its mass and present at a concentration of about 200,000 molecules per cell.[23] Spectrin is composed of two subunits, α and β, that despite many similarities are structurally distinct and are encoded by separate genes (Fig. 27-2a).[24,25] Both α and β spectrin contain homologous 106 amino acid repeats that are folded into α-helical segments containing three antiparallel helices connected by short nonhelical segments.[26,27] The presence of spectrin repeats suggests that spectrin evolved from the duplication of a single ancestral gene.[28]

The fundamental structure of the spectrin molecule is that of αβ heterodimers that align and intertwine with each other in antiparallel fashion with respect to their NH_2-termini to form flexible, rodlike molecules (Fig. 27-2a).[26,29] These dimers further self-associate to form tetramers and higher-order oligomers. These tetramers, composed of multiple repeats, provide a strong, elastic, rodlike filament that associates into multimolecular complexes capable of lending shape and resiliency to the overlying plasma membrane via formation of a lattice-like meshwork linked to integral membrane proteins.[30] Direct interactions of a weaker nature may also occur between spectrin filaments and the lipid bilayer itself. The side-to-side assembly of α- and β-spectrin chains in a zipper-like fashion begins at a defined nucleation site composed of four repeats from each chain, α19 to α22 and β1 to β4 respectively.[31,32] After tight association of complementary nucleation sites, a conformational change is initiated that promotes pairing of the remainder of the two chains. A common α-spectrin variant, α^{LELY}, interferes with normal nucleation and decreases the synthesis of functionally competent spectrin chains and may influence clinical expression of spectrin mutations (see Chap. 43).[33]

The NH_2-terminus of α spectrin and the COOH-terminus of β spectrin are the regions involved in αβ heterodimer self-association.[29] Spectrin also binds to actin and protein 4.1 via the NH_2-terminus of β spectrin and ankyrin via sites in repeats β15 and β16 near the COOH-terminus.[34-36] Other nonrepeat sequences in spectrin provide the recognition sites for binding to other modifiers, including kinases and calmodulin.

The functions of spectrin are to maintain cellular shape, regulate the lateral mobility of integral membrane proteins, and provide structural support for the lipid bilayer.[23] Defects in the αβ self-association site are associated with hereditary elliptocytosis and hereditary pyropoikilocytosis (see Chap. 43). Compound heterozygosity or homozygosity for defects outside the αβ self-association site are associated with severe, recessively inherited spherocytosis.

Ankyrin Ankyrin is an asymmetric polar protein that can be separated into three functional domains by mild proteolysis: an NH_2-terminal membrane-binding domain that contains sites for band 3 and other ligands, a central domain that contains sites for spectrin binding, and a COOH-terminal "regulatory" domain that influences ankyrin-

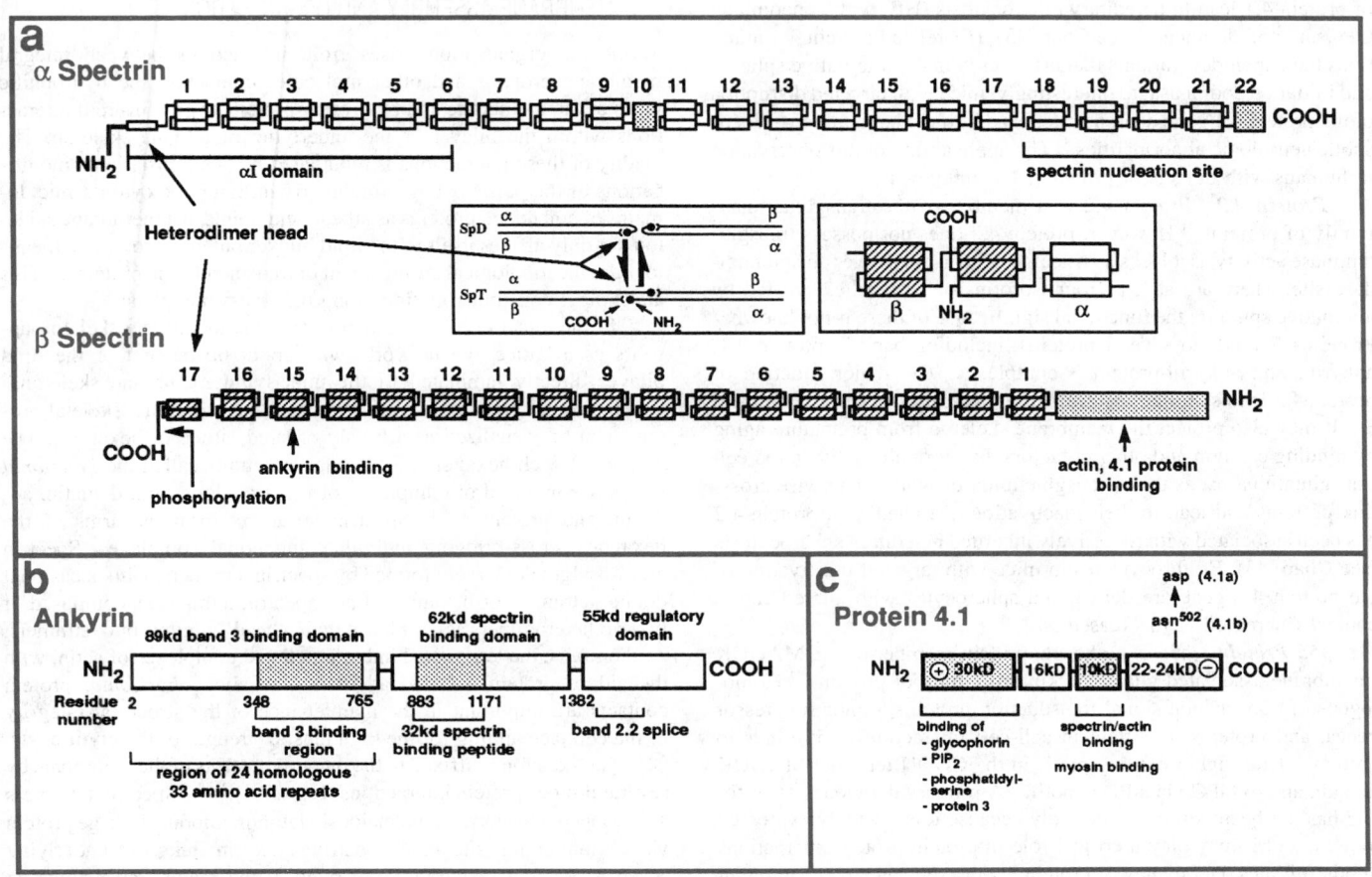

FIGURE 27-2   Spectrin, ankyrin, and protein 4.1. *(a) α and β spectrin.* Both proteins are composed of multiple homologous triple helical repetitive segments, numbered starting from the NH₂-terminus. α spectrin and β spectrin are shown in antiparallel orientation, their configuration in the spectrin heterodimer. Stippled regions represent nonhomologous segments. The αI domain (a tryptic peptide of α spectrin involved in association of α and β spectrin), the spectrin nucleation site, and the ankyrin, actin, and protein 4.1 protein-binding sites are shown. In the head region of spectrin, α and β spectrin interact to form either a heterodimer (SpD) or tetramer (SpT). The contact site between the α and β chains of a spectrin heterodimer or the opposed α and β chains of the tetramer is formed by a combined αβ triple helical segment *(insert).* *(b) Ankyrin.* The three major functional and structural domains, as defined by limited proteolytic digestion, are shown. The band 3 and spectrin-binding regions are shaded. The regulatory domain is subject to extensive alternative splicing, including the band 2.2 splice, which produces an activated form of ankyrin. *(c) Protein 4.1.* The four major functional and structural domains, as defined by limited proteolytic digestion, are shown. The regions where the 4.1 protein binds to other membrane proteins are shaded. The protein 4.1a isoform is derived from the 4.1b isoform by deamidation of aspartic acid 508 (see text for details).

protein interactions (Fig. 27-2b).[23,37,38] The membrane-binding domain contains 24 tandem repeats called *cdc10/ankyrin repeats* that contain multiple protein-binding sites.[39] Ankyrin repeats are highly conserved, L-shaped structures composed of a pair of α-helices that form an antiparallel coiled-coil, followed by an extended loop perpendicular to the helices and a β hairpin.[40] These repeats have been found in proteins with a wide variety of functions.[41,42] The regulatory domain consists of multiple isoforms generated by alternative splicing.[43,44] One of these isoforms (ankyrin 2.2) enhances ankyrin binding to band 3 and spectrin.[43]

Ankyrin provides the primary linkage between the membrane skeleton via spectrin binding and the lipid bilayer via band 3 binding (Fig. 27-1). Disruption of either of these linkages significantly decreases membrane stability. Ankyrin also appears to be involved in the local segregation of integral membrane proteins within function domains on the plasma membrane. The importance of ankyrin in the maintenance of membrane stability is underscored by the observation that abnormalities of ankyrin are the most common cause of typical hereditary spherocytosis (see Chap. 43).

Protein 4.1   Protein 4.1 is a phosphoprotein that can be separated by mild chymotryptic digestion into four proteolytic domains: 30 kDa, 16 kDa, 10 kDa, and 22 to 24 kDa (Fig. 27-2c). In red cells, two molecular weight forms are found, protein 4.1a and protein 4.1b, with protein 4.1a predominating in older erythrocytes. Protein 4.1a is derived from protein 4.1b by the gradual deamidation of two Asn residues in a nonenzymatic, age-dependent manner.[45] Alternative splicing leads to the production of a large number of tissue- and developmental stage-specific protein 4.1 isoforms,[46–50] e.g., alternatively spliced isoforms of the 10-kDa domain contain the spectrin-actin-binding site and provide erythroid and stage-specific specificity.[47–49] Protein 4.1 utilizes two different initiation codons. The upstream initiation codon encodes a protein of 135 kDa found in most nonerythroid cells.[50] The downstream initiation codon encodes the 85-kDa protein found primarily in erythrocytes.

The primary role of protein 4.1 is in the linkage of the spectrin-actin membrane skeleton to the lipid bilayer by facilitating complex formation between spectrin-actin fibers, the cytoplasmic domain of band 3, and p55/GPC (Fig. 27-1).[51] Qualitative or quantitative defects of protein 4.1 lead to hereditary elliptocytosis (HE) with concomitant GPC and p55 deficiency (see Chap. 43). HE-related protein 4.1 mutations have included variants that affect protein 4.1 alternative splicing and initiation codon usage. Interestingly, mice with targeted disruption of the protein 4.1 gene demonstrate, in addition to hematologic effects, subtle neurologic abnormalities.[52] The applicability of this observation to humans with defects of protein 4.1 is unknown.

Protein 4.2   Protein 4.2 is a member of the transglutaminase family of proteins.[53] However, protein 4.2 does not possess transglutaminase activity as it lacks a critical residue in the active transglutaminase site. There are at least four isoforms of protein 4.2 created by alternative splicing; the functional significance of these is not known.[54] Protein 4.2 binds to several proteins, including band 3, protein 4.1, ankyrin, and ankyrin-protein 3 complexes. The major function of protein 4.2 is to stabilize spectrin-actin-ankyrin association with band 3.[55] It may also protect the membrane skeleton from premature aging by binding calcium and other cofactors that normally activate red cell transglutaminases, as these transglutaminases would otherwise cross-link proteins and lead to their inactivation. Deficiency of protein 4.2 has been associated with recessively inherited hereditary spherocytosis (see Chap. 43). Erythrocytes from mice with targeted inactivation of the protein 4.2 gene are dehydrated spherocytes with altered cation content (increased K^+/decreased Na^+).[56]

p55 Protein   p55 is a phosphoprotein member of the MAGUK (membrane-associated guanylate kinase) family of proteins.[57] Homologues of p55 include signal transduction proteins, tumor suppressor genes, and proteins important in cell-cell interactions. p55 binds to protein 4.1 through a binding motif in the COOH-terminal MAGUK domain and to GPC via a PDZ motif.[58] A primary deficiency state for p55 has not been described, possibly because it is a widely expressed protein, and it may play a critical role in protein-protein interactions in other tissues. Deficiency of protein 4.1 or GPC lead to concomitant p55 deficiency. Studies of this interesting protein may shed important light on mechanisms whereby the erythrocyte membrane influences other cellular processes.

Adducin   Adducin, a calcium/calmodulin-binding phosphoprotein located at the spectrin-actin junctional complex, is composed of $\alpha\beta$ adducin heterodimers.[59] α and β adducin are structurally similar proteins encoded by separate genes.[60] Adducin contains a "MARCKS" phosphorylation domain that regulates calcium/calmodulin-regulated capping and bundling of actin filaments.[61,62] Adducin promotes the interaction of spectrin and actin and binds and bundles actin filaments.[63,64] A primary deficiency of adducin in human disease has not been described. Mice with targeted inactivation of β adducin suffer from compensated spherocytic anemia, suggesting that the adducins may be candidate genes for recessively inherited spherocytosis.[65]

Other Peripheral Membrane Proteins   Dematin (protein 4.9), tropomyosin, proteins related to troponin, and other proteins associated with actin in nonerythroid cells are found in erythrocytes. The functional roles of these proteins are now being revealed. For example, the amount of dematin present in the erythrocyte declines dramatically during erythrocyte maturation suggesting that it may play an important role in cellular maturation.

FUNCTIONS OF THE ERYTHROCYTE MEMBRANE

The roles of the erythrocyte membrane include assembling and organizing proteins of the lipid bilayer and the underlying skeleton, providing the red cell with its unique deformability and stability, participating in membrane biogenesis and aging, and providing an impermeable barrier between the erythrocyte cytoplasm and the external environment.

MEMBRANE ASSEMBLY AND ORGANIZATION

Membrane organization arises from interactions between integral membrane proteins and other molecules contacting the hydrophilic faces of the membrane and by protein-protein or protein-lipid interactions within the bilayer or the underlying membrane skeleton. The avidity of these interactions is modulated by posttranslational modifications of the participating proteins. By utilizing the cytoplasmic domains of embedded proteins as attachment points, the membrane skeleton not only affixes itself to the lipid bilayer but also provides a means to order the topological arrangement of transmembrane proteins.[66] This attachment constrains motion along the transverse plane.

In the intact erythrocyte membrane, the membrane skeleton appears as a lattice-like network, with about 60 percent of the lipid bilayer directly laminated to the underlying membrane skeleton.[67] When skeletal preparations are stretched, the individual skeletal proteins can be visualized as a highly ordered lattice of hexagons. The corners of each hexagon are globular structures called the *junctional complex* composed of complexes of F-actin, along with dematin, adducin, and protein 4.1.[68] Spectrin tetramers form the arms of the hexagons, cross-bridging individual junctional complexes. Spectrin cross-bridges are largely formed by spectrin tetramers, with occasional double tetramers or hexamers. Each spectrin tetramer is composed of two $\alpha\beta$ heterodimers assembled at their "head" regions into tetramers. At their tails, the tetramers bind to junctional complexes of actin, with the aid of protein 4.1 and adducin. The above *horizontal* protein contacts are important in the maintenance of the structural integrity of the cell, accounting for the high tensile strength of the erythrocyte.

The skeleton is affixed to the integral proteins of the membrane by several protein-protein interactions (Fig. 27-1).[23,68,69] Spectrin tetramers are connected to ankyrin, the major skeleton/membrane linkage protein via an interaction site in β spectrin. Ankyrin links the underlying spectrin skeleton to tetramers of band 3, the major transmembrane protein of the red cell. At the distal ends of spectrin tetramers, spectrin binds to the membrane via linkage to protein 4.1, which binds GPC and protein p55. In addition, both spectrin and protein 4.1 bind weakly to phosphatidylserine, which preferentially is located at the inner leaflet of the lipid bilayer. These *vertical* protein-protein and protein-lipid interactions are critical in the stabilization of the lipid bilayer, precluding its loss from the cells.

As discussed in Chap. 43, hereditary spherocytosis is characterized by defects of *vertical* interactions, which lead to uncoupling of the lipid bilayer from the skeleton and a release of membrane microvesicles.[70] In contrast, the principal defects in hereditary elliptocytosis and pyropoikilocytosis involve *horizontal* interactions of membrane skeletal proteins that maintain the two-dimensional integrity of the skeleton.

Red cell membrane proteins are subject to a variety of posttranslational modifications or other regulatory effects including phosphorylation, fatty acid acylation, methylation, glycosylation, deamidation, oxidation, and limited proteolytic cleavage.[2] With the exception of membrane protein phosphorylation, such modifications are relatively static and irreversible. In contrast, membrane protein phosphorylation represents a highly dynamic system of multiple protein kinases and phosphatases that constantly phosphorylate and dephosphorylate serine, threonine, and tyrosine residues, often in an amino-acid-specific and protein-site-specific manner, thereby tightly regulating association of membrane proteins. Additionally, membrane protein associations are influenced by a variety of intracellular factors including calcium and calmodulin, phosphoinositides, and polyanions such as 2,3-bisphosphoglycerate.

The red cell surface is negatively charged, primarily because of a high concentration of neuraminic acid residues. Ninety percent of these residues reside on glycophorin A with the remaining shared by the other glycophorins and band 3. Alterations in erythrocyte surface charge appear to have deleterious effects on the cell. For example, in sickle red cells, surface charge clustering may play a role in the adhesion of these cells to the surface of endothelial cells.

CELLULAR DEFORMABILITY AND MEMBRANE STABILITY

The most important property of red cells required for normal survival is cellular deformability.[71] *Deformability* refers to the ability of the erythrocyte to undergo distortions and deformations and then to resume its normal shape without fragmentation or loss of integrity. This is best exemplified in the wall of the splenic sinus where red cells squeeze through narrow slits among the endothelial cells that line the splenic sinus wall. The cellular deformability of erythrocytes is determined by three factors: (1) cell geometry (biconcave disc shape); (2) cytoplasmic viscosity, principally determined by the properties and the concentration of hemoglobin in the cells; and (3) intrinsic viscoelastic properties of the red cell membrane (or membrane deformability).[72] Among these factors, cell geometry as determined by the contribution of the surface-to-volume ratio is the most important, as exemplified by the cellular lesion of hereditary spherocytes. On the other hand, the intrinsic viscoelastic properties of the red cell are likely to have a relatively small effect on red cell survival. Southeast Asian ovalocytes are very rigid, yet they have a normal survival in vivo.

The cellular geometry, i.e., the biconcave disc shape of red cells, is critical for their survival. This cell surface shape provides a high ratio of surface area to cellular volume. The normal volume of the erythrocyte is about 90 μm^3; the minimum surface area that could encase this volume would be a sphere of about 98 μm^3. The surface area of a biconcave disc enclosing this volume is about 140 μm^3. Thus, shape alone provides the red cell with a considerable amount of redundant membrane and cytoskeleton. This feature provides the extra membrane surface area needed when red cells swell. More importantly, this geometric arrangement allows red cells to be stretched as they undergo deformation and distortion in response to the mechanical stress of the circulation. Loss of membrane by partial phagocytosis in immune hemolytic anemias or by fragmentation of bits of membrane from the cell in patients with cytoskeletal defects leads to elliptocytic or spherocytic shapes having greatly reduced surface area and, therefore, much less deformability.[73] The consequent reduction in tolerance of these cells to osmotic stress explains why anemias due to membrane defects are often accompanied by osmotic fragility, the basis for the clinical laboratory test. Conversely, if erythrocytes are engorged with water, they become macrospherocytic and less deformable.

Thus it is obvious that the organization of the membrane skeleton and its attachment to the plasma membrane influence the stability and deformability of the red cell. In the resting state, the folded helical segments of spectrin are highly coiled. Membrane deformation is accompanied by a rearrangement of the spectrin-actin-based membrane skeleton network with some spectrin molecules becoming uncoiled and extended, whereas others become more compressed and folded, resulting in no net change in surface area. Thus, shape changes but surface area does not. The extent to which this stretching and compression are possible determines the extent of deformability. Mutations or

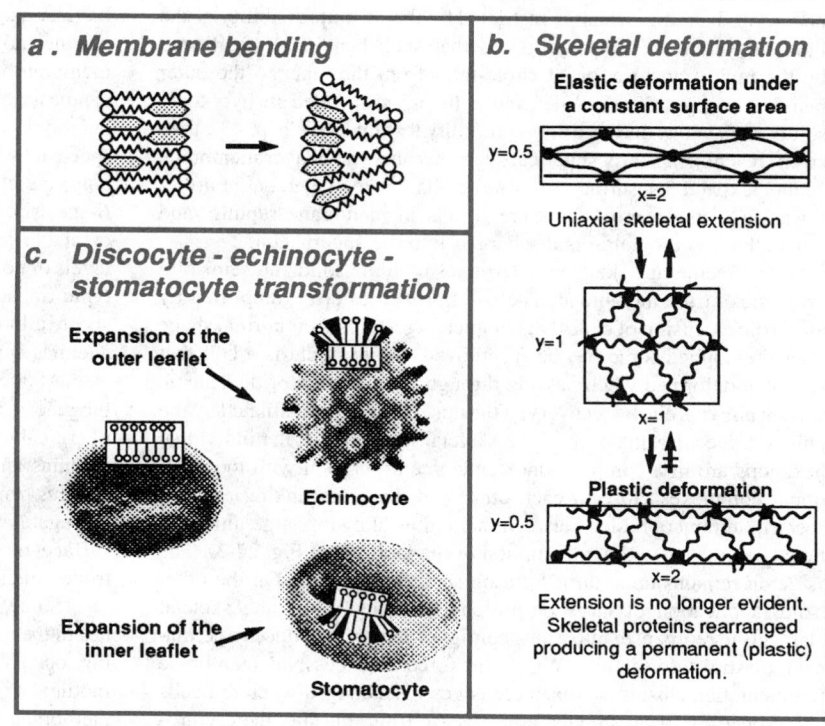

FIGURE 27-3 Material properties of the red cell membrane. *(a) Membrane bending.* The degree of membrane bending is restricted by the limited compressibility of the lipid bilayer. The rapid translocation of cholesterol (shaded diamonds) from the inner to the outer leaflet reduces the compression of the inner bilayer leaflet, thereby facilitating bending. *(b) Skeletal deformation.* While hydrophobicity of the red cell membrane lipid bilayer precludes the increase in its surface area without rupture, the membrane can undergo a large deformation under a constant surface area because of the viscoelastic properties of the membrane skeleton. During uniaxial extension, the skeleton undergoes stretching *(top rectangle).* After a cessation of an external force, a square surface area is resumed because the protein connections within this elastic skeletal network remain intact. Extensive or prolonged uniaxial extension leads to a rearrangement of the skeletal network because of a disruption of existing skeletal protein connections and a formation of new protein contacts. This leads to a permanent plastic deformation *(bottom rectangle). (c) Bilayer couple hypothesis and the stomatocyte-discocyte-echinocyte transformation.* Red cell shape reflects the ratio of the surface areas of the two hemileaflets of the lipid bilayer. The compounds *(black triangles)* that preferentially intercalate into the outer hemileaflet of the lipid bilayer produce its expansion followed by red cell crenation (echinocytosis or acanthocytosis). In contrast, expansion of the inner lipid bilayer leaflet produces a cup shape (stomatocytosis) and surface invaginations.

acquired alterations in membrane proteins that influence the spectrin-actin-based lattice of proteins leads to membrane loss with a concomitant decrease in surface area and a change in cell geometry.

Red cell viscosity is largely determined by hemoglobin content.[73] At normal intracellular concentrations (27–35g/dl), viscosity contributes very little to cellular deformability. When erythrocytes become dehydrated, the effective intracellular hemoglobin concentration rises, and viscosity increases exponentially. Membrane pumps and channels normally maintain intracellular volumes that hold hemoglobin concentrations below the level at which cytoplasmic viscosity has an impact on deformability. Inherited anomalies of pumps or channels (e.g., hereditary xerocytosis) or derangements caused by polymerized or crystallized hemoglobin (e.g., sickle cell anemia or HbC disease), lead to cellular dehydration and greatly increased red cell viscosity.

MEMBRANE MATERIAL PROPERTIES

The material properties of the membrane reflect the properties of both the lipid bilayer and the skeleton. During deformation, the membrane undergoes bending, which is restricted by the incompressibility of the lipid bilayer. It has been proposed that such bending is facilitated by the rapid translocation of cholesterol from the inner to the outer hemileaflet (Fig. 27-3). When red cells are suspended in hypotonic solutions, such as during osmotic fragility testing (see Chap. 43), they swell, reaching a nearly spherical shape because the bilayer membrane cannot expand its surface area more than 3 to 4 percent. Further lowering of the osmotic pressure results in membrane rupture, and intracellular hemoglobin is discharged into the supernatant.

The membrane skeleton determines both the solid and semisolid properties of the membrane. The solid properties are exemplified by an elastic extension of cells that completely restores their normal shape after the applied force has been removed. An example is a cell that has been deformed when passing through fenestrations of the splenic sinus wall. This elastic recovery of the normal shape is facilitated by the unique molecular anatomy of the skeletal lattice. Here the individual hexagons are in a compact, unextended configuration with the junctional complexes close to each other and the cross-linking arms of spectrin tetramers folded between them, thus allowing large unidirectional extensions without disruption of the lattice (see Fig. 27-3). The skeleton remains unperturbed during such deformation. On the other hand, application of large or prolonged forces allows the skeletal elements to reorganize into a new configuration; this produces a permanent plastic deformation. When the force is excessive, membrane fragmentation ensues. An example is vessels damaged when red cells are trapped by fibrin strands; after release from this site, the erythrocytes either are permanently deformed or are fragmented.

MEMBRANE BIOGENESIS AND AGING

Membrane protein biosynthesis occurs asynchronously during erythropoiesis. Early in erythroid development, the major proteins of the membrane skeleton (spectrin, ankyrin, and the 4.1 protein) are synthesized.[74,75] However, they turn over rapidly and do not assemble into a permanent network. At the proerythroblast stage, the synthesis of band 3 is initiated and, together with the synthesis of protein 4.1, increases up to the late erythroblast stage. During this time, mRNA levels and synthesis of spectrin and ankyrin protein decline. In contrast, the fraction of newly assembled spectrin and ankyrin protein on the membrane progressively increases, and the turnover of these proteins on the membrane declines.

Increased recruitment and stabilization of spectrin and ankyrin on the membrane in spite of the declining synthesis of these proteins is temporally related to a progressive increase in the synthesis of band 3 and protein 4.1, the principal bilayer anchors of the membrane skeleton.[76] Thus early studies suggested that the early steps of red cell membrane assembly were controlled by band 3 production where, after insertion into the membrane, it directed the assembly of stable macromolecular complexes from presynthesized pools of other proteins.[77,78] The role of band 3 in membrane assembly has been questioned by the following recent findings: (1) The organization of preformed pools of cytoskeletal elements induced by band 3 synthesis is not seen in nontransformed cells; and (2) band 3 knock-out mice exhibit normal membrane biogenesis even though their red cell membranes are unstable in the circulation.[79,80]

The biosynthesis and assembly of spectrin subunits is complex. β-spectrin biosynthesis exceeds that of α spectrin in the early erythroblasts derived from both embryonic (yolk sac) and fetal/adult (liver/spleen) origins. This ratio is preserved during later stages of erythropoiesis in embryonic cells, but not in fetal/adult-derived late erythroblasts and reticulocytes. In these latter cells, α-spectrin gene expression increases, whereas β-spectrin gene expression remains constant, resulting in a predominance of α-spectrin mRNA and protein during

the late stages, when active assembly of the actual membrane is occurring most rapidly. $\alpha\beta$-spectrin subunits are incorporated into the membrane in a 1:1 stoichiometric ratio, regardless of their rates of synthesis.[74,81,82] This point is important in the analysis of inherited hemolytic anemias. Human α-spectrin synthesis exceeds that of β-spectrin by 2:1 during the later stages of erythropoiesis, when, presumably, membrane assembly is proceeding rapidly. The availability of β-spectrin subunits therefore determines the maximum rate and amount of stable spectrin assembly. Thus, mutations reducing steady-state levels of newly synthesized β spectrin should have a far greater phenotypic impact than do mutations causing comparable decreases in α-spectrin biosynthesis. Analyses of patients with hereditary hemolytic anemias support this prediction (see Chap. 43).

At the stage of orthochromatic erythroblast, when membrane biogenesis is nearly completed, the cell membrane undergoes a series of critical remodeling steps.[83,84] The membrane surrounding the nucleus contains an actin ring that likely participates in the expulsion of the nucleus from the erythroblast.[85] At the same time, the spectrin skeleton segregates into the region of the incipient reticulocyte, while some surface receptors cluster in membrane regions surrounding the extruded nucleus.

Some synthesis of spectrin, band 3, protein 4.1, and GPC continues in the newly enucleated reticulocyte, but most membrane remodeling occurs after translation. The reticulocyte is multilobular and motile; it possesses mitochondria, polyribosomes, and numerous membrane proteins that are either absent or much less abundant in mature red cells. In addition, phospholipid composition and inside-outside lipid distribution are different. Reticulocytes are far less deformable and considerably more unstable mechanically than are mature erythrocytes. Maturation begins in the bone marrow and lasts for 2 or 3 days. It is completed in the circulation and perhaps in the spleen where it has been termed *splenic polishing*. Reticulocytes first become cup-shaped before acquiring their final biconcave disc shape. This process involves major reorganization of both membrane phospholipids and cytoskeletal and embedded proteins, as well as the loss of lipids and proteins, including receptors for transferrin, insulin, and fibronectin.

RED CELL AGING

The mechanism of red cell aging is discussed in Chap. 29.

FETAL RED CELLS

Fetal erythrocytes differ in a number of respects including activity of both glycolytic and nonglycolytic enzymes, altered ATP and phosphate metabolism, differences in methemoglobin content and oxygen affinity, and altered storage characteristics (reviewed in Gallagher[86]). These erythrocytes exhibit increased rigidity, increased mechanical fragility, and decreased life span (average 45 to 70 days) compared to adult red cells.

There are also differences in the membranes of fetal and adult erythrocytes. ABO and I antigens and the receptors for the adsorbed serum antigens of the Lewis system are incompletely expressed. Fetal membranes are more permeable to monovalent cations and contain less Na^+-K^+-ATPase activity. They contain more phospholipid and cholesterol per cell and, as a consequence, have a larger surface-to-volume ratio and are slightly more osmotically resistant than adult cells. The ratio of sphingomyelin to phosphatidylcholine is increased in fetal membranes and differences in fatty acid composition exist, but these changes evidently tend to balance each other, as membrane fluidity is normal. The protein composition of fetal red cell membrane is quantitatively normal.

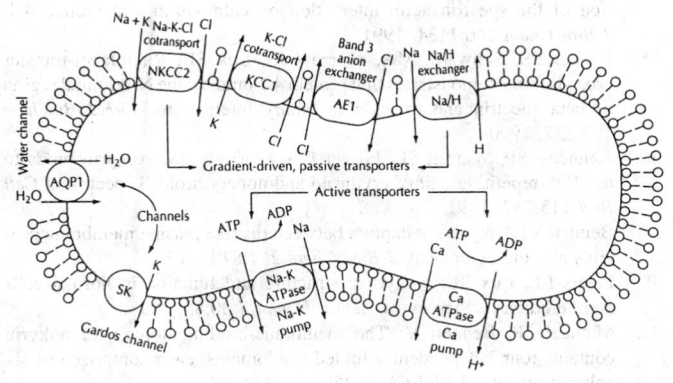

FIGURE 27-4 Principal ion transport pathways of the human erythrocyte. AE-1: band 3, the anion exchanger; AQP1: the water channel aquaporin 1; KCC-1: KCl cotransport system of the family of chloride-cation cotransporters; NKCC2: basolateral molecular form of Na-K-Cl cotransport; SK: small conductance potassium channel. Reprinted with permission from Brugnara.[87]

MEMBRANE PERMEABILITY

The normal red cell membrane is nearly impermeable to monovalent and divalent cations, thereby maintaining a high potassium, low sodium, and very low calcium content. In contrast, the red cell is highly permeable to water and anions, which are readily exchanged, and as a result erythrocytes behave as nearly perfect osmometers. Water and ion transport pathways in the red cell membrane (Fig. 27-4) include energy-driven membrane pumps, gradient-driven systems, and various channels.[87,88] An important feature of the normal red cell is its ability to maintain a constant volume. The mechanisms by which red cells "sense" changes in cell volume and activate appropriate volume regulatory pathways are unknown. Glucose is transported without the expenditure of energy utilizing a transporter, while larger charged molecules, such as ATP and related compounds, do not cross the normal red cell membrane, although phosphoenolpyruvate is an exception to this rule (Chap. 140).

The effects of disruption of the red cell permeability barrier are illustrated by complement-mediated hemolysis. Complement activation on the red cell surface leads to formation of the membrane attack complex, composed of terminal complement components embedded in the lipid bilayer. This multimolecular complex acts as a cation channel, allowing passive movements of sodium, potassium, and calcium across the membrane according to their concentration gradients. Attracted by fixed anions, such as hemoglobin, ATP, and 2,3-BPG, sodium accumulates in the cell in excess of potassium loss and in excess of the compensatory efforts of the Na^+/K^+-pump. The resulting increase in intracellular monovalent cations and water is followed by cell swelling and ultimately colloid osmotic hemolysis.

ENERGY-DRIVEN MEMBRANE PUMPS

In the red cell, two ion-motive ATPase-dependent cation pumps maintain low intracellular sodium and calcium and high potassium.[87] The ouabain inhibitable Na^+-K^+-ATPase (the sodium pump) extrudes sodium in exchange for potassium in a 3:2 stoichiometry. Ca^{++}-ATPase is a calmodulin-activated pump that extrudes calcium from the red cell and maintains a very low intracellular calcium concentration, thus protecting cells from multiple deleterious effects of calcium. Examples of such deleterious effects include echinocytosis, membrane vesiculation, calpain activation, membrane proteolysis, and cellular dehydration. Elevated intracellular calcium plays an important role in the pathophysiology of sickle cell disease, as increased levels of intracellu-

lar calcium observed during sickling are due to an increase in Ca^{++} flux and reduced activity of the Ca^{++}-ATPase. The membrane also contains an ATP-driven GSSG transporter (Chap. 26) and amino acid transport systems.

GRADIENT-DRIVEN SYSTEMS

The Na^+/K^+ gradient established by the sodium pump is used by several passive, gradient-driven systems to move ions across the red cell membrane.[87] These include the K^+Cl^+-cotransporter, band 3 (see above), the Na^+-K^+Cl^--cotransporter, and the Na^+-H^+-exchanger. The Na^+-K^+Cl^--cotransporter plays only a minor role in the red cell. The Na^+-H^+-exchanger appears to play a role primarily in early erythrocyte maturation. The K^+Cl^+-cotransporter is a typical carrier-mediated cotransporter, which is particularly active in reticulocytes.[89,90] It is activated by cell swelling, acidification, depletion of intracellular magnesium and thiol oxidation.

CHANNELS

Channels of the red cell include voltage-gated channels (mediated via Na^+K^+-ATPase), water channels (the aquaporins), and the Ca^{++}-activated K^+-channel. The Ca^{++}-activated K^+-channel, also called the *Gardos channel* after its discoverer Dr. George Gardos, causes selective loss of K^+ in response to an increase in intracellular $Ca.^{++}$[91,92] In sickle cells, increased activity of both the Gardos channel and the K^+-Cl-cotransporter leads to a net loss of K^+ and water, leading to cellular dehydration and the formation of intermediate and hyperdense erythrocytes.[93,94] Recently, pharmacologic manipulation of these two channels has been tried in attempts to improve cellular hydration of the red cell and ameliorate the clinical course of patients with sickle cell disease.[95,96]

The aquaporins are membrane channel proteins that serve as selective pores through which water crosses the plasma membrane.[97,98] Aquaporin-1, AQP1, which is expressed in many tissues including erythrocytes, contributes to the ability of the red cell to adjust rapidly to changes in osmolality. AQP1 contains the epitope for the Colton blood group system. The genetic basis of the rare Colton null phenotype has been identified as a mutation of the highly conserved NPA motif of AQP1 essential for channel function.[99] Colton null individuals exhibit no obvious clinical phenotype, although mice with targeted inactivation of AQP1 become hyperosmolar after fluid restriction.[100] Recently, evidence for the presence of AQP3 in erythrocytes has been presented.[101]

REFERENCES

1. Ways P, Hanahan DJ: Characterization and quantitation of red cell lipids in normal man. *J Lipid Res* 5:318, 1964.
2. Cohen CM, Gascard P: Regulation and post-translational modification of erythrocyte membrane and membrane-skeletal proteins. *Semin Hematol* 29:244, 1992.
3. Bevers EM, Comfurius P, Dekkers DW, Zwaal RF: Lipid translocation across the plasma membrane of mammalian cells. *Biochim Biophys Acta* 1439:317, 1999.
4. Andrews DA, Low PS: Role of red blood cells in thrombosis. *Curr Opin Hematol* 6:76, 1999.
5. Tang X, Halleck MS, Schlegel RA, Williamson P: A subfamily of P-type ATPases with aminophospholipid transporting activity. *Science* 272:1495, 1996.
6. Dekkers DW, Comfurius P, Schroit AJ, et al: Transbilayer movement of NBD-labeled phospholipids in red blood cell membranes: outward-directed transport by the multidrug resistance protein 1 (MRP1). *Biochemistry* 37:14833, 1998.
7. Kamp D, Haest CW: Evidence for a role of the multidrug resistance protein (MRP) in the outward translocation of NBD-phospholipids in the erythrocyte membrane. *Biochim Biophys Acta* 1372:91, 1998.
8. Basse F, Stout JG, Sims PJ, Wiedmer T: Isolation of an erythrocyte

membrane protein that mediates Ca^{2+}-dependent transbilayer movement of phospholipid. *J Biol Chem* 271:17205, 1996.

9. Zhou Q, Zhao J, Stout JG, et al: Molecular cloning of human plasma membrane phospholipid scramblase. A protein mediating transbilayer movement of plasma membrane phospholipids. *J Biol Chem* 272: 18240, 1997.

10. Zhao J, Zhou Q, Wiedmer T, Sims PJ: Level of expression of phospholipid scramblase regulates induced movement of phosphatidylserine to the cell surface. *J Biol Chem* 273:6603, 1998.

11. Zhou Q, Sims PJ, Wiedmer T: Identity of a conserved motif in phospholipid scramblase that is required for Ca^{2+}-accelerated transbilayer movement of membrane phospholipids. *Biochemistry* 37:2356, 1998.

12. Dekkers DW, Comfurius P, Vuist WM, et al: Impaired Ca^{2+}-induced tyrosine phosphorylation and defective lipid scrambling in erythrocytes from a patient with Scott syndrome: a study using an inhibitor for scramblase that mimics the defect in Scott syndrome. *Blood* 91:2133, 1998.

13. Stout JG, Basse F, Luhm RA, et al: Scott syndrome erythrocytes contain a membrane protein capable of mediating Ca^{2+}-dependent transbilayer migration of membrane phospholipids. *J Clin Invest* 99:2232, 1997.

14. Fairbanks G, Steck TL, Wallach DFH: Electrophoretic analysis of the major polypeptides of the human erythrocyte membrane. *Biochemistry* 10:2606, 1971.

15. Alper SL: The band 3-related anion exchanger (AE) gene family. *Annu Rev Physiol* 53:549, 1991.

16. Tanner MJ: Molecular and cellular biology of the erythrocyte anion exchanger (AE1). *Semin Hematol* 30:34, 1993.

17. Low PS: Structure and function of the cytoplasmic domain of band 3: center of erythrocyte membrane-peripheral protein interactions. *Biochim Biophys Acta* 864:145, 1986.

18. Van Dort HM, Moriyama R, Low PS: Effect of band 3 subunit equilibrium on the kinetics and affinity of ankyrin binding to erythrocyte membrane vesicles. *J Biol Chem* 273:14819, 1998.

19. Mohandas N, Winardi R, Knowles D, et al: Molecular basis for membrane rigidity of hereditary ovalocytosis. A novel mechanism involving the cytoplasmic domain of band 3. *J Clin Invest* 89:686, 1992.

20. Chasis JA, Mohandas N: Red blood cell glycophorins. *Blood* 80:1869, 1992.

21. Cartron JP, Rahuel C: Human erythrocyte glycophorins: protein and gene structure analyses. *Transfus Med Rev* 6:63, 1992.

22. Kudo S, Fukuda M: Identification of a novel human glycophorin, glycophorin E, by isolation of genomic clones and complementary DNA clones utilizing polymerase chain reaction. *J Biol Chem* 265:1102, 1990.

23. Morrow JS, Rimm DL, Kennedy SP, et al: Of membrane stability and mosaics: the spectrin cytoskeleton, in *Handbook of Physiology*, edited by J Hoffman, J Jamieson, p 485. Oxford, London, 1997.

24. Gallagher PG, Forget BG: Spectrin genes in health and disease. *Semin Hematol* 30:4, 1993.

25. Winkelmann JC, Forget BG: Erythroid and nonerythroid spectrins. *Blood* 81:373, 1993.

26. Bennett V, Lambert S: The spectrin skeleton: from red cells to brain. *J Clin Invest* 87:1483, 1991.

27. Speicher DW, Marchesi VT: Erythrocyte spectrin is comprised of many homologous triple helical segments. *Nature* 311:177, 1984.

28. Thomas GH, Newbern EC, Korte CC, et al: Intragenic duplication and divergence in the spectrin superfamily of proteins. *Mol Biol Evol* 14:1285, 1997.

29. Cherry L, Menhart N, Fung LW: Interactions of the α-spectrin N-terminal region with β spectrin. *J Biol Chem* 274:2077, 1999.

30. Grum VL, Li DN, MacDonald RI, Mondragon A: Structures of two repeats of spectrin suggest models of flexibility. *Cell* 98:523, 1999.

31. Ursitti JA, Kotula L, DeSilva TM, et al: Mapping the human erythrocyte beta-spectrin dimer initiation site using recombinant peptides and correlation of its phasing with the alpha-actinin dimer site. *J Biol Chem* 271:6636, 1996.

32. Viel A, Gee MS, Tomooka L, Branton D: Motifs involved in interchain binding at the tail-end of spectrin. *Biochim Biophys Acta* 1384:396, 1998.

33. Alloisio N, Morle L, Marechal J, et al: Sp alpha V/41: a common spectrin polymorphism at the alpha IV-alpha V domain junction. Relevance to the expression level of hereditary elliptocytosis due to alpha-spectrin variants located in trans. *J Clin Invest* 87:2169, 1991.

34. Tanaka T, Kadowski K, Lazarides E, Sobue K: Ca^{2+}- dependent regula-

35. Becker PS, Schwartz MA, Morrow JS, Lux SE: Radiolabel-transfer cross-linking demonstrates that protein 4.1 binds to the N-terminal region of beta spectrin and to actin in binary interactions. *Eur J Biochem* 193:827, 1990.

36. Kennedy SP, Warren SL, Forget BG, Morrow JS: Ankyrin binds to the 15th repetitive unit of erythroid and nonerythroid β spectrin. *J Cell Biol* 115:267, 1991.

37. Bennett V: Ankyrins. Adaptors between diverse plasma membrane proteins and the cytoplasm. *J Biol Chem* 267:8703, 1992.

38. Peters LL, Lux SE: Ankyrins: structure and function in normal cells and hereditary spherocytes. *Semin Hematol* 30:85, 1993.

39. Michaely P, Bennett V: The membrane-binding domain of ankyrin contains four independently folded subdomains, each comprised of six ankyrin repeats. *J Biol Chem* 268:22703, 1993.

40. Batchelor AH, Piper DE, de la Brousse FC, et al: The structure of GABPα/β: an ETS domain-ankyrin repeat heterodimer bound to DNA. *Science* 279:1037, 1998.

41. Bork P: Hundreds of ankyrin-like repeats in functionally diverse proteins: mobile modules that cross phyla horizontally? *Proteins* 17:363, 1993.

42. Sedgwick SG, Smerdon SJ: The ankyrin repeat: a diversity of interactions on a common structural framework. *Trends Biochem Sci* 24:311, 1999.

43. Davis LH, Davis JQ, Bennett V: Ankyrin regulation: an alternatively spliced segment of the regulatory domain functions as an intramolecular modulator. *J Biol Chem* 267:18966, 1992.

44. Gallagher PG, Tse WT, Scarpa AL, et al: Structure and organization of the human ankyrin-1 gene: basis for complexity of pre-mRNA processing. *J Biol Chem* 272:19220, 1997.

45. Inaba N, Gupta KC, Kuwabara M, et al: Deamidation of human erythrocyte protein 4.1: possible role in aging. *Blood* 79:3355, 1992.

46. Conboy J: The role of alternative pre-mRNA splicing in regulating the structure and function of skeletal protein 4.1. *Proc Soc Exper Biol Med* 220:73, 1999.

47. Gascard P, Lee G, Coulombel L, et al: Characterization of multiple isoforms of protein 4.1r expressed during erythroid terminal differentiation. *Blood* 92:4404, 1998.

48. Huang JP, Tang CJ, Kou GH, et al: Genomic structure of the locus encoding protein 4.1. Structural basis for complex combinational patterns of tissue-specific alternative RNA splicing. *J Biol Chem* 268:3758, 1993.

49. Tang TK, Qin Z, Leto T, et al: Heterogeneity of mRNA and protein products arising from the protein 4.1 gene in erythroid and nonerythroid tissues. *J Cell Biol* 110:617, 1990.

50. Chasis JA, Coulombel L, Conboy J, et al: Differentiation-associated switches in protein 4.1 expression. Synthesis of multiple structural isoforms during normal human erythropoiesis. *J Clin Invest* 91:329, 1993.

51. Marfatia SM, Leu RA, Branton D, Chishti AH: Identification of the protein 4.1 binding interface on glycophorin C and p55, a homologue of the *Drosophila* discs-large tumor suppressor protein. *J Biol Chem* 270:715, 1995.

52. Shi ZT, Afzal V, Coller B, et al: Protein 4.1R-deficient mice are viable but have erythroid membrane skeleton abnormalities. *J Clin Invest* 103:331, 1999.

53. Yawata Y: Red cell membrane protein band 4.2: phenotypic, genetic and electron microscopic aspects. *Biochim Biophys Acta* 1204:131, 1994.

54. Wada H, Kanzaki A, Yawata A, et al: Late expression of red cell membrane protein 4.2 in normal human erythroid maturation with seven isoforms of the protein 4.2 gene. *Exp Hematol* 27:54, 1999.

55. Rybicki AC, Schwartz RS, Hustedt EJ, Cobb CE: Increased rotational mobility and extractability of band 3 from protein 4.2-deficient erythrocyte membranes: evidence of a role for protein 4.2 in strengthening the band 3-cytoskeleton linkage. *Blood* 88:2745, 1996.

56. Peters LL, Jindel HK, Gwynn B, et al: Mild spherocytosis and altered red cell ion transport in protein 4.2-null mice. *J Clin Invest* 103:1527, 1999.

57. Chishti AH: Function of p55 and its nonerythroid homologues. *Curr Opin Hematol* 5:116, 1998.

58. Marfatia SM, Morais-Cabral JH, Kim AC, et al: The PDZ domain of human erythrocyte p55 mediates its binding to the cytoplasmic carboxyl terminus of glycophorin C. Analysis of the binding interface by in vitro mutagenesis. *J Biol Chem* 272:24191, 1997.

59. Li X, Bennett V: Identification of the spectrin subunit and domains

required for formation of spectrin/adducin/actin complexes. *J Biol Chem* 271:15695, 1996.

60. Joshi R, Gilligan DM, Otto E, et al: Primary structure and domain organization of human alpha and beta adducin. *J Cell Biol* 115:665, 1991.

61. Kuhlman PA, Fowler VM: Purification and characterization of an alpha 1 beta 2 isoform of CapZ from human erythrocytes: cytosolic location and inability to bind to Mg^{2+} ghosts suggest that erythrocyte actin filaments are capped by adducin. *Biochemistry* 36:13461, 1997.

62. Kuhlman PA, Hughes CA, Bennett V, Fowler VM: A new function for adducin. Calcium/calmodulin-regulated capping of the barbed ends of actin filaments. *J Biol Chem* 271:7986, 1996.

63. Li X, Matsuoka Y, Bennett V: Adducin preferentially recruits spectrin to the fast growing ends of actin filaments in a complex requiring the MARCKS-related domain and a newly defined oligomerization domain. *J Biol Chem* 273:19329, 1998.

64. Matsuoka Y, Li X, Bennett V: Adducin is an *in vivo* substrate for protein kinase C: phosphorylation in the MARCKS-related domain inhibits activity in promoting spectrin-actin complexes and occurs in many cells, including dendritic spines of neurons. *J Cell Biol* 142:485, 1998.

65. Gilligan DM, Lozovatsky L, Mohandas N, et al: Targeted disruption of the beta adducin gene (Add2) causes red blood cell spherocytosis in mice. *Proc Natl Acad Sci USA* 96:10717, 1999.

66. De Matteis MA, Morrow JS: The role of ankyrin and spectrin in membrane transport and domain formation. *Curr Opin Cell Biol* 10:542, 1998.

67. Liu SC, Derick LH, Palek J: Visualization of the hexagonal lattice in the erythrocyte membrane skeleton. *J Cell Biol* 104:527, 1987.

68. Gilligan DM, Bennett V: The junctional complex of the membrane skeleton. *Semin Hematol* 30:74, 1993.

69. Workman RF, Low PS: Biochemical analysis of potential sites for protein 4.1-mediated anchoring of the spectrin-actin skeleton to the erythrocyte membrane. *J Biol Chem* 273:6171, 1998.

70. Tse WT, Lux SE: Red blood cell membrane disorders. *Br J Haematol* 104:2, 1999.

71. Mohandas N, Chasis JA: Red blood cell deformability, membrane material properties and shape: regulation by transmembrane, skeletal and cytosolic proteins and lipids. *Semin Hematol* 30:171, 1993.

72. Hochmuth RM, Waugh RE: Erythrocyte membrane elasticity and viscosity. *Annu Rev Physiol* 49:209, 1987.

73. Narla M, Chasis JA, Shohet SB: The influence of membrane skeleton on red cell deformability, membrane material properties, and shape. *Semin Hematol* 20:225, 1983.

74. Hanspal M, Palek J: Synthesis and assembly of membrane skeletal proteins in mammalian red cell precursors. *J Cell Biol* 105:147, 1987.

75. Lazarides E: From genes to structural morphogenesis: the genesis and epigenesis of a red blood cell. *Cell* 51:345, 1987.

76. Hanspal M, Palek J: Biogenesis of normal and abnormal red blood cell membrane skeleton. *Semin Hematol* 29:305, 1992.

77. Hanspal M, Hanspal JS, Kalraiya R, Palek J: The expression and synthesis of the band 3 protein initiates the formation of a stable membrane skeleton in murine Rauscher-transformed erythroid cells. *Eur J Cell Biol* 58:313, 1992.

78. Woods CM, Boyer B, Vogt PK, Lazarides E: Control of erythroid differentiation: asynchronous expression of the anion transporter and the peripheral components of the membrane skeleton in AEV- and S13-transformed cells. *J Cell Biol* 103:1789, 1986.

79. Peters LL, Shivdasani RA, Liu SC, et al: Anion exchanger 1 (band 3) is required to prevent erythrocyte membrane surface loss but not to form the membrane skeleton. *Cell* 86:917, 1996.

80. Southgate CD, Chishti AH, Mitchell B, et al: Targeted disruption of the murine erythroid band 3 gene results in spherocytosis and severe

81. Bodine DM, Birkenmeier CS, Barker JE: Spectrin deficient inherited hemolytic anemias in the mouse: characterization by spectrin synthesis and mRNA activity in reticulocytes. *Cell* 37:721, 1984.

82. Peters LL, White RA, Birkenmeier CS, et al: Changing in cytoskeletal mRNA expression and protein synthesis patterns during murine erythropoiesis *in vivo*. *Proc Natl Acad Sci USA* 89:5749, 1992.

83. Koury MJ, Bondurant MC, Rana SS: Changes in erythroid membrane proteins during erythropoietin-mediated terminal differentiation. *J Cell Physiol* 133:438, 1987.

84. Chasis JA, Prenant M, Leung A, Mohandas N: Membrane assembly and remodeling during reticulocyte maturation. *Blood* 74:1112, 1989.

85. Takano-Ohmuro H, Mukaida M, Morioka K: Distribution of actin, myosin, and spectrin during enucleation in erythroid cells of hamster embryo. *Cell Motil Cytoskeleton* 34:95, 1996.

86. Gallagher PG: Disorders of erythrocyte metabolism and shape, in *Hematologic Problems in the Neonate*, edited by RD Christensen, p 209. Saunders, Philadephia, 1999.

87. Brugnara C: Erythrocyte membrane transport physiology. *Curr Opin Hematol* 4:122, 1997.

88. Ellory JC, Gibson JS, Stewart GW: Pathophysiology of abnormal cell volume in human red cells. *Contrib Nephrol* 123:220, 1998.

89. Lauf PK, Bauer J, Adragna NC, et al: Erythrocyte K-Cl cotransport: properties and regulation. *Am J Physiol* 263:C917, 1992.

90. Gillen CM, Brill S, Payne JA, Forbush B: Molecular cloning and functional expression of the K-Cl cotransporter from rabbit, rat, and human. A new member of the cation-chloride cotransporter family. *J Biol Chem* 271:16237, 1996.

91. Ishii TM, Silvia C, Hirschberg B, et al: A human intermediate conductance calcium-activated potassium channel. *Proc Natl Acad Sci USA* 94:11651, 1997.

92. Vandorpe DH, Shmukler BE, Jiang LW, et al: cDNA cloning and functional characterization of the mouse Ca^{++}-gated K^{+} channel, mIK1. Roles in regulatory volume decrease and erythroid differentiation. *J Biol Chem* 273:21553, 1998.

93. Brugnara C: Erythrocyte dehydration in pathophysiology and treatment of sickle cell disease. *Curr Opin Hematol* 2:132, 1995.

94. Schwartz RS, Musto S, Fabry ME, Nagel RL: Two distinct pathways mediate the formation of intermediate density cells and hyperdense cells from normal density sickle red blood cells. *Blood* 92:4844, 1998.

95. Brugnara C, Gee B, Armsby CC, et al: Therapy with oral clotrimazole induces inhibition of the Gardos channel and reduction of erythrocyte dehydration in patients with sickle cell disease. *J Clin Invest* 97:1227, 1996.

96. De Franceschi L Bachir D, Galacteros F, et al: Oral magnesium supplements reduce erythrocyte dehydration in patients with sickle cell disease. *J Clin Invest* 100:1847, 1997.

97. Lee MD, King LS, Agre P: The aquaporin family of water channel proteins in clinical medicine. *Medicine (Baltimore)* 76:141, 1997.

98. Agre P, Bonhivers M, Borgnia MJ: The aquaporins, blueprints for cellular plumbing systems. *J Biol Chem* 273:14659, 1998.

99. Chretien S, de Figueiredo M, Cartron JP: A single mutation inside the NPA motif of aquaporin 1 found in a Colton-null phenotype. *Blood* 92:5a, 1998.

100. Ma TH, Yang BX, Gillespie A, et al: Severely impaired urinary concentrating ability in transgenic mice lacking aquaporin-1 water channels. *J Biol Chem* 273:4296, 1998.

101. Roudier N, Verbavatz JM, Maurel C, et al: Evidence for the presence of aquaporin-3 in human red blood cells. *J Biol Chem* 273:8407, 1998.

haemolytic anaemia despite a normal membrane skeleton. *Nat Genet* 14:227, 1996.

STRUCTURE AND FUNCTION OF HEMOGLOBIN

HELEN M. RANNEY

VIJAY SHARMA

As a gas transport protein hemoglobin has remarkable properties, reflecting structural changes in tetrameric deoxyhemoglobin as its heme groups bind four oxygen molecules. Among the structural changes are changes in position of the heme iron and in the intersubunit hydrophobic and salt bonds of deoxyhemoglobin that are broken as ligands bind to hemoglobin. Liganded hemoglobins that do not transport oxygen, present in trace amounts normally, include methemoglobin, in which the heme iron is in the ferric (oxidized) form; carboxyhemoglobin, in which carbon monoxide is bound to the heme iron and dissociates much more slowly than oxygen; and nitrosohemoglobin, in which nitric oxide is bound to heme iron and dissociates even more slowly than carbon monoxide. Increases in methemoglobin or carboxyhemoglobin may result from toxic exposures. The many physiologic functions of nitric oxide (endothelial relaxing factor) have focused attention on the high affinity of the heme groups for nitric oxide and the potential oxygenation-linked binding of nitric oxide by the $\beta93$ cysteine residues.

Hemoglobin functions to carry oxygen from the lungs to the tissues and transport carbon dioxide from the tissues to the lungs, and it serves also to destroy the physiologically important nitric oxide molecule. It has evolved to perform its transport functions in a highly efficient manner: (1) The oxygen affinity of hemoglobin permits nearly complete saturation with oxygen in the lungs, as well as efficient oxygen unloading in the tissues; (2) Its affinity increases with oxygenation, resulting in the sigmoid shape of the oxygen dissociation curve; and (3) deoxyhemoglobin binds protons and oxyhemoglobin releases protons. The last property, expressed as the alkaline Bohr effect, also facilitates oxygen loading in the lungs and unloading in the tissues. The Perutz models of oxygenated and deoxygenated hemoglobin provide important insights into the structural basis of these three major features of the equilibria of oxygen with hemoglobin. The reader is referred to two[1,2] of the many excellent sources for a detailed analysis of structure-function relationships.

The roles of different parts of the hemoglobin molecule in its equilibria have been deduced from its amino acid sequence, its helical conformation, models derived from x-ray crystallography,[3,4] studies of the kinetics of reactions of hemoglobin with ligands,[5] and observations utilizing nuclear magnetic resonance.[6] The concentration of hemoglobin within human red cells is extraordinarily high (34 g/dl), and its efficiency as an oxygen carrier is enhanced by its packaging in flexible cells of optimal shape for the diffusion of gases.

Acronyms and abbreviations that appear in this chapter include: BPG, bisphosphoglycerate; cGMP, cyclic guanosine monophosphate; Hb, hemoglobin; HbL, liganded hemoglobin.

STRUCTURE OF HEMOGLOBIN

Normal mammalian hemoglobins contain two pairs of unlike polypeptide chains: one chain of each pair is α or α-like and the other is non-α (β, γ, or δ). The α chains of all human hemoglobins encountered after early embryogenesis are the same. The non-α chains include the β chain of normal adult hemoglobin [hemoglobin A ($\alpha_2\beta_2$)], the γ chain of fetal hemoglobin [hemoglobin F ($\alpha_2\gamma_2$)], and the δ chain of hemoglobin A_2 [hemoglobin A_2 ($\alpha_2\delta_2$)], the minor component which accounts for 2.5 percent of the hemoglobin of normal adults.

In the amino acid sequence of each polypeptide chain, certain residues appear to be critical to stability and function. Such residues are usually the same (invariant) in α or β chains. The NH_2-terminal valines of the β chains are important in 2,3-BPG interactions (bisphosphoglycerate has replaced the older term diphosphoglycerate). The C-terminal residues are important in the salt bridges that characterize the unliganded molecules. Areas of contact between chains and between heme and globin tend to contain invariant residues. Unlike many proteins, native hemoglobin contains no disulfide bonds: of its six -SH groups (cysteine residues $\alpha104$, $\beta93$, and $\beta112$), only the two $\beta93$ residues are exposed to the solvent.

PRIMARY STRUCTURE OF GLOBIN CHAINS

The non-α (β, γ, δ or ε) chains are all 146 amino acids in length; the β chain begins with valine and histidine. The C-terminal residues are Tyr $\beta145$ and His $\beta146$. The δ chain (of hemoglobin A2) differs from the β chain (of hemoglobin A) in only 10 residues. The first eight residues and the C-terminal residues (127 to 146) are the same in δ and β chains. Tetramers of β chains (hemoglobin H) may be found in α thalassemia.

The γ chain of fetal hemoglobin (hemoglobin F) differs from the β chain by 39 residues. The N-terminal residues of the γ chain and β chain are glycine and valine respectively, while the C-terminal residues, Tyr145 and His146, are the same as in γ and β chains. Appreciable quantities of free γ chains are found in the red cells of some infants with α thalassemia; free γ chains, like β chains, can form homotetramers known as hemoglobin Bart's. In addition to the different N-terminal residues, several other differences in primary structure between the γ and β chains are noteworthy: the γ chain contains isoleucine, while the β chains do not. The increased alkali resistance of hemoglobin F and hemoglobin Bart's (γ_4) has been attributed to the different amino acids at residues 112 and 130 (βCys and Tyr by γThr and Trp, respectively).

The γ genes are duplicated: one codes for glycine ($^G\gamma$) and the other for alanine ($^A\gamma$)[7] at residue 176, giving rise to two kinds of γ chains. In addition, a common polymorphism, the substitution of threonine for isoleucine, is frequently found at residue 75 of the $^A\gamma$ chain.

SECONDARY STRUCTURE

About 75 percent of the amino acids in α or β chains are in a helical arrangement. All studied hemoglobins have a similar helical content (Fig. 28-1a). Eight helical areas, lettered A to H, occur in the β chains. Hemoglobin nomenclature specifies that amino acids within helices are designated by the amino acid number and the helix letter, while amino acids between helices bear the number of the amino acid and the letters of the two helices. Thus, residue EF3 is the third residue of the segment connecting the E and F helices, while residue F8 is the eighth residue of the F helix. Alignment according to helical designation makes homology evident: residue F8 is the proximal heme-linked histidine, and the histidine on the distal side of the heme is E7.

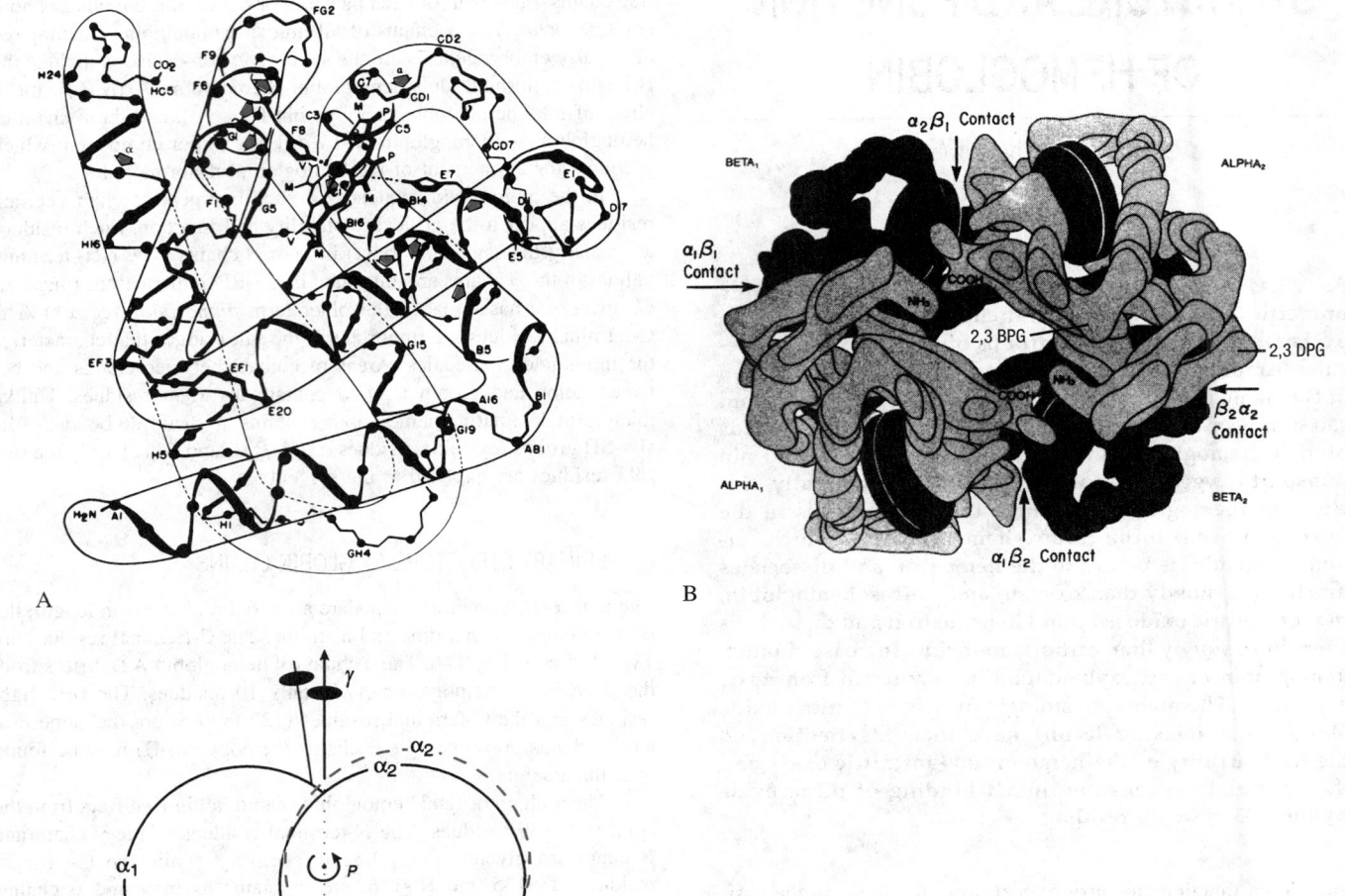

FIGURE 28-1 *(a)* The representation of the structure of β chains. Arrows indicate sites of substitutions in a number of unstable hemoglobins. *(b)* The hemoglobin molecule, as deduced from x-ray diffraction studies, shown from above. The molecule is composed of four subunits: two identical α chains *(light blocks)* and two identical β chains *(dark blocks)*. 2,3 BPG binds to the two β chains in the deoxyhemoglobin molecule. *(c)* Schematic diagram of rotation of $\alpha_2\beta_2$ dimer relative to $\alpha_1\beta_1$ in quaternary structure change from deoxyhemoglobin (solid lines) to carboxyhemoglobin (dashed lines). Modified slightly from *J Mol Biol* 129, J. Baldwin and C. Chothia, Haemoglobin: the structural changes related to ligand binding and its allosteric mechanism, page 196, 1979, by permission of authors and publisher, Academic Press Ltd., London.

TERTIARY STRUCTURE OF α AND β CHAINS[2,3]

The tertiary structure of the α and β chains is shown in Fig. 28-1*b*. The prosthetic group of hemoglobin is ferroprotoporphyrin IX. Its structure is shown in Fig. 28-2*a*. The heme group is located in a crevice between the E and F helices in each chain (Fig. 28-2*b*). The highly polar propionate side chains of the heme are on the surface of the molecule and are ionized at physiologic pH. The rest of the heme is inside the molecule, surrounded by nonpolar residues except for two histidines. The iron atom is linked by a coordinate bond to the imidazole nitrogen (N) of histidine F8; the E7 *distal* histidine, on the other side of the heme plane, is not bonded to the iron atom but is very close to the ligand-binding site.

In both types of chains there is a preponderance of nonpolar residues in the immediate vicinity of heme. On the proximal side, the important residues in contact with heme are Val FG5, Leu FG3, His F8, Leu F7, Leu H19, and Leu F4; on the distal side, important heme contacts are Phe CD4, His E7, Leu G8, Val E11, and Lys E10. The V produced by helices E and F provides the main walls of the heme pocket. Helices B, G, and H form the floor, and the segments C and CD guard the opening to this pocket. Important features of the heme pocket are as follows:

1. The hydrophobic "cage" around the heme provides the main stabilizing force for the binding of heme to the protein. The closely packed side chains that constitute the cage do not allow significant movement of the heme.

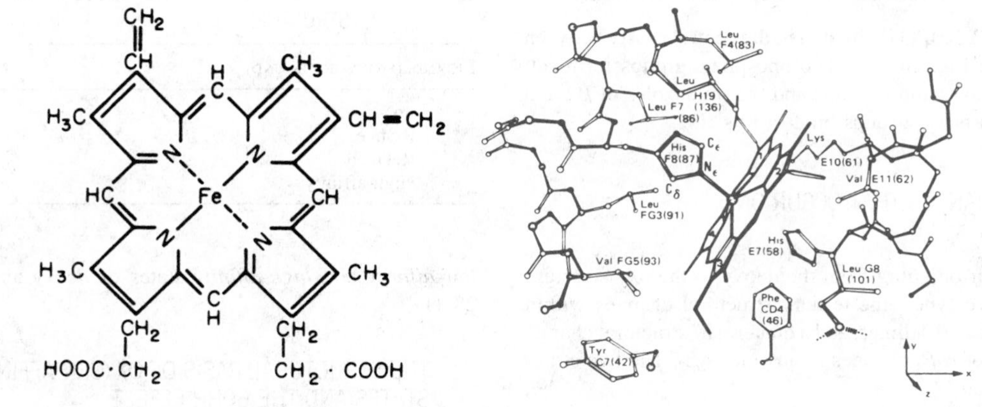

FIGURE 28-2 (a) Structure of heme (ferroprotoporphyrin IX). (b) Heme group and its environment in the unliganded α chain. Only selected side chains are shown: the heme 4-propionate is omitted (Gelin, et al[8]).

2. In a nonpolar environment it is much more difficult to oxidize Fe^{2+} to Fe^{3+}. This feature facilitates binding of oxygen without oxidation.

3. In β subunits of deoxyhemoglobin the methyl group of Val E11 is in van der Waals' contact with porphyrin. It overlaps the van der Waals radii of heme ligand(s) (O_2, CO, and NO). This steric hindrance by Val E11 is much smaller in α chains.[4]

4. Two atoms of the distal histidine (E7) are in van der Waals' contact with the porphyrin in both oxyhemoglobin and deoxyhemoglobin, and the imidazole N also overlaps with the ligand-binding site. The histidine side chain also acts as a gate to the ligand-binding site, not allowing ligand to enter or leave unless it swings out of the way.

5. The hydrophobic residues in the C and CD segments that guard the opening to the heme pocket effectively exclude polar ligands from entering the heme pocket.

6. The imidazole N of the proximal histidine is hydrogen-bonded to the carboxyl of Leu F4 and the OH of Ser F5. This hydrogen bonding and the neighboring side chains hold the proximal His F8 in position rather rigidly.

7. Both α and β hemes form about 75 contacts with 30 atoms in 16 globin residues in each heme pocket.

Although the x-ray structure of deoxyhemoglobin indicates a planar porphyrin with iron displaced 0.6 Å out of the plane in α chains and 0.63 Å in β chains, data on model compounds and considerations based on energy-minimized geometry suggest that the plane of pyrrole nitrogens might be displaced toward iron by 0.22 Å in α chains and by 0.17 Å in β chains compared with the mean plane of the porphyrin carbons. The energy difference between the domed and the planar porphyrin structure is small. The iron atom in both deoxyhemoglobins and methemoglobins is high-spin, and it has been suggested that its ionic radius is too large to fit into the plane of the porphyrin ring. Spin state of hemoglobin derivatives depends on the number of unpaired electrons in d orbitals of iron. In both subunits of deoxyhemoglobin, the imidazole ring of the proximal His F8 is in an asymmetric position with respect to the porphyrin nitrogens of the heme, such that the atom C_ϵ is closer to porphyrin $N_{(1)}$ than C_δ is to $N_{(3)}$[8] (see Fig. 28-2b).

In both the α and the β subunits of human deoxyhemoglobin, the ligand-binding site is blocked. In the α subunits a water molecule is attached to the distal His E7. There is no direct bond between the water molecule and the iron atom. In β chains, the methyl group of Val E11 lies within 1.8 Å of the ligand-binding site. Both of these

groups would have to move out of the way before the ligand could bind to iron.[4]

QUATERNARY STRUCTURE[1,2]

In the deoxy state, the hemoglobin tetramer is held together by intersubunit salt bonds and intersubunit hydrophobic contacts, in addition to a certain number of hydrogen bonds.

1. The intersubunit salt bonds (Fig. 28-3). Four of these salt bonds, involving Arg HC3(141), are between the two α chains. The two salt bonds involving His HC3(146) are between β and α chains. There are two intramolecular salt bonds in β chains.

2. The $\alpha_1\beta_1$ (or $\alpha_2\beta_2$) and $\alpha_1\beta_2$ (or $\alpha_2\beta_1$) intersubunit contacts (see Fig. 28-1b).
   a. The $\alpha_1\beta_1$ contact. This more extensive contact, between α_1 and β_1 subunits, involves 32 residues, including 126 atoms, 4 hydrogen bonds, and 1 solvent-mediated hydrogen bond.
   b. The $\alpha_1\beta_2$ contact. Slightly less extensive than the $\alpha_1\beta_1$ contacts, this contact involves 27 residues, including 107 atoms, 6 hydrogen bonds, and 3 solvent-mediated hydrogen bonds.

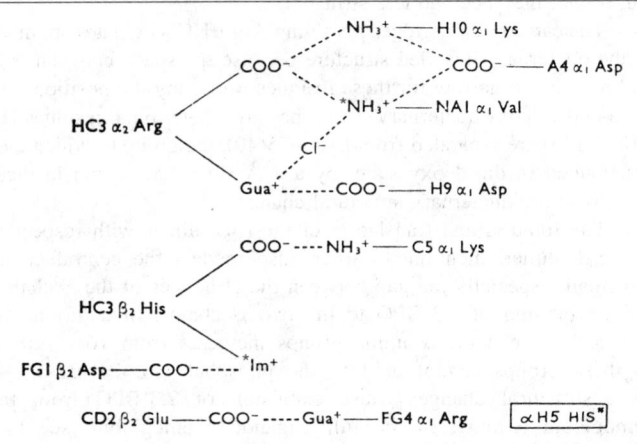

FIGURE 28-3 Salt bridges in deoxyhemoglobin (*= ionizable group less protonated at pH 9.0 than at pH 7.0). These groups account for 60 percent of the alkaline Bohr effect. The remainder is due to His αH5 (Perutz[2]).

BINDING OF 2,3-BPG TO DEOXYHEMOGLOBIN TETRAMER

In deoxyhemoglobin, 2,3-BPG is situated in the central cavity between the two β chains (see Fig. 28-1b).[9] The phosphate groups form salt bonds with β N-terminal amino groups and the imidazoles of $\beta2$ and $\beta143$ histidine; the carboxyl groups bind to Lys $\beta82$.

STRUCTURAL CHANGES THAT OCCUR ON LIGAND BINDING[10,11]

The changes that occur on going from the deoxy to the oxy structure (Fig. 28-1c) are of two types: the tertiary structural changes within the subunits of $\alpha_1\beta_1$ (or $\alpha_2\beta_2$) dimer, and a quaternary structural change in which the position of $\alpha_1\beta_1$ changes relative to $\alpha_2\beta_2$. The two structural changes are linked.

Iron-to-ligand bond formation would require moving the iron atom toward the heme plane. This would bring the C_ε atom of the proximal histidine too close to both porphyrin $N_{(1)}$ and C atoms in the pyrrole ring, producing large steric strain. The tertiary structural changes involving heme, proximal histidine, F helix, FG corner, and others all minimize the steric strain produced as a result of metal-to-ligand bond formation.

The most important of the tertiary structural changes seems to be the translation of the F helix approximately 1 Å across the heme plane, the tilting of the F helix with respect to the heme, and the movement of heme and the FG corner toward the center of the molecule. This movement of the F helix takes the proximal histidine from its asymmetric position in deoxyhemoglobin to a more symmetric position in liganded hemoglobin. The motion of β hemes removes the ligand-binding site from the vicinity of Val βE11, which may hinder ligand binding in the deoxy state. These changes in the tertiary structure are linked to the quaternary changes through the motion of FG corners. The C helices and FG corners of the $\alpha_1\beta_1$ dimer are in contact with the FG corners and C helices of $\alpha_2\beta_2$ in both quaternary structures. The contacts between α_1FG and β_2C (and α_2FG and β_1C) act as "flexible joints" and undergo only small relative motions. The contacts between α_1C and β_2FG (and α_2C and β_1FG) act as switch regions that have two different stable positions. The change between the two stable positions involves a relative movement of approximately 6 Å.

The quaternary structural change that occurs on ligand binding to hemoglobin involves rotation of the $\alpha_2\beta_2$ dimer interface relative to the $\alpha_1\beta_1$ by 14.9° and translation of 0.8 Å. The overall number of intersubunit hydrogen bonds and contacts may not change significantly, but they become less stringent.

The carboxy salt bridges involving Arg αHC3(141) are not made in the quaternary liganded structure because the space between $\alpha_1\beta_1$ and $\alpha_2\beta_2$ is too narrow for these residues to occupy the position they have in the deoxy quaternary state. The carboxy-terminal residues His βHC3(146) are separated from Lys αC5(40), the group to which they are bonded in the deoxy state, by a 7 Å shift that occurs in these regions in the quaternary structural change.

The rotation and translation of the $\alpha_2\beta_2$ dimer with respect to the $\alpha_1\beta_1$ dimer, mentioned earlier, also renders the central cavity too small, especially the gap between the H helices of the β chains, for the binding of 2,3-BPG to the two β chains. In addition, the distance between the α-amino groups increases from 16 to 20 Å, so these groups cannot bind to the phosphates of 2,3-BPG. All these structural changes cause expulsion of 2,3-BPG from the hemoglobin tetramer in the fully liganded hemoglobin (see Fig. 28-1b). The quaternary structures of unliganded and liganded hemoglobin are known as the T-state ("tense") and R-state ("relaxed") structures, respectively. Respective alternative terms are

TABLE 28-1   NOMENCLATURE OF HEMOGLOBIN QUATERNARY STRUCTURES

LIGANDED (OXYGEN BOUND)	UNLIGANDED (REDUCED)
Oxy	Deoxy
R-state	T-state
Relaxed	Tense
High-affinity	Low-affinity

low-affinity and high-affinity states or deoxy and oxy states (Table 28-1).

THE STRUCTURAL BASIS OF OXYGEN AFFINITY IN T AND R STATES AND THE BOHR EFFECT

One mechanism proposed to account for the differing oxygen affinities of the T and R states and for the Bohr effect[11] takes into account the x-ray crystallographic data and calculations of energies associated with various structural changes that might occur at the heme on ligand binding.[8,12,13] The low affinity of deoxyhemoglobin for its first ligand appears to be due to the strain induced by the steric repulsion arising from the position of the F helix and, in particular, from the position of the proximal histidine relative to the heme; the imidazole ring of each chain is tilted so that its interaction with porphyrin-ring carbons provides steric hindrance in iron-to-oxygen bond formation. Quaternary structural changes brought about by the tertiary structural changes via the changes at the intersubunit contacts (particularly at β_2FG-α_1C and β_1FG-α_2C) place the proximal histidine in R structure in a symmetric position with respect to the plane of the porphyrin ring and thus minimize the steric interaction between the imidazole (C_ε) and porphyrin $N_{(1)}$ and a carbon atom in the pyrrole-1 ring. In β subunits, an additional factor increases ligand affinities in the R state: the translational and rotational movements of β hemes remove the ligand-binding site from the vicinity of the Val E11 side chain. Both of these factors result in a much stronger iron-to-oxygen bond in R structure.

Calculations[8,13] suggest that the geometry of the heme in deoxyhemoglobin may be very similar to that in isolated heme. If this is correct, then the iron atom in deoxyhemoglobin is in its optimal position for five-coordinate high-spin Fe^{2+} ion, and there is little strain on the unliganded heme. Instead, the heme in the liganded subunit in the deoxy quaternary tetramer would be under strain.

The structural change described above also results in an altered electrostatic environment of certain protonated amino acid side chains (see Fig. 28-3), and their proton dissociation constants are increased:

$$\text{Deoxy Hb} \longleftrightarrow \text{Oxy Hb} + \text{H}^+$$

This equation forms the basis of the Bohr effect, discussed under "Oxygen Equilibria of Hemoglobin—the Oxygen Dissociation Curve," below.

THE TWO-STATE MODEL

The mechanisms of cooperative ligand binding by hemoglobin proposed by various workers must be regarded as tentative, since none of them is capable of explaining all the physicochemical properties of hemoglobin even qualitatively. It is not clear in these models at which point in ligation the transition from low-affinity (T) to high-affinity (R) structure takes place. In the most widely accepted model,[14] T and R species are considered to be in rapid equilibrium:

$$Hb_4^T \xleftrightarrow{LC^n} Hb_4^R$$

where n = number of ligands bound to Hb
$$L = [Hb_4^T]/[Hb_4^R]$$
$$C = K_R/K_T$$

and K_R and K_T are the ligand dissociation constants in the R and T states respectively. A shift in the equilibrium between T and R species with fractional saturation would then account for the cooperative ligand binding and other features of the oxygen dissociation curve. The transition point from T to R structure acquires a statistical meaning and is given by the equation

$$n_t = -\log L/\log C$$

where n_t is the number of ligands bound at the switch-over point from T to R. Depending on the experimental conditions, the value of n_t for hemoglobin lies in the range of 2.3 to 3.0.

OXYGEN EQUILIBRIA OF HEMOGLOBIN—THE OXYGEN DISSOCIATION CURVE

Important gas-transport properties of hemoglobin are evident from inspection of the oxygen dissociation curve (Fig. 28-4). The oxygen affinity increases with increasing oxygen saturation of the hemoglobin. This increasing oxygen affinity with increasing saturation is described by the sigmoid shape of the oxygen dissociation curve. The terms *heme-heme interaction* and *cooperative interactions* also describe this change in oxygen affinity as a function of saturation. The binding of more protons by deoxyhemoglobin than by oxyhemoglobin, known as the *Bohr effect,* is reflected in the left shift of oxygen dissociation curves with increasing pH. These functional properties are interdependent, or linked.[14] The oxygen affinity depends on the state of oxygenation (cooperative interactions) and on the pH (Bohr effect).

OXYGEN AFFINITY OF HEMOGLOBIN

For clinical usage, the oxygen affinity of hemoglobin is usually expressed in terms of the P_{50}, the oxygen tension at which hemoglobin is half saturated. This value is 26 torr in normal red cells or concentrated hemolysates at 37°C and plasma pH of 7.4. (The pH of the interior of the red cell is about 0.2 units lower than the pH of the plasma.) The partial pressure of oxygen in room air is about 100 torr; in the pulmonary alveoli it is about 95 torr. Oxygen diffuses passively across the alveolar capillary membrane during the time (<1 s) the red cell spends within the pulmonary vasculature. Desaturated blood from the bronchial (and other) veins returns to pulmonary veins, resulting in a P_{O_2} of about 90 torr in the left side of the heart; i.e., systemic arterial blood is almost fully saturated with oxygen. As the blood traverses the systemic capillaries, the release of oxygen is determined by the P_{O_2} of the tissues. The steep portion of the oxygen dissociation curve allows a relatively large amount of oxygen to be unloaded for a small decrement in P_{O_2}. The P_{O_2} in the capillaries of different organs varies with oxygen consumption.

The value of P_{50} is taken from the midpoint of the oxygen dissociation curve and does not reflect the shape of the curve. With increasing oxygen affinity, the value for P_{50} becomes smaller; i.e., the dissociation curve is "shifted to the left." High values for P_{50} indicate lower oxygen affinity of the hemoglobin. Since hemoglobin is nearly fully saturated with oxygen at a P_{O_2} of 85 torr, a right shift in the dissociation curve will facilitate oxygen delivery, and nearly full saturation will still occur in the lungs.

FACTORS THAT AFFECT OXYGEN AFFINITY

The three primary determinants of the value of P_{50} are temperature, pH, and red cell 2,3-BPG concentration. The increase in oxygen affinity with lower temperatures is observed in red cells or in hemoglobin solutions.

The Bohr effect is observed in red cells and hemoglobin solutions (see inset of Fig. 28-4). With increasing hydrogen ion concentration (decreasing pH), P_{50} increases; i.e., oxygen affinity declines. Protons stabilize the T state by stabilizing the intersubunit bonds and the bonds between the two β chains and 2,3-BPG; 2,3-BPG and other anions stabilize the T state by complexing preferentially with hemoglobin in this state. Both these factors shift T-to-R equilibrium toward the T (low-affinity) state.

The Bohr shift constitutes an important buffer system of the body. When blood reaches the tissues, where the oxygen tension is lower and the hydrogen ion concentration is increased by lactic acid or carbon dioxide, the Bohr shift of the dissociation curve makes more oxygen available. As the hemoglobin loses its oxygen and the unliganded form binds protons, changes in hydrogen ion concentration are minimized. The proton binding of deoxyhemoglobin provides an important part of carbon dioxide transport: Carbon dioxide diffuses into the red cell, and its conversion there to bicarbonate is catalyzed by carbonic anhydrase. The bicarbonate ion leaves the red cell, and the hydrogen ion is bound by deoxyhemoglobin. The ultimate effectiveness of this physiologic buffer system depends on the ease with which carbon dioxide or bicarbonate is retained or eliminated in the lungs and kidneys. The Bohr effect is also observed in the reactions of hemoglobin with ligands other than oxygen (e.g., carbon monoxide, ethyl isocyanide) and in the oxidation of hemoglobin to methemoglobin (the oxidation Bohr effect).

Carbon dioxide reacts with N-terminal residues of the β chains of hemoglobin to yield carbamino derivatives, a phenomenon separate from the Bohr effect. These carbamino derivatives are of minor importance in carbon dioxide transport by hemoglobins that bind organic phosphates.

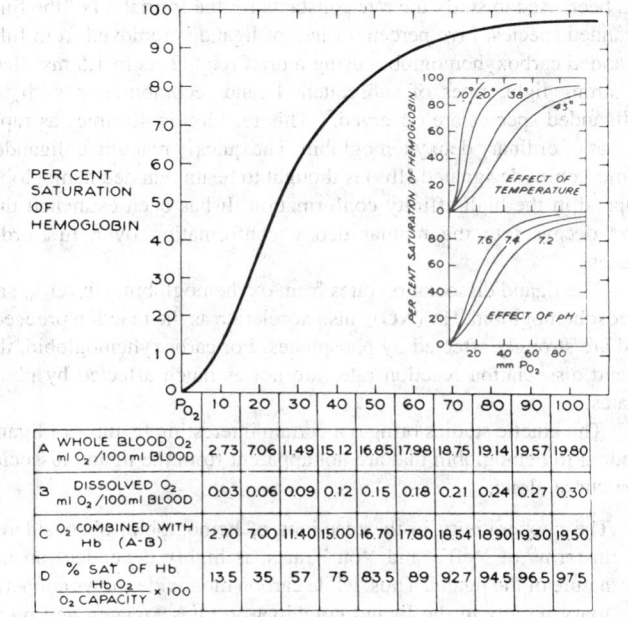

FIGURE 28-4 Oxygen dissociation curve of human hemoglobin. Inserts: Effect of temperature *(upper)* and Bohr effect *(lower)* (Comroe[15]).

EFFECTS OF 2,3-BPG ON OXYGEN EQUILIBRIA

The usual P_{50} measurements are done under standard conditions of temperature, pH, and P_{O_2}. Therefore, observed variations in the oxygen affinity are usually related to the concentration of 2,3-BPG[16] (or less commonly to the presence of structurally different hemoglobins with altered oxygen affinity). The P_{50} of whole blood or of hemoglobin solutions increases with increasing concentrations of 2,3-BPG (the normal value of 2,3-BPG is about 5 mmol/liter of packed red cells). The relationship of 2,3-BPG and P_{50} is not linear: with higher concentrations, smaller increments in P_{50} are observed. In addition to its stabilization of the deoxy form of the tetramer, 2,3-BPG, because it is a nonpermeating anion, lowers intracellular pH relative to plasma pH. Other factors, such as carbon dioxide in carbamino linkage and mean corpuscular hemoglobin concentration, probably do not much affect the oxygen affinity of normal hemoglobin under conditions encountered clinically, although the carbon dioxide effect is rather large when the P_{50} values at pH 7.2 are compared at P_{CO_2} values ranging from 0 to 40 torr. A concentration-dependent decrease of oxygen affinity in sickle hemoglobin reflects the gelation of deoxygenated hemoglobin S.

Increases in P_{50} may be observed in acidosis or in any state (anemia, hypoxia, ascent to high altitudes) in which 2,3-BPG is increased. A higher oxygen affinity (lower P_{50}) is seen in hemoglobins modified by treatment with a number of agents, including cyanate. The role of organic phosphates in regulating oxygen delivery to the tissues has provided an explanation for the finding that although the oxygen affinity of cord blood exceeds that of maternal blood, the oxygen affinity of isolated hemoglobin F does not differ greatly from that of hemoglobin A. The oxygen affinity of phosphate-free hemoglobin F is lower than that of hemoglobin A, but the effect of 2,3-BPG on the oxygen affinity of hemoglobin F is much less than that on adult hemoglobin.[1] The oxygen affinity of fetal blood is therefore higher than that of adult blood, permitting more complete placental extraction of oxygen from maternal blood.

COOPERATIVE INTERACTIONS

The physiologic advantages that derive from the sigmoid shape of the oxygen dissociation curve are obvious from the data in Fig. 28-4. A fall in P_{O_2} from 100 to 60 torr results in a decline in oxygen saturation from 97.5 to 89 percent, while a fall from 60 to 20 torr will be accompanied by a decline in oxygen saturation from 89 to 35 percent and the release of more than 10 ml oxygen per deciliter of blood to the tissues. The rather "flat" portion of the oxygen dissociation curve at P_{O_2} from 70 to 100 torr results in nearly complete saturation of hemoglobin even at the lower partial pressures of oxygen found at quite high altitudes. The advantages of decreased oxygen affinity as a compensatory mechanism in hypoxemia obtain only if the sigmoid shape of the dissociation curve is preserved.

THE HILL PLOT

The plot of log $[y/(1 - y)]$ against log P_{O_2} is known as the *Hill plot*. The Hill equation is

$$\log [y/(1 - y)] = \log K + n \log P_{O_2}$$

where y = fractional saturation with O_2

K = an empiric overall constant without physicochemical basis

The n value (the slope from the Hill plot at half saturation) is taken as a convenient measure of cooperativity. Values of n in noninteracting hemoglobins which exhibit hyperbolic oxygen dissociation curves (e.g., myoglobin and hemoglobin H) are about 1. In a normal tetrameric hemoglobin with four oxygen-reactive sites, the maximum value for n would be 4.0; however, n values of 2.7 to 3.0 rather than 4.0 are encountered in normal hemoglobin.

KINETICS OF REACTIONS WITH LIGANDS

The reactions of hemoglobin with ligands are much faster than would be needed for reaction during transit in the microvasculature. The exception to this is the slow rate of dissociation of carbon monoxide and nitric oxide from hemoglobin, which results in the extremely high affinity of these ligands for hemoglobin and prevents equilibration of carbon monoxide- or nitric oxide-containing red cells with oxygen in the lungs. The oxygen dissociation curve does not reveal certain finer details of the overall reaction between hemoglobin and ligands (i.e., O_2, CO, or NO) that can be observed when one considers the rates of ligand binding (the "on" rates) and the rates of ligand dissociation (the "off" rates) separately:

$$Hb + L \underset{\text{"off"}}{\overset{\text{"on"}}{\rightleftharpoons}} HbL$$

The stepwise binding of ligands to hemoglobin tetramer can be written in terms of the Adair four-step model.[17] Eight Adair rate constants, four stepwise "on" and four "off" for each ligand (O_2, CO, NO), and the ligand-specific equilibrium constants have been determined.[18–20] However, because of the cooperative nature of the reactions, accurate determination of the intermediate equilibrium and rate constants (steps 2 and 3) is not easy, and constants for those two steps are less certain.

The "on" reactions of oxygen, carbon monoxide, and nitric oxide with deoxyhemoglobin are strictly first-order in ligand and hemoglobin concentrations; hence, the overall reaction is second-order. The reaction rates accelerate as the reaction proceeds. The initial rates approximate the rate constant for the formation of the monoliganded species, Hb_4L.[5] Oxyhemoglobin and particularly carboxyhemoglobin are photosensitive, and each loses its ligand on exposure to light. This property has been used to study the rate constants for the formation of the fully liganded species. Five percent or less of ligand is removed from fully liganded carboxyhemoglobin using a brief (e.g., 2 μs to 1.5 ms) flash of strong light; rates of subsequent ligand recombination with the triliganded species are observed.[21] This reaction is 40 times as rapid as that of ordinary deoxyhemoglobin. The quickly reacting unliganded hemoglobin (designated Hb*) is thought to be unliganded hemoglobin trapped in the high-affinity conformation. It has been estimated that Hb* decays into the regular deoxy conformation by a first-order process.

The ligand dissociation rates from oxyhemoglobin, $Hb_4(O_2)_4$, and nitrosohemoglobin, $Hb_4(NO)_4$, also accelerate as the reaction proceeds and are strongly affected by phosphates. For carboxyhemoglobin, the ligand dissociation reaction rates are not as much affected by phosphates.

The kinetic studies bring out certain interesting features of ligand binding to hemoglobin that are not apparent from the ligand dissociation curve alone:

1. The cooperativity in the reactions of hemoglobin, if considered in terms of "off" and "on" rates, is highly dependent on the nature of the ligand. Thus, while carbon monoxide shows cooperativity *mainly* in the ligand combination rates, oxygen and nitric oxide show cooperativity in the ligand dissociation rates. These differences arise from the differences in the stereochemistry of these ligands. Oxygen prefers bent bonding (with respect to the

axis perpendicular to the heme plane) with the iron atom in heme and avoids steric interaction with the residues on the distal side of heme. The variation in ''off'' rate constants in this case mainly reflects the tension on the $Fe-O_2$ bond owing to steric and/or electronic factors originating on the proximal side of heme. This should also be true for nitric oxide. Carbon monoxide, however, prefers linear bonding with the iron atom in heme. The residues on the distal side of heme in the heme pocket—particularly His E7 and Val E11 in β chains—are situated too close to the ligand-binding site and therefore provide steric hindrance in the formation of the iron-to-ligand bond. Variations in the stepwise ''on'' rate constants for carbon monoxide therefore may reflect the variations in the steric hindrance from the distal residues, in addition to the proximal side effects discussed above. From the values of carbon monoxide ''off'' rates it is also obvious that the Fe-CO bond is too strong to respond to the same extent as the $Fe-O_2$ bond to the ''tension'' from the proximal side. It has been suggested that the heme pocket discriminates between these three ligands by electrostatic interactions with the bound ligand. Favorable electrostatic interactions stabilize the bound oxygen by a factor of about 100, nitric oxide by about 10, and carbon monoxide only by 2–3.

2. The effect of phosphates in oxyhemoglobin is due primarily to changes in the ''off'' rates rather than to changes in the ''on'' rates; species in the quaternary T state show larger enhancement in the dissociation rates.[18] Various equilibrium and kinetic studies suggest that although phosphates bind to β chains, they affect the properties of α chains more.

3. Kinetic studies indicate that α and β chains in hemoglobin tetramers have different reactivity. These differences are shown in the reactions of deoxyhemoglobin as well as in fully liganded hemoglobin.[5] The magnitude of these differences is smaller in the reactions of ferrohemoglobin than in those of ferrihemoglobin.

4. Nitric oxide binds to hemoglobin 10^5 to 10^7 times more strongly than do carbon monoxide and oxygen. The half-life for the disappearance of nitrosohemoglobin is approximately 11 h. Ligand combination rates of carbon monoxide are activation controlled; i.e., the protein has to undergo some structural change before carbon monoxide can form a covalent bond with heme. These rates therefore depend on the protein structure. The combination rates of oxygen and nitric oxide, on the other hand, are diffusion controlled; i.e., oxygen-to-heme and nitric oxide-to-hemebond formation take place prior to any major change in protein structure.

Therefore, the reaction rates of oxygen and nitric oxide depend much less on protein structure than do the rates for carbon monoxide.

LIGANDS OF HEMOGLOBIN

METHEMOGLOBIN AND SULFHEMOGLOBIN

Methemoglobin is hemoglobin in which the iron has been oxidized ($\alpha_2^{3+}\beta_2^{3+}$). This oxidized hemoglobin is no longer capable of reversibly binding oxygen. Methemoglobin is reddish brown, with an absorbance peak at 630 nm at acid pH (Fig. 28-5). The absorption spectrum of methemoglobin is strongly pH-dependent: at low pH, a water molecule is bound to the iron and occupies the space between the ferric iron and the distal histidine. At alkaline pH, hydroxyl ion is bound to the ferric iron. At an acid pH the iron atom of aquomethemoglobin is in the high-spin state and goes to a low-spin state with increasing pH. In a mixture of methemoglobin and normal ferrous hemoglobin, intermediates called valency hybrids are formed. These are tetramers in which varying numbers of hemes are in the ferrous state and the remainder are in the ferric state. These valency hybrids have been useful models for studying subunit cooperativity. In a hemoglobin solution containing oxy, deoxy, and methemoglobin species the oxygen affinity is unusual; i.e., the dissociation curve is left-shifted and P_{50} is decreased. This increase in oxygen affinity provides the explanation for the toxicity of methemoglobinemia: in addition to the nonfunctional ferric subunits, the increased oxygen affinity of ferrous hemes accompanying ferric hemes in tetramers impairs oxygen delivery. Methemoglobin solutions are believed to be equilibrium mixtures of quaternary R+T structures. Ingestion of certain drugs or accidental ingestion of oxidizing agents may lead to methemoglobinemia (see Chap. 49).

On exposure to some toxic agents, *sulfhemoglobin* is formed. Sulfhemoglobin is a curious compound in which the iron is in the ferrous state but the oxygen affinity is about 100 times lower than that of normal hemoglobin. The sulfur is not liganded to the iron but is found in the porphyrin ring (see Chap. 49).

CARBOXYHEMOGLOBIN

Carboxyhemoglobin (carbonmonoxyhemoglobin) results from the binding of carbon monoxide to the heme iron. In carboxyhemoglobin the carbon monoxide is bound at an angle different from that of oxygen relative to the plane of the heme. The rate of association of carbon

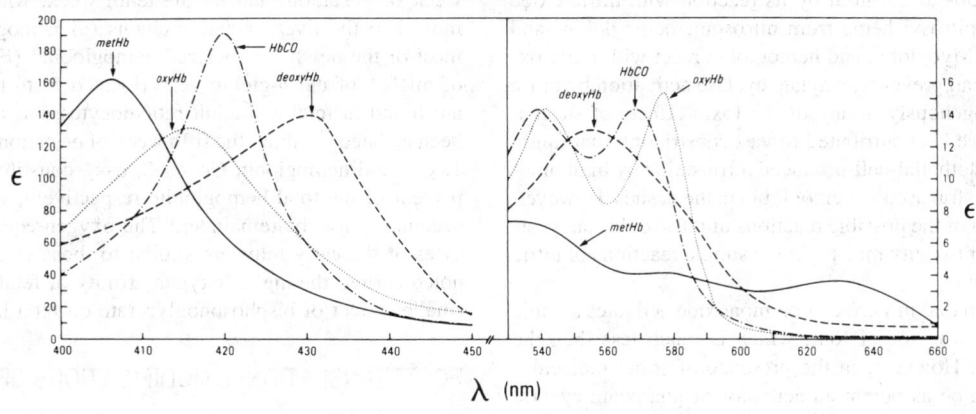

FIGURE 28-5 Spectra of some hemoglobin derivatives. Extinction coefficients plotted against wavelength (pH 7.4).

monoxide with hemoglobin is slower than that of oxygen; however, carbon monoxide dissociates much more slowly than does oxygen. Hemoglobin binds carbon monoxide about 200 times more strongly than it binds oxygen. If the partial pressure of carbon monoxide is 0.5 percent that of oxygen, the concentration of carboxyhemoglobin at equilibrium will approximately equal that of oxyhemoglobin. The symptoms of carbon monoxide poisoning result from tissue oxygen deprivation. Hemoglobin tetramers, in which some hemes are bound to oxygen and others to carbon monoxide, have high oxygen affinity. Carbon monoxide, like oxygen, binds reversibly to the heme iron of hemoglobin. However because of its slow dissociation from the heme iron, the affinity of carbon monoxide for hemoglobin is approximately 210-fold higher than the affinity of oxygen. Therefore, inhalation of carbon monoxide even at low partial pressures leads to significant levels of carboxyhemoglobin in the blood. For example, a concentration of 0.1% carbon monoxide in inspired air will result at equilibrium in 50% carboxyhemoglobin. Oxygen transport and delivery are impaired both by the unavailability of carboxyhemoglobin for oxygen transport and by the higher oxygen affinity of the mixed oxygen/carbon monoxide tetramers. In addition, carbon monoxide poisoning leads to various neurologic disorders, sometimes occurring several days after exposure. Mechanisms leading to neurologic deficits are not understood, but increased levels of reactive oxygen species, including peroxynitrite, and/or impairment of electron transfer have been suggested. At carboxyhemoglobin blood levels greater than 30–40%, dizziness, headache, and loss of consciousness occur; concentrations of carboxyhemoglobin greater than 50%–60% are usually lethal. There is no direct correlation between levels of carboxyhemoglobin and development of neurologic dysfunction; duration of unconsciousness has better correlation with outcome. The half-life of carboxyhemoglobin in vivo can be reduced by 50 percent by the administration of oxygen. In severe poisoning, the use of hyperbaric oxygen if available will reduce the levels of carboxyhemoglobin even more rapidly.

NITROSOHEMOGLOBIN AND NITROSYL HEME DERIVATIVES

Nitric oxide, another physiologic ligand of hemoglobin, has attracted interest as the production of nitric oxide and its different physiologic functions have been demonstrated in a variety of tissues.[23] Nitric oxide stimulates a cytosolic heme protein, guanylate cyclase, which catalyzes the formation of cGMP, a mediator of many biological reactions, including vascular smooth muscle relaxation, inhibition of platelet aggregation, and macrophage cytotoxicity. The activity of guanylate cyclase is increased 50- to 200-fold by its reaction with nitric oxide and by exchange of nitrosyl heme from nitrosomethemoglobin and nitrosohemoglobin.[23] Myoglobin and hemoglobin react with nitric oxide very rapidly and can prevent guanylate cyclase activation by nitric oxide produced endogenously. Many of the toxic effects of stroma-free hemoglobin[24] have been attributed to vasoconstriction that might result from loss of endothelial-cell-produced nitric oxide by tight binding of nitric oxide to extravascular hemoglobin in the tissues. However, detailed consideration of the possible reactions of nitric oxide suggests that the explanation of toxicity may not lie in simple reactions of nitric oxide with hemoglobin.

It has been shown that in vitro carbon monoxide activates soluble guanylate cyclase by a factor of four, which is much less than the effect of nitric oxide. However, in the presence of some molecules carbon monoxide can be as potent an activator of guanylate cyclase as is nitric oxide.[24] Both carbon monoxide and nitric oxide have also been shown to inhibit endothelial nitric oxide synthase. At present the physiologic significance of these in vitro observations is uncertain.

TABLE 28-2 RATE CONSTANTS FOR ASSOCIATION AND DISSOCIATION OF CARBON MONOXIDE, OXYGEN, AND NITRIC OXIDE WITH HEMOGLOBIN AT 20°C IN 0.1M PHOSPHATE BUFFER, PH 7.0*

LIGAND	$k_{ON}^{-1}(S^{-2})$	$k_{OFF}(S^{-1})$
CO	1.6×10^5	0.009
O_2	1.8×10^7	50.0
NO	2.5×10^7	1.8×10^{-5}

*Constants are for the association and dissociation of first ligand to Hb_4 and from Hb_4L_4, respectively.

Reactions of endogenously produced nitric oxide or molecules capable of releasing nitric oxide, e.g., nitroglycerine, may result in higher levels of methemoglobin, resulting from the reaction

$$HbO_2 + NO \longrightarrow Hb^+ + NO^-_3$$

The reaction is irreversible and as fast as the reaction of nitric oxide with deoxy hemoglobin (Table 28-2). Nitric oxide also reacts with Cysβ93 yielding a nitrosothiol of hemoglobin. Since Cysβ93 is exposed to solvent in the liganded structure, its nitrosation proceeds faster in oxyhemoglobin than in deoxyhemoglobin. It has been proposed that increased binding of nitric oxide to the β93 cysteine in oxyhemoglobin and its release on deoxygenation may contribute to physiologic vasodilation in response to hypoxia.[25]

The rate constants for reactions of hemoglobin with oxygen, carbon monoxide, and nitric oxide are given in Table 28-2. Data for the reaction of chloride, fluoride, azide, thiocyanate, and nitric oxide with ferric hemoglobin are not included in the table. Except for CN^- and F^-, the reactions for these ligands are very heterogeneous, reflecting different reactivities of the α and β chains. Nitric oxide and cyanide anion bind with ferric heme more strongly than do Cl^-, F^-, and SCN^-. In the case of nitric oxide, reaction with ferric heme is followed by fast reduction of ferric heme to ferro heme. Alkyl isocyanides and aromatic nitrosyl derivatives also react with deoxyhemoglobin, but at much slower rates than those of oxygen, carbon monoxide, and nitric oxide.

EMBRYONIC AND FETAL HEMOGLOBINS

The hemoglobin of the nucleated erythrocytes of the yolk sac stage of fetal development contains two embryonic polypeptide chains, the α-like ζ and β-like ε; these subunits decline rapidly after the eighth week of gestation, and by the tenth week, when erythropoiesis has moved to the liver, α and γ chains (of hemoglobin F) account for most of the newly synthesized hemoglobin[26] (Fig. 28-6). Low levels of mRNA of the θ-globin gene (located 5' to the duplicated α loci) are found in fetal and adult reticulocytes, but θ hemoglobin has not been isolated.[27] About the fifth week of gestation, hemoglobin Gower-1, $\zeta_2\varepsilon_2$ and hemoglobin Gower-2, $\alpha_2\varepsilon_2$, constitute 42 percent and 24 percent of the total hemoglobin, respectively, with fetal hemoglobin accounting for the remainder.[1] The oxygen equilibria of the erythrocytes of the early fetus are similar to those of cord blood cells.[28] As noted earlier, the higher oxygen affinity of fetal red cells reflects the smaller effect of bisphosphoglycerate on fetal hemoglobin ($\alpha_2\gamma_2$).

POSTTRANSLATIONAL MODIFICATIONS OF HEMOGLOBIN

The best known posttranslational modification of hemoglobin results from nonenzymatic glycation: a chromatographically separate component of human hemoglobin, hemoglobin A_{1c},[29] amounts to about 3 to

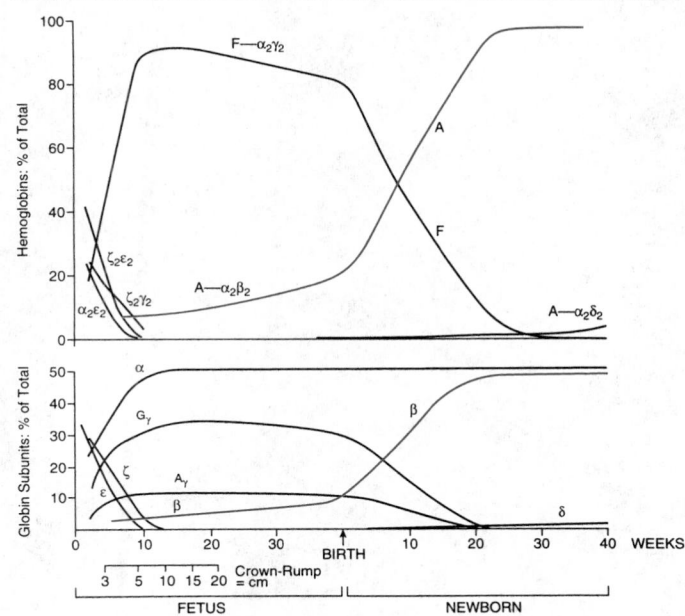

FIGURE 28-6   Changes in hemoglobin tetramers (top panel) and in globin subunits (bottom panel) during human development from embryo to early infancy. Reprinted from *Hemoglobin: Molecular, Genetic and Clinical Aspects*, HF Bunn and BG Forget,[1] p 68 by permission of authors and publisher, WB Saunders Company.

4 percent of normal hemoglobin and is increased in uncontrolled diabetes mellitus.[30–33] Hemoglobin A_{1c} results from the nonenzymatic glycation (by glucose) of the β N-terminal valine residues, in which the initial Schiff base linkage between the βNH_2 and glucose undergoes a rearrangement to form a stable ketoamine linkage.[34] The observed proportions of hemoglobin A_{1c} depend upon the concentration of glucose in the red cell during the weeks or months prior to its measurement and on the life span of the red cell.

Other posttranslational modifications of hemoglobin include acetylation of 10 to 20 percent of the γ chains of hemoglobin F,[35] resulting in a minor component designated hemoglobin F_1, which bears a more negative charge than the main fetal component. In patients with uremia the carbamylation of the N-terminal amino group of both α and β chains of hemoglobin A is attributed to the reaction with cyanate, which is increased in renal failure.[36]

REFERENCES

1. Bunn HF, Forget BG: *Hemoglobin: Molecular, Genetic and Clinical Aspects.* Saunders, Philadelphia, 1986.
2. Perutz MF, Wilkinson AJ, Paoli M, Dodson GG. The stereochemical mechanism of the cooperative effects in hemoglobin revisited. *Annu Rev Biophys Biomol Struct* 27:1, 1998.
3. Perutz MF, Rossman MG, Cullis AF, Muirhead H, Will G, North AGT: Structure of haemoglobin: A three-dimensional Fourier synthesis at 5.5 Å resolution, obtained by x-ray analysis. *Nature* 185:416, 1960.
4. Fermi G, Perutz MF, Shaanan B, Fourme R: The crystal structure of human deoxyhemoglobin at 1.74 Å resolution. *J Mol Biol* 175:159, 1984.
5. Parkhurst LJ: Hemoglobin and myoglobin ligand kinetics. *Annu Rev Phys Chem* 30:503, 1979.
6. Ho C: Proton nuclear magnetic resonance studies on hemoglobin: cooperative interactions and partially ligated species. *Adv Protein Chem.* 43:153, 1992.

7. Schroeder WA, Huisman THJ, Shelton JR, et al: Evidence for multiple structural genes for γ chains of human fetal hemoglobin. *Proc Natl Acad Sci USA* 60:537, 1968.
8. Gelin BR, Lee AW-M, Karplus M: Hemoglobin structural tertiary change on ligand binding: Its role in the cooperative mechanism. *J Mol Biol* 171:489, 1983.
9. Arnone A: X-ray diffraction study of binding of 2,3-diphosphoglycerate to human deoxyhemoglobin. *Nature* 237:146, 1972.
10. Baldwin JM: The structure of human carbonmonoxyhaemoglobin at 2.7 Å resolution. *J Mol Biol* 136:103, 1980.
11. Baldwin J, Chothia C: Haemoglobin: The structural changes related to ligand binding and its allosteric mechanism. *J Mol Biol* 129:175, 1979.
12. Eisenberger P, Shulman RG, Kincaid BM, Brown GS, Ogawa S: Extended x-ray absorption fine structure determination of iron nitrogen distances in haemoglobin. *Nature* 274:30, 1978.
13. Warshel A: Energy-structure correlations in metalloporphyrins and the control of oxygen binding by hemoglobin. *Proc Natl Acad Sci USA* 74:1789, 1977.
14. Hsia CCW: Respiratory function of hemoglobin. *N Engl J Med* 338:239 1998.
15. Comroe JH Jr: *Physiology of Respiration,* p 161. Yearbook, Chicago, 1965.
16. Benesch RE, Benesch R: Mechanisms of interaction of red cell organic phosphates with hemoglobin. *Adv Protein Chem* 28:211, 1974.
17. Adair GS: The hemoglobin system. VI. The oxygen dissociation curve of hemoglobin. *J Biol Chem* 63:529, 1925.
18. Gibson QH: The reaction of oxygen with hemoglobin and the kinetic basis of the effect of salt on binding of oxygen. *J Biol Chem* 245:3285, 1970.
19. MacQuarrie R, Gibson QH: Use of a fluorescent analogue of 2,3-diphosphoglycerate as a probe of human hemoglobin conformation during carbon monoxide binding. *J Biol Chem* 246:5832, 1971.
20. Cassoly R, Gibson QH: Conformation, co-operativity and ligand binding in human hemoglobin. *J Mol Biol* 91:301, 1975.
21. Gibson QH: The photochemical formation of a quickly reacting form of haemoglobin. *Biochem J* 71:293, 1959.
22. Sharma VS, Geibel JF, Ranney HM: "Tension" on heme by the proximal base and ligand reactivity: Conclusions drawn from model compounds for the reaction of hemoglobin. *Proc Natl Acad Sci USA* 75:3747, 1978.
23. Moncada S, Palmer RM, Higgs EA: Nitric oxide: Physiology, pathophysiology and pharmacology. *Pharmacol Rev* 43:109, 1991.
24. Friebe A, Keosling D: Mechanism of YC-1 induced activation of soluble guanyl cyclase. *Mol Pharmacol* 53: 123–127, 1998.
25. Stamler JS, Jia L, Eu JP, et al: Blood flow regulation by S-nitrosohemoglobin in the physiological oxygen gradient. *Science* 276:2034, 1997.
26. Albitar M, Peschle C, Liebhaber SA: Theta, zeta, and epsilon globin messenger RNAs are expressed in adults. *Blood* 74:629, 1989.
27. Hsu S-L, Marks J, Shaw J-P, et al: Structure and expression of the human globin gene. *Nature* 331:94, 1988.
28. Brittain T, Hofmann OM, Watmough NJ, Greenwood C, Weber RE: A two-state analysis of co-operative oxygen binding in the three human embryonic haemoglobins. *Biochem J* 326:299, 1997.
29. Holmquist WR, Schroeder WA: A new N-terminal blocking group involving a Schiff base in hemoglobin A_{1c}. *Biochemistry* 5:2489, 1966.
30. Rahbar S: An abnormal hemoglobin in red cells of diabetics. *Clin Chim Acta* 22:296, 1968.
31. Trivelli LA, Ranney HM, Lai H: Hemoglobin components in patients with diabetes mellitus. *N Engl J Med* 284:353, 1971.
32. Koenig RJ, Peterson CM, Jones RL, Saudek C, Lehrman M, Cerami A: Correlation of glucose regulation and hemoglobin A_{1c} in diabetes mellitus. *N Engl J Med* 295:417, 1976.
33. Bunn HF, Haney DN, Kamin S, Gabbay KH, Gallop PM: The biosynthesis of human hemoglobin A_{1c}: Slow glycosylation of hemoglobin in vivo. *J Clin Invest* 57:1652, 1976.
34. Koenig RJ, Blobstein SH, Cerami A: The structure of carbohydrate of hemoglobin A_{1c}. *J Biol Chem* 252:2992, 1977.
35. Schroeder WA, Cua JT, Matsuda G, Fenninger WD: Hemoglobin F_1, an acetyl-containing hemoglobin. *Biochim Biophys Acta* 63:532, 1962.
36. Fluckinger R, Harmon W, Meier W, et al: Hemoglobin carbamylation in uremia. *N Engl J Med* 304:823, 1981.

PRODUCTION AND DESTRUCTION OF ERYTHROCYTES

ERNEST BEUTLER

The volume of red cells in the body (red cell mass) can be measured by labeling a sample of erythrocytes and estimating their dilution in the circulation. The red cell mass of normal women ranges from 23 to 29 ml/kg body weight; that of normal men from 26 to 32 ml/kg. The red cell mass is maintained by the production of erythrocytes in the marrow and, after they age, their destruction by the macrophages in the spleen, liver, and marrow. Red cell production can be estimated by performing ferrokinetic studies using radioactive ^{59}Fe. The formation of red cells in the marrow is regulated largely by the hormone erythropoietin, which binds and cross-links its receptor which appears on developing erythroid cells. In the absence of erythropoietin these cells undergo apoptosis. Normal human red cells have a finite life span averaging 120 days with very little random destruction. The senescent changes in the red cell that mark it for destruction are not fully understood, but the exposure of phosphatidylserine on the membrane appears to be of major importance. The survival of red cells in the circulation can be measured by labeling with isotopes, particularly ^{51}Cr, and assessing the disappearance of radioactivity from the circulation over time, by determining the disappearance of transfused allogeneic erythrocytes using immunologic markers, and by measuring the excretion of CO, a product of heme catabolism.

THE RED CELL MASS

The red cell mass is maintained and regulated by the marrow, which under steady-state conditions precisely replaces cells lost by senescence, bleeding, or destruction. The red cell mass defines anemias and polycythemias, and the kinetics of red cell production and destruction helps to establish their pathogenesis. A number of tests have been developed to measure the three main components of red cell kinetics: the red cell mass, the rate of red cell production, and the rate of red cell destruction. Some of these are simple but indirect, such as the hematocrit, reticulocyte count, haptoglobin, lactic dehydrogenase and

This chapter is based in part on chapters in previous editions of this text by Drs. Nathaniel Berlin and Allan J. Erslev.

Acronyms and abbreviations that appear in this chapter include: ADP, adenosine diphosphate; AMP-deaminase, adenosine monophosphate-deaminase; BFU-E, burst forming units–erythroid; CFU-E, colony forming units–erythroid; CPM, counts per minute; DFP, diisopropylfluorophosphate; ELISA, enzyme-linked immunosorbent assay; EPO, erythropoietin; EPOR, EPO receptor; HIF-1, hypoxia-inducible factor-1; ICSH, International Committee on Standardization in Hematology; RCM, red cell mass.

unconjugated bilirubin concentration. Examination of the marrow allows one to assess total cellularity and the relative erythroid contribution, but it is limited in that one cannot infer the kinetics of cell production from a single static image. These tests are very useful in the aggregate, but can be supplemented by more complex but direct quantitation made possible by the use of radioisotopes.

HEMATOCRIT

The hematocrit is the fractional volume of the blood that the erythrocytes occupy. It can be measured on a sample of blood, expressed either as a percentage or as a fraction, viz., the volume occupied by the erythrocytes in a ml of blood. The total body hematocrit is the volume of red cells in the body divided by the total blood volume. The blood hematocrit is the simplest and most widely used test by which to estimate the size of the red cell mass. In most anemic patients it gives an excellent approximation of the total red cell mass and a functional estimation of the oxygen-carrying capacity and whole blood viscosity. Its main drawback is that it is an indirect measure that is influenced by changes in the plasma volume and may not reflect the size of the red cell mass in dehydrated or polycythemic patients. Dehydration is usually clinically apparent and can in most cases be taken into account when evaluating the significance of a specific hematocrit determination. When the hematocrit is moderately elevated it may also not reflect the total red cell mass, and only the direct measurement of the red cell mass can differentiate between relative and absolute polycythemia. However, when the hematocrit is above 60 percent, virtually all patients have an increase in total red cell mass.[1] The extent of the increase cannot be estimated accurately from a hematocrit measurement alone (see Fig. 30-2).

RED CELL LABELS

A more direct and accurate estimate of the size of the red cell mass is obtained from labeling a known volume of red cells and determining the dilution of this label in blood. Radioactive iron is an excellent label of red cells since it is biosynthetically incorporated into hemoglobin in vivo. In experimental animals it can be given to a donor animal and the donor's cells can be transfused into the animal whose red cell volume is being assessed. However, the radiation exposure to the donor and the hazards of transfusing allogeneic cells preclude its use in humans. Thus, currently almost all methods used clinically employ labeling of autologous red cells in vitro by any one of a number of isotopes. If studies need to be carried out in radiosensitive individuals such as pregnant women, red cell labeling can be carried out by nonradioactive chromium[2-5] or by biotin, which is then detected with streptavidin coupled to a fluorochrome.[6] Among the isotopes available, ^{51}Cr is the most widely used label, although ^{99m}Tc also is both convenient and accurate.[7] Chromium in the form of the chromate ion (CrO_2^-) readily enters the red cell and binds to globin chains. Excess isotope in the incubation mixture can be removed by washing or by using ascorbic acid to reduce the chromate ion to a nonpermeant chromic ion. About 15 min after injection of a known amount of labeled cells a sample of blood is obtained; its volume, hematocrit, and radioactivity are determined; and the total red cell volume is calculated from the equation:

$$\text{Red cell volume} = \frac{\text{cpm of isotope injected}}{\text{cpm/ml red cells in sample}}$$

Sampling time is generally 15 min. Since ^{51}Cr may also label white cells, if the white cell count is elevated (more than 25×10^9/liter) it is desirable to centrifuge and remove the buffy coat before labeling.

There is no theoretical objection to measuring the red cell mass by using labeled cells. It is independent of the hematocrit of the blood utilized to measure radioactivity, and replicate determination can be made with a coefficient of variation of approximately 1.5 percent.[8] The principal problem lies in reporting the measured red cell mass. The total red cell mass can be expressed as a volume related to body surface (ml/m²) or as a volume related to body weight (ml/kg). A committee of the International Committee on Standardization in Hematology (ICSH)[9] has extensively examined existing data and concluded that the most reproducible expressions of the red cell mass (RCM) are related to body surface area estimated from height and weight:

$$RCM_{males} = (1486 \times S) - 285$$

$$RCM_{females} = (822 \times S) + (1.06 \times age)$$

where RCM is the red cell mass, S the body surface area in square meters, and age the age in years.

These calculated values ± 25 percent included 98 percent of the measured male and 99 percent of the measured female values.[9]

Despite the ICSH recommendation, the most common method is to report red cell mass values in terms of milliliters per kilogram. This method of expression will, however, give erroneously low values in obese individuals because fat is hypovascular. A better method might be to express the red cell mass in terms of lean weight. In general lean weight is 20 percent less than actual weight in normal males and 25 percent less in normal females.[7] However, estimation of lean weight in obese individuals is most inaccurate, and from a practical point of view it is probably best to report the red cell mass in terms of actual weight and make mental adjustments based on body configuration. In general, the red cell mass of normal females ranges from 23 to 29 ml/kg body weight. In normal males it is 26 to 32 ml/kg.[9]

PLASMA LABELS

The red cell mass can also be estimated from the plasma volume. Radioactive iodine (^{125}I) is utilized to label albumin and measure its distribution volume.[10] Other radioactive isotopes of iodine as well as of ^{99m}Tc have been used, but ^{125}I has virtually supplanted all other plasma labels. Albumin labeled with radioactive iodine is commercially available, and a known amount is injected intravenously. Several blood samples are obtained within the first 15 min, centrifuged and the CPM per ml of plasma measured, plotted on semilogarithmic paper, and extrapolated to zero time. This is necessary, since in contradistinction to labeled red cells, labeled albumin is removed gradually, beginning immediately after injection. The plasma volume is calculated according to the equation:

$$Plasma\ volume = \frac{cpm\ of\ labeled\ albumin\ injected}{cpm/ml\ plasma\ at\ 0\ h}$$

The continuous exchange of intravascular with extravascular albumin is the major problem encountered when the plasma volume is measured with labeled albumin. Even with extrapolation to zero hour the plasma volume is somewhat larger than that measured with a strictly intravascular protein such as fibrinogen.[11] Consequently, if the measurement of the plasma volume is used to calculate the size of the total red cell mass, it is a less reliable measure than determining the red cell mass directly with tagged red cells. This inaccuracy is further aggravated by the fact that the venous hematocrit used to calculate the red cell mass from the measured plasma volume does not reflect accurately the distribution of plasma and red cells in the body (see below). However, from a practical point of view, the results of estimating red cell mass from plasma volume are surprisingly accurate and have been advocated on the basis of simplicity and low cost.[10,12]

TOTAL-BODY HEMATOCRIT

When the total red cell mass is measured with labeled red cells it has been found that it is about 10 percent lower than that calculated from the plasma volume and the hematocrit of the peripheral blood. In fact, it is apparent that the mean hematocrit of blood in all of the vessels (total-body hematocrit) is somewhat lower than the hematocrit determined from blood obtained from large vessels.

Generally the ratio of total-body hematocrit as estimated by direct measurements of red cell volume and plasma volume to the large-vessel hematocrit ranges from 0.89 to 0.92.[13] Consequently, when using the determined plasma volume to calculate red cell mass and total blood volume it is necessary to use a correction factor, and one of 0.90 is generally employed:

$$Corrected\ red\ cell\ mass = \frac{Hct \times plasma\ volume \times 0.90}{100 - Hct}$$

Recommended procedures for the determination and evaluation of blood volume are outlined by the International Committee for Standardization in Hematology.[14]

RED CELL PRODUCTION

Under normal circumstances most human red cells produced in the marrow live, or have the potential to live, a normal life span. Under certain conditions, however, a fraction of red cell production is ineffective, with destruction of nonviable red cells either within the marrow or shortly after the cells reach the blood.[15]

EFFECTIVE RED CELL PRODUCTION

Effective erythropoiesis is most simply estimated by determining the reticulocyte count. This count is usually expressed as the percentage of red cells that are reticulocytes, but it can also be expressed as the total number of circulating reticulocytes per unit of blood (absolute reticulocytes = reticulocyte percentage × red blood count). In order to use the reticulocyte percentage as a measure of the rate of red cell production the percentage may be corrected for the hematocrit, deriving what is designated the reticulocyte index[16]:

$$Reticulocyte\ index = reticulocyte\ \% \times \frac{actual\ Hct}{normal\ Hct}$$

Since the red cell count is readily available in any electronic blood count printout it seems more logical to use the absolute reticulocyte count as the measure. The usefulness of the absolute reticulocyte count can be enhanced by taking into account the estimated life span of the reticulocytes. The life span of the reticulocytes in blood is about one day, but when red cell production is increased under conditions of erythropoietic stress, as for example with anemia, reticulocytes are released prematurely and circulate as reticulocytes for two to four days. Accordingly, an elevated reticulocyte count may give an erroneous impression of the actual rate of red cell production. In order to take this into account when estimating the rate of red cell production in anemic patients with high reticulocyte counts, it has been suggested that dividing the absolute reticulocyte count by two gives a more accurate estimate of red cell production.[16]

INEFFECTIVE RED CELL PRODUCTION

Ineffective erythropoiesis is suspected when the reticulocyte count is normal or only slightly increased despite erythroid hyperplasia of the marrow. It was first recognized as an entity from the study of incorporation of isotopes into fecal urobilin following the administration of labeled glycine, a precursor of heme.[17] Two peaks were observed: an early one at 3 to 5 days and a late one at 100 to 120 days. It was suggested that one of the sources of the early-labeled peak was the hemoglobin of red cells that had never completed their development, having been destroyed either in the marrow or shortly after reaching the blood. Subsequent studies have revealed that in certain disorders, such as pernicious anemia, thalassemia, and sideroblastic anemia, ineffective erythropoiesis is a major component of total erythropoiesis. This component can be quantitated by measuring ^{15}N-labeled glycine incorporation into the early bilirubin peaks,[18,19] bilirubin turnover,[20] or ferrokinetics.[15] Calculated from bilirubin peaks and turnover, ineffective erythropoiesis under normal conditions amounts to about 4 to 12 percent of total erythropoiesis. Using ferrokinetic methods, ineffective erythropoiesis is calculated as the difference between total plasma iron turnover and erythrocyte iron turnover plus storage iron turnover (see below). The values estimated from such studies in normal subjects are somewhat higher, ranging from 14 to 34 percent.[15] However, these results, both the high and the low, probably are misleading, since none of the methods actually measure cell death but only the turnover of heme and iron. It is possible that there is little premature death of cells in normal subjects but that much of the early release of bilirubin and iron is derived from the rim of hemoglobin extruded during enucleation of erythroblasts (see Chap. 22).

TOTAL ERYTHROPOIESIS

Total erythropoiesis, the sum of effective and ineffective red cell production, can be estimated from a marrow examination. Films or sections from marrow aspirates are first examined for relative content of fat and hematopoietic tissue. This gives an estimate of overall hematopoietic activity within the marrow space. Then a differential count is performed with determination of the ratio between granulocytic and erythroid precursors (the M/E ratio). In a normal adult, the ratio is about 3:1 to 5:1, and it can be used to estimate whether erythropoiesis is normal, increased, or decreased (see Chap. 3). It is only an approximation of total erythroid activity, since the ratio can be altered by changing the myeloid as well as the erythroid components and an aspirate or biopsy of a small segment of the marrow may not always reflect total marrow activity. However, when used in conjunction with determination of red blood cell count and reticulocyte count, it will under most circumstances provide qualitative information about the rate and effectiveness of the production of red blood cells. A more accurate quantitation of total erythropoiesis can be made by measuring the rate of production of red cells (ferrokinetics) or, in steady-state conditions, by measuring the rate of destruction of red cells (red cell life span, bilirubin production, or carbon monoxide excretion).

FERROKINETICS

In 1950, Huff and his associates first described a method for the measurement of the rate of production of red cells utilizing a simple model of iron metabolism[21] (Fig. 29-1). In this method radioactive iron is complexed to transferrin in vitro and injected intravenously. Alternatively, ^{59}Fe can be injected directly intravenously as the gluconate without preincubation with the patient's own plasma, if enough unbound transferrin is available, since binding will be almost instantaneous. The rate of clearance of the transferrin-bound iron from the

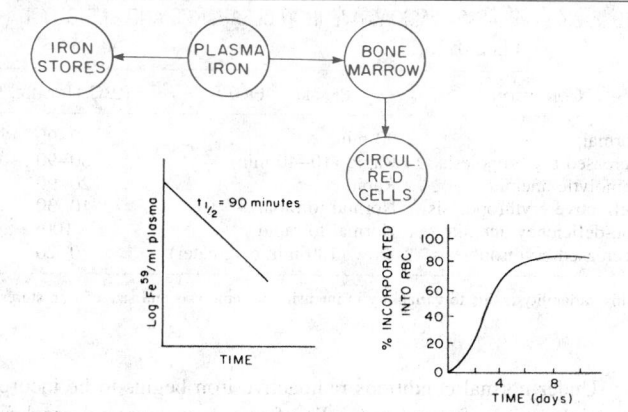

FIGURE 29-1   The single dynamic pool model of iron metabolism. Radioactive iron injected into the plasma iron pool is cleared from the plasma as a single exponential and approximately 80 percent is incorporated into circulating blood cells.

plasma (^{59}Fe plasma $T_{1/2}$) and the subsequent uptake in the red cells are measured. From these two values and from determinations of the plasma iron concentration and the plasma volume, the rate of formation of red cells can be calculated.[15]

The initial clearance of iron is exponential, and sampling during this period can be used to calculate the $T_{1/2}$. In normal individuals this averages about 90 min; it is shorter in patients with hyperplasia of the erythropoietic tissue, and longer in patients with marrow hypoplasia (Fig. 29-2). The clearance rate, however, is not a direct measurement of erythropoietic activity because it is dependent on the size of the pool of unlabeled, circulating iron. Consequently calculation of the plasma iron turnover rate must include the plasma iron concentration. The clearance is expressed in milligrams of iron and the point of reference can be hemoglobin mass, blood volume, or weight, but a commonly used expression is as μg iron per deciliters of whole blood per day.

$$\text{Plasma iron turnover rate (mg iron/dl blood/24 h)} =$$
$$\frac{\text{plasma iron (mg/dl)} \times (100 - \text{Hct})}{T_{1/2} \text{ (min)} \times 100}$$

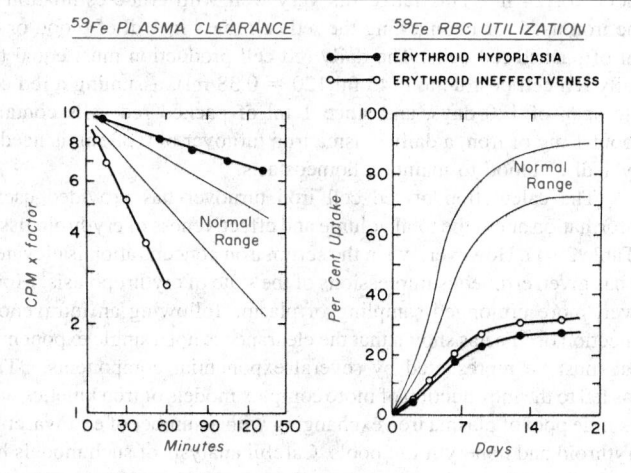

FIGURE 29-2   Iron clearance and iron utilization in normal subjects, patients with decreased effective red cell production (erythroid hypoplasia), and patients with ineffective red cell production.

TABLE 29-1   PLASMA RADIOACTIVE IRON CLEARANCE AND RED BLOOD
CELL UPTAKE

Condition	Plasma ^{59}Fe $T_{1/2}$	RBC Uptake, %
Normal	90 min	80–90
Increased erythropoiesis	Rapid (10–40 min)	80–90
Hemolytic anemia	Rapid	20–90*
Ineffective erythropoiesis	Normal to rapid	10–30
Iron-deficiency anemia	Normal to rapid	100
Decreased erythropoiesis	Slow (180 min or greater)	0–20

*This variability is due to variability in intensity of hemolysis and size of iron stores.

Under normal conditions radioactive iron begins to be incorporated into newly formed red cells after a few days and reaches a maximum at about 10 to 14 days after injection (see Fig. 29-2). The normal utilization is 70 to 90 percent on the tenth to the fourteenth day, a value that is so high that a further increase has little significance. Decreased utilization, however, is an important finding and suggests that immature red cells are destroyed in the marrow before they are released to the circulation (ineffective erythropoiesis) or that serum iron is diverted to nonerythropoietic tissues (marrow hypoplasia) because of slow marrow uptake. The shape of the red cell utilization curve is also important, since an early and steep rise (rapid marrow transit time) suggests the presence of a high erythropoietin (EPO) level. Finally, an early rise in utilization with a subsequent fall off suggests hemolysis.

In the calculation of the utilization it is necessary to know the blood volume:

$$\text{Red cell iron utilization (\%)} = \frac{\text{cpm of 1 ml blood} \times \text{blood volume} \times 100}{\text{cpm of } ^{59}\text{Fe injected}}$$

Using the plasma iron clearance and utilization of iron, the red cell turnover in milligram per deciliter blood for 24 h is calculated as follows:

$$\text{Red cell iron turnover (mg iron/dl blood/24 h)} =$$
$$\text{plasma iron turnover} \times \text{maximal red cell iron utilization}$$

The normal value of red cell iron turnover is 0.30 to 0.70 mg/dl blood for 24 h.[15] This range fits very well with crude estimation of the iron used for maintaining the red cell mass in 1 dl of blood or 45 ml of packed red cells. The daily red cell production must equal the daily red cell destruction (45 ml/120 = 0.38 ml), assuming a red cell life span of 120 days, and since 1 ml of packed red cells contains about 1 mg of iron, a daily plasma iron turnover of 0.38 mg is needed by 1 dl of blood to maintain homeostasis.

The calculation of red cell iron turnover has provided useful information about the total volume and effectiveness of erythroid tissue (Table 29-1). However, when the serum iron concentration is elevated, it has given erroneous impressions of the state of erythropoiesis. Moreover, more prolonged sampling of plasma following an intravenous injection of ^{59}Fe has shown that the clearance is not a single exponential but must be represented by several exponential components.[22] This has led to the introduction of more complex models of iron kinetics with a single pool of plasma iron exchanging with a number of extravascular erythroid and nonerythroid pools. Careful analysis of such models has generated computer-supported methods calculating the degree and effectiveness of erythroid activity.[23] Although possibly more accurate than the conventional method of calculating iron turnover, they appear to be too cumbersome for clinical use. Moreover, even these sophisticated methods may not give an accurate account of the state of erythropoiesis. It was found that despite a constant rate of red cell production, the plasma iron turnover increases with increasing plasma iron and transferrin saturation. This was first thought to be due to increased nonerythroid iron uptake and led to the introduction of various correction factors in the calculation of red cell iron turnover.[22] However, the iron in plasma is present in two pools, a diferric and a monoferric transferrin pool, and the erythroid and nonerythroid receptors have a four times greater avidity for diferric transferrin than for monoferric transferrin. Consequently, the total plasma iron turnover depends on the degree of saturation and does not necessarily reflect the number of transferrin receptors, presumably a critical measure of erythropoietic capacity.[24] In order to measure the number of these receptors, it has been proposed to adjust the plasma iron turnover equations for both nonerythroid uptake and degree of transferrin saturation and express the plasma turnover in terms of transferrin rather than iron.[25] The normal erythroid uptake of transferrin is 60 ± 12 micromoles per liter of blood per day, a value that has been found to be appropriately decreased and increased in patients with hypoplastic and hyperplastic marrow.

TRANSFERRIN RECEPTORS

Under normal conditions diferric, and to a lesser extent monoferric, transferrin is bound to transferrin receptors and internalized. After having released its iron the transferrin-transferrin receptor complex is returned to the cell surface where the receptor is reanchored. However, some of the extracellular domain of the receptors with or without bound transferrin is released into the circulating blood, and its concentration in plasma is roughly proportional to cell-bound transferrin receptors and in turn to the total amount of erythropoietic tissue.[26] Using monoclonal or polyclonal antibodies to the transferrin receptor in an ELISA technique, the normal concentration of circulating receptors is about 6-8 mg/L. It is appropriately increased in patients with hemolytic anemia and decreased in patients with hypoplastic anemia.[26,27] The advantage in using measurements of transferrin receptors in determining erythroid activity is primarily the ease with which circulating receptor concentration can be measured. Serial measurements can be carried out without the need for steady-state conditions and without the need for laborious ferrokinetic studies. The disadvantages are that it only indirectly measures or estimates the total number of cell-bound receptors, that many nonerythroid cells contribute to the number of circulating receptors,[28] and that a reduction in the intracellular concentration of iron upregulates the synthesis of transferrin receptors.[29] This latter feature is actually used to distinguish iron deficiency anemia with high receptor concentrations from the anemia of chronic disease with increased tissue iron and low receptor concentrations[29,30] (see Chaps. 38 and 41). As is true for all erythrokinetic studies, the measurement of transferrin receptors is of value in determining if the erythroid activity of a bone marrow aspirate or biopsy reflects total bone marrow activity or merely the activity of a small "hot pocket."[31] This question, however, can also be answered by a noninvasive magnetic resonance imaging of the whole skeleton.[32]

PHYLOGENY OF RED CELL PRODUCTION

Hemoglobin has been demonstrated in the most primitive animal forms, such as *Paramecium* and *Tetrahymena*, but the development of a cell especially designed to synthesize, carry, and protect respiratory pigments had to await the development of a circulatory system.[33] Until then, some crustaceans, such as the *Daphnia*, were capable of developing a fairly sophisticated oxygen transport system without circulating red cells.[34] The specific advantage derived from packaging hemoglobin in red cells is not related to viscosity, since the viscosity of blood is the same whether hemoglobin molecules are dissolved in plasma or concentrated in red cells.[35] It appears more likely that the emergence of red cells is related to the protective and regulatory effect of intracellular compounds on hemoglobin and its oxygen affinity.

Circulating nucleated erythrocytes first appear in the worms of the phylum Nemertina and in the sessile marine creatures of the phylum Phoronida. Erythropoiesis in these primitive invertebrates takes place near or on the peritoneal surface, with endothelial cells acting as stem cells.[33] In the phylum Annelida, which is considerably further up on the evolutionary scale, nonnucleated red cells are observed for the first time. However, the evolutionary advantage derived from denucleation appears to be slight, and nucleated red cells are observed in much further advanced animals, such as reptiles and birds.[36] All mammalian erythrocytes are nonnucleated, even those in the most primitive forms such as the Australian duckbilled platypus.[37]

In the premammalian species, the spleen is the fundamental erythropoietic organ. In some fish, the kidneys are also involved in red cell production,[38,39] but it is questionable if this is related to the development of a renal erythropoietic hormone. In the vertebrates, there is an evolutionary shift from the spleen to the liver and from the liver to the hollow bones. It appears that any organ with a relatively stagnant sinusoidal vascular system may serve as a site for red cell production and that the sinusoidal structure of the bone cavities in mammals renders these areas particularly well suited.[40] The homeostatic regulation of blood or hemoglobin production has been studied in *Daphnia*.[34] In these crustaceans, there is a balance between oxygen need and hemoglobin production. In the higher animals, this relationship is maintained by adjusting red cell production. Studies of birds,[41] fish,[42] and mammals[43] indicate that red cell production is controlled by a humoral substance, erythropoietin, which is capable of adjusting red cell production to the demands for oxygen in the tissues. Studies of EPO isolated from a number of mammals indicate some biochemical variability, but still a considerable biologic similarity and genetic homology.[44]

ONTOGENY OF RED CELL PRODUCTION

A number of tissues in the mammalian species can support red cell production, but the environment inside the bone apparently is optimal for cellular proliferation and maturation. However, bone cavities do not develop until the fifth fetal month, and other, presumably less favorable, sites are responsible for red cell production during early embryonic life. In the human, blood cells are first formed outside the embryo in the numerous blood islands of the yolk sac.[45] The cells formed here are very large and remain nucleated throughout their functional life span. During the second gestational month, they are slowly replaced by smaller, but still macrocytic, nonnucleated cells derived from hepatic erythropoiesis.[46] The ontogeny of the hemoglobins is discussed in Chaps. 7, 28, and 46.

During the next fetal months, the liver is the main red cell–producing organ. Splenic red cell production is presumed to be of importance between the third and the seventh fetal months. However, the spleen may sequester nucleated red cells formed elsewhere, and the presence of early erythroid cells in this organ does not conclusively indicate splenic erythropoiesis.[47]

At about the fifth fetal month, granulopoietic cells can be recognized in the central cartilaginous region of the bones, but the bone cavities only slowly become capable of supporting erythropoiesis. At the time of birth, the hepatic phase of blood cell production is finished, and all bone cavities are actively engaged in erythropoiesis. During the neonatal period, the volume of available marrow space is almost the same as the total volume of hematopoietic cells.[48] This precarious

balance continues for a few years until the growth of bones and bone cavities outstrips the growth of the hematopoietic mass. During the early years, the lack of reserve space forces reactivation of extramedullary foci in the liver and spleen whenever the hematopoietic system is challenged by blood loss, hypoxia, or hemolysis.[49]

During adult life, the expansion of marrow space continues, possibly by bone resorption, and there is a gradual increase in the amount of fatty tissue in all bone cavities. Because of the abundant marrow space, compensatory reactivation of extramedullary sites rarely takes place in later life, even during periods of prolonged and intense demand for additional blood cell formation. Extramedullary hematopoiesis during these years usually indicates inappropriate rather than compensatory blood formation.[50]

During late fetal life, the physiologic control of red cell production is probably tied to tissue hypoxia and release of EPO.[51] The fetus is under continuous hypoxic stimulation (''Everest in utero''), and EPO has been demonstrated in the amniotic fluid of mothers with erythroblastotic babies. EPO can apparently not pass the placental barrier in sheep and higher animals, and infants born of mothers with various hematologic disorders varying from severe anemia to secondary polycythemia are usually born with the same degree of normal postpartum erythrocytosis. Since bilateral nephrectomy of fetal sheep fails to alter the rate of EPO production, while hepatectomy does, it appears that during fetal life this production is primarily extrarenal and hepatic.[52] At the time of birth, there is a gradual,[53] presumably intrinsically determined[54] switch to renal production of EPO, and in the adult the kidney is responsible for 90 to 95 percent of total production.

KINETICS OF RED CELL PRODUCTION

STEM CELL AND PROGENITOR CELL POOLS

Mammalian nucleated red cells are characterized biochemically and morphologically by their continuous synthesis and accumulation of hemoglobin molecules. Because of relentless maturation, nucleated red cells must be derived from a stable compartment of cells capable of both differentiation and self-renewal. The existence of such cells, designated as stem cells, is discussed in Chap. 14.

Due to their capacity to grow luxuriously in culture, producing large bursts of hemoglobinized erythroblasts, the early progenitor cells committed to the erythroid cell line are designated as burst forming units–erythroid (BFU-E).[55] In common with other early progenitors the BFU-Es express certain surface antigens such as CD-34 and receptors for a number of growth factors and cytokines.[56] They also express a few receptors for EPO, but the mechanism of the activation of the EPO receptor (EPOR) gene that determines their commitment to the erythroid lineage is unknown.

The subsequent proliferation and maturation of the BFU-E terminate in the creation of CFU-E. This final erythroid progenitor cell receives its designation from its capacity to form a small erythroid colony consisting of 16 to 64 hemoglobinized erythroblasts.[57] It now expresses a great number of EPORs, and it appears that its survival depends on the activation of these receptors by EPO.[58]

The in vivo composition of the progenitor cell pool is quite different from that observed in an in vitro culture. When cultured in a semi-solid medium in the presence of an optimal concentration of growth factors and EPO, each BFU-E will cause the formation of about 1000 CFU-Es before each of these latter cells differentiate into small erythroid colonies. In vivo, on the other hand, the number of CFU-Es is only three to five times greater than the number of BFU-Es.[59] This suggests that stromal and accessory cells in the marrow microenvironment have a profound effect on the fertility and survival of progenitor cells. These effects of the microenvironment modulate the action of EPO and determine the number of CFU-Es available for

TABLE 29-2 ERYTHROID POOLS

| | CELL NUMBER × 10⁸ PER KG/BODY WEIGHT | |
CELL TYPE	OBSERVED*	THEORETIC MODEL (FIG. 29-1)
Proerythroblasts	1	1
Erythroblasts	49	58
Marrow reticulocytes	82	64
Blood reticulocytes	31	32
Matured red cells	3300	3800

*Adapted from Donohue et al.[60] and Finch et al.[61]

subsequent differentiation to proerythroblasts. At the level of the CFU-E, the density of EPORs is maximal and their activation becomes crucial for survival and subsequent transformation into proerythroblasts. Cross-linking of the receptor by EPO is responsible for the survival of the cell and permits it to proceed with its preordained program of proliferation and maturation into red blood cells.

PRECURSOR CELLS

The creation of a normal red cell is the end result of an orderly transformation of a proerythroblast with a large nucleus and a volume of about 900 fl to a hemoglobinized anucleated disc with a volume of about 90 fl. Although the cytoplasmic maturation is continuous, the interposed mitotic divisions cause a stepwise reduction in cytoplasmic and nuclear volume, making it quite easy morphologically to recognize proerythroblasts, basophilic erythroblasts, polychromatophilic erythroblasts, orthochromatic erythroblasts, and reticulocytes.

Direct measurements of the number of marrow erythroblasts and reticulocytes have shown that for each proerythroblast there are about 50 erythroblasts and 113 reticulocytes (Table 29-2).[60,61] This distribution would conform to the number of cells in a theoretic erythroid pyramid (Table 29-2, Fig. 29-3) in which each proerythroblast undergoes five mitotic divisions over a period of five days before it loses its nucleus and enters a three-day period of reticulocyte maturation. Undoubtedly there are some variations in the size and shape of these erythroid pyramids, but the question is if such varieties are random or play a role in the physiologic control of red cell production. When the production is suppressed, as in anemia of chronic renal disease, the erythroblastic distribution appears normal, with no morphologic or ferrokinetic evidence for the presence of ineffective erythroblasts or premature erythroblastic destruction.[15] When production is increased, as in severe anemias, the erythroblastic pyramids also appear normal, with no evidence for additional mitotic divisions. Consequently it seems likely that the rate of red cell production depends on the number of erythroid pyramids formed, not on their shape.

As the erythroblast matures, its synthetic activities increase rapidly and become targeted to the production of all of the proteins characteristic of mature red blood cells, particularly globin. Eventually 95 percent of all protein in the red cell is hemoglobin, almost all hemoglobin A ($\alpha_2\beta_2$), with only small amounts of hemoglobin F ($\alpha_2\gamma_2$) and hemoglobin A_2 ($\alpha_2\delta_2$). Hemoglobin F is unequally distributed, with certain cells, designated as F cells, containing up to 25 percent of their total hemoglobin as F hemoglobin. There is a sharp decline in the density of EPORs on early erythroblasts, and they are absent on the more mature forms. On the other hand, the number of receptors for transferrin increases sharply, reflecting the increased demands for iron in heme synthesis.

The microenvironment may be of importance for the proliferation and maturation of erythroblasts. However, in situ secreted growth factors and cytokines appear to be of less importance for precursor cells than for progenitor cells. Intercellular adhesion molecules are of course needed to secure the structural integrity of the marrow, and

fibronectin is of special importance for erythroblasts.[62] The loss of fibronectin receptors heralds the migration of reticulocytes into blood, but some reticulocytes remain sticky even after release and are temporarily sequestered by the spleen. Since erythroid colonies developed in vitro consist almost entirely of nucleated red cells, enucleation may primarily be induced by stromal or endothelial cells.

REGULATION OF RED CELL PRODUCTION

FEEDBACK CONTROLS

Under physiologic conditions, the circulating red cell mass is maintained at an optimal size by appropriate adjustments in the rate of red cell production. Red cell destruction and red cell loss may influence the size of the red cell mass, but these are not physiologic variables, and the spleen of humans,[63] unlike that of dogs and race horses,[64] does not serve as a reservoir of red cells. The feedback signals that adjust the rate of production of red cells to the need for red cells could be generated from tissues serviced by red cells (functional feedback) or from the red cells themselves (end-product feedback).

FUNCTIONAL FEEDBACK—ERYTHROPOIETIN

History   The red cell mass is a large organ designed largely for the purpose of transporting oxygen to the tissues. Thus the size of the red cell mass and the rate of red cell production must be closely related to supply and demand for oxygen in the tissues. Toward the end of the 19th century French mountaineers and physiologists had established that a low tissue tension of oxygen would stimulate the rate of red cell production.[65] However, the mode of stimulation was hotly debated. In 1906 the French Sorbonne professor, Dr. Paul Carnot, and his associate, Mademoiselle DeFlandre, suggested that hypoxia generates a humoral factor capable of stimulating red cell production.[66] On the other hand the famous biochemist, Friederich Miescher, proposed that marrow hypoxia directly stimulates red cell production.[67] Both hypotheses, unfortunately, were based on very questionable experimental data and subsequent attempts to clarify the picture brought more heat than light. Finally, in 1950, Kurt Reissmann in an ingenious study on parabiotic rats provided strong support for the existence of an indirect humoral mechanism.[68] A few years later Erslev demonstrated convincingly that the plasma from anemic rabbits and primates contains a red cell–stimulating factor.[69,70] It was appropriately named EPO, and it became generally accepted that it was involved in the regulation of red cell production. In 1957 Jacobson and coworkers[71] found that it was produced by the kidney, a finding that raised the tempting possibility that if it only could be isolated in adequate amounts it might be of therapeutic benefit to patients with renal anemia.

Structure   Purification of EPO provided some partial sequences that led to cloning of the gene and permitted mass production of the recombinant protein.[72] The EPO gene contains five exons, four introns, and functionally important 5′ and 3′ untranslated sequences.[73,74] There is 80 to 90 percent homology between the human gene and genes for mouse and monkey EPO. The cDNA codes for a chain of 193 amino acids including a 27–amino acid leader peptide. One amino acid apparently is lost during processing, leaving the mature circulating EPO with 165 amino acids. EPO and its recombinant form are heavily glycosylated α-globulins with a molecular mass of 34,000 daltons and a specific activity of about 200,000 IU/mg.[73,74] Sixty percent of the molecular weight is contributed by amino acids, while 40 percent is made up of carbohydrate. Although the recombinant form is synthesized by hamster cells, the carbohydrate structure is probably almost the same as in the natural human hormone, and so far no instances of antibody production have been observed in patients receiving recombinant EPO.

The amino acids form a single chain with two internal disulfide bonds that have been shown to be necessary for biologic activity. A

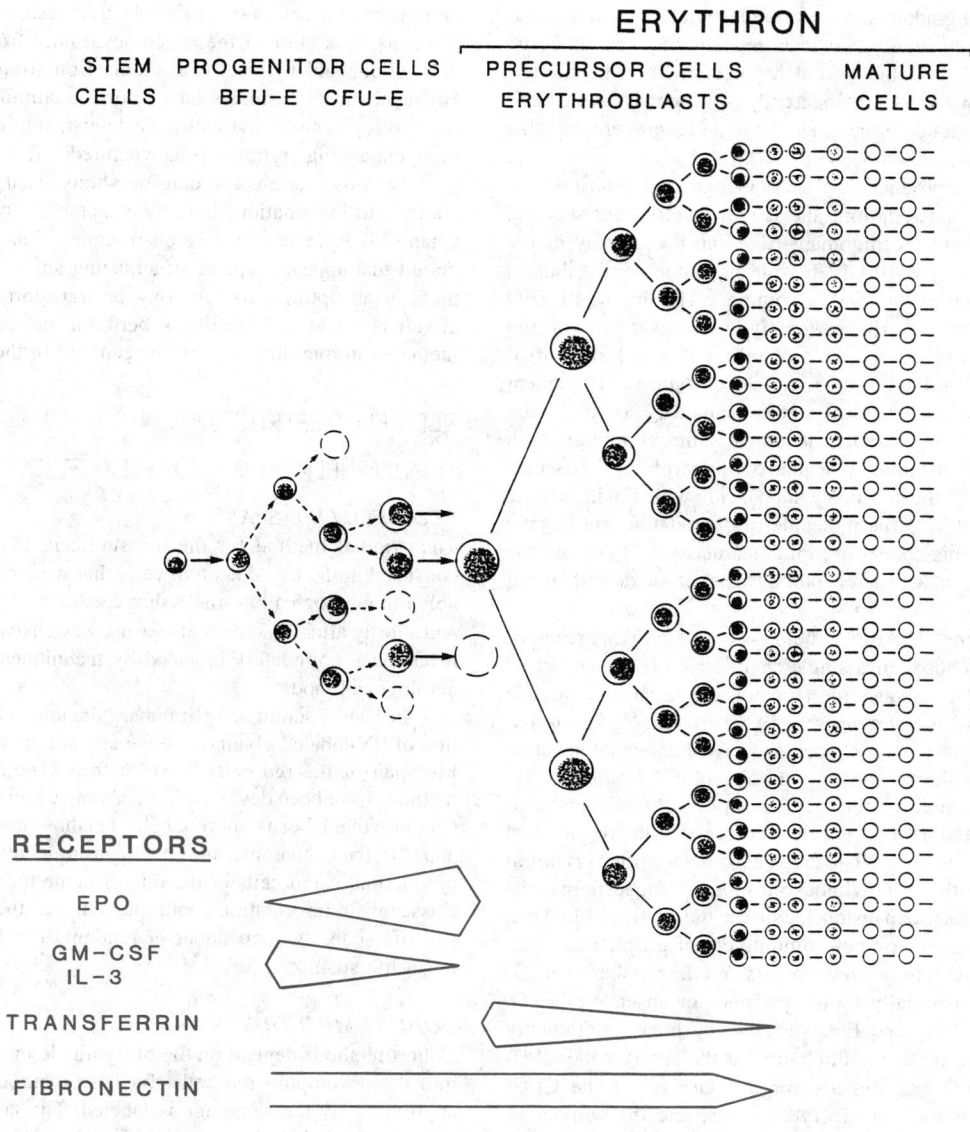

FIGURE 29-3   A theoretical model of the proliferation of the erythroid committed marrow cells, including their most important receptors.

biologically active 20–amino acid peptide has been found to be required for the cross-linking (dimerization) of the EPOR, which activates it.[75] Dimerization of the receptor with biologic activity can also be accomplished by a totally unrelated synthetic 20–amino acid cyclic peptide. Thus, the biologic effect of EPO can be mimicked by totally unrelated synthetic compounds that dimerize the receptor.[76,77] There is extensive homology among EPO from various species but also enough differences so that it is possible to raise antibodies against human EPO in rodents, antibodies vital for the performance of radioimmune assays. EPO has four linkages to carbohydrates, three to asparagine and one to serine.[73,74] The importance of the carbohydrate moiety appears to lie in its action on cellular processing and secretion. Furthermore, its terminal sialic acids prevent EPO from being incorporated and catabolized by hepatocytes in vivo. In vitro, however, sialated and desialated EPO have the same biologic activity.

Regulation   The classic study by Jacobson and coworkers in 1957 suggested strongly that the kidney was the organ of production.[71] Using molecular probes for EPO mRNA it became possible to pinpoint the synthesis to cortical interstitial cells[78,79] of endothelial or fibroblastic lineage.[80] The cells appear to function in an all-or-none fashion, with the overall production of mRNA dependent on the number of cells activated.[81]

Hypoxia is the obvious initiating cause of EPO gene activation in these cells and such activation depends on the presence of an enhancer sequence, "the hypoxic-responsive element," positioned in the 3′ tail of the gene,[82] which responds to the hypoxia-inducible factor-1 (HIF-1). HIF-1 is a heterodimer composed of α and β subunits. Its activity is primarily determined by hypoxia-induced stabilization of HIF-1α, which is otherwise rapidly degraded in oxygenated cells.[83]

Certain 5′ sequences located 6000 to 12,000 bp upstream also affect gene transcription. These sequences are not hypoxia-sensitive but appear necessary for tissue and cellular specificity.[84] Hepatic production is contributed primarily by hepatocytes but is much less than the renal production.[85] In rodents it may contribute 10 to 15 percent of total EPO circulating in plasma, but probably even less in humans. During fetal life, however, hepatic EPO production is of major importance for red cell production, and anephric fetal sheep and anephric neonatal rats produce normal amounts of EPO and red cells.[52] At the time of birth there is a gradual and irreversible switch from hepatic to renal production.[53] Interestingly, however, regenerating hepatic tissue such as that found in rats after partial hepatectomy[86] or in humans after injury caused by hepatitis apparently synthesizes more EPO than normal adult hepatic tissue.[87] Hematopoietic progenitors also produce erythropoietin.[88]

Metabolism   The production of EPO is regulated almost exclusively at the level of transcription, and it is not stored but secreted immediately.[89] Circulating recombinant EPO and presumably native EPO as well have a $T_{1/2}$ of 4 to 12 h with a volume of distribution slightly larger than that of the plasma volume.[90] The linking of EPO molecules into dimers and trimers greatly increases their $T_{1/2}$ and augments their biologic activity by >26-fold.[91] A small amount of EPO is excreted in the urine but this only can account for 10 percent of total body EPO turnover.[91] EPO may be consumed by erythropoietic tissue,[92] but the half-life of EPO is about the same in animals with marrow hypoplasia as in those with marrow hyperplasia.[93] It seems likely that removal of the terminal sialic acid, which will expose galactose residues, subjects the molecule to degradation via hepatic galactose receptors. This results in rapid clearance of EPO from the circulation via hepatic galactose receptors. However, no definite proof for this hypothesis exists.

Method of Action   The EPOR belongs to the cytokine receptor superfamily. It is composed of a single chain which is dimerized by EPO, an alteration that activates the receptor and initiates a cascade of signaling that includes activation of the JAK2 protein.[75,94] An alternatively spliced form of the receptor appears to have a dominant negative effect, i.e., it inhibits the response of the receptor.[95] Erythropoietin acts both as a mitogen and as a survival factor preventing apoptosis or premature cell death and permitting cells to proceed with programmed proliferation and maturation.[58,96] The fact that some primitive erythroid cells are produced in the EPOR knockout mouse[97] suggests that the role of EPO is that of an expansion factor for the erythroid lineage, not that of a factor that determines commitment of precursors.

The BFU-Es contain only a few EPORs and the number of BFU-Es is not influenced materially by the presence or absence of EPO. However, receptor density and EPO dependency increase gradually as the progenitor cells mature, culminating at the level of the CFU-E.[98] At that level EPO is necessary for the survival of the CFU-Es and their transformation to proerythroblasts, and the number of transformed cells determines to a great extent the number of red cells produced. The proerythroblasts also contain EPORs, which in the presence of high levels of EPO, may accelerate their entry into the first mitotic division. This may lead to a shortened marrow transit time of erythroblasts[15] and result in the release of still unfinished reticulocytes, so-called stress reticulocytes.[99] However, after having reached the stage of hemoglobin synthesis it seems unlikely that EPO will change the overall composition of each erythroblastic pyramid since, as stated before, the ratio between early and late erythroblasts is approximately the same in patients with renal disease (low EPO production) or nonrenal anemia (high EPO production).

Although EPO undoubtedly is the main regulator of red cell production, the size of the progenitor cell pool and the number and responsiveness of the EPORs must also play a role. However, it is not clear whether or how these factors are physiologically regulated.

END-PRODUCT FEEDBACK

Products released through the destruction of red cells have been thought to influence or even control the rate of red cell production. Supporting this hypothesis is the impression that anemia due to hemolysis is associated with a more pronounced erythroid hyperplasia and reticulocytosis than blood loss anemia of the same severity. Part of this difference may be related to the more chronic nature of many types of hemolytic anemia with the accompanying expansion of marrow and progenitor cell pools, to a selective destruction of nonreticulated red cells, to a shift of the reticulocyte pool from the marrow to the circulation, and to readily available iron from destroyed red cells. However, in vitro studies have shown a stimulatory effect of hemin on erythropoiesis,[100] and such a mechanism might constitute a feedback loop, enhancing erythropoiesis when red cell destruction is increased.

The observations and considerations discussed in this chapter, in addition to information about the adaptability of oxygen affinity (see Chap. 28) have led to the construction of an operational feedback circuit that appears capable of adjusting and maintaining the red cell mass at an optimal size for oxygen transport (see Fig. 40-2). This circuit is based on a feedback between the marrow and the kidney mediated in one direction by oxygen and in the opposite by EPO.

RED CELL DESTRUCTION

MEASUREMENT OF RED CELL DESTRUCTION

RED CELL LIFE SPAN

The original method for the measurement of the red cell life span consisted in the transfusion of cells that were compatible but identifiable immunologically—the Ashby technique.[101] During World War II and shortly after, this method was used extensively, but in recent years it has been completely replaced by techniques based on labeling of autologous blood.

In 1946 Shemin and Rittenberg demonstrated that the incorporation of ^{15}N-labeled glycine into heme could be utilized to measure the life span of the red cells.[102] Since then a number of other isotopic methods have been developed. These can be divided into three groups: (1) those that label a cohort of cells, (2) those that label cells randomly, and (3) those that use indirect measurements such as the rate of production of red cells or the rate of heme breakdown. The first two classes yield information about the nature of the shortening of the red cell life span, age-dependent or random. The last group yields only mean life span.

COHORT METHODS

Cohort methods depend on the biosynthetic incorporation of the label into the developing red cells. In these methods a group of cells of approximately the same age is labeled. The labels used are glycine-containing labeled nitrogen (^{15}N),[102] radioactive carbon (^{14}C),[103] or radioactive iron, either ^{55}Fe or ^{59}Fe.[104–106] The main disadvantage of cohort labeling is the need for prolonged periods of sampling, especially if the life span is only moderately reduced (Fig. 29-4). In addition, isotopes from destroyed red cells may be reutilized, making it difficult to interpret results.

RANDOM LABEL METHODS

The random label methods are the Ashby differential agglutination technique,[101] which uses an immunologic marker, and isotopic techniques employing chromium (^{50}Cr, ^{51}Cr, or ^{53}Cr)[4,107]; diisopropylfluorophosphate (DFP) labeled with ^{32}P,[108] ^{3}H,[114] or ^{14}C[109]; ^{14}C cyanate[110]; or biotin.[111,112] By far the most commonly used isotope for red cell life spans is chromium, which penetrates the red cell membrane as the chromate ion and binds to the β and γ chains of globin. Unfortunately, these bonds are not covalent and there is a continuous elution of the isotope, varying from 0.5 to 2.9 percent per day.[113] DFP, on the other hand, is irreversibly bound to red cell cholinesterase. There is some elution of unbound DFP during the first two to three days of study, but after that DFP disappearance closely matches red cell destruction.[114,115] Nevertheless, because sample preparation is somewhat complicated, this label is not commonly used.

To accurately calculate red cell life span using a random label method requires steady-state conditions or that corrections can be

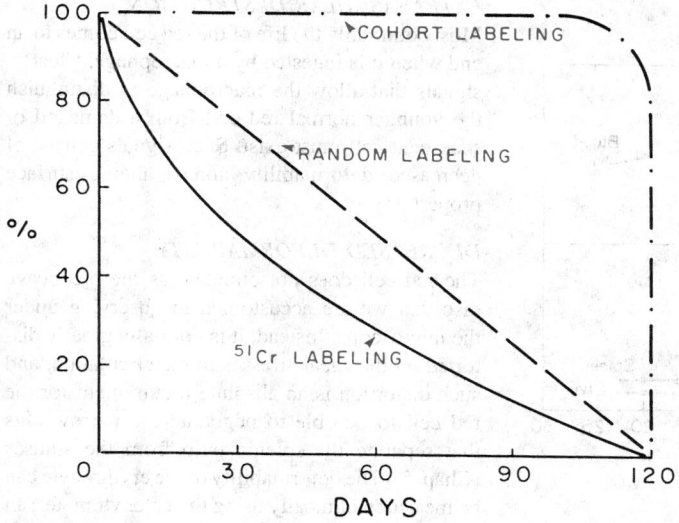

FIGURE 29-4   Red cell life span measured by cohort labeling or random labeling. When red cells are labeled randomly with ^{51}Cr there is a daily 1 percent elution which needs to be corrected for in the calculation of total red cell life span.

made for concurrent blood loss or blood transfusion. Fortunately, it is usually possible to gain an accurate estimate of red cell half-life by sampling three times a week for one to two weeks.

In the normal human the red cell life span is finite and about 120 days, with very little random destruction, i.e., loss irrespective of age (0.06 to 0.4 percent per day). In some mammalian species the amount of random destruction is much greater.[116] The survival curve of randomly labeled human red cells should consequently be nearly linear from day 0 to day 120 with a half-life of 60 days. When ^{51}Cr is used as the label, about 1 percent of label elutes per day and the survival curve becomes exponential with a half-life of about 30 days (see Fig. 29-4). For clinical use, the red cell life span is usually expressed as chromium $T_{1/2}$ and compared to the normal of 30 days.

Since merely expressing the red cell life span measured by chromium as chromium $T_{1/2}$ will not give information as to the character of destruction, senescence versus random, it has been recommended that in addition a correction factor for chromium elution be used and the data recorded using linear coordinates.[117] If the data lie on a straight line the destruction is by senescence and the life span can be calculated as twice the half-life. If the data indicate exponential disappearance and it is necessary to use a semilogarithmic paper in order to depict the data on a straight line, the destruction is random and the life span is 1.44 times half-life. One objection to this method is that the degree of chromium elution is not a constant but varies from day to day and from disease to disease.[113] Furthermore, the best fit of data is rarely linear or exponential but somewhere in between. Computer-assisted methods can resolve ambiguities, but the inherent biologic and technical variations in measuring red cell life span are such that it is better to rely on chromium $T_{1/2}$ with intuitive adjustments based on clinical findings.

INDIRECT METHODS

There are two approaches to the calculation of the red cell life span by indirect methods: from a measurement of the rate of production of red cells utilizing radioactive iron, or from a measurement of the rate of breakdown of heme to bilirubin[118] and carbon monoxide.[119] Both of these compounds are derived almost exclusively from catabolized hemoglobin, and measurements of their rate of production have provided useful information about the red cell life span. There are probably

too many variables that affect the bilirubin level to make it a reliable, quantitative measurement of red cell destruction. The measurement of CO production was formerly very tedious, but with the development of newer technology, it has become more practical. An advantage of the measurement of blood CO as an indication of the rate of red cell destruction is that it gives the rate of destruction at a single point in time.

IN SITU LOCALIZATION OF RED CELL PRODUCTION AND DESTRUCTION

As part of routine erythrokinetic studies both radioactive iron and radioactive chromium have been used for studying the localization of red cell production and red cell destruction. This is accomplished by positioning probes for external counting over the sacrum, liver, spleen, and heart and measuring the distribution of radioactivity in the body.[120]

In a normal subject ^{59}Fe injected IV is cleared rapidly from the plasma, and within 24 h about 85 percent of the radioactivity can be accounted for in the marrow. The liver and the spleen divide the remaining 15 percent. Over the next 10 days the marrow radioactivity decreases gradually due to the release into circulating blood of red cells labeled with radioactive hemoglobin. Patterns showing different uptake and distribution of the radioactive iron have been found for various hematologic disorders.[16] In hypersplenism the trapping and destruction of iron-labeled cells in the spleen will increase splenic radioactivity rapidly, and in patients with erythroid hypoplasia the distribution of radioactive iron between liver and marrow is reversed (Fig. 29-5).

More effective methods demonstrating in situ erythropoiesis involve imaging marrow, liver, and spleen with a ^{99m}Tc sulfur colloid or Indium-111.[121] Although these isotopes label primarily the monocyte-macrophage system, their uptake is similar to that of ^{59}Fe and they

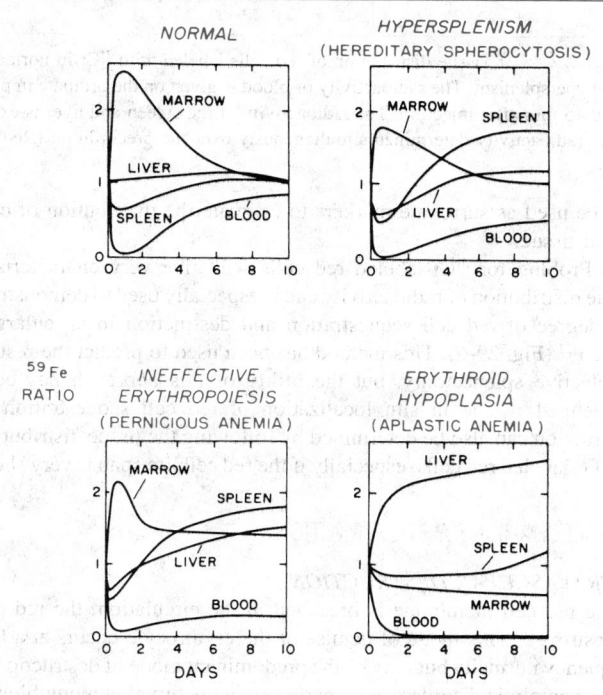

FIGURE 29-5   Tissue distribution of ^{59}Fe in normal subjects, hypersplenic patients, and anemic patients with ineffective and effective erythropoiesis. The radioactivity is expressed on the ordinate as a ratio relative to the radioactivity measured in the same organ 15 min after the intravenous administration of the isotope. (Redrawn from Hillman and Finch.[16])

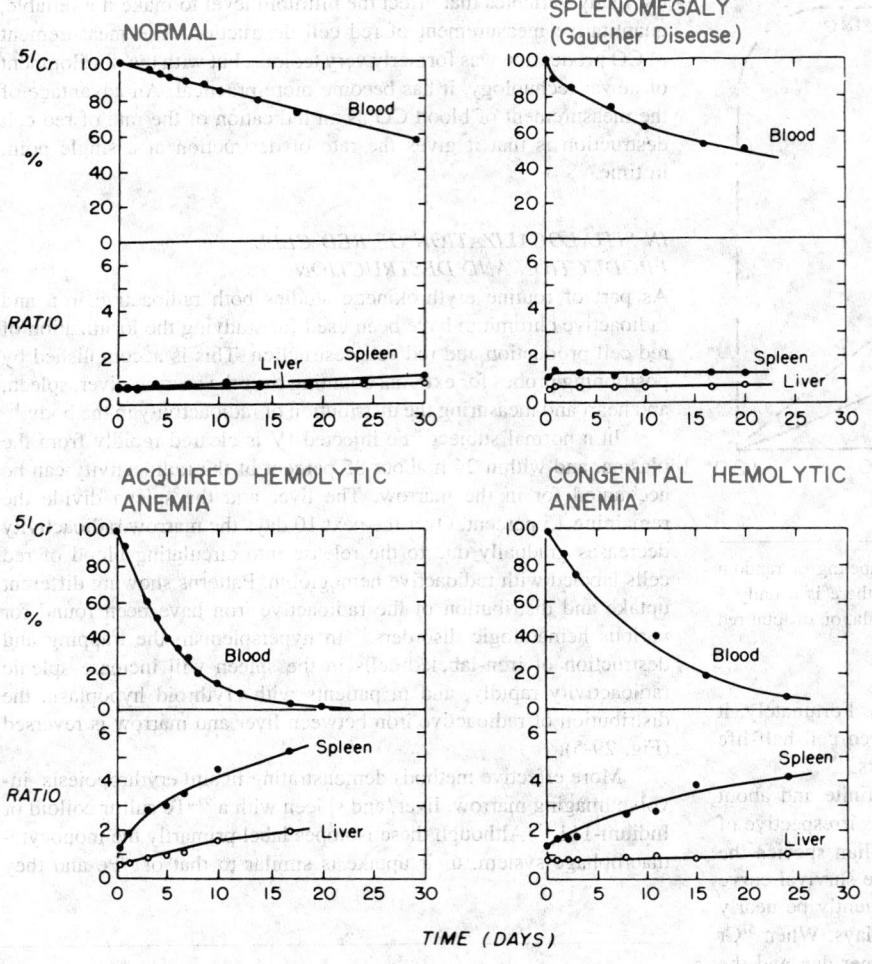

FIGURE 29-6 Tissue distribution of red cells labeled with ^{51}Cr in normal subjects and in patients with hypersplenism. The radioactivity of blood is given on the ordinate in percent of the radioactivity found 15 min after injection. The radioactivity of the spleen and liver is expressed as a ratio relative to the radioactivity determined simultaneously over the precordium. (Redrawn from Jandl et al.[122])

can be used as surrogate markers to estimate the distribution of erythroid tissue.

Probing for ^{51}Cr-labeled red cells will give very characteristic tissue distribution of radioactivity and is especially used to demonstrate the degree of red cell sequestration and destruction in an enlarged spleen[122] (Fig. 29-6). This method has been used to predict the results of elective splenectomy, but the utility of this approach has been challenged.[123] The in situ localization of red cell sequestration or destruction can also be determined by following the tissue distribution of ^{59}Fe-labeled red cells, especially if the red cell life span is very short.

MECHANISMS OF DESTRUCTION

INTRAVASCULAR DESTRUCTION

If the red cell membrane is breached in the circulation, the red cell is destroyed. This mode of demise of the erythrocyte occurs at a low frequency normally but may be the predominant mode of destruction in some hemolytic disorders, e.g., paroxysmal nocturnal hemoglobinuria (Chap. 36), where the complement complex creates holes in the red cell membrane, and in cardiac valve hemolysis (Chap. 50) and microangiopathic hemolytic anemia (Chap. 51), where the shear stress may be so strong as to break open the membrane.

EXTRAVASCULAR DESTRUCTION

Most commonly the life of the red cell comes to an end when it is ingested by a macrophage. Clearly, signals that allow the macrophage to distinguish the younger normal red cell from a damaged or senescent cell must exist. Such signals consist of decreased deformability and/or altered surface properties.

DECREASED DEFORMABILITY

The red cell does not circulate as the biconcave disc that we are accustomed to observing under the microscope. Instead, it is normally greatly distorted by the shear stresses in the circulation, and such distortion is an absolute requirement for the red cell to be able to negotiate the narrow slits that separate the splenic pulp from the sinuses (Chap. 5). The deformability of the erythrocyte can be measured clinically using the ektocytometer, an instrument which displays the diffraction pattern of a red cell suspension under shear stress.[124] The red cell membrane, a lipid bilayer, bends readily but has very little capacity to stretch. Thus, deformability is largely a function of the excess red cell membrane intrinsic to the biconcave disc shape of the cell and to some extent of the viscosity of the hemoglobin solution within the cell. As the red cell loses membrane it assumes a spherical shape and loses its ability to deform. Hereditary spherocytosis and hereditary elliptocytosis are prototypic of hemolytic anemias in which decreased deformability as a result of a decreased surface/volume ratio plays a key role in red cell destruction (Chap. 43). However, loss of membrane plays a role in many types of pathologic hemolysis, including autoimmune hemolytic anemia (Chap. 55). In sickle cell disease and hemoglobin C disease (Chap. 47) the internal viscosity of the cell is increased. Loss of water from the red cell, as may occur when the membrane is damaged and leaks potassium, as in hereditary xerocytosis (Chap. 44), also markedly impairs the deformability of the cell.

ALTERED SURFACE PROPERTIES

The surface of the red cell membrane can be altered by binding of antibodies to surface antigens, by binding of complement components, and by chemical alterations, particularly oxidation of membrane components. IgG-coated red cells[125] and red cells coated by C3[126,127] are bound and sphered by mononuclear cells in vitro, and it is likely that they are similarly damaged by macrophages in the body of patients with autoimmune hemolytic anemia (Chap. 55).

In vitro oxidation of red cells with phenylhydrazine or ADP plus iron causes clustering of band 3 protein in the membrane. Although the physiologic significance of this is far from clear, it has been suggested that the clustered proteins serve as a recognition site for the binding of IgG.[128,129] Oxidative damage to the membrane may play a role in the removal of sickle cells (Chap. 47) and thalassemic cells from the circulation (Chap. 46).

SENESCENCE OF NORMAL ERYTHROCYTES

The classical 1949 studies of London et al.[130] in which the heme in erythrocytes was labeled with ^{15}N glycine established that most red cells have a finite life span between 100 and 140 days.[131]

METHODOLOGIC CONSIDERATIONS

Labeling a cohort of human erythrocytes with ^{59}Fe and centrifuging the cells in a density gradient demonstrates that reticulocytes and young red cells are less dense than mature red cells.[132,133] However, at the end of the life span of the labeled cohort, radioactivity is fairly evenly distributed throughout red cells of all densities with only a slight tendency of the radioactivity to be concentrated in the more dense cells. Unfortunately, most studies of the properties of senescent cells in the past have been based upon the characteristics of the most dense fraction of erythrocytes, using various fractionating techniques. Although some investigators still regard density separation to be a valid way of isolating aged red cells,[134–136] there is now a large body of evidence that indicates that the most dense fraction of red cells is only slightly enriched with old erythrocytes.[137–139]

There are two animal models and one human disease model that provide cells that are truly aged. In mice, in vivo aged cells have been produced by serial transfusion, maintaining polycythemia to suppress virtually all erythropoiesis.[140] In other species, particularly the rabbit, red cells have been labeled with traces of biotin, which allows them to be recovered from the circulation.[141] The human model is transient erythroblastopenia of childhood (Chap. 32), a disorder in which there is cessation of all erythropoiesis for several months. The use of the latter model has been criticized because of the fact that this disorder is not fully understood and that the red cells in the circulation may not be entirely normal.[142] However, the results that have been obtained are consistent with those obtained in animal models and are probably reliable.

PROPERTIES OF AGED CELLS

While the activities of a large number of enzymes, including hexokinase, glucose-6-phosphate dehydrogenase, and pyruvate kinase, are higher in reticulocytes than in mature erythrocytes, they do not continue to decline during the aging of the erythrocyte.[141,143] Pyrimidine-5′-nucleotidase[144,145] and AMP-deaminase[146–148] appear to be exceptions to this rule in that there is continuing decline of enzyme activity throughout the life span of the red cell. The density and deformability of the aged cells in erythroblastopenia of childhood are normal.[137] Fluorescent sorting of NN erythrocytes transfused into humans shows that the most dense fractions are only minimally enriched with old cells,[149] and biotinylated aged cells of rabbits have been found to have only a modestly decreased surface area, volume, cell water, and density and therefore slightly decreased deformability.[138,150]

The amount of immunoglobulin on red cell membranes has been reported to increase with aging of the cells,[151,152] and it has been proposed that such accumulation of immunoglobulin mediates removal of senescent erythrocytes. However, immunoglobulin levels on aged, biotinylated rabbit cells are not increased[153] and the fact that red cell life span has never been demonstrated to be prolonged in α-gamma-globulinemic patients casts serious doubt upon the concept that immunoglobulins mediate removal of senescent red-cells.

The exposure of phosphatidylserine is one of the signals that allows macrophages to recognize apoptotic cells. It is likely that this is, indeed, the signal by which macrophages recognize senescent erythrocytes.[112,154] A model that has been developed suggests that the average time during which phosphatidylserine is exposed is only 0.3 to 0.5 days, so that few cells with increased exposure of the phospholipid are in the circulation at any time. It is not yet clear whether this is the only or even the primary signal that indicates that a cell has reached the end of its life span, but it is the only major difference between senescent and nonsenescent erythrocytes that has been documented clearly.

FATE OF DESTROYED RED CELLS

INTRAVASCULAR DESTRUCTION

Hemoglobin   When red cells are destroyed in the vascular compartment the hemoglobin escaping into the plasma is bound to haptoglobin. Each molecule of haptoglobin, a dimeric glycoprotein, can bind two hemoglobin β dimers.[155] The haptoglobin-hemoglobin complex is cleared from the plasma with a $T_{1/2}$ of 10 to 30 min.[156] After the complex is carried to the liver parenchyma[157] the heme of the hemoglobin is converted to iron and biliverdin by heme oxygenase and the biliverdin is further catabolized to bilirubin. CO is released in the course of cleavage of heme by heme oxygenase.

Free haptoglobin, in contrast to the hemoglobin-haptoglobin complex has a $T_{1/2}$ of 5 days, and when large amounts of the rapidly turned over haptoglobin-hemoglobin complex are formed the haptoglobin content of the plasma is depleted. The haptoglobin content of the plasma is diminished not only in the plasma of patients undergoing frank intravascular hemolysis but also from the plasma of patients who, like those with sickle cell disease, have accelerated red cell destruction occurring primarily within macrophages. Presumably there is either enough intravascular hemolysis in such hemolytic disorders to lower the plasma haptoglobin level or enough leakage from the phagocytic cells into the plasma to bind to haptoglobin. Thus the measurement of plasma haptoglobin levels has some usefulness in diagnosing the presence of hemolysis.

Heme   Free heme that is released into the circulation is bound in a 1:1 ratio to the plasma glycoprotein hemopexin, which is cleared from the plasma with a $T_{1/2}$ of 7 to 8 h.[158] The heme is delivered to the liver where it is converted to bilirubin. When the capacity of hemopexin to bind heme has been saturated, excess heme may bind to albumin to form methemalbumin.[159]

EXTRAVASCULAR DESTRUCTION

Red cells that are engulfed by phagocytic cells are degraded within lysosomes into lipids, protein, and heme. The proteins and lipids are reprocessed in their respective catabolic pathways, and the heme is cleaved by a microsomal heme oxygenase[160] into iron and biliverdin. The latter is catabolized to bilirubin.

BILIRUBIN EXCRETION

Regardless of the site of destruction of hemoglobin, one of the final products is bilirubin, and this is excreted through the bile into the gastrointestinal tract where it is converted to urobilinogens by bacterial reduction.[161] A small fraction of urobilinogen is reabsorbed and excreted into the urine. Thus, the fecal and urinary urobilinogen excretion have been used as an indicator of the rate of hemolysis, but is only uncommonly used for this purpose in modern practice because the collections are cumbersome and because alternatively degradative pathways detract severely from the accuracy of the estimates of the rate of heme catabolism.

REFERENCES

1. Pearson TC, Botterill CA, Glass UH, Wetherley-Mein G: Interpretation of measured red cell mass and plasma volume in males with elevated venous PCV values. *Scand J Haematol* 33:68, 1984.
2. Drysdale HC, Emerson PM, Holmes A: An improved method for the measurement of red cell survival using non-radioactive chromium. *J Clin Pathol* 32:655, 1979.
3. Heaton WAL, Hanbury CM, Keegan TE, Pleban P, Holmes S: Studies with nonradioisotopic sodium chromate: I. Development of a technique for measuring red cell volume. *Transfusion* 29:696, 1989.
4. Silver HM, Seebeck MA, Cowett RM, Patterson KY, Veillon C: Red cell volume determination using a stable isotope of chromium. *Journal of the Society For Gynecologic Investigation* 4:254, 1997.

5. Sioufi HA, Button LN, Jacobson MS, Kevy SV: Nonradioactive chromium technique for red cell labeling. *Vox Sang* 58:204, 1990.

6. Cavill I, Trevett D, Fisher J, Hoy T: The measurement of the total volume of red cells in man: a non-radioactive approach using biotin. *Br J Haematol* 70:491, 1988.

7. Jones J, Mollison PL: A simple and efficient method of labelling red cells with 99m Tc for determination of red cell volume. *Br J Haematol* 38:141, 1978.

8. Chaplin H Jr: Precision of red cell volume measurement using P^{32} labeled cells. *J Physiol* 123:22, 1954.

9. Pearson TC, Guthrie DL, Simpson J, et al: Interpretation of measured red cell mass and plasma volume in adults: Expert Panel on Radionuclides of the International Council for Standardization in Haematology. *Br J Haematol* 89:748, 1995.

10. Fairbanks VF, Klee GG, Wiseman GA, et al: Measurement of blood volume and red cell mass: Re-examination of ^{51}Cr and ^{125}I methods. *Blood Cells Mol Dis* 22:169, 1996.

11. Larson RA: Studies of the body hematocrit phenomenon: Dynamic hematocrit of large vessel and initial distribution space of albumin and fibrinogen in the whole body. *Scand J Clin Lab Invest* 22:189, 1998.

12. Fairbanks VF: Measurement of blood volume and red cell mass: Re-examination of ^{51}Cr and ^{125}I methods—Commentary. *Blood Cells Mol Dis* 22:186C, 1996.

13. Button LN, Gibson II JG, Walter CW: Simultaneous determination of the volume of red cells and plasma for survival studies of stored blood. *Transfusion* 5:143, 1965.

14. International Committee for Standardization in Haematology: Recommended methods for measurement of red-cell and plasma volume. *J Nucl Med* 21:793, 1980.

15. Finch CA, Deubelbeiss K, Cook JD, et al: Ferrokinetics in man. *Medicine (Baltimore)* 49:17, 1970.

16. Hillman RS, Finch CA: Erythropoiesis: normal and abnormal. *Semin Hematol* 4:327, 1967.

17. London IM, West R, Shemin D, Rittenberg D: On the origin of bile pigment in normal man. *J Biol Chem* 184:351, 1950.

18. Samson D, Halliday D, Nicholson DC, Chanarin I: Quantitation of ineffective erythropoiesis from the incorporation of [15N] delta-aminolaevulinic acid and [15N] glycine into early labelled bilirubin: II. Anaemic patients. *Br J Haematol* 34:45, 1976.

19. Samson D, Halliday D, Nicholson DC, Chanarin I: Quantitation of ineffective erythropoiesis from the incorporation of [15N] delta-aminolaevulinic acid and [15N] glycine into early labelled bilirubin: I. Normal subjects. *Br J Haematol* 34:33, 1976.

20. Berk PD, Blaschke TF, Scharschmidt BF, Waggoner JG, Berlin NI: A new approach to quantitation of the various sources of bilrubin in man. *J Lab Clin Med* 87:767, 1976.

21. Huff RI, Hennessey TG, Austin RE: Plasma and red cell iron turnover in normal subjects and in patients having various hematopoietic disorders. *J Clin Invest* 29:1041, 1950.

22. Cook JD, Marsaglia G, Eschbach JW, Funk DD, Finch CA: Ferrokinetics: a biologic model for plasma iron exchange in man. *J Clin Invest* 49:197, 1970.

23. Ricketts C, Cavill I, Napier JA, Jacobs A: Ferrokinetics and erythropoiesis in man: an evaluation of ferrokinetic measurements. *Br J Haematol* 35:41, 1977.

24. Bauer W, Stray S, Huebers H, Finch C: The relationship between plasma iron and plasma iron turnover in the rat. *Blood* 57:239, 1981.

25. Beguin Y: The soluble transferrin receptor: biological aspects and clinical usefulness as quantitative measure of erythropoiesis. *Haematologica* 77:1, 1992.

26. Huebers HA, Beguin Y, Pootrakul P, Einspahr D, Finch CA: Intact transferrin receptors in human plasma and their relation to erythropoiesis. *Blood* 75:102, 1990.

27. Flowers CH, Skikne BS, Covell AM, Cook JD: The clinical measurement of serum transferrin receptor. *J Lab Clin Med* 114:368, 1989.

28. Morishita Y, Kataoka T, Towatari M, et al: Up-regulation of transferrin receptor gene expression by granulocyte colony-stimulating factor in human myeloid leukemia cells. *Cancer Res* 50:7955, 1990.

29. Kuiper-Kramer PA, Huisman CMS, Van der Molen-Sinke J, Abbes A, Van Eijk HG: The expression of transferrin receptors on erythroblasts in anaemia of chronic disease, myelodysplastic syndromes and iron deficiency. *Acta Haematol (Basel)* 97:127, 1997.

30. Ferguson BJ, Skikne BS, Simpson KM, Baynes RD, Cook JD: Serum transferrin receptor distinguishes the anemia of chronic disease from iron deficiency anemia. *J Lab Clin Med* 119:385, 1992.

31. Kansu E, Erslev AJ: Aplastic anaemia with 'hot pockets.' *Scand J Haematol* 17:326, 1976.

32. Steiner RM, Mitchell DG, Rao VM, Schweitzer ME: Magnetic resonance imaging of diffuse bone marrow disease. *Radiol Clin North Am* 31:383, 1993.

33. Scott RB: Comparative hematology: the phylogeny of the erythrocyte. *Blut* 12:340, 1966.

34. Fox HM: The hemoglobin of *Daphnia*. *Proc R Soc Lond (Biol)* 135:195, 1948.

35. Schmidt-Nielsen K, Taylor CR: Red blood cells: why or why not? *Science* 162:274, 1968.

36. Andrew W: *Comparative Hematology*. Grune & Stratton, New York, 1965.

37. Bolliger A: Observations on the blood of a monotreme *Tachyglossus aculeatus*. *Aust J Sci* 22:257, 1959.

38. Jordan HE: Comparative hematology, in *Handbook of Hematology*, p 703. Hoeber-Harper, New York, 1938.

39. Iorio RJ: Some morphologic and kinetic studies of the developing erythroid cells of the common gold fish *Carassius auratus*. *Cell Tissue Kinet* 2:319, 1969.

40. Robb-Smith AHT: *The Growth of Knowledge of the Functions of the Blood*, edited by RG Macfarlane, AHT Robb-Smith. Academic Press, New York, 1961.

41. Rosse WF, Waldmann TA: Factors controlling erythropoiesis in birds. *Blood* 27:654, 1966.

42. Zanjani ED: Humoral factors influencing erythropoiesis in the fish (Blue Gourami-*Trichogaster trichopteras*). *Blood* 33:573, 1969.

43. Erslev AJ: Control of red cell production. *Ann Rev Med* 11:315, 1959.

44. Shoemaker C, Mitsock LD: Murine erythropoietin gene: Cloning expression and human gene homology. *Mol Cell Biol* 6:849, 1986.

45. Le Douarin NM: Cell migrations in embryos. *Cell* 38:353, 1984.

46. Hoyes AD, Riches DJ, Martin BGH: The fine structure of haematopoiesis in the human fetal liver. *J Anat* 115:99, 1973.

47. Rosenberg M: Fetal hematopoiesis. *Blood* 33:66, 1969.

48. Hudson G: Bone marrow volume in the human foetus and newborn. *Br J Haematol* 11:446, 1965.

49. Brannon D: Extramedullary hematopoiesis in anemia. *Bull Johns Hopkins Hosp* 41:104, 1927.

50. Erslev A: Medullary and extramedullary blood formation. *Clin Orthop* 52:25, 1967.

51. Finne PH: Erythropoietin production in fetal hypoxia and in anemic uremic patients. *Ann NY Acad Sci* 149:497, 1968.

52. Zanjani ED, Poster J, Burlington H, et al: Liver as the primary site of erythropoietin formation in the fetus. *J Lab Clin Med* 89:640, 1977.

53. Zanjani ED, Ascensao JL, McGlare PG, et al: Studies on the liver to kidney switch of erythropoietin production. *J Clin Invest* 67:1183, 1981.

54. Flake AW, Harrison MR, Adzick NS, Zanjani ED: Erythropoietin production by the fetal liver in an adult environment. *Blood* 70:542, 1987.

55. Stephenson IK, Axelrod AA, McLeod DL, Shreeve MM: Induction of hemoglobin-synthesizing cells by erythropoietin in vitro. *Proc Natl Acad Sci USA* 65:1542, 1971.

56. Civin CI, Loken MR: Cell surface antigens on human marrow cells: dissection of hematopoietic development using monoclonal antibodies and multiparameter flow cytometry. *Int J Cell Cloning* 5:267, 1987.

57. Testa NG: Structure and regulation of the erythroid system at the level of progenitor cells. *Crit Rev Oncol Hematol* 9:17, 1989.

58. Fisher JW: Erythropoietin: physiologic and pharmacologic aspects. *Proc Soc Exp Biol Med* 216:358, 1997.

59. Adamson JW, Torok-Storb B, Lin N: Analysis of erythropoiesis by erythroid colony formation in culture. *Blood Cells* 4:89, 1978.

60. Donohue DM, Reiff RH, Hanson ML, Betson Y, Finch CA: Quantitation measurement of the erythrocytic and granulocytic cells of marrow and blood. *J Clin Invest* 37:1571, 1958.

61. Finch CA, Harker LA, Cook JD: Kinetics of the formed elements of human blood. *Blood* 50:699, 1977.

62. Goltry KL, Patel VP: Specific domains of fibronectin mediate adhesion and migration of early murine erythroid progenitors. *Blood* 90:138, 1997.

63. Prankerd TAJ: The spleen and anemia. *BMJ* 2:517, 1963.

64. Baker CH, Remington JW: Role of the spleen in determining total body hematocrit. *Am J Physiol* 198:906, 1960.

65. Erslev AJ: Blood and Mountains, in *Blood, Pure and Eloquent*, edited by MM Wintrobe, p 257. McGraw-Hill, New York, 1980.

66. Carnot P, Deflandre C: Sur l'activité hématopoiétique des serum au cours de la régénaration du sang. *Acad Sci Med* 3:384, 1906.

67. Miescher F: Über die Beziehungen Zwischen Meereshohe und Beschaffenheit des Blutes. *Koresp Bltt Schweitz Aerzte* 24:809, 1893.

68. Reissmann KR: Studies on the mechanism of erythropoietic stimulation in parabiotic rats during hypoxia. *Blood* 5:372, 1950.

69. Erslev AJ: Humoral regulation of red cell production. *Blood* 8:349, 1953.

70. Erslev AJ, Lavietes PH, van Wagenen G: Erythropoietic stimulation induced by ''anemia'' serum. *Proc Soc Exp Biol Med* 83:548, 1953.

71. Jacobson LO, Goldwasser E, Fried W, Plzak L: Role of the kidney in erythropoiesis. *Nature* 179:633, 1957.

72. Lappin TR, Rich IN: Erythropoietin—the first 90 years. *Clin Lab Haematol* 18:137, 1996.

73. Jelkmann W: Erythropoietin: structure, control of production, and function. *Physiol Rev* 72:449, 1992.

74. Jelkmann W, Metzen E: Erythropoietin in the control of red cell production. *Anat Anz* 178:391, 1996.

75. Yoshimura A, Misawa H: Physiology and function of the erythropoietin receptor. *Curr Opin Hematol* 5:171, 1998.

76. Livnah O, Stura EA, Johnson DL, et al: Functional mimicry of a protein hormone by a peptide agonist: the EPO receptor complex at 2.8 A. *Science* 273:464, 1996.

77. Wrighton NC, Farrell FX, Chang R, et al: Small peptides as potent mimetics of the protein hormone erythropoietin. *Science* 273:458, 1996.

78. Koury ST, Boudurant MC, Koury MJ: Localization of erythropoietic synthesizing cells in murine kidneys by in situ hybridization. *Blood* 71:524, 1988.

79. Lacombe C, Da Silva J-L, Bruneval P, Fournier J-G: Peritubular cells are the site of erythropoietin synthesis in the murine hypoxic kidney. *J Clin Invest* 81:620, 1988.

80. Koury ST, Koury MJ, Bondurant MC, Caro J, Graber SE: Quantitation of erythropoietic-producing cells in kidneys of mice by in situ hybridization: Correlation with hematocrit, renal erythropoietin mRNA, and serum erythropoietin concentration. *Blood* 71:645, 1989.

81. Bachmann S, Le Hir M, Eckardt K-U: Co-localization of erythropoietin mRNA and Eco-5'-nucleotidase immunoreactivity in peritubular cells of rat renal cortex indicates that fibroblasts produce erythropoietin. *J Histochem Cytochem* 41:335, 1993.

82. Wenger RH, Kvietikova I, Rolfs A, Camenisch G, Gassmann M: Oxygen-regulated erythropoietin gene expression is dependent on a CpG methylation-free hypoxia-inducible factor-1 DNA-binding site. *Eur J Biochem* 253:771, 1998.

83. Huang LE, Gu J, Schau M, Bunn HF: Regulation of hypoxia-inducible factor 1alpha is mediated by an O_2-dependent degradation domain via the ubiquitin-proteasome pathway. *Proc Natl Acad Sci USA* 95:7987, 1998.

84. Semenza GL, Dureza RC, Traystman MD, Gearhart JD, Antonarakis SE: Human erythropoietin gene expression in transgenic mice: multiple transcription initiation sites and cis-acting regulatory elements. *Mol Cell Biol* 10:930, 1990.

85. Schuster SJ, Koury ST, Bohrer M, Salceda S, Caro J: Cellular sites of extrarenal and renal erythropoietin production in anaemic rats. *Br J Haematol* 81:153, 1992.

86. Naughton BA, Kaplan SM, Roy M, et al: Hepatic regeneration and erythropoietin production in the rat. *Science* 196:301, 1977.

87. Brown S, Caro J, Erslev AJ, Murray T: Spontaneous increase in erythropoietin and hematocrit value associated with transient liver enzyme abnormalities in an anephric patient undergoing hemodialysis. *Am J Med* 68:280, 1980.

88. Stopka T, Zivny JH, Stopkova P, Prchal JF, Prchal JT: Human hematopoietic progenitors express erythropoietin. *Blood* 91:3766, 1998.

89. Fandry J, Bunn HF: *In vivo* and *in vitro* regulation of erythropoietin mRNA: measurement by competitive polymerase reaction. *Blood* 81:617, 1993.

90. Flaharty KK, Caro J, Erslev A, et al: Pharmacokinetics and erythropoietic response to human recombinant erythropoietin in healthy men. *Clin Pharmacol Ther* 47:557, 1990.

91. Sytkowski AJ, Lunn ED, Davis KL, Feldman L, Siekman S: Human erythropoietin dimers with markedly enhanced in vivo activity. *Proc Natl Acad Sci USA* 95:1184, 1998.

92. Sawyer ST, Krantz SB, Goldwasser E: Binding and receptor-mediated endocytosis of erythropoietin in Friend virus-infected erythroid cells. *J Biol Chem* 262:5554, 1987.

93. Piroso E, Erslev AJ, Flaharty KK, Caro J: Erythropoietin life span in rats with hypoplastic and hyperplastic bone marrows. *Am J Hematol* 36:105, 1991.

94. Joneja B, Wojchowski DM: Mitogenic signaling and inhibition of apoptosis via the erythropoietin receptor Box-1 domain. *J Biol Chem* 272:11176, 1997.

95. Nakamura Y, Nakauchi H: A truncated erythropoietin receptor and cell death: a reanalysis. *Science* 264:588, 1994.

96. Spivak JL, Pham T, Isaacs M, Hankins WD: Erythropoietin is both a mitogen and a survival factor. *Blood* 77:1228, 1991.

97. Lin CS, Lim SK, D'Agati V, Costantini F: Differential effects of an erythropoietin receptor gene disruption on primitive and definitive erythropoiesis. *Genes Dev* 10:154, 1996.

98. Sawyer ST, Penta K: Erythropoietin cell biology. *Hematol Oncol Clin North Am* 8:895, 1994.

99. Noble NA, Xu Q-P, Hoge LL: Reticulocytes: II. Reexamination of the in vivo survival of stress reticulocytes. *Blood* 75:1877, 1990.

100. Mayeux P, Felix JM, Billat C, Jacquot R: Induction by hemin of proliferation and of differentiation of progenitor erythroid cells responsible for erythropoietin. *Exp Hematol* 14:801, 1986.

101. Ashby W: The determination of the length of life of transfused blood corpuscles in man. *J Exp Med* 29:267, 1919.

102. Shemin D, Rittenberg D: Life span of human red blood cell. *J Biol Chem* 166:627, 1946.

103. Berlin NI, Meyer LM, Lazarus M: Life span of the rat red blood cell as determined by glycine-2-C14. *Am J Physiol* 165:565, 1951.

104. Beutler E, Dern RJ, Alving AS: The hemolytic effect of primaquine: IV. The relationship of cell age to hemolysis. *J Lab Clin Med* 44:439, 1954.

105. Birgens HS, Hansen OP, Henriksen JH, Wantzin P: Quantitation of erythropoiesis in myelomatosis. *Scand J Haematol* 22:357, 1979.

106. Weinstein IM, Beutler E: The use of Cr-51 and Fe-59 in a combined procedure to study erythrocyte production and destruction in normal human subjects and in patients with hemolytic or aplastic anemia. *J Lab Clin Med* 45:616, 1955.

107. Heaton WA: Evaluation of posttransfusion recovery and survival of transfused red cells. *Transfusion Medicine Reviews* 6:153, 1992.

108. Cohen JA, Warringa MGPJ: The fate of P32 labeled diisopropyl fluorophosphonate in the human body and its use as a labeling agent in study of turnover of blood plasma and red cells. *J Clin Invest* 33:459, 1954.

109. Milner PF, Charache S: Life span of carbamylated red cells in sickle cell anemia. *J Clin Invest* 52:3161, 1973.

110. Eschbach JW, Korn D, Finch CA: 14C cyanate as a tag for red cell survival in normal and uremic man. *J Lab Clin Med* 89:823, 1977.

111. Wardrop KJ, Tucker RL, Anderson EP: Use of an in vitro biotinylation technique for determination of posttransfusion viability of stored canine packed red blood cells. *Amer J Vet Res* 59:397, 1998.

112. Boas E, Forman L, Beutler E: Phosphatidyl serine exposure and red cell viability in red cell ageing and in hemolytic anemia. *Proc Natl Acad Sci USA* 85:3077, 1998.

113. Bentley SA, Glass HI, Lewis SM, Szur L: Elution correction in 51Cr red cell survival studies. *Br J Haematol* 26:179, 1974.

114. Cline MJ, Berlin NI: Simultaneous measurement of the survival of two populations of erythrocytes with the use of labelled diisopropyl fluorophosphate. *J Lab Clin Med* 61:249, 1963.

115. McCurdy PR, Sherman AS: Irreversibly sickled cells and red cell survival in sickle cell anemia: a study with both DF32P and 51CR. *Am J Med* 64:253, 1978.

116. Eadie GS, Brown IW Jr: Red blood cell survival studies. *Blood* 8:1110, 1953.

117. International Committee for Standardization in Haematology: Recommended method for radioisotope red-cell survival studies. *Br J Haematol* 45:659, 1980.

118. Berlin NI, Berk PD: Quantitative aspects of bilirubin metabolism for hematologists. *Blood* 57:983, 1981.

119. Doyle J, Vreman HJ, Stevenson DK, et al: Does vitamin C cause hemolysis in premature newborn infants? Results of a multicenter double-blind, randomized, controlled trial. *J Pediatr* 130:103, 1997.

120. ICSH panel on diagnostic applications of radioisotopes in hematology: Recommended methods for surface counting to determine sites of red cell destruction. *Br J Haematol* 30:249, 1975.

121. Datz FL, Taylor AJ: The clinical use of radionuclide bone marrow imaging. *Semin Nucl Med* 15:239, 1985.

122. Jandl JH, Greenberg MS, Yonemoto RH, Castle WB: Clinical determination of the sites of red cell sequestration in hemolytic anemias. *J Clin Invest* 35:842, 1956.

123. Ferrant A, Cauwe F, Michaux JL, et al: Assessment of the sites of red cell destruction using quantitative measurements of splenic and hepatic red cell destruction. *Br J Haematol* 50:591, 1982.

124. Johnson RM, Ravindranath Y: Osmotic scan ektacytometry in clinical diagnosis. *J Pediatr Hematol Oncol* 18:122, 1996.

125. Lo Buglio AA, Cotran RS, Jandl JH: Red cells coated with immunoglobulin g: Binding and sphering by mononuclear cells in man. *Science* 158:1582, 1967.

126. Jandl JH, Tomlinson AS: The destruction of red cells by antibodies in man: II. Pyrogenic, leukocytic and dermal responses to immune hemolysis. *J Clin Invest* 37:1202, 1958.

127. Lutz HU, Stammler P, Kock D, Taylor RP: Opsonic potential of C3b-anti-band 3 complexes when generated on senescent and oxidatively stressed red cells or in fluid phase, in *Red Blood Cell Aging*, p 367. Plenum Press, New York, 1991.

128. Low PS, Waugh SM, Zinke K, Drenckhahn D: The role of hemoglobin denaturation and band 3 clustering in red blood cell aging. *Science* 227:531, 1985.

129. Beppu M, Mizukami A, Nagoya M, Kikugawa K: Binding of anti-band 3 autoantibody to oxidatively damaged erythrocytes. Formation of senescent antigen on erythrocyte surface by an oxidative mechanism. *J Biol Chem* 265:3226, 1990.

130. London IM, Shemin D, West R, Rittenberg D: Heme synthesis and red blood cell dynamics in normal humans and in subjects with polycythemia vera, sickle-cell anemias, and pernicious anemia. *J Biol Chem* 179:463, 1949.

131. Bratosin D, Mazurier J, Tissier JP, et al: Cellular and molecular mechanisms of senescent erythrocyte phagocytosis by macrophages. A review. *Biochimie* 80:173, 1998.

132. Borun ER, Figueroa WG, Perry SM: The distribution of Fe[59] tagged human erythrocytes in centrifuged specimens as a function of cell age. *J Clin Invest* 36:676, 1957.

133. Luthra MG, Friedman JM, Sears DA: Studies of density fractions of normal human erythrocytes labeled with iron-59 in vivo. *J Lab Clin Med* 94:879, 1979.

134. Piomelli S, Seaman C: Mechanism of red blood cell aging: Relationship of cell density and cell age. *Am J Hematol* 42:46, 1993.

135. Lutz HU, Stammler P, Fasler S, Ingold M, Fehr J: Density separation of human red blood cells on self-forming Percoll gradients: Correlation with cell age. *Biochim Biophys Acta* 1116:1, 1992.

136. Piccinini G, Minetti G, Balduini C, Brovelli A: Oxidation state of glutathione and membrane proteins in human red cells of different age. *Mech Ageing Dev* 78:15, 1995.

137. Linderkamp O, Friederichs E, Boehler T, Ludwig A: Age dependency of red blood cell deformability and density: Studies in transient erythroblastopenia of childhood. *Br J Haematol* 83:125, 1993.

138. Dale GL, Norenberg SL: Density fractionation of erythrocytes by Percoll/

139. hypaque results in only a slight enrichment for aged cells. *Biochim Biophys Acta* 1036:183, 1990.

139. Beutler E: Isolation of the aged. *Blood Cells* 14:1, 1988.

140. Ganzoni AM, Oakes R, Hillman RS: Red cell aging in vivo. *J Clin Invest* 50:1373, 1971.

141. Suzuki T, Dale GL: Senescent erythrocytes: isolation of in vivo aged cells and their biochemical characteristics. *Proc Natl Acad Sci USA* 85:1647, 1988.

142. Haram S, Carriero D, Seaman C, Piomelli S: The mechanism of decline of age-dependent enzymes in the red blood cell. *Enzyme* 45:47, 1991.

143. Zimran A, Forman L, Suzuki T, Dale GL, Beutler E: In vivo aging of red cell enzymes: Study of biotinylated red blood cells in rabbits. *Am J Hematol* 33:249, 1990.

144. Beutler E, Hartman G: Age-related red cell enzymes in children with transient erythroblastopenia of childhood and hemolytic anemia. *Pediatr Res* 19:44, 1985.

145. Beutler E: The relationship of red cell enzymes to red cell life-span. *Blood Cells* 14:69, 1988.

146. Dale GL, Norenberg SL: Time-dependent loss of adenosine 5'-monophosphate deaminase activity may explain elevated adenosine 5'-triphosphate levels in senescent erythrocytes. *Blood* 74:2157, 1989.

147. Paglia DE, Valentine WN, Nakatani M, Brockway RA: AMP deaminase as a cell-age marker in transient erythroblastopenia of childhood and its role in the adenylate economy of erythrocytes. *Blood* 74:2161, 1989.

148. Dale GL, Norenberg SL, Suzuki T, Forman L: Altered adenine nucleotide metabolism in senescent erythrocytes from the rabbit. *Prog Clin Biol Res* 319:259, 1989.

149. Clark MR, Corash L, Jensen RH: Density distribution of aging, trans-fused human red cells. *Blood* 74(Suppl 1):217a, 1989.

150. Waugh RE, Narla M, Jackson CW, et al: Rheologic properties of senescent erythrocytes: Loss of surface area and volume with red blood cell age. *Blood* 79:1351, 1992.

151. Kay MM, Marchalonis JJ, Schluter SF, Bosman G: Human erythrocyte aging: cellular and molecular biology. *Transfus Med Rev* 5:173, 1991.

152. Sheiban E, Gershon H: Recognition and sequestration of young and old erythrocytes from young and elderly human donors: in vitro studies. *J Lab Clin Med* 121:493, 1993.

153. Dale GL: Does surface bound immunoglobulin mediate erythrocyte death? Commentary. *Blood Cells* 14:36, 1988.

154. Connor J, Pak CC, Schroit AJ: Exposure of phosphatidylserine in the outer leaflet of human red blood cells. Relationship to cell density, cell age, and clearance by mononuclear cells. *J Biol Chem* 269:2399, 1994.

155. Nagel RL, Gibson QH: The binding of hemoglobin to haptoglobin and its relation to subunit dissociation of hemoglobin. *J Biol Chem* 246:69, 1971.

156. Garby L, Noyes WD: Studies on hemoglobin metabolism: I. The kinetic properties of the plasma hemoglobin pool in normal man. *J Clin Invest* 38:1479, 1959.

157. Hershko C: The fate of circulating hemoglobins. *Br J Haematol* 29:199, 1975.

158. Sears DA: Disposal of plasma heme in normal man and patients with intravascular hemolysis. *J Clin Invest* 49:5, 1970.

159. Rosen H, Sears DA: Spectral properties of hemopexinheme: The Schumm test. *J Lab Clin Med* 74:941, 1969.

160. Maines MD: The heme oxygenase system: a regulator of second messenger gases. *Annu Rev Pharmacol Toxicol* 37:517, 1997.

161. Elder G, Gray CH, Nicholson DG: Bile pigment fate in gastrointestinal tract. *Semin Hematol* 9:71, 1972.

CLINICAL MANIFESTATIONS AND CLASSIFICATION OF ERYTHROCYTE DISORDERS

ALLAN J. ERSLEV

Anemias and polycythemias are characterized, respectively by a decreased or increased size of the red cell mass. Since the anemias are associated with a decrease in the oxygen-carrying capacity of blood, they are usually expressed in terms of hemoglobin concentration and cause symptoms because of tissue hypoxia. The clinical manifestations are primarily due to hypoxia-induced compensatory features designed to prevent or ameliorate dangerous anoxia. Among these, the most important is an increase in the renal erythroid growth factor; however, almost all appear to be initiated by a single hypoxia-inducible transcription factor, HIF. The classification of anemia is evolving, since it must take into account new kinetic and molecular findings, and the classification given here is tentative and not always followed in this textbook.

The polycythemias are best expressed in terms of the hematocrit percentage, since their clinical manifestations are primarily related to the size of the red cell mass and to the viscosity of blood. The classification is less complex than that for anemias, and is based on arterial oxygen saturations, associated changes in other blood counts, and erythropoietin concentrations.

Erythrocyte disorders are traditionally divided into two groups: (1) anemia and (2) polycythemia. Although this division is based on the presence of too few red cells (erythrocytopenia) and too many red cells (erythrocytosis), anemia is functionally best characterized by a hemoglobin concentration below normal and polycythemia by a hematocrit above normal. This use of two different erythroid parameters in the characterization of anemia and polycythemia is based on clinical considerations. Anemia is a disorder in which the patient suffers from tissue hypoxia, the consequence of a low oxygen-carrying capacity of the blood. Polycythemia, on the other hand, is a disorder in which the clinical manifestations are related to increased whole blood viscosity and increased blood volume, both consequences of a high hematocrit.

ANEMIA

PATHOPHYSIOLOGY AND MANIFESTATIONS

The clinical manifestations of anemia are to some extent determined by its etiology and pathogenesis. Certain signs and symptoms, however, are general and can be attributed to a reduction in oxygen-carrying capacity. Although the red cells also carry carbon dioxide

Acronyms and abbreviations used in this chapter include: HIF-1, hypoxia inducible factor.

from the tissues to the lungs and help distribute nitric oxide throughout the body, the transport of these gases does not appear to be dependent on the number of red cells available and stays normal in anemic patients. A reduction in oxygen-carrying capacity, on the other hand, will cause tissue hypoxia and in turn mobilize a number of compensatory mechanisms designed to prevent or ameliorate destructive tissue anoxia.

Tissue hypoxia occurs when the pressure head of oxygen in the capillaries is too low to provide distant cells with enough oxygen for their metabolic needs. This may happen despite the presence of several times the needed amount of oxygen in the circulating blood. Using approximate figures for a normal adult, the red cell mass has to provide the tissues with about 250 ml/min of oxygen to support life. Since the oxygen-carrying capacity of normal blood is 1.34 ml per gram hemoglobin, or about 20 ml/dl of normal blood, and the cardiac output is about 5000 ml/min, 1000 ml/min of oxygen is available at the tissue level. The extraction of one-fourth of this amount will reduce the oxygen tension of 100 mmHg in the arterial end of the capillary to 40 mmHg in the venous end. This partial extraction will ensure the presence of sufficient diffusion pressure throughout the capillaries to provide all cells within a truncated cone segment with enough oxygen for their metabolic needs (Fig. 30-1). In anemia, the extraction of the same amount of oxygen would lead to greater hemoglobin desaturation and a lower oxygen tension at the venous end of the capillary. Since this would result in destructive cellular hypoxia or anoxia in the immediate vicinity, a number of compensatory and frequently symptomatic adjustments in the supply of blood and oxygen are initiated selectively throughout the body.

Many of these protective adjustments involve the production and stabilization of a single protein complex, HIF-1. This protein was first identified as a transcriptional factor for the erythropoietin gene[1] (see Chap. 29). Subsequent studies have shown that it is also capable of activating other genes involved in protection against hypoxia. For example, HIF-1 transcribes genes coding for many glycolytic enzymes, for growth factors controlling vessel formation, and for proteins regulating vasomotor function.[2-4] It appears that the HIF-1 complex consists of two parts, HIF-1α and HIF-1β. Both are constitutively produced, but while HIF-1β is stable, HIF-1α has a very short lifespan and is continually destroyed under normoxic conditions. However, in the absence of oxygen, it is also stable, and the HIF-1 complex becomes functional as a transcriptional protein. The oxygen-sensitive process of destruction may be controlled by a hypothetical heme protein which, when deoxygenated under hypoxic conditions, inactivates the degradation process.[4] Alternatively, degradation may be controlled by an enzyme sensitive to the presence or absence of oxygen.[5] Although HIF-1 may be present and functional in all hypoxic cells, its action varies from cell to cell. Consequently, tissue-specific and still unknown interacting factors must be present to explain the mobilization of the many compensatory mechanisms listed below that permit survival under hypoxic conditions.

DECREASED OXYGEN CONSUMPTION

The activation of genes coding for glycolytic enzymes[2] will save oxygen but at the expense of using less-efficient metabolic pathways. Actually anaerobic glycolysis is not employed extensively in chronic well-tolerated anemias,[6] and the overall consumption of oxygen in anemia may actually be 10 to 15 percent higher than normal because of the metabolic cost of cardiac and pulmonary overactivity.[7]

DECREASED OXYGEN AFFINITY

One of the earliest and least costly adjustments of oxygen delivery is a decrease in the affinity of hemoglobin for oxygen. This permits increased oxygen extraction without jeopardizing oxygen pressure[8,9] (Chap. 28). Since there is no consistent decrease in the pH of blood

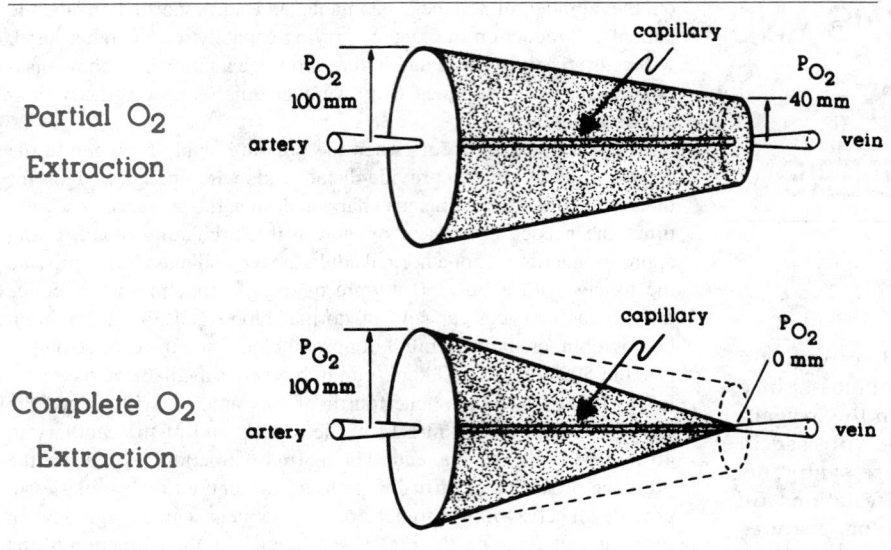

Partial O₂ Extraction

Complete O₂ Extraction

FIGURE 30-1   Theoretical tissue segment provided with oxygen from one capillary. With an arterial diffusion pressure of oxygen of 100 mmHg and partial oxygen extraction resulting in a venous oxygen pressure of 40 mmHg, one capillary can provide oxygen to cells within a truncated cone segment. With complete oxygen extraction, however, oxygen cannot be supplied to cells within a rim of tissue around the apex of the cone.

or evidence of impaired CO_2 removal from the tissues, the observed change in oxygen affinity cannot be accounted for by a simple Bohr shift to the right. However, the red cells of patients with anemia generate increased amounts of 2,3-bisphosphoglycerate,[9] and this phosphate compound has the capacity to combine with deoxygenated hemoglobin and decrease its affinity for oxygen (Chap. 28). The reason for increased synthesis of 2,3-bisphosphoglycerate in anemia is not fully understood but is related, in part, to a rise in the intracellular pH of red cells (Chap. 26). Accumulation of 2,3-bisphosphoglycerate has also been demonstrated in red cells of individuals with high-altitude hypoxemia.[10]

INCREASED TISSUE PERFUSION

The effect of a decreased oxygen-carrying capacity on the tissue tension of oxygen can be offset if, by using all potential capillary channels, the distance from tissue cells to oxygen supply is reduced. This can be accomplished via HIF-1 activation of genes regulating both vasomotor activity and angiogenesis.[2] Since in most anemias the blood volume is not changed significantly (Fig. 30-2),[11] increased tissue perfusion has to be performed selectively with blood shunted from presumably nonvital donor areas to oxygen-sensitive recipient organs. The major donor areas for the redistribution of blood in moderate acute anemia in the experimental animal are the mesenteric and iliac beds.[12] However, in chronic anemia in humans the donor areas appear to be the cutaneous tissue[13] and the kidneys.[14] Vasoconstriction and oxygen deprivation in the dermal tissue appear to be well tolerated but are in part responsible for the characteristic pallor of anemia. Whether they also are responsible for the retinal hemorrhages seen occasionally in severe anemia is unknown, but no better explanation is available.[15] Although the kidney can hardly be thought of as a nonvital area, the oxygen supply under normal conditions is in excess of oxygen demands. The arteriovenous oxygen difference in the kidney is as low as 1.4 ml/dl (compared with the myocardium, where it may be as high as 20 ml/dl), indicating that even a severe reduction in the kidney perfusion will not limit oxidative cellular metabolism. Nevertheless, enough renal hypoxia must be present to activate HIF-1 and generate

increased amounts of erythropoietin and in turn new red cells (Chap. 33). The effect on renal excretory mechanisms is slight, since the reduction in renal blood flow is offset by the high plasmacrit and, even in severe anemia with the renal blood flow reduced by almost 50 percent, the renal plasma flow is only moderately curtailed.

The benefits derived from a redistribution of blood are obvious, and the organs with the most pressing need for oxygen, such as myocardium, brain, and muscles, will to a great extent be unhampered by a moderate reduction in oxygen-carrying capacity.

INCREASED CARDIAC OUTPUT

An increase in cardiac output is an excellent but metabolically expensive compensatory device.[16,17] It will decrease the fraction of oxygen that needs to be extracted during each circulation and thereby keep the oxygen pressure high. Since the viscosity of blood in anemic patients is lower than normal, and since selective vascular dilatation will decrease peripheral resistance, a high cardiac output can be maintained without any increase in blood pressure. Nevertheless, a measurable increase in the resting cardiac output does not occur until the hemoglobin concentration is below 7 g/dl, and clinical signs of cardiac hyperactivity are usually not present until the hemoglobin concentration reaches even lower levels.[18]

Signs of cardiac hyperactivity include tachycardia, increased arterial and capillary pulsation, and many hemodynamic murmurs.[19] The cardiac murmurs are usually systolic and are heard best at the apex or at the pulmonary valve area. Diastolic murmurs are unusual, but all murmurs in an anemic patient should be considered hemodynamic until proved otherwise. Murmurs and bruits have been described in many regions, such as over the jugular vein, the closed eye, and the parietal region of the skull, and these murmurs and bruits often are sensed by the patient as roaring in the ears (tinnitus), especially at

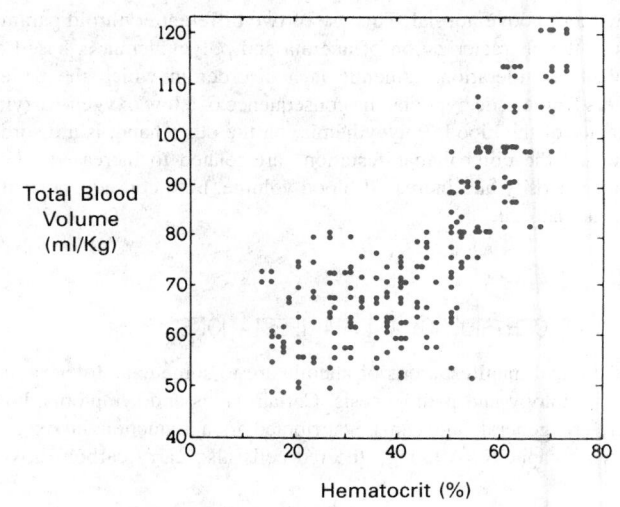

FIGURE 30-2   Relation between hematocrit and total blood volume in normal individuals and in patients with anemia and polycythemia (Huber, Lewis, and Szur[11]).

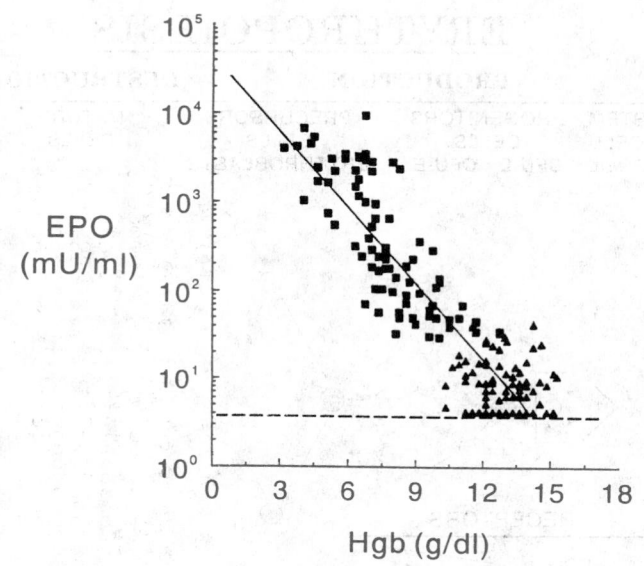

FIGURE 30-3   Erythropoietin levels in plasma of normal individuals and patients with anemia uncomplicated by renal or inflammatory disease. The lower limit of accuracy of the erythropoietin assay is 3 mU/ml and is indicated by a broken line. ■, anemias; ▲, normals.

night. Their characteristic feature is that they disappear promptly after the hemoglobin concentration has been restored to normal.[20] The normal myocardium will tolerate a prolonged period of sustained hyperactivity. However, angina pectoris and high-output failure may supervene if anemia is so extreme that it impairs coronary oxygen demands or if the patient has coronary artery disease.[21,22] Cardiomegaly, pulmonary congestion, ascites, and edema have been observed, and they require emergency treatment with oxygen, intravenous furosemide, and transfusion of packed red cells.

INCREASED PULMONARY FUNCTION
Since at sea level blood, regardless of oxygen-carrying capacity, is nearly completely oxygenated in the lungs, the oxygen pressure of arterial blood in an anemic patient should be the same as that in a normal individual, about 100 mmHg. Nevertheless, an increase in respiratory rate or vital capacity will decrease the oxygen gradient from ambient air to alveolar air and will increase the amount of oxygen available to oxygenate a greater than normal cardiac output. Consequently, exertional dyspnea and orthopnea are characteristic clinical manifestations of severe anemia.[18,19]

INCREASED RED CELL PRODUCTION
The most appropriate response to anemia is a compensatory increase in the rate of red cell production. In anemia this increase may reach 6 to 10 times normal and is powered by an increased synthesis of renal erythropoietin (see Chap. 33). The rate of synthesis of erythropoietin is inversely and logarithmically related to the hemoglobin concentration and produces an erythropoietin concentration in plasma ranging from about 10 mU/ml at normal hemoglobin concentrations to 10,000 mU or more per milliliter in severe anemia (Fig. 30-3).[24,25] The change in erythropoietin levels ensures that in most cases red cell production will balance red cell destruction or red cell loss at a hemoglobin concentration much higher than that which would be found if the rate of red cell production had stayed the same. The administration of exogenous human recombinant erythropoietin augments or replaces endogenous synthesis. Using pharmacologic amounts, the effect on

hemoglobin concentration will be most noticeable if endogenous production is subnormal due to renal failure or systemic illnesses.[26] In severe anemias in which endogenous production of erythropoietin already has increased red cell production to its utmost, no amount of recombinant erythropoietin will be of help and the patients will become transfusion-dependent. Clinically increased erythroid activity can occasionally be recognized by sternal tenderness and diffuse bone aches or pains. An increase in the number of circulating reticulocytes is the most significant laboratory reflection of accelerated red cell production. Since the erythroid transit time through the marrow is shortened, "stress reticulocytes" with increased volume and reticulum appear, and nucleated red cells may be observed.[27-29]

UNCORRECTED TISSUE HYPOXIA
Despite the mobilization of compensatory mechanisms, a certain residual degree of tissue hypoxia remains. Some of this contributes the necessary driving force to sustain cardiovascular and erythropoietic adjustments, but tissue hypoxia per se may cause disturbing and even disabling symptoms. Angina pectoris, intermittent claudication, and night cramps are muscular signs of tissue hypoxia; headache, light-headedness, and faintness are cerebral signs. A number of diffuse gastrointestinal and genitourinary symptoms have been associated with anemia, but it is uncertain whether they should be attributed to tissue hypoxia, compensatory redistribution of blood, or the underlying cause of anemia.

CLASSIFICATION

On the basis of determination of the red cell mass, both anemia and polycythemia can be classified as (1) relative or (2) absolute. *Relative anemia* and *relative polycythemia* are both characterized by a normal total red cell mass. Such conditions are usually not thought of as hematologic disorders but rather as disturbances in the regulation of the plasma volume. However, both dilution anemia and dehydration polycythemia are of considerable clinical and differential diagnostic importance for the hematologist.

The classification of the *absolute anemias* with a decreased red cell mass is difficult, since it has to take into account kinetic, morphologic, and pathophysiologic interacting criteria. Initially, all anemias should be divided into anemias caused by decreased production and anemias caused by increased destruction of red cells. This differentiation is to a great extent based on the reticulocyte count. Subsequent diagnostic breakdown can be based on either morphologic or pathophysiologic criterias.

The *morphologic classification* subdivides anemia into (1) macrocytic anemia, (2) normocytic anemia, and (3) microcytic hypochromic anemia. The main advantages of this classification are that it is simple, it is based on readily available red cell indices (MCV and MCHC), and it forces the physician always to consider the most important types of curable anemia: vitamin B_{12}, folic acid, and iron-deficiency anemias. Such practical considerations have led to a wide acceptance of this classification. However, *pathophysiologic classification* (Table 30-1) is best suited for relating disease processes to potential treatment.

An attempt will be made in this chapter to present a classification based on our present concepts of normal red cell production and red cell destruction. Figure 30-4 outlines the cascade of proliferation, differentiation, and maturation that underlies the transformation of a multipotential stem cell, first to erythroid progenitor cells, then to erythroid precursor cells, and last to mature red cells. Each of these steps can become impaired and cause an anemia, and our capacity to manage these anemias depends to a great extent on identifying the defective step. The problem with such a classification is that in most anemias the pathogenesis involves several steps. For example, a de-

TABLE 30-1   CLASSIFICATION OF ANEMIA

A. Relative
   1. Macroglobulinemia
   2. Pregnancy
   3. Athletes
   4. Postflight astronauts
B. Absolute
   1. Decreased red cell production
      a. Stem-cell failure
         (1) Aplastic anemia
         (2) Anemia of leukemia and of myelodysplastic syndromes
      b. Progenitor-cell failure
         (1) Pure red cell aplasia
         (2) Renal failure
         (3) Chronic disorders
         (4) Endocrine disorders
      c. Precursor-cell failure
         (1) Megaloblastic anemias
         (2) Iron-deficiency anemia
         (3) Thalassemia
         (4) Hemoglobinpathies
         (5) Congenital enzyme deficiencies
   2. Increased red cell destruction or loss
      a. Hereditary
         (1) Membrane defects
         (2) Globin defects
         (3) Enzyme defects
      b. Acquired
         (1) Macroangiopathic (traumatic)
         (2) Microangiopathic
         (3) Antibody-mediated
         (4) Hypersplenism
         (5) Acute blood loss

crease in the rate of production will most often result in the production of defective red cells with a shortened lifespan. Also, antibodies, cytokines growth factors, and nutritional elements usually affect several steps in the outlined cascade of production and destruction. For such reasons, the individual chapter on anemia in this textbook does not always follow this pathophysiologic classification, and the outline given here must be tentative and is provided primarily as a conceptual guide to our present understanding of the processes underlying the production and destruction of red cells.

POLYCYTHEMIA (ERYTHROCYTOSIS)

PATHOPHYSIOLGY AND MANIFESTATIONS

The production and presence of an increased number of red cells are associated with certain general and specific effects generated by changes in blood viscosity and blood volume.

At hematocrit readings higher than 50 percent, the viscosity of blood increases steeply (Fig. 30-5). The resulting decrease in blood flow will reduce the transport of oxygen, with optimal values found at hematocrit readings between 40 and 45 percent. In a study of the red cells from a number of animal species, it was found that the optimal value of oxygen transport corresponds closely to their normal hematocrits[30] and may explain the evolutionary choice of certain hematocrit levels as optimal.[30] However, before concluding that polycythemia always is a suboptimal condition, it is important to realize that it may be premature to translate viscosity readings, derived from blood tested in a rigid glass viscosimeter (Ostwald) or even in a cone-plate viscometer into blood flow through tiny distensible vessels in vivo.[32] First, the flow through these narrow channels is rapid (high shear rate), which in a non-Newtonian fluid such as blood causes a marked decrease in viscosity. Second, blood flowing through narrow channels in vivo is axial with a central core of packed red cells sliding over a

ERYTHROPOIESIS

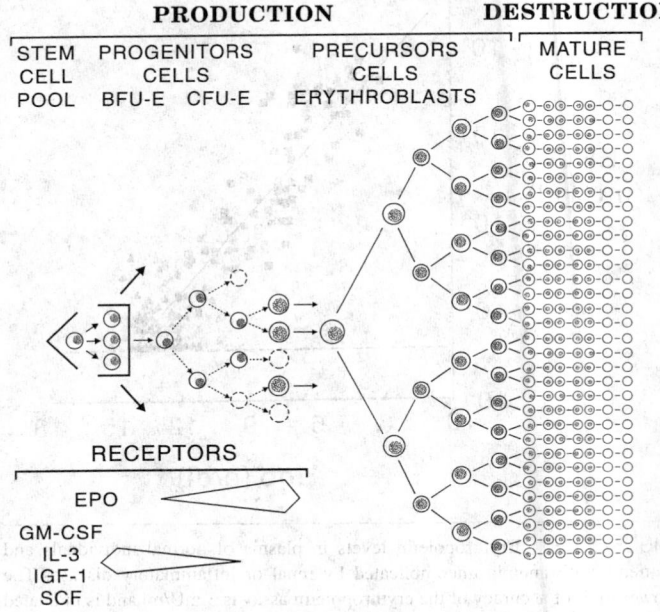

FIGURE 30-4   An outline of the process of differentiation, proliferation, and maturation underlying the production and destruction of red blood cells. The multipotential stem cells responding to a number of growth factors, granulocyte-monocyte colony-stimulating factors (GM-CSF). Interleukin-3 (IL-3), insulin growth factor (IGF-1), and stem-cell factor (SCF) among others, will differentiate to progenitor cells committed to erythroid development. The progenitor cells, burst-forming units (BFU-E), and colony-forming units (CFU-E) will proliferate under the control of erythropoietin (EPO) and finally differentiate to precursor cells (erythroblasts). In the presence of adequate amounts of nutrients, such as B_{12}, folic acid, and iron, the precursor cells will proliferate and mature into nucleated red cells, reticulocytes, and mature red blood cells. After a 120-day lifespan, these cells will age and be destroyed.

peripheral layer of lubricating low-viscosity plasma. Finally and most important, absolute polycythemia is not normovolemic but is accompanied by an increase in blood volume, which in turn enlarges the vascular bed and decreases the peripheral resistance. Since the blood pressure remains stable, the increase in blood volume must be associated with an increase in cardiac output and an increase in oxygen transport (cardiac output times hematocrit). Using measurements of cardiac output in dogs[33] and tissue oxygen tension in rats and mice,[34] it is possible to construct curves (Fig. 30-6) that relate oxygen transport to hematocrit in normovolemic and hypervolemic states. These curves show that hypervolemia per se will increase oxygen transport and that the optimum oxygen transport in these conditions is found at higher hematocrit values than in normovolemic states. Consequently, despite the increase in viscosity, a moderate increase in hematocrit is of benefit. The same may not be true of a more pronounced increase in hematocrit. Here observations in humans[35] and experimental animals[36] indicate that high viscosity causes a reduction in blood flow to most tissues and may be responsible for the cerebral and cardiovascular impairment experienced occasionally by high-altitude dwellers[37] and patients with severe polycythemia,[38,39] and also in athletes self-administering overdoses of erythropoietin (see Chap. 52).

Although the rate of red cell production is increased in erythrocytosis, changes in marrow morphology may be quite unimpressive. Under normal conditions, the rate of red cell production is adjusted to maintain the red cell mass at about 30 ml per kilogram of body weight. Since the lifespan of the red cells in polycythemia is normal, a mere doubling of the daily rate of red cell production would be adequate to maintain a red cell mass of 60 ml/kg or, in other words, to maintain a very substantial erythrocytosis. Consequently, the morphology and volume of the marrow are only moderately altered in polycythemia in comparison with the changes observed in some types of hemolytic anemia, in which the rate of red cell production may be 6 to 10 times normal. In erythrocytosis, the number of red cells destroyed daily would merely cause a slight increase in bilirubin levels and the presence of secondary gout and splenomegaly are usually signs of a myeloproliferative disorder rather than of erythrocytosis alone. Although, there is a considerable homology between erythropoietin and thrombopoietin,[40] erythropoietin-driven erythrocytosis is not associated with an increase in platelet production.

The increase in viscosity and vascular space are responsible for many of the signs and symptoms of polycythemia. The characteristic "ruddy cyanosis" in patients with polycythemia vera is caused by excessive deoxygenation of blood flowing sluggishly through dilated cutaneous vessels. Nonspecific symptoms such as headaches, dizziness, tinnitus, and a feeling of fullness of the face and head are probably also caused by a combination of increased viscosity and vascular dilatation.

Hemorrhages from the nose or stomach in patients with normal platelets and coagulation proteins can be attributed to capillary distention, but circulatory stagnation causing ischemia and necrosis may be contributory. Thromboses are common in polycythemia vera, but they also occur in erythrocytosis when aggravated by plasma loss (dehydration). Since coronary blood flow is decreased in polycythemia,[38] it has been assumed that the risk of coronary thrombosis in patients with a high hematocrit is increased, but statistical analyses have yielded equivocal results.[39,41,42] It has actually been claimed that polycythemia does not pose a risk in surgical patients.[43] Although cerebral blood flow

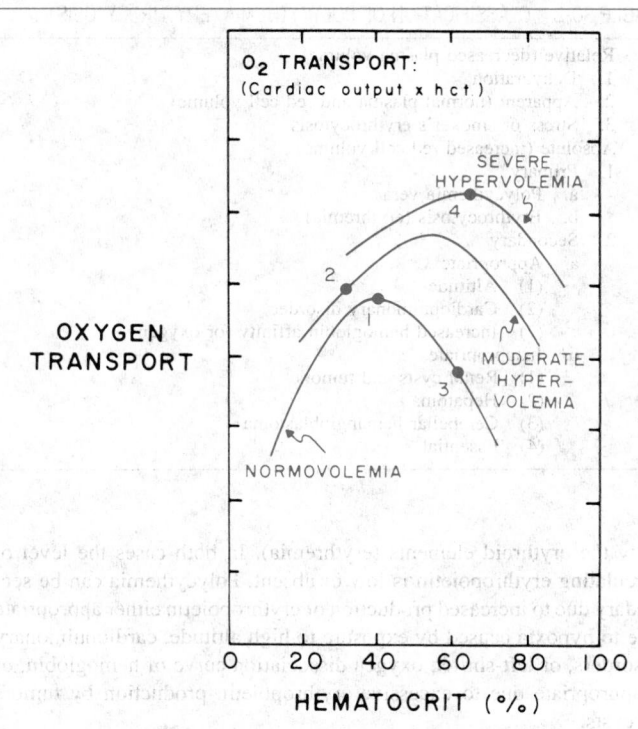

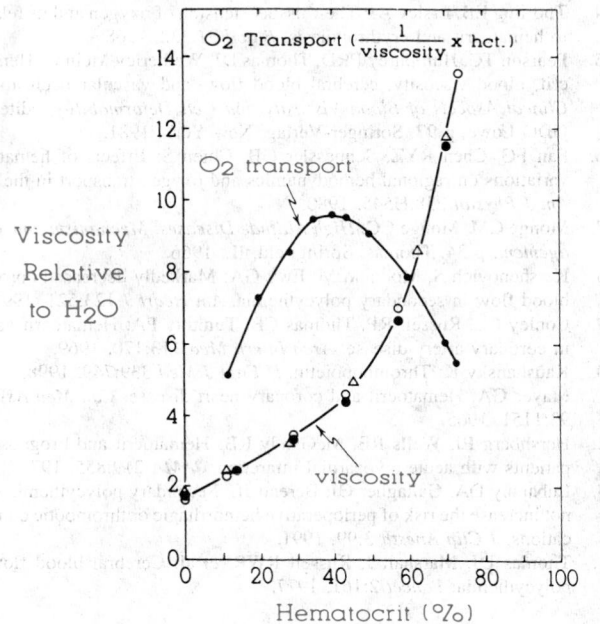

FIGURE 30-5   Viscosity of heparinized normal human blood related to hematocrit (Hct). Viscosity is measured with an Ostwald viscosimeter at 37°C and expressed in relation to viscosity of saline solution. Oxygen transport is computed from Hct and O_2 flow (1/viscosity) and is recorded in arbitrary units.

FIGURE 30-6   Oxygen transport at various hematocrit levels in normovolemic, mildly hypervolemic, and severely hypervolemic individuals. The oxygen transport is estimated by multiplying hematocrit by cardiac output. As can be seen in (1), the optimal oxygen transport for the normovolemic subjects is at a hematocrit of about 45 percent with a progressive rise in the optimal hematocrit as the blood volume increases. A suboptimal hematocrit in a hypervolemic person (anemia of pregnancy), as in (2), may be associated with a higher oxygen transport than that of a normovolemic person with normal hematocrit. However, a high hematocrit without an increase in blood volume (3) may be associated with an absolute reduction in oxygen transport and tissue hypoxia. Only high hematocrit coupled with high blood volume (4) enhances oxygen transport to the tissues. (Adapted from Murray and colleagues[33] and Thorling and Erslev.[34])

is materially reduced in patients with moderately elevated hematocrit,[44] such reductions may have little practical significance.

CLASSIFICATION

Polycythemia, or *erythrocytosis,* is defined as a condition in which the hematocrit percentage is above the upper limit of normal or in men above 51 percent and in women above 48 percent. It can be classified as relative, in which the red cell mass is normal but the plasma volume is decreased, or absolute, in which the red cell mass is increased above normal (Table 30-2). At hematocrits of less than 60 percent differentiation of absolute from relative polycythemia may, at times, be difficult. The designation of a measured red cell mass as normal is very imprecise, since it depends on the age, sex, weight, height, and body frame of the individual and since only increases above the mean greater than 25 percent are considered abnormal. This leaves a number of conditions with increased hematocrits but a "normal" red cell mass. Such conditions are usually associated with the same illnesses involved in the pathogenesis of absolute erythrocytosis. If the hematocrit is above 60 percent, the red cell mass is almost always increased.

Absolute polycythemia may be primary, representing uncontrolled overproduction of all marrow cells (polycythemia vera) or

TABLE 30-2   CLASSIFICATION OF POLYCYTHEMIA (ERYTHROCYTOSIS)

A. Relative (decreased plasma volume)
　　1. Dehydration
　　2. Apparent (normal plasma and red cell volume)
　　3. Stress or smoker's erythrocytosis
B. Absolute (increased red cell volume)
　　1. Primary
　　　　a. Polycythemia vera
　　　　b. Erythrocytosis (erythremia)
　　2. Secondary
　　　　a. Appropriate
　　　　　　(1) Altitude
　　　　　　(2) Cardiopulmonary disorder
　　　　　　(3) Increased hemoglobin affinity for oxygen
　　　　b. Inappropriate
　　　　　　(1) Renal cysts and tumors
　　　　　　(2) Hepatoma
　　　　　　(3) Cerebellar hemangioblastoma
　　　　　　(4) Essential

only the erythroid elements (erythremia). In both cases the level of circulating erythropoietin is low or absent. Polycythemia can be secondary due to increased production of erythropoietin either appropriate due to hypoxia caused by exposure to high altitude, cardiopulmonary disorders, or left-shifted oxygen dissociation curve of hemoglobin, or inappropriate due to excessive erythropoietin production by tumors or cysts.

REFERENCES

1. Semanza GL, Nejfelt MK, Chi SM, Antonarakis SE: Hypoxia-inducible nuclear factors bind to an enhancer element located 3′ to the human erythropoietin gene. *Proc Natl Acad Sci U S A* 88:5680, 1991.
2. Guillemin K, Krasnow MA: The hypoxic response: Huffing and HIFing. *Cell* 89:9, 1997.
3. Hochachka PW, Buck LT, Doll CJ, Land SC: Unifying theory of hypoxia tolerance: molecular/metabolic defense and rescue mechanisms for surviving oxygen lack. *Proc Natl Acad Sci* 93:9493, 1996.
4. Bunn HF, Gu J, Huang E, Park J-W, Zhu H: Erythropoietin: a model system for studying oxygen-dependent gene regulation. *J Exp Biol* 201:1197, 1998.
5. Srinivas V, Zhu X, Salceda S, Nakamura R, Caro J: Hypoxia-inducible Factor 1α (HIF-1α) is a non-heme iron protein. *J Biol Chem* 273:18019, 1998.
6. Robin ED: Of men and mitochondria: coping with hypoxic dysoxia. *Am Rev Respir Dis* 122:517, 1980.
7. Brannon ES, Merrill AJ, Warren JV, Stead EA, Jr: The cardiac output in patients with chronic anemia as measured by the technique of right arterial catherization. *J Clin Invest* 24:332, 1945.
8. Edwards MJ, Novy MJ, Walters CL, Metcalfe J: Improved oxygen release: an adaptation of mature red cells to hypoxia. *J Clin Invest* 47:1851, 1968.
9. Boning D, Enciso G: Hemoglobin-oxygen affinity in anemia. *Blut* 54:361, 1987.
10. Moore LG, Brewer GJ: Beneficial effect of rightward hemoglobin-oxygen dissociation curve shift for short-term high-altitude adaptation. *J Lab Clin Med* 98:145, 1981.
11. Huber H, Lewis SM, Szur L: The influence of anaemia, polycythaemia and splenomegaly on the relationship between venous haematocrit and red-cell volume. *Br J Haematol* 10:567, 1964.
12. Vatner SF: Effects of hemorrhage on regional blood flow distribution in dogs and primates. *J Clin Invest* 54:225,1974.
13. Abramson DJ, Fierst SM, Flachs K: Resting peripheral blood flow in the anemic state. *Am Heart J* 25:609, 1954.
14. Bradley SE, Bradley GP: Renal function during chronic anemia in man. *Blood* 2:192, 1947.
15. Merin S, Freund M: Retinopathy in severe anemia. *Am J Ophthalmol* 66:1102, 1968.
16. Sproule BJ, Mitchell JH, Miller WF: Cardiopulmonary physiological responses to heavy exercise in patients with anemia. *J Clin Invest* 39:378, 1960.
17. Duke M, Abelman WH: The hemodynamic response to chronic anemia. *Circulation* 39:503, 1969.
18. Sharpey-Schafer EP: Cardiac output in severe anemia. *Clin Sci* 5:125, 1944.
19. Wintrobe MM: The cardiovascular system in anemia. *Blood* 1:121, 1946.
20. Wales RT, Martin EA: Arterial bruits in anemia. *Br Med J* 2:1444, 1963.
21. Zoll PM, Wessler S, Blumgart HL: Angina pectoris: a clinical and pathologic correlation. *Am J Med* 11:330, 1951.
22. Varat MA, Adolph RJ, Fowler NO: Cardiovascular effects of anemia. *Am Heart J* 83:415, 1972.
23. Blumgart HL, Altschule MD: Clinical significance of cardiac and respiratory adjustments in chronic anemia. *Blood* 3:329, 1948.
24. Adamson JW: The erythropoietin/hematocrit relationship in normal and polycythemic man: implications of marrow regulation. *Blood* 32:597, 1968.
25. Jelkmann W: Erythropoietin: structure, control of production and function. *Physiol Rev* 72:449, 1992.
26. Erslev AJ: Erythropoietin. *N Engl J Med* 324:1339, 1991.
27. Finch CA, Deubelbeiss K, Cook JD, et al: Ferrokinetics in man. *Medicine (Baltimore)* 49:17, 1970.
28. Hillman RS, Finch CA: Erythropoiesis: normal and abnormal. *Semin Hematol* 4:327, 1967.
29. Ward HP, Halman J: The association of nucleated red cells in the peripheral smear with hypoxemia. *Ann Intern Med* 67:1190, 1967.
30. Dintenfass I: A preliminary outline of the blood high viscosity syndromes. *Arch Intern Med* 118:427, 1966.
31. Stone HO, Thompson HK Jr, Schmidt-Nielson K: Influence of erythrocytes on blood viscosity. *Am J Physiol* 221:913, 1968.
32. Erslev AJ, Caro J, Schuster SJ: Is there an optimal hemoglobin level? *Transfusion Med Rev* 3:237, 1989.
33. Murray JF, Gold P, Johnson BL Jr: The circulatory effects of hematocrit variations in normovolemic and hypervolemic dogs. *J Clin Invest* 42:1150, 1963.
34. Thorling EB, Erslev AJ: The "tissue" tension of oxygen and its relation to hematocrit and erythropoiesis. *Blood* 31:332, 1968.
35. Pearson TC, Humphrey PRD, Thomas DJ, Wetherley Mein G: Hematocrit, blood viscosity, cerebral blood flow, and vascular occlusion, in *Clincal Aspects of Blood Viscosity and Cell Deformability,* edited by GDO Lowe, p 97. Springer-Verlag, New York, 1981.
36. Fan FC, Chen RYZ, Schuessler GB, Chien S: Effects of hematocrit variations on regional hemodynamics and oxygen transport in the dog. *Am J Physiol* 238:H545, 1980.
37. Monge CM, Monge CC: *High Altitude Diseases: Mechanism and Management,* p 34. Thomas, Springfield, IL, 1966.
38. Kershenovich S, Modiano M, Ewy GA: Markedly decreased coronary blood flow in secondary polycythemia. *Am Heart J* 123:521, 1992.
39. Conley CL, Russell RP, Thomas CB, Tumulty PA: Hematocrit values in coronary artery disease. *Arch Intern Med* 113:170, 1969.
40. Kaushansky K: Thrombopoietin. *N Engl J Med* 339:749, 1998.
41. Mayer GA: Hematocrit and coronary heart disease. *Can Med Assoc J* 93:1151, 1965.
42. Hershberg PJ, Wells RE, McGandy RB: Hematocrit and prognosis in patients with acute myocardial infarction. *JAMA* 219:855, 1972.
43. Lubarsky DA, Gallagher CJ, Berend JL: Secondary polycythemia does not increase the risk of perioperative hemorrhagic or thrombotic complications. *J Clin Anesth* 3:99, 1991.
44. Thomas DJ, Marshall J, Russell RWR, et al: Cerebral blood flow in polycythemia. *Lancet* 2:161, 1977.

APLASTIC ANEMIA

RICHARD K. SHADDUCK

The term *aplastic anemia* describes a clinical syndrome in which there is a deficiency of red cells, neutrophils, and monocytes, and platelets without morphologic evidence of another marrow disorder. Marrow examination shows a near absence of hematopoietic precursor cells and fatty replacement. The disorder can be induced by toxic chemicals (e.g., benzene), specific viruses (e.g., Epstein-Barr virus), or can be inherited (e.g., Fanconi's anemia). Most cases occur without an evident incitant and are the result of autoreactive T lymphocytes that suppress or destroy hematopoietic cells. The disease may be ameliorated or sometimes cured by immunosuppressive therapy, especially antithymocyte globulin. For those with a suitable donor, allogeneic stem cell therapy is often curative. The disease, even after successful treatment with immunosuppressive agents, has a propensity to evolve into a clonal hematopoietic disorder such as paroxysmal nocturnal hemoglobinuria, oligoblastic or acute myelogenous leukemia.

DEFINITION AND HISTORY

Aplastic anemia results from a failure of blood cell production in the marrow. This results in a markedly hypocellular marrow and varying degrees of anemia, granulocytopenia, and thrombocytopenia. Most cases of aplastic anemia are acquired. The decrease in hematopoiesis may be secondary to toxic effects of offending agents on marrow stem cells; in many cases, however, the pathogenesis is the suppression of blood cell progenitor proliferation and maturation by autoreactive lymphocytes. The disease also may occur as the result of an inherited disorder, especially Fanconi anemia. A close association also exists between the clonal hemopathy, PNH, and aplastic anemia.

Aplastic anemia was first recognized by Ehrlich in 1888.[1] He described a young pregnant woman who died of severe anemia and neutropenia; autopsy examination revealed a fatty marrow with essentially no hematopoiesis. The name *aplastic anemia* was subsequently applied to this disease in 1904.[2] Over the next 30 years many conditions that caused pancytopenia were confused with aplastic anemia based on incomplete or inadequate histologic study of the patient's marrow. Marrow biopsies are required to document that a hypocellular marrow aspirate represents hypoplasia or aplasia and to exclude other conditions that may infiltrate, replace, or suppress normal marrow cells.[3]

ETIOLOGY AND PATHOGENESIS

It is unclear why some individuals who are exposed repeatedly to potential marrow toxins sustain severe and often irreversible marrow injury, whereas most have no untoward effects. It has been postulated that there is a genetic predisposition based on a high incidence of HLA class II antigens DR2[4] and DPw3[5] in patients with marrow aplasia. The disease may result from the accumulated effects of multiple noxious exposures on pluripotential stem cells. Ultimately, all stem cells sustain sufficient damage to hinder their ability to replicate. Alternatively, such exposures may induce a single abnormal cell to proliferate in a clonal fashion and to somehow hinder the growth of normal stem cells. The result in the first case would be aplastic anemia from a polyclonal injury (classical aplastic anemia) to stem cells and/or very early multipotential progenitor cells and in the latter injury to a single stem cell resulting in a monoclonal disorder (e.g., paroxysmal nocturnal hemoglobinuria—aplastic anemia syndrome). Although classic aplastic anemia and paroxysmal nocturnal hemoglobinuria are thought to be distinct clinical entities, studies suggest an overlap in these conditions. As many as 40 percent of patients with otherwise typical aplastic anemia have evidence of glycosyl-phosphatidylinositol molecule defects in leukocytes and red cells as judged by flow cytometry, analogous to that seen in PNH.[6-8] Aplastic anemia, hypoplastic myelodysplastic syndrome, and paroxysmal nocturnal hemoglobinuria each may eventually evolve into acute myelogenous leukemia.[9-13]

STEM CELLS, MICROENVIRONMENT, CYTOKINES

Potential mechanisms responsible for acquired marrow cell failure include induced defects in hematopoietic stem cells, failure of the stromal microenvironment of the marrow, impaired production or release of hemopoietic growth factors, and cellular or humoral immune suppression of the marrow. Several pathogenic abnormalities have been found in patients with aplastic anemia[14-18]; however, it is unclear whether these are inciting events or represent epiphenomena secondary to the disease. Although it is not possible to assess human totipotential stem cells in culture, their progeny are easily identified by clonal growth in vitro. The number of CFU-GM and BFU-E are reduced markedly in patients with aplastic anemia.[19-25] The more immature long-term culture initiating cells are also reduced to about 1 percent of normal values.[26] CD34-positive hematopoietic cells, in which fraction the hematopoietic stem cells reside, are also correspondingly low.[27,28] These findings suggest that reduced hematopoietic stem cells are the primary defect in the abnormal hematopoiesis. Stem cell inhibition may, however, occur by a T-cell–mediated suppressor effect. Early studies showed inhibition of colony growth by autologous marrow lymphocytes or by blood or marrow mononuclear cells from patients with aplastic anemia when cocultured with normal marrow.[20,23,29-31] In many cases the inhibition was thought to result from transfusion sensitization rather than autoimmunity.[32,33] However, culture studies in patients with aplastic anemia prior to transfusion[34] or before and after successful treatment[35,36] are highly suggestive of a T-cell–mediated suppressor cell phenomenon. Alternatively, injured hemopoietic stem cells may present neoantigens that serve as a stimulus for secondary T-cell–mediated suppression, which serves to worsen the aplasia.

Based on studies in rats, a theory of "seed" (stem cells) versus "soil" (microenvironment) abnormality was established.[37] Modest doses of irradiation to a limb lead to transient aplasia, with recovery secondary to ingress of circulating stem cells. With doses of 20 Gy (2000 rad) and greater, there is similar aplasia and recovery; however, permanent aplasia develops in this limb several months later. This appears to result from late damage to the marrow microenvironment, which may also occur in certain cases of aplastic anemia.

Pathogenetic studies have been conducted of the residual marrow damage in mice that receive busulfan.[38,39] Although blood counts are usually normal, both marrow progenitor cells and stem cells are decreased substantially. Some animals progress to chronic hypoplastic

Acronyms and abbreviations that appear in this chapter include: ALG, antilymphocyte globulin; ALS, antilymphocyte serum; ATG, antithymocyte globulin; BFU–E, erythroid burst-forming units; CFU-GM, granulocyte-macrophage colony-forming units; CMV, cytomegalovirus; EBV, Epstein-Barr virus; HHV, human herpes virus; HIV, human immunodeficiency virus; IL, interleukin; NMRI, nuclear magnetic resonance imaging; PNH, paroxysmal nocturnal hemoglobinuria; SCF, stem cell factor.

TABLE 31-1 ETIOLOGIC CLASSIFICATION OF APLASTIC ANEMIA

Acquired
  Chemicals
    Benzene
  Drugs
    Chloramphenicol
  Radiation
  Viruses
    Epstein-Barr virus; non-A, non-B, non-C hepatitis virus
  Miscellaneous
    Connective tissue disorders
    Pregnancy
Hereditary
  Fanconi anemia
  Dyskeratosis congenita
  Schwachman syndrome
Idiopathic
  About 65% of all cases

marrow failure, whereas others retain relatively normal blood counts.[38] When treated with chloramphenicol, animals exposed to busulfan have a marked decrease in progenitor cells, whereas controls are unaffected.[39] Perhaps similar repeated exposures with different agents may be necessary to induce aplastic anemia in humans.

The hematopoietic defects, macrocytic anemia, and mild hypoplasia occur in two strains of mice (WWv and Sl/Sld). WWv anemia is cured by lethal irradiation and infusion of stem cells from nonaffected litter mates, whereas the Steel (Sl) defect is not corrected by stem cell transplantation because it is the result of an abnormal microenvironment.[40] WWv cells are deficient in the proto-oncogene *kit,*[41] which encodes a tyrosine kinase receptor for the hemopoietic growth factor kit ligand[42] (see Chap. 14). Sl/Sld mice do not produce kit ligand, also called *stem cell factor* (SCF). Similar defects have not been observed in patients with aplastic anemia. Serum levels of SCF have been either moderately low or normal in several studies of aplastic anemia.[43–45] Although SCF augments the growth of hemopoietic colonies from aplastic marrows,[46] its use in patients has not led to clinical remissions. Another early acting growth factor, Flt-3 ligand, is 30- to 100-fold elevated in the serum of patients with aplastic anemia.[47] Short-term clonal assays for marrow stromal cells have shown variable defects in stromal cell function. Fibroblasts grown from patients with severe aplastic anemia have subnormal cytokine production. However, serum levels of granulocyte colony-stimulating factor,[48] erythropoietin,[49] and thrombopoietin[50] are usually high. Synthesis of IL-1, an early stimulator of hemopoiesis, is decreased in mononuclear cells from patients with aplastic anemia, but it is produced normally by cells from patients with myelodysplastic syndrome.[51] Levels of cytokines with inhibitory effects on hemopoiesis are increased in most patients with severe aplastic anemia. Increased mononuclear cell production of interferon-γ,[52,53] IL-2,[54] and tumor necrosis factor-α[55,56] has been noted spontaneously or in response to certain mitogens. Elevated serum levels of interferon-γ have been found in 30 percent of patients with aplastic anemia, and interferon-γ expression has been detected in the marrow of most patients with acquired aplastic anemia.[57] Moreover, addition of antibodies to interferon enhances in vitro colony growth of marrow cells from affected patients.[52] This suggests a potential role for interferon-γ in either the initiation or propagation of the defect in aplastic anemia.

Studies of the microenvironment have shown relatively normal stromal cell proliferation and growth factor production.[58–60] These findings, coupled with the limited response of patients with aplastic anemia to the known growth factors, suggest that cytokine deficiency is not the etiologic problem in most cases.

Potential causes for aplastic anemia are shown in Table 31-1. The disorder may follow exposure to various chemicals, drugs, radiation, or viruses. In addition, connective tissue disorders and pregnancy may be associated with marrow aplasia. Constitutional forms, particularly Fanconi anemia, develop in the setting of an underlying genetic defect. As many as 65 percent of cases of aplastic anemia, however, are idiopathic.

CHEMICALS

Benzene was the first chemical linked to aplastic anemia, based on studies in factory workers before the twentieth century.[61] Despite its known properties as a marrow toxin, benzene is still used widely as a solvent and is employed in the manufacture of chemicals, drugs, dyes, and explosives. It has been a vital chemical in the manufacture of rubber and leather goods and has been used widely in the shoe industry, leading to an increased risk for aplastic anemia and leukemia in workers in all these industries.[62–66] In China, where benzene is still used widely in industry, benzene poisoning was found in 0.5 percent of the workers; aplastic anemia among workers was sixfold higher than in the general population.[67]

The U.S. Occupational Safety and Health Administration has lowered the permissible exposure limit to benzene to 1 ppm,[68] after it was shown that exposure to 100 ppm was associated with leukopenia in about one-third of workers.[69] Other hematologic abnormalities have been observed in patients exposed to benzene, including hemolytic anemia, marrow hyperplasia, myeloid metaplasia, and acute myelogenous leukemia.[62–67,70]

There appears to be a relationship between the use of insecticides related to benzene and aplastic anemia. Chlorinated hydrocarbons and organophosphate compounds have been implicated in 280 cases reported in the literature.[71] DDT (chlorophenothane), lindane, and chlordane appear to be the most common insecticides involved. Aplastic anemia was reported following the use of lindane in home vaporizers for disinfection. This practice continued until the 1970s, when over 30 case reports of aplastic anemia led to its curtailment.[72] Occasional cases still occur following heavy exposure at industrial plants or after its use as a pesticide.[73] Lindane is metabolized in part to pentachlorophenol (PCP), another toxic chlorinated hydrocarbon that is manufactured for use as a wood preservative. Many cases of aplastic anemia and related blood disorders have been attributed to PCP over the past 25 years.[72–75] Prolonged exposures to petroleum distillates in the form of Stoddard solvent[76] and acute exposure of toluene through the practice of glue sniffing[77] have also been reported to cause aplasia. Trinitrotoluene (TNT), an explosive used extensively during World Wars I and II, is absorbed readily by inhalation and through the skin. Many fatal cases of aplastic anemia were observed in munitions workers exposed to TNT in Great Britain from 1940 to 1946.[78]

DRUGS

Chloramphenicol is a nitrobenzene compound with broad-spectrum antibiotic activity. It was introduced in 1948 and used widely during the 1950s and 1960s by various routes of administration, often for trivial indications. Reports of an association with aplastic anemia began early after its introduction.[79–81] Indiscriminant use of the drug continued, however, despite warnings to limit its use to infections caused by organisms that were resistant to other agents or for which no other drugs were available.[82] The risk of developing aplastic anemia in patients treated with chloramphenicol is about 1 in 20,000, or 10 to 50 times that of the general population.[83–85] Unfortunately, reports of fatal aplastic anemia continue to appear with topical or systemic use of the drug.[86,87]

Two adverse hematopoietic responses to the drug occur. Suppression of marrow function occurs in many individuals receiving the drug, with reduced erythroid cell production characterized by a rise in serum iron, accumulation of iron in the mitochondria, and vacuolization of marrow erythroid precursor cells.[88–91] Reticulocytes decrease and the hematocrit declines as inhibition of red cell production continues. Mild decreases in circulating neutrophils and platelets are also observed in some patients. These effects are probably the result of inhibition of mitochondrial protein synthesis and are reversible after discontinuation of the drug. There appears to be no relationship between this common, temporary inhibition of hematopoiesis and the rare, but devastating, severe aplastic anemia that ensues in a small proportion of patients. This latter reaction may occur weeks to months after treatment and does not appear related to the total drug exposure nor to the route of administration. Based on the nearly simultaneous development of aplastic anemia in identical twins given this agent,[92] it was postulated that there is a genetic defect that predisposes to this severe reaction to the drug.

With chloramphenicol, the many cases of aplastic anemia strongly established the potential for toxic effects with this drug. Owing to a lower incidence of aplastic anemia with many other drugs, however, it has often been difficult to isolate the single offending agent. Perhaps the only drug for which there is good statistical information is quinacrine (Atabrine).[93] This drug was administered to all U.S. troops in the South Pacific and Asiatic theaters of operations as prophylaxis for malaria during 1943 and 1944. The incidence of aplastic anemia was compared to army personnel in the United States and Europe who did not receive quinacrine. The incidence of aplastic anemia was 7 to 28 cases per 1,000,000 personnel per year in the prophylaxis zones, whereas nontreated soldiers had 1 to 2 cases per 1,000,000 personnel

per year. In contrast to other drugs, the aplasia occurred during administration of the offending agent and was preceded by a characteristic rash in nearly half the cases.

Many other drugs have been implicated in sporadic cases of aplastic anemia, but owing to limited reporting of information, it is possible that the spectrum of drug-induced aplastic anemia is not fully appreciated. A list of drugs that have been implicated is shown in Table 31-2. Antineoplastic drugs such as alkylating agents, antimetabolites, and certain cytotoxic antibiotics all have the potential for producing marrow aplasia. In general, this is transient, is an extension of their pharmacologic action, and resolves within several weeks of completing chemotherapy. Although unusual, severe hypoplasia can follow use of the alkylating agent busulfan and may persist for extended intervals. Patients may develop marrow aplasia 2 to 5 years after discontinuation of alkylating agent therapy. These cases often evolve into hypoplastic myelodysplastic syndromes.

Other types of drugs may be associated with occasional cases of aplastic anemia. These include analgesics as well as antiarthritic and anti-inflammatory agents. The most serious offenders in the latter group include gold salts, penicillamine, and the butazone compounds. Many nonsteroidal analgesics have been associated with sporadic cases of marrow aplasia. Anticonvulsant medications, particularly carbamazepine, are marrow suppressants. The sulfonamides and their derivatives, which include diuretics and oral hypoglycemic agents, have been associated with cases of aplastic anemia. Many of these drugs are known to induce selective cytopenias, such as agranulocytosis, which are usually reversible after discontinuation of the offending agent. These reversible reactions are not correlated with the risk of

TABLE 31-2   DRUGS ASSOCIATED WITH APLASTIC ANEMIA

Category	High Risk	Moderate Risk	Low Risk
Analgesic			Phenacetin, aspirin, salicylamide
Antiarrhythmic			Quinidine, tocainamide
Antiarthritics		Gold salts	Colchicine
Anticonvulsant		Carbamazepine, hydantoins, felbamate	Ethosuximide, phenacemide, primidone, trimethadione
Antihistamine			Chlorpheniramine, pyrilamine, tripelennamine
Antihypertensive			Captopril, methyldopa
Anti-inflammatory		Penicillamine, phenylbutazone, oxyphenbutazone	Diclofenac, ibuprofen, indomethacin, naproxen, sulindac
Antimicrobia			
Antibacterial		Chloramphenicol	Dapsone, methicillin, penicillin, streptomycin, β-lactam antibiotics
Antifungal			Amphotericin, flucytosine
Antiprotozoal		Quinacrine	Chloroquine, mepacrine, pyrimethamine
Antineoplastic drugs			
Alkylating agents	Busulfan, cyclophosphamide, melphalan, nitrogen mustard		
Antimetabolites	Fluorouracil, mercaptopurine, methotrexate		
Cytotoxic antibiotics	Daunorubicin, doxorubicin, mitoxantrone		
Antiplatelet			Ticlopidine
Antithyroid			Carbimazole, methimazole, methylthiouracil, potassium perchlorate, propylthiouracil, sodium thiocyanate
Sedative and tranquilizer			Chlordiazepoxide, chlorpromazine (and other phenothiazines), lithium, meprobamate, methyprylon
Sulfonamides and derivatives			
Antibacterial			Numerous sulfonamides
Diuretic		Acetazolamide	Chlorothiazide, furosemide
Hypoglycemic			Chlorpropamide, tolbutamide
Miscellaneous			Allopurinol, interferon, pentoxifylline

NOTE: Drugs that invariably cause marrow aplasia with high doses are termed *high risk;* drugs with 30 or more reported cases are listed as moderate risk; others are less often associated with aplastic anemia (low risk).

SOURCE: This list was compiled from the AMA Registry,[256] publications of the International Agranulocytosis and Aplastic Anemia Study,[257–261] other reviews and studies,[124,262–264] previous compilations of offending agents,[265,266] and selected reports.[267–276]

aplastic anemia, casting doubt on the effectiveness of routine monitoring of blood counts as a strategy to avoid aplastic anemia.

Since aplastic anemia remains a rare event, it may occur because of an underlying metabolic predisposition in susceptible individuals. In the case of phenylbutazone-associated aplasia, there is delayed oxidation and clearance of a related compound, acetanilide, as compared to either normal controls or those with aplastic anemia due to other causes.[94] This suggests excess accumulation of the drug as a potential mechanism for the aplasia. In some cases drug interactions or synergy may be required to induce aplasia. Cimetidine, a histamine H_2-receptor antagonist, is occasionally implicated in cytopenias and in causing aplastic anemia, perhaps owing to a direct effect on hematopoietic stem cells.[95,96] This drug accentuates the marrow-suppressive effects of the chemotherapy drug carmustine[97] and in several instances has been reported as a possible cause of aplasia when given with chloramphenicol.[87]

RADIATION

Chronic exposure to low doses of radiation or use of localized radiation for ankylosing spondylitis is associated with an increased, but delayed, risk of developing aplastic anemia and acute leukemia.[98,99] Patients who were given thorium dioxide (Thorotrast) as an intravenous contrast medium suffered numerous late complications, including malignant liver tumors, acute leukemia, and chronic aplastic anemia.[100] Chronic radium poisoning with osteitis of the jaw, osteogenic sarcoma, and aplastic anemia was seen in workers who painted watch dials with luminous paint when they moistened the brushes orally.[101]

Acute exposures to large doses of radiation are associated with the development of marrow aplasia and a gastrointestinal syndrome.[102,103] Total body exposure to between 1 and 2.5 Gy (100 to 250 rad) leads to gastrointestinal symptoms and depression of leukocyte counts, but most patients recover. A dose of 4.5 Gy leads to death in half the individuals (LD50) owing to marrow failure. Higher doses in the range of 10 Gy are universally fatal unless the patient receives extensive supportive care followed by marrow transplantation. Aplastic anemia associated with nuclear accidents was seen after the disaster that occurred at the Chernobyl nuclear power station in the Ukraine in 1986.[104–107]

VIRUSES

A striking relationship between hepatitis and the subsequent development of aplastic anemia has been the subject of a number of case reports; this association was emphasized by two major reviews in the 1970s.[108,109] In the aggregate, these reports summarized findings in over 200 cases. In many instances, the hepatitis was improving or had resolved when the aplastic anemia was noted 4 to 12 weeks later. Approximately 10 percent of cases occurred more than 1 year after the initial diagnosis of hepatitis. Most patients were young (18 to 20 years), two-thirds were male, and their survival was short (10 weeks). Although hepatitis A and B have been implicated in aplastic anemia in a small number of cases, most cases are related to non-A, non-B hepatitis.[110,111] Severe aplastic anemia developed in 9 of 31 patients who underwent liver transplantation for non-A, non-B hepatitis but in none of 1463 patients transplanted for other indications.[112] Several lines of evidence indicate there is no association with hepatitis C virus, suggesting that a hitherto unknown viral agent is involved.[113–115]

EBV has been implicated in the pathogenesis of aplastic anemia.[116,117] The onset usually occurs within 4 to 6 weeks of infection. In some cases infectious mononucleosis is subclinical, with a finding of atypical lymphocytes in the blood film and serological results consistent with a recent infection. EBV has been detected in marrow cells,[118]

but it is uncertain whether aplasia results from a direct effect or an immunologic response by the host. Some patients have recovered following therapy with antithymocyte globulin.[113,116,118]

A number of other viruses have been implicated in the pathogenesis of marrow failure. B-19 parvovirus, the cause of fifth disease, leads to transient erythroid aplasia but is not known to induce aplastic anemia.[113,119] HHV-6 has caused severe marrow aplasia subsequent to bone marrow transplantation for other disorders.[120] HIV infection is frequently associated with varying degrees of cytopenia. The marrow is often cellular, but occasional cases of aplastic anemia have been noted.[121–123] In these patients, marrow hypoplasia may result both from viral suppression and from the many drugs used to control viral replication in this disorder.

MISCELLANEOUS CAUSES

Rheumatoid arthritis is not ordinarily associated with severe aplastic anemia, but an epidemiologic study in France revealed a sevenfold increase in the incidence of aplastic anemia in patients with this disorder.[124] It is uncertain whether the aplastic anemia is related directly to rheumatoid arthritis or to the various drugs used to treat the condition (gold salts, D-penicillamine, and nonsteroidal agents). Occasional cases of aplastic anemia are seen in conjunction with systemic lupus erythematosus.[125] In vitro studies have suggested the presence of an antibody[126,127] or suppressor cell[128,129] directed against hematopoietic progenitor cells. Patients have recovered after plasmapheresis,[126,127] glucocorticoids,[129] or cyclophosphamide therapy,[128,130] suggesting a possible immune etiology.

Eosinophilic fasciitis, an uncommon connective tissue disorder with painful swelling and induration of the skin and subcutaneous tissue, has been associated with aplastic anemia on at least 14 occasions.[131–134] Although it may be antibody-mediated in some cases, it has been largely unresponsive to therapy. One patient improved with immunosuppressive therapy using ATG and cyclosporine.[133] In another case, a partial remission was achieved following therapy with ATG.

There are a number of reports of pregnancy-associated aplastic anemia, but the relationship between the two conditions is not clear.[135–141] In some patients, preexisting aplastic anemia is exacerbated with pregnancy, only to improve following termination of the pregnancy.[136,139,140] In other cases, the aplasia develops during pregnancy with recurrences during subsequent pregnancies.[136,140,141] Termination of pregnancy or delivery may improve the marrow function, but the disease may progress to a fatal outcome even after delivery.[135–141] Therapy may include elective termination of early pregnancy, supportive care, immunosuppressive therapy, or marrow transplantation after delivery.

HEREDITARY APLASTIC ANEMIA

FANCONI ANEMIA

The most common form of constitutional aplastic anemia was described in three brothers by Fanconi in 1927.[142] Since that time nearly 800 cases have been recorded, either by reports in the literature or through an International Fanconi Anemia Registry.[143–146]

Fanconi anemia is inherited as an autosomal recessive condition. It is estimated to be present in one in a million individuals, although it is more frequent in Afrikaners of European descent and in southern Italy.

At least eight gene mutations have been associated with the development of Fanconi anemia. The genes have been designated FAA through FAH. The great majority of patients have mutations of FAA or FAC. It has been proposed that the A and C gene products, which are cytoplasmic proteins, form a complex with the products of genes

B, E, F, and G, which are adaptors or phosphorylators; the complex translocates to the nucleus, where it subserves its normal function. In the presence of a mutant gene product, normal function is disturbed leading to effects in sensitive tissues, including hematopoietic cells. Mutation of the D product appears to effect tissue cells through a different mechanism, perhaps downstream from the complex.[147,148]

Blood counts and marrow cellularity are often normal until 5 to 10 years of age, when pancytopenia develops gradually over an extended interval. Thrombocytopenia may precede the development of granulocytopenia and anemia. The marrow becomes hypocellular, and in vitro colony assays reveal a decrease in CFU-GM and BFU–E.[145] It is often associated with abnormal skin pigmentation typical of *café-au-lait* lesions. Growth retardation results in short stature. Skeletal anomalies, especially dysplastic radii and thumbs, occur in half the patients. Heart, kidney, and eye defects may be present. Microcephaly and mental retardation may be present. Hypogonadism occurs. Hematologic and visceral manifestations are combined in more than a third of patients, but some may have anemia and inconspicuous somatic changes whereas others may have the anomalies with little hematopoietic disorder. A few may be virtually unaffected.[145–147] In the past, children with a similar onset of aplastic anemia without congenital abnormalities were thought to have a different disorder termed *Estren-Dameshek syndrome*.[149] These children, whose lymphocytes show sensitivity to diepoxybutane, have the same inherited disorder without skeletal abnormalities.[144]

Random chromatid breaks are present in myeloid cells, lymphocytes, and chorionic villus preparations. This chromosome damage is intensified after exposure to DNA cross-linking agents such as mitomycin C or diepoxybutane. The hypersensitivity of the chromosomes of marrow cells or lymphocytes to the latter agent is used as a diagnostic test for this condition. Cell-cycle progression is prolonged at the G2 to M transition phase of the cell mitotic cycle, and the cells are more susceptible to oxygen toxicity when cultured in vitro.[147] It is important to test the lymphocytes from pediatric patients with aplastic anemia for sensitivity to diepoxybutane, since therapy for Fanconi anemia differs from that used for idiopathic aplastic anemia.

Most patients with Fanconi anemia do not respond to ATG or cyclosporine but do improve with androgen preparations, often for as long as several years. Relapses occur gradually, with eventual death by age 10 to 20 years from progressive marrow failure or from conversion to acute myelogenous leukemia (approximately 10 percent of patients). Allogeneic stem cell transplantation is curative for this disorder.[150,277] A marked reduction in dosage of the marrow-conditioning regimen of cyclophosphamide and radiation is necessary owing to the undue sensitivity of the tissues to alkylating agents.[150]

DYSKERATOSIS CONGENITA AND SCHWACHMAN-DIAMOND SYNDROME

Dyskeratosis congenita and Schwachman-Diamond syndrome (pancreatic insufficiency with neutropenia) are two rare disorders that may also evolve into aplastic anemia. Dyskeratosis is usually inherited as a recessive X-chromosome–linked disorder although rare cases are autosomal. The disease is reflected in reticulate skin pigmentation, leukoplakia, and dystrophic nails. A variety of noncutaneous anomalies have also been observed. The skin and mucosal lesions appear in adolescence, and aplastic anemia usually develops in early adulthood.[151] Schwachman-Diamond syndrome is manifest by pancreatic insufficiency and steatorrhea. Neutropenia is present in virtually all patients and granulocytopenia and thrombocytopenia in about one-third to one-half. Thus a substantial plurality of patients have bi- or tricytopenia with hypoplastic marrows. There is a significant risk of progression to myelogenous leukemia.[152,278] Severe hematopoietic

dysfunction can be treated successfully with allogeneic stem cell transplantation.

CLINICAL FEATURES

EPIDEMIOLOGY

The incidence of aplastic anemia is estimated to be 2 to 5 cases per 1,000,000 population per year based on retrospective studies.[83] The incidence rates in Sweden (13 cases per 1,000,000 per year),[153] Israel (8 cases per 1,000,000 per year),[84] and the United States (5 to 12 new cases per 1,000,000 per year)[154,155] suggest that the rate in industrialized countries is about 5 to 10 cases per 1,000,000 per year.

SIGNS AND SYMPTOMS

The onset of aplastic anemia may be insidious, with a gradual fall in red cells leading to pallor, weakness, and fatigue, or it may be more dramatic with fever, chills, and pharyngitis or other infections resulting from neutropenia. Dependent petechiae, bruising, and bleeding secondary to thrombocytopenia are seen often and may be the initial clue to the underlying marrow disorder.

Physical examination is generally unrevealing except for evidence of infection or bleeding. Oral purpuric lesions (wet purpura) suggest a platelet count of less than $10,000/\mu l$ (10×10^9/liter), which portends a higher risk for cerebral hemorrhage. Retinal hemorrhages may be seen with severe anemia or thrombocytopenia. Lymphadenopathy or splenomegaly are not ordinarily found in aplastic anemia; such findings suggest recent infection or an alternative diagnosis such as leukemia or lymphoma.

LABORATORY FEATURES

BLOOD FINDINGS

Patients with aplastic anemia have varying degrees of pancytopenia. Anemia is associated with a low reticulocyte index.[156] The reticulocyte count is usually less than 1.0 percent and may be zero. Macrocytosis may result from the high levels of erythropoietin,[157] stimulating the few residual erythroblasts to mature more rapidly,[158] or from an abnormal clone of erythroid cells, such as is seen in myelodysplasia or paroxysmal nocturnal hemoglobinuria.[10–13] The total leukocyte count is low; the differential cell count reveals a marked decrease in neutrophils. The absolute neutrophil count is the most important prognostic feature, with a count of less than $500/\mu l$ (0.5×10^9/liter) associated with increased risk of infections and less than $200/\mu l$ (0.2×10^9/liter) associated with a dire prognosis. Lymphocyte production is thought to be normal, but patients may have mild lymphopenia. Platelets are reduced, but they function normally. On occasion, only one cell line is depressed initially, which may lead to an early diagnosis of red cell aplasia or amegakaryocytic thrombocytopenia. In such patients, other cell lines will fail shortly thereafter (days to weeks) and permit a definitive diagnosis.

MARROW FINDINGS

MORPHOLOGY

The marrow aspirate typically contains numerous spicules with empty fatty spaces and relatively few hematopoietic cells. Lymphocytes, plasma cells, macrophages, and mast cells may be prominent, but this probably reflects a lack of other cells rather than an increase in these elements. On occasion, some spicules are cellular or even hypercellular, but megakaryocytes are usually reduced. These areas of residual hematopoiesis do not appear to be of prognostic significance. Residual

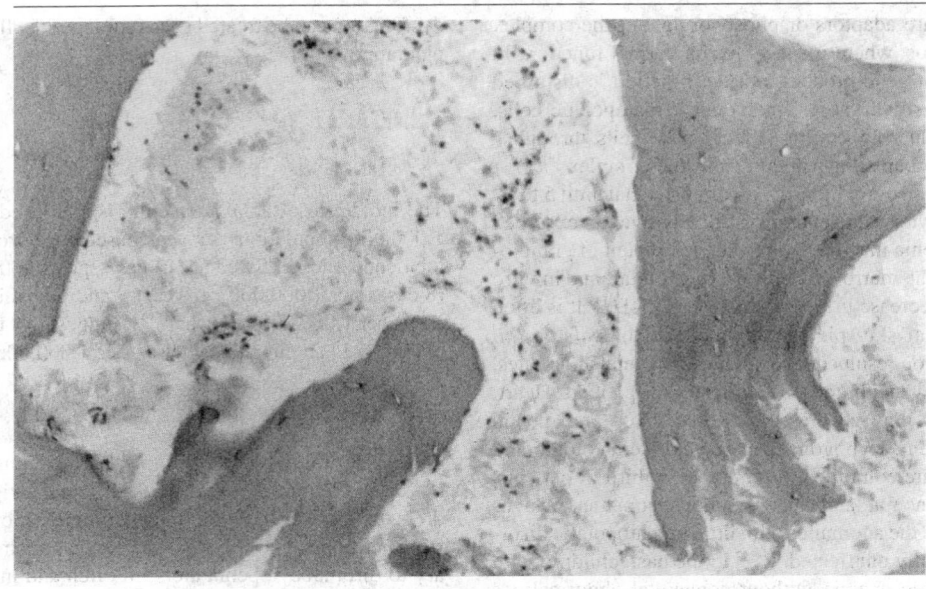

FIGURE 31-1   Marrow biopsy in aplastic anemia. The marrow is devoid of hematopoietic cells and contains only scattered lymphocytes and stromal cells.

granulocytic cells generally appear normal, but it is not unusual to see mild dysplastic or megaloblastoid features in the erythroid cells. At times they are macrocytic or macronormoblastic, presumably due to the high levels of erythropoietin. Marrow biopsy is essential to confirm the overall hypocellularity (Fig. 31-1), since a poor yield of cells is seen on marrow aspirates in a number of other hematologic disorders.

Severe aplastic anemia has been defined by the International Aplastic Anemia Study Group[159] as a marrow of less than 25 percent cellularity, or less than 50 percent cellularity with less than 30 percent hematopoietic cells, with at least two of the following: neutrophil count less than $500/\mu l$ (0.5×10^9/liter), platelet count less than 20,000/ μl (20×10^9/liter), and anemia with a corrected reticulocyte index of less than 1 percent. Those patients with a neutrophil count less than $200/\mu l$ (0.2×10^9/liter) have an extremely poor prognosis and are characterized as having very severe aplastic anemia.[160]

If a lymphocytosis is noted in the marrow or blood, a tartrate-resistant acid phosphatase determination as well as immunophenotyping should be done to exclude early cases of hairy-cell leukemia[161] or acute lymphocytic leukemia.[162]

PROGENITOR CELL GROWTH

In vitro granulocytic-monocytic (CFU-GM) and erythroid (BFU–E) colony assays reveal a marked reduction in progenitor cells.[19–25,29–35] In some instances, improvement in colony growth after incubation with anti-T-cell monoclonal antibodies may predict improvement after immunosuppressive therapy[163]; this has not, however, been a universal finding.

CYTOGENETICS

Cytogenetic analysis may be difficult to perform owing to low cellularity; thus, multiple aspirates may be required to provide sufficient cells for study. The results are often normal in aplastic anemia and abnormal in myelodysplastic syndromes; one study, however, suggested that 4 percent of patients with otherwise typical aplastic anemia had abnormalities usually seen in myelodysplasia.[164] Two of three patients with aplastic anemia and cytogenetic abnormalities who did not have marrow transplants progressed to a myelodysplastic syn-

drome, suggesting that the cytogenetic abnormalities of such patients represent or will soon evolve into a clonal (neoplastic) disorder.

RADIOLOGIC FINDINGS

NMRI can be used to distinguish between marrow fat and hematopoietic cells.[165] This may provide a better overall estimate of marrow aplasia than morphologic techniques and may differentiate hypoplastic myelodysplastic syndrome from aplastic anemia.[166,167]

PLASMA AND URINE FINDINGS

Studies should include assessment of antibodies to hepatitis A, B, and C; hepatitis B antigen; heterophile determination; and antibodies to EBV. A sucrose hemolysis test and leukocyte and red cell immunophenotyping[6–8] should be done prior to transfusions to exclude paroxysmal nocturnal hemoglobinuria (see Chap. 36).

The serum has high levels of hematopoietic growth factors, including erythropoietin, thrombopoietin, and myeloid colony-stimulating factors.[48–50]

Serum iron values are usually high, and ^{59}Fe clearance is prolonged, with decreased incorporation into circulating red cells.[168] Ferrokinetic studies or marrow scanning following injection of technetium sulfur colloid or indium chloride may be required to assess overall marrow cellularity and function.

DIFFERENTIAL DIAGNOSIS

Both marrow aspirate and biopsy are essential to show the overall marked hypocellularity and to exclude other causes of pancytopenia. Several disorders may be confused with severe aplastic anemia at the initial presentation. Approximately 10 percent of patients with myelodysplastic syndromes present with hypoplasia rather than a hypercellular marrow. This possibility is suspected if there is abnormal blood film morphology, as seen with myelodysplasia (see Chap. 92). Marrow erythroid precursors in myelodysplasia have both megaloblastoid and dysplastic features, with dumbbell and cloverleaf nuclei, Howell-Jolly bodies, and increased siderotic granules. Granulocyte precursors have reduced granulation, with abnormal blue cytoplasm in the promyelocytes and acquired Pelger-Hüet anomalies in the mature cells. Megakaryocytes may have hyperlobulation or may have a single nucleus in a small cell (unilobular micromegakaryocytes). Cytogenetic abnormalities are often found but are not essential for the diagnosis of myelodysplastic syndromes. MRI studies may be useful in differentiating severe aplastic anemia from myelodysplastic syndromes by showing a diffuse cellular pattern in the latter disorders.[165–167] Paroxysmal nocturnal hemoglobinuria is usually identified by a positive sucrose hemolysis test, or abnormal CD59 red cell membrane proteins as detected by flow cytometry.[6–8]

Acute lymphocytic leukemia may initially have a hypoplastic phase, but even then clumps of lymphocytic cells are often seen.[162] Less often, hairy-cell leukemia may be preceded by a hypoplastic phase.[161] Both conditions can be differentiated from severe aplastic anemia by use of special stains such as tartrate-resistant acid phosphatase for hairy-cell leukemia and by immunophenotyping using flow cytometry for acute lymphocytic leukemia.

TREATMENT

The median survival of untreated patients with aplastic anemia [neutrophil count $<500/\mu$l $(0.5 \times 10^9/\text{liter})$] is 3 to 6 months, with only 20 percent surviving beyond a year.[169] Very severe aplastic anemia [neutrophils $<200/\mu$l $(0.2 \times 10^9/\text{liter})$] has an extremely poor prognosis.[160] Those patients with less severe disease [i.e., neutrophils $>1000/\mu$l $(1.0 \times 10^9/\text{liter})$], who do not require red cell or platelet transfusions, may be treated conservatively with supportive care, as there are occasional cases of spontaneous recovery.

MARROW TRANSPLANTATION

Prompt and aggressive therapy is usually indicated for most patients with severe disease. The major curative approach is allogeneic marrow transplantation.[170–171] This treatment modality is described in Chap. 18. Only one-third of all patients have compatible donors. Many transplants have been performed using partially matched siblings or unrelated histocompatible donors recruited through the National Marrow Donor Program or similar organizations in other countries.[172] Umbilical cord blood may evolve as an alternative source of unrelated donors for transplantation.[173]

IMMUNOSUPPRESSIVE THERAPY

ANTILYMPHOCYTE AND ANTITHYMOCYTE GLOBULIN
Many cases of aplastic anemia may be mediated by a cellular immune reaction directed against hematopoietic stem or progenitor cells. The recovery of their own cells was observed in some recipients of mismatched allogeneic transplants after treatment with ALG.[174] Improvement occurred in benzene- or ^{32}P-induced aplastic anemia in rabbits after ALG treatment and transplantation with mismatched marrow cells.[175,176] The requirement for high-dose immunosuppressive treatment to allow engraftment in half the syngeneic transplants[170,177] also supports the concept of a cellular immune reaction. Subsequently, many investigators found evidence of T-cell–mediated suppressor mechanisms by in vitro marrow culture studies.[20,23,29,31–36] Some of these observations were undoubtedly due to transfusion sensitization, but a number of studies supported the notion of an active immune (T-lymphocyte–mediated) suppressor mechanism being responsible for the aplasia. Although ALS and ATG appear to act by reducing cytotoxic T cells, these preparations also release hematopoietic growth factors from certain T cells.[178,179]

There is about a 50 percent response rate with ALS or ATG.[180–184]

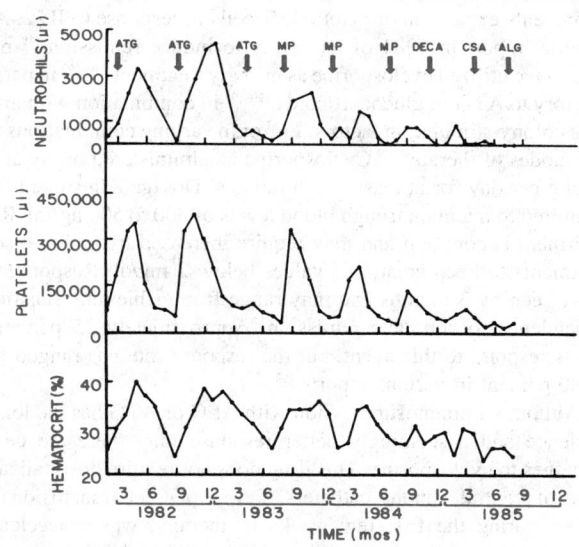

FIGURE 31-2   Responses to repeated cycles of immunosuppressive therapy. A 45-year-old woman with severe aplastic anemia had two complete responses following treatment with horse antithymocyte globulin (ATG). After an anaphylactic reaction on the third exposure, she received 1 g of methylprednisolone (MP), intravenously daily for 14 days. This led to a partial response on three occasions. She was essentially unresponsive to further treatment with nandrolone decanoate (DECA), cyclosporine (CSA), or goat antilymphocyte globulin (ALG).

Therapy is given for 4 to 10 days with doses of 15 to 40 mg/kg daily. Since the antisera are prepared in horses, it is important to perform skin tests against horse serum prior to administration.[185] If positive, pretreatment with glucocorticoids for 24 h lessens reactions. Fever and chills are common during the first day of treatment; these can be reduced with oral prednisone, 20 mg, daily. During treatment, accelerated platelet destruction is often seen. This leads to an increase in transfusion requirements over the 10-day treatment interval. Serum sickness occurs commonly 7 to 10 days from the first dose. This is characterized by spiking fevers, skin rashes, and arthralgias. The clinical manifestations of serum sickness can be prevented by increasing prednisone to 60 to 80 mg daily, from day 10 to day 17 of the treatment course.

GLUCOCORTICOIDS
Marrow recovery can occur after very high doses of glucocorticoids.[186,187] Methylprednisolone in the range of 500 to 1000 mg daily for 3 to 14 days has been successful, but the side effects can be severe. These include marked glycosuria, electrolyte disturbances, gastric distress, psychosis, increased infections, and aseptic necrosis of the hips.

Repeated responses to immunosuppressive therapy have been observed. As shown in Fig. 31-2, a 45-year-old woman with severe aplastic anemia responded completely to ATG and remained well for nearly 9 months. At relapse, she received a second course of ATG and recovered for another 6 months. She developed an anaphylactic reaction with a third exposure to ATG. There were several subsequent responses to 14-day infusions of methylprednisolone (1 g/day), but no appreciable responses to nandrolone decanoate, cyclosporine, or goat antilymphocyte globulin; she became refractory to therapy and died of fungal sepsis.

CYCLOSPORINE
Another approach to immunosuppressive therapy uses cyclosporine, a cyclic polypeptide that inhibits IL-2 production by T lymphocytes

and prevents expansion of cytotoxic T cells in response to IL-2. After the initial report in 1984 of its ability to induce remission,[188] many groups have utilized cyclosporine as primary treatment,[189–192] in patients refractory to ATG or glucocorticoids,[190–195] in combination with granulocyte colony-stimulating factors,[196,197] or in varying combinations with other modes of therapy.[198] Cyclosporine is administered orally at 3 to 7 mg/kg per day for at least 4 to 6 months. Dosage adjustments may be required to maintain trough blood levels of 300 to 500 ng/ml. Renal impairment is common and may require increased hydration or dose adjustments to keep creatinine values below 2 mg/dl. Responses are usually seen by 3 months and may range from achieving transfusion independence to complete remission. Approximately 25 percent of patients respond to this agent, but the response rate has ranged from 0 to 80 percent in various reports.[198]

Although immunosuppression with ALG or ATG has the longest experience and a seemingly better response rate, there are certain advantages to cyclosporine. This drug does not require hospitalization or use of central venous catheters. Fewer platelet transfusions are required during the first few weeks of therapy, where accelerated platelet needs are seen in patients receiving ALG or ATG. It is unclear whether cyclosporine should be considered primary therapy for most patients, with views ranging from cautious optimism to marked reservation concerning its effectiveness. A French cooperative trial showed equal effectiveness of ATG plus prednisone compared to cyclosporine.[199] In this crossover study of newly diagnosed patients, survivals of about 65 percent were observed 12 months after diagnosis. Improved in vitro tests to predict responsiveness may help tailor specific therapy for each patient in the future.[194]

COMBINATION THERAPY

Both low-dose and high-dose methylprednisolone have been used in combination with ATG and oxymethylone.[200,201] Responses and survival were similar in both groups of patients. Androgens have been used in conjunction with immunosuppressive agents in randomized trials with both negative[202] and positive results.[201,203] Nonrandomized trials suggest that coadministration of androgens with ATG or ALG improves the response rate.[204] At this time, it is unclear whether androgen preparations should be added to primary therapy; their use should be avoided in patients with posthepatitis aplastic anemia or in those with abnormal liver function tests.

Several trials have examined the effect of adding cyclosporine to basic regimens of ALG and glucocorticoids. Overall response rates increased from 47 percent to 70 percent in one study[205] and from 39 percent to 65 percent in another.[206] With combined therapy a 67 percent response rate was noted at 3 months, which improved to 78 percent at 1 year.[207] Although granulocyte colony-stimulating factor alone may be detrimental,[208] its addition to ALG, glucocorticoids, and cyclosporine appeared to improve response rates.[209] Eighty-three percent of 40 patients with very severe aplastic anemia had trilineage reconstitution and became transfusion independent within 4 months of therapy.

These encouraging results with immunosuppressive therapy are in some instances equal to the results after marrow transplantation.[210–212] The results from UCLA indicated a 49 percent survival for 146 patients treated with ATG alone.[210] This did not differ from the survival of age-matched patients that underwent bone marrow transplantation during the same time interval. However, the survival after transplants improved after 1984, from 43 percent to 72 percent, indicating better results with improved transplant protocols. Similar results were seen in Seattle,[211] where 227 patients were treated with ATG alone, and 168 received bone marrow transplants. The actuarial survival at 15 years was 38 percent following ATG therapy and 69 percent after bone marrow transplant. However, later results with combination immunosuppressive therapy showed better results. Forty-eight children treated at Memorial Sloan-Kettering between 1983 and 1992 had a 10-year survival of 76 percent for bone marrow transplantation and 74 percent for combined immunosuppressive therapy.[212] Thus, immunosuppression may be preferable for patients who are greater than 30 to 40 years of age and who may experience delay in finding a suitable donor. Marrow transplants are, however, curative for aplastic anemia, whereas many long-term sequelae have been found after immunosuppressive therapy.[213–215] Several surveys have shown a substantial rate of relapse or conversion to other stem cell disorders. Of 358 patients responding to immunosuppressive therapy, 74 relapsed after a mean of 2.1 years. The actuarial incidence was 35 percent at 10 years.[216] In the Swiss experience,[217] 29 of 129 patients treated with ALG developed myelodysplasia, leukemia, paroxysmal nocturnal hemoglobinuria, or combined disorders. This tendency to relapse and to develop clonal hematologic disorders has been reviewed by the European Cooperative Group for Bone Marrow Transplantation in 468 patients, most of whom received ATG.[218] The risk of a hematologic complication increased continuously and reached 57 percent at 8 years after immunosuppressive therapy. A further survey indicated 42 malignancies in 860 patients treated with immunosuppression, whereas only 9 malignancies were seen in 748 patients who received marrow transplants.[219] Careful morphologic review of the blood and marrow before and after therapy may distinguish those patients at risk for late hematologic complications.[220]

HIGH-DOSE CYCLOPHOSHAMIDE

High-dose cyclophosphamide has been used as a unique form of immunosuppression.[221] Although it would seem inappropriate to administer high doses of chemotherapy to patients with severe marrow aplasia, this approach was based on observations of autologous recovery after preparative therapy for allogeneic transplants.[221] Ten patients received cyclophosphamide at 45 mg/kg per day intravenously for 4 days with or without cyclosporine for an additional 100 days. Gradual neutrophil and platelet recovery ensued over 3 months. Seven patients responded completely and remain in remission 11 years after treatment.

ANDROGENS

A variety of androgenic and anabolic steroids have been used for aplastic anemia. Testosterone, methyltestosterone, testosterone enanthate, fluoxymesterone, norethandrolone, oxymetholone, nandrolone decanoate, danazol, and etiocholanolone have all been employed. These agents stimulate the production of erythropoietin, and their metabolites stimulate erythropoiesis when added to marrow cultures in vitro.[222]

Randomized trials have not shown efficacy when androgens were used as primary therapy for severe or moderately severe aplastic anemia.[159,202] However, a French study showed that high doses of androgens were superior to low doses in patients with only moderately severe aplasia.[223] Large series of patients were reported in which survival seemed improved as compared with historical controls,[224] but this could equally be attributed to better supportive care. Many physicians use androgens in those patients with moderate degrees of marrow aplasia who have failed initial treatment with immunosuppressive agents. The response of one patient who was resistant to fluoxymesterone, ATG, and cyclosporine is shown in Fig. 31-3. There was progressive marrow recovery after 5 months of treatment with etiocholanolone and nandrolone decanoate.[225]

Androgens should be continued for at least 3 to 6 months, since responses may require prolonged treatment. Nandrolone decanoate, 400 mg intramuscularly per week, is a good initial drug. Concerns about local hematomas are usually obviated by firm local pressure for 30 min following injection. Long-term survivors after androgen ther-

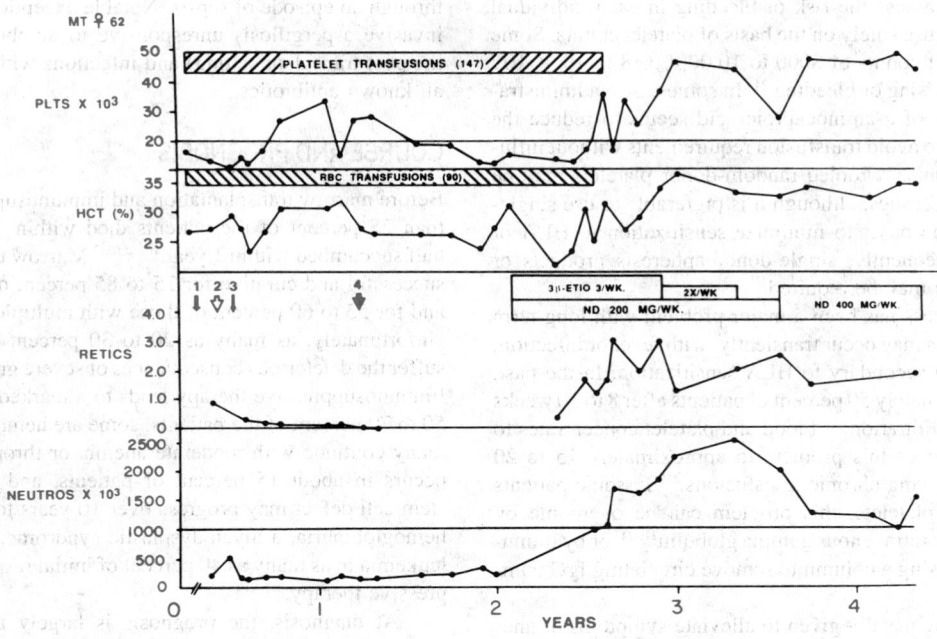

FIGURE 31-3   Response to etiocholanolone and nandrolone decanoate. A 62-year-old woman with severe aplastic anemia failed to improve after treatment with fluoxymesterone (Halotestin)(1 ↓, ×5 months), methyl-prednisolone (M Pred)(2 ↓, 14 days), antithymocyte globulin (ATG) (3 ↓, 10 days), or cyclosporine (CYS)(4 ↓, ×1 month). Marrow recovery occurred during therapy with 3-β-etiocholanolone and nandrolone decanoate. (Reproduced from Seewald et al,[225] with permission.)

apy have essentially the same progression to clonal hematologic disorders as patients treated with immunosuppressive agents.[224]

CYTOKINES

Despite their effectiveness in accelerating recovery from chemotherapy, these agents have been far less effective in achieving long-term benefits in patients with severe aplastic anemia. Daily treatment with granulocyte-macrophage colony-stimulating factor[226–228] or granulocyte colony-stimulating factor[229] has improved marrow cellularity and increased neutrophil counts approximately 1.5- to 10-fold. Unfortunately, in nearly all patients, the blood counts return to baseline within several days of cessation of therapy. Although occasional patients show evidence of trilineage marrow recovery with long-term therapy,[229–231] the vast majority do not respond. In fact, physicians have been cautioned not to use hemopoietic growth factors as primary therapy.[208] Repeated transfusions of blood and platelets while awaiting definitive therapy by bone marrow transplant or immunosuppression can reduce the chances of responding to such therapy. Therapy with myeloid growth factors is probably best reserved for instances of proved infections or as a preventive measure prior to dental work or other procedures that would compromise mucosal barriers. Doses of 250 to 300 μg daily by subcutaneous injection are easiest to administer and seem to be associated with the fewest side effects.

IL-1, a potent stimulator of marrow stromal cell production of other cytokines, and IL-3 have been ineffective in small numbers of patients with severe aplastic anemia.[233,234] These disappointing results with cytokines are not unexpected, as previous work has suggested high serum levels of growth factors in patients with aplastic anemia. Moreover, the majority of patients appear to have a stem cell defect, which may be unresponsive to factors that act on more mature progenitor cells.

OTHER THERAPY

High doses of intravenous gamma globulin have been given to small numbers of patients with severe aplastic anemia[235–237] because of its success in treating certain cases of antibody-mediated pure red cell aplasia. Some improvement was noted in four of six patients treated. Other treatments that are occasionally successful include lymphocytapheresis[238,239] and acyclovir[240] (perhaps owing to a viral etiology in some cases).

SPLENECTOMY

Removal of the spleen does not increase hematopoiesis but may increase neutrophil and platelet counts two- to threefold and improve survival of transfused red cells or platelets in highly sensitized individuals.[241] The surgical morbidity and mortality in patients with virtually no platelets makes this a questionable therapeutic procedure.

SUPPORTIVE CARE

All patients should have immediate HLA typing performed.[242] Where marrow transplant is a consideration, HLA typing of all siblings should be performed as soon as possible. Blood and platelet transfusions should be used sparingly, if at all, in potential transplant recipients to minimize sensitization. Most young adults can tolerate hemoglobin levels of 7 to 8 g/dl; platelets need to be given only for active hemorrhage or severe thrombocytopenia with platelet counts less than 10,000/μl (10 × 10⁹/liter). It is important not to transfuse patients with red cells or platelets from family members, since this may sensitize patients to minor histocompatibility antigens, increasing the risk of graft rejection after marrow transplantation. Following a marrow transplant, or in those individuals in whom transplantation is not a consideration, family members may be ideal donors for platelet apheresis products.

It is important to assess the risk of bleeding in each individual patient and not to transfuse solely on the basis of platelet counts. Some patients tolerate platelet counts of 8000 to 10,000/μl (8 to 10 $\times$ 10^9/liter) without undue bruising or bleeding.[243] In some cases, administration of 4 to 12 g daily of ε-aminocaproic acid seems to reduce the bleeding tendency and to avoid transfusion requirements without influencing the platelet counts.[244] Pooled random-donor platelets may be used until sensitization ensues, although it is preferable to use single-donor platelets from the onset to minimize sensitization to HLA or platelet antigens. Subsequently, single-donor apheresis products or HLA-matched platelets may be required.

Platelet refractoriness has been a major problem with long-term transfusion support. This may occur transiently, with fever or infection, or as a lasting problem secondary to HLA sensitization. In the past, this occurred in approximately 50 percent of patients after 8 to 10 weeks of transfusion support. Filtration of blood and platelet concentrates to remove leukocytes reduces this problem to approximately 15 to 20 percent of patients receiving chronic transfusions.[245] In some patients who are refractory to platelets, this problem can be overcome by administering high-dose intravenous gamma globulin[246,247] or by immunoabsorbent pheresis, using a column to remove circulating IgG complexes.[248]

Packed red cells are usually given to alleviate symptoms of anemia; transfusions are often indicated at hemoglobin values below 7 to 8 g/dl. These products should also be given through leukocyte-removal filters to lessen leukocyte and platelet sensitization and to reduce subsequent transfusion reactions. Since each unit of red cells provides approximately 200 to 250 mg of iron, there are long-term consequences of transfusion-induced hemosiderosis. This is not usually a major problem in patients who respond to transplantation or immunosuppressive therapy but is an issue in nonresponders who require continued support. Consideration should be given to chelation therapy with deferoxamine to avoid or reduce severe iron overload.[249]

CMV antibody titers should be obtained on admission; until these results are available, only CMV-negative blood products should be given to potential transplant recipients to minimize problems with CMV infections after transplantation. Once a patient is shown to be CMV-positive, this restriction is no longer necessary. Leukocyte-depletion filters will also decrease the risk of transmitting CMV.

Neutropenic precautions should be applied to hospitalized patients with neutrophil counts less than 1000/μl (1 $\times$ 10^9/liter). Precautions vary widely from institution to institution. One approach is to use private rooms, with requirements for face masks and hand-washing with antiseptic soap. Fresh fruits and vegetables should be avoided to prevent bacterial colonization or infection. When patients with aplastic anemia become febrile, cultures should be obtained from the blood, urine, and any suspicious lesions. Broad-spectrum antibiotics should be initiated promptly, without awaiting culture results (see Chap. 17). The choice of antibiotics depends on local practices; major organisms of concern include *Staphylococcus aureus, S. epidermidis* (in patients with venous access devices), and gram-negative organisms. Patients with persistent culture-negative fevers should receive antifungal treatment with fluconazole, itraconazole, or amphotericin.

In the past, leukocyte transfusions were used on a daily basis to reduce the short-term mortality from infections. Approximately 10^{10} leukocytes were obtained from normal donors by apheresis. However, there was generally a high proportion of mononuclear cells rather than neutrophils in these products. With a 1- to 2-h half-life in febrile patients, it was unusual to detect more than 100 to 200 neutrophils per microliter for more than a few hours after transfusion. The yield of neutrophils can be increased by administering GM-CSF or G-CSF to the donor,[250] but most physicians avoid using white cell products since present-day antibiotics are usually sufficient to carry a patient

through an episode of sepsis. Notable exceptions include documented invasive aspergillosis unresponsive to amphotericin (particularly in the post-transplant setting) and infections with organisms resistant to all known antibiotics.

COURSE AND PROGNOSIS

Before marrow transplantation and immunosuppressive therapy, more than 25 percent of the patients died within 4 months of diagnosis; half succumbed within 1 year.[169,251,252] Marrow transplantation is highly successful and curative for 75 to 85 percent of untransfused patients and for 55 to 60 percent of those with multiple previous transfusions. Unfortunately, as many as 20 to 30 percent of transplant survivors suffer the deleterious consequences of severe graft-versus-host disease. Immunosuppressive therapy leads to a marked improvement in about 50 to 70 percent of the patients; some are hematologically normal, but many continue with moderate anemia or thrombocytopenia. Relapse occurs in about 15 percent of patients, and indeed the underlying stem cell defect may progress over 10 years to paroxysmal nocturnal hemoglobinuria, a myelodysplastic syndrome, or acute myelogenous leukemia in as many as 40 percent of initial responders to immunosuppressive therapy.[213-219]

At diagnosis, the prognosis is largely related to the absolute neutrophil count and platelet count. In the past, the prognosis appeared worse when the disease followed hepatitis.[108,109,253] Recent results with immunosuppression[254] or bone marrow transplant[255] are equivalent to that seen with idiopathic or drug-induced cases. Children appear to respond better than adults, both with transplantation and with androgen therapy, especially those with mild or moderate disease. Constitutional aplastic anemia responds temporarily to androgens and glucocorticoids but is invariably fatal unless treated by transplantation.[145,150]

REFERENCES

1. Ehrlich P: Uber einen Fall von Anamie mit Bemerkungen über regenerative Veranderungen des Knochenmarks. *Charite Ann* 13:300, 1888.
2. Chauffard M: Un cas d'anémie pernicieuse aplastique. *Bull Soc Med Hop Paris* 21:313, 1904.
3. Scott JL, Cartwright GE, Wintrobe MM: Acquired aplastic anemia: an analysis of thirty-nine cases and review of the pertinent literature. *Medicine* 38:119, 1959.
4. Chapuis B, Von Fliedner VE, Jeannet M, et al: Increased frequency of DR2 in patients with aplastic anemia and increased DR sharing in their parents. *Br J Haematol* 63:51, 1986.
5. Odum N, Platz P, Morling N, et al: Increased frequency of HLA-DPw3 in severe aplastic anemia (AA). *Tissue Antigens* 20:184, 1987.
6. Scubert J, Vogt HG, Skowronek M, et al: Development of the glycosyl-phosphatidylinositol-anchoring defect characteristic for paroxysmal nocturnal hemoglobinuria in patients with aplastic anemia. *Blood* 83:2313, 1994.
7. Griscelli-Bennaceur A, Gluckman E, Scrobohaci ML, et al: Aplastic anemia and paroxysmal nocturnal hemoglobinuria: search for a pathogenetic link. *Blood* 85:1354, 1995.
8. Schrezenmeier H, Hertenstein B, Wagner B, Ragavashar A, Heimpel H: A pathogenetic link between aplastic anemia and paroxysmal nocturnal hemoglobinuria is suggested by a high frequency of aplastic anemia patients with a deficiency of phosphatidylinositol glycan anchored proteins. *Exp Hematol* 23:81, 1995.
9. Damashek W: What do aplastic anemia, paroxysmal nocturnal hemoglobinuria and hypoplastic leukemia have in common? (editorial). *Blood* 30:251, 1967.
10. Editorial: Aplasia leukaemia syndrome. *Lancet* 1:1425, 1989.
11. Marsh JCW, Geary CG: Is aplastic anaemia a preleukaemic disorder? (annotation). *Br J Haematol* 77:447, 1991.
12. Socie G: Could aplastic anaemia be considered a pre-pre-leukaemic disorder? *Eur J Haematol* 57(suppl):60, 1996.
13. Young NS: The problem of clonality in aplastic anemia: Dr. Damashek's riddle, restated (perspective). *Blood* 79:1385, 1992.

14. Camitta BM, Storb R, Thomas ED: Aplastic anemia: pathogenesis, diagnosis, treatment and prognosis. *N Engl J Med* 306:645, 712, 1982.

15. Marmont AM, Bacigalupo A: Aplastic anaemia: pathogenesis and treatment. *Haematologica* 73:133, 1988.

16. Nissen C: The pathophysiology of aplastic anemia. *Semin Hematol* 28:313, 1991.

17. Young NS: Immune pathophysiology of acquired aplastic anaemia. *Eur J Haematol* 57(suppl):55, 1996.

18. Young NS, Maciejewski J: The pathophysiology of acquired aplastic anemia. *N Engl J Med* 336:1365, 1997.

19. Kurnick JE, Robinson WA, Dickey CA: In vitro granulocytic colony-forming potential of bone marrow from patients with granulocytopenia and aplastic anemia. *Proc Soc Exp Biol Med* 137:917, 1971.

20. Kagan WA, Ascensao J, Pahwa R, et al: Aplastic anemia: presence in human bone marrow of cells that suppress myelopoiesis. *Proc Natl Acad Sci USA* 73:2890, 1976.

21. Kern P, Heimpel H, Heit W, et al: Granulocytic progenitor cells in aplastic anaemia. *Br J Haematol* 35:613, 1977.

22. Hoak HL, Goselink HM, Veenkof, et al: Acquired aplastic anaemia in adults. IV. Histological and CFU studies in transplanted and nontransplanted patients. *Scand J Haematol* 19:159, 1977.

23. Hoffman R, Zanjani ED, Lutton JD, et al: Suppression of erythroid-colony formation by lymphocytes from patients with aplastic anemia. *N Engl J Med* 296:10, 1977.

24. Hansi W, Rich I, Heimpel H, et al: Erythroid colony forming cells in aplastic anaemia. *Br J Haematol* 37:483, 1977.

25. Moriyama Y, Sato M, Kinoshita Y: Studies of hematopoietic stem cells. XI. Lack of erythroid burst-forming units (BFU-E) in patients with aplastic anemia. *Am J Hematol* 6:11, 1979.

26. Maciejewski JP, Selleri C, Sato T, Anderson S, Young NS: A severe and consistent deficit in marrow and circulating primitive hematopoietic cells (long-term culture-initiating cells) in acquired aplastic anemia. *Blood* 88:1983, 1996.

27. Maciejewski JP, Anderson S, Katevas P, Young NS: Phenotypic and functional analysis of bone marrow progenitor cell compartment in bone marrow failure. *Br J Haematol* 87:227, 1994.

28. Scopes J, Bagnara M, Gordon-Smith EC, Ball SE, Gibson FM: Haemopoietic progenitor cells are reduced in aplastic anaemia. *Br J Haematol* 86:427, 1994.

29. Ascensao J, Kagan W, Moore M, et al: Aplastic anemia: evidence for an immunological mechanism. *Lancet* 1:669, 1976.

30. Nissen C, Cornu P, Gratwohl A, Speck B: Peripheral blood cells from patients with aplastic anaemia in partial remission suppress growth of their own bone marrow precursors in culture. *Br J Haematol* 45:233, 1980.

31. Bacigalupo A, Podesta M, VanLint MT, et al: Severe aplastic anemia: correlation of in vitro tests with clinical response to immunosuppression in twenty patients. *Br J Haematol* 47:423, 1981.

32. Singer JW, Brown JE, James MC, et al: Effect of peripheral blood lymphocytes from patients with aplastic anemia on granulocyte colony growth from HLA-matched and mismatched marrows: effect of transfusion sensitization. *Blood* 52:37, 1978.

33. Torok-Storb B, Sieff C, Storb R, et al: In vitro tests for distinguishing possible immune-mediated aplastic anemia from transfusion-induced sensitization. *Blood* 55:211, 1980.

34. Singer JW, Doney KC, Thomas ED: Co-culture studies of 16 untransfused patients with aplastic anemia. *Blood* 54:180, 1979.

35. Mangan KF, Mullaney MT, Rosenfeld CS, Shadduck RK: In vitro evidence for disappearance of erythroid progenitor T suppressor cells following allogeneic bone marrow transplantation for severe aplastic anemia. *Blood* 71:144, 1988.

36. Teramura M, Kobayashi S, Iwabe K, Yoshinaga K, Mizoguchi H: Mechanism of action of antithymocyte globulin in the treatment of aplastic anaemia: *in vitro* evidence for the presence of immunosuppressive mechanism. *Br J Haematol* 96:80, 1997.

37. Knospe WH, Crosby WH: Aplastic anaemia: a disorder of the bone-marrow sinusoidal microcirculation rather than stem cell failure? *Lancet* 1:20, 1971.

38. Morley, A, Blake J: An animal model of chronic aplastic marrow failure. I. Late marrow failure after busulfan. *Blood* 44:49, 1974.

39. Morley A, Trainor K, Remes J: Residual marrow damage: possible explanation for idiosyncrasy to chloramphenicol. *Br J Haematol* 31:525, 1976.

40. Harrison DE: Use of genetic anaemia in mice as tools for haematological research. *Clin Haematol* 8:239, 1979.

41. Geissler EN, Ryan MA, Housman DE: The dominant-white spotting (W) locus of the mouse encodes the c-*kit* proto-oncogene. *Cell* 55:185, 1988.

42. Huang E, Nocka K, Beier Dr, et al: The hematopoietic growth factor KL is encoded by the Sl locus and is the ligand of the c-*kit* receptor, the gene product of the W locus. *Cell* 63:225, 1990.

43. Wodnar-Filipowicz A, Yancik S, Moser Y, et al: Levels of soluble stem cell factor in serum of patients with aplastic anemia. *Blood* 81:3159, 1993.

44. Nimer SD, Leung DHY, Wolin MJ, Golde DW: Serum stem cell factor levels in patients with aplastic anemia. *Int J Hematol* 60:185, 1994.

45. Kojima S, Matsuyama T, Kodera Y: Plasma levels and production of soluble stem cell factor by marrow stromal cells in patients with aplastic anaemia. *Br J Haematol* 99:440, 1997.

46. Wodnar-Filipowicz A, Tichelli A, Zsebo KM, Speck B, Nissen C: Stem cell factor stimulates the *in vitro* growth of bone marrow cells from aplastic anemia patients. *Blood* 79:3196, 1992.

47. Lyman SD, Seaberg M, Hanna R, et al: Plasma/serum levels of flt3 ligand are low in normal individuals and highly elevated in patients with Fanconi anemia and acquired aplastic anemia. *Blood* 86:4091, 1995.

48. Kojima S, Matsuyama T, Kodera Y, et al: Measurement of endogenous plasma granulocyte colony-stimulating factor in patients with acquired aplastic anemia by a sensitive chemiluminescent immunoassay. *Blood* 87:1303, 1996.

49. Kojima S, Matsuyama T, Kodera Y: Circulating erythropoietin in patients with acquired aplastic anaemia. *Acta Haematol* 94:117, 1995.

50. Emmons RVD, Reid DM, Cohen RL, et al: Human thrombopoietin levels are high when thrombocytopenia is due to megakaryocyte deficiency and low when due to increased platelet destruction. *Blood* 87:4068, 1996.

51. Nakao S, Matsushima K, Young N: Deficient interleukin I production by aplastic anaemia monocytes. *Br J Haematol* 71:431, 1989.

52. Zoumbos N, Gascon P, Djeu J, Young NS: Interferon is a mediator of hematopoietic suppression in aplastic anemia in vitro and possibly in vivo. *Proc Natl Acad Sci USA* 82:188, 1985.

53. Laver J, Castro-Malaspina H, Kernan NA, et al: In vitro interferon-gamma production by cultured T-cells in severe aplastic anaemia: correlation with granulomonopoietic inhibition in patients who respond to anti-thymocyte globulin. *Br J Haematol* 69:545, 1988.

54. Gascon P, Zoumbos NC, Scala G, et al: Lymphokine abnormalities in aplastic anemia: implications for the mechanism of action of antithymocyte globulin. *Blood* 65:407, 1985.

55. Hinterberger W, Adolf G, Bettelheim P, et al: Lymphokine overproduction in severe aplastic anemia is not related to blood transfusions. *Blood* 74:2713, 1989.

56. Shinohara K, Ayame H, Tanaka M, et al: Increased production of tumor necrosis factor alpha by peripheral blood mononuclear cells in the patients with aplastic anemia. *Am J Hematol* 37:75, 1991.

57. Nistico, A, Young, NS: Gamma-interferon gene expression in the bone marrow of patients with aplastic anemia. *Ann Intern Med* 120:463, 1994.

58. Marsh JC, Chang J, Testa NG, et al: In vitro assessment of marrow "stem cell" and stromal cell function in aplastic anaemia. *Br J Haematol* 78:258, 1991.

59. Kojima S, Matsuyama T, Kodera Y: Hematopoietic growth factors released by marrow stromal cells from patients with aplastic anemia. *Blood* 79:2256, 1992.

60. Holmberg LA, Seidel K, Leisenring W, Torok-Storb B: Aplastic anemia: analysis of stromal cell function in long-term marrow cultures. *Blood* 84:3685, 1994.

61. Santesson GG: Über chronische Vergiftungen mit Steinkohlenteerbenzin. vier Todesfälle. *Arch Hyg Berl* 31:336, 1897.

62. Rangau U, Snyder R: Scientific update on benzene. *Ann N Y Acad Sci* 837:105, 1997.

63. Goldstein BD: Benzene toxicity. *Occup Med* 3:541, 1988.

64. Aksoy B: Hematotoxicity and carcinogenicity of benzene. *Environ Health Perspect* 82:193, 1989.

65. Smith MT: Overview of benzene-induced aplastic anaemia. *Eur J Haematol* 60(suppl):107, 1996.

66. Paci E, Buiatti E, Costantini AS, et al: Aplastic anemia, leukemia and

other cancer mortality in a cohort of shoe workers exposed to benzene. *Scand J Work Environ Health* 15:313, 1989.

67. Yin SN, Li GL, Tain FD, et al: Leukaemia in benzene workers: a retrospective cohort study. *Br J Indust Med* 44:124, 1987.

68. Yardley-Jones A, Anderson D, Parke DV: The toxicity of benzene and its metabolism and molecular pathology in human risk assessment. *Br J Indust Med* 48:437, 1991.

69. Hamilton A: The lessening menace of benzol poisoning in American industry. *J Indust Hyg* 10:227, 1928.

70. Aksoy M, Dincol K, Akgun T, et al: Hematological effects of chronic benzene poisoning in 217 workers. *Br J Indust Med* 28:296, 1971.

71. Fleming LE, Timmeny MA: Aplastic anemia and pesticides. *JOM* 35:1106, 1993.

72. Rugman FP, Cosstick R: Aplastic anaemia associated with organochlorine pesticide: case reports and review of evidence. *J Clin Pathol* 43:98, 1990.

73. Rauch AE, Kowalsky SF, Lesar TS, et al: Lindane (Kwell)-induced aplastic anemia. *Arch Intern Med* 150:2393, 1990.

74. Sanchez-Medal L, Castanedo JP, Garcia-Rojas F: Insecticides and aplastic anemia. *N Engl J Med* 269:1365, 1963.

75. Roberts HJ: Pentachlorophenol-associated aplastic anemia, red cell aplasia, leukemia and other blood disorders. *J Fla Med Assoc* 77:86, 1990.

76. Prager D, Peters C: Development of aplastic anemia and the exposure to Stoddard solvent. *Blood* 35:286, 1970.

77. Powers D: Aplastic anemia secondary to glue sniffing. *N Engl J Med* 273:700, 1965.

78. Crawford MAD: Aplastic anaemia due to trinitrotoluene intoxication. *Br Med J* 2:430, 1954.

79. Claudon DB, Holbrook AA: Fatal aplastic anemia associated with chloramphenicol (Chloromycetin) therapy. *JAMA* 149:912, 1952.

80. Smiley RK, Cartwright GE, Wintrobe MM: Fatal aplastic anemia following chloramphenicol (Chloromycetin) administration. *JAMA* 149:914, 1952.

81. Sturgeon P: Fatal aplastic anemia in children following chloramphenicol (Chloromycetin) therapy. *JAMA* 149:918, 1952.

82. Dameshek W: Chloramphenicol (Chloromycetin) and the bone marrow (editorial). *Blood* 7:755, 1952.

83. Wallerstein RO, Condit PK, Kasper PK, et al: Statewide study of chloramphenicol therapy and fatal aplastic anemia. *JAMA* 208:2045, 1969.

84. Modan B, Segal S, Shani M, Sheba C: Aplastic anemia in Israel: evaluation of the etiological role of chloramphenicol on a community-wide basis. *Am J Med Sci* 270:441, 1975.

85. Smick K, Condit PK, Proctor RL, Sutcher V: Fatal aplastic anemia: an epidemiological study of its relationship to the drug chloramphenicol. *J Chronic Dis* 17:899, 1964.

86. Brodsky E, Zeidan Z, Biger Y, Schneider M: Topical application of chloramphenicol eye ointment followed by fatal bone marrow aplasia. *Isr J Med Sci* 25:54, 1989.

87. West BC, DeVault GA Jr, Clement JC, Williams DM: Aplastic anemia associated with parenteral chloramphenicol: review of 10 cases, including the second case of possible increased risk with cimetidine. *Rev Infect Dis* 10:1048, 1988.

88. Rubin D, Weisberger A, Botti RE, Storaasli JP: Changes in iron metabolism in early chloramphenicol toxicity. *J Clin Invest* 37:1286, 1958.

89. Saidi P, Wallerstein RO, Aggeler P: Effect of chloramphenicol on erythropoiesis. *J Lab Clin Med* 57:247, 1961.

90. Scott JL, Finegold SM, Belkin GA, Lawrence JS: A controlled double-blind study of the hematologic toxicity of chloramphenicol. *N Engl J Med* 272:1137, 1965.

91. Weisberger AS: Mechanisms of action of chloramphenicol. *JAMA* 209:97, 1969.

92. Nagao T, Mauer AM: Concordance for drug-induced aplastic anemia in identical twins. *N Engl J Med* 281:7, 1969.

93. Custer RP: Aplastic anemia in soldiers treated with Atabrine (quinacrine). *Am J Med Sci* 212:211, 1946.

94. Cunningham JL, Leyland MJ, Delamore IW, Price-Evans DA: Acetanilide oxidation in phenylbutazone-associated hypoplastic anaemia. *Br Med J* 3:313, 1974.

95. Chang HK, Morrison SL: Bone marrow suppression associated with cimetidine. *Ann Intern Med* 91:580, 1979.

96. Tonkonow B, Hoffman R: Aplastic anemia and cimetidine. *Arch Intern Med* 140:1123, 1980.

97. Volkin RL, Shadduck RK, Winkelstein A, et al: Potentiation of carmustine-cranial-irradiation-induced myelosuppression by cimetidine. *Arch Intern Med* 142:243, 1982.

98. Court-Brown WM, Doll R: Mortality from cancer and other causes after radiotherapy for ankylosing spondylitis. *Br Med J* 2:1317, 1965.

99. Darby SC, Doll R, Gill SK, Smith PG: Long term mortality after a single treatment course with x-rays in patients treated with ankylosing spondylitis. *Br J Cancer* 55:179, 1987.

100. Johnson SAN, Bateman CJT, Beard MEJ, et al: Long-term haematological complications of Thorotrast. *Q J Med* 182:259, 1977.

101. Martland HS: The occurrence of malignancy in radioactive persons: a general review of data gathered in the study of the radium dial painters, with special reference to the occurrence of osteogeneic sarcoma and the inter-relationship of certain blood diseases. *Am J Cancer* 15:2435, 1931.

102. Cronkite EP, Haley TJ: Clinical aspects of acute radiation injury, in *Manual on Radiation Haematology,* pp 169–173. International Atomic Energy Agency, Vienna, 1971.

103. Mettler FA Jr, Moseley RD Jr: *Medical Effects of Ionizing Irradiation,* pp. 1–185. Grune and Stratton, New York, 1985.

104. Gale RP: Immediate medical consequences of nuclear accidents: lessons from Chernobyl. *JAMA* 258:625, 1987.

105. Champlin RE, Kastenberg WE, Gale RP: Radiation accidents and nuclear energy: medical consequences and therapy. *Ann Intern Med* 109:730, 1988.

106. Baranov A, Gale RP, Guskova A, et al: Bone marrow transplantation after the Chernobyl nuclear accident. *N Engl J Med* 311:205, 1989.

107. Gale RP: USSR: Follow-up after Chernobyl. *Lancet* 1:401, 1990.

108. Ajlouni K, Doeblin TD: The syndrome of hepatitis and aplastic anaemia. *Br J Haematol* 27:345, 1974.

109. Hagler L, Pastore RA, Bergin JJ: Aplastic anemia following viral hepatitis: report of 2 fatal cases and literature review. *Medicine (Baltimore)* 54:139, 1975.

110. Pol S, Driss F, Devergie A, et al: Is hepatitis C virus involved in hepatitis-associated aplastic anemia? *Ann Intern Med* 113:435, 1990.

111. Hibbs JR, Frickhofen N, Rosenfeld SJ, et al: Aplastic anemia and viral hepatitis: non-A, non-B, non-C? *JAMA* 267:2051, 1992.

112. Tzakis AG, Arditi M, Whitington PF, et al: Aplastic anemia complicating orthotopic liver transplantation for non-A, non-B hepatitis. *N Engl J Med* 319:393, 1988.

113. Kurtzman G, Young N: Viruses and bone marrow failure. *Baillieres Clin Haematol* 2:51, 1989.

114. Hibbs JR, Issaragrisl S, Young NS: High prevalence of hepatitis C viremia among aplastic anemia patients and controls from Thailand. *Am J Trop Med Hyg* 46:564, 1992.

115. Brown KE, Tisdale J, Barrett AJ, Dunbar CE, Young NS: Hepatitis-associated aplastic anemia. *N Engl J Med* 336:1059, 1997.

116. Shadduck RK, Winkelstein A, Zeigler Z, et al: Aplastic anemia following infectious mononucleosis: possible immune etiology. *Exp Hematol* 7:264, 1979.

117. Lazarus KH, Baehner RL: Aplastic anemia complicating infectious mononucleosis: a case report and review of the literature. *Pediatrics* 67:907, 1981.

118. Baranski B, Armstrong G, Truman JT, et al: Epstein-Barr virus in the bone marrow of patients with aplastic anemia. *Ann Intern Med* 109:695, 1988.

119. Young N: Hematologic and hematopoietic consequences of B-19 parvovirus infection. *Semin Hematol* 25:159, 1988.

120. Rosenfeld CS, Rybka WB, Weinbaum D, et al: Late graft failure due to dual bone marrow infection with variants A and B of human Herpesvirus-6. *Exp Hematol* 23:626, 1995.

121. Vinters HV, Mah V, Mohrmann R, Wiley CA: Evidence for human immunodeficiency virus (HIV) infection of the brain in a patient with aplastic anemia. *Acta Neuropathol* 76:311, 1988.

122. Samuel D, Castaing D, Adam R, et al: Fatal acute HIV infection with aplastic anaemia, transmitted by liver graft. *Lancet* 1:1221, 1988.

123. Morales CE, Sriram I, Baumann MA: Myelodysplastic syndrome occurring as possible first manifestation of human immunodeficiency virus infection with subsequent progression to aplastic anaemia. *Int J STD AIDS* 1:55, 1990.

124. Baumelou E, Guiguet M, Mary JY, et al: Epidemiology of aplastic

anemia in France: a case control study. I. Medical history and medication use. *Blood* 81:1471, 1993.

125. Stricke RB, Shuman MA: Aplastic anemia complicating systemic lupus erythematosus: response to androgens in two patients. *Am J Hematol* 17:193, 1984.

126. Fitchen JJ, Cline MJ, Saxon A, Golde DW: Serum inhibitors of hematopoiesis in a patient with aplastic anemia and systemic lupus erythematosus: recovery after exchange plasmapheresis. *Am J Med* 66:537, 1979.

127. Bailey FA, Lilly M, Bertoli LF, Ball GV: An antibody that inhibits in vitro bone marrow proliferation in a patient with systemic lupus erythematosus and aplastic anemia. *Arthritis Rheum* 31:901, 1989.

128. Roffe C, Cahill MR, Samanta A, et al: Aplastic anaemia in systemic lupus erythematosus: a cellular immune mechanism? *Br J Rheumatol* 30:301, 1991.

129. Sumimoto S, Kawai M, Kasajima Y, Hamamoto T: Aplastic anemia associated with systemic lupus erythematosus. *Am J Hematol* 38:329, 1991.

130. Winkler A, Jackson RW, Kay DS, et al: High-dose intravenous cyclophosphamide treatment of systemic lupus erythematosus-associated aplastic anemia (letter). *Arthritis Rheum* 31:693, 1988.

131. Hoffman R, Dainiak N, Sibrack L, et al: Antibody-mediated aplastic anemia and diffuse fasciitis. *N Engl J Med* 300:718, 1979.

132. Narayanan MN, Liu Yin JA, Love EM, et al: Eosinophilic fasciitis and aplastic anaemia. *Clin Lab Haematol* 10:471, 1988.

133. Debusscher L, Bitar N, DeMaubeuge J, et al: Eosinophilic fasciitis and severe aplastic anemia: favorable response to either antithymocyte globulin or cyclosporin A in blood and skin disorders. *Transplant Proc* 20:310, 1988.

134. Blaser KU, Steiger U, Wursch A, Speck B: Eosinophilic fasciitis with aplastic anemia and Hashimoto's thyroiditis. Review of the literature and report of a typical example. *Schweiz Med Wochenschr* 119:1899, 1989.

135. Evans IL: Aplastic anaemia in pregnancy remitting after abortion. *Br Med J* 3:166, 1968.

136. Fleming AF: Hypoplastic anaemia in pregnancy. *J Obstet Gynaecol Br Commonw* 75:138, 1968.

137. Goldstein JM, Coller BS: Aplastic anemia in pregnancy: recovery after normal spontaneous delivery (letter). *Ann Intern Med* 82:537, 1975.

138. Suda T, Omine M, Tsuchiya J, Maekawa T: Prognostic aspects of aplastic anaemia in pregnancy. Experience on 6 cases and review of the literature. *Blut* 36:285, 1978.

139. Aitchison RGM, Marsh JCW, Hows JM, et al: Pregnancy associated aplastic anaemia: a report of 5 cases and review of current management. *Br J Haematol* 73:541, 1989.

140. Pajor A, Kelemen E, Szak'acs Z, Lehoczky D: Pregnancy in idiopathic aplastic anemia (report of 10 patients). *Eur J Obstet Gynecol Reprod Biol* 45:19, 1992.

141. Bourantas K, Makrydimas G, Georgiou I, Repousis P, Lolis D: Aplastic anemia: report of a case with recurrent episodes in consecutive pregnancies. *J Reprod Med* 42:672, 1997.

142. Fanconi G: Familiäre infantile pernizioásartige anämie (perniziöses blutbild und konstitution). *Jahrbuch Kinderheil* 117:257, 1927.

143. Gordon-Smith EC, Rutherford TR: Fanconi anaemia—constitutional, familial aplastic anaemia. *Baillieres Clin Haematol* 2:139, 1989.

144. Gordon-Smith EC, Rutherford TR: Fanconi anemia: constitutional aplastic anemia. *Semin Hematol* 28:104, 1991.

145. Alter BP: Fanconi's anemia: current concepts: *Am J Pediatr Hematol Oncol* 14:170, 1992.

146. Auerbach AD, Rogatko A, Schroeder-Kurth TM: International Fanconi Anemia Registry: first report, in *Fanconi Anemia: Clinical, Cytogenetic and Experimental Aspects,* edited by TM Schroeder-Kurth, AD Auerbach, G Obe, pp 3–17. Springer-Verlag, Berlin, 1989.

147. D'Apolito M, Zelante L, Savoia A: Molecular basis of Fanconi anemia. *Hematologica* 83:533, 1998.

148. Garcia-Higuera I, Kuang Y, D'Andrea AD: The molecular and cellular biology of Fanconi anemia. *Curr Opin Hematol* 6:83, 1999.

149. Estren S, Damshek W: Familial hypoplastic anemia of childhood: report of 8 cases in 2 families with beneficial effects of splenectomy in 1 case. *Am J Dis Child* 73:671, 1947.

150. Gluckman E, Auerbach A, Horowitz MM, et al: Bone marrow transplantation for Fanconi anemia. *Blood* 86:2856, 1995.

151. Dokal I: Dyskeratosis congenita: an inherited bone marrow failure syndrome. *Br J Haematol* 92:775, 1996.

152. Ginzberg H, Shin J, Ellis L, et al: Schwachman syndrome: phenotypic manifestations of sibling sets and isolated cases in a large patient cohort are similar. *J Pediatr* 135:81, 1999.

153. Bottiger LE, Westerholm B: Aplastic anemia. I. Incidence and aetiology. *Acta Med Scand* 192:315, 1972.

154. Szklo M, Sensenbrenner L, Markowitz J, et al: Incidence of aplastic anemia in metropolitan Baltimore: a population based study. *Blood* 66:115, 1985.

155. Linet MS, McCaffrey LD, Morgan WF, et al: Incidence of aplastic anemia in a three county area in South Carolina. *Cancer Res* 46:426, 1986.

156. Marsh JCW, Hows JM, Bryett KA, et al: Survival after antilymphocyte globulin for aplastic anemia depends on disease severity. *Blood* 70:1046, 1987.

157. Alexanian R: Erythropoietin excretion in bone marrow failure and hemolytic anemia. *J Lab Clin Med* 82:438, 1973.

158. Stohlman F Jr: Erythropoiesis. *N Engl J Med* 267:342, 392, 1962.

159. Camitta BM, Thomas ED, Nathan DG, et al: A prospective study of androgens and bone marrow transplantation for treatment of severe aplastic anemia. *Blood* 53:504, 1979.

160. Bacigalupo A, Hows J, Gluckman E, et al: Bone marrow transplantation (BMT) versus immunosuppression for the treatment of severe aplastic anaemia (SAA): a report of the EBMT SAA working party. *Br J Haematol* 70:177, 1988.

161. Krause JR: Aplastic anemia terminating in hairy cell leukemia. A report of 2 cases. *Cancer* 53:1533, 1984.

162. Reid MM, Summerfield GP: Distinction between a leukaemic prodrome of childhood acute lymphoblastic leukaemia and aplastic anaemia. *J Clin Pathol* 45:697, 1992.

163. Torok-Storb B, Doney K, Brown SL, Prentice RL: Correlation of two in vitro tests with clinical response to immunosuppressive therapy in 54 patients with severe aplastic anemia. *Blood* 63:349, 1984.

164. Applebaum FR, Barrall J, Storb R, et al: Clonal cytogenetic abnormalities in patients with otherwise typical aplastic anemia. *Exp Hematol* 15:1134, 1987.

165. Olson DO, Shields AF, Scheurich CJ, et al: Magnetic resonance imaging of the bone marrow in patients with leukemia, aplastic anemia, and lymphoma. *Invest Radiol* 21:540, 1986.

166. Steiner RM, Mitchell DG, Rao VM, et al: Magnetic resonance imaging of bone marrow: diagnostic value in diffuse hematologic disorders. *Magn Reson Q* 6:17, 1990.

167. Negendank W, Weissman D, Bey TM, et al: Evidence for clonal disease by magnetic resonance imaging in patients with hypoplastic marrow disorders. *Blood* 78:2872, 1991.

168. Finch CA, Duebelbeiss K, Cook JD, et al: Ferrokinetics in man. *Medicine (Baltimore)* 49:17, 1970.

169. Camitta BM, Thomas ED, Nathan DG, et al: Severe aplastic anemia: a prospective study of the effect of early marrow transplantation on acute mortality. *Blood* 48:63, 1976.

170. Storb R, Longton G, Anasetti C, et al: Changing trends in marrow transplantation for aplastic anemia. *Bone Marrow Transplant* 10(suppl 1):45, 1992.

171. Margolis DA, Cammita BM: Hematopoietic stem cell transplantation for severe aplastic anemia. *Curr Opin Hematol* 5:441, 1998.

172. Kernan NA, Bartsch G, Ash RC, et al: Analysis of 462 transplantations from unrelated donors facilitated by the National Marrow Donor Program. *N Engl J Med* 318:593, 1993.

173. Wagner JE, Rosenthal J, Sweetman R, et al: Successful transplantation of HLA-matched and HLA-mismatched umbilical cord blood from unrelated donors: analysis of engraftment and acute graft-versus-host disease. *Blood* 88:795, 1996.

174. Mathé G, Amiel JL, Schwarzenberg L, et al: Bone marrow graft in man after conditioning by antilymphocytic serum. *Br Med J* 2:131, 1970.

175. Speck B, Kissling M: Successful bone marrow grafts in experimental aplastic anemia using antilymphocytic serum for conditioning. *Eur J Clin Biol Res* 16:1047, 1971.

176. Speck B, Kissling M: Studies on bone marrow transplantation and experimental ^{31}P-induced aplastic anaemia after conditioning with antilymphocyte serum. *Acta Haematol* 50:193, 1973.

177. Champlin RE, Feig SA, Sparkes RS, Gale RP: Bone marrow transplantation from identical twins in the treatment of aplastic anaemia: implication for the pathogenesis of the disease. *Br J Haematol* 56:455, 1984.

178. Mangan KF, D'Alessandro L, Mullaney MT: Action of antithymocyte globulin on normal human erythroid progenitor cell proliferation in vitro: erythropoietic growth-enhancing factors are released from marrow accessory cells. *J Lab Clin Med* 107:353, 1986.

179. Kawano Y, Nissen C, Gratwohl A, Speck B: Immunostimulatory effects of different antilymphocyte globulin preparations: a possible clue to their clinical effect. *Br J Haematol* 68:115, 1988.

180. Speck B, Gluckman E, Haak HL, et al: Treatment of aplastic anaemia by antilymphocyte globulin with and without allogeneic bone-marrow infusions. *Lancet* 2:1145, 1977.

181. Champlin RE, Ho W, Gale RP: Antilymphocyte globulin treatment in patients with aplastic anemia. *N Engl J Med* 308:113, 1983.

182. Camitta B, O'Reilly RJ, Sensenbrenner L, et al: Antithoracic duct lymphocyte globulin therapy of severe aplastic anemia. *Blood* 62:883, 1983.

183. Young N, Griffith P, Brittain E, et al: A multi-center trial of antithymocyte globulin in aplastic anemia and related diseases. *Blood* 72:1861, 1989.

184. Camitta BM, Doney K: Immunosuppressive therapy for aplastic anemia: indications, agents, mechanisms, and results. *Am J Pediatr Hematol Oncol* 12:411, 1990.

185. Bielory L, Wright R, Nienhuis AW, et al: Antithymocyte globulin hypersensitivity in bone marrow failure patients. *JAMA* 260:3164, 1988.

186. Bacigalupo A, Van Lint MT, Cerri R, et al: Treatment of severe aplastic anemia with bolus 6-methylprednisolone and antilymphocyte globulin. *Blut* 41:168, 1980.

187. Issaragrisil S, Tangnai-Trisorana Y, Siriseriwan T, et al: Methylprednisolone therapy in aplastic anaemia: correlation of in vitro tests and lymphocyte subsets with clinical response. *Eur J Haematol* 40:343, 1988.

188. Stryckmans PA, Dumont JP, Velu T, Debusscher L: Cyclosporine in refractory severe aplastic anemia (letter). *N Engl J Med* 310:655, 1984.

189. Lazzarino M, Morra E, Canevari A, et al: Cyclosporine in the treatment of aplastic anaemia and pure red-cell aplasia. *Bone Marrow Transplant* 4(suppl 4):165, 1989.

190. Hinterberger-Fischer M, Höcker P, Lechner K, et al: Oral cyclosporin-A is effective treatment for untreated and also for previously immunosuppressed patients with severe bone marrow failure. *Eur J Haematol* 43:136, 1989.

191. Tötterman TH, Höglund M, Bengtsson M, et al: Treatment of pure red-cell aplasia and aplastic anaemia with cyclosporin: long-term clinical effects. *Eur J Haematol* 42:126, 1989.

192. Leeksma OC, Thomas LLM, van der Lelie J, van Oers MHJ, Kr.von dem Borne AEG, Goudsmit R: Effectiveness of low dose cyclosporine in acquired aplastic anaemia with severe neutropenia. *Neth J Med* 41:143, 1992.

193. Leonard EM, Raefsky E, Griffith P, et al: Cyclosporine therapy of aplastic anaemia, congenital and acquired red-cell aplasia. *Br J Haematol* 72:278, 1989.

194. Tong J, Bacigalupo A, Piaggio G, et al: Severe aplastic anemia (SAA): response to cyclosporin A (CyA) in vivo and in vitro. *Eur J Haematol* 46:212, 1991.

195. Nakao S, Yamaguchi M, Shiobara S, et al: Interferon-g gene expression in unstimulated bone marrow mononuclear cells predicts a good response to cyclosporine therapy in aplastic anemia. *Blood* 79:2531, 1992.

196. Kojima S, Fukada M, Miyajima Y, Matsuyama T: Cyclosporine and recombinant granulocyte colony-stimulating factor in severe aplastic anemia (letter). *N Engl J Med* 313:920, 1990.

197. Bertrand Y, Amri F, Capdeville R, et al: The successful treatment of two cases of severe aplastic anaemia with granulocyte colony-stimulating factor and cyclosporine A (case report). *Br J Haematol* 79:648, 1991.

198. Schrezenmeier H, Schlander M, Raghavachar A: Cyclosporin A in aplastic anemia—report of a workshop. *Ann Hematol* 65:33, 1992.

199. Gluckman E, Esperou-Bourdeau H, Baruchel A, et al: Multicenter randomized study comparing cyclosporine-A alone and antithymocyte globulin with prednisone for treatment of severe aplastic anemia. *Blood* 79:2540, 1992.

200. Doney K, Pepe M, Storb R, et al: Immunosuppressive therapy of aplastic anemia: results of a prospective, randomized trial of antithymocyte globulin (ATG), methylprednisolone and oxymetholone to ATG, very high-dose methylprednisolone, and oxymetholone. *Blood* 79:2566, 1992.

201. Bacigalupo A, Chaple M, Hows J, et al: Treatment of aplastic anaemia (AA) with antilymphocyte globulin (ALG) and methylprednisolone (MPred) with or without androgens: a randomized trial from the EBMT SAA working party. *Br J Haematol* 83:145, 1993.

202. Champlin RE, Ho WG, Feig SA, et al: Do androgens enhance the response to antithymocyte globulin in patients with aplastic anemia? A prospective randomized trial. *Blood* 66:184, 1985.

203. Kaltwasser JP, Dix U, Schalk KP, Vogt H: Effect of androgens on the response to antithymocyte globulin in patients with aplastic anaemia. *Eur J Haematol* 40:111, 1988.

204. Gluckman E, Devergie P, Poros A, et al: Results of immunosuppression in 170 cases of severe aplastic anaemia. *Br J Haematol* 51:541, 1982.

205. Park CW, Han CH, Kim CC, et al: Immunomodulation therapy for severe aplastic anemia: ALG versus ALG plus cyclosporin-A. *Korean J Intern Med* 4:28, 1989.

206. Frickhofen N, Kaltwasser JP, Schrezenmeier H, et al: Treatment of aplastic anemia with antilymphocyte globulin and methylprednisolone with or without cyclosporine. *N Engl J Med* 314:1299, 1991.

207. Rosenfeld SJ, Kimball J, Vining D, Young NS: Intensive immunosuppression with antithymocyte globulin and cyclosporine as treatment for severe acquired aplastic anemia. *Blood* 85:3058, 1995.

208. Marsh JCW, Socie G, Schrezenmeier H, et al: Haemopoietic growth factors in aplastic anaemia: a cautionary note. *Lancet* 344:172, 1994.

209. Bacigalupo A, Broccia G, Corda G, et al: Antilymphocyte globulin, cyclosporine, and granulocyte colony-stimulating factor in patients with acquired severe aplastic anemia (SAA): a pilot study of the EBMT SAA working party. *Blood* 85:1348, 1995.

210. Paquette RL, Tebyani N, Frane M, et al: Long-term outcome of aplastic anemia in adults treated with antithymocyte globulin: comparison with bone marrow transplantation. *Blood* 85:283, 1995.

211. Doney K, Leisenring W, Storb R, Appelbaum FR: Primary treatment of acquired aplastic anemia: outcomes with bone marrow transplantation and immunosuppressive therapy. *Ann Intern Med* 126:107, 1997.

212. Gillio AP, Boulad F, Small TN, et al: Comparison of long-term outcome of children with severe aplastic anemia treated with immunosuppression versus bone marrow transplantation. *Biol Blood Marrow Transplant* 3:18, 1997.

213. De Planque MM, Kluin-Nelemans HC, Van Krieken HJM, et al: Evolution of acquired severe aplastic anaemia to myelodysplasia and subsequent leukaemia in adults. *Br J Haematol* 70:55, 1988.

214. Tichelli A, Gratwohl A, Würsch A, et al: Late haematological complications in severe aplastic anaemia. *Br J Haematol* 69:413, 1988.

215. Moore MAS, Castro-Malaspina H: Immunosuppression in aplastic anemia—postponing the inevitable? *N Engl J Med* 314:1358, 1991.

216. Schrezenmeier H, Marin P, Raghavachar A, et al: Relapse of aplastic anaemia after immunosuppressive treatment: a report from the European Bone Marrow Transplantation Group SAA Working Party. *Br J Haematol* 85:371, 1993.

217. Tichelli A, Gratwohl A, Nissen C, Speck B: Late clonal complications in severe aplastic anemia. *Leuk Lymphoma* 12:167, 1994.

218. De Planque MM, Bacigalupo A, Würsch A, et al: Long-term follow-up of severe aplastic anaemia patients treated with antithymocyte globulin. *Br J Haematol* 73:121, 1989.

219. Socié G, Henry-Amar M, Bacigalupo A, et al: Malignant tumors occurring after treatment of aplastic anemia. *N Engl J Med* 319:1152, 1993.

220. Tichelli A, Gratwohl A, Nissen C, et al: Morphology in patients with severe aplastic anemia treated with antilymphocyte globulin. *Blood* 80:337, 1992.

221. Brodsky RA, Sensenbrenner LL, Jones RJ: Complete remission in severe aplastic anemia after high-dose cyclophosphamide without bone marrow transplantation. *Blood* 87:491, 1996.

222. Shahidi NT: Androgens and erythropoiesis. *N Engl J Med* 289:72, 1973.

223. French Cooperative Group for the Study of Aplastic and Refractory Anemias: Androgen therapy in aplastic anemia: a comparative study of high and low doses of 4 different androgens. *Scand J Haematol* 36:346, 1986.

224. Najean Y, Haguenauer O (for the Cooperative Group for the Study of Aplastic and Refractory Anemias): Long-term (5–20 years) evolution of non-grafted aplastic anemias. *Blood* 76:2222, 1990.

225. Seewald TR, Zeigler ZR, Gardner FH: Successful treatment of severe refractory aplastic anemia with 3-b etiocholanolone and nandrolone decanoate. *Am J Hematol* 31:216, 1989.

226. Antin JH, Smith BR, Holmes W, Rosenthal DS: Phase I/II study of

recombinant human granulocyte-macrophage colony-stimulating factor in aplastic anemia and myelodysplastic syndrome. *Blood* 72:705, 1988.

227. Vadhan-Raj S, Buescher S, Broxmeyer HE, et al: Stimulation of myelopoiesis in patients with aplastic anemia by recombinant human granulocyte-macrophage colony-stimulating factor. *N Engl J Med* 319:1628, 1988.

228. Guinan EC, Sieff CA, Oette DH, Nathan DG: A phase I/II trial of recombinant granulocyte-macrophage colony-stimulating factor for children with aplastic anemia. *Blood* 76:1077, 1990.

229. Sonoda Y, Ohno Y, Fujii H, et al: Multilineage response in aplastic anemia patients following long-term administration of filgrastim (recombinant human granulocyte colony stimulating factor). *Stem Cells* 11:543, 1993.

230. Bessho M, Jinnai I, Hirashima K, et al: Trilineage recovery by combination therapy with recombinant human granulocyte colony-stimulating factor and erythropoietin in patients with aplastic anemia and refractory anemia. *Stem Cells* 12:604, 1994.

231. Imamura M, Kobayashi M, Kobayashi S, et al: Combination therapy with recombinant human granulocyte colony-stimulating factor and erythropoietin in aplastic anemia. *Am J Hematol* 48:29, 1995.

232. Kojima S: Use of hematopoietic growth factors for treatment of aplastic anemia. *Bone Marrow Transplant* 18(suppl 3):S36, 1996.

233. Ganser A, Lindemann A, Siepelt G, et al: Effects of recombinant human interleukin-3 in aplastic anemia. *Blood* 76:1287, 1990.

234. Walsh CE, Liu JM, Anderson SM, et al: A trial of recombinant human interleukin-1 in patients with severe refractory aplastic anaemia. *Br J Haematol* 80:106, 1992.

235. Kapoor N, Hvizdala E, Good RA: High-dose intravenous gamma globulin as an approach to treatment of antibody mediated pancytopenia. *Br J Haematol* 59:98, 1988.

236. Sadowitz PD, Dubowy RL: Intravenous immunoglobulin in the treatment of aplastic anemia. *Am J Pediatr Hematol Oncol* 12:198, 1990.

237. Bodenstein H: Successful treatment of aplastic anemia with high-dose immunoglobulin (letter). *N Engl J Med* 314:1368, 1991.

238. Ito T, Haraiwa M, Ishikawa Y, et al: Lymphocytapheresis in a patient with severe aplastic anaemia. *Acta Haematol* 80:167, 1988.

239. Morales-Polanco MR, Sanchez-Valle E, Guerrero-Rivera S, Gutierrez-Alamillo L, Delgado-Marquez B: Treatment results of 23 cases of severe aplastic anemia with lymphocytapheresis. *Arch Med Res* 28:85, 1997.

240. Gómez-Almaguer D, Marfil-Rivera J, Kudish-Wersh A: Acyclovir in the treatment of aplastic anemia. *Am J Hematol* 29:172, 1988.

241. Speck B, Tichelli A, Widmer E, et al: Splenectomy as an adjuvant measure in the treatment of severe aplastic anaemia. *Br J Haematol* 92:818, 1996.

242. Nissen C, Gratwohl A, Speck B: Management of aplastic anaemia. *Eur J Haematol* 46:193, 1991.

243. Beutler E: Platelet transfusions: the 20,000/μl trigger. *Blood* 81:1411, 1993.

244. Zeigler ZR: Effects of epsilon aminocaproic acid on primary haemostasis. *Haemostasis* 21:313, 1991.

245. Sniecinski I, O'Donnell MR, Nowicki B, Hill LR: Prevention of refractoriness and HLA-alloimmunization using filtered blood products. *Blood* 71:1402, 1988.

246. Zeigler ZR, Shadduck RK, Rosenfeld CS, et al: High-dose intravenous gamma globulin improves responses to single-donor platelets in patients refractory to platelet transfusion. *Blood* 70:1433, 1987.

247. Zeigler ZR, Shadduck RK, Rosenfeld CS, et al: Intravenous gamma globulin decreases platelet associated IgG and improves transfusion responses in platelet refractory states. *Am J Hematol* 38:15, 1991.

248. Christie DJ, Howe RB, Lennon SS, Sauro SC: Treatment of refractoriness to platelet transfusion by protein A column therapy. *Transfusion* 33:234, 1993.

249. Wolfe LC, Olivieri NF, Sallan D, et al: Prevention of cardiac disease by subcutaneous deferoxamine in patients with thalassemia major. *N Engl J Med* 312:1600, 1985.

250. Caspar CB, Seger RA, Burger J, Gmür J: Effective stimulation of donors for granulocyte transfusions with recombinant methionyl granulocyte colony-stimulating factor. *Blood* 81:2866, 1993.

251. Lewis SM: Course and prognosis in aplastic anemia. *Br Med J* 1:1027, 1965.

252. Lynch RE, Williams DM, Reading JC, Cartwright GE: The prognosis in aplastic anemia. *Blood* 45:517, 1975.

253. Najean Y, Pecking A: Prognostic factors in acquired aplastic anemia. A study of 352 cases. *Am J Med* 67:564, 1979.

254. Bacigalupo A: Aetiology of severe aplastic anaemia and outcome after allogeneic bone marrow transplantation or immunosuppression therapy. *Eur J Haematol* 57(suppl):16, 1996.

255. Kiem HP, McDonald GB, Myerson D, et al: Marrow transplantation for hepatitis-associated aplastic anemia: a follow-up of long-term survivors. *Biol Blood Marrow Transplant* 2:93, 1996.

256. Best WR: Drug-associated blood dyscrasias. *JAMA* 185:286, 1963.

257. The International Agranulocytosis and Aplastic Anemia Study: Risks of agranulocytosis and aplastic anemia: a first report of their relation to drug use with special reference to analgesics. *JAMA* 256:1749, 1986.

258. Retsagi G, Kelly JP, Kaufman DW: Risk of agranulocytosis and aplastic anaemia in relation to use of antithyroid drugs: International Agranulocytosis and Aplastic Anaemia Study. *Br Med J* 297:262, 1988.

259. International Agranulocytosis and Aplastic Anemia Study: Anti-infective drug use in relation to the risk of agranulocytosis and aplastic anemia. *Arch Intern Med* 149:1036, 1989.

260. Kelly JP, Kaufman DW, Shapiro S: Risks of agranulocytosis and aplastic anemia in relation to the use of cardiovascular drugs: the International Agranulocytosis and Aplastic Anemia Study. *Clin Pharmacol Ther* 49:330, 1991.

261. Kaufmann DW, Kelly JP, Jurgelon JM, et al: Drugs in the aetiology of agranulocytosis and aplastic anemia. *Eur J Haematolo* 57(suppl):23, 1996.

262. Bithell TC, Wintrobe MM: Drug-induced aplastic anemia. *Semin Hematol* 4:194, 1967.

263. Williams DM, Lynch RE, Cartwright GE: Drug-induced aplastic anemia. *Semin Hematol* 10:195, 1973.

264. Heimpel H, Heit W: Drug-induced aplastic anaemia. *Clin Haematol* 9:641, 1980.

265. Williams DM: Pancytopenia, aplastic anemia and pure red cell aplasia, in *Wintrobe's Clinical Hematology,* 10th ed, edited by GR Lee, J Foerster, J Lukens, et al, pp 1452–1459. Williams & Wilkins, Baltimore, 1999.

266. Adamson JW, Erslev AJ: Aplastic anemia, in *Hematology,* 4th ed, edited by WJ Williams, E Beutler, AJ Erslev, MA Lichtman, pp 158–174. McGraw-Hill, New York, 1990.

267. Fernandez deSevilla T, Alegre J, Ocana I, Pahissa A: Aplastic anemia secondary to ticlopidine. *Med Clin (Barc)* 90:308, 1988.

268. Mataix R, Ojeda E, Carmen-Perez M, Jimenez S: Ticlopidine and severe aplastic anemia. *Br J Haematol* 80:125, 1992.

269. Garnier G, Taillan B, Pesce A, et al: Ticlopidine and severe aplastic anaemia. *Br J Haematol* 81:459, 1992.

270. Doney K, Storb R, Buckner CD, Thomas ED: Treatment of gold-induced aplastic anaemia with immunosuppressive therapy. *Br J Haematol* 68:469, 1988.

271. Yan A, Davis P: Gold induced marrow suppression: a review of 10 cases. *J Rheumatol* 17:47, 1990.

272. Biswas N, Ahn WH, Goldman JM, Schwartz JM: Aplastic anemia associated with antithyroid drugs (case report). *Am J Med Sci* 301:190, 1991.

273. Keisu M, Wiholm BE, Ost A, Mortimer O: Acetazolamide-associated aplastic anaemia. *J Intern Med* 228:627, 1990.

274. Mangan KF, Zidar B, Shadduck RK, et al: Interferon-induced aplasia: evidence for T-cell mediated suppression of hematopoiesis and recovery after treatment with horse anti-human thymocyte globulin. *Am J Hematol* 19:401, 1985.

275. Harousseau JL, Milpied N, Bourhis JS, et al: Lethal aplasia after treatment with alpha-interferon of recurrent chronic myeloid leukemia following allogeneic bone marrow graft (letter). *Presse Med* 17:80, 1988.

276. Kaufman DW, Kelly JP, Anderson T, Harmon DC, Shapiro S: Evaluation of case reports of aplastic anemia among patients treated with felbamate. *Epilepsia* 38:1265, 1997.

277. Guardiola Ph, Pasquini R, Dokal I, et al: Outcome of 69 allogeneic stem cell transplantations for Fanconi anemia using HLA-matched unrelated donors. *Blood* 95:422, 2000.

278. Dror Y, Freedman MH: Schwachman-Diamond Syndrome. *Blood* 94:3048, 1999.

PURE RED CELL APLASIA

ALLAN J. ERSLEV

Pure red cell aplasia is caused by a selective destruction or inhibition of erythroid progenitor or precursor cells. It is characterized by an anemia and reticulocytopenia and occurs as an acute or chronic condition. The acute pure red cell aplasia is a transient disorder and is seen primarily in childhood but can occur at all ages. When a cause is found, it usually involves a viral invasion of the erythroid progenitor cells, mostly by the parvovirus B19, but a number of drugs and chemicals have also been shown to cause a toxic or immunologic rejection of these cells. The chronic pure red cell anemias are either constitutional or acquired. The constitutional form is diagnosed in early childhood and can be inborn or inherited. It is caused by the emergence of abnormal progenitor cells, poorly responsive to the action of erythropoietin. The patients may respond to glucocorticoids, but they are rarely, if ever, cured. The acquired form of chronic pure red cell aplasia is an autoimmune disorder, occasionally associated with thymic tumors. It is either caused by T cell-mediated destruction of erythroid progenitor or precursor cells or by B cell production of antibodies to these cells. As in the case of all autoimmune disorders, the results of treatment with glucocorticoids and cytotoxic drugs or immunosuppressive agents are unpredictable, and treatment often leads to serious complications.

Pure red cell aplasia is a widely used name for an anemia caused and characterized by an isolated depletion of erythroblasts. Many terms have been applied to this marrow disorder, and names such as *erythroblast hypoplasia, erythroblastopenia, erythroid hypoplasia,* and *red cell agenesis* are all as good as *pure red cell aplasia.* Certain other names, however, such as *hypoplastic anemia* and *aregenerative anemia,* may lead to confusion, since they also are used to characterize the pancytopenia of aplastic anemia and the refractory anemia of chronic disorders, respectively. In this chapter, the term *pure red cell aplasia* has been chosen because it is vivid and descriptive. Pure red cell aplasia was first clearly separated from aplastic anemia in 1922 by Kaznelson.[1] Since then because of its intriguing relationship to autoimmunity and to thymic tumors, it has received steadily increasing attention as attested to by numerous case reports and several recent reviews.[2,3] At the present, it can be classified into three types: an acute transient type and a chronic type, either constitutional or acquired. The term *transient erythroblastopenia of childhood* has been introduced to describe a pure red cell aplasia of unknown cause that is seen in previously healthy children.[4] However, it is uncertain whether this is a distinct entity. As such, the term will not be used in this chapter.

Acronyms and abbreviations that appear in this chapter include: ADA, adenosine deaminase; BFU-E, burst forming units–erythroid; CFU-E, colony-forming units–erythroid; CFU-GM, colony forming unit–granulocyte-monocyte.

ACUTE TRANSIENT PURE RED CELL APLASIA

DEFINITION AND HISTORY

In 1942, Lyngar[5] recognized that the anemic crisis in children with hereditary spherocytosis was frequently caused by decreased production of red cells rather than by increased hemolysis. In a paper in 1948, Owren[6] employed the term *aplastic crisis* for this temporary production defect and outlined its natural history from the onset of a mild infection, through total erythroid aplasia, to recovery with rebound erythroid hyperplasia (Fig. 32-1). The following year, Gasser[7] described a similar type of self-limited erythroid aplasia in patients without hemolytic anemia. Since then, numerous instances of transient erythroid aplasia have been reported in children and adults.

ETIOLOGY AND PATHOGENESIS

PREVALENCE

Most cases of self-limited aplastic crisis have been reported in patients with chronic hemolytic disorders such as hereditary spherocytosis,[8–10] acquired hemolytic anemia,[11–13] paroxysmal nocturnal hemoglobinuria,[14] sickle cell anemia,[15,16] and others.[17–20] A brief period of erythroid aplasia in a patient with a short red cell life span will have a more rapid and noticeable effect on the hemoglobin concentration than the same period of aplasia will have in an individual with a normal red cell life span. Consequently, it can be assumed that the cases of aplastic crisis reported without underlying hemolytic disorders[21] represent merely a fraction of the actual occurrence of temporary erythroid aplasia.

INFECTIOUS ETIOLOGY

Aplastic crises are frequently preceded by a mild febrile illness, an upper respiratory infection, or gastroenteritis and may afflict several members of a family within a short period of time. When identified, the etiologic agent is usually a virus[22] including those responsible for infectious mononucleosis[23] or hepatitis.[24,25]

However, the great majority of patients experiencing an acute aplastic crisis are infected by the B19 parvovirus.[26] This DNA virus has been known to cause erythema infantosum, or fifth disease, in children. It has the capacity to invade and destroy rapidly proliferating erythroid progenitor and precursor cells. This may cause a temporary and often unnoticed erythroid aplasia[12,13,27] that is terminated by the emergence of neutralizing IgM and IgG antibodies.

Previously uninfected adults contracting a B19 parvovirus infection may develop an aplastic crisis.[28] In infected pregnant women[29,30] the virus may pass the placenta and invade the rapidly proliferating erythroid tissue of the fetus. This will in some cases result in a spontaneous abortion, and in others in hydrops fetalis similar to the condition seen in α-thalassemia.[31]

In the absence of a demonstrable parvovirus infection, humoral inhibitors of erythroid progenitor cells have been demonstrated in some and suspected in many others as the cause of acute transient pure red cell aplasia.[11,23] In one study of 12 such patients IgG inhibitors of progenitor cells, both burst forming units–erythroid (BFU-E) and colony forming units–erythroid (CFU-E), could be identified in 8 patients.[32] These inhibitors had no effect on erythroid precursor cells, erythropoietin, or myeloid progenitors. The brief and self-limited course has precluded more extensive observations on these inhibitors.

DRUG ETIOLOGY

Aplastic crises have also been related to drug toxicity,[33] and possible offenders are listed in Table 32-1.[34–71] In a carefully studied case of diphenylhydantoin-induced pure red cell aplasia it was found that the patient's serum IgG suppressed the growth of both allogeneic and autologous erythroid progenitor cells in the presence of diphenylhydan-

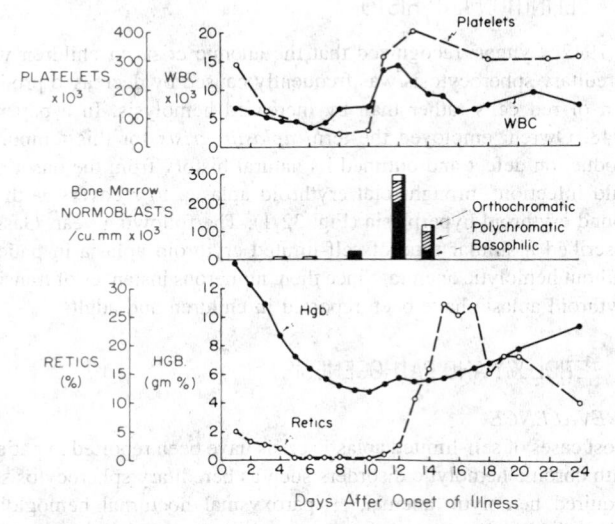

FIGURE 32-1 Erythroid parameters measured 50 years ago but still very typical of a young man with hereditary spherocytosis who developed an aplastic crisis following a brief febrile illness of unknown cause. (Case 4 in Owren.[6])

toin but had no effect on the growth of granulocyte-monocyte colony forming units (CFU-GM) in vitro.[52] The same kind of study carried out in a patient with rifampicin-induced red cell aplasia also suggested that the drug might act like a hapten.[68] In other cases the drug may act as a toxin and merely be the first manifestation of a general marrow suppression that is prevented by the immediate discontinuation of the drug.

NUTRITIONAL ETIOLOGY
Folic acid deficiency has been suspected to be a cause of aplastic crisis.[72] There is undoubtedly an increased requirement for folic acid in chronic hemolytic anemia,[73] and folic acid deficiency or resistance can produce reticulocytopenia and erythroid hypoplasia.[74,75] In the few

TABLE 32-1   DRUGS ASSOCIATED WITH THE DEVELOPMENT OF APLASTIC CRISIS

GENERIC NAME	REFERENCES
Alpha-Methyldopa (Aldomet)	34
Azathioprine	35, 36
Aztreonam	37
Sulfobromophthalein sodium (bromsulphthalein)	38
Carbamazepine	39, 40
Cephalothin	41
Chloramphenicol	42–44
Chlorpropamide	45–47
Co-trimoxazole	48, 49
D-Penicillamine	50
Diphenylhydantoin	51–55
Fenoprofen	56, 57
Lindane (gamma benzene hexachloride)	58
Gold	59
Indomethacin	60
Isoniazid	61, 62
Dapsone	63, 64
Methazolamide	65
Pentachlorophenol	66
Procainamide	67
Rifampicin	68
Sulfasalazine	69
Thiamphenicol	70
Valproic acid	71

patients treated with folic acid, however, physiologic doses were ineffective.

Deficiencies of vitamin C and riboflavin and protein malnutrition also have been implicated in the etiology of aplastic crises. Although kwashiorkor may be associated with reticulocytopenia, erythroid hypoplasia, and giant proerythroblast,[76,77] the association between nutritional deficiencies and aplastic crises is still very tenuous.

CLINICAL FEATURES

The rapid onset of listlessness and increasing pallor in a patient with a chronic, well-adjusted hemolytic process should always raise the suspicion of an aplastic crisis. Characteristically, there is a history of a recent suspected or confirmed viral illness or the use of drugs for intercurrent bacterial or inflammatory diseases. However, an aplastic crisis may occur without any preceding illness. Apart from pallor, the physical examination does not contribute any specific clues unless a careful examiner detects decreased jaundice in a patient with chronic hemolytic anemia.

LABORATORY FEATURES

The laboratory examination reveals anemia with red cell morphologic features characteristic of the underlying hematologic disorder, virtual absence of reticulocytes, and normal or low serum bilirubin. Moderate granulocytopenia and thrombocytopenia may be present, but granulocytes and platelets are usually normal or even increased in number. Because of the advanced mean age of surviving erythrocytes, the pyrimidine 5′-nucleotidase activity is uniformly diminished, but most other red cell enzyme activities are normal because of the slow decline of enzyme activity after the reticulocyte stage (see Chap. 23).[78,79] Erythrocyte adenosine deaminase (ADA) activity is also normal.

Early in the illness, the marrow is depleted of all erythroid elements. However, most patients are seen during the stage of spontaneous recovery, when the marrow may display cohorts of early erythroid cells. These cells are often erroneously interpreted as reflecting maturation arrest or megaloblastosis, but serial marrow examinations usually show a normal maturation sequence followed by a distinct reticulocytosis. Occasionally, there are large, intensely basophilic cells termed *giant proerythroblasts*.[7] There is frequently some shift to the left in the myeloid series. The morphology of megakaryocytes is not measurably changed, and they are present in normal numbers.

The rapid recovery phase may be associated with severe bone pain, presumably because of marrow expansion, and by "rebound" reticulocytosis, granulocytosis, and thrombocytosis. In splenectomized patients, or in asplenic sickle cell anemia patients, the recovery phase may be characterized by the presence in blood films of nucleated red cells. This probably reflects the absence of splenic sequestration of immature erythroid cells.

During the aplastic phase, serum ferritin and serum iron are high, with almost complete saturation of iron-binding capacity. The erythropoietin level is also high initially and decreases moderately during the recovery phase.[80]

Studies aimed at establishing a viral etiology, especially B19 parvovirus infections, are usually of retrospective rather than diagnostic value.

DIFFERENTIAL DIAGNOSIS

A sudden isolated decrease in the concentration of hemoglobin associated with a low reticulocyte count, usually less than 1.0 percent and often zero, is probably the most important clue and deserves to be followed by a bone marrow examination.[81]

THERAPY, COURSE, AND PROGNOSIS

Therapy should include discontinuation, if possible, of all drugs, maintenance of an adequate hemoglobin concentration by transfusion of red cells if needed, treatment of any associated illness, and waiting for a spontaneous remission. Folic acid and multivitamins are usually given, but their effectiveness in acute aplastic crises is at best uncertain. Recovery occurs within days or weeks and is complete.

CHRONIC PURE RED CELL APLASIA—CONSTITUTIONAL

DEFINITION AND HISTORY

A chronic form of isolated erythroid hypoplasia occurring early in childhood and believed to be congenital or inherited was first reported by Joseph[82] in 1936 and was again described 2 years later by Diamond and Blackfan.[83] Since then, many hundreds of cases have been reported of this condition, now best known as the *Diamond-Blackfan anemia.*[84,85]

ETIOLOGY AND PATHOGENESIS

PREVALENCE

In a few infants, pallor and anemia are recognized at birth, but in most reported cases, a definite diagnosis of anemia is first made between the ages of 2 weeks and 1 year.[85] There is no characteristic sex preponderance and no consistent abnormality of the pregnancy or delivery. In 10 percent of cases there is more than one affected family member, and the occasional reports of consanguinity suggest that in some cases there is an autosomal dominant or recessive inheritance[85]; however, most cases are sporadic. Also, chromosomal studies are usually normal or reveal only nonspecific breaks and inversions.[86]

Studies of erythroid colony formation have suggested that constitutional pure red cell aplasia is caused by the presence of a defective stem cell.[87] Marrow CFU-E and marrow and blood BFU-E are markedly decreased in numbers[88–90] and are also quite insensitive to the action of erythropoietin[90] or IL-3.[91] Although there is some improvement in their number and erythropoietin sensitivity after steroid-induced remissions, they remain abnormal.[92] The progeny of the presumably defective stem cells are mature but abnormal red cells. They are macrocytic, contain increased amounts of fetal hemoglobin, have little-i surface antigens, and have a fetal distribution of intracellular enzymes.[85] Although such changes could indicate a constitutional abnormality, they are also seen in normal individuals exposed to acute or chronic hematopoietic demands.[93]

The therapeutic effectiveness of steroids in constitutional pure red cell aplasia and its morphologic kinship to the acquired autoimmune cases have led to a search for an immunologic pathogenesis. Except for a few repeatedly transfused patients,[94,95] no humoral or cellular inhibition of erythropoiesis has been found. Reports of excessive anthranilic acid excretion, suggesting a metabolic defect in the utilization of tryptophan[96] for red cell production, and of high adenosine deaminase levels,[97,98] although challenging, have not led to constructive working hypotheses.

CLINICAL FEATURES

The presenting symptoms and signs can vary in severity and may reflect the prognosis of this type of anemia. Pallor, listlessness, and poor appetite are early manifestations, progressing into borderline congestive failure with breathlessness, hepatomegaly, and splenomegaly. These initial symptoms and signs respond readily to transfusions. Subsequently, however, transfusion may lead to hemosiderosis with all its problems (see Chap. 42).

A variety of minor congenital abnormalities have been reported,[85] but in contradistinction to Fanconi anemia, major abnormalities have only rarely been observed.[99] Thymic hyperplasia and thymic tumors are not manifestations of constitutional pure red cell aplasia.

LABORATORY FEATURES

Normochromic, macrocytic anemia with absolute severe reticulocytopenia is found in all cases. The white blood cell count is normal or only slightly decreased, but the platelet count is often mildly elevated. Characteristically, the marrow is cellular with a profound erythroid hypoplasia and a high myeloid/erythroid ratio. The few remaining erythroid cells are usually young and may display some nuclear changes suggestive of megaloblastosis. The morphology and maturation sequences of the myeloid cells and megakaryocytes are normal, and the plasma cells and mononuclear lymphoid cells also appear normal. Erythropoietin levels in the serum are appropriately elevated.[81]

Serum iron and serum ferritin levels are at a high normal level with increased saturation of iron-binding protein. Folic acid and vitamin B_{12} serum levels are normal. Fetal hemoglobin, distributed unevenly among the red cells, is elevated in most cases, as is the concentration of i antigen on the red cell surface.[85] Erythrocyte ADA is elevated in many, if not most, patients.[98]

DIFFERENTIAL DIAGNOSIS

The virtual absence of reticulocytes from the blood and erythroblasts from the marrow, accompanied by a near-normal concentration of neutrophils and platelets in the blood and neutrophil and megakaryocyte precursors in the marrow, are characteristics of red cell aplasia. Marrow examination is useful for a definitive diagnosis, but the absence of reticulocytes from the blood is invariably associated with marrow erythroid aplasia and separates this condition from other anemias in infancy. The absence of a sudden onset and spontaneous resolution separates it from acute pure red cell aplasia. An elevated adenosine deaminase activity[98] is useful in confirming the diagnosis.

THERAPY, COURSE, AND PROGNOSIS

Transfusions and glucocorticoids are standard therapeutic agents and can maintain many patients in nearly normal health for years. Hemosiderosis is an unavoidable complication of transfusions (see Chap. 42). Failure of growth and sexual maturity may mar an otherwise successful therapeutic regimen, and myocardial failure is frequently responsible for death.[99] Intensive iron chelation by continuous infusions of desferrioxamine may ameliorate and postpone the effect of iron overload. Splenectomy may be needed to abolish hypersplenism secondary to hepatic fibrosis. Otherwise, splenectomy would not be expected to influence erythropoietic function of the marrow. Neither would the use of recombinant human erythropoietin, but recombinant IL-3 has been reported to cause remissions.[100]

Glucocorticoids have been used extensively and have been held responsible for temporary improvements, complete remissions, and even cures.[84,85] Nevertheless, glucocorticoids do not cure but act by rendering abnormal erythroid progenitor cells more responsive to marrow growth factors, permitting them to differentiate to abnormal but functioning precursor cells. Glucocorticoids must be given in large doses, initially at 1 to 2 mg/kg of prednisone or prednisone equivalents, and the therapeutic trial should not be abandoned until the end of 4 to 6 weeks of unsuccessful therapy. At that point a trial of high doses of methylprednisolone may be justified.[101] If a reticulocyte response occurs, the dosage should be reduced appropriately. In such cases, it is frequently possible to maintain adequate red cell production with small doses of glucocorticoids. The most distressing complication has been growth retardation, muscle weakness, and osteopenia. Treatment with cyclosporine has been followed in the best of cases by only short and incomplete remissions.[102] Androgens have been used in refractory cases,[85] but their use should be undertaken with reluctance in a prepubertal child. Marrow transplantation has been used[103,104] and should be considered in patients who are refractory to therapy and have HLA-compatible siblings.

The survival data on 500 cases from the literature has been carefully analyzed[85] and shows a gratifying increase in longevity of recent cases carefully managed with glucocorticoids and cytokine factors and most recently with tranplantations.[85] Still the toll of therapy has been considerable, since most deaths are related to therapeutic complications. A few patients have developed various malignancies,[105] rarely if ever, aplastic anemia.[85]

CHRONIC PURE RED CELL APLASIA—ACQUIRED

DEFINITION AND HISTORY

Acquired chronic pure red cell aplasia is an unusual disorder characterized by an absence of or marked decrease in red cell production and occurring mostly in adults but with many links to the erythroid aplasia of childhood. In the 1930s, clinicians became aware of the association between red cell aplasia and thymomas.[106] This association led subsequently to our present concept that it mainly is a T-cell- or B-cell-derived autoimmune disorder. However, sometimes drugs or viruses may initiate and perpetuate this disorder. In some cases, it involves defective or absent progenitor cells resembling the constitutional form of pure red cell aplasia.[107,108]

ETIOLOGY AND PATHOGENESIS

In the early reports of patients with chronic pure red cell aplasia, there were almost as many with as without thymoma.[109–114] This, however, does not reflect the true prevalence of thymomas in this disease, since there undoubtedly is more of a tendency to publish cases with a challenging concurrence of two rare diseases than there is to publish cases of either disease alone. Although there still are many reports of thymomas with pure red cell aplasia,[114,115] it is comforting for hematologists who in vain have tried to find a thymoma in their patients with pure red cell aplasia to know that in a series of 37 carefully studied cases, only 2 were associated with a thymoma.[116] In patients with thymoma, the prevalence of pure red cell aplasia has been estimated to be 7 percent, probably also an unrealistically high incidence.

Nevertheless, T-cell-mediated erythroid rejection has been argued to play a major pathogenic role in eradicating erythroid progenitor cells, particularly in B-cell chronic lymphocytic leukemia.[117–125] Chronic red cell aplasia also has been found in association with numerous systemic autoimmune diseases, such as rheumatoid arthritis,[126] systemic lupus erythematosus,[127] autoimmune hemolytic anemia,[128] myasthenia gravis,[129] or Sjögren's syndrome.[130] Although in some cases autoantibodies were suspected to play a pathogenic role, it was not until 1967 that direct evidence was provided for such a mechanism.[131] Subsequently it has been found that nearly half of all patients have serum IgG autoantibodies that can suppress the in vitro growth of both allogeneic and autologous erythroid progenitor cells.[132–135] Some antibodies are complement-fixing and cytolytic, while others apparently can inhibit cell growth in the absence of complement.[135] In some cases the antibodies are directed against erythropoietin,[136,137] but in general erythropoietin levels are high and apparently unaffected. Although it has been speculated that autoantibodies directed against

erythropoietin receptors could play a pathogenic role,[138] such autoantibodies have not yet been observed in patients with this disease.

Deficient antibody production in immune compromised individuals also may cause pure red cell aplasia. In AIDS patients, for example, an infection with the B19 parvovirus will persist in the absence of neutralizing antibodies and if unchecked will continue to destroy erythroid progenitor cells.[139–141] This may also occur in pregnancy[142] and especially in patients receiving chemotherapy before organ transplantation.[143–146]

CLINICAL FEATURES

Pallor is usually the only physical finding of note on the initial examination. Some patients will have a thymoma, although such tumors are only rarely large enough to be detected on physical examination. Later on, after prolonged transfusion and glucocorticoid therapy, there may be additional findings caused by secondary hemochromatosis and steroid-induced side effects.

LABORATORY FEATURES

The anemia accompanying this disease is normochromic and normo- or macrocytic and is associated with absolute reticulocytopenia. The leukocyte and platelet counts are normal or reflect the underlying disease. The marrow is cellular but with profound erythroid hypoplasia. The remaining erythroid cells are immature but morphologically normal. In the marrow, there may be an increase in eosinophils and small mononuclear cells.

The serum iron level is elevated with almost complete saturation of the iron-binding capacity, the half-life of radioactive iron is prolonged, and the iron utilization is low, conforming to the morphologic observation of erythroid hypoplasia. The red cell life span is normal initially but may become shortened owing to transfusion-induced hemosiderosis with congestive splenomegaly or to the presence of red cell antibodies. Serum protein electrophoresis and antibody analyses reflect the underlying disorders. The metabolism of folic acid or vitamin B_{12} is usually unimpaired, although in a few cases megaloblastosis and the response to folic acid have suggested an abnormal handling or availability of this coenzyme.

Thymic enlargement, when present, is usually detected on routine chest X-ray examinations as a mass in the anterior mediastinum. However, a CT scan or MRI may be needed to demonstrate a small thymoma. In one series of 56 cases of pure red cell anemia with thymoma,[109] the thymomas in 46 cases were encapsulated and composed primarily of spindle cells. The germinal centers were absent, but there was diffuse scant infiltration with small lymphocytes. In 10 cases the thymomas were infiltrating and were considered malignant. In these cases the tissues were composed of lymphocytes and reticulum cells in a disorganized pattern. In the seven patients in this series with associated myasthenia gravis, the gross or microscopic pattern did not differ significantly from the other cases.

DIFFERENTIAL DIAGNOSIS

The diagnosis is suspected when a patient or a previously normal individual develops a sustained anemia in the presence of a severe reticulocytopenia, normal white cell total and differential count, and normal platelet count. The marrow confirms the blood findings having an absence of erythroid precursors but a normal pattern of granulocyte and megakaryocytic cells. Cytogenetic studies of marrow cells are normal. These findings distinguish erythroid aplasia from other refractory anemias, such as those that characterize the preleukemic or myelodysplastic disorders (see Chap. 92). The presence of a thymoma is helpful in establishing the diagnosis, but its absence is of little diagnostic significance. Serologic and marrow culture studies may be of importance in difficult cases.

THERAPY, COURSE, AND PROGNOSIS

TREATMENT

Transfusion   Transfusion with packed red cells is the mainstay of symptomatic therapy. A hemoglobin concentration maintained at 8 to 10 g/dl is an attainable goal in complete erythroid aplasia but demands transfusion of about 2 units of packed red cells every 2 weeks. A gradual shortening of the effective life span of transfused red cells because of hypersplenism or red cell antibodies can make this therapy increasingly frustrating and ineffective.

Erythropoietin   Recombinant human erythropoietin when given alone has occasionally been of benefit.[146,147] However, it is most often given in addition to other medications in order to enhance their effect.[148] It should initially be given in large doses such as 10,000 units, three times a week subcutaneously, with subsequent modulation of the dose according to its effect.

Thymectomy   Whenever thymic enlargement is found, it is advisable to perform a thymectomy in order to provide a diagnosis, prevent possible malignant extension, and promote reactivation of the marrow. In one series of 56 patients, 25 were treated by thymectomy, and 16 appeared to benefit from the operation.[109] The benefit derived from thymectomy could not always be related directly to surgery, and it is still difficult to assess the therapeutic effect of thymectomy alone. However, in one case a serum inhibitor of the erythroid tissue apparently disappeared after thymectomy.[149] Irradiation of the thymus was completely unsuccessful in the five patients so treated.[109] The current consensus appears to be that removing a normal-sized thymus gland without a thymoma is of no help to a patient with pure red cell aplasia.

Steroid Hormones   Glucocorticoids are frequently effective in reactivating red cell production either by blocking antibody production or action or by sensitizing abnormal erythroid progenitor cells to normal growth factors.[116] Unfortunately, rather substantial doses may be needed, and side effects often preclude the continuous employment of these drugs. When small maintenance doses are effective, however, glucocorticoid treatment can eliminate transfusion dependence and be the treatment of choice. The immunosuppressive androgen danazol[150] has also been used and may be a useful adjunct to glucocorticoid therapy.

Immunosuppressive Drugs   On the assumption that acquired red cell aplasia is an autoimmune disorder, therapy with cyclophosphamide or 6-mercaptopurine has been tried and has been successful in a number of cases.[116,148] However, the use of potentially leukemogenic drugs should always be instituted with some reluctance and after less toxic drugs have been found to be ineffective. Intravenous gamma-globulin treatment has been remarkably effective and in some cases has eradicated persistent viremia with the B19 parvovirus.[151,152] Antithymic or antilymphocyte serum has also been used with considerable success. When effective, it may cause a remission within days rather than the months needed for a remission induced in aplastic anemia.[148,153] Cyclosporine A with the addition of erythropoietin has also been used successfully.[154–156] Single reports list the potential efficacy of interferon α[157] and T3.[3]

Plasmapheresis   A good response to plasmapheresis has been reported in several patients.[158] This response may actually be long-lasting, far longer than can be explained on the basis of the temporary removal of antibodies.

Splenectomy   Splenectomy has been performed in many patients, but unless there is evidence for abnormal splenic sequestration of red cells, the therapeutic benefit derived has been minimal. Obviously, pathologic splenic red cell destruction and excessive splenic antibody formation will be eliminated by splenectomy, but the underlying disease is not dependent on splenic function and will not be helped by splenectomy.

COURSE AND PROGNOSIS

Remissions have been induced in about 25 percent of patients either with or without thymomas, but only half of these have been sustained without further therapy. In most cases, maintenance therapy with transfusions, erythropoietin, and adrenal steroids has been responsible for both symptomatic control of the disease and high mortality. In one series of 56 patients with thymomas, 17 died within 6 months of the date of diagnosis, and a total of 50 were dead at the time of the compilation of the report.[109] Of 16 cases without thymomas observed at the Mayo Clinic, 8 died 1 to 3 years after the onset of the disease.[111] The causes of death were hemosiderosis, steroid-induced hemorrhages, or infections. With the current use of immunosuppressive drugs and improved supportive care, the prognosis is no longer so grim. About 50 percent of patients enter remissions, and median survival with idiopathic disease is greater than 10 years.[116]

REFERENCES

1. Kaznelson P: Zur Enstehung der Blut Plattchen. *Verh Dtsch Ges Inn Med* 34:557, 1992.
2. Krantz SB: Pure red cell aplasia: biology and treatment, in *Clinical Disorders and Experimental Models of Erythropoietic Failure*, edited by SA Feig, MH Freedman, pp 85–124. Boca Raton, FL, CRC Press, 1993.
3. Erslev AJ, Soltan A: Pure red-cell aplasia: a review. *Blood Reviews* 10:20, 1996.
4. Cherrick I, Karayalcin G, Lanzkowsky P: Transient erythroblastopenia of childhood, prospective study of fifty patients. *Am J Pediatr Hematol/ Oncol* 16:320, 1994.
5. Lyngar E: Samtidig optreden av anemisk kriser hos 3 barn i en familie med hemolytisk ikterus. *Nord Med* 14:1246, 1942.
6. Owren PA: Congenital hemolytic jaundice: the pathogenesis of the hemolytic crisis. *Blood* 3:231, 1948.
7. Gasser C: Akute Erythroblastopenie: 10 Falle aplastischer Erythroblastenkrisen mit Riesen Proerythroblasten bei allergischtaxinen Zustands bildern. *Helv Paediatr Acta* 4:107, 1949.
8. Tsukada T, Koike T, Koike R, et al: Epidemic of aplastic crisis in patients with hereditary spherocytosis in Japan. *Lancet* 1:1401, 1985.
9. Lefrere JJ, Conronce A-M, Girot R, et al: Six cases of hereditary spherocytosis revealed by human parvovirus infection. *Br J Haematol* 62:653, 1986.
10. Takahashi M, Koike T, Moriyama Y, et al: Inhibition of erythropoiesis by human parvovirus-containing serum from a patient with hereditary spherocytosis in aplastic crisis. *Scand J Haematol* 37:118, 1986.
11. Mangan KF, Besa EC, Shadduck RK, et al: Demonstration of two distinct antibodies in autoimmune hemolytic anemia with reticulocytopenia and red cell aplasia. *Exp Hematol* 12:788, 1984.
12. Rao KRP, Patel AR, Anderson MJ, et al: Infection with parvovirus-like virus and aplastic crisis in chronic hemolytic anemia. *Ann Intern Med* 98:930, 1983.
13. Bertrand Y, Lefrere JJ, Leverger G, et al: Autoimmune hemolytic anemia revealed by human parvorvirus-linked erythroblastopenia. *Lancet* 2:382, 1985.
14. Crosby WH: Paroxysmal nocturnal haemoglobinuria: report of a case complicated by an aregenerative (aplastic) crisis. *Ann Intern Med* 39:1107, 1953.
15. Singer K, Motulsky AG, Wile SA: Aplastic crisis in sickle cell anemia: a study of its mechanism and its relationship to other types of hemolytic crisis. *J Lab Clin Med* 35:721, 1950.
16. Pattison JR, Jones SE, Hadgson J, et al: Parvovirus infections and hypoplastic crisis in sickle cell anemia. *Lancet* 1:664, 1981.
17. Duncan JR, Cappellini MD, Anderson MJ, et al: Aplastic crisis due to parvovirus infection in pyruvate kinase deficiency. *Lancet* 2:14, 1983.

18. Lefrere JJ, Conronce A-M, Girot R, et al: Human parvovirus and thalassemia. *J Infect Dis* 13:45, 1986.

19. West NC, Meigh RE, Mackie M, et al: Parvovirus infection associated with aplastic crisis in a patient with HEMPAS. *J Clin Pathol* 39:1019, 1986.

20. Solano C, Gomez-Reino F, Fernandez-Ravada JM: Pure red cell aplasia in Kala Azar. *Acta Haematol (Basel)* 72:205, 1984.

21. Shah NR, Wolff JA, Sitarz A: Transient acquired red blood cell (RBC) aplasia in children without hematologic disease. *Pediatr Res* 10:381, 1976.

22. Young NS, Mortimer PP: Viruses and bone marrow failure. *Blood* 63:729, 1984.

23. Purtilo DT, Zelkowitz L, Harada S, et al: Delayed onset of infectious mononucleosis associated with acquired agammaglobulinemia and red cell aplasia. *Ann Intern Med* 101:180, 1984.

24. Gonzalez N, Escudero A, Olmeda F, et al: Acute hepatitis and selective erythroblastopenia. *Acta Haematol (Basel)* 69:141, 1983.

25. Al-Awami Y, Sears DA, Carrum G, Udden MM, Alter BP, Conlon CL: Pure red cell aplasia associated with hepatitis C infection. *Am J Med Sci* 314:113, 1997.

26. Harris JW: Parvovirus B-19 for the hematologist. *Am J Hematol* 39:119, 1992.

27. Guillot M, Lefrere JJ, Ravenet N, et al: Acute anemia and aplastic crisis with autohemolysis in human parvovirus infection. *J Clin Pathol* 40:1264, 1987.

28. Van Horn DK, Mortimer PP, Young N, Hanson GR: Human parvovirus associated red cell aplasia in the absence of underlying hemolytic anemia. *Am J Pediatr Hematol Oncol* 8:235, 1986.

29. Picot G, Triadon P, Lacombe C, et al: Relapsing pure red cell aplasia during pregnancy. *N Engl J Med* 311:196, 1984.

30. Aitchison RGM, Marsh JCW, Hows JM, et al: Pregnancy associated aplastic anaemia: a report of five cases and review of current management. *Br J Haematol* 73:541, 1989.

31. Van Elsacke R, Niele AM, Salimans MM, et al: Fetal pathology in human parvovirus B19 infection. *Br J Obstet Gynaecol* 96:768, 1989.

32. Dessypris EN, Krantz SB, Roloff JS, et al: Mode of action of the IgG inhibitor of erythropoiesis in transient erythroblastopenia of childhood. *Blood* 59:114, 1982.

33. Thompson DF, Gales MA: Drug-induced pure red cell aplasia. *Pharmacotherapy* 16:1002, 1996.

34. Itoh K, Wong P, Asai T, et al: Pure red cell aplasia induced by alphamethyldopa. *Am J Med* 84:1088, 1988.

35. Declerck YA, Ettenger RB, Ortega JA, Pennisi AJ: Macrocytosis and pure RBC anemia caused by azathioprine. *Am J Dis Child* 134:377, 1980.

36. Old CW, Flannery EP, Grogan IM, et al: Azathioprine-induced pure red cell aplasia. *JAMA* 240:552, 1978.

37. Ferber A, Zibelli A, Konkle BA: Aztreonam induced hemolytic anemia and pure red cell aplasia. Personal communication, 1998.

38. Broccia G, Dessalvi P: Acute pure red cell aplasia following bromsulphophthalein injection in a patient with non-Hodgkin lymphoma. *Acta Haematol (Basel)* 68:680, 1983.

39. Hirai H: Two cases of erythroid hypoplasia caused by carbamazepine. *Jpn Clin Hematol* 18:33, 1977.

40. Medberry CA, Pappas AA, Ackerman BH: Carbamazepine and erythroid arrest. *Drug Intell Clin Pharm* 21:439, 1987.

41. MacCulloch D, Jackson JM, Venerys J: Drug induced red cell aplasia. *Br Med J* 4:163, 1974.

42. Vilan J, Rhyner K, Ganzoni A: Pure red cell aplasia: successful treatment with cyclophosphamide. *Blut* 26:27, 1973.

43. Yunis AA, Bloomberg GR: Chloramphenicol toxicity: clinical features and pathogenesis, in *Progress in Hematology,* edited by CB Moore, EB Brown, vol 4, p 138. Grune & Stratton, New York, 1964.

44. Ozer FL, Truax WE, Leven WC: Erythroid hypoplasia associated with chloramphenicol therapy. *Blood* 16:997, 1960.

45. Gill MJ, Ratliff DA, Harding LK: Hypoglycemic coma, jaundice, and pure RBC aplasia following chlorpropamide therapy. *Arch Intern Med* 140:714, 1980.

46. Planas AT, Kranwinkel RN, Soletsky HB, Pezzimenti JF: Chlorpropamide-induced pure RBC aplasia. *Arch Intern Med* 140:707, 1980.

47. Recker RR, Hymes HE: Pure red cell aplasia associated with chlorpropamide therapy. *Arch Intern Med* 223:445, 1969.

48. Stephens ME: Transient erythroid hypoplasia in a patient on long-term co-trimoxazole therapy. *Postgrad Med J* 50:235, 1974.

49. Unter CE, Abbott GD: Co-trimoxazole in leukemia. *Arch Dis Child* 62:85, 1987.

50. Gollan JL, Hussein S, Hoffbrand AV, Sherlock S: Red cell aplasia following prolonged D-penicillamine therapy. *J Clin Pathol* 29:135, 1976.

51. Huijgens PC, Thijs LG, Den Ottolander GJ: Pure red cell aplasia, toxic dermatitis and lymphadenopathy in a patient taking diphenylhydantoin. *Acta Haematol (Basel)* 59:31, 1978.

52. Dessypris EN, Redline S, Harris JW, Krantz SB: Diphenylhydantoin-induced pure red cell aplasia. *Blood* 65:789, 1985.

53. Pritchard KL, Quirt IC, Simpson WJ, Fleming JF: Phenytoin-associated reversible red cell aplasia. *Can Med Assoc J* 1121:1491, 1979.

54. Yune-Gill J, Jung Y, River GL: Pure RBC aplasia and diphenylhydantoin. *JAMA* 229:314, 1974.

55. Yunis AA, Arimura GK, Lutcher CL, et al: Biochemical lesion in dilantin induced erythroid aplasia. *Blood* 30:587, 1967.

56. Weinberger KA: Fenoprofen and red cell aplasia. *J Rheumatol* 6:475, 1979.

57. Reitz CL, Bohomley SS: Pure red cell aplasia associated with Fenoprofen. *Am J Med Sci* 287:62, 1984.

58. Vodopick H: Cherchez la chienne: I. Erythropoietic hypoplasia after exposure to gamma-benzene hexachloride. *JAMA* 234:850, 1975.

59. Reid G, Patterson AC: Pure red cell aplasia after gold treatment. *Br Med J* 2:457, 1977.

60. Burghuber D: Red cell aplastic anemia following Indomethacin therapy. *Acta Med Aust* 6:384, 1979.

61. Claiborne RA, Dutt AK: Isoniazide-induced pure red cell aplasia. *Annu Rev Respir Dis* 131:947, 1985.

62. Homman R, McPhedran P, Benz EJ, Duffy TP: Isoniazide pure red cell aplasia. *Am J Med Sci* 286:2, 1983.

63. Gelfand M, Froese EH: Red cell hypoplasia following Dapsone and Pyrimethamine. *Cent Afr J Med* 29:181, 1983.

64. Nicholls MD, Concannon AJ: Maloprim-induced agranulocytosis and red cell aplasia. *Med J Aust* 2:564, 1982.

65. Krivoy N, Ben-Arieh Y, Carter A, Alroy G: Methazolamide-induced hepatitis and pure RBC aplasia. *Arch Intern Med* 141:1229, 1981.

66. Roberts HJ: Aplastic anemia and red cell aplasia due to Pentochlorophenol. *South Med J* 76:45, 1983.

67. Giannone L, Kugler JW, Krantz SB: Pure red cell aplasia associated with administration of sustained-release procainamide. *Arch Intern Med* 147:1179, 1987.

68. Mariette Y, Mitjavila MT, Moulinie PR, et al: Rifampicin-induced pure red cell aplasia. *Am J Med* 87:459, 1989.

69. Dunn AM, Kerrt GD: Pure red cell aplasia associated with Sulphasalazine. *Lancet* 258:228, 1981.

70. Cornet A, Carnu P, Barbier J-Ph, et al: A case of reversible erythroblastopenia due to thiamphenicol. *Semin Hop Paris* 50:1569, 1974.

71. MacDougall LG: Pure red cell aplasia associated with sodium valproate therapy. *JAMA* 247:53, 1982.

72. Pierce LE, Rath CE: Evidence for folic acid deficiency in the genesis of anemia sickle cell crisis. *Blood* 20:19, 1962.

73. Shojania AM, Gross S: Hemolytic anemia and folic acid deficiency in children. *Am J Dis Child* 108:53, 1964.

74. Jandl JH, Greenberg MS: Bone marrow failure due to relative nutritional deficiency in Cooley's hemolytic anemia. *N Engl J Med* 260:461, 1959.

75. Gothoni G, Vuoristo M, Kontula K: High-dose folic acid treatment for red-cell aplasia. *Lancet* 345:1645, 1995.

76. Kho LK: Erythroblastemia with giant pro-erythroblasts in kwashiorkor. *Blood* 12:171, 1957.

77. Zucker JM, Tchernia G, Vuylsteke P, et al: Acute secondary and transitory erythroblastopenia in kwashiorkor under treatment. *Nouv Rev Fr Hematol* 11:131, 1971.

78. Beutler E, Hartman G: Age-related red cell enzymes in children with transient erythroblastopenia of childhood and hemolytic anemia. *Pediatr Res* 19:44, 1985.

79. Beutler E: Biphasic loss of red cell enzyme activity during in vivo aging. *Prog Clin Biol Res* 195:317, 1985.

80. Hammond D, Shore N, Movassaghi N: Production, utilization and excretion of erythropoietin. I. Chronic anemias. II. Aplastic crises. III. Erythropoietic effect of normal plasma. *Ann N Y Acad Sci* 149:516, 1968.

81. Freedman MH: Pure red cell aplasia in childhood and adolescence: pathogenesis and approach to diagnosis. *Br J Haematol* 85:246, 1993.

82. Joseph WH: Anemia of infancy and early childhood. *Medicine (Baltimore)* 15:307, 1936.

83. Diamond LK, Blackfan KD: Hypoplastic anemia. *Am J Dis Child* 56:464, 1938.

84. Diamond LK, Wang WC, Alter BP: Congenital hypoplastic anemia. *Adv Pediatr* 22:349, 1976.

85. Alter BP, Young NS: Single cytopenias—Red blood cells, in *Hematology of Infancy and Childhood,* 5th ed, edited by DG Nathan, SH Orkin, p 286. Saunders, Philadelphia, 1998.

86. Alter BP: Childhood red cell aplasia. *Am J Pediatr Hematol Oncol* 2:121, 1980.

87. Tsai PS, Arkin S, Lipton JM: An intrinsic defect in Diamond-Blackfan anemia. *Br J Haematol* 73:112, 1989.

88. McGuckin CP, Ball SE, Gordon-Smith EC: Diamond-Blackfan anaemia: three patterns of *in vitro* response to haemopoietic growth factors. *Br J Haematol* 89:457, 1995.

89. Casadevall N, Croisille, et al: Age-related alterations in erythroid and granulopoietic progenitors in Diamond-Blackfan anaemia. *Br J Haematol* 87:369, 1994.

90. Lipton JM, Kudisch M, Gross R, Nathan DG: Defective erythroid progenitor differentiation system in congenital hypoplastic (Diamond-Blackfan) anemia. *Blood* 67:962, 1986.

91. Sieff CA, Yokoyama CT, et al: The production of steel factor mRNA in Diamond-Blackfan anaemia long-term cultures and interactions of steel factor with erythropoietin and interleukin-3. *Br J Haematol* 82:640, 1992.

92. Chan HSL, Saunders EF, Freedman MH: Diamond-Blackfan syndrome: II. In vitro corticosteroid effect on erythropoiesis. *Pediatr Res* 16:477, 1982.

93. Alter BP: Fetal erythropoiesis in stress hematopoiesis. *Exp Hematol* 7:200, 1979.

94. Ortega JA, Shore NA, Dukes PP, Hammond D: Congenital hypoplastic anemia inhibition of erythropoiesis by sera from patients with congenital hypoplastic anemia. *Blood* 45:83, 1975.

95. Steinberg MH, Coleman MF, Pennebaker JB: Diamond-Blackfan syndrome: evidence for T-cell mediated suppression of erythroid development and a serum blocking factor associated with complete remission. *Br J Haematol* 41:57, 1979.

96. Altman KL, Miller G: A disturbance of tryptophan metabolism in congenital hypoplastic anaemia. *Nature* 172:868, 1953.

97. Glader BE, Backer K, Diamond LK: Elevated deaminase activity in congenital hypoplastic (Diamond-Blackfan) anemia. *N Engl J Med* 309:1486, 1983.

98. Glader BE, Backer K: Comparative activity of erythrocyte adenosine deaminase and orotidine decarboxylase in Diamond-Blackfan anemia. *Am J Hematol* 23:135, 1986.

99. Sanyal SK, Johnson W, Jayalakshmamma B, Green AA: Fatal ''iron heart'' in an adolescent: biochemical and ultrastructural aspects of the heart. *Pediatrics* 55:336, 1975.

100. Bastion Y, Bordigoni P, et al: Sustained response after recombinant interleukin-3 in Diamond Blackfan anemia. *Blood* 83:617, 1994.

101. Ozsoylu S: Oral megadose methylprednisolone for the treatment of Diamond-Blackfan anemia. *Pediatr Hematol Oncol* 11:561, 1994.

102. Raghavachar A: Pure red cell aplasia: review of treatment and proposal for a treatment strategy. *Blut* 61:47, 1990.

103. Greinix HT, Storb R, et al: Long-term survival and cure after marrow transplantation for congenital hypoplastic anaemia (Diamond-Blackfan syndrome). *Br J Haematol* 84:515, 1993.

104. Mugishima H, Gale RP, et al: Bone marrow transplantation for Diamond-Blackfan anemia. *Bone Marrow Transplant* 15:55, 1995.

105. Haupt R, Dufour C, et al: Diamond-Blackfan anemia and malignancy: a case report and a review of the literature. *Cancer* 77:1961, 1996.

106. Opsahl R: Thymus-karcinom og aplastic anemia. *Nord Med* 2:1835, 1939.

107. LaCombe C, Casadevall N, Muller O, Varet B: Erythroid progenitors in adult chronic pure red cell aplasia: relationship of in vitro erythroid colonies to therapeutic response. *Blood* 64:71, 1984.

108. Dessypris EN: The biology of pure red cell aplasia. *Semin Heamtol* 28:275, 1991.

109. Hirst E, Robertson TI: The syndrome of thymoma and erythroblastopenic anemia. *Medicine (Baltimore)* 46:225, 1967.

110. Tsai SY, Levin WC: Chronic erythrocytic hypoplasia in adults. *Am J Med* 22:322, 1957.

111. Ross JF, Finch SC, Street RB Jr, Stneder JW: The simultaneous occurrence of benign thymoma and refractory anemia. *Blood* 9:935, 1954.

112. Schmid JR, Kiely JM, Harrison EG Jr, et al: Thymoma associated with red cell agenesis: review of literature and report of cases. *Cancer* 18:216, 1965.

113. Freeman Z: Pure red cell anemia and thymoma. *Br Med J* 11:1390, 1960.

114. Masuda M, Arai Y, Okamura T, Mizoguchi H: Pure red cell aplasia with thymona: evidence of T-cell clonal disorder. *Am J Hematol* 54:324, 1997.

115. Wong KF, Chau KF, Chan JK, Chu YC, Li CS: Pure red cell aplasia associated with thymic lymphoid hyperplasia and secondary erythropoietin resistance. *Am J Clin Path* 103:346, 1995.

116. Clark DA, Dessypris EN, Krantz SB: Studies on pure red cell aplasia: XI. Results of immunosuppressive treatment of 37 patients. *Blood* 63:277, 1984.

117. Abkowitz JL, Kadin ME, Powell JS, Adamson JW: Pure red cell aplasia: lymphocyte inhibition of erythropoiesis. *Br J Haematol* 63:59, 1986.

118. Lacy MQ, Kurtin PJ, Tefferi A: Pure red cell aplasia: association with large granular lymphocyte leukemia and the prognostic value of cytogenetic abnormalities. *Blood* 87:3000, 1996.

119. Yamada O, Yun-Hua W, Motoji T, Mizoguchi H: Clonal T-cell proliferation causing pure red cell aplasia in chronic B-cell lymphocytic leukaemia: successful treatment with cyclosporine following in vitro abrogation of erythroid colony-suppressing activity. *Br J Haematol* 101:335, 1998.

120. Yamada O, Mizoguchi H, Oshimi K: Cyclophosphamide therapy for pure red cell aplasia associated with granular lymphocyte-proliferative disorders. *Br J Haematol* 97:393, 1997.

121. Mangan KF, D'Alessandro L: Hypoplastic anemia in B-cell chronic lymphatic leukemia: evolution of T-cell mediated suppression of erythropoiesis in early stage and late stage disease. *Blood* 66:533, 1985.

122. Mangan KF, Chikappa G, Scharrman WB, DesForges JF: Evidence of reduced erythroid burst (BFU-E) promoting function of T lymphocytes in the pure red cell aplasia of chronic lymphocytic leukemia. *J Exp Hematol* 9:489, 1981.

123. Hanada T, Abe T, Nakamura H, Aoki Y: Pure red cell aplasia: relationship between inhibitory activity of T cells to CFU-E and erythropoiesis. *Br J Haematol* 58:107, 1984.

124. Yoo D, Pierce LE, Lessin L: Acquired pure red cell aplasia associated with chronic lymphatic leukemia. *Cancer* 51:844, 1983.

125. Shionoya S, Amano M, Imamura Y, et al: Suppressor T cell chronic lymphocytic leukaemia associated with red cell hypoplasia. *Scand J Haematol* 33:231, 1984.

126. Dessypris EN, Baer MR, Sergent JS, Krantz SB: Rheumatoid arthritis and pure red cell aplasia. *Ann Intern Med* 100:202, 1984.

127. Kiely PD, McGuckin CP, Collins DA, Bevan DH, Marsh JC: Erythrocyte aplasia and systemic lupus erythematosus. *Lupus* 4:407, 1995.

128. Diehl LF, Ketchum LH: Autoimmune disease and chronic lymphocytic leukemia: autoimmune hemolytic anemia, pure red cell aplasia, and autoimmune thrombocytopenia. *Semin Oncol* 25:80, 1998.

129. Handa SI, Schofield KP, Sivakumaran M, Short M, Pumphrey RS: Pure red cell aplasia associated with malignant thymoma, myasthenia gravis, polyclonal large granular lymphocytosis and clonal thymic T cell expansion. *J Clin Pathol* 47:676, 1994.

130. Ibkhatra S, Jacobsson L, Manthorpe R: The association of pure red cell aplasia and primary Sjögren's syndrome. *Clin Exp Rheumatol* 15:119, 1997.

131. Krantz SB, Kao V: Studies on red cell aplasia: I. Demonstration of a plasma inhibitor to heme synthesis and an antibody to erythroblastic nuclei. *Proc Natl Acad Sci USA* 58:493, 1967.

132. Ammus SS, Yunis AA: Acquired pure red cell aplasia. *Am J Hematol* 24:311, 1987.

133. Field EO, Caughi MN, Blackett NM, Smithers DW: Marrow-suppressing factors in the blood in pure red cell aplasia, thymoma and Hodgkin disease. *Br J Haematol* 15:101, 1968.

134. Krantz SB, Moore WH, Zaentz SD: Studies on red cell aplasia: V. Presence of erythroblast cytotoxicity in γ globulin fraction of plasma. *J Clin Invest* 52:324, 1973.

135. Browman GP, Freedman MH, Blajchman MA, McBride JA: A comple-

ment independent erythropoietic inhibitor acting on the progenitor cell in refractory anemia. *Am J Med* 61:572, 1976.

136. Peschle C, Marmont AM, Marone G, et al: Pure red cell aplasia: Studies on an IgG serum inhibitor neutralizing erythropoietin. *Br J Haematol* 30:411, 1975.

137. Prabhakar SS, Muhfelder T: Antibodies to recombinant human erythropoietin causing pure red cell aplasia. *Clin Nephrol* 47:331, 1997.

138. Marmont A: Pure red cell aplasia as an autoimmune receptor disease. *Blood* 49:155, 1977.

139. Stricker RB, Goldberg B: AIDS and pure red cell aplasia. *Am J Hematol* 54:264, 1997.

140. Koduri PR, Kumapley R, Khokha ND, Patel AR: Red cell aplasia caused by parvovirus B19 in AIDS: use of i.v. immunoglobulin. *Ann Hematol* 75:67, 1997.

141. Majluf-Cruz A, Luna-Castanos G, Nieto-Cisneros L: AIDS-related pure red cell aplasia. *Am J Hematol* 51:171, 1996.

142. Baker RI, Manoharan A, DeLuca E, Begley CG: Pure red cell aplasia of pregnancy—a distinct entity. *Br J Haematol* 85:619, 1993.

143. Ahsan N, Holman MJ, Gocke CD, Groff JA, Yang HC: Pure red cell aplasia due to parvovirus B19 infection in solid organ transplantation. *Clin Transplant* 11:265, 1997.

144. Wicki J, Samii K, Cassinotti P, Voegeli J, Rochat T, Beris P: Parvovirus B-19-induced red cell aplasia in solid-organ transplant recipients. Two case reports and review of the literature. *Hematol Cell Ther* 39:199, 1997.

145. Uemura N, Ozawa K, Tani K, et al: Pure red cell aplasia caused by parvovirus B19 infection in a renal transplant recipient. *Eur J Haematol* 54:68, 1995.

146. Paltiel O, Cournoyer D, Rybka W: Pure red cell aplasia following ABO-incompatible bone marrow transplantation: response to erythropoietin. *Transfusion* 33:418, 1993.

147. Zeigler ZR, Rosenfeld CS, Shadduck RD: Resolution of transfusion dependence by recombinant human erythropoietin (rhu EPO) in acquired pure red cell aplasia (PRCA) associated with myeloid metaplasia. *Br J Haematol* 83:28, 1993.

148. Marmont AM: Therapy of pure red cell aplasia. *Semin Hematol* 28:285, 1991.

149. Al-Mondhiry H, Zanjani ED, Spivack M, et al: Pure red cell aplasia and thymoma: loss of serum inhibitor of erythropoiesis following thymectomy. *Blood* 38:576, 1971.

150. Lippman SM, Durie BGM, Harunder S, et al: Efficacy of danazol in pure red cell aplasia. *Am J Hematol* 23:373, 1986.

151. Kurtzman G, Frickhofen N, Kimball J, et al: Pure red cell aplasia of 10 years duration due to persistent parvovirus B19 injection and its cure with immunoglobulin therapy. *N Engl J Med* 321:519, 1989.

152. Ilan Y, Naparstek Y: Pure red cell aplasia associated with systemic lupus erythematosus: Remission after a single course of intravenous immunoglobulin. *Acta Haematol* 89:152, 1993.

153. Jacobs P, Wood L: Pure red cell aplasia: Stable complete remissions following antilymphocyte globulin administration. *Eur J Haematol* 40:371, 1988.

154. Leonard EM, Raefsky E, Griffith P, et al: Cyclosporine therapy of aplastic anemia, congenital and acquired red cell aplasia. *Br J Haematol* 72:278, 1989.

155. Cesana C, Carlo-Stella C, Mangoni L, et al: Response to cyclosporin A and recombinant human erythropoietin in a case of B cell chronic lymphocytic leukemia and pure red cell aplasia. *Leukemia* 10:1400, 1996.

156. Gotic M, Basara N, Rolovic Z, et al: Successful treatment of refractory pure red cell aplasia secondary to chronic lymphocytic leukaemia with cyclosporine A: correlation between clinical and in vitro effects. *Nouv Rev Fran Hematol* 36:307, 1994.

157. Martins A, Costa A, Oliveira MJ, et al: Pure red cell aplasia due to persistent B19 parvovirus infection in a patient infected with human immunodeficiency virus type 1. Recovery with alpha-interferon therapy. *Sangre* 43:67, 1998.

158. Messner HA, Fauser AA, Curtis JE, Dotten D: Control of antibody mediated pure red cell aplasia by plasmapheresis. *N Engl J Med* 304:1334, 1981.

C H A P T E R   3 3

ANEMIA OF CHRONIC RENAL FAILURE

JAIME CARO

ALLAN J. ERSLEV

Current use of recombinant human erythropoietin (EPO) to ameliorate the anemia in patients with chronic renal disease has been spectacularly successful and has shown that the primary cause of the anemia found in almost all patients with renal failure is due to a deficiency in the production of EPO. The accumulation of a number of toxic metabolic end products may also play a role in the pathogenesis of the anemia. This chapter analyzes the anemia of chronic renal disease as being caused by a failure of both renal excretory and endocrine function.

Failure of the renal excretory function causes a moderate reduction of red cell life span, the impairment of the function of blood platelets, and suppression of marrow activity. Intensive dialysis is the most effective treatment for these changes. The failure of renal endocrine function is managed by replacement treatment with EPO. If enough iron is provided, a hematocrit of 33 to 36 percent can be maintained by subcutaneous injections two to three times a week, and about 95 percent of the patients will be responsive without significant side effects.

Anemia is one of the most characteristic and visible manifestations of chronic renal failure. In 1836, Richard Bright first commented on the pallor of patients with renal disease,[1] and since then numerous observers have described and attempted to explain the underlying anemia. The degree of anemia appears to be roughly proportional to the severity of renal failure,[2] but a strict linear relationship between hematocrit and creatinine clearance does not exist. At creatinine clearances less than 20 mL/min, however, the hematocrit is almost always below 30 percent (Fig. 33-1). Infectious, neoplastic, immunologic, or metabolic disorders that may accompany renal failure may also affect the degree of anemia.

ETIOLOGY AND PATHOGENESIS

Experimental and clinical observations on the effect of intensive dialysis, bilateral nephrectomy, and EPO have clarified some of the pathophysiologic mechanisms responsible for the anemia. The main cause of the anemia of chronic renal failure is a decreased production of EPO by the failing kidney. Nevertheless, a diminished capacity to excrete potentially toxic metabolic end products aggravates the anemia by shortening the red cell life span and causing blood loss and marrow suppression.

RENAL EXCRETORY FAILURE

The life span of red cells in patients with chronic renal disease is usually shorter than normal. Since the red cells survive normally when injected into healthy recipients and since normal red cells may have a shortened life span in uremic recipients,[3,4] it appears that the metabolic or mechanical environment in uremic patients is unfavorable for normal survival of red cells.

METABOLIC RED CELL DYSFUNCTION

The presence of an erythrocyte metabolic defect is suggested by the inverse relationship that has sometimes been noted between blood urea nitrogen and red cell life span[5-7] and by the occasional normalization of the red cell life span after intensive dialysis.[7] However, most red cell enzymes show normal or increased activity in uremia, and the intracellular level of ATP is high, possibly due to a high serum phosphate concentration.[8]

The intracellular concentration of 2,3-bisphosphoglycerate is also appropriately increased in response to anemia and hyperphosphatemia,[9] with a moderate decrease in the affinity of hemoglobin for oxygen.[10] In the presence of uremic acidosis, this decrease in oxygen affinity is augmented by a shift to the right in the oxygen dissociation curve (Bohr effect). However, acidosis will also tend to decrease the concentration of intracellular organic phosphates, establishing a condition of opposing effects on the oxygen affinity of hemoglobin.[11] Intensive dialysis may initially cause a reduction in the concentration of intracellular organic phosphate compounds, possibly because of hypophosphatemia.[12] This results in increased oxygen affinity of hemoglobin and a temporary aggravation of tissue hypoxia, and may play a role in the so-called dialysis disequilibrium syndrome.[13]

Only the activity of transketolase, a hexose monophosphate shunt enzyme (see Chap. 26),[14] and ATPase, powering the Na^+-K^+ membrane pumps,[15] are decreased in uremia. The decreased response of the hexose monophosphate shunt renders the hemoglobin and red cell membrane excessively sensitive to oxidant drugs or chemicals.[16,17] For example, tap water used for hemodialysis and purified with chloramine can cause the formation of Heinz bodies and hemolytic anemia.[18] The decreased activity of the Na^+-K^+ pumps could cause changes in red cell shape and rigidity and, in turn, in red cell life span. The toxic substances responsible for these metabolic impairments are presumably dialyzable but have not been identified. Other exogenous toxins introduced by dialysis fluids, such as copper, nitrates, and formaldehyde, can also contribute to hemolysis and on occasion produce severe, even fatal, hemolytic episodes.[19] Parathyroid hormone, often increased in renal failure,[20] may also contribute to hemolysis by increasing red cell osmotic fragility.[21]

MECHANICAL RED CELL DESTRUCTION

Despite these data on a metabolic basis for hemolysis, a considerable number of investigators have failed to find a clear-cut correlation between red cell life span and degree of renal failure.[2] It has been suggested that red cell injury and premature destruction may be caused by mechanical trauma rather than by metabolic alterations.[22] Normal red cells exposed to strong shearing stress, especially at a fibrin interphase, will become deformed and vulnerable to monocyte-macrophage sequestration. In some cases of malignant hypertension, extensive red cell fragmentation occurs with severe hemolytic anemia,[23] but in most cases of chronic renal disease the hemolysis as well as the morphologic changes are moderate. At the present, it appears reasonable to relate premature destruction of red cells in uremia to mechanical disruption of metabolically impaired cells.

HEMOLYTIC UREMIC SYNDROME

The hemolytic uremic syndrome is probably a distinct entity,[24] although many of its manifestations are similar to those found in patients with

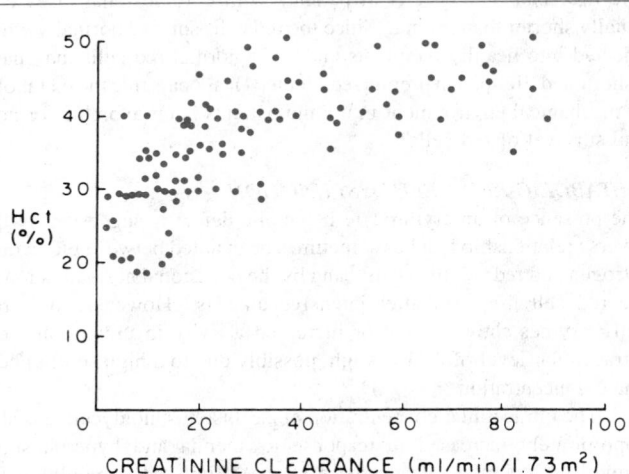

FIGURE 33-1   Relationship between hematocrit and creatinine clearance in patients with chronic renal disease. (Redrawn from Radtke et al.[2])

microangiopathic disorders (see Chap. 51) or consumptive coagulopathies (see Chap. 126). It was first described in 1955 by Gasser and coworkers,[25] who found hemolysis and uremia in infants and young children subsequent to episodes of gastrointestinal or upper respiratory infections. Since then the syndrome has been recognized in patients of all ages and associated with a variety of exogenous agents.[26] It appears to be initiated by damage to the endothelium of glomerular capillaries and renal arterioles.[27] This leads to local platelet deposition, intravascular coagulation, and ischemic renal cortical necrosis.[27] The clinical manifestations are pallor, purpura, jaundice, and oliguria, and

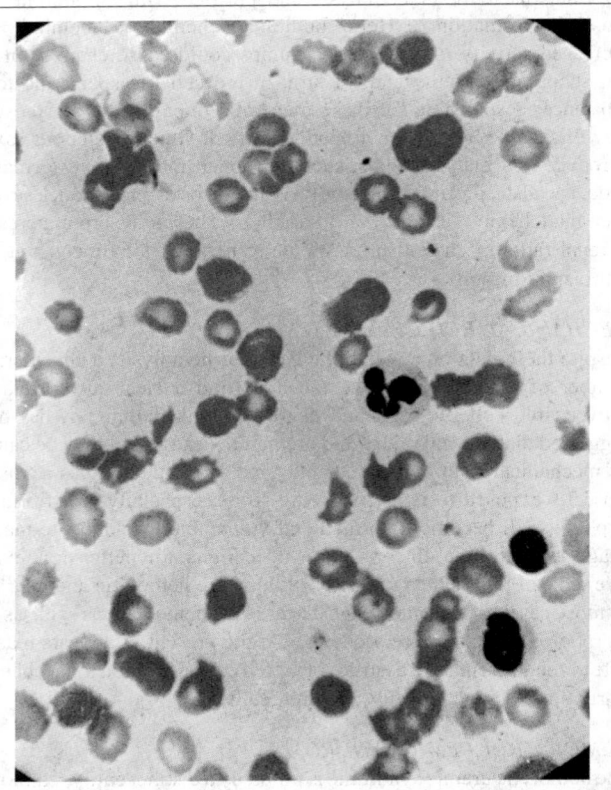

FIGURE 33-2   Blood film from a patient with the hemolytic uremic syndrome, showing fragmentation and distortion of red blood cells.

laboratory tests reveal anemia with a blood film displaying many deformed and fragmented red cells (Fig. 33-2), increased number of reticulocytes, and occasional nucleated red cells.[26,28] EPO levels are increased despite an elevated serum creatinine concentration.[29] There is thrombocytopenia and a compensatory increase in marrow megakaryocytes. In many cases it may be difficult to distinguish the hemolytic uremic syndrome from the syndrome of thrombotic thrombocytopenic purpura (see Chaps. 51 and 117). However, despite the similarity of clinical and laboratory data between these two syndromes, a basic biochemical difference has been demonstrated without, unfortunately, clarifying the pathogenesis of the hemolytic uremic syndrome. The normal cleaving of von Willebrand multimers is impaired in thrombotic thrombocytopenic purpura either due to a congenital absence of a multimer-cleaving protease or because of immunologic inactivation of this protease.[30,31] This is associated with unrestricted multimer-induced aggregation of platelets and, in turn, thrombosis and consumption of coagulation proteins. In the hemolytic uremic syndrome, however, there is no lack of this protective protease and no excessive accumulation of von Willebrand factor multimers.[30] Consequently, plasma infusions and plasmapheresis, so effective in thrombotic thrombocytopenic purpura, have been of little avail in treating patients with the hemolytic uremic syndrome. Fortunately, most milder cases of this syndrome clear spontaneously, but severe cases may cause life-threatening renal failure.

BLOOD LOSS

Purpura and gastrointestinal and gynecologic bleeding occur in one-third to one-half of all patients with chronic renal failure.[32] In addition, blood and iron are lost in laboratory testing and in discarded dialysis tubing. All this constitutes a significant loss of iron and may contribute to the development of anemia. The pathogenesis of the bleeding tendency is poorly understood. Thrombocytopenia, when present, is rarely of sufficient magnitude to explain spontaneous blood loss.[33] However, platelet or vascular function, as judged from bleeding time, platelet adhesiveness and aggregation, clot retraction, thromboxane formation, or prostacyclin production by vessel walls, is abnormal in the majority of cases and may, alone or together, account for the bleeding tendency (see Chap. 120). Dialysis has been found to correct or ameliorate both the laboratory and clinical manifestations of abnormal platelet function,[33] but the dialyzable agent responsible has not been identified. Urea or creatinine is probably not involved, but certain guanidine compounds are suspected.[34]

MARROW SUPPRESSION

Although a deficiency of EPO (see "Failure of Renal Endocrine Function") could in itself explain the development of anemia, it has been suggested that, in addition, uremic toxins may impair erythroid activity and in part be responsible for the development of anemia.[35] Older studies[36] have suggested that such uremic toxins exist, but all attempts to identify and isolate them have been unsuccessful. Spermine, an attractive candidate,[37] was found to suppress all cellular elements, and not only the erythroid tissue, when administered in toxic doses.[38] Parathyroid hormone,[39] another contender, causes general marrow suppression by inducing marrow fibrosis.[20] Exogenous EPO has been shown to be equally effective when administered to patients before and after successful kidney transplantation.[40] These observations would suggest that uremia per se does not affect normal erythroid metabolism in vivo. Nevertheless, it has also been reported[41] that the response to EPO in stable, well-dialyzed patients is about half of that in normal individuals (Fig. 33-3). Whether this decreased responsiveness is due to uremic toxins, to associated diseases, or to relative iron deficiency is not clear.

Iron may be in short supply in most patients with renal failure due to excessive blood loss (see above),[42] and iron supplementation

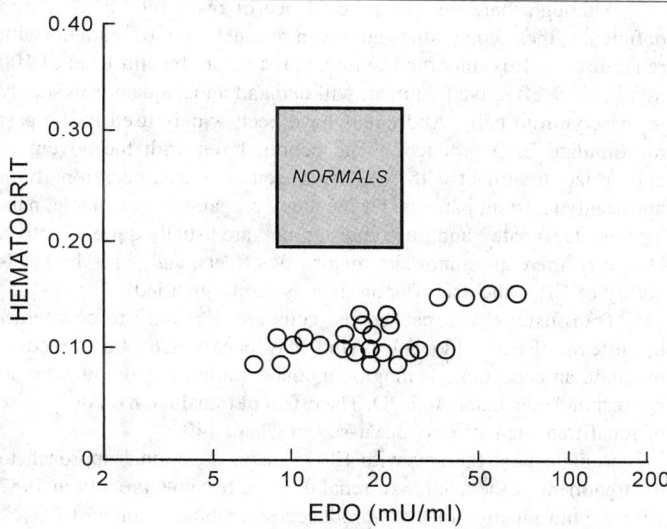

FIGURE 33-3   Rate of red cell production as related to plasma concentrations of EPO in 22 stable uremic patients (open circles). Due to their stable hematocrits, the rate of red cell production must equal the rate of red cell destruction, which was calculated by dividing red cell mass by red cell life span. The square denotes the rate of red cell production in normal individuals at normal EPO levels.[41]

in patients receiving EPO has been found to be of great importance (see below). Aluminum in dialysis water may interfere with iron incorporation in erythroid cells and cause a microcytic anemia and occasionally osteomalacia and encephalopathy.[43] In a rare case of nephrosis, the urinary loss of transferrin has been reported to cause low iron-binding capacity, with impairment in the metabolic cycling of iron.[44] Folic acid deficiency should always be suspected and prevented in patients undergoing intensive dialysis, since folic acid is dialyzable and may be lost in the dialysis bath.[45]

FAILURE OF RENAL ENDOCRINE FUNCTION

ERYTHROPOIETIN

Erythropoietin is a 34-kDa glycoprotein hematopoietic growth factor capable of controlling the rate of red cell production (see Chap. 29). In 1957, Jacobson and coworkers[46] reported that nephrectomized and uremic rats failed to respond to blood loss by releasing EPO, while ureter-ligated and equally uremic rats responded in an almost normal manner. This important observation led to the hypothesis that the kidney produces EPO. Although the role of the kidney in EPO production has not been seriously challenged, various mechanisms have been proposed, for example, that the kidney synthesizes activating enzymes or inactive precursors that, after exposure to circulating plasma proteins, produce EPO molecules.[47] In the 1970s, studies on isolated perfused kidneys supported a direct role of the kidney in EPO production.[48] However, it was not until the demonstration of EPO mRNA in renal tissue that it was finally established that the kidney is an EPO-producing organ.[49–51]

In situ hybridization studies have localized the EPO-producing cells to the cortical interstitium of mouse and rat kidneys.[52,53] These immunoelectron microscopic techniques showed that EPO-expressing cells also express the surface enzyme ecto-5′-nucleotidase,[54,55] a marker restricted to fibroblastic cells. An intriguing observation is that a number of EPO-producing cells appear to be recruited to express the gene in an all-or-none fashion, with recruitment spreading outward from the corticomedullary boundary.[56]

Hypoxia is followed within 1 h by a measurable accumulation of EPO mRNA in the kidneys and shortly afterward by an increase in circulating EPO.[51,57] The mechanism, however, by which renal hypoxia causes an activation of the EPO gene is still not clear (see Chap. 29). Extrarenal sites of EPO production exist and in adult rodents account for about 15 to 20 percent of total EPO secretion.[58] In humans, very low but still detectable levels of EPO are found in severely anemic anephric individuals (Fig. 33-4).[59] In fetal life, extrarenal production of EPO by the liver predominates, with a gradual change to renal production at time of birth.[60] In the liver, two types of cells express the EPO gene, hepatocytes and intermedullary cells,[61,62] the nonparenchymal Ito cells that are morphologically and functionally very similar to the interstitial fibroblasts in the kidneys.[63] The genomic EPO sequences that determine expression are somewhat different, with the kidney requiring a 14-kb upstream fragment not needed by the liver.[64] The inappropriate production of EPO by renal and extrarenal cysts and tumors appears to be accomplished by cells different from those responsible for normal, regulated synthesis of EPO.[54]

In patients with renal disease, the reduction in EPO production is roughly proportional to the degree of excretory impairment. However, even nonfunctioning kidneys produce some EPO and are capable of maintaining higher hemoglobin levels than those found in anephric patients (see Fig. 33-4).[59] This remaining capacity of remnant kidneys to produce EPO appears to be responsible for the polycythemia that occurs in 10 to 15 percent of patients following kidney transplantation.[65] It is also responsible for the brief but significant increase in EPO levels seen in end-stage uremic patients following episodes of acute hypoxia or blood loss.[66,67]

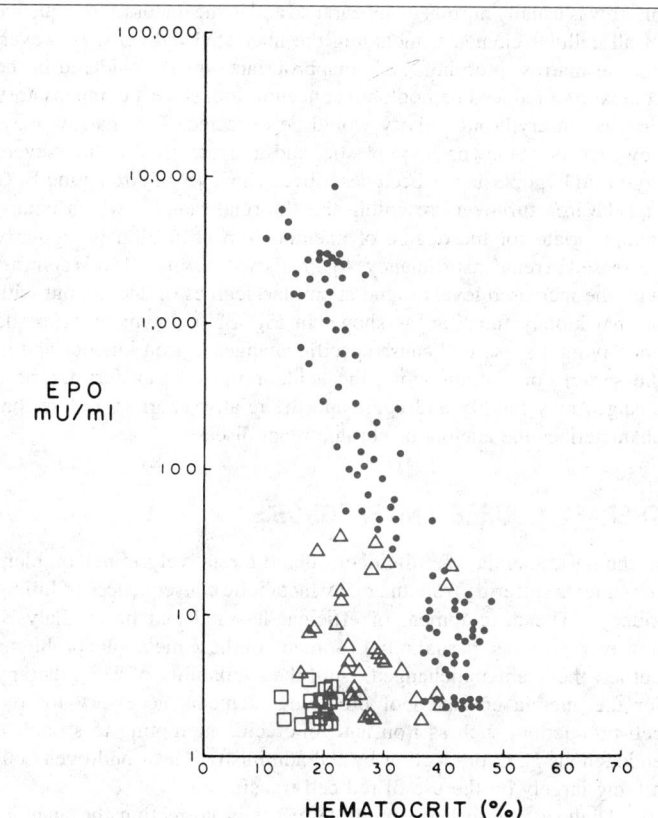

FIGURE 33-4   EPO levels in nephric and anephric uremic patients as compared to individuals with intact kidneys. Values for normal subjects and patients with simple anemia, ●; anephric patients, □; nephric patients, △. All determinations were made by bioassay of plasma concentrates in hypertransfused mice.

CLINICAL AND LABORATORY FEATURES

The symptoms and physical manifestations of renal failure depend primarily on the underlying disorder. However, pallor and anemia are almost invariably present and may become of major clinical concern.

The anemia is characteristically normocytic and normochromic and is associated with a normal or slightly decreased number of reticulocytes. A few red cells appear deformed on blood films, some with multiple tiny spicules and others with grossly abnormal contour and loss of volume. The former cells, echinocytes or burr cells, were thought to be quite characteristic of chronic renal failure.[68] However, even normal cells will undergo a reversible transformation to burr-cell–like echinocytes when exposed to a glass surface or suspended in incubated plasma.[69]

Grossly deformed cells, however, such as acanthocytes with a few large spicules or fragmented schistocytes, are undoubtedly formed in the microcirculation in vivo.[70] They are found most abundantly in the hemolytic uremic syndrome (see Fig. 33-2) but in small numbers can be recognized on blood films from most uremic patients.

The total and differential leukocyte count and the platelet count are usually normal, but, as with all other hematologic parameters, the underlying disorder plays a modifying role. Uremia and dialysis may have an effect on both leukocytes and platelets. The phagocytic activity of granulocytes may be reduced,[71] and complement activation by the hemodialysis membrane may cause pulmonary leukostasis with temporary granulocytopenia.[72] Cell-mediated immunity is also depressed, resulting in both an increased incidence of infections but also favoring prolonged graft survival.[71] Platelet function is abnormal and related to the degree of uremia and dialysis (see "Blood Loss").[73–75] The marrow is usually normal in appearance and in the maturation sequence of all cellular elements, including the nucleated red cells. However, normal marrow morphology is inappropriate when considered in the context of a reduced hemoglobin concentration, since a compensatory increase in erythroid activity would be expected. The marrow may, however, be somewhat hypoplastic, and in acute renal failure severe erythroid hypoplasia has been described. The level of circulating EPO and the iron turnover are within the "normal range," which is also inappropriate for the degree of anemia. Iron utilization is regularly decreased in renal insufficiency. Again, these "normal" levels contrast with the increased levels found at similar degrees of anemia but with normal kidney function, as shown in Fig. 33-4. In many cases the underlying disease will cause specific changes in iron kinetics and in the serum concentration of folic acid, iron, and transferrin. These changes may modify and aggravate the relative marrow failure that characterizes the anemia of chronic renal disease.

THERAPY, COURSE, AND PROGNOSIS

In the past, anemia was often considered a relatively minor problem for patients suffering from the many metabolic consequences of failing kidneys. The development of efficient hospital and home dialysis, however, provided partial relief for many of these metabolic problems but left the anemia unchanged. Until the availability of EPO, therapy for the anemia consisted of providing elements necessary for red cell production, such as iron and folic acid, attempting to stimulate endogenous EPO production by the administration of androgens but relying largely on the use of red cell transfusions.

Dialysis per se has very little effect in correcting the anemia, although a mild increase in hemoglobin concentration may occur[75] due to a decrease in bleeding tendency. For still unexplained reasons, ambulatory peritoneal dialysis tends to ameliorate and, on occasion, completely correct the anemia.[76]

Although there may be no evidence of overt folic acid or iron deficiency, these compounds are given routinely to most patients with renal disease. It is important to maintain a serum ferritin level of 100 ng/ml, since effective treatment will demand an adequate iron supply to the erythroid cells. Androgens have been widely used in the past to stimulate EPO production and action. Even with the advent of appropriate treatment with EPO, androgens are used occasionally in apparently resistant patients. Of the many preparations available, nandrolone decanoate[77] and fluoxymesterone[78] are usually quite effective. However, there are minor and major side effects, and, with the availability of EPO, the use of androgens is rarely justified.

Transfusions with packed red cells are necessary to counteract the effects of acute blood loss and may occasionally be needed to maintain an acceptable hemoglobin concentration in patients who do not respond adequately to EPO. The effect of transfusion on the course of renal transplantation is discussed in Chap. 140.

Replacement therapy with EPO, the most rational approach to the treatment of the anemia of renal disease, became a reality in 1987 with the introduction of mass-produced recombinant human EPO.[79,80] The recombinant product has the same amino acid composition as natural human EPO[81] as well as an almost identical carbohydrate composition,[82] and thus antibodies against the recombinant product have not been found in any treated patient. The results have been dramatic, and the administration of EPO has been capable of ameliorating the anemia in almost every patient treated, irrespective of the underlying cause of the renal disorder (Fig. 33-5).[80]

The National Kidney Foundation has recently published detailed guidelines for the administration of EPO to patients with the anemia of chronic renal diseases.[83] In short, the presence of an anemia with hematocrits of less than 33 percent or hemoglobins of less than 11 g/dl should first initiate a thorough search for conditions unrelated to decreased EPO production or action. Measurements of folic acid and B_{12} levels should be carried out, and it is especially important to measure iron, iron binding capacity, and ferritin levels. Determination of EPO levels is not necessary. It is important to rule out complicating chronic illnesses that, through cytokine action, can aggravate the ane-

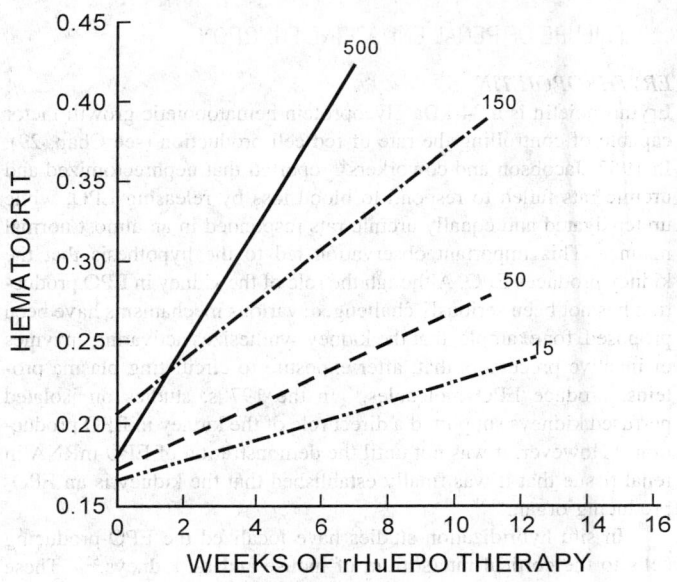

FIGURE 33-5   The slopes of hematocrit increase in uremic patients after the weekly administration of various doses of recombinant EPO. —, 500 units/kg; — · —, 150 units/kg; – – –, 50 units/kg; — · · —, 15 units/kg. (From Eschbach et al, with permission.[80])

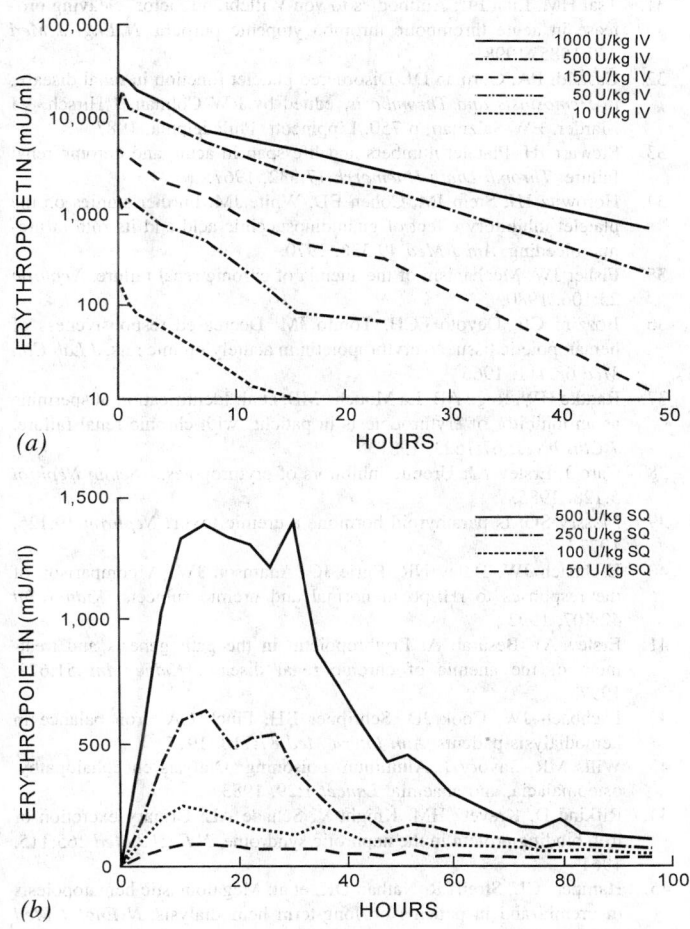

(a)

(b)

FIGURE 33-6 Pharmacokinetics of plasma EPO in normal volunteers. *(a)* Intravenous administration. *(b)* Subcutaneous administration.

mia. Although the anemia of renal disease is roughly proportional to the severity of the renal failure, renal anemia can occur with serum creatinine levels as low as 2 mg/dl.

Because of the availability of venous access in dialysis patients, EPO has been given primarily by the intravenous route. Pharmacokinetic studies in normal volunteers and in chronic renal disease patients, however, have shown that subcutaneous administration may be equally effective.[84,85] The half-life of intravenous EPO is between 6 and 9 h, with a volume of distribution slightly larger than that of the plasma volume (Fig. 33-6a).[86,87] When the subcutaneous route is employed, there are no peaks and lower plasma levels are observed, but the lower levels are more sustained throughout the course (Fig. 33-6b).[87,88] However, it appears that bioavailability after subcutaneous injections is less predictable, possibly due to erratic tissue absorption. Subcutaneous EPO administration can maintain a target hematocrit value of 30 to 33 percent with the use of about 30 percent lower doses of EPO.[89]

Based on the initial clinical trials, the U.S. Food and Drug Administration approved the clinical use of EPO in June 1989, setting the target hematocrit at 30 to 33 percent.[90] In its 1997 guidelines,[83] the National Kidney Foundation recommended an increase in the target hematocrit to 33 to 36 percent and target hemoglobin to 11 to 12 g/dl. Furthermore, they recommended that the preferred route of EPO administration be subcutaneous and that routine iron supplementation be given intravenously, rather than orally, to optimize the response. Some have advocated higher target hematocrits, close to the normal

range. However, a disappointing number of complications occur in the near-normal hematocrit group.[91]

In order to achieve the target hematocrit within 3 to 4 months of therapy,[83,92] the initial dose of EPO in adult patients should be 80 to 120 units/kg/week divided into two or three subcutaneous injections or 120 to 180 units/kg/week given as three intravenous injections. The response should be monitored by measuring the hematocrit and hemoglobin at least once every 2 weeks. Once the target hematocrit has been reached, most adult patients can be maintained by administering 50 to 100 units/kg/week in divided doses. Pediatric patients (<5 years of age) usually require higher initial and maintenance doses.

Anemia in predialysis patients can also be corrected with exogenous EPO. Such corrections will not jeopardize renal function[93,94] and may prevent the development of cardiac hypertrophy.

It is, of course, essential to maintain adequate iron stores. Although the National Kidney Foundation has expressed a preference for the use of intravenous iron, many physicians, especially when using EPO subcutaneously, will prefer the use of an oral iron preparation providing at least 100 mg of elemental iron a day.[95]

By now, large multicenter studies have shown that more than 95 percent of patients respond to EPO therapy.[83] Nevertheless, there is a small group of patients who either do not respond or first respond when larger doses are administered. The most common causes of a poor response are inadequate iron supply, intercurrent infections, or excessive splenic hemolysis.[96] Aluminum toxicity may be responsible for resistance to treatment and should be suspected in patients with microcytic red cell indices.[97]

During the initial clinical trials, most of which were uncontrolled, a number of adverse effects were reported.[98,99] Some of these have not been observed in subsequent trials, probably because of the more judicious use of the hormone.[83] However, of considerable and sustained concern have been hypertension, seizures, thrombosis of arteriovenous fistulas, and high potassium levels in treated patients.[99] Hypertension has been the most common complication. It usually represents exaggeration of a previously existing condition, but it can occur de novo. Blood pressure should be carefully monitored throughout the treatment.[83] Initiation or adjustment of antihypertensive medication and reduction of EPO dosage may be required. Also noted in the initial trials was an increased incidence of seizures. In several subsequent studies, the incidence of seizures in patients started on EPO was found to be 3 percent, with a range of 0 to 13 percent.[100] Such an incidence, however, is about the same in EPO-untreated patients.[101] It is now believed that EPO treatment is not contraindicated in patients with a previous history of seizures.

A widespread concern with the use of EPO in hemodialyzed patients is the possible effect of higher hematocrits on the native fistulas or synthetic shunts. In a review of 26 studies in which 4100 patients were enrolled, the average incidence of thrombosis of the access routes in patients on EPO was 7.5 percent.[102] This value is well within the accepted values for thrombotic episodes in dialyzed patients not receiving EPO.

Amelioration of the anemia has resulted in a variety of beneficial changes[103–105] in various systems and in general has greatly improved the quality of life of these unfortunate patients.[106,107]

REFERENCES

1. Bright R: Cases and observations, illustrative of renal disease accompanied with the secretion of albuminous urine. *Guys Hosp Rep* 1:340, 1836.
2. Radtke HW, Claussner A, Erbes PM, et al: Serum erythropoietin concentration in chronic renal failure: Relationship to degree of anemia and excretory function. *Blood* 54:877, 1979.
3. Ragen PA, Hagedorn AB, Owen CA: Radioisotope study of anemia in chronic renal disease. *Arch Intern Med* 105:518, 1960.

4. Desforges JF, Dawson JP: The anemia of renal failure. *Arch Intern Med* 101:326, 1958.

5. Joske RA, McAllister JM, Prankerd TAJ: Isotope investigations of red cell production and destruction in chronic renal disease. *Clin Sci* 15:511, 1956.

6. Adamson JW, Eschbach J, Finch CA: The kidney and erythropoiesis. *Am J Med* 44:725, 1968.

7. Berry ER, Rambach WA, Alt HL, Del Greco G: Effect of peritoneal dialysis on erythrokinetics and ferrokinetics of azotemic anemia. *Trans Am Soc Artif Intern Organs* 10:415, 1965.

8. Mansell AJ, Grimes AJ: Red and white cell abnormalities in chronic renal failure. *Br J Haematol* 42:168, 1979.

9. Chillar RK, Desforges JF: Red cell organic phosphates in patients with chronic renal failure on maintenance haemodialysis. *Br J Haematol* 26:549, 1974.

10. Mitchell TR, Pegrum GD: The oxygen affinity of haemoglobin in chronic renal failure. *Br J Haematol* 21:463, 1971.

11. Lichtman MA, Murphy MS, Whitbeck AA, Kearney EA: Oxygen binding to haemoglobin in subjects with hypoproliferative anaemia, with and without chronic renal disease: Role of pH. *Br J Haematol* 27:439, 1974.

12. Lichtman MA, Miller OR, Freeman RB: Erythrocyte adenosine triphosphate depletion during hypophosphatemia in a uremic subject. *N Engl J Med* 280:240, 1969.

13. Torrance JD, Milne FJ, Hurwitz S, et al: Changes in oxygen delivery during hemodialysis. *Clin Nephrol* 3:53, 1975.

14. Lonergan ET, Semar M, Sterzel RB, et al: Erythrocyte transketolase activity in dialyzed patients: A reversible metabolic lesion of uremia. *N Engl J Med* 284:1399, 1971.

15. Cole CH: Decreased ouabain-sensitive adenine triphosphatase activity in the erythrocyte membrane of patients with chronic renal disease. *Clin Sci* 45:775, 1973.

16. Yawata Y, Howe R, Jacob HS: Abnormal red cell metabolism causing hemolysis in uremia: A defect potentiated by tap water hemodialysis. *Ann Intern Med* 79:362, 1973.

17. Rosenwund A, Binswanger U, Straub PW: Oxidative injury to erythrocytes, cell rigidity, and splenic hemolysis in hemodialyzed uremic patients. *Ann Intern Med* 82:460, 1975.

18. Eaton JW, Kolpin CF, Swofford HS, et al: Chlorinated urban water: A cause of dialysis-induced hemolytic anemia. *Science* 181:463, 1973.

19. Orringer EP, Mattern WDL: Formaldehyde-induced hemolysis in chronic hemodialysis. *N Engl J Med* 294:416, 1976.

20. Rao DS, Shih M, Mohini R: Effect of serum PTH and bone marrow fibrosis on the response to erythropoietin in uremia. *N Engl J Med* 328:171, 1993.

21. Okmai M, Telfer N, Ansani A, et al: Erythrocyte survival in chronic renal failure: Role of secondary hyperparathyroidism. *J Clin Invest* 76:1695, 1985.

22. Brain MC: The haemolytic-uremic syndrome. *Semin Hematol* 6:162, 1969.

23. Capelli JP, Wesson LG, Erslev AJ: Malignant hypertension and red cell fragmentation syndrome. *Ann Intern Med* 64:128, 1966.

24. Kaplan BS, Drummond KN: The hemolytic-uremic syndrome is a syndrome. *N Engl J Med* 298:964, 1978.

25. Gasser C, Gautier E, Steck A, et al: Hämolytisch-urämische Syndrome: Bilaterale Nierenrindennekrosen bei akuten erworbenen hämolytischen Anämien. *Schweiz Med Wochenschr* 85:906, 1955.

26. Lieberman E, Heuser E, Donnell GN, et al: Hemolytic-uremic syndrome: Clinical and pathological considerations. *N Engl J Med* 275:277, 1966.

27. Mitra D, Jaffe EA, Weksler B, Hajjar KA, Soderland C, Laurence J: Thrombotic thrombocytopenic purpura and sporadic hemolytic-uremic syndrome plasmas induce apoptosis in restricted lineages of human microvascular endothelial cells. *Blood* 89:1224, 1997.

28. Moake JL: Haemolytic-uraemic syndrome. Basic science. *Lancet* 343:393, 1994.

29. Miller RP, Denny WF: Hemolytic anemia during acute renal failure: Observations on plasma erythropoietin levels. *South Med J* 61:29, 1968.

30. Furlan M, Robles R, Galbusera M, et al: Von Willebrand factor–cleaving protease in thrombotic thrombocytopenic purpura and the hemolytic-uremic syndrome. *N Engl J Med* 339:1578–1584, 1998.

31. Tsai HM, Lian EC: Antibodies to von Willebrand factor–cleaving protease in acute thrombotic thrombocytopenic purpura. *N Engl J Med* 339:1585, 1998.

32. Castaldi PA, Gorman DJ: Disordered platelet function in renal disease, in *Hemostasis and Thrombosis*, edited by RW Colman, J Hirsch, VJ Marder, EW Salzman, p 750. Lippincott, Philadelphia, 1987.

33. Stewart JH: Platelet numbers and life span in acute and chronic renal failure. *Thromb Diath Haemorrh* 17:532, 1967.

34. Horowitz HJ, Stein JM, Cohen BD, White JM: Further studies on the platelet inhibitory effect of guanidinosuccinic acid and its role in uremic bleeding. *Am J Med* 49:336, 1970.

35. Fisher JW: Mechanism of the anemia of chronic renal failure. *Nephron* 25:106, 1980.

36. Bozzini CE, Devoto FCH, Tomio JM: Decreased responsiveness of hematopoietic tissue to erythropoietin in acutely uremic rats. *J Lab Clin Med* 68:411, 1966.

37. Radtke HW, Rege AB, La Mouche MB, et al: Identification of spermine as an inhibitor of erythropoiesis in patients with chronic renal failure. *J Clin Invest* 67:1623, 1981.

38. Caro J, Erslev AJ: Uremic inhibitors of erythropoiesis. *Semin Nephrol* 5:128, 1985.

39. Massry SG: Is parathyroid hormone a uremic toxin? *Nephron* 19:125, 1977.

40. Eschbach JW, Haley NR, Egrie JC, Adamson JW: A comparison of the responses to rHEpo in normal and uremic subjects. *Kidney Int* 42:407, 1992.

41. Erslev AJ, Besarab A: Erythropoietin in the pathogenesis and treatment of the anemia of chronic renal disease. *Kidney Int* 51:622, 1997.

42. Eschbach JW, Cook JD, Schribner BH, Finch CA: Iron balance in hemodialysis patients. *Ann Intern Med* 87:710, 1977.

43. Wills MR, Savory J: Aluminum poisoning: Dialysis encephalopathy, osteomalacia, and anaemia. *Lancet* 1:29, 1983.

44. Rifkind D, Kravetz HM, Knight V, Schade AL: Urinary excretion of iron binding protein in the nephrotic syndrome. *N Engl J Med* 265:115, 1961.

45. Hampers CL, Streiff R, Nathan DK, et al: Megaloblastic hematopoiesis in uremia and in patients on long-term hemodialysis. *N Engl J Med* 276:551, 1967.

46. Jacobson LO, Goldwasser E, Fried W, Plazak L: Role of the kidney in erythropoiesis. *Nature* 179:633, 1957.

47. Gordon AS, Cooper GW, Zanjani E: The kidney and erythropoiesis. *Semin Hematol* 4:337, 1967.

48. Erslev AJ: In vitro production of erythropoietin by kidneys perfused with a serum-free solution. *Blood* 44:77, 1974.

49. Bondurant MC, Koury M: Anemia induces accumulation of erythropoietin mRNA in the kidney and liver. *Mol Cell Biol* 6:2731, 1986.

50. Beru N, McDonald J, Lacombe C, Goldwasser E: Expression of the erythropoietin gene. *Mol Cell Biol* 6:2571, 1986.

51. Schuster SJ, Wilson J, Erslev AJ, Caro J: Physiologic regulation and tissue localization of renal erythropoietin mRNA. *Blood* 70:316, 1987.

52. Lacombe C, DaSilva J-L, Bruneval P, et al: Peritubular cells are the site of erythropoietin synthesis in the murine hypoxic kidney. *J Clin Invest* 81:620, 1988.

53. Koury ST, Bondurant MC, Koury MJ: Localization of erythropoietin-synthesizing cells in murine kidneys by in situ hybridization. *Blood* 71:524, 1988.

54. Maxwell PH, Ferguson DJP, Nicholls LG, et al: Sites of erythropoietin production. *Kidney Int* 51:393, 1997.

55. Maxwell PH, Ratcliffe PJ: The erythropoietin-producing cells. *Exp Nephrol* 4:309, 1996.

56. Maxwell PH, Ferguson DJ, Nicholls LG, et al: The interstitial response to renal injury: Fibroblast-like cells show phenotypic changes and have reduced potential for erythropoietin gene expression. *Kidney Int* 52:715, 1997.

57. Schuster SJ, Badiavas E, Costa-Giomi P, et al: Stimulation of erythropoietin gene transcription during hypoxia and cobalt exposure. *Blood* 73:13, 1989.

58. Erslev AJ, Caro J, Kansu E, Silver R: Renal and extrarenal erythropoietin production in anemic rats. *Br J Haematol* 45:65, 1980.

59. Caro J, Brown S, Miller O, et al: Erythropoietin levels in uremic nephric and anephric patients. *J Lab Clin Med* 93:449, 1979.

60. Fried W: The liver is a source of extrarenal erythropoietin production. *Blood* 40:671, 1972.

61. Koury JT, Bondurant MC, Koury MJ, Semenza GL: Localization of cells producing erythropoietin in murine liver by in situ hybridization. *Blood* 77:2497, 1991.

62. Schuster SJ, Koury S, Borher M, et al: Cellular sites of extrarenal and renal erythropoietin production in anemic rats. *Br J Haematol* 81:153, 1992.

63. Maxwell PH, Ferguson DJ, Osmond MK, et al: Expression of a homologously recombined erythropoietin-SV40 T antigen fusion gene in mouse liver: Evidence for erythropoietin production by Ito cells. *Blood* 84:1823, 1994.

64. Köchling J, Curtis PT, Madan A: Regulation of human erythropoietin gene induction by upstream flanking sequences in transgenic mice. *Br J Haematol* 103:960, 1998.

65. Dagher FJ, Ramos E, Erslev AJ, et al: Are the native kidneys responsible for erythrocytosis in renal allorecipients? *Transplantation* 28:496, 1979.

66. Walle AJ, Wong GY, Clemons GK, et al: Erythropoietin-hematocrit feedback circuit in the anemia of end-stage renal disease. *Kidney Int* 31:1205, 1987.

67. Eckardt K-U, Druecke T, Leski M, Kurtz A: Unutilized reserves: The production capacity for erythropoietin appears to be conserved in chronic renal disease. *Contrib Nephrol* 88:18, 1991.

68. Schwartz SO, Motto SA: The diagnostic significance of "burr" red blood cells. *Am J Med Sci* 218:563, 1949.

69. Brecher G, Bessis M: Present status of spiculed red cells and their relationship to the discocyte-echinocyte transformation: A critical review. *Blood* 40:333, 1972.

70. Weed R: The red membrane in hemolytic disorders: Plenary papers. *XII Congr Int Soc Hematol,* p 81, 1968.

71. Goldblum SE, Reed WP: Host defenses and immunologic alterations associated with chronic hemodialysis. *Ann Intern Med* 93:597, 1980.

72. Craddock PR, Fehr J, Brigham KL, et al: Complement and leukocyte-mediated pulmonary dysfunction in hemodialysis. *N Engl J Med* 296:769, 1977.

73. Pasternack A, Wahlberg P: Bone marrow in acute renal failure. *Acta Med Scand* 181:505, 1967.

74. Callen JR, Limarzi LR: Blood and bone marrow studies in renal disease. *Am J Clin Pathol* 20:3, 1950.

75. Eschbach JW, Funk D, Adamson JW, et al: Erythropoiesis in patients with renal failure undergoing chronic dialysis. *N Engl J Med* 276:653, 1967.

76. Zappacosta AR, Caro J, Erslev A: The normalization of hematocrit in end-stage renal disease patients on continuous ambulatory peritonal dialysis: The role of erythropoietin. *Am J Med* 72:53, 1982.

77. Eschbach JW, Adamson JW: Improvement in the anemia of chronic renal failure with fluoxymesterone. *Ann Intern Med* 78:527, 1973.

78. Neff MS, Goldberg J, Slifkin RF, et al: A comparison of androgens for anemia in patients on hemodialysis. *N Engl J Med* 304:871, 1981.

79. Winearls CG, Oliver DO, Pippard MJ, et al: Effect of human erythropoietin derived from recombinant DNA on the anemia of patients maintained by chronic haemodialysis. *Lancet* 2:1175, 1986.

80. Eschbach JW, Egrie JC, Downing MR, et al: Correction of the anemia of end-stage renal disease with recombinant human erythropoietin. *N Engl J Med* 316:73, 1987.

81. Recny MA, Scoble HA, Kim Y: Structural characterization of natural human urinary and recombinant DNA-derived erythropoietin. *J Biol Chem* 262:17156, 1987.

82. Tsuda E, Kawanishi G, Ueda M, et al: The role of carbohydrate in recombinant human erythropoietin. *Eur J Biochem* 188:405, 1990.

83. NKF-DOA: Anemia work group: Guidelines. *Am J Kid Dis* 30:8196, 1997.

84. Besarab A, Flaharty KK, Erslev A, et al: Clinical pharmacology and economics of recombinant human erythropoietin in end stage renal disease: The case for subcutaneous administration. *J Am Soc Nephrol* 2:1405, 1992.

85. Watson A, Gimenez L, Cotton J, et al: Treatment of anemia of chronic renal failure with subcutaneous rHEpo. *Am J Med* 89:432, 1990.

86. Flaharty KK, Caro J, Erslev A, et al: Pharmacokinetics and erythropoietic response to human recombinant erythropoietin in healthy men. *Clin Pharmacol Ther* 47:557, 1990.

87. Spivak J, Cotes M: Pharmacokinetics of erythropoietin, in *Erythropoietin: Molecular, Cellular, and Clinical Biology,* edited by AJ Erslev, JW Adamson, JW Eschbach, CG Winearls, p 62. The Johns Hopkins University Press, Baltimore, 1992.

88. Newmayer H, Brockmoller J, Fritscka E, et al: Pharmacokinetics of rHEpo after sc administration and in long-term IV treatment in patients on hemodialysis. *Contrib Nephrol* 76:131, 1989.

89. Kaufman JS, Reda DJ, Fye CL, et al: Subcutaneous compared with intravenous epoietin in patients receiving hemodialysis. *N Engl J Med* 339:578, 1998.

90. Eschbach J, Adamson J: Guidelines for rHEpo therapy. *Am J Kidney Dis* 14(suppl 1):2, 1989.

91. Besarab A, Bolton WK, Browne JK, et al: The effects of normal as compared with low hematocrit values in patients with cardiac disease who are receiving hemodialysis and epoietin. *N Engl J Med* 389:584, 1998.

92. Cazzola M: How and when to use erythropoietin. *Curr Opin Hematol* 5:103, 1998.

93. Koene R, Frenken LA: Renal function of pre-dialysis patients during treatment with rHEpo. *Contrib Nephrol* 80:192, 1991.

94. Kuriyama H, Tomonari H, Yoshida H, et al: Reversal of anemia by erythropoietin therapy retards the progression of chronic renal failure, especially in non-diabetic patients. *Nephron* 77:176, 1997.

95. Sunder-Plassmann G, Horl WH: Erythropoietin and iron. *Clin Nephrol* 47:141, 1997.

96. Drueke T: Modulating factors in the hemopoietic response to erythropoietin. *Am J Kidney Dis* 18(suppl 1):87, 1991.

97. Rosenlof K, Fyhrquist F, Tenfunen R: Erythropoietin, aluminum and anemia in patients on hemodialysis. *Lancet* 335:247, 1990.

98. Casati S, Passerini P, Campise MR, et al: Benefits and risks of protracted treatment with human recombinant erythropoietin in patients having haemodialysis. *Br Med J* 295:1017, 1987.

99. Eschbach J: The anemia of chronic renal failure: Pathophysiology and the effects of rHEpo. *Kidney Int* 25:134, 1989.

100. Buccianti G, Colombi L, Battistel V: Use of recombinant human erythropoietin (rh-EPO) in the treatment of anemia in hemodialysis patients: A multicenter Italian experience. *Haematologica* 78:111, 1993.

101. Laupacis A: Changes in quality of life and functional capacity in hemodialysis patients treated with recombinant human erythropoietin. *Semin Nephrol* 10:11, 1990.

102. Bahlmann J, Schoter KH, Scigalla P, et al: Morbidity and mortality in hemodialysis patients with and without erythropoietin treatment: A controlled study. *Contrib Nephrol* 88:90, 1991.

103. Moia M, Vizotto L, Cattaneo M, et al: Improvement in the haemostatic defect of uraemia after treatment with recombinant human erythropoietin. *Lancet* 2:1227, 1987.

104. Schaefer R, Kokot F, Heidland A: Improvement of rHEpo on sexual function on hemodialyzed patients. *Contrib Nephrol* 76:273, 1989.

105. Silberberg J, Racine N, Barre P, Sniderman AD: Regression of left ventricular hypertrophy in dialysis patients following correction of anemia with recombinant human erythropoietin. *Can J Cardiol* 6:1, 1990.

106. Evans RW, Rader B, Manninen DL: The quality of life of hemodialysis recipients treated with recombinant human erythropoietin. *JAMA* 263:825, 1990.

107. Adamson JW, Eschbach JW: Erythropoietin for end-stage renal disease (editorial) *N Engl J Med* 339:625, 1998.

ANEMIA OF ENDOCRINE DISORDERS

ALLAN J. ERSLEV

The hormones released by specific endocrine organs all play a role in modulating the rate of red cell production. The mechanisms involved vary greatly, and current interest in unraveling single actions have been replaced by attempts to integrate the actions of multiple hormonal-like growth factors and cytokines on the sequential proliferation and differentiation of red cell precursors. Consequently, the discussion in this chapter of anemias caused by a deficiency of a single traditional hormone is by necessity more historic than current.

Numerous growth factors and cytokines are involved in the regulation and function of the erythropoietic tissue (see Chap. 14). Some are autocrine and released by the same cells on which they are acting, some are paracrine and released by neighboring cells, and some are endocrine and released from distant tissue and carried by blood to their target cells. The latter are traditionally designated hormones, and the effect on red cell production of altered hormone levels in blood due to endocrine tissue dysfunction is described here.[1,2] The effect of the renal hormone erythropoietin is covered in Chap. 33.

ANEMIA OF PITUITARY DEFICIENCY

Hypophysectomy in the experimental animal is regularly followed by the development of moderately severe erythroid hypoplasia and anemia.[3,4] In rats, the selective removal of the posterior or intermediate lobe does not cause anemia,[5] and it is generally assumed that the pathogenesis of the anemia is related to the absence of anterior lobe hormones, which in turn modulate renal erythropoietin production.[6] Of these, TSH is probably of most importance, since the anemia of hypophysectomy is very similar to the anemia of thyroidectomy.[7] Nevertheless, it is claimed that the rate of red cell production in hypophysectomized animals is restored to normal only if the administration of TSH is supplemented by ACTH[8] or if the administration of thyroid hormone is supplemented by both glucocorticoids and androgens.[3] It has been proposed repeatedly that the pituitary gland produces a specific erythropoietic hormone,[9,10] but the therapeutic effectiveness of target organ hormones alone is not in accord with such a possibility. Growth hormone has been shown to be capable of stimulating red cell production in vitro,[11] an effect possibly mediated by insulin-like growth factor,[12] but whether this effect is of physiologic significance remains unclear.[13] The same holds true for the hypothetical effect of the hypothalamus on red cell production. It has been claimed that hypothalamic injury may affect erythropoietin release,[14] the rate of red cell production,[15] or both,[16] and it has been proposed that these effects are mediated

via the hypophysis. However, the experimental data provided in support of this hypothesis are unimpressive.[15,16]

In human subjects, hypophyseal dysfunction or hypophyseal ablation is often associated with leukopenia and is regularly accompanied by a normochromic and normocytic anemia. The red cell life span is normal, but marrow examination and ferrokinetic studies disclose moderate hypoplasia and relative marrow failure.[17,18] Replacement therapy with a combination of thyroid, adrenal, and gonadal hormones usually corrects the anemia.[19,20] It is probable that treatment with recombinant human erythropoietin would also do so.

ANEMIA OF THYROID DYSFUNCTION

In 1881, Charcot[21] first recognized that cretins and patients with myxedema were anemic. At about the same time, the great Swiss surgeon Kocher[22] reported that thyroidectomy also is followed by a reduction in the red cell count. The character of this type of anemia has been a source of debate ever since, and it has been variously described as normocytic, microcytic, or macrocytic.[23] Studies have clarified the pathogenesis by separating the component caused by a lack of thyroid hormone from the components caused by complicating deficiencies of iron, vitamin B_{12}, or folic acid.[24–26] The rate of red cell production in experimental animals increases after the administration of thyroxin, triiodothyronine, or desiccated thyroid[27,28] and decreases after thyroidectomy.[29,30] These erythropoietic responses appear to be quite appropriate, since the need for circulating red cells depends on the cellular requirements for oxygen, which in turn are influenced by thyroid hormones.[23,31,32] Nevertheless, it has also been proposed that the thyroid hormones have a noncalorigenic effect on red cell production.[33] Studies of the influence of thyroid hormones on in vitro erythropoiesis have shown that both calorigenic T_3 and T_4 and noncalorigenic rT_3 potentiate the effect of erythropoietin on the formation of erythroid colonies[34,35] or increasing hypoxia-induced production of erythropoietin.[36] This effect appears to be mediated by burst-promoting factors released by activated lymphocytes[37] and/or by receptors with β_2-adrenergic properties.[37] Anemia observed in thyroidectomized animals conforms to both mechanisms by being normochromic and normocytic and associated with reticulocytopenia and hypoplasia of the erythropoietic tissue in the marrow. The red cell life span is normal, and ferrokinetic studies indicate the existence of a hypofunctioning but effective marrow.[38]

Anemia observed in human subjects with myxedema or other hypothyroid conditions is not always this clear-cut, since the condition may be complicated by nutritional deficiencies. However, many hypothyroid patients have a hypoplastic anemia that is unresponsive to therapy with iron, vitamin B_{12}, or folic acid and is very similar to the form of anemia observed in thyroidectomized animals.[23,24,39] The degree of anemia is mild to moderate, with a hemoglobin concentration rarely less than 8 to 9 g/dl. The corresponding decrease in erythroid marrow activity is frequently too small to be morphologically demonstrable.[40] Ferrokinetic studies show a decrease in the turnover of plasma and red cell iron, a decrease that also may be so small that it is first recognized when compared with values obtained after thyroid replacement therapy.[41,42] As in hypothyroid animals, the red cell life span and the rate of red cell utilization of iron are normal. The degree of anemia does not always reflect the reduction in marrow activity and the size of the red cell volume, since the plasma volume is decreased in hypothyroid patients.[43] This may result in a temporary aggravation of apparent anemia after thyroid replacement therapy, since the plasma volume will be restored to normal before the red cell volume. Although normochromic and normocytic anemia must be considered the characteristic form of anemia of hypothyroidism, the most frequent type of anemia observed is a microcytic, hypochromic anemia caused by iron deficiency.[23,44] In hypothyroid women, menorrhagia is a frequent

Acronyms and abbreviations that appear in this chapter include: ACTH, adrenocorticotrophic hormone; 2,3-BPG, 2,3-bisphosphoglycerate; TSH, thyroid-stimulating hormone.

complication and may explain adequately the lack of iron. However, even in men, iron is in short supply either because of the histamine-refractory achlorhydria, which is present in about 50 percent of anemic patients,[45] or possibly because of intestinal malabsorption of iron.[46,47] Macrocytosis is frequently identified with anemia of hypothyroidism.[23,39] However, when a substantial increase in the mean corpuscular volume occurs, it is usually caused by a megaloblastic erythropoiesis owing to vitamin B_{12} or folic acid deficiency.[24] In hypothyroid patients, the incidence of true pernicious anemia with gastric atrophy and intrinsic factor deficiency appears to be unusually high.[48–50] This has led to interesting but still inconclusive speculations on the effect of cross-reacting autoantibodies against thyroglobulins and intrinsic factor or gastric parietal cells.[51–53] This may be of special etiologic importance for Graves' disease and Hashimoto's thyroiditis, both autoimmune disorders. However, in a study of eight patients with coexisting megaloblastic anemia and hypothyroidism, it was concluded that all eight, rather than having vitamin B_{12} deficiency, had folic acid deficiency from either poor dietary intake of folic acid or intestinal malabsorption.[26]

Despite the direct and indirect erythropoietic effect of thyroid hormones, patients with hyperthyroidism or thyrotoxicosis rarely have elevated hemoglobin concentrations or hematocrit percentages[43,54] and may even be moderately anemic.[55,56] This absence of an expected secondary polycythemia has been explained by assuming that an increased cardiac output and rate of tissue perfusion meet the increased tissue requirements for oxygen. Conflicting data have been presented as to the effect of thyroid hormone in vitro on the intracellular concentration of 2,3-BPG and, in turn, the oxygen affinity of hemoglobin.[57] So far, however, direct studies of hyperthyroid patients do not suggest the presence of enhanced oxygen transport to the tissues.[58] It actually seems more likely that the absence of an overt secondary polycythemia is due to hemodilution. Direct measurements of the size of the red cell volume,[43] the erythroid activity of the marrow,[40] and the turnover of plasma and red cell iron[54] show them to be above normal. If it were not for the concomitant increase in plasma volume, these patients would have elevated hemoglobin and hematocrit levels. Studies of the red cell life span in patients with thyrotoxicosis suggest a moderate shortening in red cell survival,[59] possibly reflecting an autoimmune etiology with the production of anti–red-cell antibodies.[60] In a few cases, severe hyperthyroidism has been found to be associated with anemia and abnormal iron utilization, apparently reflecting ineffective red cell production,[44] or the production of erythropoietin-directed antibodies.[61] The institution of radioiodine therapy results in a reduction in the size of the red cell volume to normal but only a slight change in the hematocrit.

ANEMIA OF ADRENAL DYSFUNCTION

Adrenalectomy in experimental animals causes a mild anemia responsive to therapy with adrenal glucocorticoids or erythropoietin.[17,29,62] A similar type of normochromic, normocytic anemia has been observed in Addison's disease,[17,63] but because of the concomitant reduction in plasma volume, the hemoglobin concentration and the hematocrit percentage do not reflect the true decrease in red cell volume. The character of this type of anemia and the erythropoietic effect of physiologic amounts of ACTH or adrenal cortical hormones are still unclear, possibly because the changes involved are too small for adequate study. When administered in pharmacologic amounts, these hormones appear to cause mild erythrocytosis[64] of about the same magnitude as that observed in Cushing's disease[65,66] and occasionally in Bartter's syndrome[67] and pheochromocytoma.[68] However, whether this is mediated via release of renal erythropoietin or by direct action on the erythropoietic cells in the marrow is unknown.[69]

ANEMIA OF GONADAL DYSFUNCTION

The erythropoietic effect of androgens in both physiologic and pharmacologic dosages is well recognized and extensively utilized in the treatment of patients with various types of refractory anemia. Castration of the male experimental animal causes a decrease in the rate of red cell production until the hemoglobin concentration and the red cell volume become stabilized at levels approximately the same as those of the normal female.[70,71] In sexually mature human males, the hemoglobin level is 1 to 2 g/dl higher than the level observed in males during childhood, advanced age, orchiectomy, or gonadal hypofunction. Under those circumstances, the hemoglobin level is similar to that of the normal human female.[72–74]

In pharmacologic doses androgens have been shown to stimulate red cell production[75,76] by increasing the production of erythropoietin[77] and by enhancing the effect of erythropoietin on the marrow.[78] These actions have been attributed to two isomeric metabolites formed by the reduction of a 4-5 double bond. The 5α-H isomer is androgenic and believed to cause a release of erythropoietin from the kidney.[79] The 5β-H isomer is not androgenic or erythropoietinogenic but is believed to cause inactive marrow stem cells to enter an erythropoietin-responsive phase.[80]

Before being replaced by recombinant human erythropoietin in the treatment of anemia of renal failure, androgens were used extensively.[81,82] Even now, androgens may enhance the effect of erythropoietin and reduce the cost of such therapy.[83]

Studies on the effect of physiologic doses of estrogens suggest that these hormones cause a slight suppression of red cell production.[83] In large doses, estrogens have been shown to cause the development of moderately severe anemia,[84,85] but it has not been resolved whether this is caused by suppressed erythropoietin production[85] or by inhibition of the progenitor cell action of erythropoietin.[86] Inhibin and activin, two glycoprotein hormones released by gonadal cells in both male and female, have been shown in vitro to have an effect on human erythroid progenitor cells.[87–89] The physiologic significance of these observations is still unknown.

Human placental lactogen and sheep prolactin have been shown to have erythropoietic activity in the mouse.[90] It has been proposed that human placental lactogen is in part responsible for the stimulation of red cell production in pregnancy.[91]

ANEMIA OF PREGNANCY

Although pregnancy is not an endocrine disorder, it is associated with a mild anemia, presumably caused by changes in the hormonal environment.[92] Studies of pregnant mice have shown that, despite a progressive decrease in the hematocrit, the red cell volume, erythropoietin secretion, and rate of red cell production increase during pregnancy.[90] Placental lactogen, which is erythropoietically active in the mouse,[92] may in part be responsible for the erythropoietic stimulation, but the hormonal mechanisms underlying both the increase in red cell volume and the even more pronounced increase in plasma volume are not precisely known.

In humans, anemia in pregnancy is most often aggravated by dietary restrictions[93] and a concomitant iron deficiency.[94,95] In a smaller number of cases, folic acid deficiency may also play a pathogenetic role,[96] and it seems appropriate to give every pregnant woman preventive iron and folic acid supplements. However, even in the well-cared-for pregnant woman, anemia becomes manifest at about the eighth week of pregnancy, progresses slowly until the thirty-second to thirty-fourth week, and is then stable until it rather suddenly improves just before delivery.[97,98] It is moderate in severity, with hemoglobin concentrations rarely below 10 g/dl, and studies of the red cell volume have shown it to be a dilution anemia.[97,98] There has been an obvious reluctance to use radioactive tracers to measure red cell and plasma volume in early pregnancy. However, using a nonradioactive biotin technique,[99] it has been shown that there is a gradual increase in red cell volume beginning before the twelfth week of pregnancy. This early increase is not associated with measurable changes in the concentration of serum transferrin receptors, reticulocyte counts, or erythropoietin titers.[99,100] However, in the second and third trimester, erythrokinetic studies using both radioactive iron[101] and serum transferrin receptor concentrations[100] have shown an increased erythropoietic activity. The associated changes in reticulocyte counts, serum ferritin concentrations, and erythropoietin titers are small and difficult to detect[102] but in some studies quite significant.[103,104] Despite the increase in red cell volume, the hemoglobin concentration falls as a consequence of an even greater increase in plasma volume. The total increase in red cell volume during pregnancy is about 20 percent, while the increase in plasma volume is about 30 percent. The increase in plasma volume can probably be explained on the basis of an increase in the size of the uterine vascular bed, with a shift of fluid from extravascular to vascular space.

The induction of this hypervolemia creates a low-viscosity erythrocytosis, which promotes oxygen transport to the tissues. Although the hemoglobin concentration is decreased, the hypervolemic state ensures the pregnant uterus of an excellent blood perfusion and oxygen supply.

ANEMIA OF PARATHYROID DYSFUNCTION

Primary hyperparathyroidism is occasionally[105,106] associated with anemia that disappears after parathyroidectomy.[107,108] Similarly, it has been reported that parathyroidectomy in chronic renal disease often results in some improvement in the anemia,[109,110] and it has been suggested that the parathyroid hormone may be a toxin that can suppress normal red cell production.[111,112] However, other studies have not supported this suggestion.[112–115] These suggest that primary or secondary hyperparathyroidism, when associated with suppressed red cell production, acts by causing either renal calcification with reduction in erythropoietin formation or marrow sclerosis with reduction in erythroid proliferation.[116]

ANEMIA OF PANCREATIC DYSFUNCTION

Although insulin and the insulin-like growth factors I and II appear to be involved in expanding the red cell mass after treatment with growth hormones, there is little evidence for the notion that insulin is an erythropoietic agent.[119,120]

REFERENCES

1. Adamson JW, Popovic WJ, Brown JE: Hormonal control of erythropoiesis, in *Hematologic Cell Differentiation*, edited by DW Golde, MJ Cline, D Metcalf, pp 53–67. Academic, New York, 1978.
2. Orwoll FS, Orwoll RL: Hematologic abnormalities in patients with endocrine and metabolic disorders. *Hematol Oncol Clin North Am* 1:261, 1987.
3. Crafts RC, Meineke HA: The anemia of hypophysectomized animals. *Ann NY Acad Sci* 77:501, 1959.
4. Gordon AS: Endocrine influences upon the formed elements of blood and blood forming organs. *Prog Hormone Res* 10:339, 1954.
5. Van Dyke DC, Garcia JF, Simpson ME, et al: Maintenance of circulating red cell volume in rats after removal of the posterior and intermediate lobes of the pituitary. *Blood* 7:1017, 1952.
6. Peschle C, Rappaport IA, Magli MC, et al: Role of hypophysis in erythropoietin production during hypoxia. *Blood* 5:1117, 1978.
7. Crafts RC: The similarity between anemia induced by hypophysectomy

and that induced by a combined thyroidectomy and adrenalectomy in adult female rats. *Endocrinology* 53:465, 1953.
8. Fisher JW, Crook JJ: Influence of several hormones on erythropoiesis and oxygen consumption in the hypophysectomized rat. *Blood* 19:557, 1962.
9. Contopoulos AN, Simpson ME, Van Dyke DC, et al: The pituitary erythropoietic factor. *Anat Rec* 118:290, 1954.
10. Lindeman R, Trygstad O, Halvorsen S: Pituitary control of erythropoiesis. *Scand J Haematol* 6:77, 1969.
11. Golde DW, Bersch N, Li CH: Growth hormone: Species specific stimulation of erythropoiesis in vitro. *Science* 196:1112, 1977.
12. Merchav S, Tatarsky I, Hochberg Z: Enhancement of erythropoiesis in vitro by human growth hormone is mediated by insulin-like growth factor I. *Br J Haematol* 70:267, 1988.
13. Jepson JH, McGarry EE: Hemopoiesis in pituitary dwarfs treated with human growth hormone and testosterone. *Blood* 39:238, 1972.
14. Halvorsen S: Effect of hypothalamic stimulation on erythropoiesis and on the production of erythropoiesis-stimulating factors in intact and nephrectomized rabbits. *Ann NY Acad Sci* 149:88, 1968.
15. Feldman S, Rachmilewitz EA, Izak G: The effect of central nervous system stimulation on erythropoiesis in rats with chronically implanted electrodes. *J Lab Clin Med* 67:713, 1966.
16. Mirand EA, Grace JT, Johnston GS, Murphy GP: Effect of hypothalamic stimulation on the erythropoietic response in the rhesus monkey. *Nature* 204:1163, 1964.
17. Daughaday WH, Williams RH, Daland GA: The effect of endocrinopathies on the blood. *Blood* 3:1342, 1948.
18. Degrossi OJ, Houssay AB, Varela JE, Capalbo EE: Erythrokinetic studies in the anemia of thyroid and pituitary insufficiency, in *Advances in Thyroid Research*, edited by Pitt-Rivers R, p 410. Pergamon, New York, 1961.
19. Ferrari E, Ascari E, Bossoto PA, Barosi G: Sheehan's syndrome with complete bone marrow aplasia: Long-term results of substitution therapy with hormones. *Br J Haematol* 33:575, 1976.
20. Sanders JE, Hawley J, Levy W, et al.: Pregnancies following high-dose cyclophosphamide with or without high-dose busulfan or total-body irradiation and bone marrow transplantation. *Blood* 87:3045, 1996.
21. Charcot M: Myxedéme, cachexie pachydermique ou état cretinoide. *Gaz Hop Paris* 54:73, 1881.
22. Kocher T: Ueber Kropfexstirpation und Ihre Folgen. *Arch Klin Chir* 29:254, 1883.
23. Bomford R: Anemia in myxoedema and the role of the thyroid gland in erythropoiesis. *Q J Med* 7:495, 1938.
24. Tudhope GR, Wilson GM: Anemia in hypothyroidism: Incidence, pathogenesis and response to treatment. *Q J Med* 29:513, 1960.
25. Carpenter JT, Mohler DN Jr, Thorup OA Jr, Leavell BS: Anemia in myxedema, in *Current Concepts in Hypothyroidism,* edited by KR Crispell, p 147. Macmillan, New York, 1963.
26. Hines JD, Halsted CH, Griggs RC, Harris JW: Megaloblastic anemia secondary to folate deficiency associated with hypothyroidism. *Ann Intern Med* 68:792, 1968.
27. Donati RM, Warnecke MA, Gallagher NJ: Effect of triiodothyronine administration on erythrocyte radioiron incorporation in rats. *Proc Soc Exp Biol Med* 115:405, 1964.
28. Chalet M, Coe D, Reissmann KR: Mechanisms of erythropoietic action of thyroid hormone. *Proc Soc Exp Biol Med* 123:443, 1966.
29. Crafts RC: The effect of endocrines on the formed elements of the blood: I. The effects of hypophysectomy, thyroidectomy and adrenalectomy on the blood of the adult female rat. *Endocrinology* 29:596, 1941.
30. Gordon AS, Kadow PC, Finkelstein G, Charipper HA: The thyroid and blood regeneration in the rat. *Am J Med Sci* 212:385, 1946.
31. Jacobson LO, Goldwasser E, Gurney CW, et al: Studies on erythropoietin: The hormone regulating red cell production. *Ann NY Acad Sci* 77:551, 1959.
32. Lucarelli G, Ferrari V, Rizzoli A, et al: The effect of triiodothyronine on the erythropoiesis: Assay in the normal, starved, polycythemic and nephrectomized rat. *Biochim Biol Sper* 5:475, 1966.
33. Meineke HA, Crafts RC: Evidence for a noncalorigenic effect of thyroxin on erythropoiesis as judged by radio iron utilization. *Proc Soc Exp Biol Med* 117:520, 1964.
34. Golde DW, Bersch N, Chopra IJ, Cline MJ: Thyroid hormones stimulate erythropoiesis in vitro. *Br J Haematol* 37:173, 1977.

35. Popovic WJ, Brown JE, Adamson JW: The influence of thyroid hormones on in vitro erythropoiesis: Mediation by a receptor with beta adrenergic properties. *J Clin Invest* 60:907, 1977.

36. Fandrey J, Pagel H, Frede S, Wolff M, Jelkmann W: Thyroid hormones enhance hypoxia-induced erythropoietin production in vitro. *Exp Hematol* 22:272, 1994.

37. Daniak N, Sutter D, Kreczko S: L-triiodothyronine augments erythropoietic growth factor release from peripheral blood and bone marrow leukocytes. *Blood* 68:1289, 1986.

38. Cline MJ, Berlin NI: Erythropoiesis and red cell survival in the hypothyroid dog. *Am J Physiol* 204:415, 1963.

39. Horton L, Coburn RJ, England JM, et al: The haematology of hypothyroidism. *Q J Med* 45:101, 1975.

40. Axelrod AR, Berman L: The bone marrow in hyperthyroidism and hypothyroidism. *Blood* 6:436, 1951.

41. Kiely JM, Purnell DC, Owen CA Jr: Erythrokinetics in myxedema. *Ann Intern Med* 67:533, 1967.

42. Finch CA, Deubelbeiss K, Cook JD, et al: Ferrokinetics in man. *Medicine (Baltimore)* 49:17, 1970.

43. Muldowney FP, Crooks J, Wayne EJ: The total red cell mass in thyrotoxicosis and myxoedema. *Clin Sci* 16:309, 1957.

44. Larsson SD: Anemia and iron metabolism in hypothyroidism. *Acta Med Scand* 157:349, 1967.

45. Lerman J, Means JH: The gastric secretion in exophthalmic goiter and myxoedema. *J Clin Invest* 11:167, 1932.

46. Pirzio-Biroli G, Bothwell TH, Finch CA: Iron absorption: II. The absorption of radio iron administered with standard meal. *J Lab Clin Med* 51:37, 1958.

47. Donati RM, Fletcher JW, Warnecke MA, Gallagher NJ: Erythropoiesis in hypothyroidism. *Proc Soc Exp Biol Med* 144:78, 1973.

48. Carmel R, Spencer CA: Clinical and subclinical thyroid disorders associated with pernicious anemia. *Arch Intern Med* 142:1465, 1982.

49. Green ST, Ng JP, Chan-Lam D: Insulin dependent diabetes mellitus, myasthenia gravis, pernicious anemia, autoimmune thyroiditis and autoimmune adrenalitis in a single patient. *Scott Med J* 33:213, 1988.

50. Petite J, Rosset N, Chapnis B, Jeannet M: Genetic factors predispose to autoimmune diseases: Study of HLA antigens in a family with pernicious anemia and thyroid diseases. *Schweiz Med Wochenschr* 117:2032, 1987.

51. Irvine WJ, Davies SH, Delamore JW, Williams AW: Immunologic relationship between pernicious anemia and thyroid disease. *Br Med J* 12:454, 1962.

52. Markson JL, Moore JM: Thyroid antibodies in pernicious anemia. *Br Med J* 12:1352, 1962.

53. Ardeman S, Chanarin I, Krafchik B, Singer W: Addisonian pernicious anemia and intrinsic factor antibodies in thyroid disorders. *Q J Med* 35:421, 1966.

54. Donati RM, Warnecke MA, Gallagher NJ: Ferrokinetics in hyperthyroidism. *Ann Intern Med* 63:945, 1963.

55. Rivlin RS, Wagner HN: Anemia in hyperthyroidism. *Ann Intern Med* 70:507, 1969.

56. Perlman JA, Sternthal PM: Effect of ^{131}I on the anemia of hyperthyroidism. *J Chron Dis* 36:405, 1983.

57. Miller WW, Delivoria-Papadopoulos M, Miller LD, Oski FA: Oxygen releasing factor in hypothyroidism. *JAMA* 211:1824, 1970.

58. Zaroulis CG, Kourides JA, Valeri CR: Red cell 2,3-diphosphoglycerate and oxygen affinity of hemoglobin in patients with thyroid disorders. *Blood* 52:181, 1978.

59. McClellan JE, Donegan C, Thorup OA, Leavell BS: Survival time of the erythrocyte in myxedema and hyperthyroidism. *J Lab Clin Med* 51:91, 1958.

60. Bouchou K, Andre M, Cathebras P, et al: Pathologie thyroidienne et syndromes auto-immuns multiples: Aspects clinique et immunogenetique à-propos de 11 observations. *Rev Med Interne* 16:283, 1995.

61. Jyo-Oshiro Y, Nomura S, Fukushima T, Tamai H, Fueki H, Osawa G: Primary hyperthyroidism induced erythropoietin-resistant anemia? *Intern Med* 36:903, 1997.

62. Van Dyke DC, Contopoulos AN, Williams BS, et al: Hormonal factors influencing erythropoiesis. *Acta Haematol (Basel)* 11:203, 1954.

63. Baez-Villasenor J, Rath CE, Finch CA: The blood picture in Addison's disease. *Blood* 3:769, 1948.

64. Fisher JW: Increase in circulating red cell volume of normal rats after

65. Platz CM, Knowlton AJ, Ragan C: The natural history of Cushing's syndrome. *Am J Med* 13:597, 1952.

66. Ross EJ, Marshall-Jones P, Friedman M: Cushing's syndrome: Diagnostic criteria. *Q J Med* 35:149, 1966.

67. Erkelens DW, Statius van Eps LWS: Bartter's syndrome and erythrocytosis. *Am J Med* 55:711, 1973.

68. Shulkin BL, Shapiro B, Sisson JC: Pheochromocytoma, polycythemia and venous thrombosis. *Am J Med* 83:773, 1987.

69. Golde DW, Bersch N, Cline MJ: Potentiation of erythropoiesis in vitro by dexamethasone. *J Clin Invest* 57:57 1976.

70. Steinglass P, Gordon AS, Charipper HA: Effect of castration and sex hormones on blood of the rat. *Proc Soc Exp Biol Med* 48:169, 1941.

71. Crafts RC: Effect of hypophysectomy, castration and testosterone propionate on hemopoiesis in the adult male rat. *Endocrinology* 39:401, 1946.

72. Hawkins WW, Speck E, Leonard VG: Variation of the hemoglobin level with age and sex. *Blood* 9:999, 1954.

73. Fonseca R, Rajkumar SV, White WL, Tefferi A, Hoaglund HC: Anemia after orchiectomy. *Am J Hem* 59:230, 1998.

74. Matsumoto AM, Bremner WJ: Hypogonadism: Androgen therapy, in *Current Therapy in Endocrinology and Metabolism*, edited by DT Krieger, CW Bardin, pp 145–149. Dekker, Toronto, 1986.

75. Kennedy BJ, Gilbertsen AS: Increased erythropoiesis induced by androgenic-hormone therapy. *N Engl J Med* 256:719, 1957.

76. Shahidi NT: Androgens and erythropoiesis. *N Engl J Med* 289:72, 1973.

77. Alexanian R: Erythropoietin and erythropoiesis in anemic man following androgens. *Blood* 33:564, 1969.

78. Singer JW, Samuels AJ, Adamson JW: The effect of steroids on in vitro erythroid colony growth: Structure/activity relationships. *J Cell Physiol* 88:127, 1976.

79. Paulo LG, Fink GD, Roh BL, Fisher JW: Effects of several androgens and steroid metabolites on erythropoietin production in the isolated perfused dog kidney. *Blood* 43:39, 1974.

80. Gorshein D, Hait WN, Besa EC, et al: Rapid stem cell differentiation induced by 19-nortestosterone decanoate. *Br J Haematol* 26:215, 1974.

81. Eschbach JW, Adamson JW: Improvement in the anemia of chronic failure with fluoxymesterone. *Ann Intern Med* 78:527, 1973.

82. Neff MS, Goldberg J, Slifkin RE, et al: A comparison of androgens for anemia in patients on hemodialysis. *N Engl J Med* 30:871, 1981.

83. Gaughan WJ, Liss KA, Dunn SR, et al: A 6-month study of low-dose recombinant human erythropoietin alone and in combination with androgens for the treatment of anemia in chronic hemodialysis patients. *Am J Kidney Dis* 30:495, 1997.

84. Dukes PP, Goldwasser E: Inhibition of erythropoiesis by estrogens. *Endocrinology* 69:21, 1961.

85. Piliero SJ, Medici PT, Haber C: The interrelationships of the endocrine and erythropoietic systems in the rat with special reference to the mechanism of action of estradiol and testosterone. *Ann NY Acad Sci* 149:336, 1968.

86. Jepson JH, Lowenstein L: Inhibition of the stem-cell action of erythropoietin by estradiol. *Proc Soc Exp Biol Med* 123:457, 1966.

87. Yu J, Shao A, Lemas V, et al: Importance of FSH-releasing protein and inhibin in erythrodifferentiation. *Nature* 330:765, 1987.

88. Broxmeyer HE, Lu L, Coopers S, et al: Selective and indirect modulation of human multipotential and erythroid hematopoietic progenitor cell proliferation by recombinant human activin and inhibin. *Proc Natl Acad Sci USA* 85:9062, 1988.

89. Yu J, Shao A, Vaughan J, et al: Characterization of the potentiation effect of activin on human erythroid colony formation in vitro. *Blood* 73:952, 1989.

90. Jepson JH, Lowenstein L: Hormonal control of erythropoiesis during pregnancy in the mouse. *Br J Haematol* 14:555, 1968.

91. Berczi I, Wage E: Placental lactogen is a haemopoietic hormone. *Br J Haematol* 79:355, 1991.

92. Letsky EA: Erythropoiesis in pregnancy. *J Perinatal Med* 23:39, 1995.

93. Simmons WK, Simeon DT, Bramble D, Buffonge C, Gallagher P: Marked reduction of anemia during pregnancy over a 10-year period in Montserrat. *Bull Pan Am Health Organ* 30:18, 1996.

94. Benjamin F, Bassen FA, Meyer LM: Serum levels of folic acid, vitamin B_{12} and iron in anemia of pregnancy. *Am J Obstet Gynecol* 96:310, 1966.

95. Pritchard JA, Hunt CF: A comparison of the hematologic responses

treatment with hydrocortisone or cortico-sterone. *Proc Soc Exp Biol Med* 97:502, 1958.

following the routine prenatal administration of intramuscular and oral iron. *Surg Gynecol Obstet* 106:516, 1958.

96. Alperin JB, Hutchinson HT, Levin WC: Studies of folic acid requirements in megaloblastic anemia of pregnancy. *Arch Intern Med* 117:681, 1966.

97. Low JA, Johnston EE, McBride RL: Blood volume adjustments in the normal obstetric patient with particular reference to the third trimester of pregnancy. *Am J Obstet Gynecol* 91:356, 1965.

98. Pritchard JA: Changes in the blood volume during pregnancy and delivery. *Anesthesiology* 26:393, 1965.

99. Weiner J, Cavill I, Williams GL, et al: Red cells in pregnancy: Erythropoietin and red cell mass in a sequential cohort study. Personal communication, 1992.

100. Beguin Y, Lipscei G, Thoumsin H, Fillet G: Blunted erythropoietin production and decreased erythropoiesis in early pregnancy. *Blood* 78:89, 1991.

101. Pritchard JA, Adams RH: Erythrocyte production and destruction during pregnancy. *Am J Obstet Gynecol* 79:750, 1960.

102. Harstad TW, Mason RA, Cox SM: Serum erythropoietin quantitation in pregnancy using an enzyme-linked immunoassay. *Am J Perinatol* 9:233, 1992.

103. Howells MR, Jones SE, Napier JA, et al: Erythropoiesis in pregnancy. *Br J Haematol* 64:595, 1986.

104. Cotes PM, Canning CE, Lind T: Changes in immunoreactive erythropoietin during the menstrual cycle and normal pregnancy. *Br J Obstet Gynaecol* 90:304, 1983.

105. Malette LE, Bilezikian JP, Heath DA, Aurbach GD: Primary hyperparathyroidism: Clinical and biochemical features. *Medicine (Baltimore)* 53:127, 1974.

106. Abarca J, Trisonis C, Hamberser B, Granbers PO: Anaemia in primary hyperparathyroidism: Fantasy or reality? *Ann Chir Gynaecol* 74:74, 1985.

107. Boxer M, Ellman L, Geller R, Wang CA: Anemia in primary hyperparathyroidism. *Arch Intern Med* 13:588, 1977.

108. Falco JM, Guy JT, Smith RE, Mazzaferri EL: Primary hyperthyroidism and anemia. *Arch Intern Med* 136:887, 1976.

109. Zingraff J, Drueke T, Marie P, et al: Anemia and secondary hyperparathyroidism. *Arch Intern Med* 138:1650, 1978.

110. Kotzmann H, Abela C, Heindl J, et al: Effect of successful parathyroidectomy on hematopoietic progenitor cells and parameters of red blood cells in patients with primary hyperparathyroidism. *Horm Metab Res* 29:387, 1997.

111. Massry SG: Is parathyroid hormone a uremic toxin? *Nephron* 19:125, 1977.

112. Fujita Y, Inoue S, Horiguchi S, Kuki A: Excessive level of parathyroid hormone may induce the reduction of recombinant human erythropoietin effect on renal anemia. *Miner Electrolyte Metab* 21:50, 1995.

113. Delwiche F, Garrity MJ, Powell JS, et al: High levels of the circulating form of parathyroid hormone do not inhibit in vitro erythropoiesis. *J Lab Clin Med* 102:613, 1983.

114. Lutton JD, Solangi KB, Ibraham NG, et al: Inhibition of erythropoiesis in chronic renal failure: The role of parathyroid hormone. *Am J Kidney Dis* 3:380, 1984.

115. McGonigle RJS, Wallin JD, Husserl F, et al: Potential role of parathyroid hormone as an inhibitor of erythropoiesis in the anemia of renal failure. *J Lab Clin Med* 104:1016, 1984.

116. Slackman N, Green AA, Naiman JL: Myelofibrosis in children with chronic renal insufficiency. *J Pediatr* 87:720, 1975.

117. Ishimura E, Nishizawa Y, Okuno S, et al: Diabetes mellitus increases the severity of anemia in non-dialyzed patients with renal failure. *J Nephrol* 11:83, 1998.

118. James SH, Meyers AM: Microangiopathic hemolytic anemia as a complication of diabetes mellitus. *Am J Med Sci* 315:211, 1998.

119. Sawada K, Krantz SB, Dessypris EN, et al: Human colony-forming-units-erythroid do not require accessory cells but do require direct interaction with insulin-like growth factor I and/or insulin for erythroid development. *J Clin Invest* 83:1701, 1989.

120. Ten Have SM, van der Lely AJ, Lamberts SW: Increase in haemoglobin concentrations in growth hormone deficient adults during human recombinant growth hormone replacement therapy. *Clin Endocrinol* 47:565, 1997.

C H A P T E R 3 5

THE CONGENITAL DYSERYTHROPOIETIC ANEMIAS

ERNEST BEUTLER

The congenital dyserythropoietic anemias are a heterogeneous group of disorders characterized by anemia, the presence of multinuclear erythroid precursors in the marrow, ineffective erythropoeisis, and iron overload. Patients have been classified as type I, II, and III, but there are some patients who appear to fit into the general category of congenital dyserythropoietic anemia but do not fit into any of these three groups. Types I and II congenital dyserythropoietic anemia are inherited as autosomal recessive disorders, and type III disease is dominant. Type II congenital dyserythropoietic anemia is also known by the acronym HEMPAS, which describes characteristic serologic findings that are absent from types I and III congenital dyserythropoietic anemia.

The term *congenital dyserythropoietic anemia* applies to a group of hereditary refractory anemias characterized by ineffective erythropoiesis, erythroid multinuclearity, and accumulation of tissue iron. Anemia is characteristically first noted in infancy or childhood. The life span of circulating erythrocytes may be normal to moderately shortened, but dyserythropoiesis with a large component of intramedullary cell death is the dominant factor in pathogenesis. Ineffective erythropoiesis results in increased plasma iron turnover, diminished incorporation of tracer iron into circulating red cells, mild increases in indirect reacting bilirubin, elevated fecal stercobilin level, increased endogenous carbon monoxide production (presumably derived from heme catabolism), intense marrow erythroid hyperplasia, and normal, or at most slightly elevated, absolute reticulocyte counts. Splenomegaly, variably severe anemia, and mild increases in indirect-reacting serum bilirubin are present. Congenital dyserythropoietic anemias have been classified into three types[1] (Table 35-1). In addition, a number of cases that do not fit clearly into any of these categories have been described.

These disorders are quite uncommon. In a survey of the United Kingdom between 1994 and 1996, 47 cases were identified. Twelve had type I, 13 type II, 2 type III, and 20 had types that did not fit into this classification.[2]

CONGENITAL DYSERYTHROPOIETIC ANEMIA TYPE I

Type I dyserythropoietic anemia generally first becomes manifest in infancy, childhood, or adolescence, and is characterized by slight hyperbilirubinemia, moderate anemia (hematocrit usually 25 to 36 percent), and commonly, splenomegaly.[3–24] The mode of genetic transmission is autosomal recessive and the disorder has been documented in identical twins.[25] Linkage analysis has narrowed localization of the

gene responsible for this disorder to a 0.5 centimorgan interval in the q15.1 to q15.3 region.[24] The level of serum haptoglobin is low; that of serum iron is normal or high. The red cell morphologic picture is characterized by well-marked aniso- and poikilocytosis and slight to moderate macrocytosis. The intensely cellular erythroid marrow shows megaloblastoid features.[3–5] By light microscopy, the majority of erythroblasts have varying degrees of abnormality. In particular, three morphologic aberrations are regarded as typical: (1) very large cells containing an irregularly shaped nuclear mass with two nuclear segments suggesting incomplete nuclear division (1 to 2 percent of erythroblasts), (2) double nucleated cells in which the two nuclei differ in size, structure, and stainability (0.3 to 0.8 percent of erythroblasts), and (3) pairs of erythroblasts connected by thin chromatin bridges of different lengths (0.8 to 2.3 percent of erythroblasts).[5] Only the erythroid series shows significant abnormalities by electron and light microscopy. The pores of the nuclear envelope of the erythroid cells become abnormally numerous and wide with progressive maturation. Later the cytoplasm has invaded between the nuclear chromatin strands of many cells and there is intense clumping of the dense chromatin. In even more severely affected cells, the cytoplasm separates the chromatin fragments and gives the nucleus a spongy appearance.[5–8,10,11,13,17,21,26] The persistence of cytoplasmic microtubules has also been demonstrated.[10] Some mitochondria show deposition of ferruginous micelles, causing a loss of normal structure, but these changes are quantitatively much less severe than in the sideroblastic anemias (Chap. 63). In other studies, hypertetraploid DNA values were found in a high proportion of erythroblasts, and RNA synthesis was markedly reduced, leading to impaired hemoglobin synthesis.[11,12] Serologic abnormalities, such as occur in congenital dyserythropoietic anemia type II, have usually not been present. An increase in the α/β globin chain synthetic ratio has been reported.[13,27] An animal model of the disease has been described.[28]

No effective treatment is available, but although anemic, most subjects do not require transfusion. The latter is to be avoided if at all possible, since iron overload is often present.[14,20,29] The cautious use of phlebotomy or administration of iron-chelating agents to help prevent tissue siderosis has been suggested.[20] In one case splenectomy was noted to decrease the transfusion requirement[16] but not in two others.[14,18]

CONGENITAL DYSERYTHROPOIETIC ANEMIA TYPE II (HEMPAS)

Most commonly known as HEMPAS, a somewhat whimsical acronym for *H*ereditary *E*rythroblastic *M*ultinuclearity associated with a *P*ositive *A*cidified *S*erum test, type II congenital dyserythropoietic anemia was first described in 1962.[30,31] The unusual serologic abnormalities characterizing this disorder were defined in the late 1960s.[32] By 1975, the clinical and hematologic features of 84 patients in 55 families had been described and were reviewed.[33] A considerable number of additional patients with HEMPAS have been reported since.[27,34–43] The geographic distribution of affected patients suggests a higher frequency of the HEMPAS gene in Northwest Europe, Italy, and North Africa. Both sexes are affected; the mode of genetic transmission is autosomal recessive.[44] The gene has been localized to chromosome 20q11.2 by linkage analysis.[45]

The red cell membrane of HEMPAS patients characteristically contains abnormal complex carbohydrate patterns (Fig. 35-1). Presumably as a consequence of the abnormality in glycosylation, the electrophoretic mobilities of membrane proteins of the red cells from patients with HEMPAS deviates markedly from normal, and this could occur as a result of either genetic defect in N-acetylglucosaminyltransferase II or α-mannosidase II.[28,49,50] Targeted disruption of the α-mannosidase II gene of the mouse produces mild anemia with HEMPAS-like

TABLE 35-1   CONGENITAL DYSERYTHROPOIETIC ANEMIA, TYPES I, II, III—MARROW AND SEROLOGIC FEATURES

| | Marrow | | | |
CDA Type	Light Microscopy	Electron Microscopy	Serology	Inheritance
I	Most erythroid cells abnormal: megaloblastoid changes; large cells with incompletely divided nuclear segments; double nuclei, internuclear chromatin bridges	Widened nuclear pores, cytoplasmic invasion of nucleus, disaggregation of ribosomes, and presence of cytoplasmic microtubules	No serologic abnormalities	Autosomal Recessive
II "HEMPAS"	Late polychromatophilic and orthochromic erythroblasts often contain 2 to 7 normal-appearing nuclei	Excess endoplasmic reticulum appearing as a double cell membrane	Cells possess unique "HEMPAS" antigen and are lysed by 30% of acidified normal sera; increased agglutination by anti-i, increased lysis by anti-I	Autosomal Recessive
III	Giant erythroblasts, up to 50 μm in diameter, with up to 12 nuclei; prominent basophilic stippling	Clefts and blebs within nuclear region, autolytic areas in cytoplasm, some iron-filled mitochondria, and myelin figures	Data inadequate; a single case showed increased agglutination by anti-i and increased lysis by anti-I, but a negative acidified serum test	Autosomal Dominant

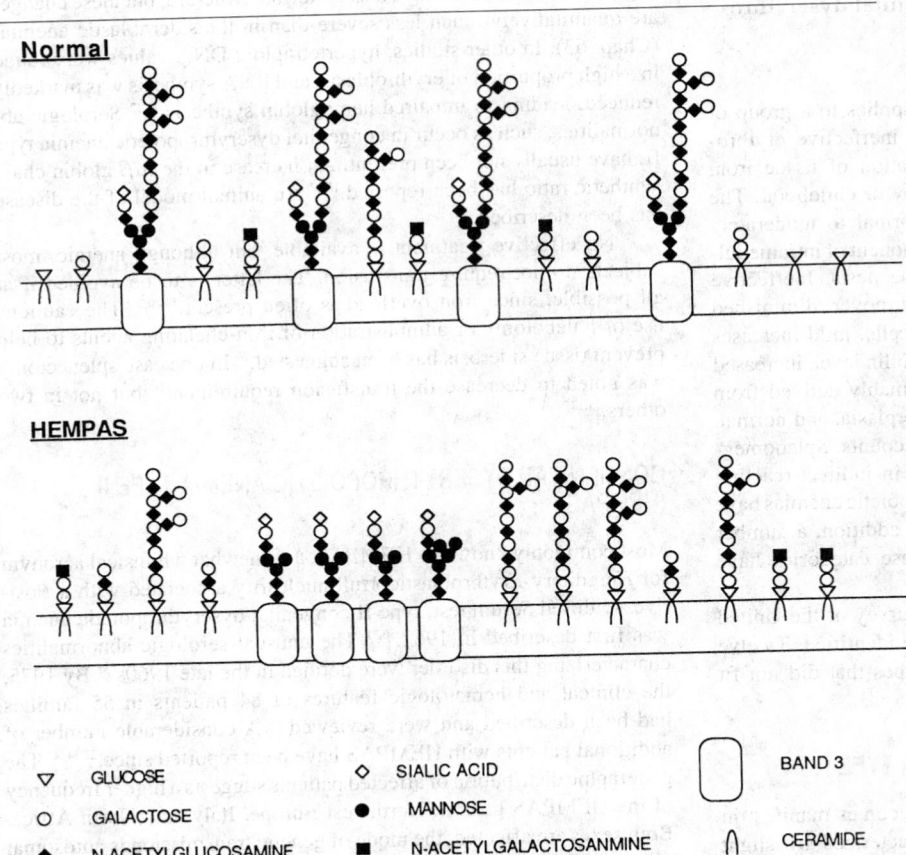

Normal

HEMPAS

▽ GLUCOSE   ◇ SIALIC ACID   ▭ BAND 3

○ GALACTOSE   ● MANNOSE

◆ N-ACETYLGLUCOSAMINE   ■ N-ACETYLGALACTOSANMINE   ∩ CERAMIDE

FIGURE 35-1   Schematic models for erythrocyte glycoproteins and glycolipids of normal, HEMPAS, and variant G.K. Band 3 glycoproteins in normal erythrocyte membranes are glycosylated by large carbohydrate chains—polylactosaminoglycans. Most glycolipids have short carbohydrate chains but have small amounts of polylactosaminylceramide. In HEMPAS erythrocytes, band 3 has truncated hybrid-type oligosaccharides and most polylactosamines shift to lipid acceptors. In variant G.K., band 3 has high mannose-type oligosaccharides and polyactosamines are not present in glycolipids either. Incompletely glycosylated band 3s in HEMPAS and variant G.K. appear to be clustered in the membranes. (Reprinted from Fukuda MN: Congenital dyserythropoietic anaemia type II (HEMPAS) and its molecular basis. *Balliere's Clinical Haematology*, Vol 6, pp 493–511, 1993. By permission of the publisher, WB Saunders Company Limited, London.[49])

changes in erythrocytes.[50] On the other hand, mapping of the gene to 20q11.2 in Italian families[45,51] ruled out both of these candidate genes as the primary defect. It is possible that in these cases, at least, the abnormality might be caused by a defect in a gene encoding a transcription factor that controls expression of both of these enzymes.

A characteristic feature of HEMPAS is the behavior of the patient's cells in serologic tests. HEMPAS cells are lysed by certain group-compatible sera at pH 6.8, resembling in this respect cells of paroxysmal nocturnal hemoglobinuria (PNH) (see Chap. 26). However, HEMPAS cells differ from those in PNH in several important respects.[44,52] The sucrose hemolysis test (see Chap. 36) is negative,[44] and the cells are not lysed by their own acidified serum. Only about 30 percent of group-compatible sera lyse HEMPAS cells. Unlike PNH cells, HEMPAS cells behave as a single population in quantitative lysis tests. The lysis of HEMPAS cells appears to be due to a naturally occurring IgM complement-binding antibody that can be removed by absorption with HEMPAS but not with normal or PNH cells. The antigen recognized by the antibody is unknown. A constant finding in HEMPAS is the strong reactivity of the red cells with anti-i autoantibodies. In this respect the red cells resemble those of newborn infants.[32,34,52] HEMPAS cells are agglutinated and lysed more readily than normal cells by cold-reacting agglutinins (anti-I and anti-i). It appears that this is largely explained by increased antibody binding rather than by increased sensitivity to complement.[53]

Multinuclearity and karyorrhexis are present in 15 to 20 percent of late erythroblasts from patients with HEMPAS, and autoradiography indicates that these cells are no longer synthesizing DNA.

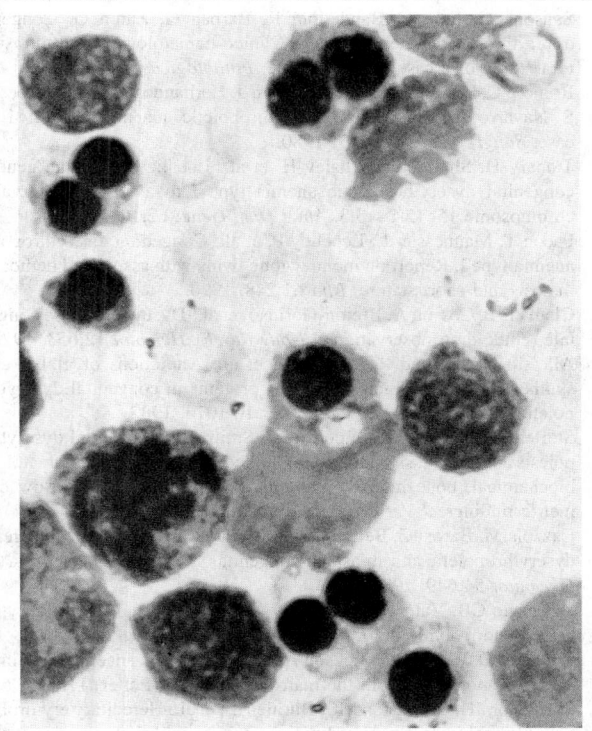

FIGURE 35-2   Multinuclearity of the erythroblasts in the marrow of a patient with HEMPAS.

The extent of anemia in different patients with HEMPAS varies widely, ranging from mild to severe. The circulating red cells exhibit moderate to marked aniso- and poikilocytosis and anisochromia. There are also a few irregularly contracted spherocytes. Ferrokinetic studies document the ineffective erythropoiesis.[32,44] Reticulocyte counts are normal or slightly elevated. Body iron stores and serum iron levels are usually increased, and the occurrence of frank hemochromatosis has been observed.[36] From 10 to 30 percent of the erythroblasts, chiefly the more mature stages, have two or more nuclei or lobulated nuclei (Fig. 35-2). Gaucher-like cells may develop due to phagocytosis of erythroblasts by macrophages. Ringed sideroblasts are not conspicuous. No satisfactory treatment is available, but partial benefit has been reported with splenectomy.[44] One patient was successfully phlebotomized, removing 1.2 g of iron, in spite of an initial hemoglobin of 7 g/dl, a level that improved in the course of phlebotomy.[43]

CONGENITAL DYSERYTHROPOIETIC ANEMIA TYPE III

A third type of congenital dyserythropoietic anemia was first described in a woman and all three of her children, in whom 16 to 22.7 percent of marrow erythroblasts were multinucleated.[54] Giant-sized erythrocytes were present in the blood, and giant erythroblasts with coarse basophilic stippling and up to 12 nuclei were present in the marrow. All patients were asymptomatic, with absent or minimal anemia. The reticulocyte count was below 3 percent. A similar, dominantly transmitted disorder has also been described in 15 members of a large Swedish family[55] under the name of hereditary benign erythroreticulosis, and other cases have been reported subsequently.

Precipitation of β chains has been observed within the abnormal erythroblasts.[66] The defect in the erythrocyte precursors is intrinsic to the stem cell: it can be reproduced in tissue culture, in which both morphologically normal and giant multinuclear erythroblasts are found.

OTHER FORMS OF CONGENITAL DYSERYTHROPOIETIC ANEMIA AND SIMILAR DISORDERS

A number of cases of congenital dyserythropoietic anemia that do not have the features of types I, II, and III have been reported,[68-80] and it has been suggested that one of these be designated as type IV.[74] The salient features of some of the earlier cases of atypical congenital dyserythropoietic anemia have been reviewed.[71] In two kindreds, congenital dyserythropoietic anemia was inherited in a dominant fashion. In some, marrow erythroid multinuclearity resembled that of HEMPAS, but the acidified serum lysis test was negative.[73,74] Long-lasting erythroblastosis occurring after splenectomy of such patients has been attributed to impairment of the denucleation of erythroblasts.[73] Unbalanced globin-chain synthesis with excess production of α chains was documented in several patients. In one such kindred, a disorder with features of both thalassemia and hereditary erythroid multinuclearity was dominantly transmitted.[70] In variant syndromes, there were also differences in the degree of agglutination by anti-i antibodies and in the concentrations of Hb F and A_2. In one case of congenital dyserythropoietic anemia, the acidified serum lysis test was positive, but erythroid multinuclearity was absent.

Still other ill-defined forms of congenital dyserythropoietic anemia undoubtedly exist. Several cases of apparently lifelong anemia, thought to be hereditary, have been described.[72] These are characterized by marked aniso- and poikilocytosis and occasional teardrop and fragmented erythrocytes in the blood. Hyperplastic marrows showed megaloblastoid features without multinuclearity or ringed sideroblasts,[72] but a case with prominent ringed sideroblasts has also been described.[77] Neutropenia is commonly present, and thrombocytopenia has been observed in some patients. Cytogenetic studies of marrow revealed no chromosomal abnormalities. The reticulocyte response to anemia was absent or inappropriately low in all. In most cases studies of parents failed to reveal abnormalities, suggesting an autosomal recessive mode of transmission. High-dose androgen therapy appeared partially to benefit two subjects.[72]

ENZYME ABNORMALITIES IN CONGENITAL DYSERYTHROPOIETIC ANEMIA

In both congenital dyserythropoietic anemia types I and II, as well as in certain less well-defined but apparently hereditary dyserythropoietic anemias, a diversity of abnormalities of individual red cell enzyme activities and of activity ratios have been identified.[72,81] Enzyme patterns differ strikingly from those of either normal red cells or reticulocyte-rich blood. They resemble closely, however, patterns observed in a variety of disorders characterized by ineffective erythropoiesis, including certain acquired and congenital sideroblastic anemias, certain preleukemic states, and certain refractory, nonsideroblastic anemias with cellular marrow.[72]

DIFFERENTIAL DIAGNOSIS

Congenital dyserythropoietic anemia may be confused with the thalassemic syndromes because of the frequent presence of marked aniso- and poikilocytosis, hypochromia, and evidence of ineffective erythropoiesis. The readily evident erythroid multinuclearity of congenital dyserythropoietic anemia type II and the marrow gigantocytes of the rarer congenital dyserythropoietic anemia type III point toward the correct diagnosis in these conditions. The marrow changes in congenital dyserythropoietic anemia type I are, however, more subtle and more easily missed. Family studies and evaluation of hemoglobin A_2 levels indicate that thalassemia is not present. The megaloblastoid marrow structure may cause some confusion with other disorders associated with abnormalities of vitamin B_{12}, folic acid, and nucleic acid metabolism. Some forms of congenital dyserythropoietic anemia also resemble some of the acquired or hereditary sideroblastic anemias, but sideroblastosis is usually not prominent and the other marrow features described earlier point to the correct diagnosis. The abnormal serologic tests observed with HEMPAS are of obvious major diagnostic importance. Otherwise, indirect hyperbilirubinemia and splenomegaly may suggest a hemolytic process, but low reticulocyte counts, the marrow features, and findings of ineffective erythropoiesis should point to the correct diagnosis.

REFERENCES

1. Wickramasinghe SN: Dyserythropoiesis and congenital dyserythropoietic anaemias. *Br J Haematol* 98:785, 1997.
2. Wickramasinghe SN, Vora AJ, Will A, et al.: Transfusion-dependent congenital dyserythropoietic anaemia with non-specific dysplastic changes in erythroblasts. *Eur J Haematol* 60:140, 1998.
3. Wendt F, Heimpel H: Kongenitale dyserythropoietische Anämie bei einem zweieiigen Zwillingsparr. *Med Klin* 62:172, 1967.
4. Heimpel H, Wendt F, Klemm D, Schubothe H, Heilmeyer L: Kongenitale dyserythropoietische Anämie. *Arch Klin Med* 215:174, 1968.
5. Heimpel H, Forteza-Vila J, Queisser W, Spiertz E: Electron and light microscopic study of the erythroblasts of patients with congenital dyserythropoietic anemia. *Blood* 37:299, 1971.
6. Keyserlingk DG, Boll I, Meuret G: Ultrastruktur der gestörten erythropäiese bei einer kongenitalen dyserythropoietischen Anämie. *Klin Wochenschr* 48:728, 1970.
7. Maldonado JE, Taswell HF: Type I dyserythropoietic anemia in an elderly patient. *Blood* 44:495, 1974.
8. Breton-Gorius J, Daniel MT, Clauvel JP, Dreyfus B: Anomalies ultrastructurales des érythroblastes et des érythrocytes dan six cas de dysérythropoiése congénitale. *Nouv Rev Fr Hematol* 13:23, 1973.
9. Faille A, Najean Y, Dresch C: Cinétique de l'érythropoiése dans 14 cas "d'erythropoiése inéfficase" avec anomalies morphologiques des érythroblastes et polynucléarité. *Nouv Rev Fr Hematol* 12:113, 1972.
10. Lewis SM, Nelson DA, Pitcher CS: Clinical and ultrastructural aspects of congenital dyserythropoietic anaemia Type I. *Br J Haematol* 23:113, 1972.
11. Meuret VG, Boll I, Keyserlingk DG, Heissmeyer H: Morphologische und kinetische Befinde bei einer kongenitalen dyserythropoietischen Anämie. *Blut* 21:341, 1970.
12. Meuret G, Tschan P, Schülter G, Graf Keyserlingk DG, Boll I: DNA-, histone-, RNA-, hemoglobin-content and DNA synthesis in erythroblasts in a case of congenital dyserythropoietic anemia type I. *Blut* 24:32, 1972.
13. Wickramasinghe SN, Pippard MJ: Studies of erythroblast function in congenital dyserythropoietic anaemia, type I; evidence of impaired DNA, RNA, and protein synthesis in unbalanced globin chain synthesis in ultrastructurally abnormal cells. *J Clin Pathol* 39:881, 1986.
14. Hanna WT, Machado EA, Montgomery RN, Lange RD: Variant of congenital dyserythropoietic anemia. *South Med J* 78:616, 1985.
15. Mori PG, Favareto F, Schenone A, et al.: Congenital dyserythropoietic anemia type I: report of a pair of siblings. *Acta Haematol (Basel)* 75:219, 1986.
16. Choudhry VP, Saraya AK, Kasturi J, Rath PK: Congenital dyserythropoietic anaemias: splenectomy as a mode of therapy. *Acta Haematol (Basel)* 66:195, 1981.
17. Conde E, Mazo E, Baro J, et al.: Transmission and scanning electron microscopy study on congenital dyserythropoietic anemia type I. *Acta Haematol (Basel)* 70:243, 1983.
18. Maeda K, Saeed SM, Rebuck JW, Monto RW: Type I dyserythropoietic anemia. A 30-year follow-up. *Am J Clin Pathol* 73:433, 1980.
19. Ghosh K, Mohanty D, Bhagwat AG, Das KC: Congenital dyserythropoietic anaemia (CDA) type I—a case report with ultrastructural study. *Folia Haematol (Leipz)* 112:716, 1985.
20. Smithson WA, Perrault J: Use of subcutaneous deferoxamine in a child with hemochromatosis associated with congenital dyserythropoietic anemia, type I. *Mayo Clin Proc* 57:322, 1982.
21. Woessner S, Pardo P, Lafuente R, Feliu E, Vives JL, Sans-Sabrefen J: Congenital dyserythropoietic anemia type I. Report of a case. *Blut* 42:47, 1981.
22. Sansone G, Intra E, Bandelloni R, Barban G, Zunin G: Congenital dyserythropoietic anemia, type I. Clinico-hematological and ultrastructural study of a case diagnosed late. *Pathologica* 79:705, 1987.
23. Romero C, Fernandez-Fuertes I, Cesar J, Hernandez-Jodra M, Woessner S, Navarro JL: Congenital dyserythropoietic anaemia, type I: a new case. *Sangre (Barc)* 25:507, 1980.
24. Tamary H, Shalmon L, Shalev H, et al.: Localization of the gene for congenital dyserythropoietic anemia type I to a <1-cM interval on chromosome 15q15.1–15.3. *Am J Hum Genet* 62:1062, 1998.
25. Facon T, Mannessier L, Lepelley P, et al.: Congenital diserythropoietic anemia type I. Report on monozygotic twins with associated hemochromatosis and short stature. *Blut* 61:248, 1990.
26. Clauvel JP, Cosson A, Breton-Gorius J, et al.: Dyséythropoiése congenitalè (etude de 6 observations). *Nouv Rev Fr Hematol* 12:653, 1972.
27. Alloisio N, Jaccoud P, Dorleac E, et al.: Alterations of globin chain synthesis and of red cell membrane proteins in congenital dyserythropoietic anemia I and II. *Pediatr Res* 16:1016, 1982.
28. Steffen DJ, Elliott GS, Leipold HW, Smith JE: Congenital dyserythropoiesis and progressive alopecia in Polled Hereford calves: hematologic, biochemical, bone marrow cytologic, electrophoretic, and flow cytometric findings. *J Vet Diagn Invest* 4:31, 1992.
29. Cazzola M, Barosi G, Bergamaschi SN, et al.: Iron loading in congenital dyserythropoietic anaemias and congenital sideroblastic anaemias. *Br J Haematol* 54:649, 1983.
30. DeLozzio CB, Valencia JI, Accame E: Chromosomal study in erythroblastic endopolyploidy. *Lancet* 1:1004, 1962.
31. Roberts PD, Wallis PG, Jackson ADM: Haemolytic anaemia with multinucleated normoblasts in the marrow. *Lancet* 1 (Letter):1186, 1962.
32. Crookston JH, Crookston MC, Burnie KL, et al.: Hereditary erythroblastic multinuclearity associated with a positive acidified-serum test: a test of congenital dyserythropoietic anaemia. *Br J Haematol* 17:11, 1969.
33. Verwilghen RL: Congenital dyserythropoietic anaemia, type II (HEMPAS), in *Congenital Disorders of Erythropoiesis, Ciba Foundation Symposium 37 (new series)*, p 151. Elsevier/Excerpta Medica/North Holland, Amsterdam, 1976.
34. Bird AR, Jacobs P, Moores P: Congenital dyserythropoietic anaemia (type II) presenting with haemosiderosis. *Acta Haematol (Basel)* 78:33, 1987.
35. Zdebska E, Anselstetter V, Pacuszka T, et al.: Glycolipids and glycopeptides of red cell membranes in congenital dyserythropoietic anaemia type II (CDA II). *Br J Haematol* 66:385, 1987.
36. Halpern Z, Rahmani R, Levo Y: Severe hemochromatosis: the predominant clinical manifestation of congenital dyserythropoietic anemia type 2. *Acta Haematol (Basel)* 74:178, 1985.
37. Ventura A, Panizon F, Soranzo MR, et al.: Congenital dyserythropoietic anaemia type II associated with a new type of G6PD deficiency (G6PD Gabrovizza). *Acta Haematol (Basel)* 71:227, 1984.
38. Faruqui S, Abraham A, Berenfeld MR, Gabuzda TG: Normal serum ferritin levels in a patient with HEMPAS syndrome and iron overload. *Am J Clin Pathol* 78:97, 1982.
39. Chrobak L, Radochova D, Smetana K, et al.: Congenital dyserythropoietic anaemia, type II (HEMPAS) in three siblings. *Folia Haematol (Leipz)* 107:628, 1980.
40. McCann SR, Firth R, Murray N, Temperley IJ: Congenital dyserythropoietic anaemia type II (HEMPAS): a family study. *J Clin Pathol* 33:1197, 1980.
41. Greiner TC, Burns CP, Dick FR, Henry KM, Mahmood I: Congenital dyserythropoietic anemia type II diagnosed in a 69-year-old patient with iron overload. *Am J Clin Pathol* 98:522, 1992.
42. Gangarossa S, Romano V, Miraglia del Giudice E, Perrotta S, Iolascon A, Schiliro G: Congenital dyserythropoietic anemia type II associated with G6PD Seattle in a Sicilian child. *Acta Haematol (Basel)* 93:36, 1995.
43. Hofmann WK, Kaltwasser JP, Hoelzer D, Nielsen P, Gabbe EE: Successful treatment of iron overload by phlebotomies in a patient with severe congenital dyserythropoietic anemia type II. *Blood* 89:3068, 1997.
44. Crookston MC: HEMPAS: Congenital dyserythropoietic anemia (type II). *Q J Med* 66:257, 1973.
45. Gasparini P, Del Giudice EM, Delaunay J, et al.: Localization of the congenital dyserythropoietic anemia II locus to chromosome 20q11.2 by genomewide search. *Am J Hum Genet* 61:1112, 1997.
46. Anselstetter V, Horstmann HJ, Heimpel H: Congenital dyserythropoietic

anaemia, types I and II: aberrant pattern of erythrocyte membrane proteins in CDA II, as revealed by two-dimensional polyacrylamide gel electrophoresis. *Br J Haematol* 35:209, 1977.

47. Fukuda MN, Klier G, Yu J, Scartezzini P: Anomalous clustering of underglycosylated band 3 in erythrocytes and their precursor cells in congenital dyserythropoietic anemia type II. *Blood* 68:521, 1986.

48. Iolascon A, D'Agostaro G, Perrotta S, Izzo P, Tavano R, Miraglia del Giudice B: Congenital dyserythropoietic anemia type II: molecular basis and clinical aspects. *Haematologica* 81:543, 1996.

49. Fukuda MN: Congenital dyserythropoietic anaemia type II (HEMPAS) and its molecular basis. *Baillieres Clin Haematol* 6:493, 1993.

50. Chui D, Oh-Eda M, Liao YF, et al.: Alpha-mannosidase-II deficiency results in dyserythropoiesis and unveils an alternate pathway in oligosaccharide biosynthesis. *Cell* 90:157, 1997.

51. Iolascon A, Miraglia del Giudice E, Perrotta S, Granatiero M, Zelante L, Gasparini P: Exclusion of three candidate genes as determinants of congenital dyserythropoietic anemia type II (CDA-II). *Blood* 90:4197, 1997.

52. Crookston JH, Crookston MC: Hereditary anemia with multinuclear erythroblasts (''HEMPAS''), in *Birth Defects, Original Article Series, Clinical Delineation of Birth Defects*, p 15. Williams & Wilkins, Baltimore, Vol. 8, 1972.

53. Lewis SM, Grammaticos P, Dacie JV: Lysis by anti-I in dyserythropoietic anaemias: role of increased uptake of antibody. *Br J Haematol* 18:465, 1970.

54. Wolff JA, von Hofe FH: Familial erythroid multinuclearity. *Blood* 6:1274, 1951.

55. Bergström I, Jacobsson L: Hereditary benign erythroreticulosis. *Blood* 19:296, 1962.

56. Wickramasinghe SN, Goudsmit R: Precipitation of beta-globin chains within the erythropoietic cells of a patient with congenital dyserythropoietic anemia, type III. *Br J Haematol* 65:250, 1987.

57. Vainchenker W, Breton-Gorius J, Guichard J, et al.: Congenital dyserythropoietic anemia type III. Studies on erythroid differentiation of blood erythroid progenitor cells (BFUE) in vitro. *Exp Hematol* 8:1057, 1980.

58. Wickramasinghe SN, Parry TE, Williams C, Bond AN, Hughes M, Crook S: A new case of congenital dyserythropoietic anaemia, type III: studies of the cell cycle distribution and ultrastructure of erythroblasts and of nucleic acid synthesis in marrow cells. *J Clin Pathol* 35:1103, 1982.

59. Goudsmit R, Beckers D, De Bruijne JI, et al.: Congenital dyserythropoietic anaemia, type III. *Br J Haematol* 23:97, 1972.

60. Goudsmit R: Congenital dyserythropoietic anaemia, type III, in *Dyserythropoiesis*, p 83. Academic, London, 1977.

61. Björksten P, Holmgren G, Roos G, Stenling R: Congenital dyserythropoietic anaemia, type III: an electron microscope study. *Br J Haematol* 38:37, 1978.

62. Jijina E, Ghosh K, Yavagal D, Pathare AV, Mohanty D: A patient with congenital dyserythropoietic anaemia type III presenting with stillbirths. *Acta Haematol (Basel)* 99:31, 1998.

63. Sandstroem H, Wahlin A, Eriksson M, et al.: Angioid streaks are part of a familial syndrome of dyserythropoietic anaemia (CDA III). *Br J Haematol* 98:845, 1997.

64. Holm T, Kildahl-Andersen O, Sjo M: Congenital dyserythropoietic anaemia type III. A case report. *Tidsskr Nor Laegeforen* 117:1898, 1997.

65. McCluggage WG, Hull D, Mayne E, Bharucha H, Wickramasinghe SN: Malignant lymphoma in congenital dyserythropoietic anaemia type III. *J Clin Pathol* 49:599, 1996.

66. Villegas A, Gonzalez L, Furio V, et al.: Congenital dyserythropoietic anemia type III with unbalanced globin chain synthesis. *Eur J Haematol* 52:251, 1994.

67. Lind L, Sandstrom H, Wahlin A, et al.: Localization of the gene for congenital dyserythropoietic anemia type III, CDAN3, to chromosome 15q21-q25. *Hum Mol Genet* 4:109, 1995.

68. McBride JA, Wilson WE, Baille N: Congenital dyserythropoietic anaemia-type IV. *Blood* 38:837, 1971.

69. Hruby MA, Mason RG, Honig GR: Unbalanced globin chain synthesis in congenital dyserythropoietic anemia. *Blood* 42:843, 1973.

70. Weatherall DJ, Clegg JB, Knox-Macaulay HH, Bunch C, Hopkins CR, Temperley IJ: A genetically determined disorder with features both of thalassemia and congenital dyserythropoietic anemia. *Br J Haematol* 24:681, 1973.

71. David G, Van Dorpe A: Aberrant congenital dyserythropoietic anaemias, in *Dyserythropoiesis*, p 93. Academic, London, 1977.

72. Valentine WN, Konrad PN, Paglia DE: Dyserythropoiesis, refractory anemia, and ''preleukemia'': metabolic features of the erythrocytes. *Blood* 41:857, 1973.

73. Bethlenfalvay NC, Hadnagy C, Heimpel H: Unclassified type of congenital dyserythropoietic anaemia (CDA) with prominent peripheral erythroblastosis. *Br J Haematol* 60:541, 1985.

74. Bird AR, Karabus CD, Hartley PS: Type IV congenital dyserythropoietic anemia with an unusual response to splenectomy. *Am J Pediatr Hematol Oncol* 7:196, 1985.

75. Ohisalo JJ, Viitala J, Lintula R, Ruutu T: A new congenital dyserythropoietic anaemia. *Br J Haematol* 68:111, 1988.

76. Pothier B, Morle L, Alloisio N, et al.: Aberrant pattern of red cell membrane and cytosolic proteins in a case of congenital dyserythropoietic anaemia. *Br J Haematol* 66:393, 1987.

77. Brien WF, Mant MJ, Etches WS: Variant congenital dyserythropoietic anaemia with ringed sideroblasts. *Clin Lab Haematol* 7:231, 1985.

78. Wickramasinghe SN, Illum N, Wimberley PD: Congenital dyserythropoietic anaemia with novel intra-erythroblastic and intra-erythrocytic inclusions. *Br J Haematol* 79:322, 1991.

79. Sansone G, Masera G, Cantu-Rajnoldi A, Terzoli S: An unclassified case of congenital dyserythropoietic anaemia with a severe neonatal onset. *Acta Haematol (Basel)* 88:41, 1992.

80. Agre P, Smith BL, Baumgarten R, et al.: Human red cell aquaporin CHIP. II. Expression during normal fetal development and in a novel form of congenital dyserythropoietic anemia. *J Clin Invest* 94:1050, 1994.

81. Valentine WN, Crookston JH, Paglia DE, Conrad P: Erythrocyte enzymatic abnormalities in HEMPAS (hereditary erythroblastic multinuclearity with a positive acidified-serum test). *Br J Haematol* 23:107, 1972.

PAROXYSMAL NOCTURNAL HEMOGLOBINURIA

ERNEST BEUTLER

Paroxysmal nocturnal hemoglobinuria is an acquired hematopoietic stem cell disease characterized by chronic hemolytic anemia, thrombotic episodes, and often pancytopenia. It is a clonal disorder, caused by a somatic mutation of the X-linked gene PIG-A, which is required for formation of the phosphatidylinositol anchor. As a result, many membrane proteins, including some inhibitors of the complement cascade, are missing from the cell surface, and the erythrocytes are usually sensitive to the hemolytic effect of complement. The disease is diagnosed provisionally with the sucrose hemolysis test and definitively by the Ham acid hemolysis test, which is being replaced by flow cytometric demonstration of a deficiency in CD55 and CD59. Treatment with glucocorticoids and/or androgenic steroids is sometimes helpful. The median survival is approximately 10 years. Stem cell transplantation is curative.

DEFINITION AND HISTORY

Although commonly regarded as a type of hemolytic anemia, paroxysmal nocturnal hemoglobinuria (PNH) is in reality a hematopoietic stem cell disorder characterized by the formation of defective platelets, granulocytes, and possibly lymphocytes as well as abnormal erythrocytes. The abnormality of the red cells predisposes them to intravascular complement-mediated lysis, which waxes and wanes in severity. The name suggests that cyclic variation in hemoglobinuria is an important feature of this disease. However, in many patients hemoglobinuria is quite irregular or occult. The classical diagnostic feature of PNH is the increased sensitivity of the red blood cells to the hemolytic action of complement.

In a scholarly historical review of PNH, Crosby[1] attributed the first definitive account of this disease to Strübing,[2] who in 1882 described a patient with hemoglobinuria after sleep. The patient's plasma was red, and Strübing suggested that the erythrocytes were being destroyed within the blood stream. He also detected in the urine a fine-grained yellowish-brown material, which must have been hemosiderin. Hijmans van den Bergh[3] demonstrated that erythrocytes from a similar patient were lysed in normal serum as well as in the patient's serum if the mixture was acidified with carbon dioxide. Marchiafava and Micheli also were early students of the disease, and for a time it was designated the Marchiafava-Micheli syndrome, an appellation that has fallen into disuse.

Because many different proteins that had in common their attachment to a phosphatidylinositol anchor are missing from the surface of blood cells in PNH, it was recognized that the underlying defect in PNH would be likely to affect this structure. The detection of the defect in an X-linked gene designated PIG-A (for phosphatidylinositol glycan class A)[4] has been the culmination of over 100 years of research into this once mysterious disorder.

ETIOLOGY AND PATHOGENESIS

In contrast to all the other intrinsic abnormalities of the erythrocyte, PNH is an acquired disorder; in a number of cases only one of a pair of identical twins was affected.[5-7] Before the basic lesion had been discovered, the expression of glucose-6-phosphate dehydrogenase alleles,[8] methylation of polymorphic restriction sites,[9] and cytogenetic studies[10] had all demonstrated the clonal nature of PNH. Thus, PNH arises, like a neoplasm, from the transformation of a single cell. The underlying defect in PNH is one or several of many different mutations in the PIG-A gene, an X-linked gene that plays a major role in the formation of the phosphatidylinositol anchor. Many different mutations have been documented in PNH patients,[11] most of them nonsense mutations or insertions or deletions producing frameshifts. It is no accident that the gene that is mutated is X-linked. In this way a single somatic mutation is enough to affect formation of the anchor. If an autosomal gene were to cause the disease, damage to both copies of the gene would be required, a statistically unlikely event. The abnormal clone appears to arise most commonly in a damaged marrow; many patients with PNH have a prior history of aplastic anemia,[12] either idiopathic or drug-induced. Cells with PIG-A mutations do not appear to have a proliferative advantage in vitro or in hybrid animal models made with PIG-A knockouts,[13] but they are resistant to apoptosis,[14,15] which may account for their survival advantage and the evolution of PNH into leukemia. Somewhat surprisingly, some patients have multiple clones, each with a distinct mutation.[16,17] This implies that mutations of the PIG-A gene may not be altogether rare, and when conditions are such that a PNH clone has a selective advantage, several independent mutational events may come to light. The PIG-A gene plays a vital role in a very early step in the conversion of N-acetylglucosamine and glucosamine-phosphoinositol into mature mannolipids.[18] Transformed lymphoblasts are unable to incorporate labeled mannose into glycosylphosphatidylinositol (GPI) anchor precursors and, when provided with uridine diphospho-N-acetyl[3H] glucosamine, there is a marked reduction in the production of anchor phospholipids. Transfection with the PIG-A cDNA corrects the defect in GPI anchor synthesis.[4]

A large number of membrane protein deficiencies have been observed in PNH. These include deficiencies of acetylcholinesterase,[19] leukocyte alkaline phosphatase,[20] the "decay accelerating factor" (DAF, CD55),[21] CD59 antigen (membrane inhibitor of reactive lysis—MIRL), homologous restriction factor (HRF, C8-binding protein),[22] CD58 (lymphocyte function–associated antigen-3—LFA-3),[23] 5'-ectonucleotidase,[24] CD16 (the low-affinity Fc receptor of granulocytes),[25] urokinase-type plasminogen activator,[26] and CD14 antigen.[27] The common denominator appears to be that all of these proteins are attached to the GPI anchor (see Chap. 27).

The classic abnormality of PNH erythrocytes is their increased sensitivity to complement-mediated lysis, whether the complement is activated by the classic or the alternative pathway (see Chap. 6). Activation of complement may be achieved by a variety of means[28]: lowering of pH, as in the acid hemolysis test; reducing ionic strength, as in the sucrose hemolysis test; treating the plasma with cobra venom; increasing the magnesium concentration; or coating the cells with antibodies such as anti-A. Using graded amounts of complement, it is possible to identify several populations of cells which have been designated PNH I, PNH II, and PNH IIIa and IIIb, manifesting progressively increasing sensitivity to complement lysis and deposition of increasing amounts of C3 on the PNH membranes.[12] The existence of multiple populations, once difficult to explain in a clonal disorder, is presumably due to the coexistence of several different clones with different mutations.[16,17]

Although several of the abnormalities involve proteins that modulate complement function, a variety of findings suggest that the absence of the CD59 antigen (MIRL) plays the most critical role in the complement sensitivity of PNH erythrocytes. Inherited deficiency of DAF is not associated with clinical hemolysis, although a weakly positive acid hemolysis test may be present,[29,30] while a hereditary deficiency of CD59 is associated with PNH.[31] Restoration in vitro of CD59 corrects the complement sensitivity of red cells more completely than restoration of DAF,[32] and PNH may occur in the absence of DAF deficiency.[33] The trimodal distribution of complement sensitivity of the red cells of some patients with PNH[19] appears to be related to the degree of deficiency of CD59 and DAF among the erythrocytes of such patients.[34,35]

Granulocytes and platelets, like red cells, show increased sensitivity to complement-mediated lysis[36] and are deficient in DAF.[37] Chemotactic responses of PNH granulocytes are also impaired.[38] Even blood lymphocytes[39] and lymphoblastoid cell lines from some patients with PNH show abnormalities in CD59 and DAF.[40]

CLINICAL FEATURES

HEMOGLOBINURIA

The nocturnal hemoglobinuria from which PNH derives its name, that is, the passage of red or brownish urine in the morning on rising, occurs in only a small proportion of the patients. When it does follow the classic cyclic pattern, the hemoglobinuria occurs during sleep regardless of the time of day.[41] It was originally believed that nocturnal hemoglobinuria was a function of a lowered blood pH during sleep, but this is not the case.[42] Hemoglobinuria may also be the result of the production of increased numbers of abnormal cells rather than of an increase in hemolytic processes.

In most patients with PNH, hemoglobinuria occurs irregularly. Bouts of hemolysis may be initiated by infections, surgery, and possibly even strenuous exercise.[43] The injection of contrast dyes, as in intravenous pyelography or myelography, may precipitate hemolysis by activating complement.[44]

CHRONIC HEMOLYSIS

Patients with PNH manifest all the clinical and laboratory signs of chronic hemolytic anemia. Weakness, dyspnea, and pallor are common, particularly when the anemia is quite severe. Splenomegaly is present in some patients, but the enlargement of the spleen is usually quite modest.

IRON DEFICIENCY

Iron deficiency is often a manifestation of PNH because of iron loss in the urine, in the form of both hemosiderin and hemoglobin. The administration of iron to patients with iron deficiency sometimes results in overt signs of hemolysis, manifested by the appearance of frank hemoglobinuria. Although this effect of iron has sometimes been attributed to its peroxidatic effect, increasing damage to the red cell membrane,[45] it seems more likely that it is due to increased production of both normal and abnormal red cells by the marrow, with the newly formed abnormal cells undergoing hemolysis.[46]

BLEEDING

Thrombocytopenia varies greatly in severity. It may be very mild and persist for years, or it may be very severe. In the latter instance extensive hemorrhagic complications may be a prominent part of the clinical presentation of patients with PNH.

THROMBOSIS

Although thrombotic complications occur in other forms of hemolytic anemia as well, they are particularly prominent and severe in PNH. The reason for this is not entirely clear, but it may be related to activation of platelets by complement,[12] the procoagulant activity of red cell membranes, or the intravascular release of adenosine diphosphate (ADP) from red cells, leading to platelet aggregation. The prevalence of factor V Leiden is not increased in PNH.[47] Venous thromboses represent one of the most frequent clinical manifestations of PNH. The Budd-Chiari syndrome, resulting from hepatic vein thrombosis, has been observed repeatedly. In one study[48] of 40 patients with Budd-Chiari syndrome, 5 were found to have PNH. Thus PNH should be a serious consideration in any patient with hepatic vein thrombosis. Budd-Chiari syndrome has an ominous prognosis when fully developed.[49,50] It may also occur in a milder, subclinical form detectable by ultrasonography,[51] and early therapy has been recommended.[48] Pain in the abdomen or in the lower part of the back also appears to be more common in patients with PNH than in those with other types of hemolytic anemia. The abdominal pain is often colicky in nature and the abdomen is tender on palpitation. Frank intestinal infarction or bleeding into the intestinal wall has sometimes been found.[52,53] Esophageal spasm has been observed in patients who are undergoing hemolysis; it has been likened to the symptoms that have occurred in patients who are receiving hemoglobin solutions as a blood substitute, symptoms that are probably related to removal of ambient nitric oxide.[12] Pulmonary hypertension has occurred and has been attributed to widespread thromboses in the pulmonary microvasculature.[54] Arterial as well as venous thrombosis has been documented.[55]

PREGNANCY

Pregnancy in PNH patients has been associated with abortion and venous thromboembolism, but the outcome is sometimes normal.[56–58] In a study of 38 pregnant patients with PNH, pregnancy was uncomplicated in one-third of the cases and life-threatening complications in mothers were uncommon.[57]

RENAL MANIFESTATIONS

A variety of abnormalities of renal function are observed. Included are hyposthenuria, abnormal tubular function, and declining creatinine clearance. Hypertension was observed in 8 of a series of 21 patients who had been followed for a long period. Radiologic findings included enlarged kidneys and cortical infarcts, cortical thinning, and papillary necrosis. Most patients have some episodes of hematuria and proteinuria distinct from hemoglobinuria.[44] Acute and chronic renal failure may occur.[44,59–61]

NEUROLOGIC MANIFESTATIONS

Severe headaches or pains in the eyes occur in patients with PNH without any objectively demonstrable neurologic abnormalities. These complications may be due to small venous occlusions. Frank cerebral venous thrombosis is a grave and fortunately uncommon complication of PNH.[62]

LABORATORY FEATURES

BLOOD

Anemia may be very severe, with hemoglobin concentrations below 5 g/dl, but in some cases the hemoglobin level is normal. A mild to moderate reticulocytosis is usually present; the reticulocyte count tends to be lower than in other patients with chronic hemolysis who manifest the same degree of anemia. A modest degree of macrocytosis commensurate with the increased reticulocyte count is usually present. However, if the patient has developed iron deficiency, the red cells may be microcytic and hypochromic. In this case, the plasma iron and ferritin levels are usually low and the iron-binding capacity elevated.

The leukocyte count is characteristically low, principally because of a diminution of the number of granulocytes. The leukocyte alkaline phosphatase activity[20] and surface urokinase receptors[63] are diminished. The platelet count is often low, but it may be 150,000/μL or more in about 20 to 50 percent of the patients.[64] Platelet survival is usually normal.[36]

MARROW

Erythroid hyperplasia is usually present in the marrow of patients with PNH. However, the marrow cellularity is generally not greatly increased, and the marrow may even be aplastic. Stainable iron is often absent.

URINE

Hemoglobin is sometimes but by no means always present in the urine. Hemoglobin casts may be present. Hemosiderinuria is one of the most constant features of the disease and is of considerable diagnostic importance.

DIFFERENTIAL DIAGNOSIS

The diagnosis of PNH should be entertained in any patient with pancytopenia of unknown origin, particularly when accompanied by reticulocytosis. Isolated defects in a single lineage, such as thrombocytopenia, may also be the presenting finding. PNH arises within the context of marrow failure states such as aplastic anemia. When such patients manifest moderate numbers of reticulocytes in the blood, tests for PNH may demonstrate that a complement-sensitive clone has appeared. A search for PNH occasionally proves rewarding in the case of patients who have repeated unexplained thrombotic episodes.

The most convenient screening tests for PNH are the sucrose hemolysis test[65] and the examination of urine for hemosiderin. Occasionally the characteristically complement-sensitive red cells cannot be demonstrated in patients with well-established PNH. This probably occurs when the production of PNH cells is relatively low and most of the PNH cells that have been made have already been destroyed either in the marrow or in the circulation. Thus a single normal sucrose hemolysis test cannot be considered strong evidence that a patient does not have PNH. Hemosiderinuria is a more constant feature of the disease and is helpful in identifying patients who may have PNH with a transiently normal sucrose hemolysis test. If the sucrose hemolysis test is positive, the diagnosis should be confirmed with fluorescent-activated cell sorting (FACS) analysis or with the complete Ham acid hemolysis test.[66] The latter test establishes that (1) hemolysis is a property of the patient's erythrocytes, (2) hemolysis requires the presence of serum, (3) the hemolytic effect of the serum is increased by acidification, (4) the hemolytic properties of serum are destroyed by heating, and (5) the hemolytic properties of heated serum are not restored by guinea pig serum. Although historically the Ham test has

been the "gold standard" for the diagnosis of PNH, it is a cumbersome and time-consuming procedure with a considerable number of potential technical pitfalls. Therefore flow cytometry of erythrocytes using anti-CD59 or of granulocytes using either anti-CD55 or anti-CD59 antibodies is rapidly replacing the older techniques once used for diagnosis[67-71] and can be regarded as a sensitive and specific diagnostic measure.

Thrombocytopenia and leukopenia are features of PNH that help to differentiate this disorder from other types of hemolytic anemia. Hemosiderinuria, a constant feature of PNH, does not usually occur in other forms of hemolytic anemia, except for those in which there is considerable intravascular destruction of erythrocytes, such as in the hemolytic anemia associated with prosthetic cardiac valves. Although HEMPAS (Hereditary Erythroblastic Multinuclearity with a Positive Acidified Serum lysis test) is characterized, as its name indicates, by a positive acidified lysis test, there should be no difficulty in distinguishing this disorder from PNH (see Chap. 35). Lysis of HEMPAS cells occurs because of the presence in normal serum of antibodies to unusual antigens on the surface of HEMPAS cells. The serum of these patients lacks the required alloantibody, and HEMPAS cells will not lyse in their own serum. Moreover, HEMPAS is a hereditary disorder and is not associated with leukopenia or thrombocytopenia.

THERAPY, COURSE, AND PROGNOSIS

TREATMENT

Treatment of PNH consists chiefly of supportive measures such as transfusion, antibiotics, and anticoagulants as may be required. Suitable patients may be cured by marrow transplantation.

TRANSFUSIONS

Transfusions with red cells are often necessary in the management of patients with severe PNH. Although washed red cells are usually recommended in order to avoid transfusing the complement contained in plasma, analysis of a large number of transfusions given to PNH patients suggests that packed red cells are equally safe.[72,73]

IRON THERAPY

The iron deficiency that often occurs in patients with PNH because of the urinary loss of iron should be treated. The oral administration of iron is usually entirely satisfactory (see Chap. 38). Although an increase in hemoglobinuria may occur during iron therapy because of increased production of PNH cells by the marrow, the net positive effect of the administration of iron may lessen the requirements for blood transfusion.

STEROIDS

Both androgens and glucocorticoids have been used in the treatment of PNH. Fluoxymesterone (Halotestin) in doses of 20 to 30 mg per day usually produces some increase in the hemoglobin concentration of the blood.[74] The administration of danazol failed to produce a therapeutic effect in two patients.[75]

The administration of glucocorticoids has also been reported to be useful in the treatment of both hemolysis and thrombotic episodes.[12] Doses ranging from 20 to 60 mg of prednisone on alternate days may be tried. In view of the potential side effects, particularly when these drugs are administered chronically, steroid therapy should be limited to those patients whose transfusion requirement is significantly decreased at well-tolerated doses.

ANTICOAGULANTS

Use of prophylactic anticoagulants in PNH has been advocated,[76] but there is no clear-cut evidence of a beneficial effect. The principal role of anticoagulants in the management of PNH is in the treatment of thrombotic complications such as the Budd-Chiari syndrome.[77] Thrombolytic therapy with streptokinase and urokinase was considered to be safe and effective in two patients with PNH.[78] Sometimes a trial of anticoagulation therapy is used in patients who have repeated episodes of abdominal and back pain, but the usefulness of this approach remains to be established. The administration of drugs associated with an increased incidence of thrombosis, particularly oral contraceptives, should be avoided in patients with PNH.

SPLENECTOMY

Generally, splenectomy is not indicated, although favorable responses have been reported in some patients. Because of the considerable risk of thromboembolic complications in patients with PNH, elective surgery of any type, including splenectomy, is best avoided. When surgery is necessary, the administration of low-dose or low-molecular-weight heparin postoperatively may be prudent because of the high risk of thrombosis.

STEM CELL TRANSPLANTATION

As in other stem cell disorders, stem cell transplantation is an effective albeit high-risk method for the treatment of PNH[79–82] (see Chap. 18). As might be expected, the abnormalities in the phosphoinositol-anchored proteins are corrected by this procedure.[83]

OTHER TREATMENTS

Erythropoietin therapy seemed to have a beneficial effect in some patients but not in others.[84,85] Hemolysis may be diminished temporarily by the infusion of a dextran solution,[86,87] but this measure does not seem to have a role in the clinical management of PNH. Some selective suppression of PNH cells was documented with 6-mercaptopurine treatment, but this did not prove to be of any clinical value.[88] Cyclosporine, sometimes in combination with granulocyte colony–stimulating factor (G-CSF), has seemed helpful in some patients.[89,90]

COURSE

The clinical course of PNH is enormously variable. In rare instances, the patient may succumb to this disease within a few months of the first onset of symptoms. Other patients experience a chronic course in which the severity of the disease may wax and wane as the normal cells and the PNH clone alternately appear to gain ascendancy. Sometimes the abnormal clone disappears altogether and the patient appears to be cured. It has been suggested that the course is more severe in children and adolescents with PNH.[91]

The development of acute leukemia is rare but well documented.[92,93] Myelodysplastic syndrome also occurs in patients with PNH.[94–96] Not surprisingly, the defect seems to arise in the PNH clone.[92]

PROGNOSIS

As with so many other diseases, initial reports on PNH tended to emphasize the more severely affected patients, so the prognosis was generally deemed to be very grave. As physicians developed a higher index of suspicion concerning this disorder, and as simplified methods for diagnosis became available, milder cases were diagnosed, and these tend to have a better long-term outlook. Nonetheless, even today the disease must be considered a very serious one, and most patients eventually succumb to its complications. The most commonly lethal complication probably is thrombotic episodes such as the Budd-Chiari syndrome, but the various complications of pancytopenia also may lead to death, and in a few patients the terminal episode has been the development of acute leukemia.[97] In a study of 220 patients with PNH

with follow-up as long as 46 years, the Kaplan-Meier survival estimate was 65 percent at 10 years and 48 percent at 15 years after diagnosis.[98] In another study of 80 consecutive patients, the outlook was similar: the median survival after diagnosis was 10 years, and 28 percent of the patients survived for 25 years.[99] Eight-year cumulative incidence rates of the main complications (pancytopenia, thrombosis, and myelodysplastic syndrome) were 15 percent, 28 percent, and 5 percent, respectively. Poor survival was associated with age over 55 years at the time of diagnosis, the occurrence of thrombosis as a complication, evolution to pancytopenia, a myelodysplastic syndrome or acute leukemia, and thrombocytopenia at diagnosis. The prognosis for patients in whom aplastic anemia antedated PNH was better than that for those in whom it did not.[98]

REFERENCES

1. Crosby WH: Paroxysmal nocturnal hemoglobinuria: A classic description by Paul Strübing in 1882, and a bibliography of the disease. *Blood* 6:270, 1951.
2. Strübing P: Paroxysmale Haemoglobinurie. *Dtsch Med Wochenschr* 8:1, 1882.
3. Hijmans van den Bergh AA: Ictère hémolytique avec crises hémoglobinuriques fragilité globulaire. *Rev Med* 31:63, 1911.
4. Takeda J, Miyata T, Kawagoe K, et al: Deficiency of the GPI anchor caused by a somatic mutation of the *PIG*-A gene in paroxysmal nocturnal hemoglobinuria. *Cell* 73:703, 1993.
5. Freman H, Hill R, Edwards AM, Wolowyk MW: Paroxysmal nocturnal hemoglobinuria in an identical twin. *Can Med Assoc J* 109:1002, 1973.
6. Endo M, Beatty PG, Vreeke TM, et al: Syngeneic bone marrow transplantation without conditioning in a patient with paroxysmal nocturnal hemoglobinuria: In vivo evidence that the mutant stem cells have a survival advantage. *Blood* 88:742, 1996.
7. Kolb HJ, Holler E, Bender-Gotze C, et al: Myeloablative conditioning for marrow transplantation in myelodysplastic syndromes and paroxysmal nocturnal haemoglobinuria. *Bone Marrow Transplant* 4:29, 1989.
8. Oni SB, Osunkoya BO, Luzzatto L: Paroxysmal nocturnal hemoglobinuria: Evidence for monoclonal origin of abnormal red cells. *Blood* 36:145, 1970.
9. Josten KM, Tooze JA, Borthwick-Clarke C, Gordon-Smith EC, Rutherford TR: Acquired aplastic anemia and paroxysmal nocturnal hemoglobinuria: Studies on clonality. *Blood* 78:3162, 1991.
10. Parlier V, Tiainen M, Beris P, et al: Trisomy 8 detection in granulomonocytic, erythrocytic and megakaryocytic lineages by chromosomal in situ suppression hybridization in a case of refractory anaemia with ringed sideroblasts complicating the course of paroxysmal nocturnal haemoglobinuria. *Br J Haematol* 81:296, 1992.
11. Luzzatto L, Bessler M: The dual pathogenesis of paroxysmal nocturnal hemoglobinuria. *Curr Opin Hematol* 3:101, 1996.
12. Rosse WF: Paroxysmal nocturnal hemoglobinuria as a molecular disease. *Medicine (Baltimore)* 76:63, 1997.
13. Rosti V, Tremml G, Soares V, et al: Murine embryonic stem cells without *PIG*-A gene activity are competent for hematopoiesis with the PNH phenotype but not for clonal expansion. *J Clin Invest* 100:1028, 1997.
14. Brodsky RA, Vala MS, Barber JP, Medof ME, Jones RJ: Resistance to apoptosis caused by *PIG*-A gene mutations in paroxysmal nocturnal hemoglobinuria. *Proc Natl Acad Sci USA* 94:8756, 1997.
15. Horikawa K, Nakakuma H, Kawaguchi T, et al: Apoptosis resistance of blood cells from patients with paroxysmal nocturnal hemoglobinuria, aplastic anemia, and myelodysplastic syndrome. *Blood* 90:2716, 1997.
16. Bessler M, Mason P, Hillmen P, Luzzatto L: Somatic mutations and cellular selection in paroxysmal nocturnal haemoglobinuria. *Lancet* 343:951, 1994.
17. Nishimura J, Inoue N, Wada H, et al: A patient with paroxysmal nocturnal hemoglobinuria bearing four independent *PIG*-A mutant clones. *Blood* 89:3470, 1997.
18. Hirose S, Ravi L, Prince GM, et al: Synthesis of mannosylglucosaminylinositol phospholipids in normal but not paroxysmal nocturnal hemoglobinuria cells. *Proc Natl Acad Sci USA* 89:6025, 1992.
19. Chow FL, Hall SE, Rosse WF, Telen MJ: Separation of the acetylcholin-

esterase-deficient red cells in paroxysmal nocturnal hemoglobinuria. *Blood* 67:893, 1986.

20. Beck WS, Valentine WN: Biochemical studies on leucocytes: II. Phosphatase activity in chronic lymphatic leukemia, acute leukemia, and miscellaneous hematologic conditions. *J Lab Clin Med* 38:245, 1951.

21. Pangburn MK, Schreiber RD, Muller-Eberhard HJ: Dysfunction of two erythrocyte membrane proteins in paroxysmal nocturnal hemoglobinuria. *Proc Natl Acad Sci USA* 80:5430, 1983.

22. Zalman LS, Wood LM, Frank MM, Muller-Eberhard HJ: Deficiency of the homologous restriction factor in paroxysmal nocturnal hemoglobinuria. *J Exp Med* 165:572, 1987.

23. Selvaraj P, Dustin ML, Silber R, Low MG, Springer TA: Deficiency of lymphocyte function–associated antigen 3 (LFA-3) in paroxysmal nocturnal hemoglobinuria. Functional correlates and evidence for a phosphatidylinositol membrane anchor. *J Exp Med* 166:1011, 1987.

24. Rosse WF: Paroxysmal nocturnal hemoglobinuria and decay-accelerating factor. *Annu Rev Med* 41:431, 1990.

25. Selvaraj P, Rosse WF, Silber R, Springer TA: The major Fc receptor in blood has a phosphatidylinositol anchor and is deficient in paroxysmal nocturnal hemoglobinuria. *Nature* 333:565, 1988.

26. Ploug M, Plesner T, Ronne E, et al: The receptor for urokinase-type plasminogen activator is deficient on peripheral blood leukocytes in patients with paroxysmal nocturnal hemoglobinuria. *Blood* 79:1447, 1992.

27. Simmons DL, Tan S, Tenen DG, Nicholson-Weller A, Seed B: Monocyte antigen CD14 is a phospholipid anchored membrane protein. *Blood* 73:284, 1989.

28. Rosse WF: Paroxysmal nocturnal hemoglobinuria. *Curr Top Microbiol Immunol* 178:163, 1992.

29. Merry AH, Rawlinson VI, Uchikawa M, et al: Studies on the sensitivity to complement-mediated lysis of erythrocytes (Inab phenotype) with a deficiency of DAF (decay accelerating factor). *Br J Haematol* 73:248, 1989.

30. Telen MJ, Green AM: The Inab phenotype: Characterization of the membrane protein and complement regulatory defect. *Blood* 74:437, 1989.

31. Yamashina M, Ueda E, Kinoshita T, et al: Inherited complete deficiency of 20-kilodalton homologous restriction factor (CD59) as a cause of paroxysmal nocturnal hemoglobinuria. *N Engl J Med* 323:1184, 1990.

32. Wilcox LA, Ezzell JL, Bernshaw NJ, Parker CJ: Molecular basis of the enhanced susceptibility of the erythrocytes of paroxysmal nocturnal hemoglobinuria to hemolysis in acidified serum. *Blood* 78:820, 1991.

33. Ono H, Kuno Y, Tanaka H, et al: A case of paroxysmal nocturnal hemoglobinuria without deficiency of decay-accelerating factor on erythrocytes. *Blood* 75:1746, 1990.

34. Shichishima T, Terasawa T, Hashimoto C, et al: Heterogeneous expression of decay accelerating factor and CD59/membrane attack complex inhibition factor on paroxysmal nocturnal haemoglobinuria (PNH) erythrocytes. *Br J Haematol* 78:545, 1991.

35. Hillmen P, Hows JM, Luzzatto L: Two distinct patterns of glycosylphosphatidylinositol (GPI) linked protein deficiency in the red cells of patients with paroxysmal nocturnal haemoglobinuria. *Br J Haematol* 80:399, 1992.

36. Devine DV, Siegel RS, Rosse WF: Interactions of the platelets in paroxysmal nocturnal hemoglobinuria with complement: Relationship to defects in the regulation of complement and to platelet survival in vivo. *J Clin Invest* 79:131, 1987.

37. Okuda K, Kanamaru A, Ueda E, Kitani T, Nagai K: Membrane expression of decay-accelerating factor on neutrophils from normal individuals and patients with paroxysmal nocturnal hemoglobinuria. *Blood* 75:1186, 1990.

38. Craddock PR, Fehr J, Jacob HS: Complement-mediated granulocyte dysfunction in paroxysmal nocturnal hemoglobinuria. *Blood* 47:931, 1976.

39. Alfinito F, Del Vecchio L, Rocco S, et al: Blood cell flow cytometry in paroxysmal nocturnal hemoglobinuria: A tool for measuring the extent of the PNH clone. *Leukemia* 10:1326, 1996.

40. Hillmen P, Bessler M, Crawford DH, Luzzatto L: Production and characterization of lymphoblastoid cell lines with the paroxysmal nocturnal hemoglobinuria phenotype. *Blood* 81:193, 1993.

41. Ham TH: Studies on destruction of red blood cells: I. Chronic hemolytic anemia with paroxysmal nocturnal hemoglobinuria: An investigation of

the mechanism of hemolysis, with observations on five cases. *Arch Intern Med* 64:1271, 1939.

42. Crosby WH: Paroxysmal nocturnal hemoglobinuria. Relation of the clinical manifestations to underlying pathogenic mechanisms. *Blood* 8:769, 1953.

43. Blum SF, Sullivan JM, Gardner FH: The exacerbation of hemolysis in paroxysmal nocturnal hemoglobinuria by strenuous exercise. *Blood* 30:513, 1967.

44. Clark DA, Butler SA, Braren V, Hartmann RC, Jenkins DE Jr: The kidneys in paroxysmal nocturnal hemoglobinuria. *Blood* 57:83, 1981.

45. Mengel CE, Kann HE Jr, O'Malley BW: Increased hemolysis after intramuscular iron administration in patients with paroxysmal nocturnal hemoglobinuria: Report of six occurrences in four patients, and speculations on a possible mechanism. *Blood* 26:74, 1965.

46. Rosse WF, Gutterman LG: The effect of iron therapy in paroxysmal nocturnal hemoglobinuria. *Blood* 36:559, 1970.

47. Nafa K, Bessler M, Mason P, et al: Factor V Leiden mutation investigated by amplification created restriction enzyme site (ACRES) in PNH patients with and without thrombosis. *Haematologica* 81:540, 1996.

48. Valla D, Dhumeaux D, Babany G, et al: Hepatic vein thrombosis in paroxysmal nocturnal hemoglobinuria: A spectrum from asymptomatic occlusion of hepatic venules to fatal Budd-Chiari syndrome. *Gastroenterology* 93:569, 1987.

49. Leibowitz AI, Hartmann RC: Annotation: The Budd-Chiari syndrome and paroxysmal nocturnal haemoglobinuria. *Br J Haematol* 48:1, 1981.

50. Wyatt HA, Mowat AP, Layton M: Paroxysmal nocturnal haemoglobinuria and Budd-Chiari syndrome. *Arch Dis Child* 72:241, 1995.

51. Birgens HS, Hancke S, Rosenklint A, Hansen NE: Ultrasonic demonstration of clinical and subclinical hepatic venous thrombosis in paroxysmal nocturnal haemoglobinuria. *Br J Haematol* 64:737, 1986.

52. Blum SF, Gardner FH: Intestinal infarction in paroxysmal nocturnal hemoglobinuria. *N Engl J Med* 274:1137, 1966.

53. Doukas MA, DiLorenzo PE, Mohler DN: Intestinal infarction caused by paroxysmal nocturnal hemoglobinuria. *Am J Hematol* 16:75, 1984.

54. Heller PG, Grinberg AR, Lencioni M, Molina MM, Roncorini AJ: Pulmonary hypertension in paroxysmal nocturnal hemoglobinuria. *Chest* 102:642, 1992.

55. Klein KL, Hartmann RC: Acute coronary artery thrombosis in paroxysmal nocturnal hemoglobinuria. *South Med J* 82:1169, 1989.

56. Jacobs P, Wood L: Paroxysmal nocturnal haemoglobinuria and pregnancy. *Lancet* 2:1099, 1986.

57. De Gramont A, Krulik M, Debray J: Paroxysmal nocturnal haemoglobinuria and pregnancy. *Lancet* 1:868, 1987.

58. Beresford CH, Gudex DJ, Symmans WA: Paroxysmal nocturnal haemoglobinuria and pregnancy. *Lancet* 2:1396, 1986.

59. Blaisdell RK, Priest RE, Beutler E: Paroxysmal nocturnal hemoglobinuria: A case report with a negative Ham presumptive test associated with serum properdin deficiency. *Blood* 13:1074, 1958.

60. Jackson GH, Noble RS, Maung ZT, et al: Severe haemolysis and renal failure in a patient with paroxysmal nocturnal haemoglobinuria. *J Clin Pathol* 45:176, 1992.

61. Zachée P, Henckens M, Van Damme B, et al: Chronic renal failure due to renal hemosiderosis in a patient with paroxysmal nocturnal hemoglobinuria. *Clin Nephrol* 39:28, 1993.

62. Hauser D, Barzilai N, Zalish M, Oliver M, Pollack A: Bilateral papilledema with retinal hemorrhages in association with cerebral venous sinus thrombosis and paroxysmal nocturnal hemoglobinuria. *Am J Ophthalmol* 122:592, 1996.

63. Olson D, Hillmen P, Luzzatto L, Blasi F: Absence of a cell surface urokinase receptor in the white blood cells of three patients with paroxysmal nocturnal hemoglobinuria. *Fibrinolysis* 6(suppl 4):89, 1992.

64. Dacie JV: *The Haemolytic Anemias*. Grune & Stratton, New York, 1967.

65. Hartmann RC, Jenkins DE Jr: The "sugar-water" test for paroxysmal nocturnal hemoglobinuria. *N Engl J Med* 275:155, 1965.

66. Ham TH, Dingle JH: Studies on destruction of red blood cells: II. Chronic hemolytic anemia with paroxysmal nocturnal hemoglobinuria: Certain immunological aspects of the hemolytic mechanism with special reference to serum complement. *J Clin Invest* 18:657, 1939.

67. Hall SE, Rosse WF: The use of monoclonal antibodies and flow cytometry in the diagnosis of paroxysmal nocturnal hemoglobinuria. *Blood* 87:5332, 1996.

68. Shichishima T, Terasawa T, Saitoh Y, et al: Diagnosis of paroxysmal

nocturnal haemoglobinuria by phenotypic analysis of erythrocytes using two-colour flow cytometry with monoclonal antibodies to DAF and CD59/MACIF. *Br J Haematol* 85:378, 1993.

69. Schubert J, Alvarado M, Uciechowski P, et al: Diagnosis of paroxysmal nocturnal haemoglobinuria using immunophenotyping of peripheral blood cells. *Br J Haematol* 79:487, 1991.

70. Guimbretière L, Bernard D, Maisonneuve H, et al: Paroxysmal nocturnal haemoglobinuria: Diagnosis aided by a monoclonal antibody directed against the decay accelerating factor glycoprotein. *Presse Med* 22:467, 1993.

71. Meletis J, Michali E, Samarkos M, et al: Detection of "PNH red cell" populations in hematological disorders using the sephacryl gel test micro typing system. *Leuk Lymphoma* 28:177, 1997.

72. Brecher ME, Taswell HF: Paroxysmal nocturnal hemoglobinuria and the transfusion of washed red cells: A myth revisited. *Transfusion* 29:681, 1989.

73. Rosse WF: Transfusion in paroxysmal nocturnal hemoglobinuria: To wash or not to wash. *Transfusion* 29:663, 1989.

74. Hartmann RC, Jenkins DE Jr, McKee LC, Heyssel RM: Paroxysmal nocturnal hemoglobinuria: Clinical and laboratory studies relating to iron metabolism and therapy with androgen and iron. *Medicine (Baltimore)* 45:331, 1966.

75. Lippman SM, Durie BG, Garewal HS, Giordano G, Greenberg BR: Efficacy of danazol in pure red cell aplasia. *Am J Hematol* 23:373, 1986.

76. Crosby WH: Paroxysmal nocturnal hemoglobinuria: Plasma factors of the hemolytic system. *Blood* 8:444, 1953.

77. Hartmann RC, Luther AB, Jenkins DE Jr, Tenorio LE, Saba HI: Fulminant hepatic venous thrombosis (Budd-Chiari syndrome) in paroxysmal nocturnal hemoglobinuria: Definition of a medical emergency. *Johns Hopkins Med J* 146:247, 1980.

78. Sholar PW, Bell WR: Thrombolytic therapy for inferior vena cava thrombosis in paroxysmal nocturnal hemoglobinuria. *Ann Intern Med* 103:539, 1985.

79. Antin JH, Ginsburg D, Smith BR, et al: Bone marrow transplantation for paroxysmal nocturnal hemoglobinuria: Eradication of the PNH clone and documentation of complete lymphohematopoietic engraftment. *Blood* 66:1247, 1985.

80. Szer J, Deeg HJ, Witherspoon RP, et al: Long-term survival after marrow transplantation for paroxysmal nocturnal hemoglobinuria with aplastic anemia. *Ann Intern Med* 101:193, 1984.

81. Kawahara K, Witherspoon RP, Storb R: Marrow transplantation for paroxysmal nocturnal hemoglobinuria. *Am J Hematol* 39:283, 1992.

82. Graham ML, Rosse WF, Halperin EC, Miller CR, Ware RE: Resolution of Budd-Chiari syndrome following bone marrow transplantation for paroxysmal nocturnal haemoglobinuria. *Br J Haematol* 92:707, 1996.

83. Perez-Oteyza J, Roldan E, Brieva JA, et al: Expression of phosphatidyl-inositol anchored membrane proteins in paroxysmal nocturnal haemoglobinuria after bone marrow transplantation. *Bone Marrow Transplant* 10:297, 1992.

84. Astori C, Bonfichi M, Pagnucco G, et al: Treatment with recombinant human erythropoietin (rHuEpo) in a patient with paroxysmal nocturnal haemoglobinuria: Evaluation of membrane proteins CD55 and CD59 with cytofluorometric assay. *Br J Haematol* 97:586, 1997.

85. Stebler C, Tichelli A, Dazzi H, et al: High-dose recombinant human erythropoietin for treatment of anemia in myelodysplastic syndromes and paroxysmal nocturnal hemoglobinuria: A pilot study. *Exp Hematol* 18:1204, 1990.

86. Stratton F, Wilkinson JF, Israels MCG: Clinical dextran for acute episodes in paroxysmal nocturnal hemoglobinuria. *Lancet* 1:831, 1958.

87. Gardner FH, Laforet MT: The use of clinical dextran in patients with paroxysmal nocturnal hemoglobinuria. *J Lab Clin Med* 55:946, 1960.

88. Beutler E, Collins Z: The effect of 6-mercaptopurine (6-MP) administration in paroxysmal nocturnal hemoglobinuria (PNH). Proceedings of the 10th Congress of the International Society of Hematology, Stockholm, August 30–September 4, 1964.

89. Schubert J, Scholz C, Geissler RG, Ganser A, Schmidt RE: G-CSF and cyclosporin induce an increase of normal cells in hypoplastic paroxysmal nocturnal hemoglobinuria. *Ann Hematol* 74:225, 1997.

90. Van Kamp H, Van Imhoff GW, de Wolf JT, et al: The effect of cyclosporine on haematological parameters in patients with paroxysmal nocturnal haemoglobinuria. *Br J Haematol* 89:79, 1995.

91. Ware RE, Hall SE, Rosse WF: Paroxysmal nocturnal hemoglobinuria with onset in childhood and adolescence. *N Engl J Med* 325:991, 1991.

92. Devine DV, Gluck WL, Rosse WF, Weinberg JB: Acute myeloblastic leukemia in paroxysmal nocturnal hemoglobinuria: Evidence of evolution from the abnormal paroxysmal nocturnal hemoglobinuria clone. *J Clin Invest* 79:314, 1987.

93. Teyssier JR, Pigeon F, Behar C, Pignon B, Blaise AM: Chromosomal subclonal evolution in paroxysmal nocturnal hemoglobinuria evolving into acute megakaryoblastic leukemia. *Cancer Genet Cytogenet* 25:259, 1987.

94. Aymard JP, Buisine J, Gregoire MJ, Janot C, Streiff F: Refractory anaemia with excess of blasts as a terminal evolution of paroxysmal nocturnal haemoglobinuria. *Acta Haematol (Basel)* 74:181, 1985.

95. Ko WS, Chen LM, Chao TY, Hwang WS: Myeloblastic leukemoid reaction in paroxysmal nocturnal hemoglobinuria associated with myelodysplasia. *Acta Haematol (Basel)* 87:75, 1992.

96. Graham DL, Gastineau DA: Paroxysmal nocturnal hemoglobinuria as a marker for clonal myelopathy. *Am J Med* 93:671, 1992.

97. Zittoun R, Bernadou A, James IM, Soria J, Bousser J: Acute myelomonocytic leukaemia: A terminal complication of paroxysmal nocturnal haemoglobinuria. *Acta Haematol (Basel)* 53:241, 1975.

98. Socie G, Mary JY, De Gramont A, et al: Paroxysmal nocturnal haemoglobinuria: Long-term follow-up and prognostic factors. *Lancet* 348:573, 1996.

99. Hillmen P, Lewis SM, Bessler M, Luzzatto L, Dacic JV: Natural history of paroxysmal nocturnal hemoglobinuria. *N Engl J Med* 333:1253, 1995.

THE MEGALOBLASTIC ANEMIAS

BERNARD M. BABIOR

Megaloblastic anemia is most commonly due to a deficiency of folate or cobalamin (vitamin B_{12}). Folate deficiency is usually nutritional in origin and may be seen in alcoholics and the elderly poor but also in patients on hyperalimentation or hemodialysis. In pregnancy, even a mild folate deficiency is associated with defects in neural tube closure in the fetus, so folate supplements should always be given to pregnant women. Diagnosis is based on measurements of folate in serum, which furnishes information about the current level of folate, and in red cells, which provides data on folate levels over the preceding 6 weeks. Nutritional folate deficiency is treated with folic acid by mouth.

Folate deficiency due to malabsorption occurs in tropical and nontropical sprue. Folate deficiency due to tropical sprue is treated with folate supplements plus antibiotics; in nontropical sprue, the treatment is folate plus a gluten-free diet.

The commonest cause of cobalamin deficiency is pernicious anemia, a condition in which the portion of gastric mucosa that contains the parietal cells is destroyed through an autoimmune mechanism. The parietal cells secrete intrinsic factor, which is essential for cobalamin absorption, and without intrinsic factor a state of cobalamin deficiency develops over the course of years. Cobalamin deficiency leads not only to megaloblastic anemia but also to a demyelinating disease that manifests itself as peripheral neuropathy, spastic paralysis with ataxia (so-called combined system disease of the spinal cord), dementia, psychosis, or a combination of the foregoing. "Subtle" cobalamin deficiency, manifested as neurologic symptoms without anemia, appears to be relatively widespread among the elderly. The incidence of gastric cancer is increased by a factor of 2 to 3 in patients with pernicious anemia. Other causes of cobalamin deficiency are gastric resection; stasis of the small intestinal contents due to blind loops, strictures, or hypomotility (seen, for example, in amyloid); or disease or resection of the terminal ileum. Patients on a vegan diet will also become cobalamin deficient. The diagnosis of cobalamin deficiency is made by measuring the level of the vitamin in the blood or by measuring serum methylmalonic acid, which accumulates in the blood stream in patients with cobalamin deficiency. The cause of the cobalamin deficiency can often be determined by the Schilling test, a measure of cobalamin absorption. In patients with nutritional megaloblastic anemia, it is of great importance to establish whether the anemia is due to folate deficiency or cobalamin deficiency, because if a patient with cobalamin deficiency is treated with folic acid, the anemia will be corrected but the neurologic abnormalities will progress. Patients with cobalamin deficiency are usually treated with parenteral cobalamin.

Megaloblastic anemia can develop as an acute disorder with rapid development of leukopenia and/or thrombocytopenia. Nitrous oxide anesthesia is responsible for some cases of acute megaloblastic anemia. It is also seen in patients with a marginal folate status in intensive care units. The condition resembles an immune cytopenia, but this can be ruled out by examining the bone marrow, which exhibits a floridly megaloblastic picture.

Other causes of megaloblastic anemia include drugs (e.g., hydroxyurea, nucleoside analogs) and certain inborn errors of metabolism. Of these inherited conditions, transcobalamin II deficiency is singled out because it causes a severe megaloblastic anemia in infants that responds completely to high-dose cobalamin; if it is not detected in time, however, irreversible neurologic complications will supervene. Finally, megaloblastic anemia is seen in refractory megaloblastic anemia, a form of the myelodysplastic syndrome, and in early stages of acute myeloblastic leukemia of the M6 type (Di Guglielmo's syndrome). The anemia of refractory megaloblastic anemia sometimes responds to pyridoxine in very high doses.

GENERAL CONSIDERATIONS

DEFINITION

Megaloblastic anemias are disorders caused by impaired DNA synthesis and characterized by the presence of megaloblastic cells, the morphologic hallmark of this group of anemias. Megaloblastic red cell precursors are larger than normal and have more cytoplasm relative to the size of the nucleus. Promegaloblasts show a blue granule-free cytoplasm and a granular chromatin that contrasts with the ground-glass texture of its normal counterpart (see Color Plate VI-4). As the cell differentiates, the chromatin condenses more slowly than normal into dark aggregates that coalesce to give the nucleus a characteristic fenestrated appearance. Condensation of the chromatin to a homogeneous mass either fails or is delayed. As the cytoplasm acquires hemoglobin, its growing maturity contrasts with the immature-looking nucleus, a feature termed *nuclear-cytoplasmic asynchrony*.

Megaloblastic granulocyte precursors are also larger than normal and show nuclear-cytoplasmic asynchrony, with cytoplasm that looks less mature than that of their normal counterparts. A characteristic cell is the *giant metamyelocyte*, with a large horseshoe-shaped nucleus, sometimes irregular in shape, containing ragged chromatin.

Megaloblastic megakaryocytes may be abnormally large, with deficient granulation of the cytoplasm. In severe megaloblastosis, the nucleus may show unattached lobes.

ETIOLOGY AND PATHOGENESIS

The causes of megaloblastic anemia are listed in Table 37-1. By far the most common of these are folate deficiency and cobalamin deficiency. Megaloblastic cells have much more cytoplasm and RNA than do their normal counterparts but have a relatively normal amount of DNA,[1,2] suggesting that cytoplasmic constituents (RNA and protein) are synthesized faster than is DNA. Supporting this conclusion is

Acronyms and abbreviations that appear in this chapter include: BFU–E, burst forming units–erythroid; CNS, central nervous system; dTMP, deoxythymidine monophosphate; dU, deoxyuracil; dUMP, deoxyuridine monophosphate; HIV, human immunodeficiency virus; IM, intramuscular; LDH, lactate dehydrogenase; MCV, mean corpuscular volume; MRI, magnetic resonance imaging; MTHFR, methylenetetrahydrofolate reductase; PA, pernicious anemia; PDW, platelet distribution width; SAH, S-adenosylhomocysteine; SAM, S-adenosylmethionine; TC, transcobalamin; UTP, uridine triphosphate.

TABLE 37-1   CLASSIFICATION OF THE MEGALOBLASTIC ANEMIAS

Folate deficiency	Acute megaloblastic anemia
Decreased intake	Nitrous oxide exposure
Poor nutrition	Severe illness with:
Old age, poverty, alcoholism	Extensive transfusion
Hyperalimentation	Dialysis
Hemodialysis	Total parenteral nutrition
Premature infants	Exposure to weak folate antagonists (e.g., trimethoprim
Children on synthetic diets	or low-dose methotrexate)
Goat's milk anemia	Drugs
Impaired absorption	Dihydrofolate reductase inhibitors
Nontropical sprue	Antimetabolites
Tropical sprue	Inhibitors of deoxynucleotide synthesis
Other disease of the small intestine	Miscellaneous
Increased requirements	Anticonvulsants
Pregnancy	Oral contraceptives
Increased cell turnover	Others
Chronic hemolytic anemia	Inborn errors
Exfoliative dermatitis	Cobalamin deficiency
Cobalamin deficiency	Imerslund-Gräsbeck disease
Impaired absorption	Congenital deficiency of intrinsic factor
Gastric causes	Transcobalamin II deficiency
Pernicious anemia	Errors of folate metabolism
Gastrectomy	Congenital folate malabsorption
Zollinger-Ellison syndrome	Dihydrofolate reductase deficiency
Intestinal causes	N^5-methyl FH_4: homocysteine methyltransferase
Ileal resection or disease	deficiency
Blind loop syndrome	Errors of cobalamin metabolism
Fish tapeworm	"Cobalamin mutant" syndromes with homocysteinuria
Pancreatic insufficiency	Others
Decreased intake	Hereditary orotic aciduria
Vegetarianism	Lesch-Nyhan syndrome
	Thiamine-responsive megaloblastic anemia
	Unexplained
	Congenital dyserythropoietic anemia
	Refractory megaloblastic anemia
	Erythroleukemia

evidence that in megaloblastic precursors maturation is retarded,[1,3] DNA synthesis is impaired,[4-6] migration of the DNA replication fork and the joining of Okazaki fragments are delayed,[7] and S phase is prolonged.[6]

The slowing of DNA replication in the megaloblastic anemias of folate and cobalamin deficiency appears to arise from a failure of the folate-dependent conversion of dUMP to dTMP (see Chap. 34). Because of this failure, and the fact that DNA polymerase has difficulty distinguishing dUTP from dTTP, dUTP instead of dTTP is incorporated into the DNA of folate-deficient cells.[8,9] Recognizing the mistake, the cells try to repair the DNA by replacing uridine with thymidine, but these attempts at repair tend to fail for the same reason that UTP was incorporated into the DNA in the first place. The result is a frustrated effort at DNA repair leading ultimately to DNA fragmentation followed by cell death.

dU normally inhibits the incorporation of tritiated thymidine into DNA, probably because it is converted via dUMP→dTMP to unlabeled dTTP that competes with the tritiated thymidine. In megaloblastic cells, this effect of dU is greatly diminished. This finding is consistent with an impairment in the dUMP→dTMP reaction in the megaloblastic cells and is the basis for the *dU suppression test* described below. This model also explains the chromosome breaks and other abnormalities that occur in megaloblastic cells.[10-13]

There is a curious group of findings suggesting that the megaloblastic line may arise from a more "primitive" precursor than is the case for the normoblastic line. Megaloblasts contain high concentrations of fetal hemoglobin[14] and the fetal isozyme of thymidine kinase.[15] Like megaloblasts, BFU-E (see Chap. 38) grown with monocyte-conditioned medium are rich in γ-globin chains and appear megalo-

blastic, but BFU-E from the same source but grown with T lymphocytes appear normal and contain the usual proportion of γ-globin chains.[16,17] The relationship between these observations and the pathogenesis of the nutritional megaloblastic anemias remains to be determined.

CLINICAL FEATURES

All megaloblastic anemias share certain general clinical features. Because the anemia develops slowly, it produces few symptoms until the hematocrit is severely depressed. When symptoms appear, they are those of anemia: weakness, palpitation, fatigue, light-headedness, and shortness of breath. Severe pallor and slight jaundice combine to produce a tell-tale lemon-yellow skin. Leukocyte and platelet counts may also be low but rarely cause clinical problems. Details of the clinical manifestations are given in the sections on the specific forms of megaloblastic anemia later in this chapter.

LABORATORY FEATURES

BLOOD CELLS

All cell lines are affected. Erythrocytes vary markedly in size and shape, are often large and oval, and in severe cases can show basophilic stippling and nuclear remnants (Howell-Jolly bodies, Cabot rings). The reticulocyte count is low. The more severe the anemia, the more pronounced the morphologic changes in the red cells. When the hematocrit is less than 20 percent, red cells with megaloblastic nuclei, including an occasional promegaloblast, may appear in the blood. The anemia is macrocytic (MCV = 100 to 150 fl or more), although coexisting iron deficiency, thalassemia trait, or inflammation can prevent macrocytosis.[18] Slight macrocytosis is often the earliest sign of megaloblastic anemia.

Neutrophil nuclei often have more than the usual three to five lobes[19] (Fig. 37-1). Typically, more than 5 percent of the neutrophils

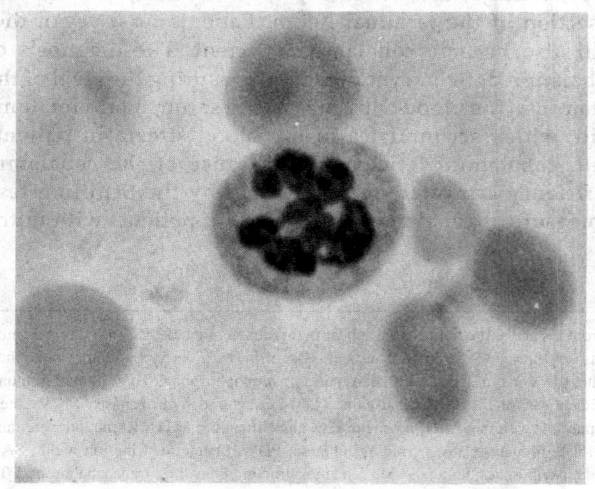

FIGURE 37-1   Megaloblastic hypersegmented neutrophil. ×1500.

have five lobes, and cells may appear containing six or more lobes, morphology never seen in normal neutrophils. In nutritional megaloblastic anemias, hypersegmented neutrophils are an early sign of megaloblastosis[19,20] and persist in the blood for many days after treatment.[21] Chromosomes are elongated and broken.[4,10,22] Specific therapy corrects these abnormalities, usually within 2 days, though some take months to disappear.[10] Platelets are slightly smaller than normal and vary more widely in size (increased PDW).[23]

MARROW

Aspirated marrow is cellular and shows striking megaloblastic changes, especially in the erythroid series. Sideroblasts are increased in number and contain increased numbers of iron granules. The ratio of myeloid to erythroid precursors (M/E ratio) falls to 1:1 or lower, and granulocyte reserves may be decreased.[24] In severe cases, promegaloblasts containing an unusually large number of mitotic figures are plentiful. Macrophage iron content is often increased.

Atypical Morphology in Megaloblastic Anemia Under certain circumstances, megaloblastic anemia may be overlooked because its characteristic morphology is imperfectly expressed.

Coexisting Microcytic Anemia. When combined with a microcytic anemia, many features of megaloblastic anemia may be masked.[25] The anemia could be normocytic or even microcytic, while the blood film may show both microcytes and macro-ovalocytes (a "dimorphic anemia") or microcytes alone if the microcytic component is sufficiently severe. The marrow may contain "intermediate" megaloblasts[26] that are smaller and less "megaloblastic"-looking than usual. In this kind of mixed anemia, the microcytic component is usually iron-deficiency anemia,[18] but it may be thalassemia minor or the anemia of chronic disease.[18,27] Even when masked by a severe microcytic anemia, however, a megaloblastic anemia will usually show hypersegmented neutrophils in the blood and giant metamyelocytes and bands in the marrow, and neutrophil myeloperoxidase levels will be high.[28]

The megaloblastic component of a mixed iron-deficiency anemia can sometimes be overlooked, and the patient may be treated only with iron. In this case the anemia will respond only partly to therapy, and megaloblastic features will emerge as iron stores fill.

Incomplete Megaloblastic Anemia. If a patient with a full-blown megaloblastic anemia receives cobalamin or folate before marrow aspiration, the anemia will persist but the megaloblastic changes may be obscured. Attenuated megaloblastic changes are also seen in patients with early megaloblastic anemia, in patients with coexisting infection, or after transfusion.

Megaloblastic Anemia Misdiagnosed as Acute Leukemia. Occasionally, very severe megaloblastic anemia may produce marrow morphology so bizarre as to be mistaken for acute leukemia, especially if the marrow lacks classical megaloblasts and displays as its principal cell type the bizarre megaloblastic white cell precursors that in a more typical morphologic background would support the diagnosis of a megaloblastic anemia. In some cases, there is no maturation of the erythroid series, and the megaloblastic pronormoblast dominates the marrow, raising the possibility of erythroid leukemia.

MEGALOBLASTIC CHANGES IN OTHER CELLS

In most forms of megaloblastic anemia, cytologic abnormalities resembling megaloblastosis may appear in other proliferating cells. Epithelial cells from the mouth, stomach, small intestine, and cervix uteri may look megaloblastic, appearing larger than their normal counterparts and containing atypical immature-looking nuclei.[28,29] It is sometimes difficult to distinguish these "megaloblastic" changes from those of malignancy.

CHEMICAL CHANGES IN BODY FLUIDS

Plasma bilirubin, iron, and ferritin levels are somewhat increased.[30] Serum LDH-1 and LDH-2 are markedly elevated, increasing with the severity of the anemia.[31] In megaloblastic anemia LDH-1 is greater than LDH-2, while in other anemias LDH-2 is greater than LDH-1.[32] Serum muramidase (lysozyme) levels are also high,[33] while serum glutamic oxaloacetic transaminase is normal.[34] Erythropoietin levels rise, but less than in other anemias of similar severity.[35] Surprisingly, the elevated erythropoietin levels fall sharply within 1 day of the beginning of treatment, an interval too short to affect the hematocrit.

CYTOKINETICS

Megaloblastic anemia is associated with two pathophysiologic abnormalities: *ineffective erythropoiesis* and *hemolysis*. Ineffective erythropoiesis causes increases in the red cell precursor/reticulocyte ratio, plasma iron turnover,[36] LDH-1 and LDH-2,[37] and "early-labeled" bilirubin.[38] Extramedullary hemolysis also occurs in megaloblastic anemia, with red cell life span decreased by 30 to 50 percent.[39]

Increased serum muramidase in megaloblastic anemia may be caused by increased granulocyte turnover,[33] possibly induced by the disintegration of granulocyte precursors in the marrow (ineffective granulopoiesis). In cobalamin deficiency, platelet production is only 10 percent of that expected from the megakaryocyte mass,[40] perhaps reflecting ineffective thrombopoiesis. Platelets in severe cobalamin deficiency are functionally abnormal.[41]

FOLIC ACID DEFICIENCY

ETIOLOGY AND PATHOGENESIS

Folate deficiency is caused by (1) dietary deficiency, (2) impaired absorption, and (3) increased requirements (see Table 37-1).

DECREASED INTAKE CAUSED BY POOR NUTRITION

An inadequate diet is the major cause of folate deficiency. Because folate reserves are small, deficiency develops rapidly in malnourished persons, typically the old, the poor, and the alcoholic. Folate deficiency can also occur during hyperalimentation[42] or hemodialysis, where folate is lost in the dialysis fluid.[43] Subclinical folate deficiency has been reported in subtotal gastrectomy.[44] Folate deficiency can occur in *premature infants,* especially with infection, diarrhea, or hemolytic anemia[45]; in children on a *synthetic diet* for inborn errors[46]; and in infants raised on *goat's milk,* which is folate-poor.[47] Destruction of folate through excessive cooking can aggravate folate deficiency (see Chap. 30).

In alcoholic cirrhosis, megaloblastic anemia is usually caused by folate deficiency.[21] In addition, alcohol may acutely depress the serum folate, even if folate stores are full,[48] and will accelerate the development of megaloblastic anemia in someone with early folate deficiency.[49–51] Alcohol causes acute marrow suppression, with declines in reticulocyte, platelet, and granulocyte levels[49,52,53]; reversible vacuolation of erythroid and myeloid precursors[54]; and dysfunction of granulocytes.[54] These changes occur even if large doses of folate are given with the alcohol.[55]

DECREASED INTAKE CAUSED BY IMPAIRED ABSORPTION

Nontropical Sprue Nontropical sprue (*celiac disease* in children) is related to the ingestion of wheat gluten.[56] Pathologically, nontropical sprue shows atrophy and chronic inflammation of the small intestinal mucosa, most severe proximally. Findings may include weight loss, glossitis (typical of folate deficiency), and other signs of a generalized vitamin deficiency, diarrhea, and the passage of light-colored, bulky stools with an unusually foul odor. Iron deficiency, hypocalcemia, osteoporosis, and osteomalacia may also occur.

Folate malabsorption occurs in most patients with this disorder.[57,58] Serum folate levels are low,[59,60] and megaloblastic anemia occurs frequently.

Tropical Sprue Tropical sprue is endemic in the West Indies, southern India, parts of southern Africa, and Southeast Asia. It can be acquired by travelers to those regions and persists for many years after they return.[61] Tropical sprue is rapidly corrected by folate therapy, even though folate deficiency does not give rise to the disease. The etiology of tropical sprue is unknown, although infection is suggested by the response of the disease to antibiotics.[62,63]

Clinically and pathologically, tropical sprue is like nontropical sprue, except that tropical sprue is more severe in the distal small intestine.[64] Therefore, tropical sprue usually leads to cobalamin deficiency[65] and should be strongly considered as a cause of cobalamin deficiency in former residents of the tropics, even though they have been away from the tropics for 20 years or more. Folate malabsorption may also occur,[66] possibly because the diseased intestine fails to deconjugate folate polyglutamates.[67] Megaloblastic anemia is therefore very common in this disease[68] and may be due to both folate and cobalamin deficiency.

Other Intestinal Disorders Malabsorption of folic acid commonly occurs in regional enteritis,[68] after extensive resections of the small intestine,[69] in lymphomatous or leukemic infiltration of the small intestine,[70] in Whipple disease,[70] in scleroderma and amyloidosis,[71] and in diabetes mellitus.[72] Systemic bacterial infections also impair folate absorption.[73]

INCREASED FOLATE REQUIREMENTS

Pregnancy[74] During pregnancy, folate requirements increase five- to tenfold because of transfer of folate to the growing fetus,[75] which will draw down maternal folate stores even in the face of severe maternal folate deficiency.[76] Further increases may result from the presence of multiple fetuses, a poor diet, infection, coexisting hemolytic anemia, or anticonvulsant medication. Lactation aggravates folate deficiency.[77] Consequently, folate deficiency is very common in pregnancy[78] and is the major cause of the megaloblastic anemia of pregnancy.[79]

Folate deficiency, however, is difficult to diagnose in pregnancy because its signs are obscured by the normal hematologic changes of pregnancy. During pregnancy, a physiologic "anemia" develops because of an increase in plasma volume that is only partly offset by an accompanying increase in red cell mass (Fig. 37-2); hemoglobin levels may fall to 10 g/dl. This anemia is associated with a physiologic macrocytosis; rises in the MCV of 20 fl occur, although the average at term is 4 fl.[80] Serum and red cell folate levels fall steadily during pregnancy even in well-nourished women.[81] All these changes are false clues that suggest folate deficiency even when folate levels are normal. Conversely, hypersegmented neutrophils, usually a reliable clue to early megaloblastic anemia, are missing in early megaloblastic anemia of pregnancy.[82] In many cases, the only finding that can reliably distinguish the physiologic anemia of pregnancy from folate deficiency is a megaloblastic marrow.

Increased Cell Turnover Because of increased marrow cell turnover, the folate requirement rises sharply in chronic *hemolytic anemia*.[83,84] During the bouts of acute hemolysis that may occur in these anemias, the marrow may become megaloblastic within days. Sometimes folate therapy is successful only if unusually large doses (up to 25 mg/day) are given.[83,84]

Folic acid deficiency may arise in chronic *exfoliative dermatitis*, in which folate losses of 5 to 20 μg/day may occur.[85] Patients with psoriasis who are treated with methotrexate have an added reason for developing signs of folate deficiency. Pretreating such patients with folate may prevent these signs without impairing the therapeutic effect of methotrexate.[85]

CLINICAL FEATURES

The clinical picture of folate deficiency includes all the nonspecific manifestations of megaloblastic anemia described above *plus* the following specific features: (1) a history and laboratory studies indicating folate deficiency, (2) absence of the neurologic signs of cobalamin deficiency (see "Cobalamin Deficiency"),* and (3) a full response to *physiologic* doses of folate.

LABORATORY FEATURES

The earliest indicator of folate deficiency is a *low serum folate*. Serum folate follows folate intake closely, so a low serum folate (below about 3 ng/ml) may indicate only a drop in folate intake over the preceding few days.[20] Similarly, a low serum folate will rise quickly on refeeding, so serum should be frozen early in case a later assay is necessary.

A better indicator of the tissue folate status is the *red cell folate*,[86] which remains relatively unchanged while a red cell is circulating and thus reflects folate turnover over the preceding 2 to 3 months. Red cell folate is usually quite low in folate-deficient megaloblastic anemia. It is also low, however, in more than 50 percent of patients with cobalamin-deficient megaloblastic anemia[87] and therefore cannot be used to distinguish between these two deficiencies. Conversely, red cell folate may be normal in the megaloblastic state that occurs, often with little accompanying anemia, in rapidly developing folate deficiency (see "Acute Megaloblastic Anemia" later in this chapter).[88]

The dU suppression test, discussed in full in "The dU Suppression Test" later in this chapter, is used in research on pathogenetic mechanisms in megaloblastic states. It adds little to the clinical evaluation of a megaloblastic anemia.

DIFFERENTIAL DIAGNOSIS

Macrocytosis occurs in alcoholism without megaloblastic anemia, liver disease, hypothyroidism, aplastic anemia, certain forms of myelodysplasia, pregnancy, and any condition associated with a reticulocytosis (e.g., autoimmune hemolytic anemia), but in these conditions the MCV rarely exceeds 110 fl.

A full hematologic response to physiologic doses of folate (i.e., 200 μg daily) distinguishes folate deficiency from cobalamin deficiency, in which a response occurs only at *pharmacologic* doses of folate (e.g., 5 mg daily).[29] This is *not* recommended as a diagnostic test, because neurologic problems may develop in cobalamin-deficient patients treated with folate alone. Cobalamin may produce a partial response in folate deficiency.[89]

The diagnosis of nontropical sprue rests on (1) the demonstration of malabsorption, (2) a jejunal biopsy showing villus atrophy, and (3) the response to a gluten-free diet. In 80 percent of patients, a gluten-free diet will gradually reverse the functional disorder, correcting folate malabsorption.[57]

NONHEMATOLOGIC EFFECTS OF FOLATE DEFICIENCY

The hematologic problems associated with folate deficiency have been recognized for decades. Recently, however, folate deficiency has been related to a number of serious disorders not involving the hematopoietic system. These disorders, moreover, are seen at folate levels usually regarded as low-normal. They include congenital anomalies, fragile site syndromes, and, most common of all, atherosclerosis.

ABNORMALITIES OF NEURAL TUBE CLOSURE

There is a close association between mild folate deficiency and congenital anomalies of the fetus, most notably defects in neural tube closure,

---

*Poorly defined neuropsychiatric abnormalities that respond to folate therapy have been reported in patients with folate deficiency.[89–91]

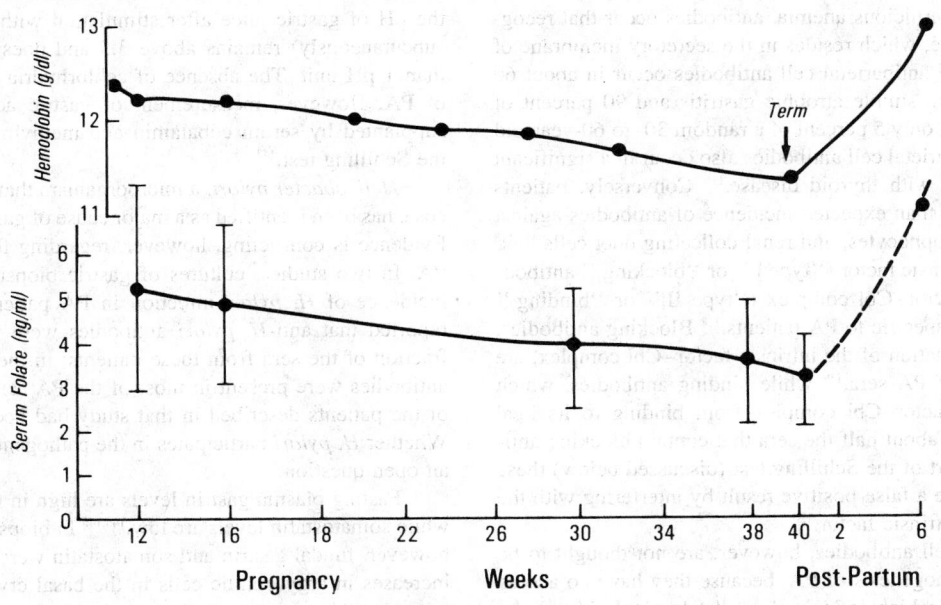

FIGURE 37-2   Hemoglobin and serum folate levels during pregnancy and the postpartum period. (Adapted from Shojania.[74])

but also abnormalities involving the heart, urinary tract, limbs, and other sites.[74,90-94] Mutations affecting enzymes of folate metabolism, especially the common 677C→T mutation of the *MTHFR* gene,[95,96] also predispose to congenital anomalies.

VASCULAR DISEASE

A mildly elevated homocysteine level is a major risk factor for atherosclerosis and venous thrombosis, possibly due to an effect on the vascular endothelium.[97-99] Homocysteine levels can be decreased with folate, cobalamin, and pyridoxine supplements, possibly reducing the risk of vascular disease.[100,101] It is curious that the 677C→T *MTHFR* mutation, which gives rise to a thermolabile enzyme, has no effect on the incidence of vascular disease.[102,103]

COLON CANCER

A large study of U.S. nurses indicated that supplementation with folate at more than 400 μg per day reduces the incidence of colon cancer by 31 percent.[104] This finding has important implications for public health. Individuals homozygous for the 677C→T methylenetetrahydrofolate reductase mutation also have a decreased incidence for colon cancer compared with 677C→T heterozygotes and normal controls.[13]

THERAPY, COURSE, AND PROGNOSIS

Folate is usually given orally at 1 to 5 mg daily, although 1 mg is usually enough. At this dose, anemia is usually corrected even in patients with malabsorption. A parenteral preparation containing 5 mg/ml of folate is also available.

Treatment for tropical sprue consists of the usual doses of folate, plus cobalamin if indicated. To prevent relapse, treatment should be maintained for at least 2 years. Broad-spectrum antibiotics are helpful adjuncts, although antibiotics alone fail to correct the condition.

It is essential that pregnant women be given at least 400 μg of folate per day.[105-107] As to the possibility of overlooking cobalamin deficiency due to folate administration, pernicious anemia in pregnancy is rare,[108] and in pregnant women at risk for cobalamin deficiency (e.g., strict vegetarians or patients with malabsorption) the deficiency

is easily prevented with 1 mg of vitamin B12 given parenterally every 3 months during the pregnancy.

Therapeutic doses of folate will partly correct the hematologic abnormalities in cobalamin deficiency, but the neurologic manifestations can progress, with disastrous results.[109] It is therefore essential to evaluate both folate status and cobalamin status early in the workup of a megaloblastic anemia. If treatment is urgent and the nature of the deficiency is unclear, both folate and cobalamin can be given after one has obtained samples for assay.

Patients who receive low-dose methotrexate therapy as an immunosuppressant may develop side effects, the worst of which is hepatotoxicity. The incidence of side effects, including hepatotoxicity, has been correlated with reduced folate levels.[110,111] These can be prevented by administration of folic or folinic acid without any reduction in the therapeutic effect of the low-dose methotrexate.

COBALAMIN DEFICIENCY

ETIOLOGY AND PATHOGENESIS

Disorders that lead to cobalamin deficiency are listed in Table 37-1.

DECREASED UPTAKE CAUSED BY IMPAIRED ABSORPTION

Cobalamin deficiency is most often a result of defective absorption, most commonly PA, a condition in which intrinsic factor production fails. There are many other causes of defective cobalamin absorption, involving the stomach, pancreas, or small intestine.

***Gastric Disorders*   Pernicious Anemia.**[*112]   Pernicious anemia is a disease of insidious onset that generally begins in middle age or later (usually after age 40). In this condition, intrinsic factor secretion fails because of gastric mucosal atrophy. Pernicious anemia is an autoimmune disease. The gastric atrophy of PA probably results from immune destruction of the acid- and pepsin-secreting portion of the gastric mucosa.

---

*The term *pernicious anemia* is sometimes used as a synonym for cobalamin deficiency, but it should be reserved for the condition resulting from defective secretion of intrinsic factor by an atrophic gastric mucosa.

In patients with pernicious anemia, antibodies occur that recognize the H^+/K^+-ATPase, which resides in the secretory membrane of the parietal cell. These antiparietal cell antibodies occur in about 60 percent of patients with simple atrophic gastritis and 90 percent of patients with PA but in only 5 percent of a random 30- to 60-year-old population.[113-115] Antiparietal cell antibodies also occur in a significant percentage of patients with thyroid disease.[116] Conversely, patients with PA have a higher than expected incidence of antibodies against thyroid epithelium, lymphocytes, and renal collecting duct cells.[117,118]

Antibodies to intrinsic factor ("type I," or "blocking," antibodies) or the intrinsic factor–Cbl complex ("type II," or "binding," antibodies) are highly specific to PA patients.[118] Blocking antibodies, which prevent the formation of the intrinsic factor–Cbl complex, are found in 70 percent of PA sera,[119] while binding antibodies, which prevent the intrinsic factor–Cbl complex from binding to its ileal receptors, are found in about half the sera that contain blocking antibody. In the second part of the Schilling test (discussed below) these antibodies may produce a false-positive result by interfering with the action of exogenous intrinsic factor.[120]

The antiparietal cell antibodies, however, are not thought to be responsible for the pathogenesis of PA, because they have no access to the H^+/K^+-ATPase, which is located on the luminal side of the parietal cell. Rather, studies in mice have suggested that the gastric atrophy in PA anemia is caused by CD4+ T cells whose receptors recognize the H^+/K^+-ATPase. Thus, thymectomized BALB/c mice develop an autoimmune atrophic gastritis similar to that seen in PA patients, and CD4+ T cells from these mice produce atrophic gastritis when injected into nude mice.[121,122]

Some findings in humans support the idea that T cells are responsible for the gastric atrophy in PA. First, lymphocytes from patients with PA are hyperresponsive to gastric antigens.[123] Second, the correlation between antiparietal cell antibodies and PA is not perfect.[114,124] Finally, the incidence of PA is higher than expected in patients with agammaglobulinemia, even though their sera contain none of the antibodies typical of PA.[125]

Other Autoimmune Diseases.   Antiparietal cell antibodies and PA are unexpectedly frequent in patients with other autoimmune diseases,[126] including autoimmune thyroid disorders (thyrotoxicosis, hypothyroidism, and Hashimoto thyroiditis),[127] type I diabetes mellitus, hypoparathyroidism,[128] Addison disease, postpartum hypophysitis,[129] ulcerative colitis,[130] vitiligo,[131] acquired agammaglobulinemia,[125] infertility in female patients under age 40,[132] and hypospermia and infertility in males.[133] The coexistence of these diseases and PA is further evidence that PA is an autoimmune disease.

Inherited Predisposition to Pernicious Anemia.   A predisposition to PA can be inherited. The disease is associated with HLA types A2, A3, B7, and B12[134] and with blood group A.[135] PA and antiparietal cell antibodies occur more frequently than expected in the families of PA patients.[136] In one study, gastric atrophy was found in more than 30 percent of the relatives of patients with PA; of these relatives, 65 percent had antiparietal cell antibodies and 22 percent had anti-intrinsic factor antibodies.[137] PA occurs relatively frequently in northern Europeans (especially Scandinavians)[137] and African Americans[124,138] but is uncommon in Asians. In African Americans, the disease tends to begin early, occurs with high frequency in women, and is often severe.[124,138]

The Stomach and Intestine in Pernicious Anemia.   Gastric manifestations in PA include achlorhydria, acquired intrinsic factor deficiency demonstrable by the Schilling test, and increases in the incidence of certain malignancies: about a twofold increase in the incidence of gastric cancer, similar increases in the incidence of certain hematologic malignancies, and an increase in the incidence of gastric carcinoid.[139,140] Achlorhydria may precede the loss of intrinsic factor secretion and the development of PA by many years.[141] It is present if the pH of gastric juice after stimulation with pentagastrin (6 μg/kg subcutaneously) remains above 3.5 and does not decrease by more than 1 pH unit. The absence of achlorhydria excludes the diagnosis of PA. However, measurement of gastric acid secretion has been supplanted by serum cobalamin and methylmalonic acid levels and the Schilling test.[142]

Helicobacter pylori, a microorganism that infects the gastric mucosa, has been identified as a major cause of gastritis and peptic ulcers. Evidence is conflicting, however, regarding the role of *H. pylori* in PA. In two studies, cultures of gastric biopsies showed a very low incidence of *H. pylori* infection in PA patients.[143,144] In one it was reported that anti-*H. pylori* antibodies were found in only a small fraction of the sera from these patients; in the other, however, these antibodies were present in most of the PA sera, indicating that most of the patients described in that study had been infected previously. Whether *H. pylori* participates in the pathogenesis of PA is at present an open question.

Fasting plasma gastrin levels are high in most patients with PA, while somatostatin levels are low.[145,146] In biopsies from PA stomachs, however, fundal gastrin and somatostatin were high, correlating with increases in argyrophilic cells in the basal crypts; antral gastrin and somatostatin were normal. Gastrin levels are also high in simple achlorhydria without PA.[147]

The stomach shows characteristic histologic abnormalities in PA (Fig. 37-3). The mucosa of the cardia and fundus is atrophic, containing few chief (i.e., pepsin-secreting) or parietal cells. The withered mucosa is infiltrated with lymphocytes[148] and plasma cells. In contrast, the antral and pyloric mucosa is normal. The gastric atrophy is partly reversible by glucocorticoid treatment, with some regeneration and return of intrinsic factor secretion, further evidence for the autoimmune nature of PA.[149]

Megaloblastic changes reversible by cobalamin are seen in the gastrointestinal epithelium. Cells recovered by lavage are large[150] and show atypical nuclei resembling early malignant change.[151] Small intestinal biopsy shows decreased mitoses in crypts, shortening of villi, megaloblastic changes in epithelial cells, and infiltration in the lamina propria.[152] These changes may account for the occasional malabsorption of D-xylose and carotene in PA.[153]

Gastrectomy Syndromes.   Gastric surgery often leads to anemia. Most common is iron-deficiency anemia, but cobalamin deficiency with megaloblastic anemia may also occur. After *total gastrectomy,* cobalamin deficiency will develop within 5 or 6 years because the operation removes the source of intrinsic factor.[154] The delay between surgery and the onset of cobalamin deficiency reflects the time needed to exhaust cobalamin stores after cobalamin absorption ceases.

After *partial gastrectomy,* few patients show frank cobalamin deficiency, but about 5 percent have intermediate megaloblastosis, approximately 25 to 50 percent have low serum cobalamin levels, and many have decreased intrinsic factor secretion (Schilling test).[155-157] Achlorhydria not present before surgery often develops some years after gastrectomy. Postgastrectomy patients with low serum cobalamin levels usually have low serum iron levels as well,[158] in contrast to the high iron levels typical of cobalamin deficiency.

Cobalamin deficiency after partial gastrectomy can be caused by mucosal atrophy in the unresected remnant of the stomach[159] or, if a gastrojejunostomy was performed, by bacterial overgrowth in the afferent loop (see "Blind Loop Syndrome"). Postgastrectomy folate deficiency from malabsorption or reduced dietary intake actually accounts for more cases of postgastrectomy megaloblastic anemia than does cobalamin deficiency. Often the two deficiencies occur together.

Zollinger-Ellison Syndrome.   In the Zollinger-Ellison syndrome, a gastrin-producing tumor, usually in the pancreas, stimulates the gastric mucosa to secrete immense amounts of HCl. The major clinical problem is a severe ulcer diathesis. Malabsorption of cobalamin occurs when the vast quantities of HCl secreted by the overactive gastric mucosa cannot be completely neutralized by the pancreatic secretions. The resulting acidification of the duodenal contents inactivates pancreatic proteases, preventing the transfer of Cbl from R binder to intrinsic factor.[160]

Intestinal Disorders   Intestinal Diseases.   A number of intestinal disorders can lead to a deficiency of cobalamin. These include (1) extensive resection of the ileum,[161] (2) regional ileitis[162] or another disease affecting the ileum (e.g., lymphoma, radiation damage[163]), (3) cobalamin malabsorption associated with hypothyroidism[164] or certain drugs (see below), (4) the effects of cobalamin deficiency itself,[155] and (5) sprue, either tropical or, less often, nontropical.[65] In each of these, exogenous intrinsic factor fails to correct an abnormal Schilling test.

Competing Intestinal Flora and Fauna: "Blind Loop Syndrome."   The *blind loop syndrome* is a state of cobalamin malabsorption with megaloblastic anemia caused by intestinal stasis from anatomic lesions (strictures, diverticula, anastomoses, surgical blind loops) or impaired motility (scleroderma, amyloid).[165] Serum cobalamin is low, but intrinsic factor secretion is normal, and the cobalamin malabsorption is not corrected by exogenous intrinsic factor. The defect in cobalamin absorption is caused by colonization of the diseased small intestine by bacteria that take up ingested cobalamin before it can be absorbed from the intestine.[166-169] Steatorrhea is also seen in the blind loop syndrome.

Another cause of cobalamin deficiency is infestation with the fish tapeworm, *Diphyllobothrium latum.* Prevalence is highest near the Baltic Sea and in Canada and Alaska. The life cycle of the worm is illustrated in Fig. 37-4. Humans are infected by eating undercooked fish or fish roe. Once ingested, the sparaganum larva becomes an adult in 5 to 6 weeks and may live for years.

Cobalamin deficiency is caused by competition between the worm and the host for ingested cobalamin.[170] The clinical picture of *D. latum* infestation ranges from no symptoms to a full-blown megaloblastic anemia with neurologic changes. Only about 3 percent of persons harboring the parasite become anemic, however.[171] The infestation is diagnosed by finding tapeworm ova in the feces.

Pancreatic Disease   In 50 to 70 percent of patients with exocrine pancreatic insufficiency, cobalamin malabsorption can be demonstrated by the Schilling test.[172,173] Cobalamin malabsorption in pancreatic insufficiency is caused by a deficiency in pancreatic proteases, resulting in a partial failure to destroy R binder-Cbl complexes, whose destruction is a prerequisite for the transfer of cobalamin to intrinsic factor. The defect in cobalamin absorption in chronic pancreatitis is corrected by oral trypsin or by presaturating the R binder with cobinamide, a cobalamin analog that is taken up by R binder but not by intrinsic factor.[174,175] Despite the high incidence of abnormal Schilling tests in pancreatic insufficiency, this disorder almost never causes clinically significant cobalamin deficiency.[176]

DIETARY COBALAMIN DEFICIENCY

Dietary cobalamin deficiency is very unusual. It occurs mainly in vegetarians who also avoid dairy products and eggs (vegans).[177-179]

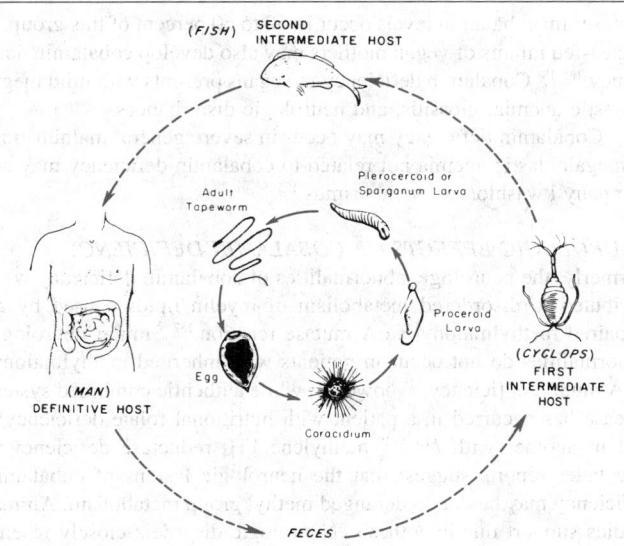

FIGURE 37-4   Life cycle of *Diphyllobothrium latum.* Inner circle represents developmental stages of parasite: (1) adult worm; (2) eggs; (3) embryonated egg (coracidium); (4) procercoid larva; (5) plerocercoid larva. Outside circle shows first intermediate host *(Cyclops),* second intermediate host (fish), and definitive host (man). (Adapted from Wirth, Farrow, Human sparganosis. *JAMA* 177:76, 1961.)

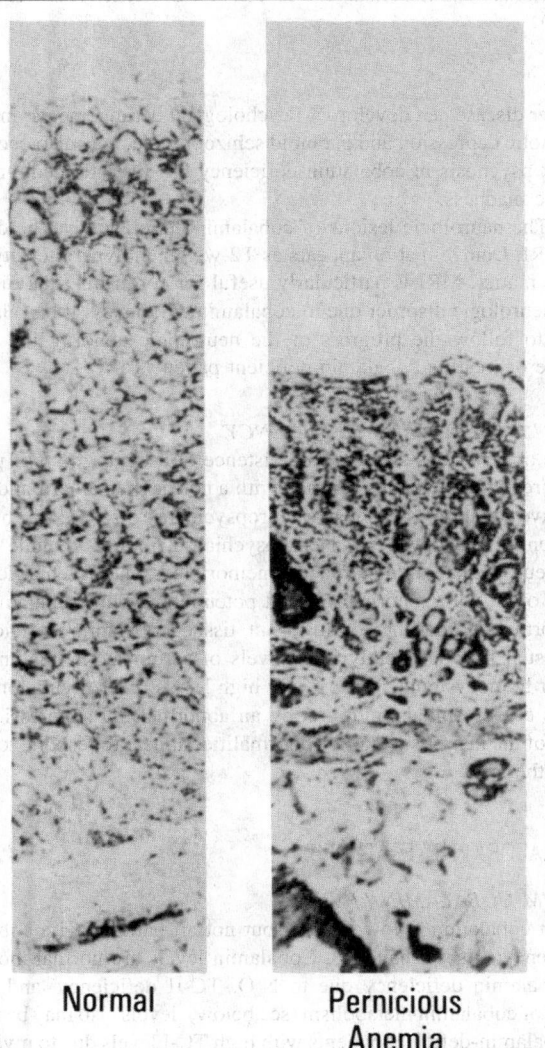

Normal   **Pernicious Anemia**

FIGURE 37-3   Gastric histology in pernicious anemia. *Left,* normal fundus. The thick mucosa is packed with gastric glands composed for the most part of chief cells and parietal cells. The mucus-secreting cells are concentrated in the necks of the glands. *Right,* fundus in pernicious anemia. Gastric glands in the atrophic mucosa are sparse and consist mainly of mucus-secreting cells; the mucosa is densely infiltrated by lymphocytes.

Low serum cobalamin levels occur in 50 to 60 percent of this group.[180] Breast-fed infants of vegan mothers may also develop cobalamin deficiency.[181–184] Cobalamin deficiency in vegans presents with mild megaloblastic anemia, glossitis, and neurologic disturbances.

Cobalamin deficiency may occur in severe general malnutrition. A megaloblastic anemia not related to cobalamin deficiency may accompany kwashiorkor or marasmus.[185,186]

NEUROLOGIC EFFECTS OF COBALAMIN DEFICIENCY

Formerly, the neurologic abnormalities of cobalamin deficiency were attributed to disordered metabolism of myelin lipids caused by an impaired methylmalonyl CoA mutase reaction.[187] Similar neurologic abnormalities do not occur in patients with inherited methylmalonyl CoA mutase deficiency,[115] however, while authentic combined system disease has occurred in a patient with nutritional folate deficiency[188] and in another with N^5,N^{10}-methylene FH$_4$ reductase deficiency.[189] The latter reports suggest that the neurologic lesions of cobalamin deficiency may be due to deranged methyl group metabolism. Animal studies support this hypothesis. Neurologic disorders closely resembling combined system disease develop in cobalamin-deficient pigs, fruit bats, and monkeys.[190,191] The development of these disorders is prevented by methionine, which is produced in a cobalamin-dependent reaction and is the precursor of the biological methylating reagent S-adenosylmethionine (SAM). Further support for a methylation defect is the finding that brains from cobalamin-deficient pigs contain increased levels of S-adenosylhomocysteine (SAH),[190] a powerful methylation inhibitor produced in SAM-dependent methylation reactions:

$$SAM + RH \rightarrow SAH + RCH_3$$

Against the methylation defect hypothesis, however, are the findings that cobalamin deficiency had no effect on S-adenosylmethionine, S-adenosylhomocysteine, or the methylation of phospholipids or myelin basic protein[192–194] in the brains of fruit bats. Are humans more like pigs or fruit bats? Possibly pigs.[195–197]

CLINICAL FEATURES

The clinical picture of cobalamin deficiency includes the nonspecific manifestations of megaloblastosis—anemia, weight loss, etc.—plus specific features caused by the lack of cobalamin, chiefly neurologic abnormalities. Because cobalamin reserves are large, years may pass between the cessation of cobalamin absorption and the appearance of deficiency symptoms. This interval is shortened in patients whose enterohepatic cobalamin cycle has been interrupted.

NEUROLOGIC ABNORMALITIES[198,199]

Cobalamin deficiency causes a neurologic syndrome that is particularly dangerous because it can develop in isolation, with no megaloblastic anemia to suggest a lack of cobalamin,[200] and because when sufficiently far advanced, it cannot be reversed by treatment. The syndrome usually begins with paresthesias in feet and fingers due to early peripheral neuropathy, together with disturbances of vibratory sense and proprioception. The earliest signs, said to precede other neurologic findings by months, are loss of position sense in the second toe and loss of vibration sense for a 256-Hz but not a 128-Hz tuning fork.[201] If untreated, the neurologic disorder progresses to spastic ataxia resulting from demyelination of the dorsal and lateral columns of the spinal cord: so-called *combined system disease* (Fig. 37-5).[202,203]

Besides the peripheral nerves and the spinal cord, the brain is affected by cobalamin deficiency. Somnolence and perversion of taste, smell, and vision with occasional optic atrophy are accompanied by slow waves on the electroencephalogram. A dementia mimicking Alz-

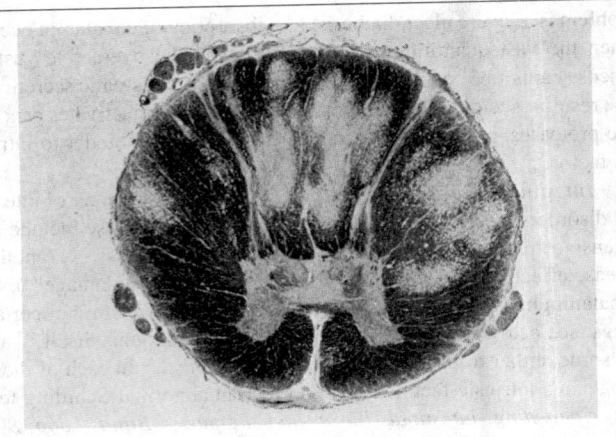

FIGURE 37-5   Degeneration of spinal cord in combined system disease. (From Harris, Kellermeyer, *The Red Cell: Production, Metabolism, Destruction: Normal and Abnormal,* rev ed, Harvard University Press, Cambridge, 1970.)

heimer disease can develop.[204] Psychological derangements, including psychotic depression and paranoid schizophrenia, may also occur.[201,205] Frank psychosis in cobalamin deficiency has been termed "megaloblastic madness."[206]

The neurologic lesions of cobalamin deficiency can be detected by MRI. Demyelination appears as T2-weighted hyperintensity of the white matter. MRI is particularly useful for confirming the diagnosis of a neurologic disorder due to cobalamin deficiency. It has also been used to follow the progress of the neurologic abnormalities in the course of treating cobalamin-deficient patients.[207–209]

SUBTLE COBALAMIN DEFICIENCY

Some observations suggest the existence of a large group of patients who are hematologically normal, with a normal hematocrit and MCV, but have cobalamin-responsive neuropsychiatric disease,[210–217] but there are conflicting views.[218,219] Neuropsychiatric findings include peripheral neuropathy, gait disturbance, memory loss, and psychiatric symptoms, often with abnormal evoked potentials. Serum cobalamin may be normal, borderline, or low, but tissue cobalamin deficiency is suggested by consistently high levels of serum methylmalonic acid and/or homocysteine,[220–224] by very high levels of methylmalonic acid in the cerebrospinal fluid, and by an abnormal dU suppression test. Most of the neuropsychiatric abnormalities appear to respond to cobalamin therapy.

LABORATORY FEATURES

SERUM COBALAMIN LEVELS

Serum cobalamin is low in most but not all patients with cobalamin deficiency[224] (see Chap. 25). Cobalamin levels are normal, however, in cobalamin deficiency due to N$_2$O, TC-II deficiency, and inborn errors of cobalamin metabolism (see below); levels also may be normal in cobalamin-deficient patients with high TC-I levels due to myeloproliferative diseases.[224,225] Conversely, serum cobalamin levels may be low in the presence of normal tissue cobalamins in vegetarians, in subjects taking megadoses of ascorbic acid,[226] in pregnancy (25 percent), in the presence of TC-I deficiency,[227] and in megaloblastic anemia due to folate deficiency (30 percent).[225] Serum folate may be higher than expected in cobalamin deficiency; patients deficient in both cobalamin and folate may show normal serum folate levels.

METHYLMALONIC ACIDURIA

Except when caused by an inborn error (see below), methylmalonic aciduria is a reliable indicator of cobalamin deficiency.[228] Normal subjects excrete only traces of methylmalonate (0 to 3.4 mg/day); in cobalamin deficiency, however, urine methylmalonate is usually elevated. Cobalamin therapy restores excretion to normal in a few days.

SERUM METHYLMALONIC ACID AND HOMOCYSTEINE

Elevated serum methylmalonic acid and homocysteine levels are indicators of *tissue* cobalamin deficiency. Their levels are high in more than 90 percent of cobalamin-deficient patients and rise before the serum cobalamin falls to subnormal levels.[220–223] Elevated serum methylmalonic acid and/or elevated homocysteine are probably the most reliable indicators of cobalamin deficiency in patients without a congenital disorder in their metabolism.

Spinal fluid methylmalonic acid levels are markedly elevated in cobalamin deficiency.[214]

THE SCHILLING TEST: ASSAYS OF COBALAMIN ABSORPTION AND INTRINSIC FACTOR

The Schilling test assays cobalamin absorption by measuring urinary radioactivity after an oral dose of radioactive cobalamin. The test can be performed even after cobalamin deficiency has been treated. After voiding, a fasting patient drinks 0.5 μCi (0.5 to 2.0 μg) of radioactive cyanocobalamin in water, and a 24-h urine collection is begun. At 2 h, 1 mg of unlabeled cyanocobalamin is given IM to saturate the circulating cobalamin-binding proteins, after which the patient may eat. The amount of radioactivity in the 24-h urine is measured. Normal subjects excrete ≥7 percent of the administered radioactivity in the first 24 h.

If excretion of radioactivity is low, the second part of the Schilling test is performed after a 5-day delay to allow intestinal megaloblastosis to be corrected by the unlabeled cobalamin given in the first part of the test.[229,230] The procedure is the same except that 60 mg of *active* hog intrinsic factor (equivalent of 1 national formulary unit) is given orally with the radioactive cobalamin. If poor excretion in the first part was due to intrinsic factor deficiency, excretion in the second part will be normal. Intrinsic factor will not correct cobalamin malabsorption due to other causes.

The Schilling test will give a false-negative result in patients who absorb free cobalamin but fail to release the vitamin from food (e.g., after partial gastrectomy[231] and vagotomy,[232] in those with a gastric ulcer,[233] and during cimetidine therapy[234]). Failure to absorb food cobalamin can be established by a modified Schilling test in which the source of the labeled vitamin is an omelet of eggs obtained from a chicken fed on radioactive cobalamin.[223] Cobalamin deficiency occasionally results from malabsorption of protein-bound cobalamin only.[235,236]

The major source of error in the Schilling test is incomplete urine collection. Completeness of collection may be assessed by measuring the creatinine in the specimen (normal >15 mg/kg per day). Renal disease may delay excretion of radioactivity, giving a false-positive Schilling test[237]; whole-body counting can be used to measure cobalamin absorption in severe renal insufficiency.[238] Other causes of a false-positive result are inadequate saturation of cobalamin-binding proteins by unlabeled cobalamin (first part of test), inactive intrinsic factor or neutralization of intrinsic factor by anti-intrinsic factor antibodies in the stomach[120] (second part), and malabsorption due to megaloblastic changes in the ileum[229,239] (second part). A false negative may be caused by isotope given with an earlier Schilling or other test.

THE DEOXYURIDINE (dU) SUPPRESSION TEST[240]

The dU suppression test is based on the finding that unlabeled dU can suppress the uptake of [³H]thymidine ([³H]Thd) into the DNA

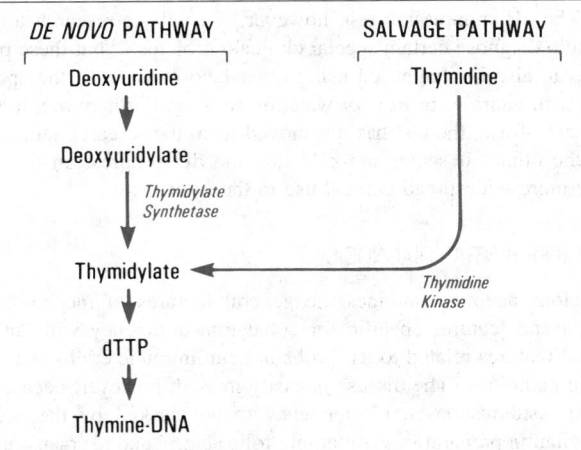

FIGURE 37-6   Incorporation of thymidine into DNA via the de novo and salvage pathways. (Adapted from Metz.[240])

of cultured lymphocytes or marrow cells.[240] Thymidine enters DNA through the dTMP pool, into which it is fed by thymidine kinase (Fig. 37-6). Deoxyuridine also enters DNA through the dTMP pool, first being phosphorylated to dUMP by thymidine kinase, then being methylated to dTMP by thymidylate synthetase. The theory of the dU suppression test is that treating normal cells with dU loads them with *unlabeled* dTMP, which competes for uptake into DNA with the *labeled* dTMP formed during a later incubation with [³H]Thd; dU thereby suppresses the uptake of [³H]Thd into DNA. If thymidylate synthetase activity is low, the conversion of dU into dTMP will be slowed, and the suppressive effect of dU on [³H]Thd uptake into DNA will be diminished. Because thymidylate synthetase uses N^5,N^{10}-methylene FH₄ as a methylating agent, its activity depends directly on folate and indirectly on cobalamin (see Chap. 30). Failure of dU suppression therefore becomes an indication of cellular folate or cobalamin deficiency. While the foregoing theory is highly oversimplified,[5,241] experience has shown that the dU suppression test can answer questions about cellular folate and cobalamin.

To perform the assay, cultured lymphocytes or marrow cells from a patient or control are incubated for an hour at 37°C with and without 0.1 μM dU. [³H]Thd is then added, and the cells are incubated for an additional 0.5 to 3.0 h. The incorporation of [³H]Thd is then determined, and dU suppression is calculated as 100× (³H incorporation in dU-treated cells/³H incorporation by control cells), expressed as a percentage. Normally, dU depresses the uptake of [³H]Thd into DNA to less than 10 percent of control values. Deoxyuridine suppression is relieved in megaloblastic anemias of nutritional origin and in certain inherited disorders of folate or cobalamin metabolism[240–242] but not in other megaloblastic states.[243] In the nutritional anemias, dU suppression can be restored with folate or cobalamin according to a pattern that depends on the nature of the deficiency (Table 37-2).[241,242] Even subclinical deficiency states can be detected by the dU suppression test.[244]

TABLE 37-2   CORRECTION OF THE dU SUPPRESSION TEST IN NUTRITIONAL MEGALOBLASTIC ANEMIA

DEFICIENCY	CORRECTED BY			
	CNCbl[a]	FOLATE	N^5-FORMYL FH₄[b]	N^5-METHYL FH₄[b]
Folate	−	+	+	+
Cobalamin	+	+	+	−

[a]CNCbl, cyanocobalamin, vitamin B₁₂.
[b]FH₄, tetrahydrofolic acid.

The dU suppression test, however, is chiefly a research tool. It can help diagnose certain special clinical problems,[240] but these problems can also be diagnosed using other laboratory tests, therapeutic trials with vitamins or iron, or watchful waiting. Furthermore, in over 25 years of use, the test has not moved from the research laboratory into the clinic. It seems unlikely that the dU suppression test will enjoy more widespread clinical use in the future.

DIFFERENTIAL DIAGNOSIS

Pernicious anemia combines the general features of megaloblastic anemia and features specific for cobalamin deficiency with unique clinical features related to its (probable) autoimmune etiology and its gastric pathology. The disease is easily missed, however, because of its (1) insidious onset, (2) tendency to be masked by the use of multivitamin preparations containing folic acid,[245] and (3) many atypical presentations,[246,247] including its presentation as a neurologic disease without hematologic findings and its tendency to be overlooked in a patient with another autoimmune disease.

Antiparietal cell and anti-intrinsic factor antibodies are rarely measured, even though the anti-intrinsic factor antibodies in particular could be of considerable diagnostic value.[88] Anti-intrinsic factor antibody is highly specific for PA (although its sensitivity is only modest), and its presence in a megaloblastic anemia makes the diagnosis of PA almost certain.

THERAPY, COURSE, AND PROGNOSIS

Treatment consists of parenteral cyanocobalamin (vitamin B_{12}) or hydroxocobalamin to replace daily losses and refill storage pools, which normally contain 2 to 5 mg of cobalamin.[248] Toxicity is nil, but doses exceeding 100 μg saturate the transcobalamins, and the excess is lost in the urine.

A typical treatment schedule consists of 1000 μg cobalamin IM daily for 2 weeks, then weekly until the hematocrit is normal, and then monthly for life. For neurologic manifestations, 1000 μg every 2 weeks for 6 months is recommended, and higher doses are given for certain inherited disorders (e.g., TC-II deficiency). Cobalamin should be given by mouth for dietary cobalamin deficiency and to patients (e.g., hemophiliac patients) who cannot take IM injections.

Transfusion is occasionally required when the hematocrit is less than 15 percent or when the patient is debilitated, infected, or in heart failure. In such instances, packed cells should be given slowly to avoid pulmonary edema. Infections can impair the response to cobalamin and must be treated vigorously.

RESPONSE TO TREATMENT

Following the parenteral administration of cobalamin to deficient patients, elevated plasma bilirubin, iron, and LDH levels fall rapidly (Fig. 37-7).[249] Decreasing plasma iron turnover and fecal urobilinogen reflect cessation of ineffective erythropoiesis. Within 12 h the marrow begins to change from megaloblastic to normoblastic, a process that is complete in 2 to 3 days. Reticulocytosis begins on day 3 to 5 and peaks on day 4 to 10.[250] The new red cells come from new normoblasts, not from the old megaloblasts, most of which die before leaving the marrow. The blood hemoglobin concentration becomes normal within 1 to 2 months; if normal values are not achieved by then, another cause of anemia should be sought.

Other changes include the following: (1) a prompt improvement in the sense of well-being; (2) normalization of the leukocyte and platelet counts, although neutrophil hypersegmentation persists for 10 to 14 days; (3) a rise in serum cobalamin and folate; and (4) a drop in serum potassium.[251] Cobalamin deficiency will not respond to a

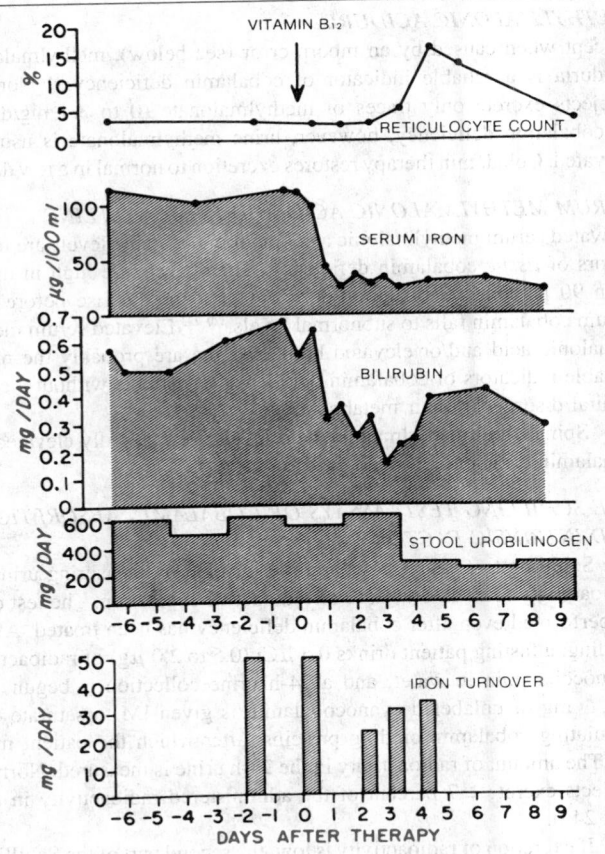

FIGURE 37-7 Effect of CNCbl on reticulocyte count, serum iron, serum bilirubin, stool urobilinogen, and plasma iron turnover. (Adapted from Finch et al.[249])

physiologic dose of folate (100 to 400 μg/day), although this dose will produce a maximal response in folate deficiency. Larger doses of folate (5 to 15 mg/day) can produce a reticulocytosis and partially correct the anemia in cobalamin deficiency.

SPECIAL CIRCUMSTANCES

After Gastrectomy   Cobalamin should always be given after total gastrectomy. Cobalamin administration is not necessary after partial gastrectomy, but these patients need to be watched for megaloblastic anemia, bearing in mind that this anemia could be masked by postgastrectomy iron deficiency.

Blind Loop Syndrome   The anemia of the blind loop syndrome can be treated by parenteral cobalamin therapy. It also responds after a week or so to oral broad-spectrum antibiotics [cephalexin monohydrate (Keflex) 250 mg qid plus metronidazole 250 mg tid for 10 days],[167] and the Schilling test becomes normal. Successful surgical correction of an anatomic lesion will cure the syndrome.

Fish Tapeworm   Treatment consists of a single 2-g dose of niclosamide.

USE OF ORAL COBALAMIN

Much interest has recently been kindled in the possibility of treating cobalamin deficiency with oral cobalamin.[253-255] Oral cobalamin can be used not only for the treatment of the dietary cobalamin deficiency that occurs in vegans and in patients with very severe general malnutrition but also for the treatment of patients with PA, provided these patients are followed carefully.[256] In patients lacking intrinsic factor, about 1 percent of an oral dose of the vitamin is forced across the intestinal epithelium by mass action. Therefore, 1000 to 2000 μg/day of oral cobalamin will supply most PA patients with their daily cobalamin requirement without the need for injections and their accompanying pain and expense.

ACUTE MEGALOBLASTIC ANEMIA

Although megaloblastic anemia is usually a chronic condition that requires weeks or months to develop, a potentially fatal megaloblastic state due to acute tissue folate or cobalamin deficiency can sometimes arise over the course of only a few days. Patients with acute megaloblastic anemia present with rapidly developing thrombocytopenia and/or leukopenia, counts sometimes falling to very low levels, but with little change in red cell levels unless another cause of anemia is present. The clinical picture can suggest an immune cytopenia. The diagnosis is made from the marrow aspirate, which is floridly megaloblastic, and confirmed by the rapid response to appropriate replacement therapy.

The most common cause of acute megaloblastic anemia is nitrous oxide (N_2O) anesthesia. N_2O rapidly destroys MeCbl,[257] leading quickly to a megaloblastic state. AdoCbl (adenosylcobalamin) is eventually lost, and S-adenosylmethionine and total folate decline as well, with an increase in the proportion of folate in the form of N^5-methyl FH$_4$.[257–259]

Clinical findings develop quickly. An impairment in dU suppression with a cobalamin-deficiency pattern (see Table 37-2) appears after 6 h of exposure, and grossly megaloblastic changes are seen in the marrow after 12 to 24 h.[260,261] Hypersegmented neutrophils do not appear until 5 days after exposure but then persist for several days.[262] Some say that the hematologic effects of N_2O can be prevented by folinic acid (30 mg at surgery and 12 h later).[261,263,264] The effects of N_2O disappear spontaneously after a few days; disappearance can be hastened by folinic acid or cobalamin.[260]

Fatalities due to N_2O-induced megaloblastosis have occurred in tetanus patients given N_2O for weeks.[265,266] Long-term recreational use of N_2O has led to psychosis[267] and to a neurologic disorder similar to combined system disease.[268,269] Operating room personnel, however, are not at risk for N_2O-induced megaloblastic anemia.[270]

Acute megaloblastic anemia also occurs in other clinical settings. A rapidly developing megaloblastic state with acute thrombocytopenia has occurred in seriously ill patients, often in intensive care units.[271–273] Especially at risk are patients transfused extensively at surgery,[274] those on dialysis or total parenteral nutrition, and those receiving weak folate antagonists such as trimethoprim.[275,276] Morphologic clues to the diagnosis (e.g., hypersegmented neutrophils) are often absent from the blood film, and both the red cell folate and the serum cobalamin may be normal, but the marrow is always megaloblastic. A rapid response to therapeutic doses of parenteral folate (5 mg/day) and cobalamin (1 mg) is the rule.

MEGALOBLASTIC ANEMIA CAUSED BY DRUGS

Drugs that cause megaloblastic anemia are listed in Table 37-3. *Aminopterin* and *methotrexate* are almost identical in structure to folic acid. After entering cells via the folate carrier[314] and acquiring a polyglutamate chain,[315] they act as very powerful inhibitors of dihydrofolate reductase.[277] By blocking the FH$_2$→FH$_4$ reaction and perhaps inhibiting other enzymes of folate metabolism, they effect the rapid withdrawal of folates from the 1-carbon fragment carrier pool, causing a fall in nucleotide (especially thymidine) biosynthesis that leads to a major derangement in DNA replication[278,279] (see Chap. 25).

Toxic effects include necrotic mouth lesions; ulcerations of the esophagus, small intestine, and colon, with abdominal pain, vomiting,

and diarrhea; megaloblastic anemia; alopecia; and hyperpigmentation. The drug is excreted by the kidney, so effects and toxicity are prolonged and enhanced if renal function is impaired.

Toxicity caused by these folate antagonists is treated with folinic acid (N^5-formyl FH$_4$). Folate itself is useless because the blocked reductase cannot convert it to the active tetrahydro form. Folinic acid, however, is already in the tetrahydro form and is therefore effective despite the reductase blockade. The usual dose of folinic acid is 3 to 6 mg/day IM. Larger doses are given in chemotherapy protocols in which folinic acid is used to rescue patients deliberately treated with otherwise fatal doses of methotrexate. Folinic acid was used intrathecally in a patient in whom a large overdose of methotrexate was accidentally delivered into the subarachnoid space.[316]

Zidovudine (azidothymidine, AZT) is used for HIV infections (AIDS) (see Chap. 89).[317] Its principal toxic effect is severe megaloblastic anemia. Anemia or neutropenia produced by zidovudine may limit the use of this drug.[290]

HIV infection itself suppresses hematopoiesis, leading to pancytopenia with myelodysplastic features (see Chap. 89). The blood film shows vacuolated monocytes. Megaloblastosis in HIV infection may be due to folate or cobalamin deficiency[318,319] or to AZT or trimethoprim toxicity.

Hydroxyurea is used at high doses to treat chronic myelogenous leukemia, polycythemia vera, and essential thrombocythemia, and at lower doses to treat psoriasis (see Chap 14). It inhibits the conversion of ribonucleotides to deoxyribonucleotides.[320] Marked megaloblastic changes are routinely found in the marrow within 1 to 2 days of initiating hydroxyurea therapy.[291,321] These changes are rapidly reversed after withdrawing the drug.

Megaloblastosis due to nitrous oxide (N_2O) is discussed under "Acute Megaloblastic Anemia."

Long-term use of *omeprazole* and presumably other H$^+$/K$^+$-ATPase inhibitors is associated with reduced serum cobalamin levels, presumably because of the ability of these drugs to inhibit parietal cell function.[309] This is not a problem when these drugs are used for short intervals.[322–325]

MEGALOBLASTIC ANEMIA IN CHILDHOOD

MALABSORPTION OF COBALAMIN

Cobalamin malabsorption occurs in five childhood conditions: (1) cobalamin malabsorption in the presence of normal intrinsic factor secretion, (2) congenital abnormality of intrinsic factor, (3) transcobalamin II deficiency, (4) congenital R-binder deficiency, and (5) true pernicious anemia of childhood. The management of cobalamin deficiency in childhood has been thoughtfully reviewed.[326]

SELECTIVE MALABSORPTION OF COBALAMIN (IMERSLUND-GRÄSBECK DISEASE)[327]

This disorder is an inherited failure of transport of the intrinsic factor-Cbl complex by the ileum, usually accompanied by proteinuria (mostly albumin).[74,328–330] It may be the most common cause of cobalamin deficiency in infancy.[115,328,331] Cobalamin deficiency is usually seen before age 2 but may appear later.[74,330,332] Both parts of the Schilling test are abnormal, but intrinsic factor and HCl secretion, TC-I and -II levels, and gastric and intestinal histology are all normal, and intrinsic factor antibodies are absent.[119,332,333] Intrinsic factor-Cbl receptors are present in some but not all patients.[334,335] The molecular defect responsible for this disease is unknown.

Patients are treated with IM cobalamin. The anemia is corrected, but proteinuria persists.

TABLE 37-3   DRUGS THAT CAUSE MEGALOBLASTIC ANEMIA

AGENTS	COMMENTS	REFERENCE
Antifolates		
Methotrexate	Very potent inhibitor of dihydrofolate reductase.	277, 279
Aminopterin	Treat overdose with folinic acid.	278
Pyrimethamine	Much weaker than methotrexate and aminopterin.	276
Trimethoprim	Treat with folinic acid or by withdrawing the drug.	275
Sulfasalazine	Can cause acute megaloblastic anemia in susceptible patients, especially those with low folate stores.	280
Chlorguanide (Proguanil)		281
Triamterine		
Purine analogs		
6-Mercaptopurine	Megaloblastosis precedes hypoplasia. Usually mild.	282
6-Thioguanine	Responds to folinic acid but not folate.	283
Azathioprine		284
Acyclovir	Megaloblastosis at high doses.	285, 286
Pyrimidine analogs		
5-Fluorouracil	Mild megaloblastosis.	287, 288
Floxuridine (5-fluorodeoxyuridine)		288
6-Azauridine	Blocks uridine monophosphate production by inhibiting orotidyl decarboxylase. Occasional megaloblastosis with orotic acid and orotidine in urine.	289
Zidovudine (AZT)	Severe megaloblastic anemia is the major side effect.	290
Ribonucleotide reductase inhibitors		
Hydroxyurea	Marked megaloblastosis within 1–2 days of starting therapy. Quickly reversed by withdrawing drug.	291, 292
Cytarabine (cytosine arabinoside)	Early megaloblastosis is routine.	293, 294
Anticonvulsants		
Phenytoin (diphenylhydantoin)	Occasional megaloblastosis, associated with low folate levels. Responds to high-dose folate	295, 296
		297, 298
Phenobarbital	(1–5 mg/day). Why anticonvulsants cause low folate	299, 300
Primidone	is not understood, though a recent study suggests that	
Carbamazepine	it relates to a drug-induced rise in cytochrome P_{450}.	301, 302
Other drugs that depress folates		
Oral contraceptives	Occasional megaloblastosis. Sometimes dysplasia of uterine cervix, corrected with folate.	303–306
Glutethimide		307
Cycloserine		308
H^+/K^+ ATPase inhibitors		
Omeprazole	Long-term use causes a fall in serum cobalamin levels.	309
Lansoprazole		
Miscellaneous		
N_2O	See ''Acute Megaloblastic Anemia'' in this chapter.	
p-Aminosalicylic acid	Causes cobalamin malabsorption with occasional mild megaloblastic anemia.	308
Metformin		310
Phenformin	Causes cobalamin malabsorption but not anemia.	
Colchicine		312
Neomycin		311
Arsenic	Causes myelodysplastic hematopoiesis, sometimes with megaloblastic changes.	313

CONGENITAL INTRINSIC FACTOR DEFICIENCY

This is an autosomal recessive disease in which parietal cells fail to produce functionally normal intrinsic factor.[336–338] Patients present with irritability and megaloblastic anemia when their cobalamin stores (<25 μg at birth) are exhausted. The disease usually presents at 6 to 24 months of age. HCl secretion and gastric histology are normal, there is no proteinuria, and anti-intrinsic factor antibodies are ab-

sent.[74,115,326,332] The abnormal Schilling test is corrected by oral intrinsic factor.[339] Treatment is with standard doses of IM cobalamin.

TRANSCOBALAMIN II (TC-II) DEFICIENCY[340]

This is an autosomal recessive disorder causing a flagrant megaloblastic anemia that generally presents in early infancy.[341] The disease is dangerously deceptive, because it results from a very severe deficiency of tissue cobalamin, usually with normal serum cobalamin levels, and if not diagnosed will cause irreversible CNS damage.[342] Patients are healthy at birth but develop signs and symptoms of cobalamin deficiency over the first few weeks of life: a rapidly progressive pancytopenia, mouth ulcers, vomiting, and diarrhea. Recurrent bacterial infections may occur.[340,343–345] Neurologic findings are not prominent in the early stages of the disease.[342]

Serum folate and cobalamin are normal (the latter because most cobalamin is carried by TC-I, not TC-II) and little homocysteine or methylmalonic acid is found in the urine,[346–348] but the marrow is megaloblastic (a few patients showed severe erythroid hypoplasia[349]). The Schilling test is usually[340] but not always[350] abnormal and is never corrected by intrinsic factor. The diagnosis is made by measuring serum TC-II.[351] Prenatal diagnosis may be possible.[352] Serum should be obtained prior to treatment, because TC-II levels in normals drop sharply after cobalamin is given.[340] TC-II deficiency is treated with doses of cobalamin large enough to force enough vitamin into the cells to allow normal function. Initial therapy can be with oral vitamin B_{12} or hydroxocobalamin, 500 to 1000 μg twice a week, or IM hydroxocobalamin, 1000 μg/week, following blood counts, symptoms, and immune function, and adjusting doses upward if necessary.

R-BINDER DEFICIENCY

Congenital R-binder deficiency has been reported in six patients,[215,227,353,354] none of whom had a clinical manifestation of cobalamin deficiency, although the patients' serum cobalamin levels were well below normal. R binders were deficient in leukocytes and saliva as well as in plasma. These patients show that the R binders are not essential for health.

TRUE JUVENILE PERNICIOUS ANEMIA

True PA, with gastric atrophy and a defect in intrinsic factor secretion, is exceedingly rare in childhood.[355,356] Patients usually present in their teens with cobalamin deficiency. Serum anti-intrinsic factor antibodies are usually present.[123] The diagnosis and treatment are the same as for PA in adults.

INBORN ERRORS OF COBALAMIN METABOLISM[357,358]

Cobalamin is converted to AdoCbl and MeCbl by a complex series of transformations involving several steps (see Chap. 34). Seven disorders affecting this cobalamin transformation pathway have been described, one for each of the steps. Since the molecular causes of these disorders have not yet been fully characterized, the disorders themselves are not named for a defective protein but instead are designated by letter, as in "cobalamin mutant class 'cobalamin A,'" or "cblA." Based on the abnormal metabolites in the patients' urine, these disorders can be grouped into three clinical syndromes (Table 37-4).

METHYLMALONIC ACIDURIA ONLY (cblA, cblB, AND cblF[359–362])

In cblA and cblB, AdoCbl production is impaired,[363,364] but MeCbl production is normal; in cblF, cobalamin export from lysosomes to cytosol is defective. Patients present in infancy with acidosis because they cannot catabolize methylmalonic acid. Symptoms include lethargy and failure to thrive, vomiting, and neurologic problems. Mental retardation is not prominent, and megaloblastic anemia is absent. Most patients respond to 1000 μg/day of OHCbl or CNCbl.[364]

HOMOCYSTINURIA ONLY (cblE AND cblG[365–367])

In these disorders, N^5-methyltetrahydrofolate-homocysteine methyltransferase is able to produce methionine but has difficulty making MeCbl. In patients with cblG, methionine synthase is missing or defective[368]; cblE is due to a failure to reactivate methionine synthase that has been inactivated by oxidation of its bound cobalamin[369] (see Chap. 34). Patients present in infancy with vomiting, mental retardation, and megaloblastic anemia. They respond well to CNCbl at 1000 μg per day or per week. Infants diagnosed prenatally and treated from birth show normal development.

METHYLMALONIC ACIDURIA AND HOMOCYSTINURIA (cblC AND cblD[365,370–372])

In these disorders, the defect in Cbl transformation affects both AdoCbl and MeCbl, probably because the reduction of the cobalt from Co^{3+} to Co^{1+} is defective. The age at initial presentation ranges from early infancy to adolescence. In addition to lethargy and failure to thrive, affected infants present with serious neurologic difficulties, while older patients present with psychological problems and progressive dementia along with motor signs and symptoms. In one fetus at risk for cblC, the diagnosis was excluded prenatally by chorionic villus sampling.[372] Megaloblastic anemia occurs in about half the cases. Patients respond partially to 1000 μg/day of OHCbl or CNCbl.

A tentative diagnosis of a cobalamin mutation can be made by demonstrating methylmalonic aciduria and/or homocystinuria in a patient with the clinical findings described above. Establishing a diagnosis requires a specialized laboratory. In a patient suspected of having a cobalamin mutation, treatment should be started while awaiting test results, because early high-dose cobalamin treatment is risk-free and may reduce the chance of damage to the central nervous system. Fetuses with these diseases have been successfully treated in utero with very large doses of cyanocobalamin given parenterally to the mother.[373,374]

TABLE 37-4 COBALAMIN MUTANT CLASS SYNDROMES

SYNDROME	METHYLMALONIC ACIDURIA	HOMOCYSTINURIA	MEGALOBLASTIC ANEMIA
CblA, CblB, CblF	+	–	–
CblE, CblG	–	+	+
CblC, CblD	+	+	±

INBORN ERRORS OF FOLATE METABOLISM[375]

Megaloblastic anemia in infancy has been described in three inherited disorders of folate metabolism.

CONGENITAL FOLATE MALABSORPTION[376,377]

Patients cannot absorb folate from the gastrointestinal tract or transport it into the cerebrospinal fluid. They present with severe megaloblastic anemia, seizures, mental retardation, and other central nervous system findings. Folate levels are low in the serum and nil in the cerebrospinal fluid. Folate given parenterally has corrected the anemia and seizures in some patients but has had no effect on other CNS symptoms or on the CSF folate level.

DIHYDROFOLATE REDUCTASE DEFICIENCY[378]

A patient postulated to have dihydrofolate reductase deficiency presented with isolated megaloblastic anemia at 6 weeks of age. His anemia responded to folinic acid but not to folic acid.

N^5-METHYL FH$_4$: HOMOCYSTEINE METHYLTRANSFERASE DEFICIENCY[379]

Decreased methyltransferase activity was found in a liver biopsy from a child with megaloblastic anemia and mental retardation. The anemia failed to respond to folate, cobalamin, or pyridoxal phosphate.

OTHER INBORN ERRORS

HEREDITARY OROTIC ACIDURIA

Hereditary orotic aciduria is an autosomal recessive disorder of pyrimidine metabolism[380–382] characterized by megaloblastic anemia, growth impairment, and excretion of orotic acid in the urine. Cobalamin and folate levels are normal.

LESCH-NYHAN SYNDROME

The Lesch-Nyhan syndrome is an X-linked disorder of purine metabolism characterized by hyperuricemia, hyperuricosuria, and a neurologic disease with self-mutilation. It is caused by a deficiency of hypoxanthine-guanine phosphoribosyltransferase. One patient had megaloblastic anemia.[383]

THIAMINE-RESPONSIVE MEGALOBLASTIC ANEMIA

Seven children have been reported with severe megaloblastic anemia, sensorineural deafness, and diabetes mellitus, all beginning in infancy.[384–386] The anemia responded to thiamine (25 to 100 mg/day). In two patients with this disorder, the marrow was reported to be myelodysplastic.[387] The gene for this puzzling disorder was recently mapped to the long arm of chromosome 1,[388] but the biochemical defect is completely unknown.

OTHER CAUSES OF MEGALOBLASTIC ANEMIA

CONGENITAL DYSERYTHROPOIETIC ANEMIA

The congenital dyserythropoietic anemias are lifelong anemias, often mild, showing dysplastic changes affecting the red cell line only, most typically multinuclearity of the normoblasts. They present as iron storage disorders. Of the three types, two (type I[389] usually and type III[390] occasionally) show megaloblastic red cell precursors (see Chap. 43).

REFRACTORY MEGALOBLASTIC ANEMIA

Refractory megaloblastic anemia is now regarded as a manifestation of myelodysplastic and sideroblastic syndromes (see Chaps. 63 and

92). The megaloblastic changes are atypical, with dysplastic features confined to the erythroid series; giant metamyelocytes and bands are absent from the marrow. The combination of a myeloproliferative disorder and true cobalamin deficiency can give rise to a confusing picture.[391,392] A few patients with refractory megaloblastic anemia respond to pharmacologic doses of pyridoxine (200 mg/day),[393] perhaps because of an effect on serine transformylase, which requires both pyridoxine and folate.

ERYTHROLEUKEMIA (DI GUGLIELMO SYNDROME)[394]

Erythroleukemia is the earliest stage of M6 acute myelogenous leukemia (see Chap. 93). Nucleated red cells appear on the blood film, and the marrow shows hyperplasia involving very bizarre-looking megaloblastic red cell precursors, often containing multiple nuclei or nuclear fragments. The disease usually evolves fairly quickly into classical acute myelogenous leukemia.

REFERENCES

1. Myhre E: Studies on megaloblasts in vitro. *Scand J Clin Invest* 16:307, 1964.
2. Bertaux O, Mederic C, Valencia R: Amplification of ribosomal DNA in the nucleolus of vtamin B_{12}-deficient *Euglena* cells. *Exp Cell Res* 195:119, 1991.
3. Rondanelli EG, Gorini P, Magliulo E, Fiori GP: Differences in proliferative activity between normoblasts and pernicious anemia megaloblasts. *Blood* 24:542, 1964.
4. Waxman S, Metz J, Herbert V: Defective DNA synthesis in human megaloblastic bone marrow: Effects of homocysteine and methionine. *J Clin Invest* 48:284, 1969.
5. Pelliniemi T-T, Beck WS: Biochemical mechanisms in the Killmann experiment: critique of the deoxyuridine suppression test. *J Clin Invest* 65:449, 1980.
6. Steinberg SE, Fonda S, Campbell CL, Hillman RS: Cellular abnormalities of folate deficiency. *Br J Haematol* 54:605, 1983.
7. Wickremasinghe RG, Hoffbrand AV: Reduced rate of DNA replication fork movement in megaloblastic anemia. *J Clin Invest* 65:26, 1980.
8. Blount BC, Mack MM, Wehr CM, et al: Folate deficiency causes uracil misincorporation into human DNA and chromosome breakage: implications for cancer and neuronal damage. *Proc Natl Acad Sci USA* 94:3290, 1997.
9. Duthie SJ, McMillan P: Uracil misincorporation in human DNA detected using single cell gel electrophoresis. *Carcinogenesis* 18:1709, 1997.
10. Das KC, Mohanty D, Garewell G: Cytogenetics in nutritional megaloblastic anaemia: prolonged persistence of chromosomal abnormalities in lymphocytes after remission. *Acta Haematol (Basel)* 76:146, 1986.
11. Titenko-Holland N, Jacob RA, Shang N, Balaraman A, Smith MT: Micronuclei in lymphocytes and exfoliated buccal cells of postmenopausal women with dietary changes in folate. *Mutat Res* 417:101, 1998.
12. Fenech MF, Dreosti IE, Rinaldo JR: Folate, vitamin B12, homocysteine status and chromosome damage rate in lymphocytes of older men. *Carcinogenesis* 18:1329, 1997.
13. Fenech M, Aitken C, Rinaldi J: Folate, vitamin B12, homocysteine status and DNA damage in young Australian adults. *Carcinogenesis* 19:1163, 1998.
14. Forni M, Meyer PR, Levy NB, et al: An immunohistochemical study of hemoglobin A, hemoglobin F, muramidase, and transferrin in erythroid hyperplasia and neoplasia. *J Clin Pathol* 80:145, 1983.
15. Ellims PH, Hayman RJ, Van Der Weyden MB: Plasma thymidine kinase in megaloblastic anemia. *Br J Haematol* 44:167, 1980.
16. Baptista LC, Reid CD: Effects of T cells and monocytes on globin chain synthesis in erythroid bursts cultured from human peripheral blood burst-forming units (BFU-e). *Exp Hematol* 3:507, 1985.
17. Reid CD, Baptista LC, Deacon R, Chanarin I: Megaloblastic change is a feature of colonies derived from an early erythroid progenitor (BFU-E) stimulated by monocytes in culture. *Br J Haematol* 49:551, 1981.
18. Spivak JL: Masked megaloblastic anemia. *Arch Intern Med* 142:2111, 1982.
19. Lindenbaum J, Nath BJ: Megaloblastic anaemia and neutrophil hypersegmentation. *Br J Haematol* 44:511, 1980.
20. Herbert V: Experimental nutritional folate deficiency in man. *Trans Assoc Am Physicians* 75:307, 1962.
21. Savage D, Lindenbaum J: Anemia in alcoholics. *Medicine* (Baltimore) 65:322, 1986.
22. Lawler SD, Roberts PD, Hoffbrand AV: Chromosome studies in megaloblastic anemia before and after treatment. *Scand J Haematol* 8:309, 1971.
23. Bessman JD, Williams LJ, Gilmer PR: Platelet size in health and hematologic disease. *Am J Clin Path* 78:150, 1982.
24. Liu YK, Sullivan LW: Marrow granulocyte reserve in pernicious anemia. *Clin Res* 14:321, 1966.
25. Fudenberg H, Estren S: The intermediate megaloblast in the differential diagnosis of pernicious and related anemias. *Am J Med* 25:198, 1958.
26. Fudenberg H, Estren S: The intermediate megaloblasts in the differential diagnosis of pernicious and related anemias. *Am J Med* 25:198, 1958.
27. Green R, Kuhl W, Jacobson R, et al: Masking of macrocytosis by alpha-globin chain deletions in blacks with pernicious anemia. *N Engl J Med* 307:1322, 1982.
28. Gulley ML, Bentley SA, Ross DW: Neutrophil myeloperoxidase measurement uncovers masked megaloblastic anemia. *Blood* 76:1004, 1990.
29. Marshall RA, Jandl HH: Responses to "physiologic" doses of folic acid in the megaloblastic anemias. *Arch Intern Med* 105:353, 1960.
30. Hussein S, Laulicht M, Hoffbrand AV: Serum ferrtin in megaloblastic anemia. *Scand J Haematol* 20:241, 1978.
31. Emerson PM, Wilkinson JH: Lactate dehydrogenase in the diagnosis and assessment of response to treatment of megaloblastic anemia. *Br J Haematol* 12:678, 1966.
32. Winston RM, Warburton FG, Scott A: Enzymatic diagnosis of megaloblastic anaemia. *Br J Haematol* 19:587, 1970.
33. Hansen NE, Karle H: Blood and bone marrow lysozyme in neutropenia: an attempt towards pathogenetic classification. *Br J Haematol* 21:261, 1971.
34. Heller P, Weinstein HG, West M, Zimmerman HJ: Glycolytic, citric acid cycle, and hexosemonophosphate shunt enzymes of plasma in megaloblastic anemia. *J Lab Clin Med* 55:425, 1960.
35. DeKlerk G, Rosengarten PC, Vet RJ, Goudsmit R: Serum erythropoietin (EST) titers in anemia. *Blood* 58:1164, 1981.
36. Myhre E: Studies on the erythrokinetics in pernicious anemia. *Scand J Clin Lab Invest* 16:391, 1964.
37. Heller P, Weinstein HG, Zimmerman HJ: Enzymes in anemia: a study of abnormalities of several enzymes of carbohydrate metabolism in the plasma and erythrocytes in patients with anemia, with preliminary observations of bone marrow enzymes. *Ann Intern Med* 53:898, 1960.
38. Lindahl J: Quantification of ineffective erythropoiesis in megaloblastic anaemia by determination of endogenous production of ^{14}CO after administration of glycine-2-^{14}C. *Scand J Haematol* 24:281, 1980.
39. Hamilton HE, Sheets RF, DeGowin EL: Studies with inagglutinable erythrocyte counts: VII. Further investigation of the hemolytic mechanism in untreated pernicious anemia and the demonstration of a hemolytic property in the plasma. *J Lab Clin Med* 51:942, 1958.
40. Harker LA, Finch CA: Thrombokinetics in man. *J Clin Invest* 48:963, 1969.
41. Aikawa R, Komuro I, Yamazaki T, et al: Oxidative stress activates extracellular signal-regulated kinases through Src and Ras in cultured cardiac myocytes of neonatal rats. *J Clin Invest* 100:1813, 1997.
42. Ballard HS, Lindenbaum J: Megaloblastic anemia complicating hyperalimentation therapy. *Am J Med* 56:740, 1974.
43. Whitehead VM, Comty CH, Posen GA, Kay M: Homeostasis of folic acid in patients undergoing maintenance hemodialysis. *N Engl J Med* 279:970, 1968.
44. Mollin DL, Hines JD: Observations on the nature and pathogenesis of anemia following partial gastrectomy. *Proc R Soc Med* 57:575, 1964.
45. Hoffbrand AV: Folate deficiency in premature infants. *Arch Dis Child* 45:441, 1970.
46. Royston NJW, Parry TE: Megaloblastic anaemia complicating dietary treatment of phenylketonuria in infancy. *Arch Dis Child* 37:430, 1962.
47. Ford JD, Scott KJ: The folic acid activity of some milk foods for babies. *J Dairy Res* 35:85, 1968.
48. Eichner ER, Hillman RS: Effect of alcohol on serum folate level. *J Clin Invest* 52:584, 1973.

49. Sullivan LW, Herbert V: Suppression of haemopoiesis by ethanol. *J Clin Invest* 43:2048, 1963.

50. Lieber CS: Metabolism and metabolic effects of alcohol. *Semin Hematol* 17:85, 1980.

51. Steinberg SE: Mechanisms of folate homeostasis. *Am J Physiol* 246:G319, 1984.

52. McFarland W, Libre EP: Abnormal leukocyte response in alcoholism. *Ann Intern Med* 59:865, 1963.

53. Post RM, Desforges JF: Thrombocytopenia and alcoholism. *Ann Intern Med* 68:1230, 1963.

54. Liu YK: Effects of alcohol on granulocyte and lymphocytes. *Semin Hematol* 17:130, 1980.

55. Lindenbaum J, Lieber CS: Hematological effects of alcohol in man in the absence of nutritional deficiency. *N Engl J Med* 281:333, 1969.

56. Trier JS: Celiac sprue. *N Engl J Med* 325:1709, 1991.

57. Kinnear DG, Johns DG, McIntosh PC: Intestinal absorption of tritium-labeled folic acid in idiopathic steatorrhea: effect of a gluten-free diet. *Can Med Assoc J* 89:957, 1963.

58. Halsted CH, Reisenauer AM, Romero JJ, et al: Jejunal perfusion of simple and conjugated folates in celiac sprue. *J Clin Invest* 59:933, 1977.

59. Dormandy KM, Waters AH, Mollin DL: Folic acid deficiency in coeliac disease. *Lancet* 1:632, 1963.

60. Hjelt K, Krasilnikoff PA: The impact of gluten on haematological status, dietary intakes of haemopoietic nutrients and vitamin B_{12} and folic acid absorption in children with coeliac disease. *Acta Paediatr Scand* 79:911, 1990.

61. Klipstein FA: Tropical sprue in New York City. *Gastroenterology* 47:457, 1964.

62. Guerra R, Wheby MS, Bayless TM: Long-term antibiotic therapy in tropical sprue. *Ann Intern Med* 63:619, 1965.

63. Klipstein FA, Schenck EA, Samloff IM: Folate repletion associated with oral tetracycline therapy in tropical sprue. *Gastroenterology* 51:317, 1966.

64. Klipstein FA: Progress in gastroenterology: tropical sprue. *Gastroenterology* 54:275, 1968.

65. Sheehy TW, Perez-Santiago E, Rubini Me: Tropical sprue and vitamin B_{12}. *N Engl J Med* 265:1232, 1961.

66. Klipstein FA: Folate in tropical sprue. *Br J Haematol* 23:119, 1972.

67. Corcino JJ, Coll G, Klipstein FA: Pteroylglutamic acid malabsorption in tropical sprue. *Blood* 45:577, 1975.

68. Chanarin I, Bennett MC: Absorption of folic acid and D-xylose as tests of small intestinal function. *Br Med J* 1:985, 1962.

69. Booth CC: Metabolic effects of intestinal resection in man. *Postgrad Med J* 37:725, 1961.

70. Pitney WR, Joske RA, Mackinnon NL: Folic acid and other absorption tests in lymphosarcoma, chronic lymphocytic leukemia and some related conditions. *J Clin Pathol* 13:440, 1960.

71. Hoskins LC, Norris TH, Gottlieb LS, Zamcheck N: Functional and morphologic alterations of the gastrointestinal tract in progressive systemic sclerosis (scleroderma). *Am J Med* 33:459, 1962.

72. Vinnik IE, Kern F, Struthers JE: Malabsorption and the diarrhea of diabetes mellitus. *Gastroenterology* 43:507, 1962.

73. Cook GC, Morgan JO, Hoffbrand AV: Impairment of folate absorption by systemic bacterial infections. *Lancet* 2:1417, 1974.

74. Shojania M: Folic acid and vitamin B_{12} deficiency in pregnancy and in the neonatal period. *Clin Perinatol* 11:2, 1984.

75. Landon MJ, Eyre DH, Hytten FE: Transfer of folate to the fetus. *Br J Obstet Gynaecol* 82:12, 1975.

76. Pritchard JA, Scott DE, Whalley PJ: Infants of mothers with megaloblastic anemia due to folate deficiency. *JAMA* 211:1982, 1970.

77. Shapiro J, Alperts HW, Welch P, Metz J: Folate and vitamin B_{12} deficiency associated with lactation. *Br J Haematol* 11:498, 1965.

78. Blot I, Papierhik F, Kaltwasser JP, et al: Influence of routine administration of folic acid and iron during pregnancy. *Gynecol Obstet Invest* 12:294, 1981.

79. Strieff RR, Little AB: Folic acid deficiency in pregnancy. *N Engl J Med* 276:776, 1967.

80. Chanarin I, McFadyen IR, Kyle R: The physiological macrocytosis of pregnancy. *Br J Obstet Gynaecol* 84:504, 1977.

81. Avery B, Ledger WJ: Folic acid metabolism in well-nourished pregnant women. *Obstet Gynecol* 35:616, 1970.

82. Giles C: An account of 335 cases of megaloblastic anemia of pregnancy. *J Clin Pathol* 19:1, 1966.

83. Jandl JH, Greenberg MS: Bone marrow failure due to relative nutritional deficiency in Cooley's hemolytic anemia. *N Engl J Med* 260:461, 1959.

84. Lindenbaum J, Klipstein FA: Folic acid deficiency in sickle cell anemia. *N Engl J Med* 269:875, 1963.

85. Hild D: Folate losses from the skin in exfoliative dermatitis. *Arch Intern Med* 123:51, 1969.

86. Hoffbrand AV, Newcombe BFA, Mollin DL: Method of assay of red cell folate activity and the value of the assay as a test for folate deficiency. *J Clin Pathol* 19:17, 1999.

87. Chanarin I: Folate in blood, cerebrospinal fluid and tissues, in *The Megaloblastic Anemias*, 2d ed, edited by I Chanarin, p 187. Blackwell, Oxford, 1979.

88. Lindenbaum J: Status of laboratory testing in the diagnosis of megaloblastic anemia. *Blood* 61:624, 1983.

89. Zalusky R, Herbert V, Castle AB: Cyanocobalamin therapy effect in folic acid deficiency. *Arch Intern Med* 109:545, 1962.

90. Kirke PN, Daly LE, Elwood JH: A randomised trial of low dose folic acid to prevent neural tube defects. *Arch Dis Child* 67:1442, 1992.

91. Scott JM, Kirke PN, Weir DG: The role of nutrition in neural tube defects. *Annu Rev Nutr* 10:277, 1990.

92. Folic acid and neural tube defects. *Lancet* 338:153, 1991.

93. MRC Vitamin Study Research Group: Prevention of neural tube defects: results of the medical research council vitamin study. *Lancet* 338: 131, 1991.

94. Hall J, Solehdin F: Folic acid for the prevention of congenital anomalies. *Eur J Pediatr* 157:445, 1998.

95. Molloy AM, Daly S, Mills JL, et al: Thermolabile variant of 5,10-methylenetetrahydrofolate reductase associated with low red-cell folates: implications for folate intake recommendations. *Lancet* 349:1591, 1997.

96. Van der Put NM, Gabreels F, Stevens EM, et al: A second common mutation in the methylenetetrahydrofolate reductase gene: an additional risk factor for neural-tube defects. *Am J Hum Genet* 62:1044, 1998.

97. Refsum H, Ueland PM, Nygård O, Vollset SE: Homocysteine and cardiovascular disease. *Annu Rev Med* 49:31, 1999.

98. Houston PE, Rana S, Sekhsaria S, Perlin E, Kim KS, Castro OL: Homocysteine in sickle cell disease: relationship to stroke. *Am J Med* 103:192, 1997.

99. Woo KS, Chook P, Lolin YI, et al: Hyperhomocyst(e)inemia is a risk factor for arterial endothelial dysfunction in humans. *Circulation* 96: 2542, 1997.

100. Ward M, McNulty H, McPartlin J, Strain JJ, Weir DG, Scott JM: Plasma homocysteine, a risk factor for cardiovascular disease, is lowered by physiological doses of folic acid. *QJM* 90:519, 1997.

101. Woodside JV, Yarnell JW, McMaster D, et al: Effect of B-group vitamins and antioxidant vitamins on hyperhomocysteinemia: a double-blind, randomized, factorial-design, controlled trial. *Am J Clin Nutr* 67:858, 1998.

102. Verhoef P, Rimm EB, Hunter DJ, Chen J, Willett WC, Kelsey K: A common mutation in the methylenetetrahydrofolate reductase gene and risk of coronary heart disease: results among U.S. men. *J Am Coll Cardiol* 32:353, 1998.

103. Schmitz C, Lindpaintner K, Verhoef P, Gaziano JM, Buring J: Genetic polymorphism of methylenetetrahydrofolate reductase and myocardial infarction—a case-control study. *Circulation* 94:1812, 1996.

104. Giovannucci E, Stampfer MJ, Colditz GA, et al: Multivitamin use, folate, and colon cancer in women in the nurses' health study. *Ann Intern Med* 129:517, 1998.

105. World Health Organization, Scientific Group on Nutritional Anemias: Nutritional anemias: report of a WHO scientific group. *WHO Tech Rep Ser* 503, 1972.

106. Rosenberg IH: Folic acid and neural-tube defects—time for action. *N Engl J Med* 327:1875, 1992.

107. Schwarz RH, Johnston RB Jr: Folic acid supplementation—when and how. *Obstet Gynecol* 88:886, 1996.

108. Hibbard ED, Spencer WS: Low serum B_{12} levels and latent Addisonian anaemia in pregnancy. *J Obstet Gynaecol Br Commonw* 77:52, 1970.

109. Vilter CF, Vilter RW, Spies TD: The treatment of pernicious and related anemias with synthetic folic acid: I. Observations on the maintenance of a normal hematologic status and on the occurrence of combined system disease at the end of one year. *J Lab Clin Med* 32:262, 1947.

110. Andersen LS, Hansen EL, Knudsen JB, Wester JU, Hansen GV, Hansen TM: Prospectively measured red cell folate levels in methotrexate treated patients with rheumatoid arthritis: relation to withdrawal and side effects. *J Rheumatol* 24:830, 1997.

111. Shiroky JB: The use of folates concomitantly with low-dose pulse methotrexate. *Rheum Dis Clin North Am* 23:969, 1997.

112. Toh BH, van Driel IR, Gleeson PA: Pernicious anemia. *N Engl J Med* 337:1441, 1997.

113. Goldberg LS, Fudenberg HH: The autoimmune aspects of pernicious anemia. *Am J Med* 46:489, 1969.

114. De Aizpurua HJ, Cosgrove LH, Ungar B, Toh BH: Autoantibodies cytotoxic to gastric parietal cells in serum of patients with pernicious anemia. *N Engl J Med* 309:625, 1983.

115. Kano K, Sakamoto S, Miura Y, Takaku F: Disorders of cobalamin metabolism. *CRC Crit Rev Oncol Hematol* 3:1, 1985.

116. Irvine WJ, Davies SH, Teitelbaum S: The clinical and pathological significance of gastric parietal cell antibody. *Ann NY Acad Sci* 124: 657, 1965.

117. Goldberg LS, Cunningham JE, Terasaki PI: Lymphocytotoxins and pernicious anemia. *Blood* 39:862, 1972.

118. Gardner PI, Heier HE: A human autoantibody to renal collecting duct cells associated with thyroid and gastric autoimmunity and possibly renal tubular acidosis. *Clin Exp Immunol* 51:19, 1983.

119. Kapadia CR, Donaldson RM: Disorders of cobalamin (vitamin B$_{12}$) absorption and transport. *Annu Rev Med* 36:93, 1985.

120. Rose MS, Chanarin I: Intrinsic-factor antibody and absorption of vitamin B$_{12}$ in pernicious anaemia. *Br Med J* 1:25, 1971.

121. Suri-Payer E, Kehn PJ, Cheever AW, Shevach EM: Pathogenesis of post-thymectomy autoimmune gastritis. Identification of the anti-H/K adenosine triphosphatase-reactive T cells. *J Immunol* 157:1799, 1996.

122. Barrett SP, Toh BH, Alderuccio F, van Driel IR, Gleeson PA: Organ-specific autoimmunity induced by adult thymectomy and cyclophosphamide-induced lymphopenia. *Eur J Immunol* 25:238, 1995.

123. Chanarin I, James D: Humoral and cell-mediated intrinsic factor antibody in pernicious anaemia. *Lancet* 1:1078, 1974.

124. Carmel R, Johnson CS: Racial patterns in pernicious anemia. *N Engl J Med* 298:647, 1978.

125. Conn HO, Binder H, Burns B: Pernicious anemia and immunologic deficiency. *Ann Intern Med* 68:603, 1968.

126. Sharpstone P, James DG: Pernicious anemia and immunologic deficiency. *Ann Intern Med* 68:603, 1968.

127. Ardeman S, Chanarin I, Krafchik B, Singer W: Addisonian pernicious anaemia and intrinsic factor antibodies in thyroid disorders. *Q J Med* 35:421, 1966.

128. Comin DB, Hines JD, Wieland RG: Coexistent pernicious anemia and idiopathic hypoparathyroidism in women. *JAMA* 207:1147, 1969.

129. Mazzone T, Kelly W, Ensinck J: Lymphocytic hypophysitis associated with antiparietal cell antibodies and vitamin B$_{12}$ deficiency. *Arch Intern Med* 143:1794, 1983.

130. Perillie PE, Nagler R: Development of pernicious anemia in a young patient with chronic ulcerative colitis. *N Engl J Med* 261:1175, 1959.

131. Howitz J, Schwartz M: Vitiligo, achlorhydria, and pernicious anaemia. *Lancet* 1:1331, 1971.

132. Jackson I, Doig WB, McDonald G: Pernicious anaemia as a cause of infertility. *Lancet* 2:1159, 1967.

133. Watson AA: Seminal vitamin B$_{12}$ and sterility. *Lancet* 2:644, 1962.

134. Ungar B, Matthews JD, Tait BD, Cowling DC: HLA-DR patterns in pernicious anaemia. *Br Med J* 282:768, 1981.

135. Hoskins LC, Loux HA, Britten A, Zamcheck N: Distribution of ABO blood groups in patients with pernicious anemia, gastric carcinoma and gastric carcinoma associated with pernicious anemia. *N Engl J Med* 273:633, 1965.

136. Wangel AG, Callender ST, Spray GH, Wright R: A family study of pernicious anaemia: I. Autoantibodies, achlorhydria, serum pepsinogen and vitamin B$_{12}$. *N Engl J Med* 273:633, 1968.

137. Varis K, Ihamaki T, Harkonen M, et al: Gastric morphology, function, and immunology in first-degree relatives of probands with pernicious anemia and controls. *Scand J Gastroenterol* 14:129, 1979.

138. Solanki DL, Jacobson RJ, Green R, et al: Pernicious anemia in blacks. *Am J Clin Path* 75:96, 1981.

139. Eriksson S, Clas L, Moquist-Olsson I: Pernicious anemia as a risk factor in gastric cancer: the extent of the problem. *Acta Med Scand* 210: 481, 1981.

140. Hsing AW, Hansson LE, McLaughlin JK, et al: Pernicious anemia and subsequent cancer. A population-based cohort study. *Cancer* 71:745, 1993.

141. Wilkinson JF: Gastric secretions in pernicious anemia. *Q J Med* 1: 361, 1932.

142. Shojania AM: Problems in the diagnosis and investigation of megaloblastic anemia. *Can Med Assoc J* 122:999, 1980.

143. Fong TL, Dooley CP, Dehesa M, et al: *Helicobacter pylori* infection in pernicious anemia: a prospective controlled study. *Gastroenterology* 100:328, 1991.

144. Karnes WE Jr, Samloff IM, Siurala M: Positive serum antibody and negative tissue staining for *Helicobacter pylori* in subjects with atrophic body gastritis. *Gastroenterology* 101:167, 1991.

145. Magnusson I, Cho JW, Ihre T, et al: Gastrin and somatostatin in plasma and gastric biopsy specimens. *Scand J Gastroenterol* 20:623, 1985.

146. Slingerland DW, Cardarelli JA, Burrows BA, Miller A: The utility of serum gastrin levels in assessing the significance of low serum B$_{12}$ levels. *Arch Intern Med* 144:1167, 1984.

147. Ganguli PC, Cullen DR, Irvine WJ: Radioimmunoassay of plasma-gastrin in pernicious anemia, achlorhydria without pernicious anemia, hypochlorhydria, and in controls. *Lancet* 1:155, 1971.

148. Kaye MD, Whorwell PJ, Wright R: Gastric mucosal lymphocyte subpopulations in pernicious anemia and in normal stomach. *Clin Immunol Immunopathol* 28:431, 1983.

149. Rodbro P, Dige-Petersen H, Schwartz M, Dalggard OZ: Effect of steriods on gastric mucosal structure and function in pernicious anemia. *Acta Med Scand* 181:445, 1967.

150. Boddington MM, Spriggs AI: The epithelial cells in megaloblastic anaemias. *J Clin Pathol* 12:228, 1969.

151. Neiburgs HE, Glass GBJ: Gastric-cell maturation disorders in atrophic gastritis, pernicious anemia, and carcinoma. *Am J Dig Dis* 8:135, 1963.

152. Foroozan P, Trier JS: Mucosa of the small intestine in pernicious anemia. *N Engl J Med* 277:553, 1967.

153. Bezman A, Kinnear DG, Zamcheck N: D-xylose and potassium iodide absorption and serum carotene in pernicious anemia. *J Lab Clin Med* 53:226, 1959.

154. MacLean LD, Sunberg RD: Incidence of megaloblastic anemia after total gastrectomy. *N Engl J Med* 254:885, 1956.

155. McLean LD: Incidence of megaloblastic anemia after subtotal gastrectomy. *N Engl J Med* 257:262, 1957.

156. Deller DJ, Witts LJ: Changes in the blood after gastrectomy with special reference to vitamin B$_{12}$, haemoglobin, serum iron, and bone marrow. *Q J Med* 31:71, 1962.

157. Gozzard DI, Dawson DW, Lewis MJ: Experiences with dual protein bound aqueous vitamin B$_{12}$ absorption test in subjects with low serum vitamin B$_{12}$ concentrations. *J Clin Pathol* 40:633, 1987.

158. Van Der Weyden MB, Rother M, Firkin BG: Megaloblastic maturation masked by iron deficiency: a biochemical basis. *Br J Haematol* 22: 299, 1973.

159. Lees F, Ganjean LC: The gastric and jejunal mucosae in healthy patients with partial gastrectomy. *Arch Intern Med* 101:943, 1958.

160. Shimoda SS, Saunders DR, Rubin CF: The Zollinger-Ellison syndrome with steatorrhea: II. The mechanism of fat and vitamin B$_{12}$ malabsorption. *Gastroenterology* 55:705, 1968.

161. Kennedy HJ, Callender ST, Truelove SC, Warner GT: Haematological aspects of life on an ileostomy. *Br J Haematol* 52:445, 1982.

162. Steinberg F: The megaloblastic anemia of regional ileitis. *N Engl J Med* 264:186, 1961.

163. Anderson CG, Walton KR, Chanarin I: Megaloblastic anaemia after pelvic radiotherapy for carcinoma of the cervix. *J Clin Pathol* 34: 151, 1981.

164. Tudhope GR, Wilson GM: Deficiency of vitamin B$_{12}$ in hypothyroidism. *Lancet* 1:703, 1962.

165. Cameron DG, Watson GM, Witts LJ: The clinical association of macrocytic anemia with intestinal stricture and anastomosis. *Blood* 4:793, 1949.

166. Donaldson RM: Role of enteric microorganisms in malabsorption. *Fed Proc* 26:1426, 1967.

167. Paalk EA Jr, Farrar WE Jr: Diverticulosis of the small intestine and megaloblastic anemia: intestinal flora and absorption before and after tetracycline administration. *Am J Med* 37:473, 1964.

168. Giannella RA, Broitman SA, Zamcheck N: Competition between bacteria and intrinsic factor for vitamin B_{12}: implications for vitamin B_{12} malabsorption in intestinal bacterial overgrowth. *Adv Intern Med* 16: 191, 1972.

169. Murphy MF, Sourial NA, Burman JF, et al: Megaloblastic anaemia due to vitamin B_{12} deficiency caused by small intestinal bacterial overgrowth: possible role of vitamin B_{12} analogues. *Br J Haematol* 62:7, 1986.

170. Nyberg W: The influence of *Diphyllobothrium latum* on the vitamin B_{12}-intrinsic factor complex: I. In vivo studies with Schilling test technique. *Acta Med Scand* 167:185, 1960.

171. Nyberg W: *Diphyllobothrium latum* and human nutrition with particular reference to vitamin B_{12} deficiency. *Proc Nutr Soc* 22:8, 1963.

172. Toskes PP, Hansel J, Cerda J, Deren JJ: Vitamin B_{12} malabsorption in chronic pancreatic insufficiency: studies suggesting the presence of a pancreatic "intrinsic factor." *N Engl J Med* 284:627, 1971.

173. Guéant JL, Champigneulle B, Gaucher P, Nicolas J-P: Malabsorption of vitamin B_{12} in pancreatic insufficiency of the adult and of the child. *Pancreas* 5:559, 1999.

174. Toskes PP, Deren JJ, Conrad ME: Trypsin-like nature of the pancreatic factor that corrects vitamin B_{12} malabsorption associated with pancreatic dysfunction. *J Clin Invest* 52:1660, 1973.

175. Allen RH, Seetharam B, Podell ER, Alpers DH: Effect of proteolytic enzymes on the binding of cobalamin to R protein and intrinsic factor: in vitro evidence that a failure to partially degrade R protein is responsible for cobalamin malabsorption in pancreatic insufficiency. *J Clin Invest* 61:47, 1978.

176. Henderson JT, Simpson JD, Warwick RRG, Shearman DJC: Does malabsorption of vitamin B_{12} occur in chronic pancreatitis? *Lancet* 2:241, 1972.

177. Chanarin I, Malkowska V, O'Hea AM, et al: Megaloblastic anaemia in a vegetarian Hindu community. *Lancet* 2:1168, 1985.

178. Bar-Sella P, Rakover Y, Ratner D: Vitamin B_{12} and folate levels in long-term vegans. *Isr J Med Sci* 26:309, 1990.

179. Gilois C, Wierzbicki AS, Hirani N: The hematological and electrophysiological effects of cobalamin: deficiency secondary to vegetarians' diets. *Ann NY Acad Sci* 669:345, 1992.

180. Ford MJ: Megaloblastic anaemia in a vegetarian. *Br J Clin Pract* 34: 222, 1980.

181. Davis JR, Goldenring J, Lubin BH: Nutritional vitamin B_{12} deficiency in infants. *Am J Dis Child* 135:566, 1981.

182. Graham SM, Arvela OM, Wise GA: Long-term neurologic consequences of nutritional vitamin B_{12} deficiency in infants. *J Pediatr* 121:710, 1992.

183. Michaud JL, Lemieux B, Ogier H, Lambert MA: Nutritional vitamin B_{12} deficiency: two cases detected by routine newborn urinary screening. *Eur J Pediatr* 151:218, 1992.

184. Monagle PT, Tauro GP: Infantile megaloblastosis secondary to maternal vitamin B_{12} deficiency. *Clin Lab Haematol* 19:23, 1997.

185. Adams EG, Scragg JN: Serum vitamin B_{12} concentrations in megaloblastic anemia associated with kwashiorkor and marasmus. *J Pediatr* 60:580, 1962.

186. Wickramasinghe SN, Akinyanju OO, Grange A, Litwinczuk RA: Folate levels and deoxyuridine suppression tests in protein-energy malnutrition. *Br J Haematol* 53:135, 1983.

187. Frenkel EP: Abnormal fatty acid metabolism in peripheral nerves of patients with pernicious anemia. *J Clin Invest* 52:1237, 1973.

188. Lever EG, Elwes RD, Williams A, Reynolds EH: Subacute combined degeneration of the cord due to folate deficiency: response to methyl folate treatment. *J Neurol Neurosurg Psychiatr* 49:1203, 1986.

189. Clayton PT, Smith I, Harding B, et al: Subacute combined degradation of the cord, dementia and Parkinsonism due to an inborn error of folate metabolism. *J Neurol Neurosurg Psychiatr* 49:920, 1986.

190. Weir DG, Keating S, Molloy A, et al: Methylation deficiency causes vitamin B_{12}-deficient monkeys with combined system disease: I. B_{12}-deficient patterns in bone marrow deoxyuridine suppression tests without morphologic or functional abnormalities. *J Neurochem* 51:1949, 1988.

191. Green R, van Tonder SV, Oettle GJ, et al: Neurologic changes in fruit bats deficient in vitamin B_{12}. *Nature* 254:148, 1975.

192. Van der Westhuyzen J, Metz J: Tissue *S*-adenosylmethionine levels in fruit bats with nitrous oxide-induced neuropathy. *Br J Nutr* 50:325, 1983.

193. McLoughlin L, Cantrill RC: Nitrous oxide induced vitamin B_{12} deficiency: Measurement of methylation reactions in the fruit bat (*Rousettus aegyptiacus*). *Int J Biochem* 18:199, 1986.

194. Deacon R, Purkiss P, Green R, et al: Vitamin B_{12} neuropathy is not due to failure to methylate myelin basic protein. *J Neurol Sci* 72:113, 1986.

195. Metz J: Pathogenesis of cobalamin neuropathy: Deficiency of nervous system *S*-adenosylmethionine? *Nutr Rev* 51:12, 1993.

196. Hyland K, Smith I, Bottiglieri T: Demyelination and decreased *S*-adenosylmethionine in 5,10-methylenetetrahydrofolate reductase deficiency. *Neurology* 38:459, 1988.

197. Surtees R, Leonard J, Austin S: Association of demyelination with deficiency of cerebrospinal-fluid *S*-adenosylmethionine in inborn errors of methyl transfer pathway. *Lancet* 388:15504, 1991.

198. Agamanolis D, Green R, Harris JW: Neuropathology of vitamin B_{12} deficiency, in *Neurobiology of the Trace Elements*, edited by IE Dreosti, RM Smith, p 293. Humana, Teaneck, NJ, 1983.

199. Beck WS: Neuropsychiatric consequences of cobalamin deficiency. *Adv Intern Med* 36:33, 1991.

200. Victor M, Lear A: Subacute combined degeneration of the spinal cord: current concepts of the disease: value of serum vitamin B_{12} determinations in clarifying some of the common clinical problems. *Am J Med* 20:896, 1956.

201. Herbert V: Biology of disease: megaloblastic anemias. *Lab Invest* 52:3, 1985.

202. Pant SS, Asbury AK, Richardson EP: The myelopathy of pernicious anemia: a neuropathologic reappraisal. *Acta Neurol Scand* 44(suppl 35):7, 1968.

203. DiLazzaro V, Restuccia D, Fogli D, et al: Central sensory and motor conduction in vitamin B_{12} deficiency. *Electroencephalogr Clin Neurophysiol Evoked Potentials* 84:433, 1992.

204. Fraser TN: Cerebral manifestations of Addisonian pernicious anemia. *Lancet* 2:258, 1960.

205. Shulman R: Psychiatric aspects of pernicious anaemia. *Br Med J* 3:266, 1967.

206. Smith ADM: Megaloblastic madness. *Br Med J* 2:1840, 1960.

207. Stojsavljevic N, Levic Z, Drulovic J, Dragutinovic G: A 44-month clinical-brain MRI follow-up in a patient with B_{12} deficiency. *Neurology* 49:878, 1997.

208. Lovblad K, Ramelli G, Remonda L, et al: Retardation of myelination due to dietary vitamin B_{12} deficiency: cranial MRI findings. *Pediatr Radiol* 27:155, 1997.

209. Karacostas D, Artemis N, Tsitourides I, Milonas I: Cobalamin deficiency: MRI detection of posterior columns involvement and posttreatment resolution. *J Neuroimaging* 8:171, 1998.

210. Karnaze DS, Carmel R: Neurologic and evoked potential abnormalities in subtle cobalamin deficiency states, including deficiency without anemia and with normal absorption of free cobalamin. *Arch Neurol* 47:1008, 1990.

211. Lindenbaum J, Healton EB, Savage DG, et al: Neuropsychiatric disorders caused by cobalamin deficiency in the absence of anemia or macrocytosis. *N Engl J Med* 318:1720, 1988.

212. Stabler SP, Allen RH, Savage DG: Clinical spectrum and diagnosis of cobalamin deficiency. *Blood* 76:871, 1990.

213. O'Brien HA, Sourial NA: Severe megaloblastic anaemia presenting as pancytopenia with red cell hypoplasia and elevated serum cobalamin and cobalamin binding proteins. *Clin Lab Haematol* 12:307, 1991.

214. Stabler SP, Allen RH, Barrett RE: Cerebrospinal fluid methylmalonic acid levels in normal subjects and patients with cobalamin deficiency. *Neurology* 41:1627, 1991.

215. Jenks J, Begley J, Howard L: Cobalamin-R binder deficiency in a woman with thalassemia. *Nutr Rev* 41:277, 1983.

216. Carmel R: Megaloblastic anemias. *Curr Opin Hematol.* 1:107, 1994.

217. Stabler SP, Lindenbaum J, Allen RH: Vitamin B_{12} deficiency in the elderly: current dilemmas. *Am J Clin Nutr* 66:741, 1997.

218. Chanarin I, Deacon R, Lumb M, et al: Cobalamin and folate: Recent developments. *J Clin Pathol* 45:277, 1992.

219. Metz J, Bell AH, Flicker L, et al: The significance of subnormal serum vitamin B_{12} concentration in older people: a case control study. *J Am Geriatr Soc* 44:1355, 1996.

220. Stabler SP, Marcell PD, Podell ER, et al: Assay of methylmalonic acid in the serum of patients with cobalamin deficiency using capillary gas chromatography-mass spectrometry. *J Clin Invest* 77:1606, 1986.

221. Stabler SP, Marcell PD, Podell ER, et al: Elevation of total homocysteine in the serum of patients with cobalamin or folate deficiency detected by capillary gas chromatography-mass spectrometry. *J Clin Invest* 81: 466, 1988.

222. Allen RH, Stabler SP, Savage DG, Lindenbaum J: Dignosis of cobalamin deficiency: I. Usefulness of serum methylmalonic acid and total homocysteine concentrations. *Am J Hematol* 34:90, 1990.

223. Lindenbaum J, Savage DG, Stabler SP, Allen RH: Diagnosis of cobalamin deficiency: II. Relative sensitivities of serum cobalamin, methylmalonic acid and total homocysteine concentrations. *Am J Hematol* 34:99, 1990.

224. Rasmussen K, Vyberg B, Pedersen KO, Brochner-Mortensen J: Methylmalonic acid in renal insufficiency: evidence of accumulation and implications for diagnosis of cobalamin deficiency. *Clin Chem* 36: 1523, 1990.

225. Malleson P: Isolated gastroduodenal Crohn's disease in a ten-year-old girl. *Postgrad Med J* 56:294, 1980.

226. Shojania AM: Physician's management of suspected vitamin B_{12} deficiency. *Can Med Assoc J* 123:1127, 1999.

227. Carmel R: R-binder deficiency: a clinically benign cause of cobalamin pseudodeficiency. *JAMA* 250:1886, 1983.

228. Kahn SB, Williams WS, Barness LA, et al: Methylmalonic acid excretion: a sensitive indicator of vitamin B_{12} deficiency. *J Lab Clin Med* 66:75, 1965.

229. Lindenbaum J, Pezzimenti JF, Shea N: Small-intestinal function in vitamin B_{12} deficiency. *Ann Intern Med* 80:326, 1974.

230. Fairbanks VF, Wahner HW, Phyliky RL: Tests for pernicious anemia: the Schilling test. *Mayo Clin Proc* 63:480, 1983.

231. Nelp WB, Wagner HN Jr, Reba RC: Renal excretion of vitamin B_{12} and its use in measurements of glomerular filtration rate in man. *J Lab Clin Med* 63:480, 1964.

232. Rath CE, McCurdy PR, Duffy BJ: Effect of renal disease on the Schilling test. *N Engl J Med* 256:111, 1956.

233. Akun SN, Miller IF, Meyer LM: Vitamin B_{12} absorption tests. *Acta Haematol* (Basel) 41:341, 1969.

234. Callender ST, Witts LJ, Warner GT, Oliver R: The use of a simple whole-body counter for haematological investigations. *Br J Haematol* 12:276, 1966.

235. Mahmud K, Ripley D, Doscherholmen A: Vitamin B_{12} absorption tests: their unreliability in postgastrectomy states. *JAMA* 216:1167, 1971.

236. Miller A, Furlong D, Burrows BA, Slingerland DW: Bound vitamin B_{12} absorption in patients with low serum B_{12} levels. *Am J Hematol* 40:163, 1992.

237. Streeter AM, Duncombe VM, Boyle R, Pheils MT: A simple method of measuring the absorption of protein-bound vitamin B_{12}. *Aust NZ J Med* 5:382, 1975.

238. Steinberg WM, King CE, Toskes PP: Malabsorption of protein-bound cobalamin but not unbound cobalamin during cimetidine administration. *Dig Dis Sci* 25:188, 1980.

239. Forshaw J: Effect of vitamin B_{12} and folic acid deficiency in small intestinal absorption. *J Clin Pathol* 22:551, 1969.

240. Metz J: The deoxyuridine suppression test. *CRC Crit Rev Clin Lab Sci* 20:205, 1984.

241. Das KC, Manusselis C, Herbert V: In vitro DNA synthesis by bone marrow cells and PHA-stimulated lymphocytes: suppression by nonradioactive thymidine of the incorporation of ^{3}H-deoxyuridine into DNA: enhancement of incorporation when inadequate vitamin B_{12} or folate is corrected. *Br J Haematol* 44:51, 1980.

242. Taheri MR, Wickremasinghe RG, Jackson BF, Hoffbrand AV: The effect of folate analogues and vitamin B_{12} on provision of thymine nucleotides for DNA synthesis in megaloblastic anemia. *Blood* 59: 634, 1982.

243. Das D, Garawal G, Mohanty D: Derangement of DNA synthesis in erythroleukaemia: normal deoxyuridine suppression and impaired thymidine incorporation in bone marrow culture. *Acta Haematol* (Basel) 64:121, 1980.

244. Carmel R, Karnaze DS: The deoxyuridine suppression test identifies subtle cobalamin deficiency in patients without typical megaloblastic anemia. *JAMA* 253:1284, 1985.

245. Ellison AB: Pernicious anemia masked by multivitamins containing folic acid. *JAMA* 173:240, 1960.

246. Smith MD, Smith DA, Fletcher M: Haemorrhage associated with thrombocytopenia in megaloblastic anemia. *Br Med J* 1:982, 1962.

247. Stefanini M, Karaca M: Acquired thrombocytopathy in patients with pernicious anemia. *Lancet* 1:400, 1966.

248. Boddy K, King P, Mervyn L, et al: Retention of cyanocobalamin, hydroxocobalamin and coenzyme B_{12} after parenteral administration. *Lancet* 2:710, 1968.

249. Finch CA, Coleman DH, Motulsky AG, et al: Erythrokinetics in pernicious anemia. *Blood* 11:807, 1956.

250. Hillman RS, Adamson J, Burka E: Characteristics of vitamin B_{12} correction of the abnormal erythropoiesis of pernicious anemia. *Blood* 31: 419, 1968.

251. Lawson DH, Murray RM, Parker JLW, Hay G: Hypokalemia in megaloblastic anaemias. *Lancet* 2:558, 1970.

252. Lawson DH, Murray RM, Parker JLW: Early mortality in megaloblastic anemias. *Q J Med* 41:1, 1972.

253. Kuzminski AM, Del Giacco EJ, Allen RH, Stabler SP, Lindenbaum J: Effective treatment of cobalamin deficiency with oral cobalamin. *Blood* 92:1191, 1998.

254. Altay C, Cetin M: Oral treatment in selective vitamin B_{12} malabsorption. *J Pediatr Hematol Oncol* 19:245, 1997.

255. Slot WB, Merkus FW, Van Deventer SJ, Tytgat GN: Normalization of plasma vitamin B_{12} concentration by intranasal hydroxocobalamin in vitamin B_{12}-deficient patients. *Gastroenterology* 113:430, 1997.

256. Lederle FA: Oral cobalamin for pernicious anemia: Medicine's best kept secret. *JAMA* 265:94, 1999.

257. Kondo H, Osborne ML, Kolhouse JF: Nitrous oxide has multiple deleterious effects on cobalamin metabolism and causes decreases in activities of both mammalian cobalamin-dependent enzymes in rats. *J Clin Invest* 67:1270, 1981.

258. Lumb M, Deacon R, Perry J: The effect of nitrous oxide inactivation of vitamin B_{12} on rat hepatic folate: implications for the methylfolate-trap hypothesis. *Biochem J* 186:933, 1980.

259. Lumb M, Sharer N, Deacon R, et al: Effects of nitrous oxide-induced inactivation of cobalamin on methionine and S-adenosylmethionine metabolism in the rat. *Biochim Biophys Acta* 756:354, 1983.

260. Kano Y, Sakamoto S, Sakuraya K, et al: Effects of leucovorin and methylcobalamin with N_2O anesthesia. *J Lab Clin Med* 104:711, 1984.

261. O'Sullivan H, Jennings F, Ward K, et al: Human bone marrow biochemical function and megaloblastic hematopoiesis after nitrous oxide anesthesia. *Anesthesiology* 55:645, 1981.

262. Skacel PO, Hewlett AM, Lewis JD, et al: Studies on the haemopoietic toxicity of nitrous oxide in man. *Br J Haematol* 53:189, 1983.

263. Skacel PO, Amess JA, Nancekievill DG, Rees GM: Prevention of nitrous oxide-induced megaloblastic changes in bone marrow using folinic acid. *Br J Anaesth* 56:103, 1984.

264. Skacel PO, Chanarin I, Hewlett A, Nunn JF: Failure to correct nitrous oxide toxicity with folinic acid. *Anesthesiology* 57:557, 1982.

265. Lassen HCA, Henriksen A, Neukirch F, Kristensen HS: Treatment of tetanus: severe bone-marrow depression after prolonged nitrous-oxide anaesthesia. *Lancet* 1:527, 1956.

266. Amess JAL, Burman JR, Rees GM: Megaloblastic haemopoiesis in patients receiving nitrous oxide. *Lancet* 2:339, 1978.

267. Brodsky L, Zuniga J: Nitrous oxide: a psychotogenic agent. *Comp Psychiatr* 16:185, 1975.

268. Sahenk Z, Mendel JR, Couri D, Nachtman J: Polyneuropathy from inhalation of N_2O cartridges through a whipped cream dispenser. *Neurology* 28:504, 1978.

269. Layzer RB, Fishman RA, Schafer JA: Neuropathy following abuse of nitrous oxide. *Neurology* 28:504, 1978.

270. Salo M, Rajamaki A, Nikoskelainen J: Absence of signs of vitamin B_{12}–nitrous oxide interaction in operating theatre personnel. *Acta Anaesthesiol Scand* 28:106, 1984.

271. Amos RJ, Amess JA, Hinds CJ, Mollin DL: Incidence and pathogenesis of acute megaloblastic bone-marrow change in patients receiving intensive care. *Lancet* 2:835, 1982.

272. Amess JA, Burman JF, Murphy MF, et al: Severe megaloblastic bone marrow change associated with unsuspected mild vitamin B_{12} deficiency. *Clin Lab Haematol* 3:231, 1981.

273. Easton DJ: Severe thrombocytopenia associated with acute folic acid deficiency and severe hemorrhage in two patients. *Can Med Assoc J* 130:418, 1984.

274. Beard ME, Hatipov CS, Hamer JW: Acute onset of folate deficiency in patients under intensive care. *Crit Care Med* 8:500, 1980.

275. Magee F, O'Sullivan H, McCann SR: Megaloglastosis and low-dose trimethoprim-sulfamethoxazole (letter). *Ann Intern Med* 95:657, 1981.

276. Chan MK, Beale D, Moorhead JF: Acute megaloblastosis due to cotrimaxazole. *Br J Clin Pract* 34:187, 1980.

277. Huennekens FM, Duffy TH, Pope LE: Biochemistry of methotrexate: teaching an old drug new tricks, in *Cancer Biology and Therapeutics*, edited by JG Corry, A Szentivanyi, p 45. Plenum, New York, 1987.

278. Matherly LH, Barlowe CK, Phillips VM, Goldman ID: The effect on 4-aminoantifolates on 5-formyltetrahydrofolate metabolism. *J Biol Chem* 262:710, 1987.

279. Kesavan V, Sur P, Doig MT: Effect of methotrexate on folates in Krebs ascites and L1210 murine leukemia cells. *Cancer Lett* 30:55, 1986.

280. Swinson CM, Perry J, Lumb M, Levi AJ: Role of sulphasalazine in the aetiology of folate deficiency in ulcerative colitis. *Gut* 22:456, 1981.

281. Boots M, Phillips M, Curtis JR: Megaloblastic anemia and pancytopenia due to proguanil inpatients with chronic renal failure. *Clin Nephrol* 18:106, 1981.

282. Bethell FH, Thompson DS: Treatment of leukemia and related disorders with 6-mercaptopurine. *Ann NY Acad Sci* 60:436, 1954.

283. Cristoph R, Pisnay D, Hartl W: Megaloblastic anaemia following treatment of rheumatoid arthritis with Imuran. *Med Welt* 46:1824, 1971.

284. Klippel JH, Decker JL: Relative macrocytosis in cyclophosphamide and azathioprine therapy. *JAMA* 229:180, 1974.

285. Allaudeen HS, Descamps J, Sehgal RK: Mode of action of acyclovir triphosphte on herpes viral and cellular DNA polymerases. *Antiviral Res* 2:123, 1982.

286. Amos RJ, Amess JA: Megaloblastic haemopoiesis due to acyclovir (letter). *Lancet* 1:242, 1983.

287. Heidelberger C, Ansfield FJ: Experimental and clinical use of fluorinated pyrimidines in cancer chemotherapy. *Cancer Res* 23:1226, 1963.

288. Reyes P, Heidelberger C: Fluorinated pyrimidines. *Mol Pharmacol* 1:14, 1963.

289. Cornell RC, Milstein HG, Fox CM: Anemia of azaribine in the treatment of psoriasis. *Arch Dermatol* 112:1717, 1976.

290. Richman DD, Fischl MA, Grieco MH, et al, The AZT Collaborative Working Group: The toxicity of azidothymidine (AZT) in the treatment of patients with AIDS and AIDS-related complex. A double-blind, placebo-controlled trial. *N Engl J Med* 317:192, 1987.

291. Krakoff JH: Clinical and physiologic effects of hydroxyurea, in *Antineoplastic and Immunosuppressive Agents*, edited by AC Sartorelli, DG Johus, p 780. Springer-Verlag, Berlin, 1975.

292. Frenkel EP, Arthur C: Induced ribotide reductive conversion by hydroxyurea and its relationship to megaloblastosis. *Cancer Res* 27:1016, 1967.

293. Cohen SS: Sponges, cancer chemotherapy and cellular aging. *Perspect Biol Med* 6:215, 1963.

294. Papac RJ: Clinical and hematologic studies with 1-β-D-arabinosylcytosine. *JNCI* 40:997, 1968.

295. Reynolds EH, Milner G, Matthews DM: Anticonvulsant therapy, megaloblastic haemopoiesis and folic acid metabolism. *Q J Med* 35:521, 1966.

296. Druskin MS, Wallen MH, Bonagura L: Anticonvulsant-associated anemia. *N Engl J Med* 267:483, 1962.

297. Rose M, Johnson I: Reinterpretation of the haematological effects of anticonvulsant treatment. *Lancet* 1:1349, 1978.

298. Gerson CD, Hepner GW, Brown N, et al: Inhibition of diphenylhydantoin of folic acid absorption in man. *Gastroenterology* 63:246, 1972.

299. Maxwell JD, Hunter J, Stewart DA, et al: Folate deficiency after anticonvulsant drugs: an effect of hepatic enzyme induction? *Br Med J* 1:297, 1972.

300. Carl GF, Smith ML, Furman GM, et al: Phenytoin treatment and folate supplementation affect folate concentrations and methylation capacity in rats. *J Nutr* 121:1214, 1991.

301. Isojarvi FI, Pakarinen AJ, Myllyla VV: Basic haematological parameters, serum gamma-glutamyl-transferase activity, and erythrocyte folate and serum vitamin B_{12} levels during carbamazepine and oxcarbazepine therapy. *Seizure* 6:207, 1997.

302. Kishi T, Fujita N, Eguchi T, Ueda K: Mechanism for reduction of serum folate by antiepileptic drugs during prolonged therapy. *J Neurol Sci* 145:109, 1997.

303. Shojania AM, Hornady G, Barnes PH: Oral contraceptives and serum-folate level. *Lancet* 1:1376, 1968.

304. Butterworth CE Jr, Hatch KD, Gore H, et al: Improvement in cervical dysplasia associated with folic acid therapy in users of oral contraceptives. *Am J Clin Nutr* 35:73, 1982.

305. Shojania AM: Oral contraceptives: effect of folate and vitamin B_{12} metabolism. *Can Med Assoc J* 126:244, 1999.

306. Lindenbaum J, Whitehead N, Reyner F: Oral contraceptive hormones, folate metabolism and cervical epithelium. *Am J Clin Nutr* 28:346, 1975.

307. Pearson D: Megaloblastic anemia due to glutethimide. *Lancet* 1:110, 1965.

308. Hainivaara O, Palva IP: Malabsorption and deficiency of vitamin B_{12} caused by treatment with para-aminosalicylic acid. *Acta Med Scand* 177:337, 1965.

309. Termanini B, Gibril F, Sutliff VE, Yu F, Venzon DJ, Jensen RT: Effect of long-term gastric acid suppressive therapy on serum vitamin B_{12} levels in patients with Zollinger-Ellison syndrome. *Am J Med* 104:422, 1998.

310. Callaghan TS, Hadden DR, Tomkin GH: Megaloblastic anaemia due to vitamin B_{12} malabsorption associated with long-term metformin treatment. *Br Med J* 280:1214, 1980.

311. Dobbins WO, Herrero BA, Mansbach CM: Morphological alterations associated with neomycin induced malabsorption. *Am J Med Sci* 255:63, 1968.

312. Webb DI, Chodos RB, Mahar CQ, Faloon WW: Mechanism of vitamin B_{12} malabsorption in patients receiving colchicine. *N Engl J Med* 279:845, 1968.

313. Lerman BB, Ali N, Green D: Megaloblastic, dyserythropoietic anemia following arsenic ingestion. *Ann Clin Lab Sci* 10:515, 1980.

314. Henderson GB, Suresh MR, Vitols KS, Huennekens FM: Transport of folate compounds in L1210 cells: kinetic evidence that folate influx proceeds via the high-affinity transport system for 5-methyltetrahydrofolate and methotrexate. *Cancer Res* 46:1639, 1986.

315. Schoo MM, Pristupa ZB, Vickers PJ, Scrimgeour KG: Folate analogues as substrates of mammalian folypolyglutamate synthetase. *Cancer Res* 46:1639, 1985.

316. Spiegel RJ, Cooper PR, Blum RH, et al: Treatment of massive intrathecal methotrexate overdose by ventriculolumbar perfusion. *N Engl J Med* 311:386, 1984.

317. Yarchoan R, Broder S: Development of antiretroviral therapy for the acquired immunodeficiency syndrome and related disorders. *N Engl J Med* 316:557, 1987.

318. Kieburtz KD, Giang DW, Schiffer RB, Vakil N: Abnormal vitamin B_{12} metabolism in human immunodeficiency virus infection: association with neurological dysfunction. *Arch Neurol* 48:312, 1991.

319. Boudes P, Zittoun J, Sober A: Folate, vitamin B_{12}, and HIV infection. *Lancet* 335:1401, 1990.

320. Krakoff IH, Brown NC, Reichard P: Inhibition of ribonucleoside diphosphate reductase by hydroxyurea. *Cancer Res* 28:1559, 1968.

321. Doll DC, Weiss RB: Chemotheraputic agents and the erythron. *Cancer Treat Rev* 10:185, 1983.

322. Hamborg B, Kittang E, Schjönsby H: The effect of ranitidine on the absorption of food cobalamins. *Scand J Gastroenterol* 20:756, 1985.

323. Walan A, Strom M: Metabolic consequences of reduced gastric acidity. *Scand J Gastroenterol* (suppl) 111:24, 1985.

324. Salom IL, Silvis SE, Doscherholmen A: Effects of cimetidine on the absorption of vitamin B_{12}. *Scand J Gastroenterol* 17:129, 1982.

325. Koop H, Bachem MG: Serum iron, ferritin, and vitamin B_{12} during prolonged omeprazole therapy. *J Clin Gastroenterol* 14:288, 1992.

326. Parry TE: The diagnosis of megaloblastic anaemia. *Clin Lab Haematol* 2:89, 1980.

327. Gräsbeck R, Gordin R, Kantero I, Kuhlback B: Selective vitamin B_{12} malabsorption and proteinuria in young people: a syndrome. *Acta Med Scand* 167:289, 1960.

328. Waters AH, Murphy MEB: Familial juvenile pernicious anaemia: a study of the hereditary basis of pernicious anaemia. *Br J Haematol* 9:1, 1963.

329. Imerslund O, Bjornstad P: Familial vitamin B_{12} malabsorption. *Acta Haematol* (Basel) 30:1, 1963.

330. Goldenberg LS, Fudenberg HH: Familial selective malabsorption of vitamin B_{12}: re-evaluation of an *in vitro* intrinsic factor inhibitor. *N Engl J Med* 279:405, 1968.

331. Zimram A, Hershko C: The changing pattern of megaloblastic anemia: megaloblastic anemia in Israel. *Am J Clin Nutr* 37:855, 1983.

332. Cooper BA, Rosenblatt DS: Inherited defects of vitamin B$_{12}$ metabolism. *Annu Rev Nutr* 7:291, 1987.

333. Chisolm JC: Selective malabsorption of vitamin B$_{12}$ and vitamin B$_{12}$-intrinsic factor complex with megaloblastic anemia in an adult. *JAMA* 77:835, 1985.

334. Mackenzie IL, Donaldson RM, Trier JS, Mathan VI: Illeal mucosa in familial selective vitamin B$_{12}$ malabsorption. *N Engl J Med* 286:1021, 1972.

335. Burman JF, Jenkins WJ, Walker-Smith JA, et al: Absent ileal uptake of IF-bound-vitamin B$_{12}$ in the Imerslund-Gräsbeck syndrome (familial B$_{12}$ malabsorption with proteinuria). *Gut* 26:311, 1985.

336. Katz M, Lee SK, Cooper BA: Vitamin B$_{12}$ malabsorption due to a biologically inert intrinsic factor. *N Engl J Med* 287:425, 1972.

337. Katz M, Mehlman CS, Allen RH: Isolation and characterization of an abnormal human intrinsic factor. *J Clin Invest* 53:1274, 1974.

338. Carmel R: Gastric juice in congenital pernicious anemia contains no immunoreactive intrinsic factor molecule: study of three kindreds with variable ages at presentation, including a patient first diagnosed in adulthood. *Am J Hum Genet* 35:66, 1983.

339. Miller DR, Bloom GE, Streiff RR, et al: Juvenile ''congenital'' pernicious anemia: clinical and immunologic studies. 275:978, 1966.

340. Hall CA: Congenital disorders of vitamin B$_{12}$ transport and their contributions to concepts: II. *Yale J Biol Med* 54:485, 1981.

341. Frater-Schröder M, Luthy R, Haurani FI, Hitzig WH: Transcobalamin II polymorphisms: Biochemische und klinische Aspecte seltener Variaten. *Schweiz Med Wochenschr* 109:1373, 1982.

342. Thomas PK, Hoffbrand AV, Smith IS: Neurological involvement in hereditary transcobalamin II deficiency. *J Neurol Neurosurg Psychiatr* 45:74, 1982.

343. Hitzig WH, Dohmann U, Pluss HJ, Vischer D: Hereditary transcobalamin II deficiency: clinical findings in a new family. *J Pediatr* 85:622, 1974.

344. Seger R, Wildfeuer A, Frater-Schröder M, et al: Granulocyte dysfunction in transcobalamin II deficiency responding to leucovorin or hydroxocobalamin-plasma transfusion. *J Inherited Metab Dis* 3:3, 1980.

345. Frater-Schröder M, Sacher M, Hitzig WH: Inheritance of transcobalamin II (TC II) in two families with TC II deficiency and related immunodeficiency. *J Inherited Metab Dis* 4:165, 1981.

346. Burman JF, Mollin DL, Sourial NA, Sladden RA: Inherited lack of transcobalamin II in serum and megaloblastic anaemia: a further patient. *Br J Haematol* 43:27, 1979.

347. Meyers PA, Carmel R: Hereditary transcobalamin II deficiency with subnormal serum cobalamin levels. *Pediatrics* 74:866, 1984.

348. Carmel R, Ravindranath Y: Congenital transcobalamin II deficiency presenting atypically with a low serum cobalamin level: studies demonstrating the coexistence of a circulating transcobalamin I (R binder) complex. *Blood* 63:598, 1984.

349. Rana SR, Colman N, Goh KO, et al: Transcobalamin II deficiency associated with usual bone marrow findings and chromosomal abnormalities. *Am J Hematol* 14:89, 1983.

350. Haurani FI, Hall CA, Rubin R: Megaloblastic anemia as a result of an abnormal transcobalamin II. *J Clin Invest* 64:1253, 1979.

351. Fernandes-Costa F, Metz J: Vitamin B$_{12}$ binders (transcobalamins) in serum. *CRC Crit Rev Clin Lab Sci* 18:1, 1983.

352. Rosenblatt DS, Hosack A, Matiaszuk N: Expression of transcobalamin II by amniocytes. *Prenat Diagn* 7:35, 1987.

353. Carmel R: A new case of deficiency of the R binder for cobalamin, with observations on minor cobalamin-binding proteins in serum and saliva. *Blood* 59:152, 1982.

354. Carmel R, Herbert V: Deficiency of vitamin B$_{12}$ alpha globulin in two brothers. *Blood* 33:1, 1969.

355. McIntyre OR, Sullivan LW, Jeffries GH, Silver RH: Pernicious anemia in childhood. *N Engl J Med* 272:981, 1965.

356. Lambert HP, Prankerd TAJ, Smellie JM: Pernicious anaemia in childhood: a report of two cases of one family and their relationship to the etiology of pernicious anemia. *Q J Med* 30:71, 1960.

357. Fowler B: Genetic defects of folate and cobalamin metabolism. *Eur J Pediatr* 157:S60, 1998.

358. Ogier de-Baulny N, Gerard M, Saudubray JM, Zittoun J: Remethylation defects: guidelines for clinical diagnosis and treatment. *Eur J Pediatr* 157:S77, 1998.

359. Matsui SM, Mahoney MJ, Rosenberg LE: The natural history of the inherited methylmalonic acidemias. *N Engl J Med* 308:857, 1983.

360. McCurley TL, Cousar JB, Graber SE, et al: Plasma cell iron—clinical and morphologic features. *Am J Clin Path* 81:312, 1984.

361. Watkins D, Rosenblatt DS: Failure of lysosomal release of vitamin B$_{12}$: a new complementation group causing methylmalonic aciduria (cb1F). *Am J Hum Genet* 39:404, 1986.

362. Rosenblatt DS, Hosack A, Matiaszuk NV: Defect in vitamin B$_{12}$ release from lysosomes: newly described inborn error of vitamin B$_{12}$ metabolism. *Science* 228:1219, 1985.

363. Mahoney MJ, Hart AC, Steen VD, Rosenberg LE: Methylmalonic acidemia: biochemical heterogeneity in defects of 5'-deoxyadenosylcobalamin synthesis. *Proc Natl Acad Sci USA* 72:2799, 1975.

364. Chalmers RA, Bain MD, Mistry J, et al: Enzymologic studies on patients with methylmalonic aciduria: basis for a clinical trial of deoxyadenosylcobalamin in a hydroxocobalamin-unresponsive patient. *Pediatr Res* 30:560, 1991.

365. Rosenblatt DS, Cooper BA, Pottier A: Altered vitamin B$_{12}$ metabolism in fibroblasts from a patient with megaloblastic anemia and homocystinuria due to a new defect in methionine biosynthesis. *J Clin Invest* 74:2149, 1984.

366. Hallam LJ, Sawyer M, Clark ACL, Van Der Weyden MB: Vitamin B$_{12}$-responsive neonatal megaloblastic anemia and homocystinuria with associated reduced methionine synthase activity. *Blood* 69:1128, 1987.

367. Rosenblatt DS, Cooper BA, Schmutz S, Zaleski WA, Casey RE: Prenatal vitamin B$_{12}$ therapy of a fetus with methylcobalamin deficiency (cobalamin E disease). *Lancet* i:1127, 1985.

368. Leclerc D, Campeau E, Goyette P, et al: Human methionine synthase: cDNA cloning and identification of mutations in patients of the *cblG* complementation group of folate/cobalamin disorders. *Hum Mol Genet* 5:1867, 1996.

369. Gulati S, Chen Z, Brody LC, Rosenblatt DS, Banerjee R: Defects in auxiliary redox proteins lead to functional methionine synthase deficiency. *J Biol Chem* 272:19171, 1997.

370. Mitchell GA, Watkins D, Malancon SB, et al: Clinical heterogeneity in cobalamin C variant of combined homocystinuria and methylmalonic aciduria. *J Pediatr* 108:410, 1986.

371. Carmel R, Bedros AA, Mace JW, Goodman SI: Congenital methylmalonic aciduria—homocystinuria with megaloblastic anemia: observations on response to hydroxocobalamin and on the effect of homocysteine and methionine on the deoxyuridine suppression test. *Blood* 55:540, 1980.

372. Zammarchi E, Lippi A, Falorni S, et al: Case report and monitoring of a pregnancy at risk by chorionic villus sampling. *Clin Invest Med* 13:139, 1980.

373. Ampola MG, Mahoney MJ, Nakamura E, Tanaka K: Prenatal therapy of a patient with vitamin B$_{12}$-responsive methylmalonic acidemia. *N Engl J Med* 293:313, 1975.

374. Van der Meer SB, Spaapen LJM, Fowler B, et al: Prenatal treatment of a patient with vitamin B$_{12}$-responsive methylmalonic acidemia. *J Pediatr* 117:923, 1990.

375. Erbe RW: Inborn errors of folate metabolism: II. *N Engl J Med* 293:807, 1975.

376. Luhby AL, Eagle FJ, Roth E, et al: Relapsing megaloblastic anemia in an infant due to a specific defect in gastrointestinal absorption of folic acid. *Am J Dis Child* 102:482, 1961.

377. Lanzkowsky P: Congenital malabsorption of folate. *Am J Med* 48:580, 1970.

378. Walters T: Congenital megaloblastic anemia responsive to N^5-formyl tetrahydrofolic acid administration. *J Pediatr* 70:686, 1967.

379. Arakawa T, Narisawa K, Tanno K, et al: Megaloblastic anemia and mental retardation associated with hyperfolic-acidemia: probably due to N^5-methyltetrahydrofolate transferase deficiency. *Tohoku J Exp Med* 93:1, 1967.

380. Huguley CM Jr, Bain JA, Rivers SL, Scoggins RB: Refractory megaloblastic anemia associated with excretion of orotic acid. *Blood* 14:615, 1959.

381. Smith LH Jr, Sullivan M, Huguley CM Jr: Pyrimidine metabolism in man: IV. Enzymatic defect of orotic aciduria. *J Clin Invest* 40:656, 1961.

382. Fox RM, Wood MH, Royse-Smith D, O'Sullivan WJ: Hereditary orotic aciduria: types I and II. *Am J Med* 55:791, 1973.

383. van der Zee SPM: Megaloblastic anemia in the Lesch-Nyhan syndrome. *Lancet* 1:1427, 1968.

384. Viana MB, Carvalho RI: Thiamine-responsive megaloblastic anemia, sensorineural deafness and diabetes mellitus: a new syndrome. *J Pediatr* 93:235, 1978.

385. Abboud MR, Alexander D, Najjar SS: Diabetes mellitus, thiamine-dependent megaloblastic anemia, and sensorineural deafness associated with deficient alpha-ketoglutarate dehydrogenase. *J Pediatr* 107:537, 1985.

386. Thiamine-responsive megaloblastic anemia. *Nutr Res* 38:374, 1980.

387. Bazarbachi A, Muakkit S, Ayas M, et al: Thiamine-responsive myelodysplasia. *Br J Haematol* 102:1098, 1998.

388. Neufeld EJ, Mandel H, Raz T, et al: Localization of the gene for thiamine-responsive megaloblastic anemia syndrome, on the long arm of chromosome 1, by homozygosity mapping. *Am J Hum Genet* 61:1335, 1997.

389. Maeda K, Saeed SM, Rebuck JW: Type I dyserythropoietic anemia. A 30-year follow-up. *Am J Clin Path* 73:433, 1980.

390. Wickramasinghe SN, Parry TE, Williams C: A new case of congenital dyserythropoietic anaemia, type III: studies of the cell cycle distribution and ultrastructure of erythroblasts and of nucleic acid synthesis in marrow cells. *J Clin Pathol* 35:1103, 1982.

391. Vogelsang GB, Spivak JL: Unusual case of acute leukemia: coexisting acute leukemia and pernicious anemia. *Am J Med* 76:1144, 1984.

392. Ahmann FR, Durie BG: Acute myelogenous leukaemia modulated by B_{12} deficiency: a case with bone marrow blast cell assay corroboration. *Br J Haematol* 58:91, 1984.

393. Najfeld V, McArthur J, Shashty GG: Monosomy 7 in a patient with pancytopenia and abnormal erythropoiesis. *Acta Haematol* (Basel) 66:12, 1981.

394. Roggli VL, Saleem A: Erythroleukemia: a study of 15 cases and literature review. *Cancer* 49:101, 1982.

IRON DEFICIENCY

VIRGIL F. FAIRBANKS
ERNEST BEUTLER

Iron deficiency and iron deficiency anemia are common nutritional and hematologic disorders in North America and worldwide, affecting an estimated 2 billion people. In infants and young children iron deficiency is most commonly due to insufficient dietary iron. In young women it is most often the result of blood loss in menstruation or as a result of pregnancy. In older adults bleeding may be from the gastrointestinal tract, as from hemorrhoids, bleeding peptic ulcer, hiatus hernia, colon cancer, or angiodysplasia. It may result from uterine leiomyomas or carcinoma, or a renal tumor. Pulmonary blood loss is usually evidenced by chronic hemoptysis due to infection, malignancy, or as a result of idiopathic pulmonary hemosiderosis. However, bloody sputum may be swallowed, and pulmonary bleeding may be mistaken for gastrointestinal bleeding. Iron deficiency has adverse effects on activity of numerous enzymes and in infants can result in impairment of growth and intellectual development. The hematologic features of iron deficiency are nonspecific and too often confused with other causes of microcytic anemia such as thalassemias, chronic disease, renal neoplasms, and other disorders. A low serum ferritin concentration is an excellent indicator of iron deficiency. Erythrocyte zinc protoporphyrin assay is a useful screening test but lacks specificity. Other laboratory tests that may prove useful include assays for serum transferrin receptor, erythrocyte ferritin concentration, or serum ferritin iron saturation. Diagnosis of iron deficiency, particularly in an adult, obliges the clinician to determine the site and cause of blood loss and to rectify that if possible. Treatment of iron deficiency with ferrous salts, in doses of 100 to 200 mg of elemental iron daily, is superior to, much safer, and far less costly than parenteral therapy. Enteric-coated and prolonged-release preparations should be avoided. Complete correction of anemia is expected in 8 to 12 weeks, depending on patient's age. If this response is not achieved, the patient and the diagnosis require reevaluation. Administration of iron should be continued for 8 months after correction of anemia or as long as bleeding continues.

DEFINITION AND HISTORY

Iron deficiency is the state in which the content of iron in the body is less than normal. It occurs in varying degrees of severity that merge imperceptibly into one another. *Iron depletion* is the earliest stage of

iron deficiency, in which storage iron is decreased or absent but serum iron concentration and blood hemoglobin levels are normal. *Iron deficiency without anemia* is a somewhat more advanced stage of iron deficiency, characterized by decreased or absent storage iron, usually low serum iron concentration and transferrin saturation, without frank anemia. *Iron deficiency anemia* is the most advanced stage of iron deficiency. It is characterized by decreased or absent iron stores, low serum iron concentration, low transferrin saturation, and low hemoglobin concentration or hematocrit value.

In certain rare disorders, such as idiopathic pulmonary hemosiderosis or paroxysmal nocturnal hemoglobinuria (see Chap. 56), iron deficiency anemia may occur without iron depletion as a result of redistribution of body iron.

The clinical manifestations of iron deficiency anemia appear to have been recognized in earliest times. A disease characterized by pallor, dyspnea, and edema was described in about 1500 BC in the *Papyrus Ebers*, a manual of therapeutics believed to be the oldest complete manuscript extant.[1] This ancient disease may have been due to chronic blood loss from hookworm infestation. Chlorosis, or "green sickness," was well known to European physicians after the middle of the sixteenth century. In France, by the middle of the seventeenth century, iron salts and other remedies (including, oddly enough, phlebotomy) were used in its treatment. Not long thereafter, iron was recommended by Sydenham as a specific remedy for chlorosis. For the 100 years preceding 1930, iron was used in the treatment of chlorosis, often in ineffective doses, although the mechanism of action of iron and the appropriateness of its use were highly controversial.

By the beginning of the twentieth century, it had been established that chlorosis was characterized by a decrease in the iron content of the blood and by the presence of hypochromic erythrocytes. Most of the fundamental work on iron metabolism and iron deficiency has been carried out during this century.[2]

ETIOLOGY AND PATHOGENESIS

ETIOLOGY

Iron deficiency may occur as a result of chronic blood loss, inadequate dietary iron intake, malabsorption of iron, diversion of iron to fetal and infant erythropoiesis during pregnancy and lactation, intravascular hemolysis with hemoglobinuria, or a combination of these factors.

BLEEDING

Gastrointestinal   In men and in postmenopausal women iron deficiency is most commonly caused by chronic bleeding from the gastrointestinal tract. A partial list of causes of such blood loss is presented in Table 38-1. In the adult the commonest causes of gastrointestinal bleeding are peptic ulcer, hiatal hernia, gastritis (including that due to alcohol or aspirin ingestion), hemorrhoids, vascular anomalies (such as angiodysplasia), and neoplasms. Helicobacter pylori infection has been associated with an increased incidence of iron deficiency, even in the absence of frank peptic ulceration.[3]

Diaphragmatic (hiatal) hernia is frequently associated with gastrointestinal bleeding. The frequency of anemia ranges from 8 to 38 percent.[4-7] Bleeding is much more likely to occur in patients with paraesophageal or large hernias than in those with sliding hernias or small ones.[4,5,8] It is likely that hemorrhage follows mucosal injury at the neck of the sac, where the herniated stomach rides to and fro over the crus of the diaphragm during respiration.[4,5,7] Mucosal changes cannot always be demonstrated by esophagoscopy or gastroscopy in patients who have had blood loss from hiatus hernia. However, a linear gastric erosion, also called a *Cameron ulcer*, commonly occurs on the crests of mucosal folds at the level of the diaphragm and appears

The following abbreviations and acronyms may be found in this chapter: MAO, monoamine oxidase; MCH, mean erythrocyte hemoglobin content; MCV, mean corpuscular volume; RDA, recommended daily allowance; RDW, red cell distribution width; TIBC, total iron-binding capacity; UIBC, unsaturated or latent iron-binding capacity.

TABLE 38-1   SOURCES OF BLOOD LOSS

Respiratory tract
  Carcinoma
  Epistaxis
  Idiopathic pulmonary hemosiderosis
  Infections
  Telangiectases
Alimentary tract
  Esophagus
    Varices

  Stomach

    Angiodysplasia
    Antrial vascular ectasia
  Carcinoma
  Gastritis
    Hemangioma
    Hiatus hernia
    Hypergastrinemia
    Leiomyoma (Ménétrier disease)

    Mucosal hypertrophy
    Ulcer
    Varices

  Small bowel
    Aberrant pancreas
    Angiodysplasia
    Carcinoma
    Helminthiasis
    Hemangioma
    Intussusception
    Leiomyoma
    Meckel diverticulum
    Polyp
    Regional enteritis
    Telangiectasia
    Ulcer
    Vascular occlusion
    Volvulus
  Genitourinary tract
    Kidney
      Hematuria
        Carcinoma
        Goodpasture disease
        Inflammatory disease
    Hemoglobinuria
    March hemoglobinuria
    Paroxysmal cold hemoglobinuria
    Paroxysmal nocturnal hemoglobinuria
    Valvular hemolysis
  Phlebotomy
  Blood donation
  Nosocomial
  Self-induced (Lasthénie de Ferjol)
  Therapeutic (e.g., in polycythemia vera)

Biliary tract
  Aberrant pancreas
  Carcinoma
  Cholelithiasis
  Intrahepatic bleeding
  Ruptured aneurysm
  Trauma

Colon
  Amebiasis
  Angiodysplasia
  Carcinoma
  Diverticulum
  Hemangioma
  Polyp
  Telangiectasia
  Ulcerative colitis

Rectum
  Angiodysplasia
  Carcinoma
  Hemorrhoids
  Ulceration

Uterus
  Adenomyomas
  Carcinoma
  Menstruation/menorrhagia

to be the site of bleeding. In a series of 109 cases of large diaphragmatic hernias, a third had such linear erosions; most of these patients were anemic.[8]

Gastritis due to drug ingestion is another common cause of bleeding. Aspirin ingestion is as likely to cause bleeding in patients without preexisting ulcer as in those with peptic ulcer.[9] Other medications (such as glucocorticoids, indomethacin, ibuprofen, or other nonsteroidal antiinflammatory drugs) may also cause bleeding by inducing gastric or duodenal ulcers or colitis.[10] Use of enteric-coated medications containing potassium chloride has led to serious bleeding from enteric ulcerations. Gastritis due to alcohol ingestion may also cause significant blood loss.

In one study of 114 outpatients referred to gastroenterologists for investigation of iron deficiency, 45 had upper gastrointestinal and 18 had colonic sources of bleeding.[11] In 100 other patients in whom the site of bleeding could not be established by any means short of laparotomy, a malignancy was found to be the cause in 10 percent.[12] Enteritis after therapeutic irradiation of abdominal viscera[12] may also be a cause of gastrointestinal bleeding leading to iron deficiency anemia. Colon cancer, colonic diverticula, periampullary tumors, leiomyomas, adenomas, and other malignant or benign neoplasms of the intestine are among the causes of chronic blood loss.[13-16]

Chronic blood loss from esophageal or gastric varices may lead to iron deficiency anemia. In hereditary hemorrhagic telangiectasia (Chap. 121 and Plate XXV-41, 42), characteristic lesions commonly occur on fingertips, nasal septum, tongue, lips, margins (helices) of ears, oral and pharyngeal mucosa, palms and soles, and other epithelial and cutaneous surfaces throughout the body. Those lesions that occur in the gastrointestinal tract are particularly likely to bleed and to cause iron deficiency to occur. Tortuous, dilated sublingual venous structures, the cherry hemangiomas commonly seen in the elderly, and the spider telangiectases of chronic liver disease are usually easily distinguished from the lesions of hereditary hemorrhagic telangiectasia. Bleeding from intestinal telangiectases has also been observed in scleroderma[17] and in Turner syndrome.[18] Cutaneous hemangiomas (blue rubber bleb nevus) may be associated with hemorrhage from intestinal hemangiomas.[19-21] Chronic blood loss is often the cause of anemia in rheumatoid arthritis (perhaps a result of the aspirin or glucocorticoid therapy), ulcerative colitis, and regional enteritis. Hemorrhoidal bleeding may lead to severe iron deficiency anemia. Chronic blood loss may result from diffuse gastric mucosal hypertrophy (Ménétrier disease).[22] Gastric ulceration and bleeding may also occur in disorders of hypergastrinemia, as in Zollinger-Ellison syndrome and pseudo-Zollinger-Ellison syndrome.[23] Polycythemia vera is typically associated with iron deficiency as a result either of spontaneous gastrointestinal hemorrhage that commonly occurs in this disorder or phlebotomy therapy, or both mechanisms.

Anemia that follows subtotal gastrectomy has usually been attributed to reduced absorption of dietary iron,[24,25] but occult intermittent gastrointestinal bleeding may also be a contributory factor. Of 8 patients whose erythrocytes were labeled with $Na_2^{51}CrO_4$ to permit precise quantitation of daily fecal blood loss,[26] 7 were shown to lose from 3.2 to 6.5 ml of blood per day. This is a very slight but significant increase in daily fecal blood loss which is normally less than 2 ml per day. Over a span of several years this could well lead to iron deficiency anemia. Chemical tests for fecal blood loss are usually insensitive to a daily loss of less than 5 to 10 ml of blood, although this depends to some extent on the site of bleeding within the gastrointestinal tract.

The lesions of angiodysplasia may occur in any part of the gastrointestinal tract but are most frequent in the cecum or ascending colon.[27] These tiny vascular anomalies may be the cause of significant blood loss. Endoscopy is usually required for diagnosis.[27-30] Vascular ectasia of the gastric antrum exhibits a characteristic endoscopic appearance ("watermelon stomach") and is another cause of blood loss.[28,31-33] Hemorrhage into the gallbladder is a rare cause of chronic iron deficiency anemia.[34]

Intestinal parasitism, particularly by hookworms, is a major cause of gastrointestinal blood loss in many parts of the world. Hemostatic defects, particularly those related to abnormal platelet function or number, may lead to gastrointestinal bleeding. Gastrointestinal bleeding is common in von Willebrand disease (Chap. 135). When a patient with a disorder of hemostasis suffers from gastrointestinal bleeding, one must consider the possibility that the bleeding may not be caused by a hemostatic defect alone and that an anatomic lesion of the gastrointestinal tract may also be present.

Ingestion of whole cow's milk may induce protein-losing enteropathy and gastrointestinal bleeding in infants,[35-39] probably on the basis of hypersensitivity or allergy. In four such cases observed endoscopically, erosive gastritis or gastroduodenitis was demonstrated as the probable source of bleeding.[37] At least during the first year of life, children should not be given whole bovine milk, either raw or pasteurized.[39] More protracted heating, as in preparation of infant formulas, eliminates this problem. Anemia itself may increase the amount of blood lost in the infant's feces, perhaps because of an adverse effect of iron deficiency on the intestinal mucosa. Intrinsic lesions of the gastrointestinal tract, such as those listed above, may cause bleeding in infants and in older children as well. In infants or small children, peptic ulcer is an uncommon cause of gastrointestinal bleeding. Meckel diverticulum usually causes gross gastrointestinal bleeding, manifested as hematochezia. Since Meckel diverticulum is usually not demonstrated by gastrointestinal x-ray examination, it is easily overlooked as a cause of gastrointestinal hemorrhage.

Respiratory Tract   Recurrent hemoptysis may lead to iron deficiency anemia. It may be due to congenital anomalies of the respiratory tract, endobronchial vascular anomalies, chronic infections, neoplasms, or valvular heart disease. Severe iron deficiency anemia is a manifestation of idiopathic pulmonary hemosiderosis and of Goodpasture syndrome (progressive glomerulonephritis with intrapulmonary hemorrhage).[40] In some of these disorders, hemoptysis may not be observed, but sufficient amounts of blood-laden sputum may be swallowed to result in positive tests for occult blood in the stools.

Genitourinary Tract   Menstrual bleeding is a very common cause of iron deficiency.[41] The amount of blood lost with menstruation varies markedly from one woman to another and is often difficult to evaluate by questioning the patient. The average menstrual blood loss is about 40 ml per cycle. Blood loss exceeds 80 ml (equivalent to about 30 mg of iron) per cycle in only 10 percent of women.[42] The volume of blood lost in the course of one menstrual cycle may be as high as 495 ml in apparently healthy, nonanemic women who do not regard their menstrual flow to be excessive. The amount of menstrual blood lost does not seem to vary markedly from one cycle to another for any given individual.[43] The use of an intrauterine coil for contraception increases menstrual blood loss,[44] especially during the first year of use. Since the absorption of 1 mg of iron per day requires a dietary intake of between 10 and 20 mg of iron, it is easy to understand why, with an average dietary iron intake of approximately 10 mg per day, iron balance in many menstruating women is precarious.

Excessive bleeding may be caused by uterine fibroids and malignant neoplasms. Neoplasms, stones, or inflammatory disease of the kidney, ureter, or bladder may cause enough chronic blood loss to produce iron deficiency.

FACTITIOUS ANEMIA

Factitious anemia due to self-inflicted bleeding may present a formidable diagnostic and therapeutic problem. This rare condition has also been called, in literary allusion to a fictitious character, *Lasthénie de Ferjol syndrome.* (In Barbey d'Aurevilly's gloomy novel, *Une Histoire Sans Nom,* Lasthénie de Ferjol was a young woman noted for extreme pallor and languor, who habitually and secretly practiced autodesanguination by thrusting needles into her heart.) Most patients are women. There is often a history of numerous blood transfusions. The anemia is chronic and may be severe, with blood hemoglobin concentration persistently as low as 5 to 6 g/dl. The site of induced blood loss is obscure. Hence, patients are subjected to numerous radiographic and endoscopic examinations, usually to no avail. The patients are usually refractory to medical advice and therapy.[45-48] The patients may be depressed and suicidal; some also suffer anorexia nervosa. Psychiatric care is needed but often is unsuccessful.

NOSOCOMIAL ANEMIA

In the course of medical care, repetitive blood sampling may result in removal of a large amount of blood,[49] and this iatrogenic phlebotomy can result in iron deficiency anemia.

ANEMIA INCIDENT TO BLOOD DONATION

Each whole blood donation removes about 200 to 250 mg of iron from the body. Lesser amounts of iron are removed in the course of donating platelets or leukocytes. Potential donors are screened in blood banks so that those with frank anemia are not phlebotomized. Yet, by the time that they are excluded from donation, blood donors are iron depleted and may readily develop iron deficiency anemia with relatively small additional blood loss.[50]

PREGNANCY

In pregnancy, the average iron loss resulting from diversion of iron to the fetus for erythropoiesis, blood loss at delivery (equivalent to an average of 150 to 200 mg of iron), and lactation is altogether about 900 mg; in terms of iron content, this is equivalent to the loss of over 2 liters of blood. Approximately 30 mg of iron may be expended monthly in lactation. Since most women begin pregnancy with low iron reserves, these additional demands frequently result in iron deficiency anemia. Iron depletion has been reported in some 85 to 100 percent of pregnant women. The incidence is lower in women who take oral iron supplementation.[51,52] Furthermore, iron-deficient mothers are likely to have babies with low iron reserves.[53] The clear implication is that all pregnant women should receive prophylactic oral iron, a practice that is often neglected by obstetricians.[54]

DIETARY IRON DEFICIENCY

In infants, iron deficiency is most often a result of the use of unsupplemented milk diets, which contain an inadequate amount of iron. During the first year of life, the full-term infant requires approximately 160 mg and the premature infant about 240 mg of iron for erythropoiesis. About 50 mg of this need is met by the destruction of erythrocytes, which occurs physiologically during the first week of life. The rest must come from the diet. Milk products are very poor sources of iron, and prolonged breast- or bottle-feeding of infants frequently leads to iron deficiency anemia unless there is iron supplementation. This is especially true of premature infants. Table 38-2 lists the iron content of several widely used infant foods. In recognition of the high prevalence of iron deficiency, and its adverse effects, when infant formula is not iron-supplemented, the American Academy of Pediatrics[55] has urged that all infant formulas be iron-fortified; unfortunately, this practice is not universal in North America.

In older children, an iron-poor diet may contribute to the development of iron deficiency anemia, but other factors, such as intestinal parasitism or bleeding gastrointestinal lesions, may be present.

Estimates of average daily iron intake for various segments of the U.S. population are shown in Table 38-3. These estimates used surveys that asked participants for 24-h recall of their food intake and then estimated the iron intake from the known content of the foods consumed. Since nearly half of the dietary iron intake of Americans is in the form of iron-fortified cereals,[56] the assimilable iron content of the diet may be considered to be approximately half of the figures shown in Table 38-3. For most persons in the United States, iron intake is approximately 5 to 7 mg/1000 cal. Children and young women are usually in precarious iron balance, their iron intake being less than 80 percent of the recommended dietary daily allowance (RDA).[57]

The RDAs for iron shown in Table 38-3 differ from those shown in Chap. 24 (Table 25-2) and in previous editions of *Hematology*. In a study of the 24-h-recall dietary data of the Second National Health

TABLE 38-2   IRON CONTENT OF INFANT FOODS

LIQUID FOOD	IRON CONTENT, mg/LITER*
Breast milk	1.1
Evaporated milk	1.8
Evaporated milk, diluted 13:19	0.7
Whole cows' milk	0.7
Similac™, "low iron"	1.3
Similac™, "with iron"	11.5
Enfamil™, "low iron"	0.45
Enfamil™, "with iron"	11.5

SEMISOLID FOOD	IRON CONTENT, mg/SERVING†
Cereal, various (Gerber)	6.75
Purees	
Vegetables	0.0–0.60
Meat and vegetable mixes	0.30–1.20

*For commercially prepared infant formulas, iron content is as stated by manufacturer, in 1999. The brand-name products shown are examples only and do not imply endorsement by the authors.

†For cereal and puree preparations, iron content was calculated from statement of the manufacturer, ambiguously expressed as "per cent of daily amount." Communication with Gerber Products, Inc., indicated that the "daily amount" is 15 mg, i.e., the old RDA that is 2.5-fold greater than the current RDA for infants. Thus, the many (Gerber) cereal products examined, whether of wheat, rice, or mixed grains, all contain (according to the manufacturer) 6.75 mg of reduced iron per 15 g of dry powder (500 ppm), that is intended to be mixed with water, milk, or formula in volume up to 250 ml, for each serving.

and Nutrition Examination Survey (NHANES II), conducted in 1976 to 1980, the estimated mean dietary iron intake of young, nonpregnant, nonlactating women was 10.7 mg (median 9.8 mg), or 56 percent of the then-stated RDA.[58] Consequently, in 1989 the Food and Nutrition Board of the National Research Council (USA) reduced the RDA from 18 to 15 mg for young, nonpregnant women, and from 15 to 6 mg for infants.[59] In the subsequent NHANES III dietary recall survey (conducted in 1988 to 1991), the estimated mean dietary iron intake of young women was 70 to 80 percent of the 1989 RDA, an *apparent* improvement in iron nutrition, although the estimates of mean iron intake were nearly identical in the two surveys.[57] With the lower 1989 RDA for infants, infant iron nutrition also appeared ample.

Iron is present in varying amounts in most foods. Liver is relatively rich in iron. Beans, peas, red meat, poultry, and fish contain smaller amounts of iron, generally not more than 1 mg of iron per ounce. All vegetables (except legumes and cruciferous vegetables such as broccoli) and nearly all fruits are either poor in iron, or, as in spinach, contain unabsorbable iron chelates. Raisins have an undeserved reputation as an iron source; simply because they are dried, the proportion by weight of all minerals is higher than in grapes. Domestic U.S. wines, beers, and other alcoholic beverages contain little iron.[60] Nearly all flour in the United States is "enriched" with

TABLE 38-4   IRON FORTIFICATION OF WHITE FLOUR, WHITE BREAD, ROLLS, AND BUNS IN THE UNITED STATES

FORM OF IRON	ABSORBABILITY	AMOUNT ADDED
Ferrous sulfate	Fair	None
Metallic ("reduced")	Poor	20 mg/lb (44.1 ppm or 0.00441% w/w)

12 mg of finely powdered metallic ("reduced") iron per pound. This provides about 36 mg of iron per kg of enriched bread, rolls, or buns. Thus, a gram of enriched bread has about the same iron content as a gram of beef. However, millers do not add ionic iron because bread made from flour enriched with ferrous salts quickly develops an unpleasant flavor. The iron added to flour is metallic iron, thus insoluble and poorly absorbed, and because flour contains phytates that chelate ionic iron, rendering it unabsorbable, the iron fortification of flour appears to have little, if any, nutritional value (Table 38-4). Microencapsulated ferrous sulfate may improve the bioavailability of iron that is added to food. Another strategy would be iron fortification of dairy products.[61,62]

The iron content of unmodified milk is no greater than that of municipal drinking water obtained from aquifers (prior to water-softening). All dairy products are similarly iron-poor. During the past 30 years there has been an extraordinary change in dietary patterns of Americans. As shown in Fig. 38-1, there has been a marked decline in consumption of red meat and a marked increase in consumption of iron-poor dairy products and snack foods. For example, in the United States, mozzarella cheese consumption has increased approximately 9 percent per year, with consumption increasing from 220 million pounds to more than 2 billion pounds annually in a 25-year interval. Pizza has become a staple in the diet of many Americans. Many secondary and primary schools have franchised commercial pizza vendors in their cafeterias. Potato chips, french fries, and packaged snack foods also now contribute substantially to the average American diet: all are high in fat and low in iron. This is a diet that is conducive to obesity, atherosclerosis, type II diabetes mellitus, and iron deficiency.

The scant iron supply of the American diet places young women and children at particular risk of negative iron balance. Since the adult male needs to absorb only about 1 mg iron daily from his diet in order to maintain normal iron balance, the iron requirements of males are very small. Therefore, iron deficiency in men is only very rarely caused by dietary iron deficiency alone. Exceptions to this rule are known, such as the case of a man who remained on a nearly iron-free diet for 27 years.[63]

TABLE 38-3   DAILY DIETARY IRON INTAKE IN THE UNITED STATES, MEAN VALUES FOR SELECTED GROUPS*

AGE AND SEX	ESTIMATED Fe INTAKE/DAY, mg	RECOMMENDED DAILY ALLOWANCE, mg	% OF RECOMMENDED DAILY ALLOWANCE
Infant, 6–11 months	11.9	6	200
Child, 1–2 years	8.4	10	84
Female, 14–30 years	10.5	15	70
Female, pregnant	14	30	47
Female, lactating	14	15	93
Female, 60–65 years	10.2	10	102
Male, 12 and older	>12	12	>100

*Modified from data obtained during the interval 1982–1984, and published in "Mineral Contents of Foods and Total Diets: The Selected Minerals in Foods Survey, 1982–1984,"[9] and from data collected during 1989–1990 in the Third National Health and Nutrition Examination Survey, NHANES-III.[6] The data obtained in these two large surveys, which were undertaken 7 years apart, provided nearly identical results. Hence, they have been combined in this table. It should be noted that in the latter survey, RDAs for iron were based on those recommended in 1989, following substantial reduction in the estimated dietary iron requirements for infants, children, and young females. Differences between ethnic groups were negligible. To simplify the table, results for all males age 12 and older were combined, since there were only minimal differences between the age groups. A similar simplification was achieved by combining data for all females in the age range 14–30 years, exclusive of those who were pregnant or lactating.

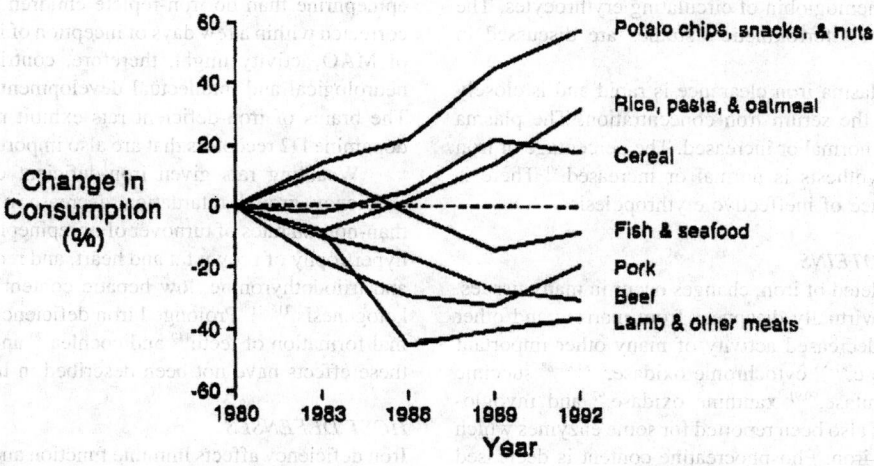

FIGURE 38-1   Changes in patterns of food consumption in the United States from 1980 to 1992, showing a marked decrease in consumption of food that has fair to moderate iron content and a marked increase in consumption of iron-poor food. (Based on data from: *Third Report on Nutrition Monitoring in the United States*, 1995.)[57]

MALABSORPTION OF IRON

Intestinal malabsorption of iron is quite an uncommon cause of iron deficiency except after gastrointestinal surgery and in malabsorption syndromes. As many as 50 percent of patients who have undergone subtotal gastric resection develop iron deficiency anemia years later. Many such patients have impaired absorption of food iron, caused in part by more rapid gastrojejunal transit and in part by partially digested food bypassing some of the duodenum as a result of the location of the anastomosis. Fortunately, medicinal iron is well absorbed in postpartial gastrectomy patients. Moreover, gastrointestinal blood loss may also play an important role in anemia following gastric resection (see section on bleeding, gastrointestinal). In malabsorption syndromes, absorption of iron may be so limited that iron deficiency anemia develops over a period of years.[64,65] Celiac disease, whether overt or occult, may be associated with iron deficiency anemia.[40]

INTRAVASCULAR HEMOLYSIS AND HEMOGLOBINURIA

Iron deficiency anemia may occur in paroxysmal nocturnal hemoglobinuria (Chap. 56) and in hemolysis resulting from mechanical erythrocyte trauma from intracardiac myoxomas,[66] valvular prostheses, or patches[67–69] (Chap. 50). In these disorders, iron is lost in the urine as hemosiderin and ferritin in diquamated tubular cells and as hemoglobin.[69]

Iron deficiency occurs frequently in athletes engaged in a variety of sports (Chap. 52), especially long-distance running but also in swimmers.[70–75] There may be mild anemia. In runners, this appears to be due to gastrointestinal bleeding. In swimmers it has been attributed to hemolysis,[73] but the existence of swimmer's anemia has been disputed.[74]

DIALYSIS TREATMENT OF CHRONIC RENAL DISEASE

The use of extracorporeal dialysis for treatment of chronic renal disease may cause iron deficiency, often superimposed upon the anemia of chronic renal disease. The retention of blood in the dialyzing equipment is the cause, and this problem usually can be avoided by returning as much blood as possible to the patient after each dialysis.[76]

CYSTIC FIBROSIS

Iron deficiency occurs in about a third of patients with cystic fibrosis, but is not related to severity of disease and may simply be due to failure to prescribe iron supplements for these children.[77]

PATHOGENESIS

Figure 38-2 shows the changes that take place in various iron compartments as iron deficiency progresses from a state of mild iron depletion to one of advanced iron deficiency anemia.[78]

ERYTHROCYTE SURVIVAL AND FERROKINETICS

Slight to moderate shortening of erythrocyte survival is characteristic of iron deficiency anemia, particularly when it is severe.[79,80] A study of the movement of iron between various iron compartments (such as plasma pool, labile pool, and hemoglobin compartment) may be performed by intravenous injection of radioactive iron (^{59}Fe) followed by measurement of the rate of clearance of ^{59}Fe from plasma and of

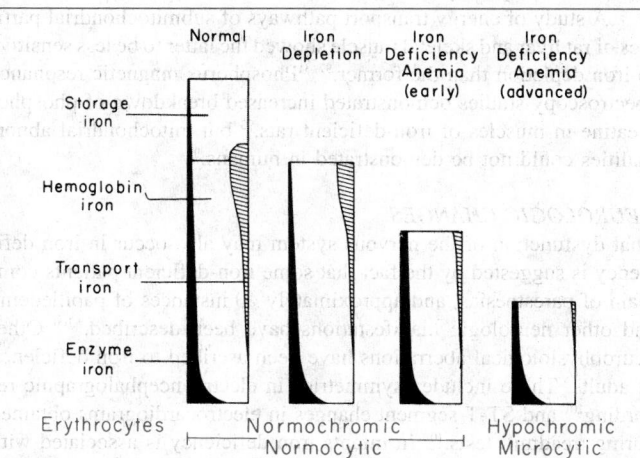

FIGURE 38-2   Stages in the development of iron deficiency. Early iron deficiency (iron depletion) is usually not accompanied by any abnormalities in blood; at this stage, serum iron concentration is occasionally below normal values and storage iron is markedly depleted. As iron deficiency progresses, development of anemia precedes appearance of morphologic changes in blood, although some cells may be smaller and paler than normal; serum iron concentration is usually low at this time, but it may be normal. With advanced iron depletion, classic changes of hypochromic, microcytic, hypoferremic anemia become manifest.

its incorporation into the hemoglobin of circulating erythrocytes. The principles underlying such "ferrokinetic" studies are discussed in Chap. 29.

In iron deficiency, plasma iron clearance is rapid and is closely inversely correlated with the serum iron concentration. The plasma iron transport rate may be normal or increased. The percentage of iron utilized in hemoglobin synthesis is normal or increased.[80] There is usually little or no evidence of ineffective erythropoiesis.

IRON-CONTAINING PROTEINS

As the body becomes depleted of iron, changes occur in many tissues. Hemosiderin and ferritin virtually disappear from marrow and other storage sites. There is a decreased activity of many other important iron proteins: cytochrome c,[81–85] cytochrome oxidase,[83,84,86–88] succinic dehydrogenase,[83–85,89] aconitase,[90,91] xanthine oxidase,[92] and myoglobin.[93] Reduced activity has also been reported for some enzymes which do not contain or require iron. Phosphocreatine content is decreased and inorganic phosphorus is increased in skeletal muscle of iron-deficient rats.[84] Many of the affected enzymes are in the oxidative glycolysis (Krebs) cycle of mitochondria. On the other hand, the activities of several mitochondrial matrix enzymes are increased in skeletal muscle of iron-deficient animals.[83,84]

MUSCULAR FUNCTION AND EXERCISE TOLERANCE

Iron-deficient rats have impaired exercise tolerance and are prone to lactic acidosis when exercised. The activity of α-glycerophosphate dehydrogenase was diminished in the skeletal muscle of iron-deficient rats, and this finding might explain the greater proclivity of iron-deficient rats to lactic acidosis[94] upon exercise. However, in skeletal muscle of iron-deficient guinea pigs, the activity of this enzyme is normal.[95] The brown fat of iron-deficient rats has lower-than-normal activities of NADH and of succinate and α-glycerophosphate oxidases.[96]

Besides these metabolic aberrations of muscle cells in iron-deficient rodents, ultrastructural studies show swollen mitochondria with distorted cristae.[85] Despite these changes, mitochondrial cytochrome c increases adaptively on repetitive electrical stimulus of muscle.[85]

A study of energy transport pathways of submitochondrial particles of rat liver and skeletal muscle showed the latter to be less sensitive to iron depletion than the former.[97] ^{31}Phosphorus magnetic resonance spectroscopy studies demonstrated increased breakdown of phosphocreatine in muscles of iron-deficient rats,[98] but mitochondrial abnormalities could not be demonstrated in humans.[99]

NEUROLOGIC CHANGES

That dysfunction of the nervous system may also occur in iron deficiency is suggested by the fact that some iron-deficient patients complain of paresthesias, and approximately 40 instances of papilledema and other neurologic manifestations have been described.[3,100] Other neurophysiological aberrations have been ascribed to iron deficiency in adults. These include asymmetries in electroencephalographic recording[101] and ST-T segment changes in electrocardiograms obtained during treadmill tests.[102] In infants iron deficiency is associated with poor attention span, poor response to sensory stimuli, and retarded behavioral and developmental achievement even in the absence of anemia.[103–109] School children with iron deficiency anemia who received iron treatment had better academic achievement than did those not so treated.[103,105,110]

Monoamine oxidase (MAO) activity was low in the liver and platelets of patients with iron deficiency.[111–114] MAO is involved in the synthesis and catabolism of important neurotransmitters such as dopamine, norepinephrine, and serotonin. Furthermore, iron-deficient children and iron-deficient rats excrete substantially more urinary nor-

epinephrine than do iron-replete children or rats, an anomaly that is corrected within a few days of inception of iron therapy.[113,114] Reduction of MAO activity might, therefore, contribute to the impairment in neurological and intellectual development of iron-deficient children. The brains of iron-deficient rats exhibit reduction in the number of dopamine D2 receptors that are also important in neurotransmission.[115]

Weanling rats given iron-deficient diets showed poor feeding efficiency, growth retardation, decrease in concentration, and greater-than-normal rates of turnover of norepinephrine in brown fat and heart, hypertrophy of brown fat and heart, and reduction in plasma thyroxine and triiodothyronine, low hepatic content of carnitine, and impaired ketogenesis.[116–118] Prolonged iron deficiency in rats also caused abnormal formation of teeth[119] and cochlea[120] and hearing loss.[121] However, these effects have not been described in humans.

HOST DEFENSES

Iron deficiency affects immune function and the susceptibility to infection.[122–124] Some studies found that iron depletion prevents growth of microorganisms and therefore protects against infections; others observed that iron deficency impairs host defenses.

GROWTH, METABOLISM, OTHER EFFECTS

Iron deficiency anemia is associated with reduction in children's height.[106,125] Impaired thermoregulation has also been demonstrated.[126,127] Iron deficiency has been proposed as a cause of atrophic rhinitis.[128,129] The evidence for this is equivocal; perhaps iron deficiency is a contributory factor.

Thus, in iron deficiency, disturbances in cellular metabolism and function occur in many tissues. Gastric secretion of hydrochloric acid is often reduced.[130–133] Histamine-fast achlorhydria has been found in as many as 43 percent of patients with iron deficiency.[17,133–135] Gastric function may improve after correction of the iron deficiency, although in persons over the age of 30 the achlorhydria is usually irreversible.[132,135–137] Furthermore, when atrophic gastritis coexists with iron deficiency, no improvement in gastric secretory function has followed iron therapy.[137]

HISTOLOGIC FINDINGS

Iron deficiency may lead to histologic changes in various organs. The rapidly proliferating cells of the upper part of the alimentary tract seem particularly susceptible to the effect of iron deficiency. There may be atrophy of the mucosa of the tongue and esophagus,[138] stomach,[139,140] and small intestine.[90,141] The epithelium of the lateral margins of the tongue is reduced in thickness despite increase in the progenitor compartment. This thinning presumably reflects accelerated exfoliation of epithelial cells.[142] Buccal mucosa has shown thinning and keratinization of epithelium and increased mitotic activity.[143,144] However, light microscopic and electron microscopic examination of exfoliated oral mucosal cells showed no aberrations in morphology of nuclei or cytoplasm of the cells of patients with iron deficiency anemia.[145] In the laryngopharynx, mucosal atrophy may lead to web formation in the postcricoid region, thereby giving rise to dysphagia (Paterson-Kelly/Plummer-Vinson syndrome).[146,147] If these alterations are of long duration, they may lead to pharyngeal carcinoma.[148] Although it has been generally thought that these changes are secondary to long-standing iron deficiency, this mechanism is not universally accepted.[149]

In iron deficiency anemia resulting from idiopathic pulmonary hemosiderosis, characteristic pathologic changes are found in the lungs, including intense deposition of iron in the littoral cells of the alveoli and interstitial fibrosis.[40] Widening of diploic spaces of bones, particularly those of the skull and hands,[150,151] may be a consequence of chronic iron deficiency beginning in infancy. In the skull, this is of the same character as in thalassemia, except that in β-thalassemia major there is maxillary hypertrophy, whereas in severe iron deficiency anemia maxillary growth and pneumatization are normal. The sella turcica may be abnormally small in iron-deficient children, and it has been suggested that this implies reduction in pituitary hormonal secretion in long-standing iron deficiency anemia.[152]

PREVALENCE

On a worldwide basis, caloric insufficiency, manifested as hunger, famine, starvation, appears to be the dominant nutritional problem. Iron deficiency affects at least a third of the world's population, or 2 billion persons, and is, therefore, second only to hunger as a major, worldwide nutritional problem. In tropical areas, where hookworm infestation is common, iron deficiency anemia has particularly high prevalence. In India, where hookworm disease is prevalent and vegetarianism is mandated by religion, iron deficiency is especially common.

In the United States, where the dominant nutritional problem is obesity, iron deficiency is also the second most common nutritional problem. It is widely believed that the prevalence of iron deficiency has declined during the past few decades, but the evidence for this is doubtful.

Progressive declines in mean hemoglobin concentration and mean hematocrit values were documented by the Centers for Disease Control and Prevention since 1959 in successive Health and Nutrition Examination Surveys. These declines were observed in every age, sex, and ethnic group examined, altogether more than 50,000 persons surveyed. They were most marked in women of ages 18 to 44 years and in African Americans of every age group, both males and females. Part of the explanation may be that the earlier surveys were performed using specimens obtained from persons sitting, and the later surveys from persons recumbent. Fluid shifts that occur with recumbency are known to reduce hemoglobin concentration and hematocrit values. Part of the explanation may be change in the anticoagulant used to collect blood specimens, a dry powder having been used in the earlier studies and a liquid anticoagulant in 0.07 ml volume/collection tube in the later studies. This droplet of anticoagulant signficantly reduces results for measurement of Hb concentration, hematocrit, and erythrocyte count, especially when the sample collection tube is not completely filled. However, differences in sampling methods are not likely to account entirely for the threefold difference in rates of decline in hemoglobin concentration and hematocrit for specimens obtained from African-Americans or white females of ages 20 to 44 as compared with those obtained from white males of ages 20 to 44. These changes may also relate to a decline in the quality of iron nutrition in the United States.

In the state of Georgia a survey showed that the prevalence of iron deficiency was 30 percent among African-American children and 33 percent among white children, although only 2 percent of the children were frankly anemic.[153] In St. Paul, Minnesota, a prosperous community with high employment, there is a high prevalence of iron deficiency anemia in infants and children of economically disadvantaged status that are eligible for the WIC (Women, Infants and Children) program of nutritional supplementation: The prevalence rates of anemia are 24 percent for white children, 22 percent for African-American children, 24 percent for Asian children (predominantly Hmong), 16 percent for Hispanic, and 7.9 percent for native American children.[154]

In Sweden, with a well-fed population and lifestyle not unlike that of middle-class white Americans, surveys have shown high prevalence rates for anemia and iron deficiency despite long-standing efforts to improve iron nutrition by addition of iron to wheat flour and bread. Since there appeared to be neither harm nor benefit from this practice, flour and bread are no longer iron-fortified in Sweden.[155-157] Elsewhere in Europe, iron fortification is not practiced.

Anemia is not a sensitive indicator of the prevalence of iron deficiency, nor is anemia due solely to iron deficiency. However, iron deficiency is by far the commonest cause of anemia. In most populations, the prevalence of iron deficiency may be estimated as being 3 or 4 times the prevalence of anemia. It may reasonably be assumed that most of the economically deprived children of St. Paul, Minnesota, are iron-deficient. Erythrocyte zinc protoporphyrin, a relatively sensitive indicator of iron deficiency (or of lead poisoning) was elevated in nearly half the white children, in nearly half the African-American children, and in nearly 80 percent of Asian children who were admitted to the WIC program in St. Paul.

Thus, poverty remains a major determinant of iron malnutrition in the United States. African-American and Hispanic children are much less likely to have sufficiency of iron nutrition. In homes with low incomes, there may be "dysfunctional nutrition," and hunger is common and iron intake is inadequate.[158]

The overall prevalence for iron deficiency anemia in the United States in the last few years of the twentieth century cannot be stated with certainty, but conservative estimates for middle class white Americans are approximately 9 percent for children of ages 1 to 2 years, 3.5 percent for children of ages 3 to 14 years, 4 percent for nonpregnant young women during the reproductive years, 30 percent for pregnant or postpartum women, 4 percent for postmenopausal women, 1 percent for males of ages 20 to 44 years, 3 percent for males of ages 45 to 70 years, and 4 percent or more for both males and females oler than 70 years.[159] The prevalence rates of iron deficiency (with or without anemia), as estimated from serum ferritin concentration, in these same age and sex groups are, respectively, 9 percent, 5 percent, 13 percent, greater than 30 percent, 2 percent, and 5 percent. African-Americans of both sexes, Mexican-Americans, native Americans, and poor people of any ethnic group have higher prevalence of iron deficiency anemia. A particularly high prevalence of iron deficiency occurs among the Inuit (Eskimo) people of Alaska and Canada.[160] From one-third to one-half of apparently healthy women of reproductive age in the United States,[161] Sweden,[162] and Japan[163] have iron depletion as assessed by marrow examination or serum ferritin or both, although 4 to 10 percent of the women are anemic.

Despite the long recognition of iron deficiency as a major nutritional problem in the United States, and limited efforts to ameliorate it, the prevalence of iron deficiency and iron deficiency anemia has remained high.

CLINICAL FEATURES

When anemia develops slowly, as in patients with chronic occult bleeding, homeostatic mechanisms provide remarkable adaptation. Patients with marked iron deficiency anemia may deny any degree of fatigue, weakness, or palpitation. However, they may recognize improved work tolerance after treatment.

There is a poor correlation between severity of symptoms and blood hemoglobin concentration.[164] Fatigue, irritability, and headaches are common complaints of patients with iron deficiency. Depletion of storage iron and, to some extent, of tissue iron precedes the appearance of anemia. These observations suggest that some of the symptoms may be caused by impaired function of iron enzymes or iron proteins other than hemoglobin. In a few studies of this problem, patients received either iron therapy or placebos in random double-blind series. In one of these investigations, patients with iron deficiency had greater symptomatic improvement with iron medication than with placebos[165]; in other studies with a somewhat different experimental design, this was not true.[166,167] Objective measurements of work performance studies using O_2 consumption as an index of work performance have also given contradictory results.[168-172] In subjects rendered iron-depleted but not anemic by repeated blood donation, iron-supplemented and untreated groups showed the same O_2 consumption during exercise.[168] However, iron-deficient, nonanemic rats exhibited diminished exercise tolerance and evidence of irritability.[94,173–175] In most studies, iron-deficient humans have demonstrated diminished maximal exercise tolerance,[176–183] although this has not been a universal finding.[168,169,184,185]

Headache, paresthesias, and a burning sensation of the tongue are symptoms of iron deficiency that are not due to anemia but seem likely to be caused by deficiency of iron within tissue cells (Chap. 35). An increase in the volume of menstrual blood loss has been considered to be a result as well as a cause of iron deficiency,[186,187] but this observation has been disputed.[188] Pica, the craving to eat unusual substances such as dirt, clay, ice, laundry starch, salt, cardboard, or hair, is a classic manifestation of iron deficiency and is usually cured promptly by iron therapy.[189–193] Restless legs, a common nocturnal problem, especially in the elderly, has been associated with iron deficiency.[194,195]

The physical findings in iron deficiency anemia include, in approximate order of frequency: pallor, glossitis (smooth, red tongue), stomatitis, and angular cheilitis. Koilonychia, once a common finding, is now encountered rarely (Fig. 38-3). Retinal hemorrhages and exudates may be seen in severely anemic patients (e.g., hemoglobin concentration of 5 g/dl or less). Proliferative retinopathy has shown rapid acceleration in patients with diabetes mellitus who have developed iron deficiency anemia.[196] The spleen is palpable in a small proportion of patients with iron deficiency anemia.

LABORATORY FEATURES

In severe uncomplicated iron deficiency anemia, the erythrocytes are hypochromic and microcytic, the plasma iron concentration is diminished, the iron-binding capacity increased, the serum ferritin concentration is low, the serum transferrin receptor and erythrocyte zinc protoporphyrin concentrations are increased, and the marrow is depleted of stainable iron. Because physicians may not always be aware of the costs of diagnostic tests, Table 38-5 compares some of the fees that were levied in 1999 for common diagnostic procedures. Unfortunately, the classic combination of laboratory findings occurs consistently only when iron deficiency anemia is far advanced, when there are no complicating factors such as infection or malignant neoplasms, and when there has not been previous therapy with transfusions or parenteral iron.

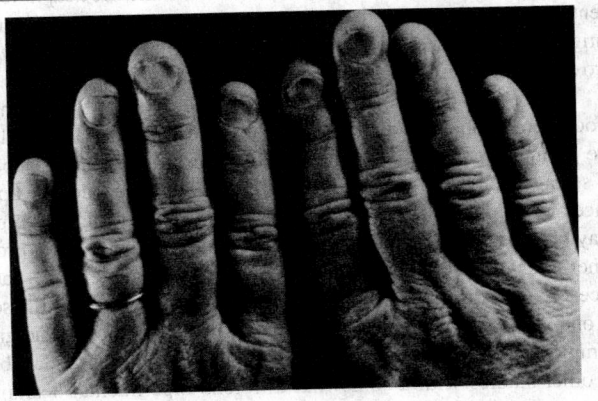

FIGURE 38-3 Koilonychia. Note the ridging, thinning, and splitting, as well as spoonlike concavity of the fingernails.

TABLE 38-5 DIAGNOSIS OF IRON DEFICIENCY, COMPARISON OF FEES OF EXAMINATIONS, $*

History and physical examination	150.00
"CBC" (excludes differential)	34.00
Serum iron and TIBC	24.50
Serum ferritin	48.00
Serum transferrin receptor	50.00
Erythrocyte zinc-protoporphyrin	24.00
Occult blood, feces (Hemoquant)	35.00
Review of blood film by physician	95.00
Chest x-ray, PA stereo	100.00
Marrow examination (with iron stain)	407.00
CT scan, abdomen	860.00
Colonoscopy	2500.00

*Approximate fees at a medical center in midwestern USA, July 1999. The fee for marrow examination includes costs of obtaining specimen, paraffin embedding, staining with Wrights stain and Perls stain for iron, and physician examination. Charge for colonoscopy includes fee for physician service plus fee for administration of Versed and for postexamination recovery room. Costs vary among institutions and between laboratories.

BLOOD CELLS

ERYTHROCYTES

Anisocytosis is the earliest recognizable morphologic change of erythrocytes in iron deficiency anemia[197] (Fig. 38-4). The anisocytosis is typically accompanied by mild ovalocytosis. As the iron deficiency worsens, there is often mild normochromic, normocytic anemia (blood hemoglobin concentration greater than 11 g/dl, mean corpuscular volume, MCV, less than 80 fl).[197–200] With further progression, hemoglobin concentration, erythrocyte count, MCV, and mean erythrocyte hemoglobin content (MCH) all decline together. In infants and children, hypochromia may occur earlier in the course of iron deficiency, and erythrocyte counts in excess of 5.5×10^{12}/liter (5,500,000/μl) are sometimes encountered. As the indices change the erythrocytes appear microcytic and hypochromic on stained blood films. Target cells may sometimes be present. Elongated hypochromic elliptocytes may be seen, in which the long sides are nearly parallel. Such cells have been called "pencil cells," although they more nearly resemble cigars in shape.

The red cell indices are consistently abnormal in adults only when iron deficiency anemia is moderate or severe (e.g., in males with hemoglobin concentrations less than 12 g/dl or in women with hemoglobin concentrations less than 10 g/dl) (Fig. 38-5). Measurement of the distribution of erythrocyte volume (e.g., red cell distribution width, or RDW) is made easy by modern cell counters. With some of these instruments the RDW is reported as the coefficient of variation (in percent) of erythrocyte volume. It has been asserted that such measurements permit discrimination between iron deficiency anemia and other microcytic anemias.[201–204] However, hemoglobinopathies and thalassemias[201,203,205–207] commonly exhibit increased RDW, as do some anemias that are due to chronic disease.[201,208–210] Highest RDWs are observed in hemolytic disorders, in which the RDW appears to reflect reticulocytosis.[206] Thus, the early expectation that RDW would permit diagnosis of iron deficiency anemia has been disappointed.

The sensitivity and specificity of erythrocyte indices for iron deficiency may be increased by use of formulae that incorporate MCV, RDW, serum ferritin concentration, and serum transferrin saturation to produce an iron index[211] or combinations of other functions.[212–214]

LEUKOCYTES

In a review of 100 cases of iron deficiency anemia observed at the Mayo Clinic, 14 percent were found to have leukocyte counts between 3.0 and 4.4×10^9/liter (3000–4400/μl). Leukopenia was unrelated

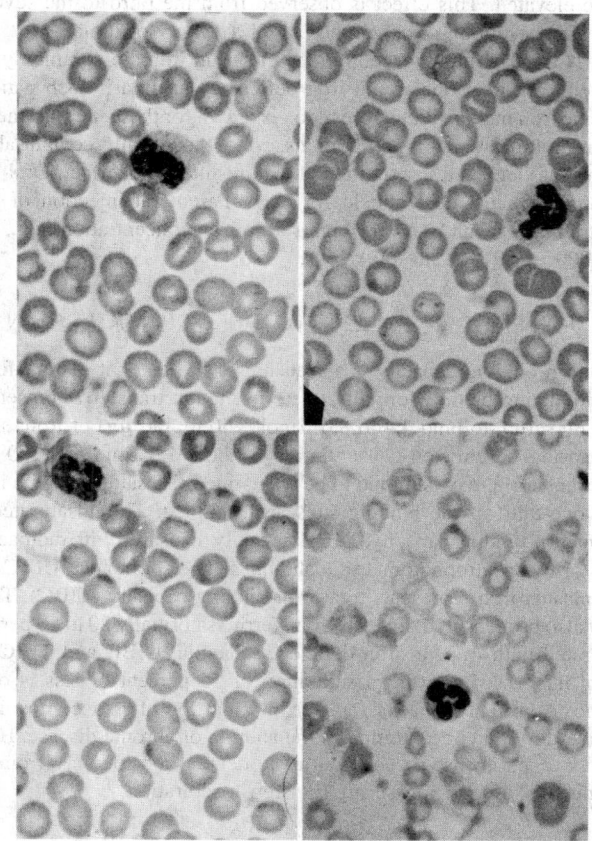

FIGURE 38-4   Variability in morphologic diagnosis of iron deficiency anemia from blood film. Interpret and compare them with those of nine experienced hematologists who reviewed the original slides. The slides were part of a coded series that contained blood films from normal subjects and from iron deficiency anemia patients in random order. The fields reproduced here were typical for each slide (X600). (From Fairbanks[200]; by permission of the J. B. Lippincott Company.) (*Upper left*) From a young woman with iron deficiency anemia due to excessive menstrual bleeding; hemoglobin 10.1 g/dl; serum iron 36 μg/dl (6.4 μmol/liter). After treatment with ferrous gluconate, hemoglobin concentration increased to 13.1 g/dl. On 13 examinations of this slide by nine hematologists, 11 opinions were that there was no evidence to suggest iron deficiency. (*Upper right*) From a normal woman. Hemoglobin 14.6 g/dl, MCHC 34%, serum iron 77 μg/dl (13.8 μmol/liter); total iron-binding capacity 300 μg/dl (53.7 μmol/liter). Three of nine hematologists who reviewed this film thought the erythrocytes were morphologically abnormal and consistent with iron deficiency anemia. (*Lower left*) From a normal young man. Hemoglobin 15.8 g/dl; MCHC 34%, serum iron 141 μg/dl (25.2 μmol/liter); total iron-binding capacity 278 μg/dl (49.8 μmol/liter). Nine hematologists made a total of 13 examinations of this slide; one examiner reported the slide as showing evidence of iron deficiency. (*Lower right*) From a 56-year-old man with anemia due to bleeding from paraesophageal hiatus hernia. Hemoglobin 4.0 g/dl; erythrocyte count 2.24% 10^{12}/liter; reticulocyte count 2.5%; serum iron 2 μg/dl (0.4 μmol/liter). Hypochromia was marked, and all observers agreed that morphologically the cells suggested iron deficiency anemia.

to severity of anemia and could not be ascribed to any other condition. In these cases, differential leukocyte counts were normal.

PLATELETS

Thrombocytopenia and thrombocytosis have both been attributed to iron deficiency. Thrombocytosis has been reported in 50 to 75 percent of adults with classic iron deficiency anemia due to chronic blood loss.[215–217] However, thrombocytosis usually occurs only in those pa-

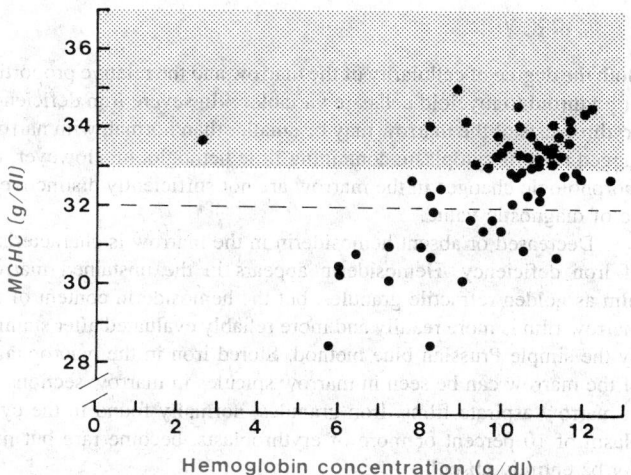

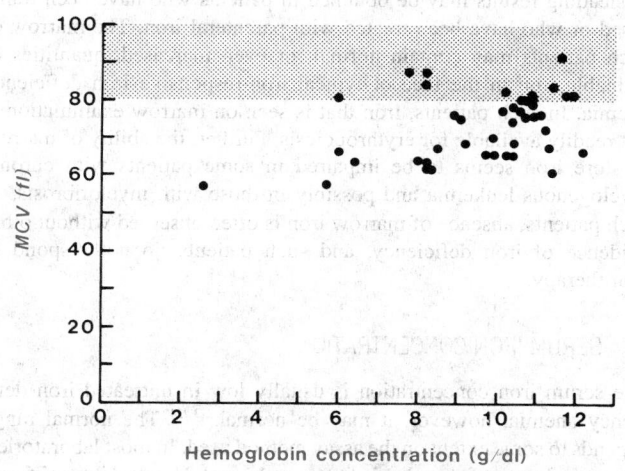

FIGURE 38-5   Erythrocyte indices in iron deficiency anemia of adults, data obtained with Coulter Counter, Model S. Normal ranges of indices observed in approximately 500 healthy adults[348] using the same instrument are indicated by stippling. The dashed line in the upper panel indicates the more widely accepted lower normal limit of MCHC stated in this text. (*Upper*) Correlation between venous blood hemoglobin concentration and mean corpuscular hemoglobin concentrations (MCHC). More than half of 62 patients with iron deficiency anemia had MCHC values clearly in the normal range. (*Lower*) Correlation between venous blood hemoglobin concentrations and MCV. Nearly 70 percent of cases exhibited distinct microcytosis. Thus when indices are determined by automated cell-counting methods, the MCV is much more sensitive than is the MCHC in detecting changes of iron deficiency. However, at least 30 percent of cases of iron deficiency anemia will be misdiagnosed if physicians rely on the erythrocyte indices. (From Beutler and Fairbanks,[349] by permission of Academic Press.)

tients who are actively bleeding.[218] In infants and children, thrombocytopenia occurs almost as frequently (28 percent) as does thrombocytosis (35 percent); thrombocytopenia is associated with more severe anemia.[219] Marked thrombocytopenia may also occur in iron-deficient adults, either as the presenting hematologic problem or early during the response to iron therapy for anemia.[210,220,221]

The reticulocyte count is usually normal or decreased in iron deficiency.

MARROW

Both the degree of cellularity of the marrow and the relative proportion of erythroid to myeloid cells are variable.[222] In severe iron deficiency, erythroblasts of the marrow may be smaller than normal, with narrow, ragged rims of cytoplasm containing little hemoglobin. However, the morphologic changes in the marrow are not sufficiently distinctive to be of diagnostic value.

Decreased or absent hemosiderin in the marrow is characteristic of iron deficiency. Hemosiderin appears in the unstained marrow film as golden refractile granules, but the hemosiderin content of the marrow film is more readily and more reliably evaluated after staining by the simple Prussian blue method. Stored iron in the macrophages of the marrow can be seen in marrow spicules in marrow sections, or in marrow aspirate films. Iron granules, normally found in the cytoplasm of 10 percent or more of erythroblasts, become rare but may not be entirely absent.

The evaluation of marrow iron stores is a sensitive and usually reliable means for the diagnosis of iron deficiency anemia. However, misleading results may be obtained in patients who have been transfused or who have been treated with parenteral iron. The marrow of such patients may contain normal, or even increased, quantities of stainable iron in the face of typical iron-responsive iron deficiency anemia. In such patients, iron that is seen on marrow examination is not readily available for erythropoiesis. Further, the ability of marrow to store iron seems to be impaired in some patients with chronic myelogenous leukemia and possibly in those with myelofibrosis. In such patients, absence of marrow iron is often observed without other evidence of iron deficiency, and such patients do not respond to iron therapy.

SERUM IRON CONCENTRATION

The serum iron concentration is usually low in untreated iron deficiency anemia; however, it may be normal.[223,224] The normal range depends to some extent on the assay method used. In most laboratories, the normal range for males is between 13 and 31 μmol/liter (75 and 175 μg/dl); for women it is about 2 μmol/liter (10 μg/dl) lower. The measurement of serum iron concentration is subject to many variables, which may introduce substantial errors into results. Such variables include inadequately processed glassware, contamination of reagents with small amounts of iron, turbidity, and entrapment of iron in plasma proteins during their precipitation. The reagents used in some techniques may not be entirely specific for iron. The presence of free hemoglobin in concentrations too small to be detected visually may give erroneously high results by the atomic absorption method unless a protein-free extract of serum is routinely used.

The serum iron concentration also is influenced by many pathologic and physiologic states. Physiologically, the serum iron concentration has a diurnal rhythm; it decreases in late afternoon and evening, reaching a nadir near 9 PM, and increases to its maximum between 7 and 10 AM.[225–227] Serum iron concentration decreases at about the time of menstrual bleeding either when menses are under normal hormonal control[228,229] or when bleeding occurs after withdrawal of oral contraceptive agents.[230,231] The serum iron concentration is reduced in the presence of either acute or chronic inflammatory processes[232–234] or malignancy[235] and following acute myocardial infarction.[236,237] The serum iron concentration under these circumstances may be decreased sufficiently to suggest iron deficiency. On the other hand, during chemotherapy of malignancy, the serum iron concentration may be quite elevated. This effect is observed from the third to the seventh day after inception of chemotherapy of a variety of tumors.[238]

Normal or high concentrations of serum iron are commonly observed even in patients with iron deficiency anemia if such patients receive iron medication before blood is drawn for these measurements. Even multiple vitamin preparations, which commonly contain about 18 mg of elemental iron per tablet, can result in this effect. Oral iron medication must be withheld for 24 h. Parenteral injection of iron dextran may result in a very high serum iron concentration (e.g., 500 to 1000 μg/dl) for several weeks.

IRON-BINDING CAPACITY AND TRANSFERRIN SATURATION

The iron-binding capacity is a measure of the amount of transferrin in circulating blood. Normally, there is enough transferrin present in 100 ml serum to bind 4.4 to 8.0 μmol (250 to 450 μg) of iron; since the normal serum iron concentration is about 1.8 μmol/dl (100 μg/dl), transferrin may be found to be about one-third saturated with iron; i.e., one-third of the binding sites are occupied. The unsaturated or latent iron-binding capacity (UIBC) is easily measured with radioactive iron or by spectrophotometric techniques. The sum of the UIBC and the plasma iron represents total iron-binding capacity (TIBC). TIBC may also be measured directly. Transferrin is normally 20 to 50 percent saturated with iron. In iron deficiency anemia, UIBC and TIBC are often increased; transferrin saturation of 15 percent or less is often found. A normal value for transferrin saturation often accompanies a low serum iron concentration in the anemia of chronic disease. However, exceptions are so common as to detract considerably from the diagnostic value of measuring transferrin saturation.[78]

SERUM FERRITIN

Serum ferritin concentration correlates with total-body iron stores, although the correlation is not as strong as has sometimes been suggested.[239–241] Serum ferritin concentrations of 10 μg/l or less are characteristic of iron deficiency anemia. For iron deficiency without anemia, serum ferritin concentration is typically in the range 10 to 20 μg/l. In one series of 73 patients marrow iron was depleted whenever the serum ferritin level was under 70 μg/l.[42] In adults older than 50 years, a serum ferritin concentration of less than 50 μg/l may be taken as evidence of iron deficiency. As noted in Chap. 25, serum ferritin predominantly consists of H monomers, which contain less iron than do L monomers; hence, serum ferritin contains relatively little iron. Moderate increase in serum ferritin concentration occurs in inflammatory disorders, such as rheumatoid arthritis, in chronic renal disease, and in malignancies.[243,244] In Gaucher disease the serum ferritin concentration is commonly in the range of thousands of μg/l. When one of these conditions coexists with iron deficiency, as they often do, the serum ferritin concentration is commonly in the normal range; interpretation of results of this assay then become difficult. In patients with rheumatoid arthritis who are anemic, concomitant iron deficiency may be suspected when the serum ferritin concentration is less than 60 μg/l.[245] Moderate increases in serum ferritin concentrations are also characteristic of some hematologic malignancies and may closely reflect remissions and relapses.[246] Marked increases in serum ferritin concentration occur in patients with hepatitis[241,247,248] and in patients with end-stage renal disease. Oral or parenteral iron administration also increases serum ferritin concentration.[249–253] This appears to be particularly a problem in infants given oral iron. In adults with iron deficiency anemia who were given oral iron in a dose of 60 mg of elemental iron thrice daily, the serum ferritin concentration remained below 10 μg/liter for 2 to 3 weeks.[250] However, for adults who have taken oral iron medication for more than 3 weeks, the serum ferritin assay would be of no value in confirming a diagnosis of iron deficiency. Parenteral administration of iron dextran results in a rise in serum ferritin concentration to normal or supranormal values within 24 h, and this effect persists for at least a month.[250] It has been proposed that measurement of the "percent saturation" of serum ferritin with iron may be a better indicator of iron deficiency or iron overload than the serum ferritin alone.[254] As yet, there has been limited experience with this test.

ERYTHROCYTE FERRITIN

Erythrocyte ferritin concentration is increased in thalassemias and sideroblastic anemias and decreased in iron deficiency. These changes appear to parallel those of serum ferritin concentration. Although it has been suggested that basic red cell ferritin was not influenced by inflammation, and could therefore detect iron deficiency when the serum ferritin concentration was normal in the elderly,[255] comparative studies show that erythrocyte ferritin and serum ferritin concentration are both elevated in chronic disease. While erythrocyte ferritin determinations appeared to have no more value than those of serum ferritin, the combination of both was more effective in the diagnosis of iron deficiency.[256]

ERYTHROCYTE ZINC PROTOPORPHYRIN

Erythrocyte protoporphyrin, principally zinc protoporphyrin, is increased in disorders of heme synthesis, including iron deficiency, lead poisoning, and sideroblastic anemias, as well as other conditions. This procedure requires small blood samples. It is quite sensitive in the diagnosis of iron deficiency[257] and practical for large-scale screening programs designed to identify children with either iron deficiency or lead poisoning. It does not differentiate among iron deficiency and chronic lead poisoning and the anemia that accompanies inflammatory or malignant processes.

SERUM TRANSFERRIN RECEPTOR

The role of transferrin receptor in transporting transferrin iron into cells is described in Chap. 24. Sensitive immunologic methods can detect about 5 mg/l of receptor in serum. The circulating receptor appears to be a truncated form of the cellular receptor, lacking the transmembrane and cytoplasmic domains of the cellular receptor. It circulates bound to transferrin. The circulating transferrin receptor apparently mirrors the amount of cellular receptor, and, since receptor synthesis is greatly increased when cells lack iron, the amount of the circulating receptor increases in iron deficiency but not in the anemia of chronic disease.[258–260] This test for iron deficiency has gradually come into clinical use but is not yet widely available. Like the serum ferritin and serum iron, serum transferrin receptor assay results may be confounded by poorly understood variations in patients with malignancies, in whom the serum transferrin receptor concentration is reduced, and in patients with rheumatoid arthritis or thalassemia trait, in whom, in the absence of iron deficiency, it is increased. Thus, to be clinically useful, separate reference ("normal") ranges need to be defined for serum transferrin receptor in these common conditions.[261–264]

RETICULOCYTE HEMOGLOBIN CONTENT

Automated hematology instruments may offer, as a new method for diagnosis of iron deficiency, an assay of hemoglobin content within reticulocytes.[265] However, preliminary data obtained with this method suggest neither a high level of specificity nor a high level of sensitivity.

^{57}CO ABSORPTION

The urinary excretion of ^{57}Co, following an oral dose, is greater in iron-deficient subjects than in normal subjects.[266,267] This appears to be a sensitive index of increased iron absorption, as occurs in iron deficiency, in iron-loading states (e.g., hemochromatosis), or following recent blood loss. It is not specific for iron deficiency.

IRON TOLERANCE TESTS

In an iron tolerance test,[268–270] the patient receives an oral dose of an inorganic iron compound, and the subsequent change in the serum iron concentration is measured. In iron deficiency, there is an increased rate of absorption of the test dose, and this is often reflected in a more rapid increase and a higher plateau than in normal subjects. However, this test has quite limited practical application.

DIFFERENTIAL DIAGNOSIS

When iron deficiency anemia is severe, it may often be easily recognized. A history of excessive blood loss is sometimes easily obtained. Pallor may be readily apparent. The blood film may display marked hypochromia, poikilocytosis, and microcytosis without polychromatophilia and other signs of erythrocyte regeneration that might suggest a different cause. Under such circumstances, it is reasonable to start iron therapy immediately and to begin a search for the site of blood loss. However, even those morphologic findings considered classic for iron deficiency anemia may occur in other conditions, particularly in chronic disease and in thalassemias: The morphologic diagnosis of iron deficiency must always be regarded as tentative and subject to confirmation by other means, including the response to therapy. The presumptive diagnosis of iron deficiency is often incorrect.[271] Early in the course of iron deficiency, changes in the blood may be imperceptible, and the differential diagnosis of anemia may then be more difficult.

DIFFERENTIATION FROM OTHER FORMS OF ANEMIA

The forms of anemia that must be distinguished from iron deficiency anemia include those of thalassemia minor, chronic inflammatory disease, malignancy, chronic liver disease, chronic renal disease, hemolytic anemia, and aplastic anemia. It is the microcytic anemias that are most likely to be confused with iron deficiency. Such anemias are summarized in Table 38-6, and each is discussed elsewhere in this

TABLE 38-6   MICROCYTIC DISORDERS THAT MAY BE CONFUSED WITH IRON DEFICIENCY

Thalassemias and hemoglobinopathies
   β-thalassemia-major
   β-thalassemia-minor
   $\delta\beta$-thalassemia-minor
   α-thalassemia-minor
   Hemoglobin Lepore trait
   Hemoglobin E trait
   Hemoglobin H disease
   Combination of above (double heterozygotes)
   Homozygous hemoglobin E
Blockade of heme synthesis caused by chemicals
   Lead
   Pyrazinamide
   Isoniazid
Disorders of obscure cause
   Sideroblastic anemias
      Hereditary sex-linked
      Idiopathic acquired
   Other
Chronic inflammatory states
Neoplasms, benign or malignant

volume. Attention will be directed here primarily to laboratory aids for differentiating iron deficiency anemia from the frequently occurring disorders that may have similar manifestations.

THALASSEMIA MINOR

In many parts of the world, and in many communities of North America, the frequency of β-thalassemia-minor is second only to that of iron deficiency as a cause of hypochromic microcytic anemia (Chap. 46). In African-Americans, homozygosity for α-thalassemia-2 (who have a pair of chromosomes each of which contain only a single α globin gene) is a common cause of microcytosis. Approximately 1 to 3 percent of African-Americans are homozygous for α-thalassemia-2.[272-274] The condition is usually not associated with anemia.[272] Heterozygotes may also have microcytosis, although usually they are hematologically normal. Among persons of Italian ancestry who appear to have thalassemia minor on the basis of erythrocyte morphology, approximately 1 of every 40 have hemoglobin Lepore trait[275,276]; probably 10,000 to 20,000 North Americans have hemoglobin Lepore trait as a cause of mild microcytosis unassociated with anemia. Among more than a million Southeast Asians resettled in the United States during the 1970s and 1980s, α-thalassemia-minor, β-thalassemia-minor, hemoglobin E trait, and iron deficiency all occur frequently. All are characterized by microcytosis, and none can be distinguished reliably from the others on the basis of erythrocyte morphology or erythrocyte indices alone. In each of these conditions there may be only mild to moderate microcytosis without any other distinctive changes. However, in the majority of patients with α- or β-thalassemia-minor, hemoglobin Lepore trait, hemoglobin E trait, the erythrocyte count is greater than 5×10^{12} per liter (5,000,000/μl), despite low hemoglobin concentration.[276,277] Homozygous hemoglobin E is also characterized by marked hypochromia, microcytosis, abundant target cells, and elevated erythrocyte count but usually not by more than minimal anemia.[278] (See Chap. 46.)

In contrast to the findings in these hemoglobinopathies, only about 3 percent of adults with iron deficiency anemia have erythrocyte counts of 5×10^{12} per liter (5,000,000/μl) or higher.[175] However, erythrocytosis may be seen in children with iron deficiency anemia or in polycythemia vera patients who have become iron deficient following hemorrhage or therapeutic phlebotomy.

The MCV is almost always reduced in α- or β-thalassemia-minor and in homozygous hemoglobin E, with values of 60 to 70 fl being the rule. Values this low are seen only in severe iron deficiency anemia. In hemoglobin Lepore trait and hemoglobin E trait, only minimal microcytosis is observed.[276-278] The widespread adoption of the routine measurement of MCV has led to proposals that criteria for differentiation of iron deficiency from thalassemia minor might be based, in part, on the values of the erythrocyte count and the MCV.[279] Some proposed rules[280] could separate iron deficiency from thalassemia minor with 90 percent reliability when groups of iron deficiency and thalassemic patients were of nearly equal numbers. However, in a population in which iron deficiency is more prevalent than thalassemia minor, use of these criteria would result in an excessive number of diagnostic errors. None of these and other proposed rules[204,214,281] seems completely reliable for distinguishing iron deficiency from thalassemia.

Because anisocytosis is an early morphologic feature of iron deficiency, measurements of variation in erythrocyte size, such as RDW, have been proposed as a means of diagnosis (see "Blood Cells," above). However, the RDW is often increased in thalassemia minor, particularly in those cases with reticulocytosis.[206] Hence, these conditions cannot be differentiated reliably by such measurements.

Mild reticulocytosis, polychromatophilia, and basophilic stippling are more likely to be encountered in β-thalassemia-minor, $\delta\beta$-thalas-

semia-minor, and hemoglobin Lepore trait than in iron deficiency anemia but may be absent in these disorders. In contrast, the serum iron concentration is usually normal or increased in thalassemic syndromes and is usually low in iron deficiency anemia. Similarly, examination of marrow iron stores helps to differentiate these disorders. The presence of thalassemia is substantiated by the demonstration of increased proportions of hemoglobin A_2 or F, or by the presence on electrophoresis of hemoglobin H or Lepore (see Chap. 46). At present the diagnosis of α-thalassemia-minor is usually made on the basis of exclusion of other causes of microcytosis, but it can be confirmed by measuring globin chain synthetic rates or by direct demonstration of mutations by DNA-based techniques.

Iron deficiency may mask concurrent thalassemia. The amounts of both hemoglobin A_2 and hemoglobin H are diminished disproportionately to the reduction in hemoglobin A in the presence of iron deficiency[282] (Chap. 46). Thus when a patient with proved iron deficiency and normal hemoglobin studies continues to exhibit microcytosis and hypochromia after adequate therapy, the concentration of hemoglobin A_2 should be measured again and electrophoresis performed to determine whether hemoglobin H is present.

ANEMIA OF CHRONIC INFLAMMATORY DISEASE AND MALIGNANCY

The anemia of chronic disease (Chap. 41) is usually normochromic and normocytic, but hypochromic microcytic anemia occurs in 20 to 30 percent of patients with chronic infections or malignancies.[233,234] Thus these disorders cannot be distinguished from iron deficiency anemia by examination of the blood film. Furthermore, the serum iron concentration is usually decreased in these disorders,[29,233,234] sometimes severely. While in iron deficiency the TIBC is usually increased, it is commonly decreased in inflammatory and neoplastic diseases. However, there is considerable overlap among TIBC values of normal subjects, those with iron deficiency anemia, and those with chronic inflammatory diseases. Among the neoplasms that may lead to erroneous diagnosis of iron deficiency, particularly to be noted are hypernephromas, atrial myxomas, and angiofollicular lymphoid hyperplasia.

In iron deficiency anemia, the transferrin saturation is usually less than 16 percent, whereas in chronic diseases it is usually greater than 16 percent. However, this widely used criterion is actually quite unreliable. Transferrin saturation may be normal in iron deficiency anemia, and conversely, low saturation is sometimes observed in chronic disease.[234] However, circulating transferrin receptors increase in iron deficiency but not in the anemia of chronic disease.[244,258-260] The serum ferritin level is usually diminished in iron deficiency, but it is generally increased in chronic inflammatory and neoplastic disorders.[242,243] Examination of the marrow for stainable iron is particularly helpful. The latter is greatly decreased in amount or absent in iron deficiency anemia and normal or increased in the other disorders.

ANEMIA OF CHRONIC LIVER DISEASE

The erythrocytes in the blood film from patients with chronic liver disease may be normochromic and normocytic, macrocytic, or hypochromic. Target cells are frequently present in large numbers. Since the blood film in iron deficiency anemia may also display these features, differential diagnosis must be based on other observations. Determination of the serum iron concentration is helpful. In acute chemically induced liver injury, and in hepatitis, the serum iron concentration is usually modestly increased,[248,283] possibly owing to release of ferritin into the plasma.[247,248] In cirrhosis, the serum iron concentration is likely to be increased unless there has been blood loss.[283] The TIBC may be normal or decreased. Thus the percentage transferrin saturation is likely to be increased. The quantity of hemosiderin is normal or increased in marrow aspirates.

ANEMIA OF CHRONIC RENAL DISEASE

Changes in small renal blood vessels may cause marked distortions in erythrocyte structure, producing schizocytes and burr cells. However, these morphologic changes, when present, are nonspecific. Unless there is distinct microcytosis and hypochromia, iron deficiency anemia cannot be differentiated from anemia resulting from chronic renal disease (Chap. 33) on the basis of the blood film. The serum iron concentration may be normal or decreased, depending on the cause of the renal disease. Measurement of the TIBC may be of no help in this circumstance. Serum ferritin concentration may be greater than 100 μg/liter, and may indeed be quite elevated despite iron deficiency. Iron deficiency may complicate the anemia of chronic renal disease in patients who are subjected to repeated extracorporeal hemodialysis, possibly as a result of loss of blood into the dialyzing apparatus.[188] When the mechanism of anemia is uncertain or appears to be complex, examination of marrow aspirates for iron content may clarify the pathogenesis.

ANEMIA OF HEMOLYTIC DISEASE

Hemolytic disease can usually be distinguished from iron deficiency anemia on the basis of the blood film. The marked poikilocytosis, polychromatophilia, and other morphologic features characteristic of hemolysis usually are not seen in iron deficiency anemia. Furthermore, reticulocytosis is usually marked in hemolytic disorders but minimal or absent in iron deficiency anemia. However, there are some outstanding exceptions to these generally valid principles.

In unstable hemoglobin disorders, such as hemoglobin H disease or hemoglobin Köln disease, erythrocytic hypochromia may be pronounced. In these disorders, there is moderate reticulocytosis, which helps to differentiate them from iron deficiency anemia. The serum iron concentration is normal or increased. Unstable hemoglobins are easily precipitated by heating or by mixing hemolysates with a buffered dilute solution of isopropanol. These measures of molecular instability are the basis of simple diagnostic tests (Chap. 48).

When there is chronic intravascular hemolysis, erythrocytes in the blood film may display marked morphologic abnormalities, such as burr cells and schizocytes. Yet, because of loss of iron in the urine, iron deficiency may be the dominant cause of the resulting anemia. Measurement of serum iron concentration or TIBC or, better, evaluation of iron content marrow aspirates may clarify the mechanism of this form of anemia. An increase in serum lactic dehydrogenase activity that is secondary to intravascular hemolysis often occurs in iron deficiency anemia. Studies of erythrocyte survival or of iron kinetics may sometimes help in investigation of the mechanism of anemia in these cases. However, these are time-consuming, expensive procedures that do not, in general, add any diagnostically useful information beyond that which can be obtained by the simpler techniques already indicated. Furthermore, iron deficiency anemia alone may result in shortened erythrocyte survival and in some degree of ineffective erythropoiesis. If bleeding occurs during studies of erythrocyte survival, the results are indistinguishable from those that are considered to be characteristic of hemolysis. Because circulating transferrin receptors reflect the erythroid mass they are increased in hemolytic anemia[258] and would not aid in distinguishing hemolysis from iron deficiency.

HYPOPLASTIC AND APLASTIC ANEMIA

In their early phases, these disorders cannot reliably be differentiated from mild iron deficiency anemia on the basis of erythrocyte morphology alone (Chap. 22). The reticulocyte count is generally less than 0.5 percent in hypoplastic or asplastic anemia. The presence of neutropenia and thrombocytopenia suggests a diagnosis of aplastic anemia, but mild neutropenia may also occur in iron deficiency anemia. The serum iron concentration is usually increased in aplastic anemia; the

percentage transferrin saturation may be high. Marrow aspiration may produce scant material for cytologic study, and marrow biopsy may be necessary: Iron stain usually reveals increased amounts of hemosiderin in aplastic or hypoplastic anemia. However, if chronic bleeding has occurred, for example, due to thrombocytopenia, iron stores may be depleted.

MYELOPROLIFERATIVE DISEASES

In polycythemia vera, erythrocytes may be small and hypochromic (Chap. 61). Even in the absence of distinctive morphologic changes in erythrocytes, the serum iron concentration is usually decreased, the TIBC is normal or increased, and marrow aspirates show little or no hemosiderin. Ferrokinetic studies show accelerated plasma iron incorporated into the hemoglobin of circulating erythrocytes.[284] These findings simply reflect iron deficiency, which is almost always present in this disease, as a result of marked expansion in total hemoglobin mass, increased gastrointestinal blood loss, or therapeutic phlebotomy. The marrow hemosiderin content is often decreased in other myeloproliferative disorders,[285] possibly due to a defect in macrophage storage of iron.

SIDEROBLASTIC ANEMIA

In this heterogeneous group of disorders (Chap. 63), the blood findings often simulate those of iron deficiency anemia. Reticulocytosis is usually absent, and the serum iron concentration is generally normal or increased. Diagnosis requires examination of films of marrow aspirates stained for iron; increased amounts of both storage and ringed sideroblasts are present.

CONGENITAL DYSERYTHROPOIETIC ANEMIA

In the rare congenital dyserythropoietic anemias, erythrocyte morphologic abnormalities may resemble those of iron deficiency or thalassemia (Chap. 35). In general, in congenital dyserythropoietic anemias, poikilocytosis is very striking and occurs with less reduction in MCV than in iron deficiency or thalassemias. Often, however, such cases are believed to be thalassemic until the marrow is examined.

MEGALOBLASTIC ANEMIA

In pernicious anemia and other types of megaloblastic anemia (Chap. 37), the blood film usually shows changes sufficiently distinctive that there is little difficulty in differential diagnosis. One potential source of error is the change in serum iron concentration that occurs after therapy. In the untreated patient with pernicious anemia or folic acid deficiency, the serum iron concentration decreases markedly as iron is utilized rapidly for hemoglobin synthesis.[286] Thus the finding of a low serum iron concentration in such circumstances should not be taken as evidence of iron deficiency. Iron deficiency anemia and anemia due to folic acid or vitamin B_{12} deficiency may coexist. During the course of treatment, with the rapid increase in the number of red cells, the typical manifestations of severe iron deficiency may develop.

ANEMIA OF MYXEDEMA

The anemia of myxedema (Chap. 34) is usually normochromic and normocytic and may be accompanied by mild-to-moderate depression of serum iron concentration. Ferrokinetic studies may show a decreased rate of plasma iron transport but normal iron utilization. Marrow examination may be required to determine whether iron deficiency is present, especially since iron deficiency often complicates myxedema because of menorrhagia, that is common in this disorder.

SPECIAL STUDIES

The physician who establishes a diagnosis of iron deficiency resulting from blood loss has the obligation to determine the site and cause of hemorrhage. Examination of the stools for the presence of blood is particularly helpful in determining what additional studies should be carried out. Specimens should be examined on several days, because bleeding may be intermittent. Occasionally, it is helpful to label the patient's erythrocytes with ^{51}Cr sodium chromate and to determine quantitatively the amount of blood lost daily. When there is reason to believe that bleeding is from the gastrointestinal tract, roentgenographic and other imaging studies and endoscopic investigation are indicated. The latter often include gastroscopy, esophagoscopy, and colonoscopy.

Percutaneous retrograde angiography of celiac or mesenteric arteries has proved valuable in localizing sites of active gastrointestinal bleeding, when rate of blood flow into the intestinal lumen is 0.5 ml/min or greater.[13,287,288] This procedure should be considered for any patient actively bleeding from the gastrointestinal tract, in whom the site of blood loss has not been established by other methods, including endoscopy, and for whom surgery is contemplated. Angiography should be carried out prior to barium contrast studies. The rate of bleeding may be increased following angiography.[288]

Meckel diverticulum is one of the most common causes of obscure gastrointestinal bleeding in children. The diverticulum often contains ectopic gastric muscosa that will concentrate pertechnetate following intravenous injection for scintigraphic study; such scintigrams have been useful in identifying Meckel diverticulum as the cause of gastrointestinal blood loss.[289–291]

In rare cases, small-bowel endoscopy by laparoscopy may detect bleeding lesions when less invasive methods have failed.[292] Rarely, exploratory laparotomy may be warranted, because some adults with unexplained occult bleeding have gastrointestinal malignancies. There may be an even stronger indication for laparotomy in children and infants with unexplained gastrointestinal bleeding, since Meckel diverticulum may not be detected otherwise.[293,294] An iron stain of sputum may reveal hemosiderin-laden macrophages when there is intrapulmonary bleeding.

THERAPEUTIC TRIAL

In the final analysis, the response to iron therapy is the proof of correctness of diagnosis of iron deficiency anemia. Furthermore, some physicians or patients may not have access to all the techniques described for diagnosis of iron deficiency anemia. In this event, the patient's response to therapy may become a primary diagnostic measure. Iron administration in such a therapeutic trial should usually be by the oral route only. A therapeutic trial under any circumstances should be followed carefully. If the cause of anemia is iron deficiency, adequate iron therapy should result in reticulocytosis with a peak occurring after 1 to 2 weeks of therapy, although if anemia is mild, the reticulocyte response may be minimal. A significant increase in the hemoglobin concentration of the blood should be evident 3 to 4 weeks later, and the hemoglobin concentration should attain a normal value within 2 to 4 months. Unless there is evidence of continued, substantial blood loss, the absence of these changes must be taken as evidence that iron deficiency is not the cause of anemia. Iron therapy should be discontinued and another mechanism sought.

THERAPY, COURSE, AND PROGNOSIS

Once it has been established that a patient is deficient in iron, replacement therapy should be instituted without further delay.

Iron may be administered in one of several forms—orally, as simple iron salts, or parenterally, as an iron-carbohydrate complex or as a blood transfusion. In general, the oral route is preferred. Iron can be administered most economically, in the highest dosage, and in the most readily assimilated form as simple iron compounds. Table 38-7 compares the cost to the patient of each grain of iron administered in each of several forms, as well as the comparative rates of response and possible toxic effects. Clearly, treatment by the oral route is safer and far less expensive than parenteral therapy. In most patients, iron deficiency anemia is a disorder of long duration and slow progression. Precipitous measures to restore a normal hemoglobin concentration overnight by transfusing the patient are never warranted and are, indeed, hazardous. There is usually time to wait for normal mechanisms of erythropoiesis to respond to the body's needs and for gradual adjustment of the cardiovascular system to reexpansion of the total circulating erythrocyte volume.

ORAL IRON THERAPY

DIETARY THERAPY

The patient should be encouraged to eat a diversified diet supplying all nutritional requirements. Nonetheless, it must be emphasized that neither meat nor any other dietary article contains enough iron to be useful therapeutically. Meat contains small amounts of myoglobin and hemoglobin (blood trapped in capillaries) and insignificant amounts of iron in other proteins. Although heme iron is better absorbed than inorganic iron, the quanitity of heme iron in meat is actually quite small. In fact, an average (3-oz) serving of steak provides only about 3 mg iron. Provision of sufficient dietary iron to permit a maximal rate of recovery from iron deficiency anemia might require a daily intake of at least 10 lb (4540 g) of steak. For these and other reasons, medicinal iron is much superior to dietary iron in the therapy of iron deficiency.

IRON PREPARATIONS

The pharmaceutical market is glutted with iron preparations in nearly every conceivable form, each promoted to appeal to physician or patient for one reason or another. The following simple principles may help the physician to find a way through this chaos.

1. Each dose of an iron preparation for an adult should contain between 30 and 100 mg elemental iron. Doses of this magnitude cause unpleasant side effects relatively infrequently.[295,296] Smaller doses have been popular in the past, but these may result in a slower recovery of the patient or no recovery at all.

2. The iron should be readily released in acidic or neutral gastric juice or duodenal juice (usually pH 5 to 6), because maximal absorption occurs when iron is presented to the duodenal mucosa. Enteric-coated and prolonged-release preparations dissolve slowly in any of these fluids. Thus with such preparations the iron that eventually is released may be presented to a portion of the intestinal mucosa in which absorption is least efficient. Some patients who have been treated unsuccessfully with enteric-coated or prolonged-release iron preparations respond promptly to the administration of non–enteric-coated ferrous salts (Fig. 38-6).

3. The iron, once released, should be readily absorbed. Iron is absorbed in the ferrous form; consequently, only ferrous salts should be used.

4. Side effects should be infrequent. This seems not to be a particular problem for any of the common commercially available iron compounds. Despite the claims of pharmaceutical companies, there is no convincing evidence that any one effective preparation is superior in this respect to any other.

5. The cost to the patient should be small.

6. The use of preparations containing several therapeutic agents is to be condemned.

TABLE 38-7   COMPARISON OF DIFFERENT METHODS OF IRON THERAPY

ORAL	IRON CONTENT (MG/G)	COST TO PATIENT ($/G FE)	PALATABILITY	EFFICACY	TOXICITY
FeSO₄	66 mg/tablet	1.65	Mediocre	Excellent	Occasional abdominal discomfort
Beefsteak	1 mg/oz	500.00	Excellent	Mediocre	Weight gain, "bloating"
Parenteral					
Transfusion (packed RBC)	1 mg/ml	1240.00*	—	Good	Fever, jaundice, AIDS, anemia, shock, death
Iron dextran	50 mg/mL	2078.00†	—	Good	Fever, rash, arthralgia, lymphadenopathy, splenomegaly, aseptic meningitis, pancytopenia, shock, death

*Based on August 1999 charges for drawing, processing, and transfusing 4 units of packed red cells at a major midwestern medical center.
†Includes estimate of fees for 20 office visits for injections, and 20 vials (2 ml each) at $41.91/vial, August 1999.

Table 38-8 compares a few of the commonly used iron preparations.

Physicians should be aware that if ferrous sulfate is prescribed generically, the choice of preparation is left to the pharmacist, who may dispense enteric-coated tablets. It is advisable to specify "nonenteric" or to prescribe by brand name a product that is not enteric-coated.

Although substances such as ascorbic acid, succinate, and fructose have been shown to enhance iron absorption, the gain is offset to a large extent by the increase in frequency of side effects or cost of therapy, or both. There is no convincing evidence to support the use of chelated forms of iron or of iron in combination with wetting agents.

Dosage   For the therapy of iron deficiency in adults, the dosage should be sufficient to provide between 150 and 200 mg elemental iron daily. The iron may be taken orally in three or four doses 1 h before meals. Infants may be given 50 to 100 mg daily in divided doses for therapy or 10 to 20 mg daily for prophylaxis of iron deficiency (Table 38-9).

Side Effects   Mild gastrointestinal side effects occur occasionally in the form of pyrosis, constipation, or loose stools. A metallic taste may be experienced. In some patients these side effects may be psychologic in origin. One should avoid suggesting to patients that adverse effects are to be expected. In truth, they are not: The majority of patients tolerate this dose of iron without the least side effect, and many tolerate much larger doses well. However, there is no doubt that some patients, perhaps 1 or 2 out of 10, experience symptoms that may be ascribed to the iron preparation and may be related in part to the size of the dose.[295,297] In such cases, reduction of the frequency of administration to one tablet a day for a few days may alleviate the symptoms; later, the patient may be able to tolerate treatment in full dosage. It may also be useful to change to another iron preparation, especially one with a different external appearance.

Carbonyl iron has been proposed as an alternative to iron salts, on the assertion that it can be given in large doses with minimal side effects. This substance is actually metallic iron powder, with a particle size less than 5 μm. Because it is insoluble, it is not absorbed until converted to the ionic form. The bioavailability of carbonyl iron has been estimated to be about 70 percent of that of an equivalent amount of ferrous sulfate,[298] but oral doses of 1 to 3 g/d may be required for optimal therapy. Oral doses as high as 600 mg three times daily did not produce toxic effects. This potentially safer form of iron is not commercially available for treatment of iron deficiency in the United States.*

During the decade of the 1990s there has been much speculation in the medical literature as to a potentially harmful effect of iron in enhancing the risk of acute myocardial infarction. However, this is not a reason for reducing the dosage of iron given to iron-deficient patients. (See also discussion in Chap. 42.)

Acute Iron Poisoning   Acute iron poisoning is usually a consequence of the accidental ingestion by infants or small children of iron-containing medications intended for use by adults. Any potent oral preparation may cause acute iron poisoning, and this serious disorder is not at all rare. For example, in the Los Angeles area alone there were 5 deaths from iron poisoning among children 11 to 18 months of age in the 7-month period following June 1992.

The earliest manifestation of iron poisoning is vomiting, usually within an hour of the ingestion. There may be hematemesis or melena. Restlessness, hypotension, tachypnea, and cyanosis may develop soon thereafter and may be followed within a few hours by coma and death. So inexorable a course is not the rule, however, and only about 1 percent of such poisonings have a fatal outcome.[299] Usually, medical aid is sought early, and, with proper treatment, most iron-poisoned children should survive. The initial treatment is prompt evacuation of the stomach. In the home this may be induced by digital stimulation of the pharyngeal gag reflex. Oral administration of a tepid solution of baking soda serves two useful purposes: it may provoke emesis,

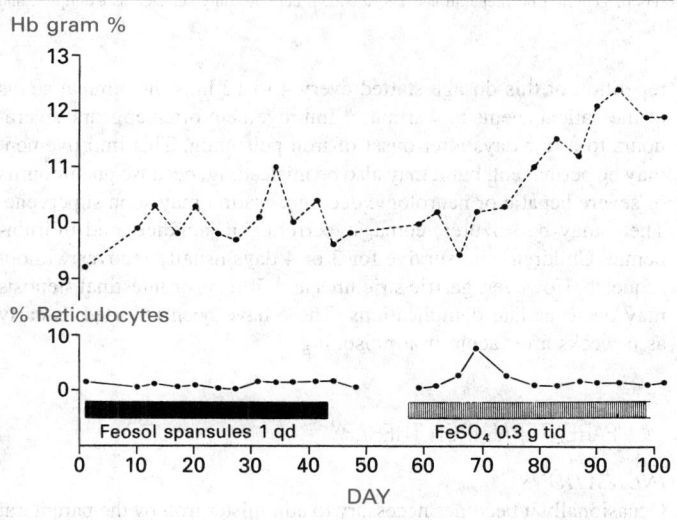

FIGURE 38-6   Rate of response of patient with iron deficiency anemia to 43 days of treatment with prolonged-release Feosol Spansules (containing 225 mg ferrous sulfate), one capsule daily, the dosage recommended by the manufacturer, followed by 43 days of treatment with nonenteric ferrous sulfate (0.3 g three times daily). Clearly, 225 mg of ferrous sulfate daily in prolonged-release form failed to elicit any significant hemopoietic response in this case. The rapid response subsequently elicited with conventional ferrous sulfate may be taken as a typical response to effect therapy in adequate dosage, whether by oral or parenteral route. (From Beutler and Meerkreebs[296]; by permission of the Massachusetts Medical Society.)

*Carbonyl iron is used in the United States in the semisolid infant foods shown in Table 38-2, although the bioavailability of iron in this form is poor.[350]

TABLE 38-8   COMPARISON OF COSTS FOR SOME IRON MEDICATIONS*

| | | | COST | |
NAME	MANUFACTURER	IRON CONTENT (mg/PILL)	$/100 PILLS	$/g IRON
Plain iron pills				
Ferrous sulfate	SK Beecham, Philadelphia, PA	66	11.16	1.69
Feosol	Goldline, Ft. Lauderdale, FL	66	7.45	0.97
Generic				
Ferrous fumarate	Kenwood	66	10.33	1.56
Generic				
Ferrous gluconate	Bayer, West Haven, CT	37	9.78	2.64
Fergon	SK Beecham	10	51.62	51.62
Simron	Schein, Florham Park, NJ	37	3.90	3.56
Generic				
Enteric-coated pills	Goldline	66	2.85	0.43
Ferrous sulfate				
"Delayed-release" pills	Lederle	50	37.32	6.46
Ferro-Sequels	SK Beecham (v.s.)	50	34.04	6.46
Feosol Spansules	Abbott	105	36.54	3.48
Fero-Gradumet				
Combination pills	SK Beecham (v.s.)	50	11.13	2.23
Geritol	Russ	90	70.16	7.8
Trinsicon	Fisons	66	16.47	2.50
Vitron-C	Upjohn	18	10.06	5.59
Unicap Plus Iron				
Femiron	Menley & James, Horsham, PA	20	2.70	1.39

Liquid Preparations

| | | | COST | |
NAME	MANUFACTURER	IRON CONTENT (mg/ml)	$/UNIT (ml)	$/g IRON
Ferrous sulfate syrup	URL	9	17.50/480	4.05
Iron dextran (InFeD)	Schein (v.s.)	50	56.55/2	565.50
Ferrous sulfate, pediatric drops		25	7.12/50	5.70
Fer-gen-sol	Goldline (v.s.)			

*Figures are based on average retail prices in the United States in 1998 (*Drug Topics Red Book*, 1998, Medical Economics, Montvale, NJ). Prices vary slightly among pharmacies. In general, a 30% retail markup has been assumed. Health Care Finance Agency (HCFA) reimbursement to providers may be at 76% of the average wholesale list price, or at approximately half the retail charge. There are numerous other iron preparations, and many other manufacturers of generic iron preparations. Those shown here are only selected as examples, and their listing does not imply endorsement.

and the bicarbonate ion complexes with the iron and retards absorption. If a child has ingested more than 60 mg of iron per kg body weight, hospital treatment is indicated.[300] In the emergency room, gastric intubation and lavage should be performed promptly, preferably with a solution containing 4 g sodium bicarbonate (or 3.6 g disodium phosphate and 0.8 g monosodium phosphate) per deciliter. Before the tube is withdrawn, a solution containing 5 to 10 g desferrioxamine, or approximately 60 ml of the bicarbonate or phosphate solution, should be introduced into the stomach. Supportive measures should be used as needed for shock or for metabolic acidosis should these develop. Desferrioxamine is the agent of choice for specific therapy of hyperferremia. It usually should be administered intramuscularly in an initial dose of 1 g, followed by 0.5 g intramuscularly 4 and 8 h later, and thereafter at 12-h intervals as the clinical status warrants. If the child is hypotensive, the dose may be administered intravenously at a rate not exceeding 15 mg/kg per hour for a total initial dose of 1 g, with

repetition of this dosage started every 4 to 12 h as the clinical status of the patient seems to warrant.[301] Improvement often appears several hours to a few days after onset of iron poisoning. This improvement may be permanent, but it may also be misleading, because pneumonitis or severe hepatic or neurologic decompensation may soon supervene. There may be seizures, coma, hyperreflexia, jaundice, and bilirubinemia. Children who survive for 3 or 4 days usually recover without sequelae. However, gastric strictures and fibrosis or intestinal stenosis may occur as late complications. These have been reported as early as 6 weeks after acute iron poisoning.[300,302-304]

PARENTERAL IRON THERAPY

INDICATIONS

Occasionally it becomes necessary to administer iron by the parenteral route. The indications are malabsorption, intolerance to iron taken orally, iron need in excess of an amount that can be taken orally, and uncooperativeness of the patient. Parenteral iron administration, together with erythropoietin, appears to alleviate the anemia that otherwise may complicate long-term dialysis treatment of patients with chronic renal disease. In rare instances, inability of the patient to follow instructions or to return for follow-up may justify use of paren-

TABLE 38-9   IRON PREPARATIONS FOR PEDIATRIC USE*

CHEMICAL DESIGNATION	IRON CONTENT. mg/ml	COMMERCIAL (PROPRIETARY) DESIGNATION	THERAPEUTIC DOSAGE
Ferrous sulfate solution, USP	8		1 p, 2 or 3 times daily
Ferrous sulfate solution, concentrated	25	Fer-In-Sol	1 ml, 3 or 4 times daily
Ferrous sulfate elixir (5% ethanol)	9	Feosol elixir	1 tsp, 2 or 3 times daily

teral iron. However, in view of the significantly greater hazards of parenteral therapy, the indications must be carefully considered.

PREPARATIONS: IRON DEXTRAN

Iron dextran and ferric saccharate are the only compounds commercially available in the United States for parenteral iron therapy. Because of as-yet-limited experience with the latter, the following discussion pertains to iron dextran.

Chemistry   Iron dextran is a colloidal suspension in which the iron-dextran complex exists as microspherules of approximately 5 nm in diameter and an average mass equivalent to 73,000 daltons. Each particle has an electron-dense ferric oxyhydroxide (FeOOH) core surrounded by a shell believed to consist of chains of dextran extending radially from the core.[305] The commercial preparation is marketed as a stable, dark brown, slightly acidic (pH 6) solution containing 50 mg elemental iron per ml.

Metabolism   After intramuscular injection iron dextran is slowly absorbed, approximately 72 h being required for 50 percent of a dose to move out of the injection site.[306,307] It is slowly cleared from plasma. Peak plasma concentrations of thousands of micrograms of iron per deciliter are found even 10 days after intramuscular injection; the plasma iron concentration decreases slowly, reaching normal values after 3 to 4 weeks.[306,308] Iron dextran is cleared from plasma by the macrophages, and ultimately the iron is used in hemoglobin synthesis. Mobilization of iron dextran from an intramuscular site is relatively slow and incomplete; 20 to 35 percent of the dose may remain at the injection site 1 month later.[309,310] Furthermore, the rate of incorporation of iron dextran into hemoglobin is somewhat slower than that for simpler ferric hydroxide colloids.[310,311] It appears that the iron dextran complex is only slowly dissociated in macrophages. At most, approximately 70 percent of the iron is readily utilized in hemoglobin synthesis, the remainder being very slowly liberated from macrophages despite persistent iron deficiency anemia.

Dosage and Route of Administration   Iron dextran is often administered in doses of 2.0 ml (100 mg) intramuscularly or intravenously. Total dose infusion has also been employed[308,312–318] and is very convenient, but this mode of administration is not included in the approved labeling of the drug in the United States. The rate of intravenous injection of undiluted iron dextran should not exceed 1 ml/min. If any adverse effect is noted, injection must be terminated at once and appropriate countermeasures taken. A syringe containing a solution of epinephrine should be immediately accessible for treatment of anaphylaxis should this occur. The manufacturer recommends intravenous test doses of 0.5 ml before therapy is started.

It is easy to estimate the amount of iron that need be given by merely remembering that 1 ml of red cells contain about 1 mg of iron. However, various formulas have been used for estimating total dose required for treatment. Since total blood volume is approximately 65 ml/kg and the iron content of hemoglobin is 0.34 percent by weight, the simplest formula for estimating the total dose required for correction of anemia only may be derived as follows:

$$D_{Fe}(g) = (D_h/100) \times W_{kg} \times 65 \times 0.0034$$
$$D_{Fe}(mg) = D_h \times W_{kg} \times 2.2$$
$$D_{Fe}(mg) = D_h \times W_{lb}$$

where D_{Fe} = total hemoglobin iron deficit
   D_h = whole blood hemoglobin deficit, g/dl
   W_{kg} = body weight, kilograms
   W_{lb} = body weight, pounds

Assuming normal mean hemoglobin concentration of 16 g/dl, a male weighing 170 lb, whose hemoglobin concentration is 7 g/dl,

would require 170% $(16 - 7) = 1530$ mg iron to correct this anemia. To this should be added a sufficient quantity of iron to replete iron stores, approximately 1000 mg for men and approximately 600 mg for women. Thus a 170-lb male with a hemoglobin concentration of 7 g/dl should receive 2530 mg iron, equivalent to 50 ml of iron dextran.

Side Effects   Intramuscular administration of iron dextran causes a moderate degree of pain at the injection site and a dark stain in the skin that may remain for as long as 1 to 2 years. "Z-track" and other techniques of injection recommended by the manufacturer reduce, but do not eliminate, the discoloration of the skin.

Intravenous administration also may cause local side effects, in the form of thrombophlebitis. This occurs most commonly when iron dextran is diluted with 5 percent glucose solution, less frequently when diluted with isotonic saline solution, and infrequently when iron dextran is injected undiluted. Thrombophlebitis at the injection site appears to be unusual with the technique of total-dose infusion, and other adverse effects appear to be no more frequent than with the intramuscular route.

The frequency of systemic reactions of iron dextran therapy has been markedly variable in different series, ranging from near 0[308,314,319] to nearly 50 percent of patients given iron dextran.[316,317,320] Dextran is a biologic product the exact structure of which is apparently difficult to control, and the frequency of adverse effects varies, probably due to variations in manufacturing techniques. Arthralgias and fever may be experienced by as many as one-third of patients. Other systemic reactions are infrequent and include hypotension, bradycardia, myalgia, headache, abdominal pain, nausea and vomiting, dizziness, lymphadenopathy, pleural effusion, and urticaria. Generalized gray discoloration of the skin has been reported following total-dose injection.[321] The discoloration persisted for 3 months. Regional lymph nodes may become enlarged and tender for a few weeks after injection. Generalized lymphadenopathy[322,323] and allergic purpura[324] have been noted. In one case,[325] fever—temperature up to 41°C (105.8°F)—persisted for 10 days and was accompanied by tachycardia, inguinal lymphadenopathy, increased erythrocyte sedimentation rate, and leukocytosis 15% 10⁹/liter (15,000/μl) with neutrophilia. Several cases have been observed in which iron dextran infusion was followed by an acute febrile illness accompanied by tender lymphadenopathy and splenomegaly lasting 10 to 14 days.[326] Pleocytosis of the cerebrospinal fluid has been observed[327] during a febrile reaction to iron dextran; in this case there was also a blood leukocyte count of 88 × 10⁹/liter (88,000/μl). In another patient meningismus without increased leukocytes in the spinal fluid but a high spinal fluid iron concentration was documented.[319] Pancytopenia may follow iron dextran therapy.[328] Acute, severe exacerbation of arthritis has been observed following iron dextran therapy in patients with rheumatoid arthritis[329–331] or ankylosing spondylitis.[332]

Intramuscular deposition of iron dextran has led to malignancy in some experimental animals.[333,334] Fibrosarcoma and undifferentiated pleomorphic sarcoma have developed at the site of injection in several human subjects following repeated or protracted iron dextran therapy.[335–337] This appears to be an extremely rare phenomenon and may in some cases have been coincidental rather than causally related.

The most dangerous complication of iron dextran therapy is anaphylactic reaction. This occurs in fewer than 1 percent of patients treated by either the intramuscular or intravenous route. It is not dose-dependent and may follow the infusion of only a few drops of diluted iron dextran solution or a fraction of a milliliter of intramuscularly injected iron dextran. This calls into question the usefulness of giving a test dose, and it is doubtful whether such a test dose serves any useful purpose. Characteristically, during the first few minutes of infusion, the patient complains of difficulty breathing, or a choking or smothering sensation, becomes sweaty and anxious, may complain of nausea, and may vomit. Respiratory stridor may be observed, followed by apnea. The blood pressure may drop abruptly; stupor and coma may quickly supervene. At the first evidence of this reaction, the infusion must be terminated, and epinephrine should immediately be injected subcutaneously (0.5 ml of 1:1000 aqueous epinephrine). Other measures to combat shock and anaphylaxis are appropriate. Most patients survive. However, at least six deaths are ascribed to iron dextran–induced anaphylactic shock,[338–342] in some cases despite appropriate treatment. Stroke or myocardial infarction may follow anaphylactic shock induced by iron dextran.[343]

Freshly opened vials of iron dextran may contain as much as 100 mg divalent iron per deciliter. Iron dextran causes hypotension when administered intravenously to cats, and the hypotensive effect correlates to some extent with the amount of divalent iron in the solution.[344] Successful administration of iron dextran after pretreatment with methylprednisolone, diphenhydramine, ephedrine, and Promit (very low molecular weight dextran) has been reported in a patient with a previous anaphylactic response,[345] and the use of glucocorticoids to prevent delayed reactions[317] had been advocated, but circumstances would need to be very unusual to justify readministration of iron dextran to a patient who had experienced a severe reaction.

Administration of iron dextran does not interfere with blood cross-matching or cause abnormalities of coagulation.[326]

COURSE

If therapy is adequate, the correction of iron deficiency anemia is usually gratifying. Symptoms such as headache, fatigue, pica, paresthesias, and burning sensation of the oropharyngeal mucosa may abate within a few days. In the blood, the reticulocyte count begins to increase after a few days, usually reaches a maximum at about 7 to 12 days, and thereafter decreases. When anemia is mild, little or no reticulocytosis may be observed. Little change in hemoglobin concentration or hematocrit value is to be expected for the first 2 weeks, but then the anemia is corrected rapidly. The hemoglobin concentration in the blood may be halfway back to normal after 4 to 5 weeks of therapy. By the end of 2 months of therapy, and often much sooner, the hemoglobin concentration should have reached a normal level. There is little difference in the rate of response whether iron is administered by the oral or the parenteral route, except in patients with intestinal malabsorption.[346]

PROGNOSIS

When the cause of the iron deficiency is a benign disorder, the prognosis is excellent, provided bleeding is controlled or can be compensated for by continual iron therapy. Too often, therapy is interrupted as soon as anemia has been corrected, and iron stores are not replenished. Such inadequately treated patients are likely to have recurrent anemia.[347] For this reason, and because iron therapy brings about replenishment of iron stores very slowly, oral therapy should be continued for at least 12 months after anemia has been corrected. If there is a benign cause of recurrent bleeding that is not an indication for surgical correction, such as hiatal hernia, menorrhagia, or hereditary hemorrhagic telangiectasia, oral iron therapy may be continued indefinitely; if the bleeding is especially brisk, supplementation with parenterally administered iron or, rarely, with transfusion may be needed. Continuous iron administration may also be required in patients with iron deficiency secondary to intravascular hemolysis with hemoglobinuria.

If the diagnosis of iron deficiency anemia is correct, anemia and other manifestations of iron deficiency will respond to adequate therapy. However, the physician is occasionally disappointed in the results of treatment of patients who seem to have iron deficiency anemia. In some cases this apparent failure of therapy is a result of treatment of patients with iron preparations that are virtually insoluble, enteric-coated, or contain iron in only minute amounts. Careful inquiry into the nature, duration, and regularity of iron therapy may reveal a reason for the failure of therapy and permit a gratifying response to be elicited with adequate therapy. Other questions that should be asked in evaluation of such a case are these: (1) Has bleeding been controlled? (2) Has the patient been on iron therapy long enough to show a response? (3) Has the dose of iron been adequate? (4) Are there other factors—inflammatory disease, neoplastic disease, hepatic or renal disease, concomitant deficiencies (vitamin B_{12}, folic acid, thyroid)—that might retard response? (5) Is the diagnosis correct?

REFERENCES

1. Bryan CP: *The Papyrus Ebers*. New York, Appleton-Century-Crofts, 1931.
2. Fairbanks VF, Fahey JL, Beutler E: *Clinical Disorders of Iron Metabolism*. New York, Grune & Stratton, 1971.
3. Choe YH, Kim SK, Son BK, Lee DH, Hong YC, Pai SH. Randomized placebo-controlled trial of Helicobacter pylori eradication for iron-deficiency anemia in preadolescent children and adolescents. *Helicobacter* 4:135, 1999.
4. Windsor CWO, Collis CL: Anaemia and hiatus hernia: Experience in 450 patients. *Thorax* 22:73, 1967.
5. Holt JM, Mayet FG, Warner GT, Callender ST, Gunning AJ: Iron absorption and blood loss in patients with hiatus hernia. *Br Med J* 3:22, 1968.
6. Moskovitz M, Fadden R, Min T, Jansma D, Gavaler J: Large hiatal hernias, anemia, and linear gastric erosion: studies of etiology and medical therapy. *Am J Gastroenterol* 87:622, 1992.
7. Weston AP: Hiatal hernia with cameron ulcers and erosions. *Gastrointest Endosc Clin North Am* 6:671, 1996.
8. Cameron AJ, Higgins JA: Linear gastric erosion. A lesion associated with large diaphragmatic hernia and chronic blood loss anemia. *Gastroenterology* 91:338, 1986.
9. Roth WA, Waldes-Dapena A, Pieses P, Buchanan E: Topical action of salicylates in gastrointestinal erosion and hemorrhage. *Gastroenterology* 44:146, 1963.
10. Faucheron JL, Parc R: Non-steroidal anti-inflammatory drug-induced colitis. *Int J Colorectal Dis* 11:99, 1996.
11. McIntyre AS, Long RG: Prospective survey of investigations in outpatients referred with iron deficiency anaemia. *Gut* 34:1102, 1993.
12. Retzlaff JA, Hagedorn AB, Bartholomew LG: Abdominal exploration for gastrointestinal bleeding of obscure origin. *JAMA* 177:104, 1961.
13. Baum S, Nusbaum M, Blakemore WS, Finkelstein AK: The preoperative radiographic demonstration of intraabdominal bleeding from the undetermined sites by percutaneous selective celiac and superior mesenteric arteriography. *Surgery* 58:797, 1965.
14. Prichard PJ, Tjandra JJ: Colorectal cancer. *Med J Aust* 169:493, 1998.
15. Swain RA, Kaplan B, Montgomery E: Iron deficiency anemia. When is parenteral therapy warranted? *Postgrad Med* 100:181, 1996.
16. Kaminski N, Shaham D, Eliakim R: Primary tumours of the duodenum. *Postgrad Med J* 69:136, 1993.
17. Holt JM, Wright R: Anaemia due to blood loss from the telangiectases of scleroderma. *Br Med J* 3:537, 1967.
18. Rosen KM, Sirota DK, Mirinoff SC: Gastrointestinal bleeding in Turner's syndrome. *Ann Intern Med* 67:145, 1967.
19. Hagood MF, Gathright JB, Jr.: Hemangiomatosis of the skin and gastrointestinal tract: Report of a case. *Dis Colon Rectum* 18:141, 1975.
20. Ohishi M, Tanaka Y, Higuchi Y, Otsuka T, Kagimoto M, Niho Y: Multiple facial hemangiomas and iron-deficiency anemia: Blue rubber-bleb nevus syndrome. *Head Neck Surg* 7:249, 1985.
21. Morris SJ, Kaplan SR, Ballan K, Tedesco FJ: Blue rubber-bleb nevus syndrome. *JAMA* 239:1887, 1978.
22. Singh AK, Cumaraswamy RC, Corrin B: Diffuse hypertrophy of gastric mucosa (Ménetrier's disease) and iron-deficiency anaemia. *Gut* 10:735, 1969.
23. Zaatar R, Younoszai MK, Mitros F: Pseudo-Zollinger-Ellison syndrome in a child presenting with anemia. *Gastroenterology* 92:508, 1987.

24. Hines JD, Hoffbrand AV, Mollin DL: The hematologic complications following partial gastrectomy: a study of 292 patients. *Am J Med* 43:555, 1967.

25. Hallberg L, Solvell L, Zederfeldt B: Iron absorption after partial gastrectomy: a comparative study on the absorption from ferrous sulphate and hemoglobin. *Acta Med Scand* 445–450:269, 1966.

26. Kimber C, Patterson JF, Weintraub LR: The pathogenesis of iron deficiency anemia following partial gastrectomy: a study of iron balance. *JAMA* 202:935, 1967.

27. Sorbi D, Conio M, Gostout CJ: Vascular disorders of the small bowel. *Gastrointest Endosc Clin North Am* 9:71, 1999.

28. Heer M, Ammann R, Bühler H: Die klinische Bedeutung der Angiodysplasien im Kolon. *Schweiz Med Wochenschr* 114:1416, 1984.

29. Meyer CT, Troncale FJ, Galloway S, Sheahan DG: Arteriovenous malformation of the bowel: an analysis of 22 cases and a review of the literature. *Medicine* 60:36, 1981.

30. Clouse RE, Costigan DJ, Mills BA, Zuckerman GR: Angiodysplasia as a cause of upper gastrointestinal bleeding. *Arch Intern Med* 145:458, 1985.

31. Jabbari M , Cherry R, Lough JO, Daly DS, Kinnear DG, Goresky CA: Gastric antral vascular ectasia: the watermelon stomach. *Gastroenterology* 87:1165, 1984.

32. Rawlinson WD , Barr GD , Lin BP: Antral vascular ectasia—the "watermelon" stomach. *Med J Aust* 144:709, 1986.

33. Kruger R, Ryan ME, Dickson KB, Nunez JF: Diffuse vascular ectasia of the gastric antrum. *Am J Gastroenterol* 82:421, 1987.

34. Fitzpatrick TJ: Hemocholecyst: a neglected cause of gastrointestinal hemorrhage. *Ann Intern Med* 55:1008, 1961.

35. Woodruff CW, Wright SW, Wright RP: The role of fresh cow's milk in iron deficiency. *Am J Dis Child* 124:26, 1972.

36. Halliday HL, Lappin RT, McClure G: Cow's milk and anemia in preterm infants. *Arch Dis Child* 60:69, 1985.

37. Coello-Ramirez P, Larrosa-Harro A: Gastrointestinal occult hemorrhage and gastroduodenitis in cow's milk protein intolerance. *J Pediatr Gastroenterol Nutr* 3:215, 1984.

38. American Academy of Pediatrics Committee on Nutrition: The use of whole cow's milk in infancy. *Pediatrics* 72:253, 1983.

39. Oski FA: Is bovine milk a health hazard? *Pediatrics* 75:182, 1985.

40. Milman N, Pedersen FM: Idiopathic pulmonary haemosiderosis. Epidemiology, pathogenic aspects and diagnosis. *Respir Med* 92:902, 1998.

41. Hallberg L, Hulthen L, Bengtsson C, Lapidus L, Lindstedt G: Iron balance in menstruating women. *Eur J Clin Nutr* 49:200, 1995.

42. Hallberg L, Högdahl AM, Nilsson L, Rybo G: Menstrual blood loss: a population study. *Acta Obstet Gynecol Scand* 45:320, 1966.

43. Hallberg L, Nilsson L: Constancy of individual menstrual blood loss. *Acta Obstet Gynecol Scand* 43:352, 1964.

44. Kivijärvi A, Timonen H, Rajamäki A, Grönroos M: Iron deficiency in women using modern copper intrauterine devices. *Obstet Gynecol* 67:95, 1986.

45. Bernard J, Najean Y, Alby N, Rain J-D: Les anémies hypochromes dues a des hémorragies volontairement provoquées: syndrome de Lasthénie de Ferjol. *Presse Med* 75:2087, 1967.

46. Boulanger JC, Delobel J, Delahousse J, Lamblin E, Hourdin J, Gross S: Le syndrome de Lasthénie de Ferjo. A propos d'une observation. *Rev Fr Gynecol Obstet* 80:279, 1985.

47. Fey MF, Radvila A: Long term follow-up of factitious anemia. *Br Med J* 296:1504, 1988.

48. Eisenfiz M, Chabolle F, Ferreri M, Meyer B, Chouard CH: Forme oropharyngée du syndrome de Lasthénie de Ferjol: A propos d'un cas. *Ann Oto-Laryngol Chir Cervicofac* 105:193, 1988.

49. Henry ML, Garner WL, Fabri PJ: Iatrogenic anemia. *Am J Surg* 151:362, 1986.

50. Guillemin C, Vigneron C, Streiff F: Serum and erythrocyte ferritin in regular blood donors. *Nouv Rev Fr Hematol* 34:259, 1992.

51. Ho CH, Yuan CC, Yeh SH: Serum ferritin levels and their significance in normal full-term pregnant women. *Int J Gynaecol Obstet* 25:291, 1987.

52. Dawson EB, McGanity WJ: Protection of maternal iron stores in pregnancy. *J Reprod Med* 32(suppl):478, 1987.

53. Milman N, Ibsen KK, Christensen JM: Serum ferritin and iron status in mothers and newborn infants. *Acta Obstet Gynecol Scand* 66:205, 1987.

54. King DE, Sobal J, Muncie HL, Jr., Alger LS, Jackson F: Prescribing postpartum iron supplementation: a survey of practicing obstetricians. *South Med J* 79:674, 1986.

55. Anonymous: Iron fortification of infant formulas. American Academy of Pediatrics. Committee on Nutrition. *Pediatrics* 104:119, 1999.

56. Gerrior SA, Zizza C: Nutrient Content of U.S. Food Supply, 1909–1990. Home Economics Research Report No. 52. Washington, DC, US Department of Agriculture, 1994.

57. Federation of American Societies for Experimental Biology LSRO: Third Report on Nutritional Monitoring in the US, Vols. 1, 2, Executive Summary. Washington, DC, US Government Printing Office, 1995.

58. Murphy SP, Calloway DH: Nutrient intakes of women in NHANES II, emphasizing trace minerals, fiber, and phytate. *J Am Diet Assoc* 86:1366, 1986.

59. Subcommittee on the Tenth Edition of the RDAs FNB: *Recommended Dietary Allowances*. 10th rev ed. Washington, DC, National Academy Press, 1989.

60. Pennington JA, Young BE, Wilson DB, Johnson RD, Vanderveen JE: Mineral content of foods and total diets: the selected minerals in food survey, 1982 to 1984. *J Am Diet Assoc* 86:876, 1986.

61. Rice WH, McMahon DJ: Chemical, physical, and sensory characteristics of mozzarella cheese fortified using protein-chelated iron or ferric chloride. *J Dairy Sci* 81:318, 1998.

62. Hekmat S, McMahon DJ: Manufacture and quality of iron-fortified yogurt. *J Dairy Sci* 80:3114, 1997.

63. Rosenbaum E, Leonard JW : Nutritional iron deficiency anemia in an adult male: report of a case. *Ann Intern Med* 60:683, 1964.

64. Meini A, Morandi L, Mora M, et al: An unusual association: celiac disease and Becker muscular dystrophy. *Am J Gastroenterol* 91:1459, 1996.

65. Corazza GR, Valentini RA, Andreani ML, et al: Subclinical coeliac disease is a frequent cause of iron-deficiency anaemia. *Scand J Gastroenterol* 30:153, 1995.

66. Vuopio P, Nikkilä EA: Hemolytic anemia and thrombocytopenia in a case of left atrial myxoma associated with mitral stenosis. *Am J Cardiol* 17:585, 1966.

67. Eyster E, Mayer K, McKenzie S: Traumatic hemolysis with iron deficiency anemia in patients with aortic valve lesions. *Ann Intern Med* 68:995, 1968.

68. Reynolds RD, Coltman CA, Jr., Beller BM: Iron treatment in sideropenic intravascular hemolysis due to insufficiency of Starr-Edwards valve prostheses. *Ann Intern Med* 66:659, 1967.

69. Sears DA, Anderson PR, Foy AL, Williams HL, Crosby WH: Urinary iron excretion and renal metabolism of hemoglobin in hemolytic diseases. *Blood* 28:708, 1966.

70. Stewart JG, Ahlquist DA, McGill DB, Ilstrup DM, Schwartz S, Owen RA: Gastrointestinal blood loss and anemia in runners. *Ann Intern Med* 100:843, 1984.

71. Magnusson B, Hallberg L, Rossander L, Swolin B: Iron metabolism and "sports anemia." I. A study of several iron parameters in elite runners with differences in iron status. *Acta Med Scand* 216:149, 1984.

72. Haymes EM, Puhl JL, Temples TE: Training for cross-country skiing and iron status. *Med Sci Sports Exerc* 18:162, 1986.

73. Selby GB, Eichner ER: Endurance swimming, intravascular hemolysis, anemia, and iron depletion. New perspective on athlete's anemia. *Am J Med* 81:791, 1986.

74. Pelliccia A, Di Nucci GB: Anemia in swimmers: Fact or fiction? Study of hematologic and iron status in male and female top-level swimmers. *Int J Sports Med* 8:227, 1987.

75. Cooper BT, Douglas SA, Firth LA, Hannagan JA, Chadwick VS: Erosive gastritis and gastrointestinal bleeding in a female runner. Prevention of the bleeding and healing of the gastritis with H2-receptor antagonists. *Gastroenterology* 92:2019, 1987.

76. Adamson JW, Eschbach J, Finch CA: The kidney and erythropoiesis. *Am J Med* 44:725, 1968.

77. Ehrhardt P, Miller MG, Littlewood JM: Iron deficiency in cystic fibrosis. *Arch Dis Child* 62:185, 1987.

78. Beutler E, Robson MJ, Buttenwiesser E: A comparison of the plasma iron, iron-binding capacity, sternal marrow iron and other methods in the clinical evaluation of iron stores. *Ann Intern Med* 48:60, 1958.

79. Loría A, Sanchez-Medal L, Lisker R, Rodriguez ED, Labardini J: Red cell life span in iron deficiency anemia. *Br J Haematol* 13:294, 1967.

80. Pollycove M: Iron metabolism and kinetics. *Semin Hematol* 3:235, 1966.

81. Beutler E: Iron enzymes in iron deficiency. I. Cytochrome C. *Am J Med Sci* 234:517, 1957.

82. Beutler E, Blaisdell RK: Iron enzymes in iron deficiency. III. Catalase in rat red cells and liver with some further observations on cytochrome C. *J Lab Clin Med* 52:694, 1958.

83. Cartier LJ, Ohira Y, Chen M, Cuddiher RW, Holloszy JO: Perturbation of mitochondrial composition in muscle by iron deficiency. Implications regarding regulation of mitochondrial assembly. *J Biol Chem* 261:13827, 1986.

84. Ohira Y, Cartier LJ, Chen M, Holloszy JO: Induction of an increase in mitochondrial matrix enzymes in muscle of iron-deficient rats. *Am J Physiol* 253:C639, 1987.

85. Harlan WR, Williams RS: Activity-induced adaptations in skeletal muscles of iron-deficient rabbits. *J Appl Physiol* 65:782, 1988.

86. Beutler E: Iron enzymes in iron deficiency. IV. Cytochrome oxidase in rat kidney and heart. *Acta Haematol* 21:371, 1959.

87. Beutler E: Iron enzymes in iron deficiency states. *Ill Med J* 116:16, 1959.

88. Masuya T: Pathophysiological studies in sideropenic symptoms: Biological consideration. *Isr J Med Sci* 1:733, 1965.

89. Beutler E, Blaisdell RK: Iron enzymes in iron deficiency. V. Succinic dehydrogenase in rat liver, kidney and heart. *Blood* 15:30, 1960.

90. Beutler E: Iron enzymes in iron deficiency. VI. Aconitase activity and citrate metabolism. *J Clin Invest* 38:1605, 1959.

91. Swarup S, Ghosh SK, Chatterjea JB: Aconitase activity in iron deficiency. *Acta Haematol* 37:53, 1967.

92. Srivastava SK, Sanwal GG, Tewari KK: Biochemical alterations in rat tissue in iron deficiency anaemia and repletion with iron. *Indian J Biochem* 2:257, 1965.

93. Celsing F, Ekblom B, Sylven C: Effects of chronic iron deficiency anaemia on myoglobin content, enzyme activity, and capillary density in the human skeletal muscle. *Acta Med Scand* 223:451, 1988.

94. Finch CA, Gollnick PD, Hlastala MP, Miller LR, Dillmann E, Mackler B: Lactic acid acidosis as a result of iron deficiency. *J Clin Invest* 64:129, 1979.

95. MacDonald VW, Charache S, Hathaway PJ: Iron deficiency anemia: Mitochondrial α-glycerophosphate dehyrdrogenase in guinea pig skeletal muscle. *J Lab Clin Med* 105:11, 1985.

96. Mackler B, Person R, Grace R: Iron deficiency in the rat: Effects on energy metabolism in brown adipose tissue. *Pediatr Res* 19:989, 1985.

97. Evans TC, Mackler B: Effects of iron deficiency on energy conservation in rat liver and skeletalmuscle submitochondrial particles. *Biochem Med* 34:93, 1985.

98. Thompson GH, Green YS, Ledingbam JG: The effect of iron deficiency on skeletal muscle submitochondrial particles. *Acta Physiol Scand* 147:85, 1993.

99. Thompson CH, Kemp GJ, Taylor DJ, Radda GK, Rajagopalan B: No evidence of mitochondrial abnormality in skeletal muscle of patients with iron-deficient anaemia. *J Intern Med* 234:149, 1993.

100. Walker JC, Selva D, Pietris G, Crompton JL: Optic disc swelling in Crohn's disease. *Aust N Z J Ophthalmol* 26:329, 1998.

101. Tucker DM, Sandstead HH, Swenson RA, Sawler BG, Penland JG: Longitudinal study of brain function and depletion of iron stores in individual subjects. *Physiol Behav* 29:740737, 1982.

102. Mehta BC, Panjwani DD, Jhala DA: Electrophysiologic abnormalities of heart in iron deficiency anemia. Effect of iron therapy. *Acta Haematol* 70:189, 1983.

103. Palti H, Meijer A, Adler B: Learning achievement and behavior at school of anemic and non-anemic infants. *Early Hum Dev* 10:217, 1985.

104. Pollitt E, Saco-Pollitt C, Leibel RL, Viteri FE: Iron deficiency and behavioral development in infants and preschool children. *Am J Clin Nutr* 43:555, 1986.

105. Soemantri AG, Pollitt E, Kim I: Iron deficiency anemia and educational achievement. *Am J Clin Nutr* 42:1221, 1985.

106. Chwang LC, Soemantri AG, Pollitt E: Iron supplementation and physical growth of rural Indonesian children. *Am J Clin Nutr* 47:496, 1988.

107. Lozoff B: Behavioral alterations in iron deficiency. *Adv Pediatr* 35:331, 1988.

108. Idjradinata P, Pollitt E: Reversal of developmental delays in iron-deficient anaemic infants treated with iron. *Lancet* 341:1, 1993.

109. Pollitt E: Iron deficiency and cognitive function. *Annu Rev Nutr* 13:521, 1993.

110. Pollitt E, Soemantri AG, Yunis F, Schrimshaw NS: Cognitive effects of iron-deficiency anemia. *Lancet* 1:158, 1985.

111. Youdim MBH, Green AR: Biogenic monoamine metabolism and functional activity in iron-deficient rats: Behavioural correlates. *CIBA Found Symp* 51:201, 1977.

112. Youdim MBH, Green AR: Iron deficiency and neurotransmitter synthesis and function. *Proc Nutr Soc* 37:173, 1978.

113. Beard J, Tobin B, Smith SM: Norepinephrine turnover in iron deficiency at three environmental temperatures. *Am J Physiol* 255:R90 (part 1), 1988.

114. Webb TE, Krill CE, Jr, Oski FA, Tsou KC: Relationship of iron status to urinary norepinephrine excretion in children 7–12 years of age. *J Pediatr Gastroenterol Nutr* 1:207, 1982.

115. Youdim MB, Ben-Shachar D: Minimal brain damage induced by early iron deficiency: modified dopaminergic neutrotransmission. *Isr J Med Sci* 23:19, 1987.

116. Bartholmey SJ, Sherman AR: Impaired ketogenesis in iron-deficient rat pups. *J Nutr* 116:2180, 1986.

117. Beard J: Feed efficiency and norepinephrine turnover in iron deficiency. *Proc Soc Exp Biol Med* 184:337, 1987.

118. Smith SM, Smith SH, Beard JL: Heart norepinephrine content in iron deficiency anemia. *J Nutr Biochem* 3:167, 1992.

119. Prime SS, MacDonald DG, Noble HW, Rennie JS: Effect of prolonged iron deficiency on enamel pigmentation and tooth structure in rat incisors. *Arch Oral Biol* 29:905, 1984.

120. Sun AH, Xiao SZ, Li BS, Wang TY, Zhang YS: Iron deficiency and hearing loss. Experimental study in growing rats. *ORL J Otorhinolaryngol Relat Spec* 49:118, 1987.

121. Sun AH, Xiao SZ, Zheng Z, Li BS, Li ZJ, Wang TY: A scanning electron microscopic study of cochlear changes in iron-deficient rats. *Acta Otolaryngol (Stockh)* 104:211, 1987.

122. Cook JD, Lynch SR: The liabilities of iron deficiency. *Blood* 68:803, 1986.

123. Kuvibidila S: Iron deficiency, cell-mediated immunity and resistance against infections—present knowledge and controversies. *Nutr Res* 7:989, 1987.

124. Jensen BM, Sando SH, Grandjean P: Screening with zinc protoporphyrin for iron deficiency in nonanemic female blood donors. *Clin Chem* 36:846, 1990.

125. Pizarro F, Olivares M, Hertrampf E, Walter T: Growth in terms of length of Chilean infants of low socioeconomic status: 1978–1992. *Arch Latinoam Nutr* 46:107, 1996.

126. Rosenzweig PH, Volpe SL: Iron, thermoregulation, and metabolic rate. *Crit Rev Food Sci Nutr* 39:131, 1999.

127. Brigham D, Beard J: Iron and thermoregulation: a review. *Crit Rev Food Sci Nutr* 36:747, 1996.

128. Bernát I, Valló J: Ozaena: the causes of its familial occurrence. *Acta Med Hung* 20:89, 1964.

129. Akhnoukh S, Saad EF: Iron deficiency in atrophic rhinits and scleroma. *Indian J Med Res* 85:576, 1987.

130. Shearman DJC, Delamore IW, Gardner DL: Gastric function and structure in iron deficiency. *Lancet* 1:845, 1966.

131. Dagg JH, Goldberg A, Gibbs WN, Anderson JR: Detection of latent pernicious anaemia in iron deficiency anaemia. *Br Med J* 2:619, 1966.

132. Voigt D, Brüschke G: Magenschleimhaut und Eisenmangel. *Dtsch Med Wochenschr* 1:1082, 1967.

133. Leonard BJ: Gastric acid in iron-deficiency anaemia. *Lancet* 2:440, 1966.

134. Jacobs A, Lawrie JH, Entwistle CC, Campbell H: Gastric acid secretion in chronic iron-deficiency anaemia. *Lancet* 2:190, 1966.

135. Stone WD: Gastric secretory response to iron therapy. *Gut* 9:99, 1968.

136. Sandstead HH, Carter JP, House FR, McConnell F, Horton KB, Vander Zwaag R: Nutritional deficiencies in disadvantaged preschool children. *Am J Dis Child* 121:455, 1971.

137. Davidson WMB, Markson JL: The gastric mucosa in iron-deficiency anaemia. *Lancet* 2:639, 1955.

138. Baird IM, Dodge OG, Palmer FJ, Wawman RJ: The tongue and oesophagus in iron-deficiency anaemia and the effort of iron therapy. *J Clin Pathol* 14:603, 1961.

139. Cheli R, Dodero M, Celle G, Vassalotti M: Gastric biopsy and secretory findings in hypochromic anaemias: comparison of the gastric mucosa with tongue and esophageal mucosa. *Acta Haematol* 22:1, 1959.

140. Lees F, Rosenthal FD: Gastric mucosal lesions before and after treatment in iron deficiency anemia. *Q J Med* 27:19, 1958.

141. Naiman JL, Oski FA, Diamond LK, Vawter GF, Shwachman H: The

gastrointestinal effects of iron-deficiency anemia. *Pediatrics* 33:83, 1964.

142. Scott J, Valentine JA, St. Hill CA, West CR: Morphometric analysis of atrophic changes in human lingual epithelium in iron deficiency anaemia. *J Clin Pathol* 38:1025, 1984.

143. Boddington MM: Changes in buccal cells in the anaemias. *J Clin Pathol* 12:222, 1959.

144. Jacobs A: The buccal mucosa in anaemia. *J Clin Pathol* 13:463, 1960.

145. Macleod RI, Hamilton PJ, Soames J: Quantitative exfoliative oral cytology in iron-deficiency and megaloblastic anemia. *Anal Quant Cytol Histol* 10:176, 1988.

146. Geerlings SE, Statius van Eps LW: Pathogenesis and consequences of Plummer-Vinson syndrome. *Clin Invest* 70:629, 1992.

147. Dantas RO, Villanova MG: Esophageal motility impairment in Plummer-Vinson syndrome. Correction by iron treatment. *Dig Dis Sci* 38:968, 1993.

148. Ahlbom HE: Simple achlorhydic anaemia, Plummer-Vinson syndrome, and carcinoma of the mouth, pharynx, and oesophagus in women: observation at Radiumhemmet, Stockholm. *Br Med J* 2:331, 1936.

149. Jacobs A, Kilpatrick GS: The Paterson-Kelly syndrome. *Br Med J* 2:79, 1964.

150. Shahidi NT, Diamond LK: Skull changes in infants with chronic iron-deficiency anemia. *N Engl J Med* 262:137, 1960.

151. Moseley JE: Skeletal changes in the anemias. *Semin Roentgenol* 9:169, 1974.

152. Reimann VF, Berker F, Gökmen E, Kücükackirlar T: Das Verhalten der Sella turcica bei jugendlichen Patienten mit schwerer Eisenmangelkrankheit. *Fortschr Rîntgenstr* 129:598, 1978.

153. Adekile AD, Yuregir TZ, Walker EL, III, Gu LH, Basal E, Huisman TH: Factors associated with hypochromia and microcytosis among high school students in the southeastern United States. *South Med J* 87:1132, 1994.

154. Moertel C, Braddock M, Henry P, Peick M, Kendrick J: The Ramsey County childhood anemia project—preliminary findings. *Blood* 88 (suppl 1):13b, 1996.

155. Hallberg L: Iron fortification ractice in Sweden. Personal communication. 1995.

156. Olsson KS, Vaisanen M, Konar J, Bruce A: The effect of withdrawal of food iron fortification in Sweden as studied with phlebotomy in subjects with genetic hemochromatosis. *Eur J Clin Nutr* 51:782, 1997.

157. Olsson KS, Safwenberg J, Ritter B: The effect of iron fortification of the diet on clinical iron overload in the general population. *Ann N Y Acad Sci* 526:290, 1988.

158. Kennedy E, Goldberg J: What are American children eating? Implications for public policy. *Nutr Rev* 53:111, 1999.

159. Expert Scientific Working Group: Summary of a report on assessment of the iron nutritional status of the United States population. *Am J Clin Nutr* 42:1318, 1985.

160. High prevalence of iron deficiency anemia among Alaskan native children. *MMWR* 37:200, 1988.

161. Scott DE, Pritchard JA: Iron deficiency in healthy young college women. *JAMA* 199:897, 1967.

162. Rybo E: Diagnosis of iron deficiency. *Scand J Haematol* 34(suppl 43):5, 1985.

163. Uchida T, Yoshida M, Sakai K, et al: Prevalence of iron deficiency in Japanese women. *Acta Haematol Jpn* 51:24, 1988.

164. Wood MM, Elwood PC: Symptoms of iron deficiency anaemia: a community survey. *Br J Prev Soc Med* 20:117, 1966.

165. Beutler E, Larsh SE, Gurney CW: Iron therapy in chronically fatigued nonanemic women: a double-blind study. *Ann Intern Med* 52:378, 1960.

166. Cochrane AL, Elwood PC: Iron deficiency without anaemia. *Lancet* 1:591, 1968.

167. Morrow JJ, Dagg JH, Goldberg A: A controlled trial of iron therapy in sideropenia. *Scott Med J* 13:78, 1968.

168. Lieden G, Adolfsson L: Physical work capacity in blood donors. *Scand J Clin Lab Invest* 34:37, 1974.

169. Vellar OD, Hermansen L: Physical performance and hernatological parameters. *Acta Med Scand* 519–525S:11, 1971.

170. Andersen HT, Barkve H: Iron deficiency and muscular work performance. *Scand J Clin Lab Invest* 114S:7, 1970.

171. Ericsson P: The effect of iron supplementation on the physical work capacity in the elderly. *Acta Med Scand* 188:361, 1970.

172. Beutler E, Larsh S, Tanzi F: Iron enzymes in iron deficiency: VII. Oxygen consumption measurements in iron-deficient subjects. *Am J Med Sci* 239:759, 1960.

173. Edgerton VR, Bryant SL, Gillespie CA, Gardner GW: Iron deficiency anemia and physical performance and activity of rats. *J Nutr* 102:381, 1972.

174. Glover J, Jacobs A: Activity pattern of iron-deficient rats. *Br Med J* 2:627, 1972.

175. Finch CA, Miller LR, Inamdar AR, Person R, Seiler K, Mackler B: Iron deficiency in the rat. Physiological and biochemical studies of muscle dysfunction. *J Clin Invest* 58:447, 1976.

176. Finch CA, Miller LR, Inamdar AR, et al: Iron deficiency anaemia and the acid-base variations of exercise. *Nutr Metab* 14:129, 1972.

177. Viteri FE, Torún B: Anaemia and physical work capacity. *Clin Haematol* 3:609, 1974.

178. Davies CTM, Chukweumeka AC, Van Haaren JPM: Iron-deficiency anaemia: its effect on maximum aerobic power and responses to exercise in African males aged 17–40 years. *Clin Sci* 44:555, 1973.

179. Davies CTM, Van Haaren JPM: Effect of treatment on physiological responses to exercise performance on East African industrial workers with iron deficiency anemia. *Br J Ind Med* 30:335, 1973.

180. Davies CTM: The physiological effects of iron deficiency anaemia and malnutrition on exercise performance in East African school children. *Acta Paediatr Belg* 28(suppl):253, 1974.

181. Gardner GW, Edgerton VR, Senewiratne B, Barnard RJ, Ohira Y: Physical work capacity and metabolic stress in subjects with iron deficiency anemia. *Am J Clin Nutr* 30:910, 1977.

182. Charlton RW, Derman D, Skikne B, et al: Anaemia, iron deficiency, and exercise. Extended studies in human subjects. *Clin Sci Mol Med* 53:537, 1977.

183. Rowland TW, Deisroth MB, Green GM, Kelleher JF: The iron therapy on the exercise capacity of nonanemic iron-deficient adolescent runners. *Am J Dis Child* 142:165, 1988.

184. Celsing F, Blomstrand E, Werner B, Pihlstedt P, Ekblom B: Effects of iron deficiency on endurance and muscle enzyme activity in men. *Med Sci Sports Med* 18:156, 1986.

185. Beard JL, Haas JD, Tufts D, Spielvogel H, Vargas E, Rodriquez C: Iron deficiency anemia and steady-state work performance at high altitude. *J Appl Physiol* 64:1878, 1988.

186. Taymor ML, Sturgis SH, Yahia C: The etiological role of chronic iron deficiency in production of menorrhagia. *JAMA* 187:323, 1964.

187. Samuels AJ: Studies in patients with functional menorrhagia: the antihemorrhagic effect of the adequate repletion of iron stores. *Isr J Med Sci* 1:851, 1965.

188. Jacobs A, Butler EB: Menstrual blood-loss in iron deficiency anemia. *Lancet* 2:407, 1965.

189. Roselle HA, Englewood NJ: Association of laundry starch and clay ingestion with anemia in New York City. *Arch Intern Med* 125:57, 1970.

190. Shapiro MD, Linas SL: Sodium chloride pica secondary to iron-deficiency anemia. *Am J Kidney Dis* 5:67, 1985.

191. Callinan V, O'Hare JA: Cardboard chewing: cause and effect of iron-deficient anernia. *Am J Med* 85:449, 1988.

192. Menge H, Lang A, Cuntze H: Pica in Germany—amylophagia as the etiology of iron deficiency anemia. *Z Gastroenterol* 36:635, 1998.

193. Phillips MR, Zaheer S, Drugas GT: Gastric trichobezoar: case report and literature review. *Mayo Clin Proc* 73:653, 1998.

194. Silber MH: Restless legs syndrome. *Mayo Clin Proc* 72:261, 1997.

195. O'Keeffe ST, Noel J, Lavan JN: Restless legs syndrome in the elderly. *Postgrad Med J* 69:701, 1993.

196. Shorb SR: Anemia and diabetic retinopathy. *Am J Ophthalmol* 100:434, 1985.

197. Bessman J, Feinstein DI: Quantitative anisocytosis as a discriminant between iron deficiency and thalassemia minor. *Blood* 53:288, 1979.

198. Conrad ME, Crosby WH: The natural history of iron deficiency induced by phlebotomy. *Blood* 20:173, 1962.

199. Beutler E: The red cell indices in the diagnosis of iron-deficiency anemia. *Ann Intern Med* 50:313, 1959.

200. Fairbanks VF: Is the peripheral blood film reliable for the diagnosis of iron deficiency anemia? *Am J Clin Pathol* 55:447, 1971.

201. Miguel A, Linares M, Miguel-Borja JM: Red cell distribution width analysis in differentiation between iron deficiency and thalassemia minor. *Acta Haematol* 80:59, 1988.

202. Bessman JB, Gilmer PR, Gardner FH: Improved classification of anemias by MCV and RDW. *Am J Clin Pathol* 80:322, 1983.

203. McClure S, Custer E, Bessman J: Improved detection of early iron deficiency in nonanemic subjects. *JAMA* 253:1021, 1985.

204. Han P, Fung KP: Discriminant analysis of iron deficiency anaemia and heterozygous thalassaemia traits: a 3-dimensional selection of red cell indices. *Clin Lab Haematol* 13:351, 1991.

205. Flynn MM, Reppun TS, Bhagavan NV: Limitations of red blood cell distribution width (RDW) in evaluaton of microcytosis. *Am J Clin Pathol* 85:445, 1986.

206. Roberts GT, El-Badawi SB: Red blood cell distribution width index in some hematologic diseases. *Am J Clin Pathol* 83:222, 1985.

207. Ghionni A, Miotti TC, Camandona U: Parametri eritrocritaro differenziali tra talassemia minor e sindromi iposideremiche. *Minerva Med* 76:1143, 1985.

208. Baynes RD, Flax H, Bothwell TH, Bezwoda WR, Atkinson P, Mendelow B: Red blood cells distribution width in anemia secondary to tuberculosis. *Am J Clin Pathol* 85:226, 1986.

209. Thompson WG, Meola T, Lipkin M, Jr., Freedman ML: Red cell distribution width, mean corpuscular volume, and transferrin saturation in the diagnosis of iron deficiency. *Arch Intern Med* 148:2128, 1988.

210. Marsh WL Jr, Bishop JW, Darcy TP: Evaluation of red cell volume distribution width (RDW). *Hematol Pathol* 1:117, 1987.

211. Charache S, Gittlelsohn AM, Allen H, et al: Noninvasive assessment of tissue iron stores. *Am J Clin Pathol* 88:333, 1987.

212. Witte DL, Kraemer DF, Johnson GF, Dick FR, Hamilton H: Prediction of bone marrow iron findings from tests performed on peripheral blood. *Am J Clin Pathol* 85:202, 1986.

213. Beck JR, Cornwell GG III, Rawnsley HM: Multivariate approach to predictive diagnosis of bone marrow iron stores. *Am J Clin Pathol* 70:665, 1978.

214. Junca J, Flores A, Roy C, Alberti R, Milla F: Red cell distribution width, free erythrocyte protoporphyrin, and England-Fraser index in the differential diagnosis of microcytosis due to iron deficiency or betathalassemia trait. A study of 200 cases of microcytic anemia. *Hematol Pathol* 5:33, 1991.

215. Schloesser LL, Kipp MA, Wenzel FJ: Thrombocytosis in iron-deficiency anemia. *J Lab Clin Med* 66:107, 1965.

216. Kasper CK, Whissel DYE, Wallerstein RO: Clinical aspects of iron deficiency. *JAMA* 191:359, 1965.

217. Kokkinos J, Levine SR: Thrombocytosis secondary to iron deficiency and recurrent central ischemia possibly improved by plateletpheresis. *Cerebrovasc Dis* 3:177, 1993.

218. Dincol K, Aksoy M: On the platelet levels in chronic iron deficiency anemia. *Acta Haematol* 41:135, 1969.

219. Gross S, Keefer V, Newman AJ: The platelets in iron-deficiency anemia. I. The response to oral and parenteral iron. *Pediatrics* 34:315, 1964.

220. Soff GA, Levin J: Thrombocytopenia associated with repletion of iron in iron-deficiency anemia. *Am J Med Sci* 295:35, 1988.

221. Berger M, Brass LF: Severe thrombocytopenia in iron deficiency anemia. *Am J Hematol* 24:425, 1987.

222. Beutler E, Drennan W, Block M: The bone marrow and liver in iron deficiency anemia: a histopathologic study of sections with special reference to the stainable iron content. *J Lab Clin Med* 43:427, 1954.

223. Ellis LD, Jensen WN, Westerman MP: Marrow iron: an evaluation of depleted stores in a series of 1,332 needle biopsies. *Ann Intern Med* 61:44, 1964.

224. Garby L, Irnell L, Werner I: Iron deficiency in women of fertile age in a Swedish community. II. Efficiency of several laboratory tests to predict the response to iron supplementation. *Acta Med Scand* 185:107, 1969.

225. Hamilton LD, Gubler CJ, Cartwright GE, Wintrobe MM: Diurnal variation in the plasma iron level of man. *Proc Soc Exp Biol Med* 61:44, 1964.

226. Hoyer K: Physiologic variations in the iron content of human blood serum. I. The variations from week to week, from day to day, and through twenty-four hours. II. Further studies of the intra diem variations. *Acta Med Scand* 119:562, 1944.

227. Speck B: Diurnal variation of serum iron and the latent iron binding capacity in normal adults. *Helv Med Acta* 34:231, 1968.

228. Zilva JF, Patston VJ: Variations in serum-iron in healthy women. *Lancet* 1:459, 1966.

229. Fujino M, Dawson EB, Holeman T, McGanity WJ: Interrelationships

230. Mardell M, Zilva JF: Effect of oral contraceptives on the variations in serum-iron during the menstrual cycle. *Lancet* 2:1323, 1967.

231. Burton JL: Effect of oral contraceptives on haemoglobin, packed-cell volume, serum-iron, and total iron-binding capacity in healthy women. *Lancet* 1:978, 1967.

232. Heilmeyer L, Plötner K: Das Serumeisen und die Eisenmangelkrankheit, in Pathogenese, Symptomatologie und Therapie, Jena, Gustav Fischer Verlag, 1937, p 92.

233. Cartwright GE: The anemia of chronic disorders. *Semin Hematol* 3:351, 1966.

234. Bainton DF, Finch CA: The diagnosis of iron deficiency anemia. *Am J Med* 37:62, 1964.

235. Banerjee RN, Narang RM: Haematological changes in malignancy. *Br J Haematol* 13:829, 1967.

236. Handjani AM, Banihashemi A, Rafiee R, Toulou H: Serum iron in acute myocardial infarction. *Blut* 23:363, 1971.

237. Syrkis I, Machtey I: Hypoferremia in acute myocardial infarction. *J Am Geriatr Soc* 21:28, 1973.

238. Follezou JY, Bizon M: Cancer chemotherapy induces a transient increase of serum-iron level. *Neoplasma* 33:225, 1986.

239. Jacobs A, Miller F, Worwood M, Beamish MR, Wardrop CA: Ferritin in the serum of normal subjects and patients with iron deficiency and iron overload. *Br Med J* 4:206, 1972.

240. Jacob RA, Sandstead HH, Klevay LM, Johnson LK: Utility of serum ferritin as a measure of iron deficiency in normal males undergoing repetitive phlebotomy. *Blood* 56:786, 1980.

241. Lipschitz DA, Cook JD, Finch CA: A clinical evaluation of serum ferritin as an index of iron stores. *N Engl J Med* 290:1213, 1974.

242. Coenen JL, van Dieijen-Visser MP, van Pelt J, et al: Measurements of serum ferritin used to predict concentrations of iron in bone marrow in anemia of chronic disease. *Clin Chem* 37:560, 1991.

243. Aulbert E, Steffens O: [Serum ferritin—a tumor marker in malignant lymphomas?]. [German]. *Onkologie* 13:102, 1990

244. Sears DA: Anemia of chronic disease. *Med Clin North Am* 76:567, 1992.

245. Hansen TM, Hansen NE: Serum ferritin as indicator of iron responsive anaemia in patients with rhemuatoid arthritis. *Ann Rheum Dis* 45:596, 1986.

246. Matzner Y, Konijn AM, Hershko C: Serum ferritin in hematologic malignancies. *Am J Hematol* 9:13, 1980.

247. Eckey VP: Die Kinetik des Serumeisenspiegels im Verlauf der Hepatitis. *Z Gesamte Inn Med* 19:433, 1964.

248. Prieto J, Barry M, Sherlock S: Serum ferritin in patients with iron overload and with acute and chronic liver disease. *Gastroenterology* 68:525, 1975.

249. Heinrich H: Serum-ferritin ungeeignet als Kontrollparameter der oralen Eisentherapie. *Dtsch Med Wochenschr* 102:1788, 1977.

250. Siimes MA, Addiego JE, Dallman PR: Ferritin in serum: diagnosis of iron deficiency and iron overload in infants and children. *Blood* 43:581, 1974.

251. Wheby MS: Effect of iron therapy on serum ferritin levels in iron-deficiency anemia. *Blood* 56:138, 1980.

252. Bodemann HH, Rieger A, Bross KJ, Schröter-Urban H, Löhr GW: Erythrocyte and plasma ferritin in normal subjects, blood donors and iron deficiency anemia patients. *Blut* 48:131, 1984.

253. Peters SW, Jacobs A, Fitzsimmons E: Erythrocyte ferritin in normal subjects and patients with abnormal iron metabolism. *Br J Haematol* 53:211, 1983.

254. Herbert V, Jayatilleke E, Shaw S: Serum ferritin iron, a new test, measures human body iron stores unconfounded by inflammation. *Stem Cells* 15:291, 1997.

255. Galan P, Sangare N, Preziosi P: Is basic red cell ferritin a more specific indiator than serum ferritin in the assessment of iron stores in the elderly? *Clin Chim Acta* 189:159, 1990.

256. Balaban EP, Sheehan RG, Demian SE, Cox JV, Frenkel EP: Evaluation of bone marrow iron stores in anemia associated with chronic disease: a comparative study of serum and red cell ferritin. *Am J Hematol* 42:177, 1993

257. Henrettig FM, Temple AR: Acute iron poisoning in children. *Emerg Med Clin North Am* 2:121, 1984.

258. Cook JD, Skikne BS, Baynes RD: Serum transferrin receptor. *Annu Rev Med* 44:63, 1993.

259. Ahluwalia N: Diagnostic utility of serum transferrin receptors measurement in assessing iron status. *Nutr Rev* 56:133, 1998.

260. Provan D: Mechanisms and management of iron deficiency anaemia. *Br J Haematol* 105(suppl)1:19, 1999.

261. Junca J, Fernandez-Aviles F, Oriol A, et al: The usefulness of the serum transferrin receptor in detecting iron deficiency in the anemia of chronic disorders. *Haematologica* 83:676, 1998.

262. Gimferrer F, Ubeda J, Remacha AF: Serum transferrin receptor levels are "physiologically high" in heterozygous beta-thalassemia. *Haematologica* 82:728, 1997.

263. North M, Dallalio G, Donath AS, Melink R, Means RT Jr: Serum transferrin receptor levels in patients undergoing evaluation of iron stores: correlation with other parameters and observed versus predicted results. *Clin Lab Haematol* 19:93, 1997

264. Pettersson T, Kivivuori SM, Siimes MA: Is serum transferrin receptor useful for detecting iron-deficiency in anaemic patients with chronic inflammatory diseases? *Br J Rheumatol* 33:740, 1994.

265. Brugnara C, Zurakowski D, DiCanzio J, Boyd T, Platt O: Reticulocyte hemoglobin content to diagnose iron deficiency in children. *JAMA* 281:225, 1999.

266. Wahner-Roedler DL, Fairbanks VF, Linman JW: Cobalt excretion test as index of iron absorption and diagnostic test for iron deficiency. *J Lab Clin Med* 85:253, 1975.

267. Flanagan PR, Haist J, Valberg LS: Comparative effects of iron deficiency induced by bleeding and a low-iron diet on the intestinal absorptive interactions of iron, cobalt, manganese, zinc, lead and cadmium. *J Nutr* 110:1754, 1980.

268. Verloop MC, Meeuwissen JET, Blokhuis EWM: Comparison of the "iron absorption test" with the determination of the iron-binding capacity of serum in the diagnosis of iron deficiency. *Br J Haematol* 4:70, 1958.

269. Wiltink WF, Ybema HJ, Leijnse B, Gerbrandy J: The iron tolerance test: measurement of absorption and utilization of a therapeutic dose of iron. *Clin Chim Acta* 13:701, 1966.

270. Crosby WH, O'Neil-Cutting MA: A small-dose iron tolerance test as an indicator of mild iron deficiency. *JAMA* 251:1986, 1984.

271. Dubeau CE, Voytovich AE, Rippey RM: Premature conclusions in the diagnosis of iron-deficiency anemia: Cause and effect. *Med Decis Making* 6:169, 1986.

272. Johnson CS, Tegos C, Beutler E: Alpha-thalassemia. Prevalence and hematologic findings in American Blacks. *Arch Intern Med* 142:1280, 1982.

273. Van der Dijs FP, van den Berg GA, Schermer JG, Muskiet FD, Landman H, Muskiet FA: Screening cord blood for hemoglobinopathies and thalassemia by HPLC. *Clin Chem* 38:1864, 1992.

274. Yorke D, Mitchell J, Clow C, et al: Newborn screening for sickle cell and other hemoglobinopathies: a Canadian pilot study. *Med Clin Exper* 15:376, 1992.

275. Gerald PS, Diamond LK: A new hereditary hemoglobinopathy (the Lepore trait) and its interaction with thalassemia trait. *Blood* 13:835, 1958.

276. Duma H, Efremov G, Sadikario A, Teodosijev D, Mladenovski B, Vlaski A, Andreeva M: Study of nine families with haemoglobin-Lepore. *Br J Haematol* 15:161, 1968.

277. Fairbanks VF, Gilchrist GS, Brimhall B, Jereb JA, Goldston EC: Hemoglobin E trait reexamined: a cause of microcytosis and erythrocytosis. *Blood* 53:109, 1979.

278. Fairbanks VF, Oliveros R, Brandabur JH, Willis RR, Fiester RF: Homozygous hemoglobin E mimics β-thalassemia minor without anemia or hemolysis: hematologic, functional, and biosynthetic studies of first North American cases. *Am J Hematol* 8:109, 1980.

279. England JM, Walford DM, Waters DAW: Reassessment of the reliability of the hematocrit. *Br J Haematol* 23:247, 1972.

280. Rose MS: Epitaph for the M.C.H.C. *Br Med J* 423:169, 1971.

281. Lin CK, Lin JS, Chen SY, Jiang ML, Chiu CF: Comparison of hemoglobin and red blood cell distribution width in the differential diagnosis of microcytic anemia. *Arch Pathol Lab Med* 116:1030, 1992.

282. Cartei G, Chisesi T, Cazzavillan M, Battista R, Barbui T, Dini E: Relationship between Hb and HbA2 concentrations in beta-thalassemia trait and effect of iron deficiency anaemia. *Biomedicine* 25:282, 1976.

283. Chiandussi I, Bianco A, Massaro A, Mazza U, Cesano L: The quantitative determination of iron Idnetics and hemoglobin synthesis in anemia of cirrhosis studied with ^{59}Fe. *Blut* 10:120, 1964.

284. Ellis LS, Westerman MP, Balcerzak SP: The effect of iron stores on ferrokinetics in polycythemia. *Br J Haematol* 13:892, 1967.

285. Cervantes F, Rozman C, Piera, C, Fernandez M-R: Decreased bone marrow iron in chronic granulocytic leukaemia: a consistent finding not reflecting iron deficiency. *Blut* 53:305, 1986.

286. Hilal H, McCurdy PR: A pitfall in the interpretation of serum iron values. *Ann Intern Med* 66:983, 1967.

287. Koehler PR, Salmon RB: Angiographic localization of unknown acute gastrointestinal bleeding sites. *Radiology* 89:244, 1967.

288. Chait A, Dann RH: G-I bleed after angiography. *N Engl J Med* 286:1418, 1972.

289. Jewett TC Jr, Duszynski DO, Allen JE: The visualization of Meckel's diverticulum with ^{99}Tc-pertechnetate. *Surgery* 68:567, 1970.

290. Kilpatrick ZM, Aseron CA Jr: Radioisotope detection of Meckel's diverticulum causing acute rectal hemorrhage. *N Engl J Med* 287:653, 1972.

291. Berquist TH, Nolan NG, Adson MA, Schutt AJ: Diagnosis of Meckel's diveriticulum by radioisotope scanning. *Mayo Clin Proc* 48:98, 1973.

292. Waye JD: Small-bowel endoscopy. *Endoscopy* 31:56, 1999.

293. Brayton D: Gastrointestinal bleeding of "unknown origin": a study of cases in infancy and childhood. *Am J Dis Child* 107:288, 1964.

294. Shandling B: Laparotomy for rectal bleeding. *Pediatrics* 35:787, 1965.

295. Hallberg L, Ryttinger L, Sölvell L: Side-effects of oral iron therapy: a double-blind study of different iron compounds in tablet form. *Acta Med Scand* 459(suppl):3, 1966.

296. Beutler E, Meerkreebs G: Doses and dosing. *N Engl J Med* 274:1152, 1966.

297. O'Sullivan DJ, Higgins PG, Wilkinson JF: Oral iron compounds: a therapeutic comparison. *Lancet* 2:482, 1955.

298. Gordeuk VR, Brittenham GM, Hughes M, Keating LJ, Opplt JJ: High-dose carbonyl iron for iron deficiency anemia: a randomized double-blind trial. *Am J Clin Nutr* 46:1029, 1987.

299. Klein-Schwartz W, Oderda GM, Gorman RL: Assessment of management guidelines. Acute iron ingestion. *Clin Pediatr* 29:316, 1990.

300. Walter T, Olivares M, Pizarro F, Munoz M: Iron, anemia and infection. *Nutr Rev* 55:111, 1997.

301. Westlin WF: Deferoxamine in the treatment of acute iron poisoning: clinical experiences with 172 children. *Clin Pediatr (Phila)* 5:531, 1966.

302. Greengard J, McEnery JT: Iron poisoning in children. *GP* 37:88, 1968.

303. Whitten CF, Brough AJ: The pathophysiology of acute iron poisoning. *Clin Toxicol* 4:585, 1971.

304. McEnery JT: Hospital management of acute iron ingestion. *Clin Toxicol* 4:603, 1971.

305. Cox JSG, Kennedy GR, King J, Marshall PR, Rutherford D: Structure of an iron-dextran complex. *J Pharm Pharmacol* 24:513, 1972.

306. Muranda M, Rivera H, Ortega F, et al: Experiencas con el uso del hierroxtran marcado con Fe-59. *Rev Med Chil* 93:134, 1965.

307. Will G: The absorption, distribution and utilization of intramuscularly administered iron-dextran: a radioisotope study. *Br J Haematol* 14:395, 1968.

308. Marchasin S, Wallerstein RO: The treatment of iron-deficiency anemia with intravenous iron dextran. *Blood* 23:354, 1964.

309. Grimes AJ, Hutt MSR: Metabolism of ^{59}Fe-dextran complex in human subjects. *Br Med J* 2:1074, 1957.

310. Garby L, Sjölin S: Some observations on the distribution kinetics of radioactive colloidal iron (Imferon and ferric hydroxide). *Acta Med Scand* 157:319, 1957.

311. Henderson PA, Hillman RS: Characteristics of iron dextran utilization in man. *Blood* 34:357, 1969.

312. Olsson KS, Weinfeld A: Availability of iron dextran for hemoglobin synthesis. *Acta Med Scand* 192:543, 1972.

313. Rhyner K, Ganzoni AM: Die therapeutische Infusion von Eisen-III-Hydroxyd-Kohlenhydrat-Komplexen. *Schweiz Med Wochenschr* 102:561, 1972.

314. Loría A, Cordourier E, Arroyo P, Piedras J, Medal L: Anémia nutricional. IV. Hierro dextran en dosis intravenosa unica en la profilaxis de la anemia hipoferrémica del embarazo. *Rev Invest Clin* 24:113, 1972.

315. Shuttleworth D, Spence C, Slade R: Meningism due to intravenous iron dextran. *Lancet* 2:453, 1983.

316. Kanakaraddi VP, Hoskatti CG, Nadig VS, Patil CK, Maiya M: Compara-

tive therapeutic study of T.D.I. and I.M. injections of iron dextran complex in anaemia. *J Assoc Physicians India* 21:849, 1973.

317. Auerbach M, Witt D, Toler W, Fierstein M, Lerner RG, Ballard H: Clinical use of the total dose intravenous infusion of iron dextran. *J Lab Clin Med* 111:566, 1988.

318. Kaisi M, Ngwalle EW, Runyoro DE, Rogers J: Evaluation of tolerance of and response to iron dextran (Imferon) administered by total dose infusion to pregnant women with iron deficiency anemia. *Int J Gynaecol Obstet* 26:235, 1988.

319. Wallerstein RO: Intravenous iron-dextran complex. *Blood* 32:690, 1968.

320. Mehta BC, Ambani LM, Pawaskar M, Patel JC: Iron-dextran total dose injection (I.V. undiluted) in the treatment of iron deficiency anemia. *Indian J Med Sci* 22:20, 1968.

321. Mehta BC, Patel JC: Iron-dextran total dose infusion in the treatment of iron deficiency anemia. *Indian J Med Sci* 22:1, 1968.

322. Theodoropoulos G, Makkous A, Constantoulakis M: Lymph node enlargement after single massive infusion of iron dextran. *J Clin Pathol* 21:492, 1968.

323. Solanki SV, Kabrawala VN: Lymphadenopathy due to parenteral iron therapy. *J Indian Med Assoc* 51:22, 1968.

324. Amitai A, Acker M: Adverse effects of intramuscular iron injection. *Acta Haematol* 68:341, 1982.

325. Helsel EV, Jr.: Severe febrile reaction to intramuscular administration of iron-dextran. *Am J Obstet Gynecol* 91:582, 1965.

326. Ruiz-Reyes G, Tamayo-Pérez R, Medoza-López M: Fiebre, adenomegalia y esplenomegalia, consecutiva a la aplicación de dosis única total de hierro-dextran en anemia por uncinariasis, *in:* Memorias de la X Jornada Anual de la Agrupación Mexicana para el Estudio de le Hematologia, Mexico DF, 1969.

327. Forristal T, Witt M: Pleocytosis after iron dextran injection. *Lancet* 1:1428, 1968.

328. Hurvitz H, Kerem E, Gross-Kieselstein E, Brand A, Branski D: Pancytopenia caused by iron-dextran. *Arch Dis Child* 61:194, 1986.

329. Reddy PS, Lewis M: The adverse effect of intravenous iron-dextran in rheumatoid arthritis. *Arthritis Rheum* 12:454, 1969.

330. Winyard PG, Blake DR, Chirico S, Gutteridge JMC, Lunec J: Mechanism of exacerbation of rheumatoid synovitis by total-dose iron-dextran infusion: in-vivo demonstration of iron-promoted oxidant stress. *Lancet* 1:69, 1987.

331. Brighton SW, de le Harpe AL: Development of an inflammatory synovitis following total-dose infusion of iron-dextran. A case report. *S Afr Med J* 62:141, 1982.

332. Cantor RL, Downs GE, Abruzzo JL: Acute exacerbation of ankylosing spondylitis after an iron dextran infusion. *Ann Intern Med* 77:933, 1972.

333. Richmond HG: Induction of sarcoma in the rat by iron-dextran complex. *Br Med J* 1:947, 1959.

334. Carter RL, Mitchley CV, Roe FJC: Induction of tumors in mice and rats with ferric sodium gluconate and iron dextran glycerol glycoside. *Br J Cancer* 22:521, 1968.

335. Robinson CEG, Bell DN, Sturdy JH: Possible association of malignant neoplasm with iron-dextran injection: a case report. *Br Med J* 2:648, 1960.

336. MacKinnon AE, Bancewicz J: Sarcoma after injection of intramuscular iron. *Br Med J* 2:277, 1973.

337. Greenberg G: Sarcoma after intramuscular iron injection. *Br Med J* 1:1508, 1976.

338. Lane RS: Intravenous infusion of iron-dextran complex for iron-deficiency anemia. *Lancet* 1:852, 1964.

339. Becker CE, MacGregor RR, Walker KS, Jandl JH: Fatal anaphylaxis after intramuscular iron-dextran. *Ann Intern Med* 65:745, 1966.

340. Clay B, Rosenberg B, Sampson N, Samuels SI: Reactions to total dose intravenous infusion of iron dextran (Imferon). *Br Med J* 1:29, 1965.

341. Callender ST, Smith MD: Intramuscular iron. *Br Med J* 2:1487 (Ltr), 1954.

342. Jacobs J: Death due to iron parenterally. *South Med J* 62:216, 1969.

343. Mitchell ABS, Gill AM: Choice of iron therapy. *Practitioner* 213:370, 1974.

344. Cox JSG, King RE: Valency investigations of iron dextran (Imferon). *Nature* 207:1202, 1965.

345. Altman LC, Petersen PE: Successful prevention of an anaphylactoid reaction to iron dextran. *Ann Intern Med* 109:346, 1988.

346. McCurdy PR: Oral and parenteral iron therapy: a comparison. *JAMA* 191:859, 1965.

347. Fry J: Clinical patterns and course of anaemias in general practice. *Br Med J* 2:1732, 1961.

348. Klee GG: ''Decision rules for accelerated hematology laboratory investigation.'' Thesis. 1974 (unpub).

349. Beutler E, Fairbanks VF: The effects of iron deficiency, in *Iron in Biochemistry and Medicine*, vol 2, edited by A Jacobs, M Worwood. Academic, New York, 1980.

350. Hallberg L, Brune M, Rossander L: Low bioavailability of carbonyl iron in man: studies on iron fortification of wheat flour. *Am J Clin Nutr* 42:59, 1986.

ANEMIA DUE TO OTHER NUTRITIONAL DEFICIENCIES

ERNEST BEUTLER

Anemia may result from nutritional deficiencies of a variety of vitamins and trace minerals. Vitamin deficiencies that have been implicated as causes of anemia in humans, in addition to folic acid and vitamin B_{12}, include vitamins A, C, and E, pyridoxine and riboflavin, members of the B group. In most instances the relationship between the hematologic abnormality and deficiency of a vitamin has been difficult to document in humans, since multiple defects are usually present in a clinical setting. Copper, as well as iron, is recognized as a mineral essential for optimal erythropoiesis; a number of different enzymes essential in the metabolism of iron are cuproenzymes. Complex nutritional disturbances such as those observed in starvation, protein-deficiency malnutrition, and alcoholism are also associated with anemia.

The anemias that result from deficiencies of vitamin B_{12}, folic acid (Chap. 38), or iron (Chap. 39) are clearly defined; they are relatively common and they exist in pure states. In contrast, the characteristics of anemias that may occur when there are deficiencies of micronutrients, such as some of the other vitamins, are poorly defined. Many of these deficiencies are relatively rare in humans, and when they exist it is not as isolated deficiencies of one vitamin or one mineral but, rather, as a combination of deficiencies. In this context it is impossible to deduce which abnormalities are due to which deficiency. Studies in experimental animals, on the other hand, may not accurately reflect the role of a micronutrient in humans. Accordingly, our knowledge of the effect of many micronutrients on hematopoiesis is fragmentary and based on clinical observations and interpretations that may well be flawed.

VITAMIN-DEFICIENCY ANEMIAS

VITAMIN A DEFICIENCY

Chronic deprivation of vitamin A results in anemia similar to that observed in iron deficiency.[1-4] Mean corpuscular volume (MCV) and mean corpuscular hemoglobin concentration (MCHC) are reduced. Anisocytosis and poikilocytosis may be present, and serum iron levels are low. Unlike iron-deficiency anemia but similar to the anemia of chronic disease, the iron stores in the liver and marrow are increased, the serum transferrin concentration is usually normal or decreased, and the administration of medicinal iron does not correct the anemia. However, it has been suggested that vitamin A may facilitate iron absorption.[5,6]

This chapter is based upon that contributed to the fifth edition by the late Frank A. Oski, M.D.

Acronyms and abbreviations that appear in this chapter include: MCHC, mean corpuscular hemoglobin concentration; MCV, mean corpuscular volume.

Nutritional surveys conducted in developing countries have demonstrated a strong relationship between serum levels of vitamin A and blood hemoglobin concentration.[7] Subjects with serum vitamin A concentrations in the range of 20 to 30 μg/dl had a mean hemoglobin concentration of 6 g/dl, compared with a mean hemoglobin level of 16 g/dl in subjects in whom the serum vitamin A concentration exceeded 60 μg/dl. Although vitamin A deficiency is recognized to occur in the United States, the relationship between it and anemia is not known.

DEFICIENCIES OF MEMBERS OF THE VITAMIN B GROUP

Isolated nutritional deficiencies of members of the vitamin B group, with the exception of folic acid and vitamin B_{12}, are apparently very uncommon in humans, and evidence linking isolated nutritional deficiencies of pyridoxine, riboflavin, pantothenic acid, and niacin to anemia in such patients is inconclusive. Deficiency states experimentally induced in animals are more commonly associated with hematologic abnormalities.

VITAMIN B_6 DEFICIENCY

Vitamin B_6 includes pyridoxal, pyridoxine, and pyridoxamine. These are converted to pyridoxal 5-phosphate, which acts as a coenzyme in the decarboxylation and transamination of amino acids and in the synthesis of δ-aminolevulinic acid, the porphyrin precursor. Vitamin B_6 deficiency induced in infants is associated with a hypochromic microcytic anemia.[8] A malnourished patient with a hypochromic anemia who failed to respond to iron therapy but subsequently responded to the administration of vitamin B_6 has also been described.[9] Occasionally, patients receiving therapy with antituberculosis agents, such as isoniazid, which interfere with vitamin B_6 metabolism, develop a microcytic anemia that can be corrected with large doses of pyridoxine.[10,11] Some patients with sideroblastic anemias (see Chap. 64) respond to the administration of pyridoxine, but these patients are not deficient in this vitamin.

RIBOFLAVIN DEFICIENCY

Riboflavin deficiency results in a decrease in red cell glutathione reductase activity, since this enzyme requires flavin adenine dinucleotide for activation. The glutathione reductase deficiency induced by riboflavin deficiency is not associated with a hemolytic anemia or increased susceptibility to oxidant-induced injury.[12] Human volunteers maintained on a semisynthetic riboflavin-deficient diet and fed the riboflavin antagonist galactoflavin develop pure red cell aplasia.[13] Vacuolated erythroid precursors are evident prior to the development of aplasia. This anemia is reversed specifically by the administration of riboflavin.

PANTOTHENIC ACID DEFICIENCY

Pantothenic acid deficiency, when artificially induced in humans, is not associated with anemia.[14]

NIACIN DEFICIENCY

Pellagra (niacin deficiency) is associated with anemia, which responds to treatment with niacin.[15] However, it is not clear whether the anemia is a direct or an indirect effect of niacin deficiency.

VITAMIN C (ASCORBIC ACID) DEFICIENCY

Although approximately 80 percent of patients with scurvy[16] are anemic, attempts to induce anemia in human volunteers by severe restriction of dietary ascorbic acid have been unsuccessful.[17] It seems that the anemia observed in subjects with scurvy is not due directly to a deficiency of ascorbic acid but, rather, due to bleeding or a deficiency of folic acid.[16] Human subjects with scurvy and megaloblastoid anemia fail to respond hematologically to vitamin C as long as they are kept on a folic acid–deficient diet. When folic acid is given to these subjects in a dose of 50 μg/day, a prompt hematologic response is observed.[18]

Ascorbic acid is required for the maintenance of folic acid reductase in its reduced, or active, form. Impaired folic acid reductase activity results in an inability to form tetrahydrofolic acid, the metabolically active form of folic acid. Patients with scurvy and megaloblastoid anemia excrete 10-formylfolic acid as the major urinary folate metabolite. Following ascorbic acid therapy, 5-methyltetrahydrofolic acid becomes the major urinary folate metabolite. This observation has led to the suggestion[19] that ascorbic acid serves to prevent the irreversible oxidation of methyltetrahydrofolic acid to formylfolic acid. Failure to synthesize tetrahydrofolic acid or protect it from oxidation ultimately results in the appearance of a megaloblastic anemia. Under these circumstances, ascorbic acid therapy will produce a hematologic response only if enough folic acid is present to interact with the ascorbic acid.[20] Dietary iron deficiency in children often occurs in association with dietary ascorbic acid deficiency. Scurvy itself may cause iron deficiency as a consequence of external bleeding. Iron balance may be further compromised by the ascorbic acid deficiency because this vitamin serves to facilitate intestinal iron absorption. Patients with scurvy, particularly children, may require both iron and vitamin C to correct a hypochromic microcytic anemia.[21]

In patients with iron overload from repeated blood transfusions, the level of vitamin C in leukocytes is often decreased because of rapid conversion of ascorbate to oxalate.[22] Deferoxamine (desferrioxamine)-induced iron excretion is diminished when stores of vitamin C are reduced, but excretion returns to expected values with vitamin C supplementation.[23,24] It has been suggested, however, that large doses of ascorbic acid may be harmful in patients with iron overload and should be given only after an infusion of desferal has been initiated (Chap. 43). The presence of scurvy in patients with iron overload may protect them from tissue damage.[25] Both in scorbutic guinea pigs and in Bantu subjects with nutritional vitamin C deficiency and dietary hemosiderosis, iron accumulates in the monocyte-macrophage system rather than in the parenchymal cells of the liver.[26,27]

VITAMIN E DEFICIENCY

Vitamin E, α-tocopherol, is a fat-soluble vitamin that appears to serve as an antioxidant in humans and not as an essential cofactor in any recognized reactions. Nutritional deficiency of vitamin E in humans is extremely uncommon because of the widespread occurrence of α-tocopherol in food. The daily requirement for adults is in the range of 5 to 7 mg of d-α-tocopherol, but the requirement varies with the polyunsaturated fatty acid content of the diet and the content of peroxidizable lipids in tissues. Hematologic manifestations of vitamin E deficiency in humans are virtually limited to the neonatal period and to pathologic states associated with chronic fat malabsorption. Low-birth-weight infants are born with low serum and tissue concentrations of vitamin E. When these infants are fed a diet unusually rich in polyunsaturated fatty acids and inadequate in vitamin E, a hemolytic anemia will develop by 4 to 6 weeks of age, particularly if iron is also present in the diet.[28] The anemia is often associated with morphologic alterations of the erythrocytes,[29] thrombocytosis, and edema of the dorsum of the feet and the pretibial area.[30] Treatment with vitamin E produces a prompt increase in hemoglobin level, a decrease in the elevated reticulocyte count, a normalization of the red cell life span, and a disappearance of the thrombocytosis and edema. Modifications of infant formulas have all but eliminated vitamin E deficiency in preterm infants.[31]

Vitamin E deficiency is common in patients with cystic fibrosis if they are not receiving daily supplements of the water-soluble form of the vitamin. Red cell life span is shortened in such patients to an average ^{51}Cr half-life of 19 days. After vitamin E therapy, the red cell half-life increases to 27.5 days.[32] Severe anemia may be present.[33]

Pharmacologic doses of vitamin E have been employed with apparent success in the absence of vitamin deficiency to compensate for genetic defects that limit the erythrocytes' defense against oxidant injury. Chronic administration of 400 to 800 units of vitamin E per day lengthened the red cell life span in some[34–36] but not all[37] studies of patients with hereditary hemolytic anemias associated with glutathione synthetase deficiency or glucose-6-phosphate dehydrogenase deficiency.

The administration of 450 units of vitamin E per day for 6 to 36 weeks to patients with sickle cell anemia has been found to produce a significant reduction in the number of irreversibly sickled erythrocytes.[38] Adult patients with sickle cell anemia have been reported to have significantly lower serum tocopherol values than do normal control subjects,[39] and in children with sickle cell anemia, those with vitamin E deficiency were found to have significantly more irreversibly sickled cells than did children without vitamin E deficiency.[40]

TRACE METAL DEFICIENCY

COPPER DEFICIENCY

Copper is present in a number of metalloproteins. Among the cuproenzymes are cytochrome c oxidase, dopamine [beta]-hydroxylase, urate oxidase, tyrosine and lysyl oxidase, ascorbic acid oxidase, and superoxide dismutase (erythrocuprein). More than 90 percent of the copper in the blood is carried bound to ceruloplasmin, an α_2-globulin with ferro-oxidase activity. Copper appears to be required for the absorption and utilization of iron. Copper, in the form of hephaestin,[41] converts and maintains iron in the Fe^{3+} state for its transport by transferrin.

Copper deficiency has been described in malnourished children[42] and in both infants and adults[43–45] receiving parenteral alimentation. It is characterized by a microcytic anemia that is unresponsive to iron therapy, hypoferremia, neutropenia, and usually the presence of vacuolated erythroid precursors in the marrow.[44,45] In infants and young children with copper deficiency, radiologic abnormalities are generally present. These abnormalities include osteoporosis, flaring of the anterior ribs with spontaneous rib fractures, cupping and flaring of long-bone metaphyses with spur formation and submetaphyseal fractures, and epiphyseal separation. These changes have frequently been misinterpreted as signs of scurvy. Copper deficiency with a resultant microcytic anemia can be produced by chronic ingestion of massive quantities of zinc. Dietary zinc in large doses leads to copper deficiency by impairing copper absorption.[46–50]

The diagnosis of copper deficiency can be established by the demonstration of a low serum ceruloplasmin or serum copper level, but the copper level is thought to be more reliable because ceruloplasmin behaves as an acute-phase protein.[44] Adequate normal values for the first 2 to 3 months have not been well defined and are normally lower than those observed later in life. Despite these limitations, a serum copper level less than 40 μg/dl or a ceruloplasmin value less than 15 mg/dl after 1 or 2 months of age can be regarded as evidence of copper deficiency. In later infancy, childhood, and adulthood, serum copper values should normally exceed 70 μg/dl. Low serum copper values may be observed in hypoproteinemic states such as exudative enteropathies and nephrosis as well as in Wilson disease. In these circumstances a diagnosis of copper deficiency cannot be established by serum measurements alone but requires an analysis of liver copper content or clinical response after a therapeutic trial of copper supplementation.

The anemia and neutropenia are quickly corrected by the administration of copper. Treatment of copper-deficient infants consist of giving about 2.5 mg of copper ($\approx$80 μg/kg/day) oral supplementation as a copper sulfate solution.[51] Intravenous bolus injection of copper chloride has also been used.[45]

ZINC DEFICIENCY

Zinc is required for a large number of zinc metalloenzymes, zinc-activated enzymes, and ''zinc finger'' transcription factors. Zinc deficiency occurs in a variety of pathologic states in humans, including hemolytic anemias such as thalassemia[52] and sickle cell anemia.[53] Zinc deficiency with or without an associated copper deficiency has been described in a patient on intensive desferrioxamine therapy[54] and in patients with decreased renal reabsorption of trace minerals.[55]

Although human zinc deficiency may produce growth retardation, impaired wound healing, impaired taste perception, immunologic abnormalities, and acrodermatitis enteropathica, there is no evidence at present that isolated zinc deficiency produces anemia.

SELENIUM DEFICIENCY

A deficiency of selenium occurs in patients who live in areas in which the selenium content of the soil is very low[56] and has been observed in patients receiving total parenteral nutrition.[57,58] Although this results in a striking decrease in the level of red cell glutathione peroxidase, there do not appear to be any adverse hematologic consequences.

ANEMIA OF STARVATION

Studies conducted during World War II among prisoners of war and conscientious objectors demonstrated that semistarvation for 24 weeks can result in a mild to moderate normocytic normochromic anemia.[59] Marrow cellularity is usually reduced and is accompanied by a decrease in the erythroid/myeloid ratio. Measurements of red cell volume and plasma volume suggest that dilution is a major factor responsible for the reduction in hemoglobin concentration.

In persons subjected to complete starvation either for experimental purposes or to treat severe obesity, anemia was not observed during the first 2 to 9 weeks of fasting.[60] Starvation for 9 to 17 weeks produced a fall in hemoglobin and marrow hypocellularity.[61] Resumption of a normal diet was accompanied by a reticulocytosis and disappearance of anemia. It has been suggested that the anemia of starvation is a response to a hypometabolic state, with its attendant decrease in oxygen requirements.[62]

ANEMIA OF PROTEIN DEFICIENCY (KWASHIORKOR)

Even strict vegetarians do not seem to develop hematologic problems related to the absence of animal proteins,[63] except for some vegans who have been reported to suffer from B$_{12}$ deficiency.[64]

In infants and children with protein-calorie malnutrition, the hemoglobin concentration may fall to 8 g/dl of blood,[65,66] but some children with kwashiorkor have normal hemoglobin levels, probably because of a decreased plasma volume. The anemia is normocytic and normochromic, but there is considerable variation in the size and shape of red cells on the blood film. The white blood cells and the platelets are usually normal. The marrow is most often normally cellular or slightly hypocellular, with a reduced erythroid/myeloid ratio. Erythroblastopenia, reticulocytopenia, and a marrow containing a few giant pronormoblasts may be found, particularly if these children have an infection. With treatment of the infection, erythroid precursors may appear in the marrow and the reticulocyte count may rise. When

nutrition is improved by giving high-protein diets (powdered milk or essential amino acids), there is reticulocytosis, a slight fall in hematocrit due to hemodilution, and then a rise in hemoglobin level, hematocrit, and red blood cell count. Improvement is very slow, however, and during the third or fourth week, when these children are clinically improved and the serum proteins are approaching normal, another episode of erythroid marrow aplasia may develop. This relapse is not associated with infection, does not respond to antibiotics, and does not remit spontaneously. It does respond either to riboflavin or to prednisone, and unless they are treated with these agents, children who develop this complication may die suddenly. It has been suggested[67] that the erythroblastic aplasia is a manifestation of riboflavin deficiency.

Although the plasma volume is reduced to a variable degree in children with kwashiorkor, the total circulating red cell volume decreases in proportion to the decrease in lean body mass as protein deprivation reduces metabolic demands. During repletion, an increase in plasma volume may occur before an increase in red cell volume, and the anemia may seem to become more severe despite reticulocytosis.

From the study of the anemia of protein deficiency in rats,[68] it was deduced that oxygen consumption and therefore erythropoietin production are reduced. Other studies confirmed this observation but related the reduction to calorie deprivation, with its associated decrease in the blood levels of T$_3$ and T$_4$.[62] As a result, erythropoiesis decreases and the reticulocyte count falls. The plasma iron turnover and red cell uptake of radioactive iron are markedly reduced, and the red cell volume gradually declines.[68] Protein deficiency also produces a maturation block at the erythroblast level and a slight decrease in the erythropoietin-sensitive progenitor cell pool.[69] If exogenous erythropoietin is provided, normal erythropoiesis is restored despite protein depletion,[70] an observation that explains the successful use of starved rats in the bioassay for erythropoietin.

ALCOHOLISM

Chronic alcohol ingestion is often associated with anemia. The anemia may be due to nutritional deficiencies, chronic gastrointestinal bleeding, hepatic dysfunction, or direct toxic effects of alcohol on erythropoiesis. Quite commonly all these factors work in concert to produce the anemia. Pyridoxal phosphate and folate deficiencies are common[71] in alcoholics. Alcohol affects not only the red cells, as described here, but also the platelets (see Chap. 119).[72,73]

Macrocytosis is common in chronic alcoholics[74] and is often associated with a megaloblastic anemia. Among hospitalized malnourished alcoholics, it is the most common type of anemia, occurring alone or in combination with ringed sideroblasts in approximately 40 percent of all patients.[75,76] In contrast, megaloblastic anemia is rarely observed in nonhospitalized chronic alcoholics or relatively well-nourished subjects admitted to the hospital for purposes of alcohol withdrawal.[77] Anemia, when associated with megaloblastic marrow changes in alcoholics, is almost always due to folate deficiency. Iron deficiency is often associated with folate deficiency in alcoholics.[77] In patients with both nutritional deficiencies, the blood film will be ''dimorphic,'' with macrocytes, hypersegmented neutrophils, and hypochromic microcytes. Although liver disease is frequently present in alcoholics with megaloblastic anemia, it is not responsible for the folate deficiency. Megaloblastic anemia occurs almost exclusively in alcoholics who have been eating poorly. It is seen more commonly in heavy drinkers of wine and whiskey, substances that contain little or no folate, than in drinkers of beer, a rich source of the vitamin. Although decreased dietary folate intake appears to be a necessary factor in the etiology of the megaloblastic anemia, ethanol itself interferes with folate metabolism (see Chap. 38).[78,79]

However, macrocytosis does not always indicate the presence of a megaloblastic anemia,[74] reticulocytosis secondary to hemolysis or bleeding, or liver disease. A so-called macrocytosis of alcoholism[80] is found in as many as 82 to 96 percent of alcoholics. In these patients the macrocytosis is usually mild, with a MCV in the range of 100 to 110 fl, and anemia is usually absent. In the blood film, the macrocytes are typically round rather than oval, and neutrophil hypersegmentation is not present. The macrocytosis persists until the patient abstains from alcohol. Even then, the MCV does not become completely normal for periods of 2 to 4 months.[79]

Alcohol ingestion for 5 to 7 days will produce vacuolization of early red cell precursors, and the formation of vacuoles can be observed in in vitro marrow cell cultures.[76,81] These changes disappear promptly when alcohol ingestion is discontinued. Vacuolization of a similar appearance occurs in subjects who are fed a phenylalanine-deficient diet, patients treated with chloramphenicol or pyrazinamide, patients in hyperosmolar coma, and individuals deficient in copper or riboflavin.[80]

A relatively rare hematologic complication of alcoholism is Zieve syndrome,[82] consisting of transient hemolytic anemia, jaundice, hyperlipidemia, and alcohol-induced liver disease.

REFERENCES

1. Blackfan KD, Wolbach SB: Vitamin A deficiency in infants: A clinical and pathological study. *J Pediatr* 3:679, 1933.
2. Vitamin A and iron. *Nutr Rev* 47: 1989.
3. Majia LA, Hodges RE, Arroyave G, Viteri F, Torun B: Vitamin A deficiency and anemia in Central American children. *Am J Clin Nutr* 30:1175, 1977.
4. Hodges RE, Sauberlich HE, Canham JE, et al: Hematopoietic studies in vitamin A deficiency. *Am J Clin Nutr* 31:876, 1978.
5. Garcia-Casal MN, Layrisse M, Solano L, et al: Vitamin A and beta-carotene can improve nonheme iron absorption from rice, wheat and corn by humans. *J Nutr* 128:646, 1998.
6. Kolsteren P, Rahman SR, Hilderbrand K, Diniz A: Treatment for iron deficiency anaemia with a combined supplementation of iron, vitamin A and zinc in women of Dinajpur, Bangladesh. *Eur J Clin Nutr* 53:102, 1999.
7. Nutrition survey of Paraguay, May–August, 1965, in *Nutrition Program, National Center for Chronic Disease Control, US Dept of Health, Education and Welfare.* US Government Printing Office, Washington, 1967.
8. Snyderman SE, Holt LE Jr, Carretero R, Jacobs KG: Pyridoxine deficiency in the human infant. *Am J Clin Nutr* 1:200, 1953.
9. Foy H, Kondi A: Hypochromic anemias of the tropics associated with pyridoxine and nicotinic acid deficiencies. *Blood* 1054, 1999.
10. McCurdy PR, Donohoe RF, Magovern M: Reversible sideroblastic anemia caused by pyrazinoic acid (pyrazinamide). *Ann Intern Med* 64:1280, 1966.
11. Frimpter GW: Pyridoxine (B₆) dependency syndromes. *Ann Intern Med* 68:1131, 1968.
12. Beutler E, Srivastava SK: Relationship between glutathione reductase activity and drug-induced haemolytic anaemia. *Nature* 226:759, 1970.
13. Lane M, Alfrey CP: The anemia of human riboflavin deficiency. *Blood* 22:811, 1963.
14. Hodges RE, Bean WB, Ohlson MA, Bleiler RE: Human pantothenic acid deficiency produced by omegamethylpantothenic acid. *J Clin Invest* 38:1421, 1959.
15. Spivak JL, Jackson DL: Pellagra: An analysis of 18 patients and a review of the literature. *Johns Hopkins Med J* 140:295, 1977.
16. Reuler JB, Broudy VC, Cooney TG: Adult scurvy. *JAMA* 253:805, 1985.
17. Hodges RE, Baker EM, Hood J, Sauberlich HE, March SC: Experimental scurvy in man. *Am J Clin Nutr* 22:535, 1969.
18. Zalusky R, Herbert V: Megaloblastic anemia in scurvy with response to 50 micrograms of folic acid daily. *N Engl J Med* 265:1033, 1961.
19. Stokes PL, Melikian V, Leeming RL, Portman-Graham H, Blair JA, Cooke WT: Folate metabolism in scurvy. *Am J Clin Nutr* 28:126, 1975.
20. Cox EV, Meynell MJ, Northam BE, Cooke WT: The anaemia of scurvy. *Am J Med* 42:220, 1967.
21. Clark NG, Sheard NF, Kelleher JF: Treatment of iron-deficiency anemia complicated by scurvy and folic acid deficiency. *Nutr Rev* 50:134, 1992.
22. Wapnick AA, Lynch SR, Krawitz P, Seftel HC, Charlton RW, Bothwell TH: Effects of iron overload on ascorbic acid metabolism. *BMJ* 3:704, 1968.
23. Wapnick AA, Lynch SR, Charlton RW, Seftel HC, Bothwell TH: The effect of ascorbic acid deficiency on desferrioxamine-induced urinary iron excretion. *Br J Haematol* 17:563, 1969.
24. Chapman RW, Hussain MA, Gorman A, et al: Effect of ascorbic acid deficiency on serum ferritin concentration in patients with beta-thalassaemia major and iron overload. *J Clin Pathol* 35:487, 1982.
25. Cohen A, Cohen IJ, Schwartz E: Scurvy and altered iron stores in thalassemia major. *N Engl J Med* 304:158, 1981.
26. Lipschitz DA, Bothwell TH, Seftel HC, Wapnick AA, Charlton RW: The role of ascorbic acid in the metabolism of storage iron. *Br J Haematol* 20:155, 1971.
27. Bothwell TH, Abrahams C, Bradlow BA, Charlton RW: Idiopathic and Bantu hemochromatosis. *Arch Pathol* 79:163, 1965.
28. Williams ML, Shoot RJ, O'Neal PL, Oski FA: Role of dietary iron and fat on vitamin E deficiency anemia of infancy. *N Engl J Med* 292:887, 1975.
29. Oski FA, Barness LA: Hemolytic anemia in vitamin E deficiency. *Am J Clin Nutr* 21:45, 1968.
30. Ritchie JH, Fish MB, McMasters V, Grossman M: Edema and hemolytic anemia in premature infants: A vitamin E deficiency syndrome. *N Engl J Med* 279:1185, 1968.
31. Zipursky A: Vitamin E deficiency anemia in newborn infants. *Clin Perinatol* 11:393, 1984.
32. Farrell PM, Bieri JG, Fratantoni JF, Wood RE, di Sant'Agnese PA: The occurrence and effects of human vitamin E deficiency: A study in patients with cystic fibrosis. *J Clin Invest* 60:233, 1977.
33. Wilfond BS, Farrell PM, Laxova A, Mischler E: Severe hemolytic anemia associated with vitamin E deficiency in infants with cystic fibrosis: Implications for neonatal screening. *Clin Pediatr (Philadelphia)* 33:2, 1994.
34. Corash L, Spielberg S, Bartsocas C, et al: Reduced chronic hemolysis during high-dose vitamin E administration in Mediterranean-type glucose-6-phosphate dehydrogenase deficiency. *N Engl J Med* 303:416, 1980.
35. Hafez M, Amar ES, Zedan M, et al: Improved erythrocyte survival with combined vitamin E and selenium therapy in children with glucose-6-phosphate dehydrogenase deficiency and mild chronic hemolysis. *J Pediatr* 108:558, 1986.
36. Eldamhougy S, Elhelw Z, Yamamah G, Hussein L, Fayyad I, Fawzy D: The vitamin E status among glucose-6-phosphate dehydrogenase deficient patients and effectiveness of oral vitamin E. *Int J Vitam Nutr Res* 58:184, 1988.
37. Johnson GJ, Vatassery GT, Finkel B, Allen DW: High-dose vitamin E does not decrease the rate of chronic hemolysis in glucose-6-phosphate dehydrogenase deficiency. *N Engl J Med* 308:1014, 1983.
38. Natta CL, Machlin LJ, Brin M: A decrease in irreversibly sickled erythrocytes in sickle cell anemia patients given vitamin E. *Am J Clin Nutr* 33:968, 1980.
39. Tangney CC, Phillips G, Bell RA, Fernandes P, Hopkins R, Wu SM: Selected indices of micronutrient status in adult patients with sickle cell anemia (SCA). *Am J Hematol* 32:161, 1989.
40. Ndombi IO, Kinoti SN: Serum vitamin E and the sickling status in children with sickle cell anaemia. *East Afr Med J* 67:720, 1990.
41. Vulpe CD, Kuo YM, Murphy TL, et al: Hephaestin, a ceruloplasmin homologue implicated in intestinal iron transport, is defective in the sla mouse. *Nature Genet* 21:195, 1999.
42. Graham GG, Cordano A: Copper depletion and deficiency in the malnourished infant. *Johns Hopkins Med J* 124:139, 1969.
43. Joffe G, Etzioni A, Levy J, Benderly A: A patient with copper deficiency anemia while on prolonged intravenous feeding. *Clin Pediatr (Philadelphia)* 20:226, 1981.
44. Spiegel JE, Willenbucher RF: Rapid development of severe copper deficiency in a patient with Crohn's disease receiving parenteral nutrition. *J Parenter Enteral Nutr* 23:169, 1999.
45. Hirase N, Abe Y, Sadamura S, et al: Anemia and neutropenia in a case of copper deficiency: Role of copper in normal hematopoiesis. *Acta Haematol (Basel)* 87:195, 1992.

46. Hoffman HN, Phyliky RL, Fleming CR: Zinc-induced copper deficiency. *Gastroenterology* 94:508, 1988.

47. Patterson WP, Winkelmann M, Perry MC: Zinc-induced copper deficiency: Megamineral sideroblastic anemia. *Ann Intern Med* 103:385, 1985.

48. Simon SR, Branda RF, Tindle BF, Burns SL: Copper deficiency and sideroblastic anemia associated with zinc ingestion. *Am J Hematol* 28:181, 1988.

49. Summerfield AL, Steinberg FU, Gonzalez JG: Morphologic findings in bone marrow precursor cells in zinc-induced copper deficiency anemia. *Am J Clin Pathol* 97:665, 1992.

50. Sandstead HH: Requirements and toxicity of essential trace elements, illustrated by zinc and copper. *Am J Clin Nutr* 61:621S, 1995.

51. Cordano A: Clinical manifestations of nutritional copper deficiency in infants and children. *Am J Clin Nutr* 67:1012S, 1998.

52. Fuchs GJ, Tienboon P, Linpisarn S, et al: Nutritional factors and thalassaemia major. *Arch Dis Child* 74:224, 1996.

53. Prasad AS, Beck FWJ, Kaplan J, et al: Effect of zinc supplementation on incidence of infections and hospital admissions in sickle cell disease (SCD). *Am J Hematol* 61:194, 1999.

54. Yuzbasiyan-Gurkan VA, Brewer GJ, Vander AJ, Guenther MJ, Prasad AS: Net renal tubular reabsorption of zinc in healthy man and impaired handling in sickle cell anemia. *Am J Hematol* 31:87, 1989.

55. De Virgiliis S, Congia M, Turco MP, et al: Depletion of trace elements and acute ocular toxicity induced by desferrioxamine in patients with thalassaemia. *Arch Dis Child* 63:250, 1988.

56. Thomson CD, Rea HM, Doesburg VM, Robinson MF: Selenium concentrations and glutathione peroxidase activities in whole blood of New Zealand residents. *Br J Nutr* 37:457, 1977.

57. Kien CL, Ganther HE: Manifestations of chronic selenium deficiency in a child receiving total parenteral nutrition. *Am J Clin Nutr* 37:319, 1983.

58. Cohen HJ, Brown MR, Hamilton D, Lyons-Patterson J, Avissar N, Liegey P: Glutathione peroxidase and selenium deficiency in patients receiving home parenteral nutrition: Time course for development of deficiency and repletion of enzyme activity in plasma and blood cells. *Am J Clin Nutr* 49:132, 1989.

59. Keys A, Brozek J, Henschel A, et al: *The Biology of Semistarvation.* University of Minnesota Press, Minneapolis, 1950.

60. Thomson TJ, Runcie J, Miller V: Treatment of obesity by total fasting for up to 249 days. *Lancet* 2:992, 1966.

61. Drenick EJ, Swendseid ME, Blahd WH, Tuttle SG: Prolonged starvation as treatment for severe obesity. *JAMA* 187:100, 1964.

62. Caro J, Silver R, Erslev AJ, Miller OP, Birgegard G: Erythropoietin production in fasted rats: Effects of thyroid hormones and glucose supplementation. *J Lab Clin Med* 98:860, 1981.

63. Lowik MR, Schrijver J, Odink J, van den BH, Wedel M: Long-term effects of a vegetarian diet on the nutritional status of elderly people (Dutch Nutrition Surveillance System). *J Am Coll Nutr* 9:600, 1990.

64. Chanarin I, Malkowska V, O'Hea AM, Rinsler MG, Price AB: Megaloblastic anaemia in a vegetarian Hindu community. *Lancet* 2:1168, 1985.

65. Adams EB, Scragg JN, Naidoo BT, et al: Observations on the aetiology and treatment of anaemia in kwashiorkor. *BMJ* 3:451, 1967.

66. Lunn PG, Morley CJ, Neale G: A case of kwashiorkor in the UK. *Clin Nutr* 17:131, 1998.

67. Foy H, Kondi A: Comparison between erythroid aplasia in marasmus and kwashiorkor and the experimentally induced erythroid aplasia in baboons by riboflavin deficiency. *Vitam Horm* 26:653, 1968.

68. Delmonte L, Aschenasy A, Eyquem A: Studies on the hemolytic nature of protein-deficiency anemia in the rat. *Blood* 24:49, 1964.

69. Naets JP, Wittek M: Effect of starvation on the response to erythropoietin in the rat. *Acta Haematol (Basel)* 52:141, 1974.

70. Ito K, Reissmann KR: Quantitative and qualitative aspects of steady state erythropoiesis induced in protein-starved rats by long-term erythropoietin injection. *Blood* 27:343, 1966.

71. Gloria L, Cravo M, Camilo ME, et al: Nutritional deficiencies in chronic alcoholics: Relation to dietary intake and alcohol consumption. *Am J Gastroenterol* 92:485, 1997.

72. Savage D, Lindenbaum J: Anemia in alcoholics. *Medicine (Baltimore)* 65:322, 1986.

73. Girard DE, Kumar KL, McAfee JH: Hematologic effects of acute and chronic alcohol abuse. *Hematol Oncol Clin North Am* 1:321, 1987.

74. Fernando OV, Grimsley EW: Prevalence of folate deficiency and macrocytosis in patients with and without alcohol-related illness. *South Med J* 91:721, 1998.

75. Colman N, Herbert V: Hematologic complications of alcoholism: Overview. *Semin Hematol* 17:164, 1980.

76. Sullivan LW, Herbert V: Suppression of hematopoiesis by ethanol. *J Clin Invest* 43:2048, 1964.

77. Eichner ER, Hillman RS: Effect of alcohol on serum folate level. *J Clin Invest* 52:584, 1973.

78. Lindenbaum J: Folate and vitamin B deficiencies in alcoholism deficiencies in alcoholism *Semin Hematol* 17:119, 1980.

79. Seppa K, Laippala P, Saarni M: Macrocytosis as a consequence of alcohol abuse among patients in general practice. *Alcohol Clin Exp Res* 15:871, 1991.

80. McCurdy PR, Rath CE: Vacuolated nucleated bone marrow cells in alcoholism. *Semin Hematol* 17:100, 1980.

81. Yeung KY, Klug PP, Lessin LS: Alcohol-induced vacuolization in bone marrow cells: Ultrastructure and mechanism of formation. *Blood Cells* 13:487, 1988.

82. Pilcher CR, Underwood RG, Smith HR: Zieve's syndrome a potential surgical pitfall? *J R Army Med Corps* 142:84, 1996.

ANEMIA ASSOCIATED WITH MARROW INFILTRATION

ALLAN J. ERSLEV

Myelophthisic anemia is a term used to describe the hematologic consequences of bone marrow infiltration. It can range from an overt leukoerythroblastic picture to the presence of a few teardrop-shaped red cells on a blood film. These changes may indicate the presence of early spread of a tumor and may herald eventual replacement of active marrow space. The traditional diagnostic bone marrow sampling has now been augmented by magnetic resonance images of bone.

DEFINITION AND HISTORY

The presence of minimal and spotty marrow infiltrations with abnormal cells or tissue components does not usually cause symptoms or hematologic changes. Such infiltrations are, however, of considerable clinical significance. In patients with an established diagnosis of cancer they indicate metastatic dissemination of the tumor. In patients treated with chemotherapy they suggest inadequate treatment. Extensive infiltration may also be well tolerated, but when associated with disruption of the normal marrow structure it may cause the development of an anemia or pancytopenia designated as a *myelophthisic anemia*.[1] Such an anemia is characterized by the presence on the blood film of schistocytes and teardrop-shaped red cells and often by prematurely released nucleated red cells, megakaryocytic fragments, and immature myeloid cells. When pronounced, this condition is referred to as *leukoerythroblastosis*.[2]

ETIOLOGY AND PATHOGENESIS

The most common causes of extensive cellular infiltration of marrow are listed in Table 40-1. In chronic leukemias the invading cells will usually not cause structural damage but live in a peaceful symbiosis with normal marrow constituents. Eventually, however, the expansion of the volume of pathologic cells and the release of suppressor cytokines will lead to anemias and other cytopenias, but without the characteristic morphologic features of myelophthisis. In myelofibrotic disorders, both agnogenic and secondary, megakaryocytes will release fibroblastic growth factors, with the subsequent reduction in available bone marrow space and disruption of its architecture (see Chap. 78). This will cause cytopenias with the production of deformed red cells, especially poikilocytes and teardrop-shaped cells, and the premature release of erythroblasts, myelocytes, and giant platelets (see Chap. 29). A similar picture can be seen when the marrow is replaced by macrophages containing indigestible lipids, as in Gaucher disease.

The invasion of metastatic cancer cells will cause the early release of suppressive and destructive cytokines, leading to the development

Acronyms and abbreviations that appear in this chapter include: MRI, magnetic resonance imaging.

of a myelophthisic blood picture even before the marrow is completely replaced.[3,4] The marrow microenvironment is second only to the lung and comparable to the liver in its susceptibility to implantation of blood-borne malignant cells. Almost all cancers can metastasize to the marrow,[5,6] but the most common are cancers of the lung, breast, and prostate. Metastatic foci in the marrow can be found in 20 to 30 percent of patients with small cell carcinoma of the lung at the time of diagnosis and in more than 50 percent at autopsy.[7] The prevalence, especially at diagnosis, is lower in patients with cancer of the breast and prostate but is still sufficiently high to make marrow biopsy an important diagnostic and prognostic procedure.[8–10] The development of frank leukoerythroblastosis occurs much less frequently,[11] and its absence should not be relied upon to indicate that marrow involvement has not occurred.

The characteristic abnormalities in hematopoiesis observed in patients with chronic myelophthisic anemia may in part be due to compensatory extramedullary blood formation. Splenic and hepatic microvasculature, especially when affected by the underlying disease, are not as effective in producing normal blood cells as is the marrow. Splenic infiltration may also result in hypersplenic sequestration and destruction of blood cells. In addition, the underlying disease, especially in metastatic malignancies, may contribute infectious and nutritional complications affecting the blood picture of patients with infiltrative disease of the marrow.

CLINICAL FEATURES

Symptoms and signs associated with infiltrative marrow disorders are usually related to the underlying disease. However, pain and tenderness of affected bones, pathologic fractures, and hypercalcemia causing nausea, symptoms of anemia, muscle weakness, or stupor may bring patients to medical attention.

LABORATORY FEATURES

The anemia is mild to moderate. The white cell and platelet counts may vary, but the most characteristic feature is the morphologic appearance of red cells on the blood film. These cells may show anisocytosis and poikilocytosis, but the presence of teardrop forms and nucleated red cells is particularly suggestive of marrow infiltration (Fig. 40-1). The combination of nucleated red cells and immature myeloid precursors constitutes the leukoerythroblastotic picture that when present is so characteristic of marrow infiltration. The leukocyte alkaline phosphatase score is normal or increased, and the karyotype of remaining normal marrow cells is intact. The presence of cancer cells on the blood film (carcinocythemia) occurs occasionally and always indicates marrow invasion.[12] Marrow biopsy is the most reliable procedure by which to make a diagnosis of marrow-infiltrative disease and should be carried out in all patients with suspected metastatic carcinoma or hematologic features of myelophthisic anemia.[13] Marrow aspirations are also of value[14] but may not provide the same yield of tumor cells and can be difficult to interpret in patients with agnogenic or secondary myelofibrosis.[15] Marrow biopsy or aspiration is best performed in areas with tender bone, and inability to aspirate marrow from such a tender bone (dry tap) leads to a high degree of suspicion of marrow replacement. Since the diagnostic marrow yield from biopsies depends on the amount of tissue examined, a single negative biopsy should be repeated. An isotopic bone scan showing a focal accumulation of radioactive tracers can be helpful in locating a suitable site for biopsy,[16] but a negative study of the area does not exclude the possibility of marrow involvement. MRI using T1-weighted images is being used with increasing frequency since it is capable of demonstrating

TABLE 40-1   MARROW INFILTRATION

Leukemic cells
  Myeloid (chronic, acute)
  Lymphoid (chronic, acute)
  Lymphomas
  Myeloma
Fibroblasts
  Agnogenic myeloid metaplasia
  Polycythemia vera
  Hairy cell leukemia
  Metastatic malignancies
Metastatic cells
  Carcinoma (lung, breast, prostate)
  Sarcoma
Inflammatory cells
  Miliary tuberculosis
  Fungal infections
Sarcoidosis
Macrophages
  Gaucher disease
Necrotic cells
  Sickle cell anemia
  Septicemia
Bone disease
  Osteopetrosis

sites of altered marrow activity, thus indicating suitable areas for biopsy.[17-19]

DIFFERENTIAL DIAGNOSIS

A myelophthisic blood picture ranging from a few teardrop-shaped red cells on the blood film to a full-blown leukoerythroblastic picture demands close attention. An underlying disease causing marrow infiltration may already have been diagnosed, but in the case of malignancies the blood picture may suggest metastatic spread and demand verification by repeated bone marrow biopsies and the use of MRI. In patients treated for a neoplastic disorder careful bone marrow examination, even in the absence of red cell changes, may also be in order to exclude foci of surviving neoplastic cells. Such an attempt may today be augmented by a sophisticated immunologic flow cytometry study using appropriate antibodies.[20] Leukoerythroblastosis may occur in conditions other than cancer metastatic to the marrow.[21] Of these, the most important are consumptive microcoagulopathy, severe blood loss, and transient hypoxia. Myelophthisic anemia with or without leukoerythroblastosis has also been described in patients with hepatitis,[22] ulcerative colitis,[23] and anorexia nervosa.[24] Idiopathic myelofibrosis, a common cause of myelophthisic anemia among the aged, may be difficult to distinguish from metastatic disease with focal reactive fibrosis[15] and should be considered in the differential diagnosis (see Chap. 29).

THERAPY, COURSE, AND PROGNOSIS

The goal of treatment is, in general, to manage the underlying disease. If the anemia is caused in part by extramedullary disease processes such as splenomegaly in idiopathic myelofibrosis, gratifying although temporary improvement can be expected after splenectomy. Patients with marrow infiltration caused by leukemia, cancer, or lymphoma should be treated appropriately, since the presence of marrow infiltration may not adversely affect the outcome. If treatment is successful there may be complete disappearance not only of the malignant cells but also of the reactive fibrosis surrounding metastatic foci. Treatment of metastatic lesions with the bone-seeking isotope strontium-89 has been tried, but usually causes unacceptable hematopoietic suppression.[25] Supplementation with recombinant erythropoietin has been found useful in infiltrative marrow disorders.[26] In hormone-refractory prostate cancer the presence of leukoerythroblastic reaction does not seem to influence survival,[27] but unfortunately in most patients with cancers metastatic to the marrow, the prognosis is for only short-term survival.

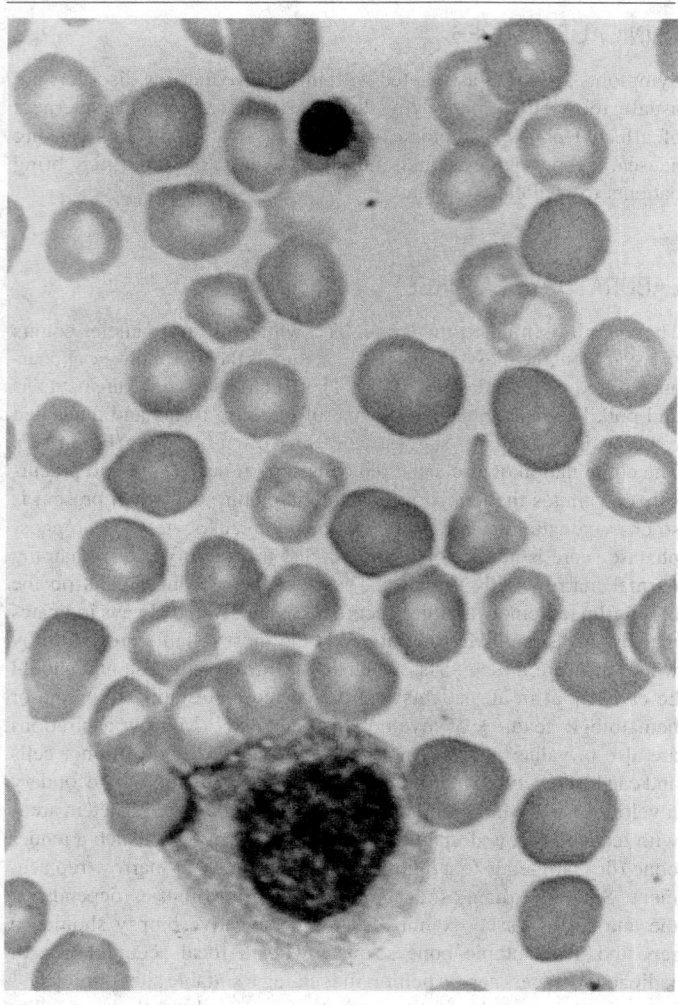

FIGURE 40-1   Blood film of a patient with prostatic adenocarcinoma metastatic to the marrow. The film shows an early myeloid cell, a nucleated red cell, and a classic teardrop-shaped red cell.

REFERENCES

1. Rundles RW, Jousson U: Metastases in the bone marrow and myelophthisic anemia from carcinoma of the prostate. *Am J Med Sci* 218:240, 1949.

2. Vaughan JM: Leuco-erythroblastic anaemia. *J Pathol Bacteriol* 42:541, 1936.

3. Abasov IT: The state of the peripheral blood in cancer metastases to bone marrow. *Haematologica (Pavia)* 2:381, 1968.

4. Laszlo J: Hematologic effects of cancer, in *Cancer Medicine,* 2d ed, edited by JF Holland, E Frei, p 1275. Lea and Febiger, Philadelphia, 1982.

5. Schwartz RA, De-Jager RL, Janniger CK, Lambert WC: Giant basal cell carcinoma with metastases and myelophthisic anemia. *J Surg Oncol* 33:223, 1986.

6. Newman HF, Howard GC, Reid PM: Metastatic oligodendroglioma presenting as a leukoerythroblastic anaemia. *Eur J Surg Oncol* 11:287, 1985.

7. Hirsch FR, Hansen HH: Bone marrow involvement in small cell ana-

plastic carcinoma of the lung: Prognostic and therapeutic aspects. *Cancer* 46:206, 1980.

8. Cohen Y, Gershoni-Baruch R, Lichtic C: Bone marrow biopsy in patients with malignant neoplasms other than lymphomas or leukemia. *Acta Haematol (Basel)* 62:181, 1979.

9. Savage RA, Hoffman GC, Shaker K: Diagnostic problems involved in detection of metastatic neoplasms by bone marrow aspirate compared with needle biopsy. *Am J Clin Pathol* 70:623, 1978.

10. Chemow B, Wallner SF: Variables predictive of bone marrow metastasis. *Cancer* 42:2373, 1978.

11. Delsol G, Guiu-Godfrin B, Guiu M, et al: Leukoerythroblastosis and cancer frequency, prognosis, and physiopathologic significance. *Cancer* 44:1009, 1979.

12. Gallivan MVE, Lokich JJ: Carcinocythemia (carcinoma cell leukemia): Report of two cases with English literature review. *Cancer* 53:1100, 1984.

13. Westerman MP: Bone marrow needle biopsy: An evaluation and critique. *Semin Hematol* 18:293, 1981.

14. Garrett TJ, Gee TS, Lieberman PH, et al: The role of bone marrow aspiration and biopsy in detecting marrow involvement by nonhematologic malignancies. *Cancer* 38:2401, 1976.

15. Kiely JM, Silverstein MN: Metastatic carcinoma simulating agnogenic myeloid metaplasia and myelofibrosis. *Cancer* 24:1041, 1969.

16. Broghamer WL Jr, Keeling MM: The bone marrow biopsy, osteoscan and peripheral blood in nonhematopoietic cancer. *Cancer* 40:836, 1977.

17. Steiner RM, Mitchell DG, Rao VM: MRI of diffuse bone marrow disease. *Radiol Clin North Am* 31:383, 1993.

18. Bollow M, Knauf W, Korfel A, et al: Initial experience with dynamic MR imaging in evaluation of normal bone marrow versus malignant bone marrow infiltration in humans. *J Magn Reson Imaging* 7:240, 1997.

19. Seto T, Imamura F, Kuriyama K, et al: Effect on prognosis of bone marrow infiltration detected by magnetic resonance imaging in small cell lung cancer. *Eur J Cancer* 33:2333, 1997.

20. Coustan-Smith E, Behm FG, Sanchez J, et al: Immunological detection of minimal residual disease in children with acute lymphoblastic leukaemia. *Lancet* 351:550, 1998.

21. Byard RW, Bormanis J, Jones TG: Leukoerythroblastosis: A much maligned phenomenon (editorial). *CMAJ* 1137:191, 1987.

22. Simon D, Gallambos JT: Leukoerythroblastosis with blasts in a patient with alcoholic hepatitis. *J Clin Gastroenterol* 9:217, 1987.

23. Chosner JM, Gozzard DJ: Ulcerative colitis complicated by a leukoerythroblastic anaemia. *Postgrad Med J* 58:662, 1982.

24. Kubanek B, Heimpel H, Paar G, et al: Hämatologische Veränderungen bei Anorexia Nervosa. *Blut* 35:115, 1977.

25. Powsner RA, Zietman AL, Foss FM: Bone marrow suppression after strontium-89 therapy and local radiation therapy in patients with diffuse marrow involvement. *Clin Nucl Med* 22:147, 1997.

26. Oster W, Herrmann F, Gamm H, et al: Erythropoietin for the treatment of anemia of malignancy associated with neoplastic bone marrow infiltration. *J Clin Oncol* 8:956, 1990.

27. Shamdas GJ, Ahmann FR, Matzner MB, Ritchie JM: Leukoerythroblastic anemia in metastatic prostate cancer: Clinical and prognostic significance in patients with hormone-refractory disease. *Cancer* 71:3594, 1993.

ANEMIA OF CHRONIC DISEASE

ALLAN J. ERSLEV

Most patients suffering from chronic infections, chronic inflammations, or various malignancies develop a mild to moderate anemia. This anemia, designated *anemia of chronic disease,* is characterized by a low serum iron level, a low to normal transferrin level, and a high to normal ferritin level. However, the anemia appears to be caused, not by these changes in iron metabolism, but, rather, by the effect of a number of suppressor cytokines. Tissues injured by infections or inflammation and neoplastic cells release cytokines, such as interleukin-1, tumor necrosis factor, and interferon gamma, known to reduce the production of erythropoietin in the kidney and impair its action in the marrow. As such, the anemia is probably caused primarily by a reduction in erythropoietin-generated red cell production. Therapeutic trials have revealed that the anemia is indeed responsive to erythropoietin, and in most cases, it can be ameliorated by the parental administration of sufficient amounts of human recombinant erythropoietin.

HISTORY AND DEFINITION

Weakness, weight loss, and pallor have been recognized as hallmarks of chronic illness as far back as we have medical and literary records. Yet, despite the preoccupation with blood and bloodlettings, it apparently was not recognized until the early nineteenth century that the common pallor of tuberculosis ("consumption") was associated with a lack of blood. In their classic review, "The Anemia of Infection,"[1] Cartwright and Wintrobe mention that French investigators in 1842 demonstrated that blood from patients with typhoid fever and smallpox contained a smaller mass of red cells than normal blood. The development of methods for the counting of red cells and for measuring hemoglobin concentration led to the realization that the common infections that ravaged the world, such as pneumonia, syphilis, tuberculosis, and typhoid fever, were associated with an anemia appropriately designated the *anemia of infection*. It is also now recognized that noninfectious disorders, such as rheumatoid arthritis, Hodgkin's disease, and metastatic carcinoma, are associated with a similar anemia, and the names *simple chronic anemia* and *anemia of chronic disorders* or *chronic disease* have been introduced.[2-5]

The reason for assuming that the anemias observed in a variety of chronic clinical disorders are related is that they have certain common features. They are usually of moderate severity with hemoglobin concentrations ranging from 7 to 11 g/dl. They are associated with a low serum iron, a low iron-binding capacity, increased tissue iron stores, and a reduced rate of red cell production. Indeed, these features are so characteristic that the name *sideropenic anemia with reticuloendothelial siderosis* has been suggested,[2] a reasonable but not a very happy addition to our collection of hematologic tongue twisters. Consequently, it appears justified to retain the name *anemia of chronic*

disease until further clarification of the pathogenesis leads to a more appropriate designation.

ETIOLOGY AND PATHOGENESIS

The spectacular change wrought by antibiotics on the ecology of disease has led to a decrease in the incidence of chronic, incapacitating infections and true anemia of infection. However, numerous past reports on tuberculosis, lung abscess, subacute bacterial endocarditis, chronic osteomyelitis, and chronic mycotic infections, as well as more recent reports of patients with AIDS, attest to the fact that almost all chronic suppurative infections are associated with anemia.[6-12] The severity of these anemias is roughly proportional to the severity of symptoms such as fever, weight loss, and general debility. It requires about 1 to 2 months of sustained infection for anemia to develop, after which time a new balance is established between red cell production and red cell destruction, and the hemoglobin level becomes stabilized.[2]

The anemia complicating chronic inflammatory diseases behaves functionally like the anemia complicating infections but has assumed greater importance because of the less effective therapies available. The collagen diseases, with rheumatoid arthritis[13-15] as the most prominent member, are regularly associated with anemia. Regional enteritis, ulcerative colitis, and a variety of poorly understood inflammatory syndromes may also be complicated by the anemia of chronic disease.[16] Of particular contemporary importance is the anemia found in patients with malignancies. This anemia, often termed *anemia of cancer,* is found not only in patients with metastatic and necrotizing carcinomas, but also frequently in patients with local and asymptomatic cancers, sarcomas, or lymphomas.[17-19]

The anemia of chronic disorders is characterized by a slightly shortened red cell life span, disturbed iron metabolism, and impaired erythropoietin-generated red cell production. Because of the moderate degree of the anemia and the modifying influence of different underlying disorders, it has been difficult to relate these observations and establish a firm pathogenetic mechanism. However, it has been suggested that the anemia is part of a "hematological stress syndrome" induced by the release of a number of cytokines in response to cellular injury, whether caused by infection, inflammation, or malignancy.[20] Such cytokines could cause excessive macrophage sequestration of iron and iron-binding protein, increased splenic destruction of red cells, and suppressed erythropoietin production in the kidneys and action in the marrow.[21] Furthermore, caloric malnutrition causing a decrease in transformation of tetraiodothyronine (T_4) to triiodothyronine (T_3) could lead to a functional hypothyroidism[22] in which the decreased demands for oxygen-carrying hemoglobin are met by a reduction in the synthesis of erythropoietin.[23]

RED CELL DESTRUCTION

A number of studies have established that the red cell life span is moderately reduced by about 20 to 30 percent in patients with chronic illnesses.[24,25] The responsible defect appears to be extracorpuscular, since red cells from patients survive normally in normal recipients.[1] It has been suggested that the activation of macrophages induced by a variety of cytokines renders these cells more phagocytic both individually and as part of the splenic filter and makes them less tolerant of minor red cell changes.[26] Such compulsive screening and removal of slightly damaged red cells have been observed in experimental infections if the red cells are coated with a few antibodies[27] or slightly damaged by heat.[28]

RED CELL PRODUCTION

IRON METABOLISM

The presence of a low serum iron level despite adequate iron stores indicates a profound disturbance of iron metabolism. See Table

TABLE 41-1   IRON METABOLISM

	NORMAL RANGE	IRON DEFICIENCY MEAN	CHRONIC DISEASE MEAN
Plasma iron, $\mu g/dl$	70–190	30	30
Iron-binding capacity, $\mu g/dl$	250–40	450	200
Percent saturation	30	7	15
Macrophage iron in marrow	2+	0	3+
Serum ferritin, $\mu g/liter$	20–200	10	150
Serum transferrin Receptors, nmol	8–28	increased	normal

41-1. This has led to the concept that the anemia is caused by a decreased availability of iron for hemoglobin synthesis.[27] However, more recent studies suggest that the presence of altered iron parameters may be of more importance for the diagnosis than for the pathogenesis of the anemia. The rate of gastrointestinal absorption of iron has been measured in a number of patients with chronic disorders, but the results have been difficult to interpret. In general, however, it appears that the intestinal absorption is moderately impaired,[2,29] as also shown in dogs with turpentine-induced abscesses.[1] Since the uptake of iron into intestinal cells and its subsequent incorporation by intracellular apoferritin are normal,[30] the defect apparently lies in the subsequent release of iron, possibly similar to the defective iron release from macrophages and hepatic cells in patients with chronic diseases.

Nevertheless, enough iron must have been released from intestinal cells to stock the iron stores, and it seems most likely that the low serum iron level is caused by impaired release of iron from macrophages to circulating transferrin or, in other words, by impaired reutilization of iron. Direct evidence for such a macrophage block was provided by experiments that showed that dogs with sterile turpentine-induced abscesses failed to reutilize iron from senescent red blood cells labeled with radioactive iron.[31] Similar studies employing both labeled red cells and labeled hemoglobin solutions revealed poor reutilization of hemoglobin iron in patients with infection, cancer, Hodgkin's disease, and rheumatoid arthritis (Fig. 41-1).[32–34] Since intact red cells are degraded in macrophages and free hemoglobin is degraded in hepatic parenchymal cells,[35] these studies suggest the presence of a common but still unexplained disturbance in the cellular mobilization of iron from ferritin or hemosiderin to circulating transferrin. This disturbance occurs rapidly after almost all kinds of infectious or inflammatory

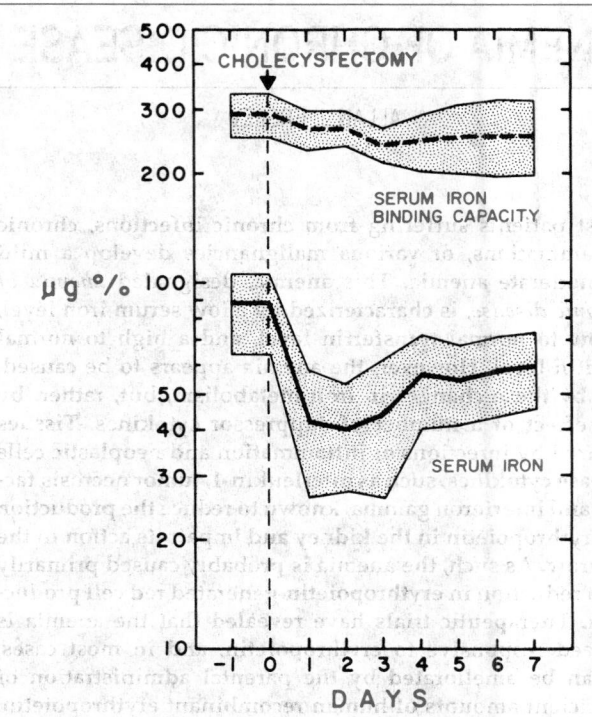

FIGURE 41-2   Mean serum iron concentration and iron-binding capacity plus or minus the standard deviation of nine patients undergoing cholecystectomy.

injuries,[36] and significant hypoferremia can be observed within 24 h after both major and minor surgery[37,38] (Fig. 41-2) and after pyrogen-induced fever.[39] Attempts to identify and rectify the cause for the low cellular iron release have not been rewarding. Since apoferritin is an acute-phase reactant and its synthesis is stimulated by the release of a number of cytokines, it has been proposed that iron is immobilized by increased intracellular concentrations of apoferritin.[40,41] Nevertheless, the relationship between the concentrations of ferritin and serum iron is not fully understood, and the search is still on for the mechanism of the iron block.

A reduced concentration of transferrin is characteristic of the anemia of chronic disorders. Turnover studies indicate a decreased rate of production,[42] but the effect of infection and inflammation on its rate of destruction is controversial and confusing.[43,44] Because of the low iron-binding capacity, the amount of saturated transferrin is

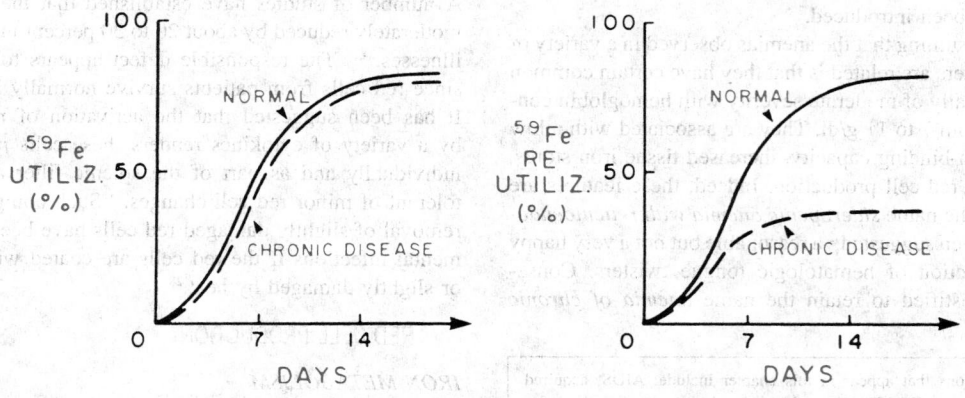

FIGURE 41-1   Utilization and reutilization of ^{59}Fe-labeled hemoglobin solution in patients with anemia of chronic disease and in normal subjects. (Adapted from Haurani et al., with permission.[34])

higher in the anemia of chronic disorders than in iron-deficiency anemia, with its elevated iron-binding capacity. Since saturated transferrin has a higher affinity for the receptors on the erythroid precursor cells than does unsaturated transferrin,[45] the transfer of iron to erythroid cells should be more efficient in chronic disorders than in iron deficiency. This may explain the fact that despite the low serum iron, the anemia of chronic disease is not an iron-deficiency anemia. The degree of anemia and the extent of hypochromia and microcytosis are rarely as pronounced as in true iron-deficiency anemia, and the serum concentration of transferrin receptors, a sensitive indicator of iron deficiency, is near normal.[46] Finally, treatment with oral iron is ineffective,[47] while treatment with recombinant erythropoietin usually is effective,[48] in sharp contrast to the observations in patients with iron-deficiency anemia.

MARROW FUNCTION

Although a normal marrow can compensate for a moderately shortened red cell life span, it needs the stimulus of erythropoietin generated by a sustained anemic hypoxia in order to do so. Consequently, an anemia may be partly but never fully compensated. In patients with chronic disease, the compensation is even less than anticipated, suggesting a decreased release of or a decreased response to erythropoietin.

Studies of the release of erythropoietin in patients with chronic disorders have produced conflicting results. In some studies erythropoietin levels have not been significantly different from those of anemic patients without chronic disorders.[49,50] However, the range is wide, and several recent studies have shown convincingly that erythropoietin production in response to moderately severe anemia, although appreciable, is blunted.[51–55] It seems likely that cytokines, such as interleukin-1 (IL-1) and tumor necrosis factor alpha (TNF-α), released by injured cells may be responsible for this blunted response. In vitro studies of erythropoietin-producing hepatoma cells have shown that these cytokines reduce the synthesis of erythropoietin.[56,57] More importantly, IL-1, when added to the perfusate of an isolated rat kidney, suppresses erythropoietin production in response to hypoxia.[57]

Studies of the response to erythropoietin have revealed the presence of a relative erythroid resistance.[58] Such studies have ranged from observations in animals with turpentine-induced abscesses[59,60] to measurements of erythroid colony formation in cultured marrow exposed to sera and cells from patients with chronic disease[61–63] or to purified cytokines and growth factors.[21] In almost all studies soluble factors released from inflammatory cells have decreased the normal erythroid response to endogenous erythropoietin or to exogenous recombinant erythropoietin.

Three factors, TNF-α, IL-1, and gamma interferons, have attracted special attention. They are all present in plasma from patients with inflammatory or neoplastic diseases, and in some, there is a direct relationship between the plasma levels and the severity of the anemia.[64–66] TNF-a is released from activated macrophages and when injected into mice it will induce a mild anemia with features characteristic of the anemia of chronic disease (low serum iron, normal ferritin, and normal white cell and platelet count).[64,67,68] In human marrow cultures it will suppress BFU-E (burst forming units—erythrocytes) and CFU-E (colony forming units—erythrocytes) colony formation.[69] Recent studies have suggested that this action may be indirect and mediated by a TNF-induced production of interferon beta from stromal cells.[70]

IL-1, released from a variety of activated cells and responsible for numerous inflammatory manifestations,[65] is also present in the sera from patients with chronic disease.[65] Similar to TNF, it has been shown to induce an anemia in rodents[71] and to suppress erythroid colony formation in human marrow cultures.[72] The latter action may also be indirect or involve the release of interferon gamma from activated

T cells.[72] That interferon may be the common denominator for the suppressive effect of TNF-α and IL-1 is suggested by studies showing a direct inhibition of human CFU-E by interferon gamma.[73,74] However, interferon can also suppress nonerythroid progenitor cells,[75] and its role in the pathogenesis of the anemia of chronic disorders is not clear.

Other factors undoubtedly play a role, but because chronic disease activates a network of interacting inflammatory cells, growth factors, precursor cells, and cytokines, the exact pathogenetic mechanisms of the anemia are far from resolved.[21]

CLINICAL AND LABORATORY FEATURES

The clinical manifestations of the mild to moderate anemia complicating chronic disorders are usually overshadowed by the symptoms of the underlying disease. Under physiologic conditions, a reduction in hemoglobin concentration to 7 to 11 g/dl, the level usually observed in the anemia of chronic disorders, need not be symptomatic. However, in patients with severe pulmonary impairment, fever, or physical debility, a moderate reduction in the oxygen-carrying capacity of the blood may aggravate preexisting symptoms. On physical examination there are no findings characteristic of this anemia, and the diagnosis hinges on the laboratory findings.

The anemia is traditionally described as normocytic and normochromic.[1] However, many patients have hypochromic red cells with a mean corpuscular hemoglobin concentration (MCHC) below 31 g/dl, and some have microcytic cells with a mean corpuscular volume (MCV) of less than 80 fl.[2]

The absolute reticulocyte count is within the normal range or slightly elevated. Changes in the white blood cell count or platelet count are not consistent and depend exclusively on the underlying disorders.

A reduction in serum iron concentration (hypoferremia) is a *sine qua non* for the diagnosis of anemia of chronic disorders (Table 41-1). It occurs promptly after the onset of an infection or injury and precedes the development of anemia. The concentration of the iron-binding protein, transferrin, is moderately decreased,[1,2] resulting in a higher iron saturation than in patients with iron-deficiency anemia (see Table 41-1). This relative ''protection'' of iron saturation may be of benefit by enhancing the transfer of iron from a reduced pool of circulating iron to immature erythroid cells.[45] The decrease in transferrin levels after injury occurs more slowly than the decrease in serum iron levels (see Fig. 41-2), presumably because of the longer half-life of transferrin (8–12 days)[76] compared to that of iron (90 min) and because of different metabolic functions.

Measurements of serum ferritin levels have been found useful in assessing marrow iron stores in patients with low serum iron concentrations.[77] In most instances there is no overlap between levels in patients with chronic disease and increased body stores of iron and patients with iron deficiency. However, depleted iron stores in patients with chronic disease may not be as readily detected by ferritin measurements, since ferritin is an acute-phase protein and fever and infections increase its synthesis and produce inappropriately high serum levels.[78] Consequently it has been suggested that only a serum ferritin level in excess of 60 μg/liter should be considered as reflecting normal or increased iron stores.[79]

Marrow aspirates may be difficult to interpret because the underlying disorders can be responsible for alterations in cellular patterns and structure. However, in general, the marrow is normal. The myeloid/erythroid ratio is about 3:1 or 4:1, and there is little evidence of compensatory erythroid hyperplasia. The most important information derived from a marrow examination pertains to its iron content. Iron in a marrow preparation can be found as storage iron in the cytoplasm of macrophages or as functional iron in nucleated red cells. In normal individuals a few Prussian blue–staining particles can be found inside or adjacent to many macrophages, and about one-third of nucleated red cells contain blue inclusion bodies and are called *sideroblasts* (Chap. 22).[80] In iron deficiency there is an absence of both sideroblasts and macrophage iron. However, in the anemia of chronic disorders only sideroblasts are decreased in number; macrophage iron is increased.[81] This increase in storage iron in the face of a decreased level of circulating iron and a decreased number of sideroblasts is characteristic of the anemia of chronic disorders and is found in no other diseases.

The results of red cell survival studies have varied, as would be expected when one considers the great diversity of the underlying disorders, but in general normal cells have displayed a moderately shortened survival when injected into patients with chronic disorders,[24,25] and red cells from such patients have had a normal survival in normal recipients.[2] These findings indicate an extracorpuscular destruction of red cells, presumably caused by infectious or inflammatory foci.

In accordance with the morphologic appearance of the marrow, measurements of plasma and red cell iron-turnover rates have disclosed a normal or only slightly increased rate of effective red cell production.[33,81] The half-life of intravenously injected radioactive iron is very short, but, when adjusted for the low level of circulating iron, the calculated plasma iron turnover is only slightly higher than normal. Since 70 percent or more of the injected radioactive iron can be accounted for in circulating red cells, erythropoiesis is mostly effective with the production and release of viable cells.[24,25] When these normal values are correlated with the fact that the marrow maintains a red cell mass of less than normal size, they support the direct measurements of a shortened red cell life span.

DIFFERENTIAL DIAGNOSIS

Most patients with chronic infections, inflammations, or neoplastic disorders are anemic, but such anemias should be designated anemias of chronic disease only if the anemia is moderate, the cellular pattern in the marrow is nearly normal, the serum iron and iron-binding capacity are low, the iron content of the marrow macrophages is normal or increased, and the serum ferritin is elevated (see Table 41-1). Since the underlying diseases can predispose the patients to many other hematologic disturbances, a final diagnosis of anemia of chronic disease should first be made after having ruled out other etiologic mechanisms. The following causes of anemia may, in particular, aggravate or obscure the anemia of chronic disease:

1. Dilution anemia. A dilution anemia has long been known to occur in patients with chronic illnesses, especially in patients with far-advanced neoplastic diseases.[82] However, it is difficult to relate plasma volume to body weight in emaciated individuals, and a true relative anemia is found rarely except in patients with myeloma or macroglobulinemia.[83]
2. Drug-induced marrow suppression or drug-induced hemolysis should always be considered. As a general rule, the serum iron level will tend to be high in marrow suppression as a reflection of reduced erythroid consumption. Reticulocyte counts, haptoglobin measurement, bilirubin determination, Coombs' test, and determination of lactic dehydrogenase activity should be done to rule out a hemolytic component.
3. Chronic blood loss will eliminate the characteristic macrophage siderosis, and one may have to rely on the levels of transferrin to distinguish between iron-deficiency anemia and the anemia of chronic disorders. Since the synthesis of transferrin receptors is

stimulated by iron deficiency, the concentration of soluble transferrin receptors is higher in iron deficiency than in chronic disease. The simplest diagnostic approach to a patient with anemia and low or absent iron in the marrow is a therapeutic trial of iron followed by reevaluation.

4. Thalassemia minor is a common cause of anemia in many parts of the world, and it may be confused at times with the anemia of chronic disease. Microcytosis is usually more severe in this group of disorders than in the anemia of chronic disease and has been present throughout the lifetime of the patient, although this has often not been documented.
5. Renal impairment causes both a shortened red cell life span and a relative marrow failure. Although the serum iron level is either normal or high in the anemia of uremia, the diagnosis rests on the finding of an increased blood urea nitrogen or creatinine level. A diagnosis of a complicating anemia of chronic disease is difficult to make in the face of overt uremia.
6. Metastatic replacement of the marrow by carcinomas or lymphomas will aggravate or mimic anemia of chronic disease. The serum iron concentration is usually normal or increased, and there may be telltale signs of marrow involvement in the peripheral blood, such as poikilocytes, teardrop-shaped red cells, normoblasts, or immature myeloid cells. Serum alkaline phosphatase determinations and X-ray or MRI studies of bone may help, but direct marrow examination usually is necessary to establish a diagnosis of myelophthisic anemia.

THERAPY, COURSE, AND PROGNOSIS

Any anemia occurring in a patient with chronic debilitating disease should be thoroughly investigated in order to rule out specific deficiencies or complications. If, after such studies, the anemia can be designated an anemia of chronic disease, it rarely demands therapy. A hemoglobin level between 7 and 11 g/dl should be of concern, but it has not been definitely shown that it is detrimental to health or impedes reparative processes. Neither has a low serum iron concentration, especially when associated with a near-normal percent saturation of transferrin. To the contrary, it has even been proposed that a low iron level may be an adaptive defense mechanism against iron-dependent bacteria.[84] Nevertheless, it still seems reasonable to believe that, if both serum iron and hemoglobin concentrations could be restored to normal, it would be of some benefit to a chronically ill patient.

Attempts to provide iron by mouth or parenterally have had little or no effect on the iron or hemoglobin concentration.[47,85] Iron dextran will release small amounts (about 1–3%) of iron directly to transferrin,[86] but the bulk of iron will be captured and retained by the monocyte-macrophage system.[87] Its release, however, is blocked in anemia of chronic disease,[88] and it has been suspected that the few patients who were helped by oral or parenteral iron had, in addition to the anemia of chronic disorders, an iron deficiency that contributed to the anemia.[2]

Cobalt chloride and androgenic steroids have been used with some effect,[89,90] but side effects render them unacceptable for a fairly benign condition. If the anemia does become symptomatic, as in patients with limited cardiovascular reserves, judicious transfusions with packed cells have been employed.

Fortunately, it seems likely in the future that the anemia can be alleviated, if not completely corrected, by treatment with erythropoietin. Recombinant erythropoietin, as expected, has been found to be dramatically effective in the correction of anemia of chronic renal disease.[91] It has now been introduced with a vengeance into the treatment of the anemia complicating chronic disease.[92] As discussed above, these anemias are caused primarily by a cytokine-induced depression of the erythroid marrow, a depression aggravated by the fact that in most patients the production of erythropoietin is blunted, with subnormal amounts of erythropoietin produced in response to anemic hypoxia.

The administration of sufficient amounts of recombinant erythropoietin should overcome this depression. The first trials in patients with rheumatoid arthritis were encouraging[94] and have been followed by numerous successful trials in anemic patients with rheumatoid arthritis,[95] AIDS,[96,97] and inflammatory bowel disease.[98] The potential use of recombinant erythropoietin for the treatment of the anemia of cancer has received special attention.[99–102] The marrow in these patients is often additionally suppressed by chemotherapy or radiation, but even here the use of sufficient amounts of recombinant erythropoietin has been gratifying in many patients.[103–105] The same is true when a chemotherapeutic agent such as cisplatin causes renal damage with a further reduction in the production of erythropoietin.[106]

The treatment should begin with the administration of adequate doses, such as 10,000 units recombinant erythropoietin three times a week intravenously or subcutaneously. An increase in the concentration of hemoglobin and/or a decrease in serum ferritin during the next 2 to 3 weeks would suggest an erythroid response and demand a continuation and final modification of the doses used. In the absence of an erythroid response during the first weeks, the dose should be increased to 20,000 units three times a week. If there is still no response, the treatment should be discontinued. However, a functional iron deficiency may abbrogate an erythroid response, and oral iron (i.e., $FeSO_4$, 300 mg tid) should be added if the ferritin concentration is less than 100 μg/liter. Significant complications have not been experienced, especially not adverse effects on blood pressure or blood coagulation. The results have varied a great deal, and attempts have been made to predict the usefulness of this expensive medication.[92] It appears that the more severe the anemia and the lower the baseline endogenous erythropoietin production, the better the results. In AIDS patients no benefit was achieved if the baseline endogenous erythropoietin level was higher than 500 mU/ml.[96] This is not surprising, since the injection of usual doses of recombinant erythropoietin will increase the level only minimally if the baseline is high. However, there are individual exceptions,[107] and in a symptomatic patient it may be worth trying a course of recombinant erythropoietin before turning to transfusions.

The goal is obviously to maintain a hemoglobin concentration at which a patient has no overt anemic symptoms and at which a sense of well-being may assist in the defense against an underlying disease.

REFERENCES

1. Cartwright GE, Wintrobe MM: The anemia of infection, in *Advances in Internal Medicine,* edited by W Dock, J Snapper, vol 5, p 165–223. Year Book, Chicago, 1952.
2. Cartwright GE: The anemia of chronic disorders. *Semin Hematol* 3:351, 1966.
3. Bentley DP: Anemia of chronic disease. *Clin Haematol* 11:465, 1982.
4. Lee GR: The anemia of chronic disease. *Semin Hematol* 20:61, 1983.
5. Wallner SF: The anemia of chronic disorders: clinical and pathological features, in *Current Concepts in Erythropoiesis,* edited by CDR Dunn, pp 209–231. Wiley, New York, 1983.
6. Glasser RM: The significance of hematologic abnormalities in patients with tuberculosis. *Arch Intern Med* 125:69, 1970.
7. Parson WB Jr, Cooper T, Scheifley CH: Anemia in bacterial endocarditis. *JAMA* 133:14, 1953.
8. Hemmeler G: *L'Anemia Infectieuse.* Benno Schwabe, Basel, 1946.
9. James GW, Riblet LA, Robinson JG, et al: Studies on prolonged suppurative infection in man. *J Lab Clin Med* 33:1607, 1948.
10. Saiti MF, Vaughan JM: The anemia associated with infection. *J Pathol Bacteriol* 56:189, 1950.
11. Vaughan JM: Anemia associated with trauma and sepsis. *Br Med J* 1:35, 1948.
12. Adams EB, Mayet FGH: Hypochromic anemia in chronic infections. *S Afr Med J* 40:738, 1966.
13. Jeffrey MR: Some observations on anemia in rheumatoid arthritis. *Blood* 8:502, 1953.
14. Roberts FD, Hagedorn AB, Slocumb CH, Owen CA: Evaluation of the anemia of rheumatoid arthritis. *Blood* 21:470, 1963.
15. Strandberg O: Anemia of rheumatoid arthritis. *Acta Med Scand (Suppl)* 454:1, 1966.
16. Ormerod TP: Observations on the incidence and cause of anaemia in ulcerative colitis. *Gut* 8:107, 1967.
17. Dall DC, Weiss RB: Neoplasia and the erythron. *J Clin Oncol* 3:429, 1985.
18. Zucker S: Anemia in cancer. *Cancer Invest* 3:249, 1985.
19. Dutcher JP: Hematologic abnormalities in patients with non-hematologic malignancies. *Hematol Oncol Clin North Am* 1:281, 1987.
20. Reizenstein P: The hematological stress syndrome. *Br J Haematol* 43:329, 1979.
21. Means RT, Krantz SB: Progress in understanding the pathogenesis of the anemia of chronic disease. *Blood* 80:1639, 1992.
22. Utiger RD: Decreased extrathyroidal triiodothyronine production in non-thyroidal illness: benefit or harm? *Am J Med* 69:807, 1980.
23. Caro J, Silver R, Erslev AJ, et al: Erythropoietin production in fasted rats. *J Lab Clin Med* 98:860, 1981.
24. Dinant HJ, deMaat CEM: Erythropoiesis and mean red-cell life span in normal subjects and in patients with the anemia of active rheumatoid arthritis. *Br J Haematol* 39:437, 1978.
25. Cavill I, Bentley DP: Erythropoiesis in the anemia of rheumatoid arthritis. *Br J Haematol* 50:583, 1982.
26. Jandl JH, Jacob HS, Daland GA: Hypersplenism due to infection: study of five cases manifesting hemolytic anemia. *N Engl J Med* 264:1063, 1961.
27. Atkinson JP, Frank MM: The effect of bacillus Calmette-Guérin–induced macrophage activation on the in vivo clearance of sensitized erythrocytes. *J Clin Invest* 53:1742, 1974.
28. Kampschmidt RF, Upchurch HF, Johnson HL: Iron transport after injection of endotoxin in rats. *Am J Physiol* 208:68, 1965.
29. Weber J, Werre JM, Julius HW, Marx JJM: Decreased iron absolution in patients with active rheumatoid arthritis with or without iron deficiency. *Ann Rheum Dis* 47: 404, 1988.
30. Schade SG: Normal incorporation of iron into intestinal ferritin in inflammation. *Proc Soc Exp Biol Med* 139:620, 1972.
31. Freireich EM, Miller A, Emerson CP, Ross JF: The effect of inflammation on the utilization of erythrocyte and transferrin-bound radio-iron for red cell production. *Blood* 12:972, 1957.
32. Noyes WD, Bothwell TH, Finch CA: The role of the reticuloendothelial cell in iron metabolism. *Br J Haematol* 6:43, 1960.
33. Haurani FI, Young K, Tocantins M: Reutilization of iron in anemia complicating malignant neoplasms. *Blood* 22:73, 1963.
34. Haurani FI, Burke W, Martinez EJ: Defective reutilization of iron in the anemia of inflammation. *J Lab Clin Med* 65:560, 1965.
35. Hershko C, Cook JD, Finch CA: Storage iron kinetics. II. The uptake of hemoglobin iron by hepatic parenchymal cells. *J Lab Clin Med* 80:624, 1972.
36. Handjani AM, Banihashemi A, Rafie R, Tolan H: Serum iron in acute myocardial infarction. *Blut* 23:263, 1971.
37. Feldthusen U, Larsen V, Lassen NA: Serum iron and operative stress. *Acta Med Scand* 147:311, 1953.
38. Erslev AJ, McKenna PJ: Effect of splenectomy on red cell production. *Ann Intern Med* 67:5, 1967.
39. Elin RJ, Wolff SM, Finch CA: Effect of induced fever on serum iron and ferritin concentrations in man. *Blood* 49:147, 1977.
40. Koniju AM, Hershko C: Ferritin synthesis in inflammation. I. Pathogenesis of impaired iron release. *Br J Haematol* 37:7, 1977.
41. Fuchs D, Zangerle R, Artner-Divorzak E, et al: Association between immune activation, changes of iron metabolism and anaemia in patients with HIV infection. *Eur J Haematol* 50:90, 1993.
42. Jarnum S, Lassen NA: Albumin and transferrin metabolism in infectious and toxic diseases. *Scand J Clin Lab Invest* 13:357, 1961.
43. Nishisato T, Aisen P: Uptake of transferrin by rat peritoneal macrophages. *Br J Haematol* 52:631, 1982.

44. Byrd TF, Horwitz MA: Regulation of transferrin receptor expression and ferritin content in human mononuclear phagocytes: coordinate upregulation by iron transferrin and down-regulation by interferon gamma. *J Clin Invest* 91:969, 1993.

45. Huebers HA, Finch CA: Transferrin: physiologic behavior and clinical implications. *Blood* 64:763, 1984.

46. Ferguson BJ, Skikine BS, Simpson KM, et al: Serum transferrin receptor distinguishes the anemia of chronic disease from iron deficiency anemia. *J Lab Clin Med* 119:385, 1992.

47. Wregdenhill G, Baltus JA, Van Eijk HG, Swaak AJ: Prediction and evaluation of iron treatment in anemic RA patients. *Clin Rheum* 8:352, 1989.

48. Pincus T, Olsen NJ, Russell IJ, et al: Multicenter study of recombinant human erythropoietin in correction of anemia in rheumatoid arthritis. *Am J Med* 89:161, 1990.

49. Birgegard G, Hallgren R, Caro J: Serum erythropoietin in rheumatoid arthritis and other inflammatory arthritides: relationship to anemia and the effect of anti-inflammatory treatment. *Br J Haematol* 65:479, 1987.

50. Nielsen OJG, Anderson LSG, Ludwigsen E, et al: Anemia of rheumatoid arthritis: serum erythropoietin concentration and red cell distribution in relation to iron status. *Ann Rheum Dis* 49:349, 1990.

51. Baer AN, Dessypris EN, Goldwasser E, Krantz SB: Blunted erythropoietin response to anaemia in rheumatoid arthritis. *Br J Haematol* 66:559, 1987.

52. Hochberg MC, Arnold CM, Hogans BB, Spivak JL: Serum immunoreactive erythropoietin in rheumatoid arthritis: imparied response to anemia. *Arthritis Rheum* 31:1318, 1988.

53. Miller CM, Jones RJ, Piantadosi S, et al: Decreased erythropoietin response in patients with the anemia of cancer. *N Engl J Med* 322:1689, 1990.

54. Spivak JL, Barnes DC, Fuchs E, Quinn TC: Serum immunoreactive erythropoietin in HIV-infected patients. *JAMA* 261:3104, 1989.

55. Boyd HK, Lappin TRJ: Erythropoietin deficiency in the anemia of chronic disorders. *Eur J Haematol* 46:198, 1991.

56. Faquin WC, Schneider TJ, Goldberg MA: Effect of inflammatory cytokines on hypoxia-induced erythropoietin production. *Blood* 79:1987, 1992.

57. Jelkmann W, Pagel H, Wolff M, Fandrey J: Monokines inhibiting erythropoietin production in human hepatoma cultures and in isolated perfused rat kidneys. *Life Sci* 50:301, 1991.

58. Krantz SB: Pathogenesis and treatment of the anemia of chronic disease. *Am J Med Sci* 307:353, 1994.

59. Lukens JN: Control of erythropoiesis in rats with adjuvant-induced chronic inflammation. *Blood* 41:37, 1973.

60. Reissmann KR, Udupa KB: Effect of inflammation on erythroid precursors (BFU-E and CFU-E) in bone marrow and spleen of mice. *J Lab Clin Med* 92:22, 1978.

61. Zanjani ED, McGlave PB, Davies SF, et al: In vitro suppression of erythropoiesis by bone marrow adherent cells from some patients with fungal infection. *Br J Haematol* 50:479, 1982.

62. Roodman GD, Horadam VW, Wright TL: Inhibition of erythroid colony formation by autologous bone marrow adherent cells from patients with the anemia of chronic disease. *Blood* 62:406, 1983.

63. Dainiak N, Hardin J, Floyd V, et al: Humoral suppression of erythropoiesis in systemic lupus erythematosus. *Am J Med* 69:537, 1980.

64. Teppo A-M, Maury CPJ: Radioimmunoassay of tumor necrosis factor in serum. *Clin Chem* 33:2024, 1987.

65. Maury CPJ, Andersson LC, Teppo A-M, et al: Mechanism of the anaemia in rheumatoid arthritis: demonstration of raised interleukin 1β concentrations in anaemic patients and of interleukin 1 mediated suppression of normal erythropoiesis and proliferation of human erythroleukemia (HEL) cells in vitro. *Ann Rheum Dis* 47:972, 1988.

66. Denz H, Fuchs D, Huber H, et al: Correlation between neopterin, interferon-gamma and haemoglobin in patients with haematological disorders. *Eur J Haematol* 44:186, 1990.

67. Johnson RA, Waddelow TA, Caro J, et al: Chronic exposure to tumor necrosis factor in vivo preferentially inhibits erythropoiesis in nude mice. *Blood* 74:130, 1989.

68. Moldawer LL, Marano MA, Wei HE, et al: Cachectin/tumor necrosis factor alters red blood cell kinetics and induces anemia in vivo. *FASEB J* 3:1637, 1989.

69. Roodman GD, Bird A, Hutzler D, Montgomery W: Tumor necrosis factor-alpha and hematopoietic progenitors: effects of tumor necrosis factor on the growth of erythroid progenitors CFU-E and BFU-E and the hematopoietic cell lines K562, HL60, and HEL cells. *Exp Hematol* 15:928, 1987.

70. Means RT, Krantz SB: Inhibition of human erythroid colony forming units by tumor necrosis factor is mediated by beta interferon. *Clin Res* 40:210a, 1992.

71. Johnson CS, Keckler DJ, Topper MI, et al: In vivo hematopoietic effects of recombinant interleukin-1α in mice: stimulation of granulocytic, monocytic, megakaryocytic, and early erythroid progenitors, suppression of late erythroid progenitors, and reversal of erythroid suppression with erythropoietin. *Blood* 73:678, 1989.

72. Means RT, Dessypris EN, Krantz SB: Inhibition of human erythroid colony-forming units by interleukin-1 is mediated by gamma interferon. *J Cell Physiol* 150:59, 1992.

73. Means RT, Krantz SS: Inhibition of human erythroid colony forming units by γ interferon can be corrected by recombinant human erythropoietin. *Blood* 78:2564, 1991.

74. Mamus SW, Beck-Schroeder S, Zanjani ED: Suppression of normal human erythropoiesis by gamma interferon in vitro: role of monocytes and T lymphocytes. *J Clin Invest* 75:1496, 1985.

75. Zoumbos NC, Djeu JY, Young NS: Interferon is the suppressor of hematopoiesis generated by stimulated lymphocytes. *J Immunol* 133:769, 1984.

76. Awai M, Brown EB: Studies of the metabolism of ^{131}I labeled human transferrin. *J Lab Clin Med* 61:363, 1963.

77. Jacobs A: Serum ferritin and iron stores. *Fed Proc* 36:2024, 1977.

78. Birgegard G, Hallgren R, Killander A, et al: Serum ferritin during infection. *Scand J Haematol* 21:333, 1978.

79. Blake DR, Waterworth RF, Bacon PA: Assessment of iron stores in inflammation by assay of serum ferritin concentrations. *Br Med J* 283:1147, 1981.

80. Cartwright GE, Deiss A: Sideroblasts, siderocytes and sideroblastic anemia. *N Engl J Med* 292:185, 1975.

81. Bush JA, Ashenbrucker H, Cartwright GE, Wintrobe MM: The anemia of infection. XX. The kinetics of iron metabolism in the anemia associated with chronic infection. *J Clin Invest* 35:89, 1956.

82. Berlin NJ, Hyde GM, Parsons RJ, Lawrence JH: The blood volume in cancer. *Cancer* 8:796, 1955.

83. Kopp WL, MacKinney AA Jr, Wasson G: Blood volume and hematocrit value in macroglobulinemia and myeloma. *Arch Intern Med* 123:394, 1969.

84. Weinberg ED: Iron and susceptibility to infectious disease. *Science* 184:952, 1974.

85. Hume R, Currie WJC, Tennant M: Anemia of rheumatoid arthritis and iron therapy. *Ann Rheum Dis* 24:451, 1965.

86. Szilagyi G, Erslev AJ: Effect of organic iron compounds on the iron uptake of reticulocytes in vitro. *J Lab Clin Med* 75:275, 1970.

87. Kornfeld S, Chipman B, Brown EB: Intracellular catabolism of hemoglobin and iron dextran by the rat liver. *J Lab Clin Med* 73:181, 1969.

88. Beamish MR: The measurement of reticuloendothelial iron release using iron dextran. *Br J Haematol* 21:617, 1971.

89. Weinsaft PP, Bernstein LHT: Cobaltous chloride in the treatment of certain refractory anemias. *Am J Med Sci* 231:246, 1955.

90. Gardner FH, Pringle JC: Androgens and erythropoiesis. *Arch Intern Med* 107:846, 1961.

91. Erslev AJ: Erythropoietin coming of age. *N Engl J Med* 316:101, 1987.

92. Erslev AJ: Erythropoietin. *N Engl J Med* 324:1339, 1991.

93. Cazzola M, Mercuriali, Brugnara C: Use of recombinant human erythropoietin outside the setting of uremia. *Blood* 89:4248, 1997.

94. Means RT, Olsen NJ, Krantz SB, et al: Treatment of the anemia of rheumatoid arthritis with recombinant human erythropoietin: clinical and in vitro results. *Blood* 70:139a, 1987.

95. Pincus T, Olsen NJ, Russell IJ, et al: Multicenter study of recombinant human erythropoietin in correction of anemia in rheumatoid arthritis. *Am J Med* 89:161, 1990.

96. Henry DH, Beall GN, Benson CA, et al: Recombinant human erythropoietin in the treatment of anemia associated with human immunodeficiency virus (HIV) infection and zidovudine therapy: overview of four clinical trials. *Ann Intern Med* 117:739, 1992.

97. Freigeiro D, Braier J, Donato H, Drelchman G, Barboni G: Double-blind multicentric randomized study of recombinant human erythropoietin in

HIV+ children with anemia treated with antiretrovirals. *Blood* 88:348a, 1996 (abstr, suppl 1).

98. Spivak JL: Recombinant human erythropoietin and the anemia of cancer. *Blood* 84:997, 1994.

99. Bunn HF: Recombinant erythropoietin therapy in cancer patients. *J Clin Oncol* 8:949, 1990.

100. Negrin RS, Stein R, Vardiman J, et al: Treatment of the anemia of myelodysplastic syndromes using recombinant human granulocyte colony stimulating factor in combination with erythropoietin. *Blood* 82:737, 1993.

101. Garton JP, Gertz MA, Witzig TE, et al: Epoetin alfa for the treatment of the anemia of multiple myeloma. *Arch Intern Med* 155:2069, 1995.

102. Cazzola M, Messinger D, Battistel V, et al: Recombinant human erythropoietin in the anemia associated with multiple myeloma or non-Hodgkin's lymphoma: dose finding and identification of predictor's of response. *Blood* 86:4446, 1995.

103. Glaspy J, Bukowski R, Steinberg D, Taylor C, Tchekmedyian S, Vadhan-Raj S for the Procrit Study Group: Impact of therapy with epoetin alfa on clinical outcomes in patients with nonmyeloid malignancies during cancer chemotherapy in community oncology practice. *J Clin Oncol* 15:1218, 1997.

104. Henry DH, Abels RI: Recombinant human erythropoietin in the treatment of cancer and chemotherapy-induced anemia: results of double-blind and open-label follow-up studies. *Semin Oncol* 21:21, 1994.

105. Dusenberry KE, McGuire WA, Holt PJ, et al: Erythropoietin increases hemoglobin during radiation therapy for cervical cancer. *Int J Radiat Oncol Biol Phys* 29:1079, 1994.

106. Cascinu S, DelFerro E, Fedeli A, Ligi M, Alessandroni P, Catalano G: Recombinant human erythropoietin treatment in elderly cancer patients with cisplatin-associated anemia. *Oncology* 52:422, 1995.

107. DaCosta NA, Hultin MB: Effective therapy of human immunodeficiency virus–associated anemia with recombinant human erythropoietin despite high endogenous erythropoietin. *Am J Hematol* 36:71, 1991.

DISORDERS OF IRON STORAGE AND TRANSPORT

VIRGIL F. FAIRBANKS

DAVID J. BRANDHAGEN

Hereditary hemochromatosis is relatively common in people of northwestern European ancestry, less common in those of southern and eastern European ancestry, and rare in other populations. It is usually due to homozygosity for a mutantant allele [845A(C282Y)] of the *HFE* gene on chromosome 6. Among Caucasians of the United States, Canada, Australia, New Zealand, Iceland, Ireland, northwestern Europe, Spain, and South Africa, approximately 5 persons per thousand are homozygous for this allele, and more than 10 percent are heterozygotes. Homozygotes are at risk for developing clinical disease; simple heterozygotes are not. The common manifestations of hereditary hemochromatosis are abdominal pains, severe fatigue, joint pains, cardiac arrhythmias or heart failure, hypothyroidism, hypogonadism, impotence, amenorrhea, diabetes mellitus, osteoporosis, hepatomegaly, splenomegaly, hepatic failure, and hyperpigmentation. These manifestations are uncommon before age 40. Diagnosis should be suspected if serum iron concentration is increased and transferrin saturation is 50 percent or greater. Confirmation may be made by testing DNA for the mutant allele, demonstrating elevated serum ferritin concentration, or liver biopsy. For many cases, liver biopsy is not warranted. Treatment requires removal of 500 ml of blood (or less in small patients) once weekly until serum ferritin concentration is 20 μg/L or less. If the diagnosis is made early and treatment is as stated, the prognosis is excellent. There is a 30 percent probability of hepatocellular carcinoma when diagnosis and treatment have been delayed and cirrhosis has developed. Siblings, parents, and children must be studied to identify other affected family members.

Other iron-overloading disorders that occur in humans include porphyria cutanea tarda, sideroblastic anemias, congenital dyserythropoietic anemias, neonatal hemochromatosis, juvenile hemochromatosis, and African hemochromatosis ("Bantu siderosis") are other iron storage disorders that have a proven or likely genetic basis. Iron overloading is rarely due to chronic excessive ingestion of iron medications. It may also rarely follow portal vein–systemic vein anastamosis. Hyperferritinemia-cataract syndrome is a disorder neither of iron transport nor of storage that may be mistaken for an iron storage disorder.

Rare disorders of iron transport include congenital atransferrinemia and congenital aceruloplasminemia.

Acronyms and abbreviations that appear in this chapter include: ALT, alanine aminotransferase; HII, hepatic iron index; IRE, iron-responsive element; MRI, magnetic resonance imaging; PCT, porphyria cutanea tarda; TSH, thyrotropin; TIBC, total iron-binding capacity.

These are also associated with excess iron in various organs in addition to anemia. Congenital atransferrinemia has many features in common with hereditary hemochromatosis. Congenital aceruloplasminemia particularly affects the basal ganglia of the brain, the pancreatic islet cells, and the retina. It is characterized by neurological features of dystonia, dysarthria, dementia, degeneration of retina, and late-onset diabetes mellitus. Paradoxically, in this disorder there is no hepatocellular injury despite marked hepatic iron overload.

DISORDERS OF IRON STORAGE

DEFINITIONS AND HISTORY

Iron overload denotes excess iron deposition in various tissues of the body. *Hemosiderosis* refers to greater than normal deposition of iron in a tissue, which may be seen microscopically as hemosiderin. Hemochromatosis is the clinical expression of iron-induced injury to cells of various organs. Table 42-1 lists many of the disorders that are associated with hemochromatosis. Among these, hereditary hemochromatosis is relatively common in people of European origin. In many of the other disorders shown in Table 42-1, the excess accumulation of iron is secondary to chronic anemia.

Hemochromatosis was first described by Trousseau[1] and Troisier[2] in France and later by von Recklinghausen,[3] who coined the term *hemochromatosis*. In 1935, Sheldon reviewed more than 300 published cases, clearly delineated the clinical and histological features, and noted the frequent association of ethanol abuse. He asserted that hemochromatosis "should be classed as an inborn error in metabolism," that "it is probably a good deal less rare than is usually believed," and that a slight increase in rate of iron absorption results, after many years, in the accumulation of a gross excess of iron which causes tissue injury, particularly of liver and pancreas.[4] Phlebotomy therapy to reduce iron stores was introduced by Davis and Arrowsmith in 1952[5] and was stressed by Finch and Finch in 1955.[6]

In 1975 it was shown that hemochromatosis is due to mutation of a gene on the short arm of chromosome 6, closely linked with the HLA locus.[7–13] It was not until 1996 that systematic examination of this region of the DNA revealed an ancestral gene, HFE, with a small number of mutations. Two of these [c.845G→A (845A;C282Y) and c.187C→G(187G;H63D)] were found to be closely associated with hemochromatosis.[14–18] The mutation primarily responsible for hemochromatosis (845A) was shown to be very common in people of northwestern European ancestry.[19–30]

HEREDITARY HEMOCHROMATOSIS

ETIOLOGY AND PATHOGENESIS

The cause of hereditary hemochromatosis is excessive tissue accumulation of iron as a result of increased rate of iron absorption beginning early in life and slowly progressive. It usually results from impaired function of a protein that is now called HFE. (See Chap. 24 and Fig. 42-1.) Normally, HFE complexes with transferrin receptor on the cell membrane and is internalized together with transferrin receptor. Within the endosome, HFE reduces the release of iron from the transferrin receptor-transferrin-Fe^{+3} complex.[31–33] The 845A(C282Y) mutation prevents the appearance HFE protein on the cell membrane; the 187G(H63D) mutation reduces the affinity of HFE for transferrin receptor. Thus, in hemochromatosis, many cells lack the normal mechanism for restricting the uptake of iron from plasma. It is unknown how alteration of the HFE-transferrin receptor interaction leads to increased iron absorption by the intestinal epithelial cells (enterocytes).

TABLE 42-1   CAUSES OF IRON OVERLOAD

HEREDITARY

Hereditary hemochromatosis
Juvenile hemochromatosis
Neonatal hemochromatosis
African hemochromatosis
Thalassemia major
Hereditary sideroblastic anemia
  Certain hereditary hemolytic anemias
    Pyruvate kinase deficiency
    Glucose-6-phosphate deficiency
Congenital dyserythropoietic anemia
Porphyria cutanea tarda
Congenital atransferrinemia
Congenital aceruloplasminemia

ACQUIRED

Chronic ingestion of medicinal iron
Transfusional iron overload
Refractory anemia with ringed sideroblasts
Shunt siderosis

The absorbed iron passes rapidly from mucosal epithelium into plasma, with no accumulation of iron in enterocytes. There is an increased expression of divalent cation transporter 1 in epithelial cells of the small intestine (enterocytes),[34] but it is not known whether this plays a role in increased iron absorption. In addition to increased iron absorption, there is also an increase in copper and cobalt absorption,[35] but this does not seem to play a role in pathogenesis.

In hemochromatosis, ferritin and hemosiderin accumulate in many tissues but especially in hepatocytes, in β-cells of the islets of Langerhans in the pancreas, in myocardium, in pituitary, and in joints.

Macrophages of blood and enterocytes are actually iron-poor. In the liver, hemosiderin first appears in Kupffer cells. Then, as iron overloading develops, deposits of hemosiderin appear in the hepatocytes. When iron is released from ferritin into the cytosol, it is as Fe^{+2}. This is converted to Fe^{+3} within the cytosol. In this process, free hydroxyl and superoxide radicals are formed. Superoxide, in turn, is converted by superoxide dismutase to hydrogen peroxide, that may injure cells by peroxidation of lipids of the membranes of microsomes, mitochondria, or other cell structures or membranes.[36,37] Although cells normally have sufficient peroxidases and catalase to dispose of the H_2O_2 that forms, harmful amounts of peroxide and active oxygen radicals may be generated when iron stores are greatly increased.

Iron is not the sole factor responsible for tissue injury in hemochromatosis. The high frequency of ethanol abuse in persons with overt hemochromatosis has been recognized for at least 60 years.[4] Those who have iron overload and who also habitually consume ethanol have a significantly higher frequency of hepatic fibrosis than do those who abstain.[38] Viral hepatitis may also be a contributing factor, as an Italian study revealed an excess frequency of hepatitis C in hemochromatosis.[39]

An iron-rich environment provides a favorable medium for bacterial growth.[40,41] Furthermore, phagocytic functions of monocytes and neutrophils are impaired in persons with iron storage disease.[42]

PATHOLOGY

Affected tissues and organs exhibit a deep brown color. The liver is enlarged and may weigh as much as 2500 g. After cirrhosis has developed, the organ becomes granular or coarsely nodular. The myocardium is thickened, and the heart is often enlarged. Testes are often atrophic. Histologic examination reveals prominent hemosiderin deposition in many tissues and organs. In the liver, hemosiderin is found primarily in hepatocytes, bile duct epithelium, and, to a lesser degree, Kupffer cells and other mesenchymal cells. Prior to the development of cirrhosis, the hemosiderin accumulates primarily in periportal hepatocytes and is less toward the central veins. The iron of cirrhotic livers is mostly in the periphery of regenerative nodules. Fibrosis begins periportally, then fibrous septa traverse the lobules. Usually, the distortion of the architecture is not as severe or as uniform as in alcoholic cirrhosis.[43-45] In patients with advanced disease the histologic features may be difficult to distinguish from those of alcoholic cirrhosis, except for the marked deposition of hemosiderin in hemochromatosis. In fact, most of the patients with much fatty change probably represent combined alcoholic cirrhosis and hemochromatosis. The pancreas also exhibits diffuse fibrotic change, with loss of islets, and intense hemosiderin deposition. In the pituitary, iron deposition is most pronounced in gonadotroph cells of the anterior lobe.[46]

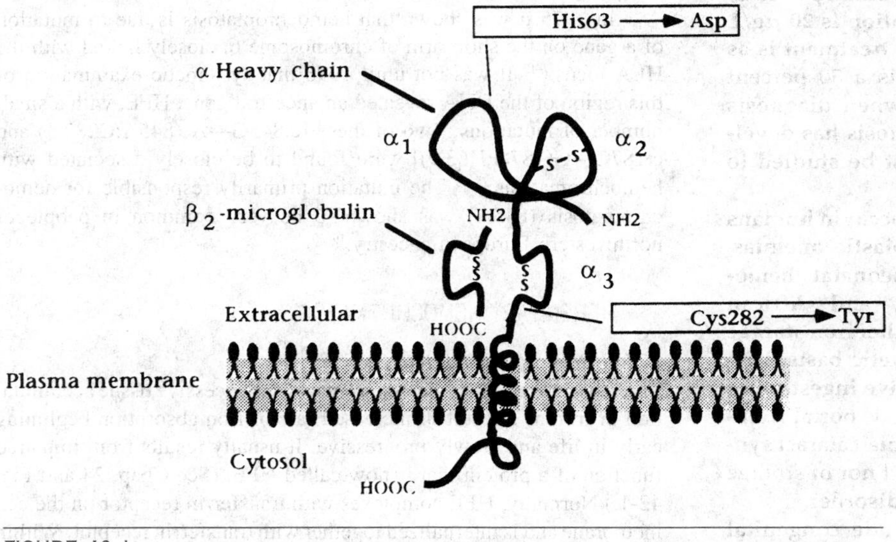

Genetics   Hemochromatosis is usually due to mutations in the *HFE* gene. Two mutations of this gene are quite prevalent in North America and in other populations derived predominantly from northwestern Europe (Fig. 42-2). The more important of these is G → A at nucleotide (nt) 845, resulting in a change from cysteine to tyrosine at amino acid position 282. Accordingly, this mutation may be designated 845A (or C282Y, where *C* represents cysteine

FIGURE 42-1   The HFE protein, as predicted from *HFE* gene sequence,[14] and later confirmed by analysis of the crystallized protein,[47] is a class I MHC-like protein that contains 321 amino acids. It spans the cell membrane. Its extracellular portion has three domains, shown as $\alpha1$, $\alpha2$, and $\alpha3$. It is closely associated with $\beta2$-microglobulin. The $\alpha1$ domain contains the binding site for transferrin receptor.[32] The major hemochromatosis mutation 845A(Cys282→Tyr, or C282Y) disrupts a disulfide bond normally present within the $\alpha3$ domain, thereby preventing expression of HFE on the cell surface, the association of HFE with $\beta2$-microglobulin, and the binding of transferrin receptor, the mechanism that normally modulates iron uptake by the cell. The mutation 187G(His63→Asp, or H63D) prevents formation of a salt bridge that is normally present within the $\alpha1$ domain and impairs the binding of transferrin receptor by HFE protein. (*From Feder and coworkers, by permission.*)[14]

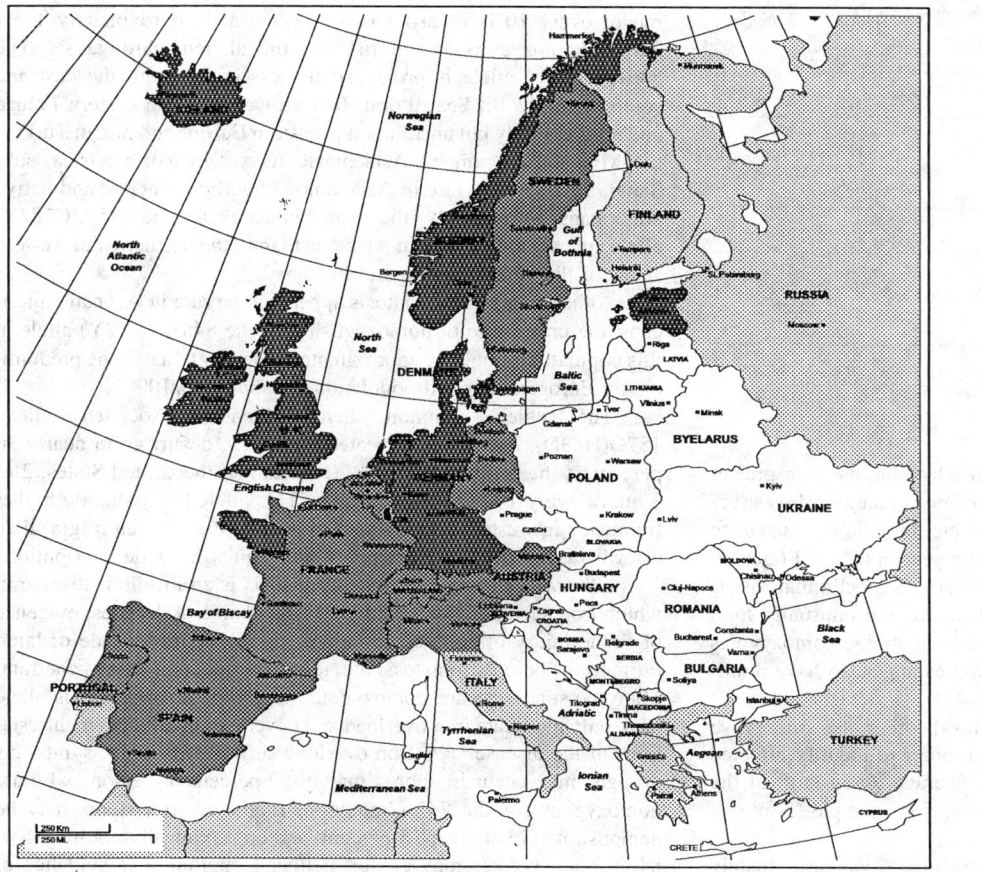

FIGURE 42-2 The approximate distribution and frequency of the major hemochromatosis allele 845A(C282Y) in Europe. The highest frequency is in the region bordering the North Sea and the North Atlantic and in populations elsewhere in the world that derive from this area of northwestern Europe.

and *Y* represents tyrosine). The other common mutation is C → G at nt 187, which results in a histidine to aspartic acid substitution at amino acid position 63. Thus, this mutation may be designated 187G (or H63D, where *H* represents histidine and *D* represents aspartic acid). Other terminology has also been used for these mutations, as shown in Tables 42-2 and 42-3. (Furthermore, some protein chemists use yet a different notational system, in which amino acid position 282 is designated 260, and position 63 is designated 41.[47] This difference depends on whether the numbering of amino acids begins with methionine at the initiation of the signal sequence or at the first amino acid of the mature protein. To avoid confusion, in this chapter reference will be made consistently to these two mutations as 845A(C282Y) and 187G(H63D). A third mutation of the *HFE* gene is nucleotide 193 A → T, corresponding to substitution of cysteine for serine at amino acid position 65. The frequency of this 193T(S65C) allele is approximately 0.025, or an approximately 5 percent prevalence (in France) of 193T(S65C) heterozygotes. It is associated with mild hemochromatosis in 845A(C282Y)/193T(S65C) compound heterozygotes.[48] A few other mutations of the *HFE* gene have been reported.

Of patients of northern European ancestry with clinically defined hereditary hemochromatosis, approximately 83 percent are homozygous for 845A(C282Y) (Table 42-3) and approximately 5 percent are compound heterozygotes, having, on one chromosome 6, the mutation 845A(C282Y) and on the other chromosome 6, 187G(H63D). Clinically significant iron overload has also been described in homozygotes for 187G(H63D), but usually such homozygotes have little or no clinical evidence of hereditary hemochromatosis. The *HFE* mutations are allelic to each other and to the wild type allele, and each *HFE* gene contains, at the most one mutation. (In a rare exception to this rule, report has appeared of a meiotic recombination event that resulted in both mutations being "in cis," that is, on the same chromosome.[49]) It is inevitable that additional mutations will be described in the future. However, up to 20 percent of patients with northern European ancestry and clinically severe hereditary hemochromatosis do not to have muta-

TABLE 42-2 NOMENCLATURE OF THE *HFE* ALLELES

	DNA NOTATION	PROTEIN NOTATION[1]	UKHC[2]
Normal (wild type)	wt	C282C, H63H (or Cys260, His41)	HC
Major hereditary hemochromatosis allele	845A	C282Y (or Cys260Tyr)	HY
Minor hereditary hemochromatosis allele	187G	H63D (or His41Asp)	DC

[1] See text for explanation of two competing systems for protein notation.
[2] United Kingdom Haemochromatosis Consortium.

TABLE 42-3 APPROXIMATE EXPECTED PREVALENCE (%) OF COMBINATION OF *HFE* ALLELES IN CAUCASIANS OF NORTH AMERICA AND NORTHWESTERN EUROPE*

HETEROZYGOTES	%
wt/845A	9.7
wt/187G	28.3
845A/187G	2.5
HOMOZYGOTES	
wt/wt	56.6
845A/845A	0.4
187G/187G	2.5

*Based on several published series. wt, wild type allele. Observed frequency of homozygotes for 187G is lower than predicted from heterozygote frequency.

tions of the *HFE* gene.[14,50] In Italy and in Alabama, an even greater proportion of patients, 35 percent, lack *HFE* gene mutations. Investigations of such patients are in progress. To date, they do not appear to have mutations of either the $\beta2$ microglobulin gene or the DCT1 gene.[51]

The mode of inheritance of hereditary hemochromatosis is autosomal recessive.[13,52–55] However, because of the unusually high 845A(C282Y) gene frequency in affected populations, homozygotes often mate with heterozygotes.[54] Such families appear to have dominant inheritance.

Because of the hereditary nature of this disorder, it is imperative that other family members be examined in order to identify affected relatives early. Within such a family, on average, one-fourth of the sibship will have the same mutant alleles, for example, homozygous 845A(C282Y).

The locus of the *HFE* gene on chromosome 6 is approximately 4 million nucleotide base pairs telomeric to that of the major histocompatibility gene *HLA-A*. Because of this relatively close proximity, the relatively recent origin of the mutation, and the fact that crossovers appear to be particularly rare in this region of the genome, linkage disequilibrium of HLA and hemochromatosis alleles exists.[10–12,55,56] The frequency of HLA-A3 antigen in the general population is approximately 28 percent, but in patients with hemochromatosis the frequency is 70 percent. The prevalence of HLA antigen B7 in patients is 50 percent, compared with 23 percent in the general population. Some series have shown increased frequency of HLA-B14.[7,8,53,57,58] The linkage disequilibrium between HLA and HFE implies an ancestral HFE mutation that occurred before the migration of Europeans to North America, Australia, New Zealand, and South Africa.[12] This mutation may have occurred 50 to 70 generations ago in northwestern Europe,[59–61] perhaps sometime between the years 500 and 700 of the common era, then become widely dispersed in this region with the migrations of Celts, Norse, and Goths. The mutation presumably conferred a selective advantage: those with this mutation would recover more quickly from blood loss than would those with only the wild type allele. Both the 845A(C282Y) and 187G(H63D) mutations have been found in Sri Lanka; haplotype analysis indicated that these occurred de novo.[62]

Prevalence The mutant genes that are responsible for hemochromatosis exhibit high frequencies in people living in the region around the North Sea and in populations that are derived from this region (Fig. 42-2, Table 42-3). Thus, the highest known gene frequencies for the 845A(C282Y) allele are in Iceland, Norway, Denmark, Sweden, the Netherlands, Germany, western France (especially the Brittany Peninsula), northern Portugal, Spain, Ireland, the United Kingdom, Australia, New Zealand, and the Caucasian populations of North America and South Africa.[19–21,23–28,30,63–69] In these populations, the gene frequency of 845A(C282Y) is 0.05 to 0.1, approximately 1 person out of every 10 is a carrier of this gene, and approximately 1 per 250 is homozygous and at risk of clinical hemochromatosis. The 845A(C282Y) allele is progressively less common to the east and south of the North Sea littoral. It is still common in eastern France and northern Italy but uncommon in eastern Europe and rare in Turkey, the Middle East, among Ashkenazic Jews,[70] in North Africa, sub-Saharan Africa, and rare in Asia, among Pacific islanders, and native Americans. Surprisingly, the gene frequency for the 845A(C282Y) allele appears to be lower in Alabama than in the northern and western states of the United States, and in Canada.[71,72]

Although hemochromatosis appears to be rare in African Americans, the prevalence of homozygosity for the 845A(C282Y) allele in this population should be approximately one-ninth that in the predominantly European-derived population, or about 0.3/1000.

The other common hemochromatosis-associated allele, 187G(H63D), has an even greater frequency, occurring in nearly 30 percent of the people of Europe, Canada, and the United States; 2 or 3 out of every 100 are homozygotes. This allele has a slightly higher frequency in western Europe (and in people of European origin) than elsewhere, but it has a more nearly uniform worldwide distribution.

Clinical Features Hemochromatosis is an insidious disease in which iron accumulation occurs over the course of decades; evidence of tissue injury often does not appear until the fifth decade or later. Further, the hemochromatosis mutations are not completely penetrant: Many persons who are homozygous for the hemochromatosis allele have only moderate iron overload and never exhibit clinical manifestations of the disease.[20,54,57] Iron overload sufficient to cause symptoms or signs may occur in approximately 50 percent of persons who are homozygous for the 845A mutation. Increased iron stores may be demonstrated in another 25 percent, and approximately one-fourth of 845A homozygotes may exhibit neither symptoms nor evidence of iron overload.[73] Thus, in large, unselected surveys, clinical expression, or penetrance, of the 845A(C282Y) allele was about 50 percent in homozygotes.[73–75] In one study of clinically unselected siblings of 99 previously identified homozygotes, 86 were found also to be homozygotes, and of these, 30 percent had clinically expressed hemochromatosis, that is, there was 30 percent penetrance. However, for homozygotes of age greater than 40 years, 50 percent had clinical manifestations, whereas for those of age less than 40 years, only 12 percent had clinical manifestations.[74] This study was later expanded to include 214 clinically unselected homozygotes in 103 kindreds that had a previously identified homozygous hemochromatosis proband.[76] Results were the same: 52 percent penetrance was observed in males of age greater than 40 years; 10 percent penetrance in women. Some studies show penetrance to be much less than 50 percent,[77,78] whereas some find penetrance to be greater than 50 percent.[79,80] Since most of the published data are based on family studies, the level of penetrance in 845A(C282Y) homozygotes of the general population will not be known until more data are available. All agree that penetrance is less for the 845A/187G (C282Y/H63D) heterozygote and much less for the 187G(H63D) homozygote.[16–18,81]

Overt disease occurs more commonly in males than in females, by a ratio of 3:1. During the reproductive years women may be protected from iron accumulation because of the iron loss attendant upon menstruation and pregnancy. Thus, women are less often affected than men, and the manifestations of hemochromatosis are uncommon prior to the menopause. However, in some women the disorder may be fully expressed in the third or fourth decade, and pituitary hypogonadism may cause amenorrhea and premature menopause. A French and Canadian study failed to demonstrate any difference between males and females with respect to time of onset or severity of clinical manifestations.[82]

In view of the high prevalence of the hemochromatosis alleles in European-derived populations, clinicians may wonder why their offices are not full of patients with this disorder. Homozygous hemochromatosis has about twice the prevalence in Caucasians as sickle cell anemia in African Americans. Both are of autosomal recessive inheritance. The hemochromatosis allele 845A(C282Y) has lower penetrance in homozygotes and often is not manifested before the age of 40 years; the Hb S mutation has 100 percent penetrance in homozygotes and is usually manifested in infancy. The recurrent, severe pain and other dramatic manifestations of sickle cell anemia demand medical care from infancy throughout the patient's life. The manifestations of hemochromatosis, late in onset and of nonspecific character, do not bring this disorder so insistently to the attention of the physician. Neither disorder is sufficiently common to fill clinicians' offices. A clinician whose patients are predominantly Caucasian should have, on average, 4 or 5 patients who are homozygous for the 845A(C282Y) allele among 1000 patients under his or her care; some have more and some have none. The manifestations of hemochromatosis in this small number of patients may be overlooked when a practice has so many patients with other complaints. "Chi non cerca, nulla trova"; he who doesn't look doesn't find.

The most frequent symptoms are abdominal pain, weakness, lethargy, loss of libido, weight loss, and arthralgia. The abdominal pain is nonspecific. Fatigue, asthenia, and mental aberrations affect at least a third of patients.[83] Fatigue may be overwhelming and disabling. Dementia is rare. The acute onset of severe adominal pain, distention, and shock is usually a fatal complication that is due to bacterial peritonitis.

The arthralgia typically involves the second and third metacarpophalangeal joints but may also involve interphalangeal joints and large joints, such as the knees.[84–87] The joints may be swollen and tender, and these manifestations may be mistakenly ascribed to rheumatoid or degenerative arthritis.

Hyperpigmentation of skin is a common manifestation. The pigment is predominantly melanin, although hemosiderin deposition also occurs in the skin. There may be a diffuse tanning or bronzing, or slate grey appearance of the skin, particularly in axillary, inguinal, and perineal areas, which are not ordinarily exposed to sunlight. Elsewhere, the appearance may be that of a perpetual suntan. Alopecia and cutaneous atrophy may also occur, especially as late manifestations.

Cardiac arrhythmias are common, particularly in young patients. Dyspnea, edema, and other manifestations of cardiac dysfunction may result from restrictive cardiomyopathy, due to impaired contractility of the iron-laden heart or may be due to dilatational cardiomyopathy.[88–90]

Coronary artery disease, as manifested by atherosclerosis or by myocardial infarction, is uncommon in patients with severe iron overload or in those who are homozygous for the 845A(C282Y) mutation.[91] Speculation about the role of iron in coronary artery disease relates to the generation of free radicals OH^- and O_2^- when Fe^{+2} is oxidized to Fe^{+3}. In eastern Finland positive correlations were observed between high normal values of serum ferritin concentration and acute myocardial infarction and also between heterozygosity for the 845A(C282Y) mutation and myocardial infarction.[92–95] However, in Helsinki, in southern Finland, a negative correlation was found between 845A(C282Y) gene heterozygosity and myocardial infarction: Heterozygotes appeared to have lower risk of coronary artery disease.[96] Most other studies in Europe and North America have shown no relationship between increased iron stores and coronary artery disease.[91,97–100]

Endocrinopathies that result from hemochromatosis include diabetes mellitus, hypothyroidism, and hypogonadotrophic hypogonadism. There is little correlation between the degree of iron overload and the severity of diabetes.[101] Peripheral neuropathy may occur secondary to diabetes.[83,102] Approximately half the patients with hemochro-

matosis have pituitary insufficiency, chiefly affecting gonadotrophins.[103–105] Ten percent of male patients have hypothyroidism, a frequency 80 times that of the general population.[106] Testicular atrophy, reduced libido, and impotence are common manifestations. Azoospermia may occur.

Hepatomegaly and splenomegaly are common. Jaundice is unusual except when there is severe cirrhosis or hepatoma. Gastrointestinal hemorrhage from esophageal varices is a late complication and is often fatal. Hepatocellular carcinoma occurs in nearly a third of persons with hepatic cirrhosis from hemochromatosis, a higher frequency than in alcoholic cirrhosis. It is quite rare in the precirrhotic phase of hemochromatosis.

Laboratory Tests   The blood hemoglobin concentration, erythrocyte count, hematocrit, erythrocyte indices, leukocyte count and differential, platelet count, and reticulocyte count are normal except late in the course of the disease, when anemia, leukopenia, and thrombocytopenia may be observed as an expression of severe liver disease. Blood glucose concentration may be increased and glucose tolerance test abnormal. The serum iron concentration exceeds the normal range for the method employed, and the transferrin saturation exceeds 50 percent. The total iron-binding capacity of serum (TIBC) is normal except when there is liver cirrhosis; then, the TIBC may be reduced.[54,57,107,108] Serum ferritin concentration exceeds 300 μg/liter and may exceed 3000 μg/liter. The serum (AST) transaminase activity is increased in approximately two-thirds of patients. Blood concentrations of pituitary gonadotrophins and androgens are usually markedly diminished. Thyrotropin (TSH) is usually increased in patients with hypothyroidism. An electrocardiogram may demonstrate arrhythmia of atrial or ventricular origin, extrasystoles, low voltage, or repolarization abnormalities of the ST and T segments. Echocardiogram and catheterization data may demonstrate dilated or restrictive cardiomyopathy. Radiographic examination of hands and wrists or of other affected joints reveals soft-tissue swelling, narrowing of the joint space, irregular articular surfaces, and decreased bone density.[84–87,109–114] Osteoporosis and subcortical cysts are also common findings.[112,113] Chondrocalcinosis or calcification of periarticular ligaments is a late manifestation of the arthropathy.[109] Synovial fluid may contain calcium pyrophosphate and hydroxyapatite crystals.[111] Chest x-ray may reveal cardiomegaly, increased pulmonary vascular markings, or pleural effusion.

Differential Diagnosis   Because hemochromatosis is a multisystem disease, it has extremely diverse manifestations and thus often masquerades as other disorders. Chronic fatigue is often ascribed to depression or neurasthenia. Impotence is also commonly considered psychological in nature. Hypothyroidism may be considered idiopathic. Palpitations that are due to arrhythmia may lead to a diagnosis of "solitary atrial fibrillation" or other cardiologic diagnosis. Cardiomegaly may be attributed erroneously to myocarditis. Arthropathy may be considered due to degenerative or rheumatoid arthritis. Elevated serum transaminases may be ascribed to ethanol indulgence or viral hepatitis. Elevation in blood glucose may lead to a diagnosis of type II, or adult-onset, diabetes mellitus. Amenorrhea or osteoporosis may be attributed to premature menopause. Hyperpigmentation is often considered due to sun exposure, even in those who have not such exposure. Thrombocytopenia, which reflects chronic liver disease, is unexplained and ignored. Pleural effusions, resulting from cirrhosis and usually accompanied by ascites, may be considered idiopathic.

Because of the diversity of clinical manifestations, and because medical specialists tend to concentrate their attention on abnormalities that are within the sphere of their specialty, the manifestations of hemochromatosis are often treated separately according to the organ system to which symptoms and signs can be related: Cardiologists treat the arrhythmias or the congestive heart failure, "depression" is treated by generalists, neurologists, or psychiatrists with antidepressive medication, urologists attempt to treat the impotence, pulmonologists drain the pleural effusions, endocrinologists treat the hypothyrodism, etc. When clinicians fail to recognize the multisystem nature of the disease, its proper diagnosis and management are delayed, often for 10 years or more, and the opportunity to provide optimal treatment is lost. Quite often, the price of diagnosis-made-too-late is cirrhosis of the liver, liver cancer, insulin-dependent diabetes mellitus, permanent joint deformities, and premature death as a result of hepatic or cardiac failure or hepatocellular carcinoma.

Prevention of organ damage to liver, pancreas, heart, pituitary, and other organs, and of hepatocellular carcinoma requires diagnosis and treatment during the precirrhotic stage, when there may be neither symptoms nor signs of iron overload. For this reason, screening tests have been recommended to ensure early diagnosis and treatment of hemochromatosis.[115–122] Analyses of costs for screening have shown a high benefit-to-cost ratio. The cost of screening per case identified has been estimated as being between $1000 and $8000.[116–118,122] By comparison, the approximate costs of screening for colon cancer, breast cancer, or for galactosemia (in neonates) are, respectively, $100,000, $70,000, and $140,000 per case identified, costs that society and third-party payers deem acceptable. With universal screening, diagnosis of hemochromatosis could be done at an overall cost of $1000 per case identified, and the average lifetime treatment cost per case should not exceed $6500; whereas, without early identification and treatment, the eventual cost of medical care, per case, would be $46,000.[122] By these estimates, universal screening, early diagnosis, and treatment would result in a net saving to society of more than $38,000 per case identified. Thus, there is a compelling financial argument for hemochromatosis screening, in addition to the ethical and humanitarian needs of reducing morbidity and early mortality. However, implementation of universal screening for hemochromatosis is being delayed because of concern over possible adverse psychologic or social effects of positive test results, such as stigmatization and difficulty obtaining life insurance and health insurance.[123–126]

Of screening tests, the most useful is the assay of serum iron, TIBC, and calculation of transferrin saturation (in percent). When the serum iron concentration is above the normal range for the method used and transferrin saturation is 50 percent or greater, there is a high probability of hemochromatosis. This presumes that other causes of elevated serum iron concentration have been excluded. A common cause for elevated serum iron concentration is exogenous iron, for example from that ingested in medication or in iron-fortified vitamin preparations. Patients often overlook providing this information; a specific inquiry about use of over-the-counter pills is necessary. Iron contamination of glassware or reagents or of the serum specimen itself is rare in a well-managed laboratory. The serum ferritin assay is not sensitive early but is only elevated when iron overload has developed. Marrow examination may or may not show increased stainable iron[127,128] and therefore is not a useful diagnostic test. Ringed sideroblasts are absent.

A liver biopsy may be appropriate, particularly in patients more than 40 years of age, who have hepatomegaly or splenomegaly, elevated serum transaminase, especially AST, and serum ferritin concentration greater than 1000 μg/L. Patients who do not meet these criteria are quite unlikely to have hepatic cirrhosis and should not undergo liver biopsy. When needed for diagnosis, liver biopsy provides a specimen for hematoxylin and eosin and Prussian blue stains and usually sufficient material as well for chemical assay of iron content. Thereby, the degree of hepatic injury may be assessed, and the amount of iron deposition estimated microscopically on a scale of 0 to 4+, in addition to the chemical assay of iron.[44,129] Microscopic estimation of iron content generally correlates well with the chemical assay. In normal liver, the iron content is estimated at 0 to 1+ histologically

and not more than 50 μmol/g (2.8 mg/g) dry weight. In persons with alcoholic liver disease, the iron content of liver is 0 to 2+ microscopically and less than 70 μmol/g (3.9 mg/g) dry weight. In hemochromatosis, liver iron content is 3 to 4+ by microscopic estimation and usually exceeds 70 μmol/g by chemical assay. Most patients with cirrhotic hemochromatosis have liver iron content of 200 μmol/g (11 mg/g) dry weight or more.[130] The *hepatic iron index* (HII) is the ratio of the hepatic iron concentration in μmol/g to the patient's age in years. This index is not greater than 1.1 in normal persons; it is usually 2.0 or more in hemochromatosis. Exceptionally, it may be as high as 24. The rationale of the HII is questionable because hepatic iron concentration has no correlation with patients' age,[131] as once thought, and since elevated HII may be observed in end-stage liver disease of any cause,[132,133] or even in patients following marrow transplant for a variety of disorders.[134]

Temporary morbidity may follow liver biopsy.[135] Serial phlebotomy provides more accurate information concerning total iron burden than does measurement of liver iron concentration. The only additional information that liver biopsy provides is whether there is cirrhosis, but this does not guide therapy. Liver biopsy is unnecessary unless the physician believes that this additional information is important for patient management. An example might be in late-stage liver disease when liver transplantation is considered.

Computed tomography is too insensitive to iron content of liver for diagnostic use. However, magnetic resonance imaging (MRI) can be used for this purpose, since the T2-weighted signal intensity is inversely proportional to iron content, and the correlation of this with iron content of liver is quite satisfactory.[136–143] MRI may not reveal early cirrhosis. As an indicator of iron overload, MRI is much more costly (in excess of $1000) than serum ferritin assay.

HLA testing, of patients or siblings, is no longer justifiable. Alcoholics who have iron overload cannot be differentiated from other persons with hereditary hemochromatosis on the basis of differences in clinical or laboratory manifestations nor in the frequencies of HLA alleles.[9,56] Thus, they have hereditary hemochromatosis complicated by ethanol abuse. On average, such persons have a slightly lower iron burden than do abstemious hemochromatotics.[56]

Treatment   Treatment is by the removal of 500 ml of blood once weekly. Less blood may be removed each week from small patients. Occasionally, when the iron burden seems very great, twice weekly phlebotomy may be worthwhile. Each phlebotomy removes 175 to 225 mg of iron. Thus, in the course of a year, 10 g of iron may be removed as a result of removal of 50 units of blood. Since the total iron burden may be 30 to 40 g, a twice weekly phlebotomy program often requires 1 to 2 years to reduce the body iron content to normal level. A program of weekly phlebotomy may require 2 to 3 years. With this program, there is an initial decline in blood hemoglobin concentration, which returns to normal value within a few weeks, as hematopoiesis is accelerated. A persistently falling blood hemoglobin concentration, after many months of phlebotomy therapy, is the best indicator that treatment has been adequate. By this time serum ferritin levels are usually below 10 ng/ml. Thereafter, 500 ml of blood should be removed every few months, in order to prevent reaccumulation of excess iron stores and to remove additional iron that was not readily available for erythropoiesis but was redistributed with time. Some patients reaccumulate iron slowly; for them, it may suffice to monitor the serum ferritin concentration annually to determine when additional phlebotomies are required.[144] In many adequately treated patients, the serum iron concentration and transferrin saturation return to elevated levels long before there is a sufficient increase in iron stores to justify repeat phlebotomy. For this reason, following completion of phlebotomy therapy, the serum ferritin concentration is the better guide to determine the need for, and the frequency of, additional phlebotomies.

Iron chelators, such as desferrioxamine, should not ordinarily be used in the treatment of hereditary hemochromatosis, because such treatment is less efficient, and far more expensive and inconvenient, than is phlebotomy.

Additional therapeutic measures include treatment of diabetes, of cardiac arrhythmias and insufficency, of variceal bleeding if it occurs, and replacement of androgens or estrogens and progesterone when clinically appropriate.

It is not practical to attempt to alter dietary intake of iron. Alcohol in excess is clearly deleterious. Complete abstinence is prudent until all excess iron has been removed. For those who have evidence of liver or other organ injury, subsequent complete avoidance of alcohol and other hepatotoxins is appropriate. Patients without evidence of organ damage should be admonished to avoid any but the most moderate alcohol indulgence. A practical guideline might be, for example, not more than 1 glass of wine (or 8 oz of beer) with dinner three times weekly. A few glasses of wine per week are probably harmless for such patients once iron stores have been depleted. For some patients complete abstinence may be easier to sustain. Patients should be advised to avoid handling or consumption of marine shellfish unless thoroughly cooked because they are peculiarly susceptible to fatal sepsis from the marine bacterium *Vibrio vulnificus*.[145,146] Peritonitis and septicemia have also been reported due to infection with *Yersinia enterocolitica* in patients with hemochromatosis or with iron overload from chronic oral ingestion or transfusion or with thalassemia major.[147,148] This organism, which causes acute febrile illness accompanied by diarrhea, mesenteric lymphadenitis, tonsillitis, and other systemic symptoms in normal persons, is more virulent in those who are iron-overloaded from any cause.

Patients in whom the diagnosis is made too late and who have advanced cirrhosis or hepatocellular carcinoma may require liver transplantation (see below).

Prognosis   Before phlebotomy was widely used as treatment for hemochromatosis, the median survival of untreated patients was estimated as approximately 2 years.[6] Subsequent studies indicate much better prognosis in treated patients[149–151] and nearly normal survival in those treated during the precirrhotic phase.[149,152] An analysis of survival data for 163 patients reported from Germany indicated a median survival, for all patients, of 20 years, compared with more than 25 years expected for matched age and sex normal persons.[149] Adverse survival factors were hepatic cirrhosis, diabetes mellitus, and inadequate iron depletion therapy (Table 42-5). This greatly improved prognosis may reflect earlier diagnosis and treatment.

Despite the improvement in survival, many problems remain for hemochromatosis patients. Adequate therapy usually has little effect on the arthritis, diabetes, hypogonadism, or sterility. Rarely, serial

TABLE 42-4   GENOTYPE FREQUENCIES FOR THE *HFE* ALLELES IN NORMAL AND HEMOCHROMATOSIS SUBJECTS*

GENOTYPES		CONTROLS No. (%)	HEMOCHROMATOSIS No. (%)
HOMOZYGOTES			
wt/wt	(C282C/C282C)	112 (58.0)	0
845A/845A	(C282Y/C282Y)	0	121 (82.3)
187G/187G	(H63D/H63D)	0	0
HETEROZYGOTES			
845A/wt	(C282C/C282Y)	27 (14.0)	2 (1.4)
187G/wt	(C282C/H63D)	52 (26.9)	6 (4.1)
845A/187G	(C282Y/H63D)	2 (1.0)	8 (5.4)

*Based on data of Beutler et al.[15] Similar results have been reported in other studies.

TABLE 42-5   SURVIVAL IN HEREDITARY HEMOCHROMATOSIS*

GROUP ANALYZED	NUMBER	MEDIAN SURVIVAL (YRS)	75% SURVIVAL (YRS)
NORMAL POPULATION[1]		>25	17
HEMOCHROMATOSIS			
All	163	20	11
Without cirrhosis	51	Not different from normal	
With cirrhosis	112	16	10
Non-diabetic	74	Not different from normal	
Diabetic	89	14	8
Depleted or iron[2]	77	Not different from normal	
Not depleted of Iron	75	13	9

[1] Age and sex matched with hemochromatosis patients.
[2] After 18 months of phlebotomy therapy.
*Based on data of Niederau, et al.[149]

biopsies may indicate regression of hepatic fibrosis. The 30 percent probability of hepatocellular carcinoma is not diminished by treatment once there is hepatic fibrosis.[153] An increased frequency of extrahepatic carcinomas, such as lung cancer, has also been reported[154] but has not been observed in other large series. Dilatational cardiomyopathy may progress despite adequate iron removal.[115] Arthritis may first appear after adequate iron depletion. Conversely, the severity of diabetes may lessen or progression of diabetes may be averted, cardiac function is usually improved by iron depletion, the cutaneous hyperpigmentation nearly always clears, and symptoms of debilitating fatigue and abdominal pains may subside. If treatment is begun before age 40, gonadal insufficiency may improve.[105,156]

Patients who have required liver transplant for late-stage hemochromatosis have a median survival of approximately 3 years, compared with median survival greater than 7 years when liver transplantation has been for other causes such as alcoholic cirrhosis.[157,158] This relatively poor posttransplant prognosis applies both to those who have hepatocellular carcinoma and to those who do not.

OTHER CAUSES OF HEMOCHROMATOSIS

CHRONIC ANEMIAS

Many chronic severe anemias are associated with iron overloading. Best recognized is that which accompanies thalassemia major. Severe iron overloading may also occur in patients with congenital dyserythropoietic anemia, pyruvate kinase deficiency anemia, or glucose-6-phosphate deficiency hemolytic anemia, even in patients who have not required transfusion. Iron overload appears to be rare in hereditary spherocytosis and unusual in thalassemia minor. Some patients with these disorders who have iron overload appear independently also to be hereditary hemochromatosis homozygotes or heterozygotes.[159–161] The clinical features of secondary hemochromatosis are the same as those of hereditary hemochromatosis, with the additional feature of anemia. Complications of hemochromatosis, are common causes of fatality. In sideroblastic anemias, iron overloading is the rule. A few such patients can be effectively treated by phlebotomy, particularly if they respond to pyridoxine administration; unfortunately, most cannot. Before erythropoeitin became available for treatment, iron overloading often followed frequent transfusions in chronic renal failure patients who received long-term dialysis therapy.[162]

Anemic patients with iron overloading may require daily infusion of 1 to 2 g (20–40 mg/kg) of desferrioxamine-B by portable battery-operated pump, for 8- to 12-h intervals, which may be overnight.[161,163] The oral administration of 100 to 500 mg of vitamin C, after each infusion has been started, enhances the rate of excretion of iron induced by chelation with desferrioxamine.[164] (See Chap. 46 for details.) An orally effective iron chelator is needed, but at this time, none of those that have been tested is safe and effective nor has any been approved for use in the United States. Patients who are not anemic, or only slightly anemic, but who have become iron overloaded as a result of chronic ingestion of iron can be treated effectively by phlebotomy, although it is unusual in nonanemic patients for enough iron to have been accumulated that such therapy is required.

AFRICAN NUTRITIONAL HEMOCHROMATOSIS (BANTU SIDEROSIS)

An endemic form of acquired hemochromatosis occurs in African people who consume a native beer brewed in iron kegs.[165,166] A liter of this beer contains 80 mg of iron, so those who drink large amounts may ingest hundreds of milligrams of iron daily. There may also be a genetic factor: In Zimbabwean villages 30 percent of the people were believed to be heterozygotes for a hemochromatosis gene that has not been identified and is not HLA-linked. Both homozygotes and heterozygotes were at risk for hemochromatosis if they consumed the native beer.[167] It is not known how widespread this gene is outside of Zimbabwe nor whether it is prevalent in African Americans.

The features of this disorder are similar to those described above for hereditary hemochromatosis except that iron deposition is predominantly in cells of the monocyte-macrophage system. However, iron is deposited in parenchymal cells of various organs, and in the synovial lining cells of joints, concurrently with the development of hepatic cirrhosis.[168]

SHUNT SIDEROSIS

Splenorenal or portal-caval shunting, in the treatment of portal hypertension, has led to astonishingly rapid iron accumulation in many reported patients.[169,170] This may occur in as many as 20 percent of patients so treated. Severe hemochromatosis has developed within 16 months of the shunting procedure, leading to death from cardiomyopathy. In rare instances the rapid development of hemochromatosis in patients with portal hypertension has been ascribed to intrahepatic shunting.[171]

PORPHYRIA CUTANEA TARDA (PCT)

PCT is a disorder with principally cutaneous manifestations which is also usually associated with iron overload that may result in hepatic cirrhosis. The underlying cause appears to be reduced activity of uroporphyrinogen decarboxylase. (See Chap. 62.) Both in humans with porphyria cutanea tarda and in mice with experimental porphyria induced by injections of iron dextran, uroporphyrin crystals and ferritin accumulate in the same hepatocytes, as demonstrated by electron microscopy.[172] Patients with the acquired form of PCT have very high prevalence of mutations of the HFE gene, 845 A in northern Europe[173–175] and 187G in southern Europe.[176] Persons with this disease have a higher frequency of hepatitis C infection than in the general population.[177] The iron overload that occurs in PCT is less than in hereditary hemochromatosis, but PCT is usually ameliorated by phlebotomy to reduce iron stores.[178,179]

NEONATAL HEMOCHROMATOSIS

A rare and usually lethal disorder of the newborn is characterized by marked iron deposition in the liver, sometimes in conjunction with giant cell hepatitis.[180–183] The cause of this disorder is unknown. No HFE mutations have been found in this disorder.[15] Because it has occurred in siblings, and in half-siblings born of two unaffected mothers, it may be conditioned by autosomal recessive inheritance.[184,185] Liver transplantation has been successful.[186]

JUVENILE HEMOCHROMATOSIS

Some patients of hereditary hemochromatosis have presented prior to age 20 with severe manifestations, especially cardiac dysfunction and hypogonadism.[184,187–192] As in the adult form, males predominate. Inheritance appears to be autosomal recessive. Juvenile hemochromatosis is an entity distinct from the commoner adult onset hereditary hemochromatosis, and it is not due to a mutation of the HFE gene.[193,194] At least in one family, the disorder has been linked to chromosome 1q.[195] Hypogonadism, in a young male, particularly when accompanied by cardiac dysfunction or arrhythmia, should alert the physician to the possibility of juvenile hemochromatosis.

DISORDERS OF IRON TRANSPORT

CONGENITAL ATRANSFERRINEMIA

In 1961, Heilmeyer and coworkers[196] described congenital atransferrinemia in a young girl with severe congenital hypochromic anemia and marked, generalized iron overload. Additional patients have been reported from Slovakia,[197–199] two (siblings) from Japan,[200–202] two (siblings) from Mexico,[203,204] one from France,[205] and one from Samoa.[206] To our knowledge, the only patient in the United States is a young woman from Illinois, who has been observed by one of the authors (VFF) for 15 years. An apparently identical disorder has been described in a strain of inbred mice.[199,207]

Atransferrinemia results in reduced delivery of iron to the marrow and reduced hemoglobin synthesis. Secondarily, there is marked increase in iron absorption by the intestinal mucosa that results in severe iron overload.

The predominant clinical features are pallor and fatigue. A systolic ejection cardiac murmur has been present in most patients. Some patients have mild hepatomegaly. Two patients died at age 7 from refractory congestive heart failure. The autopsy in both showed marked hemosiderosis and fibrosis of liver, pancreas, thyroid, myocardium, and kidneys but no iron in the marrow. Both of these patients had received numerous transfusions. Heilmeyer's patient suffered from recurrent infections, and another patient died of pneumonia.

The anemia has been of variable severity. Total iron-binding capacity has ranged from 4.1 to 14.0 μmol/liter (24 to 81 μg/dl), and transferrin concentration has been 0 to 5 μmol/liter (0 to 39 mg/dl) [normal value 25 to 40 μmol/liter (200 to 300 mg/dL)]. Measurement of transferrin in these patients has been by radial immunodiffusion method or immunoelectrophoresis. The absence or small diameter of the precipitin ring in reported patients strongly implies a quantitative deficiency of transferrin rather than a functionally abnormal protein. There may be normal to enhanced iron absorption from the gastrointestinal tract, normal to moderately accelerated plasma iron clearance, and diminished incorporation of iron into hemoglobin (ranging from 7 to 55 percent; normal 30 to 100 percent).[198,200,206] The infusion of either normal plasma or purified apotransferrin is followed in 10 to 14 days by reticulocytosis and then by a rise in hemoglobin concentration.[198,201] If this therapy is repeated once or twice monthly, the patient becomes hematologically normal within a few months, although iron stores and serum ferritin concentration remain elevated. This response permits systematic removal of excess iron by phlebotomy.

DIFFERENTIAL DIAGNOSIS

Congenital atransferrinemia may be differentiated from other causes of hypochromic anemia by low serum iron concentration together with very low total iron-binding capacity, and no transferrin in serum by immunologic test. Atransferrinemia has also been described in association with the nephrotic syndrome[208,209] and in a patient with erythroleukemia.[210] One patient has been described who had a functional disorder of transferrin due to transferrin-IgG-transferrin immune complexes,[211] clinical and laboratory features of hemochromatosis, marked elevation in serum iron concentration, and absence of stainable iron in marrow; the two latter findings distinguish this patient from congenital atransferrinemia.

TREATMENT

Good clinical reponses follow infusion of normal human plasma or of purified apotransferrin. The rise in plasma transferrin concentration does not persist beyond a week. However, the cohort of erythroblasts that take up iron during this time will mature to circulate for as long as 4 months. Therefore it may suffice to infuse normal plasma or transferrin at intervals of 2 to 4 months. The author's patient received 500 ml of plasma intravenously, from the same small group of donors, immediately preceded by a 500 ml phlebotomy, monthly for more than 10 years. After 120 phlebotomies, she was hematologically normal and completely iron depleted, with serum ferritin concentration less than 5 μg/L. However, she has hypopituitary hypogonadism requiring replacement estrogen therapy. The two Japanese patients have been given 1 to 2 g of highly purified apotransferrin intravenously every 3 to 4 months for 4 to 7 years with good effect and without the development of antitransferrin antibodies.[212] The Slovak patient was also given apotransferrin infusions and desferrioxamine to remove excess iron. This patient now has arthropathy and siderosis of synovial membranes. Use of purified transferrin reduces the risk of hepatitis that would attend infusion of whole plasma. The need for erythrocyte transfusion and the consequent long-term risk of hemochromatosis are also obviated by use of transferrin infusion. Purified transferrin is not available for therapy in the United States. However, the monthly infusion of 1 single-donor unit of normal human plasma has enabled the American patient to be treated effectively, including phlebotomies to remove excess iron, and without any complications from this treatment. It does not seem practical to treat with desferrioxamine patients who can be treated more effectively by phlebotomy.

Of the nine known patients, two died of infection, one died of cardiac failure, and one drowned while swimming. The current status of two patients is unknown. Four patients were believed to be still living in 1999. One of the Japanese patients no longer needs injections of apotransferrin.[213]

CONGENITAL ACERULOPLASMINEMIA

Several cases of congenital aceruloplasminemia have been reported from Japan and from Europe, This disorder is characterized by dementia, dystonia, dysarthria, diabetes, and degeneration of the retina.[214-219]

Ceruloplasmin converts Fe^{+2} to Fe^{+3}. In the ferrous form, iron traverses cell membranes but cannot bind to transferrin and thus it cannot be delivered efficiently to erythroblasts. Iron that is absorbed and that enters plasma as Fe^{+2} is deposited in the liver, pancreas, central nervous system, and retina. Ceruloplasmin does not cross the blood-brain barrier. However, astrocytes and other neuroglia normally contain ceruloplasmin in their cell membranes, where it oxidizes Fe^{+2} and prevents its entry into cells of the central nervous system. In aceruloplasminemia, neuroglia are unable to synthesize ceruloplasmin.[220,221]

Retinal degeneration is peripheral, where there is iron deposition and loss of photoreceptor cells but little visual impairment. Other features include late-onset diabetes mellitus, marked iron deposition in liver and pancreatic islets, loss of islet β cells, mild hypochromic, microcytic anemia, and absence of plasma ceruloplasmin. Serum copper concentration is reduced, but copper metabolism is normal, and tissue copper concentration is not increased. Increased plasma lipid peroxidation occurs.[222] Hepatocyte injury or cirrhosis are not observed.

Iron uptake in basal ganglia can be demonstrated on nuclear magnetic resonance image analysis by decreased T2-weighted signal.

Transmission is as an autosomal recessive disorder. Mutations of the ceruloplasmin gene, which resides on chromosome 3, have been described in patients with this disorder.[216,218,219,223]

Congenital aceruloplasminemia has some resemblance to Wilson disease in that both conditions are characterized by tremor and low concentrations of ceruloplasmin in serum. In Wilson disease there is usually measurable but low serum ceruloplasmin; in aceruloplasminemia there is none. Wilson disease is characterized by Kayser-Fleischer corneal ring, copper deposition in liver and hepatic cirrhosis, features lacking in aceruloplasminemia. Urinary copper excretion is increased in Wilson disease but not in aceruloplasminemia. Aceruloplasminemia is characterized by iron deficiency anemia, diabetes mellitus, and excess iron in liver and basal ganglia that can be demonstrated by MRI scan, features not found in Wilson disease. Menke disease is a disorder of copper metabolism that is also characterized by very low serum ceruloplasmin and copper concentrations and reduced copper content of liver. Menke disease is manifested in infancy by mental retardation, convulsions, abnormalities of hair, osteoporosis, and death usually within the first few years of life.

Therapy recommended for congenital aceruloplasminemia is iron chelation with desferrioxamine,[224] but the effectiveness of this therapy is as yet unknown.

RELATED CONDITIONS

CONGENITAL CATARACT WITH HYPERFERRITINEMIA

Several families have been reported in which congenital nuclear cataracts were associated with hyperferritinemia but without iron overload.[225-232] Plasma concentrations of iron, TIBC, and transferrin saturation were normal, but serum ferritin concentration values were several thousand μg/liter. The ferritin contained only the L subunit. The inheritance is autosomal dominant. Hyperferritinemia is due to mutations in the iron-responsive element (IRE) of the mRNA for apoferritin, causing unregulated apoferritin synthesis. Iron is not deposited in the lenses. However, the unregulated synthesis of a protein within the cells of the lens may have an adverse colloid osmotic effect. Other cells appear not to be adversely affected.

SUPERFICIAL HEMOSIDEROSIS OF THE CENTRAL NERVOUS SYSTEM

This condition results from recurrent subarachnoid hemorrhages, with deposition of iron in the meninges. It may be associated with ataxia and other central nervous system manifestations.[233]

HEMOCHROMATOSIS IN OTHER SPECIES

A disorder indistinguishable from human hereditary hemochromatosis has been reported from California in several members of two herds of the Saler breed of cattle[234] and also in a Channel-billed Toucan.[235] Experimental strains of mice that are homozygous for ''knockout'' deletions of the HFE gene or β2 microglobulin gene develop increased iron levels.[236-239]

REFERENCES

1. Trousseau A: Glycosurie, diabète sucré, in Clinique Médicale de l'Hôtel-Dieu de Paris, p 662. J-B Baillière, Paris, 1865.
2. Troisier E: Diabète sucré. Bull Mem Soc Anat Paris 46:231, 1871.
3. Von Recklinghausen H: Über Hämochromatose. Tageblatt der 62 Versammlung deutscher Naturforscher und Ärtzte, 1889.

4. Sheldon JH: Haemochromatosis. Oxford University Press, London, 1935.

5. Davis WD, Arrowsmith WR: The effect of repeated phlebotomies in hemochromatosis. *J Lab Clin Med* 39:526, 1952.

6. Finch SC, Finch CA: Idiopathic hemochromatosis, an iron storage disease. A. Iron metabolism in hemochromatosis. *Medicine (Baltimore)* 34:381, 1955.

7. Simon M, Pawlotsky Y, Bourel M, Fauchet R, Genetet B: Hemochromatose idiopathique: Maladie associée a l'antigène tissulaire HL-A 3? (letter to the editor). *Nouv Presse Med* 4:1432, 1975.

8. Bomford A, Eddleston ALWF, Kennedy LA, Batchelor JR, Williams R: Histocompatibility antigens as markers of abnormal iron metabolism in patients with idiopathic haemochromatosis and their relatives. *Lancet* 1:327, 1977.

9. Simon M, Bourel M, Genetet B, Fauchet R, Edan G, Brissot P: Idiopathic hemochromatosis and iron overload in alcoholic liver disease: differentiation by HLA phenotype. *Gastroenterology* 73:655, 1977.

10. Powell LW, Ferluga J, Halliday JW, Bassett ML, Kohonel-Corish M: Genetic hemochromatosis and HLA linkage. *Hum Genet* 77:55, 1987.

11. Edwards CQ, Griffen LM, Dadone MM, Skolnick MH, Kushner JP: Mapping the locus for hereditary hemochromatosis: localization between HLA-B and HLA-A. *Am J Hum Genet* 38:805, 1986.

12. Simon M, Le Mignon L, Fauchet R, et al: A study of 609 HLA haplotypes marking for the hemochromatosis gene: (1) mapping of the gene near the HLA-A focus and characters required to define a heterozygous population and (2) hypothesis concerning the underlying cause of hemochromatosis-HLA association. *Am J Hum Genet* 41:89, 1987.

13. Simon M, Brissot P: The genetics of haemochromatosis. *J Hepatol* 6:116, 1988.

14. Feder JN, Gnirke A, Thomas W, et al: A novel MHC class I-like gene is mutated in patients with hereditary haemochromatosis [see comments]. *Nature Genet* 13:399, 1996.

15. Beutler E, Gelbart T, West C, et al: Mutation analysis in hereditary hemochromatosis. *Blood Cells, Mol Dis* 22:187, 1996.

16. Beutler E: The significance of the 187G (H63D) mutation in hemochromatosis. *Am J Hum Genet* 61:762, 1997.

17. Risch N: Haemochromatosis, HFE and genetic complexity. *Nat Genet* 17:375, 1997.

18. Fairbanks VF, Brandhagen DJ, Thibodeau SN, Snow K, Wollan PC: H63D is an haemochromatosis associated allele. *Gut* 43:441, 1998.

19. Olsson KS, Ritter B, Rosen U, Heidman PA, Staugard F: Prevalence of iron overload in central Sweden. *Acta Med Scand* 213:145, 1983.

20. Borwein ST, Ghent CN, Flanagan PR, Chamberlain MJ, Valberg LS: Genetic and phenotypic expression of hemochromatosis in Canadians. *Clin Invest Med* 6:171, 1983.

21. Meyer TE, Baynes RD, Bothwell TH, et al: Phenotypic expression of the HLA-linked iron-loading gene in the Afrikaner population of the western cape. *S Afr Med J* 73:269, 1988.

22. Ballot D, Meyer TE, Bothwell TH, et al: Idiopathic haemochromatosis: family studies and results of a pilot prevalence survey. *S Afr Med J* 71:639, 1987.

23. Elliott R, Tait A, Lin BPC, Smith CI, Dent OF: Prevalence of hemochromatosis in a random sample of asymptomatic men. *Aust N Z J Med* 16:491, 1986.

24. Mercier G, Bathelier C, Lucotte G: Frequency of the C282Y mutation of hemochromatosis in five French populations. *BCMD* 24:165, 1998.

25. Baiget M, Barcelo MJ, Gimferrer E: Frequency of the HFE C282Y and H63D mutations in distinct ethnic groups living in Spain [letter]. *J Med Genet* 35:701, 1998.

26. Porto G, Vicente C, Fraga J, da Silva BM, de Sousa M: Importance of establishing appropriate local reference values for the screening of hemochromatosis: a study of three different control populations and 136 hemochromatosis family members. Hemochromatosis Clinical and Research Group. *J Lab Clin Med* 119:295, 1992.

27. Bothwell TH, Hitzeroth HW: Hereditary haemochromatosis—a South African perspective [editorial]. *S Afr Med J* 83:236, 1993.

28. Jouanolle AM, Fergelot P, Raoul ML, et al: Prevalence of the C282Y mutation in Brittany: penetrance of genetic hemochromatosis? *Ann Genet* 41:195, 1998.

29. Willis G, Jennings BA, Goodman E, Fellows IW, Wimperis JZ: A high prevalence of HLA-H 845A mutations in hemochromatosis patients and the normal population in eastern England. *Blood Cells Mol Dis* 23:288, 1997.

30. Merryweather-Clarke AT, Pointon JJ, Shearman JD, Robson KJ: Global prevalence of putative haemochromatosis mutations [see comments]. *J Med Genet* 34:275, 1997.

31. Feder JN, Penny DM, Irrinki A, et al: The hemochromatosis gene product complexes with the transferrin receptor and lowers its affinity for ligand binding. *Proc Natl Acad Sci USA* 95:1472, 1998.

32. Lebron JA, Bjorkman PJ: The transferrin receptor binding site on HFE, the class I MHC-related protein mutated in hereditary hemochromatosis. *J Mol Biol* 289:1109, 1999.

33. Roy CN, Penny DM, Feder JN, Enns CA: The hereditary hemochromatosis preotein, HFE, specifically regulates transferrin-mediated iron uptake in HeLa cells. *J Biol Chem* 274:9022, 1999.

34. Zoller H, Pietrangelo A, Vogel W, Weiss G: Duodenal metal-transporter (DMT-1), NRAMP-2) expression in patients with hereditary haemochromatosis. *Lancet* 353:2120, 1999.

35. Olatunbosun D, Corbett WE, Ludwig J, Valberg LS: Alteration of cobalt absorption in portal cirrhosis and idiopathic hemochromatosis. *J Lab Clin Med* 75:754, 1970.

36. Arstila AU, Smith MA, Trump BF: Microsomal lipid peroxidation: morphological characterization. *Science* 175:530, 1972.

37. Gutteridge JMC, Rowley DA, Griffiths E, Halliwell B: Low molecular weight iron complexes and oxygen radical reactions in idiopathic haemochromatosis. *Clin Sci* 68:463, 1985.

38. Loreal O, Deugnier Y, Moirand R, et al: Liver fibrosis in genetic hemochromatosis. Respective roles of iron and non-iron-related factors in 127 homozygous patients. *J Hepatol* 16:122, 1992.

39. Piperno A, Vergani A, Malosio I, et al: Hepatic iron overload in patients with chronic viral hepatitis: role of HFE gene mutations. *Hepatology* 28:1105, 1998.

40. Kuvibidila S: Iron deficiency, cell-mediated immunity and resistance against infection: present knowledge and controversies. *Nutr Res* 7:989, 1987.

41. Weinberg ED: Iron withholding: a defense against infection and neoplasia. *Physiol Rev* 64:65, 1984.

42. Van Asbeck BS, Marx JJM, Struyvenberg A, Verhoef J: Functional defects in phagocytic cells from patients with iron overload. *J Infect* 8:232, 1984.

43. Block M, Moore G, Wasi P, Haiby G: Histogenesis of the hepatic lesion in primary hemochromatosis: with consideration of the pseudo-iron deficient state produced by phlebotomies. *Am J Pathol* 47:89, 1965.

44. Powell LW, Kerr JFR: The pathology of the liver in hemochromatosis. *Pathol Annu* 5:317, 1975.

45. Deugnier YM, Loreal O, Turlin B, et al: Liver pathology in genetic hemochromatosis: a review of 135 homozygous cases and their bioclinical correlations. *Gastroenterology* 102:2050, 1992.

46. Kontogeorgos G, Handy S, Kovacs K, Horvath E, Scheithauer BW: The anterior pituitary in hemochromatosis. *Endo Pathol* 7:159, 1999.

47. Lebron JA, Bennett MJ, Vaughn DE, et al: Crystal structure of the hemochromatosis protein HFE and characterization of its interaction with transferrin receptor. *Cell* 93:111, 1998.

48. Mura C, Raguenes O, Ferec C: HFE mutations analysis in 711 hemochromatosis probands: evidence for S65C implication in mild form of hemochromatosis. *Blood* 93:2502, 1999.

49. Spriggs EL, Harris PE, Best LG: Hemochromatosis mutations C282Y and H63D in "cis" phase. *Am J Hum Genet* 65:A492, 1999.

50. Pietrangelo A, Montosi G, Totaro A, Garuti C, Conte D: Hereditary hemochromatosis in adults without pathogenic mutations in the hemochromatosis gene. *N Engl J Med* 341:725, 1999.

51. Lee PL, Gelbart T, West C, Halloran C, Beutler E: The human Nramp2 gene: characterization of the gene structure, alternative splicing, promoter region and polymorphisms. *BCMD* 24:199, 1998.

52. Simon M, Alexandre J-L, Fauchet R, et al: The genetics of hemochromatosis. *Prog Med Genet* 4:135, 1980.

53. Bassett ML, Halliday JW, Powell LW: HLA typing in idiopathic hemochromatosis: distinction between homozygotes and heterozygotes with biochemical expression. *Hepatology* 1:120, 1981.

54. Cartwright GE, Edwards CQ, Kravitz K, et al: Hereditary hemochromatosis: phenotype expression of the disease. *N Engl J Med* 301:175, 1979.

55. Simon M, Bourel M, Genetet B, Fauchet R: Idiopathic hemochromatosis:

demonstration of recessive transmission and early detection by family HLA typing. *N Engl J Med* 297:1017, 1977.

56. Lesage GD, Baldus WP, Fairbanks VF, et al: Hemochromatosis: genetic or alcohol-induced? *Gastroenterology* 84:1471, 1983.

57. Edwards CQ, Cartwright GE, Skolnick MH, Amos DB: Homozygosity for hemochromatosis: clinical manifestations. *Ann Intern Med* 93:519, 1980.

58. Murphy S, Curran MD, McDougall N, et al: High incidence of the Cys 282 Tyr mutation in the HFE gene in the Irish population—implications for haemochromatosis. *Tissue Antigens* 52:484, 1998.

59. Lucotte G: Celtic origin of the C282Y mutation of hemochromatosis. *BCMD* 28:433, 1998.

60. Ajioka RS, Jorde LB, Gruen JR, et al: Haplotype analysis of hemochromatosis: evaluation of different linkage-disequilibrium approaches and evolution of disease chromosomes. *Am J Hum Genet* 60:1439, 1997.

61. Thomas W, Fullan A, Loeb DB, McClelland EE, Bacon BR, Wolff RK: A haplotype and linkage disequilibrium analysis of the hereditary hemochromatosis gene region. *Hum Genet* 102:517, 1998.

62. Rochette J, Pointon JJ, Fisher CA, et al: Multicentric origin of hemochromatosis gene (HFE) mutations. *Am J Hum Genet* 64:1056, 1999.

63. Ballot D, Meyer TE, Bothwell TH, et al: Idiopathic haemochromatosis: family studies and results of a pilot prevalence survey. *S Afr Med J* 71:639, 1987.

64. MacSween RNM, Scott AR: Hepatic cirrhosis: a clinico-pathological review of 520 cases. *J Clin Pathol* 26:936, 1973.

65. De Braekeleer M, Vigneault A, Simard H: Population genetics of hereditary hemochromatosis in Saguenay Lac-Saint-Jean (Quebec, Canada). *Ann Genet* 35:202, 1992.

66. de Braekeleer M: A prevalence and fertility study of haemochromatosis in Saguenay-Lac-Saint-Jean. *Ann Hum Biol* 20:501, 1993.

67. Cardoso EM, Stal P, Hagen K, et al: HFE mutations in patients with hereditary haemochromatosis in Sweden. *J Intern Med* 243:203, 1998.

68. Phatak PD, Sham RL, Raubertas RF, et al: Prevalence of hereditary hemochromatosis in 16031 primary care patients. *Ann Intern Med* 129:954, 1998.

69. Bradley LA, Johnson DD, Palomaki GE, Haddow JE, Robertson NH, Ferrie R: Hereditary haemochromatosis mutation frequencies in the general population. *J Med Screen* 5:34, 1998.

70. Beutler E, Gelbart T: HLA-H mutations in the Ashkenazi Jewish population. *Blood Cells Mol Dis* 23:95, 1997.

71. Barton JC, Barton NH, Alford TJ: Diagnosis of hemochromatosis probands in a community hospital. *Am J Med* 103:498, 1997.

72. Barton JC, Shih WW, Sawada-Hirai R, et al: Genetic and clinical description of hemochromatosis probands and heterozygotes: evidence that multiple genes linked to the major histocompatibility complex are responsible for hemochromatosis. *Blood Cells, Mol Dis* 23:135, 1997.

73. Olynyk JK, Cullen DJ, Aquilia S, Rossi E, Summerville L, Powell LW: A population-based study of the clinical expression of the hemochromatosis gene. *N Engl J Med* 341:718, 1999.

74. Edwards CQ, Griffen LM, Kushner JP: The morbidity of hemochromatosis among clinically unselected homozygotes: preliminary report. *Adv Exp Med Biol* 356:303, 1994.

75. Adams PC, Kertesz AE, Valberg LS: Clinical presentation of hemochromatosis: a changing scene. *Am J Med* 90:445, 1991.

76. Bulaj ZJ, Edwards CQ, Ajioka RS, Phillips JD, Kushner JP: Frequency of disease related morbidity in 214 unselected hemochromatosis homozygotes. *Blood* 94 (suppl): (in press).

77. Beutler E, Felitti V, Gelbart T, Ho N: Genetics of iron storage and hemochromatosis. *Drug Metab Dispos* (in press).

78. Willis G, Wimperis JZ, Lonsdale R, Sampson MJ, Jennings BA: Low penetrance of HFE mutation in an English population. *Blood* 92 (suppl):324A, 1998.

79. Crawford DH, Jazwinska EC, Cullen LM, Powell LW: Expression of HLA-linked hemochromatosis in subjects homozygous or heterozygous for the C282Y mutation. *Gastroenterology* 114:1003, 1998.

80. Barton JC, Acton RT: Population screening for hemochromatosis: has the time finally come? *Curr Gastroenterol Rep* 2:in press, 1999.

81. Brandhagen DJ, Fairbanks VF, Baldus WP, et al: Prevalence and clinical significance of HFE gene mutations in normal blood donors and in patients with iron overload. *Gastroenterology* 114:A1214, 1998.

82. Moirand R, Adams PC, Bicheler V, Brissot P, Deugnier Y: Clinical

83. Jones HR, Jr., Hedley-Whyte ET: Idiopathic hemochromatosis (IHC): dementia and ataxia as presenting signs. *Neurology* 33:1479, 1983.

84. Hamilton E, Williams R, Barlow KA, Smith PM: The arthropathy of idiopathic haemochromatosis. *Q J Med* 37:171, 1968.

85. Hamilton EBD, Bomford AB, Laws JW, Williams R: The natural history of arthritis in idiopathic haemochromatosis: progression of the clinical and radiological features over ten years. *Q J Med* 50:321, 1981.

86. Schmacher HR Jr: Hemochromatosis and arthritis. *Arthritis Rheum* 7:41, 1964.

87. Mathews JL, Williams HJ: Arthritis in hereditary hemochromatosis. *Arthritis Rheum* 30:1137, 1987.

88. Cutler DJ, Isner JM, Bracey AW, et al: Hemochromatosis heart disease: an unemphasized cause of potentially reversible restrictive cardiomyopathy. *Am J Med* 69:923, 1980.

89. Olson LJ, Edwards WD, McCall JT, Ilstrup DM, Gersh BJ: Cardiac iron deposition in idiopathic hemochromatosis: Histologic and analytic assessment of 14 hearts from autopsy. *J Am Coll Cardiol* 10:1239, 1987.

90. Leon MB, Borer JS, Bacharach SL, et al: Detection of early cardiac dysfunction in patients with severe beta-thalassemia and chronic iron overload. *N Engl J Med* 301:1143, 1979.

91. Miller M, Hutchins GM: Hemochromatosis, multiorgan hemosiderosis, and coronary artery disease. *JAMA* 272:231, 1994.

92. Salonen JT, Tuomainen TP, Salonen R, Lakka TA, Nyyssonen K: Donation of blood is associated with reduced risk of myocardial infarction. The Kuopio Ischaemic Heart Disease Risk Factor Study. *Am J Epidemiol* 148:445, 1998.

93. Tuomainen TP, Punnonen K, Nyyssonen K, Salonen JT: Association between body iron stores and the risk of acute myocardial infarction in men. *Circulation* 97:1461, 1998.

94. Tuomainen TP, Salonen R, Nyyssonen K, Salonen JT: Cohort study of relation between donating blood and risk of myocardial infarction in 2682 men in eastern Finland [see comments]. *BMJ* 314:793, 1997.

95. Salonen JT, Nyyssonen K, Korpela H, Tuomilehto J, Seppanen R, Salonen R: High stored iron levels are associated with excess risk of myocardial infarction in eastern Finnish men. *Circulation* 86:803, 1992.

96. Manttari M, Manninen V, Huttunen JK, et al: Serum ferritin and ceruloplasmin as coronary risk factors. *Eur Heart J* 15:1599, 1994.

97. Franco RF, Zago MA, Trip MD, et al: Prevalence of hereditary haemochromatosis in premature atherosclerotic vascular disease. *Br J Haematol* 102:1172, 1998.

98. Solymoss BC, Marcil M, Gilfix BM, Gelinas F, Poitras AM, Campeau L: The place of ferritin among risk factors associated with coronary artery disease. *Coron Artery Dis* 5:231, 1994.

99. Baer DM, Tekawa IS, Hurley LB: Iron stores are not associated with acute myocardial infarction. *Circulation* 89:2915, 1994.

100. Sempos CT, Looker AC, Gillum RF, Makuc DM: Body iron stores and the risk of coronary heart disease. *N Engl J Med* 330:1119, 1994.

101. Saddi R, Feingold J: Hémochromatose idiopathique et diabète. *Rev Fr Études Clin Biol* 14:252, 1969.

102. Koerner M: Peripheral neuropathy in idiopathic hemochromatosis (letter to the editor). *Neurology* 34:843, 1984.

103. Walton C, Kelly WF, Laing I, Bu'lock DE: Endocrine abnormalities in idiopathic haemochromatosis. *Q J Med* 52:99, 1983.

104. McNeil LW, McKee LC, Jr., Lorber D, Rabin D: The endocrine manifestations of hemochromatosis. *Am J Med Sci* 285(3):7, 1983.

105. Piperno A, Rivolta MR, D'Alba R, et al: Preclinical hypogonadism in genetic hemochromatosis in the early stage of the disease: evidence of hypothalamic dysfunction. *J Endocrinol Invest* 15:423, 1992.

106. Edwards CQ, Kelly TM, Ellwein G, Kushner JP: Thyroid disease in hemochromatosis: Increased incidence in homozygous men. *Arch Intern Med* 143:1890, 1983.

107. Jenkins T, Bothwell TH, Maier G, Laidler A: Is transferrin normal in idiopathic haemochromatosis. *Br J Haematol* 51:493, 1982.

108. Milman N, Eiberg H, Thymann M, Fenger K: Transferrin subtypes in 51 Danish patients with hereditary haemochromatosis and in 847 normal subjects. *Hum Genet* 88:475, 1992.

109. Huaux JP, Geubel A, Koch MC, Malghem J, Maldauge B, Devogelaer JP: The arthritis of hemochromatosis: a review of 25 cases with special reference to chrondocalcinosis, and a comparison with patients with primary hyperparathyroidism and controls. *Clin Rheumatol* 5:317, 1986.

110. Schumacher HR Jr: Articular cartilage in the degenerative arthropathy of hemochromatosis. *Arthritis Rheum* 25:1460, 1982.

111. Adamson TC III, Resnik CS, Guerra J, Jr, Vint VC, Weisman MH, Resnick D: Hand and wrist arthropathies of hemochromatosis and calcium pyrophosphate deposition disease: distinct radiographic features. *Radiology* 147:377, 1983.

112. Askari AD, Muir WA, Rosner IA, Moskowitz RW, McLaren GD, Braun WE: Arthritis of hemochromatosis: clinical spectrum, relation to histocompatibility antigens, and effectiveness of early phlebotomy. *Am J Med* 75:957, 1983.

113. Faraawi R, Harth M, Kertesz A, Bell D: Arthritis in hemochromatosis. *J Rheumatol* 20:448, 1993.

114. Montgomery KD, Williams JR, Sculco TP, DiCarlo E: Clinical and pathologic findings in hemochromatosis hip arthropathy. *Clinical Orthopaedics and Related Research* (347):179, 1998.

115. Edwards CQ, Kushner JP: Screening for hemochromatosis. *N Engl J Med* 328:1616, 1993.

116. Phatak PD, Guzman G, Woll JE, Robeson A, Phelps CE: Cost-effectiveness of screening for hereditary hemochromatosis. *Arch Intern Med* 154:769, 1994.

117. Balan V, Baldus W, Fairbanks VF, Michels V, Burritt M, Klee GG: Screening for hemochromatosis: a cost-effectiveness study based on 12,258 patients. *Gastroenterology* 107:453, 1995.

118. Adams PC, Gregor JC, Kertesz AE, Valberg LS: Screening blood donors for hereditary hemochromatosis: decision analysis model based on a 30-year databse. *Gastroenterology* 109:177, 1995.

119. Edwards CQ: Early detection of hereditary hemochromatosis. *Ann Intern Med* 101:707, 1984.

120. Witte DL, Crosby WH, Edwards CQ, Fairbanks VF, Mitros FA: Practice guideline development task force of the College of American Pathologists. Hereditary hemochromatosis. [Review] [202 refs]. *Clin Chimica Acta* 245:139, 1996.

121. Niederau C, Niederau CM, Lange S, et al: Screening for hemochromatosis and iron deficiency in employees and primary care patients in Western Germany. *Ann Intern Med* 128:337, 1998.

122. Felitti VJ, Beutler E: New developments in hemochromatosis. *Am J Med Sci* 318:257, 1999.

123. Cogswell ME, Burke W, McDonnell SM, Franks AL: Screening for hemochromatosis. A public health perspective. [Review] [73 refs]. *Am J Prev Med* 16:134, 1999.

124. McDonnell SM, Witte DL, Cogswell ME, McIntyre R: Strategies to increase detection of hemochromatosis. [Review] [65 refs]. *Ann Intern Med* 129:987, 1998.

125. Wetterhall SF, Cogswell ME, Kowdley KV: Public health surveillance for hereditary hemochromatosis. [Review] [58 refs]. *Ann Intern Med* 129:980, 1998.

126. Cogswell ME, McDonnell SM, Khoury MJ, Franks AL, Burke W, Brittenham G: Iron overload, public health, and genetics: evaluating the evidence for hemochromatosis screening. [Review] [80 refs]. *Ann Intern Med* 129:971, 1998.

127. Herring WB, Gay RM: Absence of stainable bone marrow iron in hemochromatosis. *South Med J* 74:1088, 1981.

128. Dullman J, Wulfhekel U: The diagnostic significance of bone-marrow iron in hereditary hemochromatosis. *Ann NY Acad Sci* 526:357, 1988.

129. Ludwig J, Batts KP, Moyer TP, Baldus WP, Fairbanks VF: Liver biopsy diagnosis of homozygous hemochromatosis: a diagnostic algorithm. *Mayo Clin Proc* 68:263, 1993.

130. Bassett ML, Halliday JW, Powell LW: Value of hepatic iron measurements in early hemochromatosis and determination of the critical iron level associated with fibrosis. *Hepatology* 6:24, 1986.

131. Kowdley KV, Trainer TD, Saltzman JR, et al: Utility of hepatic iron index in American patients with hereditary hemochromatosis: a multicenter study. *Gastroenterology* 113:1270, 1997.

132. Ludwig J, Hashimoto E, Porayko MK, Moyer TP, Baldus WP: Hemosiderosis in cirrhosis: a study of 447 native livers [see comments]. *Gastroenterology* 112:882, 1997.

133. Cotler SJ, Bronner MP, Press RD, et al: End-stage liver disease without hemochromatosis associated with elevated hepatic iron index. *J Hepatol* 29:257, 1998.

134. Strasser SI, Kowdley KV, Sale GE, McDonald GB: Iron overload in bone marrow transplant recipients. *Bone Marrow Transplant* 22:167, 1998.

135. McGill DB, Rakela J, Zinsmeister AR, Ott BJ: A 21-year experience with

136. Jager HJ, Mehring U, Gotz GF, et al: Radiological features of the visceral and skeletal involvement of hemochromatosis. *Eur Radiol* 7:1199, 1997.

137. Ernst O, Sergent G, Bonvarlet P, Canva-Delcambre V, Paris JC, L'Hermine C: Hepatic iron overload: diagnosis and quantification with MR imaging. *Am J Roentgenol* 168:1205, 1997.

138. Lawrence SP, Caminer SJ, Yavorski RT, et al: Correlation of liver density by magnetic resonance imaging and hepatic iron levels. A noninvasive means to exclude homozygous hemochromatosis. *J Clin Gastroenterology* 23:113, 1996.

139. Macfarlane JD, Vreugdenhil GR, Doornbos J, van der Voet GB: Idiopathic haemochromatosis: magnetic resonance signal intensity ratios permit non-invasive diagnosis of low levels of iron overload. *Neth J Med* 47:49, 1995.

140. Gandon Y, Guyader D, Heautot JF: Hemochromatosis: diagnosis and quantification of liver iron with gradient-echo MR imaging. *Radiology* 193:533, 1994.

141. Waxman S, Eustace S, Hartnell GG: Myocardial involvement in primary hemochromatosis demonstrated by magnetic resonance imaging. *Am Heart J* 128:1047, 1994.

142. Siegelman ES, Mitchell DG, Outwater E, Munoz SJ, Rubin R: Idiopathic hemochromatosis: MR imaging findings in cirrhotic and precirrhotic patients. *Radiology* 188:637, 1993.

143. Thomsen C, Wiggers P, Ring-Larsen H, Christiansen E, Dalhoj J, Henriksen O, Christoffersen P: Identification of patients with hereditary haemochromatosis by magnetic resonance imaging and spectroscopic relaxation time measurements. [Review] [56 refs]. *Magn Reson Imaging* 10:867, 1992.

144. Adams PC, Kertesz AE, Valberg LS: Rate of iron reaccumulation following iron depletion in hereditary hemochromatosis. Implications for venesection therapy. *J Clin Gastroenterol* 16:207, 1993.

145. Blake PA, Merson MH, Weaver RE, Hollis DH, Heublein PC: Disease caused by a marine vibrio: clinical characteristics and epidemiology. *N Engl J Med* 300:1, 1979.

146. Wright AC, Simpson LM, Oliver JD: Role of iron in the pathogenesis of *Vibrio vulnificus* infections. *Infect Immun* 34:503, 1981.

147. Kruijs FJ, Tan TG: Casuïstiche Mededelingen: *Yersinia enterocolitica*-sepsis en cholecystitis bij een patiënte met primaire hemochromatose. *Ned Tijdschr Geneeskd* 128:2036, 1984.

148. Abbott M, Galloway A, Cunningham JL: Case report: haemochromatosis presenting with a double yersinia infection. *J Infect* 13:143, 1986.

149. Niederau C, Fischer R, Sonnenberg A, Stremmel W, Trampisch HJ, Strohmeyer G: Survival and causes of death in cirrhotic and in noncirrhotic patients with primary hemochromatosis. *N Engl J Med* 313:1256, 1985.

150. Williams R, Smith PM, Spicer EJF, Barry M, Sherlock S: Venesection therapy in idiopathic haemochromatosis: an analysis of 40 treated and 19 untreated patients. *Q J Med* 38:1, 1969.

151. Conte D, Piperno A, Mandelli C, et al: Clinical, biochemical and histological features of primary haemochromatosis: a report of 67 cases. *Liver* 6:310, 1986.

152. Fargion S, Mandelli C, Piperno A, et al: Survival and prognostic factors in 212 Italian patients with genetic hemochromatosis. *Hepatology* 15:655, 1992.

153. Deugnier YM, Guyader D, Crantock L, et al: Primary liver cancer in genetic hemochromatosis: a clinical, pathological, and pathogenetic study of 54 cases. *Gastroenterology* 104:228, 1993.

154. Ammann RW, Müller E, Bansky J, Schüler G, Häcki WH: High incidence of extrahepatic carcinomas in idiopathic hemochromatosis. *Scand J Gastroenterol* 15:733, 1980.

155. Westra WH, Hruban RH, Baughman KL, et al: Progressive hemochromatotic cardiomyopathy despite reversal of iron deposition after liver transplantation. *Am J Clin Pathol* 99:39, 1993.

156. Cundy T, Butler J, Bomford A, Williams R: Reversibility of hypogonadotrophic hypogonadism associated genetic haemochromatosis. *Clin Endocrinol* (Oxford) 38:617, 1993.

157. Tung BY, Farrell FJ, McCashland TM, et al: Long-term follow-up after liver transplantation in patients with hepatic iron overload. *Liver Transplant Surg* 5:369, 1999.

158. Brandhagen DJ, Alvarez W, Baldus WP, et al: Cirrhotic iron overload—

HFE genotypes and outcome after liver transplantation. *Bioiron '99* 316, 1999.

159. Mohler DN, Wheby MS: Case report: hemochromatosis heterozygotes may have significant iron overload when they also have hereditary spherocytosis. *Am J Med Sci* 292:320, 1986.

160. Young N, Henry W, Nienhuis AW: Treatment of primary hemochromatosis with deferoxamine. *JAMA* 241:1152, 1979.

161. Hakim RM, Stivelman JC, Schulman G, et al: Iron overload and mobilization in long-term hemodialysis patients. *Am J Kidney Dis* 10:293, 1987.

162. Schafer AI, Cheron RG, Dluhy R, et al: Clinical consequences of acquired transfusional iron overload in adults. *N Engl J Med* 304:319, 1981.

163. Propper RD, Cooper B, Rufo RR, et al: Continuous subcutaneous administration of deferoxamine in patients with iron overload. *N Engl J Med* 297:418, 1977.

164. O'Brien RT: Ascorbic acid enhancement of desferrioxamine-induced urinary iron excretion in thalassemia major. *Ann NY Acad Sci* 232:221, 1974.

165. Buchanan WM: Bantu siderosis—a review. *Centr Afr J Med* 15:105, 1969.

166. Walker ARP, Arvidsson B: Iron "overload" in the South African Bantu. *Trans R Soc Trop Med Hyg* 1992.

167. Isaacson C, Seftel HC, Keeley KJ, Bothwell TH: Siderosis in the Bantu: the relationship between iron overload and cirrhosis. *J Lab Clin Med* 58:845, 1961.

168. Isaacson C, Bothwell TH: Synovial iron deposits in black subjects with iron overload. *Arch Pathol Lab Med* 105:487, 1981.

169. Tisdale WA: Parenchymal siderosis in patients with cirrhosis after portasystemic-shunt surgery. *N Engl J Med* 265:928, 1961.

170. Schaefer JW, Amick CJ, Oikawa Y, Schiff L: The development of hemochromatosis following postacaval anastomosis. *Gastroenterology* 42:181, 1962.

171. Nixon DD: Spontaneous shunt siderosis. *Am J Dig Dis* 11:359, 1966.

172. Siersema PD, van Helvoirt RP, Cleton-Soeteman MI, de Bruijn WC, van Eijk HG: The role of iron in experimental porphyria and porphyria cutanea tarda. *Biol Trace Elem Res* 35(1):65, 1992.

173. Bonkovsky HL, Poh-Fitzpatrick M, Pimstone N, et al: Porphyria cutanea tarda, hepatitis C, and HFE gene mutations in North America. *Hepatology* 27:1661, 1998.

174. Stuart KA, Busfield F, Jazwinska EC, et al: The C282Y mutation in the haemochromatosis gene (HFE) and hepatitis C virus infection are independent cofactors for porphyria cutanea tarda in Australian patients. *J Hepatol* 28:404, 1998.

175. Roberts AG, Whatley SD, Morgan RR, Worwood M, Elder GH: Increased frequency of the haemochromatosis Cys282Tyr mutation in sporadic porphyria cutanea tarda. *Lancet* 349:321, 1997.

176. Sampietro M, Piperno A, Lupica L, et al: High prevalence of the His63Asp HFE mutation in Italian patients with porphyria cutanea tarda. *Hepatology* 27:181, 1998.

177. Kostler E, Pollack P, Seebacher C, Riedel H: Iron metabolism and chloroquine phosphate therapy in porphyria cutanea tarda. *Z Hautkr* 65(11):1030, 1990.

178. Kushner JP, Edwards CQ, Dadone MM, Skolnick MH: Heterozygosity for HLA-linked hemochromatosis as a likely cause of the hepatic siderosis associated with sporadic porphyia cutanea tarda. *Gastroenterology* 88:1232, 1985.

179. DiPadova C, Marchesi L, Cainelli T, et al: Effects of phlebotomy on urinary porphyrin pattern and liver histology in patients with porphyria cutanea tarda. *Am J Med Sci* 285(1):2, 1983.

180. Fienberg R: Perinatal idiopathic hemochromatosis: giant cell hepatitis interpreted as an inborn error of metabolism. *Am J Clin Pathol* 33:480, 1960.

181. Blisard KS, Bartow SA: Neonatal hemochromatosis. *Hum Pathol* 17:376, 1986.

182. Adams PC, Searle J: Neonatal hemochromatosis: a case and review of the literature. *Am J Gastroenterol* 83:422, 1988.

183. Ferrell L, Schmidt K, Sheffield V, Packman S: Neonatal hemochromatosis: genetic counseling based on retrospective pathologic diagnosis. *Am J Med Genet* 44:429, 1992.

184. Perkins KW, McInnes IWS, Blackburn SRB, Beal RW: Idiopathic haemochromatosis in children: report of a family. *Am J Med* 39:118, 1965.

185. Verloes A, Temple IK, Hubert AF, et al: Recurrence of neonatal haemochromatosis in half sibs born of unaffected mothers. *J Med Genet* 33:444, 1996.

186. Rand EB, McClenathan DT, Whitington PF: Neonatal hemochromatosis: report of successful orthotopic liver transplantation. *J Pediatr Gastroenterol Nutr* 15:325, 1992.

187. Portella A, Guida V, Valerio V: Su di un caso di emocromatosi giovanile con alterazioni endocrine. *Riforma Med* 71:1246, 1957.

188. Palacio J, Sánchez B, Hojman D, Pérez AH: Hemochromatosis: forma cardíaca juvenil. *Presna Med Argent* 47:2943, 1960.

189. Ströder U: Infantilismus und Myokardfibrose bei der Hämochromatose. *Deutsch Arch Klin Med* 189:141, 1942.

190. Charlton RW, Abrahams C, Bothwell TH: Idiopathic hemochromatosis in young subjects: clinical, pathological, and chemical findings in four patients. *Arch Pathol* 83:132, 1967.

191. Cazzola M, Ascari E, Barosi G, et al: Juvenile idiopathic haemochromatosis: a life-threatening disorder presenting as hypogonadotropic hypogonadism. *Hum Genet* 65:149, 1983.

192. Kaikov Y, Wadsworth LD, Hassall E, Dimmick JE, Rogers PC: Primary hemochromatosis in children: report of three newly diagnosed cases and review of the pediatric literature. *Pediatrics* 90:37, 1992.

193. Camaschella C, Roetto A, Cicilano M, et al: Juvenile and adult hemochromatosis are distinct genetic disorders. *Eur J Hum Genet* 5:371, 1997.

194. Kaltwasser JP, Gottschalk R, Seidl CH: Severe juvenile haemochromatosis (JH) missing HFE gene variants: implications for a second gene locus leading to iron overload [letter]. *Br J Haematol* 102:1111, 1998.

195. Roetto A, Totaro A, Cazzola M, et al: Juvenile hemochromatosis locus maps to chromosome 1q. *Am J Hum Genet* 64:1388, 1999.

196. Heilmeyer L, Keller W, Vivell O, Betke K, Wöhler F, Keiderling W: Die kongenitale Atransferrinämie. *Schweiz Med Wochenschr* 91:1203, 1961.

197. Cáp J, Lehotská V, Mayerová A: Kongenitálna atransferinémia u 11-mesacného dietata. *Cesk Pediatr* 23:1020, 1968.

198. Hromec AJ, Schwick HG: Kongenitale Atransferrinämie. Klinische Beobachtungen während einer 18 jahrigen Substitution mit Humantransferrin. *Paediat Prax* 30:633, 1989.

199. Hromec A, Payer J Jr, Killinger Z, Rybar I, Rovensky J: Congenital atransferrinemia. *Deutsche Medizinische Wochenschrift* 119:663, 1994.

200. Sakata T: A case of congenital atransferrinemia. *Shonika Shinryo* 32:1523, 1969.

201. Goya N, Miyazaki S, Kodate S, Ushio B: A family of congenital atransferrinemia. *Blood* 40:239, 1972.

202. Hayashi A, Wada Y, Suzuki T, Shimizu A: Studies on familial hypotransferrinemia: unique clinical course and molecular pathology. *Am J Hum Genet* 53:201, 1993.

203. Loperena L, Dorante S, Medrano E, et al: Atransferrinemia hereditaria. *Bol Med Hosp Infant Mex* 31:519, 1974.

204. Dorantes-Mesa S, Marquez JL, Valencia-Mayoral P: Iron overload in hereditary atransferrinemia. *Bol Med Hosp Infant Mex* 43:99, 1986.

205. Walbaum R: Déficit congénital en transferrine. *Lille Med* 16:1122, 1971.

206. Hamill RL, Woods JC, Cook BA: Congenital atransferrinemia. A case report and review of the literature. *Am J Clin Pathol* 96:215, 1991.

207. Bernstein SE: Hereditary hypotransferrinemia with hemosiderosis, a murine disorder resembling human atransferrinemia. *J Lab Clin Med* 110:690, 1987.

208. Olivia G, Dominici G, Latini P, Cozzolino G: Sindrome nefrosica atransferrinemica. *Minerva Med* 59:1297, 1968.

209. Gaston-Morata JL, Rodriquez-Cuartero A, Urbano-Jimenez F, et. al: Atransferrinemia secundaria a cirrhosis hepática, hemocromatosis y sindrome nefrótico. *Rev Esp Enferm Apar Dig* 62:491, 1960.

210. Hitzig WH, Schmid M, Betke K, Rothchild M: Erythroleukämie mit Hämoglobinopathie und Eisenstoffwechselstörung. *Helv Paediatr Acta* 15:203, 1960.

211. Westerhausen M, Meuret G: Transferrin-immune complex disease. *Acta Haematol* 57:96, 1977.

212. Sizemore DJ, Bassett ML: Monocyte transferrin-iron uptake in hereditary hemochromatosis. *Am J Hematol* 16:347, 1984.

213. Stremmel W, Riedel HD, Niederau C, Strohmeyer G: Pathogenesis of genetic haemochromatosis. *Eur J Clin Invest* 23:321, 1993.

214. Piperno A: Classification and diagnosis of iron overload. [Review] [60 refs]. *Haematologica* 83:447, 1998.

215. Harris ZL, Klomp LW, Gitlin JD: Aceruloplasminemia: an inherited neurodegenerative disease with impairment of iron homeostasis. [Review] [34 refs]. *Am J Clin Nutr* 67:972S, 1998.

216. Yazaki M, Yoshida K, Nakamura A, Furihata K, et al: A novel splicing mutation in the ceruloplasmin gene responsible for hereditary ceruloplasmin deficiency with hemosiderosis. *J Neurol Sci* 156:30, 1998.

217. Miyajima H, Takahashi Y, Shimizu H, Sakai N, Kamata T, Kaneko E: Late onset diabetes mellitus in patients with hereditary aceruloplasminemia [see comments]. *Intern Med* 35:641, 1996.

218. Takahashi Y, Miyajima H, Shirabe S, Nagataki S, Suenaga A, Gitlin JD: Characterization of a nonsense mutation in the ceruloplasmin gene resulting in diabetes and neurodegenerative disease. *Hum Mol Genet* 5:81, 1996.

219. Yoshida K, Furihata K, Takeda S, et al: A mutation in the ceruloplasmin gene is associated with systemic hemosiderosis in humans. *Nat Genet* 9:267, 1995.

220. Klomp LW, Gitlin JD: Expression of the ceruloplasmin gene in the human retina and brain: implications for a pathogenic model in aceruloplasminemia. *Hum Mol Genet* 5:1989, 1996.

221. Klomp LW, Farhangrazi ZS, Dugan LL, Gitlin JD: Ceruloplasmin gene expression in the murine central nervous system [see comments]. *J Clin Invest* 98:207, 1996.

222. Miyajima H, Takahashi Y, Serizawa M, Kaneko E, Gitlin JD: Increased plasma lipid peroxidation in patients with aceruloplasminemia. *Free Radic Biol Med* 20:757, 1996.

223. Harris ZL, Takahashi Y, Miyajima H, Serizawa M, MacGillivray RT, Gitlin JD: Aceruloplasminemia: molecular characterization of this disorder of iron metabolism. *Proc Natl Acad Sci USA* 92:2539, 1995.

224. Miyajima H, Takahashi Y, Kamata T, Shimizu H, Sakai N, Gitlin JD: Use of desferrioxamine in the treatment of aceruloplasminemia. *Ann Neurol* 41:404, 1997.

225. Girelli D, Olivieri O, DeFranceschi L, Corrocher R, Bergamaschi G, Cazzola M: A linkage between hereditary hyperferritinaemia not related to iron overload and autosomal dominant congenital cataract. *Br J Haematol* 90:931, 1995.

226. Garcia-Erce JA, Salvador-Osuna C, Cortes T, Perez-Lungmus G: [Congenital cataract syndrome and hyperferritinemia (letter)]. [Spanish]. *Med Clin* 112:398, 1999.

227. Beaumont C, Lenueve P, Devaux I, et al: Mutation in the iron responsive element of L ferritin mRNA in a family with dominant hyperferritinaemia and cataract. *Nat Genet* 11:444, 1995.

228. Martin ME, Fargion S, Brissot P, Pellat B, Beaumont C: A point mutation in the bulge of the iron-responsive element of the L ferritin gene in two families with the hereditary hyperferritinemia cataract syndrome. *Blood* 91:319, 1998.

229. McDonnell SM, Grindon AJ, Preston BL, Barton JC, Edwards CQ, Adams PC: A survey of phlebotomy among persons with hemochromatosis [see comments]. *Transfusion* 39:651, 1999.

230. Barton JC, Grindon AJ, Barton NH, Bertoli LF: Hemochromatosis probands as blood donors [see comments]. *Transfusion* 39:578, 1999.

231. Wallace DF, Dooley JS, Walker AP: A novel mutation of HFE explains the classical phenotype of genetic hemochromatosis in a C282Y heterozygote. *Gastroenterology* 116:1409, 1999.

232. Barton JC, Beutler E, Gelbart T: Coinheritance of alleles associated with hemochromatosis and hereditary hyperferritinemia-cataract syndrome [letter]. *Blood* 92:4480, 1998.

233. River Y, Honigman S, Gomori JM: Superficial hemosiderosis of the central nervous system. *Mov Disord* 9:559, 1994.

234. House JK, Smith BP, Maas J, et al: Hemochromatosis in Salers cattle. *J Vet Intern Med* 8:105, 1994.

235. Roels S, Ducatelle R, Cornelissen H: Quantitative image analysis as an alternative to chemical analysis for follow-up of liver biopsies from a toucan with hemochromatosis. A technique with potential value for the follow-up of hemochromatosis in humans. *Anal Quant Cytol Histol* 18:221, 1996.

236. Rothenberg BE, Voland JR: β_2 microglobulin knockout mice develop parenchymal iron overload: a putative role for class I genes of the major histocompatibility complex in iron metabolism. *Proc Natl Acad Sci USA* 93:1529, 1996.

237. De-Sousa M, Reimaio R, Lacerda R, Hugo P, Kaufmann S, Porto G: Iron overload in β2-microglobulin-deficient mice. *Immunol Lett* 34:105, 1994.

238. Zhou XY, Tomatsu S, Fleming RE, et al: HFE gene knockout produces mouse model of hereditary hemochromatosis. *Proc Natl Acad Sci USA* 95:2492, 1998.

239. Santos M, Schilham MW, Rademakers LHPM, Marx JJM, de Sousa M, Clevers H: Defective iron homeostatis in β2-microglobulin knockout mice recapitulates hereditary hemochromatosis in man. *J Exp Med* 184:1975, 1996.

HEREDITARY SPHEROCYTOSIS, ELLIPTOCYTOSIS, AND RELATED DISORDERS

PATRICK G. GALLAGHER
BERNARD G. FORGET

Hereditary spherocytosis (HS) is a term that refers to a group of disorders characterized by spherically shaped erythrocytes on peripheral blood smear. HS is the most common inherited anemia in individuals of northern European descent, affecting approximately 1 in 2500 individuals. The principal cellular defect in HS is loss of membrane surface area, accounting for the spherical shape and decreased deformability of the erythrocyte. Splenic destruction of nondeformable spherocytes leads to the hemolysis experienced by HS patients. Membrane loss is due to defects in several membrane proteins, including ankyrin, band 3, α spectrin, β spectrin, and protein 4.2. There is significant clinical, laboratory, biochemical, and genetic heterogeneity in HS. It may present at any age, from infancy to late in life, with signs and symptoms due to hemolytic anemia or its complications. In most patients, splenectomy is curative. With a few rare exceptions, HS is due to "private" mutations; that is, each kindred has a unique mutation. Hereditary elliptocytosis (HE) is characterized by the presence of elliptical erythrocytes on peripheral blood smear. It is common in people of African and Mediterranean ancestry and occurs in approximately 1 in 2000 individuals. The principal defect in HE erythrocytes is mechanical weakness or fragility of the membrane skeleton. This is due to abnormalities in the proteins involved in membrane skeleton interactions, including α spectrin, β spectrin, protein 4.1, or GPC. Although the clinical presentation of HE is heterogeneous, the majority of HE patients are asymptomatic, and therapy is rarely necessary. Hereditary pyropoikilocytosis (HPP) is a rare cause of severe hemolytic anemia characterized by erythrocyte morphology similar to that seen in thermal burns. There is a strong relationship between HPP and HE. Approximately one-third of family members of patients with HPP have typical HE, and many of these patients share identical biochemical and genetic defects in spectrin. A wide variety of mutations associated with HE/HPP have been identified, with a few α spectrin mutations responsible for the majority of cases.

Hemolytic anemias due to defects in the erythrocyte membrane comprise an important group of hereditary anemias. Hereditary spherocyto-

sis, HE, and HPP are the most common disorders among this group. Originally classified by their morphologic presentation, detailed studies have demonstrated considerable overlap between these disorders and significant heterogeneity in their clinical, morphologic, laboratory, and molecular characteristics (Table 43-1). Advances in molecular biology have allowed further characterization of these disorders and, in many cases, detection of the precise genetic defect (see Table 43-1). These molecular analyses have provided additional information on the pathogenesis of these disorders as well as important insights into the structure-function relationships of the proteins of the erythrocyte membrane (Chap. 27).

HEREDITARY SPHEROCYTOSIS

DEFINITION AND HISTORY

Hereditary spherocytosis is a term that refers to a group of disorders characterized by spherical, doughnut-shaped erythrocytes with increased osmotic fragility. HS occurs in all racial and ethnic groups. It is the most common inherited anemia in individuals of northern European ancestry, affecting approximately 1 in 2500 individuals in the United States and England. Clinical, laboratory, biochemical, and genetic heterogeneity characterize the spherocytosis syndromes.

Hereditary spherocytosis was first described over 100 years ago by two Belgian physicians, Vanlair and Masius. Twenty years later, the disease was rediscovered by Wilson and Minkowsky, who reported eight cases of HS in three generations of one family. The description of increased erythrocyte osmotic fragility by Chauffard, reports of correction of anemia and hemolysis by splenectomy, and the studies of Ham and Castle implicating the spleen in the conditioning of hereditary spherocytes followed. The early history of HS is elegantly reviewed by Dacie.[1]

A defect of the erythrocyte membrane was implicated when HS membranes were found to be leaky to sodium and to exhibit a loss of lipids, leading to surface area deficiency. Subsequently, abnormalities of proteins of the erythrocyte membrane have been identified as the etiology of the defect in HS.[2-5]

ETIOLOGY AND PATHOGENESIS

The hallmark of HS erythrocytes is loss of membrane surface area relative to intracellular volume, accounting for the spheroidal shape and decreased deformability of the red cell. This loss of surface area results from increased membrane fragility due to defects in proteins of the erythrocyte membrane, including ankyrin, band 3, β spectrin, α spectrin, and protein 4.2. Increased fragility leads to membrane vesiculation and surface area loss (Fig. 43-1). Splenic trapping of nondeformable spherocytes, followed by conditioning and destruction of these abnormal erythrocytes, is the cause of hemolysis experienced by HS patients. Thus the spleen plays an important role in hemolysis, secondary to the basic defect of the erythrocyte membrane.

RED CELL MEMBRANE PROTEIN DEFECTS

Study of erythrocyte membranes has revealed quantitative abnormalities of several membrane proteins.[6-8] Combined spectrin and ankyrin deficiency is most commonly observed, followed in frequency by band 3 deficiency, isolated spectrin deficiency, and protein 4.2 deficiency. Multiple genetic loci are involved. Except for a few rare exceptions, HS mutations are private, that is, each kindred has a unique mutation, implying that there is no selective advantage to mutations.

Ankyrin Ankyrin links the spectrin-based membrane skeleton to the lipid bilayer via interactions with band 3. Concomitant spectrin and ankyrin deficiency is the most common finding in HS erythrocyte membranes (Fig. 43-2a). Several mechanisms, including decreased

Acronyms and abbreviations that appear in this chapter include: 2,3-BPG, 2,3-bisphosphoglycerate; GPC, glycophorin C; GPD, glycophorin D; HE, hereditary elliptocytosis; HPP, hereditary pyropoikilocytosis; HS, hereditary spherocytosis; MCHC, mean corpuscular hemoglobin concentration; MCV, mean corpuscular volume.

TABLE 43-1   ERYTHROCYTE MEMBRANE PROTEIN DEFECTS IN INHERITED DISORDERS OF RED CELL SHAPE

PROTEIN	DISORDER	COMMENT
Ankyrin	HS	Most common cause of typical dominant HS
Band 3	HS, SAO, NIHF	"Pincered" spherocytes seen on smear presplenectomy; acanthocytosis* SAO due to 9 amino acid deletion
β spectrin	HS, HE, HPP, NIHF	"Acanthocytic" spherocytes seen on smear presplenectomy; location of mutation in β spectrin determines clinical phenotype
α spectrin	HS, HE, HPP, NIHF	Location of mutation in α spectrin determines clinical phenotype;&endline;α spectrin mutations most common cause of typical HE
Protein 4.2	HS	Primarily found in Japanese patients
Protein 4.1	HE	Found in certain European and Arab populations
GPC	HE	Concomitant protein 4.1 deficiency basis of HE in GPC defects

ABBREVIATIONS: HE, hereditary elliptocytosis; HPP, hereditary pyropoikilocytosis; HS, hereditary spherocytosis; NIHF, nonimmune hydrops fetalis; SAO, Southeast Asian ovalocytosis.
*See Chap. 45.

synthesis of ankyrin, decreased ankyrin assembly on the membrane, or assembly of an abnormal ankyrin, could lead to decreased assembly of spectrin on the membrane when spectrin binding sites on ankyrin are decreased, absent, or defective.

Genetic screening has identified a number of ankyrin gene mutations in patients and has demonstrated that ankyrin defects are the most common cause of typical, dominant HS.[9-11] The majority of ankyrin mutations are either frameshift or nonsense mutations that lead to a defective ankyrin molecule, ankyrin deficiency, or both. Missense mutations may disrupt normal ankyrin-protein interactions. One such variant, ankyrin[Waldsrode], identified in a kindred whose erythrocyte membranes were deficient in band 3 as well as ankyrin and spectrin, was due to a mutation in the band 3 binding domain of

ankyrin that decreased its affinity for band 3.[12] With one exception, all ankyrin mutations described to date have been private. The exception, ankyrin[Florianopolis], is a recurrent frameshift mutation associated with severe dominantly inherited HS.[13]

Genetic variants have been identified in the promoter of the ankyrin gene in a number of patients with recessively inherited HS.[9,14] Whether these are disease-causing mutations or are merely polymorphisms in linkage disequilibrium with the as yet unidentified mutation is unknown.

Cytogenetic studies have identified a few ankyrin-deficient HS patients with dysmorphic features, psychomotor retardation, and hypogonadism.[15] These patients suffer from a contiguous gene syndrome that includes deletion of the ankyrin gene locus at 8p11.2.

Band 3, the Anion Exchanger   Band 3 mediates interactions within the membrane skeleton via ankyrin, protein 4.1, and protein 4.2 via its NH₂-terminal cytoplasmic domain and effects anion exchange via its membrane-spanning COOH-terminal domain. A subset of patients with typical dominant HS whose red cells are approximately 20 to 40 percent deficient in band 3 and protein 4.2, but have a normal spectrin content, has been described.[4] These patients generally have mild to moderate HS and have pincered spherocytes on peripheral smears.

A variety of band 3 gene mutations associated with HS have been identified, including missense, nonsense, duplication, insertion, deletion, and RNA-processing mutations.[16-20] The missense mutations include a group of mutations that replace highly conserved arginine residues in the transmembrane domain. These mutant proteins do not

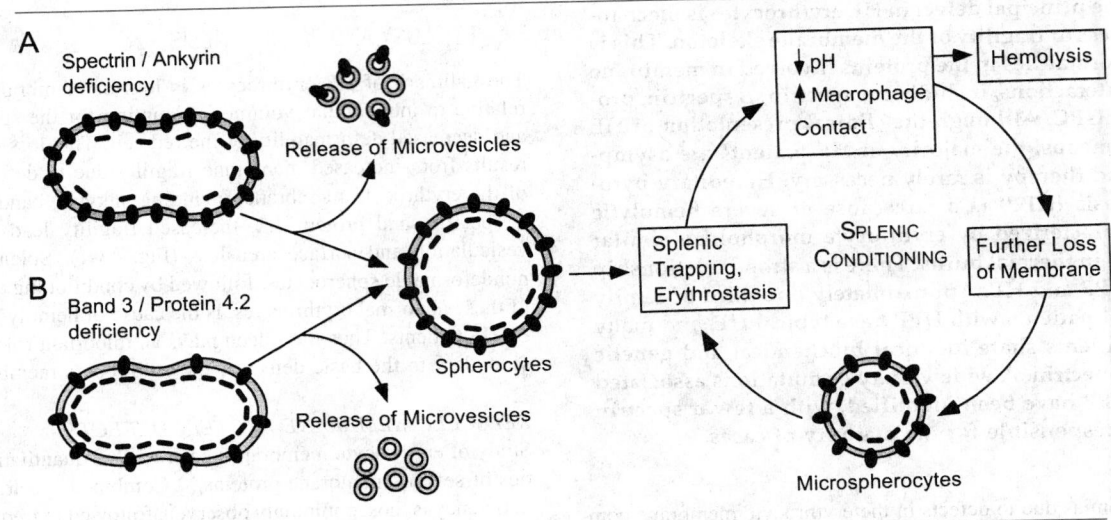

FIGURE 43-1   Pathobiology of HS. The primary defect in HS is a deficiency of membrane surface area, leading to the formation of spherocytes. Decreased surface area may be produced by two different mechanisms: (1) defects of spectrin and ankyrin lead to reduced density of the membrane skeleton, destabilizing the overlying lipid bilayer and releasing band 3-containing microvesicles; or (2) defects of band 3 or protein 4.2 lead to band 3 deficiency and loss of its lipid-stabilizing effect, resulting in the loss of band 3-free microvesicles. Both pathways result in membrane loss, decreased surface area, and formation of spherocytes with decreased deformability. These deformed erythrocytes become trapped in the hostile environment of the spleen, where splenic conditioning inflicts further membrane damage, amplifying the cycle of red cell membrane injury. (From Gallagher PG, Jarolim P: Red cell membrane disorders, in *Hematology: Basis Principles and Practice,* edited by R Hoffman, EJ Benz, Jr, SJ Shattil, et al. WB Saunders, Philadelphia, 1999. (pp. 576–610), with permission.)

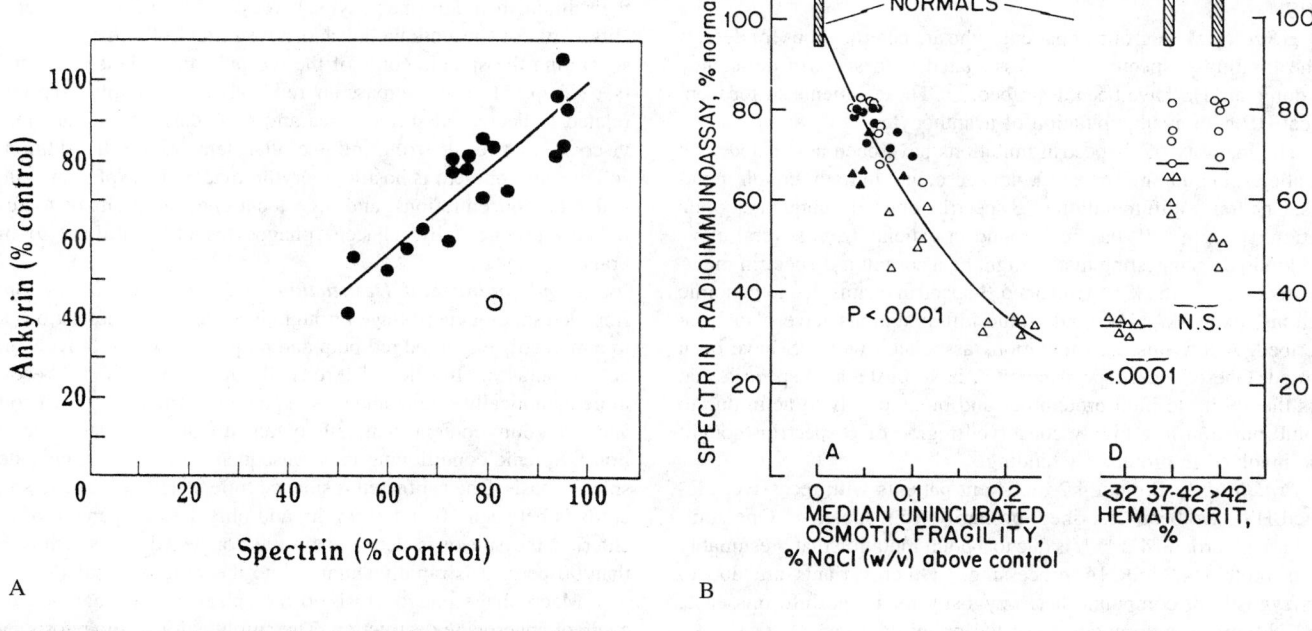

A

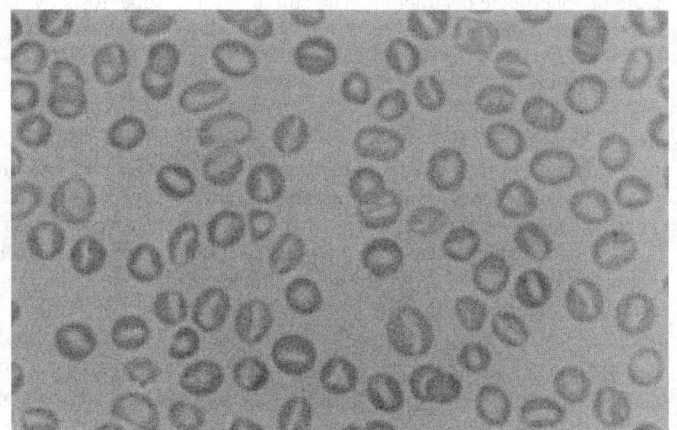

B

FIGURE 43-2 The role of ankyrin and spectrin in HS. *(a)* Correlation of spectrin and ankyrin deficiencies in 20 dominant HS kindreds. Each point, expressed as a percentage of the control (100%), represents the mean value for a kindred for both red cell spectrin and ankyrin levels. Within experimental error, the degree of spectrin and ankyrin deficiencies is essentially identical in these families with one exception (open circle), an otherwise typical family in which red cells are primarily ankyrin deficient. (From P Savvides et al,[7] with permission.) *(b)* Correlation between red cell spectrin deficiency and unincubated osmotic fragility (a measure of spheroidicity) in HS. Spectrin content, as measured by radioimmunoassay, is shown on the vertical axis; and osmotic fragility, as measured by NaCl concentration producing 50 percent hemolysis of erythrocytes, is shown on the horizontal axis. Circles represent patients with typical autosomal dominant HS, and triangles represent patients with atypical, nondominant HS. Open symbols represent patients who have undergone splenectomy. The right panel shows the hematocrit of every patient at least 4 months after splenectomy. Note that very spectrin-deficient patients have more spherical red cells and an incomplete response to splenectomy. (From P Agre et al,[22] with permission.)

fold and fail to insert into the endoplasmic reticulum and, ultimately, into the erythrocyte membrane.[17] The nonsense mutations lead to decreased band 3 mRNA accumulation, presumably due to mRNA instability.[18] In HS patients with band 3[Campinas] and band 3[Pribram], defects in band 3 mRNA processing, an unexplained renal tubular acidosis has also been observed.[19,20]

Spectrin Spectrin is composed of two subunits, α and β, which, despite the many similarities, are structurally distinct and are encoded by separate genes. The function of erythrocyte spectrin is to maintain cellular shape, regulate the lateral mobility of integral membrane proteins, and provide structural support for the lipid bilayer.[3] Erythrocytes from most patients are spectrin deficient, including both the dominant and recessive forms. The degree of spectrin deficiency correlates with the spheroidicity of erythrocytes, their ability to withstand shear stress, the degree of hemolysis, and the response to splenectomy (Fig. 43-2*b*).[21,22]

In humans, α-spectrin synthesis exceeds β-spectrin synthesis by a ratio of about three or four to one.[23] Patients who are heterozygous for an α-spectrin defect should still produce enough normal α-spectrin chains to pair with all, or nearly all, of the β-spectrin chains that are

synthesized. Thus, patients with α-spectrin defects should only be symptomatic when the defect is found in the homozygous or compound heterozygous state. In a similar manner, deficiency of the limiting β-spectrin chains due to β-spectrin defects should be expressed as a dominantly inherited trait.

α Spectrin The mechanisms of spectrin deficiency are unknown in most HS patients with recessively inherited HS. A number of patients with severe recessively inherited HS and marked spectrin deficiency have a mutant allele, α^{LEPRA} (low-expression Prague), that produces approximately one-sixth of the correctly spliced α-spectrin transcript as the normal allele, due to aberrant mRNA processing.[24] In one patient, the combination of the LEPRA allele with another defect of α spectrin *in trans,* a truncated α-spectrin chain, α^{Prague}, led to severe spectrin deficiency and severe spherocytic anemia.[25] Whether α^{LEPRA} is the etiology of many cases of α-spectrin-linked HS is yet to be determined. An amino acid substitution in the αII domain of spectrin, $\alpha^{\text{Bug Hill}}$, has been identified in many patients with spectrin-deficient, recessive HS.[26] Studies suggest that $\alpha^{\text{Bug Hill}}$ is not itself responsible for HS, but is likely a polymorphic variant that in some, but not all, cases is in linkage disequilibrium

with another uncharacterized α-spectrin gene defect that is the cause of HS.

β Spectrin   A group of patients who are heterozygous for defects in the limiting β-spectrin chain associated with spectrin deficiency and dominant HS have been described.[27–29] These patients suffer from typical HS with a subpopulation of acanthocytes.

The majority of β-spectrin mutations have been associated with null alleles, including frameshift, nonsense, and initiator codon mutations. One frameshift mutation of β spectrin, due to a single nucleotide deletion, spectrin[Houston], has been found in patients from several unrelated kindreds, suggesting that it might be a common β-spectrin mutation associated with HS.[28] Truncated β-spectrin chains due to genomic deletions, exon skipping, and frameshift mutations have also been described. A few missense mutations associated with HS have been reported. One of these, spectrin[Kissimmee], is an unstable β spectrin that lacks the ability to bind protein 4.1 and binds poorly to actin due to a point mutation in a highly conserved region of β spectrin thought to be involved in protein 4.1 binding.[27]

Protein 4.2   Protein 4.2–deficient patients with recessively inherited HS have been described, primarily from Japan.[16,30] One common variant, protein 4.2[Nippon], is due to a point mutation that presumably affects protein 4.2 mRNA processing.[30] Other variants are due to homozygosity or compound heterozygosity for frameshift, missense, or mRNA processing mutations of the protein 4.2 gene.

Deficiency of protein 4.2 has also been observed in patients with mutations in the cytoplasmic domain of band 3.[31,32] These mutations presumably involve the region of band 3-protein 4.2 interactions.

SECONDARY MEMBRANE DEFECTS

Cation Content and Membrane Permeability   Potassium and water content are diminished in HS red cells, particularly those obtained from splenic pulp. The passive permeability of HS red cells to sodium is increased, presumably secondarily to the underlying skeletal defect.[33–35] The excessive sodium influx activates Na$^+$-K$^+$-ATPase and the monovalent cation pump, and the accelerated pumping increases ATP turnover and glycolysis. The dehydration of HS red cells is likely to be inflicted, at least in part, by the adverse environment of the spleen, since spherocytes from surgically removed spleens are the most dehydrated.

The pathways causing HS red cell dehydration have not been clearly defined. One candidate is increased K-Cl cotransport, which is activated by acid pH. HS red cells, particularly from unsplenectomized subjects, have a low intracellular pH reflecting the low pH of the splenic environment (see below). The K$^+$-Cl$^-$-cotransport pathway is also activated by oxidative damage, which is likely to be inflicted by splenic macrophages. Finally, overactivity of Na$^+$-K$^+$-ATPase, triggered by increased intracellular sodium, can dehydrate red cells directly, because three sodium ions are extruded in exchange for only two potassium ions, and the loss of monovalent cations is accompanied by water.

Membrane Lipids   The principal lipid abnormality of hereditary spherocytes is a symmetrical loss of each species of membrane lipid as part of the overall loss of membrane surface, the hallmark of HS pathobiology. The relative proportions of cholesterol and the various phospholipids are normal, and the phospholipids show the usual transmembrane asymmetry, even in severe cases.

Role of the Spleen   The spleen plays a secondary but important role in the pathophysiology of HS. Splenic destruction of abnormal erythrocytes with decreased deformability is the primary cause of hemolysis. Physical entrapment of spherocytes in the splenic microcirculation and ingestion by phagocytes have been proposed as mechanisms of destruction.

Splenic Trapping of Nondeformable Spherocytes   Because of their diminished deformability, spherocytes are unable to traverse the slits between the endothelial and adventitial cells that form a wall separating the splenic cords of the red pulp from the splenic sinuses (see Chap. 5). The decrease in red cell deformability is primarily related to decreased surface area and secondarily to greater internal viscosity that results from mild cellular dehydration. In addition, the splenic environment is hostile to erythrocytes.[35] Low pH, low glucose and ATP concentrations, and high local concentrations of toxic free radicals produced by adjacent phagocytes all contribute to membrane damage.

Conditioning and Destruction of Spherocytes in the Spleen   Impeded spherocyte passage through the sinus wall fenestrations leads to a markedly engorged red pulp and pulp cords with relatively empty venous sinuses.[36] It is here that red cells are ''conditioned,'' becoming more osmotically fragile and more spherical, with a lower net sodium and potassium content than cells obtained from the systemic circulation.[37] Splenic conditioning is a consequence of multiple episodes of splenic stasis. The estimated residence time of HS erythrocytes in the cords is between 10 and 100 min, and only 1 to 10 percent of blood entering the spleen is detained by the congested cords, while more than 90 percent is rapidly shunted into the venous circulation.

Macrophage phagocytosis in the spleen is the final step in the cycle of spherocyte destruction. The stimulus for phagocytosis by the macrophage is unknown.

INHERITANCE

The genes responsible for HS include ankyrin, β spectrin, band 3 protein, α spectrin, and protein 4.2. In approximately two-thirds to three-quarters of HS patients, inheritance is autosomal dominant. In the remaining patients, dominant inheritance cannot be demonstrated. Inheritance may be autosomal recessive or due to a de novo mutation. Cases with autosomal recessive inheritance are due to defects in either α spectrin or protein 4.2. A surprising number of de novo mutations have been reported in the HS genes.[11,27,29] A few cases of ''double-dominant'' HS due to defects in band 3 or spectrin that result in fetal death or severe hemolytic anemia presenting in the neonatal period have been reported.[43,43] In general, affected individuals of the same kindred experience similar degrees of hemolysis. Rarely, members of the same kindred will experience varying degrees of hemolysis. When HS has been identified in one or more siblings whose parents have no identifiable abnormalities or when there is great variability in the clinical severity of affected HS family members, a number of explanations can be sought. These include inheritance of a modifier allele that influences the expression of a membrane protein, leading to the variability in clinical expression, variable penetrance of the genetic defect, a de novo mutation, a mild form of recessively inherited HS, or tissue-specific mosaicism of the defect.[11,27,29,38,45,46]

CLINICAL FEATURES

The clinical manifestations of the spherocytosis syndromes vary widely. The typical clinical picture of HS combines evidence of hemolysis (anemia, jaundice, reticulocytosis, gallstones, and splenomegaly) with spherocytosis (spherocytes on the blood film and increased osmotic fragility) and a positive family history. Mild, moderate, and severe forms of HS have been defined according to differences in hemoglobin, bilirubin, and reticulocyte counts (Table 43-2), which can be correlated with the degree of compensation for the hemolysis.[6,38,39] Initial assessment of a patient with suspected HS should include a family history and questions about history of anemia, jaundice, gallstones, and splenectomy. Physical examination should seek signs such as scleral icterus, jaundice, and splenomegaly.

TABLE 43-2   CLASSIFICATION OF HEREDITARY SPHEROCYTOSIS

Laboratory Findings	HS Trait or Carrier	Mild Spherocytosis	Moderate Spherocytosis	Moderately Severe Spherocytosis*	Severe Spherocytosis†
Hemoglobin, g/dl	Normal	11–15	8–12	6–8	<6
Reticulocytes, %	1–3	3–8	±8	≥10	≥10
Bilirubin	0–1	1–2	±2	2–3	≥3
Spectrin content, % of normal‡	100	80–100	50–80	40–80§	20–50
Blood film	Normal	Mild spherocytosis	Spherocytosis	Spherocytosis	Spherocytosis and poikilocytosis
Osmotic fragility					
Fresh blood	Normal	Normal or slightly increased	Distinctly increased	Distinctly increased	Distinctly increased
Incubated blood	Slightly increased	Distinctly increased	Distinctly increased	Distinctly increased	Markedly increased

*Values in untransfused patients.
†By definition, patients with severe spherocytosis are transfusion dependent.
‡Normal, 245 ± 27 × 10⁵ spectrin dimers per erythrocyte.
§The spectrin content is variable in this group of patients, presumably reflecting heterogeneity of the underlying pathophysiology.
SOURCE: Compiled from WT Tse and SE Lux,[4] A Pekrun et al,[6] and SW Eber et al.[38]

TYPICAL HEREDITARY SPHEROCYTOSIS

Hereditary spherocytosis typically presents in infancy or childhood but may present at any age. In children, anemia is the most frequent presenting complaint (50%), followed by splenomegaly, jaundice, or a positive family history.[40] No comparable data exist for adults. Two-thirds to three-quarters of HS patients have incompletely compensated hemolysis and mild to moderate anemia. The anemia is often asymptomatic except for fatigue and mild pallor or, with children, nonspecific parental complaints, such as irritability. Jaundice is seen at some time or other in about half of patients, usually in association with viral infections. When present it is acholuric, that is, unconjugated hyperbilirubinemia without detectable bilirubinuria. Palpable splenomegaly is detectable in most (75–95%) older children and adults. Typically the spleen is modestly enlarged (2–6 cm), but it may be massive. There is no proven correlation between the size of the spleen and the severity of HS; however, given the pathophysiology and the response of the disease to splenectomy, such a correlation probably exists. Typical HS is associated with both dominant and recessive inheritance. Although the recessively inherited forms tend to be more severe, there is considerable overlap.

COMPENSATED HEREDITARY SPHEROCYTOSIS

About 20 to 30 percent of HS patients have "compensated hemolysis"; that is, production and destruction are balanced, and the hemoglobin concentration of the blood is normal.[4,38] Although the erythrocyte life span may only be about 20 to 30 days, these patients adequately compensate for their hemolysis with increased marrow erythropoiesis. Since they are not anemic, they are usually asymptomatic. In some cases, diagnosis may be difficult because hemolysis, splenomegaly, and spherocytosis are unusually mild. For example, in this group of patients, reticulocyte counts are generally less than 6 percent, and spherocytes are present on smear in only about 60 percent of patients. Many of these individuals escape detection until adulthood when they are being evaluated for unrelated disorders or when complications related to anemia or chronic hemolysis occur. Hemolysis may become severe with illnesses that cause further splenomegaly, such as infectious mononucleosis, or may be exacerbated by other factors, such as pregnancy or sustained, vigorous exercise. Because of the asymptomatic course of HS in these patients, diagnosis of HS should be considered during evaluation of incidentally noted splenomegaly, gallstones at a young age, or anemia resulting from parvovirus B19 infection or other viral infections.

MODERATELY SEVERE AND SEVERE HEREDITARY SPHEROCYTOSIS

Approximately 5 to 10 percent of HS patients have moderately severe to severe anemia. Patients with "moderately severe" disease typically have a hemoglobin level of 6 to 8 g/dl, reticulocytes about 10 percent, bilirubin 2 to 3 mg/dl, and 40 to 80 percent of the normal red cell spectrin content. This category includes patients with both dominant and recessive HS and a variety of molecular defects. Patients with "severe" disease, by definition, have life-threatening anemia and are transfusion dependent. They almost always have recessive HS. Most have isolated, severe spectrin deficiency (<40%), which is thought to be due to a defect in α spectrin.[21,22,41] Patients with severe HS often have some irregularly contoured or budding spherocytes or bizarre poikilocytes in addition to typical spherocytes on blood smear. Such cells are rare prior to splenectomy in patients with moderately severe disease, but some may be seen postsplenectomy. In addition to the risks of recurrent transfusions, these patients often suffer from hemolytic and aplastic crises and may develop complications of severe uncompensated anemia including growth retardation, delayed sexual maturation, or aspects of thalassemic facies.

ASYMPTOMATIC CARRIERS

The parents of patients with recessive HS are clinically asymptomatic and do not have anemia, splenomegaly, hyperbilirubinemia, or spherocytosis on the blood films. However, most have subtle laboratory signs of HS, including slight reticulocytosis (≈2%), diminished haptoglobin levels, and slightly elevated osmotic fragility. The incubated osmotic fragility test is probably the most sensitive measure of this condition, particularly the 100 pecent lysis point, which is significantly elevated in carriers (0.43 ± 0.05 g NaCl/dl) compared to normal subjects (0.23 ± 0.07).[38] However, no single test is sufficient. Carriers can only be detected reliably by considering the results of a battery of tests.[42] It has been estimated that at least 1.4 percent of the population are silent carriers.

PREGNANCY AND HEREDITARY SPHEROCYTOSIS

Most patients do well during pregnancy.[47] Some experience anemia beyond that expected from expanded plasma volume due to increased hemolysis. A few patients are only symptomatic during pregnancy. Episodes of hemolytic crisis requiring transfusion and cases of folic acid deficiency have been described in pregnant HS patients.

HEREDITARY SPHEROCYTOSIS IN INFANCY

Anemia is the most common finding in neonates with HS, present in about 90 percent of cases.[48,49] Some infants have required blood transfusion to treat their anemia. It is interesting to note that the degree of anemia seen in the neonatal period does not predict the severity of the anemia seen in later life. Jaundice occurs in about half of HS neonates and may be severe enough to require phototherapy or exchange transfusion. Jaundice in neonates with HS may be accentuated by the coinheritance of the Gilbert syndrome UDPGT1 gene polymorphism.[50] Since kernicterus is a risk,[48] exchange transfusions may be necessary, but in most cases the jaundice can be controlled with phototherapy.

Rarely, patients may suffer from severe hemolytic anemia presenting in utero or shortly after birth, continuing through the first year of life. These patients may require regular blood transfusions and, in some cases, early splenectomy. These severe HS patients usually suffer from significant spectrin deficiency, due to presumed homozygosity or compound heterozygosity for α-spectrin gene defects. Several cases of hydrops fetalis in HS patients requiring intrauterine transfusion due to severe anemia have been reported associated with band 3 or spectrin defects.

COMPLICATIONS

Gallbladder Disease   Chronic hemolysis leads to the formation of bilirubinate gallstones, the most frequently reported complication in HS patients. Although gallstones have been detected in infancy, most appear in adolescents and young adults between 10 and 30 years of age (Fig. 43-3).[4,51] Routine management should include interval

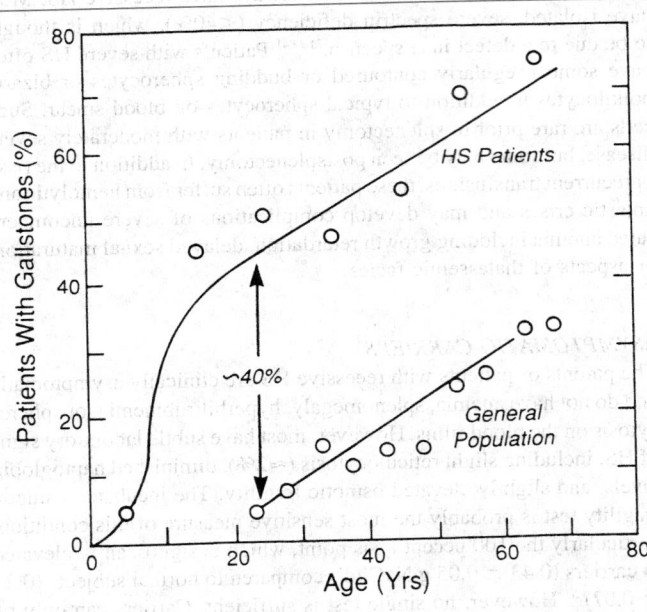

FIGURE 43-3 Proportion of normal and HS patients with gallstones as a function of age. Data are from a study of gallbladder disease in 152 consecutive HS patients seen at the Cleveland Clinic before 1952.[51] Only patients whose gallbladders were examined at surgery or by cholecystography are included. Data for the general population are from an autopsy series of patients who did not have hemolytic anemia. The prevalence of gallstones rises sharply between the ages of 10 and 30 and parallels that of the general population after 30 years. (From SE Lux and J Palek: Disorders of the red cell membrane, in *Blood: Principles and Practice of Hematology*, edited by RI Handin, SE Lux, TP Stossel. p 1701. JB Lippincott, Philadelphia, 1995, with permission. Illustration by Joy D. Marlowe.)

ultrasonography to detect gallstones, since many patients with cholelithiasis and HS are asymptomatic. This will allow prompt diagnosis and treatment and prevent complications of symptomatic biliary tract disease, including biliary obstruction, cholecystitis, and cholangitis.

Hemolytic, Aplastic, and Megaloblastic Crises   Hemolytic crises are usually associated with viral illnesses and typically occur in childhood. They are generally mild and are characterized by jaundice, increased spleen size, a drop in hematocrit, and reticulocytosis. Medical intervention is rarely necessary. When severe hemolytic crises occur, there are marked jaundice, anemia, lethargy, abdominal pain, and tender splenomegaly. Hospitalization and erythrocyte transfusion may be required.

Aplastic crises following virally induced bone marrow suppression are uncommon but may result in severe anemia with serious complications, including congestive heart failure or even death. The most common etiologic agent in these cases is parvovirus B19, the etiologic agent of erythema infectiosum. Parvovirus infection typically presents with fever, chills, lethargy, vomiting, diarrhea, myalgias, and a maculopapular rash on the face (slapped cheek syndrome), trunk, and extremities.

Parvovirus B19 selectively infects erythropoietic progenitor cells and inhibits their growth (see Chap. 32).[52] Parvovirus infections are frequently associated with mild neutropenia, thrombocytopenia, or even pancytopenia. During the aplastic phase, the hematocrit level and reticulocyte count fall, marrow erythroblasts disappear, and unused iron accumulates in the serum. Giant pronormoblasts, a hallmark of the cytopathic effects of parvovirus B19, often appear in the marrow. As production of new red cells declines, the cells that remain age, and microspherocytosis and osmotic fragility increase. Bilirubin levels may decrease as the number of abnormal red cells that can be destroyed declines. The return of marrow function is heralded by a fall in the serum iron concentration and the emergence of granulocytes, platelets, and, finally, reticulocytes.

Virally induced aplastic crisis brings many patients to medical attention, particularly asymptomatic HS patients with normally compensated hemolysis.[53] As would be expected, because parvovirus may infect multiple members of a family simultaneously, leading to aplastic crises, there have been reports of "epidemics" or "outbreaks" of HS.[54] Diagnostic confusion may arise during reemergence of marrow function, when the physician may mistake an aplastic crisis for a hemolytic one. Because aplastic crises usually last 10 to 14 days (about half the life span of HS red cells), the hemoglobin value typically falls to about half its usual level before recovery occurs. In patients with severe HS, the anemia may be profound, requiring hospitalization and transfusion.

Megaloblastic crisis occurs in HS patients with increased folate demands, such as the pregnant patient, growing children, or patients recovering from an aplastic crisis. With appropriate folate supplementation, this complication is preventable.

Other Complications   Dermatologic manifestations of HS, including skin ulceration, gouty tophi, and chronic leg dermatitis, are uncommon.[55] These dermatologic manifestations usually heal rapidly after splenectomy. The pathogenesis of these manifestations is unknown, but it has been proposed to be related to alterations in erythrocyte deformability, as has been suggested in patients with sickle cell anemia.

In some HS patients, findings attributable to extramedullary hematopoiesis have been described. These include poor growth and deformities of the hand and skull. Extramedullary tumors, particularly along the thoracic and lumbar spine or in the kidney hila, have been described in HS patients, including patients with untreated mild to moderate HS.[4,56] Biopsy may be performed, since these masses may be mistaken for a malignant tumor, but because of their composition, it may be complicated by significant hemorrhage. Magnetic resonance imaging appears to be a reliable and safer alternative diagnostic modality. Postsplenectomy, these masses involute and undergo fatty metamorphosis. However, they do not decrease in size.

It has been suggested that HS predisposes patients to hematologic malignancies, including myeloproliferative disorders, particularly multiple myeloma.[57] Chronic reticuloendothelial stimulation via splenic clearance of abnormal erythrocytes inducing the proliferation of lymphocytes, plasma cells, and macrophages has been suggested as a possible pathogenic mechanism. Thrombosis has been reported in several HS patients, usually postsplenectomy.

Iron overload has been described in untreated HS patients with coinherited hemochromatosis.[58] However, studies clearly demonstrating this association have not been performed. Several of these patients subsequently died of liver disease or hepatoma. Untreated HS may aggravate underlying heart disease, particularly in the elderly. Progressive anemia due to loss of marrow reserve may gradually worsen underlying heart failure.

Angioid streaks have been described in the optic fundi of several adult HS patients.

Nonerythroid Manifestations   In most patients with HS, the clinical manifestations are confined to the erythroid lineage. There are a few exceptions. Several HS kindreds have been reported with cosegregating nonerythroid manifestations, particularly neuromuscular abnormalities including cardiomyopathy, slowly progressive spinocerebellar degenerative disease, spinal cord dysfunction, and movement disorders.

The observation that erythrocyte ankyrin and β spectrin are also expressed in muscle, brain, and spinal cord raises the possibility that these HS patients may suffer from defects of one of these proteins.[4,35] This hypothesis is further supported by studies of ankyrin-deficient *nb/nb* mice.[59] These mice have almost no detectable ankyrin and suffer from a severe, spherocytic hemolytic anemia and a late-onset cerebellar ataxia that parallels a gradual loss of Purkinje cells. Another possibility is that another, yet to be described gene locus is causative. For example, mice that do not express the junctional complex membrane protein β adducin suffer from a spherocytic anemia and neurologic manifestations.[59,60]

A few heterozygous defects of band 3 have been described in patients with autosomal dominant distal renal tubular acidosis and normal erythrocytes. This is in contrast to most patients with heterozygous mutations of band 3, who have normal renal acidification and abnormal erythrocytes. Two kindreds with coinherited HS *and* renal acidification defects due to band 3 mRNA processing mutations, band 3[Pribram] and band 3[Campinas], have been described.[19,20]

LABORATORY FEATURES

Like the clinical presentation of HS, laboratory findings in HS are heterogeneous.

THE BLOOD FILM
Erythrocyte morphology in HS is quite variable. Typical HS patients have blood films with easily identifiable spherocytes lacking central

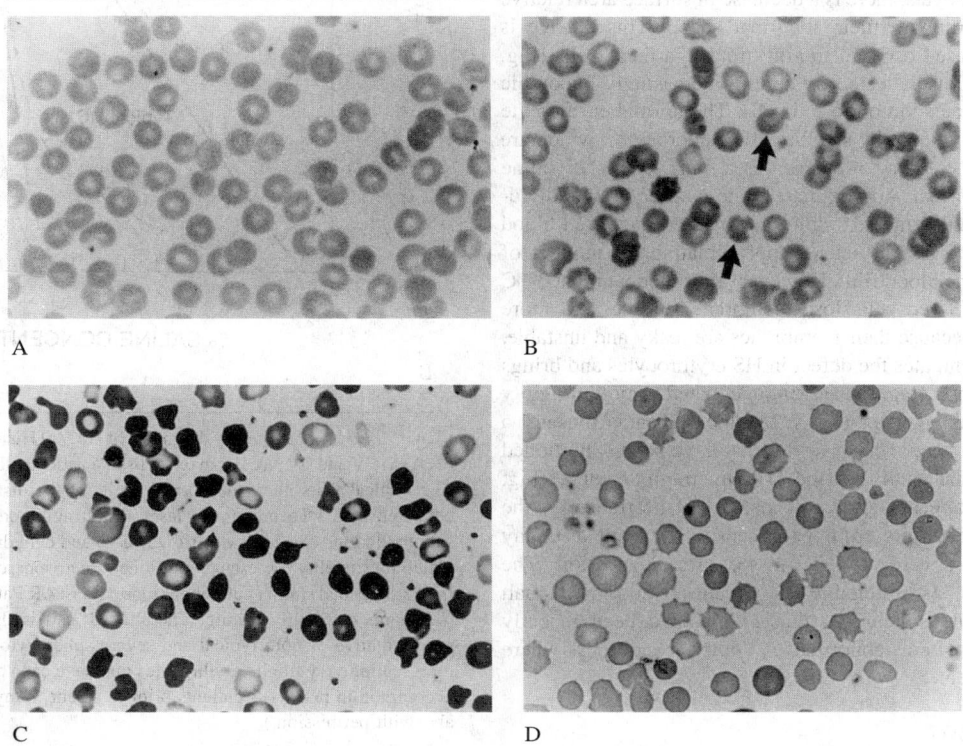

FIGURE 43-4   Peripheral blood smears from patients with HS of varying severity. *(a)* Typical HS with a mild deficiency of red cell spectrin and ankyrin. Although many cells have spheroidal shape, some of them retain a central concavity. *(b)* HS with pincered red cells (arrows), as typically seen in HS associated with band 3 deficiency. Occasionally, spiculated red cells are also present. *(c)* Severe atypical HS due to a severe combined spectrin and ankyrin deficiency. In addition to spherocytes, there are many cells with irregular contour. *(d)* HS with isolated spectrin deficiency due to a β spectrin mutation. Some of the spherocytes have prominent surface projections resembling spheroacanthocytes. (Film *d* courtesy of DL Wolfe.)

pallor (Fig. 43-4). Less commonly, patients present with only a few spherocytes on the film or, at the other end of the spectrum, with numerous small, dense spherocytes and bizarre erythrocyte morphology with anisocytosis and poikilocytosis. Rarely, spherostomatocytes may be seen. Specific morphologic findings have been identified in patients with certain membrane protein defects, such as pincered erythrocytes (band 3) or spherocytic acanthocytes (β spectrin). When examining blood from a patient with suspected spherocytosis, it is important to have a high-quality film with the erythrocytes well separated and some cells with central pallor in the field of examination, since spherocytes are a common artifact.

ERYTHROCYTE INDICES

Most patients have a mild to moderate anemia with hemoglobin in the 9- to 12-g/dl range (see Table 43-2). The MCHC is increased (between 35 and 38%) due to relative cellular dehydration in approximately 50 percent of patients, but all HS patients have some dehydrated cells. The Technicon H1 blood counter and its successors (Technicon, Tarrytown, NY) provide a histogram of MCHC that has been claimed to be accurate enough to identify nearly all HS patients (Fig. 43-5a).[61] Finally, the MCV is usually normal except in cases of severe HS, when it is slightly decreased. Typically, the MCV is relatively low for the age of the cells in most HS patients, reflecting the dehydrated state of the HS erythrocytes.

OSMOTIC FRAGILITY

In the normal erythrocyte, a redundancy of cell membrane gives the cell its characteristic discoid shape and provides it with abundant surface area. In spherocytes, there is a decrease in surface area relative to cell volume, resulting in their abnormal shape. This change is reflected in the increased osmotic fragility found in these cells (Fig. 43-5b). Osmotic fragility is tested by adding increasingly hypotonic concentrations of saline solution to red cells. The normal erythrocyte is able to increase its volume by swelling, but spherocytes, which are already at maximum volume for surface area, burst at higher saline concentrations than normal. Approximately one-quarter of HS individuals will have a normal osmotic fragility on freshly drawn red blood cells, with the osmotic fragility curve approximating the number of spherocytes seen on the blood film. However, after incubation at 37°C (98.6°F) for 24 h, HS red cells lose membrane surface area more readily than normal because their membranes are leaky and unstable. Thus, incubation accentuates the defect in HS erythrocytes and brings out the defect in osmotic fragility, making incubated osmotic fragility the standard test in diagnosing HS. When the spleen is present, a subpopulation of very fragile erythrocytes that have been conditioned by the spleen form the "tail" of the osmotic fragility curve (Fig. 43-5b). This tail disappears after splenectomy. Unfortunately, the osmotic fragility test suffers from poor sensitivity, with as many as 20 percent of mild cases of HS missed after incubation. The osmotic fragility test is unreliable in patients who have small numbers of spherocytes, including those who have been recently transfused. Its results are abnormal in other conditions where spherocytes are present.

ADDITIONAL TESTING

Other investigations, such as the autohemolysis test, the hypertonic cryohemolysis test, and the acidified glycerol test, suffer from lack of specificity, are cumbersome to perform, and are not widely used. Specialized testing is available for studying difficult cases or cases where additional information is desired. Useful tests for these purposes include structural and functional studies of erythrocyte membrane proteins, such as protein quantitation, limited tryptic digestion of spectrin, and ion transport. Membrane rigidity and fragility can be examined

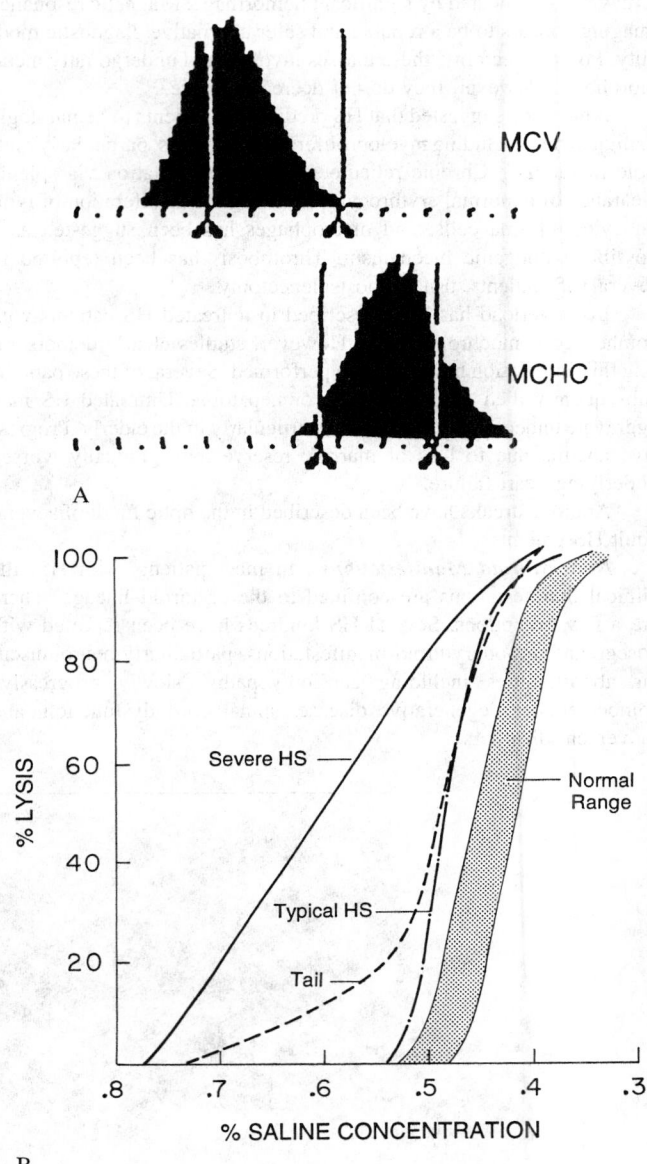

FIGURE 43-5   Laboratory diagnosis of HS. (a) Histograms of the distribution of (A) MCV and (B) MCHC in red cells of a patient with HS before splenectomy. The vertical lines mark the normal limits of the distributions. The data were collected with a Technicon H1 laser scattering blood counter. The patient has subpopulations of microcytes (low MCV) and dehydrated cells (high MCHC), which presumably represent conditioned microspherocytes. All 21 HS patients in one study had similar subpopulations. (From AR Pati et al,[61] with permission.) (b) Osmotic fragility testing. The shaded area is the normal range. Results representative of both typical and severe spherocytosis are shown. A "tail," representing very fragile erythrocytes that have been conditioned by the spleen, is common in many HS patients prior to splenectomy. (From PG Gallagher et al,[35] with permission.)

using an ektacytometer. cDNA and genomic DNA analyses are available when a molecular diagnosis is desired.

Other laboratory manifestations in HS are markers of ongoing hemolysis. Reticulocytosis, increased serum bilirubin, increased lactate dehydrogenase, increased urinary and fecal urobilinogen, and decreased serum haptoglobin reflect increased erythrocyte production or destruction. In many cases of HS, the reticulocyte count appears to be elevated disproportionately relative to the degree of anemia. This has been observed even in HS patients with normal hemoglobin levels. The etiology of this observation is unknown.

DIFFERENTIAL DIAGNOSIS

Initial laboratory investigation should include a complete blood count with a blood film, reticulocyte count, direct antiglobulin test (Coombs' test), and serum bilirubin. An incubated osmotic fragility should be obtained. Rarely, additional, specialized testing is required to confirm the diagnosis. In neonates, ABO incompatibility should be considered, but its differentiation from HS becomes clear several months after birth. Other causes of spherocytic hemolytic anemia, such as clostridial sepsis, transfusion reactions, severe burns, and bites from snakes, spiders, bees, and wasps, should be viewed in the appropriate clinical context (see Chaps. 53, 54, and 140). Occasional spherocytes are also seen in patients with a large spleen (e.g., in cirrhosis or myelofibrosis) or in patients with microangiopathic anemias (see Chap. 51), but the differentiation of these conditions from HS does not usually present diagnostic difficulties.

Hereditary spherocytosis may be obscured in disorders that increase the surface-volume ratio of erythrocytes, such as obstructive jaundice, iron deficiency, β thalassemia trait or hemoglobin SC disease, and vitamin B_{12} or folate deficiency. In obstructive jaundice, spherocytosis can be obscured by the accumulation of cholesterol and phospholipids in the membrane that characteristically accompanies this condition. While in normal subjects this process leads to target cell formation, hereditary spherocytes acquire a discoidal appearance, and their survival in the circulation is improved. Iron deficiency corrects the abnormal shape but does not improve survival of HS erythrocytes.

THERAPY AND PROGNOSIS

SPLENECTOMY

Splenic sequestration is the primary determinant of erythrocyte survival in HS patients. Thus, splenectomy cures or alleviates the anemia in the overwhelming majority of patients, reducing or eliminating the need for red cell transfusions. Elimination of the need for chronic blood transfusions has obvious implications for future iron overload and risk of end organ damage. The incidence of cholelithiasis is also decreased. Postsplenectomy, spherocytosis, and altered osmotic fragility persist, but the "tail" of the osmotic fragility curve, created by conditioning of a subpopulation of spherocytes by the spleen, disappears. Erythrocyte life span nearly normalizes, and reticulocyte counts fall to normal or near-normal levels. Changes typical of the postsplenectomy state, including Howell-Jolly bodies, target cells, siderocytes, and acanthocytes, become evident on the blood film. Postsplenectomy, patients with the most severe forms of HS still suffer from shortened erythrocyte survival and hemolysis, but their clinical improvement is striking.[21,22]

Complications of Splenectomy   Early complications of splenectomy include local infection or bleeding and pancreatitis, presumably due to injury to the tail of the pancreas incurred during removal of the spleen. In general, the morbidity of splenectomy for HS is lower than that of other hematologic disorders. The complications of splenectomy are discussed in Chap. 5.

Indications for Splenectomy   In the past, splenectomy, which has a low operative mortality, was considered routine in HS patients. However, the risk of overwhelming post-splenectomy infection (OPSI) and the recent emergence of penicillin-resistant pneumococci have led to a reevaluation of the role of splenectomy in the treatment of HS. Considering the risks and benefits, a reasonable approach would be to splenectomize all patients with severe spherocytosis and all patients who suffer from significant signs or symptoms of anemia, including growth failure, skeletal changes, leg ulcers, and extramedullary hematopoietic tumors. Other candidates for splenectomy are older HS patients who suffer vascular compromise of vital organs.

Whether patients with moderate HS and compensated, asymptomatic anemia should have a splenectomy remains controversial. Patients with mild HS and compensated hemolysis can be followed and referred for splenectomy if clinically indicated. The treatment of patients with mild to moderate HS and gallstones is also debatable, particularly since new treatments for cholelithiasis, including laparoscopic cholecystectomy, endoscopic sphincterotomy, and extracorporal choletripsy, lower the risk of this complication. If such patients have symptomatic gallstones, a combined cholecystectomy and splenectomy can be performed, particularly if acute cholecystitis or biliary obstruction has occurred. There is no evidence that performing cholecystectomy and splenectomy separately, as was done in the past, is of any benefit.

Because the risk of postsplenectomy sepsis is very high in infancy and early childhood, splenectomy should be delayed until the age of 5 to 9 years if possible and to at least 3 years if this is feasible, even if chronic transfusions are required in the interim. There is no evidence that further delay is useful, and it may be harmful, because the risk of cholelithiasis increases dramatically in children after the age of 10 years.

When splenectomy is warranted, laparoscopic splenectomy has become the method of choice in centers where there are surgeons experienced in this technique. If desired, the procedure can be combined with laparoscopic cholecystectomy. Lararoscopic splenectomy results in less postoperative discomfort, a quicker return to preoperative diet and activities, shorter hospitalization, decreased costs, and smaller scars.[65] There is an increased risk of bleeding during the operation, and about 10 percent of laparoscopic operations (for all causes) have to be converted to standard splenectomies. Even enormous spleens (>600 g) can be removed laparoscopically, since the spleen is placed in a large bag, diced, and eliminated via suction catheters.

Partial splenectomy via laparotomy has been advocated for infants and young children with significant anemia associated with erythrocyte membrane disorders.[66] The goals of this procedure are to allow for the palliation of hemolysis and anemia while maintaining some residual splenic immune function. Long-term follow-up data for this procedure are lacking.

Prior to splenectomy, patients should be immunized with vaccines against pneumococcus, *Haemophilus influenzae* type b, and meningococcus, preferably several weeks preoperatively. The use of prophylactic antibiotics postsplenectomy to prevent pneumococcal sepsis is controversial. Postsplenectomy, prophylactic antibiotics (penicillin V 125 mg orally twice daily for patients <7 years of age or 250 mg orally twice daily for those >7 years of age, including adults) have been recommended for at least 5 years postsplenectomy by some and for life by others. The optimal duration of prophylactic antibiotic therapy postsplenectomy is unknown. Presplenectomy and, in severe cases, postsplenectomy, HS patients should take folic acid (1 mg/day orally) to prevent folate deficiency.

Splenectomy Failure   Splenectomy failure is uncommon. It may be due to an accessory spleen missed during splenectomy, the development of splenunculi resulting from autotransplantation of splenic tissue during surgery, or by another intrinsic red cell defect, such as pyruvate kinase deficiency (see Chap. 45). Accessory spleens occur in 15 to 40 percent of patients and must always be sought. Recurrence of hemolytic anemia years or even decades following splenectomy should raise suspicion of an accessory spleen, particularly if Howell-Jolly bodies are no longer found on blood film. A definitive confirmation of ectopic splenic tissue can be achieved by a radiocolloid liver-spleen scan or a scan using ^{51}Cr-labeled, heat-damaged red cells.

After a patient is diagnosed with HS, family members should be examined for the presence of HS.

HEREDITARY ELLIPTOCYTOSIS, PYROPOIKILOCYTOSIS, AND RELATED DISORDERS

DEFINITION AND HISTORY

Hereditary elliptocytosis (HE) is characterized by the presence of elliptical or oval erythrocytes on the blood films of affected individuals.[67,68] The worldwide incidence of HE has been estimated at 1 in 2000 to 1 in 4000 individuals. The true incidence of HE is unknown because its clinical severity is heterogeneous and many patients are asymptomatic. It is common in individuals of African and Mediterranean descent, presumably because elliptocytes confer some resistance to malaria. The incidence of HE is 6 percent in Benin, Africa.[69] Genetic haplotyping studies suggest that one HE mutation common in Africa has a "founder effect" with origins in central Africa similar to that attributed to hemoglobin S, Benin-type.

The first description of HE in 1904 was by Dresbach, a physiologist at Ohio State University in Columbus, Ohio, who discovered the condition in a medical student during a laboratory exercise in which the students were examining their own blood.[70] This report elicited some controversy, since the student died soon thereafter, leading to speculation that the student actually suffered from pernicious anemia. The demonstration of the disease in three generations of one family by Hunter clearly established the hereditary nature of this disorder.[71] The history of HE is reviewed by Dacie.[67]

Hereditary pyropoikilocytosis (HPP) is a rare cause of anemia first described in three children with severe neonatal anemia with erythrocyte morphology similar to that seen in patients suffering severe burns.[72] The erythrocytes from these patients also exhibited increased thermal sensitivity. Subsequently, other patients, mostly of African origin, with similar clinical and laboratory findings have been described.[73-75] There is a strong relationship between HE and HPP. Approximately one-third of parents or siblings of patients with HPP have typical HE, and many of these family members share identical mutations in erythrocyte spectrin. In addition, many patients with HPP proceed to develop typical mild to moderate HE. Patients with HPP tend to experience severe hemolysis and anemia in infancy that gradually improves, evolving toward typical HE later in life.

ETIOLOGY AND PATHOGENESIS

The principal defect in HE and HPP erythrocytes is mechanical weakness or fragility of the erythrocyte membrane skeleton. As in HS, study of erythrocyte membrane proteins in these disorders has identified abnormalities of various erythrocyte membrane proteins. These include α and β spectrin, protein 4.1, and GPC. The majority of defects occur in spectrin, the principal structural protein of the erythrocyte membrane skeleton (see Chap. 27). Most spectrin defects in HE and HPP impair the ability of spectrin dimers to self-associate into tetramers and oligomers, thereby disrupting the membrane skeleton.[3,76] Structural and functional defects of protein 4.1, which share similarities in cell shape and membrane stability to abnormalities of spectrin, are primarily due to disruption of the spectrin-actin attachment to the membrane via GPC. The mechanical instability in glycophorin C (GPC) variants appear to be due to secondary protein 4.1 deficiency. In all of these defects, disruption of the membrane skeleton leads to mechanical instability sufficient to cause red cell fragmentation with hemolytic anemia under conditions of normal circulatory shear stress.[77]

The pathobiology of elliptocytic shape is less clear. Red cell precursors in common HE are round, with the cells becoming progressively more elliptical as they age in vivo. Elliptocytes and poikilocytes may become permanently stabilized in shape because weakened spectrin heterodimer contacts facilitate skeletal reorganization following axial deformation of cells from prolonged or excessive shear stress. This reorganization is likely to involve breakage of the unidirectionally stretched protein connections followed by a formation of new protein contacts that preclude the recovery of normal biconcave shape. This process accounts for the permanent deformation of irreversibly sickle cells.

SPECTRIN AND HEREDITARY ELLIPTOCYTOSIS AND HEREDITARY PYROPOIKILOCYTOSIS

Abnormalities of either α or β spectrin associated with the majority of cases of HE and HPP are due to mutations in the spectrin heterodimer self-association site.[76,78] The repeats of spectrin involved in self-association and the locations of reported mutations are shown diagrammatically in Fig. 43-6. Most of these mutations are missense mutations at or very near highly conserved residues of α spectrin. The missense mutations are primarily either α helix-breaking mutations that replace the normal residue with a proline or glycine, or charge-shift mutations. In contrast to HS, the elliptocytosis and pyropoikilocytosis syndromes, while also quite heterogeneous, have been associated with distinct spectrin mutations in persons of similar genetic backgrounds, suggesting a "founder effect" for these mutations.

HE or HPP phenotype–spectrin mutation genotype correlations are difficult to establish. There is great clinical phenotypic heterogeneity among individuals with the same spectrin mutation. This heterogeneity exists even among individuals from the same kindred. A few general phenotype-genotype correlations can be made. Mutations at the contact sites of α and β spectrin in the spectrin self-association site tend to be more severe.[73,74] For example, mutations of codon 28, which is located in this contact site region, are generally associated with phenotypically severe HE or HPP. On the other hand, a common mutation in blacks from West and Central Africa, a leucine insertion at codon 154, is phenotypically very mild, even in the homozygous state.[79] Because of the great phenotypic variability described above, the presence of low-expression modifier alleles of spectrin has been postulated (see below).

In contrast to α spectrin mutations, a variety of β spectrin mutations have been identified in HE and HPP patients, including frameshift and splicing mutations that lead to truncated β-spectrin chains lacking the spectrin self-association site.[78] Three β-spectrin mutations, spectrin[Providence], spectrin[Caligiari], and spectrin[Buffalo], [80-82] when inherited in the homozygous state, lead to severe fetal or neonatal anemia and nonimmune hydrops fetalis. Five of 6 homozygotes died; the one survivor remains transfusion dependent.

PROTEIN 4.1

Protein 4.1 defects associated with HE are much less common than spectrin defects. Protein 4.1 is a multifunctional protein that undergoes complex patterns of tissue- and stage-specific alternative splicing and contains several important functional sites, including a spectrin-actin binding domain and a GPC binding domain. Partial deficiency of protein 4.1 is associated with asymptomatic HE, while complete deficiency leads to hemolytic anemia.[77,83,84] Homozygous 4.1 ($-/-$) erythrocytes fragment more rapidly than normal at moderate sheer stresses, an indication of their intrinsic instability (Fig. 43-7). Membrane mechanical stability can be restored by reconstituting the deficient red cells with protein 4.1 or the protein 4.1-spectrin-actin binding site.[85] Homozygous protein 4.1 ($-$) erythrocytes also lack p55 and have only 30 percent of the normal content of GPC. These 4.1 ($-$) erythrocytes, as well as GPC ($-$) Leach erythrocytes (see below) demonstrate decreased invasion and growth of *Plasmodium falciparum* in vitro.[86]

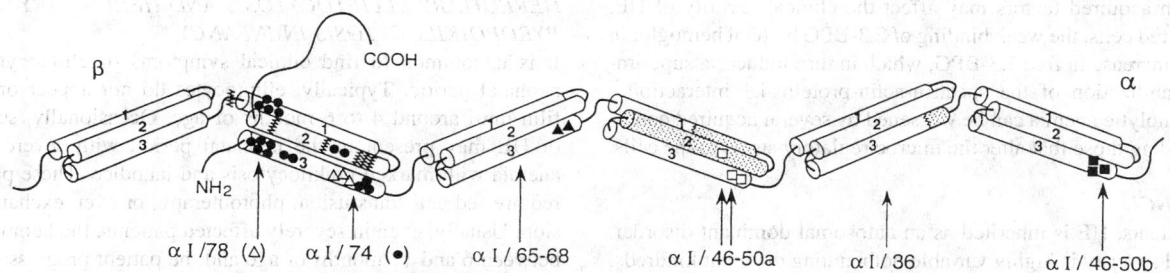

FIGURE 43-6 Defects of the spectrin self-association site in HE and HPP. A triple helical model of the spectrin repeats that constitute the spectrin self-association site is shown. The symbols denote positions of various genetic defects identified in patients with HE or HP. Limited tryptic digestion of spectrin, followed by two-dimensional gel electrophoresis, identifies abnormal cleavage sites (arrows) in spectrin associated with various mutations. (Modified from PG Gallagher et al,[68] with permission.)

Most patients with protein 4.1–associated elliptocytosis are from certain European and Arab populations. Protein 4.1 utilizes tissue-specific translation start sites, and several HE mutations have involved the downstream initiator codon.[4] In one HE mutant lacking the downstream initiator codon, because there is an erythroid stage-specific switch from the upstream initiator codon to the downstream initiator codon, the protein 4.1 HE phenotype does not develop until after the developmentally regulated switch has occurred.[87] HE-related protein 4.1 variants due to deletion or duplication of the exons involved in spectrin, actin, and protein 4.1 binding have also been described.[88,89]

GLYCOPHORIN C

Elliptocytes are present on the blood films of patients whose erythrocytes carry the Leach phenotype (i.e., lacking the Gerbich antigens, Ge-1, -2, -3, and -4) and lack both GPC and glycophorin D (GPD).[90] The Leach phenotype is usually due to a deletion of 7 kb of genomic DNA that removes exons 3 and 4 from the GPC/GPD locus.[91] A frameshift mutation due to a nucleotide deletion has also been described as the cause of this phenotype. GPC-deficient subjects are also partially deficient in the protein 4.1 and lack p55, presumably because these proteins form a complex and recruit or stabilize each other on the membrane.[92] It has been speculated that the protein 4.1 deficiency in Leach erythrocytes is the cause of the elliptocytic shape. In contrast to other forms of HE, which are dominantly inherited, heterozygous carriers are asymptomatic, with normal red blood cell morphology, while homozygous subjects have no anemia, with only mild elliptocytosis as shown on the blood film.

MOLECULAR DETERMINANTS OF CLINICAL SEVERITY

The severity of hemolysis in common HE often varies not only among different kindreds but within a given family as well. Erythrocyte spectrin content and the percentage of dimeric spectrin in crude spectrin extracts are the principal determinants of the severity of hemolysis. The percentage of dimeric spectrin in crude spectrin extracts depends on the degree of dysfunction of the mutant spectrin and by the gene dose (i.e., heterozygote versus homozygote or compound heterozygote) or the presence of other genetic defects *in trans*. Mutations in the spec-

trin self-association contact site produce a more severe defect of spectrin function and clinical phenotype than do other elliptocytogenic mutations.

The low-expression α-spectrin allele, α^LELY, is the best characterized abnormality affecting spectrin content and clinical severity. This allele is characterized by an amino acid substitution, Leu1857Val, and partial skipping of exon 46.[93] These abnormalities are located in the spectrin heterodimer nucleation site (i.e., where spectrin monomers assemble into heterodimers). Alpha-spectrin chains lacking exon 46 are poorly assembled into αβ heterodimers and are rapidly degraded.[94] Alone, the α^LELY allele is clinically silent, even when inherited in the homozygous state, because α spectrin is normally synthesized in three- to fourfold excess.[76] When it is present *in trans* to an elliptocytogenic α-spectrin mutation, it has the effect of increasing the mutant spectrin concentration and worsening the severity of the disease. Conversely, when the α^LELY allele is *in cis* to an α-spectrin mutation, it mutes the elliptocytic phenotype.

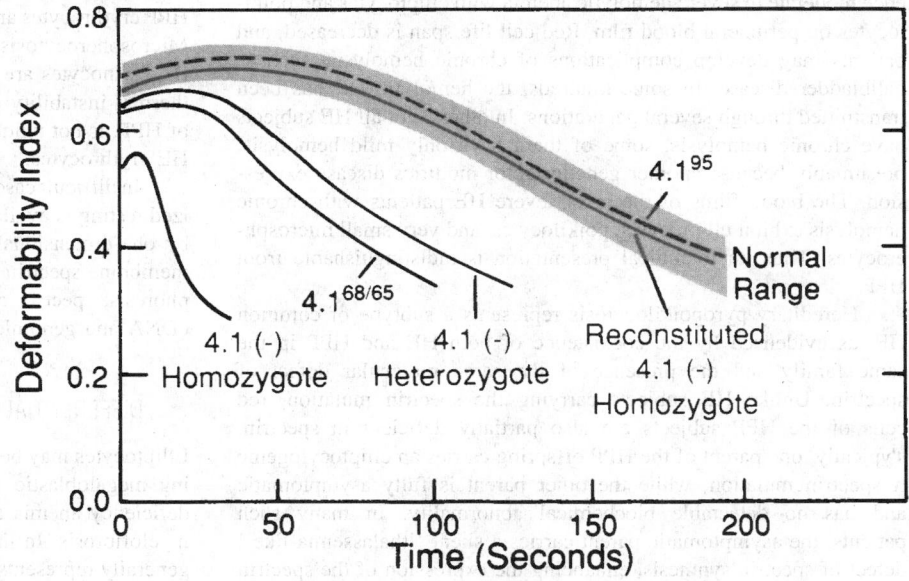

FIGURE 43-7 Erythrocyte membrane stability in defects of protein 4.1. Red cell membranes were subjected to shear stress in an ektacytometer, and deformability was measured as a function of time. A fall in deformability occurred as the membranes fragmented. Cells completely lacking protein 4.1 (−/−) have very fragile membranes, and normal fragility can be restored by reconstitution with normal protein 4.1. Heterozygous mutant cells (+/− and 68/65) have intermediate stability. (From N Mohandas and JA Chasis,[77] with permission.)

Certain acquired factors may affect the clinical severity of HE. In neonatal red cells, the weak binding of 2,3-BPG by fetal hemoglobin leads to an increase in free 2,3-BPG, which in turn induces a superimposed destabilization of the spectrin-actin-protein 4.1 interaction.[95] Finally, hemolytic anemia can be worsened by several acquired conditions, including those that alter the microcirculatory stress to the cells.

INHERITANCE

In most patients, HE is inherited as an autosomal dominant disorder. The clinical severity is highly variable both among different kindreds, reflecting heterogeneous molecular lesions, and, to a lesser extent, in a given kindred, presumably because of other genetic or acquired defects that modify disease expression. Rare cases of de novo mutation have been described,[96] as has an HE kindred with a contiguous gene syndrome inherited in an X-linked pattern.[97]

CLINICAL FEATURES

The clinical presentation of HE is heterogenous, ranging from asymptomatic carriers to patients with severe, life-threatening anemia.[73–76] The overwhelming majority of patients with HE are asymptomatic and are diagnosed incidentally during testing for unrelated conditions.

Asymptomatic carriers who possess the same molecular defect as an affected HE relative but who have normal or nearly normal blood films have been identified. The erythrocyte life span is normal, and these patients are not anemic. Asymptomatic HE patients may experience hemolysis in association with infections, hypersplenism, vitamin B_{12} deficiency, or microangiopathic hemolysis such as disseminated intravascular coagulation or thrombotic thrombocytopenic purpura. In the latter two conditions, worsening hemolysis may be due to microcirculatory damage superimposed on the underlying mechanical instability of red cells. It has been estimated that approximately 12 percent of patients with HE will become symptomatic from their anemia at some time during their lives.

Hereditary elliptocytosis patients with chronic hemolysis experience moderate to severe hemolytic anemia with elliptocytes and poikilocytes on peripheral blood film. Red cell life span is decreased, and patients may develop complications of chronic hemolysis, such as gallbladder disease. In some kindreds, the hemolytic HE has been transmitted through several generations. In others, not all HE subjects have chronic hemolysis; some of them have only mild hemolysis, presumably because another genetic factor modifies disease expression. The blood films of the most severe HE patients with chronic hemolysis exhibit elliptocytes, poikilocytes, and very small microspherocytes. Thus, their clinical presentation is indistinguishable from HPP.

Hereditary pyropoikilocytosis represents a subtype of common HE, as evidenced by the coexistence of both HE and HPP in the same family and the presence of the same molecular defect of spectrin. Unlike HE subjects carrying the spectrin mutation, red cells of the HPP subjects are also partially deficient in spectrin. Typically, one parent of the HPP offspring carries an elliptocytogenic α spectrin mutation, while the other parent is fully asymptomatic and has no detectable biochemical abnormality. In many such patients, the asymptomatic parent carries a silent ''thalassemia-like'' defect of spectrin synthesis, enhancing the expression of the spectrin mutant and leading to a superimposed spectrin deficiency in the HPP offspring. Some HPP subjects have inherited two structural variants of α spectrin. In these HPP patients, spectrin deficiency may be due to instability of the mutant spectrin. Hereditary pyropoikilocytosis is seen predominantly in subjects with African ancestry, but it has also been diagnosed in those of Arabic and European ancestry.

HEREDITARY ELLIPTOCYTOSIS AND HEREDITARY PYROPOIKILOCYTOSIS IN INFANCY

It is uncommon to find clinical symptoms of elliptocytosis in the neonatal period. Typically, elliptocytes do not appear on the blood film until around 4 to 6 months of age. Occasionally, severe forms of HE may present in the neonatal period with severe, hemolytic anemia with marked poikilocytosis and jaundice. These patients may require red cell transfusion, phototherapy, or even exchange transfusion. Usually, even in severely affected patients, the hemolysis abates between 6 and 12 months of age and the patient progresses to typical HE with mild anemia. Infrequently, patients remain transfusion-dependent beyond the first year of life and require early splenectomy. In cases of suspected neonatal HE or HPP, review of family history and analysis of blood films from the parents are usually of greater diagnostic benefit than other available studies.

A few cases of hydrops fetalis accompanied by fetal or early neonatal death due to unusually severe forms of HE have been described.[81,82] One severely affected hydropic infant salvaged by intrauterine transfusions and early exchange transfusion has remained transfusion dependent for over 2 years.[82]

LABORATORY FEATURES

The hallmark of HE is the presence of cigar-shaped elliptocytes on the blood film (Fig. 43-8). These normochromic, normocytic elliptocytes may number from few to 100 percent. The degree of hemolysis does not correlate with the number of elliptocytes present. Ovalocytes, spherocytes, stomatocytes, and fragmented cells may also be seen. The osmotic fragility is abnormal in severe HE and in HPP. The reticulocyte count generally is less than 5 percent but may be higher when hemolysis is severe. Other laboratory findings in HE are similar to those of other hemolytic anemias and are nonspecific markers of increased erythrocyte production and destruction; for example, increased serum bilirubin, increased urinary urobilinogen, and decreased serum haptoglobin reflect increased erythrocyte destruction.

In HPP, in addition to the blood film findings seen in HE, many HPP erythrocytes are bizarrely shaped, with fragmentation or budding. Microspherocytosis is common, and the MCV is usually low (50–70 fl). Pyknocytes are prominent in smears of neonates with HPP. The thermal instability of erythrocytes, originally reported as diagnostic of HPP, is not unique to this disorder and is also commonly found in HE erythrocytes.

In difficult cases or cases requiring a molecular diagnosis, specialized testing is available. This includes analysis of membrane proteins by one-dimensional gel electrophoresis, limited tryptic digestion of membrane spectrin followed by one- or two-dimensional gel electrophoresis, spectrin dimer self-association assays, ektacytometry, and cDNA and genomic DNA analyses.

DIFFERENTIAL DIAGNOSIS

Elliptocytes may be seen in association with several disorders, including megaloblastic anemias, hypochromic microcytic anemias (iron deficiency anemia and thalassemia), myelodyplastic syndromes, and myelofibrosis. In these conditions, the elliptocytosis is acquired and generally represents less than a quarter of red cells seen on peripheral smear. History and additional laboratory testing usually clarify the diagnosis of these disorders. Pseudoelliptocytosis is an artifact of blood film preparation. Pseudoelliptocytes are found only in certain areas of the film, usually near its tail, and the long axes of pseudoelliptocytes are parallel, whereas the axes of true elliptocytes are distributed randomly.

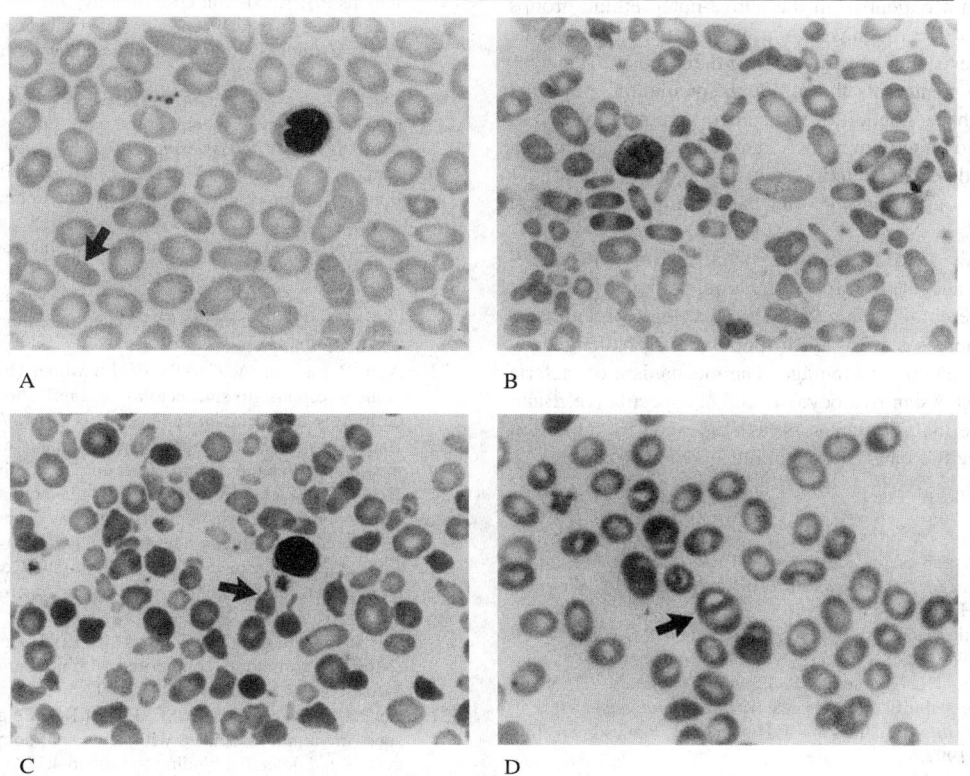

FIGURE 43-8   Blood films from patients with various forms of HE. *(a)* Simple heterozygote with mild common HE associated with an elliptogenic spectrin mutation. Note the predominant elliptocytosis, with some rod-shaped cells (arrow) and the virtual absence of poikilocytes. *(b)* Compound heterozygosity for common HE due to doubly heterozygous state for two spectrin mutations. Both parents have mild HE. There are many elliptocytes as well as numerous fragments and poikilocytes. *(c)* HPP. The patient is a compound heterozygote for an α spectrin self-association site mutation and a defect characterized by reduced synthesis of this protein. Note prominent microspherocytosis, micropoikilocytosis, and fragmentation. Only a few elliptocytes are present. Some poikilocytes are in the process of budding (arrow). *(d)* Southeast Asian (Melanesian) ovalocytosis. The majority of cells are oval, some of them containing either a longitudinal slit or a transverse ridge (arrow). See the text for further details.

THERAPY AND PROGNOSIS

Therapy is rarely needed in patients with HE. In rare cases, occasional red blood cell transfusions may be required. In cases of severe HE and HPP, splenectomy has been palliative, as the spleen is the site of erythrocyte sequestration and destruction. The same indications for splenectomy in HS can be applied to patients with symptomatic HE or HPP. Postsplenectomy, patients with HE or HPP exhibit increased hematocrits, decreased reticulocyte counts, and improvement in clinical symptoms.

Patients should be followed for signs of decompensation during acute illnesses. Interval ultrasonography to detect gallstones should be performed. Patients with significant hemolysis should receive daily folate supplementation.

SOUTHEAST ASIAN OVALOCYTOSIS

Southeast Asian ovalocytosis, also known as Melanesian elliptocytosis or stomatocytic elliptocytosis, is a dominantly inherited trait characterized by the presence of oval red cells, many of which contain one or two transverse ridges or a longitudinal slit (Fig. 43-8d). This condition is widespread in certain ethnic groups of Malaysia, Papua New Guinea, the Philippines, and Indonesia.[98] Numerous abnormalities of Southeast

Asian ovalocytosis erythrocytes have been reported, including increased red cell rigidity, decreased osmotic fragility, increased thermal stability, resistance to shape change by echinocytic agents, and a reduced expression of many red cell antigens.[4] Thus, Southeast Asian ovalocytosis red cells are unique among the elliptocytes in that they are rigid and hyperstable rather than unstable. A remarkable feature of Southeast Asian ovalocytosis erythrocytes is their resistance to in vitro invasion by several strains of malaria parasites, including *Plasmodium falciparum and Plasmodium knowlesi.*[99]

The Southeast Asian ovalocytosis phenotype is due to heterozygosity for two band 3 mutations in *cis*: the deletion of 27 bp encoding amino acids 400 to 408 located at the boundary of the cytoplasmic and membrane domains of band 3 and the amino acid substitution Lys56Glu.[100] The latter represents an asymptomatic polymorphism. It has been hypothesized that homozygosity for Southeast Asian ovalocytosis would lead to embryonic lethality.[101] Southeast Asian ovalocytosis erythrocytes exhibit increased binding of band 3 to ankyrin, increased tyrosine phosphorylation of band 3, inability to transport sulfate anions, and a markedly restricted lateral and rotational mobility of the band 3 protein in the membrane.

Clinically, the finding of 30 percent or more of oval-shaped red cells on the blood film, some containing a central slit or a transverse ridge, together with a notable absence of clinical and laboratory evidence of hemolysis in a patient from the above-noted ethnic groups is highly suggestive of the diagnosis. A useful screening test is the demonstration of the resistance of ovalocytes or their ghosts to changes in shape produced by treatments that produce spiculation in normal cells, such as overnight incubation of red cells or exposure of ghosts to salt solutions. Rapid genetic diagnosis can be made by amplifying the region containing the 27-bp deletion from genomic DNA or reticulocyte cDNA and demonstrating a shorter band compared to control after electrophoresis.

In vivo, there is evidence that Southeast Asian ovalocytosis provides some protection against all forms of malaria, particularly against heavy infections and cerebral malaria.[102,103] The prevalence of Southeast Asian ovalocytosis increases with age in populations challenged by malaria, suggesting a selective advantage. The mechanism of malaria resistance of Southeast Asian ovalocytosis cells is speculative. Band 3 serves as one of the malaria receptors, as evidenced by inhibition of invasion in vitro by the band 3–containing liposomes.

REFERENCES

1. Dacie J: The life span of the red blood cell and circumstances of its premature death, in *Blood, Pure and Eloquent*, edited by M Wintrobe, p 211. McGraw-Hill, New York, 1980.
2. Delaunay J: Genetic disorders of the red cell membrane. *Crit Rev Oncol Hematol* 19:79, 1995.
3. Morrow JS, Rimm DL, Kennedy SP, Cianci CD, Sinard JH, Weed SA: Of membrane stability and mosaics: The spectrin cytoskeleton, in *Handbook of Physiology*, edited by J Hoffman, J Jamieson, p 485. Oxford, London, 1997.
4. Tse WT, Lux SE: Red blood cell membrane disorders. *Br J Haematol* 104:2, 1999.
5. Hassoun H, Palek J: Hereditary spherocytosis: a review of the clinical and molecular aspects of the disease. *Blood Rev* 10:129, 1996.
6. Pekrun A, Eber SW, Kuhlmey A, Schröter W: Combined ankyrin and spectrin deficiency in hereditary spherocytosis. *Ann Hematol* 67:89, 1993.
7. Savvides P, Shalev O, John KM, Lux SE: Combined spectrin and ankyrin deficiency is common in autosomal dominant hereditary spherocytosis. *Blood* 82:2953, 1993.
8. Saad ST, Costa FF, Vicentim DL, Salles TS, Pranke PH: Red cell membrane protein abnormalities in hereditary spherocytosis in Brazil. *Br J Haematol* 88:295, 1994.
9. Eber SW, Gonzalez JM, Lux ML, et al: Ankyrin-1 mutations are a major cause of dominant and recessive hereditary spherocytosis. *Nature Genet* 13:214, 1996.
10. Gallagher PG, Forget BG: Hematologically important mutations: Spectrin and ankyrin variants in hereditary spherocytosis. *Blood Cell Mol Dis* 24:539, 1998.
11. Miraglia del Giudice E, Francese M, Nobili B, et al: High frequency of de novo mutations in ankyrin gene (ANK1) in children with hereditary spherocytosis. *J Pediatr* 132:117, 1998.
12. Eber SW, Pekrun A, Reinhardt D, Schröter W, Lux SE: Hereditary spherocytosis with ankyrin Walsrode, a variant ankyrin with decreased affinity for band 3. *Blood* 84:362a, 1994.
13. Gallagher PG, Ferreira JDS, Saad STO, Kerbally J, Costa FF, Forget BG: A recurring frameshift mutation of the ankyrin-1 gene associated with severe hereditary spherocytosis in Brazil. *Blood* 88:6a, 1996.
14. Basseres D, Bordin S, Costa F, Gallagher P, Saad S: A novel ankyrin promoter mutation associated with hereditary spherocytosis. *Blood* 92:8a, 1998.
15. Lux SE, Tse WT, Menninger JC, et al: Hereditary spherocytosis associated with deletion of human erythrocyte ankyrin gene on chromosome 8. *Nature* 345:736, 1990.
16. Gallagher PG, Forget BG: Hematologically important mutations: Cell band 3 and protein 4.2 variants in hereditary spherocytosis. *Blood Cell Mol Dis* 23:417, 1997.
17. Jarolim P, Rubin HL, Brabec V, et al: Mutations of conserved arginines in the membrane domain of erythroid band 3 lead to a decrease in membrane-associated band 3 and to the phenotype of hereditary spherocytosis. *Blood* 85:634, 1995.
18. Jenkins PB, Abou-Alfa GK, Dhermy D, et al: A nonsense mutation in the erythrocyte band 3 gene associated with decreased mRNA accumulation in a kindred with dominant hereditary spherocytosis. *J Clin Invest* 97:373, 1996.
19. Rysava R, Tesar V, Jirsa M Jr, Brabec V, Jarolim P: Incomplete distal renal tubular acidosis coinherited with a mutation in the band 3 (AE1) gene. *Nephrol Dial Transplant* 12:1869, 1997.
20. Lima PRM, Gontijo JAR, Lopes de Faria JB, Costa FF, Saad STO: Band 3 Campinas: A novel splicing mutation in the band 3 gene (AE1) associated with hereditary spherocytosis, hyperactivity of Na+/Li+ countertransport and an abnormal renal bicarbonate handling. *Blood* 90:2810, 1997.
21. Agre P, Casella JF, Zinkham WH, McMillan C, Bennett V: Partial deficiency of erythrocyte spectrin in hereditary spherocytosis. *Nature* 314:380, 1985.
22. Agre P, Asimos A, Casella JF, McMillan C: Inheritance pattern and clinical response to splenectomy as a reflection of erythrocyte spectrin deficiency in hereditary spherocytosis. *N Engl J Med* 315:1579, 1986.
23. Hanspal M, Palek J: Biogenesis of normal and abnormal red blood cell membrane skeleton. *Semin Hematol* 29:305, 1992.
24. Jarolim P, Wichterle H, Palek J, Gallagher PG, Forget BG: The low expression α spectrin lepra is frequently associated with autosomal recessive/non-dominant hereditary spherocytosis. *Blood* 88:4a, 1996.
25. Wichterle H, Hanspal M, Palek J, Jarolim P: Combination of two mutant alpha spectrin alleles underlies a severe spherocytic hemolytic anemia. *J Clin Invest* 98:2300, 1996.
26. Tse WT, Gallagher PG, Jenkins PB, et al: Amino acid substitution in α-spectrin commonly coinherited with nondominant hereditary spherocytosis. *Am J Hematol* 54:233, 1997.
27. Becker PS, Tse WT, Lux SE, Forget BG: Beta spectrin Kissimmee: A spectrin variant associated with autosomal dominant hereditary spherocytosis and defective binding to protein 4.1. *J Clin Invest* 92:612, 1993.
28. Hassoun H, Vassiliadis JN, Murray J, et al: Characterization of the underlying molecular defect in hereditary spherocytosis associated with spectrin deficiency. *Blood* 90:398, 1997.
29. Miraglia del Giudice E, Lombardi C, Francese M, et al: Frequent de novo monoallelic expression of β-spectrin gene (SPTB) in children with hereditary spherocytosis and isolated spectrin deficiency. *Br J Haematol* 101:251, 1998.
30. Bouhassira EE, Schwartz RS, Yawata Y, et al: An alanine-to-threonine substitution in protein 4.2 cDNA is associated with a Japanese form of hereditary hemolytic anemia (protein 4.2NIPPON). *Blood* 79:1846, 1992.
31. Rybicki AC, Qiu JJ, Musto S, Rosen NL, Nagel RL, Schwartz RS: Human erythrocyte protein 4.2 deficiency associated with hemolytic anemia and a homozygous 40 glutamic acid→lysine substitution in the cytoplasmic domain of band 3 (band 3Montefiore). *Blood* 81:2155, 1993.
32. Jarolim P, Palek J, Rubin HL, Prchal JT, Korsgren C, Cohen CM: Band 3 Tuscaloosa: Pro327-Arg327 substitution in the cytoplasmic domain of erythrocyte band 3 protein associated with spherocytic hemolytic anemia and partial deficiency of protein 4.2. *Blood* 80:523, 1992.
33. Brugnara C: Erythrocyte membrane transport physiology. *Curr Opin Hematol* 4:122, 1997.
34. De Franceschi L, Olivieri O, Miraglia del Giudice E, et al: Membrane cation and anion transport activities in erythrocytes of hereditary spherocytosis: Effects of different membrane protein defects. *Am J Hematol* 55:121, 1997.
35. Gallagher PG, Forget BG, Lux SE: Disorders of the erythrocyte membrane, in *Hematology of Infancy and Childhood*, edited by D Nathan, S Orkin, p 544. Saunders, Philadelphia, 1998.
36. Young LE, Platzer RI, Ervin DM, Izzo MJ: Hereditary spherocytosis: II. Observations on the role of the spleen. *Blood* 6:1099, 1951.
37. Emerson CJ, Shen S, Ham T, et al: Studies on the destruction of red blood cells: IX. Quantitative methods for determining the osmotic and mechanical fragility of red cells in the peripheral blood and splenic pulp: the mechanism of increased hemolysis in hereditary spherocytosis (congenital hemolytic jaundice) as related to the function of the spleen. *Arch Intern Med* 97:1, 1956.
38. Eber SW, Armbrust R, Schröter W: Variable clinical severity of hereditary spherocytosis: Relation to erythrocytic spectrin concentration, osmotic fragility, and autohemolysis. *J Pediatr* 117:409, 1990.
39. Becker P, Lux S: Disorders of the red cell membrane skeleton: Hereditary spherocytosis and hereditary elliptocytosis, in *The Metabolic Basis of*

Inherited Disease, edited by C Scriver, A Beaudet, W Sly, et al: p 529. McGraw-Hill, New York, 1995.

40. Weiss L, Tavassoli M: Anatomical hazards to the passage of erythrocytes through the spleen. *Semin Hematol* 7:372, 1970.

41. Whitfield CF, Follweiler JB, Lopresti-Morrow L, Miller BA: Deficiency of alpha-spectrin synthesis in burst-forming units-erythroid in lethal hereditary spherocytosis. *Blood* 78:3043, 1991.

42. McKinney AAJ, Morton NE, Kosower NS, et al: Ascertaining genetic carriers of hereditary spherocytosis by statistical analysis of multiple laboratory tests. *J Clin Invest* 41:554, 1962.

43. Ribeiro ML, Alloisio N, Almeida H, et al: Hereditary spherocytosis with total absence of band 3 in a baby with mutation Coimbra (V488M) in the homozygous state. *Blood* 90:265a, 1997.

44. Perrotta S, Nigro V, Iolascon A, et al: Dominant hereditary spherocytosis due to band 3 Neapolis produces a life-threatening anemia at the homozygous state. *Blood* 92:9a, 1998.

45. Alloisio N, Maillet P, Carre G, et al: Hereditary spherocytosis with band 3 deficiency: Association with a nonsense mutation of the band 3 gene (allele Lyon), and aggravation by a low-expression allele occurring in trans (allele Genas). *Blood* 88:1062, 1996.

46. Ozcan R, Kugler W, Feuring-Buske M, Schröter W, Lux SE, Eber SW: Parental mosaicism for ankyrin-1 mutations in two families with hereditary spherocytosis (HS). *Blood* 90:4a, 1997.

47. Pajor A, Lehoczky D, Szakacs Z: Pregnancy and hereditary spherocytosis: Report of 8 patients and a review. *Arch Gynecol Obstet* 253:37, 1993.

48. Burman D: Congenital spherocytosis in infancy. *Arch Dis Child* 33:335, 1958.

49. Trucco JI, Brown AK: Neonatal manifestations of hereditary spherocytosis. *Am J Dis Child* 113:263, 1967.

50. Iolascon A, Faienza MF, Moretti A, Perrotta S, Miraglia del Giudice E: UGT1 promoter polymorphism accounts for increased neonatal appearance of hereditary spherocytosis. *Blood* 91:1093, 1998.

51. Bates G, Brown C: Incidence of gallbladder disease in chronic hemolytic anemia (spherocytosis). *Gastroenterology* 21:104, 1952.

52. Brown KE, Young NS: Parvovirus B19 in human disease. *Annu Rev Med* 48:59, 1997.

53. Lefrere JJ, Courouce AM, Girot R, Bertrand Y, Soulier JP: Six cases of hereditary spherocytosis revealed by human parvovirus infection. *Br J Haematol* 62:653, 1986.

54. McLellan NJ, Rutter N: Hereditary spherocytosis in sisters unmasked by parvovirus infection. *Postgrad Med J* 63:49, 1987.

55. Lawrence P, Aronson I, Saxe N, Jacobs P: Leg ulcers in hereditary spherocytosis. *Clin Exp Dermatol* 16:28, 1991.

56. Pulsoni A, Ferrazza G, Malagnino F, et al: Mediastinal extramedullary hematopoiesis as first manifestation of hereditary spherocytosis. *Ann Hematol* 65:196, 1992.

57. Conti JA, Howard LM: Hereditary spherocytosis and hematologic malignancy. *N Engl J Med* 91:95, 1994.

58. Mohler DN, Wheby MS: Hemochromatosis heterozygotes may have significant iron overload when they also have hereditary spherocytosis. *Am J Med Sci* 292:320, 1986.

59. Peters LL, Barker JE: Spontaneous and targeted mutations in erythrocyte membrane skeleton genes: Mouse models of hereditary spherocytosis, in *Hematopoiesis*, edited by L Zon, in press. Oxford University Press, New York, 1999

60. Gilligan DM, Lozovatsky L, Gwynn B, Brugnara C, Mohandas N, Peters LL: Targeted disruption of the beta-adducin gene (Add2) causes red blood cell spherocytosis in mice. *Proc Natl Acad Sci USA* 96:10717, 1999.

61. Pati AR, Patton WN, Harris RI: The use of the Technicon H1 in the diagnosis of hereditary spherocytosis. *Clin Lab Haematol* 11:27, 1989.

62. Schilling RF: Estimating the risk for sepsis after splenectomy in hereditary spherocytosis. *Ann Intern Med* 122:187, 1995.

63. Konradsen HB, Henrichsen J: Pneumococcal infections in splenectomized children are preventable. *Acta Paediatr Scand* 80:423, 1991.

64. Robinette CD, Fraumeni JF Jr: Splenectomy and subsequent mortality in veterans of the 1939–45 war. *Lancet* 2:127, 1977.

65. Gigot JF, de Ville de Goyet J, Van Beers BE, et al: Laparoscopic splenectomy in adults and children: experience with 31 patients. *Surgery* 119:384, 1996.

66. Tchernia G, Gauthier F, Mielot F, et al: Initial assessment of the benefi-

67. Dacie J: Hereditary elliptocytosis, in *The Haemolytic Anaemias*, p 216. Churchill Livingstone, Edinburgh, 1985.

68. Gallagher PG, Tse WT, Forget BG: Clinical and molecular aspects of disorders of the erythrocyte membrane skeleton. *Semin Perinatol* 14:351, 1990.

69. Glele-Kakai C, Garbarz M, Lecomte M-C, et al: Epidemiological studies of spectrin mutations related to hereditary elliptocytosis and spectrin polymorphisms in Benin. *Br J Haematol* 95:57, 1996.

70. Dresbach M: Elliptical human red corpuscles. *Science* 19:469, 1904.

71. Hunter WC, Adams RB: Hematologic study of three generations of a white family showing elliptical erythrocytes. *Ann Intern Med* 2:1162, 1929.

72. Zarkowsky HS, Mohandas N, Speaker CB, Shohet SB: A congenital haemolytic anaemia with thermal sensitivity of the erythrocyte membrane. *Br J Haematol* 29:537, 1975.

73. Coetzer T, Palek J, Lawler J, et al: Structural and functional heterogeneity of alpha spectrin mutations involving the spectrin heterodimer self-association site: Relationships to hematologic expression of homozygous hereditary elliptocytosis and hereditary pyropoikilocytosis. *Blood* 75:2235, 1990.

74. Coetzer TL, Sahr K, Prchal J, et al: Four different mutations in codon 28 of alpha spectrin are associated with structurally and functionally abnormal spectrin alpha I/74 in hereditary elliptocytosis. *J Clin Invest* 88:743, 1991.

75. Marchesi SL, Letsinger JT, Speicher DW, et al: Mutant forms of spectrin alpha-subunits in hereditary elliptocytosis. *J Clin Invest* 80:191, 1987.

76. Delaunay J: Genetic disorders of the red cell membrane. *Crit Rev Oncol Hematol* 19:79, 1995.

77. Mohandas N, Chasis JA: Red blood cell deformability, membrane material properties and shape: Regulation by transmembrane, skeletal and cytosolic proteins and lipids. *Semin Hematol* 30:171, 1993.

78. Gallagher PG, Forget BG: Hematologically important mutations: Spectrin variants in hereditary elliptocytosis and hereditary pyropoikocytosis. *Blood Cells Mol Dis* 22:254, 1996.

79. Roux AF, Morle F, Guetarni D, et al: Molecular basis of Spα$^{1/65}$ hereditary elliptocytosis in North Africa: Insertion of a TTG triplet between codons 147 and 149 in the alpha-spectrin gene from five unrelated families. *Blood* 73:2196, 1989.

80. Gallagher PG, Weed SA, Tse WT, et al: Recurrent fatal hydrops fetalis associated with a nucleotide substitution in the erythrocyte β-spectrin gene. *J Clin Invest* 95:1174, 1995.

81. Sahr KE, Coetzer TL, Moy LS, et al: Spectrin Cagliari. An Ala→Gly substitution in helix 1 of β spectrin repeat 17 that severely disrupts the structure and self-association of the erythrocyte spectrin heterodimer. *J Biol Chem* 268:22656, 1993.

82. Gallagher PG, Petruzzi MJ, Weed SA, et al: Mutation of a highly conserved residue of βI spectrin associated with fatal and near-fatal neonatal hemolytic anemia. *J Clin Invest* 99:267, 1997.

83. Alloisio N, Dorleac E, Girot R, Delaunay J: Analysis of the red cell membrane in a family with hereditary elliptocytosis: Total or partial absence of protein 4.1. *Hum Genet* 59:68, 1981.

84. Conboy JG: Structure, function, and molecular genetics of erythroid membrane skeletal protein 4.1 in normal and abnormal red blood cells. *Semin Hematol* 30:58, 1993.

85. Takakuwa Y, Tchernia G, Rossi M, Benabadji M, Mohandas N: Restoration of normal membrane stability to unstable protein 4.1-deficient erythrocyte membranes by incorporation of purified protein 4.1. *J Clin Invest* 78:80, 1986.

86. Chishti AH, Palek J, Fisher D, Maalouf GJ, Liu SC: Reduced invasion and growth of *Plasmodium falciparum* into elliptocytic red blood cells with a combined deficiency of protein 4.1, glycophorin C, and p55. *Blood* 87:3462, 1996.

87. Conboy JG, Chasis JA, Winardi R, Tchernia G, Kan YW, Mohandas N: An isoform-specific mutation in the protein 4.1 gene results in hereditary elliptocytosis and complete deficiency of protein 4.1 in erythrocytes but not in nonerythroid cells. *J Clin Invest* 91:77, 1993.

88. Marchesi SL, Conboy J, Agre P, et al: Molecular analysis of insertion/deletion mutations in protein 4.1 in elliptocytosis: I. Biochemical identification of rearrangements in the spectrin/actin binding domain and functional characterizations. *J Clin Invest* 86:516, 1990.

89. Conboy J, Marchesi S, Kim R, Agre P, Kan YW, Mohandas N: Molecular analysis of insertion/deletion mutations in protein 4.1 in elliptocytosis: II. Determination of molecular genetic origins of rearrangements. *J Clin Invest* 86:524, 1990.

90. Reid ME, Martynewycz MA, Wolford FE, Crawford MN, Miller LH: Leach type Ge: Red cells and elliptocytosis. *Transfusion* 27:213, 1987.

91. Winardi R, Reid M, Conboy J, Mohandas N: Molecular analysis of glycophorin C deficiency in human erythrocytes. *Blood* 81:2799, 1993.

92. Marfatia SM, Lue RA, Branton D, Chishti AH: In vitro binding studies suggest a membrane-associated complex between erythroid p55, protein 4.1, and glycophorin C. *J Biol Chem* 269:8631, 1994.

93. Wilmotte R, Marechal J, Morle L, et al: Low expression allele α^{LELY} of red cell spectrin is associated with mutations in exon 40 ($\alpha^{V/41}$ polymorphism) and intron 45 and with partial skipping of exon 46. *J Clin Invest* 91:2091, 1993.

94. Wilmotte R, Harper SL, Ursitti JA, Marechal J, Delaunay J, Speicher DW: The exon 46 encoded sequence is essential for stability of human erythroid α-spectrin and heterodimer formation. *Blood* 90:4188, 1996.

95. Mentzer WC Jr, Iarocci TA, Mohandas N, et al: Modulation of erythrocyte membrane mechanical stability by 2,3-diphosphoglycerate in the neonatal poikilocytosis/elliptocytosis syndrome. *J Clin Invest* 79:943, 1987.

96. Lorenzo F, Miraglia del Giudice E, Alloisio N, et al: Severe poikilocytosis associated with a de novo α 28 Arg→Cys mutation in spectrin. *Br J Haematol* 83:152, 1993.

97. Jonsson JJ, Renieri A, Gallagher PG, et al: Alport syndrome, mental retardation, midface hypoplasia, and elliptocytosis: A new X-linked contiguous gene deletion syndrome. *Am J Med Genet* 35:273, 1997.

98. Fix AG, Baer AS, Lie-Injo LE: The mode of inheritance of ovalocytosis/elliptocytosis in Malaysian Orang Asli families. *Hum Genet* 61:250, 1982.

99. Hadley T, Saul A, Lamont G, Hudson DE, Miller LH, Kidson C: Resistance of Melanesian elliptocytes (ovalocytes) to invasion *by Plasmodium knowlesi* and *Plasmodium falciparum* malaria parasites in vitro. *J Clin Invest* 71:780, 1983.

100. Jarolim P, Palek J, Amato D, et al: Deletion in erythrocyte band 3 gene in malaria-resistant Southeast Asian ovalocytosis. *Proc Natl Acad Sci USA* 88:11022, 1991.

101. Liu SC, Jarolim P, Rubin HL, et al: The homozygous state for the band 3 protein mutation in Southeast Asian ovalocytosis may be lethal. *Blood* 84:3590, 1994.

102. Genton B, al-Yaman F, Mgone CS, et al: Ovalocytosis and cerebral malaria. *Nature* 378:564, 1995.

103. Foo LC, Rekhraj V, Chiang GL, Mak JW: Ovalocytosis protects against severe malaria parasitemia in the Malayan aborigines. *Am J Trop Med Hyg* 47:271, 1992.

ACANTHOCYTOSIS, STOMATOCYTOSIS, & RELATED DISORDERS

PATRICK G. GALLAGHER

Acanthocytes are contracted, dense cells with irregular projections from the red cell surface. They are seen in the blood films of patients with severe liver disease, abetalipoproteinemia, certain inherited neurologic disorders without abetalipoproteinemia, and in association with the inheritance of certain red cell antigen polymorphisms. Erythrocytes in these disorders are characterized by abnormal red cell membrane lipid composition with altered lipid distribution between the inner and outer leaflets of the bilayer. Typically, the hemolytic anemia associated with acanthocytosis is mild to moderate and rarely requires therapy. Stomatocytes are erythrocytes characterized by a wide transverse slit (or stoma) found in the blood films of patients with a variety of acquired and inherited red cell disorders. Stomatocytosis is commonly associated with inherited abnormalities of red cell cation permeability. These disorders are frequently associated with abnormal red cell cation content, hydration, and membrane lipids. There is great heterogeneity in the erythrocyte morphology, laboratory manifestations, and clinical course of the stomatocytosis syndromes. The etiology of these disorders of cation permeability is unknown.

ACANTHOCYTOSIS

Spiculated red cells are classified into two types, acanthocytes and echinocytes. *Acanthocytes* are contracted, dense cells with irregular projections from the red cell surface that vary in width and length. *Echinocytes* have small, uniform projections spread evenly over the circumference of the red cell. These differences are clearly seen in scanning electron micrographs (see Table 22-3)[1] but may be difficult to ascertain on standard peripheral blood smears. Acanthocytes are almost always accompanied by echinocytes, but echinocytes may be present alone. Diagnostically, the distinction is not critical, and disorders of spiculated red cells are generally classified together. Normal adults may have up to 3 percent of spiculated erythrocytes on smear, with higher levels found in patients with functional or actual splenectomy, after ingestion of alcohol or certain medications (e.g., indomethacin, salicylates, furosemide), and in premature infants (mean 5.5 percent, range 1–25 percent). Spiculated cells, particularly echinocytes, are common artifacts of blood smear preparation.

Acronyms and abbreviations that appear in this chapter include: FP, familial pseudohyperkalemia; HARP syndrome, *h*ypoprebetalipoproteinemia, *a*canthocytosis, *r*etinitis pigmentosa, and *p*allidal degeneration with iron deposition; HSt, hereditary stomatocytosis; MCHC, mean corpuscular hemoglobin concentration; MCV, mean corpuscular volume; MTP, microsomal transfer protein.

Acanthocytes are present in the blood films of patients with severe liver disease, abetalipoproteinemia, certain inherited neurologic disorders without abetalipoproteinemia, and in association with the inheritance of certain red cell antigen polymorphisms such as the McLeod blood group. Abnormal red cell membrane lipid composition and altered lipid distribution between the inner and outer leaflets of the bilayer characterize these conditions. Smaller numbers of acanthocytes (<10 percent) may be seen in patients with myelodysplasia, hypothyroidism, and anorexia nervosa. Echinocytes may be found on the blood films of patients with severe uremia, glycolytic defects, and microangiopathic hemolytic anemia, and transiently after transfusion of stored red cells.

ACANTHOCYTOSIS IN SEVERE LIVER DISEASE

DEFINITION

The anemia in patients with liver disease is of complex etiology.[2] Common causes include blood loss, iron or folate deficiency, hypersplenism, and marrow suppression from alcohol, malnutrition, hepatitis infection, or other factors. Acquired abnormalities of the red cell membrane may contribute to the anemia in these patients; one is a syndrome of hemolysis with acanthocytosis or "spur" cells, so-called spur cell anemia.[3] Although only a small number of patients with end-stage liver disease acquire spur cell anemia, the prevalence of liver disease is so high that these individuals account for the majority of cases of acanthocytosis seen in clinical practice.

ETIOLOGY AND PATHOGENESIS

Acanthocyte formation in vivo is a two-step process involving accumulation of free (nonesterified) cholesterol in the red cell membrane and remodeling of abnormally shaped red cells by the spleen.[4,5] Acanthocytes result from increased acquisition of free cholesterol from the plasma due to abnormal cholesterol/lipoprotein ratios.[4] In severe liver disease, a very high ratio of free cholesterol to phospholipids is found in lipoproteins. Free cholesterol readily partitions into the membrane, where it preferentially associates with the outer leaflet, making it less fluid. The spleen attempts to remodel the membrane leading to rigid, spherical erythrocytes with the characteristic spiculated projections[5] (Fig. 44-1). Over time, these poorly deformable cells have difficulty negotiating the narrow sinusoids of the splenic circulation and are hemolyzed (Chap. 5).

CLINICAL FEATURES

Spur cell anemia is characterized by a rapidly progressive hemolytic anemia with large numbers of acanthocytes on the blood film.[3,6,7] Splenomegaly and jaundice become more prominent accompanied by severe ascites, bleeding diatheses, and hepatic encephalopathy. Spur cell anemia is most common in patients with alcoholic liver disease, but similar clinical syndromes have been described in association with advanced metastatic liver disease, cardiac cirrhosis, Wilson disease, fulminant hepatitis, and infantile cholestatic liver disease.[8]

LABORATORY FEATURES

Most patients have moderate anemia with a hematocrit of 20 to 30 percent, marked indirect hyperbilirubinemia, and laboratory evidence of severe hepatocellular disease. Blood films reveal significant acanthocytosis (Fig. 44-1). Echinocytes, target cells, and microspherocytes, many with very fine spicules, are found in some patients.

DIFFERENTIAL DIAGNOSIS

Spur cell hemolytic anemia should be distinguished from other hemolytic syndromes associated with liver disease, including (1) chronic, mild hemolysis with occasional spherocytes seen in patients with congestive splenomegaly, (2) transient hemolysis associated with fatty

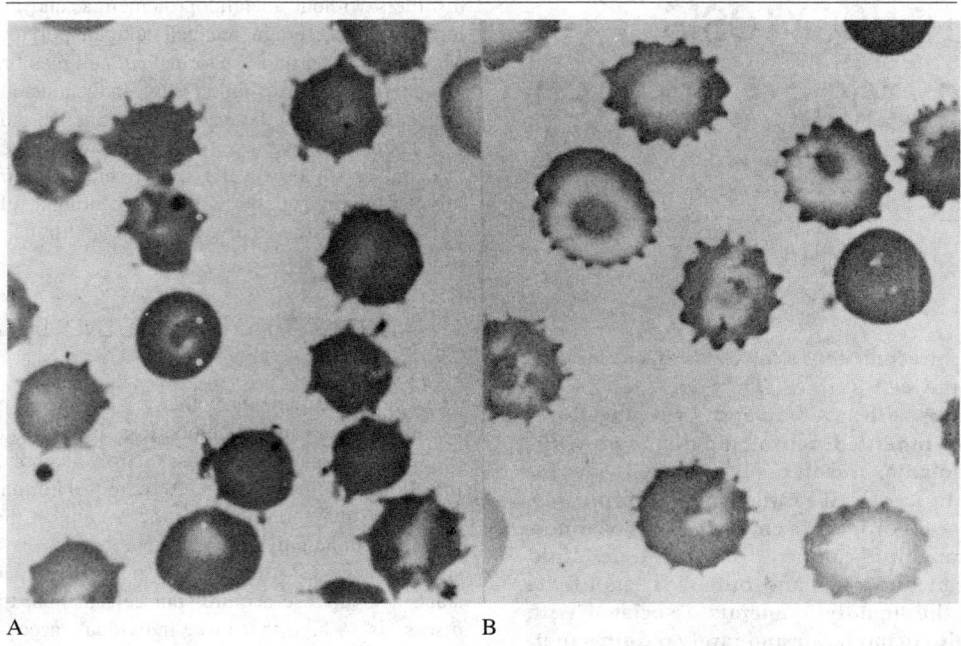

A   B

FIGURE 44-1   Blood film from a patient with liver cirrhosis and spur cell anemia. The conditioning effect of the spleen is demonstrated by the spheroidal shape of the cells and the remodeling of the spicules. *(From Cooper and coworkers[5] with permission.)*

metamorphosis of the liver and hypertriglyceridemia (which does not appear to have a causal relationship to hemolysis), (3) transient hemolytic anemia with stomatocytosis, and (4) hemolytic anemia with rigid and occasionally spiculated red cells (echinocytes) that has been reported in malnourished alcoholics with severe hypophosphatemia. Spur cell anemia appears to differ from Zieve syndrome, a poorly defined syndrome of hyperlipoproteinemia, jaundice, and spherocytic hemolytic anemia that occurs in alcoholic patients with liver disease.[9]

THERAPY, COURSE, AND PROGNOSIS

The anemia of spur cell anemia is not usually a significant clinical problem, but it can aggravate preexisting anemias, e.g., due to gastrointestinal bleeding, to the point that erythrocyte transfusion is required. The life span of spur cells is markedly decreased due to splenic sequestration, and, as would be expected, hemolysis abates after splenectomy. However, splenectomy is a dangerous and potentially fatal procedure in these critically ill patients and is generally not recommended. Spur cell anemia is an ominous clinical marker of the terminal stages of liver disease. Prior to the availability of liver transplantation, patients reaching this stage rarely lived for more than a few weeks.

ABETALIPOPROTEINEMIA (BASSEN-KORNZWEIG SYNDROME)

DEFINITION

Abetalipoproteinemia is an autosomal recessive disorder characterized by progressive ataxic neurologic disease, celiac disease, retinitis pigmentosa, and acanthocytosis found in people of diverse ethnic backgrounds.[10,11]

ETIOLOGY AND PATHOGENESIS

The primary molecular defect in this disorder is a failure to synthesize or secrete lipoproteins containing products of the apoprotein B gene.[11] In some patients, this is due to lack of microsomal transfer protein (MTP), which catalyzes the transport of triglyceride, cholesterol ester,

and phospholipid from phospholipid surfaces.[12–15] Microsomal transfer protein, a heterodimer of protein disulfide isomerase and a large 88-kDa subunit, is located in the lumen of hepatic microsomes and intestinal epithelia, the sites of lipoprotein synthesis. Other than apolipoprotein B, microsomal transfer protein is the only tissue-specific component required for secretion of apoprotein B–containing lipoproteins. All lipoproteins that contain apoprotein B are absent in plasma; consequently, preformed triglycerides are not transported from the intestinal mucosa, and plasma triglycerides are nearly absent.[11] Plasma cholesterol and phospholipid levels are markedly decreased, with a relative increase of sphingomyelin at the expense of lecithin.

In this condition, marrow red cell precursors, nucleated red cells, and reticulocytes have normal shape. Acanthocytosis becomes apparent as the red cells mature in the circulation, worsening with increasing red cell age.[16] Incubating normal red cells in abetalipoproteinemic serum does not produce acanthocytes, but normal red cells acquire acanthocytic changes when transfused into an abetalipoproteinemic recipient. Erythrocyte membrane proteins are normal, but lipids are not.[17] The cholesterol to phospholipid ratio is normal or slightly increased, reflecting changes in the distribution of plasma phospholipids and a decrease in lecithin-cholesterol acyltransferase (LCAT) activity. The phosphatidylcholine concentration is decreased, and sphingomyelin is correspondingly increased. It has been suggested that in abetalipoproteinemic acanthocytes, excess sphingomyelin is preferentially confined to the outer membrane bilayer leaflet, causing an expansion of its surface area that may be responsible for the irregularities in cell surface contour.

CLINICAL FEATURES

The disorder manifests in the first month of life by steatorrhea. Intestinal biopsy typically reveals engorgement of mucosal cells with lipid droplets. Retinitis pigmentosa, which often results in blindness, and progressive neurologic abnormalities characterized by ataxia and intention tremors develop between 5 and 10 years of age and progress to death in the second or third decade.[11]

LABORATORY FEATURES

These patients usually have a mild anemia with normal red cell indices and normal or slightly increased reticulocyte counts.[10,11,16] Acanthocytosis is prominent, ranging from about 50 to 90 percent of red cells. Despite the lipid abnormalities and frequent concomitant vitamin E deficiency, the hemolysis experienced by these patients is mild, especially when compared to patients with spur cell anemia (see above). It has been suggested that the enlarged, congested spleen in patients with portal hypertension and spur cell anemia worsens the hemolysis, whereas the spleen is normal in patients with abetalipoproteinemia.

DIFFERENTIAL DIAGNOSIS

The related disorders hypobetalipoproteinemia, normotriglyceridemic abetalipoproteinemia, and chylomicron retention disease are associated with partial production of apolipoprotein B–containing lipoproteins or with the secretion of lipoproteins containing truncated forms of apolipoprotein B.[18–20] Patients with these disorders also may experience neurologic disease and acanthocytosis, depending on the severity of the underlying defect. Even patients with heterozygous hypobetalipoproteinemia may have acanthocytosis, but typically they do not.[21]

THERAPY, COURSE, AND PROGNOSIS

Treatment includes dietary restriction of triglycerides and supplementation of vitamins A, K, D, and E.[11] Water-soluble forms of vitamin E, such as D-α-tocopherol polyethylene glycol succinate, are available for use. The role of vitamin E in the pathophysiology and clinical symptomatology of abetalipoproteinemia is unknown. It has been suggested that vitamin E deficiency is the primary stimulus for secondary manifestations of the disease such as neuropathy. This is based on the observations that vitamin E may stabilize or even improve neuromuscular and retinal abnormalities in these patients and because a similar neuropathy has been observed in patients with chronic cholestasis. Clinically evident vitamin A or D deficiencies are rarely observed.

ACANTHOCYTOSIS WITH NEUROLOGIC DISEASE AND NORMAL LIPOPROTEINS

CHOREA-ACANTHOCYTOSIS SYNDROME

Chorea-acanthocytosis is a rare autosomal recessive disorder characterized by normolipoproteinemic acanthocytosis and progressive neurodegenerative disease with onset in adolescence or adult life.[22] Chorea-acanthocytosis is characterized by progressive orofacial dyskineses with tics, limb chorea, lip and tongue biting; neurogenic muscle hypotonia and atrophy; absent or diminished reflexes; and increased serum creatine phosphokinase. Neuroimaging demonstrates abnormalities of the putamen and the head of the caudate.[23] Although variant syndromes of chorea-acanthocytosis have been described, recent linkage of chorea-acanthocytosis in 11 affected families from diverse ethnic backgrounds to a 6-cM region of 9q21 suggests a single disease locus.[24]

These patients are not anemic, and red cell survival is only slightly decreased. In some, the acanthocytosis may precede the onset of neurologic symptoms. The mechanism of acanthocytosis in chorea-acanthocytosis is unknown. Plasma and erythrocyte membrane lipids, as well as membrane fatty acid composition, are normal except for a high content of saturated fatty acids.[25] Red cell membrane fluidity is decreased, and intramembrane particles are unevenly distributed, presumably due to altered lipid fluidity. Increased proteolysis of ankyrin, band 3, and protein 4.2 and increased membrane protein phosphorylation, especially of band 3, may contribute to the cell shape change.[26] A point mutation near the COOH-terminus of band 3 has been identified in one unusual kindred with chorea-acanthocytosis.[27]

Inherited neuroacanthocytosis syndromes other than chorea-acanthocytosis have been described. These include: (1) a recessively inherited syndrome with acanthocytosis, tics, parkinsonism, and occasional motor neuron disease; (2) a mitochondrial myopathy with encephalopathy, lactic acidosis, strokelike symptoms, and acanthocytosis; (3) Hallervorden-Spatz disease (progressive dementia, dystonia, spasticity, pallidal and retinal degeneration) with acanthocytosis; and (4) HARP syndrome (hypoprebetalipoproteinemia, acanthocytosis, retinitis pigmentosa, and pallidal degeneration with iron deposition).

KELL AND LUTHERAN BLOOD GROUPS

McLeod Syndrome   The McLeod syndrome is an X-linked anomaly of the Kell blood group system characterized by a mild compensated hemolytic anemia with variable acanthocytosis and, in some patients, late-onset myopathy or chorea.[28,29] The Kell antigen consists of two major protein components: a 37-kDa protein that carries the Kx antigen, a precursor molecule necessary for the Kell antigen expression, and a 93-kDa protein that carries the Kell blood group antigen. Red cells with the McLeod phenotype have no detectable Kx antigen, and they have a marked deficiency of the 93-kDa protein that carries the Kell antigen. The *XK* gene encodes a novel 444-amino acid integral membrane transporter, and mutations of the *XK* gene have been identified in McLeod patients.[30–32] Male hemizygotes who lack Kx have 8 to 85 percent of acanthocytes on the blood film and mild, compensated hemolysis. Because of the red cell mosaicism–produced X inactivation, female heterozygote carriers may have occasional acanthocytes on the blood film,[29] and women with markedly biased X inactivation may have more severe symptoms.[31]

McLeod red cells should be distinguished from Kell null (K_o) red cells, which have a normal shape. In K_o cells, only the Kell antigen carrying 93-kDa glycoprotein is absent, while these cells have twice the amount of the Kx antigen.[33] It is important to identify patients with McLeod syndrome because if they receive transfusions they may develop antibodies that are compatible only with McLeod syndrome red cells.

The McLeod phenotype has been described in association with chronic granulomatous disease of childhood, retinitis pigmentosa, and Duchenne muscular dystrophy. These variable manifestations may be due to contiguous gene syndromes, as the genetic locus for these disorders is Xp21.[34–36] This may explain the occasional findings of either echinocytes or stomatocytes in Duchenne dystrophy or a choreiform disorder in some subjects with McLeod phenotype. Furthermore, some subjects with the McLeod phenotype exhibit laboratory features of myopathy and, later in life, a neurologic disorder that is first manifested by areflexia and, after the fifth decade, progresses to dystonia and choreiform movements.

Lutheran Blood Group   Approximately 1 in 3000 to 5000 people inherit a dominantly acting inhibitor, *In(Lu)*, that suppresses expression of Lu^a and Lu^b, the major antigens of the Lutheran blood group system. Patients with the *In(Lu)* Lu(a-b-) phenotype may have abnormally shaped red cells, including poikilocytes and acanthocytes, without evidence of anemia or hemolysis.[37] The osmotic fragility of fresh *In(Lu)* Lu(a-b-) erythrocytes is normal, but after incubation, the cells lose potassium and become osmotically resistant.[38] The identity of the inhibitor has yet to be identified.

ACANTHOCYTOSIS IN OTHER CONDITIONS

A small number of acanthocytes appear in malnutrition resulting from diverse causes, including anorexia nervosa and cystic fibrosis. The red cell shape normalizes after restoration of adequate nutritional status. Very mild acanthocytosis (0.5–2 percent) is common in 20 to 65 percent of patients with hypothyroidism.[39] Because hypothyroidism is so much more common than the other disorders that cause spiculated red cells, the finding of acanthocytes on the blood film should prompt

TABLE 44-1   HETEROGENEITY OF THE HEREDITARY STOMATOCYTOSIS SYNDROMES

| | Stomatocytosis (Hydrocytosis) | | | Intermediate Syndromes | | |
	Severe Hemolysis	Mild Hemolysis	Cryohydrocytosis	Stomatocytic Xerocytosis	Xerocytosis with High Phosphatidylcholine	Xerocytosis
Hemolysis	Severe	Mild-moderate	Moderate	Mild	Moderate	Moderate
Anemia	Severe	Mild-moderate	Mild-moderate	None	Mild	Moderate
Blood smear	Stomatocytes	Stomatocytes	Stomatocytes or normal	Stomatocytes	Targets	Targets, echinocytes
MCV (80–100 μm^3)[1]	110–150	95–130	90–105	91–98	84–92	100–110
MCHC (32–36%)	24–30	26–29	34–40	33–39	34–38	34–38
Unincubated osmotic fragility	Very increased	Increased	Normal	Decreased	Very decreased	Very decreased
RBC Na$^+$ (5–12)[2]	60–100	30–60	40–50	10–20	10–15	10–20
RBC K$^+$ (90–103)	20–55	40–85	55–65	75–85	75–90	60–80
RBC Na$^+$+K$^+$ (95–110)	110–140	115–145	100–105	87–103	93–99	75–90
Phosphatidylcholine content	Normal	± Increased	Normal	Normal	Increased	Normal
Cold autohemolysis	No	No	Yes	No	No	No
Effect of splenectomy[3]	Good	Good	Fair	?	?	? Poor
Inheritance	Autosomal dominant, ? autosomal recessive	Autosomal dominant	Autosomal dominant	Autosomal dominant	Autosomal dominant	Autosomal dominant

[1]Values in parentheses are the normal range.
[2]Values for sodium, potassium, and sodium + potassium are mEq/lRBC.
[3]Splenectomy may be contraindicated in these syndromes, see text for details. Reprinted with permission from Reference 8.

consideration of the patient's thyroid function. This association may unmask undiagnosed cases of hypothyroidism.

STOMATOCYTOSIS AND RELATED DISORDERS

Stomatocytes are erythrocytes characterized by a wide transverse slit or stoma (thus *stomatocytes*) (see Fig. 42-3).[40] There is no unifying theory to explain this morphologic abnormality which is an artifact resulting from folding of the cells during blood film preparation. Stomatocytes are seen in a variety of acquired and inherited disorders. The latter are often associated with inherited abnormalities in red cell cation permeability that may be associated with abnormal red cell hydration or membrane lipids.[41,42] Disturbances of erythrocyte hydration range from the extremes of dehydration and overhydration. These variants have been divided into provisional categories based on clinical severity, morphology, cation content, lipid and protein composition, genetics, and response to splenectomy (Table 44-1).[8]

DEHYDRATED STOMATOCYTOSIS/HEREDITARY XEROCYTOSIS

DEFINITION
Dehydrated hereditary stomatocytosis, also known as *hereditary xerocytosis* or *dessicocytosis*, is the most common form of the hereditary stomatocytosis syndromes.[40–42] The predominant phenotype associated with this disorder is an autosomal dominant hemolytic anemia with red cell dehydration and decreased osmotic fragility.[42,43] Recently, this phenotype has been recently extended to include recurrent fetal loss, hydrops fetalis, and pseudohyperkalemia (see below).

ETIOLOGY AND PATHOGENESIS
The underlying permeability defect is complex and involves a net loss of potassium from the red cells (typically about 20 percent) that is not accompanied by a proportional gain of sodium.[41,44] Consequently, the net intracellular cation content and cell water content are decreased. In some cases, erythrocytes also have increased membrane lipids, particularly phosphatidylcholine, and reduced 2,3-BPG content.[45] No quantitative abnormalities of membrane lipids and proteins have been noted, except for increased membrane-associated glyceraldehyde-3-phosphate dehydrogenase.

The precise genetic basis of this disorder remains unknown. Dehydrated hereditary stomatocytosis has been mapped to 16q23-qter.[46]

CLINICAL FEATURES
Patients may present with compensated hemolytic anemia, jaundice, splenomegaly, and gallstones. Recently, this syndrome has been extended to include recurrent fetal loss, hydrops fetalis, and familial pseudohyperkalemia (FP).[42,47] Individuals with FP present with asymptomatic hyperkalemia, attributed to an altered passive leak of potassium across the red cell membrane in vitro, similar to the one attributed to be defective in xerocytosis.[48] In approximately one third of xerocytosis patients, there is pseudohyperkalemia.[42,49] Xerocytosis, hydrops fetalis, and pseudohyperkalemia have been linked in several kindreds.[50,51] There appears to be variable penetrance in this disorder, with significant disparity in clinical symptomatology between affected individuals in the same kindred.[51] Genetic linkage analyses have mapped the FP locus to the same location as xerocytosis, supporting the hypothesis that these syndromes are due to different mutations in the same gene.[52]

LABORATORY FEATURES
The hematologic picture is that of mild to moderate hemolytic anemia with increased mean corpuscular hemoglobin concentration (MCHC), a reflection of cellular dehydration. Frequently, the mean corpuscular volume (MCV) is mildly increased, an artifact of Coulter-type electronic counters. In these counters, the conversion of pulse height (from the resistance of a cell passing through an electric field) to a cellular volume is dependent on cell shape. Xerocytes do not deform to the same degree as normal cells, which causes the MCV to be about 10 percent too high. The hematocrit is also affected because it is calculated from the MCV. Blood films do not always reveal stomatocytes, which are more prominent on wet films, but frequently target cells, dessicocytes and spiculated cells are seen (Fig. 44-2). In some of the cells, hemoglobin is concentrated ("puddled") in discrete areas on the cell periphery. Erythrocyte incubated osmotic fragility is decreased.

THERAPY, COURSE, AND PROGNOSIS
Most patients experience only mild anemia, and therapy is not required.[53] These patients should receive folate supplementation and be monitored for complications of hemolysis.

The effects of splenectomy have been variable, with many xerocytosis patients experiencing little or no improvement in their anemia. It has been suggested that xerocytes are so functionally compromised that they are detected and eliminated in other areas of the macrophage-monocyte system. Splenectomy should be carefully considered in

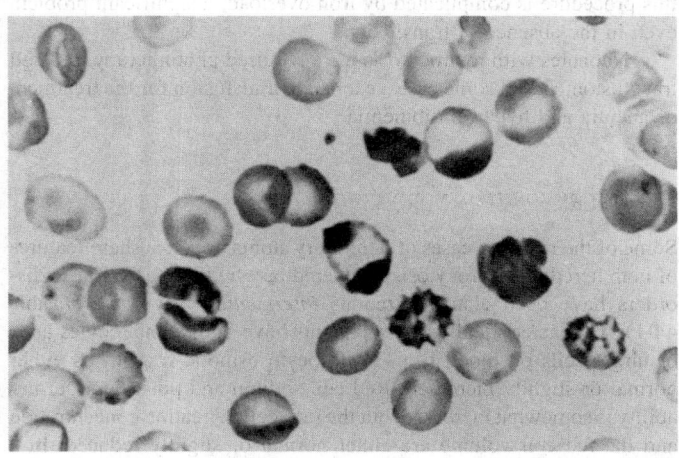

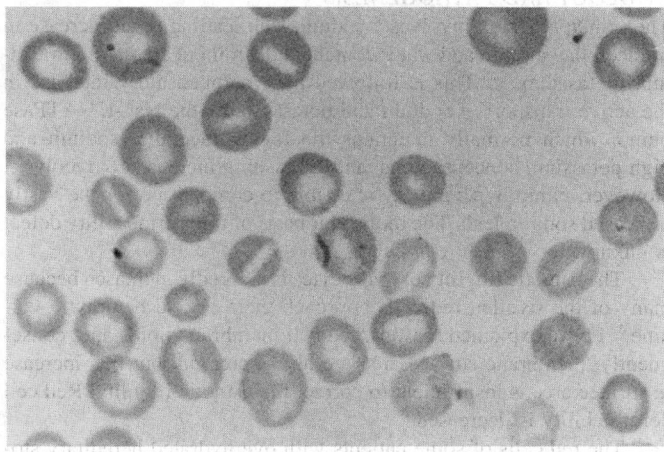

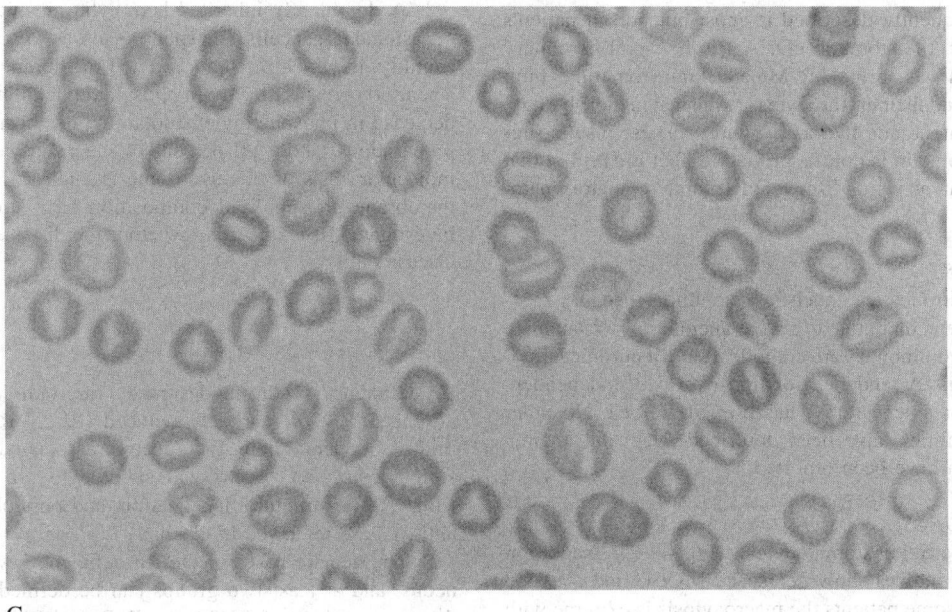

FIGURE 44-2   Stomatocytosis and variants. Peripheral blood smear from patients with hereditary xerocytosis (dessicocytosis) (*a*), stomatocytosis (hydrocytosis) (*b*), and acquired stomatocytosis due to alcoholic liver disease (*c*). *(Panels (a) and (b) reprinted with permission from Lande and Mentzer.[40])*

patients with hereditary xerocytosis. Several patients have developed hypercoagulability after splenectomy, leading to life-threatening thrombotic episodes.[43] It is important to note that all cases of thrombosis have occurred after splenectomy. In vitro, stomatocytic erythrocytes from a splenectomized xerocytosis individual demonstrated increased endothelial adherence compared to stomatocytic erythrocytes from unsplenectomized family members without hypercoagulability.[54] In one hypercoagulable xerocytosis patient, pentoxyfylline decreased red cell adherence.[54] Fortunately, the majority of hereditary stomatocytosis patients are able to maintain an adequate hemoglobin level, so that splenectomy is not required. Treatment of splenectomized patients with long-term Coumadin has had variable results. In a few severe cases, erythrocyte hypertransfusion has been beneficial. Unfortunately, this procedure is complicated by iron overload, a significant problem even in the absence of transfusion.

Neonates with xerocytosis have required phototherapy, red cell transfusion, and, in some cases, exchange transfusion, for the treatment of anemia and hyperbilirubinemia. In a few cases, in utero transfusion has been required. The presence of hydrops fetalis is not a predictor of the severity of anemia later in life, with some infants going on to experience little or no anemia later in childhood.

HEREDITARY STOMATOCYTOSIS-HYDROCYTOSIS

DEFINITION AND HISTORY
The overhydrated hereditary stomatocytosis (HSt) syndromes, also known as *hereditary hydrocytosis*, are characterized by a dominantly inherited hemolytic anemia with red cell overhydration and macrocytosis. This syndrome was first described by Lock and coworkers in a girl with dominantly inherited hemolytic anemia whose blood film contained red cells with a wide transverse slit, stomatocytes.[55] Later, abnormal cation transport and cellular overhydration, hallmarks of this disorder, were discovered by Zarkowsky and colleagues.[56]

ETIOLOGY AND PATHOGENESIS

The principal lesion involves a sodium leak leading to an increase in intracellular sodium and water content and a mild decrease in intracellular potassium.[41,44] This is followed by a compensatory increase in the active transport of sodium and potassium by the Na^+-K^+-ATPase pump, which normally maintains the low intracellular sodium and high potassium concentrations, and an ensuing increase in glycolysis. However, pump hyperactivity is unable to compensate for the vastly increased sodium leak. The molecular basis of this permeability defect is unknown.

The osmotic fragility of hydrocytes is markedly increased because many of the swollen red cells approach their critical hemolytic volume.[57] For unexplained reasons, red cell membrane lipids and, consequently, membrane surface area are also increased, but this increase in surface area is insufficient to correct the osmotic fragility. Red cell deformability is decreased.

The red cells of some patients with overhydrated hereditary stomatocytosis (HSt) were found to lack a 31-kDa integral membrane protein called *band 7.2b* or *stomatin*.[58] Varying degrees of stomatin deficiency were subsequently described in most but not all patients with HSt.[42,59] However, the stomatin cDNA from several hereditary stomatocytosis patients was normal.[60,61] Mice lacking stomatin exhibit no hemolytic anemia, and their erythrocytes are normal in morphology, cell indices, cation content, and hydration status.[62] These results suggest that a defect of stomatin is not the primary defect in HSt but that it may be involved in an as yet undiscovered volume regulatory pathway in the red cell.

CLINICAL FEATURES

The hydrocytosis syndromes are much less common than the xerocytosis disorders. There is moderate to severe anemia.[42,56,63,64] Jaundice and splenomegaly are common, as are complications of chronic hemolysis, e.g., cholelithiasis. A tendency for iron overload, independent of transfusion status or splenectomy, has been described. No other organ system abnormalities have been described. Neonatal anemia and hyperbilirubinemia have been reported.

LABORATORY FEATURES

The blood film reveals striking stomatocytosis (Fig. 44-2). In addition to the anemia, red cell indices show decreased MCHC and elevated MCV (Table 44-1). In some patients the macrocytosis is extreme with the MCV up to 150 fl. Erythrocyte osmotic fragility is markedly increased.

THERAPY, COURSE, AND PROGNOSIS

The majority of hydrocytosis patients suffer from significant lifelong anemia. Similar to patients with hereditary spherocytosis (Chap. 43), these patients should be monitored for complications of hemolysis, e.g., cholelithiasis, parvovirus infection, and should receive folate supplementation.

The results of splenectomy in this group of disorders has been variable.[8] In some patients, hemolytic anemia is improved, although often not fully corrected, by splenectomy, while in others the severity of hemolysis is unchanged. Splenectomy should be carefully considered in patients with this disorder. Like patients with xerocytosis, several hydrocytosis patients have developed hypercoagulability after splenectomy, leading to catastrophic thrombotic episodes.[43] In vivo, venous thromboemboli predominate, sometimes with complicating pulmonary or portal hypertension. This thrombotic risk is independent of postsplenectomy thrombosis, and all cases of thrombosis have occurred in splenectomized patients. Treatment of splenectomized patients with long-term Coumadin has had variable results.[43] In severe cases, erythrocyte hypertransfusion has been beneficial. Unfortunately, this procedure is complicated by iron overload, a significant problem even in the absence of transfusion.

Neonates with hydrocytosis have required phototherapy, red cell transfusion, and in some cases, exchange transfusion for the treatment of anemia and hyperbilirubinemia.

INTERMEDIATE SYNDROMES

Some of the reported cases of hereditary stomatocytosis share features of both hereditary xerocytosis and hereditary hydrocytosis. These disorders have been characterized as *intermediate syndromes* (Table 44-1).[8] Characteristically, these patients have both stomatocytes and/or target cells on blood film. Erythrocyte osmotic fragility is either normal or slightly increased. Red cell sodium and potassium permeability is somewhat increased, but the intracellular cation concentration and the red cell volume are either normal or slightly reduced. In a few patients, red cells undergo spontaneous in vitro hemolysis after storage at 5°C (41°F), hence the designation *cryohydrocytosis*.[40,65]

A dominantly inherited hemolytic anemia with stomatocytosis, occasional target cells, and spherocytes, as well as a decreased osmotic fragility, in which the main red cell membrane abnormality involved a near 50 percent increase in phosphatidylcholine and a corresponding decrease in phosphatidylethanolamine has been described.[66,67] In wet preparations, about 30 percent of the cells were stomatocytes. The molecular basis of this syndrome is unclear. Since abnormalities in membrane phospholipid composition have not been systematically investigated, it is uncertain whether the disorder represents a distinct disease entity.

RH DEFICIENCY SYNDROME

Rh deficiency syndrome designates rare individuals who have either absent (Rh$_{null}$) or markedly reduced (Rh$_{mod}$) Rh antigen expression, mild to moderate hemolytic anemia associated with the presence of stomatocytes, and occasional spherocytes on the peripheral blood film.[68,69] The structure, localization, and possible functions of the Rh antigens are reviewed in Chap. 137.

The genetic bases of the Rh deficiency syndrome are heterogeneous, and at least two groups can be defined. The *amorph type* is due to mutations of RH30, the RhD and RhE polypeptides.[70,71] The *regulatory type*, is due to mutations of RH50, a modulator of Rh gene expression.[72-76] Studies of these rare patients have provided evidence that both the Rh locus and Rh50 are required for the expression and function of Rh as a multimeric complex in the red cell membrane.

Red cells of some Rh$_{null}$ patients have increased osmotic fragility reflecting a marked reduction of membrane surface area.[77] These cells are also dehydrated, as indicated by decreased cell cation and water content and increased cell density. The potassium transport and the Na^+/K^+ pump activity are increased, possibly because of reticulocytosis. Hemolytic anemia is improved by splenectomy.

FAMILIAL DEFICIENCY OF HIGH-DENSITY LIPOPROTEINS

Severe deficiency or absence of high-density lipoproteins leads to accumulation of cholesteryl esters in many tissues, leading to clinical findings of large orange tonsils and hepatosplenomegaly. Reported hematologic manifestations include a moderately severe hemolytic anemia with stomatocytosis.[78] Membrane lipid analyses have shown a low cholesterol content leading to a decreased ratio of cholesterol to phospholipid and a relative increase in phosphatidylcholine at the expense of sphingomyelin.

ACQUIRED STOMATOCYTOSIS

Few stomatocytes (3 to 5 percent) are commonly found on blood films of normal subjects. A prospective analysis of films from a large number of hospitalized patients revealed an overall incidence of stomatocytosis (>5 percent of stomatocytes) of 2.3 percent.[79] Fifty-nine percent of these patients had 5 to 20 percent stomatocytes, 35 percent had 20 to 50 percent stomatocytes, and 6 percent had more than 50 percent stomatocytes. A wide variety of medications and diagnoses including malignant neoplasms, cardiovascular disease, hepatobiliary disease, and alcoholism were associated with stomatocytosis. Additional studies are required to determine which associations are specific and reproducible. For instance, acquired stomatocytosis is common in alcoholics, particularly those with acute alcoholism (Fig. 44-1).[80] Vinca alkaloids, e.g., vincristine and vinblastine, may induce hemolysis with increased sodium permeability and stomatocytosis in the doses used for chemotherapy of leukemias and lymphomas.[81,82] The molecular basis of stomatocytosis in these conditions is unknown; it is rarely associated with clinically significant hematologic abnormalities.

REFERENCES

1. Bessis FA: Red cell shapes: an illustrated classification and its rationale, in *Red Cell Shape: Physiology, Pathology and Ultrastructure*, edited by M Bessis, RI Weed, PF Leblond, p 1. Springer-Verlag, New York, 1973.
2. Colman N, Herbert V: Hematologic complications of alcoholism: overview. *Semin Hematol* 17:164, 1980.
3. Cooper RA: Hemolytic syndromes and red cell membrane abnormalities in liver disease. *Semin Hematol* 17:103, 1980.
4. Cooper RA, Diloy Puray M, Lando P, Greenverg MS: An analysis of lipoproteins, bile acids, and red cell membranes associated with target cells and spur cells in patients with liver disease. *J Clin Invest* 51:3182, 1972.
5. Cooper RA, Kimball DB, Durocher JR: Role of the spleen in membrane conditioning and hemolysis of spur cells in liver disease. *N Engl J Med* 290:1279, 1974.
6. Estes JW, Morley TJ, Levine IM, Emerson CP: A new hereditary acanthocytosis syndrome. *Am J Med* 42:868, 1967.
7. Silber R, Amorosi E, Lhowe J, Kayden HJ: Spur-shaped erythrocytes in Laennec's cirrhosis. *N Engl J Med* 275:639, 1966.
8. Gallagher PG, Forget BG, Lux SE: Disorders of the erythrocyte membrane, in *Hematology of Infancy and Childhood*, edited by DG Nathan, SH Orkin, p 544. Saunders, Philadelphia, 1997.
9. Zieve L: Jaundice, hyperlipemia and hemolytic anemia: a heretofore unrecognized syndrome associated with alcoholic fatty liver and cirrhosis. *Ann Intern Med* 48:471, 1958.
10. Bassen F, Kornzweig A: Malformation of the erythrocytes in a case of atypical retinitis pigmentosa. *Blood* 5:381, 1950.
11. Kane J, Havel R: Disorders of the biogenesis and secretion of lipoproteins containing the B apolipoproteins, in *The Metabolic and Molecular Bases of Inherited Disease*, edited by C Scriver, A Beaudet, W Sly, et al, p 1853. McGraw-Hill, New York, 1995.
12. Sharp D, Blinderman L, Combs KA, et al: Cloning and gene defects in microsomal triglyceride transfer protein associated with abetalipoproteinaemia. *Nature* 365:65, 1993.
13. Wetterau JR, Aggerbeck LP, Bouma ME, et al: Absence of microsomal triglyceride transfer protein in individuals with abetalipoproteinemia. *Science* 258:999, 1992.
14. Ricci B, Sharp D, O'Rourke E, et al: A 30-amino acid truncation of the microsomal triglyceride transfer protein large subunit disrupts its interaction with protein disulfide-isomerase and causes abetalipoproteinemia. *J Biol Chem* 270:14281, 1995.
15. Narcisi TM, Shoulders CC, Chester SA, et al: Mutations of the microsomal triglyceride-transfer-protein gene in abetalipoproteinemia. *Am J Hum Genet* 57:1298, 1995.
16. Simon E, Ways P: Incubation hemolysis and red cell metabolism in acanthocytosis. *J Clin Invest* 43:1311, 1964.
17. Jones JW, Ways P: Abnormalities of high density lipoproteins in abetalipoproteinemia. *J Clin Invest* 46:1151, 1967.
18. Bohlega S, Riley W, Powe J, Baynton R, Roberts G, et al: Neuroacanthocytosis and aprebetalipoproteinemia. *Neurology* 50:1912, 1998.
19. Welty FK, Hubl ST, Pierotti VR, Young SG: A truncated species of apolipoprotein B (B67) in a kindred with familial hypobetalipoproteinemia. *J Clin Invest* 87:1748, 1991.
20. Young SG, Hubl ST, Chappell DA, et al: Familial hypobetalipoproteinemia associated with a mutant species of apolipoprotein B (B-46). *N Engl J Med* 320:1604, 1989.
21. Ross RS, Gregg RE, Law SW, et al: Homozygous hypobetalipoproteinemia: a disease distinct from abetalipoproteinemia at the molecular level. *J Clin Invest* 81:590, 1988.
22. Gross KB, Skrivanek JA, Carlson KC, Kaufman DM: Familial amyotrophic chorea with acanthocytosis. New clinical and laboratory investigations. *Arch Neurol* 42:753, 1985.
23. Hardie RJ, Pullon HW, Harding AE, et al: Neuroacanthocytosis. A clinical, haematological and pathological study of 19 cases. *Brain* 114:13, 1991.
24. Rubio JP, Danek A, Stone C, et al: Chorea-acanthocytosis: genetic linkage to chromosome 9q21. *Am J Hum Genet* 61:899, 1997.
25. Critchley EM, Clark DB, Wikler A: Acanthocytosis and neurological disorder without betalipoproteinemia. *Arch Neurol* 18:134, 1968.
26. Bosman GJ, Bartholomeus IG, De Grip WJ, Horstink MW: Erythrocyte anion transporter and antibrain immunoreactivity in chorea-acanthocytosis. A contribution to etiology, genetics, and diagnosis. *Brain Res Bull* 33:523, 1994.
27. Bruce LJ, Kay MM, Lawrence C, Tanner MJ: Band 3 HT, a human redcell variant associated with acanthocytosis and increased anion transport, carries the mutation Pro-868→Leu in the membrane domain of band 3. *Biochem J* 293:317, 1993.
28. Ballas SK, Bator SM, Aubuchon JP, Marsh WL, Sharp DE, Toy EM, et al: Abnormal membrane physical properties of red cells in McLeod syndrome. *Transfusion* 30:722, 1990.
29. Wimer BM, Marsh WL, Taswell HF, Galey WR: Haematological changes associated with the McLeod phenotype of the Kell blood group system. *Br J Haematol* 36:219, 1977.
30. Ho M, Chelly J, Carter N, Harding AE, Monaco AP, et al: Isolation of the gene for McLeod syndrome that encodes a novel membrane transport protein. *Cell* 77:869, 1994.
31. Ho MF, Chalmers RM, Davis MB, et al: A novel point mutation in the McLeod syndrome gene in neuroacanthocytosis. *Ann Neurol* 39:672, 1996.
32. Shizuka M, Watanabe M, Aoki M, et al: Analysis of the McLeod syndrome gene in three patients with neuroacanthocytosis. *J Neurol Sci* 150:133, 1997.
33. Redman CM, Marsh WL, Scarborough A, Johnson CL, Rabin BI, Overbeeke M, et al: Biochemical studies on McLeod phenotype red cells and isolation of Kx antigen. *Br J Haematol* 68:131, 1988.
34. Francke U, Ochs HD, de Martinville B, et al: Minor Xp21 chromosome deletion in a male associated with expression of Duchenne muscular dystrophy, chronic granulomatous disease, retinitis pigmentosa, and McLeod syndrome. *Am J Hum Genet* 37:250, 1985.
35. Frey D, Machler M, Seger R, Schmid W, Orkin SH, et al: Gene deletion in a patient with chronic granulomatous disease and McLeod syndrome: fine mapping of the Xk gene locus. *Blood* 71:252, 1988.
36. Vasiljevic ZM, Polic DD: Morphological changes of erythrocytes in patients and carriers of Duchenne disease. *Acta Neurol Scand* 67:242, 1983.
37. Udden MM, Umeda M, Hirano Y, Marcus DM: New abnormalities in the morphology, cell surface receptors, and electrolyte metabolism of In(Lu) erythrocytes. *Blood* 69:52, 1987.
38. Ballas SK, Marcolina MJ, Crawford MN: In vitro storage and in vivo survival studies of red cells from persons with the In(Lu) gene. *Transfusion* 32:607, 1992.
39. Wardrop C, Hutchison HE: Red-cell shape in hypothyroidism. *Lancet* 1:1243, 1969.
40. Lande WM, Mentzer WC: Haemolytic anaemia associated with increased cation permeability. *Clin Haematol* 14:89, 1985.
41. Stewart GW: The membrane defect in hereditary stomatocytosis. *Baillieres Clin Haematol* 6:371, 1993.
42. Delaunay J, Stewart G, Iolascon A: Hereditary dehydrated and overhydrated stomatocytosis: recent advances. *Curr Opin Hematol* 6:110, 1999.

43. Stewart GW, Amess JA, Eber SW, et al: Thrombo-embolic disease after splenectomy for hereditary stomatocytosis. *Br J Haematol* 93:303, 1996.

44. Ellory JC, Gibson JS, Stewart GW: Pathophysiology of abnormal cell volume in human red cells. *Contrib Nephrol* 123:220, 1998.

45. Clark MR, Shohet SB, Gottfried EL: Hereditary hemolytic disease with increased red blood cell phosphatidylcholine and dehydration: one, two, or many disorders? *Am J Hematol* 42:25, 1993.

46. Carella M, Stewart G, Ajetunmobi JF, et al: Genomewide search for dehydrated hereditary stomatocytosis (hereditary xerocytosis): mapping of locus to chromosome 16 (16q23-qter). *Am J Hum Genet* 63:810, 1998.

47. Entezami M, Becker R, Menssen HD, Marcinkowski M, Versmold HT: Xerocytosis with concomitant intrauterine ascites: first description and therapeutic approach. *Blood* 87:5392, 1996.

48. Stewart GW, Corrall RJ, Fyffe JA, Stockdill G, Strong JA, et al: Familial pseudohyperkalaemia. A new syndrome. *Lancet* 2:175, 1979.

49. Coles SE, Ho MM, Chetty MC, Nicolaou A, Stewart GW, et al: A variant of hereditary stomatocytosis with marked pseudohyperkalaemia. *Br J Haematol* 104:275, 1999.

50. Grootenboer S, Schischmanoff PO, Cynober T, et al: A genetic syndrome associating dehydrated hereditary stomatocytosis, pseudohyperkalaemia and perinatal oedema. *Br J Haematol* 103:383, 1998.

51. Grootenboer S, Schischmanoff PO, Laurendeau I, et al: Pleiotropic syndrome of dehydrated hereditary stomatocytosis, pseudohyperkalemia, and perinatal edema map to 16q23-q24. *Blood* 189a, 1999.

52. Iolascon A, Stewart GW, Ajetunmobi JF, et al: Familial pseudohyperkalemia maps to the same locus as dehydrated hereditary stomatocytosis (hereditary xerocytosis). *Blood* 93:3120, 1999.

53. Nolan GR: Hereditary xerocytosis. A case history and review of the literature. *Pathology* 16:151, 1984.

54. Smith BD, Segel GB: Abnormal erythrocyte endothelial adherence in hereditary stomatocytosis. *Blood* 89:3451, 1997.

55. Lock SP, Smith RS, Hardisty RM: Stomatocytosis: a hereditary red cell anomaly associated with haemolytic anaemia. *Br J Haematol* 7:303, 1961.

56. Zarkowsky HS, Oski FA, Sha'afi R, Shohet SB, Nathan DG, et al: Congenital hemolytic anemia with high sodium, low potassium red cells. I. Studies of membrane permeability *N Engl J Med* 278:573, 1968.

57. Mentzer WC Jr, Smith WB, Goldstone J, Shohet SB: Hereditary stomatocytosis: membrane and metabolism studies. *Blood* 46:659, 1975.

58. Lande WM, Thiemann PV, Mentzer WC Jr: Missing band 7 membrane protein in two patients with high Na, low K erythrocytes. *J Clin Invest* 70:1273, 1982.

59. Kanzaki A, Yawata Y: Hereditary stomatocytosis: phenotypical expression of sodium transport and band 7 peptides in 44 cases. *Br J Haematol* 82:133, 1992.

60. Gallagher PG, Segel G, Marchesi SL, Forget BG: The gene for erythrocyte band 7.2b in hereditary stomatocytosis. *Blood* 276a, 1992.

61. Wang D, Turetsky T, Perrine S, Johnson RM, Mentzer WC, et al: Further studies on RBC membrane 7.2 B deficiency in hereditary stomatocytosis. *Blood* 80:275a, 1992.

62. Zhu Y, Paszty C, Turetsky T, et al: Stomatocytosis is absent in "stomatin"-deficient murine red blood cells. *Blood* 93:2404, 1999.

63. Nathan DG, Oski FA, Sha'afi RI, Shohet SB: Congenital hemolytic anemia with extensive cation permeability. *Blood* 28:976, 1966.

64. Oski FA, Naiman JL, Blum SF, et al: Congenital hemolytic anemia with high-sodium, low-potassium red cells. Studies of three generations of a family with a new variant. *N Engl J Med* 280:909, 1969.

65. Miller G, Townes P, MacWhinney J, et al: A new congenital hemolytic anemia with deformed erythrocytes (stomatocytes) and remarkable susceptibility of erythrocytes to cold hemolysis in vitro: I. Clinical and hematologic studies. *Pediatrics* 35:906, 1965.

66. Jaff ER, Gottfried EL: Hereditary nonspherocytic hemolytic disease associated with an altered phospholipid composition of the erythrocytes. *J Clin Invest* 47:1375, 1968.

67. Lane PA, Kuypers FA, Clark MR, et al: Excess of red cell membrane proteins in hereditary high-phosphatidylcholine hemolytic anema. *Am J Hematol* 34:186, 1990.

68. Nash R, Shojania AM: Hematological aspect of Rh deficiency syndrome: a case report and a review of the literature. *Am J Hematol* 24:267, 1987.

69. Huang CH: Molecular insights into the Rh protein family and associated antigens. *Curr Opin Hematol* 4:94, 1997.

70. Cherif-Zahar B, Matassi G, Raynal V, et al: Molecular defects of the RHCE gene in Rh-deficient individuals of the amorph type. *Blood* 92:639, 1998.

71. Huang CH, Chen Y, Reid ME, Seidl C: Rh null disease: the amorph type results from a novel double mutation in RhCe gene on D-negative background. *Blood* 92:664, 1998.

72. Cherif-Zahar B, Raynal V, Gane P, et al: Candidate gene acting as a suppressor of the RH locus in most cases of Rh-deficiency. *Nature Genet* 12:168, 1996.

73. Cherif-Zahar B, Matassi G, Raynal V, et al: Rh-deficiency of the regulator type caused by splicing mutations in the human RH50 gene. *Blood* 92:2535, 1998.

74. Huang CH: The human Rh50 glycoprotein gene. Structural organization and associated splicing defect resulting in Rh null disease. *J Biol Chem* 273:2207, 1998.

75. Huang CH, Liu Z, Cheng G, Chen Y: Rh50 glycoprotein gene and Rh$_{null}$ disease: a silent splice donor is *trans* to a Gly279→Glu missense mutation in the conserved transmembrane segment. *Blood* 92:1776, 1998.

76. Huang CH, Cheng GJ, Reid ME, Chen Y: Rh mod syndrome: A family study of the translation-initiator mutation in the Rh50 glycoprotein gene. *Am J Hum Genet* 64:108, 1999.

77. Ballas SK, Clark MR, Mohandas N, et al: Red cell membrane and cation deficiency in Rh null syndrome. *Blood* 63:1046, 1984.

78. Breslow J: Familial disorders of high-density lipoprotein metabolism, in *The Metabolic and Molecular Bases of Inherited Disease*, edited by CR Scriver, AL Beaudet, WS Sly, et al, p 2031. McGraw-Hill, New York, 1995.

79. Davidson RJ, How J, Lessels S: Acquired stomatocytosis: its prevalence of significance in routine haematology. *Scand J Haematol* 19:47, 1977.

80. Wisloff F, Boman D: Acquired stomatocytosis in alcoholic liver disease. *Scand J Haematol* 23:43, 1979.

81. Ohsaka A, Kano Y, Sakamoto S, et al: A transient hemolytic reaction and stomatocytosis following vinca alkaloid administration. *Nippon Ketsueki Gakkai Zasshi* 52:7, 1989.

82. Neville AJ, Rand CA, Barr RD, Mohan Pai KR: Drug-induced stomatocytosis and anemia during consolidation chemotherapy of childhood acute leukemia. *Am J Med Sci* 287:3, 1984.

GLUCOSE-6-PHOSPHATE DEHYDROGENASE DEFICIENCY AND OTHER RED CELL ENZYME ABNORMALITIES

ERNEST BEUTLER

Erythrocyte enzyme deficiencies may lead to hemolytic anemia and sometimes to other systemic pathology. G-6-PD deficiency is the most common of these. In some populations more than 20 percent of the population may be affected by this enzyme deficiency. In the common polymorphic forms, such as G-6-PD A−, G-6-PD Mediterranean, or G-6-PD Canton, hemolysis occurs only during the stress imposed by infection or administration of "oxidative" drugs, and in some individuals upon ingestion of fava beans. Neonatal icterus, which appears largely to be due to a defect in bilirubin conjugation, is the clinically most serious complication of G-6-PD deficiency. Patients with less common, functionally very severe, genetic variants of G-6-PD experience chronic hemolysis, a disorder designated *hereditary nonspherocytic hemolytic anemia*.

Hereditary nonspherocytic hemolytic anemia also occurs as a consequence of other enzyme deficiencies, the most common of which is pyruvate kinase deficiency. Glucosephosphate isomerase, triosephosphate isomerase, and pyrimidine-5'-nucleotidase deficiency are included among the relatively rare causes of hereditary nonspherocytic hemolytic anemia. In the case of some deficiencies, notably those of glutathione synthetase, triosephosphate isomerase, and phosphoglycerate kinase, the defect is expressed throughout the body and neurologic defects may be a prominent part of the clinical syndrome.

Diagnosis is best achieved by determining red cell enzyme activity either with a quantitative assay or a screening test. Except for the stippling of erythrocytes that is characteristic of pyrimidine-5'-nucleotidase deficiency, red cell morphology is of little or no help in differentiation of red cell enzyme deficiencies from one another. A variety of molecular lesions have been defined in most of these enzyme deficiencies. Accurate diagnosis is helpful in recommendations for treatment, since patients with some enzyme deficiencies (e.g., glucosephosphate isomerase deficiency) tend to respond more favorably to splenectomy

Acronyms and abbreviations that appear in this chapter include: AD, autosomal dominant; AMP, adenosine monophosphate; G-6-PD, glucose-6-phosphate dehydrogenase; GR, glutathione reductase; GSH, glutathione; GSSG, glutathione disulfide; HNSHA, hereditary nonspherocytic hemolytic anemia; ITP, inosine triphosphate; NAD, nicotinamide-adenine dinucleotide; NADP, nicotinamide-adenine dinucleotide phosphate; NADH, reduced nicotinamide-adenine dinucleotide; NADPH, reduced nicotinamide-adenine dinucleotide phosphate; PCR, polymerase chain reaction; PK, pyruvate kinase; TPI, triosephosphate isomerase.

than patients with other deficiencies (e.g., G-6-PD deficiency). It is also essential for genetic counseling since some of the defects, such as pyruvate kinase and glucosephosphate isomerase deficiencies, are transmitted as autosomal recessive disorders, while G-6-PD and phosphoglycerate kinase deficiencies are X-linked.

DEFINITION AND HISTORY

Deficiencies in the activities of a number of erythrocyte enzymes may lead to shortening of the red cell life span. G-6-PD deficiency was the first of these to be recognized and is the most common.

The recognition of G-6-PD deficiency was the result of investigations of the hemolytic effect of the antimalarial drug primaquine, carried out in the 1950s and described in detail elsewhere.[1-3] These early studies defined G-6-PD deficiency as a hereditary sex-linked enzyme deficiency that affected primarily the erythrocytes, older cells being more severely affected than newly formed ones. They showed that this enzyme deficiency was very prevalent in individuals of African, Mediterranean, and East Asian ethnic origins, but that it could be found in virtually any population. The common (polymorphic) forms of G-6-PD deficiency were found to be associated with anemia only under conditions of stress, such as the administration of oxidative drugs, infection, or the neonatal period.

Chronic hemolysis in the absence of a stress occurs in uncommon, functionally severe forms of G-6-PD deficiency and in patients with a variety of other red cell enzyme deficiencies. Such patients have *hereditary nonspherocytic hemolytic anemia*. Although patients fitting the description of hereditary nonspherocytic hemolytic anemia had been documented earlier, the designation was first introduced by Crosby[4] in 1950. Dacie and his colleagues[5] subsequently reported several families in which affected members manifested hemolytic anemia from an early age and in whom the osmotic fragility of the red cells was normal. The latter finding, and the fact that most of the affected individuals failed to benefit from splenectomy, distinguished this disorder from hereditary spherocytosis. Thus, defined essentially by exclusion as a hereditary hemolytic anemia that is not hereditary spherocytosis, it is not at all surprising that hereditary nonspherocytic hemolytic anemia has proven to be extremely heterogeneous, both in etiology and in clinical manifestations. Sometimes this disorder is also designated *congenital nonspherocytic hemolytic* anemia, but the name hereditary is more accurate and is therefore preferable. While hereditary ovalocytosis, pyropoikilocytosis, stomatocytosis, and even sickle cell disease and thalassemia major are hereditary hemolytic anemias that are not spherocytic, they are not included in this category. Rather, the diagnosis of hereditary nonspherocytic hemolytic anemia is reserved for those patients who have no major aberration of red cell morphology.

Although a deficiency of G-6-PD was found to be responsible for hemolysis in a few patients with hereditary nonspherocytic hemolytic anemia,[6] in the overwhelming majority of cases the cause remained obscure. In 1954 Selwyn and Dacie[7] studied autohemolysis (spontaneous lysis of red cells after sterile incubation for 24 to 48 h at 37° C) in four patients with hereditary nonspherocytic hemolytic anemia and found that in two of them lysis was only slightly increased and was prevented by glucose; these patients were designated as type 1, while the others, in whom glucose failed to correct hemolysis, were classified as type 2. Autohemolysis of the erythrocytes of type 2 patients was modified by the addition of ATP, a substance that we now recognize does not penetrate the red cell membrane. Instead, its modifying influence was probably exerted chiefly by virtue of its effect on the osmolarity and pH of the suspending solution. However, the findings suggested to De Gruchy et al[8,9] that patients with type 2 autohemolysis suffered

TABLE 45-1   RED CELL ENZYME ABNORMALITIES LEADING TO HEMATOLOGIC DISEASE

Enzyme	Clinical Features*	Inheritance*	Red Cell Morphology	Examples of Mutations Characterized at the DNA Level	Diagnosis, Reference Screening Test	Diagnosis, Reference Assay	Response to Splenectomy†	Approx. Frequency‡	References§
Hexokinase	HNSHA[1]	AR	Unremarkable	(236)	—	(237)	++	Rare	(236)
Glucose phosphate isomerase	HNSHA; neurologic abnormalities(?)	AR	Unremarkable	(238)	(237)	(237)	+++	Unusual	(197,239)
Phosphofructokinase	HNSHA and/or muscle glycogen storage disease	AR	Unremarkable	(240)	—	(237)	0	Rare	(240,241)
Aldolase	HNSHA and mild liver glycogen storage; mental retardation (?)	AR	Unremarkable	(199,242)	—	(237)	?	Very rare	(199)
Triosephosphate isomerase	HNSHA and severe neuromuscular disease	AR	Unremarkable	(243)	(237)	(237)		Rare	(196)
Phosphoglycerate kinase	HNSHA; myoglobinuria; behavioral disturbances	SL	Unremarkable	(244)	—	(237)	++	Rare	(245)
Bisphosphoglycerate mutase	HNSHA; polycythemia	AR	Unremarkable	(246)	—	(237)		Rare	(246)
Pyruvate kinase	HNSHA	AR	Usually unremarkable, occasionally contracted echinocytes	(117)	(237)	(237)	++	Unusual	(122)

Enzyme	Clinical manifestations	Inheritance*	Blood smear				Response to splenectomy†	Frequency‡	
Glucose-6-phosphate dehydrogenase	HNSHA; drug- or infection-induced hemolysis; favism	SL	Usually unremarkable; rarely "bite cells"	(106)	(237)	(237)	±	Very common	
Glutathione reductase (complete)	Drug-sensitive hemolytic anemia and favism	AR	Unremarkable		(237)	(237)	?	Very rare	(18)
γ-Glutamyl cysteine synthetase	HNSHA; drug- or infection-induced hemolysis; spinocerebellar degeneration (?)	AR	Unremarkable	(247)	(248)	(249)	?	Very rare	(60)
Glutathione synthetase	HNSHA; drug- or infection-induced hemolysis; neurologic defect and 5-oxoprolinuria in some cases	AR	Usually unremarkable	(59)	(248)	(249)	0	Rare	(60)
Pyrimidine-5'-nucleotidase	HNSHA; mental retardation in some cases (?)	AR	Prominent stippling		(250)	(251)	0	Rare	(252)
Adenosine deaminase (increased activity)	HNSHA	AD	Unremarkable		—	(237)		Rare	(253)
Adenosine deaminase (decreased activity)	Immunodeficiency	AR	Unremarkable	(254)	—	(237)		Rare	(255)
NADH-diaphorase (cytochrome b₅ reductase)	Methemoglobinemia, sometimes with mental retardation	AR	Unremarkable	(256)	(257)	(237)		Unusual	[See Chap. 49]

*AR, autosomal recessive; AD, autosomal dominant; SL, sex linked.
†On a scale of 0 to 4+ where 4+ is a complete response. In many cases data are meager.
‡Very common if incidence is >5%. Unusual if >100 cases reported. Rare if 10–100 cases reported. Very rare if <10 cases reported.
§Recent reports. Comprehensive reviews[258] may be consulted for original descriptions and other reports.
¶Hereditary nonspherocytic hemolytic anemia.

TABLE 45-2   RED CELL ENZYME ABNORMALITIES NOT LEADING TO HEMATOLOGIC DISEASE

ENZYME	CLINICAL FEATURES	INHERITANCE*	DIAGNOSIS, REFERENCE ASSAY	ESTIMATED FREQUENCY†	REFERENCE
6-Phosphogluconate dehydrogenase (complete deficiency)	None	AR	(237)	Unusual	(62)
6-Phospho-gluconolactonase (partial defect)	Probably none	AD	(259)	Unusual	(19,260)
δ-ALA dehydrase	None	AD	(261)		
Acetyl-cholinesterase	None	AR	(237)	Very rare	(14)
Adenine phosphoribosyl transferase	Kidney stones	AR	(262)	Rare	(263,264)
Adenylate kinase	HNSHA (?)	AR	(237)	Very rare	(265)
AMP deaminase	None	AR	(266)	Unusual	(267)
Carbonic anhydrase I	None	AR	(268)	Rare	(269)
Carbonic anhydrase II	Osteoporosis	AR		Rare	(270)
Catalase	Oral ulcers in some types	AR	(237)	Rare	(271,272)
Enolase	HNSHA(?)	AD (?)	(237)	Rare	(20)
Galactokinase	Cataracts	AR	(237)	Rare	(273)
Galactose-1-P-uridylyltransferase	Cataracts; mental retardation; liver disease	AR	(237)	Rare	(274)
Glutathione peroxidase (partial deficiency)	None	AR and AD	(237)	Very common	
Glutathione reductase (partial deficiency)	None	Usually not inherited	(237)	Very common	(12,275)
Glutathione-S-transferase	HNSHA	?	(237)	Very rare	(21)
Glyceraldehyde phosphate dehydrogenase (partial defect)	None	AD	(237)	Unusual	(276)
Glyoxalase I	None	AR		Rare	(277)
Hypoxanthine-guanine phosphoribosyl transferase (HGPRT)	Lesch-Nyhan syndrome (neurologic symptoms and gout)	SL	(278)	Rare	(279)
ITPase	None	AR	(269)	Rare	(280)
Lactate dehydrogenase	None	AR	(237)	Rare	(281)
NADPH diaphorase	None	AR	(237)	Rare	(282)
Phosphoglucomutase	None	AR	(237)	Rare	(283)
Uroporphyrinogen I synthase	Acute intermittent porphyria	AD	(284)	Unusual (common in selected populations)	(285)

*Very common if incidence is >5%, common if 1–5%, unusual if 0.01–1%, rare if <0.01%.
†AR, autosomal recessive; AD, autosomal dominant; SL, sex linked; ALA, δ-aminolevulinic acid; HNSHA, hereditary nonspherocytic hemolytic anemia; AMP, adenosine monophosphate; ITP, inosine triphosphate.

from a defect in ATP generation. This proposal, born of a misunderstanding of red cell biochemistry, turned out to be correct: one of the major causes of hereditary nonspherocytic hemolytic anemia proved to be a deficiency of the ATP-generating enzyme pyruvate kinase (PK),[10] but this was only the first of a large number of enzyme defects that have been shown to account for this heterogeneous syndrome.[11,12]

ETIOLOGY AND PATHOGENESIS

Red cell enzyme deficiencies that cause hemolytic anemia are hereditary. Most are inherited as autosomal recessive disorders, but G-6-PD deficiency and phosphoglycerate kinase deficiency are X-linked.

The erythrocyte enzyme deficiencies that have been shown to cause hemolytic anemia and other hematologic diseases are listed in Table 45-1. Other red cell enzyme deficiencies, listed in Table 45-2, do not appear to cause a functional abnormality of the erythrocyte.[13] For example, acatalasemia, the state in which there is a virtually total absence of red cell catalase, is devoid of hematologic manifestations. Similarly, red cells without cholinesterase[14] seem to survive normally in most cases. The lack of clinical manifestations is not always clear-cut. In some instances hemolytic anemia is reported in some individuals with a given deficiency but not in others. For example, most subjects with lactate dehydrogenase deficiency have had no anemia, but cases with hemolysis have been reported.[15] Such ambiguity could be due to

differences in environmental and genetic factors, but also to the bias of ascertainment. Erythrocyte enzyme assays are usually carried out on patients with hemolytic anemia. Thus, a benign enzyme defect may be thought mistakenly to cause hemolysis because it is found in a patient with hemolytic anemia. Deficiencies of phosphoglycerate[16,17] kinase and of glutathione synthetase are usually associated with hereditary nonspherocytic hemolytic anemia, but cases have been reported in which these deficiencies were unassociated with any hematologic manifestations. It has at times been suggested that moderate decreases in the activity of glutathione reductase and of glutathione peroxidase caused hemolytic anemia, but the best available evidence indicates that these enzymes are not ordinarily rate limiting in erythrocyte metabolism and are not associated with hemolytic anemia.[12] Even the total absence of glutathione reductase in the red cells of members of one family was associated with only rare episodes of hemolysis, possibly caused by fava beans, in otherwise hematologically normal individuals.[18] Included in Table 45-2 are deficiencies that may cause hemolytic anemia but for which a cause-and-effect relationship has not been clearly established, such as those of phosphogluconolactonase,[19] enolase,[20] glutathione-S-transferase,[21] and adenylate kinase.[22]

Patients with unstable hemoglobins (see Chap. 48) may present with the clinical picture of hereditary nonspherocytic hemolytic anemia. Hemolytic anemia due to abnormalities in the lipid composition of the red cell membrane, particularly increased phosphatidyl choline, occur rarely[23–26] (see Chapter 44).

THE MECHANISM OF HEMOLYSIS

G-6-PD DEFICIENCY AND OTHER DEFICIENCIES OF HEXOSE MONOPHOSPHATE SHUNT ENZYMES

The life span of G-6-PD-deficient red cells is shortened under many circumstances, particularly during drug administration and infection. The exact reason for this is not known.

Drug-induced Hemolysis   Drug-induced hemolysis in G-6-PD-deficient cells is generally accompanied by the formation of Heinz bodies, particles of denatured hemoglobin and stromal protein (see Chap. 22) formed only in the presence of oxygen.[27] The mechanism by which Heinz bodies are formed and become attached to red cell stroma has been the subject of considerable investigation and speculation. Exposure of red cells to certain drugs results in the formation of low levels of hydrogen peroxide as the drug interacts with hemoglobin.[28] In addition, some drugs may form free radicals that oxidize GSH without the formation of peroxide as an intermediate.[29] The formation of free radicals of GSH through the action of peroxide or by the direct action of drugs may be followed either by oxidation of GSH to the disulfide form (GSSG) or complexing of the glutathione with hemoglobin to form a mixed disulfide. Such mixed disulfides are believed to form initially with the sulfhydryl group of the β-93 position of hemoglobin.[30] The mixed disulfide of GSH and hemoglobin is probably unstable and undergoes conformational changes exposing interior sulfhydryl groups to oxidation and mixed disulfide formation. Globin chain separation into free α and β chains also occurs.[31] Phenylhydrazine-like drugs also have been shown to form a hemochromogen directly with hemoglobin, a complex forming between the iron of ferriheme and the nitrogen bound to the benzene ring of the drug.[32] Once such oxidation has occurred, hemoglobin is denatured irreversibly and will precipitate as Heinz bodies. Normal red cells can defend themselves to a considerable extent against such changes by reducing GSSG to GSH and by reducing the mixed disulfides of GSH and hemoglobin through the glutathione reductase reaction.[33] However, the reduction of these disulfide bonds requires a source of NADPH. Since G-6-PD-deficient red cells are unable to reduce NADP$^+$ to NADPH at a normal rate, they are unable to reduce hydrogen peroxide or the mixed disulfides of hemoglobin and GSH. Moreover, because catalase apparently contains tightly bound NADPH[34] that is required for activity, the lack of NADPH generation may impede an alternate pathway for the disposal of hydrogen peroxide.[35] When such cells are challenged by drugs they form Heinz bodies more readily than do normal cells. Cells containing Heinz bodies encounter difficulty in traversing the splenic pulp[36] and are eliminated relatively rapidly from the circulation. The metabolic events that may lead to red cell damage and eventually destruction are summarized in Fig. 45-1.

The formation of methemoglobin frequently accompanies the administration of drugs that have the capacity to produce hemolysis of G-6-PD-deficient cells.[37] The heme groups of methemoglobin become detached from the globin more readily than do the heme groups of oxyhemoglobin.[38] It is not clear whether methemoglobin formation plays an important role in the oxidative degradation of hemoglobin to Heinz bodies or whether formation of methemoglobin is merely an incidental side effect of oxidative drugs.[39,40]

Infection-induced Hemolysis   The mechanism of hemolysis induced by infection or occurring spontaneously in G-6-PD-deficient subjects is not well understood. It has been suggested that the generation of hydrogen peroxide by phagocytizing leukocytes may play a role in this type of hemolytic reaction.[40] Substances capable of destroying red cell GSH have been isolated from fava beans.[41] Favism occurs only in G-6-PD-deficient subjects, but not all deficient individuals in a particular family may be sensitive to the hemolytic effect of the beans. Nonetheless, some tendency toward familial occurrence has

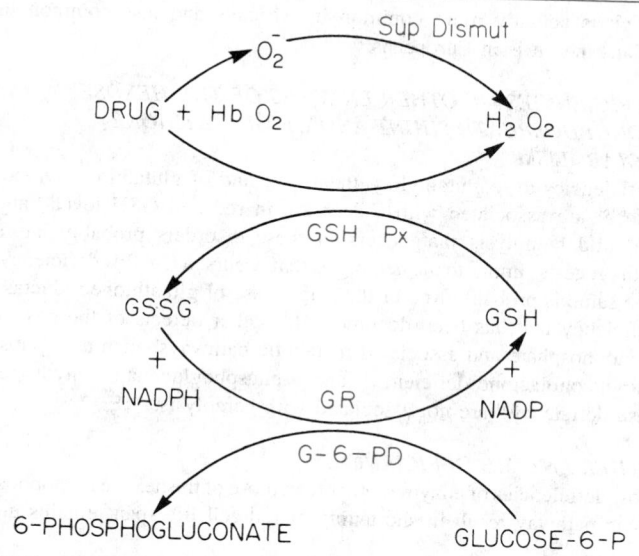

FIGURE 45-1   Reactions through which hydrogen peroxide is generated and detoxified in the erythrocyte. In G-6-PD deficiency inadequate generation of NADPH results in accumulation of GSSG and probably of H$_2$O$_2$. The accumulation of these substances leads to hemoglobin denaturation, Heinz body formation, and consequently to decreased red cell survival. GR, glutathione reductase; GSH Px, glutathione peroxide; Sup Dismut, superoxide dismutase; GSSG, glutathione disulfide (oxidized glutathione).

suggested the possibility that an additional, genetic factor may be important.[42] The observation of increased excretion of glucaric acid[43] led to the suggestion that a defect in glucuronide formation might be present. An excess of individuals with the acid phosphatase ACP_1 A/C genotype has been found and attributed to a decrease in the f isoform of this tyrosine phosphatase.[44] Immunologic factors do not seem to play a role in favism.[45] Increased levels of red cell calcium[46,47] and consequent "cross-bonding" of membranes may occur. Such bonding of the facing inner membrane surfaces[48] may play a role in the destruction of red cells.

Neonatal Jaundice   Icterus neonatorum in G-6-PD deficiency probably is due principally to inadequate processing of bilirubin by the immature liver of G-6-PD-deficient infants, although shortening of red cell life span may play a role. Anemia does not appear to be present in these infants and there is only a slight increase in CO production, signifying a minimal decrease in red cell life span.[49] Severe jaundice due to G-6-PD deficiency seems to be limited to infants who have also inherited a mutation of the uridine diphosphoglucuronate glucuronosyltransferase 1 (UDPGT-1) gene promoter,[50] the same mutation that in adults is associated with Gilbert syndrome. The limited data available on liver G-6-PD in deficient adults[51] suggest that a considerable degree of deficiency may be present. If such a deficiency also is present in infants, it may play a role in impairing the borderline ability of infant livers with the UDPGT-1 promoter defect to catabolize bilirubin. While an increased incidence of neonatal icterus has been observed in Mediterranean infants with G-6-PD deficiency and among the Chinese,[52] jaundice seems to be less common among neonates with the A— type of enzyme deficiency. Some cases have been reported in G-6-PD-deficient infants[53–55] in Africa, but in the United States the incidence of jaundice in G-6-PD A— does not appear to be increased.[56,57] The cause of the relatively low incidence of neonatal jaundice in infants with G-6-PD A— mutation is not clear. It could be due to the higher residual enzyme activity, but it does not appear to be related to the incidence of the UDPGT-1 promotor mutation, which is actually more common in Africans and less common in Asians than it is in Europeans.[58]

DEFICIENCIES OF OTHER ENZYMES OF THE HEXOSE MONOPHOSPHATE SHUNT AND OF GLUTATHIONE METABOLISM

Deficiencies of γ-glutamyl synthetase[59,60] and of glutathione synthetase[60,61] are associated with a decrease in red cell GSH levels, and the mild hemolysis that occurs in these disorders probably has a pathogenesis similar to the hemolysis that occurs in G-6-PD deficiency. The same is probably true of the single case of glutathione reductase deficiency that has been documented.[18] Other defects of the hexose monophosphate and associated metabolic pathways, such as 6-phosphogluconolactone deficiency[19] and 6-phosphogluconate dehydrogenase deficiency[62] are not associated with hemolysis.

OTHER ENZYME DEFICIENCIES

How deficiencies of enzymes other than those of the hexose monophosphate pathway result in shortening of red cell life span remains unknown, although it has been the object of much experimental work and of speculation. It is often believed that ATP depletion is a common pathway in producing damage to the cell leading to its destruction,[63] but the evidence that this is the case is not always compelling.[64] It is possible that, at least in some cases, alteration of the levels of red cell intermediate metabolites interferes with synthesis of cell components in early stages of development of the cell.

ANIMAL MODELS

G-6-PD deficiency has been encountered in rats,[65] dogs,[66] mice,[67,68] and horses.[69,70] Pyruvate kinase deficiency is polymorphic in Basenji dogs[71] and has been found in mice.[72–74] Phosphofructokinase deficiency causes hemolytic anemia in dogs,[75] and glucosephosphate isomerase deficiency has been detected in mice.[76]

BIOCHEMICAL GENETICS AND MOLECULAR BIOLOGY

GLUCOSE-6-PHOSPHATE DEHYDROGENASE

Biochemical Genetics   The "normal" enzyme is designated as G-6-PD B. It represents the most common type of enzyme encountered in all the population groups that have been studied. Many variants of G-6-PD have been detected all over the world. Before it became possible to characterize these variants at the DNA level they were distinguished from each other on the basis of biochemical characteristics, such as electrophoretic mobility, K_m for NADP and glucose-6-phosphate, ability to utilize substrate analogs, pH activity profile, and thermal stability. To facilitate comparison of variants characterized in different laboratories, international standards for the methodology were established.[77] In the case of the common G-6-PD A− and G-6-PD Mediterranean mutations, the abnormal enzyme may be synthesized at normal or near-normal rates but has decreased stability in vivo.[78] The amount of enzyme antigen in the red cells declines concurrently with enzyme activity.[79,80] This suggests that the mutant protein in these variants is rendered unusually sensitive to proteolysis in the environment of the erythrocyte.[81] Other mutations also result in the formation of enzyme molecules with decreased enzyme activity[80] and with altered kinetic properties,[82] some of which may render them functionally inadequate. For example, G-6-PD Oklahoma[83] manifests a marked decrease in its affinity for the substrates glucose-6-phosphate and NADP, and G-6-PD Manchester and G-6-PD Tripler[84] are abnormally sensitive to the inhibitory effect of NADPH. Detailed biochemical characteristics of some 400 putatively distinct G-6-PD variants have been tabulated.[85] Fig. 45-2 is a semischematic representation of the biochemical properties of two of the more common variants.

Molecular Biology   The gene for G-6-PD is over 20 kb in length, containing 13 exons. The coding sequence begins in exon 2. The intron between exons 2 and 3 is extraordinarily long, spanning 9857 base pairs.[86] Methylation of certain cytidines at the 3′ end is believed to have a regulatory function.[87] The enzyme is composed

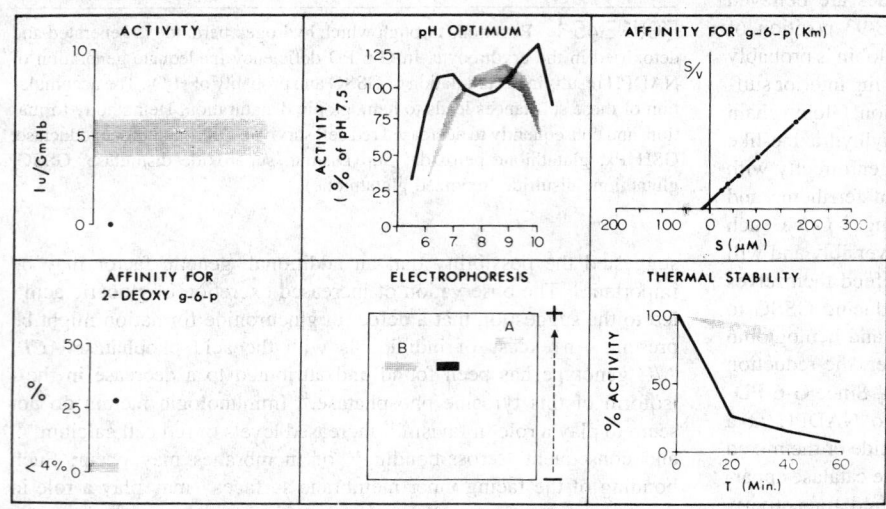

A

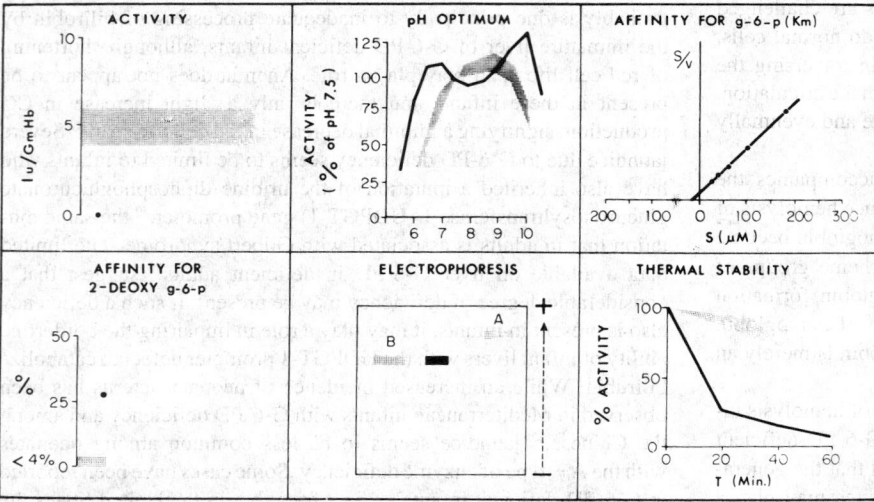

B

FIGURE 45-2   The biochemical properties of two common variants of G-6-PD. (a) The biochemical characteristics of G-6-PD A−. (b) The biochemical characteristics of G-6-PD Mediterranean. In each panel the characteristics of the normal enzyme (types A and B) are indicated by the shaded areas.

of 515 amino acids, with a calculated molecular weight of 59,256. Aggregation of the inactive monomers into catalytically active dimers and higher forms requires the presence of NADP.[88] Thus, NADP appears to be bound to the enzyme both as a structural component and as one of the substrates of the reaction.[89–91] The glucose-6-phosphate binding site has been identified at amino acid 205 by locating a lysine that is reactive in competition with glucose-6-phosphate at this position.[92,93] Examination of mutants suggested that amino acids 386 and 387 bind one of the phosphates of NADP.[94] However, the crystal structure of G-6-PD from *Leuconostoc mesenteroides*[95] is interpreted as indicating that it is actually His 201 that is the binding site, a location 36 Å distant from the 386–387 site.[95]

African Variants   Among persons of African descent a mutant enzyme with normal activity is very prevalent. Known as G-6-PD A+, it migrates electrophoretically more rapidly than the normal B enzyme. A single amino acid substitution of Asn→Asp has been identified both by peptide analysis[96] and by DNA sequencing (376 A→G).[97] G-6-PD A− is the principal deficient variant found among people of African origin. The red cells contain only 5 to 15 percent of the normal amount of enzyme activity. The mobility of the enzyme present is rapid and is indistinguishable from that of the A+ variant in conventional electrophoretic systems. The fact that these two electrophoretically rapid variants are common in African populations is not a coincidence. Sequence analysis of G-6-PD A+ and G-6-PD A− has shown that these two mutations have in common a nucleotide substitution at cDNA nucleotide 376 that produces the amino acid substitution responsible for the rapid electrophoretic mobility. Most samples with G-6-PD A− manifest an additional mutation at nucleotide 202 that accounts for its in vivo instability.[98] Apparently the interaction of the two mutations results in the deficiency.[99] Less commonly, the additional mutation is at a different site (Table 45-3). Thus, it is evident that G-6-PD A− arose in an individual who already had the G-6-PD A+ mutation. However the ancestral human sequence has been deduced to be that of G-6-PD B, both by showing that this is the sequence of the chimpanzee,[100] our nearest relative, and by analysis of linkage dysequilibrium.[101]

Variants in the Mediterranean Region Among Caucasian populations G-6-PD deficiency is most common in Mediterranean countries. The most common enzyme variant in this region is G-6-PD Mediterranean.[82] The enzyme activity of the red cells of individuals who have inherited this abnormal gene is barely detectable. Other variants are also prevalent in the Mediterranean region, including G-6-PD A− and G-6-PD Seattle (see Table 45-3).

TABLE 45-3   SOME OF THE MORE IMPORTANT G-6-PD VARIANTS THAT HAVE BEEN CHARACTERIZED AT THE DNA LEVEL*

VARIANT	NUCLEOTIDE SUBSTITUTION	WHO CLASS	AMINO ACID SUBSTITUTION	REFERENCES
Aures	143 T→C	2	48 Ile→Thr	(286)
A−	202 G→A	3	68 Val→Met	(98)
Distrito Federal				(287)
Matera				(288)
Castilla				(287)
Alabama	376 A→G		126 Asn→Asp	(Beutler E, unpublished)
Betica				(100)
Tepic				(287)
Ferrara				(289)
A	376 A→G	4	126 Asn→Asp	(97)
Santamaria	542 A→T	2	181 Asp→Val	(290)
	376 A→G		126 Asn→Asp	
Mediterranean				(288)
Dallas				(291)
Birmingham	563 C→T	2	188 Ser→Phe	(291)
Sassari				(292)
Cagliari				(292)
Panama				(Beutler E, unpublished)
Minnesota	637 G→T	1	213 Val→Leu	(215)
Marion				
Gastonia				
A−	680 G→T	3	227 Arg→Leu	(98)
	376 A→G		126 Asn→Asp	
Seattle				(292)
Lodi	844 G→C	2	282 Asp→His	(293)
Modena				(289)
Viangchan	871 G→A	2	291 Val→Met	(294)
Jammu				
A−	968 T→C	3	323 Leu→ Pro	(98)
Betica	376 A→G		126 Asn→Asp	
Selma				
Chatham	1003 G→A	3	335 Ala→Thr	(288)
Iowa	1156 A→G	1	386 Lys→Glu	(94)
Walter Reed				
Iowa City				
Springfield				
Guadalajara	1159 C→T		387 Arg→Cys	(295)
Mt. Sinai	1159 C→T	1	387 Arg→Cys	(296)
	376 A→G		126 Asn→Asp	
Beverly Hills	1160 G→A	1	387 Arg→His	(94)
Genova				(Argusti A, personal communication)
Worcester				(Beutler E, unpublished)
Nashville	1178 G→A	1	393 Arg→His	(215)
Anaheim				
Calgary				(297)
Portici				
Alhambra	1180 G→C	1	394 Val→Leu	(295)
Georgia	1284 C→A	1	428 Tyr→End	(103)
Taiwan-Hakka	1376 G→T	2	459 Arg→Leu	(298)
Gifu-like				
Agrigento-like				(299)
Canton				
Cosenza	1376 G→C	2	459 Arg→Pro	(300)
Kaiping	1388 G→A	2	463 Arg→His	(298)
Anant				
Dhon				
Petrich				
Sapporo				
Campinas	1463 G→T	1	488 Gly→Val	(108)

*See Ref. 106 for a complete tabulation.
†Class 1, nonspherocytic hemolytic anemia; class 2, severe deficiency; class 3, moderate deficiency; class 4, not deficient.

TABLE 45-4   SOME PYRUVATE KINASE MUTATIONS

DESIGNATION	cDNA nt	SUBSTITUTION	AMINO ACID #	SUBSTITUTION	REFERENCE
	391–393 del	—	131	Ile→del	(121)
Linz	394	C→T	132	Arg→Cys	(301)
Beirut	946	C→T	353	Thr→Met	(301)
Tokyo					(302)
Nagasaki					(303)
Fukushima	1261	C→A	421	Gln→Gly	(303)
Maebashi					
Common European	1529	G→A	510	Arg→Gln	(121)
Gypsy	exon 11 del				(119)

Variants in Asia   A great many different variants have been described in East Asian populations. Some of these proved to be identical at a molecular level (e.g., G-6-PD Gifu, Agrigento, Canton, and Taiwan-Hakka all have the same mutation at cDNA nt 1376), but DNA analysis has shown that over 10 different mutations are found in various East Asian populations.[102–105]

Variants Producing Hereditary Nonspherocytic Hemolytic Anemia   Some mutations of G-6-PD result in chronic hemolysis without precipitating causes. From a functional point of view these mutations are more severe than the more commonly occurring polymorphic forms of the enzyme, such as G-6-PD Mediterranean and G-6-PD A−, but the in vitro enzyme activity may actually be greater in such variants. It has been suggested that specific biochemical characteristics such as susceptibility to inhibition by NADPH might explain the chronic hemolysis that occurs in patients with such variants,[84] but no unifying principle that accounts for the clinical effects of variants has been found. On a molecular level, such variants usually are located in exon 10[94] or in the region of the glucose-6-phosphate binding site.[106] There are, however, exceptions to this rule. For example, deletion of a triplet near the 5′ end of the coding region[107] and a mutation very near the carboxy terminus of the enzyme also have been found to result in hemolysis.[108]

PYRUVATE KINASE

Pyruvate kinase deficiency, like G-6-PD deficiency, is genetically heterogeneous, with different mutations causing different kinetic and electrophoretic changes in the enzyme that is formed. Abnormalities include altered affinity for the substrate phosphoenolpyruvate (PEP) and the allosteric activator fructose 1,6-diphosphate (FDP).[109–111] There are even cases in which the activity of pyruvate kinase as measured in vitro is higher than normal but a kinetically abnormal enzyme is responsible for the occurrence of hemolytic anemia.[112] Kinetic characterization and analysis of pyruvate kinase mutants is considerably more complex, however, than analysis of G-6-PD mutants. Since two alleles are expressed in each cell, five different tetramers will be formed if the mutations are different: the two homotetramers and mixed tetramers containing different proportions of different subunits. Moreover, there are several different molecular forms of pyruvate kinase, formed from two different genes: the M, or muscle, type of enzyme, which is found in leukocytes and many other tissues, and the L, or liver, type of enzyme. Erythrocytes contain only a product of the L gene, designated the R type of enzyme. Thus, it is mutations of the pyruvate kinase L gene that cause hemolytic anemia. There has been international agreement on standard methods for characterizing pyruvate kinase variants,[113] but because of the complexities mentioned above, the biochemical information is even less robust than that obtained with G-6-PD variants. It has been suggested that some correlation exists between the quantity and biochemical characteristics of

the residual enzyme in enzyme-deficient patients and these patients' clinical course.[114]

The cDNA for human L type pyruvate kinase has been cloned,[115,116] and mutations identified in many deficient patients (Table 45-4).[117,118] The same mutations are encountered repeatedly in apparently unrelated individuals, although the existence of a common haplotype in such persons indicates that they are presumably offspring of a common ancestor.[119,120] The 1529A mutation in particular is encountered repeatedly, even in the homozygous state, in unrelated individuals.[121] Deletion of exon 11 is characteristic of the mutation found among Gypsies.[119] The nature of the mutation has relatively little predictive value with respect to the severity of the clinical course.[120,122]

OTHER ENZYME DEFICIENCIES

The mutations that cause other enzyme deficiencies have been identified in many instances. Table 45-2 provides references to some of the more recent studies in which the abnormalities in DNA sequence have been documented.

PREVALENCE, GEOGRAPHIC DISTRIBUTION, AND POPULATION GENETICS

The prevalence of G-6-PD deficiency among Caucasian populations ranges from less than 1 in 1000 among northern European populations to 50 percent of the males among Kurdish Jews. G-6-PD deficiency is also found among certain Chinese populations and in Southeast Asia but it is rare in Japan. G-6-PD deficiency of the A− type is very common in West Africa, and the prevalence among African American males is approximately 11 percent.[123] Some 16 percent of African American males carry the nondeficient G-6-PD A+ gene. The distribution of G-6-PD deficiency among various population groups has been presented in detail elsewhere.[124,125]

The high frequency of G-6-PD-deficient genes in many populations implies that G-6-PD deficiency confers a selective advantage. The suggestion[126] that resistance to malaria could account for the frequency of G-6-PD deficiency was supported by studies in heterozygotes for G-6-PD A− that showed a higher degree of infestation of G-6-PD sufficient cells than of G-6-PD-deficient cells.[127] It has been suggested that deficient cells infested with malaria parasites may be phagocytosed more efficiently than normal cells.[128]

It has been suggested[129,130] that a higher prevalence of G-6-PD deficiency in individuals with sickle cell disease than in the general African population reflects a favorable effect of the enzyme deficiency on the clinical course of the sickling disorders. However, it seems that the increased prevalence of G-6-PD deficiency in patients with sickle disease may merely result from the markedly heterogeneous genetic composition of African Americans; those with more African genes are more likely to inherit sickle hemoglobin and G-6-PD A−.[131–133] Similar factors may be responsible for the slight excess of G-6-PD deficiency observed among patients with SS hemoglobin in Arab populations.[134]

Pyruvate kinase deficiency is the most common cause of hereditary nonspherocytic hemolytic anemia. Estimates of heterozygote frequency have ranged from 0.24[135] to 3.1 percent[136] using screening techniques. More quantitative studies performed on a large number of cord blood samples have provided estimates of 1 percent in the white population and 2.4 percent in African Americans.[137] A gene frequency of about 0.005 has been deduced from study of a large number of DNA samples from subjects of the European origin. Estimates of other deficiency alleles, such as those for adenylate kinase, diphosphoglycerate mutase, enolase, triosephosphate isomerase, and phosphoglycerate kinase have also been made on large numbers of cord bloods.[137] A particularly high incidence of heterozygous TPI deficiency of over 4 percent in African Americans is supported by family studies.[138] Since it is not reflected in a correspondingly high birth incidence, the allele might be lethal in the homozygous state. It was suggested that a promoter mutation at the -5 and -8 positions created such a lethal gene,[139] but the finding of normal adult homozygotes for these mutations shows that this is not the case.[140]

In addition to the common G-6-PD mutations there are mutations in other enzymes that are repeatedly encountered in a population. Included are the 1529A mutation of pyruvate kinase,[120,121] the deletion of exon 11 found among Gypsies,[119] and the 1591 C mutation of TPI.[141] In each of these instances the existence of each mutation in the context of the same haplotype implies that there has been a *founder effect*, that is, the mutation occurred only once and all individuals now carrying it are descendants of the person who sustained the original mutation. The expansion of the mutation could represent a selective advantage for heterozygotes but may also be due to random factors or to a selective advantage provided by one or more tightly linked genes.

CLINICAL FEATURES

COMMON FORMS OF G-6-PD DEFICIENCY

Individuals who inherit the common (polymorphic) forms of G-6-PD deficiency, such as G-6-PD A− or G-6-PD Mediterranean usually have no clinical manifestations. The major clinical consequence of G-6-PD deficiency is hemolytic anemia in adults and neonatal icterus in infants. Usually the anemia is episodic, but some of the unusual variants of G-6-PD may cause hereditary nonspherocytic hemolytic disease (see below). In general, hemolysis is associated with stress, most notably drug administration, infection, and, in certain individuals, exposure to fava beans.

DRUG-INDUCED HEMOLYTIC ANEMIA
A large number of drugs and other chemicals that may have the capacity to precipitate hemolytic reactions in G-6-PD-deficient individuals are listed in Table 45-5. Some drugs, such as chloramphenicol, may induce

TABLE 45-5   DRUGS AND CHEMICALS THAT SHOULD BE AVOIDED BY PERSONS WITH G-6-PD DEFICIENCY*

AGENT	REFERENCE
Acetanilid	(27)
Dimercaptosuccinic acid†	(304)
Furazolidone (Furoxone)	(305,306)
Glibenclamide†	(308)
Isobutyl nitrite	(202,309)
Methylene blue	(310)
Nalidixic acid (NeGram)†	(311,312)
Naphthalene	(314,315)
Niridazole (Ambilhar)	(317,318)
Nitrofurantoin (Furadantin)	(319)
Phenazopyridine (Pyridium)	(320)
Primaquine	(27)
Sulfacetamide	(27)
Toluidine blue†	(307)
Sulfanilamide	(27)
Sulfapyridine	(27)
Thiazolsulfone	(27)
Trinitrotoluene (TNT)	(313)
Urate oxidase	(316)

*Further details may be found in Ref. 12.
†Single case reports. Cause and effect not certain.

mild hemolysis in a person with severe, Mediterranean-type G-6-PD deficiency[142] but not in those with the milder A− or Canton[143] types of deficiency. Drugs that are innocuous when given in normal doses (Table 45-5) may be hemolytic when given in excessive doses. A case in point is ascorbic acid, which does not cause hemolytic anemia when even as much as 40 g is given intravenously,[144] but which can produce severe, even fatal, hemolysis at doses of 80 g or more intravenously.[144-146] There appears, furthermore, to be a difference in the severity of the reaction to the same drug of different individuals with the same G-6-PD variant. For example, red cells from a single G-6-PD-deficient individual were hemolyzed in the circulation of some recipients who were given thiazolsulfone, but their survival was normal in the circulation of others.[27] Sulfamethoxazole, which was clearly hemolytic in experimental studies, does not appear to be a common cause of hemolysis in a clinical setting.[147] Undoubtedly, individual differences in the metabolism and excretion of drugs influence the extent to which G-6-PD-deficient red cells are destroyed.[148,149]

Typically, an episode of drug-induced hemolysis in G-6-PD-deficient individuals begins 1 to 3 days after drug administration is initiated.[150] Heinz bodies appear in the red cells, and the hemoglobin concentration begins to decline rapidly.[151] As hemolysis progresses Heinz bodies disappear from the circulation, presumably as they or the erythrocytes that contain them are removed by the spleen. In severe cases abdominal or back pain may occur. The urine may turn dark—even black. Within 4 to 6 days there is generally an increase in the reticulocyte count, except in instances in which the patient has received the offending drug in treatment of an active infection. Because of the tendency of infections and certain other stressful situations to precipitate hemolysis in G-6-PD-deficient individuals, many drugs have been incorrectly implicated as a cause. Other drugs, such as aspirin, have appeared on many lists of proscribed medications because very large doses could slightly reduce the red cell life span. It is important to recognize that such drugs, listed in Table 45-6, do not produce clinically significant hemolytic anemia. Advising patients not to ingest these drugs may not only deprive patients of potentially helpful medications but will also weaken their confidence in the advice that they have received. Most G-6-PD-deficient patients, after all, have taken aspirin without untoward effect and are likely to distrust an advisor who counsels them that the ingestion of aspirin would have catastrophic effects.

In the A− type of G-6-PD deficiency the hemolytic anemia is self-limited[150] because the young red cells produced in response to hemolysis have nearly normal G-6-PD levels and are relatively resistant to hemolysis.[152] The hemoglobin level may return to normal even while the same dose of drug that initially precipitated hemolysis is administered. In contrast, hemolysis is not self-limited in the more severe Mediterranean type of deficiency.[153]

HEMOLYTIC ANEMIA OCCURRING DURING INFECTION
Anemia often develops rather suddenly in G-6-PD-deficient individuals within a few days of onset of a febrile illness. The anemia is usually relatively mild, with a decline in the hemoglobin concentration of 3 or 4 g/dl. Hemolysis has been noted particularly in patients suffering from pneumonia and in those with typhoid fever. The fulminating form of the disease occurs particularly frequently among G-6-PD-deficient patients who are infected with Rocky Mountain spotted fever.[154] Jaundice is not a prominent part of the clinical picture, except where hemolysis occurs in association with infectious hepatitis.[155,156] In that case it can be quite intense. Presumably because of the effect of the infection reticulocytosis is usually absent, and recovery from the anemia is generally delayed until after the active infection has abated.

TABLE 45-6 DRUGS THAT CAN PROBABLY SAFELY BE GIVEN IN NORMAL
THERAPEUTIC DOSES TO G-6-PD DEFICIENT SUBJECTS
WITHOUT NONSPHEROCYTIC HEMOLYTIC ANEMIA*

DRUG	REFERENCE
Acetaminophen (paracetamol, Tylenol, Tralgon, hydroxyacetanilide)	(321,27)
Acetophenetidin (phenacetin)	(27)
Acetylsalicylic acid (aspirin)	(1,321)
Aminopyrine (Pyramidon)	(322)
Antazoline (Antistine)	(1)
Antipyrine	(321)
Ascorbic acid (vitamin C)	(1)
Benzhexol (Artane)	(321)
Chloramphenicol	(321,143,142)
Chlorguanidine (Proguanil, Paludrine)	(321)
Chloroquine	(321,1,323)
Colchicine	(321)
Diphenhydramine (Benadryl)	(1)
Isoniazid	(321,324)
L-Dopa	(321,325)
Menadione sodium bisulfite (Hykinone)	(326)
p-Aminobenzoic acid	(1)
p-Aminosalicylic acid	(324)
Phenylbutazone	(321)
Phenytoin	(321)
Probenecid (Benemid)	(321,326)
Procainamide hydrochloride (Pronestyl)	(1)
Pyrimethamine (Daraprim)	(321,1)
Quinine	(326)
Streptomycin	(321)
Sulfacytine	(327)
Sulfadiazine	(1,328)
Sulfaguanidine	(328)
Sulfamerazine	(1)
Sulfamethoxazole (Gantanol)	(147)
Sulfamethoxypyridazine (Kynex)	(329,330)
Sulfisoxazole (Gantrisin)	(326,327)
Tiaprofenic acid	(331)
Trimethoprim	(321)
Tripelennamine (Pyribenzamine)	(1)
Vitamin K	(56)

*Further details may be found in Ref. 12.

DIABETIC KETOACIDOSIS

Diabetic ketoacidosis has usually been considered a cause of hemolysis in G-6-PD-deficient individuals, but a review of 36 episodes of diabetic ketoacidosis in G-6-PD-deficient subjects yielded only 10 in whom hemolysis occurred, and these all were associated with infection or drug ingestion.[157] It has been suggested that hypoglycemia may precipitate hemolysis.[158]

FAVISM

Favism is potentially one of the gravest clinical consequences of G-6-PD deficiency. It occurs much more commonly in children than in adults and occurs almost exclusively in persons who have inherited variants of G-6-PD that cause severe deficiency, but rarely the disorder has been noted in patients with G-6-PD A−.[159] The onset of hemolysis may be quite sudden, having been reported to occur within the first hours after exposure to fava beans. More commonly the onset is gradual, hemolysis being noticed 1 to 2 days after ingestion of the beans.[160] The urine becomes red or quite dark, and in severe cases shock may develop within a short time. Occasionally ingestion of other foodstuffs, such as unripe peaches[161] or a spiced Nigerian barbecued meat known as red suya,[162] has been reported to precipitate hemolysis.

NEONATAL ICTERUS

Icterus neonatorum without evidence of immunologic incompatibility occurs in some infants with G-6-PD deficiency.[163] The jaundice may be quite severe and if untreated may result in kernicterus. Thus, G-6-PD deficiency is a preventable cause of mental retardation,[164,165] and this aspect of the disorder has considerable public health significance.

EFFECTS ON OTHER TISSUES

In the common variants of G-6-PD such as G-6-PD A− and G-6-PD Mediterranean, and even in most of the severely deficient variants, there is usually no demonstrated defect in leukocyte number or function.[166] However, there have been reports of isolated instances of leukocyte dysfunction associated with rare, severely deficient variants of G-6-PD.[167–169] Patients with G-6-PD deficiency do not have a bleeding tendency, and studies of platelet function have yielded conflicting results.[170,171] Occasionally, cataracts have been observed in patients with variants of G-6-PD that produce nonspherocytic hemolytic anemia.[172–174] The incidence of senile cataracts may be increased in G-6-PD deficiency,[175,176] but this remains controversial.[177] Although claims have been made that an association exists between various kinds of G-6-PD deficiency and cancer[178,179] the data are not convincing, and a detailed investigation of hematologic malignancies in patients with G-6-PD Mediterranean shows no effect.[180] Decrease in insulin release[181] and in cortisol levels after ACTH stimulation[182] have been reported to occur in G-6-PD-deficient men.

HEREDITARY NONSPHEROCYTIC HEMOLYTIC ANEMIA

Most patients with hereditary nonspherocytic hemolytic anemia manifest only the usual clinical signs and symptoms of chronic hemolysis. The degree of anemia in this group of disorders varies widely. In some cases of very severe pyruvate kinase deficiency scarcely any deficient cells survive in the circulation and only transfused cells are found, or steady-state hemoglobin levels as low as 5 g/dl may be encountered. Other patients with hereditary nonspherocytic hemolytic anemia may manifest compensated hemolysis with a normal steady-state hemoglobin concentration. Chronic jaundice is a common finding and splenomegaly is often present. Gallstones are common. As in other forms of chronic hemolytic anemia, ankle ulcers may be present.[183,184] Pregnancy has been thought to precipitate hemolysis in patients with pyruvate kinase deficiency, perhaps even in heterozygotes.[185,186]

In the case of some enzyme defects, characteristic nonhematologic systemic manifestations may be present, and these may be the only sign of the enzyme deficiency. For example, patients with phosphofructokinase deficiency may have type VII muscle glycogen storage disease. In some with this defect hemolysis is present without muscle manifestations, but in others both muscle abnormalities and hemolysis occur.[187] Glutathione synthetase deficiency may be associated with 5-oxoprolinuria and neuromuscular disturbances, and such abnormalities may occur either with[188] or without[17] hematologic abnormalities. On the other hand, some patients with glutathione synthetase deficiency manifest only the hematologic abnormalities.[60] Spinocerebellar degeneration was documented in the first case of γ-glutamylcysteine synthetase described[189,190] but was not present in subsequently investigated patients.[60,191] Patients with TPI deficiency nearly always manifest serious neuromuscular disease, and most of the patients who inherit this abnormality die in the first decade of life[192–194] but there are exceptions, since only one of two brothers with the same genotype manifested neurologic disease.[195,196] Neurologic symptoms have also been noted in a patient with glucosephosphate isomerase deficiency.[197] This enzyme seems to be identical to neuroleukin, which could explain the existence of neurologic manifestations. Myoglobinuria has been encountered in patients with phosphoglycerate kinase,[16,198] aldolase,[199] and G-6-PD deficiency.[200] The clinical features of enzyme deficiencies causing nonspherocytic hemolytic anemia are summarized in Table 45-1.

LABORATORY FEATURES

In the absence of hemolysis, the light-microscopic morphology of G-6-PD-deficient red cells appears to be normal. Differences in the texture of the stroma of the cells have, however, been observed under the electron microscope.[201]

Varying degrees of anemia and reticulocytosis are the main routine hematologic laboratory features of patients with hereditary nonspherocytic hemolytic anemia. Heinz bodies often are found in the erythrocytes of G-6-PD-deficient patients undergoing drug-induced hemolysis and in splenectomized but not in unsplenectomized patients with unstable hemoglobins. When a hemolytic drug is administered to a G-6-PD-deficient patient, Heinz bodies (see Chap. 22) develop in the erythrocytes immediately preceding and in the early phases of the hemolytic episode. If the hemolytic anemia is very severe, spherocytosis and red cell fragmentation may be seen in the stained film. Although "bite cells" have been noted in the blood of a G-6-PD-deficient patient undergoing drug-induced hemolysis,[202] such cells have also been noted in nondeficient patients.[203,204]

The presence of small, densely staining cells has often been noted in the blood films of patients with hereditary nonspherocytic hemolytic anemia with defects other than G-6-PD deficiency. Particularly when manifesting an echinocytic appearance, such cells have been thought to be common in pyruvate kinase deficiency. In one reported case[205] spectacular numbers of such cells were observed. However, cells of this type are seen in many blood films both from patients with glycolytic enzyme deficiencies and from those with other disorders, and it is hazardous to attempt to make an enzymatic diagnosis on the basis of such findings. Basophilic stippling of the erythrocytes is prominent in most patients with pyrimidine-5'-nucleotidase deficiency but may not be apparent in blood that has been collected in EDTA anticoagulant. Leukopenia occasionally is observed in patients with hereditary nonspherocytic hemolytic anemia, possibly secondary to splenic enlargement. Other laboratory stigmata of increased hemolysis may include increased levels of serum bilirubin, decreased haptoglobin levels, and increased serum lactic dehydrogenase activity.

Diagnosis of red cell enzyme deficiencies depends on the demonstration of decreased enzyme activity through either a quantitative assay or a screening test.[113,206–208] Assay of most of the enzymes generally is carried out by measuring the rate of reduction or oxidation of nicotinamide adenine nucleotides in an ultraviolet spectrophotometer, and a number of screening tests that depend upon the development or loss of fluorescence have been devised.[206]

Although detection of G-6-PD deficiency in the healthy, fully affected (hemizygous) male can be achieved readily through either assay or screening tests, difficulties arise when a patient with G-6-PD deficiency of the A− type has undergone a hemolytic episode. As the older, more enzyme-deficient cells are removed from the circulation and are replaced by young cells, the level of the enzyme begins to increase toward normal. Under such circumstances, suspicion that the patient may be G-6-PD deficient should be raised by the fact that enzyme activity is not increased even though the reticulocyte count is elevated. Centrifugation of the blood followed by testing of the most dense, reticulocyte-depleted red cells has been employed as a means for the detection of G-6-PD deficiency in persons with the A− defect who have recently undergone hemolysis.[209,210] It is helpful to carry out family studies or to wait until the circulating red cells have aged sufficiently to betray their lack of enzyme.

Even greater difficulties are encountered in attempting to diagnose heterozygotes for G-6-PD deficiency.[211] Because the gene is X-linked, a population of normal red cells coexists with the deficient cells (see Chap. 9). This may mask the enzyme deficiency when screening tests are used. Even enzyme assays carried out on erythrocytes of heterozygous females frequently may be in the normal range. Here methods that depend upon histochemical demonstration of individual red cell enzyme activity may be useful.[212,213] In addition, the ascorbate-cyanide test,[214] in which screening is carried out on a whole-cell population rather than on a lysate, may be more sensitive than the other screening procedures. However, when the nucleotide substitution is known, heterozygotes are easily detected by PCR-based analysis of the mutation.[215] Prenatal diagnosis of G-6-PD deficiency is also possible using this approach.[216]

Identifying specific G-6-PD variants on the basis of biochemical variations requires the use of relatively sophisticated techniques. The enzyme must be partially purified, and then its K_m for NADP$^+$ and glucose-6-phosphate, its utilization of substrate analogs, its pH optima, and its electrophoretic mobility must be determined in standard systems.[77] At best there is often uncertainty regarding minor differences in the characteristics of enzymes studied in this way. Detailed biochemical characterization of G-6-PD variants has therefore largely been replaced by PCR-based DNA analysis.[217,218]

DIFFERENTIAL DIAGNOSIS

Drug-induced hemolytic anemia due to G-6-PD deficiency is similar in its clinical features and in certain laboratory features to drug-induced hemolytic anemia associated with unstable hemoglobins (see Chap. 48). Other enzyme defects affecting the pentose-phosphate shunt, such as a deficiency of GSH synthetase, also may mimic G-6-PD deficiency. The diagnosis of hemoglobinopathies can be excluded by performing a hemoglobin stability test and electrophoresis. Both of these are normal in G-6-PD deficiency. Some of the screening tests, particularly the ascorbate-cyanide test,[214] may give positive results in the above-named disorders, but a G-6-PD assay or the fluorescent screening test will be positive only in G-6-PD deficiency.

Physicians often attempt to establish the cause of hereditary nonspherocytic hemolytic anemia on the basis of the appearance of red cells on a blood film and the results of the autohemolysis test. In reality, red cell morphology is helpful only in the diagnosis of pyrimidine-5'-nucleotidase deficiency, because of the characteristic stippling of the red cells that is observed in that disorder. After splenectomy, the appearance of Heinz bodies suggests the possible presence of an unstable hemoglobin. Autohemolysis tests provide no diagnostic information of value, except occasionally in the confirmation of the presence of hereditary spherocytosis.[219]

Since the laboratory diagnosis of these disorders may entail considerable expenditure of time and effort, it is prudent to perform the simplest tests for the most common causes of hereditary nonspherocytic hemolytic anemia first. Accordingly, it is useful to carry out screening tests[206,207] for G-6-PD and PK activity and an isopropanol stability test[220] to detect an unstable hemoglobin. The characteristically elevated levels of red cell 2,3-bisphosphoglycerate and of 3-phosphoglyceric acid[221] are also helpful in the diagnosis of PK deficiency. If the levels of these intermediates are normal it is extremely unlikely that the patient has PK deficiency. If prominent stippling of erythrocytes is present, examination of the ultraviolet spectrum of a perchloric acid extract of the erythrocytes may help to establish the diagnosis of pyrimidine-5'-nucleotidase deficiency.[222] Beyond these relatively simple procedures it is probably rarely profitable to pick and choose individual enzyme assays on the basis of family history or clinical manifestations. Rather, it is usually appropriate to submit a blood sample to a reference laboratory that has the capability of performing all the enzyme assays listed in Table 45-1. Prenatal diagnosis of some of the defects causing hereditary nonspherocytic hemolytic anemia has been achieved,[223] but diagnosis of pyruvate kinase deficiency in the unborn has not yet been achieved.

The estimation of the red cell membrane lipid composition and the study of membrane proteins usually are carried out only in research laboratories.

THERAPY, COURSE, AND PROGNOSIS

THERAPY OF G-6-PD DEFICIENCY

G-6-PD-deficient individuals should avoid drugs that might induce hemolytic episodes (see Table 45-5). However, it is important to realize that such patients are able to tolerate most drugs. Unfortunately, in the 1950s and 1960s a number of case reports incorrectly suggested that some drugs had hemolytic potential that subsequently were shown to be safe. Table 45-6 lists such drugs. While it is possible that some of these may be hemolytic in some patients or under some circumstances, this is unlikely, and G-6-PD-deficient patients should not be deprived of the possible benefit of these drugs.

If hemolysis occurs as a result of drug ingestion or infection, particularly in the milder A− type of deficiency, transfusion usually is not required. If, however, the rate of hemolysis is very rapid, as may occur for example in favism, transfusions of whole blood or packed cells may be useful. Good urine flow should be maintained in patients with hemoglobinuria to avert renal damage. Infants with neonatal jaundice due to G-6-PD deficiency may require exchange transfusion; in areas in which G-6-PD deficiency is prevalent, care must be taken not to give G-6-PD-deficient blood to such newborns.[224]

Patients with hereditary nonspherocytic hemolytic anemia due to G-6-PD deficiency usually do not require any therapy. Splenectomy is generally ineffective, although some improvement occasionally has been reported[12] following removal of the spleen. In most cases the anemia is not very severe, but in some instances frequent transfusions have been necessary.[225] The anti-oxidant properties of vitamin E have been tested in G-6-PD-deficient subjects, and a slight but statistically significant reduction in hemolysis was observed.[226,227] These results could not be confirmed in other studies.[228,229] It has been suggested that desferrioxamine decreases hemolysis.[230,231]

SPLENECTOMY IN NONSPHEROCYTIC HEMOLYTIC ANEMIA

The principal decision that the physician must make regarding patients with hereditary nonspherocytic hemolytic anemia is whether or not they require a splenectomy. This decision is not made easily, since the response is not predictable and some patients who fail to respond may develop serious thrombotic complications. The recommendation that is made should be based upon the following considerations: (1) severity of the disease; (2) family history of response to splenectomy; (3) the underlying defect; and (4) the need for cholecystectomy. Since it is unusual to obtain more than a partial response to splenectomy, this procedure should probably be reserved for patients whose quality of life is impaired by their anemia. The operation needs to be particularly considered for patients who need frequent transfusion and for those who require gallbladder surgery, in which splenectomy might be carried out as part of the same procedure. The best guide to the likely efficacy of splenectomy is probably the response to splenectomy of other affected family members. Unfortunately, such information is only occasionally available. The physician must therefore rely upon the experience of other patients with hereditary nonspherocytic hemolytic anemia of similar etiology to serve as a guide. However, even as

the large group of patients with hereditary nonspherocytic hemolytic anemia represents a heterogeneous population, so individuals with a single enzymatic lesion, such as pyruvate kinase deficiency, are heterogeneous. Each family is likely to be afflicted with a distinct mutant enzyme, and the various mutants may differ both with respect to clinical manifestations and with respect to response to splenectomy. Some of the available information regarding response to splenectomy of patients with hereditary nonspherocytic hemolytic anemia has been reviewed[12] and is summarized in Table 45-1. Relatively little is known of the response of patients with unstable hemoglobins to splenectomy (see Chap. 48).

GLUCOCORTICOIDS

Glucocorticoids are of no known value in this group of disorders. Folic acid is often given, as in other patients with increased bone marrow activity, but without proven hematologic benefit. In the absence of iron deficiency, iron is contraindicated. Iron overload is not a frequent complication in this group of disorders but has been reported to occur, particularly in connection with pyruvate kinase deficiency.[232]

COURSE AND PROGNOSIS

Hemolytic episodes in the A− type of deficiency are usually self-limited, even if drug administration is continued. This is not the case in the more severe Mediterranean type of deficiency. In patients with hereditary nonspherocytic hemolytic anemia due to G-6-PD deficiency, gallstones may occur, and the incidence of cholelithiasis may be increased even in patients with polymorphic forms of G-6-PD deficiency in Sardinia.[233] During periods of infections or drug administration, anemia may increase in severity. Otherwise, the hemoglobin level of affected subjects remains relatively stable.

Nearly all patients with drug- or infection-induced hemolysis recover uneventfully. Favism must be considered, by comparison, a relatively dangerous disease. Prior to the institution of modern hospital therapy, fatalities from favism were not uncommon.

In one large population study, a decreasing incidence of G-6-PD deficiency was noted with increasing age of the population,[234] but no such change was observed in another.[133] While age stratification might represent evidence of a shorter life span for individuals with the A− deficiency, other factors are more likely explanations. Examination of the health records of over 65,000 U.S. Veterans Administration males failed to reveal any higher frequency of any illness in G-6-PD-deficient compared to nondeficient subjects.[123] In view of the benign nature of the common types of G-6-PD deficiency, community-based population screening is not recommended. However, screening for G-6-PD deficiency of all patients admitted to the hospital may be useful in anticipating hemolytic reactions and in understanding them if they occur. This is particularly prudent if a drug such as dapsone, known to cause hemolysis in G-6-PD-deficient individuals, is to be given. Study of family members of patients with this X-linked enzyme deficiency can be helpful in providing appropriate counseling to affected individuals.

The diagnosis of hereditary nonspherocytic hemolytic anemia has been made as late as the seventh decade,[13] and the disease can be fatal in the first few years of life. Triosephosphate isomerase deficiency appears to have the worst prognosis of all of the known defects that cause this disorder. With few exceptions, patients with this deficiency have died by the fifth or sixth year of life, usually of cardiopulmonary failure. Pyruvate kinase deficiency, too, can be fatal in early childhood; the gene prevalent among the Amish of Pennsylvania produces particularly severe disease.[235] Unless the affected homozygous children have their spleens removed, the disorder is commonly lethal. In general, however, hereditary nonspherocytic hemolytic anemia is a relatively mild disease and most affected individuals lead a relatively normal life, apparently without much compromise of life span.

REFERENCES

1. Beutler E: The hemolytic effect of primaquine and related compounds. A review. *Blood* 14:103, 1959.
2. Beutler E: G6PD deficiency. *Blood* 84:3613, 1994.
3. Beutler E: The study of glucose-6-phosphate dehydrogenase: History and molecular biology. *Am J Hematol* 42:53, 1993.
4. Crosby WA: Hereditary nonspherocytic hemolytic anemia. *Blood* 5:233, 1950.
5. Dacie JV: The congenital anaemias, in *The Haemolytic Anaemias*, p 171. Grune & Stratton, New York, 1960.
6. Newton WA Jr, Bass JC: Glutathione sensitive chronic non-spherocytic hemolytic anemia. *Am J Dis Child* 96:501, 1958.
7. Selwyn JG, Dacie JV: Autohemolysis and other changes resulting from the incubation in vitro of red cells from patients with congenital hemolytic anemia. *Blood* 9:414, 1954.
8. Robinson MA, Loder PB, DeGruchy GC: Red-cell metabolism in nonspherocytic congenital haemolytic anaemia. *Br J Haematol* 7:327, 1961.
9. DeGruchy GC, Santamaria JN, Parsons IC, Crawford H: Nonspherocytic congenital hemolytic anemia. *Blood* 16:1371, 1960.
10. Valentine WN, Tanaka KR, Miwa S: A specific erythrocyte glycolytic enzyme defect (pyruvate kinase) in three subjects with congenital nonspherocytic hemolytic anemia. *Trans Assoc Am Physicians* 74:100, 1961.
11. Dacie JV: Life and death of the red cell, in *Blood Pure and Eloquent*, p 211. McGraw-Hill, New York, 1980.
12. Beutler E: *Hemolytic Anemia in Disorders of Red Cell Metabolism.* Plenum Press, New York, 1978.
13. Beutler E: Red cell enzyme defects as non-diseases and as diseases. *Blood* 54:1, 1979.
14. Shinohara K, Tanaka KR: Hereditary deficiency of erythrocyte acetylcholinesterase. *Am J Hematol* 7:313, 1979.
15. Wakabayashi H, Tsuchiya M, Yoshino K, Kaku K, Shigei H: Hereditary deficiency of lactate dehydrogenase H-subunit. *Intern Med* 35:550, 1996.
16. Rosa R, George C, Fardeau M, et al: A new case of phosphoglycerate kinase deficiency: PGK Creteil associated with rhabdomyolysis and lacking hemolytic anemia. *Blood* 60:84, 1982.
17. Marstein S, Jellum E, Halpern B, Eldjarn L, Perry TL: Biochemical studies of erythrocytes in a patient with pyroglutamic acidemia (5-oxoprolinemia). *N Engl J Med* 295:406, 1976.
18. Loos H, Roos D, Weening R, Houwerzijl J: Familial deficiency of glutathione reductase in human blood cells. *Blood* 48:53, 1976.
19. Beutler E, Kuhl W, Gelbart T: 6-Phosphogluconolactonase deficiency, a hereditary erythrocyte enzyme deficiency: Possible interaction with glucose-6-phosphate dehydrogenase deficiency. *Proc Natl Acad Sci USA* 82:3876, 1985.
20. Boulard-Heitzmann P, Boulard M, Tallineau C, et al: Decreased red cell enolase activity in a 40-year-old woman with compensated haemolysis. *Scand J Haematol* 33:401, 1984.
21. Beutler E, Dunning D, Dabe IB, Forman L: Erythrocyte glutathione S-transferase deficiency and hemolytic anemia. *Blood* 72:73, 1988.
22. Beutler E, Carson D, Dannawi H, et al: Metabolic compensation for profound erythrocyte adenylate kinase deficiency. *J Clin Invest* 72:648, 1983.
23. Shohet SB, Livermore BM, Nathan DG, Jaffe ER: Hereditary hemolytic anemia associated with abnormal membrane lipids: Mechanism of accumulation of phosphatidyl choline. *Blood* 38:445, 1971.
24. Lane PA, Kuypers FA, Clark MR, et al: Excess of red cell membrane proteins in hereditary high-phosphatidylcholine hemolytic anemia. *Am J Hematol* 34:186, 1990.
25. Shojania AM, Godin DV, Frohlich J: Hereditary high phosphatidylcholine hemolytic anemia: Report of a new family and review of the literature. *Clin Invest Med* 13:313, 1990.
26. Clark MR, Shohet SB, Gottfried EL: Hereditary hemolytic disease with increased red blood cell phosphatidylcholine and dehydration: One, two, or many disorders. *Am J Hematol* 42:25, 1993.
27. Dern RJ, Beutler E, Alving AS: The hemolytic effect of primaquine: V. Primaquine sensitivity as a manifestation of a multiple drug sensitivity. *J Lab Clin Med* 45:30, 1955.
28. Cohen G, Hochstein P: Generation of hydrogen peroxide in erythrocytes by hemolytic agents. *Biochemistry* 3:895, 1964.
29. Kosower NS, Song KR, Kosower EM, Correa W: Glutathione: II. Chemical aspects of azoester procedure for oxidation to disulfide. *Biochim Biophys Acta* 192:8, 1969.
30. Birchmeier W, Tuchschmid PE, Winterhalter H: Comparison of human hemoglobin A carrying glutathione as a mixed disulfide with the naturally occurring human hemoglobin A3. *Biochemistry* 12:3667, 1973.
31. Rachmilewitz EA, Harari E, Winterhalter KH: Separation of alpha- and beta-chains of hemoglobin A by acetylphenylhydrazine. *Biochim Biophys Acta* 371:402, 1974.
32. Itano HA, Hosokawa K, Hirota K: Induction of haemolytic anaemia by substituted phenylhydrazines. *Br J Haematol* 32:99, 1976.
33. Srivastava SK, Beutler E: Glutathione metabolism of the erythrocyte. The enzymic cleavage of glutathione-haemoglobin preparations by glutathione reductase. *Biochem J* 119:353, 1970.
34. Kirkman HN, Gaetani GF: Catalase: A tetrameric enzyme with four tightly bound molecules of NADPH. *Proc Natl Acad Sci USA* 81:4343, 1984.
35. Gaetani GF, Rolfo M, Arena S, et al: Active involvement of catalase during hemolytic crises of favism. *Blood* 88:1084, 1996.
36. Rifkind RA: Heinz body anemia: An ultrastructural study: II. Red cell sequestration and destruction. *Blood* 26:433, 1965.
37. Bunn HEF, Jandl JH: Exchange of heme among hemoglobin molecules. *Proc Natl Acad Sci USA* 56:974, 1966.
38. Jandl JH: The Heinz body hemolytic anemias. *Ann Intern Med* 58:702, 1963.
39. Beutler E: Abnormalities of glycolysis (HMP shunt). *Bibl Haematol* 29:146, 1968.
40. Baehner RL, Nathan DG, Castle WB: Oxidant injury of caucasian glucose-6-phosphate dehydrogenase-deficient red blood cells by phagocytosing leukocytes during infection. *J Clin Invest* 50:2466, 1971.
41. Arese P, De Flora A: Denaturation of normal and abnormal erythrocytes: II. Pathophysiology of hemolysis in glucose-6-phosphate dehydrogenase deficiency. *Semin Hematol* 27:1, 1990.
42. Stamatoyannopoulos G, Fraser GR, Motulsky AG, et al: On the familial predisposition to favism. *Am J Hum Genet* 18:253, 1966.
43. Cassimos CHR, Malaka-Zafiriu K, Tsiures J: Urinary D-glucaric acid excretion in normal and G-6-PD deficient children with favism. *J Pediatr* 84:871, 1974.
44. Bottini E, Bottini FG, Borgiani P, Businco L: Association between ACP1 and favism: a possible biochemical mechanism. *Blood* 89:2613, 1997.
45. Fiorelli G, Podda M, Corrias A, Fargion S: The relevance of immune reactions in acute favism. *Acta Haematol (Basel)* 51:211, 1974.
46. Turrini F, Naitana A, Mannuzzu L, Pescarmona G, Arese P: Increased red cell calcium, decreased calcium adenosine triphosphatase, and altered membrane proteins during fava bean hemolysis in glucose-6-phosphate dehydrogenase-deficient (Mediterranean variant) individuals. *Blood* 66:302, 1985.
47. De Flora A, Benatti U, Guida L, Forteleoni G, Meloni T: Favism: Disordered erythrocyte calcium homeostasis. *Blood* 66:294, 1985.
48. Fischer TM, Meloni T, Pescarmona GP, Arese P: Membrane cross bonding in red cells in favic crisis: A missing link in the mechanism of extravascular haemolysis. *Br J Haematol* 59:159, 1985.
49. Kaplan M, Vreman HJ, Hammerman C, et al: Contribution of haemolysis to jaundice in Sephardic Jewish glucose-6-phosphate dehydrogenase deficient neonates. *Br J Haematol* 93:822, 1996.
50. Kaplan M, Renbaum P, Levy-Lahad E, et al: Gilbert syndrome and glucose-6-phosphate dehydrogenase deficiency: A dose-dependent genetic interaction crucial to neonatal hyperbilirubinemia. *Proc Natl Acad Sci USA* 94:12128, 1997.
51. Oluboyede OA, Esan GJF, Francis TI, Luzzatto L: Genetically determined deficiency of glucose 6-phosphate dehydrogenase (type A–) is expressed in the liver. *J Lab Clin Med* 93:783, 1979.
52. Piomelli S: G6PD deficiency and hemolytic anemia: G6PD-related neonatal jaundice, in *Glucose-6-Phosphate Dehydrogenase*, p 95. Academic Press, Orlando, FL, 1986.
53. Ifekwunigwe AE, Luzzatto L: Kernicterus in G.-6-P.D.-deficiency. *Lancet* 1:667, 1966.
54. Eshaghpour E, Oski FA, Williams M: The relationship of erythrocyte glucose-6-phosphate dehydrogenase deficiency to hyperbilirubinemia in Negro premature infants. *J Pediatr* 70:595, 1967.

55. Lopez R, Cooperman JM: Glucose-6-phosphate dehydrogenase deficiency and hyperbilirubinemia in the newborn. *Am J Dis Child* 122:66, 1971.

56. Zinkham WH: Peripheral blood and bilirubin values in normal full-term primaquine-sensitive negro infants: Effect of vitamin K. *Pediatrics* 31:983, 1963.

57. Verdy E, Herve J, Boisson C, Combrisson A: Can glucose-6-phosphate dehydrogenase deficiency alone explain neonatal jaundice. *Rev Fr Transfus Immunohematol* 21:1081, 1978.

58. Beutler E, Gelbart T, Demina A: Racial variability in the UDP-glucuronosyltransferase 1 (*UGT1A1*) promoter: A balanced polymorphism for regulation of bilirubin metabolism? *Proc Natl Acad Sci USA* 95:8170, 1998.

59. Dahl N, Pigg M, Ristoff E, et al: Missense mutations in the human glutathione synthetase gene result in severe metabolic acidosis, 5-oxoprolinuria, hemolytic anemia and neurological dysfunction. *Hum Mol Genet* 6:1147, 1997.

60. Hirono A, Iyori H, Sekine I, et al: Three cases of hereditary nonspherocytic hemolytic anemia associated with red blood cell glutathione deficiency. *Blood* 87:2071, 1996.

61. Beutler E, Gelbart T, Pegelow C: Erythrocyte glutathione synthetase deficiency leads not only to glutathione but also to glutathione-S-transferase deficiency. *J Clin Invest* 77:38, 1986.

62. Parr CW, Fitch LI: Inherited quantitative variations of human phosphogluconate dehydrogenase. *Ann Hum Genet* 30:339, 1967.

63. Valentine WN, Paglia DE: The primary cause of hemolysis in enzymopathies of anaerobic glycolysis: A viewpoint. *Blood Cells* 6:819, 1980.

64. Beutler E: "The primary cause of hemolysis in enzymopathies of anaerobic glycolysis: A viewpoint." A commentary. *Blood Cells* 6:827, 1980.

65. Werth G, Mueller G: Vererbbarer Glucose-6-phosphatdehydrogenasemangel in den Erythrocyten von Ratten. *Klin Wochenschr* 45:265, 1967.

66. Smith JE, Ryer K, Wallace L: Glucose-6-phosphate dehydrogenase deficiency in a dog. *Enzyme* 21:379, 1976.

67. Pretsch W, Charles DJ, Merkle S: X-linked glucose-6-phosphate dehydrogenase deficiency in *Mus musculus*. *Biochem Genet* 26:89, 1988.

68. Sanders S, Smith DP, Thomas GA, Williams ED: A glucose-6-phosphate dehydrogenase (G6PD) splice site consensus sequence mutation associated with G6PD enzyme deficiency. *Mutat Res* 374:79, 1997.

69. Nonneman D, Stockham SL, Shibuya H, Messer NTI, Johnson GS: A missense mutation in the glucose-6-phosphate dehydrogenase gene associated with hemolytic anemia in an American saddlebred horse. *Blood* 82 (suppl 1):466a, 1993.

70. Stockham SL, Harvey JW, Kinden DA: Equine glucose-6-phosphate dehydrogenase deficiency. *Vet Pathol* 31:518, 1994.

71. Whitney KM, Goodman SA, Bailey EM, Lothrop CD Jr: The molecular basis of canine pyruvate kinase deficiency. *Exp Hematol* 22:866, 1994.

72. Kanno H, Morimoto M, Fujii H, et al: Primary structure of murine red blood cell-type pyruvate kinase (PK) and molecular characterization of PK deficiency identified in the CBA strain. *Blood* 86:3205, 1995.

73. Morimoto M, Kanno H, Asai H, et al: Pyruvate kinase deficiency of mice associated with nonspherocytic hemolytic anemia and cure of the anemia by marrow transplantation without host irradiation. *Blood* 86:4323, 1995.

74. Tsujino K, Kanno H, Hashimoto K, et al: Delayed onset of hemolytic anemia in CBA-*Pk-1^slc/Pk-1^slc* mice with a point mutation of the gene encoding red blood cell type pyruvate kinase. *Blood* 91:2169, 1998.

75. Harvey JW, Pate MG, Mhaskar Y, Dunaway GA: Characterization of phosphofructokinase-deficient canine erythrocytes. *J Inherit Metab Dis* 15:747, 1992.

76. Merkle S, Pretsch W: Glucose-6-phosphate isomerase deficiency associated with nonspherocytic hemolytic anemia in the mouse: An animal model for the human disease. *Blood* 81:206, 1993.

77. Betke K, Beutler E, Brewer GJ, et al: Standardization of procedures for the study of glucose-6-phosphate dehydrogenase. Report of a WHO scientific group. *WHO Tech Rep Ser* No. 366:1967.

78. Piomelli S, Corash LM, Davenport DD, Miraglia J, Amorosi EL: In vivo lability of glucose-6-phosphate dehydrogenase in GdA− and Gd Mediterranean deficiency. *J Clin Invest* 47:940, 1968.

79. Yoshida A, Stamatoyannopoulos G, Motulsky A: Negro variant of glucose-6-phosphate dehydrogenase deficiency (A−) in man. *Science* 155:97, 1967.

80. Kahn A, Cottreau D, Boivin P: Molecular mechanism of glucose-6-phosphate dehydrogenase deficiency. *Humangenetik* 25:101, 1974.

81. Beutler E: Selectivity of proteases as a basis for tissue distribution of enzymes in hereditary deficiencies. *Proc Natl Acad Sci USA* 80:3767, 1983.

82. Kirkman HN, Schettini F, Pickard BM: Mediterranean variant of glucose-6-phosphate dehydrogenase. *J Lab Clin Med* 63:726, 1964.

83. Kirkman HN, Riley HD Jr: Congenital nonspherocytic hemolytic anemia. *Am J Dis Child* 102:313, 1961.

84. Yoshida A: Hemolytic anemia and G-6-PD deficiency. *Science* 179:532, 1973.

85. Beutler E: Genetics of glucose-6-phosphate dehydrogenase deficiency. *Semin Hematol* 27:137, 1990.

86. Chen EY, Cheng A, Lee A, et al: Sequence of human glucose-6-phosphate dehydrogenase cloned in plasmids and a yeast artificial chromosome (YAC). *Genomics* 10:792, 1991.

87. Battistuzzi G, D'Urso M, Toniolo D, Persico GM, Luzzatto L: Tissue-specific levels of human glucose-6-phosphate dehydrogenase correlate with methylation of specific sites at the 3′ end of the gene. *Proc Natl Acad Sci USA* 82:1465, 1985.

88. Kirkman HN, Hendrickson EM: Glucose-6-phosphate dehydrogenase from human erythrocytes: II. Subactive states of the enzyme from normal persons. *J Biol Chem* 237:2371, 1962.

89. De Flora A, Morelli A, Giuliano F: Human erythrocyte glucose 6-phosphate dehydrogenase. Content of bound coenzyme. *Biochem Biophys Res Commun* 59:406, 1974.

90. De Flora A, Morelli A, Benatti U, Giuliano F, Molinari MP: Human erythrocyte glucose 6-phosphate dehydrogenase. Interaction with oxidized and reduced coenzyme. *Biochem Biophys Res Commun* 60:999, 1974.

91. Canepa L, Ferraris AM, Miglino M, Gaetani GF: Bound and unbound pyridine dinucleotides in normal and glucose-6-phosphate dehydrogenase-deficient erythrocytes. *Biochim Biophys Acta* 1074:101, 1991.

92. Camardella L, Caruso C, Rutigliano B, et al: Human erythrocyte glucose-6-phosphate dehydrogenase: Identification of a reactive lysyl residue labelled with pyridoxal 5′-phosphate. *Eur J Biochem* 171:485, 1988.

93. Jeffery J, Wood I, Macleod A, Jeffery R, Jörnvall A: Glucose-6-phosphate dehydrogenase. Characterization of a reactive lysine residue in the *Pichia jadinii* enzyme reveals a limited structural variation in a functionally significant segment. *Biochem Biophys Res Commun* 160:1290, 1989.

94. Hirono A, Kuhl W, Gelbart T, et al: Identification of the binding domain for NADP+ of human glucose-6-phosphate dehydrogenase by sequence analysis of mutants. *Proc Natl Acad Sci USA* 86:10015, 1989.

95. Naylor CE, Rowland P, Basak AK, et al: Glucose-6-phosphate dehydrogenase mutations causing enzyme deficiency in a model of the tertiary structure of the human enzyme. *Blood* 87:2974, 1996.

96. Yoshida A: A single amino acid substitution (asparagine to aspartic acid) between normal (B+) and the common negro variant (A+) of human glucose-6-phosphate dehydrogenase. *Proc Natl Acad Sci USA* 57:835, 1967.

97. Takizawa T, Yoneyama Y, Miwa S, Yoshida A: A single nucleotide base transition is the basis of the common human glucose-6-phosphate dehydrogenase variant A(+). *Genomics* 1:228, 1987.

98. Hirono A, Beutler E: Molecular cloning and nucleotide sequence of cDNA for human glucose-6-phosphate dehydrogenase variant A(−). *Proc Natl Acad Sci USA* 85:3951, 1988.

99. Town M, Bautista JM, Mason PJ, Luzzatto L: Both mutations in G6PD A− are necessary to produce the G6PD deficient phenotype. *Hum Mol Genet* 1:171, 1992.

100. Beutler E, Kuhl W, Vives-Corrons J-L, Prchal JT: Molecular heterogeneity of G6PD A−. *Blood* 74:2550, 1989.

101. Vulliamy TJ, Othman A, Town M, et al: Polymorphic sites in the African population detected by sequence analysis of the glucose-6-phosphate dehydrogenase gene outline the evolution of the variants A and A−. *Proc Natl Acad Sci USA* 88:8568, 1991.

102. Huang C-S, Hung KL, Huang MJ, et al: Neonatal jaundice and molecular mutations in glucose-6-phosphate dehydrogenase deficient newborn infants. *Am J Hematol* 51:19, 1996.

103. Xu W, Westwood B, Bartsocas CS, et al: Glucose-6 phosphate dehydrogenase mutations and haplotypes in various ethnic groups. *Blood* 85:257, 1995.

104. Saha S, Saha N, Tay JSH, et al: Molecular characterisation of red cell glucose-6-phosphate dehydrogenase deficiency in Singapore Chinese. *Am J Hematol* 47:273, 1994.

105. Tang TK, Huang C-S, Huang M-J, et al: Diverse point mutations result in glucose-6-phosphate dehydrogenase (G6PD) polymorphism in Taiwan. *Blood* 79:2135, 1992.

106. Vulliamy T, Luzzatto L, Hirono A, Beutler E: Hematologically important mutations: Glucose-6-phosphate dehydrogenase. *Blood Cells Mol Dis* 23:302, 1997.

107. MacDonald D, Town M, Mason P, et al: Deficiency in red blood cells. *Nature* 350:115, 1991.

108. Baronciani L, Tricta F, Beutler E: G6PD "Campinas": A deficient enzyme with a mutation at the far 3′ end of the gene. *Hum Mutat* 2:77, 1993.

109. Miwa S: Pyruvate kinase deficiency. *Acta Haematol Jpn* 50:1445, 1987.

110. Kahn A, Kaplan J-C, Dreyfus J-C: Advances in hereditary red cell enzyme anomalies. *Hum Genet* 50:1, 1979.

111. Johnson ML, Jones DP, Freeman JM, Wang W: Biochemical and molecular characterization of variant pyruvate kinase enzymes and genes from three patients with red blood cell pyruvate kinase deficiency. *Acta Haematol (Basel)* 86:79, 1991.

112. Beutler E, Forman L, Rios-Larrain E: Elevated pyruvate kinase activity in patients with hemolytic anemia due to red cell pyruvate kinase "deficiency." *Am J Med* 83:899, 1987.

113. Miwa S, Boivin P, Blume KG, et al: Recommended methods for the characterization of red cell pyruvate kinase variants. *Br J Haematol* 43:275, 1979.

114. Lakomek M, Neubauer B, von der Lühe A, et al: Erythrocyte pyruvate kinase deficiency: Relations of residual enzyme activity, altered regulation of defective enzymes and concentrations of high-energy phosphates with the severity of clinical manifestation. *Eur J Haematol* 49:82, 1992.

115. Tani K, Fujii H, Nagata S, Miwa S: Human liver type pyruvate kinase: complete amino acid sequence and the expression in mammalian cells. *Proc Natl Acad Sci USA* 85:1792, 1988.

116. Tani K, Fujii H, Tsutsumi H, et al: Human liver type-pyruvate kinase: cDNA cloning and chromosomal assignment. *Biochem Biophys Res Commun* 143:431, 1987.

117. Baronciani L, Bianchi P, Zanella A: Hematologically important mutations: Red cell pyruvate kinase. *Blood Cells Mol Dis* 22:85, 1996.

118. Beutler E, Baronciani L: Mutation update: Pyruvate kinase. *Hum Mutat* 7:1, 1996.

119. Baronciani L, Beutler E: Molecular study of pyruvate kinase deficient patients with hereditary nonspherocytic hemolytic anemia. *J Clin Invest* 95:1702, 1995.

120. Lenzner C, Nürnberg P, Jacobasch G, Gorth C, Thiele BJ: Molecular analysis of 29 pyruvate kinase-deficient patients from Central Europe with hereditary hemolytic anemia. *Blood* 89:1793, 1997.

121. Baronciani L, Beutler E: Analysis of pyruvate kinase-deficiency mutations that produce nonspherocytic hemolytic anemia. *Proc Natl Acad Sci USA* 90:4324, 1993.

122. Demina A, Varughese KI, Barbot J, Forman L, Beutler E: Six previously undescribed pyruvate kinase mutations causing enzyme deficiency. *Blood* 92:647, 1998.

123. Heller P, Best WR, Nelson RB, Becktel J: Clinical implications of sickle-cell trait and glucose-6-phosphate dehydrogenase deficiency in hospitalized black male patients. *N Engl J Med* 300:1001, 1979.

124. Luzzatto L, Battistuzzi G: Glucose-6-phosphate dehydrogenase, in *Advances in Human Genetics*, p 217. Plenum, New York, 1985.

125. Luzzatto L, Mehta A: Glucose 6-phosphate dehydrogenase deficiency, in *The Metabolic and Molecular Bases of Inherited Disease*, 7th ed, p 3367. McGraw-Hill, New York, 1995.

126. Motulsky AG: Metabolic metamorphisms and the role of infectious diseases in human evolution. *Hum Biol* 32:28, 1960.

127. Luzzatto L, Usanga EA, Reddy S: Glucose 6-phosphate dehydrogenase deficient red cells: Resistance to infection by malarial parasites. *Science* 164:839, 1969.

128. Cappadoro M, Giribaldi G, O'Brien E, et al: Early phagocytosis of glucose-6-phosphate dehydrogenase (G6PD)-deficient erythrocytes parasitized by *Plasmodium falciparum* may explain malaria protection in G6PD deficiency. *Blood* 92:2527, 1998.

129. Piomelli S, Reindorf CA, Arzanian MT, Corash LM: Clinical and biochemical interactions of glucose-6-phosphate dehydrogenase deficiency and sickle-cell anemia. *N Engl J Med* 287:213, 1972.

130. Lewis RA, Hathorn M: Correlation of S hemoglobin with glucose-6-phosphate dehydrogenase deficiency and its significance. *Blood* 26:176, 1965.

131. Steinberg MH, Dreiling BJ: Glucose-6-phosphate dehydrogenase deficiency in sickle cell anemia. *Ann Intern Med* 80:217, 1974.

132. Beutler E, Johnson C, Powars D, West C: Prevalence of glucose-6-phosphate dehydrogenase deficiency in sickle cell disease. *N Engl J Med* 290:826, 1974.

133. Steinberg MH, West MS, Gallagher D, Mentzer WC Jr, and the Cooperative Study of Sickle Cell Diseases: Effects of glucose-6-phosphate dehydrogenase deficiency upon sickle cell anemia. *Blood* 71:748, 1988.

134. Warsy AS: Frequency of glucose-6-phosphate dehydrogenase deficiency in sickle-cell disease. *Hum Hered* 35:143, 1985.

135. Garcia SC, Moragon AC, Lopez-Fernandez ME: Frequency of glutathione reductase, pyruvate kinase and glucose-6-phosphate dehydrogenase deficiency in a Spanish population. *Hum Hered* 29:310, 1979.

136. Abu-Melha AM, Ahmed MAM, Knox-Macaulay H, AL Sowayan SA, EL Yahia A: Erythrocyte pyruvate kinase deficiency in newborns of Eastern Saudi Arabia. *Acta Haematol (Basel)* 85:192, 1991.

137. Mohrenweiser HA: Functional hemizygosity in the human genome: direct estimate from twelve erythrocyte enzyme loci. *Hum Genet* 77:241, 1987.

138. Mohrenweiser HW, Fielek S: Elevated frequency of carriers for triosephosphate isomerase deficiency in newborn infants. *Pediatr Res* 16:960, 1982.

139. Watanabe M, Zingg BC, Mohrenweiser HA: Molecular analysis of a series of alleles in humans with reduced activity at the triosephosphate isomerase locus. *Am J Hum Genet* 58:308, 1996.

140. Schneider A, Forman L, Westwood B, et al: The relationship of the -5, -8, and -24 mutations in African-Americans to triosephosphate isomerase (TPI) enzyme activity and to TPI deficiency. *Blood* 92:2959, 1998.

141. Schneider A, Westwood B, Yim C, et al: The 1591C mutation in triosephosphate isomerase (TPI) deficiency. Tightly linked polymorphisms and a common haplotype in all known families. *Blood Cells Mol Dis* 22:115, 1996.

142. McCaffrey RP, Halsted CH, Wahab MFA, Robertson RP: Chloramphenicol-induced hemolysis in caucasian glucose-6-phosphate dehydrogenase deficiency. *Ann Intern Med* 74:722, 1971.

143. Chan TK, Chesterman CN, McFadzean AJS, Todd D: The survival of glucose-6-phosphate dehydrogenase-deficient erythrocytes in patients with typhoid fever on chloramphenicol therapy. *J Lab Clin Med* 77:177, 1971.

144. Rees DC, Kelsey H, Richards JDM: Lesson of the week: Acute haemolysis induced by high dose ascorbic acid in glucose-6-phosphate dehydrogenase deficiency. *BMJ* 306:841, 1993.

145. Mehta JB, Singhal SB, Mehta BC: Ascorbic-acid-induced haemolysis in G-6-PD deficiency. *Lancet* 336:944, 1990.

146. Campbell GD Jr, Steinberg MH, Bower JO: Ascorbic acid-induced hemolysis in G-6-PD deficiency. *Ann Intern Med* 82:810, 1975.

147. Markowitz N, Saravolatz LD: Use of trimethoprim-sulfamethoxazole in a glucose-6-phosphate dehydrogenase-deficient population. *Rev Infect Dis* 9(suppl 2):S218, 1987.

148. Magon AM, Leipzig RM, Zannoni VG, Brewer GJ: Interactions of glucose-6-phosphate dehydrogenase deficiency with drug acetylation and hydroxylation reactions. *J Lab Clin Med* 97:764, 1981.

149. Woolhouse NM, Atu-Taylor LC: Influence of double genetic polymorphism on response to sulfamethazine. *Clin Pharmacol Ther* 31:377, 1982.

150. Dern RJ, Beutler E, Alving AS: The hemolytic effect of primaquine: II. The natural course of the hemolytic anemia and the mechanism of its self-limited character. *J Lab Clin Med* 44:171, 1954.

151. Beutler E, Dern RJ, Alving AS: The hemolytic effect of primaquine: III. A study of primaquine-sensitive erythrocytes. *J Lab Clin Med* 44:177, 1954.

152. Beutler E, Dern RJ, Alving AS: The hemolytic effect of primaquine: IV. The relationship of cell age to hemolysis. *J Lab Clin Med* 44:439, 1954.

153. George JN, Sears DA, McCurdy P, Conrad ME: Primaquine sensitivity in caucasians: Hemolytic reactions induced by primaquine in G-6-PD deficient subjects. *J Lab Clin Med* 70:80, 1967.

154. Walker DH, Hawkins HK, Hudson P: Fulminant Rocky Mountain spotted fever. *Arch Pathol Lab Med* 107:121, 1983.

155. Chau TN, Lai ST, Lai JY, Yuen H: Haemolysis complicating acute viral hepatitis in patients with normal or deficient glucose-6-phosphate dehydrogenase activity. *Scand J Infect Dis* 29:551, 1997.

156. Huo TI, Wu JC, Chiu CF, Lee SD: Severe hyperbilirubinemia due to acute hepatitis A superimposed on a chronic hepatitis B carrier with glucose-6-phosphate dehydrogenase deficiency. *Am J Gastroenterol* 91:158, 1996.

157. Shalev O, Wollner A, Menczel J: Diabetic ketoacidosis does not precipitate haemolysis in patients with the Mediterranean variant of glucose-6-phosphate dehydrogenase deficiency. *BMJ* 288:179, 1984.

158. Shalev O, Eliakim R, Lugassy GZ, Menczel J: Hypoglycemia-induced hemolysis in glucose-6-phosphate dehydrogenase deficiency. *Acta Haematol (Basel)* 74:227, 1985.

159. Galiano S, Gaetani GF, Barabino A, et al: Favism in the African type of glucose-6-phosphate dehydrogenase deficiency (A−). *BMJ* 300:236, 1990.

160. Kattamis CA, Kyriazakou M, Chaidas S: Favism. Clinical and biochemical data. *J Med Genet* 6:34, 1969.

161. Globerman H, Novak T, Chevion M: Haemolysis in a G6PD-deficient child induced by eating unripe peaches. *Scand J Haematol* 33:337, 1984.

162. Williams CKO, Osotimehin BO, Ogunmola GB, Awotedu AA: Haemolytic anaemia associated with Nigerian barbecued meat (red suya). *Afr J Med Sci* 17:71, 1988.

163. Kaplan M, Hammerman C: Severe neonatal hyperbilirubinemia. *Clin Perinatol* 25:575, 1998.

164. Fok T-F, Lau S-P: Glucose-6-phosphate dehydrogenase deficiency: A preventable cause of mental retardation. *BMJ* 292:829, 1986.

165. Singh A: Glucose-6-phosphate dehydrogenase deficiency: A preventable cause of mental retardation. *BMJ* 292:397, 1986.

166. Ardati KO, Bajakian KM, Tabbara KS: Effect of glucose-6-phosphate dehydrogenase deficiency on neutrophil function. *Acta Haematol (Basel)* 97:211, 1997.

167. Vives-Corrons JL, Feliu E, Pujades MA, et al: Severe glucose-6-phosphate dehydrogenase (G6PD) deficiency associated with chronic hemolytic anemia, granulocyte dysfunction and increased susceptibility to infections. Description of a new molecular variant (G6PD Barcelona). *Blood* 59:428, 1982.

168. Gray GR, Klebanoff SJ, Stamatoyannopoulos G, et al: Neutrophil dysfunction, chronic granulomatous disease, and nonspherocytic haemolytic anaemia caused by complete deficiency of glucose-6-phosphate dehydrogenase. *Lancet* 2:530, 1973.

169. Cooper MR, DeChatelet LR, McCall CE, et al: Complete deficiency of leukocyte glucose-6-phosphate dehydrogenase with defective bactericidal activity. *J Clin Invest* 51:769, 1972.

170. Schwartz JP, Cooperberg AA, Rosenberg A: Platelet-function studies in patients with glucose-6-phosphate dehydrogenase deficiency. *Br J Haematol* 27:273, 1974.

171. Gray GR, Naiman SC, Robinson GCF: Platelet function and G-6-PD deficiency. *Lancet* 1:997, 1974.

172. Harley JD, Agar NS, Yoshida A: Glucose-6-phosphate dehydrogenase variants: Gd (+) Alexandra associated with neonatal jaundice and Gd (−) Camperdown in a young man with lamellar cataracts. *J Lab Clin Med* 91:295, 1978.

173. Harley JD, Agar NS, Gruca MA: Cataracts with a glucose-6-phosphate dehydrogenase variant. *BMJ* 2:86, 1975.

174. Westring DW, Pisciotta AV: Anemia, cataracts, and seizures in patient with glucose-6-phosphate dehydrogenase deficiency. *Arch Intern Med* 118:385, 1966.

175. Panich V, Na-Nakorn S: G6PD deficiency in senile cataracts. *Hum Genet* 55:123, 1980.

176. Orzalesi N, Sorcinelli R, Guiso G: Increased incidence of cataract in male subjects deficient in glucose-6-phosphate dehydrogenase. *Arch Ophthalmol* 99:69, 1981.

177. Bhatia RPS, Patel R, Dubey B: Senile cataract and glucose-6-phosphate dehydrogenase deficiency in Indians. *Trop Geogr Med* 42:349, 1990.

178. Zampella EJ, Bradley EL, Pretlow TA: Glucose-6-phosphate dehydrogenase; A possible clinical indicator for prostatic carcinoma. *Cancer* 49:384, 1982.

179. Sulis E: G-6-PD deficiency and cancer. *Lancet* 1:1185, 1972.

180. Ferraris AM, Broccia G, Meloni T, Forteleoni G, Gaetani GF: Glucose-6-phosphate dehydrogenase deficiency and incidence of hematologic malignancy. *Am J Hum Genet* 42:516, 1988.

181. Monte Alegre S, Saad STO, Delatre E, Saad MJA: Insulin secretion in patients deficient in glucose-6-phosphate dehydrogenase. *Horm Metab Res* 23:171, 1991.

182. Saad MJA, Monte-Alegre S, Saad STO: Cortisol levels in glucose-6-phosphate dehydrogenase deficiency. *Horm Res* 35:1, 1991.

183. Mueller-Soyano A, De Roura ET, Duke PR, et al: Pyruvate kinase deficiency and leg ulcers. *Blood* 47:807, 1976.

184. Curiel CD, Velasquez GA, Papa R: Hemolytic anemia and leg ulcers due to pyruvate kinase deficiency. Report of the second Venezuelan family. *Sangre (Barc)* 22:64, 1977.

185. Amankwah KS, Dick BW, Dodge S: Hemolytic anemia and pyruvate kinase deficiency in pregnancy. *Obstet Gynecol* 55(suppl):42S, 1980.

186. Vives Corrons J-L, García AM, Sosa AM, et al: Heterozygous pyruvate kinase deficiency and severe hemolytic anemia in a pregnant woman with concomitant, glucose-6-phosphate dehydrogenase deficiency. *Blut* 62:190, 1991.

187. Vora S: Isozymes of human phosphofructokinase: Biochemical and genetic aspects, in *Isozymes: Current Topics in Biological and Medical Research*, p 3. Liss, New York, 1983.

188. Wellner VP, Sekura R, Meister A, Larsson A: Glutathione synthetase deficiency, an inborn error of metabolism involving the gamma-glutamyl cycle in patients with 5-oxoprolinuria (pyroglutamic aciduria). *Proc Natl Acad Sci USA* 71:2505, 1974.

189. Konrad PN, Richards FI, Valentine WN, Paglia DE: Gamma-glutamyl-cysteine synthetase deficiency. *N Engl J Med* 286:557, 1972.

190. Richards FI, Cooper MR, Pearce LA, Cowan RJ, Spurr CL: Familial spinocerebellar degeneration, hemolytic anemia, and glutathione deficiency. *Arch Intern Med* 134:534, 1974.

191. Beutler E, Moroose R, Kramer L, Gelbart T, Forman L: Gamma-glutamylcysteine synthetase deficiency and hemolytic anemia. *Blood* 75:271, 1990.

192. Skala H, Dreyfus JC, Vives-Corrons JL, Matsumoto F, Beutler E: Triose phosphate isomerase deficiency. *Biochem Med* 18:226, 1977.

193. Valentine WN, Schneider AS, Baughan MA, Paglia DE, Heins HL Jr.: Hereditary hemolytic anemia with triosephosphate isomerase deficiency. *Am J Med* 41:27, 1966.

194. Schneider AS, Valentine WN, Baughan MA, et al: Triosephosphate isomerase deficiency. A multi-system inherited enzyme disorder: Clinical and genetic aspects, in *Hereditary Disorders of Erythrocyte Metabolism*, p 265. Grune & Stratton, New York, 1968.

195. Hollan S, Fujii H, Hirono A, et al: Hereditary triosephosphate isomerase (TPI) deficiency: two severely affected brothers one with and one without neurological symptoms. *Hum Genet* 92:486, 1993.

196. Hollan S, Magocsi M, Fodor E, et al: Search for the pathogenesis of the differing phenotype in two compound heterozygote Hungarian brothers with the same genotypic triosephosphate isomerase deficiency. *Proc Natl Acad Sci USA* 94:10362, 1997.

197. Kugler W, Breme K, Laspe P, et al: Molecular basis of neurological dysfunction coupled with haemolytic anaemia in human glucose-6-phosphate isomerase (GPI) deficiency. *Hum Genet* 103:450, 1998.

198. DiMauro S, Dalakas M, Miranda AF: Phosphoglycerate kinase deficiency: another cause of recurrent myoglobinuria. *Ann Neurol* 13:11, 1983.

199. Kreuder J, Borkhardt A, Repp R, et al: Brief report: Inherited metabolic myopathy and hemolysis due to a mutation in aldolase A. *N Engl J Med* 334:1100, 1996.

200. Bresolin N, Bet L, Moggio M, et al: Muscle glucose-6-phosphate dehydrogenase deficiency. *J Neurol* 236:193, 1989.

201. Danon D, Sheba C, Ramot B: The morphology of glucose 6 phosphate dehydrogenase deficient erythrocytes: Electron-microscopic studies. *Blood* 17:229, 1961.

202. Beaupre SR, Schiffman FJ: Rush hemolysis. A 'bite-cell' hemolytic anemia associated with volatile liquid nitrite use. *Arch Fam Med* 3:545, 1994.

203. Greenberg MS: Heinz body hemolytic anemia. *Arch Intern Med* 136:153, 1976.

204. Nathan DM, Siegel AJ, Bunn HF: Acute methemoglobinemia and hemolytic anemia with phenazopyridine. *Arch Intern Med* 137:1636, 1977.

205. Oski FA, Nathan DG, Sidel VW, Diamond LK: Extreme hemolysis and

red-cell distortion in erythrocyte pyruvate kinase deficiency. *N Engl J Med* 270:1023, 1964.

206. Beutler E: *Red Cell Metabolism: A Manual of Biochemical Methods.* Grune & Stratton, New York, 1984.

207. Beutler E, Blume KG, Kaplan JC, et al: International committee for standardization in haematology: Recommended methods for red-cell enzyme analysis. *Br J Haematol* 35:331, 1977.

208. Beutler E, Blume KG, Kaplan JC, et al: International committee for standardization in haematology: Recommended screening test for glucose-6-phosphate dehydrogenase (G-6-PD) deficiency. *Br J Haematol* 43:465, 1979.

209. Herz F, Kaplan E, Scheye ES: Diagnosis of erythrocyte glucose-6-phosphate dehydrogenase deficiency in the negro male despite hemolytic crisis. *Blood* 35:90, 1970.

210. Ringelhahn B: A simple laboratory procedure for the recognition of A− (African type) G6PD deficiency in acute haemolytic crisis. *Clin Chim Acta* 36:272, 1972.

211. Beutler E: X-inactivation in heterozygous G-6-PD variant females, in *Glucose-6-Phosphate Dehydrogenase,* p 405. Academic Press, Orlando, FL, 1986.

212. Beutler E: G-6-PD activity of individual erythrocytes and X-chromosomal inactivation, in *Biochemical Methods in Red Cell Genetics,* p 95. Academic Press, New York, 1969.

213. Vogels IMC, van Noorden CJF, Wolf BHM, et al: Cytochemical determination of heterozygous glucose-6-phosphate dehydrogenase deficiency in erythrocytes. *Br J Haematol* 63:402, 1986.

214. Jacob H, Jandl JH: A simple visual screening test for G-6-PD deficiency employing ascorbate and cyanide. *N Engl J Med* 274:1162, 1966.

215. Beutler E, Kuhl W, Gelbart T, Forman L: DNA sequence abnormalities of human glucose-6-phosphate dehydrogenase variants. *J Biol Chem* 266:4145, 1991.

216. Beutler E, Kuhl W, Fox M, Tabsh K, Crandall BA: Prenatal diagnosis of glucose-6-P dehydrogenase (G6PD) deficiency. *Acta Haematol (Basel)* 87:103, 1992.

217. Beutler E: Glucose-6-phosphate dehydrogenase (G6PD) deficiency: Biochemistry, molecular biology, and population genetics, in *Advances in Jewish Genetic Diseases.* Oxford University Press, New York, 1998.

218. Beutler E: Molecular biology of G6PD variants and other red cell enzyme defects. *Ann Rev Med* 43:47, 1992.

219. Beutler E: Why has the autohemolysis test not gone the way of the cephalin flocculation test? *Blood* 51:109, 1978.

220. Carrell RW, Kay R: A simple method for the detection of unstable haemoglobins. *Br J Haematol* 23:615, 1972.

221. Lestas AN, Kay LA, Bellingham AJ: Red cell 3-phosphoglycerate level as a diagnostic aid in pyruvate kinase deficiency. *Br J Haematol* 67:485, 1987.

222. Valentine WN, Paglia DE, Fink K, Madokoro G: Lead poisoning. Association with hemolytic anemia, basophilic stippling, erythrocyte pyrimidine 5′-nucleotidase deficiency, and intraerythrocytic accumulation of pyrimidines. *J Clin Invest* 58:926, 1976.

223. Beutler E: Red blood cell enzymes, in *Hematologic Contributions to Fetal Health.* Liss, New York, 1988.

224. Mimouni F, Shohat S, Reisner SH: G6PD-deficiency donor blood as a cause of hemolysis in two preterm infants. *Isr J Med Sci* 22:120, 1986.

225. Beutler E, Mathai CK, Smith JE: Biochemical variants of glucose-6-phosphate dehydrogenase giving rise to congenital nonspherocytic hemolytic disease. *Blood* 31:131, 1968.

226. Spielberg SP, Boxer LA, Corash LM, Schulman JD: Improved erythrocyte survival with high dose vitamin E in chronic hemolyzing G6PD and glutathione synthetase deficiencies. *Ann Intern Med* 90:53, 1978.

227. Corash L, Spielberg S, Bartsocas C, et al: Reduced chronic hemolysis during high-dose vitamin E administration in Mediterranean-type glucose-6-phosphate dehydrogenase deficiency. *N Engl J Med* 303:416, 1980.

228. Johnson GJ, Vatassery GT, Finkel B, Allen DW: High-dose vitamin E does not decrease the rate of chronic hemolysis in glucose-6-phosphate dehydrogenase deficiency. *N Engl J Med* 308:1014, 1983.

229. Newman JG, Newman TB, Bowie LJ, Mendelsohn J: An examination of the role of vitamin E in glucose-6-phosphate dehydrogenase deficiency. *Clin Biochem* 12:149, 1979.

230. Ekert H, Rawlinson I: Deferoxamine and favism. *N Engl J Med* 312:1260, 1985.

231. Khalifa AS, El-Alfy MS, Mokhtar G, et al: Effect of desferrioxamine B on hemolysis in glucose-6-phosphate dehydrogenase deficiency. *Acta Haematol (Basel)* 82:113, 1989.

232. Zanella A, Berzuini A, Colombo MB, et al: Iron status in red cell pyruvate kinase deficiency: Study of Italian cases. *Br J Haematol* 83:485, 1993.

233. Meloni T, Forteleoni G, Noja G, et al: Increased prevalence of glucose-6-phosphate dehydrogenase deficiency in patients with cholelithiasis. *Acta Haematol (Basel)* 85:76, 1991.

234. Petrakis NL, Wiesenfeld SL, Sams BJ, et al: Prevalence of sickle-cell trait and glucose-6-phosphate dehydrogenase deficiency. *N Engl J Med* 282:767, 1970.

235. Bowman HS, McKusick VA, Dronamraju KR: Pyruvate kinase deficient hemolytic anemia in an Amish isolate. *Am J Hum Genet* 17:1, 1965.

236. Bianchi M, Magnani M: Hexokinase mutations that produce nonspherocytic hemolytic anemia. *Blood Cells Mol Dis* 21:2, 1995.

237. Beutler E: *Red Cell Metabolism: A Manual of Biochemical Methods.* Grune & Stratton, New York, 1984.

238. Fujii H, Kanno H, Hirono A, Miwa S: Hematologically important mutations: Molecular abnormalities of glucose-6-phosphate isomerase deficiency. *Blood Cells Mol Dis* 22:96, 1996.

239. Beutler E, West C, Britton HA, Harris J, Forman L: Glucosephosphate isomerase (GPI) deficiency mutations associated with hereditary nonspherocytic hemolytic anemia (HNSHA). *Blood Cells Mol Dis* 23:402, 1997.

240. Bruno C, Minetti C, Shanske S, et al: Combined defects of muscle phosphofructokinase and AMP deaminase in a child with myoglobinuria. *Neurology* 50:296, 1998.

241. Rudolphi O, Ek B, Ronquist G: Inherited phosphofructokinase deficiency associated with hemolysis and exertional myopathy. *Eur J Haematol* 55:279, 1995.

242. Kishi H, Mukai T, Hirono A, et al: Human aldolase A deficiency associated with a hemolytic anemia: Thermolabile aldolase due to a single base mutation. *Proc Natl Acad Sci USA* 84:8623, 1987.

243. Schneider A, Cohen-Solal M: Hematologically important mutations: Triosephosphate isomerase. *Blood Cells Mol Dis* 22:82, 1996.

244. Yoshida A, Twele TW, Dave V, Beutler E: Molecular abnormality of a phosphoglycerate kinase variant (PGK-Alabama). *Blood Cells Mol Dis* 21:179, 1995.

245. Turner G, Fletcher J, Elber J, et al: Molecular defect of a phosphoglycerate kinase variant associated with haemolytic anaemia and neurological disorders in a large kindred. *Br J Haematol* 91:60, 1995.

246. Lemarchandel V, Joulin V, Valentin C, et al: Compound heterozygosity in a complete erythrocyte bisphosphoglycerate mutase deficiency. *Blood* 80:2643, 1992.

247. Beutler E, Gelbart T, Kondo T, Matsunaga AT: The molecular basis of a case of gamma-glutamylcysteine synthetase deficiency. *Blood* 94:2097, 1999.

248. Beutler E, Duron O, Kelly BM: Improved method for the determination of blood glutathione. *J Lab Clin Med* 61:882, 1963.

249. Beutler E, Gelbart T: Improved assay of the enzymes of glutathione synthesis: gamma-glutamylcysteine synthetase and glutathione synthetase. *Clin Chim Acta* 158:115, 1986.

250. Valentine WN, Fink K, Paglia DE, Harris SR, Adams WS: Hereditary hemolytic anemia with human erythrocyte pyrimidine 5′-nucleotidase deficiency. *J Clin Invest* 54:866, 1974.

251. Torrance J, West C, Beutler E: A simple rapid radiometric assay for pyrimidine-5′-nucleotidase. *J Lab Clin Med* 90:563, 1977.

252. Rees DC, Duley J, Simmonds HA, et al: Interaction of hemoglobin E and pyrimidine 5′ nucleotidase deficiency. *Blood* 88:2761, 1996.

253. Chen EH, Tartaglia AP, Mitchell BS: Hereditary overexpression of adenosine deaminase in erythrocytes: Evidence for a *cis*-acting mutation. *Am J Hum Genet* 53:889, 1993.

254. Markert ML: Molecular basis of adenosine deaminase deficiency. *Immunodeficiency* 5:141, 1994.

255. Markert ML, Hershfield MS, Wiginton DA, et al: Identification of a deletion in the adenosine deaminase gene in a child with severe combined immunodeficiency. *J Immunol* 138:3203, 1987.

256. Manabe J, Arya R, Sumimoto H, et al: Two novel mutations in the reduced nicotinamide adenine dinucleotide (NADH) cytochrome b$_5$ reductase gene of a patient with generalized type, hereditary methemoglobinemia. *Blood* 88:3208, 1996.

257. Kaplan J-C, Nicolas A, Hanlickova-Leroux A, Beutler E: A simple spot screening test for fast detection of red cell NADH-diaphorase deficiency. *Blood* 36:330, 1970.

258. Jacobasch G, Rapoport SM: Hemolytic anemias due to erythrocyte enzyme deficiencies. *Mol Aspects Med* 17:143, 1996.

259. Beutler E, Kuhl W, Gelbart T: Blood cell phosphogluconolactonase: Assay and properties. *Br J Haematol* 62:577, 1986.

260. Thorburn DR, Kuchel PW: Computer simulation of the metabolic consequences of the combined deficiency of 6-phosphogluconolactonase and glucose-6-phosphate dehydrogenase in human erythrocytes. *J Lab Clin Med* 110:70, 1987.

261. Bird TD, Hamernyik P, Nutter JY, Labbe RF: Inherited deficiency of delta-aminolevulinic acid dehydratase. *Am J Hum Genet* 31:662, 1979.

262. Kamatani N, Hakoda M, Otsuka S, Yoshikawa H, Kashiwazaki S: Only three mutations account for almost all defective alleles causing adenine phosphoribosyltransferase deficiency in Japanese patients. *J Clin Invest* 90:130, 1992.

263. Cartier P, Hamet M: Une nouvelle maladie metabolique: Le deficit complet en adenine-phosphoribosyltransferase avec lithiase de 2,8-di-hydroxyadenine. *C R Acad Sci (Paris)* 279:883, 1974.

264. Hidaka Y, Palella TD, O'Toole TE, Tarle SA, Kelley WN: Human adenine phosphoribosyltransferase. Identification of allelic mutations at the nucleotide level as a cause of complete deficiency of the enzyme. *J Clin Invest* 80:1409, 1987.

265. Lachant NA, Zerez CR, Barredo J, et al: Hereditary erythrocyte adenylate kinase deficiency: A defect of multiple phosphotransferases. *Blood* 77:2774, 1991.

266. Ogasawara N, Goto H, Yamada Y, Watanabe T: Distribution of AMP-deaminase isozymes in rat tissues. *Eur J Biochem* 87:297, 1978.

267. Yamada Y, Makarewicz W, Goto H, et al: Gene mutations responsible for human erythrocyte AMP deaminase deficiency in Poles. *Adv Exp Med Biol* 431:347, 1998.

268. Armstrong JM, Myers DV, Verpoorte JA, Edsall JT: Purification and properties of human erythrocyte carbonic anhydrases. *J Biol Chem* 241:5137, 1966.

269. Kendall AG, Tashian RE: Erythrocyte carbonic anhydrase I: Inherited deficiency in humans. *Science* 197:471, 1977.

270. Roth DE, Venta PJ, Tashian RE, Sly WS: Molecular basis of human carbonic anhydrase II deficiency. *Proc Natl Acad Sci USA* 89:1804, 1992.

271. Takahara S: Acatalasemia and hypocatalasemia in the Orient. *Semin Hematol* 8:397, 1971.

272. Aebi H, Bossi E, Cantz M, Matsubara S, Suter H: Acatalas(em)ia in Switzerland, in *Hereditary Disorders of Erythrocyte Metabolism*, p 41. Grune & Stratton, New York, 1968.

273. Gitzelmann R: Hereditary galactokinase deficiency, a newly recognized cause of juvenile cataracts. *Pediatr Res* 1:14, 1967.

274. Beutler E: Galactosemia: Screening and diagnosis. *Clin Biochem* 24:293, 1991.

275. Beutler E: Effect of flavin compounds on glutathione reductase activity: In vivo and in vitro studies. *J Clin Invest* 48:1957, 1969.

276. McCann SR, Finkel B, Cadman S, Allen DW: Study of a kindred with hereditary spherocytosis and glyceraldehyde-3-phosphate dehydrogenase deficiency. *Blood* 47:171, 1976.

277. Valentine WN, Paglia DE, Neerhout RC, Konrad PN: Erythrocyte glyoxalase II deficiency with coincidental hereditary elliptocytosis. *Blood* 36:797, 1970.

278. Johnson LA, Gordon RB, Emmerson BT: Hypoxanthine-guanine phosphoribosyltransferase: A simple spectrophotometric assay. *Clin Chim Acta* 80:203, 1977.

279. Davidson BL, Tarle SA, Palella TD, Kelley WN: Molecular basis of hypoxanthine-guanine phosphoribosyltransferase deficiency in ten subjects determined by direct sequencing of amplified transcripts. *J Clin Invest* 84:342, 1989.

280. Vanderheiden BS: Genetic studies of human erythrocyte inosine triphosphatase. *Biochem Genet* 3:289, 1969.

281. Miwa S, Nishina T, Kakehashi Y, et al: Studies on erythrocyte metabolism in a case with hereditary deficiency of H-subunit of lactate dehydrogenase. *Acta Haematol Jpn* 34:2, 1971.

282. Sass MD, Caruso CJ, Farhangi M: TPNH-methemoglobin reductase deficiency: A new red-cell enzyme defect. *J Lab Clin Med* 70:760, 1967.

283. Kaplan J-C, Alexandre Y, Dreyfus J-C: Deficit selectif d'un des loci

284. Chamberlain BR, Buttery JE: Reappraisal of the uroporphyrinogen I synthase assay, and a proposed modified method. *Clin Chem* 26:1346, 1980.

285. Strand LJ, Meyer UA, Felsher BF, Redeker AG, Marver HS: Decreased red cell uroporphyrinogen I synthetase activity in intermittent acute porphyria. *J Clin Invest* 51:2530, 1972.

286. Nafa K, Reghis A, Osmani N, et al: G6PD Aures: A new mutation (48 Ile→hr) causing mild G6PD deficiency is associated with favism. *Hum Mol Genet* 2:81, 1993.

287. Beutler E, Kuhl W, Ramirez E, Lisker R: Some Mexican glucose-6-phosphate dehydrogenase (G-6-PD) variants revisited. *Hum Genet* 86:371, 1991.

288. Vulliamy TJ, D'Urso M, Battistuzzi G, et al: Diverse point mutations in the human glucose-6-phosphate dehydrogenase gene cause enzyme deficiency and mild or severe hemolytic anemia. *Proc Natl Acad Sci USA* 85:5171, 1988.

289. Cappellini MD, Martinez di Montemuros F, Dotti C, et al: Molecular characterisation of the glucose-6-phosphate dehydrogenase (G6PD) Ferrara II variant. *Hum Genet* 95:440, 1995.

290. Beutler E, Kuhl W, Sáenz GF, Rodriguez W: Mutation analysis of G6PD variants in Costa Rica. *Hum Genet* 87:462, 1991.

291. Beutler E, Kuhl W: The NT 1311 polymorphism of G6PA: G6PD Mediterranean mutation may have originated independently in Europe and Asia. *Am J Hum Genet* 47:1008, 1990.

292. De Vita G, Alcalay M, Sampietro M, et al: Two point mutations are responsible for G6PD polymorphism in Sardinia. *Am J Hum Genet* 44:233, 1989.

293. Ninfali P, Bresolin N, Baronciani L, et al: Glucose-6-phosphate dehydrogenase Lodi844C: A study on its expression in blood cells and muscle. *Enzyme* 45:180, 1991.

294. Beutler E, Prchal JT, Westwood B, Kuhl W: Definition of the mutations of G6PD Wayne, G6PD Viangchan, G6PD Jammu and G6PD "LeJeune." *Acta Haematol (Basel)* 86:179, 1991.

295. Beutler E, Westwood B, Prchal J, et al: New glucose-6-phosphate dehydrogenase mutations from various ethnic groups. *Blood* 80:255, 1992.

296. Vlachos A, Westwood B, Lipton JM, Beutler E: G6PD Mt. Sinai. A new severe hemolytic variant characterized by dual mutations at nucleotides 376 and 1159. *Hum Mutat* 6 (suppl 1):S154, 1998.

297. Filosa S, Calabrò V, Vallone D, et al: Molecular basis of chronic non-spherocytic haemolytic anaemia: A new G6PD variant (393 Arg→His) with abnormal K_m^{GPD} and marked instability. *Br J Haematol* 80:111, 1992.

298. Chiu DTY, Zuo L, Chen E, Chang CN, Chiu DTY: Two commonly occurring nucleotide base substitutions in Chinese G6PD variants. *Biochem Biophys Res Commun* 180:988, 1991.

299. Stevens DJ, Wanachiwanawin W, Mason PJ, Vulliamy TJ, Luzzatto L: G6PD Canton a common deficient variant in South East Asia caused by a 459 Arg→Leu mutation. *Nucl Acids Res* 18:7190, 1990.

300. Calabrò V, Mason PJ, Filosa S, et al: Genetic heterogeneity of glucose-6-phosphate dehydrogenase deficiency revealed by single-strand conformation and sequence analysis. *Am J Hum Genet* 52:527, 1993.

301. Neubauer B, Lakomek M, Winkler H, et al: Point mutations in the L-type pyruvate kinase gene of two children with hemolytic anemia caused by pyruvate kinase deficiency. *Blood* 77:1871, 1991.

302. Kanno H, Fujii H, Hirono A, Miwa S: cDNA cloning of human R-type pyruvate kinase and identification of a single amino acid substitution (Thr384→Met) affecting enzymatic stability in a pyruvate kinase variant (PK Tokyo) associated with hereditary hemolytic anemia. *Proc Natl Acad Sci USA* 88:8218, 1991.

303. Kanno H, Fujii H, Hirono A, Omine M, Miwa S: Identical point mutations of the R-type pyruvate kinase (PK) cDNA found in unrelated PK variants associated with hereditary hemolytic anemia. *Blood* 79:1347, 1992.

304. Gerr F, Frumkin H, Hodgins A: Hemolytic anemia following succimer administration in a glucose-6-phosphate dehydrogenase deficient patient. *J Toxicol Clin Toxicol* 32:569, 1994.

305. Rajkondawar VL, Modi TH, Mishra SN: Drug induced acute haemolytic anaemia in glucose-6-phosphate dehydrogenase deficiency subjects. *J Assoc Physicians (India)* 16:589, 1968.

genetiques de la phosphoglucomutase dans les globules rouges. *C R Acad Sci (Paris)* 270:1060, 1970.

306. Omar MES, Wahab MFA: Treatment of typhoid and paratyphoid fever with furazolidone. *J Trop Med Hyg* 70:43, 1967.

307. Teunis BS, Leftwich EI, Pierce LE: Acute methemoglobinemia and hemolytic anemia due to toluidine blue. *Arch Surg* 101:527, 1970.

308. Meloni G, Meloni T: Glyburide-induced acute haemolysis in a G6PD-deficient patient with NIDDM. *Br J Haematol* 92:159, 1996.

309. Little C, Schacter B: Hemolytic anemia following isobutyl nitrate (IBN) inhalation in a patient with glucose-6-phosphate dehydrogenase (G-6-PD) deficiency. *Blood* 54(suppl 1):34A, 1979.

310. Rosen PJ, Johnson C, McGehee WG, Beutler E: Failure of methylene blue treatment in toxic methemoglobinemia. Association with glucose-6-phosphate dehydrogenase deficiency. *Ann Intern Med* 75:83, 1971.

311. Belton EM, Jones RV: Haemolytic anaemia due to nalidixic acid. *Lancet* 2:691, 1965.

312. Mandal BK, Stevenson J: Haemolytic crisis produced by nalidixic acid. *Lancet* 1:614, 1970.

313. Djerassi LS, Vitany L: Haemolytic episode in G6PD deficient workers exposed to TNT. *Br J Ind Med* 32:54, 1975.

314. Melzer-Lange M, Walsh-Kelly C: Naphthalene-induced hemolysis in a black female toddler deficient in glucose-6-phosphate dehydrogenase. *Pediatr Emerg Care* 5:24, 1989.

315. Todisco V, Lamour J, Finberg L: Hemolysis from exposure to naphthalene mothballs. *N Engl J Med* 325:1660, 1991.

316. Ducros J, Saingra S, Rampal M, et al: Hemolytic anemia due to G6PD deficiency and urate oxidase in a kidney-transplant patient. *Clin Nephrol* 35:89, 1991.

317. Lapierre J, Holler C, Tourte-Schaefer C, et al: Haemolytic anaemia following anti-bilharzia treatment using niridazole in a woman of caribbean origin with GPD deficiency. *Nouv Presse Med* 5:147, 1976.

318. Thomas M, Agnus D, Poirot JL, Golvan YJ: Hemolysis induced by niridazole in two patients with deficiency of G-6-PD. *Nouv Presse Med* 5:1537, 1976.

319. Chan TK, Todd D, Tso SC: Drug-induced haemolysis in glucose-6-phosphate dehydrogenase deficiency. *BMJ* 2:1227, 1976.

320. Tishler M: Phenazopyridine-induced hemolytic anemia in a patient with G-6-PD deficiency. *Acta Haematol (Basel)* 70:208, 1983.

321. Chan TK, Todd D, Tso SC: Red cell survival studies in glucose-6-phosphate dehydrogenase deficiency. *Bull Hong Kong Med Assoc* 26:41, 1974.

322. Herman J, Ben-Meir S: Overt hemolysis in patients with glucose-6-phosphate dehydrogenase deficiency. *Isr J Med Sci* 2:340, 1975.

323. Gaetani GD, Mareni C, Ravazzolo R, Salvidio E: Haemolytic effect of two sulfonamides evaluated by a new method. *Br J Haematol* 32:183, 1976.

324. McCurdy PR, Donohoe RF: Pyridoxine-responsive anemia conditioned by isonicotinic acid hydrazide. *Blood* 27:352, 1966.

325. Gaetani G, Salvidio E, Pannacciulli I, Ajmar F, Paravidino G: Absence of haemolytic effects of L-DOPA on transfused G6PD-deficient erythrocytes. *Experientia* 26:785, 1970.

326. Zail SS, Charlton RW, Bothwell TH: The haemolytic effect of certain drugs in Bantu subjects with a deficiency of glucose-6-phosphate dehydrogenase. *S Afr J Med Sci* 27:95, 1962.

327. Heinrich RA, Smith TC, Buchanan RA: A pharmacological study of a new sulfonamide in glucose-6-phosphate dehydrogenase deficient subjects. *J Clin Pharmacol* 11:428, 1971.

328. Szeinberg A, Pras M, Sheba C, Adam A, Ramot B: The hemolytic effect of various sulfonamides on subjects with a deficiency of glucose-6-phosphate dehydrogenase of erythrocytes. *Isr J Med Sci* 18:176, 1959.

329. Kellermeyer RW, Tarlov AR, Schrier SL, Alving AS: Hemolytic effect of commonly used drugs on erythrocytes deficient in glucose-6-phosphate dehydrogenase. *J Lab Clin Med* 52:827, 1958.

330. Kellermeyer RW, Tarlov AR, Brewer GJ, Carson PE, Alving AS: Hemolytic effect of therapeutic drugs. Clinical considerations of the Primaquine-type hemolysis. *JAMA* 180:388, 1962.

331. Mela Q, Perpignano G, Ruggiero V, Longatti S: Tolerability of tiaprofenic acid in patients with glucose-6-phosphate dehydrogenase (G6PD) deficiency. *Drugs* 35:107, 1988.

332. Beutler E, Gelbart T: Estimating the prevalence of pyruvate kinase deficiency from the gene frequency in the general white population. *Blood* 95:3585, 2000.

THE THALASSEMIAS

DAVID J. WEATHERALL

The thalassemias are the commonest monogenic diseases in Man. They occur at a high gene frequency throughout the Mediterranean populations, the Middle East, the Indian subcontinent, and Burma and in a line stretching from southern China through Thailand and the Malay peninsula into the island populations of the Pacific. They are also seen commonly in countries in which there has been immigration from these high-frequency populations.

There are two main classes of thalassemia, α and β, in which the α- and β-globin genes are involved, and rarer forms due to abnormalites of other globin genes. These conditions all have in common an imbalanced rate of production of the globin chains of adult hemoglobin, α chains in β thalassemia and β chains in α thalassemia. Several hundred different mutations at the α- and β-globin loci have been defined as the cause of the reduced or absent output of α or β chains.

The pathophysiology of the thalassemias can be traced to the deleterious effects of the globin-chain subunits that are produced in excess. In β thalassemia, excess α chains cause damage to the red cell precursors and red cells and lead to profound anemia. This causes expansion of the ineffective marrow, with severe effects on development, bone formation, and growth. The major cause of morbidity and mortality is the effect of iron deposition in the endocrine organs, liver, and heart, which results from increased intestinal absorption and the effects of blood transfusion. The pathophysiology of the α thalassemias is different because the excess β chains that result from defective α-chain production form β_4 molecules, or hemoglobin H, which is soluble and does not precipitate in the marrow. However, it is unstable and precipitates in older red cells. Hence, the anemia of α thalassemia is hemolytic rather than dyserythropoietic.

The clinical pictures of α and β thalassemia vary widely, and knowledge is gradually being amassed about some of the genetic factors that modify these phenotypes.

Since the carrier states for the thalassemias can be identified and affected fetuses can be diagnosed by DNA analysis after the ninth to tenth week of gestation, these conditions are widely amenable to prenatal diagnosis. Their symptomatic management is based on regular blood transfusion, iron chelation therapy, and the judicious use of splenectomy. Current experimental approaches to their management include the stimulation of fetal hemoglobin synthesis and attempts at somatic cell gene therapy.

Acronyms and abbreviations that appear in this chapter include: bp, base pairs; HPFH, hereditary persistence of fetal hemoglobin; LCR, locus control region; PCR, polymerase chain reaction; RFLP, restriction fragment length polymorphism.

DEFINITIONS AND HISTORY

A form of severe anemia occurring early in life and associated with splenomegaly and bone changes was first described by Cooley and Lee in 1925.[1] In 1932, George H. Whipple and William L. Bradford published a comprehensive account of the pathologic findings in this disease.[2] Whipple coined the phrase *thalassic anemia*,[3,4] condensing it to *thalassemia*, from $\theta\alpha\lambda\alpha\sigma\sigma\alpha$, "the sea," since early patients were all of Mediterranean background. It was only after 1940 that the true genetic character of this disorder was fully appreciated. It became clear that the disease described by Cooley and Lee is the homozygous state of an autosomal gene for which the heterozygous state is associated with much milder hematologic changes. The severe homozygous condition became known as thalassemia major, while the heterozygous states, thalassemia trait, were designated, according to their severity, thalassemia minor or minima.[3,5–8] Later, the term *thalassemia intermedia* was used to describe disorders that are milder than the major form but more severe than the traits.

More recently it has been established that thalassemia is not a single disease but a group of disorders, each of which results from an inherited abnormality of globin production.[7] These conditions form part of the spectrum of diseases known collectively as the hemoglobinopathies, which can be classified broadly into two types. First, there are those, such as sickle cell anemia, that result from an inherited structural alteration in one of the globin chains. Although such abnormal hemoglobins may be synthesized less efficiently or broken down more rapidly than normal adult hemoglobin, the associated clinical abnormalities result from the physical properties of the abnormal hemoglobin (see Chap. 48). The second major subdivision of the hemoglobinopathies, the thalassemias, is constituted by inherited defects in the rate of synthesis of one or more of the globin chains. This causes imbalanced globin chain production, ineffective erythropoiesis, hemolysis, and a variable degree of anemia.

Several monographs describe the historical aspects of thalassemia in more detail.[3,5,7]

DIFFERENT FORMS OF THALASSEMIA

Thalassemia can be defined as a condition in which a reduced rate of synthesis of one or more of the globin chains leads to imbalanced globin-chain synthesis, defective hemoglobin production, and damage to the red cells or their precursors from the effects of the globin subunits that are produced in relative excess.[3,7–9] The main varieties of thalassemia that have now been defined with certainty are summarized in Table 46-1.

The β thalassemias can be divided into two main varieties: in one form, β^0 thalassemia, there is a total absence of β-chain production, and in the other, β^+ thalassemia, there is a partial deficiency of β-chain production. The hallmark of the common forms of β thalassemia is an elevated level of hemoglobin A_2 in heterozygotes. However, there is a less common class of β thalassemias in which heterozygotes have normal levels of hemoglobin A_2. These conditions are sometimes subdivided into type 1, in which there are no hematological abnormalities and hence the condition is "silent" in the heterozygous state, and type 2, in which the hematological changes are indistinguishable from those of β-thalassemia heterozygotes with elevated hemoglobin A_2 levels.

The $\delta\beta$ thalassemias are also heterogeneous. In some cases, no δ or β chains are synthesized. Originally it was customary to classify these disorders according to the structure of the hemoglobin F produced, that is, $^G\gamma^A\gamma(\delta\beta)^0$ and $^G\gamma(\delta\beta)^0$ thalassemia. In fact, this is illogical, and these conditions are best described by the globin chains that are defectively synthesized, that is, simply into the $(\delta\beta)^+$, $(\delta\beta)^0$, and $(^A\gamma\delta\beta)^0$ thalassemias.[7,10] In the $(\delta\beta)^+$ thalassemias an abnormal

TABLE 46-1   THE THALASSEMIAS AND RELATED DISORDERS

α Thalassemia
  α^0
  α^+
      Deletion $(-\alpha)$
      Nondeletion (α^T)
β Thalassemia
  β^0
  β^+
  Normal Hb A$_2$
      Type 1 ("silent")
      Type 2
$\delta\beta$ Thalassemia
  $(\delta\beta)^+$
  $(\delta\beta)^0$
  $(^A\gamma\delta\beta)^0$
γ Thalassemia
δ Thalassemia
  δ^0
  δ^+
$\varepsilon\gamma\delta\beta$ Thalassemia
HPFH
  Deletion
      $(\delta\beta)^0$, $(^A\gamma\delta\beta)^0$
  Nondeletion
      Linked to β-globin genes
          $^G\gamma\beta^+$, $^A\gamma\beta^+$
      Unlinked to β-globin genes

hemoglobin is produced that has normal α chains combined with non-α chains that consist of the N-terminal residues of the δ chain fused to the C-terminal residues of the β chain. These fusion variants, called the Lepore hemoglobins, also show structural heterogeneity.

The δ thalassemias[7,10] are characterized by a reduced output of δ chains and hence by reduced levels of hemoglobin A$_2$ in heterozygotes and an absence of hemoglobin A$_2$ in homozygotes. They are of no clinical significance.

A disorder characterized by defective ε, γ, δ, and β-chain synthesis has been defined at the clinical and molecular level.[7,10] The homozygous state for this condition, $\varepsilon\gamma\delta\beta$ thalassemia, is presumably not compatible with fetal survival, and it has been observed only in heterozygotes.

To complete this description of the thalassemia-like mutations that involve the β-globin gene complex, we must consider hereditary persistence of fetal hemoglobin (HPFH).[7,9,10] This heterogeneous condition is characterized by persistence of fetal hemoglobin production into adult life in the absence of major hematologic changes. It is classified into deletion and nondeletion forms. The deletion forms of HPFH can be classified, like $\delta\beta$ thalassemia, as $(\delta\beta)^0$ HPFH and then further subdivided according to the particular population in which this occurs and its associated molecular defect. In effect, the deletion forms of HPFH are very similar to $\delta\beta$ thalassemia except that there is more efficient γ-chain synthesis and therefore less chain imbalance and a milder phenotype. However, the homozygous state is associated with mild thalassemic changes, and, in fact, the $\delta\beta$ thalassemias and deletion forms of HPFH form a clinical continuum. The nondeletion forms of HPFH are also heterogeneous. In some cases they are associated with mutations that involve the β-globin gene cluster and in which there is β-chain synthesis *cis* to the HPFH determinant. These conditions are subdivided into $^G\gamma\beta^+$ HPFH and $^A\gamma\beta^+$ HPFH. Again, they are often subclassified according to the population in which they occur, for example, Greek HPFH, British HPFH, and so on. Finally, there is a heterogeneous group of HPFH determinants associated with very low levels of persistent fetal hemoglobin, the genetic loci of which, at least in some cases, are not linked to the β-globin gene cluster.

Since α chains are present in both fetal and adult hemoglobins, a deficiency of α-chain production will affect hemoglobin synthesis in fetal as well as adult life. A reduced rate of α-chain synthesis in fetal life results in an excess of γ chains, which form γ_4 tetramers, or hemoglobin Bart's. In adult life, a deficiency of α chains results in an excess of β chains, which form β_4 tetramers, or hemoglobin H. Because there are two α-globin genes per haploid genome, the genetics of α thalassemia is more complicated than that of β thalassemia. There are two main groups of α-thalassemia determinants.[7,10] First, there are the α^0 thalassemias (formerly called α thalassemia 1), in which no α chains are produced from an affected chromosome. That is, both linked α-globin genes are inactivated. Second, there are the α^+ thalassemias (formerly called α thalassemia 2), in which the output of one of the linked pair of α-globin genes is defective. The α^+ thalassemias are subdivided into deletion and nondeletion types. Both the α^0 thalassemias and deletion and nondeletion forms of α^+ thalassemia are all extremely heterogeneous at the molecular level. There are two major clinical phenotypes of α thalassemia, the hemoglobin Bart's hydrops syndrome, which usually reflects the homozygous state for α^0 thalassemia, and hemoglobin H disease, which usually results from the compound heterozygous state for α^0 and α^+ thalassemia.

Since the structural hemoglobin variants and the thalassemias occur with a high frequency in some populations, the two types of genetic defect may be found in the same individual. The different genetic varieties of thalassemia and their combinations with the genes for abnormal hemoglobins produce a series of disorders known collectively as the thalassemia syndromes.[7]

ETIOLOGY AND PATHOGENESIS

GENETIC CONTROL AND SYNTHESIS OF HEMOGLOBIN[9,10]

The structure and ontogeny of the hemoglobins are reviewed in Chaps. 29 and 8, respectively, and only those aspects with particular relevance to the thalassemia problem are restated here.

Human adult hemoglobin is a heterogeneous mixture of proteins consisting of a major component, hemoglobin A, and a minor component, hemoglobin A$_2$, constituting about 2.5 percent of the total. In intrauterine life, the main hemoglobin is hemoglobin F. The structure of these hemoglobins is similar. Each consists of two separate pairs of identical globin chains. Except for some of the embryonic hemoglobins (see below), all the normal human hemoglobins have one pair of α chains: in hemoglobin A these are combined with β chains ($\alpha_2\beta_2$), in hemoglobin A$_2$ with δ chains ($\alpha_2\delta_2$), and in hemoglobin F with γ chains ($\alpha_2\gamma_2$).

Human hemoglobin shows further heterogeneity, particularly in fetal life, and this has important implications for understanding the thalassemias and for approaches to their prenatal diagnosis. Hemoglobin F is a mixture of molecular species with the formulas $\alpha_2\gamma_2^{136Gly}$ and $\alpha_2\gamma_2^{136Ala}$. The γ chains containing glycine at position 136 are designated $^G\gamma$ chains; those that contain alanine are called $^A\gamma$ chains. At birth the ratio of molecules containing $^G\gamma$ chains to those containing $^A\gamma$ chains is about 3:1; this ratio varies widely in the trace amounts of hemoglobin F present in normal adults.

Before the eighth week of intrauterine life there are three embryonic hemoglobins: hemoglobins Gower 1 ($\zeta_2\varepsilon_2$), Gower 2 ($\alpha_2\varepsilon_2$), and Portland ($\zeta_2\gamma_2$). The ζ and ε chains are the embryonic counterparts of the adult α and β and γ and δ chains, respectively. ζ-Chain synthesis persists beyond the embryonic stage of development in some of the α thalassemias; so far, persistent ε-chain production has not been found in any of the thalassemia syndromes. During fetal development there is an orderly switch from ζ to α and from ε- to γ-chain production, followed by β- and δ-chain production after birth.

The different human hemoglobins, together with the arrangement of the α-gene cluster on chromosome 16 and the β-gene cluster on chromosome 11, are shown in Fig. 46-1.

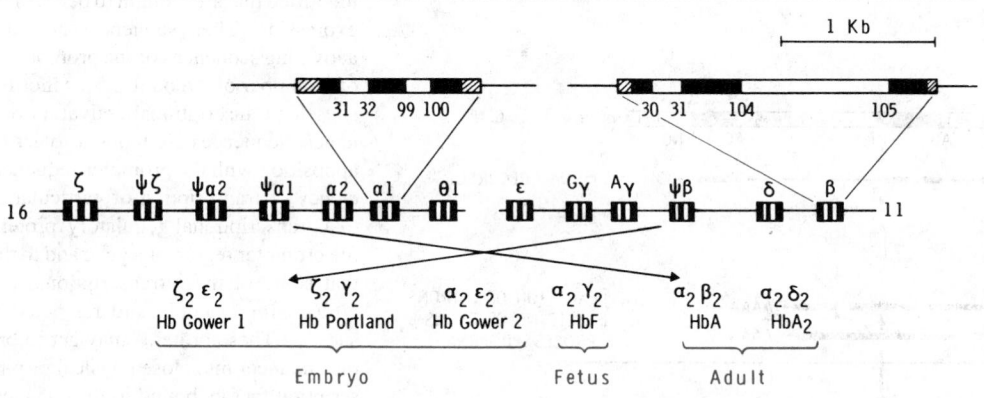

FIGURE 46-1   The genetic control of human hemoglobin. The main globin gene clusters are on chromosomes 11 and 16. At each stage of development different genes in these clusters are activated or repressed. The different globin chains directed by individual genes are synthesized independently and combine with each other in a random fashion as indicated by the arrows.

GLOBIN GENE CLUSTERS

Although there is some individual variability, the α-gene cluster usually contains one functional ζ gene and two α genes, designated α_2 and α_1. It also contains four pseudogenes: $\psi\xi_1$, $\psi\alpha_1$, $\psi\alpha_2$, and θ_1.[9,10] The latter is remarkably conserved among different species. Although it appears to be expressed in early fetal life, its function is unknown; it seems unlikely that it can produce a viable globin chain. Each α gene is located in a region of homology approximately 4 kb long, interrupted by two small nonhomologous regions.[11,13] It is thought that the homologous regions have resulted from gene duplication and that the nonhomologous segments may have arisen subsequently by insertion of DNA into the noncoding regions around one of the two genes. The exons of the two α-globin genes have identical sequences. The first intron in each gene is identical, but the second intron of α_1 is nine bases longer and differs by three bases from that in the α_2 gene.[13-15] Despite their high degree of homology, the sequences of the two α-globin genes diverge in their 3' untranslated regions 13 bases beyond the TAA stop codon. These differences provide an opportunity to assess the relative output of the genes, an important part of the analysis of the α thalassemias.[16,17] It appears that the production of α_2 messenger RNA exceeds that of α_1 by a factor of 1.5 to 3. ξ_1 and ξ_2 genes are also highly homologous. The introns are much larger than those of α-globin genes, and, in contrast to the latter, IVS-1 is larger than IVS-2. In each ξ gene, IVS-1 contains several copies of a simple repeated 14-bp sequence that is similar to sequences located between the two ξ genes and near the human insulin gene. There are three base changes in the coding sequence of the first exon of ξ_1, one of which gives rise to a premature stop codon, thus making it an inactive pseudogene.

The regions separating and surrounding the α-like structural genes have been analyzed in detail. Of particular relevance to thalassemia is the fact that this gene cluster is highly polymorphic.[18] There are five hypervariable regions in the cluster: one downstream from the α_1 gene, one between the ξ and $\psi\xi$ genes, one in the first intron of both the ξ genes, and one 5' to the cluster. These regions have been found to consist of varying numbers of tandem repeats of nucleotide sequences. Taken together with the single-base restriction fragment length polymorphisms (RFLPs), the variability of the α-globin gene cluster reaches a heterozygosity level of approximately 0.95. Thus, it is possible to identify each parental α-globin gene cluster in the majority of persons. This heterogeneity has important implications for tracing the history of the thalassemia mutations.

The arrangement of the β-globin gene cluster on the short arm of chromosome 11 is shown in Fig. 46-1. Each of the individual genes and their flanking regions have been sequenced.[19-22] Like the α_1 and α_2 gene pairs, the $^{G}\gamma$ and $^{A}\gamma$ genes share a similar sequence. In fact, the $^{G}\gamma$ and $^{A}\gamma$ genes on one chromosome are identical in the region 5' to the center of the large intron yet show some divergence 3' to that position. At the boundary between the conserved and divergent regions, there is a block of simple sequence that may be a "hot spot" for the initiation of recombination events that have led to unidirectional gene conversion.

Like the α-globin genes, the β-gene cluster contains a series of single-point RFLPs, although in this case no hypvariable regions have been identified.[23,24] The arrangement of RFLPs, or haplotypes, in the β-globin gene cluster falls into two domains. On the 5' side of the β gene, spanning about 32 kb from the ε gene to the 3' end of the $\psi\beta$ gene, there are three common patterns of RFLPs. In the region encompassing about 18 kb to the 3' side of the β-globin gene, there are also three common patterns in different populations. Between these regions there is a sequence of about 11 kb in which there is randomization of the 5' and 3' domains and hence where a relatively higher frequency of recombination may occur. The β-globin gene haplotypes are similar in most populations but differ markedly in individuals of African origin; these findings suggest that these haplotype arrangements were laid down very early during evolution, and they are consistent with data obtained from mitochondrial DNA polymorphisms that point to the early emergence of a relatively small population from Africa with subsequent divergence into other racial groups.[25] Again, they are extremely useful for analyzing the population genetics and history of the thalassemia mutations.

The regions flanking the coding regions of the globin genes contain a number of conserved sequences that are essential for their expression.[26] The first is the TATA box, which serves accurately to locate the site of transcription initiation at the CAP site, usually about 30 bases downstream, and also appears to influence the rate of transcription. In addition, there are two so-called upstream promotor elements; 70 or 80 base pairs (bp) upstream is a second conserved sequence, the CCAAT box, and further 5', approximately 80 to 100 bp from the CAP site, is a CACCC homology box that can be either inverted or duplicated.[7-26] These promotor sequences are also required for optimal transcription, and, as we shall see later, mutations in this region of the β-globin gene cause its defective expression. The globin genes also have conserved sequences in their 3' flanking regions, notably AATAAA, which is the polyadenylation signal site.

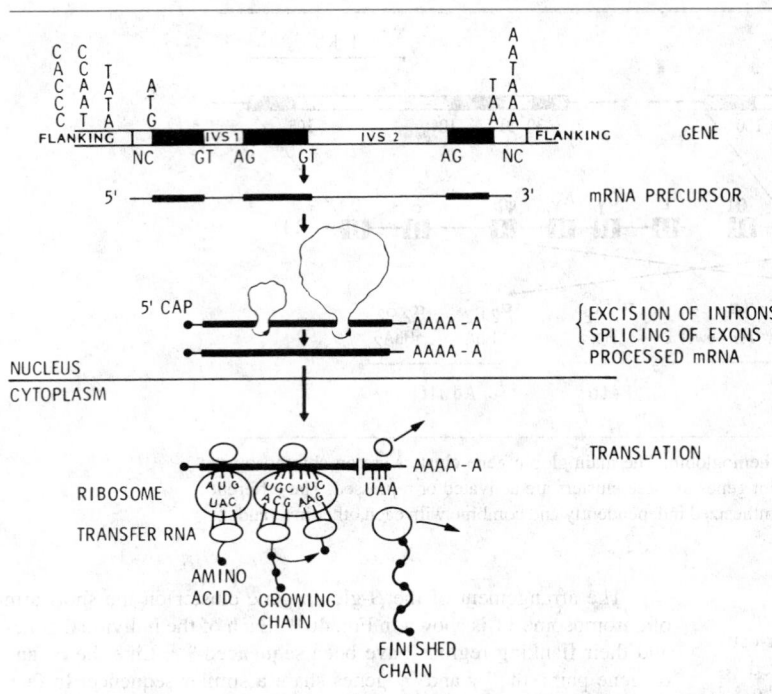

FIGURE 46-2   The expression of a human globin gene.

REGULATION OF GLOBIN GENE CLUSTERS

The mechanism of globin gene expression is summarized in detail in Fig. 46-2. In short, the primary transcript is a large mRNA precursor containing both intron and exon sequences. During its stay in the nucleus, it undergoes a good deal of processing that entails capping the 5' end and polyadenylation of the 3' end, both of which probably serve to stabilize the transcript (see Chap. 11). The intervening sequences are removed from the mRNA precursor in a complex two-stage process that relies on certain critical sequences at the intron-exon junctions.

The way in which the globin gene clusters are regulated is of major relevance to an understanding of the pathogenesis of the thalassemias. While many details remain to be worked out, studies carried out over the last few years have provided at least an outline of some of the major mechanisms of globin gene regulation.[10,26,27]

Most of the DNA within cells that is not involved in gene transcription is packaged into a compact form that is inaccessible to transcription factors and RNA polymerase. Transcriptional activity is characterized by a major change in the structure of the chromatin surrounding a particular gene. These alterations in chromatin structure can be identified by enhanced sensitivity to exogenous nucleases. Erythroid lineage–specific nuclease-hypersensitive sites are found at several locations in the β-globin gene cluster, which vary during different stages of development. In fetal life these sites are associated with the promoter regions of all four globin genes, while in adult erythroid cells the sites associated with the γ genes are absent. The methylation state of the genes also plays an important role in their ability to be expressed; in human and other animal tissues, the globin genes are extensively methylated in nonerythroid organs and are relatively undermethylated in hematopoietic tissues. The changes in chromatin configuration around the globin genes at different stages of development are reflected by alterations in their methylation state.[28]

In addition to the promoter elements mentioned earlier, several other important regulatory sequences have been identified in the globin gene clusters. For example, several enhancer sequences have been identified that are thought to be involved with tissue-specific expression. Their sequences are similar to the upstream activating sequences of the promoter elements. Both consist of a number of "modules," or motifs, that contain binding sites for transcriptional activators or repressors.[29] The enhancer sequences are thought to act by coming into spatial apposition with the promoter sequences to increase the efficiency of transcription of particular genes. It is now clear that transcriptional regulatory proteins may bind both to the promoter region of a gene and to the enhancer. It appears that some of these transcriptional proteins, GATA-1 and NFE-2, for example, are restricted to hematopoietic tissues.[30,31] These proteins may act to bring the promoter and the enhancer into close physical proximity, permitting transcription factors bound to the enhancer to interact with the transcriptional complex that forms near the TATA box. It seems likely that at least some of these hematopoietic gene transcription factors will turn out to be developmental stage specific.

Upstream from the embryonic globin genes in both the α- and β-gene clusters there is another set of erythroid-specific nuclease-hypersensitive sites. These mark the regions of particularly important control elements. In the case of the β-globin gene cluster, this region is marked by five hypersensitive sites.[32] The most 5' site (HS5) does not show tissue specificity, while HSs 1 through 4, which together form the locus control region (LCR), are largely erythroid specific. Each of the regions of the LCR contains a variety of binding sites for erythroid transcription factors. Although the precise function of the LCR is not known, it is undoubtedly required to establish a transcriptionally active domain spanning the entire globin gene cluster. The α-globin gene cluster also has a major regulatory element of this kind, in this case called HS40.[33] Its structure closely resembles HS2 of the β-globin gene cluster LCR; a 350-bp core fragment retains most of the activity and contains a duplicated NF-E2 binding site flanked by GATA-1 sites. Although deletions of this region inactivate the entire α globin gene cluster, its action must be fundamentally different from that of the β-globin LCR, since the chromatin structure of the α gene cluster is in an open conformation in all tissues.

Some forms of thalassemia result from deletions that involve these regulatory regions. In addition, the phenotypic effects of deletions of these gene clusters are strongly positional, which may reflect the relative distance of particular genes from the LCR and HS40.

DEVELOPMENTAL CHANGES IN GLOBIN GENE EXPRESSION

One aspect of the human globin genes that is of particular importance is the regulation of the switch from fetal to adult hemoglobin. Since many of the thalassemias and related disorders of the β-globin gene cluster are associated with persistent γ-chain synthesis, a full understanding of their pathophysiology must include an explanation for this important phenomenon, which plays a considerable role in modifying their phenotypic expression.

The complex topic of hemoglobin switching has been the subject of several extensive reviews.[7,9,10,34] β-Globin synthesis commences early during fetal life, at approximately 8 to 10 weeks' gestation. Subsequently, it continues at a low level, approximately 10 percent of the total non-α-globin chain production, up to about 36 weeks' gestation, after which it is considerably augmented. At the same time, γ-globin chain synthesis starts to decline so that at birth there are approximately equal amounts of γ- and β-globin chains produced. Over the first year of life there is a gradual decline in γ-chain synthesis, and by the end of the first year this amounts to less than 1 percent of the total non-α-globin chain output. In adults the small amount of hemoglobin F is confined to an erythrocyte population called F cells.

It is still not clear how this series of developmental switches is regulated. It is not organ specific but is synchronized throughout the developing hematopoietic tissues. Although environmental factors may be involved, the bulk of experimental evidence suggests that there is some form of "time clock" built into the hematopoietic stem cell. At the chromosomal level it appears that regulation occurs in a complex manner involving both developmental stage–specific *trans-*activating factors and the relative proximity of the different genes of the β-globin gene cluster to LAR. The elements involved in the stage-specific regulation of the human globin genes have not yet been identified.

Fetal hemoglobin synthesis may be reactivated at a low level in states of hematopoietic stress and occurs at higher levels in certain hematologic malignancies, notably juvenile myeloid leukemia. However, it is only in the hemoglobinopathies that high levels of hemoglobin F production are seen with any consistency in adult life.

MOLECULAR BASIS OF THE THALASSEMIAS

Once it became possible to clone and sequence the globin genes from patients with many different forms of thalassemia, it became clear that a wide spectrum of mutations underlie these conditions. A picture of remarkable heterogeneity has emerged. Indeed, it seems likely that the study of these disorders has already given us a fairly complete account of the repertoire of the types of molecular lesions that underlie human single-gene disorders. For more extensive coverage, the reader is referred to a number of recent monographs and reviews.[9,10,35,36]

β THALASSEMIA

β Thalassemia is extremely heterogeneous at the molecular level[35,36]; nearly 180 different mutations have been found in association with this phenotype. Broadly, they fall into deletions of the β-globin gene and nondeletional mutations that may affect the transcription, processing, or translation of β-globin messenger (Table 46-2 and Fig. 46-3). Each major population group has a different set of β thalassemia mutations, usually consisting of two or three that make up the bulk combined with large numbers of rare ones. Because of this pattern of distribution, only about 20 alleles account for the majority of all β thalassemia determinants.

Gene Deletions   At least seventeen different deletions affecting only the β genes have now been described.[10,36,37] With one exception, these are rare and appear to be isolated, single events; the 619-bp deletion at the 3' end of β gene is more common,[38] but even that is restricted to the Sind and Gujarati populations of Pakistan and India, where it accounts for approximately 50 percent β-thalassemia alleles.[39] The Indian 619-bp deletion removes the 3' end of the β gene but leaves the 5' end intact, while many of the other deletions remove the 5' end of the gene and leave the δ gene intact.[40–45] Homozygotes for these deletions have β° thalassemia. Heterozygotes for the Indian deletion have raised hemoglobin A2 and F levels identical to those seen in heterozygotes for the other common forms of β thalassemia. It is interesting, however, that heterozygotes for the other deletions all have unusually high hemoglobin A2 levels. The increased δ-chain production results from increased δ-gene transcription in *cis* to the deletion, possibly as a result of reduced competition from the deleted 5' β gene for transcription factors.

Transcriptional Mutations   Several different base substitutions have been found that involve the conserved sequences upstream from the β-globin gene.[35,36] In every case the phenotype is β⁺ thalassemia, although there is considerable variability in the clinical severity associated with different mutations of this type. Several of them, at positions

TABLE 46-2   MOLECULAR PATHOLOGY OF THE β THALASSEMIAS

β⁰ or β⁺ Thalassemia

Gene deletions
Promoter regions
CAP site
5'-untranslated region
Intron-exon boundaries
Splice site consensus sequences
Cryptic sites in exons
Cryptic sites in introns
Poly(A) signal
Translation of β-globin mRNA
   Initiation
   Nonsense
   Frameshift
Unstable β-globin chains

Normal Hb A2 β Thalassemia

β Thalassemia + δ thalassemia, *cis* or *trans*
"Silent" β thalassemia
   Some promoter mutations
   CAP + 1
   CAP + 33
   5'-untranslated regions
   Splice mutation IVS II 844 C to G
   Termination codon + 6

Dominant β Thalassemia

Single-base substitutions; highly unstable products
Codon deletions
Premature termination, exon 3
Frameshifts; elongated, unstable products

NOTE: A full list of mutations is given in Ref. 36.

−88 and −87 relative to the mRNA CAP site, for example,[46,47] are close to the CCAAT box, while the others lie within the ATA box homology.[48–51]

Some of the mutations upstream from the β-globin gene are associated with even more subtle alterations in phenotype. For example, a C→T substitution at position −101, which involves one of the upstream promotor elements, is associated with "silent" β thalassemia, that is, a completely normal phenotype that can be identified only by its interaction with more severe forms of β thalassemia in compound heterozygotes.[52] A single example of an A → C substitution at the CAP site (+1) was described in an Asian Indian who, despite being homozygous for the mutation, appeared to have the phenotype of the β-thalassemia trait.[53]

The upstream regulatory mutations confirm the importance of the conserved sequences in this region in their role as regulators of the transcription of the β-globin genes and provide the basis for some of the mildest forms of β thalassemia, particularly those in African populations.

RNA-Processing Mutations   One of the surprises about β-thalassemia has been the remarkable diversity of the single-base mutations that can interfere with the intranuclear processing of mRNA.

The boundaries of exons and introns are marked by invariant dinucleotides, GT at the 5' (donor) and AG at the 3' (receptor) sites. Single-base changes that involve either of these splice junctions totally abolish normal RNA splicing and result in the phenotype of β⁰ thalassemia.[36,47,50,54–58]

Surrounding the invariant dinucleotides at the splice junctions are highly conserved sequences that are involved in mRNA processing. Different varieties of β thalassemia involve single-base substitutions within the consensus sequence of the IVS-1 donor site.[36,47,50,54,55,59–61] These mutations are of particular interest because of the remarkable variability in their associated phenotypes. For example, substitution

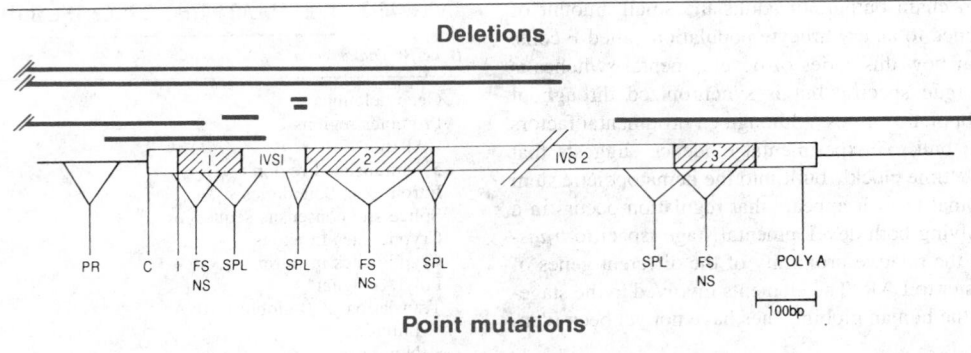

FIGURE 46-3   The classes of mutations that underlie β thalassemia. PR, promoter; C, CAP site; I, initiation site; FS, frameshift; NS, nonsense mutation; SPL, splicing mutation; POLY A, polyA addition site mutation.

of the G in position 5 of IVS-1 by C or T results in severe β⁺ thalassemia.[47] On the other hand, a T → C change at position 6, found commonly in the Mediterranean region,[62] results in a very mild form of β⁺ thalassemia. The G → C change at position 5 has also been found in Melanesia and appears to be the most common cause of β thalassemia in Papua New Guinea.[63]

RNA processing is also affected by mutations that create new splice sites within either introns or exons. Again, these lesions are remarkably variable in their phenotypic effect, depending on the degree to which the new site is utilized compared with the normal splice site. For example, the G → A substitution at position 110 of IVS-1, which is one of the most common forms of β thalassemia in the Mediterranean region, leads to only about 10 percent splicing at the normal site and hence results in a phenotype of severe β⁺ thalassemia.[64,65] Similarly, a mutation that produces a new acceptor site at position 116 in IVS-1 results in little or no β-globin mRNA production and the phenotype of β⁰ thalassemia.[66] Several mutations have been described that generate new donor sites within IVS-2 of the β-globin gene.[36,47,60]

Another interesting mechanism for abnormal splicing is the activation of donor sites within exons (Fig. 46-4). For example, within exon 1 there is a cryptic donor site in the region of codons 24 through 27. This site contains a GT dinucleotide; an adjacent substitution that alters it so that it more closely resembles the consensus donor splice site results in its activation, even though the normal site is active. Several mutations in this region can activate this site so that it is utilized during RNA processing, with the production of abnormal

mRNAs.[66–70] Three of them, A → G in codon 19, G → A in codon 26, and G → T in codon 27, result in both reduced production of β-globin mRNA and an amino acid substitution, so that the mRNA that is spliced normally is translated into protein. The abnormal hemoglobins produced are hemoglobins Malay, E, and Knossos, respectively, all of which are associated with a β-thalassemia phenotype, presumably due to the reduced overall output of normal mRNA. A variety of other cryptic splice mutations within introns and exons have been described.[35,36]

Another class of processing mutations involves the polyadenylation signal site AAUAAA in the 3′ untranslated region of β-globin mRNA.[71–73] For example, a T → C substitution in this sequence leads to the transcription of only a tenth of the normal amount of β-globin mRNA and hence in the phenotype of severe β⁺ thalassemia.[71]

Mutations That Cause Abnormal Translation of Messenger RNA   Base substitutions that change an amino acid codon into a chain termination codon, nonsense mutations, prevent translation of the mRNA and result in β⁰ thalassemia. Many substitutions of this type have been described,[36] a codon 17 mutation being common in Southeast Asia[74,75] and a codon 39 mutation occurring at a high frequency in the Mediterranean region.[76,77]

The insertion or deletion of one, two, or four nucleotides in the coding region of β-globin gene disrupts the normal reading frame and results, on translation of the mRNA, in the addition of anomalous amino acids until a termination codon is reached in the new reading frame. Several frameshift mutations of this type have been described,[36] and two, the insertion of one nucleotide between codons 8 and 9 and a deletion of four nucleotides in codons 41 and 42, are common in Asian Indians,[55] with the latter also being found frequently in different populations in Southeast Asia.[75]

Dominantly Inherited β Thalassemia   Over the past 20 years there have been sporadic reports of families in which a picture indistinguishable from moderately severe β thalassemia has segregated in Mendelian dominant fashion.[78,79] Because this condition is often characterized by the presence of inclusion bodies in the red cell precursors, it has been called inclusion body β thalassemia, although, since all severe forms of β thalassemia have inclusions in the red cell precursors, the term dominantly inherited β thalassemia is preferred.[80] Sequence analysis has shown that these conditions are heterogeneous at the molecular level

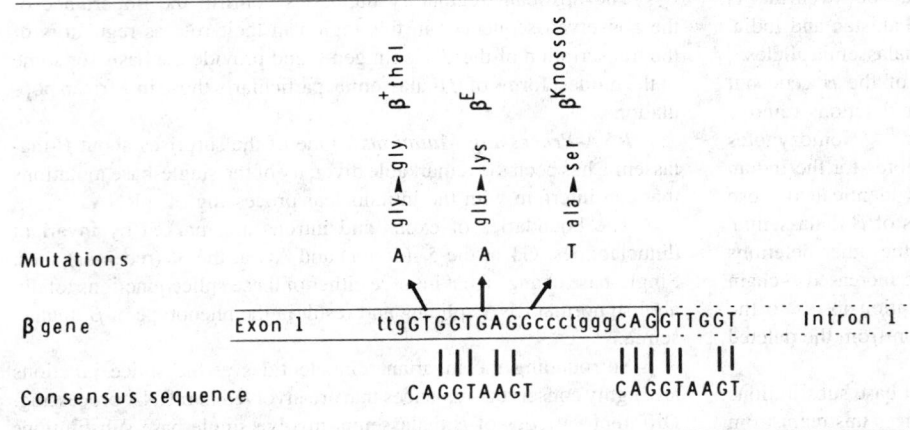

FIGURE 46-4   The activation of cryptic splice sites in exon 1 as the cause of β⁺ thalassemia, Hb E, and Hb Knossos. The similarities between the 5′ splice region of intron 1 and the cryptic splice region in exon 1 are shown in capitals.

TABLE 46-3   SOME MOLECULAR FORMS OF DOMINANT β THALASSEMIA AND STRUCTURAL VARIANTS ASSOCIATED WITH A β THALASSEMIA PHENOTYPE

MUTATION	EXON	PHENOTYPE	DESIGNATION	RACE
Dominant β Thalassemia				
Codons 128 −4 bp, +5 bp −11 bp F/S terminates codon 154	III	Thalassemia intermedia, inclusion bodies	—	Irish
Codon 121 GAA → TAA*	III	Thalassemia intermedia, inclusion bodies	—	Swiss-French, Greek-Polish
Codon 127 CAG → TAG	III	Thalassemia intermedia	—	English
Codon 114 −CT +G F/S terminates codon 15	III	Thalassemia intermedia	β Geneva	Swiss-French
Codon 126 −T F/S terminates codon 157*	III	Thalassemia intermedia, inclusion bodies	β Vercelli	Italian
Codon 94 +TG F/S terminates codon 157*	II	Severe thalassemia intermedia, inclusion bodies	β Agnana	Italian
Codon 123 −A F/S terminates codon 157	III	Thalassemia intermedia, inclusion bodies	β Makabe	Japanese
Codons 123–125 −8 bp β chain 135 residues	III	Severe thalassemia intermedia with Hb E, inclusion bodies	β Khon Kaen	Thai
Codon 127 Gln → Pro	III	Thalassemia intermedia	β Houston	British
Codons 109–110 −G F/S terminates codon 157	III	Thalassemia intermedia	β Manhattan	Ashkenazi Jew
Codons 32/34 −GGT*	II	Thalassemia intermedia	β Korea	Korean
Codon 106 Leu → Arg†	III	Thalassemia intermedia	β Terre Haute	European
Codon 28 Leu → Arg	I	Thalassemia intermedia, inclusion bodies	β Chesterfield	English
Codon 60 Val → Glu	II	Thalassemia intermedia	β Cagliari	Italian
Thalassemia Trait				
Codon 110 Leu → Pro	III	β-Thalassemia trait	β Showa-Yakushiji	Japanese
Codons 127/128 −3 bp β chain 145 residues	III	β-Thalassemia trait	β Gunma	Japanese
β132 Lys → Gln	III	β-Thalassemia trait	β K Woolwich	British
β134 Lys → Gln	III	Mild microcytosis, Hb S/β-thalassemia interaction with Hb S	Hb North Shore-Caracas	

De novo mutations.
†Originally reported as Hb Indianapolis.
ABBREVIATIONS: F/S, frameshift.
SOURCE: From THJ Huisman et al[36] and SL Thein et al.[80]

but that many of them involve mutations of exon 3 of the β-globin gene (Table 46-3). These include frameshifts, premature chain termination mutations, and complex rearrangements that lead to the synthesis of truncated or elongated and highly unstable β-globin gene products.[18–89] The most common mutation of this type is a GAA → TAA change at codon 121 that leads to the synthesis of a truncated β-globin chain.[85] Although it is unusual to demonstrate an abnormal β-chain product from loci affected by mutations of this type, many of these conditions have been designated as hemoglobin variants (see Table 46-3). As will be described in greater detail later, these β-globin products are unable to form a viable β chain and precipitate together with excess α chains in the marrow.

Unstable β-Globin Variants   Some β-globin chain variants, although highly unstable, are capable of forming a viable tetramer. The resulting unstable hemoglobins may be precipitated in the red cell precursors or in the blood and hence give rise to a spectrum of conditions ranging from dominantly inherited β thalassemia to a hemolytic anemia similar to those associated with other unstable hemoglobins. The first of these to be described, hemoglobin Indianapolis,[90] had its structure characterized by DNA analysis carried out on stored autopsy material; the original description turned out to be incorrect (see Table 46-3).[91]

Silent β Thalassemia   It is now clear that there are a number of extremely mild β thalassemia alleles that are either silent or almost unidentifiable in heterozygotes (see Table 46-2). As mentioned earlier, some of these are in the region of the promoter boxes of the β-globin gene, but others involve the CAP sites or the 5' or 3' untranslated regions.[35,36] These alleles are usually identified by the finding of a form of β thalassemia intermedia in which one parent has a typical thalassemia trait while the other appears to be normal but, in fact, is a carrier of one of these mild β-thalassemia alleles.

β-Thalassemia Mutations Unlinked to the β-Globin Gene Cluster   Although several family studies have suggested that there may

be mutations that result in the phenotype of β thalassemia that do not segregate with the β-globin genes,[92] their molecular basis has not yet been determined. The evidence for the existence of novel mutations of this type has been reviewed recently.[7,35]

Variant Forms of β Thalassemia   There are several forms of β thalassemia in which the level of hemoglobin A_2 is normal in heterozygotes.[10] In some cases these are due to "silent" β thalassemia alleles, while others reflect the coinheritance of β and δ thalassemia.

$\delta\beta$ THALASSEMIA

The ($\delta\beta$) thalassemias are classified into the ($\delta\beta$)$^+$ and ($\delta\beta$)^o thalassemias (Table 46-4). The ($\delta\beta$)^o thalassemias are further divided into those in which both the δ- and β-globin genes are deleted, ($\delta\beta$)^o thalassemia, and those in which the $^G\gamma$, δ, and β genes are deleted, ($^A\gamma\delta\beta$)^o thalassemia. Because many different deletion forms of $\delta\beta$ thalassemia have been described, they are further classified according to the country in which they were first identified (Table 46-4).

($\delta\beta$)^o and ($^A\gamma\delta\beta$)^o Thalassemia   Nearly all these conditions result from deletions that involve varying lengths of the β-globin gene cluster. Many different varieties have been described in different populations (see Table 46-4), although their heterozygous and homozygous phenotypes are very similar.[7,35,36,93] Rare forms of these conditions are due to more complex gene rearrangements. For example, one form of ($^A\gamma\delta\beta$)^o thalassemia, found in Indian populations, is not due to a simple linear deletion but, rather, it results from a complex rearrangement with two deletions, one affecting the $^A\gamma$ gene and the other the δ and β genes; the intervening region is intact but inverted.[94] Some of these conditions are illustrated in Fig. 46-5.

($\delta\beta$)$^+$ Thalassemia   The ($\delta\beta$)$^+$ thalassemias are usually associated with the production of structural hemoglobin variants called Lepore.[7,9,10] Hemoglobin Lepore contains normal α chains and non-α chains that consist of the first 50 to 80 amino acid residues of the δ chains and the last 60 to 90 residues of the normal C-terminal amino

TABLE 46-4   THE $\delta\beta$ THALASSEMIAS

($\delta\beta$)⁺ Thalassemia

Hb Lepore thalassemia
   Hb Lepore Washington-Boston
   Hb Lepore Hollandia
   Hb Lepore Baltimore
Phenocopies of ($\delta\beta$)⁺ thalassemia
   Sardinian $\delta\beta$ thalassemia
   Corfu $\delta\beta$ thalassemia
   Chinese $\delta\beta$ thalassemia
   β Thalassemia with δ thalassemia

($\delta\beta$)⁰ Thalassemia

Sicilian
Indian
Japanese
Spanish
Black
Eastern European
Macedonian
Turkish
Laotian
Thai

(${}^A\gamma\delta\beta$)⁰ Thalassemia

Indian
German
Cantonese
Turkish
Malay 2
Belgian
Black
Chinese
Yunnanese
Thai
Italian

---

acid sequence of the β chains. Thus, the Lepore non-α chain is a $\delta\beta$ fusion chain. Several different varieties of hemoglobin Lepore have been described—Washington-Boston, Baltimore, and Hollandia—in which the transition from δ to β sequences occurs at different points.[7,10] The fusion chains have probably arisen by nonhomologous crossing over between part of the δ locus on one chromosome and part of the β locus on the complementary chromosome (Fig. 46-6). This event results from misalignment of chromosome pairing during meiosis so that a δ-chain gene pairs with a β-chain gene instead of with its homologous partner.[95] As shown in Fig. 46-6, such a mechanism should give rise to two abnormal chromosomes: the first, the Lepore chromosome, will have no normal δ or β loci but simply a $\delta\beta$ fusion gene. On the opposite of the homologous pairs of chromosomes there should be an anti-Lepore ($\beta\delta$) fusion gene together with normal δ and β loci. A variety of anti-Lepore–like hemoglobins have been discovered, including hemoglobins Miyada, P-Congo, Lincoln Park, and P-Nilotic.[9,10] All the hemoglobin Lepore disorders are characterized by a severe form of $\delta\beta$ thalassemia; the output of the γ-globin genes on the chromosome with the $\delta\beta$ fusion gene is not increased sufficiently to compensate for the low output of the $\delta\beta$ fusion product. The reduced rate of production of the $\delta\beta$ fusion chains of hemoglobin Lepore presumably reflects the fact that its genetic determinant has the δ gene promoter region, which is structurally different from the β-globin gene promoter and associated with a reduced rate of transcription of its gene product.

$\delta\beta$ Thalassemia–like Disorders Due to Two Mutations in the β-Globin Gene Cluster   A heterogeneous group of nondeletion $\delta\beta$ thalassemias has been described, most of which result from two mutations in the $\varepsilon\gamma\delta\beta$-globin gene cluster (see Table 46-4). Strictly speak-

ing, they are not all $\delta\beta$ thalassemias, but because their phenotypes resemble the deletion forms of ($\delta\beta$)⁰ thalassemia, they often appear in the literature under this title. In the Sardinian form of $\delta\beta$ thalassemia, the β-globin gene has the common Mediterranean codon 39 nonsense mutation that leads to an absence of β-globin synthesis. However, there is relatively high expression of the ${}^A\gamma$ gene in cis, which gives this condition the phenotype $\delta\beta$ thalassemia; this is because there is a point mutation at position −196 upstream from the ${}^A\gamma$ gene (see "Hereditary Persistence of Fetal Hemoglobin"). The phenotypic picture, in which heterozygotes have 15 to 20 percent hemoglobin F and normal levels of hemoglobin A₂, is identical to that of $\delta\beta$ thalassemia.[96] Another condition that has the phenotype $\delta\beta$ thalassemia, with over 20 percent hemoglobin F in heterozygotes, has been described in a Chinese patient in whom defective β-globin–chain synthesis appears to be due to an A → G change in the ATA sequence in the promoter region of the β-globin gene.[97] However, the increased γ-chain synthesis, which appears to involve both ${}^G\gamma$ and ${}^A\gamma$ cis to this mutation, remains unexplained. A disorder that was originally called $\delta\beta$ thalassemia has been described in the Corfu population.[98,99] Again, this results from two mutations in the β-globin gene cluster. First, there is a 7201-bp deletion that starts in the δ-globin gene, IVS-2, position 818–822, and extends upstream to a 5′ breakpoint located 1719 to 1722 bp 3′ to the $\psi\beta$-gene termination codon. In addition there is a G → A mutation at position 5 in the donor site consensus region of IVS-1 of the β-globin gene. The output from this chromosome consists of relatively high levels of γ chains with very low levels of β chains. This condition resembles $\delta\beta$ thalassemia in the homozygous state, in which there is almost 100 percent hemoglobin F, with traces of hemoglobin A but no hemoglobin A₂; heterozygotes have only slightly elevated levels of hemoglobin F, and the phenotype is similar to "normal A₂ β thalassemia."

$\varepsilon\gamma\delta\beta$ THALASSEMIA

These rare conditions[100–106] result from long deletions that begin upstream from the β-gene complex 55 kb or more 5′ to the ε gene and terminate within the cluster (see Fig. 46-5). In two cases, designated Dutch[103,104] and English,[105] the deletions leave the β-globin gene intact, but no β-chain production occurs even though the gene is expressed in heterologous systems.

The molecular basis for the inactivation of the β-globin gene cis to these deletions was clarified by the discovery of the LCR about 50 kb upstream from the $\varepsilon\gamma\delta\beta$-globin gene cluster (see "Regulation of Globin Gene Clusters"). The removal of this critical regulatory region seems to completely inactivate the downstream globin gene complex. The Hispanic form of $\varepsilon\gamma\delta\beta$ thalassemia[106] results from a deletion that includes most of the LAR, including four of the five DNase-1–hypersensitive sites. These lesions appear to close down the chromatin domain that is usually open in erythroid tissues. They also delay the replication of the β-globin genes in the cell cycle. Thus, although they are rare, they have been of considerable importance, since it was the analysis of the Dutch deletion that first pointed to the possibility of there being a major control region upstream from the β-like–globin gene cluster and ultimately led to the discovery of the β-globin LCR.

HEREDITARY PERSISTENCE OF FETAL HEMOGLOBIN

This heterogeneous group of conditions produces phenotypes very similar to those of the $\delta\beta$ thalassemias except that defective β-chain production appears to be almost, although in some forms not completely, compensated by persistent γ-chain production. These conditions are best classified into deletion and nondeletion forms (Table 46-5). Although in the past it was customary to further classify them into pancellular and heterocellular varieties, depending on the intercellular distribution of fetal hemoglobin, this now appears to bear little

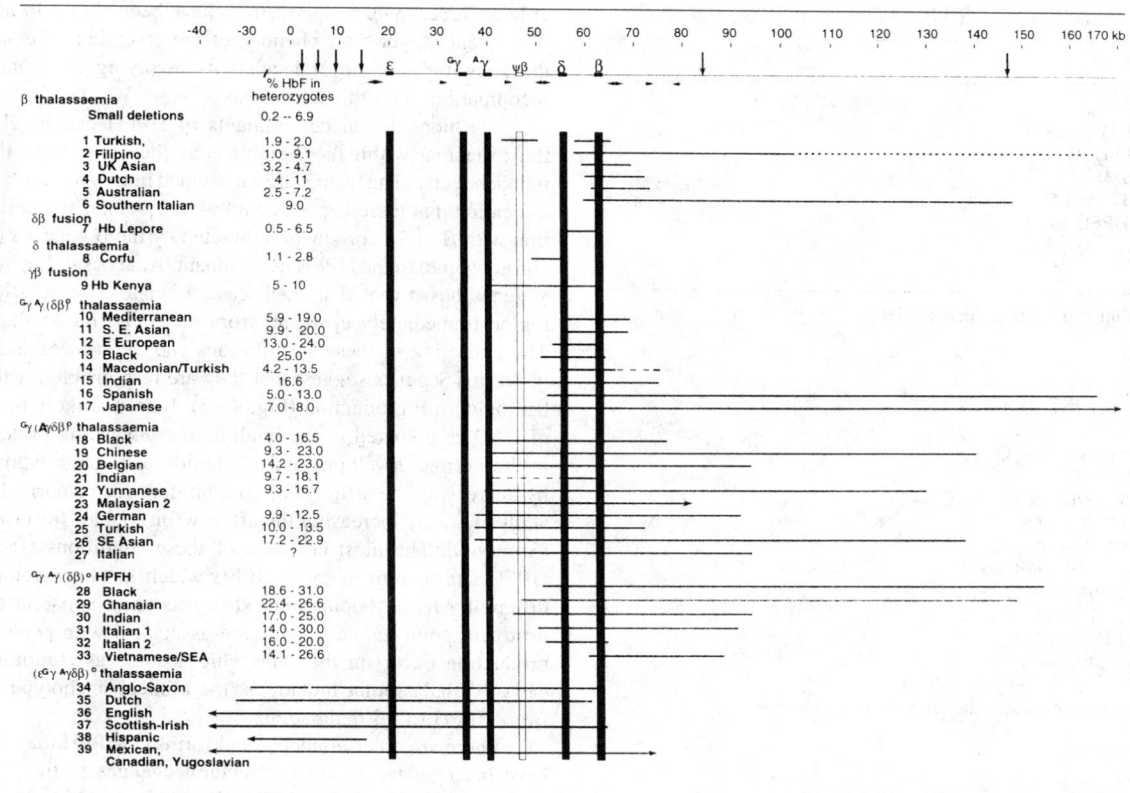

FIGURE 46-5   The various deletions that are responsible for the β and δβ thalassemias and hereditary persistence of fetal hemoglobin.

relevance to their molecular basis and probably relates more to the particular level of fetal hemoglobin and to the way in which its cellular distribution is determined.[7]

The deletion forms of HPFH are heterogeneous (see Fig. 46-5). The two African varieties are due to extensive deletions of similar length (<70 kb) but with staggered ends, differing phenotypically only in the proportions of $^G\gamma$ and $^A\gamma$ chains produced.[107] Another type of HPFH results from misalignment during crossing over between the $^A\gamma$ and β-globin genes, resulting in the production of $^A\gamma\beta$ fusion genes (see Fig. 46-6). The latter give rise to γβ fusion products that combine with α chains to form the hemoglobin variant called hemoglobin Kenya.[108,109] This is associated with an increased output of hemoglobin F, although at a lower level than the deletion forms of HPFH described above. So far, it has not been possible to develop a theory that provides an adequate explanation for the phenotypic differences between δβ thalassemia and the deletion forms of HPFH. As mentioned earlier, they form a continuum of conditions that differ only in the relative output of γ chains directed by the chromosome carrying a particular deletion. Based on the observation that as a group the HPFH deletions tend to extend farther upstream than do those that produce δβ thalassemia, attempts have been made to define putative regulatory regions in the β-globin gene cluster that may or may not be involved in their particular deletions.[98,110] For example, the 5' ends of the HPFH and δβ-thalassemia deletions that lie closest together have been ana-

lyzed in detail. It has been found that the two deletions end in a pair of Alu 1 repeats 5' to the δ gene.[98,110] The HPFH deletion ends in the 5' Alu 1 repeat of the bipolar pair, while the δβ-thalassemia deletion ends in the 3' Alu 1 repeat. Thus, the two deletions have endpoints that are within 500 nucleotides of each other; the larger deletion causes a significantly higher output of γ chains than does the smaller one.

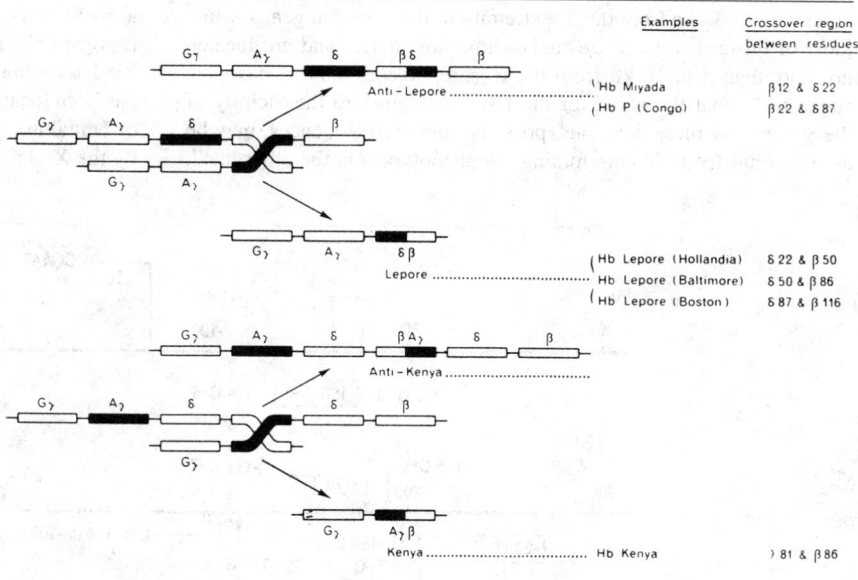

FIGURE 46-6   The mechanisms of the production of the Lepore and anti-Lepore hemoglobins and Hb Kenya.

TABLE 46-5   HEREDITARY PERSISTENCE OF FETAL HEMOGLOBIN

Deletion (Pancellular*)

$(\delta\beta)^0$
  Black (HPFH 1)
  Ghanaian (HPFH 2)
  Indian (HPFH 3)
  Italian (HPFH 4 and 5)
  Vietnamese (HPFH 6)
$^G\gamma(^A\gamma\beta)^+$ (Hb Kenya)

Nondeletion

Linked to β-globin gene cluster (pancellular*)
  $^G\gamma\beta^+$
    Black $^G\gamma$-202 C $\rightarrow$ G
    Tunisian $^G\gamma$-200+C
    Black/Sardinian $^G\gamma$-175 T $\rightarrow$ C
    Japanese $^G\gamma$-114 C $\rightarrow$ T
    Australian $^G\gamma$-114 C $\rightarrow$ G
  $^A\gamma\beta^+$
    Greek/Sardinian/Black $^A\gamma$-117 G $\rightarrow$ A
    British $^A\gamma$-198 T $\rightarrow$ C
    Black $^A\gamma$-202 C $\rightarrow$ T
    Italian/Chinese $^A\gamma$-196 C $\rightarrow$ T
    Brazilian $^A\gamma$-195 C $\rightarrow$ G
    Black $^A\gamma$-175 T $\rightarrow$ C
    Black $^A\gamma$-114 to −102 (del)
    Georgia $^A\gamma$-114 C $\rightarrow$ T
  $^G\gamma$ $^A\gamma\beta^+$
Linked to β-globin gene cluster (heterocellular*)
  Atlanta
  Czech
  Seattle
  Others (including some cases of $^G\gamma$-158 T $\rightarrow$ C)
Unlinked to β-globin gene cluster (heterocellular*)
  Chromosome 6
  Others

*The intercellular distribution of Hb F is not always reported, and there are some inconsistencies within groups.

Therefore, unless the two different phenotypes result from differences in the DNA sequences at the 3′ end of the deletions, the 5′ *Alu* 1 repeat and the nonrepetitive DNA connecting it to the 3′ *Alu* repeat must be considered to play an important regulatory role. Alternatively, it has been pointed out that the deletions that cause HPFH are situated at least 52 to 57 kb from the 3′ extremity of the β-globin genes, while most of those that cause $\delta\beta$ thalassemia are shorter and are located no more than 5 to 10 kb from the β gene. Accordingly, it has been suggested[107] that the nature of the DNA brought into the vicinity of the γ genes by these deletions, possibly enhancer sequences, may be an important factor in determining the phenotype. On the other hand,

at least three $(^A\gamma\delta\beta)^0$ thalassemias have been shown to have different 3′ sequences, yet their phenotypes are essentially the same. In fact, the phenotypes of several deletions involving this gene cluster are incompatible with this hypothesis.

The nondeletion determinants of HPFH can be classified into those that map within the β-globin gene cluster and those that segregate independently. The former are subdivided into $^G\gamma\beta^+$ and $^A\gamma\beta^+$ varieties, indicating that there is persistent $^G\gamma$- or $^A\gamma$-chain synthesis in association with β-globin production directed by the β gene *cis* (on the same chromosome) to the HPFH determinant. Analysis of the overexpressed γ genes has revealed in each case a single-base substitution in the region immediately upstream from the transcription start site.[36,111–114] The clustering of these substitutions and the lack of similar changes in normal γ genes suggest that they are responsible for the persistent hemoglobin F production (Fig. 46-7). It seems likely that this region of DNA is involved in the binding of *trans*-acting proteins involved in the normal developmental repression of γ-gene expression, either by decreasing the affinity for an inhibitory factor normally present in adult life or by increasing the affinity for a factor for promoting gene expression. The most common of these conditions are Greek $^A\gamma\beta^+$ HPFH and a form of $^G\gamma\beta^+$ HPFH which has been found in several different African populations. It is becoming apparent that, if these upstream point mutations that are associated with persistent γ-chain production occur on the same chromosome as β-globin genes that carry β^0 thalassemia mutations, the clinical phenotype is converted from HPFH to $\delta\beta$ thalassemia.

There are other nondeletional forms of HPFH that in some cases have been related to small structural changes in the β-globin gene cluster (see Table 46-4). Although strictly speaking not a true form of HPFH, since even in homozygotes it may not be associated with increased levels of hemoglobin F, the T $\rightarrow$ C polymorphism at position −158 to the $^G\gamma$-globin gene[115] may, under conditions of erythropoietic stress, be associated with an increased output of hemoglobin F.

There are other forms of HPFH characterized by the persistence of low levels of fetal hemoglobin production distributed in a heterocellular manner. In all populations studied, a small proportion of individuals have an increased amount of hemoglobin F and F cells, that is, red cells that can be detected when blood films are treated with antibodies against hemoglobin F. Although this condition was originally called the Swiss form of HPFH because it was first recognized in Swiss army recruits,[116] it has now been observed in every racial group. There is some evidence that at least one genetic determinant is responsible for determining the number of F cells is X-linked, and a putative locus has been located at Xp22.2.[117,118] However, it is clear that not all forms of hereditary persistence of low levels of hemoglobin F are encoded by the X chromosome.[119–122] In studies of a large pedigree in which a

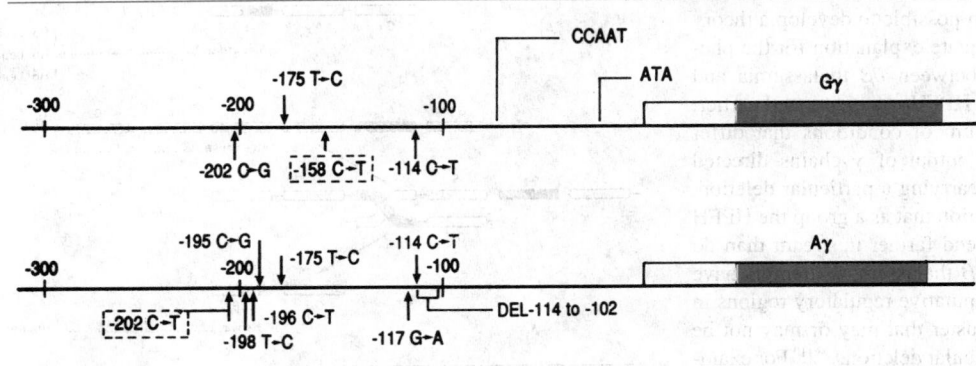

FIGURE 46-7   Some of the upstream point mutations associated with hereditary persistence of fetal hemoglobin.

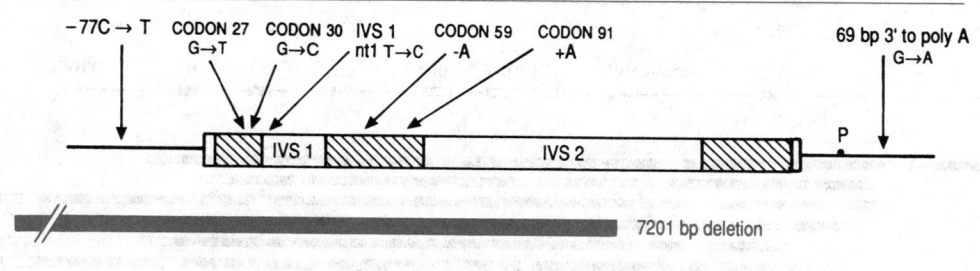

FIGURE 46-8   The molecular basis of some of the δ thalassemias (references to original descriptions in Ref. 36).

form of HPFH segregated independently from β thalassemia, the genetic determinant has been localized to chromosome 6q23.[123] However, further studies have indicated that similar forms of HPFH are not linked to chromosome 6.[124] It seems likely that these different forms of HPFH that are unlinked to the β-globin gene cluster reflect mutations of transcription factors that are involved in the switch from fetal to adult hemoglobin production. The importance of these conditions lies in the fact that, when they are inherited together with the sickle-cell or β-thalassemia genes, they may increase the output of hemoglobin F to such an extent that they modify the phenotype of the associated disorders.

δ THALASSEMIA

Several point mutations and deletions that reduce δ-globin synthesis have been described. They are summarized in Fig. 46-8.

α THALASSEMIA

The different classes of α thalassemia are summarized in Table 46-6. The α-globin gene haplotype can be written $\alpha\alpha$, indicating the α_2 and α_1 genes, respectively. A normal individual has the genotype

TABLE 46-6   CLASSES OF MUTATIONS THAT CAUSE α THALASSEMIA[+]

α^0 Thalassemia

Deletions involving α-globin gene cluster
Truncations of telomeric region of 16p
Deletions of HS40 region

α^+ Thalassemia

Deletions involving α_2 or α_1 genes
Point mutations involving α_2 or α_1 genes
  mRNA processing
    IVS 1 donor
    IVS 1 acceptor
    Poly(A) signal
  mRNA translation
    Initiation codon
    Exon I or II
    Termination codon
  Posttranslational
    Unstable α globin

α Thalassemia Mental Retardation

ATR-16
  Deletions or telomeric truncations of 16p
  Translocations
ATR-X
  Mutations of *XH2*
    Deletions
    Missense
    Nonsense
    Splice site

NOTE: Complete lists of individual mutations are found in Refs. 7, 10, and 36.

$\alpha\alpha/\alpha\alpha$. A deletion involving one $(-\alpha)$ or both $(--)$ α genes can be further classified on the basis of its size, written as a superscript; thus, $-\alpha^{3.7}$ indicates a deletion of 3.7 kb including one α gene. When the sizes of the deletions have not yet been established, a superscript describing their geographic or family origin is useful; thus, $--^{MED}$ describes a deletion of both α genes first identified in individuals of Mediterranean origin. In those thalassemia haplotypes where both genes are intact, that is, nondeletion lesions, the nomenclature $\alpha^T\alpha$ is given, the superscript T indicating that this gene is thalassemic. However, when the precise molecular defect is known, as in hemoglobin Constant Spring, for example, $\alpha^T\alpha$ can be replaced by the more informative $\alpha^{CS}\alpha$. The molecular pathology and population genetics of the α thalassemias have been the subject of several extensive reviews.[7,36,125]

α^0 Thalassemia   To date, 14 deletions that involve both α genes, and therefore abolish α-chain production from the affected chromosome, have been described (Fig. 46-9).[7,36] Several of the 3' breakpoints fall within a 6- to 8-kb region at the 3' end of the α-globin complex, suggesting that this may represent a breakpoint cluster region with a high level of recombination.[126] In at least five of the deletions, the 5' breakpoints also appear to cluster. This gives rise to a situation in which the 5' breakpoints are located approximately the same distance apart and in the same order along a chromosome as their respective 3' breakpoints. It is possible that such staggered deletions may have arisen from illegitimate recombination events that delete an integral number of chromatin loops as they pass through their nuclear attachment points during replication, a mechanism that has also been suggested to underlie some of the deletion forms of HPFH.[127] One of these deletions $(--^{MED})$ involves a more complex rearrangement that introduces a new piece of DNA bridging the two breakpoints in the α-gene cluster. This new sequence originates upstream from the α cluster and appears to have been replicated into the junction in a manner that suggests that the upstream segment of DNA also lies at the base of a replication loop. At least some of these deletions seem to have arisen by recombination events between *Alu* repeat sequences.

Several other mechanisms for the generation of α^0 thalassemia have been identified.[7,125] In some cases this condition results from a terminal truncation of the short arm of chromosome 16 to a site 50 kb distal to the α-globin genes.[128] It is interesting to note that the telomeric consensus sequence (TTAGGGG)n has been added directly to the site of the break. Since this mutation is stably inherited, it appears that telomeric DNA alone is sufficient to stabilize the broken chromosome end. This observation raises the possibility that other genetic diseases may result from chromosomal truncations.

Several deletions have now been identified that appear to downregulate the α-globin genes by removal of the α-globin locus control region (HS40).[7,129,130] In each case the α-globin genes have been left intact, although in one the 3' breakpoint is found between the ξ_2 and $\psi\xi_1$ genes, thus removing the ξ_2 gene.[129] It appears that these deletions completely inactivate the α-globin gene complex, just as deletions of the β-globin LAR inactivate the entire β-gene complex. So far, such

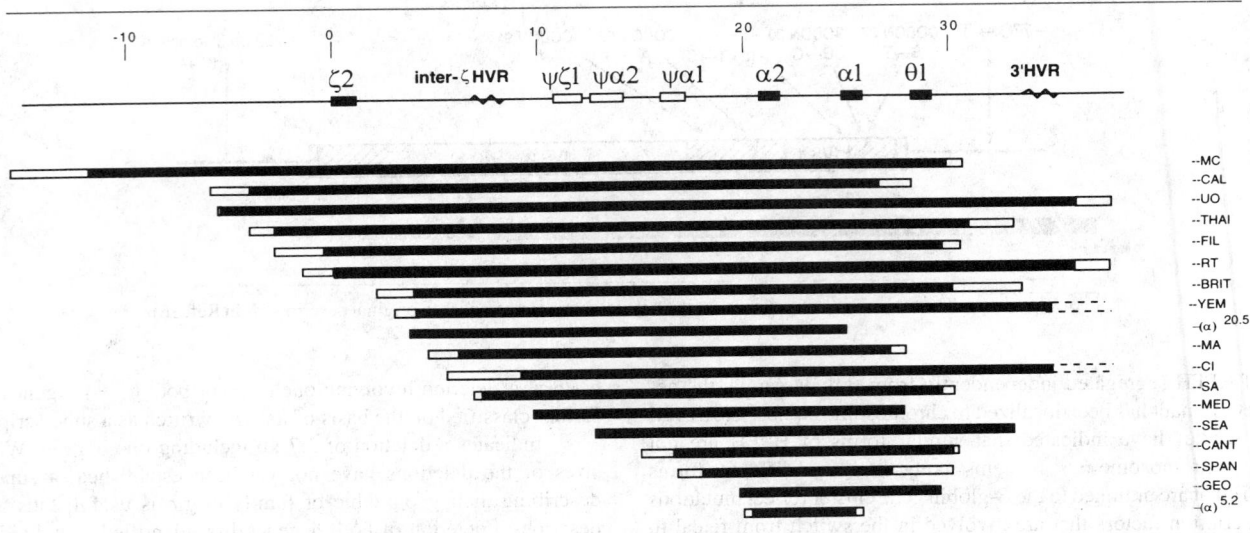

FIGURE 46-9   The deletions of the α globin gene cluster that are responsible for α° thalassemia. Deletions: MC = initials of patient; CAL = initials of patient; THAI = Thai; FIL = Filipino; CI = Conway Islands; BRIT = UK; SA = South Africa; MED = Mediterranean; SEA = Southeast Asian; SPAN = Spanish.

deletions have not been observed in the homozygous state, presumably because they would be lethal.

α⁺ Thalassemia Gene Deletions   The most common forms of α⁺ thalassemia ($\alpha^{3.7}$ and $-\alpha^{4.2}$) involve the deletion of one or the other of the duplicated α-globin genes (Fig. 46-10).

Each α gene is located within a region of homology approximately 4 kb long, interrupted by two nonhomologous regions. It is thought that the homologous regions have resulted from an ancient duplication

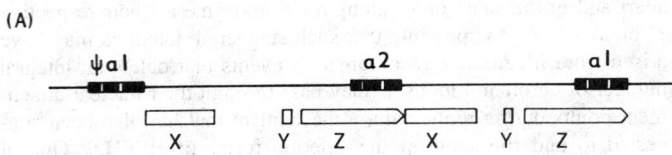

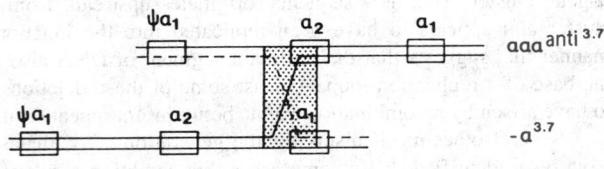

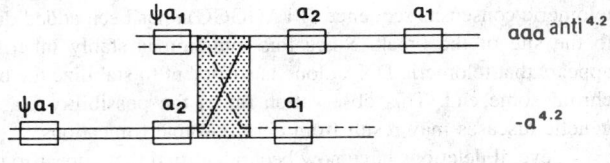

FIGURE 46-10   The mechanisms for the production of the common deletion forms of α+ thalassemia: (a) the normal α-globin gene cluster showing the homology boxes X, Y, and Z; (b) the rightward crossover through the Z bones, giving rise to the 3.7-kb deletion and a chromosome with 3 α-globin genes; (c) the leftward crossover through the Z boxes, giving rise to a 4.2-kb deletion and a chromosome containing 3 α genes.

event and that subsequently they were subdivided, presumably by insertions and deletions, to give three homologous subsegments referred to as X, Y, and Z (see Fig. 46-10). The duplicated Z boxes are 3.7 kb apart, and the X boxes are 4.2 kb apart. Misalignment and reciprocal crossover between these segments at meiosis can give rise to chromosomes with either single ($-\alpha$) or triplicated ($\alpha\alpha\alpha$) α-globin genes. Such an occurrence between homologous Z boxes deletes 3.7 kb of DNA (rightward deletion), while a similar crossover between the two X blocks deletes 4.2 kb of DNA (leftward deletion $-\alpha^{4.2}$).[131] The corresponding triplicated α-gene arrangements are referred to as $\alpha\alpha\alpha^{anti-3.7}$ and $\alpha\alpha\alpha^{anti-4.2}$.[132–134] More detailed analysis of these crossover events indicates that they occur more commonly in the Z box, and at least three different $-\alpha^{3.7}$ deletions have been found, depending on exactly where the crossover has taken place.[135] These are designated $-\alpha^{3.7I}$, $-\alpha^{3.7II}$, and $-\alpha^{3.7III}$, respectively. Other, rarer deletions of a single α gene have been observed.[7,125]

Nondeletion α Thalassemia   Since the expression of the α_2 gene is two to three times greater than that of the α_1 gene, it is not surprising that most of the nondeletion mutants discovered to date affect predominantly the expression of the α_2 gene; presumably this is ascertainment bias because of the greater phenotypic effect of these lesions. It is also possible that they have come under greater selective pressure.

Like the β-thalassemia mutations, α-thalassemia mutations[7,36,125] can be classified according to the level of gene expression they affect (see Table 46-5). Several processing mutations have been identified. For example, a pentanucleotide deletion includes the 5′ splice site of IVS-1 of the α_2-globin gene. This involves the invariant GT donor splicing sequence and thus completely inactivates the α_2 gene.[136] A second mutant of this type, found commonly in the Middle East, involves the poly-A addition signal site (AATAAA → AATAAG) and downregulates the α_2 gene by interfering with 3′ end processing.[137,138]

A second group of nondeletion α thalassemias result from mutations that interfere with the translation of mRNA.[7,36,139–142] In one case, for example, the initiation codon is inactivated by a T → C transition,[139] and, in another, efficiency of initiation is reduced by a dinucleotide deletion in the consensus sequence around the start signal.[142] Five mutations that affect termination of translation and give rise to elongated α chains have been identified: hemoglobins Constant Spring, Icaria, Koya Dora, Seal Rock, and Pakse.[7,36,143] Each specifically

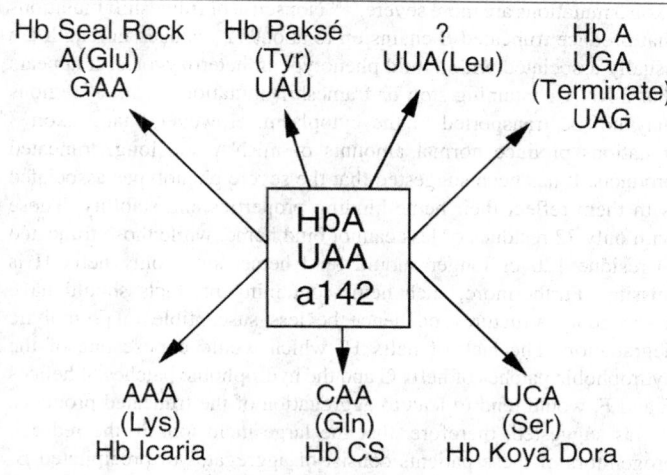

FIGURE 46-11   Point mutations in the α globin gene termination codon.

changes the termination codon TAA so that an amino acid is inserted instead of the chain terminating (Fig. 46-11). This is followed by read-through of mRNA that is not normally translated until another "in-phase" stop codon is reached. Thus, each of these variants has an elongated α chain. It seems likely that the "read-through" of α-globin mRNA that is usually not utilized somehow reduces its stability. There are several nonsense mutations, one in exon 3 of the α_2-globin gene, for example.[144] Finally, there are several mutations that cause α thalassemia by producing highly unstable α-globin chains; they include hemoglobins Quong Sze,[145] Suan Doc,[146] Petah Tikvah,[147] and Evanston.[148] A full list of nondeletion α thalassemia alleles is given in Refs. 7 and 36.

The Molecular Pathology of the α-Thalassemia–Mental Retardation Syndrome   The first descriptions of noninherited forms α thalassemia associated with mental retardation suggested that the lesions involving the α-globin gene locus might be acquired in the paternal germ cells and that their molecular pathology might help elucidate the associated developmental changes.[149] It is now clear that there are two separate syndromes of this type. In one group of patients there are long deletions involving the α-globin gene cluster and removing at least one megabase.[150] It appears that this condition can arise in several ways, including unbalanced translocation involving chromosome 16, truncation of the tip of chromosome 16, and the loss of the α-globin gene cluster and parts of its flanking regions by other mechanisms. These findings localize a region of about 1.7 Mb in band 16p13.3 proximal to the α-globin genes as being involved in mental handicap.[7,150]

The second group is characterized by defective α-globin synthesis associated with severe mental retardation and a relatively homogeneous pattern of dysmorphology.[151] Extensive structural studies have shown no abnormalities of the α-globin genes, the activity of which appears to be reduced in both *cis* and *trans*. These chromosomes direct the synthesis of normal amounts of α globin in mouse erythroleukemia cells, suggesting that the α thalassemia is due to a deficiency of a *trans*-activating factor involved in the regulation of the α-globin genes. This condition is encoded by a locus on the short arm of the X chromosome.[152] The gene involved has now been identified. It is *XH2*, a DNA helicase with many features of a DNA-binding protein.[153] Many different mutations of this gene have already been identified in different families with the ATR-X syndrome.[154] The murine homolog of this gene is widely expressed during early development. It is currently believed that the *XH2* product is a ubiquitous transcription factor that

is involved in early development, particularly of the urogenital system and brain, which also acts as a transcription factor for the α-globin genes.

Interactions of α-Thalassemia Haplotypes   Many α-thalassemia haplotypes have been described, and there are potentially over 500 interactions![7,125] Phenotypically, these result in one of four broad categories: normal, conditions in which there are mild hematologic changes but no clinical abnormality, hemoglobin H disease, and the hemoglobin Bart's hydrops fetalis syndrome. The heterozygous states for deletion or nondeletion forms of α^+ thalassemia either cause extremely mild hematologic abnormalities or are completely silent. In populations where α thalassemia is common, the homozygous state for α^+ thalassemia $(-\alpha/-\alpha)$ can produce a hematologic phenotype identical to that of the heterozygous state for α^0 thalassemia $(--/\alpha\alpha)$, that is, mild anemia with reduced MCH and MCV values.

Hemoglobin H disease usually results from the compound heterozygous state for α^0 thalassemia and either deletion or nondeletion α^+ thalassemia. It occurs most frequently in Southeast Asia $(--^{SEA}/-\alpha^{3.7})$ and the Mediterranean region (usually $--^{MED}/-\alpha^{3.7}$). Hemoglobin H disease may also result from the homozygous state for nondeletion mutants affecting the α_2 gene $(\alpha\alpha^{T\ Saudi}/\alpha\alpha^{T\ Saudi})$.[7,125]

The hemoglobin Bart's hydrops fetalis syndrome usually results from the homozygous state for α^0 thalassemia, most commonly $--^{SEA}/--^{SEA}$ or $--^{MED}/--^{MED}$. There have been a few reports of infants with this syndrome who synthesized very low levels of α chains at birth. Gene-mapping studies suggest that these cases result from the interaction of α^0 thalassemia with nondeletion mutations $(\alpha\alpha^T)$.[155] Recent studies suggest that the latter lead to the production of highly unstable α-chain variants.[156,157]

PATHOPHYSIOLOGY

It is possible to relate almost all the pathophysiologic features of the thalassemias to a primary imbalance of globin-chain synthesis. It is this phenomenon that makes them fundamentally different from all the other genetic and acquired disorders of hemoglobin production and that to a large extent explains their extreme severity in the homozygous or compound heterozygous states (Fig. 46-12).

IMBALANCED GLOBIN-CHAIN SYNTHESIS

Measurements of in vitro globin-chain synthesis in the blood or marrow of patients with different types of thalassemia,[158,159] together with family studies that enable the action of the thalassemia genes to be examined in patients who have also inherited α- or β-globin structural variants,[8] provide a clear picture of the action of the thalassemia determinants.[7] In homozygous β thalassemia, β-Globin synthesis is either absent or markedly reduced. This results in the production of an excess of α-globin chains. α-Globin chains are incapable of forming a viable hemoglobin tetramer and hence precipitate in red cell precursors. The resulting inclusion bodies can be demonstrated by both light[161] and electron microscopy.[160–162] In the marrow, precipitation can be seen in the earliest hemoglobinized precursors and through the erythroid maturation pathway.[163] These large inclusions are responsible for the intramedullary destruction of red cell precursors and hence for the ineffective erythropoiesis that characterizes all the β thalassemias. It has been calculated that a large proportion of the developing erythroblasts are destroyed within the marrow in severe cases.[164] Any red cells that are released are prematurely destroyed by mechanisms that are considered below. β-Thalassemia heterozygotes also have imbalanced globin-chain synthesis, but in this case the magnitude of the excess of α chains is much less and presumably can be dealt with

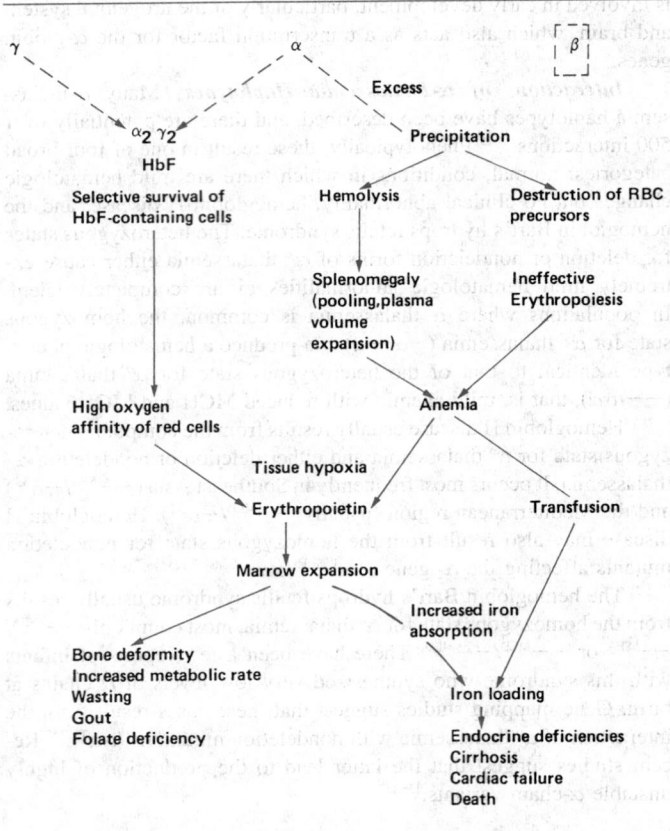

γ   α   β

Excess

α₂γ₂ HbF   Precipitation

Selective survival of HbF-containing cells   Hemolysis   Destruction of RBC precursors

Splenomegaly (pooling, plasma volume expansion)   Ineffective Erythropoiesis

High oxygen affinity of red cells   Anemia

Tissue hypoxia

Erythropoietin   Transfusion

Marrow expansion

Increased iron absorption

Bone deformity
Increased metabolic rate
Wasting
Gout
Folate deficiency

Iron loading

Endocrine deficiencies
Cirrhosis
Cardiac failure
Death

FIGURE 46-12 The pathophysiology of β thalassemia.

successfully by the proteolytic enzymes of the red cell precursors.[165] Notwithstanding, there is a mild degree of ineffective erythropoiesis.

It appears that there are two major routes to damage of the red cell membrane by the globin-chain precipitation process: the generation of hemichromes from excess α chains with subsequent structural damage to the red cell membrane, and similar damage mediated through the degradation products of excess α chains.[166–168] Membrane-bound hemichromes create a copolymer, which promotes clustering of band 3 in the membrane, first observed in sickle cell erythrocytes and later in the red cells of β thalassemics. It seems likely that these clusters are opsonized with autologous immunoglobulin G and complement, after which the cells are removed by macrophages. The products of degradation of free α chains—that is, globin, heme, hemin (oxidized heme), and free iron—also play a role in damaging red cell membranes. Excess globin chains bind to different membrane proteins and alter their structure and function. Excess iron, by generating oxygen free radicals, damages several red cell membrane components, including lipids and protein, as well as intracellular organelles. Heme and its products can catalyze the formation of a variety of reactive oxygen species which can produce damage to the red cell membrane. In β thalassemia this leads to a relatively rigid, underhydrated red cell. Damage to the red cells may also be mediated during their passage through the spleen due to the presence of rigid inclusion bodies.

While most of β-thalassemia heterozygotes are asymptomatic and have a mild hypochromic anemia, there are more severe forms that are dominantly inherited. Many of these involve mutations in exon 3 of the β-globin gene. A comparison of the lengths of abnormal gene products due to nonsense or frameshift mutations in the β-globin gene have suggested a mechanism that explains why most heterozygous forms of β thalassemia are mild, while those due to

exon 3 mutations are more severe.[80,81] Nonsense or frameshift mutations that produce truncated β chains up to about 72 residues in length are usually associated with a mild phenotype in heterozygotes. It appears that mRNA containing stop or frameshift mutations in its 5′ regions may not be transported to the cytoplasm. However, many exon 3 mutations produce normal amounts of mRNA and long, truncated products. It has been suggested that the severe phenotypes associated with them reflect their heme-binding properties and stability. Those with only 72 residues or less cannot bind heme, while those truncated to residue 120 or longer should bind heme, since only helix H is missing. Furthermore, such heme-containing products should have a secondary structure and hence be less susceptible to proteolytic degradation. The lack of helix H, which would expose one of the hydrophobic patches of helix G and the hydrophobic patches of helices E and F, would tend to lead to aggregation of the truncated products. It was suggested, therefore, that the large inclusions in the red cell progenitors of these patients consist of aggregates of precipitated β-chain products together with excess α chains, a notion that has been shown to be correct.[169] This explains the inclusion bodies in the red cell precursors and the marked degree of dyserythropoiesis that is observed in this interesting condition.

It is clear, therefore, that the anemia of β thalassemia has three major components. First and most important, there is ineffective erythropoiesis with intramedullary destruction of a variable proportion of the developing red cell precursors. Second, there is a hemolysis due to destruction of mature red cells containing α-chain inclusions. Third, because of the overall reduction in hemoglobin synthesis, the red cells are hypochromic and microcytic.

Because the primary defect in β thalassemia is in β-chain production, the synthesis of hemoglobins F and A₂ should be unaffected. Fetal hemoglobin production in utero is normal, and it is only when the neonatal switch from γ- to β-chain production occurs that the clinical manifestations of thalassemia first appear. However, fetal hemoglobin synthesis persists beyond the neonatal period in nearly all forms of β thalassemia (see Persistent Fetal Hemoglobin Production and Cellular Heterogeneity.) In β-thalassemia heterozygotes, there is an elevated level of hemoglobin A₂. This appears to reflect not only a relative decrease in hemoglobin A due to defective β-chain synthesis but also an absolute increase in the output of δ chains both *cis* and *trans* to the mutant β-globin gene.[7]

The consequences of excess non-α-chain production in the α thalassemias are quite different. Because α chains are shared by both fetal and adult hemoglobin, defective α-chain production is manifest in both fetal and adult life. In the fetus, it leads to excess γ-chain production; in the adult, to an excess of β chains. Excess γ chains form γ₄ homotetramers or hemoglobin Bart's[169]; excess β chains form β₄ homotetramers or hemoglobin H.[169] The fact that γ and β chains form homotetramers is the reason for the fundamental difference in the pathophysiology of α and β thalassemia. Because γ₄ and β₄ tetramers are soluble, they do not precipitate to any significant degree in the marrow, and therefore the α thalassemias are not characterized by severe ineffective erythropoiesis. However, β₄ tetramers precipitate as red cells age, with the formation of inclusion bodies.[171] Thus, the anemia of the more severe forms of α thalassemia in the adult is due to a shortened survival of red cells consequent to their damage in the microvasculature of the spleen as a result of the presence of the inclusions. In addition, because of the defect in hemoglobin synthesis, the cells are hypochromic and microcytic. Hemoglobin Bart's is more stable than hemoglobin H and does not form large inclusions.

It is now clear that, although, as is the case in β thalassemia, excess globin chains cause damage to the red cell membrane, the mechanisms are different in the two forms of the disease. As we saw, in the case of β thalassemia, excess α chains result in mechanical instability and oxidative damage to a variety of membrane proteins, notably protein 4.1. However, in α thalassemia the membranes are hyperstable and there is no evidence of oxidation or dysfunction of this protein. Furthermore, the state of red cell hydration is different in α thalassemia; accumulation of excess β chains results in increased hydration. These differences in the pathophysiology of membrane damage between α and β thalassemia are discussed in detail in Refs. 167 and 168.

There is another factor that exacerbates the tissue hypoxia of the anemia of the α thalassemias. Both hemoglobin Bart's and hemoglobin H show no heme-heme interaction and have almost hyperbolic oxygen dissociation curves with very high oxygen affinities. Thus, they are not able to liberate oxygen at physiologic tissue tensions and are, in effect, useless as oxygen carriers.[7,9,10]

It follows, therefore, that infants with high levels of hemoglobin Bart's have severe intrauterine hypoxia. This is the major basis for the clinical picture of homozygous α^o thalassemia, which results in the stillbirth of hydropic infants late in pregnancy or at term. Oxygen deprivation is reflected by the grossly hydropic state of the infant, presumably due to an increase in capillary permeability, and by severe erythroblastosis. Deficient fetal oxygenation is probably responsible for the enormously hypertrophied placentas, and possibly for the associated developmental abnomalities, that occur with the severe forms of intrauterine α thalassemia.[172]

PERSISTENT FETAL HEMOGLOBIN PRODUCTION AND CELLULAR HETEROGENEITY

In children with severe thalassemia, there is an increased level of hemoglobin F that persists into childhood and later[7,10]; in the β^o thalassemias, except for small amounts of hemoglobin A_2, hemoglobin F is the only hemoglobin produced. Examination of the blood using staining methods that are specific for hemoglobin F show that it is heterogeneously distributed among the red cells.[7] Persistent hemoglobin F production is not a major feature of the more severe forms of α thalassemia.

The mechanism of persistent γ-chain synthesis in the thalassemias is still incompletely understood. Normal adults have small quantities of hemoglobin F that are heterogeneously distributed among the red cells; cells with demonstrable hemoglobin F are called F cells. It is clear that one important mechanism for high levels of hemoglobin F in the blood of patients with β thalassemia is cell selection.[7,10,173,174] The major cause of ineffective erythropoiesis and shortened red cell survival in β thalassemia is the deleterious effect of excess α chains on erythroid maturation in the marrow and on the survival of red cells in the blood. It follows, therefore, that red cell precursors that produce γ chains will be at a selective advantage; excess α chains combine with γ chains to produce hemoglobin F, and therefore the magnitude of α-chain precipitation is less. Differential centrifugation experiments[174] and in vivo labeling studies[173] have shown that populations of red cells with relatively large amounts of hemoglobin F are more efficiently produced and survive longer in the blood. In fact, the blood of patients with homozygous β thalassemia shows remarkable cellular heterogeneity with respect to red cell survival; there are populations of cells that contain predominantly hemoglobin A that are destroyed very rapidly in the spleen and elsewhere, cells with a much longer survival that contain relatively more hemoglobin F, and populations of intermediate age and hemoglobin constitution.[7,10,175]

Whether cell selection of this type is the only mechanism for persistent γ-chain production in β thalassemia is uncertain. It is possible that there is also an absolute increase in hemoglobin F production; this is certainly so in some milder forms of homozygous β^o thalassemia, but in these cases there may be other genetic factors that are responsible

for the relatively high level of γ-chain synthesis (see below). However, biosynthesis studies indicate that marrow expansion and the selective survival of F-cell precursors and their progeny are the major factors in hemoglobin F production in hemoglobin E/β thalassemia.[176]

Since there is a reciprocal (see Fig. 46-9) relation between γ- and δ-chain synthesis, it follows that the red cells of β-thalassemia homozygotes that contain large amounts of hemoglobin F have relatively low levels of hemoglobin A_2.[7,10] Thus, the measured percent hemoglobin A_2 in these individuals is the average of a very heterogeneous cell population. This probably accounts for the extreme variability in the levels of hemoglobin A_2 found in homozygotes for this disorder. A further consequence of the persistence of hemoglobin F in β thalassemia is that the red cells have a high oxygen affinity.

CONSEQUENCES OF COMPENSATORY MECHANISMS FOR THE ANEMIA OF THALASSEMIA

The profound anemia of homozygous β thalassemia and the high oxygen affinity of the blood that is produced combine to cause severe tissue hypoxia. Because of the high oxygen affinity of hemoglobins Bart's and H, a similar defect in tissue oxygenation occurs in the more severe forms of α thalassemia. The major response is erythropoietin production and expansion of the dyserythropoietic marrow. This in turn leads to deformities of the skull and face and porosity of the long bones.[7] In extreme cases extramedullary hematopoietic tumors may develop. Apart from the production of severe skeletal deformities, marrow expansion may cause pathologic fractures and sinus and middle ear infection due to ineffective drainage.

Another important effect of the enormous expansion of the marrow mass is the diversion of calories required for normal development to the ineffective red cell precursors. Thus, patients severely affected by thalassemia show poor development and wasting. The massive turnover of erythroid precursors may result in secondary hyperuricemia and gout and severe folate deficiency.

The effects of gross intrauterine hypoxia in homozygous α^o thalassemia have already been described. In the symptomatic forms of α thalassemia (e.g., hemoglobin H disease) that are compatible with survival into adult life, bone changes and other consequences of erythroid expansion are seen, although less commonly than in β thalassemia.

SPLENOMEGALY: DILUTIONAL ANEMIA

The constant exposure of the spleen to red cells with inclusions consisting of precipitated globin chains gives rise to the phenomenon of "work hypertrophy." Progressive splenomegaly occurs in both α and β thalassemia and may exacerbate the anemia.[7,10,177] A large spleen acts as a sump for red cells and may sequester a considerable proportion of the red cell mass. Furthermore, splenomegaly may also cause plasma volume expansion, a complication that may be exacerbated by massive expansion of the erythroid marrow. The combination of pooling of the red cells in the spleen together with plasma volume expansion may exacerbate the anemia in both α and β thalassemia. The same process may occur in an enlarged liver, particularly after splenectomy.

ABNORMAL IRON METABOLISM

β-Thalassemia homozygotes who are anemic manifest increased intestinal iron absorption that is related to the degree of expansion of the red cell precursor population; iron absorption is decreased by blood transfusion.[10,177] Increased absorption causes a steady accumulation of iron, first in the Kupffer cells of the liver and the macrophages of the spleen and later in the parenchymal cells of the liver. Most patients homozygous for β thalassemia require regular blood transfusion, and thus transfusional siderosis adds to the iron accumulation. Iron accumulates in the endocrine glands,[7,177-180] particularly in the parathyroids, pituitary, and pancreas, as well as in the liver, and, most important, in the myocardium.[7,181] The latter leads to death either by involving the conducting tissues or by causing intractable cardiac failure. Other consequences of iron loading include diabetes, hypoparathyroidism, hypothyroidism, and abnormalities of hypopthalamic-pituitary function leading to growth retardation and hypogonadism.[7,178,180]

There is now much more accurate information about the levels of body iron, as reflected by hepatic iron, at which patients are at risk for serious complications of iron overload.[182] These studies, which extrapolate data obtained from patients with genetic hemochromatosis, suggest that patients with hepatic iron levels of approximately 80 μmol iron per gram of liver, wet weight ($\approx$15 mg iron per gram of liver, dry weight), are at an increased risk of hepatic disease and endocrine organ damage. Patients with higher body iron burdens are at particular risk of cardiac disease and early death.

Disordered iron metabolism is less common in the adult forms of α thalassemia. The reason is not clear, but the milder degree of anemia, fewer transfusions, and the less marked erythroid expansion of the marrow are the likely explanations.

There appears to be an increased susceptibility to bacterial infection in all forms of severe thalassemia.[7,10,177,183] The reason is not known. It has been suggested that the relatively high serum iron levels may favor bacterial growth. Another possible mechanism is blockade of the monocyte-macrophage system due to the increased rate of destruction of red cells. No consistent defects in white cell or immune function have been demonstrated, and it remains to be demonstrated unequivocally that high serum iron levels are an important factor. The one exception is infection with *Yersinia enterocolitica*, a normally nonvirulent pathogen that is able to produce its own siderophore and hence that thrives in iron excess.

COAGULATION DEFECTS

The increasing knowledge about the potential hypercoagulable state in some forms of thalassemia has been reviewed in detail.[166-168] There is some evidence that patients, particularly after splenectomy and with high platelet counts, may develop progressive pulmonary arterial disease due to platelet aggregation in the pulmonary circulation. Furthermore, using thalassemic red cells as a source of phospholipids, enhanced thrombin generation has been demonstrated in a thrombinase assay. The procoagulant effect of thalassemia cells appears to be due to an increased expression of anionic phospholipids on the red cell surface. Normally, neutral or negatively charged amino acids are confined to the inner leaflet of the red cell membrane, an effect that is mediated by the action of aminophospholipid translocase, an enzyme sometimes known as flipase, which, in effect, flips aminophospholipids that are diffused to the outer leaflet back to the inner leaflet (see Chap. 28). It is believed that in thalassemic red cells these aminophospholipids are moved to the outer leaflet and thus provide a surface on which coagulation can be activated. Other nonspecific changes in the coagulation pathway and its antagonists have also been observed in patients with different forms of thalassemia.

CLINICAL HETEROGENEITY

The pathophysiologic mechanisms described in the previous sections provide the basis for the remarkable diversity of the clinical findings in the thalassemia syndromes. It is apparent that all the manifestations of β thalassemia can be related to excess α-chain production. It follows that any mechanism that reduces the excess of α chains should reduce the clinical severity of the disease. An elegant ''experiment of nature'' has shown that this is so and, incidentally, has confirmed that globin-chain imbalance is the major factor in determining the severity of the thalassemias.

Coinheritance of α thalassemia can reduce the severity of the more severe forms of β thalassemia.[184-186] This effect is much more marked in individuals who are homozygotes or compound heterozygotes for different forms of β^+ thalassemia; β^0-thalassemia homozygotes who have inherited α thalassemia seem to be protected little, if at all.

Severe β thalassemia can be modified by the coinheritance of genetic determinants for enhanced production of γ chains. The interaction of the heterocellular HPFH in the amelioration of homozygous β thalassemia has already been mentioned. Other determinants may also be involved. For example, it is apparent that the inheritance of a particular RFLP haplotype in the region 5' to the β-globin gene may be an important factor.[187,188] This particular β-globin gene haplotype is associated with a single base change, C $\rightarrow$ T, at position −158 relative to the $^G\gamma$-globin gene, an alteration that creates a cleavage site for the restriction enzyme *Xmn* I.[122] There is an excess of individuals with the −158 polymorphism with the phenotype of thalassemia intermedia compared with thalassemia major in different populations.[188,189] It is still not absolutely clear, however, whether this polymorphism is the only factor in increasing hemoglobin F production in these cases. However, the association certainly points to an effect *cis* to the affected β gene as the basis for the elevated fetal hemoglobin levels in these forms of thalassemia intermedia.

Finally, some of the mutations that cause β thalassemia are associated with a mild phenotype because they result in only a modest reduction of β-chain production. For example, those at −29 and −88 have been found in association with mild β^+ thalassemia in Africans. Similarly, in Mediterranean populations particularly mild phenotypes are found commonly with a base substitution at position 6 in IVS-1 and at position −87 in the 5'-flanking region of the β-globin gene. The homozygous state for the IVS-1 position 6 mutation usually produces an extremely mild form of β thalassemia. When these ''mild'' mutations are coinherited with more severe β-thalassemia determinants, the compound heterozygous states are characterized by a more severe form of thalassemia intermedia.

Other forms of thalassemia intermedia are associated with the homozygous state for $\delta\beta$ thalassemia, the various interactions of $\delta\beta$ thalassemia with β thalassemia, and heterozygous β thalassemia of the severe variety or in association with triplicated α-gene loci.[7,10,190] These complex interactions are the subject of several extensive reviews.[190-192]

POPULATION GENETICS[7,9,10,193]

The β thalassemias are distributed widely in Mediterranean populations, the Middle East, parts of India and Pakistan, and throughout Southeast Asia (Fig. 46-13). The disease is common in the southern parts of the former USSR and in the People's Republic of China. The β thalassemias are rare in Africa, except for some isolated pockets in West Africa, notably Liberia, and in parts of North Africa. However, β thalassemia occurs sporadically in all racial groups and has been observed in the homozygous state in persons of pure Anglo-Saxon heritage. Thus, a patient's racial background does not preclude the diagnosis.

The $\delta\beta$ thalassemias have been observed sporadically in many racial groups, although no high-frequency populations have been defined. Similarly, the hemoglobin Lepore syndromes have been found in many populations, but, with the possible exceptions of central Italy,

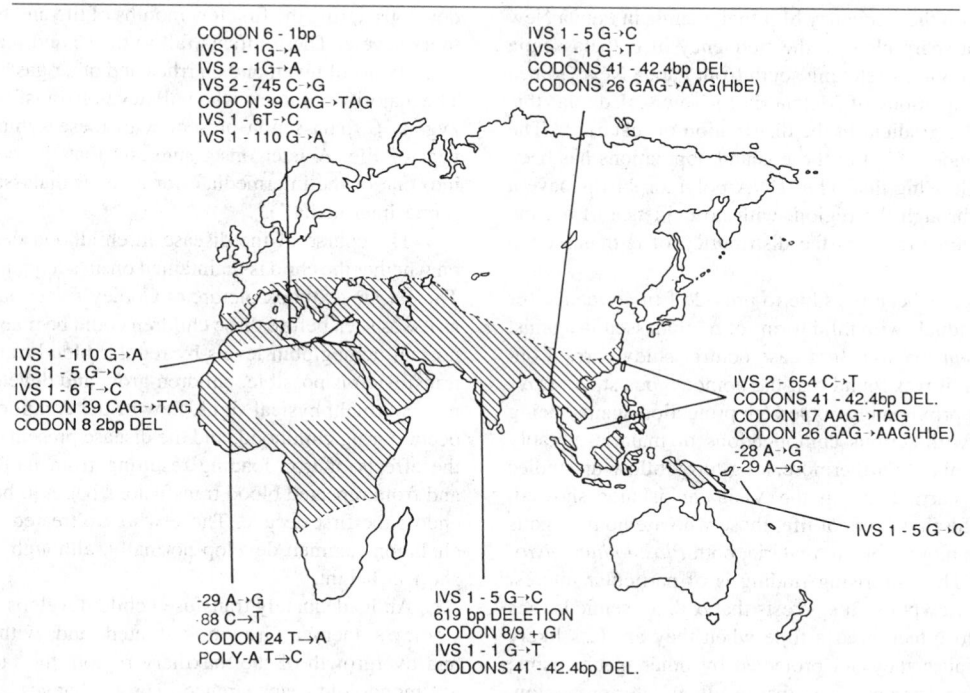

FIGURE 46-13   The world distribution of β thalassemia.

eastern Europe, and parts of Spain and Portugal, these disorders have not been found to occur with a high frequency in any particular region.

The α thalassemias occur widely throughout Africa, the Mediterranean countries, the Middle East, and Southeast Asia (Fig. 46-14). The α^0 thalassemias are found most commonly in Mediterranean and Oriental populations and are extremely rare in Africa and the Middle East. However, the deletion forms of α^+ thalassemia occur with a high frequency throughout West Africa, the Mediterranean, the Middle East, and Southeast Asia. Up to 80 percent of the population of some parts of Papua New Guinea are carriers for the deletion form of α^+ thalassemia. It is uncertain how common the nondeletion forms of α^+ thalassemia are in any particular populations, but they have been reported quite frequently in some of the Mediterranean island popula-

tions and in the Middle East and Southeast Asia. Because the hemoglobin Bart's hydrops syndrome and hemoglobin H disease require the action of an α^0-thalassemia determinant, these disorders are found at a high frequency only in Southeast Asia and in parts of the Mediterranean region. The α-chain termination mutants, such as hemoglobin Constant Spring, seem to be particularly common in Southeast Asia, and in Thailand approximately 4 percent of the population are carriers.

In 1949, J.B.S. Haldane suggested that thalassemia might have reached its high frequency in tropical regions because heterozygotes are protected against malaria.[194] Although many population studies have been carried out in order to test this hypothesis, it is only in recent years, with the advent of recombinant DNA technology, that it has been possible to elucidate some of the extremely complex population genetics that underlie polymorphic systems such as the thalassemias.

It is now apparent that in each of the high-frequency areas for the β thalassemias there are a few common mutations, together with varying numbers of rare ones (see Fig. 46-13). Furthermore, in each of these regions the pattern of mutations is different, and, even when the same mutation occurs in different populations, it is usually found together with a different arrangement of RFLPs (haplotype) in the associated β-globin gene cluster.[193,195,196] Similar observations have been made in the case of the α thalassemias (see Fig. 46-14).[193] These studies suggest that the thalassemias arose independently in different populations and then achieved their high frequency by selection. Although there may have been some movement of the thalassemia genes by drift, there is little doubt that independent mutation and selection provides the overall basis for their world distribution. Early studies in Sardinia, which showed that β thalassemia is less common in the mountainous regions where malarial transmission is low, supported Haldane's suggestion that β thalassemia might have reached its high frequency due to protection against malarial infections. For many years these data remained the only convincing evidence for such a protective effect.[197] However, more recent studies making use of malaria endemicity data together with globin-gene mapping have shown a very clear

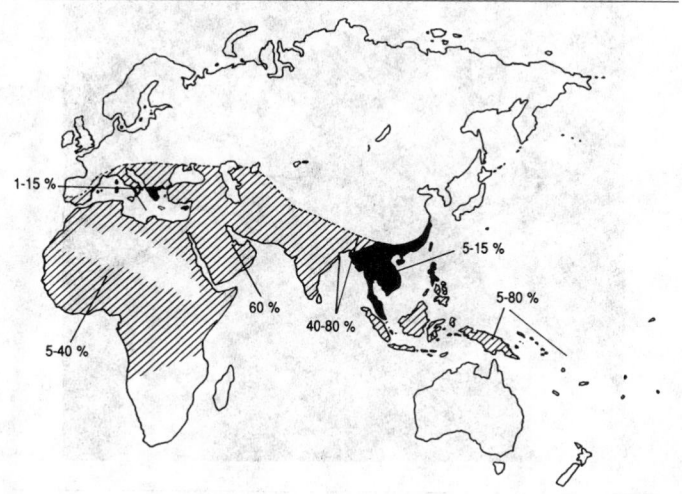

FIGURE 46-14   The world distribution of α^+ and α^0 thalassemia.

altitude-related effect on the frequency of α thalassemia in Papua New Guinea. In addition, a sharp cline in the frequency of α thalassemia has been found in the region stretching south from Papua New Guinea through the island populations of Melanesia to New Caledonia; this is mirrored by a similar gradient in the distribution of malaria.[198] The effect of drift and founder effect in these island populations has been largely excluded by showing that other DNA polymorphisms have a random distribution through the region, with no evidence of a cline similar to that which characterizes the distribution of α thalassemia and malaria.

More recently, it has been possible to provide firm evidence for the protection of individuals with mild forms of α^+ thalassemia against *Plasmodium falciparum* malaria. In a case control study carried out in Papua New Guinea, it was found that the homozygous state for α^+ thalassemia offered approximately 60 percent protection against being admitted to hospital with serious complications of malaria, notably coma or profound anemia.[199] Furthermore, long-term follow-up studies of cohorts of babies carried out in the Vanuatan islands showed, surprisingly, that, in the first years of life, those who are homozygous for α^+ thalassemia are more prone to malaria, both *Plasmodium vivax* and *P. falciparum*.[200] This surprising finding is of particular interest from the mechanistic viewpoint. It suggests that α thalassemic babies may be more prone to infection at a time when they are less likely to die of malaria because they are protected by other mechanisms; this may induce an early immunization that results in later protection. This concept is supported by the observation that these babies tend to get the mild *P. vivax* infections earlier than those due to *P. falciparum*; there is increasing evidence that there may be cross-immunization between the two species.

A great deal of work has been carried out toward understanding the reason why thalassemic red cells appear to be protective against malarial parasites. A variety of studies have failed to demonstrate any effect of the thalassemia phenotype on the rates of parasite invasion and growth.[201,202] However, parasitized α-thalassemic cells bind significantly more antibody from the serum of patients with acute *P. falciparum* malaria than do normal red cells.[203] It is not yet clear whether this reflects more efficient exposure of malarial antigens by the thalassemic cells or whether these cells expose red cell neoantigens related to senescence more effectively than do normal cells when invaded by the parasite. This phenomenon has also been observed in parasitized β-thalassemic cells, and these observations raise a new avenue of investigation for the protective effect of thalassemia against *P. falciparum* malaria. In effect, they suggest, like the population studies outlined earlier, that it may be immune mediated rather than due to the particular properties of the small thalassemic red cells themselves. Indeed, several lines of evidence now suggest that parasitized thalassemic cells may be more prone to ingestion by macrophages.[202]

CLINICAL FEATURES

β AND $\delta\beta$ THALASSEMIAS

The most clinically severe form of β thalassemia is called thalassemia major. A milder clinical picture, characterized by a later onset and either no transfusion requirement or at least fewer transfusions than are required to treat the major form of the illnesses, is designated β *thalassemia intermedia*. β *Thalassemia minor* is the term used to describe the heterozygous carrier state for β thalassemia.

β THALASSEMIA MAJOR[7,10,177]

The homozygous or compound heterozygous state for β thalassemia, thalassemia major, produces the clinical picture first described by Cooley in 1925.[1] Affected infants are well at birth. Anemia usually

develops during the first few months of life and becomes progressively more severe. These infants fail to thrive and may have feeding problems, bouts of fever, and diarrhea and other gastrointestinal symptoms. The majority of infants who will develop transfusion-dependent homozygous β thalassemia present with these symptoms within the first year of life. A later onset suggests that the condition may develop into one of the intermediate forms of β thalassemia (see "β Thalassemia Intermedia").

The course of the disease in childhood depends almost entirely on whether the child is maintained on an adequate transfusion program. The classic textbook picture of Cooley's anemia describes the disease as it was seen before these children could be maintained with relatively normal hemoglobin levels by regular blood transfusions. If adequate transfusion is possible, children grow and develop normally and have no abnormal physical signs. Few of the complications of the disorder occur during childhood, and the disease presents a problem only when the effects of iron loading resulting from ineffective erythropoiesis and from repeated blood transfusions begin to become apparent at the end of the first decade. Those who are treated with an adequate iron chelation regimen develop normally, although some of them remain short in height.

An inadequately transfused child develops the typical features of Cooley's anemia. Growth is stunted, and, with bossing of the skull and overgrowth of the maxillary region, the face gradually assumes a "mongoloid" appearance. These changes are associated with a characteristic radiologic appearance of the skull, long bones, and hands (Fig. 46-15). There is widening of the diploe, with a "hair on end" or "sun-ray" appearance and a lacy trabeculation of the long bones and phalanges, and there may be gross skeletal deformities. The liver and spleen are enlarged, and the pigmentation of the skin increases. Many features of a hypermetabolic state with fever, wasting, and hyperuricemia may develop.

The clinical course is characterized by severe anemia with frequent complications. These children are particularly prone to infection, which is a common cause of death. Because of increased folate utilization by the hypertrophied marrow, folic acid deficiency occurs fre-

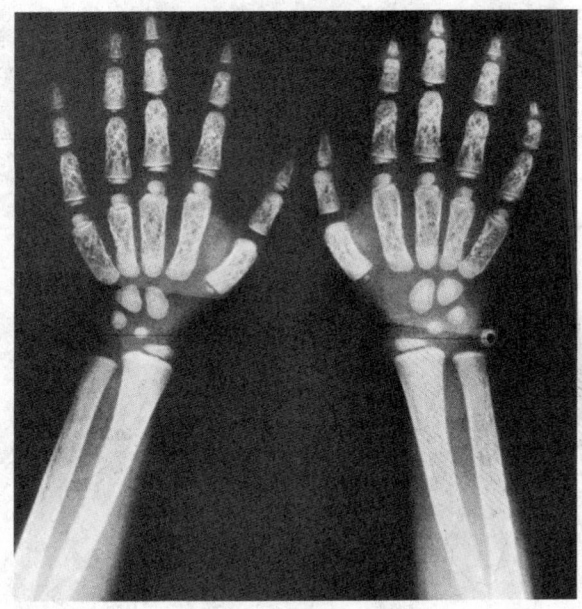

FIGURE 46-15 Radiologic appearances of the hands in homozygous β thalassemia.

quently. Spontaneous fractures occur commonly as a result of the expansion of the marrow cavities with thinning of the long bones and skull. Maxillary deformities often lead to dental problems from malocclusion. The formation of massive deposits of extramedullary hematopoietic tissue may cause neurologic complications. With the gross splenomegaly that may occur, secondary thrombocytopenia and leukopenia frequently develop, leading to a further tendency to infection and bleeding. There may be a bleeding tendency in the absence of thrombocytopenia. Epistaxis is particularly common. These hemostatic problems are associated with poor liver function in some cases. Chronic leg ulceration may occur, although this is more common in thalassemia intermedia.

Children who have grown and developed normally throughout the first 10 years of life as a result of regular blood transfusion begin to develop the symptoms of iron loading as they enter puberty, particularly if they have not received adequate iron chelation.[177] The first indication of iron loading is usually the absence of the pubertal growth spurt and a failure of the menarche. Over the succeeding years, a variety of endocrine disturbances may develop, particularly diabetes mellitus, hypogonadotrophic hypogonadism, and growth hormone deficiency; hypothyroidism and adrenal insufficiency also occur but are less common.[179] Toward the end of the second decade, cardiac complications arise, and death usually occurs in the second or third decade as a result of cardiac siderosis. This may cause an acute cardiac death with arrhythmia, or intractable cardiac failure. Both of these complications may be precipitated by intercurrent infection.

Even the adequately transfused child who has received chelation therapy may suffer a number of complications. Blood-borne infection, notably with hepatitis C[204] or HIV,[205] are extremely common in some populations, although their frequency is being reduced by the use of widespread blood-donor screening programs. Delayed puberty and growth retardation are also common and probably reflect hypogonadotrophic hypogonadism together with damage to the pituitary gland.[204,206] Osteoporosis is also being recognized increasingly and may also be, at least in part, a reflection of hypogonadism.[204]

β THALASSEMIA INTERMEDIA

The clinical phenotype of patients designated to have thalassemia intermedia is more severe than the usual asymptomatic thalassemia trait but milder than transfusion-dependent thalassemia major.[7,10,190–192] The syndrome encompasses disorders with a wide spectrum of disability. At the severe end, patients present with anemia later than is usual in the transfusion-dependent forms of homozygous β thalassemia and are just able to maintain a hemoglobin level of about 6 g/dl without transfusion. However, their growth and development are retarded, and they become seriously disabled, with marked skeletal deformities, arthritis, and bone pain; progressive splenomegaly; growth retardation; and chronic ulcerations above the ankles. At the other end of the spectrum, there are patients who remain completely asymptomatic until adult life and are transfusion-independent, with hemoglobin levels as high as 10 to 12 g/dl. All varieties of intermediate severity are observed, and some patients become disabled simply due to the effects of hypersplenism. Intensive studies of the molecular pathology of this condition have provided some guidelines about genotype-phenotype relationships that are useful for genetic counseling (Table 46-7).

β THALASSEMIA MINOR

The heterozygous state for β thalassemia is not usually associated with any clinical disability, and the abnormality is discovered only on performing a blood examination. It is most commonly discovered during periods of stress, such as pregnancy or during severe infection, when a moderate degree of anemia may be found. Some patients with thalassemia minor have increased iron stores, but often this may be

TABLE 46-7   β THALASSEMIA INTERMEDIA

Mild forms of β thalassemia
  Homozygosity for mild β^+ thalassemia alleles
  Compound heterozygosity for two mild β^+ thalassemia alleles
  Compound heterozygosity for a "silent" or mild and more severe
    β-thalassemia allele
Inheritance of α and β thalassemia
  β^+ Thalassemia with α^0 thalassemia ($--/\alpha\alpha$) or α^+ thalassemia
    ($-\alpha/\alpha\alpha$ or $-\alpha/-\alpha$)
  β^+ Thalassemia with genotype of Hb H disease ($--/-\alpha$)
  β Thalassemia with elevated γ-chain synthesis
  Homozygous β thalassemia with heterocellular HPFH
  Homozygous β thalassemia with homozygous $^G\gamma158$ T → C change
    (some cases)
  Compound heterozygosity for β thalassemia and deletion forms of HPFH
Compound heterozygosity for β thalassemia and β-chain variants
  Hb E/β thalassemia
  Other interactions with rare β-chain variants
Heterozygous β thalassemia with triplicated or quadruplicated α-chain
  genes ($\alpha\alpha\alpha$ or $\alpha\alpha\alpha\alpha$)
Dominant forms of β thalassemia
Interactions of β and $(\delta\beta)^+$ or $(\delta\beta)^0$ thalassemia

due to injudicious iron therapy started because of misdiagnosed microcytic anemia.

α THALASSEMIAS

THE HEMOGLOBIN BART'S HYDROPS FETALIS SYNDROME

This disorder is a frequent cause of stillbirth in Southeast Asia. Infants either are stillborn between 34 and 40 weeks' gestation or are born alive but die within the first few hours.[207,208] There is pallor, edema, and hepatosplenomegaly, and the clinical picture resembles hydrops fetalis due to Rh blood group incompatibility. At autopsy there is massive extramedullary hemopoiesis and enlargement of the placenta. A variety of congenital anomalies have been observed.

There have been a few reports of the rescue of infants with this syndrome by prenatal detection and exchange transfusion. These babies have grown and developed normally, although they are of course blood transfusion–dependent.[208–210]

This condition is associated with a high incidence of maternal toxemia of pregnancy and difficulties at the time of delivery because of the massive placenta.[7,207,208] The reason for placental hypertrophy is unknown, although, because a similar phenomenon is observed in hydrops infants with Rh incompatibility, it may reflect severe intrauterine hypoxia.

HEMOGLOBIN H DISEASE

Hemoglobin H disease was described independently in the United States and in Greece in 1956.[211,212] The clinical findings are variable; a few patients are almost as severely affected as patients with β thalassemia major, while most have a much milder course.[7,10,172,213] There is lifelong anemia with variable splenomegaly; bone changes are unusual.

There have been a few attempts to correlate the genotype with the phenotype of hemoglobin H disease. In general, it appears that, as might be expected, patients with a nondeletion form of α thalassemia affecting the predominant α_2 gene interacting with an α^0 thalassemia determinant ($--/\alpha^T\alpha$), $--/\alpha$ $^{Constant Spring}\alpha$, for example, have higher levels of hemoglobin H, a greater degree of anemia, and, anecdotally, a more severe clinical course than patients with the $--/-\alpha$ genotype.[214–217]

MILDER FORMS OF α THALASSEMIA, INCLUDING THE TRAITS

Because there are two α-globin genes per haploid genome, there is a wide spectrum of different conditions with overlapping phenotypes resulting from their various interactions. The carrier states for the deletion and nondeletion forms of α thalassemia, $-\alpha/\alpha\alpha$ and $\alpha^T/\alpha/\alpha\alpha$, are symptomless. Similarly, the homozygous states for the deletion forms of α^+ thalassemia, $-\alpha/-\alpha$, and the heterozygous state for α^o thalassemia, $--/\alpha\alpha$, are symptomless, although they are associated with mild anemia and red cell changes. On the other hand, the homozygous states for the nondeletion forms of α thalassemia, $\alpha^T\alpha/\alpha^T\alpha$, are associated with an extremely diverse series of phenotypes. As mentioned earlier, in the section on *Interactions of α-Thalassemia Haplotypes*, they sometimes result in the clinical picture of hemoglobin H disease, while in others they may be associated with only a mild hypochromic anemia.[7] The homozygous states for the chain termination mutants, notably hemoglobin Constant Spring, constitute a special case because they produce a particularly characteristic phenotype. In this case there is a moderate hemolytic anemia with splenomegaly and characteristic hematological findings.[218–220]

LABORATORY FEATURES

β THALASSEMIA MAJOR

Hemoglobin levels at presentation may be in the range of 2 to 3 g/dl or even lower. The red cells show marked anisopoikilocytosis, with hypochromia, target cell formation, and a variable degree of basophilic stippling (Fig. 46-16). The appearance of the blood film varies somewhat, depending on whether the spleen is intact. In nonsplenectomized patients, large poikilocytes are common, whereas after splenectomy, large, flat macrocytes and small, deformed microcytes are frequently

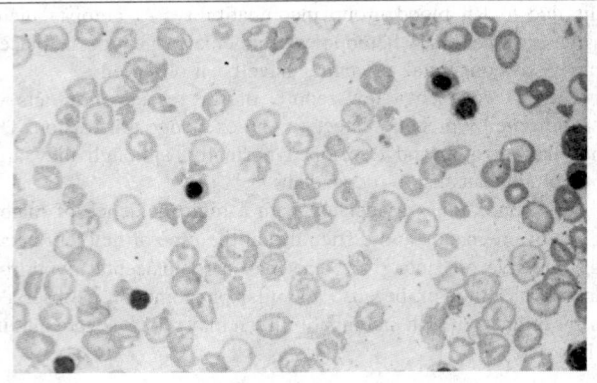

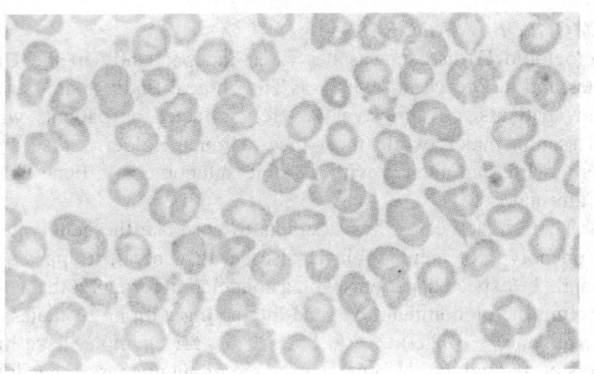

FIGURE 46-16   The peripheral blood film in homozygous β thalassemia.

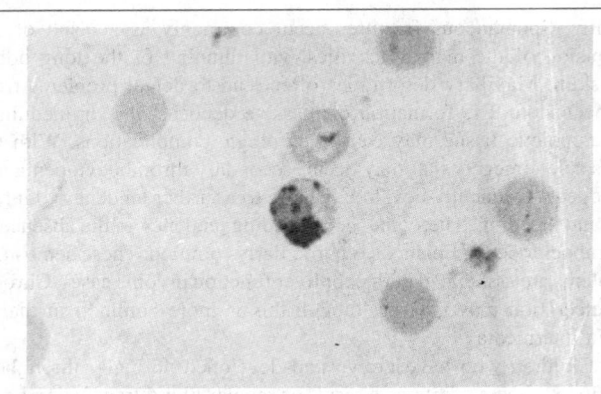

FIGURE 46-17   Red cell inclusions in peripheral blood of a homozygous β thalassemia patient (postsplenectomy).

seen. The reticulocyte count is moderately elevated, and there are nearly always nucleated red cells in the blood. These red cells may reach very high levels after splenectomy. The white cell and platelet counts are slightly elevated unless there is secondary hypersplenism. Staining of the blood with methyl violet, particularly in splenectomized subjects, reveals stippling or ragged inclusion bodies in the red cells.[160] These inclusions can nearly always be found in the red cell precursors in the marrow (Fig. 46-17). The marrow usually shows erythroid hyperplasia with morphologic abnormalities of the erythroblasts such as striking basophilic stippling and increased iron deposition. Iron kinetic studies indicate that there is markedly ineffective erythropoiesis, and red cell survival is usually shortened. There are populations of cells with very short survival and also longer-lived populations of cells; the latter contain relatively more fetal hemoglobin.[173,174] An increased level of fetal hemoglobin, ranging from less than 10 percent to over 90 percent, is characteristic of homozygous β thalassemia. In β^o thalassemia, no hemoglobin A is produced. The acid elution test shows that the fetal hemoglobin is quite heterogeneously distributed among the red cells. Hemoglobin A_2 levels in homozygous β thalassemia may be low, normal, or high. If expressed as a proportion of hemoglobin A, however, the hemoglobin A_2 level is almost invariably elevated. Differential centrifugation studies indicate some heterogeneity of hemoglobin F and A_2 distribution among thalassemic red cells, and their level in whole blood gives little indication of their total rates of synthesis.

In vitro hemoglobin synthesis studies using marrow or blood show a marked degree of globin-chain imbalance; there is always a marked excess of α over β and γ-chain production.[158,159] Other aspects of the laboratory findings in this condition, including red cell survival, iron absorption, ferrikinetics, erythrokinetics, and the consequences of iron loading, are discussed earlier (see "Pathophysiology").

β THALASSEMIA MINOR

Hemoglobin values of patients with β thalassemia minor are usually in the range of 9 to 11 g/dl. The most consistent finding is small, poorly hemoglobinized red cells, resulting in MCH values of 20 to 22 pg and MCV values of 50 to 70 fl. The red cell indices are particularly useful in screening for heterozygous carriers of thalassemia in population surveys. The marrow in heterozygous β thalassemia shows slight erythroid hyperplasia with rare red cell inclusions. Megaloblastic transformation due to folic acid deficiency occurs occasionally, particularly during pregnancy. There is a mild degree of ineffective erythropoiesis, but red cell survival is normal or nearly so. The hemoglobin A_2 level is increased to 3.5 to 7 percent. The level of fetal hemoglobin is elevated in about 50 percent of cases, usually to 1 to 3 percent and rarely to more than 5 percent.

α THALASSEMIAS

THE HEMOGLOBIN BART'S HYDROPS FETALIS SYNDROME

In infants with the hydrops fetalis syndrome, the blood film shows severe thalassemic changes with many nucleated red cells. The hemoglobin consists mainly of hemoglobin Bart's, with approximately 10 to 20 percent hemoglobin Portland. There is usually no hemoglobin A or F, although the rare cases that seem to result from the interaction of α^o thalassemia with a severe nondeletion form of α^+ thalassemia show small amounts of hemoglobin A.

HEMOGLOBIN H DISEASE

The blood film shows hypochromia and anisopoikilocytosis. The reticulocyte count is usually in the 5 percent range. Incubation of the red cells with brilliant cresyl blue results in ragged inclusion bodies in practically all the cells. These form because of precipitation of hemoglobin H in vitro as a result of redox action of the dye. After splenectomy, large, single Heinz bodies are observed in some cells (Fig. 46-18). These are formed by the in vitro precipitation of the unstable hemoglobin H molecule and are seen only after splenectomy. Hemoglobin H constitutes between 5 and 40 percent of the total hemoglobin; there may also be traces of hemoglobin Bart's, and the level of hemoglobin A_2 is usually slightly subnormal.

α^o-THALASSEMIA AND α^+-THALASSEMIA TRAITS

The α^o-thalassemia trait is characterized by the presence of 5 to 15 percent hemoglobin Bart's at birth.[7,125] This hemoglobin disappears during maturation and is not replaced by a similar amount of hemoglobin H. An occasional cell with hemoglobin H inclusion bodies may appear after incubation with brilliant cresyl blue, and this phenomenon is often used as a diagnostic test for the α-thalassemia trait. However, it is difficult to standardize and requires much experience to be useful. In adult life, the red cells of heterozygotes have morphologic changes of heterozygous thalassemia with low MCH and MCV values. The electrophoretic pattern is normal, and globin-synthesis studies show a deficit of α-chain production, with an α/β-chain production ratio of approximately 0.7.[7,125]

The α^+-thalassemia trait is characterized by minimal hematologic changes, 1 to 2 percent of hemoglobin Bart's at birth in some but not all cases, and a slightly reduced α/β-chain production ratio of approximately 0.8. This ratio can be distinguished from normal only by studying relatively large numbers of samples and comparing the mean α/β ratio with that of normal control subjects. This approach is not reliable for diagnosing individual cases of the α^+-thalassemia trait, and, unfortunately, there is no really reliable way of making the diagnosis in adults except by DNA analysis.

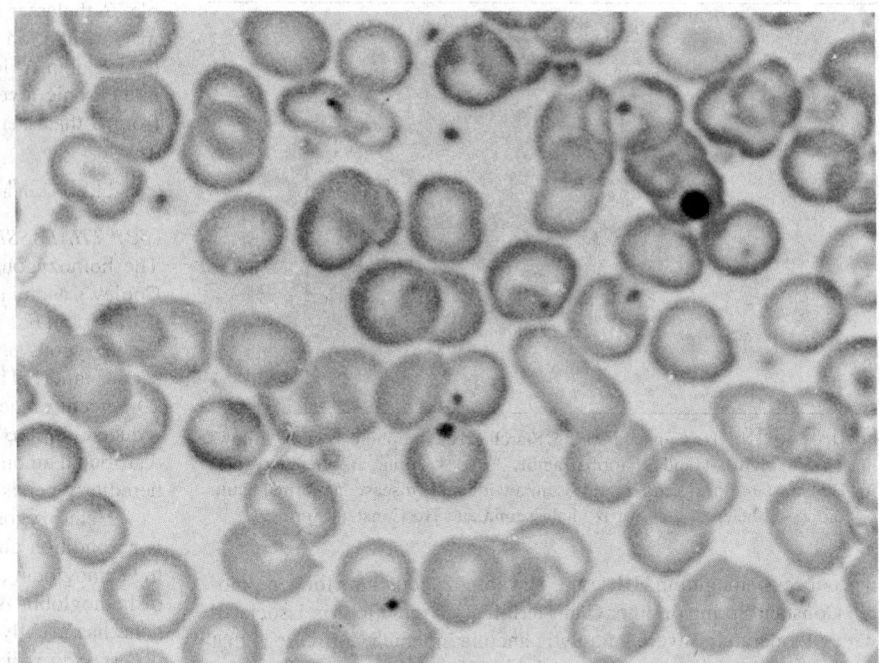

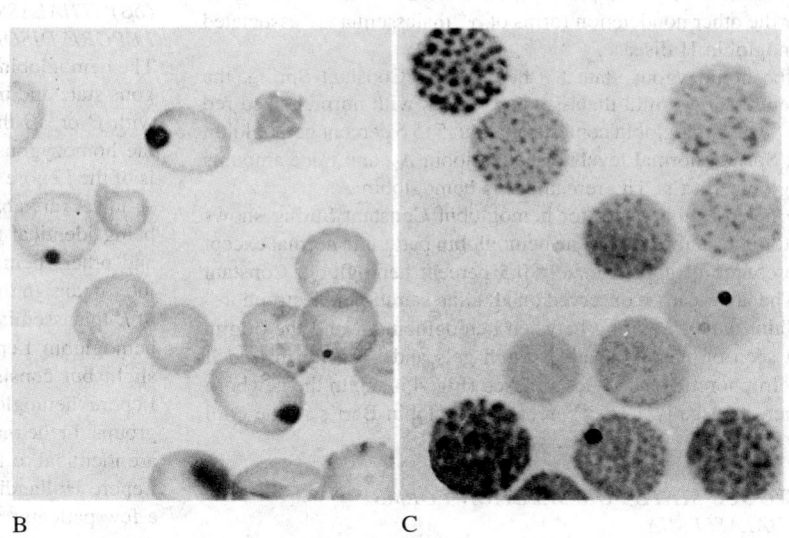

FIGURE 46-18   Hb H disease: (A) blood film; (B) preformed inclusions postsplenectomy; (C) inclusions generated by brilliant cresyl blue.

Studies using DNA analysis indicate that there is a marked overlap between the different α-thalassemia carrier states with regard to the hematologic and globin-synthesis findings (reviewed in Refs. 7 and 125). In addition, they show that many α^+-thalassemia carriers do not have elevated levels of hemoglobin Bart's at birth. These studies confirm that, short of gene-mapping analysis, there is no way to identify specific α-thalassemia carrier states with certainty.

HOMOZYGOUS STATE FOR NONDELETION TYPES OF α THALASSEMIA

The homozygous state for nondeletion forms of α thalassemia involving the dominant (α_2) globin gene causes a more severe deficit of α chains than do the deletion forms of α^+ thalassemia. In some cases

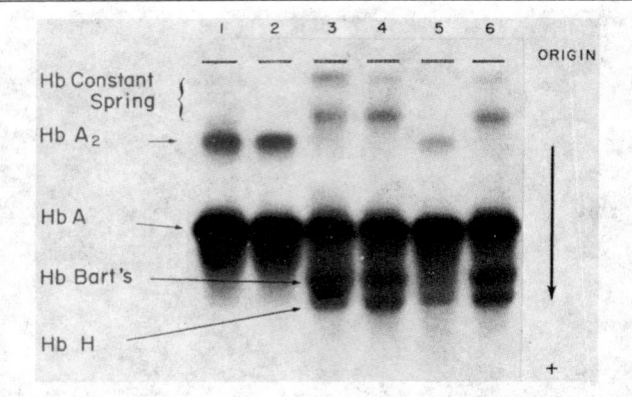

FIGURE 46-19   Hb Constant Spring. Starch gel electrophoresis of the following (left to right): 1 and 2, normal adult; 3 and 4, compound heterozygotes
for Hb Constant Spring and α^o thalassemia with Hb H disease; 5, normal adult;
6, compound heterozygote for α^o thalassemia and Hb Constant Spring.

it produces hemoglobin H disease. The homozygous state for hemoglobin Constant Spring or other chain-termination mutations is associated
with a moderately severe hemolytic anemia in which, for reasons that
are not explained, there is no hemoglobin H but there are small amounts
of hemoglobin Bart's that persist into adult life. The homozygous
states for the other nondeletion forms of α^+ thalassemia are associated
with hemoglobin H disease.

In the homozygous state for hemoglobin Constant Spring, the
blood picture shows mild thalassemic changes with normal-sized red
cells.[218–220] The hemoglobin consists of about 5 to 6 percent hemoglobin
Constant Spring, normal levels of hemoglobin A_2, and trace amounts
of hemoglobin Bart's. The remainder is hemoglobin A.

The heterozygous state for hemoglobin Constant Spring shows
no hematologic abnormality. The hemoglobin pattern is normal except
for the presence of approximately 0.5 percent hemoglobin Constant
Spring. The latter can be observed on alkaline starch-gel electrophoresis as a faint band migrating between hemoglobin A_2 and the origin.
It is best seen on heavily loaded starch gels and is easily missed if
other electrophoretic techniques are used (Fig. 46-19). In the newborn
period there is usually 1 to 3 percent hemoglobin Bart's in the cord
blood.

HOMOZYGOUS STATE FOR DELETION FORMS OF α^+ THALASSEMIA

The homozygous state for deletion forms of α^+ thalassemia is characterized by a thalassemic blood picture with 5 to 10 percent hemoglobin
Bart's at birth and hematologic findings similar to those in α^o-thalas-
semia heterozygotes in adult life.[125] In general, the $-\alpha^{4.2}$ deletion is
associated with a more severe phenotype than is the $--^{3.7}$ deletion.[221]

DIFFERENTIAL DIAGNOSIS

COMMON FORMS OF THALASSEMIA

The clinical and hematologic findings in cases of homozygous β
thalassemia and hemoglobin H disease are so characteristic that little
difficulty in diagnosis is usually encountered. A simple flowchart for
laboratory investigations of a suspected case is shown in Fig. 46-20.

In early childhood, difficulty may occasionally be encountered
in distinguishing the thalassemias from the congenital sideroblastic
anemias, but the marrow appearances in the latter are quite characteristic. Because of the high levels of hemoglobin F encountered in juvenile
chronic myelogenous leukemia, this disorder may superficially resem-

ble β thalassemia. However, the finding of primitive cells in the
marrow and, on hemoglobin electrophoresis, the absence of elevated
hemoglobin A_2 levels and the decrease in carbonic anhydrase in juvenile chronic myelogenous leukemia readily differentiate this disorder
from β thalassemia.

LESS COMMON FORMS OF THALASSEMIA

$(\delta\beta)^0$ THALASSEMIA

The homozygous state for $\delta\beta$ thalassemia is clinically milder than
Cooley's anemia and is one form of thalassemia intermedia.[222–224] Only
hemoglobin F is present, and hemoglobins A and A_2 are not produced.
Heterozygous $\delta\beta$ thalassemia is hematologically similar to β thalassemia minor.[7] The fetal hemoglobin level is higher, being in the 5 to
20 percent range, and the hemoglobin A_2 value is normal or slightly
reduced. As in β thalassemia, the fetal hemoglobin is heterogeneously
distributed among the red cells, thus distinguishing this disorder from
hereditary persistence of fetal hemoglobin (Fig. 46-21).

Heterozygosity for both β thalassemia and $\delta\beta$ thalassemia results
is a condition clinically similar to but milder than Cooley's anemia;
the hemoglobin consists largely of hemoglobin F, with a small amount
of hemoglobin A_2. This occurs because the associated β-thalassemia
gene has usually been the β^0 variety. $\delta\beta$ Thalassemia has also been
observed in individuals heterozygous for hemoglobin S or C.[7]

$(\delta\beta)^+$ THALASSEMIA AND THE HEMOGLOBIN LEPORE DISORDERS

The hemoglobin Lepore disorders have been described in the homozygous state and in the heterozygous state either alone or in association
with β or $\delta\beta$ thalassemia, hemoglobin S, or hemoglobin C.[7,10,225] In
the homozygous state, approximately 20 percent of the hemoglobin
is of the Lepore type and 80 percent is fetal hemoglobin; hemoglobins
A and A_2 are absent. The clinical picture is variable, with some cases
being identical to transfusion-dependent homozygous β thalassemia
and others being associated with the clinical picture of thalassemia
intermedia. In the heterozygous state, the findings are similar to those
of β thalassemia minor, the hemoglobin consisting of about 8 percent
hemoglobin Lepore, with a reduced level of hemoglobin A_2 and a
slight but consistent increase in the level of fetal hemoglobin. The
Lepore hemoglobins have been found sporadically in most racial
groups. In the majority of cases, chemical analysis has shown that they
are identical to hemoglobin Lepore Washington-Boston; hemoglobin
Lepore Hollandia and Lepore Baltimore have been observed in only
a few patients.[7,225]

HEREDITARY PERSISTENCE OF FETAL HEMOGLOBIN

What is known about the molelcular pathology of HPFH was described
earlier in this chapter, and the currently accepted classification and
nomenclature of this complex group of conditions are summarized in
Table 46-4. The different forms of HPFH are of very little clinical
importance except insofar as they may interact with thalassemia or
the structural hemoglobin variants.

$(\delta\beta)^0$ HPFH   Homozygotes for $(\delta\beta)^0$ HPFH have 100 percent
hemoglobin F, and their blood shows mild thalassemic changes with
reduced MCH and MCV values very similar to those observed in
heterozygous β thalassemia. Hemoglobin synthesis studies show that
such persons have imbalanced globin-chain production, with ratios
similar to those observed in β-thalassemia heterozygotes.[226] Heterozygotes have approximately 20 to 30 percent hemoglobin F with slightly
reduced hemoglobin A_2 values and completely normal blood pictures.
Thus, it appears that this condition is an extremely well compensated
form of $\delta\beta$ thalassemia in which the output γ chains almost but not
entirely compensates for the complete absence β and δ chains. The

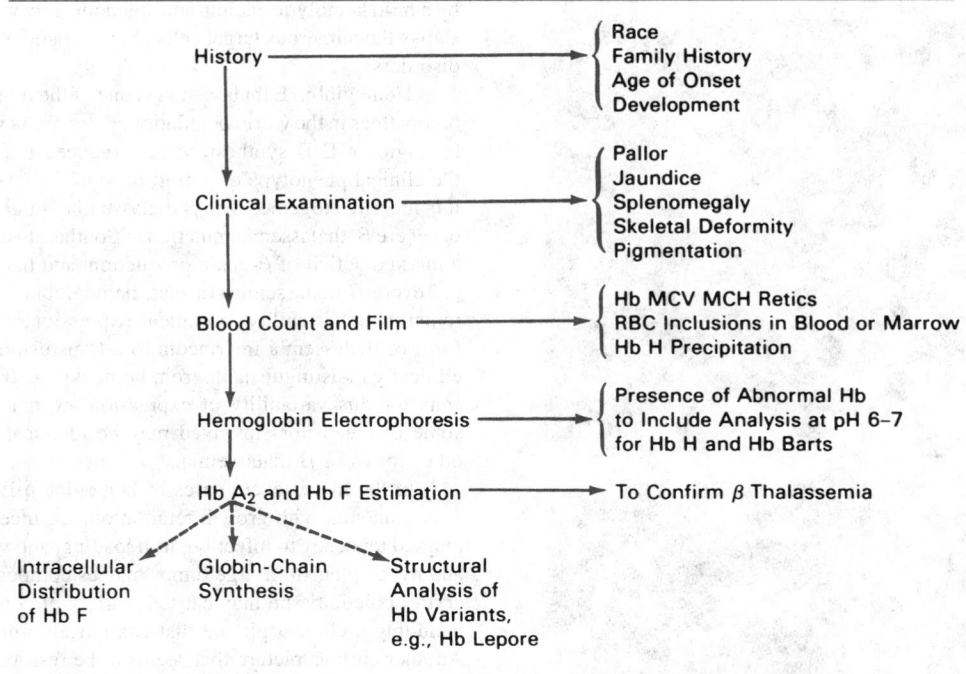

FIGURE 46-20   A flowchart showing an approach to the diagnosis of the thalassemia syndromes.

different molecular forms of this condition show no difference in phenotype except in the proportion of $^G\gamma$ chains. The African forms of $(\delta\beta)^0$ HPFH have been found in association with hemoglobins S and C or with β thalassemia. These compound heterozygous states are associated with little clinical disability.[7,9,10]

$^G\gamma(^A\gamma\beta)^+$ *HPFH and Hemoglobin Kenya*   The deletion form of HPFH associated with the production of the $^A\gamma\beta$ gene product found in hemoglobin Kenya has been observed only in heterozygotes.[108,109] Such individuals have a completely normal blood picture and, as well as having 5 to 20 percent hemoglobin Kenya, have elevated levels of hemoglobin F in the 5 to 10 percent range; only $^G\gamma$ chains are present.

Nondeletion Types of HPFH   Many nondeletion forms of HPFH associated with point mutations upstream from the γ-globin genes have been described (see Table 46-4). $^G\gamma\beta^+$ HPFH has been found in the heterozygous and compound heterozygous states with β-globin chain variants in African populations. There are no associated clinical or hematologic findings. Compound heterozygotes for $^G\gamma\beta^+$ HPFH and hemoglobins S or C produce 45 percent of the abnormal hemoglobin, 30 percent hemoglobin A, and 20 percent hemoglobin F containing only $^G\gamma$ chains.[227,228]

The most common form of nondeletion HPFH, $^A\gamma\beta^+$ HPFH, is found in Greeks.[229–231] In the homozygous state, there are no clinical or hematologic abnormalities; the hemoglobin findings are characterized by approximately 25 percent fetal hemoglobin and reduced levels of hemoglobin A_2, in the 0.8 percent range.[232] Heterozygotes, who are also hematologically normal, have 10 to 15 percent hemoglobin F, almost all of the $^A\gamma$ variety. Compound heterozygotes with β thalassemia have high levels of hemoglobin F and a clinical picture that is only slightly more severe than the β-thalassemia trait.

In the British form of $^A\gamma\beta^+$ HPFH,[233] heterozygotes have approximately 5 to 12 percent hemoglobin F, while homozygotes have approximately 20 percent. There are no associated hematologic abnormalities, although, surprisingly, in this form of nondeletion HPFH the hemoglobin F seems to be rather unevenly distributed among the red cells.

There is a heterogeneous group of conditions associated with the persistent production of small amounts of hemoglobin F in adult life. They are categorized under the general heading of heterocellular HPFH. Their clinical importance is that, when they are coinherited with different forms of β thalassemia, they may lead to a greater output of hemoglobin F and hence to a milder phenotype. This type of interaction should be suspected when one or other parent of a patient with β thalassemia intermedia has an unusually high level of hemoglobin F for the β-thalassemia trait. Similarly, it is sometimes possible to find unaffected lateral relatives or other family members with slightly elevated levels of hemoglobin F. However, until the gene loci involved in these conditions are determined, it is not possible to identify them with certainty.

β THALASSEMIA ASSOCIATED WITH β-CHAIN STRUCTURAL HEMOGLOBIN VARIANTS

The most clinically important associations of β thalassemia with β structural hemoglobin variants are sickle cell thalassemia, hemoglobin C thalassemia, and hemoglobin E thalassemia. In addition, there are many reported interactions of β thalassemia with rare structural variants.[7,9,10]

Sickle cell thalassemia[224–236] occurs in parts of Africa and in the Mediterranean population, particularly in Greece and Italy. It has also been observed in the Middle East and in parts of India. The clinical consequences of carrying one gene for hemoglobin S and one gene for β thalassemia depend entirely on the type of β-thalassemia mutation. The sickle cell–β^0 thalassemia interaction is characterized by a clinical disorder that is very similar to sickle cell anemia. Similarly, the interaction of the sickle cell gene with the more severe forms of β^+ thalassemia that are associated with a marked reduction in β-globin synthesis have a similar clinical phenotype. On the other hand, the interaction of the sickle cell gene with very mild forms of β^+ thalassemia may be quite innocuous.[7,236] The latter disorder is characterized by a mild anemia associated with splenomegaly and a hemoglobin concentration of approximately 30 percent hemoglobin S and 25 per-

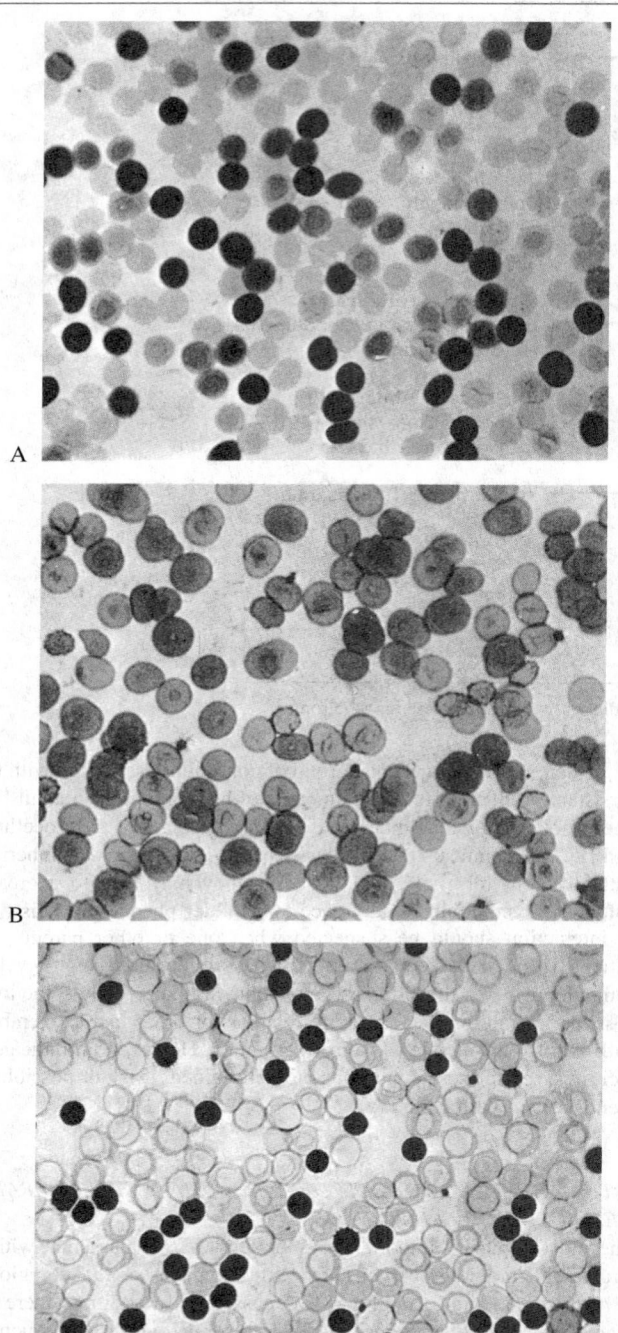

FIGURE 46-21   Acid elution preparations of blood films from the following (top to bottom): (A) $\delta\beta$ thalassemia; (B) hereditary persistence of fetal hemoglobin; (C) an artificial mixture of fetal and adult red cells.

cent hemoglobin A with an elevated level of hemoglobin A_2. In all these interactions, one parent shows the sickle cell trait, and the other the β thalassemia trait.

Hemoglobin C thalassemia is a mild hemolytic disorder associated with splenomegaly.[7,9,10] Again, the hemoglobin pattern varies depending on whether the thalassemia gene is the β^+ or β° type. This relatively innocuous condition has been recorded mainly in North Africa but is also found in West African populations. It is characterized by a mild hemolytic anemia and splenomegaly with a blood picture that shows the numerous target cells characteristic of all the hemoglobin C disorders.

Hemoglobin E thalassemia is one of the most important hemoglobinopathies in the world population.[7,9,10,237–240] As was mentioned earlier, hemoglobin E is synthesized at a reduced rate and hence produces the clinical phenotype of a mild form of β thalassemia. Hence, when it is inherited together with β thalassemia—and most often this is a β° or severe β^+ thalassemia mutation in Southeast Asia and India—there is a marked deficit of β-chain production, and hence the clinical picture of severe β thalassemia. In fact, hemoglobin E thalassemia shows a remarkable variability in clinical expression,[241] ranging from a mild form of thalassemia intermedia to a transfusion-dependent condition clinically indistinguishable from homozygous β thalassemia. The reasons for this variability of expression are not understood, although some of the factors involved may be identical to those that modify other forms of β thalassemia.

In the more severe cases of hemoglobin E thalassemia, there is severe anemia with growth retardation, leg ulcers, bone deformity, a marked tendency to infection, iron loading, and variable splenomegaly and hypersplenism. Large tumor masses composed of extramedullary erythropoietic tissue may cause a variety of compression syndromes, including a clinical picture that can closely mimic a cerebral tumor. Another curious picture that seems to be restricted to splenectomized patients is an obliterative occlusion of the pulmonary vasculature that is thought to be the result of an extremely high platelet count.[242]

The blood picture shows a typical thalassemic pattern, and the hemoglobin consists of E, F, and A_2; there is usually no hemoglobin A because the β° thalassemias are particularly common in the parts of the world where hemoglobin E is found.

β THALASSEMIA WITH NORMAL HEMOGLOBIN A_2 LEVEL

There are forms of β thalassemia in which heterozygotes have normal hemoglobin A_2 levels. Their main clinical importance is that they can be confused with the more severe forms of α thalassemia in the heterozygous state and therefore may cause difficulties for genetic counseling and prenatal diagnosis. Based on hematologic studies, there are two main classes of "normal hemoglobin A_2 β thalassemia," called types 1 and 2.[243] Type 1 is the "silent" form of β thalassemia, while type 2 is heterogeneous, many cases representing the compound heterozygous state for β thalassemia and δ thalassemia.

Normal A_2 β thalassemia type 1 is characterized by no hematologic changes in heterozygotes, and it can be identified with certainty only by globin-chain synthesis studies, which show mild chain imbalance with α/β globin-chain synthesis ratios of approximately 1.3. The condition is also called silent β thalassemia.[244] Compound heterozygotes for this condition and β thalassemia have a mild form of β thalassemia intermedia.

Normal hemoglobin A_2 β thalassemia type 2 in heterozygotes is indistinguishable from typical β thalassemia with elevated hemoglobin A_2 levels.[243] The homozygous state has not been described. The compound heterozygous state for this gene and for β thalassemia with raised hemoglobin A_2 levels is characterized by a clinical picture of severe transfusion-dependent β thalassemia. Family data obtained in Italy and Sardinia suggest that this condition usually represents the compound heterozygous state for both β thalassemia and δ thalassemia.[245,246] Most of the δ thalassemias have been observed *trans* to β thalassemia. However, the form of δ thalassemia that results from the loss of an A in codon 59 occurs on the same chromosome as the hemoglobin Knossos mutation, which is associated with a mild form of β thalassemia.[247] This explains the normal level of hemoglobin A_2 associated with this condition, which is the most common form of normal hemoglobin A_2 β thalassemia in the Mediterranean region.

Several other conditions mentioned earlier in this chapter are associated with a phenotype that is indistinguishable from normal A_2 β thalassemia. These include the heterozygous states for the Corfu form of $\delta\beta$ thalassemia, and $\varepsilon\gamma\delta\beta$ thalassemia.

OTHER UNUSUAL FORMS OF β THALASSEMIA

The clinical features of the dominant β thalassemias, the molecular pathology resembles closely that of thalassemia intermedia. There is moderate anemia and splenomegaly, together with a blood picture showing thalassemic red cell changes. The marrow shows erythroid hyperplasia with well-marked inclusion bodies in the red cell precursors; the latter may be seen in the peripheral blood after splenectomy. Hemoglobin analysis shows hemoglobins A and A_2, and the level of hemoglobin F is not usually elevated much above that seen in β-thalassemia trait. The hemoglobin A_2 levels are always raised.

Other unusual varieties of β thalassemia include those that are categorized by having unusually high hemoglobin F or A_2 levels. It is now apparent that most of these conditions result from deletions that involve the β-globin gene and its promoter region. For example, the so-called Dutch[248] form of β thalassemia is associated with unusually high levels of hemoglobin F in heterozygotes and high levels of hemoglobin A_2; several other conditions of this type, due to different-sized deletions, have been reported.

δ THALASSEMIA

δ Thalassemia causes a complete absence of hemoglobin A_2 in homozygotes and a reduction in the level of hemoglobin A_2 in heterozygotes.[249] Apart from its effect of reducing hemoglobin A_2 levels in β-thalassemia heterozygotes, it is of no clinical significance.

$\varepsilon\gamma\delta\beta$ THALASSEMIA

This heterogeneous condition has been observed only in the heterozygous state in a few families.[7,36,101-103] It is characterized by neonatal hemolysis and, in adult life, by the hematologic picture of heterozygous β thalassemia with normal hemoglobin A_2 levels.

α THALASSEMIA IN ASSOCIATION WITH α- AND β-CHAIN HEMOGLOBIN VARIANTS

Several α-globin structural variants are due to single amino acid substitutions at α-chain loci on chromosomes that carry only a single α-chain gene. Individuals who inherit variants of this type together with an α^0-thalassemia determinant have a form of hemoglobin H disease in which the hemoglobin consists of the α-chain variant hemoglobin and hemoglobin H. Well-documented examples include hemoglobin QH disease ($--/-\alpha^Q$),[250,251] hemoglobin G Philadelphia H disease ($--/-\alpha^G$),[252,253] and hemoglobin Hasharon H disease ($--/-\alpha^{Hash}$).[254] There are many examples of the coexistence of the homozygous or heterozygous states for β-chain hemoglobin variants and different α-thalassemia determinants.[7,9,10] Particularly well-characterized disorders include the various interactions of α^0 and α^+ thalassemia with hemoglobin E[7,237] and hemoglobin S.[255,256] Carriers for these hemoglobin variants who also have the α^0- or α^+-thalassemia traits have thalassemic red cell indices and unusually low levels of the abnormal hemoglobin. Individuals with sickle cell anemia who have α thalassemia show thalassemic red cell changes, more persistent splenomegaly, and lower hemoglobin F values than do those without the thalassemia genes.[255,256]

THERAPY, COURSE, AND PROGNOSIS

The only forms of treatment available for thalassemic children are regular blood transfusions, iron chelation therapy in an attempt to prevent iron overload, the judicious use of splenectomy in cases complicated by hypersplenism, and a good standard of general pediatric care. Marrow transplantation also has an important role in selected cases (see Chap. 19).

TRANSFUSION

If children with β thalassemia are maintained at a hemoglobin level of 9.5 to 14 g/dl, they grow and develop normally and develop none of the distressing skeletal complications of thalassemia.[7,257] More recent experience suggests that it may be possible to maintain a lower hemoglobin level than this without any deleterious effects on development and with the added advantage of reducing the level of iron loading. This regimen maintains a mean pretransfusion level that does not exceed 9.5 g/dl.[258] The transfusion program should not be started too early, and only when it is quite clear that the hemoglobin level is too low to be compatible with normal development. If transfusion is started too soon, thalassemia intermedia may be missed, and the child may be transfused unnecessarily. Usually blood transfusions are given every four weeks on an outpatient basis. To avoid transfusion reactions, it is important to use washed, filtered, or frozen red cells so that the majority of the white cells and plasma-protein components are removed (see Chap. 142). More ambitious programs using separated, young erythrocyte populations (''neocytes'') for transfusion, together with the removal of the patient's older cells, have been described,[229] but their use is restricted to only a few centers because of the difficulty and expense of these procedures.[257]

IRON CHELATION

Since every child maintained on a high-transfusion regimen will ultimately develop iron overload and die due to siderosis of the myocardium, it is vital, when possible, to start such children on a program of iron chelation some time within the first 2 to 3 years of life.[182] Despite extensive searches for an oral chelating agent, deferoxamine (desferrioxamine) is currently the only drug of proven value for the treatment of thalassemia. It is best administered by an 8- to 12-h overnight pump-driven infusion in the subcutaneous tissues of the anterior abdominal wall.[260,261] Chelation therapy should commence by the time the serum ferritin level has reached approximately 1000 μg/dl. In practice this is usually after the twelfth to fifteenth transfusion. It is important not to overchelate infants when the iron burden is still low in order to avoid toxicity. The initial dose is usually 20 mg/kg on 5 nights a week, with 100 mg of oral vitamin C (200 mg in older children and adults) on the days of the infusion, since this increases the level of iron excretion.[262] Higher levels of ascorbate should be avoided because of the potential for toxicity.[263] In patients who are heavily iron loaded, particularly with cardiac or endocrine complications, the body iron stores may be effectively lowered by the use of a continuous intravenous infusion of desferrioxamine at a dose of up to 50 mg/kg body weight. This usually entails the insertion of an intravenous delivery system.

It has been usual to monitor the degree of iron loading by the use of serial serum ferritin estimations. However, recent studies indicate that the relationship between hepatic iron concentration and serum ferritin is not reliable, and it is recommended that all patients on regular transfusion are monitored with hepatic iron studies (see Iron Metabolism).[257] If this is not possible, it is important to try to maintain the serum ferritin levels below 1500 μg/l.

There is extensive experience of the use of desferrioxamine and its toxic effects.[257] Apart from local erythema and painful subcutaneous nodules at the site of infusions and occasional genuine allergic reactions, there are no serious complications, and these reactions can be controlled, at least in part, by inclusion of 5 to 10 mg hydrocortisone in the infusion. Probably of greatest concern is neurosensory toxicity, which has been documented in up to 30 percent of cases. This causes high-frequency hearing loss that may sometimes become symptomatic.[264,265] In a few cases, this has not responded to discontinuation of the drug, and there has been permanent hearing loss. Ocular toxicity has also been reported.[264] This involves visual failure, with night and color blindness together with field loss. Reversal after discontinuation of the drug has been reported. Desferrioxamine may also cause bone changes and growth retardation, sometimes associated with bone pain. Body measurements characteristically show a reduced crown-pubis/pubis-heel ratio. These changes may be associated with radiological abnormalities of the vertebral column. The occurrence of these complications can be avoided by extreme care in monitoring patients receiving long-term desferrioxamine therapy. It appears that young children or individuals from whom most of the iron has been removed by chelation are at particularly high risk. It is recommended that a formal audiometry and ophthalmologic examination is carried out at 6-month intervals.

The only oral iron chelating agent that has received extensive study is 1,2-dimethyl-3-hydroxypyridin-4-one (deferiprone,L1). The current status of this drug has been reviewed recently.[257] While early studies were promising, it is now apparent that, at the dose currently used, some patients do not maintain iron balance. About 5 percent of patients develop severe neutropenia, and there have been deaths from agranulocytosis. There is also concern about the possibility that this agent may potentiate liver fibrosis. The future role of this agent is not clear, but it certainly should be used only with very close monitoring and facilities for liver biopsy.

There is increasing evidence that children maintained at a high hemoglobin level do not develop hypersplenism. However, in patients who have been kept at a lower hemoglobin level, enlargement of the spleen with increased transfusion requirements occurs commonly. Splenectomy should be carried out if there is a dramatic increase in the transfusion requirements or pain develops because of the size of the spleen. Because of the risk of overwhelming pneumococcal infections,[266,267] this should not be done in the first 5 years of life. Before it is carried out, these children should receive a pneumococcal vaccine, and then they should be placed on prophylactic oral penicillin after the operation. It is also recommended that they receive *Haemophilus influenzae* type B and meningococcal vaccines.

Children with severe thalassemia are still prone to other infections. Presentation with abdominal pain, diarrhea, and vomiting should always suggest the possibility of an infection with a member of the *Yersinia* class of bacteria. Empirical treatment should start immediately with either an aminoglycoside or a cotrimoxazole. Transfusion-transmitted virus infection is also very common in some populations. All chronically transfused patients should be tested for hepatitis C, hepatitis B, and HIV annually, and patients with serological evidence of chronic active hepatitis should be considered for treatment with interferon alpha and/or ribavirin. As mentioned earlier, there is increasing recognition of subtle endocrine deficiencies, particularly associated with growth retardation and hypogonadism. These patients require expert endocrinological assessment and, when appropriate, replacement therapy.

MARROW TRANSPLANTATION

By 1997, over 1000 marrow transplants had been performed at three centers in Italy.[268–271] Based on early experiences, it became clear that the prognosis depended very much on the adequacy of iron chelation up to the time of transplantation. Based on this history, patients were divided into three classes: class I have a history of adequate iron chelation and neither liver fibrosis nor hepatomegaly; class II are characterized by having one or two of these characteristics; and class

III have all three. Among children in class I who had undergone transplantation early in the course of the disease, disease-free survival was assessed at 90 to 93 percent, with a risk of mortality related to the procedure of 4 percent.[268] For class II patients, which form the intermediate risk group, the survival and disease-free survival rates were 86 percent and 82 percent, respectively. For what is considered to be the high-risk group, that is, class III, the survival and disease-free survival rates are 62 and 51 percent, respectively. Apart from the immediate complications of severe infection in the posttransplant period, most of the problems relate to the development of acute or chronic graft-versus-host disease. It appears that the overall frequency of mild to severe grades ranges from 30 to 27 percent.[272] The modification of preparative drug regimens has reduced the frequency of drug toxicity. The occurrence of mixed chimerism may be a risk factor for graft-versus-host disease. So far, the longest follow-up of patients after transplantation is between 15 and 20 years; no case of hematologic malignancy has been observed. A recent study suggests that it may be more effective to remove excess body iron accumulated before transplantation by venesection rather than chelation therapy.[273]

Clearly, in experienced centers, marrow transplantation now offers a genuine option for the management of different forms of thalassemia.

Apart from the measures just outlined, the management of thalassemia requires a high standard of general pediatric care. Infection should be treated early. If the diet is inadequate in folate, supplements should be given; this is probably unnecessary in children maintained on a high-transfusion regimen. Particular attention should be paid to the ear, nose, and throat because of the problem of chronic sinus infection and middle-ear diseases resulting from bone deformity of the skull. Similarly, regular dental surveillance is essential, since poorly transfused thalassemic children have a variety of deformities of the maxilla and poorly developed teeth. In the later stages of the illness, when iron loading becomes the major feature, endocrine replacement therapy may be necessary, together with symptomatic treatment for cardiac failure. It may be possible to improve cardiac function with intensive desferrioxamine therapy.

THERAPIES OF SPECIAL TYPES OF THALASSEMIA

Hemoglobin H disease usually requires no specific therapy, although splenectomy may be of value in cases associated with severe anemia and splenomegaly.[7,9,10] This may be followed by a higher incidence of thromboembolic disease than occurs in splenectomized children with β thalassemia,[7] and therefore the spleen should be removed only in cases of extreme anemia and splenomegaly. Oxidant drugs should be avoided in patients with hemoglobin H disease. The management of symptomatic sickle cell thalassemia follows the lines described for sickle cell anemia (see Chap. 48).

Thalassemia intermedia presents a particularly complex therapeutic problem. It is difficult to be certain whether a child with a steady-state hemoglobin level of 6 to 7 g/dl should be transfused. Probably the best compromise is to watch such children very closely during the first years of life, and, if they are growing and developing normally and there are no signs of bone changes, they should be maintained without transfusion. If, however, their early growth pattern is retarded or their activity is limited due to their anemia, they should be placed on a regular transfusion regimen. It is especially important to determine whether hypersplenism is playing a role in their anemia as they get older and to carry out splenectomy if this is the case. Since many of these patients have significant iron loading from the gastrointestinal tract, regular estimations of serum iron and ferritin should be carried out, and chelation therapy should be instituted when appropriate.[257]

EXPERIMENTAL APPROACHES TO TREATMENT

Two main experimental approaches are being pursued in the search for more effective therapy of the thalassemias: the reactivation or augmentation of fetal hemoglobin production and somatic gene therapy.

The main rationale for attempting to increase hemoglobin F production is based on the observation that patients recovering from cytotoxic drug therapy or during other periods of erythroid expansion may reactivate hemoglobin F synthesis. In addition, the observation that butyrate analogs might have a stimulating effect on hemoglobin F production has led to a number of studies of their potential for the management of thalassemia. A number of clinical trials have been summarized in recent reviews.[274–276] Agents that have been used have included various cytotoxic drugs, erythropoietin, and several different butyrate analogs. Overall, while these agents, used either alone or in combination, have produced some small effects on fetal hemoglobin production, the results of these trials to date have been disappointing. There have been some notable exceptions, however, particularly several cases of homozygosity or compound heterozygosity for hemoglobin Lepore in which the use of either a combination of sodium phenylbutyrate and hydroxyurea or hydroxyurea alone has produced a spectacular rise in hemoglobin F production, which, in the case of two homozygotes for hemoglobin Lepore, removed the necessity for further transfusion.[277] This raises the intriguing possibility that certain mutations, possibly deletions of the β-globin gene cluster, may be more susceptible to this type of approach. It may be that appropriate combination therapy will improve the results in other forms of thalassemia.

The other experimental approach involves somatic gene therapy. Currently this is mainly directed at gene transfer into potential hematopoietic stem cells using retroviral vectors,[278] although other approaches are being taken, including attempts at the restoration of normal splicing in cases of splicing mutations[279] or the use of trans-splicing ribozymes to correct β-globin gene transcripts.[280,281] So far, none of these methods has been developed to the scale required for human gene transfer, and it looks as though it may be some time before this is achieved.

PROGNOSIS

There is now no doubt that the prognosis for patients with severe forms of β thalassemia who are adequately treated by transfusion and chelation has improved quite dramatically over recent years. Two large studies have investigated the influence of effective long-term use of desferrioxamine on the development of cardiac disease.[282,283] In one trial, patients who had maintained sustained reduction of body iron, as estimated by a serum ferritin level of less than 2500 μg/l over 12 years of follow-up, had an estimated cardiac-disease–free survival of 91 percent, in contrast to patients in whom most determinations of serum ferritin level excluded this value, whose estimated cardiac-disease–free survival was less than 20 percent. In a second study, the relationship between survival and total body iron burden was measured directly using hepatic storage iron values. Patients who had maintained concentrations of hepatic iron equal to or exceeding 15 mg iron per gram of liver, dry weight, had a 32 percent probability of survival to the age of 25 years; no cardiac disease developed in patients who maintained hepatic iron levels below this threshold. These studies provide unequivocal evidence that adequate transfusion and chelation are now associated with longevity and a good quality of life. On the other hand, poor compliance or unavailability of chelating agents is still associated with a poor prospect of survival much beyond the second decade.

PREVENTION

In those parts of the world where the incidence is high, the economic burden placed on society by thalassemia is immense. For example, it was estimated that if all the thalassemic children who are born in Cyprus were treated by regular blood transfusions and iron chelating therapy, within 15 years the total medical budget of the island would be required to treat this single disease.[284] Clearly, this approach is not always feasible, and hence there is considerable effort toward the development of programs for prevention of the different forms of thalassemia.

There are two ways in which this can be achieved. The first is by prospective genetic counseling, that is, screening total populations while still at school and warning carriers about the potential risks of marriage to another carrier. There are few data available about the value of programs of this type; a pilot study in Greece was unsuccessful,[285] and the results of large-scale studies being carried out in parts of Italy[286] are still awaited. Because it is felt that this approach is unlikely to be very successful in many populations, considerable effort has been directed toward developing prenatal diagnosis programs.

Prenatal diagnosis for the prevention of thalassemia entails screening mothers at the first prenatal visit, screening the father in cases in which the mother is a thalassemia carrier, and offering the couple the possibility of prenatal diagnosis and termination of pregnancy if they are both carriers of a gene for a severe form of thalassemia. Currently, these programs are devoted mainly to prenatal diagnosis of the severe transfusion-dependent forms of homozygous β^+ or β° thalassemia. Considerable experience has also been gained in prenatal diagnosis of mothers at risk of having a fetus with the hemoglobin Bart's hydrops syndrome because of the distress caused by a long and difficult pregnancy and the obstetric problems that result from the birth of a hydropic infant with a massive placenta.

The first efforts at prenatal detection of β thalassemia utilized fetal blood sampling and globin-chain synthesis analysis carried out at about the eighteenth week of pregnancy. Despite the technical difficulties involved, this method was applied successfully in many countries and has resulted in a reduction in the birth rate of infants with β thalassemia.[287] It is associated with a low maternal morbidity rate, a fetal mortality rate of approximately 3 to 4 percent, and an error rate of 1 to 2 percent. Its main disadvantage is that it must be carried out relatively late in pregnancy. For this reason, efforts have turned to first-trimester prenatal diagnosis.

The application of the methods of DNA technology have made it possible to diagnose the important hemoglobin disorders in utero by fetal DNA analysis. Although this can be carried out on DNA derived from amniotic fluid, this approach has drawbacks because, again, it must be done relatively late in pregnancy, and often amniotic fluid cells have to be grown in culture to obtain enough DNA.[288] However, it is possible to obtain DNA as early as the ninth week of pregnancy by chorionic villus sampling. Although the safety of this technique remains to be fully evaluated, and it is possible that limb reduction deformities may occur when the procedure is carried out very early in pregnancy (9 or 10 weeks), enough experience has been gained to suggest that it will become the major method for the prenatal diagnosis of the thalassemias.[289–292]

The identification of thalassemia in the fetus requires different approaches, depending on the nature of the molecular pathology involved.[292] Major deletions, such as those that cause α° thalassemia and some of the β° thalassemias, can be identified directly on Southern blotting analysis of fetal DNA. About a third of the point mutations that produce β thalassemia alter restriction enzyme sites and therefore can also be identified by gene mapping. Where the mutation is known, oligonucleotide probes can be constructed to identify it directly. In families in which the mutation is not known, it is often possible to define the affected parental chromosomes by RFLP linkage analysis and then to determine whether the fetus has received both of the affected chromosomes from its parents. Experience of many hundred first-trimester prenatal diagnoses has suggested that it is possible to tell whether the fetus is affected in about 80 percent of cases.[289–292] The main difficulties arise because many potentially affected fetuses will be compound heterozygotes for a common and a rare β-thalassemia mutation or because it may not be possible to define the thalassemia chromosome by RFLP analysis.

Now that the mutations have been determined in so many different forms of α and β thalassemia, it is possible to detect them directly as the first-line approach to prenatal diagnosis. Since most racial groups have only a few common β-thalassemia mutations, it is possible in many cases to determine the mutations in the parents and then to analyze fetal DNA for their presence. The development of PCR, combined with the use of oligonucleotide probes to detect individual mutations, offers a wide variety of new approaches for facilitating the speed and accuracy of carrier detection and prenatal diagnosis.[293–296] For example, diagnoses can be made using hybridization of specific ^{32}P end-labeled oligonucleotides to an amplified region of the β-globin gene dotted onto a nylon membrane. Because the β-globin gene sequence can be amplified more than 10^6-fold, hybridization time can be limited to 1 h, and the entire procedure can be carried out in 2 h. The ARMS (see Chap. 11) also allows the diagnosis to be made in about 2 h.[297,298] Other modifications of PCR involve the use of nonradioactively labeled probes.[299,300]

The error rate using these different approaches varies, depending on a number of factors, particularly the experience of the laboratory. Low rates, less than 1 percent, have been reported from most laboratories using fetal DNA analysis. Potential sources of error include maternal contamination of fetal DNA, nonpaternity, and genetic recombination in cases where RFLP linkage analysis is used, along with other technical quirks.

The application of these approaches has caused a major reduction in the birth rate of infants with thalassemia in some populations, notably the Mediterranean islands. A number of methods are being explored to try to increase the options for prenatal detection of thalassemia. Harvesting of fetal cells from the maternal circulation is being explored, and a variety of ways are being investigated to isolate them by micromanipulation methods.[301,302] Because of the trauma of termination of pregnancy experienced by many women, preimplantation approaches are also being explored. A few preimplantation diagnoses of β thalassemia by polar body analysis have already been carried out successfully.[303]

REFERENCES

1. Cooley TB, Lee P: A series of cases of splenomegaly in children with anemia and peculiar bone changes. *Trans Am Pediatr Soc* 37:29, 1925.
2. Whipple GH, Bradford WL: Racial or familial anemia of children associated with fundamental disturbances of bone and pigment metabolism (Cooley von Jaksch). *Am J Dis Child* 44:336, 1932.
3. Weatherall DJ: Toward an understanding of the molecular biology of some common inherited anemias: The story of thalassemia, in *Blood, Pure and Eloquent*, edited by MM Wintrobe, p 373. McGraw-Hill, New York, 1980.
4. Whipple CH, Bradford WL: Mediterranean disease—thalassemia (erythroblastic anemia of Cooley): Associated pigment abnormalities simulating hemochromatosis. *J Pediatr* 9:279, 1936.
5. Bannerman RM: *Thalassemia: A Survey of Some Aspects*. Grune & Stratton, New York, 1961.
6. Chernoff AI: The distribution of the thalassemia gene: A historical review. *Blood* 14:899, 1959.
7. Weatherall DJ, Clegg JB: *The Thalassaemia Syndromes*, 4th ed. Blackwell, Oxford, 2000.
8. Ingram VM, Stretton AOW: Genetic basis of the thalassemia diseases. *Nature* 184:1903, 1959.
9. Bunn HF, Forget BG: *Hemoglobin: Molecular, Genetic and Clinical Aspects*. Saunders, Philadelphia, 1986.
10. Weatherall DJ, Clegg JB, Higgs DR, Wood WG: The hemoglobinopathies, in *The Metabolic Basis of Inherited Disease*, 8th ed, edited by CR Scriver, AL Beauder, WS Sly, D Valle. McGraw-Hill, New York, 2000. In press.
11. Orkin SH: The duplicated human α globin genes lie close together in cellular DNA. *Proc Natl Acad Sci USA* 75:5950, 1978.
12. Lauer J, Shen C-KJ, Maniatis T: The chromosomal arrangement of human α-like globin genes: Sequence homology and α-globin gene deletions. *Cell* 20:119, 1980.
13. Liebhaber SA, Goossens N, Kan YW: Homology and concerted evolution at the α_1 and α_2 loci of human α-globin. *Nature* 290:26, 1981.
14. Liebhaber SA, Goossens MJ, Kan YW: Cloning and complete nucleotide sequence of human $5'$-α-globin gene. *Proc Natl Acad Sci USA* 77:7054, 1980.
15. Proudfoot NJ, Maniatis T: The structure of a human α-globin pseudogene and its relationship to α-globin duplication. *Cell* 21:537, 1980.
16. Liebhaber SA, Kan YW: Differentiation of the mRNA transcripts originating from the α_1- and α_2-globin loci in normals and α-thalassemics. *J Clin Invest* 68:439, 1981.
17. Orkin SH, Goff SC: The duplicated human α-globin genes: Their relative expression as measured by RNA analysis. *Cell* 24:345, 1981.
18. Higgs DR, Wainscoat JS, Flint J, et al: Analysis of the human α globin gene cluster reveals a highly informative genetic locus. *Proc Natl Acad Sci USA* 83:5156, 1986.
19. Fritsch EF, Lawn RM, Maniatis T: Molecular cloning and characterization of the human β-like globin gene cluster. *Cell* 19:959, 1980.
20. Spritz RA, DeRiel JK, Forget BG, Weissman SM: Complete nucleotide sequence of the human δ-globin gene. *Cell* 21:639, 1980.
21. Baralle FE, Shoulders CC, Proudfoot NJ: The primary structure of the human ϵglobin gene. *Cell* 21:621, 1980.
22. Slightom JL, Blechl AE, Smithies O: Human $^G\gamma$- and $^A\gamma$-globin genes: Complete nucleotide sequences suggest that DNA can be exchanged between these duplicated genes. *Cell* 21:627, 1980.
23. Jeffrey AJ: DNA sequences in the $^G\gamma$-, $^A\gamma$-, δ-, and β-globin genes of man. *Cell* 18:1, 1979.
24. Antonarakis SE, Boehm CD, Giardina PVJ, Kazazian HH: Nonrandom association of polymorphic restriction sites in the β-globin gene complex. *Proc Natl Acad Sci USA* 79:137, 1982.
25. Wainscoat JS, Hill AVV, Boyce A, et al: Evolutionary relationships of human populations from an analysis of nuclear DNA polymorphisms. *Nature* 319:491, 1982.
26. Abel T, Maniatis T: Mechanisms of eukaryotic gene regulation, in *The Molecular Basis of Blood Disease*, 2nd ed, edited by G Stamatoyannopoulos, AW Nienhuis, P Leder, PW Majerus, H Varmus, p 33. Saunders, Philadelphia, 1994.
27. Evans T, Felsenfeld G, Reitman M: Control of globin gene transcription. *Annu Rev Cell Biol* 6:95, 1990.
28. Groudine M, Kohwi-Shigematsu T, Gelinas R, et al: Human fetal to adult hemoglobin switching: Changes in chromatin structure of the β-globin gene locus. *Proc Natl Acad Sci USA* 80:7551, 1983.
29. Antoniou M, DeBoer E, Habets G, Grosveld F: The human β-globin gene contains multiple regulatory regions: Identification of one promoter and two downstream enhancers. *EMBO J* 7:377, 1988.
30. Yamamoto M, Ko LJ, Leonard MW, et al: Activity and tissue specific expression of the transcription factor NF-E1 multigene family. *Gene Dev* 4:1650, 1990.
31. Whitelaw E, Tsai S-F, Hogben P, Orkin SH: Regulated expression of globin chains and the erythroid transcription factor GATA-1 during erythropoiesis in the developing mouse. *Mol Cell Biol* 10:6596, 1990.
32. Grosveld F, Blom van Assendelft G, Greaves DR, Kollias G: Position independent, high level expression of the human β globin gene in transgenic mice. *Cell* 51:975, 1987.

33. Jarman AP, Wood WG, Sharpe JA, et al: Characterization of the major regulatory element upstream of the human α globin gene cluster. *Mol Cell Biol* 11:4679, 1991.

34. Stamatoyannopoulos G, Nienhuis AW: Hemoglobin switching, in *The Molecular Basis of Blood Diseases,* 2nd ed, edited by G Stamatoyannopoulos, AW Nienhuis, P Leder, PW Majerus, H Varmus, p 107. Saunders, Philadelphia, 1994.

35. Weatherall DJ: Thalassemia, in *The Molecular Basis of Blood Diseases,* 3rd ed, edited by G Stamatoyannopoulos, AW Nienhuis, PW Majerus, H Varmus. Saunders, Philadelphia, 2000. In press.

36. Huisman THJ, Carver MFM, Baysal E: *A Syllabus of Thalassemia Mutations.* Sickle Cell Anemia Foundation, Augusta, GA, 1997.

37. Thein SL: β-Thalassaemia, in *Bailliére's Clinical Haematology. International Practice and Research: Sickle Cell Disease and Thalassaemia,* edited by GP Rodgers, p 91. Bailliére Tindall, London, 1998.

38. Orkin SH, Old JM, Weatherall DJ, Nathan DG: Partial deletion of β-globin gene DNA in certain patients with β^0-thalassemia. *Proc Natl Acad Sci USA* 76:2400, 1979.

39. Thein SL, Old JM, Wainscoat JS, Weatherall DJ: Population and genetic studies suggest a single origin for the Indian deletion β^0 thalassaemia. *Br J Haematol* 57:271, 1984.

40. Anand R, Boehm CD, Kazazian HH, Vanin EF: Molecular characterization of a β^0-thalassaemia resulting from a 1.4 kb deletion. *Blood* 72:636, 1988.

41. Gilman JG: The 12.6 kilobase DNA deletion in Dutch β^0-thalassemia. *Br J Haematol* 67:369, 1987.

42. Padanilam BJ, Felice AE, Huisman THJ: Partial deletion of the 5' β globin gene region causes β^0 thalassemia in members of an American black family. *Blood* 64:941, 1984.

43. Popovich BW, Rosenblatt DS, Kendall AG, Nishioka Y: Molecular characterization of an atypical β thalassemia caused by a large deletion in the 5' β-globin gene region. *Am J Hum Genet* 39:797, 1986.

44. Diaz-Chico JC, Yang KG, Kutlar A, et al: A 300 bp deletion involving part of the 5' β-globin gene region is observed in members of a Turkish family with β-thalassemia. *Blood* 70:583, 1987.

45. Aulehla-Scholtz C, Spielberg R, Horst J: A β-thalassemia mutant caused by a 300 bp deletion in the human β-globin gene. *Hum Genet* 81:298, 1989.

46. Orkin SH, Antonarakis SE, Kazazian HH: Base substitution at position −88 in a β-thalassemic globin gene: Further evidence for the role of the distal promoter element ACACCC. *J Biol Chem* 259:8679, 1984.

47. Orkin SH, Kazazian HH, Antonarakis SE, et al: Linkage of β-thalassaemia mutations and β-globin gene polymorphisms with DNA polymorphisms in human globin gene cluster. *Nature* 296:267, 1982.

48. Poncz M, Ballantine M, Solowiejczyk D, et al: β-Thalassemia in a Kurdish Jew. *J Biol Chem* 257:5994, 1983.

49. Orkin SH, Sexton JP, Cheng TC, et al: ATA box transcription mutation in β-thalassemia. *Nucleic Acids Res* 11:4727, 1983.

50. Antonarakis SE, Orkin SH, Cheng T-C, et al: β-Thalassemia in American blacks: Novel mutations in the TATA box and IVS-2 acceptor splice site. *Proc Natl Acad Sci USA* 81:1154, 1984.

51. Surrey S, Delgrosso K, Malladi P, Schwartz E: Functional analysis of a β-globin gene containing a TATA box mutation from a Kurdish Jew with β-thalassemia. *J Biol Chem* 260:6507, 1985.

52. Gonzalez-Redondo JH, Stoming TA, Kutlar A, et al: A C → T substitution at nt −101 in a conserved DNA sequence of the promoter region of the β-globin gene is associated with "silent" β-thalassemia. *Blood* 73:1705, 1989.

53. Wong C, Dowling CE, Saiki RK, et al: Characterization of beta-thalassemia mutations using direct genomic sequencing of amplified single copy DNA. *Nature* 330:384, 1987.

54. Treisman R, Orkin SH, Maniatis T: Specific transcription and RNA splicing defects in five cloned β-thalassemia genes. *Nature* 302:591, 1983.

55. Kazazian HH, Orkin SH, Antonarakis SE, et al: Molecular characterization of seven β-thalassaemia mutations in Asian Indians. *EMBO J* 3:593, 1984.

56. Padanilam BJ, Huisman THJ: The β^0-thalassemia in an American black family is due to a single nucleotide substitution in the acceptor splice junction of the second intervening sequence. *Am J Hematol* 22:259, 1986.

57. Atweh GF, Anagnou NP, Shearin J, Forget BG, Kaufman RE: β-Thalassemia resulting from a single nucleotide substitution in an acceptor splice site. *Nucleic Acids Res* 13:777, 1985.

58. Orkin SH, Sexton JP, Goff SC, Kazazian HH: Inactivation of an acceptor splice site by a short deletion in β-thalassemia. *J Biol Chem* 258:7249, 1983.

59. Atweh GF, Wong C, Reed R, et al: A new mutation in IVS-1 of the human β globin gene causing β thalassemia due to abnormal splicing. *Blood* 70:147, 1987.

60. Cheng T, Orkin SH, Antonarakis SE, et al: β-Thalassemia in Chinese: Use of in vivo RNA analysis and oligonucleotide hybridization in systematic characterization of molecular defects. *Proc Natl Acad Sci USA* 81:2821, 1984.

61. Gonzalez-Redondo JH, Stoming TA, Lanclos KD, et al: Clinical and genetic heterogeneity in black patients with homozygous β-thalassemia from the southeastern United States. *Blood* 72:1007, 1988.

62. Tamagnini GP, Lopes MC, Castanheira ME, et al: β^+ thalassaemia— Portuguese type: Clinical, haematological and molecular studies of a newly defined form of β thalassaemia. *Br J Haematol* 54:189, 1983.

63. Hill AVS, Bowden DK, O'Shaughnessy DF, et al: β-Thalassemia in Melanesia: Association with malaria and characterization of a common variant. *Blood* 72:9, 1988.

64. Spritz RA, Jagadeeswaran P, Choudary PV, et al: Base substitution in an intervening sequence of a β^+ thalassemic human globin gene. *Proc Natl Acad Sci USA* 78:2455, 1981.

65. Busslinger M, Moschanas N, Flavell RA: β^+ thalassemia: Aberrant splicing results from a single point mutation in an intron. *Cell* 27:289, 1981.

66. Metherall JE, Collins RS, Pan J, et al: β^0 thalassaemia caused by a base substitution that creates an alternative splice acceptor site in an intron. *EMBO J* 5:2551, 1986.

67. Orkin SH, Kazazian HH, Antonarakis SE, et al: Abnormal RNA processing due to the exon mutation of β^E-globin gene. *Nature* 300:768, 1982.

68. Goldsmith ME, Humphries RK, Bey T, et al: "Silent" nucleotide substitution in β^+ thalassemia globin gene activated splice site in coding sequence RNA. *Proc Natl Acad Sci* 88:2318, 1983.

69. Orkin SH, Antonarakis SE, Loukopoulos D: Abnormal processing of β Knossos RNA. *Blood* 64:311, 1984.

70. Yang KG, Kutlar F, George E, et al: Molecular characterization of β-globin gene mutations in Malay patients with Hb E–β-thalassemia major. *Br J Haematol* 72:73, 1989.

71. Orkin SH, Cheng T-C, Antonarakis SE, Kazazian HH: Thalassaemia due to a mutation in the cleavage-polyadenylation signal of the human β-globin gene. *EMBO J* 4:453, 1985.

72. Jankovic L, Efremov GD, Petkov G, et al: Three novel mutations leading to β thalassemia. *Blood* 74:226, 1989.

73. Rund D, Filon D, Rachmilewitz EA, et al: Molecular analysis of β-thalassemia in Kurdish Jews: Novel mutations and expression studies. *Blood* 74:821, 1989.

74. Chang JC, Kan YW: β-Thalassemia: A nonsense mutation in man. *Proc Natl Acad Sci USA* 76:2886, 1979.

75. Kazazian HH, Dowling CE, Waber PG, et al: The spectrum of β-thalassemia genes in China and Southeast Asia. *Blood* 68:964, 1986.

76. Trecartin RF, Liebhaber SA, Chang JC, et al: β Thalassemia in Sardinia is caused by a nonsense mutation. *J Clin Invest* 68:1012, 1981.

77. Rosatelli C, Leoni GB, Tuveri T, et al: β Thalassemia mutations in Sardinians: Implications for prenatal diagnosis. *J Med Genet* 24:97, 1987.

78. Weatherall DJ, Clegg JB, Knox-Macaulay HHM, et al: A genetically determined disorder with features both of thalassaemia and congenital dyserythropoietic anaemia. *Br J Haematol* 24:681, 1973.

79. Stamatoyannopoulos G, Woodson R, Papayannopoulou T, et al: Inclusion-body β-thalassemia trait: A form of β thalassemia producing clinical manifestations in simple heterozygotes. *N Engl J Med* 290:939, 1974.

80. Thein SL: Dominant β thalassemia: Molecular basis and pathophysiology. *Br J Haematol* 80:273, 1992.

81. Thein SL, Hesketh C, Taylor P, et al: Molecular basis for dominantly inherited inclusion body β thalassemia. *Proc Natl Acad Sci USA* 87:3924, 1990.

82. Beris RP, Miescher PA, Diaz-Chico JC, et al: Inclusion body β-thalassemia trait in a Swiss family is caused by an abnormal hemoglobin

(Geneva) with an altered and extended β chain carboxy-terminus due to a modification in codon 114. *Blood* 72:801, 1988.

83. Kazazian HH, Dowling CE, Hurwitz RL, et al: Thalassemia mutations in exon 3 of the β-globin gene often cause a dominant form of thalassemia and show no predilection for malarial-endemic regions of the world. *Am J Hum Genet* 45:A242, 1989.

84. Fei YJ, Stoming TA, Kutlar A, et al: One form of inclusion body β thalassemia is due to a GAA → TAA mutation at codon 121 of the β chain. *Blood* 73:1075, 1989.

85. Kazazian HH, Orkin SH, Boehm CD, et al: Characterization of a spontaneous mutation to a β-thalassemia allele. *Am J Hum Genet* 38:860, 1986.

86. Murru S, Loudianos G, Deiana M, et al: Molecular characterization of β-thalassemia intermedia in patients of Italian descent and identification of three novel β-thalassemia mutations. *Blood* 77:1342, 1991.

87. Ristaldi MS, Pirastu M, Murru S, et al: A spontaneous mutation produced a novel elongated β^0 globin chain structural variant (Hb Agnana) with a thalassemia-like phenotype. *Blood* 75:1378, 1990.

88. Fucharoen S, Kobayashi Y, Fucharoen G, et al: A single nucleotide deletion in codon 123 of the β-globin gene causes an inclusion body β-thalassaemia trait: A novel elongated globin chain β^{Makabe}. *Br J Haematol* 75:393, 1990.

89. Fucharoen G, Fucharoen S, Jetsrisuparb A, Fukumaki Y: Eight-base deletion of the β-globin gene produced a novel variant (β Khon Kaen) with an inclusion body β-thalassemia trait. *Blood* 78:537, 1991.

90. Adams JG, Steinberg MH, Boxer LA, et al: The structure of hemoglobin Indianapolis (β112 (G14) arginine): An unstable variant detectable only by isotopic labeling. *J Biol Chem* 254:3479, 1979.

91. Coleman MB, Steinberg MH, Adams JGI: Hemoglobin Terre Haute [β106 (G8) Arginine]: A posthumous correction to the original structure of Hb Indianapolis. *Blood* 76:57, 1990.

92. Thein SL, Wood WG, Wickramasinghe SN, Galvin MC: β-Thalassemia unlinked to the β-globin gene in an English family. *Blood* 82:961, 1993.

93. Wood WG: Increased HbF in adult life. *Clin Haematol* 6:177, 1993.

94. Jones RW, Old JM, Trent RJ, et al: Major rearrangement in the human β-globin gene cluster. *Nature* 291:39, 1981.

95. Baglioni C: The fusion of two peptide chains in hemoglobin Lepore and its interpretation as a genetic deletion. *Proc Natl Acad Sci USA* 48:1880, 1962.

96. Ottolenghi S, Giglioni B, Pulazzini A, et al: Sardinian $\delta\beta^0$-thalassemia: A further example of a C to T substitution at position −196 of the $^A\gamma$ globin gene promoter. *Blood* 69:1058, 1987.

97. Atweh GF, Zhu X-X, Brickner HW, et al: The β-globin gene on the Chinese $\delta\beta$-thalassemia chromosome carries a promoter mutation. *Blood* 70:1470, 1987.

98. Wainscoat JS, Thein SL, Wood WG, et al: A novel deletion in the β globin gene complex. *Ann NY Acad Sci* 445:20, 1985.

99. Kulozik A, Yarwood N, Jones RW: The Corfu $\delta\beta^0$ thalassemia: A small deletion acts at a distance to selectively β globin gene expression. *Blood* 71:457, 1988.

100. Fritsch EF, Lawn RM, Maniatis T: Characterisation of deletions which affect the expression of fetal globin genes in man. *Nature* 279:598, 1979.

101. Orkin SH, Goff SC, Nathan DG: Heterogeneity of DNA deletion in $\gamma\delta\beta$-thalassemia. *J Clin Invest* 67:878, 1981.

102. Pirastu M, Kan YW, Lin CC, et al: Hemolytic disease of the newborn caused by a new deletion of the entire β-globin cluster. *J Clin Invest* 72:602, 1983.

103. Fearon EF, Kazazian HH, Waber PG, et al: The entire β-globin gene cluster is deleted in a form of $\gamma\delta\beta$-thalassemia. *Blood* 61:1269, 1983.

104. Van Der Ploeg LHT, Konings A, Cort M, et al: $\gamma\beta$-Thalassaemia studies showing that deletion of the γ- and δ-genes influence β-globin gene expression in man. *Nature* 283:637, 1980.

105. Curtin P, Pirastu M, Kan YW, et al: A distant gene deletion affects β-globin gene function in an $\gamma\delta\beta$-thalassemia. *J Clin Invest* 76:1554, 1985.

106. Driscoll MC, Dobkin CS, Alter BP: $\gamma\delta\beta$-Thalassemia due to a de novo mutation deleting the 5' β-globin gene activation-region hypersensitive sites. *Proc Natl Acad Sci USA* 86:7470, 1989.

107. Tuan D, Feingold E, Newman M, et al: Different 3' end points of deletions causing $\delta\beta$-thalassemia and hereditary persistence of fetal hemoglobin: Implications for the control of γ-globin gene expression in man. *Proc Natl Acad Sci USA* 80:6937, 1983.

108. Kendall AG, Ojwang PJ, Schroeder WA, Huisman THJ: Hemoglobin Kenya, the product of a $\gamma\beta$ fusion gene: Studies of the family. *Am J Hum Genet* 25:548, 1973.

109. Smith DH, Clegg JB, Weatherall DJ, Gilles HM: Hereditary persistence of foetal haemoglobin associated with a $\gamma\beta$ fusion variant, haemoglobin Kenya. *Nat New Biol* 246:184, 1973.

110. Jagadeeswaran P, Tuan D, Forget BG, Weissman SM: A gene deletion ending at the midpoint of a repetitive DNA sequence in one form of hereditary persistence of fetal haemoglobin. *Nature* 296:469, 1982.

111. Collins FS, Stoeckert CJ, Serjeant GR, et al: $^G\gamma\beta^+$ hereditary persistence of fetal hemoglobin: Cosmid cloning and identification of a specific mutation 5' to the $^G\gamma$ gene. *Proc Natl Acad Sci USA* 81:4894, 1984.

112. Giglioni B, Casini C, Mantovani R, et al: A molecular study of a family with Greek hereditary persistence of fetal hemoglobin and β-thalassemia. *EMBO J* 3:2641, 1984.

113. Gelinas R, Endlich B, Pfeiffer C, et al: G to A substitution in the distal CCAAT box of the $^A\gamma$-globin gene in Greek hereditary persistence of fetal haemoglobin. *Nature* 313:323, 1985.

114. Tate VE, Wood WG, Weatherall DJ: The British form of hereditary persistence of fetal haemoglobin results from a single base mutation adjacent to an S1 hypersensitive site 5' to the $^A\gamma$ globin gene. *Blood* 68:1389, 1986.

115. Gilman JG, Huisman THJ: DNA sequence variation associated with elevated fetal $^G\gamma$ globin production. *Blood* 66:783, 1985.

116. Marti HR: *Normale und Abnormale Menschliche Haemoglobin*. Springer-Verlag, Berlin, 1963.

117. Miyoshi K, Kaneto Y, Kawai H, Huisman THJ: X-linked dominant control of F-cells in normal adult life. *Blood* 72:1854, 1988.

118. Dover GJ, Smith KD, Chang YC, et al: Fetal hemoglobin levels in sickle cell disease and normal individuals are partially controlled by an X-linked gene located at Xp22.2. *Blood* 80:816, 1992.

119. Wood WG, Weatherall DJ, Clegg JB: Interaction of heterocellular hereditary persistence of foetal haemoglobin with β thalassaemia and sickle cell anaemia. *Nature* 264:247, 1976.

120. Cappellini MD, Fiorelli G, Bernini LF: Interaction between homozygous β^0 thalassaemia and the Swiss type of hereditary persistence of fetal haemoglobin. *Br J Haematol* 48:561, 1981.

121. Jeffreys AJ, Wilson V, Thein SL, et al: DNA "fingerprints" and segregation analysis of multiple markers in human pedigrees. *Am J Hum Genet* 39:11, 1986.

122. Thein SL, Weatherall DJ: A non-deletion hereditary persistence of fetal hemoglobin (HPFH) determinant not linked to the β-globin gene complex, in *Hemoglobin Switching*, part B, *Cellular and Molecular Mechanisms*, edited by G Stamatoyannopoulos, AW Nienhuis, p 97. Liss, New York, 1989.

123. Craig JE, Rochette J, Fisher CA, et al: Dissecting the loci controlling fetal haemoglobin production on chromosomes 11p and 6q by the regressive approach. *Nat Genet* 12:58,1996.

124. Craig JE, Rochette J, Sampietro M, et al: Genetic heterogeneity in heterocellular hereditary persistence of fetal hemoglobin. *Blood* 90:428, 1997.

125. Higgs DR: α-Thalassaemia, in *Bailliére's Clinical Haematology. International Practice and Research: The Haemoglobinopathies*, edited by DR Higgs, DJ Weatherall, p 117. Bailliére Tindall, London, 1993.

126. Nicholls RB, Fischel-Ghodsian N, Higgs DR: Recombination at the human α globin gene cluster: Sequence features and topological constraints. *Cell* 49:369, 1987.

127. Vanin EF, Henthorn PS, Kioussis D, et al: Unexpected relationships between four large deletions in the human β-globin gene cluster. *Cell* 35:701, 1983.

128. Wilkie AOM, Lamb J, Harris PC, et al: A truncated human chromosome 16 associated with α thalassaemia is stabilized by addition of telomeric repeat (TTAGGG). *Nature* 346:868, 1990.

129. Hatton CSR, Wilkie AOM, Drysdale HC, et al: Alpha thalassemia caused by a large (62 kb) deletion upstream of the human α globin gene cluster. *Blood* 76:221, 1990.

130. Liebhaber SA, Griese E-U, Cash FE, et al: Inactivation of human α-globin gene expression by a de novo deletion located upstream of the α-globin gene cluster. *Proc Natl Acad Sci USA* 81:9431, 1990.

131. Embury SH, Miller JA, Dozy AM, et al: Two different molecular organizations account for the single α-globin gene of the α-thalassemia-2 genotype. *J Clin Invest* 66:1319, 1980.

132. Higgs DR, Old JM, Pressley L, et al: A novel α-globin gene arrangement in man. *Nature* 284:632, 1980.

133. Goossens M, Dozy AM, Embury SH, et al: Triplicated α-globin loci in humans. *Proc Natl Acad Sci USA* 77:518, 1980.

134. Trent RJ, Higgs DR, Clegg JB, Weatherall DJ: A new triplicated α-globin gene arrangement in man. *Br J Haematol* 49:149, 1981.

135. Higgs DR, Hill AVS, Bowden DK, Weatherall DJ: Independent recombination events between duplicated human α globin genes: Implications for their concerted evolution. *Nucleic Acids Res* 12:6965, 1984.

136. Orkin SH, Goff SC, Hechtman RL: Mutation in an intervening sequence splice junction in man. *Proc Natl Acad Sci USA* 78:5041, 1981.

137. Higgs DR, Goodbourn SEY, Lamb J, et al: α-Thalassaemia caused by a polyadenylation signal mutation. *Nature* 306:398, 1983.

138. Thein SL, Wallace RB, Pressley L, et al: The polyadenylation site mutation in the α-globin gene cluster. *Blood* 71:313, 1988.

139. Pirastu M, Saglio G, Chang JC, et al: Initiation codon mutation as a cause of α thalassemia. *J Biol Chem* 259:12315, 1984.

140. Olivieri NF, Chang LS, Poon AO, et al: An α-globin gene initiation codon mutation in a black family with Hb H disease. *Blood* 70:729, 1987.

141. Paglietti E, Galanello R, Moi P, et al: Molecular pathology of haemoglobin H disease in Sardinians. *Br J Haematol* 63:485, 1986.

142. Morle F, Lopez B, Henni T, Godet J: α-Thalassaemia associated with the deletion of two nucleotides at position −2 and −3 preceding the AUG codon. *EBMO J* 4:1245, 1985.

143. Weatherall DJ, Clegg JB: The α-chain termination mutants and their relationship to the α thalassaemias. *Philos Trans R Soc London Ser B* 271:411, 1975.

144. Liebhaber SA, Coleman MB, Adams JG, et al: Molecular basis for non-deletion α thalassemia in American blacks $\alpha_2^{116\,GAG \rightarrow UAG}$. *J Clin Invest* 80:154, 1987.

145. Liebhaber SA, Kan YW: α Thalassemia caused by an unstable α-globin mutant. *J Clin Invest* 71:461, 1983.

146. Sanguansermsri T, Matrogoon S, Changlosh L, Fletz G: Hemoglobin Suan-Dok ($\alpha_2^{109(G16)LEU \rightarrow ARG}\beta_2$): An unstable variant associated with α thalassemia. *Hemoglobin* 3:161, 1979.

147. Honig GR, Shamsuddin M, Zaizov R, et al: Hemoglobin Petah Tikvah (α110 Ala → Asp): A new unstable variant with α-thalassemia-like expression. *Blood* 57:705, 1981.

148. Honig GR, Shamsuddin M, Vida LN, et al: Hemoglogin Evanston (α14 Trp → Arg): An unstable α-chain variant expressed as α-thalassemia. *J Clin Invest* 73:1740, 1984.

149. Weatherall DJ, Higgs DR, Bunch C, et al: Hemoglobin H disease and mental retardation: A new syndrome or a remarkable coincidence? *N Engl J Med* 305:607, 1981.

150. Wilkie AOM, Buckle VJ, Harris PC, et al: Clinical features and molecular analysis of the α thalassemia/mental retardation syndromes: I. Cases due to deletions involving chromosome band 16p13.3. *Am J Hum Genet* 46:1112, 1990.

151. Wilkie AOM, Zeitlin HC, Lindenbaum RH, et al: Clinical features and molecular analysis of the α-thalassemia/mental retardation syndromes: II. Cases without detectable abnormality of the α globin complex. *Am J Hum Genet* 46:1127, 1990.

152. Gibbons RJ, Suthers GK, Wilkie AOM, Buckle VJ, Higgs DR: X-linked α thalassemia/mental retardation (ATR-X) syndrome: Localisation to Xq12-21.31 by X-inactivation and linkage analysis. *Am J Hum Genet* 51:1136, 1992.

153. Gibbons RJ, Picketts DJ, Villard L, Higgs DR: Mutations in a putative global transcriptional regulator cause X-linked mental retardation with α-thalassemia (ATR-X syndrome). *Cell* 80:837, 1995.

154. Gibbons RJ, Bachoo S, Picketts DJ, et al: Mutations in transcriptional regulator *ATRX* establish the functional significance of a PHD-like domain. *Nat Genet* 17:146, 1997.

155. Chan V, Chan TK, Liang ST, et al: Hydrops fetalis due to an unusual form of Hb H disease. *Blood* 66:224, 1985.

156. Chan V, Chan VWY, Tang M, et al: Molecular defects in Hb H hydrops fetalis. *Br J Haematol* 96:224, 1997.

157. Ko T-M, Hsieh F-J, Hsu P-M, Lee T-Y: Molecular characterization of severe α-thalassemias causing hydrops fetalis in Taiwan. *Am J Med Genet* 39:317, 1990.

158. Weatherall DJ, Clegg JB, Naughton MA: Globin synthesis in thalassemia: An in vitro study. *Nature* 208:1061, 1965.

159. Weatherall DJ, Clegg JB, Na-Nakorn S, Wasi P: The pattern of disor-

160. Fessas P: Inclusions of hemoglobin in erythroblasts and erythrocytes of thalassemia. *Blood* 21:21, 1963.

161. Bargellesi A, Pontremoli S, Menini C, Conconi F: Excess of alpha globin synthesis in homozygous beta-thalassemia and its removal from the red blood cell cytoplasm. *J Biol Chem* 3:354, 1968.

162. Wickramasinghe SN, Hughes M: Some features of bone marrow macrophages in patients with β-thalassaemia. *Br J Haematol* 38:23, 1978.

163. Yataganas X, Fessas P: The pattern of hemoglobin precipitation in thalassemia and its significance. *Ann NY Acad Sci* 165:270, 1969.

164. Finch CA, Deubelbeiss K, Cook JD, et al: Ferrokinetics in man. *Medicine (Baltimore)* 49:17, 1970.

165. Chalavelakis G, Clegg JB, Weatherall DJ: Imbalanced globin chain synthesis in heterozygous β-thalassemic bone marrow. *Proc Natl Acad Sci USA* 72:3853, 1975.

166. Rachmilewitz EA, Shinar E, Shalev O, Galili U, Schrier SL: Erythrocyte membrane alterations in beta-thalassaemia. *Clin Haematol* 14:163,1985.

167. Schrier SL: Thalassemia: Pathophysiology of red cell changes. *Ann Rev Med* 45:211, 1994.

168. Weatherall DJ: Pathophysiology of β-thalassaemia. *Clin Haematol* 11:127, 1998.

169. Ho PJ, Wickramasinghe SN, Rees DC, et al: Erythroblastic inclusions in dominantly inherited β thalassaemias. *Blood* 89:322,1997.

170. Ager JAM, Lehmann H: Observations in some "fast" haemoglobins: K, J, N and "Bart's." *Br Med J* 1:929, 1958.

171. Rigas DA, Kohler RD, Osgood EE: New hemoglobin possessing a higher electrophoretic mobility than normal adult hemoglobin. *Science* 121:372, 1955.

172. Wasi P, Na-Nakorn S, Pootrakul S: The α-thalassaemias. *Clin Haematol* 3:383, 1974.

173. Gabuzda TG, Nathan DG, Gardner FH: The turnover of hemoglobins A, F and A₂ in the peripheral blood of three patients with thalassemia. *J Clin Invest* 42:1678, 1963.

174. Loukopoulos D, Fessas P: The distribution of hemoglobin types in thalassemic erythrocyte. *J Clin Invest* 44:231, 1965.

175. Nathan DG, Gunn RB: Thalassemia: The consequences of unbalanced hemoglobin synthesis. *Am J Med* 41:815, 1966.

176. Rees DC, Porter JB, Clegg JB, Weatherall DJ: Why are hemoglobin F levels increased in Hb E/β thalassemia? *Blood* 94(9):3199, 1999.

177. Modell CB, Berdoukas VA: *The Clinical Approach to Thalassemia.* Grune & Stratton, New York, 1984.

178. De Sanctis V, Vullo C, Katz M, et al: Endocrine complications in thalassaemia major. *Prog Clin Biol Res* 309:77, 1989.

179. Italian Working Group on Endocrine Complications in Non-endocrine Diseases: Multi-centre study on prevalence of endocrine complications in thalassemia major. *Clin Endocrinol* 42:581, 1995.

180. Wonke B, Hoffbrand AV, Pouloux P, et al: New approaches to the management of hepatitis and endocrine disorders in Cooley's anemia. *Ann NY Acad Sci* 850: 232, 1998.

181. Jessup M, Manno CS: Diagnosis and management of iron-induced heart disease in Cooley's anemia. *Ann NY Acad Sci* 850:242,1998.

182. Olivieri NF, Brittenham GM: Iron-chelating therapy and the treatment of thalassemia. *Blood* 89:739, 1997.

183. Hershko C, Peto TEA, Weatherall DJ: Iron and infection. *Br Med J* 296:660, 1988.

184. Kan YW, Nathan DG: Mild thalassemia: The result of interactions of alpha and beta thalassemia genes. *J Clin Invest* 49:635, 1970.

185. Weatherall DJ, Pressley L, Wood WG, et al: The molecular basis for mild forms of homozygous β thalassaemia. *Lancet* 1:527, 1981.

186. Wainscoat JS, Old JM, Weatherall DJ, Orkin SH: The molecular basis for the clinical diversity of β thalassaemia in Cypriots. *Lancet* 1:1235, 1983.

187. Labie D, Pagnier J, Lapoumeroulie C, et al: Common haplotype dependency of high ᴳγ-globin gene expression and high Hb F levels in β-thalassemia and sickle cell anemia patients. *Proc Natl Acad Sci USA* 82:2111, 1985.

188. Thein SL, Sampietro M, Old JM, et al: Association of thalassaemia intermedia with a beta-globin gene haplotype. *Br J Haematol* 65:370, 1987.

189. Thein SL, Hesketh C, Wallace RB, Weatherall DJ: The molecular basis of thalassaemia major and thalassaemia intermedia in Asian Indians: Application to prenatal diagnosis. *Br J Haematol* 70:225, 1988.

190. Ho PJ, Hall GW, Luo LY, Weatherall DJ, Thein SL: Beta thalassaemia intermedia: Is it possible to predict phenotype from genotype? *Br J Haematol* 100:70, 1998.

191. Camaschella C, Cappellini MD: Thalassemia intermedia. *Haematologica* 80:58, 1995.

192. Rund D, Oron-Karni V, Filon D, et al: Genetic analysis of β-thalassemia intermedia in Israel: Diversity of mechanisms and unpredictability of phenotype. *Am J Hematol* 54:16, 1997.

193. Flint J, Harding RM, Boyce AJ, Clegg JB: The population genetics of the haemoglobinopathies. *Clin Haematol* 11:1, 1998.

194. Haldane JBS: The rate of mutation of human genes. *Hereditas* 35(suppl):267, 1949.

195. Orkin SH, Kazazian HH: The mutation and polymorphism of the human β-globin gene and its surrounding DNA. *Annu Rev Genet* 18:131, 1984.

196. Orkin SH, Antonarakis SE, Kazazian HH: Polymorphisms and molecular pathology of the human β-globin gene. *Prog Hematol* 13:49, 1983.

197. Siniscalco M, Bernini L, Filippi G, et al: Population genetics of haemoglobin variants, thalassaemia and glucose-6-phosphate dehydrogenase deficiency, with particular reference to malaria hypothesis. *Bull WHO* 34:379, 1966.

198. Flint J, Hill AVS, Bowden DK, et al: High frequencies of α thalassaemia are the result of natural selection by malaria. *Nature* 321:744, 1986.

199. Allen SJ, O'Donnell A, Alexander NDE, et al: α⁺-Thalassaemia protects children against disease due to malaria and other infections. *Proc Natl Acad Sci USA* 94:14736, 1997.

200. Williams TN, Maitland K, Bennett S, et al: High incidence of malaria in α-thalassaemic children. *Nature* 383:522, 1996.

201. Pasvol G, Wilson RJM: The interaction of malaria parasites with red blood cells. *Br Med Bull* 38:133, 1982.

202. Luzzatto L: Malaria and the red cell, in *Recent Advances in Haematology,* edited by AV Hoffbrand, p 109. Churchill Livingstone, Edinburgh, 1985.

203. Luzzi GA, Merry AH, Newbold CI, et al: Surface antigen expression on *Plasmodium falciparum*–infected erythrocytes is modified in α- and β-thalassaemia. *J Exp Med* 173:785, 1991.

204. Wonke B, Hoffbrand AV, Bouloux P, Jensen C, Telfer P: New approaches to the management of hepatitis and endocrine disorders in Cooley's anemia. *Ann NY Acad Sci* 850:232, 1998.

205. Girot R, Lefrére JJ, Schettini F, Kattamis C, Ladis V: HIV infection and AIDS in thalassemia, in *Thalassemia 1990: 5th Annual Meeting of the COOLEYCARE Group,* edited by P Rebulla, P Fessas, p 69. Centro Trasfusionale Ospedale Maggiore Policlinico Dio Milano, Athens, 1991.

206. Chatterjee R, Katz M, Cox TF, Porter JB: Prospective study of the hypothalmic-pituitary axis in thalassaemic patients who developed secondary amenorrhoea. *Clin Endocrinol* 39:287, 1993.

207. Liang ST, Wong VCW, So WWK, et al: Homozygous α-thalassaemia: Clinical presentation, diagnosis and management: A review of 46 cases. *Br J Obstet Gynaecol* 92:680, 1985.

208. Chui DHK, Waye JS: Hydrops fetalis caused by α-thalassaemia: An emerging health care problem. *Blood* 91:2213, 1998.

209. Beaudry MA, Ferguson DJ, Pearse K, et al: Survival of a hydropic infant with homozygous α-thalassaemia-1. *J Pediatr* 108:713, 1986.

210. Bianchi DW, Beyer EC, Stark AR, et al: Normal long-term survival with α thalassaemia. *J Pediatr* 108:716, 1986.

211. Gouttas A, Fessas P, Tsevrenis H, Xefteri E: Description d'une nouvelle variete d'anemie hemolytique congenitale. *Sang* 26:911, 1955.

212. Rigas DA, Koler RD, Osgood EE: Hemoglobin H: Clinical, laboratory, and genetic studies of a family with a previously undescribed hemoglobin. *J Lab Clin Med* 47:51, 1956.

213. Wasi P: Hemoglobinopathies in Southeast Asia, in *Distribution and Evolution of the Hemoglobin and Globin Loci,* edited by JE Bowman, p 179. Elsevier, New York, 1983.

214. Kattamis C, Tzotzos S, Kanavakis E, et al: Correlation of clinical phenotype to genotype in haemoglobin H disease. *Lancet* 1:442, 1988.

215. Galanello R, Pirastu M, Melis MA, et al: Phenotype-genotype correlation in haemoglobin H disease in childhood. *J Med Genet* 20:425, 1983.

216. Fuchareon S, Winichagoon P, Pootrakul P, et al: Differences between two types of Hb H disease, α-thalassemia 1/α-thalassemia 2 and α-thalassaemia 1/Hb Constant Spring. *Birth Defects Orig Artic Ser* 23:309, 1988.

217. Styles L, Foote DH, Kleman KM, et al: Hemoglobin H-Constant Spring disease: An underrecognized, severe form of α thalassemia. *Int J Pediatr Hematol Oncol* 4:69, 1997.

218. Lie-Injo LE, Ganesan J, Clegg JB, Weatherall DJ: Homozygous state for Hb Constant Spring (slow-moving Hb X components). *Blood* 43:251, 1974.

219. Lie-Injo LE, Ganesan J, Lopez CG: The clinical, hematological and biochemical expression of hemoglobin Constant Spring and its distribution, in *Abnormal Hemoglobins and Thalassemia,* edited by RM Schmidt, p 275. Academic, New York, 1975.

220. Derry S, Wood WG, Pippard MJ, et al: Hematologic and biosynthetic studies in homozygous hemoglobin Constant Spring. *J Clin Invest* 73:1673, 1984.

221. Bowden DK, Hill AVS, Higgs DR, et al: Different hematologic phenotypes are associated with leftward (-α⁴·²) and rightward (-α³·⁷) α⁺-thalassemia deletions. *J Clin Invest* 79:39, 1987.

222. Silvestroni E, Bianco L, Reitano G: Three cases of homozygous δβ-thalassaemia (or microcythemia) with high haemoglobin F in a Sicilian family. *Acta Hematol (Basel)* 40:220, 1968.

223. Ramot BN, Ben-Bassat I, Gafni D, Zaanoon R: A family with three δβ-thalassemia homozygotes. *Blood* 35:158, 1970.

224. Tsistrakis GA, Amarantos SP, Konkouris LL: Homozygous βδ-thalassaemia. *Acta Hematol (Basel)* 51:185, 1974.

225. Efremov GD: Hemoglobins Lepore and anti-Lepore. *Hemoglobin* 2:197, 1978.

226. Charache S, Clegg JB, Weatherall DJ: The Negro variety of hereditary persistence of fetal haemoglobin is a mild form of thalassaemia. *Br J Haematol* 34:527, 1976.

227. Huisman THJ, Miller A, Schroeder WA: A ᴳγ type of hereditary persistence of fetal haemoglobin with β chain production in *cis. Am J Hum Genet* 27:765, 1975.

228. Higgs DR, Clegg JB, Wood WG, Weatherall DJ: ᴳγδβ⁺-Type of hereditary persistence of fetal haemoglobin in association with Hb C. *J Med Genet* 16:288, 1979.

229. Fessas P, Stamatoyannopoulos G: Hereditary persistence of fetal hemoglobin in Greece: A study and a comparison. *Blood* 24:223, 1964.

230. Sofroniadou K, Wood WG, Nute PE, Stamatoyannopoulos G: Globin chain synthesis in Greek type (ᴬγ) of hereditary persistence of fetal haemoglobin. *Br J Haematol* 29:137, 1975.

231. Clegg JB, Metaxatou-Mavromati A, Kattamis C, et al: Occurrence of ᴳγ Hb F in Greek HPFH: Analysis of heterozygotes and compound heterozygotes with β thalassaemia. *Br J Haematol* 43:521, 1979.

232. Camaschella C, Oggiano L, Sampietro M, et al: The homozygous state of G to A—117 ᴬγ hereditary persistence of fetal hemoglobin. *Blood* 73:1999, 1989.

233. Weatherall DJ, Cartner R, Clegg JB, et al: A form of hereditary persistence of fetal haemoglobin characterised by uneven cellular distribution of haemoglobin F and the production of haemoglobins A and A₂ in homozygotes. *Br J Haematol* 29:205, 1975.

234. Silvestroni E, Bianco I: *La Malattia Microdrepanocitica.* Il Pensiero Scientifico, Rome, 1955.

235. Serjeant GR, Ashcroft MY, Serjeant BE, Milner PF: The clinical features of sickle-cell β thalassaemia in Jamaica. *Br J Haematol* 24:19, 1973.

236. Serjeant GR: *Sickle Cell Disease,* 2nd ed. Oxford University Press, New York, 1992.

237. Wasi P, Na-Nakorn S, Pootrakul S, et al: Alpha- and beta-thalassemia in Thailand. *Ann NY Acad Sci* 165:60,1969.

238. Rees DS, Styles J, Vichinsky EP, Clegg JB, Weatherall DJ: The hemoglobin E syndromes. *Ann NY Acad Sci* 850: 334, 1998.

239. Agarwal S, Gulati R, Singh K: Hemoglobin E-beta thalassemia in Uttar Pradesh. *Indian Pediatr* 34:287, 1997.

240. Khanh NC, Thu LT, Truc DB, et al: Beta-thalassemia/haemoglobin E disease in Vietnam. *J Trop Pediatr* 36:43, 1990.

241. Fucharoen S, Winichagoon P, Pootrakul P, et al: Variable severity of Southeast Asian β⁰-thalassemia/Hb E disease, in *Thalassemia: Pathophysiology and Management,* part A, edited by S Fucharoen, PT Rowley, NW Paul, p 241. Liss, New York, 1988.

242. Sonakul D, Suwanagool P, Sirivaidyapong P, Fucharoen S: Distribution of pulmonary thromboembolic lesions in thalassemic patients, in *Thalassemia: Pathophysiology and Management,* part A, edited by S Fucharoen, PT Rowley, NW Paul, p 375. Liss, New York, 1988.

243. Kattamis C, Metaxatou-Mavromati A, Wood WG, et al: The heterogeneity of normal Hb A₂-β thalassaemia in Greece. *Br J Haematol* 42:109, 1979.

244. Schwartz E: The silent carrier of beta thalassemia. *N Engl J Med* 281:1327, 1969.

245. Bianco I, Graziani B, Carboni C: Genetic patterns in thalassemia intermedia (constitutional microcytic anemia): Familial, hematologic and biosynthetic studies. *Hum Hered* 27:257, 1977.

246. Pirastu M, Ristaldi MS, Loudianos G, et al: Molecular analysis of atypical β-thalassemia heterozygotes. *Ann NY Acad Sci* 612:90, 1990.

247. Olds RJ, Sura T, Jackson B, et al: A novel δ⁰ mutation in *cis* with Hb Knossos: A study of different interactions in three Egyptian families. *Br J Haematol* 78:430, 1991.

248. Schokker RC, Went LN, Bok J: A new genetic variant of β-thalassaemia. *Nature* 209:44, 1966.

249. Ohta Y, Yamaoka K, Sumida I, et al: Homozygous delta-thalassemia first discovered in Japanese family with hereditary persistence of fetal hemoglobin. *Blood* 37:706, 1971.

250. Vella F, Wells RMC, Ager JAM: A haemoglobinopathy involving haemoglobin H and a new (Q) haemoglobin. *Br J Haematol* 1:752, 1958.

251. Lie-Injo LE, Pillay RP, Thuraisingham V: Further cases of Hb-Q-H disease (Hb Q-α-thalassemia). *Blood* 28:830, 1966.

252. Milner PF, Huisman THJ: Studies on the proportion and synthesis of haemoglobin G Philadelphia in red cells of heterozygotes, a homozygote, and a heterozygote for both haemoglobin G and α thalassaemia. *Br J Haematol* 34:207, 1976.

253. Rieder RF, Woodbury DH, Rucknagel DL: The interaction of α-thalassaemia and haemoglobin G Philadelphia. *Br J Haematol* 32:159, 1976.

254. Pich P, Saglio G, Camaschella C, et al: Interaction between Hb Hasharon and α thalassaemia: An approach to the problem of the number of human α loci. *Blood* 51:339, 1978.

255. Higgs DR, Aldridge BE, Lamb J, et al: The interaction of alpha-thalassemia and homozygous sickle cell disease. *N Engl J Med* 306:1441, 1982.

256. Embury SH, Dozy AM, Miller J, et al: Concurrent sickle-cell anemia and α-thalassemia. *N Engl J Med* 306:270, 1982.

257. Olivieri N: Thalassaemia: Clinical management. *Clin Haematol* 11:147, 1998.

258. Cazzola M, Borgna-Pignatti C, Locatelli F, et al: A moderate transfusion regimen may reduce iron loading in β-thalassemia major without producing excessive expansion of erythropoiesis. *Transfusion* 37:135, 1997.

259. Propper RD: Transfusion management of thalassaemia, in *Methods in Haematology: The Thalassaemias*, edited by DJ Weatherall, p 145. Churchill Livingstone, Edinburgh, 1983.

260. Propper RD, Cooper B, Rufo RR, et al: Continuous subcutaneous administration of deferoxamine in patients with iron overload. *N Engl J Med* 297:418, 1977.

261. Pippard MJ, Callender ST, Letsky EA, Weatherall DJ: Prevention of iron loading in transfusion-dependent thalassaemia. *Lancet* 1:1178, 1978.

262. Pippard MJ, Callender ST, Finch CA: Ferrioxamine excretion in iron-loaded man. *Blood* 60:288, 1982.

263. Nienhuis AW: Safety of intensive chelation therapy. *N Engl J Med* 296:114, 1977.

264. Olivieri NF, Bunic JR, Chew E, et al: Visual and auditory neurotoxicity in patients receiving subcutaneous deferoxamine infusions. *N Engl J Med* 314:869, 1986.

265. Porter JB, Jawson MS, Huehns ER, et al: Desferrioxamine ototoxicity: Evaluation of risk factors in thalassaemia patients and guidelines for safe dosage. *Br J Haematol* 73:403, 1989.

266. Smith CH, Erlandson ME, Stern G, Hilgartner MW: Postsplenectomy infection in Cooley's anemia. *Ann NY Acad Sci* 119:748, 1964.

267. Bullen AW, Losowsky MS: Consequences of impaired splenic function. *Clin Sci* 57:129, 1979.

268. Lucarelli G, Giardini C, Baronciani D: Bone marrow transplantation in β-thalassemia. *Semin Hematol* 32:297, 1995.

269. Galimberti M, Angelucci M, Baronciani D, et al: Bone marrow transplantation in thalassemia: The experience of Pesaro. *Bone Marrow Transplant* 19(suppl 2):45, 1997.

270. Di Bartolomeo P, Di Girolamo G, Olioso P, et al: The Pescara experience of allogenic bone marrow transplantation in thalassemia. *Bone Marrow Transplant* 19(suppl 2):48, 1997.

271. Argiolu F, Sanna MA, Addari MC, et al: Bone marrow transplantation in thalassemia: The experience of Cagliari. *Bone Marrow Transplant* 19(suppl 2):65, 1997.

272. Gaziev D, Polchi P, Galimberti M, et al: Graft-versus-host disease following bone marrow transplantation for thalassemia: An analysis of incidence and risk factors. *Transplantation* 63:854, 1997.

273. Angelucci E, Ripalti M, Baronciani D, et al: Phlebotomy to reduce iron overload in patients cured of thalassemia by marrow transplantation. *Bone Marrow Transplant* 19(suppl 2):123, 1997.

274. Olivieri NF: Reactivation of fetal hemoglobin in patients with β thalassemia. *Semin Hematol* 33:24, 1996.

275. Olivieri NF, Weatherall DJ: The therapeutic reactivation of fetal haemoglobin. *Hum Mol Genet* 7:1655, 1998.

276. Swank RA, Stamatoyannopoulos G: Fetal gene reactivation. *Curr Opin Genet Dev* 8:366, 1998.

277. Olivieri NF, Rees DC, Ginder GD, et al: Treatment of thalassaemia major with phenylbutyrate and hydroxyurea. *Lancet* 350:491, 1997.

278. Sadelain M: Genetic treatment of the haemoglobinopathies: Recombinations and new combinations. *Br J Haematol* 98:247, 1997.

279. Dominski Z, Kole R: Restoration of correct splicing in thalassemic pre-mRNA by antisense oligonucleotides. *Proc Natl Acad Sci USA* 90:8673, 1993.

280. Lan N, Howrey RP, Lee S-W, Smith CA, Sullenger BA: Ribozyme-mediated repair of sickle β-globin mRNAs in erythrocyte precursors. *Science* 280:1593, 1998.

281. Weatherall DJ: Gene therapy: Repairing haemoglobin disorders with ribozymes. *Curr Biol* 8:R696, 1998.

282. Brittenham GM, Griffith PM, Nienhuis AW, et al: Efficacy of deferoxamine in preventing complications of iron overload in patients with thalassemia major. *N Engl J Med* 331:567, 1994.

283. Olivieri NF, Nathan DG, MacMillan JH, et al: Survival of medically treated patients with homozygous β thalassemia. *N Engl J Med* 331:574, 1994.

284. WHO Working Group: Hereditary anemias: Genetic basis, clinical features, diagnosis and treatment. *Bull WHO* 60:543, 1982.

285. Stamatoyannopoulos G: Problems of screening and counselling in the hemoglobinopathies, in *Proceedings of the IV International Conference on Birth Defects*, p 268. Vienna, 1973.

286. Silvestroni E, Bianco I, Graziani B, Carboni C, D'Arca SU: First premarital screening of thalassaemia carriers in intermediate schools in Latium. *J Med Genet* 15:202, 1978.

287. Alter BP: Antenatal diagnosis: Summary of results. *Ann NY Acad Sci* 612:237, 1990.

288. Kazazian HH, Phillips JAI, Boehm CD, et al: Prenatal diagnosis of β-thalassemia by amniocentesis: Linkage analysis of multiple polymorphic restriction endonuclease sites. *Blood* 56:926, 1980.

289. Old JM, Ward RHT, Petrou M, et al: First trimester diagnosis for haemoglobinopathies: A report of 3 cases. *Lancet* 2:1413, 1982.

290. Old JM, Fitches A, Heath C, et al: First trimester fetal diagnosis for haemoglobinopathies: Report on 200 cases. *Lancet* 2:763, 1986.

291. Goossens M, Dumez Y, Kaplan L, et al: Prenatal diagnosis of sickle-cell anemia in the first trimester of pregnancy. *N Engl J Med* 309:831, 1983.

292. Cao A, Rosatelli MC: Screening and prenatal diagnosis of the haemoglobinopathies. *Clin Haematol* 6:263, 1993.

293. Pirastu M, Kan YW, Cao A, et al: Prenatal diagnosis of β-thalassemia: Detection of a single nucleotide mutation in DNA. *N Engl J Med* 309:284, 1983.

294. Kogan SC, Doherty M, Gitschier J: An improved method for prenatal diagnosis of genetic diseases by analysis of amplified DNA sequences: Application to hemophilia. *N Engl J Med* 317:985, 1987.

295. Chehab F, Doherty M, Cai S, et al: Detection of sickle cell anaemia and thalassaemia. *Nature* 329:293, 1987.

296. Saiki RK, Chang C-A, Levenson CH, et al: Diagnosis of sickle cell anemia and β-thalassemia with enzymatically amplified DNA and non-radioactive allele-specific oligonucleotide probes. *N Engl J Med* 319:537, 1988.

297. Old JM, Varawalla NY, Weatherall DJ: The rapid detection and prenatal diagnosis of β-thalassemia in the Asian Indian and Cypriot populations in the UK. *Lancet* 336:834, 1990.

298. Tan JAMA, Tay JSH, Lin LI, et al: The amplification refractory mutation system (ARMS): A rapid and direct prenatal diagnostic technique for β-thalassaemia in Singapore. *Prenatal Diagn* 14:1077, 1994.

299. Cai SP, Chang CA, Zhang JZ, et al: Rapid prenatal diagnosis of β-thalassemia using DNA amplification and nonradioactive probes. *Blood* 73:372, 1989.

300. Saiki RK, Walsh PS, Levenson CH, Erlich HA: Genetic analysis of

amplified DNA with immobilized sequence-specific oligonucleotide probes. *Proc Natl Acad Sci USA* 86:6230, 1989.

301. Takabayashi H, Kuwabara S, Ukita T, et al: Development of non-invasive fetal DNA diagnosis from maternal blood. *Prenatal Diagn* 15:74, 1995.

302. Cheung M-C, Goldberg JD, Kan YW: Prenatal diagnosis of sickle cell anemia and thalassemia by analysis of fetal cells in maternal blood. *Nat Genet* 14:264, 1996.

303. Kuliev A, Rechitsky S, Verlinsky O, et al: Preimplantation diagnosis of thalassemias. *J Assist Reprod Genet* 15:219, 1998.

THE SICKLE CELL DISEASES AND RELATED DISORDERS

ERNEST BEUTLER

Sickle hemoglobin is a mutant hemoglobin in which valine has been substituted for the glutamic acid normally at the sixth amino acid of the β-globin chain. This hemoglobin polymerizes and becomes poorly soluble when the oxygen tension is lowered, and red cells that contain this hemoglobin become distorted and rigid. Sickle cell disease occurs when an individual is homozygous for the sickle cell mutation or is a compound heterozygote for sickle hemoglobin and β-thalassemia, hemoglobin C, or some less common β-globin mutations. Diagnosis depends upon demonstrating the presence of the abnormal hemoglobin(s) in the red cells. The disease is characterized by hemolytic anemia and by three types of crises: painful (vasoocclusive), sequestration, and aplastic. Complications include splenic infarction and autosplenectomy, stroke, bone infarcts and aseptic necrosis of the femoral head, leg ulcers, priapism, pulmonary hypertension, and renal failure. The severity of clinical manifestations varies greatly from patient to patient and the aggressiveness of treatment needs to be modified accordingly. Early diagnosis, immunization against pneumococcal infection, and prompt treatment of infections that do occur has contributed to greatly improved survival of those born with these disorders. Stem cell transplantation, when successful, cures the disease. Treatment with hydroxyurea increases the fetal hemoglobin level and can result in amelioration of crises. Sickle trait, the heterozygous state for sickle hemoglobin, affects some eight percent of African Americans, and with rare exception is entirely benign. Hemoglobin C disease is associated with splenomegaly but minimal hematologic changes, and the rare hemoglobin D disease is essentially asymptomatic. Hemoglobin E is very common in some parts of Asia. This hemoglobin is greatly underproduced, and the homozygous state or compound heterozygous state with β-thalassemia resembles thalassemia.

DEFINITION AND HISTORY

James Herrick, the astute Chicago physician who is also credited with description of the clinical syndrome of coronary thrombosis, was the first to observe sickled cells in the blood of an anemic African graduate student[1] (Fig. 47-1). Emmel[2] demonstrated that red cells sickled when blood from such patients was sealed under glass and allowed to stand at room temperature for several days, but the fact that the transformation to sickled cells occurs in response to a fall in oxygen tension was not recognized until the classic studies of Hahn and Gillespie in 1927.[3]

Acronyms and abbreviations that appear in this chapter include: BPG, bisphosphoglycerate; G-6-PD, glucose-6-phosphate dehydrogenase; MCHC, mean corpuscular hemoglobin concentration; VLA-4, very late activation antigen-4.

In 1923 the sickling phenomenon was shown to be inherited as an autosomal dominant trait.[4] Much later, Neel[5] and Beet[6] clarified the genetic basis of sickle cell anemia by demonstrating that heterozygosity for the sickle cell gene resulted in sickle cell trait without significant clinical symptoms, while homozygosity resulted in sickle cell anemia.

In 1949 Pauling and his colleagues[7] found that all the hemoglobin in patients with sickle cell anemia showed an abnormally slow rate of migration on electrophoresis, while the parents of the these patients had normal as well as abnormal hemoglobin. Soon after, other abnormal hemoglobins were discovered by subjecting hemoglobin to electrophoresis. The biochemical nature of the defect in sickle cell anemia was elucidated by Ingram,[8] who digested hemoglobin with trypsin and separated the resulting peptides on paper by electrophoresis in one direction and chromatography in the other. This technique ("fingerprinting") demonstrated that one of the digestion products of sickle hemoglobin migrated differently from that of normal hemoglobin. Determination of the amino acid composition of this peptide indicated that sickle cell anemia was the result of the replacement of a glutamic acid residue by valine. This discovery established that the substitution of a single amino acid in a polypeptide chain can alter the function of the gene product sufficiently to produce widespread clinical effects. Conley has chronicled the fascinating history of sickle cell disease.[9]

NOMENCLATURE

After the discovery that sickle hemoglobin, or hemoglobin S (Hb S), was electrophoretically altered, additional variants were assigned letters of the alphabet—C, D, E, etc. The letters of the alphabet were rapidly exhausted, however, and subsequent abnormal hemoglobins were named after the geographic location in which they were found (e.g., hemoglobin Memphis, hemoglobin Mexico). If the hemoglobin had the electrophoretic characteristics of one previously described by a letter, the geographic designation was added as a subscript (e.g., hemoglobin $M_{Saskatoon}$). In this case M indicates an amino acid substitution resulting in a methemoglobin. In a fully characterized hemoglobin the amino acid substitution is designated by a superscript to the globin chain involved, as, for example, hemoglobin S, $\alpha_2\beta_2^{6\ Glu\rightarrow Val}$ and hemoglobin $G_{Norfolk}$, $\alpha_2^{35\ Asp\rightarrow Asn}\beta_2$. Thus, this notation indicates that hemoglobin S has a substitution of valine for glutamic acid in the sixth position of the β chain and that hemoglobin $G_{Norfolk}$ is a substitution of asparagine for aspartic acid in the thirty-fifth position of the α chain.

The term sickle cell disorder refers to states in which the red cell undergoes sickling when it is deoxygenated. The sickle cell diseases are those disorders in which sickling produces prominent clinical manifestations. Included are sickle cell–hemoglobin C disease (hemoglobin SC disease), sickle cell–hemoglobin D disease (hemoglobin SD disease), sickle cell β-thalassemia, and sickle cell anemia. The latter term is reserved for the homozygous state for the sickle cell gene.

THE SICKLE CELL DISEASES

Sickle cell anemia (SS disease) may be considered the prototype of the sickle cell diseases, and in general the clinical features and treatment of all these disorders are the same and are therefore considered together here. The homozygous state, sickle cell anemia, is the most severe of these disorders, with hemoglobin SC disease and sickle cell β-thalassemia tending to be somewhat milder, and hemoglobin SD disease being the mildest of the group. However, there is a great deal of overlap in the severity of the clinical manifestations of these disorders, and they are therefore described together here. Some patients with sickle cell thalassemia or hemoglobin SC disease may be more anemic and have more severe and frequent crises than some mildly affected patients with sickle cell anemia. A major difference among these diseases is in their laboratory diagnosis.

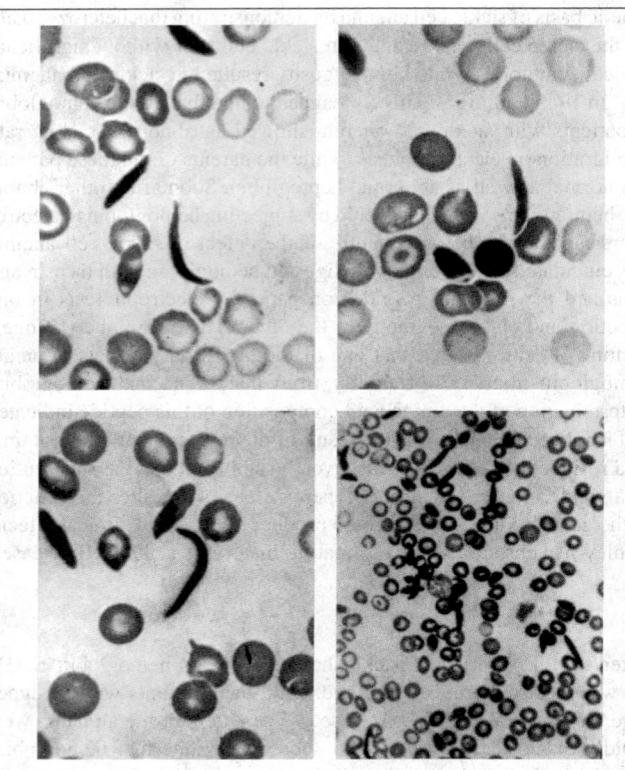

FIGURE 47-1   Peculiar elongated and sickle-shaped red corpuscles in a case of severe anemia. (Herrick,[1] by permission.)

ETIOLOGY AND PATHOGENESIS

BIOCHEMICAL BASIS OF SICKLING

There are few diseases of man whose etiology can be traced to as basic a level as sickle cell disease. Sickle cell anemia is due to the substitution of thymine for adenine in the glutamic acid DNA codon (GAG→GTG), which results, in turn, in substitution of $\beta6$ valine for glutamic acid. As discussed in Chap. 28, hemoglobin exists in two conformations, designated the oxy (relaxed, R) and deoxy (tense, T) states. Deoxygenation of hemoglobin shifts this equilibrium toward the T conformation. Molecules of deoxyhemoglobin S have a strong tendency to aggregate, and such aggregation requires the substitution of valine for glutamic acid in the $\beta6$ position, since only those hemoglobin variants with this substitution (e.g., S and Harlem) undergo sickling. Certain other structural features of the molecule are also of importance.[10,11]

Electron micrographs of deoxygenated sickle hemoglobin show the presence of multiple microtubules consisting of hemoglobin molecules stacked on top of each other (Fig. 47-2). The molecules do not lie directly over one another, so that a helical structure is formed. Fourteen strands of the fiber are organized into pairs,[12] giving rise to a fiber that is 21 nm in diameter. Most of the intermolecular contacts that give rise to this structure have been elucidated.[12,13]

The deoxygenated hemoglobin solution turns into a firm gel. The distorted sickled red cell is the visible end result of this molecular aggregation. The process is time dependent.[14] Initially there is a rate-limiting nucleation process; a few molecules of sickle hemoglobin must aggregate, forming a "seed" on which aggregation of further molecules occurs rapidly. Thus, the sickling process is characterized by a long delay that is strongly dependent on temperature and concentration.[15] The delay is inversely proportional to approximately the

thirtieth power of the hemoglobin concentration.[16] This delay is quite important in protecting the patient from even more dire consequences than might otherwise be anticipated. Even though the oxygen concentration of venous blood is sufficiently low so that at equilibrium about 85 percent of the red cells would contain sickle hemoglobin polymer, kinetic data suggest that about 80 percent of cells are prevented from sickling during their round trip through the circulation because they reach the lungs and become reoxygenated before significant polymerization has occurred.[14]

When a cell sickles and unsickles repeatedly, the membrane is affected and the cell becomes irreversibly sickled; it remains so even when the oxygen pressure is increased. These are the sickled forms seen on air-dried films. An irreversibly sickled cell has a high hemoglobin concentration and a high calcium and low potassium content, and it may be ATP-depleted.[17] These cells appear to be derived directly from reticulocytes[18] but have a short intravascular life span, and the severity of the hemolytic process is directly related to the number of these cells in a patient's circulation.[19] However, the relationship between the number of irreversibly sickled cells and the number and severity of painful crises is an inverse one.[20,21]

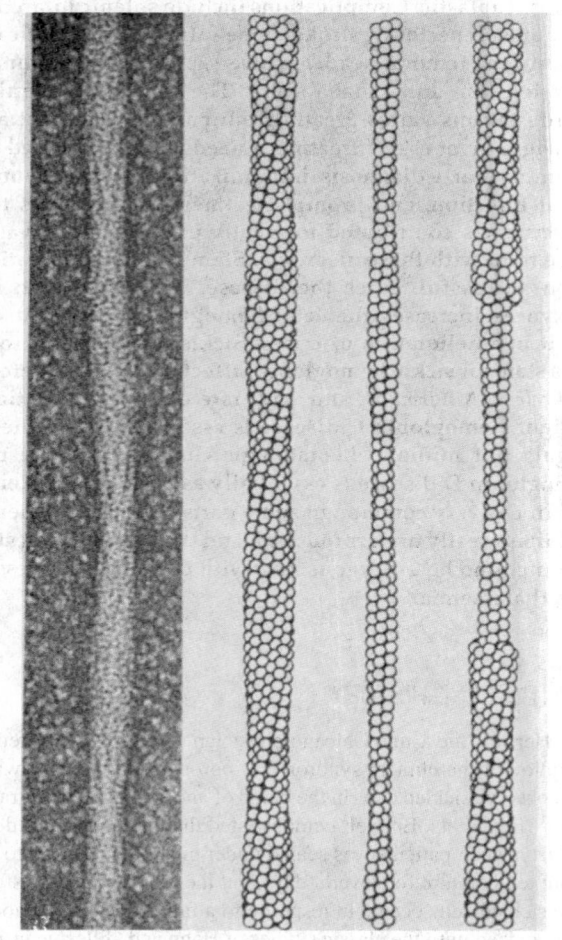

FIGURE 47-2   Electron micrograph of negatively stained fiber of hemoglobin S and the structure deduced by three-dimensional image reconstruction. The reconstructed fiber is presented as ball models, with each ball representing a hemoglobin S tetramer. The models are presented as the outer sheath (left), the inner core (center), and a combination of both inner and outer filaments (right). (Edelstein,[452] by permission.)

MEMBRANE CHANGES IN SICKLE CELLS

Although the primary defect in sickle cell disease is clearly in the hemoglobin, secondary alterations in red cell metabolism and membrane structure and function have also been described. Rapid potassium loss occurs early in the sickling process.[22] Abnormalities of sickle cell membrane phosphorylation have been documented.[23-25] The calcium pump is abnormal.[26] Although the calcium content of sickle cell membranes, particularly of those cells that are irreversibly sickled, has been found to be increased,[17,23-27] the location of the excess calcium appears to be in endocytic vacuoles, so that from a functional point of view its location is extracellular.[28,29] Increased generation of free radicals may occur in sickle cells,[30-32] and there is abnormal oxidation of thiols in sickle cells.[33] Superoxide dismutase activity of sickle cells is slightly reduced,[34] and the amount of NAD$^+$ and the NAD$^+$+NADH/NADH ratio are increased.[35] The binding of glyceraldehyde phosphate dehydrogenase to the membrane is decreased by 35 to 50 percent,[36] and there appears to be uncoupling of the lipid bilayer from the submembrane skeleton.[37] Macrophages seem to ingest sickle cells more readily than normal cells, and this could be a result of excessive auto-oxidation of membrane components with the acquisition of immuno-globulins on the cell surface[38] or to loss of membrane phospholipid asymmetry, which is a constant finding in sickle cells[39,40] and may play an important role in their clearance from the circulation as well as in activation of coagulation.

VARIABILITY IN SEVERITY OF SICKLE CELL DISEASE

Because a large number of inherited and acquired factors influence the pathogenesis of clinical symptoms, the sickle cell disorders vary in clinical severity from the virtually symptomless sickle cell trait to the potentially lethal state characteristic of sickle cell anemia. Wide variation in the severity of clinical manifestations also occurs among patients with sickle cell anemia. Some die within the first few years of life, while others have been discovered late in life as a result of a chance survey.

Both intracellular and extracellular factors influence sickling. Included are the types of hemoglobin in the cell and their concentration, the level of 2,3-bisphosphoglycerate (2,3-diphosphoglycerate; 2,3-BPG; 2,3-DPG), and the hydrogen ion concentration. Some of these factors are determined predominantly by genetic factors; others are environmentally modified. The variability of these factors as well as many others that are not understood probably accounts for the natural pattern of this group of diseases—periods of comparative well-being interspersed with periods of clinical deterioration (crises). Longitudinal studies of patients have suggested that an increase in the number of dense and poorly deformable cells precedes the development of a crisis.[41] However, calculation of the mean polymer fraction from the 2,3-BPG concentration, the MCHC, the internal pH, and the percent nonsickle hemoglobin did not make it possible to predict clinical course.[42] The precipitating circumstances responsible for the development of crises are often not clear. Of those events that appear to be associated with the appearance of crises, infections are probably among the most common.

However, it is not only the extent of sickling that is important but also the interaction of the sickled cells with the endothelium and other blood cells (see "Blood Flow in the Microvasculature," below).

Concentration of Hemoglobin S in the Red Cell   A correlation exists between the concentration of sickle hemoglobin within a red cell and the susceptibility of the cell to sickling. The red cells of the sickle cell carrier, who is virtually symptom-free, always contain less than 50 percent Hb S; the remainder is largely normal adult hemoglo-bin. The exact proportions vary from one individual to another. It was proposed many years ago that the distribution of the concentration of sickle hemoglobin in the red cells of subjects with the sickle cell trait was bimodal.[43] Subsequent studies confirmed the existence of more

than a single mode and indicated that the distribution might actually be trimodal.[44] The reason for such a discontinuous distribution has become apparent with the recognition of the very high frequency of α-thalassemia in persons of African ancestry. Individuals carrying α-thalassemic genes have a higher ratio of hemoglobin A to hemoglobin S than those who have four normal copies of the α locus.[45] Apparently the affinity of α chains for β^A chains is higher than its affinity for β^S chains,[46] possibly because of differences in the charge of the two chains.[47] Thus, when the number of α chains becomes limiting in the formation of hemoglobin tetramers, a higher proportion of $\alpha_2\beta_2{}^A$ tetramers than of $\alpha_2\beta_2{}^S$ tetramers are formed. Interaction of the α-thalassemic gene and the sickle gene also may influence the course of sickle cell disease: the lower corpuscular hemoglobin concentration in the red cells in α-thalassemia would be expected to protect against sickling. It has been suggested that such an interaction may influence the severity of sickle cell disease in African Americans[45,48,49] and that it may play an important role in producing the very mild clinical manifestation of sickle cell anemia in Saudi Arabia.[50]

The Presence of Other Hemoglobins in the Cell   Other hemo-globins present in a red cell containing sickle hemoglobin are not inert bystanders in the sickling process.[51] Some hemoglobins, such as F, Korle-Bu, and A$_2$, interact less effectively with hemoglobin S than does hemoglobin A in the sickling process. Two common abnormal hemoglobins, Hb C and Hb D, and the relatively rare hemoglobin O$_{Arab}$ become involved in the formation of the sickling tubule. The interaction of these hemoglobins with sickle hemoglobin increases the propensity of red cells to sickle. Moreover, the red cells of patients with SC disease characteristically have an increased MCHC, presum-ably due to a transport defect, and this too greatly increases sickling.[52,53]

Other hemoglobins do not appear to play an active role in the sickling process, and their presence in the red cell can greatly reduce the clinical severity of sickle cell anemia. Fetal hemoglobin, for example, protects the red cell from sickling.[54] It is distributed heterogeneously in the red cells of an SS homozygote,[55,56] and those cells with the largest amount are least susceptible to sickling.[55,56] The relatively mild clinical manifestations of patients in the Middle East with sickle cell anemia has been ascribed at least in part to the high level of fetal hemoglobin present in their red cells.[57-59] In the United States, however, no significant correlation exists between fetal hemoglobin levels and the severity of the clinical manifestations of sickle cell anemia,[60] and even in the Arab population the relationship is not always clear,[61] although it may be that the effect is obscured by a threshold phenome-non,[62] i.e., that a favorable effect of fetal hemoglobin concentration is observed only above a certain level. In adults who are heterozygotes for hemoglobin S and hereditary persistence of hemoglobin F, hemo-globin S constitutes more than 70 percent of the hemoglobin, but the high concentration of hemoglobin F inhibits sickling because the distribution is such that each cell contains a considerable amount of hemoglobin F, and the patients experience a benign clinical course.[63] The presence of the abnormal hemoglobin Memphis ($\alpha_2{}^{23Glu\rightarrow Gln}\beta_2$) also decreases the clinical severity of sickle cell disease,[64] presumably by inhibiting the formation of the sickle tubule.

Interaction of Sickling and Thalassemia   The interaction of β-thalassemia with sickling is discussed in Chap. 46, and that with α-thalassemia is considered above.

Glucose-6-Phosphate Dehydrogenase Deficiency   It has been suggested that G-6-PD deficiency may have a beneficial effect on the clinical course of sickle cell anemia,[65-68] but this correlation has not been confirmed in other studies.[69-76] It has also been proposed that hemolytic crises are more common in patients with sickle cell disease who are also G-6-PD deficient.[77] However, it seems unlikely that the G-6-PD-deficient cells of such a patient would be particularly sensitive in hemolytic stress; G-6-PD A$-$ is very age labile (Chap. 45), and because the erythrocytes are young they have relatively normal G-6-PD activity. In Jamaica,[74] the United States,[75] and Brazil[76] G-6-PD deficiency did not influence parameters of disease severity such as hemoglobin concentration, reticulocyte count, hemoglobin F concentration, irreversibly sickled cell counts, or plasma hemoglobin concentration, and there was no relationship between clinical severity and presence or absence of G-6-PD deficiency.

Pyruvate kinase deficiency is characterized by an increase of red cell 2,3-BPG levels (see Chap. 45). A patient with sickle trait who had inherited pyruvate kinase deficiency manifested sickling similar in severity to that in some patients with sickle disease.[78]

Deoxygenation   Deoxygenation for a sufficient period of time is the most important factor determining the occurrence of sickling in a red cell containing hemoglobin S. The degree of deoxygenation required to produce sickling varies with the percentage of hemoglobin S in the cells. Red cells from patients with sickle cell anemia will begin to sickle at an oxygen tension of about 40 torr.[79] Changes that impair adequate oxygenation of the blood may be deleterious to any person whose red cells contain sickle hemoglobin.

An arterial oxygen tension of about 66 torr is found at about 10,000 ft (3000 m). Hypoxemia may also result from flying in unpressurized aircraft; most commercial aircraft, however, maintain an atmospheric pressure in the cabin equivalent to that encountered at an altitude of 5000 to 7000 ft (1500 to 2100 m). Occasional patients with sickle cell anemia or hemoglobin SC disease have been reported to experience painful crises or splenic infarctions under such circumstances.[80] However, there is no evidence that a person with sickle cell trait is at risk in a pressurized airplane.[81] The oxygen content of the air may also be reduced during anesthesia or when an artificial breathing apparatus is used improperly, as in scuba diving. If pulmonary or cardiac function deteriorates (e.g., in pneumonia or in cardiac failure), any resulting reduction in arterial oxygen tension may prove hazardous to a patient with sickle cell disease.

Vascular Stasis   The P_{O_2} level producing in vitro sickling of cells containing Hb S bears only an indirect relationship to clinical measurements of arterial and venous P_{O_2}. This is because the P_{O_2} in the larger peripheral vessels does not accurately reflect the oxygen tension in areas of vascular stasis, such as the sinusoids of the spleen, in which hypoxemia is common and sickling is likely to occur. Although a period of 2 to 4 min is required for the development of marked red cell distortion[14,82] and rigidity, the red cells normally remain within the venous circulation for only about 10 to 15 s. For this reason, red cells in areas of vascular stasis are more vulnerable to sickling. Once sickling has occurred, increased blood viscosity[83] results in further vascular stasis, further sickling, possible vascular occlusion, and infarction. This course of events leads to tissue death, manifested clinically as a painful crisis.

While no organ of the body is immune to vasoocclusion due to in vivo sickling, certain sites notorious for circulatory stasis are characteristically affected. Splenic and marrow infarctions due to vascular stasis are particularly frequent, and priapism may occur in the male. The role of vascular stasis in the development of leg ulcers and of retinal and renal lesions is discussed below under "Clinical Features." Studies from Jamaica indicated that the incidence of peptic ulcer was greatly increased in patients with sickle cell disease,[84] ulceration being identified in 30.5 percent of male patients over the age of 25, but this could not be confirmed in a West African population.[85]

Temperature   Even though cold temperatures retard hemoglobin polymerization, low temperatures tend to precipitate sickle crises, presumably because of the accompanying vasoconstriction.

Acidosis   Hydrogen ions produce a right shift in the oxygen dissociation curve (the Bohr effect), presumably by displacing the equilibrium between the high-affinity oxy conformation and the low-affinity deoxy conformation toward the deoxy conformation of hemo-

globin. Since it is sickle hemoglobin in the deoxy conformation that aggregates, the lowered pH profoundly affects the sickling of red cells, even when the percent oxygenation is maintained at a constant level.[86,87] Alkalosis, on the other hand, by shifting the equilibrium toward the oxy conformation, tends to retard sickling but impairs oxygen release to tissue.

Corpuscular Hemoglobin Concentration   The tendency of hemoglobin S solutions to aggregate is proportional to the thirtieth power of the concentration.[16,88] Accordingly, sickling of red cells is markedly influenced by the concentration of sickle hemoglobin in the cells. Suspending sickle cells in a hyperosmolar medium increases the intracellular hemoglobin concentration as the cell is dehydrated. This phenomenon may account in part for sickling in renal papillae.[89,90] Conversely, any agent that causes increased red cell volume will retard the sickling process by decreasing the MCHC. Marked dehydration results in both vascular stasis and hypertonicity and can precipitate a crisis.

Blood Flow in the Microvasculature   In the last analysis, vasoocclusion is the result of a variety of factors on blood flow in the microvasculature. The factors that influence the rheologic properties of blood that contains sickle cells are extremely complex. For example, shear stresses, such as those that occur in the circulation, serve to break down gel structure.[91] However, this results in the creation of more nucleation centers and results in a decrease in the delay time. In the circulation, flow properties of blood are influenced not only by factors such as the rigidity of the erythrocytes but also by the adherence of sickle cells to the endothelium,[92] which may involve band 3,[93] and to each other.[94] Variations in such factors, modifying the rheologic consequences of the sickling process, undoubtedly play a role in determining when vasoocclusive episodes will occur. Granulocytes, too, manifest increased adherence to endothelium, and this has been attributed to increased expression of CD64.[95]

The sequence of events that leads to occlusion of blood vessels by sickle cells is thus complex.[96,97] One essential factor is the aggregation of sickle hemoglobin, with the consequent changes in the rheologic properties of the erythrocytes (see "Biochemical Basis of Sickling," above). The overall viscosity of the blood is a function of the hematocrit, and occlusion is more likely when hematocrit levels are relatively high. Adhesion of sickle cells to the vascular endothelium is an important factor and may be related to exposure of vascular endothelial adhesion molecules such as VCAM-1 (vascular cell adhesion molecule-1) and to the levels of plasma factors that enhance adhesion, including fibrinogen, factor VIII, fibronectin, von Willebrand factor, and thrombospondin. The adhesion receptors VLA-4 and CD36 are found in unusually high numbers on sickle cell reticulocytes, and they help to mediate adhesion of sickle RBC to endothelium.[98] Abnormalities in nitric oxide–induced vascular relaxation has also been indirectly implicated. Leukocytes probably also participate in this complex process, perhaps by releasing cytokines that upregulate adhesive endothelial glycoproteins, and it has been suggested that a part of the therapeutic effect of hydroxyurea may be related to reduction of the leukocyte count.[99]

Infections   It is a common clinical observation that vasoocclusive crises may be precipitated by infections. In many cases the mechanism by which infection increases sickling is easily discernible: fever, vomiting, and diarrhea may produce dehydration; lack of food intake may produce acidosis; and hypoxemia may result from pneumonia. It is quite possible that other, more subtle mechanisms may also be responsible for precipitation of crises in patients with sickle diseases with infections.

INHERITANCE

A patient with sickle cell anemia is homozygous for the gene for sickle hemoglobin and has therefore inherited one abnormal gene from

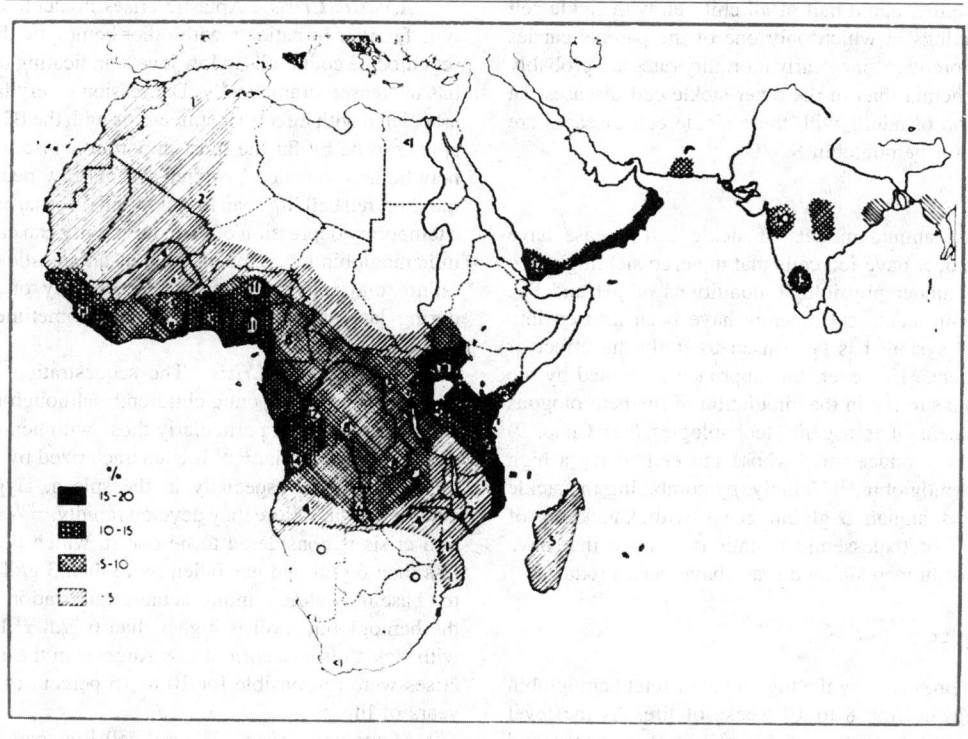

FIGURE 47-3   Distribution of sickle cell gene in Africa and Asia. (Allison,[453] by permission.)

each parent. If 7.8 percent of a population are sickle cell trait carriers,[73] as in the African American population, there is a 1:164 chance that two carriers will marry, and the chances that an offspring of such a marriage will have sickle cell anemia is 1:4. In such a population, about 1 in 650 will have sickle cell anemia.

Similarly, persons with hemoglobin SC disease must have one parent with a sickle hemoglobin gene and another with a hemoglobin C gene. Since these genes are allelic β chain mutations, persons with hemoglobin SC disease have no normal β polypeptide chain gene and therefore have no hemoglobin A. The carrier rate for hemoglobin C in African Americans is about 2.3 percent.[73] If 7.8 percent of a population carries the hemoglobin S gene, then the probability of a sickle cell trait and hemoglobin C trait mating is about 1 in 280, and therefore 1 in about 1120 newborns will inherit hemoglobin SC disease. The same principles apply for inheritance of sickle cell β-thalassemia, since the β-thalassemia gene is also allelic to the gene for sickle hemoglobin. In African Americans the frequency of β-thalassemia is approximately 0.8 percent,[100] so that the expected birth frequency of sickle cell β-thalassemia is about 1 per 3200.

Hemoglobin S occurs with greatest prevalence in tropical Africa; the heterozygote frequency is usually about 20 percent, but in some areas it reaches 40 percent. The sickle cell trait has a frequency of about 8 percent in the African American populations. The sickle cell gene is found to a lesser extent in the Middle East, in Greece, and in aboriginal tribes in India (Fig. 47-3). On occasion sickle cell disease is found in people of European extraction, especially where racial admixture has occurred over the centuries.[101]

The high prevalence of the gene for sickle hemoglobin in areas of the world where malaria has been common suggests that persons with sickle cell trait have a selective advantage over normal individuals when they contract this disease.[102] This advantage seems to be restricted to young children with sickle trait and *Plasmodium falciparum* infection. Although children with sickle cell trait are readily infected by *P. falciparum,* the parasite counts remain low. It may be that the

infected red cell is preferentially sickled and destroyed, probably in the vascular system of the liver or spleen, where oxygen tensions are low and phagocytic cells abound. Whatever the mechanism, the result is that the infection is of short duration and the incidence of cerebral malaria and death is low.

At one time one could only speculate as to whether the sickle cell mutation had arisen only once and had gradually gained a worldwide distribution or whether the same mutation had arisen independently in various populations and then been the subject of selection, presumably through a protective effect against malaria. The ability to detect mutations in nontranscribed portions of DNA adjacent to the β-globin gene (see Chap. 9) has now provided insight into this problem. Such mutations are so close to the β-globin gene that the probability of a crossover (see Chap. 9) is vanishingly small. Thus, the relationship of the two mutations to one another will persist through hundreds of generations, permitting one to trace population movements. When the β-globin gene cluster is digested with restriction endonucleases, five distinct patterns are found in association with the sickle mutation. Four of these occur in Africa and have been designated the Senegal, Benin, Bantu, and Cameroon types.[103] An additional haplotype is typical of the Indian subcontinent.[104] These findings suggest that the sickle mutation arose independently at least five times.

Hemoglobin D$_{Punjab}$, now recognized to be identical with hemoglobin D$_{Los\ Angeles}$, both having the structure $\alpha_2\beta_2^{121\ Glu\rightarrow Gln}$, also interacts with hemoglobin S in forming aggregates in the deoxy conformation. Hemoglobin SD$_{Punjab/Los\ Angeles}$ disease is a relatively severe sickle cell disease.[105] This hemoglobin is found in frequencies of approximately 3 percent in Northwest India; however, it is relatively rare in populations of African origin, and hemoglobin SD disease is therefore very uncommon.

Although we regard sickle cell anemia as the prototype of the sickle cell diseases, in the African American population only about one-half of the patients with sickle cell diseases have sickle cell anemia (homozygous SS disease). This fact is important from the point of view of genetic counseling: about half of all children with sickle cell disease arise from matings in which only one of the parents carries the sickle cell gene. Moreover, since early mortality rates are probably higher in sickle cell anemia than in the other sickle cell diseases, an even smaller proportion of adults with these sickle cell diseases are actually homozygous for hemoglobin S.

ANIMAL MODELS

No naturally occurring animal models of sickle cell disease have been described. Some deer have red cells that undergo sickling when oxygenated,[106] but not under physiologic conditions of pH and P_{O_2}. Cells from patients with sickle cell anemia have been infused into rats,[107] and this model system has been used to study the effect of various therapeutic agents. However, this approach is limited by the short time that the cells survive in the circulation of the heterologous species. The development of transgenic technologies (see Chap. 9) has made it possible to produce mice whose red cells carry a high percentage of sickle hemoglobin.[108] Notably, by combining the sickle β-globin transgene and human α-globin genes with knockouts of murine globin genes[109] or thalassemic mutations,[110] mice that have many of the features of human sickle disease have been produced.

CLINICAL FEATURES

The newborn infant is protected by the high level of fetal hemoglobin in the red cells during the first 8 to 10 weeks of life. As the level declines the clinical manifestations of sickle cell disease appear, and the hematologic manifestations of sickle disease are apparent by 10 to 12 weeks of age.[111]

CRISES

Many patients with sickle cell anemia are in reasonably good health much of the time, achieving a steady-state level of fitness. This state of relative well-being is periodically interrupted by a crisis that may have a sudden onset and occasionally a fatal outcome. The early recognition and subsequent clinical assessment of sickle crises are greatly facilitated by familiarity with the patient's steady state.

Various types of crises occur, and these may be classified as follows: vasoocclusive (painful) crisis, aplastic crisis, sequestration crisis, and hemolytic crisis.

Vasoocclusive Crisis   The vasoocclusive crisis is the most common and is the hallmark of the patient with sickle cell disease.[112] The frequency with which such crises occur varies from almost daily to less than once yearly. The vasoocclusive crises result from complex interactions between endothelium, plasma factors, leukocytes, and rigid, sickled red cells leading to the obstruction of blood vessels (see "Blood Flow in the Microvasculature," above). Tissue hypoxia occurs and ultimately leads to tissue death and localized pain. It is important to distinguish the pain of a vasoocclusive crisis from the pain caused by other, sometimes more treatable disorders. Appendicitis must sometimes be considered, but it is notable that it has been suggested that the incidence of appendicitis is lower in patients with sickle cell diseases than in the general population.[113] Fever is often present, even in the absence of demonstrable infection. Sickle cell crisis is, to a large extent, a diagnosis by exclusion.[114] Vasoocclusive crises may affect any tissue, but the pain occurs especially in bones, chest, and abdomen. Infarctions in the spleen, which may be a cause of abdominal pain, are so common in sickle cell anemia that after age 6 to 8 the spleen usually becomes very small because of scarring[111] (autosplenectomy). Myonecrosis is unusual but has been documented.[115]

Infarction of cerebral vessels, leading to stroke, is the most serious type of vasoocclusive complication (see "Other Clinical Manifestations, Central Nervous System," below).[116]

Aplastic Crisis   Aplastic crises in sickle cell disease are of the type familiar in patients with other hemolytic disorders, in which the reticulocyte count falls to low levels, indicating that red cell production has decreased dramatically. Depression of erythropoiesis is generally associated with infections. Infections with the B19 strain of *Parvovirus* appear to be by far the most important cause of such crises[117-119] and may be accompanied by extensive marrow necrosis.[120,121] Because of the short red cell life span in sickle cell disease, even in the steady state, a temporary depression of marrow activity can cause a catastrophic fall in hemoglobin level, manifesting as an aplastic crisis. Marrow output failure may also result from a deficiency of folic acid, especially during late pregnancy, and this has sometimes been designated a *megaloblastic crisis.*

Sequestration Crisis   The sequestration crisis occurs particularly in infants and young children,[122] although it may occur in adults with splenomegaly, particularly those with hemoglobin SC disease or sickle β-thalassemia.[123,124] It is characterized by sudden massive pooling of red cells, especially in the spleen. Hypovolemic shock and cardiovascular failure may develop rapidly.[122] A major acute sequestration crisis is considered to be one in which the hemoglobin level is less than 6 g/dl and has fallen more than 3 g/dl when compared with the baseline value; a minor acute sequestration crisis is one in which the hemoglobin level is higher than 6 g/dl.[125] In a study of children with sickle disease born in Los Angeles in the 1960s and 1970s, such crises were responsible for 10 to 15 percent of deaths in the first 10 years of life.[111]

Hemolytic Crisis   The red cell life span is shortened in all the varieties of sickle cell disease. It may suddenly be further reduced, probably for a variety of reasons. This increased rate of hemolysis is designated a hemolytic crisis. The resulting increase in jaundice is associated with a falling hemoglobin and an elevated reticulocyte count. Such crises are very rare; in most instances changes regarded as due to increased hemolysis represent some other complication of sickle cell disease.[126] It has been suggested that concurrent G-6-PD deficiency may be a factor leading to hemolytic crises,[77] but it seems unlikely that this is actually the case, since the young red cell population of patients with sickle cell disease has normal or near-normal G-6-PD activity even when G-6-PD deficiency is present.

An increase in the level of jaundice is not necessarily an indication of increased hemolysis (see "Other Clinical Manifestations, Liver," below). Other causes for jaundice, such as hepatitis, cirrhosis, and gallstones, should be sought. Patients with a chronic hemolytic anemia are especially likely to form bilirubin stones, which may cause extrahepatic biliary obstruction.

OTHER CLINICAL MANIFESTATIONS

Growth   Young children with sickle cell anemia tend to be shorter than normal.[127,128] Puberty is delayed, but considerable growth occurs in late adolescence, so that adults with sickle cell anemia are at least as tall as normal.[128]

Bony Abnormalities   The chronic hemolytic anemia with erythroblastic hyperplasia will result in widening of the medullary spaces, thinning of the cortices, and sparseness of the trabecular pattern.[129] Although these changes are recognizable in the skull, they are usually not as marked as the typical "hair-on-end" appearance characteristic of the patient with β-thalassemia major (see Chap. 48). The vertebral bodies may show biconcavities of the upper and lower surfaces (codfish spine). Pressure from the nucleus pulposus into an area of bone infarction may result in steplike depressions—as if a coin had been pushed into the vertebral body. This x-ray picture is highly suggestive of sickle cell disease.

Crisis with bone pain may be followed by the appearance of periosteal reaction, and irregular areas of osteosclerosis may be seen,

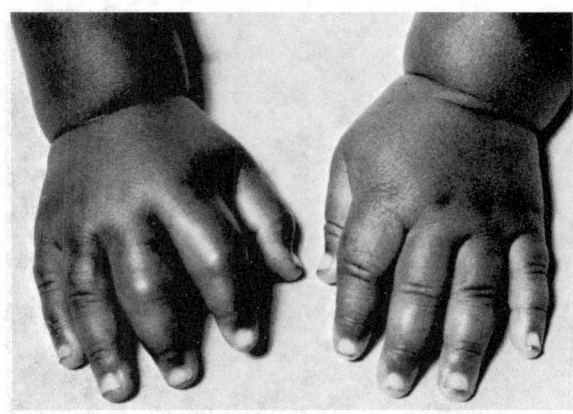

FIGURE 47-4   Sickle cell dactylitis (hand-foot syndrome). Note the swelling of the right hand involving the thumb and first and second fingers. (Diggs,[454] by permission.)

representing areas of bone infarction. Bone scans with ^{99m}Tc are not helpful in delineating areas involved in painful crisis.[130] However, magnetic resonance imaging seems more promising.[131–133]

Sickle cell dactylitis is probably due to limited avascular necrosis of marrow. Nearly one-half of children with sickle cell anemia suffer from this painful disorder, manifesting swelling of the dorsal surfaces of the hands and/or feet (Fig. 47-4). Dactylitis occurs almost entirely in the first 4 years of life, with a peak incidence at about 1 year.[134] Environmental cold is considered to be an important precipitating factor.

In later life necrosis of the head of the femur due to infarction of the nutrient artery is common and may be responsible for severe pain and serious disturbances of gait. Osteonecrosis of the head of the humerus occurs in about 5 percent of patients with sickle disease. Although the incidence in various genotypes is the same, onset tends to be earliest in those with the SS genotype, latest in those with sickle cell β-thalassemia, and intermediate in those with SC disease.[135,136] Chondrolytic arthritis has also been observed.[137] The bone manifestations of sickle cell disease may closely mimic osteomyelitis or arthritis. Ultrasonography may be helpful in making the distinction between infarction and infection.[138]

The presence of necrotic marrow may favor the development of infection, especially with *Staphylococcus aureus*[139] and *Salmonella*[140] (Fig. 47-5). Necrotic marrow may also embolize the lung, producing the "chest syndrome" or in some cases sudden death.[141]

Genitourinary System   The renal medulla is an area that is particularly susceptible to damage in sickle cell disease.[142] Its unique environment, characterized by anoxia, hyperosmolarity, and low pH, predisposes to sickling. Indeed, the kidney is highly susceptible to the effects of the sickling phenomena and is the only organ commonly affected in the generally benign sickle cell trait. The ability to concentrate urine is lost in patients with sickle cell trait as well as those with sickle cell disease.[143] Infarctions may also occur, with renal papillary necrosis (Fig. 47-6) both in patients with SS disease and patients with sickle cell trait.[144] Approximately 50 percent of patients with sickle cell anemia have enlarged kidneys as judged by radiologic examination, and calyceal abnormalities of various types are common.[145] Renal failure is a late complication of sickle cell disease.[146] In one study an increased incidence of renal carcinoma was observed in patients with sickle cell disease.[147]

Priapism is a serious complication of sickle cell disease.[148–150] It is more common in patients with the SS genotype than in other sickle

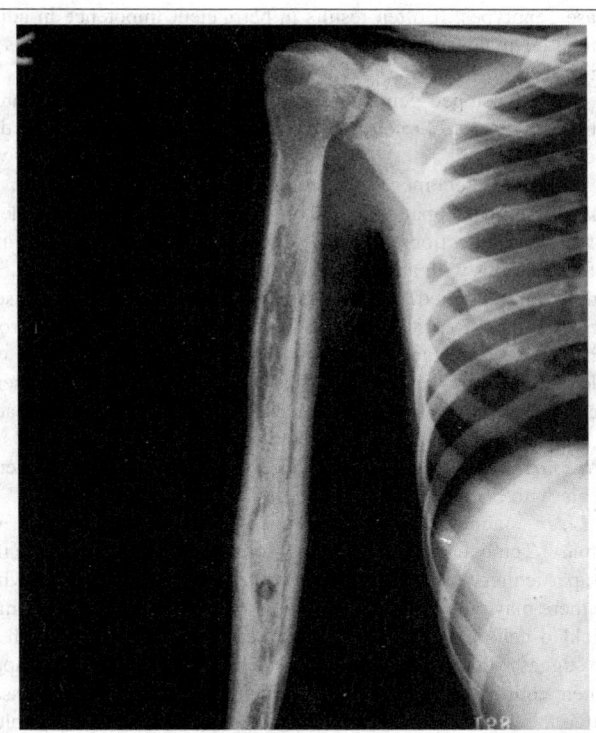

FIGURE 47-5   *Salmonella typhimurium* osteomyelitis in a patient with hemoglobin SC disease. (River et al,[455] by permission.)

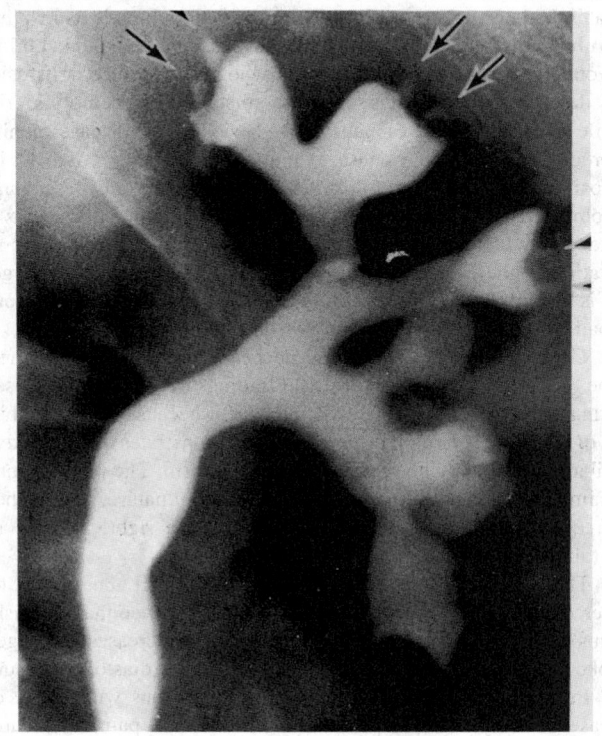

FIGURE 47-6   Renal papillary necrosis in a patient with sickle cell trait. Note the small medullary cavities in the upper three calyces of the left kidney (arrows). (Harrow et al,[456] by permission.)

disease genotypes. It often results in permanent impotence in adults. Prepubertal males have shorter episodes and a good prognosis for future erectile function.

Underdeveloped genitalia and hypogonadism may occur, and it has been suggested but not proven that this could be due to zinc deficiency.[151,152]

Spleen   Splenomegaly is prominent in early childhood, but splenic function is impaired,[153] and presumably as a result the incidence of bacteremic infections is high.[154] Infections of the splenic remnant itself, sometimes with abscess formation, have been documented.[155,156] In adults in the United States splenomegaly is uncommon because of splenic fibrosis. Repeated infarctions of the spleen lead to fibrosis, calcifications, and autosplenectomy. However, in U.S. patients with sickle cell diseases other than SS disease, i.e., sickle cell thalassemia or hemoglobin SC disease, splenomegaly commonly persists into adult life. In Africa, probably as a result of infection with organisms such as *Plasmodium,* splenomegaly is observed in almost one-quarter of patients with SS disease.[157]

Liver   Jaundice and hepatomegaly are common in sickle cell anemia.[158] The liver may be enlarged, sometimes extending to the iliac crest, particularly in young children and again in middle age, at which time there may be evidence of hepatic dysfunction. The small number of sickled cells found in the hepatic vein after passage through the liver suggests that the cells most susceptible to sickling are trapped by their rigidity and engulfed by phagocytes during their passage through the hepatic sinusoids, where the oxygen content of the blood is extremely low. The liver may transiently increase in size during a painful crisis.[159] Sickle cell intrahepatic cholestasis is a rare, catastrophic complication. Characterized by sudden onset of right upper quadrant pain, progressive hepatomegaly, and a serum bilirubin level that may rise to well over 1700 μM (100 mg/dl), its outcome is usually fatal, although recovery has been reported after exchange transfusion.[160] In sickle cell disease, excretion of urobilinogen is usually greater than normal. Some 50 to 70 percent of adult patients may have bilirubin gallstones,[161] and gallstones have also been found in children as young as 6 years of age.[162] Patients who have received transfusions may develop hepatitis that is sometimes mistaken for a hemolytic crisis. While about one-third of patients with sickle cell disease manifest liver dysfunction,[163] the cause is multifactorial.[161,163-165] Excess iron deposition is common, but frank hemochromatosis is only occasionally encountered.[164-168] Some patients with chronic jaundice that seems out of keeping with the degree of hemolysis may have inherited a common mutation in the promoter of the UDP glucuronosyl transferase gene that is known to cause Gilbert disease and increases the jaundice found in patients with thalassemia and G-6-PD deficiency.[169,170]

Cardiopulmonary System   The heart is frequently the site of some of the most prominent physical findings in sickle cell disease.[171] During crisis, striking tachycardia may occur because of the combination of fever and anemia. The precordium demonstrates the overactivity similar to that seen with marked hyperthyroidism. The point of maximal impulse is usually forceful and pounding in nature, and the heart is frequently enlarged to both the left and the right. Systolic and diastolic flow murmurs are often heard.

The blood pressure of patients with sickle cell anemia and to a lesser degree with SC disease is significantly lower than published norms for age, race, and sex, a difference that increases with age.[172] Stroke was associated with higher systolic but not diastolic pressures.

Pulmonary infarctions are common in persons with sickle cell disease and may lead to repeated episodes of chest pain, unexplained dyspnea, or "atypical pneumonia." A combination of fever, chest pain, rise in the white count, and appearance of a pulmonary infiltrate in patients with sickle diseases is referred to as the *acute chest syndrome.*[173] Age has been found to exert a marked effect on the clinical

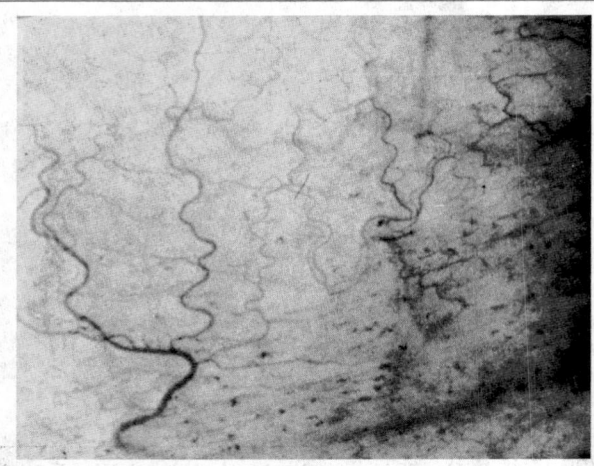

FIGURE 47-7   Lower bulbar conjunctiva in a patient with sickle cell anemia, showing many segmentations. (Paton,[457] by permission.)

picture of acute chest syndrome. In children, acute chest syndrome is milder and more likely due to infection, whereas in adults it is more likely to be severe and to be associated with pain and a higher mortality rate. The clinical and roentgenologic features observed in these patients do not aid in differentiating pulmonary infarction from pulmonary infection, but thin section CT may be more helpful.[174] Rib infarctions are commonly observed on bone scan, and it has been suggested that they may play a role in the pathogenesis of the acute chest syndrome.[175] This disorder is regarded as being multifactorial, with infection, infarction, and pulmonary fat embolism all being factors that may play a role.[176]

The combination of increased flow rate and pulmonary vascular occlusions may result in increased pulmonary pressure and eventually cor pulmonale.[177] Systemic marrow fat embolism has been associated with pulmonary hypertension.[178] However, it has been suggested that patients with recurrent episodes of the acute chest syndrome are not particularly prone to develop pulmonary hypertension.[179]

Eye   Retinal vessel obstruction is followed by neovascularization with arteriovenous aneurysms. These may eventually result in hemorrhage, scarring, retinal detachment, and blindness.[180] These changes occur at the periphery and may initially be difficult to visualize through an ophthalmoscope, even with a fully dilated pupil. At the early stage of retinal disease, vision is therefore not impaired. The retinal changes, collectively termed "sickle retinopathy" have been divided into nonproliferative and proliferative groups. Nonproliferative changes include so-called "salmon patch" hemorrhages, iridescent spots, and black sunbursts. The latter term is used to describe lesions that occur in the peripheral retina; as the retina becomes ischemic, neovascular growth starts at abnormal arterial venous anastomoses resulting from vascular occlusions. These vascular growths extend toward the periphery. Because these abnormal vascular fronds resemble the marine invertebrate *Gorgonia flabellum,* the lesions are called "sea fans."

Examination of the conjunctiva may reveal multiple short comma-shaped capillary segments that often appear isolated from the vascular network because the afferent and efferent lumens are empty. These transient sites of tightly clumped intravascular erythrocytes are found on the bulbar conjunctiva underneath the eyelids (Fig. 47-7). They occasionally disappear during the course of a lengthy examination because of the warmth of the light. Visual loss is most common in SC disease and is due principally to vitreous hemorrhage, secondary to bleeding from the neovascularized areas.

The orbital compression syndrome, consisting of fever, headache, orbital swelling, and optic nerve dysfunction, has been documented in a number of patients with sickle cell disease.[181] The most common cause appears to be orbital marrow infarctions.

Central Nervous System   Cerebrovascular accidents are one of the most devastating complications of sickle cell disease. Once thought to be due to obstruction of small blood vessels, it now appears to be due to lesions of major vessels, particularly the internal carotid and anterior and middle cerebral arteries.[116,182] Even children with no history of stroke may show evidence of infarction on MRI.[183] The prevalence of cerebrovascular accidents has been found to be 4.01 percent and the incidence 0.61 per 100 patient-years in sickle cell anemia (SS) patients, but cardiovascular accidents occur at somewhat lower frequencies in all common genotypes.[184–186] Stroke has even been reported in more than a dozen children and adults with sickle trait, but the cause-and-effect relationship must be considered unproven.[187,188] The incidence of infarctive cerebrovascular accidents is lowest in sickle cell anemia patients 20 to 29 years of age and higher in children and older patients. On the other hand, the incidence of hemorrhagic stroke in SS patients is highest among patients aged 20 to 29 years. The mortality rate was 26 percent in the 2 weeks after hemorrhagic stroke. No deaths occurred after infarctive stroke.[184] The incidence of stroke among patients with hemoglobin SC disease is significantly lower, approximately 2 percent.[184–186] Measurement of the velocity of cerebral blood flow by transcranial Doppler ultrasonography has some predictive value with respect to the probability of developing a stroke.[189] In most patients the stroke occurs without any warning, but in about one-quarter of the cases the stroke occurs in the context of some other complication, such as a painful crisis, priapism,[186] or an aplastic crisis.[190] Risk factors include low steady-state hemoglobin, previous transient ischemic attacks, occurrence of priapism,[184,191] and increased plasma homocysteine levels.[192] Preliminary studies suggest that the inheritance of the prothrombin Leiden mutation and the 677C→T mutation in the methylenetetrahydrofolate reductase (MTHFR) are not major factors in the development of strokes.[193,194] Recurrence of strokes is a prominent feature of this complication; at least 67 percent of patients who have one stroke will suffer at least one more if untreated. Such episodes are particularly common within the first 36 months after a stroke.[185]

Many other neurologic symptoms have been described, including drowsiness, coma, convulsions, headache, temporary or permanent blindness, cranial nerve palsies, and paresthesias of the extremities.[195] Multiple cerebral aneurisms appear to be more common in patients with sickle cell disease.[196,197]

Leg Ulcers   Although encountered in patients with other types of hemolytic disease, ulcers around the ankles are a particularly common feature of sickle cell disease.[198,199] They are unusual in the younger child, and stasis clearly plays some part in their formation. They usually start as a small break in the skin or a blisterlike area that breaks down and rapidly extends to form a painful, indolent ulcer. Usually the ulcers become infected, and the base is covered with a yellow, purulent layer. They may extend deeply enough to expose muscle. Once formed, leg ulcers do not heal spontaneously, and they become a major source of morbidity for affected patients.

Infections   Patients with sickle cell disease are particularly prone to develop infections, and this may be the single most common reason for hospitalization.[200] Because of functional asplenia, impaired phagocytic function,[201] and a defect in activation of the alternate complement pathway, infections may be quite hazardous, particularly so in children. The risk varies significantly from patient to patient, with some patients having very few infections. Pneumonia seems to be the most common infection encountered and often is of pneumococcal origin, particularly in children. As noted above, osteomyelitis due

to *Staphylococcus* and to *Salmonella* also is relatively common.[139] Babesiosis has been reported to occur in one patient,[202] possibly as a result of the impaired splenic function.

Pregnancy   Pregnancy in women with sickle cell anemia is accompanied by an increased incidence of pyelonephritis, pulmonary infarction, pneumonia, acute chest syndrome, antepartum hemorrhage, prematurity, and fetal death.[203] Megaloblastic anemia responsive to folic acid, especially in late pregnancy, also occurs with increased frequency. The birth weight of infants of mothers with sickle cell anemia is below average,[204,205] and the fetal wastage is high.[206,207] The cause of neonatal death is obscure, but it may sometimes result from vasoocclusion of the placenta[204]; the postmortem findings are those of intrapartum anoxia.[208] The maternal mortality in sickle cell disease was formerly prohibitively high, with rates averaging 33 percent, but is now much lower, averaging about 1.5 percent in various series.[206,207,209–213] Higher mortality rates are still observed in some parts of the world, however, with maternal mortality rates of up to 9.2 percent and a perinatal mortality of up to 19.5 percent.[210,214,215]

LABORATORY FEATURES

The steady-state hemoglobin level of patients with sickle cell anemia is usually between 5 and 11 g/dl. The anemia is normochromic and normocytic in spite of the elevated reticulocyte count.[216] In comparison with patients with similarly increased reticulocyte counts, patients with SS disease may be considered to have a "microcytic" anemia, presumably because the sickle mutation impairs the efficiency of production of hemoglobin. The range of red cell densities is increased in sickle cell anemia,[217] but the average cellular MCHC is normal. In SC disease, however, the average MCHC is increased.[217] Erythropoietin levels may be reduced relative to the degree of anemia[218] but have also been reported to be appropriate.[219] The anemia is accompanied by laboratory signs of hemolysis, with increased indirect-reacting serum bilirubin and reticulocytosis and often circulating nucleated red cells. As in any hemolytic anemia, endogenous CO production is increased[220,221] and haptoglobin absent. Sickled erythrocytes are often evident on inspection of the blood film. Target cells may be present, particularly in sickle cell–hemoglobin C disease and in sickle cell β-thalassemia. In sickle cell hemoglobin C disease, folded cells are sometimes seen (Fig. 47-8, Fig. 47-9). Examination of the red cells by inference phase-contrast microscopy reveals surface indentations, presumably resulting from splenic hypofunction, in approximately 20 percent of the cells.[153] A modest polymorphonuclear leukocytosis with a left shift is common even in the steady state[222,223] and may be due in part to redistribution of leukocytes from the marginal to the circulating granulocyte pool.[222] It does not necessarily signify an infection. Thrombocytosis is also common, but evidence of intravascular coagulation with thrombocytopenia has been noted rarely during crisis.[224]

The marrow shows erythroid hyperplasia. Immunoglobulin levels are frequently increased. IgA levels are particularly elevated in all forms of sickle cell disease. Elevations of IgG levels are also sometimes seen, while IgM levels appear to be elevated particularly in patients with sickle cell thalassemia and in individuals with other combinations such as hemoglobin SC disease.[225] A decreased number of T lymphocytes and increased B lymphocytes in the blood have been reported.[226] Activation in the alternative complement pathway has been detected in some patients[227] and is apparently a result of phosphatidylserine exposure by erythrocytes.[228] This may be responsible, in part, for increased susceptibility to infection.

Plasma tocopherol[229] and zinc[230,231] levels are often low, the latter possibly due to zincuria.[151,231] Serum ferritin levels are normal in the first two decades of life but tend to rise in older patients, and modest

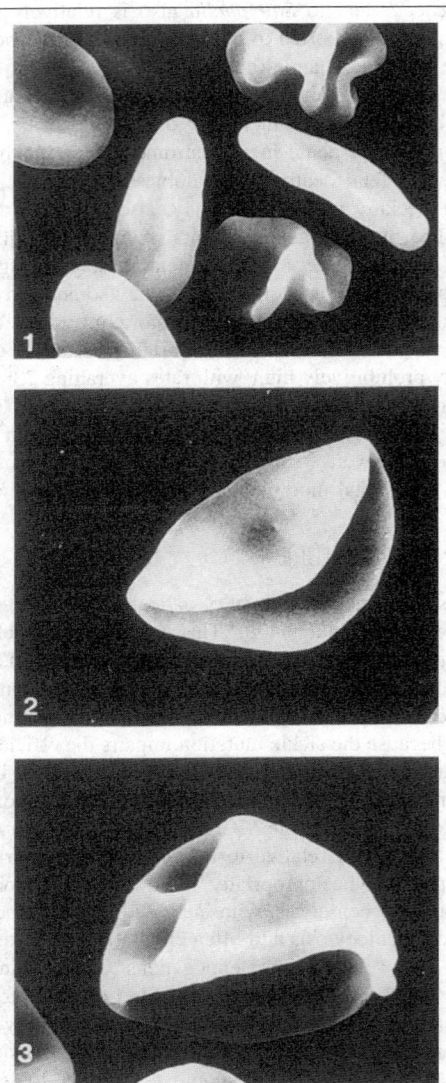

FIGURE 47-8   Scanning electron microscopy of individual SC cells: (1) multifolded cells; (2) unifolded cell resembling pita bread and most likely the same as the "fat cell" shown in Fig. 47-9; (3) tridimpled cell, also called a triangular cell. (Lawrence et al,[52] by permission.)

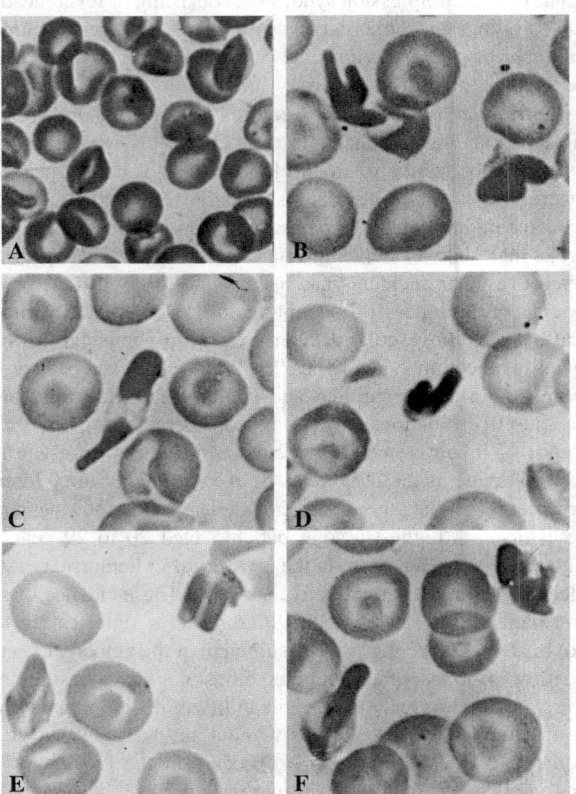

FIGURE 47-9   Bizarre-shaped erythrocytes in the blood film of patient with hemoglobin SC disease. (A) "Fat sickle cells." (B) Crescent-shaped erythrocyte with three deep-hued crystals (center left). Two bizarre condensed hemoglobin masses in a red blood cell (lower right). (C) Elongated red corpuscle with concentration of hemoglobin at each end and hemoglobin-free central area (center). (D) Red cell with two parallel, dark, crystal-like structures of different lengths, terminating in a pyramid tip (center). (E) Erythrocyte with two parallel formations separated by a clear area (upper right). Red cell with one elongated mass (lower left). (F) Erythrocyte with densely stained hemoglobin masses (upper right). Red cell with one dark, elongated, rounded bulge and one small triangular hemoglobin mass, leaving two areas relatively free of hemoglobin (lower left). (Diggs and Bell,[458] by permission.)

elevations in plasma iron content are also frequently encountered.[232] High ferritin levels and increased iron burden occurs in patients who receive chronic transfusion therapy, and such patients are often treated with desferrioxamine.[233–235] However, although the development of hemochromatosis has been reported,[165] this seems to be a relatively uncommon complication, even in extensively transfused patients. Frank iron deficiency is not rare, and overt iron deficiency with microcytosis has sometimes been observed in patients with sickle cell anemia.[236,237] Thus, the presence of microcytosis does not necessarily indicate the concurrent presence of thalassemia.

DIAGNOSIS

Diagnosis depends upon documentation of the presence of sickle hemoglobin, preferably by electrophoresis.[233] Many different media and buffers are used to distinguish different mutant hemoglobins from one another, but several relatively simple systems suffice for the differentiation of most variants from one another.[238] Rapid methods

that are less reliable for the detection of sickle hemoglobin include the observation of sickling of red cells containing sickle hemoglobin microscopically under a coverslip by suspending the cells in a droplet of a 2% solution of sodium metabisulfite[239] and solubility tests. The latter depend on the low solubility of reduced sickle hemoglobin which results in the development of turbidity under appropriate conditions.[240] However, such tests do not detect hemoglobin C or β-thalassemia and do not reliably distinguish between sickle trait and sickle disease and are therefore of limited value. With the refinement and automation of techniques it has also been possible to detect sickle hemoglobin accurately and economically by high-pressure liquid chromatography and by isoelectric focusing.[241] Use of the polymerase chain reaction to detect the sickle mutation is the method of choice for prenatal diagnosis.[242]

Because there are no normal β polypeptide chain genes, patients with sickle cell anemia or hemoglobin SC disease have no normal adult hemoglobin. In the heterozygote for the sickle cell gene and β⁰-thalassemia no hemoglobin A is found, but small amounts of normal hemoglobin are present in the compound heterozygote for the sickle cell and β⁺-thalassemia genes. The concentration of fetal hemoglobin usually is increased in sickle cell β-thalassemia and is heterogeneously distributed among the red cells. The quantitation of hemoglobin A_2 is of value in differentiating sickle cell anemia from sickle cell β^0-thalassemia; hemoglobin A_2 levels tend to be increased in the latter condition. Family studies are particularly helpful if sickle cell β^0-thalassemia is to be clearly differentiated from sickle cell anemia.

Sickle cell anemia can be diagnosed at birth by subjecting cord blood samples to electrophoresis.[243] Ideally, all babies of ethnic groups with a high frequency of the sickle cell gene should be screened at birth, because of a demonstrated decrease in mortality of very young children when the diagnosis is made.[244] The cost-effectiveness of screening depends on the composition of the target population; it has been estimated to be $206,000 per death averted in Alaska. Screening is particularly desirable if the mother has sickle cell trait.

Chorionic villus biopsy has been used extensively to obtain fetal DNA for diagnosis in the first trimester.[245] The availability of techniques for the amplification of genomic DNA makes feasible DNA-based prenatal diagnosis of sickle cell disease (see Chaps. 9 and 46). The mutant and normal sequences can be differentiated with an appropriate restriction endonuclease or by the use of synthetic oligonucleotide probes.[242,246]

THERAPY, COURSE, AND PROGNOSIS

THERAPY
An authoritative guide for the management of patients with sickle cell diseases has been published under the auspices of the Heart, Lung, and Blood Institute of the National Institutes of Health.[233]

General Measures   Since no fully satisfactory, specific treatments for the sickle cell disorders have yet become available, physicians must concentrate their therapeutic efforts in the direction of continuous and effective general medical care and appropriate management of complications as they arise.[247,248] Folic acid supplementation has been suggested, but there is little evidence that it is beneficial[249] except in pregnancy and in patients with other disorders that increase the requirement for folate. Transfusions are not usually required, except in special circumstances such as stroke, abnormal transcranial Doppler findings, leg ulcers, or intractable or frequently recurring painful crises.[250] Prophylactic transfusion does, as expected, decrease the frequency of crises,[166] but it requires administration of desferrioxamine to prevent iron overload and subjects patients to the risk of the complications of transfusion such as alloimmunization[251] and transmission of infection. A randomized double-blind study showed that conservative transfusion therapy (designed to keep the hemoglobin level over 10 g/dl) was as effective in preventing perioperative complications as more aggressive therapy (designed to maintain the hemoglobin S level under 30%) and was safer.[252] Acute neurologic symptoms have been reported to occur after partial exchange transfusion, but a cause-and-effect relationship is not established.[253] The use of neocytes (young erythrocytes; see Chap. 140) is probably not justified because of inconvenience and high cost.

Exposure to cold and high altitudes should be avoided. Special vocational training of patients with sickle cell anemia for suitable occupations is useful. It is important that patients live as normal a life as possible. Occupations that do not require heavy manual labor and in which occasional absences from work are practical may be excellent and can make these patients productive members of society.

Acute Chest Syndrome   Rapid and correct diagnosis is of paramount importance. It has been recommended that if normal flora are seen on gram-stained sputum in a patient who is not seriously ill with the acute chest syndrome, no antibiotics should be used. However, more symptomatic patients with sputum production should receive antibiotics based on the organisms found in the gram-stained sputum.

In adults, in contrast to children, such pulmonary events rarely appear to be due to infection with pneumococci.[254] Because of the life-threatening nature of the acute chest syndrome, some clinicians prefer a more aggressive approach, immediately instituting empiric antibiotic therapy including erythromycin because of the frequent involvement of bacteria such as *Chlamydia* or *Mycoplasma*.[176] Adequate hydration is important, but fluid overload resulting in pulmonary edema occurs not infrequently, and thus careful monitoring of fluid balance is required.[176] Exchange transfusion has been advocated.[255]

Infections   The administration of pneumococcal vaccine is recommended,[256] but a number of failures of the vaccine to protect children with sickle cell disease against infection with the pneumococcus have been reported, and children with sickle disease should receive pneumococcal vaccine and penicillin prophylaxis at least until the age of five.[233,257–259] Other infectious diseases against which patients with sickle diseases should be immunized include hepatitis B, diphtheria, tetanus, pertussis, poliomyelitis, and *Haemophilus influenzae*.[233] Infections should be treated vigorously with antibiotics. Because patients with sickle cell anemia are unable to concentrate urine adequately, dehydration during the course of infection represents a special risk to be avoided by adequate fluid administration.

Crises   Once a small blood vessel is totally obstructed by sickled cells in the development of a painful crisis, the obstruction is probably irreversible. Yet the function of neighboring blood vessels in the areas obstructed by rigid sickled cells may be preserved by a number of therapeutic measures. The patient should be kept warm, and adequate hydration should be maintained by the oral or intravenous route. The role of oxygen therapy in the treatment of vasoocclusive crises is poorly defined. Although the administration of oxygen was once considered to be contraindicated because of a putative negative effect on erythropoiesis, it seems doubtful that it does any harm aside from the minor discomfort incident to its administration, and it may be useful in patients with a decreased arterial oxygen saturation. Hyperbaric oxygen usually fails to benefit the patient,[260] although occasional success using this treatment has been claimed.[261]

The anticoagulants dicumarol[262] and the defibrinating enzyme Arvin[263] have been tried without success. Intravenous administration of magnesium sulfate[264] has been reported to be beneficial, although a therapeutic effect has not been confirmed.[265] Promising results of the treatment of sickle crisis with pentoxifylline, a drug reported to increase erythrocyte deformability, were reported in a double-blind study[266] but could not be confirmed.[267] Oral sodium bicarbonate or sodium citrate therapy has been tried in the treatment of an established vasoocclusive crisis, as well as in its prevention,[265] but the efficacy of this treatment could not be confirmed in a controlled study.[268]

Management with analgesics of the pain of infarctive crises represents a particularly difficult problem for the physician[233,269] and is discussed in Chap. 21. In most instances the manifestations of vasoocclusive crisis may gradually disappear over a period of hours or days on symptomatic management.

Splenic sequestration crises are a life-threatening complication that must be treated vigorously. Transfusion with red cells (exchange transfusions if there is respiratory distress) and splenectomy (see below) have been recommended.[122,125]

Strokes   Because of the high recurrence rates of strokes, special attention has been paid to this group of high-risk patients. Regular transfusion programs to maintain the sickle hemoglobin concentration at 30 percent of the total hemoglobin reduce recurrence rates.[167] Allowing no more than 50 percent of the hemoglobin to be sickle hemoglobin may provide similar protection.[270] A randomized study showed that transfusion greatly reduces the risk of a first stroke in children with sickle cell anemia who have abnormal results on transcranial Doppler ultrasonography.[183,271]

Hypersplenism and Splenectomy Because of "autosplenectomy," hypersplenism is seldom a problem in sickle cell anemia. Hypersplenism may be suspected in other forms of sickle disease if a long-term transfusion program becomes necessary to maintain life or if leukopenia and thrombocytopenia are associated with a palpable spleen. Under these circumstances splenectomy may very occasionally be warranted. It has been recommended that splenectomy be performed in all children over the age of two in which one major or two minor splenic sequestration crises have occurred because of the danger of recurrent crises.[125,233]

Cholelithiasis It is useful to examine adolescent and adult sickle cell anemia patients for the presence of gallstones. It has been suggested that elective cholecystectomy be performed when stones are present,[272] but since 50 to 70 percent of adult patients with sickle disease have been found to have gallstones,[161] gallstones that do not cause symptoms should probably not be removed. Laparoscopic cholecystectomy has been found to be safe and cost-effective in children[273] and adults.[274]

Contraception and Pregnancy Oral contraception may offer some additional hazard of thromboembolism in patients with sickle hemoglobin,[275] but the risk is probably small compared to the risk of pregnancy itself. The contraceptives medroxyprogesterone acetate (Depo-Provera®) given parenterally monthly for 3 months and then every month or levonorgestrel + ethinyl estradiol (Microgynon 30®) given daily were associated with a decrease in the number of attacks of pain in one study.[276]

Although very high maternal mortality rates have been greatly reduced with good prenatal care, pregnancy and the postpartum period are still potentially hazardous for a mother with sickle cell disease.[209] The patient should be closely supervised during pregnancy.[277] Although prophylactic blood transfusions have been given to some patients with what appear to be satisfactory results,[278–281] the effectiveness of this type of therapy is not proven.[209,282] Studies demonstrating that exchange transfusions are not required have been presented[283] and contested.[280]

Leg Ulcers Leg ulcers may respond to conservative treatment such as bed rest, elevation of the affected limb, zinc sulfate pressure dressings, or maintenance transfusion or may require surgical grafting.[199] In a study of 172 patients,[198] no difference in the rate of healing was associated with any of the different treatment modalities.

Bone and Joint Disease Joint replacement may be helpful to patients who have suffered osteonecrosis, but the number of complications and the number of revisions needed is extraordinary, so that the risk-to-benefit ratio is high.[284] Core decompression has been found to be useful in the management of early avascular necrosis of the hip.[285]

Retinal Changes Vitreous hemorrhages and subsequent blindness may be the end result of the neovascularization that follows retinal infarction. Laser photocoagulation of new vessels may help to prevent this complication.[180] When hemorrhages have occurred vitrectomy may be indicated. The administration of nifedipine seemed to improve conjunctival and retinal perfusion and color vision performance in patients with sickle cell disease.[286]

Priapism Surgical intervention is commonly practiced, particularly in postpubertal patients with priapism. However, there is no clear evidence of benefit from shunting procedures.[148] Hydration and exchange transfusions have been associated with detumescence,[150] and it has been suggested that the oral administration of the alpha-adrenergic agent etilefrine prevents recurrence of priapism.[287] Penile prostheses have been found to be useful when impotence results from priapism.[288,289]

Anesthesia and Surgery The patient with sickle cell disease is at increased risk during anesthesia. If surgery is indicated, scrupulous care is needed to avoid factors known to precipitate crisis, including hypoxemia, dehydration, circulatory stasis, acidosis, cold, and infections.[290–293]

Preoperative transfusion with packed red cells may help to avoid complications in patients with sickle cell disease undergoing major surgery.[294] Partial exchange transfusion has been advocated,[166,295] and this has the advantage of immediate removal from the circulation of sickle cells that may obstruct the microcirculation. However, this more complex procedure probably has little if any advantage over simple transfusion if surgery is elective, as might be the case with patients requiring cholecystectomy or hip replacement.[291] Exchange transfusion requires more blood to achieve an equivalent increment in the blood hemoglobin level, and therefore entails more risk than simple transfusion. Elevation of the hemoglobin level of the blood will markedly reduce the production of sickle cells by the marrow, and in view of the short life span of the patient's own circulating erythrocytes, few sickle cells will remain in the circulation after a week or two. The complication rate of patients receiving exchange transfusions is, in point of fact, no lower than that observed in patients receiving simple transfusions.[296] Exchange transfusion provides an advantage if iron overload is a concern or if removal of sickle cells is desired within a period of less than 5 to 7 days.

Transplantation Sickle cell disease is fundamentally a disease of the hematopoietic stem cell, and replacing the genetically defective cell with a normal one should cure the disease. One patient with sickle cell disease received a marrow transplant from a sib with sickle cell trait in the course of treatment of acute leukemia.[297] As expected, the sickle cell disease was cured—converted into sickle cell trait.

Subsequently a considerable number of patients with sickle cell disease have undergone marrow transplantation. Groups in France and Belgium had transplanted 42 patients by 1992, with only 1 death; the other patients were alive with follow-ups of from 1 to 75 months.[298,299] Over 90 percent of 50 patients transplanted in Belgium between April 1986 and January 1997 survived.[300,301] In the United States an increasing number of patients are undergoing transplantation, and the overall results have been quite favorable.[302] Twenty of 22 patients survived, with a median follow-up of 23.9 months (range, 10.1– 51.0), and 16 patients had stable engraftment of donor hematopoietic cells. In 1997 it was estimated that worldwide 140 patients had undergone transplantation.[303]

The decision of whether to transplant a patient with sickle cell disease is a difficult one, because the expected mortality rate for transplantation in young children with a good family donor match is still of the order of 10 percent, and the potential morbidity from chronic graft-versus-host disease needs also be taken into account. Thus, the initial focus must be upon those children with a poor prognosis, and apart from those who have already suffered a stroke, accurate prognostication is impossible.[304–306]

Agents with In Vitro Antisickling Activities For a number of years, attempts have been made to modify red cells containing hemoglobin S in a manner that will suppress the sickling process. Examples of this approach have included conversion of hemoglobin to carboxyhemoglobin[307–309] or methemoglobin[310]; acetylation of the hemoglobin molecules with aspirin,[311,312] methyl acetyl phosphate,[313] or succinyldisalicylate[314]; cross-linking hemoglobin molecules with dimethyl adipimidate[315,316]; and use of carbonic anhydrase inhibitors to reduce the formation of H_2CO_3.[317] Distilled water has been given intravenously to lower the MCHC.[318] Glutamine has been given to change the oxidative state of the cell.[319] Other antisickling agents that have been studied for a possible therapeutic effect include urea,[320] cyanate,[321] o-carbamoylsalicylates,[322] methyl acetyl phosphate,[323] lysyl-phenylalanine,[324] procaine,[325] zinc,[326] pyridoxine[327,328] and its derivatives,[329,330] phenothiazines,[331] steroids,[315] nitrogen mustard,[332] glyceraldehyde,[333] hexamethylenetetramine,[334] vitamin E,[335] lawsone,[336] substituted benzaldehydes,[337] bepridil,[338] and cetiedil.[339] The usefulness of none of these has been confirmed.

Clinical Studies of Putative Antisickling Agents   Most putative antisickling agents have been tested only with in vitro model systems, but a few have had clinical trials. The induction of methemoglobinemia[310] by the administration of sodium nitrite or p-aminopropiophenone lengthened the life span of sickle cells, and the inhalation of carbon monoxide[309] was found to have a similar effect. A patient with sickle cell anemia who was accidentally exposed to carbon monoxide levels presented with a hematocrit rising to 46 percent. A fatal outcome was attributed to extreme hyperviscosity occurring as the carboxyhemoglobin was converted to oxyhemoglobin and the cells again began to sickle.[340] Pyridoxine,[327] in contrast, did not influence red cell life span. The use of alkali to counteract the Bohr effect (the reduction of the oxygen affinity of hemoglobin at acid pH)[341] has been thought to have some therapeutic value, but no beneficial effect could be demonstrated in controlled trials.[342] The rationale for the use of urea was the ability of this chemical to dissociate hydrophobic molecular bonds and thus interfere with the sickling process. The concentration required to achieve such an effect cannot be reached in vivo, and clinical trials have proved disappointing.[220] Carbamylation of the hemoglobin molecule by cyanate increases the affinity of the hemoglobin for oxygen.[343] Because the sickling process requires the hemoglobin to be in the deoxy conformation, any agent capable of affecting the equilibrium between the oxy and deoxy conformations and thereby increasing the avidity of hemoglobin for oxygen must have an antisickling effect.[86] Unfortunately, in clinical trials cyanate provoked polyneuropathy,[344] retinal changes,[344] and cataracts[345] and therefore appears to be too toxic for systemic use. However, extracorporeal treatment with removal of excess cyanate by washing the red cells before returning them to the patient may overcome this problem.[346-348] A number of substituted benzaldehyde compounds have been given experimentally to patients, producing a left shift in the oxygen dissociation curve and suggestive evidence of a decrease in hemolysis.[337,349] It has been suggested that their effect may be due not only to stabilization of the oxy conformation of hemoglobin but also to decreasing potassium loss.[337]

Because sickling is highly concentration dependent, efforts to treat the disorder by swelling the red cells have been made. These have included the administration of distilled water intravenously[318] and the lowering of serum sodium by the administration of a long-acting vasopressin derivative and vigorous hydration.[350,351] The effectiveness and safety of the latter treatment has been questioned.[352,353] Such treatment must still be regarded as experimental.

Increasing the Level of Fetal Hemoglobin   Efforts have also been made to ameliorate the sickling process by stimulating the formation of fetal hemoglobin. Attempted originally by the administration of chorionic gonadotropin and estrogens,[310] more recent efforts have focused on 5-azacytidine, a drug that inhibits the methylation of DNA and was shown to increase fetal hemoglobin concentrations of the red cells of baboons.[354] The administration of 5-azacytidine to patients with sickle cell anemia resulted in an increased concentration of fetal hemoglobin[355,356] and in a rise in the hemoglobin concentration of the blood.[355,356] Other antineoplastic agents, including cytosine arabinoside[357,358] and hydroxyurea[357,359-361] or hydroxyurea in combination with erythropoietin,[362] and erythropoietin alone[363] also increase the fetal hemoglobin level. Butyric acid and related compounds[364-366] increase fetal hemoglobin production in progenitor cells, experimental animals, and humans. However, isobutyramide given orally was not found to be useful.[367] In vitro, interferon gamma has also been shown to increase fetal hemoglobin production.[368]

Of these agents, hydroxyurea is the one that has been tested most extensively and that has been introduced selectively into clinical practice. In a randomized study of 299 patients the median number of painful crises in patients given hydroxyurea was 2.5 per year, as compared with 4.5 per year in patients given placebo. Drug administration was started at 15 mg/kg body weight per day and was increased by 5 mg/kg/day every 12 weeks unless there were signs of marrow suppression.[369] A number of open-label studies have been conducted and have in general shown a decrease in the incidence of painful crises[370-375] without serious side effects. However, careful supervision is obviously required in the administration of a myelosuppressive agent. Compliance among children appeared to be very satisfactory in one study.[376]

Poloxamer 188, a nonionic surfactant with hemorheologic properties, has been tested in a double-blind randomized trial and found to decrease the severity of painful sickle crises.[377]

COURSE AND PROGNOSIS

For a number of years it was unclear why sickle cell anemia was relatively common in African Americans and yet appeared to be a rare disease in Central Africa. Subsequently it was recognized that the early mortality associated with sickle cell anemia in Central Africa[378,379] was responsible for its apparent rarity: the surveys of the distribution of sickle hemoglobin in Africa did not include the afflicted who had died. With good medical care, patients with sickle cell anemia usually survive to middle age.[380-382] Assessment of the overall mortality of sickle cell anemia must take into account the fact that cases first diagnosed in late childhood, adolescence, or adult life are likely to result in a preponderance of the clinically more benign patients. In the two and one-half decades after 1968, mortality rates of African American children with sickle cell disease decreased considerably.[383] In the 1–4 age group the mortality had fallen from 37 per thousand persons in those born between 1967 and 1969 to 22 per thousand among those born between 1986 and 1988. Corresponding figures for the 5–9 age group were 19 and 10 per thousand, and for the 10–14 age group 17 and 8 per thousand.[383] These improvements in survival may probably best be ascribed to newborn screening programs,[384] penicillin prophylaxis of disease caused by *Streptococcus pneumoniae*, and perhaps the use of pneumococcal vaccines. There were considerable regional differences. The mortality was considerably higher in Florida than in Maryland and Pennsylvania, probably related to the health care facilities available in different regions.[385] Astonishingly, in California and Illinois, mortality from all causes among African American children born during 1990–1994 with SC disease was slightly less than overall mortality for all African American children born in the same time period.[386]

The manifestations of sickle cell disease vary with age.[111] Acute manifestations often are associated with severe infections in childhood, while in the adult, symptoms are characteristically chronic and organ-related, albeit still potentially life threatening. Until more data on the disease in infancy become available, it is not possible to predict whether the sudden death syndrome in infants with sickle cell anemia is a common or a rare event. In the meantime, the diagnosis must be considered in cases of acute general illness and unexplained death, especially in ethnic groups where the sickle cell gene is known to occur commonly.

PREVENTION

Prevention of some of the sequelae of sickle cell diseases can be achieved by newborn screening (see "Diagnosis," above). Another form of prevention is based on prenatal diagnosis. Parents can be screened for the carrier state, and if they are carriers they can be provided with genetic counseling and educated about the options of not having children or of having pregnancies monitored for the occurrence of a sickle cell disease in the fetus. Since approximately half of the children with sickle cell diseases have only one parent with sickle hemoglobin, effective screening programs must do more than merely detect the presence of this abnormal hemoglobin. They must also use means that will permit detection of hemoglobin C and of β-thalassemia trait. Because of the benign clinical nature of β-thalassemia, hemoglobin C, and sickle cell traits, no useful purpose other than that of genetic counseling seems to be served by screening populations for these carrier states. Indeed, misunderstanding concerning the significance of the carrier states has led to unwarranted harm to individuals who are detected as carriers in screening programs.[387]

Many screening programs have been implemented and the number and background of participants have been described.[388,389,390] However, only scant data permitting assessment of the actual effect of screening programs on birth frequency of infants with sickle cell disorders are available. In Guadeloupe 62 percent of the group of mothers at risk for bearing children with sickle disease underwent prenatal diagnosis, which allowed identification of 27 SS fetuses, with an induced abortion rate of 70 percent. Such data are, of course, highly culture dependent, and very different results might be obtained elsewhere.

SICKLE CELL TRAIT

DEFINITION AND HISTORY

Sickle cell trait is the heterozygous state for the sickle cell diseases and is the most benign form of the sickling disorders.

ETIOLOGY AND PATHOGENESIS

The properties of sickle hemoglobin have been described above. In sickle cell trait less than one-half of the hemoglobin in each red cell is hemoglobin S. The abundance of normal hemoglobin A in the cell prevents sickling under most physiologic circumstances; sickle cell trait cells will sickle at an oxygen tension of about 15 torr.[79]

Sickle cell trait is inherited as an autosomal dominant disorder. It affects some 8 percent of African Americans and an even higher percentage of the population in Africa (see "Inheritance," above). Interaction between α-thalassemia and sickle cell trait to modify the amount of sickle hemoglobin has been described above.

CLINICAL FEATURES

Sickle cell trait does not produce any abnormalities of the blood counts and is an exceedingly rare cause of morbidity. Red cell life span is normal in normoxic persons with sickle cell trait.[391] Not only patients but even physicians[392] often appear to believe that sickle cell trait represents a mild type of sickle cell disease. Cerebral thrombosis, mishaps during anesthesia, and sudden death attract little notice when occurring in a person who does not have a known genetic variant, but the same occurrence in the 1 of 12 African Americans who have this trait immediately raises the question of a cause-and-effect relationship. Thus, there is a legion of anecdotal reports suggesting that sickle cell trait contributed to a patient's illness.[187,188,393,394,395,396] There may, however, be certain situations in which a risk is plausible. Thus, in severe cyanotic congenital heart diseases, such as tetralogy of Fallot, patients with sickle cell trait may show signs of hemolysis.[397] In reality, the morbidity and possible mortality associated with sickle cell trait is very low and therefore difficult to document accurately. It seems to be limited largely to renal lesions (see Fig. 47-6) leading to hematuria that is otherwise unexplained and possibly to thromboembolic episodes involving the lung. In a massive study encompassing over 65,000 consecutively admitted African American male patients in 13 U.S.

Veterans Administration hospitals,[73] slightly higher incidences only of hematuria of unspecified cause (2.5 percent versus 1.3 percent) and pulmonary embolism (2.2 percent versus 1.5 percent) were found. No age stratification was found, indicating that the life span of patients with sickle cell trait is normal. Surgical patients with sickle cell trait had no greater perioperative mortality, no longer postoperative stay, and no greater mortality than those with normal hemoglobin. Similar conclusions have been drawn in other studies.[398] It has not been possible to document any differences from normal in cardiovascular function of sickle cell trait subjects even when they were subjected to maximum exercise[399-403]; indeed, persons with sickle trait were overrepresented among champion athletes in the Ivory Coast.[404]

Sudden death resulting from rhabdomyolysis has been reported anecdotally in numerous subjects with sickle cell trait following severe exercise.[396,405-409] An extensive investigation of episodes of sudden death showed a statistically significant excess in the number of patients with sickle cell trait.[410] It is believed that the hyposthenuria (see "Other Clinical Manifestations, Genitourinary System," above) in combination with heat and extreme stress may trigger this catastrophic and usually fatal event.

Because of reports of splenic infarction in individuals thought to have sickle cell trait who were flying in unpressurized aircraft[411,412] or who ascended to very high altitudes,[413] there has been concern about the safety of permitting persons with sickle cell trait to fly. Since commercial aircraft maintain a cabin pressure equivalent to that encountered at 5000 to 7000 feet (1500 to 2100 m), this concern is unwarranted.[81] It appears that when splenic infarction does occur at high altitudes, non-African persons with sickle trait are much more likely to be affected than are Africans.[80]

LABORATORY FEATURES

The diagnosis of sickle cell trait depends upon demonstration of the presence of hemoglobin S and hemoglobin A in the affected individual. The amount of hemoglobin S is always less than the concentration of hemoglobin A. In contrast, in sickle cell β^+-thalassemia the amount of hemoglobin S exceeds that of hemoglobin A.

THERAPY, COURSE, AND PROGNOSIS

Because of its benign features, sickle cell trait does not require treatment and does not appear to affect life span.[73]

HEMOGLOBIN C DISEASE

DEFINITION AND HISTORY

Hemoglobin C was the second abnormal hemoglobin to be described, not long after the description of hemoglobin S.[414] The homozygous state (CC disease) was described independently by Spaet et al[415] and by Ranney et al[416] in 1953. Hemoglobin C trait is the heterozygous state in which hemoglobin C is inherited together with normal hemoglobin. The combination with sickle cell hemoglobin, SC disease, has been described in the discussion of sickle cell anemia, under "The Sickle Cell Diseases," above.

ETIOLOGY AND PATHOGENESIS

In hemoglobin C, glutamic acid in the sixth position from the N terminal of the β chain has been replaced by lysine.[417] Red cells containing principally hemoglobin C are more rigid than normal,[418] and their fragmentation in the circulation may result in the formation of microspherocytes. Intraerythrocytic crystals of oxygenated Hb C are found in the red cells, especially in splenectomized patients,[418,419] and the formation of crystals is inhibited by hemoglobin F.[420] The red cell life span is shortened to a mean of 30 to 35 days.[421] The rate of hemoglobin production in hemoglobin C disease has been reported to be 2.5 to 3 times normal.[422] Erythrocytes from patients with hemoglobin C disease have a low oxygen affinity, possibly due to a reduction for unknown reasons of the intracellular pH.[423] This may contribute to the mild anemia that is usually present.

Hemoglobin C is found in 17 to 28 percent of West Africans, particularly east of the Niger River in the vicinity of North Ghana.[424,425] The selective factors that account for this high prevalence are unknown at present. The prevalence among African Americans is 2 to 3 percent.[73,426] Sporadic cases also have been reported in other populations, including Italians[427] and Afrikaners.[101]

CLINICAL FEATURES

Splenomegaly is a fairly constant feature of hemoglobin C disease and may be associated with fleeting abdominal pain. However, there is little evidence for clinically significant hemodynamic disturbances.[428] Women with hemoglobin C disease appear to tolerate pregnancy well.[429] Children have mild anemia with few symptoms and normal growth.[430]

LABORATORY FEATURES

In hemoglobin C disease the hemoglobin level ranges from 8 to 12 g/dl. There is a marked increase in the number of target cells in the blood film (see Fig. 47-9). Some target cells are also present in the trait. Occasionally, intraerythrocytic hemoglobin crystals may be seen on the blood film, and these may appear in larger numbers if the red cells have been dehydrated either by drying or by suspension in a hypertonic solution (see Chap. 22). The osmotic fragility of the red cells may be decreased.

DIFFERENTIAL DIAGNOSIS

The diagnosis of homozygous hemoglobin C disease is achieved by electrophoresis, hemoglobin C moving to the same position as hemoglobin A_2, hemoglobin E, and hemoglobin O_{Arab} at an alkaline pH. Hemoglobin C is readily distinguished from other hemoglobins by acid agar gel electrophoresis.

THERAPY, COURSE, AND PROGNOSIS

No specific therapy is available or required for patients with hemoglobin C disease. Anemia may become more severe following infections, but the overall prognosis is considered to be excellent.

HEMOGLOBIN D DISEASE

DEFINITION AND HISTORY

In his early studies of the hemoglobinopathies, Itano[431] encountered a white family with an abnormal hemoglobin that migrated at the same rate as hemoglobin S but did not sickle. Its solubility in the reduced state resembled that of hemoglobin A, and this new abnormal hemoglobin was designated hemoglobin D. Subsequently, this name was given to any hemoglobin variant that manifested the same electrophoretic properties as hemoglobin S at an alkaline pH but had normal solubility properties.

ETIOLOGY AND PATHOGENESIS

With the exact chemical analysis of hemoglobin variants, it became apparent that hemoglobin $D_{Los\ Angeles}$ was identical to hemoglobin D_{Punjab}, both manifesting a substitution of glutamate for lysine at the 121st position in the β chain. Another "D" hemoglobin, $G_{Philadelphia}$, is, on the other hand, an α chain variant, with a substitution of asparagine for lysine at the sixty-eighth position.

Like the other structural mutations of hemoglobin, hemoglobin D trait is the heterozygous state for hemoglobin D and hemoglobin A, while the homozygous state for hemoglobin D is designated hemoglobin D disease. Hemoglobin D_{Punjab} is found in frequencies of approximately 3 percent in Northwest India.

CLINICAL FEATURES

The heterozygous state for hemoglobin D is entirely asymptomatic.[432] The abnormal hemoglobin constitutes between 35 and 50 percent of the total hemoglobin. Homozygous hemoglobin D disease is very rare, and some patients originally believed to be homozygous for hemoglobin D[433] subsequently were found to be heterozygous for hemoglobin D and β-thalassemia. A small number of true homozygotes have been described, however, and the clinical consequences are very mild.[434]

HEMOGLOBIN E DISEASE

DEFINITION AND HISTORY

Hemoglobin E is so prevalent that it may be the most common abnormal hemoglobin,[435] or second in prevalence only to hemoglobin S. It was first described in 1954, independently by Itano et al[436] and by Chernoff et al.[437]

ETIOLOGY AND PATHOGENESIS

Hemoglobin E is the result of a β chain mutation, $\alpha_2\beta_2^{26Glu \rightarrow Lys}$.[438] The amino acid substitution not only produces a hemoglobin that is somewhat unstable when subjected to oxidative stress,[439] perhaps because of weakening of the bonds between the monomers constituting the hemoglobin tetramer, but the nucleotide substitution also creates a new potential splicing sequence, so that some of the messenger may be spliced improperly.[440] The formation of unstable messenger accounts for the thalassemia-like nature of hemoglobin E trait and disease.

The inheritance of hemoglobin E is the same as that of the other β chain mutants. Heterozygotes for hemoglobin E and hemoglobin A have hemoglobin E trait, while homozygotes for hemoglobin E are designated as having hemoglobin E disease. Hemoglobin E, like hemoglobin S and hemoglobin C, occurs with sufficient frequency to be considered a polymorphism. The distribution of the gene for this β chain mutation is illustrated in Fig. 47-10. Decreased falciparum malaria parasitemia has been documented in patients with hemoglobin E trait,[441] and resistance to malaria may be the advantage that has led to high gene frequencies.

Hemoglobin E is found principally in Burma, Thailand, Laos, Cambodia, Malaysia, and Indonesia, and in some areas it occurs with a carrier rate of 30 percent.[442] On the other hand, it is not prevalent among the Chinese. Studies of restriction length polymorphisms in the β-globin cluster indicate that the hemoglobin E mutation has arisen several times independently.[443]

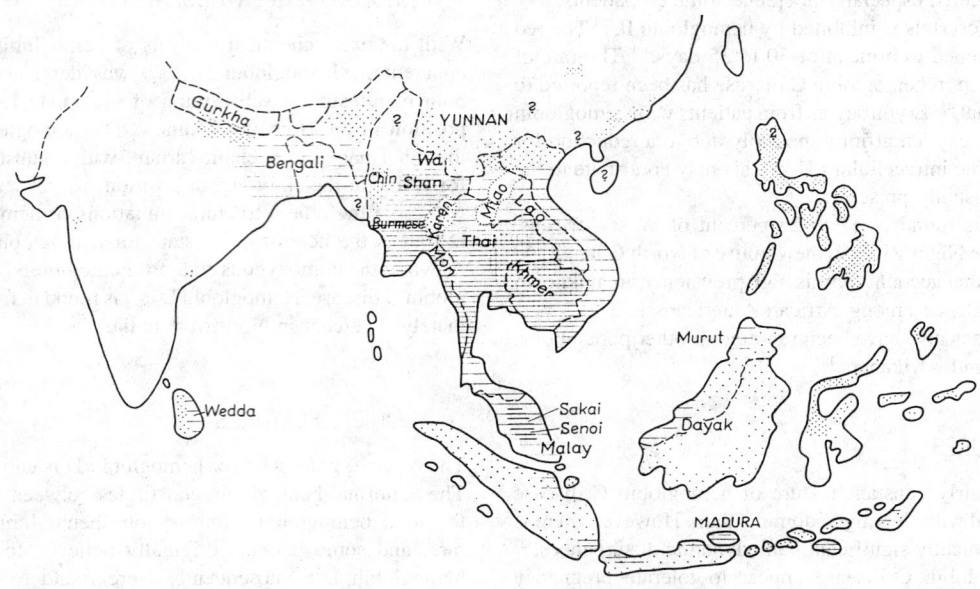

FIGURE 47-10   Distribution of hemoglobin E in Southeast Asia. Gene frequencies: cross-hatching indicates >0.2 percent; narrow hatching indicates 0.1 to 0.2 percent; wide hatching indicates 0.02 to 0.1 percent; dotted area indicates <0.02 percent and sporadic occurrence. (Flatz,[442] by permission.)

CLINICAL FEATURES

Although the prevalence of the gene for hemoglobin E is quite high in Southeast Asia (see Fig. 47-10), relatively few patients with homozygous E disease, as distinguished from hemoglobin E β-thalassemia, have been described.[444,445] When homozygous E disease is encountered, it is associated with marked microcytosis and hypochromia but little or no anemia. Splenomegaly is unusual, and the red cell life span is normal. Clinically, the state closely resembles β-thalassemia minor.

In the hemoglobin E carrier state 30 to 45 percent of the hemoglobin is hemoglobin E,[437] and such carriers are asymptomatic but do manifest microcytosis.[446]

The clinical manifestations of the heterozygous state between hemoglobin E and β-thalassemia are quite variable in severity[447] and resemble those of homozygous hemoglobin E disease, with moderate anemia and splenomegaly representing the usual manifestation.

LABORATORY FEATURES

Hemoglobin E is electrophoretically slow in an alkaline medium, comigrating with hemoglobin C and A_2. The characteristic blood change is microcytosis—mild in the trait and more severe in the homozygous state and in hemoglobin E β-thalassemia. There is a modest decrease in the α-/non-α-globin chain synthetic ratio[445] and a minimal decrease in whole blood oxygen affinity.[437,444]

TABLE 47-1   SOME REPRESENTATIVE HEMOGLOBIN VARIANTS

Amino Acid (Sequential Number)	Amino Acid Substitution	Name	Major Abnormal Property	Reference
α-CHAIN VARIANTS				
5	Ala→Asp	$J_{Toronto}$		(459)
16	Lys→Glu	I		(460)
23	Glu→Gln	Memphis		(64)
30	Glu→Gln	$G_{Honolulu}$		(461)
87	His→Arg	Iwata	(3)	(462)
β-CHAIN VARIANTS				
6	Glu→Val	S	(5)	(463)
6	Glu→Lys	C		(464)
24	Gly→Asp	Moscva	(3)(2)	(465)
62	Ala→Pro	Duarte	(3)(1)	(466)
63	His→Arg	Zürich	(3)(1)	(467)
6	Glu→Val	C_{Harlem}		(468)
73	Asp→Asn			
102	Asn→Thr	Kansas	(2)(4)	(469)
121	Glu→Gln	$D_{Los Angeles}$	(1)	(470)
*γ-CHAIN VARIANTS				
6	Glu→Lys	$F_{TexasII}$		(471)
FUSION HEMOGLOBINS				
		Lepore$_{Hollandia}$		(472)
		Lincoln Park		(473)
STOP CODON MUTATIONS				
		Constant Spring		(474)
δ-CHAIN VARIANTS				
22	Ala→Glu	A_2-Flatbush		(475)

(1) ↑ O_2 affinity; (2) ↓ O_2 affinity; (3) unstable; (4) ↑ dissociation; (5) sickling.

THERAPY, COURSE, AND PROGNOSIS

The prognosis seems to be good, although no thorough studies of the natural history of the disease have been carried out. Splenectomy increases the red cell life span and ameliorates anemia in hemoglobin E β-thalassemia,[448,449] but its role in homozygous hemoglobin E disease has not been delineated. In one family manifesting both pyrimidine 5′-nucleotidase deficiency and homozygous hemoglobin E disease, those with both defects had more severe anemia than those inheriting one alone.[450]

OTHER HEMOGLOBINOPATHIES

In comparison with hemoglobins S, C, D, and E, other abnormal hemoglobins are rare. Some, such as the unstable hemoglobins (see Chap. 48), the hemoglobins producing erythrocytosis (see Chap. 61), and those producing cyanosis (see Chap. 49), are of clinical importance. Many of the other hemoglobins do not produce significant clinical alterations but have nonetheless been important in clarifying the role of individual amino acids in the structure and function of the hemoglobin molecule. Some of the more common hemoglobin variants are summarized in Table 47-1. Complete compendia of mutations affecting hemoglobin have been published,[451] and further sources may be found at http://globin.cse.psu.edu/.

REFERENCES

1. Herrick JB: Peculiar elongated and sickle-shaped red corpuscles in a case of severe anemia. *Arch Intern Med* 6:517, 1910.
2. Emmel VE: A study of the erythrocytes in a case of severe anemia with elongated and sickle-shaped red blood corpuscles. *Arch Intern Med* 20:586, 1917.
3. Hahn EV, Gillespie EB: Report of a case greatly improved by splenectomy; experimental study of sickle cell formation. *Arch Intern Med* 39:233, 1927.
4. Taliaferro WH, Huck JG: The inheritance of sickle-cell anemia in man. *Genetics* 8:594, 1923.
5. Neel JV: The inheritance of sickle cell anemia. *Science* 110:64, 1949.
6. Beet EA: The genetics of the sickle-cell trait in a Bantu tribe. *Ann Eugen (London)* 14:279, 1949.
7. Pauling L, Itano HA, Singer SJ, Wells IC: Sickle cell anemia, a molecular disease. *Science* 110:543, 1949.
8. Ingram VM: Gene mutations in human haemoglobin: The chemical difference between normal and sickle cell haemoglobin. *Nature* 180:326, 1957.
9. Conley CL: Sickle-cell anemia. The first molecular disease, in *Blood, Pure and Eloquent*, p 319. McGraw-Hill, New York, 1980.
10. Cao Z, Liao D, Mirchev R, et al: Nucleation and polymerization of sickle hemoglobin with Leu beta 88 substituted by Ala. *J Mol Biol* 265:580, 1997.
11. Mirchev R, Ferrone FA: The structural link between polymerization and sickle cell disease. *J Mol Biol* 265:475, 1997.
12. Rodgers DW, Crepeau RH, Edelstein SJ: Pairings and polarities of the 14 strands in sickle cell hemoglobin fibers. *Proc Natl Acad Sci USA* 84:6157, 1987.
13. Watowich SJ, Gross LJ, Josephs R: Intermolecular contacts within sickle hemoglobin fibers. *J Mol Biol* 209:821, 1989.
14. Mozzarelli A, Hofrichter J, Eaton WA: Delay time of hemoglobin S polymerization prevents most cells from sickling in vivo. *Science* 237:500, 1987.
15. Samuel RE, Salmon ED, Briehl RW: Nucleation and growth of fibres and gel formation in sickle cell haemoglobin. *Nature* 345:833, 1990.
16. Eaton WA, Hofrichter J, Ross PD: Delay time of gelation: A possible determinant of clinical severity in sickle cell disease. *Blood* 47:621, 1976.
17. Eaton JW, Jacob HS, White JG: Membrane abnormalities of irreversibly sickled cells. *Semin Hematol* 16:52, 1979.
18. Bookchin RM, Ortiz OE, Lew VL: Evidence for a direct reticulocyte origin of dense red cells in sickle cell anemia. *J Clin Invest* 87:113, 1991.
19. Serjeant GR, Serjeant BE, Milner PF: The irreversibly sickled cell:

A determinant of haemolysis in sickle-cell anaemia. *Br J Haematol* 17:527, 1969.
20. Lande WM, Andrews DL, Clark MR, et al: The incidence of painful crisis in homozygous sickle cell disease: Correlation with red cell deformability. *Blood* 72:2056, 1988.
21. Ballas SK, Larner J, Smith ED, et al: Rheologic predictors of the severity of the painful sickle cell crisis. *Blood* 72:1216, 1988.
22. Tosteson DC, Carlsen E, Dunham ET: The effects of sickling on ion transport: I. Effect of sickling on potassium transport. *J Gen Physiol* 39:31, 1955.
23. Dzandu JK, Johnson RM: Membrane protein phosphorylation in intact normal and sickle cell erythrocytes. *J Biol Chem* 255:6382, 1980.
24. Beutler E, Guinto E, Johnson C: Human red cell protein kinase in normal subjects and patients with hereditary spherocytosis, sickle cell disease, and autoimmune hemolytic anemia. *Blood* 47:887, 1976.
25. Hosey MM, Tao M: Altered erythrocyte membrane phosphorylation in sickle cell disease. *Nature* 263:424, 1976.
26. Bookchin RM, Lew VL: Progressive inhibition of the Ca pump and Ca: Ca exchange in sickle red cells. *Nature* 284:561, 1980.
27. Steinberg MH, Eaton JW, Berger E, Coleman MB, Oelshlegel FJ: Erythrocyte calcium abnormalities and the clinical severity of sickling disorders. *Br J Haematol* 40:533, 1978.
28. Lew VL, Hockaday A, Sepulveda MI, et al: Compartmentalization of sickle-cell calcium in endocytic inside-out vesicles. *Nature* 315:586, 1985.
29. Williamson P, Puchulu E, Penniston JT, Westerman MP, Schlegel RA: Ca²⁺ accumulation and loss by aberrant endocytic vesicles in sickle erythrocytes. *J Cell Physiol* 152:1, 1992.
30. Hebbel RP: Auto-oxidation and a membrane-associated 'Fenton reagent': a possible explanation for development of membrane lesions in sickle erythrocytes. *Clin Haematol* 14:129, 1985.
31. Hebbel RP, Eaton JW, Balasingam M, Steinberg MH: Spontaneous oxygen radical generation by sickle erythrocytes. *J Clin Invest* 70:1253, 1982.
32. Repka T, Hebbel RP: Hydroxyl radical formation by sickle erythrocyte membranes: role of pathologic iron deposits and cytoplasmic reducing agents. *Blood* 78:2753, 1991.
33. Rank BH, Carlsson J, Hebbel RP: Abnormal redox status of membrane-protein thiols in sickle erythrocytes. *J Clin Invest* 75:1531, 1985.
34. Schacter L, Warth JA, Gordon EM, Prasad A, Klein BL: Altered amount and activity of superoxide dismutase in sickle cell anemia. *FASEB J* 2:237, 1988.
35. Zerez CR, Lachant NA, Lee SJ, Tanaka KR: Decreased erythrocyte nicotinamide adenine dinucleotide redox potential and abnormal pyridine nucleotide content in sickle cell disease. *Blood* 71:512, 1988.
36. Vasseur C, Leclerc L, Hilly M, Bursaux E: Decreased G3PDH binding to erythrocyte membranes in sickle cell disease. *Nouv Rev Fr Hematol* 34:155, 1992.
37. Liu SC, Derick LH, Zhai S, Palek J: Uncoupling of the spectrin-based skeleton from the lipid bilayer in sickled red cells. *Science* 252:574, 1991.
38. Hebbel RP, Miller WJ: Phagocytosis of sickle erythrocytes: immunologic and oxidative determinants of hemolytic anemia. *Blood* 64:733, 1984.
39. Kuypers FA, Lewis RA, Hua M, et al: Detection of altered membrane phospholipid asymmetry in subpopulations of human red blood cells using fluorescently labeled annexin V. *Blood* 87:1179, 1996.
40. Tait JF, Gibson D: Measurement of membrane phospholipid asymmetry in normal and sickle-cell erythrocytes by means of annexin V binding. *J Lab Clin Med* 123:741, 1994.
41. Ballas SK, Smith ED: Red blood cell changes during the evolution of the sickle cell painful crisis. *Blood* 79:2154, 1992.
42. Poillon WN, Kim BC, Castro O: Intracellular hemoglobin S polymerization and the clinical severity of sickle cell anemia. *Blood* 91:1777, 1998.
43. Itano HA: Qualitative and quantitative control of adult hemoglobin synthesis—A multiple allele hypothesis. *Am J Hum Genet* 5:34, 1953.
44. Huisman THJ: Sickle cell anemia as a syndrome: A review of diagnostic features. *Am J Hematol* 6:173, 1979.
45. Steinberg MH, Embury SH: Alpha-thalassemia in blacks: genetic and clinical aspects and interactions with the sickle hemoglobin gene. *Blood* 68:985, 1986.
46. Shaeffer JR, Kingston RE, McDonald MJ, Bunn HF: Competition of

normal beta chains and sickle hemoglobin beta chains for alpha chains as a post-translational control mechanism. *Nature* 276:631, 1978.

47. Bunn HF, McDonald MJ: Electrostatic interactions in the assembly of human hemoglobin. *Nature* 306:498, 1983.

48. Embury SH, Dozy AM, Miller J, et al: Concurrent sickle-cell anemia and alpha-thalassemia. Effect on severity of anemia. *N Engl J Med* 306:270, 1982.

49. Stevens MCG, Maude GH, Beckford M, et al: Alpha thalassemia and the hematology of homozygous sickle cell disease in childhood. *Blood* 67:411, 1986.

50. El-Hazmi MAF: On the nature of sickle-cell disease in the Arabian peninsula. *Hum Genet* 52:323, 1979.

51. Bookchin RM, Nagel RL: Interactions between human hemoglobins: Sickling and related phenomena. *Semin Hematol* 11:577, 1974.

52. Lawrence C, Fabry ME, Nagel RL: The unique red cell heterogeneity of SC disease: crystal formation, dense reticulocytes, and unusual morphology. *Blood* 78:2104, 1991.

53. Fabry ME, Kaul DK, Raventos-Suarez C, Chang H, Nagel RL: SC erythrocytes have an abnormally high intracellular hemoglobin concentration. Pathophysiological consequences. *J Clin Invest* 70:1315, 1982.

54. Noguchi CT, Rodgers GP, Serjeant G, Schechter AN: Levels of fetal hemoglobin necessary for treatment of sickle cell disease. *N Engl J Med* 318:96, 1988.

55. Bradley TB, Brawner JN III, Conley CL: Further observations on an inherited anomaly characterized by persistence of fetal hemoglobin. *Johns Hopkins Med J* 110:242, 1962.

56. Shepard MK, Weatherall DJ, Conley CL: Semiquantitative estimation of fetal hemoglobin in red cell populations. *Johns Hopkins Med J* 110:293, 1962.

57. Ali SA: Milder variant of sickle-cell disease in Arabs in Kuwait associated with unusually high levels of foetal haemoglobin. *Br J Haematol* 19:613, 1970.

58. Perrine RP, Pembrey ME, John P, Perrine S, Shoup F: Natural history of sickle cell anemia in Saudi Arabs. *Ann Intern Med* 88:1, 1978.

59. El-Hazmi MAF, Al-Swailem AR, Bahakim HM, AL Faleh FZ, Warsy AS: Effect of alpha thalassaemia, G-6-PD deficiency and Hb F on the nature of sickle cell anaemia in south-western Saudi Arabia. *Trop Geogr Med* 42:241, 1990.

60. Powars DR, Schroeder WA, Weiss JN, et al: Lack of influence of fetal hemoglobin levels or erythrocyte indices on the severity of sickle cell anemia. *J Clin Invest* 65:732, 1980.

61. Padmos MA, Roberts GT, Sackey K, et al: Two different forms of homozygous sickle cell disease occur in Saudi Arabia. *Br J Haematol* 79:93, 1991.

62. Powars DR, Weiss JN, Chan LS, Schroeder WA: Is there a threshold level of fetal hemoglobin that ameliorates morbidity in sickle cell anemia? *Blood* 63:921, 1984.

63. Conley CL, Weatherall DJ, Richardson SN, Shepherd MK, Charache S: Hereditary persistence of fetal hemoglobin: A study of 79 affected persons in 15 Negro families in Baltimore. *Blood* 21:261, 1963.

64. Kraus LM, Miyaji T, Iuchi I, Kraus AP: Characterization of $\alpha 23GluNH_2$ in hemoglobin Memphis. Hemoglobin Memphis/S, a new variant of molecular disease. *Biochemistry* 5:3701, 1966.

65. Lewis RA, Hathorn M: Correlation of S hemoglobin with glucose-6-phosphate dehydrogenase deficiency and its significance. *Blood* 26:176, 1965.

66. Piomelli S, Reindorf CA, Arzanian MT, Corash LM: Clinical and biochemical interactions of glucose-6-phosphate dehydrogenase deficiency and sickle-cell anemia. *N Engl J Med* 287:213, 1972.

67. El-Hazmi MAF, Warsy AS: Aspects of sickle cell gene in Saudi Arabia—interaction with glucose-6-phosphate dehydrogenase deficiency. *Hum Genet* 68:320, 1984.

68. El-Hazmi MAF, Warsy AS: The effects of glucose-6-phosphate dehydrogenase deficiency on the haematological parameters and clinical manifestations in patients with sickle cell anaemia. *Trop Geogr Med* 41:52, 1989.

69. Naylor J, Rosenthal I, Grossman A, Schulman I, Hsia DYY: Activity of glucose-6-phosphate dehydrogenase in erythrocytes of patients with various abnormal hemoglobins. *Pediatrics* 26:285, 1960.

70. Milner PF, Sergeant GR: Laboratory studies in sickle cell anaemia. *Blood* 34:729, 1969.

71. Lewis RA: Glucose-6-phosphate dehydrogenase electrophoresis in Gha-

naians with AA and SS haemoglobin. *Acta Haematol (Basel)* 50:105, 1973.

72. Beutler E, Johnson C, Powars D, West C: Prevalence of glucose-6-phosphate dehydrogenase deficiency in sickle cell disease. *N Engl J Med* 290:826, 1974.

73. Heller P, Best WR, Nelson RB, Becktel J: Clinical implications of sickle-cell trait and glucose-6-phosphate dehydrogenase deficiency in hospitalized black male patients. *N Engl J Med* 300:1001, 1979.

74. Gibbs WN, Wardle J, Serjeant GR: Glucose-6-phosphate dehydrogenase deficiency and homozygous sickle cell disease in Jamaica. *Br J Haematol* 45:73, 1980.

75. Steinberg MH, West MS, Gallagher D, Mentzer WC Jr: The cooperative study of sickle cell diseases: Effects of glucose-6-phosphate dehydrogenase deficiency upon sickle cell anemia. *Blood* 71:748, 1988.

76. Saad STO, Costa FF: Glucose-6-phosphate dehydrogenase deficiency and sickle cell disease in Brazil. *Hum Hered* 42:125, 1992.

77. Smits HL, Oski FA, Brody JI: The hemolytic crisis of sickle cell disease: The role of glucose-6-phosphate dehydrogenase deficiency. *J Pediatr* 74:544, 1969.

78. Cohen-Solal M, Préhu C, Wajcman H, et al: A new sickle cell disease phenotype associating Hb S trait, severe pyruvate kinase deficiency (PK Conakry), and an $\alpha 2$ globin gene variant (Hb Conakry). *Br J Haematol* 103:950, 1998.

79. Harris JW, Brewster HH, Ham TH, Castle WB: Studies on the destruction of red blood cells: X. The biophysics and biology of sickle-cell disease. *Arch Intern Med* 97:145, 1956.

80. Lane PA, Githens JH: Splenic syndrome at mountain altitudes in sickle cell trait. *JAMA* 253:2251, 1985.

81. Green RL, Huntsman RG, Serjeant GR: The sickle-cell and altitude. *BMJ* 2:593, 1971.

82. Charache S, Conley CL: Rate of sickling of red cells during deoxygenation of blood from persons with various sickling disorders. *Blood* 24:25, 1964.

83. Charache S, Conley CL: Factors leading to vascular occlusion in sickle cell anemia. *Prog Clin Biol Res* 1:343, 1975.

84. Serjeant GR, May H, Patrick A, Slifer ED: Duodenal ulceration in sickle cell anaemia. *Trans R Soc Trop Med Hyg* 67:59, 1973.

85. Bates I, de Caestecker J: Sickle cell disease and risk of peptic ulceration. *Trans R Soc Trop Med Hyg* 90:292, 1996.

86. Beutler E: Hypothesis: Changes in the O_2 dissociation curve and sickling: A general formulation and therapeutic strategy. *Blood* 43:297, 1974.

87. Poillon WN, Kim BC: 2,3-Diphosphoglycerate and intracellular pH as interdependent determinants of the physiologic solubility of deoxyhemoglobin S. *Blood* 76:1028, 1990.

88. Noguchi CT, Schechter AN: The intracellular polymerization of sickle hemoglobin and its relevance to sickle cell disease. *Blood* 58:1057, 1981.

89. Akinla O: Pregnancy and the skeletal complications of sickle cell disease. *Postgrad Med J* 49:255, 1973.

90. Perillie PE, Epstein FH: Sickling phenomenon produced by hypertonic solutions: A possible explanation for the hyposthenuria in sicklemia. *J Clin Invest* 42:570, 1963.

91. Briehl RW, Nikolopoulou P: Kinetics of hemoglobin S polymerization and gelation under shear: I. Shape of the viscosity progress curve and dependence of delay time and reaction rate on shear rate and temperature. *Blood* 81:2420, 1993.

92. Hebbel RP: Endothelial adhesivity of sickle red blood cells. *J Lab Clin Med* 120:503, 1992.

93. Thevenin BM, Crandall I, Ballas SK, Sherman IW, Shohet SB: Band 3 peptides block the adherence of sickle cells to endothelial cells in vitro. *Blood* 90:4172, 1997.

94. Morris CL, Rucknagel DL, Joiner CH: Deoxygenation-induced changes in sickle cell–sickle cell adhesion. *Blood* 81:3138, 1993.

95. Fadlon E, Vordermeier S, Pearson TC, et al: Blood polymorphonuclear leukocytes from the majority of sickle cell patients in the crisis phase of the disease show enhanced adhesion to vascular endothelium and increased expression of CD64. *Blood* 91:266, 1998.

96. Ballas SK, Mohandas N: Pathophysiology of vaso-occlusion. *Hematol Oncol Clin North Am* 10:1221, 1996.

97. Kaul DK, Fabry ME, Nagel RL: The pathophysiology of vascular obstruction in the sickle syndromes. *Blood Rev* 10:29, 1996.

98. Styles LA, Lubin B, Vichinsky E, et al: Decrease of very late activation

antigen-4 and CD36 on reticulocytes in sickle cell patients treated with hydroxyurea. *Blood* 89:2554, 1997.

99. Charache S, Barton FB, Moore RD, et al: Hydroxyurea and sickle cell anemia—Clinical utility of a myelosuppressive "switching" agent. *Medicine (Baltimore)* 75:300, 1996.

100. Goldstein MA, Patpongpanij N, Minnich V: The incidence of elevated hemoglobin A$_2$ levels in the American negro. *Ann Intern Med* 60:95, 1964.

101. Dunston T, Rowland R, Huntsman RG, Yawson GI: Sickle-cell haemoglobin C disease and sickle-cell beta thalassaemia in white South Africans. *S Afr Med J* 46:1423, 1972.

102. Luzzatto L: Genetics of red cells and susceptibility to malaria. *Blood* 54:961, 1979.

103. Lapouméroulie C, Dunda O, Ducrocq R, et al: A novel sickle cell mutation of yet another origin in Africa: The Cameroon type. *Hum Genet* 89:333, 1992.

104. Labie D, Srinivas R, Dunda O, et al: Haplotypes in tribal Indians bearing the sickle gene: evidence for the unicentric origin of the beta S mutation and the unicentric origin of the tribal populations of India. *Hum Biol* 61:479, 1989.

105. Kelleher JFJ, Park JO, Kim HC, Schroeder WA: Life-threatening complications in a child with hemoglobin SD-Los Angeles disease. *Hemoglobin* 8:203, 1984.

106. Taylor WJ: Sickled red cells in the Cervidae. *Adv Vet Sci Comp Med* 27:77, 1983.

107. Castro O, Roth R, Orlin J, Finch SC: Human sickle cells in a heterologous species: a model for the screening of anti-sickling agents. *Prog Clin Biol Res* 1:455, 1975.

108. Nagel RL: A knockout of a transgenic mouse—animal models of sickle cell anemia. *N Engl J Med* 339:194, 1998.

109. Ryan TM, Ciavatta DJ, Townes TM: Knockout-transgenic mouse model of sickle cell disease. *Science* 278:873, 1997.

110. Paszty C, Brion CM, Manci E, et al: Transgenic knockout mice with exclusively human sickle hemoglobin and sickle cell disease. *Science* 278:876, 1997.

111. Powars DR: Natural history of sickle cell disease—the first ten years. *Semin Hematol* 12:267, 1975.

112. Serjeant GR, Ceulaer CDE, Lethbridge R, et al: The painful crisis of homozygous sickle cell disease: Clinical features. *Br J Haematol* 87:586, 1994.

113. Antal P, Gauderer M, Koshy M, Berman B: Is the incidence of appendicitis reduced in patients with sickle cell disease? *Pediatrics* 101:E7, 1998.

114. Charache S: The treatment of sickle cell anemia. *Arch Intern Med* 133:698, 1974.

115. Mani S, Duffy TP: Sickle myonecrosis revisited. *Am J Med* 95:525, 1993.

116. Russell MO, Goldberg HI, Hodson A, et al: Effect of transfusion therapy on arteriographic abnormalities and on recurrence of stroke in sickle cell disease. *Blood* 63:162, 1984.

117. Rao SP, Miller ST, Cohen BJ: Transient aplastic crisis in patients with sickle cell disease: B19 parvovirus studies during a 7-year period. *Am J Dis Child* 29:1328, 1992.

118. Serjeant GR, Serjeant BE, Thomas PW, et al: Human parvovirus infection in homozygous sickle cell disease. *Lancet* 341:1237, 1993.

119. Pagliuca A, Hussain M, Layton DM: Human parvovirus infection in sickle cell disease. *Lancet* 342:49, 1993.

120. Anonymous: Bone-marrow aplasia and parvovirus. *Lancet* 2:21, 1983.

121. Godeau B, Galactéros F, Schaeffer A, et al: Aplastic crisis due to extensive bone marrow necrosis and human parvovirus infection in sickle cell disease. *Am J Med* 91:557, 1991.

122. Kinney TR, Ware RE, Schultz WH, Filston HC: Long-term management of splenic sequestration in children with sickle cell disease. *J Pediatr* 117:194, 1990.

123. Solanki DL, Kletter GG, Castro O: Acute splenic sequestration crises in adults with sickle cell disease. *Am J Med* 80:985, 1986.

124. Bowcock SJ, Nwabueze ED, Cook AE, et al: Fatal splenic sequestration in adult sickle cell disease. *Clin Lab Haematol* 10:95, 1988.

125. Vichinsky E, Lubin BH: Suggested guidelines for the treatment of children with sickle cell anemia. *Hematol Oncol Clin North Am* 1:483, 1987.

126. Diggs LW: Crises in sickle cell anemia. *Am J Clin Pathol* 26:1109, 1956.

127. Whitten CF: Growth status of children with sickle-cell anemia. *Am J Dis Child* 102:355, 1961.

128. Ashcroft MT, Serjeant GR, Desai P: Heights, weights, and skeletal age of Jamaican adolescents with sickle cell anaemia. *Arch Dis Child* 47:519, 1972.

129. Moseley JE: The anemias, in *Bone Changes in Hematologic Disorders (Roentgen Aspects)*, 1st ed, p 12. Grune and Stratton, New York, 1963.

130. Sain A, Sham R, Silver L: Bone scan in sickle cell crisis. *Clin Nucl Med* 3:85, 1978.

131. Rao VM, Fishman M, Mitchell DG, et al: Painful sickle cell crisis: Bone marrow patterns observed with MR imaging. *Radiology* 161:211, 1986.

132. Mankad VN, Williams JP, Harpen MD, et al: Magnetic resonance imaging of bone marrow in sickle cell disease: clinical, hematologic, and pathologic correlations. *Blood* 75:274, 1990.

133. Howlett DC, Hatrick AG, Jarosz JM, et al: The role of CT and MR in imaging the complications of sickle cell disease. *Clin Radiol* 52:821, 1997.

134. Stevens MCG, Padwick M, Serjeant GR: Observations on the natural history of dactylitis in homozygous sickle cell disease. *Clin Pediatr* 20:311, 1981.

135. Milner PF, Kraus AP, Sebes JI, et al: Osteonecrosis of the humeral head in sickle cell disease. *Clin Orthop* 289:136, 1993.

136. David HG, Bridgman SA, Davies SC, Hine AL, Emery RJA: The shoulder in sickle-cell disease. *J Bone Joint Surg [Br]* 75B:538, 1993.

137. Schumacher HR Jr, Van Linthoudt D, Manno CS, Cuckler JM, Athreya BH: Diffuse chondrolytic arthritis in sickle cell disease. *J Rheumatol* 20:385, 1993.

138. al-Umran K, al-Habdan I, al-Mulhim F: Ultrasonography: can it differentiate between vasoocclusive crisis and acute osteomyelitis in sickle cell disease? *J Pediatr Orthop* 18:552, 1998.

139. Epps CH Jr, Bryant DD III, Coles MJM, Castro O: Osteomyelitis in patients who have sickle-cell disease. Diagnosis and management. *J Bone Joint Surg [Am]* 73A:1281, 1991.

140. Hook EW, Campbell CG, Weens HS, Cooper GR: Salmonella osteomyelitis in patients with sickle-cell anemia. *N Engl J Med* 257:403, 1957.

141. Shelley WM, Curtis EM: Bone marrow and fat embolism in sickle-cell anemia and sickle-cell hemoglobin C disease. *Johns Hopkins Med J* 103:8, 1958.

142. Saborio P, Scheinman JI: Sickle cell nephropathy. *J Am Soc Nephrol* 10:187, 1999.

143. Kontessis P, Mayopoulou-Symvoulidis D, Symvoulidis A, Kontopoulou-Griva I: Renal involvement in sickle cell—beta thalassemia. *Nephron* 61:10, 1992.

144. Zadeii G, Lohr JW: Renal papillary necrosis in a patient with sickle cell trait. *J Am Soc Nephrol* 8:1034, 1997.

145. Minkin SD, Oh KS, Sanders RC, Siegelman SS: Urologic manifestations of sickle hemoglobinopathies. *South Med J* 72:23, 1979.

146. Wong WY, Elliott-Mills D, Powars D: Renal failure in sickle cell anemia. *Hematol Oncol Clin North Am* 10:1321, 1996.

147. Baron BW, Mick R, Baron JM: Hematuria in sickle cell anemia—Not always benign: Evidence for excess frequency of sickle cell anemia in African Americans with renal cell carcinoma. *Acta Haematol (Basel)* 92:119, 1994.

148. Sharpsteen JR Jr, Powars D, Johnson C, et al: Multisystem damage associated with tricorporal priapism in sickle cell disease. *Am J Med* 94:289, 1993.

149. Chakrabarty A, Upadhyay J, Dhabuwala CB, et al: Priapism associated with sickle cell hemoglobinopathy in children: Long-term effects on potency. *J Urol* 155:1419, 1996.

150. Miller ST, Rao SP, Dunn EK, Glassberg KI: Priapism in children with sickle cell disease. *J Urol* 154:844, 1995.

151. Prasad AS, Ortega J, Brewer GJ, Oberleas D, Schoomaker EB: Trace elements in sickle cell disease. *JAMA* 22:2396, 1976.

152. Abbasi AA, Prasad AS, Ortega J, Congco E, Oberleas D: Gonadal function abnormalities in sickle cell anemia. Studies in adult male patients. *Ann Intern Med* 85:601, 1976.

153. Pearson HA, McIntosh S, Ritchey AK, et al: Developmental aspects of splenic function in sickle cell diseases. *Blood* 53:358, 1979.

154. Gill FM, Sleeper LA, Weiner SJ, et al: Clinical events in the first decade in a cohort of infants with sickle cell disease. *Blood* 86:776, 1995.

155. Cavenagh JD, Joseph AE, Dilly S, Bevan DH: Splenic sepsis in sickle cell disease. *Br J Haematol* 86:187, 1994.

156. Al-Salem AH, Qaisaruddin S, Al Jam'a A, AL-Kalaf J, EL-Bashier AM: Splenic abscess and sickle cell disease. *Am J Hematol* 58:100, 1998.

157. Adekile AD, McKie KM, Adeodu OO, et al: Spleen in sickle cell anemia: Comparative studies of Nigerian and U.S. patients. *Am J Hematol* 42:316, 1993.

158. Krauss JS, Freant LJ, Lee JR: Gastrointestinal pathology in sickle cell disease. *Ann Clin Lab Sci* 28:19, 1998.

159. Green TW, Conley CL, Berthrong M: The liver in sickle cell anemia. *Johns Hopkins Med J* 92:99, 1953.

160. Sheehy TW, Law DE, Wade BH: Exchange transfusion for sickle cell intrahepatic cholestasis. *Arch Intern Med* 140:1364, 1980.

161. Schubert TT: Hepatobiliary system in sickle cell disease. *Gastroenterology* 90:2013, 1986.

162. Mintz AA, Pugh DP: Choledocholithiasis in sickle cell anemia. *South Med J* 63:1498, 1970.

163. Johnson CS, Omata M, Tong MJ, et al: Liver involvement in sickle cell disease. *Medicine (Baltimore)* 64:349, 1985.

164. Omata M, Johnson CS, Tong M, Tatter D: Pathological spectrum of liver diseases in sickle cell disease. *Dig Dis Sci* 31:247, 1986.

165. Bauer TW, Moore GW, Hutchins GM: The liver in sickle cell disease. A clinicopathologic study of 70 patients. *Am J Med* 69:833, 1980.

166. Laulan S, Bernard JF, Boivin P: Systematic blood transfusions in adult homozygous sickle-cell anaemia. *Presse Med* 19:785, 1990.

167. Miller ST, Jensen D, Rao SP: Less intensive long-term transfusion therapy for sickle cell anemia and cerebrovascular accident. *J Pediatr* 120:54, 1992.

168. Conrad ME: Sickle cell disease and hemochromatosis. *Am J Hematol* 38:150, 1991.

169. Sampietro M, Lupica L, Perrero L, et al: The expression of uridine diphosphate glucuronosyltransferase gene is a major determinant of bilirubin level in heterozygous beta-thalassaemia and in glucose-6-phosphate dehydrogenase deficiency. *Br J Haematol* 99:437, 1997.

170. Kaplan M, Renbaum P, Levy-Lahad E, et al: Gilbert syndrome and glucose-6-phosphate dehydrogenase deficiency: A dose-dependent genetic interaction crucial to neonatal hyperbilirubinemia. *Proc Natl Acad Sci USA* 94:12128, 1997.

171. Miller GJ, Sergeant GR, Sivapragasam S, Petch M: Cardiopulmonary responses and gas exchange during exercise in adults with homozygous sickle cell disease. *Clin Sci* 44:113, 1973.

172. Pegelow CH, Colangelo L, Steinberg M, et al: Natural history of blood pressure in sickle cell disease: Risks for stroke and death associated with relative hypertension in sickle cell anemia. *Am J Med* 102:171, 1997.

173. Vichinsky EP, Styles LA, Colangelo LH, et al: Acute chest syndrome in sickle cell disease: Clinical presentation and course. *Blood* 89:1787, 1997.

174. Bhalla M, Abboud MR, McLoud TC, et al: Acute chest syndrome in sickle cell disease: CT evidence of microvascular occlusion. *Radiology* 187:45, 1993.

175. Gelfand MJ, Daya SA, Rucknagel DL, Kalinyak KA, Paltiel HJ: Simultaneous occurrence of rib infarction and pulmonary infiltrates in sickle cell disease patients with acute chest syndrome. *J Nucl Med* 34:614, 1993.

176. Golden C, Styles L, Vichinsky E: Acute chest syndrome and sickle cell disease. *Curr Opin Hematol* 5:89, 1998.

177. Powars D, Weidman JA, Odom-Maryon T, Niland JC, Johnson C: Sickle cell chronic lung disease: Prior morbidity and the risk of pulmonary failure. *Medicine (Baltimore)* 67:66, 1988.

178. Castro O: Systemic fat embolism and pulmonary hypertension in sickle cell disease. *Hematol Oncol Clin North Am* 10:1289, 1996.

179. Denbow CE, Chung EE, Serjeant GR: Pulmonary artery pressure and the acute chest syndrome in homozygous sickle cell disease. *Br Heart J* 69:536, 1993.

180. To KW, Nadel AJ: Ophthalmologic complications in hemoglobinopathies. *Hematol Oncol Clin North Am* 5:535, 1991.

181. Curran EL, Fleming JC, Rice K, Wang WC: Orbital compression syndrome in sickle cell disease. *Ophthalmology* 104:1610, 1997.

182. Stockman JA, Nigro MA, Mishkin MM, Oski FA: Occlusion of large cerebral vessels in sickle-cell anemia. *N Engl J Med* 287:846, 1972.

183. Wang WC, Langston JW, Steen RG, et al: Abnormalities of the central nervous system in very young children with sickle cell anemia. *J Pediatr* 132:994, 1998.

184. Ohene-Frempong K, Weiner SJ, Sleeper LA, et al: Cerebrovascular accidents in sickle cell disease: Rates and risk factors. *Blood* 91:288, 1998.

185. Powars D, Wilson B, Imbus C, Pegelow C, Allen J: The natural history of stroke in sickle cell disease. *Am J Med* 65:461, 1978.

186. Ohene-Frempong K: Stroke in sickle cell disease: Demographic, clinical, and therapeutic considerations. *Semin Hematol* 28:213, 1991.

187. Riggs JE, Ketonen LM, Wang DD, Valanne LK: Cerebral infarction in a child with sickle cell trait. *J Child Neurol* 10:253, 1995.

188. Partington MD, Aronyk KE, Byrd SE: Sickle cell trait and stroke in children. *Pediatr Neurosurg* 20:148, 1994.

189. Adams RJ, McKie VC, Carl EM, et al: Long-term stroke risk in children with sickle cell disease screened with transcranial Doppler. *Ann Neurol* 42:699, 1997.

190. Balkaran B, Char G, Morris JS, et al: Stroke in a cohort of patients with homozygous sickle cell disease. *J Pediatr* 120:360, 1992.

191. Siegel JF, Rich MA, Brock WA: Association of sickle cell disease, priapism, exchange transfusion and neurological events: Aspen syndrome. *J Urol* 150:1480, 1993.

192. Houston PE, Rana S, Sekhsaria S, et al: Homocysteine in sickle cell disease: Relationship to stroke. *Am J Med* 103:192, 1997.

193. Andrade FL, Annichino-Bizzacchi JM, Saad ST, et al: Prothrombin mutant, factor V Leiden, and thermolabile variant of methylenetetrahydrofolate reductase among patients with sickle cell disease in Brazil. *Am J Hematol* 59:46, 1998.

194. Zimmerman SA, Ware RE: Inherited DNA mutations contributing to thrombotic complications in patients with sickle cell disease. *Am J Hematol* 59:267, 1998.

195. Baird RL: Studies in sickle cell anemia: XXI. Clinicopathological aspects of neurological manifestations. *Pediatrics* 34:92, 1964.

196. Diggs LW, Brookoff D: Multiple cerebral aneurysms in patients with sickle cell disease. *South Med J* 86:377, 1993.

197. Preul MC, Cendes F, Just N, Mohr G: Intracranial aneurysms and sickle cell anemia: multiplicity and propensity for the vertebrobasilar territory. *Neurosurgery* 42:971, 1998.

198. Koshy M, Entsuah R, Koranda A, et al: Leg ulcers in patients with sickle cell disease. *Blood* 74:1403, 1989.

199. Morgan AG: Sickle cell leg ulcers. *Int J Dermatol* 24:643, 1985.

200. Barrett-Conner E: Bacterial infection and sickle cell anemia. *Medicine (Baltimore)* 50:97, 1971.

201. Boghossian SH, Wright G, Webster AD, Segal AW: Investigations of host defence in patients with sickle cell disease. *Br J Haematol* 59:523, 1985.

202. Klein P, McMeeking AA, Goldenberg A: Babesiosis in a patient with sickle cell anemia. *Am J Med* 102:416, 1997.

203. McCurdy PR: Abnormal hemoglobins and pregnancy. *Am J Obstet Gynecol* 90:891, 1964.

204. Serjeant GR: Sickle haemoglobin and pregnancy. *BMJ* 287:628, 1983.

205. Anderson M, Went LN, MacIver JE, Dixon HG: Sickle cell disease in pregnancy. *Lancet* 2:516, 1960.

206. Poddar D, Maude GH, Plant MJ, Scorer H, Serjeant GR: Pregnancy in Jamaican women with homozygous sickle cell disease. Fetal and maternal outcome. *Br J Obstet Gynaecol* 93:727, 1986.

207. Powars DR, Sandhu M, Niland-Weiss J, et al: Pregnancy in sickle cell disease. *Obstet Gynecol* 67:217, 1986.

208. Anderson MF: The foetal risks in sickle cell anaemia. *West Indian Med J* 2:288, 1971.

209. Charache S, Scott J, Niebyl J, Bonds D: Management of sickle cell disease in pregnant patients. *Obstet Gynecol* 55:407, 1980.

210. El-Shafei AM, Dhaliwal JK, Sandhu AK: Pregnancy in sickle cell disease in Bahrain. *Br J Obstet Gynaecol* 99:101, 1992.

211. Howard RJ, Tuck SM, Pearson TC: Pregnancy in sickle cell disease in the UK: Results of a multicentre survey of the effect of prophylactic blood transfusion on maternal and fetal outcome. *Br J Obstet Gynaecol* 102:947, 1995.

212. Koshy M: Sickle cell disease and pregnancy. *Blood Rev* 9:157, 1995.

213. Smith JA, Espeland M, Bellevue R, et al: Pregnancy in sickle cell disease: Experience of the cooperative study of sickle cell disease. *Obstet Gynecol* 87:199, 1996.

214. Dare FO, Makinde OO, Faasuba OB: The obstetric performance of sickle cell disease patients and homozygous hemoglobin C disease patients in Ile-Ife, Nigeria. *Int J Gynecol Obstet* 37:163, 1992.

215. Idrisa A, Omigbodun AO, Adeleye JA: Pregnancy in hemoglobin sickle cell patients at the University College Hospital, Ibadan. *Int J Gynecol Obstet* 38:83, 1992.

216. Glader BE, Propper RD, Buchanan GR: Microcytosis associated with sickle cell anemia. *Am J Clin Pathol* 72:63, 1979.

217. Mohandas N, Johnson A, Wyatt J, et al: Automated quantitation of cell density distribution and hyperdense cell fraction in RBC disorders. *Blood* 74:442, 1989.

218. Sherwood JB, Goldwasser E, Chilcote R, Carmichael LD, Nagel RL: Sickle cell anemia patients have low erythropoietin levels for their degree of anemia. *Blood* 67:46, 1986.

219. Erslev AJ, Wilson J, Caro J: Erythropoietin titers in anemic, nonuremic patients. *J Lab Clin Med* 109:429, 1987.

220. Bensinger TA, Mahmood L, Conrad ME, McCurdy PR: The effect of oral urea administration on red cell survival in sickle cell disease. *Am J Med Sci* 264:283, 1972.

221. Solanki DL, McCurdy PR, Cuttitta FF, Schechter GP: Hemolysis in sickle cell disease as measured by endogenous carbon monoxide production. A preliminary report. *Am J Clin Pathol* 89:221, 1988.

222. Boggs DR, Hyde F, Srodes C: An unusual pattern of neutrophil kinetics in sickle cell anemia. *Blood* 41:59, 1973.

223. Buchanan GR, Glader BE: Leukocyte counts in children with sickle cell disease. Comparative values in the steady state, vaso-occlusive crisis, and bacterial infection. *Am J Dis Child* 132:396, 1978.

224. Corvelli AI, Binder RA, Kales A: Disseminated intravascular coagulation in sickle cell crisis. *South Med J* 72:23, 1979.

225. Ballas SK, Burka ER, Lewis CN, Krasnow SH: Serum immunoglobulin levels in patients having sickle cell syndromes. *Am J Clin Pathol* 73:394, 1980.

226. Glassman AB, Deas DV, Berlinsky FS, Bennett CE: Lymphocyte blast transformation and peripheral lymphocyte percentages in patients with sickle cell disease. *Ann Clin Lab Sci* 10:9, 1980.

227. Corry JM, Polhill RB Jr, Edmonds SR, Johnston RB Jr: Activity of the alternative complement pathway after splenectomy: Comparison to activity in sickle cell disease and hypogammaglobulinemia. *J Pediatr* 95:964, 1979.

228. Wang RH, Phillips G Jr, Medof ME, Mold C: Activation of the alternative complement pathway by exposure of phosphatidylethanolamine and phosphatidylserine on erythrocytes from sickle cell disease patients. *J Clin Invest* 92:1326, 1993.

229. Natta C, Machlin L: Plasma levels of tocopherol in sickle cell anemia subjects. *Am J Clin Nutr* 32:1359, 1979.

230. Karayalcin G, Lanzkowsky P, Kazi AB: Zinc deficiency in children with sickle cell disease. *Am J Pediatr Hematol Oncol* 1:283, 1979.

231. Niell HB, Leach BE, Kraus AP: Zinc metabolism in sickle cell anemia. *JAMA* 242:2686, 1979.

232. O'Brien RT: Iron burden in sickle cell anemia. *J Pediatr* 92:579, 1978.

233. Reid CD, Charache S, Lubin B, Johnson C, Ohene Frem Pong K: *Management and Therapy of Sickle Cell Disease.* Bethesda, MD, National Institutes of Health, Heart, Lung and Blood Institute, pp 96–2117, 1995.

234. Silliman CC, Peterson VM, Mellman DL, et al: Iron chelation by deferoxamine in sickle cell patients with severe transfusion-induced hemosiderosis: a randomized, double-blind study of the dose-response relationship. *J Lab Clin Med* 122:48, 1993.

235. Reed W, Vichinsky EP: New considerations in the treatment of sickle cell disease. *Annu Rev Med* 49:461, 1998.

236. Haddy TB, Castro O: Overt iron deficiency in sickle cell disease. *Arch Intern Med* 142:1621, 1982.

237. Davies S, Henthorn J, Brozovic M: Iron deficiency in sickle cell anaemia. *J Clin Pathol* 36:1012, 1983.

238. International Committee for Standardization in Haematology: Simple electrophoretic system for presumptive identification of abnormal hemoglobins. *Blood* 52:1058, 1978.

239. Daland GA, Castle WB: A simple and rapid method for demonstrating sickling of the red blood cells: The use of reducing agents. *J Lab Clin Med* 33:1082, 1948.

240. Henry RL, Nalbandian RM, Nichols BM, et al: Modified Sickledex tube test: a specific test for S hemoglobin. *Clin Biochem* 4:196, 1971.

241. Mario N, Baudin B, Aussel C, Giboudeau J: Capillary isoelectric focusing and high-performance cation-exchange chromatography compared for qualitative and quantitative analysis of hemoglobin variants. *Clin Chem* 43:2137, 1997.

242. Steinberg MH: DNA diagnosis for the detection of sickle hemoglobinopathies. *Am J Hematol* 43:110, 1993.

243. Van Baelen H, Vandepitte J, Eeckels R: Observations on sickle cell anaemia and haemoglobin Bart's in Congolese neonates. *Ann Soc Belg Med Trop* 49:157, 1969.

244. Consensus Conference: Newborn screening for sickle cell disease and other hemoglobinopathies. *JAMA* 258:1205, 1987.

245. Old JM, Fitches A, Heath C, et al: First-trimester fetal diagnosis for haemoglobinopathies: report on 200 cases. *Lancet* 2:763, 1986.

246. Conner BJ, Reyes AA, Morin C, et al: Detection of sickle cell beta(s)-globin allele by hybridization with synthetic oligonucleotides. *Proc Natl Acad Sci USA* 80:278, 1983.

247. Davies SC, Oni L: Fortnightly review—Management of patients with sickle cell disease. *BMJ* 315:656, 1997.

248. Steinberg MH: Review: Sickle cell disease: Present and future treatment. *Am J Med Sci* 312:166, 1996.

249. Rabb LM, Grandison Y, Mason K, et al: A trial of folate supplementation in children with homozygous sickle cell disease. *Br J Haematol* 54:589, 1983.

250. Wayne AS, Kevy SV, Nathan DG: Transfusion management of sickle cell disease. *Blood* 81:1109, 1993.

251. Rosse WF, Gallagher D, Kinney TR, et al: Transfusion and alloimmunization in sickle cell disease. *Blood* 76:1431, 1990.

252. Vichinsky EP, Haberkern CM, Neumayr L, et al: A comparison of conservative and aggressive transfusion regimens in the perioperative management of sickle cell disease. The Preoperative Transfusion in Sickle Cell Disease Study Group. *N Engl J Med* 333:206, 1995.

253. Rackoff WR, Ohene-Frempong K, Month S, et al: Neurologic events after partial exchange transfusion for priapism in sickle cell disease. *J Pediatr* 120:882, 1992.

254. Charache S, Scott JC, Charache P: 'Acute chest syndrome' in adults with sickle cell anemia. Microbiology, treatment, and prevention. *Arch Intern Med* 139:67, 1979.

255. Davies SC, Brozovic M: The presentation, management and prophylaxis of sickle cell disease. *Blood Rev* 3:29, 1989.

256. Ammann AJ, Addiego J, Wara DW, et al: Polyvalent pneumococcal-polysaccharide immunization of patients with sickle-cell anemia and patients with splenectomy. *N Engl J Med* 297:897, 1977.

257. Ahonkhai VI, Landesman SH, Fikrig SM, et al: Failure of pneumococcal vaccine in children with sickle-cell disease. *N Engl J Med* 301:26, 1979.

258. Penicillin prophylaxis for babies with sickle-cell disease. *Lancet* 2:1432, 1986.

259. Anglin DL, Siegel JD, Pacini DL, et al: Effect of penicillin prophylaxis on nasopharyngeal colonization with *Streptococcus pneumoniae* in children with sickle cell anemia. *J Pediatr* 104:18, 1984.

260. Laszlo J, Obenour W, Saltzman HA: Effects of hyperbaric oxygenation on sickle syndromes. *South Med J* 62:453, 1969.

261. Reynolds JDH: Painful sickle cell crisis: Successful treatment with hyperbaric oxygen therapy. *JAMA* 216:1977, 1971.

262. Henderson AB: Sickle cell disease: Studies on "in vivo" sickling and the effect of certain pharmacological agents. *Am J Med Sci* 221:628, 1951.

263. Mann JR, Deeble TJ, Breeze GR, Stuart J: Ancrod in sickle cell crisis. *Lancet* 1:934, 1972.

264. Hugh-Jones K, Lehmann H, McAlister JM: Some experiences in managing sickle cell anaemia in children and young adults, using alkalis and magnesium. *BMJ* 2:226, 1964.

265. Barreras L, Diggs LW: Sodium citrate orally for painful sickle cell crises. *JAMA* 215:762, 1971.

266. Teuscher T, Weil von der Ahe C, Baillod P, Holzer B: Double-blind randomised clinical trial of pentoxiphyllin in vaso-occlusive sickle cell crisis. *Trop Geogr Med* 41:320, 1989.

267. Billett HH, Kaul DK, Connel MM, Fabry ME, Nagel RI: Pentoxifylline (Trental) has no significant effect on laboratory parameters in sickle cell disease. *Nouv Rev Fr Hematol* 31:403, 1989.

268. Cooperative Urea Trials Group: Clinical trials of therapy for sickle cell vaso-occlusive crises. *JAMA* 228:1120, 1974.

269. Okpala I: The management of crisis in sickle cell disease. *Eur J Haematol* 60:1, 1998.

270. Cohen AR, Martin MB, Silber JH, et al: A modified transfusion program for prevention of stroke in sickle cell disease. *Blood* 79:1657, 1992.

271. Adams RJ, McKie VC, Hsu L, et al: Prevention of a first stroke by transfusions in children with sickle cell anemia and abnormal results on transcranial Doppler ultrasonography. *N Engl J Med* 339:5, 1998.

272. Solanki DL, McCurdy PR: Cholelithiasis in sickle cell anemia: A case for elective cholecystectomy. *Am J Med Sci* 277:319, 1979.

273. Jawad AJ, Kurban K, el-Bakry A, et al: Laparoscopic cholecystectomy for cholelithiasis during infancy and childhood: cost analysis and review of current indications. *World J Surg* 22:69, 1998.

274. Meshikhes AN, al-Dhurais SA, al-Jama A, et al: Laparoscopic cholecystectomy in patients with sickle cell disease. *J R Coll Surg Edinb* 40:383, 1995.

275. Greenwald JG: Stroke, sickle cell trait and oral contraceptives. *Ann Intern Med* 72:960, 1970.

276. De Abood M, De Castillo Z, Guerrero F, Espino M, Austin KL: Effect of Depo-Provera® or Microgynon® on the painful crises of sickle cell anemia patients. *Contraception* 56:313, 1997.

277. Koshy M, Burd L: Management of pregnancy in sickle cell syndromes. *Hematol Oncol Clin North Am* 5:585, 1991.

278. Morrison JC, Schneider JM, Whybrew WD, Bucovaz ET, Menzel DM: Prophylactic transfusions in pregnant patients with sickle hemoglobinopathies: Benefit versus risk. *Obstet Gynecol* 56:274, 1980.

279. Cunningham FG, Pritchard JA: Prophylactic transfusions of normal red blood cells during pregnancies complicated by sickle cell hemoglobinopathies. *Am J Obstet Gynecol* 135:994, 1979.

280. Cunningham FG, Pritchard JA, Mason R: Pregnancy and sickle cell hemoglobinopathies: Results with and without prophylactic transfusions. *Obstet Gynecol* 62:419, 1983.

281. Morrison JC, Morrison FS: Prophylactic transfusions in pregnant patients with sickle cell disease. *N Engl J Med* 320:1286, 1989.

282. Morrison JC, Foster H: Transfusion therapy in pregnant patients with sickle-cell disease: A National Institutes of Health consensus development conference. *Ann Intern Med* 91:122, 1979.

283. Koshy M, Burd L, Wallace D, Moawad A, Baron J: Prophylactic red-cell transfusions in pregnant patients with sickle cell disease: A randomized cooperative study. *N Engl J Med* 319:1447, 1988.

284. Acurio MT, Friedman RJ: Hip arthroplasty in patients with sickle-cell haemoglobinopathy. *J Bone Joint Surg [Br]* 74B:367, 1992.

285. Styles LA, Vichinsky EP: Core decompression in avascular necrosis of the hip in sickle-cell disease. *Am J Hematol* 52:103, 1996.

286. Rodgers GP, Roy MS, Noguchi CT, Schechter AN: Is there a role for selective vasodilation in the management of sickle cell disease? *Blood* 71:597, 1988.

287. Virag R, Bachir D, Lee K, Galacteros F: Preventive treatment of priapism in sickle cell disease with oral and self-administered intracavernous injection of etilefrine. *Urology* 47:777, 1996.

288. Upadhyay J, Shekarriz B, Dhabuwala CB: Penile implant for intractable priapism associated with sickle cell disease. *Urology* 51:638, 1998.

289. Monga M, Broderick GA, Hellstrom WJG: Priapism in sickle cell disease: The case for early implantation of the penile prosthesis. *Eur Urol* 30:54, 1996.

290. Ware R, Filston HC, Schultz WH, Kinney TR: Elective cholecystectomy in children with sickle hemoglobinopathies: Successful outcome using a preoperative transfusion regimen. *Ann Surg* 208:17, 1988.

291. Banerjee AK, Layton DM, Rennie JA, Bellingham AJ: Safe surgery in sickle cell disease. *Br J Surg* 78:516, 1991.

292. Derkay CS, Bray G, Milmoe GJ, Grundfast KM: Adenotonsillectomy in children with sickle-cell disease. *South Med J* 84:205, 1991.

293. Esseltine DW, Baxter MR, Bevan JC: Sickle cell states and the anaesthetist. *Can J Anaesth* 35:385, 1988.

294. Jablonska-Skwiecinska E: Unpublished, 1998.

295. Neumayr L, Koshy M, Haberkern C, et al: Surgery in patients with hemoglobin SC disease. *Am J Hematol* 57:101, 1998.

296. Bischoff RJ, Williamson A III, Dalali MJ, Rice JC, Kerstein MD: Assessment of the use of transfusion therapy perioperatively in patients with sickle cell hemoglobinopathies. *Ann Surg* 207:434, 1988.

297. Johnson FL, Look AT, Gockerman J, et al: Bone-marrow transplantation in a patient with sickle-cell anemia. *N Engl J Med* 311:780, 1984.

298. Vermylen C, Cornu G, Ferster A, Ninane J, Sariban E: Bone marrow transplantation in sickle cell disease: The Belgian experience. *Bone Marrow Transplant* 12 (suppl 1):116, 1993.

299. Bernaudin F, Souillet G, Vannier JP, et al: Bone marrow transplantation (BMT) in 14 children with severe sickle cell disease (SCD): The French experience. *Bone Marrow Transplant* 12 (suppl 1):118, 1993.

300. Kröplin T, Weyer N, Gutsche S, Iven H: Thiopurine S-methyltransferase activity in human erythrocytes: a new HPLC method using 6-thioguanine as substrate. *Eur J Clin Pharmacol* 54:265, 1998.

301. Vermylen C, Cornu G, Ferster A, et al: Haematopoietic stem cell transplantation for sickle cell anaemia: the first 50 patients transplanted in Belgium. *Bone Marrow Transplant* 22:1, 1998.

302. Walters MC, Patience M, Leisenring W, et al: Bone marrow transplantation for sickle cell disease. *N Engl J Med* 335:369, 1996.

303. Vermylen C, Cornu G: Hematopoietic stem cell transplantation for sickle cell anemia. *Curr Opin Hematol* 4:377, 1997.

304. Beutler E: Bone marrow transplantation for sickle cell anemia: Summarizing comments. *Semin Hematol* 28:263, 1991.

305. Davies SC: Bone marrow transplant for sickle cell disease—the dilemma. *Blood Rev* 7:4, 1993.

306. Platt OS, Guinan EC: Bone marrow transplantation in sickle cell anemia—The dilemma of choice. *N Engl J Med* 335:426, 1996.

307. Sirs JA: The use of carbon monoxide to prevent sickle-cell formation. *Lancet* 1:971, 1963.

308. Purugganan HB, McElfresh AE: Failure of carbonmonoxy sickle-cell haemoglobin to alter the sickle state. *Lancet* 1:79, 1964.

309. Beutler E: The effect of carbon monoxide on red cell life span in sickle cell disease. *Blood* 46:253, 1975.

310. Beutler E: The effect of methemoglobin formation in sickle cell disease. *J Clin Invest* 40:1856, 1961.

311. Paniker NV, Ben-Bassat I, Beutler E: Evaluation of sickle hemoglobin and desickling agents by falling ball viscometry. *J Lab Clin Med* 80:282, 1972.

312. Shamsuddin M, Mason RG, Ritchey JM, Honig GR, Klotz IM: Sites of acetylation of sickle cell hemoglobin by aspirin. *Proc Natl Acad Sci USA* 71:4693, 1974.

313. Ueno H, Yatco E, Benjamin LJ, Manning JM: Effects of methyl acetyl phosphate, a covalent antisickling agent, on the density profiles of sickle erythrocytes. *J Lab Clin Med* 120:152, 1992.

314. Zaugg RH, King LC, Klotz IM: Acylation of hemoglobin by succinyldisalicylate, a potential crosslinking reagent. *Biochem Biophys Res Commun* 64:1192, 1975.

315. Isaacs WA, Hayhoe FGJ: Steroid hormones in sickle cell disease. *Nature* 215:1139, 1967.

316. Waterman MR, Yamaoka K, Chuang AH, Cottam GL: Anti-sickling nature of dimethyl adipimidate. *Biochem Biophys Res Commun* 63:580, 1975.

317. Hilkowitz G: Sickle cell disease: New method for treatment: Preliminary report. *BMJ* 2:266, 1957.

318. Knochel JP: Hematuria in sickle cell trait. *Arch Intern Med* 123:160, 1969.

319. Niihara Y, Zerez CR, Akiyama DS, Tanaka KR: Oral L-glutamine therapy for sickle cell anemia: I. Subjective clinical improvement and favorable change in red cell NAD redox potential. *Am J Hematol* 58:117, 1998.

320. Nalbandian RM, Shulta G, Lusher JM, Anderson JW, Henry RL: Sickle cell crisis terminated by intravenous urea in sugar solutions a preliminary report. *Am J Med Sci* 261:309, 1971.

321. Gillette PN, Manning JM, Cerami A: Increased survival of sickle cell erythrocytes after treatment in vitro with sodium cyanate. *Proc Natl Acad Sci USA* 68:2791, 1971.

322. Parameswaran KN, Shi GY, Klotz IM: O-carbamoylsalicylates: agents for modification of hemoglobins. *J Med Chem* 30:936, 1987.

323. Ueno H, Benjamin LJ, Manning JM: Effects of methyl acetyl phosphate on hemoglobin S: a novel acetylating agent directed towards the DPG binding site. *Prog Clin Biol Res* 240:105, 1987.

324. Franklin IM, Cotter RI, Cheetham RC, et al: A potent new dipeptide inhibitor of cell sickling and haemoglobin S gelation. *Eur J Biochem* 136:209, 1983.

325. Baker R, Powars D, Haywood J: Restoration of the deformability of "irreversibly" sickled cells by procaine hydrochloride. *Biochem Biophys Res Commun* 59:548, 1974.

326. Brewer GJ, Brewer LF, Prasad AS: Suppression of irreversibly sickled erythrocytes by zinc therapy in sickle cell anemia. *J Lab Clin Med* 90:549, 1977.

327. Beutler E, Paniker NV, West CJ: Pyridoxine administration in sickle cell disease: An unsuccessful attempt to influence the properties of sickle hemoglobin. *Biochem Med* 6:139, 1972.

328. Kark JA, Tarassoff PG, Bongiovanni R: Pyridoxal phosphate as an antisickling agent in vitro. *J Clin Invest* 71:1224, 1983.

329. Kark JA, Kale MP, Tarassoff PG, et al: Inhibition of erythrocyte sickling in vitro by pyridoxal. *J Clin Invest* 62:888, 1978.

330. Benesch R, Benesch RE, Edalji R, Suzuki T: 5′-Deoxypyridoxal as a potential anti-sickling agent. *Proc Natl Acad Sci USA* 74:1721, 1977.

331. Bounameaux Y: Action inhibitrice de la nivaquine et de divers anti-histaminiques sur la formation d'hematies en faucilles dans l'anemie drepanocytaire. *C R Soc Biol (Paris)* 155:425, 1961.

332. Fung LWM, Ho C, Roth EF Jr, Nagel RL: The alkylation of hemoglobin S by nitrogen mustard: High resolution proton nuclear magnetic resonance studies. *J Biol Chem* 250:4786, 1975.

333. Nigen AM, Manning JM: Inhibition of erythrocyte sickling in vitro by DL-glyceraldehyde. *Proc Natl Acad Sci USA* 74:367, 1977.

334. Ross PD, Subramanian S: Hexamethylenetetramine: A powerful and novel inhibitor of gelation of deoxyhemoglobin S. *Arch Biochem Biophys* 190:736, 1978.

335. Natta CL, Machlin LJ, Brin M: A decrease in irreversibly sickled erythrocytes in sickle cell anemia patients given vitamin E. *Am J Clin Nutr* 33:968, 1980.

336. Clarke DT, Jones GR, Martin MM: The anti-sickling drug lawsone (2-OH-1,4-naphthoquinone) protects sickled cells against membrane damage. *Biochem Biophys Res Commun* 139:780, 1986.

337. Stone PCW, Nash GB, Stuart J: Substituted benzaldehydes (12C79 and 589C80) that stabilize oxyhaemoglobin also protect sickle cells against calcium-mediated dehydration. *Br J Haematol* 81:419, 1992.

338. Reilly MP, Asakura T: Antisickling effect of bepridil. *Lancet* 1:848, 1986.

339. Asakura T, Ohnishi ST, Adachi K, et al: Effect of cetiedil on erythrocyte sickling: New type of antisickling agent that may affect erythrocyte membranes. *Proc Natl Acad Sci USA* 77:2955, 1980.

340. Charache S, De La Monte S, MacDonald V: Increased blood viscosity in a patient with sickle cell anemia. *Blood Cells* 8:103, 1982.

341. Greenberg MS, Kass EH: Studies on the destruction of red blood cells: XIII. Observations on the role of pH in the pathogenesis and treatment of painful crisis in sickle-cell disease. *Arch Intern Med* 101:355, 1958.

342. Rhodes RS, Revo L, Hara S, Hartmann RC, Van Eys J: Therapy for sickle cell vaso-occlusive crises controlled clinical trials and cooperative study of intravenously administered alkali. *JAMA* 228:1129, 1974.

343. Kilmartin JV, Rossi-Bernardi L: The binding of carbon dioxide by horse haemoglobin. *Biochem J* 124:31, 1971.

344. Peterson CM, Tsairis P, Ohnishi A, et al: Sodium cyanate induced polyneuropathy in patients with sickle-cell disease. *Ann Intern Med* 81:152, 1974.

345. Nicholson DH, Harkness DR, Benson WE, Peterson CM: Cyanate-induced cataracts in patients with sickle-cell hemoglobinopathies. *Arch Ophthalmol* 94:927, 1976.

346. Langer EE, Stamatoyannopoulos G, Hlastala MP, et al: Extracorporeal treatment with cyanate in sickle cell disease: Preliminary observations in four patients. *J Lab Clin Med* 87:462, 1976.

347. Charache S, Dreyer R, Zimmerman I, Hsu CK: Evaluation of extracorporeal alkylation of red cells as a potential treatment for sickle cell anemia. *Blood* 47:481, 1976.

348. Diederich DA, Trueworthy RG, Gill P, Crader AM, Larsen WE: Hematologic and clinical responses in patients with sickle cell anemia after chronic extracorporeal red cell carbamylation. *J Clin Invest* 58:642, 1976.

349. Keidan AJ, White RD, Huehns ER, et al: Effect of BW12C on oxygen affinity of haemoglobin in sickle-cell disease. *Lancet* 1:831, 1986.

350. Rosa RM, Bierer BE, Thomas R, et al: A study of induced hyponatremia in the prevention and treatment of sickle-cell crisis. *N Engl J Med* 303:1138, 1980.

351. Baldree LA, Ault BH, Chesney CM, Stapleton FB: Intravenous desmopressin acetate in children with sickle trait and persistent macroscopic hematuria. *Pediatrics* 86:238, 1990.

352. Leary M, Abramson N: Induced hyponatremia for sickle-cell crisis. *N Engl J Med* 304:844, 1981.

353. Charache S, Walker WG: Failure of desmopressin to lower serum sodium or prevent crisis in patients with sickle cell anemia. *Blood* 58:892, 1981.

354. DeSimone J, Heller P, Hall L, Zwiers D: 5-Azacytidine stimulates fetal hemoglobin synthesis in anemic baboons. *Proc Natl Acad Sci USA* 79:4428, 1982.

355. Charache S, Dover G, Smith K, et al: Treatment of sickle cell anemia with 5-azacytidine results in increased fetal hemoglobin production and

356. Ley TJ, DeSimone J, Noguchi C, et al: 5-Azacytidine increases gamma-globin synthesis and reduces the proportion of dense cells in patients with sickle cell anemia. *Blood* 62:370, 1983.

357. Veith R, Galanello R, Papayannopoulou T, Stamatoyannopoulos G: Stimulation of F-cell production in Hb S patients treated with Ara-C or hydroxyurea. *N Engl J Med* 313:1571, 1985.

358. Platt OS, Orkin SH, Dover G, et al: Hydroxyurea enhances fetal hemoglobin production in sickle cell anemia. *J Clin Invest* 74:652, 1984.

359. Dover GJ, Humphries RK, Moore JG, et al: Hydroxyurea induction of hemoglobin F production in sickle cell disease: Relationship between cytotoxicity and F-cell production. *Blood* 67:735, 1986.

360. Kaufman RE: Hydroxyurea: Specific therapy for sickle cell anemia. *Blood* 79:2503, 1992.

361. Charache S, Dover GJ, Moore RD, et al: Hydroxyurea: Effects on hemoglobin F production in patients with sickle cell anemia. *Blood* 79:2555, 1992.

362. Rodgers GP, Dover GJ, Uyesaka N, et al: Augmentation by erythropoietin of the fetal-hemoglobin response to hydroxyurea in sickle cell disease. *N Engl J Med* 328:73, 1993.

363. Nagel RL, Vichinsky E, Shah M, et al: F reticulocyte response in sickle cell anemia treated with recombinant human erythropoietin: A double-blind study. *Blood* 81:9, 1993.

364. Perrine SP, Faller DV, Swerdlow P, et al: Stopping the biologic clock for globin gene switching. *Ann N Y Acad Sci* 612:134, 1990.

365. Dover GJ, Brusilow S, Samid D: Increased fetal hemoglobin in patients receiving sodium 4-phenylbutyrate. *N Engl J Med* 327:569, 1992.

366. Perrine SP, Ginder GD, Faller DV, et al: A short-term trial of butyrate to stimulate fetal-globin-gene expression in the β-globin disorders. *N Engl J Med* 328:81, 1993.

367. Saleh AW Jr, Van Goethem A, Jansen R, et al: Isobutyramide therapy in patients with sickle cell anemia. *Am J Hematol* 49:244, 1995.

368. Miller BA, Olivieri N, Hope SM, Faller DV, Perrine SP: Interferon-gamma modulates fetal hemoglobin synthesis in sickle cell anemia and thalassemia. *J Interferon Res* 10:357, 1990.

369. Charache S, Terrin ML, Moore RD, et al: Effect of hydroxyurea on the frequency of painful crises in sickle cell anemia. Investigators of the Multicenter Study of Hydroxyurea in Sickle Cell Anemia. *N Engl J Med* 332:1317, 1995.

370. El-Hazmi MAF, Al-Momen A, Warsy AS, et al: The pharmacological manipulation of fetal haemoglobin: Trials using hydroxyurea and recombinant human erythropoietin. *Acta Haematol (Basel)* 93:57, 1995.

371. Voskaridou E, Kalotychou V, Loukopoulos D: Clinical and laboratory effects of long-term administration of hydroxyurea to patients with sickle-cell/β-thalassaemia. *Br J Haematol* 89:479, 1995.

372. Jayabose S, Tugal O, Sandoval C, et al: Clinical and hematologic effects of hydroxyurea in children with sickle cell anemia. *J Pediatr* 129:559, 1996.

373. Scott JP, Hillery CA, Brown ER, Misiewicz V, Labotka RJ: Hydroxyurea therapy in children severely affected with sickle cell disease. *J Pediatr* 128:820, 1996.

374. Rogers ZR: Hydroxyurea therapy for diverse pediatric populations with sickle cell disease. *Semin Hematol* 34:42, 1997.

375. Saleh AW Jr, Velvis HJR, Gu LH, Hillen HFP, Huisman THJ: Hydroxyurea therapy in sickle cell anemia patients in Curacao, The Netherlands Antilles. *Acta Haematol (Basel)* 98:125, 1997.

376. Olivieri NF, Vichinsky EP: Hydroxyurea in children with sickle cell disease: impact on splenic function and compliance with therapy. *J Pediatr Hematol Oncol* 20:26, 1998.

377. Adams-Graves P, Kedar A, Koshy M, et al: RheothRx (poloxamer 188) injection for the acute painful episode of sickle cell disease: A pilot study. *Blood* 90:2041, 1997.

378. Lambotte-Legrand J, Lambotte-Legrand C: Le prognostic de l'anemie drepanocytaire au Congo Belge (a propos de 300 cas et de 150 deces). *Ann Soc Belg Med Trop* 35:53, 1955.

379. Trowell HC, Raper AB, Welbourn HF: The natural history of homozygous sickle cell anaemia in Central Africa. *Q J Med* 25:401, 1957.

380. Sydenstricker VP, Kemp JA, Metts JC: Prolonged survival in sickle cell disease. *Am Pract* 13:584, 1962.

is associated with nonrandom hypomethylation of DNA around the gamma-delta-beta globin gene complex. *Proc Natl Acad Sci USA* 80:4842, 1983.

381. Serjeant GR, Richards RR, Barbor PHH, Milner PF: Relatively benign sickle anaemia in 60 patients over 30 in the West Indies. *BMJ* 2:86, 1968.

382. Platt OS, Brambilla DJ, Rosse WF, et al: Mortality in sickle cell disease—Life expectancy and risk factors for early death. *N Engl J Med* 330:1639, 1994.

383. Davis H, Schoendorf KC, Gergen PJ, Moore RM: National trends in the mortality of children with sickle cell disease, 1968 through 1992. *Am J Public Health* 87:1317, 1997.

384. Powars D: Diagnosis at birth improves survival of children with sickle cell anemia. *Pediatrics* 83:830, 1989.

385. Davis H, Gergen PJ, Moore RJ: Geographic differences in mortality of young children with sickle cell disease in the United States. *Public Health Rep* 112:52, 1997.

386. Israel JB, Arias IM: Inheritable disorders of bilirubin metabolism. *Adv Intern Med* 77:21–96, 1976.

387. Beutler E, Boggs DR, Heller P, et al: Hazards of indiscriminate screening for sickling. *N Engl J Med* 285:1485, 1971.

388. Dorticos-Balea A, Martin-Ruiz M, Hechevarria-Fernandez P, et al: Reproductive behaviour of couples at risk for sickle cell disease in Cuba: a follow-up study. *Prenat Diagn* 17:737, 1997.

389. Neuenschwander H, Modell B: Audit of process of antenatal screening for sickle cell disorders at a north London hospital. *BMJ* 315:784, 1997.

390. Modell B, Petrou M, Layton M, et al: Audit of prenatal diagnosis for haemoglobin disorders in the United Kingdom: the first 20 years. *BMJ* 315:779, 1997.

391. Barbedo MMR, McCurdy PR: Red cell life span in sickle cell trait. *Acta Haematol (Basel)* 51:339, 1974.

392. Kellon DB, Beutler E: Physician attitudes about sickle cell. *JAMA* 227:71, 1974.

393. Sears DA: The morbidity of sickle cell trait. *Am J Med* 64:1021, 1978.

394. Humphries JE, Wheby MS: Case report: Sickle cell trait and recurrent deep venous thrombosis. *Am J Med Sci* 303:112, 1992.

395. Genet P, Pulik M, Lionnet F, Petitdidier C, Touahri T: Multiple spontaneous vascular infarcts in sickle-cell trait: A case report. *Am J Hematol* 51:173, 1996.

396. Gozal D, Lorey FW, Chandler D, et al: Incidence of sudden infant death syndrome in infants with sickle cell trait. *J Pediatr* 124:211, 1994.

397. Smith EW, Conley CL: Clinical manifestations of sickle-cell disease. NASNRC publ 554:276, 1958.

398. Atlas SA: The sickle cell trait and surgical complications. *JAMA* 229:1078, 1974.

399. Francis CK, Bleakley DW: The risk of sudden death in sickle cell trait: Noninvasive assessment of cardiac response to exercise. *Cathet Cardiovasc Diagn* 6:73, 1980.

400. Weisman IM, Zeballos RJ, Johnson BD: Cardiopulmonary and gas exchange responses to acute strenuous exercise at 1,270 meters in sickle cell trait. *Am J Med* 84:377, 1988.

401. Gozal D, Thiriet P, Mbala E, et al: Effect of different modalities of exercise and recovery on exercise performance in subjects with sickle cell trait. *Med Sci Sports Exerc* 24:1325, 1992.

402. Nuss R, Loehr JP, Daberkow E, Graham L, Lane PA: Cardiopulmonary function in men with sickle cell trait who reside at moderately high altitude. *J Lab Clin Med* 122:382, 1993.

403. Le Gallais D, Prefaut C, Mercier J, et al: Sickle cell trait as a limiting factor for high-level performance in a semi-marathon. *Int J Sports Med* 15:399, 1994.

404. Bilé A, Le Gallais D, Mercier J, Bogui P, Préfaut C: Sickle cell trait in Ivory Coast athletic throw and lump champions, 1956–1995. *Int J Sports Med* 19:215, 1998.

405. Jones SR, Binder RA, Donowho EM Jr: Sudden death in sickle-cell trait. *N Engl J Med* 282:323, 1970.

406. Koppes GM, Daly JJ, Coltman CA Jr, Butkus DE: Exertion-induced rhabdomyolysis with acute renal failure and disseminated intravascular coagulation in sickle cell trait. *Am J Med* 63:313, 1977.

407. Kerle KK, Nishimura KD: Exertional collapse and sudden death associated with sickle cell trait. *Milit Med* 161:766, 1996.

408. Le Gallais GD, Bile A, Mercier J, et al: Exercise-induced death in sickle cell trait: role of aging, training, and deconditioning. *Med Sci Sports Exerc* 28:541, 1996.

409. Murray MJ, Evans P: Sudden exertional death in a soldier with sickle cell trait. *Milit Med* 161:303, 1996.

410. Kark JA, Posey DM, Schumacher HR, Ruehle CJ: Sickle-cell trait as a risk factor for sudden death in physical trainees. *N Engl J Med* 317:781, 1987.

411. O'Brien RT, Pearson HA, Godley JA, Spencer RP: Splenic infarct and sickle (cell) trait. *N Engl J Med* 287:720, 1972.

412. Nichols SD: Splenic and pulmonary infarction in a Negro athlete. *Rocky Mt Med J* 65:49, 1968.

413. Rywlin AM, Benson J: Massive necrosis of the spleen with formation of a pseudocyst: Report of a case in a white man with sickle cell trait. *Am J Clin Pathol* 36:142, 1961.

414. Itano HA, Neel JV: A new inherited abnormality of human hemoglobin. *Proc Natl Acad Sci USA* 36:613, 1950.

415. Spaet TH, Alway RH, Ward G: Homozygous type "C" hemoglobin. *Pediatrics* 12:483, 1953.

416. Ranney HM, Larson DL, McCormack GH Jr: Some clinical, biochemical and genetic observations on hemoglobin C. *J Clin Invest* 32:1277, 1953.

417. Hunt JA, Ingram VM: Allelomorphism and the chemical differences of the human hemoglobins A, S, and C. *Nature* 181:1062, 1958.

418. Fabry ME, Kaul DK, Raventos C, et al: Some aspects of the pathophysiology of homozygous Hb CC erythrocytes. *J Clin Invest* 67:1284, 1981.

419. Hirsch RE, Raventos-Suarez C, Olson JA, Nagel RL: Ligand state of intraerythrocyte circulating Hb C crystals in homozygote CC patients. *Blood* 66:775, 1985.

420. Hirsch RE, Lin MJ, Nagel RL: The inhibition of hemoglobin C crystallization by hemoglobin F. *J Biol Chem* 263:5936, 1988.

421. Thomas ED, Motulsky AG, Walters DH: Homozygous hemoglobin C disease. *Am J Med* 18:832, 1955.

422. Movitt ER, Pollycove M, Mangum JF, Porter WR: Hemoglobin C disease: Quantitative determination of iron kinetics and hemoglobin synthesis. *Am J Med Sci* 247:558, 1964.

423. Murphy JR: Hemoglobin CC erythrocytes: Decreased intracellular pH and decreased O_2 affinity-anemia. *Semin Hematol* 13:177, 1976.

424. Edington GN, Lehmann H: A case of sickle cell hemoglobin C disease in a survey of hemoglobin C incidence in West Africa. *Trans R Soc Trop Med Hyg* 48:332, 1954.

425. Labie D, Richin C, Pagnier J, Gentilini M, Nagel RL: Hemoglobins S and C in Upper Volta. *Hum Genet* 65:300, 1984.

426. Schneider RG: Incidence of hemoglobin C trait in 505 normal Negroes: A family with homozygous hemoglobin C and sickle-cell trait union. *J Lab Clin Med* 44:133, 1954.

427. Diggs LW, Kraus AP, Morrison DB, Rudnicki RPT: Intraerythrocytic crystals in a white patient with hemoglobin C in the absence of other types of hemoglobin. *Blood* 9:1172, 1954.

428. Fort JA, Graham-Pole JR, Chopik J: Vasoocclusion with homozygous hemoglobin-C disease. *Am J Pediatr Hematol Oncol* 10:323, 1988.

429. Maberry MC, Mason RA, Cunningham FG, Pritchard JA: Pregnancy complicated by hemoglobin CC and C-beta-thalassemia disease. *Obstet Gynecol* 76:324, 1990.

430. Olson JF, Ware RE, Schultz WH, Kinney TR: Hemoglobin C disease in infancy and childhood. *J Pediatr* 125:745, 1994.

431. Itano HA: A third abnormal hemoglobin associated with hereditary hemolytic anemia. *Proc Natl Acad Sci USA* 37:775, 1951.

432. Chernoff AI: HgB D syndromes. *Blood* 13:116, 1958.

433. Bird GWG, Lehmann H: Haemoglobin D in India. *BMJ* 1:514, 1956.

434. Adekile AD, Kazanetz EG, Leonova JY, et al: Co-inheritance of Hb D-Punjab (codon 121; GAA→CAA) and beta (0)-thalassemia (IVS-II-1; G→A). *J Pediatr Hematol Oncol* 18:151, 1996.

435. Lachant NA: Hemoglobin E: An emerging hemoglobinopathy in the United States. *Am J Hematol* 25:449, 1987.

436. Itano HA, Bergren WR, Sturgeon P: Identification of fourth abnormal human hemoglobin. *J Am Chem Soc* 76:2278, 1954.

437. Chernoff AI, Minnich V, Na Nakorn S, et al: Studies on hemoglobin E: I. The clinical, hematologic and genetic characteristics of the hemoglobin E syndromes. *J Lab Clin Med* 47:455, 1956.

438. Hunt JA, Ingram VM: Abnormal human haemoglobins: VI. The chemical difference between haemoglobins A and E. *Biochim Biophys Acta* 49:520, 1961.

439. Frischer H, Bowman J: Hemoglobin E, an oxidatively unstable mutation. *J Lab Clin Med* 85:531, 1975.

440. Orkin SH, Kazazian HH Jr, Antonarakis SE, et al: Abnormal RNA processing due to the exon mutation of beta^E-globin gene. *Nature* 300:768, 1982.

441. Oo M, Tin-Shwe, Marlar-Than, O'Sullivan WJ: Genetic red cell disor-

ders and severity of falciparum malaria in Myanmar. *Bull World Health Organ* 73:659, 1995.

442. Flatz G: Hemoglobin E: Distribution and population dynamics. *Humangenetik* 3:189, 1967.

443. Kazazian HH Jr, Waber PG, Boehm CD, et al: Hemoglobin E in Europeans: Further evidence for multiple origins of the beta^E-globin gene. *Am J Hum Genet* 36:212, 1984.

444. Fairbanks VF, Oliveros R, Brandabur JH, Willis RR, Fiester RF: Homozygous hemoglobin E mimics beta-thalassemia minor without anemia or hemolysis: Hematologic, functional, and biosynthetic studies of first North American cases. *Am J Hematol* 8:109, 1980.

445. Wong SC, Ali MAM: Hemoglobin E diseases: Hematological, analytical, and biosynthetic studies in homozygotes and double heterozygotes for alpha-thalassemia. *Am J Hematol* 13:15, 1982.

446. Fairbanks VF, Gilchrist GS, Brimhall B, Jereb JA, Goldston EC: Hemoglobin E trait reexamined: A cause of microcytosis and erythrocytosis. *Blood* 52:109, 1979.

447. Winichagoon P, Fucharoen S, Wilairat P, Chihara K, Fukumaki Y: Role of alternatively spliced beta E-globin mRNA on clinical severity of beta-thalassemia/hemoglobin E disease. *Southeast Asian J Trop Med Public Health* 26 (suppl)1:282, 1995.

448. Ruymann FB, Popejoy LA, Brouillard RB: Splenic sequestration and ineffective erythropoiesis in hemoglobin E-beta-thalassemia disease. *Pediatr Res* 12:1020, 1978.

449. Hathirat P, Isarangkura P, Numhom S, Opasathien P, Chuansumrit A: Results of the splenectomy in children with thalassemia. *J Med Assoc Thai* 72 (suppl 1):133, 1989.

450. Rees DC, Duley J, Simmonds HA, et al: Interaction of hemoglobin E and pyrimidine 5' nucleotidase deficiency. *Blood* 88:2761, 1996.

451. Huisman THJ, Carver MFH, Efremov GD: *A Syllabus of Human Hemoglobin Variants.* The Sickle Cell Anemia Foundation, Augusta, GA, 1996.

452. Edelstein SJ: Structure of the fibers of hemoglobin S. *Tex Rep Biol Med* 81:221, 1980.

453. Allison AC: Abnormal haemoglobin and erythrocyte enzyme-deficiency traits, in *Genetical Variations in Human Populations*, p 16. 1961.

454. Diggs LW: Sickle-cell crises. *Am J Clin Pathol* 44:1, 1965.

455. River GL, Robbins AB, Schwartz SO: SC Hemoglobin: A clinical study. *Blood* 18:385, 1961.

456. Harrow BR, Sloane JA, Lieberman NC: Roentgenologic demonstration of renal papillary necrosis in sickle-cell trait. *N Engl J Med* 268:969, 1963.

457. Paton D: Conjunctival sign of sickle cell disease. *Arch Ophthalmol* 68:627, 1962.

458. Diggs LW, Bell A: Intraerythrocytic hemoglobin crystals in sickle cell hemoglobin C disease. *Blood* 25:218, 1958.

459. Crookston JH, Irvine D, Beale D, Lehmann H: A new haemoglobin, J Toronto ($\alpha^{5Ala \rightarrow Asp}$). *Nature* 208:1059, 1965.

460. Schneider RG, Alperin JB, Beale D, Lehmann H: Hemoglobin I in an American Negro family: structural and hematologic studies. *J Lab Clin Med* 68:940, 1966.

461. Schneider RG, Jim RTS: A new haemoglobin variant (the 'Honolulu type') in a Chinese. *Nature* 190:454, 1961.

462. Ohba Y, Miyaji T, Hattori Y, Fuyuno K, Matsuoka M: Unstable hemoglobins in Japan. *Hemoglobin* 4:307, 1980.

463. Ingram VM: Abnormal human haemoglobins: III. The chemical difference between normal and sickle cell haemoglobins. *Biochim Biophys Acta* 36:402, 1959.

464. Hunt JA, Ingram VM: Abnormal human haemoglobins: IV. The chemical difference between normal human haemoglobin and haemoglobin C. *Biochim Biophys Acta* 42:409, 1960.

465. Idelson LI, Didkowsky NA, Casey R, Lorkin PA, Lehmann H: New unstable haemoglobin Hb Moscva, beta 24(B6) Gly$\rightarrow$Asp found in the U.S.S.R. *Nature* 249:768, 1974.

466. Beutler E, Lang A, Lehmann H: Hemoglobin Duarte ($\alpha_2\beta_2^{62Ala \rightarrow Pro}$): A new unstable hemoglobin with increased oxygen affinity. *Blood* 43:527, 1974.

467. Muller CJ, Kingma S: Haemoglobin Zurich: $\alpha_2\beta_2^{63\,Arg}$. *Biochim Biophys Acta* 50:595, 1961.

468. Bookchin RM, Nagel RL, Ranney HM, Jacobs AS: Hemoglobin C Harlem: a sickling variant containing amino acid substitutions in two residues of the beta-polypeptide chain. *Biochem Biophys Res Commun* 23:122, 1966.

469. Bonaventura J, Riggs A: Hemoglobin Kansas, a human hemoglobin with a neutral amino acid substitution and an abnormal oxygen equilibrium. *J Biol Chem* 243:980, 1968.

470. Wasi P, Pootrakul S, Na-Nakorn S, Beale D, Lehmann H: Haemoglobin D-beta Los Angeles (D$_{Punjab}\alpha_2\beta_2^{121\,GluNH2}$) in a Thai family. *Acta Haematol (Basel)* 39:151, 1968.

471. Larkin IL, Baker T, Lorkin PA, et al: Haemoglobin F Texas II ($\alpha_2\gamma_2^{6\,Glu \rightarrow Lys}$), the second of the haemoglobin F Texas variants. *Br J Haematol* 14:233, 1968.

472. Barnabas J, Muller CJ: Haemoglobin-Lepore$_{HOLLANDIA}$. *Nature* 194:931, 1962.

473. Honig GR, Shamsuddin M, Mason RG, Vida LN: Hemoglobin Lincoln Park: a betadelta fusion (anti-Lepore) variant with an amino acid deletion in the delta chain-derived segment. *Proc Natl Acad Sci USA* 75:1475, 1978.

474. Clegg JB, Weatherall DJ, Milner PF: Haemoglobin Constant Spring—a chain termination mutant? *Nature* 234:337, 1971.

475. Jones RT, Brimhall B, Huisman TH: Structural characterization of two delta chain variants. Hemoglobin A'- 2 (B2) and hemoglobin Flatbush. *J Biol Chem* 242:5141, 1967.

HEMOGLOBINOPATHIES ASSOCIATED WITH UNSTABLE HEMOGLOBIN

ERNEST BEUTLER

Mutations that cause destabilization of the hemoglobin tetramer are an uncommon cause of hemolytic anemia. In contrast to the hemolytic anemias caused by enzyme deficiencies, a dominant mode of inheritance characterizes the unstable hemoglobins. Heinz bodies are a characteristic feature of the red cells in the blood when splenectomy has been carried out. Hemolytic anemia may be precipitated by the ingestion of oxidative drugs. The diagnosis is established by precipitating the unstable hemoglobin in a system in which the hemolysate is heated or incubated in a mixture of isopropanol and buffer. Although splenectomy has occasionally ameliorated the anemia, it should be avoided in most cases, because it has sometimes been followed by fatal thromboembolic complications.

DEFINITION AND HISTORY

The sporadic occurrence of hemolytic anemia with the appearance of inclusion bodies in the red cells was occasionally observed in the 1940s and 1950s,[1-3] but it was not until 1962[4,5] that it was recognized that such patients had abnormal hemoglobins that spontaneously denatured within the circulating red cell. The unstable hemoglobins that will be discussed in this chapter are those that result from a mutation that changes the amino acid sequence of one of the globin chains. Homotetramers of normal β chains (hemoglobin H) or normal γ chains (hemoglobin Barts) are also unstable hemoglobins. These unstable hemoglobins occur in patients with α thalassemia and are discussed in Chap. 46. *Hyperunstable hemoglobins*[6] have defects that are so severe that the globin chain is not found in the red cells, but their formation can be deduced from the DNA sequence.

ETIOLOGY AND PATHOGENESIS

The tetrameric hemoglobin molecule has evolved so that a variety of noncovalent forces maintain the structure of each subunit and bind the subunits to each other. The delicate balance that allows the molecule to change from one state to another, facilitating its oxygen-binding function while maintaining its structural integrity, has been discussed in Chap. 28. It is not surprising that a variety of amino acid substitutions or deletions will weaken the forces that maintain the structure of hemoglobin. When this occurs, the hemoglobin molecule denatures and precipitates as insoluble globins. These precipitates often attach to the cell membrane and are recognized as Heinz bodies.

Instability of hemoglobin can arise from any one of the following processes:

1. Replacement of an amino acid that contacts the heme group or produces a change in the property of the heme pocket often results in an unstable molecule with a tendency to lose heme from the abnormal globin chains. Hb$_{Hammersmith}$,[7,8] Hb$_{Sendagi}$, Hb$_{Alesha}$,[10] and Hb$_{La Roche-sur-Yon}$[11] are examples of this type of unstable hemoglobin.

2. Replacement of nonpolar by polar residues at the interior of the molecule results in gross distortion of the protein, particularly if the new polar residue remains in the interior portion of the molecule, as in Hb$_{Bristol}$[12] and Hb$_{Volga}$.[13]

3. Deletions or insertions of additional amino acids, particularly when critical helical regions of the sequence are involved, creates instability, as in Hb$_{Niteroi}$[14] and Hb$_{Montreal}$.[15]

4. Replacements at intersubunit contacts, particularly those between the α1 and β1 chain, create instability so that dissociation into monomers may occur. Hb$_{Philly}$[16] and Hb$_{Tacoma}$[17] are mildly unstable for this reason. Replacements at the contact between the α1 and β2 globin monomers usually result in hemoglobins with a high oxygen affinity.

5. If proline is introduced into an α helix beyond the third residue, distortion of the helix results in instability.[18] Variants in which proline substitution results in instability include Hb$_{Duarte}$[19] and Hb$_{Santa Ana}$.[20]

6. In areas of the hemoglobin molecule in which atoms are very tightly packed, substitution of amino acids with larger side chains for glycine may produce marked changes in stability. In particular, at the points where the B and E helices approach each other there is no room for the substitution of larger amino acids for glycine at B6 and E8. Hb$_{Riverdale-Bronx}$,[21] Hb$_{Savannah}$,[22] and Hb$_{Moscva}$[23] arise in such a fashion.

7. Replacement of a hydrophobic residue that normally fits into a hydrophobic pocket with a more hydrophilic amino acid, such as the substitution of histidine for leucine at β81 in Hb$_{La Roche-sur-Yon}$.[11]

Many unstable hemoglobins have an increased susceptibility to oxidation to methemoglobin. However, the exact sequence of events that leads to the precipitation of hemoglobin is not fully understood and very likely varies with different unstable hemoglobins. The formation of hemichromes may be involved. These are compounds in which heme has been removed from its normal binding site and has become bonded to another part of the globin molecule.[24] These pigments can be shown to form during in vitro denaturation of some abnormal hemoglobins,[25] and they are present in hemoglobin H inclusion bodies.[26] The release of activated oxygen in the form of superoxide radicals with the subsequent formation of peroxide and the hydroxyl radicals[27,28] may also play a role. The attachment of Heinz bodies to the cell membrane impairs the deformability of the erythrocyte and impedes its ability to negotiate the narrow spaces between the endothelial cells lining the splenic sinuses. The "pitting" of Heinz bodies from the erythrocyte results in loss of membrane and ultimately in destruction of the red cells. Although Heinz bodies are formed, their presence in the blood does not become a prominent feature except in patients who have been splenectomized (see "Laboratory Features"). Selected unstable hemoglobins that have been characterized are listed in Table 48-1. Detailed tabulations are available.[29]

Hyperunstable hemoglobins are characterized by β-globin formation that is so defective that no β-chains are found. However, they differ from the β-thalassemias in that inheritance is dominant, i.e., a single copy of the mutant gene is all that is required to give the clinical phenotype. They may be due to single base substitution, deletion of codons, frameshifts leading to elonged β-chains, or premature terminations.[30]

MODE OF INHERITANCE

Unstable hemoglobins are generally inherited as autosomal dominant disorders. Affected individuals are usually heterozygotes who have inherited the defect from one of their parents and who on the average

TABLE 48-1   THE UNSTABLE HEMOGLOBINS

HEMOGLOBIN	SUBSTITUTION
Torino	α43 Phe$\rightarrow$Val
Hasharon† (Sinai, Sealy)	α47 Asp$\rightarrow$His
Iwata	α87 His$\rightarrow$Arg
Petah Tikva	α100 Ala$\rightarrow$Asp
Freiburg	β23 Val deleted
Riverdale-Bronx	β24 Gly$\rightarrow$Arg
Yokohama	β31 Leu$\rightarrow$Pro
Castilla	β32 Leu$\rightarrow$Arg
Perth† (Abraham Lincoln)	β32 Leu$\rightarrow$Pro
Philly	β35 Tyr$\rightarrow$Phe
Hammersmith	β42 Phe$\rightarrow$Ser
Bucuresti† (Louisville)	β42 Phe$\rightarrow$Leu
Niteroi	β42-44 or β43-45 Phe, Glu, Ser deleted
Duarte	β62 Ala$\rightarrow$Pro
Zürich	β63 His$\rightarrow$Arg
Bristol	β67 Val$\rightarrow$Asp
Sydney	β67 Val$\rightarrow$Ala
Mizuho	β68 Leu$\rightarrow$Pro
Seattle	β70 Ala$\rightarrow$Asp
Christchurch	β71 Phe$\rightarrow$Ser
Shepherd's Bush	β74 Gly$\rightarrow$Asp
Bushwick	β74 Gly$\rightarrow$Val
Buenos Aires† (Bryn Mawr)	β85 Phe$\rightarrow$Ser
Santa Ana	β88 Leu$\rightarrow$Pro
Redondo	β92 His$\rightarrow$Asn$\rightarrow$Asp
St. Etienne† (Istanbul)	β92 His$\rightarrow$Gln
Gun Hill	β91-95 or 92-96 or 93-97 Leu, Cys, Asp, His deleted
Köln† (Ube I)	β98 Val$\rightarrow$Met
Djelfa	β98 Val$\rightarrow$Ala
Presbyterian	β108 Asn$\rightarrow$Lys
Shelby (Deaconess)	β131 Gln$\rightarrow$Lys
North Shore	β134 Val$\rightarrow$Glu
Coventry	β141 Leu deleted
Tak	Elongation of β-chain C-terminus
Cranston	Elongation of β-chain C-terminus
La Grange	γ101 Glu$\rightarrow$Lys
Poole	γ130 Trp$\rightarrow$Gly

†The parentheses indicate alternative names for these variants but are not intended to suggest that one or the other name is to be preferred.

will transmit it to one-half of their offspring. Since unstable hemoglobins produce a disease state, genes for these disorders are subjected to negative selection, and the continued existence of the unstable hemoglobinopathies in the population is the result of such new mutations. Thus, occasionally patients with an unstable hemoglobin are encountered neither of whose parents had the abnormality. The homozygous state for the unstable hemoglobins Hb$_{\text{Sun Prairie}}$[31] and Hb$_{\text{Bushwick}}$[32] have been observed, and a homozygous-like state can occur when an unstable β chain mutation is inherited together with a β^o thalassemic gene.[19,33]

Over 80 percent of unstable hemoglobins that have been characterized affect the β chain. This probably reflects the fact that the normal genome contains four copies of the α chain. The clinical effects of such mutants, affecting only one-fourth of the total hemoglobin formed, is apt to be less pronounced than those of β-chain mutants, in which one-half of the hemoglobin produced is abnormal. Thus, many α-globin mutations are likely to be overlooked.

Although most patients with unstable hemoglobins have been found to have a combination of hemoglobin A and the unstable hemoglobin in their red cells, there are a number of reports of the inheritance of unstable hemoglobins with other hemoglobinopathies.[19,34–38]

CLINICAL FEATURES

A broad spectrum of clinical manifestations can be induced by unstable hemoglobins. In most cases, hemolysis is well compensated, and some

hemoglobins that are unstable in vitro (e.g., Hb$_{\text{Muscat}}$[39]) are not associated with hemolysis at all. When an unstable hemoglobin also has a left-shifted oxygen dissociation curve, i.e., a raised O_2 affinity, the hemoglobin level may be in the upper portion of the normal range. Episodes of infection and treatment with "oxidant" drugs are likely to precipitate hemolytic episodes in persons whose anemia is well compensated under ordinary circumstances. It is at this juncture that the diagnosis is often first made. In the case of patients who have particularly unstable variants, such as Hb$_{\text{Hammersmith}}$,[7] Hb$_{\text{Bristol}}$,[12] Hb$_{\text{Santa Ana}}$,[20] or Hb$_{\text{Madrid}}$,[40] a chronic hemolytic anemia may become evident during the first year of life as γ chain production is replaced by production of the mutant β chain. In contrast, in the rare instances where the γ chain bears the abnormality,[41] the hemolytic anemia is evident at birth, and it disappears as normal β chains are formed.

Physical findings include jaundice, splenomegaly, and, when the anemia is severe, pallor. In some patients, dark urine has been observed, probably as a result of the excretion of dipyrrole pigments derived from the catabolism of free heme groups or of Heinz bodies.[42] In some instances methemoglobulinemia may develop, and cyanosis may then be evident.

LABORATORY FEATURES

The hemoglobin concentration of the blood may be normal or decreased. The mean corpuscular hemoglobin is usually diminished because of the loss of hemoglobin from the red cells as a result of its denaturation and subsequent pitting from the erythrocytes. The blood film may show slight hypochromia, and, in addition, poikilocytosis, polychromasia, anisocytosis, and some basophilic stippling may be evident. Hyperunstable hemoglobins, in particular, are associated with severe hypochromia of the erythrocytes and present clinically as dominant β-thalassemia. Reticulocytosis is often out of proportion to the severity of the anemia, particularly when the abnormal hemoglobin has a high oxygen affinity. After splenectomy many Heinz bodies may be found in the circulation. Hemoglobin F levels may be increased.[43]

Diagnosis of this disorder usually depends upon the demonstration of the presence of an unstable hemoglobin. Three tests are used for this purpose. The most convenient is the isopropanol stability test.[44] The heat stability test is also useful[45] but is somewhat more difficult to interpret. It has been found, however, that at least one unstable hemoglobin, hemoglobin Olmsted, can be detected by heat stability but not isopropanol stability.[46] Finally, incubation of blood with brilliant cresyl blue generates Heinz bodies in hemoglobin H disease.[47,48] Further identification of unstable hemoglobins is aided by procedures such as hemoglobin electrophoresis; however, the electrophoretic pattern is often normal, and the diagnosis of the hemoglobinopathy cannot be ruled out in this way. The oxygen affinity of unstable hemoglobins is often altered, and the determination of the P_{50} may help in detecting and characterizing the unstable hemoglobin. In the final analysis unstable hemoglobins can be identified only by DNA analysis[10,43,49,50] or by physical separation of the abnormal hemoglobin from the normal hemoglobin, followed by globin chain separation and peptide analysis.

DIFFERENTIAL DIAGNOSIS

The possibility that an unstable hemoglobin is present should be considered in all patients who present with the clinical picture of hereditary nonspherocytic hemolytic anemia (Chap. 45), particularly when hypochromia of the red cells is present and when the extent of the reticulocytosis is out of keeping with the degree of anemia. Not all patients with a positive test for unstable hemoglobins should be classified as having this disorder. The stability of methemoglobin, hemoglobin F, and sickle hemoglobin is appreciably less than that of hemoglobin A, and false-positive isopropanol stability tests may be obtained in patients with increased quantities of these hemoglobins. Hemoglobin H ($\beta 4$) and hemoglobin Barts ($\gamma 4$) are unstable. These fast-moving hemoglobins can be detected on electrophoresis. Patients whose red cells contain these hemoglobins are diagnosed as having α thalassemia (see Chap. 46).

Sometimes the hemoglobins are so unstable that none of the protein can be detected. Such abnormal hemoglobins have been diagnosed by DNA-based analysis.[10,43,49,50]

TREATMENT, COURSE, AND PROGNOSIS

Most patients with unstable hemoglobins follow a relatively benign course. As with other hemolytic states, gallstones are common, and cholecystectomy may be required. Hemolytic episodes may be precipitated by infection or by the ingestion of "oxidative" drugs. Sulfonamides have been particularly prominent in inducing hemolysis, and derivatives that do not produce hemolysis in G-6-PD deficiency have been shown to precipitate hemolysis in patients with some unstable hemoglobins. A few deaths that are believed to have been directly related to unstable hemoglobins have been reported. A patient with Hb_Hirosaki is thought to have died following a hemolytic crisis precipitated by a common cold.[51] Two sisters with Hb_Duarte[19] died of thromboembolic complications less than a year following splenectomy. This unstable variant has an increased oxygen affinity, and it is likely that a combination of postsplenectomy erythrocytosis and thrombocytosis led to the demise of the patients.

Treatment is not usually required. As in the case of other hemolytic disorders, folic acid in a dose of 1 mg per day is often given, but its usefulness has not been established. "Oxidant" drugs such as those listed in Table 45-5 should be avoided. In addition, the use of all sulfonamides should be eschewed, particularly in the case of those variants which have been associated with drug-induced hemolysis. Splenectomy has proved to be useful in some patients with splenomegaly and severe hemolysis,[52,53] while others have enjoyed little benefit.[46] In view of the fact that patients with high-oxygen-affinity unstable hemoglobin have died after a splenectomy[19] and that thromboembolic complications have been reported in a number of other patients,[54] it is probably best to avoid splenectomy. Preliminary results suggested that hydroxyurea therapy might be useful,[53] presumably by increasing the level of fetal hemoglobin.

REFERENCES

1. Cathie IAB: Apparent idiopathic Heinz body anaemia. *Great Ormond St J* 3:343, 1952.
2. Lange RD, Akeroyd JH: Congenital hemolytic anemia with abnormal pigment metabolism and red cell inclusion bodies: a new clinical syndrome. *Blood* 13:950, 1958.
3. Schmid R, Brecher G, Clemens T: Familial hemolytic anemia with erythrocyte inclusion bodies and a defect in pigment metabolism. *Blood* 14:991, 1959.
4. Grimes AJ, Meisler A: Possible cause of Heinz bodies in congenital Heniz-body anaemia. *Nature* 194:190, 1962.
5. Frick PG, Hitzig WH, Betke K: Hemoglobin Zurich. I. A new hemoglobin anomaly associated with acute hemolytic episodes with inclusion bodies after sulfonamide therapy. *Blood* 20:261, 1962.
6. Thein SL: Dominant beta thalassaemia: molecular basis and pathophysiology. *Br J Haematol* 80:273, 1992.
7. Dacie JV, Shinton NK, Gaffney PJ, Carrell RW, Lehmann H: Haemoglobin Hammersmith (beta-42(CD1)Phe→Ser). *Nature* 216:663, 1967.
8. Rahbar S, Feagler RJ, Beutler E: Hemoglobin Hammersmith associated with severe hemolytic anemia. *Hemoglobin* 5:97, 1981.
9. Ogata K, Ito T, Okazaki T, et al: Hemoglobin Sendagi (beta 42 Phe→Val): a new unstable hemoglobin variant having an amino acid substitution at CD1 of the beta-chain. *Hemoglobin* 10:469, 1986.
10. Molchanova TP, Postnikov YV, Pobedimskaya DD, et al: Hb Alesha or Alpha_2Beta_267(E11)Val→Met: a new unstable hemoglobin variant identified through sequencing of amplified DNA. *Hemoglobin* 17:217, 1993.
11. Wajcman H, Kister J, Vasseur C, et al: Structure of the EF corner favors deamidation of asparaginyl residues in hemoglobin: the example of Hb La Roche-sur-Yon [$\beta 81$ (EF5) Leu→His]. *Biochim Biophys Acta* 1138:127, 1992.
12. Sakuragawa M, Ohba Y, Miyaji T, Yamamoto K, Miwa S: A Japanese boy with hemolytic anemia due to an unstable hemoglobin (Hb Bristol). *Nippon Ketsueki Gakkai Zasshi* 47:896, 1984.
13. Idelson LI, Didkovsky NA, Filippova AV, et al: Haemoglobin Volga, beta 27 (B9) Ala→Asp: a new highly unstable haemoglobin with a suppressed charge. *FEBS Lett* 58:122, 1975.
14. Praxedes H, Wiltshire BG, Lehmann H: *Proceedings of the International Symposium on Standardization in Haematology and Clinical Pathology, Medical Edition Archivio, "Casa Sollievo della Sofferenza"*, 2nd ed, edited by SG Rotondo, p 11. C.I.S.M.E.L., Foggia, Italy, 1972
15. Plaseska D, Dimovski AJ, Wilson JB, et al: Hemoglobin Montreal: a new variant with an extended beta chain due to a deletion of Asp, Gly, Leu at positions 73, 74, and 75, and an insertion of Ala, Arg, Cys, Gln at the same location. *Blood* 77:178, 1991.
16. Rieder RF, Oski FA, Clegg JB: Hemoglobin Philly (beta 35 tyrosine → phenylalanine): studies in the molecular pathology of hemoglobins. *J Clin Invest* 48:1627, 1969.
17. Idelson LI, Didkovsky NA, Casey R, Lorkin PA, Lehmann H: Structure and function of haemoglobin Tacoma (beta 30 Arg→Ser) found in a second family. *Acta Haematol (Basel)* 52:303, 1974.
18. Perutz MF, Kendrew JC, Watson HC: Structure and function of haemoglobin. II. Some relations between polypeptide chain configuration and amino acid sequence. *J Mol Biol* 13:669, 1965.
19. Beutler E, Lang A, Lehmann H: Hemoglobin Duarte: ($\alpha_2\beta_2$62[E6] Ala→Pro): a new unstable hemoglobin with increased oxygen affinity. *Blood* 43:527, 1974.
20. Fairbanks VF, Opfell RW, Burgert EO: Three families with unstable hemoglobinopathies (Köln, Olmsted and Santa Ana) causing hemolytic anemia with inclusion bodies and pigmenturia. *Am J Med* 46:344, 1969.
21. Ranney HM, Jacobs AS, Udem L, Zalusky R: Hemoglobin Riverdale-Bronx, an unstable hemoglobin resulting from the substitution of arginine for glycine at helical residue B6 of the beta polypeptide chain. *Biochem Biophys Res Commun* 33:1004, 1968.
22. Huisman THJ, Brown AK, Efremov GD, et al: Hemoglobin Savannah (B6²⁴ beta glycine→valine): an unstable variant causing anemia with inclusion bodies. *J Clin Invest* 50:650, 1971.
23. Idelson LI, Didkowsky NA, Casey R, Lorkin PA, Lehmann H: New unstable haemoglobin Hb Moscva, beta 24(B6) Gly→Asp found in the U.S.S.R. *Nature* 249:768, 1974.
24. Winterbourn CC: Oxidative denaturation in congenital hemolytic anemias: the unstable hemoglobins. *Semin Hematol* 27:41, 1990.
25. Rachmilewitz EA, White JM: Haemichrome formation during the *in vitro* oxidation of haemoglobin Köln. *Nature (New Biol)* 241:115, 1973.
26. Rachmilewitz EA, Peisach J, Bradley TB, Blumberg WE: Role of haemichromes in the formation of inclusion bodies in haemoglobin H disease. *Nature* 222:248, 1969.
27. Carrell RW, Winterbourn CC, Rachmilewitz EA: Activated oxygen and haemolysis. *Br J Haematol* 30:259, 1975.
28. Winterbourn CC, McGrath BM, Carrell RW: Reactions involving superoxide and normal and unstable haemoglobins. *Biochem J* 155:493, 1976.
29. Huisman THJ, Carver MFH, Efremov GD: *A Syllabus of Human Hemoglobin Variants*, The Sickle Cell Anemia Foundation, Augusta, GA, 1996.
30. Cao A, Galanello R, Rosatelli MC: Genotype-phenotype correlations in beta-thalassemias. *Blood Rev* 8:1, 1994.
31. Ho PJ, Rochette J, Rees DC, et al: Hb Sun Prairie: diagnostic pitfalls in thalassemic hemoglobinopathies. *Hemoglobin* 20:103, 1996.
32. Srivastava P, Kaeda JS, Roper D, et al: Severe hemolytic anemia associated with the homozygous state for an unstable hemoglobin variant (Hb Bushwick). *Blood* 86:1977, 1995.
33. Loukopoulos D, Fessas P, Kister J, et al: Hemoglobin Köln occurring in association with a beta zero thalassemia: hematologic and functional consequences. *Blood* 74:496, 1989.
34. King MAR, Wiltshire BG, Lehmann H, Morimoto H: An unstable

haemoglobin with reduced oxygen affinity: haemoglobin Peterborough beta-111 (G13) valine→phenylalanine, its interaction with normal haemoglobin and haemoglobin Lepore. *Br J Haematol* 22:125, 1972.

35. Casey R, Lang A, Lehmann H, Shinton NK: Double heterozygosity for two unstable haemoglobins: Hb Sydney beta-67(E11)Val→Ala and Hb Coventry beta-141(H19) Leu deleted. *Br J Haematol* 33:143, 1976.

36. Lutcher CL, Huisman THJ: Hemoglobin Leslie, an unstable variant due to deletion of Gln beta-131 occurring in combination with beta-thalassemia, Hb S and Hb C. *Clin Res* 23:278A, 1975.

37. Beuzard Y, Basset P, Braconnier F, et al: Haemoglobin Saki alpha₂ beta₂^Leu→ProA11 structure and function. *Biochim Biophys Acta* 393:182, 1975.

38. Tentori L: Three examples of double heterozygosis: Beta-thalassemia and rare hemoglobinopathies, in *Hematologic Contributions to Fetal Health*, p 68. Istanbul, 1974.

39. Ramachandran M, Gu LH, Wilson JB, et al: A new variant, Hb Muscat [alpha 2 beta (2)32(B14)Leu→Val] observed in association with Hb S in an Arabian family. *Hemoglobin* 16:259, 1992.

40. Outeirino J, Casey R, White JM, Lehmann H: Haemoglobin Madrid beta 115 (G17) alanine→proline: an unstable variant associated with haemolytic anaemia. *Acta Haematol (Basel)* 52:53, 1974.

41. Lee-Potter JP, Deacon-Smith RA, Simpkiss MJ, Kamuzora H, Lehmann H: A new cause of haemolytic anaemia in the newborn. A description of an unstable fetal haemoglobin: F Poole, $\alpha_2{}^G\gamma_2$ 130 tryptophan to glycine. *J Clin Pathol* 28:317, 1975.

42. Kreimer-Birnbaum M, Pinkerton PH, Bannerman RM, Hutchison HE: Dipyrolic urinary pigments in congenital Heinz-body anaemia due to Hb Köln and thalassaemia. *BMJ* 2:396, 1966.

43. Keeling MM, Bertolone SJ, Baysal E, et al: Hb Mizuho or alpha 2 beta (2)68(E12)Leu→Pro in a Caucasian boy with high levels of Hb F; identification by sequencing of amplified DNA. *Hemoglobin* 15:477, 1991.

44. Carrell RW, Kay R: A simple method for the detection of unstable haemoglobins. *Br J Haematol* 23:615, 1972.

45. Dacie JV, Grimes AJ, Meisler A, et al: Hereditary Heinz-body anaemia. A report of studies on five patients with mild anaemia. *Br J Haematol* 10:388, 1964.

46. Phyliky RL, Fairbanks VF: Thromboembolic complication of splenectomy in unstable hemoglobin disorders: Hb Olmsted, Hb Koln. *Am J Hematol* 55:53, 1997.

47. Skogerboe KJ, West SF, Smith C, et al: Screening for alpha-thalassemia. Correlation of hemoglobin H inclusion bodies with DNA-determined genotype [see comments]. *Arch Pathol Lab Med* 116:1012, 10-1992.

48. Winterbourn CC, Carrell RW: Studies of hemoglobin denaturation and Heinz body formation in the unstable hemoglobins. *J Clin Invest* 54:678, 1974.

49. Girodon E, Ghanem N, Vidaud M, et al: Rapid molecular characterization of mutations leading to unstable hemoglobin β-chain variants. *Ann Hematol* 65:188, 1992.

50. Landin B, Astrom M: Unstable haemoglobin causing haemolytic anaemia: de novo mutation in Sweden identified by PCR. *J Intern Med* 233:299, 1993.

51. Ohba Y, Miyaji T, Matsuoka M, et al: Hemoglobin Hirosaki (alpha 43 (CD1) Phe→Leu): a new unstable variant. *Biochim Biophys Acta* 405:155, 1975.

52. Vichinsky EP, Lubin BH: Unstable hemoglobins, hemoglobins with altered oxygen affinity, and M-hemoglobins. *Pediatr Clin North Am* 27:421, 1980.

53. Rose C, Bauters F, Galacteros F: Hydroxyurea therapy in highly unstable hemoglobin carriers. *Blood* 88:2807, 1996.

54. Thuret I, Bardakdjian J, Badens C, et al: Priapism following splenectomy in an unstable hemoglobin: Hemoglobin Olmsted beta141 (H19) Leu→Arg. *Am J Hematol* 51:133, 1996.

METHEMOGLOBINEMIA AND OTHER CAUSES OF CYANOSIS

ERNEST BEUTLER

Cyanosis, blue discoloration of the skin and mucous membranes, is usually due to a change in the color of hemoglobin. Commonly this is due to a high concentration of deoxyhemoglobin because of cardiorespiratory failure or right-to-left shunting. Cyanosis also may indicate that an abnormal hemoglobin is present or that there is an increased concentration of a normally present hemoglobin derivative. Methemoglobin is a reversible oxidation product of hemoglobin and can be present in excess amounts either because of rapid oxidation of hemoglobin by drugs or toxic chemicals or because of a hereditary defect in the methemoglobin-reducing system. Hemoglobins M are mutant hemoglobins that cannot be adequately reduced by the enzymatic systems of the red cell. Sulfhemoglobins are irreversible denaturation products of hemoglobin which can produce cyanosis even when present in relatively low and harmless quantities.

Toxic methemoglobinemia is effectively treated by intravenous infusion of methylene blue, which links the highly efficient NADPH-reducing system to methemoglobin.

DEFINITION AND HISTORY

A bluish discoloration of the skin and mucous membranes, designated cyanosis, has been recognized since antiquity as a manifestation of lung or heart disease. Cyanosis resulting from drug administration has also been recognized since before 1890.[1] Toxic methemoglobinemia occurs when various drugs or toxic substances either oxidize hemoglobin directly in the circulation or facilitate its oxidation by molecular oxygen.

In 1912 Sloss and Wybauw reported a case of a patient with idiopathic methemoglobinemia.[2] Later Hitzenberger[3] suggested that a hereditary form of methemoglobinemia might exist, and subsequently numerous such cases were reported.[4] In 1948 Hörlein and Weber[5] described a family in which eight members over four generations manifested cyanosis. The absorption spectrum of methemoglobin was abnormal. They demonstrated that the defect must reside in the globin portion of the molecule. Subsequently Singer suggested that such abnormal hemoglobins be given the designation hemoglobin M.[6]

The existence of abnormal hemoglobins that cause cyanosis through quite another mechanism was first recognized in 1968 with the description of hemoglobin Kansas.[7] Here the cyanosis was not due to methemoglobin, as occurs in hemoglobin M, but rather to an abnormally low oxygen affinity of the mutant hemoglobin. Thus, at normal oxygen tensions a large amount of deoxygenated hemoglobin is present in the blood.

Acronyms and abbreviations that appear in this chapter include: G-6-PD, glucose-6-phosphate dehydrogenase.

The cause of still another form of methemoglobinemia that occurs independently of drug administration and without the existence of any abnormality of the globin portion of hemoglobin was first explained by Gibson,[8] who clearly pointed to the site of the enzyme defect, NADH diaphorase.

Sulfhemoglobinemia refers to the presence in the blood of hemoglobin derivatives that are defined by their characteristic absorption of light at 620 nm even in the presence of cyanide.

ETIOLOGY AND PATHOGENESIS

Methemoglobinemia decreases the oxygen-carrying capacity of blood, because the oxidized iron cannot reversibly bind oxygen. Moreover, when one or more iron atoms have been oxidized, the conformation of hemoglobin is changed so as to increase the oxygen affinity of the remaining ferrous heme groups. In this way methemoglobinemia exerts a dual effect in impairing the supply of oxygen to tissues.[9]

TOXIC METHEMOGLOBINEMIA

Hemoglobin is continuously oxidized in vivo from the ferrous to the ferric state. The rate of such oxidation is accelerated by many drugs and toxic chemicals, including sulfonamides, lidocaine and other aniline derivatives, and nitrites. A vast number of chemical substances may cause methemoglobinemia.[10–12] Some of the agents that are responsible for clinically significant methemoglobinemia in current clinical practice are listed in Table 49-1.

NADH-DIAPHORASE DEFICIENCY

NADH diaphorase catalyzes a step in the major pathway for methemoglobin reduction. This enzyme reduces cytochrome b_5, using NADH as a hydrogen donor. The reduced cytochrome b_5 reduces, in turn, methemoglobin to hemoglobin (see Chap. 26). A steady-state methemoglobin level is achieved when the rate of methemoglobin formation equals the rate of methemoglobin reduction, either through the NADH-diaphorase system or through the relatively minor auxiliary mechanisms such as direct chemical reduction by ascorbate and reduced glutathione. A NADPH-linked enzyme, NADPH diaphorase, does not play a role in methemoglobin reduction except when a linking dye such as methylene blue is supplied (see "Treatment," below). A marked diminution in the activity of NADH diaphorase will result in the accumulation of the brown pigment in circulating erythrocytes.

Accordingly, hereditary deficiency of the enzyme that reduces cytochrome b_5, NADH diaphorase (sometimes designated cytochrome b_5 reductase), is one of the causes of methemoglobinemia. A number of mutations of NADH diaphorase have been identified at the nucleotide level.[41–49]

Most of the patients with this disorder merely have methemoglobinemia, and these have been classified as having type I disease. In type II disease, deficiency also exists in nonerythroid cells, such as fibroblasts and lymphocytes.[50] Patients with this form of disease are afflicted, in addition to methemoglobinemia, with a progressive encephalopathy and with mental retardation. The finding that fatty acid elongation is defective in the platelets and leukocytes of such patients[51] may provide a clue to the type of defect that could occur in the central nervous system, where fatty acid elongation plays an important role in myelination. Occasionally patients with deficiency of NADH diaphorase in nonerythroid cells do not suffer any neurologic disorder, and it has been suggested that they be designated as having type III disease.[42,52]

A combination of both increased hemoglobin oxidation and decreased methemoglobin reduction also may occur. Since the activity of NADH diaphorase is normally low in newborn infants,[53] they are

TABLE 49-1 SOME DRUGS THAT CAUSE METHEMOGLOBINEMIA

DRUG	REFERENCE
Phenazopyridine (Pyridium)	(13) (14,15)
Sulfamethoxazole	(16)
Dapsone	(17) (18,19)
Aniline	(20) (21)
Paraquat/monolinuron	(22) 23)
Nitrate	(24) (25)
Nitroglycerin	(26) (13)
Amyl nitrite	(27)
Isobutyl nitrite	(28)
Sodium nitrite	(29) (30)
Benzocaine	(31) (32–34)
Prilocaine	(35) (36,37)
Methylene blue	(38)
EMLA creme	(39)
Clofazimine	(40)

particularly susceptible to the development of methemoglobinemia. Thus, serious degrees of methemoglobinemia have been observed in infants as a result of toxic materials, such as aniline dyes used on diapers,[54] and the ingestion of nitrate-contaminated water.[55] Bacterial action in the intestinal tract may reduce nitrates to nitrites, which in turn cause methemoglobinemia. In rural areas, fatal methemoglobinuria in infants due to wells contaminated with nitrates still occurs.[56]

Heterozygotes for NADH-diaphorase deficiency are not usually clinically methemoglobinemic. However, under the stress of administration of drugs which normally induce only slight, clinically unimportant, methemoglobinemia such persons may become severely cyanotic because of methemoglobinemia.[57]

An animal model of NADH-diaphorase deficiency has been described in the cat.[58-60]

HEMOGLOBINS M

The molecular mechanisms by which hemoglobin binds oxygen and releases it are discussed in detail in Chapter 28. Heme is held in a hydrophobic "heme pocket" between the E and F α-helices of each of the four globin chains. The iron atom in the heme forms four bonds with the pyrrole nitrogen atoms of the porphyrin ring and a fifth covalent bond with the imidazole nitrogen of a histidine residue in the nearby F α-helix (Fig. 49-1).[61] This histidine, residue 87 in the α chain and 92 in the β chain, is designated as the proximal histidine. On the opposite side of the porphyrin ring the iron atom lies adjacent to another histidine residue to which, however, it is not covalently bonded. This distal histidine occupies position 58 in the α chain and position 63 in the β chain. Under normal circumstances oxygen is occasionally discharged from the heme pocket as a superoxide anion, removing an electron from the iron and leaving it in the ferric state. The enzymatic machinery of the red cell efficiently reduces the iron to the divalent form, converting the methemoglobin to hemoglobin (see Chap. 26).

In most of the hemoglobins M, tyrosine has been substituted for either the proximal or the distal histidine. Tyrosine can form an iron-phenolate complex that resists reduction to the divalent state by the normal metabolic systems of the erythrocyte. Four hemoglobins M are a consequence of substitution of tyrosine for histidine in the proximal and distal sites of the α and β chains. As shown in Table 49-2, these four hemoglobins M have been designated by the geographic names Boston, Saskatoon, Iwate, and Hyde Park. Analogous His→Tyr substitutions in the α chain of fetal hemoglobin have also been documented and have been designated hemoglobins FM-Osaka[62] and FM-Fort Ripley.[63]

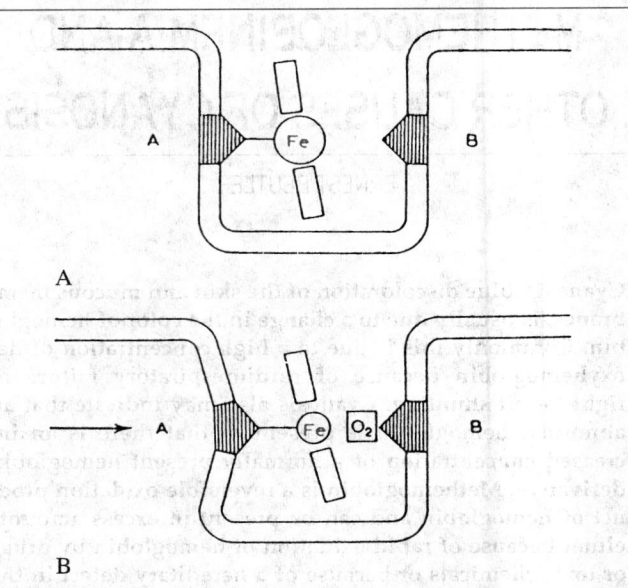

FIGURE 49-1   Diagrammatic representation of the heme group inserted into the heme pocket. A, proximal histidine; B, distal histidine. (a) In the deoxygenated form the larger ferrous atom lies out of the plane of the porphyrin ring. (b) In the oxygenated form the now smaller "ferric-like" atom can slip into the plane of the porphyrin ring. As a result, the proximal histidine and the helix F into which it is incorporated are displaced. (Lehmann and Huntsman,[61] with permission.)

Another hemoglobin M, Hb M$_{Milwaukee}$, is formed by substitution of glutamic acid for valine in the sixty-seventh residue of the β chain rather than substitution of tyrosine for histidine. The glutamic acid side chain points toward the heme group, and its γ-carboxyl group interacts with the iron atom, stabilizing it in the ferric state.

It is rare for methemoglobinemia to occur as result of hemoglobinopathies other than hemoglobin M, but hemoglobin$_{Chile}$ (β28 Leu→ Met) is such a hemoglobin. Producing hemolysis only with drug administration, this unstable hemoglobin is characterized clinically by chronic methemoglobinemia.[70]

LOW-OXYGEN AFFINITY HEMOGLOBINS

In some hemoglobin variants the deoxy conformation of the hemoglobin molecule is favored because the angle of the heme is altered from that found normally in deoxyhemoglobin. Such changes occur in Hb$_{Hammersmith}$, Hb$_{Bucuresti}$, Hb$_{Torino}$, and Hb$_{Peterborough}$. In other instances the quaternary conformation is changed by mutations involving the $\alpha_1\beta_2$ contact (Hb$_{Kansas}$, Hb$_{Titusville}$, and Hb$_{Yoshizuka}$). Properties of abnormal hemoglobins associated with low oxygen affinity are summarized in Table 49-3.

In response to the improved tissue oxygen supply brought about by a right-shifted oxygen dissociation curve, the "oxygen sensor"[73] of the body decreases the output of erythropoietin.[71] As a result, the steady state level of hemoglobin is diminished; mild anemia is characteristic of patients with hemoglobins with a decreased oxygen affinity.

SULFHEMOGLOBIN

Sulfhemoglobin derives its name from the fact that it can be produced in vitro from the action of hydrogen sulfide on hemoglobin[74] and that the feeding of elemental sulfur to dogs has been associated with sulfhemoglobinemia.[75] Sulfhemoglobin may contain one excess sulfur atom.[76-78] Sulfhemoglobinemia has been associated with the ingestion of various drugs, particularly sulfonamides, phenacetin, acetanilid, and phenazopyridine.[79,80] It also occurs independent of drug use and has been thought to be related to chronic constipation or to purging.[81] Some patients with sulfhemoglobinemia or a past history of this disorder appear to have increased levels of red blood cell GSH.[82] The reason for this increase and its relationship to sulfhemoglobinemia is not clearly understood, but it may be of significance that some of the types of drugs which have been associated with sulfhemoglobinemia cause an elevation of red cell GSH levels,[83] probably by activating the enzyme glutathione synthetase[83] or by increasing intracellular glutamate levels.[84]

MODE OF INHERITANCE

Cyanosis due to abnormal hemoglobins is inherited as an autosomal dominant disorder. In contrast, hereditary methemoglobinemia due to NADH-diaphorase deficiency is inherited in an autosomal recessive fashion. Evidence for the occurrence of hereditary sulfhemoglobinemia[85] is not convincing, and it is likely that the single family reported represents a hemoglobin M hemoglobinopathy.

CLINICAL FEATURES

Methemoglobinemia may be chronic or acute. Severe acute methemoglobinemia, usually the consequence of drug ingestion or toxic exposure, can produce symptoms of anemia, since methemoglobin lacks the capacity to transport oxygen. Acutely developing levels of methemoglobin exceeding 60 to 70 percent of the total pigment may be associated with vascular collapse, coma, and death,[24,29] although recovery was documented in one patient with a level as high as 81.5% of the total pigment.[86]

Chronic methemoglobinemia, whether due to exposure to drugs or toxins or to hereditary causes, is usually asymptomatic. In instances when the methemoglobin levels are very high (>20% of the total pigment) mild erythrocytosis is occasionally noted. Patients with hemoglobins M or with low oxygen affinity hemoglobin also manifest cyanosis. In the case of α-chain variants, the dusky color of the infants will be noted at birth, but the clinical manifestations of β-chain variants become apparent only after β-chains have largely replaced the fetal α-chains at 6 to 9 months of age. In spite of the impaired hemoglobin function, no cardiopulmonary symptoms are observed and there is no clubbing. In the case of Hb M$_{Saskatoon}$ and Hb M$_{Hyde Park}$ hemolytic anemia with jaundice may be present. The hemolytic state may be exacerbated by administration of sulfonamides.[87]

LABORATORY FEATURES

TOXIC METHEMOGLOBINEMIA

In toxic methemoglobinemia an elevated level of methemoglobin is found, but the activity of NADH diaphorase is normal.

NADH-DIAPHORASE DEFICIENCY

In hereditary methemoglobinemia due to NADH-diaphorase deficiency, between 8 and 40 percent of the hemoglobin is in the oxidized (methemoglobin) form. The blood may have a chocolate-brown color. NADH-diaphorase activity is best measured using ferricyanide as a receptor, measuring the rate of oxidation of NADH.[88,89] The residual level of enzyme activity is usually less than 20 percent of normal in patients with methemoglobinemia due to deficiency of this enzyme. An immunoassay has been described,[90] but such an assay would not detect mutants in which enzyme molecules with impaired catalytic activity are present. For unknown reasons, glutathione reductase activity is usually also diminished.[91] Cytochrome b$_5$ assays[92] may be useful if diaphorase activity is normal.

TABLE 49-2   PROPERTIES OF HEMOGLOBINS M

HEMOGLOBIN	AMINO ACID SUBSTITUTION	OXYGEN DISSOCIATION AND OTHER PROPERTIES	CLINICAL EFFECT	REFERENCE
Hb M$_{Boston}$	α58(E7)His→Tyr	Very low O$_2$ affinity, almost nonexistent heme-heme interaction, no Bohr effect	Cyanosis due to formation of methemoglobin	(64)
Hb M$_{Saskatoon}$	β63(E7)His→Tyr	Increased O$_2$ affinity, reduced heme-heme interaction, normal Bohr effect, slightly unstable	Cyanosis due to methemoglobin formation, mild hemolytic anemia exacerbated by ingestion of sulfonamides	(65)(64)
Hb M$_{Iwate}$ Hb M$_{Kankakee}$ Hb M$_{Oldenburg}$ Hb M$_{Sendai}$	α87(F8)His→Tyr	Low O$_2$ affinity, negligible heme-heme interaction, no Bohr effect	Cyanosis due to formation of methemoglobin	(64)(66)
Hb M$_{Hyde Park}$ Hb M$_{Milwaukee 2}$ Hb M$_{Akita}$	β92(F8)His→Tyr	Increased O$_2$ affinity, reduced heme interaction, normal Bohr effect, slightly unstable	Cyanosis due to formation of methemoglobin, mild hemolytic anemia	(67)
Hb M$_{Milwaukee}$	β7(E11)Val→Glu	Low O$_2$ affinity, reduced heme-heme interaction, normal Bohr effect, slightly unstable	Cyanosis due to methemoglobin formation	(68)
Hb FM$_{Osaka}$	α63His→Tyr	Low O$_2$ affinity, increased Bohr effect, methemoglobinemia	Cyanosis at birth	(62)
Hb FM$_{Fort Ripley}$	α92His→Tyr	Slightly increased O$_2$ affinity	Cyanosis at birth	(69)

TABLE 49-3   SOME ABNORMAL HEMOGLOBINS ASSOCIATED WITH LOW OXYGEN AFFINITY

HEMOGLOBIN	AMINO ACID SUBSTITUTION	OXYGEN DISSOCIATION AND OTHER PROPERTIES	CLINICAL EFFECT	REFERENCE
Hb Seattle	β70(E14)Ala→Asp	Decreased O$_2$ affinity, normal heme-heme interaction	Mild chronic anemia associated with reduced urinary erythropoietin, physiologic adaptation to more efficient oxygen release to tissues	(71)
Hb Kansas	β102(G4)Asn→Thr	Very low O$_2$ affinity, low heme-heme interaction, dissociates into dimers in ligand form	Cyanosis due to deoxyhemoglobin, mild anemia	(72)

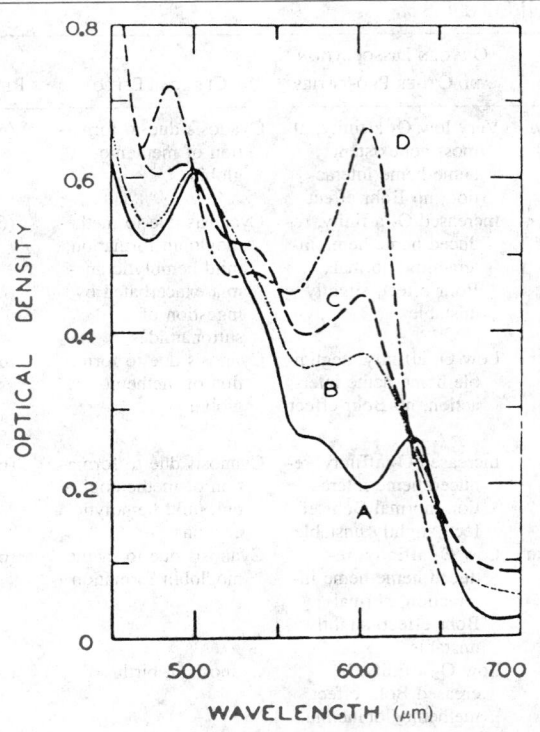

FIGURE 49-2   Absorption spectra at pH 7.0. A; B, methemoglobin A; B, methemoglobin M$_{Boston}$; C, methemoglobin M$_{Saskatoon}$; D, methemoglobin A fluoride complex. For purposes of comparison all the optical densities have been made equal to 0.61 at 500 nm. (Gerald and George,[93] with permission of the American Association for the Advancement of Science.)

ABNORMAL HEMOGLOBINS

OPTICAL SPECTRUM

The spectrum of normal methemoglobin A at pH 7.0 is illustrated in Fig. 49-2.[93] Hemoglobins M may be differentiated from methemoglobin formed from hemoglobin A by their absorption spectra in the range of 450 to 750 nm. Since only some 20 to 35 percent of the total hemoglobin will ordinarily be hemoglobin M, the mixed spectra of methemoglobin A and hemoglobin M may be difficult to interpret. Therefore, it is preferable to perform these spectral studies on purified hemoglobin M isolated by electrophoretic or chromatographic means.[61]

ELECTROPHORESIS

All hemoglobin M samples should be converted to methemoglobin so that any difference found in electrophoresis will be due to the amino acid substitution and not to the different charge of the iron atom. Electrophoresis at pH 7.1 is most useful for separation of hemoglobins M since the imidazole groups of histidine have a net positive charge at this pH, while at higher pH levels the histidines and the substituting tyrosines are both neutral.

OTHER STUDIES

The hemoglobins M differ in their reactivity to cyanide and to azide ions.[94]

SULFHEMOGLOBINEMIA

Sulfhemoglobin is detected in the lysate of blood treated with ferricyanide, cyanide, and ammonia by comparing the optical density at 620 nm with that at 540 nm.[95,96]

DIFFERENTIAL DIAGNOSIS

Cyanosis due to methemoglobinemia or sulfhemoglobinemia should be differentiated from cyanosis due to cardiac or pulmonary disease particularly when right-to-left shunting is present. In the latter instances the arterial oxygen tension will be low, while in methemoglobinemia and sulfhemoglobinemia it should be normal. One should be certain, however, that the oxygen tension was measured directly and not deduced from the percent saturation of hemoglobin. Blood from a patient with cyanosis due to arterial oxygen desaturation promptly becomes bright red upon being shaken with air. In addition, these causes of cyanosis are readily differentiated by carrying out quantitative blood methemoglobin and sulfhemoglobin levels. Because of the potential lethal nature of high levels of methemoglobin, and because prompt treatment may be life saving, a high index of suspicion is important. A patient with cyanosis whose arterial blood is brown with a P$_{O_2}$ that is found to be normal on blood gas examination is likely to have methemoglobinemia. One should not rely on the readings of a pulse oximeter, since false readings may be obtained in the presence of methemoglobin. Rapid examination of a blood sample using an automatic analyzer such as a CoOximeter is the first step in confirming the diagnosis. However, as pointed out under "Laboratory Features" above, although treatment should not be delayed, direct spectrophotometric analysis should be carried out on the pretreatment sample as soon as possible to distinguish between methemoglobinemia and sulfhemoglobinemia.

A family history is usually helpful in differentiating hereditary methemoglobinemia due to NADH-diaphorase deficiency from hemoglobin M disease. The former has a recessive mode of inheritance, the latter a dominant mode. Thus, cyanosis in successive generations suggests the presence of hemoglobin M; normal parents but possibly affected sibs implies the presence of NADH-diaphorase deficiency. Consanguinity is more common in NADH-diaphorase deficiency. In NADH-diaphorase deficiency incubation of the blood with small amounts of methylene blue will result in rapid reduction of the methemoglobin; in hemoglobin M disease such reduction does not take place. The absorption spectra of methemoglobin and its derivatives are normal in NADH-diaphorase deficiency; they are abnormal in hemoglobin M disease. In the case of toxic methemoglobinemia cyanosis is generally of relatively recent origin, and a history of exposure to drug or toxin may usually be obtained; in hereditary methemoglobinemia a history of lifelong cyanosis may usually be elicited.

THERAPY, COURSE, AND PROGNOSIS

TOXIC METHEMOGLOBINEMIA

Acute toxic methemoglobinemia may represent a serious medical emergency. Because of the loss of oxygen-carrying capacity of the blood and because of the left shift in the oxygen dissociation curve that occurs when methemoglobin is present in high concentration,[97] acute methemoglobinemia may be life threatening when the level of the pigment exceeds half of the total circulating hemoglobin.

Methylene blue is an effective treatment for patients with methemoglobinemia because NADPH formed in the hexose monophosphate pathway can rapidly reduce this dye to leukomethylene blue in a reaction catalyzed by NADPH diaphorase. Leukomethylene blue, in turn, nonenzymatically reduces methemoglobin to hemoglobin.[98] An exception to the efficacy of this treatment exists in those patients who are G-6-PD deficient (see Chap. 45). In these subjects methylene blue would not only fail to give the desired effect on methemoglobin levels but might compound the patient's difficulty by inducing an acute hemolytic episode.[99] In patients with acute toxic methemoglobinemia who are symptomatic or whose methemoglobin level is rising rapidly, the intravenous administration of 1 or 2 mg methylene blue per kg body weight over a period of 5 min is the preferred treatment because of its very rapid action.[20] Use of excessive amounts of methylene blue should be avoided: the administration of repeated doses of 2 mg methylene blue/kg body weight has produced acute hemolysis even in patients with normal G-6-PD levels.[21] The response to treatment is so rapid, with marked lowering or normalization of methemoglobin levels within an hour or two, that no other treatment is usually needed, but the patient should be observed carefully because continued absorption of a toxic substance from the gastrointestinal tract may cause recurrence of the methemoglobinemia. In patients who are in shock blood transfusion may be helpful. Cimetidine, used as a selective inhibitor of N-hydroxylation, may decrease the methemoglobinemia produced by dapsone in patients with dermatitis herpetiformis.[100]

HEREDITARY METHEMOGLOBINEMIA

The course of hereditary methemoglobinemia is benign, but patients with this disorder should be shielded from exposure to aniline derivatives, nitrites, and other agents which may, even in normal persons, induce methemoglobinemia. Hereditary methemoglobinemia due to NADH-diaphorase deficiency is readily treated by the administration of ascorbic acid, 300 to 600 mg orally daily divided into three or four doses. While intravenously administered methylene blue is very effective in correcting this type of methemoglobinemia, it is not suitable for the long-term therapy that needs to be given if the state is to be treated at all.

The iron phenolate complex which exists in the hemoglobins M prevents the reduction of ferric to ferrous iron. For these reasons the methemoglobinemia does not respond to administration of ascorbic acid or of methylene blue. No effective treatment exists for the cyanosis that is present in patients with abnormal hemoglobins with reduced oxygen affinity.

SULFHEMOGLOBINEMIA

Sulfhemoglobinemia is almost always a benign disorder. Unlike methemoglobin, sulfhemoglobin does not produce a left shift in the oxygen dissociation curve but rather decreases the affinity of hemoglobin for oxygen.[79] The disorder tends to recur repeatedly in the same persons after exposure to drugs but does not generally appear to affect their overall health. Unlike methemoglobin, sulfhemoglobin cannot be converted to hemoglobin. Thus, once sulfhemoglobinemia occurs it will persist until the erythrocytes carrying the abnormal pigment reach the end of their life span.

REFERENCES

1. Hsieh HS, Jaffe ER: The metabolism of methemoglobin in human erythrocytes, in *The Red Blood Cell*, edited by DM Surgenor, pp 799–824. Academic Press, New York, 1975.
2. Sloss A, Wybauw R: Un cas de methemoglobinemie idiopathique. *Ann Soc R Sci Med Nat Bruxettes* 70:206, 1912.
3. Hitzenberger K: Autotoxische Zyanose: Intraglobulare Methämoglobinamie. *Wien Arch Inn Med* 23:85, 1932.
4. Jaffe ER: Hereditary methemoglobinemias associated with abnormalities in the metabolism of erythrocytes. *Am J Med* 41:786, 1966.
5. Hörlein H, Weber G: Über Chronische familiare Methämoglobinamie und eine neue Modificazation des Methämoglobins. *Dtsch Med Wochenschr* 73:476, 1948.
6. Singer K: Hereditary hemolytic disorders associated with abnormal hemoglobins. *Am J Med* 18:633, 1955.
7. Bonaventura J, Riggs A: Hemoglobin Kansas, a human hemoglobin with a neutral amino acid substitution and an abnormal oxygen equilibrium. *J Biol Chem* 243:980, 1968.
8. Gibson QH: The reduction of methemoglobin in red blood cells and studies on the cause of idiopathic methemoglobinemia. *Biochem J* 42:13, 1948.
9. Sorensen PR: The influence of pH, pCO_2 and concentrations of dyshemoglobins on the oxygen dissociation curve (ODC) of human blood determined by non-linear least squares regression analysis. *Scand J Clin Lab Invest (Suppl)* 203:163–8:163, 1990.
10. Bodansky O: Methemoglobinemia and methemoglobin-producing compounds. *Pharmacol Rev* 3:144, 1951.
11. Kiese M: The biochemical production of ferrihemoglobin-forming derivatives from aromatic amines, and mechanisms of ferrihemoglobin formation. *Pharmacol Rev* 18:1091, 1966.
12. Dean BS, Lopez G, Krenzelok EP: Environmentally induced methemoglobinemia in an infant. *J Toxicol Clin Toxicol* 30:127, 1992.
13. Paris PM, Kaplan RM, Stewart RD, Weiss LD: Methemoglobin levels following sublingual nitroglycerin in human volunteers. *Ann Emerg Med* 15:171, 1986.
14. Gavish D, Knobler H, Gottehrer N, Israeli A, Kleinman Y: Methemoglobinemia, muscle damage and renal failure complicating phenazopyridine overdose. *Isr J Med Sci* 22:45, 1986.
15. Christensen CM, Farrar HC, Kearns GL: Protracted methemoglobinemia after phenazopyridine overdose in an infant. *J Clin Pharmacol* 36:112, 1996.
16. Damergis JA, Stoker JM, Abadie JL: Methemoglobinemia after sulfamethoxazole and trimethoprim. *JAMA* 249:590, 1983.
17. Trillo RA Jr, Aukburg S: Dapsone-induced methemoglobinemia and pulse oximetry. *Anesthesiology* 77:594, 1992.
18. Erstad BL: Dapsone-induced methemoglobinemia and hemolytic anemia. *Clin Pharm* 11:800, 1992.
19. Wagner A, Marosi C, Binder M, et al: Fatal poisoning due to dapsone in a patient with grossly elevated methaemoglobin levels. *Br J Dermatol* 133:816, 1995.
20. Kearney TE, Manoguerra AS, Dunford JV Jr: Chemically induced methemoglobinemia from aniline poisoning. *West J Med* 140:282, 1983.
21. Harvey JW, Keitt AS: Studies of the efficacy and potential hazards of methylene blue therapy in aniline-induced methaemoglobinaemia. *Br J Haematol* 54:29, 1983.
22. Ng LL, Naik RB, Polak A: Paraquat ingestion with methaemoglobinaemia treated with methylene blue. *BMJ* 284:1445, 1982.
23. Proudfoot AT: Methaemoglobinaemia due to monolinuron—not paraquat. *BMJ* 285:812, 1983.
24. Johnson CJ, Bonrud PA, Dosch TL, et al: Fatal outcome of methemoglobinemia in an infant. *JAMA* 257:2796, 1987.
25. Johnson CJ, Kross BC: Continuing importance of nitrate contamination of groundwater and wells in rural areas. *Am J Ind Med* 18:449, 1990.
26. Gibson GR, Hunter JB, Rabbe DS, Manjoney DL, Ittleman FP: Methemoglobinemia produced by high-dose intravenous nitroglycerin. *Ann Intern Med* 96:615, 1982.
27. Forsyth RJ, Moulden A: Methaemoglobinaemia after ingestion of amyl nitrite. *Arch Dis Child* 66:152, 1991.
28. Guss DA, Normann SA, Manoguerra AS: Clinically significant methemoglobinemia from inhalation of isobutyl nitrite. *Am J Emerg Med* 1:46, 1985.
29. Ellis M, Hiss Y, Shenkman L: Fatal methemoglobinemia caused by inadvertent contamination of a laxative solution with sodium nitrite. *Isr J Med Sci* 28:289, 1992.
30. Chan TY: Food-borne nitrates and nitrites as a cause of methemoglobinemia. *Southeast Asian J Trop Med Public Health* 27:189, 1996.
31. Collins JF: Methemoglobinemia as a complication of 20% benzocaine spray for endoscopy. *Gastroenterology* 98:211, 1990.
32. Postiglione KF, Herold DA: Benzocaine-adulterated street cocaine in association with methemoglobinemia. *Clin Chem* 38:596, 1992.
33. Guerriero SE: Methemoglobinemia caused by topical benzocaine. *Pharmacotherapy* 17:1038, 1997.
34. Cooper HA: Methemoglobinemia caused by benzocaine topical spray. *South Med J* 90:946, 1997.
35. Nilsson A, Engberg G, Henneberg S, Danielson K, de Verdier C-H: Inverse relationship between age-dependent erythrocyte activity of methaemoglobin reductase and prilocaine-induced methaemoglobinaemia during infancy. *Br J Anaesth* 64:72, 1990.
36. Duncan PG, Kobrinsky N: Prilocaine-induced methemoglobinemia in a newborn infant. *Anesthesiology* 59:75, 1983.

37. Lloyd CJ: Chemically induced methaemoglobinaemia in a neonate. *Br J Oral Maxillofac Surg* 30:63, 1992.

38. Bilgin H, Özcan B, Bilgin T: Methemoglobinemia induced by methylene blue pertubation during laparoscopy. *Acta Anaesthesiol Scand* 42:594, 1998.

39. Brisman M, Ljung BML, Otterbom I, Larsson LE, Andréasson SE: Methaemoglobin formation after the use of EMLA cream in term neonates. *Acta Paediatr* 87:1191, 1998.

40. Moreira VD, De Medeiros BC, Bonfim CMS, Pasquini R, De Medeiros CR: Methemoglobinemia secondary to clofazimine treatment for chronic graft-versus-host disease. *Blood* 92:4872, 1998.

41. Yubisui T, Shirabe K, Takeshita M, et al: Structural role of serine 127 in the NADH-binding site of human NADH-cytochrome b₅ reductase. *J Biol Chem* 266:66, 1991.

42. Katsube T, Sakamoto N, Kobayashi Y, et al: Exonic point mutations in NADH-cytochrome B5 reductase genes of homozygotes for hereditary methemoglobinemia, types I and III: putative mechanisms of tissue-dependent enzyme deficiency. *Am J Hum Genet* 48:799, 1991.

43. Shirabe K, Yubisui T, Borgese N, et al: Enzymatic instability of NADH-cytochrome b_5 reductase as a cause of hereditary methemoglobinemia type I (red cell type). *J Biol Chem* 267:20416, 1992.

44. Manabe J, Arya R, Sumimoto H, et al: Two novel mutations in the reduced nicotinamide adenine dinucleotide (NADH) cytochrome b₅ reductase gene of a patient with generalized type, hereditary methemoglobinemia. *Blood* 88:3208, 1996.

45. Shirabe K, Fujimoto Y, Yubisui T, Takeshita M: An in-frame deletion of codon 298 of the NADH-cytochrome b_5 reductase gene results in hereditary methemoglobinemia type II (generalized type). A functional implication for the role of the COOH-terminal region of the enzyme. *J Biol Chem* 269:5952, 1994.

46. Vieira LM, Kaplan J-C, Kahn A, Leroux A: Four new mutations in the NADH-cytochrome b₅ reductase gene from patients with recessive congenital methemoglobinemia type II. *Blood* 85:2254, 1995.

47. Jenkins MM, Prchal JT: A novel mutation found in the 3′ domain of NADH-cytochrome B5 reductase in an African-American family with type I congenital methemoglobinemia. *Blood* 87:2993, 1996.

48. Shirabe K, Landi MT, Takeshita M, et al: A novel point mutation in a 3′ splice site of the NADH-cytochrome b₅ reductase gene results in immunologically undetectable enzyme and impaired NADH-dependent ascorbate regeneration in cultured fibroblasts of a patient with type II hereditary methemoglobinemia. *Am J Hum Genet* 57:302, 1995.

49. Higasa K, Manabe J, Yubisui T, et al: Molecular basis of hereditary methaemoglobinaemia, types I and II: two novel mutations in the NADH-cytochrome b₅ reductase gene. *Br J Haematol* 103:922, 1998.

50. Tanishima K, Tomoda A, Yoneyama Y, Ohkuwa H: Three types of hereditary methemoglobinemia due to NADH-cytochrome b₅ reductase deficiency. *Adv Clin Enzymol* 5:81, 1987.

51. Takeshita M, Tamura M, Kugi M, et al: Decrease of palmitoyl-CoA elongation in platelets and leukocytes in the patient of hereditary methemoglobinemia associated with mental retardation. *Biochem Biophys Res Commun* 148:384, 1987.

52. Tanishima K, Tanimoto K, Tomoda A, et al: Hereditary methemoglobinemia due to cytochrome b₅ reductase deficiency in blood cells without associated neurologic and mental disorders. *Blood* 66:1288, 1985.

53. Lo SC-L, Agar NS: NADH-methemoglobin reductase activity in the erythrocytes of newborn and adult mammals. *Experientia* 42:1264, 1986.

54. Graubarth J, Bloom CJ, Coleman FC, Solomon HN: Dye poisoning in the nursery: a review of seventeen cases. *JAMA* 128:1155, 1945.

55. Lukens JN: The legacy of well-water methemoglobinemia. *JAMA* 257:2793, 1987.

56. Hanukoglu A, Danon PN: Endogenous methemoglobinemia associated with diarrheal disease in infancy. *J Pediatr Gastroenterol Nutr* 23:1, 1996.

57. Cohen RJ, Sachs JR, Wicker DJ, Conrad ME: Methemoglobinemia provoked by malarial chemoprophylaxis in Vietnam. *N Engl J Med* 279:1127, 1968.

58. Hegesh E, Hegesh J, Kaftory A: Congenital methemoglobinemia with a deficiency of cytochrome b₅. *N Engl J Med* 314:757, 1986.

59. Mansouri A, McClellan JL: Congenital methemoglobinemia with cytochrome b₅ deficiency. *N Engl J Med* 315:893, 1986.

60. Tauber AI, Blanchard RA: Congenital methemoglobinemia with cytochrome b₅ deficiency. *N Engl J Med* 315:894, 1986.

61. Lehmann H, Huntsman RG: *Man's Haemoglobins*, p 213. Lippincott, Philadelphia, 1974.

62. Hayashi A, Fujita T, Fujimura M, Titani K: A new abnormal fetal hemoglobin, Hb FM-Osaka ($\alpha_2\gamma_2^{63His}\rightarrow^{Tyr}$). *Hemoglobin* 4:447, 1980.

63. Priest JR, Watterson J, Jones RT, Faassen AE, Hedlund BE: Mutant fetal hemoglobin causing cyanosis in a newborn. *Pediatrics* 83:734, 1989.

64. Gerald PS, Efron ML: Chemical studies of several varieties of Hb M. *Proc Natl Acad Sci USA* 47:1758, 1961.

65. Staven P, Strome J, Lorkin PA, Lehmann H: Haemoglobin M Saskatoon with slight constant haemolysis, markedly increased by sulphonamides. *Scand J Haematol* 9:566, 1972.

66. Hayashi N, Motokawa Y, Kikuchi G: Studies on relationships between structure and function of hemoglobin M Iwate. *J Biol Chem* 241:79, 1966.

67. Hutt PJ, Pisciotta AV, Fairbanks VF, Thibodeau SN, Green MM: DNA sequence analysis proves Hb M-Milwaukee-2 is due to beta-globin gene codon 92 (CAC→TAC), the presumed mutation of Hb M-Hyde Park and Hb M-Akita. *Hemoglobin* 22:1, 1998.

68. Horst J, Schafer R, Kleihauer E, Kohne E: Analysis of the Hb M Milwaukee mutation at the DNA level. *Br J Haematol* 54:643, 1983.

69. Hain RD, Chitayat D, Cooper R, et al: Hb FM-Fort Ripley: confirmation of autosomal dominant inheritance and diagnosis by PCR and direct nucleotide sequencing. *Hum Mutat* 3:239, 1994.

70. Hojas-Bernal R, McNab-Martin P, Fairbanks VF, et al: Hemoglobin Chile beta 28(B10)Leu→met: an unstable hemoglobin associated with chronic methemoglobinemia and sulfonamide or methylene blue-induced hemolytic anemia. *Hemoglobin* 23:125, 1999.

71. Stamatoyannopoulos G, Parer JT, Finch CA: Physiologic implication of a hemoglobin with decreased oxygen affinity (hemoglobin Seattle). *N Engl J Med* 281:915, 1969.

72. Reissmann KR, Ruth WE, Namura T: A human hemoglobin with lowered oxygen affinity and impaired heme-heme interactions. *J Clin Invest* 40:1826, 1971.

73. Beutler E: "A shift to the left" or "a shift to the right" in the regulation of erythropoiesis. *Blood* 33:496, 1969.

74. Lemberg R, Legge JW: Hematin Compounds and Bile Pigments, Interscience Publishers, New York, 1949.

75. Harrop GA, Jr., Waterfield RL: Sulphemoglobinemia. *JAMA* 95:647, 1930.

76. Nichol AW, Hendry I, Morell DB: Mechanism of formation of sulphhaemoglobin. *Biochim Biophys Acta* 156:97, 1968.

77. Berzofsky JA, Peisach J, Horecker BL: Sulfheme proteins. IV. The stoichiometry of sulfur incorporation and the isolation of sulfhemin, the prosthetic group of sulfmyoglobin. *J Biol Chem* 247:3783, 1972.

78. Berzofsky JA, Peisach J, Blumberg WE: Sulfheme proteins. II. The reversible oxygenation of ferrous sulfmyoglobin. *J Biol Chem* 246:7366, 1971.

79. Park CM, Nagel RL: Sulfhemoglobinemia. Clinical and molecular aspects. *N Engl J Med* 310:1579, 1984.

80. Halvorsen SM, Dull WL: Phenazopyridine-induced sulfhemoglobinemia: inadvertent rechallenge. *Am J Med* 91:315, 1991.

81. Discombe G: Sulphaemoglobinaemia and glutathione. *Lancet* 2:371, 1960.

82. McCutcheon AD, Melb MD, Flack EH: Sulphaemoglobinaemia and glutathione. *Lancet* 2:240, 1960.

83. Paniker NV, Beutler E: The effect of methylene blue and diaminodiphenylsulfone on red cell reduced glutathione synthesis. *J Lab Clin Med* 80:481, 1972.

84. Smith JE, Mahaffey E, Lee M: Effect of methylene blue on glutamate and reduced glutathione of rabbit erythrocytes. *Biochem J* 168:587, 1977.

85. Miller AA: Congenital sulfhemoglobinemia. *J Pediatr* 51:233, 1957.

86. Caudill L, Walbridge J, Kuhn G: Methemoglobinemia as a cause of coma. *Ann Emerg Med* 19:677, 1990.

87. Dacie JV, Lewis SM: Chemical and physico-chemical methods of haematological importance, in *Practical Haematology*. pp 476–524. Grune and Stratton, New York, 1998.

88. Beutler E: *Red Cell Metabolism: A Manual of Biochemical Methods*. Grune and Stratton, New York, 1984.

89. Board PG: NADH-ferricyanide reductase, a convenient approach to the evaluation of NADH-methaemoglobin reductase in human erythrocytes. *Clin Chim Acta* 109:233, 1981.

90. Lan FH, Tang YC, Huang CH, Wu YS, Zhu ZY: Antibody-based spot

test for NADH-cytochrome b$_5$ reductase activity for the laboratory diagnosis of congenital methemoglobinemia. *Clin Chim Acta* 273:13, 1998.

91. Das Gupta A, Vaidya MS, Bapat JP, et al: Associated red cell enzyme deficiencies and their significance in a case of congenital enzymopenic methemoglobinemia. *Acta Haematol (Basel)* 64:285, 1980.

92. Kaftory A, Hegesh E: Improved determination of cytochrome b$_5$ in human erythrocytes. *Clin Chem* 30:1344, 1984.

93. Gerald PS, George P: A second spectroscopically abnormal methemoglobin associated with hereditary cyanosis. *Science* 129:393, 1959.

94. Carrell RW, Kay R: A simple method for the detection of unstable haemoglobins. *Br J Haematol* 23:615, 1972.

95. Evelyn KA, Malloy HT: Microdetermination of oxyhemoglobin, methemoglobin, and sulfhemoglobin in a single sample of blood. *J Biol Chem* 126:655, 1938.

96. Beutler E: Carboxyhemoglobin, methemoglobin, and sulfhemoglobin determinations, in *Williams Hematology*, 5th ed, edited by E Beutler, MA Lichtman, BS Coller, TJ Kipps, p L50. McGraw-Hill, New York, 1995.

97. Darling RC, Roughton FJW: The effect of methemoglobin on the equilibrium between oxygen and hemoglobin. *Am J Physiol* 137:56, 1942.

98. Beutler E, Baluda MC: Methemoglobin reduction. Studies of the interaction between cell populations and of the role of methylene blue. *Blood* 22:323, 1963.

99. Rosen PJ, Johnson C, McGehee WG, Beutler E: Failure of methylene blue treatment in toxic methemoglobinemia. Association with glucose-6-phosphate dehydrogenase deficiency. *Ann Intern Med* 75:83, 1971.

100. Coleman MD, Rhodes LE, Scott AK, et al: The use of cimetidine to reduce dapsone-dependent methaemoglobinaemia in dermatitis herpetiformis patients. *Br J Clin Pharmacol* 34:244, 1993.

TRAUMATIC CARDIAC HEMOLYTIC ANEMIA

ALLAN J. ERSLEV

The abrasive effect on red cells of arteriosclerotic or stenotic cardiac valves is usually minimal, resulting at most in a mild, often compensated hemolytic anemia. However, the introduction of artificial valves was initially associated with marked red cell destruction and the development of an overt hemolytic anemia. Recently, the design of the artificial valves and the use of more compatible plastics or biologic materials have greatly reduced their traumatic effects and minimized hemolysis. Actually, the potential thrombogenic effect of artificial valves far outstrips their destructive effect on red cells, and cardiac hemolytic anemia is now an almost nonexistent problem.

In the 1950s cardiac corrective surgery became possible, and it was almost immediately observed that patients in whose aorta a Hufnagel valve was inserted developed anemia.[1] This anemia was shown to be caused by mechanical injury and fragmentation of red cells impacted at high speed on a foreign surface.[2,3] Since then the prevention of such injury has been a challenge in the construction of prosthetic valves and surfaces, and successful innovations have led to a decreased incidence of valve-related traumatic cardiac hemolytic anemia. Currently, hemolytic anemia is considered a minor complication in reviews of large series of patients[4-8] and is mainly relegated to case reports of patients with old or dysfunctional prosthetic valves.[9-14]

ETIOLOGY AND PATHOGENESIS

In aqueous suspension the red cell membrane can withstand shear-producing stress of up to 15,000 dyne/cm^2.[15] Such a stress is rarely encountered in vivo, but determination of red cell survival, serum haptoglobin level, and serum lactic dehydrogenase concentration in patients with valvular disorders suggests that some hemolysis takes place. This hemolysis, however, is mild and rarely causes overt hemolytic anemia except in patients with severe aortic[16] or subaortic[17] stenosis generating pressure gradients across the valve of more than 50 torr.[18] The abnormalities that have been found to produce hemolytic anemia are summarized in Table 50-1.

All prosthetic cardiac valves have an orifice size smaller than that of the natural valve, and after implantation this orifice is further reduced by tissue ingrowth and endothelialization.[19] The Starr-Edwards cage ball valve has a slightly smaller aperture than the more commonly used tilting disc valve (Bjork-Shiley or St. Jude), but the hemodynamic differences between well-functioning prosthetic valves and natural valves are small. Several complications, however, may cause turbulence in the blood flowing around or through a prosthetic valve and expose the red cells to very high shear stresses. The blood may flow around the valve through openings created by improper positioning or by spontaneous separation of the valve from the annular ring.[20,21] It may also flow through a constricted outlet in the Starr-Edwards model because of "ball variance," in which the plastic ball takes up lipids, swells, and fails to move freely in the cage.[22,23]

Nevertheless, the turbulence and shear stresses encountered in patients with artificial valves are rarely much higher than those in patients with uncorrected aortic stenosis or mitral regurgitation. Consequently, the severe red cell destruction seen in some patients with artificial valves cannot be caused only by hemodynamic turbulence but requires that this turbulence occur in a space enclosed or bordered by a foreign surface. Studies of red cells in a cone-plate viscosimeter show that hemolysis occurs when shear forces at plastic interfaces exceed 2000 dyne/cm^2 (Fig. 50-1).[24] Such shear forces are encountered across artificial prosthetic devices that are coated with various plastic compounds or constructed of carbon or metallic material. These coatings are eventually covered by a layer of endothelial cells. Unfortunately, this covering is not firmly bonded to the materials, and if it is denuded, red cells in rapidly flowing blood will become damaged by contact with the artificial surface. This damage will result in mild, usually compensated anemia,[25] but severe hemolytic anemia may occur.[26] Of more clinical importance is the fact that nonendothelialized surfaces are thrombogenic and may cause platelet activation, thrombus formation, and distant embolization (see Chap. 130). In patients undergoing artificial heart transplantation, the hemolysis, although significant and requiring transfusion replacement, is overshadowed by complications from thrombosis and embolization.[27,28] When blood is exposed to foreign surfaces under less turbulent conditions, as in an oxygenator,[7] dialysis tubing,[29] or endocardic[30] or aortofemoral prostheses,[31] hemolysis may occur but is rarely pronounced. In such cases it has been proposed that the hemolysis is due in part to complement activation.[32]

Largely to overcome these thromboembolic problems, nonthrombogenic bioprosthetic valves have been developed. These can be allografts, derived from human aortic leaflets, or xenographs (Carpenter-Edwards or Hancock's), derived from porcine aortic leaflets.[19] The valvular orifice is slightly smaller than in the ball or disc artificial valve, but overt hemolysis does not occur unless the stitching fails and permits perivalvular leakage.[13,14] The valves usually have a potentially thrombogenic Teflon sewing ring, but since it becomes endothelialized within a few months, permanent anticoagulant therapy is not needed. Unfortunately, these valves are less durable than mechanical prosthetic valves and may need replacement 5 to 10 years after insertion.[19] In order to limit the need for anticoagulation, bioprosthetic material has been preferred for valve replacement in the elderly, in whom long-term durability may be of lesser concern. In the future such considera-

TABLE 50-1   CAUSES OF MACROANGIOPATHIC HEMOLYTIC ANEMIA

A. Without surgery
 1. Aortic stenosis
 2. Ruptured sinus of Valsalva
 3. Ruptured chordae tendineae
 4. Coarctation of aorta
 5. Aortic aneurysm
B. Following surgery
 1. Complement activation in oxygenator or hemodialysis tubing
 2. "Patching" operations
  a. Ostium primum repair, especially if mitral regurgitation present
  b. Aortic aneurysm repair (aortofemoral bypass)
 3. Valvular replacement
  a. Uncomplicated
   (1) Outflow too small
   (2) Large area of exposed plastic
   (3) Cloth-covered struts
   (4) Two or more valves replaced
  b. Complicated
   (1) Ball variance
   (2) Regurgitation around seating of valve
   (3) Rupture of cloth-covered strut

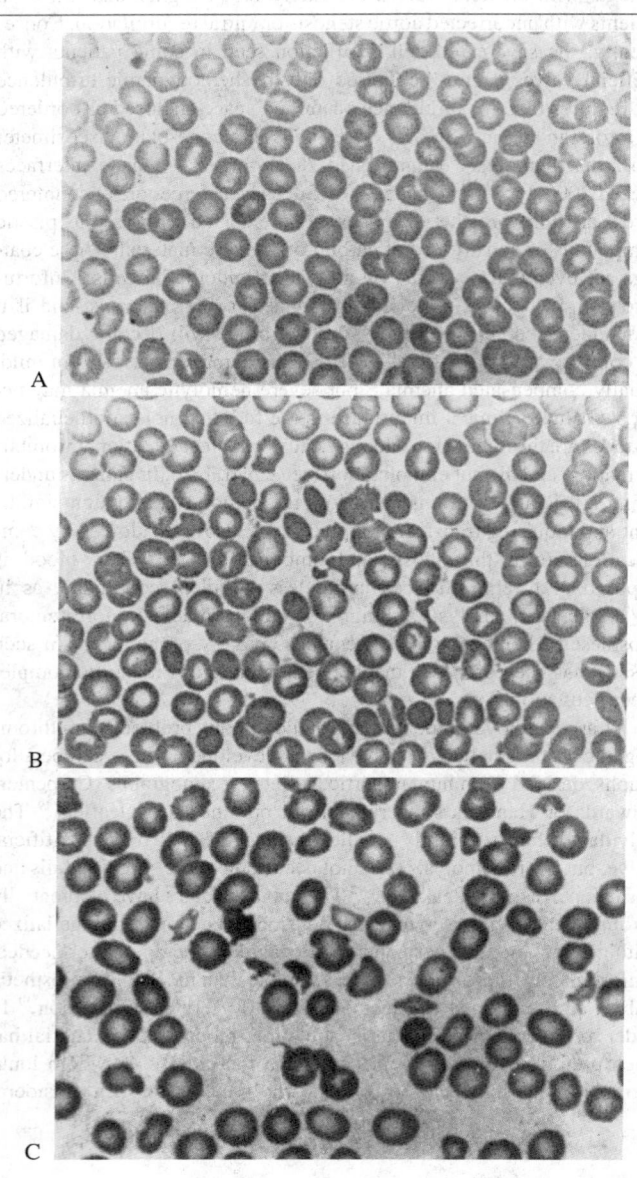

FIGURE 50-1   (a) Normal human erythrocytes. (b) Human erythrocytes subjected to shearing stress of 2616 dyne/cm². (c) Erythrocytes from a patient with a hemolytic anemia associated with a malfunctioning prosthetic aortic valve. Each blood film stained with Wright stain. (From Nevaril et al.[24])

tions may be less important, since improved design appears to have rendered bioprosthetic valves as durable as mechanical valves.[33]

CLINICAL FEATURES

The severity of the anemia is highly variable in patients with heart valve prostheses. Mild compensated hemolysis is usually present, but overt anemia is unusual, and only in a rare individual will the anemia be severe enough to require transfusions. However, since patients with cardiac diseases generally have less capacity to adapt to an anemia, even a mild reduction in hemoglobin concentration may cause angina or congestive heart failure.

LABORATORY FEATURES

Even when the hemoglobin level is almost normal, the reticulocyte count is usually elevated, as is the serum lactic acid dehydrogenase activity. Blood films display helmet cells, triangular cells, and other fragmented red cell forms having characteristically sharp points.

The plasma hemoglobin level may be elevated, and the haptoglobin concentration may be diminished, resulting in hemosiderinuria,[34] and occasionally there is a significant loss of iron in the urine, with reduced serum ferritin levels and, not uncommonly, with frank iron deficiency.[35]

The white cell count may be normal or slightly elevated. The platelet count may be decreased, suggesting intravascular consumption of platelets on the foreign surfaces.[36]

DIFFERENTIAL DIAGNOSIS

The diagnosis is usually straightforward and is based on the presence of fragmented red cells and evidence of chronic hemolysis in a patient with an artificial valve. The use of transesophageal electrocardiography may be useful in identifying paravalvular regurgitation.[37] It is, of course, important to remember that even patients with artificial valves may have unrelated autoimmune or nutritional deficiency anemias.

THERAPY, COURSE, AND PROGNOSIS

If the anemia is sufficiently severe, the most effective treatment consists of replacement of the prosthesis. In most cases, however, the anemia is very mild or completely compensated, and it is merely necessary to ensure good erythropoietic activity in order to maintain this compensation. For that purpose it is recommended to replace urinary iron loss with 300 mg/day of ferrous sulfate orally. Folic acid, 1 mg/day, may also be beneficial. Recombinant erythropoietin has also been successful in alleviating the anemia in a few transfusion-dependent patients.[38]

REFERENCES

1. Ross JC, Hufnagel CA, Fries ED, et al: The hemodynamic alterations produced by plastic valvular prosthesis for severe aortic insufficiency in man. *J Clin Invest* 33:891, 1954.
2. Sayed HM, Dacie JV, Handley DA, et al: Haemolytic anaemia of mechanical origin after open heart surgery. *Thorax* 16:356, 1961.
3. Marsh GW, Lewis SM: Cardiac haemolytic anaemia. *Semin Hematol* 6:133, 1969.
4. Starr A: Ball valve prostheses: a perspective after 22 years, in *Advances in Cardiac Valves,* edited by ME DeBakey, pp 1–13. Yorke Medical Books, New York, 1983.
5. DeBakey ME, Lawrie GM, Morris GC, et al: Experience with 366 St. Jude valve prostheses in 346 patients, in *Advances in Cardiac Valves,* edited by ME DeBakey, pp 14–21. Yorke Medical Books, New York, 1983.
6. Thompson ME, Lewis JH, Porkolab FL, Hasiba U, Spero JA: Indexes of intravascular hemolysis, quantification of coagulation factors and platelet survival in patients with porcine heterograft valves. *Am J Cardiol* 51:489, 1983.
7. Arom K: Aortic valve replacement: long-term results with various mechanical prostheses. *Asian Cardiovasc Thorac J* 1:39, 1993.
8. Aoyagi S, Oryoji A, Nishi Y, Tanaka K, Kosuga K, Oishi K: Long-term results of valve replacement with the St. Jude medical valve. *J Thorac Cardiovasc Surg* 108:1021, 1994.
9. Schaer DH, Cheng TO, Aaron BL: Hemolytic anemia and acute mitral regurgitation caused by a torn cusp of a porcine mitral prosthetic valve 7 years after its implantation. *Am Heart J* 113:404, 1987.
10. Kutsche LM, Alexander JA, VanMierop LH: Hemolytic anemia secondary to erosion of a Silastic band into the lumen of the pulmonary trunk. *Am J Cardiol* 55:1438, 1985.

11. Barmada H, Starr A: Clinical hemolysis with the St. Jude heart valve without paravalvular leak. *Med Prog Technol* 20:191, 1994.

12. Kihara S, Kasegawa H, Kobayashi N, et al: Severe hemolysis due to artificial chordae displacement. *J Heart Valve Dis* 6:69, 1997.

13. Amidon TM, Chou TM, Rankin JS, Ports TA: Mitral and aortic paravalvular leaks with hemolytic anemia. *Am Heart J* 125:266, 1993.

14. Formolo JM, Reyes P: Refractory hemolytic anemia secondary to perivalvular leak diagnosed by transesophageal echocardiography. *J Clin Ultrasound* 23:185, 1995.

15. Blackshear PL Jr, Dorman FD, Steinbach JH, Maybach EJ, Singh A, Collingham RE: Shear wall interaction and hemolysis. *Trans Am Soc Artif Intern Organs* 12:113, 1966.

16. Miller DS, Mengel CE, Kremer WB, et al: Intravascular hemolysis in a patient with valvular heart disease. *Ann Intern Med* 65:210, 1966.

17. Solanski DL, Sheikh MU: Fragmentation and hemolysis in idiopathic hypertrophic subaortic stenosis. *South Med J* 71:599, 1978.

18. Jacobson AJ, Rath CE, Perloff SK: Intravascular hemolysis and thombocytopenia in left ventricular outflow obstruction. *Br Heart J* 35:49, 1973.

19. Braunwald E: Artificial cardiac valves, in *Heart Disease,* 5th ed, edited by E Braunwald, pp 1061–1076. Saunders, Philadelphia, 1997.

20. Kastor JA, Akburian M, Buckley MJ: Paravalvular leaks and hemolytic anemia following Starr-Edwards aortic and mitral valves. *J Thorac Cardiovasc Surg* 56:279, 1968.

21. Viner ED, Frost W: Hemolytic anemia due to a Teflon aortic valve prosthesis. *Ann Intern Med* 63:295, 1965.

22. Eyster E: Traumatic hemolysis with hemoglobinuria due to ball variance. *Blood* 33:391, 1969.

23. Stohlman F Jr, Sarnoff SJ, Case RB, Ness AT: Hemolytic syndrome following the insertion of a Lucite ball valve prosthesis into the cardiovascular system. *Circulation* 13:586, 1956.

24. Nevaril CG, Lynch EC, Alfrey CP, Hellums JD: Erythrocyte damage and destruction induced by shearing stress. *J Lab Clin Med* 71:784, 1968.

25. Brodeur MTH, Sutherland DW, Koler RD, et al: Red blood cell survival in patients with aortic valvular disease and ball valve prostheses. *Circulation* 32:570, 1965.

26. Marsh GW: Intravascular haemolytic anemia after aortic-valve replacement. *Lancet* 2:986, 1964.

27. Kormos RL, Borovetz HS, Griffith BP, Huns TC: Rheologic abnormalities in patients with the Jarvik-7 total artificial heart. *Trans Am Soc Artif Intern Organs* 33:413, 1987.

28. DeVries WC: The permanent artificial heart: four case reports. *JAMA* 259:849, 1988.

29. Francos GC, Burke JF Jr, Besarab A, Baumer LH, Paek SU, Sebening F: An unsuspected cause of acute hemolysis during hemodialysis. *Trans Am Soc Artif Intern Organs* 29:140, 1983.

30. Sigler AT, Forman EN, Zinkham WH, Neill CA: Severe intravascular hemolysis following surgical repair of endocardial cushion defects. *Am J Med* 35:407, 1963.

31. Manny J, Manny N, Abu-Dallo K, et al: Traumatic hemolysis after aortofemoral bypass. *Isr J Med Sci* 13:50, 1977.

32. Salama A, Hugo P, Heinrich D, et al: Deposition of terminal C5b-9 complement complexes on erythrocytes and leukocytes during cardiopulmonary bypass. *N Engl J Med* 318:408, 1988.

33. Holper K, Wottke M, Lewe T, et al: Bioprosthetic and mechanical valves in the elderly: benefits and risks. *Ann Thorac Surg* 60:S443, 1995.

34. Slater SD, Rahman M, Lindsay RM: Renal function in chronic intravascular haemolysis associated with prosthetic cardiac valves. *Clin Sci* 44:511, 1973.

35. Heilman E, Bender F, Gulker H, Bonke J: Investigations of iron and folate levels in serum after implantation of heart valve prostheses. *Herz* 4:298, 1979.

36. Harker LA, Slichter SJ: Studies of platelet and fibrinogen kinetics in patients with prosthetic heart valves. *N Engl J Med* 283:1302, 1970.

37. Garcia MJ, Vandervoort P, Stewart WJ, et al: Mechanisms of hemolysis with mitral prosthetic regurgitation study using transesophageal echocardiography and fluid dynamic simulation. *J Am Coll Cardiol* 27:399, 1996.

38. Kornowski R, Schwartz D, Jaffe A, Pines A, Aderka D, Levy Y: Erythropoietin therapy obviates the need for recurrent tranfusions in a patient with severe hemolysis due to prosthetic valves. *Chest* 102:315, 1992.

MICROANGIOPATHIC HEMOLYTIC ANEMIA

JOSE MARTINEZ

The term *microangiopathic hemolytic anemia* refers to a group of clinical disorders characterized by the fragmentation of red cells as they pass through the platelet-fibrin mesh present in microthrombi which are deposited in capillaries and arterioles. Since platelet-fibrin clot deposition in the small vessels is the main pathogenic mechanism, this disorder has also been referred to as thrombotic microangiopathy. The formation of arteriolar microthrombi can be caused by a variety of mechanisms, including activation of the coagulation system as occurs in disseminated intravascular coagulation, or by the formation of platelet aggregates induced by the release of very large von Willebrand factor multimers as in thrombotic thrombocytopenic purpura (TTP). In addition, antineoplastic and immunosuppressive agents as well as radiation therapy and bacterial toxins may induce endothelial cell injury leading to the formation of microthrombi in the affected vessels. Identification of the microangiopathic process and its specific etiology can help the clinician to institute prompt and appropriate treatment that frequently improves the hemolytic process and reverses end-organ failure.

Microangiopathic hemolytic anemia, first described in 1962,[1] refers to a group of clinical disorders that are characterized by fragmentation of the red cells within the circulatory system, leading to intravascular hemolysis. The common pathogenic mechanism is extracorpuscular and involves red cell fragmentation as a result of passage of the red cell through abnormal arterioles. Since deposition of platelets and fibrin is the most frequent cause of the microvascular lesion, this type of anemia has also been named *thrombotic microangiopathic hemolytic anemia*[2] or simply *thrombotic microangiopathy*.[2,3]

ETIOLOGY AND PATHOGENESIS

Thrombus formation inside blood vessels can play a major role in the disruption of red cells, as it can be directly observed when the red cells are forced through a loose fibrin clot formed inside a slide chamber.[4] The cells, after attaching to the fibrin, fold around the strands and are either released or fragmented by the force of the flowing blood. Some of the cell fragments reseal their membranes and acquire different shapes that are dependent upon the position and plane in which the red cell attaches and upon the distribution of membrane and hemoglobin within each fragment (Fig. 51-1). Fragmentation of the red cells induced by shear stress from interaction with platelet-fibrin deposits in the vascular bed may not be the only explanation. It is also possible that young erythrocytes may attach to endothelial cells via the association of red cell integrins with endothelial cells expressing adhesion molecules such as vascular cell adhesion molecule-1 (VCAM-1).[5] Other mechanisms for the attachment of red cells to the endothelium may include the interaction of large von Willebrand factor multimers as bridges between integrins present in the membrane of both young red cells and endothelial cells.[6] The attached red cells are then fragmented by the high shear stress present in microvessels. In vivo studies have also demonstrated the role of fibrin in the pathogenesis of microangiopathic hemolytic anemia. For example, snake venoms injected into rabbits induce a rapid defibrination syndrome that is associated with morphological alterations of the red cell, hemoglobinemia, and thrombus formation in several organs. The degree of hemoglobinemia correlates with the intensity of defibrination, and the hemolytic process is aggravated by treating the rabbits with fibrinolytic inhibitors.[7] Injection of endotoxin or thrombin into rabbits can also lead to intravascular coagulation with thrombosis of the renal vascular bed, resulting in the fragmentation of the red cells and intravascular hemolysis.[8] This experimental model resembles the microangiopathic hemolytic anemia and vascular occlusion found in some patients with sepsis, mainly induced by gram-negative bacteria,[9] or purpura fulminans.[10] Gastrointestinal infections with *Shigella dysenteria* or with *Escherichia coli*, mainly the serotype *E. coli* O157:H7, can induce a syndrome which is similar to either the uremic hemolytic syndrome or thrombotic thrombocytopenic purpura. Both *Shigella* and *E. coli* produce exotoxins that cause endothelial cell injury and platelet-fibrin microthrombi formation.[11,12] Microangiopathic hemolysis due to thrombotic thrombocytopenic purpura and uremic hemolytic syndrome is also associated with HIV infection, and the clinical and hematological manifestations of this group of patients respond as well to plasma exchange as non-HIV infected individuals.[13,14]

UNDERLYING DISORDERS

CANCER

Patients with invasive carcinoma may have a microangiopathic hemolytic anemia as described in one of the first reports of this syndrome.[1] It occurs in approximately 5 percent of cases, and its presence in patients with cancer suggests the presence of disseminated disease.[15–17] Thrombocytopenia, leukocytosis, with a shift to the left, and nucleated red blood cells in the blood film may also be present in this group of patients. The hemolytic process is most likely caused by fibrin deposition inside the blood vessels, but vascular disruption by malignant cells and secretion of cytokines that cause endothelial cell injury may also play a role.[15–17] In some instances, the diagnosis of intravascular coagulation can be made by finding a decrease in the concentration of specific clotting factors and detection of fibrin degradation products (see Chap. 126).[16] Mucin-producing tumors are more frequently associated with intravascular coagulation,[16] possibly due to the release of tissue factor and of a cysteine protease that is capable of activating factor X directly.[18]

PREGNANCY

Intravascular hemolysis can accompany certain complications of pregnancy, most notably preeclampsia, eclampsia, and abruptio placentae.[19,20] Intravascular coagulation is thought to play a role in the pathogenesis of the hemolytic process present in preeclampsia and eclampsia. This is supported by the presence of a small number of schistocytes, thrombocytopenia, high levels of fibrinopeptide A, and the deposition of fibrin in the kidney and liver.[19–21] These manifestations are most prominent in a subset of patients with severe preeclampsia, known as the HELLP syndrome, which is characterized by *h*emolysis, *e*levated *l*iver enzymes, and *l*ow *p*latelets.[19,22] However, hemolysis due to red cell fragmentation is also associated with malignant hypertension,[1] and it is possible that the severe hypertension which occurs in most of these patients contributes to the disruption of the red cell. The cause of the hemolysis is obscure, but narrowing and hardening of the arterioles along with endothelial cell swelling probably contrib-

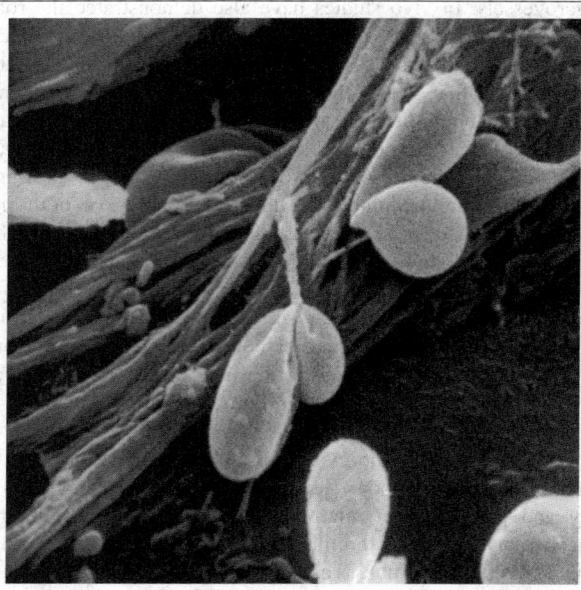

FIGURE 51-1   Hanged red cell. Dense fibrin band in background was formed from accumulations of finer strands, some of which are still evident. It is only these denser, more amorphous structures that typically persist postmortem. ×5200 in vitro model, scanning electron microscope. [From BS Bull, Kuhn IN: The production of schistocytes by fibrin strands (a scanning electron microscope study). *Blood* 35:104, 1970, with permission.]

utes to the mechanical destruction of the erythrocyte. Moreover, hemolysis may subside following normalization of the blood pressure.[23]

TTP AND UREMIC HEMOLYTIC SYNDROME

Two related clinical entities, thrombotic thrombocytopenic purpura and uremic hemolytic syndrome, are prototypical of microangiopathic hemolysis, which is accompanied by thrombocytopenia and by thrombosis of the small blood vessels of several organs, mainly the central nervous system and/or the kidneys[24] (see Chap. 117). Moreover, these microthrombi are mainly formed by platelet aggregates containing small amounts of fibrin(ogen).[25] In TTP the platelet thrombi appear to be formed by the binding of large multimers of von Willebrand factor to platelets under high shear stress.[26,27]

DRUGS

Certain drugs, especially antineoplastic agents, can cause clinical disorders that resemble uremic hemolytic syndrome or, less frequently, thrombotic thrombocytopenic purpura[17,28] (see Chap. 117). Mitomycin, given alone or in combination with other agents, is the drug most frequently associated with this disorder. However, bleomycin, daunorubicin in combination with cytosine arabinoside, and regimens containing cisplatin also have been implicated.[17,28] The clinical manifestations of uremic hemolytic syndrome following mitomycin therapy frequently do not become apparent until several weeks or months after discontinuation of the drug.[17,28] Although the pathogenesis of the hemolytic uremic syndrome is unclear, in some patients the disease is stable while in others the malignant process is in remission at the time of diagnosis, suggesting that mitomycin is, at least in part, responsible for the hematological abnormalities and for the lesions seen in the kidneys.[17,28] It is unclear whether mitomycin directly induces endothelial damage of the renal vascular bed or the lesions are induced by the deposition of immune complexes.[17] The pathological lesions

consist of arteriolar microthrombi similar to those described in idiopathic uremic hemolytic syndrome, and these patients frequently die from renal failure.[17,28] The recognition of this entity is important, since these patients can develop severe complications following the transfusion of blood products, whereas they may improve following extracorporeal immunoadsorption of their plasma on columns of staphyloccocal protein A.[28,29] Paradoxically, ticlopidine, a drug that inhibits platelet function, can cause severe thrombotic thrombocytopenic purpura leading to the demise of about one-third of the affected individuals.[30,31] The mechanism by which ticlopidine, or one of its metabolites, induces the thrombotic disorder is unknown, but the early recognition of this disorder is important, since plasma exchange reduces the mortality substantially.[31]

TRANSPLANTATION

Patients who have undergone kidney or liver transplantation occasionally develop microangiopathic hemolysis, thrombocytopenia, and impaired kidney function.[32] Multiple pathogenic mechanisms may be involved in this group of patients, including vascular damage induced by tissue rejection, the formation of immune complexes, and immunosuppressive therapy. These factors may lead to the formation of microthrombi in the small vessels of the kidney.[32,33] Among the immunosuppressive agents, cyclosporine is the drug most frequently associated with the hemolytic syndrome in this group of patients, and reduction of the dose or discontinuation of the drug followed by plasma exchange can reverse this pathologic process.[34,35] Hemolytic uremic syndrome can also occur after allogeneic and autologous marrow transplants, and it seems that total body irradiation, rather than chemotherapy, given to ablate the bone marrow is the responsible agent for the appearance of the uremic hemolytic syndrome.[32,33]

VASCULITIS

Patients with generalized vasculitis associated with immunological disorders (e.g., systemic lupus erythematosus, polyarteritis nodosa, Wegener's granulomatosis, and scleroderma) may also develop intravascular hemolysis due to microangiopathic hemolytic anemia.[36] The deposition of immune complexes in the arterioles may lead to local activation of the coagulation factors and fibrin formation. Damaged endothelium together with fibrin deposition are responsible for the fragmentation of the red cells.[36]

LOCALIZED VASCULAR ABNORMALITIES

Although the majority of cases of microangiopathic hemolytic anemia are due to disorders involving the vascular bed of several organs, occasionally fragmentation of the red cells occurs due to localized vascular abnormalities. Patients with cutaneous cavernous hemangiomas and with hemangioendotheliomas of the liver can sometimes develop microangiopathic hemolytic anemia associated with intravascular coagulation induced by the vascular malformation.[37,38]

CLINICAL FEATURES

The clinical manifestations of microangiopathic hemolytic anemia are the consequence of the primary process and may also reflect the organ affected by the intravascular deposition of platelets and fibrin (e.g., neurological manifestations of thrombotic thrombocytopenic purpura). Severe anemia and kidney failure may contribute to the constitutional symptoms in these patients. The physical findings can also reflect those expressed by the clinical entity causing the microangiopathic hemolytic anemia.

LABORATORY FINDINGS

The most prominent laboratory findings in microangiopathic hemolytic anemia are the alteration in the shape of the red blood cell, such as helmet cells, and formation of fragments termed *schistocytes*. Increases in the number of schistocytes to more than 3 per 5000 red cells should be considered abnormal, and a cause for this abnormality should be sought.[39] The typical schistocyte can be recognized by the presence of one to three sharp spicules (see Chap. 22). Microspherocytosis is also commonly seen. The alteration in the morphology of the red cell is similar to that seen in traumatic cardiac hemolytic anemia (see Chap. 50 and Fig. 50-1). The reticulocyte count is usually elevated, while the degree of thrombocytopenia is variable depending on the intensity of the consumption of platelets and on the capacity of the bone marrow to compensate for this process.

Another pertinent laboratory finding is a decrease in the concentration of haptoglobin, and some patients with marked hemolysis also have increased levels of plasma hemoglobin and hemoglobinuria. High levels of lactic dehydrogenase is almost a constant finding in microangiopathic hemolysis, and the level of this enzyme correlates with the activity of the disease. Coagulation abnormalities due to consumption coagulopathy can be seen in this group of patients. In patients with overt disseminated intravascular coagulation, factors V, VIII, antithrombin III, and fibrinogen are usually depleted. In addition, the levels of fibrinogen and fibrin degradation products are elevated, reflecting increased fibrinolytic activity. In other patients, the coagulation abnormalities are rather subtle, and immunological assays of fibrinopeptide A or of fibrin D dimer are useful in establishing the diagnosis. In several of the clinical entities associated with microangiopathic hemolysis like TTP, the formation of microthrombi is mainly due to platelet aggregates rather than fibrin deposition secondary to the activation of the coagulation system, and these cases show minimal or no evidence of intravascular coagulation.[24,25]

DIFFERENTIAL DIAGNOSIS

Microangiopathic hemolytic anemia should be differentiated from other types of intravascular hemolysis, for example, certain forms of autoimmune hemolytic anemia or paroxysmal nocturnal hemoglobinuria. However, the presence of schistocytes in the blood film, thrombocytopenia, negative Coombs' test combined with the detection of intravascular coagulation, and identification of the primary process are characteristic of microangiopathic hemolytic anemia. The causes of the anemia can be multifactorial; iron and/or folate deficiency, hemorrhage, and marrow involvement due to infiltrative processes can contribute to the anemia. The most common causes of microangiopathic hemolytic anemia are listed in Table 51-1.

THERAPY, COURSE, AND PROGNOSIS

The treatment of this disorder should be directed toward the management of the underlying process that is responsible for the microangiopathic hemolysis. Frequently, patients require red cell transfusions to maintain an adequate level of hemoglobin. In cases presenting bleeding manifestations and thrombocytopenia, platelet transfusions can help to arrest the bleeding. The clinical management of thrombotic thrombocytopenic purpura and uremic hemolytic syndrome is discussed in detail in Chap. 117.

Although intravascular coagulation is commonly a pathogenic mechanism in microangiopathic hemolytic anemia, the use of anticoagulants is controversial. In a few selected cases, heparin therapy seems to improve this process,[40] but the use of anticoagulants does not seem to be efficacious in the majority of patients[40] (Chap. 126). In the

TABLE 51-1   CLASSIFICATION OF MICROANGIOPATHIC HEMOLYTIC ANEMIA

Primary
Thrombotic thrombocytopenic purpura[1–3,24–27]
Hemolytic uremic syndrome[1–3,24–27]
Secondary
Associated with disseminated intravascular coagulation
  Infections[8–10]
  Shiga type toxins[11,12]
  HIV[13,14]
  Snake venoms[7,36]
  Abruptio placentae[19,20]
Associated with hypertension
  Malignant hypertension[1,23]
  Preeclampsia, eclampsia, HELLP syndrome[19–22]
Associated with malignancy
  Adenocarcinomas: gastrointestinal, breast, lung[1,15–17]
Associated with drugs and/or radiation
  Antineoplastic agents[16,17,28,29]
  Radiation nephritis and chemotherapy in organ transplantation[32–35]
  Ticlopidine[30,31]
Associated with immunological disorders
  Acute glomerulonephritis[36]
  Polyarteritis nodosa[36]
  Scleroderma[36]
Associated with congenital malformations
  Cavernous hemangioma (Kasabach-Merritt syndrome)[37]
  Hemangioendothelioma of the liver[38]

particular case of uremic hemolytic syndrome associated with mitomycin C, immunoadsorption of patient plasma by staphylococcal protein A can normalize the platelet count and stabilize the serum creatinine.[29]

REFERENCES

1. Brain MC, Dacie JV, Hourihane DO: Microangiopathic haemolytic anaemia: the possible role of vascular lesions in pathogenesis. *Br J Haematol* 8:358, 1962.
2. Symmers WC: Thrombotic microangiopathic haemolytic anaemia. *Br Med J* 2:897, 1952.
3. Kwaan HC: Introduction: thrombotic microangiopathy. *Semin Hematol* 24:69, 1987.
4. Bull BS, Rubenberg ML, Dacie JV, Brain MC: Microangiopathic haemolytic anaemia: mechanisms of red cell fragmentation in vitro studies. *Br J Haematol* 14:643, 1968.
5. Swerlick RA, Eckman JR, Kumar A, Jeitler M, Wick TM: $\alpha_4\beta_1$-integrin expression on sickle reticulocytes: vascular cell adhesion molecule-1-dependent binding to endothelium. *Blood* 82:1891, 1993.
6. Wick TM, Moake JL, Udden MM, McIntire LV: Unusually large von Willebrand factor multimers preferentially promote young sickle and nonsickle erythrocyte adhesion to endothelial cells. *Am J Haematol* 42:284, 1993.
7. Rubenberg ML, Regoeczi E, Bull BS, Dacie JV, Brain MC: Microangiopathic haemolytic anaemia: the experimental production of haemolysis and red cell fragmentation by defibrination in vivo. *Br J Haematol* 14:627, 1968.
8. Brain MC: Microangiopathic hemolytic anemia. *Ann Rev Med* 21:133, 1970.
9. Kreger BE, Craven DE, McCabe WR: Gram-negative bacteremia: IV. Re-evaluation of clinical features and treatment in 612 patients. *Am J Med* 68:344, 1980.
10. Hollingsworth JH, Mohler DN: Microangiopathic hemolytic anaemia caused by purpura fulminans. *Ann Intern Med* 68:1310, 1968.
11. Keusch GT, Acheson DWK: Thrombotic thrombocytopenic purpura associated with Shiga toxins. *Semin Hematol* 34:106, 1997.
12. Boyce TG, Swerdlow DL, Griffin PM: *Escherichia coli* O157:H7 and the hemolytic-uremic syndrome. *N Engl J Med* 333:364, 1995.
13. Thompson CE, Damon LE, Ries CA, Linker CA: Thrombotic microangiopathies in the 1980s: clinical features, response to treatment, and the impact of the human immunodeficiency virus epidemic. *Blood* 80:1890, 1992.

14. Hymes KB, Karpatkin S: Human immunodeficiency virus infection and thrombotic microangiopathy. *Semin Hematol* 34:117, 1997.

15. Antman KH, Skarin AT, Mayer RJ, Hargreaves HK, Canellos GP: Microangiopathic hemolytic anemia and cancer: a review. *Medicine* 58:377, 1979.

16. Murgo AJ: Thrombotic microangiopathy in the cancer patient including those induced by chemotherapeutic agents. *Semin Hematol* 24:161, 1987.

17. Gordon LI, Kwaan HC: Cancer- and drug-associated thrombotic thrombocytopenic purpura and hemolytic uremic syndrome. *Semin Hematol* 34:140, 1997.

18. Rickles FR, Edwards RL: Activation of blood coagulation in cancer: Trousseau's syndrome revisited. *Blood* 62:14, 1983.

19. McCrae KR, Cines DB: Thrombotic microangiopathy during pregnancy. *Semin Hematol* 34:148, 1997.

20. Pritchard JA, Brekken AL: Clinical and laboratory studies on severe abruptio placentae. *Am J Obstet Gynecol* 97:681, 1967.

21. Vassalli P, Morris RH, McCluskey RT: The pathogenic role of fibrin deposition in the glomerular lesions of toxemia of pregnancy. *J Exp Med* 118:467, 1963.

22. Weinstein L: Syndrome of hemolysis, elevated liver enzymes, and low platelet count: a severe consequence of hypertension in pregnancy. *Am J Obstet Gynecol* 142:159, 1982.

23. Capelli JP, Wesson LG Jr, Erslev AJ: Malignant hypertension and red cell fragmentation syndrome. *Ann Intern Med* 64:128, 1966.

24. Kwaan HC: Clinicopathologic features of thrombotic thrombocytopenic purpura. *Semin Hematol* 24:71, 1987.

25. Asada Y, Sumiyoshi A, Hayashi T: Immunohistochemistry of the vascular lesion in thrombotic thrombocytopenic purpura, with special reference to factor VIII related antigen. *Thromb Res* 38:469, 1985.

26. Tsai H-M, Lian E C-Y: Antibodies to von Willebrand factor-cleaving protease in acute thrombotic thrombocytopenic purpura. *N Engl J Med* 339:1585, 1998.

27. Furlan M, Robles R, Galbusera M, et al: von Willebrand factor-cleaving protease in thrombotic thrombocytopenia purpura and the hemolytic-uremic syndrome. *N Engl J Med* 339:1578, 1998.

28. Doll DC, Yarbro JW: Vascular toxicity associated with antineoplastic agents. *Semin Oncol* 19:580, 1992.

29. Snyder HW Jr, Mittelman A, Oral A, et al: Treatment of cancer chemotherapy-associated thrombotic thrombocytopenic purpura/hemolytic uremic syndrome by protein A immunoadsorption of plasma. *Cancer* 71:1882, 1993.

30. Page Y, Tardy B, Zeni F, Comtet C, Terrana R, Bertrand JG: Thrombotic thrombocytopenic purpura related to ticlopidine. *Lancet* 337:774, 1991.

31. Bennett CL, Weinberg PD, Rozenberg-Ben-Dror K, Yarnold PR, Kwaan HC, Green G: Thrombotic thrombocytopenic purpura associated with ticlopidine: a review of 60 cases. *Ann Int Med* 128:541, 1998.

32. Schriber JR, Herzig GP: Transplantation-associated thrombotic thrombocytopenic purpura and hemolytic uremic syndrome. *Semin Hematol* 34:126, 1997.

33. Rabinowe SN, Soiffer RJ, Tarbell NJ, et al: Hemolytic-uremic syndrome following bone marrow transplantation in adults for hematologic malignancies. *Blood* 77:1837, 1991.

34. Buturovic J, Kandus A, Malovrh M, Bren A, Drinovec J: Cyclosporine-associated hemolytic uremic syndrome in four renal allograft recipients: resolution without specific therapy. *Transplant Proc* 22:1726, 1990.

35. Venkat KK, Tkach D, Kupin W, et al: Reversal of cyclosporine-associated hemolytic-uremic syndrome by plasma exchange with fresh-frozen plasma replacement in renal transplant recipients. *Transplant Proc* 23:1256, 1991.

36. Kwaan HC: Miscellaneous secondary thrombotic microangiopathy. *Semin Hematol* 24:141, 1987.

37. Propp RP, Scharfmann WB: Hemangioma-thrombocytopenia syndrome associated with microangiopathic hemolytic anemia. *Blood* 28:623, 1966.

38. Alpert LI, Benisch G: Hemangioendothelioma of the liver associated with microangiopathic hemolytic anemia. *Am J Med* 48:624, 1970.

39. Chou C, Jajeh A, Shiomoto G, Shah P: Schistocytes in normal individuals. *Blood* 92:4b, 1998.

40. Feinstein DI: Diagnosis and management of disseminated intravascular coagulation: the role of heparin therapy. *Blood* 60:284, 1982.

MARCH HEMOGLOBINURIA, SPORTS ANEMIA, AND SPACE ANEMIA

ALLAN J. ERSLEV

Strenuous activities may cause traumatic damage to red cells, with subsequent hemolysis and hemoglobinuria or metabolic changes leading to an expanded plasma volume and dilution anemia. In astronauts, the effect of microgravity leads to changes in blood volume, with relative erythrocytosis when in space and mild anemia after reentry to Earth's gravitational field.

Individuals involved in strenuous physical activities and astronauts following spaceflights are frequently found to be mildly anemic.[1-3] The causes are complex and controversial but appear to involve hemolysis and blood loss as well as induced alterations in plasma volume and red cell mass. In marchers and runners, traumatic hemolysis may cause hemoglobinuria and anemia, while in athletes and astronauts, a change in blood volume appears to be the major cause.

ETIOLOGY AND PATHOGENESIS

MARCH HEMOGLOBINURIA

The first clue to the pathogenesis of hemoglobinuria and anemia in individuals participating in long marches was provided in 1861 by an army physician who studied a young German soldier who had complained of passing dark urine following strenuous field marches.[4] He found that the urine contained hemoglobin and that the condition clearly differed from the well-described paroxysmal hemoglobinuria due to cold. During the next 80 years, many additional cases of hemoglobinuria following long-distance running were reported,[5,6] but it was not until 1964 that Davidson provided a logical explanation.[7] He noticed that two track runners who complained of dark urine after games had a particularly forceful stamping gait, and he proposed that red cells were destroyed in the soles of the feet during running. After some ingenious preparatory studies the runners were encouraged to change their stride and especially to wear soft linings in their shoes, and the hemoglobinuria disappeared. The beneficial effect of better footwear has been noticed in many subsequent studies of athletes,[8] but even with well-designed, padded insoles there is still some traumatic disruption of red cells by pressure on the soles during running and walking.[9] Similar traumatic red cell destruction with hemoglobinuria has been reported after beating the head against a wall,[10] hand-strengthening exercises in a practitioner of karate,[11] and playing the conga drums.[12]

SPORTS ANEMIA

The effects of intravascular hemolysis on hemoglobin concentration in athletes may be augmented by gastrointestinal blood loss, which occurs in about 20 percent of long-distance runners during strenuous races[13,14] and by occasional traumatic renal blood loss.[15] These effects, however, should be easily compensated for by healthy individuals and would not be expected to cause a measurable anemia.[16] Furthermore, hemoglobinuria and gastrointestinal blood loss have only been observed in runners, not in swimmers or bicyclists, and those endurance athletes also have a reduction in hemoglobin concentration.[17] It is also unlikely that the associated loss of iron would result in an iron-deficiency state. Nevertheless, the serum ferritin has been found to be decreased in many studies of athletes in training.[18-20] The cause is obscure but may indicate a greater than anticipated loss of iron in sweat[21] or even the rapid turnover of iron-containing compounds active in muscular oxidative metabolism.[22] It could also be caused by a shift of iron from tissues to the red cell mass if, despite the slight anemia, there is an increase in the size of the red cell mass. That this may actually be the case is suggested by measurements of the red cell and plasma volumes in athletes in active training.[23] It appears that elite runners have an increase in both plasma volume and red cell mass,[24-26] but the gain in plasma volume always exceeds the gain in red cell mass. The results should in theory be of considerable benefit, since the circulatory advantage of an increased red cell mass and blood volume are augmented by an increase in blood fluidity.[27]

SPACE ANEMIA

Astronauts are moderately anemic when tested several days after reentry. The cause of this anemia has been related to the redistribution of blood volume that occurs during weightlessness.[28] At blast-off, there is acute redistribution of blood from the extremities to the torso, resulting in an acute hypervolemia in the upper part of the body. This induces a diuretic response, which reduces the plasma volume and local hypervolemia but results in an increase in the hematocrit. This causes a reduction in the erythropoietin level and the rate of red cell production. After 8 to 10 days in space, the red cell mass is reduced by 10 to 15 percent, and the astronaut will continue the flight with a normal hematocrit but a reduced red cell mass. At reentry into a normal gravitational field, the plasma and blood volumes are restored rapidly to normal, but the hematocrit, now reflecting the low red cell mass, decreases until an increase in the rate of red cell production restores both hematocrit and red cell mass to normal.

The relatively rapid changes in the size of the red cell mass in space and after reentry have been difficult to explain, since erythrokinetic studies have failed to show dramatic changes in iron turnover or erythropoietin titers.[29] The absence of overt hemolysis of red cells labeled by ^{51}Cr before the spaceflight has led to the hypothesis that newly created red cells depend on erythropoietin for their survival and will be selectively destroyed during spaceflight.[30] However, the lack of marked changes in erythropoietin levels during and after spaceflight fail to explain both the traditional and the new explanation for the acute changes in red cell mass.

CLINICAL AND LABORATORY FEATURES

In march hemoglobinuria and sports anemia, traumatic hemolysis and blood loss play a role in the mild reduction in the hemoglobin concentration; the anemia is usually associated with a slight increase in reticulocyte count and occasionally the presence of echinocytes.[31] Immediately after a period of physical exertion, the urine may contain hemoglobin, hemoglobin casts, and hemosiderin. Serum iron and iron-binding capacity are usually normal, but the ferritin may be lower than before the physical exertion. In space anemias, the only finding is a moderate lowering of hemoglobin and hematocrit for a few weeks after reentry.

DIFFERENTIAL DIAGNOSIS

The history is, of course, of primary importance and leaves little to the imagination. Nevertheless, a reduction in hemoglobin in any young, healthy individual should be investigated further if not easily explained by the history.

The widespread use by athletes of erythropoietin to augment hemoglobin concentration and in turn oxygen transport to muscles has been difficult to diagnose. However, a high hematocrit in a competing athlete should raise suspicion of such misuse, since intense training would tend to lower the hematocrit.

THERAPY, COURSE, AND PROGNOSIS

No treatment is necessary, but if hemolysis is severe enough to cause hemoglobinuria, good footwear and a reduction in physical activities may be recommended.

REFERENCES

1. Londemann R: Low hematocrits during basic training: athlete's anemia. *N Engl J Med* 299:1191, 1978.
2. Eichner ER: The anemias of athletes. *Phys Sports Med* 14:122, 1986.
3. Leach CS, Johnson PC: Influence of spaceflight on erythrokinetics in man. *Science* 225:216, 1984.
4. Fleischer R: Uber eine neue Form von Hämoglobinurie beim Menschen. *Berlin Klin Wochenschr* 18:691, 1881.
5. Gilligan DR, Blumgart HL: March hemoglobinuria: studies of the clinical characteristics, blood metabolism and mechanisms with observations on three new cases and review of literature. *Medicine (Baltimore)* 20:314, 1941.
6. Gilligan DR, Altschule MD, Katersky EM: Psychologic intravascular hemolysis of exercise: hemoglobinemia and hemoglobinuria following cross-country runs. *J Clin Invest* 22:859, 1943.
7. Davidson RJL: Exertional hemoglobinuria: a report on three cases with studies on the haemolytic mechanism. *J Clin Pathol* 17:536, 1964.
8. Buckle RM: Exertional (march) hemoglobinuria: reduction of haemolytic episodes by use of sorbo-rubber insoles in shoes. *Lancet* 1:1136, 1965.
9. Eichner ER: Runner's macrocytosis: a clue to footstrike hemolysis. Runner's anemia as a benefit versus runner's hemolysis as a detriment. *Am J Med* 78:321, 1985.
10. Ensor CW, Barnett JOW: Paroxysmal hemoglobinuria of traumatic origin. *Med-Chir Trans* 86:165, 1903.
11. Streeton JA: Traumatic haemoglobinuria caused by karate exercises. *Lancet* 2:191, 1967.
12. Furie B, Penn AS: Pigmenturia from conga drumming: hemoglobinuria and myoglobinuria. *Ann Intern Med* 80:727, 1974.
13. Buckman MT: Gastrointestinal bleeding in long distance runners. *Ann Intern Med* 101:127, 1984.
14. Mechrefe A, Wexler B, Feller E: Sports anemia and gastrointestinal bleeding in endurance athletes. *Med Health* 80:216, 1997.
15. Abarbanel J, Benet AE, Lask D, Kimche D: Sports hematuria. *J Urol* 143:887, 1990.
16. Hallberg L, Magnusson B: The etiology of "sports anemia." *Acta Med Scand* 216:145, 1984.
17. Clement DB, Asmundson RC, Medhurst CW: Hemoglobin values: comparative study of the 1976 Canadian Olympic Team. *Can Med Assoc J* 117:614, 1977.
18. Magnuson B, Hallberg L, Rossander L, Swolin B: Iron metabolism and "sports anemia": I and II. *Acta Med Scand* 216:149, 1984.
19. Newhouse J, Clement D: Iron status in athletes: an update. *Sports Med* 5:337,1988.
20. Roberts D, Smith DJ: Training at moderate altitude: iron status of elite male swimmers. *J Lab Clin Med* 120:387, 1992.
21. Pauley P, Jordal R, Strandberg Pedersen N: Dermal excretion of iron in intensely training athletes. *Clin Chem Acta* 127:19, 1983.
22. Holloszy J, Coyle EF: Adaptations of skeletal muscle to endurance exercise and their metabolic consequences. *J Appl Physiol* 56:831, 1984.
23. Fellmann N: Hormonal and plasma volume alterations following endurance exercise. *Sports Med* 13:37, 1992.
24. Brotherhood J, Brogovic B, Pugh LGC: Haematological status of middle- and long-distance runners. *Clin Sci Mol Med* 48:139, 1975.
25. Dressendorfer RH, Wade CE, Amsterdam EA: Development of pseudoanemia in marathon runners during a 20-day road race. *JAMA* 246:1215, 1981.
26. Schmidt W, Maasen N, Trost R, Boening D: Training-induced effects on blood volume, erythrocyte turnover, and hemoglobin oxygen properties. *Eur J Appl Physiol* 57:490, 1988.
27. Thorling EB, Erslev AJ: The "tissue" tension of oxygen and its relation to hematocrit and erythropoiesis. *Blood* 31:332, 1968.
28. Udden MM, Driscoll TB, Pickett MH, Leach-Huntoon CS, Alfrey CP: Decreased production of red blood cells in human subjects exposed to microgravity. *J Lab Clin Med* 125:442, 1995.
29. Alfrey CP, Udden MM, Leach-Huntoon C, Driscoll T, Pickett MH: Control of the red blood cell mass in spaceflight. *J Appl Physiol* 81:98, 1996.
30. Alfrey CP, Rice L, Udden MM, Driscoll TB: Neocytosis: physiological down-regulator of red-cell mass. *Lancet* 349:1389, 1997.
31. Selby GB, Frame DC, Eichner LK, Eichner ER: Athlete's echinocytes: new cause of exertional hemolysis? *Blood* 70(suppl):56a, 1987.

HEMOLYTIC ANEMIA DUE TO CHEMICAL AND PHYSICAL AGENTS

ERNEST BEUTLER

Arsenic, lead, copper, chlorates, and a variety of other chemicals can cause severe red cell destruction, and hemolytic anemia is a part of the clinical syndrome associated with intoxication by these substances. Arsenic may cause hemolysis by interacting with sulfhydryl groups. Lead inhibits a variety of red cell enzymes, including several enzymes of porphyrin metabolism and pyrimidine-5′-nucleotidase. The anemia that it produces is usually not primarily hemolytic in nature. Copper inhibits a number of red cell enzymes and catalyses the oxidation of intracellular GSH. Chlorates produce methemoglobin and Heinz bodies. There are many drugs that have appeared to cause hemolytic anemia, usually by unknown or poorly defined mechanisms. Animal toxins, such as those elaborated by insects, spiders, and snakes, may also cause hemolytic anemia. Hemolytic anemia is a common accompaniment of severe burns, probably as a result of direct damage to erythrocytes by heat.

Many drugs and a variety of toxins have been associated with red cell destruction. Hemolysis that results when certain drugs are administered to patients deficient in glucose-6-phosphate dehydrogenase or with unstable hemoglobins is discussed in Chaps. 45 and 48. Immune mechanisms may also play a role in drug- or toxin-induced hemolytic anemias. Such hemolytic anemias are discussed in Chap. 57. Microangiopathic hemolytic anemias (Chap. 51) may also be caused by drugs such as mitomycin.

The present chapter deals with drugs, toxins, and other physical agents that can cause red cell destruction by other mechanisms, or by mechanisms that are not understood at present.

ARSENIC HYDRIDE

The inhalation of arsine gas (arsenic hydride, AsH_3) is a well-recognized cause of hemolytic anemia.[1,2] Arsine is formed during many industrial processes. Most commonly it results from the reaction of nascent hydrogen, generated by the action of acid on metal, with arsenic compounds. The arsenic is usually present as a contaminant of either the acid or the metal, so that the contact with arsenic compounds may not be apparent from the history. Exposure to sufficient amounts of the gas will lead to severe anemia, jaundice, and hemoglobinuria. The mechanism of hemolysis is not clearly understood, al-

though the well-known reactions of arsenic compounds with sulfhydryl groups in the cell membrane may play an important role.

LEAD

Lead poisoning (plumbism) has been recognized since antiquity. The ingestion of beverages containing lead leached from highly soluble lead glazes or earthenware containers has been blamed for the decline and fall of the Roman aristocracy and is even now an occasional cause of lead intoxication.[3] The distillation of alcohol in leaded flasks is another rare cause of plumbism in certain areas, although the practice was prohibited in 1723 by the Massachusetts Bay Colony after it was noticed that consumption of rum so distilled resulted in abdominal pain known as the "dry gripes."[3] Among the earliest published descriptions of lead poisoning is a letter written in 1786 by Benjamin Franklin[4,5] who had learned as a printer that working over small furnaces of melted metal or drying racks of wet type in front of a fire might cause pain in the hands. Today, lead intoxication in children generally results from ingestion of flaking lead paint or from chewing lead-painted articles. In adults, it occurs primarily as the result of inhalation of lead compounds used or produced in industrial processes[6] as in battery manufacture,[7] but poisoning may occur as a result of leaching from pottery or dishes that come in contact with food.[8,9] Restoring tapestries and producing pottery and tiles[10,11] have also caused lead poisoning. Most patients with lead poisoning manifest some degree of anemia, although anemia is only rarely the predominant clinical manifestation.[12] However, examination of the blood often provides the key diagnostic clue, and thus the hematologic findings are of special interest. Modest shortening of red cell life-span is a relatively constant feature of the disorder.[13,14] In vitro treatment of red cells with lead produces measurable membrane damage: lead interferes with the cation pump,[15,16] possibly in inhibiting membrane ATPase.[17,18] It is not at all clear, however, that the hemolysis observed in lead poisoning is due to these changes. In some children with lead poisoning, an electrophoretically fast moving hemoglobin indistinguishable from hemoglobin A_3 comprises approximately 15 percent of the total pigment.[19]

The anemia of lead intoxication is not usually due primarily to hemolysis. Lead apparently interferes with the normal production of erythrocytes, probably through a combination of mechanisms. Heme synthesis is markedly abnormal in patients with lead poisoning. Several enzymes of heme synthesis are inhibited, including δ-aminolevulinic acid (ALA) synthetase, ALA dehydrase, heme synthetase, porphyrinogen deaminase, uroporphyrinogen decarboxylase, and coproporphyrinogen oxidase.[12,13] ALA dehydrase has been considered particularly sensitive to inhibition, showing decreased activity in erythrocytes at blood lead levels in the upper portions of the normal range,[17] but its sensitivity at low blood lead levels has been questioned.[20] Increased amounts of δ-aminolevulinic acid and coproporphyrin are found in the urine,[21] and the free protoporphyrin levels[22] of the erythrocytes are strikingly increased, presumably as a result of inhibition of the heme biosynthetic enzymes. Marked inhibition of the enzyme pyrimidine 5′-nucleotidase is also observed.[23,24] In the absence of this enzyme, pyrimidine nucleotides accumulate in the red cells and normal depolymerization of reticulocyte ribosomal RNA does not occur. In hereditary pyrimidine 5′-nucleotidase deficiency, basophilic stippling of erythrocytes is a characteristic finding (Chap. 45), and it has been suggested that inhibition of pyrimidine-5′-nucleotidase by lead may be responsible for the basophilic stippling of erythrocytes that occurs in plumbism (see below). Inhibition of activity of the hexose monophosphate shunt has been documented.[25] Synthesis of α- and β-globin chains seems to be defective in lead poisoning,[26] and this may play a contributory role in the anemia of lead poisoning.

Acronyms and abbreviations that appear in this chapter include: ALA, aminolevulinic acid; EDTA, ethylenediaminetetraacetic acid; GR, glutathione reductase; GSH, reduced glutathione; G-6-PD, glucose-6-phosphate dehydrogenase; NADPH, reduced nicotinamide-adenine dinucleotide phosphate.

Remarkably complete observations of the acute hematologic changes occurring after the intravenous injection of lead in an attempt to treat malignant disease were published in 1928.[27] Distortion of red cells was observed both in blood films and in wet preparations made immediately after infusion of lead. This was characterized by a "folding" that made the cells appear as semicircles, clumping, and the presence of "bite cells." The anemia of chronic lead poisoning is usually mild in the adult but is frequently more severe in children. A relatively close relationship exists between blood lead levels and the hematocrit.[28] The red cells are normocytic and slightly hypochromic. The hypochromia may be due to coexisting iron deficiency.[29] Basophilic stippling of the erythrocytes may be fine or coarse, and the number of granules seen in each cell may be quite variable. When blood is collected in ethylenediaminetetraacetic acid (EDTA; "purple top" tube), as is commonly done, the stippling may disappear.[30] Young polychromatophilic cells are most likely to be stippled. Electron microscopic studies[31] have demonstrated that the basophilic granules represent abnormally aggregated ribosomes. In the marrow, ringed sideroblasts (Chap. 22) are frequently found. Iron-laden mitochondria are present[31] but do not appear to contribute to the basophilic stippling that is observed on light microscopy. It may be presumed that iron entering the developing erythroblast fails to be incorporated into heme at a normal rate, either because of lead-induced impairment of heme synthesis or because of the direct effect of lead on mitochondria.

Meso 2,3-dimercaptosuccinic acid, an orally administered chelating agent has been used to treat lead poisoning.[32,33]

COPPER

Hemolysis has also resulted from ingestion of copper sulfate in suicide attempts and from accumulation of toxic amounts from hemodialysis fluid contaminated by copper pipes.[34,35] Hemolysis in Wilson disease has been attributed to the elevated plasma copper levels characteristic of that disorder,[36-38] and hemolytic anemia may be the presenting symptom.[39,40] The pathogenesis of this hemolytic anemia may be related to oxidation of intracellular GSH, hemoglobin, and NADPH and inhibition of glucose-6-phosphate dehydrogenase (G-6-PD) by copper.[41] However, the amount of copper required to inhibit G-6-PD is large, and copper in much lower concentrations inhibits pyruvate kinase,[42] hexokinase, phosphogluconate dehydrogenase, phosphofructokinase, and phosphoglycerate kinase.[43] Plasma exchange has been used successfully to treat the hemolytic anemia of Wilson disease.[44]

CHLORATES

Sodium and potassium chlorate are oxidative drugs which have been known to produce methemoglobinemia, Heinz bodies, and hemolytic anemia. While it might be presumed that the mechanism of hemolysis is similar to that resulting from other oxidative drugs, no cases have been observed in patients deficient in G-6-PD. The rare instances of chlorate poisoning that have been reported usually resulted from prescription errors in which sodium chlorate was dispensed instead of sodium chloride.[45] Hemolytic anemia with Heinz body formation has also occurred in patients undergoing dialysis when the tap water used contained a substantial amount of chloramines. Oxidative damage of the red cells of these patients was demonstrated by the presence of Heinz bodies, a positive ascorbate-cyanide test, and methemoglobinemia.[46,47] Leaching of formaldehyde from plastic used in a water filter employed for hemodialysis is also a cause of hemolytic anemia. It was suggested that the effect of the low levels of formaldehyde found in the water were not mediated through its fixative effect but rather by inducing metabolic changes in the red cells.[48]

TABLE 53-1   DRUGS AND CHEMICALS THAT HAVE BEEN REPORTED TO CAUSE CLINICALLY SIGNIFICANT HEMOLYTIC ANEMIA

CHEMICALS

Aniline[49]
Apiol[50]
Dichlorprop (herbicide)[51]
Formaldehyde[48]
Hydroxylamines[52]
Lysol[53]
Mineral spirits[54]
Nitrobenzene[55]
Resorcin[56]

DRUGS

Amyl nitrite[57]
Mephenesin[58]
Methylene blue[59,60]
Omeprazole[61]
Pentachlorophenol[62]
Phenazopyridine (Pyridium)[63,64]
Salicylazosulfapyridine (Azulfidine)[65,66]

MISCELLANEOUS DRUGS AND CHEMICALS

There are also isolated reports of hemolytic anemia occurring after the administration of a variety of other substances, listed in Table 53-1.

Hemolytic anemia produced by phenazopyridine is often associated with "bite cells" and "blister cells."[67] When large amounts of distilled water gain access to the systemic circulation, either by intravenous injection or when used as an irrigating solution during surgery, hemolysis will occur.[68] Severe hemolysis may also result from water inhalation in near-drowning.[69]

OXYGEN

Hemolytic anemia has been observed in astronauts exposed to 100 percent oxygen; a reduction of red cell volume also occurs when the O_2 tension is maintained at normal atmospheric levels, and this is believed to be due in some unknown way to weightlessness.[70] In at least one patient, hyperbaric oxygenation was associated with acute hemolysis.[71] It was suggested that hemolysis in this instance may have been due to abnormal peroxidation of lipids in the erythrocytes, but evidence supporting this view was indirect and equivocal.

INSECT, SPIDER, AND SNAKE VENOMS

Bee[72] and wasp[73-75] stings have been associated with severe hemolysis, and spider or scorpion bites have occasionally been followed by hemolytic anemia and hemoglobinuria.[76-81] The spiders usually thought to be responsible are *Loxosceles loeta* and *Loxosceles reclusus*. It is unknown why some patients suffer hemolysis after insect bites whereas others do not. Although snake venom may cause hemolysis in vitro by converting lecithin to lysolecithin (see Chap. 27), hemolysis does not often result from snake bites,[82] and when it does occur, it may represent microangiopathic hemolytic anemia associated with coagulation abnormalities induced by the venom.[83]

HEAT

It has been known for over a hundred years that heating blood to temperatures above 47°C (117°F) rapidly produces visible damage to erythrocytes. The sequence of events has been defined in detail.[84] Cells damaged by heating not only show morphologic changes and increases in osmotic and mechanical fragility but are also removed rapidly after reinjection into the circulation.[85] These observations explain the severe hemolytic anemia which occurs in patients with extensive burns. Spherocytosis and increased osmotic fragility are found in many patients, and blood films may show fragmentation, budding, spherocytosis, and severe microspherocytosis. These changes are particularly evident if films are made promptly after the burn occurs. Gross hemoglobinemia was observed in 11 of 40 patients with second- and third-degree burns involving 15 to 65 percent of the body surface.[86] It seems likely that the acute hemolytic anemia occurring within the 24 h following a burn is due to the direct effect of heat on circulating erythrocytes. Hemolysis occurring more than 24 h after the burn may sometimes be due to the infusion of isoagglutinins (particularly anti-A) in pooled plasma, when this has been administered to the patient as part of treatment,[87] or be the result of infection or coagulation disorders that are common complications of extensive burn injury.

RADIATION

Although reduced red cell survival is a part of the complex series of events occurring after administration of large doses of total body radiation,[88] erythrocytes appear to be very resistant to the direct effects of radiation.[89] Such shortened red cell survival as may occur after radiation is probably related largely to red cell loss through internal bleeding and to various secondary events such as infection.

REFERENCES

1. Phoon WH, Chan MO, Goh CH, et al: Five cases of arsine poisoning. *Ann Acad Med Singapore* 13(2, suppl):394, 1984.
2. Romeo L, Apostoli P, Kovacic M, Martini S, Brugnone F: Acute arsine intoxication as a consequence of metal burnishing operations. *Am J Ind Med* 32:211, 1997.
3. Klein M, Namer R, Harpur E, Corbin R: Earthenware containers as a source of fatal lead poisoning. *N Engl J Med* 283:669, 1970.
4. *The Complete Works of Benjamin Franklin*, edited by J Bigelow, Putnam, New York, 1888.
5. Andreasen NJC: Benjamin Franklin: Physicus et medicus. *JAMA* 236:57, 1976.
6. Staudinger KC, Roth VS: Occupational lead poisoning. *Am Fam Physician* 57:719, 1998.
7. Froom P, Kristal-Boneh E, Benbassat J, Ashkanazi R, Ribak J: Predictive value of determinations of zinc protoporphyrin for increased blood lead concentrations. *Clin Chem* 44:1283, 1998.
8. Autenrieth T, Schmidt T, Habscheid W: Lead poisoning caused by a Greek ceramic cup. *Dtsch Med Wochenschr* 123:353, 1998.
9. Kakosy T, Hudak A, Naray M: Lead intoxication epidemic caused by ingestion of contaminated ground paprika. *J Toxicol Clin Toxicol* 34:507, 1996.
10. Fischbein A, Wallace J, Sassa S, et al: Lead poisoning from art restoration and pottery work: unusual exposure source and household risk. *J Environ Pathol Toxicol Oncol* 11:7, 1992.
11. Vahter M, Counter SA, Laurell G, et al: Extensive lead exposure in children living in an area with production of lead-glazed tiles in the Ecuadorian Andes. *Int Arch Occup Environ Health* 70:282, 1997.
12. Harris JW, Kellermeyer RW: Acquired abnormality: Porphyrinuria, in *The Red Cell*, p 35. Harvard University Press, Cambridge, 1970.
13. Waldron HA: The anaemia of lead poisoning: A review. *Br J Ind Med* 23:83, 1966.
14. Westerman MP, Pfitzer E, Ellis LD, Jensen WN: Concentrations of lead in bone in plumbism. *N Engl J Med* 273:1246, 1965.
15. Khalil-Manesh F, Tartaglia-Erler J, Gonick HC: Experimental model of lead nephropathy. IV. Correlation between renal functional changes and hematological indices of lead toxicity. *J Trace Elem Electrolytes Health Dis* 8:13, 1994.
16. Vincent PC, Blackburn CRB: The effects of heavy metal ions on the human erythrocyte. I. Comparisons of the action of several heavy metals. *Aust J Exp Biol Med Sci* 36:471, 1958.

17. Hernberg S, Nikkanen J: Enzyme inhibition by lead under normal urban conditions. *Lancet* 1:63, 1970.
18. Hasan J, Vihko V, Hernberg S: Deficient red cell membrane Na$^+$ + K$^+$-ATPase in lead poisoning. *Arch Environ Health* 14:313, 1967.
19. Charache S, Weatherall DJ: Fast hemoglobin in lead poisoning. *Blood* 28:377, 1966.
20. Chalevelakis G, Bouronikou H, Yalouris AG, et al: delta-Aminolaevulinic acid dehydratase as an index of lead toxicity. Time for a reappraisal? *Eur J Clin Invest* 25:53, 1995.
21. Goldberg A: Annotation. Lead poisoning and haem biosynthesis. *Br J Haematol* 23:521, 1972.
22. McElvaine MD, Orbach HG, Binder S, et al: Evaluation of the erythrocyte protoporphyrin test as a screen for elevated blood lead levels. *J Pediatr* 119:548, 1991.
23. Paglia DE, Valentine WN, Dahlgren JG: Effects of low-level lead exposure on pyrimidine 5'-nucleotidase and other erythrocyte enzymes. *J Clin Invest* 56:1164, 1975.
24. Aly MH, Kim HC, Renner SW, et al: Hemolytic anemia associated with lead poisoning from shotgun pellets and the response to Succimer treatment. *Am J Hematol* 44:280, 1993.
25. Lachant N, Tomoda A, Tanaka KR: Inhibition of the pentose phosphate shunt by lead: A potential mechanism for hemolysis in lead poisoning. *Blood* 63:518, 1984.
26. White JM, Harvey DR: Defective synthesis of alpha and beta globin chains in lead poisoning. *Nature* 236:71, 1972.
27. Brookfield RW: Blood changes occurring during the course of treatment of malignant disease by lead, with special reference to punctate basophilia and the platelets. *J Pathol* 31:277, 1928.
28. Schwartz J, Landrigan PJ, Baker EL, Jr., Orenstein WA, von Lindern IH: Lead-induced anemia: dose-response relationships and evidence for a threshold. *Am J Public Health* 80:165, 1990.
29. Clark M, Royal J, Seeler R: Interaction of iron deficiency and lead and the hematologic findings in children with severe lead poisoning. *Pediatrics* 81:247, 1988.
30. White JM, Selhi HS: Lead and the red cell. *Br J Haematol* 30:133, 1975.
31. Jensen WN, Moreno GD, Bessis MC: An electron microscopic description of basophilic stippling in red cells. *Johns Hopkins Med J* 25:933, 1965.
32. Berlin CMJ: Lead poisoning in children. *Curr Opin Pediatr* 9:173, 1997.
33. Miller AL: Dimercaptosuccinic acid (DMSA), a non-toxic, water-soluble treatment for heavy metal toxicity. *Altern Med Rev* 3:199, 1998.
34. Klein WJ Jr, Metz EN, Price AR: Acute copper intoxication. A hazard of hemodialysis. *Arch Intern Med* 129:578, 1972.
35. Manzler AD, Schreiner AW: Copper-induced acute hemolytic anemia. A new complication of hemodialysis. *Ann Intern Med* 73:409, 1970.
36. McIntyre N, Clink HM, Levi AJ, Cumings JN, Sherlock S: Hemolytic anemia in Wilson's disease. *N Engl J Med* 276:439, 1967.
37. Deiss A, Lee GR, Cartwright GE: Hemolytic anemia in Wilson's disease. *Ann Intern Med* 73:413, 1970.
38. Hansen PB: Wilson's disease presenting with severe haemolytic anaemia. *Ugeskr Laeger* 150:1229, 1988.
39. Shimono N, Ishibashi H, Ikematsu H, et al: Fulminant hepatic failure during perinatal period in a pregnant woman with Wilson's disease. *Gastroenterol Jpn* 26:69, 1991.
40. Jain S, Nur AM, Ghosh K: Acute hemolytic anemia and biliary colic as presenting manifestations of Wilson's disease. *Am J Gastroenterol* 85:476, 1990.
41. Fairbanks VF: Copper sulfate-induced hemolytic anemia. *Arch Intern Med* 120:428, 1967.
42. Blume KG, Hoffbauer RW, Löhr GW, Rüdiger HW: Genetische und biochemische Aspekte der Pyruvatkinase menschlicher Erythrozyten (E.C.2.7.1.40). *Verh Dtsch Ges Inn Med* 75:450, 1969.
43. Boulard M, Blume K, Beutler E: The effect of copper on red cell enzyme activities. *J Clin Invest* 51:459, 1972.
44. Kiss JE, Berman D, Van Thiel D: Effective removal of copper by plasma exchange in fulminant Wilson's disease. *Transfusion* 38:327, 1998.
45. Jackson RC, Elder WJ, McDonnell H: Sodium-chlorate poisoning complicated by acute renal failure. *Lancet* 2:1381, 1961.
46. Eaton JW, Kolpin CF, Swofford HS, Kjellstrand CM, Jacob HS: Chlorinated urban water: A cause of dialysis-induced hemolytic anemia. *Science* 181:463, 1973.
47. Caterson RJ, Savdie E, Raik E, Coutts D, Mahony JF: Heinz-body

haemolysis in haemodialysed patients caused by chloramines in Sydney tap water. *Med J Aust* 2:367, 1982.

48. Orringer EP, Mattern WD: Formaldehyde-induced hemolysis during chronic hemodialysis. *N Engl J Med* 294:1416, 1976.

49. Lubash GD, Phillips RE, Shields JD, Bonsnes RW: Acute aniline poisoning treated by hemodialysis. *Arch Intern Med* 114:530, 1964.

50. Lowenstein L, Ballew DH: Fatal acute haemolytic anaemia, thrombocytopenic purpura, nephrosis and hepatitis resulting from ingestion of a compound containing apiol. *Can Med Assoc J* 78:195, 1958.

51. Schroder C, Kruger E, Abel J: Acute poisoning caused by the herbicide dichlorprop (preparation SYS 67 PROP). *Kinderarztl Prax* 59:81, 1991.

52. Martin H, Woerner W, Rittmeister B: Hämolytische Anämie durch Inhalation von Hydroxylaminen. *Klin Wochenschr* 42:725, 1964.

53. Fisher B: The significance of Heinz bodies in anemias of obscure etiology. *Am J Med Sci* 143, 1955.

54. Nierenberg DW, Horowitz MB, Harris KM, James DH: Mineral spirits inhalation associated with hemolysis, pulmonary edema, and ventricular fibrillation. *Arch Intern Med* 151:1437, 1991.

55. Hunter D: Industrial toxicology. *Q J Med* 12:185, 1943.

56. Gasser VC: Perakute hämolytische Innenkörperanamie mit Methämoglobinamie nach Behandlung eines Säuglingsekzems mit Resorcin. *Helv Paediatr Acta* 9:285, 1954.

57. Brandes JC, Bufill JA, Pisciotta AV: Amyl nitrite-induced hemolytic anemia. *Am J Med* 86:252, 1989.

58. Pugh JI, Enderby GEH: Haemoglobinuria after intravenous myanesin. *Lancet* 2:387, 1947.

59. Poinsot J, Guillois B, Margis D, et al: Neonatal hemolytic anemia after intra-amniotic injection of methylene blue. *Arch Fr Pediatr* 45:657, 1988.

60. Sills MR, Zinkham WH: Methylene blue-induced Heinz body hemolytic anemia. *Am J Dis Child* 148:306, 1994.

61. Davidson S, Seldon M, Jones B: Omeprazole and Heinz-body haemolytic anaemia. *Aust N Z J Med* 27:441, 1997.

62. Hassan AB, Seligmann H, Bassan HM: Intravascular hemolysis induced by pentachlorophenol. *BMJ* 291:21, 1985.

63. Adams JG, Heller P, Abramson RK, Vaithianathan T: Sulfonamide-induced hemolytic anemia and hemoglobin Hasharon. *Arch Intern Med* 137:1449, 1977.

64. Greenberg MS: Heinz body hemolytic anemia. *Arch Intern Med* 136:153, 1976.

65. Kaplinsky N, Frankl O: Salicylazosulphapyridine-induced Heinz body anemia. *Acta Haematol (Basel)* 59:310, 1978.

66. Ward PCJ, Schwartz BS, White JG: Heinz-body anemia: "Bite cell" variant—A light and electron microscopic study. *Am J Hematol* 15:135, 1983.

67. Yoo D, Lessin LS: Drug-associated "bite cell" hemolytic anemia. *Am J Med* 92:243, 1992.

68. Landsteiner EK, Finch CA: Haemoglobinuria after intravenous myanesin. *N Engl J Med* 237:310, 1947.

69. Rath CE: Drowning hemoglobinuria. *Blood* 8:1099, 1953.

70. Tavassoli M: Anemia of spaceflight. *Blood* 60:1059, 1982.

71. Mengel CE, Kann HE Jr, Heyman A, Metz E: Effects of in vivo hyperoxia on erythrocytes. II. Hemolysis in a human after exposure to oxygen under high pressure. *Blood* 25:822, 1965.

72. Dacie JV: *The Haemolytic Anaemias.* Grune & Stratton, New York, 1967.

73. Monzon C, Miles J: Hemolytic anemia following a wasp sting. *J Pediatr* 96:1039, 1980.

74. Schulte KL, Kochen MM: Haemolytic anaemia in an adult after a wasp sting. *Lancet* 2:478, 1981.

75. Vachvanichsanong P, Dissaneewate P, Mitarnun W: Non-fatal acute renal failure due to wasp stings in children. *Pediatr Nephrol* 11:734, 1997.

76. Nance WE: Hemolytic anemia of necrotic arachnidism. *Am J Med* 31:801, 1961.

77. Madrigal GC, Ercolani RL, Wenzl JE: Toxicity from a bite of the brown spider (Loxosceles Reclusus): skin necrosis, hemolytic anemia, and hemoglobinuria in a nine-year-old child. *Clin Pediatr* 11:641, 1972.

78. Chadha JS, Leviav A: Hemolysis, renal failure, and local necrosis following scorpion sting. *JAMA* 241:1038, 1979.

79. Barretto OCO, Cardoso JL, De Cillo D: Viscerocutaneous form of loxoscelism and erythrocyte glucose-6-phosphate deficiency. *Rev Inst Med trop Sao Paulo* 27:264, 1985.

80. Wasserman GS, Siegel C: Loxoscelism (brown recluse spider bites): A review of the literature. *Clin Toxicol* 14:353, 1979.

81. Wright SW, Wrenn KD, Murray L, Seger D: Clinical presentation and outcome of brown recluse spider bite. *Ann Emerg Med* 30:28, 1997.

82. Reid HA: Cobra-bites. *BMJ* 2:540, 1964.

83. Gillissen A, Theakston RD, Barth J, et al: Neurotoxicity, haemostatic disturbances and haemolytic anaemia after a bite by a Tunisian saw-scaled or carpet viper (Echis 'pyramidum'-complex): failure of anti-venom treatment. *Toxicon* 32:937, 1994.

84. Ham TH, Shen SC, Fleming EM, Castle WB: Studies on the destruction of red blood cells. IV. *Blood* 3:373, 1948.

85. Wagner HN, Jr., Razzak MA, Gaertner RA, Caine WP, Jr., Feagin OT: Removal of erythrocytes from the circulation. *Arch Intern Med* 110:90, 1962.

86. Shen SC, Ham TH, Fleming EM: Studies on the destruction of red blood cells. III. Mechanism and complications of hemoglobinuria in patients with thermal burns: Spherocytosis and increased osmotic fragility of red blood cells. *N Engl J Med* 229:701, 1943.

87. Topley E, Bull JP, Maycock WDA, Mourant AE, Parkin D: The relation of the isoagglutinins in pooled plasma to the haemolytic anaemia of burns. *J Clin Pathol* 16:79, 1963.

88. Stohlman F, Jr., Brecher G, Schneiderman M, Cronkite EP: The hemolytic effect of ionizing radiations and its relationship to the hemorrhagic phase of radiation injury. *Blood* 12:1061, 1957.

89. Jin YS, Anderson G, Mintz PD: Effects of gamma irradiation on red cells from donors with sickle cell trait. *Transfusion* 37:804, 1997.

HEMOLYTIC ANEMIA DUE TO INFECTIONS WITH MICROORGANISMS

ERNEST BEUTLER

Hemolytic anemia is a prominent part of the clinical presentation of patients infected with organisms, such as the malaria parasites, *Babesia*, and *Bartonella*, that directly invade the erythrocyte. Malaria is probably the most common cause of hemolytic anemia on a worldwide basis, and much has been learned about how the parasite enters the erythrocyte. Falciparum malaria, in particular, can cause severe and sometimes fatal hemolysis (blackwater fever). Other organisms cause hemolytic anemia by producing a hemolysin (e.g., *Clostridium welchii*), by stimulating an immune response (e.g., *Mycoplasma pneumoniae*), by enhancing macrophage recognition and hemophagocytosis, or by as yet unknown mechanisms. The many different infections that have been associated with hemolytic anemia are tabulated, and references to the original studies provided.

Shortening of erythrocyte life span occurs commonly in the course of inflammatory and infectious diseases. This may occur particularly in patients with glucose-6-phosphate dehydrogenase (G-6-PD) deficiency (Chap. 45), splenomegaly (Chap. 60), and the microvascular fragmentation syndrome (Chaps. 41 and 126). In some infections, however, rapid destruction of erythrocytes represents a prominent part of the overall clinical picture (Table 54-1). This chapter deals only with the latter states.

Several distinct mechanisms may lead to hemolysis during infections.[1] These include direct invasion of erythrocytes by the infecting organism, as in malaria, babesiosis, and bartonellosis; elaboration of hemolytic toxins, as by *Clostridium perfringens*; development of antibodies or autoantibodies against red cell antigens; or deposition of microbial antigens or immune complexes on erythrocytes.[2]

MALARIA

Known since antiquity, malaria is the world's most common cause of hemolytic anemia.[3] After the host is bitten by an infected female *Anopheles* mosquito, the sporozoites invade the liver and possibly other internal organs in the asymptomatic tissue stage of malaria. Merozoites, emerging at first from the tissues and later from previously parasitized red cells, bind to glyocophorin A and B by means of a 175-kD protein that has been designated the erythrocyte-binding antigen.[4–6] A complex series of events, not yet fully understood, eventuates in invasion of the interior of the red cell by the parasite.[4] Having entered the erythrocyte, the parasite grows intracellularly, nourished by

Acronyms and abbreviations that appear in this chapter include: CMV, cytomegalovirus; G-6-PD, glucose-6-phosphate dehydrogenase; HIV, human immunodeficiency virus; ICAM, intercellular adhesion molecule; VCAM, vascular cell adhesion molecule.

the cell's contents. Erythrocytes infected with *Plasmodium falciparum* develop surface knobs[7,8] that contain receptors, especially the *P. falciparum* erthrocyte membrane protein 1, for endothelial proteins. All parasites bind to CD36 antigen and thrombospondin found on endothelial surfaces, while some bind to the intercellular adhesion molecule 1(ICAM-1), and a few bind to vascular cell adhesion molecule (VCAM)[9–13] and mediate the adherence of parasitized cells to endothelium. Rosetting of parasitized cells with unparasitized cells also occurs through another undefined mechanism.[4] One of the membrane proteins of the *P. falciparum* binds specifically to the spectrin on the inner surface of the red cell membrane.[14] A large number of genetic polymorphisms that interfere with invasion of erythrocytes by parasites and their proliferation have developed in areas where malaria has been a leading cause of death for many generations.[15] These include G-6-PD deficiency, Southeast Asian ovalocytosis, thalassemias, and hemoglobinopathies.

The degree to which anemia develops often seems to be out of proportion to the number of cells infected with the parasite; the reason for this apparent destruction of uninvaded cells is not clear. Osmotic fragility is increased in nonparasitized cells as well as cells containing plasmodia.[16] The erythrocyte cation permeability is altered in monkeys with malaria.[17] Positive Coombs' test results have been reported, but the role of antibodies in the etiology of the anemia is not clear.[18] It has been suggested that oxidative damage to red cell lipids occurs[19,20] and that there is an abnormality in the phosphorylation of membranes of parasitized red cells.[21] *Plasmodium falciparum*–infected red cells have a highly irregular surface defect. This may be produced by the intracellular growth of the plasmodium, or it could represent the site of parasite entry. Nonparasitized cells often have similar surface defects,[22] suggesting a phenomenon known to occur in simian malaria,[23] the ''pitting'' of parasites from an infected cell.

Destruction of parasitized red cell appears to occur largely in the spleen, and splenomegaly is typically present in chronic malarial infection. The ''pitting'' of parasites from infected erythrocytes may also occur in the spleen.[24] The fever associated with malaria is characteristically cyclic, varying in frequency according to the malaria type. Although classic periodicity is often absent, febrile paroxysms of *Plasmodium vivax* malaria tend to occur every 48 h, those of *Plasmodium malariae* infection every 72 h, and those of *P. falciparum malaria* daily. Falciparum malaria is occasionally associated with particularly severe hemolysis and may result in the passage of dark, almost black, urine. This disorder, also called blackwater fever, is no longer common. At one time it was seen frequently among Europeans in Africa and in India, usually after quinine was given to treat malaria. The relative roles of the malarial infection and of the drug have never been clarified.[25]

Diagnosis of malaria depends upon demonstration of the parasites on the blood film[26] (Plate I-11,22) or demonstration of the appropriate DNA sequences in the blood.[27,28] The morphological distinction of *P. falciparum* from other forms of malaria, principally *P. vivax*, is clinically important, since *P. falciparum* infection may constitute a clinical emergency. If more than 5 percent of the red cells infected contain parasites, the infection is almost certainly with *P. falciparum*. In an infection with this organism, rings are practically the only form of parasite evident on the blood film. The finding of two or more rings within the same red cells is regarded as pathognomic of *P. falciparum*.[28]

Eradication of blood forms is achieved with quinine, chloroquine, or various sulfones or sulfonamides given together with pyrimethamine. Tissue stages of vivax malaria are effectively treated with primaquine. This drug, as well as certain sulfones used in the treatment of malaria, produces severe hemolysis in patients with G-6-PD deficiency (see Chap. 45).

When acute, unusually severe hemolysis occurs in the course of falciparum malaria (blackwater fever), the physician should be certain

TABLE 54-1   ORGANISMS CAUSING HEMOLYTIC ANEMIA

Aspergillus[57]
Babesia microti and *Babesia divergens*[38]
Bartonella bacilliformis[29,31]
Campylobacter jejuni[64,65]
Clostridium welchii[47]
Coxsackie virus[54]
Cytomegalovirus[66]
Diplococcus pneumoniae[67]
Epstein-Barr virus[60,68]
Escherichia coli[67,69,70]
Haemophilus influenzae[51,67]
Hepatitis A virus[71,72]
Hepatitis B virus[72,73]
Herpes simplex virus[54]
Human immunodeficiency virus (Chap. 89)
Influenza A virus[54]
Leishmania donovani[59]
Leptospira ballum and/or *Leptospira butembo*[74]
Mumps virus[75]
Mycobacterium tuberculosis[67]
Mycoplasma pneumoniae[58]
Neisseria intracellularis (meningococci)[67]
Parvovirus B19[76]
Plasmodium falciparum[3]
Plasmodium malariae[3]
Plasmodium vivax[3]
Rubella virus[77]
Rubeola virus[54]
Salmonella[67]
Shigella[61,62]
Streptococcus[67,78,79]
Toxoplasma[67]
Trypanosoma brucei[80]
Varicella virus[54]
Vibrio cholerae[67]
Yersinia enterocolitica[81]

that a hemolytic drug is not being administered to a G-6-PD–deficient individual. Transfusions may be needed with severe hemolysis, and if renal failure occurs, extracorporeal dialysis may be required. With early institution of therapy, the prognosis in malaria is excellent. However, when treatment is delayed or the strain is resistant to the administered agent, falciparum malaria may follow a rapid fatal course.

BARTONELLOSIS

In 1885, Daniel A. Carrón, a medical student, inoculated himself with blood obtained from a verrucous node of the skin of a patient with verruca peruviana. He developed a fatal hemolytic anemia with the characteristics of Oroya fever, a disease that had first been observed some years earlier among workers in a railroad construction project near the city of Oroya in the Peruvian Andes. This fatal self-experiment established the identity of the verrucous form and the hemolytic phase of human bartonellosis, an infection that now bears the name Carrión's disease.[29] Human bartonellosis is transmitted by the sand fly. The red blood cells become infected with *Bartonella bacilliformis*. It is believed that the organism does not grow within the red cell but, rather, adheres to its exterior surface: when infected red cells are washed with citrated plasma, free organisms are found but the red cells are not hemolyzed. In hanging-drop cultures, masses of organisms are clearly seen outside the erythrocytes, while the cells themselves are intact.[30] The osmotic fragility of the red cells is normal.[29] They are rapidly removed from the circulation, apparently both by liver and spleen. Normal red cells transfused into patients with bartonellosis

meet a similar fate.[31] A 130-kD bartonella protein that causes erythrocytes to acquire trenches, indentations, and invaginations has been purified from culture broths and has been called deformin.[32] In addition, two *B. bacilliformis* genes, designated *ialA* and *ialB*, predicted to code for polypeptides of 170 amino acids (20.1 kDa) and 186 amino acids (19.9 kDa), respectively, have been shown to greatly enhance the ability of *Escherichia coli* to invade erythrocytes.[33]

As demonstrated by Carrión's experiment, bartonellosis has two clinical stages. The acute hemolytic anemia, Oroya fever, represents the early, invasive stage of a chronic granulomatous disorder, the late stage of which is designated verruca peruviana. Most patients manifest no clinical symptoms during the Oroya fever phase, but when anemia does occur, its onset is dramatic. Red counts as low as $750,000/\mu l$ have been documented.[34] In addition to symptoms of anemia, patients manifest thirst, anorexia, sweating, and generalized lymphadenopathy. Spleen and liver enlargement is unusual. Large numbers of nucleated red cells appear in the blood smear, and reticulocytosis is often striking. The white cell count is variable. Diagnosis is established by demonstrating the presence of the organism *B. bacilliformis* on the erythrocytes. Giemsa-stained blood films reveal red-violet rods varying in length from 1 to 3 μm and in width from 0.25 to 0.2 μm.

The mortality rate among untreated patients is very high, but those who do survive undergo a sudden transitional period in which the bartonellae change from an elongated to a coccoid form, the number of parasitized cells decreases, and the red cell count increases. Lymphocytosis and a right shift in the granulocyte series are observed with disappearance of the fever and abatement of other symptoms. Oroya fever responds well to treatment with penicillin, streptomycin, chloramphenicol, and the tetracyclines. The second stage of *Bartonella* infection, verruca peruviana, is a nonhematologic disorder characterized by an eruption over the face and extremities developing into bleeding warty tumors.

BABESIOSIS

Babesia are intraerythrocytic protozoa known as piroplasms transmitted by ticks that may infect many species of wild and domestic animals. Humans occasionally become infected with *Babesia microti* or *Babesia divergens*, species that normally parasitize rodents and cattle, respectively.[35] Other babesia-like piroplasms, such as WA1, first isolated from a patient in the state of Washington, are also becoming recognized.[36,37] Once thought to be rare, babesiosis is being recognized with increasing frequency.[38] The disease is usually tick-borne in man but has apparently also been transmitted by transfusion.[37,39,40] Presumably because of the distribution of the vector, in the United States the disease is most common in the northeastern coastal region, where it became known as "Nantucket fever," but it has also been encountered in the Midwest.[41] Infections with *B. divergens* usually occur in splenectomized patients, but this is not the case with *B. microti* infections.[38]

The disease generally has a gradual onset with malaise, anorexia, and fatigue, followed by fever, sweats, and muscle and joint pains. Parasites can be seen in the red cells in Giemsa-stained thin blood films (Plate I-10). Serologic tests for antibodies to *Babesia* have been described,[42] and PCR-based diagnostic tests are also available.[38] It has responded to chemotherapy with clindamycin and quinine,[43] but failure to respond to antibiotics has also been encountered.[40] Whole-blood exchange was used with a marked improvement.[39]

CLOSTRIDIUM WELCHII

Clostridium perfringens (*welchii*) sepsis is most likely to occur in patients who have undergone septic abortion. It has also been observed following acute cholecystitis.[44] The α toxin of *C. welchii* is a lecithinase that may react with lipoprotein complexes at cell surfaces, liberating potent hemolytic substances, lysolecithins (see Chap. 38). It has also been suggested that erythrocyte membrane proteolysis plays an important role in hemolysis.[45] Severe, often fatal hemolysis occurs in patients with *C. welchii* septicemia. Striking hemoglobinemia and hemoglobinuria occur. The serum may become a brilliant red, and the urine is a dark-brown mahogany color. The high plasma hemoglobin level may produce a marked dissociation between the blood hemoglobin and hematocrit levels. Microspherocytosis is prominent, and leukocytosis with a left shift and thrombocytopenia are often present. Acute renal and hepatic failure usually develop, and the prognosis is grave; more than half of the patients die, even with extensive treatment (see Chap. 126).[46,47] Therapy consists of high-dose penicillin and surgical debridement.[48]

OTHER INFECTIONS

A variety of other infections have occasionally been associated with hemolytic anemia. The mechanisms involved vary. Some organisms, among them such common pathogens as *Haemophilus influenzae*, *E. coli*, and *Salmonella* species, can produce red cell agglutination in vitro, but it is not known whether this phenomenon is important in initiating in vivo hemolysis.[49] Bacteria may also produce destruction of red cells indirectly when bacterial polysaccharides are adsorbed onto erythrocytes. Action of an antibody directed against the antigen-coated cells results in their agglutination[50] or in complement-mediated lysis.[51] The unmasking of T-type antigens by bacteria renders the cell polyagglutinable. This may be a rare cause of hemolysis occurring in the course of bacterial infections.[52,53]

Many different types of microorganisms may play a role in precipitating autoimmune hemolytic disease (see Chap. 63). In one study of 234 patients,[54] 55 were found to have an antecedent bacterial infection, 18 of these exhibiting an ''unequivocal etiologic relationship'' of infection to anemia. However, the principal evidence for such a relationship was a temporal one. A number of viral agents, including measles, cytomegalovirus (CMV), varicella, herpes simplex, influenza A and B, Epstein-Barr, human immunodeficiency virus (HIV), and coxsackievirus, have also been associated with immune hemolytic disease.[54,55] Various mechanisms have been postulated, including absorption of immune complexes and complement, cross-reacting antigen, and a true autoimmune state with possible loss of tolerance secondary to the infectious organism.[54] Histopathologic and sometimes virologic evidence of infection with cytomegalovirus has been reported in a high percentage of children with lymphadenopathy and hemolytic anemia.[56] A positive antiglobulin reaction was demonstrated in some of these patients, and it has been suggested that some cases of ''idiopathic autoimmune hemolytic anemia'' are in reality due to cytomegalovirus infection.[56]

The high cold agglutinin titer that sometimes develops in the course of *Mycoplasma pneumoniae* pneumonia (see Chap. 56) may occasionally result in hemolytic anemia[57,58] or compensated hemolysis, although most patients with high cold agglutinin titers do not become anemic. The red cells of a number of patients with kala-azar were found to be agglutinated with anticomplement and anti–non-γ-globulin serum.[59] Both splenic and hepatic sequestration of red cells appears to occur in this disease.[60]

Microangiopathic hemolytic anemia is discussed in detail in Chap. 51. This disorder may be triggered by a variety of infections, some of which are caused by well-characterized organisms, such as species of *Shigella*,[61,62] *Campylobacter*,[63] and *Aspergillus*.[57]

REFERENCES

1. Berkowitz FE: Hemolysis and infection: Categories and mechanisms of their interrelationship. *Rev Infect Dis* 13:1151, 1991.
2. Seitz RC, Buschermohle G, Dubberke G, Herbrand R, Maiwald M, Hellwege HH: The acute infection-associated hemolytic anemia of childhood: Immunofluorescent detection of microbial antigens altering the erythrocyte membrane. *Ann Hematol* 67:191, 1993.
3. White NJ: The treatment of malaria. *N Engl J Med* 335:800, 1996.
4. Pasvol G, Clough B, Carlsson J: Malaria and the red cell membrane. *Blood Rev* 6:183, 1992.
5. Orlandi PA, Klotz FW, Haynes JD: A malaria invasion receptor, the 175-kilodalton erythrocyte binding antigen of *Plasmodium falciparum* recognizes the terminal Neu5Ac(alpha 2-3)Gal- sequences of glycophorin A. *J Cell Biol* 116:901, 1992.
6. Sim BKL, Chitnis CE, Wasniowska K, Hadley TJ, Miller LH: Receptor and ligand domains for invasion of erythrocytes by *Plasmodium falciparum*. *Science* 264:1941, 1994.
7. Nakamura K, Hasler T, Morehead K, Howard RJ, Aikawa M: *Plasmodium falciparum*-infected erythrocyte receptor(s) for CD36 and thrombospondin are restricted to knobs on the erythrocyte surface. *J Histochem Cytochem* 40:1419, 1992.
8. Aikawa M, Kamanura K, Shiraishi S, et al: Membrane knobs of unfixed *Plasmodium falciparum*–infected erythrocytes: New findings as revealed by atomic force microscopy and surface potential spectroscopy. *Exp Parasitol* 84:339, 1996.
9. Newbold C, Warn P, Black G, et al: Receptor-specific adhesion and clinical disease in *Plasmodium falciparum*. *Am J Trop Med Hyg* 57:389, 1997.
10. Baruch DI, Ma XC, Singh HB, Bi X, Pasloske BL, Howard RJ: Identification of a region of PfEMP1 that mediates adherence of *Plasmodium falciparum*–infected erythrocytes to CD36: Conserved function with variant sequence. *Blood* 90:3766, 1997.
11. Pasloske BL, Howard RJ: Malaria, the red cell, and the endothelium. *Annu Rev Med* 45:283, 1994.
12. Udomsangpetch R, Taylor BJ, Looareesuwan S, White NJ, Elliott JF, Ho M: Receptor specificity of clinical *Plasmodium falciparum* isolates: Nonadherence to cell-bound E-selectin and vascular cell adhesion molecule-1. *Blood* 88:2754, 1996.
13. McCormick CJ, Craig A, Roberts D, Newbold CI, Berendt AR: Intercellular adhesion molecule-1 and CD36 synergize to mediate adherence of *Plasmodium falciparum*–infected erythrocytes to cultured human microvascular endothelial cells. *J Clin Invest* 100:2521, 1997.
14. Herrera S, Rudin W, Herrera M, et al: A conserved region of the MSP-1 surface protein of *Plasmodium falciparum* contains a recognition sequence for erythrocyte spectrin. *EMBO J* 12:1607, 1993.
15. Nagel RL: Innate resistance to malaria: The intraerythrocytic cycle. *Blood Cells* 16:321, 1990.
16. George JN, Wicker DJ, Fogel BJ, Shields CE, Conrad ME: Erythrocytic abnormalities in experimental malaria. *Proc Soc Exp Biol Med* 124:1086, 1967.
17. Overman RR: Reversible cellular permeability alterations in disease: In vivo studies on sodium, potassium and chloride concentrations in erythrocytes of the malarious monkey. *Am J Physiol* 152:113, 1948.
18. Lefrancois G, Bras JL, Simonneau M, Bouvet E, Vroklans M, Vachon F: Anti-erythrocyte autoimmunisation during chronic falciparum malaria. *Lancet* 1:661, 1981.
19. Clark IA, Hunt NH: Evidence for reactive oxygen intermediates causing hemolysis and parasite death in malaria. *Infect Immun* 39:1, 1983.
20. Stocker R, Cowden WB, Tellan RL, Weidemann MJ, Hunt NH: Lipids from *Plasmodium vinckei*–infected erythrocytes and their susceptibility to oxidative damage. *Lipids* 22:51, 1987.
21. Yuthavong Y, Limpaiboon T: The relationship of phosphorylation of membrane proteins with the osmotic fragility and filterability of *Plasmodium berghei*–infected mouse erythrocytes. *Biochim Biophys Acta* 929:278, 1987.
22. Balcerzak SP, Arnold JD, Martin DC: Anatomy of red cell damage by *Plasmodium falciparum* in man. *Blood* 40:98, 1972.
23. Conrad ME: Pathophysiology of malaria: Hematologic observations in human and animal studies. *Ann Intern Med* 70:134, 1969.
24. Angus BJ, Chotivanich K, Udomsangpetch R, White NJ: In vivo removal

of malaria parasites from red blood cells without their destruction in acute falciparum malaria. *Blood* 90:2037, 1997.

25. Zuckerman A: Autoimmunization and other types of indirect damage to host cells as factors in certain protozoan diseases. *Exp Parasitol* 15:138, 1964.

26. Anthony RL, Bangs MJ, Anthony JM, Purnomo: On-site diagnosis of *Plasmodium falciparum*, *P. vivax*, and *P. malariae* by using the quantitative buffy coat system. *J Parasitol* 78:994, 1992.

27. Weiss JB: DNA probes and PCR for diagnosis of parasitic infections. *Clin Microbiol Rev* 8:113, 1995.

28. Oliveira DA, Holloway BP, Durigon EL, Collins WE, Lal AA: Polymerase chain reaction and a liquid-phase, nonisotopic hybridization for species-specific and sensitive detection of malaria infection. *Am J Trop Med Hyg* 52:139, 1995.

29. Ricketts WE: *Bartonella bacilliformis* anemia (Oroya fever): A study of thirty cases. *Blood* 3:1025, 1948.

30. Aldana L: Bacteriologia de la enfermedad de Carrión. *Cronica Med* 46:235, 1929.

31. Reynafarje C, Ramos J: The hemolytic anemia of human bartonellosis. *Blood* 17:562, 1961.

32. Xu YH, Lu ZY, Ihler GM: Purification of deformin, an extracellular protein synthesized by *Bartonella bacilliformis* which causes deformation of erythrocyte membranes. *Biochim Biophys Acta* 1234:173, 1995.

33. Mitchell SJ, Minnick MF: Characterization of a two-gene locus from *Bartonella bacilliformis* associated with the ability to invade human erythrocytes. *Infect Immun* 63:1552, 1995.

34. Weinman D: Human *Bartonella* infection and African sleeping sickness. *Bull NY Acad Med* 22:647, 1946.

35. Ruebush TK, II, Cassaday PB, Marsh HJ, et al: Human babesiosis on Nantucket island. *Ann Intern Med* 86:6, 1977.

36. Thomford JW, Conrad PA, Telford SR3, et al: Cultivation and phylogenetic characterization of a newly recognized human pathogenic protozoan. *J Infect Dis* 169:1050, 1994.

37. Herwaldt BL, Kjemtrup AM, Conrad PA, et al: Transfusion-transmitted babesiosis in Washington State: First reported case caused by a WA1-type parasite. *J Infect Dis* 175:1259, 1997.

38. Pruthi RK, Marshall WF, Wiltsie JC, Persing DH: Human babesiosis. *Mayo Clin Proc* 70:853, 1995.

39. Jacoby GA, Hunt JV, Kosinski KS, et al: Treatment of transfusion-transmitted babesiosis by exchange transfusion. *N Engl J Med* 303:1098, 1980.

40. Smith RP, Evans AT, Popovsky M, Mills L, Spielman A: Transfusion-acquired babesiosis and failure of antibiotic treatment. *JAMA* 256:2726, 1986.

41. Steketee RW, Eckman MR, Burgess EC, et al: Babesiosis in Wisconsin: A new focus of disease transmission. *JAMA* 253:2675, 1985.

42. Chisholm ES, Sulzer AJ, Ruebush TK, II: Indirect immunofluorescence test for human *Babesia microti* infection: Antigenic specificity. *Am J Trop Med Hyg* 35:921, 1986.

43. Wittner M, Rowin KS, Tanowitz HB, et al: Successful chemotherapy of transfusion babesiosis. *Ann Intern Med* 96:601, 1982.

44. Clancy MT, OBriain S: Fatal *Clostridium welchii* septicaemia following acute cholecystitis. *Br J Surg* 62:518, 1975.

45. Simpkins H, Kahlenberg A, Rosenberg A, Tay S, Panko E: Structural and compositional changes in the red cell membrane during *Chlostridium welchii* infection. *Br J Haematol* 21:173, 1971.

46. Mahn HE, Dantuono LM: Postabortal septicotoxemia due to *Clostridium welchii*. *Am J Obstet Gynecol* 70:604, 1955.

47. Rogstad B, Ritland S, Lunde S, Hagen AG: *Clostridium perfringens* septicemia with massive hemolysis. *Infection* 21:54, 1993.

48. Moustoukas NM, Nichols RL, Voros D: Clostridial sepsis: Unusual clinical presentations. *South Med J* 78:440, 1985.

49. Neter E: Bacterial hemagglutination and hemolysis. *Bacteriol Rev* 20:166, 1956.

50. Ceppellini R, De Gregorio M: Crisi emolitica in animali batterio-immuni transfusi con sangue omologo sensibilizzato in vitro mediante l'antigene batterico specifico. *Boll Ist Sieroter Milan* 32:445, 1953.

51. Shurin SB, Anderson P, Zollinger J, Rathbun RK: Pathophysiology of hemolysis in infections with *Hemophilus influenzae* type B. *J Clin Invest* 77:1340, 1986.

52. Dausset J, Moullec J, Bernard J: Acquired hemolytic anemia with poly-

agglutinability of red blood cells due to a new factor. *Blood* 14:1079, 1959.

53. Klein PJ, Vierbuchen M, Roth B, et al: Hemolytic anemia in infections caused by neuraminidase-producing bacteria. *Verh Dtsch Ges Pathol* 67:415, 1983.

54. Pirofsky B: Infectious disease and autoimmune hemolytic anemia, in *Autoimmunization and the Autoimmune Hemolytic Anemias*, p 147. Waverly Press, Baltimore, 1969.

55. McGinniss MH, Macher AM, Rook AH, Alter HJ: Red cell autoantibodies in patients with acquired immune deficiency syndrome. *Transfusion* 26:405, 1986.

56. Zuelzer WW, Stulberg CS, Page RH, Teruya J, Brough AJ: The Emily Cooley lecture: Etiology and pathogenesis of acquired hemolytic anemia. *Transfusion* 6:438, 1966.

57. Robboy SJ, Salisbury K, Ragsdale B, Bobroff M, Jacobson BM, Colman RW: Mechanism of *Aspergillus*-induced microangiopathic hemolytic anemia. *Arch Intern Med* 128:790, 1971.

58. Fiala M, Myhre BA, Chinh LT, Territo M, Edgington TS, Kattlove H: Pathogenesis of anemia associated with *Mycoplasma pneumoniae*. *Acta Haematol (Basel)* 51:297, 1974.

59. Woodruff AW, Topley E, Knight R, Downie CGB: The anaemia of kala azar. *Br J Haematol* 22:319, 1972.

60. Tonkin AM, Mond HG, Alford FP, Hurley TH: Severe acute haemolytic anaemia complicating infectious mononucleosis. *Med J Aust* 2:1048, 1973.

61. Ullis KC, Rosenblatt RM: Shiga bacillus dysentery complicated by bacteremia and disseminated intravascular coagulation. *J Pediatr* 83:90, 1973.

62. Chesney R, Kaplan BS: Hemolytic-uremic syndrome with shigellosis. *J Pediatr* 84:312, 1974.

63. Dickgiesser A: *Campylobacter* infection and the hemolytic-uremic syndrome. *Immun Infect* 11:71, 1983.

64. Smith MA, Shah NR, Lobel JS, Hamilton W: Methemoglobinemia and hemolytic anemia associated with *Campylobacter jejuni* enteritis. *Am J Pediatr Hematol Oncol* 10:35, 1988.

65. Damani NN, Humphrey CA, Bell B: Haemolytic anaemia in *Campylobacter* enteritis. *J Infect* 26:109, 1993.

66. van Spronsen DJ, Breed WP: Cytomegalovirus-induced thrombocytopenia and haemolysis in an immunocompetent adult. *Br J Haematol* 92:218, 1996.

67. Dacie JV: Secondary or symptomatic hemolytic anemias, in *The Haemolytic Anaemias*, part III, edited by JV Dacie, p 908. Grune & Stratton, New York, 1967.

68. Whitelaw F, Brook MG, Kennedy N, Weir WR: Haemolytic anaemia complicating Epstein-Barr virus infection. *Br J Clin Pract* 49:212, 1995.

69. Ludwig K, Ruder H, Bitzan M, Zimmermann S, Karch H: Outbreak of *Escherichia coli* O157:H7 infection in a large family. *Eur J Clin Microbiol Infect Dis* 16:238, 1997.

70. Pennings CM, Seitz RC, Karch H, Lenard HG: Haemolytic anaemia in association with *Escherichia coli* O157 infection in two sisters. *Eur J Pediatr* 153:656, 1994.

71. Gundersen SG, Bjoerneklett A, Bruun JN: Severe erythroblastopenia and hemolytic anemia during a hepatitis A infection. *Scand J Infect Dis* 21:225, 1989.

72. Kanematsu T, Nomura T, Higashi K, Ito M: Hemolytic anemia in association with viral hepatitis. *Nippon Rinsho* 54:2539, 1996.

73. Gurgey A, Yuce A, Ozbek N, Kocak N: Acute hemolysis in association with hepatitis B infection in a child with beta-thalassemia trait. *Turk J Pediatr* 36:259, 1994.

74. Trowbridge AA, Green JB, III, Bonnett JD, Shohet SB, Ponnappa BD, McCombs WB, III: Hemolytic anemia associated with leptospirosis: Morphologic and lipid studies. *Am J Clin Pathol* 76:493, 1981.

75. Ozen S, Damarguc I, Besbas N, Saatci U, Kanra T, Gurgey A: A case of mumps associated with acute hemolytic crisis resulting in hemoglobinuria and acute renal failure. *J Med* 25:255, 1994.

76. Chambers LA, Rauck AM: Acute transient hemolytic anemia with a positive Donath-Landsteiner test following parvovirus B19 infection. *J Pediatr Hematol Oncol* 18:178, 1996.

77. Moriuchi H, Yamasaki S, Mori K, Sakai M, Tsuji Y: A rubella epidemic in Sasebo, Japan, in 1987, with various complications. *Acta Paediatr Jpn* 32:67, 1990.

78. Lersch C, Gain T, von Siemens M, Hagenmuller F, Classen M: Toxic shock-like syndrome due to severe hemolytic group A streptococcal infection. *Klin Wochenschr* 68:523, 1990.

79. Inada T, Shirono K, Tsuda H: Hemolytic anemia in a patient with subacute bacterial endocarditis due to *Streptococcus sanguis. Acta Haematol (Basel)* 94:95, 1995.

80. Wéry M, Mulumba PM, Lambert PH, Kazyumba L: Hematologic manifestations, diagnosis, and immunopathology of African trypanosomiasis. *Semin Hematol* 19:83, 1982.

81. Von Knorring J, Pettersson T: Haemolytic anaemia complicating *Yersinia enterocolitica* infection: Report of a case. *Scand J Haematol* 9:149, 1972.

ACQUIRED HEMOLYTIC ANEMIA DUE TO WARM-REACTING AUTOANTIBODIES

CHARLES H. PACKMAN

Autoimmune hemolytic anemia (AHA) is characterized by shortened red cell survival and the presence of autoantibodies directed against autologous red blood cells (RBC). A positive direct antiglobulin reaction (Coombs' test) is important for the diagnosis. Most patients with AHA (80 percent) exhibit warm-reactive antibodies of the IgG isotype. Most of the remainder exhibit cold-reactive autoantibodies of the IgM class, labeled cold agglutinins because they directly agglutinate RBC in vitro. The direct antiglobulin reaction may detect IgG, proteolytic fragments of complement (mainly C3), or both on the RBC of patients with warm-antibody AHA. In cold-antibody AHA, only complement is detected because the antibody dissociates from the RBC during washing of the cells. About half of patients with AHA have no underlying associated disease; these cases are termed idiopathic. Secondary cases are associated with underlying autoimmune, malignant, or infectious diseases or with ingestion of certain drugs. The etiology of AHA is unknown.

The symptoms of AHA are those of anemia. The usual laboratory features include anemia, reticulocytosis, and a positive direct antiglobulin reaction. The blood film exhibits polychromasia and spherocytosis, the latter a hallmark of the disease. Indirect hyperbilirubinemia, increased urinary urobilinogen and serum lactate dehydrogenase (LDH), and decreased serum haptoglobin are variably present but not necessary for the diagnosis.

Although most patients do not require transfusion of RBC, transfusion should not be withheld from those with symptomatic anemia. Glucocorticoids are effective in slowing the rate of hemolysis. Splenectomy is indicated for patients who require an unacceptably high maintenance dose or prolonged administration of glucocorticoids. Intravenous immunoglobulin may provide short-term control of hemolysis, and immunosuppressive drugs and danazol have been used with success in refractory cases.

DEFINITION AND HISTORY

The two main features of AHA are (1) shortened RBC survival in vivo and (2) evidence of host antibodies reactive with autologous

RBC, most frequently demonstrated by a positive direct antiglobulin reaction (Coombs' test).

The antiglobulin test was introduced in 1945. Previously, it was recognized that the sera of some patients with AHA could directly agglutinate saline suspensions of normal or autologous human RBC. These serum factors, later shown to be specific antibodies (largely of the IgM class), were termed direct or saline agglutinins. In a smaller proportion of cases, the patients' sera could mediate lysis of the test RBC in the presence of fresh serum as a complement source. The heat-stable factors (antibodies) necessary for such in vitro complement-mediated lysis were called hemolysins. However, in the majority of cases of AHA, neither direct agglutinins nor hemolysins could be demonstrated in the patients' sera. In 1945, Coombs, Mourant, and Race[1] reported that RBC coated with nonagglutinating Rh antibodies (now known to be of the IgG isotype) could be agglutinated by rabbit antiserum to human γ-globulin. That is, the rabbit antiglobulin serum cross-linked IgG antibody–coated RBC to produce visible agglutination. Subsequently, it was found that addition of rabbit antiglobulin serum to a suspension of washed RBC isolated from patients with suspected AHA produced agglutination in many cases, including those lacking saline agglutinins or hemolysins.[2,3] This procedure is now termed the direct antiglobulin (Coombs') test. Subsequent studies established that positive direct antiglobulin reactions in AHA are attributable to coating of the RBC with immunoglobulins (mainly IgG) and/or complement proteins. When the RBC are coated chiefly with complement proteins, a positive direct antiglobulin test is dependent upon the presence of anticomplement (principally anti-C3) in the antiglobulin reagent.

CLASSIFICATION

Autoimmune hemolytic anemia may be classified in two complementary ways (Table 55-1). The majority of cases (80 to 90 percent in adults) are mediated by warm-reactive autoantibodies[4-6] or antibodies displaying optimal reactivity with human RBC at 37°C (98.6°F). A smaller proportion is attributable to autoantibodies exhibiting greater affinity for RBC at temperatures below 37°C (cold-reactive autoantibodies; see Chap. 56). This distinction is important, not only because of differences in the pathophysiology of RBC injury, but also in the therapeutic approaches required. An even smaller proportion of patients with AHA exhibit both cold-reactive and warm-reactive autoantibodies,[7,8] which apparently recognize different antigens on the RBC membrane.[9] Red blood cell destruction is generally more severe in such mixed cases.

It is also useful to classify AHA based on the presence or absence of underlying diseases (see Table 55-1). When no recognizable underlying disease is present, the AHA is termed primary or idiopathic. When AHA appears to be a manifestation or complication of an underlying disorder, the term *secondary AHA* is applied. Lymphocytic malignancies, particularly chronic lymphocytic leukemia (CLL) and lymphomas, account for about half of secondary AHA cases (see Chaps. 98 and 103). Systemic lupus erythematosus (SLE) and other autoimmune diseases account for a lesser but considerable proportion of secondary AHA cases. A large proportion of patients with mixed cold and warm autoantibodies have SLE.[7,8] Infectious mononucleosis and *Mycoplasma pneumoniae* occasionally are associated with cryopathic AHA (see Chap. 90). In spite of the frequent occurrence of immune thrombocytopenia in patients infected with the human immunodeficiency virus (HIV), AHA is relatively rare in these patients (see Chap. 89).[10,11] Other associated diseases, less commonly reported, are listed in Table 55-1. The etiologic and pathogenic significance of these associations is poorly understood, but most of these associated diseases are recognized to involve components of the immune system, either by neoplasia or by aberrant immunopathologic responses.

TABLE 55-1 CLASSIFICATION OF AUTOIMMUNE HEMOLYTIC ANEMIA

I. On basis of serologic characteristics of involved autoimmune process
A. Warm-autoantibody type: autoantibody maximally active at body temperature, 37°C
B. Cold-autoantibody type: autoantibody active at temperatures below 37°C
C. Mixed cold and warm autoantibodies
II. On basis of presence or absence of underlying or significantly associated disorder
A. Primary or idiopathic AHA
B. Secondary AHA
1. Associated with lymphoproliferative disorders (e.g., Hodgkin disease, lymphoma)
2. Associated with the rheumatic disorders, particularly SLE
3. Associated with certain infections
4. Associated with certain nonlymphoid neoplasms (e.g., ovarian tumors)
5. Associated with certain chronic inflammatory diseases (e.g., ulcerative colitis)
6. Associated with ingestion of certain drugs (e.g., α-methyldopa)

EPIDEMIOLOGY

Estimates of the frequency of primary (idiopathic) AHA vary from 20 to 80 percent of all types of AHA, depending on the referral patterns of the reporting center.[4,6,12,13] In general, AHA may be considered secondary (1) when AHA and the underlying disease occur together with greater frequency than can be accounted for by chance alone; (2) when the AHA reverses simultaneously with correction of the associated disease; or (3) when AHA and the associated disease are related by evidence of immunologic aberration.[4] Using these criteria, the frequency of primary AHA is probably closer to 50 percent of all cases. Careful follow-up of patients with "primary" AHA is essential, since hemolytic anemia may be the presenting finding in a patient who subsequently develops overt evidence of underlying lymphoproliferative disorder or SLE.

ETIOLOGY AND PATHOGENESIS

ETIOLOGY

The etiology of warm-antibody AHA is unknown. Warm-antibody AHA is the most common type of AHA and is the focus of the remainder of this chapter. The autoantibodies that mediate RBC destruction are predominantly (but not exclusively) IgG globulins possessing relatively high binding affinity for human RBC at 37°C. As a result, the major share of autoantibodies is commonly bound to the patient's circulating erythrocytes. Eluates prepared from the patient's washed, autoantibody-coated RBC constitute a very important source of purified autoantibody for investigation of specificity, immunoglobulin structure, or other properties. In addition, sera from patients with warm AHA often are used in blood banks for cross-matching and for general screening of antibody specificity. The quantity of such autoantibody in serum may be low and in some cases may not reflect the full spectrum of anti-RBC specificity revealed in concurrently prepared RBC eluates.[14]

Autoimmune hemolytic anemia has been diagnosed in people of all ages, from infants to the elderly. The majority of patients are over age 40, with peak incidence around the seventh decade. This age distribution probably reflects, in part, the increased frequency of lymphoproliferative malignancies in the elderly, resulting in an age-related increase in the frequency of secondary AHA. Although multiple cases occasionally are observed in families,[15–17] most cases of primary AHA arise sporadically. Development of AHA does not have an apparent association with any particular HLA haplotype or other genetic factor.

In patients with primary AHA, erythrocyte autoantibodies are the only recognizable immunologic aberration. Furthermore, the autoantibodies of any one patient often are specific for only a single RBC membrane protein (see "Serologic Features"). The narrow spectrum of autoreactivity suggests that the mechanism underlying the development of AHA in such patients is not secondary to a generalized defect in immune regulation. Rather, it appears that these patients may develop warm-antibody AHA through an aberrant immune response to a self-antigen or to an immunogen that mimics a self-antigen.

In patients with secondary AHA, the disease may be associated with a fundamental disturbance in the immune system; for example, when it appears in the setting of lymphoma, CLL, SLE, primary agammaglobulinemia (common variable immunodeficiency), or hyper-IgM immunodeficiency syndrome. In these settings, warm-antibody AHA most likely arises through an underlying defect in immune regulation, although the contribution of an aberrant immune response to self-antigen cannot be excluded. Autoimmune hemolytic anemia seems especially frequent in patients with low-grade lymphoma or CLL treated with fludarabine[18] or 2-chlorodeoxyadenosine (cladribine).[19] The T lymphocytopenia induced by these drugs may exacerbate the preexisting tendency of these patients to form autoantibodies.

A still unexplained observation is that certain drugs, such as α-methyldopa, can induce warm-reacting IgG anti-RBC autoantibodies in otherwise normal persons. The autoantibodies induced by α-methyldopa have Rh-related serologic[20] and immunochemical[21] specificity similar to that of autoantibodies arising in many patients with "spontaneous" AHA (see below and Chap. 57). A critical difference is that the drug-associated autoantibodies subside when the drug is discontinued, suggesting (1) that the latent potential to form this type of anti-RBC autoantibody is present in many immunologically normal individuals and (2) that the steps required to generate such autoantibodies do not necessarily create a sustained autoimmune state. The maintenance of chronic idiopathic AHA, on the other hand, either may be secondary to a continuing (but unknown) stimulus or may be induced by a short stimulus to which the patient continues to respond.

To be sure, normal subjects may be found to be Coombs-positive when they volunteer to donate blood.[22–24] The positive direct antiglobulin test in these normal donors often is due to warm-reacting IgG autoantibodies, similar in serologic specificity[14] and in IgG subclass[23] to those occurring in AHA. Although many of these donors remain Coombs-positive without developing overt hemolytic anemia, a few have been documented to develop AHA.[23,24] The incidence of positive direct antiglobulin tests in normal blood donors is roughly 1 in 10,000.[22,23] This figure is higher than the reported incidence of AHA itself (1 to 2 cases per 100,000).[4,5] Since blood donation per se is not likely to contribute to an increased risk of developing autoantibodies, the 1-in-10,000 proportion may be the approximate frequency of positive direct antiglobulin tests in the entire population. It may be that a substantial proportion of patients who present with clinically overt primary AHA are from a subset of those asymptomatic individuals who are innately Coombs-positive. This concept, however, is not established.

Several concepts have been developed to explain immunologic tolerance to self-antigens.[25–27] Relevant to AHA, membrane-bound antigens expressed in a multivalent array at high concentration may induce tolerance by effecting clonal deletion of autoreactive B cells.[28] Both the Rh-related and the non-Rh types of RBC antigens that are targeted by AHA autoantibodies (see "Serologic Features") are expressed normally by human fetal erythrocytes, as early as 10 to 12 weeks of life.[29] However, because new B cells develop daily in the marrow throughout life and because B cells may somatically mutate their Ig receptors (see Chap. 83), self-tolerance in the B-cell compartment is never assured. It has been suggested by analogy to observations in NZB mice[30,31] that the peritoneal cavity may be a privileged compartment that could shelter autoreactive B cells from host RBC, allowing them to escape deletion, later to produce anti-RBC autoantibodies with appropriate T-cell help.[32] The strong predominance of IgG antibodies in AHA suggests B-cell isotype switching, which is consistent with the idea of an antigen-driven process. Moreover, since T-cell help is necessary for inducing B-cell isotype switching, the pathway or pathways to autoantibody induction in AHA also may involve an abnormal or unique mode of antigen presentation to T cells.[33]

PATHOGENESIS

Erythrocyte autoantibodies in AHA are pathogenic. In contrast to autologous RBC, labeled RBC lacking the antigen targeted by the autoantibodies may survive normally in patients with warm-antibody AHA.[5,34,35] On the other hand, transplacental passage of IgG anti-RBC autoantibodies from a mother with AHA to the fetus can induce intrauterine or neonatal hemolytic anemia.[36] Finally, despite notable exceptions and differences relating to IgG subclass of the autoantibody, there is, in general, an inverse relationship between the quantity of RBC-bound IgG antibody and RBC survival when serial studies are made on a given patient.[37-42]

In AHA, the patient's RBC typically are coated with IgG autoantibodies with or without complement proteins. Autoantibody-coated RBC are trapped by macrophages in the Billroth cords of the spleen and, to a lesser extent, by Kupffer cells in the liver (see Chap. 5).[34,37,38,40-44] This process leads to sphering, fragmentation, and ingestion of the antibody-coated RBC.[45,46] The macrophage has surface receptors for the Fc region of IgG, with preference for the IgG_1 and IgG_3 subclasses,[47,48] and surface receptors for opsonic fragments of C3 (C3b and C3bi) and C4b.[49-51] When present together on the RBC surface, IgG and C3b/C3bi appear to act cooperatively as opsonins to enhance trapping and phagocytosis.[40,41,50-54] Although RBC sequestration in warm-antibody AHA occurs primarily in the spleen,[34,41-43] very large quantities of RBC-bound IgG[37,39,44] or the concurrent presence of C3b on the RBC[37,40,41] may favor trapping in the liver as well.

Interaction of a trapped RBC with splenic macrophages may result in phagocytosis of the entire cell. More commonly, a type of partial phagocytosis occurs that results in the formation of spherocytes. As RBC adhere to macrophages via the Fc receptors, portions of RBC membrane are internalized by the macrophage. Since membrane is lost in excess of contents, the noningested portion of the RBC assumes a spherical shape, the shape with the lowest ratio of surface area to volume.[45,46,55] Spherical RBC are more rigid and less deformable than normal RBC. As such, spherical RBC are fragmented further and/or destroyed in future passages through the spleen. Spherocytosis is a consistent and diagnostically important hallmark of AHA,[56] and the degree of spherocytosis correlates well with the severity of hemolysis.[5]

Direct complement-mediated hemolysis with hemoglobinuria is unusual in warm-antibody AHA, despite the fact that many warm autoantibodies fix complement. The failure of C3b-coated RBC to be hemolyzed by the terminal complement cascade (C5–C9) has been attributed, at least in part, to the ability of complement regulatory proteins (factors I and H) in plasma and C3b receptors on the RBC surface to alter the hemolytic function of cell-bound C3b and C4b.[57] Glycosylphosphatidylinositol-linked erythrocyte membrane proteins, such as decay-accelerating factor (CD55)[58] and homologous restriction factor,[59] may limit the action of autologous complement on autoantibody-coated RBC.

In addition, cytotoxic activities of macrophages and lymphocytes may play a role in the destruction of RBC in warm-antibody AHA. Monocytes can lyse IgG-coated RBC in vitro independently of phagocytosis.[60,61] Cell-bound complement is neither necessary nor sufficient for such cytotoxicity, but bound C3b/C3d can potentiate the effects of IgG.[61] In one study,[60] cytotoxicity, but not phagocytosis, was inhib-ited by hydrocortisone in vitro. Lymphocytes also are able to lyse IgG antibody–coated RBC in vitro.[62-64] The relative contribution of antibody-dependent monocyte- and lymphocyte-mediated cytotoxicity to RBC destruction in patients with warm-antibody AHA is not known.

CLINICAL FEATURES

Presenting complaints of warm-antibody AHA usually are referable to the anemia itself, although occasionally jaundice is the immediate cause for seeking medical advice. Symptoms are usually slow and insidious in onset over several months, but occasionally a patient may have sudden onset of symptoms of severe anemia and jaundice over a period of a few days. In secondary AHA, the symptoms and signs of the underlying disease may overshadow the hemolytic anemia and associated features.

In idiopathic AHA with only mild anemia, the physical examination may be normal. Even patients with relatively severe hemolytic anemia may have only modest splenomegaly. However, in very severe cases, particularly those of acute onset, patients may present with fever, pallor, jaundice, hepatosplenomegaly, hyperpnea, tachycardia, angina, or heart failure.

Clinical warm-antibody AHA may be aggravated or first become apparent during pregnancy.[36,65,66] Most cases are mild, however, and the prognosis for the fetus is generally good, provided the mother is treated early.[65]

LABORATORY FEATURES

GENERAL FEATURES

By definition, patients with AHA present with anemia, the severity of which can range from life-threatening to very mild. Patients with AHA may present with hematocrit levels below 10 percent. On the other hand, some AHA patients may have compensated hemolytic anemia and a near-normal hematocrit. For these patients, the predominant laboratory features are an increased reticulocyte count and a positive direct Coombs' test. Occasionally, however, the patient may have leukopenia and neutropenia.[5,72] Platelet counts are typically normal. Rarely, severe immune thrombocytopenia is associated with warm-antibody AHA. This constellation is termed Evans syndrome.[73] In this syndrome, the RBC and platelet antibodies are apparently distinct.[74]

Evaluation of the blood film can reveal several features related to AHA. Polychromasia indicates a reticulocytosis, reflecting an increased rate of reticulocyte egress from the marrow. Spherocytes are seen in patients with moderate to severe hemolytic anemia (see Color Plate II-8). Unless hereditary spherocytosis cannot be excluded, this finding suggests an immune hemolytic process. Red blood cell fragments, nucleated RBC, and, occasionally, erythrophagocytosis by monocytes may be seen in severe cases. Most patients have mild leukocytosis and neutrophilia.

The reticulocyte count usually is elevated. Nevertheless, early in the course of the disease, over one-third of all patients may have transient reticulocytopenia despite having a normal or hyperplastic erythroid marrow.[67-70] The mechanism for this is unknown, although it has been speculated that autoantibodies reactive against antigens on reticulocytes may lead to their selective destruction.[71] One unusual patient with AHA, reticulocytopenia, and marrow erythroid aplasia had a serum antibody that inhibited erythroid colony formation in vitro.[71] The aplastic crisis remitted after the serum IgG level was lowered by immunoadsorption. Reticulocytopenia also may be seen in patients with marrow function compromised by an underlying disease, parvovirus infection, toxic chemicals, or nutritional deficiency. Marrow examination usually reveals erythroid hyperplasia and also may provide evidence of an underlying lymphoproliferative disorder.

Hyperbilirubinemia (chiefly unconjugated) is highly suggestive of hemolytic anemia, although its absence does not exclude the diagnosis. Total bilirubin is only modestly increased, up to 5 mg/dl, and, with rare exceptions, the conjugated (direct) fraction constitutes less than 15 percent of the total. Urinary urobilinogen is increased regularly, but bile is not detected in the urine unless serum conjugated bilirubin is increased. Usually, serum haptoglobin levels are low, and LDH levels are elevated. Hemoglobinuria is encountered in rare patients with hyperacute hemolysis who develop significant hemoglobinemia.

SEROLOGIC FEATURES

DIRECT ANTIGLOBULIN TEST PATTERN

The diagnosis of AHA requires the demonstration of immunoglobulin and/or complement bound to the patient's RBC. As a screening procedure, it is customary to use a "broad-spectrum" antiglobulin (Coombs') reagent, that is, one that contains antibodies directed against human immunoglobulin as well as complement components (principally C3). If agglutination is noted with a broad-spectrum reagent, antisera reacting selectively with IgG (the "gamma" Coombs') or with C3 (the "nongamma" Coombs') are used to define the specific pattern of RBC sensitization. Monospecific antisera to IgM or IgA also have been used in selected cases.

There are three *major* patterns of direct antiglobulin reaction in warm-antibody AHA: (1) RBC coated with only IgG, (2) RBC coated with IgG and complement components, and (3) RBC coated with complement components without detectable immunoglobulin.[5,75–77] In patterns 2 and 3, the complement components most readily detected are C3 fragments (mainly C3dg). Each pattern has been associated with accelerated RBC destruction. Positive antiglobulin reactions with anti-IgA or anti-IgM are encountered less commonly, often in association with bound IgG and/or complement.[78–84]

FREE VERSUS BOUND AUTOANTIBODY

The autoantibody molecules in patients with warm-antibody AHA exist in a reversible, dynamic equilibrium between RBC and plasma.[85,86] In addition to the major portion of autoantibody bound to the patient's RBC (detected by the direct antiglobulin test, DAT), "free" autoantibody may be detected in the plasma or serum of these patients by means of the indirect antiglobulin test (IAT). In the IAT, the patient's serum or plasma is incubated with normal donor erythrocytes at the appropriate temperature (in this case, 37°C). The cells are washed, suspended in saline solution, and then tested for agglutination by antiglobulin serum. The presence of such unbound autoantibody in plasma depends upon the total amount of antibody being produced and the binding affinity of the antibody for RBC antigens. In general, patients with heavily sensitized RBC are more likely to exhibit plasma autoantibody. Protease-modified RBC are more sensitive than native RBC in detecting plasma autoantibody, but such data must be interpreted with caution, since alloantibodies, naturally occurring antibodies to cryptic antigens, and other serum components may interact with enzyme-modified RBC. Patients with a positive IAT due to a warm-reactive autoantibody should also have a positive DAT. A patient with a serum anti-RBC antibody (positive IAT) and a negative DAT probably has, not an autoimmune process, but, rather, an alloantibody stimulated by prior transfusion or pregnancy.

QUANTITY OF RBC-BOUND AUTOANTIBODY

Figure 55-1 relates the intensity of the direct antiglobulin reaction, using specific anti-IgG serum, to the number of IgG molecules bound per RBC. The latter was determined by a sensitive antibody-consump-

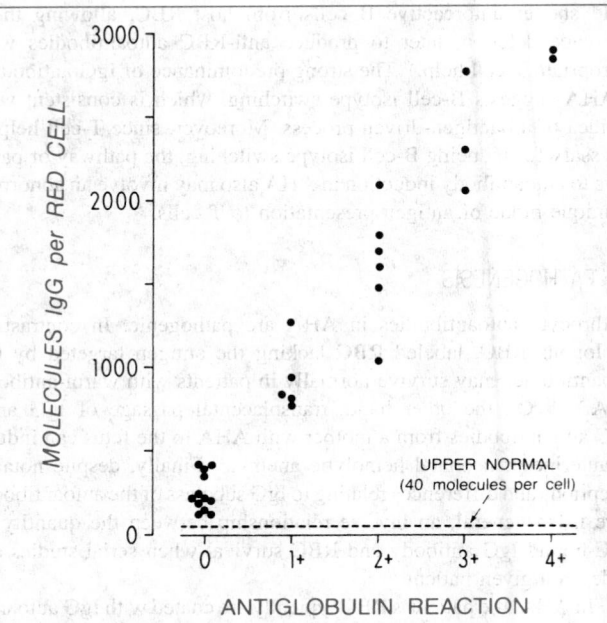

FIGURE 55-1   Comparison of direct antiglobulin reactions (with anti-IgG serum) with molecules of red cell–bound IgG determined by a quantitative antibody consumption assay (method in Ref. 87). The two assays were conducted concurrently on the same blood specimen. The antiglobulin reactions were performed manually and read macroscopically.

tion method.[87] A trace-positive antiglobulin reaction (read macroscopically) detects 300 to 400 molecules of IgG per cell.[87,88] In another laboratory, a trace-positive antiglobulin reaction with anti-C3 was obtained with 60 to 115 molecules C3 per cell.[87]

More sensitive methods of quantifying RBC-bound IgG allow the identification of AHA patients who have all the usual hallmarks of warm-antibody AHA but a negative DAT with anti-immunoglobulin and anticomplement reagents.[87–89] In many such patients, the RBC are coated with quantities of IgG autoantibody that are too low to give a positive antiglobulin reaction (subthreshold IgG). However, the specialized methods (e.g., anti-IgG consumption assays, automated enhanced agglutination techniques, enzyme-linked and radioimmunoassays) do detect very small quantities of cell-bound IgG. In such cases, studies with highly concentrated RBC eluates confirm that these IgG molecules are warm-reacting anti-RBC autoantibodies.[87] These patients generally have relatively mild hemolysis and often respond favorably to glucocorticoid therapy. By these specialized methods, subthreshold IgG also may be detected in a significant number of patients who exhibit the "complement alone" pattern of direct antiglobulin reaction in the absence of drug sensitivity or cold agglutinins. In such cases, studies with concentrated RBC eluates have suggested that these subthreshold quantities of bound IgG antibodies are capable of fixing much larger quantities of C3 to the cell membrane.[87]

NATURE OF THE AUTOANTIBODIES AND RBC TARGET ANTIGENS

In any series of warm-antibody AHA patients, the correlation between the strength of the antiglobulin reaction (IgG molecules per RBC) and the rate of RBC destruction is variable. The IgG subclass of warm autoantibodies apparently influences the degree to which these antibodies shorten RBC survival. IgG$_1$ is the most commonly encountered subclass, either alone or in combination with other IgG subclasses.[78,90] IgG$_1$ and IgG$_3$ autoantibodies appear to be more effective in decreasing

RBC life span than do those of the IgG$_2$ or IgG$_4$ subclass.[78,91] This difference may be due to the greater affinity of macrophage Fc receptors for IgG$_1$ and IgG$_3$ [47,48] and the higher complement-fixing activity of IgG$_1$ or IgG$_3$ antibodies relative to that of IgG$_2$ or IgG$_4$ antibodies.[57]

The autoantibodies eluted from patients' RBC or present in their plasma typically bind to all the common types of human RBC represented in test panels used by blood banks and thus might appear to be nonspecific. However, the antibodies of any one patient typically recognize one or more antigenic determinants (epitopes) that are common to virtually all human RBC, that is, "public" antigens. These antibodies have been useful for evaluating RBC membrane structures and for identifying rare RBC phenotypes, namely, RBC that lack a common blood group antigen or antigens. Nearly half of all AHA patients have autoantibodies specific for epitopes on Rh proteins.[4,5,14,92–94] The autoantibodies of such patients commonly do not react with human RBC of the rare Rh$_{null}$ phenotype, lacking expression of the Rh complex. Occasionally, the anti-Rh autoantibodies have anti-e, anti-E, or anti-c (or, more rarely, anti-D) specificity. Patients who have autoantibodies with selective specificity (e.g., anti-e) nearly always have other autoantibodies reactive with all human RBC, except Rh$_{null}$. Autoantibodies with such specificity have been designated collectively as Rh related.[21,94]

The remaining patients with warm-antibody AHA have IgG autoantibodies that are fully reactive with Rh$_{null}$ RBC.[4,5,14,92–94] The exact specificity of the autoantibodies for many of these patients is undefined. In other instances, autoantibody specificity for serologically defined blood group antigens outside the Rh system have been defined using RBC of appropriate antigen-deficient phenotype: anti-Wr^b,[14] anti-En^a,[95] anti-LW,[96] anti-U,[97] anti-Ge,[83,98] anti-Sc1,[99] or antibodies to Kell blood group antigens.[100] For ease of reference, this entire group of autoantibodies is designated non–Rh related.[21,94]

Immunochemical studies indicate that the autoantibodies from almost any AHA patient react with individual membrane proteins. The major target of the Rh-related autoantibodies is a 32- to 34-kDa nonglycosylated polypeptide lacking on Rh$_{null}$ RBC.[21,101] This polypeptide is similar, if not identical, to the polypeptide expressing the Rh(e) alloantigen. Many α-methyldopa–induced autoantibodies also react with this polypeptide.[21] Autoantibodies with non-Rh serologic specificity have been found that react with the band 3 anion transporter[21,102] or with both band 3 and glycophorin A.[21] The latter autoantibodies may react with an epitope formed through the interaction of these two proteins on the RBC membrane.[103] It is interesting to note that anti-RBC autoantibodies in NZB mice exhibit anti–band 3 specificity.[104] Furthermore, naturally occurring anti–band 3 IgG autoantibodies are found in essentially all humans.[105–107] These autoantibodies may play a role in the clearance of senescent RBC by reacting with neoantigens formed on these cells by proteolytic alteration[105] or aggregation[106] of band 3 proteins. Such neoantigens are not found on younger RBC. An important but unanswered question concerns the possible relationship between the naturally occurring and pathologic anti–band 3 autoantibodies.

DIFFERENTIAL DIAGNOSIS

Several nonautoimmune diseases also may result in spherocytic anemia, such as hereditary spherocytosis (HS), Zieve's syndrome, clostridial sepsis, and the hemolytic anemia that precedes Wilson's disease. Among the hereditary hemolytic anemias, HS can resemble acquired AHA most closely. This is because the spherocytic anemia associated with HS may be detected first in adulthood (see Chap. 43). In addition, splenomegaly may be prominent in both HS and AHA. Family studies of patients with HS, however, usually can identify other affected individuals. Most important, the RBC of patients with congenital hemolytic anemia do not have a positive DAT.

In hemolytic anemia accompanied by a positive DAT, serologic characterization of the autoantibody may distinguish warm-antibody AHA from cold-reacting autoantibody syndromes (see Chap. 56). Diagnosis of a drug-related immune hemolytic anemia depends upon a history of appropriate drug intake supported by compatible serologic findings (see Chap. 57). In patients who recently have been transfused, a positive direct antiglobulin reaction may in reality reflect the binding of a newly formed alloantibody to donor RBC in the patient's circulation. This could lead to a false impression of an autoimmune process.

Recent recipients of organ transplants may develop an alloimmune hemolytic anemia that mimics AHA. The problem is seen in kidney, liver, or marrow transplants and usually occurs when an organ from a blood group O donor is transplanted into a blood group A recipient. It is thought that B lymphocytes present in the donated organ or marrow form *allo*antibodies against recipient RBC.[108–112] Patients of blood group O who receive a marrow transplant from a donor of blood group A or B may develop a transiently positive DAT and hemolysis of RBC made by the marrow graft, due to temporary persistence of previously synthesized host anti-A or anti-B.[113] Furthermore, some group O marrow transplant recipients exhibit mixed hematopoietic chimerism with persistence of host B lymphocytes that can make alloantibodies directed against RBC made by the marrow graft.[113] In these settings, the findings of hemolysis and a positive DAT due to anti-A and anti-B are probably diagnostic of an alloimmune process, since *auto*antibodies directed against the major blood group antigens A and B are extremely rare.

Other acquired types of hemolytic anemia are less easily confused with AHA because spherocytes are not prominent on the blood film and the DAT is negative. Patients with paroxysmal nocturnal hemoglobinuria (PNH) may complain of dark urine (hemoglobinuria). This finding is unusual in patients with warm-antibody AHA but can occur in patients with the cold-antibody syndromes (see Chap. 56). Both the acidified serum test and the sucrose hemolysis test are usually positive in PNH but negative in AHA. Microangiopathic hemolytic disorders, such as thrombotic thrombocytopenic purpura and hemolytic uremic syndrome, can be distinguished from AHA by examining the blood film. In the former diseases, the blood smear displays marked RBC fragmentation and minimal spherocytosis. In addition, microangiopathic hemolytic anemia more frequently is associated with thrombocytopenia than is warm-antibody AHA.

THERAPY, COURSE, AND PROGNOSIS

THERAPY

TRANSFUSION

The clinical consequences of AHA are related to the severity of the anemia and acuity of its onset. Most patients with AHA develop anemia over a period sufficient to allow for cardiovascular compensation and hence do not require RBC transfusions. However, RBC transfusions may be necessary for an AHA patient who has an underlying disease complicating the anemia, such as symptomatic coronary artery disease, or who rapidly develops severe anemia with signs and/or symptoms of circulatory failure.

Transfusion of RBC in AHA presents two difficulties: one is the problem of cross-matching, and the other is the short half-life of the transfused RBC. It is nearly always impossible to find truly serocompatible donor blood except in rare cases when the autoantibody is found specific for a defined blood group antigen (see "Serologic Features"). Otherwise, one must choose donor RBC that are least incompatible with the patient's serum in cross-match testing. Before transfusing an incompatible unit, it is important to test the patient's serum carefully for an alloantibody that could cause a severe hemolytic transfusion reaction against donor RBC, especially in patients with a history of pregnancy or prior transfusion.[94,114,115]

Once selected, the packed RBC should be administered slowly. During the transfusion, the patient should be monitored for signs of a hemolytic transfusion reaction (see Chap. 140). The transfused cells may be destroyed as fast as the patient's own cells or perhaps even faster. However, the increased oxygen-carrying capacity provided by the transfused cells may be sufficient to maintain the patient during the acute interval required for other modes of therapy to become effective.

GLUCOCORTICOIDS

Therapy with glucocorticoids has reduced the mortality associated with severe idiopathic warm-antibody AHA. First used for this disorder almost 50 years ago,[116] glucocorticoids can cause dramatic cessation or marked slowing of hemolysis in about two-thirds of patients.[4,5,76,117,118] About 20 percent of treated patients with warm-antibody AHA achieve complete remission. About 10 percent show minimal or no response to glucocorticoids. The best responses are seen in idiopathic cases or in those related to SLE.

Most patients should be treated with oral prednisone at an initial daily dose of 60 to 100 mg. Critically ill patients with rapid hemolysis may receive intravenous methylprednisolone, 100 to 200 mg in divided doses over the first 24 h. High doses of prednisone may be required for 10 to 14 days. When the hematocrit stabilizes or begins to increase, the prednisone dose may be decreased in rapid-step dose reductions to approximately 30 mg/day. With continued improvement, the prednisone dose may be further decreased at a rate of 5 mg/day every week, to a dose of 15 to 20 mg/day. These doses should be administered for 2 to 3 months after the acute hemolytic episode has subsided, after which the patient may be weaned from the drug over 1 to 2 months or treatment switched to an alternate-day therapy schedule (e.g., 20 to 40 mg every other day). Alternate-day therapy reduces glucocorticoid side effects but should be attempted only after the patient has achieved stable remission on daily prednisone in the range of 15 to 20 mg/day. Therapy should not be stopped until the DAT becomes negative. Although many patients achieve full remission of their first hemolytic episode, relapses may occur after the glucocorticoids are discontinued. Therefore, these patients should be followed for at least several years after treatment. A relapse may require repeat glucocorticoid therapy, splenectomy, or immunosuppression.

Occasionally, patients who present with only a positive DAT, minimal hemolysis, and stable hematocrit may require no treatment. However, these patients should be observed for clinical deterioration, since the rate of RBC destruction may increase spontaneously.

Glucocorticoids may influence hemolysis in warm-antibody AHA by several mechanisms. Earlier investigators noted that hematologic improvement was often, but not always, accompanied by reduction in the strength of the DAT.[5] The subsequent observation of a decrease in cell-bound and/or free serum autoantibody during stable glucocorticoid-induced remission suggested that improved RBC survival following treatment with glucocorticoids resulted from a decrease in synthesis of anti-RBC autoantibodies.[39,85] However, this cannot explain why the glucocorticoid-treated patients often improve within 24 to 72 h, a time much shorter than the half-life of anti-RBC autoantibody. Rather, glucocorticoids may suppress RBC sequestration by splenic macrophages.[41,42,53,119] A quantitative decrease in one of the three known classes of Fcγ receptors[47,48] has been observed in the blood monocytes of AHA patients during glucocorticoid therapy.[120]

SPLENECTOMY

Nearly one-third of patients with warm-antibody AHA may require prednisone chronically in doses greater than 15 mg/day to maintain an acceptable hemoglobin concentration. These patients are candidates for splenectomy.

Splenectomy removes the primary site of RBC trapping. Investigations in human[39] and other animal[41] subjects confirm that maintenance of a given rate of RBC destruction requires 6 to 10 times as much RBC-bound IgG in splenectomized subjects than in nonsplenectomized subjects. The continuation of hemolysis after splenectomy is partly related to persisting high levels of autoantibody, favoring RBC destruction in the liver by hepatic Kupffer cells.[39,41,44]

Several investigators have noted the amount of RBC-bound autoantibody to decrease in AHA patients following splenectomy.[5,117,121] However, a significant proportion of patients show no change in cell-bound autoantibody following splenectomy. The processes that determine the rate of autoantibody production are poorly understood. The beneficial effect of splenectomy may be related to several factors interacting in complex fashion.[122]

A patient's clinical data currently constitute the best selection criteria for splenectomy. Attempts to select potential responders by ^{51}Cr RBC sequestration studies have been disappointing.[5,117,123] In most cases, it is reasonable to continue glucocorticoids for 1 to 2 months while waiting for a maximal response. However, if there is no response at all within 3 weeks, the patient's condition deteriorates, or the anemia is very severe, splenectomy should be done sooner.

Results of splenectomy are variable. Approximately two-thirds of AHA patients will have a partial or complete remission following splenectomy.[117,122,124] The relapse rate, however, is disappointingly high. Many patients require further glucocorticoid therapy to maintain acceptable hemoglobin levels, although often at a lower dose than they required prior to splenectomy.[5,76,117] Alternate-day therapy is preferable to daily therapy in these cases if adequate control of the anemia can be achieved.

The immediate mortality and morbidity from splenectomy depends upon the presence of underlying disease and the preoperative clinical status. In general it is quite low.[125] Following splenectomy, children, more than adults, have an increased risk for developing sepsis due to encapsulated organisms.[126] Vaccination against *Haemophilus influenzae* type b and pneumococcal and meningicoccal organisms is recommended prior to surgery.[127]

IMMUNOSUPPRESSIVE DRUGS

Cytotoxic drugs such as cyclophosphamide, 6-mercaptopurine, azathioprine, or 6-thioguanine have been given to patients with AHA to suppress synthesis of autoantibody. Direct evidence of such an effect is lacking. Although immunosuppressive therapy has not received universal acceptance, beneficial responses to immunosuppressive drugs have been observed in some patients who failed to respond to glucocorticoids.[128,129] It must be emphasized that the majority of patients with warm-antibody AHA respond to glucocorticoids and/or splenectomy and are usually not candidates for immunosuppressive therapy. At present, immunosuppressive therapy should be reserved primarily for those patients who fail to respond to glucocorticoids and splenectomy or for those patients who are poor surgical risks.[128]

The drugs of choice are cyclophosphamide 60 mg/m^2 or azathioprine 80 mg/m^2, given daily. If the patient tolerates the drug, it is reasonable to continue treatment for up to 6 months while waiting for a response. When response occurs, the patient may be slowly weaned from the drug. If there is no response, the alternative drug may be tried. Because of the ability of cyclophosphamide or azathioprine to suppress erythropoiesis, blood counts must be monitored with extra care during therapy. Treatment with either agent increases the risk of subsequent neoplasia. In addition, cyclophosphamide may cause severe hemorrhagic cystitis.

OTHER THERAPIES

Plasma exchange or plasmapheresis has been used in patients with warm-antibody AHA. Improvement has been reported in a few cases, but its use is controversial.[130,131] Thymectomy has been reported as being useful in a few children who were refractory to glucocorticoids and splenectomy.[128] Selective injury to splenic macrophages by administration of vinblastine-loaded, IgG-sensitized platelets has been reported as successful in a few patients.[132] There are several anecdotal reports and a case series reporting short-term successful treatment of patients with AHA using high-dose intravenous γ-globulin.[133–137] Danazol, a nonvirilizing androgen, may be useful in patients with AHA, based on uncontrolled studies.[138,139] Danazol may eliminate the need for splenectomy when combined with prednisone and may allow for a shorter duration of prednisone therapy.[139] Some patients with ulcerative colitis and AHA unresponsive to glucocorticoids and splenectomy may respond to colectomy.[140] In patients with AHA associated with an ovarian dermoid cyst, removal of the cyst produced remission of the hemolysis.[141] Finally, patients with refractory AHA may be treated effectively with the purine analog 2-chlorodeoxyadenosine (cladribine).[142]

COURSE AND PROGNOSIS

Patients with idiopathic warm-antibody AHA have unpredictable clinical courses characterized by relapses and remissions. No particular feature of the illness has been a consistent predictor of outcome. In spite of a rather high initial rate of response to glucocorticoids and splenectomy, the overall mortality rate was significant (up to 46 percent) in several older series but much lower in more recent studies.[4,5,117,143,144] The actuarial survival at 10 years is reported to be 73 percent.[143] Thromboembolic episodes in the form of deep-vein thrombosis or splenic infarcts are relatively common during active phases of the disease.[117] Pulmonary emboli, infection, and cardiovascular collapse are causes of death. The prognosis in secondary warm-antibody AHA is largely dependent on the course of the underlying disease.

In children, warm-antibody AHA frequently follows an acute infection or immunization.[121,145,146] Most of these patients exhibit a self-limited course and respond rapidly to glucocorticoids. Children with chronic AHA tend to be older.[146,147] Those who recover from the initial hemolytic episode have a good prognosis and are unlikely to relapse, although exceptions are known. The overall mortality rate is lower than in adults, ranging from 10 to 30 percent,[121,145-149] with higher mortality rates in those with chronic AHA[121,149] and in those with associated autoimmune thrombocytopenia (Evans syndrome).[150]

REFERENCES

1. Coombs RRA, Mourant AE, Race EE: A new test for the detection of weak and incomplete Rh agglutinins. *Br J Exp Pathol* 26:255, 1945.
2. Boorman KE, Dodd BE, Loutit JF: Haemolytic icterus (acholuric jaundice), congenital and acquired. *Lancet* 1:812, 1946.
3. Loutit JF, Mollison PL: Haemolytic icterus (acholuric jaundice), congenital and acquired. *J Pathol Bacteriol* 58:711, 1946.
4. Petz LD, Garratty G: *Acquired Immune Hemolytic Anemias.* Churchill Livingstone, London, 1980.
5. Dacie JV: *The Haemolytic Anaemias, vol 3, The Autoimmune Haemolytic Anaemias,* 3d ed. Churchill Livingstone, New York, 1992.
6. Sokol RJ, Hewitt S, Stamps BK: Autoimmune haemolysis: An 18 year study of 865 cases referred to a regional transfusion centre. *Br Med J* 282:2023, 1981.
7. Sokol RJ, Hewitt S, Stamps BK: Autoimmune haemolysis: Mixed warm and cold antibody type. *Acta Haematol* 69:266, 1983.
8. Shulman IA, Branch DR, Nelson JM, et al: Autoimmune hemolytic anemias with both cold and warm autoantibodies. *JAMA* 253:1746, 1985.
9. Kajii E, Miura Y, Ikemoto S: Characterization of autoantibodies in mixed-type autoimmune hemolytical anemia. *Vox Sang* 60:45, 1991.
10. Telen MJ, Roberts KB, Bartlett JA: HIV-associated autoimmune hemolytic anemia: Report of a case and review of the literature. *J Acquir Immune Defic Syndr* 3:933, 1990.
11. Rapoport AP, Rowe JM, McMican A: Life-threatening autoimmune hemolytic anemia in patient with acquired immune deficiency syndrome. *Transfusion* 28:190, 1988.
12. Dacie JV: *The Haemolytic Anemias, Congenital and Acquired.* Vol. 3 *Secondary or Symptomatic Haematolytic Anaemias,* 2d ed. Grune & Stratton, New York, 1967.
13. Chaplin H, Avioli LV: Autoimmune hemolytic anemia. *Arch Intern Med* 137:346, 1977.
14. Issitt PD, Pavone BG, Goldfinger D, et al: Anti-Wr^b and other autoantibodies responsible for positive direct antiglobulin test in 150 individuals. *Br J Haematol* 34:5, 1976.
15. Pirofsky B: Hereditary aspects of autoimmune hemolytic anemia: A retrospective analysis. *Vox Sang* 14:334, 1968.
16. Dobbs CE: Familial auto-immune hemolytic anemia. *Arch Intern Med* 116:273, 1965.
17. Cordova MS, Baez-Villasenor J, Mendez JJ, Campos E: Acquired hemolytic anemia with positive antiglobulin (Coombs' test) in mother and daughter. *Arch Intern Med* 117:692, 1966.
18. Gonzalez H, Leblond V, Azar N, et al: Severe autoimmune hemolytic anemia in eight patients treated with fludarabine. *Hematol Cell Ther* 40:113, 1998.
19. Chasty RC, Myint H, Oscier DG, et al: Autoimmune haemolysis in patients with B-CLL treated with chlorodeoxyadenosine (CDA). *Leuk Lymphoma* 29:391, 1998.
20. Worlledge SM: Immune drug-induced haemolytic anaemias. *Semin Hematol* 6:181, 1969.
21. Leddy JP, Falany JL, Kissel GE, et al: Erythrocyte membrane proteins reactive with human (warm-reacting) anti-red cell autoantibodies. *J Clin Invest* 91:1672, 1993.
22. Worlledge SM: The interpretation of a positive direct antiglobulin test. *Br J Haematol* 39:157, 1978.
23. Gorst DW, Rawlinson VI, Merry AH, Stratton F: Positive direct antiglobulin test in normal individuals. *Vox Sang* 38:99, 1980.
24. Bareford D, Langster G, Gilks L, Demick-Torey LA: Follow-up of normal individuals with a positive antiglobulin test. *Scand J Haematol* 35:348, 1985.
25. Nossal GJV: B-cell selection and tolerance. *Curr Opin Immunol* 3:193, 1991.
26. Basten A, Brink R, Peake P, et al: Self-tolerance in the B-cell repertoire. *Immunol Rev* 122:5, 1991.
27. Kroemer G, Martinez-A C: Mechanisms of self-tolerance. *Immunol Today* 13:401, 1992.
28. Hartley SB, Crosbie J, Brink R, et al: Elimination from peripheral lymphoid tissue of self-reactive B lymphocytes recognizing membrane bound antigens. *Nature* 353:765, 1991.
29. Leddy JP: Reactivity of human γG erythrocyte autoantibodies with fetal, autologous and maternal red cells. *Vox Sang* 17:525, 1969.
30. Okamoto M, Murakami M, Shimizu A, et al: A transgenic model of autoimmune hemolytic anemia. *J Exp Med* 175:71, 1992.
31. Murakami M, Tsubata T, Okamoto M et al: Antigen-induced apoptotic death of Ly-1 B cells responsible for autoimmune disease in transgenic mice. *Nature* 357:77, 1992.
32. Leddy JP: Immune hemolytic anemia, in *Clinical Immunology: Principles and Practice* edited by RR Rich et al, p 1273. Mosby, St Louis, 1996.
33. Lin RH, Mamula MJ, Hardin JA, Janeway CA: Induction of autoreactive B cells allows priming of autoreactive T cells. *J Exp Med* 173:1433, 1991.
34. Mollison PL: Measurement of survival and destruction of red cells in haemolytic syndromes. *Br Med Bull* 15:59, 1959.
35. Holländer L: Erythrocyte survival time in a case of acquired haemolytic anaemia. *Vox Sang* 4:164, 1954.
36. Chaplin H, Cohen R, Bloomberg G, et al: Pregnancy and idiopathic autoimmune haemolytic anaemia: A prospective study during 6 months gestation and 3 months ''post-partum.'' *Br J Haematol* 24:219, 1973.
37. Mollison PL, Crome P, Hughes-Jones NC, Rochna E: Rate of removal from the circulation of red cells sensitized with different amounts of antibody. *Br J Haematol* 11:461, 1965.
38. Mollison PL, Hughes-Jones NC: Clearance of Rh-positive red cells by low concentration of Rh antibody. *Immunology* 12:63, 1967.
39. Rosse WF: Quantitative immunology of immune hemolytic anemia: II.

The relationship of cell-bound antibody to hemolysis and the effect of treatment. *J Clin Invest* 50:734, 1971.

40. Schreiber AD, Frank MM: Role of antibody and complement in the immune clearance and destruction of erythrocytes: I. In vivo effects of IgG and IgM complement-fixing sites. *J Clin Invest* 51:575, 1972.

41. Atkinson JP, Schreiber AD, Frank MM: Effects of corticosteroids and splenectomy on the immune clearance and destruction of erythrocytes. *J Clin Invest* 52:1509, 1973.

42. Atkinson JP, Frank MM: Complement independent clearance of IgG sensitized erythrocytes: Inhibition by cortisone. *Blood* 44:629, 1974.

43. Jandl JH, Richardson-Jones A, Castle WB: The destruction of red cells by antibodies in man: I. Observations on the sequestration and lysis of red cells altered by immune mechanisms. *J Clin Invest* 36:1428, 1957.

44. Jandl JH, Kaplan ME: The destruction of red cells by antibodies in man: III. Quantitative factors influencing the pattern of hemolysis in vivo. *J Clin Invest* 39:1145, 1960.

45. Abramson N, LoBuglio AF, Jandl JH, Cotran RS: The interaction between human monocytes and red cells: Binding characteristics. *J Exp Med* 132:1191, 1970.

46. LoBuglio AF, Cotran RS, Jandl JH: Red cells coated with immunoglobulin G: Binding and sphering by mononuclear cells in man. *Science* 158:1582, 1967.

47. Anderson CL, Looney RJ: Human leukocyte IgG Fc receptors. *Immunol Today* 7:264, 1986.

48. Ravetch JV, Kinet J-P: Fc receptors. *Annu Rev Immunol* 9:457, 1991.

49. Gigli I, Nelson RA: Complement-dependent immune phagocytosis: I. Requirements of C1, C4, C2, C3. *Exp Cell Res* 51:45, 1968.

50. Lay WF, Nussenzweig V: Receptors for complement on leukocytes. *J Exp Med* 128:991, 1968.

51. Ross GD: Opsonization and membrane complement receptors, in *Immunobiology of the Complement System*, edited by GD Ross, p 87. Academic, Orlando, FL, 1986.

52. Fischer JT, Petz LD, Garratty G, Cooper NR: Correlations between quantitative assay of red cell bound C3, serologic reactions, and hemolytic anemia. *Blood* 44:359, 1974.

53. Schreiber AD, Parsons J, McDermott P, Cooper RA: Effect of corticosteroids on the human monocyte IgG and complement receptors. *J Clin Invest* 56:1189, 1975.

54. Ehlenberger AG, Nussenzweig V: The role of membrane receptors for C3b and C3d in phagocytosis. *J Exp Med* 145:357, 1977.

55. Rosse WF, de Boisfleury A, Bessis M: The interaction of phagocytic cells and red cells modified by immune reactions: Comparison of antibody and complement coated red cells. *Blood Cells* 1:345, 1975.

56. Dameshek W, Schwartz SO: Acute hemolytic anemia (acquired hemolytic icterus, acute type). *Medicine* 19:231, 1940.

57. Leddy JP, Rosenfeld SI: Role of complement in hemolytic anemia and thrombocytopenia, in *Immunobiology of the Complement System*, edited by GD Ross, p 213. Academic, Orlando, FL, 1986.

58. Nicholson-Weller A, Burge J, Fearon DT, et al: Isolation of a human erythrocyte membrane glycoprotein with decay-accelerating activity for C3 convertases of the complement system. *J Immunol* 129:184, 1982.

59. Lachmann PJ: The control of homologous lysis. *Immunol Today* 12:312, 1991.

60. Fleer A, Van Schaik MLJ, von dem Borne AEG Kr, Engelfriet CP: Destruction of sensitized erythrocytes by human monocytes in vitro: Effects of cytochalasin B, hydrocortisone and colchicine. *Scand J Immunol* 8:515, 1978.

61. Kurlander RJ, Rosse WF, Logue WL: Quantitative influence of antibody and complement coating of red cells on monocyte-mediated cell lysis. *J Clin Invest* 61:1309, 1978.

62. Urbaniak SJ: Lymphoid cell dependent (K-cell) lysis of human erythrocytes sensitized with rhesus alloantibodies. *Br J Haematol* 33:409, 1976.

63. Handwerger BS, Kay NW, Douglas SD: Lymphocyte-mediated antibody-dependent cytolysis: Role in immune hemolysis. *Vox Sang* 34:276, 1978.

64. Milgrom H, Shore SL: Lysis of antibody-coated human red cells by peripheral blood mononuclear cells: Altered effector cell profile after treatment of target cells with enzymes. *Cell Immunol* 39:178, 1978.

65. Sokol RJ, Hewitt S, Stamps BK: Erythrocyte autoantibodies, autoimmune haemolysis and pregnancy. *Vox Sang* 43:169, 1982.

66. Issaragrisil S, Kruatrachue M: An association of pregnancy and autoimmune haemolytic anaemia. *Scand J Haematol* 31:63, 1983.

67. Liesveld JL, Rowe JM, Lichtman MA: Variability of the erythropoietic response in autoimmune hemolytic anemia: Analysis of 109 cases. *Blood* 69:820, 1987.

68. Hegde UM, Gordon-Smith EC, Worlledge SM: Reticulocytopenia and absence of red cell autoantibodies in immune haemolytic anaemia. *Br Med J* 2:1444, 1977.

69. Conley CL, Lippman SM, Ness P: Autoimmune hemolytic anemia with reticulocytopenia: A medical emergency. *JAMA* 244:1688, 1980.

70. Greenberg J, Curtis-Cohen M, Gill FM, Cohen A: Prolonged reticulocytopenia in autoimmune hemolytic anemia of childhood. *J Pediatr* 97:784, 1980.

71. Mangan KF, Besa EC, Shadduck RK, et al: Demonstration of two distinct antibodies in autoimmune hemolytic anemia with reticulocytopenia and red cell aplasia. *Exp Hematol* 12:788, 1984.

72. Evans RS, Duane RT: Acquired hemolytic anemia: I. The relation of erythrocyte antibody production to activity of the disease. II. The significance of thrombocytopenia and leukopenia. *Blood* 4:1196, 1949.

73. Evans RS, Takahashi K, Duane RT, et al: Primary thrombocytopenic purpura and acquired hemolytic anemia: Evidence for a common etiology. *Arch Intern Med* 87:48, 1951.

74. Pegels JG, Helmerhorst FM, vanLeeuwen EF, et al: The Evans syndrome: Characterization of the responsible autoantibodies. *Br J Haematol* 51:445, 1982.

75. Leddy JP: Immunological aspects of red cell injury in man. *Semin Hematol* 3:48, 1966.

76. Eyster ME, Jenkins DE Jr: Erythrocyte coating substances in patients with positive direct antiglobulin reactions: Correlation of γG globulin and complement coating with underlying diseases, overt hemolysis and response to therapy. *Am J Med* 46:360, 1969.

77. Engelfriet CP, von dem Borne AEG Kr, Vander Giessen M, et al: Autoimmune haemolytic anaemias: I. Serological studies with pure anti-immunoglobulin reagents. *Clin Exp Immunol* 3:605, 1968.

78. Engelfriet CP, von dem Borne AEG Kr, Beckers D, van Loghem JJ: Autoimmune haemolytic anaemia: Serological and immunochemical characteristics of the autoantibodies: Mechanisms of cell destruction. *Ser Haematol* 7:328, 1974.

79. Suzuki S, Amano T, Mitsunaga M, et al: Autoimmune hemolytic anemia associated with IgA autoantibody. *Clin Immunol Immunopathol* 21:247, 1981.

80. Wolf CF, Wolf DJ, Peterson P: Autoimmune hemolytic anemia with predominance of IgA autoantibody. *Transfusion* 22:238, 1982.

81. Szymanski IO, Teno R, Rybak ME: Hemolytic anemia due to a mixture of low-titer IgG lambda and IgM lambda agglutinins reacting optimally at 22°C. *Vox Sang* 51:112, 1986.

82. Reusser P, Osterwalder B, Burri H, Speck B: Autoimmune hemolytic anemia associated with IgA: Diagnostic and therapeutic aspects in a case with long-term follow-up. *Acta Haematol* 77:53, 1987.

83. Göttsche B, Salama A, Mueller-Eckhardt C: Autoimmune hemolytic anemia associated with an IgA autoanti-Gerbich. *Vox Sang* 58:211, 1990.

84. Girelli G, Perrone MP, Adorno G, et al: A second example of hemolysis due to IgA autoantibody with anti-c specificity. *Haematologica* 75:182, 1990.

85. Evans RS, Bingham M, Boehni P: Autoimmune hemolytic disease: Antibody dissociation and activity. *Arch Intern Med* 108:338, 1961.

86. Evans RS, Bingham M, Turner E: Autoimmune hemolytic disease: Observations of serological reactions and disease activity. *Ann NY Acad Sci* 124:422, 1965.

87. Gilliland BC, Leddy JP, Vaughan JH: The detection of cell-bound antibody on complement-coated human red cells. *J Clin Invest* 49:898, 1970.

88. Gilliland BC, Baxter E, Evans RS: Red cell antibodies in acquired hemolytic anemia with negative antiglobulin serum tests. *N Engl J Med* 285:252, 1971.

89. Gilliland BC: Coombs-negative immune hemolytic anemia. *Semin Hematol* 13:267, 1976.

90. Sokol RJ, Hewitt S, Booker DJ, Bailey A: Erythrocyte autoantibodies, subclasses of IgG and autoimmune haemolysis. *Autoimmunity* 6:99, 1990.

91. von dem Borne AE Kr, Beckers D, van der Meulen W, Engelfriet CP: IgG4 autoantibodies against erythrocytes, without increased hemolysis: A case report. *Br J Haematol* 37:137, 1977.

92. Weiner W, Vos GH: Serology of acquired hemolytic anemia. *Blood* 22:606, 1963.

93. Vos GH, Petz L, Funenberg HH: Specificity of acquired haemolytic anaemia autoantibodies and their serological characteristics. *Br J Haematol* 19:57, 1970.

94. Leddy JP, Peterson P, Yeaw MA, Bakemeier RF: Patterns of serologic specificity of human γG erythrocyte autoantibodies. *J Immunol* 105:677, 1970.

95. Bell CA, Zwicker H: Further studies on the relationship of anti-En^a and anti-Wr^b in warm autoimmune hemolytic anemia. *Transfusion* 18:572, 1978.

96. Celano MJ, Levine P: Anti-LW specificity in autoimmune acquired hemolytic anemia. *Transfusion* 7:265, 1967.

97. Marsh WL, Reid ME, Scott EP: Autoantibodies of U blood group specificity in autoimmune haemolytic anaemia. *Br J Haematol* 22:625, 1972.

98. Shulman IA, Vengelen-Tyler V, Thompson JC, et al: Autoanti-Ge associated with severe autoimmune hemolytic anemia. *Vox Sang* 59:232, 1990.

99. Owen I, Chowdhury V, Reid ME, et al: Autoimmune hemolytic anemia associated with anti-Sc1. *Transfusion* 32:173, 1992.

100. Marsh WL, Oyen R, Alicea E, et al: Autoimmune hemolytic anemia and the Kell blood groups. *Am J Hematol* 7:155, 1979.

101. Barker RN, Casswell KM, Reid ME, et al: Identification of autoantigens in autoimmune haemolytic anaemia by a non-radioisotope immunoprecipitation method. *Br J Haematol* 82:126, 1992.

102. Victoria EJ, Pierce SW, Branks MJ, Masouredis SP: IgG red blood cell autoantibodies in autoimmune hemolytic anemia bind to epitopes on red blood cell membrane band 3 glycoprotein. *J Lab Clin Med* 115:74, 1990.

103. Telen JM, Chasis JA: Relationship of the human erythrocyte Wr^b antigen to an interaction between glycophorin A and band 3. *Blood* 76:842, 1990.

104. Barker RN, de la Sa Oliveira GG, Elson CJ, et al: Pathogenic autoantibodies in the NZB mouse are specific for erythrocyte band 3 protein. *Eur J Immunol* 23:1723, 1993.

105. Kay MMB, Marchalonis JJ, Hughes J, et al: Definition of a physiologic aging autoantigen by using synthetic peptides of membrane protein band 3: Localization of the active antigenic sites. *Proc Natl Acad Sci USA* 87:5734, 1990.

106. Turrini F, Mannu F, Arese P, et al: Characterization of autologous antibodies that opsonize erythrocytes with clustered integral membrane proteins. *Blood* 181:3146, 1993.

107. Lutz HU, Bussolino F, Flepp R, et al: Naturally occurring anti-band 3 antibodies and complement together mediate phagocytosis of oxidatively stressed human erythrocytes. *Proc Natl Acad Sci USA* 84:7368, 1987.

108. Lundgren G, Asaba H, Bergström J, et al: Fulminating anti-A autoimmune hemolysis with anuria in a renal transplant recipient: A therapeutic role of plasma exchange. *Clin Nephrol* 16:211, 1981.

109. Ramsey G, Nusbacher J, Starzl TE, Lindsay GD: Isohemagglutinins of graft origin after ABO-unmatched liver transplantation. *N Engl J Med* 311:1167, 1984.

110. Mangal AK, Growe GH, Sinclair M, et al: Acquired hemolytic anemia due to "auto"-anti-a or "auto"-anti-b induced by group O homograft in renal transplant recipients. *Transfusion* 24:201, 1984.

111. Hazlehurst GR, Brenner MK, Wimperis JZ, et al: Haemolysis after T-cell depleted bone marrow transplantation involving minor ABO incompatibility. *Scand J Haematol* 37:1, 1986.

112. Solheim BG, Albrechtsen D, Egeland T, et al: Auto-antibodies against erythrocytes in transplant patients produced by donor lymphocytes. *Transplant Proc* 6:4520, 1987.

113. Sniecinski IJ, Oien L, Petz LD, Blume KG: Immunohematologic consequences of major ABO-mismatched bone marrow transplantation. *Transplantation* 45:530, 1988.

114. Issitt PD: Autoimmune hemolytic anemia and cold hemagglutinin disease: Clinical disease and laboratory findings. *Prog Clin Pathol* 7:137, 1978.

115. Wallhermfechtel MA, Pohl BA, Chaplin H: Alloimmunization in patients with warm autoantibodies: A retrospective study employing three donor alloabsorptions to aid in antibody detection. *Transfusion* 24:482, 1984.

116. Dameshek W, Rosenthal MC, Schwartz SO: The treatment of acquired hemolytic anemia with adrenocorticotrophic hormone (ACTH). *N Engl J Med* 244:117, 1951.

117. Allgood JW, Chaplin H Jr: Idiopathic acquired autoimmune hemolytic anemia: A review of forty-seven cases treated from 1955 to 1965. *Am J Med* 43:254, 1967.

118. Meyer O, Stahl D, Beckhove P, Huhn D, Salama A: Pulsed high-dose dexamethasone in chronic autoimmune haemolytic anaemia of warm type. *Br J Haemotal* 98:860, 1997.

119. Greendyke RM, Bradley EB, Swisher SN: Studies of the effects of administration of ACTH and adrenal corticosteroids on erythrophagocytosis. *J Clin Invest* 44:746, 1965.

120. Fries LF, Brickman CM, Frank MM: Monocyte receptors for the Fc portion of IgG increase in number in autoimmune hemolytic anemia and other hemolytic states and are decreased by glucocorticoid therapy. *J Immunol* 131:1240, 1983.

121. Habibi B, Homberg JC, Schaison G, Salmon C: Autoimmune hemolytic anemia in children. A review of 80 cases. *Am J Med* 56:61, 1974.

122. Christensen BE: The pattern of erythrocyte sequestration in immunohaemolysis: Effects of prednisone treatment and splenectomy. *Scand J Haematol* 10:120, 1973.

123. Parker AC, MacPherson AIS, Richmond J: Value of radiochromium investigation in autoimmune haemolytic anaemia. *Br Med J* 1:208, 1977.

124. Bowdler AJ: The role of the spleen and splenectomy in autoimmune hemolytic disease. *Semin Hematol* 13:335, 1976.

125. Schwartz SI, Bernard RP, Adams JT, Bauman AW: Splenectomy for hematologic disorders. *Arch Surg* 101:338, 1970.

126. Eichner ER: Splenic function: Normal, too much and too little. *Am J Med* 66:311, 1979.

127. Centers for Disease Control and Prevention: Recommendations of the Advisory Committee on Immunization Practices (ACIP): Use of vaccines and immune globulins in persons with altered immunocompetence. *MMWR* 42:1, 1993.

128. Murphy S, LoBuglio AF: Drug therapy of autoimmune hemolytic anemia. *Semin Hematol* 13:323, 1976.

129. Skinner MD, Schwartz RS: Immunosuppressive therapy. *N Engl J Med* 287:221, 1972.

130. Shumak KH, Rock GA: Therapeutic plasma exchange. *N Engl J Med* 310:762, 1984.

131. Council Report: Current status of therapeutic plasmapheresis and related techniques. *JAMA* 253:819, 1985.

132. Ahn YS, Harrington WJ, Byrnes JJ, et al: Treatment of autoimmune hemolytic anemia with vinca-loaded platelets. *JAMA* 249:2189, 1983.

133. Leickly FE, Buckley RH: Successful treatment of autoimmune hemolytic anemia in common variable immunodeficiency with high-dose intravenous gamma globulin. *Am J Med* 82:159, 1987.

134. Oda H, Honda A, Sugita K, et al: High-dose intravenous intact IgG infusion in refractory autoimmune hemolytic anemia (Evans syndrome). *J Pediatr* 107:744, 1985.

135. Bussel JB, Cunningham-Rundles C, Abraham C: Intravenous treatment of autoimmune hemolytic anemia with very high dose gammaglobulin. *Vox Sang* 41:264, 1986.

136. Besa EC: Rapid transient reversal of anemia and long-term effects of maintenance intravenous immunoglobulin for autoimmune hemolytic anemia in patients with lymphoproliferative disorders. *Am J Med* 84:691, 1988.

137. Flores G, Cunningham-Rundles C, Newland AC, Bussel JB: Efficacy of intravenous immunoglobulin in the treatment of autoimmune hemolytic anemia: Results in 73 patients. *Am J Hematol* 44:237 1993.

138. Ahn YS, Harrington WJ, Mylvaganam R, et al: Danazol therapy for autoimmune hemolytic anemia. *Ann Intern Med* 102:298, 1985.

139. Pignon J-M, Poirson E, Rochant H: Danazol in autoimmune haemolytic anaemia. *Br J Haematol* 83:343, 1993.

140. Shashaty GG, Rath CE, Britt EJ: Autoimmune hemolytic anemia associated with ulcerative colitis. *Am J Hematol* 3:199, 1977.

141. Payne D, Muss HB, Homesley HD: Autoimmune hemolytic anemia and ovarian dermoid cysts: Case report and review of the literature. *Cancer* 48:721, 1981.

142. Beutler E: New chemotherapeutic agent: 2-Chlorodeoxyadenosine. *Semin Hematol* 31:40, 1994.

143. Silverstein MN, Gomes MR, Elveback LR, et al: Idiopathic acquired hemolytic anemia: Survival in 117 cases. *Arch Intern Med* 129:85, 1972.

144. Dausset J, Colombani J: The serology and the prognosis of 128 cases of autoimmune hemolytic anemia. *Blood* 14:1280, 1959.

145. Buchanan GR, Boxer LA, Nathan DG: The acute and transient nature of idiopathic immune hemolytic anemia in childhood. *J Pediatr* 88:780, 1976.

146. Zupanska B, Lawkowicz W, Gorska B, et al: Autoimmune haemolytic anemia in children. *Br J Haematol* 34:511, 1976.

147. Heisel MA, Ortega JA: Factors influencing prognosis in childhood auto-immune hemolytic anemia. *Am J Pediatr Hematol Oncol* 5:147, 1983.

148. Carapella de Luca E, Casadei AM, diPero G, et al: Autoimmune haemolytic anemia in childhood: Follow-up in 29 cases. *Vox Sang* 36:13, 1979.

149. Sokol RJ, Hewitt S, Stamps BK, Hitchen PA: Autoimmune haemolysis in childhood and adolescence. *Acta Haematol* 72:245, 1984.

150. Wang WC: Evans syndrome in childhood: Pathophysiology, clinical course and treatment. *Am J Pediatr Hematol Oncol* 10:330, 1988.

CHAPTER 56

CRYOPATHIC HEMOLYTIC SYNDROMES

CHARLES H. PACKMAN

Cryopathic hemolytic syndromes are caused by autoantibodies that bind optimally to red blood cells (RBC) at temperatures below body temperature. The ability of these antibodies to injure RBC is directly related to their ability to fix complement. Two types of cold-reactive autoantibodies to RBC are recognized: cold agglutinins and cold hemolysins. Both may be idiopathic, without an underlying disease, or may occur as a secondary form, usually associated with B-lymphoproliferative disorders or with certain infections. With both types of cold-reactive autoantibody, there is potential for intravascular hemolysis. Warm autoantibodies, on the other hand, usually cause extravascular hemolysis. Cold agglutinins are generally of IgM isotype, while cold hemolysins are usually of IgG isotype. In both types, the direct antiglobulin test result is positive for complement. Cold-agglutinin disease is associated with high-titer RBC agglutinating activity in the serum, more active at 4°C (39.2°F) than at 37°C (98.6°F). Cold hemolysins are detected by the biphasic Donath-Landsteiner test. Therapy consists mainly of keeping the patient warm and controlling the underlying disorder in secondary forms.

Cryopathic hemolytic syndromes are autoimmune disorders caused by autoantibodies that bind RBC optimally at temperatures below 37°C (98.6°F) and usually below 31°C (87.8°F). There are two major types of "cold antibody" that may produce autoimmune hemolytic anemia (Table 56-1). One is mediated by cold agglutinins. The other, paroxysmal cold hemoglobinuria, is mediated by an autoantibody (the Donath-Landsteiner antibody) that is not an agglutinin but a potent hemolysin (for discussion of these terms, see the introductory section of Chap. 55). Chronic cold-agglutinin–mediated autoimmune hemolytic anemia is extremely rare in children. Conversely, acute hemolytic anemia due to Donath-Landsteiner antibody accounts for a substantial proportion of autoimmune hemolytic anemia in children but is very rare in adults. Either of these disorders is encountered less commonly than autoimmune hemolytic anemia due to warm autoantibodies. In both cryopathic syndromes, the complement system plays a major role in RBC injury, and there is a much greater potential for direct intravascular hemolysis than in warm-antibody–mediated autoimmune hemolytic anemia.

COLD-AGGLUTININ–MEDIATED AUTOIMMUNE HEMOLYTIC ANEMIA

DEFINITION AND HISTORY

Cold agglutinins were first described by Landsteiner in 1903.[1] However, recognition of the connection among cold agglutinins, hemolytic

---

Acronyms and abbreviations that appear in this chapter include: DAF, decay-accelerating factor; HRF, homologous restriction factor; RBC, red blood cell.

---

anemia, and Raynaud-like peripheral vascular phenomena evolved slowly. In 1918, Clough and Richter detected cold agglutinins in a patient with pneumonia.[2] In 1925 and 1926, Iwai and Mei-Sai[3,4] reported two patients with cold agglutinins and Raynaud's phenomenon and showed that flow of blood through capillary tubes in vitro or in superficial capillaries in vivo was impeded at low temperatures. During the late 1940s and early 1950s, the observations of many workers gradually established the pathogenic importance of cold agglutinins in RBC injury. Schubothe introduced the term cold-agglutinin disease in 1953 and clearly distinguished this disorder from other acquired hemolytic syndromes.[5]

In current usage, cold-agglutinin disease pertains to patients with chronic autoimmune hemolytic anemia in which the autoantibody directly agglutinates human RBC at temperatures below body temperature, maximally at 0 to 5°C (32 to 41°F). Fixation of complement to a patient's RBC by cold agglutinins in vivo occurs at higher temperatures, but generally below 37°C (98.6°F). Cold agglutinins typically are IgM, although occasionally they may be globulins of other isotypes. Those occurring in chronic cold-agglutinin disease generally are monoclonal. Most cold agglutinins have specificity for oligosaccharide antigens (I or i) of the RBC (see "Origin of Cold Agglutinins," below).

Cold-agglutinin disease traditionally has been classified as being either primary (idiopathic) or secondary (see Table 56-1). The latter is most commonly seen in adolescents or young adults as a self-limited process associated with Mycoplasma pneumoniae infections or infectious mononucleosis and, rarely, in children with chickenpox. The term also has been used to describe a chronic disorder occurring in older patients with known malignant lymphoproliferative diseases. On the other hand, idiopathic (primary) chronic cold-agglutinin disease has its peak incidence after age 50. This disorder, with its characteristic monoclonal IgM cold agglutinins, may be considered a special form of monoclonal gammopathy. As with other "essential" or idiopathic monoclonal gammopathies, some cases in this group gradually develop features of a B-cell lymphoproliferative disorder that resembles Waldenström's macroglobulinemia. Thus, the distinction between primary and secondary types of chronic cold-agglutinin disease is not absolute.

ETIOLOGY AND PATHOGENESIS

ORIGIN OF COLD AGGLUTININS

A high proportion of monoclonal IgM cold agglutinins with either anti-I or anti-i specificity have heavy-chain variable regions encoded by V_H4–34, formerly designated $V_H4.21$.[6-8] This V_H gene encodes a distinct idiotype identified by a rat monoclonal antibody, 9G4. This idiotype is expressed both by the cold agglutinins themselves and on the surface immunoglobulin of B cells synthesizing cold agglutinins or related immunoglobulins possessing V_H4–34 sequences.[9] Using the 9G4 monoclonal antibody as a probe, this idiotype was found, not only in a very high proportion of circulating B cells and marrow lymphoplasmacytoid cells of patients with lymphoma-associated chronic cold-agglutinin disease, but also in a smaller proportion of B cells in the blood and lymphoid tissues of normal adult donors and in the spleens of 15-week human fetuses.[9] These data suggest that B cells expressing the V_H4–34 gene (or a closely related sequence) are present throughout ontogeny. Chronic cold-agglutinin disease, therefore, may represent a marked, unregulated expansion of a subset (clone) of such B cells.

Light-chain V-region gene use in anti-I cold agglutinins is also highly selective; there is a strong bias toward use of the kappa III variable region subgroup (V_κ-III).[7,10] Light-chain selection among anti-i cold agglutinins, however, is much more variable and includes those of type lambda.[7,11]

These observations that pathologic cold agglutinins are synthesized with distinct and highly selected V-region sequences must be

TABLE 56-1 CRYOPATHIC HEMOLYTIC SYNDROME

I. Mediated by cold agglutinins
   A. Idiopathic (primary) chronic cold-agglutinin disease
   B. Secondary cold-agglutinin hemolytic anemia
      1. Postinfectious (e.g., *Mycoplasma pneumoniae* or infectious mononucleosis)
      2. Associated with preexisting malignant B-cell lymphoproliferative disorder
II. Mediated by cold hemolysins
   A. Idiopathic (primary) paroxysmal cold hemoglobinuria—very rare
   B. Secondary
      1. Donath-Landsteiner hemolytic anemia, usually associated with an acute viral syndrome in children—relatively common
      2. Congenital or tertiary syphilis in adults—very rare

viewed against the background of two other subsequent observations. First, V_H4–34 or related V_H genes also may encode the heavy-chain variable regions of other types of antibodies, such as rheumatoid factor autoantibodies and alloantibodies to a variety of blood group antigens, including polypeptide determinants such as Rh.[12] Second, normal human antibodies to an exogenous carbohydrate antigen, *Haemophilus influenzae* type b capsular polysaccharide, also are encoded by a restricted set of V_H genes[13] and Ig light-chain V genes.[14] Thus, the regulation of Ig gene use for the production of anti-I or anti-i cold agglutinins may not differ fundamentally from normal antibody formation to other carbohydrate antigens.

In the setting of B-cell lymphoma or Waldenström's macroglobulinemia, cold agglutinins may be produced by the malignant clone itself. Two patients with lymphoma and monoclonal cold agglutinin were each identified to have a karyotypically abnormal B-cell clone that produced a cold agglutinin identical to that found in their sera.[15,16] Trisomy 3 has been the most frequently observed karyotypic abnormality in patients with non-Hodgkin's lymphoma and cold agglutinins.[15–17]

Normal human sera generally have naturally occurring cold agglutinins in low titer (usually 1/32 or less). Otherwise healthy persons may develop elevated titers of cold agglutinins specific for I/i antigens during certain infections (e.g., *M. pneumoniae*, Epstein-Barr virus, or cytomegalovirus). In contrast to other forms of cold-agglutinin disease, the hyperproduction of these postinfectious cold agglutinins is transient. There is some evidence that such postinfectious cold agglutinins may be less clonally restricted than those occurring in chronic cold-agglutinin disease,[18] but this is not a universal finding.[19] Whether V_H4–34 also encodes most heavy-chain variable regions of all naturally occurring or postinfectious cold agglutinins remains to be determined.

The increased production of cold agglutinins in response to infection with *M. pneumoniae* may be secondary to the fact that the oligosaccharide antigens of the I/i type serve as specific *Mycoplasma* receptors.[20] This may lead to altered antigen presentation involving a complex between a self-antigen (I/i) and a non–self-antigen (*Mycoplasma*). Alternatively, the anti-i cold agglutinins may arise as a consequence of polyclonal B-cell activation, as occurs in infectious mononucleosis (see Chap. 90).

PATHOGENIC EFFECTS OF COLD AGGLUTININS
Most cold agglutinins are unable to agglutinate RBC at temperatures above 30°C (86°F). The highest temperature at which these antibodies cause detectable agglutination is termed the thermal amplitude. This value may vary considerably from one patient to another. Generally, patients with cold agglutinins of higher thermal amplitudes have a greater risk for cold-agglutinin disease.[5] Active hemolytic anemia, for example, has been observed in patients with cold agglutinins of modest titer (e.g., 1:256) that have high thermal amplitudes.[21]

The pathogenicity of a cold agglutinin is dependent upon its ability to bind host RBC and to activate complement.[22–28] This process

is called complement fixation. Although in vitro agglutination of the RBC may be maximal at 0 to 5°C (32 to 41°F), complement fixation by these antibodies may occur optimally at 20 to 25°C (68 to 77°F) and may be significant at even higher physiologic temperatures.[21–23] Agglutination is not required for this process. The great preponderance of cold-agglutinin molecules are IgM pentamers, but small numbers of IgM hexamers with cold-agglutinin activity are found in patients with cold-agglutinin disease. Hexamers fix complement and lyse RBC more efficiently than do pentamers, suggesting that hexameric IgM may play a role in the pathogenesis of hemolysis in these patients.[29]

Cold agglutinins may bind to RBC in superficial vessels of the extremities, where the temperature generally ranges between 28 and 31°C (82.4 and 87.8°F), depending upon ambient temperature.[24] Cold agglutinins of high thermal amplitude may cause RBC to aggregate at this temperature, thereby impeding RBC flow and producing acrocyanosis. In addition, the RBC-bound cold agglutinin may activate complement via the classical pathway. Once activated complement proteins are deposited onto the RBC surface, it is no longer necessary for the cold agglutinin to remain bound to the RBC for hemolysis to occur. Instead, the cold agglutinin may dissociate from the RBC at the higher temperatures in the body core and again be able to bind another RBC at the lower temperatures in the superficial vessels. As a result, patients with high–thermal-amplitude cold agglutinins tend to have a sustained hemolytic process and acrocyanosis.[30]

Patients with antibodies of lower thermal amplitude require significant chilling to initiate complement-mediated injury of RBC. This sequence may result in a burst of hemolysis with hemoglobinuria.[30] Combinations of these clinical patterns also occur. Cold agglutinins of the IgA isotype, an isotype that does not fix complement, may cause acrocyanosis but not hemolysis.[31] Thus, the relative degree of hemolysis or impeded RBC flow is influenced significantly by the properties and quantity of the cold agglutinins in a given patient.

Complement fixation may effect RBC injury by two major mechanisms: (1) direct lysis and (2) opsonization for hepatic and splenic macrophages. Both mechanisms probably operate to varying degrees in any one patient. Direct lysis requires propagation of the full C1-to-C9 sequence on the RBC membrane. If this occurs to a significant degree, the patient may experience intravascular hemolysis leading to hemoglobinemia and hemoglobinuria. Intravascular hemolysis of this severity is relatively rare. More commonly, the complement sequence on many RBC is completed only through the early steps, leaving opsonic fragments of C3 (C3b/C3bi) and C4 (C4b) on the cell surface. These fragments provide only a weak stimulus for phagocytosis by monocytes in vitro.[32,33] However, activated macrophages may ingest C3b-coated particles avidly.[34] Accordingly, a RBC heavily coated with C3b (and/or C3bi) may be removed from the circulation by macrophages either in the liver or, to a lesser extent, the spleen.[23,26,35,36] The trapped RBC may be ingested entirely or released back into the circulation as a spherocyte after losing some of its plasma membrane.

In vivo studies of the fate of ^{51}Cr-labeled C3b-coated RBC[23,26,27,37] indicate that many of the erythrocytes trapped in the liver or spleen gradually may reenter the circulation. Such released cells generally are coated with the opsonically inactive C3 fragment, C3dg. Conversion of cell-bound C3b or C3bi to C3dg results from the action of the naturally occurring complement inhibitor, factor I, in concert with factor H or CR1 receptors.[38] These surviving C3dg-coated RBC circulate with a near-normal life span[23,26,27,37,39] and are resistant to further uptake of cold agglutinins or complement.[23,26,40] However, C3dg-coated RBC also may react in vitro with anticomplement (anti-C3) serum in the direct antiglobulin test. In fact, most of the antiglobulin-positive RBC of patients with cold agglutinin disease are coated with C3dg.

Progression of the complement cascade on many RBC generally does not go beyond the formation of C3b. Phosphatidylinositol-linked RBC membrane proteins protect against injury by autologous complement components. These proteins include decay-accelerating factor (DAF, or CD55; see Chap. 13) and homologous restriction factors (HRF). DAF inhibits the formation and function of cell-bound C3-converting enzyme,[41] thus indirectly limiting formation of C5-converting enzyme. HRF, on the other hand, impedes C9 binding and formation of the C5b–9 membrane attack complex.[42]

PREVALENCE

Cold-agglutinin disease is less common than warm-antibody autoimmune hemolytic anemia, accounting for only 10 to 20 percent of all cases of autoimmune hemolytic anemia.[22,43,44] Women are affected more commonly than men.[22,43] No genetic or racial factors are known to contribute to the pathogenesis of this disease.

Although the majority of patients with mycoplasma pneumonia have significant cold-agglutinin titers, they only infrequently develop clinical hemolytic anemia.[45–47] However, subclinical RBC injury may occur. In one series of *M. pneumoniae* infections, weakly positive direct antiglobulin reactions and/or mild reticulocytosis were noted in the absence of anemia in a substantial number of cases.[45] Cold agglutinins occur in over 60 percent of patients with infectious mononucleosis but, again, hemolytic anemia is rare.[48–50]

CLINICAL FEATURES

Most patients with cold-agglutinin hemolytic anemia have chronic hemolytic anemia with or without jaundice. In others, the principal feature is episodic, acute hemolysis with hemoglobinuria induced by chilling (see the discussion of thermal amplitude under "Pathogenic Effects of Cold Agglutinins," above.) Combinations of these clinical features may occur. Acrocyanosis and other cold-mediated vasoocclusive phenomena affecting the fingers, toes, nose, and ears are associated with sludging of RBC in the cutaneous microvasculature. Skin ulceration and necrosis are distinctly unusual. Hemolysis occurring in *M. pneumoniae* infections is acute in onset, typically appearing as the patient is recovering from pneumonia and coincident with peak titers of cold agglutinins. The hemolysis is self-limited, lasting 1 to 3 weeks.[43] Hemolytic anemia in infectious mononucleosis develops either at the onset of symptoms or within the first 3 weeks of illness.[49]

Other physical findings are variable, depending upon the presence of an underlying disease. Splenomegaly, a characteristic finding in lymphoproliferative diseases or infectious mononucleosis, also may be observed in idiopathic cold-agglutinin disease.

LABORATORY FEATURES

GENERAL

In classic chronic cold-agglutinin disease, the anemia is mild to moderate and fairly stable. However, patients may develop hemoglobin levels as low as 5 to 6 g/dl. In addition to polychromasia, the blood film also may show spherocytosis. However, these features are generally less marked than in typical cases of warm-antibody autoimmune hemolytic anemia. RBC autoagglutination may be noted on the blood film. Autoagglutination also may be evident in anticoagulated blood at room temperature. This phenomenon may be intensified by cooling the blood to 4°C (39.2°F) and reversed by warming to 37°C (98.6°F). This property distinguishes cold autoagglutination from rouleaux formation. Mild to moderate leukocytosis is often seen during active hemolysis, for example, following exposure of the patient to chilling. The platelet count is usually normal. Mild hyperbilirubinemia is common.

SEROLOGIC FEATURES

Cold agglutinins are distinguished by their ability to agglutinate saline-suspended human RBC at low temperature, maximally at 0 to 5°C

(32 to 41°F). This reaction is reversible by warming. In chronic cold-agglutinin disease, the serum titers are commonly 1:10,000 or higher and may reach 1:1,000,000 or more. As noted above, cold agglutinins are characteristically IgM. IgA or IgG cold agglutinins have been reported in a few cases,[31,43,51] sometimes in combination with IgM.[52] Occasionally, warm-reactive IgG autoantibodies are found in association with IgM cold agglutinins.[53] Mixed warm- and cold-antibody autoimmune hemolytic anemia is discussed in Chap. 55.

The direct antiglobulin test result, as noted above, is positive with anticomplement reagents. The antibody itself, however, is not detected by the antiglobulin test using antisera to human immunoglobulins. This is because the cold agglutinins readily dissociate from the RBC both in vivo and during the washing steps of the standard antiglobulin procedure. In contrast, C4b and C3b are covalently bound to target RBC via thioester linkages. In one unusual case, it was possible to detect a low-titer IgG cold agglutinin by washing the patient's RBC in ice-cold saline solution and performing the direct antiglobulin test at 4°C (39.2°F).[51]

As noted earlier, the majority of cold agglutinins are reactive with oligosaccharide antigens of the I/i system, which are precursors of the ABH and Lewis blood group substances.[54–56] The I/i determinants are bound to erythrocyte membrane glycoprotein (band 3 anion transporter) or to glycolipids.[55,56] Anti-I and anti-i have been reported to bind solubilized RBC glycoproteins at 37°C (98.6°F), suggesting that the temperature dependence of cold agglutination of intact RBC may be a function of temperature-induced conformational effects on the cell surface.[57,58]

I antigens are expressed strongly on adult RBC but weakly on neonatal (cord) RBC. The converse is true of i antigens, indicating that I/i antigen expression is developmentally regulated.[55] These differences between adult and cord blood RBC allow evaluation of the serologic specificity of cold agglutinins.[22,31,43] I/i antigens, or structurally related analogs, occur in human saliva, milk, amniotic fluid, or hydatid cyst fluid[31] and are expressed on human lymphocytes, neutrophils, and monocytes.[59]

Anti-I is the predominant specificity of cold agglutinins in idiopathic cold-agglutinin disease, in patients with *M. pneumoniae*, and in some cases of lymphoma. Cold agglutinins with anti-i specificity are found in patients with infectious mononucleosis and in some patients with lymphoma. A small percentage of cold agglutinin–containing sera react equally well with adult and neonatal RBC. These antibodies recognize antigens outside the I/i system, including Pr antigens, consisting of carbohydrate epitopes of glycophorins that are inactivated by protease treatment,[31] and, less commonly, the M or P blood group antigens.[60,61] Most cold agglutinins associated with chickenpox exhibit anti-Pr specificity; a single case with anti-I specificity has been observed as well.[62] Hemolysis due to a cold agglutinin with anti-Pr specificity occurred following an allogeneic marrow transplant.[63]

In hemolytic anemia associated with infectious mononucleosis, the patient's serum may contain IgM anti-i cold agglutinins or cold-reactive nonagglutinating IgG anti-i along with IgM cold-reactive anti-IgG antibodies ("rheumatoid factors") that may cross-link the IgG-coated red cells to produce agglutination.[64]

DIFFERENTIAL DIAGNOSIS

The clinical and laboratory features of chronic cold-agglutinin disease are sufficiently distinctive that the diagnostic possibilities are limited. In general, a high-titer cold agglutinin (>1:10,000) together with a direct antiglobulin test result that is positive with anticomplement serum (but not with anti-IgG) is consistent with cold-agglutinin disease. In many instances of drug-induced immune hemolytic anemia, the direct antiglobulin test result is also positive only for complement.

The drug history and a low (or absent) cold agglutinin titer, however, help to distinguish this from cold-agglutinin disease. If the patient has elevated cold agglutinins and a positive direct antiglobulin test result with both anti-IgG and anti-C3, then the patient may have a mixed-type autoimmune hemolytic anemia (see Chap. 55). Warm-antibody autoimmune hemolytic anemia, congenital hemolytic disorders, and paroxysmal nocturnal hemoglobinuria should be excluded in cases exhibiting primarily a chronic hemolytic anemia. The pattern of the antiglobulin reaction, family history, and the acid or sucrose hemolysis test provides additional help in difficult cases. When the hemolysis is episodic in nature, one also should consider paroxysmal cold hemoglobinuria (see "Paroxysmal Cold Hemoglobinuria," below) and march hemoglobinuria, as well as paroxysmal nocturnal hemoglobinuria. When cold-induced peripheral vasoocclusive symptoms are predominant, the differential diagnosis should include cryoglobulinemia and Raynaud's phenomenon, with or without an associated rheumatic disease. Infectious mononucleosis, *M. pneumoniae* infection, or lymphoma may be considered in appropriate clinical settings.

THERAPY

It is important to keep the patient warm, particularly the extremities. This is moderately effective in providing symptomatic relief. This may be the only measure required in patients with mild chronic hemolysis. Therapy with chlorambucil or cyclophosphamide may be helpful for patients with chronic cold-agglutinin disease of greater severity.[5,22,43,65,66] A patient treated with interferon-α experienced rapid resolution of acrocyanosis and hemolytic anemia, associated with a marked decrease in cold agglutinin titer.[67] Treatment with interferon-α also has proven beneficial in patients with type II cryoglobulinemia involving monoclonal IgM anti-IgG.[68] The results from splenectomy[22,43,69] or use of glucocorticoids[22,43] generally have been disappointing, although exceptions have been reported,[21,22,51,52] particularly in atypical cases. There is experimental[35] and clinical[21] basis for considering very high doses of glucocorticoids in seriously ill patients. An elderly woman with a B-lymphoproliferative disease and severe refractory hemolysis mediated by cold agglutinins was successfully treated with the anti-CD20 monoclonal antibody, rituximab.[70] RBC transfusions generally are reserved for those patients with severe anemia of rapid onset who are in danger of cardiorespiratory complications.[51] Washed RBC often are used to avoid replenishing depleted complement components and reactivating the hemolytic process. In critically ill patients, plasma exchange (with replacement by albumin-containing saline solution) may provide transient amelioration of hemolysis.[71–73]

COURSE AND PROGNOSIS

Patients with idiopathic cold-agglutinin disease often have a relatively benign course and survive for many years.[5,22,43,66] Occasionally, death results from infection or severe anemia or, in the case of secondary cold-agglutinin disease, from an underlying lymphoproliferative process.

The postinfectious forms of cold-agglutinin disease typically are self-limited. Recovery generally occurs in a few weeks. A few cases with massive hemoglobinuria have been complicated by acute renal failure, requiring temporary hemodialysis.

PAROXYSMAL COLD HEMOGLOBINURIA

DEFINITIONS AND HISTORY

Paroxysmal cold hemoglobinuria is a very rare form of autoimmune hemolytic anemia in adults characterized by recurrent episodes of massive hemolysis following cold exposure.[22,43] A related form of hemolytic anemia occurs much more commonly in children (or young adults) as an acute, self-limited hemolytic process following several types of viral syndromes (see Table 56-1).[22,74–78]

In 1904, Donath and Landsteiner first described the cold-reactive autoantibody that is responsible for the complement-mediated hemolysis. The disease was recognized during the latter half of the nineteenth century, when it probably was more common because of its association with congenital or tertiary syphilis. With the advent of effective therapy for syphilis, this cause of paroxysmal cold hemoglobinuria has virtually disappeared. Now, recurrent paroxysmal cold hemoglobinuria occurs very rarely in a chronic idiopathic form.[22,43] An increasing proportion of Donath-Landsteiner autoantibody–mediated hemolytic anemias occurs as a single postviral episode in children, without recurrent attacks (paroxysms). The prognosis for such cases is excellent. Thus, rather than paroxysmal cold hemoglobinuria, it has been proposed that this entity be termed Donath-Landsteiner hemolytic anemia.[75,76] However, this term has not gained widespread acceptance.

ETIOLOGY AND PATHOGENESIS

The mechanism or mechanisms whereby dissimilar infectious agents (e.g., spirochetes and several types of virus) induce the immune system to produce Donath-Landsteiner antibodies with specificity for the human P blood group antigen (see Serologic Features below) is not known. The mechanism of hemolysis, however, probably parallels in vitro events described below. During severe chilling, blood flowing through skin capillaries is exposed to low temperatures. The Donath-Landsteiner antibody and early-acting complement components are presumed to bind to RBC at these lowered temperatures. Upon return of the cells to 37°C (98.6°F) in the central circulation, the cells are lysed by propagation of the terminal complement sequence through C9.

The Donath-Landsteiner antibody itself dissociates from the RBC at 37°C (98.6°F). However, prior to dissociation, it initiates the classical pathway of complement. Erythrocyte membrane proteins that restrict C5b–9 assembly (e.g., homologous restriction factors) may be, for some reason, less effective in controlling Donath-Landsteiner antibody–initiated complement activation than that initiated by cold agglutinins (see section on Cold Agglutinins).

PREVALENCE

Medical centers that receive many referrals report that paroxysmal cold hemoglobinuria constitutes 2 to 5 percent of all cases of autoimmune hemolytic anemia.[22,43] Among children, however, Donath-Landsteiner hemolytic anemia accounted for 32.4 percent of 68 immune hemolytic syndromes diagnosed over a 4-year period.[77] Most commonly, the diagnosis is missed because of lack of physicians' awareness or failure to perform the proper serologic studies (see Serologic Features below).[74,77] Thus, the true incidence actually may be higher. Although familial occurrence has been reported, there are no known racial or genetic risk factors.[22] As noted, most childhood cases follow either specific viral infections or upper respiratory infections of undefined etiology.[22,43,74–77]

CLINICAL FEATURES

Constitutional symptoms are prominent during a paroxysm. A few minutes to several hours after cold exposure, the patient develops aching pains in the back or legs, abdominal cramps, and perhaps headaches. Chills and fever usually follow. The first urine passed after onset of symptoms typically contains hemoglobin. The constitutional symptoms and hemoglobinuria generally last a few hours. Raynaud's phenomenon and cold urticaria sometimes occur during an attack, and jaundice may follow.

LABORATORY FEATURES

GENERAL

Hemoglobinuria is an expected finding if the patient is seen early in the attack. The urine may be dark red or brown due to the presence of hemoglobin or methemoglobin, respectively. The blood hemoglobin level often drops rapidly during a severe attack. Reticulocytosis, hemoglobinemia, and hyperbilirubinemia (mainly unconjugated) may be present, depending on when the patient is assessed. Serum complement titers usually are depressed during an acute episode because of rapid consumption. Spherocytosis and erythrophagocytosis by monocytes and neutrophils may be found on the blood film during an attack. Leukopenia often is seen early in the attack, followed by neutrophilic leukocytosis.

SEROLOGIC FEATURES

The direct antiglobulin reaction is usually positive during and briefly following an acute attack. The positive reaction is due to the coating of surviving RBC with complement, primarily C3dg fragments. The Donath-Landsteiner antibody is a nonagglutinating IgG that binds RBC only in the cold. It readily dissociates from the RBC at room temperature. In those adults subject to recurring episodes in association with cold exposure, the direct antiglobulin test result remains negative between attacks. The antibody is detected by the biphasic Donath-Landsteiner test, in which the patient's fresh serum is incubated with RBC initially at 4°C (39.2°F) and the mixture is then warmed to 37°C (98.6°F).[43] Intense hemolysis occurs. It may be necessary to add fresh guinea pig serum or ABO-compatible human serum to serve as a source of fresh complement if the patient's serum has been stored or is complement depleted. Antibody titers rarely exceed 1:16. The Donath-Landsteiner antibody typically has specificity for the P blood group antigen, a glycosphingolipid structure.[56] The P antigen has been reported to occur also on lymphocytes and skin fibroblasts.[78] The latter finding might be related in some way to the occurrence of cold urticaria in paroxysmal cold hemoglobinuria, a phenomenon that may be transferred passively by serum to normal skin.[22] Antibody specificities for RBC antigens other than the P blood group also have been noted.[79]

DIFFERENTIAL DIAGNOSIS

Paroxysmal cold hemoglobinuria must be distinguished from the subset of cases of chronic cold-agglutinin disease that manifests episodic hemolysis and hemoglobinuria. This distinction is made primarily in the laboratory. In general, patients with paroxysmal cold hemoglobinuria lack high titers of cold agglutinins. Furthermore, the Donath-Landsteiner antibody is a potent in vitro hemolysin, in contrast to most cold agglutinins, which are weak hemolysins. Warm-antibody autoimmune hemolytic anemia, march hemoglobinuria, myoglobinuria, and paroxysmal nocturnal hemoglobinuria may be distinguished through the history and appropriate laboratory studies.

THERAPY

Most contemporary cases of paroxysmal cold hemoglobinuria are self-limited. Acute attacks in both chronic and transient forms of paroxysmal cold hemoglobinuria may be prevented by avoiding exposure to cold. Glucocorticoid therapy and splenectomy have not been useful. When paroxysmal cold hemoglobinuria is associated with syphilis, effective treatment of the infection may result in a complete remission.

Antihistaminic and adrenergic agents may relieve symptoms of cold urticaria.

COURSE AND PROGNOSIS

Postinfectious forms of paroxysmal cold hemoglobinuria terminate spontaneously within a few days to weeks after onset,[74–77] although the Donath-Landsteiner antibody may persist in low titer for several years.[22] Most patients with chronic idiopathic paroxysmal cold hemoglobinuria survive for many years in spite of occasional paroxysms of hemolysis.

REFERENCES

1. Landsteiner K: Uber Beziehungen zwischen dem Blutserum und den Körperzeller. *Munch Med Wochenschr* 50:1812, 1903.
2. Clough MC, Richter IM: A study of an autoagglutinin occurring in a human serum. *Johns Hopkins Hosp Bull* 29:86, 1918.
3. Iwai S, Mei-Sai N: Etiology of Raynaud's disease: A preliminary report. *Jpn Med World* 5:119, 1925.
4. Iwai S, Mei-Sai N: Etiology of Raynaud's disease. *Jpn Med World* 6:345, 1926.
5. Schubothe H: The cold hemagglutinin disease. *Semin Hematol* 3:27, 1966.
6. Silverman GJ, Carson DA: Structural characterization of human monoclonal cold agglutinins: Evidence for a distinct primary sequence-defined V_H4 idiotype. *Eur J Immunol* 20:351, 1990.
7. Silberstein LE, Jefferies LC, Goldman J, et al: Variable region gene analysis of pathologic human autoantibodies to the related i and I red blood cell antigens. *Blood* 78:2372, 1991.
8. Pascual V, Victor K, Spellerberg M, et al: V_H restriction among human cold agglutinins: The V_H4-21 gene segment is required to encode anti-I and anti-i specificities. *J Immunol* 149:2337, 1992.
9. Stevenson FK, Smith GJ, North J, et al: Identification of normal B-cell counterparts of neoplastic cells which secrete cold agglutinins of anti-I and anti-i specificity. *Br J Haematol* 72:9, 1989.
10. Silverman GJ, Chen PP, Carson DA: Cold agglutinins: Specificity, idiotypy and structural analysis, in *Idiotypes in Biology and Medicine: Chemistry and Immunology*, vol 48, edited by DA Carson, PP Chen, TJ Kipps, p 109. Karger, Basel, 1990.
11. Feizi T: Lambda chains in cold agglutinins. *Science* 156:111, 1987.
12. Thompson KM, Sutherland J, Barden G, et al: Human monoclonal antibodies against blood group antigens preferentially express a V_H4-21 variable region gene-associated epitope. *Scand J Immunol* 34:509, 1991.
13. Adderson EE, Shackelford PG, Quinn A, et al: Restricted immunoglobulin VH usage and VDJ combinations in the human response to *Haemophilus influenzae* type b capsular polysaccharide: Nucleotide sequences of monospecific anti-*Haemophilus* antibodies and polyspecific antibodies cross-reacting with self-antigens. *J Clin Invest* 91:2734, 1993.
14. Adderson EE, Shackelford PG, Insel RA, et al: Immunoglobulin light chain variable region gene sequences for human antibodies to *Haemophilus influenzae* type b capsular polysaccharide are dominated by a limited number of V_κ and V_λ segments and VJ combinations. *J Clin Invest* 89:729, 1992.
15. Silberstein LE, Robertson GA, Hannam-Harris AC, et al: Etiologic aspects of cold agglutinin disease: Evidence of cytogenetically defined clones of lymphoid cells and the demonstration that an anti-Pr cold autoantibody is derived from an aberrant B cell clone. *Blood* 67:1705, 1986.
16. Gordon J, Silberstein LE, Moreau L, Nowell PC: Trisomy 3 in cold agglutinin disease. *Cancer Genet Cytogenet* 46:89, 1990.
17. Michaux L, Dierlamm J, Wlodarska I, et al: Trisomy 3q11-q29 is recurrently observed in B-cell non-Hodgkin's lymphomas associated with cold agglutinin syndrome. *Ann Hematol* 76:201, 1998.
18. Harboe M, Lind K: Light chain types of transiently occurring cold haemagglutinins. *Scand J Haematol* 3:269, 1966.
19. Feizi T: Monotypic cold agglutinins in infection by *Mycoplasma pneumoniae*. *Nature* 215:540, 1967.
20. Loomes LM, Uemura K, Childs RA, et al: Erythrocyte receptors for *Mycoplasma pneumoniae* are sialylated oligosaccharides of Ii antigen type. *Nature* 307:560, 1984.

21. Schreiber AD, Herskovitz BS, Goldwein M: Low-titer cold-hemaggluti-nin disease. *N Engl J Med* 296:1490, 1977.

22. Dacie J: *The Haemolytic Anaemias*, vol 3, *The Auto-Immune Haemolytic Anaemias*, 3d ed, p 210. Churchill Livingstone, New York, 1992.

23. Evans RS, Turner E, Bingham M, Woods R: Chronic hemolytic anemia due to cold agglutinins: II. The role of C' in red cell destruction. *J Clin Invest* 47:691, 1968.

24. Logue GL, Rosse WF, Gockerman JP: Measurement of the third compo-nent of complement bound to red blood cells in patients with the cold agglutinin syndrome. *J Clin Invest* 52:493, 1973.

25. Fischer JT, Petz LD, Garratty G, Cooper NR: Correlations between quantitative assay of red cell bound C3, serologic reactions and hemolytic anemia. *Blood* 44:359, 1974.

26. Jaffe CH, Atkinson JP, Frank MM: The role of complement in the clearance of cold agglutinin-sensitized erythrocytes in man. *J Clin Invest* 58:942, 1976.

27. Atkinson JP, Frank MM: Studies on in vivo effects of antibody: Interac-tion of IgM antibody and complement in the immune clearance and destruction of erythrocytes in man. *J Clin Invest* 54:339, 1974.

28. Kirschfink M, Fritze H, Roelcke D: Complement activation by cold agglutinins. *Vox Sang* 63:220, 1992.

29. Hughey CT, Brewer JW, Colosia AD, Rosse WF, Corley RB: Production of IgM hexamers by normal and autoimmune B cells: Implications for the physiologic role of hexameric IgM. *J Immunol* 161:4091, 1998.

30. Evans RS, Turner E, Bingham M: Studies with radioiodinated cold agglutinins of ten patients. *Am J Med* 38:378, 1965.

31. Roelcke D: Cold agglutination: Antibodies and antigens. *Clin Immunol Immunopathol* 2:266, 1974.

32. Mantovani B, Rabinovitch M, Nussenzweig V: Phagocytosis of immune complexes by macrophages: Different roles of the macrophage receptor sites for complement (C3) and for immunoglobulin (IgG). *J Exp Med* 135:780, 1972.

33. Ehlenberger AG, Nussenzweig V: The role of membrane receptors for C3b and C3d in phagocytosis. *J Exp Med* 145:357, 1977.

34. Silverstein SC, Steinman RM, Cohn ZA: Endocytosis. *Annu Rev Bio-chem* 46:669, 1977.

35. Atkinson JP, Schreiber AD, Frank MM: Effects of corticosteroids and splenectomy on the immune clearance and destruction of erythrocytes. *J Clin Invest* 52:1509, 1973.

36. Brown DL, Nelson DA: Surface microfragmentation of red cells as a mechanism for complement-mediated immune spherocytosis. *Br J Haematol* 24:301, 1973.

37. Schreiber AD, Frank MM: Role of antibody and complement in the immune clearance and destruction of erythrocytes: I. In vivo effects of IgG and IgM complement-fixing sites. *J Clin Invest* 51:575, 1972.

38. Ross GD: Opsonization and membrane complement receptors, in *Immu-nobiology of the Complement System*, edited by GD Ross, p 87. Aca-demic, Orlando, FL, 1986.

39. Lewis SM, Dacie JV, Szur L: Mechanism of haemolysis in the cold-haemagglutinin syndrome. *Br J Haematol* 6:154, 1960.

40. Evans RS, Turner E, Bingham M: Chronic hemolytic anemia due to cold agglutinins: I. The mechanism of resistance of red cells to C' hemolysis by cold agglutinins. *J Clin Invest* 46:1461, 1967.

41. Nicholson-Weller A, Burge J, Fearon DT, et al: Isolation of a human erythrocyte membrane glycoprotein with decay-accelerating activity for C3 convertases of the complement system. *J Immunol* 129:184, 1982.

42. Lachmann PJ: The control of homologous lysis. *Immunol Today* 12:312, 1991.

43. Petz LD, Garratty G: *Acquired Immune Hemolytic Anemias*. Churchill Livingstone, New York, 1980.

44. Eyster ME, Jenkins DE Jr: Erythrocyte coating substances in patients with positive direct antiglobulin reactions: Correlation of γG globulin and complement coating with underlying diseases, overt hemolysis and response to therapy. *Am J Med* 46:360, 1969.

45. Feizi T: Cold agglutinins, the direct Coombs' test and serum immuno-globulins in *Mycoplasma pneumoniae* infection. *Ann NY Acad Sci* 143:801, 1967.

46. Jacobson LB, Longstreth GF, Edington TS: Clinical and immunologic features of transient cold agglutinin hemolytic anemia. *Am J Med* 54:514, 1973.

47. Murray HW, Masur H, Senterfit LB, Roberts RB: The protean manifesta-tions of *Mycoplasma pneumoniae* infection in adults. *Am J Med* 58:229, 1975.

48. Rosenfield RE, Schmidt PJ, Calvo RC, McGinniss MH: Anti-i, a frequent cold agglutinin in infectious mononucleosis. *Vox Sang* 10:631, 1965.

49. Worlledge SM, Dacie JV: Haemolytic and other anaemias in infectious mononucleosis, in *Infectious Mononucleosis*, edited by RL Carter, HG Penman, p 82. Blackwell Scientific, Oxford, 1969.

50. Hossaini AA: Anti-i in infectious mononucleosis. *Am J Clin Pathol* 53:198, 1970.

51. Curtis BR, Lamon J, Roelcke D, Chaplin H: Life-threatening, antiglobu-lin test-negative, acute autoimmune hemolytic anemia due to a non-complement-activating IgG 1k cold antibody with Pr_a specificity. *Trans-fusion* 30:838, 1990.

52. Silberstein LE, Berkman EM, Schreiber AD: Cold hemagglutinin disease associated with IgG cold reactive antibody. *Ann Intern Med* 106:238, 1987.

53. Sokol RJ, Hewitt S, Stamps BK: Autoimmune hemolysis: Mixed warm and cold antibody type. *Acta Haematol* 69:266, 1983.

54. Feizi T, Kabat EA, Vicari G, et al: Immunochemical studies on blood groups: XLVII. The I antigen complex precursors in the A, B, H, Le^a and Le^b blood group system: Hemagglutination inhibition studies. *J Exp Med* 133:39, 1971.

55. Hakomori S: Blood group ABH and Ii antigens of human erythrocytes: Chemistry, polymorphism, and their developmental change. *Semin He-matol* 18:39, 1981.

56. Marcus DM: A review of the immunogenic and immunomodulatory properties of glycosphingolipids. *Mol Immunol* 21:1083, 1984.

57. Rosse WF, Lauf PK: Reaction of cold agglutinins with I antigen solubi-lized from human red cells. *Blood* 36:777, 1970.

58. Lauf PK, Rosse WF: The reactivity of red blood cell membrane glyco-phorin with "cold-reacting" antibodies. *Clin Immunol Immunopathol* 4:1, 1975.

59. Pruzanski W, Shumak KH: Biologic activity of cold-reacting autoanti-bodies. *N Engl J Med* 297:583, 1977.

60. Chapman J, Murphy MF, Waters AH: Chronic cold hemagglutinin dis-ease due to an anti-M-like autoantibody. *Vox Sang* 42:272, 1982.

61. von dem Borne AEG Kr, Mol JJ, Joustra-Maas N, et al: Autoimmune hemolytic anemia with monoclonal IgM (K) anti-P cold autohemolysins. *Br J Haematol* 50:345, 1982.

62. Terada K, Tanaka H, Mori R, Kataoka N, Uchikawa M: Hemolytic anemia associated with cold agglutinin during chickenpox and a review of the literature. *J Pediatr Hematol Oncol* 20:149, 1998.

63. Tamura T, Kanamori H, Yamazaki E, et al: Cold agglutinin disease following allogeneic bone marrow transplantation. *Bone Marrow Trans-plant* 13:321, 1994.

64. Capra JD, Dowling P, Cook S, Kunkel HG: An incomplete cold-reactive λ-G antibody with i specificity in infectious mononucleosis. *Vox Sang* 16:10, 1969.

65. Hippe E, Jensen KB, Olesen H, et al: Chlorambucil treatment of patients with cold agglutinin syndrome. *Blood* 35:68, 1970.

66. Evans RS, Baxter E, Gilliland BC: Chronic hemolytic anemia due to cold agglutinins: A 20-year history of benign gammopathy with response to chlorambucil. *Blood* 42:463, 1973.

67. O'Connor BM, Clifford JS, Lawrence WD, Logue GL: Alpha-interferon for severe cold agglutinin disease. *Ann Intern Med* 111:255, 1989.

68. Nydegger UE, Kazatchkine MD, Miescher PA: Immunopathologic and clinical features of hemolytic anemia due to cold agglutinins. *Semin Hematol* 28:66, 1991.

69. Bell CA, Zwicker H, Sacks HJ: Autoimmune hemolytic anemia. *Am J Clin Pathol* 60:903, 1973.

70. Lee EJ, Kueck B: Rituxan in the treatment of cold agglutinin disease [letter]. *Blood* 92:3490, 1998.

71. Taft EG, Propp RP, Sullivan SA: Plasma exchange for cold agglutinin hemolytic anemia. *Transfusion* 17:173, 1977.

72. Brooks BD, Steane EA, Sheehan RG, Frenkel EP: Therapeutic plasma exchange in the immune hemolytic anemias and immunologic thrombo-cytopenic purpura. *Prog Clin Biol Res* 106:317, 1982.

73. Silberstein LE, Berkman EM: Plasma exchange in antoimmune hemo-lytic anemia (AIHA). *J Clin Apheresis* 1:238, 1983.

74. Nordhagen R, Stensvold K, Winsnes A, et al: Paroxysmal cold hemoglo-

binuria. The most frequent autoimmune hemolytic anemia in children? *Acta Paediatr Scand* 73:258, 1984.

75. Wolach B, Heddle N, Barr RD, et al: Transient Donath-Landsteiner hemolytic anemia. *Br J Haematol* 48:425, 1981.

76. Sokol RJ, Hewitt S, Stamps BK: Autoimmune hemolysis associated with Donath-Landsteiner antibodies. *Acta Haematol* 68:268, 1982.

77. Gottsche B, Salama A, Mueller-Eckhardt C: Donath-Landsteiner autoim-mune hemolytic anemia in children: A study of 22 cases. *Vox Sang* 58:281, 1990.

78. Fellous M, Gerbal A, Tessier C, et al: Studies on the biosynthetic pathway of human P erythrocyte antigens using somatic cells in culture. *Vox Sang* 26:518, 1974.

79. Shirey RS, Park K, Ness PM, et al: An anti-i biphasic hemolysin in chronic paroxysmal cold hemoglobinuria. *Transfusion* 26:62, 1986.

DRUG-RELATED IMMUNE HEMOLYTIC ANEMIA

CHARLES H. PACKMAN

Drugs may cause immune injury of RBC by three mechanisms. These types of injury are classified by the effector mechanisms of hemolysis, since the induction mechanisms of antibody formation are poorly understood. (1) The hapten/drug adsorption mechanism involves covalent binding of drug to RBC membrane and attachment of antidrug antibody to the membrane-bound drug, which opsonizes the cells for destruction by splenic macrophages. (2) The ternary complex mechanism is characterized by formation of a trimolecular immune complex consisting of drug, RBC membrane antigen, and an antibody that recognizes the compound neoantigen formed by drug and membrane antigen. RBC destruction occurs intravascularly, by activation of the whole complement sequence. The antibodies involved in hapten/drug adsorption- and ternary complex-mediated hemolysis are said to be drug-dependent, since the drug must be present with RBC and antibody in vivo or in vitro for the antibody to cause RBC injury. (3) In sharp contrast, some drugs induce formation of true autoantibodies indistinguishable from the autoantibodies seen in autoimmune hemolytic anemia, perhaps by T-lymphocyte immuno-modulation. In these cases, presence of the drug is not necessary for RBC injury to occur.

Hemolysis with drug-related immune mechanisms is generally mild, but severe and sometimes fatal hemolysis may be seen in cases mediated by the ternary complex mechanism and in patients with chronic lymphocytic leukemia with autoantibodies induced by purine analogs. These latter cases often respond to prednisone therapy, whereas in most other cases, withdrawal of the offending drug is usually the only treatment required.

DEFINITIONS AND HISTORY

The first example of drug-related immune blood cell destruction was Ackroyd's description of Sedormid purpura in 1949.[1] In 1953, Snapper and coworkers described a case of immune hemolysis and pancytopenia in a patient treated with mephenytoin (Mesantoin).[2] The hemolysis ceased upon withdrawal of the drug. In 1956, Harris reported what are now classical studies of a patient who developed immune hemolytic anemia during a second course of stibophen for schistosomiasis.[3] Since then, many drugs have been implicated in the production of positive direct antiglobulin tests and accelerated red cell destruction. Table 57-1 lists important drugs or classes of drugs implicated in immune red cell injury.

Acronyms and abbreviations that appear in this chapter include: CLL, chronic lymphocytic leukemia; RBC, red blood cell.

ETIOLOGY AND PATHOGENESIS

Three general mechanisms of drug-mediated immunologic injury to red cells are recognized (Table 57-2 and Fig. 57-1). This classification is based on the effector mechanism of red cell injury, since the induction mechanism for formation of drug-related red cell antibodies is unknown. Two of these mechanisms, hapten/drug adsorption and ternary complex formation, involve drug-dependent antibodies, while in the third mechanism the drugs in question appear to induce formation of true autoantibodies capable of reacting with human red cells in the absence of the inciting drug. Distinguishing among these mechanisms is not always possible, and some cases involve a combination of mechanisms. In addition, drug-related nonimmunologic protein adsorption by red cells may result in a positive direct antiglobulin test without actual red cell injury. This phenomenon should be distinguished from the other three forms of drug-induced immune red cell injury.

HAPTEN OR DRUG ADSORPTION MECHANISM

This mechanism applies to drugs that can bind firmly to proteins, including red cell membrane proteins. The classic setting is very high dose penicillin therapy,[4-10] which is encountered less commonly today than in previous decades.

Most individuals who receive penicillin develop IgM antibodies directed against the benzylpenicilloyl determinant of penicillin, but this antibody plays no role in penicillin-related immune injury to red cells. The antibody responsible for hemolytic anemia is of the IgG class, occurs less frequently than the IgM antibody, and may be directed against the benzylpenicilloyl[7] or, more commonly, nonbenzylpenicilloyl determinants.[4-6,8] Other manifestations of penicillin sensitivity usually are not present.

Patients receiving high doses of penicillin develop substantial coating of their red cells with penicillin. This penicillin coating itself is not injurious. If the dose of penicillin is very high (10×10^6 to 30×10^6 units per day, or less in the setting of renal failure) and if the patient has an IgG antipenicillin antibody, the antibody binds to the red cell–bound penicillin molecules, and the direct antiglobulin test with anti-IgG becomes positive[5,7,8,23,78] (see Fig. 57-1a). Antibodies eluted from such patients' red cells, or present in their sera, react (in indirect antiglobulin tests) only against penicillin-coated red cells. This is a critical step in distinguishing these drug-dependent antibodies from true autoantibodies.

Significantly, not all patients receiving high-dose penicillin develop a positive direct antiglobulin reaction or hemolytic anemia, since only a small proportion of such individuals produce the requisite antibody. Destruction of red cells coated with penicillin and IgG antipenicillin antibody occurs mainly through sequestration by splenic macrophages.[6,79] In some patients with penicillin-induced immune hemolytic anemia, blood monocytes, and presumably splenic macrophages, may lyse the IgG-coated red cells without phagocytosis.[80] Hemolytic anemia due to penicillin typically occurs only after the patient has received the drug for 7 to 10 days and ceases a few days to 2 weeks after discontinuing the drug.

Low-molecular-weight substances, such as drugs, generally are not immunogenic in their own right. Induction of antidrug antibody is thought to require firm chemical coupling of the drug (as a hapten) to a protein carrier. In the case of penicillin, the carrier protein involved in antibody induction need not be the same as the erythrocyte membrane protein to which penicillin is coupled in the effector phase, i.e., when the IgG antipenicillin antibodies bind to penicillin-coated red cells. In contrast to growing evidence concerning the ternary complex mechanism (see below), there is no present evidence that the drug-dependent antibodies responsible for red cell injury in this hapten/

TABLE 57-1   ASSOCIATION BETWEEN DRUGS AND POSITIVE DIRECT ANTIGLOBULIN TESTS*

DRUGS	REFERENCES	DRUGS	REFERENCES
HAPTEN OR DRUG ADSORPTION MECHANISM			
Penicillins	4–10	Carbromal	18
Cephalosporins	11–15	Tolbutamide	19, 20
Tetracycline	16, 17	Cianidanol	21
TERNARY COMPLEX MECHANISM			
Stibophen	3	Probenecid	32
Quinine	22	Nomifensine	33–35
Quinidine	23, 24	Cephalosporins	13–15, 36
Chlorpropamide	25, 26	Diethylstilbestrol	37
Rifampicin	27, 28	Amphotericin B	38
Antazoline	29	Doxepin	39
Thiopental	30	Diclofenac	40
Tolmetin	31		
AUTOANTIBODY MECHANISM			
Cephalosporins	15	Cianidanol	21
Tolmetin	31	Latamoxef	52
Nomifensine	33	Glafenine	52
α-methyldopa	41–44	Procainamide	53
l-Dopa	45–49	Diclofenac	40, 54
Mefenamic acid	50, 51	Pentostatin	55
Teniposide	52	Fludarabine	56
		Chlorodeoxyadenosine	57
NONIMMUNOLOGIC PROTEIN ADSORPTION			
Cephalosporins	58, 59	Cisplatin	60
UNCERTAIN MECHANISM OF IMMUNE INJURY			
Mesantoin	2	Streptomycin	68
Phenacetin	22	Ibuprofen	69
Insecticides	61	Triamterene	70
Chlorpromazine	62	Erythromycin	71
Melphalan	63	5-Fluorouracil	72
Isoniazid	64	Nalidixic acid	73
p-Aminosalicylic acid	65	Sulindac	74
Acetaminophen	66	Omeprazol	75
Thiazides	67	Temafloxacin	76
		Carboplatin	77

* See text for explanation of mechanisms. It is not always possible to infer the mechanism of immune injury induced by a drug. Moreover, some drugs can act by more than one mechanism. In cases of uncertain mechanism, the cited drug use is coincident with the hemolytic anemia, and causality is inferred, not established experimentally. These cases are included so that the reader may be aware of these potential associations.

drug adsorption mechanism also recognize native erythrocyte membrane structures.

Cephalosporins have antigenic cross-reactivity with penicillin[81–83] and also bind firmly to red cell membranes, as do semisynthetic penicillins.[9,10] Hemolytic anemia similar to that seen with penicillin has been ascribed to cephalosporins[11–15] and some semisynthetic penicillins.[9,10] Tetracycline[16,17] and tolbutamide[19,20] also may cause hemolysis by this mechanism. Carbromal causes positive IgG antiglobulin reactions by a similar mechanism,[18] but hemolytic anemia has not been described.

TERNARY COMPLEX MECHANISM: DRUG-ANTIBODY–TARGET CELL COMPLEX

Many drugs can induce immune injury not only of red cells but also of platelets or granulocytes by a process that differs in several ways from the mechanism of hapten/drug adsorption. First, drugs in this group (see Table 57-1) exhibit only weak direct binding to blood cell membranes. Second, a relatively small dose of drug is capable of triggering destruction of blood cells. Third, cellular injury appears to be mediated chiefly by complement activation at the cell surface. The cytopathic process induced by such drugs previously has been termed the *immune complex mechanism*. This reflected the prevailing notion

that, in vivo, drug-antidrug complexes formed first and then became secondarily bound to target blood cells as "innocent bystanders," either nonspecifically or possibly via membrane receptors (e.g., Fcγ receptors on platelets or C3b receptors on red cells), with the potential for subsequent activation of complement by bound complexes.

The "immune complex" and "innocent bystander" terminology now seems less appropriate because of models developed from research on analogous drug-dependent platelet injury[84–86] (see Chap. 117), together with a series of relevant serologic observations on drug-mediated immune hemolytic anemia. These studies suggest that blood cell injury actually is mediated by a cooperative interaction among three reactants to generate a ternary complex (see Fig. 57-1b) involving (1) the drug (or drug metabolite in some cases), (2) a drug-binding membrane site on the target cell, and (3) antibody. For example, several patients were found to possess drug-dependent antibodies that exhibited specificity for red cells bearing defined alloantigens such as those of the Rh, Kell, or Kidd blood groups. That is, those antibodies were selectively nonreactive with human red cells lacking the alloantigen in question even in the presence of drug.[30,52,87–89] In each of these cases, high-affinity drug binding to cell membrane could not be demonstrated. The drug-dependent antibody may bind, through its Fab domain, to a compound neoantigen consisting of loosely bound drug and a blood group antigen intrinsic to the red cell membrane. Elegant studies on quinidine- or quinine-induced immune thrombocytopenia have demonstrated that the IgG antibodies implicated in this disorder bind through their Fab domains, not by their Fc domains to platelet Fcγ receptors.[90,91]

These data elucidate how one patient with quinidine sensitivity may have selective destruction of platelets and another may have selective destruction of red cells. This is because the pathogenic antibody recognizes the drug only in combination with a particular membrane structure of the red cell (e.g., a known alloantigen) or of the platelet [e.g., α domain of the glycoprotein Ib (GPIb) complex]. Therefore, at least in these cases, the target cell does not appear to be purely an innocent bystander. Binding of the drug itself to the target cell membrane is weak until stabilized by the attachment of the antibody to *both* drug and cell membrane. Yet the binding of the antibody is drug-dependent. Such a three-reactant interdependent "troika" is unique to this mechanism of immune cytopenia.

The foregoing discussion depicting drugs as creating a "self+ nonself" neoantigen on the target cell applies to the effector phase of the process. The same drug-binding membrane protein appears to be involved in some way in forming the immunogen that induces the antibody, as evidenced by those drug-dependent antibodies exhibiting selective reactivity with defined red cell alloantigens (carrier specificity).[30,52,87–89] How this is accomplished in the absence of evidence for strong, covalent binding of the drugs in this group to a host membrane protein remains to be elucidated.

Red cell destruction by this mechanism may occur intravascularly after completion of the whole complement sequence, resulting in he-

TABLE 57-2   MAJOR MECHANISMS OF DRUG-RELATED HEMOLYTIC ANEMIA

	HAPTEN/DRUG ADSORPTION	TERNARY COMPLEX FORMATION	AUTOANTIBODY BINDING	NONIMMUNOLOGIC PROTEIN ADSORPTION
Prototype drug	Penicillin	Quinidine	α-Methyldopa	Cephalothin
Role of drug	Binds to red cell membrane	Forms ternary complex with antibody and red cell membrane component	Induces formation of antibody to native red cell antigen	Possibly alters red cell membrane
Drug affinity to cell	Strong	Weak	None demonstrated to intact red cell but binding to membranes reported	Strong
Antibody to drug	Present	Present	Absent	Absent
Antibody class predominating	IgG	IgM or IgG	IgG	None
Proteins detected by direct antiglobulin test	IgG, rarely complement	Complement	IgG, rarely complement	Multiple plasma proteins
Dose of drug associated with positive antiglobulin test	High	Low	High	High
Presence of drug required for indirect antiglobulin test	Yes (coating test red cells)	Yes (added to test medium)	No	Yes (added to test medium)
Mechanism of red cell destruction	Splenic sequestration of IgG-coated red cells	Direct lysis by complement plus splenic-hepatic clearance of C3b-coated red cells	Splenic sequestration	None

moglobinemia and hemoglobinuria. Some destruction of intact C3b-coated red cells may be mediated by splenic and liver sequestration via the C3b/C3bi receptors on macrophages. The direct antiglobulin test is positive usually only with anticomplement reagents, but exceptions occur. Sometimes, however, the drug-dependent antibody itself can be detected on the red cell if the offending drug (or its metabolites) is included in all steps of the antiglobulin test, including red cell washing.[92]

AUTOANTIBODY MECHANISM

A variety of drugs have been reported to induce the formation of autoantibodies reactive with autologous (or homologous) red cells in the absence of the instigating drug (see Table 57-1). The most important drug in this category has been αmethyldopa.[41-44] Levodopa and several unrelated drugs also have been incriminated.[15,21,31,33,40,45-54] Patients with chronic lymphocytic leukemia (CLL) treated with pento-

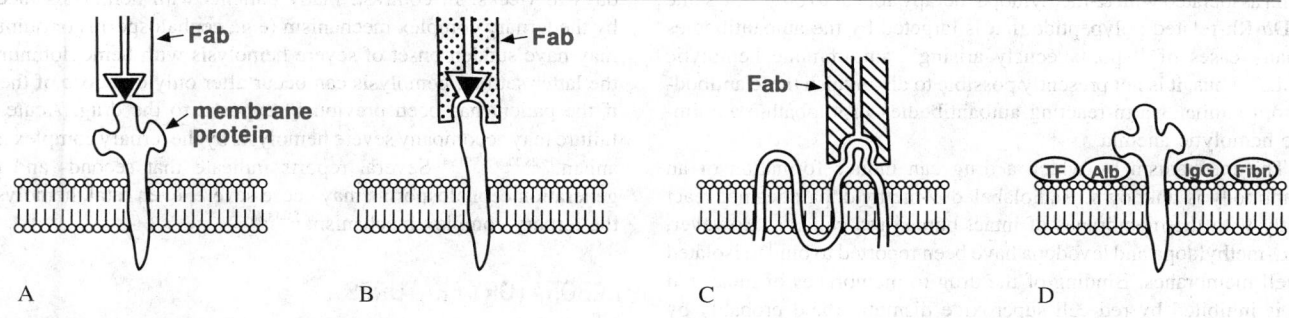

FIGURE 57-1   These figures show the effector mechanisms by which drugs mediate a positive direct antiglobulin test, demonstrating the relationships of drug, antibody-combining site, and red cell membrane protein. Only a single immunoglobulin Fab region (bearing one combining site) is shown in panels A, B, and C. (A) Drug adsorption/hapten mechanism. The drug (▼) binds avidly to an unknown red cell membrane protein in vivo. Antidrug antibody (usually IgG) binds to the protein-bound drug. So far as is known, the membrane protein is not part of the epitope recognized by the antidrug antibody. The direct antiglobulin test (with anti-IgG) detects IgG antidrug antibody on the patient's circulating (drug-coated) red cells. The indirect antiglobulin test detects antibody in the patent's serum only when the test red cells have been precoated with the drug by incubation in vitro. (B) Ternary complex mechanism. Drug binds loosely or in undetectable amounts to red cell membrane. However, in the presence of appropriate antidrug antibody, a stable trimolecular (ternary) complex is formed among drug, red cell membrane protein, and antibody. In general, the antibody-combining site (Fab) recognizes both drug and membrane protein components but binds only weakly to either drug or protein unless both are present in the reaction mixture. In this mechanism, the direct antiglobulin test typically detects only red cell–bound complement components (e.g., C3 fragments) that are bound covalently and in large number to the patient's red cells in vivo. The antibody itself escapes detection, possibly due to its low concentration but also because washing of the red cells (in the antiglobulin test procedure) apparently dissociates antibody and drug from the cells, leaving only the covalently bound C3 fragments. The indirect antiglobulin test also detects complement proteins on the test red cells when both antibody (patient serum) and a complement source (fresh patient serum or fresh normal serum) are present in the reaction mixture together with the drug. (C) Autoantibody induction. Some drug-induced antibodies can bind avidly to red cell membrane proteins (usually Rh proteins) in the absence of the inducing drug and are indistinguishable from the anti–red cell autoantibodies of patients with autoimmune hemolytic anemia (see Chap. 55). The direct antiglobulin test detects the IgG antibody on the patient's red cells. The indirect antiglobulin test usually detects antibody in the serum of patients with active hemolysis. (D) Drug-induced nonimmunologic protein adsorption. Certain drugs cause plasma proteins to attach to the red cell membrane nonspecifically. The direct antiglobulin test detects nonspecifically bound IgG and complement components. If special antiglobulin reagents are used, other plasma proteins, such as transferrin, albumin, and fibrinogen, may be detected as well. In contrast to the other mechanisms of drug-induced red cell injury, this mechanism does not shorten red cell survival in vivo.

statin,[55] fludarabine,[56] or chlorodeoxyadenosine[57] are particularly predisposed to autoimmune hemolysis which is usually severe and sometimes fatal.

Positive direct antiglobulin reactions (with anti-IgG reagents) in patients taking α-methyldopa vary in frequency from 8 to 36 percent. Patients taking higher doses of the drug develop positive reactions with greater frequency.[41,43,44] There is a lag period of 3 to 6 months between the start of therapy and development of a positive antiglobulin test. The delay is not shortened when the drug is administered to patients who previously had positive antiglobulin tests while taking α-methyldopa.[43]

In contrast to the frequent observation of positive antiglobulin reactions, less than 1 percent of patients taking α-methyldopa exhibit hemolytic anemia.[42] Development of hemolytic anemia does not depend on drug dosage. The hemolysis is usually mild to moderate and occurs chiefly by splenic sequestration of IgG-coated red cells. It has been proposed that αmethyldopa suppresses splenic macrophage function in some patients, and that normal survival of antibody-coated red cells in such patients may be related, in part, to this effect of the drug.[93]

The direct antiglobulin reaction is usually positive only for IgG.[94,95] Occasionally, weak anticomplement reactions are encountered as well.[95] Patients with immune hemolytic anemia due to α-methyldopa therapy typically have strongly positive direct antiglobulin reactions as well as serum antibody, evidenced by the indirect antiglobulin reaction.[95] (See Chap. 137 for explanation of direct and indirect antiglobulin tests.) Antibodies in the serum or eluted from red cell membranes react optimally at 37°C (98.6°F) with unaltered autologous or homologous red cells in the absence of drug[42,44,96] (see Fig. 57-1c). The antibodies frequently are reactive with determinants of the Rh complex.[42,44,96] The autoantibodies of some patients with hemolytic anemia associated with α-methyldopa therapy appear to target the same 34-kDa Rh-related polypeptide that is targeted by the autoantibodies in many cases of "spontaneously arising" autoimmune hemolytic anemia.[97] Thus, it is not presently possible to distinguish these antibodies from similar warm-reacting autoantibodies in idiopathic autoimmune hemolytic anemia.

The mechanism by which a drug can induce formation of an autoantibody is unknown. Radiolabeled α-methyldopa does not react directly with the membranes of intact human red cells.[44,98] However, both α-methyldopa and levodopa have been reported to bind to isolated red cell membranes. Binding of the drug to membranes of intact red cells is inhibited by red cell superoxide dismutase and probably by hemoglobin.[98,99] Although not formally demonstrated, these drugs probably bind to membrane antigens of cells that are relatively hemoglobin-free, for example, cells at the early proerythroblast stage or red cell stroma. In any case, the resulting altered membrane antigens then may induce autoantibodies. The concept that a drug-membrane compound neoantigen could lead to production of an autoantibody is supported by studies of patients receiving drugs unrelated to α-methyldopa. These patients simultaneously developed a drug-dependent antibody and an autoantibody, both of which showed specificity for the same red cell alloantigen.[52] It also has been hypothesized that α-methyldopa may interact with human T-lymphocytes, resulting in loss of suppressor cell function.[100] However, subsequent studies have failed to demonstrate any evidence for such a mechanism.[101]

Uncommonly, patients with CLL treated with the purine analogs fludarabine or chlorodeoxyadenosine develop autoimmune hemolysis.[56,57] Risk factors for autoimmune hemolysis include prior therapy with a purine analog, a positive direct antiglobulin test prior to therapy, and hypogammaglobulinemia. Purine analogs are potent suppressors of T-lymphocytes. These drugs may accelerate the pre-existing T-cell immune suppression that normally occurs during progression of CLL,

exacerbating the underlying tendency to autoimmunity in CLL. However the degree of depletion of T-cell subsets is similar in those patients who develop hemolysis and in those who do not.

NONIMMUNOLOGIC PROTEIN ADSORPTION

Fewer than 5 percent of patients receiving cephalosporin antibiotics develop positive antiglobulin reactions[95] due to nonspecific adsorption of plasma proteins to their red cell membranes.[58,59,102] This may occur within a day or two after the drug is instituted. Multiple plasma proteins, including immunoglobulins, complement, albumin, fibrinogen, and others, may be detected on red cell membranes in such cases.[102,103] Hemolytic anemia due to this mechanism has not been reported. The clinical importance of this phenomenon is its potential to complicate cross-match procedures unless the drug history is taken into account. As noted above, cephalosporin antibiotics also may induce red cell injury by the hapten mechanism or by the ternary complex mechanism. These latter reactions are more serious but apparently occur less frequently than the nonimmunologic reaction.

CLINICAL FEATURES

A careful history of drug exposure should be obtained in all patients with hemolytic anemia and/or a positive direct antiglobulin test. As in idiopathic autoimmune hemolytic anemia (see Chaps. 55 and 56), the clinical picture in drug-related immune hemolytic anemia is quite variable. The severity of symptoms is largely dependent upon the rate of hemolysis. In general, patients with hapten/drug adsorption (e.g., penicillin) and autoimmune (e.g., α-methyldopa) types of drug-induced hemolytic anemia exhibit mild to moderate red cell destruction, with insidious onset of symptoms developing over a period of days to weeks. In contrast, many patients with hemolysis mediated by the ternary complex mechanism (e.g., cephalosporins or quinidine) may have sudden onset of severe hemolysis with hemoglobinuria. In the latter setting, hemolysis can occur after only one dose of the drug if the patient has been previously exposed to the drug. Acute renal failure may accompany severe hemolysis by the ternary complex mechanism.[15,28,30,34,35,54,94] Several reports indicate that second- and third-generation cephalosporins may cause severe, even fatal, hemolysis by the ternary complex mechanism.[13–15,36]

LABORATORY FEATURES

The hematologic findings are similar to those described for spontaneously occurring autoimmune hemolytic anemia (see Chaps. 55 and 56). Most patients exhibit anemia and reticulocytosis. Leukopenia and thrombocytopenia may be noted in cases of ternary complex–mediated hemolysis. The appearance of hemoglobinemia or hemoglobinuria suggests the ternary complex mechanism. The serologic features are summarized in Table 57-2.

DIFFERENTIAL DIAGNOSIS

Immune hemolysis due to drugs should be distinguished from (1) the warm- or cold-antibody types of idiopathic autoimmune hemolytic anemia, (2) congenital hemolytic anemias such as hereditary spherocytosis, and (3) drug-mediated hemolysis due to disorders of red cell metabolism, such as glucose-6-phosphate dehydrogenase deficiency. Patients with drug-related immune hemolytic anemia have a positive direct antiglobulin test. This feature generally makes it easy to distinguish this group from those with inherited red cell defects.

In the hapten/drug adsorption mechanism of immune injury associated with cephalosporins or penicillin, the patient's drug-coated red cells bind drug-specific IgG antibody and exhibit positive direct anti-globulin reactions with anti-IgG. Rarely, both anti-IgG and anti-C3d antisera produce positive antiglobulin reactions. Such cases could have superficial resemblance to warm-antibody autoimmune hemolytic anemia. The key serologic difference is that in this form of drug-induced immune hemolytic anemia the antibodies in the patient's serum or eluted from the patient's red cells react *only* with drug-coated red cells. In contrast, the IgG antibodies in warm-type autoimmune hemolytic anemia react with unmodified human red cells and may show preference for certain known blood groups (e.g., within the Rh complex). Such serologic distinction plus the history of exposure to high blood levels of penicillin or a cephalosporin should be decisive.

In hemolysis mediated by the ternary complex mechanism, the direct antiglobulin test is positive with anticomplement serum. Immunoglobulins are only rarely detectable on the patient's red cells. This pattern is similar to that encountered in autoimmune hemolytic anemia mediated by cold agglutinins. Moreover, the brisk type of hemolysis in the ternary complex mechanism also is seen in certain cases of cold-antibody autoimmune hemolytic anemia (see Chap. 56). In the drug-induced cases, however, the cold agglutinin titer and the Donath-Landsteiner test are normal, and the demonstration of serum antibody acting on human red cells is dependent upon the presence of the drug in the test system. For example, the indirect antiglobulin reaction with anticomplement serum may be positive if the incubation mixture permits the interaction of (1) normal red cells; (2) antidrug antibody from the patient's serum; (3) the relevant drug, either still in the patient's serum or added in vitro in appropriate concentration; and (4) a source of complement, that is, fresh normal serum or the patient's own serum if freshly obtained. A negative result does not necessarily absolve the suspected drug because the critical determinant may be a metabolite of the drug in question. In some cases, the use of urine or serum (of the patient or a volunteer taking the drug) as a source of drug metabolite has permitted successful demonstration of a drug-dependent mechanism.[33,88,92,104]

In patients with autoimmune hemolytic anemia due to α-methyldopa, the direct antiglobulin reaction is strongly positive for IgG, but only rarely is complement detected on the patient's red cells. Anti–red cell autoantibody is regularly present in the serum of those patients and mediates a positive indirect antiglobulin reaction with unmodified human red cells, often showing specificity related to the Rh complex. There is, however, no presently available specific serologic test to separate idiopathic warm-reacting IgG autoantibodies with Rh-related specificities from those induced by α-methyldopa administration. The evidence must be circumstantial, with the helpful knowledge that discontinuation of αmethyldopa, without any form of immunosuppressive therapy, has consistently permitted a slow recovery from anemia and a gradual disappearance of anti–red cell antibodies.

In recently transfused patients, a positive "direct" antiglobulin test may reflect the binding of newly formed alloantibodies to transfused donor red cells. Neither the drugs the patient is receiving nor autoantibodies may be involved.

Drugs not now known to cause immune red cell injury will be implicated in the future. In any patient with a clinical picture compatible with drug-related immune hemolysis it is reasonable to stop any drug that is suspect while serologic studies are being obtained. The patient should be monitored for improvement in hematocrit level, decrease in reticulocytosis, and gradual disappearance of the positive antiglobulin reaction. Repeat challenge with the suspected drug may confirm the diagnosis, but this measure is seldom necessary in patient management and may be unsafe. Therefore, rechallenge to exclude the possibility that a suspected drug-caused hemolytic anemia in a patient should be undertaken only for compelling reasons, such as the need to use that drug in particular for the patient's illness.

THERAPY, COURSE, AND PROGNOSIS

THERAPY

Discontinuation of the offending drug is often the only treatment needed. This measure is essential and may be life-saving in patients with severe hemolysis mediated by the ternary complex mechanism.

If high-dose penicillin is the treatment of choice in a life-threatening infection and alternative antibiotic regimens are clearly inferior to penicillin, the drug need not be discontinued because of a positive direct antiglobulin reaction alone. A change in therapy is indicated only in the presence of overt hemolytic anemia. Lowering the penicillin dose, for example, by coadministering other antibiotics, may allow continuation of drug in some cases, particularly if hemolysis is not severe.

In patients taking α-methyldopa in the absence of hemolysis, a positive direct antiglobulin test is not necessarily an indication for stopping the drug, although it may be prudent to consider alternative antihypertensive therapy.

Glucocorticoids are generally unnecessary, and their efficacy is questionable. However prednisone is effective in patients with CLL and autoimmune hemolysis caused by purine analogs.[56,57] Transfusions should be given in the unusual circumstance of severe, life-threatening anemia. Problems with cross-matching, similar to those encountered in warm-antibody autoimmune hemolytic anemia, may occur in patients with a strongly positive indirect antiglobulin test, for example, in α-methyldopa-related cases. Patients with hemolytic anemia due to the hapten/drug adsorption mechanism should have a compatible cross-match, because the serum antibody reacts only with the drug-coated cells. However, if therapy with the offending drug is still in progress, transfused cells may be destroyed at an increased rate as they become coated with drug in vivo.

Several cases of transfusion-associated graft-versus-host disease have been reported in CLL patients transfused for hemolysis due to purine analogs.[57,105,106] Such patients should receive irradiated blood products.

COURSE AND PROGNOSIS

Immune hemolysis due to drugs is usually mild, and the prognosis good. Occasional episodes of exceptionally severe hemolysis with renal failure or death have been reported, usually due to drugs operating through the ternary complex mechanism or due to purine analogs in patients with CLL.[15,28,30,34–37,39,54,73,74,94] In hemolysis due to ternary complex or hapten/drug adsorption mechanisms, the direct antiglobulin test becomes negative within a short time after the drug is discontinued, that is, soon after the drug is cleared from the circulation. In addition, the hemolysis associated with α-methyldopa-induced autoantibodies ceases promptly after cessation of the drug. However, a positive direct antiglobulin test of gradually diminishing intensity may remain for weeks or months.

REFERENCES

1. Ackroyd JF: The pathogenesis of thrombocytopenic purpura due to hypersensitivity to Sedormid (allylisopropyl-acetylcarbamide). *Clin Sci* 7:249, 1949.
2. Snapper I, Marks D, Schwartz L, Hollander L: Hemolytic anemia secondary to Mesantoin. *Ann Intern Med* 39:619, 1953.
3. Harris JW: Studies on the mechanism of drug-induced hemolytic anemia. *J Lab Clin Med* 47:760, 1956.
4. VanArsdel PP Jr, Gilliland BC: Anemia secondary to penicillin treatment: Studies on two patients with non-allergic serum hemagglutinins. *J Lab Clin Med* 65:277, 1965.

5. Petz LD, Fudenberg HH: Coombs-positive hemolytic anemia caused by penicillin administration. *N Engl J Med* 274:171, 1966.

6. Swanson MA, Chanmougan D, Schwartz RS: Immuno-hemolytic anemia due to antipenicillin antibodies. *N Engl J Med* 274:178, 1966.

7. Levine B, Redmond A: Immunochemical mechanisms of penicillin-induced Coombs positivity and hemolytic anemia in man. *Int Arch Allergy Appl Immunol* 1:594, 1967.

8. White JM, Brown DL, Hepner GW, Worlledge SM: Penicillin-induced hemolytic anaemia. *Br Med J* 3:26, 1968.

9. Seldon MR, Bain B, Johnson CA, Lennox CS: Ticarcillin-induced immune haemolytic anaemia. *Scand J Haematol* 28:459, 1982.

10. Tuffs L, Manoharan A: Flucloxacillin-induced haemolytic anaemia. *Med J Aust* 144:559, 1986.

11. Gralnick HR, McGinnis MH, Elton W, McCurdy P: Hemolytic anemia associated with cephalothin. *JAMA* 217:1193, 1971.

12. Branch DR, Berkowitz LR, Becker RL, et al: Extravascular hemolysis following the administration of cefamandole. *Am J Hematol* 18:213, 1985.

13. Chambers LA, Donovan BA, Kruskall MS: Ceftazidime-induced hemolysis patient with drug-dependent antibodies reactive by immune complex and drug adsorption mechanisms. *Am J Clin Pathol* 95:393, 1991.

14. Gallagher NI, Schergen AK, Sokol-Anderson ML, et al: Severe immune-mediated hemolytic anemia secondary to treatment with cefotetan. *Transfusion* 32:266, 1992.

15. Garratty G, Nance S, Lloyd M, Domen R: Fatal immune hemolytic anemia due to cefotetan. *Transfusion* 32:269, 1992.

16. Wenz B, Klein RL, Lalezari P: Tetracycline-induced immune hemolytic anemia. *Transfusion* 14:265, 1974.

17. Simpson MB, Pryzbylik J, Innis B, Denham MA: Hemolytic anemia after tetracycline therapy. *N Engl J Med* 312:840, 1985.

18. Steanini M, Johnson NL: Positive antihuman globulin test in patients receiving carbromal. *Am J Med Sci* 259:49, 1970.

19. Bird GWG, Ecles GH, Litchfield JA, et al: Haemolytic anaemia associated with antibodies to tolbutamide and phenacetin. *Br Med J* 1:728, 1972.

20. Malacarne P, Castaldi G, Bertusi M, Zavagli G: Tolbutamide-induced hemolytic anemia. *Diabetes* 26:156, 1977.

21. Salama A, Mueller-Eckhardt C: Cianidanol and its metabolites bind tightly to red cells and are responsible for the production of auto- and/or drug-dependent antibodies against these cells. *Br J Haematol* 66:263, 1987.

22. Muirhead EE, Halden ER, Granes M: Drug-dependent Coombs (antiglobulin) test and anemia: observations on quinine and acetophenetidine (phenacetin). *Arch Intern Med* 101:827, 1958.

23. Croft JD Jr, Swisher SN, Gilliland BC, et al: Coombs test positivity induced by drugs: mechanisms of immunologic reactions and red cell destruction. *Ann Intern Med* 68:176, 1968.

24. Freedman AL, Barr PS, Brody E: Hemolytic anemia due to quinidine: observations on its mechanism. *Am J Med* 20:806, 1956.

25. Logue GL, Boyd AE, Rosse WF: Chlorpropamide-induced immune hemolytic anemia. *N Engl J Med* 283:900, 1970.

26. Kopicky JA, Packman CH: The mechanisms of sulfonylurea-induced immune hemolysis. Case report and review of the literature. *Am J Hematol* 23:283, 1986.

27. Lakshminarayan S, Sahn SA, Hudson LD: Massive hemolysis caused by rifampicin. *Br Med J* 2:282, 1973.

28. Pereira A, Sanz C, Cervantes F, Castillo R: Immune hemolytic anemia and renal failure associated with rifampicin-dependent antibodies with anti-I specificity. *Ann Hematol* 63:56, 1991.

29. Bengtsson U, Staffan A, Aurell M, Kaijser B: Antazoline-induced immune hemolytic anemia, hemoglobinuria and acute renal failure. *Acta Med Scand* 198:223, 1975.

30. Habibi B, Basty R, Chodez S, Prunat A: Thiopental-related immune hemolytic anemia and renal failure. *N Engl J Med* 312:353, 1985.

31. Squires JE, Mintz PD, Clark S: Tolmetin-induced hemolysis. *Transfusion* 25:410, 1985.

32. Sosler SD, Behzad V, Garratty G, et al: Immune hemolytic anemia associated with probenecid. *Am J Clin Pathol* 84:391, 1985.

33. Salama A, Mueller-Eckhardt C: Two types of nomifensine-induced immune haemolytic anaemias: drug-dependent sensitization and/or autoimmunization. *Br J Haematol* 64:613, 1986.

34. Habibi B, Cartron JP, Bretagne M, et al: Anti-nomifensine antibody causing immune hemolytic anemia and renal failure. *Vox Sang* 40:79, 1981.

35. Fulton JD, Briggs JD, Dominiczak AF, et al: Intravascular haemolysis and acute renal failure induced by nomifensine. *Scott Med J* 31:242, 1986.

36. Garratty G, Postoway N, Schwellenbach J, McMahill PC: A fatal case of ceftriaxone (Rocephin)-induced hemolytic anemia associated with intravascular immune hemolysis. *Transfusion* 31:176, 1991.

37. Rosenfeld CS, Winters SJ, Tedrow HE: Diethylstilbestrol-associated hemolytic anemia with a positive direct antiglobulin test result. *Am J Med* 86:617, 1989.

38. Salama A, Burger M, Mueller-Eckhardt C: Acute immune hemolysis induced by a degradation product of amphotericin B. *Blut* 58:59, 1989.

39. Wolf B, Conradty M, Grohmann R, et al: A case of immune complex hemolytic anemia, thrombocytopenia, and acute renal failure associated with doxepin use. *J Clin Psychiatry* 50:99, 1989.

40. Salama A, Kroll H, Wittmann G, Mueller-Eckhardt C: Diclofenac-induced immune haemolytic anaemia: simultaneous occurrence of red blood cell autoantibodies and drug-dependent antibodies. *Br J Haematol* 95:640, 1996.

41. Carstairs KC, Breckenridge A, Dollery CT, Worlledge SM: Incidence of a positive direct Coombs test in patients on alpha-methyldopa. *Lancet* 2:133, 1966.

42. Worlledge SM, Carstairs KC, Dacie JV: Autoimmune haemolytic anaemia associated with æmethyldopa therapy. *Lancet* 2:135, 1966.

43. Breckenridge A, Dollery CT, Worlledge SM, et al: Positive direct Coombs tests and antinuclear factors in patients treated with methyldopa. *Lancet* 2:1265, 1967.

44. Lo Buglio AF, Jandl JH: The nature of alpha-methyldopa red cell antibody. *N Engl J Med* 276:658, 1967.

45. Cotzias GC, Papavasiliou PS: Autoimmunity in patients treated with levodopa. *JAMA* 207:1353, 1969.

46. Henry RE, Goldberg LS, Sturgeon P, Ansel RD: Serologic abnormalities associated with *l-dopa therapy*. *Vox Sang* 20:306, 1971.

47. Joseph C: Occurrence of positive Coombs test in patients treated with levodopa. *N Engl J Med* 286:1400, 1972.

48. Gabor EP, Goldberg LS: Levodopa-induced Coombs positive haemolytic anaemia. *Scand J Haematol* 11:201, 1973.

49. Territo MC, Peters RW, Tanaka KR: Autoimmune hemolytic anemia due to levodopa therapy. *JAMA* 226:1347, 1973.

50. Scott GL, Myles AB, Bacon PA: Autoimmune haemolytic anaemia and mefenamic acid therapy. *Br Med J* 3:543, 1968.

51. Robertson JH, Kennedy CC, Hill CM: Haemolytic anaemia associated with mefenamic acid. *Irish J Med Sci* 140:226, 1971.

52. Habibi B: Drug-induced red blood cell autoantibodies co-developed with drug-specific antibodies causing a hemolytic anaemia. *Br J Haematol* 61:139, 1985.

53. Kleinman S, Nelson R, Smith L, Goldfinger D: Positive direct antiglobulin tests and immune hemolytic anemia in patients receiving procainamide. *N Engl J Med* 311:809, 1984.

54. Kramer MR, Levene C, Hershko C: Severe reversible autoimmune haemolytic anaemia and thrombocytopenia associated with diclofenac therapy. *Scand J Haematol* 36:118, 1986.

55. Byrd JC, Hertler AA, Weiss RB, et al: Fatal recurrence of autoimmune hemolytic anemia following pentostatin therapy in a patient with a history of fludarabine-associated hemolytic anemia. *Ann Oncol* 6:300, 1995.

56. Gonzalez H, Leblond V, Azar N, et al: Severe autoimmune hemolytic anemia in eight patients treated with fludarabine. *Hematol Cell Ther* 40:113, 1998.

57. Chasty RC, Myint H, Oscier DG, et al: Autoimmune haemolysis in patients with B-CLL treated with chlorodeoxyadenosine (CDA). *Leuk Lymphoma* 29:391, 1998.

58. Gralnick HR, Wright LD, McGinnis MH: Coombs' positive reactions associated with sodium cephalothin therapy. *JAMA* 199:725, 1967.

59. Molthan L, Reidenberg MM, Eichman MF: Positive direct Coombs' tests due to cephalothin. *N Engl J Med* 277:123, 1967.

60. Zeger G, Smith L, McQuiston D, Goldfinger D: Cisplatin-induced non-immunologic adsorption of immunoglobulin by red cells. *Transfusion* 28:493, 1988.

61. Muirhead EE, Groves M, Guy R, et al: Acquired hemolytic anemia, exposures to insecticides and positive Coombs' test dependent on insecticide preparations. *Vox Sang* 4:277, 1959.

62. Lindberg LG, Norden A: Severe hemolytic reaction to chlorpromazine. *Acta Med Scand* 170:195, 1961.

63. Eyster ME: Melphalan (Alkeran) erythrocyte agglutinin and hemolytic anemia. *Ann Intern Med* 66:573, 1967.

64. Robinson MG, Foadi M: Hemolytic anemia with positive Coomb's test. Association with isoniazid therapy. *JAMA* 208:656, 1969.

65. Mueller-Eckhardt C, Kretschmer V, Coburg KH: Allergic, immunohemolytic anemia due to para-aminosalicylic acid (PAS). Immunohematologic studies of three cases. *Dtsch Med Wochenschr* 97:234, 1972.

66. Manor E, Marmor A, Kaufman S, Leiba H: Massive hemolysis caused by acetaminophen. *JAMA* 236:2777, 1976.

67. Vilal JM, Blum L, Dosik H: Thiazide-induced immune hemolytic anemia. *JAMA* 236:1723, 1976.

68. Letona JM-L, Barbolla L, Frieyro E, et al: Immune haemolytic anaemia and renal failure induced by streptomycin. *Br J Haematol* 35:561, 1977.

69. Korsager S, Sorensen H, Jensen OH, Falk JV: Antiglobulin tests for determination of autoimmunohaemolytic anaemia during long-term treatment with ibuprofen. *Scand J Rheumatology* 10:174, 1981.

70. Takahashi H, Tsukada T: Triamterine-induced immune hemolytic anemia with acute intravascular hemolysis and acute renal failure. *Scand J Haematol* 23:169, 1979.

71. Wong KY, Boose GM, Issitt CH: Erythromycin-induced hemolytic anemia. *J Pediatr* 98:647, 1981.

72. Sandvei P, Nordhagen R, Michaelsen TE, Wolthuis K: Fluorouracil (5-FU) induced acute immune haemolytic anaemia. *Br J Haematol* 65:357, 1987.

73. Tafani O, Mazzoli M, Landini G, Alterini B: Fatal acute immune haemolytic anaemia caused by nalidixic acid. *Br Med J* 285:936, 1982.

74. Angeles ML, Reid ME, Yacob UA, Cash KL, Fetten JV: Sulindac-induced immune hemolytic anemia. *Transfusion* 34:255, 1994.

75. Marks DR, Joy JV, Bonheim NA: Hemolytic anemia associated with the use of omeprozole. *Am J Gastroenterol* 86:217, 1991.

76. Blum MD, Graham DJ, McCloskey CA: Temafloxacin syndrome: review of 95 cases. *Clin Infect Dis* 18:946, 1994.

77. Marani TM, Trich MB, Armstrong KS, et al: Carboplatin-induced immune hemolytic anemia. *Transfusion* 36:1016, 1996.

78. Kerr RO, Cardamone J, Dalmasso AP, Kaplan ME: Two mechanisms of erythrocyte destruction in penicillin-induced hemolytic anemia. *N Engl J Med* 287:1322, 1972.

79. Nesmith LW, Davis JW: Hemolytic anemia caused by penicillin. *JAMA* 203:27, 1968.

80. Yust I, Frisch B, Goldsher N: Simultaneous detection of two mechanisms of immune destruction of penicillin-treated human red blood cells. *Am J Hematol* 13:53, 1982.

81. Brandriss MW, Smith JW, Steinman HG: Common antigenic determinants of penicillin G, cephalothin and 6-aminopenicillanic acid in rabbits. *J Immunol* 94:696, 1965.

82. Abraham GN, Petz LD, Fudenberg HH: Immuno-hematological cross-allergenicity between penicillin and cephalothin in humans. *Clin Exp Immunol* 3:343, 1968.

83. Petz LD: Immunologic cross reactivity between penicillins and cephalosporins: a review. *J Infect Dis* 137:S74, 1978.

84. Kunicki TJ, Russell N, Nurten AT, et al: Further studies of the human platelet receptor for quinine- and quinidine-dependent antibodies. *J Immunol* 126:398, 1981.

85. Christie DJ, Aster RH: Drug-antibody-platelet interaction in quinine- and quinidine-induced thrombocytopenia. *J Clin Invest* 70:989, 1982.

86. Berndt MC, Chong BH, Bull HA, et al: Molecular characterization of quinine/quinidine drug-dependent antibody platelet interaction using monoclonal antisera. *Blood* 66:1292, 1985.

87. Sosler SD, Behzad O, Garratty G, et al: Acute hemolytic anemia associated with a chlorpropamide-induced apparent auto-anti-Jk$_a$. *Transfusion* 24:206, 1984.

88. Salama A, Mueller-Eckhardt C: Rh blood group-specific antibodies in immune hemolytic anemia induced by nomifensine. *Blood* 68:1285, 1986.

89. Salama A, Mueller-Eckhardt C: On the mechanisms of sensitization and attachment of antibodies to RBC in drug-induced immune hemolytic anemia. *Blood* 69:1006, 1987.

90. Christie DJ, Mullen PC, Aster RH: Fab-mediated binding of drug-dependent antibodies to platelets in quinidine- and quinine-induced thrombocytopenia. *J Clin Invest* 75:310, 1985.

91. Smith ME, Reid DM, Jones CE, et al: Binding of quinine- and quinidine-dependent drug antibodies to platelets is mediated by the Fab domain of immunoglobulin G and is not Fc dependent. *J Clin Invest* 29:912, 1987.

92. Salama A, Mueller-Eckhardt C: The role of metabolite-specific antibodies in nomifensine-dependent immune hemolytic anemia. *N Engl J Med* 313:469, 1985.

93. Kelton JG: Impaired reticuloendothelial function in patients treated with methyldopa. *N Engl J Med* 313:596, 1985.

94. Worlledge SM: Immune drug-induced hemolytic anemias. *Semin Haematol* 10:327, 1973.

95. Petz LD, Garratty G (eds): *Acquired Immune Hemolytic Anemia.* Churchill Livingstone, New York, 1980.

96. Bakemeier RF, Leddy JP: Erythrocyte autoantibody associated with alpha-methyldopa: heterogeneity of structure and specificilty. *Blood* 32:1, 1968.

97. Leddy JP, Falany JL, Kissel GE, et al: Erythrocyte membrane proteins reactive with human (warm-reacting) anti-red cell autoantibodies. *J Clin Invest* 91:1672, 1993.

98. Green FA, Jung CY, Rampal A, Lorusso DJ: Alpha-methyldopa and the erythrocyte membrane. *Clin Exp Immunol* 40:554, 1980.

99. Green Fa, Jung CY, Hui H: Modulation of alpha-methyldopa binding to the erythrocyte membrane by superoxide dismutase. *Biochem Biophys Res Commun* 95:1037, 1980.

100. Kirtland HH III, Mohler DN, Horwitz DA: Methyldopa inhibition of suppressor-lymphocyte function. A proposed cause of autoimmune hemolytic anemia. *N Engl J Med* 302:825, 1980.

101. Garratty G, Arndt P, Prince HE, Schulman IA: The effect of methyldopa and procainamide on suppressor cell activity in relation to red cell autoantibody production. *Br J Haematol* 84:310, 1993.

102. Spath P, Garratty G, Petz LD: Studies on the immune response to penicillin and cephalothin in humans. II. Immunohematologic reactions to cephalothin administration. *J Immunol* 107:860, 1971.

103. Garratty G, Petz L: Drug-induced hemolytic anemia. *Am J Med* 58:398, 1975.

104. Salama A, Santoso S, Mueller-Eckhardt C: Antigenic determinants responsible for the reactions of drug-dependent antibodies with blood cells. *Br J Haematol* 78:535, 1991.

105. Zulian GB, Roux E, Tiercy J-M, et al: Transfusion-associated graft-versus-host disease in a patient treated with cladribine (2-chlorodeoxyadenosine): demonstration of exogenous DNA in various tissue extracts by PCR analysis. *Br J Haematol* 89:83, 1995.

106. Briz M, Cabrera R, Sanjuan I: Diagnosis of transfusion-associated graft-versus-host disease by polymerase chain reaction fludarabine-treated B-chronic lymphocytic leukaemia. *Br J Haematol* 91:409, 1995.

ALLOIMMUNE HEMOLYTIC DISEASE OF THE NEWBORN

JAYASHREE RAMASETHU

NAOMI L.C. LUBAN

Hemolytic disease of the newborn occurs as a result of sensitization of the mother's immune system to red cell antigens of the fetus. This sensitization results in the transplacental passage of maternal IgG antibodies that bind to the fetal red cells, causing hemolysis, and as a consequence of the hemolytic process, anemia, extramedullary hematopoiesis, and neonatal hyperbilirubinemia, sometimes with devastating morbidity for the fetus and newborn infant. This chapter discusses the pathophysiology, the recent developments in diagnostic methods, and the preventive and therapeutic strategies that have contributed to a dramatic decrease in the incidence and severity of hemolytic disease of the newborn.

DEFINITION AND HISTORY

Alloimmune hemolytic disease of the newborn is a disorder in which the life span of fetal and/or neonatal red cells is shortened due to the binding of transplacentally transferred maternal IgG antibodies on fetal red cell antigens foreign to the mother, inherited by the fetus from the father.

Although the condition was described in newborn infants as early as the 1600s, it was not until 1932 that Diamond, Blackfan, and Baty recognized that the clinical syndromes of stillbirth with unusual erythroblastic activity in the extramedullary sites and blood, fetal hydrops, anemia in the newborn, and "icterus gravis neonatorum" were closely related and were probably due to the same underlying disturbance of the hematopoietic system.[1] The discovery of the Rh factor by Landsteiner and Weiner[2] in 1940 led to further elucidation of the condition by Levine,[3] who established that erythroblastosis fetalis was caused by the red blood cells from immunization of an Rh-negative mother by an Rh-positive fetus. Antibodies produced by the sensitized mother crossed the placenta and coated the fetal Rh-positive cells, leading to hemolysis and thus to anemia, hydrops, and severe neonatal jaundice secondary to hemolysis. Over the next decade, neonatal mortality from Rh hemolytic disease of the newborn was reduced considerably by exchange transfusion techniques for correction of severe anemia and prevention of the extreme hyperbilirubinemia.[4] However, severely affected infants continued to die in utero before 34 weeks' gestation. In 1961, Liley demonstrated the prognostic value of amniotic fluid spectrophotometry to identify these infants and then showed that intrauterine transfusions could prevent fetal deaths.[5] The most dramatic reduction in the incidence of Rh hemolytic disease of the newborn was achieved in the sixties and seventies with the development of postpartum and antepartum anti-D prophylaxis to prevent Rh sensitization.[6] Progress in the diagnosis and management of both the fetus and the affected newborn infant and prevention of Rh hemolytic disease of the newborn has resulted in a hundred-fold drop in deaths due to Rh hemolytic disease of the newborn in the past century.[7] However, the disease has not disappeared, and cases of hemolytic disease of the newborn due to red cell antibodies directed toward antigens other than the Rh blood group system are being increasingly recognized.[8–10]

ETIOLOGY AND PATHOGENESIS

CAUSATIVE ANTIBODIES

When considering the specificity of alloantibodies that can cause maternal isoimmunization, it is useful to group them into the following three categories: (1) antibodies directed against the D antigen in the Rh blood group system, (2) antibodies directed against the A and B antigens, and (3) antibodies directed against the remaining red cell antigens. Hemolytic disease of the newborn due to the various antibody systems may differ among races, resulting in differences in clinical severity and outcome.

RH HEMOLYTIC DISEASE

GENETICS

The D antigen in the Rh blood group system is the most important of the three pairs of Rh antigens Cc, Dd, and Ee. Every individual inherits a set of each of the three pairs of antigens from each parent. The presence or absence of D determines the Rh-positive or Rh-negative status of the individual. A mutation deleting the D locus is responsible for the d- or Rh-negative phenotype. Many D-positive individuals are homozygous for D (DD), having inherited the D antigen from both parents. Other D-positive individuals are heterozygous for D (Dd), having inherited a D-containing set from one parent and a non-D-containing set of Rh antigens from the other parent. Therefore, it is evident that all the offspring of a homozygous Rh-positive (DD) man and an Rh-negative (dd) woman will be Rh- or D-positive (Dd), whereas a fetus produced by a heterozygous Rh-positive (Dd) father with an Rh-negative mother (dd) could be either Rh-positive (Dd) or Rh-negative (dd). The probable Rh genotype of the father may be deduced from phenotyping studies, based on gene frequencies in various populations.[11] There is considerable racial variability in the prevalence of Rh-negativity. About 15 percent of Caucasians are Rh negative,[11] compared to 7 to 8 percent of American blacks, 5 percent of Asian Indians,[12] and 0.3 percent of the Chinese.[13]

IMMUNIZATION

Since the mandatory institution of Rh-matched blood transfusions, isoimmunization of Rh-negative women by Rh-positive transfusions is now rare. The potential for immunization of the mother is determined by the existence of maternal-fetal blood group incompatibility and by the extent of feto-maternal hemorrhage. Asymptomatic transplacental passage of fetal red cells occurs in 75 percent of pregnant women at some time during pregnancy or during labor and delivery.[14] The incidence of fetomaternal transfusion increases with advancing gestation: from 3 percent in the first trimester, 12 percent in the second trimester, and 45 percent in the third trimester to 64 percent after delivery. The volume of fetal red cells that enters the maternal circulation also increases as pregnancy progresses. The average volume of fetal blood in the maternal circulation following delivery is about 0.1 ml in most women and less than 1 ml in 96 percent of women,[15] but intrapartum fetomaternal hemorrhage of more than 30 ml may occur in up to 1 percent of pregnancies.[16] Fetomaternal transfusion can result from

Acronyms and abbreviations that appear in this chapter include: DAT, direct antiglobulin test; ΔOD_{450}, change in optical density at 450 nm; IgG, immunoglobulin G; IVT, intravascular fetal transfusion.

obstetric procedures such as chorionic villus sampling,[17] amniocentesis,[18] funipuncture,[19] therapeutic abortion, cesarean section and manual removal of the placenta,[20] and pathologic conditions such as abdominal trauma, spontaneous abortion, or ectopic pregnancy.

The presence of D-positive red cells in the D-negative mother initially provokes a primary immune response that is weak and slow and consists of IgM antibodies that do not cross the placenta. Subsequently, anti-D IgG antibodies capable of crossing the placenta are produced. In the absence of Rh immunoglobulin prophylaxis, sensitization occurs in 7 to 16 percent of women at risk within 6 months after delivery of the first Rh-positive ABO-compatible fetus and in 2 percent after delivery of an ABO-incompatible fetus.[21] Fetomaternal ABO incompatibility offers some protection against primary Rh immunization because incompatible fetal red cells are destroyed rapidly by maternal anti-A and anti-B antibodies, reducing the maternal exposure to Rh D antigenic sites. Repeated exposure to Rh-positive fetal red blood cells, as in a second Rh-positive pregnancy in a sensitized Rh-negative woman, produces a secondary immune response that is marked by the rapid production of large amounts of anti-D IgG antibody. ABO incompatibility confers no protection against the secondary immune response once sensitization has occurred.[22] The volume of blood required to cause sensitization is often minuscule. Primary sensitization has been reported in 80 percent of individuals injected with 0.5 ml of Rh-positive cells; secondary immune responses may occur with as little as 0.03 ml of Rh-positive cells. Repetitive exposure to D-positive cells in D-negative intravenous-drug–abusing women who share needles with Rh- positive partners has lead to severe Rh sensitization.[23]

The reason why most women at risk for development of anti-D do not appear to be sensitized is unclear. Several theories proposed include active T-cell suppression, tolerance induction by small amounts of antigen, and the possibility that low-titer anti-D may not be detected by current diagnostic methods.

HEMOLYSIS

The binding of transplacentally transferred maternal anti-D IgG antibodies to D-antigen sites on the fetal red cell membrane is followed by adherence of the coated red cells to the Fc receptors of macrophages with rosette formation, leading to extravascular noncomplement-mediated phagocytosis and lysis, predominantly in the spleen.[24] Although Rh antigens are found on fetal cells as early as the seventh week of gestation, the active transport of IgG across the placenta is slow until 24 weeks of gestation. The degree of hemolysis may be influenced by the functional immaturity of the fetal reticuloendothelial system prior to 20 weeks of gestation, maternal IgG levels, the IgG subclass, and the rate of transplacental transfer.[25] Antibodies of the IgG1 and IgG3 subclasses, often produced in Rh alloimmunization, have a high affinity for Fcγ receptors and are associated with severe disease, while maternal antibodies with specificity for allogeneic monocytes, which block Fcγ receptors on mononuclear phagocytic cells, may result in unexpectedly mild hemolytic disease of the newborn.[24]

Fetal anemia secondary to hemolysis results in compensatory extramedullary hematopoiesis in the liver, spleen, kidneys, and adrenal glands and is associated with an outpouring of immature nucleated red blood cells into the circulation. Increased fetal plasma erythropoietin levels have been reported with severe fetal anemia.[26] The marked increase in erythropoiesis in fetuses with hemolytic anemia is accompanied by a down-modulation of platelet as well as neutrophil production.[27] Extensive extramedullary hemopoiesis in the liver and spleen may lead to portal and umbilical venous hypertension. Placental function is diminished as a result of trophoblastic hypertrophy and placental edema. Ascites and pleural effusions develop, probably secondary to portal and umbilical venous hypertension.[28] Hypoproteinemia due to

liver dysfunction results in generalized edema. When the edema and ascites become extreme (anasarca), the fetus is at risk for inadequate placental oxygen exchange. This situation, known also as hydrops fetalis, is postulated to be secondary to cardiac failure and elevated venous pressures together with increased capillary permeability and impaired lymphatic clearance.[29] In the final stages of hydrops fetalis, there is hydrothorax, with compression of the lungs, resulting in pulmonary hypoplasia. Prior to the institution of intrauterine transfusions, most of these infants died in utero or soon after birth.

Although fetal bilirubin levels are elevated secondary to hemolysis,[32] the placenta effectively transports most of the lipid-soluble unconjugated fetal bilirubin, so the infant is not clinically jaundiced at birth. In severe cases, bilirubin secreted from the fetal trachea stains the amniotic fluid, umbilical cord, and vernix caseosa.

Some infants with hemolytic disease develop anemia beyond the immediate neonatal period lasting up to 8 to 12 weeks of age. Delayed anemia is related to continuing hemolysis due to persistence of maternal antibodies[30] and a hyporegenerative component with decreased red cell production, associated with low serum concentrations of erythropoietin.[31]

ABO HEMOLYTIC DISEASE

ABO hemolytic disease of the newborn is limited to mothers who are blood group type O and whose babies are group A or B. Although ABO incompatibility exists in 15 percent of O group pregnancies, ABO hemolytic disease is estimated to occur only in about 3 percent of all births. Although far more common than Rh hemolytic disease of the newborn, ABO hemolytic disease of the newborn is usually mild and rarely responsible for fetal deaths. A higher incidence and greater severity is reported in southeast Asians, Latin Americans, Arabs, and South African and American blacks,[33–36] but even in these populations the clinical phenomenon is early neonatal jaundice requiring phototherapy or exchange transfusions. Severe fetal anemia and hydrops has been rarely reported (Table 58-1).[37,38]

There are many reasons for the low incidence and severity of ABO hemolytic disease of the newborn despite considerable fetomaternal ABO incompatibility. Most anti-A and anti-B antibodies are of

TABLE 58-1   COMPARISON OF RH AND ABO INCOMPATIBILITY

CHARACTERISTIC	Rh	ABO
Blood groups		
Mother	Negative	O
Infant	Positive	A or B
Type of antibody	IgG1 and/or IgG3	IgG2
Clinical aspects		
Occurrence in firstborn	5%	40–50%
Predictable severity in subsequent pregnancies	Usually	No
Stillbirth and/or hydrops	Frequent	Rare
Severe anemia	Frequent	Rare
Degree of jaundice	+++	+
Hepatosplenomegaly	+++	+
Laboratory findings		
Maternal antibodies	Always present	Not clear-cut
Direct antiglobulin test (infant)	+	+ or −
Spherocytes	0	+
Treatment		
Antenatal measures	Yes	No
Exchange transfusion frequency	$\approx \frac{2}{3}$	$\approx \frac{1}{10}$
Donor blood type	Rh negative, group specific when possible	Group O only
Incidence of late anemia	Common	Rare

the IgM type and do not cross the placenta. A small number of group O women produce anti-A and anti-B antibodies of the IgG type that can cross the placenta. The severity of the disease in the infant may relate in part to the level of IgG anti-A or anti-B in the mother and the IgG subclass. IgG2 constitutes a significant component of anti-A and anti-B antibody; this subclass of IgG is transported less readily across the placenta than are IgG1 or IgG3 and is a less efficient mediator of macrophage-induced red cell clearance.[11] There are a small number of fully developed A or B antigen sites on fetal red blood cells. IgG anti-A and anti-B are absorbed onto other tissues bearing these surface antigens, thereby diluting their effect. In addition, individuals of the type O blood group have different lymphocyte precursor frequencies, resulting in different titers of anti-A and anti-B, than do individuals of A, B, or AB blood groups.[39]

Unlike Rh disease, ABO hemolytic disease of the newborn occurs with the same frequency in the first as in subsequent pregnancies, since maternal anti-A and anti-B antibodies are present normally, probably secondary to sensitization against A or B substances in food or bacteria. Anti-A and anti-B IgG antibodies do not bind complement on the fetal red cell membrane[40]; hemolysis occurs by noncomplement-mediated phagocytosis of Ig-coated red cells, similar to Rh hemolytic disease of the newborn. The blood film in ABO hemolytic disease of the newborn is marked by the presence of microspherocytes, a feature not seen in Rh hemolytic disease of the newborn.[41] The spherocytosis is postulated to be due to loss of membrane surface area when the spleen removes antigen-antibody complexes from the affected cell. Increased osmotic fragility and autohemolysis, similar to hereditary spherocytosis, may be demonstrated in ABO hemolytic disease of the newborn, but, unlike hereditary spherocytosis, the autohemolysis in ABO hemolytic disease of the newborn is not corrected by the addition of glucose.

HEMOLYTIC DISEASE DUE TO OTHER RED CELL ANTIBODIES

Antenatal screening programs detect clinically significant antibodies in 0.24 to 1 percent of pregnant women.[8-10] Despite the success of Rh prophylaxis, anti-D antibodies still constitute a large proportion of the antibodies detected. When D and ABO are excluded, non-D Rh antibodies (c, C, e, E, cc, and Ce) and those belonging to the Kell, Duffy, Kidd, and MNS systems are most frequently involved (Table 58-2). Although the list of antibodies reported to cause hemolytic disease of the newborn includes IgG specific for virtually any known red cell antigen, some specificities are seen more frequently in severe cases. Anti-c, anti-Kell, and anti-E may cause hemolytic disease of the newborn as severe as that seen in anti-D hemolytic disease of the newborn.[42]

Kell hemolytic disease accounts for 10 percent of the cases of antibody-mediated severe fetal anemia.[43] The Kell blood group system is composed of at least 24 discrete antigens. The Kell antigen (also called KEL1 or K1) is expressed by erythroid progenitor cells and mature erythroid cells, but in only 9 percent of individuals. Alloimmunization in Kell-negative women is often the result of blood transfusion rather than sensitization by fetomaternal hemorrhage from a Kell-positive fetus.[44-46] Kell hemolytic disease is rare in alloimmunized pregnancies because fetal anemia due to transplacentally transmitted antibodies can occur only in a Kell-positive fetus. The partners of Kell-negative women are likely to be Kell positive only in 10 percent of pregnancies, and only half of these pregnancies are likely to be incompatible because of paternal heterozygosity. Published results on the outcome of maternal Kell alloimmunization indicate that between 2.5 and 10 percent of Kell-immunized pregnancies end in the delivery of affected infants,[44,47,48] with about half the infants requiring intervention. Unlike anti-D alloimmunized pregnancies, maternal antibody

TABLE 58-2   RED BLOOD CELL ANTIBODY SEROPREVALENCE IN WOMEN IN THREE STUDIES

Antibody	Sweden[10] 1980–1991 (12 Years)	New York[8] 1993–1995 (2.5 Years)	Mersey and North Wales[9] 1993–1994 (1 Year)
D	159 (19.0%)	101 (18.4%)	100 (40.9%)
E	51 (6.1%)	77 (14.0%)	29 (11.9%)
C	36 (4.3%)	26 (4.7%)	15 (6.1%)*
C^w	10 (1.2%)	1 (0.2%)	
c	38 (4.5%)	32 (5.8%)	28 (11.5%)†
e	1 (0.1%)		1 (0.4%)
Kell	48 (5.7%)	121 (22%)	42 (17.2%)
Duffy	26 (3.1%)	31 (5.6%)	9 (3.7%)
MNS	35 (4.2%)	26 (4.7%)	10 (4.1%)
Kidd	10 (1.2%)	8 (1.5%)	10 (4.1%)
Lutheran	13 (1.6%)	7 (1.3%)	
P₁	48 (5.7%)	1 (0.2%)	
Le^a, Le^b	241 (28.8%)	113 (20.5%)	
I		5 (0.9%)	
Others	120 (14.4%)	1 (0.2%)	
Total antibodies	836	550	244
Blood samples	110,765	37,506‡	22,264

*Includes C^w.
†Includes c plus e.
‡Racial distribution of this population: caucasian 70%, black 20%, other 10%.

titers and amniotic fluid readings in Kell-alloimmunized pregnancies fail to reflect the severity of the disease in the affected fetus.[48] Affected fetuses also have inappropriately low levels of circulating reticulocytes and normoblasts for the degree of anemia, secondary to specific suppression of erythropoiesis at the progenitor cell level by anti-Kell antibodies.[49]

CLINICAL FEATURES

Anemia, jaundice, and hepatosplenomegaly are the hallmarks of hemolytic disease of the newborn. The clinical spectrum of affected infants is highly variable. In Rh hemolytic disease of the newborn, half of the infants have very mild disease and do not require intervention. One-quarter of affected infants are born at term with moderate anemia and develop severe jaundice. In the days prior to intrauterine intervention, hydrops developed in utero in the remaining one-quarter, with half becoming hydropic prior to 34 weeks' gestation. In Kell hemolytic disease of the newborn, the clinical spectrum of hemolytic disease of the newborn is less predictable, ranging from limited clinical stigmata to frank hydrops. Anemia, jaundice, and hepatosplenomegaly are also seen in ABO hemolytic disease of the newborn, but the disease is usually milder than is Rh hemolytic disease of the newborn.

ANEMIA

Infants with mild hemolytic disease of the newborn have cord blood hemoglobin concentrations slightly lower than the age-related normal range. Hemoglobin values usually begin to fall during the first 24 h of life, and hemolysis continues until all incompatible red cells and/or circulating maternal alloantibody is eliminated from the circulation. Since the alloantibodies are IgG, the half-life is approximately 3 weeks. Physical examination in infants with moderate to severe anemia will reveal pallor, tachypnea, and tachycardia. Signs of cardiovascular collapse and tissue hypoxia appear when anemia is severe (hemoglobin <4 g/dl, hematocrit 15%).

JAUNDICE

Most infants with hemolytic disease are not jaundiced at birth. In untreated patients with mild disease, the serum-indirect bilirubin peaks by the fourth or fifth day and then declines slowly. Premature infants may have greater levels of serum bilirubin due to lower activity of hepatic glucuronyl transferase activity. The umbilical cord and vernix caseosa may be stained with bilirubin from the amniotic fluid in severely affected infants. Clinical icterus usually develops during the first day of life, often in the first few hours of life, in such infants, progressing in a cephalopedal direction with rising bilirubin levels. Infants who have received intrauterine transfusions may have marked conjugated hyperbilirubinemia at birth.

An important complication of significantly elevated serum levels of indirect bilirubin in the neonate is the development of bilirubin encephalopathy.[50] This disorder, also termed kernicterus, is caused by bilirubin pigment deposition, leading to neuronal necrosis in the basal ganglia and cerebellum. Bilirubin encephalopathy is initially marked by lethargy, poor feeding, and hypotonia. With increasing severity, the infant develops a high-pitched cry, fever, hypertonia progressing to frank opisthotonos, and irregular respiration; 50 percent of affected term infants die at this stage. The hypertonia becomes less pronounced in surviving infants, who then develop any or all of the classic sequelae of choreoathetoid cerebral palsy, upward gaze palsy, sensorineural hearing loss, and mental retardation. Presentation in preterm infants is less characteristic, but the mortality is higher. Occasionally, infants may have subclinical bilirubin encephalopathy in the neonatal period, manifesting later with the development of mild motor or cognitive dysfunction.

Infants with hemolytic disease of the newborn, particularly those with alloimmune hemolytic disease of the newborn, are at higher risk for kernicterus than are other infants with the same bilirubin level. There are several possible explanations for this finding. Heme pigments might inhibit bilirubin-albumin binding. Alternatively, the complex in utero physiology of erythroblastosis with acidosis and cerebral hypoxia may compromise the blood-brain barrier. Other factors that predispose to kernicterus include hypothermia, hypoglycemia, sepsis, hemolysis, and prematurity. Many of these conditions are present in severely affected infants.

OTHER CLINICAL FEATURES

Hepatosplenomegaly is usually present, and the degree usually correlates with severity of the disease. For those infants who survive, no laboratory evidence of liver disease is evident. The most marked hepatosplenomegaly is seen in infants with hydrops fetalis, who also have peripheral edema and ascites. Respiratory distress may be present due to pulmonary hypoplasia or pleural and/or pericardial effusions or may be due to surfactant deficiency. Purpura associated with thrombocytopenia is commonly seen in severely affected infants and may be a bad prognostic sign. The placenta is thickened, enlarged, and pale.

OBSTETRIC HISTORY

The course and outcome of prior pregnancies is of paramount importance in the initial evaluation of an alloimmunized pregnancy. The history of early fetal deaths or hydrops is ominous. In Rh alloimmunization, the severity of hemolytic disease of the newborn either remains the same or worsens in subsequent affected pregnancies. Hydrops recurs in 90 percent of affected pregnancies, often at an earlier gestation. Jaundice due to hemolysis is also likely to recur to the same degree of severity in subsequent affected pregnancies. The history of prior blood transfusions is important in sensitization to antibodies other than D, particularly Kell alloimmunization. The establishment of paternity for each pregnancy is particularly relevant in both Rh and Kell alloimmunization, since the fetus is at risk only if the father is positive for the antigen in question. ABO hemolytic disease of the newborn may affect the first-born ABO-incompatible infant. Although rare, severe ABO hemolytic disease of the newborn may also recur in subsequent ABO-incompatible pregnancies.[37]

LABORATORY FEATURES

MATERNAL

The aims of antenatal serological testing are to identify Rh-negative women for whom anti–D immunoglobulin prophylaxis will be required, to identify maternal alloimmunization, and to ascertain the risk to the fetus from alloimmune hemolytic disease. Every obstetric patient should have ABO and Rh-D typing and be tested for irregular serum antibodies, irrespective of Rh type, at the initial prenatal visit, preferably by 12 to 16 weeks' gestation. Women who initially test as Rh negative should be tested for the weak-D phenotype, also termed as D^u or D^{+w}. Tests with enzyme-treated red cells or polyspecific antiglobulin sera are not recommended, since they may detect clinically insignificant antibodies. The current American Association of Blood Banks standards for blood banks and transfusion testing recommend repeat Rh testing only in women undergoing delivery, abortion, or an invasive obstetric procedure, or if there is a request for red blood cell transfusion. Antibody screening is repeated at 28 to 30 weeks' gestation only in Rh-negative women, while in Britain and Canada all women undergo repeated screening for irregular antibodies regardless of Rh type.[51] A weakly reactive anti-D (titer of 4 or less) may be demonstrated in women who have received antenatal Rh immunoglobulin and should not be mistaken for sensitization.[52]

If the mother is found to be alloimmunized, the specificity of the antibody and its ability to cause hemolytic disease of the newborn need to be determined. Antibody quantification is usually performed by titration using the indirect antiglobulin test, with different laboratories establishing "critical titers" varying from 8 to 32 for Rh-D antibodies. Specimens are frozen, and successive titration is performed using the same methods. The trend in sequential antibody levels, together with the previous obstetric history, is considered more important than any isolated level in predicting disease severity.[51,53,55] Serological tests in alloimmunized women may be measured every 2 to 4 weeks from 18 weeks' gestation, with rapidly rising levels or a critical titer or level dictating further investigation. The significance of titer levels for antibodies other than D have not been defined. Maternal anti-Kell titers, in particular, correlate poorly with fetal outcome.[43]

The imperfect predictive value of serological tests has led to the development of functional cellular assays that measure the ability of maternal antibodies to cause red cell destruction. In these assays, red blood cells sensitized with maternal antibodies are incubated with effector cells carrying Fcγ receptors, such as lymphocytes or monocytes. Cellular interaction, such as binding, phagocytosis, or cytotoxic lysis, is measured by different techniques.[24,54,56]

TESTING FOR FETOMATERNAL HEMORRHAGE

The standard 300-μg dose of anti-Rh immunoglobulin (RhIg) affords protection against 30 mL of Rh-positive blood. However, fetomaternal hemorrhage in excess of 30 mL may occur in women without predisposing risk factors.[16] All Rh-negative nonimmunized women should have blood tested approximately 1 h after delivery of an Rh-positive baby for fetomaternal hemorrhage. During the antenatal period, testing is indicated after 20 weeks' gestation if clinical circumstances suggest the possibility of excessive transplacental hemorrhage (e.g., abdominal trauma or abruptio placentae). Both a rosette test[57] and an enzyme-linked antiglobulin test[58] are recommended methods of screening for excessive fetomaternal hemorrhage at delivery. If the rosette test result is positive, the number of fetal red cells should be determined. The Kleihauer-Betke test,[59] the standard test in use in most laboratories, permits quantification of fetal hemoglobin-containing red cells in a maternal blood sample. The test is based on the resistance of fetal hemoglobin, unlike adult hemoglobin, to acid elution. False-positive results may be obtained in conditions that are associated with increased fetal hemoglobin, such as hereditary persistence of fetal hemoglobin, sickle cell disease, or sickle cell trait. Flow cytometric methods appear to offer increased accuracy and reliability.[60,61]

FETAL

DETERMINATION OF FETAL BLOOD TYPE

The child of an Rh-negative mother and a heterozygous Rh-positive father has a 50 percent chance of being Rh negative and thus being unaffected by prior maternal Rh alloimmunization. When the father is heterozygous or when paternal zygosity is unknown, the determination of fetal blood type early in pregnancy allows the early institution of monitoring and therapy in Rh-D–positive fetuses who are at risk and the avoidance of invasive procedures if the fetus is Rh negative. Early diagnosis also allows for termination of pregnancy in women who are unwilling to undergo the frequent invasive procedures often necessary for the salvage of severely affected fetuses. Fetal blood sampling for serologic blood typing is associated with a 40 percent risk of fetomaternal hemorrhage and worsening maternal sensitization, and up to 2 percent risk of fetal loss.[19] Rh-D–positive fetal cells may be detected rapidly in chorionic villus samples by flow cytometry.[62] Cloning of the human Rh-D gene[63] has facilitated fetal Rh-D genotyping from small samples of fetal cells obtained by chorionic villus sampling or amniocentesis by the use of polymerase chain reaction techniques.[64] The risks of augmenting maternal sensitization and fetal loss even by these procedures have been eliminated by noninvasive methods of prenatal diagnosis of fetal Rh-D status, through the use of fetal cells isolated from the maternal blood,[65–67] and by using fetal DNA extracted from maternal plasma early in the second trimester of pregnancy.[68]

Prenatal determination of the Kell genotype, necessary for analyzing the possible risk to the fetus in Kell alloimmunization, may be performed either by flow cytometry,[62] by DNA amplification of fetal tissue[69] obtained by chorionic villus sampling, or from amniocytes.[70]

AMNIOTIC FLUID SPECTROPHOTOMETRY

In 1961, Liley reported that the spectrophotometric analysis of amniotic fluid for bilirubin was useful in predicting the severity of fetal anemia from 27 weeks to term. Elevations of optical density at 450 nm (ΔOD_{450}) reflect the concentration of amniotic fluid bilirubin derived from fetal tracheal and pulmonary secretions. The change in optical density is quantified by measuring the elevation of the optical density at 450 nm above a line connecting the optical density values obtained at 375 and 550 nm, and then plotting it against gestational age. Contamination of amniotic fluid samples with blood or meconium make ΔOD_{450} readings impossible. Liley defined three zones, with readings in zone 3, the upper zone, indicating severe fetal disease with hydrops or impending fetal death; zone 1, the lowest zone, indicating mild or no hemolytic disease with a 10 percent risk of needing a postnatal exchange transfusion; and zone 2, indicating moderate disease. Serial determinations of ΔOD_{450} can achieve a sensitivity of 95 percent in detecting the severity of fetal anemia in the third trimester of pregnancy[42] but are unreliable during the second trimester.[71] Modifications of the Liley zones before 25 weeks' gestation[48,72] may help to

determine whether fetal blood sampling is indicated for definitive diagnosis and treatment. Ultrasound-guided amniocentesis carries a 2.5 percent risk of fetomaternal hemorrhage with the possibility of worsening alloimmunization.[18]

REAL-TIME ULTRASONOGRAPHY

Ultrasonography is noninvasive, can be performed serially, and may be combined with other diagnostic studies to assess the fetal condition, to estimate the need for further aggressive management, and to obtain a biophysical profile of the fetus to determine fetal well-being. Hepatosplenomegaly, ascites, edema, or frank hydrops can be detected. The earliest ultrasound signs of cardiac decompensation are a small pericardial effusion and dilatation of the cardiac chambers. In the absence of hydrops, ultrasonographic parameters such as intra- and extrahepatic vein diameters, abdominal and head circumference, head–abdominal circumference ratio, and intraperitoneal volume have been unreliable in distinguishing mild from severe fetal anemia.[73] Fetal splenic circumference is a sensitive indicator of severe anemia in nonhydropic cases without prior transfusion.[74] Preliminary data show that Doppler monitoring of flow velocity indices in the middle cerebral artery and umbilical vein may also be useful noninvasive techniques.[75,76]

PERCUTANEOUS UMBILICAL BLOOD SAMPLING

Percutaneous umbilical blood sampling allows for direct measurement of blood indices to specifically evaluate the degree of severity of fetal hemolytic disease as early as 17 to 18 weeks' gestation.[77] Specimens of fetal blood are obtained for direct measurement of complete blood count, reticulocyte count, red cell antigen phenotyping, direct antiglobulin test, bilirubin, blood gases, and lactate to assess acid-base status. To exclude maternal blood contamination, fetal blood should be examined using a number of fetal-specific markers, such as red cell size, hemoglobin F, and/or expression of the i red-cell antigen.[78] Indications for perimumblical blood sampling in alloimmunized pregnancies include fetal Rh typing, ΔOD_{450} measurement in Liley zone III or rising through zone II, when an anterior placenta precludes amniocentesis in a fetus where maternal history or antibody titers indicate high fetal risk, or ultrasonographic evidence of early or frank hydrops.[79] For a woman with a previous alloimmunized pregnancy, umbilical blood sampling with transfusion should be timed 10 weeks before the time of the earliest previous fetal or neonatal death, fetal transfusion, or birth of a severely affected baby, but not before 18 weeks' gestation unless hydrops is evident. The use of management protocols can reduce the need for multiple invasive procedures while providing specific information about fetal status.[80] Fetal blood samples with reticulocyte counts greater than the 97.5 percentile for gestation, a strongly positive direct Coombs test result, or a mild anemia (hematocrit >30% but <2.5 percentile for gestation) predict fetuses at high risk of having significant antenatal anemia, thus requiring frequent ultrasonographic monitoring and repeated cordocentesis at 1- to 2-week intervals to determine whether intrauterine transfusion is warranted.[81] Complications of fetal blood sampling include fetal loss, with procedure-related rates ranging from 0 to 4.9 percent, umbilical cord bleeding, fetal bradycardia, chorioamnionitis, and a significant risk of fetomaternal hemorrhage with anamnestic maternal sensitization.[82]

NEONATAL

A sample of cord blood should be collected at the time of delivery from all newborns. However, specific testing of cord blood samples is performed only if the mother is Rh negative, if when the maternal serum contains red cell alloantibodies of potential clinical significance, or if the neonate develops signs of hemolytic disease. Tests should include ABO and Rh typing and a direct antiglobulin test (DAT).

Occasionally, high titers of maternal antibody may block Rh-antigenic sites on the neonatal red cells, leading to false-negative Rh typing.

Antepartum RhIG given to the mother may result in a weakly positive DAT result in the infant at birth.[52] Contamination of the cord blood sample with Wharton's jelly during collection can result in a false-positive DAT result. Although the antiglobulin test usually is positive in all forms of hemolytic disease of the newborn, it cannot predict reliably the degree of clinical severity. This is especially true for cases due to ABO sensitization. Elution of maternal antibody from the infant's red cells, followed by tests to determine the specificity of the antibody in the eluate may be useful, particularly when several antibodies are present in the maternal serum.

Cord blood hemoglobin and indirect bilirubin determinations more closely reflect disease severity. Most infants with cord hemoglobin levels within the age-adjusted normal range do not require exchange transfusion. In these infants, determination of cord-indirect bilirubin is more valuable. Usually, a cord hemoglobin level of less than 11 g/dl and/or a cord-indirect bilirubin level of greater than 4.5 to 5 mg/dl warrants exchange transfusion. Early exchange transfusion may also be indicated if the rate of rise of bilirubin, measured every 4 to 6 h, exceeds 0.5 mg/dl/h.

The reticulocyte count is usually more than 6 percent and may approach 30 to 40 percent in severe Rh disease.[41] The peripheral blood smear is characterized by increased nucleated red blood cell counts, polychromasia, and anisocytosis. Severely affected infants may develop thrombocytopenia with platelet counts below 30,000/ml. Spherocytosis is usually seen only in ABO hemolytic disease. Low reticulocyte counts disproportionate to the low hematocrit are evident in Kell hemolytic disease of the newborn.

Hypoglycemia, secondary to hyperinsulinemia, is also seen in severely affected infants. Arterial blood gas analysis may reveal metabolic acidosis and/or respiratory decompensation. Hypoalbuminemia is often present.

Cardiomegaly and pleural and pericardial effusions may be evident on radiological investigation. Cardiac hypertrophy with disproportionate septal hypertrophy has been noted in severely affected infants by echocardiography.[83]

Infants who have received intrauterine transfusions may have mild or moderate anemia with little reticulocytosis. Since most of their circulating red cells are transfused antigen-negative cells, the direct antiglobulin test result may be negative, but the indirect antiglobulin test result will be strongly positive.

DIFFERENTIAL DIAGNOSIS

Hydrops fetalis may be secondary to cardiac anomalies or arrhythmias, fetal genetic or metabolic disorders, intrauterine infections such as syphilis or toxoplasmosis, or any of a multitude of causes that lead to severe derangements in fetal homeostasis. These disorders may be classified as nonimmune hydrops and are differentiated from anasarca secondary to hemolytic disease of the newborn by the absence of any clinically significant red cell alloantibodies in the mother's blood. Parvovirus B19 infection of the mother at any point in gestation can cause nonimmune hydrops, profound fetal anemia, and death.

Neonatal anemia due to intrinsic red cell defects such as hereditary spherocytosis, red cell enzyme deficiencies, and specific hemoglobinopathies can give a similar clinical picture to hemolytic disease of the newborn. The absence of maternal red cell alloantibodies, a negative direct antiglobulin test result, and the detection of the specific defect determining the disorder will clarify the diagnosis.

Disorders of bilirubin metabolism, either indirect, direct, or a combination of both pigments, usually are not associated with anemia. Also, hepatitis or obstructive biliary diseases may present with hyper-

bilirubinemia. The direct antiglobulin test result is negative except in those cases that happen to be from ABO-incompatible pregnancies. In these instances, a positive direct antiglobulin test result usually does not reflect associated hemolytic disease of the newborn.

THERAPY, COURSE, AND PROGNOSIS

THERAPY

FETUS

Intrauterine Fetal Transfusion　Intraperitoneal fetal transfusion has been largely replaced by direct intravascular fetal transfusion (IVT) by funipuncture. Other techniques of fetal transfusion reported include intrahepatic venous puncture, combinations of intravascular with intraperitoneal transfusions, and even intracardiac transfusion as a last resort.[84] Intraperitoneal fetal transfusion was performed when serial amniotic fluid spectrophotometric measurements rose into upper zone II before 30 weeks' gestation or into zone III before 32 to 34 weeks' gestation. Intraperitoneal transfusions may be necessary when intravascular access is difficult, as in early pregnancy when the umbilical vessels are narrow or later when increased fetal size prevents access to the umbilical cord. The intravascular technique offers precise diagnostic evaluation of the fetal status (see Percutaneous Umbilical Blood Sampling, above) and is effective even in hydropic fetuses by circumventing the problem of erratic and often poor absorption of red blood cells from the peritoneal cavity in such fetuses. The relative merits of direct simple intravascular transfusion versus intravascular exchange transfusion have been debated, but the shorter procedure time with direct simple IVT has made it the procedure of choice at most centers.

The first umbilical blood sampling with transfusion ideally should be performed when the fetus is anemic but before hydrops has developed. Transfusions are performed at hematocrit levels of 25 to 30 percent or less. Generally, the hematocrit drops by 1 to 2 percent per day in the transfused hydropic fetus; the fall in hematocrit is rapid in fetuses with severe hemolytic disease, necessitating a second transfusion within 7 to 14 days; the interval between subsequent transfusions is usually 21 to 28 days. Very low pretransfusion fetal hematocrit levels, rapid large increases in posttransfusion hematocrit level, and increases in umbilical venous pressure during IVT are associated with fetal death post-transfusion.[85,86]

Freshly packed O-negative red blood cells that are antigen negative for any other identified antibody, cytomegalovirus seronegative or leukodepleted, irradiated, and cross-matched against the mother's blood are used.[87] Fetuses are at risk for both posttransfusion cytomegalovirus and graft-versus-host disease. Blood that is washed free of the anticoagulant citrate and other additives and that has maximal in vivo survival is advocated. Acidosis is to be avoided so that the hemoglobin oxygen affinity is not reduced due to a shift in the hemoglobin dissociation curve. Blood is prepared to increase the fetal hematocrit to between 40 and 45 percent. The blood should be as fresh as possible, warmed, and packed to a hematocrit of 70 to 85 percent in a volume calculated based on estimated fetal placental blood volume, fetal hematocrit, and hematocrit of donor blood.

Delivery　The decision as to when to deliver the fetus is based on gestational age, fetal weight and lung maturity, fetal response to the transfusions, and the ease of performing the transfusion combined with the antenatal ultrasound and Doppler studies. Transfusions are provided up to 33 to 34 weeks, with delivery as soon as lung maturity is achieved by antenatal steroid therapy. Less severely affected fetuses may be allowed to proceed to term before delivery.

Immunomodulation　Other treatments used in Rh-sensitized pregnancies include intravenous IgG, plasmapheresis, plasmapheresis combined with intravenous immunoglobulin, glucocorticoids, oral enteric-coated D-positive erythrocytes, and promethazine hydrochloride.[88] Each of these modalities attempts a different kind of immune modulation or suppression to reduce antibody response to antigen and may have an adjunctive role in the treatment of severe isoimmunization.[89]

NEONATE

Results of antenatal monitoring and obstetric interventions during pregnancy, together with the history of the outcome of previous pregnancies, allows the neonatal team to anticipate the needs of the infant born with hemolytic disease. In infants with severe hemolytic disease, severe anemia and hydrops are the immediate life-threatening concerns and are often accompanied by perinatal asphyxia, surfactant deficiency, hypoglycemia, acidosis, and thrombocytopenia. The prevention of kernicterus and neurotoxicity due to severe unconjugated hyperbilirubinemia is the next pressing problem. Phototherapy and exchange transfusions are the main treatment modalities.

The resuscitation and stabilization of hydropic infants is often difficult and involves prompt intubation and positive-pressure ventilation with oxygen. Drainage of pleural effusions and ascites may be required to facilitate gas exchange. Metabolic acidosis and hypoglycemia should be corrected. A partial exchange transfusion may be performed using packed red cells to improve hemoglobin levels and oxygenation; a double-volume exchange transfusion is contemplated only after the initial stabilization.

Infants who have received multiple intrauterine transfusions are delivered closer to term and often require less phototherapy and fewer exchange transfusions in the neonatal period.[90,91] However, some still have significant hemolytic anemia at birth, requiring aggressive intervention, and many require additional simple transfusions for severe and prolonged hyporegenerative anemia secondary to suppression of fetal erythropiesis.[92]

Exchange Transfusion Exchange transfusion removes sensitized red blood cells, bilirubin, and free maternal antibody in the plasma; corrects anemia; and, when a double blood volume exchange is performed (calculated as 2×80 ml/kg), replaces 90 percent of the infant's blood volume with antigen-negative red blood cells that should have normal in vivo survival.

The indications for early exchange transfusions, performed within 9 to 12 h of birth, although debated, have remained essentially unchanged over the last 40 years, with minor modifications. Cord hemoglobin levels ≤ 110 g/liter, cord bilirubin levels ≥ 5.5 mg/dl, and rapidly rising bilirubin levels ≥ 0.5 mg/dL/hr despite phototherapy are commonly used criteria for early exchange transfusions ≥ 0. "Late" exchange transfusions are performed when serum bilirubin levels threaten to exceed 20 mg/liter in term infants, the level at which the risk of kernicterus is approximately 10 percent. Exchange transfusions are performed at lower bilirubin levels in premature infants, particularly those with hypoxemia, acidosis, and hypothermia (see Table 58-2). Conjugated or direct bilirubin values are not subtracted from total bilirubin levels when considering levels for exchange transfusions, unless the direct reacting portion exceeds 50 percent of the total bilirubin.

A double volume exchange should eliminate more than 50 percent of the intravascular bilirubin removed. However, the amount of bilirubin is often less, reflecting the equilibrating tissue-bound pool. The use of albumin prior to exchange transfusion in an effort to mobilize tissue bilirubin is controversial. Equilibration of extravascular and intravascular bilirubin and continued breakdown of sensitized and newly formed red cells by persisting maternal antibodies result in a rebound of bilirubin following initial exchange transfusion, often necessitating repeated exchange transfusions in severe hemolytic dis-

ease. In infants with ABO hemolytic disease, single-volume exchange transfusions have been shown to be comparable to double volume exchange transfusions.

Blood chosen for the exchange should be ABO compatible, Rh negative, negative for the antigen responsible for the hemolytic disease, and cross-matched against the mother's blood. Irradiated citrate-phosphate-dextrose blood is prepared as whole blood or reconstituted whole blood (red cells suspended in saline solution, albumin, or plasma) with a hematocrit of 40 to 50 percent warmed through a temperature-controlled in-line blood warmer.[93] Hypoxemic or acidotic infants should receive blood known to lack hemoglobin S. Additive solution anticoagulants are avoided, but the blood should be as fresh as possible (<7 days) to maximize the in vivo survival of the transfused red cells.

Exchange transfusions may be performed by the traditional push-pull method with a single vascular access, usually the umbilical vein, or by isovolumetric techniques utilizing two access sites for simultaneous removal of the infant's blood and administration of new blood.[94] Aliquots of 5 to 20 ml, with a maximum of 5 ml/kg, are withdrawn or infused in the discontinuous method at a rate not exceeding 5 ml/kg every 3 min to avoid rapid fluctuations in arterial pressure, which are accompanied by changes in intracranial pressure. When an isovolumetric exchange is being done, volumes to be removed or reinfused should not exceed 2 ml/kg/min. The duration of the exchange is usually 1 to 2 h.

Potential complications of exchange transfusion include hypocalcemia, hyper- or hypoglycemia, thrombocytopenia, dilutional coagulopathy, neutropenia, disseminated intravascular coagulation, umbilical venous and/or arterial thrombosis, necrotizing enterocolitis, and infection. Despite advances in the management of critically ill newborn infants, morbidity and mortality associated with exchange transfusions remains high, particularly in infants who are premature or sick or both. The risk of death or permanent serious sequelae has been estimated to be as high as 12 percent in sick infants, compared with less than 1 percent in healthy infants in a recent study.[95] Careful clinical judgment is required in balancing the potential risk of adverse events from exchange transfusion with the risk of bilirubin encephalopathy in ill infants.

Phototherapy The exposure of bilirubin to light results in structural and configurational isomerization and photo-oxidation of bilirubin to less toxic and less lipophilic products that are excreted efficiently without hepatic conjugation. Phototherapy is the prime treatment for unconjugated hyperbilirubinemia, with the aim of treatment being prevention of bilirubin neurotoxicity.

Intensive phototherapy has been found to effectively reduce bilirubin levels and decrease the need for exchange transfusions for hyperbilirubinemia in ABO and Rh hemolytic disease of the newborn.[96–98] Earlier protocols called for the early institution of phototherapy in all infants with hemolytic disease, resulting in the unnecessary, albeit usually benign, treatment of large numbers of infants with mild hemolytic disease whose bilirubin levels would not have risen to nonphysiologic levels even without treatment. Early and intensive phototherapy should be initiated in infants with moderate or severe hemolysis or in infants with rapidly rising bilirubin levels (>0.5 mg/dl/h). Phototherapy is indicated at lower levels for preterm or sick infants (Table 58-3). The effectiveness of phototherapy may be influenced by the wavelength and irradiance of light, the surface area of exposed skin, and the duration of exposure.

Other Treatments Preliminary studies with high-dose intravenous immunoglobulin have shown reduced bilirubin levels and decreased need for exchange transfusions in infants with hemolytic disease.[99,100] The decrease in bilirubin levels in IVIG-treated infants is attributed to reduction in hemolysis, probably secondary to blockade of reticuloendothelial Fc receptors. There is increasing interest in the

TABLE 58-3   GUIDELINES FOR THE MANAGEMENT OF HYPERBILIRUBINEMIA BASED ON THE GESTATIONAL AGE AND RELATIVE HEALTH OF THE NEWBORN

	TOTAL SERUM BILIRUBIN LEVEL, mg/dl			
	UNCOMPLICATED COURSE		COMPLICATED COURSE	
WEIGHT	PHOTOTHERAPY	EXCHANGE TRANSFUSION	PHOTOTHERAPY	EXCHANGE TRANSFUSION
Premature				
<1000 g	5–7	Variable	4–6	Variable
1001–1500 g	7–10	Variable	6–8	Variable
1501–2000 g	10–12	Variable	8–10	Variable
2001–2500 g	12–15	Variable	10–12	Variable
Term				
>2500 g	15–18	20–25	12–15	18–20

SOURCE: From LP Halamek and DK Stevenson,[110] with permission.

use of synthetic heme analogs. By competitively inhibiting the activity of heme oxygenase, the rate-limiting enzyme in the catabolism of heme to biliverdin, such analogs can suppress bilirubin production. Sn-protoporphyrin, a potent heme oxygenase inhibitor, has been shown to blunt the postnatal rise and peak bilirubin levels in term newborns with ABO hemolytic disease.[101] Further documentation of safety and effectiveness of these treatment modalities will be required before they are widely used. Recombinant human erythropoietin decreases the need for postnatal transfusions in infants with late hyporegenerative anemia of Rh hemolytic disease.[102]

PREVENTION

The use of RhIg has dramatically decreased the incidence of hemolytic disease of the fetus and newborn. The mechanism by which RhIg prevents sensitization to the D antigen is not understood. One of the theories proposed is that passively administered anti-D attaches to the D-antigen sites on Rh-positive red blood cells in the circulation and interferes with the host's primary immune response to the foreign antigen. RhIg also may inhibit antigen-induced B-cell responsiveness

TABLE 58-4   DOSAGE OF RH IMMUNOGLOBULIN

INDICATION	ROUTE OF ADMINISTRATION	DOSE
Pregnancy termination <12 weeks' gestation	IM	50 μg
Abortion, miscarriage, ectopic pregnancy, or other pregnancy complications >12 weeks' gestation	IM, IV	300 μg
Amniocentesis or chorionic villus sampling >34 weeks' gestation	IM	300 μg[1]
	IV	300 μg
Amniocentesis, chorionic villus sampling, or other manipulation during pregnancy >34 weeks' gestation	IM	300 μg[2]
	IV	120 μg[2]
Obstetrical complication (e.g., abruptio placentae or placenta previa)	IM, IV	300 μg
Antepartum, 28 weeks' gestation	IM, IV	300 μg
Postpartum[3]	IM	300 μg[4]
	IV	120 μg[4]
Transfusion of Rh-positive blood	IM	20 μg/ml RBCs
	IV	18 μg/ml RBCs

ABBREVIATIONS: RBC, red blood cell; IM, intramuscular; IV, intravenous.
SOURCE: From EA Hartwell,[52] with permission.
[1]To be repeated at 12-week intervals until delivery
[2]Same dose should be administered if procedure is repeated >21 days after first dose.
[3]Infant should be Rh positive
[4]Dose should be adjusted for fetaomaternal hemorrhage >15 ml.

by stimulating an increase in suppressor T cells. The postpartum administration of RhIg to all nonsensitized Rh-negative women who deliver an Rh-positive infant decreases the incidence of Rh isoimmunization from 12 to 13 percent to approximately 2 percent. However about 1.8 percent of Rh-negative women are apparently sensitized during pregnancy from small asymptomatic transplacental hemorrhages. Further reduction in the incidence of Rh-isoimmunization to 0.1 percent has been achieved by antepartum RhIg prophylaxis at 28 to 30 weeks' gestation.[52] Although the cost-effectiveness of routine antepartum prophylaxis is questioned, it has been recommended in the United States since 1981 and was recently endorsed in the United Kingdom.[103] The standard dose in the United States, 300 μg RhIg (1500 IU), affords protection against a fetomaternal transfusion of 15 ml of Rh-positive red blood cells or 30 ml of Rh-positive whole blood. Recommendations for the routine prophylactic dose vary around the world.[104,105] Table 58-4 indicates the recommended dosage of RhIg for prevention of sensitization in the United States.[52] Testing with the Kleihauer-Betke test is recommended as a routine in the postpartum period and antenatally if clinical circumstances suggest the possibility of excessive fetomaternal hemorrhage, to determine if additional doses of RhIg are indicated. The failure to implement current recommendations is estimated to be responsible for almost 40 percent of recent cases of Rh isoimmunization.[9,105] Despite appropriate Rh prophylaxis, about 0.1 percent of Rh-negative women may be sensitized prior to 28 weeks' gestation.

Monoclonal anti-RhIg, currently in phase I trials,[106] may replace polyclonal RhIg derived from human plasma from immunized volunteer donors in the future.

Prophylaxis similar to RhIg does not yet exist for alloimmunization to antigens other than D. Transfusion of blood compatible with not only the D antigen but also Kell and other Rh antigens has been advocated for premenopausal women to prevent alloimmunization.[8,9]

PROGNOSIS

In Manitoba, Canada, perinatal mortality from hemolytic disease dropped from 100 per year in the 1940s in a population of 1 million to 1 every 3 years in the mid 1990s.[7] Similar reductions have been described in the United States and United Kingdom. There is little doubt that Rh immunoprophylaxis played a critical role in the decline of perinatal mortality due to Rh hemolytic disease. Changes in birth-order distribution and improvements in the quality of perinatal care have also been important factors.[107] Prior to the development of treatment measures in the 1940s, almost half of all newborn infants with Rh hemolytic disease died or were severely handicapped. Perinatal survival rates of over 90 percent have been achieved with intrauterine transfusions in nonhydropic fetuses with severe Rh hemolytic disease.[84] The survival rate for hydropic fetuses is lower, at 74 percent, despite intrauterine transfusions, but still remarkable considering nearly all would have perished in the 1960s.

The neurodevelopmental outcome for infants saved by intrauterine transfusion has generally been excellent, with more than 90 percent of survivors being free of disability.[90,108] Perinatal asphyxia and lower cord hemoglobin level at birth have been associated with an increased risk of neurologic abnormalities. Neurologic abnormality due to extreme indirect hyperbilirubinemia secondary to alloimmune hemolytic disease has virtually disappeared in the United States and Canada but is still seen in countries with more limited resources.[109]

REFERENCES

1. Diamond LK, Blackfan KD, Baty JM: Erythroblastosis fetalis and its association with universal edema of the fetus, icterus gravis neonatorum and anemia of the newborn. *J Pediatr* 1:269, 1932.

2. Landsteiner K, Wiener AS: An agglutinable factor in human blood recognized by immune sera for Rhesus blood. *Proc Soc Exp Biol Med* 43:223, 1940.

3. Levine P, Katzin EM, Burnham L: Isoimmunization in pregnancy: Its possible bearing on the etiology of erythroblastosis fetalis. *JAMA* 116:825, 1941.

4. Diamond LK, Allen FH Jr, Thomas WO Jr: Erythroblastosis fetalis: VII. Treatment with exchange transfusion. *N Engl J Med* 244:39, 1951.

5. Liley AW: The use of amniocentesis and fetal transfusion in erythroblastosis fetalis. *Pediatrics* 35:836, 1965.

6. Wegmann A, Gluck R: The history of Rhesus prophylaxis with anti-D (classical article). *Eur J Pediatr* 155:835, 1996.

7. Bowman J: The management of hemolytic disease in the fetus and newborn. *Semin Perinatol* 21:39, 1997.

8. Geifman-Holtzman O, Wojtowycz M, Kosmas E, Artal R: Female alloimmunization with antibodies known to cause hemolytic disease. *Obstet Gynecol* 89:272, 1997.

9. Howard H, Martlew V, McFadyen I, et al: Consequences for fetus and neonate of maternal red cell alloimmunization. *Arch Dis Child Fetal Neonatal Ed* 78;F62, 1998.

10. Filbey D, Hanson U, Wesstrom G: The prevalence of red cell antibodies in pregnancy correlated to the outcome of the newborn. *Acta Obstet Gynecol Scand* 74:687, 1995.

11. Issit PD, Anstee DJ: *Applied Blood Group Serology,* 4th ed. Montgomery Scientific Publications, Durham, 1998.

12. Joseph KS: Controlling Rh haemolytic disease of the newborn in India. *Br J Obstet Gynaecol* 98:369, 1991.

13. Mak KH, Yan KF, Cheng SS, Yuen MY: Rh phenotypes of Chinese blood donors in Hong Kong, with special reference to weak D antigens. *Transfusion* 33:348, 1993.

14. Bowman JM, Pollack JM, Penston LE: Fetomaternal transplacental hemorrhage during pregnancy and after delivery. *Vox Sang* 51:117, 1986.

15. Sebring ES, Polesky HF: Fetomaternal hemorrhage: Incidence, risk factors, time of occurrence, and clinical effects. *Transfusion* 30:344, 1990.

16. Ness PM, Baldwin ML, Niebyl JR: Clinical high-risk designation does not predict excess fetomaternal hemorrhage. *Am J Obstet Gynecol* 156:154, 1987.

17. Jansen MWJC, Brandenburg H,Wildshut HIJ, et al: The effect of chorionic villus sampling on the number of fetal cells isolated from maternal blood and on maternal serum alpha-fetoprotein levels. *Prenatal Diagnosis* 17:953, 1997.

18. Bowman JM, Pollack JM: Transplacental fetal hemorrhage after amniocentesis. *Obstet Gynecol* 66:749, 1985.

19. Bowman JM, Pollock JM, Peterson LE, Harman CR, Manning FA, Menticoglou SM: Fetomaternal hemorrhage following funipuncture: Increase in severity of maternal red-cell alloimmunization. *Obstet Gynecol* 84:839, 1994.

20. Zipursky A, Pollack J, Chown B, Israels LG: Transplacental fetal hemorrhage after placental injury during delivery or amniocentesis *Lancet* 2:493, 1963.

21. Bowman JM: Immune hemolytic disease, in *Nathan and Oski's Hematology of Infancy and Childhood,* 5th ed, edited by DG Natan, SH Orkin, p 53. Saunders, Philadelphia, 1998.

22. Bowman JM: Fetomaternal ABO incompatibility and erythroblastosis fetalis. *Vox Sang* 50:104, 1986.

23. Bowman J, Harman C, Manning F, Menticoglou S, Pollock J: Intravenous drug abuse causes Rh immunization. *Vox Sang* 61:96, 1991.

24. Engelfriet CP, Overbeeke MAM, Dooren MC, Ouwehand WH, von dem Borne AEG Jr: Bioassays to determine the clinical significance of red cell alloantibodies based on Fc receptor-induced destruction of red cells sensitized by IgG. *Transfusion* 34:617, 1994.

25. Palfi M, Hilden J, Gottvall T, Selbing A: Placental transport of maternal immunoglobulin G in pregnancies at risk of Rh(D) hemolytic disease of the newborn. *Am J Reprod Immunol* 39:323, 1998.

26. Thilaganathan B, Salvesan D, Abbas A, et al: Fetal plasma erythropoietin concentration in red blood cell–isoimmunized pregnancies. *Am J Obstet Gynecol* 167:1292, 1992.

27. Koenig JM, Christensen RD: Neutropenia and thrombocytopenia in infants with Rh hemolytic disease. *J Pediatr* 114:625, 1989.

28. Nicolaides KH: Studies in fetal physiology and pathophysiology in Rhesus disease. *Semin Perinatol* 13:328, 1989.

29. Phibbs RH: Hydrops fetalis and other causes of neonatal edema and ascites, in *Fetal and Neonatal Physiology,* 2nd ed, edited by RA Polin, WW Fox, p 1730. Saunders, Philadelphia, 1998.

30. Hayde M, Widness JA, Pollack A, Kohlhauser-Vollmuth C, Vreman HJ, Stevenson DK: Rhesus isoimmunization: Increased hemolysis during early infancy. *Pediatr Res* 41:716, 1997.

31. Koenig JM, Ashton D, DeVore GR, Christensen RD: Late hyporegenerative anemia in Rh hemolytic disease. *J Pediatr* 115:315, 1989.

32. Weiner CP: Human fetal bilirubin levels and fetal hemolytic disease. *Am J Obstet Gynecol* 166:1449, 1992.

33. Lin M, Broadberry RE: ABO Hemolytic disease of the newborn is more severe in Taiwan than in white populations. *Vox Sang* 68:136, 1995.

34. Cariani L, Romano EL, Martinez N, et al: ABO-haemolytic disease of the newborn (ABO-HDN): Factors influencing its severity and incidence in Venezuela. *J Trop Pediatr* 41:14, 1995.

35. Vos GH, Adhikari M, Coovadia HM: A study of ABO incompatibility and neonatal jaundice in black South African newborn infants. *Transfusion* 21:744, 1981.

36. Bucher KA, Patterson AM Jr, Elston RC, Jones CA, Kirkman HN Jr: Racial difference in incidence of ABO hemolytic disease. *Am J Public Health* 66:854, 1976.

37. Stiller RJ, Herzlinger R, Siegel S, Whetham JCG: Fetal ascites associated with ABO incompatibility: Case report and review of the literature. *Am J Obstet Gynecol* 175:1371, 1996.

38. McDonnell M, Hannam S, Devane SP: Hydrops fetalis due to ABO incompatibility. *Arch Dis Child Fetal Neonatal Ed* 78:F220, 1998.

39. Conger JD, Chan MM, DePalma L: Analysis of the repertoire of human B lymphocytes specific for the types A and B blood group terminal trisaccharide epitopes. *Transfusion* 33:200, 1993.

40. Brouwers HA, Overbeeke MA, Huiskes E, et al: Complement is not activated in ABO-hemolytic disease of the newborn. *Br J Hematol* 68:363, 1988.

41. Oski FA, Naiman JL: Erythroblastosis fetalis, in *Hematologic Problems in the Newborn,* 4th ed, p 283. Saunders, Philadelphia, 1982.

42. Bowman JM, Maternal blood group immunization: Hemolytic disease (erythroblastosis fetalis), in *Maternal-Fetal Medicine: Principles and Practice,* 4th ed, edited by RK Creasy, R Resnick, p 711. Saunders, Philadelphia, 1994.

43. Vaughan JI, Warwick R, Letsky E, Nicolini U, Rodeck CH, Fisk NM: Erythropoietic suppression in fetal anemia because of Kell alloimmunization. *Am J Obstet Gynecol* 171:247, 1994.

44. Caine ME, Mueller-Heubach E: Kell sensitization in pregnancy. *Am J Obstet Gynecol* 154:85, 1986.

45. Wenk RE, Goldstein P, Felix JK: Kell alloimmunization, hemolytic disease of the newborn and perinatal management. *Obstet Gynecol* 66:473, 1985.

46. Mayne KM, Bowell PJ, Pratt GA: The significance of anti-Kell sensitization in pregnancy. *Clin Lab Haematol* 12:379, 1990.

47. Leggat HM, Gibson JM, Barron SL, Reid MM: Anti-Kell in pregnancy. *Br J Obstet Gynecol* 98:162, 1991.

48. Bowman JM, Pollack JM, Manning FA, Harman CR, Menticoglou S: Maternal Kell blood group alloimmunization. *Obstet Gynecol* 79:239, 1992.

49. Vaughan JI, Manning M, Warwick RM, Letsky EA, Murray NA, Roberts IAG: Inhibition of erythroid progenitor cells by anti-Kell antibodies in fetal alloimmune anemia. *N Engl J Med* 338:798, 1998.

50. Connolly AM, Volpe VJ: Clinical features of bilirubin encephalopathy. *Clin Perinatol* 17:371, 1990.

51. Duguid JKM: Antenatal serological testing and prevention of hemolytic disease of the newborn. *J Clin Pathol* 50:193, 1997.

52. Hartwell EA: Use of Rh immune globulin: ASCP practice parameter. *Am J Clin Pathol* 110:281, 1998.

53. Management of isoimmunization in pregnancy. *ACOG Educational Bulletin* no 227, August 1996.

54. Engelfriet CP, Reesink HW: International forum: Laboratory procedures for the prediction of the severity of hemolytic disease of the newborn. *Vox Sang* 69:61, 1995.

55. van Dijk BA, Dooren MC, Overbeeke AM: Red cell antibodies in pregnancy: There is no critical titre. *Transfusion Med* 4:199, 1995.

56. Zupanska B: Assays to predict the clinical significance of blood group antibodies. *Curr Opin Hematol* 5:412, 1998.

57. Sebring ES, Polesky HG: Detection of fetal maternal hemorrhage in Rh immune globulin candidates: A rosetting technique using enzyme-treated Rh_2Rh_2 indicator erythrocytes. *Transfusion* 22:468, 1982.

58. Riley JZ, Ness PM, Taddie SJ, et al: Detection and quantitation of fetal maternal hemorrhage utilizing an enzyme-linked antiglobulin test. *Transfusion* 22:472, 1982.

59. Kleihauer E, Braun H, Betki K: Demonstration von fetalem Hämoglobin in den Erythrocyten eines Blutausstrichs. *Klin Wochenschr* 35:637, 1957.

60. Bromilow IM, Duguid JKM: Measurement of fetomaternal haemorrhage: A comparative study of three Kleihauer techniques and two flow cytometry methods. *Clin Lab Haematol* 19:137, 1997.

61. Nelson M, Zarkos K, Popp H, Gibson J: A flow-cytometric equivalent of the Kleihauer test. *Vox Sang* 75:234, 1998.

62. Nelson M, Forsyth C, Popp H, Gibson J: Rapid detection of Rh-D- or K-positive fetal red cells in chorionic villus samples by a flow cytometric technique. *Trans Med* 4:297, 1994.

63. Le Van Kim C, Mouro I, Cherif-Zahar B, et al: Molecular cloning and primary structure of the human blood group Rh-D polypeptide. *Proc Natl Acad Sci USA* 89:10925, 1992.

64. Bennett PR, Le Van Kim C, Colin Y, et al: Prenatal determination of fetal Rh-D type by DNA amplification. *N Engl J Med* 329:607, 1993.

65. Lo YMD, Bowell PJ, Selinger M, et al: Prenatal determination of fetal Rh-D status by analysis of peripheral blood of rhesus negative mothers. *Lancet* 341:1147, 1993.

66. Geifman-Holtzman O, Bernstein IM, Berry SM, et al: Fetal Rh-D genotyping in fetal cells flow sorted from maternal circulation. *Am J Obstet Gynecol* 174:818,1996.

67. Sekizawa S, Watanabe A, Kimura KT, Saito H, Yanaihara T, Sato T: Prenatal diagnosis of the fetal Rh-D blood type using a single fetal nucleated erythrocyte from maternal blood. *Obstet Gynecol* 87:501, 1996.

68. Lo YMD, Hjelm NM, Fidler C, et al: Prenatal diagnosis of fetal Rh-D status by molecular analysis of maternal plasma. *N Engl J Med* 339:1734, 1998.

69. Spence WC, Maddalena A, Demers DB, Bick DP: Prenatal determination of genotypes Kell and Cellano in at-risk pregnancies. *J Reprod Med* 42:353, 1997.

70. Lipitz S, Many A, Mitrani-Rosenbaum S, Carp H, Frenkel Y, Achiron R: Obstetric outcome after Rh-D and Kell testing. *Human Reprod* 13:1472, 1998.

71. Nicolaides KH, Rodeck CH, Mibashan RS, Kemp JR: Have Liley charts outlived their usefulness? *Am J Obstet Gynecol* 155:90, 1986.

72. Queenan JT, Tomai TP, Ural SH, King JC: Deviation in amniotic fluid optical density at a wavelength of 450 nm in Rh-immunized pregnancies from 14 to 40 weeks' gestation: A proposal for clinical management. *Am J Obstet Gynecol* 168:1370, 1993.

73. Nicolaides KH, Fontanarosa M, Gabbe SG, Rodeck CH: Failure of ultrasonographic parameters to predict the severity of fetal anemia in rhesus isoimmunization. *Am J Obstet Gynecol* 158:920, 1988.

74. Bahado-Singh R, Oz U, Mari G, Jones D, Paidas M, Onderoglu L: Fetal splenic size in anemia due to Rh-alloimmunization. *Obstet Gynecol* 92:828, 1998.

75. Mari G, Adrignolo A, Abuhamad AZ, et al: Diagnosis of fetal anemia with Doppler ultrasound in the pregnancy complicated by maternal blood group immunization. *Ultrasound Obstet Gynecol* 5:400, 1995.

76. Iskaros J, Kingdom J, Morrison JJ, Rodeck C: Prospective noninvasive monitoring of pregnancies complicated by red cell alloimmunization. *Ultrasound Obstet Gynecol* 11:432, 1998.

77. Daffos F, Capella-Pavlovsky M, Forestier F: Fetal blood sampling during pregnancy with use of a needle guided by ultrasound: A study of 606 consecutive cases. *Am J Obstet Gynecol* 153:655, 1985.

78. Forestier F, Cox WL, Daffos F, Rainaut M: The assessment of fetal blood samples. *Am J Obstet Gynecol* 158:1184, 1988.

79. Gollin YG, Copel JA: Management of the Rh-sensitized mother. *Clin Perinatol* 22:545, 1995.

80. Reece EA, Copel JA, Scioscia AL, et al: Diagnostic fetal umbilical blood sampling in the management of isoimmunization. *Am J Obstet Gynecol* 159:1057, 1988.

81. Weiner CP, Williamson RA, Wenstrom RD, et al: Management of fetal hemolytic disease by cordocentesis: I. Prediction of fetal anemia. *Am J Obstet Gynecol* 165:546, 1991.

82. Ghidini A, Sepulveda W, Lockwood CJ, Romero R: Complications of fetal blood sampling. *Am J Obstet Gynecol* 168:1339, 1993.

83. Carter BS, DiGiacomo JE, Balderston SM, Wiggins JW, Merenstein GB: Disproportionate septal hypertrophy associated with erythroblastosis fetalis. *Am J Dis Child* 144:1225, 1990.

84. Schumacher B, Moise KJ Jr: Fetal transfusion for red blood cell alloimmunization in pregnancy. *Obstet Gynecol* 88:137, 1996.

85. Radunovic N, Lockwood CJ, Alvarez M, Plecas D, Chitkara U, Berkowitz RL: The severely anemic and hydropic isoimmune fetus: Changes in fetal hematocrit associated with intrauterine death. *Obstet Gynecol* 79:390, 1992.

86. Hallak M, Moise KJ, Hesketh DE, et al: Intravascular transfusion of fetuses with rhesus incompatibility: Prediction of fetal outcome by changes in umbilical venous pressure. *Obstet Gynecol* 80:286, 1992.

87. Chambers LA, Luban NC: Neonatal and intrauterine transfusion, in *Transfusion Therapy: Clinical Principles and Practice,* edited by PD Mintz. AABB Press, Bethesda, MD, 1999.

88. Gibble JW, Ness PM: Maternal immunity to red cell antigens and fetal transfusion. *Clin Lab Med* 12:553, 1992.

89. Porter TF, Silver RM, Jackson M, Branch DW, Scott JR: Intravenous immune globulin in the management of severe Rh-D hemolytic disease. *Obstet Gynecol Survey* 52:193, 1997.

90. Janssens HM, deHaan MJJ, vanKamp IL, Brand R, Kanhai HHH, Veen S: Outcome for children treated with fetal intravascular transfusions because of severe blood group antagonism. *J Pediatr* 131:373,1997.

91. Weiner CP, Williamson RA, Wenstrom KD et al: Management of fetal hemolytic disease by cordocentesis. II. Outcome of treatment. *Am J Obstet Gynecol* 165:1302, 1991.

92. Millard DD, Gidding SS, Socol ML, et al: Effects of intravascular intrauterine transfusion on prenatal and postnatal hemolysis and erythropiesis in severe fetal isoimmunization. *J Pediatr* 117:447, 1990.

93. Luban NLC: Massive transfusion in the neonate. *Transfusion Med Rev* 10:200, 1995.

94. Edwards MC, Fletcher MA: Exchange transfusions, in *Atlas of Procedures in Neonatology,* 2nd ed, edited by Fletcher MA, MacDonald MG. p363. JB Lippincott, Philadelphia 1993.

95. Jackson JC: Adverse events associated with exchange transfusion in healthy and healthy and ill newborns. *Pediatrics* 99: p. e7, 1997.

96. Sisson TRC, Kendall N, Glaucer SC, Knutson S, Bunyaviroch E: Phototherapy of jaundice in newborn infants: I. ABO blood group incompatibility. *J Pediatr* 79:904, 1971.

97. Tan KL, Lim GC, Boey KW: Phototherapy for ABO haemolytic hyperbilirubinemia. *Biol Neonate* 61:358, 1992.

98. Ebbesen F: Superiority of intensive phototherapy—blue double light—in Rhesus haemolytic disease. *Eur J Pediatr* 130:279, 1979.

99. Hammerman C, Vreman HJ, Kaplan M, Stevenson DK: Intravenous immune globulin in neonatal immune hemolytic disease: Does it reduce hemolysis? *Acta Paediatr* 85:1351, 1996.

100. Voto LS, Sexer H, Ferreiro G, et al: Neonatal administration of high-dose intravenous immunoglobulin in rhesus hemolytic disease. *J Perinatal Med* 23:443, 1995.

101. Kappas A, Drummond GS, Manola T, Petmezaki S, Valaes T: Sn-protoporphyrin use in the management of hyperbilirubinemia in term newborns with direct Coombs-positive ABO incompatibility. *Pediatrics* 81:485, 1988.

102. Ovali F, Samanchi N, Dagoglu T: Management of late anemia in Rhesus hemolytic disease: Use of recombinant human erythropoietin (a pilot study). *Pediatr Res* 39:831, 1996.

103. Urbaniak SJ: Consensus conference on anti-D prophylaxis, April 7 and 8, 1997: Final consensus statement. Royal College of Physicians of Edinburgh/Royal College of Obstetricians and Gynaecologists. *Transfusion* 38:97, 1998.

104. James D: Anti-D prophylaxis in 1997: The Edinburgh consensus statement. *Arch Dis Child Fetal Neonatal Ed* 78:F161, 1998.

105. Robson SC, Lee D, Urbaniak S: Anti-D immunoglobulin in Rh-D prophylaxis. *Br J Obstet Gynaecol* 105:129, 1998.

106. Kumpel BM: Monoclonal anti-D for prophylaxis of Rh-D haemolytic disease of the newborn. *Transfusion Clin Biol* 4:351, 1997.

107. Joseph KS, Kramer MS: The decline in Rh hemolytic disease: Should Rh prophylaxis get all the credit. *Am J Public Health* 88:209, 1998.

108. Hudon L, Moise KJ Jr, Hegemier SE, et al: Long-term neurodevelopmental outcome after intrauterine transfusion for the treatment of fetal hemolytic disease. *Am J Obstet Gynecol* 179:858, 1998.

109. Wolf MJ, Beunen G, Casaer P, Wolf B: Extreme hyperbilirubinemia in Zimbabwean neonates: Neurodevelopmental outcome at 4 months. *Eur J Pediatr* 156:803, 1997.

110. Halamek LP, Stevenson DK: Neonatal jaundice and liver disease, in *Neonatal Perinatal Medicine: Diseases of the Fetus and Infant,* 6th ed, edited by AA Fanaroff, RJ Martin, p 1345. Mosby Year Book, St Louis, 1997.

ACUTE BLOOD LOSS ANEMIA

ROBERT S. HILLMAN

CHAIM HERSHKO

> The clinical manifestations of acute blood volume loss reflect adjustments in cardiac output and vascular tone that help prevent circulatory collapse and maintain oxygen supply to vital organs. The first requirement in the management of a patient with acute hemorrhage is to maintain an adequate blood volume and prevent shock. This can be accomplished by intravenous infusion of crystalloid solutions or, when available, whole blood. When blood loss is relatively slow and the total blood volume is maintained by natural or artificial means, anemia becomes a problem. The importance of this problem depends on a number of variables, including the patient's general condition, the nature of the complicating illness, the ability of the cardiovascular system to compensate, and the flow characteristics of vital vascular pathways. A decision on blood transfusion is not based on any specific hemoglobin level but rather on a thoughtful evaluation of the anemic individual. Preexisting cardiac or pulmonary disease, advanced age, hypertension, a history of heavy smoking, or the use of beta-adrenergic antagonists may all indicate increased morbidity risk and justify a more liberal approach to blood transfusion. Once hemorrhage has ceased, the recovery of the red cell mass to normal is usually accomplished gradually by increased red cell production.

A hemorrhage of major proportions represents a double threat to the homeostasis of the organism. First, acute severe blood loss can decrease the blood volume to a point of cardiovascular collapse, irreversible shock, and death. In this situation, the loss of circulating red cells is of far less importance than the sudden depletion of the blood volume. Second, when blood loss is more gradual, the circulating red cell mass may be so depleted as to impair oxygen delivery to vital organs. The response to these threats involves a number of physiologic mechanisms, including adjustments in cardiovascular dynamics, blood volume, red cell production, and oxygen transport by erythrocytes.[1]

VOLUME LOSS AND REPLACEMENT

CLINICAL MANIFESTATIONS

The clinical manifestations of acute blood volume loss reflect adjustments in cardiac output and vascular tone that help prevent circulatory collapse and maintain oxygen supply to vital organs. As outlined in Table 59-1, a normal person can rapidly lose up to 20 percent of the blood volume without signs or symptoms of anemia or cardiovascular collapse. If the hemorrhage exceeds 20 percent, signs of cardiovascular distress appear. At first, this is limited to tachycardia with exercise and postural hypotension. When the blood loss exceeds 30 to 40 percent of the blood volume, there is a fall in cardiac output and the gradual onset of shock: The patient becomes immobile and exhibits air hunger; a rapid, thready pulse; and cold, clammy skin. Unless further hemorrhage is prevented and effective therapy is begun, organ damage and death ensue. A very rapid blood loss that exceeds 50 percent of the patient's blood volume carries a high mortality rate unless immediate volume replacement therapy is initiated. With acute hemorrhage, the hemoglobin or hematocrit will not reflect the quantity of blood lost.

With more gradual blood loss, sufficient restoration of plasma volume can occur to permit losses of even larger volumes of blood without the onset of shock. However, unless the physician intercedes with volume replacement therapy, plasma volume expansion is a relatively slow process. Following a sudden loss of 20 percent of the total volume, it requires 20 to 60 h to restore a normal blood volume by endogenous plasma replacement.[2,6,7] In humans, this is accomplished acutely by mobilizing albumin-containing fluid from extracellular sites.[7] For this reason, the hematocrit falls gradually over a period of 2 to 3 days after a sudden, single hemorrhage (Fig. 59-1). At the same time, normal individuals can produce enough albumin to tolerate chronic blood losses of 1000 ml or more each week.

REPLACEMENT THERAPY

The first requirement in the management of a patient with acute hemorrhage is to maintain an adequate blood volume and prevent shock. This can be accomplished by intravenous infusion of crystalloid (electrolyte) solutions; colloid solutions of plasma protein, albumin, or hydroxyethyl starch; or, when available, whole blood. The choice of solution depends on the clinical setting, including such factors as the severity and rate of hemorrhage, the patient's age and cardiovascular status, and the duration of hypotension. With hemorrhagic shock of short duration, losses are primarily from the intravascular space, with little change in extracellular and intracellular fluid compartments. In this situation, the infusion of a crystalloid solution can rapidly restore blood volume and circulation. With more prolonged hypotension, extracellular fluid shifts into both the intravascular and the intracellular fluid spaces. The latter reflects a failure of the active ATPase-dependent membrane sodium pump, with a resultant increase in intracellular levels of sodium, chloride, and water, and by an increase in extracellular potassium.[8,9] To adequately resuscitate a patient suffering from severe hemorrhagic shock, large volumes of crystalloid and colloid solutions must be given quickly to replete both intravascular and exracellular fluid compartments and restore circulation to the point where cellular membrane transport can recover.

Based on this scenario, a crystalloid solution—isotonic saline or Ringer's lactate—is the first choice in the emergency treatment of an acutely hemorrhaging patient.[10] Since crystalloid solutions are rapidly distributed between the intravascular and extravascular compartments, they need to be infused in a volume of two to four times the estimated blood loss. In patients with relatively normal cardiovascular status, this will quickly return hemodynamic parameters toward normal, including the mean arterial pressure, cardiac output, systemic vascular resistance, and tissue oxygen consumption. When large volumes of crystalloid are given to elderly patients, or patients with heart disease, there is a risk of fluid overload and pulmonary edema. However, it is still debatable whether colloid solutions are any better than crystalloid solutions in supporting the blood volume.[11] In pathologic states such as respiratory distress syndrome, capillary membrane integrity is altered, resulting in increased permeability of fluids with leakage of albumin into the pulmonary interstitial space. Consequently, in such patients the administration of colloidal fluids may result in the development of pulmonary edema.[12]

When the volume of blood lost is very large, it may be necessary to treat with a colloid solution such as 5% albumin or hydroxyethyl starch.[13] Both 5% albumin in isotonic saline and a comparable product, "purified protein fraction," provide volume-for-volume expansion in hypovolemic patients. Neither product has been found to transmit hepatitis B, hepatitis C, or HIV. An infusion of a 6% solution of

TABLE 59-1   REACTION TO ACUTE BLOOD LOSS OF INCREASING SEVERITY

Volume Lost Up To		
%TBV*	ml†	Clinical Signs
10	500	None. Rarely seen, vasovagal syncope in blood bank donors.[1]
20	1000	With the patient at rest it is still impossible to detect volume loss. Tachycardia is usual with exercise, and a slight postural drop in blood pressure may be evident.[2,3]
30	1500	Neck veins are flat when supine. Postural hypotension and exercise tachycardia are generally present, but the resting, supine blood pressure and pulse still can be normal.
40	2000	Central venous pressure, cardiac output, and arterial blood pressure are below normal even when the patient is supine and at rest.[4,5] The patient usually demonstrates air hunger; a rapid, thready pulse; and cold, clammy skin.
50	2500	Severe shock, death.

*TBV, total blood volume.
†For a normal 70-kg person with a 5000-ml total blood volume.

hydroxyethyl starch produces a volume expansion slightly larger than the volume infused and maintains its effect as long as 24 to 36 h. The starch polymer solution contains a spectrum of molecules with different molecular weights, the smaller of which are rapidly excreted in the urine, while larger molecules require molecular degradation. The half-life of hydroxyethyl starch is 17 days, and traces of the material can be detected in the circulation for many months.[14] Hydroxyethyl starch solutions are used frequently in surgery when patients undergo elective cardiac procedures and as a volume replacement fluid in pheresis therapy. Acute reactions to the starch polymer are unusual, and volumes of 2 to 3 liters of 6% hydroxyethyl starch can be administered with only minor impact on platelet function and coagulation. For the emergency situation, it is a reliable, readily available colloid expander and is relatively inexpensive.

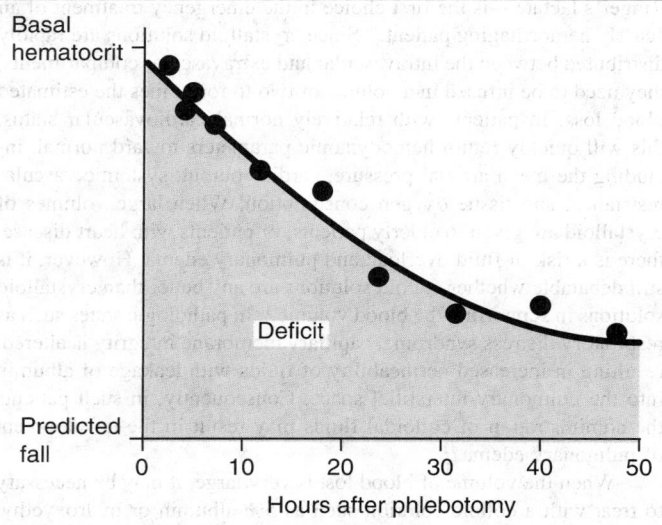

FIGURE 59-1   After a sudden loss of whole blood, the fall in hematocrit is a gradual process that depends on the rate of mobilization of albumin from extravascular sites.[7] Full expansion of the blood volume and the lowest hematocrit value may not be appreciated for up to 72 h.

Reliance on whole blood or packed red cells plus fresh frozen plasma for the emergency treatment of acute blood loss should be discouraged. Its use would require that large amounts of type O Rh-negative whole blood or type-specific blood be constantly available. If typing and cross-match procedures are required prior to transfusion, an unnecessary and possibly dangerous delay in therapy is introduced. In addition, whole blood cannot always be relied upon to produce adequate volume expansion. A reaction to allergenic substances within the plasma or to the cells in whole blood can interfere with volume expansion and even produce plasma volume contraction.[15] Therefore, transfusion of whole blood or red blood cells should be reserved for specific treatment of a low red cell mass where tissue hypoxia is a potential threat.

RED CELL LOSS AND REPLACEMENT

CLINICAL MANIFESTATIONS

With precipitous hemorrhage the immediate effects of volume depletion are more important than the loss of circulating red blood cells. Only when blood loss is relatively slow and the total blood volume is maintained by natural or artificial means does anemia become a problem. How much of a problem depends on a number of variables, including the patient's general physical condition, the nature of the complicating illness, the ability of the cardiovascular system to compensate, and the flow characteristics of vital vascular pathways.[1]

While the change in hematocrit after hemorrhage occurs relatively slowly, there can be a rapid increase in the numbers of circulating leukocytes and platelets during the bleeding episode. The leukocyte count can rise to levels between 10,000 and 30,000/μl (10 and 30 × 10^9/liter) within a few hours as a result of a shift of marginated leukocytes into the circulation and a release of white cells from the marrow. The platelet count can rise to levels approaching 1,000,000/μl (1000 × 10^9/liter). In severe hemorrhage accompanied by shock and tissue hypoxia, immature elements—metamyelocytes, myelocytes, and nucleated red blood cells—may enter the circulation.

As there is no ready reserve of mature red cells to replace the lost red cell mass, oxygen supply to tissues is initially maintained by a shift in the hemoglobin oxygen dissociation curve and adjustments in cardiovascular dynamics. With sudden blood volume loss, there is reflex arteriolar constriction in oxygen-insensitive areas such as skin and kidneys and a decrease in vascular resistance in sensitive organs where oxygen delivery is essential. At the tissue level, changes in pH result in a shift of the oxygen dissociation curve to the right, the Bohr effect, and a greater release of oxygen. Over the next several hours and days, red cell levels of 2,3-bisphosphoglycerate (2,3-BPG) increase to sustain the shift in the curve. Although this mechanism may be of importance in chronic anemias,[16] its effectiveness as a compensatory mechanism immediately after a hemorrhage remains to be defined. Plasma levels of erythropoietin also increase according to the severity of the anemia; a linear fall in the hemoglobin is accompanied by a logarithmic rise in plasma erythropoietin.[17] This hormone is responsible for the subsequent increase in red cell production by the erythroid marrow (see Chap. 29).

ERYTHROPOIETIC RESPONSE

Replacement of the red cell mass by increased red cell production is a gradual process. In response to erythropoietin stimulation, marrow progenitor cells must first proliferate and then mature over a period of 2 to 5 days prior to their delivery to the circulation as adult red cells. There is, therefore, a considerable time lag before red cell production can appreciably increase the red cell mass.

Erythropoietin has a specific effect on the progenitor cells, and a rising tide of erythropoietin initiates proliferation and maturation of early erythroblasts. The response of the erythroid marrow may be recognized as early as the second day by examination of a marrow aspirate. A surge in erythropoietin also appears to cause premature delivery of marrow reticulocytes to the circulation.[18–20] The latter event may be detected within 6 to 12 h of the onset of a hemorrhagic anemia by an increase in reticulocyte counts.[20] A full level of marrow production as estimated from the absolute reticulocyte count occurs only after 8 to 10 days, at which time the erythroid hyperplasia of the marrow and the absolute reticulocyte count are increased to the same extent.[21]

The severity of the anemia is important in determining the degree of marrow response. As long as the marrow structure is intact and iron supply to the red cell precursors is not rate-limiting, the observed increase in red cell production will usually reflect the severity of the anemia. However, damage to the kidneys, inflammation, or a hypometabolic state can markedly interfere with the response.[22,23] A normal individual with an intact erythropoietin mechanism will increase marrow production by a factor of two to three times normal when the hematocrit falls below 30 percent. With progressively more severe anemia, plasma erythropoietin levels rise even higher, and marrow production can increase to levels of three to five times normal if iron supply is sufficient.[21]

In the majority of individuals where marrow structure and erythropoietin response mechanisms are normal, the amount of iron available to the erythroid marrow is the prime determinant of the level of marrow production (Fig. 59-2).[21–23] With increasing anemia, the level of marrow response directly reflects the number of available iron supply pools and the rate of iron delivery from those pools.[21] For example, following a gastrointestinal hemorrhage, a normal individual is able to deliver sufficient iron to support a marrow production level of no greater than three times normal despite increasingly severe anemia. This reflects the maximum rate of mobilization and delivery of storage iron from the monocyte-macrophage system. Furthermore, if these iron stores are exhausted, as is often seen with chronic blood loss, the subject is unable to increase red cell production even to this level, and the proliferative response of the marrow is severely restricted. This effect on marrow production is the earliest sign of absolute iron deficiency. It antedates by weeks or months the typical microcytosis and hypochromia of long-standing iron deficiency. In contrast, when additional iron supply pools are available, as in a subject who bleeds internally and can mobilize iron from the degraded red cells, marrow production may attain levels of four to five times normal. When large numbers of red cells are destroyed in the monocyte-macrophage system, as with a hemolytic anemia, the iron recovered from the degraded hemoglobin is even more rapidly returned to the erythroid marrow so as to permit marrow production levels exceeding five times normal. These characteristics of marrow production must be recognized in order to predict the rate of recovery of the patient's hematocrit and plan proper therapy.

THERAPY

The primary objective of red blood cell transfusions is the restoration of normal oxygen delivery to tissues.[24] However, the hemoglobin level is only one of several variables determining oxygen delivery (Fig. 59-3). The addition of oxygen to inhaled respiratory gases and an increase in cardiac output achieved by optimizing cardiopulmonary hemodynamics with fluid therapy or pharmacologic intervention can compensate for acute blood loss. These interventions and the subsequent evaluation of therapeutic response should precede the decision to transfuse blood.

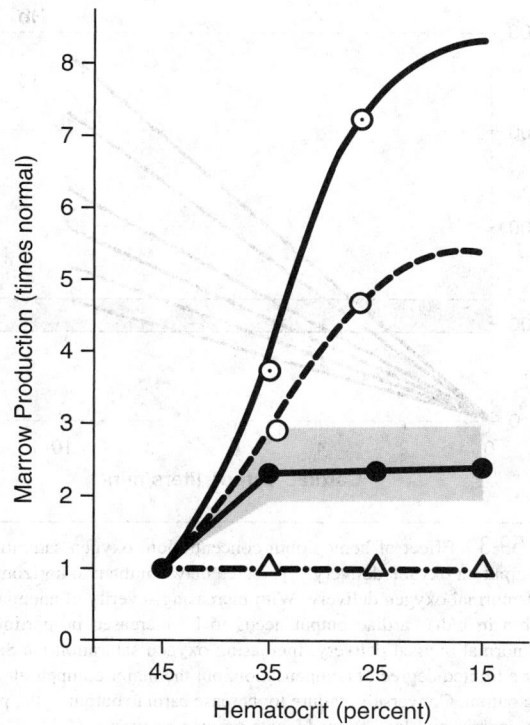

FIGURE 59-2   The rate of red blood cell production after hemorrhage reflects both the severity of the anemia and the rate of iron delivery from various sources. With red cell mass depletions of 20 percent or less, marrow production will increase to two to three times normal regardless of the source of iron. However, at lower hematocrit levels, production reflects the type of iron supply. A normal individual who must rely on hemosiderin stores in the monocyte-macrophage system is unable to increase production further (solid circles, shaded area). In contrast, in patients with a hemolytic process (circled dots) or with more than one source of iron supply (open circles), production can increase to levels of four to seven times normal when the hematocrit falls to 25 percent. Iron-deficient patients fail to show a marrow production increase at either hematocrit level (triangles).

HOMOLOGOUS BLOOD TRANSFUSION

The level of hemoglobin at which a blood transfusion is justified is flexible. The traditional practice of transfusing blood preoperatively when hemoglobin concentration is lower than 10 g/dl or hematocrit less than 30 percent can no longer be supported. An expert NIH panel has proposed a "transfusion trigger" of less than 7.0 g/dl with recommendations for more liberal transfusion criteria in patients at increased risk of suffering damage from decreased oxygen-carrying capacity.[25] Indeed, in resting healthy subjects, isovolemic reductions of blood hemoglobin concentration to 5.0 g/dl produce no evidence of inadequate oxygen delivery because of effective compensation by a shift in the hemoglobin oxygen dissociation curve, a decrease in systemic vascular resistance, and increases in heart rate and stroke volume.[26]

However, patients presenting with acute blood loss are not healthy resting subjects. Hence, a decision on blood transfusion cannot be based on any specific hemoglobin level but rather on a thoughtful evaluation of the anemic individual. Preexisting cardiac or pulmonary disease, advanced age, hypertension, a history of heavy smoking, or the use of beta-adrenergic antagonists may all indicate increased morbidity risk and justify a more liberal approach to blood transfusion.[27] Similarly, increased temperature, heart rate, sympathetic activ-

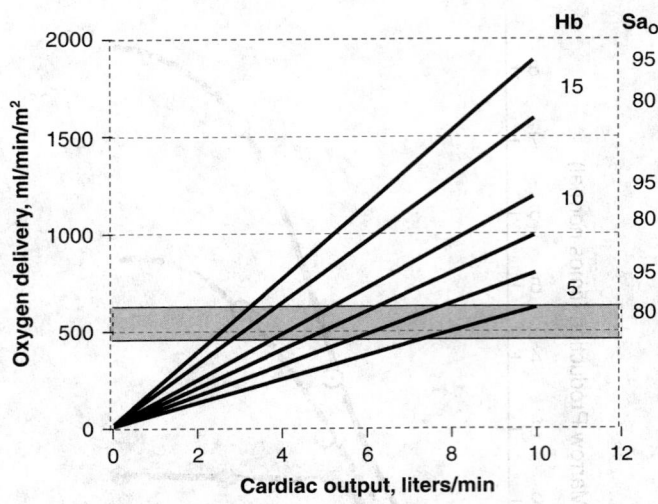

FIGURE 59-3   Effect of hemoglobin concentration, oxygen saturation, and cardiac output on oxygen delivery.[24] The area between the two horizontal lines represents normal oxygen delivery. With increasing severity of anemia (Hb = hemoglobin in g/dl) cardiac output needs to be increased proportionally to maintain normal oxygen delivery. Increasing oxygen saturation (% Sa_{O_2}) will also offer a limited degree of compensation, but the major compensatory force is cardiac output. Conversely, failure to increase cardiac output in the presence of severe anemia will lead to inadequate oxygen delivery.

ity, or metabolic state may alter the balance between oxygen delivery and oxygen consumption, resulting in an increased transfusion requirement.[28]

Packed red blood cells are the preferred component for restoring oxygen-carrying capacity in patients with a normal coagulation status and a stable blood volume. Each unit contains about 200 ml of red blood cells with a hematocrit of about 70 to 80 percent. The infusion of one unit should raise the average-sized adult's hematocrit by 2 to 3 percent. Packed red cells do not provide significant amounts of coagulation factors or platelets.

For massive transfusion therapy, whole blood or packed red cells together with fresh frozen plasma and platelets is preferable to packed red blood cells alone. In emergency situations, large volumes of blood may be administered rapidly by using large-bore intravenous catheters, multiple infusion sites, and infusion under pressure. The rate of infusion may be further increased by mixing red blood cells with normal saline. When transfusing large volumes of blood, careful hemodynamic monitoring and frequent hematocrit measurements are mandatory.[29] Hypothermia during massive blood transfusion can be prevented by warming the blood to 37°C using high-flow blood-warming devices. Citrate intoxication may occur when massive amounts of blood are given; it can be prevented by the infusion of calcium gluconate (Chap. 140). The impact of homologous blood transfusion on survival in general and in surgical patients in particular has been eloquently demonstrated by a major study of survival in 1958 surgical patients who declined blood transfusion for religious reasons.[30] The 30-day postoperative mortality was 1.3 percent in patients with a hemoglobin of 12 g/dl or greater, and 33.3 percent in patients with a hemoglobin of less than 6 g/dl. The adjusted odds ratio for mortality by cardiovascular disease according to preoperative hemoglobin showed only a modest increase in patients without cardiovascular disease with hemoglobin levels decreasing from 12 to 6 g/dl but increasing 16-fold in patients with cardiovascular disease defined by a history of angina, myocardial infarction, congestive heart failure, or peripheral vascular disease. This study illustrates the importance of identifying patients at risk in whom the ability to compensate for anemia by increased cardiac output is limited, and in whom the correction of anemia by blood transfusion may be life-saving.

Refusal of a patient on religious grounds to receive blood transfusion may result in an apparent conflict between the right of a person not to accept a service and the professional values of the physician involved in his or her management. It is useful to remember, however, that if surgical blood loss is limited to less than 500 ml, low hemoglobin levels may be well tolerated.[31] Likewise, minimizing perioperative diagnostic phlebotomies, effective use of combined iron and erythropoietin treatment to correct anemia preoperatively, and the use of intraoperative blood salvage methods (see below) may limit significantly the risks of "bloodless surgery."[32] Finally, if a patient insists on avoiding transfusion after being informed of the possible consequences of such refusal, as in the case of severe anemia in a patient with cardiovascular disease, a physician is not obligated to violate his or her own professional and moral values, and arrangements can be made to transfer responsibility to another physician who is more comfortable with the patient's decision.[33,34]

MAXIMIZING RED CELL OUTPUT

Every effort should be made to evaluate the adequacy of the patient's marrow production response and institute appropriate therapy to maximize red cell output. Primarily, this involves an evaluation of iron supply and the use of oral or parenteral iron preparations when indicated. In selected patients, for example, individuals with an impaired erythropoietin response due to renal disease or chronic inflammation (the anemia of chronic disease), treatment with recombinant erythropoietin can speed recovery.[35]

Studies of the rate of hemoglobin regeneration in iron-deficient patients given either oral or parenteral iron have shown no significant advantage for either form of iron.[36,37] Marrow production studies[21,38] do show a greater increase in red cell production immediately after intravenous infusions of large amounts of iron dextran than is seen with oral iron. However, this is sustained for only 10 to 14 days; the major portion of the injected iron dextran is made available by the action of macrophages at a rate no greater than the level of iron absorbed from four oral iron tablets containing 60 mg of elemental iron each per day. Therefore, in the final analysis a single source of iron, whether normal macrophage storage iron, oral iron, or parenteral iron injections, will provide approximately the same iron supply, enough for a maximum red cell production level of three times normal. In order to exceed this limit, it is necessary to provide several sources of iron at one time. Thus, a combination of an oral iron supplement and macrophage or parenchymal iron deposits may improve iron delivery and permit marrow production to increase to levels of four to five times normal.

Once hemorrhage has ceased, the recovery of the red cell mass to normal is usually accomplished gradually without inconvenience to the patient. Serious attempts at increasing iron supply by combination therapy should therefore be reserved for those situations where a rapid maximum response is essential, as in preparation of a patient for surgery or in the treatment of prolonged, continuous hemorrhage. Blood transfusion should be reserved for those instances where normal response mechanisms and iron supplementation are insufficient to sustain an adequate red cell mass or the acuteness of the situation demands an immediate response.

REFERENCES

1. Finch CA, Lenfant G: Oxygen transport in man. *N Engl J Med* 286:407, 1972.
2. Ebert RV, Stead EA Jr, Gibson JG: Response of normal subjects to acute blood loss. *Arch Intern Med* 68:578, 1941.
3. Theyl RA, Tuohy GF: Hemodynamics and blood volume during operation with ether anesthesia and unreplaced blood loss. *Anesthesiology* 25:6, 1964.
4. Howarth S, Sharpey-Schafer EP: Low blood pressure phases following hemorrhage. *Lancet* 1:19, 1947.
5. Tovey GH, Lennon GG: Blood volume studies in accidental hemorrhage. *J Obstet Gynecol Br Commonw* 5:749, 1962.
6. Lister J, McNeill IF, Marshall VC, et al: Transcapillary refilling after hemorrhage in normal man: basal rates and volumes; effect of norepinephrine. *Ann Surg* 158:698, 1963.
7. Adamson J, Hillman RS: Blood volume and plasma protein replacement following acute blood loss in normal man. *JAMA* 205:609, 1968.
8. Gann DS, Carlson DE, Brynes GJ: Impaired restitution of blood volume after large hemorrhage. *J Trauma* 21:598,1981.
9. Shires GT, Cunningham JN, Barker CRF: Alterations in cellular membrane function during hemorrhagic shock in primates. *Ann Surg* 176:288, 1972.
10. Maier RV, Carrico CJ: Developments in the resuscitation of critically ill surgical patients. *Adv Surg* 19:271, 1986.
11. Shine KI, Kuhn M, Young LS, Tillisch JH: Aspects of the management of shock. *Ann Intern Med* 93:723, 1980.
12. Velanovich VIC: Crystalloid vs colloid fluid resuscitation: a metaanalysis of mortality. *Surgery* 105:65, 1989.
13. Lamke LO, Liljedal SO: Plasma volume changes after infusion of various plasma expanders. *Resuscitation* 5:93,1977.
14. Thompson WL, Fukishima T, Rutherford RB, Walton RP: Intravascular persistence, tissue storage, and excretion of hydroxyethyl starch. *Surg Gynecol Obstet* 131:965, 1970.
15. Hutchison JK, Freedman JO, Richards BA, Burgen ASV: Plasma volume expansion and reactions after infusion of autologous and nonautologous plasma in man. *J Lab Clin Med* 56:734, 1960.
16. Torrance J, Jacobs P, Restrepo A, et al: Intraerythrocytic adaptation to anemia. *N Engl J Med* 283:165, 1970.
17. Erslev AJ: Erythropoietin. *N Engl J Med* 324:1339, 1991.
18. Hillman RS: Characteristics of marrow production and reticulocyte maturation in normal man in response to anemia. *J Clin Invest* 48:443, 1969.
19. Hillman RS, Finch CA: Erythropoiesis: Normal and abnormal. *Semin Hematol* 4:327, 1967.
20. Hillman RS, Finch CA: *Red Cell Manual*, 7th ed. Davis, Philadelphia, 1997.
21. Hillman RS, Henderson PA: Control of marrow production by the level of iron supply. *J Clin Invest* 48:454, 1969.
22. Hillman RS: The importance of iron supply in thalassemic erythropoiesis. *Ann NY Acad Sci* 165:100, 1969.
23. Erslev AJ, McKenna PJ: Effect of splenectomy on red cell production. *Ann Intern Med* 67:990, 1967.
24. Greenburg AG: A physiologic basis for red blood cell transfusion decision. *Am J Surg* 170:6A(suppl)44S, 1995.
25. NIH Consensus Conference: Perioperative red blood cell transfusion. *JAMA* 260:2700, 1988.
26. Weiskopf RB, Viele MK, Feiner J, et al: Human cardiovascular and metabolic response to acute, severe isovolemic anemia. *JAMA* 279:217, 1998.
27. Carson JL: Morbidity risk assessment in the surgically anemic patient. *Am J Surg* 170:32S, 1995.
28. Strauss RG, Weiskopf RB, AuBuchon JP: Physiology and practice of red blood cell transfusions for surgical patients, in *Hematology 1998*, edited by JR McArthur, GP Schechter, SL Schrier, p 454. American Society of Hematology Education Program Book. Miami Beach, 1998.
29. Reiner AP: Massive transfusion, in *Perioperative Transfusion Medicine*, edited by BD Spiess, RB Counts, SA Gould, p 351. Williams & Wilkins, Baltimore, 1995.
30. Carson JL, Duff A, Poses RM, et al: Effect of anaemia and cardiovascular disease on surgical mortality and morbidity. *Lancet* 348:1055, 1996.
31. Spence RK, Carson JA, Poses R, et al: Elective surgery without transfusion: influence of preoperative hemoglobin level and blood loss on mortality. *Am J Surg* 159:320, 1990.
32. Rosengart TK, Helm RE, deBois WJ, et al: Open heart operations without transfusion using a multimodality blood conservation strategy in Jehovah's witness patients: implications for a "bloodless" surgical technique. *J Am Coll Surg* 184:618, 1997.
33. Goldman EB: Legal considerations for allogeneic blood transfusion. *Am J Surg* 170:27S, 1995.
34. Alving BM, Spivak JL, DeLoughery TG: Consultative hematology: hemostasis and transfusion issues in surgery and critical care medicine, in *Hematology 1998*, edited by JR McArthur, GP Schechter, SL Schrier, p 320. American Society of Hematology Education Program Book. Miami Beach, 1998.
35. Watanabe Y, Fuse K, Naruse Y, et al: Subcutaneous use of erythropoietin in heart surgery. *Ann Thorac Surg* 54:479, 1992.
36. Cope W, Gillhespy RO, Richardson RW: Treatment of iron-deficiency anemia: comparisons of methods. *Br Med J* 2:638, 1956.
37. Bothwell TH, Charlton RW, Cook JD, Finch CA: *Iron Metabolism in Man*. Blackwell Scientific, Oxford, 1979.
38. Henderson PA, Hillman RS: Characteristics of iron dextran utilization in man. *Blood* 24:357, 1969.

HYPERSPLENISM AND HYPOSPLENISM

ALLAN J. ERSLEV

The normal spleen shares with other tissues a number of functions, such as the formation, storage, and destruction of blood cells and the production of antibodies, but the spleen has one unique function, that of filtering blood and removing abnormal or foreign material. From an evolutionary point of view, this latter function is no longer vital, but it determines the clinical consequences of hyper- or hyposplenism.

Hypersplenism occurs when the size of the spleen is increased by cells or tissue components or by vascular engorgement. This augments its filtering function, and even normal blood cells experience a delayed transit and temporary sequestration. The sequestration of granulocytes and platelets causes neutropenia and thrombocytopenia, but these cells appear to tolerate their prolonged stay in the spleen. The trapped red cells on the other hand are usually destroyed causing a hemolytic anemia. Splenectomy is called for if the hypersplenic cytopenias are severe enough to demand intervention or if the enlarged spleen causes pain and discomfort. To eliminate the surgical trauma and maintain some splenic functions, partial destruction of the spleen by embolization can be accomplished by the intraarterial infusion of gel particles.

Hyposplenism occurs when splenic function is reduced in certain illnesses or eliminated by splenectomy. It may be well tolerated but demands prevention or vigorous treatment of all suspected bacterial infections.

HYPERSPLENISM

HISTORY AND DEFINITION

The size and function of the spleen have intrigued physicians and philosophers since ancient times.[1] Many mysterious powers have been assigned to the spleen, but it was not until the turn of the century that it was related to destruction of blood cells. In 1899, Chauffard proposed that increased splenic activity causes hemolysis.[2] This proposal provided the impetus for therapeutic splenectomy, which was carried out first in 1910 by Sutherland and Burghard[3] in a patient with hereditary spherocytosis and then in 1916 by Kaznelson[4] in a patient with idiopathic thrombocytopenic purpura. Since then, normal and abnormal functions of the spleen have been identified and assigned to two basic mechanisms: filtration and macrophage surveillance of blood in the red pulp and antibody synthesis in the white pulp (see Chap. 5).

Hypersplenism occurs when these functions are appropriately increased (as in hereditary spherocytosis or idiopathic thrombocytopenic purpura) or inappropriately increased (as in portal hypertension).[5] As enunciated by Dameshek,[6] hypersplenism is usually associated with splenomegaly, causes cytopenias with compensatory marrow hyperplasia, and is most often corrected by splenectomy.

ETIOLOGY AND PATHOGENESIS

The normal spleen is an important component of the mononuclear phagocyte system and participates in antigen processing and antibody synthesis. Speculation exists that the spleen is the principal producer of autoantibodies aimed at circulating blood cells, but firm support for this proposal exists only for antiplatelet antibodies.[9] The main mission of the spleen, however, is to serve as a filter, retaining defective blood cells and foreign particles in a bed of phagocytic cells.[10] This is accomplished by having part of the splenic blood supply (about 5 to 10 percent) diverted into the red pulp, where it slowly percolates through a nonendothelialized mesh studded with macrophages.[11] The blood then reenters the circulation through narrow slits, measuring 1 to 3 microns, in the endothelium of the venous sinuses. The bulk of the blood supply is rapidly channeled through regular endothelialized vessels, linking the arterioles with the venous sinuses and is not filtered or modified.[12] In many animals, such as the dog and the horse, the red pulp serves as a reservoir for red cells, and splenic contraction can provide the red cell volume with a functionally important boost.[13] In humans, however, the splenic capsule is poorly contractile and red cells are not stored to any significant degree in the spleen.[14] On the other hand, a large fraction of the circulating neutrophil pool is marginated in the spleen,[14] and about one-third of platelets are sequestered temporarily by this organ.[15]

The slow transit of blood through the red pulp permits the macrophages to recognize and destroy antibody- or complement-coated cells and microorganisms and to poorly deformable cells or particles retained mechanically by the narrow exit slits in the venous sinuses (see Chap. 5).

This appropriate filtration and elimination of aged and defective cells becomes excessive and harmful in patients with hereditary abnormalities of the red cell membranes or with antibody-coated blood cells. These cells may be functionally intact, but, since they are retained and destroyed in the spleen, symptomatic cytopenias may ensue. The spleen becomes moderately enlarged due to overwork hypertrophy and may, in addition to the elimination of the abnormal cells, sequester and destroy normal blood cells.

Splenomegaly due to a variety of causes usually increases the proportion of blood channeled through the red pulp, causing inappropriate hypersplenic sequestration of both normal and abnormal blood cells.[16] The causes of such splenomegaly are many and various (Table 60-1), with a few diseases associated with massive splenic enlargement (Table 60-2). However, the increase in the size of the filtering bed is more pronounced when the splenomegaly is caused by congestion (as in portal hypertension) than when it is caused by cellular infiltration (as in leukemias, thalassemias, or amyloidosis). Nevertheless, even infiltrative disorders such as Gaucher disease and myelofibrosis may be associated with severe hypersplenic sequestration of normal cells.

The platelets are especially likely to be sequestered by an enlarged spleen, and up to 90 percent of the total number of platelets in blood may be found there.[15] However, both sequestered white cells and platelets survive almost normally in the spleen and may be available, although slowly, when needed to combat infections or vascular damage.[14,15,17] The red cells, on the other hand, are metabolically less self-sufficient and may be destroyed prematurely in the red pulp.[18]

It has been proposed that anemia in patients with splenomegaly is in part due to dilution of red cells in an expanded plasma volume.[19] However, it appears that this expansion, as measured by radiolabeled albumin or fibrinogen, is due more to an increase in the splenic pool of protein rather than to an increase in circulating plasma volume.[20]

The increased blood flow from an enlarged spleen tends to overload the splanchnic vasculature and increase portal pressure. This initiates a vicious cycle, with portal hypertension causing splenomegaly, which in turn increases portal pressure. In a few cases splenectomy has alleviated some of the problems of portal hypertension.[21]

TABLE 60-1   CLASSIFICATION AND THE MOST COMMON CAUSES OF SPLENOMEGALY WITH HYPERSPLENISM

SPLENOMEGALY WITH APPROPRIATE HYPERSPLENISM	SPLENOMEGALY WITH INAPPROPRIATE HYPERSPLENISM
Hereditary hemolytic anemias	Congestion (Band syndrome)
Hereditary spherocytosis	Cirrhosis of the liver
Hereditary elliptocytosis	Portal vein thrombosis
Thalassemia	Splenic vein obstruction
Sickle cell anemia (infants)	Budd-Chiari syndrome
	Congestive heart failure
Autoimmune cytopenias	
Idiopathic thrombocytopenia	Infiltrative disease
Essential neutropenia	Leukemias, chronic and acute
Acquired hemolytic anemia	Lymphomas
	Polycythemia vera
Infections and inflammations	Agnogenic myeloid metaplasia
Infectious mononucleosis	Gaucher disease
Subacute bacterial endocarditis	Niemann-Pick disease
Miliary tuberculosis	Glycogen storage disease
Rheumatoid arthritis (Felty syndrome)	Amyloidosis
Lupus erythematosus	
Sarcoidosis	
Brucellosis	
Leishmaniasis	
Schistosomiasis	
Malaria	

CLINICAL FEATURES

A slight to moderate enlargement of the spleen is usually asymptomatic and is first found during a routine examination of the abdomen. Even massive splenomegaly can be well tolerated, but the patients may complain of abdominal discomfort, early satiety, and trouble sleeping on one or the other side. Pleuritic-like pain in the left upper quadrant with or without a rub may accompany a splenic infarct. In children with sickle cell anemia or malaria and in adults with red cell abnormalities such as spherocytosis, the spleen may become acutely enlarged and painful due to a sudden increase in red cell pooling and sequestration. These hemolytic or sequestration crises often follow infections and are characterized by a sudden aggravation of the anemia.

The size of an enlarged spleen is difficult to assess by manual palpation. Youngsters and thin patients with low diaphragms may have a palpable spleen tip without splenomegaly.[22] In general, however, a palpable spleen signifies splenomegaly and is measured by the number of centimeters it protrudes below the costal margin. Such an enlargement can be verified and more accurately measured by abdominal scanning after the injection of colloid particles labeled with radioactive technetium or of heat-damaged red cells tagged with radioactive chromium. However, these tests have almost all been replaced by the use of ultrasound for the assessment of splenic size. CT scans and magnetic resonance imaging are used primarily to provide structural information in order to identify cysts, tumors, and infarcts.[23]

TABLE 60-2   CAUSES OF MASSIVE SPLENOMEGALY*

Chronic myeloid leukemia
Idiopathic and secondary myelofibrosis
Malignant lymphoma
Hairy-cell leukemia
Gaucher disease
Thalassemia major
Leishmaniasis (kala azar)
Malaria

*The spleen extends into one or both lower quadrants of the abdomen.

LABORATORY FEATURES

Cytopenia associated with splenomegaly and hyperplasia of the corresponding cellular element in the marrow constitute the characteristic triad of hypersplenism. The cellular morphology is usually normal, although a few spherocytes may be present due to metabolic conditioning of red cells during the slow transit through the red pulp.[24] A compensatory increase in red cell production usually is evident by an increase in the reticulocyte count. However, since the spleen preferentially sequesters reticulocytes, the reticulocytosis may not be as prominent as otherwise expected. The presence of a compensatory increase in granulocyte or platelet production is more difficult to identify, and tests such as the epinephrine mobilization tests have been used to distinguish sequestration from ineffective cellular production. Epinephrine will release neutrophils and platelets from the spleen, but since it also will release the cells from marginal pools, the test may be difficult to interpret.[25]

THERAPY, COURSE, AND PROGNOSIS

TOTAL SPLENECTOMY

Total splenectomy is indicated as an emergency procedure after abdominal trauma and partial rupture of the spleen. It is also indicated when splenic size or infarcts causes sustained left upper abdominal pain or discomfort. Splenectomy also is considered when there is pathologic splenic sequestration of circulating blood cells resulting in potentially dangerous cytopenias (see Table 60-1). In such circumstances, splenectomy may result in dramatic restoration of blood counts to normal levels within weeks after surgery.

Hereditary spherocytosis and idiopathic thrombocytopenic purpura are the most common responsive causes, but other congenital or autoimmune cytopenias frequently are treated with splenectomy. The hemolytic anemia of thalassemia major is usually aggravated and complicated by hypersplenic cytopenias. In such cases, splenectomy may improve the response to transfusion. Patients with sickle cell anemia may benefit if repeated sequestration crises and abdominal pains occur before autosplectomy renders the spleen inactive.[27] In autoimmune neutropenias and acquired hemolytic anemias, splenectomy may not only remove an inappropriate sequestration site but also decrease the production of autoantibodies.

Since splenectomy will reduce the volume of blood flowing into the portal circulation, it often is used to alleviate portal hypertension.[28] However, since intra- or extrahepatic portal-systemic shunts can reduce both excessive blood flow and congestive hypersplenic sequestration, they may be preferable.[29–32]

In patients with infiltrative splenomegaly and hypersplenism, it is often difficult to decide what to do. In some diseases, such as

TABLE 60-3   HYPOSPLENISM

Normal infants	Gastrointestinal disorders
Congenital asplenia	Celiac disease
Old age	Regional enteritis
Repeated sequestration crises	Ulcerative colitis
Sickle hemoglobinopathies	Dermatitis herpetiformis
Essential thrombocytosis	Tumors and cysts
Malaria	Amyloidosis
Thrombosis of splenic artery	Splenic irradiation
or vein	Postsplenectomy
Autoimmune disorders	
Glomerulonephritis	
Systemic lupus erythematosus	
Rheumatoid arthritis	
Graft-versus-host disease	
Sarcoidosis	

Gaucher disease, the spleen serves a useful function as a sink for indigestible glycocerebosides. In others such as agnogenic myeloid metaplasia or chronic leukemias, it participates in not only the destruction but also the production of blood cells. Various tests have been designed to evaluate how much splenic enlargement is due to cellular sequestration versus useful cellular production.[33] However, such tests have had limited clinical utility. Partial splenectomy has become popular because it may minimize the risks for immediate postsplenectomy surges in the platelet count or systemic infections due to complete absence of protective splenic filtering.[34-36]

PARTIAL SPLENECTOMY

Partial surgical removal of the spleen[37] often is performed with ligation of some of the splenic arteries[38] or the intra-arterial infusion of gel-foam particles.[39] These latter procedures result in the induction of large splenic infarcts and a reduction in the active splenic mass. These procedures can be performed percutaneously or transvascularly, but the patients have to be observed closely for a number of days to weeks to detect signs of intra-abdominal rupture of the splenic infarcts. The results have been encouraging as testified by a number of long-term follow-ups.[40-44]

Partial ablation by X-ray radiation, especially in poor surgical risk patients, is a popular alternative to more invasive procedures.[45] Although supported by some enthusiastic reports, the results have not been too encouraging.

HYPOSPLENISM

DEFINITION

Hyposplenism occurs when splenic functions are reduced by disease or are absent after splenectomy.[7] It may or may not be associated with a reduction in splenic size. Impaired filtering function usually causes a mild thrombocytosis and an increased risk of severe bloodstream infections.[8] The filtering and immunogenic functions of the spleen are reduced to a varying degree in a number of illnesses (Table 60-3) and of course are absent after splenectomy.[26]

ETIOLOGY AND PATHOGENESIS

The normal neonate[46,47] as well as the aged individual[48,49] may demonstrate findings suggestive of impaired splenic function. These include occasional Howell-Jolly bodies and erythrocyte pits (see "Laboratory Features,"). However, the clinical significance of such functional hyposplenism is uncertain.

Congenital asplenia may be found in infants with situs inversus and other developmental abnormalities.[50] Autoimmune disorders, such as glomerulonephritis,[51] systemic lupus erythematosus,[52-54] or rheumatoid arthritis,[54] have been associated with both laboratory evidence (Howell-Jolly bodies and erythrocyte pits, increased white cell and platelet counts) and the clinical manifestations (impaired clearance of sensitized cells, overwhelming sepsis with encapsulated bacteria) of functional hyposplenism. The same is true for chronic graft-versus-host disease,[56,57] sarcoidosis,[58] alcoholic liver cirrhosis,[59,60] or hepatic amyloidosis.[61,62] Hyposplenism occurs in 30 to 50 percent of patients with celiac disease[63,64] and also commonly occurs in inflammatory bowel disease.[65,66] The mechanisms for this are unknown.

The presence of space-occupying lesions such as cysts or tumors may cause hyposplenism. However, in many cases compensatory hypertrophy of the remaining normal tissue prevents this complication. Splenic replacement by neoplastic cells, as in lymphomas and leukemias, does not usually cause hyposplenism, although splenic sequestration may be less than anticipated in view of the extent of splenic enlargement. Splenic irradiation[67] and vascular obstruction[68] also may lead to functional hyposplenism. However, among all these possibilities, sickle cell anemia and surgical splenectomy are the most common causes of clinically significant hyposplenism.

Although the presence of an enlarged spleen usually suggests hypersplenism, the size of the spleen is not a reliable index of splenic function. Complete splenic replacement by cysts, neoplastic tissues, or amyloid is an example of hyposplenic splenomegaly.[69] In addition, acute sequestration crises, which occur occasionally in patients with malaria[70] and essential thrombocythemia[71] and regularly in infants with sickle hemoglobinopathies,[72] may clog the red cell pulp with cellular debris and result in hypersplenic sequestration being replaced temporarily or permanently by hyposplenism.

CLINICAL FEATURES

In most patients with hyposplenism, reductions in the filtering of blood and immunologic handling of antigens are of little or no clinical consequence, and the diagnosis when made is based exclusively on laboratory findings.

If the spleen is totally destroyed or removed, however, serious infections may ensue. Since the spleen is a major component of the mononuclear phagocyte system, hyposplenism or splenectomy will reduce antibody synthesis at least temporarily. This rarely causes a problem and may actually be beneficial in autoimmune disorders. However, the removal of an efficient filtering bed in which opsonized organisms are exposed to macrophages may lead to an overwhelming sepsis. The responsible organism is usually an encapsulated bacterium, such as *Pneumococcus* or *Haemophilus influenzae*. Unrestrained in vivo proliferation of such microorganisms may cause fatal septicemia.[73-75] The risk is greatest among the very young whose general immunologic tolerance has not matured enough to counteract bacterial infections. For this reason, splenectomy in young children should be deferred until after the fourth year of life. The risk is lower in adults, but even healthy adults whose normal spleens have been removed after accidental rupture are at increased risk.

LABORATORY FEATURES

The reduction or absence of normal splenic function can be recognized by certain hematologic changes. Some of these are nonspecific, such as a slight to moderate increase in the white cell count and platelet count. However, the finding of Howell-Jolly bodies, pitted erythrocytes, and target cells in the blood smear is of greater diagnostic significance. For still unknown reasons the red cell surface area is increased, causing buckling and target cell formation.[76] Nuclear fragments that normally are removed in the spleen are present in circulating red cells and are termed *Howell-Jolly bodies*.[77] They are almost always present in the asplenic state, but only 1 of 100 to 1000 red cells is affected.[77] A sensitive indication of hyposplenism is the appearance of pits or pocks on the cell surface.[78,79] They consist of submembraneous vacuoles and can be seen only in wet preparations of red cells using direct interference-contrast microscopy.

Oxidative drugs may produce Heinz bodies even in normal individuals, but those red cell inclusions are effectively removed by the spleen. After splenectomy they may be observed in supravitally stained blood films. Nucleated red cells are, on the other hand, only rarely seen on blood films after splenectomy (except in patients with hemolytic disorders, in whom their number may increase dramatically). The reticulocyte count remains within normal values, and the life span of red cells is unchanged as other organs take up the function of removing senescent red cells.

Ultrasound, MRI, or CT scan can measure the actual size of the spleen. The clearance of ^{51}Cr-labeled heat-damaged red cells has been used as a measure of splenic function, but this is a difficult test to evaluate. Technetium ^{9m}Tc sulfur colloid particles are now more commonly used for scanning, a reliable measure of the capacity of the spleen to clear particulate matter from the bloodstream.[80]

THERAPY, COURSE, AND PROGNOSIS

Immunization with a polyvalent pneumococcal vaccine[81] should be carried out in all patients with hyposplenism, preferably before splenectomy.[82] No revaccination is needed according to present recommendations. In children, a vaccine against *H. influenzae* should also be administered. Some pediatricians prescribe penicillin as prophylaxis for every asplenic child.[83] Other physicians advise all asplenic patients that no febrile infection should be considered trivial. They instruct these patients to take penicillin upon the onset of symptoms and not to wait for office visits or culture results. Also, dental work, especially tooth extraction, should always be covered with broad-spectrum antibiotics, such as clindamycin or amoxicillin.

REFERENCES

1. Crosby WH: The spleen, in *Blood, Pure and Eloquent*, edited by MM Wintrobe, pp 96–138. McGraw-Hill, New York, 1980.
2. Chauffard AME: Des hepatites d'origine splenique. *Semin Med* 19:177, 1899.
3. Sutherland GA, Burghard FF: The treatment of splenic anaemia by splenectomy. *Lancet* 2:1819, 1910.
4. Kaznelson P: Verschwinden der hamorrhagischen Diathesis bei einen falle von "Essentieller Thrombopenia." *Wien Klin Wochesnchr* 29:1451, 1916.
5. Crosby WH: Hypersplenism. *Annu Rev Med* 13:127, 1962.
6. Dameshek W: Hypersplenism. *Bull NY Acad Sci* 31:113. 1955.
7. Crosby WH: Hyposplenism. *Annu Rev Med* 14:349, 1963.
8. Ferguson A: Hazards of hyposplenism. *Br Med J* 285:1375, 1982.
9. Karpatkin S: The spleen and thrombocvtopenia. *Clin Haematol* 12:591, 1983.
10. Rosse WF: The spleen as a filter (editorial). *N Engl J Med* 317:704, 1987.
11. Weiss L: The reticuloendothelial basis of the clearance of blood by the spleen, in *Disorders of the Spleen: Pathophysiology and Management*, edited by C Pochedly, R Sills, A Schwartz, p 431. Marcel Dekker, New York, 1989.
12. Peters AM: Splenic blood flow and blood cell kinetics. *Clin Haematol* 12:421, 1983.
13. Areas Elenas N, Ewald R, Crosby WH: The reservoir function of the spleen and its relation to postsplenectomy anemia of the dog. *Blood* 24:299, 1964.
14. Wadenvik H, Kutti J: The spleen and pooling of blood cells. *Eur J Haematol* 41:1, 1988.
15. Aster RH: Pooling of platelets in the spleen: role in the pathogenesis of "hypersplenic thrombocytopenia." *J Clin Invest* 45:645, 1966.
16. Bowdler AJ: Splenomegaly and hypersplenism. *Clin Haematol* 12:467, 1983.
17. Brubaker LH. Johnson CA: Correlation of splenomegaly and abnormal neutrophil pooling (margination). *J Lab Clin Med* 92:508, 1978.
18. Christensen BE: Quantitative determination of splenic red cell blood destruction in patients with splenomegaly. *Scand J Haematol* 14:295, 1975.
19. Hess CE, Ayers CR, Sandusky WR, et al: Mechanism of dilutional anemia in massive splenomegaly. *Blood* 47:629, 1976.
20. Zhang B, Lewis SM: Splenic hematocrit and the splenic plasma pool. *Br J Haematol* 66:97, 1987.
21. Williams R, Condon RE, Williams HS, Blendis LM, Kreel L: Splenic blood flow in cirrhosis portal hypertension. *Clin Sci* 34:441, 1968.
22. McIntyre OR, Ebaugh FA: Palpable spleens in college freshmen. *Ann Intern Med* 66:301, 1967.
23. Sty JR, Wells RG: Imaging the spleen, in *Disorders of the Spleen:*

Pathophysiology and Management, edited by C Pochedly, RH Sills, AD Schwartz, p 355. Marcel Dekker, New York, 1989.
24. Jandl JH, Aster RH: Increased splenic pooling and the pathogenesis of hypersplenism. *Am J Med Sci* 253:383, 1967.
25. Joyce RA, Boggs DR, Hasiba U, Srodes CH: Marginal neutrophil in the pool size in normal subjects as measured by epinephrine infusion. *J Lab Clin Med* 88:614, 1976.
26. Pochedly C, Sills RH, Schwartz A (eds): *Disorders of the Spleen: Pathophysiology and Management*. Marcel Dekker, New York, 1989.
27. Al-Salem AH, Qaisaruddin S, Nasserallah Z, al Dabbous I, al Jam'a A: Splenectomy in patients with sickle-cell disease. *Am J Surg* 172:254, 1996.
28. Shah SH, Hayes PC, Allan PL, Nicoll J, Finlayson ND: Measurement of spleen size and its relation to hypersplenism and portal hemodynamics in portal hypertension due to hepatic cirrhosis. *Am J Gastroenterol* 91:2580, 1996.
29. Pursnani KG, Sillin LF, Kaplan DS: Effect of transjugular intrahepatic portosystemic shunt on secondary hypersplenism. *Am J Surg* 173:169, 1997.
30. Alvarez OA, Lopera GA, Patel V, Encarnacion CE, Palmaz JC, Lee M: Improvement of thrombocytopenia due to hypersplenism after transjugular intrahepatic portosystemic shunt placement in cirrhotic patients. *Am J Gastroenterol* 91:134, 1996.
31. Sanyal AJ, Freedman AM, Purdum PP, Shiffman ML, Luketic VA: The hematologic consequences of transjugular intrahepatic portosystemic shunts. *Hepatology* 23:32, 1996.
32. Jalan R, Redhead DN, Simpson KJ, Elton RA, Hayes PC: Transjugular intrahepatic portosystemic stent-shunt (TIPSS): long term follow-up. *QJM* 87:565, 1994.
33. Beguin Y, Fillet G, Bury J, Fairon Y: Ferrokinetic study of splenic erythropoiesis: Relationships among clinical diagnosis, myelofibrosis, splenomegaly, and extramedullary erythropoiesis. *Am J Hematol* 32:123, 1989.
34. Brevit R Herer B. Fremaux A, et al: Fatal postsplenectomy pneumococcal sepsis despite postsplenectomy pneumococcal vaccine and penicillin prophylaxis. *Lancet* 2:356, 1984.
35. Reynafarje C, Ramos J: The hemolytic anemia of human bartonellosis. *Blood* 17:562, 1961.
36. Reubush TK 2nd, Cassaday PB, Marsh HJ, et al: Human babesiosis on Nantucket Island: clinical features. *Ann Intern Med* 86:6, 1977.
37. Banani SA: Partial dearterialization of the spleen in thalassemia major. *J Pediatr Surg* 33:449, 1998.
38. Bar-Moor JA: Partial splenectomy in Gaucher's disease. *J Pediatr Surg* 28:686, 1993.
39. Shah R, Mahour GH, Ford EG, Stanley P: Partial splenic embolization: an effective alternative to splenectomy. *Am Surg* 56:774, 1990.
40. Murata K, Shiraki K, Takase K, Nakano T, Tameda Y: Long term follow-up for patients with liver cirrhosis after partial splenic embolization. *Hepatogastroenterology* 43:1212, 1996.
41. Stanley P, Shen TC: Partial embolization of the spleen in patients with thalassemia. *J Vasc Interv Radiol* 6:137, 1995.
42. Muguerza MR, Lassaletta L, Vasquez J, et al: Partial splenic embolizaiton in the treatment of hypersplenism. Long-term results. *Cir Pediatr* 8:11, 1995.
43. Sangro B, Bilbao I, Herrero I, et al: Partial splenic embolization for the treatment of hypersplenism in cirrhosis. *Hepatology* 21:1203, 1995.
44. Watanabe Y, Todani T, Noda T: Changes in splenic volume after partial splenic embolization in children. *J Pediatr Surg* 31:241, 1996.
45. Paulino AC, Reddy AC: Splenic irradiation in the palliation of patients with lymphoproliferative and myeloproliferative disorders. *Am J Hosp Palliat Care* 13:32, 1996.
46. Freedman RM, Johnston D, Mahoney MJ, et al: Development of splenic reticuloendothelial function in neonates. *J Pediatr* 96:466, 1980.
47. Padmanabhan J, Risemberg HM, Rome RD: Howell-Jolly bodies in the peripheral blood of full-term and premature neonates. *Johns Hopkins Med J* 132:146, 1973.
48. Markus HS, Toghill PJ: Impaired splenic function in elderly people. *Age Ageing* 20:287, 1991.
49. Ravaglia G, Forti P, Biagi F, Maioli F, Boschi F, Corazza GR: Splenic function in old age. *Gerontology* 44:91, 1998.
50. Hickman MP, Lucas D, Novak Z, et al: Preoperative embolization of

the spleen in children with hypersplenism. *J Vasc Intervent Radiol* 3:647, 1992.

51. Lawrence S E, Pussell BA, Charlesworth JA: Splenic function in primary glornerulonephritis. *Adv Exp Med Biol* 1–55:641, 1982.

52. Webster J, Williams BD, Smith AP, et al: Systemic lupus erythematosus presenting as pneumococcal septicemia and septic arthritis. *Ann Rheum Dis* 49:181, 1990.

53. Liote F, Angle J, Gilmore N, Osterland CK: Asplenism and systemic lupus erythematosus. *Clin Rheumatol* 14:220, 1995.

54. Childs JC, Adelizzi RA, Dabrow MB, Freed N: Splenic hypofunction in systemic lupus erythematosus. *J Am Osteopath Assoc* 94:414, 1994.

55. Jarolim DR: Asplenia and rheumatoid arthritis (letter). *Ann Intern Med* 97:61,6. 1982.

56. Kalhs P, Panzer S, Kletter K, et al: Functional asplenia after bone marrow transplantation. *Ann Intern Med* 109:461, 1988.

57. Cuthbert RJ, Iqbal A, Gates A, Toghill PJ, Russell NH: Functional hyposplenism following allogeneic bone marrow transplantation. *J Clin Pathol* 48:257, 1995.

58. Stone RW, McDaniel WR, Armstrong EM, et al: Acquired functional asplenia. in sarcoidosis. *J Natl Med Assoc* 77:930, 1985.

59. Muller AF, Toghill PJ: Splenic function in alcoholic liver disease.. *Gut* 33:1386, 1992.

60. Muller AF, Toghill PJ: Functional hyposplenism in alcoholic liver disease: a toxic effect of alcohol? *Gut* 35:679, 1994.

61. Gertz MA, Kyle RA: Hepatic amyloidosis (primary [AL], immunoglobulin light chain): the natural history in 80 patients. *Am J Med* 85:73, 1988.

62. Powsner RA, Simms RW, Chudnovsky A, Lee VW, Skinner M: Scintigraphic functional hyposplenism in amyloidosis. *J Nucl Med* 39:221, 1998.

63. Robinson PJ, Bullen AW, Hall R, et al: Splenic size and functions in adult coeliac disease. *Br J Radiol* 53:532, 1980.

64. O'Grady JG, Stevens FM, Harding B, et al: Hyposplenism and gluten-sensitive enteropathy. *Gastroenteroldgy* 87:1316, 1984.

65. Palmer KR, Sherriff SB, Holdsworth CD et al: Further experience of hyposplenism in inflammatory bowel disease. *Q J Med* 50:461, 1981.

66. Muller AF, Toghill PJ: Hyposplenism in gastrointestinal disease. *Gut* 36:165, 1995.

67. Dailey MO, Coleman CN, Kaplan HS: Radiation-induced splenic atrophy in patients with Hodgkin disease and non-Hodgkin lymphoma. *N Engl J Med* 302:215, 1990.

68. Spencer RP, Sgiklas JJ, Turner JW: Functional obstruction of splenic blood vessel adults: a radiocolloid study. *Int J Nucl Med Biol* 9:208, 1982.

69. Steinberg MH, Gatling RR, Tavassoli M: Evidence of hyposplenism in the presence of splenomegaly. *Scand J Haematol* 31:437, 1983.

70. Looareesuwan S, Ho M, Wallanagoon. Y, et al: Dynamic alteration in splenic function during acute falciparum malaria. *N Engl J Med* 317:675, 1987.

71. Jandl JH: Case records of the Massachusetts General Hospital. *N Engl J Med* 318:691, 1988.

72. Emond AM, Callis R, Darvill D, et al: Acute splenic sequestration in homozygous sickle cell disease: natural history and management. *J Pediatr* 107:201, 1985.

73. Torres, J, Bisno AL: Hyposplenism and pneumococcemia. *Am J Med* 55:851, 1973.

74. Cavenagh JD, Joseph AE, Dilly S, Bevan DH: Splenic sepsis in sickle cell disease. *Br J Haematol* 86:187, 1994.

75. Gopal V, Bisno AL: Fulminant pneumococcal infections in "normal" asplenic hosts. *Arch Intern Med* 137:1526, 1977.

76. Singer K, Miller EB, Dameshek W: Hematologic changes following splenectomy in man with particular reference to target cells. *Am J Med Sci* 202:171, 1941.

77. Corazza GR, Ginaldi L, Zoli G, et al: Howell-Jolly body counting as a measure of splenic function: a reassessment. *Clin Lab Haematol* 12:269, 1990.

78. Holroyde CP, Oski FA, Gardner FH: The "pocked" erythrocytes. *N Engl J Med* 281:516, 1969.

79. Reinhart WH, Chien S: Red cell vacuoles: their size and distribution under normal conditions and after splenectomy. *Am J Hematol* 27:265, 1988.

80. Rutland MD: Correlation of splenic function with the splenic uptake rate of Tc-colloids. *Nucl Med Commun* 13:843, 1992.

81. Amman AJ, Addiego J, Wara DW, et al: Polyvalent pneumococcal-polysaccharide immunization of patients with sickle cell anemia and patients with splenectomy. *N Engl J Med* 297:987, 1977.

82. Hosea SW, Burch CG, Brown EJ et al: Impaired immune response of splenectomized patients to polyvalent pneumococcal vaccine. *Lancet* 1:804, 1981.

83. Gaston MM, Verter JJ, Woods G, et al: Prophylaxis with oral penicillin in children with sickle cell anemia: a randomized trial. *N Engl J Med* 314:1593, 1986.

POLYCYTHEMIA

ERNEST BEUTLER

Polycythemia is characterized by an increase of the total body red cell volume. It exists in the primary form, polycythemia rubra vera, a clonal neoplastic disorder, and in secondary forms due to appropriate or inappropriate increases in levels of EPO. Such increases may occur, for example, in persons residing at high altitudes, in heavy smokers, in patients with cardiopulmonary disease, and in patients who inherit abnormal, high-affinity hemoglobins. Although primary and secondary polycythemia are entirely different disorders, they are discussed together here because the patients' presentations may be quite similar, and the correct diagnosis is of great importance. Primary polycythemia is characterized by increases not only of the numbers of red cells but also of granulocytes and platelets and by splenomegaly. These findings are not usually present in secondary polycythemia. Control of both types of polycythemia can be achieved by phlebotomy. Myelosuppression is usually used only in primary polycythemia, where drugs such as hydroxyurea, busulfan, chlorambucil, interferon, and anagralide may be useful in controlling not only the hemoglobin levels of blood but also the concentration of other formed elements.

DEFINITION AND HISTORY

The term *polycythemia,* denoting an increased amount of blood, has traditionally been applied to those conditions in which the number of erythrocytes is increased. Primary polycythemia, *polycythemia rubra vera* (polycythemia vera), is an abnormality of the hematopoietic stem cell characterized by uncontrolled proliferation of erythroid, granulocytic, and megakaryocytic cells. *Secondary polycythemia,* more appropriately *secondary erythrocytosis,* refers to those conditions in which only the erythrocytes are increased in number and volume. Although the term *secondary erythrocytosis* is more descriptive of this group of disorders, secondary polycythemia is a time-honored name and will be used interchangeably with secondary erythrocytosis. A classification of these disorders is presented in Table 61-1.

Polycythemia vera was first described in 1892 by Vaquez.[1] In 1903 Osler reviewed four cases of his own and an additional five from the literature. He wrote, "The condition is characterized by chronic cyanosis, polycythemia, and moderate enlargement of the spleen. The chief symptoms have been weakness, prostration, constipation, headache, and vertigo."[2] The increased proliferation of granulocyte precursors and megakaryocytes was first described by Türk in 1904.[3]

Acronyms and abbreviations that appear in this chapter include: BFU-E, burst forming unit–erythroid; 2,3-BPG, 2,3-bisphosphoglycerate; CFU-E, colony forming unit–erythroid; COPD, chronic obstructive pulmonary disease; EPO, erythropoietin.

This chapter is based, in part, on Chapter 70 "Secondary polycythemia (erythrocytosis)" by Dr. Allan J. Erslev in the 5th edition of this text.

Secondary polycythemia is a term that describes a group of disorders characterized by an increased red cell mass brought about by enhanced stimulation of red cell production. Secondary polycythemia may be subdivided into *appropriate polycythemia* in which the erythron is responding normally to hypoxia and *inappropriate polycythemia* in which erythropoiesis is being stimulated by the aberrant production of or response to erythropoietin. In his famous monograph on barometric pressure published in 1878,[4] Paul Bert showed that the physiologic impairment observed at high altitude was due to a reduction in the oxygen content of air. A few years earlier his friend and mentor Dennis Jourdanet had observed an increase in the number of red corpuscles in the blood of the highlanders of Mexico,[5] and Bert recognized that such an increase would tend to ameliorate the effect of atmospheric hypoxia. However, neither he nor Jourdanet suspected a cause-effect relationship. It was actually not until Viault[6] in 1890 observed a prompt increase in the number of his own red corpuscles after having traveled from Lima, Peru, at sea level to Morococha at 4570 m (15,000 ft) above sea level that altitude erythrocytosis was accepted as a compensatory adaptation to hypoxia.[7] At about the same time, it was observed that many patients with cyanosis were also polycythemic. Both the *cardiacos negros*[8] with severe pulmonary failure and arterial oxygen desaturation and the children with *morbus caeruleus,* or right-to-left shunt through a congenital cardiac malformation, were found to have increased red cell counts.[9] Mechanical or neurogenic hypoventilation as a cause of cyanosis and polycythemia was first popularized in 1956 with the classic description of the Pickwickian syndrome by Burwell and colleagues.[10,11] More recently, there has been an increasing interest in the polycythemia associated with arterial hypoxemia due to smoking and with tissue hypoxia due to inherited abnormal hemoglobins with high oxygen affinity. The erythrocytosis associated with abnormal hemoglobins with an increased affinity to oxygen also represents an appropriate response to hypoxia first noted by Charache and coworkers[12] in 1966 when they described hemoglobin Chesapeake.

Inappropriate polycythemia may occur as a result of aberrant erythropoietin production by the kidney, by certain tumors, or by the ingestion of cobalt. *Familial erythrocytosis* is a rare autosomal dominant or a recessive form of inappropriate polycythemia.

In addition to appropriate and inappropriate secondary polycythemia there are some patients with mild erythrocytosis in which neither the cause or the clinical significance is clear. These patients do not have an increased red cell mass and their erythrocytosis is the result of a decreased plasma volume. The disorder is therefore not a true erythrocytosis and is designated *apparent, spurious,* or *relative polycythemia.* As long ago as 1905, Gaisbock reported that a number of hypertensive patients had plethora and an elevated red cell count but no splenomegaly, a condition he termed *polycythemia hypertonica* and that is now sometimes called *Gaisbock syndrome.*[13,14] In 1952 direct measurement of the blood volume in patients with polycythemia led Lawrence and Berlin to identify a subgroup of patients with a normal red cell volume but a reduced plasma volume. Although some members of this group were hypertensive, the authors were more impressed by their tense and anxious behavior and coined the term *stress polycythemia.*[14]

ETIOLOGY AND PATHOGENESIS

POLYCYTHEMIA VERA

Polycythemia vera arises from transformation of a single stem cell into a cell that has a selective growth advantage and that then gradually becomes the predominant source of marrow precursors. The clonal origin of polycythemia vera has been demonstrated in women heterozy-

TABLE 61-1 CLASSIFICATION OF POLYCYTHEMIA AND ERYTHROCYTOSES

Polycythemia vera (primary polycythemia)
  Pure erythrocytosis
Secondary polycythemia (secondary erythrocytosis)
  Appropriate
    High-altitude
    Cardiopulmonary disease
    Smoker's
    Abnormal hemoglobin
    Red cell enzyme deficiencies
    Chemicals (cobalt)
  Inappropriate
    Familial
    Renal disease
    Tumors
      Myomas
      Brain tumors
      Hepatoma
      Endocrine disorders
    Neonatal
Apparent (spurious)

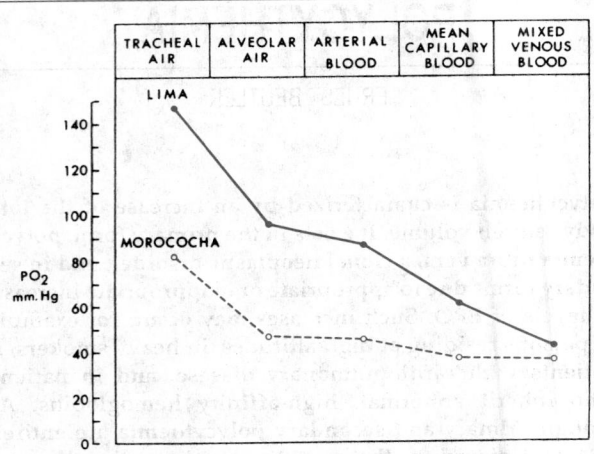

FIGURE 61-1 The oxygen gradient from atmospheric air to the tissues in individuals living at sea level and in Morococha, Peru, at 4540 m (14,900 ft) above sea level.

gous for a polymorphic X-chromosome marker, glucose-6-phosphate dehydrogenase.[15] (see Chap. 9) In each case all hematopoietic cell lineages express either the enzyme encoded by the maternal or paternal X chromosome, whereas nonhematopoietic cells are a mosaic of both enzyme types.

Examination of marrow-derived colonies from patients with polycythemia vera indicates that BFU-Es with normal EPO sensitivity coexist in the marrows of patients along with cells that are EPO-independent or hyperresponsive.[16-19] The latter cells are the hallmark of the neoplastic change that results in uncontrolled production of erythrocytes. Other abnormalities that have been described include impaired thrombopoietin-mediated platelet tyrosine phosphorylation[20] expression of Bcl-x, an inhibitor of apoptosis in an increased proportion of erythroid precursors,[21] and increased expression of protein tyrosine phosphatase activity by red cell precursors.[22] The fibroblasts that accumulate in the marrow of patients with polycythemia vera as the disease progresses are not a part of the abnormal clone. Rather they seem to be a response to the proliferating marrow cells, perhaps to the platelet-derived fibroblast growth factor elaborated by megakaryocytes.[23]

About a quarter of the patients have karyotypic abnormalities at diagnosis,[24,25] and the incidence rises as the disease progresses.[25] It is very likely that a somatic mutation is responsible for the disorder, but its nature is currently unknown. Since most patients have a normal karyotype at the time of diagnosis, gross genetic rearrangements do not seem to be the cause of the disease. There do appear to be genetic factors in susceptibility to polycythemia vera. Although most patients with polycythemia vera do not have a family history of the disorder, there are a number of reports of familial incidence,[26] but the mode of inheritance is unclear. The disease appears to be more common in Jews of European extraction[27] than in most non-Jewish populations. Indeed, of Osler's four original patients, two were Jewish.[2] The incidence of polycythemia was reported to be 6.7/1,000,000 in Israel[28] and 4.9/1,000,000 in Baltimore.[29] However, a higher incidence, increasing from 10 in 1950 to 1959 to 26 per million in 1980 to 1984 has been reported from Malmo, Sweden.[30]

SECONDARY POLYCYTHEMIA

APPROPRIATE POLYCYTHEMIA

High-Altitude Polycythemia The adaptive adjustments of humans living at high altitude involve a series of steps that reduce the steepness of the oxygen gradient between the atmosphere and the mitochondria[31] (Fig. 61-1). The initial oxygen gradient between atmospheric and alveolar air can be reduced by an increase in respiratory rate and volume. Since dead space and water vapor pressure are

constant and acclimatized individuals do not ventilate excessively, the normal sea level gradient of about 60 torr is only reduced to about 40 torr at Morococha at 4540 m (14,900 ft) above sea level.[31] Further reduction can be achieved, and at the top of Mount Everest extreme hyperventilation reduces the gradient to less than 10 torr. A shift in the oxygen dissociation curve to the right may be of benefit for short-term high-altitude acclimatization,[32] but its usefulness for chronic acclimatization has probably been exaggerated.[33] In the unacclimatized subject exposed acutely to high altitude, hyperventilation alkalosis leads initially to a shift of the oxygen dissociation curve to the left and to additional tissue hypoxia. The alkalosis and the hypoxia will in turn promote red cell synthesis of 2,3-bisphosphoglycerate (2,3-BPG) and ATP and cause the oxygen dissociation curve to shift back to a normal or even a right-shifted position (Chap. 26). In chronic acclimatization, the blood pH slightly increased, and when this is taken into account the dissociation curve is shifted approximately normal.[34] It actually seems very questionable if a shift to the right would be to the advantage of high-altitude dwellers.[35]

Cardiac and Pulmonary Disease Degrees of arterial hypoxia comparable to those observed in individuals at high altitudes are observed in patients with right-to-left shunting due to cardiac or intrapulmonary shunts or to ventilation defects as in chronic obstructive pulmonary disease (COPD). Patients with right-to-left shunting develop a degree of erythrocytosis that is quite comparable to that observed with similar degrees of desaturation at high altitudes,[36] but many patients with COPD with severe cyanosis are not polycythemic. This has been attributed to the infection that is often present in the lungs of these patients and to an increase in plasma volume. COPD is frequently associated with cyanosis, clubbing, and arterial oxygen desaturation.[37,38] The sleep apnea syndrome[39] can, if severe, cause arterial hypoxemia and hypercapnia, somnolence, and secondary polycythemia.[40] Central alveolar hypoventilation due to an impaired respiratory center has been reported following cerebral thrombosis, parkinsonism, encephalitis, and barbiturate intoxication.[41] Peripheral alveolar hypoventilation due to mechanical impairment of the chest may be seen in patients with myotonic dystrophy, poliomyelitis, or severe spondylitis.[42-44] In the colorful Pickwickian syndrome,[11] characterized by extreme obesity and somnolence, the associated erythrocytosis appears to be caused by a combination of central and peripheral hypoventilation. Eisenmenger syndrome, characterized by elevated pulmonary vascular resistance and right-to-left shunting of blood, is usually accompanied by erythrocytosis.[45]

Smoker's Polycythemia   Heavy smoking will result in the formation of carboxyhemoglobin, which does not transport oxygen and also causes an increase in oxygen affinity of the remaining normal hemoglobin. This leads to tissue hypoxia, erythropoietin production, and stimulation of red cell production.[46] Smoking may also cause a reduction in plasma volume,[47] and these two effects could easily explain the rise in the hematocrit without significant changes from normal in the red cell or plasma volumes. Chronic carbon monoxide poisoning is an important but generally unappreciated cause of mild polycythemia.[48]

Polycythemia Secondary to Abnormal (High-Affinity) Hemoglobins   Hemoglobinopathies with certain amino acid substitutions may result in an increased affinity for oxygen, producing tissue hypoxia and a compensatory erythrocytosis. Mutations affecting the amino acids of the $\alpha_1\beta_2$-globin chain contact affect normal rotation within the molecule and impair the rate of deoxygenation. Changes in the carboxy terminal and penultimate amino acids will also impair intramolecular motions and tend to keep the molecules in a high-affinity state. Alterations in the amino acids lining the central cavity will destabilize the binding of 2,3-BPG in this cavity and lead to increased oxygen affinity. Finally, heme pocket mutations may in some cases interfere with deoxygenation; however, most hemoglobins with mutations involving amino acids in the heme pocket are unstable and associated with hemolytic anemia and cyanosis. The inheritance of these hereditary disorders is autosomal dominant. An up-to-date listing that includes such hemoglobin variants may be found on the internet at the following addresses: http://www.ncbi.nlm.nih.gov/htbin-post/Omim/dispmim?141900#VariantList; http://www.ncbi.nlm.nih.gov/htbin-post/Omim/dispmim?141800; and http://www.ncbi.nlm.nih.göv/htbin-post/Omim/dispmim?141850.

Polycythemia Secondary to Red Cell Enzyme Deficiencies   Deficiencies of red cell enzymes in early steps of glycolysis sometimes cause marked decreases in the levels of 2,3-BPG. This results in an increased oxygen affinity of hemoglobin and, in some cases, polycythemia. Polycythemia is particularly likely to occur in bisphosphoglyceromutase deficiency[49] and in phosphofructokinase deficiency.[50] Polycythemia has also been observed in the "high ATP syndrome" associated with an abnormality of pyruvate kinase.[51] Occasionally mild erythrocytosis occurs in patients with methemoglobinemia due to cytochrome b_5 reductase (methemoglobin reductase) deficiency[36] (see Chap. 49).

Chemically Induced Tissue Hypoxia   A number of chemicals have been suspected of causing histotoxic anoxia and secondary polycythemia, but the only chemical with a predictable capacity to cause erythrocytosis is cobalt. Cobalt administration will increase the oxygen tension in subcutaneous air pockets in rats[36] as well as increase erythropoietin production[36]; it seems likely that it acts by inhibiting oxidative metabolism. This erythropoietic effect has led to the therapeutic administration of 60 to 150 mg of cobalt chloride to patients with refractory anemias such as the anemias of chronic infection, cancer, or uremia.[52] Consequently, in the treatment of anemias, an agent that causes histotoxic anoxia is not much better than a trip to the top of Pikes Peak.

INAPPROPRIATE POLYCYTHEMIA

Familial Erythrocytosis   Most patients with familial erythrocytosis have been shown to have mutations of the EPO receptor. The mutations are usually ones that cause truncations of the carboxy terminal of the receptor,[53–57] resulting in constitutive activity of the receptor or hypersensitivity to EPO. The disorder is inherited in an autosomal dominant manner.

An endemic form of erythrocytosis occurs in the population of the Chuvash Autonomous Republic, located on the west bank of the Volga River in the central part of European Russia.[58] There is no abnormality in the EPO receptor in these patients, and there seems to be no linkage with the EPO gene. Unlike the patients who have lesions of their EPO receptors, genetic transmission seems to be autosomal recessive.

A child with hypersecretion of EPO without any evident cause has been studied.[59] It was suggested that an abnormality in the pathway that regulates EPO levels may have been present in this patient.

Renal Polycythemia   Absolute erythrocytosis has been observed in a considerable number of patients with solitary renal cysts, polycystic renal disease, or hydronephrosis.[60] In most of these cases erythropoietin assays on cyst fluid, serum, or urine have disclosed the presence of erythropoietin.[61] In general, it appears that patients with polycystic disease have a hematocrit value slightly higher than normal and definitely higher than would have been expected of patients with uremia. In some patients on prolonged dialysis treatment cystic transformation occurs in the native kidneys. This acquired cystic disease is occasionally associated with marked erythrocytosis.[62] It has been estimated that about 1 to 3 percent of all patients with hypernephromas have erythrocytosis.[63] In many of these, erythropoietin assays of serum and urine have disclosed higher-than-normal levels, and the erythrocytosis is most likely caused by excessive erythropoietin secretion. This assumption has been supported by the presence of erythropoietin mRNA in tumor cells.[64] Wilms' tumors[65] and metanephric adenomas[66] are also occasionally associated with an erythrocytosis.

Post–renal transplantation erythrocytosis occurs in about 10 percent of patients[67] but is usually mild and time-limited and in many cases may have been caused by excessive use of diuretics. In some cases this erythrocytosis is associated with an increase in erythropoietin production and has been treated successfully in a few patients with theophylline or captopril, both believed to attenuate erythropoietin production.[68–70] A role of insulin growth factor-1 has also been proposed in the erythrocytosis that occurs after transplantation,[71] and the effect of angiotensin-activating enzyme in controlling the erythrocytosis[72] may be due to suppression of this growth factor. Studies of venous effluents have determined that the native rather than the transplanted kidneys are the source of the inappropriate production of erythropoietin,[73] and removal of the native kidneys has led to rapid restoration of normal hematocrit values.[74]

Successful extirpation of renal lesions in patients with erythrocytosis has in many cases been followed by hematologic remission.[60] Subsequent relapses have been described in patients developing metastatic recurrence of the tumors in the contralateral kidney.[75]

A partial obstruction of the renal artery would be expected to cause renal tissue hypoxia and a physiologic stimulation of erythropoietin production. Nevertheless, it has proved quite difficult to induce an erythrocytosis in laboratory animals by inserting a Goldblatt clamp on the renal arteries.[76] Only a few of the many patients who have arteriosclerotic narrowing of the renal arteries have been reported to have been polycythemic.[77]

Polycythemia with Connective Tissue Tumors   Occasionally there is an association of erythrocytosis with large uterine myomas[78] and rarely with cutaneous leiomyomas.[79] Usually the tumor has been huge, and extirpation has routinely been followed by a hematologic "cure." It has been suggested that the tumor may interfere with pulmonary ventilation, but arterial gas findings have been normal in the few patients so studied. Another possible mechanism is that the large abdominal mass causes mechanical interference with the blood supply to the kidneys, resulting in renal hypoxia and erythropoietin production. Inappropriate erythropoietin secretion by smooth muscle cells has been demonstrated both in uterine myomas and in one case of cutaneous leiomyoma.[78,79] Isolated instances of polycythemia attributed to a myxoma of the atrium,[80] hamartoma of the liver,[81] and focal hyperplasia of the liver[82] have been documented.

Brain Tumors   Erythrocytosis and inappropriate secretions of erythropoietin may be found in about 15 percent of patients with cerebellar hemangiomas.[83,84] In adequately studied patients the arterial gas tensions have been normal. That the tumors are directly responsible for the polycythemia can be surmised from the identification of erythropoietin in cyst fluid and stromal cells and from a case in which erythropoietin mRNA was present in the tumor.[85]

Hepatoma   In 1958, McFadzean and coworkers reported that almost 10 percent of patients in Hong Kong with hepatocarcinoma developed erythrocytosis.[86] Since then, this association has been recognized as an important clinical clue in the diagnostic consideration of patients with liver disease.[87] The cause of erythrocytosis is probably inappropriate production of erythropoietin by the neoplastic cells.[88] Normal hepatocytes and to a lesser degree nonparenchymal liver cells produce small amounts of erythropoietin both constitutively and in response to hypoxia.

Endocrine Disorders   Pheochromocytomas,[89] aldosterone-producing adenomas,[90] Bartter syndrome,[91] and dermoid cyst of the ovary[92] have been described in association with erythrocytosis. Erythropoietin levels were found elevated in the serum and returned to normal after extirpation of the tumors. A number of pathogenetic mechanisms have been suggested, including mechanical interference with renal blood supply; hypertensive damage to renal parenchyma; functional interaction between aldosterone, renin, and erythropoietin; and inappropriate secretion of erythropoietin by the tumors. The mild polycythemia frequently observed in patients with Cushing syndrome may be caused by an excessive release of glucocorticoids.

The erythropoietic effect of androgens is of considerable practical importance. For many years, it was assumed that the higher red cell count in males was caused by androgens, but it was not until pharmacologic doses of testosterone were administered to women with carcinoma of the breast that the erythropoietic potency of androgens was appreciated.[93] Since then various androgen preparations have been used in the treatment of refractory anemias,[94,95] occasionally causing dramatic overshoots into the polycythemic range (Fig. 61-2).

The erythropoietic effect of androgens appears to be caused both by their capacity to stimulate erythropoietin production[96] and by their capacity to induce differentiation of marrow stem cells directly. These two effects have specific structural requirements. Androgens with the 5α-H configuration stimulate renal and extrarenal erythropoietin production, while androgens with the 5β-H configuration enhance the differentiation of stem cells.[96]

Neonatal Erythrocytosis   Erythrocytosis at birth is a normal physiologic response to intrauterine hypoxia and to the high oxygen affinity of fetal red cells (see Chaps. 7 and 28). However, it may become excessive and even symptomatic, especially in infants of diabetic mothers or if the clamping of the cord is delayed, permitting placental blood to boost the blood volume of the infant.[97] Since it is difficult to recognize symptoms of hyperviscosity in the neonate, many pediatricians perform a partial exchange transfusion if the venous hematocrit is above 65 percent at birth.[98]

APPARENT POLYCYTHEMIA

Some believe that apparent polycythemia is merely a mild absolute polycythemia accentuated by a compensatory reduction in plasma volume. Others suggest that it is caused by a primary reduction in plasma volume and have associated it with hypertension, obesity, and stress. Its clinical significance has also been disputed. The high hematocrit with its associated high viscosity is believed by some to be a risk factor heralding cerebral and cardiac complications, while others believe it is merely a well-tolerated blemish. Because the designation *apparent polycythemia*[99] is noncommittal, it is used here.

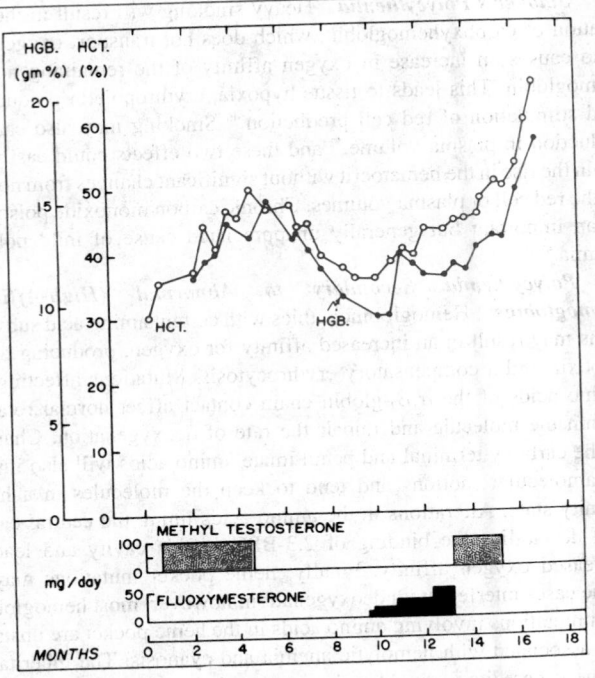

FIGURE 61-2   Erythropoietic response to testosterone derivatives in a patient with myelofibrosis.

The main clinical associations with apparent polycythemia are obesity, hypertension, and smoking. In obese patients the finding of a normal red cell volume may be spurious, since if the volume is expressed in terms of lean body weight, some of these patients would have a significant increase in red cell mass. In hypertensive patients there is no adequate explanation for the apparent increase in red cell production or decrease in plasma volume. Sleep apnea (common in patients with congestive failure), excessive production of atrial natriuretic factor, increased adrenal activation, decreased aldosterone secretion, and hypoxic vasoconstriction are all factors that have been invoked,[100–102] but with little enthusiasm. Chronic administration of diuretics to treat hypertension may be a more likely cause.[102]

CLINICAL FEATURES

POLYCYTHEMIA VERA

ONSET

Polycythemia vera usually has an insidious onset, most commonly during the sixth decade of life, although the onset may occur in childhood or in old age.[103] Presenting symptoms include headache, plethora, pruritus, thrombosis, and gastrointestinal bleeding, but some patients are diagnosed simply because abnormal blood counts are found on routine screening. Symptoms reported by at least 30 percent of patients with polycythemia, in approximate decreasing order of frequency, are headache, weakness, pruritus, dizziness, and sweating.[103]

THROMBOSIS AND HEMORRHAGE

Thrombotic episodes are the most common complications of polycythemia vera, occurring in about one-third of the patients.[104] These can be very serious, including episodes of hepatic vein thrombosis (Budd-Chiari syndrome), occurring in 10 percent of 140 patients in one series.[105] Over a period of 10 years, 40 to 60 percent of patients develop at least one thrombotic event, the annual incidence being approximately equal throughout this period.[106,107] The most common serious complication is a cerebrovascular accident, which accounts for about one-third of the thrombotic events, followed in frequency by myocardial infarction, deep-vein thrombosis, and pulmonary embolism.[106]

Bleeding and bruising, too, are common complications, being observed in about one-quarter of the patients.[104] While such episodes are usually minor, such as gingival bleeding or easy bruising, serious thrombotic complications with a fatal outcome also occur.

CUTANEOUS
Pruritus occurs in approximately 40 percent of patients.[108] It is usually aggravated by bathing or showering and may be so severe as to markedly compromise the quality of life of the patient. Its cause is unclear, and it has been attributed to increased numbers of mast cells in the skin[109] and to elevated histamine levels.[110]

GASTROINTESTINAL
The occurrence of Budd-Chiari syndrome has been noted above. Portal hypertension and varices are not uncommon.[111] The incidence of peptic ulcer is four to five times as great as in the general population.[112]

CARDIOVASCULAR
Cardiovascular symptoms include angina, myocardial infarction, and congestive heart failure.

NEUROLOGICAL
Neurological symptoms, such as dizziness are very common.[113] Neurological complications such as chorea[114] or the POEMS (polyneuropathy, organomegaly, endocrinopathy, M protein, and skin changes) syndrome (see Chap. 108)[115] have been reported in single cases. Spinal cord compression secondary to extramedullary hematopoiesis has been documented.[116]

OTHER ORGAN SYSTEMS
The increased nucleic acid turnover that results from the excessive proliferation of marrow cells often leads to an increase in blood uric acid concentration, and gout is a frequent complication. Several patients have developed the dermatological disorder, acute febrile neutrophilic dermatosis (Sweet syndrome).[117,118]

SURGERY
Over 75 percent of patients with uncontrolled polycythemia vera develop complications during or after major surgery because both bleeding and thrombosis are common.[119]

ASSOCIATION WITH OTHER DISEASES
Patients with both polycythemia vera and chronic lymphocytic leukemia[120,121] appear to have a relatively mild clinical course. An increased incidence of lymphocytic lymphomas has been documented.[106]

SECONDARY POLYCYTHEMIA

APPROPRIATE POLYCYTHEMIA
Tolerance to high altitudes varies greatly, but most normal individuals have no discomfort at altitudes of up to 2130 m (7000 ft). Above this level and especially if the ascent is rapid, some manifestations of cerebral hypoxia are common. Headaches, sleeplessness, and palpitations are frequently encountered, and weakness, nausea, vomiting, and mental dullness may be present. More severe manifestations include pulmonary and cerebral edema. Cheyne-Stokes respiration commonly

occurs, especially during sleep. These symptoms constitute the syndrome of *acute mountain sickness.*[122]

Ruddy cyanosis and physiologic emphysema are the two characteristic features of humans living at high altitudes. Venous and capillary engorgement can be observed readily in the conjunctiva, mucous membranes, and skin and may contribute to the remarkable capacity of Sherpas to walk barefoot and sleep on ice and snow.[123] Asymptomatic retinal hemorrhages are seen frequently at high altitudes but rarely at altitudes of 3000 m (9000 ft) or less.[124] Splenomegaly and jaundice are unusual, although the sustained erythrocytosis is associated with an increased rate of red cell destruction and bilirubin generation.

The polycythemia associated with smoking is generally asymptomatic, but there may be an increase in thrombotic events.[125]

INAPPROPRIATE POLYCYTHEMIA
Familial Erythrocytosis   Erythrocytosis may be very severe with hemoglobin levels of more than 20 g/dl. Headaches are commonly present. Hypertension, coronary artery disease, and strokes have been reported to occur[55] but are not a constant feature of the disorder.[57]

Renal Polycythemia   The erythrocytosis that occurs with renal polycythemia can be very severe with red counts as high as 8×10^{12}/liter having been reported and associated with hypertension and congestive failure.[126]

Tumors   The erythocytosis that occurs with tumors is generally mild,[85] and the predominating clinical manifestations are those of the tumor itself. Even moderate elevations to a hematocrit of 64 percent have been encountered without symptoms referable to the polycythemia.[82]

Neonatal   Of 55 infants with neonatal polycythemia, 85 percent had signs and symptoms attributed to this disorder. These included "feeding problems" (21.8%), plethora (20.0%), lethargy (14.5%), cyanosis (14.5%), respiratory distress (9.1%), jitteriness (7.3%), and hypotonia (7.3%). Other findings included hypoglycemia (40.0%) and hyperbilirubinemia (21.8%). In a larger group of nearly 1000 infants, 6 had an intracranial hemorrhage.[97]

LABORATORY FEATURES

POLYCYTHEMIA VERA

MARROW
The marrow is characteristically hypercellular, with involvement of all lineages. There are no characteristic cytogenetic findings, but occasional clonal abnormalities are observed (Chap. 10).

ERYTHROCYTES
The erythrocyte count is usually increased, and in patients who have undergone phlebotomy or who have had gastrointestinal bleeding episodes it may be increased out of proportion to the increase in the hemoglobin and hematocrit, since there will be marked hypochromia and microcytosis. The plasma iron in such patients is decreased, the iron binding capacity increased, and plasma ferritin levels are low. The red cell mass is usually increased in proportion to the hematocrit value (Fig. 61-3).

In late stages of the disease the morphologic changes that are characteristic of myelofibrosis are present, with marked aniso- and poikilocytosis and abundant tear-drop cells (dacrocytes) (see Chap. 22). Alterations in red cell glycolytic metabolism have been documented[127,128] but are not unique nor of any diagnostic value.

The P_{O_2} of the arterial blood is often lower than normal, and levels as low as 63 torr were encountered in more than 10 percent of patients, and the percent saturation with oxygen was accordingly slightly reduced.[129]

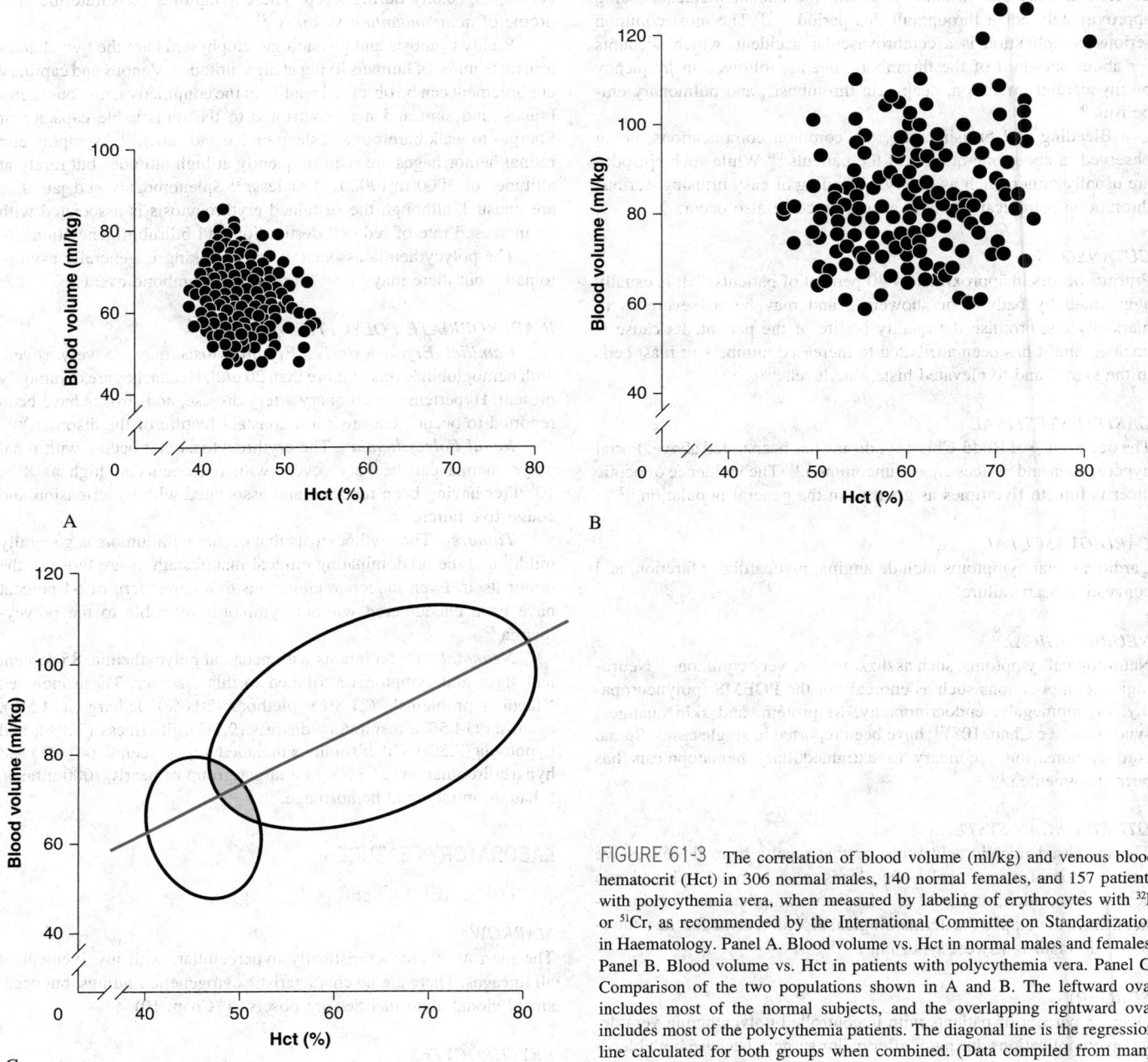

FIGURE 61-3   The correlation of blood volume (ml/kg) and venous blood hematocrit (Hct) in 306 normal males, 140 normal females, and 157 patients with polycythemia vera, when measured by labeling of erythrocytes with ^{32}P or ^{51}Cr, as recommended by the International Committee on Standardization in Haematology. Panel A. Blood volume vs. Hct in normal males and females. Panel B. Blood volume vs. Hct in patients with polycythemia vera. Panel C. Comparison of the two populations shown in A and B. The leftward oval includes most of the normal subjects, and the overlapping rightward oval includes most of the polycythemia patients. The diagonal line is the regression line calculated for both groups when combined. (Data compiled from many sources by Fairbanks, et al.[192-195])

LEUKOCYTES

An absolute neutrophilia occurs in about two-thirds of the patients.[103] Occasional myelocytes and metamyelocytes are often present in the blood, and considerable degrees of immaturity are often present in patients with long-standing, advanced disease. Basophilia occurs in about two-thirds of patients with uncontrolled disease.[130] Serum lysozyme levels are slightly increased in some patients,[131] and because of the increased leukocyte turnover, levels of vitamin B_{12} are usually increased.[132] The leukocyte alkaline phosphate level is elevated in about 70 percent of patients with polycythemia vera.[103] Selective abnormalities in granulocyte chemoluminescent response to some agonists, e.g., leukotriene B_2, but not to others, e.g., phorbol myristate acetate, have been reported,[133] but there is no indication that patients with the disease have increased susceptibility to infection.

PLATELETS

The platelet count is increased in about one-half of patients at the time of diagnosis, and in about 10 percent it is over $1,000,000/\mu l$.[103] In contrast to normal individuals, where phlebotomy results in an increase in the platelet count, platelet levels are not affected by phlebotomy of patients with polycythemia vera.[134] There are no consistent abnormalities of thrombopoietin levels.[135]

Qualitative abnormalities of the platelets have been described. Patients with polycythemia vera, essential thrombocythemia, and other myeloproliferative disorders have a very unusual, nearly pathognomic defect in the primary wave of platelet aggregation induced by epinephrine.[136] In contrast there is increased platelet thromboxane A_2 generation[137] and increased excretion of thromboxane metabolites,[138] even though the response to thromboxane A_2 may be subnormal.[139] Platelet factor 4 levels are elevated,[140] and platelet survival is normal[141] or shortened.[134,140] Fibrinogen binding after stimulation with platelet activating factor is diminished,[142] and there is reduced expression of the thrombopoietin receptor.[20]

The prothrombin time, partial prothrombin time, and fibrinogen level are usually normal, but fibrinogen turnover may, at times, be increased.[143]

SECONDARY POLYCYTHEMIA

Characteristically only the numbers of erythrocytes in the blood are increased. Increase in the leukocyte count may be present as another feature of the underlying disease, e.g., the pulmonary infection in chronic obstructive lung disease. In patients with appropriate polycythemia the underlying defect is usually demonstrable. Arterial hypoxia can be demonstrated in most cases. However, some obese patients who, like Mr. Wardle's proverbial boy, Joe, are always half asleep, will be very much awake when exposed to arterial punctures and ventilatory testing, and their apprehensive hyperventilation will cause the disappearance of all abnormalities in arterial gas composition. As soon as they return to bed, however, they will go to sleep again and display the characteristic somnolent cyanosis. In inappropriate polycythemia the laboratory findings will be those of the underlying defect.

DIFFERENTIAL DIAGNOSIS

Polycythemia vera must be distinguished from secondary polycythemia and from apparent polycythemia. Some of the differences are summarized in Table 61-2.

POLYCYTHEMIA VERA

The most important diagnostic features of polycythemia vera are *erythrocytosis, leukocytosis, thrombocytosis,* and *splenomegaly*. Frequently only two or three of these features are found at presentation and if sufficiently pronounced suffice to establish the diagnosis. In some patients only one of these features is found initially, most commonly the erythrocytosis, but occasionally only thrombocytosis, leukocytosis, or splenomegaly. Such patients represent more difficult diagnostic challenges. A subset of patients with erythrocytosis as the only manifestation of unregulated proliferation of the erythron do not develop the other features of polycythemia vera, even after they have been followed for many years.[144,145] Such patients have been designated as manifesting *pure erythrocytosis* or *idiopathic erythrocytosis*.[146] Some patients who are classified in this way eventually develop typical polycythemia vera; this seems to be true in about one-half of the patients after several years. However, some patients have been observed for periods as long as 8 or 10 years without a change in their clinical state.[145–147] Studies of red cell precursors suggest that patients who have been diagnosed as having pure erythrocytosis can be divided into two groups of about equal size, those with EPO-independent BFU-E and those without such precursors.[145,147] It is possible that pure erythrocytosis is a distinct entity but that some of the patients who meet the criteria for this diagnosis actually have polycythemia vera.

Other clinical features that may be helpful in arriving at a diagnosis include the presence of elevated vitamin B_{12} levels, elevated serum uric acid levels, normal or near-normal arterial oxygen saturations, and pruritus.

TABLE 61-2   TYPICAL LABORATORY FINDINGS IN PATIENTS WITH POLYCYTHEMIA VERA, SECONDARY POLYCYTHEMIA, AND RELATIVE POLYCYTHEMIA

FINDINGS*	POLYCYTHEMIA VERA	SECONDARY POLYCYTHEMIA	APPARENT POLYCYTHEMIA
Splenomegaly	Present	Absent	Absent
Leukocytosis	Present	Absent	Absent
Thrombocytosis	Present	Absent	Absent
Abnormal primary wave of epinephrine-induced platelet aggregation	Present	Absent	Absent
Red blood cell volume	Increased	Increased	Normal
Arterial oxygen saturation	Normal	Decreased or normal	Normal
Serum vitamin B_{12}	Increased	Normal	Normal
Leukocyte alkaline phosphatase	Increased	Normal	Normal
Marrow	Panhyperplasia	Erythroid hyperplasia	Normal
EPO level	Decreased	Increased	Normal
Endogenous CFU-E growth	Present	Absent	Absent

*The differences listed are not present in all patients.

Since polycythemia is distinguished by the fact that erythroid cells proliferate even in the absence of substantial levels of EPO, one would expect that at high hematocrit levels the production of EPO would be inhibited and the serum levels consequently reduced. Overlapping values are frequently observed.[148,149] With more sensitive assay methods it has been reported that quite reliable differentiation of polycythemia vera from secondary and relative polycythemia can be achieved.[150–152] Another potential approach to diagnosis is to demonstrate the presence of a population of erythroid progenitors that proliferates in the absence of EPO.[18,147,153–155] There are occasional cases in which such colonies do not form, particularly when blood rather than marrow is examined[156] and when cytotoxic treatment has been administered.[147]

The Polycythemia Vera Study Group has employed the direct determination of the red cell mass as the *sine qua non* of the diagnosis of polycythemia vera in patients entered into their studies.[106] It has been suggested that even in the routine clinical setting, this procedure should be performed on all patients to establish this diagnosis.[106] Unfortunately, the determination of the red cell mass is expensive and, when performed by the inexperienced, often inaccurate.[157] It is not useful in distinguishing polycythemia vera from secondary polycythemia, the differentiation that is usually needed, because red cell mass is increased in both disorders. The principal value of a red cell mass determination might then be to distinguish apparent or spurious polycythemia from polycythemia vera and secondary polycythemia. Fortunately, in most cases the diagnosis of polycythemia vera can be established with confidence without measuring the red cell volume.

SECONDARY POLYCYTHEMIA

Patients with secondary polycythemia, like those with polycythemia vera, have a genuine increase in the number of circulating erythrocytes and of the red cell mass. However, in secondary polycythemia the increase in the red cell mass is a response to the stimulation of the marrow by EPO or the abnormal functioning of a mutant EPO receptor. Such patients do not have the increase in the platelet count and leukocyte count or the splenomegaly that is characteristic of polycythemia vera, and it is the lack of involvement of other formed elements in hematopoietic proliferation that should arouse suspicion that the patient may have secondary polycythemia. In patients in whom the cause of the secondary polycythemia is lung or cardiac disease, clubbing is often present. In some cases determining the arterial oxygen saturation will often clarify the diagnosis, but modest arterial oxygen saturation may also be present in polycythemia vera.[36,129] Imaging of the kidneys may reveal a neoplasm or cyst in some patients. Determining the oxygen dissociation curve will detect abnormalities related to increased oxygen affinity, either because of 2,3-BPG depletion, as in phosphoglyceromutase deficiency (see Chap. 45) or because of inheritance of a high-affinity hemoglobin. The nature of the polycythemia in such patients is also sometimes apparent because of the familial nature of the disorder; polycythemia due to a high-affinity hemoglobin is inherited as an autosomal dominant disorder. It may also be useful to determine the carboxyhemoglobin level of the blood if smoker's polycythemia is suspected. Sequence analysis of the EPO receptor will define the defect in most patients with hereditary erythrocytosis.

SPURIOUS POLYCYTHEMIA

The erythrocytosis observed in patients with spurious polycythemia (apparent polycythemia, stress polycythemia) is a consequence of a decrease in the plasma volume.[99] The erythrocytosis that is observed does not represent a true increase in the red cell mass. Usually the increase in the hematocrit is very modest. Such patients do not have an increased white blood count, thrombocytosis, or splenomegaly. The arterial oxygen saturation is normal. The estimation of the red cell mass is required to establishing a diagnosis of spurious polycythemia, but it must be recognized that during the natural history of patients who develop primary or secondary polycythemia their red cell mass is, at some point, within the normal range while it is rising to abnormal values.

THERAPY, COURSE, AND PROGNOSIS

POLYCYTHEMIA VERA

Polycythemia vera usually remains in a plethoric phase for many years, after which a "spent" phase characterized by falling red cell counts and progressive splenomegaly supervenes.

THE PLETHORIC PHASE

The treatment of patients in the plethoric phase of the disease is aimed at ameliorating symptoms and decreasing the risk of thrombosis or bleeding by reducing the blood counts. The red count and hematocrit can be controlled in some patients by periodic phlebotomy, while the administration of drugs that suppress marrow activity is required also to control the platelet count and white count. In most patients both treatment modalities are used. The advantages and disadvantages of various forms of therapy are summarized in Table 61-3.

TABLE 61-3　TREATMENT OF POLYCYTHEMIA VERA

TREATMENT	ADVANTAGES	DISADVANTAGES
Phlebotomy	Low Risk. Simple to perform.	Does not control thrombocytosis or leukocytosis.
Hydroxyurea	Controls leukocytosis and thrombocytosis. Low leukemogenic risk.	Continuous therapy required.
Busulfan	Easy to administer. Prolonged remissions. Risk of leukemogenesis probably not high.	Overdose produces prolonged marrow suppression. Risks of leukemogenesis, long-term pulmonary and cutaneous toxicity.
^{32}P	Patient compliance not required. Prolonged control of thrombocytosis and leukocytosis.	Expensive and relatively inconvenient. Moderate leukemogenic risk.
Chlorambucil	Easy to administer. Good control of thrombocytosis and leukocytosis.	High risk of leukemogenesis.
Interferon	Low leukemogenic potential. Effect on pruritus.	Inconvenient, costly, frequent side effects.
Anagrelide	Selective effect on platelets.	Selective effect on platelets.

Phlebotomy　The initial treatment for most patients is phlebotomy. The hematocrit may be reduced to normal or near-normal values by the removal of 450 to 500 ml of blood at intervals of 2 to 4 days for the average-size patients, with smaller amounts being removed from patients who weigh less than 50 kg. The shorter interval is appropriate for patients with hematocrits that are over 64 percent, while less energetic bleeding suffices for those who have only a modest increase in their hematocrit. Patients with impaired cardiovascular functions are better treated with smaller phlebotomies at more frequent intervals.

The immediate effect of phlebotomies is to reduce the hematocrit, which results in improvement of symptoms such as headaches. It neither reduces the leukocyte or platelet count nor affects symptoms such as pruritus or gout. Iron deficiency is the usual consequence of repeated phlebotomy. The deficient state helps to control the hematocrit; when iron is administered to polycythemia vera patients who have been rendered iron deficient by phlebotomy, a dramatic rise of the hemoglobin level and hematocrit usually occurs. The iron deficiency that results from repeated phlebotomies causes striking microcytosis, but the viscosity of the blood is a function of the hematocrit and appears to be independent of the number of red cells,[158] and the deformability of iron-deficient erythrocytes appears to be normal[159]; phlebotomy clearly is an effective way in which to normalize the viscosity of the blood of patients with polycythemia vera.

A randomized study[106,160] comparing phlebotomy alone with treatment with ^{32}P and with chlorambucil indicated that the life span of patients treated only with phlebotomy is better than that of patients treated with chlorambucil and no worse than the life span of those given ^{32}P. Early in their course patients undergoing phlebotomy suffered more thrombotic episodes, but this was balanced by a lower incidence of leukemia late in their course. Surprisingly, there was no correlation between the level of the platelet count and the development of thrombotic complications. Apparently many patients can be well controlled by phlebotomy alone during much or all of their course, and the role of myelosuppressive therapy in the treatment of polycythemia vera has sometimes been questioned.[161] It has been suggested that patients under the age of 50 who have no prior history of thrombosis might be treated with phlebotomy alone.[162]

Myelosuppression　Although treatment with myelosuppressive agents appears to increase the incidence of leukemic transformation of patients with polycythemia vera, patients are usually treated with such drugs when the platelet count rises to levels of higher than 800,000 to 1,000,000/μl. Platelet counts at these levels usually cause concern about the risk of bleeding and thrombosis. Myelosuppressive therapy is also considered when thrombotic or bleeding complications occur, when the patient requires phlebotomy at intervals exceeding one every month or two, and in patients with severe pruritus.

Hydroxyurea (Hydrea)　Hydroxyurea is probably the most commonly used myelosuppressive agent used in the treatment of polycythemia vera. Its suppressive effect is of short duration. Thus, continuous rather than intermittent therapy is required. Because hydroxyurea is short-acting, it is relatively safe to use; when excessive marrow suppression occurs, the blood counts rise within a few days or weeks of discontinuing the drug. Moreover, because it is not an alkylating agent, it is believed to have much less potential for causing leukemic transformation than other myelosuppressive agents. When used in conjunction with phlebotomy, the incidence of thrombotic complications appeared to be decreased, and after about 7 years' maximum follow-up the incidence of leukemia was slightly higher than that in patients treated with phlebotomy alone, but not significantly so.[163] Experience in the use of hydroxyurea in the treatment of essential thrombocythemia has suggested a leukemogenic risk of about 3.5 percent.[164,165]

Busulfan (Myleran)   The administration of busulfan is a convenient and effective means for the treatment of polycythemia vera. Marrow suppression produced by this drug is long-lasting, and as a consequence it can be given intermittently. The administration of 2 or 4 mg daily over a period of several weeks is usually sufficient to normalize the blood counts; the counts continue to fall for several weeks after drug administration is discontinued. The counts may then remain normal for many months or even years. In one large study the median first remission duration of busulfan-treated patients was 4 years.[166]

The prolonged depression of marrow activity that is brought about by busulfan is its major advantage in the treatment of polycythemia vera, but it also poses a hazard. If therapy is continued too long or given at too high a dose, the marrow suppression that results may persist for many months or even a year. For this reason it is safer not to exceed a daily dose of 4 mg but to extend the period of treatment rather than to increase the daily dose. The incidence of transformation to acute leukemia in patients treated intermittently with busulfan is relatively low. Of 145 patients followed from 2 to 11 years, only 3 developed acute leukemia.[166]

Radioactive Phosphorus ^{32}P therapy was one of the first effective modes of treatment used. Extensive investigations of the long-term outcome of treatment with ^{32}P have been documented.[106,167] Good control of the disease usually can be achieved with initial doses of 2 to 4 mC of ^{32}P given intravenously, followed in 6 to 8 weeks by doses that are based upon the response to the first dose. ^{32}P treatment is associated with a moderate increase in the incidence of leukemic transformation, similar in magnitude to that observed with busulfan.[166] Since the treatment is administered directly by a physician, it is more suitable than busulfan for patients who cannot be relied upon to take their medication as prescribed. However, the logistics of ^{32}P administration have made it an inconvenient and expensive mode of therapy. Consultation with a radiotherapist is usually required, and each dose must be ordered especially for the patient. It is largely for this reason and because it is generally supposed that the leukemogenic potential of hydroxyurea is lower than that of radioactive phosphorus, that the latter has been used less frequently. Some investigators, however, consider radioactive phosphorus the treatment of choice, especially among older patients.[168,169]

Interferon   Administration of recombinant interferon α (rIFN-α) at a starting dose of 3 million units given 3 times weekly, produces a therapeutic response in 50 percent[170] or more[171,172] of patients with polycythemia vera. A decrease in the red cell mass, the leukocyte count, and the platelet count has been documented, and it seems effective in ameliorating the pruritus that is common in polycythemia vera. Indeed, the amelioration of the pruritus does not seem directly related to the hematologic response.[172] It is not clear whether this treatment, which requires frequent injections of a drug that causes toxicity that is troublesome to the patients, has any advantage over less costly, more convenient therapies. However, the possibility exists that the incidence both of leukemia and myelofibrosis may be lower in interferon-treated patients.[172]

Pipobroman (Vercyte)   Although it was described in the early 1960s and appears to be effective in controlling polycythemia vera, pipobroman has not been used as frequently as has ^{32}P, busulfan, or hydroxyurea. However, it remains in active use in some countries.[173,174] Hematologic remission is achieved in over 90 percent of previously untreated patients[175,176] and is maintained for long periods of time. Gastrointestinal intolerance can be a problem.[137,174] The risk of leukemia is relatively high, being observed in 6 percent and 9 percent of patients at 5 and 7 years of treatment and in 27 percent at 14 years in one study.[174]

Anagrelide (Agrelin)   Among 113 patients with polycythemia vera who had thrombocytosis, administration of anagrelide produced a platelet response in 85 (75%).[177] It was suggested that the higher rates of response might be expected when the drug was administered by those more skilled in its use. The starting dose was 0.5 or 1.0 mg given four times daily, and a response was noted in most patients within a week. The average dose required to control the platelet count was 2.4 mg per day. Adverse events included headache, palpitations, diarrhea, and fluid retention and were occasionally sufficiently severe to require discontinuation of the treatment.

Symptomatic Therapy   Many of the symptoms of polycythemia are controlled either by phlebotomy or by controlling the number of circulating blood cells with myelosuppressive therapy. Pruritus is a frequent exception. It tends to be more severe when the disease is active and becomes milder or disappears when control is achieved by myelosuppression. Nonetheless, in some patients it becomes a nearly intolerable annoyance. Since the itching is usually intensified by bathing or showering, often the best advice that can be offered is to bathe less frequently.

Photochemotherapy with psoralens and ultraviolet light has been found to be helpful.[178] Antihistamines are usually not very effective. Aspirin[179] and cyproheptadine[130] have each been recommended. Interferon alpha has been helpful in some patients.[170,171,180]

Since thromboembolic episodes represent a major source of morbidity and mortality in patients with polycythemia, attempts using aspirin and dipyridamole to prevent such episodes have been made. The results of early trials using 300 mg of aspirin daily have been an increase in the incidence of bleeding without a favorable impact on the incidence of thrombotic episodes.[181] The administration of low-dose aspirin has been suggested in patients who have a vascular occlusion.[182] A pilot controlled trial showed that low-dose aspirin was well tolerated by polycythemia vera patients,[183] but the efficacy of this approach has not been shown in any controlled studies.

Since dehydration may be a precipitating factor for thrombosis, patients should be kept well hydrated when they develop intercurrent gastrointestinal disorders.

THE SPENT PHASE

Ultimately, sometimes after only a few years and sometimes after 20 or more, the erythrocytosis of patients with polycythemia who have not succumbed to other complications gradually abates, and anemia develops. During this ''spent'' phase of the disease, marrow fibrosis becomes more marked, and the spleen often becomes greatly enlarged. Instead of phlebotomies, transfusions now may be required. The platelet count may remain high or may decline, even to thrombocytopenic levels. Marked leukocytosis may occur with the appearance of immature granulocytes in the blood. Treatment of this phase of the disease is almost entirely symptomatic. Irradiation of the spleen is usually not helpful, and the use of chemotherapy with busulfan or hydroxyurea is precluded by the advancing thrombocytopenia. Occasionally splenectomy may be warranted, particularly if there is severe thrombocytopenia, if the transfusion requirement becomes very high, or if a greatly enlarged spleen produces severe physical discomfort.[184] Usually periodic transfusions are the only possible treatment, although a few younger patients have undergone marrow transplantation.[185]

PROGNOSIS

Polycythemia vera is a disease that is compatible with normal or near-normal life for many years. However, ultimately leukemia may develop or the disease enters the spent phase. Leukemia occurs even in patients who have been treated only by phlebotomy, although its incidence is increased somewhat by the various forms of cytotoxic therapy that have been employed (Table 61-3). While acute myeloid leukemia is most common, acute lymphoid leukemia[186] and neutrophilic leukemia[187] have been documented as well.

The Polycythemia Vera Study Group[106] found that the median survival from the beginning of treatment was 13.9 years for those treated by phlebotomy alone, 11.8 years for ^{32}P-treated patients, and 8.9 years for chlorambucil-treated patients. Thrombosis was the most common cause of death, accounting for 31 percent of the fatalities. Nineteen percent of the patients died of acute leukemia, 15 percent from other neoplasms, and about 5 percent each from hemorrhage or the development of the spent phase. Similarly a large French study revealed a median survival of 13.5 years of polycythemia vera patients initially treated with ^{32}P, only slightly less than the 15.2 years of age-matched controls.[172]

SECONDARY POLYCYTHEMIA

The clinical course of secondary polycythemia is largely a function of the severity of the erythrocytosis. This can be quite marked with hemoglobin levels in excess of 20 g/(dl) in patients with dominant familial erthrocytosis secondary to mutations of the HFE gene, and in such patients hypertension, coronary artery disease, and strokes have been reported,[55] although not in all series.[57] The apparently recessive erythrocytosis that is endemic in Chuvashia is characterized by elevations of the hemoglobin level to a mean of 22.6 with a standard deviation of 1.4 g/dl.[58] Most of the patients are symptomatic with headache and fatigue and with signs including clubbing, thrombosis, and peptic ulcer. Eleven of the 103 patients died at ages ranging from 16 to 58 years of age during a 10-year period. The milder erythrocytosis that is associated with abnormal hemoglobins and with tumors is often asymptomatic or associated with only mild symptoms.

The morbidity that attends marked erythrocytosis is presumably related to the increase in blood viscosity.[188] The blood viscosity increases very rapidly as levels rise beyond 50 percent (see Fig. 30-2). Therefore, lowering the hematocrit to a normal or near-normal level by phlebotomy is the usual treatment.[59,189] The appropriate level is that at which the patient becomes asymptomatic.[45,190] Although cytotoxic agents are sometimes used for this purpose, phlebotomy is preferred because of the leukemogenic risk of the agents that are used in polycythemia vera. Theophylline and enalapril have been used to lower the hematocrit of patients with polycythemia following renal transplantation,[68–70] and theophylline has been given to patients with chronic obstructive lung disease.[191] These drugs apparently exert their beneficial effect by lowering erythropoietin levels.

When erythrocytosis is secondary to a renal tumor or cyst, to a myoma, or to a brain tumor, removal of the neoplasm has usually resulted in disappearance of the erythrocytosis.

REFERENCES

1. Vaquez MH: Sur une forme spéciale de cyanose s'accompagnant d'hyperglobulie excessive et persistante. *CR Soc Biol* 44:384, 1892.
2. Osler W: Chronic cyanosis, with polycythemia and enlarged spleen: a new clinical entity. *Am J Med Sci* 126:187, 1903.
3. Türk W: Beitrage zur Kenntnis des Symptomenbildes Polycythamie mit Milztumor und Zyanose. *Wien Klin Wochenschr* 17:153, 1904.
4. Bert P: La Pression Barometrique. Paris, Masson, 1878.
5. Jourdanet D: *De l'anemie des altitudes et de l'anemie en general dans ses rapports avec la pression l'atmosphere*, Bailliere, Paris, 1863.
6. Viault F: Sur l'augmentation considerable du nombre des globules rouges dans le sang chez les habitants des hauts plateaux de l'Amrique du Sud. *CR Acad Sci* 111:917, 1890.
7. Erslev AJ: Blood and mountains, in *Blood, Pure and Eloquent*, p 257. McGraw-Hill, New York, 1980.
8. Leopold SS: The etiology of pulmonary arteriosclerosis (Ayerza's syndrome). *Am J Med* 219:152, 1950.
9. Abbott ME: *Atlas of Congenital Heart Disease*. American Heart Association, New York, 1936.
10. Burwell CS, Robin ED, Whaley RD, Bickelman AG: Extreme obesity associated with alveolar hypoventilation: A Pickwickian syndrome. *Am J Med* 21:811, 1956.
11. Kuhl W: History of clinical research on the sleep apnea syndrome. The early days of polysomnography. *Respiration* 1:5–10:5, 1997.
12. Charache S, Weatherall DJ, Clegg JB: Polycythemia associated with a hemoglobinopathy. *J Clin Invest* 45:813, 1966.
13. El-Yousef MK, Bakewell WEJ: The Gaisbock syndrome. *JAMA* 220:864, 1972.
14. Lawrence JH, Berlin NI: Relative polycythemia—the polycythemia of stress. *Yale J Biol Med* 24:498, 1952.
15. Adamson JW, Fialkow PJ, Murphy S, Prchal JF, Steinmann L: Polycythemia vera: Stem-cell and probable clonal origin of the disease. *N Engl J Med* 295:913, 1976.
16. Prchal JF, Adamson JW, Murphy S, Steinmann L, Fialkow PJ: Polycythemia vera. The in vitro response of normal and abnormal stem cell lines to erythropoietin. *J Clin Invest* 61:1044, 1978.
17. Eaves CJ, Eaves AC: Erythropoietin (Ep) dose-response curves for three classes of erythroid progenitors in normal human marrow and in patients with polycythemia vera. *Blood* 52:1196, 1978.
18. Reid CD, Fidler J, Kirk A: Endogenous erythroid clones (EEC) in polycythaemia and their relationship to diagnosis and the response to treatment. *Br J Haematol* 68:395, 1988.
19. Dai CH, Krantz SB, Dessypris EN, Means RT Jr., Horn ST, Gilbert HS: Polycythemia vera: II. Hypersensitivity of bone marrow erythroid, granulocyte-macrophage, and megakaryocyte progenitor cells to interleukin-3 and granulocyte-macrophage colony-stimulating factor. *Blood* 80:891, 1992.
20. Moliterno AR, Hankins WD, Spivak JL: Impaired expression of the thrombopoietin receptor by platelets from patients with polycythemia vera. *N Engl J Med* 338:572, 1998.
21. Silva M, Richard C, Benito A, Sanz C, Olalla I, Fernandez-Luna JL: Expression of Bcl-x in erythroid precursors from patients with polycythemia vera. *N Engl J Med* 338:564, 1998.
22. Sui X, Krantz SB, Zhao Z: Identification of increased protein tyrosine phosphatase activity in polycythemia vera erythroid progenitor cells. *Blood* 90:651, 1997.
23. Groopman JE: The pathogenesis of myelofibrosis in myeloproliferative disorders. *Ann Intern Med* 92:857, 1980.
24. Wurster-Hill D, Whang-Peng J, McIntyre OR, et al: Cytogenetic studies in polycythemia vera. *Semin Hematol* 13:13, 1976.
25. Diez-Martin JL, Graham DL, Petitt RM, Dewald GW: Chromosome studies in 104 patients with polycythemia vera. *Mayo Clin Proc* 66:287, 1991.
26. Miller RL, Purvis JD, Weick JK: Familial polycythemia vera. *Cleve Clin J Med* 56:813, 1989.
27. Chaiter Y, Brenner B, Aghai E, Tatarsky I: High incidence of myeloproliferative disorders in Ashkenazi Jews in northern Israel. *Leuk Lymphoma* 7:251, 1992.
28. Modan B, Kallner H, Zemer D, Yoran C: A note on the increased risk of polycythemia vera in Jews. *Blood* 37:172, 1971.
29. Modan B: An epidemiological study of polycythemia vera. *Blood* 26:657, 1965.
30. Berglund S, Zettervall O: Incidence of polycythemia vera in a defined population. *Eur J Haematol* 48:20, 1992.
31. Hurtado A: Acclimatization of high altitudes, in *Physiological Effects of High Altitude*, edited by WH Weihe, p 1. Macmillan, New York, 1964.
32. Moore LG, Brewer GJ: Beneficial effect of rightward hemoglobin-oxygen dissociation curve shift for short-term high-altitude adaptation. *J Lab Clin Med* 98:145, 1981.
33. Finch CA, Lenfant C: Oxygen transport in man. *N Engl J Med* 286:407, 1972.
34. Winslow RM, Monge CC, Statham NJ, et al: Variability of oxygen affinity of blood: human subjects native to high altitude. *J Appl Physiol* 51:1411, 1981.

35. Eaton JW, Skelton TD, Berger E: Survival at extreme altitude: protective effect of increased hemoglobin-oxygen affinity. *Science* 183:743, 1974.

36. Murray JF: Classification of polycythemic disorders. With comments on the diagnostic value of arterial blood oxygen analysis. *Ann Intern Med* 64:892, 1966.

37. Flenley DC: Chronic obstructive pulmonary disease. *Dis Mon* 34:537, 1988.

38. Limthongkul S, Wongthim S, Udompanich V, Charoenlap P, Nuchprayoon C: Chronic obstructive pulmonary disease at Chulalongkorn Hospital: an analysis of 400 episodes. *J Med Assoc Thai* 74:639, 1991.

39. Block AJ, Boysen PG, Wynne JW, Hunt LA: Sleep apnea, hypopnea and oxygen desaturation in normal subjects. A strong male predominance. *N Engl J Med* 300:513, 1979.

40. Moore-Gillon JC, Treacher DF, Gaminara EJ, Pearson TC, Cameron IR: Intermittent hypoxia in patients with unexplained polycythaemia. *Br Med J (Clin Res Ed)* 293:588, 1986.

41. Rodman T, Close HP: The primary hypoventilation syndrome. *Am J Med* 26:808, 1959.

42. Fishman AP, Turino GO, Bevgofsky EF: The syndrome of alveolar hypoventilation. *Am J Med* 23:233, 1957.

43. Alexander JK, Amad KH, Cole VW: Observations on some clinical features of extreme obesity with particular reference to cardio-respiratory effects. *Am J Med* 32:512, 1962.

44. Hsu AA, Staats BA: "Postpolio" sequelae and sleep-related disordered breathing. *Mayo Clin Proc* 73:216, 1998.

45. Vongpatanasin W, Brickner ME, Hillis LD, Lange RA: The Eisenmenger syndrome in adults. *Ann Intern Med* 128:745, 1998.

46. Smith JR, Landaw A: Smokers' polycythemia. *N Engl J Med* 298:6, 1978.

47. Stonesifer LD: How carbon monoxide reduces plasma volume [letter]. *N Engl J Med* 299:311, 1978.

48. Aitchison R, Russell N: Smoking—a major cause of polycythemia. *J Roy Soc Med* 81:89, 1998.

49. Galactéros F, Rosa R, Prehu M-O, Najean Y, Calvin M-C: Deficit en diphosphoglycerate mutase: Nouveaux cas associés à une polyglobulie. *Nouv Rev Fr Hematol* 26:69, 1984.

50. Vora S, Corash L, Engel WK, Durham S, Seaman C, Piomelli S: The molecular mechanism of the inherited phosphofructokinase deficiency associated with hemolysis and myopathy. *Blood* 55:629, 1980.

51. Roos D, van Zwieten R, Wijnen JTh, et al: Molecular basis and enzymatic properties of glucose-6-phosphate dehydrogenase Volendam, leading to chronic nonspherocytic anemia, granulocyte dysfunction and increased susceptibility to infections. *Blood* 94:2955, 1999.

52. Gardner FH: The use of cobaltous chloride in the anemia associated with chronic renal disease. *N Engl J Med* 41:56, 1998.

53. Sokol L, Luhovy M, Guan Y, Prchal JF, Semenza GL, Prchal JT: Primary familial polycythemia: a frameshift mutation in the erythropoietin receptor gene and increased sensitivity of erythroid progenitors to erythropoietin. *Blood* 86:15, 1995.

54. Kralovics R, Indrak K, Stopka T, Berman BW, Prchal JF, Prchal JT: Two new EPO receptor mutations: truncated EPO receptors are most frequently associated with primary familial and congenital polycythemias. *Blood* 90:2057, 1997.

55. Kralovics R, Sokol L, Prchal JT: Absence of polycythemia in a child with a unique erythropoietin receptor mutation in a family with autosomal dominant primary polycythemia. *J Clin Invest* 102:124, 1998.

56. Furukawa T, Narita M, Sakaue M, et al: Primary familial polycythaemia associated with a novel point mutation in the erythropoietin receptor. *Br J Haematol* 99:222, 1997.

57. Arcasoy MO, Degar BA, Harris KW, Forget BG: Familial erythrocytosis associated with a short deletion in the erythropoietin receptor gene. *Blood* 89:4628, 1997.

58. Sergeyeva A, Gordeuk VR, Tokarev YN, Sokol L, Prchal JF, Prchal JT: Congenital polycythemia in Chuvashia. *Blood* 89:2148, 1997.

59. Manglani MV, DeGroff CG, Dukes PP, Ettinger LJ: Congenital erythrocytosis with elevated erythropoietin level: an incorrectly set "erythrostat"? *J Pediatr Hematol Oncol* 20:560, 1998.

60. Bailey RR, Shand BI, Walker RJ: Reversible erythrocytosis in a patient with a hydronephrotic horseshoe kidney. *Nephron* 70:104, 1995.

61. Hammond D, Winnick S: Paraneoplastic erythrocytosis and ectopic erythropoietins. *Ann N Y Acad Sci* 230:219–27:219, 1974.

62. Navarro J, Aguilera A, Liano F, Pascual J, Ortuno J: Phlebotomy for polycythemia associated with acquired cystic renal disease in a patient on hemodialysis. *Nephron* 62:110, 1992.

63. Thorling EB: Paraneoplastic erythrocytosis and inappropriate erythropoietin production. A review. *Scand J Haematol* suppl 17:1, 1972.

64. Da Silva JL, Lacombe C, Bruneval P, et al: Tumor cells are the site of erythropoietin synthesis in human renal cancers associated with polycythemia. *Blood* 75:577, 1990.

65. Lal A, Rice A, al Mahr M, Kern IB, Marshall GM: Wilms tumor associated with polycythemia: case report and review of the literature. *J Pediatr Hematol Oncol* 19:263, 1997.

66. Grignon DJ, Eble JN: Papillary and metanephric adenomas of the kidney. *Semin Diagn Pathol* 15:41, 1998.

67. Wickre CG, Norman DJ, Bennison A, Barry JM, Bennett WM: Postrenal transplant erythrocytosis: a review of 53 patients. *Kidney Int* 23:731, 1983.

68. Bakris GL, Sauter ER, Hussey JL, Fisher JW, Gaber AO, Winsett R: Effects of theophylline on erythropoietin production in normal subjects and in patients with erythrocytosis after renal transplantation. *N Engl J Med* 323:86, 1990.

69. Islam MS, Bourbigot B, Codet JP, Songy B, Fournier G, Cledes J: Captopril induces correction of postrenal transplant erythremia. *Transpl Int* 3:222, 1990.

70. Mazzali M, Filho GA: Use of aminophylline and enalapril in posttransplant polycythemia. *Transplantation* 65:1461, 1998.

71. Morrone LF, Di Paolo S, Logoluso F, et al: Interference of angiotensin-converting enzyme inhibitors on erythropoiesis in kidney transplant recipients: role of growth factors and cytokines. *Transplantation* 64:913, 1997.

72. Navarro JF, Garcia J, Macia M, et al: Effects of losartan on the treatment of posttransplant erythrocytosis. *Clin Nephrol* 49:370, 1998.

73. Thevenod F, Radtke HW, Grutzmacher P, et al: Deficient feedback regulation of erythropoiesis in kidney transplant patients with polycythemia. *Kidney Int* 24:227, 1983.

74. Friman S, Nyberg G, Blohme I: Erythrocytosis after renal transplantation; treatment by removal of the native kidneys. *Nephrol Dial Transplant* 5:969, 1990.

75. Murphy GP, Kenny GM, Mirand EA: Erythropoietin levels in patients with renal tumors or cysts. *Cancer* 26:191, 1970.

76. Fisher JW, Samuels AI: Relationship between renal blood flow and erythropoietin production in dogs. *Proc Soc Exp Biol Med* 125:482, 1967.

77. Beebe HG, Chesebro K, Merchant F, Bush W: Results of renal artery balloon angioplasty limit its indications. *J Vasc Surg* 8:300, 1988.

78. LevGur M, Levie MD: The myomatous erythrocytosis syndrome: a review. *Obstet Gynecol* 86:1026, 1995.

79. Venencie PY, Puissant A, Boffa GA, Sohier J, Duperrat B: Multiple cutaneous leiomyomata and erythrocytosis with demonstration of erythropoietic activity in the cutaneous leiomyomata. *Br J Dermatol* 107:483, 1982.

80. Levinson JP, Kinkaid OW: Myxoma of the right atrium associated with polycythemia. Report of successful excision. *N Engl J Med* 264:1187, 1961.

81. Josephs BN, Robbins G, Levine A: Polycythemia secondary to hamartoma of the liver. *JAMA* 179:867, 1961.

82. Sandler A, Rivlin L, Filler R, Freedman M, Ky AJ: Polycythemia secondary to focal nodular hyperplasia. *J Pediatr Surg* 32:1386, 1997.

83. Sharma RR, Cast IP, O'Brien C: Supratentorial haemangioblastoma not associated with Von Hippel Lindau complex or polycythaemia: case report and literature review. *Br J Neurosurg* 9:81, 1995.

84. Constans JP, Meder F, Maiuri F, Donzelli R, Spaziente R, de Divitiis E: Posterior fossa hemangioblastomas. *Surg Neurol* 25:269, 1986.

85. Trimble M, Caro J, Talalla A, Brain M: Secondary erythrocytosis due to a cerebellar hemangioblastoma: demonstration of erythropoietin mRNA in the tumor. *Blood* 78:599, 1991.

86. McFadzean AJS, Todd D, Tsang KC: Polycythemia in primary carcinoma of the liver. *Blood* 13:427, 1958.

87. Davidson CS: Hepatocellular carcinoma and erythrocytosis. *Semin Hematol* 13:115, 1976.

88. Muta H, Funakoshi A, Baba T, et al: Gene expression of erythropoietin in hepatocellular carcinoma. *Intern Med* 33:427, 1994.

89. Shulkin BL, Shapiro B, Sisson JC: Pheochromocytoma, polycythemia, and venous thrombosis. *Am J Med* 83:773, 1987.

90. Mann DL, Gallagher NI, Donati RM: Erythrocytosis and primary aldosteronism. *Ann Intern Med* 66:335, 1967.

91. Erkelens DW, Statius VEL: Bartter's syndrome and erythrocytosis. *Am J Med* 55:711, 1973.

92. Ghio R, Haupt E, Ratti M, Boccaccio P: Erythrocytosis associated with a dermoid cyst of the ovary and erythropoietic activity of the tumour fluid. *Scand J Haematol* 27:70, 1981.

93. Gardner FH, Nathan DG, Piomelli S, Cummins JF: The erythrocythaemic effects of androgen. *Br J Haematol* 14:611, 1968.

94. Piedras J, Hernandez G, Lopez-Karpovitch X: Effect of androgen therapy and anemia on serum erythropoietin levels in patients with aplastic anemia and myelodysplastic syndromes. *Am J Hematol* 57:113, 1998.

95. Gardner FH, Pringle JC Jr: Androgens and erythropoiesis: II. Treatment of myeloid metaplasia. *N Engl J Med* 264:103, 1961.

96. Besa EC: Hematologic effects of androgens revisited: an alternative therapy in various hematologic conditions. *Semin Hematol* 31:134, 1994.

97. Wiswell TE, Cornish JD, Northam RS: Neonatal polycythemia: frequency of clinical manifestations and other associated findings. *Pediatrics* 78:26, 1986.

98. Black VD, Lubchenco LO, Koops BL, Roland RL, Powell DP: Neonatal hyperviscosity: randomized study of effect of partial plasma exchange transfusion on long-term outcome. *Pediatrics* 75:1048, 1985.

99. Pearson TC: Apparent polycythaemia. *Blood Rev* 5:205, 1991.

100. Chrysant SG, Frolich SG, Adamopoulos PN, et al: Pathologic significance of "stress" or relative polycythemia in essential hypertension. *Am J Cardiol* 37:1069, 1976.

101. Isbister JP: The contracted plasma volume syndromes (relative polycythemias) and their haemorheological significance. *Baillieres Clin Haematol* 1; 1987.

102. Leth A: Changes in plasma and extracellular fluid volumes in patients with essential hypertension during long-term treatment with hydrochlorothiazide. *Circulation* 42:479, 1970.

103. Berlin NI: Diagnosis and classification of the polycythemias. *Semin Hematol* 12:339, 1975.

104. Wehmeier A, Daum I, Jamin H, Schneider W: Incidence and clinical risk factors for bleeding and thrombotic complications in myeloproliferative disorders. A retrospective analysis of 260 patients. *Ann Hematol* 63:101, 1991.

105. Anger BR, Seifried E, Scheppach J, Heimpel H: Budd-Chiari syndrome and thrombosis of other abdominal vessels in the chronic myeloproliferative diseases. *Klin Wochenschr* 67:818, 1989.

106. Berk PD, Goldberg JD, Donovan PB, Fruchtman SM, Berlin NI: Therapeutic recommendations in polycythemia vera based on Polycythemia Vera Study Group protocols. *Semin Hematol* 23:132, 1986.

107. Starzl TE, Demetris AJ, Trucco M, et al: Chimerism after liver transplantation for type IV glycogen storage disease and type 1 Gaucher's disease. *N Engl J Med* 328:745, 1993.

108. Murphy S: Polycythemia vera. *Disease-a-Month* 38:158, 1992.

109. Jackson N, Burt D, Crocker J, Boughton B: Skin mast cells in polycythaemia vera: relationship to the pathogenesis and treatment of pruritus. *Br J Dermatol* 116:21, 1987.

110. Steinman HK, Kobza-Black A, Lotti TM, Brunetti L, Panconcsi E, Greaves MW: Polycythaemia rubra vera and water-induced pruritus: blood histamine levels and cutaneous fibrinolytic activity before and after water challenge. *Br J Dermatol* 116:329, 1987.

111. Wanless IR, Peterson P, Das A, Boitnott JK, Moore GW, Bernier V: Hepatic vascular disease and portal hypertension in polycythemia vera and agnogenic myeloid metaplasia: a clinicopathological study of 145 patients examined at autopsy. *Hepatology* 12:1166, 1990.

112. Tinney WS, Hall BE, Giffin HZ: Polycythemia vera and peptic ulcer. *Mayo Clin Proc* 18:24, 1943.

113. Newton LK: Neurologic complications of polycythemia and their impact on therapy. *Oncology (Williston Park)* 4:59, 1990.

114. Cohen AM, Gelvan A, Yarmolovsky A, Djaldetti M: Chorea in polycythemia vera: a rare presentation of hyperviscosity. *Blut* 58:47, 1989.

115. Schulz W, Domenico D, Nand S: POEMS syndrome associated with polycythemia vera. *Cancer* 63:1175, 1989.

116. Jackson A, Burton IE: Retroperitoneal mass and spinal cord compression due to extramedullary haemopoiesis in polycythaemia rubra vera. *Br J Radiol* 62:944, 1989.

117. Furukawa T, Takahashi M, Shimada H, Moriyama Y, Shibata A, Katsumi S: Polycythaemia vera with Sweet's syndrome. *Clin Lab Haematol* 11:67, 1989.

118. Cox NH, Leggat H: Sweet's syndrome associated with polycythemia rubra vera. *J Am Acad Dermatol* 23:1171, 1990.

119. Wasserman LR, Gilbert HS: Surgical bleeding in polycythemia vera. *Ann N Y Acad Sci* 115:122, 1964.

120. Jacobsen N, Theilade K, Videbaek A: Two additional cases of coexisting polycythemia vera and chronic lymphocytic leukaemia. *Scand J Haematol* 29:405, 1982.

121. Botelho de Sousa A, Gouveia J: Coexistent chronic lymphocytic leukemia and polycythemia vera requiring no treatment. *Med Oncol Tumor Pharmacother* 6:239, 1989.

122. Zafren K, Honigman B: High-altitude medicine. *Emerg Med Clin North Am* 15:191, 1997.

123. Bishop BC: Wintering in the high Himalayas. *Natl Geographic* 122:503, 1962.

124. Botella DM, Martinez-Costa R: High altitude retinal hemorrhages in the expeditions to 8,000-meter peaks. A study of 10 cases. *Med Clin (Barc)* 110:457, 1998.

125. Doll DC, Greenberg BR: Cerebral thrombosis in smokers' polycythemia. *Ann Intern Med* 102:786, 1985.

126. Stefenelli T, Silberbauer K, Ulrich W, Sommeregger K, Zechner O: Cardiac decompensation caused by hypertension and polyglobulia associated with multiple renal oncocytomas. *Clin Nephrol* 23:307, 1985.

127. Arnaud J, Pris J, Brun H, Constans J: Consequences of moderate hypoxia on red cell glycolytic metabolism in polycythemia rubra vera. *Ann Biol Clin (Paris)* 49:9, 1991.

128. Avissar N, Farkash Y, Shaklai M: Erythrocyte enzymes in polycythemia vera: a comparison to erythrocyte enzyme activities of patients with iron deficiency anemia. *Acta Haematol (Basel)* 76:37, 1986.

129. Lertzman M, Frome BM, Israels LG, Cherniack RM: Hypoxia in polycythemia vera. *Ann Intern Med* 60:409, 1964.

130. Gilbert HS, Warner RRP, Wasserman LR: A study of histamine in myeloproliferative disease. *Blood* 28:795, 1966.

131. Binder RA, Gilbert HS: Muramidase in polycythemia vera. *Blood* 36:228, 1970.

132. Gilbert HS, Krauss S, Pasternack B, Herbert V, Wasserman LR: Serum vitamin B_{12} content and unsaturated vitamin B_{12}-binding capacity in myeloproliferative disease. Value in differential diagnosis and as indicators of disease activity. *Ann Intern Med* 71:719, 1969.

133. Samuelsson J, Berg A: Further studies of the defective stimulus-response coupling for the oxidative burst in neutrophils in polycythemia vera. *Eur J Haematol* 47:239, 1991.

134. Kutti M, Weinfield A: Platelet survival in active polycythaemia vera with reference to the haematocrit level. An experimental study before and after phlebotomy. *Scand J Haematol* 8:405, 1971.

135. Cerutti A, Custodi P, Duranti M, Noris P, Balduini CL: Thrombopoietin levels in patients with primary and reactive thrombocytosis. *Br J Haematol* 99:281, 1997.

136. Yamamoto K, Sekiguchi E, Takatani O: Abnormalities of epinephrine-induced platelet aggregation and adenine nucleotides in myeloproliferative disorders. *Thrombos Haemostas* 52:292, 1984.

137. Mehta P, Mehta J, Ross M, Ostrowski N, Player D: Decreased platelet aggregation but increased thromboxane A2 generation in polycythemia vera. *Arch Intern Med* 145:1225, 1985.

138. Landolfi R, Ciabattoni G, Patrignani P, et al: Increased thromboxane biosynthesis in patients with polycythemia vera: evidence for aspirin-suppressible platelet activation in vivo. *Blood* 80:1965, 1992.

139. Ushikubi F, Ishibashi T, Narumiya S, Okuma M: Analysis of the defective signal transduction mechanism through the platelet thromboxane A2 receptor in a patient with polycythemia vera. *Thromb Haemost* 67:144, 1992.

140. Berild D, Hasselbalch H, Knudsen JB: Platelet survival, platelet factor-4 and bleeding time in myeloproliferative disorders. *Scand J Clin Lab Invest* 47:497, 1987.

141. Harker LA, Finch CA: Thrombokinetics in man. *J Clin Invest* 48:963, 1969.

142. Le Blanc K, Lindahl T, Rosendahl K, Samuelsson J: Impaired platelet binding of fibrinogen due to a lower number of GPIIB/IIIA receptors in polycythemia vera. *Thromb Res* 91:287, 1998.

143. Boughton BJ, Dallinger KJC: [125]I fibrinogen turnover in polycythaemia: the effect of phlebotomy. *Br J Haematol* 53:97, 1983.

144. Najean Y, Triebel F, Dresch C: Pure erythrocytosis: Reappraisal of a study of 51 cases. *Am J Hematol* 10:129, 1981.

145. Clement S, Eberlin A, Najean Y, Chedeville A: Two different in vitro growth patterns for erythroid precursors in 18 patients with pure erythrocytosis. *Scand J Haematol* 29:319, 1982.

146. Pearson TC, Wetherley-Mein G: The course and complications of idiopathic erythrocytosis. *Clin Lab Haematol* 1:189, 1979.

147. Shih LY, Lee CT, See LC, et al: In vitro culture growth of erythroid progenitors and serum erythropoietin assay in the differential diagnosis of polycythaemia. *Eur J Clin Invest* 28:569, 1998.

148. Egli F, Niemoller UM, Rhyner K: Serum erythropoietin levels: a new diagnostic tool? *Schweiz Rundsch Med Prax* 78:551, 1989.

149. Cotes PM, Dore CJ, Yin JA, et al: Determination of serum immunoreactive erythropoietin in the investigation of erythrocytosis. *N Engl J Med* 315:283, 1986.

150. Birgegard G, Wide L: Serum erythropoietin in the diagnosis of polycythaemia and after phlebotomy treatment. *Br J Haematol* 81:603, 1992.

151. Carneskog J, Kutti J, Wadenvik H, Lundberg PA, Lindstedt G: Plasma erythropoietin by high-detectability immunoradiometric assay in untreated and treated patients with polycythaemia vera and essential thrombocythaemia. *Eur J Haematol* 60:278, 1998.

152. Remacha AF, Montserrat I, Santamaria A, Oliver A, Barcelo MJ, Parellada M: Serum erythropoietin in the diagnosis of polycythemia vera. A follow-up study. *Haematologica* 82:406, 1997.

153. Marsh JC, Hibbin J, Marsh GW: Primary proliferative polycythaemia without splenomegaly: a diagnostic problem. *Clin Lab Haematol* 9:123, 1987.

154. Lemoine F, Najman A, Baillou C, et al: A prospective study of the value of bone marrow erythroid progenitor cultures in polycythemia. *Blood* 68:996, 1986.

155. Casadevall N, Lacombe C, Varet B: Erythroid cultures and erythropoietin assay. Clinical and diagnostic value. *Nouv Rev Fr Hematol* 32:77, 1990.

156. Weinberg RS, Worsley A, Gilbert HS, Cuttner J, Berk PD, Alter BP: Comparison of erythroid progenitor cell growth in vitro in polycythemia vera and chronic myelogenous leukemia: only polycythemia vera has endogenous colonies. *Leuk Res* 13:331, 1989.

157. Beutler E: Polycythemia. *Med Grand Rounds* 3:142, 1984.

158. Van De Pette JEW, Guthrie DL, Pearson TC: Whole blood viscosity in polycythaemia: The effect of iron deficiency at a range of haemoglobin and packed cell volumes. *Br J Haematol* 63:369, 1986.

159. Reinhart WH: The influence of iron deficiency on erythrocyte deformability. *Br J Haematol* 80:550, 1992.

160. Berlin NI, Wasserman LR: Polycythemia vera: a retrospective and reprise. *J Lab Clin Med* 130:365, 1997.

161. Nand S, Messmore H, Fisher SG, Bird ML, Schulz W, Risher RI: Leukemic transformation in polycythemia vera: analysis of risk factors. *Am J Hematol* 34:32, 1990.

162. Hocking WG, Golde DW: Polycythemia: evaluation and management. *Blood Rev* 3:59, 1989.

163. Kaplan ME, Mack K, Goldberg JD, Donovan PB, Berk PD, Wasserman LR: Long-term management of polycythemia vera with hydroxyurea: a progress report. *Semin Hematol* 23:167, 1986.

164. Sterkers Y, Preudhomme C, Lai JL, et al: Acute myeloid leukemia and myelodysplastic syndromes following essential thrombocythemia treated with hydroxyurea: high proportion of cases with 17p deletion. *Blood* 91:616, 1998.

165. Liu TC, Suri R: Multiple factors in the transformation of essential thrombocythemia to acute leukemia or myelodysplastic syndrome. *Blood* 92:1465, 1998.

166. Treatment of polycythaemia vera by radiophosphorus or busulphan: a randomized trial. "Leukemia and Hematosarcoma" Cooperative Group, European Organization for Research on Treatment of Cancer (E.O.R.T.C.). *Br J Cancer* 44:75, 1981.

167. Randi ML, Fabris F, Varotto L, Rossi C, Maeri C, Girolami A: Haematological complications in polycythaemia vera and thrombocythaemia patients treated with radiophosphorus (^{32}P). *Folia Haematol (Leipz)* 117:461, 1990.

168. Balan KK, Critchley M: Outcome of 259 patients with primary proliferative polycythaemia (PPP) and idiopathic thrombocythaemia (IT) treated in a regional nuclear medicine department with phosphorus-32—a 15 year review. *Br J Radiol* 70:1169, 1997.

169. Roberts BE, Smith AH: Use of radioactive phosphorus in haematology. *Blood Rev* 11:146, 1997.

170. Foa P, Massaro P, Caldiera S, et al: Long-term therapeutic efficacy and toxicity of recombinant interferon-alpha 2a in polycythaemia vera. *Eur J Haematol* 60:273, 1998.

171. Ozturk A, Gunay A, Uskent N: Therapeutic efficacy of recombinant interferon-alpha in polycythaemia vera. *Acta Haematol (Basel)* 99:89, 1998.

172. Silver RT: Interferon alfa: effects of long-term treatment for polycythemia vera. *Semin Hematol* 34:40, 1997.

173. Petti MC, Spadea A, Avvisati G, et al: Polycythemia vera treated with pipobroman as single agent: low incidence of secondary leukemia in a cohort of patients observed during 20 years (1971–1991). *Leukemia* 12:869, 1998.

174. Najean Y, Rain JD: Treatment of polycythemia vera: the use of hydroxyurea and pipobroman in 292 patients under the age of 65 years. *Blood* 90:3370, 1997.

175. Brusamolino E, Salvaneschi L, Canevari A, Bernasconi C: Efficacy trial of pipobroman in polycythemia vera and incidence of acute leukemia. *J Clin Oncol* 2:558, 1984.

176. Najman A, Stachowiak J, Parlier Y, Gorin NC, Duhamel G: Pipobroman therapy of polycythemia vera. *Blood* 59:890, 1982.

177. Petitt RM, Silverstein MN, Petrone ME: Anagrelide for control of thrombocythemia in polycythemia and other myeloproliferative disorders. *Semin Hematol* 34:51, 1997.

178. Swerlick RA: Photochemotherapy treatment of pruritus associated with polycythemia vera. *J Am Acad Dermatol* 13:675, 1985.

179. Bircher AJ: Water-induced itching. *Dermatologica* 181:83, 1990.

180. De Wolf JT, Hendriks DW, Egger RC, Esselink MT, Halie MR, Vellenga E: Alpha-interferon for intractable pruritus in polycythaemia vera. *Lancet* 337:241, 1991.

181. Tartaglia A, Goldberg J, Berk P, Wasserman L: Adverse effects of antiaggregating platelet therapy in the treatment of polycythemia vera. *Semin Hematol* 23:172, 1986.

182. Willoughby S, Pearson TC: The use of aspirin in polycythaemia vera and primary thrombocythaemia. *Blood Rev* 12:12, 1998.

183. Landolfi R, Marchioli R: European collaboration on low-dose aspirin in polycythemia vera (ECLAP): a randomized trial. *Semin Thromb Hemost* 23:473, 1997.

184. Rosenthal DS: Clinical aspects of chronic myeloproliferative diseases. *Am J Med Sci* 304:109, 1992.

185. Anderson JE, Sale G, Appelbaum FR, Chauncey TR, Storb R: Allogeneic marrow transplantation for primary myelofibrosis and myelofibrosis secondary to polycythaemia vera or essential thrombocytosis. *Br J Haematol* 98:1010, 1997.

186. Camos M, Cervantes F, Montoto S, Hernandez Boluda JC, Villamor N, Montserrat E: Acute lymphoid leukemia following polycythemia vera. *Leuk Lymphoma* 32:395, 1999.

187. Higuchi T, Oba R, Endo M, et al: Transition of polycythemia vera to chronic neutrophilic leukemia. *Leuk Lymphoma* 33:203, 1999.

188. Chetty KG, Light RW, Stansbury DW, Milne N: Exercise performance of polycythemic chronic obstructive pulmonary disease patients. Effect of phlebotomies. *Chest* 98:1073, 1990.

189. Piccirillo G, Fimognari FL, Valdivia JL, Marigliano V: Effects of phlebotomy on a patient with secondary polycythemia and angina pectoris. *Int J Cardiol* 44:175, 1994.

190. Thorne SA: Management of polycythaemia in adults with cyanotic congenital heart disease. *Heart* 79:315, 1998.

191. Oren R, Beeri M, Hubert A, Kramer MR, Matzner Y: Effect of theophylline on erythrocytosis in chronic obstructive pulmonary disease. *Arch Intern Med* 157:1474, 1997.

192. Fairbanks VF, Klee GG, Wiseman GA, et al: Measurement of blood volume and red cell mass: re-examination of ^{51}Cr and ^{125}I methods. *Blood Cells Mol Dis* 22:169, 1996.

193. Berlin NI, Lawrence JH, Gartland J: Blood volume in polycythemia as determined by P^{32} labeled red blood cells. *Am J Med* 9:747, 1950.

194. Huber H, Lewis SM, Szur L: Die Indikation zur Bestimmung von blutvolumen und zirkulierender Erythrozytenmenge bei Polycythaemia vera und Polyglobulien. *Acta Haematol (Basel)* 34:116, 1965.

195. Najean Y, Dresch C, Rain J, Chomienne C: Radioisotope investigations for the diagnosis and follow-up of polycythemic patients, in *Polycythemia Vera and the Myeloproliferative Disorders*, edited by LR Wasserman, PD Berk, NI Berlin, p 361. Saunders, Philadelphia, 1995.

THE HEMATOLOGIC ASPECTS OF PORPHYRIA

SHIGERU SASSA

The porphyrias are both inherited and acquired disorders in which the activities of the enzymes of the heme biosynthetic pathway are partially or almost totally deficient. There are eight enzymes involved in the synthesis of heme and, with the exception of the first enzyme, an enzymatic defect at every step leads to tissue accumulation and excessive excretion of porphyrins and/or their precursors such as δ-aminolevulinic acid (ALA) and porphobilinogen (PBG). While heme, the final product of the biosynthetic pathway, is biologically important, porphyrins and their precursors are not only useless but also toxic.

Porphyrias can be classified as either photosensitive or neurological, depending on the type of their symptoms, but some have both symptoms. Alternatively, they can be classified either hepatic or erythropoietic, depending on the principal site of expression of the specific enzymatic defect, but some also show overlapping expression. The tissue-specific expression of porphyrias is largely due to the tissue-specific control of heme pathway gene expression.

Congenital erythropoietic porphyria (CEP), though rare, is a major erythropoietic porphyria in its expression and severity. It is inherited in an autosomal recessive fashion and is characterized by marked skin photosensitivity and hemolytic anemia. The genetic defect is a marked deficiency of uroporphyrinogen III cosynthase activity. The hemolytic anemia is photosensitive in nature, usually manifests at birth, and is due to massive accumulation of isomer I uro- and coproporphyrin in erythrocytes. Increased erythropoietic activity serves as a further stimulus for increased porphyrin production in the bone marrow. Hemolysis may improve after splenectomy. The clinical symptoms of CEP are indistinguishable from those of hepatoerythropoietic porphyria (HEP), hence it is possible that some hepatoerythropoietic porphyria may be confused with CEP.

Erythropoietic protoporphyria (EPP), another erythropoietic porphyria, is inherited in an autosomal dominant fashion. In contrast to CEP, EPP is relatively common. EPP is due to a 30 to 50 percent deficiency of ferrochelatase activity, which results in an excessive accumulation of protoporphyrin in erythrocytes and massive excretion of protoporphyrin into the stool. The disease is characterized by mild to moderate photosensitivity; there are no hematologic manifestations. Clinical expression is highly variable,

such that some carriers have only mildly elevated red cell protoporphyrin levels but no skin photosensitivity. EPP is generally a mild disease, but some patients may develop porphyrin-rich gall stones and hepatic failure, resulting in death.

In contrast to CEP and EPP, δ-aminolevulinate dehydratase deficiency porphyria (ADP) is an acute hepatic porphyria characterized by severe neurological disturbances; it may involve the gastrointestinal and respiratory systems but does not produce skin photosensitivity. ADP is due to a marked deficiency of δ-aminolevulinate dehydratase activity, and patients with ADP excrete a large amount of ALA, but not PBG, into urine. It is the least frequent form of porphyria, and only four well-documented cases have been reported to date.

Acute intermittent porphyria (AIP) is the most common and important acute hepatic porphyria. It is inherited in an autosomal dominant fashion, but disease expression is very variable. Both clinically affected and asymptomatic carriers of AIP have about a 50 percent deficiency of porphobilinogen deaminase activity, but only clinically affected individuals excrete a large amount of ALA and PBG into urine. Many heterozygotes (about 90 percent) are asymptomatic throughout their lives. Patients present with severe neurological symptoms but never develop cutaneous photosensitivity. AIP is almost always latent before puberty, and symptoms are more frequent in females than in males. Hormonal, drug, and nutritional factors may aggravate the disease, probably by inducing hepatic ALA synthase, the rate-limiting enzyme in the heme biosynthetic pathway.

Hereditary coproporphyria (HCP) is also an acute hepatic porphyria, and its symptoms are similar to but generally milder than ADP and AIP. In contrast, HCP patients may additionally display skin photosensitivity. The underlying genetic defect in HCP is an approximately 50 percent deficiency of coproporphyrinogen oxidase activity, which is inherited in an autosomal dominant fashion. Patients excrete an excessive amount of ALA, PBG, and coproporphyrin into their urine and coproporphyrin into their stool. Harderoporphyria is a variant form of HCP, which produces harderoporphyrin III rather than coproporphyrin III. Neonatal hemolytic anemia has been reported with harderoporphyria. Clinical expression of HCP is dependent upon the same metabolic and chemical factors that influence expression of the gene defect in AIP.

Variegate porphyria (VP) has been recognized in many populations but is most common in South African whites, and thus it is also called the South African porphyria. The underlying defect is an approximately 50 percent deficiency of protoporphyrinogen oxidase, which is inherited in an autosomal dominant fashion. Clinical expression and symptoms are similar to HCP but often more severe. Patients with VP excrete a large amount of ALA and PBG into their urine and protoporphyrin into their stool. The same spectrum of factors that activate other acute hepatic porphyrias also induce VP. In South Africa, many patients with VP have the same R59W mutation of the protoporphyrinogen oxidase gene. Clinical management of VP is the same as that for other acute hepatic porphyrias.

Porphyria cutanea tarda (PCT) is the most common form of porphyria and usually begins in middle or late adult life. It is neither an erythropoietic nor an acute hepatic porphyria; instead, it is a chronic hepatic porphyria. Most

---

Acronyms and abbreviations that appear in this chapter include: ADP, δ-aminolevulinate dehydratase deficiency porphyria; AIP, acute intermittent porphyria; ALA, aminolevulinic acid; ALAS-E, erythroid-specific ALA synthase; ALAS-N, nonspecific ALA synthase; CEP, congenital erythropoietic porphyria; CRIM, cross-reactive immunological material; EPP, erythropoietic protoporphyria; HCP, hereditary coproporphyria; HEP, hepatoerythropoietic porphyria; PBG, porphobilinogen; PCT, porphyria cutanea tarda; VP, variegate porphyria.

PCT occurs as an acquired disease, while some occurs as an inherited disease. A deficiency of hepatic uroporphyrinogen decarboxylase activity is present in all patients with PCT. PCT patients have mild to severe photosensitivity and often have overt liver disease but no neurological symptoms. PCT patients excrete a large amount of 8- and 7-carboxylated porphyrins into their urine and isocoproporphyrin into their stool, but not ALA or PBG. Alcohol, estrogens, and hepatic siderosis are common aggravating factors in PCT. Some PCT patients also coinherit the hemochromatosis gene. PCT can be successfully treated by phlebotomy, which reduces hepatic iron stores. Polyhalogenated aromatic hydrocarbons have been associated with development of acquired PCT both in man and in animals.

Homozygous deficiency of uroporphyrinogen decarboxylase is known as hepatoerythropoietic porphyria (HEP), and patients with this condition are characterized by severe photosensitivity, which is indistinguishable from that of CEP. While both PCT and HEP are due to the same uroporphyrinogen decarboxylase deficiency, the heterozygous defect in PCT leads to a chronic hepatic porphyria, whereas the homozygous defect in HEP results in a hepatic and erythropoietic porphyria.

Molecular analysis of the gene defects in the porphyrias has demonstrated that there are numerous types of mutations for each porphyria. Many clinically "homozygous" porphyrias are in reality due to heteroallelic mutations, i.e., compound heterozygosity for two distinct mutations. The existence of rare homozygous (or compound heterozygous) deficiencies has also been recognized in all dominantly inherited forms of porphyrias. Porphyrias occur not only as inherited diseases but also as acquired diseases due to exposure to environmental chemicals or in association with other defects. Clinically unaffected gene carriers of porphyrias may also be at a greater risk than normal subjects for infertility and for intoxication by environmental chemicals, such as lead or dioxin.

DEFINITION AND HISTORY

The porphyrias are metabolic diseases due to deficiencies, usually of a genetic nature, in the activity of specific enzymes in the heme biosynthetic pathway. The intermediates of this pathway, i.e., porphyrinogens, porphyrins, and their precursors such as δ-aminolevulinic acid or porphobilinogen, are produced in excess and accumulate in tissues resulting in neurological, photocutaneous, or both types of symptoms. These disorders are classified as either *erythropoietic* or *hepatic*, depending on the principal site of expression of the specific enzymatic defect. Erythropoietic porphyrias include congenital erythropoietic porphyria and erythropoietic protoporphyria. Hepatic porphyrias are further classified into *acute* and *chronic* forms. *Acute hepatic porphyrias* refer to a condition which exhibits acute attacks, mostly neurological, related to deranged porphyrin biosynthesis in the liver; they are represented by ALA dehydratase deficiency porphyria, acute intermittent porphyria, hereditary coproporphyria, or variegate porphyria. In contrast, chronic hepatic porphyrias are characterized by chronic skin photosensitivity due to overproduction of porphyrins, but without acute attacks, as represented by porphyria cutanea tarda. Hepatoerythropoietic porphyria is an intermediate form expressing the defect both in the liver and erythroid cells. There are eight enzymes involved in the synthesis of heme and, with the exception of the first enzyme, i.e., ALA synthase, each enzymatic defect is associated with

TABLE 62-1　THE PORPHYRIAS AND THEIR ENZYMATIC DEFECTS

ENZYME DEFICIENCY	PORPHYRIA	PRINCIPAL SITE OF EXPRESSION	MODE OF TRANSMISSION
ALA dehydratase	ADP	Liver	Recessive
PBG deaminase	AIP	Liver	Dominant
Uro'gen cosynthase	CEP	Bone marrow	Recessive
Uro'gen decarboxylase	PCT	Liver	
	type I		Acquired
	type II		Dominant
	type III		Dominant
	HEP	Liver and bone marrow	Recessive
Copro'gen oxidase	HCP	Liver	Dominant
Proto'gen oxidase	VP	Liver	Dominant
Ferrochelatase	EPP	Bone marrow	Dominant

a specific form of porphyria (Table 62-1 and Fig. 62-1). In this chapter, the genetic defect or disturbances of heme biosynthesis is described for *erythropoietic porphyrias, acute hepatic porphyrias*, and *chronic hepatic porphyrias*. The major clinical and laboratory features of the porphyrias are summarized in Table 62-2, and hematological features of the porphyrias are summarized in Table 62-3.

Perhaps, the first published case of the acute hepatic porphyria was an elderly woman described by Stokvis in 1889. She excreted dark red urine and later died after taking sulphonal.[1] Subsequently, two brothers, 23 and 26 years old respectively, who most likely had CEP, were described by T. McCall Anderson in 1898.[2] These patients suffered from early childhood from attacks of *hydroa aestivale*, a cutaneous vesicular eruption associated with pruritus and burning that occurs on skin surfaces exposed to the sun, which recurred during each summer. The urine of the younger brother was persistently red, while that of the elder was said to be normal in color during the intervals between the attacks of hydroa. Their skin was extensively scarred in regions exposed to light, and there was loss of substance of their ears and noses. F. Harris[3] demonstrated that the urine of both patients contained substance related to the hematoporphyrin group. Although the characterization of the nature of porphyrins was understandably primitive, other descriptions match perfectly with those of CEP or HEP. In a monograph published in 1911, Hans Günther classified porphyrias into four different groups, i.e., (1) those which have an acute onset without association with drug ingestion, (2) those which are due to sulphonal or trional, (3) hematoporphyria congenita, and (4) chronic hematoporphyria.[4] These groups probably correspond to (1) drug-unrelated relapse of acute hepatic porphyrias (ALA dehydratase deficiency porphyria, acute intermittent porphyria, hereditary coproporphyria, or variegate porphyria), (2) drug-induced relapse (ALA dehydratase deficiency porphyria, acute intermittent porphyria, hereditary coproporphyria, or variegate porphyria), (3) congenital erythropoietic porphyria (or hepatoerythropoietic porphyria), and (4) porphyria cutanea tarda (or hepatoerythropoietic porphyria), respectively. In 1923, Archibald Garrod proposed the term *inborn errors of metabolism* for a group of inherited metabolic disorders that included porphyrias.[5]

ETIOLOGY AND PATHOGENESIS

HEME

Heme is essential for the function of all aerobic cells. In addition to hemoglobin, heme serves as the prosthetic group of hemeproteins such as myoglobin, mitochondrial and microsomal cytochromes, catalase, peroxidase, tryptophan pyrrolase, and nitric oxide synthase. Heme

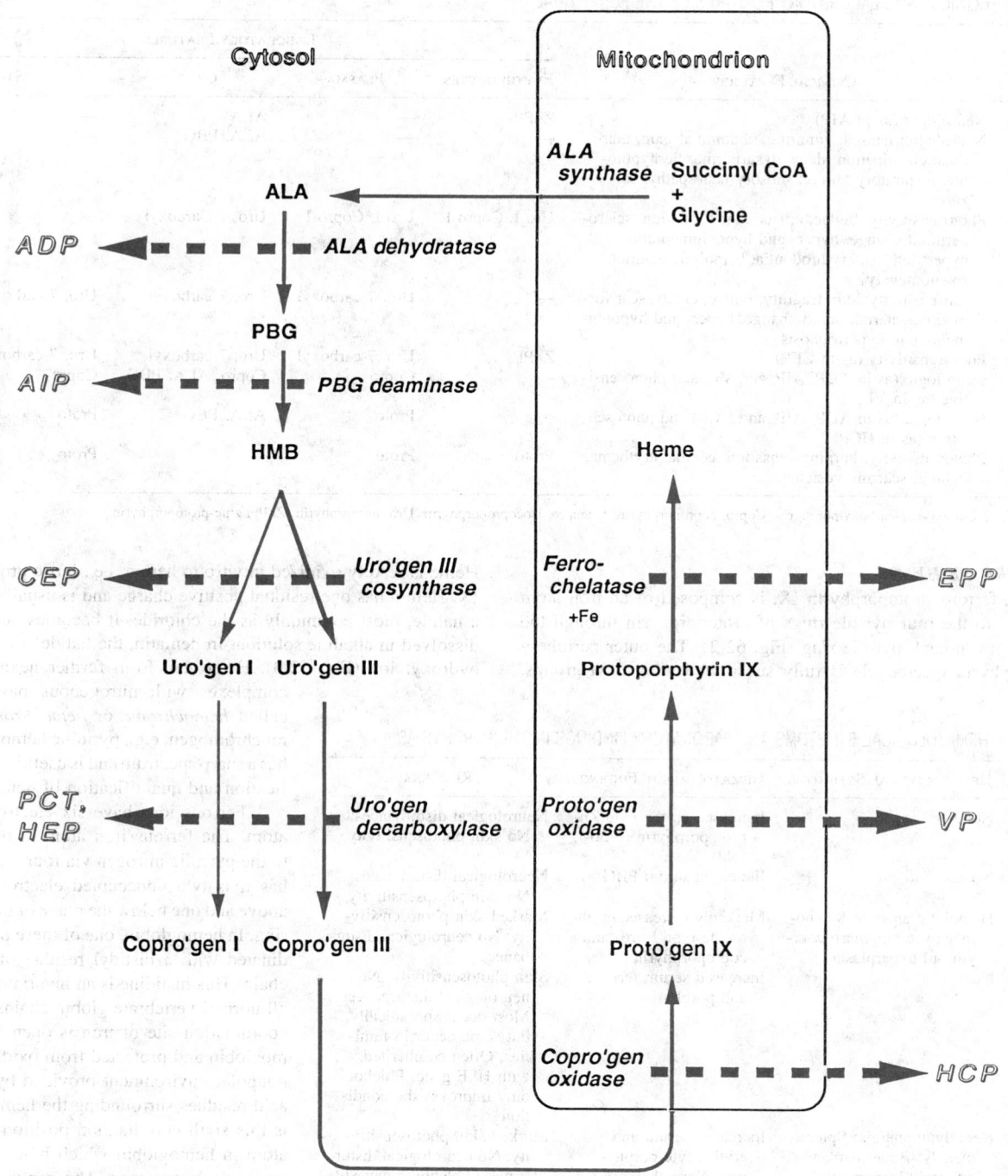

FIGURE 62-1 The enzymatic defects in the porphyrias. The enzymatic defect in each porphyria is shown by a broken line. In patients, the substrate for the defective enzymatic step accumulates in the tissue, e.g., erythrocytes, and plasma, and is excreted in large excess into urine and/or stool. In addition, the excretion of porphyrin precursors, i.e., ALA and PBG, may be increased in patients with acute hepatic porphyrias as a result of derepression of ALA synthase activity in the liver.

proteins are involved in the transport of oxygen and electrons, in the oxidative metabolism of various endogenous and exogenous chemicals, in the decomposition of hydrogen peroxide and organic peroxides, and in the oxidation of tryptophan. Most organisms have the ability to synthesize heme and apohemeproteins. Exogenously administered heme can also be incorporated into certain heme proteins such as hemoglobin[6] and cytochrome P450.[7] There is approximately 500 to 700 g of hemoglobin (of which 3.8 percent is heme) in a normal man with 70 kg body weight.[8] Approximately 85 percent of heme is synthesized in the erythropoietic marrow, while the remainder is synthesized largely by the liver.[9] In the liver, the majority of heme synthesized is incorporated into microsomal cytochrome P450s that perform important biotransformations of a variety of chemicals, including carcinogens, steroids, vitamins, fatty acids, and prostaglandins.[10]

TABLE 62-2   CLINICAL AND LABORATORY FEATURES OF THE PORPHYRIAS

		LABORATORY FEATURES			
PORPHYRIA	CLINICAL FEATURES	ERYTHROCYTES	PLASMA	URINE	STOOL
ADP	Neurologic (as in AIP)	ZnPP	—	ALA	—
AIP	Neurologic: nausea, vomiting, abdominal pain, diarrhea, constipation, ileus, dysuria, muscle hypotonia, respiratory failure, sensory neuropathy, seizures	—	—	ALA, PBG	—
CEP	Photosensitivity: bullae, crusts, scar formation, sclerodermoid change, hyper- and hypopigmentation, hypertrichosis, erythrodontia, hemolytic anemia, splenomegaly	Uro I, Copro I	Uro I, Copro I	Uro, 7-Carboxyl	—
PCT	Photosensitivity: skin fragility, bullae, crusts, scar formation, sclerodermoid change, hyper- and hypopigmentation, hypertrichosis	—	Uro, 7-carboxyl	Uro, 7-carboxyl	Uro, 7-carboxyl, Isocopro
HEP	Photosensitivity (as in CEP)	ZnPP	Uro, 7-carboxyl	Uro, 7-carboxyl	Uro, 7-carboxyl, Isocopro
HCP	Neurologic (as in ADP, AIP, and VP) and photosensitive (as in VP)	—	Copro	Copro, ALA, PBG	Copro
VP	Neurologic (as in ADP, AIP, and HCP) and photosensitive (as in HCP)	—	Proto	ALA, PBG	Proto
EPP	Photosensitivity: burning sensation, edema, erythema, itching, scarring vesicles	Proto	Proto	—	Proto

ABBREVIATIONS: 7-Carboxyl, 7-carboxylporphyrin; Copro, coproporphyrin; Isocopro, isocoproporphyrin; Uro, uroporphyrin; ZnPP, zinc-protoporphyrin.

STRUCTURE OF HEME

Heme, i.e., ferrous protoporphyrin IX, is composed of an iron atom coordinated to the four pyrrole rings of protoporphyrin through the nitrogen atom in each pyrrole ring (Fig. 62-2). The outer periphery of the porphyrin macrocycle is fully substituted with alkyl groups.

TABLE 62-3   HEMATOLOGICAL SYMPTOMS AND LABORATORY FINDINGS IN THE PORPHYRIAS

PORPHYRIA	HEMATOLOGICAL SYMPTOMS	HEMATOLOGICAL FINDINGS	REMARKS
ADP	None	Increased erythrocyte Zn-protoporphyrin (~30-fold)	Neurological disturbances; No skin photosensitivity
AIP	None	Increased serum PBG	Neurological disturbances; No skin photosensitivity
CEP	Hemolytic anemia; Splenomegaly; Bone marrow erythroid hyperplasia	Markedly increased erythrocyte type I uro- and coproporphyrin	Marked skin photosensitivity; No neurological disturbances
PCT	None	Increased serum ferritin and porphyrin	Skin photosensitivity; No neurological disturbances; Most occur sporadically, but some occur in families; Often coinherited with HFE gene; Phlebotomy improves the condition
HEP	Hemolytic anemia; Splenomegaly; Bone marrow erythroid hyperplasia	Increased serum and erythrocyte porphyrins; Normal serum ferritin concentration	Marked skin photosensitivity; No neurological disturbances; Phlebotomy has little effect
HCP	None	Increased serum coproporphyrin	Skin photosensitivity and neurological disturbances; Neonatal hemolytic anemia was associated with harderoporphyria, a variant form of HCP
VP	None	Increased serum protoporphyrin	Skin photosensitivity and neurological disturbances; Rare homozygous variants are known which are associated with malformation, and/or growth retardation, but without anemia
EPP	None	Increased erythrocyte free protoporphyrin	Skin photosensitivity; No neurological disturbances

Heme is readily oxidized in vitro to hemin, i.e., ferric protoporphyrin IX. Hemin has one residual positive charge and is usually isolated as a halide, most commonly as the chloride. It becomes hematin when dissolved in alkaline solution. In hematin, the halide is replaced by a hydroxyl ion (Fig. 62-3). Heme can form further hexacoordinated complexes with nitrogenous bases that are called *hemochrome* or *hemochromogen*. Hemochromogen, e.g., pyridine hemochromogen, has a sharp spectrum and is useful for the identification and quantification of heme proteins.

Ferrous ions have six electron pairs per atom. The ferrous iron atom in heme, bound to the pyrrolic nitrogen via four electron pairs, has thus two unoccupied electron pairs, one above and one below the plane of the porphyrin ring. In hemoglobin, one of these pairs is coordinated with a histidyl residue of the globin chain. This histidine is an invariable feature of all normal vertebrate globin chains. The other coordination site of iron is open in deoxyhemoglobin and protected from oxidation by the nonpolar environment provided by the amino acid residues surrounding the heme moiety. It is this sixth coordination position of the iron atom in hemoglobin which binds the oxygen molecule for transport. The iron in hemoglobin must be in the ferrous state in order to be able to reversibly bind oxygen. Although oxidized hemoglobin, i.e., methemoglobin, is generated in erythrocytes, it is continuously reduced to ferrous hemoglobin in the cell by the NADH-cytochrome b_5 reductase-cytochrome b_5-system (see Chap. 26).

BIOSYNTHESIS OF HEME

The steps involved in heme biosynthesis are illustrated in Fig. 62-4. In eukaryote cells, the first step and the last three steps take place in mitochondria; the four intermediate steps

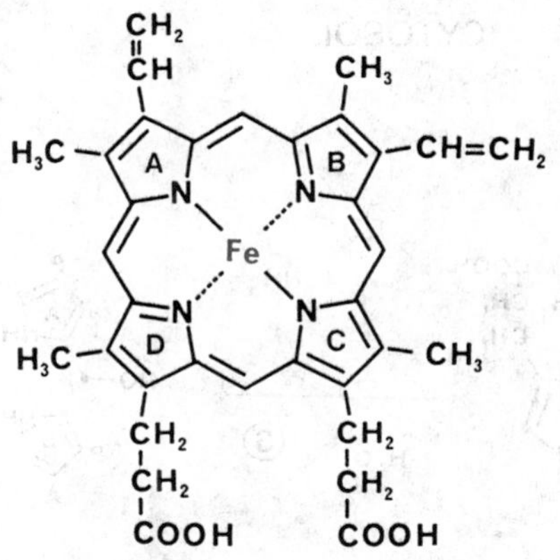

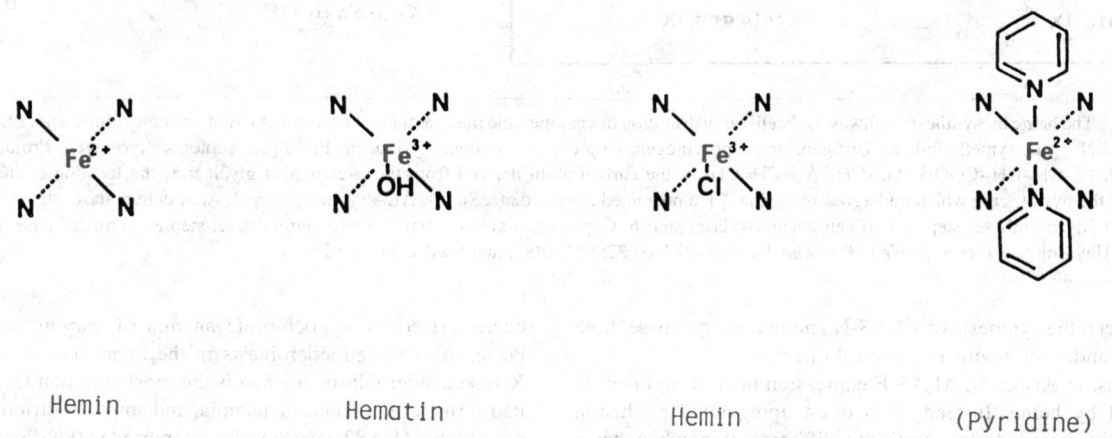

FIGURE 62-2   Structure of heme. Each ring is labeled with the Roman alphabet.

occur in the cytosol. The two major organs involved in heme synthesis are the bone marrow and the liver. In the bone marrow, heme is made in erythroblasts and reticulocytes, which contain mitochondria, while circulating erythrocytes lack the ability to form heme. The first intermediate of the heme biosynthetic pathway is δ-aminolevulinic acid, a 5-carbon aminoketone, which is formed by the condensation of glycine and succinyl CoA. Two molecules of ALA are combined to form the monopyrrole PBG; four molecules of PBG are then combined to form uroporphyrinogen, a cyclic tetrapyrrole. Uroporphyrinogen is converted to coproporphyrinogen and subsequently to protoporphyrin IX. Finally, ferrous ion is inserted into protoporphyrin IX to form heme. Protoporphyrin IX is the immediate precursor of the various hemes and also of the chlorophylls.

Step 1. Formation of δ-Aminolevulinic Acid [δ-Aminolevulinate Synthase (Succinyl CoA: Glycine C-Succinyl Transferase) (Decarboxylating) (EC 2.3.1.37)]   The first enzyme in the heme biosynthetic pathway is ALA synthase. ALA synthase catalyzes the condensation of glycine and succinyl CoA to form ALA (Fig. 62-4, step 1). In mammalian cells, the enzyme is localized in the inner membrane of the mitochondria.[11] The enzyme reaction requires pyridoxal 5′-phosphate as a cofactor. The enzyme is synthesized as a precursor

protein in the cytosol and transported into mitochondria. There are two separate ALA synthase genes, i.e., ALAS1 and ALAS2, encoding nonspecific (ALAS-N) and erythroid-specific (ALAS-E) isoforms, respectively.[12,13] The human ALAS-E gene encodes a precursor of 587 amino acids, with a M_r of 64,600. Nucleotide sequences for the ALAS-E and the ALAS-N isoforms are about 60 percent similar; there is no homology in the amino-terminal region, while there is a high homology (about 73 percent) after the hepatic residue 197.[14] The two human ALA synthase genes appear to have evolved by duplication of a common ancestral gene which encoded a primitive catalytic site, with subsequent addition of DNA sequences encoding variable functions, mostly at the amino termini.[15] The gene locus for the human ALAS-N is at 3p.21, while that for the erythroid ALA synthase is at Xp11.2.[13]

The promoter in the human ALAS-E gene contains several putative erythroid-specific *cis*-acting elements including both a GATA-1 and an NF-E2 binding site[15]; both GATA-1 and NF-E2 are erythroid transcription factors that also bind to multiple DNA sites such as the promoter of the human β-globin gene and the erythroid porphobilinogen deaminase gene.[16] These findings suggest that ALAS-E gene expression is likely to be under the regulatory influence of erythroid transcription factors such as GATA-1. Additionally, ALAS-E mRNA contains an iron-responsive element (IRE) in its 5′-untranslated region,[15] similar to mRNAs encoding ferritin[17] and transferrin receptor[18] (see Chap. 24). Gel retardation analysis showed that the IRE in ALAS-E mRNA is functional and suggests that translation of the erythroid-specific mRNA can be upregulated by the availability of iron, or heme, in erythroid cells.[19]

The ALAS-N level in the liver is under positive and negative controls by porphyrogenic chemicals and hemin, respectively.[20] Its level increases dramatically when the liver needs to make more heme in response to various chemical treatments. The enzyme synthesis is also derepressed in heme deficiency during the relapse of acute hepatic porphyrias. Stimuli that increase hepatic heme demands, such as (1) induction of cytochrome P450 by various drugs and/or hormones, or (2) induction of heme oxygenase by stress or fever, are usually associated with clinical aggravation of these disorders. In contrast, administration of hemin,[21] or inhibitors of heme oxygenase activity,[22] induces clinical remission. At heme concentrations much higher than those that repress the synthesis of the enzyme, heme induces microsomal heme oxygenase, resulting in its enhanced catabolism.[23] Thus it can be visualized that the hepatic heme concentration is maintained by a

FIGURE 62-3   Forms of iron protoporphyrin IX. The nitrogen atom indicates the pyrrolic nitrogen.

Hemin   Hematin   Hemin (chloride)   (Pyridine) Hemochrome

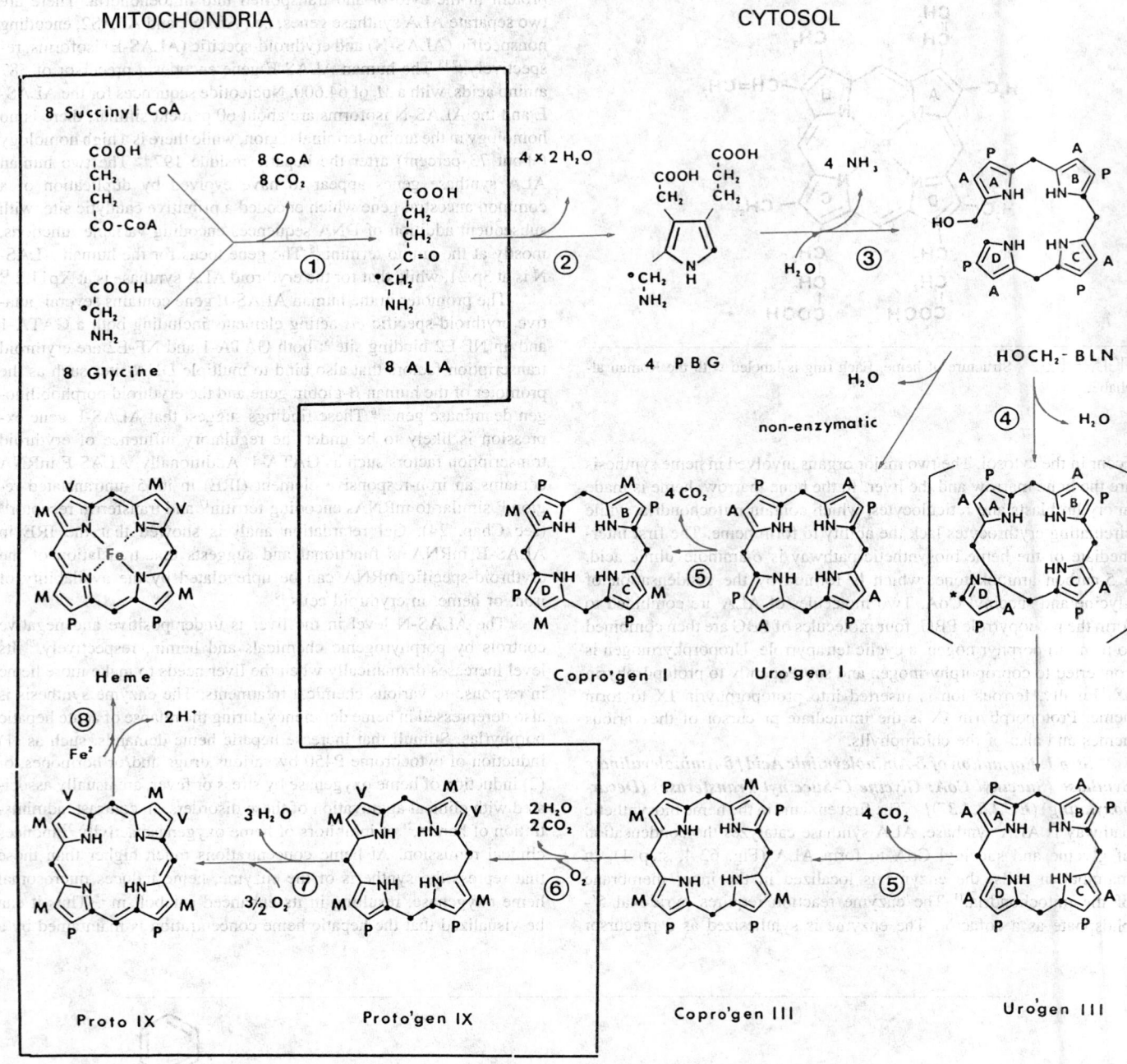

FIGURE 62-4   The heme biosynthesis pathway. Subcellular distribution of enzymes and intermediates are shown. ALA, δ-aminolevulinic acid; PBG, porphobilino-gen; HOCH$_2$-BLN, hydroxymethylbilane; Uro'gen, uroporphyrinogen; Copro'gen, coproporphyrinogen; Proto'gen, protoporphyrinogen; Proto, protoporphyrin. A, -CH$_2$COOH; P, -CH$_2$-CH$_2$-COOH; M, -CH$_3$; V, -CH=CH$_2$; •, the carbon atom derived from the α-carbon of glycine; *, the location of the α-carbon atom from glycine in the pyrrole ring which undergoes reversion; [ ], a presumed intermediate. Step 1, ALA synthase; step 2, ALA dehydratase; step 3, PBG deaminase; step 4, Uro'gen III cosynthase; step 5, Uro'gen decarboxylase; step 6, Copro'gen oxidase; step 7, Proto'gen oxidase; step 8, Ferrochelatase. [This figure was modified after Hayashi N, *Protein, Nucleic Acid and Enzyme (Tokyo)* 32:797, 1987, and used with permission.]

balance between the synthesis of ALAS-N and heme oxygenase, both of which are under the regulatory control of heme.

In contrast to ALAS-N, ALAS-E expression in erythroid cells is not repressed by heme. Instead, it is often upregulated by hemin treatment or increased during erythroid differentiation when heme synthesis is increased.[24,25] Thus the regulation of heme synthesis in erythroid cells is distinct from that in the liver.[26]

The sideroblastic anemias are a heterogeneous group of disorders

characterized by hypochromic anemia of varying severity and the presence of ringed sideroblasts in the bone marrow (see Chap. 63). X-linked sideroblastic anemia is the most common form of the inherited forms of sideroblastic anemia, and some 20 different point mutations of the ALAS2 gene have been reported in this disorder. Mutations frequently, but not necessarily, are in exon 9 of the ALAS2 gene, which contains the binding site for pyridoxal 5'phosphate (K391), the essential cofactor for ALA synthase.

Step 2. Formation of Porphobilinogen [δ-Aminolevulinate Dehydratase; δ-Aminolevulinate Hydrolase (EC 4.2.1.24)]   ALA dehydratase is a cytosolic enzyme that catalyzes the condensation of two molecules of ALA to form a monopyrrole, PBG, with the removal of two molecules of water (Fig. 62-4, step 2). The human ALA dehydratase gene is located at chromosome 9q.[27] ALA dehydratase activity requires an intact sulfhydryl group and a zinc atom in the enzyme. The enzyme activity is inhibited by sulfhydryl reagents[28] or by lead, which displaces zinc.[29] Patients with lead poisoning show marked inhibition of ALA dehydratase activity in erythrocytes, excrete excessive amounts of ALA into urine, and exhibit various neurological symptoms which often mimic those of acute hepatic porphyria[30] (see Chap. 53). The most potent inhibitor of the enzyme activity is 4,6-dioxoheptanoic acid (succinylacetone). This compound, which is found in urine and blood of patients with hereditary tyrosinemia,[31] is a substrate analogue and a potent inhibitor of the enzyme.[32,33] Patients with tyrosinemia show little ALA dehydratase activity in blood and in the liver and present symptoms similar to acute hepatic porphyria.[31,33]

The human ALA dehydratase is encoded by mRNA with an open-reading frame of 990 bp, corresponding to a protein with an M_r of 36,274, and has a high degree of homology to the rat enzyme.[34,35] There are sequences essential for enzymatic activity, i.e., those for the active lysine residue, and for the cysteine- and histidine-rich zinc binding sites.[36] The gene for human ALA dehydratase is localized at chromosome 9p34.[27]

Unlike ALA synthase, there is no known tissue-specific isozyme for ALA dehydratase. However, it is known that ALA dehydratase mRNA occurs in housekeeping (1A) and erythroid-specific (1B) forms, and there is a significant tissue-specific control of these transcripts. Namely, both GATA-1 and ALA dehydratase 1B mRNA are significantly upregulated during erythroid differentiation in mice.[37] This finding may be accounted for by the fact that, in both man and mouse, the promoter region upstream of exon 1B contains GATA-1 sites.[37]

Human ALA dehydratase is a polymorphic enzyme,[38] with two common alleles (allele 1 and allele 2), which result in three distinct charge isozyme phenotypes, i.e., 1-1, 1-2, and 2-2. The allele 2 sequence is different from the allele 1 sequence only by a G to C transversion of nucleotide 177 in the coding region.[39] This base substitution results in the replacement of lysine by asparagine, an amino acid change consistent with the more electronegative charge of the allele 2 subunit.

Step 3. Formation of Uroporphyrinogen I [Porphobilinogen Deaminase; Porphobilinogen Ammonia-Lyase (Polymerizing) (EC 4.3.1.8)]   Porphobilinogen deaminase catalyzes the condensation of four molecules of PBG to yield a linear tetrapyrrole, hydroxymethylbilane[40] (Fig. 62-4, step 3). In the absence of the subsequent enzyme in the pathway, uroporphyrinogen III cosynthase, the bilane spontaneously forms a ring structure, uroporphyrinogen I. The type I porphyrinogen isomers do not produce any useful metabolites, while the type III isomers are the precursor for heme synthesis. Although PBG deaminase used to be referred to as *uroporphyrinogen I synthase*, this is incorrect as it does not form uroporphyrinogen I. It should be called either *PBG deaminase* or *hydroxymethylbilane synthase*, since the enzyme furnishes hydroxymethylbilane by deamination of four PBG molecules.

The gene locus encoding human PBG deaminase is at chromosome 11q23→11qter.[41] The human PBG deaminase gene is split into 15 exons spread over 10 kb of DNA.[42] There are two distinct molecular forms of PBG deaminase, i.e., the erythroid- and the nonspecific isoforms.[43] The two distinct mRNAs are produced through alternative splicing of two primary transcripts arising from two promoters. The upstream promoter is active in all tissues, and thus the enzyme encoded by the larger transcript is termed the *nonspecific*, or the *housekeeping*,

PBG deaminase. The size of the human housekeeping isoform predicted from its cDNA is 344 amino acids, with an M_r of 37,627.[44] The other promoter, located about 3 kb downstream, is active only in erythroid cells. Erythroid-specific *trans*-acting factors, e.g., GATA-1 and NF-E2, recognize sequences in the PBG deaminase erythroid promoter.[16] There is a 1320-bp stretch of perfect identity between the erythroid and the nonerythroid PBG deaminase, but with a mismatch in the first exon at their 5′ extremities. The additional 17 amino acid residues at the N-terminus of the nonerythropoietic isoform are accounted for by an additional in-frame AUG codon present at 51 bp upstream from the initiating codon of the erythropoietic cDNA.

Step 4. Formation of Uroporphyrinogen III (Uroporphyrinogen III Cosynthase)   Uroporphyrinogen III cosynthase, a cytosolic enzyme, catalyzes the formation of uroporphyrinogen III from hydroxymethylbilane. This involves an intramolecular rearrangement which affects only ring D of the porphyrin macrocycle[40] (Fig. 62-4, step 4). The protein predicted from a human uroporphyrinogen III cosynthase cDNA, which has an open-reading frame of 798 bp, consists of 263 amino acid residues, with a M_r of 28,607.[45] The amino acid compositions of the hepatic uroporphyrinogen III cosynthase and the purified erythrocyte enzyme are essentially identical, suggesting that the enzyme in the liver and in erythroid cells is identical.

Step 5. Formation of Coproporphyrinogen [Uroporphyrinogen Decarboxylase (EC 4.1.1.37)]   A cytosolic enzyme, uroporphyrinogen decarboxylase, catalyzes the sequential removal of the four carboxylic groups of the carboxymethyl side chains in uroporphyrinogen to yield coproporphyrinogen (Fig. 62-4, step 5). The single enzyme catalyzes four successive decarboxylation reactions yielding 7-, 6-, 5-, and 4-carboxylated porphyrinogens, and the occurrence of all these intermediates has been identified in urine and stool. The enzyme activity in the liver can be inhibited by environmental chemicals such as polyhalogenated aromatic hydrocarbons. Human uroporphyrinogen decarboxylase is a 42-kDa polypeptide encoded by a single gene, containing 10 exons that are spread over 3 kb.[46] The gene has been mapped to chromosome 1p34. Although it contains two initiation sites, both sites are used with the same frequencies in all tissues, and the gene is transcribed into a unique mRNA.[47]

Step 6. Formation of Protoporphyrinogen IX (Coproporphyrinogen Oxidase)   Coproporphyrinogen oxidase in mammalian cells is a mitochondrial enzyme that catalyzes the removal of the carboxyl group and two hydrogens from the propionic groups of pyrrole rings A and B of coproporphyrinogen III to form vinyl groups at these positions, yielding protoporphyrinogen IX (Fig. 62-4, step 6). The gene for human coproporphyrinogen oxidase has been assigned to chromosome 3q12, spans approximately 14 kb, and consists of seven exons and six introns[48]; cDNA cloning for this enzyme has been reported in mouse erythroleukemia cells.[49] The predicted protein comprises 354 amino acid residues (M_r 40,647), with a putative leader sequence of 31 amino acid residues, the result of being a mature protein of 323 amino acid residues (M_r 37,225).[49] There are potential regulatory elements in the GC-rich promoter region on the gene, such as six Sp1, four GATA, and one CACCC sites. Coproporphyrinogen oxidase mRNA is known to increase during erythroid cell differentiation.[50]

Step 7. Formation of Protoporphyrin IX [Protoporphyrinogen Oxidase (EC 1.3.3.4)]   The penultimate step in heme biosynthesis, i.e., the oxidation of protoporphyrinogen IX to protoporphyrin IX, is mediated by a mitochondrial enzyme, *protoporphyrinogen oxidase*, that catalyzes the removal of six hydrogen atoms from the porphyrinogen nucleus (Fig. 62-4, step 7). Human protoporphyrinogen oxidase cDNA has been cloned.[51] The gene is present as a single copy per haploid genome, at chromosome 1q22.[52] Protoporphyrinogen oxidase consists of 477 amino acids with a M_r 50,800. The deduced protein

TABLE 62-4　TISSUE-SPECIFIC REGULATION OF ENZYMES IN THE HEME BIOSYNTHETIC PATHWAY

ENZYME	ERYTHROID CELLS	LIVER	REMARKS	REFERENCE
ALA synthase	ALAS2 mRNA, ALAS2 protein	ALAS1 mRNA, ALAS1 protein	ALAS1 and ALAS2 are two separate gene products. ALAS1 expression is suppressed, while ALAS2 expression is upregulated by heme.	174
ALA dehydratase	ALAD1B mRNA	ALAD1A mRNA	While their protein product is identical, ALAD1A and 1B mRNA are subject to tissue-specific regulation.	37
PBG deaminase	PBGD-E mRNA, PBGD-E protein	PBGD-N mRNA, PBGD-N protein	Two mRNAs are the result of alternate splicing arising from two promoters. PBGD-E expression is controlled by GATA-1 and NF-E2.	16
Uroporphyrinogen cosynthase	The same enzyme is expressed in these tissues.		No tissue-specific regulation.	
Uroporphyrinogen decarboxylase	The same enzyme is expressed in these tissues.		Uroporphyrinogen decarboxylase mRNA is known to increase during erythroid cell differentiation, though its mechanism is unknown.	175
Coproporphyrinogen oxidase	The same enzyme is expressed in these tissues.		There is potential distinct regulation between the two tissues by tissue-specific *trans*-acting factors.	
Protoporphyrinogen oxidase	The same enzyme is expressed in these tissues.		No tissue-specific regulation.	
Ferrochelatase	The same enzyme is expressed in these tissues.		Ferrochelatase mRNA is known to increase during erythroid cell differentiation, though its mechanism is unknown.	176

exhibits a high degree of homology over its entire length to the amino acid sequence of protoporphyrinogen oxidase encoded by the *HEMY* gene of *Bacillus subtilis*. Protoporphyrinogen oxidase is a monomer with no apparent transport-specific leader sequence but is ultimately localized in mitochondria.[51]

Step 8. Formation of Heme [Ferrochelatase; Protoheme-Ferrolyase (EC 4.99.1.1)]　The final step of heme biosynthesis is the insertion of iron into protoporphyrin IX. This reaction is catalyzed by a mitochondrial enzyme, *ferrochelatase* (Fig. 62-4, step 8). Unlike other enzymatic steps in the heme biosynthetic pathway, ferrochelatase utilizes protoporphyrin IX as substrate, rather than its reduced form. However, ferrous, not ferric ion, is utilized for insertion into protoporphyrin IX.[53] The gene encoding human ferrochelatase has been assigned to chromosome 18q.[54,55] There are two ferrochelatase mRNA species, about 2.5 kb and about 1.6 kb in size, which are derived from the utilization of two alternative polyadenylation sites in the mRNA. The human ferrochelatase gene contains a total of 11 exons and has a minimum size of about 45 kb.[54] A major site of transcription initiation is at an adenine, 89 bp upstream from the translation-initiating ATG. The promoter region contains a potential binding site for several transcription factors, Sp1, NF-E2, and GATA-1, but not a typical TATA or CAAT sequence. The transcripts are identical in all tissues examined.

Recently, crystal structure of *Bacillus subtilis* ferrochelatase has been determined at 1.9A resolution.[56] Ferrochelatase seems to have a structurally conserved core region that is common to the enzyme from bacteria, plants, and mammals, and the porphyrin and the metal appear to bind in the identical cleft.

CONTROL OF HEME SYNTHESIS IN THE LIVER AND ERYTHROID CELLS

The rate of heme synthesis in the liver is largely regulated by the level of ALAS-N activity. The synthesis of ALAS-N is in turn under feedback control by heme. Compounds that increase hepatic cytochrome P450 synthesis, accelerate the destruction of heme, or inhibit heme formation induce ALAS-N. Regulation of ALAS-N by heme is known to occur at least at four different levels; (1) transcription, (2) translation, (3) transfer into mitochondria, and (4) enzyme inhibition.

The last mechanism appears least important, while all the other mechanisms may play an important role in regulating ALAS-N levels.

ALAS-E is not inducible by drugs that induce ALAS-N.[57] Unlike ALAS-N, the synthesis of ALAS-E is uninfluenced, or often upregulated, by hemin treatment, both at the transcriptional and the translational level.[19,24,58] While hemin treatment of rats strongly inhibits the synthesis of hepatic cytochrome P450,[59] the same treatment of marrow cultures increases erythroid-colony forming units.[60] Thus the mode of regulation of ALA synthases in these two major heme-synthesizing organs is distinct. Other aspects of tissue-specific regulation of heme biosynthesis are summarized in Table 62-4.

ERYTHROPOIETIC PORPHYRIAS

CONGENITAL ERYTHROPOIETIC PORPHYRIA (CEP)

DEFINITION AND HISTORY
CEP is an erythropoietic porphyria, inherited in an autosomal recessive fashion. The primary abnormality is an almost total deficiency of uroporphyrinogen III cosynthase activity which results in accumulation and massive excretion of type I porphyrins (Table 62-1 and Fig. 62-1). After the first two cases of CEP described by Anderson in 1898,[2] about 130 cases have been reported,[61] but some of these individuals may really have had HEP. Patients with CEP suffer from symptoms due to phototoxic reactions including cutaneous lesions and hemolytic anemia.

PATHOPHYSIOLOGY
There is remarkable molecular heterogeneity of the uroporphyrinogen III cosynthase defects in CEP. To date, 18 different mutations of the uroporphyrinogen cosynthase gene have been reported in CEP. They include deletions, insertions, rearrangements, splicing abnormalities, and both missense and nonsense mutations. Six of these are found in exon 4, four in exon 10, and three in both exons 2 and 9.[62] Of the twelve single base substitutions, four (T228M, G225S, A66V, and A104V) were hot spot mutations, occurring at CpG dinucleotides. With the exception of V82F, all CEP missense mutations occurred in amino acid residues that are conserved in both the mouse and the human uroporphyrinogen cosynthase.

Genotype-phenotype comparison of the uroporphyrinogen cosynthase was studied using the prokaryotic expression of mutant cDNAs. Mean activities of the mutant enzymes ranged from zero to 36 percent of the activity expressed in *E. coli* by the normal cDNA. The majority of the mutant cDNAs expressed polypeptides with null enzyme activity, while only V82F, A66V, A104V, and V99A showed 36, 15, 8, and 6 percent enzyme activity, respectively, as compared with the normal control. A66V and V82F were thermodynamically unstable mutants.[62] Homoallelism for C73R, the most common mutation, was found in five patients and is associated clinically with the most severe phenotype, hydrops fetalis, and/or transfusion dependency from birth.

PATHOGENESIS OF THE CLINICAL FINDINGS

Most marrow normoblasts display fluorescence, principally in the nuclei.[63] Marrow-derived porphyrins become distributed throughout the body and account for the multiple pathologies of the integument. Splenomegaly is frequently observed in CEP and is presumed to be secondary to the hemolytic process. Hemolysis of erythrocytes may also result from photolysis as porphyrin-laden cells are exposed to light in the dermal capillaries.

CLINICAL FEATURES

Early onset of cutaneous photosensitivity exacerbated by exposure to sunlight is characteristic. Subepidermal bullous lesions progress to crusted erosions which heal with scarring and either hyperpigmentation or hypopigmentation. Hypertrichosis and alopecia are common, and erythrodontia (with red porphyrin fluorescence under ultraviolet light) is virtually pathognomonic of CEP. Hemolytic anemia may be accompanied by splenomegaly and porphyrin-rich gallstones. Compensatory expansion of the marrow may result in pathological fractures, vertebral compression or collapse, shortness of stature, and, rarely, osteolytic and sclerotic lesions in the skeleton.

DIAGNOSIS

CEP can be recognized in utero by dark brownish amniotic fluid enriched in porphyrins. The diagnosis of CEP in infants can be made by pink to dark brown staining of the diapers, due to large amounts of urinary porphyrins. Severe cutaneous photosensitivity in infancy (or rarely in adults) should suggest the diagnosis of CEP. Urinary porphyrin levels are always elevated 20-to 60-fold above normal. Uroporphyrin levels are increased more than those of coproporphyrin; type I isomers of uro- and coproporphyrin series predominate, but the levels of type III isomers are also elevated. Fecal porphyrin excretion is usually increased and is predominantly coproporphyrin I. Anemia may be present, and erythrocytes may exhibit polychromasia, poikilocytosis, anisocytosis, and basophilic stippling. Demonstration of elevated urinary and fecal porphyrins of type I isomers, and free erythrocyte uro- and coproporphyrins are diagnostic of CEP. HEP may also present as photosensitivity in childhood, and porphyrin excretion is also elevated, but elevated fecal levels of isocoproporphyrin and 5-carboxylic porphyrins in this condition distinguish it from CEP.

THERAPY

Patients should be advised to avoid sunlight, trauma to the skin, and infections. Topical sunscreens may be of some help as may oral treatment with β-carotene.[64] Transfusions with packed erythrocytes transiently decrease hemolysis and its attendant drive to increased erythropoiesis.[65] Splenectomy has been performed on many patients but with only short-term reductions in hemolysis, porphyrin excretion, and skin manifestations. Treatment with charcoal for 9 months in a man with CEP was reported to have lowered porphyrin levels in plasma and skin and resulted in complete clinical remission during therapy.[66]

Oral administration of the free radical scavenger ascorbic acid and α-tocopherol has been reported to be effective in improving anemia.[61]

ERYTHROPOIETIC PROTOPORPHYRIA

DEFINITION AND HISTORY

EPP is characterized by a partial deficiency of ferrochelatase activity, and the disease is generally inherited in an autosomal dominant fashion with a variable degree of clinical expression (Table 62-1 and Fig. 62-1). This defect results in massive accumulations of protoporphyrin in erythrocytes, plasma, and feces. Clinically, the disease is characterized by the childhood onset of cutaneous photosensitivity in light-exposed areas, but skin lesions are milder and less disfiguring than those seen in CEP, PCT, HEP, and VP. EPP is the most common form of erythropoietic porphyria. By 1976, some 300 case reports had been published.[67] There is no racial or sexual predilection, and onset is typically in childhood.

PATHOPHYSIOLOGY

Molecular analysis of the ferrochelatase gene in patients with EPP has revealed missense mutations, splicing mutations, intragenic deletions, and possible nonsense mutations associated with functional deficiency of ferrochelatase.[68] Splicing mutations are most common. In a proband's family, typically one parent is classified as a carrier of the disease because of elevated erythrocyte and stool protoporphyrin levels. In many cases, the mode of inheritance is autosomal dominant, but it is often vague or with a variable degree of penetrance. Parent-to-offspring transmission of the clinical disease is less than 10 percent.[69] In addition to the typical dominant inheritance, a few cases of EPP with recessive inheritance have been confirmed.[70] Disease expression is also influenced by other factors, including pregnancy.[71] These findings suggest that EPP is a heterogeneous disorder.

PATHOGENESIS OF THE CLINICAL FINDINGS

Histological examinations of skin biopsies from EPP patients show thickened capillary walls in the papillary dermis surrounded by amorphous hyalinelike deposits, immunoglobulin, complement, and PAS-positive mucopolysaccharides.[72] Basement membrane abnormalities are observed in EPP but are quantitatively less marked than in other forms of porphyria.[73] Thus EPP may be suggested, but not positively identified, from skin biopsies. Light-excited porphyrins are known to generate free radicals and singlet oxygen,[74] which then leads to peroxidation of lipids[75] and cross-linking of membrane proteins.[76] Marrow reticulocytes may display fluorescence, but protoporphyrin content and fluorescence of circulating reticulocytes is nonuniform and decreases with age.[77] Erythrocyte protoporphyrin in EPP is free and not complexed with zinc, unlike other conditions associated with increased erythrocyte protoporphyrin content. The content of free protoporphyrin in these cells declines much more rapidly with red cell age than it does in conditions in which erythrocyte zinc protoporphyrin is increased.[77a] In lead poisoning and iron deficiency the excess erythrocyte zinc protoporphyrin is bound to hemoglobin and persists in the red cell as long as it circulates, whereas free protoporphyrin in EPP binds less readily to hemoglobin and diffuses more rapidly into the plasma. Interestingly, free protoporphyrin, but not zinc protoporphyrin, is released from erythrocytes following irradiation, which may explain why lead intoxication and iron deficiency, which are associated with elevated erythrocyte zinc protoporphyrin levels, are not associated with photosensitivity.[78] Skin irradiation in EPP patients leads to complement activation and polymorphonuclear chemotaxis, and this event may also contribute to the pathogenesis of skin lesions in EPP.[79]

Light and electron microscopic examination of liver biopsies from EPP patients have revealed a wide variability in findings ranging

TABLE 62-5   COMMON CLINICAL FEATURES OF ERYTHROPOIETIC PROTOPORPHYRIA FROM A SERIES OF 32 CASES[67]

SYMPTOMS AND SIGNS	INCIDENCE
	% of total
Burning	97
Edema	94
Itching	88
Erythema	69
Scarring	19
Vesicles	3
Anemia	27
Cholelithiasis	12
Abnormal liver function results	4

from complete normality to periportal fibrosis and severe cirrhosis. Abnormally elevated, sometimes massive, accumulations of protoporphyrin have been detected as brown pigment in hepatocytes, Kupffer cells, and biliary cannaliculae and are doubly refractive under polarizing lenses.[80] Some 20 patients with EPP have developed hepatic failure resulting in death, presumably secondary to protoporphyrin damage. A high ratio of protoporphyrin to bile acids in bile may be indicative of those patients with EPP who have advanced liver disease.[81]

CLINICAL FEATURES

The most common symptoms in a series of 32 patients with EPP are shown in Table 62-5. Symptoms are usually worse during spring and summer and occur in light-exposed areas, especially of the face and hands. Within 1 h of exposure to the sun, stinging or painful burning sensations occur in the skin and are followed several hours later by erythema and edema. Petechiae, or more rarely, purpura, vesicles, and crusting may develop and persist for several days after sun exposure. Some patients experience burning sensations in the absence of objective signs of cutaneous phototoxicity. Artificial lights may also cause photosensitivity.[82] Severe exposure to the sun may result in onycholysis, leathery hyperkeratotic skin over the dorsae of the hands, and mild scarring. Bullae, skin fragility, hypertrichosis, hyperpigmentation, severe scarring, and mutilation are unusual in EPP. Gallstones, sometimes presenting at an unusually early age, are fairly common, and hepatic disease, although unusual, may be severe and associated with significant morbidity. Anemia is uncommon. There are no known precipitating factors and no neurovisceral manifestations. Conversely, pregnancy is known to lower erythrocyte protoporphyrin levels and increase tolerance to sunlight.[71]

DIAGNOSIS

Photosensitivity should suggest the diagnosis which can be confirmed by the demonstration of elevated concentrations of free protoporphyrin in erythrocytes, plasma, and stool, in association with normal urinary porphyrins. The presence of protoporphyrin in both plasma and erythrocytes is specific for EPP. Fluorescent reticulocytes on examination of peripheral blood smear also suggest the diagnosis. Evidence tends to favor the marrow and the newly released reticulocytes or erythrocytes as the major source of elevated protoporphyrin concentrations.[77] Mild anemia with hyperchromia and microcytosis may also occur. Mild hypertriglyceridemia occurs with increased frequency in patients with EPP.

THERAPY

Avoidance of the sun and use of topical sunscreen agents may be helpful. Oral administration of β-carotene may afford photoprotection, resulting in improved, but highly variable, tolerance to the sun. The recommended serum β-carotene level of 600 to 800 μg/dl[83] is usually achieved with oral doses of 120 mg to 180 mg daily, and beneficial effects are typically seen 1 to 3 months after the onset of therapy; β-carotene probably quenches activated oxygen radicals.[84] Hypertransfusion therapy has also been advocated to suppress erythropoiesis,[85] but the potential hazards of transfusion are a drawback. Cholestyramine has been reported to improve photosensitivity and reduce hepatic protoporphyrin content.[86] Several patients who developed hepatic failure have been treated by liver transplantation, with only temporary relief of deranged liver function and accumulation of protoporphyrin in the liver.[87]

HEPATIC PORPHYRIAS

ACUTE HEPATIC PORPHYRIAS

ALA DEHYDRATASE DEFICIENCY PORPHYRIA

Definition and History   ADP is an autosomal recessive disorder resulting from an almost complete deficiency of ALA dehydratase activity (Table 62-1 and Fig. 62-1). This is the rarest form of the porphyrias; only four well-documented cases have been reported.[88] Two cases were German males with onset in their teens,[89] the third case was a Swedish infant with severe acute hepatic porphyria,[90] and the fourth was a Belgian male with a late onset.[91]

Pathophysiology   The molecular defect of ALA dehydratase in the first German patient has been demonstrated to be compound heterozygosity for two distinct point mutations of the ALA dehydratase gene, one at each allele.[92] One, termed G2, was a base substitution of A for G at nucleotide 820, which resulted in an amino acid change, Ala274→Thr, and the other, termed G1, was a C to T transition at nucleotide 718, resulting in an amino acid change, Arg240→Trp.[93] The G1 mutation was located within the substrate binding site, while the G2 mutation was present downstream of this site. Expression of the G1 cDNA in Chinese hamster ovary cells produced ALA dehydratase protein with little activity; the G2 cDNA produced the enzyme with about 50 percent normal enzyme activity. Pulse-labeling studies demonstrated that the G1 enzyme had a normal half-life, while the G2 enzyme had a markedly decreased half-life. These findings demonstrated that the proband was a compound heterozygote for two separate point mutations in each ALA dehydratase allele and accounted for the almost complete lack of enzymatic activity in the proband's cells and the half-normal activity in cells from the family members.

The molecular defect in the Swedish infant with ADP was also reported.[94] A maternal G to A transition at nucleotide 397 predicted a Gly133→Arg change, which occurred at the carboxyl end of the zinc binding site in the enzyme. The paternal mutation was a G to A transition at nucleotide 823, resulting in an amino acid change, Val275→Met. The four distinct point mutations in two pedigrees suggest a marked heterogeneity in the mutations in this disorder.[88]

Clinical Features   The symptomatology is similar to that seen in AIP. The two German male patients with onset in their teens were characterized by vomiting, pain in the legs, and neuropathy. In one patient this was also accompanied by abdominal pain.[89] Later, the second patient developed paralysis of the arms, legs, and respiratory muscles. Both patients displayed clinical exacerbation following stress, decreased food intake, or alcohol ingestion. Despite these problems, the two patients fared well even 20 years after the onset of the disease.[95] The Swedish infant was diagnosed at the age of 2 and had a stormy course characterized by general muscle hypotonia, respiratory insufficiency, and bilateral paralysis of the legs.[90] The Belgian patient developed porphyria-related symptoms for the first time at the age of 63. This patient had additionally a myeloproliferative disorder.[91]

Diagnosis   Definitive diagnosis of ADP is dependent on the demonstration of markedly deficient erythrocyte ALA dehydratase activity and the enzyme protein in the proband and intermediate decreases in the proband's relatives. Supportive evidence for the diagnosis includes massive elevations in urinary ALA and substantial elevation of porphyrins in urine and erythrocytes; in contrast, urinary PBG excretion is within the normal range. Urinary and erythrocyte porphyrins, predominantly coproporphyrin III and protoporphyrin IX, respectively, are markedly elevated (about 100-fold); no satisfactory explanation has been forwarded to account for this observation. Erythrocyte ALA dehydratase activity is markedly decreased (less than 2 percent of normal) in the proband, and intermediately decreased (about 50 percent of normal) in the parents' erythrocytes.

Lead poisoning can be differentiated by increased blood lead and zinc protoporphyrin, excessive urinary excretion of ALA and coproporphyrin, and markedly inhibited ALA dehydratase activity in erythrocytes, which, however, can be restored to normal by the addition of reduced glutathione, or dithiothreitol in vitro. There is no reduction in the ALA dehydratase protein in lead poisoning,[96] which differentiates it from ADP.[88]

Hereditary tyrosinemia I is due to an inherited deficiency of fumaryl acetoacetate hydrolase.[31] Patients with this condition excrete large amounts of ALA into urine, but not PBG. Diagnosis of tyrosinemia can be made by demonstrating succinylacetone in urine, as for example, by showing inhibition of ALA dehydratase activity of normal blood by the addition of a patient's urine. There is no reduction in the amount of ALA dehydratase protein in this disease.[97]

Therapy   The clinical similarities of ADP to AIP suggest that clinical guideline for treatment of ADP probably should follow that of AIP. However, the reported responses to treatment of the four cases varied greatly. One German patient responded to intravenous glucose, while the Swedish child failed to respond to glucose or to intravenous hematin. This child finally required liver transplantation at the age of 7, which did not suppress urinary ALA excretion but improved the patient's condition to withstand several porphyrogenic challenges.[98]

ACUTE INTERMITTENT PORPHYRIA (AIP)

Definition and History   An autosomal dominant disorder resulting from a partial deficiency of PBG deaminase activity (Table 62-1 and Fig. 62-1), AIP is the major porphyria both in its incidence and severity. In the majority of patients (more than 85 percent) the deficient enzyme activity (about 50 percent of normal) is found in all tissues, including erythrocytes. This is consistent with a heterozygous enzyme deficiency in affected individuals. The first case of porphyria described in 1889 by Stokvis[1] was probably a sulfonal-induced AIP. Since then, many cases of AIP, with or without drug ingestion, have been described. The prevalence of AIP was estimated to be 1 to 2 per 100,000 in Europe,[99] or 2.4 per 100,000 in Finland.[100] A cluster of AIP is known to exist in northern Sweden (1 per 1500[101]). The frequency of low PBG deaminase activity, which additionally includes latent gene carriers of AIP, is, however, as high as 1 per 500 in the general population of Finland.[102] In France, based on molecular defect analysis, the minimal prevalence of the AIP gene has been calculated to be 1:1675.[103]

Pathophysiology   More than 90 different abnormalities of the PBG deaminase gene have been reported in AIP since 1989.[104] The prevalence of specific defective alleles among AIP families appears to vary depending on the population studied. Founder effects are likely to account for a high frequency of a single mutation in Finland and, to a lesser extent, in Holland, while many other mutations have only been found once, each of them in a single family. Both negative and positive types of cross-reactive immunological material (CRIM) were reported among AIP patients. Based on these findings, AIP can be classified into three subtypes, which are summarized in Table 62-6.

TABLE 62-6   CLASSIFICATION OF AIP

	ACTIVITY	MASS	MASS/ACTIVITY	CRIM
Type I	50	50	1	Negative
Type II	100	100	1	Negative
Type IIIa	50	85	1.7	Positive
IIIb	50	280	5.7	Superpositive

Type I.   Patients with this subtype are characterized by a *CRIM-negative* mutation of PBG deaminase. Namely, patients exhibit both intermediately reduced enzyme activity and protein content (about 50 percent of normal). The mutations include single base substitutions, deletions that result in either changes in a single amino acid change or truncated proteins produced by splicing defects or frameshift mutations.

Type II.   Patients with type II AIP (less than 5 percent of all AIP) are characterized by a partially decreased PBG deaminase activity in nonerythroid cells, but by *normal erythrocyte PBG deaminase activity*. A G→A transition was reported in a Dutch family at the first position of the first intron of the PBG deaminase gene. This modified the normal splice consensus sequence CGGTGAGT to CGATGAGT. A single base substitution (CG→CT) which resulted in a splicing defect at the last position of exon 1 was found in a Finnish family. Both mutations had no consequence on the expression of PBG deaminase in erythroid cells, since transcription of the gene in this cell type starts downstream of the site of mutation.

Type III.   Patients with type III AIP are characterized by a *CRIM-positive mutation*, i.e., decreased activity with the presence of a structurally abnormal enzyme protein.[105] Within this type, there are patients with moderately increased CRIM (type IIIa)[106] and those with markedly increased CRIM (type IIIb)[107] (Table 62-6).

Pathogenesis of the Clinical Findings   The symptomatology of AIP is principally due to neurological dysfunction. Postmortem findings are, however, nonremarkable, suggesting their metabolic nature. Various theories have been put forth for the pathogenesis of neuropathy in AIP: (1) PBG deaminase deficiency in the nervous system tissues could limit the synthesis of heme for brain heme proteins; (2) deficiency in heme synthesis in the liver may adversely influence heme protein formation in the brain; (3) heme pathway intermediates, such as ALA, PBG, or their metabolites, may be toxic to nerve cells; and (4) in acute attacks, hepatic heme deficiency may lead to decreased activity of hepatic tryptophan pyrrolase, resulting in enhanced plasma levels and brain uptake of tryptophan, and ultimately to increased synthesis of 5-hydroxytryptamine, a neurotransmitter.

Precipitating Factors   It should be recognized that up to 90 percent of individuals with documented deficiencies of PBG deaminase activity remain asymptomatic throughout their lifetimes. Some individuals with PBG deaminase deficiency may, however, have acute attacks precipitated by various endogenous or exogenous factors. There are at least five different classes of precipitating factors.

Inducers of Hepatic ALA Synthase.   Most precipitating factors are inducers of nonspecific hepatic ALA synthase, ALAS-N. An increase in the metabolic demand for hepatic heme synthesis leads to an induction of ALAS-N and an overproduction of ALA. The partial deficiency of PBG deaminase activity (about 50 percent of normal) then becomes rate-limiting.

Endocrine Factors.   Hormonal factors play a major role in the induction of ALAS-N activity. Clinical expression of AIP is virtually absent before puberty. The clinical disease is more common in women, especially at the time of menses; a subset of female patients experiences regular perimenstrual exacerbation of their disease. Synthetic estrogens and progesterone are known to induce porphyria.

Caloric Intake. Reducing caloric intake leads to exacerbation of AIP; conversely, carbohydrate-rich diets decrease PBG excretion and suppress clinical attacks.[108]

Drugs and Foreign Chemicals. Many chemicals, particularly barbiturates, exacerbate AIP. They are inducers of hepatic cytochrome P450 and result in enhanced demand for de novo heme synthesis, also leading to derepression of hepatic ALA synthase activity.

Stress. Various forms of stress, including intermittent illnesses, infections, alcoholic excess, and surgery may contribute to the genesis of an acute attack, via induction of hepatic heme oxygenase, which then results in heme depletion.

Clinical Features   The clinical findings from three large series of AIP patients (417 was the total number[109-111]) are summarized in Table 62-7. The course of an acute attack of AIP is highly variable, with attacks lasting from a few days to several months. Abdominal pain is almost always present and is often the initial symptom of an acute attack. It may be generalized or localized. In severe cases the pain mimics an acute surgical abdomen and may lead to inappropriate laparotomy. Chest, back, and limb pain may also occur. Pains are usually intermittent, but they may also be chronic, and the severity may fluctuate. Gastrointestinal features are common which may include nausea, vomiting, constipation or diarrhea, abdominal distention, and ileus. The incidence of hepatocellular carcinoma is increased.[112] Urinary incontinence, dysuria, frequency, and urinary retention may occur. The urine may appear "port-wine red" due to the high content of porphobilin, an auto-oxidation product of PBG and some porphyrins which are formed by nonenzymatic cyclization of PBG.

Neuropathy, particularly of the motor type, is a common feature of AIP, but any type of neuropathy may also occur. Motor neuropathy may involve the cranial nerves (most commonly the seventh and tenth) or lead to bulbar paralysis, respiratory impairment, and death; rarely, AIP may present as respiratory failure.[113] Acute attacks of AIP are often accompanied by seizures, especially in patients with hyponatremia due to vomiting, inappropriate fluid therapy, or the syndrome of inappropriate antidiuretic hormone release.

Diagnosis   Diagnosis can be established by the demonstration of reduced PBG deaminase activity (about 50 percent of normal) in erythrocytes, except in the case of type II AIP patients who show normal erythrocyte PBG deaminase activity. PBG deaminase activity in type II patients is, however, reduced in nonerythroid cells such as fibroblasts or lymphocytes.[114,115] The distinction among (1) silent gene carriers, (2) clinically latent but biochemically manifest carriers, and (3) clinically and biochemically fully expressed patients is dependent

on demonstration of elevated urinary excretion of PBG and ALA and on the history of the individual subject. Patients with the clinically expressed disease, as well as some latent gene carriers, excrete increased amounts of ALA and PBG in the urine, often even during clinical remission. The onset of an acute attack is accompanied by further massive increases in excretion of these precursors (ALA 25 to 100 mg/day; PBG 50 to 200 mg/day).[116] The Watson-Schwartz test[117] is widely used as a screening test for urinary PBG. The column method of Mauzerall and Granick[118] should be used to quantify the amount of ALA and PBG in urine. Elevated levels of ALA and PBG may also be seen in HCP and VP. Urinary and stool porphyrin assays differentiate these conditions from AIP. Patients with ADP show elevated ALA in urine, but not PBG.[88]

Therapy   The treatment of AIP as well as ADP, HCP, and VP is essentially identical. Treatment between attacks comprises adequate nutritional intake, avoidance of drugs known to exacerbate porphyria, and prompt treatment of other conditions, e.g., starvation, intermittent diseases, or infections. Unresponsive cases should be admitted to the hospital and intravenous administration of carbohydrate initiated with dextrose to provide a minimum of 300 g of carbohydrate per day. The use of intravenous hematin is now considered the treatment of choice. It curtails urinary excretion of ALA and PBG, acute attacks, and perhaps the severity of neuropathy. Nasal or subcutaneous administration of long-acting agonists of LHRH inhibits ovulation and greatly reduces the incidence of perimenstrual attacks of AIP in such women.[119] Pain, which is invariably present and severe, can be treated with frequent regular doses of narcotic analgesics.

HEREDITARY COPROPORPHYRIA

Definition   HCP is a disease caused by a partial deficiency of coproporphyrinogen oxidase activity (about 50 percent of normal) which is inherited in an autosomal dominant manner (Table 62-1 and Fig. 62-1). Clinically expressed HCP is much less common than is clinically expressed AIP. In Denmark, the incidence of HCP has been estimated to be 2 per 1,000,000.[120] However, with the recent improvement of laboratory techniques such as quantitative HPLC of porphyrins and a radioactive assay of coproporphyrinogen oxidase activity, more gene carriers for this condition have been recognized.

Pathophysiology   Clinically, the disease is similar to ADP, or AIP, although it is often milder; additionally, HCP may be associated with photosensitivity due to accumulation of coproporphyrin in the tissue. Expression of the disease is variable and influenced by the same precipitating factors responsible for the exacerbation of AIP. Very rarely, homozygous deficiency of this enzyme may occur and is associated with a more severe form of the disease.[121]

Clinical Features   The principal symptoms of HCP are neurological dysfunctions which are indistinguishable from those of ADP, AIP, and VP. Abdominal pain, vomiting, constipation, neuropathy, and psychiatric manifestations are common. Approximately 30 percent of patients with HCP accompany photocutaneous symptoms. Clinical attacks can be precipitated by pregnancy, the menstrual cycle, and contraceptive steroids, but the most common precipitating factor is administration of drugs, such as phenobarbital.

Diagnosis   The diagnosis of HCP should be suspected in patients with the signs, symptoms, and clinical course characteristic of the acute hepatic porphyria but in whom erythrocyte PBG deaminase activity is normal. Urinary excretion of porphyrin precursors is simi-

TABLE 62-7   SIGNS AND SYMPTOMS OF AIP

SYMPTOMS & SIGNS	WALDENSTRÖM 321 CASES[109]	GOLDBERG 50 CASES[110]	STEIN & TSCHUDY 46 CASES[111]
	% of total	% of total	% of total
Abdominal pain	85	94	95
Vomiting	59	88	43
Constipation	48	84	48
Diarrhea	9	12	5
Limb, head, neck, or chest pain	—	52	50
Muscle weakness	42	68	60
Sensory loss	9	38	26
Convulsions	10	16	20
Respiratory paralysis	14	10	9
Mental symptoms	55	58	40
Hypertension	40	54	36
Tachycardia	28	64	80
Fever	37	14	9

lar in HCP and VP, but the predominance of coproporphyrin III is highly suggestive of HCP. Fecal coproporphyrin concentrations are also markedly elevated. Excessive excretion of ALA, PBG, and uroporphyrin into the urine is common during acute attacks, but, in contrast to AIP, these findings generally normalize between attacks. Rarely, two variant forms of HCP have been described. One is harderoporphyria, which is due to a homozygous defect of a structurally altered coproporphyrinogen oxidase, and the other is homozygous HCP, which is due to a homozygous deficiency of the normal enzyme. Fecal or urinary predominance of harderoporphyrin, with greatly reduced coproporphyrinogen oxidase activity, indicates harderoporphyria. Interestingly, harderoporphyria with K404E substitution in the coproporphyrinogen oxidase gene, either in the homozygous or compound heterozygous state, associated with a mutation leading to the absence of functional mRNA or protein, has been found to be responsible for neonatal hemolytic anemia.[122]

Therapy The identification and avoidance of precipitating factors is essential. Treatment of acute attacks is similar to the treatment of AIP.

VARIEGATE PORPHYRIA

Definition and History VP is caused by a partial deficiency in protoporphyrinogen oxidase activity and is inherited in an autosomal dominant manner (Table 62-1 and Fig. 62-1). The incidence of VP is particularly high in South Africa, i.e., 3 per 1000. In 1980, it was estimated that there were 10,000 affected individuals in South Africa,[123] and evidence suggests that they are all descendants of a single Dutch settler in 1680.[124] However, the disease is also recognized worldwide, and with the exception of South Africa, there is probably no racial or geographical predilection. Incidence in Finland is reported at 1.3 per 100,000.[125]

Pathophysiology Patients with this disorder may show neurovisceral symptoms, photosensitivity, or both, due to a partial deficiency in protoporphyrinogen oxidase activity.[126] Disease expression is highly influenced by factors similar to those which precipitate the acute attack of AIP.

Clinical Features The neurovisceral symptomatology is indistinguishable from that of ADP, AIP, and HCP. Photosensitivity is more common, and cutaneous symptoms tend to be more chronic in VP than in HCP. Lesions are clinically and histologically indistinguishable from PCT, and in the absence of neurovisceral symptoms, the diagnosis of VP is easily overlooked. Skin manifestations are less frequently observed in cold climates (e.g., 45 percent in a series from Finland[127]) than in hot climates (e.g., 85 percent in a series from South Africa[123]). The same spectrum of factors which activate ADP, AIP, and HCP also induce VP.

Diagnosis VP should be considered in the differential diagnosis of acute hepatic porphyria, i.e., ADP, AIP, and HCP. If PBG deaminase activity is normal in a patient with an acute hepatic porphyria syndrome, it is particularly important to evaluate VP and type II AIP. Characteristic plasma porphyrin fluorescence is usually seen in VP.[128] The differentiation of VP from HCP is usually possible by fecal porphyrin analysis. In patients with only cutaneous manifestations, the demonstration of urinary 8- and 7-carboxylic porphyrins and isocoproporphyrin is usually sufficient for differentiation of PCT from VP. If protoporphyrinogen oxidase assay is not available, screening of family members is best achieved by measuring fecal porphyrin concentrations and profiles.

Four homozygous cases of VP have been described. Parents of these patients had about 50 percent protoporphyrinogen oxidase activity but without clinical symptoms. Clinical features of these patients were severe photosensitivity, growth and mental retardation, and marked neurological abnormalities in two cases; onset was in child-

hood in all cases. None of the patients were anemic, suggesting that the principal site of protoporphyrinogen oxidase deficiency occurs in the liver, not erythroid cells.

Therapy Identification and avoidance of precipitating factors is essential. Photosensitivity can be minimized by protective clothing, and canthaxanthin (a β-carotene analogue) may be of some help.[129] Treatment of neurovisceral symptoms is identical to that described for AIP.

CHRONIC HEPATIC PORPHYRIAS

PORPHYRIA CUTANEA TARDA

Definition PCT is due to a partial deficiency of uroporphyrinogen decarboxylase activity (Table 62-1 and Fig. 62-1). PCT is the most common of all the porphyrias—genetic and acquired combined—but its exact incidence is not clear. The disease is recognized worldwide, and there is no racial predilection except among the Bantus in South Africa, secondary to their high incidence of hemosiderosis. Previously, PCT was more common in men than in women, in part due to higher alcohol intake in men, but the incidence in women has recently approached that of men, perhaps due to increased use of contraceptive steroids, postmenopausal estrogens, and alcohol. PCT can be classified into three subtypes (Table 62-8). The hallmark of all types of PCT is cutaneous photosensitivity due to increased accumulation of uroporphyrin and 7-carboxylic porphyrin.

Pathophysiology *Type I.* Patients with type I PCT are characterized by the lack of family history and by normal erythrocyte uroporphyrinogen decarboxylase activity and concentrations, but with decreased enzyme activity in the liver. Type I PCT typically presents in adults, either spontaneously, or more commonly, in conjunction with precipitating environmental factors such as alcohol, estrogen, drug use, iron overload, or in association with other disorders.

Type II. In type II PCT patients, the catalytic activity and the concentration of uroporphyrinogen decarboxylase are both about 50 percent of normal in all tissues, and the enzyme deficiency segregates as an autosomal dominant trait in the patient's pedigree.

Type III. Patients with type III PCT are characterized by normal erythrocyte uroporphyrinogen decarboxylase activity and concentrations, but with decreased hepatic uroporphyrinogen decarboxylase activity, and this abnormality is found in more than one member in the same family.

Pathogenesis of the Clinical Findings. The initial event in bullous formation is the appearance of membrane-limited vacuoles in the superficial dermis. Porphyrin biosynthesis in the skin of PCT patients is increased compared to normal controls. Thus phototoxic porphyrins in the skin may be derived from both the liver and locally from the skin. Activation of the complement system after irradiation has been demonstrated in PCT patients both in vivo and in vitro in sera[130] and is thought to result from generation of reactive oxygen species. Bullous fluid contains prostaglandin E_2, and photoactivation of uroporphyrin damages lysosomes; inflammation and autolysis may be attributable to these factors.

TABLE 62-8   CLASSIFICATION OF PCT

		URO'GEN DECARBOXYLASE ACTIVITY	
TYPE	FAMILIAL OCCURRENCE	ERYTHROCYTES	LIVER
I	−	Normal	Decreased
II	+	50% of normal	50% of normal
III	+	Normal	50% of normal

Liver biopsy specimens from patients with PCT, particularly those with type I, almost invariably display siderosis. Red autofluorescence and needlelike cytoplasmic inclusion bodies, representing crystallized porphyrins, have also frequently been recognized. Most cases of type I PCT have evidence of cirrhosis at autopsy. The incidence of hepatocellular carcinoma in PCT is greater than normal.[131] Rarely, primary hepatomas may secrete porphyrins and simulate PCT.[132]

Precipitating Factors. Sporadic PCT is often triggered by exposure to environmental factors, such as alcohol, estrogens, iron, and polychlorinated aromatic hydrocarbons. Ethanol has long been known to exacerbate PCT, and the incidence of heavy alcohol intake has been reported to range from 25 to 100 percent. The mechanisms by which alcohol exacerbates PCT are unclear, but alcohol has been reported to increase iron uptake,[133] which subsequently may contribute to the aggravation of the disease.

Estrogen administration has been associated with clinical relapse of PCT.[134] Pregnancy may also aggravate PCT.[135] PCT has been associated with the hyperestrogenic condition, Klinefelter's syndrome.[136]

Iron plays an important role in the pathogenesis of PCT. Serum iron and ferritin concentrations are frequently elevated in PCT patients,[137] and iron absorption and its turnover have been reported either normal or elevated. Hemosiderosis is seen in about 80 percent of liver biopsy specimens from patients with PCT.[137] Phlebotomy induces clinical remission, while iron supplementation may lead to relapse of PCT.[138] Addition of iron to in vitro systems has been reported either to inhibit[139] or to stimulate uroporphyrinogen decarboxylase activity.[140]

The cause of the hepatic siderosis and mild iron overload in PCT, however, remains elusive. An association between HLA-linked hereditary hemochromatosis and PCT has been suggested, but also contested. Recently, a new histocompatibility-complex (MHC) class I-like gene, *HFE*, has been identified,[141] and two missense variants, 845 G6A (C282Y) and 187 C6G (H63D), were found in the majority of unselected patients with hereditary hemochromatosis (see Chap. 42). It has also been shown that there is a high prevalence of the C282Y mutation in patients with PCT,[142,143] suggesting the involvement of the *HFE* gene in the pathogenesis of PCT.

Polyhalogenated aromatic hydrocarbons have been associated with development of PCT in man and in laboratory animals; 2,3,7,8-tetrachlorodibenzo-*p*-dioxin (TCDD) was reported to cause PCT in 11 chemical factory workers in Czechoslovakia.[144] Three cases of PCT were reported from a factory manufacturing the herbicides 2,4-dichloro- and trichlorophenoxyacetic acid,[145] and one janitor developed PCT after accidental exposure to polychlorinated biphenyls (PCB) in a disinfectant.[146] A massive outbreak of about 4000 cases of PCT occurred following the ingestion of hexachlorobenzene-contaminated wheat in Turkey from 1956 to 1961.[147,148] A number of studies on the porphyrinogenic effects of TCDD, hexachlorobenzene, and PCB suggest that metabolic activation of the compounds (probably by cytochrome P450) is required to decrease uroporphyrinogen decarboxylase activity.

PCT has been observed in association with hemodialysis,[149] systemic lupus erythematosus, Sjögren syndrome,[150] rheumatoid arthritis,[151] diabetes mellitus,[152] viral hepatitis,[153] Wilson disease,[154] striopallidodentate calcinosis (Fahr disease),[155] tumors and reticulosis,[156] thalassemia minor and hemophilia.[157,158] PCT has also been reported to develop after treatment with cyclophosphamide[159] and bone marrow transplantation for chronic myelogenous leukemia.[160] Recently an increasing number of patients with PCT in association with HIV infection has been reported, and positive links between PCT and AIDS have been suggested.[161]

Clinical Features Sporadic PCT (type I) almost exclusively presents in adults, while types II and III PCT may occur also in childhood. Patients have increased skin fragility; minor trauma results in erosions from shearing of the skin. Sun exposure may lead to the formation of vesicles and bullae, which crust over, take weeks to heal, and leave a scar. Milia may develop in the skin where bullae have healed. Hyperpigmentation, melanosis, and violaceous-brownish discolorations may develop on light-exposed areas. Facial hypertrichosis slowly develops and is most noticeable in women. Alopecia may develop in sites of repeated trauma or bullous formation. Hypopigmented indurated plaques of skin may develop and may appear as scleroderma-like changes.

Diagnosis The clinical picture of PCT is fairly specific, and its diagnosis is usually not difficult. However, it is necessary to differentiate it from other cutaneous photosensitivity syndromes. Clinical suspicion of PCT should lead to examination of the urine for fluorescence under an ultraviolet light and to quantitation of porphyrins. Uroporphyrin greater than coproporphyrin favors PCT; the reverse favors VP or HCP and may be associated with elevations in urinary ALA and PBG concentrations. Plasma porphyrins are invariably elevated in PCT and in other photosensitizing porphyrias. Isocoproporphyrin in feces represents the most important diagnostic criterion for PCT (Table 62-2).[162] In the presence of uroporphyrinogen decarboxylase deficiency, 5-carboxylate porphyrinogen III accumulates and undergoes metabolism by coproporphyrinogen oxidase to yield dehydroisocoproporphyrinogen. This product also accumulates because its conversion to harderoporphyrinogen is impaired by the decarboxylase deficiency. Isocoproporphyrins are then generated by the auto-oxidation of the dehydro compound. Measurement of erythrocytic and hepatic uroporphyrinogen decarboxylase activity is usually a research procedure and decreased erythrocyte enzyme activity identifies only those patients with type II PCT.

Therapy The first line of treatment is the identification and avoidance of precipitating factors. Phlebotomy reduces urinary porphyrin concentrations and induces clinical remissions. There is strong evidence that the beneficial effects of phlebotomy result from a diminution in the stores of body iron. Typically, 450 ml of blood is withdrawn at each phlebotomy, and this is initially repeated 1 to 2 times per week. Remission is usually achieved after withdrawal of a total of about 4 to 10 liters of blood. The best objective indices of progress are the serum iron, or preferably the ferritin levels, which should be reduced to the lower limit of normal.

If phlebotomy is contraindicated by the presence of other diseases such as anemia or cardiopulmonary disorders, chloroquine therapy may be considered. Low-dose chloroquine (125 mg twice weekly) and high-dose therapy (500 mg daily) in refractory cases have been beneficial. Both treatment regimens transiently induce increases in plasma and urinary porphyrin concentrations and in liver transaminases. Continued therapy eventually leads to a reduction in porphyrin excretion, and clinical improvement, or remission, may occur typically in 6 to 9 months.

HEPATOERYTHROPOIETIC PORPHYRIA

Definition and History HEP is a rare form of porphyria resulting from a homozygous defect in uroporphyrinogen decarboxylase activity (see Table 62-1 and Fig. 62-1). Clinically, HEP is indistinguishable from CEP and is characterized by childhood onset of severe photosensitivity and skin fragility. HEP is extremely rare; after the first report of HEP by Günther in 1967,[163] only some 20 cases have been reported worldwide to date.[164]

Pathophysiology The uroporphyrinogen decarboxylase mutation in the first patient studied consisted of an 860 G→A change in the cDNA sequence which led to a Gly281→Glu change in the amino acid sequence. In vitro experiments showed that the cDNA with this mutation encoded a polypeptide that was very rapidly degraded in the presence of cell lysates. Two other point mutations were recognized.

One was the replacement of Glu167→Lys which produced a protein with an unstable phenotype.[165] The other mutation was a Arg292→Gly change.[166] It should be noted that the majority of the mutations found in familial PCT and HEP are distinct.

The molecular defect in familial PCT is heterogeneous. A Gly281→Val substitution with unstable phenotype,[167] a splice-site mutation,[168] and exon 6 deletion (unstable phenotype) have been described.[168] The exon 6 deletion has been found in 5 of 22 pedigrees examined and is the only mutation that has been found in more than one pedigree with PCT. HEP patients represent individuals with homozygous or compound heterozygous deficiency of uroporphyrinogen decarboxylase, which is, however, stable enough to meet the requirements for heme synthesis.[167] In contrast, patients with familial PCT who are heterozygous for uroporphyrinogen decarboxylase deficiency may carry mutations with little enzyme activity or with a very unstable protein. One patient with HEP was heteroallelic for Val134→Gln substitution which was due to three sequential point mutations (T417G418T419→CCA) and His220→Pro substitution due to A677→C.[169] Interestingly, the same Val134→Gln substitution was also found in another pedigree, however, as familial PCT.[170]

Clinical Features   The clinical findings are similar to those seen in CEP; pink urine, severe photosensitivity leading to scarring and mutilation of sun-exposed areas of skin, sclerodermoid changes, hypertrichosis, erythrodontia, anemia (often hemolytic), and hepatosplenomegaly. Unlike PCT, onset of HEP is usually in early infancy or childhood,[164] but occasional adult onset has also been described.[171] Curiously, some of the cases with onset in childhood have shown spontaneous resolution of their photosensitivity,[172] and others have experienced relatively mild symptoms from onset despite markedly elevated urinary porphyrin concentrations.[164] In contrast to PCT, serum iron concentrations have usually been normal in HEP patients, and phlebotomy has little effect in improving symptoms. Elevated erythrocyte protoporphyrin level and occasional fluorescent normoblasts suggest the bone marrow as a source of porphyrins.[173]

Diagnosis   The diagnosis must be considered in patients with severe photosensitivity, such as CEP. Diagnostic criteria include elevated levels of fecal or urinary isocoproporphyrin and erythrocyte zinc-protoporphyrin. Patients with EPP, who also show elevated erythrocyte protoporphyrin, can be distinguished from HEP, since they excrete normal amounts of urinary porphyrins. EPP is also clinically milder than HEP. Measurement of erythrocyte or fibroblast uroporphyrinogen decarboxylase activities typically shows reductions to 2 to 10 percent of normal control values with intermediate reductions of uroporphyrinogen decarboxylase activities in family members. As in the case of PCT, isocoproporphyrin concentrations equal to or greater than coproporphyrin is the characteristic of HEP. Elevated erythrocyte protoporphyrin (usually zinc protoporphyrin) has also been a feature of several cases of HEP. In contrast to PCT, serum iron is usually normal.

Therapy   Avoidance of the sun and the use of topical sunscreens is all that can be offered to these patients at present. Patients with HEP do not respond to phlebotomy.[164]

REFERENCES

1. Stokvis BJ: Over Twee Zeldsame Kleuerstoffen in Urine van Zicken. *Nederlands Tijdschr Geneeskunde* 13:409, 1889.
2. Anderson TM: Hydroa aestivale in two brothers, complicated with the presence of haematoporphyrin in the urine. *Br J Dermatol* 10:1, 1898.
3. Harris DF: Haematoporphyrinuria and its relations to the source of urobilin. *J Anat Physiol* 31:383, 1897.
4. Günther H: Die Hämatoporphyrie. *Deutsches Archiv f.klin.Medizin* 105:89, 1911.
5. Garrod AE: *Inborn Errors of Metabolism*. London, Hodder & Stoughton, 1923.

6. Granick JL, Sassa S: Hemin control of heme biosynthesis in mouse Friend virus-transformed erythroleukemia cells in culture. *J Biol Chem* 253:5402, 1978
7. Correia MA, Farrell GC, Schmid R, Ortiz de Monetellano PR, Yost GS, Mico BA: Incorporation of exogenous heme into hepatic cytochrome P-450 in vivo. *J Biol Chem* 254:15, 1979
8. Berk PD, Howe RB, Berlin NI: Disorders of bilirubin metabolism, in Bondy PK, Rosenberg LE (eds): *Duncan's Diseases of Metabolism*. Philadelphia, WB Saunders, 1974, p 825.
9. Granick S, Sassa S: δ-aminolevulinic acid synthetase and the control of heme and chlorophyll synthesis, in Vogel HJ (ed): *Metabolic Regulation*. New York, Academic, 1971, p 77.
10. Sassa S, Kappas A: Genetic, metabolic, and biochemical aspects of the porphyrias, in Harris H, Hirschhorn K (eds): *Advances in Human Genetics*. New York, Plenum Publsh. Corp., 1981, p 121.
11. McKay R, Druyan R, Getz GS, Rabinowitz M: Intramitochondrial localization of δ-aminolevulinate synthase and ferrochelatase in rat liver. *Biochem J* 114:455, 1969.
12. Riddle RD, Yamamoto M, Engel JD: Expression of δ-aminolevulinate synthase in avian cells: Separate genes encode erythroid-specific and nonspecific isozymes. *Proc Natl Acad Sci USA* 86:792, 1989.
13. Bishop DF, Astrin KH, Ioannou YA: Human δ-aminolevulinate synthase: Isolation, characterization, and mapping of house-keeping and erythroid-specific genes. *Am J Hum Genet* 45:A176, 1989.
14. Bishop DF: Two different genes encode δ-aminolevulinate synthase in humans: nucleotide sequences of cDNAs for the housekeeping and erythroid genes. *Nucl Acids Res* 18:7187, 1990.
15. Cox TC, Bawden MJ, Martin A, May BK: Human erythroid 5-aminolevulinate synthase: promoter analysis and identification of an iron-responsive element in the mRNA. *EMBO J* 10:1891, 1991.
16. Mignotte V, Eleouet JF, Raich N, Romeo P-H: *Cis*- and *trans*-acting elements involved in the regulation of the erythroid promotor of the human porphobilinogen deaminase gene. *Proc Natl Acad Sci USA* 86:6548, 1989.
17. Aziz N, Munro HN: Iron regulates ferritin mRNA translation through a segment of its 5' untranslated region. *Proc Natl Acad Sci* 84:8478, 1987.
18. Casey JL, Di Jeso B, Rao K, Rouault TA, Klausner RD, Harford JB: The promoter region of the human transferrin receptor gene. *Ann NY Acad Sci* 526:54, 1988.
19. Melefors O, Goossen B, Johansson HE, Stripecke R, Gray NK, Hentze MW: Translational control of 5-aminolevulinate synthase mRNA by iron-responsive elements in erythroid cells. *J Biol Chem* 268:5974, 1993.
20. Elferink CJ, Srivastava G, Maguire DJ, Borthwick IA, May BK, Elliott WH: A unique gene for 5-aminolevulinate synthase in chickens. Evidence for expression of an identical messenger RNA in hepatic and erythroid tissues. *J Biol Chem* 262:3988, 1987.
21. Bonkowsky HL, Tschudy DP, Collins A, Doherty J, Bossenmaier I, Cardinal R, Watson CJ: Repression of the overproduction of porphyria precursors in acute intermittent porphyria by intravenous infusions of hematin. *Proc Natl Acad Sci USA* 68:2725, 1971.
22. Galbraith RA, Kappas A: Pharmacokinetics of tin-mesoporphyrin in man and the effects of tin-chelated porphyrins on hyperexcretion of heme pathway precursors in patients with acute inducible porphyria. *Hepatology* 9:882, 1989.
23. Kitchin KT: Regulation of rat hepatic δ-aminolevulinic acid synthetase and heme oxygenase activities: evidence for control by heme and against mediation by prosthetic iron. *Int J Biochem* 15:479, 1983.
24. Fujita H, Yamamoto M, Yamagami T, Hayashi N, Sassa S: Erythroleukemia differentiation. Distinctive responses of the erythroid-specific and the nonspecific δ-aminolevulinate synthase mRNA. *J Biol Chem* 266:17494, 1991.
25. Dandekar T, Stripecke R, Gray NK, et al: Identification of a novel iron-responsive element in murine and human erythroid δ-aminolevulinic acid synthase mRNA. *EMBO J* 10:1903, 1991.
26. Sassa S: Heme stimulation of cellular growth and differentiation. *Semin Hematol* 25:312, 1988.
27. Potluri VR, Astrin KH, Wetmur JG, Bishop DF, Desnick RJ: Human 5-aminolevulinate dehydratase: Chromosomal localization to 9q34 by in situ hybridization. *Hum Genet* 76:236, 1987.
28. Sassa S: δ-Aminolevulinic acid dehydratase assay. *Enzyme* 28:133, 1982.
29. Tsukamoto I, Yoshinaga T, Sano S: The role of zinc with special refer-

ence to the essential thiol groups in δ-aminolevulinic acid dehydratase of bovine liver. *Biochem Biophys Acta* 570:167, 1979.

30. Granick JL, Sassa S, Kappas A: Some biochemical and clinical aspects of lead intoxication, in *Advances in Clinical Chemistry*, edited by O Bodansky, AL Latner, pp 287–339. New York, Academic Press, 1978.

31. Lindblad B, Lindstedt S, Steen G: On the genetic defects in hereditary tyrosinemia. *Proc Natl Acad Sci USA* 74:4641, 1977.

32. Tschudy DP, Hess RA, Frykholm BD: Inhibition of δ-aminolevulinic acid dehydratase by 4,6-dioxoheptanoic acid. *J Biol Chem* 256:9915, 1981.

33. Sassa S, Kappas A: Hereditary tyrosinemia and the heme biosynthetic pathway. Profound inhibition of δ-aminolevulinic acid dehydratase activity by succinylacetone. *J Clin Invest* 71:625, 1983.

34. Bishop TR, Cohen PJ, Boyer SH, Noyes AN, Frelin LP: Isolation of a rat liver δ-aminolevulinate dehydratase (ALAD) cDNA clone: Evidence for unequal ALAD gene dosage among inbred mouse strains. *Proc Natl Acad Sci USA* 83:5568, 1986.

35. Wetmur JG, Bishop DF, Ostasiewicz L, Desnick RJ: Molecular cloning of a cDNA for human δ-aminolevulinate dehydratase. *Gene* 43:123, 1986.

36. Gibbs PN, Jordan PM: Identification of lysine at the active site of human 5-aminolaevulinate dehydratase. *Biochem. J* 236:447, 1986.

37. Bishop TR, Miller MW, Beall J, et al: Genetic regulation of delta-aminolevulinate dehydratase during erythropoiesis. *Nucl Acids Res* 24:2511, 1996.

38. Wetmur JB, Bishop DF, Cantelmo C, Desnick RJ: Human δ-aminolevulinate dehydratase: nucleotide sequence of a full length cDNA clone. *Proc Natl Acad Sci USA* 83:7703, 1986.

39. Wetmur JG, Kaya AH, Plewinska M: Molecular characterization of the human δ-aminolevulinate dehydratase 2 (ALAD2) allele: implications for molecular screening of individuals for genetic susceptibility to lead poisoning. *Am J Hum Genet* 49:757, 1991.

40. Battersby AR, Fookes CJR, Matcham GWJ, McDonald E: Order of assembly of the four pyrrole rings during biosynthesis of the natural porphyrins. *J Chem Soc Chem Commun* 539, 1979.

41. Wang AL, Arrendondo-Vega FX, Giampietro PF, Smith M, Anderson WF, Desnick RJ: Regional gene assignment of human porphobilinogen deaminase and esterase A4 to chromosome 11q23−11qter. *Proc Natl Acad Sci USA* 78:5734, 1981.

42. Chretien S, Dubart A, Beaupain D, et al: Alternative transcription and splicing of the human porphobilinogen deaminase gene result either in tissue-specific or in housekeeping expression. *Proc Natl Acad Sci USA* 85:6, 1988.

43. Grandchamp B, Beaumont C, de Verneuil H, Walter O, Nordmann Y: Genetic expression of porphobilinogen deaminase and uroporphyrinogen decarboxylase during the erythroid differentiation of mouse erythroleukemic cells, in *Porphyrins and Porphyrias,* edited by Y Nordmann, pp 35. London, John Libbey, 1986.

44. Raich N, Romeo P-H, Dubart A, Beaupain D, Cohen Solal M, Goosens M: Molecular cloning and complete primary sequence of human erythrocyte porphobilinogen deaminase. *Nucl Acids Res* 14:5955, 1986.

45. Tsai SF, Bishop DF, Desnick RJ: Human uroporphyrinogen III synthase: molecular cloning, nucleotide sequence, and expression of a full-length cDNA. *Proc Natl Acad Sci USA* 85:7049, 1988.

46. Romana M, Dubart A, Beaupain D, Chabret C, Goossens M, Romeo PH: Structure of the gene for human uroporphyrinogen decarboxylase. *Nucl Acids Res* 15:7343, 1987.

47. Romeo P-H, Raich N, Dubart A, et al: Molecular cloning and nucleotide sequence of a complete human uroporphyrinogen decarboxylase cDNA. *J Biol Chem* 261:9825, 1986.

48. Cacheux V, Martasek P, Fougerousse F, et al: Localization of the human coproporphyrinogen oxidase gene to chromosome band 3q12. *Hum Genet* 94:557, 1994.

49. Kohno H, Furukawa T, Yoshinaga T, Tokunaga R, Taketani S: Coproporphyrinogen oxidase: purification, molecular cloning, and induction of mRNA during erythroid differentiation. *J Biol Chem* 268:21359, 1993.

50. Conder LH, Woodard SI, Dailey HA: Multiple mechanisms for the regulation of haem synthesis during erythroid cell differentiation. Possible role for coproporphyrinogen oxidase. *Biochem J* 275:321, 1991.

51. Nishimura K, Taketani S, Inokuchi H: Cloning of a human cDNA for protoporphyrinogen oxidase by complementation in vivo of a hemG mutant of *Escherichia coli*. *J Biol Chem* 270:8076, 1995.

52. Taketani S, Inazawa J, Abe T, et al: The human protoporphyrinogen oxidase gene (PPOX): organization and location to chromosome 1. *Genomics* 29:698, 1995.

53. Porra RJ, Jones OTG: Studies on ferrochelatase 1. Assay and properties of ferrochelatase from a pig liver mitochrondrial extract. *Biochem J* 87:181, 1963.

54. Taketani S, Inazawa J, Nakahashi Y, Abe T, Tokunaga R: Structure of the human ferrochelatase gene: Exon/intron gene organization and location of the gene to chromosome 18. *Eur J Biochem* 205:217, 1992.

55. Whitcombe DM, Carter NP, Albertson DG, Smith SJ, Rhodes DA, Cox TM: Assignment of the human ferrochelatase gene (FECH) and a locus for protoporphyria to chromosome 18q22. *Genomics* 11:1152, 1991.

56. Al-Karadaghi S, Hansson M, Nikonov S, Jonsson B, Hederstedt L: Crystal structure of ferrochelatase: the terminal enzyme in heme biosynthesis. *Structure* 5:1501, 1997.

57. Wada O, Sassa S, Takaku F, Yano Y, Urata G, Nukao K: Different responses of the hepatic and erythropoietic δ-aminolevulinic acid synthetase of mice. *Biochim Biophys Acta* 148:585, 1967.

58. Ross J, Sautner D: Induction of globin mRNA accumulation by hemin in cultured erythroleukemic cells. *Cell* 8:513, 1976.

59. Marver HS: The role of heme in the synthesis and repression of microsomal protein, in *Microsomes and Drug Oxidations*, edited by JR Gillette, AH Conney, GJ Cosmides, et al, pp 495–515. New York, Academic, 1969.

60. Porter PN, Meints RH, Mesner K: Enhancement of erythroid colony growth in culture by hemin. *Exp Hematol* 7:11, 1979.

61. Fritsch C, Bolsen K, Ruzicka T, Goerz G: Congenital erythropoietic porphyria. *J Am Acad Dermatol* 36:594, 1997.

62. Desnick RJ, Glass IA, Xu W, Solis C, Astrin KH: Molecular genetics of congenital erythropoietic porphyria. *Semin Liver Dis* 18:77, 1998.

63. Watson CJ, Perman V, Spurrel FA, Hoyt HH, Schwartz S: Some studies of the comparative biology of human and bovine porphyria erythropoietia. *Trans Assoc Am Physicians* 71:196, 1958.

64. Seip M, Thune PO, Eriksen L: Treatment of photosensitivity in congenital erythropoietic porphyria (CEP) with beta-carotene. *Acta Derm. Venereol* (Stockh) 54:239, 1974.

65. Haining RG, Cowger ML, Labbe RF, Finch CA: Congenital erythropoietic porphyria: II. The effects of induced polycythemia. *Blood* 36:297, 1970.

66. Pimstone NR, Gandhi SN, Mukerji SK: Therapeutic efficacy of oral charcoal in congenital erythropoietic porphyria. *N Engl J Med* 316:390, 1987.

67. DeLeo VA, Poh-Fitzpatrick MB, Mathews-Roth MM, Harber LC: Erythropoietic protoporphyria. 10 years experience. *Am J Med* 60:8, 1976.

68. Cox TM, Alexander GJ, Sarkany RP: Protoporphyria. *Semin Liver Dis* 18:85, 1998.

69. Went LN, Klasen EC: Genetic aspects of erythropoietic protoporphyria. *Ann Hum Genet* 48:105, 1984.

70. Lamoril J, Boulechfar S, de Verneuil H, Grandchamp B, Nordmann Y, Deybach JC: Human erythropoietic protoporphyria: two point mutations in the ferrochelatase gene. *Biochem Biophys Res Commun* 181:594, 1991.

71. Poh-Fitzpatrick MB: Human protoporphyria: reduced cutaneous photosensitivity and lower erythrocyte porphyrin levels during pregnancy. *J Am Acad Dermatol* 36:40, 1997.

72. Ryan EA: Histochemistry of the skin in erythropoietic protoporphyria. *Br J Dermatol* 78:43, 1966.

73. Poh-Fitzpatrick MB: The erythropoietic porphyrias. *Dermatol Clin* 4:291, 1986.

74. Spikes JD: Porphyrins and related compounds as photodynamic sensitizers. *Ann NY Acad Sci* 244:496, 1975.

75. Goldstein BD, Harber LC: Erythropoietic protoporphyria: Lipid peroxidation and red cell membrane damage associated with photohemolysis. *J Clin Invest* 51:892, 1972.

76. Schothorst AA, van Steveninck J, Went IN, Suurmond D: Photodynamic damage of the erythrocyte membrane caused by protoporphyrin in protoporphyria and in normal red blood cells. *Clin Chim Acta* 39:161, 1972.

77. Bottomley SS, Tanaka M, Everett MA: Diminished erythroid ferrochelatase activity in protoporphyria. *J Lab Clin Med* 86:126, 1975.

77a. Piomelli S, Lamola AA, Poh-Fitzpatrick MF, Seaman C, Harbe R: Erythropoietic protoporphyria and lead intoxication: the molecular basis for difference in cutaneous photosensitivity. I. Different rates of disappearance of protoporphyrin from the erythrocytes, both in vivo and in vitro. *J Clin Invest* 56: 1519, 1975.

78. Sandberg S, Brun A, Hovding G, Bjordal M, Romslo I: Effect of zinc on protoporphyrin induced photohaemolysis. *Scan J Clin Lab Invest* 40(2):185, 1980.

79. Lim HW, Poh-Fitzpatrick MB, Gigli I: Activation of the complement system in patients with porphyrias after irradiation in vivo. *J Clin Invest* 74:1961, 1984.

80. Bloomer JR, Enrichez R: Evidence that hepatic crystalline deposits in a patient with protoporphyria are composed of protoporphyrin. *Gastroenterology* 82:569, 1982.

81. Morton KO, Schneider F, Weimer MK, Straka JG, Bloomer JR: Hepatic and bile porphyrins in patients with protoporphyria and liver failure. *Gastroenterology* 94:1488, 1988.

82. Mooney B, Tennant F: Operating theatre lights as hazard in photosensitive patients. *Br Med J* 287:1028, 1983.

83. Mathews-Roth MM: Systemic photoprotection. *Dermatol Clin* 4:335, 1986.

84. Mathews-Roth MM, Pathak MA, Fitzpatrick TB, Harber LH, Kass EH: Beta carotene therapy for erythropoietic protoporphyria and other photosensitivity diseases. *Arch Dermatol* 113:1229, 1977.

85. Bechtel MA, Bertolone SJ, Hodge SJ: Transfusion therapy in a patient with erythropoietic protoporphyria. *Arch Dermatol* 117:99, 1981.

86. Bloomer JR: Pathogenesis and therapy of liver disease in protoporphyria. *Yale J Biol Med* 52:39, 1979.

87. Samuel D, Boboc B, Bernuau J, Bismuth H, Benhamou JP: Liver transplantation for protoporphyria. Evidence for the predominant role of the erythropoietic tissue in protoporphyrin overproduction. *Gastroenterology* 95:816, 1988.

88. Sassa S: ALAD porphyria, in *Seminars in Liver Disease*, edited by PD Berk. Thieme, New York, 1998, p 95.

89. Doss M, von Tiepermann R, Schneider J, Schmid H: New type of hepatic porphyria with porphobilinogen synthase defect and intermittent acute clinical manifestation. *Klin Wochenschr* 57:1123, 1979.

90. Thunell S, Holmberg L, Lundgren J: Aminolevulinate dehydratase porphyria in infancy. A clinical and biochemical study. *J Clin Chem Clin Biochem* 25:5, 1987.

91. Hassoun A, Verstraeten L, Mercelis R, Martin J-J: Biochemical diagnosis of an hereditary aminolaevulinate dehydratase deficiency in a 63-year-old man. *J Clin Chem Clin Biochem* 27:781, 1989.

92. Ishida N, Fujita H, Noguchi T, Doss M, Kappas A, Sassa S: Message amplification phenotyping of an inherited δ-aminolevulinate dehydratase deficiency in a family with acute hepatic porphyria. *Biochem Biophys Res Commun* 172:237, 1990.

93. Ishida N, Fujita H, Fukuda Y, et al: Cloning and expression of the defective genes from a patient with δ-aminolevulinate dehydratase porphyria. *J Clin Invest* 89:1431, 1992.

94. Plewinska M, Thunell S, Holmberg L, Wetmur JG, Desnick RJ: δ-aminolevulinate dehydratase deficient porphyria: identification of the molecular lesions in a severely affected homozygote. *Am J Hum Genet* 49:167, 1991.

95. Gross U, Sassa S, Deybach JC, Nordmann Y, Frank M, Doss MO: 5-Aminolevulinic acid dehydratase deficiency porphyria: a twenty-year clinical and biochemical follow up. *Clin Chem* 44 (9):1892, 1998

96. Fujita H, Sato K, Sano S: Increase in the amount of erythrocyte δ-aminolevulinic acid dehydratase in workers with moderate lead exposure. *Int Arch Occup Environ Health* 50:287, 1982.

97. Sassa S, Fujita H, Kappas A: Succinylacetone and δ-aminolevulinic acid dehydratase in hereditary tyrosinemia: immunochemical study of the enzyme. *Pediatrics* 86:84, 1990.

98. Thunell S, Henrichson A, Floderus Y, et al: Liver transplantation in a boy with acute porphyria due to aminolaevulinate dehydratase deficiency. *Eur J Clin Chem Clin Biochem* 30:599, 1992.

99. Goldberg A, Moore MR, McColl KEL, Brodie MJ: Porphyrin metabolism and the porphyrias, in *Oxford Textbook of Medicine*, edited by JGG Ledingham, DA Warrell, DJ Weatherall, pp 9.136–9.145. Oxford University Press, Oxford, 1987.

100. Mustajoki P, Koskelo P: Hereditary hepatic porphyrias in Finland. *Acta Med Scand* 200:171, 1976.

101. Wetterberg L: A neuropsychiatric and genetical investigation of acute intermittent porphyria. Ph.D. thesis. Stockholm, Scandinavian University Books, 1967.

102. Mustajoki P, Kauppinen R, Lannfelt L, Koistinen J: Frequency of low porphobilinogen deaminase activity in Finland. *J Intern Med* 231:389, 1992.

103. Nordmann Y, Puy H, Da SV, et al: Acute intermittent porphyria: prevalence of mutations in the porphobilinogen deaminase gene in blood donors in France. *J Intern Med* 242:213, 1997.

104. Grandchamp B: Acute intermittent porphyria. *Semin Liver Dis* 18:17, 1998.

105. Grandchamp B, Picat C, de Rooij F, et al: A point mutation G→A in exon 12 of the porphobilinogen deaminase gene results in exon skipping and is responsible for acute intermittent porphyria. *Nucl Acids Res* 17:6637, 1989.

106. Desnick RJ, Ostasiewicz LT, Tishler PA, Mustajoki P: Acute intermittent porphyria: Characterization of a novel mutation in the structural gene for porphobilinogen deaminase. Demonstration of noncatalytic enzyme intermediates stabilized by bound substrate. *J Clin Invest* 76:865, 1985.

107. Wilson JHP, de Rooij FWM, Te Velde K: Acute intermittent porphyria in the Netherlands: Heterogeneity of the enzyme porphobilinogen deaminase. *Neth J Med* 29:393, 1986.

108. Welland FH, Hellman ES, Gaddis EM, Collins A, Hunter GW, Jr: Factors affecting the excretion of porphyrin precursors by patients with acute intermittent porphyria: I. The effects of diet. *Metabolism* 13:232, 1964.

109. Waldenström J: The porphyrias as inborn errors of metabolism. *Am J Med* 22:758, 1957.

110. Goldberg A: Acute intermittent porphyria: a study of 50 cases. *Q J Med* 28:183, 1959.

111. Stein JA, Tschudy DP: Acute intermittent porphyria: a clinical and biochemical study of 46 patients. *Medicine* 49:1, 1970.

112. Kauppinen R, Mustajoki P: Acute hepatic porphyria and hepatocellular carcinoma. *Br J Cancer* 57:117, 1988.

113. Greenspan GH, Block AJ: Respiratory insufficiency associated with acute intermittent porphyria. *South Med J* 74:954, 1981.

114. Sassa S, Solish G, Levere RD, Kappas A: Studies in porphyria: IV. Expression of the gene defect of acute intermittent porphyria in cultured human skin fibroblasts and amniotic cells: prenatal diagnosis of the porphyric trait. *J Exp Med* 142:722, 1975.

115. Sassa S, Zalar GL, Kappas A: Studies in porphyria: VII. Induction of uroporphyrinogen-I synthase and expression of the gene defect of acute intermittent porphyria in mitogen-stimulated human lymphocytes. *J Clin Invest* 61:499, 1978.

116. Granick S, van den Schreieck HG: Porphobilinogen and δ-aminolevulinic acid in acute porphyria. *Proc Soc Exp Biol Med* 88:270, 1955.

117. Watson CJ, Schwartz S: A simple test for urinary porphobilinogen. *Proc Soc Exp Biol Med* 47:393, 1941.

118. Gorschein A: Determination of delta-aminolaevulinic acid in biological fluids by gas-liquid chromatography with electron-capture detection. *Biochem J* 219:883, 1984.

119. Anderson KE, Spitz IM, Sassa S, Bardin CW, Kappas A: Prevention of cyclical attacks of acute intermittent porphyria with a long-acting agonist of luteinizing hormone-releasing hormone. *N Engl J Med* 311:643, 1984.

120. With TK: Hereditary coproporphyria and variegate porphyria in Denmark. *Dan Med Bull* 30:106, 1983.

121. Grandchamp B, Phung N, Nordmann Y: Homozygous case of hereditary coproporphyria [letter]. *Lancet* 2:1348, 1977.

122. Lamoril J, Puy H, Gouya L, et al: Neonatal hemolytic anemia due to inherited harderoporphyria: clinical characteristics and molecular basis. *Blood* 91:1453, 1998.

123. Eales L, Day RS, Blekkenhorst GH: The clinical and biochemical features of variegate porphyria: an analysis of 300 cases studied at Groote Schuur Hospital, Cape Town. *Int J Biochem* 12:837, 1980.

124. Dean G: *The Porphyrias. A Study of Inheritance and Environment*. London, Pitman Medical, 1971.

125. Mustajoki P: Variegate porphyria. Twelve years' experience in Finland. *Q J Med* 194:191, 1980.

126. Kappas A, Sassa S, Galbraith RA, Nordmann Y: The porphyrias, in *The Metabolic and Molecular Basis of Inherited Disease*, edited by CR Scriver, AL Beaudet, WS Sly, D Valle, pp 2103–2159. McGraw-Hill, New York, 1995.

127. Morris AJ, Liang K: Interaction of globin and heme during hemoglobin biosynthesis. *Arch Biochem Biophys* 125:468, 1968.

128. Longas MO, Poh-Fitzpatrick MB: A tightly bound protein-porphyrin complex isolated from the plasma of a patient with variegate porphyria. *Clin Chim Acta* 118:219, 1982.

129. Eales L: The effects of canthaxanthin on the photocutaneous manifestations of porphyrias. *S Afr Med J* 54:1050, 1978.

130. Pigatto PD, Polenghi MM, Altomare GF, Giacchetti A, Cirillo R, Finzi AF: Complement cleavage products in the phototoxic reaction of porphyria cutanea tarda. *Br J Dermatol* 114:567, 1986.

131. Pierach C: Porphyria and hepatocellular carcinoma. *Br J Cancer* 55:111, 1987.

132. Tio TH, Leijnse B, Jarrett A, Rimington C: Acquired porphyria from a liver tumor. *Clin Sci Mol Med* 16:517, 1959.

133. Felsher BF, Kushner JP: Hepatic siderosis and porphyria cutanea tarda: relation of iron excess to the metabolic defect. *Semin Hematol* 14:243, 1977.

134. Domonkos AN: Porphyria cutanea tarda induced by estrogen therapy. *Arch Derm* 102:229, 1970.

135. Lamon JM, Frykholm BC: Pregnancy and porphyria cutanea tarda. *Johns Hopkins Med J* 145:235, 1979.

136. Saced-Uz-Zafar M, Gronewald WR, Bluhm GB: Co-existent Klinefelter's syndrome, acquired cutaneous hepatic porphyria and systemic lupus erythematosus. *Henry Ford Hosp Med J* 18:227, 1970

137. Grossman ME, Bickers DR, Poh-Fitzpatrick MB, DeLeo VA, Harber LC: Porphyria cutanea tarda: Clinical features and laboratory findings in forty patients. *Am J Med* 67:277, 1979.

138. Lundvall O: The effect of replenishment of iron stores after phlebotomy therapy in porphyria cutanea tarda. *Acta Med Scand* 189:51, 1971.

139. Kushner JP, Steinmuller DP, Lee GR: The role of iron in the pathogenesis of porphyria cutanea tarda: II. Inhibition of uroporphyrinogen decarboxylase. *J Clin Invest* 56:661, 1975.

140. Blekkenhorst GH, Eales L, Pimstone NR: Activation of uroporphyrinogen decarboxylase by ferrous iron in porphyria cutanea tarda. *S Afr Med J* 56:918, 1979.

141. Feder JN, Gnirke A, Thomas W, et al: A novel MHC class I-like gene is mutated in patients with hereditary haemochromatosis. *Nature Genet* 13:399, 1996.

142. Stuart KA, Busfield F, Jazwinska EC, et al: The C282Y mutation in the haemochromatosis gene (HFE) and hepatitis C virus infection are independent cofactors for porphyria cutanea tarda in Australian patients. *J Hepatol* 28:404, 1998.

143. Roberts AG, Whatley SD, Morgan RR, et al: Increased frequency of the haemochromatosis Cys282Tyr mutation in sporadic porphyria cutanea tarda. *Lancet* 349:321, 1997.

144. Buckberg AM, Kinniburgh AJ: Induction of liver apolipoprotein A-IV mRNA in porphyric mice. *Nucl Acids Res* 13:1953, 1985.

145. Poland AP, Smith D, Metter G, Possick P: A health survey of workers in a 2,4-D and 2,4,5-T plant. *Arch Environ Health* 22:316, 1971.

146. Lynch RE, Lee GR, Kushner JP: Porphyria cutanea tarda associated with disinfectant misuse. *Arch Intern Med* 135:549, 1975.

147. Cam C, Nigogoysan G: Acquired toxic porphyria cutanea tarda due to hexachlorobenzene. *JAMA* 183:88, 1963.

148. Schmid R: Cutaneous porphyria in Turkey. *N Engl J Med* 263:397, 1960.

149. Goldsman CI, Taylor JS: Porphyria cutanea tarda and bullous dermatoses associated with chronic renal failure: a review. *Cleve Clin Q* 50:151, 1983.

150. Ramasamy R, Kubik MM: Porphyria cutanea tarda in association with Sjogren's syndrome. *Practitioner* 226:1297, 1982.

151. Nyman CR: Porphyria cutanea tarda, carcinoma of the lung, rheumatoid arthritis, right hydronephrosis. *Proc Roy Soc Med* 65:688, 1972.

152. Franks AG, Pulini M, Bickers DR, Rayfield EJ, Harber LC: Carbohydrate metabolism in porphyria cutanea tarda. *Am J Med Sci.* 277:163, 1979.

153. Coburn PR, Coleman JC, Cream JJ, Hawk JLM, Lamb SGS, Murray-Lyon IM: Porphyria cutanea tarda and porphyria variegata unmasked by viral hepatitis. *Clin Exp Dermatol* 10:169, 1985.

154. Chesney TM, Wardlaw LL, Kapalna RJ, Chow JF: Porphyria cutanea tarda complicating Wilson's disease. *J Am Acad Dermatol* 4:64, 1981.

155. Beall SS, Patten BM, Mallette L, Jankovic J: Abnormal systemic metabolism of iron, porphyrin, and calcium in Fahr's syndrome. *Ann Neurol* 26:569, 1989.

156. Grossman ME, Bickers DR: Porphyria cutanea tarda. A rare cutaneous manifestation of hepatic tumors. *Cutis* 21:782, 1978.

157. Burnett JW, Lamon JM, Levin J: Haemophilia, hepatitis and porphyria. *Br J Dermatol* 97:453, 1977.

158. Chapman RWG: Porphyria cutanea tarda and beta-thalassaemia minor with iron overload in mother and daughter. *Br Med J* 280(6226): 1255, 1980.

159. Manzione NC, Wolkoff AW, Sassa S: Development of porphyria cutanea tarda after treatment with cyclophosphamide. *Gastroenterology* 95:1119, 1988.

160. Guyotat D, Nicolas JF, Augey F, Fiere D, Thivolet J: Porphyria cutanea tarda after allogeneic bone marrow transplantation for chronic myelogenous leukemia. *Am J Hematol* 34:69, 1990.

161. Wissel PS, Sordillo P, Anderson KE, Sassa S, Savillo RL, Kappas A: Porphyria cutanea tarda associated with the acquired immune deficiency syndrome. *Am J Hematol* 25:107, 1987.

162. Elder GH: The metabolism of porphyrins of the isocoproporphyrin series. *Enzyme* 17:61, 1974.

163. Günther WW: The porphyrias and erythropoietic protoporphyria: an unusual case. *Australas J Dermatol* 9:23, 1967.

164. Toback AC, Sassa S, Poh-Fitzpatrick MB, et al: Hepatoerythropoietic porphyria: clinical, biochemical, and enzymatic studies in a three-generation family lineage. *N Engl J Med* 316:645, 1987.

165. Romana M, Grandchamp B, Dubart A, et al: Identification of a new mutation responsible for hepatoerythropoietic porphyria. *EurJ Clin Invest* 21:225, 1991.

166. De Verneuil H, Bourgeois F, de Rooij F, et al: Characterization of a new mutation (R292G) and a detection at the human uroporphyrinogen decarboxylase locus in two patients with hepatoerythropoietic porphyria. *Hum Genet* 89:548, 1992.

167. Garey JR, Hansen JL, Harrison LM, Kennedy JB, Kushner JP: A point mutation in the coding region of uroporphyrinogen decarboxylase associated with familial porphyria cutanea tarda. *Blood* 73:892, 1989.

168. Garey JR, Harrison LM, Franklin KF, Metcalf KM, Radisky ES, Kushner JP: Uroporphyrinogen decarboxylase: a splice site mutation causes the deletion of exon 6 in multiple families with porphyria cutanea tarda. *J Clin Invest* 86:1416, 1990.

169. Meguro K, Fujita H, Ishida N, et al: Molecular defects of uroporphyrinogen decarboxylase in a patient with mild hepatoerythropoietic porphyria. *J Invest Dermatol* 102:681, 1994.

170. McManus JF, Begley CG, Ratnaike IS: A mutation previously described in hepatoerythropoietic porphyria observed in a patient diagnosed with familial porphyria cutanea tarda. *Proceedings of the International Symposium on Porphyrins and Heme Related Disorders: Molecular Basis, Diagnostic, and Clinical Aspects.* 144, 1995 (abstr) Forssan Kirjapaino Oy, Forssa, Finland.

171. Simon N, Berko GY, Schneider I: Hepatoerythropoietic porphyria presenting as scleroderma and acrosclerosis in a sibling pair. *Br J Dermatol* 96:663, 1977.

172. Czarnecki DB: Hepatoerythropoietic porphyria. *Arch Dermatol* 116:307, 1980.

173. Pinol-Aguade J, Herrero C, Almeida J, et al: Porphyrie hepatoerythrocytaire. Une nouvelle forme de porphyrie. *AnnDerm Syphil* 102:129, 1975.

174. Sassa S, Nagai T: The role of heme in gene expression. *Int J Hematol* 63, 167, 1996.

175. Romana M, Le Boulch P, Romeo PH: Rat uroporphyrinogen decarboxylase cDNA: nucleotide sequence and comparison to human uroporphyrinogen decarboxylase. *Nucl Acids Res* 15:7211, 1987.

176. Fukuda Y, Fujita H, Taketani S, Sassa S: Haem is necessary for a continued increase in ferrochelatase mRNA in murine erythroleukaemia cells during erythroid differentiation. *Br J Haematol* 85:670, 1993.

HEREDITARY AND ACQUIRED SIDEROBLASTIC ANEMIAS

ERNEST BEUTLER

Sideroblastic anemias are characterized by the presence of ring sideroblasts in the marrow. These cells are erythroid precursors that have accumulated abnormal amounts of mitochondrial iron. A variety of abnormalities of porphyrin metabolism have been documented. Hereditary sideroblastic anemias are usually X-linked, the result of mutations in the erythroid form of D-ALA synthase. Inherited autosomal and mitochondrial forms (Pearson syndrome) are also occasionally seen. Acquired sideroblastic anemias can occur as a result of the ingestion of drugs, alcohol, or toxins such as lead or zinc. Ring sideroblasts are also a feature of myelodysplastic states, discussed in Chap. 92. Patients with sideroblastic anemia may respond to pharmacologic doses of pyridoxine, which is often given together with folic acid. Iron loading is common in the sideroblastic anemias, and can be treated by phlebotomy when the anemia is mild or with desferal when it is more severe.

DEFINITION AND HISTORY

Sideroblastic anemias are a heterogeneous group of disorders that have as common features the presence of large numbers of ringed sideroblasts in the marrow (Plate 3), ineffective erythropoiesis, increased levels of tissue iron, and varying proportions of hypochromic erythrocytes in the blood. They may be acquired or hereditary (Table 63-1).

Acquired sideroblastic anemia may be a neoplastic disease, i.e. a clonal disorder that can progress to acute leukemia. This subject is considered in Chap. 92, in which clonal, preleukemic disorders are discussed. Sideroblastic anemia may also develop as a result of the administration of certain drugs, exposure to toxins, or coincident to neoplastic or inflammatory disease. Hereditary sideroblastic anemias include X-chromosome–linked, autosomally linked, and mitochondrial entities. Occasionally a patient with apparently familial disease has developed a myelodysplastic syndrome later,[1,2] but with these rare exceptions the disorders are distinct and do not coexist or evolve one from the other.

Although the perinuclear distribution of siderotic granules in the nucleated red cells of patients with various types of anemia was described in 1947,[3,4] the concept of sideroblastic anemia as a generic designation was not generally accepted until the publications of Björkman,[5] Dacie et al,[6] Heilmeyer et al,[7,8] Bernard et al,[9] and Mollin.[10] After description of the primary adult form of refractory sideroblastic anemia,[5,6] similarity to the morphologic and erythrokinetic changes in hereditary (sex-linked) hypochromic anemia was recognized. Cooley[11] described a patient with an anemia with ovalocytosis, who was shortly thereafter shown to have a hereditary sex-linked disorder[12] which we

now know to be due to a ALA synthase mutation.[13] Autosomally inherited cases were also described,[14] and prominent sideroblastic changes of the marrow were found in Pearson's marrow-pancreas syndrome, a disorder that is associated with mutations of the mitochondrial DNA.[15-19] Subsequently, it became evident that similar abnormalities were associated with a wide variety of diseases,[20] therapy with antituberculosis drugs,[21,22] and lead intoxication.[23-26] In some patients the anemia responded to large doses of pyridoxine and was designated "pyridoxine-responsive anemia."[10,27-29] These "secondary" acquired disorders were then incorporated into the classification.

ETIOLOGY AND PATHOGENESIS

MORPHOLOGIC ASPECTS. THE SIDEROBLASTS

Sideroblasts are erythroblasts containing aggregates of nonheme iron appearing as one or more Prussian blue positive granules on light microscopy.[30] The morphology of these cells in normal and abnormal states is discussed in detail in Chap. 22. In normal subjects, 30 to 50 percent of marrow erythroblasts contain such granules, which, when viewed by electron microscopy, are seen to be neither within mitochondria nor associated with other cytoplasmic organelles.[31] In contrast to the normal cytoplasmic location of siderotic granules, the pathologic sideroblasts in the sideroblastic anemias exhibit large amounts of iron deposited as dust or plaque-like ferruginous micelles between the cristae of mitochondria (Fig. 34-3).[32] The iron-loaded mitochondria are distorted and swollen, their cristae are indistinct, and the identification of mitochondria may itself be difficult. In humans, the mitochondria of the erythroblast are distributed perinuclearly,[23] and this accounts for the distinctive "ringed" sideroblast identified by Prussian blue staining when mitochondrial iron overload is present (Fig. 33-3 and Plate XVIII-7). The morphologic features that characterize pathologic sideroblasts in various disorders have been summarized.[33]

PATHOGENESIS

The pathogenesis of most of the sideroblastic anemias is not well understood. It is not clear whether the basic mechanism by which abnormal accumulations of intra-mitochondrial iron occur are the same in inherited and acquired forms of the disease. However, it seems appropriate, given the present state of knowledge, to discuss both forms together. The pathogenesis of the disorder may be viewed from two standpoints: the underlying biochemical lesions and the mechanism(s) of the anemia itself.

BIOCHEMICAL LESIONS AND GENETICS
In the search for the biochemical lesions responsible for the development of sideroblastic anemia, attention has been focused upon an intramitochondrial defect in heme synthesis and on possible disturbances in pyridoxine metabolism.

Heme Synthesis The possible role of defects in heme biosynthesis have occupied center stage since the early studies of Garby et al[34] who postulated that such a defect might exist and demonstrated that the level of free erythrocyte protoporphyrin was decreased and that of coproporphyrin was increased. Subsequently, a variety of abnormalities of the levels of precursors and of their rate of incorporation into heme was documented.[35-40] However, the findings have not all been consistent, since levels of free erythrocyte protoporphyrin have often been increased,[41,42] not diminished. The role of mitochondria in the etiology of sideroblastic anemia gained further credence when mutations of the mitochondrial genome were found in patients with Pearson's syndrome.[15-19]

Sideroblastic anemia with deficiency of ALA synthase of marrow erythroid cells has been documented in subjects both with the congeni-

---

Acronyms and abbreviations that appear in this chapter include: ALA, aminolevulinic acid.

TABLE 63-1   CLASSIFICATION OF SIDEROBLASTIC ANEMIAS

I. Acquired
   A. Primary sideroblastic anemia (myelodysplastic syndromes) (see Chap. 92)
   B. Sideroblastic anemia secondary to:
      1. isoniazid[74]
      2. pyrazinamide[22,75]
      3. cycloserin[22,75]
      4. chloramphenicol[22,56,101,102]
      5. ethanol[122,103–108]
      6. lead[23,24,25,26,110]
      7. chronic neoplastic and inflammatory disease[10,20,22,69,71,111]
      8. triethylene tetramine dihydrochloride[112,113]
      9. zinc[114–117]
     10. D-penicillamine[118]
     11. progesterone[119]
II. Hereditary
   A. X chromosome-linked
      1. pyridoxine-responsive[12,82,83,92–94]
      2. pyridoxine-refractory[7,34,42]
   B. Autosomal: pyridoxine-refractory[120]
   C. Mitochondrial: Pearson's marrow-pancreas syndrome[91,121,122]

tal disorder and the acquired disease.[43–45] Identification of the defect at the DNA level in the X-linked gene for erythroid-specific ALA synthase (*ALAS2*) establishes that hereditary X-linked cases are due to structural mutations in this enzyme.[45–51] Hereditary sideroblastic anemia with spinocerebellar degeneration is an X-linked syndrome that appears to be distinct from the other forms of sideroblastic anemia.[52,53] Although it has been mapped to a region close to the erythroid ALA synthase gene, no changes in the restriction pattern of the ALA synthetase gene was observed,[53] as might have been anticipated if the neurologic and hematologic manifestations were due to a small deletion from the X-chromosome. An X-linked ATP-binding cassette has been identified as a candidate gene for this rare disorder.[54] Rare autosomal forms of inherited sideroblastic anemia have been reported.[55]

In one or more additional patients with sideroblastic anemia a deficiency of uroporphyrinogen decarboxylase,[56,57] and heme synthetase,[36,37,58–60] enzymes also necessary for the synthesis of heme (see Chap. 62), has been identified, but the defect in heme synthetase could simply be due to the inhibitory effect of mitochondrial iron overload on enzyme activity.[37] The suggestion[34] that a defect in coproporphyrinogen oxidase might be responsible for sideroblast formation could not be confirmed by direct measurement.[61] Increased levels of uroporphyrinogen 1 synthase are commonly encountered.[40] Alcohol, a common cause of secondary sideroblastic anemia, inhibits heme synthesis at several steps.[39] In many instances, no abnormalities in the protoporphyrin synthetic pathway have been demonstrable.[62]

No single defect in heme synthesis accounts for sideroblast formation in this heterogeneous group of disorders. Moreover, a simple defect in heme synthesis fails to explain certain commonly encountered features such as megaloblastoid and other dyserythropoietic features, the frequently low serum folate levels, and, at times, partial responses to folate administration.

Pyridoxine Metabolism   The belief in a possible role for pyridoxine has been fostered by the clear demonstration that pyridoxine deficiency in animals is a prototype of sideroblastic anemia.[32] Sideroblastic anemia can be induced by drugs that reduce the level of pyridoxal phosphate in blood and decrease the δ-aminolevulinic acid (ALA) synthetase activity in normoblasts.[21,38] Moreover, certain sideroblastic disorders, though clearly not due to pyridoxine deficiency in a conventional sense, are nonetheless responsive to pharmacologic doses of pyridoxine.[45,63–65] Pyridoxal phosphate is a necessary coenzyme for the initial reaction of protoporphyrin synthesis, the condensation of glycine and succinyl CoA to form ALA, a reaction mediated

by ALA synthetase (see Chap. 62). Furthermore, pyridoxal phosphate is a factor in the enzymatic conversion of serine to glycine (see Chap. 25). This reaction generates a form of folate coenzyme necessary for the formation of thymidylate, an important step in DNA synthesis. Pyridoxal 5'-phosphate, the active form of the coenzyme, must itself be enzymatically synthesized from pyridoxine. Deficiencies in its biosynthesis have also been invoked as the possible cause of certain sideroblastic anemias,[29,66] but direct measurements of pyridoxal kinase have failed to confirm that the postulated lesion was present.[67] There are additional abnormalities that are difficult to rationalize in terms of defects in heme synthesis or abnormalities of pyridoxine metabolism. Sideroblastic anemia has been found in a patient with apparent antibody-mediated red cell aplasia.[68] Dramatically altered activity ratios of a wide diversity of enzymes[69,70] have been described. There are alterations in red cell antigen patterns frequently with an increase of i and a loss of A_1,[71] and, in some instances, a variety of metabolic abnormalities. Similar findings occur in certain hereditary and acquired refractory anemias with cellular marrows but without ringed sideroblasts.[69] Such dyscrasias are also characterized by ineffective erythropoiesis, and except for the lack of ringed sideroblasts, may in some instances be virtually indistinguishable from their sideroblastic counterparts.[72]

MECHANISM OF ANEMIA[73]

The dominant factor producing anemia is ineffective erythropoiesis; the rate of red cell destruction is usually near-normal or only moderately accelerated to levels for which a normally functioning marrow could easily compensate. The half-time of disappearance of intravenously injected tracer doses of radioactive iron may be normal, but it usually is rapid (25 to 50 min; normal mean, 90 to 100 min). The plasma iron turnover tends to be increased (1.5 to 5.9 mg per dl of whole blood per day; normal, approximately 0.6 to 0.2 mg) but incorporation of radioactive iron into heme and its delivery to the blood as newly synthesized hemoglobin are depressed (15 to 30 percent of tracer dose; normal, 70 to 90 percent). Red cell survival, as determined by the ^{51}Cr technique, varies from a half-time of 15 days to normal, corresponding to a mean erythrocyte life-span of approximately 40 to 120 days. As in other kinds of anemia characterized by ineffective erythropoiesis, the total fecal stercobilin excreted per day may be greater than can be accounted for by the daily catabolism of circulating hemoglobin.

CLINICAL AND LABORATORY FEATURES

PRIMARY ACQUIRED SIDEROBLASTIC ANEMIA

The features of primary acquired sideroblastic anemia are described in Chap. 92.

SECONDARY ACQUIRED SIDEROBLASTIC ANEMIA

The administration of certain drugs and the ingestion of alcohol may cause sideroblastic anemia. The drugs that are most commonly associated with this type of anemia are isonicotinic acid hydrazide,[74] pyrazinamide,[21,22,75] and cycloserine,[21,22,75] all pyridoxine antagonists. Although plasma pyridoxal phosphate levels are often low in alcoholic patients, there is no correlation between these levels and the appearance of ringed sideroblasts in the marrow.[76]

Anemia secondary to drugs may be quite severe, even necessitating transfusion,[21] but characteristically the anemia improves rapidly when the patient is given pyridoxine and/or when administration of the offending drug is discontinued. The red cells are hypochromic and commonly there is a dimorphic appearance of the erythrocytes in the blood film, i.e. two populations of red cells can be distinguished. The reticulocyte count is low or normal.[77] In rare instances a sideroblastic anemia first observed during the course of drug administration has progressed in the face of discontinuing the putative offending drug. In such cases the patient presumably was suffering from an underlying myelodysplastic disorder.

Heteroplasmic point mutations in subunit 1 of the mitochondrial cytochrome oxidase have been documented in two patients with sideroblastic anemia.[78]

HEREDITARY SIDEROBLASTIC ANEMIA

Hereditary sideroblastic anemia is very uncommon. More instances of the X-chromosome–linked varieties than of apparently autosomally inherited cases have been documented.[79] The disorder is heterogeneous. In some of the cases of hereditary iron loading anemia that are cited below either the presence of the sideroblasts in the marrow or the hereditary nature of the disorder is presumed; it has not been clearly documented in each case.

Anemia is usually apparent during the first few months[80] or years[34,35] of life; it may even occur prenatally.[81] However, two remarkable patients, in whom microcytic anemia first became evident in the eighth and ninth decade of life, were found to have a microcytic, pyridoxine-responsive anemia apparently related to inherited mutations of the ALAS2 gene.[82]

Pallor is the most prominent physical finding; splenomegaly may be present[44] but not universally so.[34,80] The anemia is characteristically microcytic and hypochromic and prominent dimorphism of the red cell population has been noted in carrier females of the sex-linked form of the anemia.[12,80,83] This has been regarded as evidence of X-inactivation affecting the locus responsible for this disorder,[35,80,83,84] but it is notable that marked dimorphism sometimes is seen in the red cells of affected males as well,[12,34] and in autosomal forms of the disease.[85] The degree of aniso- and poikilocytosis is usually striking. Sometimes the anemia can be macrocytic,[1,86] especially in mitochondrial forms of the disease. The red cells show marked heterogeneity with respect to resistance to osmotic lysis: a flattened curve indicates that cells with both increased and decreased resistance to lysis are present.[34,87] The white cell count is usually normal or slightly decreased, unless splenectomy has been performed. Then it may be greatly elevated.[88] Splenomegaly is present in most cases.[88] In one family a platelet function abnormality resembling a storage pool defect was noted,[89] but this could have been an independently inherited disorder.

Pearson marrow-pancreas syndrome is a refractory sideroblastic anemia with vacuolization of marrow precursors and exocrine pancreatic dysfunction occurring during infancy.[90,91] Most patients die in infancy, although there is considerable phenotypic variation, presumably depending upon the number of mitochondria affected and their tissue distribution.

TREATMENT

Most patients with hereditary sideroblastic anemia appear to have some response to treatment with pyridoxine in doses of 50 to 200 mg per day,[12,80,83,88,92–94] but failures have also been observed.[7,34,42] Some patients have responded to doses as low as 2.5 mg/day.[88] An additional effect may be achieved by the administration of folic acid.[80] Very rarely patients have been reported to respond to a crude liver extract, and it has been suggested that tryptophane may be an active principle, enhancing the effect of pyridoxine.[95,96] Responses to pyridoxine may result in an increase in the steady-state hemoglobin level of the blood or a decrease in the transfusion requirement, but normalization of the

hemoglobin level does not usually occur, and the anemia relapses when pyridoxine administration is discontinued.

Iron overloading regularly accompanies this disorder and may be the cause of death[42] (Chap. 42). Iron storage may be enhanced when the mutations of hereditary hemochromatosis are co-inherited.[97] If the anemia is not too severe, or if it can be partially corrected by the administration of pyridoxine, phlebotomy may be used to diminish the iron burden.[98,99] Otherwise it may be advisable to attempt to decrease the amount of body iron by the use of desferrioxamine (Chap. 42).

One child with a hereditary form of the disease has been treated successfully by marrow transplantation.[100]

REFERENCES

1. Tuckfield A, Ratnaike S, Hussein S, Metz J: A novel form of hereditary sideroblastic anaemia with macrocytosis. *Br J Haematol* 97:279, 1997.
2. Kardos G, Veerman AJ, de Waal FC, van Oudheusden LJ, Slater R: Familial sideroblastic anemia with emergence of monosomy 5 and myelodysplastic syndrome. *Med Pediatr Oncol* 26:54, 1996.
3. Dacie JV, Doniach I: The basophilic property of the iron-containing granules in siderocytes. *J Pathol Bacteriol* 59:684, 1947.
4. McFadzean AJS, Davis LJ: Iron-staining erythrocyte inclusions with special reference to acquired haemolytic anaemia. *Glasgow Med J* 28:237, 1947.
5. Björkman SE: Chronic refractory anemia with sideroblastic bone marrow: a study of four cases. *Blood* 11:250, 1956.
6. Dacie JV, Smith MD, White JC, Mollin DL: Refractory normoblastic anaemia: a clinical and haematologic study of seven cases. *Br J Haematol* 5:56, 1959.
7. Heilmeyer L, Keiderling W, Bilger R, Bernauer H: Über chronische refractare Anämien mit sideroblastischen Knochenmark (anaemia refractoria sideroblastica). *Folia Haematol (Frankfurt)* 2:49, 1958.
8. Heilmeyer L, Emmrich J, Hennemann HH, et al: Über eine chronische hypochrome Anämie bei zwei Gerschwistern auf der Grundlage einer Eisenverwertungs-störung (anaemia hypochromica sideroachrestica hereditaria). *Folia Haematol (Frankfurt)* (N.F.) 2:61, 1958.
9. Bernard J, Lortholary P, Levy JP, et al: Les Anémies normochromes sidéroblastiques primitives. *Nouv Rev Fr Hematol* 3:723, 1963.
10. Mollin DL: Sideroblasts and sideroblastic anaemia. *Br J Haematol* 11:41, 1965.
11. Cooley TB: A severe type of hereditary anemia with elliptocytosis. Interesting sequence of splenectomy. *Am J Med Sci* 209:561, 1945.
12. Rundles RW, Falls HF: Hereditary (sex-linked) anemia. *Am J Med Sci* 211:641, 1946.
13. Cotter PD, Rucknagel DL, Bishop DF: X-linked sideroblastic anemia: identification of the mutation in the erythroid-specific δ-aminolevulinate synthase gene (ALAS2) in the original family described by Cooley. *Blood* 84:3915, 1994.
14. Kasturi J, Basha HM, Smeda SH, Swehli M: Hereditary sideroblastic anaemia in 4 siblings of a Libyan family–autosomal inheritance. *Acta Haematol (Basel)* 68:321, 1982.
15. Gürgey A, Rötig A, Gümrük F, et al: Pearson's marrow-pancreas syndrome in 2 Turkish children. *Acta Haematol (Basel)* 87:206, 1992.
16. McShane MA, Hammans SR, Sweeney M, et al: Pearson syndrome and mitochondrial encephalomyopathy in a patient with a deletion of mtDNA. *Am J Hum Genet* 48:39, 1991.
17. Rötig A, Cormier V, Blanche S, et al: Pearson's marrow-pancreas syndrome. A multisystem mitochondrial disorder in infancy. *J Clin Invest* 86:1601, 1990.
18. Cormier V, Rötig A, Quartino AR, et al: Widespread multi-tissue deletions of the mitochondrial genome in the Pearson marrow-pancreas syndrome. *J Pediatr* 117:599, 1990.
19. Jakobs C, Rotig A, Munnich A, Veerman AJ: Pearson's syndrome: a multi-system disorder based on a mt-DNA deletion. *Tijdschr Kindergeneeskd* 59:196, 1991.
20. MacGibbon BH, Mollin DL: Sideroblastic anaemia in man: observations on seventy cases. *Br J Haematol* 11:59, 1965.
21. Verwilghen R, Reybrouck G, Callens L, Cosemans J: Antituberculous drugs and sideroblastic anaemia. *Br J Haematol* II:92, 1965.

22. Hines JD, Grasso JA: The sideroblastic anemias. *Semin Hematol* 7:86, 1970.

23. Bessis MC, Jensen WN: Sideroblastic anaemia, mitochondria and erythroblastic iron. *Br J Haematol* 11:49, 1965.

24. Jensen WN, Moreno G: Les Ribosomes et les ponctuations basophiles des érythrocytes dans l'intoxication par le plomb. *C R Acad Sci (Paris)* 258:3596, 1964.

25. Jensen WN, Moreno GD, Bessis MC: An electron microscopic description of basophilic stippling in red cells. *Johns Hopkins Med J* 25:933, 1965.

26. Griggs RC: Lead poisoning: hematologic aspects, in *Progress in Hematology*, p 117. Grune & Stratton, New York, vol 4, 1964.

27. Harris JW, Whittington RM, Weisman RJ, Horrigan DL: Pyridoxine responsive anemia in the human adult. *Proc Soc Exp Biol Med* 91:427, 1956.

28. Horrigan DL, Harris JW: Pyridoxine-responsive anemia in man, in *Vitamins and Hormones, Advances in Research and Applications, Vol. 26*, p 549. Academic, New York, 1968.

29. Gehrmann G: Pyridoxine responsive anaemias. *Br J Haematol* 11:86, 1965.

30. Cartwright GE, Deiss A: Sideroblasts, siderocytes, and sideroblastic anemia. *N Engl J Med* 292:185, 1975.

31. Bessis MC: *Living Blood Cells and Their Ultrastructure*, translated by R.I. Weed. Springer-Verlag, New York, 1973.

32. Hammond E, Deiss A, Carnes WH, Cartwright GE: Ultrastructural characteristics of siderocytes in swine. *Lab Invest* 21:292, 1969.

33. Koc S, Harris JW: Sideroblastic anemias: variations on imprecision in diagnostic criteria, proposal for an extended classification of sideroblastic anemias. *Am J Hematol* 57:1, 1998.

34. Garby L, Sjölin S, Vahlquist B: Chronic refractory hypochromic anaemia with disturbed haem-metabolism. *Br J Haematol* 3:55, 1957.

35. Lee GR, MacDiarmid WD, Cartwright GE, Wintrobe MM: Hereditary, X-linked, sideroachrestic anemia. The isolation of two erythrocyte populations differing in Xga blood type and porphyrin content. *Blood* 32:59, 1968.

36. Konopka L, Hoffbrand AV: Haem synthesis in sideroblastic anaemia. *Br J Haematol* 42:73, 1979.

37. Vogler WR, Mingioli ES: Porphyrin synthesis and heme synthetase activity in pyridoxine-responsive anemia. *Blood* 32:979, 1968.

38. Tanaka M, Bottomley SS: Bone marrow delta-aminolevulinic acid synthetase activity in experimental sideroblastic anemia. *J Lab Clin Med* 84:92, 1974.

39. McColl KEL, Thompson GG, Moore MR, Goldberg A: Acute ethanol ingestion and haem biosynthesis in healthy subjects. *Eur J Clin Invest* 10:107, 1980.

40. Pasanen AVO, Vuopio P, Borgström GH, Tenhunen R: Haem biosynthesis in refractory sideroblastic anaemia associated with the preleukaemic syndrome. *Scand J Haematol* 27:35, 1981.

41. Kuschner JP, Lee GR, Wintrobe MM, Cartwright GE: Idiopathic refractory sideroblastic anemia: clinical and laboratory investigation of 17 patients and review of the literature. *Medicine (Baltimore)* 50:139, 1971.

42. Heilmeyer L: *Disturbances in Heme Synthesis*. Charles C. Thomas, Springfield, Ill., 1966.

43. Aoki Y, Urata G, Wada O, Takaku F: Measurement of delta aminolevulinic acid synthetase activity in human erythroblasts. *J Clin Invest* 53:1326, 1974.

44. Buchanan GR, Bottomly SS, Nitschke R: Bone marrow delta-aminolaevulinate synthase deficiency in a female with congenital sideroblastic anemia. *Blood* 55:109, 1980.

45. Cotter PD, Baumann M, Bishop DF: Enzymatic defect in ''X-linked'' sideroblastic anemia: molecular evidence for erythroid δ-aminolevulinate synthase deficiency. *Proc Natl Acad Sci USA* 89:4028, 1992.

46. Cox TC, Bottomley SS, Wiley JS, et al: X-linked pyridoxine-responsive sideroblastic anemia due to a Thr[388]-to-Ser substitution in erythroid 5-aminolevulinate synthase. *N Engl J Med* 330:675, 1994.

47. Edgar AJ, Wickramasinghe SN: Hereditary sideroblastic anaemia due to a mutation in exon 10 of the erythroid 5-aminolaevulinate synthase gene. *Br J Haematol* 100:389, 1998.

48. Furuyama K, Fujita H, Nagai T, et al: Pyridoxine refractory X-linked sideroblastic anemia caused by a point mutation in the erythroid 5-aminolevulinate synthase gene. *Blood* 90:822, 1997.

49. May A, Bishop DF: The molecular biology and pyridoxine responsiveness of X-linked sideroblastic anaemia. *Haematologica* 83:56, 1998.

50. Bottomley SS, Healy HM, Brandenburg MA, May BK: 5-Aminolevulinate synthase in sideroblastic anemias: mRNA and enzyme activity levels in bone marrow cells. *Am J Hematol* 41:76, 1992.

51. Edgar AJ, Vidyatilake HMS, Wickramasinghe SN: X-linked sideroblastic anaemia due to a mutation in the erythroid 5-aminolaevulinate synthase gene leading to an arginine[170] to leucine substitution. *Eur J Haematol* 61:55, 1998.

52. Pagon RA, Bird TD, Detter JC, Pierce I: Hereditary sideroblastic anaemia and ataxia: an X linked recessive disorder. *J Med Genet* 22:267, 1985.

53. Raskind WH, Wijsman E, Pagon RA, et al: X-linked sideroblastic anemia and ataxia: linkage to phosphoglycerate kinase at Xq13. *Am J Hum Genet* 48:335, 1991.

54. Shimada Y, Okuno S, Kawai A, et al: Cloning and chromosomal mapping of a novel ABC transporter gene (hABC7), a candidate for X-linked sideroblastic anemia with spinocerebellar ataxia. *J Hum Genet* 43:115, 1998.

55. Jardine PE, Cotter PD, Johnson SA, et al: Pyridoxine-refractory congenital sideroblastic anaemia with evidence for autosomal inheritance: exclusion of linkage to ALAS2 at Xp11.21 by polymorphism analysis. *J Med Genet* 31:213, 1994.

56. Goodman JR, Hall SG: Accumulation of iron in mitochondria of erythroblasts. *Br J Haematol* 13:335, 1967.

57. Kuschner JP, Barbuto AJ: Decreased activity of hepatic uroporphyrinogen decarboxylase (Urodecarb) in porphyria cutanea tarda (PCT). *Clin Res* 22:178, 1974.

58. Lee GR, Cartwright GE, Wintrobe MM: The response of free erythrocyte protoporphyrin to pyridoxine therapy in a patient with sideroachrestic (sideroblastic) anemia. *Blood* 27:557, 1966.

59. Chauhan MS, Dakshinamurti K: Fluorometric assay of b6 vitamers in biological material. *Clin Chim Acta* 109:159, 1981.

60. Pasanen AVO, Salmi M, Vuopio P, Tenhunen R: Heme biosynthesis in sideroblastic anemia. *Int J Biochem* 12:969, 1980.

61. Pasanen AVO, Eklöf M, Tenhunen R: Coproporphyrinogen oxidase activity and porphyrin concentrations in peripheral red blood cells in hereditary sideroblastic anaemia. *Scand J Haematol* 34:235, 1985.

62. Vavra JD, Poff SA: Heme and porphyrin synthesis in sideroblastic anemia. *J Lab Clin Med* 69:904, 1967.

63. Murakami R, Takumi T, Gouji J, Nakamura H, Kondou M: Sideroblastic anemia showing unique response to pyridoxine. *Am J Pediatr Hematol Oncol* 13:345, 1991.

64. Barton JR, Shaver DC, Sibai BM: Successive pregnancies complicated by idiopathic sideroblastic anemia. *Am J Obstet Gynecol* 166:576, 1992.

65. Breton-Gorius J, Bachir D, Rochant H: Congenital sideroblastic anemia without clinical iron overload. A case report. *Am J Hematol* 32:298, 1989.

66. Mason DY, Emerson PM: Primary acquired sideroblastic anaemia: response to treatment with pyridoxal-5-phosphate. *BMJ* 1:389, 1973.

67. Chillar RK, Johnson CS, Beutler E: Erythrocyte pyridoxine kinase levels in patients with sideroblastic anemia. *N Engl J Med* 295:881, 1976.

68. Ritchey AK, Hoffman R, Dainiak N, McIntosh S, Weininger R, Pearson HA: Antibody-mediated acquired sideroblastic anemia: response to cytotoxic therapy. *Blood* 54:734, 1979.

69. Valentine WN, Konrad PN, Paglia DE: Dyserythropoiesis, refractory anemia, and ''preleukemia'': metabolic features of the erythrocytes. *Blood* 41:857, 1973.

70. Nishibe H, Yamagata K, Gotoh H: A case of sideroblastic anaemia associated with marked elevation of erythrocytic arginase activity. *Scand J Haematol* 15:17, 1975.

71. Rochant H, Dreyfus B, Bouguerra M, Hoi Tant-Hot: Hypothesis: refractory anemias, preleukemic conditions, and fetal erythropoiesis. *Blood* 39:721, 1972.

72. Geschke W, Beutler E: Refractory sideroblastic and nonsideroblastic anemia. A review of 27 cases. *West J Med* 127:85, 1977.

73. Singh AK, Shinton NK, Williams JDF: Ferrokinetic abnormalities and their significance in patients with sideroblastic anaemia. *Br J Haematol* 18:67, 1970.

74. Lowe JG, Johnston RN: Anti-tuberculous drugs and sideroblastic anaemia. *Br J Clin Pract* 44:706, 1990.

75. Harris EB, MacGibbon BH, Mollin DL: Experimental sideroblastic anemia. *Br J Haematol* 11:99, 1965.

76. Pierce HI, McGuffin RG, Hillman RS: Clinical studies in alcoholic sideroblastosis. *Arch Intern Med* 136:283, 1976.

77. McCurdy PR, Donohoe RF: Pyridoxine-responsive anaemia conditioned by isonicotinic acid hydrazide. *Blood* 27:352, 1966.

78. Gattermann N, Retzlaff S, Wang YL, et al: Heteroplasmic point mutations of mitochondrial DNA affecting subunit I of cytochrome c oxidase in two patients with acquired idiopathic sideroblastic anemia. *Blood* 90:4961, 1997.

79. Nusbaum NJ: Concise review: genetic bases for sideroblastic anemia. *Am J Hematol* 37:41, 1991.

80. Weatherall DJ, Pembrey ME, Hall EG, et al: Familial sideroblastic anaemia: problem of Xg and X chromosome inactivation. *Lancet* 2:744, 1970.

81. Andersen K, Kaad PH: Congenital sideroblastic anaemia with intrauterine symptoms and early lethal outcome. *Acta Paediatr Scand* 81:652, 1992.

82. Cotter PD, May A, Fitzsimons EJ, et al: Late-onset X-linked sideroblastic anemia. *J Clin Invest* 96:2090, 1995.

83. Prasad AS, Tranchida L, Konno ET, et al: Hereditary sideroblastic anemia and glucose-6-phosphate dehydrogenase deficiency in a negro family. *J Clin Invest* 47:1415, 1968.

84. Beutler E: The distribution of gene products among populations of cells in heterozygous humans. *Cold Spring Harb Symp Quant Biol* 29:261, 1964.

85. van Waveren Hogervorst GD, van Roermund HP, Snijders PJ: Hereditary sideroblastic anaemia and autosomal inheritance of erythrocyte dimorphism in a Dutch family. *Eur J Haematol* 38:405, 1987.

86. Fitzsimons EJ, May A: The molecular basis of the sideroblastic anemias. *Curr Opin Hematol* 3:167, 1996.

87. Seip M, Gjessing LR, Lie SO: Congenital sideroblastic anaemia in a girl. *Scand J Haematol* 8:505, 1971.

88. Horrigan DL, Harris JW: Pyridoxine-responsive anemia: Analysis of 62 cases. *Adv Intern Med* 12:103, 1964.

89. Soslau G, Brodsky I: Hereditary sideroblastic anemia with associated platelet abnormalities. *Am J Hematol* 32:298, 1989.

90. Smith OP, Hann IM, Woodward CE, Brockington M: Pearson's marrow/pancreas syndrome: haematological features associated with deletion and duplication of mitochondrial DNA. *Br J Haematol* 90:469, 1995.

91. Seneca S, De Meirleir L, De Schepper J, et al: Pearson marrow pancreas syndrome: a molecular study and clinical management. *Clin Genet* 51:338, 1997.

92. Bishop RC, Bethell FH: Hereditary hypochromic anemia with transfusion siderosis treated with pyridoxine. *N Engl J Med* 261:486, 1959.

93. Harris JW, Horrigan DL: Pyridoxine responsive anemia: The prototype and variations on the theme. *Vitam Horm* 22:721, 1964.

94. Vogler WR, Mingioli ES: Heme synthesis in pyridoxine responsive anemia. *N Engl J Med* 273:347, 1965.

95. Horrigan DL: Pyridoxone-responsive anemia: Influence of tryptophane on pyridoxine responsiveness. *Blood* 42:187, 1973.

96. Albahary C, Boiron M: Anémie primitive réfractaire avec hypersidérose sanguine médullaire et hépatique—(cas féminin). *Acta Med Scand* 163:429, 1959.

97. Yaouanq J, Grosbois B, Jouanolle AM, Goasguen J, Leblay R: Haemochromatosis Cys282Tyr mutation in pyridoxine-responsive sideroblastic anaemia. *Lancet* 349:1475, 1997.

98. Weintraub LR, Conrad ME, Crosby WH: Iron-loading anemia. Treatment with repeated phlebotomies and pyridoxine. *N Engl J Med* 275:169, 1966.

99. French TJ, Jacobs P: Sideroblastic anaemia associated with iron overload treated by repeated phlebotomy. *S Afr Med J* 50:594, 1976.

100. Urban C, Binder B, Hauer C, Lanzer G: Congenital sideroblastic anemia successfully treated by allogeneic bone marrow transplantation. *Bone Marrow Transplant* 10:373, 1992.

101. Beck EA, Ziegler G, Schmid R, Lüdin H: Reversible sideroblastic anemia caused by chloramphenicol. *Acta Haematol (Basel)* 38:1, 1967.

102. Firkin FC: Mitochondrial lesions in reversible erythropoietic depression due to chloramphenicol. *J Clin Invest* 51:2085, 1972.

103. Hines JD: Reversible megaloblastic and sideroblastic marrow abnormalities in alcoholic patients. *Br J Haematol* 16:87, 1969.

104. Hines JD, Cowan DH: Studies on the pathogenesis of alcohol-induced sideroblastic bone-marrow abnormalities. *N Engl J Med* 283:441, 1970.

105. Eichner ER, Hillman RS: The evolution of anemia in alcoholic patients. *Am J Med* 50:218, 1971.

106. Anderson BB, Fulford-Jones CE, Child JA, Beard EJ, Bateman CJT: Conversion of vitamin B_6 compounds to active forms in the red blood cell. *J Clin Invest* 50:1901, 1971.

107. Hines JD: Altered phosphorylation of vitamin B_6 in alcoholic patients induced by oral administration of alcohol. *J Lab Clin Med* 74:882, 1969.

108. Lumeng L, Li TK: Vitamin B6 metabolism in chronic alcohol abuse. Pyridoxal phosphate levels in plasma and the effects of acetaldehyde on pyridoxal phosphate synthesis and degradation in human erythrocytes. *J Clin Invest* 53:693, 1974.

109. Dacie JV, Mollin DL: Siderocytes, sideroblasts, and sideroblastic anaemia. *Acta Med Scand* 179 (Suppl.)445:237, 1966.

110. Goldberg A: Lead poisoning as a disorder of heme synthesis. *Semin Hematol* 5:424, 1968.

111. Hayhoe FGJ, Quaglino D: Refractory sideroblastic anaemia and erythremic myelosis: possible relationship and cytochemical observations. *Br J Haematol* 6:381, 1960.

112. Condamine L, Hermine O, Alvin P, et al: Acquired sideroblastic anaemia during treatment of Wilson's disease with triethylene tetramine dihydrochloride. *Br J Haematol* 83:166, 1993.

113. Perry AR, Pagliuca A, Fitzsimons EJ, Mufti GJ, Williams R: Acquired sideroblastic anaemia induced by a copper-chelating agent. *Int J Hematol* 64:69, 1996.

114. Greist A, Tricot G, Hoffman R: Excessive zinc ingestion. A reversible cause of sideroblastic anemia and bone marrow depression. *JAMA* 264:1441, 1990.

115. Schwartz J, Landrigan PJ, Baker EL, Jr., Orenstein WA, von Lindern IH: Lead-induced anemia: dose-response relationships and evidence for a threshold. *Am J Public Health* 80:165, 1990.

116. Ramadurai J, Shapiro C, Kozloff M, Telfer M: Zinc abuse and sideroblastic anemia. *Am J Hematol* 42:227, 1993.

117. Fiske DN, McCoy HE, III, Kitchens CS: Zinc-induced sideroblastic anemia: report of a case, review of the literature, and description of the hematologic syndrome. *Am J Hematol* 46:147, 1994.

118. Ramselaar AC, Dekker AW, Huber-Bruning O, Bijlsma JW: Acquired sideroblastic anaemia after aplastic anaemia caused by D-penicillamine therapy for rheumatoid arthritis. *Ann Rheum Dis* 46:156, 1987.

119. Brodsky RA, Hasegawa S, Fibach E, et al: Acquired sideroblastic anaemia following progesterone therapy. *Br J Haematol* 87:859, 1994.

120. Cottom HB, Harris JW: Familial pyridoxine-responsive anemia. *J Clin Invest* 41:1352, 1962.

121. Muraki K, Goto Y, Nishino I, et al: Severe lactic acidosis and neonatal death in Pearson syndrome. *J Inherit Metab Dis* 20:43, 1997.

122. Santorelli FM, Barmada MA, Pons R, Zhang LL, DiMauro S: Leigh-type neuropathology in Pearson syndrome associated with impaired ATP production and a novel mtDNA deletion. *Neurology* 47:1320, 1996.

PART VI

NEUTROPHILS, EOSINOPHILS, BASOPHILS, AND MAST CELLS

MORPHOLOGY OF NEUTROPHILS, EOSINOPHILS, AND BASOPHILS

DOROTHY FORD BAINTON

Early in precursor development in the marrow, cells destined to be leukocytes of the granulocytic series, neutrophils, eosinophils, and basophils, synthesize proteins and store them as cytoplasmic granules. The synthesis of primary or azurophilic granules defines the conversion of the myeloblast, a virtually agranular, primitive cell that is the earliest granulocyte precursor identifiable by light microscopy into the promyelocyte, which is rich in azurophilic granules. Synthesis and accumulation of secondary or specific granules follows. The appearance of specific granules marks the progression of the promyelocyte to neutrophilic, eosinophilic, or basophilic myelocytes. Thereafter, the cell continues maturation into an amitotic cell with a segmented nucleus, capable of ameboid motility, phagocytosis and microbial killing. The mature granulocytes also develop cytoplasmic and surface structures that permit them to attach to and penetrate the wall of venules. The mature granulocytes enter the blood from the marrow, circulate briefly, and move to the tissues to carry out their major function of host defense. The neutrophil is highly phagocytic and can kill a variety of microorganisms. The eosinophil and basophil are specialized to participate in allergic inflammatory responses. The stages of maturation from promyelocyte to mature cell can be recognized on a stained film of marrow using a light microscope. Further details of granulocyte structure and inherited and acquired abnormalities of neutrophil granules are portrayed and reviewed in this chapter.

NEUTROPHILS

In the normal adult human, the life of neutrophils is spent in three environments: marrow, blood, and tissues. Marrow is the site of differentiation of stem cells into neutrophil progenitors and of proliferation and terminal maturation of neutrophilic granulocytes (myeloblast to segmented neutrophils)[1-4] (Fig. 64-1). Precursor cell proliferation, consisting of approximately five divisions, takes place only during the first three stages of neutrophil maturation (blast, promyelocyte, and myelocyte). After the myelocyte stage, the cells are no longer capable of mitosis and enter a large marrow storage pool. After five days, they are released into the blood, where they circulate for a few hours before entering tissues.[5,6]

Acronyms and abbreviations that appear in this chapter include: AGEs, advanced glycation end products; AML, acute myelogenous leukemia; CML, chronic myelogenous leukemia; ECF-A, eosinophil chemotactic factor of anaphylaxis; HLA, human leukocyte antigens; LAMPs, lysozomal-associated membrane proteins; LAP, leukocyte alkaline phosphatase; MLC, multilaminar compartment; MVB, multivesicular bodies; PAS, periodic acid-Schiff; SRS-A, slow-reacting substance of anaphylaxis; VEGF/VPF, vascular endothelial growth factor/vascular permeability factor

LIGHT MICROSCOPY AND PEROXIDASE HISTOCHEMISTRY

Figure 64-1 is a diagrammatic representation of the stages of neutrophil maturation.[1,2] The myeloblast is an immature cell with a large, oval nucleus, sizable nucleoli, and few or no granules. The cell, derived from progenitor cells, matures into the promyelocyte. In the promyelocyte stage, large peroxidase-positive granules that stain metachromatically (reddish-purple) with a polychromatic stain such as Wright's stain, the azurophilic or primary granules, are formed. During the next, or myelocyte, stage of maturation the specific or secondary granules, which are peroxidase-negative, are formed. The metamyelocyte and band neutrophils are nonproliferating cells that precede the development of the mature neutrophil. The mature, segmented neutrophilic cells contain primary, peroxidase-positive granules and specific peroxidase-negative granules in a one to two ratio. The nucleus of the circulating neutrophil is segmented, usually into two to four interconnected lobes.

During the myelocyte stage, the larger, metachromatic, azurophilic granules lose their intense staining properties and are no longer evident by light microscopy of stained blood films. This diminution of the metachromatic staining results from an increase in acid mucin-containing molecules that form complexes with basic proteins of the azurophilic granules.[7] However, the presence of large (about 500 nm), peroxidase-positive, azurophilic granules in mature neutrophils is evident by electron microscopy.[2] Thus, the violet-colored granules seen with light microscopy in mature neutrophils on Wright's-stained blood films are azurophilic granules whose staining characteristics have altered during maturation. Therefore, with light microscopy, the most reliable method for identifying azurophilic granules on blood films is to stain the cells for peroxidase. Most of the peroxidase-negative granules are in a size range (about 200 nm; see below) at the limit of resolution of the light microscope; they cannot be distinguished individually, but are responsible for the pink background color of neutrophil cytoplasm during and after the myelocyte stage.

The purpose of the nuclear segmentation is not known. Fluorescence in situ hybridization with chromosome-specific probes has shown that chromosomes are randomly distributed among the nuclear lobes.[8] Some mature neutrophils in women have drumstick- or club-shaped nuclear appendages. These appendages contain the inactivated X chromosome. An X chromosome-specific nucleic-acid probe has confirmed the position of the X chromosomes in the drumstick structure of leukocyte nuclei by in situ hybridization.[9]

ELECTRON MICROSCOPY AND PEROXIDASE CYTOCHEMISTRY

The peroxidase reaction has become a key tool with which to study the formation of the azurophilic granule. The dense product of the peroxidase reaction serves as a marker of azurophilic granules in human marrow and blood cells for electron as well as light microscopy.[2]

THE MYELOBLAST

The earliest precursor in the evolution of the neutrophil from the colony-forming unit is an immature cell with a large nucleus and multiple nucleoli. The nucleolus is the site of assembly of ribosomal proteins and rRNA and is a prominent feature of early maturing cells. The scant cytoplasm contains reaction product for peroxidase within the rough-surfaced endoplasmic reticulum and Golgi cisternae and, sometimes, in early developing azurophilic granules.

THE PROMYELOCYTE

As shown in Fig. 64-2, the promyelocyte produces and accumulates a large population of peroxidase-positive granules. Most of these granules are spherical and have a diameter of 500 nm, but there are also

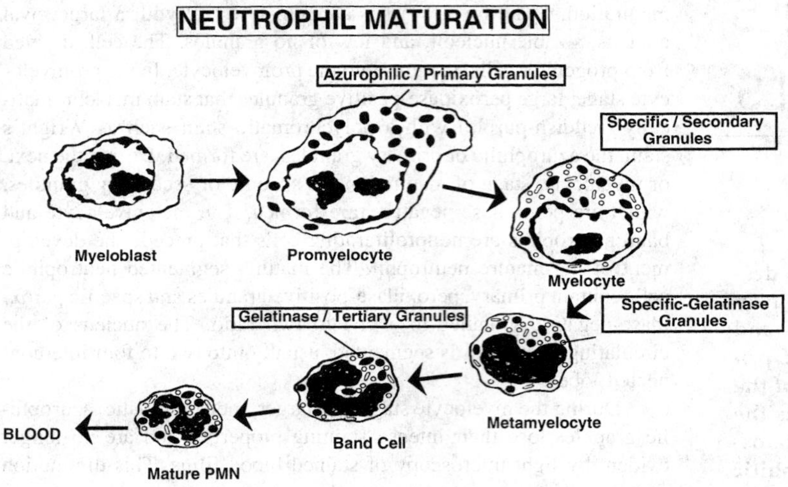

NEUTROPHIL MATURATION

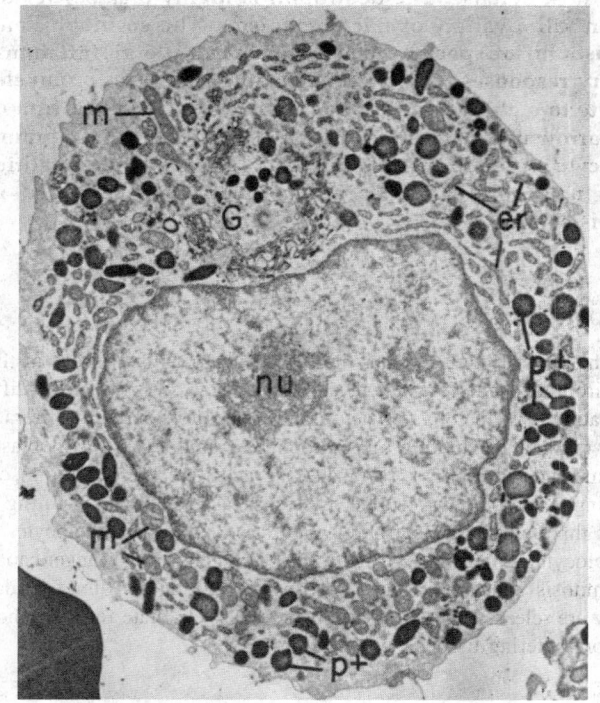

FIGURE 64-1   Diagrammatic representation of neutrophil [polymorphonuclear neutrophil (PMN)] life-span and stages of maturation. For discussion, see text. Out of every 100 nucleated cells in marrow, 0.5 percent are myeloblasts, 5 percent are promyelocytes, 12 percent are myelocytes, 22 percent are metamyelocytes and bands, and 20 percent are maturing and mature neutrophilic cells, yielding a total of ~60 percent developing neutrophils in normal human marrow. The azurophilic (primary) granules, which are peroxidase-positive, are shown as solid black dots; the other granules are shown as open dots and are discussed in more detail in the text. Basically, the peroxidase-negative granules may be divided into specific/secondary granules and gelatinase/tertiary granules based on their relative content of lactoferrin and gelatinase. (Modified from Bainton et al.[2])

ellipsoid, crystalline forms, as well as small granules connected by filaments.[10] As with other secretory cells, peroxidase is present throughout the secretory apparatus of the promyelocyte, for example, in cisternae of the rough endoplasmic reticulum, in all Golgi cisternae, in some vesicles, and in all developing granules.[2]

THE NEUTROPHILIC MYELOCYTE
At the end of the promyelocyte stage, peroxidase abruptly disappears from rough endoplasmic reticulum and Golgi cisternae and the production of azurophilic granules ceases. The myelocyte stage begins with the production of the peroxidase-negative specific granules.

As shown in Fig. 64-3, the only peroxidase-positive elements at this stage are the azurophilic granules. The specific granules are formed by the Golgi complex (Fig. 64-4). They vary in size and shape but are typically spherical (about 200 nm) or rod-shaped (130 × 1000 nm). About three cell divisions occur at this stage of maturation. Mitoses can be observed (Fig. 64-5) and the two types of granules appear to be distributed to the daughter cells in fairly equal numbers.

THE METAMYELOCYTE, BAND, AND MATURE NEUTROPHIL
The late stages of maturation consist of non-dividing cells that can be distinguished by their nuclear morphology, mixed granule populations, small Golgi regions, and accumulations of glycogen particles. On the average, an electron micrograph of a neutrophil will display 200 to 300 granules and about one-third will be peroxidase-positive (Fig. 64-6).

The peroxidase-negative granules are more numerous than peroxidase-positive granules during the myelocyte stage because peroxidase granule formation ceases after the promyelocyte stage, the number of peroxidase-positive granules per cell is reduced by mitoses, and peroxidase-negative granules continue to be produced by each myelocyte generation.[1]

OTHER CYTOPLASMIC CHANGES DURING MATURATION

MICROPEROXISOMES
Microperoxisomes are present from the promyelocyte stage through the development of mature neutrophils.[11] These organelles are small membrane-bound vesicles that contain catalase. Although this enzyme is known to destroy H_2O_2, it can also act as a peroxidase; its exact function in neutrophils has yet to be determined.

SURFACE MARKERS AND CYTOSKELETON
Changes in cell surface carbohydrates, glycoproteins, glycolipids, and HLA antigens occur during maturation (reviewed in Ref. 12). For example, the densities of membrane HLA-A, B, and C antigens decrease with granulocyte maturation. Some surface antigens appear during neutrophil maturation. The development of chemotactic and recognition capabilities parallels the acquisition of certain membrane receptors.[13,14] Fc receptors are not present, or are poorly expressed, on progenitors younger than myelocytes, whereas over 90 percent of mature neutrophils have Fc receptors. Mature neutrophils possess at least two classes of receptors for fragments of the complement component C3, called CRI and CR3. Other maturational changes occur in cytoskeletal elements, such as microtubules,[15] and in biophysical features such as deformability and surface charge.[12,16] During early myeloid development, direct inter-

FIGURE 64-2   Electron micrograph of a neutrophilic promyelocyte reacted for peroxidase from normal human marrow. This cell is the largest of the neutrophilic series. It has a sizable, slightly indented nucleus with a nucleolus (nu), a prominent Golgi region (G), and cytoplasm packed with dense peroxidase-positive (p+) azurophilic granules of varying shapes and sizes. Peroxidase reaction product is visible in less concentrated form within all compartments of the secretory apparatus—endoplasmic reticulum (er), perinuclear cisterna, and Golgi cisternae (G). No reaction product is apparent in the cytoplasmic matrix or mitochondria (m). X8000

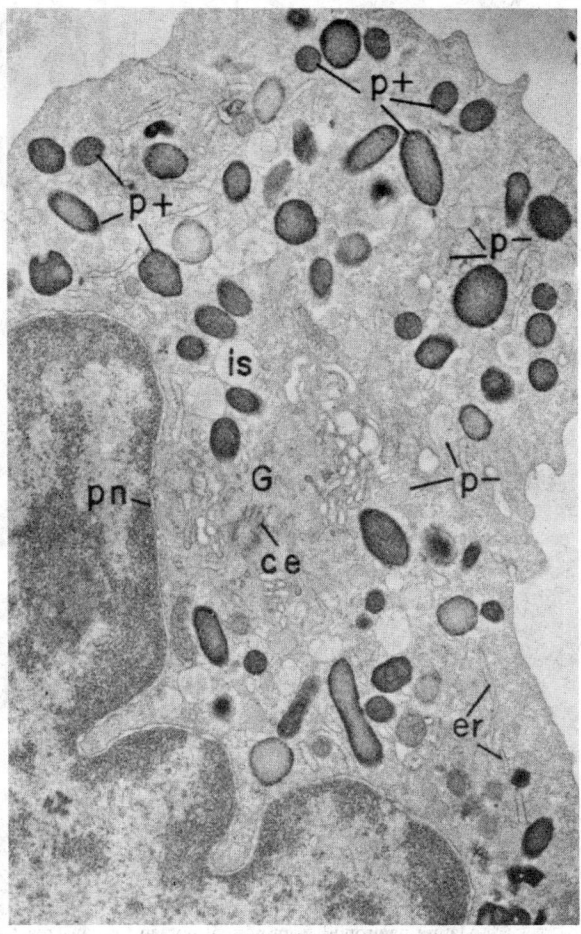

FIGURE 64-3   Neutrophilic myelocyte reacted for peroxidase. At this stage, the cell is smaller than the promyelocyte, the nucleus is more indented, and the cytoplasm contains two different types of granules: (a) large, peroxidase-positive azurophilic granules (p+) and (b) the generally smaller specific granules (p−), which do not stain for peroxidase. A number of immature specific granules (is)—larger, less compact, and more irregular in contour than mature granules—appear in the Golgi region (G). Note that peroxidase reaction product is present only in azurophilic granules and not in the rough surfaced endoplasmic reticulum (er), perinuclear cisterna (pn), or Golgi cisternae (G). This is in keeping with the fact that azurophilic granule production has ceased and only peroxidase-negative specific granules are produced during the myelocyte stage. (ce, centriole.) X20,000

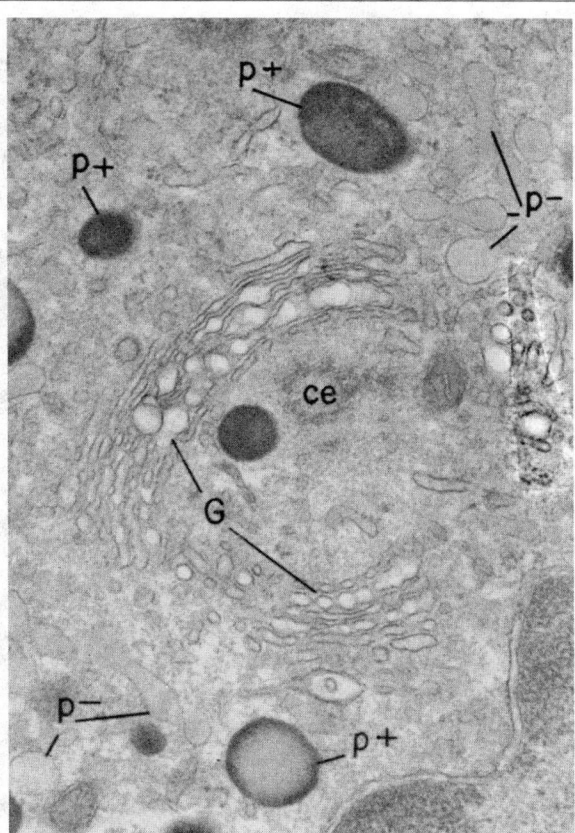

FIGURE 64-4   Golgi region of a neutrophilic myelocyte reacted for peroxidase. As in the preceding figure, peroxidase reaction product is found in azurophilic granules (p+), but not in specific granules (p−). The stacked, smooth-surfaced Golgi cisternae (G) are oriented around the centriole (ce). X43,000

actions must occur between hematopoietic cells and the components of the marrow microenvironment, both cellular and extracellular matrix.[17-25] Most of the known matrix protein receptors belong to the β_1 integrin family. On CD34+ marrow cells, $\alpha 4b_1$ and $\alpha 5b_1$ are expressed. During myeloid differentiation $\alpha 5b_1$ is lost at the myelocytic-metamyelocyte stage, before the loss of $\alpha 4b_1$ at the band stage.[21] ICAM-1, a member of the immunoglobulin superfamily, is detected on blasts and promyelocytes, but is lost at later stages of myeloid maturation.[21] One of the members of the new adhesion molecule family of selectins, L-selectin, can be detected as early as the colony-forming unit for granulocytes and monocytes,[24] through the mature neutrophil stage, until it is shed within minutes after activation.[25]

EXPRESSION OF mRNA TRANSCRIPTS

During granulocytic maturation, numerous genes that encode proteins important for the specific functions of mature cells are expressed.[26,27]

Myeloperoxidase and elastase mRNA transcripts are found almost exclusively at the promyelocyte stage, but myeloperoxidase mRNA disappears earlier than elastase mRNA.[28] Lactoferrin mRNA transcripts are detected later in neutrophil maturation, marking the beginning of the myelocyte stage[28] (see Fig. 64-7). Mature neutrophils are capable of synthesizing and secreting interleukin-1 as well as tumor necrosis factor α.[29] In addition, bacterial infection induces nitric oxide synthase in human neutrophils.[30]

APOPTOSIS

Programmed cell death, or apoptosis, is a physiologic phenomenon associated with the elimination of mature cells. Apoptosis is characterized biochemically by internucleosomal DNA fragmentation, and morphologically by nuclear and cytoplasmic condensation, and it plays an important role in cell removal.[31,32] There is evidence that senescent neutrophils and eosinophils undergo apoptosis. One of the key features of programmed cell death in many tissues is the phagocytosis of apoptotic cells by macrophages. Ingestion of intact apoptotic granulocytes by macrophages may prevent the release of their toxic intracellular contents extracellularly, thereby promoting resolution of inflammation.

CONTENTS OF NEUTROPHIL GRANULES

Initially, the granules were classified into two major types, based on their content of peroxidase. It is now recognized that granules can be

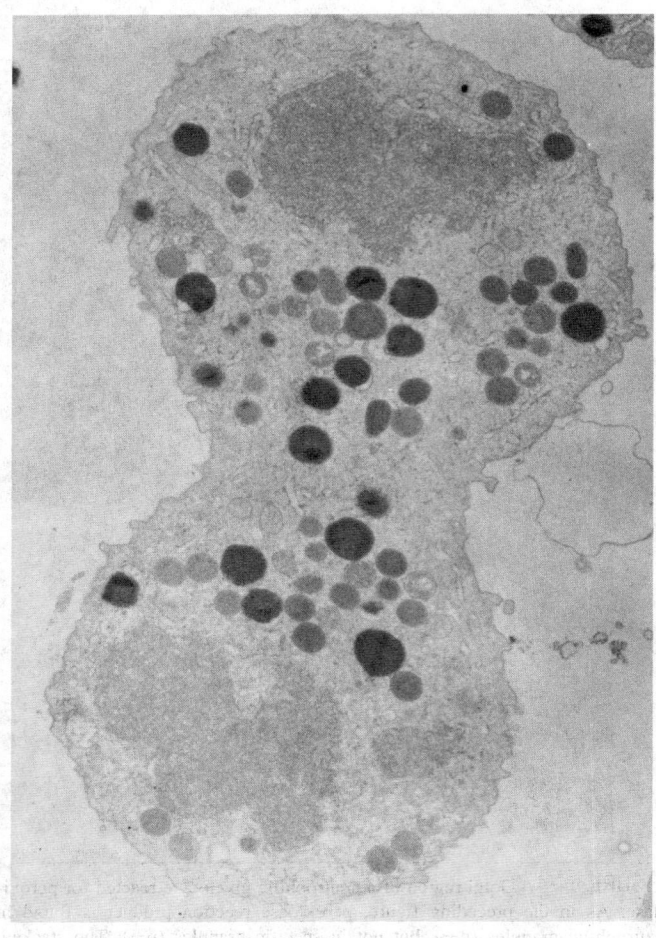

FIGURE 64-5 Myelocyte in the late stage of mitosis, from rabbit marrow. This myelocyte is in telophase. Note that the granules are being relatively equally distributed to the daughter cells. X15,000

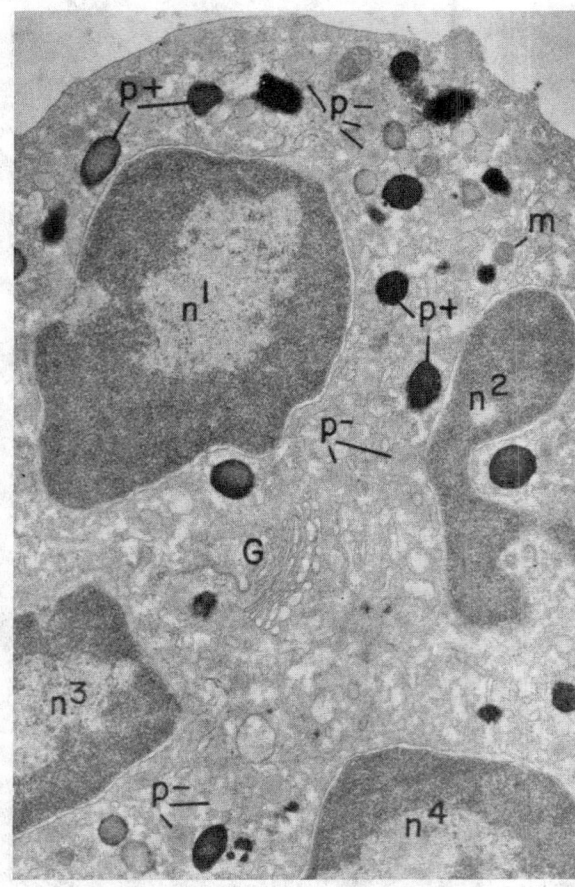

FIGURE 64-6 Mature neutrophil from normal human marrow, reacted for peroxidase. The cytoplasm is filled with granules of the two basic types: the smaller, pale, peroxidase-negative granules (p−) and the large, dense, peroxidase-positive granules (p+). The nucleus is condensed and lobulated (n^1−n^4), the Golgi region (G) is small and without any forming granules, the endoplasmic reticulum is scant, and mitochondria (m) are few. X21,000

further subdivided on the basis of other granular and membrane proteins (see Fig. 64-8).

The components of human neutrophilic granules have been analyzed by both cytochemical and fractionation procedures[2,28,33–98] and are extensively covered in Chap. 68.

PRIMARY OR AZUROPHILIC GRANULES

In addition to myeloperoxidase, the azurophilic granule contains numerous lysosomal enzymes. Elastase,[64–66] proteinase 3,[66,67] and α-1 antitrypsin[78] co-localize with some peroxidase-positive granules. Bactericidal factors such as defensins,[46,56,59,71,98] azurophil-derived bactericidal factors,[42] and bactericidal permeability-increasing protein,[48] which were previously called cationic proteins, have been found in some azurophilic granules.[52] Lysozyme has been found in both azurophilic and specific granules.[68–70]

Of the ten antimicrobial proteins of known sequence in the human azurophil granules,[55] two have unique primary structures (lysozyme and bactericidal permeability-increasing protein), while the remaining eight fall into two families of four members each: the defensins (which compromise 30 to 50 percent of granule proteins) on the one hand, and cathepsin G, elastase, proteinase-3, and azurocidin on the other. These latter four proteins can be termed ''serprocidins,'' to denote that they are closely related to serine proteases with microbicidal activity.[55] Very little is known about the limiting membrane of azuro-

philic granules, but CD63[80,92] and CD68[79] are present. We had anticipated that the lysosomal-associated membrane proteins (LAMPs) would be found there, but such was not the case.[77,93] Rather, LAMPs were absent in all identified granule populations, but were consistently found in the membranes of vesicles, multivesicular bodies (MVB), as well as in multilaminar compartments (MLC), which are identified by their content of concentric arrays of internal membranes.[93]

SECONDARY OR SPECIFIC GRANULES

The specific or secondary granule, which, by definition, does not contain peroxidase, contains lactoferrin, lysozyme, B12 binding proteins, and other proteins.[28,89] These peroxidase-negative granules vary greatly in size, shape, electron-lucency, isopycnic density and granule content. However, they can be loosely categorized by the distribution of two proteins, lactoferrin and gelatinase. Approximately 16 percent of the peroxidase-negative granules contain only lactoferrin, 24 percent only gelatinase, and 60 percent contain both marker enzymes. Thus, based on ultrastructure alone, three types of peroxidase-negative granules can be identified: peroxidase-negative granules, containing gelatinase but no lactoferrin, peroxidase-negative granules, containing lactoferrin but no gelatinase, and peroxidase-negative granules, containing both lactoferrin and gelatinase.[88] This heterogeneity may be a result of overlapping synthesis and packaging of different granule proteins during granulopoiesis and is functionally significant as the gelatinase-containing granules are released from the cells by certain inflammatory mediators more readily than those containing lactoferrin.[28]

SECRETORY VESICLES

These vesicles are distinct from the azurophilic or specific granules and have been defined as intracellular organelles that contain CD35 and latent alkaline phosphatase.[28,83,88,89] The latter enzyme is located on the luminal side of the vesicle membrane and can therefore be identified, in the presence of detergent, as latent alkaline phosphatase. This localization was also demonstrated by enzyme cytochemistry.[73] Further, these secretory vesicles contain plasma proteins, such as albumin, that are not synthesized by the cells, but are endocytosed from plasma. These represent a specialized form of endocytic vesicle. Secretory vesicles are transported to the cell surface after the stimulus of formyl methionyl-leucyl phenylalanine or certain cytokines.[89]

Other proteins found in neutrophil granules are discussed in Chap. 67, reviews[28,89] and other papers.[32–98] Two membrane adhesion proteins have been found on the tips of neutrophil microvilli in resting neutrophils, L-selectin, and P-selectin glycoprotein-1.[94–96]

PATHOLOGIC ALTERATIONS OF GRANULES

Leukemic cells can be shown to contain chemical properties unique for a given normal cell line, and thus are considered to be of that particular cell lineage. This has been particularly helpful in subdividing the acute leukemias. For example, peroxidase is recognized as one of the earliest synthetic products of granulocytic precursor cells. Production of this enzyme by leukemic cells has been the hallmark for distinguishing acute lymphocytic from myelogenous leukemia.[99] Chloroacetate esterases appear early in maturation, and are used to detect the origin of the immature cells in granulocyte sarcomas. The substrate used for this incubation, naphthyl AS-D chloroacetate, is a general substrate of neutrophil proteinases. Lactoferrin is recognized as a marker of specific granules.

Pathologic neutrophil granulations can be classified as a selective abnormality of a granule type.[100,101] Pathologic granules in hereditary or acquired disease states can be classified as either abnormalities of azurophilic granules or specific granules (Table 64-1).

ABNORMALITIES OF AZUROPHILIC GRANULES

Quantitative   Neutrophils sometime contain either smaller- or larger-than-normal numbers of azurophilic granules, or the azurophilic granule population may be missing. Some mature neutrophils lack azurophilic granules in acute myelogenous leukemia (AML)[102,103] or in the blast crisis of chronic myelogenous leukemia (CML).[104] Children with severe congenital neutropenia and repeated life-threatening infections have neutrophilic abnormalities that include: (1) defective synthesis or degeneration of azurophilic (primary) granules, (2) an absence or marked deficiency of specific (secondary) granules, and (3) autophagia. This rare disease has been called congenital dysgranulopoietic neutropenia.[105]

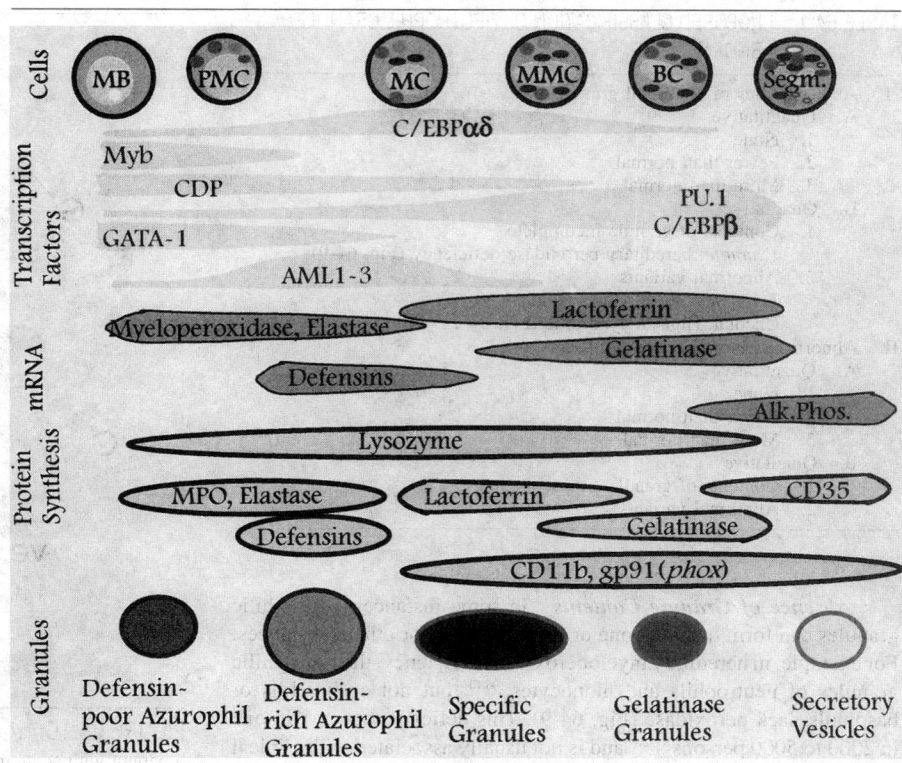

FIGURE 64-7   Granules defined by timing of biosynthesis of their characteristic proteins. The granules formed at any given stage of maturation of neutrophil precursors will be composed of the granule proteins synthesized at that time. MB, myeloblast; PMC, promyelocyte; MC, myelocyte; MMC, metamyelocyte; BC, band cell; Segm., segmented cell. (Reproduced with permission from Borregaard and Cowland.[28])

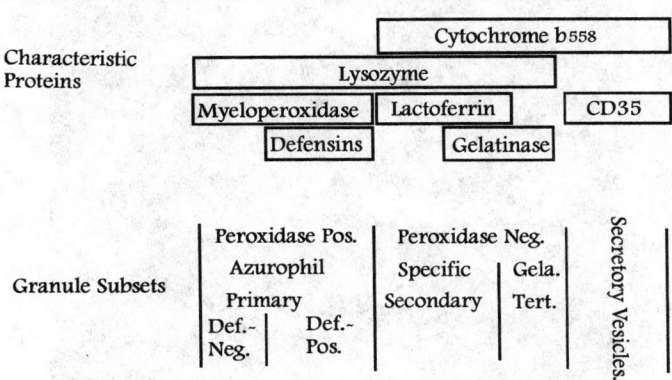

FIGURE 64-8   Classification of granules in neutrophils. Peroxidase-positive (azurophilic or primary) granules are characterized by their content of myeloperoxidase and may be further divided based on their content of defensins into large, defensin-rich granules and the smaller defensin-poor granules. The peroxidase-negative granules may be divided into specific (secondary) granules and gelatinase (tertiary) granules on the basis of their relative content of lactoferrin and gelatinase. All granules contain lysozyme. Secretory vesicles share some of their membrane proteins with peroxidase-negative granules, whereas others are unique to secretory vesicles. Def., defensins; Gela., gelatinase; Tert., tertiary. (Reproduced with permission from Borregaard and Cowland.[28])

TABLE 64-1   PROPOSED CLASSIFICATION OF NEUTROPHIL GRANULE
ABNORMALITIES

I. Abnormalities of azurophil granules
   A. Quantitative
      1. None
      2. Fewer than normal
      3. More than normal
   B. Qualitative
      1. Contents of granule incomplete
         Example: hereditary peroxidase deficiency (Fig. 64-9)
      2. Abnormal variants
         Examples: Auer bodies (Fig. 64-10)
         Chédiak-Higashi syndrome (Fig. 64-11)
II. Abnormalities of specific granules
   A. Quantitative
      1. None
      2. Fewer than normal
      3. More than normal
   B. Qualitative
      1. Contents of granule are incomplete
      2. Abnormal variants

Absence of Granule Contents   In some instances, azurophilic
granules can form that lack one or more enzymes or other substances.
For example, in hereditary myeloperoxidase deficiency, the azurophilic
granules of neutrophils and monocytes,[106,107] but not eosinophils or
basophils, lack peroxidase (Fig. 64-9). This deficiency occurs in one
in 2000 to 5000 persons[108,109] and is not usually associated with clinical
abnormalities. Although not detectable with enzyme assays, peroxidase

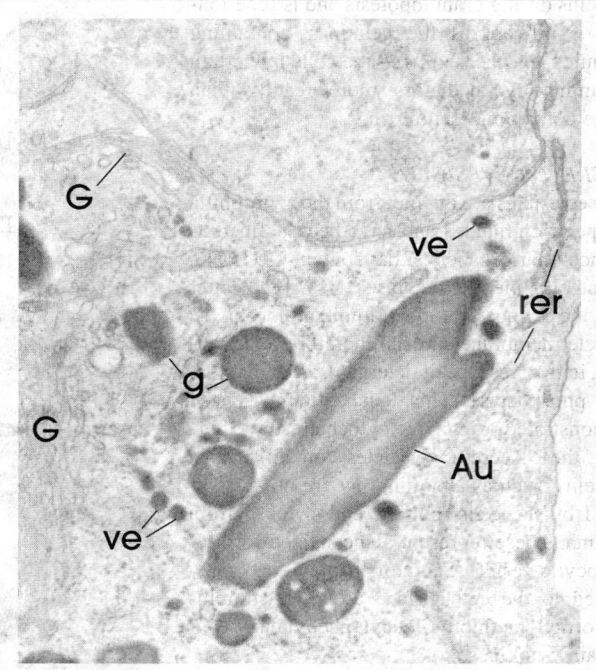

FIGURE 64-10   Peroxidase localization in an abnormal immature cell from
a patient with acute myelogenous leukemia. Note the Auer body (Au) with its
crystalline inclusion and a matrix containing peroxidase. (G, Golgi cisternae;
ve, vesicles, rer, RER.) X40,000

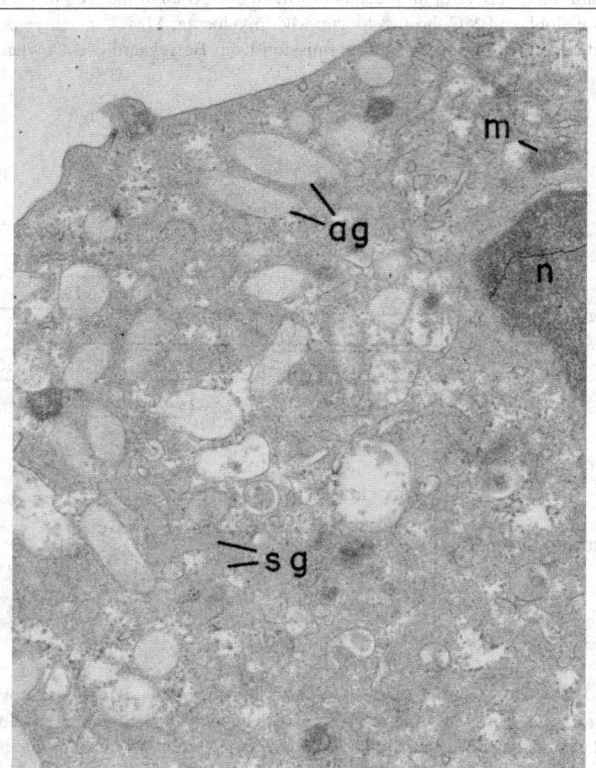

FIGURE 64-9   Neutrophil reacted for peroxidase, from the blood of a patient
with hereditary peroxidase deficiency. Note that both types of granules are
present, the large azurophilic granules (ag), pale because of the absence of
peroxidase, and the small specific granules (sg). (m, mitochondria; n, nucleus.) X19,000

can be revealed by immunologic methods in the neutrophils of persons
with the deficiency.[110] Molecular analysis of cells from family members
with this deficiency has revealed mutations of the gene(s) that resides
on chromosome 17 and encodes a protein that is incapable of posttranslational processing and thus is enzymatically inactive.[111,112] Peroxidase deficiency has also been observed in refractory anemia,[113] in
preleukemia,[114,115] and in the blast crisis of CML.[104] In all these examples of peroxidase deficiency, both types of granules are present and
apparently normal; only the enzyme is missing. In the hereditary
deficiency, all the neutrophils are peroxidase-negative, whereas in the
refractory anemias and leukemias,[116,117] the percentage of peroxidase-
negative neutrophils varies. Neutrophils lacking peroxidase are observed in AML and in the case of blast cell transformation of CML.[104]
This abnormality, when present, affects 8 to 70 percent of the circulating neutrophils. The deficient neutrophils may originate from the
leukemic precursors. A high neutrophil peroxidase activity is present
in the neutrophils of patients with megaloblastic anemia.[118] Finally,
immunologic techniques for peroxidase were found to be useful in
the diagnosis of minimally differentiated acute myeloid leukemia
(AML-M0).[119]

   Abnormal Variants   Auer bodies, found in the immature cells of
some patients with AML, are abnormally large, elongated, azurophilic
granules, containing peroxidase, lysosomal enzymes, and large crystalline inclusions.[99,103,120–122] Although similar to normal azurophilic granules in content and staining properties, Auer bodies are "abnormal"
because they are so large (Fig. 64-10). Furthermore, Auer body formation in leukemic blasts and promyelocytes differs markedly from the
normal secretory process of azurophilic granule formation in that Golgi
cisternae contain very little peroxidase.[103,119] More Auer bodies can be
detected on marrow and blood films from patients with AML when
special stains, e.g., peroxidase, chloroacetate esterase, acid phosphatase, or Sudan black, are applied than when the Romanovsky stain is

used. Not all Auer bodies exhibit all of these staining characteristics at the same time. Auer rod formation may be an occasional but normal phenomenon in fetal hematopoiesis.[123] Auer rod-like inclusions can also be seen at the light microscopic level in certain B-cell neoplasms, but they are peroxidase-negative.[124]

The Chédiak-Higashi anomaly or syndrome, a rare autosomal recessive disease, is characterized clinically by oculocutaneous albinism and increased susceptibility to infection, and microscopically by the presence of abnormally large lysosome-like organelles in most granule-containing cells (see Chap. 72). The large inclusions in the neutrophils of persons with Chédiak-Higashi syndrome are enormous abnormal azurophilic granules.[125,126] Early in neutrophil maturation, normal azurophilic granules form, but they then fuse together to form megagranules. Later, during the myelocyte stage, normal specific granules form. The mature neutrophils contain both the abnormal azurophilic and the normal specific granules (Fig. 64-11). The contents of specific granules can be present in the megagranules,[127] presumably because of limited fusion with megagranules. There is an absence of elastase and cathepsin G, along with defensin content, in patients with Chédiak-Higashi syndrome.[128] The syndrome results from a mutation of the gene, *LYST*, which encodes a protein with multiple phosphorylation sites.[129]

Giant peroxidase-positive granules have been observed in the neutrophils of a patient with neutrophil dysfunction.[130,131] These granules were structurally similar to those seen in Chédiak-Higashi syndrome, but the neutrophils were biochemically different in that there was defective activation of the respiratory burst.

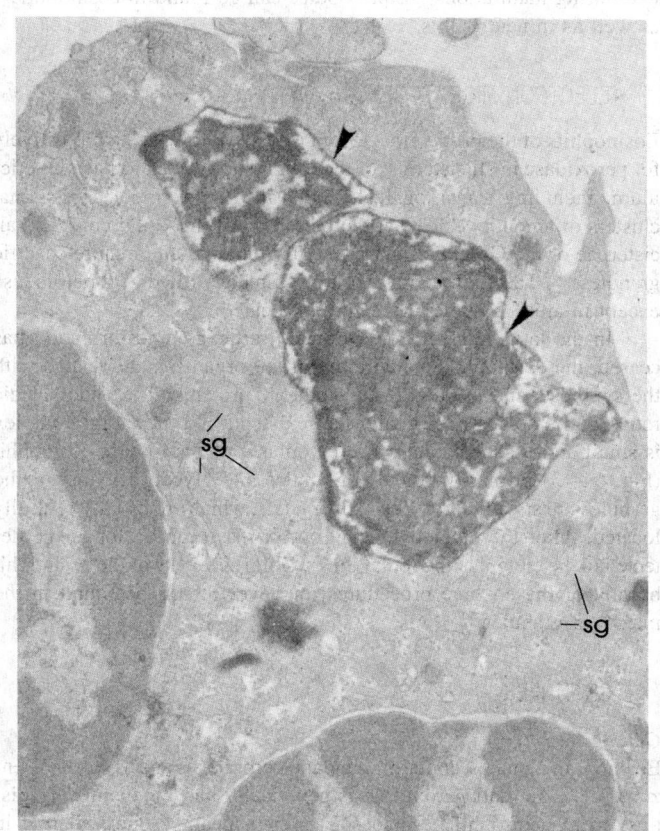

FIGURE 64-11   Peroxidase localization in a neutrophil from a patient with Chédiak-Higashi syndrome. Note that the large megagranules are peroxidase-positive (arrows), whereas the specific granules appear normal (sg). X26,000

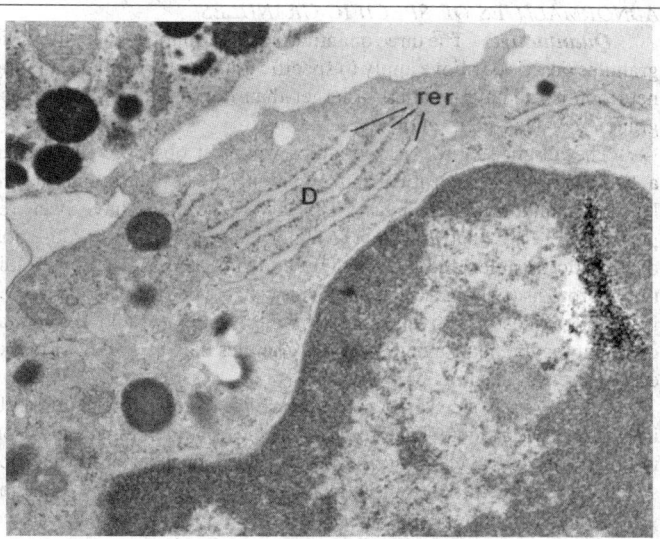

FIGURE 64-12   A portion of a neutrophil depicts a Döhle body (D): it consists of three stacks of rough endoplasmic reticulum (rer). It stains blue by light microscopy because of the concentration of ribosomes.

Giant round granules have been observed in Wright's-stained cells from patients with acute myelomonocytic leukemia.[132] This acquired abnormality closely mimicked the giant-round granules seen in the Chédiak-Higashi syndrome, and is termed the *pseudo-Chédiak-Higashi anomaly*.[133,134] In marrow from patients with AML, one may observe enormous round pink inclusions that resemble ingested erythrocytes in blasts and promyelocytes. Electron microscopy and peroxidase cytochemistry show that these inclusions are homogeneous large, membrane-bound, peroxidase-positive granules that correspond to the abnormal granules seen in the pseudo-Chédiak-Higashi anomaly. Like the Auer rods also seen in AML, these granules are an abnormal variant of peroxidase-positive azurophils. Their lack of azurophilic staining is due to the absence of sulfated glycosaminoglycans.[135]

In certain inflammatory disorders, morphologic changes occur in blood neutrophils. The best-known alteration is the "shift to the left," which denotes the presence of bands, metamyelocytes, and sometimes myelocytes in the blood. The mature neutrophil can also display cytoplasmic modifications, including: (1) "toxic" granules, which stain more prominently than those of normal neutrophils; (2) light-blue, amorphous inclusions called Döhle bodies; and (3) vacuoles. Toxic granules are azurophilic granules that have an abnormal staining pattern when viewed with the light microscope[136] but are indistinguishable from normal azurophilic granules when viewed by electron microscopy. Döhle bodies are not granules; rather, they have been defined as several rows of rough endoplasmic reticulum. They stain as blue bodies in the cytoplasm because of the ribosomes bound to the membrane of the reticulum (Fig. 64-12). Toxic neutrophils have decreases in chemotaxis and in phagocytic and intracellular bactericidal activities.[137,138] Increased numbers of lipid bodies have been observed in inflammatory reactions[139] and other inclusion bodies can be seen in certain hereditary conditions.[140–142]

An acquired azurophil granule abnormality occurs in neutrophils of patients with amiodarone pulmonary toxicity.[143] Some of the peroxidase-positive azurophil granules contain lamellar inclusions. The target antigen of anticytoplasmic antibodies in patients with Wegener's granulomatosis is proteinase 3, located in azurophilic granules.[66,67,144–146]

ABNORMALITIES OF SPECIFIC GRANULES

Quantitative The three quantitative abnormalities of azurophilic granules described above apply to specific granules as well: circulating neutrophils can have smaller- or larger-than-normal quantities of these granules or lack them entirely.

The absence of specific granules was first observed in 1974 in a 14-year-old boy with recurrent infection whose neutrophils lacked leukocyte alkaline phosphatase (LAP).[147] More cases have been reported.[148–155] These patients have an abnormality that affects production of specific granules and their protein contents, and at least two additional proteins (gelatinase and defensins).[148–155] There are abnormalities in the peroxidase-positive granules of these patients.[152] In congenital dysgranulocytic neutropenia, specific granules may be absent or markedly decreased in number.[105]

This absence of certain normal organelles from mature neutrophils in patients with acute leukemia has been documented by electron microscopic and cytochemical studies. There can be an absence of specific granules in neutrophils from patients with AML.[103] This absence or paucity of specific granules in the more mature segmented neutrophils in certain leukemic patients results from a cessation of cytoplasmic development after the promyelocytic stage, whereas nuclear maturation progresses in a fairly normal fashion. These abnormal neutrophils are frequent in AML with maturation (i.e., the M2 variety) and in myelodysplastic syndromes. After treatment of acute promyelocyte leukemia with all-trans retinoic acid, aberrant peroxidase-positive granules, including Auer rod, have become normal, although the neutrophils lacked the specific (secondary) peroxidase-negative population.[156] Furthermore, neutrophils in patients with AML can be deficient in all granules.[157]

Absence of Granule Contents There are no well-documented examples in this category. The specific granules are present in normal numbers in all neutrophils of patients with CML.[158] The low leukocyte alkaline phosphatase score seen in most CML is associated with undetectable levels of mRNA, so the protein is not being synthesized.[159] Two major antibacterial proteins, lysozyme and lactoferrin, can specifically bind glucose-modified proteins bearing advanced glycation end products (AGEs).[160] Exposure to AGE-modified proteins inhibits the enzymatic and bacterial activity of lysozyme, and blocks the bacterial agglutination and bacterial killing activities of lactoferrin.

Abnormal Variants Morphologically abnormal variants of specific granules have not been reported. Other granule abnormalities[161] that cannot be subclassified include the Alder-Reilly anomaly, in which the cytoplasm of neutrophils contains prominent granules that stain a deep lilac color (see color plate in Ref. 161). The inheritance pattern of this disorder is not clear, but it may be part of a general metabolic disorder of polysaccharides. The May-Hegglin anomaly is an autosomal dominant disorder characterized by leukopenia, and the presence of abnormally large basophilic bodies in neutrophils, eosinophils, basophils, monocytes, and giant platelets. There are marked differences between these large inclusions and the Döhle bodies, which develop with infection. In the May-Hegglin anomaly the blue area is occupied by rods and small granules, which may be ribosomes.[162]

OTHER CELLULAR ABNORMALITIES

The *Pelger-Huët anomaly*, an inherited disorder, is characterized by abnormal lobe development in granulocytes; neutrophils can have a monolobed (homozygote) or bilobed (heterozygote) appearance. This abnormality can be mimicked in the neutrophils of patients with AML (acquired Pelger-Huët anomaly).[161] *Hypersegmentation* of neutrophils is a characteristic of folate and vitamin B_{12} deficiencies, but it can also be seen after hydroxyurea or glucocorticoid therapy.[163] In patients suffering from severe alcoholism, *ring-shaped nuclei* may be seen in granulocytes.[164] Peculiar *fibrillary inclusions* of both the cytoplasm and

nuclei may be seen by ultrastructural examination in the neutrophils of human renal allograft recipients who have serious infections.[165] Neutrophils of patients with infection may show nuclear pyknosis, degranulation, and vacuolation[166] in addition to *toxic granulation* and *Döhle bodies*. Döhle bodies may also be found in the neutrophils of pregnant women for unexplained reasons.[167] Multiple persistent vacuoles can be seen in neutrophils, eosinophils, monocytes, and their precursors in *familial Jordan's anomaly*.[168] Döhle bodies and inclusions of *May-Hegglin anomaly* have also been reported in the *Fechtner syndrome*, which includes nephritis, deafness, congenital cataracts, and macrothrombocytopenia.[140] Abnormal neutrophil granules consisting of large membranous whirls have been observed after chloroquine therapy[169] and amiodarone toxicity.[143]

EOSINOPHILS

LIGHT MICROSCOPY OF EOSINOPHILS IN MARROW AND BLOOD FILMS

The earliest identifiable form of an eosinophilic leukocyte is as a late myeloblast or early promyelocyte. This cell is about 15 μm in diameter, has a large nucleus with nucleoli, and a few blue or azurophilic granules in intensely basophilic cytoplasm. The later eosinophilic promyelocyte and myelocyte contain mostly acidophilic granules. The fully mature eosinophilic leukocyte has a bilobed nucleus and its cytoplasm is filled with large eosinophilic granules whose rims stain for peroxidase and Sudan black. Multilobed nuclei, comparable to those of neutrophils, are rare.[170] Eosinophils are susceptible to mechanical damage during the preparation of blood films. Eosinophilic precursors may degranulate during maturation.[171] Lipid bodies can be found in eosinophils[172] as well as in neutrophils.

ELECTRON MICROSCOPY AND CYTOCHEMISTRY

Eosinophils of the promyelocyte and myelocyte stages stain positively for peroxidase in all cisternae of the rough-surfaced endoplasmic reticulum, including transitional elements and the perinuclear cisterna; clusters of smooth vesicles at the periphery of the Golgi complex, all cisternae of the Golgi complex, and all immature and mature specific granules.[3,173] The mature granules are completely filled with peroxidase except in areas occupied by centrally located crystals.

In the later stages of development, after granule formation has ceased, the eosinophils contain few of the organelles associated with the synthesis and packaging of secretory proteins. The endoplasmic reticulum is sparse or virtually non-existent, and the Golgi complex is small and inconspicuous. The cytoplasm of the mature eosinophil (Fig. 64-13) primarily contains granules and glycogen. Most of the granules are specific granules with crystals, which are usually centrally located. After the myelocyte stage, peroxidase can no longer be detected in the endoplasmic reticulum or Golgi elements of the eosinophil by any of the enzyme procedures; however, it can be found in the matrix of granules.[3,173]

GRANULES

CONTENTS

Eosinophil granules contain abundant peroxidase and lysosomal enzymes.[3] Eosinophil peroxidase is genetically and biochemically distinct from neutrophil peroxidase, and it appears to play no role in the eosinophil's bactericidal activity.[174] Eosinophils have much less bactericidal activity than do neutrophils.[175] The specific granules of eosinophils are true peroxisomes in that they also contain catalase,[176] two enzymes of peroxisomal lipid β-oxidation (enoyl-CoA hydratase

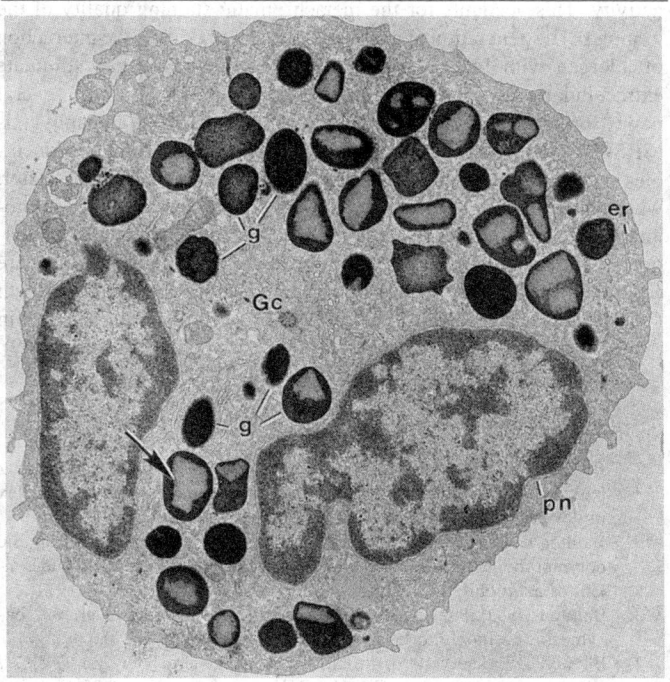

FIGURE 64-13   Human mature eosinophil incubated for peroxidase. Reaction product is present only in granules (g). The rough endoplasmic reticulum (er), including the perinuclear cisterna (pn) and the Golgi cisternae (Gc), does not contain reaction product. Most of the granules (arrow) contain the distinctive crystalline bar. X8000 (Reproduced with permission from Bainton.[4])

and ketoacyl-CoA thiolase[177]), and a flavoprotein, (acyl-CoA oxidase[178]). All of these substances have been found in the matrix, but not the crystalloid, of the granule. Lectins have also been identified in eosinophil granules, most heavily in the crystalloids.[179] The eosinophil granule is also known to contain several basic proteins: a major basic protein, eosinophil cationic protein, and eosinophil-derived neurotoxin.[180–185] More than half of the granule protein is the major basic protein, which constitutes the crystalline core of the granule. It is cytotoxic to parasites as well as normal mammalian cells and induces histamine release from basophils and mast cells.[184] The other two cationic proteins are found in the matrix of the granule.[180–182] Eosinophil cationic protein can cause the formation of transmembrane pores and may thereby cause membrane damage.[184] The amino-acid sequence of eosinophil cationic protein is homologous with that of eosinophil-derived neurotoxin, and both sequences show striking homology with that of ribonuclease.[185,186] Eosinophils also contain proteoglycans,[187] interleukin-6,[188] tumor necrosis factor-α,[189] transforming growth factor-α,[190] and granulocyte-macrophage colony-stimulating factor.[191]

Charcot-Leyden crystals, bipyramidal crystals observed in fluids in association with eosinophilic inflammatory reactions, possess lysophospholipase activity and comprise 7 to 10 percent of total eosinophil protein.[192–195] The ultrastructural localization of this protein is in a large, crystal-free granule and supports the presence of a distinct primary granule population ($\approx 5\%$) in mature eosinophils.[3,194,195]

ABNORMALITIES

Inherited Abnormalities of Eosinophils   There are four inherited abnormalities of eosinophils: (1) The absence of peroxidase and phospholipids in eosinophils is an autosomal-recessive defect that produces no signs of disease;[196,197] (2) In Chédiak-Higashi syndrome,[125] almost all granulated cells, including eosinophils, contain large abnor-

mal granules; (3) A family was found to have gray inclusions in eosinophils and basophils; this abnormality was autosomal dominant and had no clinical effects. Electron microscopy revealed cytoplasmic crystals and curved lamellar bodies in the cells;[198] (4) Neutrophil-specific granule deficiency, previously described, also involves eosinophils.[150]

Several acquired gross morphologic or cytochemical abnormalities of eosinophils have been observed in leukemias or in association with benign eosinophilias (see below).

Cytochemistry of Abnormalities in Leukemias   In a cytochemical study of eosinophils in acute leukemia,[199] the cells were considered normal when they did not show toluidine blue metachromasia or positivity for alkaline phosphatase, chloroacetate esterase, Astra blue, or periodic acid-Schiff (PAS), but did show positivity for peroxidase and Sudan black, and moderate reactivity with naphthol-AS or alpha-naphthyl esterase. The observation of chloroacetate esterase activity in some abnormal eosinophils is of particular interest in view of the subsequent finding that abnormal marrow eosinophils in acute myelomonocytic leukemia are associated with the inversion of chromosome 16.[200] Most of the patients studied had a higher than normal percentage of immature eosinophils containing a mixture of eosinophilic and basophilic granules. The eosinophilic granules showed abnormal reactivity for chloroacetate esterase and periodic acid Schiff. None of the granules had well-formed central crystalloids.

An abnormality seen in patients with CML is the presence of basophilic and eosinophilic granules in eosinophilic myelocytes and, occasionally, in mature eosinophils.[201] Eosinophilic and basophilic granules are mutually exclusive markers of the respective granulocytic

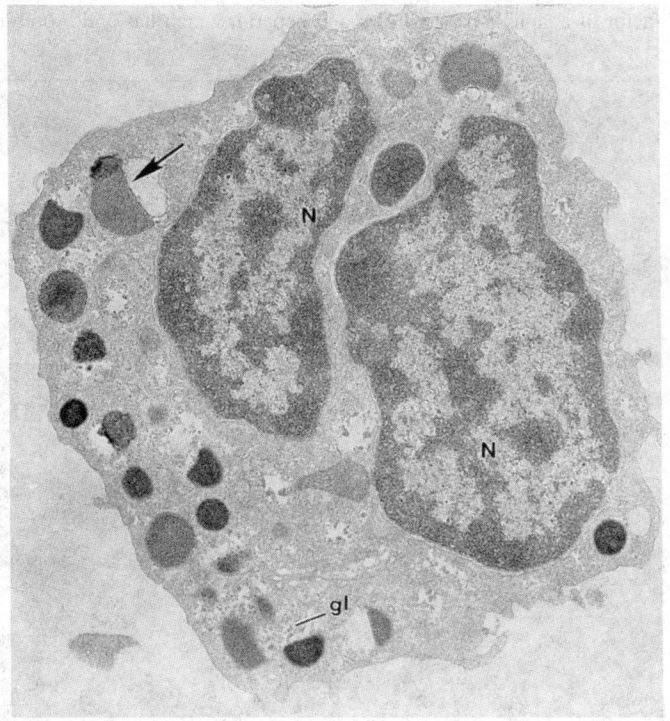

FIGURE 64-14   Mature basophil from human blood, reacted for peroxidase. Note unusually large nucleus (n) and scattered glycogen particles (gl). Human basophil granules contain peroxidase, as illustrated by their density (due to the presence of reaction product) in this type of preparation. They are usually spherical, difficult to fix, and may be speckled in appearance (arrow). X17,000 (Reproduced with permission from Bainton.[4])

lineages; the presence of both markers in CML cells is a sign of lineage infidelity.

Degranulated and light density eosinophils are associated with eosinophilia.[181,202,203] There is an expanding clinical spectrum of multisystem diseases associated with eosinophilia[204] (see Chap. 68).

Intranuclear Crystals Associated With Abnormal Granules
Eosinophils with abnormal granules and intranuclear crystalloids were observed in a 2-year-old girl with chronic benign neutropenia.[205] The father had the same morphologic abnormality, but was asymptomatic and had normal leukocyte counts.

ACQUIRED EOSINOPHIL PSEUDO-PELGER-HUËT ANOMALY
Incomplete segmentation of the nucleus of mature eosinophils is seen in AML[206] and myelodysplasia.[207] Eosinophil accumulation, activation, fate, and apoptosis have recently been reviewed.[208–210]

BASOPHILS AND MAST CELLS

Basophils and mast cells are distinct cell lines, although they have many functional similarities.[211–217] The granules of both cell types stain metachromatically, but they are distinct[218–220] when examined by electron microscopy (Figs. 64-14 and 64-15). The cells can phagocytose sensitized red cells but are less active phagocytes than the other granulocytes and lack significant amounts of antibacterial or lysosomal enzymes. Basophils are found in small numbers in blood (0.5%) and can be seen in tissues in which inflammation resulting from hypersensitivity to proteins, contact allergy, or skin-allograft rejection is present.

Mast cells are normal residents of connective tissue throughout the body. Mast-cell granules contain various substances,[211–217] including several preformed biologically active substances such as histamine, which causes increased vascular permeability; eosinophil chemotactic factor of anaphylaxis (ECF-A); and heparin, which has antithrombin

activity. This accounts for the metachromatic staining quality of the granules. The generation of anaphylatoxin (C3a, C5a) or the interaction of allergen with IgE receptors of plasma membrane can stimulate extracellular release of these granule contents as well as of several newly formed substances, e.g., slow-reacting substance of anaphylaxis (SRS-A), a leukotriene, which causes contraction of human bronchioles and increased vascular permeability; and platelet-activating factor, which causes platelet aggregation and the subsequent release of serotonin. This phenomenon is called IgE-mediated mast cell degranulation.[213] Mast cells have also been implicated in various diseases that are accompanied by neovascularization, and vascular endothelial growth factor/vascular permeability factor (VEGF/VPF) has been detected in secretory granules of isolated human skin mast cells[221] (see Chap. 69).

REFERENCES

1. Bainton DF, Farquhar MG: Origin of granules in polymorphonuclear leukocytes: Two types derived from opposite faces of the Golgi complex in developing granulocytes. *J Cell Biol* 28:277, 1966.
2. Bainton DF, Ullyot JL, Farquhar MG: The development of neutrophilic polymorphonuclear leukocytes in human bone marrow: Origin and content of azurophil and specific granules. *J Exp Med* 134:907, 1971.
3. Bainton DF, Farquhar MG: Segregation and packaging of granule enzymes in eosinophilic leukocytes. *J Cell Biol* 45:54, 1970.
4. Bainton DF: The cells of inflammation: A general view, in *The Cell Biology of Inflammation*, edited by G Weissman, vol 2, pp 1-25. Elsevier, North-Holland/New York, 1980.
5. Cronkite EP, Vincent PC: Granulocytopoiesis. *Ser Haematol* 2:3, 1969.
6. Jamuar MP, Cronkite EP: The fate of granulocytes. *Exp Hematol* 8:884, 1980.
7. Hardin JH, Spicer SS: Ultrastructural localization of dialyzed iron-reactive mucosubstance in rabbit heterophils, basophils, and eosinophils. *J Cell Biol* 48:368, 1971.
8. Sanchez AJ, Karni RJ, Wangh LJ: Fluorescent in situ hybridization (FISH) analysis of the relationship between chromosome location and nuclear morphology in human neutrophils. *Chromosoma* 106(3): 168, 1997.
9. Hochstenbach PF, Scheres JM, Hustinx TW, Wieringa B: Demonstration of X chromatin in drumstick-like nuclear appendages of leukocytes by in situ hybridization on blood smears. *Histochem* 84:383, 1986.
10. Pryzwansky KB, Breton-Gorius J: Identification of a subpopulation of primary granules in human neutrophils based upon maturation and distribution: Study by transmission electron microscopy cytochemistry and high voltage electron microscopy of whole cell preparations. *Lab Invest* 53:664, 1985.
11. Breton-Gorius J, Coquin Y, Guichard J: Cytochemical distinction between azurophils and catalase-containing granules in leukocytes. *Lab Invest* 38:21, 1978.
12. Wallace PJ, Packman CH, Lichtman MA: Maturation-associated changes in the peripheral cytoplasm of human neutrophils: A review. *Exp Hematol* 15:34, 1987.
13. Sullivan R, Griffin JD, Malech HL: Acquisition of formyl peptide receptors during normal human myeloid differentiation. *Blood* 70:1222, 1987.
14. Berger M, Wetzler EM, Welter E, et al: Intracellular sites for storage and recycling of C3b receptors in human neutrophils. *Proc Natl Acad Sci USA* 88:3019, 1991.
15. Rothwell SW, Nath J, Wright DG: Interactions of cytoplasmic granules with microtubules in human neutrophils. *J Cell Biol* 108:2313, 1989.
16. Cramer EB: Cell biology of phagocyte migration from the bone marrow, out of the bloodstream, and across organ epithelia, in *Inflammation: Basic Principles and Clinical Correlates*, edited by JI Gallin, IM Goldstein, R. Snyderman pp 341-351. Raven Press Ltd., New York, 1992.
17. Long MW: Review: Blood cell cytoadhesion molecules. *Exp Hematol* 20:288, 1992.
18. Soligo D, Schirò R, Luksch R, et al: Expression of integrins in human bone marrow. *Br J Haematol* 76:323, 1990.
19. Liesveld JL, Winslow JM, Frediani KE, et al: Expression of integrins

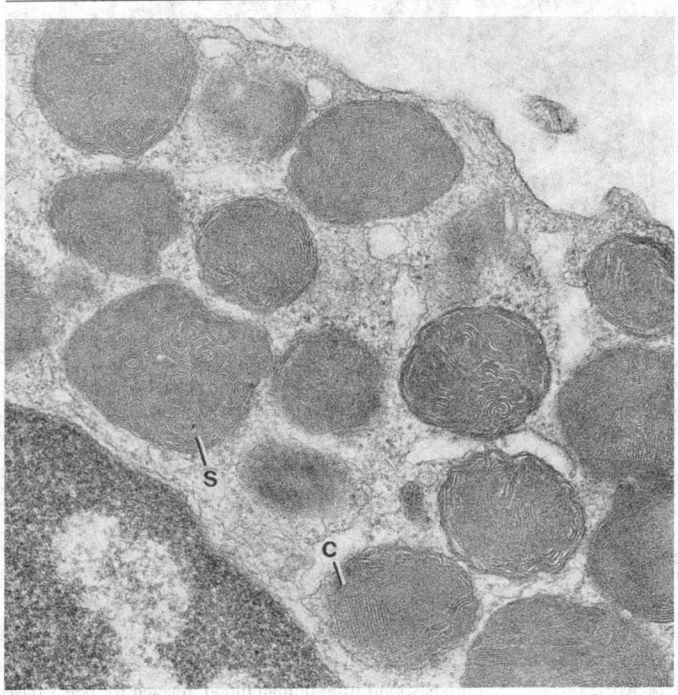

FIGURE 64-15   Portion of a mast cell from human bone marrow. Note that the granules are filled with scroll-like (s) and crystal (c) images and are distinct from human basophil granules (see Fig. 64-14) in fine-structural morphology. (X50,000.) (Reproduced with permission from Bainton.[4])

and examinations of their adhesive function in normal and leukemic hematopoietic cells. *Blood* 81:112, 1993.

20. Verfaillie CM, Hurley R, Zhao RCH, Prosper F, Delforge M, Bhatia R: Pathophysiology of CML: Do defects in integrin function contribute to the premature circulation and massive expansion of the BCR/ABL positive clone? *J Lab Med* 129 (6):584, 1997.

21. Kerst JM, Sanders JB, Slaper-Cortenbach ICM, et al: Alpha 4 beta 1 and alpha 5 beta 1 are differentially expressed during myelopoiesis and mediate the adherence of human CD34+ cells to fibronectin in an activation-dependent way. *Blood* 81:344, 1993.

22. Arkin S, Naprstek B, Guarini L, Ferrone S, Lipton JM: Expression of intercellular adhesion molecule-1 (CD-54) on hematopoietic progenitors. *Blood* 77:948, 1991.

23. Williams DA, Rios M, Stephens C, Patel VP: Fibronectin and VLA-4 in haematopoietic stem cell-microenvironment interactions. *Nature* 352:438, 1991.

24. Griffin JD, Spertini O, Ernst TJ, et al: Granulocyte-macrophage colony-stimulating factor and other cytokines regulate surface expression of the leukocyte adhesion molecule-1 on human neutrophils, monocytes, and their precursors. *J Immunol* 145:576, 1990.

25. Kishimoto TK, Jutila MA, Berg EL, Butcher EC: Neutrophil Mac-1 and MEL-14 adhesion proteins inversely regulated by chemotactic factors. *Science* 245:1238, 1989.

26. Berliner N: Molecular biology of neutrophil differentiation. *Curr Opin Hematol* 5:49, 1998.

27. Clarke S, Gordon S: Myeloid-specific gene expression. *J Leukoc Biol* 63:153, 1998.

28. Borregaard N, Cowland BJ: Granules of the human neutrophilic polymorphonuclear leukocyte. *Blood* 89:3503, 1997.

29. Dubravec DB, Spriggs DR, Mannick JA, Rodrick ML: Circulating human peripheral blood granulocytes synthesize and secrete tumor necrosis factor alpha. *Proc Natl Acad Sci USA* 87:6758, 1990.

30. Wheeler MA, Smith SD, Garcia-Cardena G, Nathan CF, Weiss RM, Sessa WC: Bacterial infection induces nitric oxide synthase in human neutrophils. *J Clin Invest* 99:110, 1997.

31. Shi J, Fujieda H, Kokubo Y, Wake K: Apoptosis of neutrophils and their elimination by Kupffer cells in rat liver. *Hepatology* 5:1256, 1996.

32. Homburg CHE, Roos D: Apoptosis of neutrophils. *Curr Opin Hematol* 3:94, 1996.

33. Klebanoff SJ, Clark RA: *The Neutrophil: Function and Clinical Disorders.* Elsevier/North Holland Biomedical Press, Amsterdam, 1978. p. 556.

34. Bendix-Hansen K: Annotation: Enzyme cytochemistry of neutrophil granulocytes. *Br J Haematol* 65:127, 1987.

35. Bretz U, Baggiolini M: Biochemical and morphological characterization of azurophil and specific granules of human neutrophilic polymorphonuclear leukocytes. *J Cell Biol* 63:251, 1974.

36. Spitznagel JK, Dalldorf FG, Leffell MS, et al: Character of azurophil and specific granule purified from human polymorphonuclear leukocytes. *Lab Invest* 30:774, 1974.

37. West BC, Rosenthal AS, Gelb NA, Kimball HR: Separation and characterization of human neutrophil granules. *Am J Pathol* 77:41, 1974.

38. Kane SP, Peters TJ: Analytical subcellular fractionation of human granulocytes with reference to the localization of vitamin B12-binding proteins. *Clin Sci Mol Med* 49:171, 1975.

39. Borregaard N, Heiple JM, Simons ER, Clark RA: Subcellular localization of the b-cytochrome component of the human neutrophil microbicidal oxidase: Translocation during activation. *J Cell Biol* 97:52, 1983.

40. Ringel EW, Soter NA, Austen KF: Localization of histaminase to the specific granule of the human neutrophil. *Immunology* 52:649, 1984.

41. O'Shea JJ, Brown EJ, Seligmann E, Metcalf JA, Frank MM, Gallin JI: Evidence for distinct intracellular pools of receptors for C3b and C3bi in human neutrophils. *J Immunol* 134:2580, 1985.

42. Gabay JE, Heiple JM, Cohn ZA, Nathan CF: Subcellular location and properties of bactericidal factors from human neutrophils. *J Exp Med* 164:1407, 1986.

43. Heiple JM, Ossowski L: Human neutrophil plasminogen activator is localized in specific granules and is translocated to the cell surface by exocytosis. *J Exp Med* 164:826, 1986.

44. Rice WG, Kinkade JM, Parmley RT: High resolution of heterogeneity

45. Bjerrum OW, Bjerrum OJ, Borregaard N: Beta 2-microglobulin in neutrophils: An intragranular protein. *J Immunol* 138:3913, 1987.

46. Rice WG, Ganz T, Kinkade JM Jr, Selsted ME, Lehrer RI, Parnley RT: Defensin-rich dense granules of human neutrophils. *Blood* 70:757, 1987.

47. Stevenson KB, Nauseef WM, Clark RA: The neutrophil glycoprotein Mo1 is an integral membrane protein of plasma membranes and specific granules. *J Immunol* 139:3759, 1987.

48. Weiss J, Olsson I: Cellular and subcellular localization of the bactericidal/permeability-increasing protein of neutrophils. *Blood* 69:652, 1987.

49. Yoon PS, Boxer LA, Mayo LA, Yang AY, Wicha WS: Human neutrophil laminin receptors: Activation-dependent receptor expression. *J Immunol* 138:259, 1987.

50. Lacal P, Pulido R, Sanchez-Madrid F, Mollinedo F: Intracellular location of T200 and Mo1 glycoproteins in human neutrophils. *J Biol Chem* 263:9946, 1988.

51. Bjerrum OW, Borregaard N: Dual granule localization of the dormant NADPH oxidase and cytochrome b559 in human neutrophils {published erratum appears in *Eur J Haematol* [1989]8:270}. *Eur J Haematol* 43:67, 1989.

52. Gabnay JE, Scott RW, Campanelli D: Antibiotic proteins of human polymorphonuclear leukocytes. *Proc Natl Acad Sci USA* 86:5610, 1989.

53. Singer II, Scott S, Kawka DW, Kazazis DM: Adhesomes: Specific granule containing receptors for laminin, C3bi/fibrinogen, fibronectin, and vitronectin in human polymorphonuclear leukocytes and monocytes. *J Cell Biol* 109:3169, 1989.

54. Borregaard N, Christensen L, Bejerrum OW, Birgens HS, Clemmensen I: Identification of a highly mobilizable subset of human neutrophil intracellular vesicles that contains tetranectin and latent alkaline phosphatase. *J Clin Invest* 85:408, 1990.

55. Campanelli D, Detmers PA, Nathan CF, Gabay JE: Azurocidin and a homologous serine protease from neutrophils. *J Clin Invest* 85:904, 1990.

56. Lehrer RI, Ganz T: Antimicrobial polypeptides of human neutrophils. *Blood* 76:2169, 1990.

57. Pereira HA, Spitznagel JK, Winton EF, et al: The ontogeny of a 57-Kd cationic antimicrobial protein of human polymorphonuclear leukocytes: Localization to a novel granule population. *Blood* 76:825, 1990.

58. Spitznagel JK: Antibiotic proteins of human neutrophils. *J Clin Invest* 86:1381, 1990.

59. Lehrer RI, Ganz T, Selsted ME: Defensins: Endogenous antibiotic peptides of animal cells. *Cell* 64:229, 1991.

60. Cramer E, Pryzwansky KB, Villeval J-L, Testa U, Breton-Gorius J: Ultrastructural localization of lactoferrin and myeloperoxidase in human neutrophils by immunogold. *Blood* 65:423, 1985.

61. Bainton DF, Miller LJ, Kishimoto TK, Springer TA: Leukocyte adhesion receptors are stored in peroxidase-negative granules of human neutrophils. *J Exp Med* 166:1641, 1987.

62. Hibbs MS, Bainton DF: Human neutrophil gelatinase is a component of specific granules. *J Clin Invest* 84:1395, 1989.

63. Esaguy N, Aguas AP, Silva MT: High-resolution localization of lactoferrin in human neutrophils: Labeling of secondary granules and cell heterogeneity. *J Leukoc Biol* 46:51, 1989.

64. Damiano VV, Kucich U, Murer E, Laudenslager N, Weinbaum G: Ultrastructural quantitation of peroxidase- and elastase-containing granules in human neutrophils. *Am J Pathol* 131:235, 1988.

65. Cramer EM, Beesley JE, Pulford KA, Breton-Gorius J, Mason DY: Colocalization of elastase and myeloperoxidase in human blood and bone marrow neutrophils using a monoclonal antibody and immunogold. *Am J Pathol* 134:1275, 1989.

66. Calafat J, Goldschmeding R, Ringeling PL, Janssen H, van der Schoot CE: In situ localization by double-labeling immunoelectron microscopy of anti-neutrophil cytoplasmic autoantibodies in neutrophils and monocytes. *Blood* 75:242, 1990.

67. Csernok E, Lüdemann J, Gross WL, Bainton DF: Ultrastructural localization of proteinase 3, the target antigen of anti-cytoplasmic antibodies circulating in Wegener's granulomatosis. *Am J Pathol* 137:1113, 1990.

68. Cramer EM, Breton-Gorius J: Ultrastructural localization of lysozyme in human neutrophils by immunogold. *J Leukoc Biol* 41:242, 1987.

69. Livesey SA, Beuscher ES, Krannig GL: Human neutrophil granule heterogeneity: Immunolocalization studies using cryofixed, dried and embedded specimens. *Scanning Microsc* 3:231, 1989.

70. Mutasa HC: Combination of diaminobenzidine staining and immunogold labeling: A novel technical approach to identify lysozyme in human neutrophil cells. *Europ J Cell Biol* 49:319, 1989.

71. Ganz T, Selsted ME, Szklarek D, et al: Defensins: Natural peptide antibiotics of human neutrophils. *J Clin Invest* 76:1427, 1985.

72. Dewald B, Bretz U, Baggiolini M: Release of gelatinase from a novel secretory compartment of human neutrophils. *J Clin Invest* 70:518, 1982.

73. Robinson JM, Kobayashi TA: Novel intracellular compartment with unusual secretory properties in human neutrophils. *J Cell Biol* 113:743, 1991.

74. Rotrosen D, Gallin JI, Spiegel AM, Malech HL: Subcellular localization of Gi alpha in human neutrophils. *J Biol Chem* 263:10958, 1988.

75. Ginsel LA, Onderwater JJM, Fransen JAM, et al: Localization of the low-Mr subunit of cytochrome b558 in human blood phagocytes by immunoelectron microscopy. *Blood* 76:2105, 1990.

76. Jesaitis AJ, Buescher ES, Harrison D, et al: Ultrastructural localization of cytochrome b in the membranes of resting and phagocytosing human granulocytes. *J Clin Invest* 85:821, 1990.

77. Bainton DF, August JT: Multivesicular bodies of human neutrophils (PMN) not granules, immunolabile with the two major lysosomal membrane glycoproteins hLAMP-1 and hLAMP-2. *J Histochem Cytochem* 36:953, 1988.

78. Mason DY, Cramer EM, Massé J-M, Crystal R, Bassot JM, Breton-Gorius J: Alpha1-antitrypsin is present within the primary granules of human polymorphonuclear leukocytes. *Am J Pathol* 139:623, 1991.

79. Saito N, Pulford KA, Breton-Gorius J, Massé JM, Mason DY, Cramer EM: Ultrastructural localization of the CD68 macrophage-associated antigen in human blood neutrophils and monocytes. *Am J Pathol* 139:1053, 1991.

80. Kuijpers TW, Tool ATJ, van der Schoot DE, et al: Membrane surface antigen expression on neutrophils: A reappraisal of the use of surface markers for neutrophil activation. *Blood* 78:1105, 1991.

81. VanWinkle BW: Lectinocytochemical specificity in human eosinophils and neutrophils: A reexamination. *J Histochem Cytochem* 39:1157, 1991.

82. Jost CR, Gaillard ML, Fransen JA, Daha MR, Ginsel LA: Intracellular localization of glycosyl-phosphatidylinositol-anchored CD67 and FcRIII (DC16) in affected neutrophil granulocytes of patients with paroxysmal nocturnal hemoglobinuria. *Blood* 78:3030, 1991.

83. Borregaard N, Kjeldsen L, Rygaard K, et al: Stimulus-dependent secretion of plasma proteins from human neutrophils. *J Clin Invest* 90:86, 1992.

84. Matzner Y, Vlodavsky I, Bar-Ner M, Ishaï-Michaeli R, Tauber AI: Subcellular localization of heparanase in human neutrophils. *J Leukoc Biol* 51:519, 1992.

85. Figueroa CD, Henderson LM, Kaufmann J, et al: Immunovisualization of high (HK) and low (LK) molecular weight kininogens on isolated human neutrophils. *Blood* 79:754, 1992.

86. Suchard SJ, Burton MJ, Stoehr SJ: Thrombospondin receptor expression in human neutrophils coincides with the release of a subpopulation of specific granules. *Biochem J* 284:513, 1992.

87. Ducker TP, Skubitz KM: Subcellular localization of CD66, CD67, and NCA in human neutrophils. *J Leukoc Biol* 52:11, 1992.

88. Kjeldsen L, Bainton DF, Sengelov H, Borregaard N: Structural and functional heterogeneity among peroxidase negative granules in human neutrophils: Identification of a distinct gelatinase containing granule subset by combined immunocytochemistry and subcellular fractionation. *Blood* 82:3183, 1993.

89. Borregaard N, Lollike K, Kjeldsen L, et al: Human neutrophil granules and secretory vesicles. *Eur J Haematol* 51:187, 1993.

90. Egesten A, Breton-Gorius J, Guichard J, Gullberg U, Olsson I: The heterogeneity of azurophil granules in neutrophil promyelocytes: Immunogold localization of myeloperoxidase, cathepsin G, elastase, proteinase 3, and bactericidal/permeability increasing protein. *Blood* 83:2985, 1994.

91. Peretz R, Shaft D, Yaari A, Nir E: Distinct intracellular lysozyme content in normal granulocytes and monocytes: A quantitative immunoperoxidase and ultrastructural immunogold study. *J Histochem Cytochem* 42:1471, 1994.

92. Cham BP, Gerrard JM, Bainton DF: Granulophysin is located in the membranes of azurophilic granules in human neutrophil and mobilizes to the plasma membrane following cell stimulation. *Am J Pathol* 144:1369, 1994.

93. Cieutat A-M, Lobel P, August JT, et al: Azurophilic granules of human neutrophilic leukocytes are deficient in lysosome-associated membrane proteins but retain the mannose 6-phosphate recognition. *Blood* 91:1044, 1998.

94. Borregaard N, Kjeldsen L, Sengelov H, et al: Changes in subcellular localization and surface expression of L-selectin, alkaline phosphatase, and Mac-1 in human neutrophils during stimulation with inflammatory mediators. *J Leukoc Biol* 56:80, 1994.

95. Moore KL, Patel KD, Bruehl RE, et al: P-selectin glycoprotein ligand-1 mediates rolling of human neutrophils on P-selectin. *J Cell Biol* 128:661, 1995.

96. Bruehl RE, Moore KL, Lorant DE, et al: Leukocyte activation induces surface redistribution of P-selectin glycoprotein ligand-1. *J Leukoc Biol* 61:489, 1997.

97. Le Cabec V, Cowland JB, Calafat J, Borregaard N: Targeting of proteins to granule subsets is determined by timing and not by sorting: The specific granule protein NGAL is localized to azurophil granules when expressed in HL-60 cells. *Proc Natl Acad Sci USA* 93:6454, 1996.

98. Ganz T, Lehrer RI: Antimicrobial peptides of vertebrates. *Curr Opin Immunol* 10:41, 1998.

99. Beckstead JH, Halverson PS, Ries CA, Bainton DF: Enzyme histochemistry and immunohistochemistry on biopsy specimens of pathologic human bone marrow. *Blood* 57:1088, 1981.

100. Bainton DF: Selective abnormalities of azurophil and specific granules of human neutrophilic leukocytes. *Fed Proc* 40:1443, 1981.

101. Zucker-Franklin D, Greaves MF, Grossi CE, Marmont AM: *Atlas of Blood Cells: Function and Pathology*, Lea & Febiger, Philadelphia, 191, 1988.

102. Bainton DF: Abnormal neutrophils in acute myelogenous leukemia: Identification of subpopulations based on analysis of azurophil and specific granules. *Blood Cells* 1:191, 1975.

103. Bainton DF, Friedlander LM, Shohet SB: Abnormalities in granule formation in acute myelogenous leukemia. *Blood* 49:693, 1977.

104. Ullyot JL, Bainton DF: Azurophil and specific granules of blood neutrophils in chronic myelogenous leukemia: An ultrastructural and cytochemical analysis. *Blood* 44:469, 1974.

105. Parmley RT, Crist WM, Ragab AH, et al: Congenital dysgranulopoietic neutropenia. Clinical, serologic, ultra-structural, and in vivo proliferative characteristics. *Blood* 56:465, 1980.

106. Lehrer RI, Cline MJ: Leukocyte myeloperoxidase deficiency and disseminated candidiasis: The role of myeloperoxidase in resistance to *Candida* infection. *J Clin Invest* 48:1478, 1969.

107. Breton-Gorius J, Coquin MY, Guichard J: Activités péroxydasiques de certaines granulations des neutrophils dans deux cas de déficit congénital en myélopéroxidase. *C.R. Acad Sci Paris (D)* 280:1753, 1975.

108. Kitahara M, Eyre HJ, Simonian Y: Hereditary myeloperoxidase deficiency. *Blood* 57:888, 1981.

109. Parry MF, Root RK, Metcalf JA, Delaney KK, Kaplow LS, Richar WJ: Myeloperoxidase deficiency. *Ann Intern Med* 95:293, 1981.

110. Ross DW, Kaplow LS: Myeloperoxidase deficiency: Increased sensitivity for immunocytochemical compared to cytochemical detection of enzyme. *Arch Pathol Lab Med* 109:1005, 1985.

111. Nauseef WM, Brigham S, Cogley M: Hereditary myeloperoxidase deficiency due to a missense mutation of arginine 569 to tryptophan. *J Biol Chem* 269:1212, 1994.

112. Nauseef WM, Cogley M, McCormick S: Effect of R569W missense mutation on the biosynthesis of myeloperoxidase. *J Biol Chem* 271:9546, 1996.

113. Lehrer RI, Goldberg LS, Apple MA, Rosenthal NP: Refractory megaloblastic anemia with myeloperoxidase and deficient neutrophils. *Ann Intern Med* 76:447, 1972.

114. Breton-Gorius J, Houssay D, Dryfux B: Partial myeloperoxidase deficiency in a case of preleukemia. *Br J Haematol* 30:273, 1975.

115. Davey FR, Erber WN, Gatter KC, Mason DY: Abnormal neutrophils in acute myeloid leukemia and myelodysplastic syndrome. *Hum Pathol* 19:454, 1988.

116. Catovsky D, Galton DAG, Robinson J: Myeloperoxidase-deficient neutrophils in acute myeloid leukaemia. *Scand J Haematol* 9:142, 1972.

117. Elghetany MT, Peterson B, MacCallum J, et al: Deficiency of neutrophilic granule membrane glycoproteins in the myelodysplastic syndromes: A common deficiency in 216 patients studied by the Cancer and Leukemia Group B. *Leukemia Res* 21(9):801, 1997.

118. Gulley ML, Bentley SA, Ross DW: Neutrophil myeloperoxidase measurement uncovers masked megaloblastic anemia. *Blood* 76:1004, 1990.

119. Venditti A, Del Poeta G, Buccisano F, et al: Minimally differentiated acute myeloid leukemia (AML-M0): Comparison of 25 cases with other French-American-British subtypes, *Blood* 89(2):621, 1997.

120. Breton-Gorius J, Houssay D: Auer bodies in acute promyelocytic leukemia: Demonstration of their fine structure and peroxidase localization. *Lab Invest* 28:135, 1973.

121. Tulliez M, Breton-Gorius J: Three types of Auer bodies in acute leukemia. *Lab Invest* 41:419, 1979.

122. Hassan HT, Rees JKH: Auer bodies in acute myeloid leukemia patients. *Path Res Pract* 186:293, 1990.

123. Newburger PE, Novak TJ, McCaffrey RP: Eosinophilic cytoplasmic inclusions in fetal leukocytes: Are Auer bodies a recapitulation of fetal morphology? *Blood* 61:593, 1983.

124. Juneja HS, Rajaraman S, Alperin JB, Bainton DF: Auer rod-like inclusions in prolymphocytic leukemia. *Acta Haematol* 77:115, 1987.

125. Davis WC, Douglas SD: Defective granule formation and function in the Chediak-Higashi syndrome in man and animals. *Semin Hematol* 9:431, 1972.

126. Oliver C, Essner E: Formation of anomalous lysosomes in monocytes, neutrophils, and eosinophils from bone marrow of mice with Chediak-Higashi syndrome. *J Lab Invest* 32:17, 1975.

127. Rausch PG, Pryzwansky KB, Spitznagel JK: Immunocytochemical identification of azurophilic and specific granule markers in the giant granules of Chediak-Higashi neutrophils. *N Engl J Med* 298:694, 1978.

128. Ganz T, Metcalf JA, Gallin JI, Boxer LA, Lehrer RI: Microbicidal/cytotoxic proteins of neutrophils are deficient in two disorders: Chediak-Higashi syndrome and "specific" granule deficiency. *J Clin Invest* 82:552, 1988.

129. Barbosa MD, Nguyen QA, Tchernev VT, et al: Identification of the homologous beige and Chediak-Higashi syndrome genes. *Nature* 382:262, 1996.

130. Gale PF, Parkin JL, Quie PG, Pettit RE, Nelson RP, Brunning RD: Leukocyte granulation abnormality associated with normal neutrophil function and neurologic impairment. *Am J Clin Path* 86:33, 1986.

131. Newburger PE, Robinson JM, Pryzwansky KB, Rosoff PM, Greenberger JS, Tauber AI: Human neutrophil dysfunction with giant granules and defective activation of the respiratory burst. *Blood* 61:1247, 1983.

132. VanSlyck EJ, Rebuck JW: Pseudo-Chediak-Higashi anomaly in acute leukemia: A significant morphologic corollary? *Am J Clin Path* 62:673, 1974.

133. Gorman AM, O'Connell LG: Pseudo-Chediak-Higashi anomaly in acute leukemia. *Am J Clin Path* 65:1030, 1976.

134. Efrati P, Nir E, Kaplan H, Dvilanski A: Pseudo-Chediak-Higashi anomaly in acute myeloid leukaemia: An electron microscopical study. *Acta Haematol* (Basel) 61:264, 1979.

135. Dittman WA, Kramer RJ, Bainton DF: Electron microscopic and peroxidase cytochemical analysis of pink pseudo-Chediak-Higashi granules in acute myelogenous leukemia. *Cancer Res* 40:4473, 1980.

136. McCall CE, Katayama I, Cotran RS, Finland M: Lysosomal ultrastructural changes in human "toxic" neutrophils during bacterial infection. *J Exp Med* 129:267, 1969.

137. McCall CE, Caves J, Cooper R, DeChatelet L: Functional characteristics of human toxic neutrophils. *J Infect Dis* 124:68, 1971.

138. McCall CE, DeChatelet LR, Cooper MR, Shannon C: Human toxic neutrophils. III. Metabolic characteristics. *J Infect Dis* 127:26, 1973.

139. Weller PF, Ackerman SJ, Nicholson-Weller A, Dvorak A: Cytoplasmic lipid bodies of human neutrophilic leukocytes. *Am J Pathol* 135:947, 1989.

140. Peterson LC, Rao KV, Crosson JT, White JG: Fechtner syndrome—a variant of Alport's syndrome with leukocyte inclusions and macrothrombocytopenia. *Blood* 65:397, 1985.

141. Heynen MJ, Blockmans D, Verwilghen RL, Vermylen J: Congenital macrothrombocytopenia, leukocyte inclusions, deafness and proteinuria: Functional and electron microscopic observations on platelets and megakaryocytes. *Br J Haematol* 70:441, 1988.

142. Greinacher A, Mueller-Eckhardt C: Hereditary types of thrombocytopenia with giant platelets and inclusion bodies in the leukocytes. *Blut* 60:54, 1990.

143. Dake MD, Madison JM, Montgomery CK, et al: Electron microscopic demonstration of lysosomal inclusion bodies in lung, liver, lymph nodes, and blood leukocytes of patients with amiodarone pulmonary toxicity. *Am J Med* 78:506, 1985.

144. Burkholder L, Bainton DF: Auto-antigens in Wegener's granulomatosis. *Blood* 75:1588, 1990.

145. Stummann WA, Kjeldsen L, Borregaard N, Ullman S, Jacobsen S, Halberg P: The diversity of perinuclear antineutrophil cytoplasmic antibodies (pANCA) antigens. *Clin Exp Immunol* 101:Suppl 1:15, 1995.

146. Gilligan HM, Bredy B, Brady HR, et al: Antineutrophil cytoplasmic autoantibodies interact with primary granule constituents on the surface of apoptotic neutrophils in the absence of neutrophil priming. *J Exp Med* 184:6:2231, 1996.

147. Strauss RG, Bove KE, Jones JF, Mauer AM, Fulginiti VA: An anomaly of neutrophil morphology with impaired function. *N Engl J Med* 290:478, 1974.

148. Komiyama A, Morosawa H, Nakahata T, Miyagawa Y, Akabane T: Abnormal neutrophil maturation in a neutrophil defect with morphologic abnormality and impaired function. *J Pediatr* 94:19, 1979.

149. Breton-Gorius J, Mason DY, Buriot D, Vilde JL, Griscelli C: Lactoferrin deficiency as a consequence of a lack of specific granules in neutrophils from a patient with recurrent infections: Detection by immunoperoxidase staining for lactoferrin and cytochemical electron microscopy. *Am J Pathol* 99:413, 1980.

150. Rosenberg HF, Gallin JI: Neutrophil-specific granule deficiency includes eosinophils. *Blood* 82:268, 1993.

151. Malech HL, Gallin JI: Current concepts: Immunology. Neutrophils in human diseases. *N Engl J Med* 317:687, 1987.

152. Parmley RT, Gilbert CS, Boxer LA: Abnormal peroxidase-positive granules in "specific granule" deficiency. *Blood* 73:838, 1989.

153. Lomax KJ, Gallin JI, Rotrosen D, et al: Selective defect in myeloid cell lactoferrin gene expression in neutrophil specific granule deficiency. *J Clin Invest* 83:514, 1989.

154. Johnson JJ, Boxer LA, Berliner N: Correlation of messenger RNA levels with protein defects in specific granule deficiency. *Blood* 80:2088, 1992.

155. Holland SM, Gallin JI: Evaluation of the patient with recurrent bacterial infections. *Ann Rev Med* 49:185, 1998.

156. Miyauchi J, Ohyashiki K, Inatomi Y, Toyama K: Neutrophil secondary-granule deficiency as a hallmark of all-trans retinoic acid-induced differentiation of acute promyelocytic leukemia cells. *Blood* 90:2:803, 1997.

157. Repine JE, Clawson CC, Brunning RD: Abnormal pattern of bactericidal activity of neutrophils deficient in granules, myeloperoxidase, and alkaline phosphatase. *J Lab Clin Med* 88:788, 1976.

158. Thiele J, Timmer J, Jansen B, Zankovich R, Fischer R: Ultrastructure of neutrophilic granulopoiesis in the bone marrow of patients with chronic myeloid leukemia (CML). A morphometric study with special emphasis on azurophil (primary) and specific (secondary) granules. *Virchows Archiv B, Cell Pathol* 59:125, 1990.

159. Rambaldi A, Terao M, Bettoni S: Differences in the expression of alkaline phosphatase mRNA in chronic myelogenous leukemia and paroxysmal nocturnal hemoglobinuria polymorphonuclear leukocytes. *Blood* 73:1113, 1989.

160. Li YM, Tan AX, Vlassara H: Antibacterial activity of lysozyme and lactoferrin is inhibited by binding of advanced glycation-modified proteins to a conserved motif. *Nature Med* 1:10:1057, 1995.

161. Brunning RD: Morphologic alternations in nucleated blood and marrow cells in genetic disorders. *Hum Pathol* 1:99, 1970.

162. Cawley JJ, Hayhoe FGJ: The inclusions of the May-Hegglin anomaly and Döhle bodies of infection: An ultrastructural comparison. *Br J Haematol* 22:491, 1972.

163. Eichacker P, Lawrence C: Steroid-induced hypersegmentation in neutrophils. *Am J Hematol* 18:41, 1985.

164. Knecht H, Eichhorn P, Streuli RA: Granulocytes with ring-shaped nuclei in severe alcoholism. *Acta Haematol* 73:184, 1985.

165. Valenzuela R, McMahon JT, Deodhar SD, Braun WE: Ultrastructural study of tissue and peripheral blood neutrophils in human renal allograft recipients. A clinicopathological description of an unusual abnormality discovered in three cases. *Hum Pathol* 12:355, 1981.

166. Malcolm ID, Flegel KM, Katz M: Vacuolization of the neutrophil in bacteremia. *Arch Intern Med* 139:675, 1979.

167. Abernathy MR: Döhle bodies associated with uncomplicated pregnancy. *Blood* 27:380, 1966.

168. Ulukutlu L, Koc ON, Tasyurekli M, et al: Persistent vacuoles in leukocytes: Familial Jordans anomaly. *Acta Paediatrica Japonica* 37(2): 177, 1995.

169. Fedorko M: Effect of chloroquine on morphology of cytoplasmic granules in maturing human leukocytes: An ultrastructural study. *J Clin Invest* 46:1932, 1967.

170. Archer RK: *The Eosinophil Leucocytes.* Blackwell Scientific Publications, Oxford, 1963.

171. Butterfield JH, Ackerman SJ, Scott RE, Pierre RV, Gleich GJ: Evidence for secretion of human eosinophil granule major basic protein and Charcot-Leyden crystal protein during eosinophil maturation. *Exp Hematol* 12:163, 1984.

172. Weller PF, Monahan-Earley RA, Dvorak HF, Dvorak AM: Cytoplasmic lipid bodies of human eosinophils. *Am J Pathol* 138:141, 1991.

173. Bainton DF: Developmental biology of neutrophils and eosinophils, in *Inflammation: Basic Principles and Clinical Correlates,* edited by JI Gallin and R Snyderman, Chapter 65, Raven Press, Ltd., New York, in press, 1999.

174. Bujak JS, Root RK: The role of peroxidase in the bactericidal activity of human blood eosinophils. *Blood* 43:727, 1974.

175. Yazdanbakhsh M, Eckmann CM, Bot AA, Roos D: Bactericidal action of eosinophils from normal human blood. *Infect Immun* 53:192, 1986.

176. Iozzo RV, MacDonald GH, Wight TN: Immunoelectron microscopic localization of catalase in human eosinophilic leukocytes. *J Histochem Cytochem* 30:697, 1982.

177. Yokota S, Deimann W, Hashimoto T, Fahimi HD: Immunocytochemical localization of two peroxisomal enzyme of lipid beta-oxidation in specific granules of rat eosinophils. *Histochem* 78:425, 1983.

178. Yokota S, Deimann W, Hashimoto T, Fahimi HD: Specific granules of rat eosinophils contain peroxisomal acyl-CoA oxidase: Possible involvement in production of H_2O_2. *Histochem J* 16:573, 1984.

179. Eguchi M, Ozawa T, Suda J, Sugita K, Furukawa T: Lectins for electron microscopic distinction of eosinophils from other blood cells. *J Histochem Cytochem* 37:743, 1989.

180. Peters MS, Rodriguez M, Gleich GJ: Localization of human eosinophil granule major basic protein, eosinophil cationic protein, and eosinophil-derived neurotoxin by immunoelectron microscopy. *Lab Invest* 54:656, 1986.

181. Popken-Harris P, Checkel J, Loegering D, et al: Regulation and processing of a precursor form of eosinophil granule major basic protein (ProMBP) in differentiating eosinophils. *Blood* 92 (2):623, 1998.

182. Adolphson CR, Gleich GJ: Eosinophils, in *Allergy,* edited by ST Holgate, MK Church, p 6.1-6.12. Gower Medical Publishing, London, 1993.

183. McGrogan M, Simonsen C, Scott R, et al: Isolation of a complementary DNA clone encoding a precursor to human eosinophil major basic protein. *J Exp Med* 168:2295, 1988.

184. Young JD-E, Peterson CGB, Venge P, Cohn ZA: Mechanism of membrane damage mediated by human eosinophil cationic protein. *Nature* 321:613, 1986.

185. Gleich GJ, Loegering DA, Bell MP, Checkel JL, Ackerman SJ, McKean DJ: Biochemical and functional similarities between human eosinophil-derived neurotoxin and eosinophil cationic protein: Homology with ribonuclease. *Proc Natl Acad Sci USA* 83:3146, 1986.

186. Rosenberg HF, Ackerman SJ, Tenen DG: Human eosinophilationic protein: Molecular cloning of a cytotoxin and helminthotoxin with ribonuclease activity. *J Exp Med* 170:163, 1989.

187. Rothenberg ME, Pomerantz JL, Owen WF, Jr, et al: Characterization of a human eosinophil proteoglycan and augmentation of its biosynthesis and size by interleuken 3, interleukin 5, and granulocyte/macrophage colony stimulating factor. *J Biol Chem* 263:13901, 1988.

188. Hamid Q, Barkans J, Meng Q, et al: Human eosinophils synthesize and secrete interleukin-6, in vitro. *Blood* 80:1496, 1992.

189. Waltraud JB, Weller PF, Tzizik DM, Galli SJ, Dvorak AM: Ultrastructural immunogold localization of tumor necrosis factor-α to the matrix compartment of eosinophil secondary granules in patients with idiopathic hypereosinophilic syndrome. *J Histochem Cytochem* 41:1611, 1993.

190. Egesten A, Calafat J, Knol EF, Janssen H, Walz TM: Subcellular local-ization of transforming growth factor-α in human eosinophil granulocytes. *Blood* 87:3910, 1996.

191. Levi-Schaffer F, Lacy P, Severs NJ, et al: Association of granulocyte-macrophage colony-stimulating factor with the crystalloid granules of human eosinophils. *Blood* 85:2579, 1995.

192. Weller PF, Bach DS, Austen KF: Biochemical characterization of human eosinophil Charcot-Leyden crystal protein (lysophospholipase). *J Biol Chem* 259:15100, 1984.

193. Zhou Z, Tenen DG, Dvorak AM, Ackerman SJ: The gene for human eosinophil Charcot-Leyden crystal protein directs expression of lysophospholipase activity and spontaneous crystallization in transiently transfected COS cells. *J Leukoc Biol* 52:587, 1992.

194. Dvorak AM, Letourneau L, Login GR, Weller PF, Ackerman SJ: Ultrastructural localization of the Charcot-Leyden crystal protein (lysophospholipase) to a distinct crystalloid-free granule population in mature human eosinophils. *Blood* 72:150, 1988.

195. Dvorak AM, Ackerman SJ, Weller PF: Subcellular morphological and biochemistry of eosinophils, in *Blood Cell Biochemistry, Megakaryocytes, Platelets, Macrophages, and Eosinophils,* edited by JR Harris, Vol 2. Plenum Press, New York and London, 1990.

196. Presentey B: Ultrastructure of human eosinophils genetically lacking peroxidase. *Acta Haematol* 71:334, 1984.

197. Zabucchi G, Soranzo MR, Menegazzi R, et al: Eosinophil peroxidase deficiency: Morphological and immunocytochemical studies of the eosinophil-specific granules. *Blood* 80:2903, 1992.

198. Tracey R, Smith H: An inherited anomaly of human eosinophils and basophils. *Blood Cells* 4:291, 1978.

199. Liso V, Troccoli G, Specchia G, Magno M: Cytochemical "normal" and "abnormal" eosinophils in acute leukemias. *Am J Hematol* 2:123, 1977.

200. LeBeau MM, Larson RA, Bitter MA, Vardiman JW, Golomb HM, Rowley JD: Association of an inversion of chromosome 16 with abnormal marrow eosinophilis in acute myelomonocytic leukemia. A unique cytogenetic-clinicopathology association. *N Engl J Med* 309:630, 1983.

201. Mlynek M-L, Leder L-D: Lineage infidelity in chronic myeloid leukemia: Demonstration and significance of hybridoid leukocytes. *Virchows Archiv Cell Pathol,* 51:107, 1986.

202. Fauci AS: In the idiopathic hypereosinophilic syndrome: Clinical pathophysiologic, and therapeutic considerations. *Ann Intern Med* 97:78–92, 1982.

203. Caulfield JP, Hein A, Rothenberg ME, et al: A morphometric study of nomodense and hypodense human eosinophils that are derived in vivo and in vitro. *Am J Pathol* 137:27, 1990.

204. Kaufman LD, Gleich GJ: The expanding clinical spectrum of multisystem disease associated with eosinophilia (editorial comment). *Arch Dermatol* 133:2:225, 1997.

205. Parmley RT, Crist WM, Roper M, Takagi M, Austin RL: Intranuclear crystalloids associated with abnormal granules in eosinophilic leukocytes. *Blood* 58:1134, 1981.

206. Chilosi M, Fossaluzza V, Tosato F: Eosinophilic acquired Pelger-Huét anomaly in acute myeloblastic leukemia. *Acta Haematol (Basel)* 61:198, 1979.

207. Fossaluzza V, Tosato F: Acquired Pelger-Huét anomaly limited to eosinophils. *Acta Haematol (Basel)* 63:295, 1980.

208. Walsh GM: Mechanisms of human eosinophil survival and apoptosis. *Clin Exp Allergy,* 27:5:482, 1997.

209. Walsh GM: Human eosinophils: Their accumulation, activation and fate. *Br J Haematol* 97:701, 1997.

210. Rollins BJ: Chemokines. *Blood* 90:909, 1997

211. Galli SJ: New concepts about the mast cell. *N Engl J Med* 328:257, 1993.

212. Valent P: Mast cell differentiation antigens: Expression in normal and malignant cells and use for diagnostic purposes. *Eur J Clin Invest* 25:715, 1995.

213. Costa JJ, Weller PF, Galli SJ: The cells of the allergic response: Mast cells, basophils, and eosinophils. *JAMA* 278:1815, 1997.

214. Marone G, Casolaro V, Patella V, Florio G, Triggiani M: Molecular and cellular biology of mast cells and basophils. *Int Arch Allergy Immunol* 114:207, 1997.

215. Dvorak AM: New aspects of mast cell biology. *Int Arch Allergy and Immunol* 114:1, 1997.

216. Hogan AD, Schwartz LB: Markers of mast cell degranulation. *Methods* 13:43, 1997.

217. Metcalfe DD, Baram D, Mekori YA: Mast cells. *Physiol Rev* 77:1033, 1997.

218. Calafat J, Janssen H, Knol EF, Weller PF, Egesten A: Ultrastructural localization of Charcot-Leyden crystal protein in human eosinophils and basophils. *Eur J Haematol* 58:56, 1997.

219. Dvorak AM, MacGlashan DW, Warner JA, et al: Localization of Charcot-Leyden crystal protein in individual morphological phenotypes of human basophils stimulated by f-met peptide. *Clin Exp Allergy* 27:452, 1997.

220. Denburg JA: Basophil and mast cell lineages in vitro and in vivo. *Blood* 79:846, 1992.

221. Grützkau A, Krüger-Krasagakes S, Baumeister H, et al: Synthesis, storage, and release of vascular endothelial growth factor/vascular permeability factor (VEGF/VPF) by human mast cells: Implications for the biological significance of VEGF$_{206}$. *Mol Biol Cell* 9:875, 1998.

COMPOSITION AND METABOLISM
OF NEUTROPHILS

ERNEST BEUTLER

Neutrophils are highly specialized differentiated cells, and details of their specialized metabolic pathways are given in Chaps. 67 and 72. This chapter deals with the composition of granulocytes, their content of water, electrolytes, carbohydrates, amino acids, peptides, proteins, lipids, nucleic acids, vitamins, and cofactors. The housekeeping metabolic pathways of neutrophils for aerobic and anaerobic energy metabolism, and DNA, nucleotide, and lipid metabolism are also reviewed.

COMPOSITION OF NEUTROPHILS

Many of the measurements of the composition of leukocytes were performed at a time when those carrying out the analyses did not appreciate that the white cells of the blood were heterogeneous in origin and function. Thus, many of the data pertain to leukocytes as a whole, not to isolated neutrophils. Often, granulocytes were studied rather than neutrophils. In many cases, however, the content of analytes is similar in neutrophils and other white blood cells, and the best data available are presented here and expressed as values in neutrophils, recognizing that in some cases the values may be distorted by the presence of other leukocytes in the mixtures analyzed.

WATER AND ELECTROLYTES

Approximately 82 percent of the leukocyte weight is water.[1] There is a remarkable paucity of data regarding the electrolyte content of neutrophils. The often quoted 1929 study of Endres and Herget[1] was carried out on mixed leukocytes from the blood of horses obtained at a slaughterhouse. They found an average of 2610 mg (113 mmol) sodium, 889 mg (22.7 mmol) potassium, 72 mg (1.8 mmol) calcium, 10.3 mg (0.18 mmol) iron, 2487 mg (70.2 mmol) chloride, and 299 mg (9.65 mmol) inorganic phosphate per liter of leukocytes. The copper content of neutrophils has been reported to average 4.69 nmol/10^9 cells,[2] zinc 109.2 nmol/10^9 cells[2] and 50.16 nmol/10^9 cells,[3] and magnesium 3.11 fmol/cell.[4] There is little selenium in neutrophils, the median concentration having been reported as less than 0.0075 μmol/10^9 cells.[5] Otherwise, electrolyte determinations on

Acronyms and abbreviations that appear in this chapter include: ATP, adenosine triphosphate; cAMP, cyclic adenosine monophosphate; cGMP, cyclic guanosine monophosphate; GM-CSF, granulocyte-macrophage colony-stimulating factor; 5-HETE, 5-hydroxyeicosatetraenoic acid; 5-HPETE, 5-hydroxyperoxy-6,8,11,14-eicosatetraenoic acid; 15-HPETE, 15-hydroperoxy-5,8,11,13-eicosatetraenoic acid; LAP, leukocyte alkaline phosphatase; LTA4, leukotriene A4; PAF, platelet-activating factor; SE, standard error; SRS, slow-reactivity substance.

human leukocytes appear to have been limited to leukemic cells and to pus.[6]

CARBOHYDRATES

The rate of metabolism of glucose by neutrophils is affected by insulin in diabetics but not in normal subjects.[7,8] The neutrophil is particularly rich in glycogen. The concentration of this complex polysaccharide has been reported to average 7.36 mg/10^9 cells.[9–11]

AMINO ACIDS, PEPTIDES, AND PROTEINS

The concentrations of most amino acids are higher in neutrophils than is the surrounding plasma.[12] The amino acid concentration in neutrophils is summarized in Table 65-1. The reduced glutathione content of neutrophils is 9.8 nmol per 10^7 cells.[13]

The protein content of the neutrophil is 74.2 ± 3.1 (mean ± 1 SE) mg/10^9 cells.[14] These proteins include those of the structural matrix of the neutrophil; proteins required for its locomotion, chemotactic properties, and adhesiveness; and the many granule proteins with bactericidal, hydrolytic, and inflammatory functions. These proteins are described in detail in Chaps. 64, 67, and 72.

LIPIDS

As in other cells, the plasma membrane and the membranes of the intracellular organelles are rich in lipids. Five percent of the wet weight of neutrophils is lipid, which is distributed among various classes, as shown in Table 65-2.[15–19] The rare polyphosphoinositides are of special interest as sources of inositol 1,4,5-trisphosphate (a calcium-releasing mediator) and diacylglycerol (which activates protein kinase C).[20,21] The main glycolipid of neutrophils is lactosylceramide.[22]

NUCLEOTIDES AND NUCLEIC ACIDS

The levels of nucleotides in the neutrophils are summarized in Table 65-3.[23,24]

Neutrophils contain all the forms of RNA needed for protein synthesis: transfer RNA, ribosomal RNA, and messenger RNA.[27,28] The DNA content of neutrophils is identical to that of all other haploid cells, at 0.7 pg DNA phosphorus per cell.[29]

VITAMINS AND COFACTORS

The average folic acid content of packed leukocytes of normal subjects was 0.1 μg/ml of packed leukocytes, and about 20 percent of this was free and the remainder conjugated.[30] The cocarboxylate content is 340 μg/10^{11} cells,[31] pyridoxal phosphate 0.24–0.38 ng/10^6 cells,[32] thiamine 67.5 ± 4.1 μg/100 ml,[33] ascorbic acid 16.5 ± 5.1 mg/100 ml,[34] and folate 92 ng/ml.[35]

METABOLISM OF NEUTROPHILS

CARBOHYDRATE METABOLISM

GLYCOLYSIS

The Main Glycolytic (Embden-Meyerhoff) Pathway The main energy-producing pathway in the neutrophil is glycolysis, resulting in the conversion of glucose to lactate.[36–38] When intact or homogenized leukocytes are incubated with glucose uniformly labeled with ^{14}C, about 80 percent of the radioactivity is recovered in lactic acid. Glycolysis is inhibited by cortisol.[7] The activities of the glycolytic enzymes of neutrophils are summarized in Table 65-4[39–41]; in some cases the conditions under which the neutrophils are disrupted have a significant

TABLE 65-1　UNBOUND AMINO ACID CONCENTRATIONS IN LEUKOCYTES (LYMPHOCYTES INCLUDED)

Amino Acid	μMol/kg Water*
Alanine	2881 ± 256
Arginine	<290
Ergothioneine	<300
Ethanolamine	<250
Glutamic acid	2745 ± 251
Glutamine	2650 ± 251
Histidine	762 ± 70
Leucine plus isoleucine	1999 ± 195
Lysine	2111 ± 216
Methionine	391 ± 54
O-phosphoethanolamine	2651 ± 389
Ornithine	1767 ± 113
Phenylalanine	647 ± 105
Proline	862 ± 79
Serine plus glycine	13,021 ± 1480
Taurine	28,683 ± 2726
Threonine	2345 ± 174
Tryptophan	222 ± 31
Tyrosine	480 ± 97
Valine	1335 ± 132

*Mean ± 1 standard deviation.
SOURCE: From RH McMenamy et al.[12]

effect on the activities measured.[40] Hexokinase is the rate-limiting enzyme of glycolysis in normal neutrophils.[37] The rate of glycolysis is not altered during phagocytosis,[38] but ATP levels, normally 1.9 nmol/10[6] cells, fall to 0.8 nmol/10[6] cells. Both the glycogen stores of neutrophils and the glucose of the plasma can serve as the source of glucose. Galactose, mannose, and fructose can also be metabolized by leukocytes.[43]

The Hexose Monophosphate Shunt Pathway　Neutrophils also metabolize glucose by way of the hexose monophosphate shunt,[44–46] and this accounts for some of the oxygen consumption of the cells. In resting cells, the amount of glucose metabolized via this route amounts to only 2 to 3 percent of the total glucose consumed by the cell.[45–47] The operation of the hexose monophosphate shunt, however, is of special importance to the neutrophil, because it is this pathway that provides the NADPH needed for the generation of microbicidal oxidants (see Chap. 67).

Glycogen Metabolism　Neutrophils contain a large quantity of glycogen (see above), arising mostly from glucose; there is little net synthesis from substrates at the triose phosphate level. Glycogen

TABLE 65-2　LIPID COMPOSITION OF NEUTROPHILS

Lipid	Content, %
Phospholipid	
Phosphatidylcholine	12
Phosphatidylethanolamine	12
Sphingomyelin	6.5
Phosphatidylserine	1.5
Phosphatidylinositol	1.5
Phosphatidic acid	1.5
Total	35
Triglyceride	20
Glycolipid	16
Cholesterol	10

SOURCE: From EL Gottfried.[15]

TABLE 65-3　NUCLEOTIDES IN LEUKOCYTES (LYMPHOCYTES INCLUDED)

Nucleotide	nmol/10[9] Cells (Mean ± SE)
NAD	32 ± 2.0[24]
NADH	25 ± 2.3[24]
NADP	8 ± 1.5[24]
NADPH	24 ± 39[25]
ATP	8800[26]
ADP	1600[26]
AMP	6100[26]

turnover increases when these cells are deprived of glucose, especially if they are engaged in phagocytosis, but resynthesis occurs when adequate glucose is added.[38,48,49] During phagocytosis by glucose-starved cells, glycogen phosphorylase activity rises, but phosphorylase kinase and glycogen synthase levels remain unchanged.[48] Glycogen first appears in myelocytes and increases with cell maturation.[50]

OXIDATIVE METABOLISM

Neutrophils consume 0.15 μmol oxygen per 10[7] cells in the absence of glucose and 0.015 μmol oxygen per 10[7] cells in the presence of glucose.[51] Oxygen consumption by neutrophils is influenced by a wide variety of physiologic and pathologic stimuli.[52] In addition to phagocytosis (see Chap. 67), these include thyroid hormone, CO_2 tension,[53] glucose concentration,[54] serum,[55] pyrogens,[56] complement components, chemotactic peptides, and immune complexes.[57] A number of chemicals depress neutrophil respiration, including saponin, thiouracil, chloramphenicol, cyanide, fluoroacetate, malonate, and p-hydroxymercuribenzoate. Other compounds, such as ascorbic acid and dinitrophenol, increase O_2 consumption.[52]

Few mitochondria are found in mature neutrophils,[58] and mitochondrial respiration accounts for only 5 percent of the glucose consumed by the neutrophil.[59,60] Because of the efficiency of mitochondrial ATP synthesis, however, it furnishes nearly half the ATP generated by the cell. The following Krebs cycle enzymes have been detected in leukocytes: isocitric dehydrogenase, aconitase, fumarase, and malic dehydrogenase.[61,62] In addition, the metabolically related enzymes glutamate-oxaloacetate aminotransferase and glutamate-pyruvate aminotransferase are also found in neutrophils.[63] The four enzymes necessary for gluconeogenesis were not detected in leukocytes.

DNA AND RNA METABOLISM

DNA polymerase is most active in early neutrophil precursors.[64] Activity diminishes with cell maturation and is barely detectable in mature cells. Consistent with this finding, the myelocyte is the most mature neutrophil precursor that can still incorporate thymidine into DNA and undergo mitosis.[65,66] Like other cells, neutrophils synthesize RNA using DNA as a template.[67,68] Earlier studies using the incorporation of [^{14}C]uridine into RNA as a measure of RNA synthesis were difficult to interpret because they were carried out with mixed populations of cells.[67] However, Northern blotting has indicated unequivocally that neutrophils have the capacity to synthesize specific messenger RNA.[69,70]

PROTEIN

Mature neutrophils and neutrophil precursors incorporate labeled amino acids into proteins[68,71–74] and have been shown to synthesize fibronectin.[70] Protein synthesis also seems to play a role in receptor recycling by neutrophils.[75] Once proteins are synthesized, they undergo extensive posttranslational modification and are sorted into the appropriate organelle.[76]

NUCLEOTIDE METABOLISM

BIOSYNTHESIS

Many of the studies on nucleotide biosynthesis have been conducted in mixed cell populations. Conclusions from such studies regarding nucleotide biosynthesis in neutrophils must be regarded as provisional. Leukocytes are capable of de novo biosynthesis of pyrimidines. The enzymes of pyrimidine biosynthesis (aspartate carbamyltransferase, dihydroorotase, dihydroorotic dehydrogenase, and orotidylic decarboxylase) are found in normal leukocytes (predominantly neutrophils).[77] The failure to demonstrate ^{14}C-glycine incorporation into the acid-insoluble nucleotide pool in normal leukocytes suggested that, in contradistinction to their ability to carry on pyrimidine biosynthesis de novo, these cells are incapable of the earlier steps of purine synthesis.[78] In addition to de novo pyrimidine synthesis, ribo- and deoxyribonucleotides can also be formed via the "salvage" pathway through the kinase-catalyzed interaction of ATP with nucleosides and deoxynucleosides (cytidine, uridine, deoxycytidine, deoxyuridine, and thymidine).[79–84] The enzyme that catalyzes the conversion of ribonucleotides to deoxyribonucleotides, however, has not been detected in normal neutrophils.

CATABOLISM

The presence of ribonuclease and deoxyribonuclease in lysosomal granules of leukocytes[85,86] suggests that these organelles are involved in the breakdown of exogenous and/or endogenous nucleic acids. Ribonuclease activity is 10 times higher in mature neutrophils than in blast forms.[87] In addition, nucleotidases,[88] several isoenzymes of acid phosphatase,[89] and a nucleoside deaminase have been described.[83] Mature neutrophils, however, contain only very low levels of 5'-nucleotidase and adenosine deaminase.

One of the most extensively investigated neutrophil enzymes is LAP. Leukocyte alkaline phosphatase is a zinc-containing phosphomonoesterase with a pH optimum near 10 that catalyzes the hydrolysis of a wide variety of phosphoester substrates.[90,91] The activity of LAP, which is limited to the neutrophilic series, first appears in myelocytes and rapidly increases with maturation of the cell to the segmented polymorphonuclear neutrophil.[92] Glucocorticoids markedly increase the activity in normal leukocytes, probably by induction of the enzyme, which may explain the high LAP activity observed during infections.[93] Although the in vivo function of LAP remains uncertain, the assay of this activity has found many clinical applications. Marked changes in LAP activity are observed in chronic myelocytic leukemia and other myeloproliferative disorders, as well as in certain other conditions, including idiopathic thrombocytopenic purpura, infectious mononucleosis, aplastic anemia, and sarcoidosis.[94–97]

TABLE 65-4   GLYCOLYTIC AND RELATED ENZYME ACTIVITIES IN NEUTROPHILS

ENZYME	ACTIVITY AT 37°C IN NEUTROPHILS*	ACTIVITY AT 30°C IN NEUTROPHILS†	ACTIVITY AT 25°C IN MIXED LEUKOCYTES‡
Hexokinase	78 ± 14	39.6 ± 27.3	—
Phosphofructokinase	36 ± 2	—	—
Aldolase	76 ± 7	118.7 ± 27.4	123
Glucosephosphate isomerase	4930 ± 716	—	—
Triosephosphate isomerase	7853 ± 323	—	2189
Glyceraldehyde P dehydrogenase	3683 ± 124	—	242
Monophosphoglycerate mutase	508 ± 35	—	—
Phosphoglycerate kinase	3744 ± 197	—	890
Enolase	136 ± 17	—	734
Pyruvate kinase	173 ± 11	4125 ± 549	976
Lactate dehydrogenase	1128 ± 51	2981 ± 893	1165
Glucose-6-phosphate dehydrogenase	517 ± 11	596 ± 116.6	176
6-Phosphogluconate dehydrogenase	287 ± 5	—	—
Glutathione reductase	63 ± 7	—	—
Glutathione peroxidase	17 ± 3	—	—
Glutamic oxaloacetic transaminase	25 ± 2	—	43
Adenylate kinase	32 ± 2	163 ± 9.9	149
α-Glycerophosphate dehydrogenase	—	—	23
Isocitric dehydrogenase	—	—	47
Fructose 1,6-diphosphatase	—	0.76 ± 0.18	—
Isocitrate dehydrogenase	—	44.1 ± 6.4	—
Citrate synthase	—	32.0 ± 5.4	—
Malate dehydrogenase	—	482 ± 62.6	—
Transketolase	—	0.99 ± 0.27	—
Phosphorylase A	—	9.60 ± 2.66	—
Lipoamide dehydrogenase	—	29.7 ± 13.8	—
Ca++ ATPase	—	—	28
Mg++ ATPase	—	—	30

*IU/mg protein.[42]
†IU/liter.[40]
‡IU/mg protein, recalculated from Bücher units/10[11] leukocytes,[26] assuming a protein content of 7.4 mg/10 leukocytes.

CYCLIC NUCLEOTIDES

Cyclic 3',5'-cAMP is present in the human neutrophil.[98] This "second messenger" is involved in the activation of leukocyte glycogen phosphorylase. The synthesis of cAMP is catalyzed by adenyl cyclase and its degradation by cAMP phosphodiesterase, both of which are found in normal neutrophils.[89] The accumulation of cAMP in the leukocyte is stimulated by epinephrine, prostaglandin E, and adenyl cyclase.[99,100] A transient rise in cAMP levels (duration 2–5 min) is also seen after exposure of neutrophils to inflammatory agonists such as formylated oligopeptides or immune complexes, but the cyclic nucleotide appears to have only a minor effect on neutrophil function.[101] The cytosol of neutrophils contains a protein kinase that is stimulated by cAMP.[102] These cells also contain histone phosphatases, which dephosphorylate the product of the protein kinase reaction.[103] A reduced responsiveness of β-receptor function for isoproterenol (Isuprel) in leukocytes of patients suffering from acute bronchial asthma has been reported.[104,105] In asthmatic patients in remission, this response was within normal limits.[106]

There has been little study of cGMP in neutrophils; exposure of neutrophils to inflammatory mediators caused no change in their levels of cGMP.[101]

LIPID METABOLISM

Early studies revealed that lipid biosynthesis, as measured by the incorporation of [14C]acetate, takes place in neutrophils. Two-thirds of the radioactivity was incorporated into neutral lipids and the remainder into phospholipids.[107] Neutrophils also incorporated [2-14C]acetate

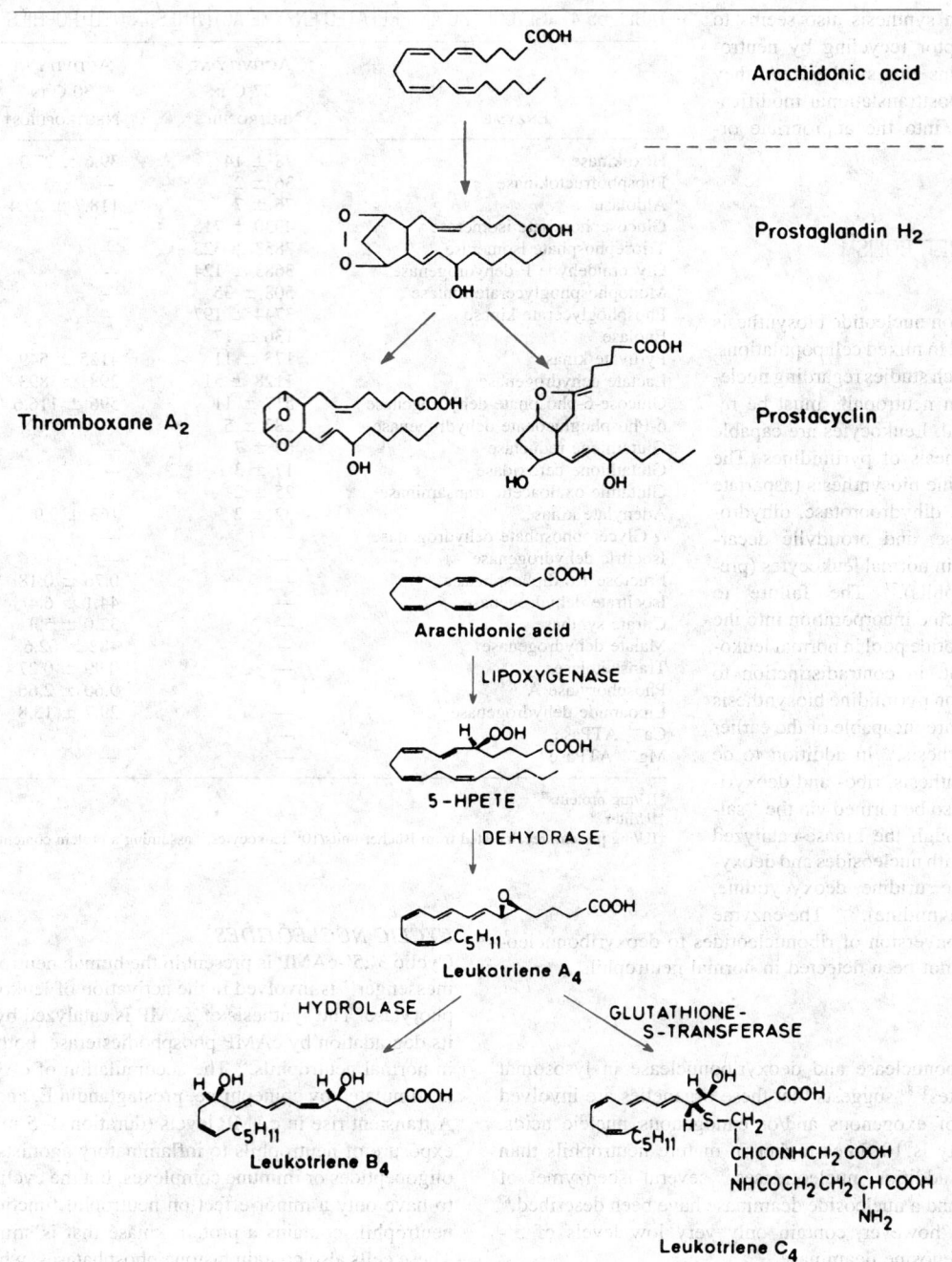

FIGURE 65-1   Production of lipid mediators from arachidonic acid. Above, production of thromboxane A2 and prostacyclin. Below, production of leukotrienes A4, B4, and C4.

and [2-14C]mevalonate into squalene but not into sterols.[108] Younger neutrophils, as found in infection, had lower rates of incorporation of labeled acetate into lipids.[109]

The phosphatidic acid pathway incorporating fatty acids into neutral lipids is operative in these cells.[110] The incorporation of fatty acids into lysophospholipids also occurs in neutrophils, leading to the formation of diacylglyceryl phosphocholine and diacylglyceryl phosphoethanolamine.[111] Phagocytosis is accompanied by a threefold increase in the acylation of exogenous lysolecithin, leading to a net

increase in phospholipid. PAF is synthesized by replacing the 2-acyl group (usually arachidonate) in 1-alkyl-2-acylglycerol phosphocholine with acetate.[112]

Acetyl CoA carboxylase, the first enzyme required for the synthesis of long-chain fatty acids, has been found in myeloblasts but not in mature neutrophils. The latter cells, however, retain the capability of elongating the chains of preformed fatty acids.[113]

A number of lipolytic activities are present in human neutrophils. One of these, a triacylglycerol acylhydrolase acting on lipoprotein and chylomicron substrates, has been purified.[114] A cholesterylesterase activity is also associated with this enzyme. Fatty acid ester hydrolases have been described.[115] Several phospholipases are found in neutrophils.[116,117] Their activation occurs upon stimulation of the neutrophil, leading to the production of signal-transducing chemicals and lipid mediators.

Arachidonic acid is the precursor of a group of lipid mediators that play important roles in the regulation of a wide range of biological responses.[118] It is released from phospholipids by phospholipase A2,[119] activated by the exposure of neutrophils to such stimuli as opsonized zymosan, calcium ionophore, or chemotactic factors.[119-121] Lipid mediators are then produced from the liberated arachidonic acid by either a cyclooxygenase- or a lipoxygenase-catalyzed oxidation (Fig. 65-1). In the neutrophil, oxidation by lipoxygenase exceeds that by cyclooxygenase,[112,119,122,123] and it may be that the arachidonic acid activates the lipoxygenase.[124]

Cyclooxygenase (prostaglandin synthetase) catalyzes the conversion of arachidonic acid into the cyclic endoperoxides PGG2 and PGH2, which in turn are isomerized into the prostaglandins PGE2, PGD2, and PGF2.[118] PGE2 is a major mediator of the inflammatory process, dilating and permeabilizing small blood vessels to give rise to edema and erythema.[104] PGH2 may also be converted to the unstable vasoconstrictor thromboxane A2, which rapidly hydrolyzes to thromboxane B2,[125] which is vasoinactive but chemotactic.

The most important lipoxygenase in neutrophils is 5-lipoxygenase.[126,127] This enzyme catalyzes the oxidation of arachidonic acid to 5-HPETE and its subsequent conversion to leukotriene A4 (LTA4), the unstable parent compound of the leukotrienes, a group of lipid mediators with major effects on the inflammatory process (Fig. 65-2). LTA4 may add glutathione to form LTC4,[128] whose peptide bonds may subsequently be successively hydrolyzed to yield LTD4, containing a cysteine-glycine dipeptide, and LTE4, containing cysteine only. Together, leukotrienes C4, D4, and E4 constitute the activity known formerly as the SRS of anaphylaxis.[129-132]

Alternatively, LTA4 may be hydrolyzed to generate LTB4,[133,134] a potent chemotactic factor and neutrophil activator.[135,136] LTB4 production by neutrophils is induced by a number of stimuli[137-140] whose effects on its production are further regulated by the growth factor GM-CSF.[138-141] LTB4 is inactivated by neutrophil P$_{450}$ cytochrome(s), which catalyze successive oxidations at the x omega position to yield 20-OH-LTB4, LTB4-20-carboxaldehyde, and finally LTB4-20-carboxylic acid.[142-144]

The enzymes responsible for leukotriene production can also oxidize C20-D3 (c-linolenic) and C20-D5 fatty acids, leading to the LTA3 and A5 series of leukotrienes. Because they are less potent than the A4 series of leukotrienes, the A3 and A5 leukotrienes can act as anti-inflammatory agents, partially antagonizing the effects of the A4 series.[145,146]

The hydroperoxyl group of 5-HPETE is sometimes reduced to a hydroxyl group before conversion to LTA4 can take place. This reduction yields a major product, 5-HETE,[147] and a minor product, 12-HETE (an isomer of 12,L-hydroxy-5,8,10,14-eicosatetraenoic acid). Both 5- and 12-HETE have chemotactic properties and stimulate the release of lysozyme from neutrophils.[148]

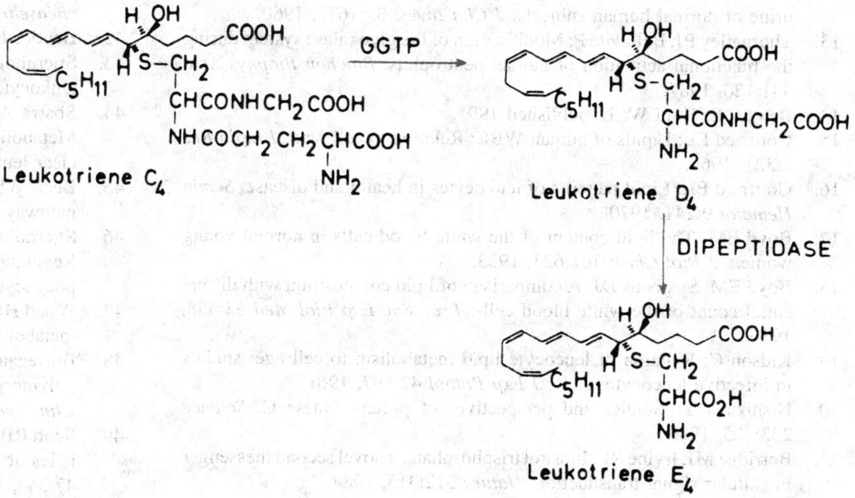

FIGURE 65-2   Structure and formation of the cysteinyl leukotrienes. Leukotriene C4, produced by the reaction of glutathione with leukotriene A4, as shown in Fig. 65-1, is converted to leukotrienes D4 and E4 by the successive removal of the terminal amino acids from the peptide chain. GGTP, γ-glutamyl tripeptidase.

Neutrophils also contain a 15-lipoxygenase that converts arachidonic acid to 15-HPETE.[126] Subsequent oxidation of 15-HPETE by 5-lipoxygenase followed by hydrolysis of the resulting epoxide gives rise to the lipoxins, a family of C-20 fatty acids containing four conjugated double bonds and three hydroxyl groups.[128,148] These, too, are inflammatory mediators, with effects that are similar in general but different in particular from those of the leukotrienes.

REFERENCES

1. Endres G, Herget L: Mineralzusammensetzung der Bluplättchen und weissen Blutkörperchen. Z Biol 88:451, 1929.
2. Williams NR, Rajput-Williams J, West JA, Nigdikar SV, Foote JW, Howard AN: Plasma, granulocyte and mononuclear cell copper and zinc in patients with diabetes mellitus. Analyst 120:887, 1995.
3. Prasad AS, Mantzoros CS, Beck FW, Hess JW, Brewer GJ: Zinc status and serum testosterone levels of healthy adults. Nutrition 12:344, 1996.
4. Loun B, Astles R, Copeland KR, Sedor FA: Intracellular magnesium content of mononuclear blood cells and granulocytes isolated from leukemic, infected, and granulocyte colony-stimulating factor-treated patients. Clin Chem 41:1768, 1995.
5. Rukgauer M, Zeyfang A, Uhland K, Kruse-Jarres JD: Isolation of corpuscular components of whole blood for the determination of selenium in blood cells. J Trace Elem Med Biol 9:130, 1995.
6. Rigas DA: Electrolyte nitrogen and water content of human leukemic leukocytes: Relation to cell maturity. J Lab Clin Med 58:234, 1961.
7. Rauch HC, Loomis ME, Johnson ME, Favour CB: In vitro suppression of polymorphonuclear leukocyte and lymphocyte glycolysis by cortisol. Endocrinology 68:375, 1961.
8. Martin SP, McKinney GR, Green R, Becker C: The influence of glucose, fructose, and insulin on the metabolism of leukocytes of healthy and diabetic subjects. J Clin Invest 32:1171, 1953.
9. Scott RB, Cooper LW: Glycogen in human peripheral blood leukocytes: I. Characteristics of the synthesis and turnover of glycogen in vitro. J Clin Invest 47:344, 1968.
10. Scott RB, Still WJS, Cooper LW: Glycogen in human peripheral blood leukocytes: II. The macromolecular state of leukocyte glycogen. J Clin Invest 47:353, 1968.
11. Esman V: The glycogen content of WBC from diabetic and nondiabetic subjects. Scand J Lab Invest 13:134, 1961.
12. McMenamy RH, Lund CC, Neville GJ, Wallach DFH: Studies of un-

bound amino acid distributions in plasma, erythrocytes, leukocytes and urine of normal human subjects. *J Clin Invest* 39:1675, 1960.

13. Thornalley PJ, Bellavite P: Modification of the glyoxalase system during the functional activation of human neutrophils. *Biochim Biophys Acta* 931:120, 1987.

14. Beutler E, Kuhl W: Unpublished 1991.

15. Gottfried EL: Lipids of human WBC: Relation to cell type. *J Lipid Res* 8:321, 1967.

16. Gottfried EL: Lipid patterns of leukocytes in health and disease. *Semin Hematol* 9:241, 1970.

17. Boyd EM: The lipid content of the white blood cells in normal young women. *J Biol Chem* 101:623, 1933.

18. Boyd EM, Stephens DJ: A comparison of lipid composition with differential count of the white blood cells. *Proc Soc Exp Biol Med* 33:558, 1936.

19. Kidson C: Relation of leucocyte lipid metabolism to cell age: studies in infective leucocytosis. *Br J Exp Pathol* 42:597, 1961.

20. Nishizuka Y: Studies and perspectives of protein kinase C. *Science* 233:305, 1986.

21. Berridge MJ, Irvine RF: Inositol trisphosphate, a novel second messenger in cellular signal transduction. *Nature* 312:315, 1984.

22. Symington FW, Murray WA, Bearman SI, Hakomori S-I: Intracellular localization of lactosylceramide, the major human neutrophil glycophingolipid. *J Biol Chem* 262:11356, 1987.

23. Willoughby HW, Waisman HA: Nucleic acid precursors and nucleotides in normal and leukemic blood: I. Comparison of formic acid chromatograms. *Cancer Res* 17:942, 1957.

24. Silber R, Gabrio BW, Huennekens FM, Albrecht M: Studies on normal and leukemic leukocytes: III. Pyridine nucleotides. *J Clin Invest* 41:230, 1962.

25. Noyes BE, Mevarech M, Stein R, Agarwal KL: Detection and partial sequence analysis of gastrin mRNA by using an oligodeoxynucleotide probe. *Proc Natl Acad Sci USA* 76:1770, 1979.

26. Löhr GW, Waller HD: Zellstoffwechsel und Zellalterung. *Klin Wochenschr* 37:833, 1959.

27. Silber R, Unger KW, Ellman L: RNA metabolism in normal and leukaemic WBC: Further studies on RNA synthesis. *Br J Haematol* 14:261, 1968.

28. Tryfiates GP, Laszlo J: Human leukemic polyribosomes. *Proc Soc Exp Biol Med* 124:1125, 1967.

29. Garcia AM, Iorio R: Studies on DNA in WBC and related cells of mammals: V. The fast green histone and the fuelgen-DNA content of rat WBC. *Acta Cytol* 12:46, 1968.

30. Swendseid ME, Bethell FH, Bird OD: The concentration of folic acid in leukocytes. Observations on normal subjects and persons with leukemia. *Cancer Res* 11:864, 1951.

31. Smits G, Florijn E: The aneurinpyrophosphate content of red and white blood corpuscles in the rat and in man, in various states of aneurin provision and in disease. *Biochim Biophys Acta* 3:44, 1949.

32. Boxer GE, Pruss MP, Goodhart RS: Pyridoxal-5-phosphoric acid in whole blood and isolated leukocytes of man and animals. *J Nutr* 63:623, 1957.

33. Burch HB, Bessey OA, Love RH, Lowry OH: The determination of thiamine and thiamine phosphates in small quantities of blood and blood cells. *J Biol Chem* 198:477, 1952.

34. Barkhan P, Howard AN: Distribution of ascorbic acid in normal and leukaemic human blood. *Biochem J* 70:163, 1958.

35. Hoffbrand AV, Newcombe BFA: Leucocyte folate in vitamin B12 and folate deficiency and in leukaemia. *Br J Haematol* 13:954, 1967.

36. Beck WS, Valentine WN: The aerobic metabolism of leukocytes in health and leukemia: I. Glycolysis and respiration. *Cancer Res* 12:818, 1952.

37. Beck WS: A kinetic analysis of the glycolytic rate and certain glycolytic enzymes in normal and leukemic leukocytes. *J Biol Chem* 216:333, 1955.

38. Borregaard N, Herlin T: Energy metabolism of human neutrophils during phagocytosis. *J Clin Invest* 70:550, 1982.

39. Lane TA, Beutler E, West C, Lamkin GE: Glycolytic metabolism of stored granulocytes. *Transfusion* 21:717, 1981.

40. Fauth U, Schlechtriemen T, Heinrichs W, Puente-Gonzalez I, Halmagyi M: The measurement of enzyme activities in the resting human polymorphonuclear leukocyte—Critical estimate of a method. *Eur J Clin Chem Clin Biochem* 31:5, 1993.

41. Löhr GW, Waller HD: Zellstoffwechsel und Zellalterung. *Klin Wochenschr* 37:833, 1959.

42. Beutler E, West C: Unpublished, 1993.

43. Stjernholm RL, Burns CP, Hohnadel JH: Carbohydrate metabolism by leukocytes. *Enzyme* 13:7, 1972.

44. Sbarra AJ, Karnovsky ML: The biochemical basis of phagocytosis: I. Metabolic changes during the ingestion of particles by polymorphonuclear leukocytes. *J Biol Chem* 234:1355, 1959.

45. Beck WS: Occurrence and control of the phosphogluconate oxidation pathway in normal and leukemic leukocytes. *J Biol Chem* 232:271, 1958.

46. Stjerholm R, Manek RC: Carbohydrate metabolism in leukocytes: XIV. Regulation of pentose cycle activity and glycogen metabolism during phagocytosis. *J Reticuloendothel Soc* 8:550, 1970.

47. Wood HG, Katz J, Landau BR: Estimation of pathways of carbohydrate metabolism. *Biochem J* 338:809, 1963.

48. Borregaard N, Juhl H: Activation of the glycogenolytic cascade in human polymorphonuclear leucocytes by different phagocytic stimuli. *Eur J Clin Invest* 11:257, 1981.

49. Scott RB: Glycogen in human peripheral blood leukocytes: I. Characteristics of the synthesis and turnover of glycogen *in vitro*. *J Clin Invest* 47:344, 1968.

50. Wachstein M: The distribution of histochemically demonstrable glycogen in human blood and bone marrow cells. *Blood* 4:54, 1949.

51. Martin SP, McKinney GR, Green R: The metabolism of human polymorphonuclear leukocytes. *Ann NY Acad Sci* 59:996, 1955.

52. Cline MJ: *The White Cell*, Harvard, Cambridge, 1975.

53. Bicz W: The influence of carbon dioxide tension on the respiration of normal and leukemic leukocytes: I. Influence on endogenous respiration. *Cancer Res* 20:184, 1960.

54. McKinney GR, Martin SP, Rundles RW, Green R: Respiration and glycolytic activities of human leukocytes *in vitro*. *J Appl Physiol* 5:355, 1953.

55. McLeod J, Rhoads C: Metabolism of leukocytes in Ringer-phosphate and in serum. *Proc Soc Exp Biol Med* 41:268, 1939.

56. Cline MJ, Melmon KL, Davis WC, Williams HE: Mechanism of endotoxin interaction with human leukocytes. *Br J Haematol* 15:539, 1968.

57. Strauss BS, Stetson CA Jr: Studies on the effect of certain macromolecular substances on the respiratory activity of the leucocytes of peripheral blood. *J Exp Med* 112:652, 1960.

58. Bessis M: *Cytology of the Blood and Blood-Forming Organs*, Grune & Stratton, New York, 1956.

59. Foster JM, Terry ML: Studies on the energy metabolism of human leukocytes: I. Oxidative phosphorylation by human leukocyte mitochondria. *Blood* 30:168, 1967.

60. Cheson DB, Curnutte JT, Babior BM: The oxidative killing mechanisms of the neutrophil, in *Progress in Clinical Immunology*, vol 3, p 1. Grune & Stratton, New York, 1977.

61. Tanaka KR, Valentine WN: Aconitase activity of human leukocytes. *Acta Haematol* 26:12, 1961.

62. Tanaka KR, Valentine WN: Fumarase activity of human leukocytes and erythrocytes. *Blood* 17:328, 1961.

63. Belfiore F, Borzi V, LoVecchio L, Napoli E, Rabuazzo AM: Enzyme activities of NADPH forming metabolic pathways in normal and leukemic leukocytes. *Clin Chem* 21:880, 1925.

64. Rabinowitz Y: DNA polymerase and carbohydrate metabolizing enzyme content of normal leukemic glass column separated leukocytes. *Blood* 27:470, 1966.

65. Bond VP, Fliedner TM, Cronkite EP, Rubine JR, Brecher G, Schork PK: Proliferative potentials of bone marrow and blood cells studied by *in vitro* uptake of H³-thymidine. *Acta Haematol* 21:1, 1959.

66. Rubine JR, Cronkite EP, Bond VP, Fliedner TM: The metabolism and fate of tritiated thymidine in man. *J Clin Invest* 39:909, 1960.

67. Cline MJ: Isolation and characterization of RNA from human leukocytes. *J Lab Clin Med* 68:33, 1966.

68. Torelli V, Torelli G, Cadossi R: Double stranded ribonucleic acid in human blast cells. *Eur J Cancer* 11:117, 1975.

69. Ezekowitz RAB, Orkin SH, Newburger PE: Recombinant interferon gamma augments phagocyte superoxide production and X-chronic granulomatous disease gene expression in X-linked variant chronic granulomatous disease. *J Clin Invest* 80:1009, 1987.

70. La Fleur M, Beaulieu AD, Kreis C, Poubelle P: Fibronectin gene expres-

sion in polymorphonuclear leukocytes. Accumulation of mRNA in inflammatory cells. *J Biol Chem* 262:2111, 1987.

71. Weisberger AS, Suhrland LS, Griggs RC: Incorporation of radioactive L-cystine and L-methionine by leukemic leukocytes *in vitro. Blood* 9:1095, 1954.

72. Weisberger AS, Levine B: Incorporation of radioactive L-cystine by normal and leukemic leukocytes *in vivo. Blood* 9:1082, 1954.

73. Baker WH, Zamecnik PC, Stephenson ML: *In vitro* incorporation of C^{14}-DL-leucine into normal and leukemic white cells. *Blood* 12:822, 1957.

74. Granelli-Piperno A, Vassalli JD, Reich E: RNA and protein synthesis in human peripheral blood polymorphonuclear leukocytes. *J Exp Med* 149:284, 1979.

75. Woodman RC, Curnutte JT, Babior BM: Evidence that *de novo* protein synthesis participates in a time-dependent augmentation of the chemotactic peptide-induced respiratory burst in neutrophils: Effects of recombinant human colony stimulating factors and dihydrocytochalasin B. *Free Radical Biol Med* 5:355, 1988.

76. Gullberg U, Andersson E, Garwicz D, Lindmark A, Olsson I: Biosynthesis, processing and sorting of neutrophil proteins: insight into neutrophil granule development. *Eur J Haematol* 58:137, 1997.

77. Smith LH Jr, Baker FA: Pyrimidine metabolism in man: I. The biosynthesis of orotic acid. *J Clin Invest* 38:798, 1959.

78. Scott JL: Human leukocyte metabolism *in vitro:* I. Incorporation of adenine-8-C^{14} and formate-C^{14} into the nucleic acids of leukemic leukocytes. *J Clin Invest* 41:67, 1962.

79. Wilmanns W: Thymidine kinase in normal and leukemic myeloid cells [translated]. *Klin Wochenschr* 45:505, 1967.

80. Bianchi PA: Thymidine phosphorylation and deoxyribonucleic acid synthesis in human leukaemia cells. *Biochim Biophys Acta* 55:547, 1962.

81. Marsh JC, Perry S: Thymidine catabolism by normal and leukemic human leukocytes. *J Clin Invest* 43:267, 1964.

82. Silber R, Gabrio BW, Huennekens FM: Studies on normal and leukemic leukocytes: VI. Thymidylate synthetase and deoxycytidylate deaminase. *J Clin Invest* 42:1913, 1963.

83. Silber R: Regulatory mechanism in human leukocyte: I. Feedback control of deoxycytidylate deaminase. *Blood* 29:896, 1967.

84. Coleman CN, Stoller RG, Chabner BA: Properties of cytidine kinase enzyme from human leukemic granulocytes. *Blood* 46:791, 1975.

85. Barnes JM: The enzymes of lymphocytes and polymorphonuclear leucocytes. *Br J Exp Pathol* 21:261, 1940.

86. Cohn ZA, Hirsch JG: The isolation and properties of specific cytoplasmic granules of rabbit polymorphonuclear leukocytes. *J Exp Med* 112:983, 1960.

87. Silber R, Unger KW, Keller J, Bertino JR: RNA metabolism of normal and leukemic leukocytes: II. Ribonuclease. *Blood* 29:57, 1967.

88. Swenseid ME, Wright PD, Bethell FH: Variations in nucleotidase activity of leukocytes in normal and pathologic conditions. *J Lab Clin Med* 40:515, 1952.

89. Li CY, Yam LT, Lam KW: Acid phosphatase isoenzyme in human leukocytes in normal and pathologic conditions. *J Histochem Cytochem* 18:473, 1970.

90. Follette JH, Valentine WN, Hardin EB, Lawrence JS: A comparison of human phosphate activity toward sodium beta-glycerophosphate, adenosine 5′-phosphate, and glucose-1-phosphate. *Blood* 14:415, 1959.

91. Trubowitz S, Feldman D, Morgenstern SW, Hunt VM: The isolation, purification and properties of the alkaline phosphatase of human leukocytes. *Biochem J* 80:369, 1961.

92. Valentine WN, Beck WS: Biochemical studies on leukocytes: I. Phosphatase activity in health, leukocytosis, and myelocytic leukemia. *J Lab Clin Med* 38:39, 1951.

93. Valentine WN, Follette JH, Solomon DH, Reynolds J: The relationship of leukocyte alkaline phosphatase to "stress," to ACTH, and to adrenal 17-OH-corticosteroids. *J Lab Clin Med* 49:723, 1957.

94. Wachstein M: Alkaline phosphatase activity in normal and abnormal human blood and bone marrow. *J Lab Clin Med* 31:1, 1946.

95. Cline MJ: Metabolism of the circulating leukocyte. *Physiol Rev* 45:674, 1965.

96. Hayhoe FGJ, Quaglino D, Doll R: *The Cytology and Cytochemistry of Acute Leukemias.* HM Stationery Office, London, 1964.

97. Garg S, Silber R: Decreased leukocyte alkaline phosphatase in monocytic leukemia. *Am J Clin Pathol* 58:668, 1972.

98. Mittal CK: Measurements of cyclic adenosine monophosphate and cyclic guanosine monophosphate levels in polymorphonuclear leukocytes. *Methods Enzymol* 132:428, 1986.

99. Scott RE: Effects of prostaglandins, epinephrine and NaF on human leukocyte, platelet and liver adenyl cyclase. *Blood* 35:514, 1970.

100. Ishitoya J, Takenawa T: Potentiation of PGE1-induced increase in cyclic AMP by calmodulin-dependent processes. *J Immunol* 138:1201, 1987.

101. Smolen JE, Korchak HM, Weissmann G: Increased levels of cyclic adenosine-3′,5′-monophosphate in human polymorphonuclear leukocytes after surface stimulation. *J Clin Invest* 65:1077, 1980.

102. Huang CK, Mackin WM, Bormann BJ, Becker EL: Cyclic AMP receptor protein and cyclic AMP-dependent protein kinase activity in rabbit peritoneal neutrophils. *J Reticuloendothel Soc* 34:413, 1983.

103. Tsung PK, Sakamoto T, Weissmann G: Protein kinase and phosphatases from human polymorphonuclear leukocytes. *Biochem J* 145:437, 1975.

104. Parker CW, Baumann ML, Huber MG: Alterations in cyclic AMP metabolism in human bronchial asthma: II. Leukocyte and lymphocyte responses to prostaglandins. *J Clin Invest* 52:1336, 1973.

105. Parker CW, Huber MG, Baumann ML: Alterations in cyclic AMP metabolism in human bronchial asthma: III. Leukocyte and lymphocyte responses to steroids. *J Clin Invest* 52:1342, 1973.

106. Alston WC, Patel KR, Kerr JW: Response of leukocyte adenyl cyclase to isoprenaline and effects of alpha blocking drugs in extrinsic bronchial asthma. *Br Med J* 1:90, 1974.

107. Marks PA, Gellhorn A, Kidson C: Lipid synthesis in human leukocytes, platelets, and erythrocytes. *J Biol Chem* 235:2579, 1960.

108. Fogelman AM, Seager J, Edwards PA, Hokom M, Popjak G: Cholesterol biosynthesis in human lymphocytes, monocytes, and granulocytes. *Biochem Biophys Res Commun* 76:167, 1977.

109. Chanock SJ, Faust LR, Barrett D, et al: O$_2^-$ production by B lymphocytes lacking the respiratory burst oxidase subunit of p47-*phox* after transfection with an expression vector containing a p47-*phox* cDNA. *Proc Natl Acad Sci USA* 89:10174, 1992.

110. Elsbach P: Lipid metabolism by phagocytes. *Semin Hematol* 9:227, 1972.

111. Wang P, Waite M, Dechatelet LR: Membrane lipid metabolism of bacillus Calmette-Guérin-induced rabbit alveolar macrophages. *Biochim Biophys Acta* 487:163, 1977.

112. Nieto ML, Velasco S, Sanchez Crespo M: Modulation of acetyl-Coa: 1-alkyl-2-lyso-sn-glycero-3-phosphocholine (lyso-PAF) acetyltransferase in human polymorphonuclears: The role of cyclic AMP-dependent and phospholipid-sensitive, calcium-dependent protein kinases. *J Biol Chem* 263:4607, 1988.

113. Majerus PW, Lastra R: Fatty acid biosynthesis in human leukocytes. *J Clin Invest* 46:1596, 1967.

114. Elsbach P, Kayden HJ: Chylomicron lipid-splitting activity in homogenates of rabbit polymorphonuclear leukocytes. *Am J Physiol* 209:765, 1965.

115. Dienstle F, Sailer S, Sandhager F, Braunsteiner H: Lipid activity in leucocytes and macrophages. *Blood* 24:607, 1964.

116. Elsbach P, Weiss J: *Lipid Metabolism by Phagocytic Cells in the Reticulendothelial System,* edited by AJ Sbarra, RR Strauss. Plenum, New York, 1980, p. 91.

117. Pai J-K, Siegel MI, Egan RW, Billah MM: Phospholipase D catalyzes phospholipid metabolism in chemotactic peptide-stimulated HL-60 granulocytes. *J Biol Chem* 263:12472, 1988.

118. Samuelsson B, Goldyne M, Granstrom E, Hamberg M, Hammarstrom S, Malmsten C: Prostaglandins and thromboxanes. *Annu Rev Biochem* 47:997, 1978.

119. Walsh CE, Waite BM, Thomas MJ, Dechatelet LR: Release and metabolism of arachidonic acid in human neutrophils. *J Biol Chem* 256:7228, 1981.

120. Sellmayer A, Strasser T, Weber PC: Differences in arachidonic acid release, metabolism and leukotriene B$_4$ synthesis in human polymorphonuclear leukocytes activated by different stimuli. *Biochim Biophys Acta* 927:417, 1987.

121. Godfrey RW, Manzi RM, Clark MA, Hoffstein ST: Stimulus-specific induction of phospholipid and arachidonic acid metabolism in human neutrophils. *J Cell Biol* 104:925, 1987.

122. Borgeat P, Samuelsson B: Transformation of arachidonic acid by rabbit polymorphonuclear leukocytes. Formation of a novel dihydroxyeicosatetraenoic acid. *J Biol Chem* 254:2643, 1979.

123. Bokoch GM, Reed PW: Stimulation of arachidonic acid metabolism in

the polymorphonuclear leukocytes by an N-formylated peptide. Comparison with ionophore A23187. *J Biol Chem* 255:10223, 1980.

124. Dusi S, Poli G, Berton G, Catalano P, Fornasa CV, Peserico A: Chronic granulomatous disease in an adult female with granulomatous cheilitis. Evidence for an X-linked pattern of inheritance with extreme lyonization. *Acta Haematol* 84:49, 1990.

125. Moncada S, Ferreira SH, Vane JR: Prostaglandins, aspirin-like drugs and the oedema of inflammation. *Nature* 246:217, 1978.

126. Samuelsson B, Dahlen S-E, Lingren J-A, Rouzer CA, Serhan CN: Leukotrienes and lipoxins: Structures, biosynthesis, and biological effects. *Science* 237:1171, 1987.

127. Rouzer CA, Samuelsson B: On the nature of the 5-lipoxygenase reduction in human leukocytes: Enzyme purification and requirement for multiple stimulatory factors. *Proc Natl Acad Sci USA* 82:6040, 1985.

128. Samuelsson B, Dahlen S-E, Lindgren J-A, Rouzer CA, Serhan CN: Leukotrienes and lipoxins: Structures, biosynthesis and biological effects. *Science* 237:1171, 1987.

129. Orning L, Hammarstrom S, Samuelsson B: Leukotriene D: A slow reacting substance from rat basophilic leukemia cells. *Proc Natl Acad Sci USA* 77:2014, 1980.

130. Bach MK, Brashler JR, Hammarstrom S, Samuelsson B: Identification of leukotriene C-1 as a major component of slow reacting substance from rat mononuclear cells. *J Immunol* 125:115, 1980.

131. Bach MK, Brashler JR, Hammarstrom S, Samuelsson B: Identification of a component of rat mononuclear cell SRS as leukotriene D. *Biochem Biophys Res Commun* 93:1121, 1980.

132. Samuelsson B, Hammarstrom S, Murphy RC, Borgeat P: Leukotrienes and slow-reacting substance of anaphylaxis (SRS-A). *Allergy* 35:375, 1980.

133. Radmark O, Malmsten C, Samuelsson B, Goto G, Marfat A, Corey EJ: Leukotriene A. Isolation from human polymorphonuclear leukocytes. *J Biol Chem* 255:11828, 1980.

134. Evans JF, Dupuis P, Ford-Hutchinson AW: Purification and characterization of leukotriene A4 hydrolase from rat neutrophils. *Biochim Biophys Acta* 840:43, 1985.

135. Ford-Hutchinson AW, Bray MA, Cunningham FM, Davidson EM, Smith MJH: Isomers of leukotriene B4 possess different biological potencies. *Prostaglandins* 21:143, 1981.

136. Goldman DW, Gifford LA, Olson DM, Goetzl EJ: Transduction by leukotriene B4 receptors of increases in cytosolic calcium in human polymorphonuclear leukocytes. *J Immunol* 135:525, 1985.

137. Dahinden CA, Zingg J, Maly FE, de Weck AL: Leukotriene production in human neutrophils primed by recombinant human granulocyte/macrophage colony-stimulating factor and stimulated with the complement component C5A and FMLP as second signals. *J Exp Med* 167:1281, 1988.

138. Fitzharris P, Cromwell O, Moqbel R, et al: Leukotriene B4 generation by human neutrophils following IgG-dependent stimulation. *Immunology* 61:449, 1987.

139. Roubin R, Elsas PP, Fiers W, Dessein AJ: Recombinant human tumour necrosis factor (rTNF)2 enhances leukotriene biosynthesis in neutrophils and eosinophils stimulated with the Ca^{2+} ionophore A23187. *Clin Exp Immunol* 70:484, 1987.

140. Weisbart RH, Kwan L, Golde DW, Gasson JC: Human GM-CSF primes neutrophils for enhanced oxidative metabolism in response to the major physiological chemoattractants. *Blood* 69:18, 1987.

141. Kelleher D, Bloomfield FJ, Lenehan T, Griffin M, Geighery C, McCann SR: Chronic granulomatous disease presenting as an oculomucocutaneous syndrome mimicking Beheçt's syndrome. *Postgrad Med J* 62:489, 1986.

142. Marcus AJ: The eicosanoid in biology and medicine. *J Lipid Res* 25:1511, 1984.

143. Soberman RJ, Harper TW, Murphy RC, Austen KF: Identification and functional characterization of leukotriene B4 20-hydroxylase of human polymorphonuclear leukocytes. *Proc Natl Acad Sci USA* 82:2292, 1985.

144. Sumimoto J, Takeshige K, Minakami S: Characterization of human neutrophil leukotriene B4 omega-hydroxylase as a system involving a unique cytochrome P-450 and NADPH-cytochrome P-450 reductase. *Eur J Biochem* 172:315, 1988.

145. Lee TH, Hoover RL, Williams JD, et al: Effect of dietary enrichment with eicosapentaenoic and docosahexaenoic acids on *in vitro* neutrophil and monocyte leukotriene generation and neutrophil function. *N Engl J Med* 312:1217, 1985.

146. Payan DG, Wong MY, Chernov-Rogan T, et al: Alterations in human leukocyte function induced by ingestion of eicosapentaenoic acid. *J Clin Immunol* 6:402, 1986.

147. Borgeat P, Hamberg M, Samuelsson B: Transformation of arachidonic acid and homo-gamma-linoleic acid by rabbit polymorphonuclear leukocytes: Monohydroxy acids from novel lipoxygenases. *J Biol Chem* 251:7816, 1976.

148. Stenson WF, Parker SW: Monohydroxyeicosatetraenoic acids (HETEs) induce degranulation of human neutrophils. *J Immunol* 124:2100, 1980.

149. Serhan CN, Fiore S, Levy BD: Cell-cell interactions in lipoxin generation and characterization of lipoxin A4 receptors. *Ann N Y Acad Sci* 744:166, 1994.

PRODUCTION, DISTRIBUTION, AND FATE OF NEUTROPHILS

BERNARD M. BABIOR
DAVID W. GOLDE

The neutrophil count in the blood is maintained in a normal steady state by the balance among neutrophilopoiesis in the marrow, the distribution of neutrophils between the marginated pool in the microvasculature and the freely circulating pool in the blood, and the rate of egress from blood to tissues. Marrow production is regulated by three principal glycoprotein hormones, or cytokines: interleukin-3, granulocyte-monocyte, and granulocyte colony-stimulating factors. The latter two cytokines are available as recombinant pharmaceutical products that can be administered therapeutically to ameliorate certain causes of neutropenia. Neutrophil interaction with endothelium is mediated by selectins, polypeptides that contain sugar-binding sites and enter tissues in response to inflammatory mediators by the up-regulation and exposure of integrins on the neutrophil and endothelial cell, which permits firm attachment to endothelium and emigration into tissues through intercellular junctions under the influence of chemoattractant chemicals. Neutrophils migrate from blood to tissues in an age-independent (random) manner, with a half-disappearance time of about 7 h. This process can be accelerated when inflammation is present and highlights the need for a sustained rate of production to maintain a normal blood neutrophil count. The pathogenesis of neutropenia is more complex to analyze kinetically than anemia or thrombocytopenia because at least four compartments are involved: marrow storage pool, circulating pool, marginated pool, and tissue pool. The latter is particularly difficult to assay. Measurements can be further complicated in the nonsteady state, when dramatic increases in turnover rates and distribution among the four principal pools are in disequilibrium, such as during acute inflammatory states.

Neutrophils are produced in the marrow, where they arise from progenitor and precursor cells by a process of cellular proliferation and maturation. They differentiate from the pluripotential stem cell[1,2] through a series of more and more narrowly committed progenitor, or colony-forming units (CFU), including the CFU for granulocytes and monocytes (CFU-GM) and the CFU for granulocytes (CFU-G), which give rise to neutrophils.[3] These early progenitor cells cannot

Acronyms and abbreviations that appear in this chapter include: CFU, colony-forming unit; CFU-GM, colony forming unit–granulocyte-monocyte; CSF, colony-stimulating factor; $DF^{32}P$, diisopropyl fluorophosphate; G-CSF, granulocyte colony stimulating factor; GM-CSF, granulocyte-monocyte colony stimulating factor; [³H]TdR, tirtiated thymidine; ICAM-1, intracellular adhesion molecule-1; IL, interleukin; M_r, relative molecular mass; NTR, neutrophil turnover rate; PECAM-1, platelet–endothelial cell adhesion molecule-1; PMN, polymorphonuclear neutrophil; $T_{1/2}$, half-time; TBNP, total blood neutrophil pool.

be recognized under the microscope but can be identified by marrow culture (see Chap. 14). The earliest microscopically recognizable neutrophil precursor is the myeloblast. From there, the formal sequence of precursor development is myeloblast → promyelocyte → myelocyte → metamyelocyte → band neutrophil → segmented neutrophil (see Chap. 64). The term *granulocyte* is often loosely used to refer to neutrophils but strictly speaking includes eosinophils and basophils as well. Eosinophilic and basophilic granulocytes develop from progenitors in a manner analogous to the neutrophils, although commitment to neutrophilic, eosinophilic, or basophilic development is probably established at an early progenitor stage.

The normal human neutrophil production rate is 0.85 to 1.6 × 10⁹ cells per kilogram per day. The mature neutrophils are stored in the marrow before release into the blood. They leave the circulation randomly, with a half-disappearance time of about 6 h. These cells then enter the tissues and probably function for a day or two before their death or loss into the gastrointestinal tract through mucosal surfaces.

The neutropoietic system has a high production volume, and yet it is finely modulated in the steady state and has a great capacity to increase production in response to inflammatory stimuli. This chapter outlines current concepts of neutrophil production, distribution, and survival. For detailed data and methods, the reader is referred to primary articles and reviews on neutropoiesis and neutrophil kinetics.[4-14]

REGULATION OF NEUTROPHILIC GRANULOPOIESIS

Although the primary cellular manifestation of commitment is the expression of receptors for lineage-specific hematopoietins, the "decision" for a stem cell to self-renew or differentiate may in part be a random or stochastic event.[1,15] On the other hand, stromal elements, collectively referred to as the *hematopoietic microenvironment*, release short-range signals that regulate the process of commitment from multipotential stem cell pools. Although the details of hematopoietic stem cell regulation are poorly understood, much is now known regarding the interaction of hematopoietic hormones with committed granulocyte progenitor cells and their mature progeny.[16-20]

HUMORAL REGULATORS

The humoral regulators involved in granulopoiesis have been defined by in vitro culture systems.[16,17] Originally identified by their ability to stimulate colony formation from marrow progenitor cells, the hemopoietins came to be called *colony-stimulating factors* (CSF). With regard to neutrophil production, at least four human CSF have been defined. GM-CSF is a 22,000-M_r glycoprotein that stimulates the production of neutrophils, monocytes, and eosinophils. G-CSF has an M_r of 20,000 and stimulates only the production of neutrophils. Interleukin-3 (IL-3), or multi-CSF, also has an M_r of 20,000 and acts relatively early in hemopoiesis, affecting multipotential stem cells. Finally, stem cell factor (also known as c-*kit* ligand or steel factor), with an M_r of 28,000, acts in combination with IL-3 or GM-CSF to stimulate the proliferation of the early hematopoietic precursor cells. In addition to their effects on neutrophil precursors, both G-CSF and GM-CSF act directly on the neutrophil to enhance its function. These hemopoietins therefore are important in regulating the production, survival, and functional activity of neutrophils.[17,18,21-23] The mature neutrophil lacks IL-3 receptors and thus is not affected by IL-3. IL-3 receptors are present, however, on mature eosinophils and monocytes. IL-3 is produced by activated T lymphocytes and thus would be expected to have a physiologic role in circumstances of cell-mediated immunity. GM-CSF is also produced by activated lymphocytes, but, like G-CSF, it is also elaborated by mononuclear phagocytes and endothelial and mesenchymal cells when these cell types are stimulated by certain cytokines, including IL-1 and tumor necrosis factor, or bacterial products, such as endotoxin.[24–26] Stem cell factor is secreted by a variety of cells, including marrow stromal cells,[27] and affects the development of several kinds of tissues.[28–30] (see Chaps. 4 and 14).

The activities of exogenously administered biosynthetic (recombinant) human G-CSF and GM-CSF in humans are well documented.[18,31] G-CSF administration rapidly induces neutrophilia, whereas GM-CSF causes an increase in neutrophils, eosinophils, and monocytes. GM-CSF cannot be detected easily in normal plasma, and thus its role as a day-to-day, long-range modulator of neutrophil production is uncertain. Mice in whom the GM-CSF gene is "knocked out" have generally normal hematopoiesis but show macrophage abnormalities, pulmonary alveolar proteinosis, and decreased resistance to microbial challenge.[32–35]

G-CSF, however, appears to be a critical regulator of neutrophilopoiesis, since giving an animal an antibody to G-CSF leads to profound neutropenia.[36] The G-CSF knockout mouse shows severe neutropenia.[37] Also, neutropenia that results from a production disturbance, such as exposure to cytotoxic drugs, is associated with high circulating serum concentrations of G-CSF.[38] As part of an inflammatory response, macrophages and T lymphocytes are activated. They release CSF and also produce cytokines that cause endothelial and mesenchymal cells to release CSF. These CSF stimulate marrow neutrophil production. When the microorganism is contained and eliminated, the stimulus for CSF gene expression is removed and neutrophil production returns to baseline.

Many biologic systems employ negative feedback mechanisms whereby the end product of a process has an inhibitory effect on its further production. Tissue-specific inhibitors are referred to as *chalones*, and a granulocytic chalone elaborated by mature neutrophils has been reported.[39,40] The role of other inhibitors, such as lactoferrin and acidic isoferritins, is uncertain.[41,42]

NEUTROPHIL KINETICS

Methods used to study granulocyte kinetics may be listed under the following categories: (1) neutrophil depletion or destruction to determine the size and rate of mobilization of reserves and the level of compensatory neutropoiesis; (2) the use of radioactive tracers to study neutrophil distribution, production rates, and survival times; (3) mitotic indices of marrow granulocytic cells to assess proliferative activity and cell cycle times; and (4) induced inflammatory lesions to study cell movement into the tissues. Of these categories, the most popular has been the use of radioactive tracers.

Neutrophilopoiesis and neutrophil kinetics are usually analyzed by describing neutrophil movement through a number of interconnected compartments. These compartments may be arranged in three major groups: the marrow, the blood, and the tissue (Fig. 66-1).

THE MARROW

Marrow neutrophils may be divided into the mitotic, or proliferative, compartment and the maturation-storage compartment (see Fig. 66-1). Myeloblasts, promyelocytes, and myelocytes are capable of replication and constitute the mitotic compartment. Earlier progenitor cells are few in number, not morphologically identifiable, and usually neglected in kinetic studies. Metamyelocytes, bands, and mature neutrophils, none of which replicate, constitute the maturation-storage compartment (see Color Plate VII).

The number of cell divisions from the myeloblast to the myelocyte stage in the proliferative compartment has been estimated at between four and five.[43] Data obtained using radioactive diisopropyl fluorophosphate (DF[32]P) suggest that there are three divisions at the

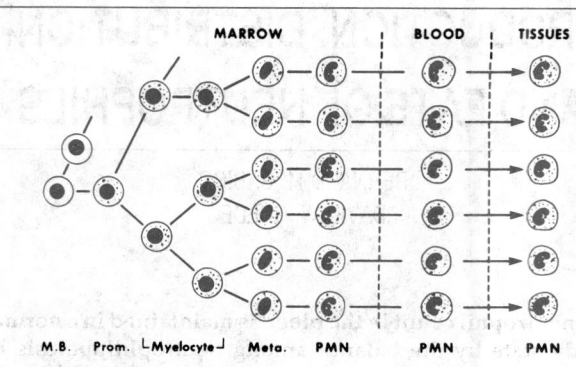

FIGURE 66-1   A scheme of maturation of neutrophil precursor cells. The myeloblast (MB) is the first recognizable precursor of neutrophils. Myeloblasts undergo division and maturation into promyelocytes (Prom) and thereafter into neutrophilic myelocytes (Myelocyte), after which stage mitotic capability is lost. The major compartments of precursor proliferation and distribution are indicated across the top of the figure: marrow, blood, and tissues. The marrow precursor compartment is made up of the proliferating compartment (myeloblasts through myelocytes) and the maturation and storage compartment [metamyelocytes (Meta) to mature polymorphonuclear neutrophils (PMN)]. Under normal conditions, there is no return of cells from the tissue compartment to the blood or marrow.

myelocyte stage, but the number of cell divisions at each step may not be constant. The major increase in neutrophil number probably occurs at the myelocyte level, since the myelocyte pool is at least four times the size of the promyelocyte pool. Because of the difficulties in measuring human intramarrow neutrophil kinetics, a precise model of the dynamics of the mitotic compartment is not available. Estimates of the sizes of the marrow neutrophil compartments and the transit times and cell cycle stages of the cells in the various compartments are given in Table 66-1. Precise studies have measured a postmitotic pool of $(5.59 \pm 0.9) \times 10^9$ cells per kilogram and a mitotic pool (promyelocytes and myelocytes) of $(2.11 \pm 0.36) \times 10^9$ cells per kilogram. These studies have led to a calculated normal marrow neutrophil production of 0.85×10^9 cells per kilogram per day. Radioautographic studies with [³H]thymidine support the concept of an orderly progression from metamyelocytes to mature PMN within the maturation-storage compartment. These studies also suggest a "first in, first out" pattern for cells leaving this compartment and entering the blood. Several labeling techniques indicate that the myelocyte-to-blood transit time is 5 to 7 days.[11,44] Previous studies with DF[32]P gave a range of 8 to 14 days.[8,43] During infections, however, the myelocyte-to-blood transit time may be as short as 48 h.[45]

It is not known with certainty whether the production of neutrophils in the mitotic compartment exactly equals the neutrophil turnover rate. Studies in dogs have suggested that some immature neutrophils die in the marrow ("ineffective neutrophilopoiesis").[46] Ineffective neutrophilopoiesis has not been shown in normal humans, however,[13,47] although ineffective neutrophilopoiesis occurs in some pathologic states. In the preleukemic syndromes[48] there is probably substantial intramedullary cell death, as may occur also in myelofibrosis and perhaps some of the idiopathic neutropenic disorders. At present, however, there is no convenient means to quantitate ineffective neutrophilopoiesis.

On completion of maturation, the neutrophils are stored in the marrow and are referred to as the *mature neutrophil reserve*. This reserve contains many more cells than are normally circulating in the blood. Comparative data on the characteristics of the maturation-storage compartment are given in Table 66-2. Under stress, maturation time may be shortened, divisions may be skipped, and release into the blood may occur prematurely.

THE BLOOD

Neutrophils leave the marrow storage compartment and enter the blood without significant reentry into the marrow. The total blood neutrophil pool consists of all the neutrophils in the vascular spaces. Some of these neutrophils are free in the circulation (the circulating pool), while others roll along the endothelium of small vessels (the marginated pool). Cells in the two pools are freely exchangeable. When neutrophils labeled with DF^{32}P are injected into normal subjects, approximately half can be accounted for in the circulating pool; the remainder enter the marginated pool.[4-6] Neutrophils shift from the marginated to the circulating pool with exercise, epinephrine injection, or stress but eventually leave the blood and enter the tissues. Once they have entered the tissues, they do not normally return to the blood; the flow of cells is unidirectional.

The behavior of neutrophils in the blood appears to be controlled by two classes of membrane-bound adhesion proteins: selectins and integrins. Selectins are polypeptides containing a sugar-binding site, while integrins are heterodimers composed of a large α subunit ($M_r \approx 150,000$) and a smaller β subunit ($M_r \approx 95,000$).[49-51] Two selectins have been found to participate in the interaction between neutrophils and endothelial cells: L-selectin, a protein also found on lymphocytes and monocytes, and E-selectin, also found on endothelial cells. The ligand for L-selectin has not been identified, although heparan sulfates on the luminal surface of endothelial cells are candidates.[52] For E-selectin, ligands include certain sialylated fucosylated glycolipids that are expressed by neutrophils. Through interactions between these selectins and their ligands, circulating neutrophils attach reversibly to the endothelium, where they retain their spherical shape and roll with the flowing blood.[53,54] These endothelium-associated neutrophils exchange freely with circulating neutrophils and probably constitute the marginated pool.

Exposure to inflammatory mediators causes L-selectin to be shed and neutrophil integrins to be activated.[55-57] The principal neutrophil integrins are $\alpha_L\beta_2$ (CD11a/CD18) and $\alpha_M\beta_2$ (CD11b/CD18). These interact with ICAM-1, an integrin counterligand that is displayed on the luminal surfaces of endothelial cells exposed to inflammatory mediators.[58,59] [A third neutrophil integrin, $\alpha_X\beta_2$ (CD11c/CD18), interacts with complement-coated particles but has little to do with the binding of neutrophils to endothelial cells.] As a result of the interaction between the neutrophil integrins and ICAM-1, the neutrophils flatten onto the endothelial surface, to which they are now attached irreversibly.[60] Migration of the neutrophils into the tissues now begins. Neutrophils leave the blood vessels by crawling between the endothelial cells. This process depends on the phosphorylation of an endothelial cell protein called platelet-endothelial cell adhesion molecule (PECAM-1), also known as CD31. PECAM-1 phosphorylation occurs in response to molecules such as endotoxin[61] and platelet-activating factor,[62] which are known to stimulate the egress of neutrophils from the circulation into the tissues.

DF^{32}P-labeled neutrophils disappear from the circulation with a half-time ($T_{1/2}$) of 6.7 h.[6,63,64] These data are supported by the finding that over one-half of Pelger-Huët cells infused into a normal individual disappeared after 6 to 8 h.[65] (Data obtained with ^{51}Cr-labeled neutrophils give substantially longer half-times.[66]) The exponential disap-

pearance of cells from the blood suggests that they leave in a random manner. Thus, neutrophils newly released from the marrow are as likely to leave the blood as are neutrophils that have been circulating for several hours. Certain senescent neutrophils, however, may be eliminated in a nonrandom fashion, perhaps by programmed cell death induced by growth factor deficiency,[67] and are probably disposed of by the macrophage system.[45]

Assuming a random loss of neutrophils from the blood, the neutrophil turnover rate (NTR) can be calculated from the half-time and the total blood neutrophil pool (TBNP): NTR = 0.693 × TBNP/$T_{1/2}$. In the steady state, the neutrophil turnover rate measures the rate of effective neutrophilopoiesis. Definitions and calculations related to blood neutrophil kinetics are given in Table 66-3 and data for normal humans in Table 66-4. The high production rate of neutrophils under normal conditions is remarkable, especially since it may increase severalfold in response to inflammatory stimuli.

Glucocorticoids increase the total blood neutrophil pool by increasing influx from the marrow and decreasing efflux from the circulation. Five hours after a pharmacologic dose of glucocorticoid, the neutrophil count increases by about 4000/μl due to release from the marrow, demargination, and prolongation of the $T_{1/2}$ to approximately 10 h.[68-70] Consistent with the increase in the $T_{1/2}$, prednisone reduces the accumulation of neutrophils at induced sites of skin inflammation.[71] (Dexamethasone has been reported to produce a contrary effect.[72]) With alternate-day, single-dose prednisone, neutrophil counts and kinetics are normal 24 h after administration and during the day off.[71] Endotoxin causes a prompt neutropenia as a result of cell margination and sequestration, followed in 2 to 4 h by a rebound neutrophilia as a result of cell release from the marrow. The size of the neutrophilic response correlates with the functional marrow reserves.[73-76] After administration of epinephrine, a peak leukocytosis occurs in 5 to 10 min and rarely lasts more than 20 min. This reflects a shift of cells from the marginated to the circulating pool.

TABLE 66-1   MARROW NEUTROPHIL KINETICS

	FRACTION IN MITOSIS (MITOTIC INDEX)	FRACTION IN DNA SYNTHESIS (S PHASE)	TRANSIT TIME RANGE, h	TOTAL CELLS × 10^9/kg
Mitotic compartment				
Myeloblast	0.025	0.85	23	0.14
Promyelocyte	0.015	0.65	26–78	0.51
Myelocyte	0.011	0.33	17–126	1.95
Maturation-storage compartment				
Metamyelocyte			8–108	2.7
Band			12–96	3.6
PMN			0–120	2.5

SOURCE: Cronkite and Fliedner[10] and Donohue et al.[12]

TABLE 66-2   COMPARATIVE DATA ON MARROW MATURATION-STORAGE COMPARTMENT

SIZE, CELLS × 10^9/kg	TRANSIT TIME, DAYS	MEASUREMENT TECHNIQUE	REFERENCES
6.5–13	4–8	[^{3}H]thymidine, in vitro DF^{32}P	4
3–23	8–14	In vivo and in vitro DF^{32}P	43
5.6	6.6	^{59}Fe and neutrophil/erythroid ratio	13

TABLE 66-3 DEFINITIONS AND CALCULATIONS RELATING TO BLOOD NEUTROPHIL KINETICS

Circulating neutrophil pool (CNP)	=	blood neutrophil concentration × blood volume
Total blood neutrophil pool (TBNP)	=	all neutrophils in the circulation
Marginal neutrophil pool (MNP)	=	total blood neutrophil pool less circulating pool (MNP = TBNP − CNP)
Blood clearance half-time ($T_{1/2}$)	=	the disappearance time of half the labeled neutrophils from circulation
Neutrophil turnover rate (NTR)	=	$\dfrac{0.693 \times \text{TBNP}}{T_{1/2}}$

THE TISSUES

The migration of neutrophils into areas of inflammation has been widely studied, but little is known of the fate of these cells in normal tissues. Neutrophils normally migrate into the lung, oral cavity, gastrointestinal tract, liver, and spleen.[77] They may be lost from mucosal surfaces or die in the tissues and be degraded by macrophages. The average life span of the mature neutrophil is thought to be very short, although an individual cell may survive for as long as 2 weeks.[78] The neutrophil life span is further shortened if it takes in bacteria or other particles. Chemotactic stimuli, such as C5a and IL-8, draw neutrophils to areas of infection, where they may die in large numbers.

EVALUATION OF ADEQUACY OF NEUTROPHIL PRODUCTION

NEUTROPHIL RESERVES

THE WHITE CELL COUNT AND MARROW CELLULARITY

The white cell and absolute neutrophil counts are the most widely used guides to the status of neutrophil production. They are useful in evaluating the effects of cytotoxic chemotherapy, although they do not provide quantitative information as to the rate of neutrophil production or destruction, the status of marrow reserves, or the presence of abnormalities in cell distribution.

Gauging neutropoiesis by the appearance of marrow films, clot sections, or biopsies also suffers from the limitations of sampling error and relatively poor correlation with kinetics, as measured by other techniques.[64] For example, the morphologic findings in the marrow of a "maturation arrest," with little neutrophil development beyond the promyelocyte or myelocyte stage, does not distinguish between a true defect in cellular maturation and rapid mobilization of cells from the marrow. Similarly, it is often difficult to distinguish by purely morphologic means neutropenic conditions due to ineffective neutropoiesis from those caused by peripheral destruction of neutrophils. However, despite these limitations, when the absolute neutrophil count and marrow cellularity are used together, they provide a useful guide in most clinical settings. If the absolute neutrophil count is less than $1000/\mu l$ (1.0×10^9/liter) and multiple marrow aspirations and/or biopsies are hypocellular, the patient almost invariably has impaired production of neutrophils. Very low neutrophil counts predispose to infections by bacteria and certain fungi (e.g., *Candida* and *Aspergillus*). Such infections become especially troublesome as the neutrophil count falls below $500/\mu l$ (0.5×10^9/liter). Unfortunately, the converse is not true; the finding of a cellular marrow and a neutrophil count above $1000/\mu l$ ($>1.0 \times 10^9$/liter) does not mean that production is normal. Nevertheless, when marrow cellularity and absolute neutrophil count are considered together, they provide the most clinically useful assessment of neutrophil production.

FUNCTIONAL EVALUATION

Several agents that stimulate neutrophil production, including glucocorticoids, endotoxin, and etiocholanolone, have been used in the past to evaluate neutrophil reserves in a clinical setting. These have now been supplanted by recombinant human G-CSF, a remarkably nontoxic cytokine that, when given in therapeutic doses (5 to 8 μg/kg), increases the blood neutrophil count by stimulating neutropoiesis and accelerating neutrophil release from the marrow storage compartment (see also Chap. 15). The increase in neutropoiesis results from a threefold increase in the number of cell divisions in the mitotic compartment, together with a shortening of the maturation time from myelocyte to neutrophil from 4 to 5 days to less than 1 day.[79,80] Thus, as a byproduct of its therapeutic action, the administration of G-CSF directly tests an individual's capacity to produce neutrophils. This effect of G-CSF makes most of the older methods for evaluating neutrophil compartments obsolete.

G-CSF, however, does not test the distribution of neutrophils between the marginated and circulating pools. On the rare occasions when such information is desirable, epinephrine stimulation can be used to assess this distribution. For this purpose, 0.1 mg of epinephrine is infused intravenously over 5 min, and blood for white counts is obtained before and 1, 3, and 5 min after completion of the epinephrine infusion. Normally the neutrophils should increase by approximately 50 percent after epinephrine infusion.[81]

DNA MEASUREMENT: TRITIATED THYMIDINE AND MICROFLUORIMETRY

Tritiated thymidine ([³H]TdR) is selectively incorporated into the DNA of dividing cells and has the advantages of rapid degradation of unincorporated material, low reutilization of label released by cell death, and weak β-particle emission that is ideal for radioautography.[82,83] This DNA marker is used to label S-phase cells (i.e., cells engaged in DNA synthesis) in the mitotic compartment. Labeled cells can be followed as they progress to more mature compartments. For example, this technique showed that myelocytes are the most mature cells of the neutrophil series that are capable of division.

In vivo administration of [³H]TdR to humans is no longer permitted. In vitro studies, however, provide useful information about initial pulse labeling and generation times of neutrophil precursors. Cell proliferation in vitro may not be equivalent to that in the intact subject but may be useful in acute leukemia, where such data may be of therapeutic and prognostic significance.

Microfluorimetry measures the DNA content of individual cells stained with a fluorescent DNA-binding dye. It can provide rapid information on the cell cycle distribution and proliferative status of normal and leukemic cells.[84,85]

TABLE 66-4 DATA FOR HUMAN BLOOD NEUTROPHIL KINETICS

POOL	MEAN POOL SIZE × 10^7 kg	95% LIMITS
TBNP	70	14–160
CNP	31	11–46
MNP	39	0–85

	MEAN VALUE	95% LIMITS
Blood clearance $T_{1/2}$	6.7 h	4–10 h
NTR	163×10^7 kg/day	$50–340 \times 10^7$ kg/day

SOURCE: Athens et al.[4–6]
NOTE: For abbreviations, see Table 66-3.

MITOTIC INDEX

The mitotic index for any morphologically homogeneous cell pool (e.g., the promyelocyte pool) is the ratio of cells in mitosis to total cells in the pool. Used alone, the mitotic index provides little information on cell kinetics; when combined with [^{3}H]TdR-labeling studies, however, it can give valuable information on neutrophil precursor proliferation.[11,44,86] Determining a mitotic index is laborious, and interpretation is somewhat uncertain because of the variability of the mitotic index in humans (7 to 43 per 1000 nucleated marrow cells) and the limitations in defining the morphologic pool.

TRACER TECHNIQUES FOR STUDYING NEUTROPHIL KINETICS IN HUMANS

The kinetics of neutrophil production and use in humans were worked out many years ago using radioactively labeled tracers. Materials formerly used for these in vivo studies included [^{3}H]thymidine, DF^{32}P, and radioactive chromium (^{51}Cr^{3+}). For reasons related to safety and technical difficulties, these tracers have been replaced for in vivo studies by lipophilic complexes of radioactive indium (^{111}In): ^{111}In-oxime and ^{111}In-tropolone.[87] To study neutrophil behavior in vivo using an ^{111}In-labeled tracer, the leukocytes are isolated, incubated with the ^{111}In complex, washed, and reinfused into the subject. Leukocyte life span can be determined by measuring the disappearance of ^{111}In from the blood, while the distribution of the labeled leukocytes can be evaluated by imaging. ^{111}In-labeled leukocytes are sometimes used clinically to locate abscesses and other sites of bacterial infection.[87]

LYSOZYME AND TRANSCOBALAMIN I

Lysozyme (muramidase) is an enzyme found in the granules of neutrophils but not of eosinophils or basophils. Measurements of serum and marrow lysozyme have been used to assess neutrophil production.[88,89] Unfortunately, the correlation with cell kinetics is disappointing, and it is not useful in assessing neutrophil production.[90] The clearance of the enzyme from the serum is also variable, depending primarily on the proximal renal tubule cells. Serum lysozyme is almost invariably elevated in monocytic leukemia, and serial measurements may be useful in the disease.[88,91]

Transcobalamin I is a B$_{12}$-binding protein found in the specific (secondary) granules of neutrophils. It is present in cells as immature as myelocytes but is more abundant in mature cells.[88,92] Serum levels tend to be high in patients with chronic myelogenous leukemia, polycythemia vera, or inflammatory leukocytosis.[92] At extremely high neutrophil counts there is a reasonable correlation with serum concentration of this protein. Measurement of total B$_{12}$-binding capacity in combination with serum lysozyme determination can provide useful information, particularly in myeloproliferative disorders.[88]

ACCUMULATION IN INFLAMMATORY SITES

The Rebuck window technique, utilizing the adherence of leukocytes to sterile cover slips overlying areas of superficially abraded skin, was introduced in 1955.[93] Because this method is qualitative and does not assess nonadherent cells, attempts have been made to introduce more quantitative techniques by producing and examining skin blisters[94] and skin chambers.[95] None of these methods, however, is wholly satisfactory, and all are at best semiquantitative.

IN VITRO MARROW CULTURE

The CFU-GM is the cell that forms a mixed colony containing neutrophils and macrophages in semisolid agar culture. This cell is usually regarded as the committed progenitor of these cell lines. The number of colonies formed in agar from marrow aspirates should therefore reflect the number of CFU-GM in vivo. Unfortunately, in human subjects the technique can give information only about the relative concentration of CFU-GM among all the nucleated marrow cells; it does not give data about the total number of these progenitors. The technique therefore suffers from problems with sampling and determining absolute cell numbers. Total circulating CFU-GM can be quantified in blood, but this determination may reflect distribution more than production.[96] The in vitro culture method does permit assessment of abnormalities of granulocytic development in various hematologic disorders and may be of particular use in preleukemia (see Chap. 92) and the acute leukemias (see Chap. 93).[97] Inhibition of CFU-GM growth has also been used to identify antineutrophil antibodies.[98,99]

REFERENCES

1. Morrison SJ, Uchida N, Weissman IL: The biology of hematopoietic stem cells. *Ann Rev Cell Gen Biol* 11:35, 1995.
2. Spangrude GJ: Biological and clinical aspects of hematopoietic stem cells. *Ann Rev Med* 45:93, 1994.
3. Metcalf D: Control of granulocytes and macrophages: molecular, cellular, and clinical aspects. *Science* 254:529, 1991.
4. Athens JW: Neutrophilic granulocyte kinetics and granulopoiesis, in Gordon AS (ed): *Regulation of Hematopoiesis*. New York, Appleton-Century-Crofts, 1970, p 1143.
5. Athens JW, Raab SO, Haab OP, et al: Leukokinetic studies: III. The distribution of granulocytes in the blood of normal subjects. *J Clin Invest* 40:159, 1961.
6. Athens JW, Haab OP, Raab SO, et al: Leukokinetic studies: IV. The total blood, circulating and marginal granulocyte pools and the granulocyte turnover rate in normal subjects. *J Clin Invest* 40:989, 1961.
7. Boggs DR: The kinetics of neutrophilic leukocytes in health and in disease. *Semin Hematol* 4:359, 1967.
8. Cartwright GE, Athens JW, Boggs DR, Wintrobe MM: The kinetics of granulopoiesis in normal man. *Ser Haematol* 1:1, 1965.
9. Cronkite EP: Kinetics in granulocytopoiesis. *Clin Haematol* 8:351, 1979.
10. Cronkite EP, Fliedner TM: Granulocytopoiesis. *N Engl J Med* 270:1347, 1964.
11. Vincent PC: The measurement of granulocyte kinetics. *Br J Haematol* 36:1, 1977.
12. Donohue DM, Reiff RH, Hanson ML, Betson Y, et al: Quantitative measurement of the erythrocytic and granulocytic cells of the marrow and blood. *J Clin Invest* 37:1511, 1958.
13. Dancey JT, Deubelbeiss KA, Harker LA, Finch CA: Neutrophil kinetics in man. *J Clin Invest* 58:705, 1978.
14. Dresch C, Faille A, Rain JD, Najean Y: Granulopoièse: étude comparative de différentes méthodes de mesure de la production et de la richesse médullaire. *Nouv Rev Fr Hematol* 15:31, 1975.
15. Ogawa M: Differentiation and proliferation of hematopoietic stem cells. *Blood* 81:2844, 1993.
16. Metcalf D: Hematopoietic regulators. *Blood* 82:3515, 1993.
17. Metcalf D, Nicola NA: *The Hemopoietic Colony Stimulating Factor*. Cambridge, UK, Cambridge University Press, 1995.
18. Lieschke GJ, Burgess AW: Granulocyte colony-stimulating factor and granulocyte-macrophage colony-stimulating factor. *N Engl J Med* 327:99, 1992.
19. Kaushansky K, Karplus PA: Hemopoietic growth factors. *Blood* 82:3229, 1993.
20. Groopman JE, Molina J-M, Sandden DT: Hematopoietic growth factors. *N Engl J Med* 321:1449, 1989.
21. Welte K, Gabrilove J, Bronchud MH, Platzer E, Morstyn G: Filgrastim (r-metHuG-CSF): the first 10 years. *Blood* 88:1907, 1996.
22. Anderlini P, Przepiorka D, Champlain R, Köling M: Biologic effects of granulocyte colony stimulating factor in normal individuals. *Blood* 88:2819, 1996.
23. Lopez AF, Williamson DJ, Gamble JR, et al: Recombinant human granulocyte-macrophage colony-stimulating factor stimulates in vitro mature human neutrophil and eosinophil function, surface receptor expression, and survival. *J Clin Invest* 78:1220, 1986.

24. Munker R, Gasson J, Ogawa M, Koeffler HP: Recombinant human tumor necrosis factor induces production of granulocyte-monocyte colony-stimulating factor mRNA and protein from lung fibroblasts and vascular endothelial cells in vitro. *Nature* 323:79, 1986.

25. Zucali JR, Dinarello CA, Oblon DJ, et al: Interleukin-1 stimulates fibroblasts to produce granulocyte-macrophage colony-stimulating activity and prostaglandin E2. *J Clin Invest* 77:1857, 1986.

26. Metcalf D, Nicola NA, Mifsud S, Di Rago L: Receptor clearance obscures the magnitude of granulocyte-macrophage colony-stimulating factor responses in mice to endotoxin or local infections. *Blood* 93:1579, 1999.

27. Aye MT, Hashemi S, Leclair B, et al: Expression of stem cell factor and c-kit mRNA in cultured endothelial cells, monocytes and cloned human bone marrow stromal cells (CFU-RF). *Exp Hematol* 20:523, 1992.

28. Williams DE, de Vries P, Namen AE, Widmer MB, Lyman SD: The steel factor. *Dev Biol* 151:368, 1992.

29. Lyman SD, Williams DE: Biological activities and potential therapeutic uses of steel factor: a new growth factor active on multiple hematopoietic lineages. *Am J Pediatr Hematol Oncol* 14:1, 1992.

30. Dolci S, Williams DE, Ernst MK, et al: Requirement for mast cell growth factor for primordial germ cell survival in culture. *Nature* 352:809, 1991.

31. Anderlini P, Przepiorka D, Champlin R, Korbling M: Biologic and clinical effects of granulocyte colony-stimulating factor in normal individuals. *Blood* 88:2819, 1996.

32. Le Vine AM, Reed JA, Kurak KE, Cianciolo E, Whitsett JA: GM-CSF-deficient mice are susceptible to pulmonary group B streptococcal infection. *J Clin Invest* 103:563, 1999.

33. Dranoff G, et al: Involvement of granulocyte-macrophage colony-stimulating factor in pulmonary homeostasis. *Science* 264:713, 1994.

34. Stanley E, Lieschke GJ, Grail D, et al: Granulocyte/macrophage colony-stimulating factor-deficient mice show no major perturbation of hematopoiesis but develop a characteristic pulmonary pathology. *Proc Natl Acad Sci U S A* 91:5592, 1994.

35. Huffman JA, Hull WM, Dranoff G, Mulligan RC, Whitsett JA: Pulmonary epithelial cell expression of GM-CSF corrects the alveolar proteinosis in GM-CSF-deficient mice. *Proc Natl Acad Sci U S A* 91:5592, 1996.

36. Hammond W, Csiba E, Canin A, et al: Chronic neutropenia: a new canine model induced by human granulocyte colony-stimulating factor. *J Clin Invest* 87:704, 1991.

37. Lieschke GJ, Grail D, Hodgson G, et al: Mice lacking granulocyte colony-stimulating factor have chronic neutropenia, granulocyte and macrophage progenitor cell deficiency, and impaired neutrophil mobilization. *Blood* 84:1737, 1994.

38. Mempel K, Pietsch T, Menzel T, Zeidler C, Welte K: Increased serum levels of granulocyte colony-stimulating factor in patients with severe congenital neutropenia. *Blood* 77:1919, 1991.

39. Axelrod A: Some hemopoietic negative regulators. *Exp Hematol* 18:143, 1990.

40. Guigon M, Bonnet D: Inhibitory peptides in hematopoiesis. *Exp Hematol* 23:477, 1995.

41. Pelus LM, Broxmeyer HE, Kurland JI, Moore MAS: Regulation of macrophage and granulocyte proliferation: specificities of prostaglandin E and lactoferrin. *J Exp Med* 150:277, 1979.

42. Breton-Gorius J, Mason DY, Buriot D, et al: Lactoferrin deficiency as a consequence of a lack of specific granules in neutrophils from a patient with recurrent infections. *Am J Pathol* 99:413, 1980.

43. Warner HR, Athens JW: An analysis of granulocyte kinetics in blood and bone marrow. *Ann N Y Acad Sci* 113:523, 1964.

44. Dresch C, Faille A, Bauchet J, Najean Y: Granulopoïèse: comparison de différentes méthodes d'étude de la durée de maturation et des réserves médullaires. *Nouv Rev Fr Hematol* 13:5, 1973.

45. Fliedner TM, Cronkite EP, Robertson JS: Granulocytopoiesis: I. Senescence and random loss of neutrophilic granulocytes in human beings. *Blood* 24:402, 1964.

46. Patt HM, Maloney MA: Kinetics of neutrophil balance, in Stohlman F Jr (ed): *The Kinetics of Cellular Proliferation.* New York, Grune and Stratton, 1959, p 201.

47. Cronkite EP: Enigmas underlying the study of hemopoietic cell proliferation. *Fed Proc* 23:649, 1964.

48. Koeffler HP, Golde DW: Human preleukemia. *Ann Intern Med* 93:347, 1980.

49. Ruoslahti E: Integrins. *J Clin Invest* 87:1, 1991.

50. Hynes RO: Integrins: versatility, modulation, and signaling in cell adhesion. *Cell* 69:11, 1992.

51. Bevilacqua MP, Nelson RM: Selectins. *J Clin Invest* 91:379, 1993.

52. Varki A: Selectin ligands: will the real ones please stand up? *J Clin Invest* 99:158, 1997.

53. Lawrence MB, Springer TA: Leukocyte roll on a selectin at physiologic flow rates: distinction from and prerequisite for adhesion through integrins. *Cell* 65:859, 1991.

54. Lawrence MB, Smith CW, Eskin SG, McIntire LV: Effect of venous shear stress on CD18-mediated neutrophil adhesion to cultured endothelium. *Blood* 75:227, 1990.

55. Berg M, James SP: Human neutrophils release the Leu-8 lymph node homing receptor during cell activation. *Blood* 76:2381, 1990.

56. Detmers PA, Powell DE, Walz A, Clark-Lewis I, Baggiolini M, Cohn ZA: Differential effects of neutrophil-activating peptide 1/IL-8 and its homologues on leukocyte adhesion and phagocytosis. *J Immunol* 147:4211, 1991.

57. Vedder NB, Harlan JM: Increased surface expression of CD11b/CD18 (Mac-1) is not required for stimulated neutrophil adherence to cultured endothelium. *J Clin Invest* 81:676, 1988.

58. Kuijpers TW, Hakkert BC, Hoogerwerk M, Roos D: Role of endothelial leukocyte adhesion molecule-1 and platelet-activating factor in neutrophil adherence to IL-1 prestimulated endothelial cells: endothelial leukocyte adhesion molecule-1-mediated CD18 activation. *J Immunol* 147:1367, 1991.

59. Bochner BS, Friedman B, Krishnaswami G, et al: Episodic eosinophilia-myalgia-like syndrome in a patient without L-tryptophan use: association with eosinophil activation and increased serum levels of granulocyte-macrophage colony-stimulating factor. *J Allergy Clin Immunol* 88:629, 1991.

60. Butcher EC: Leukocyte-endothelial cell recognition: three (or more) steps to specificity and diversity. *Cell* 67:1033, 1991.

61. Shen Y, Sultana C, Arditi M, Kim KS, Kalra VK: Endotoxin-induced migration of monocytes and PECAM-1 phosphorylation are abrogated by PAF receptor antagonists. *Am J Physiol* 275:E479, 1998.

62. Kalra VK, Shen Y, Sultana C, Rattan V: Hypoxia induces PECAM-1 phosphorylation and transendothelial migration of monocytes. *Am J Physiol Heart Circ Physiol* 271:H2025, 1996.

63. Mauer AM, Athens JW, Ashenbrucker H, et al: Leukokinetic studies: II. A method for labeling granulocytes in vitro with radioactive diisopropylfluorophosphate (DFP32). *J Clin Invest* 39:1481, 1960.

64. Bishop CR, Rothstein G, Ashenbrucker HE, Athens JW: Leukokinetic studies: XIV. Blood neutrophil kinetics in chronic, steady-state neutropenia. *J Clin Invest* 50:1678, 1971.

65. Rosse WF, Gurney CW: The Pelger-Huet anomaly in three families and its use in determining the disappearance of transfused neutrophils from the peripheral blood. *Blood* 14:170, 1959.

66. Dresch C, Najean Y, Bauchet J: Kinetic studies of ^{51}Cr and DF^{32}P labelled granulocytes. *Br J Haematol* 29:67, 1975.

67. Colotta F, Re F, Polentarutti N, Sozzani S, Mantovani A: Modulation of granulocyte survival and programmed cell death by cytokines and bacterial products. *Blood* 80:2012, 1992.

68. Bishop CR, Athens JW, Boggs DR, et al: Leukokinetic studies: XIII. A nonsteady-state kinetic evaluation of the mechanism of cortisone-induced granulocytosis. *J Clin Invest* 47:249, 1968.

69. Dale DC, Fauci AS, Guerry ID, Wolff SM: Comparison of agents producing a neutrophilic leukocytosis in man: hydrocortisone, prednisone, endotoxin and etiocholanolone. *J Clin Invest* 56:808, 1975.

70. Stausz I, Barcsak J, Kekes E, Szebeni A: Prednisone-induced acute changes in circulating neutrophil granulocytes: I. In cases of normal granulocyte reserves. *Haematologia* 1:319, 1993.

71. Dale DC, Fauci AS, Wolff SM: Alternate-day prednisone: leukocyte kinetics and susceptibility to infections. *N Engl J Med* 291:1154, 1974.

72. Peters WJ, Holland JF, Senn H, et al: Corticosteroid administration and localized leukocyte mobilization in man. *N Engl J Med* 286:342, 1972.

73. Craddock CG, Perry S, Ventyke L, Lawrence JS: Evaluation of marrow granulocyte reserves in normal and disease states. *Blood* 15:840, 1960.

74. Marsh JC, Perry S: The granulocyte response to endotoxin in patients with hematologic disorders. *Blood* 23:581, 1964.

75. DeConti RC, Kaplan SR, Calabresi P: Endotoxin stimulation in patients with lymphoma: correlation with the myelosuppressive effects of alkylating agents. *Blood* 39:602, 1972.

76. Korbitz BC, Toren FA, Davis HL, et al: The Piromen test: a useful assay of bone marrow granulocyte reserves. *Curr Ther Res* 11:491, 1969.

77. Osgood EE: Number and distribution of human hemic cells. *Blood* 9:1141, 1954.

78. Buescher ES, Gallin JI: Leukocyte transfusions in chronic granulomatous disease: persistence of transfused leukocytes in sputum. *N Engl J Med* 307:800, 1982.

79. Lord BI, Bronchud MH, Owens S, et al: The kinetics of human granulopoiesis following treatment with granuloycte colony-stimulating factor in vivo. *Proc Natl Acad Sci U S A* 86:9499, 1989.

80. Lord BI, Gurney H, Chang J, Thatcher N, Crowther D, Dexter TM: Haemopoietic cell kinetics in humans treated with rGM-CSF. *Int J Cancer* 50:26, 1992.

81. Buchanan MR, Crowley CA, Rosin RE, Gibrone MA Jr, Babior BM: Studies on the interaction between GP-180-deficient neutrophils and vascular endothelium. *Blood* 60:160, 1982.

82. Cleaver JE: *Thymidine Metabolism and Cell Kinetics.* New York, Wiley, 1967.

83. Hughes WL, Bond UP, Brecher G, et al: Cellular proliferation in the mouse as revealed by autoradiography with tritiated thymidine. *Proc Natl Acad Sci U S A* 44:476, 1958.

84. Hillen H, Wessels J, Haanen C: Bone-marrow-proliferation patterns in acute myeloblastic leukemia determined by pulse cytophotometry. *Lancet* 1:609, 1975.

85. Anonymous: Pulse cytophotometry. *Lancet* 1:435, 1975.

86. LoBue J: Analysis of normal granulocyte production and release, in Gordon AS (ed): *Regulation of Hematopoiesis.* New York, Appleton-Century-Crofts, 1970, p 1167.

87. Peters AM, Saverymuttu SH: The value of indium-labelled leucocytes in clinical practice. *Blood Rev* 1:65, 1987.

88. Catovsky D, Galton DAG, Griffin C, Hoffbrand AV, et al: Serum lysozyme and vitamin B_{12} binding capacity in myeloproliferative disorders. *Br J Haematol* 21:661, 1971.

89. Hansen NE: The relationship between the turnover rate of neutrophilic granulocytes and plasma lysozyme levels. *Br J Haematol* 25:771, 1973.

90. Levi JA, Macqueen A, Vincent PC: Assessment of the value of lysozyme assay in neutropenia. *Br J Haematol* 25:757, 1973.

91. Ohta H, Nagase H: Serial estimation of serum, urine, and leukocyte muramidase (lysozyme) in monocytic leukemia. *Acta Haematol (Basel)* 46:257, 1971.

92. Rachmilewitz B, Rachmilewitz M, Moshkowitz B, Gross J: Serum transcobalamin in myeloid leukemia. *J Lab Clin Med* 78:276, 1971.

93. Rebuck JW, Crowley JH: A method of studying leukocyte functions in vivo. *Ann N Y Acad Sci* 59:757, 1955.

94. Boggs DR, Athens JW, Cartwright GE, Wintrobe MM: The effect of glucocorticosteroids upon the cellular composition of inflammatory exudates. *Am J Pathol* 44:763, 1964.

95. Mass MF, Dean PB, Weston WL, Humbert JR: Leukocyte migration in vivo: a new method of study. *J Lab Clin Med* 86:1040, 1975.

96. Socinski MA, Cannistra SA, Elias A, Antman KH, et al: Granulocyte-macrophage colony stimulating factor expands the circulating haemopoietic progenitor cell compartment in man. *Lancet* 1:1194, 1988.

97. Metcalf D: In vitro cloning techniques for hemopoietic cells: clinical applications. *Ann Intern Med* 87:483, 1977.

98. Kelton JG, Huang AT, Mold N, et al: The use of in vitro technics to study drug-induced pancytopenia. *N Engl J Med* 301:621, 1979.

99. van Brummelen P, Willemz R, Tan WD, Thompson J: Captopril-associated agranulocytosis. *Lancet* 1:150, 1980.

FUNCTIONS OF NEUTROPHILS

JAMES E. SMOLEN

LAURENCE A. BOXER

Neutrophils protect the host against pyogenic infections. Their function is closely related with that of lymphocytes and macrophages, cells that are also involved in the response to infection. Chemotactic factors or chemotaxins, which are generated by the interaction of plasma proteins with antigens or pathogens, attract neutrophils from the blood to sites of infection. The diffusion of these factors creates a chemical gradient that directs the migration of neutrophils, with the cells moving toward the source of the chemotactic factor. Plasma, in addition to elaborating chemical attractants, provides antibodies and complement that coat microorganisms. This process of antibody and complement coating has been called opsonization, from the Greek word for "providing victuals." The pathogenicity of microorganisms often results from their ability to prevent opsonization. Neutrophils ingest the opsonized microorganisms by surrounding them with moving pseudopodia, which fuse to enclose the microbe within a vesicle called the phagosome. The cytoplasmic granules of the neutrophil fuse with the phagosome and discharge their contents into it, a process called degranulation. The neutrophil reduces molecular oxygen enzymatically to generate "activated" metabolites such as superoxide and hydrogen peroxide that, together with material discharged into the phagosome from the granules, can kill ingested microbes. Granule contents and oxygen metabolites may leak from the neutrophil into extracellular fluid, where they can injure tissue as well as microbes. This leakage results from both direct secretion as well as from partially closed phagosomes (Fig. 67-1). This side effect of the attack of neutrophils against antigens or pathogens may be an important cause of tissue inflammation and in certain locations may be detrimental to the host.

Acronyms and abbreviations that appear in this chapter include: ADP, adenosine diphosphate; ARF, ADP-ribosylation factor; ATP, adenosine triphosphate; ATPase, adenosinetriphosphatase; BPI, bactericidal/permeability-increasing protein; BPB, bromophenacyl bromide; cAMP, cyclic adenosine monophosphate; cGMP, cyclic guanosine monophosphate; DAG, diacylglycerol; DAGK, diacylglycerol kinase; EGTA, ethylene glycol-bis(β-aminomethyl ether)-N,N-tetraacetic acid; ERK, extracellular signal-related protein kinase; FAD, flavin prosthetic group; fMet-Leu-Phe, formyl-methionyl-leucyl-phenylalanine; FMLP, formyl-methionyl-leucyl-phenylalanine; GPI, glycosylphosphatidylinositol; GTP, guanosine triphosphate; CGD, chronic granulomatous disease; HETEs, hydroxyeicosatetraenoic acids; ICAM-1, intercellular adhesion molecule-1; IL-1, interleukin-1; IL-8, interleukin-8; IP$_3$, inositol trisphosphate; LAD I, leukocyte adhesion deficiency type I; LAD II, leukocyte adhesion deficiency type II; LTB$_4$, leukotriene B$_4$; LFA-1, leukocyte function-associated antigen-1; LPS, lipopolysaccharide; MAPK, microtubule-associated protein kinases; MPO, myeloperoxidase; NADPH, nicotinamide adenine dinucleotide phosphate; NEM, N-ethyl maleimide; NSF, NEM-sensitive fusion protein; PA, phosphatidic acid; PAF, platelet activating factor; PC, phosphatidylcholine; PIP$_1$, phosphatidyl inositol-4-monophosphate; PIP$_2$, phosphatidylinositol-4,5-bisphosphate; PKA, protein kinase A; PKC, protein kinase C; PLA$_2$, phospholipase A$_2$; PLC, phospholipase C; PLD, phospholipase D; PMA, phorbol 12-myristate 13-acetate; PPH, phosphatidic acid phosphohydrolase; PT, pertussis toxin; SCAMP, secretory carrier membrane protein; SNAP, soluble NSF-attachment proteins; SNAREs, SNAP-receptors; TNF, tumor necrosis factor; VAMP-2, vesicle associated membrane protein-2

The primary function of neutrophils is to protect the host against bacterial infections. Exposure of human neutrophils to a variety of particulate and soluble stimuli evokes a series of responses, including chemotaxis, phagocytosis, degranulation, hexose monophosphate shunt stimulation, generation of reactive derivatives of oxygen, release of membrane-bound calcium, and reorganization of the cytoskeleton. All of these responses and the signal transduction processes mediating them are of considerable scientific and clinical interest. In this chapter, we will focus on the above mentioned responses, with special emphasis on stimulus-response coupling.

CHEMOTAXIS AND MOTILITY

The similarity between neutrophil locomotion and that of amebas was noted long ago.[1] Neutrophils can respond to spatial gradients of chemotaxins with differences in concentration of chemotaxin of as little as 1 percent,[2] although there has been contention as to whether chemotaxis also requires temporal, as well as spatial, sensing.[3] Even with populations of cells as "homogenous" as neutrophils, a broad range of responsiveness is found.[4] During locomotion toward a chemotactic source, these cells acquire a characteristic asymmetric shape (Figs. 67-1 and 67-2). In the front of the cell is a pseudopodium that advances before the body of the cell containing the nucleus and the cytoplasmic granules. At the rear of the moving cell is a knoblike tail. The anterior pseudopodium undulates or "ruffles" as the neutrophil moves, at a rate of up to 50 μm/min. The membrane lipids also flow during locomotion,[5] and enhanced cytosolic Ca^{2+} is observed along the membrane margin.[6,7] The pseudopodium, which is very thin, forms immediately when the cell encounters a gradient of chemotactic factor. As the cell moves, the cytoplasm behind the anterior pseudopodium streams forward, almost obliterating the pseudopodium. At this point some granules appear to contact the cell periphery, and the release of granule contents, a recognized response to chemotactic agents,[8] can occur. The pseudopodium extends again and the process repeats itself. A flow of cortical materials, composed particularly of actin filaments, has been proposed to account for chemotaxis as well as other cellular movements.[9] This may also account for changes in cell viscosity.[10]

INGESTION

When a neutrophil comes in contact with a particle, the pseudopodium flows around the particle, its extensions fuse, and it thereby encompasses the particle within the phagosome.[1] The ingestion phase can be said to extend from recognition to the end of pseudopodium fusion. The particle thus becomes enclosed within a phagosome into which granules are rapidly discharged, as illustrated in Fig. 67-2. As with locomotion, phagocytosis results in Ca^{2+} being released in the vicinity of the active membranes.[6] The number of ingested particles may be eventually limited by the availability of plasma membrane.[11] Locomotion is not a prerequisite for ingestion: if neutrophils collide with a particle not secreting a chemotactic substance, pseudopodia form abruptly at the contact point and envelop the particle. Ingested particles gradually move toward the cell interior, where they tumble about with the nucleus and cytoplasmic granules as the cell moves off. A small number of the phagocytosed particles are actually expelled.[12]

The formation of a pseudopodium is essential for neutrophil locomotion. The interior cytoplasm is squeezed in the direction of the lamellopodium, possibly by the peripheral cytoplasm in the rear of the cell. The pseudopodium is also required for ingestion. When dissolution of the pseudopodium occurs, the interior contents of the cell are allowed to contact the cell membrane. Granule discharge may occur. Fusion of membranes is a common feature of (1) ingestion, where pseudopodia fuse; (2) degranulation, where granules fuse with the phagosome; and possibly (3) locomotion, where some granules

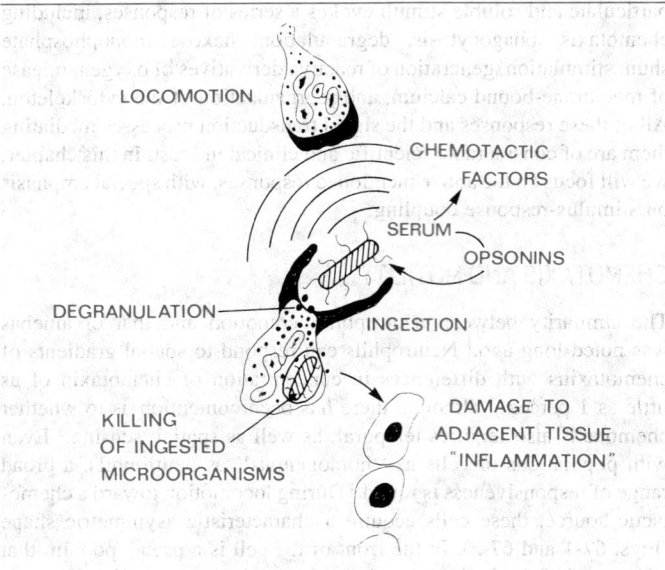

FIGURE 67-1   Activities of the neutrophil.

may fuse with the plasma membrane. Pseudopodia form whether neutrophils are suspended in liquid medium or are attached to a surface, but the cell can only move translationally when fixed to a surface[13]; thus it crawls but does not swim.[14] Such "stickiness" is also a phase of ingestion. The neutrophil membrane adheres firmly to particles they ingest,[15] presumably to provide the frictional force needed to move pseudopodia around the particles. Thus, the formation of pseudopodia, membrane fusion, and membrane adhesiveness are all characteristics associated with the functional responses of neutrophils.

ADHESION MOLECULES

Neutrophils circulate in the blood in a nonadherent state. Upon activation, the neutrophil becomes more adhesive, enabling receptor-medi-

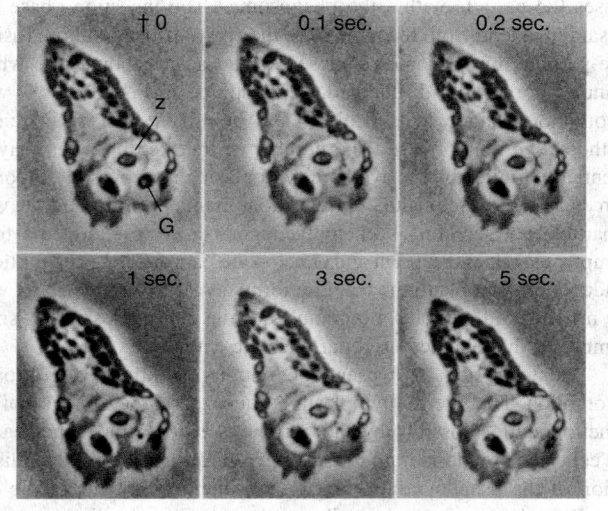

FIGURE 67-2   Cinemicrophotographic observation of granule lysis of a chicken neutrophil following phagocytosis of zymosan particles. Note the lysis of the cytoplasmic granule (G) against one of two ingested zymosan particles (Z). The dense body of the granule disappears from view in the interval of 5 s (x1200). (From JG Hirsch. *J Exp Med* 116:827,1962, with permission.)

ated margination to the vasculature and subsequent chemotaxis and phagocytosis.[16] A number of surface proteins, most notably the β_2 integrins and the L-selectins, have been identified as mediators of adherence.[17-19] The bonding properties of these adherence molecules seem to govern the transient tethering of neutrophils to venules, with characteristic "rolling."[17] Adherent cells are often "primed" or sensitized, and can have substantially different functional properties as compared to cells in suspension.[20] When neutrophils are in suspension, they aggregate if stimulated with chemotactic factors, a process that is distinct from adherence in many respects.[21]

A sequence of molecular and biophysical events leading to neutrophil activation and increased adherence during the acute inflammatory response in vivo is shown in Fig. 67-3. An activated neutrophil enters post-capillary venules adjacent to inflammatory foci and develops transient adhesive interactions with inflamed endothelium via specific classes of adhesion molecules that include the selectins.[22] Endothelial cell selectins (E-selectin and P-selectin) are inducibly expressed by endothelial cells following exposure to inflammatory cytokines such as tumor necrosis factor (TNF) and interleukin-1 (IL-1) (products of endotoxin-stimulated mononuclear phagocytes)[22] (Fig. 67-3b). Specific oligosaccharide moieties expressed on neutrophil membranes serve as counter-receptors for E-selectin and P-selectin (sialyl Lewis X and Lewis X, respectively). In conjunction with neutrophil membrane L-selectin, which recognizes oligosaccharide moieties expressed by endothelial cells, they promote transient neutrophil-endothelial binding under flow conditions, termed neutrophil "rolling."[17,22]

Neutrophil rolling is a prerequisite for the transition to an interaction with the inflamed endothelium that is more resistant to shear stress.[17,18,23] Firm adhesion is mediated by a separate class of molecules whose expression level and functional affinity are increased by high local concentrations of inflammatory stimuli.[17] Specifically, on endothelial cells the ICAM-1 (CD54) glycoprotein is induced by cytokines that include TNF and IL-1. ICAM-1 serves as a recognition target for neutrophil β_2 integrin counter-receptors Mac-1 (CD11b/CD18) and LFA-1 (CD11a/CD18). The relative affinity of Mac-1 and LFA-1 for ICAM-1 is increased by exposure of neutrophils to numerous stimuli, including C5a, N-formylated bacterial peptides (FMLP), IL-8 (synthesized by inflamed endothelium), and LTB$_4$.[18,22] (Figs. 67-3c and d). High-affinity sticking between neutrophils and endothelial cells, dependent upon β_2 integrin, promotes subsequent transendothelial migration through the basement membrane. This migration continues into the extracellular matrix in response to local gradients of chemotactic factors[18,24] (Fig. 67-3d). During neutrophil activation, there is a reciprocal relationship on the plasma membrane between the expression of L-selectin and the β_2 integrin Mac-1. L-selectin, which initially has a high basal expression, is shed upon exposure to chemotactic stimuli. Mac-1 receptor sites are initially at a low basal expression and affinity, but increase ten- to twentyfold after stimulation.[19] The changes in affinity and surface expression occur over seconds to minutes following stimulation.[25]

The CD11/CD18 integrins are vital to firm adherence and transmigration. Complete inhibition of CD18, the common β_2 chain of the leukocyte integrins, profoundly reduces emigration of neutrophils at sites of inflammation but leads to a severe immunodeficiency syndrome termed leukocyte adhesion deficiency type I (LAD I).[26] Patients with LAD I have mutations in CD18 that lead to a severe or total deficiency of the CD11/CD18 integrins from the cell surface, which include CD11a/CD18 (LFA-1, α_{L2}), CD11b/CD18 (Mac-1, CR3, α_{M2}), CD11c/CD18 (p150,95, α_{x2}), and CD11d/CD18 (α_{d2}). Another type of deficiency, LAD II, is related to defects in synthesis of the glycoprotein ligands for adhesion molecules.[27]

Neutrophil-mediated inflammatory injury that is dependent upon these adhesive events can occur by one of several mechanisms: (a) activation of integrin-dependent neutrophil hyperadherence promotes

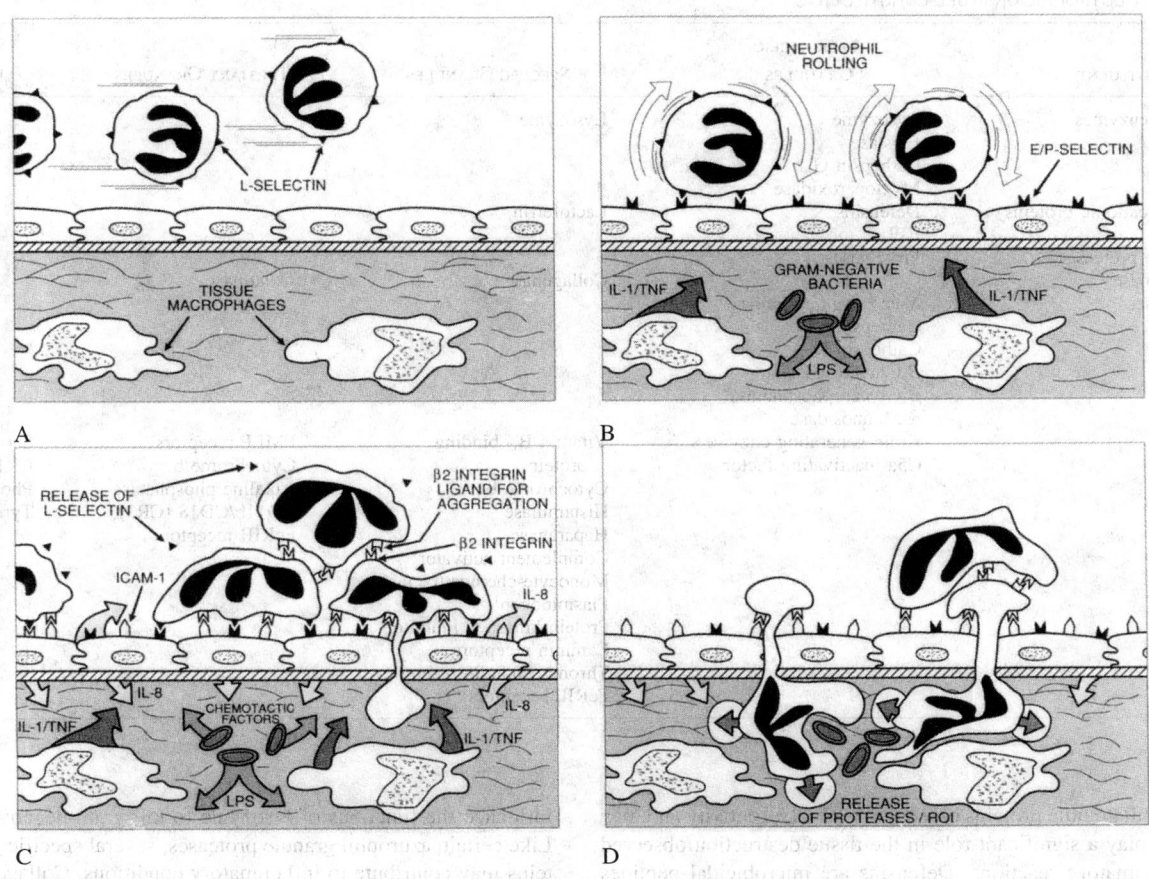

FIGURE 67-3   The neutrophil-mediated inflammatory response. (A) Unstimulated neutrophils (expressing L-selectin) entering a postcapillary venule. (B) Invasion of gram-negative bacteria with release of lipopolysaccharide stimulates tissue macrophages to secrete inflammatory monokines, IL-1 and TNF, which, in turn, activate endothelial cells to express E- and P-selectins. E- and P-selectins serve as counter-receptors for neutrophil L-selectin to cause low-avidity neutrophil rolling. (C) Activated endothelial cells express ICAM-1, which serves as a counter- receptor for neutrophil β_2 integrin molecules leading to high-avidity leukocyte spreading and the start of transendothelial migration. Transendothelial migration of activated neutrophils is stimulated by chemotactic factors such as endothelial cell-derived IL-8 and formylated bacterial factors. Chemoattractants promote neutrophil activation with the release of L-selectin and an increase in β_2 integrin affinity for ICAM-1 and for other counter-receptors promoting intravascular neutrophil aggregation. (D) Neutrophil invasion through the vascular basement membrane with the release of proteases and reactive oxidative intermediates that cause local destruction of the extracellular matrix.

homotypic aggregation (mediated by CD11b/CD18) that may result in plugging of microvessels and resultant distal ischemia[28]; (b) high concentrations of inflammatory stimuli cause neutrophil degranulation and the release of a variety of proteases (see below) that may cause destructive proteolysis of the subadjacent extracellular matrix; and (c) the NADPH oxidase-dependent generation of oxidative metabolites from neutrophils, primed by endotoxins, inflammatory cytokines, and/ or substrate adhesion and stimulated by other activating factors, may promote direct endothelial cell injury or promote the destructive effects of secreted proteases either by activating latent metalloproteinases or by deactivating oxidant-sensitive antiproteinases.[29]

GRANULES

TYPES OF GRANULES

PRIMARY GRANULES

Neutrophil granules serve as reservoirs for digestive and hydrolytic enzymes prior to delivery into the phagosome. Based on their biochem-

ical and morphological properties and time of appearance during cell maturation, three major granule populations have been described (Table 67-1). Azurophil or primary granules are synthesized first during granulocytopoiesis, with secondary and tertiary granules being developed at succeeding times. It has been reported that the contents of granules are determined by the timing of their expression, rather than by signal sequences.[30] Thus, granule contents become packaged into the type of granule being formed at the time they are synthesized.

Azurophil granules contain myeloperoxidase, neutral proteases (elastase, cathepsin G, cathepsin D), protease inhibitors, acid hydrolases (β-glucuronidase, acid phosphatase, α-mannosidase, N-acetyl-glucosaminidase), and cationic proteins.[31–33] Two subpopulations of azurophil granules have been identified and differ in their distribution of several lysosomal enzymes.[32,34] Elastase can be preferentially released from a denser subpopulation,[34] suggesting that these granule subpopulations may be under separate regulatory control. Recent studies have shown substantial heterogeneity of azurophil granule contents.[35]

TABLE 67-1   NEUTROPHIL GRANULE CONSTITUENTS

Constituent	Azurophilic Granules	Specific Granules	Tertiary Granules	Secretory Granules
Microbicidal enzymes	Lysozyme Elastase Cathepsin G Myeloperoxidase	Lysozyme		
Antibacterial cationic proteins	Defensins BPI	Lactoferrin		
Neutral serine proteases	Proteinases			
Metalloproteinases		Collagenase	Gelatinase	
Acid hydrolases	N-acetyl-glucuronidase Cathepsin B Cathepsin D β-Glucuronidase β-Glycerophosphatase α-Mannosidase			
Others	Kinin-generating enzyme C5a-inactivating factor	Vitamin B_{12} binding protein Cytochrome b Histaminase Heparanase Complement activator Monocyte-chemoattractant Plasminogen Protein kinase C inhibitor Laminin receptors Thrombospondin receptors FcRIII receptors	FMLP receptors Cytochrome b Alkaline phosphatase CD11b/CD18 (CR3) FcRIII receptors	Serum albumin CR1 Phospholipases Tyrosine kinases

Azurophil granule proteins possess microbicidal activity and may additionally play a significant role in the tissue destruction observed during inflammatory reactions. Defensins are microbicidal peptides that are found in these granules.[31,36] These proteins are released concomitantly with other azurophil granule constituents following stimulation.[37] Bactericidal/permeability-increasing protein (BPI), a cationic protein that lyses gram-negative bacteria and inhibits endotoxin, is also found in these granules.[38] Myeloperoxidase (MPO) reacts with H_2O_2 and a halide to produce hypochlorous acid (HOCl), a potent oxidant (Clorox) believed to significantly contribute to the killing of microorganisms.[39] MPO may also play a modulating role in degranulation secondary to its ability to inactivate chemotactic factors[40] and inhibit the mechanisms underlying the respiratory burst and phagocytosis.[41]

With respect to the tissue destruction observed during inflammatory reactions, the most important azurophil constituents are the proteases. Three of these proteases have been well characterized. The serine protease, elastase, hydrolyzes typical pancreatic elastase substrates and a variety of elastin preparations from several sources.[42] Cathepsin G is a chymotrypsin-like neutral protease that hydrolyzes proteoglycans and insoluble collagen.[43] Finally, cathepsin D can cleave leukokinogens to generate pharmacologically active leukokinins.[44] It is also active against proteoglycans. Working in concert, these proteases can exacerbate existing inflammatory reactions by generating chemotactic factors from C5.[45]

SPECIFIC GRANULES
Specific or secondary granules are synthesized later during granulocytopoiesis. As shown in Table 67-1, proteins packaged within these granules (in human neutrophils) include lysozyme, collagenase, vitamin B_{12}-binding protein, heparanase, and lactoferrin.[46–49] Lysozyme hydrolyzes cell wall proteoglycan of some bacterial species and is also found in azurophil granules. Lactoferrin is an iron-binding protein that appears to be necessary for hydroxyl radical formation[50] and can

influence the functions of lysozyme to kill gram-negative bacteria.[51] Like certain azurophil granule proteases, several specific granule proteins may contribute to inflammatory conditions. Collagenase, in the presence of a neutral protease, hydrolyzes collagen fibrils; this enzyme may also be activated by oxidative metabolism.[52] Heparanase, a heparan sulfate-degrading endoglycosidase, may be involved in extravasation of neutrophils through the subendothelial basement membrane.[49] In addition, these granules also contain activators of the complement cascade.[53] A modulatory role for these granules in cell locomotion is suggested by the observation that specific granule membranes contain receptors for chemoattractants, extracellular matrix proteins, and adhesion molecules.[54–59] These granule membranes also possess FAD-containing cytochrome b[60–62] that translocates to the plasma membrane upon cell stimulation, suggesting a potential for regulation of the respiratory burst. Individuals whose neutrophils are lacking in specific granule contents are susceptible to repeated staphylococcal skin and respiratory infections,[63] emphasizing the importance of these proteins in host defense mechanisms (see Chap. 82). Neutrophils from these patients have impaired chemotaxis and adherence.[64] The finding that these cells also do not increase expression of chemotactic receptors following activation is consistent with a role for specific granules in locomotion and may underlie their defective chemotactic response.

TERTIARY GRANULES
Tertiary granules contain gelatinase,[65,66] an enzyme which bears many similarities to neutrophil collagenase,[29] and heparanase.[66] Tertiary granule membranes appear to contain a pool of membrane glycoproteins that participates in cell adhesion.[67,68] The C3bi receptor is essential to cell adhesiveness[69] and there is evidence to suggest that it is partially localized in tertiary granules.[68] A tertiary granule localization has also been reported for the oxidase cytochrome b.[70] Finally, the tertiary granules (like the secondary granules) constitute important intracellular pools for neutrophil adhesion molecules.[66,71]

PHOSPHASOMES AND SECRETORY GRANULES

As improved methods have become available for the isolation and characterization of granules and their constituents, other granule populations have been identified. For instance, "phosphasomes," which contain alkaline phosphatase, have recently been isolated from neutrophils.[72,73] These granules are lighter in density than specific granules, but do not contain gelatinase. Another granule type that has been reported is the "secretory" granule, which contains plasma proteins.[74] These granules are highly labile and are most readily released in response to stimuli[75]; their membrane components are also rapidly recovered into vesicles.[75] Secretory granules also contain complement receptor I,[76] tyrosine kinases,[77] and phospholipases.[78]

FUNCTION OF GRANULES

Granule contents play very important roles in nonoxidative mechanisms of immunity and inflammation. Secondary granules are readily mobilized to the extracellular environment in response to many stimuli, such as N-formylated peptides released by bacteria, complement proteins, and leukotriene products.[29,79,80] At sites of inflammation, the neutrophils ingest microorganisms or other particles, as well as discharge granules by exocytosis.[80] To a large extent, the extracellular release of specific and azurophil granules remains under separate control.[79,81] Chemoattractants and other substances can be used to selectively release specific granules under conditions wherein azurophilic granule enzymes are not discharged.[81,82] On the other hand, stimuli for azurophilic granule release also stimulate concomitant exocytosis of specific granules,[83] with rare exceptions.[84] The resistance of azurophil granules to secretion may be due to a requirement for a biochemical signal in addition to Ca^{2+}.[85] Tertiary and secretory granules are more readily discharged than specific granules during cell stimulation; thus, their contents are available to modify the response of the cell to stimuli as well as to affect function.[65,68,75]

Studies of the function of granule contents have depended upon the isolation and characterization of granule proteins and upon evaluation of the behavior of neutrophils with abnormal granules. For instance, the function of tertiary granules is best illustrated by patients who are deficient in a group of neutrophil membrane glycoproteins, namely the β_2 integrins discussed earlier. One of these crucial integrins is CD11b/CD18, also known as Mac-1, Mo-1, or the C3bi receptor (CR3), which is normally found on neutrophil plasma membranes, specific granules, tertiary granules, and secretory granule membranes.[67,71,86] Patients with a complete lack of CD18 (and hence the family of β_2 integrins) present with recurrent and severe bacterial and fungal infections, impaired wound healing, diminished pus formation, and persistent neutrophilia (see Chap. 82). The severity of the clinical manifestation directly relates to the degree of deficiency of adhesive glycoproteins on the membrane.[26,86] CD11b/CD18 is one of these molecules responsible for neutrophil adhesiveness.[69] CD11b/CD18 is stored in gelatinase-bearing tertiary granules[68] and in secretory granules.[71]

Release of specific granules is crucial in mobilizing mediators of inflammation, since these granules contain activators of the complement cascade, leading to the generation of the chemoattractant C5a and the opsonin C3b.[53] Lactoferrin can both attenuate granulopoiesis[87] and alter the functions of mature cells.[88] The release of lactoferrin during degranulation diminishes the negative surface charge of cells, which may be important in sustaining cell adhesiveness.[89] Lactoferrin also facilitates the generation of a highly reactive product of oxygen metabolism, namely hydroxyl radical.[50] The flavoprotein cytochrome b is an important constituent of the electron transport chain for the NADPH oxidase. It is also found in specific granules and is translocated[60-62,90] to the plasma membrane during cell activation, perhaps playing a key role in amplifying the respiratory burst. Recent publica-

tions have reported the presence of b cytochrome in tertiary[70] and secretory[91] granules as well. In addition, there is considerable evidence that the membranes of specific granules contain receptors for chemoattractants and ECM proteins.[54,56-58,67] Thus, translocation of chemoattractant receptors from the granule membrane to the leading edge of the plasma membrane may be essential for cell orientation by providing fresh receptors at the leading edge of the cell during margination and diapedesis.[92] In addition, membranes of specific granules contain an inhibitor of protein kinase C, which in turn may serve to dampen ongoing neutrophil activation.[93,94]

Azurophilic granules contain potent digestive and microbicidal enzymes. Elastase, together with the specific granule component collagenase, may facilitate the penetration of cells through extracellular matrix.[95] Other lysosomal proteases serve to degrade ingested material. Lysozyme, cationic proteins, and defensins have bactericidal activity.[36,96] Myeloperoxidase, a heme-containing protein, has both cytotoxic and anti-bacterial activities, through its ability to interact with halides and hydrogen peroxide to generate hydroxyl radical and hypochlorous acid, and can oxidize chemoattractant peptides and neutrophil secretory products.[40,50,97] Other azurophilic granule proteins inactivate chemoattractants. Thus, the azurophilic granules mediate target cell death and modulate the inflammatory response.

STIMULUS-RESPONSE COUPLING

Secretion by neutrophils has been the subject of intense research for many years. This work has been fruitful in illuminating some of the underlying causes of defects in cell activation. Studies of neutrophil degranulation and oxidative metabolism have also revealed transduction mechanisms common to a wide variety of other important secretory cell types, thereby greatly expanding the relevance of this work. The techniques employed by researchers in this field have been extensively reviewed elsewhere.[98] This review will now discuss in considerably more depth our current understanding of the activation process, which is shown schematically in Fig. 67-4.

RECEPTOR-LIGAND INTERACTIONS

FORMYL PEPTIDE RECEPTOR

Neutrophil responses can be evoked by a variety of particulate and soluble stimuli. Opsonized particles, immune complexes and chemotactic factors produced during the inflammatory process activate neutrophils by binding to specific cell surface receptors. Of the neutrophil chemotactic receptors, the N-formyl peptide receptor is the best characterized. N-Formyl peptides, the synthetic analogs of bacterial products, induce a variety of neutrophil responses and have been extensively employed as activating stimuli. Specific receptors for the chemotactic peptide, N-formyl-methionyl-leucyl-phenylalanine (fMet-Leu-Phe), have been identified on the neutrophil surface,[99] and binding of the formyl peptide to its receptor correlates with its ability to induce chemotaxis and degranulation.[100] The fMet-Leu-Phe receptor is stereospecific,[100] has multiple affinity states,[101] and has an apparent molecular mass of 50 to 70 kDa.[102] An intracellular storage location has also been suggested for the fMet-Leu-Phe receptor, since neutrophil activation results in enhanced fMet-Leu-Phe binding in normal cells,[103] but not in egranulated neutrophil cytoplasts.[104] These receptors have been identified on the membranes of tertiary and secretory granules[105] and are biochemically similar to those on the plasma membrane,[106,107] suggesting that they are mobilized to the cell surface following stimulation and may thus serve a modulatory role. The formyl peptide receptor has been cloned and sequenced[108,109] and belongs to a family of seven membrane-spanning domain proteins typical of G-protein coupled receptors. The receptor occurs in several forms,[110] is physically associated

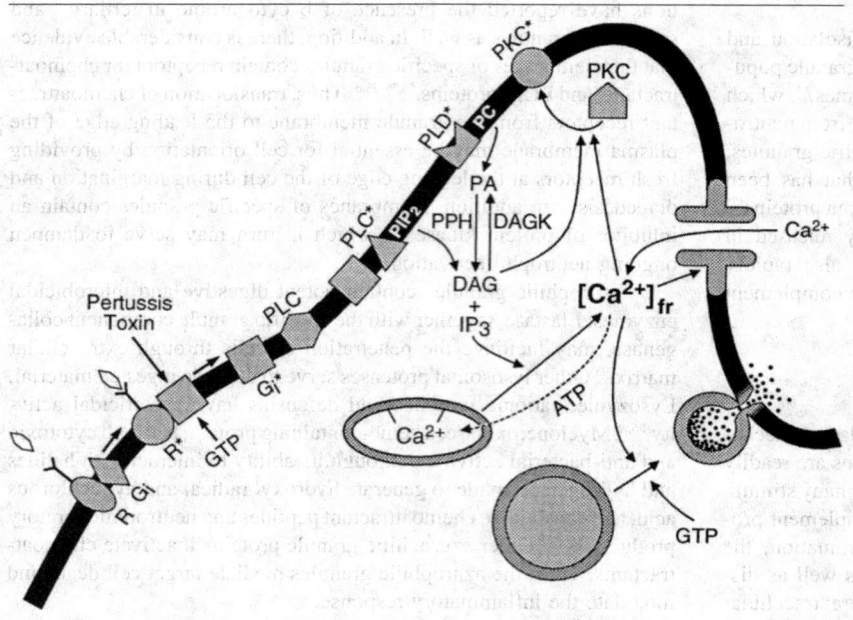

FIGURE 67-4   Model of stimulus-response coupling in the neutrophil leading to degranulation. The signal transduction mechanisms alluded to in the text are schematically illustrated in this figure. The resting state of the cell is represented in the lower left side by an unoccupied cell surface receptor (R) coupled with an inactive G_i-like guanine nucleotide binding protein (G_i). Binding of a specific ligand to this receptor leads to conformational changes in this protein (R*) and activation of the accompanying G-protein (square figure). Activation of this G-protein is blocked by pertussis toxin and involves the binding of GTP, leading to an activated G-protein (G_i*). This G-protein then interacts with a polyphosphatidylinositol-specific phospholipase C (PLC, hexagon) leading to the activation of this enzyme (PLC*, triangle). PLC* cleaves an endogenous lipid, namely phosphatidylinositol bisphosphate (PIP_2), yielding diacylglycerol (DAG) and inositol trisphosphate (IP_3). IP_3 is known to liberate calcium from bound intracellular stores leading to a rise in intracellular free calcium (Ca^{2+}_{fr}). The increase in intracellular Ca^{2+}_{fr} is augmented by an influx from the extracellular space (right side of figure). Increased DAG, in consort with elevated Ca^{2+}_{fr}, and activated protein kinase C (PKC, pentagon) leads to translocation of this enzyme to membranous sites (PKC*). In addition, phospholipase D can be activated (PLD*) by PKC*, G_i*, or Ca^{2+}_{fr} (details currently under investigation), converting phosphatidylcholine (PC) to phosphatidic acid (PA). PA and DAG can be interconverted through the actions of phosphatidic acid phosphohydrolase (PPH) and diacylglycerol kinase (DAGK). Elevations in intracellular Ca^{2+}_{fr} alone are known to induce the secretion of granule constituents to the extracellular space (lower right side) by fusion of granule membranes with the plasma membranes. This process is augmented by the presence of GTP. These transduction mechanisms are discussed in greater detail in the text.

with guanine nucleotide binding proteins (G-proteins)[108,111–113] and the cytoskeleton[111,114,115] (see Ref. 116 for review).

C5A RECEPTOR

Activation of the complement system generates C5a, a derivative of C5 and the most potent of the chemotactic proteins. C5a induces neutrophil chemotaxis,[117] degranulation,[118] and superoxide generation.[119] In turn, it has been suggested that a C5a inhibitor may play a role in the regulation of inflammatory processes and that its deficiency, which is familial, may explain the attacks of sterile inflammation characteristic of Mediterranean fever.[120] Responses to C5a result from interactions with specific receptors on the cell surface.[121] The receptor was identified as a single polypeptide in the plasma membrane with an apparent molecular mass of 40 to 48 kDa.[122] Binding studies have shown that there are 50,000 to 113,000 receptor sites per cell with a dissociation constant (Kd) of 2×10^{-9} M. Strong interactions between the C5a receptor and G-proteins has been reported.[123] Like the FMLP receptor, C5a receptors have been isolated and cloned.[124,125] There is

some heterogeneity in both of these receptors,[126] which are 20 to 35 percent identical in their amino acid sequences. The C5a receptor also belongs to the diverse class of receptors that features seven membrane-spanning domains. Expression of these receptors in other cells has been used to explore their common means of signal transduction.[124,127,128]

C3 RECEPTORS

Neutrophils also express receptors for the complement-derived chemotactic factors C3b and C3bi. Receptors for C3b and C3bi (also known as CR1 and CR3, respectively) are sparse on resting neutrophils but significantly increase in number following activation with several stimuli.[129] Like formyl peptide receptors, the stimulus-induced increase in surface expression of C3b and C3bi receptors appears to result from the mobilization of intracellular pools,[130] although the subcellular locations for these receptors appear to be distinct.[54] Indeed, CR3, which is of the β_2-integrin family (CD11b/CD18), may be located in tertiary granules[68,131] and may be functionally linked to the cytoskeleton[132] (see below). The C3b receptor (CR1) is a glycoprotein with a molecular weight of 205 kDa[133] and appears to be located in secretory granules.[76,134]

INTEGRINS

CD11/CD18 integrins also play an important role in cell signaling. The adhesion of cells to surfaces or to other cells can either activate neutrophils directly or "prime" them for an enhanced response to other stimuli. For example, the oxidative burst of neutrophils is very different in cells that are suspended versus those that are adherent to surfaces.[135] H_2O_2 production in response to chemotaxins has been shown to be influenced by monoclonal antibodies to CD11b, but not CD11a.[136] Yet CD11a-dependent adhesion of canine neutrophils can alone trigger H_2O_2 production in the absence of other stimuli.[137]

Integrins are involved in both outside-in and inside-out signaling that induces conformational changes regulating the affinity of ligand binding.[138–140] In addition to traditional trans-acting receptors, there is also evidence that CD11b and CD11c can serve as cis-acting receptors that transduce signals from glycosylphosphatidylinositol (GPI)-linked receptors[138] (see below).

FC RECEPTORS

Neutrophils possess three different receptors for immunoglobulins. Unstimulated cells express FcγRII and FcγRIII, also known as CD32 and CD16, respectively. Functionally, the most important of the two could be FcγRIII,[141] which is attached to the membrane by a GPI linkage. This linkage is relatively labile, so the amount of FcγRIII on the membrane reflects a balance between shedding and mobilization from intracellular stores.[56,58,142] FcγRII is a conventional protein that spans the plasma membrane.[143] Interestingly, the signal transduction pathways initiated by FcγRIII can cross-talk with the formyl peptide receptor,[144] with CR3,[145] and even with each other.[146] Both FcγRII and FcγRIII produce Ca^{2+} transients,[147] although this has been disputed.[148] The Fc receptors also signal through a variety of kinases, including tyrosine kinases,[149] phosphatidyl inositol kinases,[150] and MAP kinases.[151] Finally, cytokine-stimulated neutrophils express yet another receptor FcγRI, or CD64,[152] which is beginning to be understood.[153] FcγRI can signal through Fcγ RIIIA.[154]

RECEPTOR "CROSS-TALK"

Several lines of evidence suggest that CD11b participates in FcγR-mediated functions. First, neutrophils from patients with LAD I have impaired IgG-dependent phagocytosis and cytolysis.[69] Also, antibodies to CD11b inhibit the phagocytosis of Ig-coated substrates.[155] A direct physical linkage between CD11b and FcγRIIIB has been demonstrated by experiments in which capping of one receptor results in co-capping a substantial fraction of the other receptor.[156] CD11b can also interact with the transmembrane FcγRII, and both of these molecules can modify each other's signals.[157] Finally, the uroplasminogen activator receptor (uPAR, CD187) is a GPI-anchored glycoprotein present on neutrophils with which CD11b can interact directly, but reversibly.[158] In summary, although CD11b and CD11c do not directly participate in antibody-dependent recognition, these integrins provide a novel mechanism for a GPI-anchored receptor to transduce signals leading to effector responses in neutrophils.

OTHER RECEPTORS

Three other important receptors are for platelet activating factor (PAF), IL-8, and leukotriene B$_4$ (LTB$_4$). PAF and IL-8 receptors have been cloned[124,127,159] and belong to the seven-transmembrane domain family. Their intracellular stores and signal transduction mechanisms are largely similar to those used by similar receptors (e.g., FMLP).[123,127] IL-8 has two related receptors, for which slightly different signal transduction pathways have been detected.[160,161] The LTB$_4$ receptor undergoes cycling,[162] as do the IL-8 receptors,[163] and preliminary steps toward purification have been accomplished.[164] The LTB$_4$ receptor also signals through G-proteins.[165]

G-PROTEINS

Recent data strongly suggest that receptors for the chemotactic stimuli fMet-Leu-Phe, C5a, LTB$_4$, and PAF are coupled to cellular responses through a guanine nucleotide binding protein similar to the inhibitory protein, Gi, of the adenylate cyclase system. Evidence linking a G-protein to these receptors has been provided by studies demonstrating that guanine nucleotides can regulate receptor affinity.[166] A high-affinity GTPase located in neutrophil plasma membranes is stimulated by these same receptor-mediated stimuli, but not by the phorbol ester, PMA.[167] This enzymatic activity is likely to be involved in terminating the activation of the guanine nucleotide binding protein. Also, direct linkages between receptors and G-proteins have been observed.[108,111–113,123,162]

Studies using pertussis toxin have proven instrumental in the understanding of G-protein involvement in the proposed stimulus-response coupling pathway. Pertussis toxin ADP-ribosylates the α-subunit of Gi of the adenylate cyclase system and also a 40- to 41-kDa protein in neutrophil plasma membranes.[168] Initial studies demonstrated a strong correlation between the ability of the toxin to catalyze the ADP-ribosylation of the membrane protein and its ability to affect cellular responses initiated by surface receptors. However, pertussis toxin does not alter intracellular cyclic AMP levels, suggesting that the G-protein involved is distinct from G$_i$ of the adenylate cyclase system.[169] More recently, purification and characterization of a guanine nucleotide binding protein in neutrophils have shown that this protein differs both structurally and immunochemically from previously reported guanine nucleotide binding proteins.[168,170–172]

Not only can neutrophil responses be abolished by pertussis toxin, but stable guanine nucleotides can directly stimulate permeabilized neutrophils.[173–176] In other cells, heterotrimeric G-proteins may also play a tonic inhibitory role in degranulation.[177] While PT inhibits fMet-Leu-Phe-induced secretion from intact cells, it does not inhibit degranulation in response to guanine nucleotides, PMA, and Ca^{2+} in the permeabilized cell system, suggesting that a second G-protein is involved at distal sites in secretion.[174] Potential candidates in this role are the family of small G-proteins (with Mw of 20-30 kDa) that has been reported in neutrophils.[171,178,179] Some of these proteins are components of the bactericidal NADPH oxidase system[180] that will be discussed later. Another study suggests that G-proteins sensitive to botulinum toxins C3 and D are involved in degranulation.[181] Perhaps related to this, rho proteins have been shown to be involved in adhesion[182] and rab5 proteins (that are probably involved in vesicular traffic) have been reported to translocate from cytosol to granules following neutrophil stimulation.[183]

PHOSPHOLIPID METABOLISM

The next step in signal transduction can be attributed to interactions of receptor-activated G-proteins and tyrosine kinases with phospholipases.[172,176,184–186] Of primary importance, a membrane-associated phosphoinositide-specific phospholipase is activated upon stimulation with chemotactic stimuli. In particular, phospholipase C hydrolyzes phosphatidylinositol-4,5-bisphosphate (PIP$_2$) and phosphatidyl inositol-4-monophosphate (PIP$_1$)[184,187] to the putative second messenger products inositol 1,4,5-trisphosphate (IP$_3$) and 1,2-diacylglycerol (DAG).[184] In permeabilized neutrophils, IP$_3$ has been shown to interact with a specific intracellular receptor[188] and stimulate the release of Ca^{2+}.[189,190] Evidence has been presented that the Ca^{2+} is not derived from either the mitochondria[189] or the endoplasmic reticulum,[191] but rather from a distinct organelle which has been termed "calcisome." Receptor stimulation also elicits the production of inositol 1,3,4-tris-phosphate and inositol 1,3,4,5-tetrakisphosphate, but these compounds do not appear to have significant functional consequences with regard to Ca^{2+} release.[192]

Other pathways pertinent to signaling and cell activation are also involved. It has been proposed that phospholipase D, which preferentially uses phosphatidylcholine (PC) to produce phosphatidic acid (PA),[172,193,194] is involved in neutrophil activation of the respiratory burst. The evidence is growing that PA generated by this enzyme is critical in cellular responses.[5,193,195] Activation of PLD appears to be mediated by *rho* and/or ADP-ribosylation factor (ARF) along with a higher Mw factor.[196,197] The evidence is growing that PA generated by this enzyme is critical in cellular responses, and particularly degranulation.[176,193,195,198] Furthermore, it appears that the bulk of the DAG generated in stimulated neutrophils may be derived from the action of phosphatidate phosphohydrolase on this PA, rather than from the PLC pathway.[195] The hallmark of these DAGs, which are ultimately derived from PC, is the presence of 1-*O*-alkyl linkages. In addition, it now appears that PA can also be synthesized de novo, from glucose.[199] It has also been reported that the PA generated by the action of PLD, in combination with annexin I, promotes the Ca^{2+}-dependent apposition of membranes.[200]

Fatty acids are also important in signaling and fusion. Phospholipase A$_2$ (PLA$_2$), found in the cytosol, membrane, and granule fractions of neutrophils,[201,202] is activated during neutrophil stimulation,[203] yielding arachidonic acid as a major product. The cytosolic PLA$_2$ is important to intracellular signaling and is activated by phosphorylation[204,205] and by PLD.[206] Although the cytosolic enzyme per se is not Ca^{2+}-dependent, the increases in intracellular Ca^{2+} occurring during cell activation result in translocation to the membrane[203,204] and overall enhancement of arachidonic acid release.[176,207] The role of arachidonic acid and its metabolites will be covered later in this review.

Recently, sphingolipid turnover in neutrophils has been under considerable study. Products of sphingolipid metabolism variously stimulate or inhibit cellular functions,[208] including degranulation.[209] The place of sphingolipid metabolism in the signal transduction scheme is now being elucidated.[210,211]

CALCIUM

The importance of Ca^{2+} as an effector of cellular function has received widespread attention in recent years. Like other cell types, the intracellular Ca^{2+} concentration in resting neutrophils is maintained at submicromolar levels by a plasma membrane-bound Ca^{2+}-ATPase pump.[212,213] There is substantial evidence that intracellular Ca^{2+} levels rise in stimulated neutrophils and that these increments may directly or indirectly bring about cell responses. Studies employing the fluorescent Ca^{2+} probes quin-2 and fura-2 indicate that following surface stimulation, intracellular Ca^{2+} rises almost immediately from a resting level of 0.1 μM to 1 μM.[6,214,215] It is likely that local intracellular Ca^{2+} levels can reach far higher levels. Due to a variety of methodologic problems, including kinetic, spatial, and chemical limitations, conventional indicators underestimate those local subplasmalemmal Ca^{2+} concentrations that are the actual determinants of cellular responses.[216,217] In excitable cells, it has been reported that these local concentrations could exceed 100 μM.[216,217] Studies in neutrophils with new, more sensitive techniques demonstrate that local Ca^{2+} levels reach 1 to 5 μM,[218–220] considerably higher than previously supposed.

There are two separate mechanisms involved in the stimulus-induced rise in intracellular Ca^{2+} levels; there is an initial IP_3-mediated mobilization of Ca^{2+} from intracellular depots followed by an influx of extracellular Ca^{2+}. It should also be noted that individual cells undergo periodic oscillations in intracellular Ca^{2+}, which may be related to responsiveness.[221]

As discussed above, the mechanism by which Ca^{2+} is released following cell activation appears to involve the breakdown of membrane phosphatidylinositols[222,223] that are in turn maintained by specialized enzymes.[224] In permeabilized neutrophils, IP_3 binds to a specific, saturable receptor[188] and induces the specific release of intracellular Ca^{2+}.[189] The storage pool contributing to observed increases in Ca^{2+} is currently being characterized.[225,226] A useful pharmacologic tool for these studies is thapsigargin, an inhibitor that blocks filling and maintenance of the storage pool.[227,228] In subcellular fractions of neutrophil homogenates, IP_3 stimulates Ca^{2+} release only from microsomes.[191] Further separation of microsomal components suggests that neither the plasma membrane nor the endoplasmic reticulum is involved in sequestering IP_3-sensitive Ca^{2+}.[191] Intracellular Ca^{2+} is sequestered in an organelle termed a "calciosome."[229] Ca^{2+} is stored in these sites by binding to a high-affinity calreticulin.[229] However, nonmobilizable intracellular pools also exist.[227]

The initial mobilization of intracellular Ca^{2+} liberated in response to IP_3 appears to directly regulate the permeability changes to Ca^{2+} across the plasma membrane.[225,230] The repletion state of the storage pool and a soluble factor, rather than the production of inositol phosphates, are actually responsible for triggering Ca^{2+} influx.[230–232] These findings are consistent with the previously reported observation that enhanced Ca^{2+} permeability during activation is dependent on mobilization of intracellular Ca^{2+}.[233] However, cell responses are not blocked by EGTA, suggesting that extracellular Ca^{2+} and a Ca^{2+} influx are not absolute requirements.[234]

In an effort to directly demonstrate Ca^{2+}-dependent secretion, neutrophils have been permeabilized by a variety of means, including cholesterol-complexing agents (saponin,[235] digitonin,[166,189,236] and streptolysin O[237]), Sendai virus,[174] and high-voltage electric fields,[175,238] and then exposed to Ca^{2+} in EGTA-containing media. With some excep-

tions,[235] these studies have shown that micromolar levels of Ca^{2+} alone are sufficient to induce the release of both specific and azurophil granule constituents.[174,175,202,236] Specific granules require lower Ca^{2+} concentrations for secretion. The implication that azurophil and specific granule exocytosis differ in their Ca^{2+} requirements is supported by intact cell studies using quin-2 and ionomycin to establish the desired intracellular Ca^{2+} concentrations.[85,239] While secretion can be modulated by both guanine and adenine nucleotides as well as by PKC activation, it appears that the primary intracellular trigger for exocytosis is Ca^{2+}.[240,241] Other aspects of neutrophil function require Ca^{2+} to various extents.[242]

The mechanistic significance of stimulus-induced elevations in intracellular Ca^{2+} is not absolutely established at present. Several investigators have reported that inducing optimal increments in intracellular Ca^{2+} levels is an ineffective measure for evoking some neutrophil responses.[214,243] In addition, a number of responses take place independently of rises in intracellular Ca^{2+}.[244,245] These observations indicate that Ca^{2+} is not a sufficient or mandatory signal in some activation pathways. Elucidation of the role of this cation in signal transduction awaits further investigation.

PROTEIN KINASES

The phorbol ester, phorbol 12-myristate 13-acetate (PMA), has been used extensively as an activating stimulus to investigate the signal transduction pathways operative in neutrophils. The phosphorylation state of a wide variety of intracellular proteins changes upon stimulation with PMA.[246] These changes occur in parallel with the induction of neutrophil functional responses and have also been observed with chemotactic peptide stimulation,[247] suggesting the involvement of a protein kinase in the activation pathway. The ability of PMA to elicit neutrophil responses has been attributed to the activation of a Ca^{2+}-sensitive, phospholipid-dependent protein kinase (protein kinase C or PKC). High levels of PKC have been detected in neutrophils,[248] and the enzyme binds phosphatidyl serine.[249] PKC is present as several isozymes,[94,250] of which β and γ are the most common[250,251] in neutrophils. In neutrophils, PKC is located in the cytoplasm of resting cells and is redistributed to the plasma membrane following cell activation, as monitored by PMA binding, enzymatic, and immunologic activities.[252]

While implicated in neutrophil signal transduction, protein kinases play an undetermined role in responses. A strong case can be made for protein kinase C (PKC), since this enzyme can be activated by DAGs derived from the hydrolysis of phospholipids.[184,222] This is consistent with the observation that synthetic DAGs also activate neutrophils by interacting with the same intracellular receptor as PMA.[253] The close correlation between the activation of PKC and neutrophil functions, and the synergy between PKC agonists and other stimuli, have suggested a role for this enzyme in stimulus-response coupling.[254]

The inability of PKC inhibitors[255,256] to block neutrophil activation in response to several physiologic stimuli suggests that PKC activation is not a necessary requirement for cell activation. In permeabilized neutrophils, no definitive role for PKC has been found with respect to degranulation.[257,258] A direct role for PKC in degranulation can be excluded under certain circumstances.[257] Indeed, neutrophils contain other kinases that may be involved in cell activation.[259,260] There is growing evidence for the involvement of proteolytically modified PKC,[261] cGMP-dependent kinases,[262] tyrosine kinases,[194,263–265] H4 histone kinases,[266] and phosphatases[259,264,265] in signal transduction. In addition, there is evidence that DAGs, particularly the 1-O-alkyl variety formed from PC, have other properties,[267] independent of PKC activation, that can lead to cell stimulation.

Other kinases activated by low molecular weight G-proteins, particularly *src* and p21, are also involved in stimulus-response coupling.[268,269] The JAK-STAT sequence, common to other cells of immune import, has recently been reported.[270] However, the greatest concentration of research has revolved around the microtubule-associated protein kinases (MAPK) and the multiple kinases in that cascade.[271,272] Such kinases have been implicated in adhesion-related signaling,[273] particularly through L-selectins.[272] Adhesive function in signaling through integrins has been shown to involve *src* kinases,[274] *syk*,[275] and tyrosine phosphorylation.[276] Of particular interest to this topic is the finding that neutrophil stimulation leads to phosphorylation of PLA_2.[204] This enzyme appears to be regulated by the p42/p44 MAPK pathway.[205,277] In macrophages, both MAPK and Ca^{2+} regulate PLA_2 activation in response to most stimuli.[278] It is likely that phosphorylation and activation of enzymes such as PLA_2 are vital in regulating degranulation and membrane fusion.

ARACHIDONATE METABOLISM

In addition to their participation as putative second messenger products in the stimulus-response coupling pathway, many lipid metabolites may be released from stimulated neutrophils and in turn modulate cell function by interacting with receptors on other neutrophils. Phospholipase A_2, present on both the granules and plasma membranes of neutrophils[279] as well as the cytosol,[280] is activated during neutrophil stimulation,[185] yielding arachidonic acid as one of the major end products. Arachidonic acid is not only released from stimulated neutrophils,[281] but also serves as a regulator of PLA_2 activity[282] and as a stimulus for these cells.[283] Sensitivity of the cells to stimuli (priming) can be obtained with arachidonic acid and other long-chain fatty acids.[284] Recently, arachidonic acid has been reported to be a mediator in the stimulation of a H^+ pump that is associated with NADPH oxidase.[285] This fatty acid can regulate other aspects of signal transduction, such as intracellular Ca^{2+} handling.[284,286]

In addition to directly affecting cell function, metabolites of arachidonic acid, generated through either the cyclooxygenase or lipoxygenase pathways, may also stimulate neutrophils. The most potent cyclooxygenase product of activated neutrophils is thromboxane B_2, which, in addition to its vasoconstrictor activity, may also enhance neutrophil chemotaxis,[287] aggregation,[288] and adhesiveness.[289]

Arachidonic acid can also be metabolized by the lipoxygenase pathway to produce hydroxyeicosatetraenoic acids (HETEs), including 5-HETE, 12-HETE, and 5,12-diHETE.[290,291] These compounds have also been shown to induce several neutrophil responses.[292,293] Stimulated neutrophils also produce the diHETE LTB_4 through the lipoxygenase pathway. LTB_4 and other leukotrienes can be released in response to a variety of stimuli.[294] Receptors for LTB_4 have been partially purified,[164,295] and their activation serves as a potent stimulus for degranulation,[296] chemotaxis[297] and adherence.[297]

Another potent mediator of inflammation produced by stimulated neutrophils is 1-*O*-alkyl-2-acetyl-*sn*-glyceryl-3-phosphoryl choline, also known as platelet-activating factor (PAF).[298] Not only is PAF synthesized by neutrophils and activated endothelial cells,[22] but it has been shown to induce degranulation,[299,300] aggregation[299] and superoxide generation.[300]

CYTOSKELETON

The role played by microfilaments in degranulation is suggested by the observation that in resting neutrophils, the granules are separated from the plasma membrane by filament-rich hyaline ectoplasm.[301] As already discussed, surface stimulation of the cell leads to an increased mobilization of Ca^{2+}, particularly in the periphery[6,302]; this increase in

cytosolic Ca^{2+} would be expected to activate gelsolin, thereby shortening actin filaments and decreasing the viscosity in this area.[303] Indeed, it has long been observed that stimulation leads to such rearrangements of microfilaments and their regulatory proteins.[304–306] A decrease in viscosity of the hyaline ectoplasm could permit the granules to have access to the inner surface of the plasma membrane, thereby facilitating degranulation. The well-known ability of cytochalasins to enhance secretion[307] and block locomotion[308] is consonant with this model, since these alkaloids can split actin filaments.[309]

The enhanced turnover of microfilaments following stimulation of neutrophils is also manifested biochemically. The amount of actin associated with detergent-insoluble cytoskeleton fractions increases,[305,310] as does the amount of filamentous actin (F-actin).[311] This cytoskeletal network has been visualized with high-voltage electron microscopy.[312] When a chemotactic peptide is used as the stimulus, these changes in cytoskeletal actin may be associated with the clearance of receptor-ligand complexes,[132,310,313] probably by endocytosis. Using techniques suitable for monitoring short-term kinetics, it was shown that polymerization commences within the first few seconds following stimulation and may thus conceivably play some role in stimulus-response coupling.[314,315]

Recent observations indicate that this response by microfilaments is one of the earliest and most fundamental of neutrophil reactions to surface stimuli. Cell shape and F-actin content oscillate in individual neutrophils,[314,316–318] as does intracellular Ca^{2+},[221] suggesting that the two responses are closely connected. Other evidence supports this conclusion.[319] Yet compelling studies have shown that F-actin and intracellular Ca^{2+} can be completely dissociated.[244,320,321]

Also, while actin assembly is generally mediated through G-proteins,[322,323] fewer active G-proteins are required for F-actin assembly than for most other responses.[316,324] Other recent investigations have focused on various pools of intracellular actins,[303,325] regulatory interactions with actin-binding proteins,[303,323,325–327] and the relationship of actin assembly to other neutrophil responses,[328] particularly phosphatidylinositol metabolism.[329] There is increasing evidence that polyphosphoinositides are involved in anchoring microfilaments to the plasma membrane as well as in regulating their integrity.[330,331] Also, stimulation of cell surface receptors often leads to subsequent interactions of these receptors and signal transduction proteins with elements of the cytoskeleton.[269,332] The possible role of other cytoskeletal proteins, such as fodrin,[333] vinculin,[327] and vimentin,[262] are now being appreciated. While microtubules have long been studied in neutrophils, their roles are not clear, although research continues.[334,335]

CYCLIC NUCLEOTIDES

Exposure of neutrophils to phagocytizable particles results in a rapid doubling of cyclic adenosine 3′,5′-monophosphate (cAMP) levels.[336–338] This increment is prompt (maximal within 15 s) and brief (returning to basal levels in 1–2 min). Such a rapid response, which is comparable to the earliest changes in neutrophil biochemistry and physiology, could possibly play a role in stimulus-response coupling. During the same time interval, no changes in cGMP levels are observed.[336,337] The observations that changes in cAMP levels correlate closely with chemotaxis and degranulation,[338] display specific desensitization after repeated exposures to the same stimulus, and that this desensitization is accompanied by a parallel decrease in O_2^- generation,[339] suggest that changes in cyclic nucleotide levels are of mechanistic significance. However, a number of lines of evidence suggest that changes in cAMP are neither necessary[340] nor sufficient[82,336,338] for neutrophil responses in suspension. These findings seem to rule out cAMP in a second messenger role. However, redistribution of cAMP (without concomitant elevated levels) could still be of mechanistic significance, as immunochemical observations of cAMP show it to be localized near forming phagosomes.[341]

Recent work has uncovered the biochemistry leading to these rapid increases in cAMP content. Stimulated neutrophils release adenosine, which can bind to cell surface purine receptors, and which amplify adenylate cyclase activity.[342] Thus, this response is outside of the mainstream of signal transduction pathways. But cAMP produced within the cells can still modulate other cellular responses and signals,[343-346] particularly those mediated by phospholipases.[344,345] cAMP-dependent protein kinase (PKA) appears to regulate a number of responses, including the respiratory burst,[347] motility,[348] and apoptosis.[349] Signal transduction steps, such as PKC and tyrosine kinases,[347,350] interact with PKA as well. Finally, there is growing evidence that cGMP-dependent protein kinases can modulate the neutrophil cytoskeleton.[351]

DEGRANULATION AND MEMBRANE FUSION

In stimulated cells, the signal transduction cascade activates G-proteins, followed by enhanced intracellular Ca^{2+}, lipid remodeling, and protein kinase activation. These events culminate in secretion. This ultimate event, the fusion of granule membranes with phagosomes or the plasma membrane (with the accompanying discharge of granule contents and expression of granule membrane components on the cell surface), is coming under increased scrutiny because of its scientific and clinical importance. Degranulation is very rapid[352] and apparently highly efficient, since intracellular liberation of granule contents has not been reported. This efficiency and rapidity have not yet been demonstrated with in vitro systems, hindering our comprehension of degranulation.

CALCIUM

As discussed above, the importance of elevated free Ca^{2+} levels in degranulation has been directly demonstrated in permeabilized neutrophils.[174,175,235,352,353] How might this divalent cation mediate fusion? At the most primitive level, Ca^{2+} may promote membrane fusion intracellularly through its interactions with the negatively charged head groups of membrane phospholipids.[354,355] Other metal cations and polylysine have been shown to induce aggregation and fusion of phospholipid vesicles in a pH-dependent fashion.[354,355] The pH-dependence of fusion may be related to the ability of hydrogen ions to provide a charge-neutralizing effect.[356] Thus, Ca^{2+} may change the physical properties of granules and membranes in such a way as to allow them to come into close apposition.[357] Ca^{2+} may likewise interact with proteins to regulate fusion. As outlined above, Ca^{2+} can activate phospholipase A_2[278] (which can liberate membrane-fluidizing fatty acids). Alternatively, Ca^{2+} may regulate the interactions of annexins with phospholipids.

ANNEXINS

Annexins, which include synexin and the lipocortins, are defined functionally as Ca^{2+}-dependent, phospholipid-binding proteins and structurally as proteins that share a conserved four-repeat, 70 amino acid sequence. Several annexins have been detected in neutrophils[358-360] that also have Ca^{2+}-dependent aggregating and fusion-promoting activity.[359-361] These annexins bind neutrophil membranes and granules.[200,362,363] Lipocortins I and II promote fusion of liposomes.[361] By themselves, these annexins require high (millimolar) concentrations of Ca^{2+} to promote fusion. But they need not work alone, and it has been shown that annexin I functions synergistically with phospholipases to promote membrane apposition and fusion.[200] Peptides derived from the N-terminus of annexin I also inhibit degranulation,[364] suggesting a critical role for this protein. Others attempted to deplete annexins

from permeabilized neutrophils.[365] However, 41 percent of annexin I and 12 percent of annexin III were retained within the cells, along with most of the ability to degranulate. Restoration of these annexins also restored additional degranulation, suggesting that annexins I and III are important in secretion.

LIPIDS

Many of the lipid products that have been linked to degranulation in stimulated neutrophils are known to be fusogenic. For example, incubating Ca^{2+}- and PLA_2-treated chromaffin cell plasma membrane with chromaffin granules causes the release of granule contents,[366] and cis-unsaturated fatty acids have been shown to induce the fusion of chromaffin granules aggregated by synexin and Ca^{2+}.[367] Of considerable interest are reports that DAGs, produced in stimulated neutrophils, can affect fusion.[368] Furthermore, fusion may be modulated by asymmetric transmembrane distributions of phospholipids.[369] The radii of curvature associated with the individual lipid components may also be important in progressing from semi-fused states (hemi-fusion) to complete fusion.[370] Finally, sphingolipid metabolites are proving to have profound effects of liposome leakage and fusion.[371] These data show that the physicochemical properties of lipids can greatly influence membrane fusion.

Phospholipase A_2 may be particularly important in degranulation. It was reported in 1980 that the PLA_2 inhibitor BPB blocks degranulation by neutrophils.[372] Inhibition of this enzyme also arrests phagocytosis and disrupts vesicle trafficking in monocytes.[373] While inhibitor studies must be interpreted with caution, these data suggest that PLA_2 might be involved in membrane fusion. Indeed, PLA_2 greatly enhances fusion of liposomes constructed to resemble biological membranes, lowering Ca^{2+} thresholds for fusion over 100-fold.[374] PLA_2 also augments fusion of these plasma membrane-like liposomes with each other and with specific granules isolated from neutrophils.[374] Thus, there is good evidence for a vital role of PLA_2 in neutrophil degranulation.

FUSION PROTEINS

Over the past decade, the SNARE hypothesis has become the reigning paradigm for fusion of biomembranes. Thanks to the early development of unambiguous contents-mixing assays, researchers studying a number of fusion systems (such as endosomes, Golgi, and synaptosomes) were able to readily identify and reconstitute the vital components. These systems are widespread, being found virtually complete in a wide range of species and tissues. They are centered around a protein that is sensitive to N-ethyl maleimide (designated ''NEM-sensitive fusion protein'' or NSF), several soluble NSF-attachment proteins (SNAP), and ''SNAP-receptors'' (SNAREs) on the participating membranes. The SNAREs are termed the v-SNAREs and t-SNAREs—v-SNAREs being found on vesicles or granules and the t-SNAREs being found on the target plasma membranes. This SNARE system has been the subject of many excellent reviews,[375] and will not be described in detail here.

The SNARE hypothesis has proven to have great predictive value, as the constellation of fusion proteins and their interactions appears in almost all species and tissues. However, it has gradually become apparent that some cell types possess incomplete sets of proteins; indeed, it has been proposed that such an incomplete set (called SNAREpins and consisting of VAMP, syntaxin, and SNAP-25) might be functionally sufficient.[376] There is increasing evidence that the fusion proteins operating in cells of the myeloid lineage are substantially different from those in neurons. For example, vesicle-associated membrane protein-2 (VAMP-2) has been detected in neutrophils and HL-60 cells using molecular techniques.[377] VAMP-2 in addition to syntaxin-4 and secretory carrier membrane protein (SCAMP) were detected in neutrophils by Western blot.[378] Syntaxin-4 and SCAMP are nonneuronal. These investigators also reported that they were unable to find the classical neuronal components syntaxin-1, VAMP-1, SNAP-25, synaptophysin, and cellubrevin. Another research group did find SNAP-25 protein, but it was on the "wrong" vesicle (granule membrane rather than plasma membrane).[379] Human neutrophils and HL-60 cells have been reported to have two forms of SNAP-23,[380] based on molecular studies. SNAP-23 is nonneuronal, and these researchers found that mRNA for this protein, unlike VAMP-2,[377] increased during differentiation of HL-60 cells. Interestingly, those components that have been detected in neutrophils and HL-60 cells, namely VAMP-2, syntaxin-4, and SNAP-23,[25] are homologues of the SNAREpin set.[376] Thus, the proteins and lipids responsible for degranulation in neutrophils are yet to be elucidated.

BACTERICIDAL MECHANISMS

NONOXIDATIVE MECHANISMS

From the information presented in Section III, it should be apparent that neutrophil granules contain a wide variety of materials that possess bacterial activity. Such compounds include the degradative enzymes, lipases, proteases, and glycosidases as well as the more specialized antibacterial defensins and cationic proteins.[381] Indeed, crude preparations of neutrophil granules themselves have been shown to possess substantial bactericidal activity in vitro.[382] The bactericidal armamentarium is sufficiently broad to permit relatively efficient killing in the absence of an oxidative burst, such as is found under anaerobic conditions[383] or in cells from patients with chronic granulomatous disease.[384,385] The effects of cationic proteins on ingested bacteria are enhanced by increases in phagosomal acidity[386]; this decline in pH following phagocytosis[387] may be due to both the acidity of the fusing azurophil granules[387-389] and to ion pumps. Many cationic proteins and defensins involved in killing have been isolated and cloned.[390-394] Proteases on the surface membrane, as well as those found in the granules, may be involved in cytolysis.[395]

Lysozyme, which hydrolyzes cell wall proteoglycan of some bacterial species, and lactoferrin, which sequesters the iron required for bacterial growth, must be considered as part of the nonoxidative arsenal of neutrophils.[51] These agents, along with the cationic proteins found primarily in azurophil granules, would be expected to be most potent when confined to the phagolysosome. However, it is also likely that such compounds, even when released from dead neutrophils, could perform as systemic antibiotics. Furthermore, cationic proteins could function as opsonins in the extracellular space.[396] The next three sections describe general classes of these microbicidal proteins.

DEFENSINS

Of the various cationic antibacterial proteins found in neutrophils, the defensins are the most common and of the lowest molecular weight. These proteins are less than 4 kDa in weight, consisting of 29-33 amino acids, and constitute from 5 to 8 percent of the total cellular protein.[31,33,36] The defensins have attracted much research interest, and the major forms have been isolated and cloned[391,397]; the precursor molecules have also been investigated.[398] Like other azurophil granule constituents, they can be released to the extracellular space following stimulation.[37,399] If released into the cytoplasm of the cell, the defensins could modify signal transduction by inhibiting PKC[400] and by inhibiting NADPH oxidase.[401] The defensins have an unusual cyclic structure and appear to kill bacteria by disrupting their outer membranes[402]; however, they can also induce single-strand DNA breaks in target cells.[403] There are even reports that defensins are chemotactic for phagocytes.[404]

CAP37 FAMILY

This group of neutrophil cationic proteins, which includes cathepsin G and azurocidin in addition to CAP37, shares considerable sequence homology to other inflammatory proteases.[33,392,405,406] CAP37 is both bactericidal and chemotactic.[33,405,407] An azurophil granule localization also appears likely for this protein.[407] Once outside the neutrophil, it can stimulate PKC activity in endothelial cells.[408] However, it has been reported that acidification of the phagolysosome can promote the antimicrobial action of CAP37.[386] The antimicrobial and chemotactic activities of the CAP37 family are becoming better defined.[409]

BPI FAMILY

Bactericidal/permeability-increasing protein (BPI), a cationic protein that lyses gram-negative bacteria, belongs to a family that includes CAP57 and lipopolysaccharide binding protein.[33] These activities have been localized to particular populations of the azurophil granules.[38,393,410] The activity of BPI has been shown to reside in the amino terminus of the molecule[411,412]; this region is both cationic and amphipathic.[390] Like the defensins, members of the BPI family have been shown to disrupt the bacterial membranes.[413] Most members of this family have also been isolated and cloned.[390,414] BPI itself has been shown to bind LPS, and may hence serve to buffer the serum concentration of this potent inflammatory mediator.[410,411] Furthermore, the activity of BPI itself is modulated by some low molecular weight proteins (p15s) that are themselves antimicrobial.[394,415]

ADDITIONAL ANTIBACTERIAL PROTEINS

A number of novel microbicidal agents have recently been reported in neutrophils. Bactonectin, a dodecapeptide antibiotic, has been isolated and described.[416,417] In addition to its bactericidal activity, indolicin features five tryptophan residues out of 13 amino acids,[418] giving it the highest observed mole concentration among known protein sequences. A proline/arginine-rich antibacterial (and chemotactic) peptide related to PR39 has been recently described.[419] Some additional low molecular weight proteins have been found in guinea pig cells.[420]

Most interesting of all is an extremely abundant, cytosolic, Ca^{2+}-binding protein known as L1 or MRP8/MRP14[421,422] that is a major component of pus. Initially, its very low molecular weight subunit structure hindered its detection by investigators. Its antimicrobial activity has led to the name calprotectin.[421] As a cytosolic protein, MRP8/MRP14 is subject to the action of PKC[423] and is translocated to the plasma membrane and cytoskeleton following stimulation.[424]

OXIDATIVE METABOLISM

OXIDATIVE BACTERICIDAL ACTIVITY

Activated neutrophils produce several antimicrobial oxygen metabolites, including superoxide anion (O_2^-), H_2O_2, hydroxyl radicals (OH·), hypochlorous acid (HOCl), and singlet oxygen. Even chlorine gas has been detected.[425] Substantial evidence indicates that these reactive metabolites are generated by a nicotinamide adenine dinucleotide phosphate (NADPH)-dependent oxidase, located on the plasma membrane, which reduces molecular oxygen to O_2^- (Fig. 67-5). The oxidase is quiescent in resting neutrophils and is stimulated following neutrophil activation. The importance of the NADPH-oxidase to the bactericidal capacity of the cell is demonstrated in individuals with chronic granulomatous disease (CGD) whose neutrophils fail to generate O_2^- and related metabolites. This is a genetic disorder in which neutrophils and monocytes ingest, but do not kill, catalase-positive microorganisms. Neutrophils of CDG patients do kill pneumococci or streptococci, which do not contain catalase; these organisms generate enough H_2O_2 which, together with myeloperoxidase delivered into the phagosomes by degranulation, kills them. *Staphylococcus aureus* is

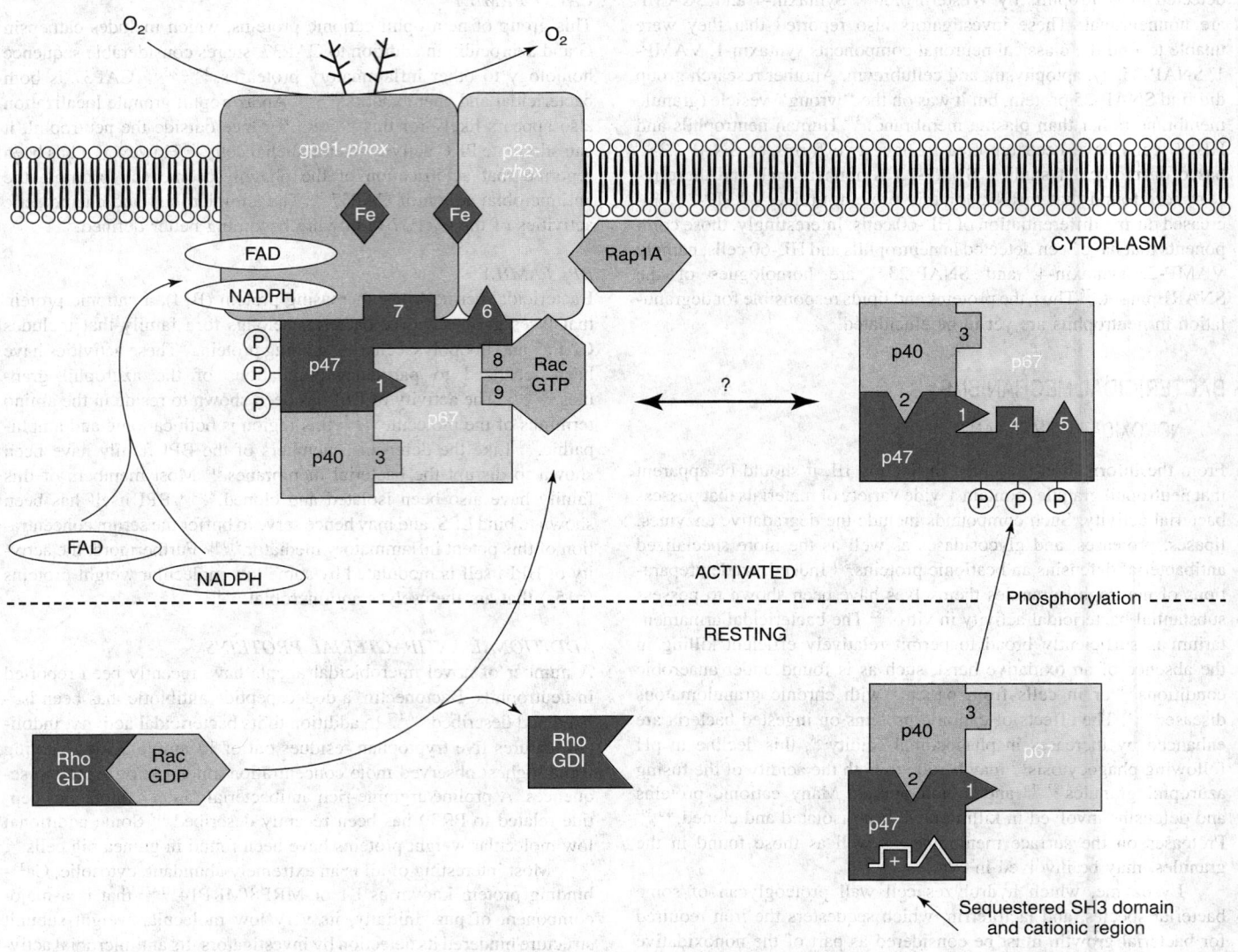

FIGURE 67-5   Possible mechanisms for the production of superoxide anion in polymorphonuclear leukocytes. Oxygen is reduced to superoxide (O_2^-) by an NADPH oxidase. The oxidase appears to be a composite of (1) a 47-kDa cytosolic protein (p47); (2) a 67-kDa cytosolic protein (p67); (3) a 40-kDa cytosolic protein (p40); (4) one or more low molecular weight cytosolic G-proteins, such as Rac1 and Rap1A; and (5) a membrane-bound cytochrome b-558. Cytochrome b consists of a 22 kDa protein subunit and a 91-kDa glycoprotein subunit, both of which contain heme. The gp91 subunit is an FAD-dependent flavoprotein which contains the NADPH binding site and ultimately shuttles electrons to molecular oxygen, forming O_2^-. The cytosol components have also been reported to translocate to the membrane and may serve to alter the tertiary structure of cytochrome b, to permit the flow of electrons from NADPH to O_2. The p47 subunit can be phosphorylated to various extents, but the significance of this phosphorylation is unclear. The low molecular weight G-protein is also important in stabilizing the oxidase complex. (This figure is reproduced with permission from DeLeo, F.R. and Quinn, M.T. Assembly of the phagocyte NADPH oxidase: Molecular interaction of oxidase proteins. *J Leukocyte Biol* 60(6):677–691, 1996.)

the most common pathogen in this disorder, although any catalase-positive organism may be involved. Chap. 82 provides a more complete review of the disorders of neutrophil function.

THE CELL-FREE NADPH-DEPENDENT OXIDASE SYSTEM

Considerable attention has been given to the molecular factors underlying activation of the NADPH-oxidase, and multiple pathways appear to exist. Stimulation of the oxidase enzyme results in the generation of O_2^- after a lag period of several seconds,[426] thus allowing sufficient time for the intervention of many of the aforementioned biochemical events in the activation pathway. Studies conducted in intact cells have been extended to broken cells. Cell-free oxidase activity was first reported in homogenates from resting guinea pig peritoneal macro-

phages.[427] Activation of the NADPH-oxidase from macrophages requires both particulate and soluble fractions and certain unsaturated fatty acids or anionic detergents.[428] Cell-free oxidase activity has also been obtained from neutrophil homogenates and appears to have similar requirements.[429] The oxidase has also recently been fully solubilized from neutrophil membranes and displays kinetic properties similar to the oxidase of intact cells.[430] In some forms of autosomal recessive CGD, one or another of the cytosolic factors has been found to be defective.[431] Studies employing this system proved valuable in characterizing the mechanism(s) underlying activation of the NADPH-dependent oxidase.[432] The next section will detail the advances made in understanding the oxidase, advances that are directly attributable to the development of the in vitro assay system.

COMPONENTS OF THE NADPH-DEPENDENT OXIDASE

The biochemistry of the NADPH oxidase has come under intense scrutiny in recent years. The oxidase appears to be a composite of (1) a 47-kDa cytosolic protein, termed "p47-*phox*," where "*phox*" refers to "phagocyte oxidase"[433-435]; (2) a 67-kDa cytosolic protein, termed "p67-*phox*"[433,435]; (3) two low molecular weight cytosolic G-proteins, identified variously as *rac*1/2 (rac2 in human neutrophils) and *rap*1A[436,437]; (4) a 40-kDa protein, termed "p40-*phox*"[438]; and (5) a membrane-bound cytochrome b-558,[439-441] which is an FAD-dependent flavoprotein.[440,442] (The designation "b-558" is based on spectral properties. The cytochrome is also termed "b-245" on the basis of electrochemical potential.) The cytosolic constituents are believed to activate an electron transport chain in cytochrome b, which serves to ferry electrons from NADPH at the binding site, through a flavin prosthetic group (FAD), and finally to molecular oxygen, forming superoxide.[443,444] NADPH is subsequently regenerated through the hexose monophosphate shunt (Fig. 67-5).[445] That these constituents may indeed be intrinsic to the oxidase has been recognized in studies utilizing neutrophils from individuals with the genetic disorder CGD. Patients with the X-linked form of the disease lack cytochrome b[442,445-447] and contain reduced levels of flavoprotein.[442,445,446] Levels of both oxidase components are normal in patients with the autosomally transmitted form,[442,446] but the enzyme cannot be activated[448,449] due to dysfunctions of either p47-*phox* or p67-*phox*.

The subcellular localization of the NADPH-oxidase as well as its mechanism of activation have been disputed. Cytochrome b consists of a 22-kDa protein subunit and a 91-kDa glycoprotein subunit,[447,450,451] both of which contain heme.[452] The 91-kDa subunit is missing in X-linked CGD, and the 22-kDa subunit is missing in a very rare form of autosomal recessive CGD.[447,453] The well-known flavoprotein component[454,455] and NADPH binding site have recently been attributed to the b cytochrome.[60,61,455] This cytochrome has been reported to be distributed between the plasma membrane and the membranes of cytoplasmic granules in resting cells.[62,70,439,456-458] Stimulation results in the translocation of the cytochrome from granule fractions to the plasma membrane.[62,457,459] Based on these observations, several investigators have advanced the hypothesis that the granules are involved in activation of the oxidase.[445,458,459] However, the relevance of the translocation phenomenon to oxidase activation is obscure.[457,458] The cytosol components have also been reported to translocate to the membrane[460,461] and may serve to alter the tertiary structure of cytochrome b, to permit the flow of electrons from NADPH to O_2. Following assembly, the entire oxidase complex is associated with the cytoskeleton.[462]

The oxidase components assemble in a sequential fashion. Using the b cytochrome on the membrane as a nucleus, the oxidase complex assembles first with p47-*phox*.[460,461] The p67-*phox* then binds to the p47-*phox* moiety,[460] which then alters the cytochrome b to allow binding of NADPH.[61] The low molecular weight G-protein rac2 serves to stabilize this complex.[461,463-465] Another low molecular weight G-protein, rap1A, appears to be associated with the b cytochrome.[437,464,466] Other soluble oxidase components are also suspected[467]; however, these other components can only play modulatory roles since the oxidase has been reconstituted using recombinant p47-*phox*, p67-*phox*, b cytochrome, and *rac*1[436,468] or *rac*2 (in humans).[465] Absence of either p47-*phox* or p67-*phox* leads to CGD (see Chap. 82). An accessory role is likely for p40-*phox*, which associates with both p47-*phox* and p67-*phox* via SH3 and PC motifs.[438,469,470] The role of protein kinases in oxidase activation is still unclear. On one hand, in whole neutrophils[471] and in the reconstituted system,[472] several PKC inhibitors are ineffective in abolishing stimulus-induced activation of the oxidase. Furthermore, the "requirement" for ATP noted by some investigators actually reflects the GTP requirement for the low molecular weight G-protein.[473] On the other hand, p47-*phox* can be phosphorylated to various ex-

tents,[474] and the amount of phosphorylation is correlated with translocation of the oxidase components[475-477] and with oxidase activity[476,478,479]; however, in some cases, hyperphosphorylation results in inhibition.[480] A variety of protein kinases[481] may be involved in phosphorylating p47-*phox*, including PKC,[482,483] PKA,[483] MAP kinase,[483] p38,[484] ERK,[484] proline-directed kinases,[485] and other novel kinases.[486,487] In fact, the in vitro oxidase system can be activated by PKC[488] or by a phosphatidic acid–regulated protein kinase.[489] The various phosphorylation sites on p47-*phox* have been extensively mapped and the essential serine residues identified.[479,490] Even p67-*phox* is phosphorylated during neutrophil activation, by both PKC and other enzymes.[491] Phosphorylation of the *rap*1A oxidase protein can actually inhibit activity.[466] The b cytochrome may also be phosphorylated,[492] but the significance of this is unclear. Finally, there also appears to be a role for phosphatidic acid and diacylglycerols in oxidase assembly.[493,494]

A final aspect of the oxidase is its ubiquity. Components of the phagocyte oxidase, or their homologues, can be found in a wide variety of tissues. For example, the full oxidase complex can be found in B lymphocytes[495] and the only reason for low enzymatic activity in those cells is a transcriptional block in the synthesis of B cytochrome.[496] A fully active oxidase complex has also been found in fibroblasts[497] and keratinocytes.[498] Even plants can generate H_2O_2 and have proteins immunologically related to p47-*phox* and p67-*phox*.[499]

REFERENCES

1. Mudd J, McCutcheon M, Lucke B: Phagocytosis. *Physiol Rev* 14:210, 1934.
2. Zigmond SH: Ability of polymorphonuclear leukocytes to orient in gradients of chemotactic factors. *J Cell Biol* 75:606, 1977.
3. Foxman EF, Campbell JJ, Butcher EC: Multistep navigation and the combinatorial control of leukocyte chemotaxis. *J Cell Biol* 139:1349, 1997.
4. Quitt M, Torres M, McGuire W, et al: Neutrophil chemotactic heterogeneity to *N*-formyl-methionyl-leucyl-phenylalanine detected by the under-agarose assay. *J Lab Clin Med* 115:159, 1990.
5. Lee J, Gustafsson M, Magnusson K-E, Jacobson K: The direction of membrane lipid flow in locomoting polymorphonuclear leukocytes. *Science* 247:1229, 1990.
6. Marks PW, Maxfield FR: Local and global changes in cytosolic free calcium in neutrophils during chemotaxis and phagocytosis. *Cell Calcium* 11:181, 1990.
7. Stendahl O, Krause K-H, Krischer J, et al: Redistribution of intracellular Ca^{2+} stores during phagocytosis in human neutrophils. *Science* 265:1439, 1994.
8. Kuijpers TW, Hoogerwerf M, Roos D: Neutrophil migration across monolayers of resting or cytokine-activated endothelial cells: Role of intracellular calcium changes and fusion of specific granules with the plasma membrane. *J Immunol* 148:72, 1992.
9. Bray D, White JG: Cortical flow in animal cells. *Science* 239:883, 1988.
10. Frank RS: Time-dependent alterations in the deformability of human neutrophils in response to chemotactic activation. *Blood* 76:2606, 1990.
11. Simon SI, Schmid Schonbein GW: Biophysical aspects of microsphere engulfment by human neutrophils. *Biophys J* 53:163, 1988.
12. Berlin RD, Fera JP, Pfeiffer FR: Reversible phagocytosis in rabbit polymorphonuclear leukocytes. *J Clin Invest* 63:1137, 1979.
13. Furie MB, Tancinco MCA, Smith CW: Monoclonal antibodies to leukocyte integrins CD11a/CD18 and CD11b/CD18 or intercellular adhesion molecule-1 inhibit chemoattractant-stimulated neutrophil transendothelial migration in vitro. *Blood* 78:2089, 1991.
14. Schmalstieg FC, Rudloff HE, Hillman GR, Anderson DC: Two-dimensional and three-dimensional movement of human polymorphonuclear leukocytes: two fundamentally different mechanisms of location. *J Leuk Biol* 40:677, 1986.
15. Wright SD, Silverstein SC: Phagocytosing macrophages exclude proteins from the zones of contact with opsonized targets. *Nature* 309:359, 1984.
16. Henricks PAJ, Van der Tol ME, Verhoef J: Aggregation of human

polymorphonuclear leucocytes during phagocytosis of bacteria. *Immunology* 52:671, 1984.

17. Lawrence MB, Springer TA: Leukocytes roll on a selectin at physiologic flow rates: distinction from and prerequisite for adhesion through integrins. *Cell* 65:859, 1991.

18. Smith CW, Marlin SD, Rothlein R, et al: Cooperative interactions of LFA-1 and Mac-1 with intercellular adhesion molecule-1 in facilitating adherence and transendothelial migration of human neutrophils in vitro. *J Clin Invest* 83:2008, 1989.

19. Kishimoto TK, Jutila MA, Berg EL, Butcher EC: Neutrophil Mac-1 and MEL-14 adhesion proteins inversely regulated by chemotactic factors. *Science* 245:1238, 1989.

20. Mrowietz U, Schroder J-M, Brasch J, Christophers E: Infiltrating neutrophils differ from circulating neutrophils when stimulated with C5a, NAP-1/IL-8, LTB₄ and FMLP. *Scand J Immunol* 35:71, 1992.

21. Fehr J, Huber A: Complement-induced granulocyte adhesion and aggregation are mediated by different factors: evidence for non-equivalence of the two cell functions. *Immunology* 53:583, 1984.

22. Zimmerman GA, Prescott SM, McIntyre TM: Endothelial cell interactions with granulocytes: tethering and signaling molecules. *Immunol Today* 13:93, 1992.

23. Hammer DA, Apte SM: Simulation of cell rolling and adhesion on surfaces in shear flow: General results and analysis of selectin-mediated neutrophil adhesion. *Biophys J* 63:35, 1992.

24. Huber AR, Kunkel SL, Todd RF III, Weiss SJ: Regulation of transendothelial neutrophil migration by endogenous interleukin-8. *Science* 254:99, 1991.

25. Simon SI, Chambers JD, Butcher E, Sklar LA: Neutrophil aggregation is β₂-integrin- and L-selectin-dependent in blood and isolated cells. *J Immunol* 149:2765, 1992.

26. Kishimoto TK, Hollander N, Roberts RM, et al: Heterogeneous mutations in the B subunit common to the LFA-1, Mac-1 and p150,95 glycoproteins cause leukocyte adhesion deficiency. *Cell* 50:193, 1987.

27. Karsan A, Cornejo CJ, Winn RK, et al: Leukocyte adhesion deficiency Type II is a generalized defect of de novo GDP-fucose biosynthesis. Endothelial cell fucosylation is not required for neutrophil rolling on human nonlymphoid endothelium. *J Clin Invest* 101:2438, 1998.

28. Anderson DC, Miller LJ, Schmalstieg FC, et al: Contributions of the Mac-1 glycoprotein family to adherence-dependent granulocyte functions: Structure-function assessments employing subunit-specific monoclonal antibodies. *J Immunol* 137:15, 1986.

29. Weiss SJ: Tissue destruction by neutrophils. *N Engl J Med* 320:365, 1989.

30. Le Cabec V, Cowland JB, Calafat J, Borregaard N: Targeting of proteins to granule subsets is determined by timing and not by sorting: The specific granule protein NGAL is localized to azurophil granules when expressed in HL-60 cells. *Proc Natl Acad Sci USA* 93:6454, 1996.

31. Selsted ME, Harwig SSL, Ganz T, et al: Primary structures of three human neutrophil defensins. *J Clin Invest* 76:1436, 1985.

32. West BC, Rosenthal AS, Gelb NA, Kimball HR: Separation and characterization of human neutrophil granules. *Am J Pathol* 77:41, 1974.

33. Spitznagel JK: Antibiotic proteins of human neutrophils. *J Clin Invest* 86:1381, 1990.

34. Garcia RC, Peterson CG, Segal AW, Venge P: Elastase in the different primary granules of the human neutrophil. *Biochem Biophys Res Comm* 132:1130, 1985.

35. Egesten A, Breton-Gorius J, Guichard J, et al: The heterogeneity of azurophil granules in neutrophil promyelocytes: Immunogold localization of myeloperoxidase, cathepsin G, elastase, proteinase 3, and bactericidal/permeability increasing protein. *Blood* 83:2985, 1994.

36. Ganz T, Selsted ME, Szklarek D, et al: Defensins. Natural peptide antibiotics of human neutrophils. *J Clin Invest* 76:1427, 1985.

37. Ganz T: Extracellular release of antimicrobial defensins by human polymorphonuclear leukocytes. *Infect Immun* 55:568, 1987.

38. Weiss J, Olsson I: Cellular and subcellular localization of the bactericidal/permeability-increasing protein of neutrophils. *Blood* 69:652, 1987.

39. Tauber AI, Borregaard N, Simons E, Wright J: Chronic granulomatous disease: A syndrome of phagocyte oxidase deficiencies. *Medicine* 62:286, 1983.

40. Clark RA: Chemotactic factors trigger their own oxidative inactivation by human neutrophils. *J Immunol* 129:2725, 1982.

41. Stendahl O, Coble BI, Dahlgren C, et al: Myeloperoxidase modulates the phagocytic activity of polymorphonuclear neutrophil leukocytes. Studies with cells from a myeloperoxidase-deficient patient. *J Clin Invest* 73:366, 1984.

42. Ohlsson K: Granulocyte collagenase and elastase and their interactions with alpha₁-antitrypsin and alpha₂-macroglobulin, in *Proteases and Biological Control,* edited by D Reich, DB Rifkin, E Shaw, pp 591–602. Cold Spring Harbor Lab, Cold Spring Harbor, NY, 1975.

43. Virca GD, Metz G, Schnebli HP: Similarities between human and rat leukocyte elastase and cathepsin G. *Eur J Biochem* 144:1, 1984.

44. Movat HZ, Steinberg SG, Flavio M, et al: Demonstration of a kinin-generating enzyme in the lysosomes of human polymorphonuclear leukocytes. *Lab Invest* 29:669, 1973.

45. Ward PA, Hill JH: C5 chemotactic fragments produced by an enzyme in lysosomal granules of neutrophils. *J Immunol* 104:535, 1970.

46. Murphy G, Reynolds JJ, Bretz U, Baggiolini M: Collagenase as a component of the specific granules of human neutrophil leukocytes. *Biochem J* 162:195, 1977.

47. Kane SP, Peters TJ: Analytical subcellular fractionation of human granulocytes with reference to the localization of vitamin B₁₂-binding proteins. *Clin Sci Molec Med* 49:171, 1975.

48. Leffell MS, Spitznagel JK: Association of lactoferrin with lysozyme in granules of human polymorphonuclear leukocytes. *Infect Immun* 6:761, 1972.

49. Matzner Y, Vlodavsky I, Bar-Ner M, et al: Subcellular localization of heparanase in human neutrophils. *J Leukocyte Biol* 51:519, 1992.

50. Ambruso DR, Johnston RB Jr: Lactoferrin enhances hydroxyl radical production by human neutrophils, neutrophil particulate fractions, and an enzymatic generating system. *J Clin Invest* 67:352, 1981.

51. Ellison RT III, Giehl TJ: Killing of gram-negative bacteria by lactoferrin and lysozyme. *J Clin Invest* 88:1080, 1991.

52. Burkhardt H, Hartmann F, Schwingel ML: Activation of latent collagenase from polymorphonuclear leukocytes by oxygen radicals. *Enzyme* 36:221, 1986.

53. Wright DG, Gallin JI: A functional differentiation of human neutrophil granules: generation of C5a by a specific (secondary) granule product and inactivation of C5a by azurophil (primary) granule products. *J Immunol* 119:1068, 1977.

54. O'Shea JJ, Brown EJ, Seligmann BE, et al: Evidence for distinct intracellular pools of receptors for C3b and C3bi in human neutrophils. *J Immunol* 134:2580, 1985.

55. Stevenson KB, Nauseef WM, Clark RA: The neutrophil glycoprotein Mo1 is an integral membrane protein of plasma membranes and specific granules. *J Immunol* 139:3759, 1987.

56. Jost CR, Huizinga TWJ, De Goede R, et al: Intracellular localization and de novo synthesis of FcRIII in human neutrophil granulocytes. *Blood* 75:144, 1990.

57. Suchard SJ, Burton MJ, Stoehr SJ: Thrombospondin receptor expression in human neutrophils coincides with the release of a subpopulation of specific granules. *Biochem J* 284:513, 1992.

58. Tosi MF, Zakem H: Surface expression of Fcτ receptor III (CD16) on chemoattractant-stimulated neutrophils is determined by both surface shedding and translocation from intracellular storage compartments. *J Clin Invest* 90:462, 1992.

59. Buyon JP, Philips MR, Merrill JT, et al: Differential phosphorylation of the β₂ integrin CD11b/CD18 in the plasma and specific granule membranes of neutrophils. *J Leukocyte Biol* 61:313, 1997.

60. Rotrosen D, Yeung CL, Leto TL, et al: Cytochrome b₅₅₈: The flavin-binding component of the phagocyte NADPH oxidase. *Science* 256:1459, 1992.

61. Segal AW, West I, Wientjes F, et al: Cytochrome b₋₂₄₅ is a flavocytochrome containing FAD and the NADPH-binding site of the microbicidal oxidase of phagocytes. *Biochem J* 284:781, 1992.

62. Jesaitis AJ, Buescher ES, Harrison D, et al: Ultrastructural localization of cytochrome b in the membranes of resting and phagocytosing human granulocytes. *J Clin Invest* 85:821, 1990.

63. Breton-Gorius J, Mason DY, Buriot D, et al: Lactoferrin deficiency as a consequence of a lack of specific granules in neutrophils from a patient with recurrent infections. Detection by immunoperoxidase staining for lactoferrin and cytochemical electron microscopy. *Am J Pathol* 99:413, 1980.

64. Gallin JI, Fletcher MP, Seligmann BE, et al: Human neutrophil-specific granule deficiency: A model to assess the role of neutrophil-specific

granules in the evolution of the inflammatory response. *Blood* 59:1317, 1982.

65. Mollinedo F, Pulido R, Lacal PM, Sanchez-Madrid F: Mobilization of gelatinase-rich granules as a regulatory mechanism of early functional responses in human neutrophils. *Scand J Immunol* 34:33, 1991.

66. Mollinedo F, Nakajima M, Llorens A, et al: Major co-localization of the extracellular-matrix degradative enzymes heparanase and gelatinase in tertiary granules of human neutrophils. *Biochem J* 327:917, 1997.

67. Todd RF III, Arnaout MA, Rosin RE, et al: Subcellular localization of the large subunit of Mo1, a surface glycoprotein associated with neutrophil adhesion. *J Clin Invest* 74:1280, 1984.

68. Petrequin PR, Todd RF III, Devall LJ, et al: Association between gelatinase release and increased plasma membrane expression of the Mo1 glycoprotein. *Blood* 69:605, 1987.

69. Anderson DC, Schmalstieg FC, Arnaout MA, et al: Abnormalities of polymorphonuclear leukocyte function associated with a heritable deficiency of high molecular weight surface glycoproteins (GP138): Common relationship to diminished cell adherence. *J Clin Invest* 74:536, 1984.

70. Mollinedo F, Gajate C, Schneider DL: Cytochrome *b* co-fractionates with gelatinase-containing granules in human neutrophils. *Mol Cell Biochem* 105:49, 1991.

71. Sengelov H, Kjeldsen L, Diamond MS, et al: Subcellular localization and dynamics of Mac-1 ($\alpha_m\beta_2$) in human neutrophils. *J Clin Invest* 92:1467, 1993.

72. Smith GP, Sharp G, Peters TJ: Isolation and characterization of alkaline phosphatase-containing granules (phosphasomes) from human polymorphonuclear leucocytes. *J Cell Sci* 76:167, 1985.

73. Sengelov H, Nielsen MH, Borregaard N: Separation of human neutrophil plasma membrane from intracellular vesicles containing alkaline phosphatase and NADPH oxidase activity by free flow electrophoresis. *J Biol Chem* 267:14912, 1992.

74. Borregaard N, Kjeldsen L, Rygaard K, et al: Stimulus-dependent secretion of plasma proteins from human neutrophils. *J Clin Invest* 90:86, 1992.

75. Tapper H, Grinstein S: Fc receptor-triggered insertion of secretory granules into the plasma membrane of human neutrophils—Selective retrieval during phagocytosis. *J Immunol* 159:409, 1997.

76. Sengelov H, Kjeldsen L, Kroeze W, et al: Secretory vesicles are the intracellular reservoir of complement receptor 1 in human neutrophils. *J Immunol* 153:804, 1994.

77. Möhn H, Le Cabec V, Fischer S, Maridonneau-Parini I: The *src*-family protein-tyrosine kinase p59^hck is located on the secretory granules in human neutrophils and translocates towards the phagosome during cell activation. *Biochem J* 309:657, 1995.

78. Morgan CP, Sengelov H, Whatmore J, et al: ADP-ribosylation-factor-regulated phospholipase D activity localizes to secretory vesicles and mobilizes to the plasma membrane following *N*-formylmethionyl-leucyl-phenylalanine stimulation of human neutrophils. *Biochem J* 325:581, 1997.

79. Bainton DF: Sequential degranulation of the two types of polymorphonuclear leukocyte granules during phagocytosis of microorganisms. *J Cell Biol* 58:249, 1973.

80. Wright DG, Gallin JI: Secretory responses of human neutrophils: exocytosis of specific (secondary) granules by human neutrophils during adherence *in vivo* and during exudation *in vivo*. *J Immunol* 123:285, 1979.

81. Niessen HWM, Verhoeven AJ: Differential up-regulation of specific and azurophilic granule membrane markers in electropermeabilized neutrophils. *Cell Signal* 4:501, 1992.

82. Smolen JE, Weissmann G: Stimuli which provoke secretion of azurophil granules induce increments in adenosine cyclic 3',5'-monophosphate. *Biochim Biophys Acta* 672:197, 1981.

83. Estensen RD, White JG, Holmes B: Specific degranulation of human polymorphonuclear leukocytes. *Nature* 248:347, 1974.

84. Fittschen C, Henson PM: Selective secretion of azurophil granule contents induced by monovalent cation ionophores in human neutrophils: Evidence for direct ionophore effects on the granule membrane. *J Leukocyte Biol* 50:517, 1991.

85. Niessen HW, Kuijpers TW, Roos D, Verhoeven AJ: Release of azurophilic granule contents in fMLP-stimulated neutrophils requires two activa-

tion signals, one of which is a rise in cytosolic free Ca^{2+}. *Cell Signal* 3:625, 1991.

86. Anderson DC, Schmalsteig FC, Finegold MJ, et al: The severe and moderate phenotypes of heritable Mac-1, LFA-1 deficiency: Their quantitative definition and relation to leukocyte dysfunction and clinical features. *J Infec Dis* 152:668, 1985.

87. Broxmeyer HE, DeSousa M, Smithyman A, et al: Specificity and modulation of the action of lactoferrin, a negative feedback regulator of myelopoiesis. *Blood* 55:324, 1980.

88. Gahr M, Speer CP, Damerau B, Sawatzki G: Influence of lactoferrin on the function of human polymorphonuclear leukocytes and monocytes. *J Leukocyte Biol* 49:427, 1991.

89. Gallin JI: Degranulating stimuli decrease the negative surface charge and increase adhesiveness of human neutrophils. *J Clin Invest* 65:298, 1980.

90. Johansson A, Jesaitis AJ, Lundqvist H, et al: Different subcellular localization of cytochrome *b* and the dormant NADPH-oxidase in neutrophils and macrophages: Effect on the production of reactive oxygen species during phagocytosis. *Cell Immunol* 161:61, 1995.

91. Calafat J, Kuijpers TW, Janssen H, et al: Evidence for small intracellular vesicles in human blood phagocytes containing cytochrome b_{558} and the adhesion molecule CD11b/CD18. *Blood* 81:3122, 1993.

92. English D, Graves V: Simultaneous mobilization of Mac-1 (CD11b/CD18) and formyl peptide chemoattractant receptors in human neutrophils. *Blood* 80:776, 1992.

93. Balazovich KJ, Smolen JE, Boxer LA: Endogenous inhibitor of protein kinase C: association with human peripheral blood neutrophils but not with specific granule-deficient neutrophils or cytoplasts. *J Immunol* 137:1665, 1986.

94. Balazovich KJ, McEwen EL, Lutzke ML, et al: Purification of PKC-I, an endogenous protein kinase C inhibitor, and types II and III protein kinase C isoenzymes from human neutrophils. *Biochem J* 284:399, 1992.

95. Weiss SJ, Regiani S: Neutrophils degrade subendothelial matrices in the presence of alpha-1-proteinase inhibitor. Cooperative use of lysosomal proteinases and oxygen metabolites. *J Clin Invest* 73:1297, 1984.

96. Spitznagel JK, Shafer WM: Neutrophil killing of bacteria by oxygen-independent mechanisms: A historical summary. *Rev Infec Dis* 7:398, 1985.

97. Clark RA, Borregaard N: Neutrophils autoinactivate secretory products by myeloperoxidase-catalyzed oxidation. *Blood* 65:375, 1985.

98. Smolen JE: Secretion from neutrophils: A critique of modern *in vitro* techniques, in *In Vitro Methods for Studying Secretion*. 3rd ed, edited by AM Poisner, JM Trifaro, pp 29–43. Elsevier, Amsterdam, 1987.

99. Williams LT, Snyderman R, Pike MC, Lefkowitz RJ: Specific receptor sites for chemotactic peptides on human polymorphonuclear leukocytes. *Proc Natl Acad Sci (USA)* 74:1204, 1977.

100. Schiffmann E, Aswanikumar S, Venkatasubramanian K, et al: Some characteristics of the neutrophil receptor for chemotactic peptides. *FEBS Lett* 117:1, 1980.

101. Sklar LA, Mueller H, Omann G, Oades Z: Three states for the formyl peptide receptor on intact cells. *J Biol Chem* 264:8483, 1989.

102. Allen RA, Jesaitis AJ, Sklar LA, et al: Physicochemical properties of the *N*-formyl peptide receptor on human neutrophils. *J Biol Chem* 261:1854, 1986.

103. Van Epps DE, Simpson S, Bender JG, Chenoweth DE: Regulation of C5a and formyl peptide receptor expression on human polymorphonuclear leukocytes. *J Immunol* 144:1062, 1990.

104. Gallin JI, Metcalf JA, Roos D, et al: Organelle-depleted human neutrophil cytoplasts used to study fMet-Leu-Phe receptor modulation and cell function. *J Immunol* 133:415, 1984.

105. Sengelov H, Boulay F, Kjeldsen L, Borregaard N: Subcellular localization and translocation of the receptor for *N*-formylmethionyl-leucyl-phenylalanine in human neutrophils. *Biochem J* 299:473, 1994.

106. Gardner JP, Melnick DA, Malech HL: Characterization of the formyl peptide chemotactic receptor appearing at the phagocytic cell surface after exposure to phorbol myristate acetate. *J Immunol* 136:1400, 1986.

107. Fletcher MP, Gallin JI: Human neutrophils contain an intracellular pool of putative receptors for the chemoattractant *N*-formyl-methionyl-leucyl-phenylalanine. *Blood* 62:792, 1983.

108. Boulay F, Tardif M, Brouchon L, Vignais P: The human *N*-formylpeptide receptor. Characterization of two cDNA isolates and evidence for a new subfamily of G-protein-coupled receptors. *Biochemistry* 29:11123, 1990.

109. Murphy PM, Tiffany HL, McDermott D, Ahuja SK: Sequence and

organization of the human *N*-formyl peptide receptor-encoding gene. *Gene* 133:285, 1993.

110. Hoffman JF, Linderman JJ, Omann GM: Receptor up-regulation, internalization, and interconverting receptor states. Critical components of a quantitative description of *N*-formyl peptide-receptor dynamics in the neutrophil. *J Biol Chem* 271:18394, 1996.

111. Painter RG, Zahler Bentz K, Dukes RE: Regulation of the affinity state of the *N*-formylated peptide receptor of neutrophils: Role of guanine nucleotide-binding proteins and the cytoskeleton. *J Cell Biol* 105:2959, 1987.

112. Schreiber RE, Prossnitz ER, Ye RD, et al: Domains of the human neutrophil *N*-formyl peptide receptor involved in G protein coupling. Mapping with receptor-derived peptides. *J Biol Chem* 269:326, 1994.

113. Bommakanti RK, Dratz EA, Siemsen DW, Jesaitis AJ: Extensive contact between G_{i2} and *N*-formyl peptide receptor of human neutrophils: Mapping of binding sites using receptor-mimetic peptides. *Biochemistry* 34:6720, 1995.

114. Klotz K-N, Krotec KL, Gripentrog J, Jesaitis AJ: Regulatory interaction of *N*-formyl peptide chemoattractant receptors with the membrane skeleton in human neutrophils. *J Immunol* 152:801, 1994.

115. Sarndahl E, Bokoch GM, Boulay F, et al: Direct or C5a-induced activation of heterotrimeric G_{i2} proteins in human neutrophils is associated with interaction between formyl peptide receptors and the cytoskeleton. *J Biol Chem* 271:15267, 1996.

116. Prossnitz ER, Ye RD: The *N*-formyl peptide receptor: A model for the study of chemoattractant receptor structure and function. *Pharmacol Ther* 74:73, 1997.

117. Webster RO, Zanolari B, Henson PM: Neutrophil chemotaxis in response to surface-bound C5a. *Exp Cell Res* 129:55, 1980.

118. Chenoweth DE, Hugli TE: Human C5a and C5a analogs as probes of the neutrophil C5a receptor. *Mol Immunol* 17:151, 1980.

119. McPhail LC, Snyderman R: Activation of the respiratory burst enzyme in human polymorphonuclear leukocytes by chemoattractants and other soluble stimuli. Evidence that the same oxidase is activated by different transductional mechanisms. *J Clin Invest* 72:192, 1983.

120. Matzner Y, Partridge RE, Levy M, Babior BM: Diminished activity of a chemotactic inhibitor in synovial fluids from patients with familial Mediterranean fever. *Blood* 63:629, 1984.

121. Chenoweth DE, Hugli TE: Demonstration of specific C5a receptor on intact human polymorphonuclear leukocytes. *Proc Natl Acad Sci USA* 75:3943, 1978.

122. Rollins TE, Springer MS: Identification of the polymorphonuclear leukocyte's C5a receptor. *J Biol Chem* 260:7157, 1985.

123. Amatruda TT III, Gerard NP, Gerard C, Simon MI: Specific interactions of chemoattractant factor receptors with G-proteins. *J Biol Chem* 268:10139, 1993.

124. Murphy PM, Gallin EK, Tiffany HL: Characterization of human phagocytic cell receptors for C5a and platelet activating factor expressed in *Xenopus* oocytes. *J Immunol* 145:2227, 1990.

125. Alvarez V, Coto E, Setién F, et al: Molecular evolution of the *N*-formyl peptide and C5a receptors in non-human primates. *Immunogenetics* 44:446, 1996.

126. Remes JJ, Petaja-Repo UE, Rajaniemi HJ: Rat and human neutrophil *N*-formyl-peptide chemotactic receptors. Species difference in the glycosylation of similar 35–38 kDa polypeptide cores. *Biochem J* 277:67, 1991.

127. Didsbury JR, Uhing RJ, Tomhave E, et al: Receptor class desensitization of leukocyte chemoattractant receptors. *Proc Natl Acad Sci USA* 88:11564, 1991.

128. Pease JE, Burton DR, Barker MD: Generation of chimeric C5a/formyl peptide receptors: Towards the identification of the human C5a receptor binding site. *Eur J Immunol* 24:211, 1994.

129. Berger M, O'Shea J, Cross AS, et al: Human neutrophils increase expression of C3bi as well as C3b receptors upon activation. *J Clin Invest* 74:1566, 1984.

130. Berger M, Wetzler EM, Welter E, et al: Intracellular sites for storage and recycling of C3b receptors in human neutrophils. *Proc Natl Acad Sci USA* 88:3019, 1991.

131. Brown GE, Reed EB, Lanser ME: Neutrophil CR3 expression and specific granule exocytosis are controlled by different signal transduction pathways. *J Immunol* 147:965, 1991.

132. Zhou M-J, Poo H, Todd RF III, Petty HR: Surface-bound immune complexes trigger transmembrane proximity between complement receptor type 3 and the neutrophil's cortical microfilaments. *J Immunol* 148:3550, 1992.

133. Fearon DT: Identification of the membrane glycoprotein that is the C3b receptor of the human erythrocyte, polymorphonuclear leukocyte, B lymphocyte, and monocyte. *J Exp Med* 152:20, 1980.

134. Kumar A, Wetzler E, Berger M: Isolation and characterization of complement receptor type 1 (CR1) storage vesicles from human neutrophils using antibodies to the cytoplasmic tail of CR1. *Blood* 89:4555, 1997.

135. Nathan CF: Neutrophil activation on biological surfaces. Massive secretion of hydrogen peroxide in response to products of macrophages and lymphocytes. *J Clin Invest* 80:1550, 1987.

136. Shappell SB, Toman C, Anderson DC, et al: Mac-1 (CD11b/CD18) mediates adherence-dependent hydrogen peroxide production by human and canine neutrophils. *J Immunol* 144:2702, 1990.

137. Lu HF, Smith CW, Perrard J, et al: LFA-1 is sufficient in mediating neutrophil emigration in Mac-1-deficient mice. *J Clin Invest* 99:1340, 1997.

138. Todd RF III, Petty HR: β2(CD11/CD18) integrins can serve as signaling partners for other leukocyte receptors. *J Lab Clin Med* 129:492, 1997.

139. Simon SI, Burns AR, Taylor AD, et al: L-Selectin (CD62L) cross-linking signals neutrophil adhesive functions via the Mac-1 (CD11b/CD18) β2-integrin. *J Immunol* 155:1502, 1995.

140. Zhou M, Brown EJ: CR3 (Mac-1, $\alpha_M\beta_2$, CD11b/CD18) and FcγRIII cooperate in generation of a neutrophil respiratory burst: Requirement for FcγRII and tyrosine phosphorylation. *J Cell Biol* 125:1407, 1994.

141. Hundt M, Schmidt RE: The glycosylphosphatidylinositol-linked Fcγ receptor III represents the dominant receptor structure for immune complex activation of neutrophils. *Eur J Immunol* 22:811, 1992.

142. Huizinga TWJ, De Haas M, Van Oers MHJ, et al: The plasma concentration of soluble Fc-gamma RIII is related to production of neutrophils. *Br J Haematol* 87:459, 1994.

143. Leeuwenberg JFM, Van de Winkel JGJ, Jeunhomme TMAA, Buurman WA: Functional polymorphism of IgG FcRII (CD32) on human neutrophils. *Immunology* 71:301, 1990.

144. Kew RR, Grimaldi CM, Furie MB, Fleit HB: Human neutrophil FcγRIIB and formyl peptide receptors are functionally linked during formyl-methionyl-leucyl-phenylalanine-induced chemotaxis. *J Immunol* 149:989, 1992.

145. Sehgal G, Zang K, Todd RF III, et al: Lectin-like inhibition of immune complex receptor-mediated stimulation of neutrophils. Effects on cytosolic calcium release and superoxide production. *J Immunol* 150:4571, 1993.

146. Kocher M, Siegel ME, Edberg JC, Kimberly RP: Cross-linking of Fcγ receptor IIa and Fcγ receptor IIIb induces different proadhesive phenotypes on human neutrophils. *J Immunol* 159:3940, 1997.

147. Edberg JC, Moon JJ, Chang DJ, Kimberly RP: Differential regulation of human neutrophil FcγRIIa (CD32) and FcγRIIIb (CD16)-induced Ca^{2+} transients. *J Biol Chem* 273:8071, 1998.

148. Lang ML, Glennie MJ, Kerr MA: Human neutrophil FcαR and FcγRIIa but not FcγRIIIb generate intracellular calcium signals which trigger the respiratory burst. *Biochem Soc Trans* 25:333S, 1997.

149. Zhou M, Lublin DM, Link DC, Brown EJ: Distinct tyrosine kinase activation and Triton X-100 insolubility upon FcγRII or FcγRIIIB ligation in human polymorphonuclear leukocytes. Implication for immune complex activation of the respiratory burst. *J Biol Chem* 270:13553, 1995.

150. Vossebeld PJM, Homburg CHE, Schweizer RC, et al: Tyrosine phosphorylation-dependant activation of phosphatidylinositide 3-kinase occurs upstream of Ca^{2+}-signaling induced by Fcγ receptor cross-linking in human neutrophils. *Biochem J* 323:87, 1997.

151. Trotta R, Kanakaraj P, Perussia B: FcγR-dependent mitogen-activated protein kinase activation in leukocytes: A common signal transduction event necessary for expression of TNF-α and early activation genes. *J Exp Med* 184:1027, 1996.

152. Cassatella MA, Flynn RM, Amezaga MA, et al: Interferon gamma induces in human neutrophils and macrophages expression of the mRNA for the high affinity receptor for monomeric IgG (Fc gamma R-I or CD64). *Biochem Biophys Res Commun* 170:582, 1990.

153. Bovolenta C, Gasperini S, McDonald PP, Cassatella MA: High affinity receptor for IgG (FcgammaRI/CD64) gene and STAT protein binding

to the IFN-gamma response region (GRR) are regulated differentially in human neutrophils and monocytes by IL-10. *J Immunol* 160:911, 1998.

154. Indik ZK, Hunter S, Huang MM, et al: The high affinity Fcγ receptor (CD64) induces phagocytosis in the absence of its cytoplasmic domain: The γ subunit of FcγRIIIA imparts phagocytic function to FcγRI. *Exp Hematol* 22:599, 1994.

155. Arnaout MA, Todd RF III, Dana N, et al: Inhibition of phagocytosis of complement C3 or immunoglobulin G coated particles and of C3bi binding by monoclonal antibodies to a monocyte-granulocyte membrane glycoprotein (Mo1). *J Clin Invest* 72:171, 1983.

156. Zhou M, Todd RF III, Van de Winkel JGJ, Petty HR: Cocapping of the leukoadhesin molecules complement receptor type 3 and lymphocyte function-associated antigen-1 with Fcγ receptor III on human neutrophils: Possible role of lectin-like interactions. *J Immunol* 150:3030, 1993.

157. Worth RC, Mayo-Bond L, Van de Winkel JGJ, et al: CR3 ($\alpha_m\beta_2$; CD11b/CD18) restores IgG-dependent phagocytosis in transfectants expressing a phagocytosis-defective FcγRIA (CD32) tail-minus mutant. *J Immunol* 157:5660, 1996.

158. Kindzelskii AL, Laska ZO, Todd RF III, Petty HR: Urokinase-type plasminogen activator receptor reversibly dissociates from complement receptor type 3 ($\alpha_M\beta_2$, CD11b/CD18) during neutrophil polarization. *J Immunol* 156:297, 1996.

159. Nakamura M, Honda Z, Izumi T, et al: Molecular cloning and expression of platelet-activating factor receptor from human leukocytes. *J Biol Chem* 266:20400, 1991.

160. Damaj BB, McColl SR, Neote K, et al: Diverging signal transduction pathways activated by interleukin 8 (IL-8) and related chemokines in human neutrophils—IL-8 and Gro-α differentially stimulate calcium influx through IL-8 receptors A and B. *J Biol Chem* 271:20540, 1996.

161. Jones SA, Wolf M, Qin SX, et al: Different functions for the interleukin 8 receptors (IL-8R) of human neutrophil leukocytes: NADPH oxidase and phospholipase D are activated through IL-8R1 but not IL-8R2. *Proc Natl Acad Sci USA* 93:6682, 1996.

162. Sherman JW, Mendelson MA, Boggs JM, et al: Ligand-induced formation of the leukotriene B$_4$ receptor-G protein complex of human polymorphonuclear leukocytes. *J Cell Biochem* 48:367, 1992.

163. Soejima K, Fujishima S, Nakamura H, et al: Downmodulation of IL-8 receptors, type A and type B, on human lung neutrophils in vivo. *Am J Physiol Lung Cell Mol Physiol* 273:L618, 1997.

164. Goldman DW, Gifford LA, Young RN, et al: Affinity labeling of the membrane protein-binding component of human polymorphonuclear leukocyte receptors for leukotriene B$_4$. *J Immunol* 146:2671, 1991.

165. Yokomizo T, Izumi T, Chang K, et al: A G-protein-coupled receptor for leukotriene B$_4$ that mediates chemotaxis. *Nature* 387:620, 1997.

166. Sklar LA, Bokoch GM, Button D, Smolen JE: Regulation of ligand-receptor dynamics by guanine nucleotides. Real-time analysis of inter-converting states for the neutrophil formyl peptide receptor. *J Biol Chem* 262:135, 1987.

167. Pelz C, Matsumoto T, Molski TFP, et al: Characterization of the membrane-associated GTPase activity: Effects of chemotactic factors and toxins. *J Cell Biochem* 39:197, 1989.

168. Bokoch GM, Bickford K, Bohl BP: Subcellular localization and quantitation of the major neutrophil pertussis toxin substrate, G$_n$. *J Cell Biol* 106:1927, 1988.

169. Cronstein BN, Haines KA, Kolasinski S, Reibman J: Occupancy of G$_{\alpha s}$-linked receptors uncouples chemoattractant receptors from their stimulus-transduction mechanisms in the neutrophil. *Blood* 80:1052, 1992.

170. Goldsmith P, Gierschik P, Milligan G, et al: Antibodies directed against synthetic peptides distinguish between GTP-binding proteins in neutrophil and brain. *J Biol Chem* 262:14683, 1987.

171. Bokoch GM, Parkos CA: Identification of novel GTP-binding proteins in the human neutrophil. *FEBS Lett* 227:66, 1988.

172. Kanaho Y, Kanoh H, Nozawa Y: Activation of phospholipase D in rabbit neutrophils by fMet-Leu-Phe is mediated by a pertussis toxin-sensitive GTP-binding protein that may be distinct from a phospholipase C-regulating protein. *FEBS Lett* 279:249, 1991.

173. Smolen JE, Stoehr SJ: Guanine nucleotides reduce the free calcium requirement for secretion of granule constituents from permeabilized human neutrophils. *Biochim Biophys Acta* 889:171, 1986.

174. Barrowman MM, Cockcroft S, Gomperts BD: Two roles for guanine nucleotides in the stimulus-secretion sequence of neutrophils. *Nature* 319:504, 1986.

175. Smolen JE, Sandborg RR: Ca^{2+}-induced secretion by electroperme-abilized human neutrophils. The roles of Ca^{2+}, nucleotides and protein kinase C. *Biochim Biophys Acta* 1052:133, 1990.

176. Cockcroft S: G-protein-regulated phospholipases C, D and A$_2$-mediated signalling in neutrophils. *Biochim Biophys Acta Rev Biomembr* 1113:135, 1992.

177. Ohnishi H, Ernst SA, Yule DI, et al: Heterotrimeric G-protein G$_{q/11}$ localized on pancreatic zymogen granules is involved in calcium-regulated amylase secretion. *J Biol Chem* 272:16056, 1997.

178. Philips MR, Abramson SB, Kolasinski SL, et al: Low molecular weight GTP-binding proteins in human neutrophil granule membranes. *J Biol Chem* 266:1289, 1991.

179. Maridonneau-Parini I, De Gunzburg J: Association of rap1 and rap2 proteins with the specific granules of human neutrophils. Translocation to the plasma membrane during cell activation. *J Biol Chem* 267:6396, 1992.

180. Dagher MC, Fuchs A, Bourmeyster N, et al: Small proteins and the neutrophil NADPH oxidase. *Biochimie* 77:651, 1995.

181. Nath J, Powledge A, Wright DG: Involvement of a botulinum toxin-sensitive 22-kDa G protein in stimulated exocytosis of human neutrophils. *J Immunol* 152:1370, 1994.

182. Laudanna C, Campbell JJ, Butcher EC: Role of Rho in chemoattractant-activated leukocyte adhesion through integrins. *Science* 271:981, 1996.

183. Vita F, Soranzo MR, Borelli V, et al: Subcellular localization of the small GTPase Rab5a in resting and stimulated human neutrophils. *Exp Cell Res* 227:367, 1996.

184. Cockcroft S, Baldwin JM, Allan D: The Ca^{2+}-activated polyphosphoino-sitide phosphodiesterase of human and rabbit neutrophil membranes. *Biochem J* 221:477, 1984.

185. Ando M, Furui H, Suzuki K, et al: Direct activation of phospholipase A$_2$ by GTP-binding protein in human peripheral polymorphonuclear leukocytes. *Biochem Biophys Res Commun* 183:708, 1992.

186. Dusi S, Donini M, Della Bianca V, Rossi F: Tyrosine phosphorylation of phospholipase C-γ2 is involved in the activation of phosphoinositide hydrolysis by Fc receptors in human neutrophils. *Biochem Biophys Res Commun* 201:1100, 1994.

187. Fruman DA, Gamache DA, Ernest MJ: Changes in inositol 1,4,5-tris-phosphate mass in agonist-stimulated human neutrophils. *Agents Actions* 34:16, 1991.

188. Spat A, Bradford PG, McKinney JS, et al: A saturable receptor for ^{32}P-inositol-1,4,5-trisphosphate in hepatocytes and neutrophils. *Nature* 319:514, 1986.

189. Prentki M, Wollheim CB, Lew PD: Ca^{2+} homeostasis in permeabilized human neutrophils. Characterization of Ca^{2+}-sequestering pools and the action of inositol 1,4,5-trisphosphate. *J Biol Chem* 259:13777, 1984.

190. Favre CJ, Lew DP, Krause K-H: Rapid heparin-sensitive Ca^{2+} release following Ca^{2+}-ATPase inhibition in intact HL-60 granulocytes. Evidence for Ins(1,4,5)P$_3$-dependent Ca^{2+} cycling across the membrane of Ca^{2+} stores. *Biochem J* 302:155, 1994.

191. Krause KH, Lew PD: Subcellular distribution of Ca^{2+} pumping sites in human neutrophils. *J Clin Invest* 80:107, 1987.

192. Bradford PG, Rubin RP: Quantitative changes in inositol 1,4,5-trisphos-phate in chemoattractant-stimulated neutrophils. *J Biol Chem* 261:15644, 1986.

193. Agwu DE, McPhail LC, Chabot MC, et al: Choline-linked phosphoglyc-erides. A source of phosphatidic acid and diglycerides in stimulated neutrophils. *J Biol Chem* 264:1405, 1989.

194. Uings IJ, Thompson NT, Randall RW, et al: Tyrosine phosphorylation is involved in receptor coupling to phospholipase D but not phospho-lipase C in the human neutrophil. *Biochem J* 281:597, 1992.

195. Billah MM, Eckel S, Mullmann TJ, et al: Phosphatidylcholine hydrolysis by phospholipase D determines phosphatidate and diglyceride levels in chemotactic peptide-stimulated human neutrophils. Involvement of phosphatidate phosphohydrolase in signal transduction. *J Biol Chem* 264:17069, 1989.

196. Houle MG, Kahn RA, Naccache PH, Bourgoin S: ADP-ribosylation factor translocation correlates with potentiation of GTPgammaS-stimu-lated phospholipase D activity in membrane fractions of HL-60 cells. *J Biol Chem* 270:22795, 1995.

197. Kwak JY, Lopez I, Uhlinger DJ, et al: RhoA and a cytosolic 50-kDa

factor reconstitute GTPgammaS-dependent phospholipase D activity in human neutrophil subcellular fractions. *J Biol Chem* 270:27093, 1995.

198. English D, Cui Y, Siddiqui RA: Messenger functions of phosphatidic acid. *Chem Phys Lipids* 80:117, 1996.

199. Rossi F, Grzeskowiak M, Della Bianca V, Sbarbati A: *De novo* synthesis of diacylglycerol from glucose. A new pathway of signal transduction in human neutrophils stimulated during phagocytosis of beta-glucan particles. *J Biol Chem* 266:8034, 1991.

200. Blackwood RA, Smolen JE, Transue AT, et al: Phospholipase D activity facilitates Ca^{2+}-induced aggregation and fusion of complex liposomes. *Am J Physiol* 272:C1279, 1997.

201. Smith DM Jr, Waite M: Phospholipid metabolism in human neutrophil subfractions. *Arch Biochem Biophys* 246:263, 1986.

202. Cockcroft S: Relationship between arachidonate release and exocytosis in permeabilized human neutrophils stimulated with formylmethionyl-leucyl-phenylalanine (fMetLeuPhe), guanosine 5′-[γ-thio]triphosphate (GTP[S]) and Ca^{2+}. *Biochem J* 275:127, 1991.

203. Durstin M, Durstin S, Molski TFP, Becker EL, Sha'afi RI: Cytoplasmic phospholipase A_2 translocates to membrane fraction in human neutrophils activated by stimuli that phosphorylate mitogen-activated protein kinase. *Proc Natl Acad Sci USA* 91:3142, 1994.

204. Nahas N, Waterman WH, Sha'afi RI: Granulocyte-macrophage colony-stimulating factor (GM-CSF) promotes phosphorylation and an increase in the activity of cytosolic phospholipase A_2 in human neutrophils. *Biochem J* 313:503, 1996.

205. Stewart A, Jackson CG, Wakelam MJO: The regulation by phosphorylation of 'priming’ of phospholipase A_2 activity in the neutrophil model system, differentiated HL60 cells. *Br J Pharmacol* 122:13, 1997.

206. Bauldry SA, Wooten RE: Induction of cytosolic phospholipase A_2 activity by phosphatidic acid and diglycerides in permeabilized human neutrophils: Interrelationship between phospholipases D and A_2. *Biochem J* 322:353, 1997.

207. Balsinde J, Diez E, Schuller A, Mollinedo F: Phospholipase A_2 activity in resting and activated human neutrophils. Substrate specificity, pH dependence, and subcellular localization. *J Biol Chem* 263:1929, 1988.

208. Nakamura T, Abe A, Balazovich KJ, et al: Ceramide regulates oxidant release in adherent human neutrophils. *J Biol Chem* 269:18384, 1994.

209. Wilson E, Rice WG, Kinkade JM Jr, et al: Protein kinase C inhibition by sphingoid long-chain bases: Effects on secretion in human neutrophils. *Arch Biochem Biophys* 259:204, 1987.

210. Wong K, Kwan-Yeung L: Sphingosine mobilizes intracellular calcium in human neutrophils. *Cell Calcium* 14:493, 1993.

211. Mullmann TJ, Siegel MI, Egan RW, Billah MM: Sphingosine inhibits phosphatidate phosphohydrolase in human neutrophils by a protein kinase C-independent mechanism. *J Biol Chem* 266:2013, 1991.

212. Perianin A, Snyderman R: Analysis of calcium homeostasis in activated human polymorphonuclear leukocytes. Evidence for two distinct mechanisms for lowering cytosolic calcium. *J Biol Chem* 264:1005, 1989.

213. Scharff O, Foder B: Delayed activation of plasma membrane Ca^{2+} pump in human neutrophils. *Cell Calcium* 16:455, 1994.

214. Korchak HM, Vienne K, Rutherford LE, et al: Stimulus response coupling in the human neutrophil: II. Temporal analysis of changes in cytosolic calcium and calcium influx. *J Biol Chem* 259:4076, 1984.

215. Sage SO, Pintado E, Mahaut-Smith MP, Merritt JE: Rapid kinetics of agonist-evoked changes in cytosolic free Ca^{2+} concentration in fura-2-loaded human neutrophils. *Biochem J* 265:915, 1990.

216. Llinás R, Sugimori M, Silver RB: Microdomains of high calcium concentration in a presynaptic terminal. *Science* 256:677, 1992.

217. Klingauf J, Neher E: Modeling buffered Ca^{2+} diffusion near the membrane: Implications for secretion in neuroendocrine cells. *Biophys J* 72:674, 1997.

218. Davies EV, Hallett MB: Near membrane Ca^{2+} changes resulting from store release in neutrophils: Detection by FFP-18. *Cell Calcium* 19:355, 1996.

219. Omann GM, Axelrod D: Membrane-proximal calcium transients in stimulated neutrophils detected by total internal reflection fluorescence. *Biophys J* 71:2885, 1996.

220. Pettit EJ, Hallett BM: Temporal and spatial resolution of Ca^{2+} release and influx in human neutrophils using a novel confocal laser scanning mode. *Biochem Biophys Res Commun* 229:109, 1996.

221. Jaconi MEE, Rivest RW, Schlegel W, et al: Spontaneous and chemo-attractant-induced oscillations of cytosolic free calcium in single adherent human neutrophils. *J Biol Chem* 263:10557, 1988.

222. Dougherty RW, Godfrey PP, Hoyle PC, et al: Secretagogue-induced phosphoinositide metabolism in human leucocytes. *Biochem J* 222:307, 1984.

223. Krause KH, Schlegel W, Wollheim CB, et al: Chemotactic peptide activation of human neutrophils and HL-60 cells. Pertussis toxin reveals correlation between inositol trisphosphate generation, calcium ion transients, and cellular activation. *J Clin Invest* 76:1348, 1985.

224. Stephens L, Jackson T, Hawkins PT: Synthesis of phosphatidylinositol 3,4,5-trisphosphate in permeabilized neutrophils regulated by receptors and G-proteins. *J Biol Chem* 268:17162, 1993.

225. Demaurex N, Schlegel W, Varnai P, et al: Regulation of Ca^{2+} influx in myeloid cells. Role of plasma membrane potential, inositol phosphates, cytosolic free $[Ca^{2+}]$, and filling state of intracellular Ca^{2+} stores. *J Clin Invest* 90:830, 1992.

226. Montero M, Garcia-Sancho J, Alvarez J: Activation by chemotactic peptide of a receptor-operated Ca^{2+} entry pathway in differentiated HL60 cells. *J Biol Chem* 269:29451, 1994.

227. Rotnes JS, Iversen JG: Thapsigargin reveals evidence for fMLP-insensitive calcium pools in human leukocytes. *Cell Calcium* 13:487, 1992.

228. Geiszt M, Káldi K, Szeberényi JB, Ligeti E: Thapsigargin inhibits Ca^{2+} entry into human neutrophil granulocytes. *Biochem J* 305:525, 1995.

229. Van Delden C, Favre C, Spat A, et al: Purification of an inositol 1,4,5-trisphosphate-binding calreticulin-containing intracellular compartment of HL-60 cells. *Biochem J* 281:651, 1992.

230. Demaurex N, Monod A, Lew DP, Krause K-H: Characterization of receptor-mediated and store-regulated Ca^{2+} influx in human neutrophils. *Biochem J* 297:595, 1994.

231. Alvarez J, Montero M, Garcia-Sancho J: Agonist-induced Ca^{2+} influx in human neutrophils is not mediated by production of inositol polyphosphates but by emptying of the intracellular Ca^{2+} stores. *Biochem Soc Trans* 22:809, 1994.

232. Davies EV, Hallett MB: A soluble cellular factor directly stimulates Ca^{2+} entry in neutrophils. *Biochem Biophys Res Commun* 206:348, 1995.

233. Korchak HM, Rutherford LE, Weissmann G: Stimulus response coupling in the human neutrophil: I. Kinetic analysis of changes in calcium permeability. *J Biol Chem* 259:4070, 1984.

234. Smolen JE, Korchak HM, Weissmann G: The roles of extracellular and intracellular calcium in lysosomal enzyme release and superoxide anion generation by human polymorphonuclear leukocytes. *Biochim Biophys Acta* 677:512, 1981.

235. Smolen JE, Stoehr SJ: Micromolar concentrations of free calcium provoke secretion of lysozyme from human neutrophils permeabilized with saponin. *J Immunol* 134:1859, 1985.

236. Smolen JE, Stoehr SJ, Boxer LA: Human neutrophils permeabilized with digitonin respond with lysosomal enzyme release when exposed to micromolar levels of free calcium. *Biochim Biophys Acta* 886:1, 1986.

237. Stutchfield J, Cockcroft S: Guanine nucleotides stimulate polyphosphoinositide phosphodiesterase and exocytotic secretion from HL60 cells permeabilized with streptolysin O. *Biochem J* 250:375, 1988.

238. Grinstein S, Furuya W: Receptor-mediated activation of electropermeabilized neutrophils. Evidence for a Ca^{2+}- and protein kinase C-independent signaling pathway. *J Biol Chem* 263:1779, 1988.

239. Lew PD, Monod A, Waldvogel FA, et al: Quantitative analysis of the cytosolic free calcium dependency of exocytosis from three subcellular compartments in intact human neutrophils. *J Cell Biol* 102:2197, 1986.

240. Nüsse O, Lindau M: The calcium signal in human neutrophils and its relation to exocytosis investigated by patch-clamp capacitance and Fura-2 measurements. *Cell Calcium* 14:255, 1993.

241. Merritt JE, Moores KE, Evans AT, et al: Involvement of calcium in modulation of neutrophil function by phorbol esters that activate protein kinase C isotypes and related enzymes. *Biochem J* 289:919, 1993.

242. Foyouzi-Youssefi R, Petersson F, Lew DP, et al: Chemoattractant-induced respiratory burst: Increases in cytosolic Ca^{2+} concentrations are essential and synergize with a kinetically distinct second signal. *Biochem J* 322:709, 1997.

243. Pozzan T, Lew DP, Wollheim CB, Tsein RY: Is cytosolic ionized calcium regulating neutrophil activation? *Science* 221:1413, 1983.

244. Al-Mohanna FA, Hallett MB: Actin polymerization in neutrophils is triggered without a requirement for a rise in cytoplasmic Ca^{2+}. *Biochem J* 266:669, 1990.

245. Seetoo KF, Schonhorn JE, Gewirtz AT, et al: A cytosolic calcium transient is not necessary for degranulation or oxidative burst in immune complex-stimulated neutrophils. *J Leukocyte Biol* 62:329, 1997.

246. Andrews PC, Babior BM: Endogenous protein phosphorylation by resting and activated human neutrophils. *Blood* 61:333, 1983.

247. Schneider C, Zanetti M, Romeo D: Surface-reactive stimuli selectively increase protein phosphorylation in human neutrophils. *FEBS Lett* 127:4, 1981.

248. Helfman DM, Applebaum BD, Volger WR, Kuo JF: Phospholipid-sensitive Ca^{2+}-dependent protein kinase and its substrates in human neutrophils. *Biochem Biophys Res Comm* 111:847, 1983.

249. Wolf M, Baggiolini M: Identification of phosphatidylserine-binding proteins in human white blood cells. *Biochem J* 269:723, 1990.

250. Majumdar S, Rossi MW, Fujiki T, et al: Protein kinase C isotypes and signaling in neutrophils. Differential substrate specificities of a translocatable, calcium- and phospholipid-dependent β-protein kinase C and a novel calcium-independent, phospholipid-dependent protein kinase which is inhibited by long chain fatty acyl coenzyme A. *J Biol Chem* 266:9285, 1991.

251. Stasia MJ, Strulovici B, Daniel-Issakani S, et al: Immunocharacterization of β- and zeta-subspecies of protein kinase C in bovine neutrophils. *FEBS Lett* 274:61, 1990.

252. Deli E, Kiss Z, Wilson E, et al: Immunocytochemical localization of protein kinase C in resting and activated human neutrophils. *FEBS Lett* 221:365, 1987.

253. O'Flaherty JT, Schmitt JD, Wykle RL, et al: Diacylglycerols and mezerein activate neutrophils by a phorbol myristate acetate-like mechanism. *J Cell Physiol* 125:192, 1985.

254. Salamino F, Sparatore B, De Tullio R, et al: Respiratory burst in activated neutrophils is directly correlated to the intracellular level of protein kinase C. *Eur J Biochem* 200:573, 1991.

255. Wright CD, Hoffman MD: The protein kinase C inhibitors H-7 and H-9 fail to inhibit human neutrophil activation. *Biochem Biophys Res Comm* 135:749, 1986.

256. Combadiere C, Hakim J, Giroud J-P, Perianin A: Staurosporine, a protein kinase inhibitor, up-regulates the stimulation of human neutrophil respiratory burst by *N*-formyl peptides and platelet activating factor. *Biochem Biophys Res Commun* 168:65, 1990.

257. Smolen JE, Stoehr SJ, Bartone D: Protein kinase C is not involved in secretion by permeabilized human neutrophils. *Cell Signal* 1:471, 1989.

258. Niessen HWM, Verhoeven AJ: Role of protein phosphorylation in the degranulation of electropermeabilized human neutrophils. *Biochim Biophys Acta Mol Cell Res* 1223:267, 1994.

259. Tsung PK, Sakamoto T, Weissmann G: Protein kinase and phosphatases from human polymorphonuclear leukocytes. *Biochem J* 145:437, 1975.

260. Huang CK, Hill JM Jr, Bormann BJ, et al: Endogenous substrates for cyclic AMP-dependent and calcium-dependent protein phosphorylation in rabbit peritoneal neutrophils. *Biochim Biophys Acta* 760:126, 1983.

261. Pontremoli S, Michetti M, Melloni E, et al: Identification of the proteolytically activated form of protein kinase C in stimulated human neutrophils. *Proc Natl Acad Sci USA* 87:3705, 1990.

262. Wyatt TA, Lincoln TM, Pryzwansky KB: Vimentin is transiently colocalized with and phosphorylated by cyclic GMP-dependent protein kinase in formyl-peptide-stimulated neutrophils. *J Biol Chem* 266:21274, 1991.

263. Berkow RL, Dodson RW, Kraft AS: Human neutrophils contain distinct cytosolic and particulate tyrosine kinase activities: Possible role in neutrophil activation. *Biochim Biophys Acta* 997:292, 1989.

264. Steinbeck MJ, Hegg GG, Karnovsky MJ: Arachidonate activation of the neutrophil NADPH-oxidase. Synergistic effects of protein phosphatase inhibitors compared with protein kinase activators. *J Biol Chem* 266:16336, 1991.

265. Grinstein S, Furuya W, Lu DJ, Mills GB: Vanadate stimulates oxygen consumption and tyrosine phosphorylation in electropermeabilized human neutrophils. *J Biol Chem* 265:318, 1990.

266. Huang C-K, Laramee GR, Yamazaki M, Sha'afi RI: Stimulation of a histone H4 protein kinase in Triton X-100 lysates of rabbit peritoneal neutrophils pretreated with chemotactic factors: Lack of requirements of calcium mobilization and protein kinase C activation. *J Cell Biochem* 44:221, 1990.

267. Bass DA, McPhail LC, Schmitt JD, et al: Selective priming of rate and duration of the respiratory burst of neutrophils by 1,2-diacyl and 1-*O*-alkyl-2-acyl diglycerides. Possible relation to effects on protein kinase C. *J Biol Chem* 263:19610, 1988.

268. Knaus UG, Morris S, Dong H-J, et al: Regulation of human leukocyte p21-activated kinases through G protein-coupled receptors. *Science* 269:221, 1995.

269. Yan SR, Fumagalli L, Berton G: Activation of *SRC* family kinases in human neutrophils. Evidence that p58$^{C\text{-}FGR}$ and p53/56^{LYN} redistributed to a Triton X-100-insoluble cytoskeletal fraction, also enriched in the caveolar protein *Caveolin*, display an enhanced kinase activity. *FEBS Lett* 380:198, 1996.

270. Brizzi MF, Aronica MG, Rosso A, et al: Granulocyte-macrophage colony-stimulating factor stimulates JAK2 signaling pathway and rapidly activates p93^{fes}, STAT1 p91, and STAT3 p92 in polymorphonuclear leukocytes. *J Biol Chem* 271:3562, 1996.

271. Krump E, Sanghera JS, Pelech SL, et al: Chemotactic peptide *N*-formyl-Met-Leu-Phe activation of p38 mitogen-activated protein kinase (MAPK) and MAPK-activated protein kinase-2 in human neutrophils. *J Biol Chem* 272:937, 1997.

272. Waddell TK, Fialkow L, Chan CK, et al: Signaling functions of L-selectin. Enhancement of tyrosine phosphorylation and activation of MAP kinase. *J Biol Chem* 270:15403, 1995.

273. Pillinger MH, Feoktistov AS, Capodici C, et al: Mitogen-activated protein kinase in neutrophils and enucleate neutrophil cytoplasts. Evidence for regulation of cell-cell adhesion. *J Biol Chem* 271:12049, 1996.

274. Lowell CA, Fumagalli L, Berton G: Deficiency of Src family kinases p59/61^{hck} and p58$^{c\text{-}fgr}$ results in defective adhesion-dependent neutrophil functions. *J Cell Biol* 133:895, 1996.

275. Fernandez R, Suchard SJ: Syk activation is required for spreading and H_2O_2 release in adherent human neutrophils. *J Immunol* 160:5154, 1998.

276. Fuortes M, Jin W, Nathan C: β2 integrin-dependent tyrosine phosphorylation of paxillin in human neutrophils treated with tumor necrosis factor. *J Cell Biol* 127:1477, 1994.

277. Hazan I, Dana R, Granot Y, Levy R: Cytosolic phospholipase A_2 and its mode of activation in human neutrophils by opsonized zymosan—Correlation between 42/44 kDa mitogen-activated protein kinase, cytosolic phospholipase A_2 and NADPH oxidase. *Biochem J* 326:867, 1997.

278. Qiu ZH, Gijón MA, De Carvalho MS, et al: The role of calcium and phosphorylation of cytosolic phospholipase A_2 in regulating arachidonic acid release in macrophages. *J Biol Chem* 273:8203, 1998.

279. Diez E, Balsinde J, Mollinedo F: Subcellular distribution of fatty acids, phospholipids and phospholipase A_2 in human neutrophils. *Biochim Biophys Acta Lipids Lipid Metab* 1047:83, 1990.

280. Ramesha CS, Ives DL: Detection of arachidonoyl-selective phospholipase A_2 in human neutrophil cytosol. *Biochim Biophys Acta Lipids Lipid Metab* 1168:37, 1993.

281. Walsh CE, Waite MB, Thomas MJ, DeChatelet LR: Release and metabolism of arachidonic acid in human neutrophils. *J Biol Chem* 256:7228, 1981.

282. Winkler JD, Sung C-M, Hubbard WC, Chilton FH: Influence of arachidonic acid on indices of phospholipase A_2 activity in the human neutrophil. *Biochem J* 291:825, 1993.

283. Naccache PH, Showell HJ, Becker EL, Sha'afi RI: Arachidonic acid induced degranulation of rabbit peritoneal neutrophils. *Biochem Biophys Res Comm* 87:292, 1979.

284. Hardy SJ, Robinson BS, Ferrante A, et al: Polyenoic very-long-chain fatty acids mobilize intracellular calcium from a thapsigargin-insensitive pool in human neutrophils. The relationship between Ca^{2+} mobilization and superoxide production induced by long- and very-long-chain fatty acids. *Biochem J* 311:689, 1995.

285. Suszták K, Mócsai A, Ligeti E, Kapus A: Electrogenic H$^+$ pathway contributes to stimulus-induced changes of internal pH and membrane potential in intact neutrophils: Role of cytoplasmic phospholipase A_2. *Biochem J* 325:501, 1997.

286. Alonso-Torre SR, García-Sancho J: Arachidonic acid inhibits capacitative calcium entry in rat thymocytes and human neutrophils. *Biochim Biophys Acta Bio-Membr* 1328:207, 1997.

287. Kitchen EA, Root JR, Dawson W: Chemotactic activity of thromboxane B_2, prostaglandins and their metabolites for polymorphonuclear leukocytes. *Prostaglandins* 16:239, 1978.

288. Tahamont MV, Gee MH, Flynn JT: Aggregation and thromboxane syn-

thesis and release in isolated sheep neutrophils and lymphocytes in response to complement stimulation. *Prost Leukotr Med* 16:181, 1984.

289. Spagnuolo PJ, Ellner JJ, Hassid A, Dunn MJ: Thromboxane A₂ mediates augmented polymorphonuclear leukocyte adhesiveness. *J Clin Invest* 66:406, 1980.

290. Borgeat P, Hamberg M, Samuelsson B: Transformation of arachidonic acid and homo-gamma-linoleic acid by rabbit polymorphonuclear leukocytes. Monohydroxy acids from novel lipoxygenases. *J Biol Chem* 251:7816, 1976.

291. Borgeat P, Samuelsson B: Transformation of arachidonic acid by rabbit polymorphonuclear leukocytes. Formation of a novel dihydroxyeicosate-traenoic acid. *J Biol Chem* 254:2643, 1979.

292. Stenson WF, Parker CW: Monohydroxytetraenoic acids (HETEs) induce degranulation of human neutrophils. *J Immunol* 124:2100, 1980.

293. Naccache PH, Sha'afi RI, Borgeat P, Goetzl EJ: Mono- and dihydroxy-eicosatetraenoic acids alter calcium homeostasis in rabbit neutrophils. *J Clin Invest* 67:1584, 1981.

294. Palmer RMJ, Salmon JA: Release of leukotriene B₄ from human neutrophils and its relationship to degranulation induced by *N*-formyl-methionyl-leucyl-phenylalanine, serum-treated zymosan and the iono-phore A23187. *Immunology* 50:65, 1983.

295. Goldman DW, Goetzl EJ: Heterogeneity of human polymorphonuclear leukocyte receptors for leukotriene B₄. Identification of a subset of high affinity receptors that transduce the chemotactic response. *J Exp Med* 159:1027, 1984.

296. Prescott SM, Zimmerman GA, Seeger AR: Leukotriene B₄ is an incomplete agonist for the activation of human neutrophils. *Biochem Biophys Res Comm* 122:535, 1984.

297. Palmblad J, Malmsten CL, Uden AM, et al: Leukotriene B₄ is a potent and stereospecific stimulator of neutrophil chemotaxis and adherence. *Blood* 58:658, 1981.

298. Sugiura T, Onuma Y, Sekiguchi N, Waku K: Ether phospholipids in guinea pig polymorphonuclear leukocytes and macrophages. Occurrence of high levels of 1-O-alkyl-2-acyl-*sn*-glycero-3-phosphocholine. *Biochim Biophys Acta* 712:515, 1982.

299. O'Flaherty JT, Wykle RL, Miller CH, et al: 1-O-alkyl-*sn*-glyceryl-3-phosphorylcholines. A novel class of neutrophil stimulants. *Am J Pathol* 103:70, 1981.

300. Jouvin-Marche E, Poitevin B, Benveniste J: Platelet-activating factor (PAF-acether), an activator on neutrophil functions. *Agents Actions* 12:716, 1982.

301. Stossel TP: On the crawling of animal cells. *Science* 260:1086, 1993.

302. Hoffstein ST: Ultrastructural demonstration of calcium loss from local regions of the plasma membrane of surface stimulated human granulocytes. *J Immunol* 123:1395, 1979.

303. Watts RG, Howard TH: Evidence for a gelsolin-rich, labile F-actin pool in human polymorphonuclear leukocytes. *Cell Motil Cytoskeleton* 21:25, 1992.

304. Hoffstein S, Weissmann G: Microfilaments and microtubules in calcium ionophore-induced secretion of lysosomal enzymes from human polymorphonuclear leukocytes. *J Cell Biol* 78:769, 1978.

305. Fechheimer M, Zigmond SH: Changes in cytoskeletal proteins of polymorphonuclear leukocytes induced by chemotactic peptides. *Cell Motility* 3:349, 1983.

306. Howard TH, Oresajo CO: The kinetics of chemotactic peptide-induced change in F-actin content, F-actin distribution, and the shape of neutrophils. *J Cell Biol* 101:1078, 1985.

307. Zurier RB, Hoffstein S, Weissmann G: Cytochalasin B: effect on lysosomal enzyme release from human leukocytes. *Proc Natl Acad Sci USA* 70:844, 1973.

308. Howard TH, Casella J, Lin S: Correlation of the biologic effects and binding of cytochalasins to human polymorphonuclear leukocytes. *Blood* 57:399, 1981.

309. Maruyama K, Hartwig JH, Stossel TP: Cytochalasin B and the structure of actin gels. II. Further evidence for the splitting of F-actin by cytochalasin B. *Biochim Biophys Acta* 626:494, 1980.

310. Jesaitis AJ, Tolley JO, Painter RG, et al: Membrane-cytoskeleton interactions and the regulation of chemotactic peptide-induced activation of human granulocytes: the effects of dihydrocytochalasin B. *J Cell Biochem* 27:241, 1985.

311. Wallace PJ, Wersto RP, Packman CH, Lichtman MA: Chemotactic peptide-induced changes in neutrophil actin conformation. *J Cell Biol* 99:1060, 1984.

312. Pryzwansky KB, Schliwa M, Porter KR: Comparison of the three-dimensional organization of unextracted and Triton-extracted human neutrophilic polymorphonuclear leukocytes. *Eur J Cell Biol* 30:112, 1983.

313. Jesaitis AJ, Tolley JO, Bokoch GM, Allen RA: Regulation of chemoat-tractant receptor interaction with transducing proteins by organizational control in the plasma membrane of human neutrophils. *J Cell Biol* 109:2783, 1989.

314. Wymann MP, Kernen P, Bengtsson T, et al: Corresponding oscillations in neutrophil shape and filamentous actin content. *J Biol Chem* 265:619, 1990.

315. Wang DH, Berry K, Howard TH: Kinetic analysis of chemotactic peptide-induced actin polymerization in neutrophils. *Cell Motil Cytoskeleton* 16:80, 1990.

316. Omann GM, Porasik-Lowes MM: Graded G-protein uncoupling by pertussis toxin treatment of human polymorphonuclear leukocytes. *J Immunol* 146:1303, 1991.

317. Ehrengruber MU, Coates TD, Deranleau DA: Shape oscillations: A fundamental response of human neutrophils stimulated by chemotactic peptides. *FEBS Lett* 359:229, 1995.

318. Omann GM, Rengan R, Hoffman JF, Linderman JJ: Rapid oscillations of actin polymerization depolymerization in polymorphonuclear leukocytes stimulated by leukotriene B₄ and platelet-activating factor. *J Immunol* 155:5375, 1995.

319. Bengtsson T: Correlation between chemotactic peptide-induced changes in chlorotetracycline fluorescence and F-actin content in human neutrophils: A role for membrane-associated calcium in the regulation of actin polymerization. *Exp Cell Res* 191:57, 1990.

320. Downey GP, Chan CK, Trudel S, Grinstein S: Actin assembly in electropermeabilized neutrophils: Role of intracellular calcium. *J Cell Biol* 110:1975, 1990.

321. Elsner J, Dichmann S, Dobos GJ, Kapp A: Actin polymerization in human eosinophils, unlike human neutrophils, depends on intracellular calcium mobilization. *J Cell Physiol* 167:548, 1996.

322. Bengtsson T, Sarndahl E, Stendahl O, Andersson T: Involvement of GTP-binding proteins in actin polymerization in human neutrophils. *Proc Natl Acad Sci USA* 87:2921, 1990.

323. Heringdorf DMZ, Liedel K, Kaldenberg-Stasch S, et al: Translocation of microfilament-associated inhibitory guanine-nucleotide-binding proteins to the plasma membrane in myeloid differentiated human leukemia (HL-60) cells. *Eur J Biochem* 235:670, 1996.

324. Brennan PJ, Zigmond SH, Schreiber AD, et al: Binding of IgG containing immune complexes to human neutrophil FcγRI and FcγRII induces actin polymerization by a pertussis toxin-insensitive transduction pathway. *J Immunol* 146:4282, 1991.

325. Cano ML, Lauffenburger DA, Zigmond SH: Kinetic analysis of F-actin depolymerization in polymorphonuclear leukocyte lysates indicates that chemoattractant stimulation increases actin filament number without altering the filament length distribution. *J Cell Biol* 115:677, 1991.

326. Howard T, Chaponnier C, Yin H, Stossel T: Gelsolin-actin interaction and actin polymerization in human neutrophils. *J Cell Biol* 110:1983, 1990.

327. Yuruker B, Niggli V: α-Actinin and vinculin in human neutrophils: Reorganization during adhesion and relation to the actin network. *J Cell Sci* 101:403, 1992.

328. Sheikh S, Gratzer WB, Pinder JC, Nash GB: Actin polymerisation regulates integrin-mediated adhesion as well as rigidity of neutrophils. *Biochem Biophys Res Commun* 238:910, 1997.

329. Eberle M, Traynor-Kaplan AE, Sklar LA, Norgauer J: Is there a relationship between phosphatidylinositol trisphosphate and F-actin polymerization in human neutrophils. *J Biol Chem* 265:16725, 1990.

330. DiNubile MJ, Huang S: High concentrations of phosphatidylinositol-4,5-bisphosphate may promote actin filament growth by three potential mechanisms: Inhibiting capping by neutrophil lysates, severing actin filaments and removing capping protein-β₂ from barbed ends. *Biochim Biophys Acta Mol Cell Res* 1358:261, 1997.

331. Niggli V, Keller H: The phosphatidylinositol 3-kinase inhibitor wortmannin markedly reduces chemotactic peptide-induced locomotion and increases in cytoskeletal actin in human neutrophils. *Eur J Pharmacol* 335:43, 1997.

332. Yan SR, Fumagalli L, Dusi S, Berton G: Tumor necrosis factor triggers redistribution to a Triton X-100-insoluble, cytoskeletal fraction of β_2 integrins, NADPH oxidase components, tyrosine phosphorylated proteins, and the protein tyrosine kinase p58^{fgr} in human neutrophils adherent to fibrinogen. *J Leukocyte Biol* 58:595, 1995.

333. Fujimoto T, Ogawa K: Fodrin in the human polymorphonuclear leucocyte: redistribution induced by the chemotactic peptide. *J Cell Sci* 96:477, 1990.

334. Rothwell SW, Nath J, Wright DG: Rapid and reversible tubulin tyrosination in human neutrophils stimulated by the chemotactic peptide, fMet-Leu-Phe. *J Cell Physiol* 154:582, 1993.

335. Ding M, Robinson JM, Behrens BC, Vandré DD: The microtubule cytoskeleton in human phagocytic leukocytes is a highly dynamic structure. *Eur J Cell Biol* 66:234, 1995.

336. Smolen JE, Korchak HM, Weissmann G: Increased levels of cyclic adenosine-3′,5′-monophosphate in human polymorphonuclear leukocytes after surface stimulation. *J Clin Invest* 65:1077, 1980.

337. Simchowitz L, Fischbein LC, Spilberg I, Atkinson JP: Induction of a transient elevation in intracellular levels of adenosine-3′,5′-monophosphate by chemotactic factors: an early event in human neutrophil activation. *J Immunol* 124:1482, 1980.

338. Naef A, Damerau B, Keller HU: Relationship between the transient cAMP increase, exocytosis from specific and azurophil granules and chemotaxis in neutrophil granulocytes. *Agents Actions* 14:63, 1984.

339. Simchowitz L, Atkinson JP, Spilberg I: Stimulus-dependent deactivation of chemotactic factor-induced cyclic AMP response and superoxide generation by human neutrophils. *J Clin Invest* 66:736, 1980.

340. Simchowitz L, Spilberg I, Atkinson JP: Evidence that the functional responses of human neutrophils occur independently of transient elevations in cyclic AMP levels. *J Cyc Nucl Prot Phos Res* 9:35, 1983.

341. Pryzwansky KB, Steiner AL, Spitznagel JK, Kapoor CL: Compartmentalization of cyclic AMP during phagocytosis of human neutrophilic granulocytes. *Science* 211:407, 1981.

342. Iannone MA, Wolberg G, Zimmerman TP: Ca^{2+} ionophore-induced cyclic adenosine-3′,5′-monophosphate elevation in human neutrophils. A calmodulin-dependent potentiation of adenylate cyclase response to endogenously produced adenosine: Comparison to chemotactic agents. *Biochem Pharmacol* 42(Suppl):S105, 1991.

343. Smolen JE, Stoehr SJ, Kuczynski B: Cyclic AMP inhibits secretion from electroporated human neutrophils. *J Leuk Biol* 49:172, 1991.

344. Tyagi SR, Olson SC, Burnham DN, Lambeth JD: Cyclic AMP-elevating agents block chemoattractant activation of diradylglycerol generation by inhibiting phospholipase D activation. *J Biol Chem* 266:3498, 1991.

345. Agwu DE, McCall CE, McPhail LC: Regulation of phospholipase D-induced hydrolysis of choline-containing phosphoglycerides by cyclic AMP in human neutrophils. *J Immunol* 146:3895, 1991.

346. Ahmed MU, Hazeki K, Hazeki O, et al: Cyclic AMP-increasing agents interfere with chemoattractant induced respiratory burst in neutrophils as a result of the inhibition of phosphatidylinositol 3-kinase rather than receptor-operated Ca^{2+} influx. *J Biol Chem* 270:23816, 1995.

347. Savitha G, Salimath BP: Cross-talk between protein kinase C and protein kinase A down-regulates the respiratory burst in polymorphonuclear leukocytes. *Cell Signal* 5:107, 1993.

348. Ydrenius L, Molony L, Ng-Sikorski J, Andersson T: Dual action of cAMP-dependent protein kinase on granulocyte movement. *Biochem Biophys Res Commun* 235:445, 1997.

349. Parvathenani LK, Buescher ES, Chacon-Cruz E, Beebe SJ: Type I cAMP-dependent protein kinase delays apoptosis in human neutrophils at a site upstream of caspase-3. *J Biol Chem* 273:6736, 1998.

350. Asahi M, Tanaka Y, Qin S, et al: Cyclic AMP-elevating agents negatively regulate the activation of p72^{syk} in N-formyl-methionyl-leucyl-phenylalanine receptor signaling. *Biochem Biophys Res Commun* 212:887, 1995.

351. Pryzwansky KB, Wyatt TA, Lincoln TM: Cyclic guanosine monophosphate-dependent protein kinase is targeted to intermediate filaments and phosphorylates vimentin in A23187-stimulated human neutrophils. *Blood* 85:222, 1995.

352. Smolen JE, Stoehr SJ, Traynor AE, Sklar LA: The kinetics of secretion from permeabilized human neutrophils: release of elastase and correlations with other granule constituents and right angle light scatter. *J Leuk Biol* 41:8, 1987.

353. Smolen JE, Todd RF III, Boxer LA: Expression of a granule membrane marker on the surface of neutrophils permeabilized with digitonin. Correlations with Ca^{2+}-induced degranulation. *Am J Pathol* 124:281, 1986.

354. Walter A, Steer CJ, Blumenthal R: Polylysine induces pH-dependent fusion of acidic phospholipid vesicles: a model for polycation-induced fusion. *Biochim Biophys Acta* 861:319, 1986.

355. Ohki S, Duax J: Effects of cations and polyamines on the aggregation and fusion of phosphatidylserine membranes. *Biochim Biophys Acta* 861:177, 1986.

356. Duzgunes N, Straubinger RM, Baldwin PA, et al: Proton-induced fusion of oleic acid-phosphatidylethanolamine liposomes. *Biochemistry* 24:3091, 1985.

357. Morris SJ, Gibson CC, Smith PD, et al: Rapid kinetics of Ca^{2+}-induced fusion of phosphatidylserine/phosphatidylethanolamine vesicles. The effect of bilayer curvature on leakage. *J Biol Chem* 260:4122, 1985.

358. Stoehr SJ, Smolen JE, Suchard SJ: Lipocortins are major substrates for protein kinase C in extracts of human neutrophils. *J Immunol* 144:3936, 1990.

359. Ernst JD, Hoye E, Blackwood RA, Jaye D: Purification and characterization of an abundant cytosolic protein from human neutrophils that promotes Ca^{2+}-dependent aggregation of isolated specific granules. *J Clin Invest* 85:1065, 1990.

360. Francis JW, Balazovich KJ, Smolen JE, et al: Human neutrophil annexin I promotes granule aggregation and modulates Ca^{2+}-dependent membrane fusion. *J Clin Invest* 90:537, 1992.

361. Blackwood RA, Ernst JD: Characterization of Ca^{2+}-dependent phospholipid binding, vesicle aggregation and membrane fusion by annexins. *Biochem J* 266:195, 1990.

362. Meers P, Mealy T, Tauber AI: Annexin I interactions with human neutrophil specific granules: Fusogenicity and coaggregation with plasma membrane vesicles. *Biochim Biophys Acta Bio-Membr* 1147:177, 1993.

363. Sjölin C, Movitz C, Lundqvist H, Dahlgren C: Translocation of annexin XI to neutrophil subcellular organelles. *Biochim Biophys Acta Bio-Membr* 1326:149, 1997.

364. Perretti M, Wheller SK, Choudhury Q, et al: Selective inhibition of neutrophil function by a peptide derived from lipocortin 1 N-terminus. *Biochem Pharmacol* 50:1037, 1995.

365. Rosales JL, Ernst JD: Calcium-dependent neutrophil secretion: Characterization and regulation by annexins. *J Immunol* 159:6195, 1997.

366. Izumi F, Yanagihara N, Wada A, et al: Lysis of chromaffin granules by phospholipase A2-treated plasma membranes. A cell-free model for exocytosis in adrenal medulla. *FEBS Lett* 196:349, 1986.

367. Creutz CE: *cis*-Unsaturated fatty acids induce fusion of chromaffin granules aggregated by synexin. *J Cell Biol* 91:247, 1981.

368. Siegel DP, Banschbach J, Alford D, et al: Physiological levels of diacylglycerols in phospholipid membranes induce membrane fusion and stabilize inverted phases. *Biochemistry* 28:3703, 1989.

369. Wu H, Zheng LX, Lentz BR: A slight asymmetry in the transbilayer distribution of lysophosphatidylcholine alters the surface properties and poly(ethylene glycol)-mediated fusion of dipalmitoylphosphatidylcholine large unilamellar vesicles. *Biochemistry* 35:12602, 1996.

370. Chernomordik L, Chanturiya A, Green J, Zimmerberg J: The hemifusion intermediate and its conversion to complete fusion: Regulation by membrane composition. *Biophys J* 69:922, 1995.

371. Ruiz-Argüello MB, Basáñez G, Goñi FM, Alonso A: Different effects of enzyme-generated ceramides and diacylglycerols in phospholipid membrane fusion and leakage. *J Biol Chem* 271:26616, 1996.

372. Smolen JE, Weissmann G: Lysosomal enzyme release from human granulocytes is inhibited by indomethacin, ETYA, and BPB, in *Advances in Prostaglandin and Thromboxane Research*, 8th ed, edited by B Samuelsson, P Ramwell and R Paoletti, pp 1695–1700. Raven Press, New York, 1980.

373. Lennartz MR, Yuen AFC, Masi SM, et al: Phospholipase A$_2$ inhibition results in sequestration of plasma membrane into electronlucent vesicles during IgG-mediated phagocytosis. *J Cell Sci* 110:2041, 1997.

374. Blackwood RA, Transue A, Harsh DM, et al: PLA$_2$ promotes fusion between PMN specific granules and complex liposomes. *J Leuk Biol* 59:663, 1996.

375. Augustine GJ, Burns ME, DeBello WM, et al: Exocytosis: Proteins and perturbations. *Annu Rev Pharmacol Toxicol* 36:659, 1996.

376. Weber T, Zemelman BV, McNew JA, et al: SNAREpins: Minimal machinery for membrane fusion. *Cell* 92:759, 1998.

377. Smolen JE, Hessler RJ, Nauseef WM, et al: Identification and cloning of the fusion protein VAMP-2 in HL-60 cells and human neutrophils. *Mol Biol Cell* 8:295a, 1997. (Abstract)

378. Brumell JH, Volchuk A, Sengelov H, et al: Subcellular distribution of docking/fusion proteins in neutrophils, secretory cells with multiple exocytic compartments. *J Immunol* 155:5750, 1995.

379. Nabokina S, Egea G, Blasi J, Mollinedo F: Intracellular location of SNAP-25 in human neutrophils. *Biochem Biophys Res Commun* 239:592, 1997.

380. Mollinedo F, Lazo PA: Identification of two isoforms of the vesicle-membrane fusion protein SNAP-23 in human neutrophils and HL-60 cells. *Biochem Biophys Res Commun* 231:808, 1997.

381. Spitznagel JK: Nonoxidative antimicrobial reactions of leukocytes. *Contemporary Top Immunobiol* 14:283, 1984.

382. Gabay JE, Heiple JM, Cohn ZA, Nathan CF: Subcellular location and properties of bactericidal factors from human neutrophils. *J Exp Med* 164:1407, 1986.

383. Weiss J, Kao L, Victor M, Elsbach P: Oxygen-independent intracellular and oxygen-dependent extracellular killing of *Escherichia coli* S15 by human polymorphonuclear leukocytes. *J Clin Invest* 76:206, 1985.

384. Kharazmi A, Jepsen S, Valerius NH: Polymorphonuclear leucocytes defective in oxidative metabolism inhibit *in vitro* growth of *Plasmodium falciparum*. Evidence against an oxygen-dependent mechanism. *Scand J Immunol* 20:93, 1984.

385. Segal AW, Harper AM, Garcia RC, Merzbach D: The action of cells from patients with chronic granulomatous disease on *Staphylococcus aureus. J Med Microbiol* 15:441, 1982.

386. Shafer WM, Martin LE, Spitznagel JK: Late intraphagosomal hydrogen ion concentration favors the *in vitro* antimicrobial capacity of a 37-kilodalton cationic granule protein of human neutrophil granulocytes. *Infect Immun* 53:651, 1986.

387. Bassoe CF, Laerum OD, Glette J, et al: Simultaneous measurement of phagocytosis and phagosomal pH by flow cytometry: role of polymorphonuclear neutrophilic leukocyte granules in phagosome acidification. *Cytometry* 4:254, 1983.

388. Smolen JE, Korchak HM, Weissmann G: The kinetics of lysosomal degranulation of human neutrophils as measured by 9-aminoacridine quenching. *Biochim Biophys Acta* 762:145, 1983.

389. Styrt B, Klempner MS: Internal pH of human neutrophil lysosomes. *FEBS Lett* 149:113, 1982.

390. Gray PW, Flaggs G, Leong SR, et al: Cloning of the cDNA of a human neutrophil bactericidal protein. Structural and functional correlations. *J Biol Chem* 264:9505, 1989.

391. Wilde CG, Griffith JE, Marra MN, et al: Purification and characterization of human neutrophil peptide 4, a novel member of the defensin family. *J Biol Chem* 264:11200, 1989.

392. Pereira HA, Spitznagel JK, Pohl J, et al: CAP 37, a 37-kD human neutrophil granule cationic protein shares homology with inflammatory proteinases. *Life Sci* 46:189, 1990.

393. Pereira HA, Spitznagel JK, Winton EF, et al: The ontogeny of a 57-kD cationic antimicrobial protein of human polymorphonuclear leukocytes: Localization to a novel granule population. *Blood* 76:825, 1990.

394. Ooi CE, Weiss J, Levy O, Elsbach P: Isolation of two isoforms of a novel 15-kDa protein from rabbit polymorphonuclear leukocytes that modulate the antibacterial actions of other leukocyte proteins. *J Biol Chem* 265:15956, 1990.

395. Pontremoli S, Melloni E, Michetti M, et al: Cytolytic effects of neutrophils: role for a membrane-bound neutral proteinase. *Proc Natl Acad Sci USA* 83:1685, 1986.

396. Ginsburg I: Cationic polyelectrolytes: A new look at their possible roles as opsonins, as stimulators of respiratory burst in leukocytes, in bacteriolysis, and as modulators of immune-complex diseases. (A review hypothesis). *Inflammation* 11:489, 1987.

397. Linzmeier R, Michaelson D, Liu L, Ganz T: The structure of neutrophil defensin genes. *FEBS Lett* 321:267, 1993.

398. Harwig SSL, Park ASK, Lehrer RI: Characterization of defensin precursors in mature human neutrophils. *Blood* 79:1532, 1992.

399. Rice WG, Ganz T, Kinkade JM Jr, et al: Defensin-rich dense granules of human neutrophils. *Blood* 70:757, 1987.

400. Charp PA, Rice WG, Raynor RL, et al: Inhibition of protein kinase C by defensins, antibiotic peptides from human neutrophils. *Biochem Pharmacol* 37:951, 1988.

401. Tal T, Michaela S, Irit A: Cationic proteins of neutrophil azurophilic granules: protein-protein interaction and blockade of NADPH oxidase activation. *J Leukocyte Biol* 63:305, 1998.

402. Viljanen P, Koski P, Vaara M: Effect of small cationic leukocyte peptides (defensins) on the permeability barrier of the outer membrane. *Infect Immun* 56:2324, 1988.

403. Gera JF, Lichtenstein A: Human neutrophil peptide defensins induce single strand DNA breaks in target cells. *Cell Immunol* 138:108, 1991.

404. Territo MC, Ganz T, Selsted ME, Lehrer R: Monocyte-chemotactic activity of defensins from human neutrophils. *J Clin Invest* 84:2017, 1989.

405. Morgan JG, Sukiennicki T, Pereira HA, et al: Cloning of the cDNA for the serine protease homolog CAP37/azurocidin, a microbicidal and chemotactic protein from human granulocytes. *J Immunol* 147:3210, 1991.

406. Pereira HA: CAP37, a neutrophil-derived multifunctional inflammatory mediator. *J Leukocyte Biol* 57:805, 1995.

407. Pereira HA, Shafer WM, Pohl J, et al: CAP37, a human neutrophil-derived chemotactic factor with monocyte specific activity. *J Clin Invest* 85:1468, 1990.

408. Pereira HA, Moore P, Grammas P: CAP37, a neutrophil granule-derived protein stimulates protein kinase C activity in endothelial cells. *J Leukocyte Biol* 60:415, 1996.

409. Elferink JGR: Captopril-induced enhancement of fMet-Leu-Phe-activated enzyme secretion from neutrophils. *Agents Actions* 38(Suppl C): C136, 1993.

410. Marra MN, Wilde CG, Collins MS, et al: The role of bactericidal/permeability-increasing protein as a natural inhibitor of bacterial endotoxin. *J Immunol* 148:532, 1992.

411. Ooi CE, Weiss J, Doerfler ME, Elsbach P: Endotoxin-neutralizing properties of the 25 kD N-terminal fragment and a newly isolated 30 kD C-terminal fragment of the 55–60 kD bactericidal/permeability-increasing protein of human neutrophils. *J Exp Med* 174:649, 1991.

412. Capodici C, Weiss J: Both N- and C-terminal regions of the bioactive N-terminal fragment of the neutrophil granule bactericidal/permeability-increasing protein are required for stability and function. *J Immunol* 156:4789, 1996.

413. in't Veld G, Mannion B, Weiss J, Elsbach P: Effects of the bactericidal/permeability-increasing protein of polymorphonuclear leukocytes on isolated bacterial cytoplasmic membrane vesicles. *Infect Immun* 56:1203, 1988.

414. Ooi CE, Weiss J, Elsbach P: Structural and functional organization of the human neutrophil 60 kDa bactericidal/permeability-increasing protein. *Agents Actions* 34:274, 1991.

415. Zarember K, Elsbach P, Shin-Kim K, Weiss J: p15s (15-kD antimicrobial proteins) are stored in the secondary granules of rabbit granulocytes: Implications for antibacterial synergy with the bactericidal/permeability-increasing protein in inflammatory fluids. *Blood* 89:672, 1997.

416. Storici P, Del Sal G, Schneider C, Zanetti M: cDNA sequence analysis of an antibiotic dodecapeptide from neutrophils. *FEBS Lett* 314:187, 1992.

417. Cowland JB, Johnsen AH, Borregaard N: hCAP-18, a cathelin/pro-bactenecin-like protein of human neutrophil specific granules. *FEBS Lett* 368:173, 1995.

418. Selsted ME, Novotny MJ, Morris WL, et al: Indolicidin, a novel bactericidal tridecapeptide amide from neutrophils. *J Biol Chem* 267:4292, 1992.

419. Huang HJ, Ross CR, Blecha F: Chemoattractant properties of PR-39, a neutrophil antibacterial peptide. *J Leukocyte Biol* 61:624, 1997.

420. Nagaoka I, Tsutsumi-Ishii Y, Yomogida S, Yamashita T: Isolation of cDNA encoding guinea pig neutrophil cationic antibacterial polypeptide of 11 kDa (CAP11) and evaluation of CAP11 mRNA expression during neutrophil maturation. *J Biol Chem* 272:22742, 1997.

421. Steinbakk M, Naess-Andresen C-F, Lingaas E, et al: Antimicrobial actions of calcium binding leucocyte L1 protein, calprotectin. *Lancet* 336:763, 1990.

422. Hessian PA, Edgeworth J, Hogg N: MRP-8 and MRP-14, two abundant Ca²⁺-binding proteins of neutrophils and monocytes. *J Leukocyte Biol* 53:197, 1993.

423. Bengis-Garber C, Gruener N: Calcium-binding myeloid protein (P8,14) is phosphorylated in fMet-Leu-Phe-stimulated neutrophils. *J Leukocyte Biol* 54:114, 1993.

424. Roth J, Burwinkel F, Van den Bos C, et al: MRP8 and MRP14, S-100-

like proteins associated with myeloid differentiation, are translocated to plasma membrane and intermediate filaments in a calcium-dependent manner. *Blood* 82:1875, 1993.

425. Hazen SL, Hsu FF, Mueller DM, et al: Human neutrophils employ chlorine gas as an oxidant during phagocytosis. *J Clin Invest* 98:1283, 1996.

426. Cohen HJ, Chovaniec ME: Superoxide generation by digitonin-stimulated guinea pig granulocytes. A basis for a continuous assay for monitoring superoxide production and for the study of the activation of the generating system. *J Clin Invest* 61:1081, 1978.

427. Bromberg Y, Pick E: Unsaturated fatty acids stimulate NADPH-dependent superoxide production by cell-free system derived from macrophages. *Cell Immunol* 88:213, 1984.

428. Tanaka T, Makino R, Iizuka T, et al: Activation by saturated and monounsaturated fatty acids of the O_2-generating system in a cell-free preparation from neutrophils. *J Biol Chem* 263:13670, 1988.

429. McPhail LC, Shirley PS, Clayton CC, Snyderman R: Activation of the respiratory burst enzyme from human neutrophils in a cell-free system. Evidence for a soluble cofactor. *J Clin Invest* 75:1735, 1985.

430. Curnutte JT, Kuver R, Babior BM: Activation of the respiratory burst oxidase in a fully soluble system from human neutrophils. *J Biol Chem* 262:6450, 1987.

431. Curnutte JT, Berkow RL, Roberts RL, et al: Chronic granulomatous disease due to a defect in the cytosolic factor required for nicotinamide adenine dinucleotide phosphate oxidase activation. *J Clin Invest* 81:606, 1988.

432. Gallin JI, Leto TL, Rotrosen D, et al: Delineation of the phagocyte NADPH oxidase through studies of chronic granulomatous diseases of childhood. *Curr Opin Immunol* 4:53, 1992.

433. Curnutte JT, Scott PJ, Mayo LA: Cytosolic components of the respiratory burst oxidase: Resolution of four components, two of which are missing in complementing types of chronic granulomatous disease. *Proc Natl Acad Sci USA* 86:825, 1989.

434. Volpp BD, Nauseef WM, Donelson JE, et al: Cloning of the cDNA and functional expression of the 47-kilodalton cytosolic component of human neutrophil respiratory burst oxidase. *Proc Natl Acad Sci USA* 86:7195, 1989.

435. Leto TL, Garrett MC, Fujii H, Nunoi H: Characterization of neutrophil NADPH oxidase factors p47-*phox* and p67-*phox* from recombinant baculoviruses. *J Biol Chem* 266:19812, 1991.

436. Abo A, Boyhan A, West I, et al: Reconstitution of neutrophil NADPH oxidase activity in the cell-free system by four components: p67-*phox*, p47-*phox*, p21*rac*1, and cytochrome b_{-245}. *J Biol Chem* 267:16767, 1992.

437. Gabig TG, Crean CD, Mantel PL, Rosli R: Function of wild-type or mutant Rac2 and Rap1a GTPases in differentiated HL60 cell NADPH oxidase activation. *Blood* 85:804, 1995.

438. Sathyamoorthy M, De Mendez I, Adams AG, Leto TL: p40[phox] downregulates NADPH oxidase activity through interactions with its SH3 domain. *J Biol Chem* 272:9141, 1997.

439. Cross AR, Higson FK, Jones OTG, et al: The enzymic reduction and kinetics of oxidation of cytochrome b_{-245} of neutrophils. *Biochem J* 204:479, 1982.

440. Light DR, Walsh C, O'Callaghan AM, et al: Characteristics of the cofactor requirements for the superoxide-generating NADPH oxidase of human polymorphonuclear leukocytes. *Biochemistry* 20:1468, 1981.

441. Gabig TG, Schervish EW, Santinga JT: Functional relationship of the cytochrome b to the superoxide-generating oxidase of human neutrophils. *J Biol Chem* 257:4114, 1982.

442. Cross AR, Jones OTG, Garcia R, Segal AW: The association of FAD with the cytochrome b_{-245} of human neutrophils. *Biochem J* 208:759, 1982.

443. Segal AW: The electron transport chain of the microbicidal oxidase of phagocytic cells and its involvement in the molecular pathology of chronic granulomatous disease. *J Clin Invest* 83:1785, 1989.

444. Green TR, Pratt KL: Detection and isolation of the NADPH-binding protein of the NADPH:O_2 oxidoreductase complex of human neutrophils. *J Biol Chem* 265:19324, 1990.

445. Borregaard N: The respiratory burst of phagocytosis: Biochemistry and subcellular localization. *Immunol Lett* 11:165, 1985.

446. Ohno Y, Buescher ES, Roberts R, et al: Reevaluation of cytochrome b and flavin adenine dinucleotide in neutrophils from patients with chronic granulomatous disease and description of a family with probable autoso-

mal recessive inheritance of cytochrome b deficiency. *Blood* 67:1132, 1986.

447. Parkos CA, Dinauer MC, Jesaitis AJ, et al: Absence of both the 91kD and 22kD subunits of human neutrophil cytochrome b in two genetic forms of chronic granulomatous disease. *Blood* 73:1416, 1989.

448. Segal AW, Jones OTG: Absence of cytochrome b reduction in stimulated neutrophils from both female and male patients with chronic granulomatous disease. *FEBS Lett* 110:111, 1980.

449. Segal AW, Cross AR, Garcia RC, et al: Absence of cytochrome b_{-245} in chronic granulomatous disease. A multicenter European evaluation of its incidence and relevance. *N Engl J Med* 308:245, 1983.

450. Segal AW: Absence of both cytochrome b_{-245} subunits from neutrophils in X-linked chronic granulomatous disease. *Nature* 326:88, 1987.

451. Kleinberg ME, Mital D, Rotrosen D, Malech HL: Characterization of a phagocyte cytochrome b_{558} 91-kilodalton subunit functional domain: Identification of peptide sequence and amino acids essential for activity. *Biochemistry* 31:2686, 1992.

452. Quinn MT, Mullen ML, Jesaitis AJ: Human neutrophil cytochrome *b* contains multiple hemes. Evidence for heme associated with both subunits. *J Biol Chem* 267:7303, 1992.

453. Dinauer MC, Pierce EA, Erickson RW, et al: Point mutation in the cytoplasmic domain of the neutrophil p22-*phox* cytochrome *b* subunit is associated with a nonfunctional NADPH oxidase and chronic granulomatous disease. *Proc Natl Acad Sci USA* 88:11231, 1991.

454. Green TR, Pratt KL: Purification of the solubilized NADPH:O_2 oxidoreductase of human neutrophils. Isolation of its catalytically inactive cytochrome b and flavoprotein redox centers. *J Biol Chem* 263:5617, 1988.

455. Yoshida LS, Chiba T, Kakinuma K: Determination of flavin contents in neutrophils by a sensitive chemiluminescence assay: Evidence for no translocation of flavoproteins from the cytosol to the membrane upon cell stimulation. *Biochim Biophys Acta Mol Cell Res* 1135:245, 1992.

456. Ohno Y, Seligmann BE, Gallin JI: Cytochrome b translocation to human neutrophil plasma membranes and superoxide release. Differential effects of *N*-formylmethionylleucylphenylalanine, phorbol myristate acetate, and A23187. *J Biol Chem* 260:2409, 1985.

457. Parkos CA, Cochrane CG, Schmitt M, Jesaitis AJ: Regulation of the oxidative response of human granulocytes to chemoattractants. No evidence for stimulated traffic of redox enzymes between endo and plasma membranes. *J Biol Chem* 260:6541, 1985.

458. Bjerrum OW, Borregaard N: Dual granule localization of the dormant NADPH oxidase and cytochrome b559 in human neutrophils. *Eur J Haematol* 43:67, 1989.

459. Borregaard N, Heiple JM, Simons ER, Clark RA: Subcellular localization of the b cytochrome component of the human neutrophil microbicidal oxidase: translocation during activation. *J Cell Biol* 97:52, 1983.

460. Heyworth PG, Curnutte JT, Nauseef WM, et al: Neutrophil nicotinamide adenine dinucleotide phosphate oxidase assembly. Translocation of p47-*phox* and p67-*phox* requires interaction between p47-*phox* and cytochrome b_{558}. *J Clin Invest* 87:352, 1991.

461. Raj Tyagi S, Neckelmann N, Uhlinger DJ, et al: Cell-free translocation of recombinant p47-phox, a component of the neutrophil NADPH oxidase: Effects of guanosine 5′-*O*-(3-thiotriphosphate), diacylglycerol, and an anionic amphiphile. *Biochemistry* 31:2765, 1992.

462. Woodman RC, Ruedi JM, Jesaitis AJ, et al: Respiratory burst oxidase and three of four oxidase-related polypeptides are associated with the cytoskeleton of human neutrophils. *J Clin Invest* 87:1345, 1991.

463. Abo A, Pick E, Hall A, et al: Activation of the NADPH oxidase involves the small GTP-binding protein p21[rac1]. *Nature* 353:668, 1991.

464. Quinn MT, Mullen ML, Jesaitis AJ, Linner JG: Subcellular distribution of the Rap1A protein in human neutrophils: Colocalization and cotranslocation with cytochrome b_{559}. *Blood* 79:1563, 1992.

465. Dorseuil O, Reibel L, Bokoch GM, et al: The Rac target NADPH oxidase p67[phox] interacts preferentially with Rac2 rather than Rac1. *J Biol Chem* 271:83, 1996.

466. Bokoch GM, Quilliam LA, Bohl BP, et al: Inhibition of Rap1A binding to cytochrome b_{558} of NADPH oxidase by phosphorylation of Rap1A. *Science* 254:1794, 1991.

467. Someya A, Yomogida S, Nagaoka I, et al: Purification of the 28.5 kDa cytosolic protein involved in the activation of NADPH oxidase from guinea pig neutrophils. *FEBS Lett* 302:69, 1992.

468. Radeke HH, Cross AR, Hancock JT, et al: Functional expression of NADPH oxidase components (alpha- and beta-subunits of cytochrome

b_{558} and 45-kDa flavoprotein) by intrinsic human glomerular mesangial cells. *J Biol Chem* 266:21025, 1991.

469. Nakamura R, Sumimoto H, Mizuki K, et al: The PC motif: A novel and evolutionarily conserved sequence involved in interaction between p40^{phox} and p67^{phox}, SH3 domain-containing cytosolic factors of the phagocyte NADPH oxidase. *Eur J Biochem* 251:583, 1998.

470. Fuchs A, Dagher MC, Fauré J, Vignais PV: Topological organization of the cytosolic activating complex of the superoxide-generating NADPH-oxidase. Pinpointing the sites of interaction between p47phox, p67phox and p40phox using the two-hybrid system. *Biochim Biophys Acta Mol Cell Res* 1312:39, 1996.

471. Seifert R, Schachtele C: Studies with protein kinase C inhibitors presently available cannot elucidate the role of protein kinase C in the activation of NADPH oxidase. *Biochem Biophys Res Comm* 152:585, 1988.

472. Clark RA, Leidal KG, Pearson DW, Nauseef WM: NADPH oxidase of human neutrophils. Subcellular localization and characterization of an arachidonate-activatable superoxide-generating system. *J Biol Chem* 262:4065, 1987.

473. Peveri P, Heyworth PG, Curnutte JT: Absolute requirement for GTP in activation of human neutrophil NADPH oxidase in a cell-free system: Role of ATP in regenerating GTP. *Proc Natl Acad Sci USA* 89:2494, 1992.

474. Sozzani S, Sallusto F, Luini W, et al: Migration of dendritic cells in response to formyl peptides, C5a, and a distinct set of chemokines. *J Immunol* 155:3292, 1995.

475. Dusi S, Della Bianca V, Grzeskowiak M, Rossi F: Relationship between phosphorylation and translocation to the plasma membrane of p47phox and p67phox and activation of the NADPH oxidase in normal and Ca^{2+}-depleted human neutrophils. *Biochem J* 290:173, 1993.

476. Rotrosen D, Leto TL: Phosphorylation of neutrophil 47-kDa cytosolic oxidase factor. Translocation to membrane is associated with distinct phosphorylation events. *J Biol Chem* 265:19910, 1990.

477. Park J-W, Ahn SM: Translocation of recombinant p47^{phox} cytosolic component of the phagocyte oxidase by *in vitro* phosphorylation. *Biochim Biophys Res Commun* 211:410, 1995.

478. Curnutte JT, Erickson RW, Ding J, Badwey JA: Reciprocal interactions between protein kinase C and components of the NADPH oxidase complex may regulate superoxide production by neutrophils stimulated with a phorbol ester. *J Biol Chem* 269:10813, 1994.

479. Inanami O, Johnson JL, McAdara JK, et al: Activation of the leukocyte NADPH oxidase by phorbol ester requires the phosphorylation of p47^{PHOX} on serine 303 or 304. *J Biol Chem* 273:9539, 1998.

480. Yamaguchi M, Saeki S, Yamane H, et al: Hyperphosphorylated p47-phox lost the ability to activate NADPH oxidase in guinea pig neutrophils. *Biochem Biophys Res Commun* 216:203, 1995.

481. Yamaguchi M, Saeki S, Yamane H, et al: Involvement of several protein kinases in the phosphorylation of p47-phox. *Biochem Biophys Res Commun* 220:891, 1996.

482. Huang C-K, Coleman H, Stevens T, Liang L: Rapid modification of ribosomal S6 kinase II (S6KII) in rabbit peritoneal neutrophils stimulated with chemotactic factor fMet-Leu-Phe. *J Leukocyte Biol* 55:430, 1994.

483. el Benna J, Faust LP, Johnson JL, Babior BM: Phosphorylation of the respiratory burst oxidase subunit p47^{phox} as determined by two-dimensional phosphopeptide mapping—Phosphorylation by protein kinase C, protein kinase A, and a mitogen-activated protein kinase. *J Biol Chem* 271:6374, 1996.

484. el Benna J, Han JH, Park JW, et al: Activation of p38 in stimulated human neutrophils: Phosphorylation of the oxidase component p47^{phox} by p38 and ERK but not by JNK. *Arch Biochem Biophys* 334:395, 1996.

485. el Benna J, Faust LP, Babior BM: The phosphorylation of the respiratory burst oxidase component p47^{phox} during neutrophil activation. Phosphorylation of sites recognized by protein kinase C and by proline-directed kinases. *J Biol Chem* 269:23431, 1994.

486. Ding J, Badwey JA: Stimulation of neutrophils with a chemoattractant activates several novel protein kinases that can catalyze the phosphorylation of peptides derived from the 47-kDa protein component of the phagocyte oxidase and myristoylated alanine-rich C kinase substrate. *J Biol Chem* 268:17326, 1993.

487. Prigmore E, Ahmed S, Best A, et al: A 68-kDa kinase and NADPH oxidase component p67^{phox} are targets for Cdc42Hs and Rac1 in neutrophils. *J Biol Chem* 270:10717, 1995.

488. Park JW, Babior BM: Activation of the leukocyte NADPH oxidase subunit p47^{phox} by protein kinase C. A phosphorylation-dependent change in the conformation of the C-terminal end of p47^{phox}. *Biochemistry* 36:7474, 1997.

489. Waite KA, Wallin R, Qualliotine-Mann D, McPhail LC: Phosphatidic acid-mediated phosphorylation of the NADPH oxidase component p47^{phox}. Evidence that phosphatidic acid may activate a novel protein kinase. *J Biol Chem* 272:15569, 1997.

490. Faust LP, el Benna J, Babior BM, Chanock SJ: The phosphorylation targets of p47^{phox}, a subunit of the respiratory burst oxidase—Functions of the individual target serines as evaluated by site-directed mutagenesis. *J Clin Invest* 96:1499, 1995.

491. el Benna J, Dang PMC, Gaudry M, et al: Phosphorylation of the respiratory burst oxidase subunit p67^{phox} during human neutrophil activation—Regulation by protein kinase C-dependent and independent pathways. *J Biol Chem* 272:17204, 1997.

492. Garcia RC, Segal AW: Phosphorylation of the subunits of cytochrome b$_{-245}$ upon triggering of the respiratory burst of human neutrophils and macrophages. *Biochem J* 252:901, 1988.

493. Bellavite P, Corso F, Dusi S, et al: Activation of NADPH-dependent superoxide production in plasma membrane extracts of pig neutrophils by phosphatidic acid. *J Biol Chem* 263:8210, 1988.

494. Burnham DN, Uhlinger DJ, Lambeth JD: Diradylglycerol synergizes with an anionic amphiphile to activate superoxide generation and phosphorylation of p47^{phox} in a cell-free system from human neutrophils. *J Biol Chem* 265:17550, 1990.

495. Morel F, Cholley LCT, Brandolin G, et al: The O$_2^-$ generating oxidase of B lymphocytes: Epstein-Barr virus-immortalized B lymphocytes as a tool for the identification of defective components of the oxidase in chronic granulomatous disease. *Biochim Biophys Acta Mol Basis Dis* 1182:101, 1993.

496. Chetty M, Thrasher AJ, Abo A, Casimir CM: Low NADPH oxidase activity in Epstein-Barr-virus-immortalized B-lymphocytes is due to a post-transcriptional block in expression of cytochrome b$_{558}$. *Biochem J* 306:141, 1995.

497. Meier B, Jesaitis AJ, Emmendörffer A, et al: The cytochrome *b*-558 molecules involved in the fibroblast and polymorphonuclear leucocyte superoxide-generating NADPH oxidase systems are structurally and genetically distinct. *Biochem J* 289:481, 1993.

498. Goldman R, Moshonov S, Zor U: Generation of reactive oxygen species in a human keratinocyte cell line: Role of calcium. *Arch Biochem Biophys* 350:10, 1998.

499. Dwyer SC, Legendre L, Low PS, Leto TL: Plant and human neutrophil oxidative burst complexes contain immunologically related proteins. *Biochim Biophys Acta Gen Subj* 1289:231, 1996.

EOSINOPHILS AND THEIR DISORDERS

A.J. WARDLAW

A. BARRY KAY

As a result of their potential role in asthma, eosinophils have received considerable attention from the research community in the last decade. The concept of the eosinophil as a cell that has protective effects against helminthic parasite infection but can cause tissue damage when inappropriately activated remains intact, although the evidence for both these roles remains circumstantial.

Eosinophil production and function are profoundly influenced by interleukin-5 (IL-5), and thus eosinophilia is associated with diseases characterized by Th2-mediated immune responses, including helminthic parasite infections and extrinsic asthma. However, eosinophilia also occurs in diseases not associated with Th2 dominance such as intrinsic asthma, hypereosinophilic syndrome (HES), and inflammatory bowel disease. It is clear that IL-5 and other eosinophil mediators can be generated in various types of inflammatory response.

The eosinophil, like other leukocytes, can generate proinflammatory mediators. Eosinophil-specific granule proteins are toxic for a range of mammalian cells and parasitic larvae. Eosinophils, like mast cells, produce sulfidopeptide leukotrienes, as well as other lipid mediators such as platelet-activating factor (PAF). Cytokine production by eosinophils broadens their potential functions, for example in wound healing through the generation of transforming growth factor (TGF)-α. Synthesis of TGF-β may explain the propensity of eosinophils to be associated with fibrotic reactions such as endomyocardial fibrosis, characteristic of HES, and fibrosing alveolitis.

Considerable effort has gone into trying to unravel the molecular basis of eosinophil tissue recruitment. The selective accumulation of eosinophils is due to a concerted and integrated series of events involving marrow egress, adhesion to endothelium, selective chemotaxis, and prolonged survival in tissues. These events are controlled, either directly or indirectly, by production of IL-4, IL-5, and IL-13. Understanding these events may lead to novel therapies that will help treat diseases caused by eosinophils without inhibiting their potentially beneficial roles.

Acronyms and abbreviations that appear in this chapter include: ECF-A, eosinophil chemotactic factor of anaphylaxis; ECP, eosinophil cationic protein; EDN, eosinophil-derived neurotoxin; EPO, eosinophil peroxidase; GM-CSF, granulocyte-monocyte colony stimulating growth factor; HES, hypereosinophilic syndrome; IL, interleukin; mAbs, monoclonal antibodies; PAF, platelet-activating factor; TGF, transforming growth factor.

EOSINOPHIL PRODUCTION

Eosinophils are nondividing, end-stage cells that, like other leukocytes, differentiate from the hematopoietic stem cell in the marrow. Eosinophils migrate into the blood, where they circulate with a half-life of about 18 h before entering the tissues. Eosinophils are primarily tissue-dwelling cells, and it has been estimated that there are about 100 tissue eosinophils for each eosinophil in the blood, although relatively few studies have been performed on eosinophil kinetics and even fewer have compared eosinophil turnover in health and disease.[1] Normal human adult marrow contains about 3 percent eosinophils of which one-third are mature and two-thirds are precursors. Eosinophilic myelocytes are large cells with a single-lobed nucleus, expanded Golgi, and extensive dilated cisterns of rough endoplasmic reticulum. The myelocytes become identifiable when they develop the core-containing specific granules, which initially are interspersed with large numbers of homogeneous dense granules[2] (Fig. 68-1) (see Chap. 64).

The massive increase in eosinophils associated with helminthic parasitic infection is T-cell dependent. The eosinophilia in rodents infected with helminths is abolished by thymectomy, thoracic duct drainage, or administration of antilymphocyte antiserum.[3,4] This effect is mediated by soluble factors released from sensitized lymphocytes.[5] Three T-cell–derived cytokines promote eosinophil growth and differentiation, IL-3, IL-5, and GM-CSF. Of these only human IL-5 promotes terminal maturation of eosinophils. It is also a basophil maturation factor.[6] Eosinophils and basophils are closely related. Eosinophil and basophil colonies appear together in marrow cell colony-forming assays.[7] IL-5 is a disulfide-linked homodimeric glycoprotein of 40–45/kD consisting of 115 amino acids.[8,9] The dimers are aligned in a head-to-tail fashion, and dimerization is essential for function.[10] IL-5 has a two-domain structure; the formation of each domain requires the participation of both chains. There is similarity between the domains in IL-5 and the cytokine-fold of other growth factors such as GM-CSF.[11,12] Transgenic mice with increased amounts of IL-5 have a marked blood and tissue eosinophilia and increased numbers of eosinophil precursors in their marrow suggesting that IL-5 is the rate-limiting step in eosinophil proliferation and maturation.[13,14] Despite a marked eosinophilia, these mice have no obvious pathological abnormalities. Both IL-3 and GM-CSF induce eosinophil colony formation in human cord blood culture[15] and eosinophilia after administration in vivo, although the increase in eosinophils is modest.[16] In humans, the genes for IL-3, IL-4, IL-5, IL-9, IL-13, and GM-CSF are clustered on the long arm of chromosome 5.[17] IL-4 and IL-5 are expressed by Th2 but not Th1 lymphocytes.[18] The receptors for IL-3, IL-5, and GM-CSF are structurally similar.[19] They consist of homologous α chains that bind their respective cytokines with low affinity, with a kD of approximately 10/nM. There is a common β chain that is noncovalently associated with core of the α chains at the cell surface and transforms the receptor into one of high affinity (kD150/pM). The β chain is required for signal transduction. Both the α and β chains are members of the type 1 hematopoietin cytokine receptor family. The α chains are between 60 and 80 kD and the β chain 12kD. Unlike the α chains of IL-3 and GM-CSF, the α chain of the IL-5R can bind IL-5 with relatively high affinity (kD 250–590/pM).[20,21] Blood eosinophils and HL-60 cell lines with eosinophilic features express IL-5 receptors with kDs of 170 to 330 and 10 to 50/pM, respectively.[22] Expression of the IL-5 alpha chain is down regulated by exposure to IL-5, IL-3, and GM-CSF, thus constituting a negative feedback loop.[23]

EOSINOPHIL HETEROGENEITY

Blood eosinophils from normal individuals are relatively dense cells which can be separated from other leukocytes by density-gradient centrifuge. For many years these differences were the basis for the

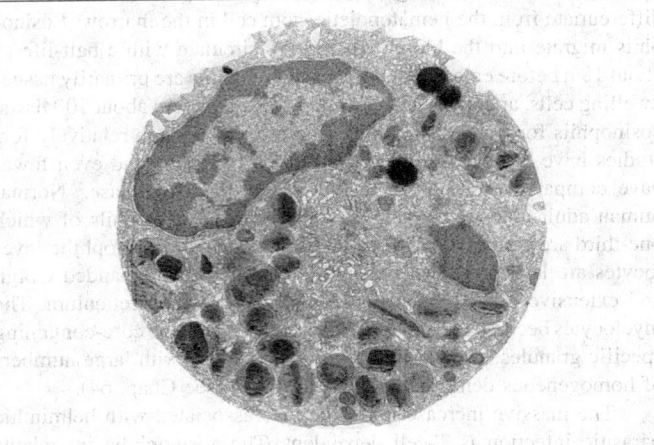

FIGURE 68-1   Transmission electron micrograph of an eosinophil showing the characteristic specific granules with their electron dense core (×10,000; courtesy of Dr. A Dewar, National Heart and Lung Institute).

standard method of purifying eosinophils. This has now been largely superseded by negative immunomagnetic selection based on the expression of the low affinity (FcγRIII, CD16) IgG receptor by neutrophils but not eosinophils. This latter technique has the advantage of improved purity and cell yields as well as enabling purification of eosinophils from individuals with low eosinophil counts.[24] A proportion of eosinophils from individuals with elevated eosinophil counts are less dense than eosinophils from normal subjects.[25] So-called hypodense eosinophils appear to be vacuolated and contain smaller granules, although in equal numbers to normal-density eosinophils.[26] The mechanism for this heterogeneity is unclear, although a correlation with eosinophil activation has been a favored hypothesis.[27] The evidence to support this hypothesis, however, is contradictory.[28]

MOLECULAR BASIS FOR EOSINOPHIL TISSUE ACCUMULATION

A striking feature of many eosinophilic diseases is the selective accumulation of these cells in the tissue in the absence of increased numbers of tissue neutrophils. The factors controlling this selective migration have been the subject of intensive study for over three decades, stimulated by the hope of identifying targets for treatment of diseases thought to be caused by eosinophil-mediated tissue damage. In asthma there is an approximately 100-fold enrichment of eosinophils over neutrophils in the bronchial mucosa compared to normal mucosa.[29] Historically this was thought to be due to a selective chemoattractant. A factor, termed *eosinophil chemotactic factor of anaphylaxis* (ECF-A), which appeared to be selectively chemotactic for eosinophils, was detected in supernatants from guinea-pig lung during anaphylaxis.[30] ECF-A was subsequently found to consist of leukotriene (LT)B$_4$, which is active on guinea-pig eosinophils but less so on human eosinophils, and 15-hydroxyeicosateraenoicacid (15-HETE).[31] ECF-A from human lung, composed of two tetrapeptides, Val-Gly-Ser-Glu and Ala-Gly-Ser-Glu, was identified later.[32] However in comparison to PAF these peptides were found to have negligible activity.[33] The role of chemokines as selective chemoattractants has also been studied. Selective tissue accumulation of eosinophils is probably not the result of any single event but rather due to selective pressure at every stage in the life-cycle of the eosinophil including eosinophilopoiesis, egress from the marrow, endothelial cell adhesion, chemotaxis, and prolonged survival in tissues under the influence of locally generated growth factors.

EOSINOPHILOPOIESIS AND EGRESS FROM THE MARROW

Eosinophil growth factors such as IL-5 generated at sites of allergic inflammation act to increase eosinophil production. There is on average about a fourfold increase compared with normal subjects in the number of circulating eosinophils in allergic individuals, and in other diseases this increase can be much greater. There are increased numbers of eosinophil precursors in the blood of allergic patients, and there is an increase in marrow progenitors expressing the IL-5α receptor (IL-5αR) (presumably eosinophil precursors) 24 h after allergen challenge.[34] This increase is the consequence of both increased production and increased egress from the marrow. IL-5 selectively promotes the egress of eosinophils from the marrow.[35] This egress is enhanced by eotaxin, an eosinophil-selective chemokine, and controlled by the integrin adhesion receptor α$_4$β$_1$ (CD CD49a; VLA-4), inhibition of which accelerates egress, and αMβ2 (CD16/CD18) and Mac, the inhibition of which prevents egress.[36]

ADHESION

The receptors and ligands involved in eosinophil adhesion are listed in Table 68-1.[37] Eosinophils adhere with up to tenfold greater avidity to nasal polyp endothelium (a model of eosinophilic inflammation) compared to neutrophils, suggesting that adhesion can account for a substantial part of the selective accumulation of eosinophils. Eosinophils can preferentially bind to P-selectin under flow conditions compared to neutrophils, especially at low levels of expression of this receptor, whereas neutrophils preferentially bind to E-selectin.[38,39] The reasons for these differences in adhesion are unclear although possibly related to differences in the glycosylation of the P-selectin receptor PSGL-1 between the two cell types. Endothelial P-selectin expression is increased by the Th2-related cytokines IL-4 and IL-13, although not by IL-1 or TNF-α.[40] Treatment of endothelial cells with these cytokines results in constitutive expression of low levels of P-selectin, which is sufficient to support eosinophil but not neutrophil binding to endothelial cells under flowing conditions.[41,42] In support of a role for P-selectin in eosinophil adhesion is the observation that eosinophil migration is reduced in a P-selectin gene-deleted mouse.[43] IL-4 and IL-13 can also induce low levels of VCAM-1 expression on endothelial cells, which supports P-selectin–mediated eosinophil tethering under flowing conditions. VLA-4/VCAM-1 also support se-

TABLE 68-1   EOSINOPHIL ADHESION RECEPTORS

	LIGAND	
RECEPTOR	ENDOTHELIAL	MATRIX PROTEIN
Integrins		
α4β1(VLA-4)	VCAM-1	Fibronectin
α4β6		Laminin
α4β7	MAdCAM-1	Fibronectin
LFA-1(αΛβ2)	ICAM-1-3	
Mac-1(αMβ2)	ICAM-1	
P150,95(αxβ2)		
αdβ2	VCAM-1(ICAM-3?)	
Selectins and Ligands		
PSGL-1	P-selectin(E-selectin)	
L-selectin	Gly-CAM-1,CD34,Podocalyxin	
Other		
CD44		Hyaluronate
ICAM-3		
PECAM	PECAM	
Siglec-8		Sialic Acid

ABBREVIATIONS: VCAM-1, vascular cell adhesion molecule; ICAM, intercellular cell adhesion molecule; MAdCAM-1, mucosal addressin cell adhesion molecule; PECAM: platelet endothelial cell adhesion molecule; PSGL-1: P-selectin glycoprotein 1.

lective transmigration through endothelial cells, and animal models have shown that eosinophil migration into the lung is inhibited by anti-$\alpha_4\beta1$ mAbs. Eosinophils express all four members of the $\beta2$ integrin family (CDa-d/CD18), and $\alpha M\beta2$ and $\alpha L\beta2$ are both important in mediating eosinophil transmigration.[44] The newest member of this family, $\alpha D\beta2$, appears to be a ligand for VCAM-1,[45] although the physiological relevance of this remains unclear.

CHEMOTAXIS

Most known eosinophil chemoattractants, such as PAF and C5a, are also active on other cell types. Members of the chemokine family, in particular C-C chemokines, are also involved in selective eosinophil recruitment. Eosinophils express CCR3 and low levels of expression of CCR1 have been detected on the eosinophils of some donors. Eosinophils from eosinophilic donors, but not normal subjects, migrate in response to IL-8, although eosinophils do not appear to express IL-8 receptors.[46] Expression of CCR3 is restricted to eosinophils, basophils, and a small subset of Th2 T cells, so it is a potential therapeutic target for inhibition of eosinophil migration.[47] Chemokines that bind to CCR3, including RANTES, eotaxin, and MCP-4, are highly effective eosinophil chemoattractants both in vitro and in vivo (Table 68-2).[48,49] IL-5 enhances the response of eosinophils to chemoattractants, including eotaxin.[50] In an IL-5–deficient mouse, eosinophils are unresponsive to eotaxin.[51] A number of CC chemokines have been shown to be expressed in increased amounts in allergic disease. Mouse models of eosinophilic lung disease, generally utilizing peritoneal sensitization with ovalbumin, have also been informative. Increases in eotaxin and RANTES expression parallel eosinophil migration, and blockade of eotaxin reduces eosinophil accumulation by half.[52] Blockade of both eotaxin and RANTES partially reduced eosinophil infiltration and bronchial hyperresponsiveness.[53] mRNA expression of eotaxin, but not RANTES, is increased in pulmonary eosinophilia, and eotaxin expression is T-cell dependent.[54] Chemokines seem to function as eosinophil chemoattractants, although they can also enhance eosinophil adhesion to endothelial cells and purified adhesion receptors. Chemokines do not appear to trigger mediator release.

PROLONGED SURVIVAL

Eosinophils rapidly undergo apoptosis in the absence of eosinophil growth factors such as IL-5, GM-CSF, and IL-3, which are all generated in the tissue during eosinophilic inflammation. Anti-IL-5 antibodies caused rapid loss of eosinophils from cultured explants of nasal polyps.[55] Thus cytokine generation is an important mechanism for selective eosinophil accumulation.

SYNTHESIS AND RELEASE OF EOSINOPHIL MEDIATORS

Eosinophils have the capacity to generate and/or release a number of potent inflammatory mediators (Fig. 68-2). These include basic proteins stored in eosinophil granules, lipid mediators (newly formed

TABLE 68-2   CHEMOKINES ACTIVE ON EOSINOPHILS

RECEPTOR	CHEMOKINE
CCR1*	Mip-1a; RANTES
CCR3	Eotaxin1; Eotaxin 2; MCP2–4; RANTES
CXCR1 & 2	IL-8†

*Only expressed on eosinophils from some donors.
†Only active on in vivo activated or cytokine-primed eosinophils (may be indirect effect via neutrophils).

after eosinophil activation), cytokines, eosinophil proteases, and components of the oxygen burst, including superoxide and hydrogen peroxide.

LIPID MEDIATORS

Eosinophils generate an array of lipid mediators, principally eicosanoids and PAF.[56] Eosinophils can generate relatively large amounts of the sulfidopeptide leukotriene LTC_4, after stimulation with the calcium ionophore via activation of the enzyme 5 lipoxygenase, but only negligible amounts of LTB_4.[57] This is in contrast to neutrophils which produce large amounts of LTB_4 but little, if any, LTC_4. LTC_4 generation by human eosinophils also occurs after stimulation with opsonized zymosan and beads coated with IgG.[58] Eosinophils can also generate substantial quantities of 15-HETE via 15-lipoxygenase. Eosinophils also generate PAF after stimulation with either calcium ionophore or IgG-coated beads.[59] Eosinophils can also generate mediators of the cyclooxygenase pathway, including prostaglandins E_1 and E_2, and thromboxane B_2 (TXB_2). The principal sites of eicosanoid formation in eosinophils are the lipid bodies which contain large amounts of arachidonic acid and enzymes required for eicosanoid synthesis, including 5-lipoxygenase, LTC_4 synthase, and cyclooxygenase.[60]

EOSINOPHIL GRANULE PROTEINS

MAJOR BASIC PROTEIN
Major basic protein (MBP) has a molecular mass of 13.8 kDa and a pI of 10.9. Its 17 arginine residues account for its basicity. It is initially synthesized as an acidic proprotein which is stored in the eosinophil granule[61]; MBP becomes toxic only after it is released and processed into its final form. Purified MBP is cytotoxic for the schistosomula of *S. mansoni,* and adherence of eosinophils to IgG-coated schistosomula results in the secretion of MBP onto the tegument of the larvae, resulting in loss of viability.[62] MBP at concentrations as low as 10 μg/ml has also been shown to be toxic for both guinea pig and human respiratory epithelial cells, as well as for rat and human pneumocytes.[63] The mechanism of action of MBP on epithelial cells appears to be mediated through inhibition of ATPase activity. The inhalation of MBP, albeit at high concentrations (1 mg/ml), produced increased bronchial hyperresponsiveness in monkeys.[64] MBP and eosinophil peroxidase (EPO) are strong agonists for platelet activation as well as activation of mast cells, basophils, and neutrophils.[65] The mechanisms of action of MBP is likely to be related to its hydrophobicity and strong negative charge. Basophils also contain MBP but only about 2 percent that of eosinophils.

EOSINOPHIL PEROXIDASE
This compound is a heme-containing protein that is synthesized as a single protein and then cleaved into 14- and 58-kD subunits.[66] The molecule shares a 68 percent identity in amino acid sequence with human neutrophil myeloperoxidase as well as other peroxidase enzymes. The substance is toxic for parasites, respiratory epithelium, and pneumocytes, either alone, or (more potently) when combined with H_2O_2 and halide, the preferred ion in vivo being bromide.

EOSINOPHIL CATIONIC PROTEIN
Eosinophil cationic protein (ECP) is an arginine-rich protein. The cDNA encodes for a 27 amino acid leader sequence and a 133 amino acid mature polypeptide with a molecular mass of 15.6 kDa. ECP has 66 percent amino acid sequence homology with eosinophil-derived neurotoxin (EDN) and 31 percent homology with human pancreatic ribonuclease,[67] but it has low ribonuclease activity compared to EDN.

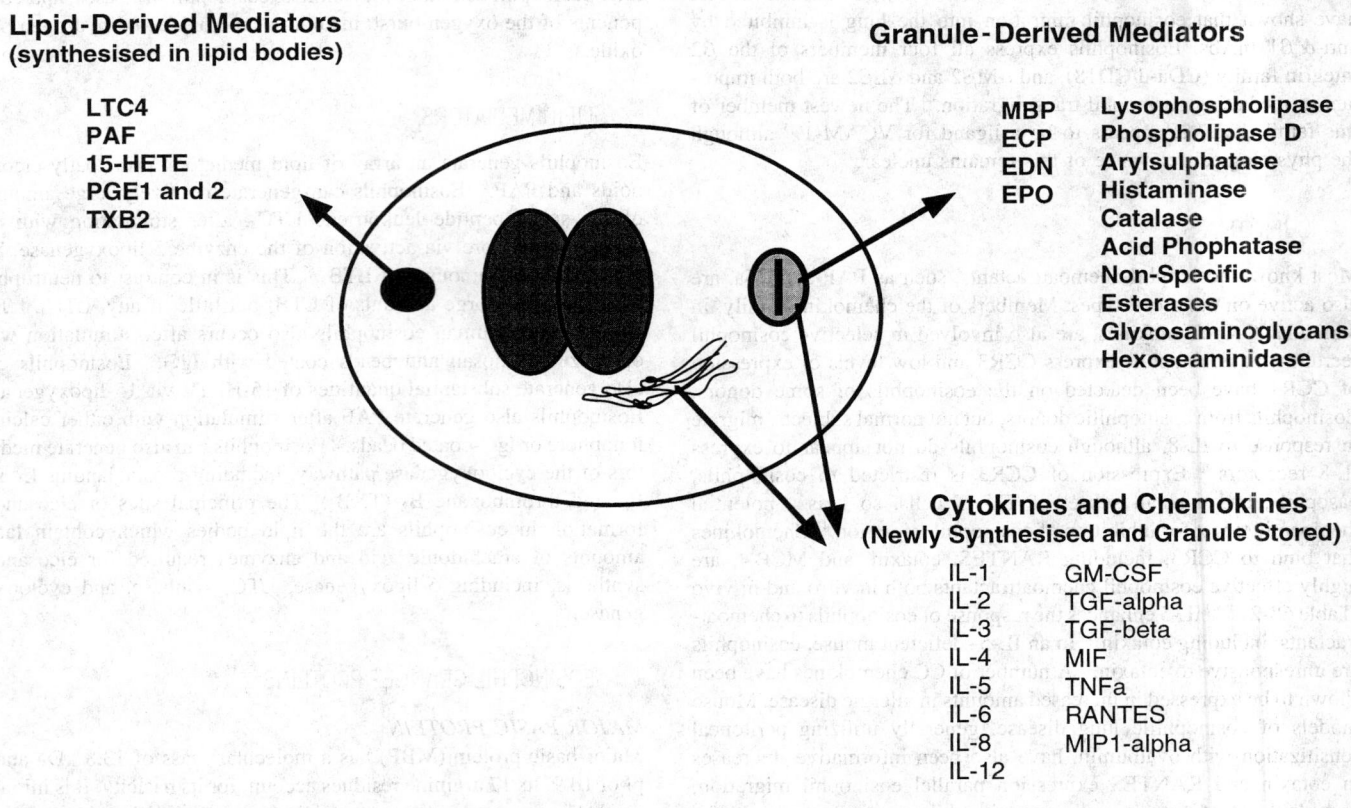

Lipid-Derived Mediators
(synthesised in lipid bodies)

LTC4
PAF
15-HETE
PGE1 and 2
TXB2

Granule-Derived Mediators

MBP	Lysophospholipase
ECP	Phospholipase D
EDN	Arylsulphatase
EPO	Histaminase
	Catalase
	Acid Phophatase
	Non-Specific
	Esterases
	Glycosaminoglycans
	Hexoseaminidase

Cytokines and Chemokines
(Newly Synthesised and Granule Stored)

IL-1	GM-CSF
IL-2	TGF-alpha
IL-3	TGF-beta
IL-4	MIF
IL-5	TNFa
IL-6	RANTES
IL-8	MIP1-alpha
IL-12	

FIGURE 68-2   Schematic representation of eosinophil-derived mediators. MBP, major basic protein; ECP, eosinophil cationic protein; EDN, eosinophil-derived neurotoxin; EPO, eosinophil-derived peroxidase; GM-CSF, granulocyte-monocyte colony stimulating factor; TGF, transforming growth factor; MIF, macrophage inhibition factor; TNF, tumor necrosis factor; MIP, macrophage inhibitory protein; PAF, platelet activating factor. LTC, leukotriene C; HETE, hydroxyeicosatetraenoic acid; PGE, prostaglandin E; TXB, thromboxane B.

ECP is toxic for helminthic parasites, isolated myocardial cells, and guinea pig tracheal epithelium. ECP also inhibits lymphocyte proliferation in vitro. Both ECP and EDN produce neurotoxicity (the Gordon phenomenon) when injected into the cerebrospinal fluid of experimental animals. ECP may damage cells by a colloid osmotic process, as it can induce non–ion-selective pores in both cellular and synthetic membranes.[68] The secreted form of ECP differs structurally and antigenically from the stored form.[69]

EOSINOPHIL-DERIVED NEUROTOXIN
EDN, also called *EPX*, is a 16-kD, glycosylated protein possessing marked ribonuclease activity. The cDNA predicts a 134 amino acid, mature polypeptide that is identical to human urinary ribonuclease. Like ECP, it is a member of a ribonuclease multigene family.[70] EDN expression is not restricted to eosinophils, as it is found in mononuclear cells and possibly neutrophils. It is also probably secreted by the liver. It does not appear to be toxic to parasites or mammalian cells, and its only known effect, other than its ribonuclease activity, is neurotoxicity.

A major constituent of eosinophil is CLC protein, which is a lysophospholipase. It constitutes up to 10 percent of eosinophil protein and is also found in large quantities in basophils.[71] Its precise function is unknown.

CYTOKINES

The first report that eosinophils were cytokine-producing cells was in 1990 when they were shown to generate transforming growth factor alpha (TGF-α).[72] This was of particular interest because of the possible

role of eosinophils in wound healing. Since then there has been an ever increasing list of cytokines and chemokines produced by eosinophils.[73] These include the eosinophil growth factors IL-3, IL-5, and GM-CSF, and the eosinophil cytokine IL-4. The cytokines can act on eosinophils themselves in an autocrine fashion, and, since they are produced in relatively low concentrations, this may be their primary function.[74] More recently eosinophils have been shown to generate IL-12, showing that they are not exclusively linked to Th2-mediated inflammatory responses,[75] and macrophage migration inhibitory factor (MIF), which could have a role in the adult respiratory distress syndrome as well as asthma.[76]

OTHER EOSINOPHIL-DERIVED MEDIATORS

Vasoactive intestinal peptide (VIP) has been detected in eosinophils in granulomas from mice infected with schistosomes,[77] and the eosinophil contains a number of granule-stored enzymes, whose roles in eosinophil function are not clear.[78] These enzymes include acid phosphatase, collagenase, arylsulfatase B, histaminase, phospholipase D, catalase, nonspecific esterases, vitamin B_{12}–binding proteins, and glycosaminoglycans. Eosinophils can undergo a respiratory burst with release of superoxide ion and H_2O_2 in response to stimulation with both particulate stimuli such as opsonized zymosan, and soluble mediators, such as leukotriene and phorbolmyrisate acetate. Eosinophils are twice as chemoluminescent as neutrophils.

EOSINOPHIL SECRETION AND ACTIVATION

The observation that eosinophils kill schistosomulae of *S. mansoni* led to the hypothesis that the role of eosinophils is in host defense against helminthic parasites.[79] Eosinophils can only kill schistosomes after they have been opsonized with IgG, IgE, or complement. Eosinophils, activated by a wide range of inflammatory mediators, are more effective at killing schistosomula than resting eosinophils. Schistosomula killing involves an initial adherence stage, which is quite rapid, followed by close attachment of the eosinophil to the tegument. Over about a three-hour period, the eosinophil secretes its proteins onto the surface of the larvae; after the tegument is breached, the eosinophil appears to crawl under it and strip the tegument away.[80] It has been suggested that eosinophils prefer to secrete their mediators onto a large target rather than engulf them and secrete their toxic mediators into intracellular phagolysosomes as is generally the case with neutrophils and macrophages. Neutrophils can also kill schistosomula after opsonization with IgG but less effectively than eosinophils. In contrast, monocytes and neutrophils are much more effective than eosinophils in engulfing antibody-coated erythrocytes.[81] A further illustration of the target specificity of granulocyte killing is that eosinophils are more effective at killing sensitized Daudi lymphoma cells than are neutrophils.[82]

A striking feature of eosinophil-rich inflammatory reactions is the high concentration of granule proteins, often in the presence of relatively small numbers of intact eosinophils. Mediator secretion can be triggered physiologically by engagement of immunoglobulin Fc receptors, especially after eosinophil activation has been primed with soluble mediators such as PAF and IL-5.[83] The eosinophil expresses receptors for IgG, IgA, and IgD (Table 68-3). The eosinophil also binds IgE, and eosinophils can undertake a number of IgE-dependent functions, including killing of schistomsomes opsonized with specific IgE.[84] It was thought that the eosinophil IgE receptor was related to the low-affinity IgE receptor found on B-lymphocytes, platelets, and macrophages—FcεRIII (CD23).[85] However, blood eosinophils inconsistently express messenger RNA (mRNA) for CD23 and do not stain with a panel of mAbs directed against this receptor. Eosinophils express the IgE binding protein Mac-2, but so do neutrophils, which lack IgE-dependent functions.[86] Blood eosinophils express weakly the high-affinity IgE receptor FcεR1,[87] although it may be expressed at higher levels on tissue eosinophils.[88] The extent to which this receptor is involved in triggering eosinophil degranulation in allergic disease is still unclear.

Three receptors for IgG have been described: the high-affinity receptor FcγR1 (CD64), and two low-affinity receptors FcγRII (CDw32) and FcγRIII (CD16).[89] CD16 is expressed both as a transmembrane form and a form with a phosphotidylinositol anchor, transcribed from two distinct genes. Only FcγRII is constitutively expressed by eosinophils to any significant degree.[90] A number of eosinophil functions are mediated via this receptor, including schistosomula killing, phagocytosis, secretion of granule proteins, and generation of newly formed, membrane-derived lipid mediators such as PAF and LTC$_4$. After stimulation for 2 days in vitro with IFN-γ, eosinophils express CD16 and CD64 as well as CD32.[91] Perhaps the most potent stimulus for eosinophil degranulation is cross-linking of IgA receptors,

especially when the cells have been primed with growth factors.[92] Consistent with the preference of eosinophils to secrete their mediators onto a large surface, Fc-mediated degranulation is enhanced if the eosinophils are adherent to a protein-coated surface via αMβ2.[93]

The killing of schistosomula opsonized with nonimmune serum is presumed to be mediated via the complement receptors, CR3, CR1, and CR3. Incubation of eosinophils with serum-coated beads results in the release of 15 percent of ECP.[94] Similarly, opsonized zymosan interacts with eosinophils, causing generation of hydrogen peroxide and the phagocytosis of the zymosan.[95] Soluble mediators such as PAF, LTB$_4$, and 5-oxo-eicosatetraenoate can elicit the direct secretion of both granule proteins and lipid mediators, although only with highly activated eosinophils or when used in conjunction with cytochalasin B, which inhibits microtubule assembly.[96] Stimulus-specific differential secretion of granule proteins has been reported. IgG complexes induce the secretion of ECP but not EPO, whereas IgE complexes induce secretion of EPO but not ECP.[97] However, secretion is low in both instances. Eosinophils release their granule components by exocytosis, with individual granules fusing with the plasma membrane. This process involves a GTP-binding protein and is modulated by the intracellular calcium concentration.[98]

EOSINOPHIL SURVIVAL AND APOPTOSIS

IL-5, besides being a growth and maturation factor for eosinophils, also selectively stimulates a number of eosinophil functions, including survival, cytotoxicity toward helminth targets, and increased adhesion to vascular endothelium.[99] IL-3 and GM-CSF have similar, though less selective, activities. IFN-γ stimulates eosinophil cytotoxicity, prolongs eosinophil survival, and stimulates expression of mRNA for GM-CSF.[100,101] TNF-α stimulates eosinophil cytotoxicity toward endothelium.[102] IL-3, IL-5, and GM-CSF have both short-term priming effects on eosinophils, which are maximal within an hour, and long-term effects, which depend on protein synthesis and include increased receptor expression. One of their most profound effects is to prolong eosinophil survival by delaying the onset of apoptosis. In inflammatory responses, these cytokines are generated by several cell types, and eosinophils may themselves generate GM-CSF after interaction with extracellular matrix.[103]

Complex signaling pathways determine eosinophil survival.[104] IL-5 signaling involves Lyn, Jak 2, Raf 1, and MAP kinases. Treatment of eosinophils with antisense to Lyn and Raf 1 resulted in inhibition of the survival-enhancing effects of IL-5, as did inhibition of tyrosine phosphorylation of Jak 2 using tyrphostin. However, Lyn and Jak 2 kinases are not involved in the IL-5–induced upregulation of the integrin receptor subunit αM, whereas Raf-1 kinase is.[105] Triggers of eosinophil apoptosis include TGFb, cross-linking of CD69, and cross-linking of Fas which is expressed by eosinophils.[106–108] Fas-induced eosinophil apoptosis is blocked by nitric oxide (NO), which may explain the relative resistance of eosinophils from allergic donors to Fas-induced apoptosis. Fas-induced apoptosis is mediated through activation of caspases, is amplified by the sphingomyelinase:ceramide signaling pathway, and is resistant to IL-5.[109] A clear link between growth-factor-induced prolongation of survival and expression of the Bcl-2 family proteins has not yet been made. Eosinophils express Bcl-2 weakly, the survival enhancing Bcl-xL to a greater degree, and large amounts of the death-inducing Bax. Expression of these proteins is not closely correlated with IL-5–induced survival. The phosporylation status of Bad, mediated through phosphorylation of Raf-1, may be responsible for the IL-5 effects.[110,111]

EOSINOPENIA AND EOSINOPHILIA

Eosinophils can be enumerated in the blood either by "wet counts" in modified Neubauer chambers, differential counts on dried films, or

TABLE 68-3   MAJOR EOSINOPHIL RECEPTORS (OTHER THAN ADHESION RECEPTORS)

Immunoglobulin receptors: Fcγ R11 (CD32); Fcα R; Fcε R1
Receptors for mediators: CCR3*; CCR1; PAF-R; LTC4/D4/E4-R; LTB4-R; C5a; C3a; IL-5*; IL-3; IL-4; IL-13
Receptors induced by cytokine stimulation: Fcγ RIII (CD16); Fcγ R1; (CD69:)HLA-DR; ICAM-1; CD25; CD4
Well expressed miscellaneous receptors: CD9;CD45;CR1; CD154 (CD40 ligand); CD95 (Fas)

*Expression relatively restricted to eosinophils.

by automated cell counting by flow cytometry.[112] Automated counting that uses detection of eosinophil peroxidase is the most accurate method, followed by counting in a cell chamber. Counting on films is least accurate because of the tendency for eosinophils to congregate at the margins of the slide. Common wet stains for eosinophils include eosin in acetone, phloxin, and Kimura's stain, which was originally developed to stain basophils.[113] Many stains, including May Grunewald/Giemsa, Romanowsky's stain, Chromotrope 2R, and Bierbrich scarlet, will identify eosinophils in blood films, cytospin preparations, or tissues.

The eosinophil count should be evaluated in absolute numbers rather than as a percentage of white cells, as the latter will depend on the total cell count. The normal eosinophil count is generally taken as less than 0.4×10^9/liter, although healthy medical students in the United States had a range of 0.015 to 0.65×10^9/liter.[114] Eosinophil counts are higher in neonates.[115] The eosinophil count varies with age, time of day, exercise status, and environmental stimuli, particularly allergen exposure. Blood eosinophil counts undergo diurnal variation, being lowest in the morning and highest at night. This effect results in a greater than 40 percent variation[116] and may be related to the reciprocal diurnal variation in cortisol levels, which are highest in the morning. The factors that control blood eosinophil counts in health are imperfectly understood. Concentrations of eosinophil growth factors are likely to be important, but other factors may be involved. Normal counts vary by up to fortyfold, and, in populations where eosinophilia is common, such as endemically parasitized areas, there are marked variations in the blood eosinophil level, independent of the degree of infection. This variation is comparable to variations in IgE levels. There are no differences between ethnic groups in eosinophil counts.[117]

CAUSES OF AN EOSINOPHILIA

The causes of eosinophilia can be classified according to the degree and frequency of occurrence (Table 68-4). Division of eosinophil counts is arbitrary, but a mild eosinophilia could be regarded as less than 1.5×10^9/liter, a moderate elevation as 1.5 to 5.0×10^9/liter, and a high count as greater than 5.0×10^9/liter. The most common cause of an eosinophilia worldwide is infection with helminthic parasites, which can often result in a very high eosinophil count. The most common cause of an eosinophilia in industrialized countries is the atopic allergic diseases, seasonal and perennial rhinitis, atopic dermatitis, and asthma. Allergic disease generally results in only a mild increase in eosinophil counts. A moderate or high eosinophil count in asthma raises the possibility of a complication such as Churg-Strauss syndrome or allergic bronchopulmonary aspergillosis.

MECHANISMS OF EOSINOPHILIA

Eosinophilia is largely T-cell-dependent through the actions of growth factors, especially IL-5. Increased IL-5 production occurs in many conditions associated with increases in eosinophils, including asthma,[118] parasitic disease,[119] IL-2 therapy,[120] HES,[121] and eosinophilia/myalgia syndrome.[122] IL-5 mRNA has been detected in Reed Sternberg cells in Hodgkin's disease with an eosinophilia.[123] Antibodies against IL-5 abolish the eosinophilia in parasitized animals.[124] Although IL-5 has been detected in mast cells and eosinophils,[125] T lymphocytes are the principal source of this cytokine. Eosinophils are closely associated with the Th2 immune response and the production of IL-4 and IL-5 by Th2 cells, as opposed to IFNγ and IL-2 by Th1 cells.[126] A Th2 profile of cytokine gene expression has been described in allergic inflammation,[127] whereas a Th1 profile is a feature of cell-mediated reactions to tuberculin.[128] T-cell clones from atopic individu-

als specific for D pterynissimus release IL-4, whereas T-cell clones from nonatopic donors or from atopic donors against tetanus toxoid produce IFN-γ and IL-2.[129] There is, therefore, good evidence that the eosinophilia of allergic and parasitic disease is due to a specific type of T-cell response to certain types of antigen. Eosinophils, however, are not invariably associated with production of specific IgE, as for example in intrinsic asthma. Drug-induced eosinophilia may be due to the drug acting as a hapten for a Th2 response.

The mechanism for the Th1/Th2 polarization is still unclear but may relate to the cytokine mileu at the time of sensitization, genetically regulated transcriptional control of IL-4, or the route of sensitization and the way in which the antigen is presented.[130] The nature of the antigen may also be important. Many allergens have now been purified and sequenced. No common structural features have been established that can explain their allergenicity,[131] although many are proteases, which could influence their immunogenicity.[132] The HLA haplotype of individuals responsive to certain allergens has also been investigated. A degree of restriction has been observed, particularly to more simple allergens, with, for example, the phenotype DR2.2 being overrepresented in individuals atopic to the ragweed allergen Amb a V.[133] However, with the majority of allergens, no clear pattern has emerged. While HLA haplotypes may influence responses to individual allergens, it is unlikely to provide a universal explanation for Th2 type responsiveness.

EOSINOPHILS AND DISEASE

THE ROLE OF EOSINOPHILS

For years eosinophils were thought to ameliorate inflammatory responses; now they are believed to cause tissue damage in some situations.[134,135] Eosinophils are a potentially important source of a range of cytokines.[136] The observation that eosinophils secrete TGF-α together with studies showing increased numbers of eosinophils at the edges of healing wounds suggests that they may be important in wound healing.[137] Cytokine-stimulated eosinophils secrete IL-1, express HLA Class II receptors, and can present antigen to T cells in vitro, suggesting they may be important as accessory cells in T-cell–mediated reactions. There is evidence that eosinophils slow the rate of progression of solid tumors, presumably by being cytotoxic to tumor cells.[138] Eosinophils can cause severe tissue damage under certain circumstances. Chronically high eosinophil counts from many causes including drug reactions, parasitic infections, eosinophilic leukemia, and HES, are associated with endomyocardial fibrosis.[139] The observation in the mid-1970s that eosinophils could kill parasite targets led to the hypothesis that the principal role of eosinophils was to counter parasitic infection.[140] The realization that eosinophils could release proinflammatory mediators such as PAF and eicosanoids, and the observation that eosinophil basic proteins are toxic for airway epithelium, has led to a consensus that eosinophils are a major effector cell for tissue damage in asthma and could cause many of the pathological features of the disease.[141] Eosinophils are therefore associated with a number of different types of pathological and reparative processes ranging from the permanent tissue damage seen in hypereosinophilic syndromes, the partly reversible tissue damage seen in asthma and pulmonary eosinophilia, and tissue repair characteristic of wound healing. The factors that determine which role the eosinophil adopts are unclear.

EOSINOPHILS AND ASTHMA

Large numbers of eosinophils and mononuclear cells are found in and around the bronchi of patients who have died of asthma, and their bronchial tissue contains large amounts of MBP.[142] Slight increases in blood eosinophils may occur in both atopic and nonatopic chronic asthma. In one study of glucocorticoid-dependent patients, eosinophil

TABLE 68-4   CAUSES OF AN EOSINOPHILIA

Disease	Frequency of Cause of Eosinophilia	Usual Degree of Eosinophilia	Comment
Infections			
Parasitic disease	Common worldwide	Moderate to high	
Bacterial	Rare		Usually cause eosinopenia, though serum ECP levels may be raised, suggesting eosinophil involvement in tissue.
Mycobacterial	Rare		More often secondary to drug therapy.
Fungal	Rare		Apart from allergic reactions and coccidiomycosis, in which as many as 88% of patients have an eosinophilia.
Rickettsial infections	Rare		
Yeast	Rare		Cryptococcus reported as causing CSF eosinophilia.
Viral infections	Rare		Occasional case reports of an eosinophilia in a variety of viral infections, including herpes and HIV infection.
Allergic diseases			
Allergic rhinitis	Common worldwide	Mild	
Atopic dermatitis	Common especially children	Mild	
Urticaria/angioedema	Common	Variable	Eosinophils seen in skin even with normal count.
Asthma	Common	Mild	Syndrome of intrinsic asthma, nasal polyps, and aspirin intolerance associated with higher-than-usual eosinophil counts.
Drug reactions			
Many drugs	Uncommon	Mild to high	Count usually returns to normal on stopping drug.
Neoplasms			
Eosinophil leukemia	Rare	High	100 cases reported by 1988; important to distinguish from hypereosinophilic syndrome (HES).
Myeloid leukemia	Uncommon	Moderate to high	Raised eosinophil counts often seen in chronic myeloid leukemia.
Lymphomas	Uncommon	Moderate	Often intense tissue eosinophilia with moderate blood eosinophil count; Hodgkin disease commonest type.
Histiocytosis X	Rare	Mild	Intense tissue eosinophilia in eosinophilic granuloma but blood eosinophilia unusual.
Solid tumors	Uncommon	Mild to high	Many different tumors reported.
Musculoskeletal			
Rheumatoid arthritis	Rare	Mild to high	Occasional case reports. More usually secondary to therapy.
Fasciitis	Rare	High	
Gastrointestinal			
Eosinophilic gastroenteritis	Rare	Mild to moderate	As with many GI diseases there is often a marked tissue eosinophilia with only a mild or absent blood eosinophilia.
Coeliac disease	Uncommon	Normal	Tissue eosinophilia.
Inflammatory bowel disease			Eosinophils seen in biopsies in both Crohn and UC but blood eosinophilia unusual.
Allergic gastroenteritis	Rare	Mild to high	Young children
Respiratory tract (for *asthma* see *allergic diseases*)			
Churg-Strauss syndrome	Rare	Moderate to high	Syndrome of eosinophilic vasculitis and asthma.
Pulmonary eosinophilia	Uncommon	Mild to high	Syndrome of eosinophilia and CXR shadowing. Apart from ABPA usually of unknown cause.
Bronchiectasis/CF	Uncommon	Mild	Often associated with asthma or ABPA.
Skin diseases (for *atopic dermatitis* see *allergic diseases*)			
Bullous pemphigoid	Uncommon	Moderate	
Miscellaneous causes			
IL-2 therapy	Rare	Moderate to high	For renal cell carcinoma.
HES	Rare	High	
Endomyocardial fibrosis	Rare	High	Secondary to any cause of a high eosinophil count.
Hyper IgE syndrome	Rare	Moderate to high	
Eosinophilia/myalgia and toxic oil syndrome	Rare	High	Two related conditions, one caused by poisoning with contaminated cooking oil in Spain and the other by a batch of tryptophan.

counts correlated with the degree of airflow obstruction.[143] Bronchial hyperreactivity inversely correlated with the blood eosinophil count in patients developing a late-phase response after antigen challenge.[144]

Antigen Challenge Studies in Humans and Animal Models
Inhaled antigen in sensitized asthmatics causes an early fall in forced expiratory volume, thought to be due to the bronchoconstricting media-tors from mast cells and a late response that consists of an influx of inflammatory cells, including large numbers of eosinophils, thereby mimicking the pathology of asthma.[145] Twenty-four hours after antigen challenge administered through a bronchoscope, up to 50 percent of the cells obtained by bronchial lavage are eosinophils.[146] An increase in airway neutrophils may also occur, although this is less dramatic.

Similar events have been observed after challenge with agents that cause occupational asthma.[147,148] Eosinophil recruitment is accompanied by increased numbers of activated T cells and monocytes, and similar findings have been observed in the skin and nose.[149,150] Antigen challenge in animal models, many involving gene-deleted mice, have generally provided support for the hypothesis that asthma is an eosinophil-mediated disease driven by Th2-associated cytokines IL-4, IL-5, and IL-13.[151–154] However, there has not been a clear correlation between the presence of an airway eosinophilia and bronchial hyperresponsiveness, the latter a marker of an asthma phenotype, in all studies.

Clinical Asthma   An increase in the number of eosinophils, detected either by bronchoscopy or examination of sputum, is observed in the airways of asthmatics, if the patient is not using inhaled steroids.[155] The eosinophil count in induced sputum is increasingly being used to aid in the diagnosis of asthma and monitor response to treatment.[156] Airway eosinophils in asthma are activated,[157,158] eosinophil infiltration is accompanied by increased numbers of activated CD25-positive T lymphocytes (which have a Th2-like profile of cytokine secretion),[159] and there is evidence of bronchial epithelial desquamation.[160] Increased eosinophils are also present in the airways of patients with intrinsic and occupational asthma.[161,162] An airway eosinophilia is also a feature of some patients with an exacerbation of smoking-related airflow obstruction,[163] and an increase in eosinophils in BAL fluid is seen in pulmonary eosinophilia and fibrosing alveolitis.[164] There is a general correlation between the numbers of airway eosinophils and the severity of asthma.[165] However, this is not a close relationship, and subjects with marked eosinophilia may have mild asthma and airway hyperresponsiveness, and many severe asthmatics may have minimal airway eosinophilia. Inhibition of airway eosinophilia by DSCG[166] or, more effectively, glucocorticoids,[167,168] is associated with an improvement in bronchial hyperresponsiveness, asthmatic symptoms, and lung function. Although glucocorticoids do induce eosinophil apoptosis at very high concentrations, their primary mechanism of action is probably inhibition of Th2 cytokine production. For eosinophils to cause tissue damage in the airways, they need to be actively secreting their mediators. Measurements of eosinophilic basic proteins may, therefore, be a better guide to the degree of eosinophilic inflammation than eosinophil numbers. For example, inhaled glucocorticoids may have little effect on the number of airway eosinophils but markedly reduce the amount of ECP in lavage fluid.[169]

EOSINOPHILS AND PARASITIC DISEASE

The most common helminthic causes of an eosinophilia are summarized in Table 68-5.[170–172] Eosinophils have been shown to be able to kill a number of opsonized parasites including newborn larvae of *Trichinella. spiralis,* larvae of *Nippostrongylus brasiliensis*, a gut parasite in the rat, and larvae of *Fasciola hepatica*, as well as shistosomulae of *S. mansoni*.[173] In vivo, parasite larvae become opsonized with both specific IgG and IgE antibodies and components of the complement cascade such as C3bi, which can promote adhesion and activation of eosinophils. Dead larvae of *S. haematobium* and other parasites have been detected in the skin surrounded by eosinophils and eosinophil granule products.[174] Adult worms both in vitro and in vivo appear resistant to eosinophil-mediated damage. Despite the circumstantial evidence of eosinophils being involved in host defense against parasites, there remains some doubt about their role. Except for one study in the Gambia,[175] there is no obvious correlation between the degree of eosinophilia and protection against infection or reinfection. Moreover, treatment of mice infected with *N. brasiliensis* or *S. mansoni* with neutralizing anti-IL-5 mAb's abolished the eosinophilia without modulating the disease process.[176] IL-5 transgenic mice were, however, protected from infection with *N. brasiliensis* but not *T. canis*.[177] The mechanism of eosinophilia in parasitic disease is thought to be similar

TABLE 68-5   HELMINTHIC CAUSES OF AN EOSINOPHILIA

PARASITE	COMMENT
Nematodes	
Ascariasis	Higher eosinophil counts in children. Larvae migrate from intestine to lungs where they cause Loeffler syndrome, a form of pulmonary eosinophilia.
Toxocara canis	Infective eggs are present in feces of puppies and pregnant bitches. Larvae in hosts such as chicken. Eosinophilia seen mainly in children under 9 years. Can migrate to eye and cause blindness. Serological evidence suggests infection not uncommon in industrialized countries.
Filiriasis	Common. Invariably result in marked eosinophilia, especially Loa Loa infection. Filiriasis is the cause of tropical pulmonary eosinophilia due to migration of adult worms to lung, elephantiasis due to involvement of lymphatics (*Wuchereria bancrofti* and *Brugia malayi*) and river blindness (*Onchocerca volvulus*). Treatment can result in systemic reaction called *Mazzotti reaction,* possibly due to massive eosinophil degranulation.
Ancyclostomiasis	Hookworm infection. *Ancyclostoma duodenale* and *Necator americanus.* One of the main causes of eosinophilia in patients returning from tropical countries. Counts in region of 2×10^9/liter.
Strongyloidiasis	Subclinical infection can persist for over 20 years. Stool examinations often negative. Cause of eosinophilia in ex-servicemen who spent time in tropics. If strongyloides infection is not considered and these patients are given steroids for suspected HES or as trial of therapy, they can develop disseminated disease.
Trichinosis	Caused by ingestion of encysted muscle larvae of *Trichinella spiralis.* Most prominent eosinophilia seen during early stages of infection when larvae migrating into striated muscle via the blood. Fatal cases reported of which only 20% were noted to have an eosinophilia.
Others	Other nematodes that can cause eosinophilia include *Trichuris trichuria, Capillaria* and *Gnathostomiasis.* The thread worm *Enterobius vermicularis* occasionally causes an eosinophilia when they invade tissues.
Trematodes	
Schistosomiasis (Bilharzia)	Infection with one of the *Schistosoma* (blood flukes), *S mansoni, S haematobium* and *S japonicum,* is perhaps the commonest causes of a moderate to high eosinophilia worldwide with 200 million people being infected. Infection is nearly always associated with an eosinophilia.
Fascioliasis	Adult worms of *F. hepatica* reside in the bile ducts, where they are associated with abnormal liver function tests and an eosinophilia.
Cestodes	
Echinococcus	Eosinophilia occurs in 25–50% of patients with hydatid disease.

to allergic disease, with a Th2-type response to helminthic antigens resulting in increased production of eosinophil growth factors, in particular IL-5.[178] The more pronounced eosinophilia in parasitic disease is presumably due to the systemic nature of the disease compared to the localized, single-organ nature of asthma and allergic disease. Helminthic parasites also secrete eosinophil chemotactic factors.[179,180] Mast cell degranulation as a result of larval migration through tissue, especially the skin, may contribute to the local tissue eosinophilia. The similarities in the immune responses seen in allergic disease and infection with helminths has led to speculation about the relationship between the two conditions.[181] There is limited evidence that the atopic state protects against parasitic infection.[182,183] In addition it is possible that parasitic infection could protect against allergic symptoms by increasing the amount of nonallergenic IgE bound to mast cells,[184] although epidemiological evidence for this hypothesis is lacking.

HYPEREOSINOPHILIC SYNDROMES

Idiopathic Hypereosinophilic Syndrome   *Definition and History.*   The sporadic occurrence of striking eosinophilia without apparent cause and with a predisposition to cardiac and neurologic injury[185] was identified as a syndrome by Hardy and Anderson in 1968.[186] Subsequent reports have referred to it as the *hypereosinophilic syndrome.*[187,188]

Etiology and Pathogenesis.   The cause of the disorder is unknown. Some cases are manifestations of a polyclonal and others of a monoclonal proliferations of eosinophils. The latter is a primary disturbances in myelopoiesis.[189,190] Other cases may be a reflection of polyclonal or monoclonal expansion of T lymphocytes that elaborate eosinophilopoietic cytokines.[191–193,256,257] The organ damage is thought to be largely a result of noxious effects of eosinophil granule contents in certain tissues, especially the heart and nervous system.[194,195] Damage to tissues is mediated by eosinophilic secretory products, especially cationic proteins, peroxidase, and neurotoxin. Analysis of patterns of X-chromosome inactivation in the hypereosinophilic syndrome using HUMARA analysis showed a clonal pattern in some patients suggesting that in these patients this syndrome is a neoplastic disorder.[196]

Clinical Features.   The onset is often marked by anorexia, weight loss, fatigue, nausea, abdominal pain, diarrhea, non-productive cough, pruritic rash, and fever accompanied by night sweats. Hepatic and splenic enlargement is common, as is dependent edema.[188] Virtually all patients have cardiac involvement and most have clinical evidence of congestive heart failure, new heart murmurs, or electrocardiographic abnormalities, including conduction defects or arrhythmias.[195,197] Interstitial pulmonary infiltrates and pleural effusion may occur.[198] Nervous system dysfunction may be profound, including confusion, delirium, coma, and signs of dementia. Blurred vision, slurred speech, or a peripheral neuritis may be present.[199] Erythematous or papular rashes can occur in a minority of patients. A predisposition to venous thrombosis may be present.

Laboratory Features.   The hematocrit is below normal in most patients, and the anemia mimics that of chronic inflammation. The platelet count is usually normal but may be decreased. The key finding is a leukocytosis with a striking eosinophilia, usually greater than 1500 eosinophils/μl (1.5×10^9/liter), occasionally as high as 100,000 eosinophils/μl (100×10^9/liter). Marrow examination shows eosinophilia with few other specific findings. Eosinophilia may be progressive, with eosinophil counts of 50,000 cells/μl (50×10^9/liter) or more occurring in over half the patients during the course of the illness.[190] Circulating immune complexes, elevated IgE, or hypergammaglobulinemia occur frequently.[188]

Differential Diagnosis.   When the condition is fully expressed, the diagnosis is evident because of the absence of other causes of extreme hypereosinophilia with tissue injury. In more subtle forms, determining that another cause of eosinophilia is not present may require a longer period of observation. In geographic areas in which parasitic infestation is common, the differential diagnosis requires good microbiological diagnostic facilities. The distinction from eosinophilic leukemia, a very rare disorder, is made principally by determining the presence or absence of leukemic blast cells in the marrow (and blood). The presence of a clonal cytogenetic abnormality and progressive anemia and thrombocytopenia also indicates that leukemia is more likely the correct diagnosis. Another condition to consider

is familial eosinophilia.[200] This is an autosomal dominant disorder characterized by peripheral hypereosinophilia of unidentifiable cause with or without other organ involvement. The disorder has been mapped to the cytokine gene cluster on chromosome 5q31-q33, although it doesn't appear to involve any of the known eosinophil growth factors in this region.[201] A rare condition characterized by hypereosinophilia and immunodeficiency is Omenn syndrome, which is due to mutations in the Rag 1 or Rag 2 genes that control genomic rearrangement of the T-cell antigen receptor.[202]

Therapy, Course, and Prognosis.   The disease is chronic, sometimes indolent, but more often progressive, and can be rapidly fatal. Although symptoms may remit and relapse, the organ damage is usually steadily progressive, with cardiac failure resulting from endomyocardial fibrosis that often involves the valve leaflets. Central nervous system dysfunction is commonly progressive, leading to encephalopathy, polyneuropathy, or stroke. Episodes of venous thrombosis may complicate the course. In one series, over three-quarters of the patients died after three years of observation, despite therapy with glucocorticoids or cytotoxic agents.[203] In occasional patients with mild disease without apparent progression, no therapy may be advisable. Careful observation is important, however, since patients with an apparently indolent course may be having tissue damage. Symptomatic or progressive disease requires therapy. Glucocorticoids and hydroxyurea have been the mainstays of treatment and have been used with apparent success in some patients. Prednisone 60 mg/day, orally, for one week followed by 60 mg every other day for three months is one suggested regimen. Glucocorticoid-unresponsive patients have responded to hydroxyurea at 1 to 2 g/day orally so as to decrease the white cell count to about 5000/μl (5×10^9/liter). Responses to other cytostatic agents (e.g., methotrexate, cyclophosphamide) have been very infrequent. Etoposide has been used successfully in a glucocorticoid- and hydroxyurea-resistant patient.[204] Interferon-α may be a very useful agent in some patients with this disorder; occasional dramatic responses having been recorded,[205–207] although this treatment may on occasion cause renal damage.[208] Cladribine has been useful in some patients (258). Leukapheresis[209] and marrow transplantation have also been used.[210]

Surgical replacement of severely damaged heart valves has been accomplished successfully.[211,212]

Troleandamycin and methylprednisolone have also been successful in one patient. The former antibiotic has a glucocorticoid-sparing effect on methylprednisolone.[213] Occasional patients may evolve into overt malignancy, either hemopoietic[214,215] or lymphocytic,[216,217] and it is unclear whether the eosinophilia is the most striking early reaction to a clonal lymphocytic disorder. In certain cases the primary tissue involved may be T lymphocytes that elaborate IL-5, with the eosinophilic hyperplasia being a secondary phenomenon.

Eosinophilia-Myalgia Syndrome   This disorder was first described in 1989 in New Mexico.[218] Over 1500 cases were reported over the next 2 years, with over 30 deaths.[219] The syndrome was caused by the ingestion of L-tryptophan and is thought to be the result of a contaminant, possibly 1,1′-ethylidenebis (tryptophan). The syndrome is characterized histologically by a perivascular lymphocytic and eosinophilic infiltrate in the dermis, fascia, and skeletal muscle, with a pulmonary vasculitis and alveolitis mimicking eosinophilic fasciitis.

Severe myalgias and an eosinophil count greater than 1000 cells/μl (1×10^9/liter) are constant features. Arthralgias, cough, shortness of breath, dependent edema, and hair loss are very common. A significant proportion of patients, perhaps 50 percent, develop parasthesias, peripheral neuropathy, and/or sclerodermalike skin changes. A high proportion of patients have symptoms and signs one year after onset of the disease.[220–222]

Glucocorticoid or nonsteroidal anti-inflammatory therapy has had little effect on the course of the disease, although some improvement may occur in symptoms. Cytotoxic drug therapy has also had little effect on symptoms or the course of the disease.[223]

Toxic Oil Syndrome In 1981, more than 20,000 cases of a syndrome manifested by fever, cough, dyspnea and leukocytosis, neutrophilia, and an eosinophil count greater than 750 cells/μl (0.75 × 10^9/liter) were reported in Spain.[225] Occasionally, the eosinophil count rose above normal only after the onset of the pulmonary symptoms. Pulmonary infiltrates were evident on X-rays of the chest. Pleural effusion was common, and hypoxemia was frequent. There were over 300 deaths (about 1.5 percent of affected subjects). About half the patients went on to a chronic course that mimicked the eosinophilia-myalgia syndrome, with myalgias, eosinophilia, peripheral neuritis, sclerodermalike skin lesions, hair loss, and a sicca syndrome. Most patients improved from the acute or chronic symptoms and signs, but some residual nerve, muscle, or skin damage persisted. Endothelial cell proliferation, mononuclear cell infiltrates around blood vessels (vasculitis), and perineural inflammatory infiltrates were identified histopathologically. Glucocorticoid therapy may have decreased the pulmonary symptomatology. The disease was thought to be a response to an unlabeled food oil, aniline-denatured rapeseed oil, marketed as pure olive oil.[226]

Reactive Hypereosinophilia and Neoplasms Exaggerated eosinophilia has been reported in association with a variety of lymphoid[227,228] and solid tumors.[229,230] In these cases, the eosinophilia is thought to be the result of an increase to IL-5 and other cytokines or chemokines (259) elaborated by the tumor cells, although the expression by eosinophils of receptors of the TNF-α family suggest that they could regulate tumor growth.[231] The eosinophilia may precede the clinical diagnosis of the tumor but is usually manifested concomitantly. In some cases successful treatment of the tumor is associated with amelioration of the eosinophilia. Angiolymphoid hyperplasia also has been associated with eosinophilia.[232,233]

Eosinophilic Leukemia This rare disorder is described in Chap. 93.

Eosinophilia, Angiitis, and Asthma A group of related diseases, including polyarthritis nodosa and allergic granulomatosis (Churg-Strauss angiitis), are associated with a prominent eosinophilia.[234,235] In a review of subjects with asthma and necrotizing angiitis, all patients had anemia and hypereosinophilia, with a mean blood eosinophil count over 8000 cells/μl (8 × 10^9/liter).[238] Remission can be achieved in about 90 percent of patients. About 10 percent of patients die of the vasculitis.[239] In subjects with asthma and exaggerated eosinophilia, the development of multiorgan signs (skin, nervous system, kidney, joints, lung, heart, gastrointestinal tract) should lead to consideration of this disorder.

Eosinophilic Fasciitis This syndrome may occur at any age in both sexes and is characterized by stiffness, pain, and swelling of the arms, forearms, thighs, legs, hands, and feet in descending order of frequency.

Malaise, fever, weakness, and weight loss also occur.[240,241] Eosinophilia greater than 1000 cells/μl (1 × 10^9/liter) is present in most patients but may be intermittent. A biopsy, usually required for the diagnosis, shows inflammation, edema, thickening, and fibrosis of the fascia. Synovial tissue may show similar changes. Aplastic anemia, isolated cytopenias, pernicious anemia, and leukemia have been associated with eosinophilic fasciitis.[242,243]

Eosinophiluria and Eosinophilorrhachia The urinary excretion of eosinophils is seen in several inflammatory disorders of the kidney but most often in urinary tract infection or acute interstitial nephritis.[244,245] Hansel stain is superior to Wright stain in identifying eosinophils in a stained urinary sediment. Cerebrospinal fluid eosinophilia may occur with infection, shunts, and allergic reactions involving the meninges.[246,247] Eosinophilic meningoencephalitis with cerebrospinal fluid eosinophilia, but no blood eosinophilia, can occur in Hodgkin's disease.[248]

EOSINOPENIA

The eosinophil count in hospitalized patients is less than 10 cells/μl (0.01 × 10^9/liter) in only 0.1 percent of patients, and in virtually all patients the eosinopenia can be ascribed to glucocorticoids or to disease.[115] Acute infection, or treatment with glucocorticoids or adrenaline, decreases eosinophil counts.[249,250] In contrast, beta blockers inhibit adrenaline-induced eosinopenia and can cause a rise in the eosinophil count.

There have been several isolated case reports of patients with absent eosinophils in the blood and marrow.[251] Several patients without eosinophils were reported as having asthma and allergic symptoms.[252] In one case, it occurred after drug-induced agranulocytosis,[253] and in another there was a serum inhibitor of eosinophil colony formation.[254] A rare disorder, eosinophil peroxidase deficiency, may be brought to light by automatic counting that uses detection of EPO to count eosinophils. EPO deficiency does not have any adverse clinical consequences.[255]

REFERENCES

1. Spry CJF: The natural history of eosinophils, in *The Immunopharmacology of Eosinophils*, edited by H Smith and RM Cook, pp 1–9. Academic, London, 1993.
2. Saito H, Hatake K, Dvorak AM, et al: Selective differentiation and proliferation of hematopoietic cells induced by recombinant human interleukins. *Proc Natl Acad Sci USA* 85:2288, 1988.
3. Baston A, Beeson PB: Mechanism of eosinophilia. II: Role of the lymphocyte. *J Exp Med* 131:1288, 1970.
4. Hsu CK, Hsu SH, Whitney RA, Hansen CT: Immunopathology of schistosomiasis in athymic mice. *Nature* 262:397, 1976.
5. Colley D: Lymphokine-related eosinophil responses. *Lymphokine Research* 1:133, 1980.
6. Bischoff SC, Brunner T, De Weck AL, Dahinden CA: Interleukin 5 modifies histamine release and leukotriene generation by human basophils in response to diverse agonists. *J Exp Med* 172:1577, 1990.
7. Leary AG, Ogawa M: Identification of pure and mixed basophil colonies in culture of human peripheral blood and marrow cells. *Blood* 64:78, 1984.
8. Kinashi T, Harada N, Severinson E, et al: Cloning of a complementary DNA encoding T cell replacement factor and identity with B cell growth factor II. *Nature* 324:70, 1986.
9. Campbell HD, Sanderson CJ, Wang Y, et al: Molecular cloning, nucelotide sequence and expression of the gene encoding human eosinophil differentiation factor (interleukin 5). *Proc Natl Acad Sci USA* 84:6629, 1987.
10. McKenzie ANJ, Ely B, Sanderson CJ: Mutated interleukin-5 monomers are biologically inactive. *Mol Immunol* 28:155, 1991.
11. Milburn MV, Hassell AM, Lambert MH, et al: A novel dimer configuration revealed by the crystal structure at 2.4A resolution of human interleukin-5. *Nature* 363:172, 1993.
12. Sanderson CJ, Campell HD, Young IG: Molecular and cellular biology of eosinophil differentiation factor (IL-5) and its effects on human and mouse B cells. *Immunol Rev* 102:29, 1988.
13. Tominaga A, Takaki S, Koyama N, et al: Transgenic mice expressing a B cell growth and differentiation factor gene (interleukin 5) develop eosinophilia and autoantibody production. *J Exp Med* 173:429, 1991.
14. Dent LA, Strath M, Mellor AL, Sanderson CJ: Eosinophilia in transgenic mice expressing interleukin 5. *J Exp Med* 172:1425, 1990.
15. Saeland S, Caux C, Favre C, et al: Combined and sequential effects of human IL-3 and GM-CSF on the proliferation of CD34+ hematopoietic cells from cord blood. *Blood* 73:1195, 1989.
16. Ottman OG, Ganser A, Seipelt G, et al: Effects of recombinant human

interleukin 3 on human hematopoietic progenitor and precursor cells in vivo. *Blood* 76:1494, 1990.

17. Van-Leeuwen BH, Martinson ME, Webb GC, Young IG: Molecular organization of the cytokine gene cluster, involving the human IL-3, IL-4 IL-5 and GM-CSF genes on human chromosomes. *Blood* 73:1142, 1989.

18. Mossman TR, Coffman RL: Th1 and Th2 cells:different patterns of lymphokine secretion lead to different functional properties. *Annu Rev Immunol* 7:145, 1989.

19. Miyajima A, Kitamura T, Harada N, et al: Cytokine receptors and signal transduction. *Annu Rev Immunol* 10:295, 1992.

20. Tavernier J, Devos R, Cornelis S, et al: A human high affinity interleukin-5 receptor (IL-5R) is composed of an IL-5-specific a chain and a b chain shared with the receptor for GM-CSF. *Cell* 66:1175, 1991.

21. Murata Y, Takaki S, Migita M, et al: Molecular cloning and expression of the human interleukin 5 receptor. *J Exp Med* 175:341, 1992.

22. Plaetinck G, der Heyden JV, Tavernier J, et al: Characterization of interleukin 5 receptors on eosinophilic sublines from human promyelocytic leukemia (HL60) cells. *J Exp Med* 172:683, 1990.

23. Wang P, Wu P, Cheewatrakoolpong B, Myers JG, Egan RW, Billah MM: Selective inhibition of IL-5 receptor alpha-chain gene transcription by IL-5, IL-3 and granulocyte-macrophage colony stimulating factor in human eosinophils. *J Immunol* 160:4427, 1998.

24. Hansel TT, Braunstein JB, Walker C: An improved immunomagnetic procedure for the isolation of highly purified human blood eosinophils. *J Immunol Methods* 145:105, 1991.

25. Bass DA, Grover WH, Lewis JC, et al: Comparison of human eosinophils from normals and patients with eosinophilia. *J Clin Invest* 66:1265, 1980.

26. Caulfield JP, Hein A, Rothenburg ME, et al: A morphometric study of normodense and hypodense human eosinophils that are derived in vivo and in vitro. *Am J Pathology* 137:27, 1991.

27. Fukuda T, Makino S: Heterogeneity and activation, in *Eosinophils Biological and Clinical Aspects*, edited by T Fukuda and S Makino, pp 156–170. CRC, Boca Raton, FL, 1993.

28. Wardlaw AJ: Eosinophil density: What does it mean? *Clin Exp Allergy* 25:1145, 1995.

29. Azzawi M, Bradley B, Jeffery PK, et al: Identification of activated T lymphocytes and eosinophils in bronchial biopsies in stable atopic asthma. *Am Rev Respir Dis* 142:1407, 1990.

30. Kay AB, Stechschulte DJ, Austen KF: An eosinophil leukocyte chemotactic factor of anaphylaxis. *J Exp Med* 133:602, 1971.

31. Sehmi R, Cromwell O, Taylor GW: Identification of guinea pig eosinophil chemotactic factor of anaphylaxis as leukotriene B$_4$ and 8(S),15(S)-dihydroxy-5,9,11,13 (Z,E Z,E)-eicosatetranoic acid. *J Immunol* 147:2276, 1991.

32. Goetzl EJ, Austen KF: Purification and synthesis of eosinophilotactic tetrapeptides of human lung. Identification as eosinophil chemotactic factor of anaphylaxis. *Proc Natl Acad Sci USA* 72:4123, 1975.

33. Wardlaw AJ, Moqbel R, Cromwell O, Kay AB: Platelet activating factor is a potent chemotactic and chemokinetic factor for human eosinophils. *J Clin Invest* 78:1701, 1986.

34. Sehmi R, Wood LJ, Watson R, et al: Allergen induced increases in IL-5 receptor alpha subunit expression on bone marrow derived CD34+ cells from asthmatic subjects. A novel marker of progenitor cell committment towards eosinophilic differentiation. *J Clin Invest* 100:2466, 1997.

35. Collins PD, Marleau S, Griffiths-Johnson DA, et al: Co-operation between interleukin 5 and the chemokine eotaxin to induce eosinophil accumulation in vivo. *J Exp Med* 182:1169, 1995.

36. Palframan RT, Collins PD, Severs NJ, et al: Mechanisms of acute eosinophil mobilization from the bone marrow stimulated by inerleukin 5: the role of specific adhesion molecules and phosphotidylinositol 3-kinase. *J Exp Med* 188:1621, 1998.

37. Wardlaw AJ, Symon FA, Walsh GM: Eosinophil adhesion in allergic inflammation. The role of basophils and eosinophils in human disease. *J Allergy Clin Immunol* 94(pt 2):1163, 1994.

38. Symon FA, Lawrence MB, Walsh GM, et al: Characterisation of the eosinophil P-selectin ligand. *J Immunol* 157:1711, 1996.

39. Sriramarao P, Norton CR, Borgstrom P, et al: E-selectin preferentially supports neutrophil but not eosinophil rolling under conditions of flow in vitro and in vivo. *J Immunol* 157:4672, 1996.

40. Yao L, Pan J, Setiadi H, et al: Interleukin 4 or Oncostatin M induces a prolonged increase in P-selectin mRNA and protein in human endothelial cells. *J Exp Med* 184:81, 1996.

41. Patel KD: Eosinophil tethering to interleukin-4-activated endothelial cells requires both p-selectin and vascular cell adhesion molecule-1. *Blood* 92:3904, 1998.

42. Woltmann G, McNulty CA, Dewson G, et al: IL-13 induces eosinophil but not neutrophil binding to HUVECs via PSGL-1. *Blood* 95:3146, 2000.

43. Reinhardt PH, Kubes P: Differential leukocyte recruitment from whole blood via endothelial adhesion molecules under shear conditions. *Blood* 92:4691, 1998.

44. Bochner BS, Luskinsas FW, Gimbrone MA: Adhesion of human basophils, eosinophils and neutrophils to interleukin-1 activated human vascular endothelial cells: contribution of endothelial cell adhesion molecules. *J Exp Med* 173:1553, 1991.

45. Grayson MH, Van der Vieren M, Sterbinsky SA, et al: Alpha d beta 2 integrin is expressed on human eosinophils and functions as an alternative ligand for vascular cell adhesion molecule 1 (VCAM-1). *J Exp Med* 188:2187, 1998.

46. Petering H, Gotze O, Kimmig D, et al: The biologic role of interleukin-8: Functional analysis and expression of CXCR1 and CXCR2 on human eosinophils. *Blood* 93:694, 1999.

47. Kitaura M, Nakajima T, Imai T, et al: Molecular cloning of human eotaxin, an eosinophil-selective CC chemokine and identification of a specific eosinophil eotaxin receptor, CC chemokine receptor 3. *J Biol Chem* 271:7725, 1996.

48. Kita H, Gleich GJ: Chemokines active on eosinophils. Potential roles in allergic inflammation. *J Exp Med* 183:2421, 1996.

49. Uguccioni M, Loetscher P, Forsmann U, et al: Monocyte chemotactic protein 4 (MCP-4) a novel structural and functional analogue of MCP-3 and eotaxin. *J Exp Med* 183:2379, 1996.

50. Collins PD, Marleau S, Grifiths-Johnson DA, et al: Co-operation between interleukin 5 and the chmeokine eotaxin to induce eosinophil accumulation in vivo *J Exp Med* 182:1169, 1995.

51. Mould AW, Matthaei KI, Young IG, et al: Relationship between interleukin-5 and eotaxin in regulating blood and tissue eosinophilia in mice. *J Clin Invest* 99:1064, 1997.

52. Gonzalo JA, Lolyd CM, Kremer L, et al: Eosinophil recruitment to the lung in a murine model of allergic inflammation. The role of T cells, chemokines and adhesion receptors. *J Clin Invest* 98:2332, 1996.

53. Gonzalo JA, Lloyd CM, Wen D, et al: The co-ordinated action of CC chemokines in the lung orchestrates allergic inflammation and airway hyperresponsiveness. *J Exp Med* 188:157, 1998.

54. MacLean JA, Ownbey R, Luster AD: T cell-dependent regulation of eotaxin in antigen-induced pulmonary eosinophilia. *J Exp Med* 184:1461, 1996.

55. Simon H-U, Yousefi S, Schranz C, Schapowal A, Bachert C, Blaser K: Direct demonstration of delayed eosinophil apoptosis as a mechanism causing tissue eosinophilia. *J Immunol* 158:3902, 1997.

56. Weller PF: Eicosanoids, cytokines and other mediators elaborated by eosinophils, in *Eosinophils, Biological and Clinical Aspects*, edited by S Makino, T Fukuda, pp 125–154. CRC, Boca Raton, FL, 1993.

57. Weller PF, Lee CN, Foster DW, et al: Generation and metabolism of 5-lipoxygenase pathway leukotrienes by human eosinophils; predominant production of leukotriene C4. *Proc Natl Acad Sci USA* 80:7625, 1983.

58. Shaw RJ, Walsh GM, Comwell O, et al: Activated human eosinophils generate SRS-A leukotrienes following physiological (IgG dependent) stimulation. *Nature* 316:150, 1985.

59. Cromwell O, Wardlaw AJ, Champion A, et al: IgG-dependent generation of platelet activating factor by normal and low density eosinophils. *J Immunol* 145:3862, 1990.

60. Bozza PT, Yu W, Penrose JF, Morgan ES, Dvorak AM, Weller PF: Eosinophil lipid bodies: specific, inducible intracellular sites for enhanced eicosanoid formation. *J Exp Med* 186:909, 1997.

61. Barker RL, Gleich GJ, Pease LR: Acidic precursor revealed in human eosinophil granule major basic protein cDNA. *J Exp Med* 168:1493, 1988.

62. Butterworth AE, Wassom DL, Gleich GJ, Loegering DA, David JR: Damage to schistosomula of *S. manson* induced directly by eosinophil major basic protein. *J Immunol* 122:221, 1979.

63. Gleich GJ: The eosinophil and bronchial asthma: current understanding. *J Allergy Clin Immunol* 85:422, 1986.

64. Gundel RH, Letts LG, Gleich GJ: Human eosinophil major basic protein induces airway constriction and airway hyperresponsiveness in primates. *J Clin Invest* 87:1470, 1991.

65. Rohrbach MS, Wheatley CL, Slifman NR, Gleich GJ: Activation of platelets by eosinophil granule proteins. *J Exp Med* 172:1271, 1990.

66. Ten RM, Pease LR, McKean DJ, Bell MP, Gleich GJ: Molecular cloning of the human eosinophil peroxidase. *J Exp Med* 169:1757, 1989.

67. Rosenburg HF, Ackerman SJ, Tenen DG: Human eosinophil cationic protein. Molecular cloning of a cytotoxin and helminthotoxin with ribonuclease activity. *J Exp Med* 170:163, 1989.

68. Young JDE, Peterson CGB, Venge P, Cohn ZA: Mechanism of membrane damage mediated by human eosinophil cationic protein. *Nature* 321:613, 1986.

69. Tai PC, Spry CJF, Peterson C, Venge P, Olsson I: Monoclonal antibodies distinguish between storage and secreted forms of eosinophil cationic protein. *Nature* 309:182, 1984.

70. Rosenburg HF, Tenen DG, Ackerman SJ: Molecular cloning of the human eosinophil-derived neurotoxin: a member of the ribonuclease gene family. *Proc Natl Acad Sci USA* 86:4460, 1989.

71. Weller PF, Goetzl EJ, Austen KF: Identification of human eosinophil lysophospholipase as the constituent of Charcot-Leyden crystals. *Proc Natl Acad Sci USA* 77:7440, 1980.

72. Wong DT, Weller PF, Galli SJ, et al: Human eosinophils express transforming growth factor α. *J Exp Med* 172:673, 1990.

73. Wardlaw AJ, Moqbel R, Kay AB: Eosinophils: biology and role in disease. *Adv Immunol* 80:151, 1995.

74. Elovic AE, Ohyama H, Sauty A, et al: IL-4 dependent regulation of TGF-alpha and TGF-beta expression in human eosinophils. *J Immunol* 160:6121, 1998.

75. Grewe M, Czech W, Morita A, et al: Human eosinophils produce biologically active IL-12: implications for control of T cell responses. *J Immunol* 161:415, 1998.

76. Rossi AG, Haslett C, Hirani N, et al: Human circulating eosinophils secrete macrophage migration inhibitory factor (MIF). Potential role in asthma. *J Clin Invest* 101:2869, 1998.

77. Weinstock JV: Production of neuropeptides by inflammatory cells within granulomas of murine schistosomiasis mansoni. *Eur J Clin Invest* 21:145, 1991.

78. Spry C: *Eosinophils*, p 29. Oxford and London: Oxford University Press, 1988.

79. Butterworth AE, Sturrock RF, Houba V, et al: Eosinophils as mediators of antibody-dependent damage to schistosomula. *Nature* 256:727, 1975.

80. McLaren DJ, Mackenzie CD, Ramahlo-Pinto FJ: Ultrastructural observations on the in vitro interaction between rat eosinophils and some parasitic helminths (*Schistosoma mansoni, Trichinella spiralis* and *Nippostongylus brasiliensis*). *Clin Exp Immunol* 30:105, 1977.

81. Fanger MW, Shen L, Graziano RF, Guyre P: Cytotoxicity mediated by human Fc receptors for IgG. *Immunol Today* 10:92, 1989.

82. Valerius T, Repp R, Kalden JR, Platzer E: Effects of interferon g on human eosinophils in comparison with others cytokines. *J Immunol* 145:2950, 1990.

83. Kita H, Weiler DA, Abu-Ghazaleh R, et al: Release of granule proteins from eosinophils cultured with IL-5. *J Immunol* 149:629, 1992.

84. Capron M, Capron A, Dessaint J-P, et al: Fc receptors for IgE on human and rat eosinophils. *J Immunol* 126:2087, 1981.

85. Capron M, Jouault T, Prin L, et al: Functional study of a monoclonal antibody to IgE Fc receptor (Fc R2) of eosinophils, platelets and macrophages. *J Exp Med* 164:72, 1986.

86. Capron M, Troung M-J, Desreumaux P, et al: Eosinophil membrane receptors: Function of IgE and IgA binding molecules, in *Eosinophils: Immunological and Clinical Aspects,* Edited by GJ Gleich, AB Kay. Marcel Dekker, New York, in press.

87. Gounni AS, Lamkhioued B, Ochiai K, et al: High affinity IgE receptor on eosinophils is involved in defense against parasites. *Nature* 367:183, 1994.

88. Ying S, Barata LT, Meng O, et al: High affinity immunoglobulin E receptor (Fc epsilon R1–bearing eosinophils, mast cells, macrophages and langerhans cells in allergen induced late-phase cutaneous reactions in atopic subjects. *Immunology* 93:281, 1998.

89. Unkeless JC, Scigliano E, Freedman VH: Structure and function of human and murine receptors for IgG. *Annu Rev Immunol* 6:251, 1988.

90. Hartnell A, Moqbel R, Walsh GM, et al: Fcg and CD11/CD18 receptor

91. Hartnell A, Kay AB, Wardlaw AJ: IFN-g induces expression of FcgRIII(CD16) on human eosinophils. *J Immunol* 148:1471, 1992.

92. Abu-Ghazaleh RI, Fujisawa T, Mestecky J, et al: IgA-induced eosinophil degranulation. *J Immunol* 142:2393, 1989.

93. Kaneko M, Horie S, Kato M, et al: A crucial role for beta 2 integrins in the activation or eosinophils stimulated by Ig. *J Immunol* 155:2631, 1995.

94. Winquist I, Olofsson T, Olofsson I: Mechanisms for eosinophil degranulation. Release of the eosinophil granule protein. *Immunology* 51:1, 1984.

95. Yazdanbakhsh M, Eckmann CM, Roos D: Characterization of the interaction of human eosinophils and neutrophils with opsonized particles. *J Immunol* 135:1378, 1985.

96. O'Flaherty JTO, Kuroki M, Nixon AB, et al: 5-Oxo-Eicosatetraenoate is a broadly active eosinophil selective stimulus for human granulocytes. *J Immunol* 157:336, 1996.

97. Khaliffe J, Capron M, Cesbron JY, et al: Role of specific IgE antibodies in peroxidase (EPO) release from human eosinophils. *J Immunol* 137:1659, 1986.

98. Nusse O, Lindau M, Cromwell O, Kay AB, Gomperts BD: Intracellular application of guanosine-5′-O-(3-thiotriphosphate) induces exocytic granule fusion in guinea pig eosinophils. *J Exp Med* 171:775, 1990.

99. Roboz GJ, Rafii S: Interleukin-5 and the regulation of eosinophil production. *Curr Opin Hematol* 6:148, 1999.

100. Hartnell A, Kay AB, Wardlaw AJ: IFNg induces expression of FcgRIII(CD16) on human eosinophils. *J Immunol* 142:2393, 1992.

101. Moqbel R, Hamid Q, Sun Y, et al: Expression of mRNA and immunoreactivity for the granulocyte macrophage colony stimulating factor (GM-CSF) in activated human eosinophils. *J Exp Med* 174:749, 1991.

102. Slungard A, Vercellotti GM, Walker G, et al: Tumor necrosis factor α/ cachectin stimulates eosinophil oxidant production and toxicity towards human endothelium. *J Exp Med* 171:2025, 1990.

103. Walsh GM, Symon FA, Wardlaw AJ: Human eosinophils preferentially survive on tissue compared with plasma fibronectin. *Clin Exp Allergy* 25:1128, 1995.

104. Simon H-U, Alam R: Regulation of eosinophil apoptosis: transduction of survival and death signals. *Int Arch Allergy Immunol* 118:7, 1999.

105. Padrak K, Olszewska-Pazdrak B, Stafford S, et al: Jak 2 and Raf-1 kinases are critical for the antiapoptotic effect of interleukin 5, whereas only Raf-1 kinases is essential foe eosinophil activation and degranulation. *J Exp Med* 188:421, 1998.

106. Alam R, Forsythe P, Stafford S, Fukuda Y: Transforming growth factor β abrogates the effects of hematopoietins on eosinophils and induces their apoptosis. *J Exp Med* 179:1041, 1994.

107. Walsh GM, Williamson MS, Symon FA, et al: Ligation of CD69 induces apoptosis and cell death in human eosinophils cultured with GM-CSF. *Blood* 87:2815, 1996.

108. Matsumoto K, Schleimer RP, Saito H, et al: Induction of apoptosis in human eosinophils by anti-Fas antibody treatment in vitro. *Blood* 86:1437, 1995.

109. Hebestreit H, Dibbert B, Balatti B, et al: Disruption of Fas receptor signaling by nitric oxide in eosinophils. *J Exp Med* 187:415, 1998.

110. Dibbert B, Daigle I, Braun D, et al: Role for Bcl-XL in delayed eosinophil apoptosis mediated by grnaulocyte-macrophage colony stimulating factor and interleukin-5. *Blood* 92:778, 1998.

111. Dewson G, Walsh GM, Wardlaw AJ: Expression of Bcl-2 and its homologues in human eosinophils: Modulation by interleukin-5. *Am J Resp Cell Mol Biol* 20:720, 1999.

112. Laviolette S, Bosse M, Boulet L-P, et al: Identification and analysis of eosinophils by flow cytometry using the depolarized side scatter-saponin method. *Cytometry* 29:197, 1997.

113. Kimura I, Moritani Y, Tanizaki Y: Basophils in bronchial asthma with reference to reagin-type allergy. *Clin Allergy* 3:195, 1973.

114. Krause JR, Boggs DR: Search for eosinophilia in hospitalized patients with normal blood leukocyte concentration. *Am J Haematol* 24:55, 1987.

115. Matheson A, Rosenblum A, Glazer R, Dacanay E: Local tissue and blood eosinophils in newborn infants. *J Pediatr* 51:502, 1957.

116. Winkel P, Statland BE, Saunders AM, et al: Within day physiologic variation of leukocyte types in healthy subjects as assayed by two automated leukocyte differential analyzers. *Am J Clin Pathol* 75:693, 1981.

117. Bain BJ, Seed M, Godsland I: Normal values for peripheral blood white

cell counts in women of four different ethnic origins. *J Clin Pathol* 37:188, 1984.

118. Hamid Q, Azzawi M, Sun Ying, et al: Expression of mRNA for interleukin-5 in mucosal bronchial biopsies from asthma. *J Clin Invest* 87:1541, 1991.

119. Limaye AP, Abrams JS, Silver JE, et al: Regulation of parasite induced eosinophilia: selectively increased interleukin 5 production in helminth-infected patients. *J Exp Med* 172:399, 1990.

120. Enokihara H, Furusawa S, Nakakubo H: T cells from eosinophilic patients produce interleukin 5 with interleukin 2 stimulation. *Blood* 73:1809, 1989.

121. Owen WF, Rothenberg ME, Peterson J: Interleukin 5 and phenotypically altered eosinophils in the blood of patients with the idiopathic hypereosinophilic syndrome. *J Exp Med* 170:343, 1989.

122. Owen WF, Peterson J, Sheff DM: Hypodense eosinophils and interleukin 5 activity in the blood of patients with the eosinophilia-myalgia syndrome. *Proc Natl Acad Sci USA* 87:8647, 1990.

123. Samoszuk M, Nansen L: Detection of interleukin-5 messenger RNA in Reed-Sternberg cells of Hodgkins disease with eosinophlia. *Blood* 75:13, 1990.

124. Coffman RL, Seymour BW, Hudak S, Jackson J, Rennick D: Antibody to interleukin-5 inhibits helminth-induced eosinophilia in mice. *Science* 245:308, 1989.

125. Desreumaux P, Janin A, Colombel JF, et al: Interleukin 5 messenger RNA expression by eosinophils in the intestinal mucosa of patients with coeliac disease. *J Exp Med* 175:293, 1992.

126. Mossman R, Coffman RL: Th1 and Th2 cells: different patterns of lymphokine secretion lead to different functional properties. *Annu Rev Immunol* 7:145, 1989.

127. Kay AB, Sun Ying, Varney V: Messenger mRNA expression of the cytokine gene cluster, IL-3, IL-4, IL-5 and GM-CSF in allergen-induced late-phase cutaneous reactions in atopic subjects. *J Exp Med* 173:775, 1991.

128. Tsicopolous A, Hamid Q, Varney V, et al: Preferential mRNA expression of Th1-type cells (IFNgamma+,IL-2+) in classical delayed-type hypersentivity reactions in human skin. *J Immunol* 148:2085, 1992.

129. Wierenga EA, Snoek M, De Groot C: Evidence for compartmentalization of functional subsets of CD4+ T lymphocytes in atopic patients. *J Immunol* 144:4651, 1990.

130. Kirman J, Le Gros G: Which is the true regulator of Th2 cell development in allergic immune responses? *Clin Exp Allergy* 28:908, 1998.

131. King T-P: Immunochemical properties of antigens that cause atopic diseases, in *Bronchial Asthma, Mechanisms and Therapeutics*, 3d ed, edited by EB Weiss, M Stein, pp 4349. Little, Brown, Boston, 1993.

132. Hewitt CRA, Horton H, Jones RM, Pritchard DI: Heterogeneous proteolytic specificity and activity of the house dust mite proteinase allergen. *Clin Exp Allergy* 27:201, 1997.

133. Marsh DG, Hsu SH, Roebber M: HLA-Dw2: a genetic marker for human immune response to short ragweed pollen allergen Ra5.1. Response resulting primarily from natural antigenic exposure. *J Exp Med* 155:1439, 1982.

134. Weller PF, Goetzl EJ: The regulatory and effector roles of eosinophils. *Adv Immunolgy* 27:339, 1979.

135. Rothenberg ME: Eosinophilia. *N Engl J Med* 338:1592, 1998.

136. Kita H: The eosinophil: a cytokine producing cell? *J Allergy Clin Immunol* 97:966, 1996.

137. Todd R, Donoff BR, Chiang T: The eosinophil as a cellular source of transforming growth factor alpha in healing cutaneous wounds. *Am J Pathol* 138:1307 1991.

138. Lowe D, Jorizzo J, Hutt MSR: Tumor associated eosinophilia, a review. *J Clin Path* 34:1343, 1981.

139. Weller PF: The idiopathic hypereosinophilic syndrome. *Blood* 83:2759, 1994.

140. Butterworth AE: Cell mediated damage to helminths. *Adv Parasitology* 23:143, 1984.

141. Seminario C, Gleich GJ: Role of the eosinophil in asthma. *Curr Opinion Immunol* 6:860, 1994.

142. Filley WV, Holley KE, Kephart GM, Gleich GJ: Identification by immunofluorescence of eosinophil granule major basic protein in lung tissue of patients with bronchial asthma. *Lancet* 2:11, 1982.

143. Horn BR, Robin ED, Theodore J, Van Kessel A: Total eosinophil counts in the management of bronchial asthma. *N Engl J Med* 292:1152, 1975.

144. Durham SR, Kay AB: Eosinophils, bronchial hyperreactivity and late-phase asthmatic reactions. *Clin Allergy* 15:411, 1985.

145. De Monchy JGR, Kauffman HF, Venge P, et al: Bronchoalveolar eosinophilia during allergen-induced late asthmatic reactions. *Am Rev Respir Dis* 139:1383, 1985.

146. Metzger WJ, Zavala D, Richerson HB, et al: Local allergen challenge and bronchoalveolar lavage of allergic asthmatic lungs: description of the model and local airway inflammation. *Am Rev Respir Dis* 135:433, 1987.

147. Lam S, LeRichie J, Phillips D, et al: Cellular and protein changes in bronchial lavage fluid after late asthmatic reaction in patients with red cedar wood asthma. *J Allergy Clin Immunol* 80:44, 1987.

148. Fabbri LM, Boschetto P, Zocca E: Bronchoalveolar neutrophilia during late asthmatic reactions induced by toluene diisocyanate. *Am Rev Respir Dis* 136:36, 1987.

149. Frew AJ, Kay AB: The relationship between infiltrating CD4+ lymphocytes, activated eosinophils and the magnitude of the allergen induced late-phase response in man. *J Immunol* 141:4158, 1988.

150. Bentley AM, Jacobson MR, Cumberworth V, et al: Immunohistology of the nasal mucosa in seasonal allergic rhinitis: increase in activated eosinophils and epithelial mast cells. *J Allergy Clin Immunol* 89:877, 1992.

151. Hogan SP, Mould AW, Young JM, et al: Cellular and molecular regulation of eosinophil trafficking to the lung. *Immunol Cell Biol* 76:454, 1998.

152. Akimoto T, Numato F, Tamura M, et al: Abrogation of bronchial eosinophilic inflammation and airway hyperreactivity is signal transducers and activators of transcription (STAT) 6-deficient mice. *J Exp Med* 187:1537, 1998.

153. Gonzalo JA, Lloyd CM, Wen D, et al: The co-ordinated action of CC chemokines in the lung orchestrates allergic inflammation and airway hyperresponsiveness. *J Exp Med* 188:157, 1998.

154. Gonzalo JA, Lloyd CM, Kremer L, et al: Eosinophil recruitment to the lung in a murine model of allergic inflammation. The role of T cells, chemokines and adhesion receptors. *J Clin Invest* 98:2332, 1996.

155. Wardlaw AJ, Dunnette S, Gleich GJ, et al: Eosinophils and mast cells in bronchoalveolar lavage fluid and mild asthma: relationship to bronchial hyperreactivity. *Am Rev Respir Dis* 137:62, 1988.

156. Pavord ID, Pizzichini MM, Pizzichini E, Hargreave FE: The use of induced sputum to investigate airway inflammation. *Thorax* 52:498, 1997.

157. Azzawi M, Bradley B, Jeffery PK, et al: Identification of activated T lymphocytes and eosinophils in bronchial biopsies in stable atopic asthma. *Am Rev Respir Dis* 142:1407, 1990.

158. Hartnell A, Robinson DS, Kay AB, Wardlaw AJ: CD69 is expressed by human eosinophils activated *in vivo* in asthma and *in vitro* by cytokines. *Immunology* 80:281, 1993.

159. Robinson DS, Hamid Q, Sun Ying: Evidence for a predominant Th2-type bronchoalveolar lavage T lymphocyte population in atopic asthma. *N Engl J Med* 326:298, 1992.

160. Jeffery PK, Wardlaw AJ, Nelson FC, Collins JV, Kay AB: Bronchial biopsies in asthma: an ultrastructural, quantitative study and correlation with hyperreactivity. *Am Rev Respir Dis* 140:1745, 1990.

161. Bentley AM, Maestrelli P, Saetta M, et al: Activated T lymphocytes and eosinophils in the bronchial mucosa in isocyanate-induced asthma *J Allergy Clin Immunol* 89:821, 1992.

162. Bentley AM, Menz G, Storz CHR, et al: Identification of T lymphocytes, macrophages and activated eosinophils in the bronchial mucosa in intrinsic asthma: relationship to symptoms and bronchial responsiveness. *Am Rev Respir Dis* 146:500, 1992.

163. Jeffery PK: Structural and inflammatory changes in COPD: a comparison with asthma. *Thorax* 53:129, 1998.

164. Allen JN, Davis WB, Pacht ER: Diagnostic significance of increased bronchoalveolar lavage fluid eosinophils. *Am Rev Respir Dis* 142:642, 1990.

165. Bousquet J, Chanez P, Lacoste JY, et al: Eosinophilic inflammation in asthma. *N Engl J Med* 323:1033, 1990.

166. Diaz P, Galleguillos FR, Gonzales MC, et al: Bronchoalveolar lavage in asthma: the effect of disodium cromoglycate (cromolyn) on leukocyte counts, immunoglobulins and complement. *J Allergy Clin Immunol* 74:41, 1984.

167. Schleimer RP, Bochner BS: The effects of glucocorticoids on human eosinophils. *J Allergy Clin Immunol* 94:1202, 1994.

168. Juniper EF, Kline PA, Vanzieleghem A, Ramsdale H, O'Byrne PM,

Hargreave FE: Effect of long term treatment with an inhaled corticosteroid (budesonide) on airway hyperresponsiveness and clinical asthma in nonsteroid dependent asthmatics. *Am Rev Respir Dis* 142:832, 1990.

169. Adelroth E, Rosenhall L, Johansson S, Linden M, Venge P: Inflammatory cells and eosinophilic activity in asthma investigated by bronchoalveolar lavage. The effects of anti-asthmatic treatment with budesonide or terbutaline. *Am Rev Respir Dis.* 142:91 1990.

170. Kojima S: Eosinophils in parasitic diseases, in *Eosinophils, Biological and Clinical Aspects*, edited by S Makino, T Fukuda, pp 391–402. CRC, Boca Raton, FL, 1993.

171. Spry CJF: *Eosinophils*, Chap. 10, p 136. Oxford University, Oxford, 1988.

172. Butterworth AE, Thorne KJI: Eosinophils and parasitic diseases, in *Immunopharmacology of Eosinophils,* edited by H Smith, RM Cook, p 119. Academic, London, 1993.

173. Gleich GJ, Adolphson CR: The eosinophil leukocyte: structure and function. *Adv Immunol* 39: 177, 1986.

174. Kephart GM, Gleich GJ, Connor DH, et al: Deposition of eosinophil granule major basic protein onto micofilariae of *Onchocerca volvulus* in the skin of patients treated with diethylcarbamazine. *Lab Invest* 50:51, 1984.

175. Hagan P, Wilkins HA, Blumenthal UJ, et al: Eosinophilia and resistance to *Schistosoma haematobium* in man. *Parasite Immunol* 7:625, 1985.

176. Sher A, Coffman RL, Hieny S, Cheever AW: Ablation of eosinophil and IgE responses with anti-IL-5 and anti-IL-4 antibodies fails to affect immunity against *Schistosoma mansoni* larvae in the mouse. *J Immunol* 145:3911, 1990.

177. Dent LA, Daly CM, Mayrhofer G, et al: Interleukin-5 transgenic mice show enhanced resistance to primary infections with *Nippostrongylus brasiliensis* but not primary infections with *Toxocara canis*. *Infection Immunity* 67: 989, 1999.

178. Limaye AP, Abrams JS, Silver JE, et al: Regulation of parasite-induced eosinophilia: selectively increased interleukin 5 production in helminth-infected patients. *J Exp Med* 172:399, 1990.

179. Tanaka J, Torisu M: Ascaris and the eosinophil II: isolation and characterization of eosinophil chemotactic factor and neutrophil chemotactic factor of parasite in Ascaris antigen. *J Immunol* 122:302, 1979.

180. Owashi M, Ishii K: Purification and characterization of a high molecular weight eosinophil chemotactic factor from *Schistosoma japonicum* eggs. *J Immunol* 129:2226, 1982.

181. Moqbel R: *Allergy and Immunity to Helminths: Common Mechanisms or Divergent Pathways*? Taylor and Francis, London, 1992.

182. Grove DI: What is the relationship between asthma and worms? *Allergy* 37:139, 1982.

183. Van Dellen RG, Thompson JH: Absence of intestinal parasites in asthma. *N Engl J Med* 285:146, 1971

184. Turton JA: IgE, parasites and allergy. *Lancet* ii:686, 1976.

185. Engfeldt B, Zetterstrom R: Disseminated eosinophilic "collagen disease." *Acta Med Scand* 153:337:1956.

186. Hardy WR, Anderson RE: The hyperesoniophilic syndromes. *Ann Intern Med* 68:1220, 1968.

187. Resnick M, Myerson RM: Hypereosinophilic syndromes. *Am J Med* 51:560, 1971.

188. Weller PF, Bubley GJ: The idiopathic hypereosinophilic syndrome. *Blood* 83:2759, 1994.

189. Chang H-W, Leong K-H, Koh D-R, Leen S-H: Clonality of isolated eosinophils in the hypereosinophilic syndrome. *Blood* 93:1651, 1999.

190. Luppi M, Marasca R, Morselli M, et al: Clonal nature of hypereosinophilic syndrome. *Blood* 84:349, 1994.

191. Raghavachar A, Fleischer S, Frickhoven N: T lymphocyte control of human eosinophil granulopoiesis. *J Immunol* 139:3753, 1987.

192. Owen WF, Rothenberg ME, Peterson J, et al: Interleukin 5 and phenotypically altered eosinophils in the blood of patients with the idiopathic hypereosinophilic syndrome. *J Exp Med* 170:343, 1989.

193. Cogan E, Shandene L, Crusiaux A, et al: Clonal proliferation of type 2 helper cells in a man with hypereosinophilic syndrome. *N Engl J Med* 330:535, 1994.

194. Shah AM, Brutsaert DL, Menlemans AL, et al: Eosinophils from hypereosinophilic patients damage endocardium of isolated feline heart muscle preparations. *Circulation* 81:1081, 1990.

195. Olsen EG, Spry CJ: Relations between eosinophilia and endomyocardial disease. *Prog Cardiovasc Dis* 27:241, 1985.

196. Chang HW, Leon KH, Koh DR, Lee SH: Clonality of isolated eosinophils in the hypereosinophilic syndrome. *Blood* 93:1651, 1999.

197. Parillo JE, Borerts WL, Henry WL, et al: The cardiovascular manifestations of hypereosinophilic syndrome. *Am J Med* 67:572, 1979.

198. Schooley RT, Flaum MA, Gralnick HR, Fauci AS: A clinicopathologic correlation of the idiopathic hypereosinophilic syndrome. II: Clinical manifestations. *Blood* 58:1021, 1981.

199. Moore PM, Harley JB, Fauci AS: Neurologic dysfunction in the idiopathic hypereosinophilic syndrome. *Ann Intern Med* 102:109, 1985.

200. Lin AY, Nutman TB, Kasow D, et al: Familial eosinophilia: clinical and laboratory results on a US Kindred. *Am J Med Genet* 76:229, 1998.

201. Rioux JD, Stone VA, Daly MJ, et al: Familial eosinophilia maps to the cytokine gene cluster on human chromosomal region 5q31-q33. *Am J Hum Genet* 63:1086, 1998.

202. Villa A, Santagata S, Bozzi F, et al: Partial V9D)J recombination activity leads to Omenn syndrome. *Cell* 93:885, 1998.

203. Parillo JE, Fauci AS, Wolff SM: Therapy of the hypereosinophilic syndrome. *Ann Intern Med* 87:167, 1978.

204. Smit AJ, Van Essen LH, de Vries EGE: Successful long term control of idiopathic hypereosinophilic syndrome with etoposide. *Cancer* 67: 2820, 1991.

205. Murphy PT, Fennelly DF, Stuart M, O'Donnell JR: Alpha interferon in a case of hypereosinophilic syndrome. *Br J Haematol* 75:6189, 1990.

206. Zielinski RM, Lawrence WD: Interferon-alpha for the hypereosinophilic syndrome. *Ann Intern Med* 113:716, 1990.

207. Butterfield JH, Gleich GJ: Interferon-α treatment of six patients with the idiopathic hypereosinophilic syndrome. *Ann Intern Med* 121:648, 1994.

208. Nassar GM, Pedro P, Remmers RE, et al: Reversible renal failure in a patient with the hypereosinophilia syndrome during therapy with alpha interferon. *Am J Kidney Dis* 31:121, 1998.

209. Ellman L, Miller L, Rappeport J: Leukapheresis therapy of a hypereosinophilic disorder. *JAMA* 230:1004, 1974.

210. Esteva-Lorenzo F, Meehan KR, Spitzer TR, Mazumeder A: Allogenic bone marrow transplantation in a patient with hypereosinophilic syndrome. *Am J Hematol* 51:164, 1996.

211. Smith MD, Metcalfe M, DeMaria AN, et al: Hypereosinophilic syndrome resulting in aortic and mitral stenosis. A case requiring double valve replacement. *Am Heart J* 117:475, 1989.

212. Boustang CW, Murphy GW, Hicks GL Jr: Mitral valve replacement in idiopathic hypereosinophilic syndrome. *Ann Thorac Surg* 51:1007, 1991.

213. Edwards D, Wald JA, Dobozen BS, et al: Troleandomycin and methylprednisolone for treatment of the hypereosinophilic syndrome. *N Engl J Med* 317:573, 1987.

214. Betran JD, Rowley JD, Plapp F, et al: Chromosomal aneuploidy in a patient with hypereosinophilic syndrome. *Am J Med* 63:1010, 1977.

215. Owen J, Scott C: Transition of hypereosinophilic syndrome to myelomonocytic leukemia. *Can Med Assoc J* 121:1489, 1979.

216. Prin L, Legeurn M, Ameissen JC, et al: HTLV-1 and malignant hypereosinophilic syndrome. *Lancet* 2:569, 1988.

217. Keidan AJ, Catovsky D, DeCastro JT, et al: Hypereosinophilic syndrome preceding T cell lymphblastic lymphoma. *Clin Lab Haematol* 7:83, 1985.

218. Eosinophilia-myalgia syndrome—New Mexico. *MMWR* 38:765, 1989.

219. Eosinophilia-myalgia syndrome and L-tryptophan containing products—New Mexico, Minnesota, Oregon and New York. *MMWR* 38: 785, 1989.

220. Culpeper RC, Williams RG, Mease PJ, et al: Natural history of the eosinophilia-myalgia syndrome. *Ann Intern Med* 115:437, 1991.

221. Belonga EA, Mayeno AN, Gleich GJ, et al: An investigation of the cause of the eosinophilia-myalgia syndrome associated with tryptophan use. *N Engl J Med* 323:357, 1990.

222. Varga J, Witts J, Jiminez SA: The cause and pathogenesis of the eosinophilia-myalgia syndrome. *Ann Intern Med* 116:140, 1992.

223. Belonga EA, Mayeno AN, Gleich GJ, Kita H: Eosinophilia-myalgia syndrome, in *Eosinophils, Biological and Clinical Aspects*, edited by S Makino, T Fukado, pp 421–440. CRC, Boca Raton, FL, 1993.

224. Kilbourne EM, Posada de la Paz M, Borda IA, et al: Toxic oil syndrome. *J Am Coll Cardiol* 18:711, 1991.

225. Kilbourne EM, Posada de la Paz M, Borda IA, et al: Toxic oil syndrome. *J Am Coll Cardiol* 18:711, 1991.

226. Kilbourne EM, Rigau Perez JG, Health CW Jr, et al: Clinical epidemiology of toxic oil syndrome. *N Engl J Med* 309:1408, 1983.

227. Spitzer C, Carson OM: Lymphoblastic leukaemia with marked eosinophilia. *Blood* 42:377, 1973.

228. Vukelja SJ, Weiss RB, Perry DJ, Longo DL: Eosinophilia associated with adult T-cell leukaemia/lymphoma. *Cancer* 62:1527, 1988.

229. Slumgaard A, Ascensao J, Zanjani E, Jacobs HS: Pulmonary carcinoma with eosinophila. *N Engl J Med* 309:778, 1983.

230. Stefanini M, Claustro JC, Motos RA, Bendigo LL: Blood and marrow eosinophilia in malignant tumors. *Cancer* 68:543, 1991.

231. Pinto A, Aldinucci D, Gloghini A, et al : The role of eosinophils in the pathobiology of Hodgkin's disease. *Ann Oncol* 8:(suppl 2) s89, 1997.

232. Sharp JF, Rodgers MJC, MacGregor FB, et al: Angiolymphoma hyperplasia with eosinophilia. *J Laryngol Otol* 104:977, 1990.

233. Hallam LA, MacKinlay GA, Wright AMA: Angiolymphoid hyperplasia with eosinophilia. *J Clin Pathol* 42:944, 1989.

234. Nazum JW Jr, Nuzum JW: Polyarteritis nodosa: statisitical review of on one hundred and seventy five cases from the literature and report on one typical case. *Arch Intern Med* 94:942, 1954.

235. Lhote F, Guillevin L: Polyarteritis nodosa, microscopic polyangiitis and Churg Strauss syndrome. *Sem Resp Crit Care Med* 191:27, 1998.

236. Churg J, Strauss L: Allergic granulomatosis, allergic angiitis and periarteritis nodosa. *Am J Pathol* 27:277, 1951.

237. Fauci AS: Vasculitis. *J Allergy Clin Immunol* 72:211, 1983.

238. Guillevin L, Guittard T, Bletry O, et al: Systemic necrotizing angiitis with asthma. Causes and precipitating factors in 43 cases. *Lung* 165:165, 1987.

239. Guillevin L, Cohen P, Gayraud M, et al: Churg-Strauss syndrome. Clinical study and long term follow up of 96 patients. *Medicine* (Baltimore) 78:26, 1999.

240. Abeleles M, Belin DC, Zurier AB: Eosinophilic fasciitis. *Arch Intern Med* 139:586, 1979.

241. Lakhanpal S, Ginsburg WW, Michet CJ, et al: Eosinophilic fasciitis: clinical spectrum and therapeutic responses in 52 cases. *Semin Arthritis Rheum* 17:221, 1988.

242. Doyle JA, Ginsburg WW: Eosinophilic fasciitis. *Med Clin North Am* 73:1157, 1989.

243. Bidula LP, Myers AR: Eosinophilic fasciitis associated with hematologic disorders. *Clin Rheumatol Pract* 3:117, 1985.

244. Corwin HL, Bray RA, Haber MH: The detection and interpretation of urinary eosinophils. *Arch Pathol Lab Med* 113:1256, 1989.

245. Nolan CR III, Anger MS, Kelleher SP: Eosinophilia—a new method of detection and definition of the clinical spectrum. *N Engl J Med* 315:1516, 1986.

246. Bosch I, Oehmichen M: Eosinophilic granulocytes in cerebrospinal fluid specimens and review of the literature. *J Neurol* 219:93, 1978.

247. Weingarten JS, O'Shea SF, Margolis WS: Eosinophilic meningitis and the hypereosinophilic syndrome. *Am J Med* 78:674, 1985.

248. Calame JJ, Von’t Woret JW, VanDijk JG, Botsgth AM: A case of eosinophilic meningoencephalitis accompanied by eosinophilic inflammation of the myenteric plexus in Hodgkin's disease. *Histopathology* 10:535, 1986.

249. Beeson PB, Bass DA: Mechanisms of Eosinopenia, in *The Eosinophil,* edited by PB Beeson, DA Bass, p 92. WB Saunders, Philadelphia, 1977.

250. Bass DA, Gonwa TA, Szejda P, et al: Eosinopenia of acute infection. *J Clin Invest* 65:1265, 1980.

251. Juhlin L, Michaelsson G: A new syndrome characterized by absence of eosinophils and basophils. *Lancet* i:1233, 1977.

252. Juhlin L, Venge P: Total absence of eosinophils in a patient with chronic urticaria and vitiligo. *Eur J Haematol* 40:368, 1987.

253. Telerman A, Amson RB, Delforge A, et al: A case of chronic aneosinocytosis. *Am J Hematol* 12:187, 1982.

254. Nakahata T, Spicer SS, Leary AG, et al: Circulating eosinophil colony-forming cells in pure eosinophil aplasia. *Ann Intern Med* 101:321, 1984.

255. Joshua H, Zucker A, Presentey B: Peroxidase and phospholipid deficiency in eosinophil granulocytes among Arabs of the Nazareth district. *Isr J Med Sci* 12:71, 1976.

256. Brugnoni D, Airò P, Rossi G, et al: A case of hypereosinophilic syndrome is associated with the expansion of a CD3⁻CD4⁺ T-cell population able to secrete large amounts of interleukin-5. *Blood* 87:1416, 1996.

257. Roufosse F, Schandené L, Sibille C, et al: T-cell receptor-independent activation of clonal Th2 cells associated with chronic hypereosinophilia. *Blood* 94:994, 1999.

258. Ueno NT, Zhaos S, Robertson LE, et al: 2-chlorodeoxyadenosine therapy for idiopathic hypereosinophilic syndrome. *Leukemia* 11:1386, 1997.

259. Teroya-Feldstein J, Jaffe ES, Burd PR, et al: Differential chemokine expression in tissues involved by Hodgkin's disease: Direct correlation of eotaxin expression and tissue eosinophilia. *Blood* 93:2463, 1999.

BASOPHILS AND MAST CELLS AND THEIR DISORDERS

STEPHEN J. GALLI

DEAN D. METCALFE

ANN M. DVORAK

Although basophils and mast cells share certain biochemical and functional characteristics, they are not identical. In humans, basophils are the least frequent of the three granulocytes, typically accounting for less than 0.5 percent of blood leukocytes. Basophils circulate as mature cells and can be recruited into tissues, particularly at sites of immunological or inflammatory responses, but they ordinarily do not reside in tissues. By contrast, mast cells typically are derived from blood precursors that lack many of the characteristic features of the mature cells and complete their maturation in the tissues. The mature mast cells can reside in tissues for long periods of time. Mast cells are particularly abundant near blood vessels and nerves and in connective tissues beneath surfaces that are exposed to the external environment, such as the skin, gastrointestinal, and urogenital tracts and the respiratory system. Tissue mast cell numbers can increase at sites of parasite infection, certain chronic allergic diseases, or other forms of pathology, by the recruitment and local maturation of blood precursors and the proliferation of resident mast cells.

Mast cells and basophils express the high-affinity receptor for IgE ($Fc_\varepsilon RI$) on their surface, and both types of cells can be triggered to release potent mediators in response to activation via the $Fc_\varepsilon RI$, e.g., when their cell-bound IgE recognizes bi- or multivalent allergens. Accordingly, mast cells and basophils have long been regarded as important effector cells in asthma, hay fever, and other allergic disorders. Indeed, it is thought that the cells' cytoplasmic granule-associated preformed mediators, including histamine and certain proteases, their lipid mediators (such as prostaglandin D2 and leukotriene C4), which are generated upon activation of the cells, and their cytokines, contribute to many of the characteristic signs and symptoms of these diseases. However, several lines of evidence indicate that mast cells and basophils also contribute to protective host responses that are associated with IgE production, especially those directed against parasites, and for mast cells in innate immune responses to certain bacterial infections. Through cytokine production and other mechanisms, mast cells and basophils may also execute immunoregulatory functions.

While a variety of systemic disorders have been associated with changes in the numbers of blood basophils, and many pathological processes can be associated with changes in the numbers of tissue mast cells, patients with primary deficiencies in basophils appear to be exceedingly rare (if they exist at all), and there have been no reports of patients with a primary deficiency of tissue mast cells. By contrast, neoplastic processes can affect both of these lineages. Increased numbers of basophils may be present in association with myeloproliferative disorders and several forms of myelogenous or promyelocytic leukemias, and increased numbers of basophils, sometimes to levels of 20 to 90 percent of blood leukocytes, occur in virtually all patients with chronic myelogenous leukemia. It is thought that the basophils associated with cases of leukemia are themselves neoplastic. The management of patients with "basophilic leukemia" can be complicated by shock due to the massive release of histamine and other mediators in association with acute cytolysis.

Disorders of mast cell hyperplasia/neoplasia include solitary mastocytomas, the pathogenesis of which is uncertain, the spectrum of disorders encompassed in the term *mastocytosis*, in which significantly increased numbers of mast cells occur in the skin and/or other organs, and mast cell leukemia. The most common form of mastocytosis (category I or *indolent mastocytosis*), typically presents with urticaria pigmentosa involving the skin, although other organs may also be involved; patients with indolent mastocytosis have the best prognosis and can expect a normal life-span. The prognosis of category II disease (*mastocytosis with an associated hematological disorder*) depends on the course of the associated disease. Patients with category III disease (*aggressive mastocytosis*) have a guarded prognosis because of complications arising from rapid increases in tissue mast cell numbers. And patients with mast cell leukemia (category IV disease), who often present with large numbers of immature mast cells in the peripheral blood at the time of diagnosis, have a fulminant and rapidly fatal course. Many, if not all, adult patients with mastocytosis have gain-of-function mutations affecting c-kit, which encodes the receptor for the major mast cell growth factor, stem cell factor (also known as *kit ligand* and *mast cell growth factor*). Some pediatric patients with mastocytosis have been reported to have the same Asp816Val gain-of-function c-kit mutation that is observed in adult patients, others have a dominant inactivating c-kit mutation, whereas others appear to lack c-kit mutations entirely.

DISTINGUISHING FEATURES OF BASOPHILS AND MAST CELLS

BASOPHILS

Despite certain striking similarities in biochemistry and function, mammalian basophils and mast cells are not identical, [1-5] a distinction appreciated by Paul Ehrlich, who described the histochemical staining characteristics of both of these cells in the late nineteenth century. Many lines of evidence indicate that basophils share a common precursor with other granulocytes and monocytes. [1-5] Basophils have a short life-span [6] and retain granulocytic features even after emigrating into tissues (Fig. 69-1).

The human basophil is the least common blood granulocyte, with a prevalence of about 0.5 percent of total leukocytes and about 0.3 percent of nucleated marrow cells. [7] Although the basophil's prominent metachromatic cytoplasmic granules allow unmistakable identification

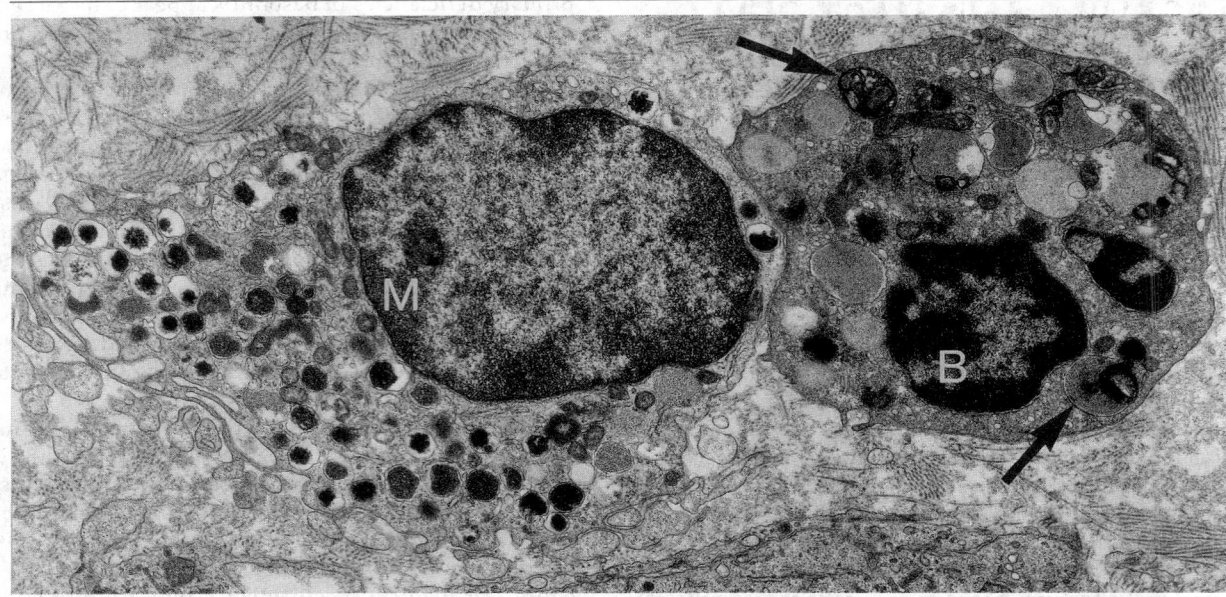

FIGURE 69-1   Mast cell (M) and basophil (B) in the ileal submucosa of a patient with Crohn's disease. The mast cell is a larger, mononuclear cell with a more complex plasma membrane surface and cytoplasmic granules that are smaller and more numerous than those of the basophil. In this section plane, the basophil exhibits two nuclear lobes. Several basophil cytoplasmic granules contain whorls of membranes (arrows). Osmium collidine uranyl en bloc processing. (Source: Dvorak and coworkers[37] with permission.)

in Wright-Giemsa–stained films of blood or marrow, accurate basophil determinations require absolute counting methods.[8] Differential counts of blood films yield valid results only if the percentage of basophils is substantially elevated or if many thousands of leukocytes are counted.

Interleukin-3 (IL-3) promotes the production and survival of human basophils in vitro[3,9] and can induce basophilia in vivo.[10] Findings in IL-3 −/− mice indicate that IL-3 is not necessary for the development of normal numbers of bone marrow or blood basophils but is very important for the bone marrow and blood basophilia associated with certain Th2 cell-associated immunological responses.[11,12] Basophils also express receptors for several other cytokines (Table 69-1). IL-3 and some of these other cytokines can modulate basophil function, e.g., by inducing mediator release directly and/or by augmenting the cells' ability to release mediators in response to challenge with IgE and specific antigen.[3,10,13,14]

MAST CELLS

Mast cells normally reside in the connective tissue, particularly beneath epithelial surfaces and around blood vessels and, in some species, in serous cavities.[1,2,4,5,15–17] Mast cells are derived from hemopoietic precursors,[15,18] but, except for a numerically minor population of mast cells that resides in the marrow,[7] this lineage completes its program of maturation in the tissues.[1,2,4,15–18] Unlike basophils, mast cells are long-lived cells, and at least some mast cells can locally proliferate in the tissues during a variety of inflammatory or reparative processes.[1,2,4,15–17]

Studies in murine rodents, nonhuman primates, and humans indicate that many aspects of mast cell development are critically regulated by SCF, the ligand for the c-kit tyrosine growth factor receptor.[11,16–20] SCF is produced in both membrane-associated and soluble forms, both of which are biologically active.[17,21] In addition to promoting the migration, survival, proliferation, and maturation of cells in the mast cell lineage, SCF also can directly promote mast cell mediator re-

lease[20,22–26] and, at even lower concentrations, can augment mast cell mediator release in response to stimulation by IgE and antigen.[23–25] Abnormalities affecting the c-kit receptor are involved in the pathogenesis of certain examples of mastocytosis (see below). Moreover, it is likely that alterations in the production of SCF by fibroblasts and other cells can contribute to the changes in mast cell numbers that occur during many chronic inflammatory conditions and other pathological responses.[16,17,19,27]

MAST CELL AND BASOPHIL HETEROGENEITY

Variation in the morphologic, biochemical, and/or functional characteristics of mast cells from different anatomic locations or from the same organ or site has been reported in several mammalian species, including humans.[1,2,5,15,17,28–30] This phenomenon, often referred to as *mast cell heterogeneity,* raises the possibility that mast cells of different phenotype may express different functions in health or disease and may also exhibit different sensitivities to pharmacologic manipulation. At least four mechanisms may account for phenotypic variation in mast cell populations: (1) factors promoting branching within the mast cell lineage; (2) factors influencing differentiation/maturation (within single pathways or, if they occur, within multiple pathways); (3) factors modulating mast cell function; and (4) factors influencing local concentrations of exogenous substances not derived from mast cells but taken up and stored in mast cell granules. Of these four mechanisms, experimental evidence has been obtained for all but the first.[29] Basophils can also exhibit some variation in phenotypic characteristics, such as immunoreactivity for tryptase, chymase, and carboxypeptidase A.[31]

RELATIONSHIP BETWEEN BASOPHILS AND MAST CELLS

Mature basophils and mast cells differ in morphology, natural history, tissue distribution, mediator production, cell surface phenotype, growth factor requirements, and responses to drugs (see Fig. 69-1 and Table 69-1).[1–5] Nevertheless, the two cells do exhibit a number of

TABLE 69-1   NATURAL HISTORY, MAJOR MEDIATORS, AND SURFACE MEMBRANE STRUCTURES OF HUMAN MAST CELLS AND BASOPHILS

Characteristics	Basophils	Mast Cells
Natural history		
Origin of precursor cells	Marrow	Marrow
Site of maturation	Marrow	Connective tissue (a few in marrow)
Mature cells in circulation	Yes (usually <1% of blood leukocytes)	No
Mature cells recruited into tissues from circulation	Yes (during immunologic, inflammatory responses)	No
Mature cells normally residing in connective tissues	No (not detectable by microscopy)	Yes
Proliferative ability of morphologically mature cells	None reported	Yes (limited; under certain circumstances)
Life-span	Days (like other granulocytes)	Weeks to months (according to studies in rodents)
Major growth factor	IL-3	Stem cell factor (SCF)
Mediators		
Major mediators stored performed in cytoplasmic granules	Histamine, chondroitin sulfates, tryptase*, chymase*, carboxypeptidase A*, neutral protease with bradykinin-generating activity, β-glucuronidase, elastase, cathepsin G-like enzyme, major basic protein, Charcot-Leyden crystal protein	Histamine, heparin, and/or chondroitin sulfates; neutral proteases (chymase and/or tryptase), many acid hydrolases, cathepsin, carboxypeptidases
Major lipid mediators produced on appropriate activation	Leukotriene C_4	Prostaglandin D_2, leukotriene C_4, platelet-activating factor
Cytokines released on appropriate activation	IL-4, IL-13	TNF-α, macrophage inflammatory protein-1α, VPF/VEGF, IL-13, IL-16 (mouse and perhaps human mast cells many more—see text)
Surface structures		
Ig receptors	Fc$_\varepsilon$RI, Fc$_\gamma$RII (CDw32)	Fc$_\varepsilon$RI
Cytokine or growth factor receptors for:	IL-1, IL-2 (CD25), IL-3, -4, -5, and -8; Chemokine and Interferon receptors; SCF (some basophils express low numbers of c-KIT receptors)	SCF (c-KIT receptor)
Cell adhesion structures (structures in italics are apparently expressed on just one of the two cell types)	P24 (CD09), *LFA-1α chain (CD11a), C3bi receptor/Mac-1α (CD11b)*, LFA-1β chain, β2 & β1 (CD18 & 29), *PECAM (CD31)*, leukosialin (CD43), Pgp-1 (CD44), VLA-4α, β1 (CD49d), VLA-5α, β1 (CD49e), ICAM-3 (CD50), ICAM-1 (CD54), CD58 (LFA-3), ICAM-2 (CD102)	CD09, CD29, CD43, CD44, CD49d, CD49e, CD50, *VNRα, β3 (CD51)*, CD54, CD58, *LFA-1β chain, β3 (CD61)*, CD102 ($\pm$)

*Basophil content of these (and perhaps other) mediators apparently can vary, e.g., in association with certain allergic diseases.[31]
ABBREVIATIONS: IL, interleukin; SCF, stem cell factor; LFA, lymphocyte function–associated antigen; VLA, very late antigen; ICAM, intercellular adhesion molecule; VNR, vitronectin receptor.
SOURCE: Modified after Galli[2] with permission; data regarding CD antigens are from analyses of blood basophils and lung or uterine mast cells.[3] Note: Expression of these and other surface structures, including chemokine receptors, can vary in different in vitro- or in vivo-derived basophil or mast cell populations.

striking similarities. These similarities, taken together with evidence from murine rodents indicating that tissue mast cells are derived from circulating marrow-derived precursors,[15,18] have suggested to some investigators that basophils might represent the circulating precursor of mast cells. Although this hypothesis has not formally been excluded, current evidence greatly favors the view that mature basophils represent terminally differentiated granulocytes and not circulating mast cell precursors. In addition to the morphologic evidence discussed below, the latter position is supported by the following observations: (1) no actual evidence has been presented, in any species, indicating that mature circulating basophils are capable either of mitosis or of differentiation into mast cells; (2) the rare reports of patients with hereditary or acquired abnormalities affecting basophil numbers or morphology indicate that eosinophils may also be affected in these disorders but not mast cells[32–34]; (3) morphologically identifiable human tissue mast cells can exhibit mitotic activity,[35] indicating that this cell lineage is capable of replication independent of a stage resembling that of circulating basophils.

MORPHOLOGY OF BASOPHILS AND MAST CELLS

Routine methods of tissue fixation and processing are poorly suited for demonstration of basophils and mast cells (See Plate VII); optimal visualization is achieved in appropriately prepared 1-μm sections or with an ultrastructural approach.[1,4] Ultrastructurally, human basophils

are 5 to 7 μm in spherical diameter, exhibit a segmented or, in some cases, unsegmented nucleus with marked condensation of nuclear chromatin, and contain round or oval cytoplasmic granules; these granules are surrounded by a membrane and contain a substructure of dense particles, less dense matrix, and, in some granules, membrane whorls and Charcot-Leyden crystals[1,4] (see Fig. 69-1). A second, minor population of small, uniform granules is characteristically located close to the nucleus.[36] The cytoplasm of mature human basophils also contains glycogen particles, mitochondria, free ribosomes, and small membrane-bound vesicles; lipid bodies are rarely present. Other organelles are inconspicuous.

In tissue sections, mast cells typically appear as either round or elongated cells, usually with a nonsegmented nucleus with moderate condensation of nuclear chromatin, and contain prominent cytoplasmic granules; mast cell granules are smaller, more numerous, and generally more variable in appearance than in basophils and contain scroll-like structures, particles, and crystals, alone or in combination.[1,4] In contrast to the irregularly spaced blunt surface projections of basophils, mast cells are covered by uniformly distributed thin surface processes. Mast cells also differ from basophils in that they have many more cytoplasmic filaments and lack cytoplasmic glycogen deposits. Human mast cells can also contain numerous cytoplasmic lipid bodies. Figure 69-1 is an electron micrograph showing a human basophil adjacent to a human mast cell in the same tissue, the ileal submucosa.

BIOCHEMISTRY AND ROLE IN IgE-ASSOCIATED IMMUNE RESPONSES

MEDIATORS

The cytoplasmic granules of basophils and mast cells contain proteoglycans, consisting of sulfated glycosaminoglycans covalently linked to a protein core.[38,39] Under appropriate conditions, these substances stain metachromatically with basic dyes. In humans and murine species, individual mast cell populations can contain variable mixtures of heparin and chondroitin sulfate proteoglycans.[15,29,38,39] Although the sulfated glycosaminoglycans of normal human blood basophils have not yet been characterized, two studies of the proteoglycans synthesized by blood leukocytes (containing 10 to 75 percent basophils) of 5 patients with myelogenous leukemia indicate that such cells may produce entirely chondroitin sulfates[40] or a mixture of chondroitin sulfates (50 to 84 percent) and heparin (8 to 43 percent).[41] Normal guinea pig basophils synthesize predominantly (85 percent) chondroitin sulfates, with the remainder characterized as heparan sulfate rather than heparin.[42] While the biological functions of basophil and mast cell proteoglycans are not yet fully understood, in mice, heparin is required for normal packaging of certain neutral proteases in mast cell cytoplasmic granules.[43,44] Both human mast cells and basophils synthesize and store histamine.[1,31,38] Basophils represent the source of most (if not all) of the histamine present in normal human blood.[45] Studies in mice indicate that mast cells represent the source of virtually all the histamine stored in normal tissues, with the notable exceptions of the glandular stomach and parts of the central nervous system.[46]

In addition to proteoglycans and histamine, basophils and mast cells generate many other mediators that can influence the course of inflammatory processes[1–3,5,38,47] (see Table 69-1). These substances are either preformed and granule-associated (e.g., histamine, neutral proteases, proteoglycans) or produced during activation of the cell [e.g., prostaglandin D2, leukotrienes ("slow-reacting substances of anaphylaxis") and other metabolites of arachidonic acid, and platelet-activating factor]. Appropriately, stimulated mouse or human mast cells can release the cytokine TNF-α,[2,5,48–50] and mouse and perhaps human mast cells,[2,5,50,51] and human basophils,[5,52] can produce IL-4. Work with mouse and human mast cells indicates that mast cells may also represent a potential source of many additional cytokines with effects on inflammation, immunity, hematopoiesis, tissue remodeling, and many other biological processes.[5,50,53–56] By contrast, the spectrum of basophil-derived cytokines appears to be more limited but includes IL-4 and IL-13.[5,52,57]

ROLE IN ACUTE REACTIONS

Basophils and mast cells have specific, high-affinity plasma membrane receptors for the Fc region of homocytotropic immunoglobulins; in humans this is largely IgE.[58–60] When IgE antibodies bound to the basophil or mast cell surface are bridged by specific di- or multivalent antigens, anaphylactic degranulation is triggered.[1,2,5,38,39,58–60] The critical signal in this event is the bridging of IgE receptors (Fc$_\varepsilon$RI) on the plasma membrane, and antibodies to the receptors may substitute for IgE and antigen to initiate degranulation in vitro.[58–60] Antigen binding is independent of divalent cations. However, later steps in degranulation require both calcium and physiologic temperatures.[31,58–60] Morphologically, anaphylactic degranulation involves the fusion of plasma membranes with the membranes delimiting individual cytoplasmic granules or with groups of granules whose membranes have undergone fusion, leading to rapid noncytolytic release of granule contents, such as histamine and other preformed mediators.[1,4] The complex sequence of biochemical events associated with anaphylactic

degranulation and the rationale of their pharmacologic manipulation have been reviewed.[31,38,59–61]

The sudden, massive release of mediators from basophils and mast cells is thought to provoke many of the clinical manifestations of acute immediate hypersensitivity reactions in such disorders as certain forms of bronchial asthma; urticaria; allergic rhinitis; and anaphylaxis to foods, drugs, insect stings, and other antigens.[1,2,31,38,61] Other diverse stimuli, including certain complement fragments (anaphylatoxins), neutrophil lysosomal proteins, a variety of basic peptides and peptide hormones, components of insect venoms, radiocontrast solutions, cold, calcium ionophores, and certain drugs such as narcotics and muscle relaxants, may also initiate rapid release of mediators from basophils and mast cells, independently of IgE.[5,31,38,61] The clinical reactions provoked by these agents can closely mimic those of immediate hypersensitivity. Finally, certain agents, including protein Fv (pFv), a sialoprotein found in normal liver and released into the intestinal tract in patients with viral hepatitis, can interact with the VH3 domain of IgE and thereby induce histamine release from human basophils and mast cells and IL-4 release from human basophils.[62] The extent to which this proposed "endogenous superallergen" function of pFv is important in host defense or in the pathogenesis of viral infections remains to be determined.[62]

ROLE IN LATE-PHASE AND CHRONIC ALLERGIC REACTIONS

ROLE IN LATE-PHASE REACTIONS AND THE MAST CELL–LEUKOCYTE CYTOKINE CASCADE

In addition to their roles in classic acute immediate hypersensitivity responses, such as anaphylaxis, mast cells and basophils also can contribute to late-phase reactions. Late-phase reactions occur when antigen challenge is followed, hours after initial IgE-dependent mast cell activation, by the recurrence of signs (e.g., cutaneous edema) and symptoms (e.g., bronchoconstriction).[61,63] It is widely believed that much of the morbidity associated with chronic allergic conditions, such as allergic asthma, reflects the actions of leukocytes that are recruited to sites of late-phase reactions.[61,63] Studies in mast cell knockin mice (see below) indicate that mast cells are responsible for virtually all of the vascular permeability changes and leukocyte infiltration associated with cutaneous late-phase reactions and that TNF-α importantly contributes to these responses.[64] It is likely that mast cell TNF-α production also helps to initiate late-phase reactions in humans[2,5,49,50] and that basophils, eosinophils, and other leukocytes that are recruited to these reactions produce cytokines and other mediators that regulate the further development and, ultimately, the resolution of these reactions.[2,5,50] This sequence of events in the pathogenesis of late-phase reactions is termed the *mast cell–leukocyte cytokine cascade.*[2,5,50]

IGE-DEPENDENT UPREGULATION OF FC$_\varepsilon$RI EXPRESSION AND FC$_\varepsilon$RI-DEPENDENT FUNCTION

Notably, as plasma levels of IgE increase (as typically occurs in subjects with allergic diseases or parasite infections), levels of Fc$_\varepsilon$RI expression on the surface of basophils and mast cells also increase.[65,66] Compared with cells with low "baseline" levels of Fc$_\varepsilon$RI expression, such cells can bind more IgE, release mediators in response to lower concentrations of allergens, and produce significantly larger amounts of preformed and lipid mediators and cytokines.[54,65–68] Thus, basophils and mast cells in subjects with high levels of IgE may be significantly enhanced in their ability to express IgE-dependent and/or immunoregulatory functions.[61]

ROLES IN T-CELL-DEPENDENT RESPONSES NOT INVOLVING IgE

Mast cell activation, and/or infiltration of affected tissues with circulating basophils, also can occur during a variety of T-cell-dependent immunological responses in both humans and experimental animals.[1,69] However, genetically mast-cell-deficient mice can express certain apparently unimpaired T-cell-dependent responses.[2,16,70] Accordingly, the specific roles of mast cells and basophils in such responses remain to be determined.

BIOLOGICAL FUNCTIONS OF BASOPHILS AND MAST CELLS

ROLES IN HOST DEFENSE

It is likely that basophils and mast cells have critical roles in the expression of host resistance to certain parasites. Whether the basophil or the mast cell represents the major effector cell type in these responses appears to vary according to such factors as species of parasite, species of host, and site of infection. Thus, in the guinea pig, basophils appear to be required for the expression of immune resistance to infestation of the skin by larval ixodid *Amblyomma americanum* ticks,[69,71,72] whereas expression of IgE-dependent immune resistance to the cutaneous infestation of larval *Haemaphysalis longicornis* ticks in mice is dependent on mast cells.[72] Findings such as these support the notion that basophils and mast cells may express similar or complementary functions in host defense against parasites and other agents.

Studies in "mast cell knock-in mice" (see below) have shown that mast cells can also contribute to "innate immunity" to host defense against some bacterial infections.[73] This role of the mast cell in "natural immunity" is due in part to complement-dependent activation of mast cells and in part to TNF-α production by mast cells.[73]

OTHER FUNCTIONS AND MAST CELL KNOCK-IN MICE

Factors capable of inducing basophil infiltration, mast cell proliferation, and/or basophil or mast cell degranulation are generated during a wide variety of immunological or pathological processes, in addition to immune responses to parasites.[1,11,29,31,61,69] As a result, there has been considerable speculation that basophils and mast cells may express critical roles in diverse biological responses. On the other hand, the precise functions of basophils and mast cells in most of the biological responses in which the cells have been implicated are obscure.[16,46] In the mouse, mutant animals virtually devoid of mast cells and the congenic normal mice may be used to define and quantify the contributions of mast cells to many different biological responses.[2,15,16,46,73,74] A particularly useful approach is to transfer cultured mast cells derived from the bone marrow of normal (WBB6F1-+/+) mice (or mast cells derived from precursors with spontaneous or targeted mutations that affect mast cell development or function) into the skin or other tissues of WBB6F1-*W/W*^{v} mice, which lack mast cells because of mutations at the *W/c-kit* locus.[16,17,73,74] After sufficient time has been allowed to permit the transferred mast cells to acquire phenotypic characteristics appropriate for their anatomical location, biological responses can be elicited at the sites where the mast cell deficiency has been locally and selectively repaired and at paired ("control") mast-cell–deficient sites.

Studies employing such mast cell knock-in mice have shown that mast cells are essential for certain IgE-dependent acute- or late-phase reactions in the skin,[2,65] gastrointestinal tract,[75] or respiratory system,[76] that they significantly augment innate immunity to certain bacterial infections,[73] and that they contribute to certain other immunologically nonspecific acute inflammatory reactions.[2,16] However, no human patients devoid of mast cells have yet been identified. Nor is it easy to interpret the clinical findings in those rare patients who have been found to express a deficiency of basophils. Thus, one human patient with a profound basopenia experienced persistent and severe infestation with scabies,[32] a finding that might be viewed as consistent with the role of basophils in resisting ectoparasites in humans. But that patient also had eosinopenia, IgA deficiency, and multiple other clinical problems.[32] A second basophil-deficient patient had a history of recurrent bacterial and viral infections.[34] However, this patient also had a deficiency of eosinophils, hypogammaglobulinemia, abnormal suppressor T-cell function in vitro, and a thymoma.[34]

BLOOD BASOPHIL COUNT

The normal blood basophil count is difficult to define precisely, but two studies place the normal range between 20 and 80/μl (0.020 and 0.080 × 10^9/liter).[7,8,47,77] The blood basophil count has been reported to vary by age,[78] gender,[78] and season.[79]

BASOPHILOPENIA

Because numbers of blood basophils can be very low even in apparently normal individuals,[7,8,47,77] it can be difficult to determine whether examples of *basophilopenia* reflect pathological processes as opposed to normal variation. Nevertheless, reduced numbers of circulating basophils have been reported in several disorders (Table 69-2). Basophilopenia has been recorded in association with urticaria and anaphylaxis,[80,81] but the extent to which this finding represents a loss of metachromatic staining of circulating degranulated cells rather than a true decrease in the number of cells is undetermined. Basophilopenia occurs in conditions that are also associated with eosinophilopenia; these conditions are often associated with increased secretion of adrenal glucocorticoids.[47,77,82,83] Basophil counts may diminish, sometimes

TABLE 69-2   CONDITIONS ASSOCIATED WITH ALTERATIONS IN NUMBERS OF BLOOD BASOPHILS[47,77,82]

Decreased numbers (basopenia)
  Hereditary absence of basophils (very rare)
  Elevated levels of glucocorticoids
  Hyperthyroidism or treatment with thyroid hormones
  Ovulation
  Hypersensitivity reactions
    Urticaria
    Anaphylaxis
    Drug-induced reactions
  Leukocytosis (in association with diverse disorders)
Increased numbers (basophilia)
  Allergy or inflammation
    Ulcerative colitis
    Drug, food, inhalant hypersensitivity
    Erythroderma, urticaria
    Juvenile rheumatoid arthritis
  Endocrinopathy
    Diabetes mellitus
    Estrogen administration
    Hypothyroidism (myxedema)
  Infection
    Chickenpox
    Influenza
    Smallpox
    Tuberculosis
  Iron deficiency
  Exposure to ionizing radiation
  Neoplasia
    "Basophilic leukemia" (see text)
  Myeloproliferative diseases (especially chronic myelogenous leukemia; also
    polycythemia vera, idiopathic myelofibrosis, primary thrombocythemia)
    Carcinoma

markedly, during leukocytosis accompanying infection, inflammatory states, immunological reactions, neoplasia, or hemorrhage.[82] Also, basophil counts are diminished in thyrotoxicosis or after pharmacologic administration of thyroid hormones, and, conversely, basophil counts may be increased in myxedema or after ablation of thyroid function.[47,82] A rapid and significant drop of up to 50 percent in blood basophil levels has been documented at ovulation.[84] A few patients with an apparent total lack of basophils have been reported.[32,34]

A morphologic abnormality expressed in the majority of eosinophils and basophils but not in other leukocytes or mast cells, has been described as an autosomal dominant condition affecting four members of a family.[33] Cytoplasmic inclusions and crystals in basophils resembling the May-Hegglin anomaly have occurred in healthy individuals.

BASOPHILIA

Conditions associated with increased numbers of blood basophils (*basophilia*) are presented in Table 69-2.

INFLAMMATORY/IMMUNOLOGICAL RESPONSES

An increase in the number of basophils is commonly associated with hypersensitivity disorders of the IgE-associated "immediate" type. This is often accompanied by increased levels of IgE. While serum IgE levels and basophil numbers are not directly related,[85] increased levels of IgE are associated with increased expression of $Fc_\epsilon RI$ on the surfaces of both basophils and mast cells.[66,67,86] Moreover, basophils can be recruited into tissues at sites of IgE-associated and other immunological responses.[1,5,31,61,69] Basophil levels may be elevated in ulcerative colitis[87] and juvenile rheumatoid arthritis,[88] whereas many inflammatory conditions that cause a leukocytosis are associated with basophilopenia. Basophilia can also occur in subjects exposed to ionizing radiation.[89]

HEMATOPOIETIC STEM CELL DISEASES

Chronic Myeloproliferative Diseases The concentration of blood basophils is slightly increased in many patients with polycythemia vera (see Chap. 61), idiopathic myelofibrosis (see Chap. 95), and thrombocythemia (see Chap. 118), and a slight increase in the absolute basophil count may be a useful early sign of a myeloproliferative disease. An increase in absolute basophil count occurs in virtually all patients with CML,[90–92] and, in some, basophils can represent 20 to 90 percent of blood leukocytes (see Chap. 94). Exaggerated basophilia of this type is a poor prognostic sign and may herald transformation to the accelerated phase of CML.[93] The basophil in myeloproliferative diseases is generally thought to be derived from the malignant clone, and in CML can contain the Ph chromosome[94] and presumably also the breakpoint cluster gene rearrangement on chromosome 22. The basophils in CML exhibit a variety of ultrastructural and biochemical abnormalities,[95,96] in some cases obscuring some of the typical distinctions between basophils and mast cells.[97–100] Release of basophil-associated histamine can lead to episodes of flushing, pruritus, and hypotension in occasional patients with basophilic CML,[101,102] and severe peptic ulcer of the stomach and duodenum can occur in association with hypersecretion of gastric acid and pepsin.[103,104] Ph chromosome–positive acute basophilic leukemia may be a presenting manifestation of CML.[105]

Basophilic Leukemias The literature includes many reports of *basophilic leukemias*. However, the basis for designating some cases as basophilic leukemias as opposed to examples of myelogenous leukemia with an associated pronounced basophilia is not always clear. Accordingly, we have referred to these conditions herein as *leukemias associated with basophilia*. The leukemias associated with basophilia

TABLE 69-3　LEUKEMIAS ASSOCIATED WITH BASOPHILIA

Chronic myelogenous leukemia with exaggerated basophilia[94,101–104]
Acute basophilic transformation of chronic myelogenous leukemia[101,109]
Ph chromosome–positive "acute basophilic leukemia"[105]
Acute myelogenous leukemia with t(6;9), t(3;6), or inv(16), and marrow basophilia[112–115]
Acute promyelocytic leukemia with basophilic maturation[116–118]
"Acute basophilic leukemia"[106–111]

are listed in Table 69-3. In addition to extreme basophilia in chronic phase CML, or as a manifestation of the accelerated phase of CML, acute basophilic leukemia apparently can rarely occur de novo.[106–111] A form of acute myelogenous leukemia (AML) in which the blast cells contain a translocation between chromosomes 6 and 9, t(6;9), is associated with marrow basophilia (see Chap. 93),[112,113] although basophilia can also occur in cases of AML with other translocations or inversions.[114,115] Finally, basophilic maturation of leukemic cells may be observed in cases of acute promyelocytic leukemia.[116–118]

While the clinical and pathological features of acute basophilic leukemia are largely similar to those of myelogenous leukemia, affected patients occasionally exhibit symptoms that result from release of mediators (especially histamine) derived from degranulating or dying basophils.[47,101,102,111,119] Remission induction therapy is similar to that used for other types of AML (see Chap. 93), but management can be complicated by shock due to massive release of histamine and other mediators associated with acute cytolysis.

DISORDERS AFFECTING MAST CELLS

NORMAL MAST CELL LEVELS

Mast cells cannot be identified in the blood of healthy individuals by standard techniques. However, mast cells can be observed in the blood of monkeys that have been treated chronically with large amounts of the c-kit ligand, stem cell factor,[19] and in the blood of some patients with systemic mastocytosis.[120] Increases in tissue mast cells can occur by a combination of enhanced progenitor influx and proliferation of resident mast cells in tissues.[5,15,121] Human mast cells have been classified according to their content of neutral proteases: MC_T, so designated because its granules contain tryptase but not detectable chymase, and MC_{TC}, whose secretory granules contain both enzymes.[30] The former mast cell type ordinarily predominates in lung and gastrointestinal mucosal tissues and the latter type in dermis and submucosal tissues.[122–124] Mast cells that express chymase but little or no tryptase (MC_C) also have been described.[125]

SECONDARY CHANGES IN MAST CELL NUMBERS

Although long-term treatment with glucocorticoids (particularly topical treatment of the skin) can result in diminished mast cell numbers,[126] there has been no report of a clinical disorder whose primary feature is a reduction in levels of tissue mast cells. Studies of small numbers of patients indicate that certain mast cell populations, namely the MC_T mast cells in the gastrointestinal mucosa, can be strikingly reduced in numbers in subjects with genetically determined or acquired (HIV-induced) immunodeficiency.[127]

A number of disorders are associated with small to up to several-fold increases in mast cell numbers in or near the tissues affected by the disorder (Table 69-4). Tissues at sites of recurrent allergic reactions often exhibit increases in mast cell numbers, to levels as high as approximately fourfold normal.[122,128] Small increases in mast cell numbers have been observed at sites of pathology in rheumatoid arthritis, psoriatic arthritis, scleroderma, and systemic lupus erythematosus.[129,130]

TABLE 69-4 CONDITIONS ASSOCIATED WITH SECONDARY CHANGES IN MAST CELL NUMBERS

Decreased numbers
  Long-term treatment with glucocorticoids
  Primary or acquired immunodeficiency disorders (certain mast cell populations, see text and ref. 135)
Increased numbers
  IgE-associated "immediate hypersensitivity" reactions
    Rhinitis
    Asthma
    Urticaria
  Connective tissue disorders
    Rheumatoid arthritis
    Psoriatic arthritis
    Scleroderma
    Systemic lupus erythematosus
  Infectious diseases
    Tuberculosis
    Syphilis
    Parasitic diseases
  Neoplastic disorders
    *Lymphoproliferative diseases (Waldenström macroglobulinemia, lymphoma, chronic lymphocytic leukemia)
    *Hematopoietic stem cell diseases (acute or chronic myelogenous leukemias, preleukemia, idiopathic refractory sideroblastic anemia)
    Lymph nodes draining areas of tumor growth
  *Osteoporosis
  *Chronic liver disease
  *Chronic renal disease

*Can include increases in numbers of mast cells in the bone marrow.

Mast cells have been reported to be increased in osteoporosis,[131] but it is unclear to what extent this may reflect decreases in other cell types and/or a decrease in bone matrix. Numbers of marrow mast cells can be increased in patients with chronic liver or renal diseases.[132] Increases in mast cells have also been documented in infectious diseases, particularly at sites of infection with parasites such as *Strongyloides*, in which a greater than fourfold increase in mast cell numbers can occur.[133] In such settings, mast cell numbers can return toward normal upon resolution of the infection. Finally, mast cell numbers can be increased several-fold in lymph nodes draining areas of tumor growth,[132,134] and in subjects with stem cell diseases and lymphoproliferative diseases, including lymphoma in the bone marrow, as well as in association with chronic myelogenous leukemia.[132,135–137]

DISORDERS OF MAST CELL HYPERPLASIA/NEOPLASIA

DEFINITION AND HISTORY

A group of systemic disorders associated with significant increases in mast cell numbers in the skin and internal organs have been brought together under the term *mastocytosis*. The first report[138] of a primary mast cell disorder was probably that of Unna in 1887, who found that the skin lesions of UP[139,140] contained numerous mast cells. But it was not until 1949 that Ellis[141] recognized the systemic nature of this disorder. In addition to the systemic disorders classified as mastocytosis, apparently localized cutaneous aggregates of mast cells, ranging from *mast cells nevuses* and *mastocytomas* in infants and children to multiple nodules in older children have also been reported.[142,143] Solitary mastocytomas generally present before 6 months of age and usually involute spontaneously, although in rare cases they have been followed by urticaria pigmentosa.[143] The pathogenesis of such lesions has not yet been elucidated. Accordingly, the remainder of this section will focus on mastocytosis.

It should be emphasized that the clinical patterns of disease in mastocytosis, and their prognosis, can vary substantially from one patient to the next (see "Course and Prognosis," below). To address

this issue, and to provide guidelines regarding prognosis and treatment, a consensus classification for mastocytosis was developed[144] that is now widely used (Table 69-5). Patients in Category I (*indolent mastocytosis*), comprising the great majority of subjects with mastocytosis, can expect a normal life-span. Patients with Category II disease have a prognosis determined by the associated hematologic disorder, and patients with Category III disease (*aggressive mastocytosis*) generally have a 3- to 5-year survival. Mastocytic leukemia (Category IV disease, see "Mast Cell Leukemia," below) is usually rapidly fatal.

ETIOLOGY AND PATHOGENESIS

Activating mutations in c-*KIT*, which encodes the receptor for stem cell factor, recently have been identified in patients with mastocytosis, and several lines of evidence indicate that such mutations can be involved in the pathogenesis of this disease. The most common of these mutations (Asp816Val), which results in ligand-independent activation of the c-KIT receptor, was first identified in a long-term cell line derived from a patient with mast cell leukemia.[145] It was then detected in mononuclear cells in the peripheral blood of patients with mastocytosis who had an associated hematologic disorder,[146] as a somatic mutation in lesional tissue obtained from one patient with an aggressive form of mastocytosis and from a second patient with an indolent form of urticaria pigmentosa,[147] and in the skin, but not the bone marrow and peripheral blood, of an 11-month-old child with mastocytosis.[148]

Taken together, these findings suggest that the mutation may occur initially in a mast cell progenitor and that, as the clone expands, it first becomes detectable in mastocytosis skin lesions. In patients with more severe disease, and thus with a larger clonal expansion, it can also be identified in circulating cells. The Asp816Val mutation, or similar 816 activating mutations that result in the substitution of valine or tyrosine for aspartate, are now believed to occur in all adult patients with mastocytosis, in whom the mutation can be readily identified in the skin lesions of urticaria pigmentosa.[149] Mutations at codon 816 (valine, tyrosine, or phenylalanine for aspartate) have also been identified in a small subset of pediatric patients, whereas other pediatric patients exhibit a dominant inactivating c-*KIT* mutation, in which lysine is substituted for glutamic acid in position 839, the site of a potential salt bridge.[149]

The extent to which the presence of various c-kit mutations, and the anatomical distribution of the affected cells, can be used to predict prognosis or disease severity in patients with mastocytosis largely remains to be determined. Notably, some pediatric patients with mastocytosis appear to lack any c-*KIT* mutations.[149] Perhaps additional "gain-of-function" mutations of c-*KIT* in human subjects with mastocytosis remain to be characterized. In dogs, a species in which up to 20 percent of all neoplasms are mast cell tumors, 5 of 11 analyzed mast cell tumors exhibited tandem duplications involving exons 11 and 12 of c-*KIT*.[150] Analysis of a dog mastocytoma cell line indicates that such mutations, which affect the juxtamembrane portion of the cytoplasmic domain of the c-KIT receptor, result in ligand-independent

TABLE 69-5 MASTOCYTOSIS CLASSIFICATION*

Category I:	Indolent mastocytosis (can occur as primarily cutaneous disease, e.g., urticaria pigmentosa, with involvement of both skin and other organs, or, more rarely, without skin involvement)
Category II:	Mastocytosis with an associated hematologic disorder (usually a myeloproliferative or myelodysplastic disease)
Category III:	Aggressive mastocytosis (also known as *lymphadenopathic mastocytosis with eosinophilia*)
Category IV:	Mastocytic leukemia (also known as *mast cell leukemia*)

*Modified after ref. 144.

activation of the receptor.[150] Gain-of-function mutations of c-*KIT* have also been reported in gastrointestinal stromal tumors,[151] in one pedigree as a germ line mutation.[152] However, in these subjects, it is not yet clear whether mast cell numbers are increased.

CLINICAL FEATURES

The organs that are most frequently involved in systemic mastocytosis are the skin, lymph nodes, liver, spleen, marrow, and gastrointestinal tract.

The Skin   The usual presenting lesion of cutaneous mast cell disease is UP. UP lesions appear as small yellowish-tan to reddish-brown macules or slightly raised papules (Fig. 69-2), which can exhibit the Darier sign, that is, urticaria after mild friction of the skin.[120,153] The palms, soles, face, and scalp generally remain free of lesions. In many cases, UP can develop before the age of 2 and can subside by puberty; in adults with UP, extracutaneous involvement by mastocytosis is common.[120,153-155] However, some patients, particularly those with mastocytosis and an associated hematologic disorder, may entirely lack cutaneous lesions. In such cases, other organs must be biopsied to make the diagnosis (see below). Diffuse cutaneous mastocytosis is an unusual manifestation of mastocytosis[143,155] The skin appears yellowish-brown and is thickened. Young children with cutaneous disease may have bullous eruptions with hemorrhage.[143] Some adult patients develop prominent vascularity in association with the skin lesions, a condition termed *telangiectasia macularis eruptiva perstans.*[143]

Lymph Nodes   In one series, peripheral lymphadenopathy occurred in 26 percent and central lymphadenopathy in 19 percent of patients at diagnosis.[156] Lymphadenopathy tends to be most prominent in patients with Category II or III disease. Mast cell infiltrates are observed in the paracortex, follicles, medullary cords, and sinuses. Additional findings can include prominent infiltrates of eosinophils (accounting for the alternative term for aggressive mastocytosis:

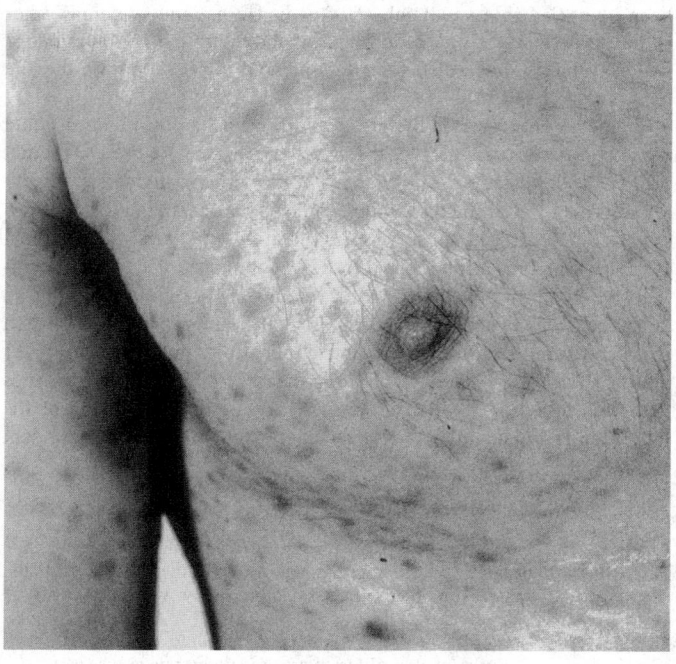

FIGURE 69-2   Urticaria pigmentosa in an adult man with indolent systemic mastocytosis. Multiple pigmented macules are present, and if local pressure were to be applied to the skin, individual lesions would show urtication and become raised, pruritic, and erythematous.

lymphadenopathic mastocytosis with eosinophilia), blood vessel proliferation in association with mast cells in the paracortical areas, and extramedullary hematopoiesis. In routine H&E, stained sections, mast cell infiltrates in the lymph nodes may resemble T-cell lymphomas in their pericortical distribution, in the clear cytoplasm that is sometimes exhibited by the mast cells, and in the associated vascular proliferation and eosinophilia.[156] Alternatively, when mast cells replace lymphoid follicles, the pattern may resemble follicular hyperplasia or follicular lymphoma.[156]

Liver   Patients with mastocytosis frequently exhibit infiltration of the liver with mast cells. While many of these individuals have some associated liver pathology, severe liver disease is uncommon. When it does occur, it typically affects those with mastocytosis (Category II or III disease) and an associated hematologic disorder or aggressive mastocytosis. In one series of 41 patients, 61 percent had some liver disease.[157] Elevated alkaline phosphatase aminotransamidases, 5′ nucleotidase, or GGTP was detected in the serum of approximately half of the patients. Hepatomegaly, prominent infiltration of the liver with mast cells, and hepatic fibrosis are positively correlated with elevated levels of alkaline phosphatase and were observed more frequently in patients with aggressive disease, and ascites or portal hypertension occurred in some of these individuals. Portal fibrosis was observed in 68 percent and was positively correlated with hepatic inflammation and mast cells infiltrates. Venopathy and associated veno-occlusive disease was observed in four patients, all of whom had an associated hematologic disorder.

Spleen   Splenic involvement at diagnosis has been reported in approximately half of the patients with systemic disease.[156,158] Mast cells most commonly occurred in a paratrabecular distribution, followed by perifollicular, follicular, and diffuse infiltrates. Trabecular and capsular fibrosis and eosinophilic infiltration were also observed, and extramedullary hematopoiesis was documented in the majority of biopsies. On H&E sections, the infiltrates of mast cells produced lesions that resembled those of T-cell lymphoma, follicular hyperplasia, follicular lymphoma, Kaposi sarcoma, myeloproliferative disorder, hairy cell leukemia, or a granulomatous process. Splenomegaly was also noted to occur in the absence of infiltration of the spleen by mast cells.[159] Increased splenic weights of greater than 700 g generally occurred in patients within unfavorable categories of mastocytosis.

Marrow   More than 90 percent of adults with systemic mast cell disease have focal mast cell lesions in the marrow,[158,160-163] which typically appear as foci of spindle-shaped mast cells in a fibrotic background (Fig. 69-3), sometimes with associated eosinophils and lymphocytes. These collections of cells can occur in perivascular, paratrabeuclar, and intertrabecular locations. There may be an increase in reticulin staining, and Masson trichome staining may reveal collagen deposition. In specimens that are extensively involved by mast cell lesions, the bony trabeculae may be moderately to markedly thickened.

In H&E stained sections, the mast cells typically exhibit a spindle-shaped or oval nucleus, and fine eosinophilic granules are apparent in the cytoplasm at high-power magnification (Fig. 69-3A). Mast cells with bilobed nuclei also may be seen in these lesions; and this finding is associated with a poor prognosis.[158] Wright-Giemsa and toluidine blue stains can be employed, especially with nondecalcified, plastic-embedded specimens, for a more definitive visualization of mast cells. Unfortunately, these stains are less effective on EDTA-decalcified, paraffin-embedded material. Mast cells also stain positively for chloracetate esterase and aminocaproate esterase, and, in suitably processed specimens, for mast cell tryptase by immunohistochemistry (Fig. 69-3B). Aspirate films or clot sections alone cannot be used to diagnose mast cell disease in the marrow. While increased numbers of mast cells may be present in bone marrow aspirate films of patients with systemic mast cell diseases, similar findings have been reported in

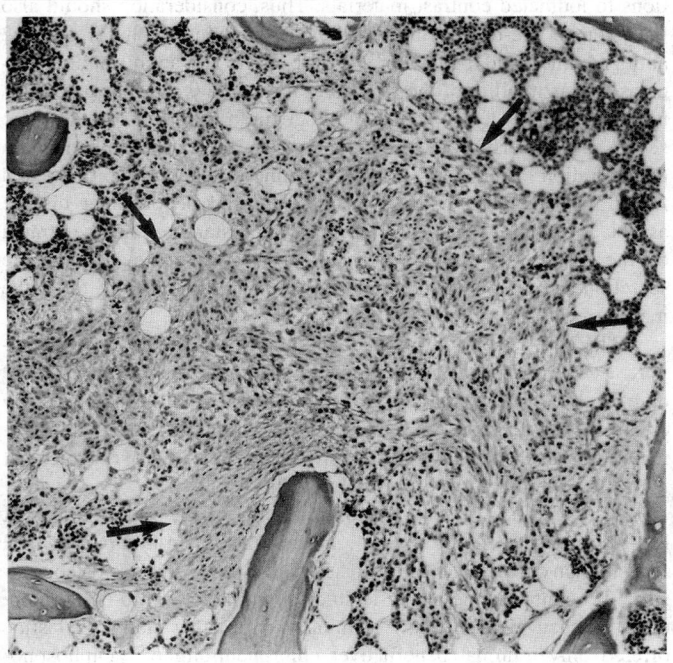

A

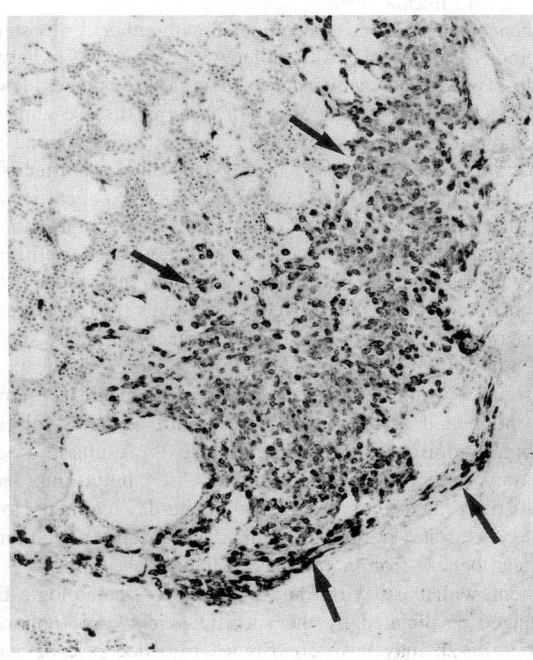

B

FIGURE 69-3   Bone marrow biopsy from an adult with indolent systemic mastocytosis showing characteristic collections of mast cells, some of which appear spindle-shaped; different areas of the specimen were stained by H&E; (A) or with an antibody to human mast cell tryptase (B) (X100). Areas that contain many mast cells are depicted with arrows in A and B.

patients without mast cell disorders or when there is a reactive increase in marrow mast cells.

Marrow involvement appears to be much less common in children. In a study[163] of 17 children with cutaneous or disseminated mast cell disease, small focal mast cell lesions were observed in marrow

biopsies in 10 individuals, and increased mast cells in bone marrow aspirate smears were noted in 5. Moreover, the focal lesions found in children were uniformly small and perivascular.

The progression of marrow involvement in systemic mast cell disease is variable. Many adults with indolent disease appear to have stable, or even decreasing, marrow involvement over time.[158] In contrast, a progressive increase in focal mast cell lesions is more commonly observed in patients with more aggressive patterns of disease.

CLINICAL PRESENTATION

Even though they may differ in the specific pathogenesis of their disease, all patients within a given category of mastocytosis generally exhibit similar clinical features. Manifestations of the disease largely reflect the local and systemic consequences of mediator release from tissue mast cells. There also may be effects due to the disruption of normal structures by local collections of mast cells.

At presentation, patients with mastocytosis may complain of vague and nonspecific constitutional symptoms such as fatigue, weakness, flushing, and musculoskeletal pain; some experience fever and/or weight loss.[120,155] A subset may present with recurrent episodes of unexplained anaphylaxis.[164] However, most patients with indolent mastocytosis and a hematologic disorder are usually diagnosed on the basis of bone marrow biopsy findings, during the investigation of their hematologic disease.[155,158] Those with aggressive disease often present with unexplained lymphadenopathy and splenomegaly and/or hepatomegaly.

Gastrointestinal disease and associated symptoms are also commonly associated with systemic mastocytosis, either at presentation or as the disease progresses.[155,165] Findings include nausea, vomiting, abdominal pain, and diarrhea. Peptic ulcer disease, which is thought to reflect, at least in part, the promotion of gastric acid secretion by elevated histamine levels, occurs in up to 50 percent of those with systemic disease.[165] With progressive disease, patients may develop mild malabsorption.[165]

If systemic involvement is already advanced at the time of diagnosis, patients may also exhibit lymphadenopathy, hepatomegaly, and splenomegaly during the initial evaluation.[120,155] Because osteoporosis may accompany systemic disease, rare patients present with pathological fractures.[166]

LABORATORY FEATURES

When mastocytosis is suspected following the history and physical examination, a routine workup in adults should consist of a gross and microscopic examination of the skin, a bone marrow biopsy, and aspirate[120,144,155]; and serum for alpha and beta tryptase levels (Table 69-6)[26] (two forms of tryptase, a protease that is produced abundantly by most if not all human mast cells, but which also may be found in

TABLE 69-6   DIAGNOSTIC EVALUATION OF MASTOCYTOSIS

Routine
  Examine skin—gross and microscopic*
  Bone marrow biopsy and aspiration
  Serum for mast cell alpha and beta tryptase
Additional studies†
  Bone scan
  Skeletal survey
  Gastrointestinal workup
  Upper gastrointestinal series
  Small-bowel radiography
  Endoscopy
  Computed tomography

*An increase in numbers of dermal mast cells above 10 times normal, in the absence of other pathology that could account for this, generally is diagnostic of mastocytosis.
†Performed if indicated by clinical findings.

at least some human basophils).[31,167] Additional studies, as suggested by the need to assess the extent of disease or to evaluate pain, may include a bone scan and a skeletal survey. A gastrointestinal evaluation, involving radiographic studies of the upper gastrointestinal tract and small intestines, a computed tomography scan of the abdomen, and endoscopy may also be justified. The requirements for the diagnosis of mastocytosis remain the presence of substantial increases in mast cell numbers in one or more tissues. Slight increases (e.g., up to fourfold) in mast cell numbers in target tissues, such as the skin, gastrointestinal tract, or bone marrow, are not diagnostic because they may only reflect normal variation or inflammatory or reactive processes. In skin biopsies of sites that lack other causes of increased numbers of mast cells, such as chronic inflammatory processes, a tenfold increase in mast cells numbers is generally considered diagnostic of mastocytosis.[20,128,143,155] Mast cell aggregates or the presence of confluent infiltrates of mast cells are required for the diagnosis of bone marrow involvement. In patients with advanced Category II or III disease, mast cells may be detectable in the peripheral blood, and rare patients can progress to mast cell leukemia (see below).[155,158,168–171]

Plasma or urinary histamine levels are frequently increased in systemic mastocytosis.[172] However, the isolated findings of increased levels of histamine or histamine metabolites may reflect any of a number of other situations, including anaphylaxis. Further, the accuracy of laboratory measurement of histamine depends on the assay used. Urine histamine levels may be falsely elevated as result of bacterial contamination, pharmacologic agents and their metabolites excreted in the urine, or diets rich in histamine or histamine precursors. Similarly, serum beta tryptase may be elevated after anaphylaxis. Alpha tryptase is more specific for mastocytosis but may sometimes be normal, even in patients with a diagnostic bone marrow biopsy.[167] Thus, no single laboratory test is diagnostic of mastocytosis. Rather, the demonstration of mast cell mediators in blood or urine should prompt the clinician to investigate further for the presence of mastocytosis.

DIFFERENTIAL DIAGNOSIS

The differential diagnosis of systemic mastocytosis includes several disorders which may produce a similar clinical presentation, such as allergic diseases, the hyper-IgE syndrome, hereditary or acquired angioneurotic edema, idiopathic flushing or anaphylaxis, carcinoid tumor, and idiopathic capillary leak syndrome. When episodic hypertension is a major finding, pheochromocytoma must be considered. Significant unexplained gastroduodenal ulcer disease requires that a Zollinger-Ellison gastrinoma syndrome be ruled out. *Helicobacter pylori* infection should be considered in all patients with ulcer disease, even those diagnosed with mastocytosis.

THERAPY, COURSE, AND PROGNOSIS

Therapy There currently is no cure for mastocytosis.[173] There also is no evidence that symptomatic therapy significantly alters the course of the underlying disease.[173] Management of mastocytosis includes instruction on the avoidance of factors that may trigger symptoms (presumably by the direct or indirect activation of mast cell mediator production); these can include temperature extremes, physical exertion, or, in some unusual cases, the ingestion of ethanol, nonsteroidal anti-inflammatory drugs, or opiate analgesics.[155,173] Anaphylaxis may sometimes follow insect stings, even in the absence of evidence of allergic sensitivity. For these reasons, consideration should be given to providing epinephrine-filled syringes to all patients. Patients with mast cell disease and a history of anaphylaxis clearly should be advised to carry epinephrine-filled syringes and taught to self-medicate. These patients may also benefit from the concurrent use of H1 and H2 antihistamines prophylactically. Patients may experience severe reactions to iodinated contrast materials. Thus, consideration should also be given to pre-medicating mastocytosis patients with H1 and H2 antihistamines and prednisone. Nonsedative H1 antihistamines decrease the irritability of the skin and pruritus.[155,173–175] More potent H1 blockers, such as hydroxyzine and doxepin,[176] may be useful in more severe cases. Pruritis may also be relieved by approaches that maintain the hydration of the skin. H2 antihistamines, including ranitidine and famotidine, are used to treat the gastritis and peptic ulcer disease associated with mastocytosis.[155,173,177] H2 antihistamines may be titrated on the basis of symptom control or to a particular level of gastric secretion. Proton pump inhibitors (omeprazole) are also useful in the management of gastric hypersecretion.[155,173]

The oral administration of disodium cromoglycate has been reported to be useful in the treatment of gastrointestinal cramping and diarrhea.[178,179] This agent has also been reported to be of benefit in cutaneous mast cell disease in children and infants.[180] Other symptoms, including headache, have also been reported to improve somewhat with the administration of cromolyn sodium.

Ketotifen has been widely used outside of the United States. It has been reported to be effective in the relief of pruritus and wheal formation in cutaneous mastocytosis[181] and even to improve osteoporosis.[182] By contrast, one pediatric study found ketotifen to be no more effective than hydroxyzine.[183] Similarly, in another study, azelastine offered only minimal benefit over chlorpheniramine.[184] Diphosphonates have been reported to be useful in the treatment of the osteopenia associated with mastocytosis.[185]

Cutaneous lesions have been treated with either corticosteroids[186] or 8-methoxypsoralen plus ultraviolet A (PUVA),[187,188] largely to reduce pruritus or for cosmetic improvement. There is no evidence that such approaches alter the progression of systemic disease, and relapses 3 to 6 months after cessation of PUVA therapy are common. Patients may also experience a decrease in the intensity of lesions after exposure to natural sunlight. Repeated or extensive application of corticosteroids may result in cutaneous atrophy or adrenocortical suppression.[186]

Nonsteroidal anti-inflammatory agents have been useful in some patients whose primary manifestations are recurrent episodes of flushing or syncope, or both.[173] However, these agents may also exacerbate ulcer disease. Patients with a history of aspirin sensitivity should not be placed on this therapy, unless they first undergo desensitization.

Systemic corticosteroids are employed to decrease significant malabsorption and ascites[189] in patients with advanced disease. In adults, oral prednisone (40–60 mg/day) usually results in a decrease in symptoms over a 2- to 3-week period. After initial improvement, steroids usually may be tapered to an alternate-day regimen. However, with time, the ascites frequently recurs. It has been reported that such patients can benefit from a portacaval shunt.[189]

Patients with mastocytosis and an associated hematologic disorder are managed as dictated by the specific hematologic abnormality. Interferon-alfa-2b may have contributed to a decrease in mast cell infiltration in one patient with mastocytosis and an associated hematologic disorder,[190] but a subsequent study reported that interferon-alfa-2b was of no benefit in three patients,[191] and there is a report of an anaphylactic-like syndrome after treatment with interferon.[192]

A small number of patients with mastocytosis may have a syndrome resembling non-Hodgkin's lymphoma, an aggressive myeloproliferative disease, or rarely an overt nonlymphocytic leukemia.[193] Two patients have been reported with systemic mast cell disease associated with primary mediastinal germ cell tumor.[194,195] In such patients, traditional chemotherapy directed toward the neoplastic process may be appropriate. Chemotherapy with cyclophosphamide, vincristine, and prednisone has been used in some mastocytosis patients whose clinical picture is that of a non-Hodgkin's lymphoma, although the response to chemotherapy was variable.[193] Radiotherapy has been used in a limited number of patients to control local disease.[196] One patient with a myelodysplastic syndrome of recent onset, a leukemic spread of immature mast cells, and hyperfibrinolysis, possibly related to mast-cell–derived tissue plasminogen activator, responded well to remission-induction polychemotherapy followed by two cycles of consolidation with intermediate-dose ARA-C.[197]

Splenectomy has been performed on patients with severe aggressive mastocytosis, in an attempt to improve their limiting cytopenias.[198] Based on comparisons to historical controls, splenectomy increased survival by an average of 12 months. Patients who had undergone splenectomy also appeared to be better able to tolerate chemotherapy. Splenectomy is of no value in the management of indolent mast cell disease.[198]

Course and Prognosis   The prognosis of adult patients with mast cell disorders is related to the disease category. The vast majority of patients who present with UP and are found to have indolent (Category I) disease have a chronic protracted course that responds to symptomatic medical management. A normal life-span is the expectation, and few of these cases progress to more severe forms of the disease; some patients may even experience a diminution in the severity of skin lesions in later years.[155,158,199] However, elevated serum lactate dehydrogenase levels, a late age of onset, and, in Category II patients, presence of a significant hematologic abnormality (such as a myeloproliferative or myelodysplastic disorder or, more rarely, overt leukemia) are indicators of a poor prognosis and shortened survival.[158] Indeed, the prognosis for patients in Category II (mastocytosis with an associated hematologic disorder) depends on the course of the associated hematologic disorder.[158] Patients with Category III disease (aggressive mastocytosis) have a guarded prognosis due to complications arising from rapid and profound increases in mast cell numbers; these patients usually have a 3- to 5-year survival.[158] Patients with mast cell leukemia (Category IV disease) typically die within approximately 6 months of diagnosis.[169]

Mast Cell Leukemia   This rapidly fatal disorder develops in a small minority of patients with Category II or III disease[168–171] but can also represent the initial clinical presentation of the mast cell disorder.[169,200,201] Patients with mast cell leukemia may have fever, anorexia, and weight loss, fatigue, severe abdominal cramping, nausea, vomiting, diarrhea, flushing, hypotension, pruritus, or bone pain. Peptic ulcer and gastrointestinal bleeding are frequent findings, as are hepatomegaly, splenomegaly, and lymph node enlargement. Anemia is a constant feature, and thrombocytopenia is nearly always present.[169,200,201] The total leukocyte count varies from 10,000 to 150,000 μl (10 to 150 $\times$ 10^9/liter), and mast cells make up 10 to 90 percent of the leukocytes. Marrow biopsy invariably shows a striking increase in mast cells, sometimes up to 90 percent of marrow cells, although the leukemic mast cells are often hypogranular or agranular. Leukemic mast cells are stained with Sudan black and alcian blue; they are positive for chloracetate esterase and acid phosphatase and are negative in the peroxidase and α-naphthylesterase reactions.[169,200] Electron microscopy may show the characteristic scroll-like ultrastructural features of the mast cell granule.

Mast Cell Sarcoma   This apparently is a exceedingly rare tumor, characterized by nodules at various cutaneous and mucosal sites.[132] Subsequently, almost every organ becomes involved by extensive mast cell infiltration. Terminally, the blood cells are nearly all immature mast cells with monocytoid appearance.

REFERENCES

1. Galli SJ, Dvorak AM, Dvorak HF: Basophils and mast cells: morphological insights into their biology, secretory patterns, and function. *Prog Allergy* 34:1, 1984.
2. Galli SJ: New concepts about the mast cell. *N Engl J Med* 328:257, 1993.
3. Valent P: Immunophenotypic characterization of human basophils and mast cells. *Chem Immunol* 61:34, 1995.
4. Dvorak AM: Blood cell biochemistry, vol 4: *Basophil and Mast Cell Degranulation and Recovery.* Plenum, New York, 1991.
5. Costa JJ, Galli SJ: Mast cells and basophils, in *Clinical Immunology: Principles and Practice* 1st ed, edited by RR Rich, editor-in-chief and TA Fleisher, BD Schwartz, WT Shearer, W Strober, p 408. Mosby, St. Louis, Missouri, 1996.
6. Murakami I, Ogawa M, Amo H, Ota K: Studies of kinetics of human leukocytes in vivo with 3H-thymidine autoradiography. II. Eosinophils and basophils. *Acta Hamatol Jpn* 32:384, 1969.
7. Juhlin L: Basophil leukocyte differential in blood and bone marrow. *Acta Haematol* 29:89, 1963.
8. Gilbert HS, Ornstein L: Basophil counting with a new staining method using alcian blue. *Blood* 46:279, 1975.
9. Ishizaka T, Dvorak AM, Conrad DH, et al: Morphological and immunological characterization of human basophils developed in cultures of cord blood mononuclear cells. *J Immunol* 134:532, 1985.
10. Ganser A, Lindemann A, Seipelt G, et al: Effects of recombinant human interleukin-3 in patients with normal hemopoiesis and in patients with bone marrow failure. *Blood* 76:666, 1990.
11. Lantz CS, Boesiger J, Song CH, et al: Role for interleukin-3 in mast-cell and basophil development and immunity to parasites. *Nature* 293:445, 1998.
12. Lantz CS, Song CH, Dranoff G, Galli SJ: Interleukin-3 (IL-3) is required for blood basophilia, but not for increased IL-4 production, in response to parasite infection in mice. *FASEB J* 13:A325, 1999 (Abstr. No. 255.18).
13. Kurimoto Y, de Weck AL, Dahinden CA: The effect of interleukin 3 upon IgE-dependent and IgE-independent basophil degranulation and leukotriene generation. *Eur J Immunol* 21:361, 1991.
14. Alam R, Welter JB, Forsythe PA, et al: Comparative effect of recombinant IL-1, -2, -3, -4, and -6, IFN-γ, granulocyte-macrophage-colony-stimulating factor, tumor necrosis factor-α, and histamine-releasing factors on the secretion of histamine from basophils. *J Immunol* 142:3431, 1989.
15. Kitamura Y: Heterogeneity of mast cells and phenotypic changes between subpopulations. *Annu Rev Immunol* 7:59, 1989.
16. Galli SJ, Geissler EN, Wershil BK, et al: Insights into mast cell development and function derived from analyses of mice carrying mutations at beige, W/c-kit or Sl/SCF (c-kit ligand) loci, in *The Role of the Mast Cell in Health and Disease*, edited by MA Kaliner, DD Metcalfe, p 129. Marcel Dekker, New York, 1992.
17. Galli SJ, Zsebo KM, Geissler EN: The c-kit ligand, stem cell factor. *Adv Immunol*, 55:1, 1994.
18. Rodewald H-R, Dressing M, Dvorak AM, Galli SJ: Identification of a committed precursor for the mast cell lineage. *Science* 87:326, 1996.
19. Galli SJ, Iemura A, Garlick DS, et al: Reversible expansion of primate mast cell populations in vivo by stem cell factor. *J Clin Invest* 91:148, 1993.
20. Costa JJ, Demetri GD, Harrist TJ, et al: Recombinant human stem cell factor (kit ligand) promotes human mast cell and melanocyte hyperplasia and functional activation in vivo. *J Exp Med* 183:2681, 1996.
21. Broudy VC: Stem cell factor and hematopoiesis. *Blood* 90:1345, 1997.
22. Wershil BK, Tsai M, Geissler EN, et al: The rat c-kit ligand, stem cell factor, induces c-kit receptor-dependent mouse mast cell activation in vivo: evidence that signaling through the c-kit receptor can induce expression of cellular function. *J Exp Med* 175:245, 1992.
23. Columbo M, Horowitz EM, Botana LM, et al: The human recombinant c-kit receptor ligand, rhSCF, induces mediator release from human cutaneous mast cells and enhances IgE-dependent mediator release from both skin mast cells and peripheral blood basophils. *J Immunol* 149:599, 1992.
24. Coleman JW, Holliday MR, Kimber I, et al: Regulation of mouse peritoneal mast cell secretory function by stem cell factor, IL-3 or IL-4. *J Immunol* 150:556, 1993.
25. Bischoff SC, Dahinden CA: c-kit ligand: a unique potentiator of mediator release by human lung mast cells. *J Exp Med* 175:237, 1992.
26. Gargari E, Tsai M, Lantz CS, Fox LG, Galli SJ: Differential release of mast cell interleukin-6 via c-kit. *Blood* 89:2654, 1997.
27. Finotto S, Mekori YA, Metcalfe DD: Glucocorticoids decrease tissue mast cell number by reducing the production of the c-kit ligand, stem

cell factor, by resident cells. In vitro and in vivo evidence in murine systems. *J Clin Invest* 99:1721, 1997.

28. Enerbäck L: Mast cell heterogeneity: The evolution of the concept of a specific mucosal mast cell, in *Mast Cell Differentiation and Heterogeneity*, edited by AD Befus, J Bienenstock, JA Denburg, p 1. Raven, New York, 1986.

29. Galli SJ: New insights into ''the riddle of the mast cells'': microenvironmental regulation of mast cell development and phenotypic heterogeneity. *Lab Invest* 62:5, 1990.

30. Irani AA, Schechter NM, Craig SS, et al: Two human mast cell subsets with different neutral protease composition. *Proc Natl Acad Sci USA* 83:4464, 1986.

31. Li L, Li Y, Reddel SW, et al: Identification of basophilic cells that express mast cell granule proteases in the peripheral blood of asthma and drug-reactive patients. *J Immunol* 161:5079, 1998.

32. Juhlin L, Michäelsson G: A new syndrome characterized by absence of eosinophils and basophils. *Lancet* 1:1233, 1977.

33. Tracey R, Smith H: An inherited anomaly of human eosinophils and basophils. *Blood Cells* 4:291, 1978.

34. Mitchell EB, Platts-Mills TAE, Pereira RS, et al: Basophil and eosinophil deficiency in a patient with hypogammaglobulinemia associated with thymoma, in *Primary Immunodeficiency Diseases, Birth Defects*. Original Article Series, vol 19, no 3, edited by RJ Wedgewood, FS Rosen, NW Paul, p 331. Liss, New York, 1983.

35. Dvorak AM, Mihm MC Jr, Dvorak HF: Morphology of delayed-type hypersensitivity reactions in man. II. Ultrastructural alterations affecting the microvasculature and the tissue mast cells. *Lab Invest* 34:179, 1976.

36. Hastie RI: A study of the ultrastructure of human basophil leukocytes. *Lab Invest* 31:223, 1974.

37. Dvorak AM, Monahan RA, Osage JE, Dickersin GR: Crohn's disease: Transmission electron microscope studies. II. Immunologic inflammatory responses: alterations of mast cells, basophils, eosinophils, and the microvasculature. *Human Pathol* 11:606, 1980.

38. Schwartz LB, Austen KF: Structure and function of the chemical mediators of mast cells. *Prog Allergy* 34:271, 1984.

39. Stevens RL, Austen KF: Recent advances in the cellular and molecular biology of mast cells. *Immunol Today* 10:381, 1989.

40. Metcalfe DD, Bland CE, Wasserman SI: Biochemical and functional characterization of proteoglycans isolated from basophils of patients with chronic myelogenous leukemia. *J Immunol* 132:1943, 1984.

41. Rothenberg ME, Caulfield JP, Austen KF, et al: Biochemical and morphological characterization of basophilic leukocytes from two patients with myelogenous leukemia. *J Immunol* 138:2616, 1987.

42. Orenstein NS, Galli SJ, Dvorak AM, et al: Sulfated glycosaminoglycans of guinea pig basophilic leukocytes. *J Immunol* 121:586, 1978.

43. Humphries DE, Wong GW, Friend DS, et al: Heparin is essential for the storage of specific granule proteases in mast cells. *Nature* 400:769, 1999.

44. Forsberg E, Pejler G, Ringvall M, et al: Absence of heparin and altered mast cell mediator content in NDST-2 deficient mice. *Nature* 400:773, 1999.

45. Porter JF, Mitchell RGL: Distribution of histamine in human blood. *Physiol Rev* 52:361, 1972.

46. Galli SJ, Kitamura Y: Genetically mast-cell-deficient *W/W^v* and *Sl/Sl^d* mice. Their value for the analysis of mast cells in biological responses in vivo. *Am J Pathol* 127:191, 1987.

47. Parwaresch MR: *The Human Blood Basophil*. Springer-Verlag, New York, 1976.

48. Gordon JR, Galli SJ: Mast cells as a source of both preformed and immunologically inducible TNF-α/cachectin. *Nature* 346:274, 1990.

49. Walsh LJ, Trinchieri G, Waldorf HA, et al: Human dermal mast cells contain and release tumor necrosis factor α, which induces endothelial leukocyte adhesion molecule 1. *Proc Natl Acad Sci USA* 88:4220, 1991.

50. Galli SJ, Gordon JR, Wershil BK: Cytokine production by mast cells and basophils. *Curr Opin Immunol* 3:865, 1991.

51. Bradding P, Feather IH, Howarth PH, et al: Interleukin 4 is localized to and released by human mast cells. *J Exp Med* 176:1381, 1992.

52. Brunner T, Heusser CH, Dahinden CA: Human peripheral blood basophils primed by interleukin 3 (IL-3) produce IL-4 in response to immunoglobulin E receptor stimulation. *J Exp Med* 177:605, 1993.

53. Burd PR, Rogers HW, Gordon JR, et al: Interleukin 3-dependent and -independent mast cells stimulated with IgE and antigen express multiple cytokines. *J Exp Med* 170:245, 1989.

54. Yano K, Yamaguchi M, de Mora F, et al: Production of macrophage inflammatory protein-1α by human mast cells: increased anti-IgE-dependent secretion after IgE-dependent enhancement of mast cell IgE-binding ability. *Lab Invest* 77:185, 1997.

55. Pawankar R, Okuda M, Yssel H, Okumura K, Ra C: Nasal mast cells in perennial allergic rhinitics exhibit increased expression of the FcεRI, CD40L, IL-4, and IL-13, and can induce IgE synthesis in B cells. *J Clin Invest* 99:1492, 1997.

56. Rumsaeng V, Cruikshank WW, Foster B, et al: Human mast cells produce the CD4+ T lymphocyte chemoattractant factor, IL-16. *J Immunol* 159:2904, 1997.

57. Li H, Sim TC, Alam R: IL-13 released by and localized in human basophils. *J Immunol* 156:4833, 1996.

58. Ishizaka T, Ishizaka K: Activation of mast cells for mediator release through IgE receptors. *Prog Allergy* 34:188, 1984.

59. Kinet J-P: The high affinity IgE receptor (FcεRI) from physiology to pathology. *Annu Rev Immunol* 17:931, 1999.

60. Beavan MA, Metzger H: Signal transduction by Fc receptors: the FcαRI case. *Immunol Today* 14:222, 1993.

61. Galli SJ, Lantz CS: Allergy, in *Fundmental Immunology*, 4th ed, edited by WE Paul, p 1137. Lippincott-Raven, Philadelphia, 1999.

62. Patella V, Giuliano A, Bouvet JP, Marone G: Endogenous superallergen protein Fv induces IL-4 secretion from human FcεRI cells through interaction with the VH3 region of IgE. *J Immunol* 161:5647, 1998.

63. Lemanske RF Jr, Kaliner MA: Late phase allergic reactions, in *Allergy: Principles and Practice*, 4th ed, edited by E Middleton Jr, CE Reed, EF Ellis, et al, p 320. Mosby, St Louis, 1993.

64. Wershil BK, Wang Z-S, Gordon JR, Galli SJ: Recruitment of neutrophils during IgE-dependent cutaneous late phase responses in the mouse is mast cell-dependent: partial inhibition of the reaction with antiserum against tumor necrosis factor-alpha. *J Clin Invest* 87:446, 1991.

65. Yamaguchi M, Lantz CS, Oettgen HC, et al: IgE enhances mouse mast cell FcεRI expression in vitro and in vivo. Evidence for a novel amplification mechanism in IgE-dependent reactions. *J Exp Med* 185:663, 1997.

66. MacGlashan DW Jr., Bochner BS, Adelman DC, et al: Down-regulation of FcεRI expression on human basophils during in vivo treatment of atopic patients with anti-IgE antibody. *J Immunol* 158:1438, 1997.

67. Boesiger J, Tsai M, Maurer M, et al: Mast cells can secrete VPF/VEGF and exhibit enhanced release after IgE-dependent upregulation of FcεRI expression. *J Exp Med* 188:1135, 1998.

68. Yamaguchi M, Sayama K, Yano K, et al: IgE Enhances Fcε receptor I expression and IgE-dependent release of histamine and lipid mediators from human umbilical cord blood-derived mast cells: Synergistic effect of IL-4 and IgE on human mast cell Fcε receptor I expression and mediator release. *J Immunol* 162:5455, 1999.

69. Galli SJ, Askenase PW: Cutaneous basophil hypersensitivity, in *The Reticuloendothelial System: A Comprehensive Treatise*, vol 9, edited by P Abramoff, SM Phillips, NR Escobar, p 321. Plenum, New York, 1986.

70. Galli SJ, Hammel I: Unequivocal delayed hypersensitivity in mast cell-deficient and beige mice. *Science* 226:710, 1984.

71. Brown SJ, Galli SJ, Gleich GJ, Askenase PW: Ablation of immunity to *Amblyomma americanum* by anti-basophil serum: cooperation between basophils and eosinophils in expression of immunity to extoparasites (ticks) in guinea pigs. *J Immunol* 129:790, 1982.

72. Matsuda H, Watanabe N, Kiso Y, et al: Necessity of IgE antibodies and mast cells for manifestation of resistance against larval *Haemaphysalis longicornis* ticks in mice. *J Immunol* 144:259, 1990.

73. Galli SJ, Maurer M, Lantz CS. Mast cells as sentinels of innate immunity. *Curr Opinion Immunol* 11:53, 1999.

74. Nakano T, Sonoda T, Hayashi C, et al: Fate of bone-marrow derived cultured mast cells after intracutaneous, intraperitoneal and intravenous transfer into genetically mast cell-deficient *W/W^v* mice. Evidence that cultured mast cells can give rise to both connective tissue-type and mucosal mast cells. *J Exp Med* 162:1025, 1985.

75. Wershil BK, Furuta GT, Wang Z-S, Galli SJ: Mast cell-dependent neutrophil and mononuclear cell recruitment in immunoglobulin E-induced gastric reactions in mice. *Gastroenterology* 110:1482, 1996.

76. Martin TR, Takeishi T, Katz HR, Austen KF, Drazen JM, Galli SJ: Mast cell activation enhances airway responsiveness to methacholine in the mouse. *J Clin Invest* 91:1176, 1993.

77. Shelley WB, Parnes HM: The absolute basophil count. *JAMA* 192:108, 1965.

78. Thonnard-Neumann E: Studies of basophils. Variations with age and sex. *Acta Haematol* 30:221, 1963.

79. Chavance M, Herbeth B, Kauffmann F: Seasonal patterns of circulating basophils. *Int Arch Allergy Appl Immunol* 86:462, 1988.

80. Shelley WB, Juhlin L: New test for detecting anaphylactic sensitivity: basophil reaction. *Nature* 191:1056, 1961.

81. Shelley WB: Circulating basophil as indicator of hypersensitivity in man. *Arch Dermatol* 88:759, 1963.

82. Juhlin L: Basophil and eosinophil leukocytes in various internal disorders. *Acta Med Scand* 174:249, 1963.

83. Juhlin L: The effects of corticotropin and corticosteroids on the basophil and eosinophil granulocytes. *Acta Haematol* 29:157, 1963.

84. Mettler L, Shirwani D: Direct basophil count for timing ovulation. *Fertil Steril* 25:718, 1974.

85. Malveaux FJ, Conroy MC, Adkinson NF, Lichtenstein LM: IgE receptors on human basophils. Relationship to serum IgE concentration. *J Clin Invest* 62:176, 1978.

86. Lantz CS, Yamaguchi M, Oettgen HC, et al: IgE regulates mouse basophil FcεRI expression in vivo. *J Immunol* 158:2517, 1997.

87. Juhlin L: Basophil leukocytes in ulcerative colitis. *Acta Med Scand* 173:351, 1963.

88. Athreya BH, Moser G, Raghavan TES: Increased circulating basophils in juvenile rheumatoid arthritis. *Am J Dis Child* 129:935, 1975.

89. Fredericks RE, Moloney WC: The basophilic granulocyte. *Blood* 14:571, 1959.

90. Spiers ASD, Bain BJ, Turner JE: The peripheral blood in chronic granulocytic leukemia: a study of 50 untreated Philadelphia positive cases. *Scand J Haematol* 18:25, 1977.

91. Kamada N, Uchino H: Chronologic sequence in appearance of clinical and laboratory findings characteristic of chronic myelocytic leukemia. *Blood* 51:843, 1978.

92. Drewinko B, Bollinger P, Brailas C, et al: Flow cytotechnical patterns of white blood cells in human hemopoietic malignancies. *Br J Haematol* 67:157, 1987.

93. Denburg JA, Browman G: The chronic myeloid leukemia study group: prognostic implications of basophilic differentiation in chronic myeloid leukemia. *Am J Hematol* 27:110, 1988.

94. Goh KO, Anderson FW: Cytogenetic studies in basophilic chronic myelocytic leukemia. *Arch Pathol Lab Med* 103:288, 1979.

95. Denburg JA, Wilson WEC, Goodacre R, Bienenstock J: Chronic myeloid leukemia—evidence for basophil differentiation and histamine synthesis from cultured peripheral blood cells. *Br J Haematol* 45:13, 1980.

96. Parkin JL, McKenna RW, Brunning RD: Philadelphia chromosome-positive blastic leukemia: ultrastructural and ultracytochemical evidence of basophil and mast cell differentiation. *Br J Haematol* 52:633, 1982.

97. Zucker-Franklin D: Ultrastructural evidence for the common origin of human mast cells and basophils. *Blood* 56:534, 1980.

98. Soler J, O'Brien M, Travares de Castro J, et al: Blast crisis of chronic granulocytic leukemia with mast cell and basophilic precursors. *Am J Clin Pathol* 83:254, 1985.

99. Weitt SC, Hrisinko MA: A hybrid eosinophilic-basophilic granulocyte in chronic granulocytic leukemia. *Am J Clin Pathol* 87:66, 1987.

100. Gabriel LC, Escribano LM, Marie JP, et al: Peroxidase activity in circulating mast cells in blast crisis of chronic granulocytic leukemia. *Am J Clin Pathol* 86:212, 1986.

101. Youman JD, Taddeini L, Cooper T: Histamine excess symptoms in basophilic chronic granulocytic leukemia. *Arch Intern Med* 131:560, 1973.

102. Rosenthal S, Schwartz JH, Canellos GP: Basophilic chronic granulocytic leukemia with hyperhistaminemia. *Br J Haematol* 36:367, 1977.

103. Valimaki M, Vuopio P, Salaspuro M: Plasma histamine and serum pepsinogen 1 concentration in chronic myelogenous leukaemia. *Acta Med Scand* 217:89, 1985.

104. Anderson W, Helman CA, Hirschowitz BI: Basophilic leukemia and the hypersecretion of gastric acid and pepsin. *Gastroenterology* 95:195, 1988.

105. Kue Y, Gus Y, Lu D, et al: A case of basophilic leukemia bearing simultaneous translocations t(8;21) and t(9;22). *Cancer Genet Cytogenet* 51:215, 1991.

106. Cecio A, Dini E, Quattrin N: Preliminary observations with the electron microscope of two cases of acute basophilic leukemia. *Boll Soc Ital Biol Sper* 46:459, 1970.

107. Lertprasertsuke N, Tsutsumi Y: An unusual form of chronic myeloproliferative disorder. *Acta Pathol Jpn* 41:473, 1991.

108. Wick MR, Li CY, Pierre RV: Acute nonlymphocytic leukemia with basophilic differentiation. *Blood* 60:38, 1982.

109. Peterson LC, Parkin JL, Arthur DC, Brunning RD: Acute basophilic leukemia. *Am J Clin Pathol* 96:160, 1991.

110. Dvorak AM, Dickersin GR, Connell A, Carey RW, Dvorak HF: Degranulation mechanisms in human leukemic basophils. *Clin Immunol Immunopathol* 5:235, 1976.

111. Quattrin N: Follow up of sixty-two cases of acute basophilic leukemia. *Biomedicine* 28:72, 1978.

112. Pearson MG, Vardiman JW, LeBeau MM, et al: Increased numbers of marrow basophils may be associated with t(6;9) in ANLL. *Am J Hematol* 18:393, 1985.

113. Horsman DE, Kalousek DK: Acute myelomonocytic leukemia (AML-M4) and translocation t(6;9)(p23;q34): Two additional patients with prominent myelodysplasia. *Am J Hematol* 26:77, 1987.

114. Hoyle CF, Sherrington P, Hayhoe FG: Translocation (3;6)(q21;p21) in acute myeloid leukemia with abnormal thrombopoiesis and basophilia. *Cancer Genet Cytogenet* 30:261, 1988.

115. Matsura Y, Sato N, Kimura F, et al: An increase in basophils in a case of acute myelomonocytic leukaemia associated with marrow eosinophilia and inversion of chromosome 16. *Eur J Haematol* 39:457, 1987.

116. Moir DJ, Pearson J, Buckle VJ: Acute promyelocytic transformation in a case of acute myelomonocytic leukemia. *Cancer Genet Cytogenet* 12:359, 1984.

117. Umeda M, Nojima Z, Yamaguchi R, et al: Two cases of acute promyelocytic leukemia with marked basophilia--a variant type of APL with the capability of differentiating into basophils. *Rinsho Ketsueki* 28:2004, 1987.

118. Gotoh H, Murakami S, Oku N, et al: Translocations t(15;17) and t(9;14)(q34;q22) in a case of acute promyelocytic leukemia with increased number of basophils. *Cancer Genet Cytogenet* 36:103, 1988.

119. Lewis RA, Goetzl EJ, Wasserman SI, et al: The release of four mediators of immediate hypersensitivity from human leukemic basophils. *J Immunol* 114:87, 1975.

120. Travis WD, Li C-Y, Bergstralh EF, et al: Systemic mast cell disease. Analysis of 58 cases and literature review. *Medicine* (Baltimore) 67:345, 1988.

121. Tsai M, Shih L-S, Newlands GFJ, et al: The rat c-kit ligand, stem cell factor, induces the development of connective tissue-type and mucosal mast cells in vivo. Analysis by anatomical distribution, histochemistry and protease phenotype. *J Exp Med* 174:125, 1991.

122. Irani AA, Garriga MM, Metcalfe DD, Schwartz LB: Mast cells in cutaneous mastocytosis: accumulation of the MCtc type. *Clin Exp Allergy* 20:52, 1990.

123. Schwartz LB, Metcalfe DD, Miller JS, et al: Tryptase levels as an indicator of mast-cell activation in systemic anaphylaxis and mastocytosis. *N Engl J Med* 316:1622, 1987.

124. Weidner N, Horan RF, Husten KF: Mast-cell phenotype in indolent forms of mastocytosis. *Am J Pathol* 140:847, 1992.

125. Weidner N, Austen KF. Heterogeneity of mast cells at multiple body sites. Fluorescent determination of avidin binding and immunofluorescent determination of chymase, tryptase, and carboxypeptidase content. *Pathol Res Pract* 189:156, 1993.

126. Lavker RM, Schechter NM, Robertson CR: Cutaneous mast cell depletion result from topical corticosteroid usage. *J Invest Dermatol* 82:414, 1984.

127. Irani AA, Golzar N, DeBlois G, Elson CO, Schechter NM, Schwartz LB: Deficiency of the tryptase-positive, chymase-negative mast cell type in gastrointestinal mucosa of patients with defective T lymphocyte function. *J Immunol* 138:4338, 1987.

128. Garriga MM, Friedman MM, Metcalfe DD: A survey of the number and distribution of mast cells in the skin of patients with mast cell disorders. *J Allergy Clin Immunol* 82:425, 1988.

129. Malone DG, Irani AA, Schwartz LB, Barrett KE, Metcalfe DD: Mast cell numbers and histamine levels in synovial fluids from patients with diverse arthritides. *Arthritis Rheum* 29:956, 1986.

130. Malone DG, Wilder RL, Saavedra-Delgado AM, Metcalfe DD: Mast cell numbers in rheumatoid synovial tissues. *Arthritis Rheum* 30:130, 1987.

131. Frame B, Nixon RK: Bone marrow mast cells in osteoporosis of aging. *N Engl J Med* 279:626, 1968.

132. Lennert K, Parwaresch MR: Mast cells and mast cell neoplasia—a review. *Histopathology* 3:349, 1979.

133. Barrett KE, Neva FA, Gam AA, et al: The immune response to nematode parasites: modulation of mast cell numbers and function during *Strongyloides stercoralis* infections in nonhuman primates. *Am J Trop Med Hyg* 30:574, 1988.

134. Bowers HM, Mahapatro RC, Kennedy JW: Numbers of mast cells in the axillary lymph nodes of breast cancer patients. *Cancer* 43:568, 1979.

135. Yoo D, Lessin LS, Jensen WN: Bone marrow mast cells in lymphoproliferative disorders. *Ann Intern Med* 88:753, 1978.

136. Yoo D, Lessin LS: Bone marrow mast cell content in preleukemic syndrome. *Am J Med* 73:539, 1982.

137. Fohlmeister I, Reber T, Fischer R: Bone marrow mast cell reaction in preleukemic myelodysplasia and in aplastic anemia. *Virchows Arch* [A] 405:503, 1985.

138. Unna PG: Beitrage zur anatomic und pathogenese der urticaria simplex und pigmentosa. *Mscch Prakt Dermatol, Suppl Dermatol Stud* 3:9, 1887.

139. Nettleship E, Tay W: Rare forms of urticaria. *Br Med J* 2:323, 1869.

140. Sangster A: An anomalous mottled rash, accompanied by pruritus, factious urticaria and pigmentation, "urticaria pigmentosa (?)." *Trans Clin Soc London* 11:161, 1878.

141. Ellis JM: Urticaria pigmentosa: a report of a case with autopsy. *Arch Pathol* 48:426, 1949.

142. Fine JD: Mastocytosis (review). *Int Soc Trop Dermatol* 19:117, 1980.

143. Soter NA: The skin in mastocytosis. *J Invest Dermatol* 3:32S, 1991.

144. Metcalfe DD: Clinical advances in mastocytosis—conclusions. *J Invest Dermatol* 96:64S, 1991.

145. Furitsu T, Tsujimura T, Tono T, et al: Identification of mutations in the coding sequences of the proto-oncogene c-kit in a human mast cell leukemia cell line causing ligand independent activation of c-kit product. *J Clin Invest* 92:1736, 1993.

146. Nagata H, Worobec AS, Oh CK, et al: Identification of a point mutation in the catalytic domain of the proto-oncogene c-kit in the peripheral blood mononuclear cells of patients with mastocytosis. *Proc Natl Acad Sci USA* 92:10560, 1995.

147. Longley BJ, Tyrell L, Lu SZ, et al: Somatic c-KIT activating mutation in urticaria pigmentosa and aggressive mastocytosis: establishment of clonality in a human mast cell neoplasm. *Nat Genet* 12:312, 1996.

148. Nagata H, Okada T, Worobec AS, Semere T, Metcalfe DD: c-Kit mutation in a population of patients with mastocytosis. *Int Arch Allergy Immunol* 113:184, 1997.

149. Longley BJ, Metcalfe DD, Tharp M, et al: Activating and dominant inactivating c-kit catalytic domain mutations in distinct clinical forms of human mastocytosis. *Proc Natl Acad Sci USA* 96:1609, 1999.

150. London CA, Galli SJ, Yuuki T, Hu Z-Q, Helfland SC, Geissler EN: Spontaneous canine in mast cell tumors express tandem duplications in the proto-oncogene c-kit. *Exp Hematol* 27:689, 1999.

151. Hiroto S, Isozaki K, Moriyami Y, et al: Gain-of-function mutations of c-kit in human gastrointestinal stromal turmors. *Science* 279:577, 1998.

152. Nishida T, Hirota S, Taniguchi M, et al: Familial gastrointestinal stromal tumors with germline mutation of the KIT gene. *Nat Genet* 19:323, 1998.

153. Czarnetzki BM, Behrendt H: Urticaria pigmentosa: clinical picture and response to oral disodium cromoglycate. *Br J Dermatol* 105:563, 1981.

154. Tharp MD: The spectrum of mastocytosis. *Am J Med Sci* 289:117, 1985.

155. Kirshenbaum AS, Metcalfe DD: The biology and therapy of mastocytosis, in *Mast Cell and Basophil Differentiation and Function in Health and Disease*, edited by SJ Galli, KF Austen, p 317. Raven, New York, 1989.

156. Travis WD, Li C-Y: Pathology of the lymph node and spleen in systemic mast cell disease. *Mod Pathol* 1:4, 1988.

157. Mican JM, DiBisceglie AM, Fong T-L, et al: Hepatic involvement in mastocytosis: clinicopathologic correlations in 41 cases. *Hepatolgy* 22:1163, 1995.

158. Lawrence JB, Friedman GB, Travis WD, et al: Hematologic manifestations of systemic mast cell disease: a prospective study of laboratory and morphologic features and their relation to prognosis. *Am J Med* 91:612, 1991.

159. Horny H-P, Ruck MT, Kaiserling E: Spleen findings in generalized mastocytosis. *Cancer* 70:459, 1992.

160. Horny H-P, Parwaresch MR, Lennart K: Bone marrow findings in systemic mastocytosis. *Hum Pathol* 16:808, 1985.

161. Ridell B, Olafsson JH, Roupe G, et al: The bone marrow urticaria pigmentasa in systemic mastocytosis. *Arch Dermatol* 122:422, 1986.

162. Parker RI: Hematologic aspects of mastocytosis I: bone marrow pathology in adult and pediatric systemic mast cell disease. *J Invest Dermatol* 96:47S, 1991.

163. Kettlehut BV, Parker RI, Travis WD, Metcalfe DD: Hematopathology of the bone marrow in pediatric cutaneous mastocytosis: a study of 17 patients. *Am J Clin Pathol* 91:558, 1989.

164. Roberts LJ, Fields JP, Oats JA: Mastocytosis without urticaria pigmentosa: a frequently unrecognized cause of recurrent syncope. *Trans Assoc Am Physicians* 95:36, 1982.

165. Cherner JA, Jensen RT, Dubois A, et al: Gastrointestinal dysfunction in systemic mastocytosis. *Gastroenterology* 95:657, 1988.

166. Rafü M, Birooznia H, Colimbu C, Balthazar E: Pathologic fracture in systemic mastocytosis. *Clin Orthop* 180:260, 1983.

167. Schwartz LB, Sakai K, Bradford TR, et al: The α form of human tryptase is the predominant type present in blood at baseline in normal subjects and is elevated in those with systemic mastocytosis. *J Clin Invest* 96:2702, 1995.

168. Joachim G: Über mastzellenleukämie. *Dtsch Arch Klin Med* 87:437, 1906.

169. Travis WD, Li C-Y, Hoaglan HC, et al: Mast cell leukemia: report of a case and review of the literature. *Mayo Clin Proc* 61:957, 1986.

170. Torrey E, Simpson K, Wilbur S, et al: Malignant mastocytosis with circulating mast cells. *Am J Med* 34:283, 1990.

171. Lennert K, Koster E, Martin H: Über die Mastzellen-leukaemie. *Acta Haematol* 16:255, 1956.

172. Friedman BS, Steinberg S, Meggs WJ, et al: Analysis of plasma histamine levels in patients with mast cell disorders. *Am J Med* 87:649, 1989.

173. Metcalfe DD: The treatment of mastocytosis: an overview. *J Invest Dermatol* 96:5S, 1991.

174. Frieri M, Alling DW, Metcalfe DD: Comparison of the therapeutic efficacy of cromolyn sodium with that of combined chlorpheniramine and cimetidine in systemic mastocytosis. *Am J Med* 78:9, 1985.

175. Roberts LJ II, Marney SR Jr, Oates JA: Blockade of the flush associated with metastatic gastric carcinoid by combined histamine H1 and H2 receptor-antagonists. *N Engl J Med* 300:236, 1979.

176. Sullivan TJ: Pharmacologic modulation of the whealing response to histamine in human skin: identification of doxepin as a potent in vivo inhibitor. *J Allergy Clin Immunol* 69:260, 1982.

177. Hirschowitz BI, Broarke JF: Effect of cimetidine on gastric hypersecretion and diarrhea in systemic mastocytosis. *Ann Intern Med* 90:769, 1979.

178. Soter NA, Austen KF, Wasserman ST: Oral disodium cromoglycolate in the treatment of systemic mastocytosis. *N Engl J Med* 310:465, 1979.

179. Frieri M, Alling DW, Metcalfe DD: Comparison of the therapeutic efficacy of cromolyn sodium with that of combined chlopheniramine and cimetidine in systemic mastocytosis: results of double-blind clinical trial. *Am J Med* 78:9, 1985.

180. Welch EA, Alper JC, Boggars H, Farrell DS: Treatment of bullous mastocytosis with disodium cromoglycolate. *J Am Acad Dermatol* 9:349, 1983.

181. Czarnetzki BM: A double-blind cross-over study of the effect of ketotifen in urticaria pigmentosa. *Dermatologica* 166:44, 1983.

182. Graves L III, Stechschulty DJ, Morris DC, Lukert BP: Inhibition of mediator release in systemic mastocytosis is associated with reversal of bone changes. *J Bone Mineral Res* 5:113, 1990.

183. Kettlehut BV, Berkebile C, Bradely D, Metcalfe DD: A double-blind placebo controlled trial of ketotifen verses hydroxyzine in the treatment of pediatric mastocytosis. *J Allergy Clin Immunol* 83:866, 1989.

184. Friedman BS, Santiago ML, Berkebile C, Metcalfe DD: Comparison of azelastine and chlorpheniramine in the treatment of mastocytosis. *J Allergy Clin Immunol* 92:520, 1993.

185. Cundy T, Beneton MNC, Darby AJ, et al: Osteopenia in systemic mastocytosis: natural history and responses to treatment with inhibitors of bone resorption. *Bone* 8:149, 1987.

186. Barton J, Lauker RM, Schecter NM, Lazarus GS: Treatment of urticaria pigmentosa with corticosteroids. *Arch Dermatol* 121:1516, 1985.

187. Czarnetzki PM, Rosenbach T, Kolde G, Frosch PJ: Phototherapy of urticaria pigmentosa: clinical response and changes of cutaneous reactivity, histamine and chemotactic leukotrienes. *Arch Dermatol* 227:105, 1985.

188. Kolde G, Frosch PJ, Czarnetzki BM: Responses of cutaneous mast cells

to PUVA in patients with urticaria pigmentosa: histomorphometric, ultrastructural and biochemical investigations. *J Invest Dermatol* 83:175. 1984.

189. Reisberg IR, Oyakawa S: Mastocytosis with malabsorption, myelofibrosis, and massive ascites. *Am J Gastroenterol* 82:54, 1987.

190. Klunin-Nelemans HC, Jansen JH, Breukelman H, et al: Response to interferon alfa-2b in a patient with systemic mastocytosis. *N Engl J Med* 326:619, 1992.

191. Worobec AS, Kirshenbaum AS, Schwartz L: Treatment of three patients with systemic mastocytosis with interferon alpha-2b. *Leuk Lymphoma* 18:179, 1995.

192. Pardini S, Bosincu L, Bonfigli S, et al: Anaphylactic-like syndrome in systemic mastocytosis treated with alpha-2-interferon. *Acta Haematol* 85:220, 1991.

193. Hutchinson RM: Mastocytosis and co-existent Non-Hodgkin's lymphoma and myeloproliferative disorders. *Leuk Lymphoma* 7:29, 1992.

194. Chariot P, Monnet I, LeLong F, et al: Systemic mast cell disease associated with primary mediastinal germ cell tumor. *Am J Med* 90:381, 1991.

195. Chariot P, Monnet I, Guarland P, et al: Systemic mastocytosis following mediastinal germ cell tumor: an association confirmed. *Hum Pathol* 24:111, 1993.

196. Johnstone PA, Mican JM, Metcalfe DD, Delaney TF: Radiotherapy of refractory bone pain due systemic mast cell disease. *Am J Clin Oncol* 17:328, 1994.

197. Wimazal F, Sperr WR, Horny HP, et al: Hyperfibrinolysis in a case of myelodysplastic syndrome with leukemic spread of mast cells. *Am J Hematol* 61:66, 1999.

198. Friedman B, Darling G, Norton J, et al: Splenectomy in the management of systemic mast cell disease. *Surgery* 107:94, 1990.

199. Horan RF, Austen KF: Systemic mastocytosis: a retrospective view of a decade's clinical experience at the Brigham and Women's Hospital. *J Invest Dermatol* 96:55, 1991.

200. Coser P, Quaglino D, DePasquale A, et al: Cytobiological and clinical aspects of tissue mast cell leukemia. *Br J Haematol* 45:5, 1980.

201. Dalton R, Chan L, Batten E, Eridani S: Mast cell leukemia: evidence for bone marrow origin of the pathological clone. *Br J Haematol* 64:397, 1984.

CLASSIFICATION AND CLINICAL MANIFESTATIONS OF NEUTROPHIL DISORDERS

MARSHALL A. LICHTMAN

Neutrophil disorders can be grouped into deficiencies, or neutropenia, and excesses, or neutrophilia. The former can have the severe consequence of predisposing to infection, whereas the latter is usually a manifestation of an underlying inflammatory or neoplastic disease: the neutrophilia, per se, having no specific consequences. Neutropenia may reflect an inherited disease that is usually evident in childhood (such as congenital neutropenia), but it is more often acquired. The most common cause for neutropenia is the adverse effect of the use of a drug. Some cases of neutropenia have no evident cause. The health consequence of neutropenia is a function of the severity of the decrease in the blood neutrophil count and the abruptness and duration of the decrease. Qualitative disorders of neutrophils may lead to infection as a result of defective chemotaxis to an inflammatory site or defective microbial killing. Table 70-1 provides a comprehensive categorization of neutrophil disorders.

CLASSIFICATION

Table 70-1 lists disorders that result from a primary deficiency in neutrophil numbers or function. Neutropenia or neutrophilia may also occur as part of a disorder that affects multiple blood cell lineages, such as occurs in infiltrative diseases of the marrow or after cytotoxic drug therapy, but these are not included in this classification and are discussed in other parts of this text. In this classification, and in this section of the text, we consider diseases resulting from neutrophil deficiencies in which the neutrophil is either the only cell type affected or is the dominant cell type affected.

A pathophysiologic classification of neutrophil disorders has proved elusive. Techniques to measure mechanisms of impaired production or accelerated destruction of neutrophils are more difficult and complex than those used for red cells or platelets. The low concentration of blood neutrophils, accentuated in neutropenic states, makes radioactive labeling techniques to study the kinetics of autologous cells in neutropenic subjects technically difficult or not possible. The two compartments of neutrophils in the blood, the random disappearance of neutrophils from the circulation, the extremely short circulation time of neutrophils, the absence of techniques to measure the size of the tissue neutrophil compartment, and the disappearance of neutrophils by death or excretion from the tissue compartment also make multicompartment kinetic analysis exceedingly difficult. Also, neutropenic disorders are uncommon, and few laboratories are able, or prepared, to undertake the studies necessary to define the mechanisms of their development in sporadic cases. Therefore, efforts to understand the pathophysiology of neutropenia have had limited success. Hence, the classification of neutrophil disorders is partly pathophysiologic

and partly descriptive (see Table 70-1). Although imperfect, classification does provide a language for communication and a basis for rectification as knowledge of the cause and mechanism of disease advances.

The classification is self-explanatory except in two areas. First, certain childhood syndromes have been listed under decreased neutrophilic granulopoiesis. They could have been listed under chronic hypoplastic or chronic idiopathic neutropenia; however, they seem to hold a special interest, and their pathogenesis is still disputed. Three childhood syndromes, although associated with neutropenia, are omitted because the neutropenia is part of a more global suppression of hemopoiesis: Pearson syndrome,[1,2] Fanconi syndrome,[3,4] and dyskeratosis congenita.[5,6]

A second area requiring explanation is the chronic idiopathic neutropenias. This group includes: (1) cases with normocellular marrows but an inadequate compensatory increase in granulopoiesis for the degree of neutropenia and (2) cases with hyperplastic granulopoiesis that is apparently ineffective. Unlike hypoplastic neutropenias in which the granulocyte precursors are markedly reduced or absent, precursors are present in the marrow in the idiopathic neutropenias, but the extent of effective granulopoiesis is probably low.

Qualitative disorders of neutrophils affect their ability to enter inflammatory exudates, to ingest microorganisms, or to kill ingested microorganisms (see Chap. 72).

CLINICAL MANIFESTATIONS

The clinical manifestations of decreased concentrations or abnormal function of neutrophils are principally the result of infection.

The combined deficit of neutrophils and monocytes characteristic of aplastic anemia, hairy-cell leukemia, and cytotoxic therapy leads to susceptibility to a broader spectrum of infectious agents. Increased concentrations of normal neutrophils per se have not been associated with clinical manifestations, although increased concentrations of leukemic neutrophil precursors can produce clinical manifestations of microcirculatory leukostasis (see Chap. 91).

NEUTROPENIA

The lower limit of the normal neutrophil count is about $1800/\mu l$ (1.8×10^9/liter) in subjects of European descent and $1400/\mu l$ (1.4×10^9/liter) in subjects of African descent.[148-154] This finding is especially striking in Yemenite Jews, another ethnic group with very low "normal" neutrophil counts.[155] A decrement in neutrophil concentration to $1000/\mu l$ (1.0×10^9/liter) usually poses little threat in the otherwise healthy individual. If the neutrophil count drops further, the risk of infection increases, and subjects chronically neutropenic as a result of a production abnormality with counts less than 500 neutrophils/μl (0.5×10^9/liter) are at risk of developing recurrent infections.[156]

The relationship of frequency or type of infection to neutrophil concentration is an imperfect one. The cause of the neutropenia, the coincidence of monocytopenia or lymphopenia, concurrent use of alcohol or glucocorticoids, and other factors can influence the likelihood of infection.

Infections in neutropenic subjects, not otherwise compromised, are most likely to result from gram-positive cocci and usually are superficial, involving skin, oropharynx, bronchi, anal canal, or vagina. However, any site may become infected, and gram-negative organisms, viruses, or opportunistic organisms may be involved.

A decrease in neutrophil count can occur abruptly or gradually (see Chap. 71). One type of drug-induced neutropenia is distinguished by the rapidity of onset. This abrupt-onset neutropenia is more likely to be severe and lead to symptoms. If the neutrophil count approaches

TABLE 70-1   CLASSIFICATION OF NEUTROPHIL DISORDERS

I. Quantitative disorders of neutrophils
    A. Neutropenia
        1. Decreased neutrophilic granulopoiesis
            a. Congenital neutropenias (Kostmann syndrome and related disorders[7–12]
            b. Reticular dysgenesis (congenital aleukocytosis)[13,14]
            c. Neutropenia and exocrine pancreas dysfunction (Schwachman-Diamond syndrome)[15–17]
            d. Neutropenia and immunoglobulin abnormality[18–20]
            e. Neutropenia and disordered cellular immunity (cartilage-hair hypoplasia)[21,22]
            f. Mental retardation, anomalies, and neutropenia (Cohen syndrome)[23,24]
            g. X-linked cardioskeletal myopathy and neutropenia (Barth syndrome)[25,26]
            h. Myelokathexis[27,28]
            i. Congenital neutropenia with dysgranulopoiesis[29]
            j. Neonatal neutropenia and maternal hypertension[30,31]
            k. Chronic hypoplastic neutropenia
                (1) Drug-induced[32–35]
                (2) Cyclic
                     (a) Sporadic[36–40]
                     (b) Familial[41–43]
                (3) Idiopathic
                     (a) Sporadic[44]
                     (b) Familial[44]
                (4) Branched-chain aminoacidemia[45]
            l. Acute hypoplastic neutropenia
                (1) Drug-induced[32–35]
                (2) Infectious[46,47]
            m. Chronic idiopathic neutropenia
                (1) Benign
                     (a) Familial[48]
                     (b) Sporadic[49–54]
                (2) Symptomatic[55,56]
        2. Accelerated neutrophil destruction
            a. Alloimmune neonatal neutropenia[57,58]
            b. Autoimmune neutropenia[59,60]
                (1) Idiopathic[61–63]
                (2) Drug-induced[32,33]
                (3) Felty syndrome[64–66]
                (4) Systemic lupus erythematosus[66]
                (5) Other autoimmune diseases[67,68]
                (6) Complement activation–induced neutropenia[69,70]
                (7) Pure white cell aplasia[71,72]
        3. Maldistribution of neutrophils
            a. Pseudoneutropenia[73]
    B. Neutrophilia
        1. Increased neutrophilic granulopoiesis
            a. Hereditary neutrophilia[74]
            b. Chronic idiopathic neutrophilia[75]
                (1) Asplenia[76]
            c. Neutrophilic leukemoid reactions[77]
                (1) Inflammation[77,176]
                (2) Infection[78,176]
                (3) Cancer[79,176,177]
                (4) Drugs (e.g., glucocorticoids, lithium, G- or GM-CSF)[80,81,178,179]
                (5) Exercise[180]
            d. Sweet's syndrome[82]
            e. Cigarette smoking[83]
        2. Decreased neutrophil circulatory egress
            a. Drugs (e.g., glucocorticoids)[40,179]
        3. Maldistribution of neutrophils
            a. Pseudoneutrophilia[84]
            b. Membrane CD11/18 deficiency[85]

TABLE 70-1   CLASSIFICATION OF NEUTROPHIL DISORDERS (CONTINUED)

II. Qualitative disorders of neutrophils[86–88]
    A. Defective adhesion of neutrophils
        1. Cell adhesion protein deficiency[89–92]
        2. Drug-induced[93]
    B. Defective locomotion and chemotaxis[94,95]
        1. Lazy leukocyte syndrome[96]
        2. Actin polymerization abnormalities[97,98]
        3. Juvenile periodontitis[99]
        4. Neonatal neutrophils[100]
        5. Leiner disease[88]
        6. High-dose interleukin-2[101]
    C. Defective phagocytosis[86,87]
    D. Defective microbial killing[102,103]
        1. Chronic granulomatous disease[102–104]
        2. Myeloperoxidase deficiency[104–106]
        3. Hyperimmunoglobulin E (Job) syndrome[107]
        4. Glucose-6-phosphate dehydrogenase deficiency[108]
        5. Extensive burns[109]
        6. Glycogen storage disease Ib[110,111]
        7. Ethanol toxicity[112]
        8. End-stage renal disease[113]
    E. Multiple or mixed disorders[86]
    F. Abnormal structure of the nucleus or of an organelle
        1. Hereditary macropolycytes[114]
        2. Hereditary hypersegmentation[115]
        3. Specific granule deficiency[116,117]
        4. Pelger-Huët anomaly[118]
        5. Alder-Reilly anomaly[119]
        6. May-Hegglin anomaly[120]
        7. Chédiak-Higashi disease[121,122]
III. Neutrophil-induced vascular or tissue damage[123–147]

broad-spectrum antibiotics, severe, sustained neutropenia or agranulocytosis is a serious illness with a high fatality rate.

There is a decrease in the formation of pus in patients with severe neutropenia.[160,161] This failure to suppurate can mislead the clinician and delay identification of the site of infection because minimal physical or radiographic findings develop. For example, lack of pneumonic consolidation is characteristic of pneumonia in granulocytopenic subjects. Exudate, swelling, heat, and regional adenopathy are much less prevalent in granulocytopenic patients. Fever is common, and local pain, tenderness, and erythema are nearly always present despite a marked reduction in neutrophils.[162–164]

The mechanism of neutropenia, as well as the severity of the deficiency of cells, plays a role in clinical manifestations. *Chronic idiopathic (benign) neutropenia* is associated with normal granulopoiesis in the marrow and is asymptomatic even when present for prolonged periods, sometimes in the face of neutrophil counts approaching zero.[49] Presumably the delivery of neutrophils from marrow to tissues is sufficient to prevent infection despite the low blood pool size.[50,51] Monocyte counts are normal, and this may also aid in host defenses, since these cells are effective phagocytes.

Chronic idiopathic (symptomatic) neutropenia is often associated with pyoderma and otitis media in children.[55] The former is usually caused by *Staphylococcus aureus*, *Escherichia coli*, and *Pseudomonas* spp., and the latter is usually the result of infection by pneumococci or *Pseudomonas aeruginosa*. Unexplained chronic gingivitis also may be a manifestation of chronic neutropenia.[165] Pneumonia, lung abscesses, stomatitis, hepatic abscesses, or infections in other sites may occur.[56]

Chronic cyclic neutropenia is characterized by periodic oscillations in the number of neutrophils, with the nadir occurring at about 3-week intervals.[36,166] During neutropenia, patients develop malaise, fever, and buccal, labial, or lingual ulcers, and cervical adenopathy. Furuncles, carbuncles, cellulitis, infected cuts with lymphangitis, chronic gingivitis, and abscesses of the axilla or groin also may occur.

zero (agranulocytosis), high fever; chills; necrotizing, painful oral ulcers (agranulocytic angina); and prostration may occur, presumably as a result of sepsis.[157–159] As the disease progresses, headache, stupor, and rash may develop. In the preantibiotic era, persistent agranulocytosis had a fatality rate approaching 100 percent. Even with bactericidal,

Although severe infections may lead to fatality, life-threatening complications are uncommon (see Chap. 71).

Some individuals may have neutropenia because a larger proportion of their blood neutrophils is in the marginal rather than in the circulating pool. The total blood neutrophil pool is normal, and infections do not result from this atypical distribution of neutrophils.[167] This type of alteration has been called *pseudoneutropenia.*

QUALITATIVE NEUTROPHIL ABNORMALITIES

Neutrophil function depends on the ability of neutrophils to adhere to endothelium, move, respond to chemotactic gradients, ingest microorganisms, and kill ingested pathogens. Loss of any of these functions can predispose to infection (see Chap. 72). Defects in each step of the neutrophil's participation in the inflammatory response have been identified.[168,169] Defects in cytoplasmic contractile proteins, granule synthesis or contents, or intracellular enzymes may underlie a movement, ingestion, or killing defect. These defects may be congenital or acquired. Chronic granulomatous disease[102,103] and Chédiak-Higashi disease[121] are two examples of the former. Among the acquired disorders are those extrinsic to the cell, such as in the movement, chemotactic, or phagocytic defects of diabetes mellitus,[168–171] alcohol abuse,[172,173] or glucocorticoid excess.[174] Acquired intrinsic disorders are usually manifestations of stem cell disorders like preleukemia[175] (see Chap. 91).

Severe defects in bacterial killing, such as occur in chronic granulomatous disease, result in *S. aureus, Klebsiella-Aerobacter, E. coli,* and other catalase-positive bacterial infections. Suppurative lymphadenitis, pneumonia, dermatitis, hepatic abscesses, osteomyelitis, and stomatitis occur, and chronic granulomatous reactions in these sites give the disease its name. Fatality rates have been high. Functional disorders may be severe, as in chronic granulomatous disease. Mild functional disorders predispose to infections that are relatively infrequent and that respond readily to antibiotics. Severe functional disorders result in suppurative lesions because neutrophil influx into inflammatory foci is not impaired, whereas agranulocytosis is associated with non-suppurative lesions.

NEUTROPHILIA

An overabundance of neutrophils has not been shown to result in specific clinical manifestations. Neutrophils can transiently occlude capillaries, as determined by supravital microscopy, and such occlusions may reduce local blood flow transiently and contribute to the development of ischemia.[124] Impairment of reperfusion of the coronary microcirculation has been thought to be dependent, in part, on neutrophil plugging of myocardial capillaries.[123]

NEUTROPHIL-INDUCED VASCULAR OR TISSUE DAMAGE

Neutrophil products may contribute to the pathogenesis of inflammatory skin, bowel, synovial, glomerular, and bronchial and interstitial pulmonary diseases.[124–138] In addition, these products may act as mediators of tissue injury in myocardial infarction.[139–142] Also, highly reactive oxygen products of neutrophils may be mutagens that increase the risk of neoplasia.[144,145] This action may explain, for example, the development of carcinoma of the bowel in patients with chronic ulcerative colitis and the relationship between elevated leukocyte count and the occurrence of lung cancer, independent of the effect of cigarette usage.[146] The oxidants, especially hypochlorous acid and chloramines, released by the neutrophil are extremely short lived and may play a role in tissue injury by inactivating several protease inhibitors in tissue fluids, permitting proteases, especially elastase, collagenase, and gela-

tinase, to cause tissue injury.[129] Thrombogenesis has also been ascribed to leukocyte products.[143]

REFERENCES

1. Pearson HA, Lobel JS, Kocoshis SA, et al: A new syndrome of refractory sideroblastic anemia with vacuolization of marrow precursors and exocrine pancreatic dysfunction. *J Pediatr* 95:976, 1979.
2. van de Corput MP, van den Ouweland JM, Dirks RW, et al: Detection of mitochondrial DNA deletions in human skin fibroblasts of patients with Pearson's syndrome by two-color fluorescence in situ hybridization. *J Histochem Cytochem* 45:55, 1997.
3. Gordon-Smith EC, Rutherford TR: Fanconi anemia. *Ballières Clin Haematol* 2:139, 1989.
4. d'Appolito M, Zelante L, Savoia A: Molecular basis of Fanconi anemia. *Haematologica* 83:533, 1998.
5. Srinavin C, Trowbridge A: Dyskeratosis congenita: Clinical features and genetic aspects. *J Med Genet* 12:339, 1975.
6. Dokal I: Severe aplastic anemia including Fanconi's anemia and dyskeratosis congenita. *Curr Opin Hematol* 3:453, 1996.
7. Kostmann R: Infantile genetic agranulocytosis. *Acta Pediatr Scand* 64:362, 1975.
8. Tidow N, Pilz C, Teichmann B, et al: Clinical relevance of point mutations in the cytoplasmic domain of granulocyte colony-stimulating factor receptor gene in patients with severe congenital neutropenia. *Blood* 89:2369, 1997.
9. Rappeport JM, Parkman R, Newburger P, et al: Correction of infantile agranulocytosis (Kostmann's syndrome) by allogeneic transplantation. *Am J Med* 68:605, 1980.
10. Kyds U, Pietsch T, Welte K: Expression of receptors for granulocyte colony-stimulating factor on neutrophils from patients with severe congenital neutropenia and cyclic neutropenia. *Blood* 79:1144, 1992.
11. Bonilla MA, Gillio AP, Ruggeiro M, et al: Effects of recombinant human granulocyte colony-stimulating factor on neutropenia in patients with congenital agranulocytosis. *N Engl J Med* 320:1574, 1989.
12. Weston B, Todd RF III, Axtell R, et al: Severe congenital neutropenia: Clinical effects and neutrophil function during treatment with granulocyte colony-stimulating factor. *J Lab Clin Med* 117:282, 1991.
13. Haas RJ, Niethammer D, Goldmann SF, et al: Congenital immunodeficiency and agranulocytosis (reticular dysgenesis) *Acta Paediatr Scand* 66:279, 1977.
14. Levinsky RJ, Tiedman K: Successful bone-marrow transplantation for reticular dysgenesis. *Lancet* 1:671, 1983.
15. Saunders EF, Gall G, Freedman MH: Granulopoiesis in Schwachman's syndrome (pancreatic insufficiency and bone marrow dysfunction). *Pediatrics* 64:515, 1979.
16. Woods WG, Roloff JS, Lukens JN: The occurrence of leukemia in patients with Schwachman syndrome. *J Pediatr* 99:425, 1981.
17. Azzarà A, Carulli G, Ceccarelli M, et al: In vivo effectiveness of lithium on impaired neutrophil chemotaxis in Schwachman-Diamond syndrome. *Acta Haematol* 85:100, 1991.
18. Lonsdale D, Doedhar SD, Mercer RD: Familial granulocytopenia associated with immunoglobulin abnormality. *J Pediatr* 71:760, 1967.
19. Wetzler M, Talpaz M, Kleinerman ES, et al: A new familial immunodeficiency disorder characterized by severe neutropenia, a defective marrow release mechanism, and hypogammaglobulinemia. *Am J Med* 89:663, 1990.
20. Kozlowski C, Evans DIK: Neutropenia associated with X-linked agammaglobulinemia. *J Clin Pathol* 44:388, 1991.
21. Lux SE, Johnston RB Jr, August CS, et al: Chronic neutropenia and abnormal cellular immunity in cartilage-hair hypoplasia. *N Engl J Med* 282:231, 1970.
22. Trojak JE, Polmar SH, Winkelstein JA: Immunologic studies of cartilage-hair hypoplasia in the Amish. *Johns Hopkins Med J* 148:157, 1981.
23. Norio R, Raitta C, Lindahl E: Further delineation of the Cohen syndrome. *Clin Genet* 25:1, 1984.
24. Warburg M, Pedersen SA, Hønlyk H: The Cohen syndrome. *Ophthalmic Pediatr Genet* II:7, 1990.
25. Barth PG, Scholte HR, Berden JA, et al: An X-linked mitochondrial disease affecting cardiac muscle, skeletal muscle and neutrophil leukocytes. *J Neurol Sci* 62:327, 1983.
26. Bohurs PA, Hensels GW, Hulsebos TJM, et al: Mapping of the locus

for the X-linked cardioskeletal myopathy with neutropenia and abnormal mitochondria (Barth syndrome) to Xq28. *Am J Hum Genet* 48:481, 1991.

27. Bassan R, Viero P, Minetti B, et al: Myelokathexis: A rare form of chronic benign neutropenia. *Br J Haematol* 58:115, 1984.

28. Wetzler M, Talpaz M, Kellagher MJ, et al: Myelokathexis. *JAMA* 267:2179, 1992.

29. Lightsey AL, Parmley RT, Marsh WL, et al: Severe congenital neutropenia with unique features of dysgranulopoiesis. *Am J Hematol* 18:59, 1985.

30. Koenig JM, Christensen RD: Incidence, neutrophil kinetics and natural history of neonatal neutropenia associated with maternal hypertension. *N Engl J Med* 321:557, 1989.

31. Koenig JM, Christensen RD: The mechanism responsible for diminished neutrophil production in neonates delivered of women with pregnancy-induced hypertension. *Am J Obstet Gynecol* 165:467, 1991.

32. Hartl PW: Drug-induced agranulocytosis, in *Blood Disorders Due to Drugs and Other Agents,* edited by RH Girdwood, pp 147–186. Excerpta Medica, Amsterdam, 1974.

33. Hine LK, Gerstman BB, Wise RP, Tsang Y: Mortality resulting from blood dyscrasias in the United States, 1984. *Am J Med* 88:151, 1990.

34. Pisciotta AV: Drug-induced agranulocytosis peripheral destruction of polymorphonuclear leukocytes and their marrow precursors. *Blood Rev* 4:226, 1990.

35. Julia A, Olona M, Bueno J, et al: Drug-induced agranulocytosis. *Br J Haematol* 79:366, 1991.

36. Wright DG, Dale DC, Fauci AS, Wolff SM: Human cyclic neutropenia. *Medicine* 60:13, 1981.

37. Tefferi A, Solberg LA, Petett RM, Willis LG: Adult-onset cyclic bicytopenia. *Am J Hematol* 30:181, 1989.

38. Loughran TP Jr, Clark EA, Hammond WP: Adult-onset cyclic neutropenia is associated with increased large granular lymphocytes. *Blood* 68:1082, 1986.

39. Hammond WP, Price TH, Souza LM, Dale DC: Treatment of cyclic neutropenia with granulocyte colony-stimulating factor. *N Engl J Med* 320:1306, 1989.

40. Marinone G, Roncoli B, Marinone MG: Pure white cell aplasia. *Semin Hematol* 28:298, 1991.

41. Morley AA, Carew JP, Baikie AG: Familial cyclic neutropenia. *Br J Haematol* 13:719, 1967.

42. Hammond WP, Chatta GS, Andrews RG, Dale DC: Abnormal responsiveness of granulocyte-committed progenitor cells in cyclic neutropenia. *Blood* 79:2536, 1992.

43. Dale DC, Hammond WP: Cyclic neutropenia: A clinical review. *Blood Rev* 2:178, 1988.

44. Spaet TH, Dameshek W: Chronic hypoplastic neutropenia. *Am J Med* 13:35, 1952.

45. Hutchinson R, Bunnell K, Thorne J: Suppression of granulopoietic progenitor cell proliferation by metabolites of the branched-chain amino acids. *J Pediatr* 106:62, 1985.

46. Murdock JMC, Smith CC: Haematologic aspects of systemic disease—infection. *Clin Haematol* 1:619, 1972.

47. Olson JP, Lichtman MA: Neutropenia, in *Hematology for Practitioners,* edited by MA Lichtman, pp 105–120. Little, Brown, Boston, 1978.

48. Cutting HO, Lange JE: Familial-benign chronic neutropenia. *Ann Intern Med* 61:876, 1964.

49. Kyle RA: Natural history of chronic idiopathic neutropenia. *N Engl J Med* 302:908, 1970.

50. Wright DG, Meierovics AI, Foxley JM: Assessing the delivery of neutrophils to tissues in neutropenia. *Blood* 67:1023, 1986.

51. Mant MJ, Gordon PA, Akabotu JJ: Bone marrow granulocyte reserve in chronic benign idiopathic neutropenia. *Clin Lab Haematol* 9:281, 1987.

52. Logue GL, Shastri KA, Laughlin M, et al: Idiopathic neutropenia: Anti-neutrophil antibodies and clinical correlations. *Am J Med* 90:211, 1991.

53. Jonsson OG, Buchanan GR: Chronic neutropenia during childhood. *Am J Dis Child* 145:232, 1991.

54. Jakubowski AA, Souza L, Kelly F, et al: Effects of human granulocyte colony-stimulating factor in a patient with idiopathic neutropenia. *N Engl J Med* 320:38, 1989.

55. Pincus SH, Boxer LA, Stossel TP: Chronic neutropenia in childhood. *Am J Med* 61:849, 1976.

56. Dale DC, Guerry D IV, Wewerka JR, et al: Chronic neutropenia. *Medicine* 58:128, 1979.

57. Lalezari P: Alloimmune neonatal neutropenia, in *Clinical Immunology and Allergy,* edited by CP Engelfriet, AEG VondemBorne, p 423. Balliére Tindall, London, 1987.

58. Fromont P, Bettaieb A, Skouri H, et al: Frequency of the polymorphonuclear neutrophil Fc receptor III deficiency in the French population and its involvement in the development of neonatal alloimmune neutropenia. *Blood* 79:2131, 1992.

59. Shastri KA, Logue GL: Autoimmune neutropenia. *Blood* 81:1984, 1993.

60. Bux J, Behrens G, Jaeger G, Welte K: Diagnosis and clinical course of autoimmune neutropenia in infancy: Analysis of 240 cases. *Blood* 91:181, 1998.

61. Boxer LA, Greenberg MS, Boxer GJ, Stossel TP: Autoimmune neutropenia. *N Engl J Med* 293:748, 1975.

62. Hadley AG, Holdurn AM, Bunch C, Chapel H: Antigranulocyte opsonic activity and autoimmune neutropenia. *Br J Haematol* 63:581, 1986.

63. Hartman KR, Wright DG: Identification of autoantibodies specific for the neutrophil adhesion glycoproteins CD116/CD18 in parents with autoimmune neutropenia. *Blood* 78:1096, 1991.

64. Starkebaum G, Loughran TP Jr, Gaur LK, et al: Immunogenetic similarities between patients with Felty's syndrome and those with clonal expansion of large granular lymphocytes in rheumatoid arthritis. *Arthr Rheum* 40:624, 1997.

65. Mason C, Perroux-Goummy L, Audran M: Felty's syndrome, pseudo-Felty's syndrome, monoclonal or polyclonal CD3 lymphocytosis of undetermined significance. *Rev Rhumat* 63:5, 1996.

66. Gross WL, Schmitt WH, Csernok E: ANCA and associated diseases: immunodiagnostic and pathogenic aspects. *Clin Exp Immunol* 91:1, 1993.

67. Yamato E, Fujioka Y, Masugi F, et al: Autoimmune neutropenia with anti-neutrophil autoantibody associated with Sjögren's syndrome. *Am J Med Sci* 300:102, 1990.

68. Stevens C, Peppercorn MA, Grand RJ: Crohn's disease associated with autoimmune neutropenia. *J Clin Gastroenterol* 13:328, 1991.

69. Zachee P, Daeleans R, Pollaris P, et al: Neutrophil adhesion molecules in chronic hemodialysis patients. *Nephron* 68:192, 1994.

70. Knudsen F, Nielsen AH, Pedersen JO, et al: Adult respiratory distress-like syndrome during hemodialysis: relationship between activation of complement, leukopenia, and release of granulocyte elastase. *Int J Artif Organs* 8:187, 1985.

71. Firkin FC, Prewett EJ, Nicholls K, Moran J: Antithymocyte globulin therapy for pure white cell aplasia. *Am J Hematol* 25:101, 1987.

72. Mathieson PW, O'Neill JH, Durrant STS, et al: Antibody-mediated pure neutrophil aplasia, recurrent myasthenia gravis and previous thymoma. *Q J Med* 74:57, 1990.

73. Joyce RA, Boggs DR, Hasiba U, Srodes CH: Marginal neutrophil pool size in normal subjects and neutropenic patients as measured by epinephrine infusion. *J Lab Clin Med* 88:614, 1976.

74. Herring WB, Smith LG, Walker RI, Herion JC: Hereditary neutrophilia. *Am J Med* 56:729, 1974.

75. Ward HN, Reinhard EH: Chronic idiopathic leukocytosis. *Ann Intern Med* 75:193, 1971.

76. Joyce RA, O'Donnell J, Sanghvi J, Westerman MP: Asplenia and abnormal neutrophil kinetics in chronic idiopathic neutrophilia. *Am J Med* 69:633, 1980.

77. Hilts SV, Shaw CC: Leukemoid blood reactions. *N Engl J Med* 149:343, 1953.

78. Marsh JC, Boggs DR, Cartwright GE, Wintrobe MM: Neutrophil kinetics in acute infection. *J Clin Invest* 46:1943, 1967.

79. McKee LC: Excess leukocytosis (leukemoid reactions) associated with malignant diseases. *South Med J* 78:1475, 1985.

80. Bishop CR: Leukokinetic studies: XIII. A non-steady state kinetic evaluation of the mechanism of cortisone-induced granulocytosis. *J Clin Invest* 47:249, 1968.

81. Murphy DL, Goodwin FK, Bunney WE: Leukocytosis during lithium treatment. *Am J Psychiatry* 127:135, 1971.

82. Huang W, McNeely MC: Neutrophilic tissue reactions. *Adv Dermatol* 13:33, 1998.

83. Petitti DB, Kipp H: The leukocyte count: association with intensity of smoking and persistence of effect after quitting. *Am J Epidemiol* 123:89, 1986.

84. Athens JW, Haab OP, Raab SO, et al: Leukokinetic studies: IV. The total

blood, circulating and marginal granulocyte pools and the granulocyte turnover rate in normal subjects. *J Clin Invest* 40:989, 1961.

85. Arnaout MA, Pitt J, Cohen HJ, et al: Deficiency of membrane glycoprotein (gp 150) in a boy with recurrent bacterial infections. *N Engl J Med* 306:693, 1982.

86. Rotrosen D, Gallin JI: Disorders of phagocyte function. *Annu Rev Immunol* 5:127, 1987.

87. Klebanoff SJ, Clark RA: *The Neutrophil: Function and Clinical Disorders.* North-Holland, Amsterdam, 1978.

88. Yang KD, Hill HR: Neutrophil function disorders: Pathophysiology, prevention and therapy. *J Pediatr* 119:343, 1991.

89. Gallin J: Leukocyte adherence-related glycoproteins LFA-1, Mo-1, and p 150,95: A new group of monoclonal antibodies, a new disease and a possible opportunity to understand the molecular basis of leukocyte adherence. *J Infect Dis* 152:661, 1985.

90. Anderson DC, Springer TA: Leukocyte adhesion deficiency: An inherited defect in Mac-1, LFA-1, and p150,95 glycoproteins. *Annu Rev Med* 38:175, 1987.

91. Etzioni A, Frydman M, Pollock S, et al: Recurrent severe infections caused by a novel leukocyte adhesion deficiency. *N Engl J Med* 327:1789, 1992.

92. Davies KA, Toothill VJ, Savill J, et al: A 19-year-old man with leukocyte adhesion deficiency. *Clin Exp Immunol* 84:223, 1991.

93. MacGregor RR, Spagnulo PJ, Lentnek AL: Inhibition of granulocyte adherence by ethanol, prednisone, and aspirin, measured with an assay system. *N Engl J Med* 291:642, 1974.

94. Clark RA: Disorders of granulocyte chemotaxis: An analytical review. *Clin Immunol Immunopathol* 15:52, 1980.

95. Rotrosen D, Gallen JI: Disorders of phagocyte function. *Annu Rev Immunol* 5:127, 1987.

96. Miller ME, Oski FA, Harris MB: Lazy-leucocyte syndrome. A new disorder of neutrophil function. *Lancet* 1:665, 1971.

97. Boxer LA, Hedley-White ET, Stossel TP: Neutrophil actin dysfunction and abnormal neutrophil behavior. *N Engl J Med* 291:1043, 1974.

98. Coates TD, Torkildson JC, Torres M, et al: An inherited defect of neutrophil motility and microfilamentous cytoskeleton associated with abnormalities in 47-Kd and 89-Kd proteins. *Blood* 78:1338, 1991.

99. Meyle J: Leukocyte adhesion deficiency and prepubertal periodontitis. *Periodontology* 2000:6,1994.

100. Hill HR, Augustine NH, Jaffe HS: Human recombinant interferon gamma enhances neonatal PMN activation and movement increases free intracellular calcium. *J Exp Med* 173:767, 1991.

101. Klempner MS, Noring R, Meir JW, Atkins MB: An acquired chemotactic defect in neutrophils from patients receiving interleukin-2 immunotherapy. *N Engl J Med* 322:959, 1990.

102. Meischi C, Roos D: The molecular basis of chronic granulomatous disease. *Springer Sem Immunopathol* 19:417, 1998.

103. Segal AW: Biochemistry and molecular biology of chronic granulomatous disease. *J Inherited Metab Dis* 15:683, 1992.

104. Bogomolski-Yahalom V, Matzner Y: Disorders of neutrophil function. *Blood Reviews* 9:183, 1995.

105. Lehrer RI, Cline MJ: Leukocyte myeloperoxidase deficiency and disseminated candidiasis: The role of myeloperoxidase in resistance to *Candida* infection. *J Clin Invest* 48:1478, 1989.

106. Gerber CE, Kuci S, Zipfel M, et al: Phagocytic activity and oxidative burst of granulocytes in persons with myeloperoxidase deficiency. *Eur J Clin Chem Clin Biochem* 34:901, 1996.

107. Jeppson JD, Jaffe HW, Hill HR: Use of recombinant human interferon gamma enhances neutrophil chemotactic responses in Job syndrome of hypergammaglobulin E and recurrent infections. *J Pediatr* 118:383, 1991.

108. Cooper MR, DeChatelet LR, McCall CE, et al: Complete deficiency of leukocyte glucose-6-phosphate dehydrogenase with defective bactericidal activity. *J Clin Invest* 51:769, 1972.

109. Bjerknes R, Vindenes H, Pitkänen J, et al: Altered polymorphonuclear neutrophilic granulocyte functions in patients with large burns. *J Trauma* 29:847, 1989.

110. Couper R, Kapellushnik J, Griffiths AM: Neutrophil dysfunction in glycogen storage disease Ib: Association with Crohn's-like colitis. *Gastroenterology* 100:549, 1991.

111. Schroten H, Wendel U, Burdach S, et al: Colony-stimulating factors for neutropenia in glycogen storage disease Ib. *Lancet* 337:736, 1991.

112. Tamura DY, Moore EE, Patrick DA, et al: Clinically relevant concentrations of ethanol attenuate primed neutrophil bacteriocidal activity. *J Trauma* 44:320, 1998.

113. Porter CJ, Burden RP, Morgan AG, et al: Impaired bacterial killing and hydrogen peroxide production by polymorphonuclear neutrophils in end-stage renal failure. *Nephron* 77:479, 1997.

114. Davidson WM, Milner RDG, Lawlor SD: Giant neutrophil leukocytes: An inherited anomaly. *Br J Haematol* 6:339, 1960.

115. Undritz VE: Eine neue Sippe mit Erblich—Konstitutioneller Hochsegmentierung der Neutrophilenkerne. *Schweiz Med Wochenschr* 94:1365, 1964.

116. Falloon J, Gallin JI: Neutrophil granules in health and disease. *J Allergy Clin Immunol* 77:653, 1986.

117. Lomax KJ, Gallin JI, Benz EJ Jr, et al: Neutrophil specific granule deficiency likely results from an abnormality of expression of a subset of secretory protein genes. *Blood* 70(suppl 1):93a, 1988.

118. Rebuck JW, Barth CL, Petz AJ: New leucocytic dysfunction at the inflammatory sites in Hegglines, Hurler's and Pelger-Huët anomalous states. *Fed Proc* 22:427, 1963.

119. Reilly WA, Lindsay S: Gargoylism (lipochondrodystrophy): A review of clinical observations in eighteen cases. *Am J Dis Child* 75:595, 1948.

120. Oski FA, Naiman JL, Allen DM, Diamond LK: Leukocytic inclusions—Döhle bodies-associated with platelet abnormality (the May-Hegglin anomaly): Report of a family and review of the literature. *Blood* 20:657, 1962.

121. Bara KY: Chédiak-Higashi syndrome. *Scand J Haematol* 37:1627, 1987.

122. Ganz T, Metcalf JA, Gallin JI, et al: Microbicidal/cytotoxic proteins of neutrophils are deficient in two disorders: Chédiak-Higashi syndrome and specific granule deficiency. *J Clin Invest* 82:552, 1988.

123. Dahlgren MD, Petersen MA, Engler RL, Schmid-Schönbein GW: Leukocyte rheology in cardiac ischemia, in *White Cell Mechanics: Basic Science and Clinical Aspects,* edited by H Meiselman, MA Lichtman, PL La Celle, pp 271–283. Liss, New York, 1984.

124. Schmid-Schönbein GN: Leukocyte kinetics in the microcirculation. *Biorheology* 24:139, 1987.

125. Gallin JI: Neutrophil specific granules: A fuse that ignites the inflammatory response. *Clin Res* 32:320, 1984.

126. Janoff A: Elastase in tissue injury. *Annu Rev Med* 36:207, 1985.

127. Smedly LA, Tonnesen MG, Sandhaus RA, et al: Neutrophil-mediated injury to endothelial cells: Enhancement by endotoxin and essential role of neutrophil elastase. *J Clin Invest* 77:1233, 1986.

128. Malech HL, Gallin JI: Neutrophils in human diseases. *N Engl J Med* 317:687, 1987.

129. Weiss SJ: Tissue destruction by neutrophils. *N Engl J Med* 320:365, 1989.

130. Meiselman H, Lichtman MA, La Celle PL (eds): *White Cell Mechanics: Basic Science and Clinical Aspects.* Liss, New York, 1984.

131. Swank DW, Moore SB: Roles of the neutrophil and other mediators in adult respiratory distress syndrome. *Mayo Clin Proc* 64:1118, 1989.

132. MacNee W, Wiggs B, Balzberg AS, Hogg JC: The effect of cigarette smoking on neutrophil kinetics in human lungs. *N Engl J Med* 321:924, 1989.

133. Parker CW: Neutrophil mechanisms. *Am Rev Resp Dis* 143:559, 1991.

134. Martin TR, Pistorese BP, Hudson LD, Maunder RJ: The function of lung and blood neutrophils in patients with the adult respiratory distress syndrome. Implication for the pathogenesis of lung infections. *Am Rev Resp Dis* 144:254, 1991.

135. Godek JE: Adverse effects of neutrophils on the lung. *Am J Med* 92(suppl 6A):27S, 1992.

136. Palmgren MS, deShazo RO, Cater RM, et al: Mechanisms of neutrophil damage to human alveolar extracellular matrix: The role of serine and metalloproteases. *J Allergy Clin Immunol* 89:905, 1992.

137. Boventre JV, Colvin RB: Adhesion molecules in renal disease. *Curr Opin Nephrol Hypertension* 5:254,1996.

138. Weiss ST, Segal MR, Sparrow D, Wager C: Relation of FEV1 and peripheral blood leukocyte count to total mortality. *Am J Epidemiol* 142:493, 1995.

139. Bednar M, Smith B, Pinto A, Mullane KM: Nafazatrom-induced salvage of ischemic myocardium in anesthetized dogs is mediated through inhibition of neutrophil function. *Circ Res* 57:131, 1985.

140. Allan G, Bhattacherjee P, Brook CD, et al: Myeloperoxidase activity as a quantitative marker of polymorphonuclear leukocyte accumulation

into an experimental myocardial infarct—the effect of ibuprofen on infarct size and polymorphonuclear leukocyte accumulation. *J Cardiovasc Pharmacol* 7:1154, 1985.

141. Ranjadayalan K, Umachandran V, Daviews SW, et al: Thrombolytic treatment in acute myocardial infarction: Neutrophil activation, peripheral leucocyte responses, and myocardial injury. *Br Heart J* 66:10, 1991.

142. Welbourn CRB, Goldman G, Paterson IS, et al: Pathophysiology of ischaemia reperfusion injury: Central role of the neutrophil. *Br J Surg* 78:651, 1991.

143. Schaub RG, Yamashita A, Simmons CA, et al: Leukocyte-mediated large vein injury and thrombosis: Pharmacologic intervention with lipoxygenase inhibitors, in *Leukocyte Emigration and Its Sequelae,* edited by HZ Morat, pp 62–68. Karger, Basel, 1987.

144. Weitzman SA, Weitburg AB, Clark EP, Stossel TP: Phagocytes as carcinogens: Malignant transformation produced by human neutrophil. *Science* 227:1231, 1985.

145. Trush MA, Seed JL, Kensler TW: Oxidant-dependent metabolic activation of polycyclic aromatic hydrocarbons by phorbol ester–stimulated human polymorphonuclear leukocytes: Possible link between inflammation and cancer. *Proc Natl Acad Sci USA* 82:5194, 1985.

146. Phillips AN, Neaton JD, Cook DG, et al: The leukocyte count and risk of lung cancer. *Cancer* 69:680, 1992.

147. Fadlon E, Vordermeier S, Pearson TC, et al: Blood polymorphonuclear leukocytes from the majority of sickle cell patients in the crisis phase of the disease show adhesion to vascular endothelium and increased expression of CD64. *Blood* 91:266, 1998.

148. Orfanakis NG, Ostlund RE, Bishop CR, Athens JW: Normal blood leukocyte concentration values. *Am J Clin Pathol* 53:649, 1970.

149. Rumke CL, Brezemer PD, Kuik DJ: Normal values and least significant differences for differential leukocyte counts. *J Chronic Dis* 28:661, 1975.

150. England JM, Bain BJ: Total and differential leukocyte count. *Br J Haematol* 33:1, 1976.

151. Broun GO, Herbeg FK, Hamilton JR: Leukopenia in Negroes. *N Engl J Med* 275:1410, 1966.

152. Rippey JJ: Leukopenia in West Indians and Africans. *Lancet* 2:44, 1967.

153. Karakyalcin G, Rosner F, Saurtsky A: Pseudoneutropenia in Negroes. *NY State J Med* 72:1815, 1972.

154. Reed WW, Diehl LF: Leukopenia, neutropenia, and reduced hemoglobin levels in healthy American blacks. *Arch Intern Med* 151:501, 1991.

155. Shoenfeld Y, Weinberger A, Avishar R, et al: Familial leukopenia among Yemenite Jews. *Isr J Med Sci* 14:1271, 1978.

156. Bodey GP, Buckley M, Sathe YS: Quantitative relationships between circulating leukocytes and infection in patients with acute leukemia. *Ann Intern Med* 64:328, 1966.

157. Kracke RR: Recurrent agranulocytosis. *Am J Clin Pathol* 1:385, 1931.

158. Gorlin RJ, Chaudhry AP: The oral manifestations of cyclic (periodic) neutropenia. *Arch Dermatol* 82:344, 1960.

159. Levine S: Neutropenia with marked periodontal lesions. *Oral Surg* 12:310, 1959.

160. Boggs DR: The cellular composition of inflammatory exudates in human leukemia. *Blood* 15:466, 1960.

161. Dale DC, Wolff SM: Skin window studies of the acute inflammatory responses of neutropenic patients. *Blood* 38:138, 1971.

162. Sickles EA, Green WH, Wiernick PH: Clinical presentation of infection in granulocytopenic patients. *Arch Intern Med* 135:715, 1975.

163. Russin SJ, Fillipo BH, Adler AG: Neutropenia in adults. *Postgrad Med* 88:209, 1990.

164. Welte K, Boxer LA: Severe chronic neutropenia; pathophysiology and therapy. *Sem Hematol* 34:267, 1997.

165. Kyle RA, Linman JW: Gingivitis and chronic idiopathic neutropenia. *Mayo Clin Proc* 45:494, 1970.

166. Wright DG, Dale DC, Fauci AS, Wolff SM: Human cyclic neutropenia: Clinical review and long-term follow-up of patients. *Medicine* 60:1, 1981.

167. Joyce RA, Boggs DR, Hasiba U, Srodes CH: Marginal neutrophil pool size in normal subjects and neutropenic patients as measured by epinephrine infusion. *J Lab Clin Med* 88:614, 1976.

168. Baehner RL: Neutrophil dysfunction associated with states of chronic and recurrent infection. *Pediatr Clin North Am* 27:377, 1980.

169. Gallin JI, Wright DG, Malech HL, et al: Disorders of phagocyte chemotaxis. *Ann Intern Med* 92:520, 1980.

170. Mowat AG, Baum J: Chemotaxis of polymorphonuclear leukocytes from patients with diabetes mellitus. *N Engl J Med* 284:621, 1971.

171. Tan JS, Anderson JL, Watanakunakorn C, et al: Neutrophil dysfunction in diabetes mellitus. *J Lab Clin Med* 85:26, 1975.

172. Brayton RG, Stokes PE, Schwartz MS, Louria DB: Effect of alcohol and various diseases on leukocyte mobilization, phagocytosis, and intracellular killing. *N Engl J Med* 282:123, 1970.

173. Liu YK: The effect of alcohol on granulocytes and lymphocytes. *Semin Hematol* 17:130, 1980.

174. Dale DC, Fauci AS, Dupont G IV, Wolff SM: Comparison of agents producing a neutrophilic leukocytosis in man: Hydrocortisone, prednisone, endotoxin and etiocholanolone. *J Clin Invest* 56:808, 1975.

175. Breton-Gorius J: Abnormalities of granulocytes and megakaryocytes in preleukemic syndromes, in *Preleukemia,* edited by F Schmalzl, K-P Helbriegel, p 24. Springer-Verlag, Berlin, 1979.

176. Reding MT, Hibbs JR, Morrison VA, et al: Diagnosis and outcome of 100 consecutive patients with extreme granulocytic leukocytosis. *Amer J Med* 104:12, 1998.

177. Watanabe M, Ono K, Ozeki Y, et al: Production of granulocyte-macrophage colony-stimulating factor in a patient with metastatic chest wall large cell carcinoma. *Jap J Clin Oncol* 28:559, 1998.

178. Salloum E, Stoessel KM, Cooper DL: Hyperleukocytosis and retinal hemorrhages after chemotherapy and filgrastim administration for peripheral blood progenitor cell mobilization. *Bone Marrow Transpl* 21:835, 1998.

179. Crockard AD, Boylan MT, Droogan AG, et al: Methylprednisolone-induced neutrophil leukocytosis-down-modulation of neutrophil L-selectin and Mac-1 expression and induction of colony-stimulating factor. *Inter J Clin Lab Invest* 28:110, 1998.

180. Ceddia MA, Price EA, Kohlmeier CK, et al: Differential leukocytosis and lymphocyte mitogenic response to acute maximal exercise in the young and old. *Med Sci Sport Exer* 31:829, 1999.

NEUTROPENIA AND NEUTROPHILIA

DAVID C. DALE

Neutropenia designates a blood absolute neutrophil count that is less than two standard deviations below the normal population mean. Certain geographic areas contain population groups, such as those of African descent, in which the normal blood concentration of neutrophils is lower than in persons of European descent. Neutropenia results from diseases that decrease the normal rate of production of these cells in the marrow or from processes that accelerate neutrophil destruction, sequestration, or egress from the circulation. Some diseases spare erythrocyte and platelet production or survival and result in "isolated" neutropenia, such as chronic idiopathic neutropenia or drug-induced neutropenia. In some cases, other cell lineages are mildly affected but the neutropenia is severe, such as Felty syndrome. Neutropenia can be inherited or acquired. In some patients with either type of neutropenia, continuous cytokine therapy with granulocyte colony-stimulating factor can improve or restore the neutrophil count. Apparent neutropenia can occur as a result of a greater than normal proportion of neutrophils that are marginated in microvascular beds and not measured in the blood count; this condition does not lead to an increased risk of infection. Neutropenia may be an indicator of an underlying disease, such as early vitamin B_{12} deficiency or drug reaction. If severe, neutropenia increases the likelihood of contracting a bacterial or fungal infection and impairs the resolution of such infections.

Neutrophilia is an increase in the absolute neutrophil count to a concentration greater than two standard deviations above the normal population mean value. The most frequent causes of such an increase in count are inflammation or infection, but solid tumors occasionally may engender such a reaction. When the neutrophil count is very high, it may be referred to as a leukemoid reaction. The rare neutrophilic variants of chronic myeloid leukemia may also result in striking neutrophilia. Bacterial infections usually produce neutrophilia, whereas viral infections may not do so or the rise in neutrophil count may be slight. Demargination of neutrophils or rapid release of neutrophils from a large marrow pool may increase the blood neutrophil count transiently. Sustained increases require an increase in production of these cells. Neutrophilia facilitates the inflammatory response and antimicrobial action.

NEUTROPENIA

Neutropenia refers to an absolute blood neutrophil count (total leukocyte count per microliter × percent of neutrophils) that is less than two standard deviations below the normal mean of the population. The terms *leukopenia,* a reduced total white blood cell count, and *granulocytopenia,* reduced numbers of blood granulocytes (neutrophils, eosinophils, and basophils), sometimes are imprecisely used as synonyms for neutropenia. *Agranulocytosis* literally means a complete absence of blood granulocytes, but this term often is used to indicate severe neutropenia, i.e., less than $0.5 \times 10^3/\mu l$ ($0.5 \times 10^9/liter$).

The concentration of neutrophils in blood is influenced by age, activity, and genetic and environmental factors (see Chap. 2). For children from 1 month to 10 years old, neutropenia is defined as a blood neutrophil count of less than $1.5 \times 10^3/\mu l$ ($1.5 \times 10^9/liter$). For individuals over age 10, neutropenia is less than about $1.8 \times 10^3/\mu l$ ($1.8 \times 10^9/liter$) (see Chap. 7 regarding newborns). Healthy older persons have the same blood neutrophil counts as younger individuals (see Chap. 8). Some racial and ethnic groups, such as Africans, African Americans, and Yemenite Jews, have lower mean neutrophil counts than Americans of European ancestry. These mean differences in neutrophils are modest ($800-1000/\mu l$) and have no recognized health consequences.[1,2]

Neutropenia is a predisposing factor for infections, usually with the organisms normally found on the skin, in the nasopharynx, and as part of the intestinal flora. The risk of infections is inversely related to the severity of the neutropenia (see Chap. 17). Individuals with neutrophil counts of $1.0-1.8 \times 10^3/\mu l$ ($1.0-1.8 \times 10^9/liter$) are at little risk. In general, between 0.5×10^3 and $1.0 \times 10^3/\mu l$ ($0.5-1.0 \times 10^9/liter$) neutrophils, the risk is moderate. Individuals with neutrophil counts of less than $0.5 \times 10^3/\mu l$ ($0.5 \times 10^9/liter$) are at substantially greater risk, but the frequency of infections varies considerably, depending on the cause and duration of neutropenia. Severe acute neutropenia (i.e., developing over a few hours or days) is usually associated with greater risk of infection than severe chronic neutropenia (usually present for months or years). Neutropenia due to disorders of production, affecting early hematopoietic precursor cells (e.g., aplastic anemia, severe congenital neutropenia) results in a greater susceptibility to infections than conditions with adequate neutrophil precursors in the marrow and neutropenia attributed to accelerated turnover in the blood (e.g., rheumatoid arthritis, autoimmune neutropenia). For patients made severely neutropenic by cancer chemotherapy, the risk is greater when the neutrophils are decreasing than with similar counts when neutrophils are increasing. Neutropenia accompanied by monocytopenia, lymphocytopenia, or hypogammaglobulinemia is more serious than solitary neutropenia. Other factors, e.g., the integrity of the skin and mucous membranes, the vascular supply to tissues, and the nutritional status of the patient, also influence the risk of infections.

PATHOPHYSIOLOGIC MECHANISMS

GENERAL MECHANISMS

Neutropenia occurs because of reduced or ineffective production, accelerated utilization or turnover, shifts of cells from the circulating to the marginal blood pools, or a combination of these mechanisms (Fig. 71-1). Some production disorders are due to intrinsic abnormalities of hematopoietic progenitor cells (see Chaps. 14 and 91). Other disorders in cell production are caused by extrinsic factors, including changes in the marrow environment, e.g., tumor infiltration, fibrosis, or irradiation. Cytotoxic drugs usually cause more severe neutropenia earlier than anemia or thrombocytopenia because of the higher fractional turnover rate of neutrophils in the blood. Production is defined as ineffective when, under a steady state of hematopoiesis, there is a relative abundance of early neutrophil precursors and a paucity of late-maturing cells.

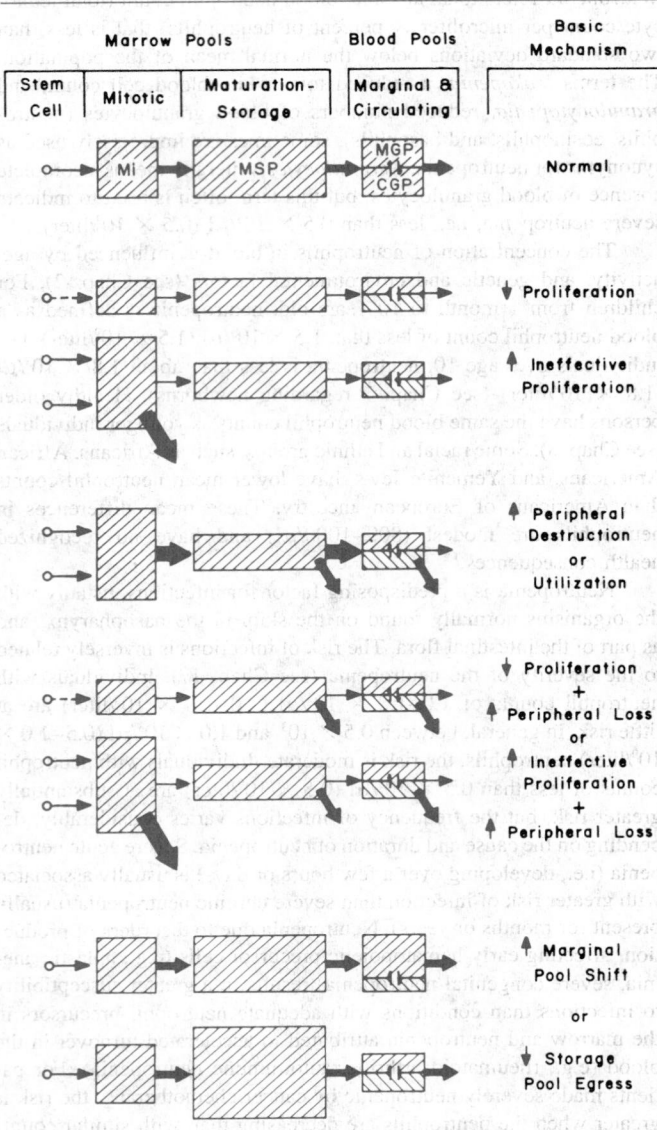

FIGURE 71-1　The mechanisms of neutropenia are shown schematically. The size of each pool is represented by the size of the cross-hatched areas. The rate of flow of cells through each compartment is represented by the size of the arrows. Mi, mitotic; MSP, maturation (marrow storage) pool; MGP, marginated granulocyte (neutrophil) pool; CGP, circulating granulocyte (neutrophil) pool.

Accelerated neutrophil utilization occurs with autoimmune neutropenia and acute bacterial infections. When there is both rapid neutrophil utilization and impaired production, acute severe neutropenia often develops. This is illustrated by the abrupt and sustained fall in neutrophils when an alcoholic patient develops pneumococcal pneumonia. Alcohol suppresses the marrow, and the infection consumes the available neutrophil supply. The abrupt fall in blood neutrophils at the onset of infection in patients recently given cancer chemotherapy reflects a similar mechanism. With idiosyncratic drug-induced neutropenia, the counts may fall abruptly because both blood and marrow cells are simultaneously damaged. When acute neutropenia develops because of a shift of blood neutrophils from the circulating to the marginal pool, i.e., increased margination (for example, after injection

of endotoxin, with exposure of blood to dialysis membranes, or after intravenous G-CSF or GM-CSF), it is usually a transient event.

CELLULAR AND MOLECULAR MECHANISMS OF NEUTROPENIA

Our understanding of the mechanisms of neutropenia at the cellular and molecular level is increasing rapidly, due to advances in molecular genetics and cell biology. For several diseases associated with neutropenia, such as the congenital immunodeficiency syndromes, the abnormal genetic loci have been identified, but the precise cellular mechanisms for failure to produce and maintain normal neutrophil levels is not yet known. In Kostmann syndrome, a form of congenital neutropenia, a cellular mechanism—namely, an abnormality of the G-CSFR receptor—has been identified in some, but not all, patients.[3] How this mutation leads to neutropenia is still unclear. Neutropenia can develop because of a failure of cell survival, i.e., apoptotic loss, due to acquired or congenital intrinsic defects, that is, to vitamin B_{12} deficiency,[4] myelodysplasia,[5] or myelokathexis.[6] Neutrophilia can be depleted from both the blood and the marrow due to extrinsic factors such as antibodies to specific neutrophil surface antigens, as in immune neutropenia. Some disorders that cause neutropenia also perturb neutrophil function, such as glycogen storage disease type 1b[7] and HIV infection.[8] The susceptibility to infection in these conditions relates to the combination of defects.

CAUSES OF NEUTROPENIA

Causes of neutropenia are classified physiologically as disorders of production, distribution, or turnover. Not every condition fits neatly into this scheme, but it provides a framework for understanding these diverse disorders.

DISORDERS OF PRODUCTION

Cytotoxic drugs given for cancer chemotherapy and as immunosuppressive agents regularly cause neutropenia by decreasing cell production (see Chap. 16). These drugs are probably now the most frequent cause for neutropenia in the United States. Neutropenia due to impaired production is a common feature of several diseases affecting hematopoietic stem cells, e.g., leukemia, aplastic anemia, and the myelodysplastic (preleukemic) syndromes. The selective causes for impaired production, progressing from disorders of early precursors to disorders presumed to involve defective maturation (ineffective production), are described briefly as follows.

Congenital Disorders　*Kostmann Syndrome and Related Disorders.*　In 1956, Kostmann described congenital neutropenia (agranulocytosis) as an autosomal recessive disease of families in northern Sweden.[9,10] Symptoms and signs of otitis, gingivitis, pneumonia, enteritis, peritonitis, and bacteremia usually begin in the first month of life. Often the neutrophil count is less than $0.2 \times 10^3/\mu l$ ($0.2 \times 10^9/$ liter). Eosinophilia, monocytosis, and splenomegaly may be present. Characteristically the marrow shows early neutrophil precursors (myeloblasts, promyelocytes) but few or no myelocytes or mature neutrophils. Marrow eosinophilia is common. In vitro marrow culture studies show that the number of colonies composed of granulocytes and monocytes (CFU-GM) and the response to some growth factors may be reduced.[11] Blood lymphocyte numbers are normal, immunoglobulin levels are usually normal or increased, and lymphocyte functions are intact. Some patients have abnormalities of the receptor for G-CSF; most frequently this is a truncation of the distal portion of the cytoplasmic domain of this receptor.[12] Patients' capacity for G-CSF and GM-CSF production appears to be normal.[13] Because there is no specific diagnostic test for this disorder, it may be difficult to distinguish isolated cases of Kostmann syndrome from other severe causes of neutropenia (agranulocytosis) of early childhood.

G-CSF is now recognized to be a very effective therapy in increasing the neutrophil count in patients with Kostmann syndrome.[14] However, patients with Kostmann syndrome and some other congenital neutropenia, including patients on long-term G-CSF treatment, have developed acute myelogenous leukemia, frequently in association with acquired abnormalities of the G-CSF receptor, monosomy 7, and Ras mutations, at a rate of about two percent per year.[15] No other cytokines are of proven efficacy; bone marrow transplantation is the alternative therapy for patients with a suitable donor.

Congenital Immunodeficiency Diseases.   Neutropenia is a feature of the congenital immunodeficiency diseases and a contributing factor to susceptibility to infection in many, but not all, patients (see Chap. 88). In X-linked agammaglobulinemia, which is attributed to defective B-cell development and a mutation in a cytoplasmic (Bruton) tyrosine kinase (Btk), severe neutropenia is present in approximately 25 percent of patients.[16] Children with common variable immunodeficiency often have neutropenia associated with thrombocytopenia and hemolytic anemia.[17] Neutropenia occurs in almost half of the patients with the X-linked hyper-IgM syndrome, a disorder caused by a mutation in the gene that encodes the CD-40 ligand.[18,19] With SCID, neutropenia is variably present.[20] The neutropenia also varies over time in individual patients. Neutropenia is particularly prominent in the rarest of the immunodeficiencies, reticular dysgenesis.[20,21] Neutropenia is a less common feature of adenosine deaminase deficiency, the $T-B+$, $T-B-$, and Omenn syndromes.[20] Case reports indicate that G-CSF therapy is effective in patients with neutropenia associated with immunodeficiencies, except that it appears to be ineffective in reticular dysgenesis.[22-27]

Cartilage-Hair Hypoplasia Syndrome.   In this rare autosomal recessive syndrome, short-limbed dwarfism is associated with hyperextensible digits, very fine hair, neutropenia, lymphopenia, and recurrent infections.[28] The degree of neutropenia is variable, ranging from 0.1 to $2.0 \times 10^3/\mu l$. It contributes to the recurrent respiratory infections of some patients. An accompanying defect in T-cell proliferation, with a defect in the transition from the G_0 to the G_1 of the lymphocyte miotic cycle, makes patients susceptible to viral respiratory infections[29]; the mechanism for neutropenia is not yet known.

Shwachman-Diamond Syndrome.   This autosomal recessive disorder combines short stature, pancreatic exocrine deficiency, and neutropenia beginning early in the neonatal period. The patients are malnourished, but the neutropenia is not corrected by improving their nutritional status. Thrombocytopenia and anemia may also be severe and evolution to myelodysplastic syndrome and acute myeloid leukemia occurs.[30,31]

Diamond-Blackfan Syndrome.   Neutropenia is a rare complication of congenital hypoplastic anemia; other features include congenital anomalies of the head and upper limbs. The varying severity of neutropenia may reflect genetic heterogeneity among patients with this diagnosis. The mechanism for neutropenia is not known.[32,33]

Gracelli Syndrome.   This rare autosomal recessive disorder is characterized by pigmentary dilution, variable degrees of cellular immunodeficiency, and an acute phase of uncontrolled lymphocyte and macrophage activation leading rapidly to death unless bone marrow transplantation is successful.[34-36] In the skin, there is accumulation of diffuse pigmentation due to melanosome accumulation in the patient's melanocytes. The pigmentation occurs because of an abnormal transfer of the cellular granules from the melanocytes to the keratinocytes. The mutation is in a gene on chromosome 15 at q21 that encodes a member of the myosin protein family. The neutropenia is relatively mild and associated with pancytopenia. Evolution to myelodysplasia has been reported.[37]

Chédiak-Higashi Syndrome.   This rare autosomal recessive disorder is characterized by partial oculocutaneous albinism, abnormal giant granules in many cells (including granulocytes, monocytes, and lymphocytes), neutropenia, and recurrent infections (see Chap. 72). The neutropenia is usually mild, and susceptibility to infection is attributed to both neutropenia and defective microbicidal activity of the phagocytes[38] (see Chap. 70).

Myelokathexis and Related Syndromes.   Myelokathexis is a rare autosomal dominant disorder in which patients have severe neutropenia and lymphocytopenia, with total white blood cell counts less than $1.0 \times 10^3/\mu l$, although the marrow has abundant precursors and developing neutrophils. Morphologic abnormalities in the marrow and blood include hypersegmentation and severely pyknotic nuclei, as well as cytoplasmic vacuoles. These morphologic changes and some molecular studies suggest cell loss in the marrow and blood by accelerated apoptosis.[6,39] Favorable responses to G-CSF and GM-CSF occur, as well as evolution to the myelodysplastic syndrome.[40,41] A myelokathexis-like variant of myelodysplastic syndrome has also been reported.[42] In the 1970s a condition called the "lazy leukocyte syndrome" was described in which the neutrophils accumulated in the marrow. The neutrophils were morphologically normal. The neutropenia was attributed to defective chemotaxis of cells in the marrow to the blood.[43] No genetic or molecular mechanism has yet been identified.

Glycogen Storage Diseases.   These autosomal recessive disorders are characterized by hypoglycemia, hepatosplenomegaly, seizures, and failure to thrive in infants. Neutropenia develops in glycogen storage disease type 1b, but not in other types. The marrow appears normal despite a severe reduction in blood neutrophils. The neutrophils have a reduced oxidative burst and defective chemotaxis.[44] The genetic defect maps to chromosome 11q23 and is attributed to an intracellular transport protein defect for glucose.[45] Treatment with G-CSF is effective for both correcting the neutropenia and improving the associated inflammatory bowel disease.[46,47]

Cyclic Neutropenia.   Cyclic neutropenia, an autosomal dominant or sporadically occurring disease, is characterized by regularly recurring episodes of severe neutropenia, usually every 21 days. It is diagnosed in young children, especially when there is a family history of this condition.[48,49] The neutropenic periods last for 3 to 6 days and are accompanied by malaise, anorexia, fever, lymphadenopathy, and ulcerations of the mucous membranes. There are also regular oscillations of other white blood cells, reticulocytes, and platelets. There is also an acquired syndrome in adults, some of whom have an associated clonal proliferation of large granular lymphocytes.[48]

Pathophysiologic studies in humans and in gray collie dogs, which have a very similar disorder, indicate that cycling is due to a defect in the regulation of hemopoietic stem cells.[50] Serial marrow culture studies show cyclical fluctuations in the number of granulocyte colonies, generally with fewer colonies forming from samples taken during the period of maximum neutrophilia.[51] Oscillations in colony-stimulating factors have been measured, but these changes probably are secondary to the recurrent inflammation which occurs with the neutropenic periods.

The diagnosis of cyclic neutropenia can be made only by serial differential counts, at least two or three times per week for a minimum of 6 weeks. Most affected children survive to adulthood; the symptoms are often milder after puberty. Fatal clostridial bacteremia has been reported in several cases, and careful observation is warranted with each neutropenic period in untreated patients. Treatment with granulocyte colony-stimulating factor is very effective.[52] It does not abolish cycling, but it shortens the neutropenic periods sufficiently to avoid symptoms and infections.[53]

Neutropenia Due to Genetic Defects of Folate, Cobalamin, and Transcobalamin II.   A variety of congenital disorders lead to disturbed function of the two cobalamin-requiring enzymes, methylmalo-nyl CoA mutase and methionine synthetase. Each of these disorders causes neutropenia, as well as anemia and thrombocytopenia, as a result of ineffective hematopoiesis[54,55] (see Chap. 25).

Chronic Idiopathic Neutropenia Several disorders, some congenital and some acquired, cause selective neutropenia in both children and adults. Childhood cases have been called familial (severe) neutropenia (probably autosomal dominant), familial benign neutropenia (probably autosomal dominant), chronic benign neutropenia of childhood (usually a negative family history), and chronic idiopathic neutropenia in adults (usually considered to be an acquired disease or occasionally, the case of affected children escaping detection until adulthood).[56-59]

Patients with these diverse syndromes share several characteristics: normal or near-normal erythrocyte, reticulocyte, lymphocyte, and platelet counts and normal or increased blood monocyte counts and immunoglobulin levels. The spleen is normal or only minimally enlarged. They have no chromosomal abnormalities or other evidence of myelodysplasia. Marrow examinations show a spectrum of abnormalities, from normal cellularity to selective hypoplasia of the neutrophilic series.[60,61] In most cases, quantitative marrow studies show that the ratio of immature to mature cells is increased, suggesting the loss of cells during the maturation process, that is, ineffective granulocytopoiesis. This suggests the presence of an intrinsic defect in the developing neutrophils or immunological mediated cell injury. In these cases, however, antineutrophil antibodies are not detected and tests for other autoantibodies, including antinuclear or antimitochondrial, are negative.[62]

The clinical course of individual patients usually can be predicted based on the level of the blood neutrophils, marrow examination, and the prior history of fevers and infections.[63] In general, patients with the lowest levels of blood neutrophils and the fewest neutrophil precursors in the marrow will have the most frequent problems. Long-term observations have shown, however, that some patients can have very low blood neutrophil levels with few or no infections. Evolution to acute leukemia or aplastic anemia generally does not occur. G-CSF will increase neutrophils in most patients and is a useful therapy for those with recurrent fever and infections.[64]

Acquired Disorders of Neutrophil Production *Neutropenia in Neonates of Hypertensive Mothers.* Hypertensive women often have low-birth weight infants with low neutrophil counts, attributed to decreased production.[65,66] The neutropenia is often severe with a high risk of infection, particularly during the first few weeks of life. The neutropenia usually resolves within a few weeks. G-CSF will elevate the neutrophils in this form of neonatal neutropenia, but the clinical benefit of treatment remains to be determined.[67]

Neutropenia Due to Nutritional Deficiencies. Neutropenia is an early and consistent feature of megaloblastic anemias due to vitamin B_{12} or folate deficiency, although when present it is usually accompanied by macrocytic anemia and mild thrombocytopenia (see Chap. 25). Copper deficiency can cause neutropenia in patients on total parenteral nutrition[68] and in malnourished children.[69] Mild neutropenia can occur in some patients with anorexia nervosa but is generally not a feature of kwashiorkor or marasmus.[70]

Neutropenia Due to Immune Suppression of Production. Pure white cell aplasia is a rare acquired disorder with severe selective neutropenia and a marrow devoid or nearly devoid of neutrophils and their precursors.[71] Some cases have been attributed to ibuprofen, chlorpropamide, excessive zinc, and various infectious and inflammatory diseases.[72-75] An autoimmune mechanism is suggested by presence of antibodies in the plasma of patients that bind to the human promyelocytic cell line HL-60.[76] Immunosuppressive therapy with antithymocyte globulin, corticosteroids, and cyclosporine has been used in individual cases.

DISORDERS AFFECTING NEUTROPHIL UTILIZATION AND TURNOVER

Mechanisms of Immune Neutropenia Neutropenia due to alterations of the distribution of cells in the blood and accelerated turnover is usually attributable to immunologic mechanisms. Antineutrophil antibodies are known to cause transfusion reactions, alloimmune neonatal neutropenia, and autoimmune neutropenia. Antigen-antibody complexes and autoantibodies are thought to be involved in the neutropenia of systemic lupus erythematosus and Felty syndrome. The association of neutropenia with increased numbers of circulating large granular lymphocytes has suggested that cellular as well as humoral immune mechanisms may be involved (see Chap. 85).

Neutrophils share surface antigens with other tissues including the i-I antigens and HLA antigens. They also have some specific antigens, including NA-1, NA-2 (now recognized as isotypes of Fcγ RIII or CD-16), NB-1, NC-1, and 9a.[77,78] A number of other antigens can be identified on neutrophils and neutrophil precursors with monoclonal antibodies. The clearest associations of autoantibodies and neutropenia are with NA-1 and NA-2.[77,78]

Several tests are available for detecting antineutrophil antibodies, including agglutination and microagglutination, cytotoxicity, direct and indirect immunofluorescence, direct and indirect antiglobulin assays, and tests involving the binding of staphylococcal protein A to immunoglobulins on the surface of cells.[78] The agglutination tests are the oldest methods and depend on the propensity of immunoglobulin-coated cells to aggregate. Immunofluorescence tests utilize anti–human gamma globulin tagged with a fluorescein label. These tests can be adapted for quantitative studies with a flow cytometer. Immunofluorescence and staphylococcal protein A–binding tests also can be adapted for examining immunoglobulins bound to single cells, including marrow cells. *Direct* methods are used to detect the antibodies on the patient's neutrophils. *Indirect* methods are used to test the patient's plasma or serum against panels of normal cells. The use of paraformaldehyde to expose antigens and to preserve the neutrophils for multiple tests has been especially helpful. Appropriate controls are essential for proper interpretation of these studies.

Causes of Immune Mediated Neutropenia *Alloimmune (Isoimmune) Neonatal Neutropenia.* Newborn infants may have neutropenia for a variety of reasons. In some cases it is due to the transplacental passage of maternal IgG antibodies that bind to the infant's neutrophil-specific antigens, usually the Fcγ RIII isotype inherited from the infant's father.[78,79] This disorder occurs in approximately one in 2000 neonates. It usually lasts for 2 to 4 months.

Alloimmune (isoimmune) neonatal neutropenia may be severe or relatively mild. It is often not recognized until bacterial infections occur in an otherwise healthy infant. The hematologic picture usually consists of severe neutropenia with normal to increased lymphocytes and normal monocytes, erythrocytes, and platelets. Marrow cellularity is normal or increased, with reduced numbers of mature neutrophils. Alloimmune neonatal neutropenia may be confused with neonatal sepsis, since the latter condition also causes severe neutropenia. The diagnosis of alloimmune neutropenia is usually made with neutrophil agglutination or immunofluorescence tests. Treatment should be conservative; antibiotics are used only when necessary. Exchange transfusions to decrease antibody titers or neutrophil transfusions from the patient's mother are rarely needed.

Autoimmune Neutropenia. It has been thought for years that neutrophil autoantibodies can decrease neutrophil survival and impair neutrophil production. It has proved difficult, however, to distinguish cases of autoimmune neutropenia unequivocally from cases of chronic idiopathic neutropenia.[80,81] Patients diagnosed as having autoimmune neutropenia usually have one or more positive tests for antineutrophil antibodies. They also usually have normal numbers of erythrocytes, platelets, and other leukocytes. Marrow morphology, colony-forming cells, and other tests are similar to those in cases of chronic idiopathic neutropenia. In general, therapy should be conservative and expectant. Intravenous gamma globulin may increase neutrophils but is generally not a satisfactory therapy. The response to glucocorticoid therapy is unpredictable. Daily or alternate day G-CSF is effective but should be reserved for patients with recurrent infections. Spontaneous remissions sometimes occur.

Systemic Lupus Erythematosus. Total leukocyte counts between 2 and 5 × 10³/μl (2–5 × 10⁹/liter) occur in about 60 percent of patients with systemic lupus erythematosus.[82,83] Mild neutropenia is often accompanied by monocytopenia and lymphocytopenia, anemia, thrombocytopenia, and mild degrees of splenomegaly. There is an increased amount of IgG on the surface of neutrophils, and immune complexes are increased within the neutrophils.[84] The marrow cellularity and maturation of cells is usually normal. Most patients with lupus do not have neutropenia severe enough to increase their susceptibility to infections, unless they are treated with immunosuppressive drugs (glucocorticoids, cytotoxic agents). G-CSF and GM-CSF have now been used to elevate neutrophils in many patients with SLE, including patients on immunosuppressive therapies.[85]

Rheumatoid Arthritis, Sjögren Syndrome, and Felty Syndrome. Leukopenia is unusual in association with rheumatoid arthritis, occurring in less than three percent of large series of patients. About one percent of patients with rheumatoid arthritis develop additional features of Felty syndrome (splenomegaly, deforming rheumatoid arthritis, and leukopenia).[86] Usually, these patients have had active, deforming arthritis and very high rheumatoid factor titers. The neutropenia may be moderate to severe; occasionally patients are seen with no circulating neutrophils. The incidence of bacterial infections in patients with Felty syndrome is low until the neutrophil count is under 0.2 × 10³/μl (0.2 × 10⁹/liter), which suggests that neutrophils are made but that their blood kinetics are altered. There is no clear relationship between spleen size and the neutrophil count. High levels of circulating and intracellular immune complexes and IgG on the surface of neutrophils have been observed. The marrow is usually normal or hypercellular, but occasionally it is hypocellular. Granulopoiesis is usually marked by sufficient precursors but few band or segmented neutrophils.

In Sjögren syndrome about 30 percent of patients have moderate leukopenia; the total leukocyte count is usually 2 to 5 × 10³/μl (2–5 × 10⁹/liter) with a normal differential count.[87,88] Rarely, severe neutropenia occurs associated with recurrent bacterial infections.

Therapeutic options include methotrexate, glucocorticoids, G-CSF, GM-CSF, and splenectomy. Results with these therapies are unpredictable.[89,90] Weekly methotrexate is preferred by many rheumatologists. G-CSF or GM-CSF can increase neutrophils but also may exacerbate arthralgias.[85] Splenectomy is followed by a rapid increase in counts in about two-thirds of cases, but about two-thirds of those who respond to splenectomy have a recurrence of neutropenia. A subset of patients with Felty syndrome has a high blood concentration of large granular lymphocytes with a phenotype characteristic of immature natural killer cells. These patients tend to respond poorly to all therapies directed toward increasing neutrophil levels.[91] Several factors in addition to neutropenia predispose these patients to infections, including monocytopenia, hypocomplementemia, circulating immune complexes, and treatment with glucocorticoids or cytotoxic drugs. In general, treatments to correct neutropenia should be reserved for patients with documented infections.

Other Causes of Neutropenia Associated With Splenomegaly In 1942 Wiseman and Doan described a disorder that they called *primary splenic neutropenia.*[92] Since that time it has been recognized that a variety of diseases also may cause this type of neutropenia, or pseudoneutropenia. Diseases associated with splenomegaly and neutropenia include sarcoidosis, lymphoma, tuberculosis, malaria,

kala-azar, and Gaucher disease. Usually there is thrombocytopenia and anemia as well. In patients with inflammatory diseases, immune mechanisms similar to those observed in patients with lupus erythematosus and Felty syndrome may be operative. In others, the sluggish blood flow through the spleen with passive trapping of neutrophils in the congested red pulp probably is the primary cause. For the most part the neutropenia in these patients is not sufficiently severe to be of clinical consequence. Removal of the spleen to raise the neutrophil count is rarely indicated.

DRUG-INDUCED NEUTROPENIA

Idiosyncratic drug reactions cause neutropenia with an estimated annual frequency of three cases per million population.[93] In 1922 Schultz reported six cases of severe sore throat and prostration with absent blood neutrophils, which led rapidly to sepsis and death.[94] A few years later this syndrome was associated with the coal tar-derived drug aminopyrine.[95] Over the past 50 years scores of other drugs have been recognized to cause this syndrome.

Two main types of idiosyncratic drug-induced neutropenia are recognized.[96,97] One type is a dose-related toxicity due to interference of the drug with protein synthesis or cell replication. This effect is often nonselective. It can involve the pluripotential hematopoietic stem cells and highly proliferative cells in other organs such as the epithelial cells of the gastrointestinal tract. Prototype drugs for this type of reaction include phenothiazines, antithyroid drugs, chloramphenicol, and clozapine.[98,99] Similar effects on marrow cells may also be mediated through free radicals and drug metabolites. Patients receiving multiple drugs and patients having high plasma concentration of drugs due, for example, to the dose administered, to slow metabolism, or to renal impairment are more prone to develop these reactions.[100]

A second type of drug-induced neutropenia may not be dose related. It is thought to be allergic or immunologic in origin, similar to drug-induced skin reactions and drug-initiated, antibody-mediated erythrocyte destruction. These reactions occur with an even broader array of drugs.[101–103] Large studies suggest that women are affected more often than men, that older patients are affected more frequently than younger ones, and that patients with a history of allergies, including allergies to other drugs, are affected more often than individuals without the allergies. Neutropenia may occur at any time but tends to occur relatively early in the course of treatment with drugs to which the patient has been previously exposed.

Our basic understanding of drug-induced neutropenia is limited, in part because of the unpredictable occurrence of cases, the myriad agents involved, and the lack of good animal models for research. Clinical studies suggest that the rate of recovery can be roughly predicted from the degree of marrow hypoplasia found when neutropenia is discovered. Once the offending drug is stopped, patients with sparse marrow neutrophils but normal-appearing precursor cells (promyelocytes and myelocytes) will have neutrophils reappear in the blood in about 4 to 7 days. Often an increase in the blood monocyte count heralds marrow recovery, and an "overshoot" with marked neutrophilia will follow. When early precursor cells are severely depleted, recovery may take considerably longer.

Patients with drug-induced neutropenia usually present with fever, myalgia, and sore throat; they usually do not have a rash or evidence of allergy elsewhere. The blood examination shows few or absent neutrophils. There may be mild lymphopenia, but other cell counts are usually normal. A high level of suspicion and careful clinical history are critical to identifying the offending drug. The differential diagnosis includes acute viral infections, particularly infectious mononucleosis and infectious hepatitis, and acute bacterial sepsis. If other hematologic abnormalities are also present, acute leukemia and aplastic anemia should be considered. Treatment usually consists of supportive care, including broad spectrum antibiotics for febrile patients. The benefit of hematopoietic growth factors in this setting has not been established in randomized trials.[104,105]

Table 71-1 lists some of the drugs frequently implicated in neutropenia. With the rapidity of introduction of new agents, when questions arise it is often useful to consult the manufacturer, a drug information center, or a poison control center to learn if a drug may cause neutropenia.

NEUTROPENIA WITH INFECTIOUS DISEASES

Neutropenia can result from acute or chronic bacterial, viral, parasitic, or rickettsial diseases. Several mechanisms are involved. Certain viral infections, e.g., infectious mononucleosis, infectious hepatitis, parvovirus B-19, Kawasaki disease, and human immunodeficiency virus (HIV) infection, may cause severe or protracted neutropenia and pancytopenia due to infection of hematopoietic precursor cells. Other agents, e.g., *Rickettsia* and *Bartonella*, can infect endothelial cells. They may cause leukopenia, neutropenia, thrombocytopenia, and anemia as part of a generalized vasculitic process. In dengue, measles,

and other viral infections, increased neutrophil adherence to altered endothelial cells may occur. With severe gram-negative bacterial infections, neutropenia is probably due to increased adherence to the endothelium as well as increased utilization at the site of infection. Some chronic infections causing splenomegaly, e.g., tuberculosis, brucellosis, typhoid fever, malaria, and kala-azar, probably cause neutropenia because of splenic sequestration and marrow suppression.

A CLINICAL APPROACH TO THE PATIENT PRESENTING WITH NEUTROPENIA

Ordinarily, patients with the acute onset of severe neutropenia present with fever, sore throat, and evidence of inflammation beneath the skin or mucous membranes. This is an urgent clinical situation requiring prompt microbial cultures, the institution of intravenous fluids, antibiotics, and other supportive measures. In the absence of recent hospitalization and antibiotic exposure, infections in this situation usually are caused by surface bacteria sensitive to numerous agents. Immediate investigation should include a careful history with particular attention to drugs and a physical examination with careful attention to the presence of bone tenderness and the size of the lymph nodes and spleen. The blood and marrow film should be studied thoroughly for atypical lymphocytes and abnormal cells. The marrow may show fibrosis, selective or nonselective hypoplasia, excessive blasts, or atypical cells. With this information in hand and supportive care started, further diagnostic tests can be considered, including measurements of antineutrophil antibodies, studies of in vitro marrow progenitor cell-proliferative activity, and studies of possible mechanisms for drug-induced neutropenia.

Chronic neutropenia usually is discovered as a chance finding with a routine examination or during the course of investigation of a patient with recurrent fevers and infections. It is useful to know if the neutropenia is chronic or cyclic and the mean level of the blood cell counts when the patient is afebrile and relatively well. Other hematologic and immunologic data that are important include the absolute monocyte, lymphocyte, eosinophil, and platelet counts; hematocrit or hemoglobin determination; and immunoglobulin levels. Patients with hypergammaglobulinemia usually have chronic and recurrent inflammation; patients with hypogammaglobulinemia and neutropenia usually are very susceptible to recurrent infections. Morphologic examination of the blood and marrow can identify some causes of benign neutropenia in children, the Chédiak-Higashi syndrome, and myelokathexis. The marrow examination is most useful to rule out leukemia and myelodysplastic disorders and to assess the severity of the marrow defect.

In patients with chronic neutropenia, it may be useful to measure antinuclear antibodies (ANA) and rheumatoid factor titers and to perform other serologic tests for autoimmune diseases. Usually, neutropenia associated with

---

TABLE 71-1   CLASSIFICATION OF WIDELY USED DRUGS ASSOCIATED WITH IDIOSYNCRATIC NEUTROPENIA

Analgesics and Anti-inflammatory Agents
  Indomethacin*
  Gold salts
  Pentazocine
  *Para-*aminophenol derivatives*
    Acetaminophen
    Phenacetin
  Pyrazolone derivatives*
    Aminopyrine
    Dipyrone
    Oxyphenbutazone
    Phenylbutazone
Antibiotics
  Cephalosporins
  Chloramphenicol*
  Clindamycin
  Gentamicin
  Isoniazid
  *Para-*aminosalicylic acid
  Penicillins and semisynthetic penicillins*
  Rifampin
  Streptomycin
  Sulfonamides*
  Tetracyclines
  Trimethoprim-sulfamethoxazole
  Vancomycin
Anticonvulsants
  Carbamazepine
  Mephenytoin
  Phenytoin
Antidepressants
  Amitriptyline
  Amoxapine
  Desipramine
  Doxepin
  Imipramine
Antihistamines—H₂ blockers
  Cimetidine
  Ranitidine

Antimalarials
  Amodiaquine
  Chloroquine
  Dapsone
  Pyrimethamine
  Quinine
Antithyroid Drugs
  Carbimazole
  Methimazole
  Propylthiouracil
Cardiovascular Drugs
  Captopril
  Disopyramide
  Hydralazine
  Methyldopa
  Procainamide
  Propranolol
  Quinidine
  Tocainide
Diuretics
  Acetazolamide
  Chlorthalidone
  Chlorothiazide
  Ethacrynic acid
  Hydrochlorothiazide
Hypoglycemic Agents
  Chlorpropamide
  Tolbutamide
Hypnotics and Sedatives
  Chlordiazepoxide and other benzodiazepines
  Meprobamate
Phenothiazines
  Chlorpromazine
  Phenothiazines
Other Drugs
  Allopurinol
  Clozapine
  Levamisole
  Penicillamine
  Ticlopidine

*More frequently reported to cause neutropenia in epidemiologic studies.
NOTE: Documentation of the role of specific drugs in the causation of neutropenia is dependent on: (1) the frequency of the occurrence among patients; (2) the timing of the event in relationship to drug use; (3) the absence of alternative explanations; or (4) the inadvertent or intentional reuse of the drug (rechallenges) with a similar response. Readers who require supplementary lists of putative drugs involved in the development of neutropenia or wish to read original references for these interactions are referred to: The International Agranulocytosis and Aplastic Anemia Study, Risks of agranulocytosis and aplastic anemia, *JAMA* 256:1749, 1986; HP Roeser, Drug-bone marrow interactions, *Med J Australia* 146:145, 1987; Hemopoietic System, in *Meyler's Side Effects of Drugs,* 10th ed, edited by MNG Dukes, pp 951–953, Elsevier, New York, 1984; DW Kaufman, Drugs in the aetiology of agranulocytosis and aplastic anaemia, *Eur J Haematol Suppl* 60:23, 1996.

these disorders occurs in patients with obvious and severe disease, but occasionally patients are seen with occult splenomegaly, high ANA and rheumatoid factor titers, and a few other symptoms. Examination of the blood and marrow for large granular lymphocytes also may be helpful. Infectious and nutritional causes for chronic neutropenia are rare and rarely difficult to recognize. In adults, the most difficult differentiation may be between chronic idiopathic neutropenia and the myelodysplastic syndromes. Abnormalities in other cell lines (e.g., anemia, poikilocytosis and thrombocytopenia, pseudo-Pelger-Huët cells), atypical cells in the marrow, and chromosomal abnormalities suggest myelodysplasia, particularly in older patients. Investigations of the mechanism of neutropenia with marrow and blood kinetic studies, in vitro marrow cultures, measurements of marrow granulocyte reserves, and indirect measurements of marrow-proliferative activity may be useful to define mechanisms of neutropenia but are not widely available.

NEUTROPHILIA

Neutrophilia is defined as an increase in the absolute blood neutrophil count to a level greater than two standard deviations above the mean value for normal individuals. For children 1 month or older and adults of all ages this level is about $7.5 \times 10^3/\mu l$ (7.5×10^9/liter) bands and mature neutrophils (see Chap. 2). At birth the mean neutrophil count is $12 \times 10^3/\mu l$ (12×10^9/liter), and counts as high as $26 \times 10^3 \ \mu l$/liter (26×10^9/liter) are regarded as normal (see Chap. 7).

Several terms are used almost synonymously with neutrophilia, including *neutrophilic leukocytosis, polymorphonuclear leukocytosis,* and *granulocytosis. Leukocytosis* is used because an elevation of the number of neutrophils is the most frequent cause for an increase in the total white cell count. *Granulocytosis* is less specific than neutrophilia, since granulocytes include eosinophils and basophils as well as neutrophils. Extreme neutrophilia is often referred to as a *leukemoid reaction* because the height of the white cell count may suggest leukemia. This exaggerated reaction may be the result of segmented neutrophils or may be associated with band neutrophils, metamyelocytes, and myelocytes in smaller proportions.

In normal individuals, neutrophil counts follow a diurnal pattern of variation, with peak counts in the late afternoon. Neutrophil counts also rise slightly after meals, with erect posture, and with emotional stimuli. Ordinarily these changes are not sufficient to cause neutrophilia.[108]

MECHANISMS OF NEUTROPHILIA

Under normal circumstances neutrophils follow an orderly progression from the marrow through the blood to tissue sites of utilization.[1,2] Neutrophilia may occur by several mechanisms: increased cell production, accelerated release of cells from the marrow into the blood, shift within the circulation from the marginal to the circulating pool, reduced egress of neutrophils from the blood to tissues, or a combination of these mechanisms. The time required for these events varies substantially. Shifts between the marginal and circulating pools take only a few minutes. Shifts of neutrophils from the marrow to the blood occur within a few hours. Increases in the production of neutrophils, even with intense stimulation, may take at least a few days (Fig. 71-2).

ACUTE NEUTROPHILIA

Pseudoneutrophilia (Demargination)   Vigorous exercise and acute physical and emotional stress can substantially increase the number of blood neutrophils within a few minutes.[109,110] This response is mimicked by the infusion of epinephrine and other catecholamines that increase heart rate and cardiac output.[111] It is caused by a shift of cells from the marginal to the circulating pool; hence it is frequently referred to as *demargination*. In humans this response is dependent partially on release of neutrophils from the spleen,[112] but redistribution from other vascular beds, particularly the pulmonary capillaries,[113] is quantitatively more important. The increase in lymphocytes and monocytes, in addition to neutrophils, that occurs with demargination may be helpful in distinguishing this type of neutrophilia from the response to infections, protracted stress, or glucocorticoid administration. With these conditions, neutrophil counts are elevated but lymphocyte and monocyte counts generally are depressed.

Marrow Storage Pool Shift   Acute neutrophilia also occurs as a consequence of release of neutrophils from the marrow storage pool, the *marrow neutrophil reserves.*[114] This mechanism produces acute neutrophilia in response to inflammation and infections. The marrow reserve pool consists principally of segmented neutrophils and bands; metamyelocytes are not released to the blood except under extreme circumstances. The postmitotic marrow neutrophil pool is approximately ten times the size of the blood neutrophil pool, and about one-half of these cells are band and segmented neutrophils.[107] In neutrophil production disorders, in chronic inflammatory diseases and malignancies, and with cancer chemotherapy, the size of this pool is reduced and the capacity to develop neutrophilia is impaired. Exposure of blood to foreign surfaces, such as hemodialysis membranes, activates the complement system and causes transient neutropenia followed by neutrophilia due to release of marrow neutrophils.[115] Colony-stimulating factors (i.e., G-CSF and GM-CSF), cause acute and chronic neutrophilia by mobilizing cells from the marrow reserves and stimulate neutrophil production.[116,117]

CHRONIC NEUTROPHILIA

Chronic neutrophilia follows a prolonged stimulus to proliferation of neutrophil precursors. It can be studied experimentally with repeated doses of endotoxin, glucocorticoids, or colony-stimulating factors. Although the details of the mediators and mechanisms for the development of chronic neutrophilia are not understood fully, a general scheme for this response is now widely accepted (see Fig. 71-2). Expansion of cell production follows stimulation of cell divisions within the mitotic precursor pool, that is, divisions of promyelocytes and myelocytes. Subsequently, the size of the *postmitotic pool* increases. These changes cause an increase in the marrow granulocytic-to-erythroid ratio. In humans the neutrophil production rate increases severalfold with chronic infections; even greater increases may occur in polycythemia vera, chronic myelogenous leukemia, and leukemoid reactions in response to nonhematologic malignancies[118] and in response to exogenously administered hematopoietic growth factors such as G-CSF,[116,117] with a maximum response taking at least a week to develop.

Neutrophilia due to decreased egress from the vascular compartment occurs infrequently. A prototype disorder illustrating this mechanism occurs in patients with the neutrophil cell membrane defect CD11a/CD18 deficiency.[119] The neutrophils do not adhere to the capillary endothelium normally, but cell production and marrow release are apparently normal. Because these patients cannot mobilize neutrophils to sites of inflammation when they develop infections, extreme neutrophilia is observed (see Chap. 72). Glucocorticoids may produce a functionally similar state, with neutrophils accumulating in the blood, at least transiently, after each dose is administered.[120,121] In patients recovering from infections, as the "tissue demand" for neutrophils diminishes, the persistence of neutrophilia may be attributed to this same mechanism. In chronic myelogenous leukemia, accumulation of neutrophils with a longer than normal half-life in the blood is a partial explanation for the extreme neutrophilia.[122]

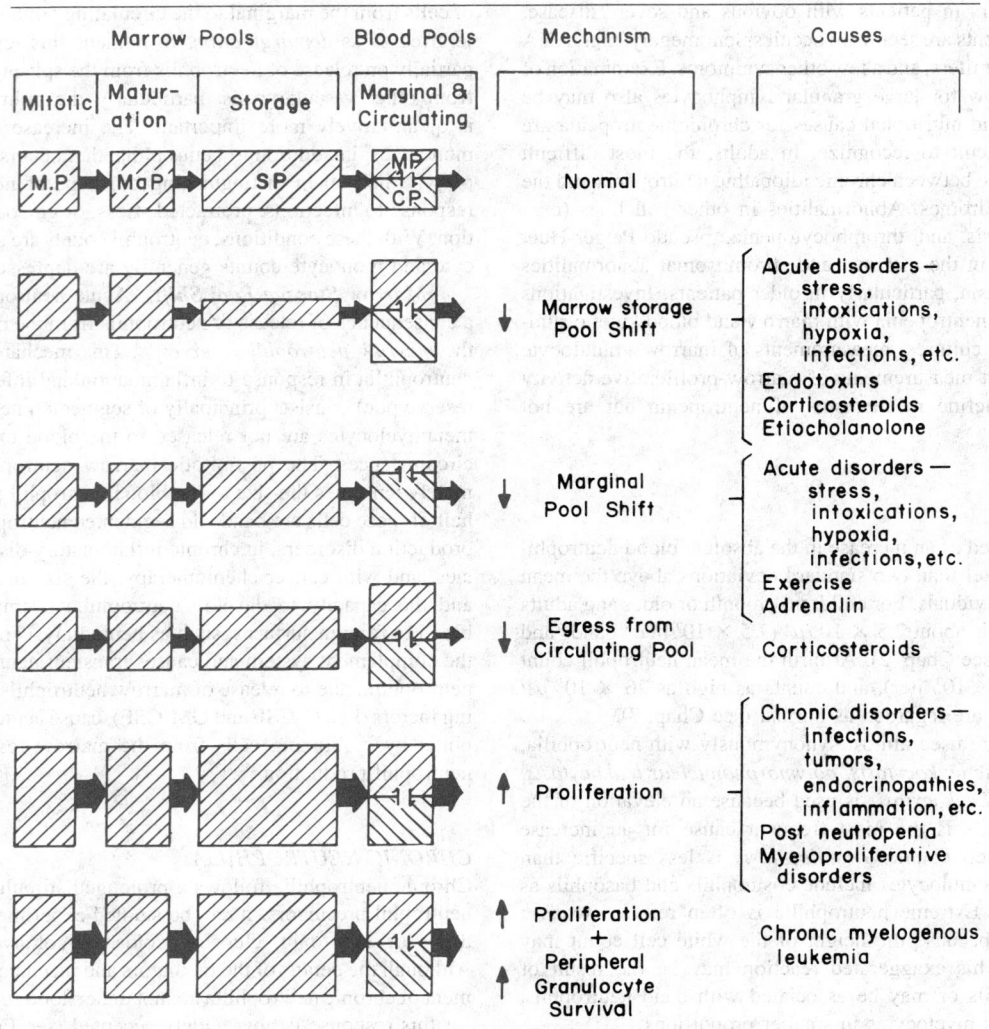

FIGURE 71-2   The mechanisms of neutrophilia are shown schematically. The rate of flow of cells through each compartment is represented by the size of the arrows. M.P., mitotic pool; MaP, maturation (postmitotic) pool; SP, storage pool (marrow reserves); MP, marginated neutrophil pool; CP, circulating neutrophil pool.

DISORDERS ASSOCIATED WITH NEUTROPHILIA

Neutrophilia in Response to Inflammation and Stress The categories and causes of acute and chronic neutrophilia are listed in Table 71-2. Probably the most frequent causes for acute neutrophilia are exercise, emotional stress, or any other circumstance that raises endogenous epinephrine, norepinephrine, or cortisol levels. Acute neutrophilia also occurs in pregnant patients and may be especially notable at the time of entering labor; with induction of general or epidural anesthesia; with all types of surgery; and with other acute events such as seizures, gastrointestinal hemorrhage, subarachnoid hemorrhage, or other internal bleeding.

Neutrophilia occurs with many acute bacterial infections. It occurs less predictably with infections caused by viruses, fungi, and parasites. Many aspects of the complex interactions of microbes with the infected host are not yet fully understood. Most patients with gram-positive infections, e.g., pneumococcal pneumonia, staphylococcal abscesses, or streptococcal pharyngitis, have neutrophilia. Infections caused by gram-negative bacteria, particularly those resulting in bacteremia or septic shock, may cause neutropenia or extreme neutrophilia.[123] Increased circulating levels of activated complement components, G-CSF, tumor necrosis factor, and the interleukins IL-1, IL-6, and

IL-8 may cause this response. Bacterial infections that have an insidious onset and cause splenomegaly, such as typhoid fever and brucellosis, characteristically do not show neutrophilia except in the initial or disseminated phases. Miliary tuberculosis is an important cause of leukemoid reactions. With viral infections, neutrophilia is far less common. In general, neutrophilia is seen in those infections producing substantial tissue injury, evoked by toxins produced by the infecting organisms. Damage to host tissues is also the presumed mechanism of neutrophilia in thermal burns, electric shock, myocardial infarction, pulmonary embolism, sickle cell crisis, and systemic vasculitis.

There are many chronic noninfectious conditions causing neutrophilia. Probably the most frequent cause is cigarette smoking.[124] Neutrophil counts of smokers are increased in proportion to the amount of exposure. Neutrophil counts of smokers inhaling two packs per day are on average twice the normal levels. Chronic inflammatory diseases, including dermatitis, bronchitis, rheumatoid arthritis, ulcerative colitis, and gout, may cause a persistent neutrophilia. Sweet syndrome is an unusual dermatologic condition with intense neutrophil accumulation in the skin and persistent neutrophilia.[125]

Neutrophilia in Association With Cancer or Heart Disease Neutrophilia is associated with many nonhematologic malignancies, e.g., lung and gastrointestinal malignancies, particularly when they metastasize to the liver and lung.[118,126] In some cases tumor cells have been found to produce colony-stimulating factors that presumably cause the neutrophilia by direct marrow stimulation.[127,128] Tumor necrosis and superinfections are other possible mechanisms. Neutrophilia is unusual in brain tumors, melanoma, prostate cancer, and lymphocytic malignancies.[126]

Neutrophilia is a marker for both the occurrence and severity of a variety of illnesses. Neutrophilia is associated with an increased incidence and severity of coronary heart disease independent of smoking status.[129–131] Similarly, elevated white cell counts have been associated with increased cancer mortality independent of smoking history.[132] In patients with cancer, subarachnoid hemorrhage, and other serious inflammatory conditions, neutrophilia portends a less favorable prognosis.[133]

Neutrophilia as a Manifestation of an Hematologic Disorder.   In addition to the myeloproliferative syndromes including chronic neutrophilic leukemia and neutrophilic chronic myelogenous leukemia (see Chap. 94), several unusual hematologic conditions may be associated with neutrophilia. The mechanisms for most of these disorders remain obscure. In Down syndrome, transient neonatal leukemoid reactions may occur that resemble chronic myelogenous leukemia.[134] This type of neutrophilia may be related to a defect in regulation of neutrophil production caused by the chromosome 21 trisomy, but the precise mechanism is unknown. Idiopathic neutrophilic leukocytosis with a negative family history and a similar condition of hereditary neutrophilia with an autosomal dominant pattern of inheritance have been reported[135,136] but are very rare conditions. Careful clinical examination and follow-up will almost always result in an explanation for neutrophilia.

Neutrophilia Associated With Drugs   Many drugs cause neutropenia, but neutrophilia in response to drugs is uncommon except for the well-known effects of epinephrine, other catecholamines, and glucocorticoids. Lithium salts cause sustained neutrophilia.[137] The counts return to normal when the drug is discontinued. The drug increases levels of colony-stimulating factor. Cases of neutrophilia have been reported with ranitidine and quinidine therapy, but such reactions are very uncommon.

CLINICAL APPROACH TO PATIENTS WITH NEUTROPHILIA

In most instances the finding of neutrophilia, band neutrophils, and toxic granules in the mature cells can be related to an obvious ongoing inflammatory condition. Often the finding of neutrophilia helps to secure the diagnosis of appendicitis, cholecystitis, or bacterial pharyngitis. When the cause of neutrophilia is not readily apparent, especially if the neutrophilia is associated with fever or other signs of inflammation, more subtle infections such as tuberculosis or osteomyelitis should be considered. In addition, a history of smoking, along with evidence for a chronic anxiety state or an occult malignancy, should be sought. If neutrophilia is accompanied by myelocytes and promyelocytes, increased basophils, and unexplained splenomegaly, the diagnosis of a myeloproliferative disease (e.g., chronic myelogenous leukemia, idiopathic myelofibrosis, or polycythemia vera) should be

TABLE 71-2   MAJOR CAUSES OF NEUTROPHILIA

ACUTE NEUTROPHILIA	CHRONIC NEUTROPHILIA
Physical Stimuli Cold, heat, exercise, convulsions, pain, labor, anesthesia, surgery *Emotional Stimuli* Panic, rage, severe stress, depression	*Infections* Persistence of infections that cause acute neutrophilia *Inflammation* Most acute inflammatory reactions, such as colitis, dermatitis, drug-sensitivity reactions, gout, hepatitis, myositis, nephritis, pancreatitis, periodontitis, rheumatic fever, rheumatoid arthritis, vasculitis, thyroiditis, Sweet syndrome *Tumors* Gastric, bronchogenic, breast, renal, hepatic, pancreatic, uterine, and squamous cell cancers; rarely Hodgkin's disease, lymphoma, brain tumors, melanoma, and multiple myeloma
Infections Many localized and systemic acute bacterial, mycotic, rickettsial, spirochetal, and certain viral infections	
Inflammation or Tissue Necrosis Burns, electric shock, trauma, infarction, gout, vasculitis, antigen-antibody complexes, complement activation *Drugs, Hormones, and Toxins* Colony-stimulating factors, epinephrine, etiocholanolone, endotoxin, glucocorticoids, smoking tobacco, vaccines, venoms	*Drugs, Hormones, and Toxins* Continued exposure to many substances that produce acute neutrophilia, lithium; rarely as a reaction to other drugs *Metabolic and Endocrinologic Disorders* Eclampsia, thyroid storm, overproduction of ACTH *Hematologic Disorders* Rebound from agranulocytosis or therapy of megaloblastic anemia, chronic hemolysis or hemorrhage, asplenia, myeloproliferative disorders, chronic idiopathic leukocytosis *Hereditary and Congenital Disorders* Down syndrome, congenital

considered. Measurement of the leukocyte alkaline phosphatase activity can be a useful screening test in cases of moderate neutrophilia (15 to 25 × 10³ neutrophils/μl [15–25 × 10⁹ neutrophils/liter]). Ordinarily the values are elevated with inflammation of any cause and in subjects receiving glucocorticoid therapy. The values are low in chronic myelogenous leukemia and variable with other myeloproliferative disorders. Serum vitamin B_{12} levels and B_{12}-binding proteins are elevated in both benign neutrophilia and chronic myelogenous leukemia. In unexplained neutrophilia, testing for the cytogenetic alterations and the BCR gene rearrangement is important in the diagnostic evaluation. The diagnosis of chronic myelogenous leukemia and of other myeloproliferative disorders with prominent neutrophilia are considered in Chapter 94.

Except for the epidemiologic associations of neutrophilia with adverse effects of smoking, coronary artery disease, and malignancies, there is no known direct adverse effect of an elevated circulating neutrophil count. In some inflammatory diseases, glucocorticoids and immunosuppressive therapies are used to reduce inflammation; a part of their mechanism is to reduce production and deployment of neutrophils and other leukocytes. For instance, glucocorticoids usually suppress the inflammation of the skin in Sweet syndrome.[125] Otherwise, specific therapy to reduce the neutrophil counts generally is not indicated.

REFERENCES

1. Sahr F, Hazra PK, Grillo TA: White blood cell count in healthy Sierra Leoneans. *West Afr J Med* 14:105, 1995.

2. Weingarten MA, Pottick-Schwartz EA, Brauner A: The epidemiology of benign leukopenia in Yemenite Jews. *Isr J Med Sci* 29:297, 1993.

3. Tidow N, Pilz C, Teichmann B, et al: Clinical relevance of point mutations in the cytoplasmic domain of the granulocyte colony-stimulating

factor receptor gene in patients with severe congenital neutropenia. *Blood* 90:2839, 1997.

4. Bunting RW, Selig MK, Dickersin GR: Apoptotic cells in peripheral blood from patients with low serum cobalamin. *J Submicrosc Cytol Pathol* 29:223, 1997.

5. Bouscary D, DeVos J, Guesnu M, et al: Fas/Apo-1 (CD95) expression and apoptosis in patients with myelodysplastic syndromes. *Leukemia* 11:839, 1997.

6. Liles WC, Park JR, Chi EY, Dale DC: Myelokathexis—a congenital form of neutropenia characterized by accelerated apoptosis and defective expression of BCL-X in neutrophil precursors. *Blood* 86:259a, 1995.

7. Gitzelman R, Bosshard NU: Defective neutrophil and monocyte functions in glycogen storage disease type Ib: a literature review. *Eur J Pediatr* 152:S33, 1993.

8. Pitrak DL, Bak PM, DeMarais P, et al: Depressed neutrophil superoxide production in human immunodeficiency virus infection. *J Infect Dis* 167:1406, 1993.

9. Kostmann R: Infantile genetic agranulocytosis. *Acta Paediatr Scand* 105:1(suppl), 1956.

10. Kostmann R: Infantile genetic agranulocytosis. *Acta Paediatr Scand* 64:362, 1975.

11. Hestdal K, Welte K, Lie SO, et al: Severe congenital neutropenia: abnormal growth and differentiation of myeloid progenitors to granulocyte colony-stimulating factor (G-CSF) but normal response to G-CSF plus stem cell factor. *Blood* 82:2991, 1993.

12. Dong F, Hoefsloot LH, Schelen AM, et al: Identification of a nonsense mutation in the granulocyte colony-stimulating factor receptor in severe congenital neutropenia. *Proc Natl Acad Sci U S A* 91:4480, 1994.

13. Bernhardt TM, Burchardt ER, Welte K: Assessment of G-CSF and GM-CSF mRNA expression in peripheral blood mononuclear cells from patients with severe congenital neutropenia and in human myeloid leukemic cell lines. *Exp Hematol* 21:163–168, 1993.

14. Welte K, Boxer LA: Severe chronic neutropenia: pathophysiology and therapy. *Semin Hematol* 34:267, 1997.

15. Freedman MH: Safety of long-term administration of granulocyte colony-stimulating factor for severe chronic neutropenia. *Curr Opin Hematol* 4:217, 1997.

16. Farrar JE, Rohrer J, Conley ME: Neutropenia in X-linked agammaglobulinemia. *Clin Immunol Immunopathol* 81:271, 1996.

17. Conley ME, Park CL, Douglas SD: Childhood common variable immunodeficiency with autoimmune disease. *J Pediatr* 108:915, 1986.

18. Allen RC, Armitage RJ, Conley ME, et al: CD40 ligand gene defects responsible for X-linked hyper-IgM syndrome. *Science* 259:990, 1993.

19. Levy J, Espanol-Boren T, Thomas C, et al: Clinical spectrum of X-linked hyper-IgM syndrome. *J Pediatr* 131:47, 1997.

20. Stephan JL, Vlekova V, LeDeist F, et al: Severe combined immunodeficiency: a retrospective single-center study of clinical presentation and outcome in 117 patients. *J Pediatr* 123:564, 1993.

21. Buckley RH, Schiff RI, Schiff SE, et al: Human severe combined immunodeficiency: genetic, phenotypic, and functional diversity in one hundred eight infants. *J Pediatr* 130:378, 1997.

22. Bujan W, Ferster A, Sariban E, Friedrich W: Effect of recombinant human granulocyte colony-stimulating factor in reticular dysgenesis. *Blood* 82:1684, 1993.

23. Azcona C, Alzina V, Barona P, Sierrases'umaga L, Villa-El'izaga I: Use of recombinant human granulocyte-macrophage colony-stimulating factor in an infant with reticular dysgenesis. *Eur J Pediatr* 153:164, 1994.

24. Niehus T, Schwarz K, Schneider M, et al: Severe combined immunodeficiency (SCID) associated neutropenia: a lesson from monozygotic twins. *Arch Dis Child* 74:340, 1996.

25. Ostenstad B, Giliani S, Mellbye OJ, et al: A boy with X-linked hyper-IgM syndrome and natural killer cell deficiency. *Clin Exp Immunol* 107:230, 1997.

26. Wang WC, Cordoba J, Infante AJ, Conley ME: Successful treatment of neutropenia in the hyper-immunoglobulin M syndrome with granulocyte colony-stimulating factor. *Am J Pediatr Hematol Oncol* 16:160, 1994.

27. Calhoun DA, Christensen RD: Recent advances in the pathogenesis and treatment of nonimmune neutropenias in the neonate. *Curr Opin Hematol* 5:37, 1998.

28. Lux SE, Johnston RB Jr, August CS, et al: Chronic neutropenia and abnormal cellular immunity in cartilage-hair hypoplasia. *N Engl J Med* 282:231, 1970.

29. Kooijman R, van der Burgt CJ, Weemaes CM, et al: T cell subsets and T cell function in cartilage-hair. *Scand J Immunol* 46:209, 1997.

30. Smith OP, Hann IM, Chessells JM, et al: Haematological abnormalities in Shwachman-Diamond syndrome. *Br J Haematol* 94:279, 1996.

31. Welte K, Boxer LA: Severe chronic neutropenia: pathophysiology and therapy. *Semin Hematol* 34:267, 1997.

32. Schofield KP, Evans DI: Diamond-Blackfan syndrome and neutropenia. *J Clin Pathol* 44:742, 1991.

33. Krijanovski OI, Sieff CA: Diamond-Blackfan anemia. *Hematol Oncol Clin North Am* 11:1061, 1997.

34. Mancini AJ, Chan LS, Paller AS: Partial albinism with immunodeficiency: Griscelli syndrome: report of a case and review of the literature. *J Am Acad Dermatol* 38:295, 1998.

35. Pastural E, Barrat FJ, Dufourcq-Lagelouse R, et al: Griscelli disease maps to chromosome 15q21 and is associated with mutations in the myosin-Va gene. *Nat Genet* 16:289, 1997.

36. Gogus S, Topcu M, Kucukali T, et al: Griscelli syndrome: report of three cases. *Pediatr Pathol Lab Med* 15:309, 1995.

37. Cetin M, Hicsonmez G, Gogus S: Myelodysplastic syndrome associated with Griscelli syndrome. *Leuk Res* 22:859, 1998.

38. Malech HL, Nauseef WM: Primary inherited defects in neutrophil function: etiology and treatment. *Semin Hematol* 34:279, 1997.

39. Hord JD, Whitlock JA, Gay JC, Lukens JN: Clinical features of myelokathexis and treatment with hematopoietic cytokines; a case report of two patients and review of the literature. *J Pediatr Hematol Oncol* 19:443, 1997.

40. Weston B, Axtell RA, Todd RF 3d, et al: Clinical and biologic effects of granulocyte colony-stimulating factor in the treatment of myelokathexis. *J Pediatr* 118:229, 1991.

41. Wetzler M, Talpaz M, Kellagher MJ, et al: Myelokathexis: normalization of neutrophil counts and morphology by GM-CSF. *JAMA* 267:2179, 1992.

42. Sheridan BL, Pinkerton PH, Curtis JE, et al: The myelokathexis-like variant of the myelodysplastic syndrome—a second example. *Clin Lab Haematol* 13:81, 1991.

43. Patrone F, Dallegri F, Rebora A, Sacchetti C: Lazy leukocyte syndrome. *Blut* 39:265, 1979.

44. Garty BZ, Douglas SD, Danon YL: Immune deficiency in glycogen storage disease type 1B. *Isr J Med Sci* 32:1276, 1996.

45. Annabi B, Hiraiwa H, Mansfield BC, et al: The gene for glycogen-storage disease type 1b maps to chromosome 11q23. *Am J Hum Genet* 62:400, 1998.

46. McCawley LJ, Korchak HM, Douglas SD, et al: In vitro and in vivo effects of granulocyte colony-stimulating factor on neutrophils in glycogen storage disease type 1B: granulocyte colony-stimulating factor therapy corrects the neutropenia and the defects in respiratory burst activity and Ca^{2+} mobilization. *Pediatr Res* 35:84, 1994.

47. Zuccotti GV, Longhi R, Flumine P, et al: Effect of granulocyte colony-stimulating factor in glycogen storage disease type 1b. *J Int Med Res* 21:276, 1993.

48. Dale DC, Hammond WP: Cyclic neutropenia: a clinical review. *Blood Rev* 2:178, 1988.

49. Palmer SE, Stephens K, Dale DC: Genetics, phenotype, and natural history of autosomal dominant cyclic hematopoiesis. *Am J Med Gen* 66:413, 1996.

50. Haurie C, Dale DC, Mackey MC: Cyclical neutropenia and other periodic hematological disorders: a review of mechanisms and mathematical models. *Blood* 92:2629, 1998.

51. Migliaccio AR, Migliaccio G, Dale DC, Hammond WP: Hematopoietic progenitors in cyclic neutropenia: effect of granulocyte colony stimulating factor *in vivo*. *Blood* 75:1951, 1990.

52. Hammond WP, Price TH, Souza LM, Dale DC: Treatment of cyclic neutropenia with granulocyte colony stimulating factor. *N Engl J Med* 320:1306, 1989.

53. Welte K, Dale DC: Pathophysiology and treatment of severe chronic neutropenia. *Ann Hematol* 72:158, 1996.

54. Fowler B: Genetic defects of folate and cobalamin metabolism. *Eur J Pediatr* 157:S60, 1998.

55. Monagle PT, Tauro GP: Long-term follow up of patients with transcobalamin II deficiency. *Arch Dis Child* 72:237, 1995.

56. Dale DC: Immune and idiopathic neutropenia. *Curr Opin Hematol* 5:33, 1998.

57. Pincus SH, Boxer LA, Stossel TP: Chronic neutropenia in childhood. Analysis of 16 cases and a review of the literature. *Am J Med* 61:849, 1976.

58. Dale DC, Guerry D, Werwerka JR, et al: Chronic neutropenia. *Medicine* 58–128, 1979.

59. Kyle RA: Natural history of chronic idiopathic neutropenia. *N Engl J Med* 302:908, 1980.

60. Price TH, Lee MY, Dale DC, Finch CA: Neutrophil kinetics in chronic neutropenia. *Blood* 54:581, 1979.

61. Dancey JT, Brubaker LH: Neutrophil marrow cellularity in neutropenia. *Am J Hematol* 12:309, 1982.

62. Logue GL, Shastri KA, Laughlin M, et al: Idiopathic neutropenia: antineutrophil antibodies and clinical correlations. *Am J Med* 90:211, 1991.

63. Bernini JC: Diagnosis and management of chronic neutropenia during childhood. *Pediatr Clin North Am* 43:773, 1996.

64. Welte K, Dale DC: Pathophysiology and treatment of severe chronic neutropenia. *Ann Hematol* 72:158, 1996.

65. Doran M, Makhlouf R, Katz V, et al: Increased incidence of sepsis at birth in neutropenic infants of mothers with preeclampsia. *J Pediatr* 125:452, 1994.

66. Koenig J, Christensen R: The mechanism responsible for diminished neutrophil production in neonates delivered of women with pregnancy-induced hypertension. *Am J Obstet Gynecol* 165:467, 1989.

67. Kocherlakota P, LaGamma E: Recombinant human granulocyte colony-stimulating factor (rhG-CSF) increased the absolute neutrophil count (ANC) and decreased the incidence of infections in persistent preeclampsia-associated-neutropenia in VLBW neonates. *Pediatr Res* 41:937A, 1997.

68. Percival SS: Neutropenia caused by copper deficiency: possible mechanisms of action. *Nutr Rev* 53:59, 1995.

69. Olivares M, Uauy R: Copper as an essential nutrient. *Am J Clin Nutr* 63:791S, 1996.

70. Devuyst O, Lambert M, Rodhain J, et al: Haematological changes and infectious complications in anorexia nervosa: a case-control study. *Q J Med* 86:791, 1993.

71. Marinone G, Roncoli B, Marinone MG Jr.: Pure white cell aplasia. *Semin Hematol* 28:298, 1991.

72. Mamus SW, Burton JD, Groat JD, et al: Ibuprofen-associated pure white cell aplasia. *N Engl J Med* 314:624, 1986.

73. Levitt LJ: Chlorpropamide-induced pure white cell aplasia. *Blood* 69:394, 1987.

74. Forsyth PD, Davies JM: Pure white cell aplasia and health food products. *Postgrad Med J* 71:557, 1995.

75. Marinone GM, Roncoli B: Selective myeloid aplasia: a long-lasting presentation of an unusual hairy cell leukemia variant? *Haematologica* 78:239, 1993.

76. Currie MS, Weinberg JB, Rustagi PK, Logue GL: Antibodies to granulocyte precursors in selective myeloid hypoplasia and other suspected autoimmune neutropenias: use of HL-60 cells as targets. *Blood* 69:529, 1987.

77. Lalezari P, Radel E: Neutrophil-specific antigens: immunology and clinical significance. *Semin Hematol* 11:281, 1974.

78. Bux J, Chapman J: Report on the second international granulocyte serology workshop. *Transfusion* 37:977, 1997.

79. Bux J, Stein EL, Bierling P, et al: Characterization of a new alloantigen (SH) on the human neutrophil Fc gamma receptor IIIb. *Blood* 89:1027, 1997.

80. Bux J, Behrens G, Jaeger G, Welte K: Diagnosis and clinical course of autoimmune neutropenia in infancy: analysis of 240 cases. *Blood* 91:181, 1998.

81. Bux J: Challenges in the determination of clinically significant granulocyte antibodies and antigens. *Transfus Med Rev* 10:222, 1996.

82. Nossent JC, Swaak AJ: Prevalence and significance of haematological abnormalities in patients with systemic lupus erythematosus. *Q J Med* 80:605, 1991.

83. Sibley JT, Haga M, Visram DA, Mitchell DM: The clinical course of Felty's syndrome compared to matched controls. *J Rheumatol* 18:1163, 1991.

84. Starkebaum G, Price TH, Lee MY, Arend WP: Autoimmune neutropenia in systemic lupus erythematosus. *Arthritis Rheum* 21:504; 1978.

85. Starkebaum G: Use of colony-stimulating factors in the treatment of neutropenia associated with collagen vascular disease. *Curr Opin Hematol* 4:196, 1997.

86. Campion G, Maddison PJ, Goulding N, et al: The Felty syndrome: a case-matched study of clinical manifestations and outcome, serologic features, and immunogenetic associations. *Medicine* 69:69, 1990.

87. Bloch KJ, Buchanan WW, Wohl MJ, Bunim JJ: Sjögren's syndrome. *Medicine* 44:187, 1965.

88. Starkebaum G, Dancey JT, Arend WP: Chronic neutropenia: possible association with Sjögren's syndrome. *J Rheumatol* 21:504, 1978.

89. Wassenberg S, Herborn G, Rau R: Methotrexate treatment in Felty's syndrome. *Br J Rheumatol* 37:908, 1998.

90. Rashba EJ, Rowe JM, Packman CH: Treatment of the neutropenia of Felty syndrome. *Blood Rev* 10:177, 1996.

91. Bowman SJ, Geddes GC, Corrigall V, et al: Large granular lymphocyte expansions in Felty's syndrome have an unusual phenotype of activated CD45RA+ cells. *Br J Rheumatol* 35:1252, 1996.

92. Wiseman BK, Doan CA: A newly recognized granulopenic syndrome caused by excessive splenic leukolysis and successfully treated by splenectomy. *Ann Intern Med* 16:1097, 1942.

93. Kaufman DW, Kelly JP, Jurgelon JM, et al: Drugs in the aetiology of agranulocytosis and aplastic anaemia. *Eur J Haematol Suppl* 60:23, 1996.

94. Schulz W: Ueber eigenartige Halserkrankungen. *Dtsch Med Wockenschr* 48:1495, 1922.

95. Kracke RR: Relation of drug therapy to neutropenic states. *JAMA* 111:1255, 1938.

96. Uetrecht JP: Reactive metabolites and agranulocytosis. *Eur J Haematol Suppl* 60:33, 1996.

97. Claas FH: Immune mechanisms leading to drug-induced blood dyscrasias. *Eur J Haematol Suppl* 60:64, 1996.

98. Parent-Massin DM, Sens'eb'e L, L'eglise MC, et al: Relevance of in vitro studies of drug-induced agranulocytosis. Report of 14 cases. *Drug Saf* 9:463, 1993.

99. Frimat B, Gressier B, Odou P, Brunet C, et al: Metabolism of clozapine by human neutrophils: evidence for a specific oxidation of clozapine by the myeloperoxidase system with inhibition of enzymatic chlorination cycle. *Fundam Clin Pharmacol* 11:267, 1997.

100. Mauri MC, Rudelli R, Bravin S, et al: Clozapine metabolism rate as a possible index of drug-induced granulocytopenia. *Psychopharmacology (Berl)* 137:341, 1998.

101. Heit W, Heimpel H, Fischer A, Frickhofen N: Drug-induced agranulocytosis: evidence for the commitment of bone marrow haematopoiesis. *Scand J Haematol* 35:459, 1985.

102. Juli'a A, Olona M, Bueno J, et al: Drug-induced agranulocytosis: prognostic factors in a series of 168 episodes. *Br J Haematol* 79:366, 1991.

103. D'Antonio D, Iaacone A, Fioritoni G, et al: Patterns of infection in 41 patients with idiosyncratic drug-induced agranulocytosis. *Ann Hematol* 63:84, 1991.

104. Sprikkelman A, deWolf JT, Vellenga E: The application of hematopoietic growth factors in drug-induced agranulocytosis: a review of 70 cases. *Leukemia* 8:2031, 1994.

105. Wickramanayake PD, Scheid C, Josting A, et al: Use of granulocyte colony-stimulating factor (filgrastim) in the treatment of non-cytotoxic drug-induced agranulocytosis. *Eur J Med Res* 1:153, 1995.

106. Athens JW, Haab OP, Raab SO, et al: Leukokinetic studies. IV. The total blood, circulating and marginal granulocyte pools and the granulocyte turnover rate in normal subjects. *J Clin Invest* 40:989, 1961.

107. Dancey JT, Deubelbeiss KA, Harker LA, Finch CA: Neutrophil kinetics in man. *J Clin Invest* 58:705, 1976.

108. Garrey WE, Bryan WR: Variations in white blood cell counts. *Physiol Rev* 15:597, 1935.

109. Moyna NM, Acker GR, Weber KM, et al: The effects of incremental submaximal exercise on circulating leukocytes in physically active and sedentary males and females. *Eur J Appl Physiol* 74:211, 1996.

110. Foster NK, Martyn JB, Rangna RE, et al: Leukocytosis of exercise: role of cardiac output and catecholamines. *J Appl Physiol* 61:2218, 1986.

111. Benschop RJ, Rodriguez-Feuerhahn M, Schedlowski M: Catecholamine-induced leukocytosis: early observations, current research, and future directions. *Brain Behav Immun* 10:77, 1996.

112. Toft P, Helbo-Hansen HS, Tonnesen E, et al: Redistribution of granulocytes during adrenaline infusion and following administration of cortisol in healthy volunteers. *Acta Anaesthesiol Scand* 38:254, 1994.

113. Hogg JC, Doerschuk CM: Leukocyte traffic in the lung. *Ann Rev Physiol* 57:97, 1995.

114. Dale DC, Fauci AS, Gerry D IV, Wolff SM: Comparison of agents producing a neutrophilic leukocytosis in man. *J Clin Invest* 56:808, 1975.

115. Craddock PR, Fehr J, Dalmasso AP, et al: Hemodialysis leukopenia. Pulmonary vascular leukostasis resulting from complement activation by dialyzer cellophane membranes. *J Clin Invest* 59:879, 1977.

116. Price TH, Chatta GS, Dale DC: The effect of recombinant granulocyte colony-stimulating factor on neutrophil kinetics in normal young and elderly humans. *Blood* 88:335,1996.

117. Dale DC, Liles WC, Llewellyn C, Price TH: The effects of granulocyte macrophage colony-stimulating factor (GM-CSF) on neutrophil kinetics and function in normal human volunteers. *Am J Hematol* 57:7–15, 1998.

118. Reding MT, Hibbs JR, Morrison VA, et al: Diagnosis and outcome of 100 consecutive patients with extreme granulocytic leukocytosis. *Am J Med* 104:12, 1998.

119. Kuijpers TW, Van Lier RA, Hamann D, et al: Leukocyte adhesion deficiency type 1 (LAD-1)/variant. A novel immunodeficiency syndrome characterized by dysfunctional beta2 integrins. *J Clin Invest* 100:1725, 1997.

120. Bishop CR, Athens JW, Boggs DR, et al: Leukokinetic studies. XIII. A non-steady-state kinetic evaluation of the mechanism of cortisone-induced granulocytosis. *J Clin Invest* 47:249, 1968.

121. Crockard AD, Boylan MT, Droogan AG, et al: Methylprednisolone-induced neutrophil leukocytosis—down-modulation of neutrophil L-selectin and Mac-1 expression and induction of granulocyte colony-stimulating factor. *Int J Clin Lab Res* 28:110, 1998.

122. Cartwright GE, Athens JW, Haab OP, et al: Blood granulocyte kinetics in conditions associated with granulocytosis. *Ann N Y Acad Sci* 11:963, 1964.

123. Deulofeu F, Cervell'o B, Capell S, et al: Predictors of mortality in patients with bacteremia: the importance of functional status. *J Am Geriatr Soc* 46:14, 1998.

124. Parry H, Cohen S, Schlarb JE, et al: Smoking, alcohol consumption, and leukocyte counts. *Am J Clin Pathol* 107:64, 1997.

125. Su WP, Fett DL, Gibson LE, Pittelkow MR: Sweet syndrome: acute febrile neutrophilic dermatosis. *Semin Dermatol* 14:173, 1995.

126. Shoenfeld Y, Tal A, Berliner S, Pinkhas J: Leukocytosis in nonhematological malignancies—a possible tumor-associated marker. *J Cancer Res Clin Oncol* 111:54, 1986.

127. Katoh Y, Nakamura M, Ohnishi Y, et al: Autonomous production of granulocyte-colony-stimulating factor in tumour xenografts associated with leukocytosis. *Br J Cancer* 68:715, 1993.

128. Horii A, Shimamura K, Honjo Y, et al: Granulocyte colony-stimulating factor-producing tongue carcinoma. *Head Neck* 19:351, 1997.

129. Zalokar JB, Richard JL, Claude JR: Leukocyte count, smoking, and myocardial infarction. *N Engl J Med* 304:465, 1981.

130. Green SM, Vowels J, Waterman B, Rothrock SG, Kuniyoshi G: Leukocytosis: a new look at an old marker for acute myocardial infarction. *Acad Emerg Med* 3:1034, 1996.

131. Bovill EG, Bild DE, Heiss G, et al: White blood cell counts in persons aged 65 years or more from the Cardiovascular Health Study. Correlations with baseline clinical and demographic characteristics. *Am J Epidemiol* 143:1107, 1996.

132. Ascensao JL, Oken MM, Ewing SL, et al: Leukocytosis and large cell lung cancer. A frequent association. *Cancer* 60:903, 1987.

133. Grimm RH, Neaton JD, Ludwig W: Prognostic importance of the white blood cell count for coronary, cancer, and all-cause mortality. *JAMA* 254:1932, 1985.

134. Kwong YL, Cheng G, Tang TS, et al: Transient myeloproliferative disorder in a Down's neonate with rearranged T-cell receptor beta gene and evidence of in vivo maturation demonstrated by dual-colour flow cytometric DNA ploidy analysis. *Leukemia* 7:1667, 1993.

135. Ward HN, Reinhard EH: Chronic idiopathic leukocytosis. *Ann Intern Med* 75:193, 1971.

136. Herring WB, Smith LB, Walker RI, Herion JC: Hereditary neutrophilia. *Am J Med* 56:729, 1974.

137. Joyce RA: Sequential effects of lithium on haematopoiesis. *Br J Haematol* 56:307, 1984.

138. Gelwan JS, Schmitz RL, Pellecchia C: Ranitidine and leukocytosis. *Am J Gastroenterol* 81:685, 1986.

139. Bedell SE, Kang JL: Leukocytosis and left shift associated with quinidine fever. *Am J Med* 77:345, 1984.

NEUTROPHIL DISORDERS: QUALITATIVE ABNORMALITIES OF THE NEUTROPHIL

LAURENCE A. BOXER

The differential diagnosis for a patient presenting recurrent infections is formidable, given the complexity of the immune system. The clinical presentation of a patient who has a qualitative neutrophil abnormality may be similar to that of one who has an antibody or complement disorder. In general, evaluation for phagocyte cell disorders (Table 72-1) should be initiated among those patients who have at least one of the two following clinical features: (1) two or more systematic bacterial infections; (2) frequent, serious respiratory infections, such as pneumonia or sinusitis, or frequent bacterial infections such as cellulitis, draining otitis media, or lymphadenitis; (3) infections present at unusual sites (liver or brain abscess); and (4) infections associated with unusual pathogens (e.g., *Aspergillus* pneumonia, disseminated candidiasis, or infections with *Serratia marcescens, Nocardia* species, and *Burkholderia cepacia*).

CLASSIFICATION

Neutrophils serve as the first line of defense against most bacterial pathogens. This function requires that the host have sufficient numbers of neutrophils that respond to chemotactic stimuli and ingest and kill bacteria. Chronic granulomatous disease (CGD) of childhood was the first qualitative neutrophil abnormality described. In this disorder, neutrophils are capable of ingesting but not killing certain microorganisms.

Neutrophil dysfunction may arise from (1) absence of antibodies or complement components required to opsonize microorganisms, an interaction that provides a chemotactic signal; (2) abnormalities of cytoplasmic movement that alter the chemotactic response or that result in abnormalities of the plasma membrane affecting the cell's intrinsic capability to modulate movement; or (3) defects in microbicidal capability. Other comprehensive reviews of these syndromes are available to the interested reader.[1-4]

ABNORMALITIES OF THE SIGNAL MECHANISM AS A RESULT OF ANTIBODY OR COMPLEMENT DEFECTS

Since the synergistic action of immunoglobulins and complement proteins creates the opsonins that coat microorganisms and stimulate the

Acronyms and abbreviations that appear in this chapter include: cAMP, cyclic adenosine monophosphate; CDP, CCAAP displacement protein; CGD, chronic granulomatous disease; CHS, Chédiak-Higashi syndrome; EBV, Epstein-Barr virus; FMF, familial Mediterranean fever; GDP, glucose diphosphate; G-6-PD, glucose-6-phosphate dehydrogenase; HLA, human leukocyte antigen; Ig, immunoglobulin; INF, interferon; LAD, leukocyte adhesion deficiency; LFA-1, lymphocyte function-associated antigen 1; MBP, mannose-binding protein; NADPH, reduced nicotinamide adenine dinucleotide phosphate; NBT, nitroblue tetrazolium; PCR, polymerase chain reaction; *phox*, phagocyte oxidase; rINF, recombinant interferon; SGD, specific granule deficiency; SH3, *SRC* homology 3.

development of chemotactic factors, a deficiency of either one may result in impaired neutrophil function. The most profound disturbances arise from abnormalities in C3, since this protein is the focal point for generation of opsonins and chemotactic factors (see Chap. 5).[5,6] Activation of C3 can occur in the absence of either antibody or the classical complement components, C1, C4, and C2; thus, disorders of these molecules result in less severe clinical conditions. C3 deficiency is inherited as an autosomal recessive disorder.[5] Homozygotes have undetectable serum levels of C3 and suffer from recurrent severe pyogenic infections, while asymptomatic heterozygotes have half the normal values.

A functional deficiency in C3 protease resulting in severe pyogenic infections also is seen in patients with a deficiency in C3b inactivator, a protein inhibitor of the alternative complement pathway. Unchecked activation of this pathway leads to hypercatabolism of C3 and factor B.[7] Properidin deficiency also results in a functional deficiency in C3.[8] Properidin is a serum protein that belongs to the alternative complement pathway; it is involved in the stabilization of the enzyme complex $C3b_22Bb$. The protein is a multimeric glycoprotein with a subunit M_r of 56,000, the gene for which has now been cloned.[9] Absence of properidin is associated with severe, often fatal pyogenic infection, often with meningococci.

Approximately 5 percent of the population have low serum levels of mannose-binding protein (MBP).[10] It is a serum lectin secreted by the liver that binds mannose sugars present on the surface of bacteria, fungi, and some viruses. Mannose-binding protein is one of the collectin-soluble effector proteins that contribute to the basic armamentarium of nonclonal immunity. Mannose-binding protein can function as an opsonin when bound to surfaces by activating the complement cascade. A deficiency of MBP has been reported in infants with frequent unexplained infections, chronic diarrhea, and otitis media.[10] Deficiency of MBP in adults with recurrent infections has also been associated with autosomal dominant inheritance of point mutations of MBP polypeptide, which leads to the failure of MBP to activate complement.[11-13] It is possible that the adults expressing the defective MBP are lacking the ability to produce anticarbohydrate antibodies, which further predisposes them to recurrent infections.

Because of the large number of chemoattractants generated during inflammation, it is difficult to establish the relative significance of a given individual component. Furthermore, chemotactic factors and opsonins are involved in the activity of both neutrophils and mononuclear phagocytes. Therefore, it is not clear whether the clinical consequences of disorders involving these substances are unique to one or the other of these phagocytic cells. Patients with antibody- or complement-deficiency syndromes suffer mainly from infections with encapsulated pathogens such as *Haemophilus influenzae*, pneumococci, streptococci, and meningococci.[14] Furthermore, splenectomized individuals, deprived of an organ rich in mononuclear phagocytes, have a small but finite risk of sepsis due to these same microorganisms.[15] Encapsulated pathogens characteristically are not associated with neutropenic states. Antibody coating of encapsulated organisms facilitates their ingestion by mononuclear phagocytes but may be less important for their ingestion by neutrophils.

ABNORMALITIES OF THE CELLULAR RESPONSES AS A RESULT OF DEFECTS IN CYTOPLASMIC MOVEMENT

DEGRANULATION ABNORMALITIES

THE CHÉDIAK-HIGASHI SYNDROME

Definition and History This rare autosomal recessive disease was initially recognized as one in which neutrophils, monocytes, and lymphocytes contained giant cytoplasmic granules (Fig. 72-1). Chédiak-Higashi syndrome (CHS) is now recognized as a disorder of

TABLE 72-1   NEUTROPHIL DYSFUNCTION

DISORDER	ETIOLOGY	IMPAIRED FUNCTION	CLINICAL CONSEQUENCE
Degranulation abnormalities: Chédiak-Higashi syndrome	Autosomal recessive; disordered coalescence of lysosomal granules. Responsible gene found at 1q 42-45. The encoded protein has structural features homologous to a vascular sorting protein.	Decreased neutrophil chemotaxis, degranulation and bactericidal activity; platelet storage pool defect; impaired NK function, failure to disperse melanosomes.	Neutropenia; recurrent pyogenic infections, propensity to develop marked hepatosplenomegaly in the accelerated phase; pigment dilution in skin and fundus.
Specific granule deficiency	Autosomal recessive; abnormal regulation of various myeloid granule genes by a transacting factor.	Impaired chemotaxis and bactericidal activity; biolebed nuclei in neutrophils; reduced content of neutrophil defensins, gelatinase, collagenase, vitamin B12-binding protein, lactoferrin.	Recurrent deep-seated abscesses.
Adhesion abnormalities: Leukocyte adhesion deficiency	Autosomal recessive; absences of CD11/CD18 surface adhesive glycoprotein (β_2 integrins) on leukocyte membranes most commonly arising from failure to express CD18 mRNA.	Decreased binding of C3bi to neutrophils and impaired adhesion to ICAM1 and ICAM2.	Neutrophilia; recurrent bacterial infection associated with a lack of pus formation.
Leukocyte adhesion deficiency type 2	Autosomal recessive (?); absence of neutrophil sialyl-Lewis X.	Decreased adhesion to activated endothelium expressing ELAM.	Neutrophilia; recurrent bacterial infection without pus.
Neutrophil actin dysfunction	Altered polymerization of neutrophil cytoplasmic actin; perhaps arising from the presence of an inhibitor to F-actin formation.	Impaired neutrophil adhesion, chemotaxis, and bacterial killing.	Neutrophilia; recurrent bacterial infections without pus.
Disorders of cell motility: Enhanced motile responses: Familial Mediterranean Fever (FMF)	Autosomal recessive gene responsible for FMF on chromosome 16 which encodes for a protein called "pyrin." Pyrin may modify neutrophil activation.	Excessive accumulation of neutrophils at inflamed sites which may be the result of the neutrophil to inhibit C5a activity.	Recurrent fever, peritonitis, pleuritis, arthritis, and amyloidosis.
Depressed motile responses: Defects in the generation of chemotactic signals	IgG deficiencies; C3 and properdin deficiency can arise from genetic or acquired abnormalities; Mannose binding protein deficiency predominantly in neonates.	Deficiency of serum chemotaxis and opsonic activities.	Recurrent pyogenic infections.
Intrinsic defects of the neutrophil, e.g. leukocyte adhesion deficiency, Chédiak-Higashi syndrome, specific granule deficiency, neutrophil actin dysfunction, neonatal neutrophils	In the neonatal neutrophil there is diminished ability to express β_2-integrins and there is a qualitative impairment in β_2-integrin function.	Diminished chemotaxis.	Propensity to develop pyogenic infections.
Direct inhibition of neutrophil mobility, e.g. drugs	Ethanol, glucocorticoids, cyclic AMP.	Impaired locomotion and ingestion. Impaired adherence.	Possible cause for frequent infections; neutrophilia seen with epinephrine is the result of cyclic AMP release from endothelium.
Immune complexes	Bind to Fc receptors on neutrophils in patients with rheumatoid arthritis, systemic lupus erythematosus, other inflammatory states.	Impaired chemotaxis.	Recurrent pyogenic infections.
Hyperimmunoglobulin E syndrome	Autosomal dominant; variable expression of a soluble inhibitor from mononuclear cells affecting neutrophil chemotaxis; high levels of antistaphylococcal IgE.	Impaired chemotaxis at times; impaired IgG opsonization of *Staphylococcal aureus.*	Recurrent skin and senopulmonary infections.
Defects of microbicidal activity: Chronic granulomatous disease	X-linked and autosomal recessive; failure to express functional gp91^{phox} in the phagocyte membrane in p22^{phox} (autosomal recessive). Other autosomal recessive forms of CGD arise from failure to express protein p47^{phox} or p67^{phox}.	Failure to activate neutrophil respiratory burst leading to failure to kill catalase-positive microbes.	Recurrent pyogenic infections with catalase-positive microorganisms.
G-6-PD deficiency	Less than 5% of normal activity of G-6-PD.	Failure to activate NADPH-dependent oxidase.	Infections with catalase-positive microorganisms.
Myeloperoxidase deficiency	Autosomal recessive; failure to process modified precursor protein arising from missense mutation.	H_2O_2-dependent antimicrobial activity not potentiated by myeloperoxidase.	None.
Deficiencies of glutathione reductase and glutathione synthetase	Failure to detoxify H_2O_2.	Excessive formation of H_2O_2.	Minimal problems with recurrent pyogenic infections.

NOTE: X, X-linked; AR, autosomal recessive; G-6-PS, glucose 6-phosphate dehydrogenase; CGD, chronic granulomatous disease; CD, cluster designation; ICAM, intracellular adhesion molecule; NK, natural killer; C, complement; FMF, Familial Mediterranean Fever.

generalized cellular dysfunction characterized by increased fusion of cytoplasmic granules.[16] Pigmentary dilution affecting the hair, skin, and ocular fundi results from pathologic aggregation of melanosomes and is associated with a failure of decussation of the optic and auditory nerves (Table 72-1).[17] Patients with this syndrome exhibit an increased susceptibility to infection, which can be explained at least in part through defects in neutrophil chemotaxis, degranulation, and bactericidal activity. The presence of giant granules in the neutrophil interferes with their ability to traverse narrow passages between endothelial cells. Other features of the disease include neutropenia, thrombocytopathy, natural killer cell abnormalities, and peripheral neuropathies.[18] Similar genetic syndromes have been described in mice, mink, cats, rats, cattle, and killer whales.[19]

Etiology and Pathogenesis   Although the basic mechanism underlying CHS is unknown, alterations in membrane fusion probably play an important role.[16,20–22] It appears CHS is caused by a fundamental defect in granule morphogenesis that results in abnormally large granules in multiple tissues. Giant granules are seen in Schwann cells, leukocytes, and macrophages of the liver and spleen, and certain cells of the pancreas, gastric mucosa, kidney, adrenal gland, and pituitary gland. Giant melanosomes form and prevent the even distribution of melanin, which results in pigmentary dilution of the hair, skin, iris, and optic fundus. In the early stages of myelopoiesis some of the normal-size azurophil granules coalesce to form giant granules that result in large secondary lysosomes that contain reduced content of hydrolytic enzymes, including proteinases, elastase, and cathepsin G.[16,23–26] Many of the myeloid precursors die in the marrow, resulting in a moderate neutropenia, with white cell counts of about 2500/μl (2.5 × 10⁹/liter).[27] In spite of the normal ingestion of particles and active oxygen metabolism, these neutrophils kill microorganisms relatively slowly. This delay reflects a slow and inconsistent delivery of diluted amounts of hydrolytic enzymes from the giant granules into the phagosomes, which may predispose the host to bacterial infection.[16,20] In this syndrome, monocytes have the same functional derangements as neutrophils.[16]

The CHS blood cell membranes are more fluid than cells of normal individuals,[16,22] and the altered membrane structure could lead to defective regulation of membrane activation. Conceivably, changes in membrane fluidity may affect cell function by altering expression of membrane receptors. This, in turn, could result in elevated levels of intracellular cyclic adenosine monophosphate, disordered assembly of microtubules, and the defective interaction of microtubules with lysosome membranes, which occur in this disorder and are reflected in the reduced chemotactic responses.[16]

The gene for CHS, known as *LYST,* has been cloned based on its homology to the murine gene responsible for mouse CHS (beige phenotype).[28] The gene was recognized by the presence of *LYST* mutations. The gene is localized on chromosome 1q42–q44 and has structural features homologous to a vacuolar sorting protein called VPS15 in yeast. The CHS protein may be associated with vacuolar transport and mediate protein-protein associations that integrate cellular signal response coupling.

Clinical Features   Characteristically patients with CHS have light skin and silvery hair. They frequently complain of solar sensitivity and photophobia. Other signs and symptoms vary considerably. Infec-

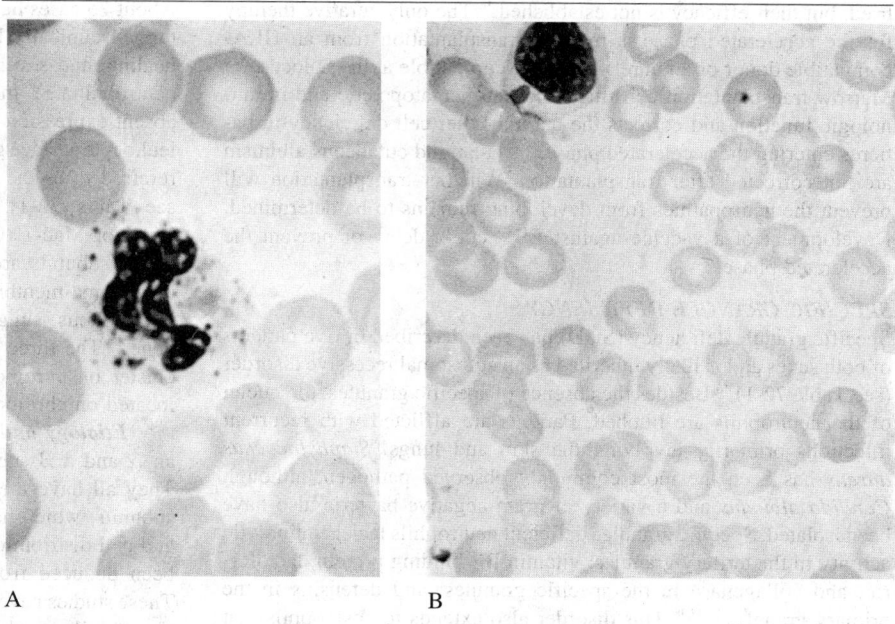

FIGURE 72-1   Blood films of patients with the Chédiak-Higashi syndrome. (*a*) The granulocyte contains large amorphic cytoplasmic granulations. (*b*) A large inclusion is easily seen in a lymphocyte.

tions and neuropathy are common. The infections involve the mucous membranes, skin, and respiratory tract. They are susceptible to both gram-positive and gram-negative bacteria as well as fungi, with *Staphylococcus aureus* being the most common infecting organism. The neuropathy may be sensory or motor in type, and ataxia may be a prominent feature.

Patients with CHS have prolonged bleeding times with normal platelet counts, resulting from impaired platelet aggregation associated with a deficiency of the storage pools of adenosine diphosphate and serotonin.[29] Natural killer cell function also is impaired.[16,30] The diagnosis is established by the presence of large inclusions in all nucleated blood cells. These can be seen on Wright-stained blood films but are accentuated by peroxidase stains.

The accelerated phase of CHS is characterized by lymphocytic proliferation in the liver, spleen, and bone marrow. The accelerated phase may occur at any age. Typically the patient develops hepatosplenomegaly and high fever in the absence of bacterial sepsis. The pancytopenia becomes worse at this stage, producing hemorrhage and an increased susceptibility to infection. The onset of the accelerated phase may be related to the inability of these patients to contain and control the Epstein-Barr virus (EBV) and leads to features simulating viral-mediated hemophagocytic syndrome (see Chap. 5).[31,32] The lymphocyte proliferation is associated with recurrent bacterial and viral infections, fever, and prostration, usually resulting in death. At autopsy, the lymphohistiocytic infiltrates in the liver, spleen, and lymph nodes are extensive, but not neoplastic by histopathologic criteria.[16,30] Occasionally, giant lysosomes resembling those of CHS may be observed in acute myelogenous leukemia.[33]

Therapy, Course, and Prognosis   High-dose ascorbic acid (200 mg/day for infants, 2 g/day for adults) has been found to improve the clinical status of some patients in the stable phase.[16,34] Although there is controversy regarding the efficacy of ascorbic acid, given the safety of the vitamin it is reasonable to administer it to all patients. The CHS presents a therapeutic dilemma, particularly when the accelerated phase begins. Prophylactic antibiotics do not prevent infections. Treatment regimens with glucocorticoids and vincristine therapy have been tried, but their efficacy is not established.[16] The only curative therapy for the accelerated phase is marrow transplantation from an HLA-compatible donor or an unrelated donor compatible at the D locus.[35,36] Marrow transplantation constitutes normal hematopoietic and immunologic function and corrects the natural killer cell deficiency in patients entering the accelerated phase.[36] Ocular and cutaneous albinism are not corrected after transplantation. Whether transplantation will prevent the neuropathies from developing remains to be determined. Development of a vaccine against EBV could delay or prevent the accelerated phase.

SPECIFIC GRANULE DEFICIENCY

Specific granule deficiency (SGD) has been described in five patients of both sexes and is likely inherited as an autosomal recessive disorder (see Table 72-1).[16] Besides the absence of specific granules, the nuclei of the neutrophils are bilobed. Patients are afflicted with recurrent infections primarily involving the skin and lungs. *Staphylococcus aureus* has been the most commonly observed pathogen, although *Candida albicans* and a variety of gram-negative bacteria also have been isolated. Specific granule–deficient neutrophils lack gelatinolytic activity in the tertiary granules; vitamin B_{12}-binding protein, lactoferrin, and collagenase in the specific granules; and defensins in the primary granules.[25,37,38] This disorder also extends to eosinophils that lack the characteristic eosinophil granule proteins, major basic proteins, eosinophilic cationic proteins, and eosinophil-derived neurotoxins (see Chap. 68).[39] Thus, the disorder is a global defect in phagocytic granules rather than limited to specific granules, as suggested by its name. Neutrophils from these patients have abnormal chemotaxis, possibly related to the absence of the intracellular pool of leukocyte adhesion molecules that normally reside in the specific granules,[40–43] and a mild defect in bactericidal activity, possibly related to the deficiency of the granule constituents lactoferrin and defensins.[25,40] The impairment in granule protein synthesis affecting the granulocytic cells likely reflects a primary defect in gene expression, possibly in a shared transcription factor common to the affected subset of proteins.[38] Such a transcription factor might be the CCAAP displacement protein (CDP) that binds to a specific region of both the lactoferrin and the collagenase promoter.[44,45] This protein is the first identified transcription factor that is a candidate for mediating the shared regulation of neutrophil-specific granule protein genes. Overexpression of CDP leads to the coordinate loss of specific granule protein expression; thus, an abnormality in expression of CDP could account for the biochemical phenotype seen in SGD. Alternatively in one patient a five-basepair deletion in the transcription factor CCAAT/enhancer binding protein (C/EBP) epsilon, which is a factor known to regulate myeloid granule formation, was found.[45] The defect is restricted to blood cells, since normal lactoferrin secretion has been demonstrated in the nasal secretions of a SGD patient despite the abnormality demonstrated in his neutrophils.[37]

The diagnosis of SGD is suggested by the presence of neutrophils devoid of specific granules but containing azurophilic granules on the blood film.[16] Electron microscopy reveals small peroxidase-negative vesicles presumably representing empty specific granules.[46] The diagnosis can be confirmed by demonstrating a severe deficiency in either lactoferrin or vitamin B_{12}-binding protein. An acquired form of SGD can be observed in thermally injured patients or in individuals with myelodysplasia.[16,47] Treatment of SGD is symptomatic, with the administration of parenteral antibiotics for acute infections and surgical drainage of refractory infections.[16] With aggressive medical management, patients may survive into their adult years.

ADHESION ABNORMALITIES

LEUKOCYTE ADHESION DEFICIENCY

Definition and History   Leukocyte adhesion deficiency type I (LAD 1) is a rare autosomal recessive disorder of leukocyte function.

About 75 cases have been reported worldwide. The disease is characterized clinically by recurrent soft-tissue infections, delayed wound healing, and severely impaired pus formation despite striking blood neutrophilia.[3,48] Individuals with this disorder have a decreased or absent expression of a family of structurally and functionally related leukocyte surface glycoproteins designated CD11/CD18 complex (also referred to as the β_2-integrin family of leukocyte adhesive proteins; see Table 72-1). These proteins include LFA-1 (CD11a/CD18), Mo-1 or Mac-1 (CD11b/CD18), and p150,95 (CD11c/CD18).[48] The CD11 subunits are integral membrane glycoproteins, each spanning the plasma membrane only once. They are approximately 40 percent homologous, suggesting that they arise from a common primordial gene.[48] The three distinct genes encoding the α subunits occur in a cluster on chromosome 16, whereas the gene for the β subunit is located on chromosome 21.[49]

Etiology and Pathogenesis   Each of these molecules contains an α and a β subunit noncovalently associated in an $\alpha\beta$ structure. They all have the same β subunit and are distinguished by their α subunits, which have different isoelectric points, molecular weights, and cell distribution (Table 72-2).[48] The structure of CD11/CD18 has been deduced from molecular cloning of the various subunits.[50–52] These studies have established that CD11/CD18 are members of a large gene family involved in cell-cell and cell-matrix adhesion (integrins).[53] Several subfamilies of integrins have been described and classified according to the type of their highly homologous β subunits.[54] The α subunits are also homologous to each other, but to a lesser degree than are the associated β subunits. Within each subfamily, a single β subunit usually is shared by several α subunits. Certain α subunits often share more than one β subunit, which alters their specificity for various ligands.[54] The molecular defect involves all three members of the CD11 integrin subfamily. In the patients with LAD I who have been evaluated at the molecular level, absent, diminished, or structurally abnormal β subunits (CD18) have been identified. A heterogeneous group of mutations that are confined to the gene on chromosome 21q22.3 have been identified.[55] Many patients have point mutations that result in single amino acid substitutions in CD18, which predominantly reside between amino acids 111 and 361.[56–62] This peptide domain is highly conserved among all β subunits and appears to be important for interaction with the α subunit. Several affected individuals are compound heterozygotes for two different mutant alleles, whereas others are homozygotes for a single mutant allele. Messenger RNA splicing abnormalities described in two kindreds can result in either deletion or insertion of amino acids in the conserved extracellular domain of CD18.[63] Small deletions within the coding sequences of the CD18 gene disrupting the reading frame or a nucleotide substitution resulting in a premature termination signal has been described.[57,62,65] Mutations in CD18 disrupt the association in the $\alpha\beta$ subunits so that maturation, intracellular transport, and cell surface assembly of functionally active $\alpha\beta$ molecules fail to occur.[48] Approximately half of patients exhibit a low level of CD11/CD18 cell surface molecules and moderate disease, with the remainder having totally absent surface expression of these proteins, which accounts for a profound impairment of neutrophil and monocyte adherence and adhesion-dependent functions in vitro, including cell migration, phagocytosis, and complement- or antibody-dependent cytotoxicity.[66,67]

Besides the requirement for surface expression of the CD11/CD18, the molecules must undergo posttranslational modification during leukocyte activation.[68] In one patient with LAD, the integrin molecules were expressed on the surface of the neutrophil but failed to undergo high-avidity ligand binding.[69] The resulting neutrophil functional abnormalities resulted in a moderate clinical disorder in the patient. The bulk of the neutrophil Mac-1 glycoprotein is stored inside the cell in the membrane of neutrophil-specific gelatinase and secretory granules.[70–72] Exposure of neutrophils to degranulating stimuli results

TABLE 72-2   BIOLOGICAL AND CLINICAL FEATURES OF LEUKOCYTE ADHERENCE DEFICIENCY

THE CD11/CD18 FAMILY	LEUKOCYTE FUNCTIONAL ABNORMALITIES[a]	CLINICAL FEATURES[a]
Mac-1 (CD11b/CD18): molecular mass of α chain 170 kD; found on monocytes; neutrophils, NK cells; receptor for C3bi (CR3) function, i.e., adherence, and antibody-dependent cellular cytotoxicity LFA-1 (CD11a/CD18): molecular mass of α chain 170 kD; found on all human leukocytes; adhesion-promoting molecule for leukocytes; facilitates NK binding, cytolytic T-lymphocyte-mediated killing, and helper T-cell response p150,95 (CD11c/CD18): molecular mass of α chain 150 kD; found on monocytes and neutrophils; promotes neutrophil and monocyte adhesion.	Neutrophils: adherence, spreading, aggregation, chemotaxis receptor CR3 activities (C3bi-binding phagocytosis, respiratory burst and degranulation in response to C3bi-coated particles) antibody-dependent cellular cytotoxicity. Monocytes: adherence, CR3 activities Lymphocytes: cytotoxic T-lymphocytes activities, NK activities, blastogenesis	Autosomal recessive; delayed umbilical cord separation, neutrophilia, defective neutrophil mobilization, recurrent bacterial infection without pus, impaired wound recurrent bacterial (sometimes life-threatening) bacterial infections.

[a]These functional abnormalities and clinical features are a consequence of lack of the CD11/CD18 complex, which includes CD11a, CD11b, CD11c markers of three different α chains and the common β chain CD18 of molecular mass 95 kD.

in a five- to tenfold increase in the number of Mac-1 molecules on the cell surface, which parallels the fusion of granules to the plasma membrane.[71] Neutrophils from these patients fail to augment their surface adhesive glycoproteins, since the defect in β-subunit synthesis affects both membrane and granule pools of Mac-1.[73] In contrast to Mac-1 and p150,95, lymphocyte function-associated antigen 1 (LFA-1) is predominantly confined to the neutrophil plasma membrane. Consequently, the cell surface levels of LFA-1 are not enhanced by neutrophil degranulation.

Lymphocytes deficient in CD11/CD18 are able to adhere to endothelial surfaces via the expression on lymphocytes of very late activation 4 (VLA-4) integrin receptors, which bind to the vascular cell adhesion molecule 1 (VCAM-1), found on the endothelial cells[74]; this residual adhesion may account for the paucity of clinical symptoms related to lymphocyte function.

The failure of the leukocyte adhesion–deficient neutrophils to migrate to the sites of inflammation outside of the lung and peritoneum is due to their inability to adhere firmly to surfaces and undergo transendothelial migration from venules.[75–77] Failure of CD11/CD18-deficient neutrophils to undergo transendothelial migration occurs because β_2-integrins bind to intercellular adhesion molecules 1 and 2 (CD54 and ICAM-2) expressed on inflamed endothelial cells.[48,78] The neutrophils that do arrive at inflammatory sites in the lung and peritoneum by CD11/CD18-independent processes fail to recognize microorganisms coated with the opsonic complement fragment C3bi (an important stable opsonin formed by the cleavage of C3b by C3b inactivator).[48,53] Other neutrophil functions such as degranulation and oxidative metabolism normally triggered by C3bi binding are also diminished and markedly compromised in neutrophils from LAD 1.[48] Similarly, the urokinase-plasminogen activator-receptor and the FcγRIII receptors, both phosphatidylinositol-linked proteins, are defective in their functions because these receptors transduce their signals through CD11/CD18.[79,80] Monocyte function is also impaired. Monocytes of affected individuals have poor fibrinogen-binding function, an activity promoted by the CD11/CD18 complex[48,81]; consequently, such cells are not able to participate effectively in wound healing. Thus, impairment in neutrophil function underlies the propensity to have recurrent infections, which is the clinical expression of this disease. Similar genetic syndromes have been discovered in a dog and Holstein cattle.[82,83] A CD11/CD18-deficient mouse with 2 to 6 percent of normal β_2-integrin expression has been produced by gene targeting.[75,84]

Clinical Features   Activated leukocytes of patients with the most severe clinical form express less than 0.3 percent of the normal amount of the β_2-integrins, whereas those of patients with the moderate

phenotype may express 2 to 7 percent of normal numbers of β_2-integrin molecules.[48] The severely affected patients suffer from recurrent and chronic or even gangrenous soft-tissue infections (subcutaneous tissues or mucous membranes), generally by bacterial or fungal microorganisms such as *Staph. aureus, Pseudomonas* spp. and other gram-negative enteric rods, or *Candida* spp. Patients with the moderate phenotype have fewer and less severe infections. Infectious susceptibility and impaired wound healing are related to diminished or delayed infiltration of neutrophils and monocytes into extravascular inflammatory sites. In all patients surviving infancy, severe progressive generalized periodontitis is present. Individuals who are clinically well but are heterozygous carriers of LAD have been identified. Their stimulated neutrophils express approximately 50 percent of the normal amount of the Mac-1 α subunit and the common β subunit.[48]

The diagnosis of LAD is suggested by one or more clinical features, including recurrent cutaneous, periodontal, or other soft-tissue infections, as well as delayed wound healing and delayed umbilical cord severance and/or infections, especially in the setting of persistent neutrophilia.

Laboratory Features   The diagnosis is made most readily by flow cytometric measurement of surface CD11b in stimulated and unstimulated neutrophils using monoclonal antibodies directed against CD11b (Fig. 72-2). Assessment of neutrophil and monocyte adherence, aggregation, chemotaxis, C3bi-mediated phagocytosis, and cytotoxicity generally will demonstrate striking abnormalities that are directly related to the molecular deficiency. Delayed-type hypersensitivity reactions are normal, and most individuals have normal specific antibody synthesis. The ability of lymphocytes to generate specific antibodies explains the self-limited course of varicella or viral respiratory infections. However, some patients have impaired T-lymphocyte–dependent antibody responses, for example, to repeat vaccination with tetanus toxoid, diphtheria toxoid, and polio virus.

Patients with LAD I usually have blood neutrophil counts of 15 to 60×10^9/liter. However, during infectious episodes, they commonly have neutrophil counts in excess of 100×10^9/liter and sometimes as high as 160×10^9/liter. Granulocytic hyperplasia is a feature of the marrow examination. Despite elevated blood counts, there is a paucity of neutrophils in inflammatory skin windows and biopsies of infected tissues.

Differential Diagnosis   Two patients have been described who had neutrophilia, recurrent bacterial infections, and an inability to form pus.[85] Both patients also had the Bombay blood phenotype and were the progeny of consanguineous parents, suggesting an autosomal recessive inheritance pattern. Functionally, the neutrophils were unable to adhere to E-selectin or cytokine-activated endothelial cells and

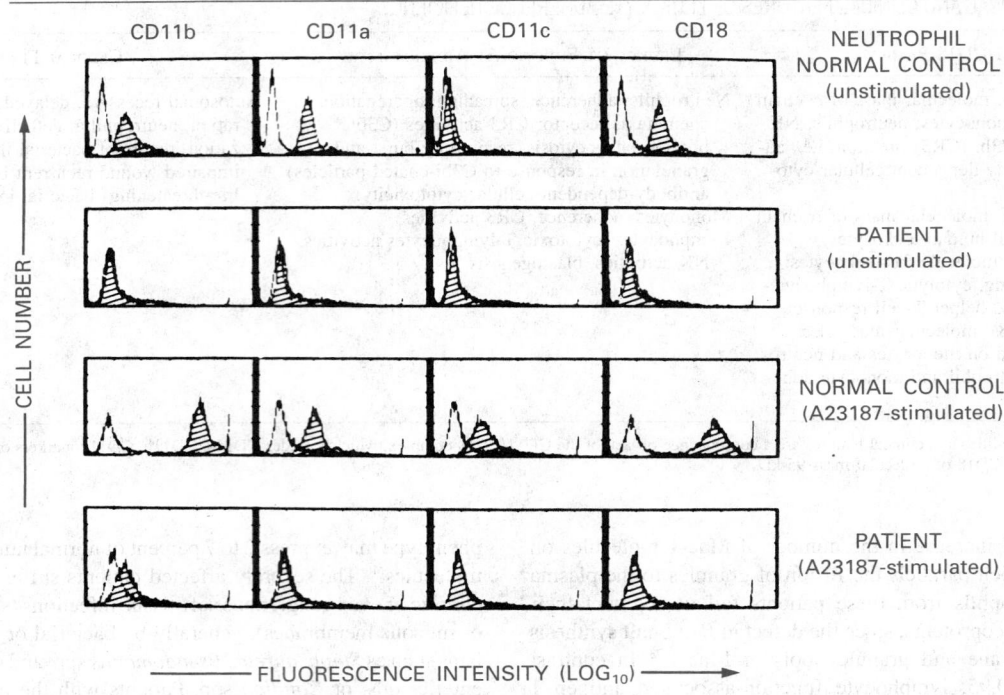

FIGURE 72-2   Specific diagnosis of CD11/CD18 glycoprotein deficiency by indirect immunofluorescence flow cytometric analysis. Blood neutrophils of a pediatric patient suspected of having CD11/CD18 glycoprotein deficiency and those of an abnormal individual were subjected to immunofluorescence staining for the expression of the CD11b, CD11a, CD11c, and CD18 epitope (cross-hatched histogram) as compared with the background immunofluorescence staining by isotype-identical negative-control antibodies (open histograms). Neutrophils were either stained immediately after purification by Ficoll-Hypaque density centrifugation (unstimulated) or after exposure to calcium ionophore A23187 (1 mM) for 15 min at 37°C (A23187-stimulated). A23187 stimulation causes significant increase in CD11b and CD18 epitope staining (surface MO1 expression) by normal neutrophils as compared with unstimulated normal cells. A23187 stimulation also causes a small increase in the CD11b-epitope expression of patient cells (the CD11b cross-hatched histogram becomes distinguishable from background staining after A23187 stimulation), suggesting that this patient has a "moderate" form of the disorder (capable of expressing small but detectable quantities of CD11/CD18 glycoproteins). Flow cytometric analysis was performed on a Coulter Electronics EPICS F C Flow Cytometer with a logarithmic amplifier. (From Todd and Freyer,[202] with permission.)

exhibited impaired chemotaxis and an inability to roll on postcapillary venules in vivo. The patients also exhibited distinctive facial appearance, were short in stature, had severe mental retardation, and were secretor-negative and Lewis antigen–negative. These patients are now classified as having LAD II. In contrast to LAD I, the patient's natural killer cell activity was normal.[86] The LAD II neutrophils expressed normal levels of CD18 integrins but were deficient in the carbohydrate structure sialyl–Lewis X, which renders the cells unable to roll on activated endothelial cells expressing E-selectin. Thus, the neutrophils from the patients categorized as having LAD II are unable to tether to inflamed venules, which is necessary for subsequent activation (see Chap. 66). The basis for LAD II cells appears to be a defect in the de novo pathway of glucose diphosphate (GDP)-fucose biosynthesis, which leads to deficient formation of Fucα1phosphate → 2 Gal linkages in ABO blood group core antigen, thereby accounting for the Bombay phenotype, whereas the Lewis antigen–negative phenotype arises from failure to synthesize Fucα1phosphate → 4 GlcNAc and Fucα1phosphate → 3 GlcNAc moieties.[85,87]

Therapy, Course, and Prognosis   Treatment of this disorder is largely supportive.[4,48,73] Patients with a history of recurrent infections can be maintained on prophylactic trimethoprim-sulfamethoxazole. Marrow transplantation with HLA-compatible siblings or parental do-

nors has resulted in engraftment and restoration of neutrophil function[88] and remains the treatment of choice for patients with a severe phenotype.

The restoration of CD11/CD18 expression in CD34 peripheral stem cells from LAD I following transduction with a retrovirus bearing CD18 and induced to differentiate into neutrophils with growth factors indicates that LAD I is caused by defective CD18 gene and provides a basis for somatic gene therapy.[89] Not only did the neutrophils express the integrins, but the cells demonstrated improvement in their functional responses, such as adhesion and the respiratory burst when challenged with ligands for CD11/CD18. These results indicate that ex vivo of the transfer gene for CD18 into LAD I CD34+ cells followed by reinfusion of the transfused cells may represent a therapeutic approach to LAD.

The severity of infectious complications correlates with the degree of β_2 deficiency.[73] Patients with severe deficiency may die in infancy, and those surviving infancy have a susceptibility to severe life-threatening systemic infections. In patients with moderate deficiency, life-threatening infections are infrequent and survival relatively long.[73] Fetal blood sampling and flow cytometric analysis for expression of CD11/CD18 integrins can be used for prenatal diagnosis of LAD I.[90] However, contamination of the sample by maternal blood can complicate the interpretation of the analysis.

NEUTROPHIL ACTIN DYSFUNCTION

These infants, like patients with LAD, have recurrent pyogenic infection from birth as a result of defective chemotactic and phagocytic response (see Table 72-1). In one patient, actin isolated from blood neutrophils did not polymerize under conditions that fully polymerized the actin of neutrophils from normal individuals.[91] Subsequent studies on the index patient's family confirmed that partial actin dysfunction was present in the parents and one sister.[92] One of the parents was found to be a heterozygote for LAD, but the other was not.[93] Further studies established that LAD is not generally associated with defective actin filament assembly.[94] The basis of the defective polymerization of actin in the index patient remains unknown, but this disorder of phagocytes is distinct from LAD.

Defective actin polymerization has been described in a 2-month-old infant with severe recurrent bacterial infections associated with impaired chemotaxis and phagocytic response.[95] This patient's neutrophils showed increased expression of CD11b, distinguishing the patient's clinical problem from LAD I. Morphologically the neutrophils display thin, filamentous projections of membrane with an underlying abnormal cytoskeletal structure. Subsequently a 47-kD protein was purified that inhibited actin polymerization in vitro.[96] Further biochemical studies revealed a markedly defective actin polymerization in the patient's neutrophils along with a severe deficiency of an 89-kD protein and an elevated level of the 47-kD protein. The 47-kD protein has been identified as LSP-1 (the lymphocyte-specific protein–1), which is an actin-binding protein present in normal neutrophils. Overexpression of the LSP-1 has resulted in bundling of actin in cells, leading to an abnormal cytoskeletal structure and motility defects.[97] Because actin dysfunction is lethal, treatment requires restoration of normal neutrophil function by marrow replacement from a normal donor. Bone marrow transplantation was attempted in both infants. In the first infant it was unsuccessful, whereas in the patient with the neutrophil actin dysfunction associated with overexpression of the 47-kD protein, bone marrow transplantation was successful.[95,98]

DISORDERS OF NEUTROPHIL MOTILITY

FAMILIAL MEDITERRANEAN FEVER

Definition and History   Familial Mediterranean fever (FMF) is an autosomal recessive disease that primarily affects populations surrounding the Mediterranean basin. The disease is characterized by acute limited attacks of fever often accompanied by pleuritis, peritonitis, arthritis, pericarditis, inflammation of the tunica vaginalis of the testes, and erysipelas-like skin disease (see Table 72-1).

Etiology and Pathogenesis   The pathologic findings in FMF are those of nonspecific acute inflammation affecting serosal tissues such as the pleura, peritoneum, and synovium. Neutrophilic infiltration predominates in the affected tissues. Physical and emotional stress, menstruation, and a high-fat diet may trigger the attacks.[99]

There is a lack of a C5a inhibitor activity in joints and peritoneal fluid in FMF, and since C5a is a highly potent chemotattractant for neutrophils, it has been suggested that lack of the inhibitor might account for the acute attacks of inflammation.[100] This hypothesis has not been confirmed. The observation that FMF has clinical manifestations similar to those of systemic lupus erythematosus suggests the possibility of an underlying autoimmune disorder. However, FMF does not respond to steroids and autoantibodies have not been found.[99,101]

The gene responsible for FMF has been identified to be located on chromosome 16. It encodes for a 781–amino acid protein called pyrin.[102,103] Homology searches indicate that pyrin is a new member of the *RETRO* gene family and suggests that pyrin itself may be a transcription factor, presumably regulating the expression of target genes, at least some of which are likely involved in the suppression of inflammation. The gene is expressed in neutrophils, but not other leukocytes. Pyrin has been designated as the gene for FMF because missense mutations have been identified in exon 10 in most of the affected patients, but not in normal subjects. Additional mutations in exon 2 of the gene have recently been detected in several families from various ethnic groups.[99] These mutations have not been found in all patients, indicating that other mutations are likely to be discovered. It is possible that pyrin may be involved in attenuating neutrophil activation by chemotactic factors. A puzzle, however, remains as to why the serosal tissues are the main targets of inflammation in FMF.

Clinical Features   The duration and frequency of attacks may vary considerably even in the same patient.[99] Acute attacks frequently last 24 to 48 h and recur once or twice a month. In some patients, attacks may recur as frequently as several times a week or as infrequently as once a year, and symptoms may persist as long as a week during individual episodes. Some patients experience spontaneous remission that persists for years followed by recurrence of frequent attacks. Peritonitis due to FMF may resemble an acute abdomen, thereby leading to potential uncertainties about the clinical management of the acute abdominal episode. Attacks of pleuritic pain occur in about 25 to 80 percent of patients. Symptoms of pleuritis may sometimes precede abdominal pain, and some patients experience pleuritic attacks without abdominal symptoms. Recurrent pericarditis has been reported, rarely. The course of peritonitis in FMF is similar to attacks at other serosal sites; however, it tends to appear at a late stage of the disease. Mild arthralgia is a common feature of febrile attacks, and monoarticular or oligoarticular arthritis may occur. Arthritis usually affects large joints, the knees in particular, and effusions are common. As many as one-third of the patients experience transient erysipelas-like skin lesions that appear typically on the lower leg, ankle, or dorsum of the foot. These lesions are circumscribed, painful, erythematous areas of swelling, which usually subsides within 24 to 48 h.

In about 25 percent of affected patients a form of renal amyloidosis develops in which the amyloid derives from a normal serum protein called serum amyloid A (amyloidosis of the AA type; see Chap. 105). The amyloidosis progresses over a period of years to renal failure in almost all cases, and the cause of death in patients with FMF is usually attributed to this complication.

Laboratory Features   Laboratory findings in FMF are nonspecific. During acute attacks leukocytosis (up to 30,000/ml) is present, and the erythrocyte sedimentation is increased. Between attacks the leukocyte count is normal.[100]

The cloning of the FMF gene now allows a reliable diagnostic test. By employing a set of polymerase chain reaction (PCR) primers, it is possible to identify the mutations responsible for the disease. Three major mutations are present in 85 percent of FMF carrier chromosomes. If the carrier gene frequency is 1 in 8, 98 percent of FMF patients will carry one or two of these mutations, and only 2 percent will bear an unidentified mutation.[99]

Therapy, Course, and Prognosis   Colchicine treatment is effective in FMF and may prevent the development of amyloidosis.[100] Prophylactic colchicine, 0.6 mg orally, two to three times a day, prevents or substantially reduces the acute attacks of FMF in most patients. Some patients can abort attack with intermittent doses of colchicine beginning at the onset of attacks (0.6 mg orally every hour for 4 h, then every 2 h for four doses, and then every 12 h for 2 days). In general, patients who benefit from intermittent colchicine therapy are those who experience a recognizable prodrome before developing fever and clear-cut acute symptoms.

The prognosis for normal longevity for patients has been excellent since the recognition of colchicine efficacy in this disease. Most patients can be maintained almost entirely symptom free. However, if amyloidosis develops, it may be followed by the nephrotic syndrome or uremia. Unless the patient receives a renal transplant, the likelihood of eventual death from renal failure is high.

OTHER DISORDERS OF NEUTROPHIL MOTILITY

The directed migration of neutrophils from the circulation to an inflammatory site is a consequence of chemotaxis and leads to the accumulation of an exudate. For normal chemotaxis to occur, a complex series of events must be coordinated. Chemotactic factors must be generated in sufficient quantities to establish a chemotactic gradient. The neutrophils must have receptors for the chemotactic agents and mechanisms for discerning the direction of the chemotactic gradient. Depressed neutrophil chemotaxis has been observed in a wide variety of clinical conditions (see Table 72-1).[1] These can be stratified as follows: (1) defects in the generation of chemotactic signals; (2) intrinsic defects of the neutrophil; and (3) direct inhibitors of neutrophil motility in response to chemotactic factors.

Older patients with chemotactic disorders may be infected by a variety of microorganisms, including fungi and gram-positive or gram-negative bacteria.[1] *Staphylococcus aureus* is the most frequent bacterial offender. Typically, the skin, gingival mucosa, and regional lymph nodes are involved. Respiratory tract infections are frequent, but sepsis is rare. Delayed or inappropriate signs and symptoms of inflammation are common. Although the cells move slowly in Boyden chambers or other chemotactic assays, they do accumulate in sufficient numbers in inflammatory sites to produce pus. However, detection of patients with neutrophils that have profound defects in chemotaxis usually is accomplished through other phagocytic assays.

Patients with the hereditary deficiency of complement factors C3, C5, or properidin exhibit an increased incidence of bacterial infections because they are unable to form the chemotactic peptide C5a.[104] The degree to which defective chemotaxis plays a role in C3 deficiency is unclear because opsonization and ingestion rates also are abnormal in these disorders. Frequently, chemotactic disorders are associated with other impaired neutrophil functions. For instance, both glycogen storage disease type 1b and myelokathexis are chemotactic disorders frequently associated with an absolute neutrophil count below 0.5×10^9/liter.[105,106] Following restoration of a normal neutrophil count with granulocyte colony stimulating factor, the patients no longer are predisposed to recurrent bacterial infections in spite of a persistent chemotactic defect. Thus, a chemotactic defect observed in vitro does not correlate invariably with decreased resistance to bacterial infections in vivo.

Among the impaired defense mechanisms of the neonate is neutrophil chemotaxis, as demonstrated by the in vitro response of neonatal neutrophils to a variety of chemotactic factors.[76] The impaired motility of the neonatal neutrophils in part arises from the diminished ability to mobilize neutrophil β_2-integrins following neutrophil activation.[107] Additionally, the neonatal neutrophil may have a qualitative defect in β_2-integrin function, resulting in impaired neutrophil transendothelial migration for up to 1 month after birth.

DRUGS AND EXTRINSIC AGENTS THAT IMPAIR NEUTROPHIL MOTILITY

Although many pharmacologic agents can influence neutrophil function, few drugs used in clinical medicine affect neutrophil behavior in vivo. Ethanol in concentrations that occur in human blood can inhibit neutrophil locomotion and ingestion.[108] Glucocorticoids, especially at high and sustained doses, inhibit neutrophil locomotion, ingestion, and degranulation.[109] Administration of glucocorticoids on alternate days does not interfere with neutrophil movement.[110] Epinephrine does not have a direct affect on neutrophil adhesion.[111] Cyclic adenosine

monophosphate (cAMP), which is released from endothelial cells following exposure to epinephrine, can depress neutrophil adherence. Similarly, elevated cAMP levels following epinephrine administration may impair neutrophil adherence, leading to diminished neutrophil margination and apparent neutrophilia. Immune complexes, as seen in patients with rheumatoid arthritis or other autoimmune diseases, also can inhibit neutrophil movement by binding to neutrophil Fc receptors.[1]

HYPERIMMUNOGLOBULIN E SYNDROME

DEFINITION AND HISTORY

The hyperimmunoglobulin E syndrome is a disorder characterized by markedly elevated serum IgE levels, chronic dermatitis, and serious recurrent bacterial infections.[112] The skin infections in these patients are remarkable for their absence of surrounding erythema, leading to the formation of "cold abscesses." The neutrophils and monocytes from patients with this syndrome exhibit a variable but at times profound chemotactic defect that appears extrinsic to the neutrophil.

ETIOLOGY AND PATHOGENESIS

Approximately 150 patients have been reported with this disorder. Both males and females have been affected. A familial occurrence in successive generations is suggestive of an autosomal dominant form of inheritance. The molecular basis for this syndrome remains unknown. Some believe that the immunologic basis of hyperimmunoglobulin E arises from insufficient suppressor T cells, which is manifested in part by reduced production of interferon (IFN)-α and tumor necrosis factor (TNF).[113] The proposed T-cell defect could explain the hyperproduction of IgE and the abnormal antibody responses that have been documented in some patients in response to various vaccines.[114] The predisposition to bacterial infections may arise from production of a chemotactic inhibitor released by mononuclear cells that inhibits normal neutrophil chemotaxis.[115] Another mechanism thought to predispose patients to recurrent bacterial infections is that the generation of excessive amounts of IgE directed against *Staph. aureus* and other varieties of bacterial and fungal antigens may be at the expense of the generation of protective IgE antibodies against the same organisms.[114]

CLINICAL FEATURES

Hyperimmunoglobulin E may begin as early as 1 to 8 weeks of age. The syndrome is characterized by chronic eczematoid rashes, which are typically papular and pruritic.[112] The rash generally involves the face and extensor surfaces of arms and legs; skin lesions are frequently sharply demarcated and usually lack surrounding erythema. By 5 years of age all patients have had a history of recurrent skin abscess formation and recurrent pneumonias, along with chronic otitis media and sinusitis. Patients may also develop septic arthritis, cellulitis, or osteomyelitis. The major offending pathogen is generally *Staph. aureus*. Other associated features include coarse facial features, manifested by a broad nasal bridge, prominent nose, and irregularly proportional cheeks and jaw. Growth retardation is also found in a minority of patients and appears related to the presence of chronic illness. Occasionally osteoporosis complicated by recurrent bone fractures has been noted as well as conjunctivitis complicated by corneal ulcerations.

LABORATORY FEATURES

All patients have serum IgE levels exceeding 2500 IU/ml. Unlike atopic patients who may also have similarly elevated IgE levels, patients with hyperimmunoglobulin E syndrome have their serum IgE antibody directed to *Staph. aureus*.[112] Usually the patients have normal concentrations of IgG, IgA, and IgM; pronounced blood and sputum eosinophilia; abnormally low anamnestic antibody response; and poor antibody and cell-mediated responses to neoantigens.[116] At variable times the neutrophils and monocytes of patients have a profound chemotactic defect. Sera from some, but not all, patients also have been demonstrated to inhibit chemotaxis of normal control neutrophils.

THERAPY, COURSE, AND PROGNOSIS

No known therapy is curative, and management decisions are based on the clinical findings. Prophylactic trimethoprim-sulfamethoxazole is effective in reducing infections with *Staph. aureus*.[112] Type and route of antibiotic therapy are dictated by the results of the Gram stain and culture in patients with acute bacterial infections. Incision and drainage are essential for the management of abscesses, including superinfected pneumatoceles. Eczematoid dermatitis can be controlled with topical glucocorticoids to reduce inflammation and antihistamines to control pruritus. Plasmapheresis has been reported to be effective in patients who fail more conservative approaches.

The use of recombinant IFN-α improves the in vitro chemotactic response of neutrophils.[117] In five patients treated with recombinant IFNα, their blood mononuclear cells decreased their spontaneous in vitro IgE production with no change in IgG and IgM.[118] Clinical trials are now needed to test the efficacy of IFN-γ in patients with the syndrome.

DEFECTS IN MICROBICIDAL ACTIVITY

CHRONIC GRANULOMATOUS DISEASE

DEFINITION AND HISTORY

Chronic granulomatous disease (CGD) is a genetic disorder affecting 4 to 5 in 1 million humans in which the neutrophils and monocytes ingest but do not kill catalase-positive microorganisms because of an inability to generate antimicrobial oxygen metabolites (see Table 72-1). It is caused by mutations involving one of several genes encoding a component of the reduced nicotinamide adenine dinucleotide phosphate (NADPH)-oxidase.[119,120]

ETIOLOGY AND PATHOGENESIS

Several laboratory tests are used to classify forms of CGD and aid in understanding its pathogenesis (Table 72-3). The diagnosis is usually made using the nitroblue tetrazolium (NBT) test, in which the yellow water-soluble tetrazolium dye is reduced to a blue insoluble formazan pigment by superoxide anion generated by activated normal phagocytes. Patients with CGD may have a heterogeneous array of symptoms and severity, depending on which subunit is defective and on the nature of the genetic mutation.[121]

NADPH-Oxidase Function Engulfment of microbes by phagocytic cells is associated with a burst of oxygen consumption that is important for microbicidal killing and digestion. The respiratory burst is accompanied, not by mitochondrial respiration, but by a unique electron transport chain called the NADPH-oxidase (see Chap. 66). Prior to stimulation, the components of the oxidase are physically separated into two major subcellular locations. The membrane-bound portion of the NADPH-oxidase contains a heterodimeric cytochrome b_{558} composed of a large, heavily glycosylated subunit with a M_r of 91 kD, known as a gp91^{phox} (91-kD glycoprotein of the phagocyte oxidase), and a 22-kD protein known as p22^{phox}.[122] The heavy chain of cytochrome b contains sites for heme binding, FAD groups, and NADPH binding.[123-126] The three-dimensional structure of cytochrome b_{558} is not known for certain, but there is a likely cytoplasmic globular domain in the carboxyl terminus half of the peptide that contains consensus sequences for flavin and NADPH binding.[127] Current models are also consistent with three transmembrane domains within the amino terminus half of the molecule, which contains the histidines that coordinate heme binding.[128] The p22^{phox} also contains a site for heme binding.[123] The synthesis of the p22^{phox} peptide is absolutely required for stability of gp91^{phox} and for oxidase activity in the membrane.[3] The p22^{phox} contains proline-rich regions that have consensus structure for binding SH3 (*SRC* homology 3–type domains) found in p47^{phox}.[129] Three other proteins vital to the function of this oxidase system have been identified and determined to reside in the cytosol of the resting phagocyte. Upon stimulation, translocation of p47^{phox} takes place. Phosphorylated p47^{phox} together with two other cytoplasmic components of the oxidase, p67^{phox} and a low-molecular-weight guanosine triphosphate *rac* 2, translocate to the membrane, where they interact with cytoplasmic domains of the transmembrane cytochrome b_{558} to form the active oxidase.[130,131] Both p47^{phox} and p67^{phox} contain two SH3 domains that may participate in intramolecular and intermolecular binding with consensus proline-rich regions in p47^{phox}.[132] Phosphorylation, which occurs on serines in the cationic C-terminal region of p47^{phox}, might serve to disrupt this intermolecular interaction, making the SH3 regions available for binding to p22^{phox}. Another cytoplasmic component with homology to p47^{phox} has been identified to be p40^{phox}, which appears to interact with p67^{phox} before and during oxidase assembling.[133] An inhibitory role for the p40^{phox} in regulating oxidase activation has been suggested.[134]

The cell-free system for activating the oxidase has permitted the dissection of the enzyme system into its components and the evaluation of the function of each unit.[135-141] Both cytosolic and membrane proteins

TABLE 72-3   DIAGNOSTIC CLASSIFICATION OF CHRONIC GRANULOMATOUS DISEASE.

MALE/FEMALE RATIO 6:1

AFFECTED COMPONENT	INHERITANCE	SUBTYPE*	CYTOCHROME B SPECTRUM	NBT POSITIVITY	RELATIVE FREQUENCY (%)	IMMUNOBLOT LEVELS gp91	p22	p47	p67	ACTIVITY IN CELL-FREE SYSTEM MEMBRANE	CYTOSOL
gp91-^{phox}	X	X91°	0	0	50	0	0	N	N	0	N
		X91$^-$	low	80–100 (weak)	3	low	low	N	N	Trace	N
		X91$^+$	N	0	3	N	N	N	N	0	N
p22-^{phox}	A	A22	0	0	5	0	0	N	N	0	N
		A22$^+$	N	0	1	N	N	N	N	0	0
p47-^{phox}	A	A47°	N	0	33	N	N	0	N	N	0
p67-^{phox}	A°	A67°	N	0	5	N	N	N	0	N	0

*In this nomenclature, the first letter represents the mode of inheritance [X-linked (X) or autosomal recessive (A)] while the number indicates the phox component which is genetically affected. The superscript symbols indicate whether the level of protein of the affected component is undetectable (o), diminished (−), or normal (+) as measured by immunoblot analysis employing component-specific antibodies. X, X-linked; A, autosomal recessive inheritance; N, normal level of protein; 0, undetectable level of protein activity; NBT, nitroblue tetrazolium. The classification is taken from reference 99 with permission.

are required for oxidase activation, and all patients with CGD have defects involving cytochrome b or the cytosolic components p47^{phox} or p67^{phox}.[142] The membrane and cytosol interaction for oxidase activation in the cell-free system defines the genetic heterogeneity of CGD.[142] Table 72-3 illustrates this point. The neutrophil membrane fractions from patients with XO (X-linked, cytochrome b–negative) and AO (autosomal recessive, cytochrome b–negative) CGD do not support oxidase activation even upon addition of normal cytosol, while the corresponding patient's cytosols function normally.[142] The membrane defect in both these types of CGD is due to the absence of cytochrome b. In the case of A+ CGD (autosomal recessive, cytochrome b–positive), the membrane fraction is normal, whereas the cytosol is severely defective.

Genetic Alterations Affecting Cytochrome b   The most frequent form of CGD occurs in two-thirds of patients and is caused by mutations in the gp91^{phox} gene located on chromosome Xp21.1.[119,120] These mutations lead to the X-linked form. Large interstitial deletions causing other X-linked disorders, such as retinitis pigmentosa, Duchenne muscular dystrophy, McLeod hemolytic anemia, and ornithine transcarbamylase deficiency, have been reported in a few patients with X-linked CGD.[121,143–145] Mutation analysis of the gene encoding gp91^{phox} and a large group of X-linked CGD kindreds has documented many distinct defects, including point mutations, inversions, deletions, or insertions that disrupt the reading frame and nonsense mutations that create a premature stop codon.[119,120,146] Some splice site defects have also been identified. In this situation, short deletions in gp91^{phox} mRNA are caused by point mutations that produce partial or complete exon skipping during mRNA splicing.[147] This abnormality is a common cause of X-linked CGD. In the remaining patients, point mutations have been identified that generate either premature stop codons or amino acid substitutions that apparently disrupt protein stability or function and lead to a complete lack of detectable cytochrome b$_{558}$ protein in phagocytic cells in most patients with X-linked CGD.[148] In some situations, low levels of functional cytochrome b are present, whereas in others, normal levels of dysfunctional cytochrome b$_{558}$ occur.[148] In the latter situation there is some clustering of defects in regions of known function, such as the NADPH- or flavin-binding consensus regions.[120,146]

A similar array of mutations has been identified in the rare CGD patients who have abnormalities in the p22^{phox} gene located on chromosome 16q24.[120,149] In this autosomal disorder, mutations in the p22^{phox} gene result in deletions, frameshifts, and/or missense mutations.[120] Two patients have been identified as homozygous for missense mutations due to consanguineous heritage. Patients with a defective p22^{phox} gene do not express the other cytochrome unit polypeptide.[150] In one patient, a point mutation in p22^{phox} peptide was associated with normal amounts of cytochrome b with normal heme spectrum, but p47^{phox} translocation membrane did not occur and there was no oxidase activation.[151] The mutation affected a proline-rich region thought to mediate binding to one of the SH3 domains of p47^{phox}.[132] In gp91^{phox}-deficient patients, p22^{phox} mRNA is present, but it is not translated, which is consistent with the notion that either cytochrome subunit polypeptide is dependent upon the stable expression of the other subunit.[121]

Genetic Alterations Affecting Cytosolic Proteins   Two other proteins have been identified as being vital to the function of the NADPH-oxidase system. Their absence results in the syndrome of CGD.[152] These proteins have molecular masses of 47 kD and 67 kD, respectively, and are located in the cytosol of resting cells. Defects in the genes for p47^{phox} found on chromosome 7q11 are responsible for one-fourth of all cases of CGD, whereas inherited defects for the gene for neutrophil p67^{phox} account for a small subgroup of autosomal recessive CGD.[120] The function of p47^{phox} and p67^{phox} in regulating the respiratory burst oxidase is thought to involve activation of the electron transport function of cytochrome b$_{558}$. The mutation analysis in patients with p47^{phox}-deficient forms of CGD reveals an unusual pattern, in that more than 90 percent of mutant alleles have guanine-thymine dinucleotide deletion at the start of exon 2, resulting in frameshift and premature stop.[120,153] The truncated protein is unstable, in that it cannot be detected immunologically. The majority of patients appear to be homozygous for this mutation without any history of consanguinity.[154] The p47^{phox} gene occurs in an area of chromosome 7 that has a high degree of evolutionary duplication in normal individuals because a pseudogene highly homologous to the normal p47^{phox} gene exists in the normal genome in this region of duplication. The pseudogene contains the same GT deletion associated with most cases of p47^{phox} CGD. This implies that recombination of the normal gene and pseudogene with conversion of the normal gene to partial pseudotype sequence in that region may be responsible for the high relative rate of this specific mutation in diverse racial groups.

A second rare form of CGD is caused by mutations in the gene for the p67^{phox} cytosolic component.[120] The p67^{phox} gene, which has been mapped to the long arm of chromosome 1, spans 37 kb and contains 16 exons. The mutations identified in p67^{phox}-deficiency CGD have included missense mutations and spliced junction mutations affecting mRNA processing, which led to nondetectable p67^{phox} protein by immunological means.[120]

The conversion of oxygen to superoxide anion and hydrogen peroxide by the neutrophils is described in Chap. 66. Complex signal transduction pathways serve to link membrane surface receptors with the activation of the respiratory burst oxidase. Cytochrome b is involved in the function of NADPH oxidase.[121,141] Cytochrome b has a very low midpoint potential, which makes it thermodynamically feasible for the cytochrome to function as an electron carrier in the oxidase.[155] Based on the midpoint potential for cytochrome b, electrons could theoretically be passed from NADPH to a flavin prosthetic group in the oxidase (FAD), then to the heme prosthetic group or cytochrome, and finally to molecular oxygen to form O$_2^-$. Indeed, the heavy chain of cytochrome b has been found to bind NADPH and FAD and to contain one of the heme prosthetic groups.[127,128] As indicated above, mutations in the gene for cytochrome b$_{558}$ or the cytosolic factors involved in activating the cytochrome have been associated with the CGD phenotype.

Predisposition to Infection   The manner in which the metabolic deficiency of the CGD neutrophil predisposes the host to infection is shown schematically in Fig. 72-3. Normal neutrophils accumulate hydrogen peroxide and other oxygen metabolites in the phagosomes containing ingested microorganisms. Myeloperoxidase is delivered to the phagosome by degranulation, and in this setting hydrogen peroxide acts as a substrate for myeloperoxidase to oxidize halide to hypochlorous acid and chloramines, which kill the microbes. The quantity of hydrogen peroxide produced by the normal neutrophils is sufficient to exceed the capacity of catalase, a hydrogen peroxide-catabolizing enzyme produced by many aerobic microorganisms, including *Staph. aureus,* most gram-negative enteric bacteria, *C. albicans,* and *Aspergillus* spp. In contrast, hydrogen peroxide is not produced by CGD neutrophils, and any generated by the microbes themselves may be destroyed by their own catalase. Thus, catalase-positive microbes can multiply inside CGD neutrophils, where they are protected from most circulating antibiotics, and can be transported to distant sites and released to establish new foci of infection.[156] Activation of the oxidase also has a pronounced effect on the pH within the phagocytic vacuole.[157] Activation of the respiratory burst is associated with an alkaline phase produced by the pumping of electrons and accompanied by protons along the wall of the phagosome. The alkaline phase is important for the antimicrobial and digestive functions of the neutral hydrolases released from the cytoplasmic granules into the vacuole upon phagocytosis. In CGD, the phagocytic vacuoles remain acidic and the bacteria are not digested properly. In hematoxylin-eosin-stained sections from patients, macrophages may contain a golden pigment, which reflects this abnormal accumulation of ingested material and also contributes to the diffuse granulomata that give CGD its descriptive name.[152] On the other hand, when CGD neutrophils ingest pneumococci or streptococci, these organisms generate enough hydrogen peroxide to result in a microbicidal effect.

CLINICAL FEATURES

Although the clinical presentation is variable, several clinical features suggest the diagnosis of CGD.[156,158] Any patient with recurrent lymphadenitis should be considered to have CGD. Additionally, patients with bacterial hepatic abscesses, osteomyelitis at multiple sites or in the small bones of the hands and feet, a family history of recurrent infections, or unusual catalase-positive microbial infections all require clinical evaluation for this disorder. The most common clinical disorders that afflict CGD patients are listed in Table 72-4.

The onset of clinical signs and symptoms may occur from early infancy to young adulthood. The attack rate and severity of infections are exceedingly variable. The most common pathogen is *Staph. aureus,* although any catalase-positive microorganism may be involved. Infection with *Serratia marcescens, Pseudomonas cepacia, Aspergillus* spp., or *C. albicans* occurs frequently. Infections are characterized by microabscesses and granuloma formation. The presence of pigmented histiocytes is helpful in establishing the diagnosis. Patients may suffer from the sequelae of chronic infection, including the anemia of chronic disease, lymphadenopathy, hepatosplenomegaly, chronic purulent dermatitis, restrictive lung disease, gingivitis, hydronephrosis, and gastroenteral narrowing. Pneumonias, lymphadenitis, and skin infections are the most common infections encountered. Pneumonias caused by *Aspergillus* or *Nocardia,* recurrent lymphadenitis, perirectal abscesses, and recurrent skin infections including folliculitis, cutaneous granulomata, and discoid lupus erythematosus should alert the physician to the possibility of CGD.

Several mothers of patients in whom X-linked inheritance was established had an illness resembling systemic lupus erythematosus.[159] Both X-linked and autosomal recessive patients with CGD also have a similar disorder.[160,161] It may be that these mothers' and patients' cells are unable to clear immune complexes sufficiently, which is a characteristic feature of CGD cells in vitro.[162]

LABORATORY FEATURES

The defect in the respiratory burst is best determined by measuring superoxide or hydrogen peroxide production in response to both soluble and particulate stimuli. A test that is being employed is the use of flow cytometry using dihydrorhodamine 123 fluorescence.[163] Dihydrorhodamine fluorescence detects oxidant production because it increases fluorescence upon oxidation. In most cases there is no detectable superoxide or hydrogen peroxide generation with either type of stimulus. In the variant form of CGD, on the other hand, superoxide may be produced at rates between 0.5 and 10 percent of control.[164]

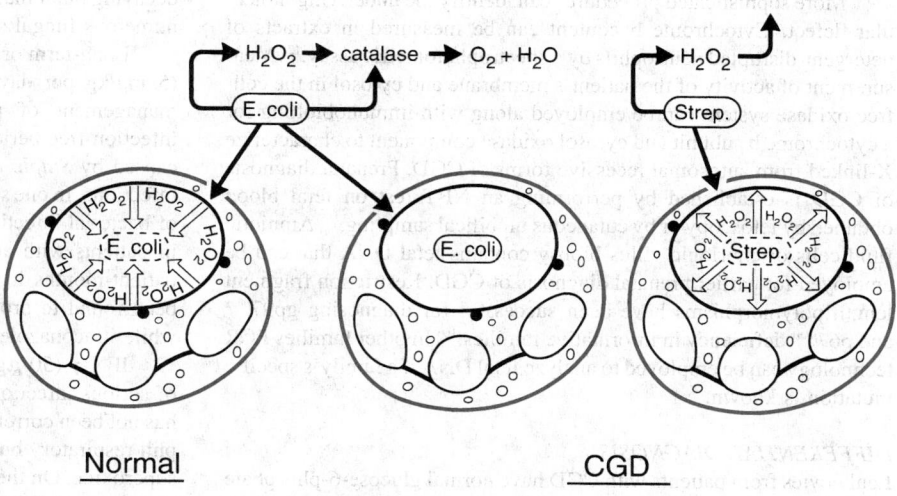

FIGURE 72-3 The pathogenesis of chronic granulomatous disease. The manner in which the metabolic deficiency of the CGD neutrophil predisposes the host to infection is shown schematically. Normal neutrophils accumulate hydrogen peroxide in the phagosome containing ingested *Escherichia coli.* Myeloperoxidase is delivered to the phagosome by degranulation, as indicated by the closed circles, and in this setting, hydrogen peroxide acts as a substrate for myeloperoxidase to oxidize halide to hypochlorous acid and chloramines, which kill the microbes. The quantity of hydrogen peroxide produced by the normal neutrophils is sufficient to exceed the capacity of catalase, a hydrogen peroxide–catabolizing enzyme of many aerobic microorganisms, including most gram-negative enteric bacteria, *Staph. aureus, C. albicans,* and *Aspergillus* spp. When organisms such as *E. coli* gain entry into the CGD neutrophils, they are not exposed to hydrogen peroxide because the neutrophils do not produce it, and the hydrogen peroxide generated by microbes themselves is destroyed by their own catalase. When CGD neutrophils ingest streptococci or pneumococci, these organisms generate enough hydrogen peroxide to result in a microbicidal effect. On the other hand, as indicated in the middle figure, catalase-positive microbes, such as *E. coli,* can survive within the phagosome of the CGD neutrophil.

An alternative method for measuring respiratory burst activity is the NBT test. This assay is performed by microscopically assessing the ability of individual cells to reduce NBT to purple formazan crystals following stimulation. Commonly there is no NBT reduction with most forms of CGD. In some of the variant forms, however, a high percentage of cells may contain some formazan, a finding indicative of a greatly diminished respiratory burst in most of the neutrophils. This test also permits detection of the carrier state in X-linked CGD when as few as 5 to 10 percent of the cells are NBT-negative.[121]

TABLE 72-4   CLINICAL MANIFESTATION OF CHRONIC GRANULOMATOUS DISEASE

Incidence	1:1,000,000
Male/female ratio	6:1
Clinical disorders	Pneumonitis (77%)
	Dermatitis (68%)
	Lymphadenitis (60%)
	Hepatic abscess (39%)
	Osteomyelitis (32%)
	Persistent diarrhea (18%)
	Septicemia/meningitis (17%)
	Persistent rhinitis (15%)
	Perianal abscess (14%)
	Stomatitis (14%)
	Gastric antral narrowing (rare) and pyelonephritis secondary to ureteral (rare) obstruction, pericarditis (rare).

The clinical disorders are based on data taken from ref 120 with permission. The number in parenthesis represents the percentage of patients affected.

More sophisticated procedures can identify the underlying molecular defect. Cytochrome b content can be measured in extracts of detergent-disrupted neutrophils by a spectrophotometric assay.[121] Measurement of activity of the patient's membrane and cytosol in the cell-free oxidase system can be employed along with immunoblotting for a cytochrome b subunit and cytosol oxidase component to characterize X-linked from autosomal recessive forms of CGD. Prenatal diagnosis of CGD is established by performing an NBT test on fetal blood obtained by fetoscopy or by cutaneous umbilical sampling.[165] Amniotic fluid cells or chorionic villus biopsy contains fetal DNA that can be employed for earlier prenatal diagnosis of CGD. Restriction fragment length polymorphisms have been successful for diagnosing gp97^{phox} and p67^{phox} deficiency in informative families.[166] In other families PCR technology can be employed to analyze fetal DNA if a family's specific mutation is known.

DIFFERENTIAL DIAGNOSIS

Leukocytes from patients with CGD have normal glucose-6-phosphate dehydrogenase (G-6-PD) activity. However, a few individuals with apparent CGD have been described that have neutrophils that lack or almost lack in G-6-PD activity.[167–169] The erythrocytes of these patients also lack the enzyme, and the patients have chronic hemolysis. In the cases of severe neutrophil G-6-PD deficiency, an attenuated respiratory burst progressively decreases due to the depletion of intracellular NADPH, the primary substrate for the respiratory burst oxidase. CGD and G-6-PD deficiency can be distinguished from each other by the hemolytic anemia seen in the latter disorder and by the fact that erythrocyte G-6-PD activity is normal in CGD and markedly reduced in G-6-PD deficiency.[148]

THERAPY, COURSE, AND PROGNOSIS

Because marrow transplantation is the only known cure for CGD, vigorous supportive care along with the use of rIFN-γ continues to be the foundation of treatment.[148,156,170,171] Cultures must be obtained as soon as infection is suspected, as unusual organisms are commonly the source of infection and may grow promptly in vitro. Most abscesses will require surgical drainage for therapeutic and diagnostic purposes, and prolonged use of antibiotics is often required. If fever occurs, it is advisable to obtain certain studies that aid in the management of septic episodes. These include roentgenograms of the chest and skeleton and a CT scan of the liver because of the frequency of pneumonia, osteomyelitis, and liver abscesses.[172,173] Arrangements should be made for prompt medical attention at the first signs of infection. With early intervention, many lesions can be managed by conservative medical means. For example, enlarging lymph nodes often regress when treated with local heat and orally administered antistaphylococcal antibiotics. More serious events require hospitalization and a diagnostic and therapeutic approach applicable to any patient with severe infection. In general, antibiotic therapy for the offending organisms is indicated and purulent masses should be drained. The cause of fever and prostration cannot always be established, and empiric treatment with broad-spectrum parenteral antibiotics is required. Often it is necessary to treat with antibiotics for a prolonged time until the initial sedimentation rate approaches normal values.[172] Aspergillus spp. infection requires treatment with amphotericin B or, in refractory cases, with granulocyte transfusions.[172] Glucocorticoids also may be useful in the treatment of patients with antral and urethral obstruction.[174,175] The risk of Aspergillus infection can be reduced by avoiding marijuana smoke and decaying plant material, such as mulch and hay, both of which contain numerous fungal spores.[176]

Long-term oral prophylaxis with trimethoprim-sulfamethoxazole (5 mg/kg per day of trimethoprim) is an accepted practice in the management of patients with CGD.[177] Patients have prolonged infection-free periods, which result from the prevention of infections caused by Staph. aureus, without increasing the incidence of fungal infections. In one series this regimen resulted in a diminished incidence of bacterial infection from 7.1 to 2.4 per one hundred patient-months in patients with autosomal CGD and from 15.8 to 6.9 per hundred patient-months in X-linked patients.[177] Use of ketoconazole has not been found to provide any protection against Aspergillus infections, while itraconazole may prove to be efficacious in this regard.[178]

IFN-γ (50 $\mu g/m^2$, three times per week) can reduce the number of serious infections.[179] IFN-γ–enhanced neutrophil function in vitro has not been correlated with improvement in the activity of the neutrophil respiratory burst in patients totally lacking the ability to generate superoxide. On the other hand, its use increases the neutrophil expression of the high-affinity Fcγ receptor 1 as well as monocyte expression of FcγRI, FcγRII, FcγRIII, CD11/CD18, and HLA-DR.[180] The IFN-γ protective effect in patients with CGD may involve improved microbial clearance, as suggested by the enhanced phagocytic activity by neutrophils of opsonized Staph. aureus. In rare X-linked CGD patients able to generate some superoxide, IFN-γ programs granulocyte cells to increase their expression of cytochrome b, which results in normal superoxide generation.[181] With the use of current prophylactic treatments, the mortality in CGD has been reduced to two patient deaths per year per hundred patients followed.[3]

Mutations in CGD that result in 5 to 10 percent of normal functioning amounts of NADPH have a mild phenotype and better clinical prognosis than that of patients with complete absence of any NADPH oxidase activity.[182,183] Similarly, female carriers of X-linked CGD who have only 3 to 5 percent oxidase-normal neutrophils rarely get serious infections suggestive of the CGD clinical phenotype.[184] Thus, even low levels or partial correction by gene therapy of CGD are likely to provide clinical benefits. In support of that hypothesis, mouse models of X-linked and p47^{phox}-deficient CGD have been developed by gene targeting.[185,186] Studies have shown in the gp91^{phox}- and the p47^{phox}-deficient mouse models of CGD that retrovirus-mediated gene therapy targeting of marrow progenitor cells ex vivo can result in the correction of defects in oxidant production in vivo in peripheral blood neutrophils after radiation conditioning and transplantation of the transduced marrow stem cells.[187,188] Protection from infection challenge occurred even when the oxidase-corrected cells comprised less than 10 percent of circulating neutrophils. These promising results have suggested that somatic gene therapy can be employed to correct defective phagocyte oxidase function in selected patients with CGD. In a phase I clinical trial, gene therapy for p47^{phox}-deficiency CGD, five adult patients received intravenous infusions of autologous blood stem cells that were ex vivo transduced using a retrovirus encoding normal p47^{phox}.[189] Although conditioning therapy was not given prior to the stem cell infusion, functionally corrected neutrophils were detectable in peripheral blood 3 to 6 weeks after the single infusion and ranged from 0.004 to 0.05 percent of total blood neutrophils. The corrected cells were detectable for as long as 6 months after infusion in some patients. These results indicate a promise for gene therapy in the future to correct phagocytic oxidase function in selected patients with CGD.

FIGURE 72-4 Algorithm for the workup patients with recurrent infections. Abbreviations: CBC, complete blood count; G-6-PD, glucose-6-phosphate dehydrogenase; Ig, immunoglobulin; LAD, leukocyte adhesion deficiency. (Modified from Curnutte JT, Boxer LA: Clinically significant phagocytic cell defects, in *Current Clinical Topics in Infectious Diseases,* 6th ed, edited by JS Remington, MN Swartz, p 144. McGraw-Hill, New York, 1985.)

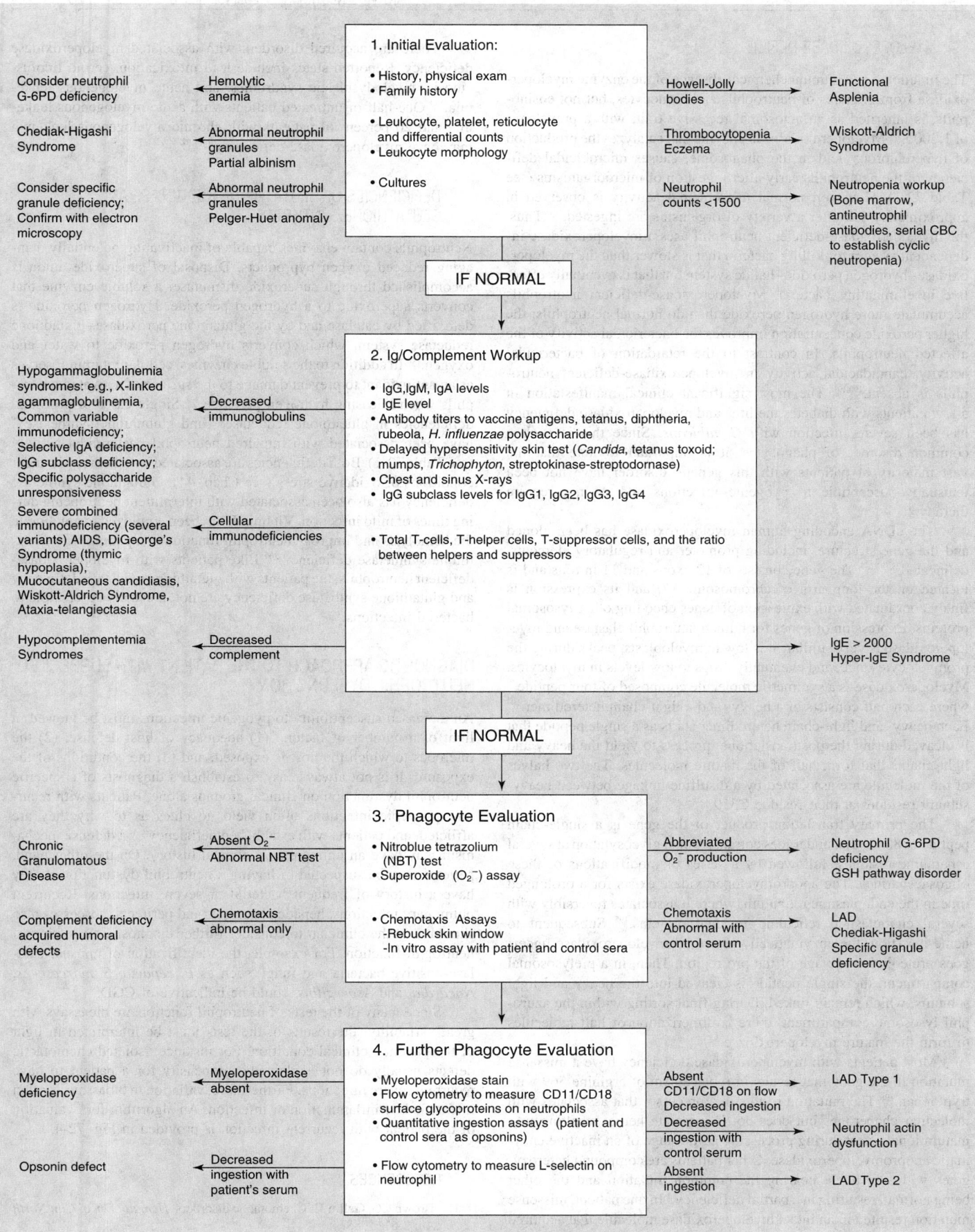

1. Initial Evaluation:

- History, physical exam
- Family history

- Leukocyte, platelet, reticulocyte and differential counts
- Leukocyte morphology

- Cultures

Consider neutrophil G-6PD deficiency ← Hemolytic anemia

Chediak-Higashi Syndrome ← Abnormal neutrophil granules / Partial albinism

Consider specific granule deficiency; Confirm with electron microscopy ← Abnormal neutrophil granules / Pelger-Huet anomaly

Howell-Jolly bodies → Functional Asplenia

Thrombocytopenia Eczema → Wiskott-Aldrich Syndrome

Neutrophil counts <1500 → Neutropenia workup (Bone marrow, antineutrophil antibodies, serial CBC to establish cyclic neutropenia)

IF NORMAL

2. Ig/Complement Workup

- IgG,IgM, IgA levels
- IgE level
- Antibody titers to vaccine antigens, tetanus, diphtheria, rubeola, *H. influenzae* polysaccharide
- Delayed hypersensitivity skin test (*Candida*, tetanus toxoid; mumps, *Trichophyton*, streptokinase-streptodornase)
- Chest and sinus X-rays
- IgG subclass levels for IgG1, IgG2, IgG3, IgG4

- Total T-cells, T-helper cells, T-suppressor cells, and the ratio between helpers and suppressors

Hypogammaglobulinemia syndromes: e.g., X-linked agammaglobulinemia, Common variable immunodeficiency; Selective IgA deficiency; IgG subclass deficiency; Specific polysaccharide unresponsiveness ← Decreased immunoglobulins

Severe combined immunodeficiency (several variants) AIDS, DiGeorge's Syndrome (thymic hypoplasia), Mucocutaneous candidiasis, Wiskott-Aldrich Syndrome, Ataxia-telangiectasia ← Cellular immunodeficiencies

Hypocomplementemia Syndromes ← Decreased complement

IgE > 2000 Hyper-IgE Syndrome →

IF NORMAL

3. Phagocyte Evaluation

- Nitroblue tetrazolium (NBT) test
- Superoxide (O₂⁻) assay

- Chemotaxis Assays
  -Rebuck skin window
  -In vitro assay with patient and control sera

Chronic Granulomatous Disease ← Absent O_2^- / Abnormal NBT test

Complement deficiency acquired humoral defects ← Chemotaxis abnormal only

Abbreviated O_2^- production → Neutrophil G-6PD deficiency GSH pathway disorder

Chemotaxis Abnormal with control serum → LAD Chediak-Higashi Specific granule deficiency

4. Further Phagocyte Evaluation

- Myeloperoxidase stain
- Flow cytometry to measure CD11/CD18 surface glycoproteins on neutrophils
- Quantitative ingestion assays (patient and control sera as opsonins)

- Flow cytometry to measure L-selectin on neutrophil

Myeloperoxidase deficiency ← Myeloperoxidase absent

Opsonin defect ← Decreased ingestion with patient's serum

Absent CD11/CD18 on flow Decreased ingestion → LAD Type 1

Decreased ingestion with control serum → Neutrophil actin dysfunction

Absent ingestion → LAD Type 2

MYELOPEROXIDASE DEFICIENCY

The functional and immunochemical absence of the enzyme myeloperoxidase from granules of neutrophils and monocytes, but not eosinophils, is inherited as an autosomal recessive trait, with a prevalence of 1:2000.[190] Myeloperoxidase, an enzyme that catalyzes the production of hyperchlorous acid in the phagosome, causes microbicidal deficiency of the neutrophils early after ingestion of microorganisms (see Table 72-1). However, normal microbicidal activity is observed in approximately 1 h after a variety of organisms are ingested.[191] Thus, the myeloperoxidase-deficient neutrophil uses a myeloperoxidase-independent system for killing bacteria that is slower than the myeloperoxidase–hydrogen peroxide–halide system but that is eventually effective in eliminating bacteria. Myeloperoxidase-deficient neutrophils accumulate more hydrogen peroxide than do normal neutrophils; the higher peroxide concentration improves the bactericidal activity of the affected neutrophils. In contrast to the retardation of bactericidal activity, candidacidal activity in myeloperoxidase-deficient neutrophils is absent.[190,191] The most significant clinical manifestation in a few patients with diabetes mellitus and myeloperoxidase deficiency has been severe infection with *C. albicans*. Since this is such a common disorder of phagocytes, it is important to note that the vast majority of patients with this genetic disorder have not been unusually susceptible to pyogenic infections and do not require therapy.

The cDNA encoding human myeloperoxidase has been cloned and the gene structure, including promoter and regulatory elements, delineated.[3,192,193] The gene consists of 12 exons and 11 introns and is located on the long arm of chromosome 17, and its expression is finely coordinated with expression of genes encoding other lysosomal proteins. Expression of genes for human neutrophil elastase and myeloperoxidase is very similar; it is low in myeloblasts, peaks during the promyelocyte stage, and eventually drops to low levels in myelocytes. Myeloperoxidase is a symmetric molecule composed of four peptides, where each half consists of a heavy- and a light-chain heterodimer.[194] Each heavy- and light-chain heterodimer starts as a single peptide that is cleaved during the posttranslational process to yield the heavy and light chains that form half of the mature molecules. The two halves of the molecule are associated by a disulfide linkage between heavy-subunit residues at their residue C319.

The primary translation product of the gene is a single-chain peptide of 80 kD that undergoes cotranslational glycosylation at several asparagine residues, followed by a series of modifications of these oligosaccharides. The apopromyeloperoxidase exists for a prolonged time in the endoplasmic reticulum, where it associates reversibly with several endoplasmic reticulum–resident proteins.[195] Subsequent to heme insertion, the enzymatically active promyeloperoxidase undergoes proteolytic cleavage of the pro region. Then, in a prelysosomal compartment, the single peptide is cleaved into the heavy and light subunits, which remain linked. During final sorting within the azurophil lysosome compartment, there is dimerization of half-molecules to form the mature myeloperoxidase.[3]

Most patients with myeloperoxidase deficiency have a missense mutation in the gene that results in replacement of arginine 569 with tryptophan.[196] The mutation results in a precursor that associates with molecular chaperones but does not incorporate heme, resulting in a maturational arrest during processing at the stage of an inactive enzymatic apopromyeloperoxidase. Other patients are compound heterozygotes with one allele bearing the common mutation and the other being normal, resulting in a partial deficiency.[3] In one patient, missense mutation resulted in an intact myeloperoxidase molecule that acquired heme but failed to undergo proteolytic processing to a mature molecule.[197]

There are acquired disorders with associated myeloperoxidase deficiency. Reported states include lead intoxication, ceroid lipofuscinosis, myelodysplastic syndromes, and acute myelogenous leukemia.[190] One-half of untreated patients with acute myelogenous leukemia and 20 percent of patients with chronic myelogenous leukemia may have myeloperoxidase deficiency.[190,191]

DEFICIENCIES OF GLUTATHIONE REDUCTASE AND GLUTATHIONE SYNTHETASE

Neutrophils contain enzymes capable of inactivating potentially damaging reduced oxygen byproducts. Disposal of superoxide anion is accomplished through superoxide dismutase, a soluble enzyme that converts superoxide to a hydrogen peroxide. Hydrogen peroxide is detoxified by catalase and by the glutathione peroxidase–glutathione reductase system, which converts hydrogen peroxide to water and oxygen.[198] In addition to the soluble enzymes, cellular vitamin E serves as an antioxidant to prevent damage to the surface of activated neutrophils when releasing hydrogen peroxide.[198] Single cases of profound deficiencies in glutathione reductase[199] and glutathione synthetase[199] have been associated with impaired neutrophil bactericidal activity (see Table 72-1). Both deficiencies are associated with hemolysis under conditions of oxidative stress (see Chap. 44). Glutathione synthetase deficiency has also been associated with intermittent neutropenia during times of mild infection. Vitamin E has been employed to ameliorate the hemolysis and improve neutrophil function in a patient with glutathione synthetase deficiency.[200] Like patients with myeloperoxidase-deficient neutrophils, the patients with glutathione reductase deficiency and glutathione synthetase deficiency are not unusually susceptible to bacterial infections.

DIAGNOSTIC APPROACH TO THE PATIENT WITH SUSPECTED NEUTROPHIL DYSFUNCTION

An increased susceptibility to pyogenic infections must be viewed in light of a number of factors: (1) adequacy of host defense, (2) the microbes to which the host is exposed, and (3) the conditions of the exposure. It is not always easy to establish a diagnosis of a specific neutrophil dysfunction on clinical grounds alone. Patients with recurrent pyogenic infections often yield no clues as to why they are afflicted, and patients with established deficiency of a defense mechanism may have an unimpressive clinical history. On the other hand, patients may be suspected of having a neutrophil dysfunction if they have a history of frequent bacterial or severe infections. Recurrent pulmonary infections, hepatic abscesses, and perirectal abscesses also should alert the clinician to consider further diagnostic evaluation of neutrophil function. For example, the identification of unusual catalase-positive bacteria and fungi, such as *P. cepacia, S. marcescens, Nocardia,* and *Aspergillus,* could be indicative of CGD.

Since many of the tests of neutrophil function are bioassays with great variability, the results of the tests must be interpreted in light of the patient's clinical condition. For instance, isolated chemotactic defects usually do not explain the propensity for a patient to have recurrent severe infections. Furthermore, variation in bioassays is often intensified by inflammation or infection. An algorithm for evaluation of the patient with recurrent infection is provided in Fig. 72-4.

REFERENCES

1. Brown CC, Gallin JI: Chemotactic disorders. *Hematol Oncol Clin North Am* 2:61, 1988.
2. Leung DYM, Geha RS: Clinical and immunologic aspects of the hyperimmunoglobulin syndrome. *Hematol Oncol Clin North Am* 2:81, 1988.

3. Malech HL, Nauseef WA: Primary inherited defects in neutrophil function: Etiology and treatment. *Semin Hematol* 34:279, 1997.

4. Dinauer MC: The phagocyte-system and disorders of granulopoiesis and granulocyte function, in *Hematology of Infancy and Childhood*, 5th ed, edited by DG Nathan, SH Orkin, p 889. Saunders, Philadelphia, 1998.

5. Botto M, Fong KY, So AK, Walport MJ: Molecular basis of hereditary C3 deficiency. *J Clin Invest* 86:1158, 1990.

6. Walport MJ: Inherited complement deficiency: Clues to the physiological activity of complement in vivo. *Q J Med* 86:355, 1993.

7. Alper CA, Abramson W, Johnston RB Jr, et al: Studies in vivo and in vitro on an abnormality in the metabolism of C3 in a patient with increased susceptibility to infection. *J Clin Invest* 49:1975, 1970.

8. Densen P, Weiler JM, Griffiss JM, et al: Familial properidin deficiency and fatal meningococcemia. *N Engl J Med* 316:922, 1987.

9. Nolan KF, Schwaeble FW, Kaluz S, et al: Molecular cloning of the cDNA coding for properidin, a positive regulator of the alternative pathway of human complement. *Eur J Immunol* 21:771, 1991.

10. Super M, Thiel S, Lu J, et al: Association of low levels of mannan-binding protein with a common defect of opsonization. *Lancet* 2:1236, 1989.

11. Turner MW, Lipscombe RJ, Levinsky RJ, et al: Mutations in the human mannose binding protein gene: Their frequencies in three distinct populations and relationship to serum levels of the protein. *Immunodeficiency* 4:285, 1993.

12. Epstein J, Eichbaum Q, Sheriff S, Ezekowitz RAB: The collectins in innate immunity. *Curr Opin Immunol* 8:29, 1996.

13. Summerfield JA, Ryder S, Sumiya M, et al: Mannose binding protein gene mutations associated with unusual and severe infections in adults. *Lancet* 345:886, 1995.

14. Buckley RH: Immunodeficiency states. *JAMA* 268:2797, 1992.

15. Bisno Al, Freeman JC: The syndrome of asplenia, pneumococcal sepsis, and disseminated intravascular coagulation. *Ann Intern Med* 72:389, 1970.

16. Boxer LA, Smolen JE: Neutrophil granule constituents and their release in health and disease. *Hematol Oncol Clin North Am* 2:101, 1988.

17. Creel D, Boxer LA, Fauci AS: Visual and auditory anomalies in Chédiak-Higashi syndrome. *Electroencephal Clin Neurophys* 5:252, 1983.

18. Haliotis T, Roder J, Klein M, et al: Chédiak-Higashi gene in humans: I. Impairment of natural-killer function. *J Exp Med* 151:1039, 1980.

19. Nishimura M, Inoue M, Nakano T, et al: Beige rat: A new animal model of Chédiak-Higashi syndrome. *Blood* 74:270, 1989.

20. White JG, Clawson CC: The Chédiak-Higashi syndrome: The nature of the giant neutrophil granules and their interactions with cytoplasm and foreign particulates, *Am J Pathol* 98:151, 1980.

21. Ostlund RE Jr, Tucker RW, Leung JT, et al: The cytoskeleton in Chédiak-Higashi syndrome fibroblasts. *Blood* 56:806, 1980.

22. Ingraham LM, Burns C, Boxer LA, et al: Fluidity properties and lipid composition of erythrocyte membranes in Chédiak-Higashi syndrome. *J Cell Biol* 89:510, 1981.

23. Strausbauch P, Sehgal N: Three-dimensional reconstruction of anomalous beige mouse macrophage lysosomes. *J Leuk Biol* 46:441, 1989.

24. Rausch PG, Pryzwansky KB, Spitznagel JK: Immunocytochemical identification of azurophilic and specific granulocyte markers in the giant granules of Chédiak-Higashi neutrophil. *N Engl J Med* 298:693, 1978.

25. Ganz T, Metcalf JA, Gallin JI, et al: Microbicidal/cytotoxic proteins of neutrophils are deficient in two disorders: Chédiak-Higashi syndrome and ''specific'' granule deficiency. *J Clin Invest* 82:552, 1988.

26. Takeuchi KH, Swank RT: Inhibitors of elastase and cathepsin G in Chédiak-Higashi (beige) neutrophils. *J Biol Chem* 264:7431, 1989.

27. Blume RS, Bennet JM, Yankee RA, Wolff SM: Defective granulocyte regulation in the Chédiak-Higashi syndrome. *N Engl J Med* 279:1009, 1968.

28. Nagle DL, Karim MA, Woolf EA, et al: Identification and mutation analysis of the complete gene for Chédiak-Higashi syndrome. *Nature Genet* 14:307, 1996.

29. Boxer GJ, Holmsen H, Robkin L, et al: Abnormal platelet function in Chédiak-Higashi syndrome. *Br J Haematol* 35:521, 1977.

30. Merino F, Henle W, Ramirez Duque P: Chronic active Epstein-Barr virus infection in patients with Chédiak-Higashi syndrome. *J Clin Immunol* 6:299, 1986.

31. Rubin CM, Burke BA, McKenna RW, et al: The accelerated phase of Chédiak-Higashi syndrome: An expression of the virus-associated hemophagocytic syndrome. *Cancer* 56:524, 1985.

32. Nair MPN, Gray, RH, Boxer LA, Schwartz S: Deficiency of inducible suppressor cell activity in the Chédiak-Higashi syndrome. *Am J Hematol* 26:55, 1987.

33. Aonuma K, Komiyama A, Akabone T: Pseudo-Chédiak-Higashi anomaly in acute myeloid leukemia (M2) of childhood. *Acta Paediatr Jpn* 32:651, 1990.

34. Weening RS, Shoorel ER, Roos D, et al: Effect of ascorbate on abnormal neutrophil, platelet and lymphocyte function in a patient with Chédiak-Higashi syndrome. *Blood* 57:856, 1981.

35. Virelizier JL, Lagrue A, Durandy A, et al: Reversal of natural killer defect in a patient with Chédiak-Higashi syndrome after bone marrow transplantation. *N Engl J Med* 306:1055, 1982.

36. Haddad E, LeDeist F, Blanche S, et al: Treatment of Chédiak-Higashi syndrome by allogenic bone marrrow transplantation: Report of 10 cases. *Blood* 85:3328, 1995.

37. Lomax KJ, Gallin JI, Rostrosen D, et al: A selective defect in myeloid cell lactoferrin gene expression in neutrophil specific granule deficiency. *J Clin Invest* 83:514, 1989.

38. Johnston JJ, Boxer LA, Berliner N: Correlation of mRNA levels with protein defects in specific granule deficiency. *Blood* 80:2088, 1992.

39. Rosenberg HF, Gallin JI: Neutrophil specific granule deficiency includes eosinophils. *Blood* 82:268, 1993.

40. Gallin JI, Fletcher MP, Seligmann BE, et al: Human neutrophil-specific granule deficiency: A model to assess the role of neutrophil-specific granules in the evolution of the inflammatory response. *Blood* 59:1317, 1982.

41. Boxer LA, Coates TD, Haak RA, et al: Lactoferrin deficiency associated with altered granulocyte function. *N Engl J Med* 307:404, 1982.

42. Yoon PS, Boxer LA, Mayo LA, et al: Human neutrophil laminin receptors: Activation dependent receptor expression. *J Immunol* 183:259, 1987.

43. Petrequin PR, Todd RF III, Smolen JE, Boxer LA: Expression of specific granule markers on the cell surface of neutrophil cytoplasts. *Blood* 67:1119, 1986.

44. Lawson ND, Khanna-Gupta A, Berliner N: Isolation and characterization of the cDNA for mouse neutrophil collagenase: Demonstration of shared negative regulatory pathways for neutrophil secondary granule protein gene expression. *Blood* 91:2517, 1998.

45. Sigurdsson F, Khanna-Gupta A, Lawson N, et al: Control of late neutrophil-specific gene expression: Insights into regulation of myeloid differentiation. *Semin Hematol* 34:303, 1997.

46. Parmley RT, Tzeng DY, Baehner RL, Boxer LA: Abnormal distribution of complex carbohydrates in neutrophils of a patient with lactoferrin deficiency. *Blood* 62:538, 1983.

47. Kuriyama K, Tomonaga M, Matsuo T, et al: Diagnostic significance of detecting pseudo-Pelger-Huet anomalies and micro-megakaryocytes in myelodysplastic syndrome. *Br J Haematol* 63:665, 1986.

48. Arnaout MA: Leukocyte adhesion molecule deficiency: Its structural basis, pathophysiology and implications for modulating the inflammatory response. *Immunol Rev* 114:145, 1990.

49. Corbi AL, Larson RS, Kishumoto TK, et al: Chromosome location of the genes encoding the leukocyte adhesion receptors LFA-1, Mac-1 and p150,95: Identification of a gene cluster involved in cell adhesion. *J Exp Med* 167:159, 1988.

50. Corbi HL, Kishimoto TK, Miller LJ, Springer TA: The human leukocyte adhesion glycoprotein Mac-1 (complement receptor type 3, CD11b) α subunit. *J Biol Chem* 263:12403, 1988.

51. Law SKA, Gagnon J, Hildreth JEK, et al: The primary structure of the beta subunit of the cell surface adhesion glycoproteins LFA-1, CR3 and p150,95 and its relationship to the fibronectin receptor. *EMBO J* 6:915, 1988.

52. Arnaout MA, Remold-O'Donnell E, Pierce MW, et al: Molecular cloning of the human and guinea pig alpha subunit of leukocyte adhesion glycoprotein, Mol: Chromosomal localization and homology to the alpha subunits of the integrins. *Proc Natl Acad Sci USA* 85:2776, 1988.

53. Arnaout MA: Dynamics and regulation of leukocyte-endothelial cell interactions. *Curr Opin Hematol* 1:113,1993.

54. Cheresh DA, Smith JW, Cooper M II, Quaranta V: A novel vitronectin receptor integrin ($\alpha_4\beta_4$) is responsible for distinct adhesive properties of carcinoma cells. *Cell* 57:59, 1989.

55. Marlin SO, Morton CC, Anderson DC, et al: LFA-1 immunodeficiency disease: Definition of the genetic defect and chromosome mapping of alpha and beta subunits by complementation in hybrid cells. *J Exp Med* 164:855, 1986.

56. Ohashi Y, Yambe T, Tsuchiya S, et al: Familial genetic defect in a case of leukocyte adhesion deficiency. *Hum Mutat* 2:458, 1993.

57. Back AL, Kerkering M, Baker D, et al: A point mutation associated with leukocyte adhesion deficiency type 1 of moderate severity. *Biochem Biophys Res Commun* 193:912, 1993.

58. Corbi AL, Vara A, Ursa A, et al: Molecular basis for a severe case of leukocyte adhesion deficiency. *Eur J Immunol* 22:1877, 1992.

59. Arnaout MA, Dana N, Gupta SK, et al: Point mutations impairing cell surface expression of the common β subunit CD18 in a patient with Leu-CAM deficiency. *J Clin Invest* 85:977, 1990.

60. Wardlaw AJ, Hibbs ML, Stacker SA, Springer TA: Distinct mutations in two patients with leukocyte adhesion deficiency and their functional correlates. *J Exp Med* 172:335, 1990.

61. Matsuura S, Kishi F, Tsukahara M, et al: Leukocyte adhesion deficiency: Identification of novel mutations in two Japanese patients with a severe form. *Biochem Biophys Res Commun* 184:1460, 1992.

62. Sligh JE Jr, Hurwitz MY, Zhu C, et al: An initiation codon mutation in CD18 in association with moderate phenotype of leukocyte adhesion deficiency. *J Biol Chem* 267:714, 1992.

63. Kishimoto TK, O'Connor K, Springer TA: Leukocyte adhesion deficiency: Aberrant splicing of a conserved integrin sequence causes a moderate deficiency phenotype. *J Biol Chem* 264:3588, 1989.

64. Nelson C, Rabb H, Arnaout MA: Genetic cause of leukocyte adhesion molecule deficiency: Abnormal splicing and a missense mutation in a conserved region of CD18 impairs cell surface expression of 2 integrins. *J Biol Chem* 267:3351, 1992.

65. Rodriquez CL, Nueda A, Grospierre B, et al: Characterization of two new C18 alleles causing severe leukocyte adhesion deficiency. *Eur J Immunol* 23:2792, 1995.

66. Springer TA, Thompson WS, Miller LJ, et al: Inherited deficiency of the Mac-1, LFA-1, p150,95 glycoprotein and its molecular basis. *J Exp Med* 160:1901, 1984.

67. Anderson DC, Schmalsteig FC, Finegold MJ, et al: The severe and moderate phenotypes of heritable Mac-1, LFA-1, p150,95 deficiency: Their quantitative dysfunction and clinical features. *J Infect Dis* 152:668, 1985.

68. Larson RS, Springer TA: Structure and function of leukocyte integrins. *Immunol Rev* 114:118, 1990.

69. Kuiyers TW, VanLier RA, Hamann D, et al: Leukocyte adhesion deficiency type 1 (LAD-1)/variant: A novel immunodeficiency syndrome characterized by dysfunctional beta 2 integrins. *J Clin Invest* 100:1725, 1997.

70. Arnaout MA, Spits H, Terhost C, et al: Deficiency of a leukocyte surface glycoprotein (LFA-1) in two patients with Mo1 deficiency: Effects of cell activation on Mo1/LFA-1 surface expression in normal and deficient leukocytes. *J Clin Invest* 74:1291, 1984.

71. Petrequin PR, Todd RD III, Devall LJ, et al: Association between tertiary granule release and increased plasma membrane expression of the MO1 glycoprotein. *Blood* 69:605, 1987.

72. Kjeldsen L, Senrgelov H, Lollike K, et al: Granular and secretory vesicles in human neonatal neutrophils. *Pediatr Res* 40:120, 1996.

73. Anderson DC, Springer TA: Leukocyte adhesion deficiency: An inherited defect in the Mac-1, LFA-1, and p150,95 glycoproteins. *Ann Rev Med* 38:175, 1987.

74. Schwartz BR, Wayner EA, Carlos TM, et al: Identification of surface proteins mediating adherence of CD11/CD18-deficient lymphoblastoid cells to cultured human endothelium. *J Clin Invest* 85:2019, 1990.

75. Mizgerd JP, Kubo H, Kutkoski GJ, et al: Neutrophil emigration in the skin, lungs and peritoneum: Different requirements for CD11/CD18 revealed by CD18-deficient mice. *J Exp Med* 186:1357, 1997.

76. Anderson DC, Rothlein R, Marlin DS, et al: Imparied transendothelial migration by neonatal neutrophils: Abnormalities of Mac-1 (CD11b/CD18)-dependent adhesive reactions. *Blood* 76:2613, 1990.

77. Mulligan MS, Varani J, Dome MK, et al: Role of endothelial-leukocyte adhesion molecule 1 (ELAM-1) in neutrophil mediated lung injury in rats. *J Clin Invest* 88:1396, 1991.

78. Wertheimer SJ, Myers CL, Wallace RW, Parks TP: Intercellular adhesion molecule-1 gene expression in human endothelial cells: Differential regulation by tumor necrosis factor-α and phorbol myristate acetate. *J Biol Chem* 267:12030, 1992.

79. Sehgal G, Zang K, Todd RF III, et al: Lectin-like inhibition of immune complex receptor-mediated stimulation of neutrophils: Effects on cytosolic calcium release and superoxide production. *J Immunol* 150:226, 1993.

80. Cas D, Mizukami LF, Garni-Wagner BA, et al: Human urokinase-type plasminogen activator primes neutrophils for superoxide anion release: Possible roles of complement receptor type 3 and calcium. *J Immunol* 154:1817, 1995.

81. Altieri DC, Barder R, Mannucci PM, Edginton TS: Oligospecificity of the cellular adhesion receptor Mac-1 encompasses an inducible recognition specificity for fibrinogen. *J Cell Biol* 107:1893, 1988.

82. Giger U, Boxer LA, Simpson PJ, et al: Deficiency of leukocyte surface glycoproteins Mo1, LFA1, and Leu M5 in a dog with recurrent bacterial infections: An animal model. *Blood* 69:1622, 1987.

83. Shuster DE, Kehrli ME, Ackerman MR, Gilbert RO: Identification and prevalence of a genetic defect that causes leukocyte adhesion deficiency in Holstein cattle. *Proc Natl Acad Sci USA* 89:9225, 1992.

84. Wilson RW, Ballantyne CM, Smith CW, et al: Gene targeting yields a CD18-mutant mouse for study of inflammation. *J Immunol* 151:1571, 1993.

85. Etzioni A, Frydman M, Polack S, et al: Brief report: Recurrent severe infections caused by a novel leukocyte adhesion deficiency. *N Engl J Med* 3 27:1789, 1992.

86. Etzioni A: Adhesion molecules: Their role in health and disease. *Pediatr Res* 39:191, 1996.

87. Karsan A, Cornejo CJ, Winn RK, et al: Leukocyte adhesion deficiency type II is a generalized defect of *de novo* GDP-fucose biosynthesis: Endothelial cell fucosylation is not required for neutrophil rolling on human non-lymphoid endothelium. *J Clin Invest* 101:2438, 1998.

88. Fischer A, Lisowska-Cirospierre B, Anderson DC, Springer TA: Leukocyte adhesion deficiency: Molecular basis and functional consequences. *Immunodefic Rev* 1:39, 1988.

89. Bauer TR, Schwartz BR, Liles C, et al: Retroviral-mediated gene transfer of the leukocyte integrin CD18 into peripheral blood CD34+ cells derived from a patient with leukocyte adhesion deficiency type 1. *Blood* 91:1520, 1998.

90. Kral V, Bartunkova J, Svorc K, et al: The first case of leukocyte integrin deficiency syndrome in the Czech Republic and successful prenatal diagnosis in the affected family. *Cas Lek Cesk* 135:154, 1996.

91. Boxer LA, Hedley-Whyte ET, Stossel TP: Neutrophil actin dysfunction and abnormal neutrophil behavior. *N Engl J Med* 291:1093, 1974.

92. Southwick FS, Dabiri GA, Stossel TP: Neutrophil actin dysfunction is a genetic disorder associated with partial impairment of neutrophil actin assembly in three family members. *J Clin Invest* 82:1525, 1988.

93. Southwick FS, Holbrook T, Howard T, et al: Neutrophil actin dysfunction is associated with a deficiency of Mo1. *Clin Res* 34:533A, 1986.

94. Southwick FS, Howard TH, Holbrook T, et al: The relationship between CR3 deficiency and neutrophil actin assembly. *Blood* 73:1793, 1989.

95. Coates TD, Torkildson JC, Torres M, et al: An inherited defect of neutrophil motility and microfilamentous cytoskeleton associated with abnormalities in 47-kD and 89-kD proteins. *Blood* 78:1338, 1991.

96. Howard T, Li Y, Torres M, et al: The 47-kD protein increased in neutrophil actin dysfunction with 47- and 89-kD protein abnormalities is lymphocyte-specific protein. *Blood* 83:231, 1994.

97. Howard TH, Hartwig J, Cunningham C: Lymphocyte-specific protein 1 expressed in eukaryotic cells reproduces the morphologic and motile abnormality of NAD 47/89 neutrophils. *Blood* 91:4786, 1998.

98. Camitta BM, Quesenberry PJ, Parkman R, et al: Bone marrow transplantation for a syndrome of neutrophil dysfunction. *Exp Hematol* 5:109, 1977.

99. Ben-Chetrit E, Levy M: Familial Mediterranean fever. *Lancet* 51:659, 1998.

100. Matzner Y: Acquired neutrophil dysfunction and diseases with an inflammatory component. *Semin Hematol* 34:291, 1997.

101. Swissa M, Schul V, Korish S, et al: Determination of autoantibodies in patients with familial Mediterranean fever and their first degree relative. *J Rheumatol* 18:606, 1991.

102. The International FMF Consortium: Ancient missense mutations in a new member of the RoRet gene family are likely to cause familial Mediterranean fever. *Cell* 90:797, 1997.

103. The French FMF Consortium: A candidate gene for familial Mediterranean fever. *Nature Genet* 17:25, 1997.

104. Shur PH: Inherited complement component abnormalities. *Ann Rev Med* 37:333, 1986.

105. Wang WC, Crist WN, Ihle JN, et al: Granulocyte colony stimulating factor corrects the neutropenia associated with glycogen strorage disease type 1b. *Leukemia* 5:347, 1991.

106. Weston BW, Axtell RA, Todd RF III, et al: Clinical and biologic effects of granulocyte-colony stimulating factor in the treatment of myelokathexis. *J Pediatr* 188:229, 1991.

107. Jones DH, Schmalstieg FC, Dempsey K, et al: Subcellular distribution and mobilization of Mac-a (CD11b/CD18) in neonatal neutrophils. *Blood* 74:848, 1990.

108. Brayton RG, Stokes PE, Schwartz MS, Louria DB: Effect of alcohol and various diseases on leukocyte mobilization, phagocytosis, and intracellular killing. *N Engl J Med* 282:123, 1970.

109. Oseas RS, Allen J, Yang HH, et al: Mechanism of dexamethasone inhibition of chemotactic factor induced granulocyte aggregation. *Blood* 59:265, 1982.

110. Dale DC, Fauci AS, Wolff SM: Alternate-day prednisone: Leukocyte kinetics and susceptibility to infections. *N Engl J Med* 291:1154, 1974.

111. Boxer LA, Allen JM, Baehner RL: Diminished polymorphonuclear leukocyte adherence: Function dependent on release of cyclic AMP by endothelial cells after stimulation of β-receptors by epinephrine. *J Clin Invest* 66:268, 1980.

112. Leung DYM, Geha RS: Clinical and immunologic aspects of the hyperimmunoglobulin E syndrome. *Hematol Oncol Clin North Am* 2:81, 1988.

113. DelPrete G, Tiri A, Maggi E, et al: Defective *in vitro* production of gamma interferon and tumor necrosis factor-alpha by circulating T cells from patients with the hyperimmunoglobulin E syndrome. *J Clin Invest* 84:1830, 1989.

114. Sheerin KA, Buckley RH: Antibody responses to protein, polysaccharide, and pili X174 antigens in the hyperimmunoglobulin E (hyper-IgE) syndrome. *J Allergy Clin Immunol* 87:803, 1991.

115. Donabedian H, Gallin JI: Two inhibitors of neutrophil chemotaxis are produced by hyperimmunoglobulin E recurrent infection syndrome mononuclear cells exposed to heat-killed staphylococci. *Infect Immun* 40:1030, 1983.

116. Burkley RH: Immunodeficiency diseases. *JAMA* 268: 2797, 1992.

117. Jeppson JD, Jaffe HS, Hill HR: Use of recombinant human interferon gamma to enhance neutrophil chemotactic responses in Job syndrome of hyperimmunoglobulin E and recurrent infections. *J Pediatr* 3:383, 1991.

118. King CL, Gallin JI, Malech HL, et al: Regulation of immunoglobulin production in hyperimmunoglobulin E recurrent-infection syndrome by interferon gamma. *Proc Natl Acad Sci USA* 86:10085, 1989.

119. Heyworth PG, Curnutte JT, Noack D, Cross AR: Hematologically important mutations: X-linked chronic granulomatous disease—an update. *Blood Cells Mol Dis* 23:443, 1997.

120. Roos D, deBoer M, Kuribayashi F, et al: Mutations in the X-linked and autosomal recessive forms of chronic granulomatous disease. *Blood* 87:1663, 1996.

121. Curnutte J: Chronic granulomatous disease: The solving of a clinical riddle at the molecular level. *Clin Immunol Immunopathol* 67:52, 1993.

122. Parkos CA, Allen RA, Cochrane CG, Jesaitis AJ: Purified cytochrome b from human granulocyte plasma membrane is comprised of two polypeptides with relative molecular weights of 91,000 and 22,000. *J Clin Invest* 80:732, 1987.

123. Quinn MT, Mullen ML, Jesaitis AJ: Human neutrophil cytochrome b contains multiple hemes: Evidence for heme associated with both subunits. *J Biol Chem* 167:7303, 1992.

124. Rotrosen D, Yeung CL, Leto TL, et al: Cytochrome b$_{558}$: The flavin-binding component of the phagocyte NADPH oxidase. *Science* 256:1459, 1992.

125. Segal AW, West I, Wientjes F, et al: Cytochrome b$_{245}$ is a flavocytochrome containing FAD and the NADPH-binding site of the microbicidal oxidase of phagocytes. *Biochem J* 284:781, 1992.

126. Sumimato H, Sakamoto N, Nazaki M, et al: Cytochrome b$_{558}$, a component of the phagocyte NADPH oxidase, is a flavoprotein. *Biochem Biophys Res Commun* 186:1368, 1992.

127. Zhen L, Yu L, Denauer MC: Probing the role of the carboxyl terminus of the gp91^{phox} subunit of neutrophil flavocytochrome b$_{558}$ using site-directed mutagenesis. *J Biol Chem* 273:6575, 1998.

128. Shatwell KP, Dancis A, Cross AR, et al: The FRE1 ferric reductase of *Saccharomyces cerevisiae* is a cytochrome b similar to that of NADPH oxidase. *J Biol Chem* 271:14240, 1996.

129. deMendez I, Homayoumpour N, Leto TL: Specificity of p47^{phox} SH3 domain interactions in NADPH oxidase assembly and activation. *Mol Cell Biol* 17:2177, 1997.

130. DeLeo FR, Quinn MT: Assembly of the phagocyte NADPH oxidase: Molecular interaction of oxidase proteins. *J Leuk Biol* 60:677, 1996.

131. Segal AW: The NADPH oxidase and chronic granulomatous disease. *Mol Med Today* 2:129, 1996.

132. Leto TL, Adams AG, deMendez I: Assembly of the phagocyte NADPH oxidase: Binding of Src homology 3 domain to proline-rich targets. *Proc Natl Acad Sci USA* 91:10650, 1994.

133. Wientjes FB, Hsuaii JJ, Totty NF, et al: p40^{phox} a third cytosolic component of the activation complex of the NADPH oxidase to contain Src homology 3 domains. *J Biochem* 296:557, 1993.

134. Sathyamoorthy M, deMendez I, Adams AG, et al: p40 (phox) down-regulates NADPH oxidase activity through interactions with its SH3 domain. *J Biol Chem* 272:9141, 1997.

135. Abo A, Boyhan A, West I, et al: Reconstitution of neutrophil NADPH oxidase activity in the cell-free system by four components: p67^{phox}, p47^{phox}, p21 rac1, and cytochrome b$_{245}$. *J Biol Chem* 267:16767, 1992.

136. Clark RA, Volpp BD, Leidal KG, Nauseef WM: Two cytosolic components of the human neutrophil respiratory burst oxidase translocate to the plasma membrane during cell activation. *J Clin Invest* 85:714, 1990.

137. Heyworth PG, Curnutte JT, Nauseef WM, et al: Neutrophil nicotinamide adenine dinucleotide phosphate oxidase assembly: Translocation of p47^{phox} and p67^{phox} requires interaction between p47^{phox} and cytochrome b$_{558}$. *J Clin Invest* 87:352, 1991.

138. Knaus UG, Heyworth PG, Evans T, et al: Regulation of phagocyte oxygen radical production of the GTP-binding protein Rac-2. *Science* 254:1512, 1991.

139. Bromberg Y, Pick E: Unsaturated fatty acids stimulate NADPH-dependent superoxide production by cell-free system derived from macrophages. *Cell Immunol* 88:213, 1984.

140. Curnutte JT: Activation of human neutrophil nicotinamide adenine dinucleotide phosphate reduced (triphosphopyridine nucleotide reduced) oxidase by arachidonic acid in a cell-free system. *J Clin Invest* 75:1740, 1985.

141. McPhail LC, Shirley PS, Clatyon CC, Snyderman R: Activation of the respiratory burst enzyme from human neutrophils in a cell-free system. *J Clin Invest* 75:1735, 1985.

142. Curnutte JT: Molecular basis of the autosomal recessive forms of chronic granulomatous disease. *Immunodefic Rev* 3:149, 1992.

143. Francke U, Ochs HD, DeMartinville B, et al: Minor Xp21 chromosome deletion in a male associated with expression of Duchenne muscular dystrophy, chronic granulomatous disease, retinitis pigmentosa, and McLeod syndrome. *Am J Hum Genet* 37:250, 1985.

144. Royer-Pokora B, Kunkel LM, Monaco AP, et al: Cloning the gene for an inherited human disorder—chronic granulomatous disease—on the basis of its chromosomal location. *Nature* 322:32, 1986.

145. Frey D, Machler M, Seger R, et al: Gene deletion in a patient with chronic granulomatous disease and McLeod syndrome: Fine mapping of the Xk gene locus. *Blood* 71:252, 1988.

146. Roos D: X-CGD base: A database of X-CGD causing mutations. *Immunol Today* 17:517, 1996.

147. deBoer M, Bolscher BGJM, Dinauer MC, et al: Splice site mutations are a common cause of X-linked chronic granulomatous disease. *Blood* 80:1553, 1992.

148. Curnutte J, Orkin S, Dinauer M: Genetic disorders of phagocyte function, in *The Molecular Basis of Blood Diseases*, 2nd ed, edited by G Stamnatoyannopoulos, p 493. Saunders, Philadelphia, 1994.

149. Dinauer MC, Pierce EA, Bruns GAP, et al: Human neutrophil cytochrome-b light chain (p22^{phox}): Gene structure, chromosomal location, and mutations in cytochrome-negative autosomal recessive chronic granulomatous disease. *J Clin Invest* 86:1729, 1990.

150. Parkos CA, Dinauer MC, Jesaitis AJ, et al: Absence of both the 91-kD and 22-kD subunits of human neutrophil cytochrome b in two genetic forms of chronic granulomatous disease. *Blood* 73:1416, 1989.

151. Dinauer MC, Pierce EH, Erickson RW, et al: Point mutation in the cytoplasmic domain of the neutrophil p22^{phox} cytochrome b subunit is associated with a nonfunctional NADPH oxidase and chronic granulomatous disease. *Proc Natl Acad Sci USA* 88:11231, 1991.

152. Segal AW: Biochemistry and molecular biology of chronic granulomatous disease. *J Inher Metab Dis* 15:683, 1992.

153. Casmir CM, Bu-Ghanium HR, Rodaway AR, et al: Autosomal recessive chronic granulomatous disease caused by deletion at a dinucleotide repeat. *Proc Natl Acad Sci USA* 88:2753, 1991.

154. Gorlach A, Lee PL, Roesler J, et al: A p47^{phox} pseudogene carrier is the

most common mutation causing p47^{phox}-deficient chronic granulomatous disease. *J Clin Invest* 100:1907, 1977.

155. Cross AR, Jones OTG, Harper AM, Segal AW: Oxidation-reduction properties of the cytochrome b found in the plasma-membrane fraction of human neutrophils. *Biochem J* 194:599, 1981.

156. Forrest CB, Forehand JR, Axtell RA, et al: Clinical features and current management of chronic granulomatous disease. *Hematol Oncol Clin North Am* 2:253,1988.

157. Segal AW, Gerson M, Garcia R, et al: The respiratory burst of phagocytic cells is associated with a rise in vacuolar pH. *Nature* 290:406, 1982.

158. Weening RS, Adriaansz LH, Weemaes CMR, et al: Clinical differences in chronic granulomatous disease in patients with cytochrome b-negative or cytochrome b-positive neutrophils. *J Pediatr* 107:102, 1985.

159. Manzi S, Urbach AH, McCune AB, et al: Systemic lupus erythematosus in a boy with chronic granulomatous disease: Case report and review of the literature. *Arthritis Rheum* 34:101, 1991.

160. Stalder JF, Dreno B, Bureau B, Hakim J: Discoid lupus erythematosus-like lesions in an autosomal form of chronic granulomatous disease. *Br J Dermatol* 114:251, 1986.

161. Smitt JHS, Bos JD, Weening RS, Krieg SR: Discoid lupus erythematosus-like skin changes in patients with autosomal recessive chronic granulomatous disease. *Arch Dermatol* 126:1656, 1990.

162. Petty HR, Francis JW, Boxer LA: Deficiency in immune complex uptake by chronic granulomatous disease neutrophils. *J Cell Sci* 135:1, 1988.

163. Crockard AD, Thompson JM, Boyd NA, et al: Diagnosis and carrier detection of chronic granulomatous disease in five families by flow cytometry. *Int Arch Allergy Immunol* 114:144, 1997.

164. Newburger PE, Luscinska FW, Ryan T, et al: Variant chronic granulomatous disease: Modulation of the neutrophil by severe infection. *Blood* 68:914, 1986.

165. Newburger P, Cohen HJ, Rothchild SB, et al: Prenatal diagnosis of chronic granulomatous disease. *N Engl J Med* 300:178, 1979.

166. Pelham A, O'Reilly M-AJ, Malcolm S, et al: RFLP and deletion analysis for X-linked chronic granulomatous disease using the cDNA probe: Potential for improved prenatal diagnosis and carrier determination. *Blood* 76:820, 1990.

167. Cooper MR, DeChatelet LR, McCall CE, et al: Complete deficiency of leukocyte glucose-6-phosphate dehydrogenase with defective bactericidal activity. *J Clin Invest* 51:769, 1979.

168. Mamlok RJ, Mamlock V, Mills GC, et al: Glucose-6-phosphate dehydrogenase deficiency, neutrophil dysfunction and *Chromobacterium violaceum* sepsis. *J Pediatr* 111:852, 1987.

169. Vives Corrons JL, Feliu E, Pujades MA, et al: Severe glucose-6-phosphate dehydrogenase (G6PD) deficiency associated with chronic hemolytic anemia, granulocyte dysfunction, and increased susceptibility to infection: Description of a new molecular variant (G6PD Barcelona). *Blood* 59:428, 1982.

170. Bemiller LS, Roberts DH, Starko KM, Curnutte JT: Safety and effectiveness of long-term interferon gamma therapy in patients with chronic granulomatous disease. *Blood Cells Mol Dis* 21:239, 1995.

171. Klempner MS, Malech HL: Phagocytes: Normal and abnormal host defenses, in *Infectious Diseases,* edited by SL Gorbach, JG Bartlett, NR Blacklow. Saunders, Philadelphia, 1997.

172. Gallin JL, Buescher ES, Seligimann BE, et al: Recent advances in chronic granulomatous disease. *Ann Intern Med* 99:657, 1983.

173. Sponseller PD, Malech HL, McCarthy EF Jr: Skeletal involvement in children who have chronic granulomatous disease. *J Bone Joint Surg* 73:37, 1991.

174. Chin TW, Stiehm ER, Falloon J, Gallin JI: Corticosteroids in the treatment of obstructive lesions of chronic granulomatous disease. *J Pediatr* 111:349, 1987.

175. Walther MM, Malech H, Berman A, et al: The urological manifestations of chronic granulomatous disease. *J Urol* 174:1314, 1992.

176. Chused MJ, Gelfand JA, Nutter C, Fauci AS: Pulmonary aspergillosis inhalation of contaminated marijuana smoke, chronic granulomatous disease. *Ann Intern Med* 82:682, 1975.

177. Margolis DM, Melnick DA, Alling DW, Gallin JI: Trimethoprim-sulfamethoxazole prophylaxis in the management of chronic granulomatous disease. *J Infect Dis* 162:723, 1990.

178. Moury R, Fischer A, Vilmer E, et al: Incidence, severity and prevention of infections in chronic granulomatous disease. *J Pediatr* 114:555, 1989.

179. International Chronic Granulomatous Disease Study Group: A controlled study of interferon gamma to prevent infections in chronic granulomatous disease. *N Engl J Med* 324:509, 1991.

180. Schiff DE, Martin TR, Davis BH, Curnutte JT: Increased phagocyte Fc gamma R1 expression and improved Fc gamma-receptor-mediated phagocytosis after in vivo recombinant human interferon-gamma treatment of normal human subjects. *Blood* 90:3187, 1997.

181. Woodman RC, Erickson RW, Rae J, et al: Prolonged recombinant interferon-gamma therapy in chronic granulomatous disease: Evidence against enhanced neutrophil oxidase activity. *Blood* 79:1558, 1992.

182. Seeger RA, Tiefenauer L, Matsunaga T, et al: Chronic granulomatous disease due to granulocytes with abnormal NADPH oxidase activity and deficient cytochrome-b. *Blood* 61:423, 1983.

183. Styrt B, Klempner MS: Late-presenting variant of chronic granulomatous disease. *Pediatr Infect Dis* 3:556, 1984.

184. Malech HL, Bauer TR Jr, Hickstein DD: Prospects for gene therapy of neutrophil defects. *Semin Hematol* 34:355, 1997.

185. Pollock JD, Williams DA, Gifford MAC, et al: Mouse model of X-linked chronic granulomatous disease: An inherited defect in phagocyte superoxide production. *Nature Genet* 9:202, 1995.

186. Jackson SH, Gallin JI, Holland SM: The p47^{phox} mouse knockout model of chronic granulomatous disease. *J Exp Med* 182:751, 1995.

187. Marding M 3rd, Jackson SH, Spratl SK, et al: Enhanced host defense after gene transfer in the murine p47^{phox}-deficient model of chronic granulomatous disease. *Blood* 89:2268, 1997.

188. Bjorgvinsdattir H, Ding C, Peck N, et al: Retroviral-mediated gene transfer of gp91^{phox} into bone marrow cells rescues defect in host response after *Aspergillus fumigatus* in murine X-linked chronic granulomatous disease. *Blood* 89:41, 1997.

189. Malech HL, Maples PB, Whiting-Theobald N, et al: Prolonged production of NADPH oxidase-corrected granulocytes after gene therapy of chronic granulomatous disease. *Proc Natl Acad Sci USA* 94:12133, 1997.

190. Nauseef WM: Myeloperoxidase deficiency. *Hematol Pathol* 4:165, 1990.

191. Nauseef WM: Myeloperoxidase deficiency. *Hematol Oncol Clin North Am* 2:135, 1988.

192. Austen GE, Zhao WG, Zhang W, et al: Identification and characterization of the human myeloperoxidase promoter. *Leukemia* 9:848, 1995.

193. Morisha K, Tsuchiya M, Asano S, et al: Chromosomal gene of human myeloperoxidase and regulation of its expression by granulocyte colony-stimulating factor. *J Biol Chem* 262:15208, 1987.

194. Zeng J, Fenna RE: X-ray crystal structure of canine myeloperoxidase at 3 Angstrom resolution. *J Mol Biol* 226:185, 1992.

195. Nauseef WM, McCormick SJ, Clark RA: Calreticulin functions as a molecular chaperone in the biosynthesis of myeloperoxidase. *J Biol Chem* 270:4741, 1995.

196. Nauseef WM, Brigham S, Cogley M: Hereditary myeloperoxidase deficiency due to a missense mutation of arginine 569 to tryptophan. *J Biol Chem* 269:1212, 1994.

197. DeLeo FR, Goedkren M, McCormick SJ, Nauseef WM: A novel form of hereditary myeloperoxidase deficiency linked to ER/proteasome degradation. *J Clin Invest* 101:2900, 1998.

198. Boxer LA: The role of antioxidants in modulating neutrophil functional responses, in *Advances in Experimental Medicine,* edited by A Bendich, M Phillips, P Tengedy, vol 262, pp 19–34. Plenum Press, New York, 1990.

199. Roos D, Weeining RS, Voetman AA, et al: Protection of phagocytic leukocytes by endogenous glutathione: Studies in a family with glutathione reductase deficiency. *Blood* 53:851, 1979.

200. Boxer LA, Oliver JM, Spielberg SP, et al: Protection of granulocytes by vitamin E in glutathione synthetase deficiency. *N Engl J Med* 301:901, 1979.

201. Lekstrom-Himes JA, Dorman SE, Kopar P, et al: Neutrophil-specific granule deficiency results from a novel mutation with loss of function of the transcription factor CCAAT/enhancer protein E. *J Exp Med* 189:1847, 1999.

202. Todd RF III, Freyer DR: The CD11/CD18 leukocyte glycoprotein deficiency. *Hem-Oncol Clin No Amer* 2:13, 1988.

PART VII

MONOCYTES
AND
MACROPHAGES

MORPHOLOGY OF MONOCYTES AND MACROPHAGES

STEVEN D. DOUGLAS
WEN-ZHE HO

The monocyte is a spherical cell with prominent surface ruffles and blebs when examined by scanning electron microscopy. When reconstructed from sections examined under transmission electron microscopy, the monocyte has a reniform nucleus containing a small nucleolus. The cytoplasm has many mitochondria, microtubules, and microfilaments. The Golgi apparatus is well developed and has neighboring centrioles. Numerous microvilli and microcytotic vesicles are evident at or near the cell surface. The cytoplasm contains scattered granules, akin to lysosomes. The granule contents share features with the primary granules of neutrophils, although, in contrast to the neutrophil, the monocyte granule is characterized by fluoride-inhibitable esterases. As the monocyte enters the tissue and differentiates into a macrophage, there is an increase in cell volume and number of cytoplasmic granules. The cell shape varies depending on the tissue type in which the macrophage resides (e.g., lung, liver, spleen, brain, etc.). A characteristic feature of macrophages is their prominent electron-dense membrane-bound lysosomes that can be seen fusing with phagosomes to form secondary lysosomes. The latter contain ingested cellular and noncellular material in stages of degradation. A broad range of surface receptors for many ligands, including the Fc portion of immunoglobulin, complement proteins, cytokines, chemokines, lipoproteins, and others are on the cell surface. Macrophages differ in appearance, biochemistry, and function based on the environment in which they mature from monocytes. These differences are exemplified by the diversity among dendritic cells of lymph nodes, histiocytes of connective tissue, osteoclasts of bone, Kupffer cells of liver, microglia of the central nervous system, and macrophages of the serosal surfaces, each fashioned to meet the local needs of the mononuclear phagocyte system.

MONONUCLEAR PHAGOCYTE SYSTEM

Modern study of mammalian phagocytes began with Metchnikoff in the nineteenth century. An understanding of the ontogeny, kinetics, and function of phagocytic cells in animals has led to the concept of

Acronyms and abbreviations that appear in this chapter include: ADCC, antibody-dependent cellular cytotoxicity; CR1, complement receptor 1; CR3, complement receptor 3; FcR, Fc receptors; GM-CSF, granulocyte-monocyte colony stimulating factor; HIV-1, human immunodeficiency virus; HLA, human leukocyte antigens; IL-4, interleukin-4; IMP, intramembrane particles; LFA-1, lymphocyte function-associated antigen; LPS, lipopolysaccharide; MHC, major histocompatibility complex; PAS, periodic acid–Schiff; TEM, transmission electron microscopy.

the mononuclear phagocyte system.[1,2] The system consists of marrow monoblasts and promonocytes, blood monocytes, and both free and fixed-tissue macrophages. Vascular endothelium, reticular cells, and dendritic cells of lymphoid germinal centers are not usually included in the mononuclear phagocyte system, although the now-obsolete term *reticuloendothelial system*[3] denoted these cells as playing some complementary part with mononuclear phagocytes. Studies indicate that monocytes can differentiate into dendritic cells in vitro.[4] Monocytes and macrophages comprise the functional system formerly thought to be the reticuloendothelial system. Tissue macrophages share many functional characteristics such as phagocytic and microbial killing capabilities and adherence to glass or plastic surfaces in vitro. Kinetic studies indicate that macrophages are transformed monocytes and that the monocyte is derived from the differentiation of the hematopoietic stem cell.

The blood monocyte is a medium to large motile cell that can marginate along vessel walls and has a propensity for adherence to surfaces. Monocytes respond to inflammation and chemotactic stimuli by active diapedesis across vessel walls into inflammatory foci, where they can mature into macrophages, with greater phagocytic capacity and increased content of hydrolytic enzymes. Free macrophages also are present in mammary glands, alveolar spaces, pleura, peritoneum, and synovia. The somewhat less motile fixed-tissue macrophages are found in different tissues and serous cavities (Table 73-1). The functions of mononuclear phagocytes include the following: phagocytosis and digestion of microorganisms, particulate material, or tissue debris; secretion of chemical mediators and regulators of the inflammatory response; interaction with antigen and lymphocytes in the generation of the immune response; cytotoxicity, such as killing of some tumor cells; and other functions specific for macrophages of particular tissues.

The development of techniques to isolate monocytes from blood of adult subjects has led to the discovery that monocytes are heterogeneous with regard to cell volumes. Isolation of purified monocytes by adherence to glass substrates or to gelatin-coated flasks or by centrifugal elutriation reveals distinct populations of monocytes.[1,2] In addition to the usual 12- to 15-μm diameter monocyte, a somewhat smaller cell has been identified that is less active than its larger, more mature counterpart. This cell is referred to as a small immature monocyte, yet its functional significance is not clear.

Monocytes continuously emigrate from the blood into peripheral tissue, with a half-life in the blood of about 1 day in mice.[5] Nondividing monocytes can be induced to differentiate into dendritic-like cells in vitro. However, this requires culture of the cells for 7 to 10 days with exogenous cytokines, typically interleukin-4 (IL-4) and granulocyte-monocyte colony stimulating factor (GM-CSF).[6] In the presence of endothelial cells grown on an extracellular matrix, monocytes differentiate along two distinct pathways, toward dendritic cells or macrophages. Monocytes that migrate across endothelium in an abluminal to luminal direction differentiate into dendritic cells. In contrast, monocytes that remain in the subendothelial matrix differentiate into macrophages.

MORPHOLOGY OF MONOCYTE PRECURSORS

The monoblasts and promonocytes are the precursors of the monocytes, bearing finely dispersed nuclear chromatin and nucleoli when observed in the stained film of the blood or marrow. The monoblast is a very low prevalence marrow cell, indistinguishable by light microscopy from the myeloblast.

In animal studies, a small percentage of marrow cells are phagocytic, synthesize DNA, adhere to glass surfaces, and contain nonspecific esterases.[7] These have been referred to as *promonocytes* and considered to be intermediate between monoblasts and the monocytes of the blood.[7] Cytochemical studies identify the promonocyte in normal

TABLE 73-1   DISTRIBUTION OF MONONUCLEAR PHAGOCYTES

Marrow	Tissues
Monoblasts	Liver (Kupffer cells)
Promonocytes	Lung (alveolar macrophages)
Monocytes	Connective tissue (histiocytes)
Macrophages	Spleen (red pulp macrophages)
Blood	Lymph nodes
Monocytes	Thymus
Body cavities	Bone (osteoclasts)
Pleural macrophages	Synovium (type A cells)
Peritoneal macrophages	Mucosa-associated lymphoid tissue
Inflammatory tissues	Gastrointestinal tract
Epithelioid cells	Genitourinary tract
Exudate macrophages	Endocrine organs
Multinucleate giant cells	Central nervous system (microglia
	Skin (histiocyte/dendritic cells)

SOURCE: Adapted from Angen and Ross, in Lewis and McGee,[2] with permission. Refer to References 7, 60, 61.

human marrow. These cells have deeply indented and irregularly shaped nuclei and bundled and scattered single filaments in the cytoplasm; these morphologic features distinguish the promonocyte from the progranulocyte.[8,9] Peroxidase is present throughout the cell secretory apparatus in all cisternae of the rough-surfaced endoplasmic reticulum, the Golgi complex, associated vesicles, and all immature and mature granules. Cytochemical reaction products for acid phosphatase and arylsulfatase are also deposited throughout the secretory apparatus of the promonocyte.

MORPHOLOGY OF MONOCYTES

LIGHT MICROSCOPY

The morphology of the monocytes has been investigated by light and phase-contrast optics,[10] scanning and transmission electron microscopy, and freeze-fracture and freeze-etch procedures.[11]

In the stained blood film, the monocyte has a diameter of 12 to 15 μm. Its nucleus occupies about half the area of the cell and is usually eccentrically placed. The nucleus is most often reniform but may be round or irregular. It contains a characteristic chromatin net with fine strands bridging small chromatin clumps. Chromatin aggregates are arranged along the internal aspect of the nuclear membrane. The nuclear chromatin pattern has been called "raked" because of its fine-stranded appearance. The cytoplasm is spread out, stains grayish-blue with Wright stain, and contains a variable number of fine, pink-purple granules, which at times are sufficiently numerous to give the entire cytoplasm a pink hue. Clear cytoplasmic vacuoles and a variable number of larger azurophilic granulations are often encountered in these cells.

PHASE MICROSCOPY

The monocyte nucleus has a distinct chromatin pattern on a cloudy background when examined by phase-contrast microscope. The cytoplasm is clear gray. Mitochondria are extremely fine and on occasion form a small, juxtanuclear rosette surrounding the centrosome. The phase-dense cytoplasmic granules, varying in number, are generally at the limit of resolution of light microscopy and appear as fine intracytoplasmic dust. Monocytes contain several types of cytoplasmic vacuoles. Characteristic of the monocyte are its reniform nucleus with a juxtanuclear depression filled by a centrosome and its active undulating movement similar to that of other leukocytes. The locomotion of the monocyte has the same pattern of undulating cytoplasmic veils seen in macrophages. The monocyte generally assumes a triangular shape as it moves, with one point trailing behind and the other two points

advancing before the cell. Blood monocytes undergo adherence and cytoplasmic spreading following attachment to glass surfaces.[12] The extent of spreading is increased in the presence of antigen-antibody complexes, certain divalent metals, and proteolytic enzymes.[12,13] The spread form of the monocyte reveals that the nucleus and granules are located centrally and the abundant hyaloplasm is in the periphery of the cell, terminating in a fringed border that displays undulating movement. The small monocyte may be difficult to distinguish from the large lymphocyte when examined by phase-contrast microscopy.

A striking feature on phase-contrast microscopy is the ruffled plasma membrane that forms prominent phase-dense folds at the cell surface and edges. Some cells have a dense thickening at the edge of the cytoplasm, with microextensions on the thickened edge.

SCANNING ELECTRON MICROSCOPY

The monocyte surface has very prominent ruffles and small surface blebs.[14,15] Extensive ruffling on the monocyte plasma membrane is of functional significance. The monocyte is both motile and phagocytic, and these functions require physical contact with particles or cell surfaces. Reduction in the radius of curvature of the cell surface by formation of ruffles or microvilli may reduce repulsive forces when surface negative-charge groups on the cell approach and contact a negatively charged substratum or cell. Also, redundancy of the cell membrane may provide reserve membrane required for locomotion and for phagocytosis.

TRANSMISSION ELECTRON MICROSCOPY (TEM)

The nucleus of the monocyte contains one or two small nucleoli surrounded by nucleolar-associated chromatin (Fig. 73-1).[16] The cytoplasm contains a relatively small quantity of endoplasmic reticulum and a variable quantity of ribosomes and polysomes. The mitochondria are numerous, small, and elongated. The Golgi complex is well developed and is situated about the centrosome within the nuclear indentation. Centrioles and filamentous centriolar satellites are often visualized in this region. Microtubules are numerous, and microfibrils are found in bundles surrounding the nucleus. In cultured macrophages collections of microfilaments are present underneath the plasma membrane near sites of cell attachment either to a substratum or to phagocytizable particles.[17] The cell surface is characterized by numerous microvilli and vesicles of micropinocytosis. The cytoplasmic granules resemble the small granules found in the granulocytic series, measuring approximately 0.05 to 0.2 μm in diameter. They are dense and homogeneous and are surrounded by a limiting membrane. These granules, as with the lysosomal granules of other leukocytes, are packaged by the Golgi apparatus after their enzymatic content has been produced by the ribosomal complex of the cell.[7,8,18] These cytoplasmic granules contain acid phosphatase and arylsulfatase and are therefore primary lysosomes. After endocytosis, lysosomes fuse with the phagosome, forming secondary lysosomes. Some monocyte granules stain positive for peroxidase, whereas others are peroxidase-negative.[7,8]

FREEZE-FRACTURE MICROSCOPY

In this technique a cell suspension is frozen, placed in a high-vacuum chamber, and struck with a blunt edge so as to produce a fracture that is propagated through the frozen specimen. The utility of the procedure comes from the remarkable finding that when the fracture encounters a cell, it tends to propagate along the interior of the plasma membrane and thus split the lipid bilayer in half. After fracture, the specimen is coated with platinum, which is electron-dense when viewed with TEM. All cell types examined thus far by the freeze-fracture technique reveal

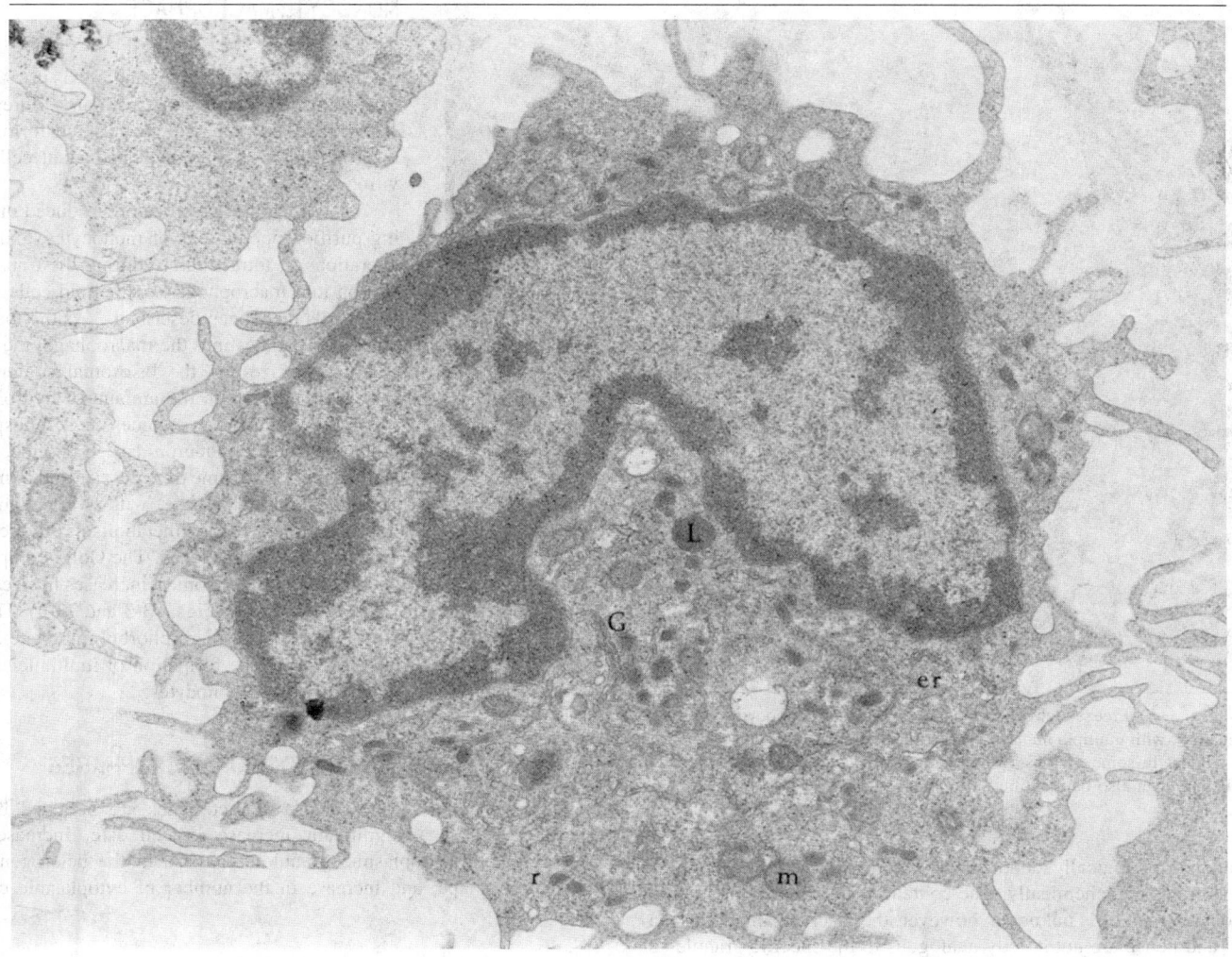

FIGURE 73-1   Transmission electron micrograph of a monocyte. The eccentric reniform nucleus has a thinly dispersed chromatin pattern. The Golgi complex (G) is in a juxtanuclear position. Small electron-dense granules can be seen evolving in the Golgi complex. A small amount of rough endoplasmic reticulum (er) and polyribosomes (r) are present, particularly about the cell periphery. Mitochondria (m) are concentrated in the region of the Golgi apparatus and are scattered in the cell periphery as well. Lysosomes (L) are small, electron-dense granules surrounded by a limiting membrane. The irregular ruffled cell margin is apparent with numerous microprojections. ×24,000.

intramembrane particles (IMP) as the predominant feature of the topography of the interior of the bilayer. Studies of the erythrocyte have shown that at least some particles may contain intercalated membrane proteins, and this has been assumed to be the case with nucleated cells as well. The distribution of IMP is dramatically altered in a number of cell systems by physiologic stimuli, for example, hormonal stimulation.

Profound changes in the distribution of IMP on mononuclear phagocytes occur following binding of antibody-coated erythrocytes.[11] Since redistribution of IMP also occurs in some nonphagocyte Fc receptor-bearing cells[11] and after exposure to aggregated IgG, this alteration in IMP presumably reflects interaction with the Fc receptor. Freeze-etch electron micrographs of the monocyte show nuclear pores traversing both lamellae of the nuclear membrane and contours of cytoplasmic lysosomes and mitochondria (Fig. 73-2).

HISTOCHEMISTRY OF MONOCYTES

Hydrolytic enzyme contents of monocytes, neutrophils, and lymphocytes are compared in Table 73-2. Monocytes also give a weak but positive periodic acid–Schiff (PAS) reaction (for polysaccharides) and Sudan black B reaction (for lipids).

Nonspecific esterase[19–21] is frequently used as a marker for monocytes. Monocyte esterases are inhibited by sodium fluoride, whereas the esterases of the granulocytic series are not. The nonspecific esterase reaction is positive in promyelocytes and myelocytes, and therefore analysis of fluoride inhibition is necessary to distinguish marrow monocytes from early myelocytes. Monocyte granules, although heterogeneous in size (0.3 to 0.6 μm), are not separable into populations by routine electron microscopic criteria (except in the rat).[22] Identification of monocyte granule populations has depended on subcellular localization of monocyte enzymes by electron microscopic cytochemistry.[8] Human marrow promonocytes and blood monocytes contain granules that comprise two functionally distinct populations.[8,9] One population contains the enzymes acid phosphatase, arylsulfatase, and, in the human (but not in the rabbit), also peroxidase; these granules are therefore modified primary lysosomes and are analogous to the azurophil granules of the neutrophil. The monocyte azurophil granule population is heterogeneous in cytochemical reactivity for peroxidase, acid phosphatase, and arylsulfatase.[23,24] Moreover, primary granules

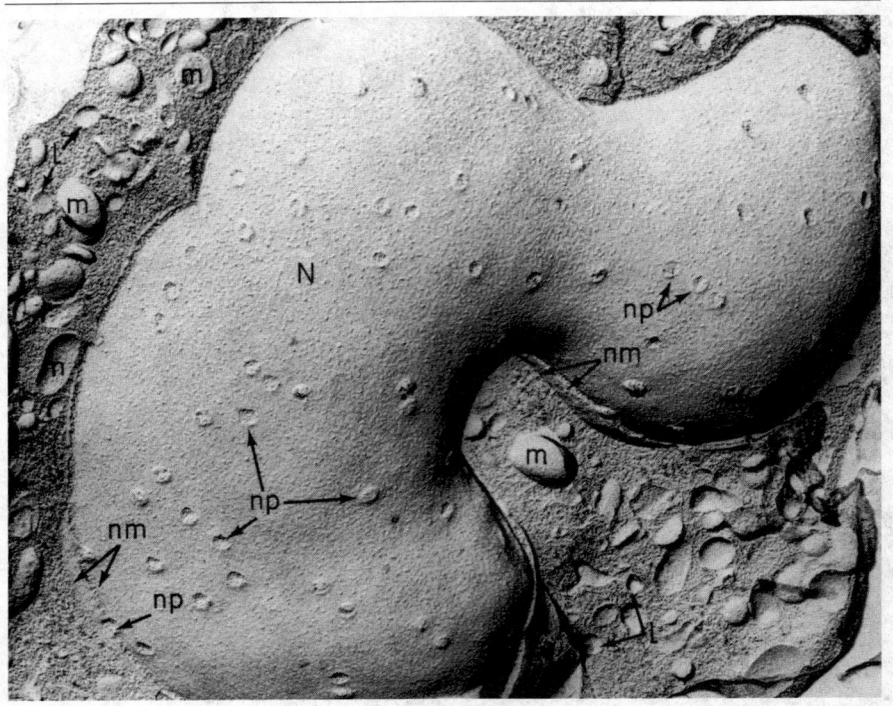

FIGURE 73-2   Freeze-etch electron micrograph of a monocyte. Fracture plane displays the large nucleus (N), with multiple nuclear pores (np) and the two lamellae of the fractured nuclear membrane (nm) evident in some regions. Membrane and cleaved surfaces of mitochondria (m) and lysosomal granules (L) can also be identified in the cytoplasm.

that are morphologically identical with other vesicles may be identified as lysosomes cytochemically. The content of the other population of monocyte granules is unknown; however, they lack alkaline phosphatase[23] and hence are not strictly analogous to the specific granules of neutrophils. The lysosomes have a digestive function, whereas the function of the second population is unknown.

About 10 percent of granules in normal human blood monocytes stain with reagents that identify complex acid carbohydrates, or "acid mucosubstances."[25] These substances are found in leukemic monocyte granules as well as in granules of normal neutrophils, and their function is unknown.

TABLE 73-2   CYTOCHEMICAL REACTIONS OF LEUKOCYTE ENZYMES

CHEMICAL	MONOCYTES	NEUTROPHILS	LYMPHOCYTES
Acid phosphatase	++	+	+
β-Glucuronidase	++	+	0 to +
Sulfatase	+	+	0
N-Acetylglucosaminidase	++	++	0
Lysozyme*	++	++	0
Naphthylamidase	++	+	0 to +
α-Naphthyl butyrate esterase[†]	++	0 to +	0
Naphthol AS-D chloroacetate esterase	0 to +	++	0
Peroxidase	+	++	0
Alkaline phosphatase	0	0 to +	0

*Most lysozyme produced by mononuclear phagocytes is secreted rather than stored intracellularly.
[†]α-Naphthyl acetate and α-naphthyl butyrate esterase activities may appear in human T lymphocytes under certain conditions.
SOURCE: Modified from Braunsteiner and Schmalzl[20] and Li et al.[21]

MONOCYTE-MACROPHAGE DIFFERENTIATION

The classic studies of Lewis and Lewis in 1926,[26] Maximow in 1932,[27] and Ebert and Florey in 1939[28] have shown that monocytes transform into macrophages and multinucleated giant cells in vitro.

These studies have been reproduced utilizing purified populations of monocytes, and the alterations of ultrastructure during the transformation into macrophages, epithelioid cells, and giant cells have been described.[16] As the monocyte differentiates into the macrophage, the cell enlarges in size and the lysosomal content is increased, along with the amount of hydrolytic enzymes within the lysosomes (e.g., phosphatases, esterases, β-glucuronidase, lysozyme, arylsulfatase). At the same time the size and number of mitochondria increase, with a concomitant increase in their energy metabolism. Production of lactate is also increased. The Golgi complex, which packages lysosomes, increases in size and vesicle complexity (Figs. 73-3 and 73-4). There are several stimuli (e.g., phorbol myristate acetate) which induce formation of multinucleated giant cells from monocytes.[29]

MORPHOLOGY OF MACROPHAGES

Macrophage characteristics are heralded by a significant increase in cell size, increase in the number of cytoplasmic granules, increase in the heterogeneity of the cell shape, and increase in the number of cytoplasmic clear vacuoles.

MOTILITY

An effective monocyte response to infection is predicated upon the ability to migrate and accumulate at an infection site. Monocytes are capable of both random and directed movement. Random migration is nondirected movement that occurs in the absence of attracting substances. Directed movement, or chemotaxis, refers to monocyte migration that occurs in response to chemotactic factors or stimuli and that is mediated by different types of receptors on phagocyte cell surfaces.[30] A number of different methods have been used to study macrophage movement both in vivo[31] and in vitro.[32]

LIGHT AND PHASE-CONTRAST MICROSCOPY

In vitro culture of monocytes purified from adult human blood has provided an opportunity to observe the maturation of these cells into mature macrophages.

The macrophages of the pulmonary alveoli, peritoneal and pleural cavities, and inflammatory exudates are hypermature cells that have undergone in vivo stimulation and maturation. This results in enhanced bactericidal activity[1,2] due to augmentation of the number of lysosomes and acid hydrolase content.

Macrophages display attributes of morphologic specialization specific to their location and function. The fixed macrophages of the spleen (littoral cells) are involved in the sequestration and destruction of effete or abnormal red cells and exhibit stages of erythrophago-

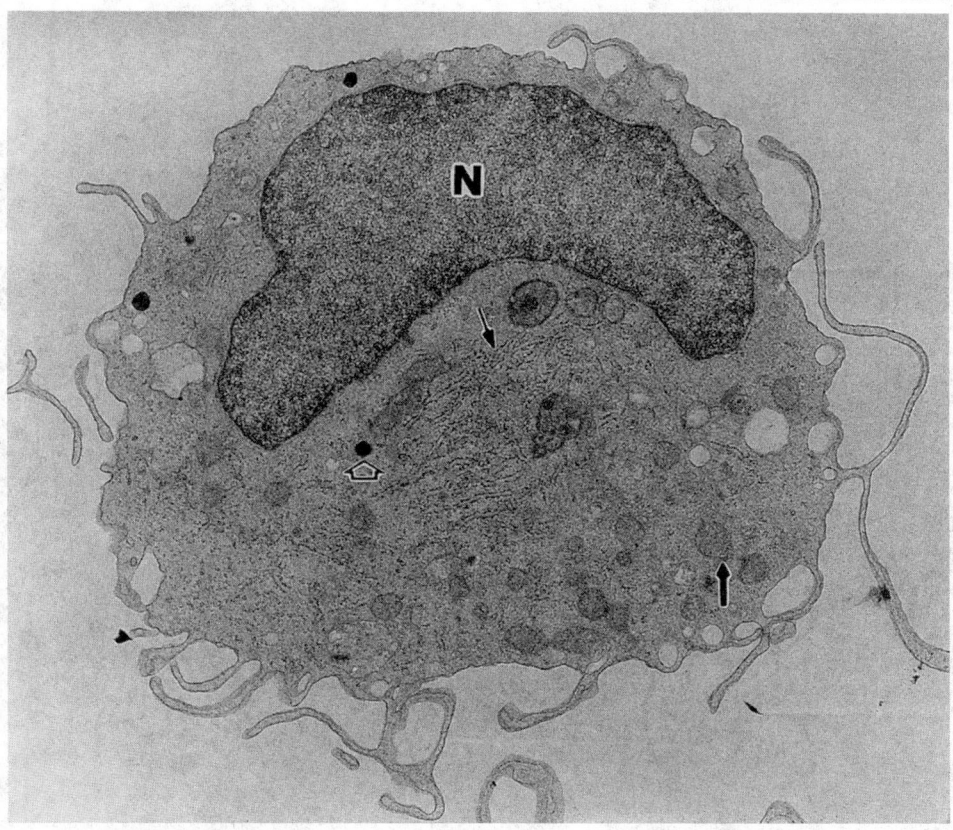

FIGURE 73-3   Electron micrograph of monocytes in vitro for 2 days. Nucleus (N), endoplasmic reticulum (thin arrow), mitochondria (thick arrow), lysosomes (empty arrow).

cytosis and intracytoplasmic aggregates of ferritin (see Chap. 5). The macrophages of the marrow, the ''nurse cells'' of the erythroblastic island, play a similar role in erythrophagocytosis and iron storage and transfer (see Chap. 4). Hepatic macrophages (Kupffer cells), found in liver sinusoids, also phagocytize red cells and other cellular elements and are important sites of iron storage. Macrophages of the pulmonary alveoli, the lamina propria of the gastrointestinal tract, and the peritoneal and pleural fluids reflect in their morphology a specific function of phagocytosis of microorganisms, cells, and cellular and noncellular debris, characteristic of the specific organ location.

On Wright-stained films, most macrophages are 25 to 50 μm in diameter. They have an eccentrically placed reniform or fusiform nucleus with one or two distinct nucleoli and finely dispersed, loosely stranded nuclear chromatin that tends to clump in the nuclear interior and along the internal aspect of the nuclear membrane. A juxtanuclear clear zone (Golgi complex) is well defined. The cytoplasm shows fine granules and multiple pink-purple, large azurophil granules. The cytoplasmic borders are irregularly serrated. Cytoplasmic vacuoles are present near the cell periphery, reflecting the active pinocytosis in these cells.

On phase-contrast microscopy, living macrophages are large cells with a propensity to adhere to and spread on glass surfaces, leaving the cell organelles concentrated within the central portion of the cell and clear veils of hyaloplasm spreading about the cell, with intense ruffling of the membrane borders. Vesicles and contractile vacuoles are seen about the cell periphery and in the cell interior. The juxtanuclear clear zone bearing the centrosome and the Golgi complex is particularly dynamic and displays an undulating motion.

ELECTRON MICROSCOPY

Macrophages show a variable degree of differentiation, nuclear ''maturity,'' ribosomes, mitochondria, and lysosome content. In thin sections, the nucleus varies from horseshoe-shaped to fusiform. The heterochromatin is disposed in fine clumps in the interior of the nucleus and along the internal aspect of the nuclear membrane. Clear spaces between membrane-fixed chromatin aggregates mark the sites of nuclear pores that are relatively abundant in freeze-etch electron micrographs of macrophages as well as monocytes (see Fig. 73-2). Polyribosomes and scant smooth and rough endoplasmic reticulum are seen about the cell periphery. A well-developed Golgi complex is in a juxtanuclear location. It is often multicentric and contains a concentration of vesicles, some with dense inclusions that mark them as early lysosomes. A relatively constant feature of cells engaged in endocytosis is the large number of microvilli at the cell surface, forming the equivalent of a ''brush border.'' The degree of development of this surface adaptation is related to the phagocytic activity of the cell and its rate of pinocytosis.

The number and size of the mitochondria vary with the phagocytic and hence metabolic activity of the cell. Mitochondria tend to be grouped about the region of the Golgi complex, although several are usually seen dispersed about the cell periphery, presumably supplying energy for the active endocytic processes occurring there.

The most constant and characteristic ultrastructural features of the macrophages are the electron-dense membrane-bound lysosomes that can often be seen fusing with phagosomes to form secondary lysosomes. Within the secondary lysosomes, ingested cellular, bacte-

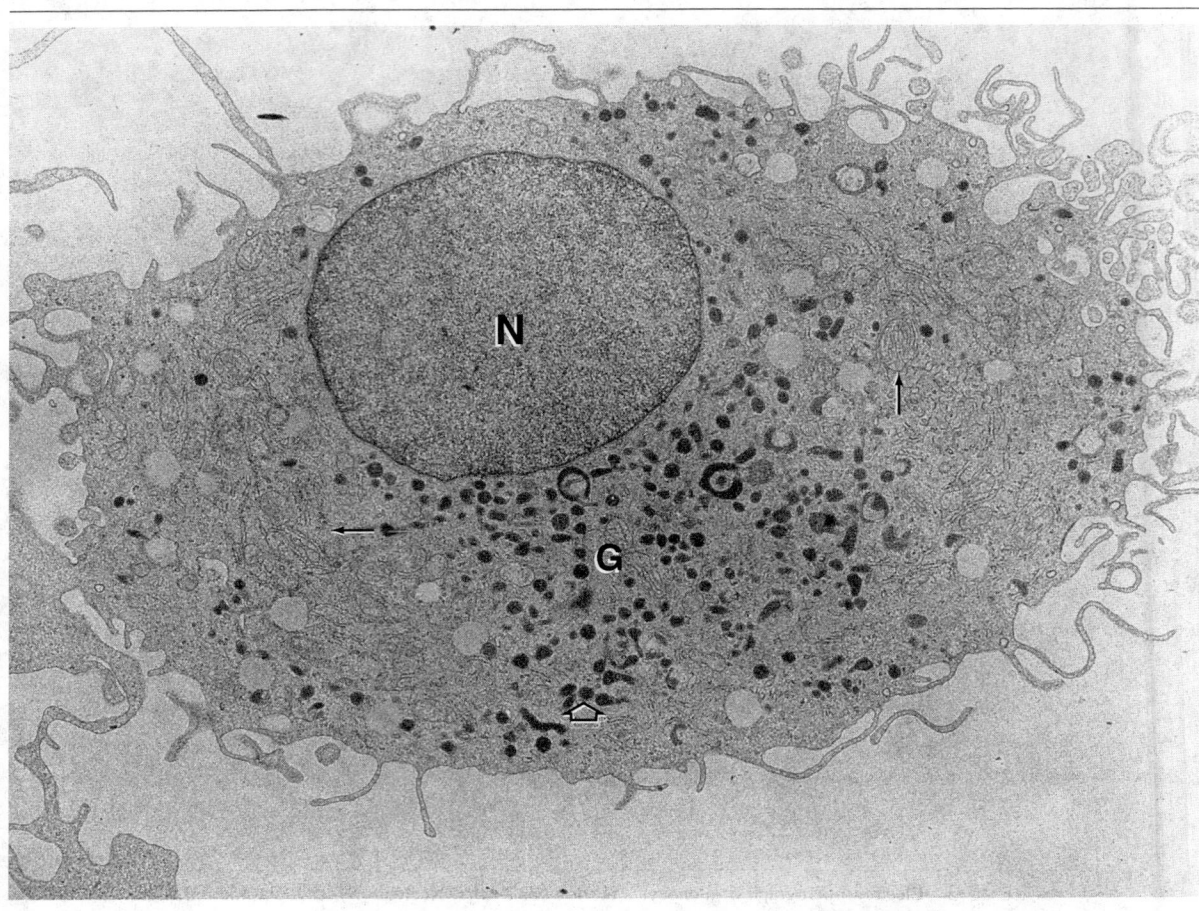

FIGURE 73-4   Electron micrograph of monocyte-derived macrophage in vitro for 9 days. Nucleus (N), endoplasmic reticulum (thin arrow), Golgi zone (G), mitochondria (thick arrow), lysosomes (empty arrow). ×7,600.

rial, and noncellular material can be seen in various stages of degradation, often recognizable as degenerating mitochondria or nuclear material. These secondary lysosomes also contain partially degraded material from the late stages of the endocytic process, often appearing as multilamellar lipid bodies.

Microtubules and microfilaments are prominent in macrophages, and actin- and myosin-like proteins have been isolated from monocytes and partially characterized.

Resting macrophages have irregular cell borders and pseudopodia pushed out in all directions. Their cytoplasm has rough endoplasmic reticulum and Golgi complex in the perinuclear area. Lipid globules, primary lysosomes, and mitochondria are characteristically prominent. Activated monocytes/macrophages are motile cells that extend a leading pseudopod as they move forward.[33]

MONOCYTE-MACROPHAGE SURFACE RECEPTORS

Monocyte-macrophage cells have surface receptors that have been characterized by their binding to specific monoclonal antibodies. These receptors (Table 73-3) are markers for origin, growth, differentiation,[34] activation, recognition, migration, and function of the monocyte-macrophage.

RECEPTORS FOR PEPTIDES AND SMALL MOLECULES

Fc RECEPTORS (FcR)

Fc receptors for IgG are expressed on the surface of mononuclear cells, macrophages, granulocytes, and platelets.[35,36] There are three

distinct classes of FcR: FcRI, FcRII, and FcRIII. These receptors have broad ranges of expression on different cells. The first, FcRI (CD64), is a receptor found on monocytes, macrophages, and activated neutrophils. This receptor binds monomeric IgG through the Fc portion of the molecule. This immunoglobulin receptor has increased expression on activated monocytes and macrophages. CD64 allows for receptor-mediated endocytosis of IgG-antigen complexes for presentation to T cells, can trigger release of cytokines and reactive oxygen intermediates, and can play a role in granulocyte-mediated antibody-dependent cytotoxicity. The second IgG receptor, FcRII (CD32), is a widely distributed receptor present on many cell types, including monocytes, platelets, neutrophils, B cells, some T cells, and some capillary endothelium. This receptor can bind complexed IgG rather than monomeric IgG. This Fc receptor regulates B cell function when coengaged with the B cell receptor for antigen, namely surface Ig. It also can induce mediator release from myeloid cells and phagocytosis of Ig-coated particles in vitro. Finally, this Fc receptor also can target antigen into presenting pathways. The third IgG receptor, FcRIII (CD16) is expressed by neutrophils, natural killer cells, and tissue macrophages.[37] This receptor can bind Ig in immune complexes and Ig bound to cell surface membranes and is the main Fc receptor responsible for antibody-dependent cellular cytotoxicity (ADCC). All three FcR specifically bind the human IgG subclasses IgG_1 and IgG_3 (see Chap. 83). The interaction of the FcR on macrophages with immune complexes results in cell "activation," with an increase in phagocytosis, superoxide production, and prostaglandin and leukotriene release.

TABLE 73-3   SURFACE RECEPTORS OF MONOCYTES AND MACROPHAGES

Fc receptors
  IgG2a, IgG2b/IgG1, IgG3, IgA, IgE
Complement receptors
  C3b, C3bi, C5a, C1q
Cytokine receptors
  MIF, MAF, LIF, CF, MFF, IL-1, IL-2, IL-3, IL-4
  INF-α, INF-β, INF-γ, GM-CSF, MCSF/CSF-1
Chemokine receptors
  CCR1, CCR2A, CCR2B, CCR3, CXCR4, CCR5
Receptors for peptides and small molecules
  H$_1$, H$_2$, 5-HT
  1,2,5-Dihydroxy vitamin D$_3$
  N-Formylated peptides
  Enkephalins/endorphins
  Substance P
  Arg-vasopressin
Hormone receptors
  Insulin
  Glucocorticoids
  Angiotensin
Transferrin and lactoferrin receptors
Lipoprotein lipid receptors
  Anionic low-density lipoproteins
  PGE$_2$, LTB$_4$, LTC$_4$, PAG
  Apolipoproteins B and E (chylomicron remnants, VLDL)
Receptors for coagulants and anticoagulants
  Fibrinogen/fibrin
  Coagulation factor VII
  α_1-Antithrombin
  Heparin
Fibronectin receptors
Laminin receptors
Mannosyl, fucosyl, galactosyl residue
α_2-Macroglobulin-proteinase complex receptors
Others
  Cholinergic agonists
  α_1-Adrenergic agonists
  β_2-Adrenergic agonists

NOTE: Ig, immunoglobulin; C, complement; MIF, macrophage inhibitory factor; MAF, macrophage-activating factor; LIF, leukocyte migration inhibition factor; MFF, macrophage fusion factor; IL, interleukin; INF, interferon; GM, granulocyte macrophage; H$_1$, histamine; 5-HT, 5-hydroxytryptamine; PG, prostaglandin; LT, leukotriene; PAG, platelet-activating factor; VLDL, very low density lipoprotein.

SOURCE: Adapted from Angen and Ross, in Lewis and McGee,[2] with permission. Refer to References 62 to 67.

COMPLEMENT RECEPTORS

Activation of the complement system results in the liberation of numerous ligands that bind to specific receptors on mononuclear phagocytes (Chap. 6). Four receptors have been identified that bind fragments of the complement component C3.[38] Complement receptor 1 (CR1, or CD35) binds dimeric C3bi and is found on both monocytes and macrophages. Complement receptor 3 (CR3, or CD11b) binds the complement fragment C3b. CR3 is a heterodimeric glycoprotein that is composed of two noncovalently linked polypeptides. The α chain of the polypeptide has an M_r of 185,000, and the β subunit an M_r of 95,000. This receptor, along with the leukocyte antigens LFA-1 (lymphocyte function-associated antigen, CD11a) and alpha-X integrin chain (CD11c), compose a family of heterodimers that share a common β subunit (CD18).[39] This family is designated the *leukocyte integrin* (β_2) *subfamily*.[40] These heterodimers are involved in cell-to-cell interactions, in the binding of opsonized particles and plasma proteins, and in attachment to various substrates. They may also modulate intercellular adhesion.

MONOCYTE-MACROPHAGE SURFACE ANTIGENS

HLA CLASS II RECEPTORS

Monocytes and macrophages serve an important function as antigen-presenting cells: They bear the class II glycoproteins of the major histocompatibility gene complex, HLA-DR, -DP, and -DQ. There is a wide variation in expression of MHC class II antigens on macrophages from different tissues. While spleen macrophages contain a high percentage of HLA-DR-positive cells (50 percent), peritoneal macrophages have relatively few (10 to 20 percent)[41]; the percentage of Ia-positive alveolar macrophages is only about 5 percent.[42] Lymphokines, primarily interferon-γ, can induce macrophages to express higher levels of MHC class II antigens,[43] while prostaglandin E, alpha-fetoprotein, and glucocorticoids[44] downregulate the HLA-DR antigen expression on macrophages.

CD11 RECEPTORS

CD11 defines a family of three accessory adhesion surface glycoproteins: CD11a, CD11b, and CD11c. These proteins are distinct α subunits for three heterodimeric surface glycoproteins, each sharing a common β subunit, designated CD18. The α subunits have different isoelectric points, molecular weights, and cell distribution[45] (see Chap. 14). Whereas CD11a is expressed on all leukocytes, CD11b or CD11c is expressed predominantly on monocytes and macrophages, a minor subset of B lymphocytes, and most polymorphonuclear leukocytes. CD11b is expressed on more than 95 percent of fresh human monocytes and macrophages but declines rapidly on cells maintained in vitro. Antibodies specific for CD11b, such as OKM1 or Mo1, may block this complement receptor's ability to bind to CD3bi.[46] Accordingly, these antibodies strongly inhibit complement receptor-mediated rosetting of erythrocyte-IgM antibody-complement complexes.

CD14 AND CD68 RECEPTORS

The CD14 molecule is one of the most characteristic surface antigens of the monocyte lineage. It is a polypeptide of 356 amino acids that is anchored to the plasma membrane by a phosphoinositol linkage.[47] It is expressed strongly on the surface of monocytes and weakly on the surface of granulocytes and most tissue macrophages. It also can be detected on some nonmyeloid cells (e.g., hepatocytes and some epithelial cells). CD14 functions as a receptor for endotoxin (LPS). LPS binds to a serum protein, LPS-binding protein, that facilitates the binding of LPS to CD14. When LPS binds to CD14 expressed by monocytes or neutrophils, the cells become activated and release cytokines such as tumor necrosis factor and upregulate cell surface molecules, including adhesion molecules. In vitro, soluble CD14 binds to LPS and the complex stimulates cells that do not express CD14 to secrete cytokines and coregulate adhesion molecules.[48]

The CD68 antigen is a specific marker of monocytes and macrophages. Antibodies against the antigen label macrophages and other members of the mononuclear phagocyte lineage in routinely processed tissue sections and have been used to stain a range of lymphoid, histiocytic, and myelomonocytic proliferation.[49]

CD4 RECEPTORS

T lymphocytes express several surface receptors, with the surface antigen CD4 expressed exclusively in T-helper lymphocytes (see Chap. 95). CD4 and its corresponding mRNA have been demonstrated on monocytes, macrophages, and monocyte-like cell line, U-937.[50] Although CD4 is present at low concentrations in blood monocytes, the percentage of cells that display this plasma membrane determinant ranges from fewer than 5 percent to 90 percent. Several monoclonal antibodies have been described that react with different epitopes of the CD4 antigen.[51] The CD4 molecule is involved in the induction of T-lymphocyte helper functions (T4) and T-proliferative responses to antigen stimulation; however, its role in the function of monocyte-macrophages has not yet been determined. An important aspect of the monocyte-macrophage phenotype is the presence of CD4 molecules on the surface of monocytes that can act as the receptors for the human immunodeficiency virus (HIV-1). HIV-1 utilizes the CD4 receptors as an entry pathway for the infection of monocyte-macrophages.[52]

CHEMOKINE RECEPTORS

Chemokines mediate their activities by binding to target cell surface chemokine receptors that belong to a large family of G protein-coupled, seven transmembrane domain receptors. Human monocytes/macrophages express several chemokine receptors (Table 73-3). The chemokine receptor, CCR5, has been implicated in HIV infection of monocytes/macrophages.[53–57] CCR5 is a major coreceptor on monocytes/macrophages for M-tropic HIV infection. A 32-nucleotide deletion within the CCR5 gene has a highly protective role against acquisition of HIV.[58,59]

REFERENCES

1. van Furth R (ed): *Mononuclear Phagocytes: Characteristics, Physiology and Function.* Martinus Nijhoff, Dordrecht, 1985.
2. Lewis CE, McGee JO'D (eds): *The Macrophage.* Oxford University Press, New York, 1992.
3. Aschoff L: Das reticulo-endotheliale System. *Ergeb Inn Med Kinderheilkd* 26:1, 1924.
4. Randolph GJ, Beaulieu S, Lebecque S, et al: Differentiation of monocytes into dendritic cells in a model of transendothelial trafficking. *Science* 282:480, 1998.
5. van Furth R, Cohn ZA: The origin and kinetics of mononuclear phagocytes. *J Exp Med* 128:415, 1968.
6. Sallusto F, Lanzavecchia A: Efficient presentation of soluble antigen by cultured human dendritic cells is maintained by granulocyte/macrophage colony-stimulating factor plus interleukin 4 and downregulated by tumor necrosis factor-α. *J Exp Med* 179:1109, 1994.
7. van Furth R: Phagocytic cells: Development and distribution of mononuclear phagocytes in normal steady state and inflammation, in *Inflammation: Basic Principles and Clinical Correlates,* 2d ed, edited by JI Gallin, R Snyderman. Raven, New York, 1992.
8. Nichols BA, Bainton DF, Farquahr MG: Differentiation of monocytes: Origin, nature and fate of their azurophil granules. *J Cell Biol* 50:498, 1971.
9. Nichols BA, Bainton DF: Differentiation of human monocytes in bone marrow and blood: Sequential formation of two granule populations. *Lab Invest* 29:27, 1973.
10. Ploem JS: Reflection contrast microscopy as a tool in investigations of the attachment of living cells to a glass surface, in *Mononuclear Phagocytes in Immunity, Infection, and Pathology,* edited by R van Furth, p 405. Blackwell, Oxford, 1975.
11. Douglas SD: Alterations in intramembrane particle distribution during interaction of erythrocyte-bound ligands with immunoprotein receptors. *J Immunol* 120:151, 1978.
12. Rabinovitch M, DeStefano MJ: Macrophage spreading in vitro: I. Inducers of spreading. *Exp Cell Res* 77:323, 1973.
13. Douglas SD: Human monocyte spreading in vitro: Inducers and effects on Fc and C3 receptors. *Cell Immunol* 21:344, 1976.
14. Ackerman SK, Douglas SD: Purification of human monocytes on microexudate-coated surfaces. *J Immunol* 120:1372, 1978.
15. Zuckerman SH, Ackerman SK, Douglas SD: Long-term peripheral blood monocyte cultures: Establishment and morphology of primary human monocyte-macrophage cell culture. *Immunology* 38:401, 1979.
16. Sutton JS, Weiss L: Transformation of monocytes in tissue culture into macrophages, epithelioid cells and multinucleated giant cells. *J Cell Biol* 29:303, 1966.
17. Reaven EP, Axline SG: Subplasmalemmal microfilaments and microtubules in resting and phagocytizing cultivated macrophages. *J Cell Biol* 29:303, 1966.
18. Cohn ZA, Benson B: The differentiation of mononuclear phagocytes: Morphology, cytochemistry, and biochemistry. *J Exp Med* 121:153, 1965.
19. Wachstein M, Wolf G: The histochemical demonstration of esterase activity in human blood and bone marrow smears. *J Histochem Cytochem* 6:457, 1958.
20. Braunsteiner H, Schmalzl F: Cytochemistry of monocytes and macrophages, in *Mononuclear Phagocytes,* edited by R van Furth, p 62. Blackwell, Oxford, 1970.
21. Li CY, Lam KW, Yam LT: Esterases in human leukocytes. *J Histochem Cytochem* 21:1, 1973.
22. van der Rhee HJ, de Winter CPM, Daems WT: Fine structure and peroxidative activity of rat blood monocytes. *Cell Tissue Res* 185:1, 1977.
23. Bodel PT, Nichols BA, Bainton DF: Appearance of peroxidase reactivity within the rough ER of blood monocytes after surface adherence. *J Exp Med* 145:264, 1977.
24. Nichols BA, Bainton DF: Ultrastructure and cytochemistry of mononuclear phagocytes, in *Mononuclear Phagocytes in Immunity, Infection and Pathology,* edited by R van Furth, p 17. Blackwell, Oxford, 1975.
25. Parmley RT, Spicer SS, O'Dell RF: Ultrastructural identification of acid complex carbohydrate in cytoplasmic granules of normal and leukemic human monocytes. *Br J Haematol* 39:33, 1978.
26. Lewis MR, Lewis WH: Transformation of mononuclear blood-cells into macrophages, epithelioid cells, and giant cells in hanging-drop blood-cultures from lower vertebrates. Carnegie Institute of Washington, Pub 96. *Contrib Embryol* 18:95, 1926.
27. Maximow AA: The macrophages or histiocytes, in *Special Cytology: The Form and Functions of the Cell in Health and Disease,* 2d ed, edited by EV Cowdry, vol II, sec 19, p 711. Hoeber-Harper, New York, 1932.
28. Ebert RH, Florey HW: The extravascular development of the monocyte observed in vitro. *Br J Exp Pathol* 20:341, 1939.
29. Hassan NF, Kamani N, Messaros M, Douglas SD: Induction of multinucleated giant cell formation from human blood-derived monocytes by phorbol myristate acetate in *in vitro* culture. *J Immunol* 143:2179, 1989.
30. Snyderman R, Pike MC: Structure and function of monocytes and macrophages, in McCarty DJ (ed): *Arthritis and Allied Conditions.* Philadelphia, Lea & Febiger, p.306, 1989.
31. Rebuck JW, Crowley JH: A method of studying leukocytic functions in vivo. *Ann N Y Acad Sci* 59:757, 1955.
32. Boyden S: The chemotactic effect of mixtures of antibody and antigen on polymorphonuclear leukocytes. *J Exp Med* 115:453, 1962.
33. Fawcett DW, Raviola E: *Bloom and Fawcett: A Textbook of Histology,* p 150–156. Chapman and Hall, New York, 1994.
34. Russell SW, Gordon S: *Macrophage Biology and Activation.* Springer-Verlag, New York, 1992.
35. Metzger H: *Fc Receptors and the Action of Antibodies.* American Society for Microbiology, Washington, DC, 1990.
36. Anderson CL, Guyre PM, Whitin JC, et al: Monoclonal antibodies to Fc receptors for IgG on human mononuclear phagocytes. *J Biol Chem* 261:12856, 1986.
37. Looney RJ, Abraham GN, Anderson CL: Human monocytes and U-937 cells bear two distinct Fc receptors for IgG. *J Immunol* 136:1641, 1986.
38. Wright SD, Griffin FM Jr: Activation of phagocytic cells' C3 receptors for phagocytosis. *J Leukoc Biol* 38:327, 1985.
39. Kishimoto TK, Hollander N, Roberts TM, et al: Heterogenous mutations in the β subunit common to the LFA-1, Mac-1, and p150,95 glycoproteins cause leukocyte adhesion deficiency. *Cell* 50:193, 1987.
40. Hynes RO: Integrins: A family of cell surface receptors. *Cell* 48:549, 1987.
41. Cowing C, Schwartz BD, Dickler HB: Macrophage Ia antigens: I. Macrophage populations differ in their expression on Ia antigens. *J Immunol* 120:378, 1978.
42. Unanue ER, Allen PM: The basis for the immunoregulatory role of macrophages and other accessory cells. *Science* 236:551, 1987.
43. Belle ID: Functional significance of the regulation of macrophage Ia expression. *Eur J Immunol* 14:138, 1984.
44. Snider DD, Ulnae ER: Corticosteroids inhibit murine macrophages, Ia expression and interleukin-1 production. *J Immunol* 129:1803, 1982.
45. Sanchez-Madrid F, Nagy JA, Robbins E, et al: A human leukocyte differentiation antigen family with distinct alpha subunits and a common beta subunit: The lymphocyte-function associated antigen (LFA-1). The C3bi complement receptor (OKM1/Mac) and the p150,95 molecule. *J Exp Med* 158:1785, 1983.
46. Beller DI, Springer TA, Schreiber RD: Anti-Mac-1 selectively inhibits

the mouse and human type three complement receptor. *J Exp Med* 156:1000, 1982.

47. Kazazi F, Mathijs J-M, Foley P, Cunningham AL: Variations in CD4 expression by human monocytes and macrophages and their relationship to infection with the human immunodeficiency virus. *Gen Virol* 70:2661, 1989.

48. Yu B, Hailman E, Wright SD: Lipopolysaccharide binding protein and soluble CD14 catalyze exchange of phospholipid. *J Clin Invest* 99:315, 1997.

49. Collman R, Godfrey B, Cutilli J, et al: Macrophage-tropic strains of human immunodeficiency virus type 1 utilize the CD4 receptor. *J Virol* 64:4468, 1990.

50. Haziot A, Chen S, Ferrero E, et al: The monocyte differentiation antigen, CD14, is anchored to the cell membrane by a phospatidylinositol linkage. *J Immunol* 141:547, 1988.

51. Schneider EM, Lorenz I, Kogler G, Wernet P: Modulation of monocyte function by CD14-specific antibodies in vitro, in *Leukocyte Typing,* edited by W Knapp et al., vol IV, p 794. Oxford University Press, New York, 1989.

52. Warnke RA, Pulford KAF, Pallensen G, et al: Diagnosis of myelomonocytic and macrophage neoplasms in routinely processed tissue biopsies with monoclonal antibody KP1. *Am J Pathol* 135:1089, 1989.

53. Alkhatib G, Combadiere C, Broder CC, et al: ckr5: a rantes, mip-1a, receptor as a fusion cofactor for macrophage-tropic HIV. *Science* 272:1955, 1996.

54. Hill CM, Littman DR: Natural resistance to HIV. *Nature* 382:668, 1996.

55. Deng HK, Liu F, Ellmeier W, et al: identification of a major co-receptor for primary isolates of HIV. *Nature* 381:661, 1996.

56. Huang Y: The role of a mutant CCR5 allele in HIV transmission and disease progression. *Nat Med* 2:1240, 1996.

57. Dragic T, Litwin V, Allaway GP, et al: HIV entry into CD4 cells is mediated by the chemokine receptor CC-CKR-5. *Nature* 381:667, 1996.

58. Samson M, Libert F, Doranz BJ, et al: Resistance to HIV infection in Caucasian individuals bearing mutant alleles of the CCR-5 chemokine receptor gene. *Nature* 382:722, 1996.

59. Liu R, Paxton WA, Choe S, et al: Homozygous defect in HIV-1 co-receptor accounts for resistance of some multiply-exposed individuals to HIV-1 infection. *Cell* 86:367, 1996.

60. Gordon S, Fraser I, Nath D, et al: Macrophages in tissues and in vitro. *Curr Opin Immunol* 4:25, 1992.

61. Lasser AP: The mononuclear phagocyte system: A review. *Hum Pathol* 14:1080, 1983.

62. Fogelman AM, Van Lenten BJ, Warden C, et al: Macrophage liproprotein receptors. *J Cell Sci* 9(suppl):135, 1988.

63. Adams DO, Hamilton TA: Phagocytic cells. Cytotoxic activities of macrophages, in *Inflammation. Basic Principles and Clinical Correlates,* 2d ed, edited by JI Galin, IM Goldstein, R Snyderman, p 471. Raven, New York, 1992.

64. Werb Z, Goldstein IM: Phagocytic cells: Chemotactic and effector functions of macrophages and granulocytes, in *Basic and Clinical Immunology,* 7th ed, edited by DP Stites, AI Terr, p 96. Appleton and Lange, Norwalk, 1991.

65. Papadimitriou JM, Ashman RB: Macrophages: Current views on their differentiation, structure and function. *Ultrastruct Pathol* 13:343, 1989.

66. Gordon S, Perry H, Rabinowitz S, et al: Plasma membrane receptors of the mononuclear phagocyte system. *J Cell Sci* 9(suppl):1, 1988.

67. Law SKA: C3 receptors on macrophages. *J Cell Sci* 9(suppl):67, 1988.

BIOCHEMISTRY AND FUNCTION
OF MONOCYTES AND
MACROPHAGES

ROBERT I. LEHRER

TOMAS GANZ

Mononuclear phagocytes play central roles in resistance to many infectious diseases, including tuberculosis, leishmaniasis, typhoid fever, and systemic mycoses. Highly specialized mononuclear cells called *dendritic cells* excel in presenting antigens to T cells, a critical step in initiating the adaptive immune response. Unlike short-lived neutrophils, macrophages can survive within tissues for weeks and even months. They exhibit a prodigious capacity for macromolecular synthesis, secrete numerous bioactive molecules, and are highly responsive to the internal milieu. Macrophages possess receptors for cytokines, including interferon gamma and tumor necrosis factor alpha, allowing their functional state to be modulated by such molecules. Additional surface receptors enhance their phagocytic properties by recognizing various host-derived factors, including immunoglobulins, complement, and integrins. Macrophage receptors have been identified that recognize molecular motifs characteristic of microbial membranes and cell walls, including lipopolysaccharide, mannans, and (lipo)teichoic acids. The antimicrobial mechanisms of macrophages are mediated largely, but not exclusively, by various oxidants produced by their NADPH oxidase and/or inducible nitric oxide synthase (iNOS) systems. Macrophages also exhibit cytotoxic and cytostatic properties in vitro, although attempts to harness these activities have not yet been successfully applied to humans.

Mononuclear phagocytes (monocytes and macrophages) are relatively large phagocytic cells with abundant cytoplasm and a round to reniform nucleus (see Chap. 73). Macrophages that depart from this appearance can bear eponyms, such as *Gaucher* or *Kupffer cells,* or have pseudonyms, such as *foam* (lipid-laden) or epithelioid cells. Mononuclear

Acronyms and abbreviations that appear in this chapter include: ADCC, antibody-dependent cellular cytotoxicity; BPI, bactericidal/permeability enhancing factor; CGD, chronic granulomatous disease; CSF-1, colony-stimulating factor 1; FGF, fibroblast growth factor; G-CSF, granulocyte colony-stimulating factor; GM-CSF, granulocyte-monocyte colony-stimulating factor; ICAMs, intercellular adhesion molecules; iNOS or NOS2, inducible nitric oxide synthase; IRF-1, interferon regulatory factor 1; LBP, lipopolysaccharide binding protein; LDL, low-density lipoprotein; LPS, lipopolysaccharide; M-CSF, macrophage colony-stimulating factor; MHC, major histocompatibility complex; MPO, myeloperoxidase; NADPH, nicotinamide adenine dinucleotide phosphate (reduced form); NO, nitric oxide; Nramp, natural resistance-associated macrophage protein; O2−, superoxide; ONOO−, peroxynitrite; PDGF, platelet-derived growth factor; RANTES, *r*egulated upon *a*ctivation, *n*ormal T-cell *e*xpressed and presumably *s*ecreted; SR-A, type A scavenger receptor; TGF-β, transforming growth factor β.

phagocytes combine prodigious biosynthetic and secretory abilities with an ability to vary their output in response to local conditions and chemical mediators. Although cells of the monocyte-macrophage lineage may undergo malignant transformation or exuberant proliferation (Chap. 78), most often their routine duties—host defense, antigen presentation, and removal of detritus—are performed away from the spotlight of disease.

Although human blood monocytes can be obtained readily, most other human macrophage populations are less accessible. Consequently, much of our information about macrophages is derived from in vivo experiments on mice or from in vitro experiments with cultured blood monocytes or cell lines. This chapter will review selected aspects of the biology of mononuclear phagocytes, including their endocytic and phagocytic behavior, receptors, secretory properties, and microbicidal and cytotoxic mechanisms. Production, distribution, and fate of monocytes and macrophages are discussed in Chap. 75.

DENDRITIC CELLS

Dendritic cells are widely distributed, HLA-DR/DQ–positive, migratory marrow–derived cells that are specialized for antigen capture and T-cell stimulation, rather than for phagocytosis and direct host defense.[1] Antigen-presenting cells are important because, rather than recognizing intact protein antigens directly, T-cell receptors recognize peptide fragments that are bound to cell surface, major histocompatibility complex (MHC) molecules. Class I MHC molecules normally bind peptides, such as viral coat components, that are derived from intracellular proteins. MHC class II molecules typically present peptides derived from extracellular antigens.

Unlike macrophages, dendritic cells lack receptors for immunoglobulin, complement, and colony-stimulating factor 1 (CSF-1).[2] They are only weakly phagocytic and take up exogenous antigens principally by fluid-phase endocytosis and adsorptive pinocytosis. After these internalized antigens are partially degraded and bound to MHC class II molecules, the antigens return to the dendritic cell's surface as a MHC II peptide complex. Recognition of this complex by antigen receptors on CD4-positive T-helper cells generates one signal for these cells. Full T-cell activation requires a second, costimulatory signal from the antigen-presenting cell. Although the mechanisms that convey this second signal are incompletely known, dendritic cells excel in providing it, perhaps aided by specific chemokines.[3] In addition to their MHC class II molecules, dendritic cells express multiple surface adhesion molecules, including LFA-1 (CD11a/CD18), LFA-3 (CD58), ICAM-1(CD54), and ICAM-2. By promoting close associations with T lymphocytes, such adhesion molecules can enhance the dendritic cell's ability to signal T-cell receptors.

Dendritic cells constitute approximately 0.1 to 1 percent of the blood's mononuclear cell.[2] Their dynamic, veil-like or branching cytoplasmic processes provide a large surface area for interactions with T cells. GM-CSF and certain interleukins, including IL-4 or IL-13, promote in vitro differentiation of functional dendritic cells from blood monocytes[4] or CD 34+ bone marrow or blood progenitor cells.[5-7] Other dendritic cell populations include migratory veiled cells in afferent lymph, interdigitating cells in thymic medulla, and interstitial cells in the lung and heart. The Langerhans cells of skin are dendritic cells that express MHC class II antigens constitutively. Dendritic cells can pick up local antigens or haptens and migrate via the lymphatics to enter T-dependent, paracortical areas of regional lymph nodes.

MOTILITY AND CHEMOTAXIS

Many mononuclear phagocytes are present in the lamina propria of organs regularly exposed to microbes, including the intestinal and genitourinary tracts, skin, and lungs. Local tissue populations of macrophages are rapidly augmented by entry of blood monocytes responding to various signals that arise during infection and inflammation. Macrophage motility depends on the contractile properties of actin and myosin, regulated by many additional proteins, including profilin, gelsolin, acumentin, tropomyosin, actin-binding protein, and calmodulin.[8]

Chemotaxis refers to the ability of cells to orient in and move along a chemical gradient. Many molecules that are generated during infection or injury are recognized by the surface receptors of monocytes and macrophages and trigger chemotactic responses. Such substances include N-formylated peptides produced by bacteria,[9,10] complement component C5a,[11] leukotriene B4 and other eicosanoids,[12,13] collagen and elastin fragments,[14,15] thrombin,[16] platelet factor 4, platelet-derived growth factor (PDGF),[17] and at least two neutrophil proteins, cathepsin G and azurocidin.[18]

Chemokines (i.e., chemotactic cytokines) are important mediators of chemotactic and migratory behavior. These 8- to 10-kDa molecules contain four conserved cysteines that are linked by disulfide bonds. They have been divided into two groups, based on their homology and the spacing of their first two cysteine residues. CXC chemokines, also called *α-chemokines,* have an amino acid interposed between these cysteines. In CC chemokines, also called *β*-chemokines, these cysteines are adjacent. The genes for CXC and CC chemokines are clustered on human chromosomes 4 and 17, respectively.[18] Whereas CXC chemokines such as IL-8 act primarily on neutrophils, CC chemokines such as MCP 1–4, MIP-1α, MIP-β, and RANTES are potent activators of monocytes and T lymphocytes.[18,19]

Multiple, structurally related receptors for chemokines have been identified. Typically, these receptors have seven transmembrane domains and signal through heterotrimeric GTP-binding proteins. Chemokines and their receptors vary with respect to binding specificity. Many chemokines bind to more than one receptor, and most chemokine receptors bind more than one chemokine. Expression of chemokine receptors is regulated by the ambient cytokine environment, thereby allowing complex and graded responses.

Certain chemokine receptors have been subverted by pathogens in ways detrimental to the host. For example, CCR5, the macrophage receptor for RANTES, MIP-1α, and MIP-1β, is used by monocyte/macrophage-tropic strains of HIV-1 as a coreceptor for intracellular entry.[20] Additionally, many members of the poxvirus, herpesvirus, and retrovirus families have captured genes encoding cytokine or chemokine receptors and modified them in ways that enhance viral pathogenicity.[21–23] For example, molluscum contagiosum virus secretes a modified CC chemokine that interferes with the chemotactic response of human leukocytes to multiple CC and CXC chemokines, thereby blunting the in vivo inflammatory response to the virus.[24] Human herpesvirus 8, a Kaposi's sarcoma–associated herpesvirus, appears to use similar strategies to deliver signals that initiate inappropriate growth or transformation.[25]

ENERGETICS AND ENDOCYTOSIS

Mononuclear phagocytes derive most of their metabolic energy from glycolytic metabolism. In alveolar macrophages, this is augmented substantially by oxidative phosphorylation. Macrophages imbibe extracellular fluid continually by a process known as *pinocytosis* (literally, "cell drinking"). Their fluid uptake occurs in several types of vesicles, including macropinosomes that are larger than 0.2 μm in diameter, clathrin-coated vesicles, and small uncoated vesicles. Receptor-mediated endocytosis takes place principally via clathrin-coated vesicles.[26] Exposure of macrophages to M-CSF promptly induces active cell ruffling and enhanced macropinosome formation.[27]

The content of degradative enzymes in macrophages increases after they take up digestible substances by endocytosis or phagocytosis.

Although proteins retained within the lysosomal apparatus emerge only after extensive degradation, endocytic mechanisms specialized for antigen presentation allow partially degraded antigens to be displayed on the macrophage cell membrane, bound to MHC molecules.[28]

SECRETION

Certain secretory products of macrophages, such as lysozyme, are produced regularly and in large amounts. Most others are produced and released in a highly controlled fashion, determined by the functional state of the cell and its exposure to regulatory stimuli. In addition to many cytokines (e.g., IL-1α and β, IL-6, TNF-α, and interferons α, β, and γ) and chemokines, macrophages produce numerous growth factors, including G-CSF, GM-CSF, erythroid colony potentiating factor, transforming growth factor (TGF)-β, PDGF, and fibroblast growth factor (FGF).[29] By secreting classical and alternative pathway complement factors,[30] macrophages can augment local tissue concentrations of these host-defense molecules. Macrophages release various enzymes (e.g., plasminogen activator, elastase, collagenases, and acid hydrolases) that participate in tissue remodeling and wound healing. They also produce matrix proteins such as fibronectin, thrombospondin, proteoglycans, and diverse lipid mediators, including prostaglandins (PGE$_2$, PGF$_{2α}$), prostacyclin, and various lipoxygenase products.[31]

RECEPTORS

Receptors allow mononuclear phagocytes to recognize and respond to other cells. They also permit macrophages to adhere to extracellular matrix, bind and ingest microorganisms, and respond to various cytokines and growth factors. Expression of membrane receptors varies according to the macrophage's functional state and reflects its prior exposure to cytokines.[31] When receptor-ligand binding events occur, this is communicated to the intracellular machinery by transduction pathways that ultimately impinge on molecules that regulate transcription. These include NF-κB, NF-IL6, PU.1, interferon regulatory factor 1 (IRF-1), Egr-1, and Stat-1.

ADHESINS

Macrophages can adhere reversibly to various surfaces, including endothelial cells and extracellular matrix proteins. This property allows them to migrate on such surfaces and is imparted by adhesive plasma membrane glycoprotein receptors called *adhesins*. At least three families of adhesins participate in these processes—selectins, integrins, and intercellular adhesion molecules (ICAMs). The integrin superfamily is composed of heterodimeric molecules with noncovalently associated α and β chains. Several β$_2$-integrins are prominent in macrophages, including LFA-1 (CD11a/CD18), MAC-1 (CD11b/CD18), and p150/95 (CD 11c/CD18). The ligands (often called *counterreceptors*) of these adhesins include ICAMS-1, -2, and -3 (LFA-1); fibrinogen and fibronectin (MAC-1); and iC3b (p150,95). Several β$_1$-integrins (VLA-4, −5, and −6) expressed by monocytes are fibronectin receptors that may promote recruitment of monocytes to inflammatory foci.[32] Leukocyte adhesion deficiency—a complex inherited disorder that results from a marked deficiency of β$_2$-integrins[33]—is associated with frequent and severe infections, poor wound healing, and diminished accrual of leukocytes at sites of infection.

Mononuclear phagocytes and other leukocytes contain "homing receptors" called *L-selectins* or *LECAMs*. These adhesive, lectinlike molecules mediate an initial, low-affinity rolling type of adhesion between leukocytes and their counterreceptors on vascular endothelium, before stronger connections are made via integrins.[34]

RECEPTORS INVOLVED IN PHAGOCYTOSIS

The surface membranes of mononuclear phagocytes contain specific receptors for immunoglobulins, including IgG$_1$ and other IgG subtypes, IgA, and IgE. IgG binds organisms via its Fab sites and binds the macrophage's Ig receptors via its Fc portion. IgG receptors promote both attachment and ingestion of immunoglobulin-coated particles. Macrophages also display receptors for several complement components, including C3b, C3bi, C3a, and C5a. The C3b receptor (also called *CR1* and *CD35*) is also found on neutrophils. It recognizes opsonized particles and accelerates C3b breakdown by factor I. CR1 mediates attachment without ingestion unless small amounts of IgG are present[35] or the macrophages are otherwise stimulated.[36] The C3bi receptor (also called *CR3, Mac1,* and *CD 11b/CD18*) recognizes an Arg-Gly-Asp (RGD) triplet in its ligand, C3bi,[37] as well as in fibrinogen and fibrin. CR3 binds many other ligands, including molecules found on bacteria, fungi, and protozoans as well as ICAM-1 and other ligands of endothelial cells.[38] The contact sites of the C3bi receptor for several such ligands have been shown to partially overlap.[39] IgG and C3b receptors allow macrophages to recognize microorganisms opsonized (tagged for phagocytosis) by the deposition of immunoglobulin and/or complement on their surface. In vivo administration of interferon-γ to normal subjects significantly increases the expression of Ig receptors (Fc gammaRI, Fc gammaRII, Fc gammaRIII), integrins (CD11a/CD18, CD11b/CD18), and HLA-DR by monocytes.[40]

Certain macrophage receptors recognize molecules or molecular arrays that are typically found on microbes and can be classified as "pattern recognition receptors."[41] A well-studied example is the macrophage mannose receptor—a 180-kDa transmembrane protein with eight tandem carbohydrate recognition domains.[42] Two of these domains interact with linear or branched-chain mannosyl and fucosyl residues, allowing the mannose receptor to recognize a wide variety of bacteria, mycobacteria, yeasts, and parasites and initiate phagocytic, endocytic, or antigen capture responses. Mannose receptors are also expressed on dendritic cells.[43]

Several macrophage receptors can recognize lipopolysaccharide (LPS), an abundant glycolipid that occupies most of a gram-negative bacterium's outer membrane surface.[44] These receptors include CD 14, a GPI-anchored glycoprotein; the CD11/18 family of β$_2$-integrins; and the macrophage's type A scavenger receptor (SR-A). Binding of LPS to CD14 is enhanced by lipopolysaccharide binding protein (LBP), a 65-kDa plasma protein homologous to bactericidal/permeability enhancing factor (BPI). CD14-deficient mice are markedly resistant to shock induced by LPS or gram-negative bacterial challenge.[45] After exposure to LPS, normal monocytes produce and release many inflammatory mediators, including reactive oxygen and nitrogen intermediates, prostaglandins, and various proinflammatory cytokines, including TNF-α, IL-1β, IL-6, and IL-8.

SCAVENGER RECEPTORS

Macrophages contain several receptors that recognize various negatively charged macromolecules. Among these are the trimeric, macrophage type I and type II scavenger receptors, which bind oxidized and acetylated low-density lipoproteins (LDLs) and mediate their endocytic uptake. These receptors contribute to cholesterol deposition in atherosclerotic foam cells in humans and mice.[46,47] Types I and II scavenger receptors have a collagenlike domain, and the type I receptor also has a cysteine-rich domain common to several other receptors. Type I and type II scavenger receptors also mediate adhesion and bind lipopolysaccharide,[48] lipoteichoic acids from gram-positive bacteria,[49] and advanced glycation protein end products. Additional macrophage scavenger receptors include CD36 and CD68 (macrosialin). CD36 can

bind apoptotic cells, *Plasmodium falciparum*-infected erythrocytes, long-chain fatty acids, and oxidized LDL.[50]

Other macrophage receptors allow these cells to recognize regulatory molecules such as macrophage colony-stimulating factor (M-CSF), hormones, leukotrienes, other eicosanoids, coagulation factors, transport proteins, antiproteases, and many other bioactive molecules.[51]

RESISTANCE TO INFECTION

By subjecting inbred mice differing in resistance to infection by different microbes to detailed genetic analysis, Nramp1 (natural resistance-associated macrophage protein)—a macrophage protein that contributes substantially to innate resistance to intracellular infections—was identified. Nramp1 is a hydrophobic, integral membrane protein that is encoded by the *Lsh/Ity/Bcg* gene, which regulates resistance to *Leishmania, Salmonella,* and *Mycobacteria.* The expression of Nramp1 in mice is restricted to macrophages and is enhanced by treatment with interferon-γ and lipopolysaccharide. Nramp1 is also found in late endosomal and lysosomal vesicular compartments of the macrophage. The protein may enhance vacuolar acidification and endosome-phagosome fusion[52] or act to influence transport of iron or other trace metals needed for microbial growth.[53] Intracellular pathogens, such as mycobacteria, can interfere with phagosome-lysosome fusion, thereby preventing vacuolar acidification and reducing the delivery of Nramp1 to phagosomes.[54]

ANTIMICROBIAL MECHANISMS

Experimental studies of murine listeriosis were instrumental in developing the concept of "activated macrophages."[55] In this model, bacterial numbers increased logarithmically in the liver and spleen for 3 days after intravenous inoculation of *L. monocytogenes.* Thereafter, net bacterial growth ceased, and viable bacteria declined sharply in numbers, disappearing by the next week. These beneficial changes were accompanied by the appearance of delayed hypersensitivity. An altered phenotype was evident in the peritoneal macrophages, which enlarged, became more phagocytic, and more effectively resisted in vitro challenge by *L. monocytogenes.* Similar changes were noted after mice were infected with *Brucella abortus, Salmonella typhimurium,* or *Mycobacterium bovis.*[55] The antimicrobial efficacy of these macrophages was nonspecific, since infection by any one of these intracellular pathogens engendered macrophages with an enhanced ability to inhibit intracellular replication by all of them. Although such activated macrophages reverted to their basal state after 1 to 2 weeks, the phenotypic changes recurred within 24 h after a challenge by the same organism that had initiated the original infection. In vivo resistance was not transferred from immune to naive mice by serum, but the transfer of splenic T lymphocytes conferred protection.

During the past decade, much has been learned about the events responsible for these phenomena. Mononuclear phagocytes possess multiple mechanisms that allow them to kill ingested microorganisms or restrict their replication. Ingested microbes are sequestered within membrane-bounded compartments, called *phagocytic vacuoles* or *phagosomes,* which can be acidified to a pH of approximately 4.5. Within such phagosomes, the microbes are exposed to a mixture of lysolipids, macrophage-derived enzymes and proteins, and various oxidants. Moreover, microbial access to micronutrients, especially iron, that are essential for their growth is limited. Although entrapment within phagolysosomes is a lethal event for most microbes, successful pathogens have developed stratagems that allow them to survive and even thrive in this environment. Some, such as *Listeria monocytogenes,* escape from phagosomes and enter the cytoplasmic compartment,[56] where they co-opt the host cell's actin and use it to propel themselves into adjacent cells.[57,58] Other pathogens modulate their phagosomal microenvironments by inhibiting vacuolar acidification[59] or phagolysosomal fusion[60] or by undergoing phenotypic changes that enhance their resistance.[61,62]

REACTIVE OXYGEN INTERMEDIATES

Macrophages with enhanced antimicrobial or cytotoxic activity generally show an increased production of reactive oxygen intermediates.[63] To generate these oxidants, phagocytes, including monocytes and macrophages, contain multiple protein components that, when assembled and activated, form an NADPH oxidase complex that transfers electrons to molecular oxygen from intracellular NADPH. Activation of NADPH oxidase is triggered by protein kinases[64] and involves translocation to the plasma membrane of several cytosolic components, including p67^{phox}, p47^{phox}, p40^{phox}. The fully active NADPH oxidase complex also includes several small GTP-binding proteins.[65] In the plasma membrane, the several cytosolic components interact via proline-rich and SH3 domains with a flavo-hemoprotein, cytochrome b$_{558}$, that is composed of large and small subunits called gp91^{phox} and p22^{phox}, respectively. Superoxide (O$_2^-$) anions generated by NADPH oxidase are unstable and undergo various reactions, including dismutation to form hydrogen peroxide (H$_2$O$_2$) and oxygen.

Chronic granulomatous disease (CGD) refers to a group of uncommon disorders associated with defective activation and assembly of NADPH oxidase by neutrophils and mononuclear phagocytes. The neutrophils and monocytes of children with CGD fail to produce superoxide and H$_2$O$_2$ and show markedly impaired antimicrobial activity against many bacteria and fungi in vitro. The most common variant of CGD is transmitted with X-linked inheritance and affects male children only.[66] It results from the absence or abnormality of gp91^{phox}, whose gene is located on the X chromosome, at Xp21.1. Defects in p47^{phox} (chromosome 7q11.23) are transmitted autosomally and account for about 30 percent of total CGD cases, affecting males and females equally. Primary genetic defects involving p22^{phox}, p67^{phox}, and gp91 have also been described and account for the remaining cases of CGD. Children affected by CGD sustain repeated infections, most often caused by *Staphylococcus aureus* but caused also by bacteria and fungi of limited pathogenic potential (e.g., *Serratia marcescens, Burkholderia cepacia,* and *Aspergillus fumigatus*). Prophylactic administration of antibiotics, such as trimethoprim-sulfamethoxazole, and of interferon-γ,[67] decreases the frequency and severity of infections in patients with all forms of CGD (See Chap. 72).

MYELOPEROXIDASE

Like neutrophils, blood monocytes contain myeloperoxidase (MPO) and use it to convert H$_2$O$_2$ into microbicidal oxidants.[68] Their MPO is lost when monocytes differentiate into macrophages. Hereditary deficiency of MPO is relatively common, perhaps affecting as many as 1 in 2000 individuals.[69] Neutrophils and monocytes of affected individuals lack MPO and are unable to convert the H$_2$O$_2$ produced by the dismutation of superoxide into more potent oxidants such as hypochlorite or chloramines. Neutrophils and monocytes from subjects with hereditary MPO deficiency show selectively impaired microbicidal activity in vitro, and several such patients (typically with additional predisposing factors, such as diabetes mellitus) have developed disseminated *C. albicans* infections. Although other abnormalities can also cause MPO-deficiency, R569W missense mutations occur in the MPO genes of many affected subjects, often associated with some other abnormality of the allelic gene.[70,71]

NITRIC OXIDE

Nitric oxide (NO) and other reactive nitrogen intermediates play important roles in restricting the growth of many pathogenic organisms in mice and in murine macrophages.[72,73] NO is both diffusible and unstable. It reacts with oxygen and water to yield equimolar amounts of nitrite and nitrate and reacts with other molecules to form *S*-nitrosothiols. NO and superoxide (O$_2^-$) can interact to form peroxynitrite (ONOO$^-$), a potent oxidant that may also mediate antimicrobial activity.

Distinct NO synthase enzymes are responsible for the constitutive and inducible production of nitric oxide.[74] In murine macrophages, stimulation by lipopolysaccharide or cytokines such as interferon γ leads to the expression of an inducible nitric oxide synthase, called *NOS2* or *iNOS*. This heme-containing enzyme converts L-arginine to citrulline + NO , using NADPH and oxygen as additional substrates and FAD, FMN, calmodulin, and tetrahydrobiopterin as cofactors.[74] iNOS itself may mediate production of superoxide in L-arginine-depleted murine macrophages.[75]

Pathogens whose susceptibility to rodent macrophages can be attributed to NO production include *Cryptococcus neoformans, Francisella tularensis, Leishmania major,* and *Schistosoma mansoni*[73,76]; iNOS knockout mice show increased susceptibility to acute infection by many, but not all, organisms.[77,78] For example, macrophages from knockout mice deficient in interferon regulatory factor 1 (IRF-1) efficiently controlled *Listeria monocytogenes* despite failing to produce iNOS and NO,[79] and mice deficient in NF-IL6 were highly susceptible to *Listeria* despite a normal iNOS response.[80] The role of NO in human host defense is less certain but is under intense study.[81] Human lung macrophages from patients with tuberculosis express iNOS,[82] and inflammatory human macrophages have been induced to express iNOS in vitro.[83]

CYTOSTATIC AND CYTOCIDAL ACTIVITY

Activation of macrophage cytostatic or cytocidal activity usually requires the delivery of two signals, one that "primes" and the other that "triggers." Priming signals often derive from T cells and can include molecules such as interferon γ, IL-2, IL-4 , G-CSF, and GM-CSF or combinations thereof.[84] The cytostatic properties of activated macrophages[85] arise from both oxygen-independent and oxygen-dependent mechanisms. The former are mediated by cytotoxic molecules, including TNF-α and enzymes (e.g., cytolytic proteases or arginase). The latter are mediated by reactive chemical intermediates formed by NADPH oxidase or inducible nitric oxide synthase.

Macrophage-mediated cellular cytotoxicity has been divided into four basic categories: rapid antibody-dependent cellular cytotoxicity (ADCC), slow ADCC, antibody-independent tumor cytolysis, and cytostasis.[86] All require macrophage activation, and all but cytostasis required intimate physical contact between the macrophage and its target cell. Just as many pathogenic microbes can subvert the microbicidal actions of macrophages, tumors may also release cytokines and other regulatory factors that suppress macrophage-mediated cytotoxicity.[87]

ANTIBODY-DEPENDENT CELLULAR CYTOTOXICITY

ADCC can occur rapidly (within 4 to 6 h) or slowly (over 24 to 48 h) after macrophage–target cell contact occurs. Such contact can be induced by antibody and is promoted by adhesive glycoproteins of the integrin/selectin group. IgG$_1$, IgG$_{2a}$, IgG$_{2b}$, or IgG$_3$ isotype antibodies impart immunologic specificity to the process—with IgG2$_a$ perhaps being most efficient.[88] ADCC against antibody-coated erythrocytes can contribute to erythrocyte destruction in autoimmune hemolytic anemias, and ADCC directed toward surface-bound gliadin may contribute to the pathogenesis of celiac disease.[89]

ANTIBODY-INDEPENDENT TUMOR CYTOLYSIS

This process, reportedly specific for neoplastic or transformed cells, lyses a wide range of syngeneic, allogeneic, and xenogeneic targets, while sparing their normal counterparts. The macrophage delivers the fatal blow at close quarters, using molecular weaponry that includes TNF-α, reactive oxygen intermediates, and nitric oxide.[31,90]

CYTOSTASIS

Unlike ADCC, macrophage-mediated cytostasis is neither target specific nor contact-dependent. It affects proliferation of a broad range of normal and neoplastic targets and results from release of various macrophage-derived molecules, including prostaglandins, arginase, nitric oxide, and cytokines, including interferons, TNF-α or IL-1α, and -1β.[31]

CYTOTOXIC MECHANISMS

Production of reactive oxygen intermediates by NADPH oxidase, discussed above with reference to antimicrobial activity, also contributes to the ability of macrophages to destroy tumor cells[91,92] and to lyse antibody-coated erythrocyte targets.[93]

Cytostasis caused by NO or peroxynitrite (OONO) results from oxidation or nitrosylation of cytoplasmic enzymes, such as ribonucleotide reductase,[94] and mitochondrial enzymes with iron-sulfur centers, such as aconitase and succinate-ubiquinone oxidoreductase.[95] Damage of these vital enzymes inhibits the target cell's energy metabolism and its production of deoxyribonucleotides.[96] Expression of iNOS has been demonstrated in tumor-associated macrophages that infiltrate human breast and gastric cancers[97]; iNOS production in human macrophages is regulated by an interplay between membrane CD23, a low-affinity receptor for IgE FCε, and the cytokine IL-10.[98]

CYTOTOXIC PROTEINS AND PEPTIDES

Although activated murine macrophages secrete a cytotoxic serine protease,[99] and rabbit alveolar macrophages contain potentially cytotoxic peptide defensins,[100] a contribution by human homologues of these molecules to macrophage-mediated cytotoxicity has not been shown. The cytotoxicity of cytolytic protease[99] and defensins[101] is enhanced by otherwise nontoxic concentrations of hydrogen peroxide.

TNF-α was originally identified in the circulation of LPS-treated animals and received its alternative original name, "cachexin," from its ability to inhibit lipoprotein lipase and induce wasting in mice.[102,103] A 26-kDa TNF-α precursor is displayed on the plasma membrane,[104] and proteolytic processing trims this to a monomeric, 17-kDa form, which can form trimers.[105] The cytotoxic properties of TNF-α are enhanced by concomitant production of nitric oxide by macrophages.[106] Lymphocytes also produce TNF-α, as well as a closely related lymphotoxin molecule called TNF-β.[107]

TNF-α mediates most of its varied effects on cells via a specific 75-kDa receptor[108] which also circulates in a soluble form. In addition to killing certain tumor cells in vitro and in vivo, TNF-α causes fever, leukopenia followed by leukocytosis, neutrophil priming and activation, T-cell activation, increased serum levels of IL-6, and an enhanced procoagulatory state.[109] These effects resemble those of IL-1 and include many responses seen typically with acute inflammation and infection.

REFERENCES

1. Kamperdijk EWA, Nieuwenhuis P, Hoefsmit ECM: *Dendritic Cells in Fundamental and Clinical Immunology*, p 1. Plenum Press, New York, 1993.
2. Freudenthal PS, Steinman RM: The distinct surface of human blood dendritic cells, as observed after an improved isolation method. *Proc Natl Acad Sci USA* 87:7698, 1990.
3. Adema GJ, Hartgers F, Verstraten R, et al: A dendritic-cell-derived C-C chemokine that preferentially attracts naive T cells. *Nature* 387:713, 1997.
4. Chapuis F, Rosenzwajg M, Yagello M, et al: Differentiation of human dendritic cells from monocytes in vitro. *Eur J Immunol* 27:431, 1997.
5. Szabolcs P, Ciocon DH, Moore MA, Young JW: Growth and differentiation of human dendritic cells from CD34+ progenitors. *Adv Exp Med Biol* 417:15, 1997.
6. Brossart P, Grunebach F, Stuhler G, et al: Generation of functional human dendritic cells from adherent peripheral blood monocytes by CD40 ligation in the absence of granulocyte-macrophage colony-stimulating factor. *Blood* 92:4238, 1998.
7. Rosenzwajg M, Camus S, Guigon M, Gluckman JC: The influence of interleukin (IL)-4, IL-13, and Flt3 ligand on human dendritic cell differentiation from cord blood CD34+ progenitor cells. *Exp Hemat* 26:63, 1998.
8. Stossel TP: On the crawling of animal cells. *Science* 260:1086, 1993.
9. Marasco WA, Phan SH, Krutzsch H: Purification and identification of formylmethionyl-leucyl-phenylalanine as the major peptide neutrophil chemotactic factor produced by *Escherichia coli*. *J Biol Chem* 259:5430, 1984.
10. Snyderman R, Pike MC, Edge S, Lane B: A chemoattractant receptor on macrophages exists in two affinity states regulated by guanine nucleotides. *J Cell Biol* 98:444, 1984.
11. Shang XZ, Issekutz AC: Beta 2 (CD18) and beta 1 (CD29) integrin mechanisms in migration of human polymorphonuclear leucocytes and monocytes through lung fibroblast barriers: shared and distinct mechanisms. *Immunology* 92:527, 1997.
12. Malmsten CL, Palmblad J, Uden AM, et al: A highly potent stereospecific factor stimulates migration of polymorphonuclear leukocytes. *Acta Physiol Scand* 110:449, 1980.
13. Sozzani S, Zhou D, Locati M, et al: Stimulating properties of 5-oxo-eicosanoids for human monocytes: synergism with monocyte chemotactic protein-1 and -3. *J Immunol* 157:4664, 1996.
14. Hunninghake GW, Davison JM, Rennard S, et al: Elastin fragments attract macrophage precursors to diseased sites in pulmonary emphysema. *Science* 212:925, 1981.
15. Uemura Y, Okamoto K: Elastin-derived peptide induces monocyte chemotaxis by increasing intracellular cyclic GMP level and activating cyclic GMP dependent protein kinase. *Biochem Mol Biol Int* 41:1085, 1997.
16. Naldini A, Sower L, Bocci V, et al: Thrombin receptor expression and responsiveness of human monocytic cells to thrombin is linked to interferon-induced cellular differentiation. *J Cell Physiol* 77:76, 1998.
17. Deuel TF, Senior RM, Huang JS, Griffin GL: Chemotaxis of monocytes and neutrophils to platelet-derived growth factor. *J Clin Invest* 69:1046, 1982.
18. Baggiolini M, deWald B, Moser B: Human chemokines: an update. *Ann Rev Immunol* 15:675, 1997.
19. Boulay F, Naik N, Giannini E, et al: Phagocyte chemoattractant receptors. *Ann NY Acad Sci* 832:69, 1997.
20. Dragic T, Litwin V, Allaway GP, et al: HIV-1 entry into CD4+ cells is mediated by the chemokine receptor CC-CKR-5. *Nature* 381:667, 1996.
21. Guo HG, Browning P, Nicholas J, et al: Characterization of a chemokine receptor-related gene in human herpesvirus 8 and its expression in Kaposi's sarcoma. *Virology* 228:371, 1997.
22. McFadden G, Lalani A, Everett H, et al: Virus-encoded receptors for cytokines and chemokines. *Semin Cell Dev Biol* 9:359,1998.
23. Rucker J, Edinger AL, Sharron M, et al: Utilization of chemokine receptors, orphan receptors, and herpesvirus-encoded receptors by diverse human and simian immunodeficiency viruses. *J Virol* 71:8999, 1997.
24. Damon I, Murphy PM, Moss B: Broad spectrum chemokine antagonistic activity of a human poxvirus chemokine homolog. *Proc Nat Acad Sci USA* 95:6403, 1998.

25. Geras-Raaka E, Arvanitakis L, Bais C, et al: Inhibition of constitutive signaling of Kaposi's sarcoma-associated herpesvirus G protein-coupled receptor by protein kinases in mammalian cells in culture. *J Exp Med* 187:801,1998.

26. Mukherjee S, Ghosh RN, Maxfield FR: Endocytosis. *Physiol Rev* 77: 759, 1997.

27. Racoosin EL, Swanson JA: M-CSF-induced macropinocytosis increases solute endocytosis but not receptor-mediated endocytosis in mouse macrophages. *J Cell Science* 102:867, 1992.

28. Unanue ER: Antigen presenting function of the macrophage. *Annu Rev Immunol* 2:395, 1984.

29. Nathan CF: Secretory products of macrophages. *J Clin Invest* 79:319, 1987.

30. Ezekowitz RAB, Sim RB, MacPherson GG, Gordon S: Interaction of human monocytes, macrophages, and polymorphonuclear leukocytes with zymosan in vitro. Role of type 3 complement receptors and macrophage-derived complement. *J. Clin Invest* 76:2368, 1985.

31. Adams DO, Hamilton TA: Macrophages as destructive cells in host defense, in *Inflammation, Basic Principles and Clinical Correlates*, 2d ed, edited by JI Gallin, IM Goldstein, R Snyderman, p 637. Raven, New York, 1992.

32. Hemler ME: VLA proteins in the integrin family: Structures, functions, and their role on leukocytes. *Annu Rev Immunol* 8:365, 1990.

33. Mazzone A, Ricevuti G: Leukocyte CD11/CD18 integrins: biological and clinical relevance. *Haematologica* 80:161, 1995.

34. VanAndvian U, Chambers J, McEvoy L, et al: Two-step model of leukocyte-endothelial cell interaction inflammation: distinct roles for LECAM-I and the leukocyte beta 2 integrins in vivo. *Proc Natl Acad Sci USA* 88:7538, 1991.

35. Ehlenberger AG, Nussenzweig V: The role of membrane receptors for C3b and C3d in phagocytosis. *J Exp Med* 145:357, 1977.

36. Griffin FMJ, Griffin JA: Augmentation of macrophage complement receptor function in vitro: II. Characterization of the effects of a unique lymphokine upon the phagocytic capabilities of macrophages. *J Immunol* 125:844, 1980.

37. Wright SD, Reddy PA, Jong MTC, Erickson BW: C3bi receptor (complement receptor type 3) recognizes a region of complement protein C3 containing the sequence Arg-Gly-Asp. *Proc Natl Acad Sci USA* 84:1965, 1987.

38. Wright SD: Receptors for complement and the biology of phagocytosis, in *Inflammation, Basic Principles and Clinical Correlates*, 2d ed, edited by JI Gallin, IM Goldstein, R Snyderman, p 477. Raven, New York, 1992.

39. Zhang L, Plow EF: Overlapping, but not identical, sites are involved in the recognition of C3bi, neutrophil inhibitory factor, and adhesive ligands by the alpha M beta 2 integrin. *J Biol Chem* 271:18211, 1996.

40. Schiff DE, Rae J, Martin TR, et al: Increased phagocyte Fc gammaRI expression and improved Fc gamma-receptor-mediated phagocytosis after in vivo recombinant human interferon-gamma treatment of normal human subjects. *Blood* 90:3187, 1997.

41. Janeway CA: The immune system evolved to discriminate infectious nonself from noninfectious self. *Immunol Today* 13:11, 1992.

42. Stahl PD, Ezekowitz RAB: The mannose receptor is a pattern recognition receptor involved in host defense. *Curr Opin Immunol* 10:50, 1998.

43. Reis e Souza C, Stahl PD, Austyn JM: Phagocytosis of antigens by Langerhans cells in vitro. *J Exp Med* 178:509, 1993.

44. Fenton MJ, Golenbock DT: LPS-binding proteins and receptors. *J Leuk Biol* 64:25, 1998.

45. Haziot A, Ferrero E, Kontgen F, et al: Resistance to endotoxin shock and reduced dissemination of gram-negative bacteria in CD14-deficient mice. *Immunity* 4:407, 1996.

46. Brown MS, Goldstein JI: Lipoprotein metabolism in the macrophage: implications for cholesterol deposition in atherosclerosis. *Annu Rev Biochem* 52:223, 1983.

47. Yla-Herttuala S: Expression of lipoprotein receptors and related molecules in atherosclerotic lesions. *Curr Opin Lipidol* 7:292, 1996.

48. Hampton RY, Goklenbock DT, Penman M, et al: Recognition and plasma clearance of endotoxin by scavenger receptors. *Nature* 352: 342, 1991.

49. Dunne DW, Resnick D, Greenberg J, et al: The type I macrophage scavenger receptor binds to gram-positive bacteria and recognizes lipoteichoic acid. *Proc Nat Acad Sci USA* 91:1863, 1994.

50. Daviet L, McGregor JL: Vascular biology of CD36: roles of this new adhesion family molecule in different disease states. *Thromb Haemostasis* 78:65, 1997.

51. Fraser I, Gordon S: An overview of receptors of MPS cells, in *Blood Cell Biochemistry*, vol 5, *Macrophages and Related Cells*, edited by MA Horton, p 1. Plenum, New York, 1993.

52. Hackam DJ, Rotstein OD, Zhang W, et al: Host resistance to intracellular infection: mutation of natural resistance-associated macrophage protein 1 (Nramp1) impairs phagosomal acidification. *J Exp Med* 188: 351, 1998.

53. Searle S, Bright NA, Roach TIA, et al: Localization of Nramp1 in macrophages: modulation with activation and infection. *J Cell Sci* 111:2855, 1998.

54. Sturgill-Koszycki S, Schaible U, Russell DG: *Mycobacterium*-containing phagosomes are accessible to early endosomes and reflect a transitional state in the normal phagosome biogenesis. *EMBO J* 15:6960, 1996.

55. Mackaness GB: Reflections on the history of the macrophage, in *Mononuclear Phagocytes in Cell Biology*, edited by G Lopez-Berestein, J Klostergaard, p 1. CRC, Boca Raton, FL, 1993.

56. Portnoy DA: Innate immunity to a facultative intracellular bacterial pathogen. *Curr Opin Immunol* 4:20, 1992.

57. Southwick FS, Purich DL: Dynamic remodeling of the actin cytoskeleton: lessons learned from *Listeria* locomotion. *Bioessays* 16:885, 1994.

58. Smith GA, Portnoy DA: How the *Listeria monocytogenes* ActA protein converts actin polymerization into a motile force. *Trends Microbiol* 5:272, 1997.

59. Sibley LD, Weidner E, Krahenbuhl JL: Phagosome acidification is blocked by intracellular *Toxoplasma gondii*. *Nature* 315:416, 1985.

60. Horwitz MA: The legionnaire's disease bacterium (*Legionella pneumophila*) inhibits phagosome-lysosome fusion in human monocytes. *J Exp Med* 158:2108, 1983.

61. Alpuche A, Swanson JA, Loomis WP, Miller SI: *Salmonella typhimurium* activates virulence gene transcription within acidified macrophage phagosomes. *Proc Natl Acad Sci USA* 89:10079, 1992.

62. Rathman M, Sjaastad MD, Falkow S: Acidification of phagosomes containing *Salmonella typhimurium* in murine macrophages. *Infect Immun* 64:2765, 1996.

63. Nathan CF: Secretion of oxygen intermediates: Role in effector functions of activated macrophages. *Fed Proc* 41, 2206, 1982.

64. El Benna J, Faust RP, Johnson JL, Babior BM: Phosphorylation of the respiratory burst oxidase subunit p47phox as determined by two-dimensional phosphopeptide mapping. Phosphorylation by protein kinase C, protein kinase A, and a mitogen-activated protein kinase. *J Biol Chem* 271:6374, 1996.

65. Meischl C, Roos D: The molecular basis of chronic granulomatous disease. *Springer Semin Immunopathol* 19:417, 1998.

66. Roos D: X-CGDbase: a database of X-CGD-causing mutations. *Immunol Today* 17:517, 1996.

67. Gallin JI, Malech HL, Meinick DA: A controlled trial of interferon gamma to prevent infection in chronic granulomatous disease. The International Chronic Granulomatous Disease Study Group. *New Engl J Med* 324:509, 1991.

68. Klebanoff SJ: Oxygen metabolites from phagocytes, in *Inflammation, Basic Principles and Clinical Correlates*, 2d ed, edited by Jl Gallin, IM Goldstein, R Snyderman, p 541. Raven, New York, 1992.

69. Nauseef WM, Root RK, Malech HL: Biochemical and immunologic analysis of hereditary myeloperoxidase deficiency. *J Clin Invest* 71:1297, 1983.

70. DeLeo FR, Goedken M, McCormick SJ, Nauseef WM: A novel form of hereditary myeloperoxidase deficiency linked to endoplasmic reticulum/proteasome degradation. *J Clin Invest* 101:2900, 1998.

71. Nauseef WM, Cogley M, Bock S, Petrides PE: Pattern of inheritance in hereditary myeloperoxidase deficiency associated with the R569W missense mutation. *J Leuk Biol* 63:264, 1998.

72. James S: Role of nitric oxide in parasitic infections. *Microb Rev* 59:533, 1995.

73. Fang FC: Mechanisms of nitric oxide-related antimicrobial activity. *J Clin Invest* 99:2818, 1997.

74. Nathan C, Xie Q: Nitric oxide synthases: roles, tolls and controls. *Cell* 78:915, 1994.

75. Xia Y, Zweier JL: Superoxide and peroxynitrite generation from inducible nitric oxide synthase in macrophages. *Proc Nat Acad Sci USA* 94:6954, 1997.

76. Granger DL, Cameron ML, Lee-See K, Hibbs JB Jr: Role of macrophage-derived nitrogen oxides in antimicrobial function, in *Mononuclear Phagocytes in Cell Biology*, edited by G Lopez-Berestein, J Klostergaard, p 7, CRC, Boca Raton, FL, 1993.

77. MacMicking JD, Nathan C, Hom G, et al: Altered responses to bacterial infection and endotoxic shock in mice lacking inducible nitric oxide synthase. *Cell* 81:641, 1995.

78. Sharton-Kersten T, Yap G, Magram J, Sher A: Inducible nitric oxide is essential for host control of persistent but not acute infection with the intracellular pathogen *Toxoplasma gondii*. *J Exp Med* 185:1261, 1997.

79. Fehr T, Schoedon G, Odermatt B, et al: Crucial role of interferon consensus sequence binding protein, but neither of interferon regulatory factor 1 nor of nitric oxide synthesis for protection against murine listeriosis. *J Exp Med* 185:921, 1997.

80. Tanaka T, Akira S, Yoshida K, et al: Targeted disruption of the NF-IL6 gene discloses its essential role in bacteria killing and tumor cytotoxicity by macrophages. *Cell* 80:353, 1995.

81. Nathan C: Inducible nitric oxide synthase: what difference does it make? *J Clin Invest* 100:2417, 1997.

82. Nicholson S, Bonecini-Almeida M Da G, Lapa e Silva JR, et al: Inducible nitric oxide synthase in pulmonary alveolar macrophages from patients with tuberculosis. *J Exp Med* 183:2293, 1996.

83. Nozaki Y, Hasegawa Y, Ichiyama S, et al: Mechanism of nitric-oxide dependent killing of *Mycobacterium* BCG in human alveolar macrophages. *Infect Immun* 65:3644, 1997.

84. Hamilton TA, Ohmori Y, Narumi S, Tannenbaum CS: Regulation of diversity of macrophage activation, in *Mononuclear Phagocytes in Cell Biology*, edited by G Lopez-Berestein, J Klostergaard, pp 48–70. CRC, Boca Raton, FL, 1993.

85. Krahenbuhl JL, Remington JS: The role of activated macrophages in specific and nonspecific cytostasis of tumor cells. *J Immunol* 113:507, 1974.

86. Adams DO, Hamilton TA: Destruction of tumor cells by mononuclear phagocytes. Models for analyzing effector mechanisms and regulation of macrophage activation, in *Mechanisms of Host Resistance to Infectious Agents, Tumors, and Allografts*, edited by RM Steinman, RJ North, pp 185–204. Rockefeller University, New York, 1986.

87. Elgert KD, Alleva DG, Mullins DW: Tumor-induced immune dysfunction: the macrophage connection. *J Leuk Biol* 64:275, 1998.

88. Kipps TJ, Parham P, Punt J, Herzenberg AL: Importance of immunoglobulin isotype in human antibody-dependent cell-mediated cytotoxicity directed by murine monoclonal antibodies. *J Exp Med* 161:1, 1985.

89. Saalman R, Wold AE, Dahlgren UI, et al: Antibody-dependent cell-mediated cytotoxicity to gliadin-coated cells with sera from children with coeliac disease. *Scand J Immunol*, 47:37, 1998.

90. Keller R, Keist R, Wechsler A, et al: Mechanisms of macrophage-mediated tumor cell killing: a comparative analysis of the roles of reactive nitrogen intermediates and tumor necrosis factor. *Int J Cancer* 46:682, 1990.

91. Nathan CF: Reactive oxygen intermediates in lysis of antibody-coated tumor cells, in *Macrophage-Mediated Antibody-Dependent Cellular Cytotoxicity*, edited by HS Koren, pp 199–215. Marcel Dekker, New York, 1983.

92. Cohen MS, Taffet SM, Adams DO: The relationship between competence for secretion of H_2O_2 and completion of macrophage cytotoxicity by BCG-elicited murine macrophages. *J Immunol* 128:1781, 1982.

93. Fleer A, Roos D, von den Borne EG Jr, Engelfriet CP: Cytotoxic activity of human monocytes toward sensitized red cells is not dependent on the generation of reactive oxygen species. *Blood* 54:407, 1979.

94. Lepoivre M, Chenais B, Yapo A, et al: Alterations of ribonucleotide reductase activity following induction of the nitrite-generating pathway in adenocarcinoma cells. *J Biol Chem* 265:14143, 1990.

95. Darpier JC, Hibbs JB Jr: Murine cytotoxic activated macrophages inhibit aconitase in tumor cells: inhibition involves the iron-sulfur prosthetic group and is reversible. *J Clin Invest* 78:790, 1986.

96. Keller R, Geiges M, Keist R: Arginine dependent reactive nitrogen intermediates as mediators of tumor cell killing by activated macrophages. *Cancer Res* 50:1421, 1990.

97. Thomsen LT, Miles DW: Role of nitric oxide in tumour progression: lessons from human tumours. *Cancer Metastasis Rev* 17:107, 1998.

98. Dugas N, Palacios-Calender M, Dugas B, et al: Regulation by endogenous interleukin-10 of the expression of nitric oxide synthase induced after ligation of CD23 in human macrophages. *Cytokine* 10:680, 1998.

99. Adams DO, Hamilton TA: The cell biology of macrophage activation. *Annu Rev Immunol* 2:283, 1984.

100. Lehrer RI, Lichtenstein AK, Ganz T: Antimicrobial and cytotoxic peptides of mammalian cells. *Annu Rev Immunol* 11:105, 1993.

101. Lichtenstein AK, Ganz T, Selsted ME, Lehrer RI: Synergistic cytolysis mediated by hydrogen peroxide combined with peptide defensins. *Cell Immunol* 114:104, 1988.

102. Beutler B, Cerami A: Cachectin: more than a tumor necrosis factor. *N Engl J Med* 316:379, 1987.

103. Beutler B (ed): *Tumor Necrosis Factors: The Molecules and Their Emerging Role in Medicine*. Raven, New York, 1992.

104. Chaudhri G: Differential regulation of biosynthesis of cell surface and secreted TNF-alpha in LPS-stimulated murine macrophages. *J Leuk Biol* 62:249, 1997.

105. Jones EY, Stuart DI, Walker NPC: Structure of tumor necrosis factor. *Nature* 338:225, 1989.

106. Higuchi M, Higashi N, Taki H, Osawa T: Cytolytic mechanisms of activated macrophages. Tumor necrosis factor and L-arginine dependent mechanisms act synergistically as the major cytolytic mechanisms of activated macrophages. *J Immunol* 144:1425, 1990.

107. Nedwin GE, Naylor SI, Sakaguchi AY: Human lymphotoxin and tumor necrosis factor genes: structure, homology and chromosomal localization. *Nucleic Acids Res* 13:6361, 1985.

108. Dembric Z, Loetscher H, Gubler U: Two human TNF receptors have similar extracellular but distinct intracellular domain sequences. *Cytokine* 2:231, 1990.

109. Dinarello CA: Role of interleukin-1 and tumor necrosis factor in systemic responses to infection and inflammation, in *Inflammation, Basic Principles and Clinical Correlates*, 2d ed, edited by JI Gallin, IM Goldstein, R Snyderman, pp 211–232. Raven, New York, 1992.

PRODUCTION, DISTRIBUTION, AND FATE OF MONOCYTES AND MACROPHAGES

TOMAS GANZ

ROBERT I. LEHRER

Macrophages are ancient, mesoderm-derived host defense cells. During embryogenesis, they appear first in the yolk sac, then in the liver, and finally in the marrow—a sequence that recapitulates the phylogeny of blood-forming tissues in vertebrates. Large populations of tissue macrophages exist in the small intestine, liver (Kupffer cells), and lungs. Tissue macrophages can replicate sufficiently to sustain steady-state macrophage populations. Blood monocytes arise in the marrow from precursor cells (monoblasts) that are derived from the differentiation of multipotential progenitors. Blood monocytes rapidly enter into inflamed or infected tissues, where they can mature into macrophages and substantially augment resident macrophage populations. Monocytes can also mature into dendritic cells that efficiently present antigen to T cells.

IDENTIFICATION AND KINETIC STUDIES OF MONOCYTES AND MACROPHAGES

Monocytes and macrophages are recognized outside the marrow as smaller (spread diameter of 10 to 18 μm) and larger (20 to 80 μm) cells that are mononuclear and phagocytic (see Chap. 73). Among the histochemical markers characteristic of mammalian monocytes and macrophages, "lipase" (a nonspecific esterase usually detected by its hydrolysis of α-naphthyl butyrate) and myeloperoxidase (detected by the peroxidation of diaminobenzidine) have been the most useful. Human monocytes and macrophages both express lipase activity, but only the monocytes and immature macrophages contain granules that react with peroxidase substrates. Marrow macrophages and monocytes are morphologically and histochemically similar to their extramyeloid counterparts. Myeloid lineage-specific genes that encode transcription factors regulate macrophage development. A transcription factor PU.1 encoded by an *ETS* family gene appears to be central in macrophage development. Transcription factor gene expression is probably induced by exogenous cytokine stimulation, especially by M-CSF, interacting with GM-CSF, and IL-3.[43] Promonocytes, monocyte precursors in the marrow, are weakly phagocytic mononuclear cells 10 to 20 μm in diameter that contain cytoplasmic filaments visible under electron microscopy and a small number of peroxidase-positive cytoplasmic granules.[1,2] Monoclonal antibodies and lectins variably specific for monocytes and macrophages have been developed.[3]

Acronyms and abbreviations that appear in this chapter include: FIM, factor increasing monocytopoiesis; GM-CSF, granulocyte-monocyte colony stimulating factor; IL-1, interleukin-1; M-CSF, monocyte colony-stimulating factor; TNF, tumor necrosis factor.

Monocytes or macrophages can be isolated from body fluids, labeled with lipophilic dyes or radioactive compounds, then reinfused and their fate followed by repeated sampling of blood or tissues. Alternatively, genetic markers can be employed to follow the fate of infused monocytes, macrophages, or marrow cells. Concerns have been raised about the effects of in vitro handling on the fate of reinfused cells. The kinetics of monocytes and macrophages after marrow transplantation also may be altered from normal by the effects of radiation and conditioning drugs on the recipient.[4]

Experimental animals treated with a brief infusion of ³H-thymidine incorporate the radioactive nucleotide into cells undergoing DNA replication. The labeled cells and their descendants can be detected by overlaying tissue sections, imprints, or thin films with photographic emulsions where the beta particles emitted by tritium cause black "grains" to develop. Cells that have divided more than once after incorporating ³H-thymidine are less radioactive, since each division splits the labeled DNA equally between the daughter cells. The films or tissue sections can be conventionally stained to allow the classification of the labeled cells according to their morphologic and staining characteristics. When a nondividing population arises only by maturation of a dividing precursor cell population, most of the precursors incorporate tritiated thymidine abundantly but the mature descendants incorporate comparatively little. As the precursors mature, the number of labeled precursors decreases while their labeled descendants increase. Quantitative analysis can yield kinetic models of traffic between various cell populations and their rates of proliferation. Since macrophages are labeled both directly (dividing macrophages) and indirectly (macrophages arising from dividing earlier marrow precursors), the interpretation of the experimental data can be complex and has led to controversy.[4,5]

Dual in vivo labeling of macrophage populations is largely avoided by using parabiotic animals,[4] whose blood circulations are joined by a permanent cutaneous connection. The skin tunnel between the two animals can be clamped to temporarily separate their circulations while only one animal is infused with tritiated thymidine. When labeling is complete, cross-circulation is allowed to resume. In this case, the macrophages of the recipient animal that was not injected with tritiated thymidine are labeled only if they develop from labeled donor-derived circulating cells.

PHYLOGENY AND ONTOGENY OF MACROPHAGES

Large mononuclear phagocytic cells of mesodermal origin (macrophages) are the principal host defense cells in invertebrates[6] (e.g., mollusks, crustaceans, or insects), where they are usually referred to as *amebocytes* or *hemocytes*. The premyeloid phylogenetic origin of macrophages may be mirrored during embryonic development. Primitive (weakly phagocytic) macrophages with an ameboid shape that react with the monocyte-macrophage lineage-specific monoclonal antibody F4/80 are found in the developing yolk sac when blood vessels and blood cells first appear.[7-9] Promonocytes and monocyte-like cells appear subsequently. Before hematopoiesis shifts from the yolk sac to the liver, macrophages become more phagocytic, develop lysosomal structures, display lipase activity, and divide rapidly as indicated by incorporation of tritiated thymidine into DNA. At the same time, macrophages identified morphologically and by staining with *Griffonia simplicifolia* isolectin B4 are already present in the developing liver, brain, and lungs and persist there throughout embryonic development.[8,9] It is not clear whether these tissue macrophages are of yolk sac origin or arise independently. Normal tissue macrophage populations can undergo prominent expansion in response to postnatal influences. For example, rabbit alveolar macrophages exposed to ambient microbes, their products, and various particulates proliferate rapidly during the first 2 weeks of life.[10]

TISSUE DISTRIBUTION OF MONOCYTES AND MACROPHAGES

In the adult, the major macrophage populations are found in the lamina propria of the small intestine, in the liver (Kupffer cells), the lungs (alveolar and interstitial macrophages), the spleen, the lymph nodes, the bone marrow, the serosal cavities (peritoneal and pleural), the kidney and endocrine glands, and in the brain (microglia).[11,46] The heart and the muscles are relatively macrophage-poor. Additional cells thought to be closely related to macrophages functionally, antigenically, and developmentally are found in the skin (Langerhans or dendritic cells) and in the bone (osteoclasts). The precise lineage relationship of the latter two cells to monocytes is complex.[47,48,51] Dendritic cells arise from both myeloid and lymphoid progenitors,[51,53] and osteoclasts may develop from myeloid progenitors at an early stage.[48] In the absence of inflammation, monocytes are found principally in the marrow and blood. Monocytes migrate from blood into inflammatory lesions, where they differentiate into typical macrophages.[12-15] Macrophages, whether resident or inflammatory, assume different morphologic and functional features depending on their location in organs and tissues. The determinants of this tissue-specific differentiation are not known.

THE DEVELOPMENT OF MONOCYTES IN THE MARROW

Blood monocytes arise from progenitor cells in the marrow,[15,16] since they do not incorporate tritiated thymidine into their DNA, do not undergo mitosis while in blood, and carry the genotype of the donor after marrow transplantation. Labeled monocytes do not appear in blood for 13 to 24 h after intravenous injection of tritiated thymidine,[17] indicating that blood monocytes arise from precursors that divided at least 13 h previously. Since blood monocytes have myeloperoxidase-containing granules, monocyte precursors in the marrow were sought among dividing cells that synthesized myeloperoxidase and resembled monocytes morphologically. The immediate monocyte precursors, promonocytes, were identified by intense thymidine labeling, peroxidase staining of rough endoplasmic reticulum and Golgi, and the presence of cytoplasmic filaments and cleft nuclei.[1,2,18] Although similar to myelocytes under light microscopy, they could be distinguished from the latter under electron microscopy: Promonocyte cell membranes displayed many fingerlike projections, cytoplasmic filaments, and contained many fewer and smaller granules than did the myelocytes. The putative precursors of promonocytes, termed *monoblasts,* were recognized in macrophage-forming colonies as smaller dividing cells that contained large nuclei, scant cytoplasm, and few peroxidase-positive granules.[19] Monoblasts probably develop from multipotential granulocyte-monocyte progenitors.[20] A model of monocyte development has been proposed in which each monoblast gives rise to two promonocytes, each of which then divides into two monocytes.[21]

KINETICS OF MONOCYTES IN CIRCULATION AND IN INFLAMMATORY LESIONS

Human monocytes appear in the circulation 13 to 26 h after the last round of promonocyte DNA synthesis, followed by mitotic division. They leave the circulation at random times with a half-life that has been estimated at 8 to 70 h.[17,22,23] The shorter half-lives were obtained in experiments in which monocytes were removed from blood, labeled, and reinfused, manipulations that may have shortened the half-life of labeled cells. The longer half-life was seen after labeling monocytes in vivo.[17] The calculated basal monocyte output is approximately 9.4 $\times$ 10^8 cells per day for the average adult. In rabbits there is a large pool of monocytes transiently trapped in the lung vasculature, but it is not known whether human monocytes are similarly marginated. Within a few hours of the onset of infection or inflammation, monocytes migrating from the bloodstream are found in the lesions, although they are initially much less numerous than neutrophils. In model lesions, monocytes begin to predominate over neutrophils after 12 h.[24] Endothelial transmigration is mediated by platelet/endothelial cell adhesion molecule-1 (PECAM-1) and other surface molecules.[49] In rats, hematogenous infection with *Salmonella enteritidis* elicits transient monocytopenia followed by prolonged monocytosis.[25] The monocytosis is a combined effect of the release of immature monocytes into the circulation, shortened monocyte generation time, and an expanded monocyte precursor pool. In this model of infection, the half-life of monocytes in blood is shortened to 50 percent of normal, probably due to more rapid efflux into tissues.

The interleukins IL-3 and IL-6 and the colony-stimulating factors GM-CSF and M-CSF, all cytokines (see Chap. 22), and a less extensively characterized protein named *factor increasing monocytopoiesis* (FIM) induce monocytosis in experimental animals,[5,26-29] but the role of these factors in the physiologic regulation of monocyte and macrophage production and kinetics is not yet fully understood. Release of cytokines and hematopoietic growth factors by macrophages engaged in host defense contributes to the increase in monocyte/macrophage production during infections (Fig. 75-1). Pharmacologic doses of glucocorticoids induce monocytopenia and diminish monocyte recruitment into test skin lesions.[30]

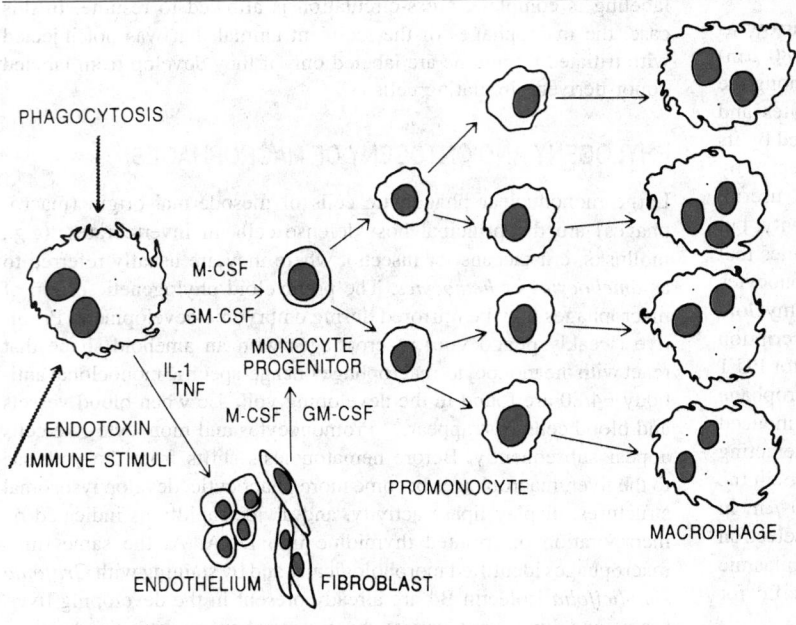

FIGURE 75-1 Autoregulation of mononuclear phagocyte production in response to host defense stimuli. Macrophages exposed to microbial or immune stimuli release hematopoietic growth factors GM-CSF and M-CSF that increase the proliferation of monocyte/macrophage precursors. Additionally, by releasing interleukin-1 (IL-1) and tumor necrosis factor (TNF), activated macrophages induce GM-CSF and M-CSF production by endothelial cells and fibroblasts. Prostaglandin E produced by macrophages may act as a negative regulator of monocyte production.

DIFFERENTIATION OF MONOCYTES INTO MACROPHAGES

Monocytes in cell culture[12] and in tissues[31] spontaneously transform into macrophages, and it is well established that monocytes migrating into inflamed tissues give rise to most of the reactive macrophage population[13,16,32] Nevertheless, macrophages are capable of cell division, and resident (noninflammatory) macrophage populations may be largely self-sustaining.[4] Serial analysis of gene expression during cytokine-induced maturation of human blood monocytes to macrophages has found a high frequency of expressed genes involved in lipid metabolism.[50] In human marrow transplant recipients, alveolar and liver macrophages (Kupffer cells) are eventually replaced by donor-derived cells,[33,34] occurring in the case of alveolar macrophages over a period of about 100 days. It is not certain whether the influx of donor-derived cells results from tissue inflammation or from damage to resident macrophages caused by radiation or cytotoxic therapy or reflects the natural dynamics of macrophage populations. The former possibilities are supported by studies on parabiotic mice and rats, wherein macrophage replacement from the cross-circulating monocytes is not seen unless inflammation is induced.[4,35,36] In human liver transplant recipients, liver macrophages (Kupffer cells) were replaced by recipient-derived cells over a period of several months.[37] It is likely that the migration of macrophage precursors into donor tissue was stimulated by the inflammation associated with low-grade transplant rejection.

MULTINUCLEATED GIANT CELLS

Multinucleated giant cells are phagocytic and microbicidal cells found in areas of chronic tissue inflammation. They arise from macrophages either by cell fusion or perhaps by a process in which nuclear division occurs without cell division. In vitro, transformation of macrophages to giant cells occurs by fusion after about 1 to 2 weeks of culture[12] and is stimulated by interferon-γ or IL-3 or macrophage adherence to surfaces.[38]

DENDRITIC CELLS AND THEIR RELATIONSHIP TO MONOCYTES AND MACROPHAGES

Dendritic cells are found in peripheral tissues where they take up proteins and particulates, process them, then migrate into lymph nodes where they present antigenic fragments to T lymphocytes.[39,40] Their ability to present antigen very efficiently and their characteristic morphology have been used as the defining characteristics of this cell type. In vivo, dendritic cells are especially important during primary immunization. "Veiled cells" are dendritic cells that migrate in lymph vessels to lymph nodes. Studies in animals pulsed with ^{3}H-thymidine show that these cells arose from precursors that last divided a few days before. This time course can be reproduced in an in vitro model, where maturation of monocytes into dendritic cells takes place within 48 h after exposure to particles or microorganisms followed by a signal from endothelial cells during transmigration of monocytes from the luminal surface to the subendothelial matrix.[41] In the absence of the second signal, monocytes develop into macrophages. Slower differentiation of marrow precursors or blood monocytes to dendritic cells occurs under the influence of mixtures of cytokines, typically including GM-CSF with IL-4 or TNF-α.[42–45,52,53] Using different mixtures of cytokines not including GM-CSF, dendritic cells can also be generated in vitro from lymphoid cells.[47,51] Dendritic cells of lymphoid origin are abundant in the thymus and may participate in lymphocyte selection.[51,53]

THE FATE OF MONOCYTES AND MACROPHAGES

The fate of monocytes under noninflammatory conditions is not known with certainty. Some may develop into macrophages, while others may be destroyed in as yet unknown disposal sites. Alveolar macrophages leave the body in swallowed mucus from the airways, and other macrophages may migrate to local lymph nodes.[42] However, the ultimate destination of the majority of senescent macrophages is not known. The lymph nodes appear to be the principal final destination of dendritic cells.[39–41]

REFERENCES

1. Van Furth R, Hirsch JG, Fedorko ME: Morphology and peroxidase cytochemistry of mouse promonocytes, monocytes, and macrophages. *J Exp Med* 132:794, 1970.
2. Nichols BA, Bainton DF: Differentiation of human monocytes in bone marrow and blood. *Lab Invest* 29:27, 1973.
3. Lawson GL, Rabinowitz PR, Morris L, Perry VH: Antigen markers of macrophage differentiation in murine tissues. *Curr Top Microbiol Immunol* 181:1, 1992.
4. Volkman A: Disparity in origin of mononuclear phagocyte populations. *J Reticuloend Soc* 19:249, 1976.
5. Van Furth R: Production and migration of monocytes and kinetics of macrophages, in *Mononuclear Phagocytes,* edited by R van Furth, pp 3–12. Kluwer, Netherlands, 1992.
6. Metchnikoff E: *Immunity in Infective Diseases.* University Press, Cambridge, 1905.
7. Sorokin SP, Hoyt RF, Blunt DG, McNelly NA: Macrophage development: II. Early ontogeny of macrophage populations in brain, liver, and lungs of rat embryos as revealed by a lectin marker. *Anat Rec* 232:527, 1992.
8. Sorokin SP, McNelly NA, Hoyt RF: CFU-rAM, the origin of lung macrophages, and the macrophage lineage. *Am Physiol Soc* 263:L299, 1992.
9. Takahashi K, Yamamura F, Naito M: Differentiation, maturation, and proliferation of macrophages in the mouse yolk sac: a light-microscopic, enzyme-cytochemical, immunohistochemical, and ultrastructural study. *J Leukoc Biol* 45:87, 1989.
10. Evans MJ, Sherman MP, Campbell LA, Shami SG: Proliferation of pulmonary alveolar macrophages during postnatal development of rabbit lung. *Am Rev Respir Dis* 136:384, 1987.
11. Hume DA, Robinson AP, Macpherson GC, Gordon S: The mononuclear phagocyte system of the mouse defined by immunohistochemical localization of antigen F4/80. *J Exp Med* 158:1522, 1983.
12. Sutton JS, Weiss L: Transformation of monocytes in tissue culture into macrophages, epithelioid cells, and multinucleated giant cells. *J Cell Biol* 28:303, 1966.
13. Van Furth R, Diesselhoff-den Dulk MMC, Mattie H: Quantitative study on the production and kinetics of mononuclear phagocytes during an acute inflammatory reaction. *J Exp Med* 138:1314, 1973.
14. Volkman A: The origin and turnover of mononuclear cells in peritoneal exudates in rats. *J Exp Med* 124:241 1966.
15. Van Furth R, Cohn ZA: The origin and kinetics of mononuclear phagocytes. *J Exp Med* 128:415 1968.
16. Volkman A, Gowans JL: The production of macrophages in the rat. *Br J Exp Pathol* 46:50 1965.
17. Whitelaw DM: Observations on human monocyte kinetics after pulse labeling. *Cell Tissue Kinet* 5:311, 1972.
18. Van der Meer JWM, Beelen RHJ, Fluitsma DM, van Furth R: Ultrastructure of mononuclear phagocytes developing in liquid bone marrow cultures. *J Exp Med* 149:17, 1979.
19. Van der Meer JWM, van de Gevel JS, Beelen RHJ, et al: Culture of human bone marrow in the Teflon culture bag: identification of the human monoblast. *J Reticuloend Soc* 32:355, 1982.
20. Metcalf D, Burgess AW: Clonal analysis of progenitor cell commitment to granulocyte or macrophage production. *J Cell Physiol* 111:275, 1982.
21. Van Furth R, Diesselhoff-den Dulk MMC: The kinetics of promonocytes and monocytes in the bone marrow. *J Exp Med* 132:813, 1970.
22. Meuret G, Batara E, Fürste HO: Monocytopoiesis in normal man: pool

size, proliferation activity and DNA synthesis time of promonocytes. *Acta Haematol* 54:261, 1975.

23. Meuret G, Hoffmann G: Monocyte kinetic studies in normal and disease states. *Br J Haematol* 24:275, 1973.

24. Issekutz TB, Issekutz AC, Movat HZ: The in vivo quantitation and kinetics of monocyte migration into acute inflammatory tissue. *Am J Pathol* 103:47, 1981.

25. Volkman A, Collins FM: The cytokinetics of monocytosis in acute salmonella infection in the rat. *J Exp Med* 139:264, 1974.

26. Ulich TR, del Castillo J, Watson LR, et al: In vivo hematologic effects of recombinant human macrophage colony-stimulating factor. *Blood* 75:846, 1990.

27. Andrews RG, Knitter GH, Bartelmez SH, et al: Recombinant human stem cell factor, a *c-kit* ligand, stimulates hematopoiesis in primates. *Blood* 78:1975, 1991.

28. Ulich TR, del Castillo J, Busser K, et al: Acute in vivo effects of IL-3 alone and in combination with IL-6 on the blood cells in circulation and bone marrow. *Am J Pathol* 135:663, 1989.

29. Ulich TR, del Castillo J, McNiece I, et al: Hematologic effects of recombinant murine granulocyte-macrophage colony-stimulating factor on the peripheral blood and bone marrow. *Am J Pathol* 137:369, 1990.

30. Dale DC, Fauci AS, Wolff SM: Alternate-day prednisone. Leukocyte kinetics and susceptibility to infection. *N Engl J Med* 291:1154, 1993.

31. Ryan GB, Spector WG: Macrophage turnover in inflamed connective tissue. *Proc R Soc Lond* 175:269, 1970.

32. Van Furth R, Nibbering PH, van Dissel JT, Diesselhoff-den Dulk MMC: The characterization, origin, and kinetics of skin macrophages during inflammation. *J Invest Dermatol* 85:398, 1985.

33. Thomas ED, Ramberg RE, Sale GE, et al: Direct evidence for a bone marrow origin of the alveolar macrophage in man. *Science* 192:1016, 1976.

34. Gale RP, Sparkes RS, Golde DW: Bone marrow origin of hepatic macrophages (Kupffer cells) in humans. *Science* 201:937, 1978.

35. Sawyer RT: The ontogeny of pulmonary alveolar macrophages in parabiotic mice. *J Leukoc Biol* 40:347, 1986.

36. Collins FM, Auclair LK: Mononuclear phagocytes within the lungs of unstimulated parabiotic rats. *J Reticuloend Soc* 27:429, 1980.

37. Porter KA: Origin of Kupffer cells and endothelial cells in long-surviving human hepatic homografts, in *Experience in Hepatic Transplantation,* edited by TE Starzl, pp 464–465. Saunders, Philadelphia, 1969.

38. Enelow RI, Sullivan GW, Carper HT, Mandell GL: Induction of multinucleated giant cell formation from in vitro culture of human monocytes with interleukin-3 and interferon-gamma: comparison with other stimulating factors. *Am J Respir Cell Mol Biol* 6:57, 1992.

39. Hart DN: Dendritic cells: unique leukocyte populations which control the primary immune response. *Blood* 90:3245, 1997.

40. Shortman K, Maraskovsky E: Developmental options. *Science* 282:424, 1998.

41. Randolph GJ, Beaulieu S, Lebecque S, Steinman RM, Muller WA: Differentiation of monocytes into dendritic cells in a model of transendothelial trafficking. *Science* 282: 480, 1998.

42. Lauweryns JW, Baert JH: Alveolar clearance and the role of the pulmonary lymphatics. *Am Rev Respir Dis* 115:625, 1977.

43. Valledor AF, Borràs FE, Cullell-Young M, Celada A: Transcription factors that regulate monocyte/macrophage differentiation. *J Leuk Biol* 63:405, 1998.

44. Lane PJ, Brocker T: Developmental regulation of dendritic cell function. *Curr Opin Immunol* 11:308, 1999.

45. Banyer JL, Hapel AJ: Myb-transformed hematopoietic cells as a model for monocyte differentiation into dendritic cells and macrophages. *J Leuk Biol* 66:217, 1999.

46. Kennedy DW, Abkowitz JL: Kinetics of central nervous system microglial and macrophage engraftment: analysis using a transgenic bone marrow transplantation model. *Blood* 90:986, 1997.

47. Anjùere F, Martinez del Hoyo G, Martin P, Ardavín : Langerhans cells develop from a lymphoid-committed precursor. *Blood* 96:1633, 2000.

48. Muguruma Y, Lee MY: Isolation and characterization of murine clonogenic osteoclast progenitors by cell surface phenotype analysis. *Blood* 91:1272, 1998.

49. Muller WA, Randolph GJ: Migration of leukocytes across endothelium and behond: molecules involved in the transmigration and fate of monocytes. *J Leuk Biol* 66:698, 1999.

50. Hashimoto S-i, Suzuki T, Dong H-Y, et al: Serial analysis of gene expression in human monocytes and macrophages. *Blood* 94:837, 1999.

51. Young JW: Dendritic cells: expansion and differentiation in the hematopoietic growth factors. *Curr Opin Hematol* 6:135, 1999.

52. Steinman R, Inaba K: Myeloid dendritic cells. *J Leuk Biol* 66:205, 1999.

53. Santiago-Schwarz F: Positive and negative regulation of the myeloid dendritic cell lineage. *J Leuk Biol* 66:209, 1999.

CLASSIFICATION AND CLINICAL MANIFESTATIONS OF DISORDERS OF MONOCYTES AND MACROPHAGES

MARSHALL A. LICHTMAN

Disorders that result in abnormalities of monocytes exclusively are uncommon and are referred to as histiocytoses. These disorders may be inherited, such as familial hemophagocytic lymphohistiocytosis; inflammatory, such as infectious hemophagocytic syndrome; neoplastic, such as Langerhans cell histiocytosis; or they may result from exaggerated storage of macromolecules, such as Gaucher's disease. Some cases of myelogenous leukemia have progenitor cells that mature preferentially into leukemic monocytes. Certain acquired diseases that affect hematopoiesis result in a severe depression of blood monocytes (along with other blood types). Inherited disorders affecting white cells may result in impaired monocyte function, such as Chédiak-Higashi syndrome. Table 76-1 categorizes the qualitative and quantitative abnormalities of monocytes and macrophages.

CLASSIFICATION

Classification of monocytic disorders is difficult because few abnormalities result solely in a disturbance of monocytes or macrophages. However, the presence of monocytopenia or monocytosis may be an important diagnostic feature or contribute to the functional abnormality in the patient.

The terms *histiocyte* and *macrophage* have been synonymous. The latter term is customary when discussing the biology of the cells of the mononuclear phagocyte system, which is the total pool of marrow, blood, and tissue monocytes and macrophages (formerly referred to as the *reticuloendothelial system*). In disease nosology, the terms *histiocytosis* and *histiocyte* continue to be used for diseases that principally involve cells derived from blood monocytes, i.e., macrophages.

It is important that the physician consider the absolute count and not the percent of cells that are monocytes when evaluating the differential blood cell count before concluding that there is an inappropriate content of blood monocytes (see Chap. 77).

Table 76-1 contains a classification of monocyte and macrophage disorders.

MONOCYTOPENIA

Two striking examples of disorders accompanied by severe monocytopenia are aplastic anemia and hairy cell leukemia. In both conditions pancytopenia is usual, but the predisposition to serious infection is heightened by the deficiency in monocyte production.

MONOCYTOSIS AND HISTIOCYTOSIS

Monocytosis is often the manifestation of an inflammatory or a neoplastic disease (see Chap. 91). Certain hemopoietic tumors, especially acute and chronic monocytic leukemia, have as their principal manifestation a predominance of monocytic cells in blood and marrow. Occasionally, chronic monocytosis can precede the onset of acute myelogenous leukemia. Dendritic cell variants of acute myelogenous leukemia have also been discovered since immunophenotyping and genotyping of acute leukemias have become frequent.

Histiocytic lymphoma was so named because it was thought to be a tumor of malignant macrophages involving lymph nodes, based on microscopic examination of lymph node cell appearance. Now, as a result of immunophenotyping, it is recognized as a malignancy usually of large T or occasionally B lymphocytes (see Chap. 78). In very infrequent cases the tumors have a histiocytic (macrophagic) phenotype. These cases are referred to as malignant histiocytosis or histiocytic sarcoma (see Chap. 78). In some cases of monocytic leukemia, the malignant clone does not appear to include precursors of red cells and platelets and thus is not likely to be the result of a mutation in the stem cell. Progenitor cell monocytic leukemia and malignant histiocytosis support the concept that primitive monocyte cells, committed to the monocyte-macrophage lineage, can undergo malignant transformation.

Several uncommon types of histiocytoses are serious systemic diseases and may mimic malignant disease; however, the cytopathologic changes in monocytes or macrophages are not indicative of a malignant transformation and are presumably not clonal in origin. Familial and sporadic hemophagocytic lymphohistiocytosis, infection-induced hemophagocytic syndromes, and sinus histiocytosis with massive lymphadenopathy are among such disorders (see Chap. 78).

QUALITATIVE DISORDERS OF MONOCYTES

Inherited abnormalities of macrophages can result in ineffective function of these cells. In these situations the abnormality is usually shared by other cells, as in chronic granulomatous disease, which results from a defect in oxygen-dependent microbial killing, and in Chédiak-Higashi disease, which results from an abnormality of the membranes of cell granules (see Chap. 72). An indomethacin-sensitive monocyte killing defect in children has been associated with a predisposition to atypical mycobacterial disease (see Table 76-1). Also, enzyme deficiencies can result in accumulation of undegraded macromolecules in macrophages, leading to various types of storage diseases. A classic example is Gaucher disease, a disorder that results from deficiency of the enzyme glucocerebrosidase (see Chap. 79).

Acquired functional abnormalities of monocytes have been reported in a variety of diseases and circumstances (see Table 76-1, especially ''Monocyte and Macrophage Dysfunction''). For example, the output of prostaglandin E_2 is elevated and interleukin-2 synthesis is depressed in monocytes for several weeks after an individual suffers major trauma. Interferon-γ synthesis by mitogen-stimulated lymphocytes is depressed concomitantly. These changes may play a role in posttraumatic immunosuppression.

Monocyte dysfunction may also be acquired in patients with solid tumors. This dysfunction is correlated with decreased monocyte expression of HLA-DR antigens and lower than expected production of interleukin-1β and tumor necrosis factor-α.

CLINICAL MANIFESTATIONS OF MONOCYTE DISORDERS

MONOCYTOPENIA OR MONOCYTE DYSFUNCTION

Isolated monocytopenia does not occur. Thus, the manifestations of such a clinical state must be inferred. Neutrophils, endothelial cells,

TABLE 76-1   DISORDERS OF MONOCYTES AND MACROPHAGES

1. Monocytopenia (see Chap. 77)
   A. Aplastic anemia[1]
   B. Hairy cell leukemia[2,3]
   C. Glucocorticoid therapy[4]
2. Monocytosis (see Chap. 77)
   A. Benign
      (1) Reactive monocytosis[5]
   B. Clonal monocytosis
      Indolent
      (1) Chronic idiopathic monocytosis[6]
      (2) Oligoblastic leukemia (myelodysplasia)[7]
      Progressive
      (1) Acute monocytic leukemia[8]
      (2) Terminal deoxynucleotide transferase-positive acute monocytic leukemia[9]
      (3) Dendritic cell leukemia[10,11]
      (4) Progenitor cell monocytic leukemia[12]
      (5) Chronic myelomonocytic leukemia[13]
      (6) Chronic monocytic leukemia[14]
3. Macrophage Deficiency
   A. Osteopetrosis (isolated osteoclast deficiency)[15,16]
4. Inflammatory Histiocytosis (see Chap. 78)
   A. Primary hemophagocytic lymphohistiocytosis
      (1) Familial[17–19]
      (2) Sporadic[20]
   B. Infectious hemophagocytic histiocytosis[21,22]
   C. Tumor-associated hemophagocytic histiocytosis[23]
   D. Drug-associated hemophagocytic histiocytosis[23]
   E. Disease-associated hemophagocytic histiocytosis[24,25]
   F. Xanthogranuloma[26]
      (1) Juvenile
      (2) Adult
   G. Sinus histiocytosis with massive lymphadenopathy[27,28]
5. Storage Histiocytosis (see Chap. 79)
   A. Gaucher disease[29]
   B. Niemann-Pick disease[30]
   C. Gangliosidosis[31]
   D. Sea-blue histiocytosis syndrome[32]
   E. Erdheim-Chester disease[33]
   F. Other
6. Clonal (Neoplastic) Histiocytosis (see Chap. 78)
   A. Langerhans cell histiocytosis[34–36]
      (1) Localized
      (2) Systemic
   B. Malignant histiocytosis (histiocytic sarcoma)[37,38]
7. Monocyte and Macrophage Dysfunction[39–41]
   A. Alpha₁-proteinase inhibitor deficiency[42]
   B. Chédiak-Higashi syndrome[43]
   C. Chronic granulomatous disease[44]
   D. Disseminated mucocutaneous candidiasis[45,46]
   E. Glucocorticoid therapy[47]
   F. Kawasaki disease[48]
   G. Malakoplakia[49]
   H. Mycobacteriosis syndrome[50–53]
   I. Posttraumatic[54–56]
   J. Septic shock induced[57]
   K. Solid tumors[58,59]
   L. Tobacco smoking[60,61]
   M. Whipple's disease[62,63]
8. Thrombogenesis[64]

and other cell types can substitute in part for some monocyte functions. Monocytes have antibacterial, antiviral, antifungal, and antiparasitic capabilities. They are effective phagocytes that are involved in the ingestion of organisms such as mycobacteria, *Listeria, Brucella,* trypanosomes, and other granuloma-producing organisms. Thus, their deficiency or functional abnormality predisposes to such infections. Macrophages can serve as a reservoir for the human immunodeficiency virus and is the principal locus for the virus in brain and neural tissue.

Deficiency in a specific subset of macrophages, the osteoclasts,

results in *osteopetrosis*, an imbalance in bone metabolism that favors accretion; osteoclasts play a key role in bone resorption.

Macrophages process and present antigens and play a role in immune regulation. In complex systems, such as that of antibody production, abnormal macrophages might lead to faulty modulation of antibody synthetic rates. Activated monocytes secrete over 50 chemical mediators or monokines. The absence of monocytes from the inflammatory response and the failure to elaborate or the inappropriate elaboration of monokines such as IL-1, α_1-proteinase inhibitor, prostaglandins, leukotrienes, plasminogen activator, elastase, tumor necrosis factor, IL-6, IL-12, and others may cause or contribute to disease manifestations. A deficiency or impairment of monocytes has the potential of influencing several functions and systems because monocytes are such important sources of cytokines.

Monocytopenia and decreased monocyte entry into inflammatory sites occur after glucocorticoid administration. This may explain why patients treated with glucocorticoids are predisposed to infections in which monocytes play a protective role, such as those resulting from fungi, mycobacteria, and other opportunistic organisms. Dysfunctional monocytes, incapable of killing ingested microorganisms, are present in chronic granulomatous disease (see Chap. 72), as well as in hematopoietic stem cell diseases such as acute myelogenous leukemia.

MONOCYTOSIS

Benign monocytosis is not associated with specific clinical manifestations. All forms of myelogenous leukemia with a predominance of monocytes are associated with a predisposition to troublesome tissue infiltrates, especially in the skin, gingiva, lymph nodes, meninges, and anal canal. The higher the proportion of leukemic monocytes and the higher the monocyte count, the more prevalent is tissue infiltration. Release of procoagulants leading to intravascular coagulation also occurs in myelogenous leukemia with a high proportion of monocytes (see Chap. 93).

HISTIOCYTOSIS

This term usually refers to the accumulation of activated macrophages (histiocytes) in tissue sites. The cells may become cytophagocytic; ingestion of red cells and occasionally of leukocytes, platelets, erythroblasts in marrow or cells in other tissue sites is an important feature of certain inflammatory histiocytosis (see Chap. 78). Because morphology has been misleading, the diagnosis of histiocytosis requires identification of specific cell markers. Histiocytoses may be inflammatory (polyclonal) or neoplastic (clonal). Because tissue macrophages can take on highly specialized phenotypes and localize in different tissues, histiocytoses are further defined by whether they carry markers of these cell types (e.g., Langerhans cells, dendritic cells).

REFERENCES

1. Twomey JJ, Douglas CC, Sharkey O Jr: The monocytopenia of aplastic anemia. *Blood* 41:187, 1973.
2. Golomb HM, Catovsky D, Golde DW: Hairy cell leukemia: A clinical review based on 71 cases. *Ann Intern Med* 89:667, 1978.
3. Paoletti M, Bitter MA, Vardiman JW: Hairy cell leukemia: morphologic, cytochemical, and immunologic features. *Clin Lab Med* 8:179, 1988.
4. Fauci AS, Dale DC: The effect of in vivo hydrocortisone on subpopulations of human lymphocytes. *J Clin Invest* 53:240, 1974.
5. Maldonado GE, Hanlon DG: Monocytosis. *Mayo Clin Proc* 40:248, 1965.
6. Jaworkowsky LI, Solovey DY, Rhausova LY, Udris OY: Monocytosis as a sign of subsequent leukemia in patients with cytopenias (preleukemia). *Folia Hematol* 110:395, 1983.
7. Rigolin GM, Cuneo A, Roberti MG, et al: Myelodysplastic syndrome

with monocytic component: hematologic and cytologic characterization. *Haematologica* 82:25, 1997

8. Fung H, Shepherd JD, Naiman SC, et al: Acute monocytic leukemia. *Leuk Lymphoma* 19:259, 1995

9. Cuttner J, Seremetis S, Najfeld V, et al: TDT-positive acute leukemia with monocytoid characteristics. *Blood* 64:237, 1984.

10. Santiago-Schwartz F, Coppock DL, Hindenberg AA, Kern J: Identification of a malignant counterpart of the monocytic-dendritic cell progenitor in an acute myeloid leukemia. *Blood* 84:3054, 1994.

11. Srivastava HI, Srivistava A, Srivastava MD: Phenotype, genotype and cytokine production in acute leukemia involving progenitors of dendritic Langerhans' cell. *Leuk Res* 18:499, 1994.

12. Ferraris AM, Broccia G, Meloni T, et al: Clonal origin of cells restricted to monocytic differentiation in acute nonlymphocytic leukemia. *Blood* 64:817, 1984.

13. Cambier N, Baruchel A, Schlageter MH, et al: Chronic myelomonocytic leukemia: from biology to therapy. *Hematol Cell Ther* 39:41, 1997.

14. Bearman RM, Kjeldsberg CR, Pangalis GA, Rapoport H: Chronic monocytic leukemia in adults. *Cancer* 48:2239, 1981.

15. Teitelbaum SI: The osteoclast and osteopetrosis. *Mt Sinai J Med* 63:399, 1996.

16. Felix R, Hofstetter W, Cecchini MG: Recent developments in the understanding of the pathophysiology of osteopetrosis. *Eur J Endocrinol* 134:143, 1966.

17. Filipovich AH: Hemophagocytic lymphohistiocytosis. *J Pediatr* 130:337, 1997.

18. Jabado N, de Graeff-Meeder ER, Cavazzana-Calvo M, et al: Treatment of familial hemophagocytic lymphohistiocytosis with bone marrow transplantation from genetically nonidentical donors. *J Pediatr* 108:267, 1986.

19. Arico M, Janka G, Fischer A, et al, for the FHL Study Group of the Histiocyte Society: Hemophagocytic lymphohistiocytosis. Report of 122 children from the international registry. *Leukemia* 10:197, 1996.

20. Winkelmann RK, Bowie EJW: Hemorrhagic diathesis associated with benign histiocytic, cytophagic panniculitis and systemic histiocytosis. *Arch Intern Med* 140:1460, 1980.

21. Imashuku S: Differential diagnosis of hemophagocytic syndrome: underlying disorders and selection of the most effective treatment. *Int J Hematol* 66:135, 1997.

22. Tsuda H: Hemophagocytic syndrome (HPS) in children and adults. *Int J Hematol* 65:215, 1997.

23. Reiner AP, Spivak JL: Hematophagic histiocytosis. *Medicine* 67:369, 1988.

24. Stephan JL, Zeller J, Hubert P, et al: Macrophage activation syndrome and rheumatic diseases in childhood. *Clin Exp Rheumatol* 11:451, 1993.

25. Favara BE, Feller AC, Pauli M, et al: Contemporary classification of histiocytic disorders. *Med Pediatr Oncol* 29:157, 1997.

26. Zelger B, Cerio R, Orchard G, Wilson-Jones E: Juvenile and adult xanthogranuloma. A histological and immunohistological comparison. *Am J Surg Pathol* 18: 126, 1994.

27. Foucar E, Rosai J, Dorfman RF: Sinus histiocytosis with massive lymphadenopathy. *Cancer* 54:1834, 1984.

28. Pauli M, Bergamashi G, Tonon L, et al: Evidence of a polyclonal nature of the cell infiltrate in sinus histiocytosis with massive lymphadenopathy (Rosai-Dorfman disease). *Br J Haematol* 91:415, 1995.

29. Balicki D, Beutler E: Gaucher disease. *Medicine* 74:305, 1995.

30. Weisz B, Spirer Z, Reif S: Niemann-Pick disease: newer classification based on genetic mutation of the disease. *Adv Pediatr* 41:415, 1994

31. Lysosomal enzymes (Part 12), in *The Metabolic and Molecular Bases of Inherited Disease*, 6th ed, edited by CR Scriver, AL Beaudet, WS Sly, D Valle, pp 2427–2882. McGraw-Hill, New York, 1995.

32. Hirayama Y, Kohada K, Andoh M, et al: Syndrome of the sea-blue histiocyte. *Intern Med* 35:419, 1996.

33. Eble JN, Rosenberg AE, Young RH: Retroperitoneal xanthogranuloma in a patient with Erdheim-Chester disease. *Am J Surg Pathol* 18:843, 1994.

34. Leavey P, Varughese M, Breatnach F, O'Meara A: Langerhans cell histiocytosis—a 31 year review. *Ir J Med Sci* 160:271, 1991.

35. Willman CL, Busque L, Griffith BB, et al: Langerhans'-cell histiocytosis (histiocytosis X)—a clonal proliferative disease. *N Engl J Med* 331:154, 1994.

36. Egeler RM, Nesbit ME: Langerhans cell histiocytosis and other disorders of monocyte-histiocyte lineage. *Crit Rev Oncol Hematol* 18:9, 1995.

37. Wilson MS, Weiss LM, Gatter KC, et al: Malignant histiocytosis. *Cancer* 66:530, 1990.

38. Hsu S-M, Ho Y-S, Hsu P-L: Lymphoma of true histiocytic origin. *Am J Pathol* 138:1389, 1991.

39. Lopez-Berestein G, Klostergaard J (eds): *Mononuclear Phagocytes in Cell Biology*, pp 1–239. CRC Press, Boca Raton, FL, 1993.

40. Cline MJ: Histiocytes and histiocytosis. *Blood* 84:2840, 1994.

41. Asherson GL, Zembala M: Monocyte abnormalities in disease, in *Human Monocytes*, edited by M Zembala, GL Asherson, pp 395–415. Academic Press, London, 1989.

42. Perlmutter DH, Travis J, Punsal PI: Elastase regulates the synthesis of its inhibitor, alpha 1-proteinase inhibitor and exaggerates the defect in homozygous pizz alpha 1 PI deficiency. *J Clin Invest* 81:1774, 1998.

43. Dinauer MC: The phagocyte system and disorders of granulopoiesis and granulocyte function, in *Nathan and Oski's Hematology of Infancy and Childhood*, 5th ed, edited by DG Nathan and SH Orkin, pp 826–828. Saunders, Philadelphia, 1998.

44. Davis WC, Huber H, Douglas SD, Fudenberg HH: A defect in circulating mononuclear phagocytes in chronic granulomatous disease of childhood. *J Immunol* 101:1093, 1968.

45. Snyderman R, Altman LC, Frankel A, Blaese RM: Defective mononuclear leukocyte chemotaxis. *Ann Intern Med* 78:509, 1973.

46. Komiyama A, Ichikawa M, Kanda H, et al: Defective interleukin 1 production in a familial monocyte disorder with a combined abnormality of mobility and phagocytosis-killing. *Clin Exp Immunol* 73:500, 1988.

47. Rinehart JJ, Sagone AL, Balcerzak SP, et al: Effects of corticosteroid therapy on human monocyte function. *N Engl J Med* 292:236, 1975.

48. Furukawa S, Matsubara T, Jujok K, et al: Peripheral blood monocytes/macrophages and serum tumor necrosis factor in Kawasaki Disease. *Clin Immunol Immunopathol* 48:27, 1988.

49. Qualman SJ, Gupta PK, Mendelsohn G: Intracellular *Escherichia coli* in urinary malakoplakia, a reservoir of infection and its therapeutic implication. *Am J Clin Pathol* 81:35, 1984.

50. Uchiyama N, Green GR, Warren BJ, Morzumi PA, et al: Possible monocyte killing defect in familial mycobacteriosis. *J Pediatr* 98:785, 1981.

51. Mason UG III, Greenberg LE, Yen SS, Kirkpatrick CH: Indomethacin-responsive mononuclear cell dysfunction in "atypical" mycobacteriosis. *Cell Immunol* 71:54, 1982.

52. Ridgeway D, Wolff LJ, Wall M, Bouzy MS, et al: Indomethacin-sensitive monocyte killing defect in a child with disseminated atypical mycobacterial disease. *J Clin Immunol* 11:357, 1991.

53. Onwubalili JK: Defective monocyte chemotactic responsiveness in patients with active tuberculosis. *Immunol Lett* 16:39, 1987.

54. Farst E, Mewes A, Strasser T, Walz A, et al: Alteration of monocyte function following major injury. *Arch Surg* 123:287, 1988.

55. Miller-Graziano CL, Szabo G, Kodys K, Guffery K: Aberration in post-trauma monocyte (MO) subpopulation: Role in septic shock syndrome. *J Trauma* 30:586, 1990.

56. Farst E, Ertel W, Mewes A, et al: Mediators and the trauma induced cascade of immunologic defects. *Prog Clin Biol Res* 308:495, 1989.

57. Calandra T, Baumgartner J-D, Grau GE, et al: Prognostic value of tumor necrosis factor/cachectin, interleukin-1, interferon and interferon-8 in the serum of patients with septic shock. *J Infect Dis* 161:982, 1990.

58. Anastosopoulos E, Reclos GJ, Boxevanis CN, Gutzapis AD, et al: Monocyte disorders associated with T cell defects in patients with solid tumors. *Anticancer Res* 12:489, 1992.

59. Elgert KD, Alleva DG, Mullins DW: Tumor-induced immune dysfunction: the macrophage connection. *J Leukoc Biol* 64:275, 1998.

60. Green GM, Carolin D: The depressant effect of cigarette smoke on the in vitro antibacterial activity of alveolar macrophages. *N Engl J Med* 276:421, 1967.

61. Hubbard RC, Ogushi F, Fells GA, et al: Oxidants spontaneously released by alveolar macrophages of cigarette smokers can inactivate the active site of alpha 1-antitrypsin, rendering it ineffective as an inhibitor of neutrophil elastase. *J Clin Invest* 80:1289, 1988.

62. Silva MT, Macedo PM, Moura Nunes JF: Ultrastructure of bacilli and the bacillary origin of the macrophagic inclusions in Whipple's disease. *J Gen Microbiol* 131:1001, 1985.

63. Bjerknes R, Laerum OP, Degaards S: Impaired bacterial degradation of monocytes and macrophages from a patient with treated Whipple's disease. *Gastroenterology* 89:1139, 1985.

64. Spillent CR, Lazaro EJ: Contribution of the monocyte to thrombotic potential. *Agents Actions* 34:28, 1991.

MONOCYTOSIS AND MONOCYTOPENIA

MARSHALL A. LICHTMAN

The blood monocyte is in transit between the marrow and tissues, where it transforms into a macrophage. It participates in virtually all inflammatory and immune disorders, and thus its concentration may be increased in many such conditions, including autoimmune diseases, gastrointestinal disorders, sarcoidosis, and several viral and bacterial infections. Monocytosis may occur in some patients with cancer and several unrelated conditions, such as partuition, depression, and exogenous cytokine administration. The inconsistency and unpredictability in the monocyte response is a function of its relatively small blood pool size, the dampening effect of a large tissue pool, and the ability to expand macrophage numbers by local mitosis in tissues. The most striking increases in blood monocyte concentration occur with hematopoietic malignancies, especially monocytic or myelomonocytic leukemia. The reader is referred to Table 77-1 for a comprehensive list of causes of monocytosis. Monocytopenia is notable in patients with aplastic anemia or hairy-cell leukemia. Although other cytopenias accompany the monocytopenia, the latter is of particular functional importance and, often, in hairy-cell leukemia an aid to diagnosis.

The blood monocyte is a cell in transit from marrow to tissues.[1-3] There are two populations of blood monocytes: one is thought to represent a less mature stage, has a higher buoyant density, is smaller in volume, lacks Fc receptors, and has greater tumoricidal activity; the second is thought to represent a more mature stage, has a lower buoyant density, is larger in volume, displays Fc receptors, and has less tumoricidal activity.[3] Thus, this heterogeneity is analogous to that of the blood band and segmented neutrophil.[4] About 90 percent of blood monocytes strongly express CD14 (lipopolysacchride receptor) and do not express CD16 (Fcγ receptor III), while 10 percent of blood monocytes have weak expression of CD14 and strong expression of CD16.[5-7]

In tissues, the monocyte is capable of transformation, under the influence of local environmental factors, into a macrophage. The monocyte plays an important role in acute and chronic inflammatory reactions, including granulomatous inflammation; immunologic reactions, including those involved in delayed hypersensitivity; tissue repair and reorganization; atheroma formation; and the reaction to neoplasia and allografts. Because of the monocyte's key role in a variety of pathophysiologic reactions, a modest elevation in blood monocyte count can occur in many disparate conditions. In addition, in circumstances in which large increases in the number of macrophages are required in tissue sites, the demand may be met by local proliferation

Acronyms and abbreviations that appear in this chapter include: M-CSF, macrophage colony-stimulating factor.

of macrophages and not be reflected either in increased transit of monocytes through the blood compartment from marrow to tissue or in an increased concentration of blood monocytes.[8] Thus, unlike the case of neutrophils, increased tissue needs can be met locally. Occasionally, T-cell clones release only macrophage colony-stimulating factor (M-CSF), and their conditioned medium stimulates growth only of macrophage colonies, providing a hypothetical model for local control of macrophage proliferation.[9]

NORMAL BLOOD MONOCYTE CONCENTRATION

Monocytes constitute 1 to 9 percent of blood leukocytes.[10] In the first 2 weeks of life, the average absolute blood monocyte count is about $1000/\mu l$ $(1 \times 10^9/\text{liter})$.[10,11] There is a gradual decline in the normal monocyte count to a mean of $400/\mu l$ $(0.4 \times 10^9/\text{liter})$ in adulthood. Monocytosis is present when the absolute count exceeds $800/\mu l$ $(0.8 \times 10^9/\text{liter})$ in adults.[10,12] Men tend to have slightly higher monocyte counts than women.[12] Increments in the number of blood monocytes correlate directly with increases in the total blood monocyte pool and the monocyte turnover rate.[13] The blood monocyte count cycles with a periodicity of 5 days.[14]

DISORDERS ASSOCIATED WITH MONOCYTOSIS

Table 77-1 outlines the diseases reported to be associated with monocytosis. In one review, hematologic disorders represented more than 50 percent, collagen vascular diseases about 10 percent, and malignant disease about 8 percent of cases of monocytosis.[15]

HEMATOLOGIC DISORDERS

About one-quarter of patients with myelodysplastic states have an increase in the absolute monocyte count.[16-18] Occasionally, patients may have monocytic leukemoid reactions with the absolute monocyte count as high as $30,000/\mu l$ $(30 \times 10^9/\text{liter})$.[18,19] Chronic monocytosis may be the principal feature of a clonal hemopathy (preleukemic syndrome) and precede by years the development of acute leukemia.[20,21] The number of promonocytes and monocytes may be increased in patients with acute myelogenous leukemia of the myelomonocytic[17] or monocytic type.[21-23] Patients with chronic myelogenous leukemia may have an increased proportion of monocytes in the blood, and in variants of chronic myelogenous leukemia the monocytosis may be striking. Such cases have been classified as subacute or chronic myelomonocytic[25-31] or monocytic leukemia.[32] In some cases the monocytes are immature and have features of monoblasts or promonocytes, but in many cases they are indistinguishable by light microscopy from blood monocytes.

Monocytosis occurs in a number of neutropenic states: cyclic neutropenia,[33] chronic granulocytopenia of childhood,[34] familial benign chronic neutropenia,[35] infantile genetic agranulocytosis,[36,37] and chronic hypoplastic neutropenia.[38] Transient elevations of the monocyte count have been reported in the acute phases of drug-induced agranulocytosis.[39,40] Monocytosis characteristically appears later in the recovery phase of agranulocytosis.[41,42] Several reports[39,41,42] have indicated that a normal or increased number of monocytes is a harbinger of recovery from agranulocytosis, but a few studies found monocyte counts to be of no prognostic value.[35,43] Monocytosis has also been noted to precede agranulocytosis due to chlorpromazine use.[44] A rare form of agranulocytosis with an accompanying monocytosis has been described as leukopenic infectious monocytosis.[45]

Monocytosis can occur with lymphomas and can increase with exacerbation of disease activity.[46] Monocytosis has been noted in about 25 percent of cases of Hodgkin disease, although it does not correlate with prognosis.[47-49] Blood monocytosis is likely to occur in diseases

TABLE 77-1   DISORDERS ASSOCIATED WITH MONOCYTOSIS

Hematologic disorders	**Inflammatory and immune disorders**
Hemopoietic stem cell disorders	Collagen diseases
Preleukemia[17–22]	Rheumatoid arthritis[58]
Acute myelogenous leukemia	Systemic lupus erythematosus[53,59]
Monocytic type[21–23]	Temporal arteritis[15]
Myelomonocytic type[25]	Myositis[15]
Chronic myelogenous leukemia	Polyarteritis nodosa[15]
Myelomonocytic type[26–31]	Gastrointestinal disorders
Monocytic type[32]	Alcoholic liver disease[92]
Polycythemia vera[15]	Ulcerative colitis[83]
Lymphocytic tumors	Regional enteritis[83]
Chronic lymphocytic leukemia[107]	Sprue[15]
Lymphoma[46,47,57]	Sarcoidosis[84,85]
Hodgkin disease[48,49]	Infections
Macroglobulinemia[56]	Cytomegalovirus infection[81]
Multiple myeloma[54,55]	Varicella zoster virus[82]
Histiocytosis[50]	Subacute bacterial endocarditis[66–67]
Hemolytic anemia[15]	Syphilis[79,80]
Idiopathic thrombocytopenic	Nonhemopoietic malignancies[86,87]
purpura[15]	
Tuberculosis[62–64]	**Miscellaneous conditions**
Chronic neutropenias	Tetrachlorethane poisoning[93]
Familial benign[35]	Langerhan's cell histiocytosis[94]
Cyclic[33]	Glucocorticoid administration[99,100]
Infantile genetic[36,37]	Parturition[97,98]
Hypoplastic[38–44]	Drug related[39–41]
Postsplenectomy state[51–53]	Depression[102,103]
	Exogenous cytokine adminis-
	tration[88–91]
	Myocardial infarction[118]

associated with histiocytic proliferation, such as the rare cases of true malignant histiocytosis.[50] Monocytosis may also occur in individuals who have had splenectomy.[51–53] A statistically significant increase in blood monocyte concentration has been reported in multiple myeloma[54,55] and has been correlated with the presence of γ light chains–containing monoclonal antibody.[55] Rarely, cases of M-CSF–secreting lymphoid tumors have been associated with monocytosis.[56,57]

INFLAMMATORY AND IMMUNE DISORDERS

Collagen vascular disease, including rheumatoid arthritis,[58] systemic lupus erythematosus, temporal arteritis, myositis, and periarteritis nodosa, may be associated with monocytosis, although monocytosis is not common in these diseases. The usual alterations of the white cell count of systemic lupus erythematosus, for example, are neutropenia and lymphopenia,[59] but 10 percent of patients have a mild monocytosis.[60]

Infectious disease is an uncommon cause of monocytosis. Only a few instances of infection were noted in a comprehensive review of causes of monocytosis, including tonsillitis, dental infection, recurrent liver abscesses, candidiasis, and one instance of tuberculous peritonitis.[15] Tuberculosis was once a leading cause of monocytosis, because of the role of monocytes in granuloma (tubercle) formation,[61] and monocytic leukemoid reactions have been reported in the disease.[62] Neither the monocyte count nor the ratio of monocytes to lymphocytes correlates with the stage or activity of tuberculosis.[63,64]

Monocytosis is found in 15 to 20 percent of patients with subacute bacterial endocarditis[65,66] but is not correlated with the presence of blood macrophages, which may be present in this disease.[67] Rarely, in acute bacterial infections, blood monocytes can

exceed 20,000/μl (20 × 10⁹/liter), and an increase in monocytes and monocyte precursors in the marrow can mimic acute monocytic leukemia.[68]

A number of infections formerly thought to be associated with monocytosis have been found not to be, when examined systematically. These include rickettsial diseases,[69–72] brucellosis,[73] leishmaniasis,[74] typhoid fever,[75] malaria,[76] and disseminated candidiasis.[77]

A monocytosis in the resolution phase of acute infections has been noted,[78] and monocytosis appears in neonatal, primary, and secondary syphilis.[79] Occasionally, cases of neonatal syphilis have been associated with monocytic leukemoid reactions.[80] Certain viruses, especially cytomegalovirus and varicella zoster virus, induce an increase in blood monocytes.[81,82]

Sprue, ulcerative colitis, and regional enteritis have been associated with monocytosis.[15,83] Elevation of the blood monocyte count occurs in sarcoidosis[84] and is inversely related to a reduction in circulating T lymphocytes.[85] A similar correlation has also been noted in patients with malignant disease.[86]

NONHEMATOPOIETIC MALIGNANCIES

Sixty percent of patients with nonhematologic malignancy exhibit a monocytosis that is independent of the presence or absence of metastatic disease.[87] Thus, unexplained monocytosis should raise the possibility of a malignancy.

EXOGENOUS CYTOKINE ADMINISTRATION

The administration of granulocyte-macrophage colony-stimulating factor[88] or interleukin-10[89] may result in mild increases in blood monocyte counts. Administration of M-CSF[89–91] results in an invariable increase in blood monocyte counts. At doses of 40 to 120 μg/kg/day, the peak increase, which may reach three-to fourfold baseline, is reached at about 8 days.

MISCELLANEOUS CONDITIONS

Other disorders associated with monocytosis include alcoholic liver disease,[92] tetrachloroethane poisoning,[93] and Langerhans cell histiocytosis.[94] Increased monocyte counts do not occur in Niemann-Pick disease[95] or Gaucher disease.[96] Monocytosis is a frequent finding at the time of parturition.[97,98] An increase in blood monocytes occurs in healthy volunteers[99,100] or, rarely, in preleukemic patients[101] given moderately high, therapeutic-level doses of glucocorticoids. Psychiatric depression is associated with a conjoint increase in neutrophils and monocytes.[102,103]

Spurious elevations of the blood monocyte count can occur when blood is obtained from the fingertips of patients who have peripheral vascular disease, such as Raynaud syndrome.[104]

DISORDERS ASSOCIATED WITH MONOCYTOPENIA

Although monocytopenia may occur in any hematopoietic stem cell disease associated with pancytopenia (e.g., myelogenous leukemia), a decrease in monocytes is notable and constant in aplastic anemia as part of the global decrease in production of blood cells.[105] It is also a constant and important feature of hairy-cell leukemia, in which monocytopenia can be a helpful diagnostic clue and also a contributor to the predisposition to infection, which is an important morbid feature of the disease.[106] Monocytopenia occurs in a small proportion of patients with chronic lymphocytic leukemia, and these patients may have a higher frequency of infections, especially by viruses.[107] Cyclic neutropenia is also notable for intermittent periods of monocytopenia. Severe thermal injuries also can result in monocytopenia.[108] Rare cases of conjoint severe neutropenia and monocytopenia occur.[109,110]

Automated blood cell counts in large numbers of subjects have demonstrated that decreased absolute monocyte counts are frequent in patients with rheumatoid arthritis,[111] systemic lupus erythematosus,[112] and human immunodeficiency virus infection.[113]

Glucocorticoid hormones produce a monocytopenia transiently about 6 h after administration to human volunteers[114] or to patients.[99,115] Administration of interferon α and tumor necrosis factor α may also cause monocytopenia.[116] Monocytopenia may follow radiotherapy.[117]

REFERENCES

1. Zembala M, Asherson GL: *Human Monocytes.* Academic Press, London, 1989.
2. Metcalf D: Control of granulocytes and macrophages: Molecular, cellular and clinical aspects. *Science* 254:529, 1991.
3. Turpin JA, Lopez-Berestein G: Differentiation, maturation, and activation of monocytes and macrophages: Functional activity is controlled by a continuum of activation, in *Mononuclear Phagocytes in Cell Biology*, edited by G. Lopez-Berestein, J Klostergaard, p 71. CRC Press, Boca Raton, FL, 1993.
4. Andreesen R, Bross KJ, Osterhok J, Emmrich F: Human macrophage maturation and heterogeneity: Analysis with a newly generated set of monoclonal antibodies to differentiation antigens. *Blood* 67:1257, 1986.
5. Passlick B, Flieger D, Ziegler-Hertbrock L: Identification and characterization of a novel monocyte subpopulation in human peripheral blood. *Blood* 74:2527, 1989.
6. Zeigler-Heitbrock HWL, Strobel M, Fingerlo G, et al: Small (CD14+/CD16+) monocytes and regular monocytes in human blood. *Pathology* 59:127, 1991.
7. Zeigler-Heitbrock HW: Heterogeneity of human blood monocytes: The CD14+ CD16+ subpopulation. *Immunol Today* 17:424, 1996.
8. Meuret G, Detel U, Kilz HP, et al: Human monocytopoiesis in acute and chronic inflammation. *Acta Haematol* 54:328, 1975.
9. Griffin JD, Meuer SC, Schlossman SF, Reinherz EL: T-cell regulation of myelopoiesis: Analysis at a clonal level. *J Immunol* 133:1863, 1984.
10. Miale JB: Leukocytes, in *Laboratory Medicine Hematology*, p 658. Mosby, St. Louis, 1982.
11. Nathan DG, Orkin SH: Appendix 28, in *Hematology of Infancy and Childhood*, 5th ed, edited by DG Nathan, SH Orkin, p xv. Saunders, Philadelphia, 1998.
12. Munan L, Kelly A: Age-dependent changes in blood monocyte 2 populations in man. *Lin Exp Immunol* 35:161, 1979.
13. Meuret G, Hoffman G: Monocyte kinetic studies in normal and disease states. *Br J Haematol* 24:275, 1973.
14. Meuret G, Bremer C, Bammert J, Ewen J: Oscillation of blood monocyte counts in healthy individuals. *Cell Tissue Kinet* 7:223, 1974.
15. Maldonado JE, Hanlon DG: Monocytosis: A current appraisal. *Mayo Clin Proc* 40:248, 1965.
16. Rigolin GM, Cuneo A, Roberti MG, et al: Myelodysplastic syndromes with monocytic component: Hematologic and cytogenetic characterization. *Haematologia* 82:25, 1997.
17. Economopoulus T, Stathakis N, Marasayannis Z, et al: Myelodysplastic syndrome: Clinical and prognostic significance of the monocyte count, degree of blastic infiltration and ring sideroblasts. *Acta Haematol* 65:97, 1981.
18. Cunningham I, MacCallum SJ, Nicholls MD, et al: The myelodysplastic syndromes: An analysis of prognostic factors in 226 cases from a single institution. *Br J Haematol* 90:602, 1995.
19. Weitberg AB: A monocytic leukemoid reaction in a patient with myelodysplasia. *CA* 35:308, 1985.
20. Pretlow TG II: Chronic monocytic dyscrasia culminating in acute leukemia. *Am J Med* 46:130, 1969.
21. Jaworkowsky LI, Solovey DY, Rhausova LY, Udris OY: Monocytosis as a sign of subsequent leukemia in patients with cytopenias (preleukemia). *Folia Hematol* 110:395, 1983.
22. Janvier M, Tobelem G, Daniel MT et al: Acute monoblastic leukaemia:

Clinical, biological data and survival in 45 cases. *Scand J Haematol* 32:385, 1984.
23. Scott CS, Stark AN, Limbert HJ, et al: Diagnostic and prognostic factors in acute monocytic leukaemia. *Br J Haematol* 69:247, 1988.
24. Odom LF, Lampkin BC, Tannous R, et al: Acute monoblastic leukemia. *Leuk Res* 14:1, 1990.
25. Sexauer J, Kass L, Schnitzer B: Subacute myelomonocytic leukemia. *Am J Med* 57:853, 1974.
26. Storniolo AM, Moloney WC, Rosenthal DS, et al: Chronic myelomonocytic leukemia. *Leukemia* 4:766, 1990.
27. Kantarjiam HM, Keating MJ, Walters RS, et al: Clinical and prognostic features of Philadelphia chromosome-negative chronic myelogenous leukemia. *Cancer* 58:2023, 1986.
28. Heyll A, Derigs G: Chronic myelomonocytic leukemia: Clerical data, morphological features and outcome in 56 patients. *Hematol Blood Transfus* 33:387, 1990.
29. Group Francais de Cytogénétique Hematologique: Chronic myelomonocytic leukemia: Single entity or heterogeneous disorder? *Cancer Genet Cytogenet* 55:57, 1991.
30. Owen G, Lewis IJ, Morgan M, et al: Prognostic factors in juvenile chronic granulocytic leukaemia. *Br J Cancer* 66(suppl XVIII):568, 1992.
31. Emanuel PD, Bates LJ, Zhu S-W, et al: The role of monocyte-derived hemopoietic growth factors in the regulation of myeloproliferation in juvenile chronic myelogenous leukemia. *Exp Hematol* 19:1017, 1991.
32. Bearman RM, Kjeldsberg CR, Pangalis GA, Rappaport H: Chronic monocytic leukemia in adults. *Cancer* 48:2239, 1981.
33. Wright D, Dale DC, Fauci AS, Wolff SM: Human cyclic neutropenia: Clinical review and long-term follow-up of patients. *Medicine* 60:1, 1981.
34. Zuelzer WW, Bajoghli M: Chronic granulocytopenia in childhood. *Blood* 23:359, 1964.
35. Cutting HO, Lang JE: Familial benign chronic neutropenia. *Ann Intern Med* 61:876, 1964.
36. Krill CE, Mauer AM: Congenital agranulocytosis. *J Pediatr* 68:361, 1966.
37. Lang JE, Cutting HO: Infantile genetic agranulocytosis. *Pediatrics* 35:596, 1965.
38. Spaet TH, Dameshek W: Chronic hypoplastic neutropenia. *Am J Med* 13:35, 1952.
39. Cassileth PA: Monocytosis in chlorpromazine-associated agranulocytosis: Termination in acute leukemia. *Am J Med* 43:471, 1967.
40. Graf M, Tarlov A: Agranulocytosis with monohistiocytosis associated with ampicillin therapy. *Ann Intern Med* 69:91, 1968.
41. Reznikoff P: The etiologic importance of fatigue and the prognostic significance of monocytosis in neutropenia (agranulocytosis). *Am J Clin Pathol* 6:205, 1936.
42. Rosenthal N, Abel HA: The significance of the monocytes in agranulocytosis (leukopenic infectious agranulocytosis). *Am J Clin Pathol* 6:205, 1936.
43. Pretty HM, Gosselin G, Colprian G, Long LA: Agranulocytosis: A report of 30 cases. *Can Med Assoc J* 93:1058, 1965.
44. Lutz EG: Monocytosis, blood dyscrasia and chlorpromazine toxicity. *Int J Neuropsychiatry* 1:76, 1965.
45. Stone GE, Redmond AJ: Leukopenic infectious monocytosis: Report of a case closely simulating acute monocytic leukemia. *Am J Med* 34:541, 1963.
46. Hurst DW, Meyer OO: Giant follicular lymphoblastoma. *Cancer* 14:753, 1961.
47. Wiseman BK: The blood pictures in the primary diseases of the lymphatic system: Their character and significance. *JAMA* 107:2016, 1936.
48. Levinson G, Walter BA, Wintrobe MM, et al: A clinical study of Hodgkin's disease. *Arch Intern Med* 99:519, 1957.
49. Ultmann JE: Clinical features and diagnosis of Hodgkin's disease. *Cancer* 9:297, 1966.
50. Hsu S-M, Ho Y-S, Hsu P-L: Lymphomas of true histiocytic origin. *Am J Pathol* 138:1389, 1991.
51. McBride JA, Dacie JV, Shapley R: The effect of splenectomy on the leucocyte count. *Br J Haematol* 14:225, 1968.
52. Durig M, Landmann RMA, Harder F: Lymphocyte subsets in human peripheral blood after splenectomy and autotransplantation of splenic tissue. *J Lab Clin Med* 104:110, 1984.
53. Lanng Nielson J, Romer FK, Ellegaard J: Serum angiotensin-converting

enzyme and blood monocytes in splenectomized individuals. *Acta Haematol* 67:132, 1982.

54. Sewell RL: Lymphocyte abnormalities in myeloma. *Br J Haematol* 36:545, 1977.

55. Blom J, Nielsen H, Larsen SO, et al: A study of certain functional parameters of monocytes from patients with multiple myeloma: Comparison with monocytes from healthy individuals. *Scand J Haematol* 33:425, 1984.

56. Nakajima H, Mori S, Takeuchi T, et al: Monocytosis and high serum macrophage colony-stimulating factor in Waldenström's macroglobulinemia. *Blood* 86:2863, 1995.

57. Tokioka T, Shimamoto Y, Motoyoshi K, Yamaguchi M: Clinical significance of monocytosis and human monocytic colony-stimulating factor in patients with adult T-cell leukaemia/lymphoma. *Haematologia* 26:1, 1994.

58. Buchan GS, Palmer DG, Gibbins BL: The response of human peripheral blood mononuclear phagocytes to rheumatoid arthritis. *J Leukocyte Biol* 37:221, 1985.

59. Budman DR, Steinberg AD: Hematologic aspects of systemic lupus erythematosus: Current concepts. *Ann Intern Med* 86:220, 1977.

60. Michael SR, Vural IL, Bassen FA, et al: The hematologic aspects of disseminated (systemic) lupus erythematosus. *Blood* 6:1059, 1951.

61. Groopman JE, Golde DW: The histiocytic disorders: A pathophysiologic analysis. *Ann Intern Med* 94:95, 1981.

62. Gibson A: Monocytic leukemoid reaction associated with tuberculosis and a mediastinal teratoma. *J Pathol Bacteriol* 58:469, 1946.

63. Flinn JW: A study of the differential blood count in 1000 cases of active pulmonary tuberculosis. *Ann Intern Med* 2:622, 1929.

64. Stobie W, England NJ, McMenemy WH: The interpretation of haemograms in pulmonary tuberculosis. *Am Rev Tuberc* 46:1, 1942.

65. Daland GA, Gottlieb L, Wallerstein RO, et al: Hematologic observations in bacterial endocarditis. *J Lab Clin Med* 48:827, 1956.

66. Hill RW, Bayrd ED: Phagocytic reticuloendothelial cells in subacute bacterial endocarditis with negative cultures. *Ann Intern Med* 52:310, 1960.

67. Dameshek W: The appearance of histiocytes in the peripheral blood. *Arch Intern Med* 47:968, 1931.

68. Myhre EB, Braconier JH, Sjögren U: Automated cytochemical differential leukocyte count in patients hospitalized with acute bacterial infections. *Scand J Infect Dis* 17:201, 1985.

69. Horsfall FL Jr, Tamm I: *Viral and Rickettsial Diseases of Man*, 4th ed. Lippincott, Philadelphia, 1965.

70. Harrel GT, Aikawa JK, Kelsey WM: Rocky Mountain spotted fever. *Am Pract* 1:425, 1947.

71. Morgan HR, Neva FA, Fahey RJ, et al: Brill's disease: Report of two serologically proved cases of typhus fever in Irish-born residents of Boston. *N Engl J Med* 238:87, 1948.

72. Murray ES, Baehr G, Shwartzman G, et al: Brill's disease: I. Clinical and laboratory diagnosis. *JAMA* 142:1059, 1950.

73. Spink WW: *The Nature of Brucellosis*. University of Minnesota Press, Minneapolis, 1956.

74. Cartwright GE, Chung HL, Chang A: Studies on the pancytopenia of kalazar. *Blood* 3:249, 1948.

75. Dubos RJ, Hirsch JC: *Bacterial and Mycotic Infections*, 4th ed. Lippincott, Philadelphia, 1965.

76. Vryonis G: Blood studies in malaria. *Am J Med Sci* 200:809, 1940.

77. Louria DB, Stiff DP, Bennett B: Disseminated moniliasis in the adult. *Medicine* 41:307, 1962.

78. Hickling RA: The monocytes in pneumonia: A clinical and hematologic study. *Arch Intern Med* 40:594, 1927.

79. Rosahn PD, Pearce L: The blood cytology in untreated and treated syphilis. *Am J Med Sci* 187:88, 1934.

80. Karyalcin G, Khanijou A, Kim KY, et al: Monocytosis in congenital syphilis. *Am J Dis Child* 131:782, 1977.

81. Klemola E: Cytomegalovirus infection in previously healthy adults. *Ann Intern Med* 79:267, 1973.

82. Tsukahara T, Yogushi A, Horiuchi Y: Significance of monocytosis in varicella herpes zoster. *J Dermatol* 19:94, 1992.

83. Mees AS, Berney J, Jewell DP: Monocytes in inflammatory bowel disease: Absolute monocyte counts. *J Clin Pathol* 33:917, 1980.

84. Goodwin JS, DeHaratius R, Israel H, et al: Suppressor cell function in sarcoidosis. *Ann Intern Med* 90:169, 1979.

85. Daniele RP, Dauber JH, Rossman MD: Immunologic abnormalities in sarcoidosis. *Ann Intern Med* 92:406, 1980.

86. Wood GW, Neff JE, Stephens R: Relationship between monocytosis and T-lymphocyte function in human cancer. *J Natl Cancer Inst* 63:587, 1979.

87. Barrett O'N Jr: Monocytosis in malignant disease. *Ann Intern Med* 73:991, 1970.

88. Schmitz LL, McClure JS, Litz CE, et al: Morphologic and quantitative changes in blood and marrow cells following growth factor therapy. *Am J Clin Pathol* 101:67, 1994.

89. Chernoff AE, Granowitz EV, Shapiro L, et al: A randomized controlled trial of IL-10 in humans. *J Immunol* 154:5492, 1995.

90. Weiner LM, Li W, Holmes M, et al: Phase I trial of recombinant macrophage colony-stimulating factor and recombinant gamma-interferon: Toxicity, monocytosis, and clinical effects. *Cancer Res* 54:4084, 1994.

91. Minasian LM, Yao TJ, Steffens TA, et al: A phase I study of anti-GD3 ganglioside monoclonal antibody R24 and recombinant human macrophage colony-stimulating factor in patients with metastatic melanoma. *Cancer* 75:2251, 1995.

92. McKeever UM, O'Mahoney C, Lawlor E, et al: Monocytosis: A feature of alcoholic liver disease. *Lancet* 2:1492, 1983.

93. Minot GR, Smith LW: The blood in tetrachlorethane poisoning. *Arch Intern Med* 28:687, 1921.

94. Avioli LV, Lasersohn JT, Lopresti JM: Histiocytosis X (Schüller-Christian disease): A clinico-pathological survey, review of ten patients and the results of prednisone therapy. *Medicine* 42:119, 1963.

95. Crocker AC, Farber S: Niemann-Pick disease: A review of eighteen patients. *Medicine* 37:1, 1958.

96. Reich C, Seife M, Kessler BJ: Gaucher's disease: A review and discussion of twenty cases. *Medicine* 30:1, 1951.

97. Siegal I, Gleichner N: Peripheral white blood cells alterations in early labor. *Diagn Gynecol Obstet* 3:123, 1981.

98. Buchan GS, Gibbins BL, Griffin JFT: The influence of parturition on peripheral blood mononuclear phagocyte subpopulation in pregnant women. *J Leuk Biol* 37:231, 1985.

99. Rinehard JJ, Sagone AL, Balcerzak SP, et al: Effects of corticosteroid therapy on human monocyte function. *N Engl J Med* 292:236, 1975.

100. Shoenfeld Y, Gurewich Y, Gallant LA, et al: Prednisone-induced leukocytosis. *Am J Med* 71:773, 1981.

101. Morales M, Wilkes J, Lowder JN: Monocytic leukemoid reaction, glucocorticoid therapy, and myelodysplastic syndrome. *Cleveland Clin J Med* 6:571, 1990.

102. Maes M, Van Der Planken M, Stevens WJ, Peeters D, et al: Leukocytosis, monocytosis and neutrophilia: Hallmarks of severe depression. *J Psychiatr Res* 26:125, 1992.

103. Maes M, Lambrechts J, Suy E, et al: Absolute number and percentage of circulating natural killer, non-MHC-restricted T cytotoxic, and phagocytic cells in unipolar depression. *Neuropsychobiology* 29:157, 1994.

104. Czazkes JW, Dreyfuss F: Discrepancy of fingertip and ear lobe leukocyte counts in Raynaud's disease. *Am J Med Sci* 234:325, 1957.

105. Twormey JJ, Douglas CC, Sharkey O Jr: The monocytopenia of aplastic anemia. *Blood* 41:187, 1973.

106. Den Ottolander GJ, Van Der Burgh FJ, Lopes Cardozo P, et al: The Hemalog D automated differential counter in the diagnosis of hairy cell leukemia. *Leuk Res* 7:309, 1983.

107. DeRossi G, Mauro FR, Ialongo P, et al: Monocytopenia and infections in chronic lymphocytic leukemia (CLL). *Eur J Haematol* 46:119, 1991.

108. Peterson V, Hensbrough J, Buerk C, et al: Regulation of granulopoiesis following severe thermal injury. *J Trauma* 23:19, 1983.

109. Adams WH, Liu YK: Periodic neutropenia and monocytopenia. *Am J Hematol* 13:73, 1982.

110. Marinone G, Roncoli B, Marinone MG Jr: Pure white cell aplasia. *Semin Hematol* 28:298, 1991.

111. Isenberg DA, Martin P, Hajirousou V, et al: Haematological reassessment of rheumatoid arthritis using an automated method. *Br J Rheumatol* 25:152, 1986.

112. Isenberg DA, Patterson KG, Todd-Pokropek A, et al: Haematological aspects of systemic lupus erythematosus: A reappraisal using automated methods. *Acta Haematol* 67:242, 1982.

113. Treacy M, Lai L, Costello C, et al: Peripheral blood and bone marrow abnormalities in patients with HIV related disease. *Br J Haematol* 65:289, 1987.

114. Steer JH, Vuong Q, Joyce DA: Suppression of human monocyte tumor necrosis factor-alpha release by glucocorticoid therapy: Relationship to systemic monocytopaenia and cortisol suppression. *Br J Clin Pharmacol* 43:383, 1997.

115. Fauci AS, Dale DC: Monocytopenia after prednisone. *N Engl J Med* 292:928, 1975.

116. Aulitzky WE, Tilg H, Vogel W, Aulitz W, et al: Acute hematologic effects of interferon alpha, interferon gamma, tumor necrosis factor alpha and interleukin 2. *Ann Hematol* 62:25, 1991.

117. Rotman M, Ansley H, Rogow L, et al: Monocytosis: A new observation during radiotherapy. *Int J Radiat Oncol Biol Phys* 2:117, 1977.

118. Meisel SR, Pauzner H, Shechter M, Zeidan Z, David D: Peripheral monocytosis following myocardial infarction. *Cardiology* 90:52, 1998.

INFLAMMATORY AND MALIGNANT HISTIOCYTOSIS

MARSHALL A. LICHTMAN
CAMILLE N. ABBOUD

Clinical disorders that are the consequence of a primary proliferation of histiocytes (macrophages) may result from a metabolic, inflammatory, or neoplastic pathogenetic mechanism. This chapter deals with the latter two and Chap. 79 with the former.

Three principal inflammatory disorders of macrophages affect the marrow or lymph nodes and are relevant to hematologists. The first is familial hemophagocytic histiocytosis, usually a disease of infancy; about two-thirds of cases occur in siblings. Fever, anorexia, hepatosplenomegaly, and lymphadenopathy are common. Jaundice and ascites may develop. Anemia and thrombocytopenia are frequent, and a marrow or splenic aspirate will show macrophages phagocytizing blood cells or precursors. Stem cell transplantation is the most successful form of treatment. The second disorder is infectious hemophagocytic histiocytosis, an infrequent but severe and dramatic reaction to a viral, bacterial, fungal, or protozoal infection. Fever, myalgias, lethargy, and hepatosplenomegaly are often present. Bi- or pancytopenia is common. Activated macrophages ingesting blood cells or precursors are abundant in the marrow specimen. The disorder produces a severe systemic illness but may resolve in weeks if the underlying infection is treated successfully or resolves. The third relevant disorder is sinus histiocytosis with massive lymphadenopathy, which usually manifests itself by massive, painless cervical lymph node enlargement. Other nodes or extranodal sites are involved in many patients. Biopsy of an involved area will show engorgement of sinuses or tissue by activated, phagocytic macrophages. The disease is usually self-limited and regresses spontaneously in several months. Progressive disease can be treated with glucocorticoids or chemotherapy.

Clonal histiocytic disorders include Langerhans' cell histiocytosis and malignant histiocytosis. Langerhans' cell histiocytosis can be localized to skin, bone, or other sites or be widespread, involving almost any organ. In the latter form, diabetes insipidus is common. The diagnosis requires localization of S-100 protein and CD 1a on the histiocytic cells in the infiltrate and identification of Langerhans' cell (Birbeck) granules by electron microscopy. In the localized form, excisional biopsy, observation, or local treatment may suffice. In the progressive or disseminated form, multidrug chemotherapy or stem cell transplantation may be required. Malignant histiocytosis is an uncommon tumor that had been over-diagnosed before stringent criteria, including absence of evidence for immunoglobulin or T-lymphocyte receptor–chain gene rearrangement, were required to eliminate masquerading lymphoma. The disease is usually disseminated, involving marrow, lymph nodes, liver, and spleen, and requires multidrug chemotherapy.

Diseases associated with the proliferation of histiocytes can be grouped into three categories: inflammatory disorders, neoplastic (clonal) disorders, and storage diseases (Table 78-1). The storage diseases are described in Chap. 79. This chapter describes disorders that may be evaluated by hematologists. The large number of histiocytoses that affect principally the skin are not discussed.[1]

The terms *macrophage* and *histiocyte* have been synonyms. The former designation is favored for discussions of the cell biology and pathophysiology of the mature cell found in tissues in the monocyte-macrophage system. In the medical literature, the terms *histiocyte* and *histiocytosis* are used to describe histopathological lesions of macrophage disorders. Macrophages can subsume varied and highly distinctive phenotypes, and these specialized cells localize to specific tissues (e.g., Langerhans' cells of the skin, dendritic cells of the lymph node, etc.: see Chaps. 73–75). Histiocytic diseases may reflect these distinctions, making specific diagnosis complex, requiring careful assessment of cell phenotype and genotype. More recently, it has been suggested that the term *histiocyte* be used as a designation to encompass macrophages that process antigen and dendritic cells that present antigen, focusing solely on the role of these cells in the immune system.[2] Such a proposal may be difficult to implement, given the extensive and long-standing more general use of the term.

Considerable confusion existed in the classification of disorders of histiocytes when morphologic characterization of pathological specimens using light microscopy was the principal basis for diagnosis. The use of electron microscopy to identify the specific granules in Langerhans' cells (Birbeck bodies) (Fig. 78-1) and the development of a series of antibodies and immunocytochemical techniques that recognize cluster of differentiation (CD) sites present on monocytes or macrophages or their intracellular features has helped substantially in the classification and diagnosis of these diseases. These tools, coupled with molecular genetic studies of T and B lymphocyte gene rearrangements to exclude diseases of lymphocytes that are phenocopies of histiocytic disorders, have lead to improvement in diagnostic accuracy. In addition, refined phenotyping has permitted discernment of disorders of dendritic histiocytes, for example, Langerhans' cell histiocytosis, and macrophages involved in the secondary hemophagocytic syndromes.

INFLAMMATORY DISORDERS OF HISTIOCYTES

FAMILIAL AND SPORADIC HEMOPHAGOCYTIC HISTIOCYTOSIS

DEFINITION AND HISTORY

Familial hemophagocytic histiocytosis was first described in 1952 and also has been referred to as familial reticulosis and familial erythrophagocytic lymphohistiocytosis. The disease affects neonates and infants, and 90 percent of patients are symptomatic by 2 years of age. The annual incidence in Sweden is about 1 per million children, or 1 per 50,000 births.[3] Males and females are equally affected. Over two-thirds of cases occur in siblings.[4-6] Parents of patients are consanguineous in about one-quarter of cases, suggesting autosomal recessive inheritance. The disease, if untreated, is usually lethal.

CLINICAL FINDINGS

The most prevalent signs in infants are fever, anorexia, vomiting, and irritability. Hepatic or splenic enlargement is present in virtually every

Acronyms and abbreviations that appear in this chapter include: CD, cluster of differentiation; GM-CSF, granulocyte-monocyte colony-stimulating factor; HLA, human leukocyte antigens; IL, interleukin; M-CSF, monocyte colony-stimulating factor; TGF-β, transforming growth factor β; TNF-α, tumor necrosis factor α.

TABLE 78-1   HISTIOCYTIC DISORDERS

Hemophagocytic histiocytosis
• Familial hemophagocytic histiocytosis
• Infectious hemophagocytic histiocytosis (e.g., viral, bacterial, fungal, protozoal)
• Tumor-associated hemophagocytic histiocytosis (e.g., lymphoma, carcinoma)
• Drug-associated hemophagocytic histiocytosis (e.g., phenytoin)
Sinus histiocytosis with massive lymphadenopathy (Rosai-Dorfman disease)
Clonal histiocytosis
• Langerhans' cell histiocytosis
• Malignant histiocytosis (histiocytic sarcoma)
Storage diseases (see Chap. 79)

NOTE: The disorders listed are those most likely to be related to hematology as a diagnostic and therapeutic discipline. Histiocytic disorders that do not usually involve lymph nodes, blood, or marrow are not considered.

case. As the condition progresses, lymphadenopathy, jaundice, ascites, and edema can occur. The spleen can become greatly enlarged.[3-7]

LABORATORY FINDINGS
Anemia, reticulocytopenia, and thrombocytopenia are present in most patients. Leukopenia and neutropenia are less common. With progression of the disease, pancytopenia is the rule.

Marrow examination may be normal and erythrophagocytic histiocytes inconspicuous, but later in the course it often shows decreased numbers of normal precursors and increased numbers of macrophages ingesting blood cells (hemophagocytic histiocytes).[7] Fine-needle aspiration of the spleen shows swollen histiocytes engorged with erythrocytes and other blood cells, often when hemophagocytosis is less prominent in the marrow. Liver and lymph node sinuses and alveolar spaces are often congested with macrophages engorged with erythroid cells and other blood cells (e.g., neutrophils, lymphocytes, or platelets).

Central nervous system signs of meningitis, seizures, hemiplegia, and coma may ensue. The cerebrospinal fluid frequently has an in-

creased concentration of mononuclear cells, sometimes including macrophages. The spinal fluid total protein level is elevated in most children.[8]

Serum glutamic-oxaloacetic transaminase, glutamate pyruvate transaminase, and bilirubin levels may be elevated. The serum ferritin and triglyceride concentrations frequently are elevated. The serum albumin and fibrinogen levels are often low, and overt disseminated intravascular coagulation can be present.[5-7]

Increased serum concentrations of interferon-γ, tumor necrosis factor α(TNFα), soluble interleukin-2 (IL-2) receptor, soluble FAS ligand, and soluble CD8 are evident in most affected children, and increased IL-6 occurs in one-third of children. These alterations indicate that there is a close correlation of the disease manifestations with cytotoxic T-cell and natural killer cell activation and their exaggerated elaboration of inflammatory cytokines.[9-12]

The diagnosis of the clinical syndrome in infants is supported by biopsies showing a lymphohistiocytic infiltrate in the liver, spleen, lymph nodes, or marrow. The macrophages do not have the cytologic features of malignant cells but are engorged with phagocytosed erythrocytes and occasionally neutrophils, lymphocytes, platelets, or erythroblasts. Early in the disease, histiocytes are prominent in the T-cell zones and sinuses of lymph nodes. Later, lymphoid depletion in the paracortex of lymph nodes and the white pulp of the spleen is characteristic.[6,7,13]

THERAPY
Treatment has not been studied systematically.

Etoposide, tenoposide, vinca alkaloids, glucocorticoids, and methotrexate have been used as single or multiple agents with or without intrathecal methotrexate followed by cranial irradiation to treat central nervous system disease. Remissions have occurred in a very small proportion of patients.[6] Stem cell transplantation from an appropriate donor can result in sustained remissions.[6,14,15] Splenectomy, plasmapheresis, plasma exchange transfusion, cyclosporine A, and antithymocyte globulin have been used in individual patients with occasional reports of improvement or remission.[16] The efficacy of high-dose dexamethasone, etoposide, cyclosporine A, and intrathecal methotrexate, if the latter is indicated, is currently being assessed.[16]

COURSE
The disease, if untreated, is rapidly fatal, although temporary improvement can occur with the varying interventions noted above. Unless successful treatment, usually with stem cell transplantation, is instituted, infection, hemorrhage, or central nervous system abnormalities eventually result in death. Results from stem cell transplantations have been encouraging, and the estimated 5-year survival rate for patients treated with chemotherapy (≈10%) compared to that for stem cell transplantation (≈65%) in uncontrolled studies, highlights the value of the latter modality.[6]

INFECTION, DISEASE, OR DRUG-INDUCED HEMOPHAGOCYTIC HISTIOCYTOSIS

ETIOLOGY
Since the mid-1970s, a syndrome of exaggerated histiocytic proliferation and activation has been

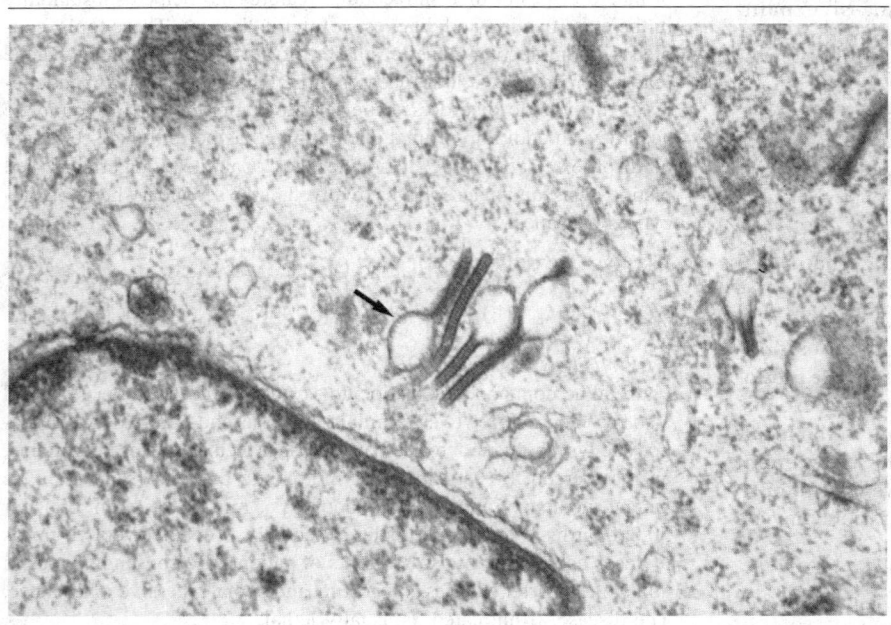

FIGURE 78-1   Transmission electron micrograph of a pathologic Langerhans' cell from a bone lesion. The cell contains typical cytoplasmic Langerhans' granules (Birbeck bodies; *arrow*). The latter have a characteristic racquet shape. (From BE Favara and ER Jaffe, *Hematol Oncol Clin North Am* 1:75, 1987, with permission.)

defined that is usually associated with systemic viral infection,[17,18] especially with Epstein-Barr virus,[19–23] and occasionally occurs with bacterial, fungal, or protozoal infections.[24–27] The disease affects children and adults, and Epstein-Barr virus, herpes simplex virus, cytomegalovirus, varicella zoster virus, adenovirus, human immunodeficiency virus, dengue virus, parvovirus, enteric bacteria, streptococcus, staphylococcus, rickettsia, mycobacteria, *Candida, Histoplasma, Cryptococcus,* leishmania, and *Babesia* have been implicated.[17–42]

Hemophagocytic histiocytosis also can occur during the accelerated phase of Chédiak-Higashi syndrome.[43] A similar syndrome can occur in patients with a variety of malignancies, perhaps as a result of the enhanced susceptibility to infection of the immunosuppressed state associated with cancer, chemotherapy, radiotherapy, and inanition.[29,33,44–56] The syndrome can occur with lymphomas as a result of cytokines released by lymphoma cells that stimulate histiocyte proliferation and phagocytosis.[39,49,51,57] The syndrome has developed in patients with lupus erythematosus;[58] other autoimmune diseases,[59] including Still's disease;[60] after phenytoin administration;[61] and in association with other, miscellaneous disorders.[62]

PATHOGENESIS

The manifestations of the disorder are thought to be mediated by inflammatory cytokines, including interferon-γ, TNF-α, soluble IL-2 receptor, FAS ligand, granulocyte-monocyte colony-stimulating factor (GM-CSF) and monocyte colony-stimulating factor (MCSF), and perhaps others.[10–12,49,51,63] Agents like Epstein-Barr virus activate T lymphocytes, resulting in cytokine release.[63,64] Elevated levels of TNF-α, soluble IL-2 receptor, IL-1, and FAS ligand are associated with the severity of the manifestations.[10–12] Soluble IL-2 receptor is thought to contribute to immune impairment by negating the effect of IL-2. Endothelial cell activation and capillary leakage coupled with hepatic injury from histiocyte infiltration, bile acids, and the FAS/FAS ligand pathway may combine to account for hypoalbuminemia and hypofibrinogenemia. Endothelial cell injury may induce microvascular thrombosis and consumption of labile coagulation factors, which contributes to the fibrinogenopenia and coagulopathy. Cytopenias may result from the effects of elevated concentrations of interferon-γ, TNF-α, or transforming growth factor β (TGF-β)–mediated suppression of the marrow and M-CSF–mediated accelerated clearance of platelets by histiocytes.[65,66]

CLINICAL FINDINGS

The signs and symptoms of this disease include fever, severe malaise, myalgias, lethargy, and often hepatic and splenic enlargement.[17,18,32,33,64] The last two findings are less prevalent in adults. Children may also have prominent lymphadenopathy. Pulmonary infiltrates can develop occasionally.

LABORATORY FINDINGS

Severe anemia (<9.0 g/dl), leukopenia [(<2500/μl) <2.5 $\times$ 10^9/liter], and thrombocytopenia [(<50,000/μl) <50 $\times$ 10^9/liter], or a combination of two cytopenias can be seen in nearly all cases.[17,18,27,33,67] A careful search may uncover macrophages in the blood film. The marrow is often hypocellular, and granulopoiesis and erythropoiesis, in particular, are markedly decreased. The number of megakaryocytes in the marrow and platelet counts are normal or reduced slightly.

An increase in marrow macrophages is a constant finding. The macrophages may range from being slightly more prominent to replacing hematopoietic tissue.[17,18,27,33,67] They are often vacuolated, with ingested cellular material in varying stages of digestion. Ingestion of erythrocytes and erythroblasts is usual, but phagocytosis of platelets

and, rarely, neutrophils also can occur (Fig. 78-2). A lymph node biopsy contains increased hemophagocytic histiocytes, but lymph node architecture is not effaced. Occasionally, histiocytic proliferation may involve the meninges, gastrointestinal tract, lung, or other sites.

During the acute phase of the illness, the plasma concentrations of inflammatory cytokines and acute-phase reactants are elevated. Interferon-γ, TNF-α, and IL-6 levels are often markedly elevated, as is soluble IL-2 receptor. Soluble IL-2 receptor and CD3+, HLA-DR+ cells in the blood are elevated notably in Epstein-Barr virus–induced hemophagocytic syndrome. Hypertriglyceridemia, hyperferritinemia, and elevated serum phenylalanine levels are frequent. Plasma fibrinogen and plasminogen activator inhibitor-1 levels are often very low, and these changes may reflect consumptive coagulopathy.[40]

TREATMENT AND COURSE

Patients with this unusual, exaggerated histiocytic inflammatory reaction to infection, although severely ill, often recover in weeks as a result of antimicrobial therapy or natural resolution. Complete disappearance of the histopathologic evidence of histiocytosis follows in months.[17,33,42,49] In patients in whom disease- or drug-induced immunodeficiency is present, such as renal transplant patients, immunosuppressive therapy should be decreased or stopped until the viral infection subsides.[18] Treatment with cyclosporine A,[21,60] antithymocyte globulin,[68] gamma globulin,[69–71] or etoposide[72] has resulted in striking improvement of Epstein-Barr virus–associated hemophagocytic syndrome.

The disease severity has been correlated with older age, lower hemoglobin and platelet concentrations, and elevated plasma ferritin, β_2 microglobulin, or serum bilirubin concentration.[67]

The disease can be distinguished from malignant histiocytosis by clinical and serologic evidence of an antecedent viral infection, the clinical setting in which the disease occurs, the absence of cytologic evidence of malignant histiocytes (see "Malignant Histiocytosis"), and the absence of effacement of lymph node architecture.

SINUS HISTIOCYTOSIS WITH MASSIVE LYMPHADENOPATHY (ROSAI-DORFMAN SYNDROME)

DEFINITION AND HISTORY

Sinus histiocytosis with massive lymphadenopathy is usually a self-limited disorder of unknown etiology described in 1969 by Rosai and Dorfman[73] that principally occurs in the first two decades of life but can occur at any age. The disease can be recurrent or progressive and can lead to death in some patients.[73,74]

CLINICAL FINDINGS

Signs and Symptoms The typical presentation is characterized by massive bilateral, painless cervical lymphadenopathy, which may be isolated or associated with generalized adenopathy. Early, the nodes may be discrete, but they often progress to adherent, multinodular masses. Axillary and inguinal adenopathy may develop in about half the patients. Fever is frequent, and weight loss may occur. Extranodal involvement is present in nearly one-half of patients, especially in the head and neck region, involving the skin, soft tissue, orbit, eye lids, uvea, lacrimal glands, paranasal sinuses, salivary glands, thyroid, or oral cavity. The respiratory tract, breast, mediastinum, thymus, heart, liver, kidneys, testes, synovia, bone, meninges, and spinal cord may also be involved.[74]

LABORATORY FINDINGS

Patients frequently have signs of chronic inflammation: anemia, neutrophilia, elevated erythrocyte sedimentation rate, hypoalbuminemia, and polyclonal hypergammaglobulinemia. Marrow examination is usu-

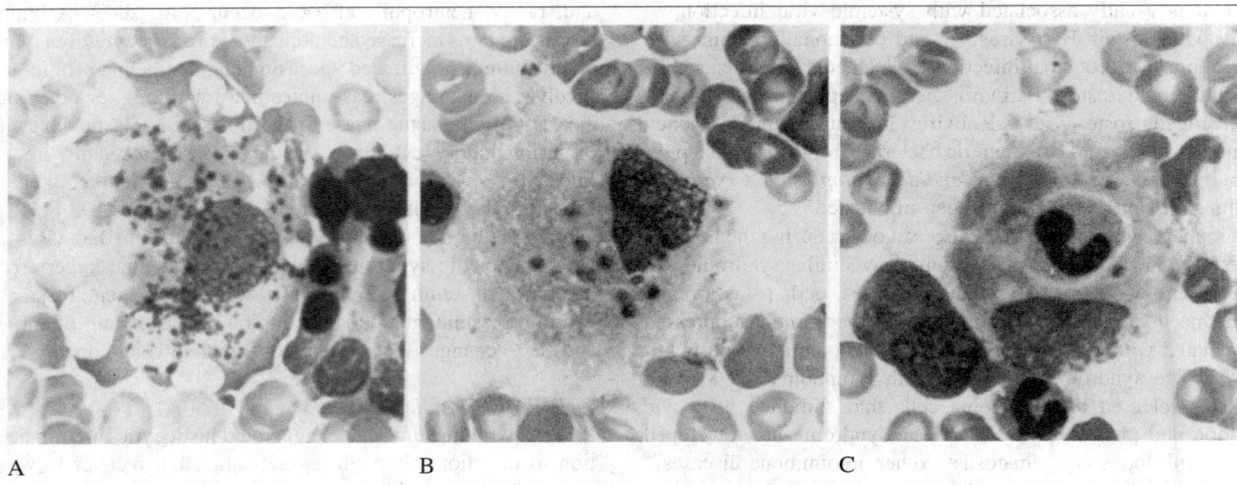

A   B   C

FIGURE 78-2   A composite showing macrophages from a patient with histiocytosis. These macrophages show *(a)* erythrophagocytosis, *(b)* platelet phagocytosis, and *(c)* band neutrophil (and erythro) phagocytosis.

ally uninformative, and histiocytic proliferation is usually not present.[74] Efforts to find an etiologic infectious agent have been unsuccessful. Epstein-Barr virus and human herpes virus-6 have been detected in some cases but not others.[75,76]

DIFFERENTIAL DIAGNOSIS

Excisional biopsy or needle aspiration of a lymph node or an extranodal site can provide specimens for diagnostic study.[74,77] The histopathologic features in the lymph node biopsy are usually diagnostic: marked fibrosis in the capsular and pericapsular areas and distention and engorgement of medullary and subcapsular sinusoids by phagocytic histiocytes. Lymphophagocytosis and erythrophagocytosis by histiocytes in the lymph node sinus are characteristic.[74] The active phagocyte is a histiocyte that is positive for S-100 protein, CD11c, CD14, CD33, CD68, acid phosphatase, and nonspecific esterase.[74,77–79] Lymphocytes and plasma cells are prominent in the intersinal spaces. Eosinophils are absent or rare. Later in the disease, continued proliferation can lead to effacement of the node. The histiocytic proliferation is polyclonal.[80] The histopathological appearance of extranodal biopsies is strikingly similar to that of lymph nodes.

COURSE AND PROGNOSIS

The course of the disease is influenced by the degree of immune impairment or dysfunction that coexists. A significant number of cases appear in children with underlying immunologic disorders, including Wiskott-Aldrich syndrome, autoimmune hemolytic disease, polyarthritis, glomerulonephritis, or severe pneumonia.[74,81,82] In other cases, no specific immune abnormality characterizes the disease.

The lymph node enlargement usually progresses for weeks to months, reaches a maximum, and then gradually recedes, so that most patients have little or no residual evidence of disease 9 to 18 months after onset.[74] Some patients have persistent lymphadenopathy but stable disease, and others have progressive disease and may have a fatal outcome. The latter patients usually have an accompanying immunologic disease and/or widespread nodal involvement that may encroach on vital organs.[74,82]

THERAPY

Other than excisional biopsy for diagnosis, many patients require no therapy, since the disease will run its course and abate. Glucocorticoids, cytoxic agents, radiotherapy, and antibiotics have had no consistent

effect on the duration of the disease.[74,83] In patients with severe or progressive disease, there have been reports of successful treatment with acyclovir,[84] glucocorticoids,[85,86] interferon-α,[87,88] thalidomide,[89] or combination chemotherapy.[83,90,91]

CLONAL HISTIOCYTOSIS

LANGERHANS' CELL HISTIOCYTOSIS

DEFINITION AND HISTORY

Langerhans' cells are macrophages with an irregularly shaped nucleus. They are normally present in the epidermis, oral and vaginal mucosa, and the lungs.[92,93] They are derived from the hematopoietic stem cells in marrow, as are all other types of macrophages.[94,95] Langerhans' cells differ from other tissue cells in their racquet-shaped ultrastructural inclusions (Birbeck bodies;[96] their content of the β chain of the neuroprotein S-100,[93,97] neuronal-specific enolase,[99] and cell surface CD 1a immunoreactivity (Table 78-2).[100,101]

TABLE 78-2   FEATURES OF LANGERHANS' CELLS

Ultrastructural marker
Birbeck bodies*
Histochemical markers
α-Naphthyl acetate esterase
α-Naphthyl butyrate esterase
Acid phosphatase
Adenosine triphosphatase*
Adenosine diphosphatase*
α-D-Mannosidase*
Immunologic markers
HLA-DR
Fc receptors
C3b receptors
CD1*
MT1, KP1, Mac
Peanut lectin receptor*
Protein markers
S-100 beta subunit*
Neuronal-specific enolase*
Fascin*

*Specific markers for Langerhans' cells. Monocytes and macrophages are positive for 5′-nucleotidase, peroxidase, and lysozyme, but Langerhans' cells are not.

The Langerhans' cell is a macrophage that is specialized to be a component of the immune accessory cell system. It processes antigens, migrates from the skin to the lymph nodes, transforms to a dendritic phenotype, and presents antigen to paracortical T cells. The antigen-presenting cells partially degrade antigen and express peptides on the cell surface in association with HLA molecules, making them recognizable to T-lymphocytes.[92,93,101,102] The veiled cell of afferent lymphatics may represent a Langerhans' cell in transit. After antigen presentation, the Langerhans' cell may alter its phenotype to an interdigitating dendritic cell.[92,93,101]

The cell was described in the epidermis by Paul Langerhans in 1868.[103] In 1973 it was recognized that the macrophages of "histiocytosis X" have the characteristics of epidermal Langerhans' cells.[104] The preferred term *Langerhans' cell histiocytosis* should be used for all the eponymic diseases Lichtenstein embraced with the term *histiocytosis X*,[105] including eosinophilic granuloma, Abt-Letterer-Siwe disease, and Hand-Schüller-Christian disease, as well as several added since the time of his writing, including self-healing histiocytosis, eosinophilic xanthomatous granuloma, pure cutaneous histiocytosis, Langerhans' cell granulomatosis, type II histiocytosis, Hashimoto-Pritzker syndrome, eosinophilic xanthomatosis of the normocholesterolemic type, and nonlipid reticuloendotheliosis.[106]

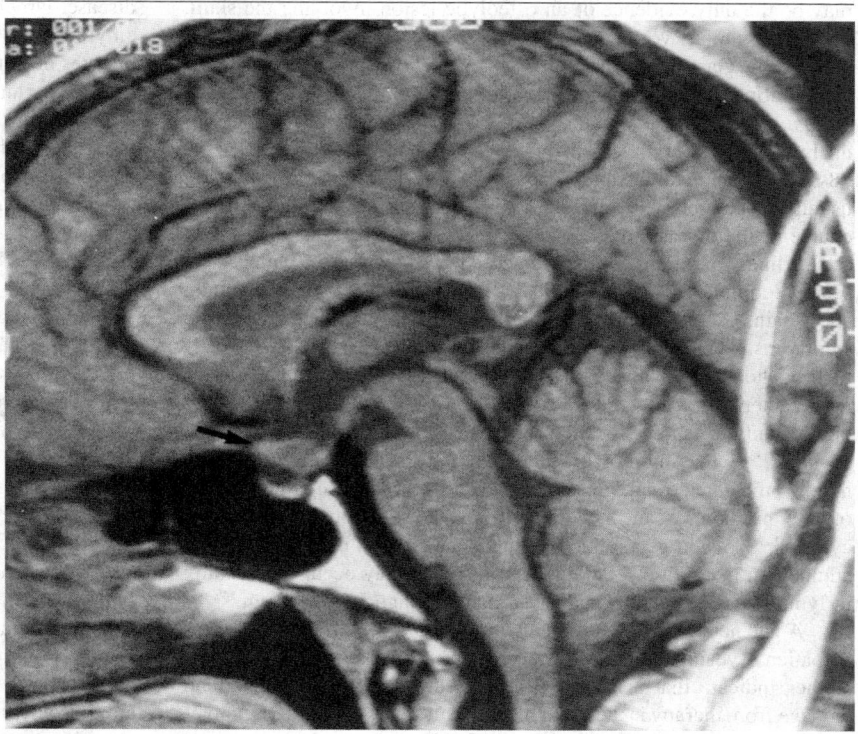

FIGURE 78-3   Magnetic resonance imaging study demonstrating hypothalamic involvement by Langerhans' cell histiocytosis. The arrow indicates the anterior pole of the greatly enlarged hypothalamic region, expanded by the tumor mass.

ETIOLOGY AND PATHOGENESIS

The etiology and nature of Langerhans' cell histiocytosis have been enigmatic. The syndrome was thought to be inflammatory, with granulomatous, xanthomatous, or fibrotic elements being observed during the evolution of the histopathologic lesions. These cellular changes were thought to be the manifestation of an autoimmune process. The cells do not appear malignant, although a high mitotic index is not uncommon. An infectious etiology has not been identified.

A neoplastic etiology was suggested in 1940 based on the x-ray appearance of bone lesions[107] and in 1986, when aneuploidy was demonstrated by flow cytometric study of the DNA content of cutaneous Langerhans' cells from a patient.[108] These speculations were proved when molecular studies indicated that the proliferating histiocytes represent a monoclonal population, and this is the case whether the lesions examined are localized or widespread.[109] Thus, the disorder appears to be a neoplasm, which can be localized and non-progressive or disseminated and progressive and which often behaves like a chronic inflammatory disease, perhaps because the cells involved can secrete a variety of inflammatory cytokines inappropriately,[109] leading to autocrine stimulation, especially by GM-CSF and TNF-α.[110] The loss of E-cadherin expression in Langerhans' cells has been associated with dissemination from the skin.[111]

Initially the lesions contain abundant numbers of pathologic Langerhans' cells. Macrophages, eosinophils, and lymphocytes frequently participate in the formation of granulomatous lesions. The masses proliferate and can be destructive. Later in the course of the disease, the lesions may become less cellular, xanthomatous, and fibrotic.[101,112,113]

The lesions usually involve bone, especially the flat bones of the skull, face, ribs, and pelvis, and the skin, lungs, liver, marrow, lymph nodes, spleen, thymus, central nervous system, and pituitary gland. Occasionally, the gastrointestinal tract is involved.[112,113]

Mode of Inheritance and Epidemiology   The disease has been reported in siblings and identical twins, but most cases are sporadic, and a strong genetic influence is not apparent, consistent with the presumptive neoplastic pathogenesis.[250]

The incidence of Langerhans' cell histiocytosis is estimated to be 1 per 200,000 children. Seventy-five percent of patients are diagnosed before age 10 years, and 90 percent before age 30. Males are more frequently (3:1) affected by limited or non-progressive disease. Females and males are affected equally by chronic progressive or fatal disease. About 90 percent of cases with multisystem involvement occur before the age of 20 years.[113–116]

CLINICAL FINDINGS

Symptoms and Signs   Lesions fulfill common histopathologic criteria, but the extent of disease and the clinical features vary.[112,113,117] The disease may be localized to a bone or to a soft-tissue site, multifocal involving only bone, or multifocal involving bone and other sites.[118–120]

The expression of the disease is correlated frequently with the age of the patient at onset. Infants may present with fever, otitis media, or mastoiditis.[121] Enlargement of the liver, spleen, and lymph nodes is frequent, as is dermatitis. A self-limited syndrome, benign cephalic histiocytosis, can occur during the first year of life. Papules and macules, which when biopsied reveal a histiocytic infiltrate, occur on forehead, ears, and cheeks and later elsewhere, and resolve spontaneously in weeks to months.[122]

Skin lesions can resemble seborrheic, eczematoid, pustular, or nodular dermatitis and often involve the scalp in infants. Tumors limited to the skin can be the sole manifestation of the disease.[123,124] Lesions of the bones or soft tissues of the head and neck are present in over 75 percent of children.[125,126] In children and adolescents, pain, tenderness, and swelling in the head, face, leg, back, chest, or groin may be the only evidence of an osteolytic lesion involving the skull, orbit, jaw, femur, vertebra, rib, or pelvis.[118–120] Protrusion of the eye may occur. Gastrointestinal tract involvement in children can result in vomiting, diarrhea, and ulceration and bleeding.[127,128] Hepatic involvement is very uncommon.[129,130] Polyuria and polydipsia can signal hypothalamic involvement and the onset of diabetes insipidus (Fig. 78-3).[131–134] Diabetes insipidus occurs in about one-quarter of cases, usually in patients with multisystem disease and usually during the course of the disease, but not as an initial manifestation.[113,117]

Primary pulmonary involvement, which is rare in children, is seen predominately in male adults.[135,136] Chronic nonproductive cough, chest pain, shortness of breath, and wheezing are the most common symptoms. The presence of more than 5 percent CD1a-positive cells in bronchoalveolar lavage fluid is evidence that favors pulmonary involvement by Langerhans' cell histiocytosis.[137] The radiographic picture initially shows a reticular pattern but can progress to cystic changes.[138–142] Pneumothoraces tend to occur and recur, especially when honeycomb changes are present on the chest x-ray. A high prevalence of other pulmonary cancers has been associated with pulmonary histiocytosis.[143] Isolated generalized lymphadenopathy is more common in adults than in children.[144,145] Langerhans' cells may occur incidentally in lymphomatous lesions and thus create a diagnostic problem.[146,147]

A late neurologic syndrome that includes cerebellar ataxia occurs in patients years after they appeared to be disease-free.[148] Autopsy studies indicate that active disease of neurologic tissue rather than damage from therapy is the usual mechanism. Dentate nuclear involvement is often prominent. Rare cases of diffuse cerebral involvement occur, although intracranial involvement is usually limited to the hypothalamus.[149]

Involvement of the female genital tract usually occurs in young women, but may occur in childhood. The ovary, endometrium, cervix, vagina, or vulva may be involved.[150,151] The disease may be localized or represent one site of multicentric involvement. Pregnancy presents special problems in women with Langerhans' cell histiocytosis.[152] The most common complication is the onset or exacerbation of diabetes insipidus. Involvement of the vagina, vulva, or pelvic bones may interfere with a normal vaginal delivery. Reactivation of the disease after years of remission has been reported during pregnancy. Reduced fecundity can occur, possibly from hypothalamic-pituitary axis involvement, resulting in decreased gonadotropins and elevated prolactin levels.

The disease, when it affects adults, involves principally the skin, lungs, bone, pituitary, and lymph nodes, and diabetes insipidus is common.[153,154]

LABORATORY FINDINGS

Neutrophilia, increased sedimentation rate, and increased serum alkaline phosphatase levels may occur. The diagnosis is based on a biopsy of involved organs, especially skin, bone, liver, or lymph node, whichever is most involved and most accessible.[101,113] Imaging studies of bone lesions can be strongly suggestive of the disease. The key diagnostic feature is the presence of pathologic Langerhans' cells, which may be abundant in proliferative lesions or scarce in fibrotic, hypocellular lesions. Giant cells with multiple nuclei resembling osteoclasts are features of the lesion, but they are not derived from Langerhans' cells. Marker studies for the presence of S-100, CD1a, peanut lectin binding, and adenosinetriphosphatase, and ultrastructural studies for Birbeck bodies are used to identify the Langerhans' cells conclusively.[93,98,100,101,105,112,113,117]

DIFFERENTIAL DIAGNOSIS

The differential diagnosis in adult patients depends on the site of involvement and can include a chronic infectious (granulomatous)

disease, lymphoma, collagen- vascular disease, pneumoconiosis, and amyloidosis.[113,117,154] Several diseases associated with proliferative histiocytes need to be differentiated from Langerhans' cell histiocytosis, including xanthogranuloma,[155] histiocytic necrotizing lymphadenitis (Kikuchi's disease),[156] and Erdheim-Chester disease.[157,158] Biopsy specimens from these entities are usually distinguishable by an experienced pathologist.

Langerhans' cells may be present in the biopsies of patients with solid tumors, Hodgkin disease, lymphoma, or chronic lymphocytic leukemia.[159–166] The focal nature of Langerhans' cell lesions and their absence from most other cancers suggest that they are a reaction to the lymphoma.[160]

Langerhans' cells also have been found in a thymus removed for the treatment of myasthenia gravis[167] and in a variety of dermatologic disorders.[168]

TREATMENT

Spontaneous fluctuations and remissions are features of the disease.[101,113,117,169] Treatment should be considered in patients with symptomatic localized or progressive multifocal disease.

Localized disease may be managed by local means. Isolated lymph node disease may be treated by excisional biopsy. Patients with bone lesions should be assessed for the possibility of pathologic fractures. Curettage, excision,[170] or intralesional glucocorticoids[171] or non-steroidal anti-inflammatory agents can be used, depending on circumstances. Physical exertion may have to be restricted in individuals with vertebral or other lesions who are at risk for pathologic fractures. Radiation therapy needs to be individualized according to the size, number, severity, and location of bone lesions.[172–174] Radiotherapy can be used for bone lesions that are painful, are inaccessible, or compromise vital organs or for large lesions in weight-bearing bones.[118,119,169] The dose employed is usually between 400 and 800 cGy. Grafts may be required also for large lesions in weight-bearing bones. Extension from a vertebra to the spinal cord requires the urgent use of radiation therapy.

Skin disease, if localized, may be treated by excisional biopsy, often required for diagnosis. If mild, skin lesions may respond to topical or interlesional therapy. Use of an aqueous solution of mustine hydrochloride (nitrogen mustard) can be very effective and is especially useful in outpatients.[175,176] Psoralen coupled with ultraviolet A light treatment may be the most consistently effective treatment.[177] Intradermal interferon-β has been associated with resolution of skin lesions.[178,179] Glucocorticoids, although frequently used in the past, are of modest, short-term benefit usually. High-potency preparations are required for the best results. Radiation therapy should be restricted to local, obstinate lesions, especially if they result in a sinus tract from an underlying visceral lesion. Etoposide, isotretinoin, trimethoprim-sulfamethoxazole, and thalidomide may be very useful for skin lesions but require further study. The former may be particularly useful for progressive, multiple sites of skin involvement.[180]

Chemotherapy may be useful for patients with progressive, multisystem disease.[169,181–183] Many agents have been used alone, but few systematic studies of single agents are available. Vinca alkaloids, alkylating agents, purine or pyrimidine antagonists, anthracycline antibiotics, epipodophyllotoxins, adenosine deaminase inhibitors, cyclosporine, and others may be useful as single agents. The distribution of the disease, threat to organ function, rate of progression, and age of the patient should be considered in deciding on the best approach to therapy. Etoposide can suppress multisystem disease and may have a special role in the treatment of disease in the skin or central nervous system.[169] For progressive multisystem disease, various combinations of three- or four-drug therapy, given at regular intervals for about 6 to 9 months, have been used in a manner akin to treatment of higher-

TABLE 78-3 DRUGS USED FOR PROGRESSIVE—LANGERHANS' CELL HISTIOCYTOSIS

Cladrabine[184–187]
Cyclosporine[188,189]*
Deoxycoformycin[190]
Etoposide[191–195]
Interferon-α[196]
Thalidomide[197–199]
Vinblastine[195]
Vinblastine, etoposide, prednisone and mercaptopurine or methotrexate[200]
Vincristine, cytarabine, prednisone[201]
Prednisone, etoposide, cyclosporine[202]

*Other drugs added in some cases.

risk lymphomas.[169,182,183] Table 78-3 lists drugs and drug combinations that have been used to ameliorate this disorder.[184–202]

In older children and adults, multisystem Langerhans' cell histiocytosis often has a relapsing and remitting course and may regress. The decision to use systemic multidrug cytotoxic therapy requires integration of the extent and progression of disease with the potential adverse effects.

There is controversy as to whether fully established diabetes insipidus requiring desmopressin therapy can be reversed by means of radiotherapy.[203,204] Early partial diabetes insipidus associated with a mass lesion seen by computed tomography or magnetic resonance imaging may be kept from advancing by treatment with radiotherapy, but reversal of fully developed diabetes insipidus, although reported, is felt to be improbable, and symptomatic therapy with desmopressin is required in virtually all cases.[251]

Blood-component therapy may be required in patients with marrow involvement and cytopenia. If the spleen is grossly enlarged, splenectomy may be useful in patients who require frequent red cell transfusions. Since this complication usually occurs in younger patients, the risk of post-splenectomy infection should be weighed against the risks of long-term, frequent red cell transfusions.

Marrow transplantation has resulted in benefit in some patients with severe multisystem disease.[205,206] Progressive hepatic failure has been treated by liver transplantation.[207,208] Pulmonary failure has been treated with lung transplantation.

COURSE AND PROGNOSIS

The following factors are associated with a poor prognosis: disease onset during the first 2 years of life, fever not explained by infection, failure to thrive in infants, blood cytopenias, abnormalities of liver function test results, and splenic enlargement. A salutory response of multisystem disease to combination chemotherapy within 6 weeks identifies patients who are likely to have a good long-term response to therapy. Isolated skin or bone lesions point to a good prognosis. The mortality rate in patients with multisystem disease, especially in those under 2 years, remains in the 25 percent range despite therapy. Some patients achieve resolution of disease, and some show marked regression ($\approx$50%). Others have an intermediate response, with some improvement of existing sites but with new sites developing. Long-term results await the follow-up of ongoing clinical trials.[169]

There may be an association between Langerhans' cell histiocytosis and acute lymphocytic leukemia and retinoblastoma.[166] The high frequency of other cancers in patients may be the consequences of chemotherapy.

MALIGNANT HISTIOCYTOSIS

DEFINITION AND HISTORY

In 1939, Scott and Robb-Smith[209,210] reported cases of a rapidly fatal disease associated with jaundice, lymphadenopathy, refractory anemia, leukopenia, and often hepatic and splenic enlargement that they called histiocytic medullary reticulosis. However, the suspected histiocytic cell proliferation could not be established beyond visual impression. Israels[211] expanded on the clinical description and histopathology and referred to the disease as giant-cell reticulosis, based on the use of the term *reticulum cells* for large malignant cells that are found to be either lymphocytes or histiocytes when assessed by more specific immunocytochemical techniques. In 1966, Rappaport[212] introduced the term *malignant histiocytosis* and focused on the nature of the malignant process, which he believed to be an invasive, progressive proliferation of neoplastic histiocytes, again based principally on the proliferating cells resembling histiocytes by light microscopy.

The introduction of techniques to characterize specific markers of macrophages and the requirement for the absence of immunoglobulin gene and T-lymphocyte receptor–chain gene rearrangements have resulted in the reclassification of most cases of malignant histiocytosis as anaplastic large T-cell (CD 30+) lymphoma or, less frequently, B-cell lymphoma or a tumor without definitive markers.[213–220] It is estimated that about 1 case in 200 to 300 lymphomas is a histiocytic malignancy, based on appropriate criteria.[216,217] Malignant histiocytosis is referred to in some reports as histiocytic sarcoma or true histiocytic lymphoma. Although there are precedents for the use of *sarcoma* with hematopoietic tumors (i.e., granulocytic sarcoma), the term usually refers to tumors derived from cells in connective tissue or muscle. The term *histiocytic lymphoma* reflects a chimeric term of two distinct tissues (macrophages and lymphocytes) and should be discarded.

CLINICAL FINDING

Only recent case studies have verified meticulously the phenotype of the cellular infiltrate in this disease using specific and sensitive markers for lymphoid and macrophagic cells. Thus, uncommon clinical correlates await the accumulation of additional cases. Moreover, in some otherwise well-studied cases, which report the absence of lymphocytic markers and the presence of macrophage markers on tumor cells, immunoglobulin and T-cell receptor–chain gene rearrangement studies have not been done, making conclusions about the diagnosis uncertain.

EPIDEMIOLOGY

The disease affects all age groups, and, in three studies totaling 18 patients, the age range was 2 to 74 years. The disease occurs more often in men than in women.[216,219,221]

SIGNS AND SYMPTOMS

Fever, headache, weakness, weight loss, dyspnea, and sweating occur commonly in most patients who have generalized disease.[219,221,222] Splenomegaly, hepatomegaly, and lymphadenopathy are very frequent.[219,221,222] Skin, central nervous system, and lung involvement may accompany the aforementioned findings. Localized presentation in the skin, a lymph node group, or especially the intestines may occur.[219,220,223–229] The appearance of malignant histiocytosis on a background of prior lymphoma may represent a biological predisposition to progress to other hematolymphoid tumors or reflect a therapy-induced event.[226,227]

LABORATORY FINDINGS

Anemia and thrombocytopenia are very common (>90% of cases), and neutropenia occurs in the majority of cases, although the white cell count can be elevated. Marrow examination may show infiltration with histiocytic cells, and cytophagocytosis by histiocytes may be evident. Cytophagocytosis was thought to be an infrequent feature of malignant histiocytosis, but this may have been a reflection of the lack of specific diagnostic criteria; most cases were actually lymphomas. The serum lactic dehydrogenase and serum bilirubin levels are often elevated, but liver-derived serum enzyme levels are not. It is significant that renal function is not disturbed.[221] Elevated serum levels of TNF, IL-6, IL-1α receptor, lysozyme, α_1-antitrypsin, and angiotensin-converting enzyme may be found.[221]

DIFFERENTIAL DIAGNOSIS

The diagnosis of malignant histiocytosis requires biopsy of a tumor mass in lymph node, skin, liver, intestine, marrow, or other involved site and immunohistochemical verification of a macrophagic phenotype including expression of some or most of the following: CD11b, CD11c, CD14, CD15, CD33, CD36, CD68, and MAC-387. The presence of cellular enzymes, including lysozyme, α_1-antitrypsin, and α_1-antichymotrypsin, are supporting markers but not sufficient in and of themselves for diagnosis. The cells in air-dried specimens of blood, marrow, or touch preparations of tissue react for non-specific esterase but not peroxidase. The cells should not express multiple T- or B-lymphocyte markers and should not show rearrangement of lymphoid lineage genes (immunoglobulin or T-receptor chains).[230,231]

The principal diseases that can mimic malignant histiocytosis include anaplastic and other large-cell lymphomas,[216–218,220,232] Hodgkin disease,[229] malignant fibrous histiocytoma (a myofibroblastic tumor),[229] hemangiopericytoma,[229] and inflammatory pseudotumor of lymph nodes.[229]

It seems probable that malignant histiocytosis is related closely to other clonal stem-cell or progenitor-cell disorders that express a monocytic or macrophagic phenotype, analogous to the spectrum of lymphoma to lymphocytic leukemia. Indeed, variants such as Langerhans' cell sarcoma, follicular dendritic cell tumors,[225,226] tumors derived from fixed as compared to free histiocytes,[233] and leukemic presentation[234,235–237] or progression[238] of malignant histiocytosis have been described, as have localized malignant histiocytomas.[239]

TREATMENT, COURSE, AND PROGNOSIS

No systematic multicenter clinical trials have been yet reported using stringent diagnostic criteria. The infrequency of this tumor makes single-center studies of limited value. Four-drug combinations, such as cyclophosphamide, doxorubicin, vincristine, and prednisone; lomustine, vincristine, bleomycin, and prednisone; or mechlorethamine hydrochloride, procarbazine, prednisone, and either vincristine or teniposide given at monthly intervals have been used for patients with generalized disease.[221] The disease is often very rapidly progressive, and most patients have not had a sustained remission of long duration. Remissions are not infrequent, however, and a remission duration of beyond 7 years has been reported in two patients.[221] Stem cell transplantation in younger patients with appropriate donors may be useful.[240] Most patients who have received transplantation prior to the development of specific diagnostic criteria probably had lymphomas.

Localized follicular dendritic cell tumors may be excised with or without the use of either local irradiation or chemotherapy.[228,229] Whether such additional therapy is beneficial is unclear.

MALIGNANT FIBROUS HISTIOCYTOMA AND GIANT-CELL TUMOR OF THE BONE

The precise cell of origin of malignant fibrous histiocytoma and giant-cell tumor of the bone has been the subject of dispute. A monocyte-macrophage and a fibroblast are the two principal cell types that have been thought to undergo malignant transformation in both tumors.[241] Current evidence points to the fibroblast or, occasionally, the myoblast, and both types of malignancy are usually fibrosarcomas or myosarcomas, not a type of malignant histiocytosis.[242–247] The histiocytic cells present in the tumor are considered reactive and may appear as a result of the release by the tumor cells of cytokines that recruit monocyte.[248,249]

REFERENCES

1. Moschella SL: An update of the benign proliferative monocyte-macrophage and dendritic cell disorders. *J Dermatol* 23:805, 1996.
2. Favara BE, Feller AC, Pauli M, et al: Contemporary classification of histiocytic disorders. *Med Pediatr Oncol* 29:157, 1997.
3. Henter JI, Söder O, Öst Ä, Elinder G: Incidence and clinical features of familial hemophagocytic lymphohistiocytosis in Sweden. *Acta Paediatr Scand* 80:428, 1991.
4. Janka GE: Familial hemophagocytic lymphohistiocytosis. *Eur J Pediatr* 140:221, 1983.
5. Favara BE: Hemophagocytic lymphohistiocytosis: A hemophagocytic syndrome. *Semin Diagn Pathol* 9:63, 1992.
6. Arico M, Janka G, Fischer A, et al: Hemophagocytic lymphohistiocytosis: Report of 122 children from the international registry. *Leukemia* 10:197, 1996.
7. Henter J-I, Elinder G, Ost A, et al: Diagnostic guidelines for hemophagocytic lymphohistiocytosis. *Semin Oncol* 18:29, 1991.
8. Haddad E, Sulis M-L, Jabado N, et al: Frequency and severity of central nervous system lesions in hemophagocytic lymphohistiocytosis. *Blood* 89:794, 1997.
9. Henter JI, Elinder G, Söder O, Hansson M, et al: Hypercytokinemia in familial hemophagocytic lymphohistiocytosis. *Blood* 78:2918, 1991.
10. Hagasagawa D, Kojima S, Tatusumi E, et al: Elevation of the serum Fas ligand in patients with the hemophagocytic syndrome and Diamond-Blackfan anemia. *Blood* 91:2793, 1998.
11. Imashuka S, Hibi S, Sako M, et al: Soluble interleukin-2 receptor: A useful prognostic factor for patients with hemophagocytic histiocytosis. *Blood* 86:4706, 1995.
12. Fujimara F, Hibi S, Imashuku S: Hypercytokinemia in hemophagocytic syndrome. *Am J Pediatr Hematol Oncol* 15:92, 1993.
13. Soffer D, Okon E, Rosen N, Stark B: Familial hemophagocytic lymphohistiocytosis in Israel: II. Pathologic findings. *Cancer* 54:2423, 1984.
14. Jabado N, de Graeff-Meeder ER, Cavazzana-Calvo M, et al: Treatment of familial hemophagocytic lymphohistiocytosis with bone marrow transplantation from HLA genetically non-identical donors. *Blood* 90:4743, 1997.
15. Baher KS, De Laat CA, Steinbush M, et al: Successful correction of hemophagocytic lymphohistiocytosis with related or unrelated bone marrow. *Blood* 89:3857, 1997.
16. Henter J-I, Arico M, Egeler RM, et al: HLH-94: A treatment protocol for hemophagocytic lymphohistiocytosis. *Med Pediatr Oncol* 28:342, 1997.
17. Risdall RJ, McKenna RW, Nesbit ME, et al: Virus associated hemophagocytic syndrome: A benign histiocytic proliferation distinct from malignant histiocytosis. *Cancer* 44:993, 1979.
18. Grateau G, Bachmeyer C, Blanche P, et al: Haemophagocytic syndrome in patients infected with the human immunodeficiency virus: Nine cases and a review. *J Infect* 34:219, 1997.
19. Sullivan JL, Woda BA, Herrod HG, et al: Epstein-Barr virus–associated hemophagocytic syndrome: Virological and immunological studies. *Blood* 65:1097, 1985.
20. Su I-J, Wang C-H, Cheng A-L, Chen R-L: Hemophagocytic syndrome in Epstein-Barr virus-associated T-lymphoproliferative disorders: Disease spectrum, pathogenesis, and mangement. *Leuk Lymph* 19:401, 1995.
21. Bird G, Peel D, McCarthy K, Williams H: Epstein-Barr virus–induced virus-associated hemophagocytic syndrome and monoclonal TCR-beta rearrangement: A case report. *Hematol Oncol* 15:47, 1997.
22. Chen JS, Tzeng CC, Tsao CJ, et al: Clonal karyotype abnormalities in EBV-associated hemophagocytic syndrome. *Haematologica* 82:572, 1997.
23. Kikuta H, Sakiyama Y, Matsumoto S, et al: Fatal Epstein-Barr–associated hemophagocytic syndrome. *Blood* 82:3259, 1993.
24. Risdall RJ, Brunning RD, Hernandez JL, et al: Bacteria-associated hemophagocytic syndrome. *Cancer* 54:2968, 1984.
25. Abbott KC, Vukelja SJ, Smith CE, et al: Hemophagocytic syndrome: A cause of pancytopenia in human Ehrlichiosis. *Am J Hematol* 38:230, 1991.
26. Auerbach M, Haubenstock A, Soloman G: Systemic babesiosis. *Am J Med* 80:301, 1986.
27. Wong KF, Chan JK: Reactive hemophagocytic syndrome: A clinicopathologic study of 40 patients in an oriental population. *Am J Med* 93:177, 1992.
28. Kawaguchi H, Miyashita T, Herbst H, et al: Epstein-Barr virus–infected

T lymphocytes in Epstein-Barr-virus–associated hemophagocytic syndrome. *J Clin Invest* 92:1444, 1993.

29. Tsuda H: Hemophagocytic syndrome (HPS) in children and adults. *Int J Hematol* 65:215, 1997.

30. Goldberg J, Nezelof C: Lymphohistiocytosis: A multifactorial syndrome of macrophagic activation: Clinico-pathologic study of 38 cases. *Hematol Oncol* 4:275, 1986.

31. Weintraub M, Siegman-Igra Y, Josiphov J, et al: Histiocytic hemophagocytosis in military tuberculosis. *Arch Intern Med* 144:2055, 1984.

32. Chandra P, Chaudhery SA, Rosner F, Kagen M: Transient histiocytosis with striking phagocytosis of platelets, leukocytes and erythrocytes. *Ann Intern Med* 135:989, 1975.

33. Reiner AP, Spivak JL: Hematophagic histiocytosis. *Medicine* 67:369, 1988.

34. Chen R-L, Su I-J, Lin K-H, et al: Fulminant childhood hemophagocytic syndrome mimicking histiocytic medullary reticulosis. *Am J Clin Pathol* 96:171, 1991.

35. Ross CW, Schnitzer B, Weston BW, Hanson CA: Chronic active Epstein-Barr virus infection and virus-associated hemophagocytic syndrome. *Arch Pathol Lab Med* 115:470, 1991.

36. Potter MN, Foot ABM, Oakhill A: Influenza A and the virus-associated haemophagocytic syndrome. *J Clin Pathol* 44:297, 1991.

37. Yufu Y, Matsumoto M, Miyamura T, et al: Parvovirus B19-associated haemophagocytic syndrome with lymphadenopathy resembling histiocytic necrotizing lymphadenitis (Kikuchi's disease). *Br J Haematol* 96:868, 1997.

38. Wong KF, Chan JKC, Chan JCW, et al: Dengue virus infection-associated hemophagocytic syndrome. *Am J Hematol* 38:339, 1991.

39. Dreyer ZE, Dowell BL, Chen H, et al: Infection-associated hemophagocytic syndrome. *Am J Pediatr Hematol Oncol* 13:476, 1991.

40. Smith KJ, Skelton HG, Yaeger J, et al: Cutaneous histopathologic immunohistochemical and clinical manifestations in patients with hemophagocytic syndrome. *Arch Dermatol* 128:193, 1992.

41. Grateau G, Bachmeyer C, Blanche P, et al: Haemophagocytic syndrome in patients infected with the human immunodeficiency—virus: Nine cases and review. *J Infect* 34:219, 1997.

42. Woda BA, Sullivan JL: Reactive histiocytic disorders. *Am J Clin Pathol* 99:459, 1993.

43. Rubin CM, Burke BA, McKenna RW, et al: The accelerated phase of Chédiak-Higashi syndrome: An expression of the virus associated hemophagocytic syndrome? *Cancer* 56:524, 1985.

44. Stark R, Manoharan A: Haemophagocytic syndrome complicating acute lymphoblastic leukaemia. *Postgrad Med J* 65:249, 1989.

45. Chan JKC, Ng CS, Law CK, et al: Reactive hemophagocytic syndrome: A study of 7 fatal cases. *Pathology* 19:43, 1987.

46. Jaffe ES, Costa J, Fauci AS, et al: Malignant lymphoma and erythrophagocytosis simulating malignant histiocytosis. *Am J Med* 75:741, 1983.

47. Ng CS, Chan JKC, Cheng PNM, Szeto SC: Nasal T cell lymphoma associated with hemophagocytic syndrome. *Cancer* 58:67, 1986.

48. Yin JAL, Kimaran TO, Marsh GW, et al: Complete recovery of histiocytic medullary reticulosis-like syndrome in a child with acute lymphoblastic leukemia. *Cancer* 51:200, 1983.

49. Imashuku S: Differential diagnosis of hemophagocytic syndrome: Underlying disorders and selection of most effective treatment. *Int J Hematol* 66:135, 1997.

50. Hassinger SL, Schiffer CA, Sun C-C: Acute myeloblastic leukemia with extensive erythrophagocytosis mimicking malignant histiocytosis. *Am J Clin Pathol* 92:696, 1989.

51. Ishii E, Ohga S, Aoki T, et al: Prognosis of children with virus-associated hemophagocytic syndrome and malignant histiocytosis: Correlation with levels of serum interleukin-1 and tumor necrosis factor. *Acta Haematol* 85:93, 1991.

52. Sun T, Brody J, Susin M, et al: Extranodal T-cell lymphoma mimicking malignant histiocytosis. *Am J Hematol* 35:269, 1990.

53. Okuda T, Sakamoto S, Deguchi T, et al: Hemophagocytic syndrome associated with aggressive natural killer cell leukemia. *Am J Hematol* 38:321, 1991.

54. Chan EYT, Pi D, Chan GTC, et al: Peripheral T-cell lymphoma presenting as hemophagocytic syndrome. *Hematol Oncol* 7:275, 1989.

55. Myers TJ, Kessimian N, Schwartz S: Mediastinal germ cell tumor associated with the hemophagocytic syndrome. *Ann Intern Med* 110:504, 1988.

56. deGremoux H, Monnet I, Fleury J, Chloq C: Histiocytic medullary reticulosis occurring with small cell lung carcinoma. *Eur Respir J* 4:122, 1991.

57. Noguchi M, Kawano Y, Sato N, Oshimi K: T-cell lymphoma of CD3+ CD4+ CD56+ granular lymphocytes with hemophagocytic syndrome. *Leuk Lymph* 26:349, 1997.

58. Wong K-F, Hui P-K, Chan JKC, et al: The acute lupus hemophagocytic syndrome. *Ann Intern Med* 114:387, 1991.

59. Kumakura S, Ishikura H, Umegae N, et al: Autoimmune-associated hemophagocytic syndrome. *Am J Med* 102:113, 1997.

60. Quesnel B, Catteau B, Aznar V, et al: Successful treatment of juvenile rheumatoid arthritis associated haemophagocytic syndrome by cyclosporin A with transient exacerbation by conventional-dose G-CSF. *Br J Haematol* 97:508, 1997.

61. Pecero VMGR, Marquez RL, Lerchundi MAA, Jurado AF: Phenytoin-induced hemocytophagic histiocytosis indistinguishable from malignant histiocytosis. *South Med J* 84:649, 1991.

62. Chin CS, Hui PK: Reactive hemophagocytic syndrome and Hodgkin's disease. *Am J Hematol* 55:49, 1997.

63. Watson HG, Goulden NJ, Manson ML, et al: Virus associated hemophagocytic syndrome: Further evidence for a T-cell related disorder. *Br J Haematol* 86:213, 1994.

64. Lay JD, Tsao CJ, Chen JY, et al: Upregulation of tumor necrosis factor-alpha gene by Epstein-Barr virus and activation of macrophages in Epstein-Barr virus–infected T cells in the pathogenesis of hemophagocytic syndrome. *J Clin Invest* 100:1069, 1997.

65. Baker GR, Levin J: Transient thrombocytopenia produced by administration of macrophage colony-stimulating factor: Investigations of the mechanism. *Blood* 91:89, 1998.

66. Chapoval AI, Kamdar SJ, Kremlev SG, Evans R: CSF-1 (M-CSF) differentially sensitizes mononuclear phagocyte subpopulations to endotoxin in vivo: A potential pathway that regulates the severity of gram-negative infections. *J Leuk Biol* 63:245, 1998.

67. Kaito K, Kobayashi M, Ktayama T, et al: Prognostic factors of hemophagocytic syndrome in adults: Analysis of 34 cases. *Eur J Hematol* 59:247, 1997.

68. Perel Y, Alos N, Ansoborlo S, Carrere A, Guillard JM: Dramatic efficacy of antithymocyte globulins in childhood EBV-associated haemophagocytic syndrome. *Acta Paediatr* 86:911, 1997.

69. Baldwin CL, Noris P, Loni C, Aiosa C: Hemophagocytic syndrome responding to high-dose gammaglobulin as presenting feature of sarcoidosis. *Am J Hematol* 54:88, 1997.

70. Freeman B, Rathore MH, Salman E, et al: Intravenously administered immune globulin for treatment of infection-associated hemophagocytic syndrome. *J Pediatr* 124:332, 1994.

71. Gill DS, Spencer A, Cobcroft RG: High-dose gamma-globulin therapy in the reactive haemophagocytic syndrome. *Br J Haematol* 88:204, 1994.

72. Hanai M, Takei M, Yamazaki T, et al: Successful treatment with intermittent administration of etoposide for an adult case with recurrent hemophagocytic syndrome, developed in association with chronic EB virus related lymphoid hyperplasia in the small intestine. *Rinsho Ketsueki* 38:682, 1997.

73. Rosai J, Dorfman RF: Sinus histiocytosis with massive lymphadenopathy: A newly recognized benign clinicopathologic entity. *Arch Pathol* 87:63, 1969.

74. Foucar E, Rosai J, Dorfman R: Sinus histiocytosis with massive lymphadenopathy (Rosai-Dorfman disease): Review of the entity. *Semin Diagn Pathol* 7:19, 1990.

75. Levine PH, Jahan N, Murari P, et al: Detection of human herpesvirus 6 in tissues involved by sinus histiocytosis with massive lymphadenopathy (Rosai-Dorfman disease). *J Infect Dis* 166:291, 1992.

76. Scheel MM, Rady PL, Tyring SK, Pandya AG: Sinus histiocytosis with massive lymphadenopathy: Presentation as giant granuloma annulare and detection of human herpesvirus 6. *J Am Acad Dermatol* 37:643, 1997.

77. Stastny JF, Wilkerson ML, Hamati HF, Kornstein MJ: Cytologic features of sinus histiocytosis with massive lymphadenopathy. *Acta Cytol* 41:871, 1997.

78. Eisen RN, Buckley PJ, Rosai J: Immunophenotypic characterization of sinus histiocytosis with massive lymphadenopathy. *Semin Diagn Pathol* 7:74, 1990.

79. Paulli M, Rosso R, Kindl S, et al: Immunophenotypic characterization

of the cell infiltrate in five cases of sinus histiocytosis with massive lymphadenopathy (Rosai-Dorfman disease). *Hum Pathol* 23:647, 1992.

80. Paulli M, Bergamaschi G, Tonon L, et al: Evidence for a polyclonal nature of the cells infiltrate in sinus histiocytosis with massive lymphadenopathy. *Br J Haematol* 91:415, 1995.

81. Maennle DL, Grierson HL, Gnarra DG, Weissenburger DD: Sinus histiocytosis with massive lymphadenopathy: A spectrum of disease associated with immune dysfunction. *Pediatr Pathol* 11:399, 1991.

82. Foucar E, Rosai J, Dorfman RF: Sinus histiocytosis with massive lymphadenopathy: An analysis of 14 deaths occurring in a patient registry. *Cancer* 54:1834, 1984.

83. Komp DM: The treatment of sinus histiocytosis with massive lymphadenopathy. *Semin Diagn Pathol* 7:83, 1990.

84. Baildam EM, D'Souza SW, Stevens RF: Sinus histiocytosis with massive lymphadenopathy (Rosai-Dorfman disease): Response to acyclovir. *JR Soc Med* 85:179, 1992.

85. Sita G, Guffanti A, Colombi M, et al: Rosai-Dorfman syndrome with extranodal localizations and response to glucocorticoids: A case report. *Haematologica* 81:165, 1996.

86. Antonius JI, Farid SM, Baez-Giangreco A: Steroid responsive Rosai-Dorfman disease. *Pediatr Hematol Oncol* 13:563, 1996.

87. Lohr HF, Godderz W, Wolfe T, et al: Long-term survival in a patient with Rosai-Dorfman disease treated with interferon-alpha. *Eur J Cancer* 31A:2427, 1995.

88. Palomera L, Domingo JM, Olave T, et al: Sinus histiocytosis with massive lymphadenopathy: Complete response to low-dose interferon-alpha. *J Clin Oncol* 15:2176, 1997.

89. Viraben R, Dupre A, Gourget B: Pure cutaneous histiocytosis resembling sinus histiocytosis. *Clin Exp Dermatol* 13:197, 1988.

90. Colleoni M, Gaion F, Perasole A, et al: Evidence of responsiveness to chemotherapy in aggressive Rosai-Dorfman disease. *Eur J Cancer* 31A:424, 1995.

91. Horneff G, Jurgens H, Hort W, et al: Sinus histiocytosis with massive lymphadenopathy (Rosai-Dorfman disease): Response to methotrexate and mercaptopurine. *Med Pediatr Oncol* 27:187, 1996.

92. Foucar K, Foucar E: The mononuclear phagocyte and immunoregulatory effector (M-PIRE) system: Evolving concepts. *Semin Diagn Pathol* 7:4, 1994.

93. Chu T, Jaffe R: The normal Langerhans cell and the LCH. *Br J Cancer* 70:S4, 1994.

94. Ishii E, Watanabe S: Biochemistry and biology of the Langerhans cell. *Hematol Oncol Clin North Am* 1:99, 1987.

95. Reid CDL, Fryer PR, Clifford C, et al: Identification of hematopoietic progenitors of macrophages and dendritic Langerhans cells (DL-CFU) in human bone marrow and peripheral blood. *Blood* 76:1139, 1990.

96. Birbeck MS, Breathnach AS, Eversall JD: An electron microscope study of basal melanocytes and high-level clear cells (Langerhans cells) in vitiligo. *J Invest Dermatol* 37:51, 1961.

97. Nakajima T, Watanabe S, Sato Y, et al: S-100 protein in Langerhans cells, interdigitating reticulum cells and histiocytosis X cells. *Gan* 73:429, 1982.

98. Ross R, Ross XL, Schwing J, et al: The actin-bundling protein fascin is involved in the formation of dendritic processes in maturing epidermal Langerhans cells. *J Immunol* 160:3776, 1998.

99. Kanitakis J, Fantini F, Pincelli C, et al: Neuron-specific enolase as a marker of cutaneous Langerhans cell histiocytosis. *Anticancer Res* 11:635, 1991.

100. Emile JF, Wechsler J, Brousse N, et al: Langerhans cell histiocytosis: Definitive diagnosis with the use of the monoclonal antibody 010 on routine paraffin-embedded samples. *Am J Surg Pathol* 19:626, 1995.

101. Favara BE: Langerhans cell histiocytosis: Pathobiology and pathogenesis. *Semin Oncol* 18:3, 1991.

102. Hance AJ: Accessory cell-lymphocyte interactions, in *The Lung: Scientific Foundations,* edited by RG Crystal, JB West, p 483. Raven, New York, 1991.

103. Langerhans P: Ueber die nerven der menschlichen Haut. *Virchows Arch [A]* 44:325, 1868.

104. Nezelof C, Basset F, Rousseau MF, et al: Histiocytosis X: Histogenetic arguments for a Langerhans' cell origin. *Biomedicine* 18:365, 1973.

105. Hashimoto K, Nagetsu N, Tamguchi Y, et al: Immunohistochemistry and electron microscopy in Langerhans cell histiocytosis confined to skin. *J Am Acad Dermatol* 25:1044, 1991.

106. Lichtenstein L: Histiocytosis X: Integration of eosinophilic granuloma of bone, "Letterer-Siwe disease" and "Schuller-Christian disease" as

related manifestations of a single nosologic entity. *Arch Pathol Lab Med* 56:84, 1953.

107. Otani S, Ehrlich J: Solitary granuloma of bone simulating primary neoplasm. *Am J Pathol* 16:479, 1940.

108. Goldberg NS, Bauer K, Rosen ST, et al: Histiocytosis X: Flow analysis. *Arch Dermatol* 122:446, 1986.

109. Willman CL, McClain KL: An update on clonality, cytokines, and viral etiology in Langerhans cell histiocytosis. *Hematol Oncol Clin North Am* 12:407, 1998.

110. deGraaf JH, Egeler RM: New insights into the pathogenesis of Langerhans cell histiocytosis. *Curr Opin Pediatr* 9:46, 1997.

111. Geissman F, Emile JF, Andig P, et al: Lack of expression of E-cadherin is associated with dissemination of Langerhan's cell histiocytosis and poor outcome. *J Pathol* 181:301, 1997.

112. Schmitz L, Favara BE: Nosology and pathology of Langerhans cell histiocytosis. *Hematol Oncol Clin North Am* 12:221, 1998.

113. Komp DM: Langerhans cell histiocytosis. *N Engl J Med* 316:747, 1987.

114. Carstensen H, Ornvold K: The epidemiology of LCH in Denmark: 1975–1989. *Med Pediatr Oncol* 21:387, 1993.

115. Broadbent V, Egeler RM, Nesbit ME: Langerhans cell histiocytosis: Clinical and epidemiological aspects. *Br J Cancer* 70(suppl):S11, 1994.

116. Bhatia S, Nesbit ME, Egeler RM, et al: Epidemiologic study of Langerhans cell histiocytosis in children. *J Pediatr* 130:774, 1997.

117. Arico M, Egeler RM: Clinical aspects of Langerhans cell histiocytosis. *Hematol Oncol Clin North Am* 12:247, 1998.

118. Berry DH, Gresik M, Maybee D, Marcus R: Histiocytosis X in bone only. *Med Pediatr Oncol* 18:292, 1990.

119. Bollini G, Jouve JL, Gentet JC, et al: Bone lesions in histiocytosis X. *J Pediatr Orthop* 11:469, 1991.

120. David R, Orio RA, Kumar R, et al: Radiology features of eosinophilic granuloma of bone. *A J R* 153:1021, 1989.

121. Cunningham MJ, Curtin HD, Jaffe R, Stool SE: Otologic manifestations of Langerhans cell histiocytosis. *Arch Otolaryngol Head Neck Surg* 115:807, 1989.

122. deLuna ML, Flikin I, Golberg J, et al: Benign cephalic histiocytosis. *Pediatr Dermatol* 6:198, 1989.

123. Santhosh-Kumar CR, Almomen A, Ajarim DSS, et al: Unusual skin tumors in Langerhans cell histiocytosis. *Arch Dermatol* 126:1617, 1990.

124. Camacho-Martinez F: Unusual skin tumors in Langerhans cell histiocytes. *Arch Dermatol* 127:1237, 1991.

125. DiNardo LJ, Wetmore RF: Head and neck manifestations of histiocytosis X in children. *Laryngoscope* 99:721, 1989.

126. DeVaney RO, Putzi MJ, Forlito A, Rinaldo A: Head and neck Langerhans cell histiocytosis. *Ann Otorhinolaryngol* 106:526, 1997.

127. Egeler RM, Schipper MEI, Heymans HSA: Gastrointestinal involvement in Langerhans cell histiocytosis (histiocytosis X). *Eur J Pediatr* 149:325, 1990.

128. Lee RG, Brozial RM, Stenzel P: Gastrointestinal involvement in Langerhans cell histiocytosis. *Mod Pathol* 3:154, 1990.

129. Radin DR: Langerhans cell histiocytosis of the liver: Imaging findings. *AJR* 159:63, 1992.

130. Heyn RM, Hamoudi A, Newton WA Jr: Pretreatment liver biopsy in 20 children with histiocytosis X. *Med Pediatr Oncol* 18:110, 1990.

131. Dunger DB, Broadbent V, Yeoman E, et al: The frequency and natural history of diabetes insipidus in children with Langerhans cell histiocytosis. *N Engl J Med* 321:1157, 1989.

132. O'Sullivan RM, Sheehan M, Poskett KJ, et al: Langerhans cell histiocytosis of hypothalamus and optic chiasm: CT and MR studies. *J Comput Assist Tomogr* 15:52, 1991.

133. Tabarin A, Corcuff J-B, Dautheribes M, et al: Histiocytosis X of the hypothalamus. *J Endocrinol Invest* 14:139, 1991.

134. MacCumber MW, Hoffman PN, Wand GS, et al: Ophthalmic involvement in aggressive histiocytosis X. *Ophthalmology* 97:22, 1990.

135. Nondahl SR, Finlay JL, Farrell PM, et al: A case report and literature review of "primary" pulmonary histiocytosis X of childhood. *Med Pediatr Oncol* 14:57, 1986.

136. Smith M, McCormack LJ, VanOrstran HS, Mercer RD: Primary pulmonary histiocytosis X. *Chest* 65:176, 1974.

137. Auerswald U, Barth J, Magnussen H: Value of CD-1 positive bronchoalveolar lavage fluid for the diagnosis of pulmonary histiocytosis. *Lung* 169:305, 1991.

138. Brauner MW, Granier P, Mouelki MM, et al: Pulmonary histiocytosis X: Evaluation of high-resolution CT. *Radiology* 172:255, 1989.

139. Brambilla E, Fontaine E, Pison CM, et al: Pulmonary histiocytosis X

with mediastinal lymph node involvement. *Am Rev Respir Res* 142:1216, 1990.

140. Moore ADA, Godwin JD, Muller NC, et al: Pulmonary histiocytosis X: Comparison of radiographic and CT findings. *Radiology* 172:249, 1989.

141. Soler P, Kambouchner M, Valeyre D, Hance AJ: Pulmonary Langerhans cell granulomatosis. *Ann Rev Med* 43:105, 1992.

142. Ha SY, Helms P, Fletcher M, et al: Lung involvement in Langerhans' cell histiocytosis: Prevalence, clinical features, and outcome. *Pediatrics* 89:466, 1992.

143. Tomashefski JF, Khiyami A, Kleinerman J: Neoplasms associated with eosinophilic granuloma. *Arch Pathol Lab Med* 115:499, 1991.

144. Motoi M, Helbron D, Kaiserling E, Lennert K: Eosinophilic granuloma of lymph nodes: A variant of histiocytosis X. *Histopathology* 4:585, 1980.

145. Williams JW, Dorfman RF: Lymphadenopathy as the initial manifestation of histiocytosis X. *Am J Surg Pathol* 3:405, 1979.

146. Neumann MP, Fizzera G: The coexistence of Langerhans's cell granulomatosis and malignant lymphoma may take different forms. *Hum Pathol* 17:1060, 1986.

147. Adornato BT, Eil C, Head GL, Lorioux DL: Cerebellar involvement in multifocal eosinophilic granuloma: Demonstration by computerized tomographic scanning. *Ann Neurol* 7:125, 1980.

148. Ragland RL, Moss DS, Duffis AW, et al: CT and MR findings in diffuse cerebral histiocytosis. *AJNR* 12:525, 1991.

149. Burn DJ, Watson JDG, Roddie M, et al: Langerhans' cell histiocytosis and the nervous system. *J Neurol* 239:345, 1992.

150. Axiotis CA, Merino MJ, Duray PH: Langerhans cell histiocytosis of the female genital tract. *Cancer* 67:1650, 1991.

151. Otis CN, Fischer RA, Johnson N, et al: Histiocytosis X of the vulva: A case report and review of the literature. *Obstet Gynecol* 75:555, 1990.

152. Ogburn PL, Cefalo RC, Nagel T, Okagahi T: Histiocytosis X and pregnancy. *Obstet Gynecol* 58:513, 1981.

153. Malpas JS: Langerhans cell histiocytosis in adults. *Hematol Oncol Clin North Am* 12:259, 1998.

154. McLelland J, Chu AC: Multisystem Langerhans-cell histiocytosis in adults. *Clin Exp Dermatol* 15:79, 1990.

155. Nascimento AG: A clinicopathologic and immunohistochemical comparative study of cutaneous and intramuscular forms of juvenile xanthogranuloma. *Am J Surg Pathol* 2:645, 1997.

156. Kumar BN, Walsh RM, Walter NN, Little JT: Histiocytic necrotizing lymphadenitis (Kikuchi's disease) of the cervical lymph nodes. *ORL J* 59:176, 1997.

157. Kambouchner M, Colby TV, Domenge C, et al: Erdheim-Chester disease with prominent pulmonary involvement associated with eosinophilic granuloma of mandibular bone. *Histopathology* 30:353, 1997.

158. Mullans EA, Helm TN, Taylor JS, et al: Generalized non-Langerhans cell histiocytosis: Spectrum of disease. *Int J Dermatol* 14:106, 1995.

159. Burns BF, Colby TV, Dorfman RF: Langerhans' cells granulomatosis (histiocytosis X) associated with malignant lymphomas. *Am J Surg Pathol* 7:529, 1983.

160. Almanaseer IY, Kosova L, Pellettiere EV: Composite lymphoma with immunoblastic features and Langerhans's cell granulomatosis (histiocytosis X). *Am J Clin Pathol* 85:111, 1986.

161. Colby TV, Hoppe RT, Warnke RA: Hodgkin disease: A clinicopathologic study of 659 cases. *Cancer* 49:1848, 1981.

162. Bonetti F, Knowles DM, Chilosi M, et al: A distinctive cutaneous malignant neoplasm expressing the Langerhans's cell phenotype: Synchronous occurrence of B-chronic lymphocytic leukemia. *Cancer* 55:2417, 1985.

163. Favara BE, Jaffe R: The histopathology of Langerhans cell histiocytosis. *Br J Cancer* 70(suppl XXIII):S17, 1994.

164. Shin MS, Buchalter SE, Kang-Jey H: Langerhans histiocytosis associated with Hodgkins disease. *J Natl Med Assoc* 86:65, 1994.

165. Egeler RM, Neglia JP, Pucetti DM, et al: Association of Langerhans histiocytosis with malignant neoplasms. *Cancer* 71:865, 1993.

166. Egeler RM, Neglia JP, Arico M, et al: The relationship of Langerhans cell histiocytosis to acute leukemia, lymphomas, and other solid tumors. *Hematol Oncol Clin North Am* 12:369, 1998.

167. Bramwell NH, Burns BF: Histiocytosis X of the thymus in association with myasthenia gravis. *Am J Clin Pathol* 86:224, 1986.

168. Goldberg NS: Histiocytosis X. *Arch Dermatol* 122:446, 1986.

169. Broadbent V, Gadner H: Current therapy for Langerhans cell histiocytosis. *Hematol Oncol Clin North Am* 12:327, 1998.

170. Greis PE, Hanken FM: Eosinophilic granuloma: The management of solitary lesions of bone. *Clin Orthop* 257:204, 1990.

171. Wirtschafter JD, Nesbit M, Anderson P, et al: Intralesion methylprednisoline for Langerhans cell histiocytosis of the orbit and cranium. *J Pediatr Ophthalmol Strabismus* 24:194, 1987.

172. El-Sayed S, Brewin TB: Histiocytosis X: Does radiotherapy still have a role? *Clin Oncol* 4:27, 1992.

173. Minehan KJ, Chen MG, Zimmerman D, et al: Radiation therapy for diabetes insipidus caused by Langerhans cell histiocytosis. *Int J Radia Oncol Biol Phys* 23:519, 1992.

174. Gramatovici R, D'Angio GJ: Radiation therapy in soft-tissue lesions in histiocytosis X (Langerhans cell histiocytosis). *J Med Pediatr Oncol* 16:259, 1988.

175. Hadfield PJ, Birchall MA, Albert DM: Otitis externa in Langerhans cell histiocytosis: The successful use of topical nitrogen mustard. *Int J Pediatr Otorhinolaryngol* 30:143, 1994.

176. Sheehan MP, Atherton DJ, Broadbeat V, et al: Topical nitrogen mustard: An effective treatment for cutaneous Langerhans cell histiocytosis. *J Pediatr* 119:317, 1991.

177. Sahai H, Ibe M, Takahashi H, et al: Satisfactory remission achieved by PUVA therapy in Langerhans cell histiocytosis in an elderly patient. *J Dermatol* 23:42, 1996.

178. Matsushima Y, Baba T: Resolution of cutaneous lesions of histiocytosis X by intralesional injections of interferon beta. *Int J Dermatol* 30:373, 1991.

179. Jakobson AM, Kreuger A, Harberg H, Sundstrome C: Treatment of Langerhans cell histiocytosis with alpha-interferon. *Lancet* 26:1520, 1987.

180. Munn S, Chu AC: Langerhans histiocytosis of the skin. *Hematol Oncol Clin North Am* 12:269, 1998.

181. Arceci RJ, Brenner MK, Pritchard J: Controversies and new approaches to Langerhans cell histiocytosis. *Hematol Oncol Clin North Am* 12:339, 1998.

182. Ceci A, de Terlizzi M, Collela R, et al: Langerhans cell histiocytosis in childhood: Results from the Italian cooperative AIEOP-CNR-HX83 study. *Med Pediatr Oncol* 21:265, 1993.

183. Gadner H, Heitger A, Grois N, et al: Treatment strategy for disseminated Langerhans cell histiocytosis. *Med Pediatr Oncol* 23:72, 1994.

184. Saven A, Burian C: Cladrifine activity in adult Langerhans-cell histiocytosis. *Blood* 93:4125, 1999.

185. Stine KC, Saylors RL, Williams LL, Becton DL: 2-Chlorodeoxyadenosine (2-CA) for the treatment of refractory Langerhans cell histiocytosis (LCH) in pediatric patients. *Med Pediatr Oncol* 29:288, 1997.

186. Carrera CJ, Terai C, Lotz M, et al: Potent toxicity of 2-chlorodeoxyadenosine toward human monocytes in vitro and in vivo: A novel approach to immunosuppressive therapy. *J Clin Invest* 86:1480, 1990.

187. Gorski A, Grieb P, Korczak-Kowalski G, et al: Cladribine (2-chlorodeoxyadenosine, CDA): An inhibitor of human B and T cell activation in vitro. *Immunopharmacology* 26:197, 1993.

188. Mahmound HH, Wang WC, Murphy SB: Cyclosporine therapy for advanced Langerhans cell histiocytosis. *Blood* 77:721, 1991.

189. Arico M, Colella R, Conter V, et al: Cyclosporine therapy for refractory Langerhans cell histiocytosis. *Med Pediatr Oncol* 25:12, 1995.

190. McCowage GB, Frush DP, Kurtzberg J: Successful treatment of two children in the Langerhans cell histiocytosis with 2-deoxycoformycin. *J Pediatr Hematol Oncol* 18:154, 1996.

191. Tsele E, Thomas DM, Chu AC: Treatment of adult Langerhans cell histiocytosis with etoposide. *J Am Acad Dermatol* 27:61, 1992.

192. Viana MB, Oliveria BM, Silva CM, Leite VHR: Etoposide in the treatment of six children with Langerhans cell histiocytosis (histiocytosis X). *Med Pediatr Oncol* 19:289, 1991.

193. Broadbent V, Pritchard J, Yeomans E: Etoposide (VP16) in the treatment of multisystem Langerhans cell histiocytosis (histiocytosis X). *Med Pediatr Oncol* 17:97, 1989.

194. Mayou SC, Chu AC, Munro DD, et al: Langerhans cell histiocytosis: Excellent response to etoposide. *Clin Exp Dermatol* 16:292, 1991.

195. Ladisch S, Gadner H, Arico M, et al: LCH-I: A randomized trial of etoposide versus vinblastine in disseminated Langerhans cell histiocytosis. *Med Pediatr Oncol* 23:107, 1994.

196. Bellmunt J, Albanell J, Salud A, et al: Interferon and disseminated Langerhans cell histiocytosis. *Med Pediatr Oncol* 20:336, 1992.

197. Thomas L, Ducros B, Secchi T, et al: Successful treatment of adult's Langerhans cell histiocytosis with thalidomide. *Arch Dermatol* 129:1261, 1993.

198. Misery L, Larbe B, Lyonnet S, et al: Remission of Langerhans cell histiocytosis with thalidomide treatment [letter]. *Clin Exp Dermatol* 18:48, 1993.

199. Meunier L, March Y, Ribeyre L, et al: Adult cutaneous Langerhans cell histiocytosis: Remission with thalidomide treatment [letter]. *Br J Dermatol* 132:168, 1995.

200. Gadner H, Heitger A, Grois N, et al: Treatment strategy for disseminated Langerhans cell histiocytosis. *Med Pediatr Oncol* 23:72, 1994.

201. Egeler RM, Kraher J, Voûte PA: Cytosine-arabinoside, vincristine, and prednisone in the treatment of children with disseminated Langerhans cell histiocytosis in the organ dysfunction: Experience at a single institution. *Med Pediatr Oncol* 21:265, 1993.

202. Körholz D, Jansen G, Göbel U: Treatment of relapse Langerhans cell histiocytosis by cyclosporine combined with etoposide and prednisone. *Pediatr Hematol Oncol* 14:443, 1997.

203. Minehan KJ, Chen MG, Zimmerman D, et al: Radiation therapy for diabetes insipidus caused by Langerhans cell histiocytosis. *Int J Radia Oncol Biol Phys* 23:519, 1992.

204. Broadbent V, Pritchard J: Diabetes insipidus associated with Langerhans cell histiocytosis. *Med Pediatr Oncol* 28:289, 1997.

205. Storb R, Sanders JE, Petersen FB: Marrow transplantation for treatment of multisystem progressive Langerhans cell histiocytosis. *Bone Marrow Transplant* 10:39, 1992.

206. Morgan G: Myeloablative therapy and bone marrow transplantation for Langerhans cell histiocytosis. *Br J Cancer* 70(suppl XXIII):S52, 1994.

207. Mahmoud H, Gaber O, Wang W, et al: Successful orthotopic liver transplantation in a child with Langerhans cell histiocytosis. *Transplantation* 51:278, 1991.

208. Concepcion W, Esquirel CO, Terry A, et al: Liver transplantation in Langerhans cell histiocytosis. *Semin Oncol* 18:24, 1991.

209. Scott RB, Robb-Smith AHT: Histiocytic medullary reticulosis. *Lancet* ii:194, 1939.

210. Robb-Smith AHT: Before our time: Half a century of histiocytic medullary reticulosis: A T-cell teaser? *Histopathology* 17:279, 1990.

211. Israels MCG: The reticuloses: A clinicopathologic study. *Lancet* ii:526, 1953.

212. Rappoport H: Tumors of the hemopoietic system, in *Atlas of Tumor Pathology*, p 49. Armed Forces Institute of Pathology, Washington, D.C., 1966.

213. Weiss LM, Trela MJ, Cleary ML, et al: Frequent immunoglobulin and T cell receptor rearrangements in "histiocytic" neoplasms. *Am J Pathol* 121:369, 1985.

214. Wright DH: Histiocytic malignancies, in *Malignant Lymphomas*, edited by JA Habeshaw, I Lauder, p 217. Churchill-Livingstone, Edinburgh, 1988.

215. Cattoretti G, Villa A, Vezzoni P, et al: Malignant histiocytosis: A phenotypic and genotypic investigation. *Am J Pathol* 136:1009, 1990.

216. Wilson MS, Weiss LM, Gatter KC, et al: Malignant histiocytosis: A reassessment of cases reported in 1975 based on paraffin section immunophenotyping studies. *Cancer* 66:530, 1990.

217. Aozasa K, Ohsawa M, Saeki K, et al: Histiocytic neoplasms: Immunohistochemical evaluation of their frequencies among malignant lymphoma and related conditions in Japan. *J Surg Oncol* 47:215, 1991.

218. Ornvold K, Carstensen H, Junge J, et al: Tumors classified as "malignant histiocytosis" in children are T-cell neoplasms. *APMIS* 100:558, 1992.

219. Lauritzen AF, Delsol G, Hansen NE, et al: Histiocytic sarcomas and monoblastic leukemias. *Am J Clin Pathol* 102:45, 1994.

220. Egeler RM, Schmitz L, Sonneveld P, et al: Malignant histiocytosis: A reassessment of cases formerly classified as histiocytic neoplasms and review of the literature. *Med Pediatr Oncol* 25:1, 1995.

221. Sonneveld P, VanLom K, Kappers-Klunne M, et al: Clinicopathological diagnosis and treatment of malignant histiocytosis. *Br J Haematol* 75:511, 1990.

222. Kemelow OW, Gocke CD, Kell DL, et al: True histiocytic lymphoma: A study of 12 cases based on current definition. *Leuk Lymph* 18:81, 1995.

223. Milchgrub S, Kamel OW, Wiley E, et al: Malignant histiocytic neoplasms of the small intestines. *Am J Surg Pathol* 16:11, 1992.

224. Patrizi A, Pileri S, Rivano MT, Di Lernia V: Malignant histiocytosis presenting as erythroderma. *Int J Dermatol* 29:214, 1990.

225. Hollowood K, Stamp G, Zouvani I, Fletcher CD: Extranodal follicular dendritic cell sarcoma of the gastrointestinal tract. *Am J Clin Pathol* 103:90, 1995.

226. Chan JK, Tsang WY, Ng CS, et al: Follicular dendritic cell tumors of the oral cavity. *Am J Surg Pathol* 18:148, 1994.

227. Miettinen M, Fletcher CDM, Lasota J: True histiocytic lymphoma of the small intestines. *Am J Clin Pathol* 100:285, 1993.

228. Osborne BM, Mackay B: True histiocytic lymphoma with multiple skin nodules. *Ultrastround Pathol* 18:241, 1994.

229. Fonesca R, Tefferi A, Strickler JG: Follicular dendritic cell sarcoma mimicking diffuse large cell lymphoma: A case report. *Am J Hematol* 55:148, 1997.

230. Soslow RA, Davis RE, Warnke RA, et al: True histiocytic lymphoma following therapy for lymphoblastic neoplasms. *Blood* 87:5207, 1996.

231. Rodilla CM, Acenero JF, Mayor LP, Carmona AA: True histiocytic lymphoma as a second neoplasm in a follicular centroblastic-centrocytic lymphoma. *Pathol Res Pract* 193:319, 1997.

232. Bucksky P, Favera B, Feller AC, et al: Malignant histiocytosis and large cell anaplastic (Ki-1) lymphoma in childhood: Guidelines for differential diagnosis. Report of the Histiocyte Society. *Med Pediatr Oncol* 22:200, 1994.

233. Hsu S-M, Ho Y-S, Hsu P-L: Lymphomas of true histiocytic origin. *Am J Pathol* 138:1389, 1991.

234. Laurencet FM, Chapuis B, Roux-Lombard P, et al: Malignant histiocytosis in the leukaemic stage: A new entity (M5c-AML) in the FAB classification? *Leukemia* 8:502, 1994.

235. Santiago-Schwartz F, Coppock DL, Hindenberg AA, Kern J: Identification of a malignant counterpart of the monocytic-dendritic cell progenitor in an acute myeloid leukemia. *Blood* 84: 3054, 1994.

236. Srivastava HI, Srivastava A, Srivastava MD: Phenotype, genotype and cytokine production in acute leukemia involving progenitors of dendritic Langerhans' cells. *Leuk Res* 18:499, 1994.

237. Ohno T, Sugiyama T, Furukawa H, et al: Malignant histiocytosis associate with autoimmune thrombocytopenia. *Am J Hematol* 45:244, 1994.

238. Esteve J, Rozman M, Campo E, et al: Leukemia after true histiocytic lymphoma: Another type of acute monocytic leukemia with histiocytic differentiation (AML-M5c)? *Leukemia* 9:1389, 1995.

239. Lauritzen AF, Ralfkiaer E: Histiocytic sarcoma. *Leuk Lymph* 18:73, 1995.

240. Kao W-Y, Hwang W-S: Bone marrow transplantation for malignant histiocytosis. *Transplant Proc* 24:1524, 1992.

241. Genberg M, Mark J, Hakelius L, et al: Origin and relationship between different cell types in malignant fibrous histiocytoma. *Am J Pathol* 135:1185, 1989.

242. Roholl PJM, Kleynen J, VanBasten CDH, et al: A study to analyze the origin of tumor cells in malignant fibrous histiocytoma: A multiparametric characterization. *Cancer* 56:2809, 1985.

243. Wood GS, Turner RR, Shiurba RA, et al: Human dendritic cells and macrophages: In situ immunophenotypic definition of subsets that exhibit specific morphologic and microenvironmental characteristics. *Am J Pathol* 10:323, 1985.

244. Goldring SR, Roelke MS, Petrison KK, Bhan AK: Human giant cell tumors of bone: Identification and characterization of cell types. *J Clin Invest* 79:483, 1987.

245. Roessner A, vonBassewitz DB, Schalke W, et al: Biologic characterization of human bone tumors: III. Giant cell tumor of bone. *Pathol Res Pract* 178:431, 1984.

246. Martorell M, Calaburg C, Peydro-Olaya A, et al: Fibroblast and myofibroblast participation in malignant fibrous histiocytoma of bone. *Pathol Res Pract* 184:582, 1989.

247. Fletcher CDM: Angiomatoid malignant fibrous histiocytoma. *Hum Pathol* 22:563, 1991.

248. Mantovani A: The interplay between primary and secondary cytokines: Cytokines involved in the regulation of monocyte recruitment. *Drugs* 54 (suppl 1):15, 1997.

249. Abboud CN, Rush S, Landesberg RL, et al: Characterization of the human mesenchymal GCT cell line: A model for stromal haematopoietic cell interactions. *Mol Biol Hematol* 2:321, 1992.

250. Arico M, Nichols K, Whitlock JA, et al: Familial clustering of Langerhans cell histiocytosis. *Br J Haematol* 107:883, 1999.

251. Katsas GA, Fowles TB, Evanson J, et al: Hypothalamic-pituitary abnormalities in adult patients with Langerhans cell histiocytosis. *J Clin Endocrin Metabol* 85:1370, 2000.

LIPID STORAGE DISEASES

ERNEST BEUTLER

Gaucher disease and Niemann-Pick disease are the two lipid storage disorders that are most likely to be encountered by the hematologist, because both may cause splenomegaly and cytopenias. Gaucher disease is the most common of the lipid storage diseases. It occurs among Ashkenazi Jews, the population in which it is most prevalent, at a rate of about 1 birth per 1000. Deficiency of the enzyme glucocerebrosidase results in accumulation of the glycolipid glucocerebroside in the cells of the macrophage-monocyte system. Patients with the common type 1 disease have no neurologic symptoms, but the central nervous system is involved in type 2 and type 3 disease. Diagnosis of Gaucher disease depends upon demonstration of a deficiency of glucocerebrosidase, an acid β-glucosidase, or of mutations of the glucocerebrosidase gene. Most patients with type 1 disease do not require treatment, but for those who have sufficiently severe disease manifestations, the replacement of the missing enzyme by infusions given once weekly or more frequently is a very effective but very costly therapy. Splenectomy corrects the thrombocytopenia that commonly occurs in Gaucher disease. The prognosis for patients with type I disease is usually excellent. Niemann-Pick disease is a heterogeneous group of disorders. Types A and B disease are due to deficiency of the enzyme sphingomyelinase, while types C, D, and E are due to a mutation in the NPC1 gene, a gene of unknown function which, however, appears to be involved with cholesterol transport, since not only sphingomyelin but also cholesterol accumulates in these disorders. Type A disease is associated with severe neurologic disease and patients general die during the first few years of life. Type B disease has a later onset and neurologic disease is usually absent. Type C disease is associated with neurologic symptoms as well has hepatosplenomegaly. Types D and E are probably variants of type C disease. There is currently no treatment for Niemann-Pick disease, but some patients have benefitted from liver transplantation. The sea-blue histiocyte syndrome is a heterogeneous group of disorders, characterized by the presence in the marrow of macrophages that contain granules that stain a bright blue color. These cells are found in some patients with Niemann-Pick disease, and are occasionally seen in a variety of hematologic disorders.

DEFINITIONS AND HISTORY

The lipid storage diseases are hereditary disorders in which one or more tissues become engorged with a lipid. The type of lipid and its distribution have a characteristic pattern in each disorder; this chapter will deal only with those disorders in which lipid storage in the macrophages causes major clinical manifestations. These disorders are Gaucher disease, in which glucocerebroside is stored, and Niemann-Pick disease, where the storage material is sphingomyelin and/or cholesterol.

GAUCHER DISEASE

HISTORY

Gaucher disease was first described by Philippe Gaucher, who thought that the peculiar large cells in the spleen were evidence of a primary neoplasm.[1] Although it was believed at one time that the glycolipid that accumulated in Gaucher disease was a galactocerebroside, it was shown in 1934 that actually glucocerebroside accumulated.[2] In 1965, the primary defect was recognized as the inability to degrade glucocerebroside.[3,4]

ETIOLOGY AND PATHOGENESIS

ENZYMATIC BASIS OF LYSOSOMAL STORAGE DISEASES

In the course of normal growth, development, and senescence, parts of cells or whole cells are continually replaced in all tissues. Breakdown of the complex constituents of cells requires sequential, enzymatic degradation. Such degradation takes place largely in secondary lysosomes, organelles formed by the fusion of primary lysosomes with the phagocytic vacuole containing the ingested material.

Gaucher disease is the result of a hereditary deficiency in the activity of one of the lysosomal enzymes required for glycolipid degradation, viz. glucocerebrosidase. The parent substance is either a globoside or a ganglioside (Fig. 79-1). In the degradation of globosides and gangliosides it is necessary for the carbohydrate portion to be removed before hydrolysis of the sphingosine-fatty acid complex, ceramide. Removal of carbohydrate always proceeds from the free end of the polysaccharide chain: the distal glycosidic linkage must be cleaved with removal of the terminal sugar before the other glycosidic linkages can be enzymatically hydrolyzed. In the glycolipid storage diseases, the hereditary lack of a lysosomal enzyme required for hydrolysis of one of the glycosidic bonds results in the accumulation of the glycolipid that serves as a substrate for the missing enzyme. As shown in Fig. 79-1, the absence of the β-glucosidase that cleaves glucocerebroside (glucocerebrosidase) will result in accumulation of glucocerebroside. Storage of this glycolipid results in Gaucher disease.

While Gaucher disease is almost always characterized by a deficiency of the lysosomal β-glucosidase, glucocerebrosidase,[5] in very rare instances a severe neuronopathic form of the disease occurs as a result of a deficiency of saposin, a heat-stable glucocerebrosidase cofactor.[6]

GENETIC BASIS OF GAUCHER DISEASE

The glucocerebrosidase gene is located on chromosome 1. A pseudogene has been identified about 16 kb downstream from the functional gene. Well over 100 mutations causing Gaucher disease have been described[7] [see williamshematology.com]. Most of these are point mutations, but one very common mutation represents the insertion of a single guanine at nucleotide (nt) 84 of the cDNA. Deletions, gene fusion events, and gene conversions involving the pseudogene also have been documented. In the Ashkenazi Jewish population the predominant mutation is at cDNA nucleotide 1226, where it causes an Asp→Ser substitution at amino acid 370. This mutation accounts for about 75 percent of the mutant alleles in Jewish patients and about 30 percent of the alleles in non-Jewish patients. It is relatively mild, both with respect to the amount of residual enzyme that can be detected in cells of affected individuals and in its phenotypic effect. A frameshift mutation resulting in the insertion of a guanine nucleotide at nt 84 is also common in the Jewish population and is phenotypically much more severe. The five most common mutations account for about 97 percent of the alleles in the Jewish population, but only for about 75 percent of the alleles in the non-Jewish population.[8–10] The common mutation in the Norrbottnian population (see Incidence) is at nt 1448,

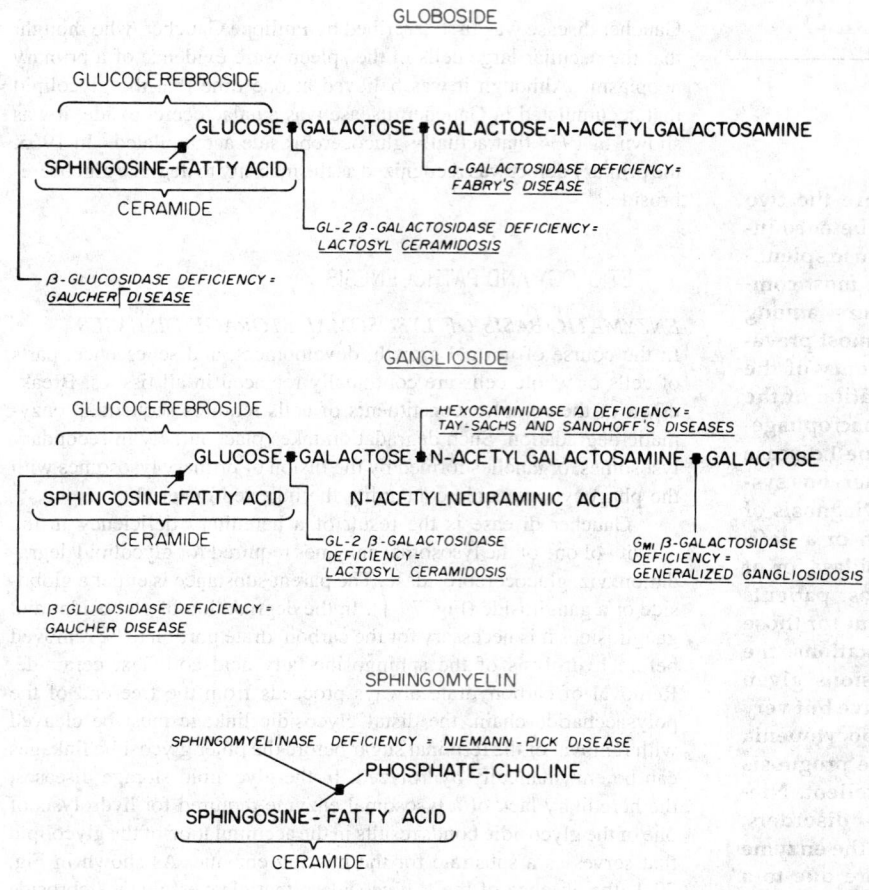

FIGURE 79-1 The structure of some of the lipids involved in lipid storage diseases. The solid squares indicate the bonds that fail to be cleaved in the diseases specified. The globosides are sometimes designated GL-1, GL-2, and so on, the number designating the number of sugar residues attached to ceramide. There are many systems of nomenclature for the gangliosides; the designation G_{M2} is commonly applied to the ganglioside that accumulates in Tay-Sachs disease.

and this mutation, which represents the normal pseudogene sequence, is also common in other ethnic groups.

INCIDENCE

Gaucher disease is inherited as an autosomal recessive disorder. It is most common in the Ashkenazi Jewish population where the gene frequency is 0.034.[9] Thus, about 6.8 percent of the Jewish population is heterozygous for Gaucher disease and the expected birth frequency is 1:1000. Gaucher disease is also relatively common in a population isolated in Norrbottnia in Northern Sweden.[11]

Gaucher disease, Niemann-Pick disease, and Tay-Sachs disease all occur with elevated frequencies among Ashkenazi Jews. The high frequency of these genes is almost certainly the result of some advantage enjoyed by heterozygotes, analogous to that found in sickle cell anemia and glucose-6-phosphate dehydrogenase deficiency among African and Mediterranean peoples. The basis for such a possible heterozygote advantage in Gaucher disease is unknown.

CLINICAL FEATURES

Three major types of Gaucher disease have been differentiated clinically.[5] All types are characterized by a deficiency of glucocerebrosidase and accumulation of glucocerebroside, but they are genetically and clinically quite distinct. Type 1 ("adult") Gaucher disease occurs

in children as well as in adults, but is clearly differentiated from types 2 (acute infantile neuronopathic) and 3 disease by the absence of neurologic symptoms. Type 2 disease is exceedingly rare, does not occur predominantly in Jewish families, and is characterized by rapid neurologic deterioration and early death. Type 3 (juvenile) Gaucher disease is a less well defined subacute neuronopathic disorder with later onset of neurologic symptoms and a better prognosis than the acute infantile neuronopathic type. The prototype of this type of the disease is the Norrbottnian form of the disorder.[11] Type 3 disease has been subdivided into three further subtypes, a, b, and c (see "Clinical Features").

The clinical manifestations of Gaucher disease are produced by the accumulation of Gaucher cells (Fig. 79-2), glucocerebroside-laden macrophages, in spleen, liver, and marrow. In type 2 and type 3 disease storage of glycolipid also occurs in the brain.

There is enormous variability in the severity of all types of Gaucher disease. Type 1 disease may be entirely asymptomatic, discovered in the course of a population survey[9] or accidentally in the course of investigation of an unrelated hematologic disorder. In those patients who do have clinical manifestations the spleen may be barely palpable or it may be massively enlarged and produce symptoms, both as a result of its great bulk and by sequestering formed elements of the blood. Chronic fatigue is a common complaint. Hepatic enlargement, like splenic enlargement, may cause mechanical symptoms and liver fibrosis accompanied by functional abnormalities and varices may develop. In children, growth retardation is common. Severe pulmonary disease with cyanosis and clubbing occurs in some patients with advanced liver involvement, probably because of shunting through the lung secondary to the liver disease. Direct involvement of the lungs with Gaucher cells also has been observed.[12,13] Pulmonary hypertension occurs in some patients and has been noted particularly after enzyme replacement therapy has been initiated.[14-18]

Skeletal lesions are often widespread. Patchy areas of bone demineralization and areas of infarction are found, and widening of the distal femur gives rise to a typical "Erlenmeyer flask" deformity (Fig. 79-3). Bone pain is probably the most troublesome clinical manifestation of Gaucher disease. Pain may occur anywhere. It generally has a deep, somewhat dull character and may be very severe. Bone pain may occur in areas with no involvement detectable by x-ray examination. It may last for weeks or months but usually subsides spontaneously, only to reappear later in the same or in another location. Aseptic necrosis of the femoral heads and vertebral collapse are particularly common, crippling complications.[19,20]

Many organs other than the liver, spleen, and bones may be affected. Brownish masses of Gaucher cells have been reported to occur at the corneoscleral limbus of the eye.[21] Gaucher cells have been found in a colonic polyp[22] and the maxillary sinus.[23] Fever may occur in patients in whom a meticulous search fails to reveal evidence of infection often[24,25] but not always[26] in connection with bone crises,[24,25] and hypermetabolism has been documented.[27] Severe neonatal ichthyosis ("collodion babies") has been described in infants with acute neuronopathic Gaucher disease.[28]

Neurologic symptoms are the hallmark of type 2 and type 3 disease. Particularly notable are oculomotor abnormalities, hypertonia of the neck muscles with extreme arching of the neck (opistotonus), bulbar signs, limb rigidity, seizures, and sometime choreoathetoid movements. Patients with type 3a[29] disease have progressive neurologic disease dominated by myoclonus and dementia; those with 3b[29] disease have aggressive visceral and skeletal disease, but with neurologic manifestations largely limited to horizontal supranuclear gaze palsy; those with type 3c disease[30-34] have neurologic manifestations largely limited to horizontal supranuclear gaze palsy, corneal opacities, and cardiac valve calcification, but generally have little visceral disease.

Neoplastic disorders are somewhat more common in patients with Gaucher disease than in the general population.[35] Especially notable are lymphoproliferative diseases including chronic lymphocytic leukemia,[24,36-38] multiple myeloma,[39-43] lymphoma,[44] and Hodgkin disease.[45,46] The existence of monoclonal immunoglobulin spikes in the serum also has been documented in a high proportion of patients with Gaucher disease who are more than 50 years of age.[47-50] Cohort control studies showed that the risk of hematologic neoplasms in Gaucher disease patients was 14.7 (confidence limits 5.2–41.7) times that of control subjects.[51]

LABORATORY FEATURES

THE BLOOD

The blood of patients with Gaucher disease may be normal or may manifest effects of hypersplenism. A normocytic, normochromic anemia is frequently present, but hemoglobin levels only uncommonly fall below 8 g/dl. A modest reticulocytosis is often present in anemic patients. The white cell count may be decreased to levels as low as $1000/\mu l$, although milder degrees of leukopenia are much more

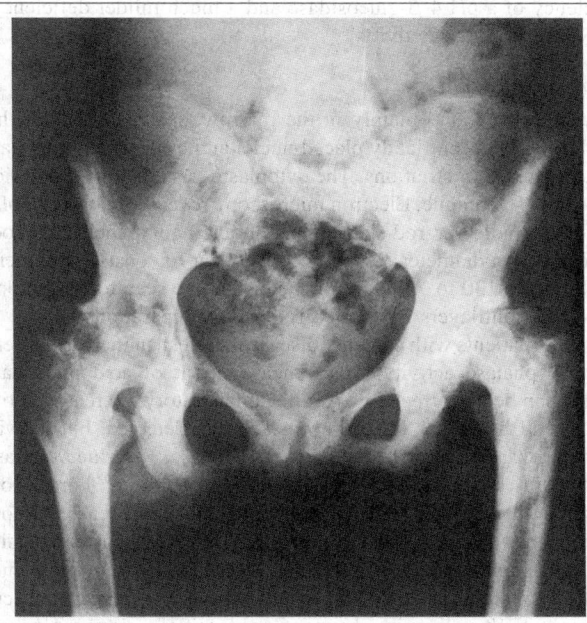

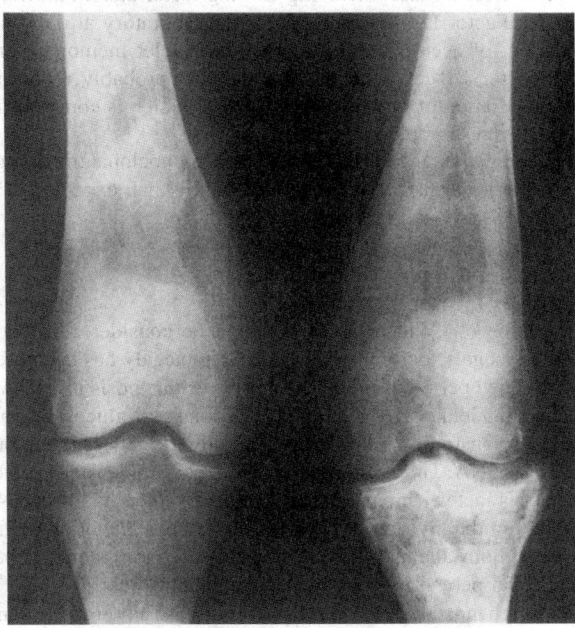

FIGURE 79-3   X-rays of distal femora and pelvis of a 27-year-old woman with Gaucher disease. The distal femur shafts are flared with thinning bone trabeculae, scattered sclerotic zones, and bone infarcts. The most extensive changes are seen in the left tibia proximally. The pelvis and upper femurs demonstrate extensive cystic and sclerotic changes with collapse of both femoral heads and of the right acetabulum. (X-rays courtesy of Dr. Hyman Gildenhorn, City of Hope Medical Center.)

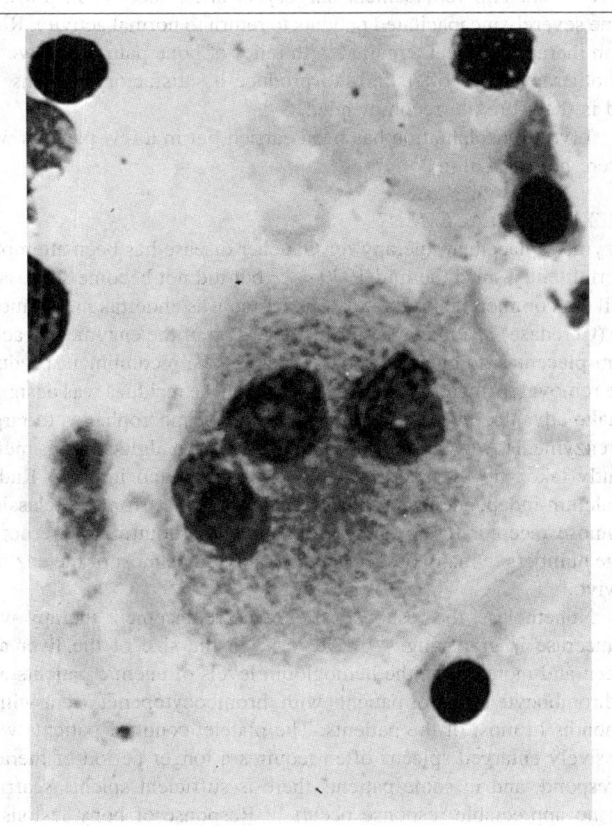

FIGURE 79-2   A Gaucher disease cell from the marrow (×915).

common. The differential count is normal, but a defect of leukocyte chemotaxis[52] that is corrected by enzyme replacement therapy[53] has been reported. Thrombocytopenia may become quite severe. If splenectomy has been carried out, severe anisocytosis and poikilocytosis occur, with many target cells, some nucleated red cells, and Howell-Jolly bodies usually being present. In splenectomized patients the white cell count and platelet count may be higher than normal. Biochemical examination of leukocytes for β-glucosidase activity shows a severe deficiency of a pH 4 β-glucosidase and a much milder deficiency of pH 5 β-glucosidase activity.[54,55]

GAUCHER CELLS

Gaucher cells, found mainly in the marrow, spleen, and liver, have small, usually eccentrically placed nuclei and cytoplasm with characteristic crinkles or striations. The cytoplasm is stained by the periodic acid–Schiff technique. Electron microscopy reveals that the cytoplasm contains spindle- or rod-shaped, membrane-bound inclusion bodies 0.6 to 4 μm in diameter. These bodies appear to consist of numerous small tubules 130 to 750 Å in diameter that are seen to be composed of twisted multilayers in negatively stained preparations.[56,57]

Most patients with Gaucher disease manifest an increase in serum acid phosphatase activity. Since measurement of acid phosphatase activity can be performed in any clinical laboratory, increased activity of this acid hydrolase is the one most often detected, but activities of other hydrolases such as β-hexosaminidase,[58] β-glucuronidase,[58] angiotensin-converting enzyme,[61] and chitotriosidase[59,60] are also increased in the serum of most patients with Gaucher disease. Although it has been suggested that the latter may be a particularly sensitive indicator of disease activity, side-by-side comparison with angiotensin-converting enzyme and acid phosphatase shows it to have no particular advantage.[62] When liver involvement is extensive, various biochemical stigmata of liver disease, including clotting factor abnormalities, may be present. Factor IX deficiency may be a laboratory artifact related to the effect of accumulated lipid on the platelet membrane on the assay.[63] Factor XI deficiency is common but probably represents a chance association of two disorders, each of which is common in the Ashkenazi Jewish population.[64]

In older patients with Gaucher disease, monoclonal immunoglobulins are found in the plasma more frequently than expected.[47,48]

DIFFERENTIAL DIAGNOSIS

DIAGNOSIS

The diagnosis of Gaucher disease should be considered in patients with splenomegaly, particularly if the splenomegaly has been present for an extended period of time. The definitive diagnosis is established by determining leukocyte[54] or cultured fibroblast[65] β-glucosidase activity or by demonstrating the presence of known Gaucher mutations in the patient's DNA. The latter method of diagnosis can usually establish the diagnosis in Jewish patients, but cannot exclude it: if the DNA is examined for the five most common mutations, mutations will be detected on both alleles in about 97 percent of the patients,[8] but in only about 55 percent of the non-Jewish patients.[66,67]

Although most patients with Gaucher disease have readily demonstrable Gaucher cells in their marrow, and the diagnosis has often been established by performing a marrow examination, determination of the β-glucosidase activity is the preferred method of diagnosis.[66] The number of these cells may be relatively small, and thorough examination of the marrow film under a low-power objective may be required to find them. Cells indistinguishable by light microscopy from typical Gaucher cells are also found in patients with hematologic abnormalities, including those with chronic myelogenous leukemia,[68,69] Hodgkin disease,[70] multiple myeloma,[71] and AIDS.[72] These patients do not lack the capacity to catabolize glucocerebroside,[73] but the great inflow of globoside into phagocytic cells exceeds their normal capacity to hydrolyze this glycolipid. Prenatal diagnosis of Gaucher disease may be established by examining cultured amniocentesis cells for their β-glucosidase activity[65] and examining the DNA for mutations.

Measurement of serum acid phosphatase activity and angiotensin converting activity are useful in confirming the diagnosis of Gaucher disease.

HETEROZYGOTE DETECTION

Heterozygotes for Gaucher disease have neither Gaucher cells in their marrow nor other stigmata of the disease. Existence of a carrier state can be established in many cases by assaying leukocytes[54,74,75] or fibroblasts[65] for β-glucosidase activity and demonstrating the reduction in the activity of the enzyme to about one-half of normal. However, regardless of the method used, there is an overlap between the measured enzyme activity in heterozygous individuals and the normal range. Definitive diagnosis of the heterozygous state can only be established by DNA analysis.

THERAPY

SYMPTOMATIC TREATMENT

Thrombocytopenia and leukopenia in Gaucher disease are more frequently the consequence of hypersplenism than of marrow replacement by Gaucher cells. These cytopenias respond very satisfactorily to splenectomy. However, the pathophysiology of Gaucher disease suggests that splenectomy be avoided as long as possible. The body must continue to metabolize all of the globoside that is formed; after the spleen has been removed, the glucocerebroside that accumulates as the result of incomplete globoside metabolism is deposited in the liver and marrow. Bone lesions may progress more rapidly following surgical removal of the spleen,[76–78] but this impression is difficult to quantitate and cannot be verified experimentally, and no worsening of bone lesions after splenectomy could be documented in one study.[35] Conservatism is advised, however, in recommending splenectomy. Partial splenectomy has been introduced in an attempt to preserve a glycolipid-sequestering site.[79] The results of such surgery have been reported in a number of patients[80–89] without conclusive data being obtained regarding the merits of the procedure.[90]

When bone lesions result in fractures, orthopedic procedures may be required. Hip replacement surgery is often successful, allowing some severely incapacitated patients to return to normal activity. Radiation therapy has been credited with relief of bone pain.[91,92] However, radiotherapy more often fails to produce a satisfactory response[93,94] and is therefore not recommended.

Liver transplantation has been carried out in a few patients with severe hepatic failure.[95–98]

ENZYME REPLACEMENT

Enzyme replacement therapy for Gaucher disease has been attempted intermittently since the mid-1970s[99–102] but did not become successful until the commercial production of enzyme was undertaken. Alglucerase (Ceredase) is a mannose-terminated form of the enzyme extracted from placenta. Imiglucerase (Cerezyme) is the recombinant product. The removal of sugars to expose inner mannose residues was designed to take advantage of the mannose receptor of macrophages to target the enzyme. However, it has been established that alglucerase is inefficiently taken up by macrophages both in vivo and in vitro. Rather a calcium-independent mannose receptor, distinct from the classical mannose receptor found on macrophages, is ubiquitously present in large numbers in many tissues and probably binds most of the enzyme in vivo.[103]

Nonetheless, the response to enzyme replacement therapy with alglucerase is gratifying.[104–111] Decrease in the size of the liver and spleen and increases in the hemoglobin levels of anemic patients and of thrombocyte levels of patients with thrombocytopenia occur within 6 months in most of the patients. The platelet count of patients with massively enlarged spleens often requires a longer period of therapy to respond, and in some patients there is sufficient splenic scarring that no appreciable response occurs.[112] Response of bony lesions is much slower than that of visceral lesions, but improvement may be evident after treatment for about 2 years, regardless of the dose that is used.[62,107,113–115] However, the expense of the preparation is daunting, particularly when administered by the high-dose/low-frequency schedule (60 units/kg every 2 weeks) recommended by the manufacturer and by some investigators.[116] Enzyme alone, given on this schedule to an average adult, costs one-half million dollars per year. Giving enzyme infusions one to three times weekly requires much less enzyme and is therefore much more economical. One unit per kilogram every day or 2.3 units/kg three times weekly has been shown to be fully as effective as a dose more than four times as large given every 2 weeks.[117] This greater effectiveness of small doses is expected for a preparation for which a few high-affinity and many lower-affinity receptors compete. Moreover, the intracellular life span of alglucerase is very short, so that infrequent administration provides therapeutic levels for only a very small proportion of the time. Even one-half of this dose was found to be fully effective in most or all patients.[118,119] The practicality and effectiveness of frequent administration of alglucerase has been questioned,[120,121] but the results obtained have been amply confirmed,[107–109,122,123] and home therapy with alglucerase has been shown to be feasible and safe.[124]

In view of the very high cost of alglucerase and imiglucerase, the fact that experience with the preparation is, as yet, somewhat limited with unknown risks, and because anaphylaxis has occurred in at least one patient, use of the preparation should be reserved for patients with relatively severe disease. These would include patients with marked organomegaly, severe or moderately severe cytopenias, or patients with extensive skeletal involvement. At present, alglucerase therapy of the many patients who have clinically mild disease cannot be endorsed, even though it is recognized that some of these patients may develop aseptic necrosis of the femoral head in an unpredictable fashion. The normal starting dose for patients who do need treatment is 3.75 to 7.5 units/kg body weight given weekly.

MARROW TRANSPLANTATION

Because the macrophage is a descendant of the hematopoietic stem cell, allogeneic marrow transplantation might be expected to cure Gaucher disease. This has, indeed, been accomplished several times.[11,60,125–131] Although some enthusiasm has been expressed for this approach,[127] the very considerable short-term risk of marrow transplantation markedly limits the number of patients who might be suitable candidates for this therapeutic approach. The availability of effective enzyme replacement therapy further limits the appropriateness of marrow transplantation. However, because of its lower cost and the potential for cure, transplantation may occasionally be considered for the management of severe Gaucher disease.

GENE THERAPY

Autologous transplantation after gene transfer into hematopoietic cells has received considerable attention as a possible alternative form of therapy.[132–136] Despite some exaggerated claims, there is no credible evidence of benefit to any patient; in vivo studies showed that, at best, 1:2000 cells carried the transgene.

OTHER THERAPIES

Decreasing globoside inflow by repeated phlebotomy has not yielded clinically significant results,[137] probably because most of the glucocerebroside is formed from sequestered white cells. Splenic transplantation was attempted in one patient, without success.[138] The possibility that inhibitors of ceramide formation in experimental animals might be effective treatment has been suggested,[139–141] but no clinical trials have been conducted.

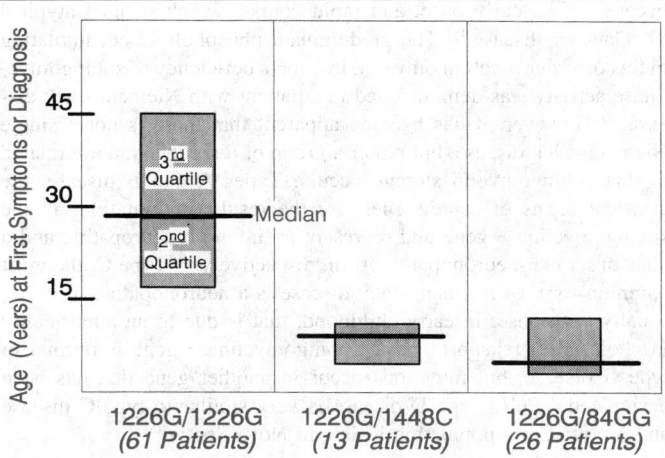

FIGURE 79-4   The median and second and third quartiles of the distribution of the age of first symptoms of diagnosis of Gaucher disease in patients with three different genotypes. (Permission from *Science*. Beutler E: Gaucher disease: New molecular approaches to diagnosis and treatment. *Science* 256:794–799, 1992)

COURSE AND PROGNOSIS

The age of onset, severity of clinical manifestations, and degree of progression are related to the genotype of the patient. Patients with the 1226G/1226G genotype tend to have late-onset disease (Fig. 79-4), relatively mild manifestations, and virtually no progression of disease during adult life. In contrast, patients who have the 1226G/84GG, 1226G/1448C, 1226G/IVS2(+1) genotypes tend to have much earlier onset of disease, usually in the first decade of life, and show gradual progression even during adult life.[62,142] Patients who are homozygous for the 1448C mutations generally develop neurologic symptoms, but some possible exceptions have been noted.[143,144]

Although the genotype of the patient does provide a guide to the prognosis, there is, unfortunately, much variability among patients with the same genotype, even between sibs. Other, as yet unknown, genetic or environmental factors are important in determining the actual course of the disease in an individual patient. However, it is important to understand that, whatever the genotype, the severity of the disease does not change after early childhood.[62,142,145] Progression, when it does occur, is gradual, except of course, insofar that complications such as aseptic necrosis and collapse of vertebrae may represent acute events.

In severely affected patients with type 1 disease or those with type 3 disease, death may occur as a result of liver disease, bleeding, or sepsis. In type 2 disease death usually is due to the neurologic manifestations and occurs in the first or second year of life. This type of disease can be fatal in the perinatal period.[146] The fact that no patient homozygous for the 84GG mutation has ever been encountered, in spite of the relative high frequency with which this mutation occurs in the Jewish population suggests that a total lack of glucocerebrosidase may not be compatible with extrauterine life. This deduction is supported by the fact that a "knockout" mouse that has been deprived of a gene for glucocerebrosidase is not capable of extrauterine life.[147]

NIEMANN-PICK DISEASE

HISTORY AND CLASSIFICATION

Niemann, a Berlin pediatrician, reported the case of an infant who died at 18 months of age with a disorder that seemed to be unique because of its early onset and rapid course, which seemed atypical for Gaucher disease.[148] The predominant phospholipid accumulating in this disorder is sphingomyelin. In 1966 a deficiency of sphingomyelinase activity was demonstrated in a patient with Niemann-Pick disease.[149] However, it has become apparent that there is not a single Niemann-Pick disease, but rather a group of disorders that are related in that sphingomyelin storage occurs. Types A and B disease, the classical forms of the disorder, are the results of mutations in the sphingomyelinase gene and represent an infantile neuropathic and a later-onset non-neuronopathic form, respectively.[150] Type C, the most common form of Niemann-Pick disease is a neuronopathic disorder, usually with onset in early childhood, that is due to an abnormality in cholesterol transport.[151] The sphingomyelinase gene is normal in type C disease, but mutations occur in another gene that has been designated *NPC1*. Type D disease is very similar to type C disease and is found in a population isolate in Nova Scotia.[151]

ETIOLOGY AND PATHOGENESIS

Types A and B disease are autosomal recessive diseases caused by mutations of the gene for sphingomyelinase[152,153] required to cleave the bond between ceramide and phosphorylcholine (see Fig. 79-1). Nonsense mutations seem to cause the more severe type A disease while missense mutations are found in the milder type B disorder.[152] Although sphingomyelinase is believed to be a part of an apoptosis-signaling pathway by generating ceramide from sphingomyelin,[154] no relationship between the disease manifestations and this pathway has been established.

Types C and D disease also show autosomal recessive inheritance and are caused by mutations in a gene that has been designated *NPC1*,[155] the function of which is not fully understood, but that presumably plays a role in cholesterol transport and homeostasis.[156] A naturally occurring murine model of the disease exists.[157]

PATHOLOGY AND CLINICAL MANIFESTATIONS

The most characteristic histopathologic feature of the various forms of Niemann-Pick disease is the presence of foam histiocytes (Fig. 79-5). These cells are found mainly in lymphoid tissues, but they may be present throughout the body. The foam cells contain largely sphingomyelin and cholesterol, the storage of cholesterol being more prominent in type C disease.

Type A Niemann-Pick disease is an affliction of infancy. During the first months of life, affected infants gain weight poorly, the abdomen enlarges, and development is delayed. They usually do not learn to sit and lose those capabilities already achieved. They may become blind and deaf. Some infants have a protracted course of jaundice of unknown cause. During the second year of life, the child lies still with nearly flaccid hyporeflexic extremities, an abdomen enlarged with enormous spleen and liver, mild lymphadenopathy, and often a fine xanthomatous rash. Bone lesions may be present but are less prominent than in Gaucher disease. Patients with type B disease generally present in the first decade of life with hepatosplenomegaly, but in mild cases abnormalities may not be noted until adult life. Neurologic manifestations are usually absent; pulmonary infiltrates are common. Sea-blue histiocytes are sometimes found in the marrow, and a number of patients have been diagnosed as having sea-blue histiocytosis before a deficiency in sphingomyelinase was demonstrated to be present.[158] Patients with type C disease often have neonatal jaundice, develop normally in early childhood, and then develop dementia, ataxia, dysarthria, dystonia, and seizures. Hepatosplenomegaly is often, but not always, present.[151]

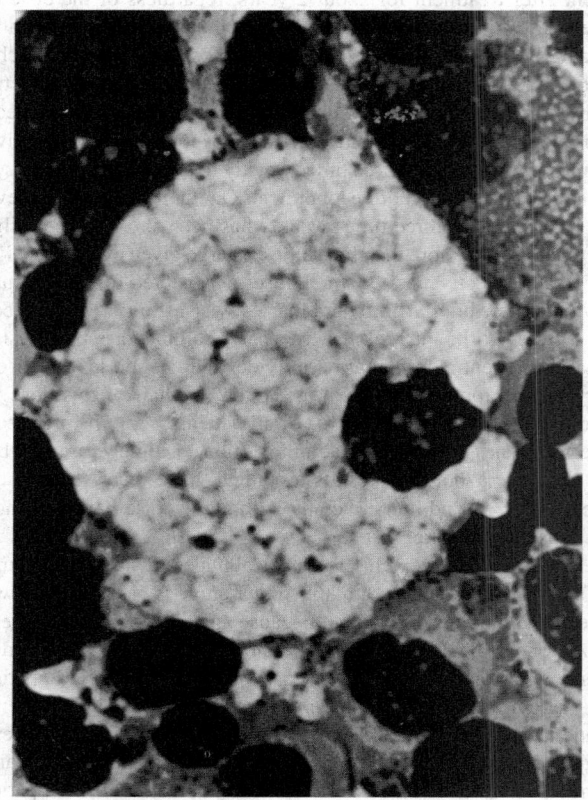

FIGURE 79-5   A foam cell from the marrow of a patient with Niemann-Pick disease (×875).

LABORATORY FEATURES AND DIFFERENTIAL DIAGNOSIS

The hemoglobin concentration of the blood may be normal, or mild anemia may be present. Typically, approximately 75 percent of the blood lymphocytes contain one to nine vacuoles. These measure approximately 2 μm in diameter. Electron microscopy reveals that these vacuoles are lipid-filled lysosomes.[159]

The marrow contains typical foam cells ranging in size from 20 to 100 μm in diameter and containing small droplets throughout the cytoplasm (Fig. 79-5). The cytoplasm of these cells stains only very faintly with the periodic acid–Schiff reagent. Phase microscopy of unstained preparations clearly reveals droplets in the cytoplasm of Niemann-Pick foam cells that distinguishes them from Gaucher cells. In polarized light the droplets may be birefringent, and in ultraviolet light they manifest a greenish-yellow fluorescence.[160] Foam cells resembling those seen in Niemann-Pick disease also are observed in generalized gangliosidosis, and foamy histiocytes, primarily involving the bone, are seen in the rare Erdheim-Chester disease, a non-Langerhans form of histiocytosis.[161] Occasionally the storage cells in Gaucher disease may present a somewhat vacuolated appearance and thereby be misinterpreted. The occurrence of sea-blue histiocytes in the spleen and marrow has been documented.[158,162-164]

Types A and B Niemann-Pick disease can be distinguished from other disorders by identification of the lipid as sphingomyelin and by demonstration of sphingomyelinase deficiency in leukocytes or in cultured fibroblasts. Heterozygotes may be detected by measurement of sphingomyelinase activity of cultured fibroblasts.[165] Prenatal diagnosis by amniocentesis has been achieved.[165,166] An artificial substrate that is very useful for the measurement of sphingomyelinase activity has been introduced.[167,168] In type C disease studies of cholesterol uptake by cultured fibroblasts is diagnostic[169] but cumbersome and not readily available. The identification of the *NPC1* gene,[155] the diagnosis of this type of disease, should be facilitated.

TREATMENT

There is no effective treatment for Niemann-Pick disease. Splenectomy is only rarely required, because death usually occurs from other manifestations of the disease before hypersplenism becomes clinically important. Liver transplantation was carried out with encouraging results.[97] Repeated implantations of amniotic epithelial cells as a source of exogenous sphingomyelinase has been claimed to be associated with clinical improvement.[170]

COURSE AND PROGNOSIS

The prognosis in type A Niemann-Pick disease is very poor; death nearly always occurs before the third year of life.[150] Patients with type B disease may survive into childhood or adult life.[150] Patients with type C disease usually die in the second decade of life.[151]

SEA-BLUE HISTIOCYTE SYNDROME

HISTORY

According to Sawitsky et al,[171] Moeschlin, in his 1947 book on splenic puncture, described a 29-year-old man with unexplained splenomegaly whose spleen contained macrophages with closely packed granules colored deep azure blue with May-Grünwald stain. He named these *blauen pigmentmakrophagen* (blue pigment macrophages). These cells have subsequently been found in marrow as well as spleen, and in 1954 Sawitsky et al[172] suggested that two cases they observed and Moeschlin's might represent a syndrome.

ETIOLOGY AND PATHOGENESIS

Although sea-blue histiocytes are found in Niemann-Pick disease, presumably and particularly in the type B disorder, sea-blue histiocytes are also found in patients who do not have any well-defined disorder. They have been reported in the marrow of patients with immune thrombocytopenic purpura,[173] in patients receiving parenteral nutrition,[174] and in patients with chronic myelogenous leukemia,[175] as well as patients with Niemann-Pick disease.[162–164,176]

CLINICAL FEATURES

In patients without other underlying disorders, the sea-blue histiocyte syndrome is often characterized by hepatosplenomegaly and thrombocytopenia and usually by a mild chronic course. Most patients are below the age of 40 when diagnosed, and there is usually not a clear family history.[171]

THERAPY, COURSE, AND PROGNOSIS

There is no treatment except that which can be offered for the underlying disease. In cases associated with parenteral nutrition, there has been improvement when the dose was decreased. In those cases in which there is no known cause the course is generally a chronic, stable one.[171]

REFERENCES

1. Gaucher PCE: De l'epithelioma primitif de la rate, hypertrophie idiopathique del la rate san leucémie. *Thesis, Paris* 1882.

2. Aghion H: *La maladie de Gaucher dans l'enfance. PhD thesis,* Paris, 1934.

3. Brady RO, Kanfer JN, Shapiro D: Metabolism of glucocerebrosides: II. Evidence of an enzymatic deficiency in Gaucher's disease. *Biochem Biophys Res Commun* 18:221, 1965.

4. Patrick AD: Short communications: A deficiency of glucocerebrosidase in Gaucher's disease. *Biochem J* 97:17C, 1965.

5. Beutler E, Grabowski G: Gaucher disease, in Scriver CR, et al. *The Metabolic and Molecular Bases of Inherited Disease,* 8th ed, McGraw-Hill, New York, 2000.

6. Schnabel D, Schröder M, Sandhoff K: Mutation in the sphingolipid activator protein 2 in a patient with a variant of Gaucher disease. *FEBS Lett* 284:57, 1991.

7. Beutler E, Gelbart T: Hematologically important mutations: Gaucher disease. *Blood Cell Mol Dis* 24:2, 1998.

8. Beutler E, Gelbart T, Kuhl W, Zimran A, West C: Mutations in Jewish patients with Gaucher disease. *Blood* 79:1662, 1992.

9. Beutler E, Nguyen NJ, Henneberger MW, et al: Gaucher disease: Gene frequencies in the Ashkenazi Jewish population. *Am J Hum Genet* 52:85, 1993.

10. Beutler E, Gelbart T: Gaucher disease mutations in non-Jewish patients. *Br J Haematol* 85:401, 1993.

11. Svennerholm L, Erikson A, Groth CG, Ringdén O, Månsson J-E: Norrbottnian type of Gaucher disease: Clinical, biochemical and molecular biology aspects: Successful treatment with bone marrow transplantation. *Dev Neurosci* 13:345, 1991.

12. Smith RL, Hutchins GM, Sack GH Jr, Ridolfi RL: Unusual cardiac, renal and pulmonary involvement in Gaucher's disease. Interstitial glucocerebroside accumulation, pulmonary hypertension and fatal bone marrow embolization. *Am J Med* 65:352, 1978.

13. Schneider EL, Epstein CJ, Kaback MJ, Brandes D: Severe pulmonary involvement in adult Gaucher's disease. *Am J Med* 63:475, 1977.

14. Belmatoug N, Launay O, Carbon C, Comité Évaluat Traitement Malad Gaucher: Pulmonary hypertension in type 1 Gaucher's disease. *Lancet* 352:240, 1998.

15. Elstein D, Klutstein MW, Lahad A, et al: Echocardiographic assessment of pulmonary hypertension in Gaucher's disease. *Lancet* 351:1544, 1998.

16. Harats D, Pauzner R, Elstein D, et al: Pulmonary hypertension in two patients with type I Gaucher disease while on alglucerase therapy. *Acta Haematol (Basel)* 98:47, 1997.

17. Dawson A, Elias DJ, Rubenson D, et al: Development of pulmonary hypertension after alglucerase therapy in two patients with hepatopulmonary syndrome complicating type 1 Gaucher disease. *Ann Intern Med* 125:901, 1996.

18. Kerem E, Elstein D, Abrahamov A, et al: Pulmonary function abnormalities in type I Gaucher disease. *Eur Respir J* 9:340, 1996.

19. Elstein D, Itzchaki M, Mankin HJ: Skeletal involvement in Gaucher's disease. *Baillieres Clin Haematol* 10:793, 1997.

20. Lachiewicz PF: Gaucher's disease. *Orthop Clin North Am* 15:765, 1984.

21. Petrohelos M, Tricoulis D, Kotsiras I, Vouzoukos A: Ocular manifestations of Gaucher's disease. *Am J Ophthalmol* 80:1006, 1975.

22. Henderson JM, Gilinsky NH, Lee EY, Greenwood MF: Gaucher's disease complicated by bleeding esophageal varices and colonic infiltration by Gaucher cells. *Am J Gastroenterol* 86:346, 1991.

23. Schwartz MR, Weycer JS, McGavran MH: Gaucher's disease involving the maxillary sinuses. *Arch Otolaryngol Head Neck Surg* 114:203, 1988.

24. Amstutz HC, Carey EJ: Skeletal manifestations and treatment of Gaucher's disease. *J Bone Joint Surg [Am]* 48:670, 1966.

25. Draznin SZ, Singer K: Legg-Perthes' disease: A syndrome of many etiologies? With clinical and roentgenographic findings in a case of Gaucher's disease. *Am J Roentgenol* 60:490, 1948.

26. Billings AA, Post M, Shapiro CM: Febrile reaction of Gaucher's disease. *Ill Med J* 145:222, 1973.

27. Barton DJ, Ludman MD, Benkov K, Grabowski GA, LeLeiko NS: Resting energy expenditure in Gaucher's disease type 1: Effect of Gaucher's cell burden on energy requirements. *Metabolism* 38:1238, 1989.

28. Fujimoto A, Tayebi N, Sidransky E: Congenital ichthyosis preceding neurologic symptoms in two sibs with type 2 Gaucher disease. *Am J Med Genet* 59:356, 1995.

29. Patterson MC, Horowitz M, Abel RB, et al: Isolated horizontal supranu-

clear gaze palsy as a marker of severe systemic involvement in Gaucher's disease. *Neurology* 43:1993, 1993.

30. Uyama E, Takahashi K, Owada M, et al: Hydrocephalus, corneal opacities, deafness, valvular heart disease, deformed toes and leptomeningeal fibrous thickening in adult siblings: A new syndrome associated with beta-glucocerebrosidase deficiency and a mosaic population of storage cells. *Acta Neurol Scand* 86:407, 1992.

31. Abrahamov A, Elstein D, Gross-Tsur V, et al: Gaucher's disease variant characterised by progressive calcification of heart valves and unique genotype. *Lancet* 346:1000, 1995.

32. Chabas A, Cormand B, Grinberg D, et al: Unusual expression of Gaucher's disease: Cardiovascular calcifications in three sibs homozygous for the D409H mutation. *J Med Genet* 32:740, 1995.

33. Beutler E, Kattamis C, Sipe J, Lipson M: The 1342C mutation in Gaucher's disease. *Lancet* 346:1637, 1995.

34. Mistry PK: Genotype/phenotype correlations in Gaucher's disease. *Lancet* 346:982, 1995.

35. Lee RE: The Pathology of Gaucher Disease, in *Gaucher Disease: A Century of Delineation and Research*, p 177. Alan R. Liss, New York, 1982.

36. Chang-Lo M, Yam LT, Rubenstone AI, Schwartz SO: Gaucher's disease associated with chronic lymphocytic leukaemia, gout and carcinoma. *J Pathol* 116:203, 1975.

37. Mark T, Dominguez C, Rywlin AM: Gaucher's disease associated with chronic lymphocytic leukemia. *South Med J* 75:361, 1982.

38. Kaufman S, Rozenfeld V, Yona R, Varon M: Gaucher's disease associated with chronic lymphocytic leukaemia. *Clin Lab Haematol* 8:321, 1986.

39. Garfinkel D, Sidi Y, Ben-Bassat M, et al: Coexistence of Gaucher's disease and multiple myeloma. *Arch Intern Med* 142:2229, 1982.

40. Lamon J, Miller W, Tavassoli M, Longmire R, Beutler E: Specialty conference: Multiple myeloma complicating Gaucher's disease. *West J Med* 136:122, 1982.

41. Ruestow PC, Levinson DJ, Catchatourian R, et al: Coexistence of IgA myeloma and Gaucher's disease. *Arch Intern Med* 140:1115, 1980.

42. Benjamin D, Joshua H, Djaldetti M, Hazaz B, Pinkhas J: Nonsecretory IgD-kappa multiple myeloma in a patient with Gaucher's disease. *Scand J Haematol* 22:179, 1979.

43. Gal R, Gukovsky-Oren S, Floru S, Djaldetti M, Kessler E: Sequential appearance of breast carcinoma, multiple myeloma and Gaucher's disease. *Haematologica (Pavia)* 73:63, 1988.

44. Paulson JA, Marti GE, Fink JK, et al: Richter's transformation of lymphoma complicating Gaucher's disease. *Hematol Pathol* 3:91, 1989.

45. Bruckstein AH, Karanas A, Dire JJ: Gaucher's disease associated with Hodgkin's disease. *Am J Med* 68:610, 1980.

46. Cho SY, Sastre M: Coexistence of Hodgkin's disease and Gaucher's disease. *Am J Clin Pathol* 65:103, 1976.

47. Shoenfeld Y, Berliner S, Pinkhas J, Beutler E: The association of Gaucher's disease and dysproteinemias. *Acta Haematol (Basel)* 64:241, 1980.

48. Pratt PW, Estren F, Kochwa S: Immunoglobulin abnormalities in Gaucher's disease: Report of 16 cases. *Blood* 31:633, 1968.

49. Turesson I, Rausing A: Gaucher's disease and benign monoclonal gammopathy: A case report with immunofluorescence study of bone marrow and spleen. *Acta Med Scand* 197:507, 1975.

50. Liel Y, Hausmann MJ, Mozes M: Case report: Serendipitous Gaucher's disease presenting as elevated erythrocyte sedimentation rate due to monoclonal gammopathy. *Am J Med Sci* 301:393, 1991.

51. Shiran A, Brenner B, Laor A, Tatarsky I: Increased risk of cancer in patients with Gaucher disease. *Cancer* 72:219, 1993.

52. Aker M, Zimran A, Abrahamov A, Horowitz M, Matzner Y: Abnormal neutrophil chemotaxis in Gaucher disease. *Br J Haematol* 83:187, 1993.

53. Zimran A, Abrahamov A, Aker M, Matzner Y: Correction of neutrophil chemotaxis defect in patients with Gaucher disease by low-dose enzyme replacement therapy. *Am J Hematol* 43:69, 1993.

54. Beutler E, Kuhl W: The diagnosis of the adult type of Gaucher's disease and its carrier state by demonstration of deficiency of beta-glucosidase activity in peripheral blood leukocytes. *J Lab Clin Med* 76:747, 1970.

55. Beutler E: Gaucher disease: New developments, in Fairbanks VF (ed): *Current Hematology and Oncology*, p 1–25. Year Book Medical Publishers, Chicago, 1988.

56. Brady RO, King FM: Gaucher's disease, in *Lysosomes and Storage Diseases*, p 381. Academic Press, New York, 1973.

57. Naito M, Takahashi K, Hojo H: An ultrastructural and experimental study on the development of tubular structures in the lysosomes of Gaucher cells. *Lab Invest* 58:590, 1988.

58. Öckerman PA, Köhlin P: Acid hydrolases in plasma in Gaucher's disease. *Clin Chem* 15:61, 1969.

59. Aerts JM, Hollak CE: Plasma and metabolic abnormalities in Gaucher's disease. *Baillieres Clin Haematol* 10:691, 1997.

60. Young E, Chatterton C, Vellodi A, Winchester B: Plasma chitotriosidase activity in Gaucher disease patients who have been treated either by bone marrow transplantation or by enzyme replacement therapy with alglucerase. *J Inherit Metab Dis* 20:595, 1997.

61. Lieberman J, Beutler E: Elevation of serum angiotensin-converting enzyme in Gaucher's disease. *N Engl J Med* 294:1442, 1976.

62. Beutler E, Demina A, Laubscher K, et al: The clinical course of treated and untreated Gaucher disease. A study of 45 patients. *Blood Cell Mol Dis* 21:86, 1995.

63. Boklan BF, Sawitsky A: Factor IX deficiency in Gaucher disease. An in vitro phenomenon. *Arch Intern Med* 136:489, 1976.

64. Berrebi A, Malnick SDH, Vorst EJ, Stein D: High incidence of factor XI deficiency in Gaucher's disease. *Am J Hematol* 40:153, 1992.

65. Beutler E, Kuhl W, Trinidad F, Teplitz R, Nadler H: Beta-glucosidase activity in fibroblasts from homozygotes and heterozygotes for Gaucher's disease. *Am J Hum Genet* 23:62, 1971.

66. Beutler E, Saven A: Misuse of marrow examination in the diagnosis of Gaucher disease. *Blood* 76:646, 1990.

67. Beutler E: Modern diagnosis and treatment of Gaucher's disease. *Am J Dis Child* 147:1175, 1993.

68. Rosner F, Dosik H, Kaiser SS, Lee SL, Morrison AN: Gaucher cell in leukemia. *JAMA* 209:935, 1969.

69. Hopfner C, Potron G, Adnet JJ, Caulet AT, Boy J: Histiocytes bleus et ''cellules de Gaucher'' avec surcharges splenique et ganglionnaire au cours d'une leucemie myeloide chronique. *Nouv Rev Fr Hematol* 14:607, 1974.

70. Zidar BL, Hartsock RJ, Lee RE, et al: Pseudo-Gaucher cells in the bone marrow of a patient with Hodgkin's disease. *Am J Clin Pathol* 87:533, 1987.

71. Scullin DC Jr, Shelburne JD, Cohen HJ: Pseudo-Gaucher cells in multiple myeloma. *Am J Med* 67:347, 1979.

72. Solis OG, Belmonte AH, Ramaswamy G, Tchertkoff V: Pseudo-Gaucher cells in *Mycobacterium avium intracellulare* infections in acquired immune deficiency syndrome (AIDS). *Am J Clin Pathol* 85:233, 1986.

73. Kattlove HE, Williams JC, Gaynor E, et al: Gaucher cells in chronic myelocytic leukemia: An acquired abnormality. *Blood* 33:379, 1969.

74. Beutler E, Kuhl W, Matsumoto F, Pangalis G: Acid hydrolases in leukocytes and platelets of normal subjects and in patients with Gaucher's and Fabry's disease. *J Exp Med* 143:975, 1976.

75. Raghavan SS, Topol J, Kolodny EH: Leukocyte beta-glucosidase in homozygotes and heterozygotes for Gaucher disease. *Am J Hum Genet* 32:158, 1980.

76. Silverstein MN, Kelly PJ: Osteoarticular manifestations of Gaucher's disease. *Am J Med Sci* 253:569, 1967.

77. Ashkenazi A, Zaizov R, Matoth Y: Effect of splenectomy on destructive bone changes in children with chronic (type I) Gaucher disease. *Eur J Pediatr* 145:138, 1986.

78. Shiloni E, Bitran D, Rachmilewitz E, Durst AL: The role of splenectomy in Gaucher's disease. *Arch Surg* 118:929, 1983.

79. Beutler E: Newer aspects of some interesting lipid storage diseases: Tay-Sachs and Gaucher's diseases. *West J Med* 126:46, 1977.

80. Stellin GP, Lilly JR, Githens JH: On partial splenectomy in Gaucher's disease. *Pediatrics* 77:618, 1986.

81. Rubin M, Yampolski I, Lambrozo R, Zaizov R, Dintsman M: Partial splenectomy in Gaucher's disease. *J Pediatr Surg* 21:125, 1986.

82. Rodgers BM, Tribble C, Joob A: Partial splenectomy for Gaucher's disease. *Ann Surg* 205:693, 1987.

83. Guzzetta PC, Connors RH, Fink J, Barranger JA: Operative technique and results of subtotal splenectomy for Gaucher disease. *Surg Gynecol Obstet* 164:359, 1987.

84. Morgenstern L, Phillips EH, Fermelia D, Weinstein IM: Near-total splenectomy for massive splenomegaly due to Gaucher disease: A new surgical approach. *Mt Sinai J Med* 53:501, 1986.

85. Kyllerman M, Conradi N, Månsson J-E, Percy AK, Svennerholm L: Rapidly progressive type III Gaucher disease: Deterioration following partial splenectomy. *Acta Paediatr Scand* 79:448, 1990.

86. Guzzetta PC, Ruley EJ, Merrick HFW, Verderese C, Barton N: Elective subtotal splenectomy: Indications and results in 33 patients. *Ann Surg* 211:34, 1990.

87. Thomas WEG, Winfield DA: Partial splenectomy for massive splenomegaly secondary to Gaucher's disease. *Postgrad Med J* 67:1072, 1991.

88. Zer M, Freud E: Subtotal splenectomy in Gaucher's disease: Towards a definition of critical splenic mass. *Br J Surg* 79:742, 1992.

89. Cohen IJ, Katz K, Freud E, Zer M, Zaizov R: Long-term follow-up of partial splenectomy in Gaucher's disease. *Am J Surg* 164:345, 1992.

90. Zimran A, Elstein D, Schiffmann R, et al: Outcome of partial splenectomy for type I Gaucher disease. *J Pediatr* 126:596, 1995.

91. Amstutz HC: The hip in Gaucher's disease. *Clin Orthop* 90:83, 1973.

92. Davies FWT: Gaucher's disease in bone. *J Bone Joint Surg [Br]* 34B:454, 1952.

93. Schein AJ, Arkin AM: The classic: Hip-joint involvement in Gaucher's disease. *Clin Orthop* 90:4, 1973.

94. Moore M Jr, Coley BL: Bone lesions in Gaucher's disease. *J Tenn Med Assoc* 40:101, 1947.

95. Carlson DE, Busuttil RW, Giudici TA, Barranger JA: Orthotopic liver transplantation in the treatment of complications of type I Gaucher disease. *Transplantation* 49:1192, 1990.

96. DuCerf C, Bancel B, Caillon P, et al: Orthotopic liver transplantation for type 1 Gaucher's disease. *Transplantation* 53:1141, 1992.

97. Smanik EJ, Tavill AS, Jacobs GH, et al: Orthotopic liver transplantation in two adults with Niemann-Pick and Gaucher's diseases: Implications for the treatment of inherited metabolic disease. *Hepatology* 17:42, 1993.

98. Starzl TE, Demetris AJ, Trucco M, et al: Chimerism after liver transplantation for type IV glycogen storage disease and type 1 Gaucher's disease. *N Engl J Med* 328:745, 1993.

99. Brady RO, Pentchev PG, Gal AE, Hibbert SR, Dekaban AS: Replacement therapy for inherited enzyme deficiency: Use of purified glucocerebrosidase in Gaucher's disease. *N Engl J Med* 291:989, 1974.

100. Beutler E, Dale GL: Enzyme replacement therapy, in Atkinson D, Fox CF (eds): *Covalent and Non-covalent Modulation of Protein Function*, p 449. Academic Press, Inc., New York, 1979.

101. Beutler E, Dale GL, Guinto E, Kuhl W: Enzyme replacement therapy in Gaucher's disease: Preliminary clinical trial of a new enzyme preparation. *Proc Natl Acad Sci USA* 74:4620, 1977.

102. Belchetz PE, Crawley JCW, Braidman IP, Gregoriadis G: Treatment of Gaucher's disease with liposome-entrapped glucocerebroside: Beta-glucosidase. *Lancet* 2:116, 1977.

103. Sato Y, Kuhl W, Beutler E: Binding, internalization and degradation of mannose-terminated glucocerebrosidase by macrophages. *Blood* 80 (suppl 1):100a, 1992.

104. Barton NW, Brady RO, Dambrosia JM, et al: Replacement therapy for inherited enzyme deficiency: Macrophage-targeted glucocerebrosidase for Gaucher's disease. *N Engl J Med* 324:1464, 1991.

105. Beutler E, Kay A, Saven A, et al: Enzyme replacement therapy for Gaucher disease. *Blood* 78:1183, 1991.

106. Zimran A, Elstein D, Kannai R, et al: Low-dose enzyme replacement therapy for Gaucher's disease: Effects of age, sex, genotype, and clinical features on response to treatment. *Am J Med* 97:3, 1994.

107. Elstein D, Hadas-Halpern I, Itzchaki M, et al: Effect of low-dose enzyme replacement therapy on bones in Gaucher disease patients with severe skeletal involvement. *Blood Cell Mol Dis* 22:104, 1996.

108. Beutler E: Enzyme replacement therapy for Gaucher disease. *Baillieres Clin Haematol* 10:711, 1997.

109. Elstein D, Abrahamov A, Hadas-Halpern I, Meyer A, Zimran A: Low-dose low-frequency imiglucerase as a starting regimen of enzyme replacement therapy for patients with type I Gaucher disease. *Q J Med* 91:483, 1998.

110. Petrides PE: Mobus Gaucher: Aktueller Stand der Therapie. *Arzneimitteltherapie* 2:49, 1998.

111. McCabe ERB, Fine BA, Golbus MS, et al: Gaucher disease—Current issues in diagnosis and treatment. *JAMA* 275:548, 1996.

112. Krasnewich D, Dietrich K, Bauer L, et al: Splenectomy in Gaucher Disease: New management dilemmas. *Blood* 91:3085, 1998.

113. Beutler E: Effect of low-dose enzyme replacement therapy on bones in Gaucher disease patients with severe skeletal involvement—[commentary]. *Blood Cells Mol Dis* 22:113, 1996.

114. Rosenthal DI, Doppelt SH, Mankin HJ, et al: Enzyme replacement therapy for Gaucher disease: Skeletal responses to macrophage-targeted glucocerebrosidase. *Pediatrics* 96 (part 1):629, 1995.

115. Cohen IJ, Katz K, Kornreich L, et al: Low-dose high-frequency enzyme replacement therapy prevents fractures without complete suppression of painful bone crises in patients with severe juvenile onset type I Gaucher disease. *Blood Cells Mol Dis* 24:296, 1998.

116. Barton NW, Brady RO, Murray GJ, et al: Enzyme-replacement therapy for Gaucher's disease: Reply. *N Engl J Med* 325:1811, 1991.

117. Figueroa ML, Rosenbloom BE, Kay AC, et al: A less costly regimen of alglucerase to treat Gaucher's disease. *N Engl J Med* 327:1632, 1992.

118. Hollak CEM, Aerts JMFG, Goudsmit R, et al: Individualised low-dose alglucerase therapy for type 1 Gaucher's disease. *Lancet* 345:1474, 1995.

119. Beutler E: Treatment regimens in Gaucher's disease. *Lancet* 346:581, 1995.

120. Barton NW, Brady RO, Dambrosia JM: Treatment of Gaucher's disease. *N Engl J Med* 328:1564, 1993.

121. Moscicki RA, Taunton-Rigby A: Treatment of Gaucher's disease. *N Engl J Med* 328:1564, 1993.

122. Zimran A, Hadas-Halpern I, Zevin S, Levy-Lahd E, Abrahamov A: Low dose high frequency enzyme replacement therapy for very young children with Gaucher disease. *Br J Haematol* 85:783, 1993.

123. Hollak CEM, Aerts JMFG, van Oers MHJ: Treatment of Gaucher's disease. *N Engl J Med* 328:1565, 1993.

124. Zimran A, Hollak CEM, Abrahamov A, et al: Home treatment with intravenous enzyme replacement therapy for Gaucher disease: An international collaborative study of 33 patients. *Blood* 82:1107, 1993.

125. Rappeport JM, Ginns EI: Bone-marrow transplantation in severe Gaucher disease. *N Engl J Med* 311:84, 1984.

126. Groth CG, Ringden O: Transplantation in relation to the treatment of inherited disease. *Transplantation* 38:319, 1984.

127. Hobbs JR, Shaw PJ, Jones KH, Lindsay I, Hancock M: Beneficial effect of pre-transplant splenectomy on displacement bone marrow transplantation for Gaucher's syndrome. *Lancet* 1:1111, 1987.

128. Tsai P, Lipton JM, Sahdev I, et al: Allogenic bone marrow transplantation in severe Gaucher disease. *Pediatr Res* 31:503, 1992.

129. Gluckman E, Esperou H, Devergie A, et al: Pediatric bone marrow transplantation for leukemia and aplastic anemia: Report of 222 cases transplanted in a single center. *Nouv Rev Fr Hematol* 31:111, 1989.

130. Ringén O, Groth CG, Erikson A, et al: Ten years' experience of bone marrow transplantation for Gaucher disease. *Transplantation* 59:864, 1995.

131. Chan KW, Wong LTK, Applegarth D, Davidson AGF: Bone marrow transplantation in Gaucher's disease: Effect of mixed chimeric state. *Bone Marrow Transplant* 14:327, 1994.

132. Takiyama N, Mohney T, Swaney W, et al: Comparison of methods for retroviral mediated transfer of glucocerebrosidase gene to CD34+ hematopoietic progenitor cells. *Eur J Haematol* 61:1, 1998.

133. Schuening F, Longo WL, Atkinson ME, Zaboikin M: Retrovirus-mediated transfer of the cDNA for human glucocerebrosidase into peripheral blood repopulating cells of patients with Gaucher's disease. *Hum Gene Ther* 8:2143, 1997.

134. Dunbar C, Kohn D, Karlsson S, et al: Retroviral mediated transfer of the cDNA for human glucocerebrosidase into hematopoietic stem cells of patients with Gaucher disease: A phase I study. *Hum Gene Ther* 7:231, 1996.

135. Nolta JA, Sender LS, Barranger JA, Kohn DB: Expression of human glucocerebrosidase in murine long-term bone marrow cultures after retroviral vector-mediated transfer. *Blood* 75:787, 1990.

136. Sorge J, Kuhl W, West C, Beutler E: Gaucher disease: Retrovirus-mediated correction of the enzymatic defect in cultured cells. *Cold Spring Harbor Symp Quant Biol* 60:1041, 1986.

137. Beutler E, Southgate MT: Clinical pathological conference: Hepato-splenomegaly, abdominal pain, anemia, and bone lesions. *JAMA* 224:502, 1973.

138. Groth CG, Dreborg S, Öckerman PA, et al: Splenic transplantation in a case of Gaucher's disease. *Lancet* 1:1260, 1971.

139. Lev M, Sundaram KS: Gaucher's disease. *N Engl J Med* 317:572, 1987.

140. Platt FM, Neises GR, Reinkensmeier G, et al: Prevention of lysosomal

141. Radin NS: Treatment of Gaucher disease with an enzyme inhibitor. *Glycoconjugate J* 13:153, 1996.

142. Balicki D, Beutler E: Gaucher disease. *Medicine (Baltimore)* 74:305, 1995.

143. Sidransky E, Tsuji S, Martin BM, Stubblefield B, Ginns EI: DNA mutation analysis of Gaucher patients. *Am J Med Genet* 42:331, 1992.

144. Masuno M, Tomatsu S, Sukegawa K, Orii T: Non-existence of a tight association between a 444leucine to proline mutation and phenotypes of Gaucher disease: High frequency of a NciI polymorphism in the non-neuronopathic form. *Hum Genet* 84:203, 1990.

145. Zimran A, Kay AC, Gelbart T, et al: Gaucher disease: Clinical, laboratory, radiologic and genetic features of 53 patients. *Medicine (Baltimore)* 71:337, 1992.

146. Ginsburg SJ, Groll M: Hydrops fetalis due to infantile Gaucher's disease. *J Pediatr* 82:1046, 1973.

147. Tybulewicz VLJ, Tremblay ML, LaMarca ME, et al: Animal model of Gaucher's disease from targeted disruption of the mouse glucocerebrosidase gene. *Nature* 357:407, 1992.

148. Niemann A: Ein unbekanntes Krankheitsbild. *Jahr Kinderheilkd* 79:1, 1914.

149. Brady RO, Kanfer JN, Mock MB, Fredrickson DS: The metabolism of sphingomyelin II. Evidence of an enzymatic deficiency in Niemann-Pick disease. *Proc Natl Acad Sci USA* 55:366, 1966.

150. Schuchman EH, Desnick RJ: Niemann-Pick disease types A and B: Acid sphingomyelinase deficiencies, in Scriver, et al. *The Metabolic and Molecular Bases of Inherited Disease,* 7th ed, p 2601. McGraw-Hill, New York, 1995.

151. Pentchev PG, Vanier MT, Suzuki K, Patterson MC: Niemann-Pick disease type C: A cellular cholesterol lipidosis, in Scriver et al, *The Metabolic and Molecular Bases of Inherited Disease,* 7th ed, p 2625. McGraw-Hill, New York, 1995.

152. Takahashi T, Suchi M, Desnick RJ, Takada G, Schuchman EH: Identification and expression of five mutations in the human acid sphingomyelinase gene causing types A and B Niemann-Pick disease. Molecular evidence for genetic heterogeneity in the neuronopathic and non-neuronopathic forms. *J Biol Chem* 267:12552, 1992.

153. Ida H, Rennert OM, Maekawa K, Eto Y: Identification of three novel mutations in the acid sphinogomyelinase gene of Japanese patients with Niemann-Pick disease type A and B. *Hum Mutat* 7:65, 1996.

154. De Maria R, Rippo MR, Schuchman EH, Testi R: Acidic sphingomyelinase (ASM) is necessary for fas-induced GD3 ganglioside accumulation and efficient apoptosis of lymphoid cells. *J Exp Med* 187:897, 1998.

155. Carstea ED, Morris JA, Coleman KG, et al: Niemann-Pick C1 disease gene: homology to mediators of cholesterol homeostasis. *Science* 277:228, 1997.

156. Liscum L, Klansek JJ: Niemann-Pick disease type C. *Curr Opin Lipidol* 9:131, 1998.

157. Loftus SK, Morris JA, Carstea ED, et al: Murine model of Niemann-Pick C disease: mutation in a cholesterol homeostasis gene. *Science* 277:232, 1997.

158. Golde DW, Schneider EL, Bainton EL, et al: Pathogenesis of one variant of sea-blue histiocytosis. *Lab Invest* 33:371, 1975.

159. Lazarus SS, Vethamany VG, Schneck L, Volk B: Fine structure and histochemistry of peripheral blood cells in Niemann-Pick disease. *Lab Invest* 17:155, 1967.

160. Brady RO: Sphingomyelin lipidoses: Niemann-Pick disease, in Stanbury, et al (eds): *The Metabolic Bases of Inherited Disease,* 5th ed, p 831. McGraw-Hill, New York, 1983.

161. Veyssier-Belot C, Cacoub P, Caparros-Lefebvre D, et al: Erdheim-Chester disease: Clinical and radiologic characteristics of 59 cases. *Medicine (Baltimore)* 75:157, 1996.

162. Landas S, Foucar K, Sando GN, Ellefson R, Hamilton HE: Adult Niemann-Pick disease masquerading as sea blue histiocyte syndrome: Report of a case confirmed by lipid analysis and enzyme assays. *Am J Hematol* 20:391, 1985.

163. Briere J, Calman F, Lageron A, et al: Maladie de Niemann-Pick de l'adulte suivie de la naissance a l'age de 26 ans: Forme viscerale pure avec surcharge en sphingomyeline et deficit en sphingomyelinase. *Nouv Rev Fr Hematol* 16:185, 1976.

164. Dewhurst N, Besley GTN, Finlayson NDC, Parker AC: Sea blue histiocytosis in a patient with chronic non-neuropathic Niemann-Pick disease. *J Clin Pathol* 32:1121, 1979.

165. Brady RO, King FM: Niemann Pick disease, in Hers HG, Van Hoof F (eds): *Lysosomes and Storage Diseases,* p 439. Academic Press, New York, 1973.

166. Epstein CJ, Brady RO, Schneider EL, Bradley RM, Shapiro D: In utero diagnosis of Niemann-Pick disease. *Am J Hum Genet* 23:533, 1971.

167. Gal AE, Brady RO, Hibberg SR, Pentchev PG: A practical chromogenic procedure for the detection of homozygotes and heterozygous carriers of Niemann-Pick disease. *N Engl J Med* 293:632, 1975.

168. Levade T, Salvayre R, Douste-Blazy L: Sphingomyelinases and Niemann-Pick disease. *J Clin Chem Clin Biochem* 24:205, 1986.

169. Roff CF, Goldin E, Comly ME, et al: Niemann-Pick type-C disease: Deficient intracellular transport of exogenously derived cholesterol. *Am J Med Genet* 42:593, 1992.

170. Bembi B, Comelli M, Scaggiante B, et al: Treatment of sphingomyelinase deficiency by repeated implantations of amniotic epithelial cells. *Am J Med Genet* 44:527, 1992.

171. Sawitsky A, Rosner F, Chodsky S: The sea-blue histiocyte syndrome, a review: genetic and biochemical studies. *Semin Hematol* 9:285, 1972.

172. Sawitsky A, Hyman GA, Hyman JB: An unidentified reticuloendothelial cell in bone marrow and spleen: Report of two cases with histochemical studies. *Blood* 9:977, 1954.

173. Baumgartner C, Bucher U: Blaue Pigmentmakrophagen (sea blue histiocytes) und Gaucher-aehnliche Zellen. Vorkommen und Bedeutung. *Blut* 30:309, 1975.

174. Bigorgne C, Le Tourneau A, Vahedi K, et al: Sea-blue histiocyte syndrome in bone marrow secondary to total parenteral nutrition. *Leuk Lymphoma* 28:523, 1998.

175. Kelsey PR, Geary CG: Sea-blue histiocytes and Gaucher cells in bone marrow of patients with chronic myeloid leukaemia. *J Clin Pathol* 41:960, 1988.

176. Zelingher J, Shouval D: Liver failure and the sea-blue histiocyte/adult Niemann-Pick disease: Case report and review of the literature. *J Clin Gastroenterol* 2:146, 1992.

PART VIII

LYMPHOCYTES AND PLASMA CELLS

MORPHOLOGY OF LYMPHOCYTES AND PLASMA CELLS

STEPHEN M. BAIRD

Lymphocytes are a heterogeneous collection of cells that can be distinguished easily from other leukocytes by their characteristic morphology. However, this morphology is shared by all three major blood lymphocyte subsets, namely T cells, B cells, and natural killer (NK) cells. Although B cells can differentiate into plasma cells that have a distinctive morphology, most changes that occur in morphology during differentiation or activation are not unique to any one of the three major subgroups. Instead, other means are required to distinguish the major subsets and sub-subsets of lymphocytes. This has been achieved through the advent of monoclonal antibodies and the characterization of surface membrane antigens that are distinctive for each lymphocyte subset. This chapter describes the morphologic features that distinguish lymphocytes from other leukocytes and the membrane antigens that most commonly are used to distinguish the major lymphocyte subsets.

DEFINITION AND HISTORY

Lymphocytes and plasma cells first were described morphologically in 1774 and 1875, respectively.[1,2] Investigations of these cells from then until the 1960s primarily were to further define their morphology. Subsequently, lymphocytes were found to make immunoglobulins and to be necessary for cell-mediated immunity.[3-7] With the advent of monoclonal antibodies and flow cytometry, the refinement of in vitro functional assays, and the application of molecular techniques, there have been major advances in the understanding of lymphocytes. Membrane antigens have been identified that assist in the designation of lymphocyte subsets and function. Three major blood lymphocyte subsets have been identified: T lymphocytes, B lymphocytes, and NK cells. Further, there are small numbers of circulating hematopoietic stem cells that resemble lymphocytes and that are capable of differentiating into any one of the various lymphocyte subsets.

MICROSCOPY AND HISTOCHEMISTRY OF NORMAL BLOOD LYMPHOCYTES

LIGHT MICROSCOPY

Classic studies of blood and tissues have demonstrated populations of spherical and/or ovoid cells that are from 6 to 15 μm in diameter when flattened on glass slides.[4] Some of these studies described small

Acronyms and abbreviations that appear in this chapter include: ADCC, antibody-dependent cell-mediated cytotoxicity; CD, clusters of differentiation; LFA-3, lymphocyte-function–associated antigen-3; MHC, major histocompatibility complex; N-CAM, neural adhesion protein; NK, natural killer; PAS, periodic acid–Schiff; TCR, T-cell antigen receptor.

lymphocytes, which are 6 to 9 μm in diameter, and large lymphocytes, which have a diameter of 9 to 15 μm. There are increased numbers of circulating large lymphocytes in patients with acute viral illnesses and in certain genetic immunologic deficiencies, particularly the Wiskott-Aldrich syndrome. Normal adults have a mean absolute number of circulating small lymphocytes of 2.5×10^9/liter (range of 1.5 to 4.0), or 35 percent of the total leukocytes (with a range of 20 to 50 percent).

The typical small lymphocyte as observed with Romanovsky polychromatic stains (e.g., Giemsa or Wright) has an ovoid or kidney-shaped nucleus that stains purple, has densely packed nuclear chromatin, and occupies about 90 percent of the cell area (see Plate XX-4). There is a small rim of cytoplasm that stains light blue. Although nucleoli rarely are observed in Giemsa-stained films, they can be demonstrated with methyl green-pyronine stains. Cytoplasmic basophilia is related to RNA content. The cytoplasm of some lymphocytes, particularly large lymphocytes, contains a number of coarse pink granules, usually 5 to 15 per cell, and occasional clear vacuoles. Cytoplasmic glycogen is detected with periodic acid–Schiff (PAS) and methenamine-silver techniques. A number of enzymes, including phosphorylase, acid hydrolases, nucleases, and mitochondrial enzymes, are in the lymphocyte cytoplasm.[8] Peroxidase reactions are negative in lymphocytes.[9]

In a normal adult about 3 percent of blood lymphocytes are large granular lymphocytes[10] (see Plate XX-3). These cells are a mixed population consisting of NK cells and some of the CD8 subset of mature T cells. The majority of mature T lymphocytes, however, show a localized "dot" staining pattern for acid phosphatase, acid and neutral nonspecific esterases, β-glucuronidase, and N-acetyl-β-glucosaminidase.[11-13] B lymphocytes either lack esterase and acid phosphatase or show scattered granular staining.

Enzymes in the purine salvage pathways are expressed differently in lymphocyte subsets. The enzyme 5′-nucleotidase is detectable on plasma membranes of both B and T cells. In contrast, more adenosine deaminase and purine nucleoside phosphorylase are present in the cytoplasm of T cells than in the cytoplasm of B cells.[14,15] Terminal deoxynucleotidyl transferase is present in cortical thymocytes, undifferentiated stem cells, and the malignant cells of acute lymphoid leukemias.[16,17]

PHASE-CONTRAST MICROSCOPY

Active movement of lymphocytes is studied by phase-contrast, or interference-contrast, microscopy. Lymphocytes move slowly with a "hand mirror" appearance. Cytoplasmic spreading does not occur. However, during cell movement a thickening occurs in the cytoplasmic rim (the *Hof* region), a region that houses most of the cell's organelles, including the Golgi. Lymphocytes from patients with chronic lymphocyte leukemia have decreased movement.[18]

TRANSMISSION ELECTRON MICROSCOPY AND CYTOCHEMISTRY

As visualized by transmission electron microscopy,[19-22] the circulating lymphocyte measures about 5 μm in diameter. The nucleus has an abundance of electron-dense, condensed heterochromatin, a feature characteristic of nonproliferating cells. The nucleoli are round in section, about 1.0 to 1.5 μm in diameter, and composed of three distinct and concentrically arranged structural units: the central region or agranular zone; the middle, fibrillar region; and the granular zone, which contains intranucleolar chromatin. The lymphocyte's nuclear membrane contains nuclear pores and a perinuclear space.

The cytoplasmic organelles of the lymphocytes are characteristic of eukaryotic cells.[19-22] Some organelles, like the Golgi zone, are

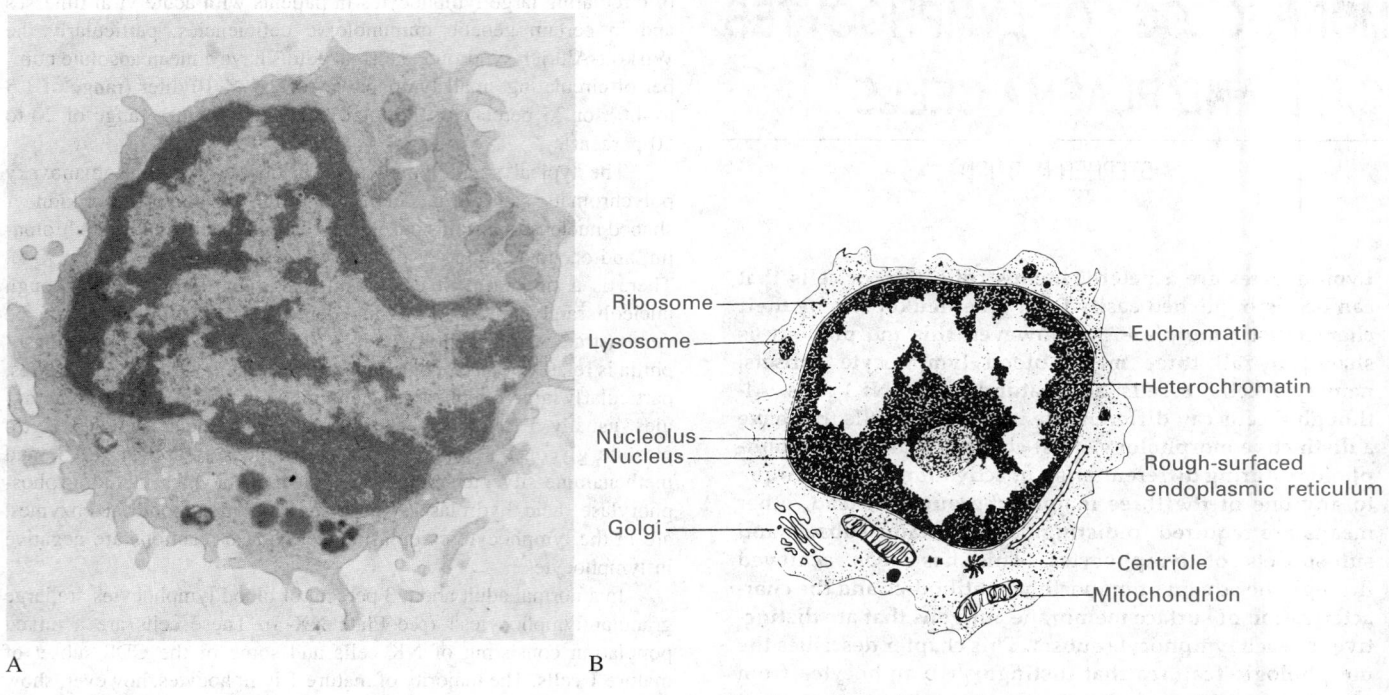

FIGURE 80-1   (A) Electron micrograph of normal human blood lymphocytes. Organelles are labeled in (B). (×12,000) (b) Diagrammatic representation of normal blood lymphocyte.

poorly developed. The cytoplasm contains free ribosomes, occasional ribosome clusters, and strands of rough-surfaced endoplasmic reticulum (Fig. 80-1). Centrioles, mitochondria, microtubules (diameter of approximately 0.25 μm), and microfilaments (diameter of about 0.07 μm) are present in the cytoplasm adjacent to the cell membrane. The cytoplasm also contains lysosomes, which are about 0.4 μm in diameter, are electron-opaque, and contain classic lysosomal enzymes (e.g., acid phosphatase, β-glucuronidase, and acid ribonuclease).[8] The lymphocyte plasma membrane stains with colloidal iron, a marker for membrane sialic acid. Lymphocyte cell membranes and cell coat glycoproteins are shown with other electron-dense markers including phosphotungstic acid, lanthanum colloid, and ruthenium red.

SCANNING ELECTRON MICROSCOPY

Scanning electron microscopy provides three-dimensional information.[23] However, the resolution achieved with scanning electron microscopy, about 0.1 μm, is considerably less than that possible with transmission electron microscopy, generally 0.002 to 0.0039 μm. Normal blood lymphocytes, washed and collected onto silver membranes and fixed in glutaraldehyde, have a spherical topography with varying numbers of stubby or fingerlike microvilli (Fig. 80-2).[24,25] In contrast, monocytes are much larger, have few microvilli, and display ruffled membranes and ridgelike profiles. T lymphocytes have smaller numbers of microvilli than B lymphocytes.[24,25] However, the surface morphology of B lymphocytes is heterogeneous. Many B cells have moderate to markedly villous surfaces, but about 10 to 20 percent of B cells are smooth with few microvilli and thus are indistinguishable from most T lymphocytes.[26] Furthermore, human blood lymphocytes fixed in suspension appear uniformly covered with short microvilli, and no differences between T and B cells are demonstrable.

MORPHOLOGIC CHANGES ASSOCIATED WITH ACTIVATION

Lymphocyte stimulation is associated with a complex sequence of morphologic and biochemical events, culminating in the transformation of small lymphocytes into blast or plasmacytoid cells (Figs. 80-3 and 80-4). Plant lectins, bacterial products, polymeric substances, and enzymes stimulate lymphocyte mitosis. Such agents are called *mitogens*. Some mitogens are specific for either B cells or T lymphocytes, whereas others stimulate both. The responses of specific lymphocyte subpopulations to various mitogens are complex.[33] Nucleolar changes become evident as early as 4 h after exposure to phytomitogens

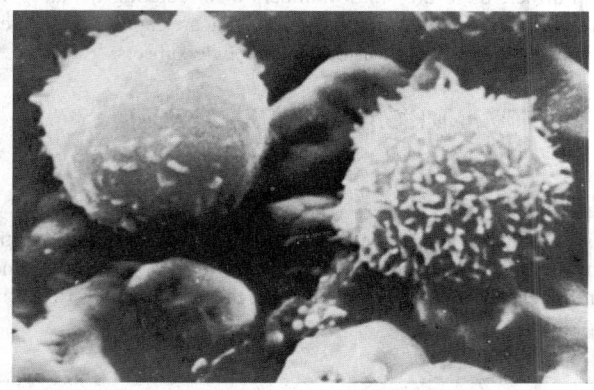

FIGURE 80-2   Scanning electron micrograph of normal blood lymphocytes separated by the Ficoll-Hypaque method. Cells show varying numbers of microvilli. (×5000) (Figs. 80-2, 80-4, and 80-5 provided by Dr. Aaron Polliack of the Department of Hematology, Hebrew University Hadassah Medical School, Jerusalem, Israel.)

(e.g., phytohemagglutinin, which stimulates T cells). These morphologic changes consist of increases in nucleolar size and in the number and concentration of granules in the granular zone. This is followed by an increase in fibrillar zones and increased intranucleolar chromatin. Nucleolar chromatin becomes more electron-lucent or dispersed. Electron microscopic autoradiography demonstrates that tritiated thymidine, incorporated into newly synthesized DNA, is spread throughout the nucleoplasm but is most concentrated at the nuclear membrane. From 48 to 72 h following the addition of phytohemagglutinin there is an increase in size of the cytoplasm. In addition, the cytoplasm contains an increase in the number of ribosomal clusters and more rough-surfaced endoplasmic reticulum. The transformed cell (lymphoblast) has increased numbers of lysosomes and a larger Golgi complex with more components.[19–22] Under some circumstances (e.g., cultures of human lymphocytes stimulated for 7 to 10 days with pokeweed mitogen), some cells may form well-developed Golgi and plasmacytoid features.[34] Similar plasmacytoid cells are observed in antigen-stimulated lymph nodes, during graft rejection in vivo, and in some in vitro systems, including the mixed lymphocyte culture.

Following stimulation with antigen or mitogens the lymphocyte enters the cell cycle. The cell-cycle phases and accompanying genetic or morphologic changes are summarized in Fig. 80-5. These parallel genetic and morphologic alterations are necessary correlates of the cell-cycle phases. The fate and function of lymphocytes that traverse the cell cycle may be divided into two pathways. Some lymphocytes may undergo several mitotic cycles and then return to the G_o phase, indistinguishable in morphology from the original nonactivated cells. A separate subset of lymphocytes may become memory cells, programmed to remember the stimulating antigen and thus more rapidly respond to reexposure to the original antigen. Finally a small number

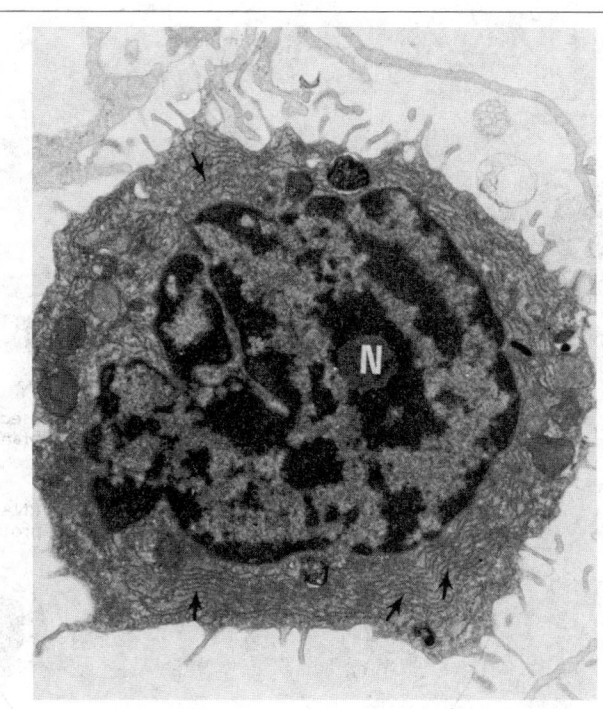

FIGURE 80-4   Transmission electron micrograph of plasmacytoid cell present in culture of lymphocytes from a patient with chronic lymphocytic leukemia incubated with pokeweed mitogen for 7 days. The nucleolus (*N*) and rough-surfaced endoplasmic reticulum (*arrows*) are evident. (×9000) (From Cohnen, Douglas, Konig, et al: Pokeweed mitogen response of lymphocytes in chronic lymphocytic leukemia. *Blood* 42:591, 1973, with permission.)

of lymphocytes are destined to become terminally differentiated lymphocytes, such as plasma cells or cytotoxic T cells.

MICROSCOPY AND HISTOCHEMISTRY OF PLASMA CELLS

MORPHOLOGIC STUDIES

Plasma cells derive from small B lymphocytes after antigenic stimulation and T-cell help. Several sequential mitotic divisions occur during cellular differentiation from the resting lymphocyte to the plasmablast to the immature plasma cell. Immature plasma cells also can undergo successive waves of mitosis in the medullary cords of lymph nodes in response to antigen.[37] Cell transfer experiments demonstrated that these transformed cells later mature into antibody-producing plasma cells.[38]

Pokeweed mitogen induces B lymphocytes to transform into plasma cells after 7 to 10 days' culture.[39] These plasma cells infrequently contain large electron-dense inclusions, which may measure 2 to 3 μm in diameter (Russell bodies) (Fig. 80-6).[40] Russell bodies, cytoplasmic immunoglobulin in the endoplasmic reticulum, sometimes are dissolved during the Giemsa staining procedure. They usually occur in pathologic states but may be found in normal lymph nodes or marrow. When cytoplasmic immunoglobulin becomes detectable, the same immunoglobulin isotype is present in the cytoplasm as on the cell membrane.

LIGHT MICROSCOPY, HISTOCHEMISTRY, AND ELECTRON MICROSCOPY

When treated with a polychrome stain, the mature plasma cell has a characteristic basophilic cytoplasm and an eccentric nucleus. The nu-

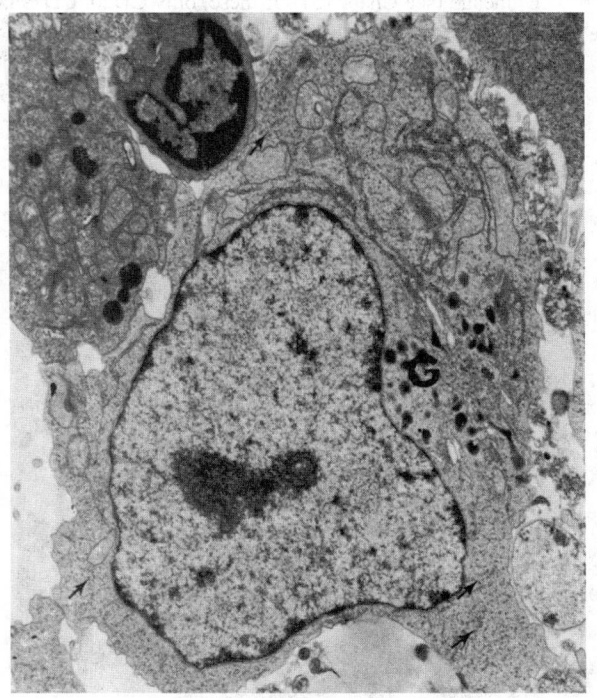

FIGURE 80-3   Transmission electron micrograph of lymphocyte from normal individual incubated with PHA for 3 days. The transformed cell has a large Golgi zone (*G*) and many ribosomal aggregates (*arrows*), and the nucleus is euchromatic. (×7500)

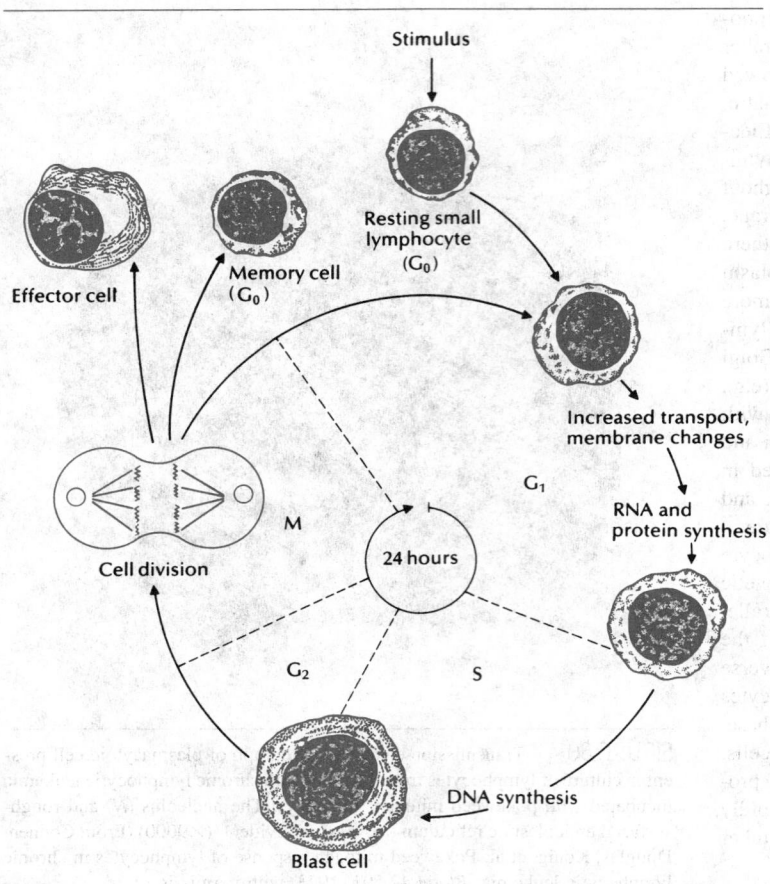

FIGURE 80-5   This is a diagram of lymphocyte activation that displays the relationship of cell-cycle phases (G_0, G_1, S, and M) with changes in cell metabolism and cell function. A lymphocyte may become an effector cell or a memory cell in G_0 after having traversed the cell cycle. (Klein, *Immunology*, p 40. Blackwell, Cambridge, MA, 1990, with permission.)

clear polarity is attributable to a large paranuclear zone, which corresponds to the Golgi apparatus. The typical mature plasma cell spread on a slide is usually round or oval and has a diameter from 9 to 20 μm, with a mean cell diameter of 14.4 μm and a mean nuclear diameter of 8.5 μm[27] (see Plate XXI-1). The nuclear heterochromatin is coarse and distributed in a pattern that, in paraffin sections, sometimes resembles the spokes of a wheel (cartwheel nucleus). Plasma cells with two or more nuclei occasionally may be seen in the marrow of normal individuals. The nucleus stains blue-green with methyl green. The cytoplasm is characterized by its intense affinity for cationic dyes. The cytoplasm, basophilic due to ribonucleoprotein, stains selectively with methyl green-pyronine; it stains red with pyronine due to its high content of ribonucleoprotein (pyroninophilia). The cytoplasm also stains with several basic dyes, including toluidine blue and azures.

Plasma cells that are found in patients with certain diseases may have different histochemical properties. These cells may have a larger size and contain cytoplasmic inclusions that may be observed with PAS stains.[28] In hemochromatosis and hemosiderosis, plasma cells may contain hemosiderin when examined by electron microscopy.[29] Other cytochemical features include absence of peroxidase and nonspecific esterase. Plasma cells are strongly positive for β-glucuronidase and for mitochondrial enzyme markers.[30] Plasma cell size and morphology may be altered substantially in multiple myeloma and macroglobulinemia (see Plates XXI-4–XXI-9). Cells with 2 or 3 nuclei may be seen, even in adults without plasma cell dyscrasias. Under some

circumstances amyloid inclusions have been detected by electron microscopy in plasma cells.[31]

By electron microscopy the plasma cell is packed with a rough-surfaced endoplasmic reticulum that has numerous attached ribosomes. There is a large circumscribed Golgi zone that forms a paranuclear halo when observed by light microscopy. The nucleus has dense areas of heterochromatin. The Golgi zone contains lamellae, vesicles, vacuoles, and a number of granules. Between the strands of endoplasmic reticulum there are mitochondria (Fig. 80-7).[32]

ANTIGENS OF HUMAN LYMPHOCYTES

Human blood lymphocytes possess an array of different membrane antigens. Standardization of monoclonal antibody reagents by identifying *clusters of differentiation* (CD) and the advent of flow cytometry have facilitated detection of lymphocyte subsets (see Chap. 13). The following sections list those surface antigens and morphologic features that help define the major human lymphocyte subsets.

B-LYMPHOCYTE ANTIGENS

Table 80-1 summarizes the expression of CD antigens on cells of the B-lymphocyte lineage, including committed progenitor B cells and pre-B cells. These cells, and the maturation stages that they represent, are discussed in Chap. 82. Also presented in Table 80-1 are antigens that are expressed or are increased upon B-cell activation. The physiology, structure, and distribution of each of the CD antigens listed in Table 80-1 are presented in Chap. 13 (see Table 13-1).

Of the B cell-associated antigens listed in the first column of Table 80-1, only a few are restricted to cells of the B lineage (see Chap. 13). Of these, only CD20, CD79a, and CD79b are not found on other cell types. The latter two antigens associate with Ig to facilitate surface Ig expression

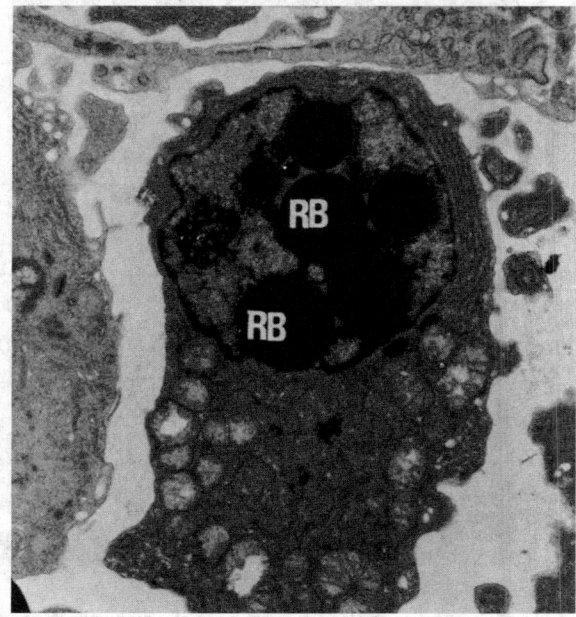

FIGURE 80-6   Intranuclear electron-dense bodies (Russell bodies) (RB) in plasma cell from the marrow of a patient with multiple myeloma. (×7000)

and surface-Ig–mediated signal transduction and are expressed only by cells that produce Ig, an exclusive function of B lymphocytes and plasma cells (see Chaps. 15 and 83). CD19 is restricted mostly to B cells but may be expressed weakly by follicular dendritic cells. This antigen, however, is expressed by B cells at all stages of maturation, including the committed B-cell progenitor. As such, it is the best-defined pan-B cell surface antigen. Cytoplasmic CD22 is perhaps the broadest mature B-cell marker.

In addition to the CD antigens, B cells express the three major histocompatibility complex (MHC) class II antigens (DR, DP, DQ). These antigens are heterodimers of α heavy chains and β light chains that are encoded by genes within the D complex of the HLA complex (see Chap. 138).

B-1 B CELLS

A subset of normal B cells express CD5,[45] a 67-kDa transmembrane glycoprotein[46] that is expressed by T cells (see Chap. 13). These cells are designated CD5 B cells, or, more recently, *B-1 B cells*.[47] B-1 B cells do not express other T-cell markers but do express all other pan-B-cell surface antigens.[48] B-cell expression of CD5 can be modulated by various agents.[49,50] B-1 B cells are found in umbilical cord blood,[51] adult blood, the pleura and peritoneum, and all major secondary lymphoid organs but are rare in the marrow.[52] These cells apparently are enriched for cells that spontaneously produce polyreactive autoantibodies.[53-55] They are the cells that are clonally expanded in chronic lymphocytic leukemia (see Chap. 98).

PLASMA CELLS

Most B-cell differentiation antigens are not expressed by the mature plasma cell, including surface immunoglobulin and HLA class II antigens[56] (see Table 80-1). Of the cells of the B lineage, plasma cells are distinctive in that they express CD28 and PCA-1. CD28 is found on marrow plasma cells and myeloma cell lines.[57] PCA-1 also is found on human plasma cells[58] and may function as a threonine-specific protein kinase.[59] This latter function may assist in phosphorylation of secretory proteins. PCA-1 also is present at low density on granulocytes and monocytes. In contrast to mature B lymphocytes, plasma cells do not bear surface Ig but express CD38 and very high levels of CD43 and CD85 (see Table 80-1).

T-LYMPHOCYTE ANTIGENS

CD1

CD1 is a family of three membrane glycoproteins, CD1a, CD1b, and CD1c, of 49, 45, and 43 kDa, respectively, that is found on all cortical thymocytes (see Chap. 13). CD1 also can be expressed on monocytes following activation and on Langerhans cells.[60] CD1 has a structural relationship to HLA class I and class II proteins. This structural association suggests that CD1 is involved in T-cell interaction with accessory/antigen-presenting cells, perhaps presenting hydrophobic antigens such as lipids.

CD2

This T-cell antigen is expressed early in T-cell development. It is a 50-kDa surface glycoprotein that facilitates T-lymphocyte target cell interactions and T-lymphocyte activation.[61] Lymphocyte-function-associated antigen-3 (LFA-3) (CD58) is a ligand for CD2 (see Chaps. 13 and 84). Cross-linking CD2 may activate T cells through a pathway that is distinct from that used by the T-cell receptor for antigen. This may result in augmentation of the immune response in the absence of additional antigenic stimulation. Since anti-CD2 monoclonal antibodies activate early T-lymphocyte progenitors, CD2 antigen probably

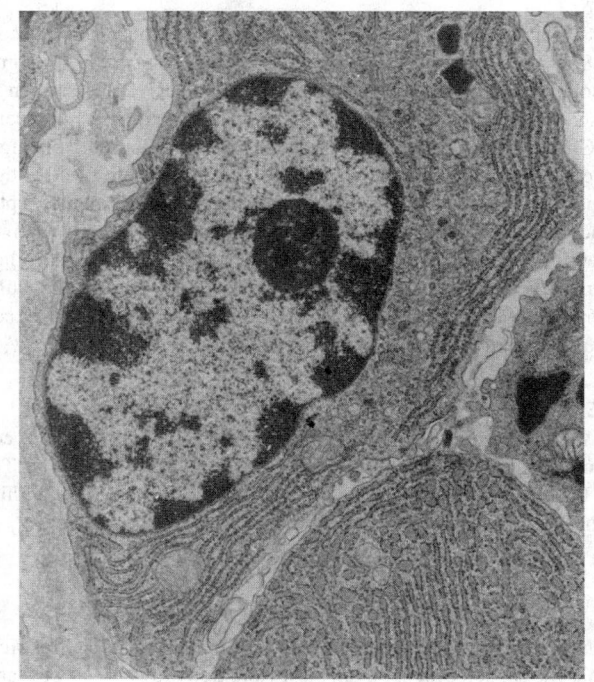

A

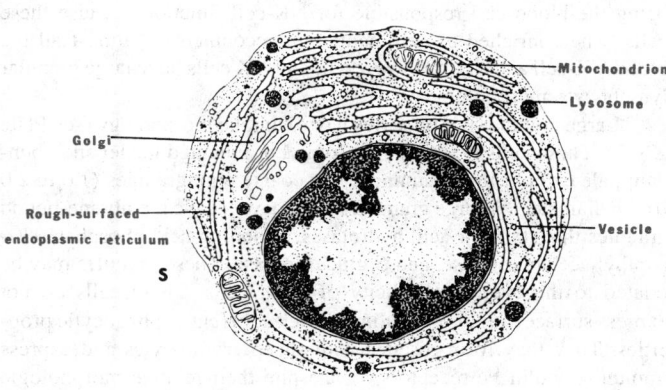

B

FIGURE 80-7   (A) Electron micrograph of mature plasma cells in normal human lymph node. (×9000) (B) Diagrammatic representation of normal plasma cell labeling the organelles.

TABLE 80-1   B-LYMPHOCYTE ANTIGENS USED IN CLINICAL MEDICINE

CELL TYPE	ANTIGEN
Committed progenitor	CD34, CD19, CD40, CD72
Pre B cell	CD10, CD19, CD20, cytoplasmic μ chain, terminal deoxynucleotidyl transferase (TdT)
Mature B cell	CD10 (weak and only on germinal center B cells), CD19, CD20, CD21, CD22 (α and β isoforms), CD5 (B-1 B-cell subset, weak), and CD11c (subset)
Activated B cells[2]	CD23 (usually germinal center B cells), CD38, CD39
Plasma cell	CD38, PCA-1, BB4, cytoplasmic immunoglobulin

In the diagram labels:
- Mitochondrion
- Lysosome
- Golgi
- Rough-surfaced endoplasmic reticulum
- Vesicle
- S

is a receptor used in the activation of thymocytes prior to appearance of a functional T-cell receptor.[62]

CD3

CD3 is expressed by early thymocytes and mature T cells.[63] It is tightly linked to the T-cell receptor (see Chap. 84). The CD3 molecule serves as a signal transduction unit after T-cell receptor activation. In addition, this antigen frequently is expressed on T-cell acute lymphoblastic leukemia.

CD5

CD5 is found on all T cells. It appears early in T-lymphocyte ontogeny.[64] CD5 also may be detected on a subset of blood and cord B cells.

CD7

CD7 is a 40-kDa glycoprotein that is expressed very early in T-cell ontogeny.[65] The antigen is lost during the terminal stage of T-cell maturation. The function of CD7 is not known. CD7 also is expressed on monocytes or natural killer cells.[66]

CD4 AND CD8

CD4 is first expressed on thymocytes along with CD8 (see Chaps. 82 and 84). CD4, a member of the immunoglobulin supergene family, is a single-chain transmembrane glycoprotein.[67] CD8 is a homodimeric transmembrane glycoprotein of 34 kDa.[68] Each molecule also is associated with the T-cell–specific tyrosine kinase p56.[69] CD4 and CD8 act as coreceptors during T-cell activation by antigen (see Chap. 84). CD4 also is a coreceptor for the human immunodeficiency virus[70] (see Chap. 89), along with CCR5 or CXCR4.

CD25

CD25 originally was defined as a component of the interleukin-2 receptor (IL-2R).[71] This antigen is expressed on activated T and B cells. CD25 also is found on thymocytes and monocytes. The IL-2 receptor is made of three distinct proteins [α chain (CD25), β chain (CD122), and γ chain, also a component of the receptors for IL-4, 7, and 9]. When bound to the α chain alone, IL-2 binds with higher affinity to the IL-2R β chain. This then results in formation of a high-affinity complex of IL-2 bound to both IL-2R α and β chains.[73] The γ chain is involved in signaling to the cell after IL-2 binding. IL-2 binding to the high-affinity receptor signals T cells to proliferate and differentiate into specific effector T cells (e.g., helper T or cytotoxic T cells).

CD45

CD45 is tyrosine-specific phosphatase.[74] It is expressed by virtually all hematopoietic cells. However, different isoforms exist due to alternative splicing of the CD45 transcript and differential glycosylation.[75] These different isoforms of CD45 are expressed differentially by different cell subsets (see Chap. 84). CD4+ helper T cells can be divided into functionally disparate subsets based on their expression of the different CD45 isoforms and CD29 (the VLA β chain). Naive CD4+ helper T cells are CD45RA+ and express low levels of CD29. These CD4+ T cells can induce CD8+ T cells to downregulate B-cell IgG synthesis.[76] After activation, T-cell expression of CD45RA is diminished, but that of CD29 and CD45RO (a lower-molecular-weight isoform of CD45) is enhanced.[77] CD4+ CD45RO+ CD29 high-affinity T cells are called *memory-helper T cells,* in that they apparently facilitate induction of B-cell IgG synthesis in response to secondary challenge with antigen. In addition, CD45 is necessary for activation of either CD4+ T cells or CD8+ T cells. T cells that lack expression of CD45 do not respond well to various activation stimuli.[77]

CD28

CD28 is a 44-kDa homodimer that is expressed on resting T cells. CD28 is a surface receptor for a cyclosporine-resistant T-cell signal-transduction pathway.[78] CD28 binds the CD80 (B7/BB1) antigen expressed by activated B cells and professional antigen-presenting cells[79] (see Chap. 84). This interaction provides a second costimulatory signal to T cells that are activated by the cross-linking of their T-cell antigen receptors in response to specific interactions with antigenic peptide bound to the major histocompatibility antigens expressed by antigen-presenting cells.[80,81] Without this second costimulatory signal, the T cell may be induced into anergy.[82] In this state the T cells fail to respond to the antigen(s) presented by the antigen-presenting cell because of a block in IL-2 gene expression.[83]

T-CELL RECEPTOR

The T-cell antigen receptor (TCR) is present on all mature T cells and on developing immature thymocytes (see Chap. 84). The TCR may have unique determinants that are found on all T cells within a given T-cell clone. It is expressed by most T-cell lymphomas.

NATURAL KILLER CELLS

The NK cell is defined as an effector cell that is not MHC-restricted and has the capacity for spontaneous cytotoxicity toward various target cells (see Chap. 85). The large granular lymphocyte was identified as being the blood cell responsible for NK-cell function because these cells, when enriched by sedimentation, accounted for almost all the blood NK-cell activity.[84] However, not all NK cells have large granular lymphocyte morphology.

Large granular lymphocytes have a unique morphology (see Plate XX-3). These cells typically have round or indented nuclei and abundant pale cytoplasm containing a few coarse pink granules (1.0 to 2.0 μm in diameter).[85] Large granular lymphocytes have membrane-bound granules that stain for acid hydrolases, including acid phosphatase, α napthyl acetate esterase, and β glucuronidase. These granules may be related to the cytolytic capacity of these cells. These cells do not express surface immunoglobulin and lack adherent or phagocytic properties. They may form rosettes with sheep erythrocytes and express immunoglobulin Fc receptors.[25,86] Despite their relative morphologic homogeneity, they comprise several subpopulations with distinct phenotypes. NK cells express class I but not class II antigens of the MHC. Human NK cells characteristically express CD16 (FcγRIII) and CD56, but not CD3.[87,88] CD16 (FcγRIII) is a low-affinity receptor that binds to IgG that is bound specifically to antigens present on cells targeted for destruction in antibody-dependent cell-mediated cytotoxicity (ADCC). CD16 is expressed on all NK cells, neutrophils, and tissue macrophages. CD56 is the neural adhesion protein (N-CAM) and is seen on most NK cells, albeit at low density.[89] This 200-kDa protein is expressed at higher levels following activation.

NK cells have some T-cell antigens on their cell membrane, including CD8, found on approximately 30 to 50 percent of NK cells; CD2, present on about half of all NK cells; and CD38, present at low density on most NK cells. However, NK cells do not express CD4.[90] Upon activation, NK cells express increased levels of CD25, CD56, and class II antigens of the MHC. Three cytokines that can activate NK cells are IL-2, interferon-alpha, and IL-12. IL-2 also can induce NK cells and some T cells to differentiate into lymphokine-activated killer cells in vitro (see Chap. 85).

REFERENCES

1. Hewson W, Johnson J: No. 72, Pauls Church Yard London, 1774, in

Lymphatics, Lymph and Lymphomyeloid Complex, 3d ed, edited by JM Yoffey, FC Courtice, p. 3. Harvard, Cambridge, MA, 1970.

2. Ramon Y Cajal S: *Manual de Anatomia Pathologica General.* Intr. de la Casa provincial de Caridad, Barcelona, 1890.

3. Everett NB, Caffey RW, Rieke WO: Recirculation of lymphocytes. *Ann NY Acad Sci* 113:887, 1964.

4. Ford WL, Gowans JL: The traffic of lymphocytes. *Semin Hematol* 6:67, 1969.

5. Nossal GJV, Makela O: Elaboration of antibodies by single cells. *Ann Rev Microbiol* 16:53, 1962.

6. Miller RG: Physical separation of lymphocytes in the lymphocyte structure and function, in *Immunology Series,* edited by JJ Marchalonis, vol 5, p 205. Dekker, New York, 1977.

7. Ackerman GA: Structural studies of the lymphocyte and lymphocyte development, in *Regulation of Hematopoiesis,* edited by AS Gordon, vol 2, p 1297. Appleton Century Crofts, New York, 1970.

8. Brottinger G, Hirschhorn R, Douglas SD, Weissmann G: Studies on lysosomes: XI. Characterization of a hydrolase-rich fraction from human lymphocytes. *J Cell Biol* 37:394, 1968.

9. Yam LT, Li CY, Crosby WH: Cytochemical identification of monocytes and granulocytes. *Am J Clin Pathol* 55:283, 1971.

10. Timonen T, Ortaldo JR, Herberman RB: Characteristics on human large granular lymphocytes and relationship to natural killer and K cells. *J Exp Med* 153:569, 1981.

11. Bevan A, Burns GF, Gray L, Cawley JC: Cytochemistry of human T-cell subpopulations. *Scand J Immunol* 11:223, 1980.

12. Basso G, Cocito MG, Semenzato G, et al: Cytochemical study of thymocytes and T lymphocytes. *Br J Haematol* 44:577, 1980.

13. Machin GA, Halper JP, Knowles DM: Cytochemically demonstrable β-glucuronidase activity in normal and neoplastic human lymphoid cells. *Blood* 56:1111, 1980.

14. Tung R, Silber R, Quagliata F, et al: ADA activity in chronic lymphocytic leukemia—relationship to B- and T-cell subpopulations. *J Clin Invest* 57:756, 1976.

15. Rowe M, deGast GG, Platts-Mills TA, et al: 5'-nucleotidase of B and T lymphocytes isolated from human peripheral blood. *Clin Exp Immunol* 36:97, 1979.

16. Greenwood MF, Coleman MS, Hutton JJ, et al: Terminal deoxynucleotidyl transferase distribution in neoplastic and hematopoietic cells. *J Clin Invest* 59:889, 1977.

17. Bollum FJ: Terminal deoxynucleotidyl transferase as a hematopoietic cell marker. *Blood* 54:1203, 1979.

18. Cohen HJ: Human lymphocyte surface immunoglobulin capping: normal characteristics and anomalous behavior of chronic lymphocytic leukemic lymphocytes. *J Clin Invest* 55:84, 1975.

19. Douglas SD: Human lymphocyte growth in vitro: morphologic, biochemical and immunologic significance. *Int Rev Exp Pathol* 10:42, 1971.

20. Tanaka Y, Goodman JR: *Electron Microscopy of Human Blood Cells.* Harper & Row, New York, 1972.

21. Douglas SD: Electron microscopic and functional aspects of human lymphocyte response to mitogens. *Transplant Rev* 11:39, 1972.

22. Douglas SD, Cohnen G, Brittinger G: Ultrastructural comparison between phytomitogen transformed normal and chronic lymphocytic leukemic lymphocytes. *J Ultrastruct Res* 44:11, 1973.

23. Hayes TL: Scanning electron microscope techniques in biology, in *Advanced Techniques in Biological Electron Microscopy,* edited by JK Koehler, p 153. Springer, New York, 1973.

24. Polliack A, Lampen N, Clarkson BD, et al: Identification of human B and T lymphocytes by scanning electron microscopy. *J Exp Med* 138:607, 1973.

25. Polliack A, Fu SM, Douglas SD, et al: Scanning electron microscopy of human lymphocyte sheep erythrocyte rosettes. *J Exp Med* 140:146, 1974.

26. Polliack A, Hammerling V, Lampen N, DeHarven E: Surface morphology of murine B and T lymphocytes: a comparative study by scanning electron microscopy. *Eur J Immunol* 5:32, 1975.

27. Sachetti D: Le plasmacellule nel midollo osseo delluomo nella norma e nella pathologia: Richerche quantitative citometriche et auxologiche. *Haematologica (Pavia)* 35:13, 1951.

28. Quaglino D, Torelli V, Sauli S, Mauri C: Cytochemical and autoradiographic investigations on normal and myelomatous plasma cells. *Acta Haematol (Basel)* 38:79, 1967.

29. Lerner RG, Parker JW: Dysglobulinemia and iron in plasma cells: ferrokinetics and electron microscopy. *Arch Intern Med* 121:284, 1968.

30. Suzuki A, Shibata A, Onodera S, et al: Histochemical study on plasma cells. *Tohoku J Exp Med* 97:1, 1969.

31. Franklin EC, Zucker-Franklin D: Current concepts on amyloid. *Adv Immunol* 15:249, 1972.

32. Bessis MC: Ultrastructure of lymphoid and plasma cells in relation to globulin and antibody formation. *Lab Invest* 10:1040, 1961.

33. Handwerger BS, Douglas SD: The cell biology of blastogenesis, in *Handbook of Inflammation,* edited by G. Weissman, vol 2, pp 609–706. Elsevier-North Holland, Amsterdam, 1980.

34. Douglas SD, Fudenberg HH: In vitro development of plasma cells from lymphocytes following pokeweed mitogen stimulation: a fine structural study. *Exp Cell Res* 54:277, 1969.

35. Fagraeus A: Antibody production in relation to the development of plasma cells. In vivo and in vitro experiments. *Acta Med Scand* 130:1, 1948.

36. Nossal CJV, Makela O: Autoradiographic studies on the immune response: I. The kinetics of plasma cell proliferation. II. DNA synthesis amongst single antibody producing cells. *J Exp Med* 115:209, 1962.

37. Sainte-Marie G: Study on plasmocytopoiesis: description of plasmocytes and of their mitoses in the mediastinal lymph nodes of ten-week-old rats. *Am J Anat* 114:207, 1964.

38. Sainte-Marie G, Coons AH: Studies on antibody production: X. Mode of formation of plasmocytes in cell transfer experiments. *J Exp Med* 119:742, 1964.

39. Parkhouse RME, Janossy G, Greaves MF: Selective stimulation of IgM synthesis in mouse B lymphocytes by pokeweed mitogen. *Nature (New Biol)* 235:21, 1972.

40. Welsh RA: Electron microscopic localization of Russell bodies in the human plasma cell. *Blood* 16:1307, 1960.

41. Shands JW, Peavy DL, Smith RT: Differential morphology of mouse spleen cells stimulated in vitro by endotoxin, phytohemagglutinin, pokeweed mitogen and staphylococcal enterotoxin B. *Am J Pathol* 70:1, 1973.

42. Andersson J, Buxbaum J, Citronbaum R, et al: IgM-producing tumors in the Balb/c mouse: a model for B-cell maturation. *J Exp Med* 140:742, 1974.

43. Weiss L: *The Cells and Tissues of the Immune System: Structure, Functions, Interactions.* Foundations of Immunology Series, Prentice-Hall, Englewood Cliffs, NJ, 1972.

44. Murphy MJ, Hay JB, Morris B, Bessis MC: An ultrastructural analysis of antibody synthesis in cells from lymph and lymph nodes. *Am J Pathol* 66:25, 1972.

45. Gobbi M, Caligaris-Cappio F, Janossy G: Normal equivalent of cells of B cell malignancies: analysis with monoclonal antibodies. *Br J Haematol* 54:393, 1983.

46. Jones NH, Clabby MI, Dialynas DP, et al: Isolation of complementary DNA clones encoding the human lymphocyte glycoprotein T1/Leu-1. *Nature* 323:346, 1986.

47. Allison A, Alt F, Arnold L, et al: A new nomenclature for B cells. *Immunol Today* 12:383, 1991.

48. Kipps TJ: The CD5 B cell. *Adv Immunol* 47:117, 1989.

49. Freedman AS, Boyd AW, Beiber FR, et al: Normal cellular counterparts of B cell chronic lymphocytic leukemia. *Blood* 70:418, 1987.

50. Defrance T, Vanbervliet B, Durand I, Banchereau J: Human interleukin 4 down-regulates the surface expression of CD5 on normal and leukemic B cells. *Eur J Immunol* 19:293, 1989.

51. Durandy A, Thuillier L, Forveille M, Fischer A: Phenotype and functional characteristics of human newborns' B lymphocytes. *J Immunol* 144:60, 1990.

52. Caligaris-Cappio F, Gobbi M, Bofill M, Janossy G: Infrequent normal B lymphocytes express features of B-chronic lymphocytic leukemia. *J Exp Med* 155:623, 1982.

53. Casali P, Prabhakar BS, Notkins AL: Characterization of multireactive autoantibodies and identification of LEU-1+ B lymphocytes as cells making antibodies binding multiple self and exogenous molecules. *Int Rev Immunol* 3:17, 1988.

54. Hayakawa K, Hardy RR, Honda M, et al: Ly-1 B cells: functionally distinct lymphocytes that secrete IgM autoantibodies. *Proc Natl Acad Sci USA* 81:2494, 1984.

55. Stoegher ZM, Wakai M, Tse DB, et al: Production of autoantibodies by

CD5-expressing B lymphocytes from patients with chronic lymphocytic leukemia. *J Exp Med* 169:255, 1989.

56. Halper J, Fu SM, Kunkel HG: Patterns of expression of human "Ia-like" antigens during the terminal stages of B cell development. *J Immunol* 120:1480, 1978.

57. Kozbor D, Moretta A, Messner HA, et al: Tp44-molecules involved in antigen-independent T-cell activation are expressed on human plasma cells. *J Immunol* 138:4128, 1987.

58. Anderson KC, Park EK, Bates MP, et al: Antigens on human plasma cells identified by monoclonal antibodies. *J Immunol* 130:1132, 1983.

59. Rebbe NF, Tong BD, Finley EM, Hickman S: Identification of nucleotide pyrophosphatase/alkaline phosphodiesterase I activity associated with the mouse plasma cell differentiation antigen PC-1. *Proc Natl Acad Sci USA* 88:5192, 1991.

60. Fithian E, Kuag P, Goldstein G, et al: Receptivity of Langerhans cells with hybridoma antibody. *Proc Natl Acad Sci USA* 78:2541, 1988.

61. Siciliano R, Pratt JC, Schmidt RE, et al: Activation of cytolytic T lymphocyte and natural killer cell function through the T11 sheep erythrocyte binding protein. *Nature* 317:428, 1985.

62. Fox DA, Hussey RE, Fitzgerald KA, et al: Activation of human thymocytes via the 50-kD T11 sheep erythrocyte binding protein induces the expression of interleukin 2 receptors on both T3+ and T3− populations. *J Immunol* 134:330, 1985.

63. Reinherz EL, Schlossman SF: The characterization and function of human immunoregulatory T lymphocyte subsets. *Immunol Today* 2:69, 1981.

64. Link M, Warnke R, Finlay J, et al: A single monoclonal antibody identifies T-cell lineage of childhood lymphoid malignancies. *Blood* 2:722, 1983.

65. Haynes BF, Martin ME, Kay HH, Kuntzborg J: Early events in human T cell ontogeny. *J Exp Med* 168:1061, 1988.

66. Chabannon C, Wood P, Torak-Storg B: Expression of CD7 normal human myeloid progenitors. *J Immunol* 149:2110, 1992.

67. Madden PJ, Littman DR, Godfrey M, et al: The isolation and nucleotide sequence of a cDNA encoding the T cell surface protein T4: a new member of the immunoglobulin gene family. *Cell* 42:93, 1985.

68. Snow PM, Terhorst C: The T8 antigen is a multimeric complex of two distinct subunits as human thymocytes but consists of homomultimeric forms on peripheral blood T lymphocytes. *J Biol Chem* 258:14675, 1983.

69. Luo K, Sefton BM: Cross linking of T cell surface molecules CD4 and CD8 stimulates phosphorylation of the lck tyrosine phosphorylation kinase at the autophosphorylation site. *Mol Cell Biol* 10:5305, 1990.

70. Dalgleish AG, Beverley PCL, Clapham PR, et al: The CD4(T4) antigen is an essential component of the receptor for the AIDS retrovirus. *Nature* 312:763, 1984.

71. Greene WC, Leonard WJ: The human interleukin-2 receptor, in *Annual Review of Immunology,* edited by WE Paul, CG Fathman, H Metzger, vol 4, pp 69–96. Annual Reviews, Palo Alto, CA, 1986.

72. Teshigawara K, Wang HM, Kato K: Interleukin-2 high affinity receptor expression requires two distinct binding proteins. *J Exp Med* 165:223, 1987.

73. Arima N, Kamio M, Okuma M, et al: The IL-2 receptor α-chain alters the binding of IL-2 to the β-chain. *J Immunol* 147:3396, 1991.

74. Tonks NK, Charbonneau H, Diltz CD, et al: Demonstration that the leucocyte common antigen (CD45) is a protein tyrosine phosphatase. *Biochemistry* 27:8695, 1989.

75. LeFrancois L, Thomas ML, Beran MJ, Trowbridge IS: Different classes of T lymphocytes have different mRNAs for the leucocyte-common antigen T200. *J Exp Med* 163:1337, 1986.

76. Sugita K, Hirose T, Rothstein DM: CD27, a member of the nerve growth factor receptor family, is preferentially expressed on CD45RA+ CD4 T cell clones and involved in distinct immuno-regulatory functions. *J Immunol* 149:3208, 1992.

77. Janeway CA: The T cell receptor as a multicomponent signalling machine: CD4/CD8 coreceptors and CD45 in T cell activation. *Annu Rev Immunol* 10:645, 1992.

78. van Lier RA, Brouwer M, Aarden LA: Signals involved in T cell activation. T cell proliferation through the synergistic action of anti-CD28 and anti-CD2 monoclonal antibodies. *Eur J Immunol* 18:167, 1988.

79. Linsley PS, Brady W, Grosmaire L, et al: Binding of the B cell activation antigen B7 to CD28 costimulates T cell proliferation and interleukin 2 mRNA accumulation. *J Exp Med* 173:721, 1991.

80. Koulova L, Clark EA, Shu G, Dupont B: The CD28 ligand B7/BB1 provides costimulatory signal for alloactivation of CD4+ T cells. *J Exp Med* 173:759, 1991.

81. Gimmi CD, Freeman GJ, Gribben JG, et al: B-cell surface B7 provides a costimulatory signal that induces T cells to proliferate and secrete interleukin 2. *Proc Natl Acad Sci USA* 88:6575, 1991.

82. Linsley PS, Wallace PM, Johnson J, et al: Immunosuppression in vivo by a soluble form of the CTLA-4 T cell activation molecule. *Science* 257:792, 1992.

83. Kang S-M, Beverly B, Tran A-C, et al: Transactivation by AP-1 is a molecular target of T cell clonal anergy. *Science* 257:1134, 1992.

84. Timonen T, Jaksela E: Isolation of human natural killer cells by density gradient centrifugation. *J Immunol Methods* 36:285, 1980.

85. Grossi CE, Ferrarini M: Morphology and cytochemistry of human large granular lymphocytes, in *NK Cells and Other Natural Effector Cells,* edited by RB Herberman, p 1. Academic, New York, 1982.

86. West WH, Cannon GB, Kay HD, et al: Natural cytotoxic reactivity of human lymphocytes against a myeloid cell line: characterization of effector cells. *J Immunol* 118:355, 1977.

87. Lanier LL, Phillips JH, Hackett J, et al: Opinion and natural killer cells: definition of a cell type rather than a function. *J Immunol* 137:2735, 1986.

88. Hercend T, Griffin JD, Bensussan A, et al: Generation of monoclonal antibodies to a human natural killer clone: characterization of two natural killer associated antigens, NKH1a and NKH2, expressed on subsets of large granular lymphocytes. *J Clin Invest* 75:932, 1985.

89. Lanier LL, Le AM, Phillips JH, et al: Subpopulations of human natural killer cells defined by expression of the Leu7 (HNK-1) and Leu11 (NK-15) antigens. *J Immunol* 131:1789, 1983.

90. Hercend T, Schmidt RE: Characteristics and uses of natural killer cells. *Immunol Today* 9:292, 1988.

91. Steinman R: The dendritic cell system and its role in immunogenicity. *Annu Rev Immunol* 9:271, 1991.

COMPOSITION AND BIOCHEMISTRY OF LYMPHOCYTES AND PLASMA CELLS

THOMAS J. KIPPS

DENNIS A. CARSON

Mature lymphocytes can be divided into several functional types and subtypes. The major classes of lymphocytes are the T cells, B cells, and natural killer (NK) cells. T lymphocytes are derived from the thymus (see Chaps. 5 and 82) and are responsible for cell-mediated cytotoxic reactions and for delayed hypersensitivity responses (see Chap. 84). They also produce the cytokines that regulate immune responses and provide helper activity for B cells. The B lymphocytes concentrate and present antigens to T cells and are the precursors of immunoglobulin-secreting plasma cells (see Chap. 83). NK cells account for innate immunity against infectious agents and transformed cells that have altered expression of transplantation antigens (see Chap. 85). This chapter describes methods for isolating lymphocytes and discusses their physical and biochemical properties. In addition, this chapter also provides insight into mechanisms that may account for the activity of purine deoxynucleoside analogs, ionizing radiation, or glucocorticoids against resting normal or neoplastic lymphocytes.

ISOLATION OF LYMPHOCYTES

LYMPHOCYTE DENSITY

Lymphocytes can be isolated from the whole blood using density gradient centrifugation. Most commonly, this is performed using a step gradient composed of a mixture of the carbohydrate polymer Ficoll and the dense iodine-containing compound sodium metrizoate.[1] This technique takes advantage of the low density of lymphocytes (1.07 gm/ml) relative to that of erythrocytes (1.09–1.10 gm/ml), granulocytes (1.08–1.09 gm/ml), or monocytes (1.08 gm/ml).

A Ficoll solution adjusted to a density of 1.077 gm/ml is ideal for isolating human lymphocytes. Whole blood is layered onto a cushion of Ficoll-sodium metrizoate prior to centrifugation at $400 \times g$ for 30 min. The denser red blood cells and granulocytes will sediment to the bottom of the tube, and the monocytes will enter into the Ficoll cushion. The lymphocytes can be collected from the interface formed between the Ficoll-sodium metrizoate cushion and the plasma above, which contains the lighter-density platelets (1.04–1.06 gm/ml). This layer contains lymphocytes along with some monocytes that can be removed by plating the cells in culture flasks and harvesting the lymphocytes that are not adherent to plastic.

LYMPHOCYTE SURFACE ANTIGENS

Lymphocyte subsets generally cannot be distinguished from one another by morphology. Most resting lymphocytes appear as small round cells with a dense nucleus and little cytoplasm (see Chap. 80). However, this homogeneous appearance is deceptive, as these cells comprise many functionally distinct subpopulations.

These subsets can be distinguished through the differential expression of cell-surface proteins. The advent of monoclonal antibody technology has allowed for the generation of virtually unlimited quantities of antibodies, each specific for a particular surface protein or molecule. Coupled with the biochemical analyses of the surface molecules that are recognized by these each of these antibodies, many lymphocyte surface antigens have been defined (see Chap. 13).

Typically, it is necessary to monitor for co-expression of two or more cell-surface proteins to define a functional subset of lymphocytes. The same cell-surface protein is often expressed by more than one cell subset. For example, both helper and cytotoxic T cells express CD3, the proteins associated with the T-cell receptor for antigen (see Chap. 84). Expression of both CD3 and CD4 helps to distinguish mature helper T cells from cytotoxic T cells that express CD3 and CD8, and from other cells, such as dendritic cells, that express CD4 but lack expression of CD3.[2] As such, it is the expression of a characteristic constellation of surface molecules, rather than any one particular surface marker, that generally helps to distinguish one subset of lymphocytes from another (see Chap. 13).

FLOW CYTOMETRY

The flow cytometer is a highly effective tool for defining these lymphocyte subsets.[3] This instrument is based on the principle of fluorescence, or the emission of light resulting from the release of energy gained through the absorption of light at a different wavelength. Monoclonal antibodies specific for desired cell-surface proteins can each be coupled to a fluorescent dye, called a *fluorochrome*, that will fluoresce with a defined spectrum of light when excited by light at a certain wavelength.[4] The flow cytometer can detect cells labeled with such fluorochrome-conjugated antibodies as they pass in a liquid stream through a beam of laser light of defined wavelength. As each cell passes through the laser beam, the laser light is scattered and excites any dye molecules bound to the cell, causing it to fluoresce. Sensitive photomultiplier tubes can detect the scattered light and the fluorescence emissions, respectively providing information on each cell's granularity and extent to which it bound a given fluorescence dye. This is the most common means used for distinguishing the lymphocyte subsets from one another.

The flow cytometer also can be used to isolate lymphocytes that express selected surface antigens. This requires a *fluorescence activated cell sorter*, or *FACS*. With this instrument, the fluorescence signals of cells passing through the laser light are passed back to a computer. This in turn triggers an electric charge that passes from the nozzle through the liquid stream at the precise time the stream is breaking up into droplets containing the desired cell.[5] Such droplets therefore will have a positive or negative charge, allowing for their deflection from the main stream of droplets as they pass between plates of opposite charge. In this way, two different subsets of cells

Acronyms and abbreviations that appear in this chapter include: ADP, adenosine 5′-diphosphate; ATP, adenosine 5′-triphosphate; apaf-1, apoptosis activating factor 1; Btk, Bruton tyrosine kinase; cAMP, adenosine 3′,5′-cyclic phosphate; DHEA, dehydroepiandrosterone; DPPI, dipeptidyl peptidase I; FACS, fluorescence activated cell sorter; GPI, glycerol phosphatidylinositol; lck, leukocyte tyrosine kinase; NAD, nicotinamide adenine dinucleotide; NK, natural killer; TACE, tumor necrosis factor alpha converting enzyme.

can be isolated from each other and from the unsorted cells in nondeflected droplets.

OTHER SEPARATION TECHNIQUES

An effective way of isolating lymphocyte subpopulations is to expose them to paramagnetic beads coated with a monoclonal antibody specific for the distinguishing surface molecule.[6] The tube of cells then is placed in a strong magnetic field, thereby attracting the cells that are attached to the beads. The cells attached to the beads are retained, allowing for decanting of the cells that lack the desired surface molecule. The decanted cells lacking the surface molecule are designated as being isolated via *negative selection*. Bead-bound cells can be harvested and released from the magnetic beads by adding an antibody that reacts with the antibody attached to the magnetic beads, thereby displacing the cells that are bound to the magnetic-bound antibody. The released cells are said to have been isolated via *positive selection*.

Lymphocyte subsets also can be isolated by binding the cells to plates that are coated with antibodies to a selected surface antigen, a technique known as *panning*. Alternatively, cells binding a specific complement-fixing antibody can be lysed with complement, leaving behind those cells that lack expression of the targeted surface antigen. All these techniques can be used to enrich for a selected cell subset or to deplete an undesired subset, prior to sorting using the fluorescence-activated cell sorter.

COMPOSITION OF LYMPHOCYTES

Unfortunately, few studies of the composition and biochemistry of lymphocytes have used purified lymphocyte subpopulations. Since mature helper T cells are the predominant blood lymphocyte of normal adults, many reported biochemical parameters are most relevant to this population.

ION AND WATER CONTENT

The resting blood lymphocyte has a mean cell volume of 200 μm^3 and contains 71 $\pm$ 1.2 percent by weight of water.[7] The total lymphocyte cation content is 35 fentamole per cell, of which 22 to 28 fentamole per cell is potassium, and 7.9 $\pm$ 3.2 fentamole per cell is sodium.[8] Lymphocyte membranes have both voltage-gated and calcium-activated potassium channels that regulate cell volume. Pharmacological inhibition of these channels blocks T-cell activation. The calcium content of resting lymphocytes has been estimated at 580 to 800 pmol/10^6 cells.[9] Cytosolic free calcium concentrations are relatively low in resting lymphocytes (approximately 10^{-7} M) but increase several-fold after activation.[10]

LYMPHOCYTE MEMBRANE

The lymphocyte plasma membrane is composed of equal parts of weight of protein and lipid and 6 percent by weight of carbohydrate.[11] The molar ratio of cholesterol to phospholipid is approximately 0.5.[12,13] Phosphatidylcholine is the predominant phospholipid in the lymphocyte plasma membrane, but phosphatidylethanolamine, phosphatidylinositol, phosphatidylserine, and sphingomyelin are also present. Approximately half the membrane fatty acids are saturated. The membrane proteins are usually glycosylated.

EXTRACELLULAR MEMBRANE-ASSOCIATED ENZYMES

Exposed on the exterior surface of lymphocytes are several enzymes (Table 81-1). Generally, the number of surface enzyme molecules is low compared with that of other surface molecules, such as those involved in lymphocyte adhesion (see Chap. 13). This probably reflects

TABLE 81-1   SURFACE MOLECULES AND THEIR ENZYMATIC ACTIVITIES

SURFACE MOLECULES WITH EXTRACELLULAR ENZYMATIC ACTIVITY	ENZYMATIC ACTIVITY
CD10	Neutral endopeptidase, EC 3.4.24.11
CD13	Aminopeptidase N, EC 3.4.11.2
CD26	Dipeptidylpeptidase IV, EC 3.4.14.5
CD38	ADP-ribosyl cyclase, EC 3.4.14.5
CD39	Ecto (Ca2+, Mg2+)-apyrase (ecto-ATPase)
CD73	Ecto-5′-nucleotidase
PC-1	5′-nucleotidase phosphodiesterase I, EC 3.1.4.1, and nucleotide pyrophosphatase, EC 3.6.1.9

the fact that these molecules are catalytic and have a higher functional specific activity than do molecules involved in adhesion events, where multiple interactions over large surface areas are required. As such, it is possible that many more enzymes are present than the ones currently recognized because they are expressed at levels that are not detectable by conventional methods using monoclonal antibodies and flow cytometry.

Some of the surface enzymes are involved in nucleotide metabolism (Table 81-1). For example, CD73 is an ecto-5′-nucleotidase that catalyzes the 5′ dephosphorylation of purine and pyrimidine ribo- and deoxyribonucleoside monophosphates to nucleosides that can be taken up by transport systems. This ecto-5′-nucleotidase is attached to the plasma membrane by a glycerol phosphatidylinositol (GPI) anchor (see Chap. 13). In addition, lymphocytes express a membrane-associated adenosine deaminase, the levels of which are increased after activation.[14] The shedding of adenosine deaminase by stimulated cells may explain why plasma levels of this enzyme are increased in early HIV infection and in other diseases associated with immune activation.[15]

The ectoenzymes of nucleotide metabolism may regulate lymphocyte and granulocyte function at sites of inflammation. Activated T lymphocytes can release ATP, which in turn can bind to specific plasma membrane ATP receptors.[15] In addition, CD38 can catalyze the transient formation of cyclic ADP-ribose, a new second messenger molecule directly involved in the control of calcium homeostasis by means of receptor-mediated release of calcium from ryanodine-sensitive intracellular stores.[16] The consequent increase in calcium mobilization and phospholipid breakdown can provoke activation or death, depending on the target cell. Subsequently, the dephosphorylation of ATP generates adenosine, which can interact with A2 receptors on the plasma membranes of neutrophils, monocytes, and lymphocytes. The engagement of A2 receptors elevates cAMP levels, counteracting the effects of ATP on cell activation.[17] The deamination of adenosine permits the cycle to begin anew.

The ectodomains of several other surface antigens can possess proteolytic activity. For example, CD10 (or CALLA) also has neutral endopeptidase activity, and CD26 has dipeptidyl peptidase IV activity.[18] These enzymes may play a role in modulating the binding of lymphocytes to other cells and to the extracellular matrix. In addition, inhibition of the catalytic activity of CD26 can provoke many cellular effects, including induction of tyrosine phosphorylation and p38 MAP kinase activation, as well as suppression of DNA synthesis and reduced production of various cytokines. As such, these ectoenzymes may play an important role in lymphocyte activation.

Some membrane-bound proteases have a disintegrin and a metalloprotease domain, termed *ADAMs*.[19,20] One such member of this family of proteins is the *tumor necrosis factor alpha converting enzyme*, or *TACE*, otherwise known as ADAM17. These enzymes cleave other surface molecules, such as tumor necrosis factor, thereby releasing the soluble active cytokine.[21] In addition, they may play an important role in modifying the activity of cytokines or other cell-surface molecules that are present in the vicinity of the plasma membrane.

INTRACELLULAR MEMBRANE-ASSOCIATED ENZYMES

Transmembrane proteins that have cytoplasmic regions with kinase or phosphatase activities are common in biology although relatively few of these are restricted to lymphocytes. Nevertheless, many cytoplasmic domains of transmembrane proteins interact directly with enzymes that are restricted or preferentially expressed by lymphocytes or lymphocyte subsets (see Chap. 15). B lymphocytes, for example, selectively express *Lyn, Syk,* and *Bruton tyrosine kinase,* commonly termed *Btk,* receptor-protein tyrosine kinases that associate with B-cell-receptor–associated proteins and play a critical role in signal transduction.[22] Moreover, mutations that disrupt the function of these kinases can impair B-cell development, leading to dysregulated B-cell function or immune deficiency.[23,24] T-cell development and function, on the other hand, rely heavily on receptor-protein tyrosine kinases such as *ZAP-70* or *leukocyte tyrosine kinase,* and *lck.*[25,26] ZAP-70 interacts with the T-cell receptor for antigen, whereas the latter enzyme, lck, is a Src-family tyrosine kinase that interacts with cytoplasmic domains of CD2,[27] CD4,[28] CD8,[28] CD44,[29] CD50,[30] and CD137.[31] Through such interactions, these receptor-protein-tyrosine kinases play important roles in signal transduction following immune recognition and/or cognate intercellular immune interactions.

In addition, lymphocytes possess an important class of intracellular molecules known collectively as *adapter proteins* that have no intrinsic enzymatic activity.[32–34] Instead, these molecules couple proximal biochemical events initiated by surface-receptor ligation with more distal signaling pathways by recruiting other cytosolic proteins (see Chap. 15).

CYTOMATRIX

Beneath the lymphocyte's plasma membrane is a fully developed cytomatrix with several different structural and mechanical proteins, including tubulin, actin, myosin, tropomyosin, α-actinin, filamin, and a spectrinlike molecule. These are arranged into typical microfilaments, microtubules, and intermediate filaments.[35] Lymphocyte activation by antigens or mitogens can lead to changes in the interaction of membrane components with the cytoskeleton, allowing for antigen processing, immunoglobulin secretion, or cell-mediated cytotoxic reactions.

ORGANELLES

In large part the composition and metabolism of long-lived blood T lymphocytes reflects their resting state. The T cells have a high nuclear-to-cytoplasmic ratio, few ribosomes or mitochondria, and scant endoplasmic reticulum. Glycogen stores are meager. The DNA content of the resting small lymphocyte, 8 pg per cell, is the same amount in other diploid cells. In contrast, the RNA content averages 2.5 pg per cell, yielding an RNA/DNA ratio of approximately 0.32.[36] This value is less than in most other human cells, due to the small amount of ribosomal RNA in lymphocytes.

In contrast to most lymphocytes, however, plasma cells have a high RNA/DNA ratio. These cells are the end products of B-cell differentiation and are committed to the synthesis, assembly, and secretion of immunoglobulin. Accordingly, these cells have a well-developed rough endoplasmic reticulum and Golgi apparatus but lack many of the surface receptors found on lymphocytes. Mature plasma cells are probably terminally differentiated and have a low rate of DNA synthesis and abundant RNA, reflecting the plasma cell's high-level synthesis of immunoglobulin protein.

LYSOSOMES

The few lysosomes in blood lymphocytes contain several different acid hydrolases including acid phosphatase, β glucuronidase, β galactosidase, β hexosaminidase, α arabinosidase, α galactosidase, α mannosidase, α glucosidase, and β glucosidase.[37] Acid hydrolase activities are generally higher in T cells than in non-T lymphocytes. Lysosomal acid esterase, assayed histochemically with α-naphthyl acetate as substrate, has a characteristic punctate appearance in mature T lymphocytes.[38]

CYTOTOXIC LYMPHOCYTES

In contrast to other lymphocytes, cytotoxic T lymphocytes and natural killer cells possess abundant cytoplasmic granules. These contain a pore-forming proteolytic enzyme, termed *perforin,* and a series of serine proteinases with specific proapoptotic activity, called *granzymes.*[39] To protect against possible autolysis by granule contents, cytotoxic lymphocytes possess serine-proteinase inhibitors, termed *serpins.*[40] As an additional safeguard, the granzymes of resting lymphocytes are stored as inactive proenzymes.

Cytotoxic lymphocytes rely primarily on the perforin/granzyme system to kill their targets.[41,42] Upon contact with its target cell, the cytotoxic lymphocyte converts the granzymes into active forms by a lysosomal cysteine protease called *dipeptidyl peptidase I* (DPPI).[43] Then perforin introduces a pore in the membrane, allowing the activated granzymes and other granule contents to pass into the cytoplasm and then the nucleus of the cell targeted for destruction.[44,45] In vitro studies indicate that granzyme nuclear import is independent of ATP, cannot be inhibited by nonhydrolysable GTP analogues, and involves binding within the nucleus, unlike conventional signal-dependent nuclear protein import. The perforin-dependent nuclear entry of granzymes precedes the nuclear events of apoptosis, such as DNA fragmentation and breakdown of the nuclear envelope (see Chap. 11).

LYMPHOCYTE METABOLISM

FATTY ACID AND LIPID SYNTHESIS

Normal lymphocytes synthesize phospholipids from acetate. The cells contain phospholipases A1, A2, C, and D, and the enzymes of the inositol phosphate metabolic cycle.[46]

In contrast to monocytes, small lymphocytes probably do not synthesize prostaglandins or leukotrienes; however, small lymphocytes may contain prostaglandin receptors. Prostaglandins synthesized by macrophages inhibit lymphocyte function and may be partially responsible for the impaired immunity associated with chronic inflammatory states such as in Hodgkin's disease or systemic fungal infections.[47] Certain natural fatty acid precursors of prostaglandins, such as gamma-linoleic acid, suppress immune function, and may be useful for the treatment of autoimmune disorders.[48] However, some prostaglandins may facilitate immunoglobulin class switching and synthesis of selected cytokines or cytokine receptors.[49]

CARBOHYDRATE METABOLISM

Quiescent blood lymphocytes have few or no insulin receptors, although these appear following activation. The rate of glucose metabolism is limited by the rate of entry of glucose into the cells by facilitated diffusion. Lymphocytes contain all the enzymes of the glycolytic pathway and the tricarboxylic acid cycle. Although resting lymphocytes consume only small amounts of oxygen in vitro, their mitochondria have typically coupled electron transport chains.

The resting lymphocyte requires energy to maintain its ionic milieu, to replace degraded proteins and lipids, and for active locomotion.[50,51] The recirculation of long-lived lymphocytes through the vascular space to the interstitial tissues and back from the lymphatic drainage system requires directed cell movement and utilizes considerable amounts of ATP. Lymphocytes treated with nonlethal concentrations of drugs that specifically inhibit mitochondrial respiration, but not with agents that inhibit glycolysis, recirculate sluggishly. This suggests that the energy for lymphocyte locomotion is derived largely from oxidative phosphorylation.[51]

The enzymes of the pentose-phosphate pathway account for only a small fraction of energy production in resting lymphocytes.[52] As in other cell types, the pathway provides lymphocytes with phosphorylated ribose derivatives necessary for purine and pyrimidine synthesis and with a source of reducing energy in the form of NADPH.

PROTEIN SYNTHESIS AND AMINO ACID METABOLISM

Human blood lymphocytes actively incorporate radioactive amino acids into protein. The protein synthesis is necessary for survival, and inhibition with cycloheximide or puromycin leads to the rapid death of lymphocytes.

The metabolic pathways for the synthesis of two normally nonessential amino acids, L-cysteine and L-asparagine, are inadequate in thymic lymphocytes, and probably in blood T cells.[53,54] A similar L-asparagine requirement among certain null and T-cell leukemias is responsible for the L-asparaginase sensitivity of these neoplasms.

NUCLEIC ACID SYNTHESIS AND REPAIR

RNA SYNTHESIS

Blood lymphocytes incorporate radioactive uridine into RNA at a slow but measurable rate. The cells contain the heterogeneous ribonucleoprotein particles that are important for RNA transport and splicing. In B cells, different species of RNA direct the synthesis of immunoglobulin light and heavy chains that are either inserted into the plasma membrane or secreted.[55] It is the former that predominate in nonstimulated B cells. These RNA species undergo extensive processing in the cytoplasm prior to translation, including the generation of 5′-terminal cap structures, internal methylations, and the selective removal of intervening sequences.[55]

NUCLEOTIDE METABOLISM

The enzymes for the early pathways of *de novo* purine and pyrimidine synthesis have very low activity in blood lymphocytes, consistent with the small nucleotide requirements of these nondividing cells. The lymphocytes also have minimal ribonucleotide reductase activity and a concomitantly low rate of deoxyribonucleotide synthesis. In contrast, enzymes for purine and pyrimidine intraconversion are easily detectable, with the exception of xanthine oxidase and guanase, which are absent in lymphocytes. The lymphocytes have the capacity to utilize preformed purines and pyrimidines in the plasma, when these are available. However patients with genetic deficiencies of the purine salvage enzymes hypoxanthine-guanine phosphoribosyltransferase (the Lesch-Nyhan syndrome) and adenine phosphoribosyltransferase have normal numbers of lymphocytes and adequate immune function. Hence, the purine salvage pathways are not absolutely necessary for lymphocyte survival.

Genetic deficiencies in two enzymes of purine metabolism, adenosine deaminase and purine nucleoside phosphorylase, are associated with a specific impairment of the development and function of the lymphoid system.[56] The primary function of these enzymes is the catabolism of the potentially toxic nucleosides deoxyadenosine and deoxyguanosine. In adenosine deaminase- and purine nucleoside phosphorylase-deficient patients, phosphorylated derivatives of deoxyadenosine and deoxyguanosine may accumulate in lymphocytes. When

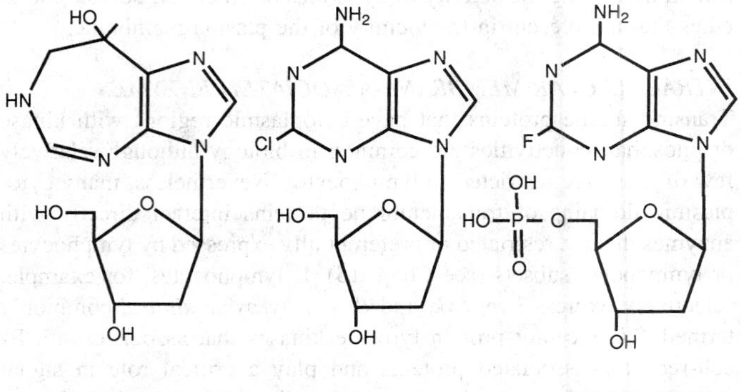

FIGURE 81-1   Structures of 2′-deoxycoformycin (*left*), 2-chlorodeoxyadenosine (*middle*), and fludarabine (*right*).

compared with other cell types, the lymphocytes have high levels of deoxycytidine kinase, for which the purine deoxyribonucleosides are alternative substrates, and low levels of cytoplasmic deoxynucleotidase.

DEOXYADENOSINE ANALOGS

Appreciation of the pathways involved in lymphocyte metabolism of nucleosides prompted development of three antilymphocyte agents, 2-chlorodeoxyadenosine (cladribine), 2-fluoroadenine arabinoside 5′-monophosphate (fludarabine), and 2′-deoxycoformycin (pentostatin) (Fig. 81-1). The two former agents are substrate analogs of 2′-deoxyadenosine that are resistant to adenosine deaminase.[57,58] They accumulate selectively in lymphocytes and inhibit both DNA replication and repair. In addition, 2′-deoxycoformycin is a tight-binding inhibitor of adenosine deaminase that prevents degradation of endogenously generated deoxyadenosine.

2-Chlorodeoxyadenosine and 2′-deoxycoformycin induce sustained remissions in the majority of patients with hairy cell leukemia[59] (see Chap. 99). Fludarabine and 2-chlorodeoxyadenosine also exert beneficial effects in chronic lymphocytic leukemia patients (see Chap. 98). The ratio of deoxycytidine kinase to 5′-nucleotidase in chronic lymphocyte leukemia cells has an apparent relationship to the clinical responsiveness of patients to 2-chlorodeoxyadenosine.[60] Leukemia lymphocytes with a high ratio respond best, probably because they selectively accumulate the toxic 5′-triphosphate metabolite.

Although the 5′-triphosphate metabolites can be incorporated into the DNA to interfere with its synthesis, these metabolites probably exert other effects to kill normal and leukemic lymphocytes. Other nucleoside analogs that are incorporated into DNA and cause chain termination, such as gemcitabine or cytosine arabinoside, do not kill blood lymphocytes.[61] Also, it is unlikely that these metabolites kill lymphocytes through adenine nucleotide depletion, since intracellular ATP levels generally are far higher than the Km values for most vital ATP-dependent enzymes.

Instead, the deoxyadenosine analogs probably exert direct effects on the machinery governing programmed cell death, or *apoptosis* (see Chap. 11). Various stimuli of apoptosis lead to the activation in the cytoplasm of cysteine proteases with specificity for aspartic acid residues, referred to as *caspases*.[62,63] The activated caspases can cleave structural proteins and enzymes necessary for the survival of both proliferating and resting cells.[64] In addition, caspases have been shown to activate the endonuclease responsible for the internucleosomal cleavage of genomic DNA, a hallmark of apoptosis. Activation of the caspase cascade in a cell-free HeLa system, depleted of endogenous low-molecular-weight compounds, requires dATP.[65] The dATP interacts with a homologue of the *C. elegans* death protein *ced4*, which was designated *apoptosis activating factor 1*, or *apaf-1*. In the presence of dATP, apaf-1 forms multimers that combine both with cytochrome c, released from "damaged" mitochondria, and procaspase-9.[66,67] This complex induces procaspase-9 processing to generate an active protease that cleaves the "executioner" caspase-3 and perhaps other caspases, with resultant activation of several enzymes that mediate cell death.[68] Inactivation of apaf-1 or caspase-9 can substitute for loss of p53 in promoting the oncogenic transformation of cells that overexpress the *MYC* oncogene.[69]

As such, adenine nucleotides may play an important role in the modulation of apoptotic and necrotic cell death signals, although different experimental models have yielded conflicting results.[70] In the cell-free system, ADP was a good inhibitor of apaf-1-dependent caspase activation, with a K_i of 133 μM. However, to understand the role of ATP and ADP in the regulation of apoptosis, one must measure changes in the concentrations of both nucleotides.

Normal lymphocytes and chronic lymphocytic leukemia cells have been reported to have average cell volumes of 160 to 200 Fl and ADP contents of 1000 to 1200 pmols/10^7 cells, respectively.[71,72] These values yield an estimated ADP concentration of about 400 μM, threefold higher than the K_i of ADP as an inhibitor of caspase activation. Taken together, the data indicate that ADP may work as a physiological intracellular inhibitor of the cytochrome c and apaf-1–mediated caspase pathway.

The positive relationship between the clinical efficacy of the purine deoxynucleosides and the capacities of their corresponding 5′-triphosphate derivatives to activate the caspase pathway underscores the relevance of these effects in the therapy of indolent lymphoproliferative diseases. However, the potency of nucleotides as activators of apaf-1 does not fully explain their diverse activities against chronic lymphocytic leukemia and hairy cell leukemia cells. Cladribine is more toxic than fludarabine when tested in purified chronic lymphocytic leukemia cells, and the in vivo dosage of fludarabine is approximately five times higher than cladribine. In contrast, 5′-triphosphate metabolite of fludarabine, F-Ara-ATP, is more effective than that of cladribine in activating caspases. Therefore, there must be additional mechanisms involved in the nucleoside cytotoxicity toward chronic lymphocytic leukemia cells.

One contributing parameter may be DNA strand break formation, which triggers the consumption of adenine nucleotide pools for poly(ADP-ribose) synthesis and reduces ADP constraints on caspase activation. In addition, various adenine deoxynucleotide analogs may interfere with mitochondrial function, perhaps fostering the release of cytochrome c. Thus, purine deoxynucleotides may be able to modulate three different components of the intrinsic apoptosis pathway: (1) DNA damage (2) mitochondrial function, and (3) apaf-1 activation, thus accounting for their activity in inducing apoptosis of resting normal or neoplastic lymphocytes.

DNA REPAIR

Nonreplicating blood T lymphocytes are capable of DNA excision/repair and contain exonucleases, endonucleases, DNA polymerases, and DNA ligase(s). These enzymes play critical roles in the rearrangement and expression of lymphocyte antigen receptors. Mutations in the DNA ligase I gene are a rare cause of an immunodeficiency with a phenotype similar to that of Bloom's syndrome.[73,74] Mice with mutations in the gene encoding the Ku antigen have a defect in repair of double-stranded DNA breaks.[75] These animals are not able to effectively repair the double-stranded DNA breaks that occur during rearrangement of immunoglobulin variable region genes and T-cell re-

ceptor genes, resulting in impaired lymphocyte development and a severe combined immunodeficiency disease (see Chap. 88). Cortical thymocytes and normal marrow B-lymphocyte precursors contain DNA polymerase γ, a DNA-template independent terminal deoxynucleotidyl transferase.[76] The enzyme adds new purine and pyrimidine bases at sites of immunoglobulin and T-cell receptor gene rearrangements, during early lymphocyte development.[77] As a developmentally restricted enzyme, DNA polymerase γ is a useful marker for the classification of acute leukemias.[78]

The variable, diversity, and joining genes segments for immunoglobulin heavy and light chains, and for the T-cell receptors for antigen, are assembled by lymphocyte-specific recombinases, designated *RAG-1* and *RAG-2* (see Chap. 83). Mutations that disrupt either of these genes impair lymphocyte development in mice[79] and humans.[80] Mutations that impair but do not completely abolish the function of RAG-1 and RAG-2 in humans can result in *Omenn syndrome*, a combined immune deficiency characterized by oligoclonal, activated T lymphocytes with a skewed Th2 profile.[81]

Despite their resting state, interphase lymphocytes are among the most sensitive cells in the body to the cytotoxic effects of ionizing radiation and ultraviolet light.[82] The reasons for their hypersensitivity are not entirely clear. Contributing factors may include the minute pools of deoxynucleotide triphosphates that limit the rate of DNA repair and the presence of abundant endonucleases that degrade DNA at sites of single- or double-strand breaks in the double helix. In addition, the activation of the nuclear enzyme poly(ADP-ribose) polymerase by DNA strand breaks may exhaust the lymphocyte's minimal NAD stores, leading to a block in oxidation-reduction reactions.[83]

HORMONES AND VITAMINS

Lymphocytes have receptors for several biologically active peptides, including ACTH, corticotrophin-releasing hormone, calcitonin, calcitonin-gene–related peptide, melatonin, endorphins, enkephalins, vasopressin, oxytoxin, thyrotropin, the tachykinins, bombesin, prolactin, growth hormone, prolactin, somatostatin, vasoactive intestinal peptide, and chemokines.[84–87] The various neuropeptides can deliver both positive and negative activation signals to lymphocytes. For example, the tachykinin substance P, which is released by peripheral nerves at sites of injury or inflammation, enhances lymphocyte activation by monocytes.[88] Immune function is inhibited by the dopamine D2 receptor-agonist bromocriptine, which causes hypoprolactinemia. Antibodies against prolactin block lymphocyte mitogenesis.[85] In general, the receptor density for peptide hormones on lymphocytes increases markedly following activation of the cells.

Glucocorticoids in pharmacological concentrations have a unique lympholytic effect that is not dependent upon cell division, and they are potent immunosuppressive agents.[89] Among normal lymphocyte subsets, immature T cells in the thymus are most sensitive. Lymphocytes contain high-affinity receptors for glucocorticoids that may direct and enhance immune functions when they interact with glucocorticoids at physiologic concentrations.[90] The glucocorticoid-receptor complexes bind to specific DNA sequences and induce mRNA for proteins that inhibit glucose transport and phospholipid hydrolysis.[91] Exposure of lymphocytes to high concentrations of glucocorticoids causes endonuclease activation and DNA fragmentation.[92–95] Glucocorticoids also profoundly inhibit the synthesis of interleukin 2 by activated T cells, and of interleukin 1 by monocytes.[96] The latter two effects offer an attractive explanation for the immunosuppressive effects of the hormones.

Lymphocytes presumably have receptors for androgens and estrogens, since the sex hormones can modulate immune function.[97] The incidence of many autoimmune diseases is higher in females than in males. Androgen therapy may benefit some women with systemic lupus erythematosus but frequently causes unacceptable masculinizing side effects. The androgens may inhibit the formation of proinflammatory cytokines by lymphocytes and monocytes, either directly or through the release of transforming growth factor $\beta1$.

The natural adrenal steroid dehydroepiandrosterone (DHEA) stimulates lymphocyte function in old mice, perhaps by interaction with a DHEA receptor complex on T cells.[98] Plasma levels of DHEA in people decline with age.[99] Whether DHEA supplementation can enhance immune responses in aged humans is still not known.

REFERENCES

1. Bøyum A: Isolation of mononuclear cells and granulocytes from human blood. Isolation of mononuclear cells by one centrifugation, and of granulocytes by combining centrifugation and sedimentation at 1 g. *Scand J Clin Lab Invest* 97 (suppl):77, 1968.
2. O'Doherty U, Steinman RM, Peng M, et al Dendritic cells freshly isolated from human blood express CD4 and mature into typical immunostimulatory dendritic cells after culture in monocyte-conditioned medium. *J Exp Med* 178:1067, 1993.
3. Jennings CD, Foon KA: Recent advances in flow cytometry: application to the diagnosis of hematologic malignancy. *Blood* 90:2863, 1997.
4. Cunningham RE: Overview of flow cytometry and fluorescent probes for cytometry. *Methods Mol Biol* 115:249, 1999.
5. Orfao A, Ruiz-Arguelles A: General concepts about cell sorting techniques. *Clin Biochem* 29:5, 1996.
6. Thiel A, Scheffold A, Radbruch A: Immunomagnetic cell sorting—pushing the limits. *Immunotechnology* 4:89, 1998.
7. Segel GB, Cokelet GR, Lichtman MA: The measurement of lymphocyte volume: importance of reference particle deformability and counting solution tonicity. *Blood* 57:894, 1981.
8. Segel GB, Simon W, Lichtman MA: Regulation of sodium and potassium transport in phytohemagglutinin-stimulated human blood lymphocytes. *J Clin Invest* 64:834, 1979.
9. Lichtman AH, Segel GB, Lichtman MA: An ultrasensitive method for the measurement of human leukocyte calcium: lymphocytes. *Clin Chim Acta* 97:107, 1979.
10. Komada H, Nakabayashi H, Nakano H, et al: Measurement of the cytosolic free calcium ion concentration of individual lymphocytes by microfluorometry using quin 2 or fura-2. *Cell Struct Funct* 14:141, 1989.
11. Crumpton MJ, Snary D: Preparation and properties of lymphocyte plasma membrane. *Contemp Top Mol Immunol* 3:27, 1974.
12. Goppelt M, Eichhorn R, Krebs G, Resch K: Lipid composition of functional domains of the lymphocyte plasma membrane. *Biochim Biophys Acta* 854:184, 1986.
13. Johnson SM, Robinson R: The composition and fluidity of normal and leukaemic or lymphomatous lymphocyte plasma membranes in mouse and man. *Biochim Biophys Acta* 558:282, 1979.
14. Kameoka J, Tanaka T, Nojima Y, Schlossman SF, Morimoto C: Direct association of adenosine deaminase with a T cell activation antigen, CD26. *Science* 261:466, 1993.
15. Apasov S, Redegeld F, Sitkovsky M: Cell-mediated cytotoxicity: contact and secreted factors. *Curr Opin Immunol* 5:404, 1993.
16. De Flora A, Guida L, Franco L, Zocchi E: The CD38/cyclic ADP-ribose system: a topological paradox. *Int J Biochem Cell Biol* 29:1149, 1997.
17. Jacobson KA, van Galen PJ, Williams M: Adenosine receptors: pharmacology, structure-activity relationships, and therapeutic potential. *J Med Chem* 35:407, 1992.
18. Kahne T, Lendeckel U, Wrenger S, Neubert K, Ansorge S, Reinhold D: Dipeptidyl peptidase IV: a cell surface peptidase involved in regulating T cell growth. *Int J Mol Med* 4:3, 1999.
19. Arribas J, Coodly L, Vollmer P, Kishimoto TK, Rose-John S, Massagué J: Diverse cell surface protein ectodomains are shed by a system sensitive to metalloprotease inhibitors. *J Biol Chem* 271:11376, 1996.
20. Yamamoto S, Higuchi Y, Yoshiyama K, et al: ADAM family proteins in the immune system. *Immunol Today* 20:278, 1999.
21. Blobel CP: Metalloprotease-disintegrins: links to cell adhesion and cleavage of TNF alpha and notch. *Cell* 90:589, 1997.
22. Kurosaki T: Genetic analysis of B cell antigen receptor signaling. *Annu Rev Immunol* 17:555, 1999.
23. Rawlings DJ: Bruton's tyrosine kinase controls a sustained calcium signal essential for B lineage development and function. *Clin Immunol* 91:243, 1999.
24. Harnett M: Syk deficiency—a knockout for B-cell development. *Immunol Today* 17:4, 1996.
25. Chu DH, Morita CT, Weiss A: The Syk family of protein tyrosine kinases in T-cell activation and development. *Immunol Rev* 165:167, 1998.
26. Elder ME: ZAP-70 and defects of T-cell receptor signaling. *Semin Hematol* 35:310, 1998.
27. Bell GM, Fargnoli J, Bolen JB, Kish L, Imboden JB: The SH3 domain of p56lck binds to proline-rich sequences in the cytoplasmic domain of CD2. *J Exp Med* 183:169, 1996.
28. Zamoyska R: The CD8 coreceptor revisited: one chain good, two chains better. *Immunity* 1:243, 1994.
29. Taher TE, Smit L, Griffioen AW, Schilder-Tol EJ, Borst J, Pals ST: Signaling through CD44 is mediated by tyrosine kinases. Association with p56lck in T lymphocytes. *J Biol Chem* 271:2863, 1996.
30. Juan M, Viñas O, Pino-Otín MR, et al: CD50 (intercellular adhesion molecule 3) stimulation induces calcium mobilization and tyrosine phosphorylation through p59fyn and p56lck in Jurkat T cell line. *J Exp Med* 179:1747, 1994.
31. Kim YJ, Pollok KE, Zhou Z, et al: Novel T cell antigen 4-1BB associates with the protein tyrosine kinase p56lck1. *J Immunol* 151:1255, 1993.
32. Clements JL, Boerth NJ, Lee JR, Koretzky GA: Integration of T cell receptor-dependent signaling pathways by adapter proteins. *Annu Rev Immunol* 17:89, 1999.
33. Wollscheid B, Wienands J, Reth M: The adaptor protein SLP-65/BLNK controls the calcium response in activated B cells. *Curr Top Microbiol Immunol* 246:283, 1999.
34. Rudd CE: Adaptors and molecular scaffolds in immune cell signaling. *Cell* 96:5, 1999.
35. Braun J, Unanue ER: The lymphocyte cytoskeleton and its control of surface receptor functions. *Semin Hematol* 20:322, 1983.
36. Glen AC: Measurement of DNA and RNA in human peripheral blood lymphocytes. *Clin Chem* 13:299, 1967.
37. Pangalis GA, Kuhl W, Waldman SR, Beutler E: Acid hydrolases in normal B and T blood lymphocytes. *Acta Haematol* 59:285, 1978.
38. Kulenkampff J, Janossy G, Greaves MF: Acid esterase in human lymphoid cells and leukaemic blasts: a marker for T lymphocytes. *Br J Haematol* 36:231, 1977.
39. Smyth MJ, O'Connor MD, Trapani JA: Granzymes: a variety of serine protease specificities encoded by genetically distinct subfamilies. *J Leukoc Biol* 60:555, 1996.
40. Bird PI: Regulation of pro-apoptotic leucocyte granule serine proteinases by intracellular serpins. *Immunol Cell Biol* 77:47, 1999.
41. Shresta S, Pham CT, Thomas DA, Graubert TA, Ley TJ: How do cytotoxic lymphocytes kill their targets? *Curr Opin Immunol* 10:581, 1998.
42. Kajino K, Kajino Y, Greene MI: Fas- and perforin-independent mechanism of cytotoxic T lymphocyte. *Immunol Res* 17:89, 1998.
43. Pham CT, Ley TJ: Dipeptidyl peptidase I is required for the processing and activation of granzymes A and B in vivo. *Proc Natl Acad Sci USA* 96:8627, 1999.
44. Spaeny-Dekking EH, Hanna WL, Wolbink AM, et al: Extracellular granzymes A and B in humans: detection of native species during CTL responses in vitro and in vivo. *J Immunol* 160:3610, 1998.
45. Blink EJ, Trapani JA, Jans DA: Perforin-dependent nuclear targeting of granzymes: a central role in the nuclear events of granule-exocytosis-mediated apoptosis? *Immunol Cell Biol* 77:206, 1999.
46. Morimoto K, Kanoh H: The role of the de novo synthetic pathway in forming molecular species of phospholipids in resting lymphocytes from human tonsils. *Biochim Biophys Acta* 617:51, 1980.
47. Olding LB, Papadogiannakis N, Barbieri B, Murgita RA: Suppressive cellular and molecular activities in maternofetal immune interactions; suppressor cell activity, prostaglandins, and alpha-fetoproteins. *Curr Top Microbiol Immunol* 222:159, 1997.
48. Callegari PE, Zurier RB: Botanical lipids: potential role in modulation of immunologic responses and inflammatory reactions. *Rheum Dis Clin North Am* 17:415, 1991.
49. Phipps RP, Stein SH, Roper RL: A new view of prostaglandin E regulation of the immune response. *Immunol Today* 12:349, 1991.
50. Segel GB, Androphy EJ, Lichtman MA: Increased ouabain-sensitive

glycolysis of lymphocytes treated with phytohemagglutinin: relationship to potassium transport. *J Cell Physiol* 97:407, 1978.

51. Freitas AA, Bognacki J: The role of locomotion in lymphocyte migration. *Immunology* 36:247, 1979.

52. Hedeskov CJ: Early effects of phytohaemagglutinin on glucose metabolism of normal human lymphocytes. *Biochem J* 110:373, 1968.

53. Miller HK, Krakoff IH, Salser JS, Balis ME: Sensitivity to L-asparaginase and amino acid metabolism. *J Natl Cancer Inst* 44:1129, 1970.

54. Kamatani N, Carson DA: Differential cyst(e)ine requirements in human T and B lymphoblastoid cell lines. *Int Arch Allergy Appl Immunol* 68:84, 1982.

55. Harriman W, Völk H, Defranoux N, Wabl M: Immunoglobulin class switch recombination. *Annu Rev Immunol* 11:361, 1993.

56. Carson DA, Carrera CJ: Immunodeficiency secondary to adenosine deaminase deficiency and purine nucleoside phosphorylation deficiency. *Semin Hematol* 27:260, 1990.

57. Beutler E: Cladribine (2-chlorodeoxyadenosine). *Lancet* 340:952, 1992.

58. Feldman EJ, Keating MJ: Fludarabine in the treatment of lymphoproliferative malignancies. *Cancer Invest* 11:314, 1993.

59. Cheson BD: New antimetabolites in the treatment of human malignancies. *Semin Oncol* 19:695, 1992.

60. Kawasaki H, Carrera CJ, Piro LD, Saven A, Kipps TJ, Carson DA: Relationship of deoxycytidine kinase and cytoplasmic 5′-nucleotidase to the chemotherapeutic efficacy of 2-chlorodeoxyadenosine. *Blood* 81:597, 1993.

61. Plunkett W, Huang P, Searcy CE, Gandhi V: Gemcitabine: preclinical pharmacology and mechanisms of action. *Semin Oncol* 23:3, 1996.

62. Rathmell JC, Thompson CB: The central effectors of cell death in the immune system. *Annu Rev Immunol* 17:781, 1999.

63. Los M, Wesselborg S, Schulze-Osthoff K: The role of caspases in development, immunity, and apoptotic signal transduction: lessons from knockout mice. *Immunity* 10:629, 1999.

64. Salvesen GS, Dixit VM: Caspase activation: the induced-proximity model. *Proc Natl Acad Sci USA* 96:10964, 1999.

65. Liu X, Kim CN, Yang J, Jemmerson R, Wang X: Induction of apoptotic program in cell-free extracts: requirement for dATP and cytochrome c. *Cell* 86:147, 1996.

66. Pan G, O'Rourke K, Dixit VM: Caspase-9, Bcl-XL, and Apaf-1 form a ternary complex. *J Biol Chem* 273:5841, 1998.

67. Zhou P, Chou J, Olea RS, Yuan J, Wagner G: Solution structure of Apaf-1 CARD and its interaction with caspase-9 CARD: a structural basis for specific adaptor/caspase interaction. *Proc Natl Acad Sci USA* 96:11265, 1999.

68. Zou H, Li Y, Liu X, Wang X: An APAF-1 cytochrome c multimeric complex is a functional apoptosome that activates procaspase-9. *J Biol Chem* 274:11549, 1999.

69. Soengas MS, Alarcón RM, Yoshida H, et al: Apaf-1 and caspase-9 in p53-dependent apoptosis and tumor inhibition. *Science* 284:156, 1999.

70. Eguchi Y, Srinivasan A, Tomaselli KJ, Shimizu S, Tsujimoto Y: ATP-dependent steps in apoptotic signal transduction. *Cancer Res* 59:2174, 1999.

71. Liebes LF, Krigel RL, Conklyn M, Nevrla DR, Silber R: Ribonucleotide content of mononuclear cells from normal subjects and patients with chronic lymphocytic leukemia: increased nicotinamide adenine dinucleotide concentration in chronic lymphocytic leukemia lymphocytes. *Cancer Res* 43:5608, 1983.

72. Kuse R, Schuster S, Schübbe H, Dix S, Hausmann K: Blood lymphocyte volumes and diameters in patients with chronic lymphocytic leukemia and normal controls. *Blut* 50:243, 1985.

73. Webster AD, Barnes DE, Arlett CF, Lehmann AR, Lindahl T: Growth retardation and immunodeficiency in a patient with mutations in the DNA ligase I gene. *Lancet* 339:1508, 1992.

74. Bentley D, Selfridge J, Millar JK, et al: DNA ligase I is required for fetal liver erythropoiesis but is not essential for mammalian cell viability. *Nat Genet* 13:489, 1996.

75. Chu G: Role of the Ku autoantigen in V(D)J recombination and double-strand break repair. *Curr Top Microbiol Immunol* 217:113, 1996.

76. Coleman MS, Yang B, Sorscher D: Regulation of terminal deoxynucleotidyl transferase gene expression in mice and men. *Crit Rev Eukaryot Gene Expr* 2:237, 1992.

77. Gilfillan S, Benoist C, Mathis D: Mice lacking terminal deoxynucleotidyl transferase: adult mice with a fetal antigen receptor repertoire. *Immunol Rev* 148:201, 1995.

78. Hammer RD, Collins RD, Ebrahimi S, Casey TT: Rapid immunocytochemical analysis of acute leukemias. *Am J Clin Pathol* 97:876, 1992.

79. Mombaerts P, Iacomini J, Johnson RS, Herrup K, Tonegawa S, Papaioannou VE: RAG-1-deficient mice have no mature B and T lymphocytes. *Cell* 68:869, 1992.

80. Schwarz K, Gauss GH, Ludwig L, et al: RAG mutations in human B cell-negative SCID. *Science* 274:97, 1996.

81. Villa A, Santagata S, Bozzi F, Imberti L, Notarangelo LD: Omenn syndrome: a disorder of Rag1 and Rag2 genes. *J Clin Immunol* 19:87, 1999.

82. Anderson RE, Warner NL: Ionizing radiation and the immune response. *Adv Immunol* 24:215, 1976.

83. Carson DA, Seto S, Wasson DB, Carrera CJ: DNA strand breaks, NAD metabolism, and programmed cell death. *Exp Cell Res* 164:273, 1986.

84. Goetzl EJ, Adelman DC, Sreedharan SP: Neuroimmunology. *Adv Immunol* 48:161, 1990.

85. Clevenger CV, Freier DO, Kline JB: Prolactin receptor signal transduction in cells of the immune system. *J Endocrinol* 157:187, 1998.

86. Baird AM, Gerstein RM, Berg LJ: The role of cytokine receptor signaling in lymphocyte development. *Curr Opin Immunol* 11:157, 1999.

87. Cyster JG, Ngo VN, Ekland EH, Gunn MD, Sedgwick JD, Ansel KM: Chemokines and B-cell homing to follicles. *Curr Top Microbiol Immunol* 246:87, 1999.

88. Lotz M, Vaughan JH, Carson DA: Effect of neuropeptides on production of inflammatory cytokines by human monocytes. *Science* 241:1218, 1988.

89. Cupps TR, Gerrard TL, Falkoff RJ, Whalen G, Fauci AS: Effects of in vitro corticosteroids on B cell activation, proliferation, and differentiation. *J Clin Invest* 75:754, 1985.

90. Wilckens T, De Rijk R: Glucocorticoids and immune function: unknown dimensions and new frontiers. *Immunol Today* 18:418, 1997.

91. Miller AH, Pariante CM, Pearce BD: Effects of cytokines on glucocorticoid receptor expression and function. Glucocorticoid resistance and relevance to depression. *Adv Exp Med Biol* 461:107, 1999.

92. Cohen JJ, Duke RC: Glucocorticoid activation of a calcium-dependent endonuclease in thymocyte nuclei leads to cell death. *J Immunol* 132:38, 1984.

93. Evans-Storms RB, Cidlowski JA: Regulation of apoptosis by steroid hormones. *J Steroid Biochem Mol Biol* 53:1, 1995.

94. Montague JW, Cidlowski JA: Glucocorticoid-induced death of immune cells: mechanisms of action. *Curr Top Microbiol Immunol* 200:51, 1995.

95. Scudeletti M, Lanza L, Monaco E, et al: Immune regulatory properties of corticosteroids: prednisone induces apoptosis of human T lymphocytes following the CD3 down-regulation. *Ann NY Acad Sci* 876:164, 1999.

96. Northrop JP, Crabtree GR, Mattila PS: Negative regulation of interleukin 2 transcription by the glucocorticoid receptor. *J Exp Med* 175:1235, 1992.

97. Grossman CJ, Roselle GA, Mendenhall CL: Sex steroid regulation of autoimmunity. *J Steroid Biochem Mol Biol* 40:649, 1991.

98. Meikle AW, Dorchuck RW, Araneo BA, et al: The presence of a dehydroepiandrosterone-specific receptor binding complex in murine T cells. *J Steroid Biochem Mol Biol* 42:293, 1992.

99. Orentreich N, Brind JL, Rizer RL, Vogelman JH: Age changes and sex differences in serum dehydroepiandrosterone sulfate concentrations throughout adulthood. *J Clin Endocrinol Metab* 59:551, 1984.

LYMPHOCYTE ONTOGENY

TUCKER W. LEBIEN

FRED E. BERTRAND

The functional mammalian immune system consists of three major lymphocyte populations with different antigen recognition systems: thymus-derived (T) cells; bursal, or marrow-derived, (B) cells; and natural killer (NK) cells. The three populations mediate complex and distinct immune effector functions. The development and manifestation of immune effector functions reflect differences in patterns of gene expression in T, B, and NK cells. Of primary importance in T and B cells are receptor complexes that mediate antigen recognition: the T-cell receptor (TCR) on T cells and the B-cell receptor (BCR) on B cells. NK cells do not express antigen-specific receptors; rather, specificity of NK cell recognition is provided by inhibitory signals transduced by receptors recognizing class I major histocompatibility complex molecules.[1] The differences in effector functions and organ distribution can be traced to differences in early ontogeny. This chapter reviews lymphocyte ontogeny. We emphasize the genesis, gene expression, developmental options, and growth requirements of T, B, and NK cells. A more extensive discussion of B-cell, T-cell, and NK-cell function can be found in Chaps. 83, 84, and 85, respectively.

LYMPHOCYTE DEVELOPMENT FROM PLURIPOTENTIAL STEM CELLS

Lymphocytes are derived from pluripotential stem cells (PSC), also called hematopoietic stem cells. Pluripotential stem cells have the capacity to give rise to all cellular components of the blood and are discussed in greater detail in Chap. 14. Two terms used to describe the potential fate of PSC are *self-renewal* and *differentiation*. Self-renewal refers to the capacity of a cell to divide and give rise to two daughter cells that exhibit an indistinguishable pattern of gene expression. Differentiation refers to the genetically programmed sequence of events wherein cells undergo orderly changes in gene expression, culminating in a precursor-progeny relationship. The closer two cells are in a developmental pathway, the subtler are the differences in gene expression.

For many years the embryonic yolk sac (i.e., tissue outside the embryo proper) was considered to be the reservoir of self-renewing PSC that contribute to life-long lymphohematopoiesis.[2] That concept has been seriously challenged by studies in murine embryos indicat-

Acronyms and abbreviations that appear in this chapter include: B, marrow derived; BCR, B-cell receptor; CD, cluster of differentiation; CS-1, connecting segment 1; DC, dendritic cell; DP, double positive; FL, flt-3 ligand; Ig, immunoglobulin; IL, interleukin; KIR, killer inhibitory receptors; NK, natural killer; PSC, pluripotential stem cells; RAG, recombination activating gene; ψLC, surrogate light chain; SP, single positive; T, thymus derived; TCR, T-cell receptor; TdT, terminal deoxynucleotidyl transferase; TREC, TCR rearrangement excision circle; TRI, trilineage; VCAM-1, vascular adhesion molecule-1.

ing that intraembryonic tissue encompassing paraaortic splanchnopleura and derived aorta-gonad-mesonephros harbor PSC prior to the fetal liver.[3,4] Furthermore, lymphoid precursors were identified in the paraaortic splanchnopleura prior to the onset of circulation.[3,5] Human hematopoiesis initiates in the yolk sac at week 3 of gestation and shifts to fetal liver circa week 5.[6,7] Two studies employing human embryonic tissue addressed whether an intraembryonic source of definitive human PSC exists. The cell surface sialomucin CD34, a widely used marker for human PSC (see Chap. 14), was used to identify candidate stem cells. In one study, highly proliferating CD34+ stem cells were identified in 5-week human embryonic tissue devoid of yolk sac and liver anlage.[8] In a second study, clusters of CD34+ hematopoietic-like cells were detected in the ventral aortic endothelium.[9] CD34+ hematopoietic cells clustered in the ventral aortic endothelium were analyzed by the technique of in situ hybridization and were shown to express transcription factors and growth factor receptors important in early hematopoiesis.[10] It is conceivable, however, that CD34+ PSC migrate from the yolk sac or ventral aortic endothelium to the fetal liver and differentiate into lymphoid progenitors with multilymphoid lineage potential.

Landmark studies in the mouse employing chromosomal markers[11] and transfected gene markers[12] were instrumental in defining the relationship between PSC and cells committed to the T, B, and NK lineages. Antibodies to specific cell-surface antigens and fluorescence-activated cell sorting were used to purify mouse PSC.[13] Mouse PSC express cell-surface Sca-1 and low levels of Thy-1 but are negative for lineage-specific antigens. Cells with this phenotype constitute less than 0.05 percent of adult mouse marrow. Fewer than 100 of these cells injected into an irradiated mouse can reconstitute the entire lymphohematopoietic system, including B and T cells.[13,14]

The development of T, B, and NK cells from PSC is well accepted, but the existence of a common lymphoid progenitor that is restricted to developing into T, B, or NK cells, but not myeloid and erythroid cells, has been controversial. Data from the study of alterations in the hypoxanthine guanine phosphoribosyl-transferase gene in blood mononuclear cells from an atomic bomb survivor suggest that T, B, and NK cells are derived from a common progenitor.[15] However, it is not clear whether the progenitor characterized in this study was truly lymphoid restricted or whether it also harbored the capacity to differentiate into nonlymphoid (i.e., myeloid and erythroid) blood cells. Two recent reports have provided fresh evidence supporting the existence of a common lymphoid progenitor in humans and mice. Fluorescence-activated cell sorting was used to isolate a rare population of CD10+/CD19− lymphoid progenitors from human adult and fetal marrow.[16] These CD10+/CD19− cells were capable of developing into T, B, NK, or lymphoid dendritic cells, but not myeloid or erythroid cells.[16] A second study used fluorescence-activated cell sorting to isolate a rare population of mouse marrow lymphoid cells expressing the interleukin-7 (LI-7) receptor and demonstrated that a single one of these cells could generate at least T and B cells, but not myeloid cells.[17] However, single cell plating of individual fetal liver-derived mouse stem cells in vitro has suggested the existence of bipotential precursors with the capacity to mature into myeloid or B lineage cells.[14] Thus, more work is necessary to fully characterize the common lymphoid progenitors and the signaling events (e.g., cytokines or stromal-cell–associated molecules) that regulate survival, growth, and apoptosis of these cells. Figure 82-1 shows the existence of common lymphoid progenitors in the marrow and the developmental potential of this progenitor. It is important to emphasize that the existence of this cell is based on a single study.[16] The cell designated common lymphoid progenitors-TRI (for *trilineage*) is a candidate progenitor that migrates to the thymus (see below), but experimental evidence that this cell exists is lacking.

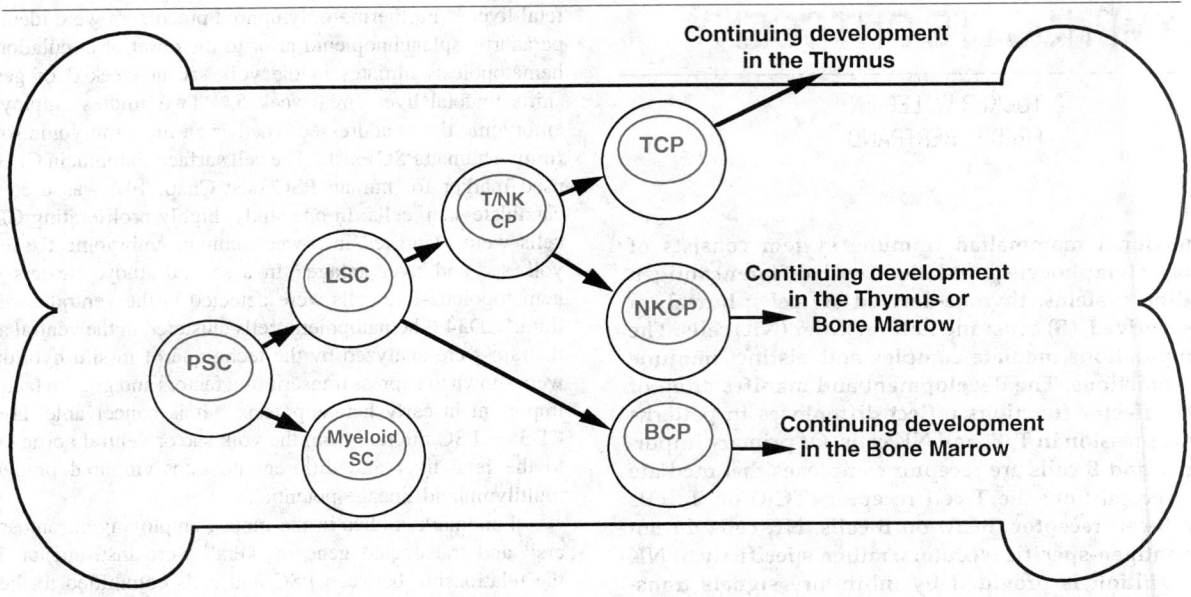

FIGURE 82-1   Developmental relationship among PSC, common lymphoid progenitors, and T, B, NK, and lymphoid DC lineages. The common lymphoid progenitors-TRI progenitor is proposed to be distinct from the common lymphoid progenitors by virtue of the inability of common lymphoid progenitors-TRI to develop into the B lineage. The two pathways shown for common lymphoid progenitors-TRI development in the thymus are based on a review of the literature discussed by Spits and colleagues.[102] The NK/DC dual progenitor shown in pathway 2 is based on studies by Márquez et al.[106] The dashed line underneath the PSC indicates the capacity to undergo self-renewal. The arrows with parallel slashes indicate that several stages of development between a progenitor (e.g., a pro-B cell) and a mature lymphocyte (e.g., a B cell) have been deleted for simplicity. Completed pathways for B, T, and NK development are shown in Figs. 82-2, 82-3, and 82-4.

B-CELL DEVELOPMENT

The defining characteristic of a mature B cell is the expression of cell surface immunoglobulin (Ig). The cell-surface Ig consists of mu (μ), delta (δ), gamma (γ), alpha (α), or epsilon (ε) heavy chains disulfide-linked to kappa (κ) or lambda (λ) light chains (see Chap. 83). The cell surface Ig and associated signaling molecules (see below) are often referred to as the BCR. Precursor (pre-) B cells are generally defined by the presence of cytoplasmic μ heavy chains in the absence of cell surface Ig. Progenitor (pro-) B cells are generally defined by the absence of cytoplasmic and surface μ heavy chains. This minimalist definition of pro-B, pre-B, and B cells[18,19] forms the basis of the present detailed model of human B-cell development. B-cell development can be divided into two stages: an antigen-independent stage that occurs primarily in fetal liver and fetal and adult marrow, and an antigen-dependent stage that occurs primarily in secondary lymphoid tissue, such as spleen and lymph node.

ORGANS INVOLVED IN B-CELL DEVELOPMENT

Human fetal liver and omentum are the main sites of B-cell development from 8 to 14 weeks' gestation. Fetal omentum is a thin, vascularized, membranous fold of peritoneum and has been considered part of the lymphoid system because it contains aggregates of lymphoid cells called milk spots. Pre-B cells can be detected in fetal liver at 7 to 8 weeks' gestation[18] and in fetal omentum at 10 weeks' gestation.[20] Second-trimester B-cell development is multifocal, since pro-B, pre-B, and immature B cells can be detected in the marrow and liver and, to a lesser extent, the lung and kidney.[21] From the end of the second trimester throughout adult life, marrow is the exclusive site of B-cell development. The frequency of early B-lineage cells as a percentage of the total nucleated lymphohematopoietic cell pool is much higher in fetal than in adult marrow.[21,22]

IMMUNOGLOBULIN GENE REARRANGEMENT AND EXPRESSION

The hallmark of marrow B-cell development is the ordered rearrangement of gene segments that encode the variable portion of the antibody molecule (see Chap. 83 for additional detail). This process typically begins with germ-line transcription of the μ heavy-chain locus, followed by the joining of one of 30 D_H segments to one of six J_H segments.[23] Once this DJ_H join is completed, one of approximately 130 upstream V_H gene segments[24] can join to form a completed VDJ_H rearrangement.[23] If the VDJ_H rearrangement is "in frame," meaning that it is capable of encoding a functional μ heavy-chain protein, VDJ rearrangement ceases. This process is termed allelic exclusion. Experiments in mice demonstrated that allelic exclusion depends on the presence of μ heavy chain,[25] but the mechanism or mechanisms of allelic exclusion is unknown. If the initial VDJ_H rearrangement is nonfunctional (i.e., the rearrangement does not encode a μ heavy-chain protein), then rearrangement can proceed to the other heavy-chain allele. If a nonfunctional VDJ_H rearrangement occurs on both alleles, the cell undergoes apoptosis and is phagocytized by marrow macrophages.

Following completion of a functional μ heavy-chain rearrangement, recombination at the light-chain locus proceeds in a similar fashion.[23] This usually begins with germ-line transcription of the κ locus followed by the rearrangement of a V_κ to J_κ. If an initial VJ_κ rearrangement is functional, the light-chain locus also undergoes allelic exclusion. If not, rearrangement proceeds to the other κ allele.

It is generally thought that, should recombination at both κ alleles fail to result in a functional rearrangement, the λ light-chain locus will rearrange.[23] An alternative model proposes that light-chain rearrangement begins at the κ and λ loci simultaneously.[26] Due to a difference in recombination rate, the κ locus usually finishes recombining first, potentially explaining the high ratio of κ- to λ-expressing B cells in the mouse.[26]

Heavy- and light-chain Ig gene rearrangement encompasses multiple stages of human B-cell development, shown in Fig. 82-2. DJ$_H$ rearrangements initially occur in a CD10+/CD34+/CD19− progenitor designated the early B cell.[27,28] CD19+/CD34+ pro-B cells harbor VDJ$_H$ rearrangements,[27] and a functional VDJ$_H$ rearrangement results in differentiation to the pre-BI cell stage. The pre-BI compartment is enriched for cells in cycle that express the pre-BCR (see below). The subsequent pre-BII compartment undergoes V to Jκ light-chain rearrangement, and pre-BII cells with functional light-chain rearrangements differentiate into immature B cells expressing μ/κ or μ/λ BCR. Ig gene rearrangement generally proceeds through an ordered progression, beginning with the μ heavy-chain gene and proceeding through κ and (if necessary) λ light-chain genes.[29] Alternative pathways have been described in which light-chain rearrangement precedes heavy-chain rearrangement[30] and λ light-chain rearrangement precedes κ light-chain rearrangment.[31]

At the pro-B to pre-B transition, μ heavy-chain encoded by a functional VDJ rearrangement associates with a complex called the surrogate light chain (ψLC).[32] ψLC is a heterodimeric protein complex consisting of the $\lambda5$ and VpreB gene products.[33,34] ψLC genes exhibit significant homology with conventional λ light chains but do not undergo gene rearrangement. The μ-ψLC receptor associates with the Igα and Igβ signaling molecules (see below) to form the pre-BCR.[32] The VpreB protein is expressed in the cytoplasm of CD19− early B cells prior to the expression of μ heavy chain.[35] However, surface expression of the μ-ψLC pre-BCR is restricted to a subset of large pre-BI and small pre-BII cells.[35,36]

The importance of the ψLC in B-cell development was first demonstrated in mice with a targeted disruption in the $\lambda5$ locus.[37] $\lambda5$-deficient mice exhibit a block in B-cell development at the pro-B to pre-B transition, presumably because the cells fail to receive a positive selection signal in the absence of a functional pre-BCR.[37] Patients with mutations in the $\lambda5$ gene exhibit a profound block in pro-B to pre-B cell differentiation,[38] confirming the importance of the μ-ψLC in human B-cell development as well.

Pre-B cells undergo a type of positive selection by virtue of pre-BCR expression. That is, pre-BCR expression is a requisite for pre-B cell survival and differentiation. A ligand for the pre-BCR has never been identified, and the molecular basis for this positive selection is unknown. However, recent studies in the mouse provide a clue. Some nascent μ heavy chains can physically pair with ψLC, whereas others cannot. Pre-B cells expressing μ heavy chains that can pair with ψLC to form a pre-BCR will survive and differentiate into immature B cells.[39,40]

EXPRESSION OF RECOMBINATION-ASSOCIATED GENES

Two genes, designated recombination activating gene-1 (RAG-1) and recombination activating gene-2 (RAG-2), are necessary and essential for Ig and TCR gene rearrangements.[41] Mice deficient in either RAG-1 or RAG-2 have severe disruptions in early B-cell development.[42,43]

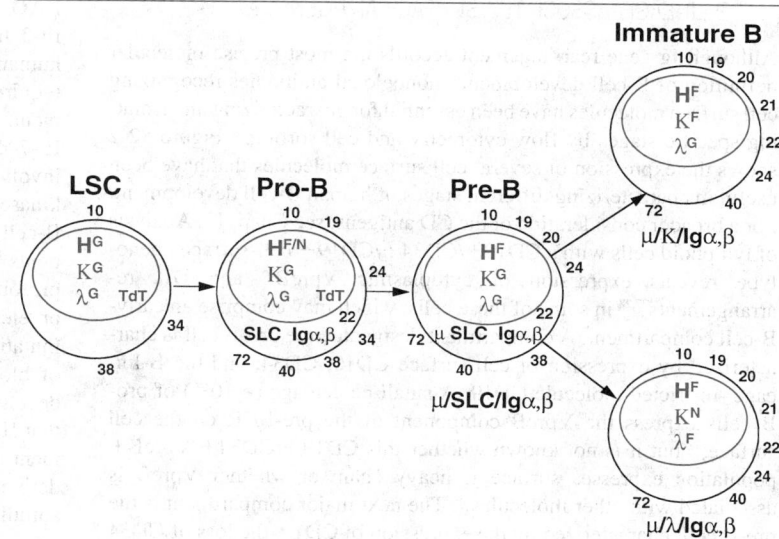

FIGURE 82-2   B-cell development in human marrow. The common lymphoid progenitors correspond to the common lymphoid progenitors in Fig. 82-1 with multilymphoid lineage developmental potential. The TdT, RAG, VpreB, Igα, and μ designations within the cells indicate nuclear (TdT and RAG) and cytoplasmic (VpreB, Igα, and μ) expression of these proteins. The shaded areas indicate active Ig gene rearrangement at that stage of development. *Marrow stromal cells* is a generic phrase encompassing several different nonlymphohematopoietic cell types in the marrow microenvironment.

Furthermore, mutations in the RAG genes have been identified in some patients with severe combined immunodeficiency.[44] In vitro studies have shown that the RAG gene products bind to recombination signal sequences and introduce double-stranded DNA breaks during initiation of the recombination cleavage reaction.[45] In humans, RAG-1 and RAG-2 are expressed from the early-B-cell stage through the pre-B stage of development (Fig. 82-2). Once a cell has successfully completed heavy- and light-chain rearrangement, RAG gene expression generally ceases. In B cells with autoreactive BCR specificity, RAG expression can be reactivated by a process called receptor editing.[46,47] Little is known about how expression of RAG genes is regulated. Some investigators have reported that levels of RAG transcription vary as a function of B-cell development.[29] In addition, the RAG-2 protein is regulated in a cell-cycle-dependent fashion through phosphorylation.[48] The promoters for human RAG-1 and RAG-2 have been identified.[49] Although the promoter sequences will drive transcription of each gene, they are not sufficient to confer lineage and stage specificity to RAG transcription.

Terminal deoxynucleotidyl transferase (TdT) is not required for the recombination reaction but is necessary for the generation of antigen-receptor diversity. TdT inserts non–template-encoded nucleotides (so-called N-region insertions) at the D$_H$ to J$_H$ and V$_H$ to DJ$_H$ junctions of heavy chains.[50] The N-region insertions serve to increase the diversity of the antigen-receptor repertoire to encode more than 1×10^8 different specificities. A limited number of κ light-chain rearrangements contain TdT N-region insertions.[51] Mice bearing a targeted deletion of the TdT gene lack characteristic N-region insertions at the D$_H$ to J$_H$ and V$_H$ to DJ$_H$ heavy-chain boundaries.[52,53] TdT protein is initially expressed in common lymphoid progenitors.[15,54] As shown in Fig. 82-2, the CD19+/CD34+ pro-B–cell population is TdT+, but expression is turned off in the pre-B cell.[29,55,56] Reduction in TdT expression at the pro-B to pre-B transition explains why light-chain gene rearrangements have so few N-region insertions.

B-LINEAGE–ASSOCIATED SURFACE ANTIGENS

Although Ig gene rearrangement accords the most precise molecular definition of B-cell development, monoclonal antibodies recognizing cell surface molecules have been essential for characterizing and isolating specific stages by flow cytometry and cell sorting.[57] Figure 82-2 shows the expression of several cell surface molecules that have been useful in characterizing different stages of human B-cell development. For a broader consideration of the CD antigens, see Chap. 13. Analysis of lymphoid cells with a CD10+/CD34+/CD19– cell-surface phenotype reveals expression of cytoplasmic VpreB[35] and DJ_H rearrangements[27,28] in some of these cells, which may comprise an early-B-cell compartment. A compartment designated the pro-B cell is characterized by expression of cell surface CD10, CD34, and the B-lineage–restricted molecule CD19. A small percentage ($\approx$10%) of pro-B cells express the VpreB component of the pre-BCR on the cell surface,[35] but it is not known whether this CD19+/CD34+/VpreB+ population expresses surface μ heavy chain or whether VpreB is associated with other molecules.[58] The next major compartment is the pre-B cell, characterized by the expression of CD19, the loss of CD34 and TdT, and the acquisition of μ heavy chain in more than 90 percent of the cells.[29,55,56] The pre-B–cell population can be subdivided into large cycling cells and small noncycling cells based on cell cycle analysis.[29] A subset of pre-B cells expresses the μ-ψLC pre-BCR[29,35] in association with a heterodimer designated Igα/CD79a and Igβ/CD79b. The Igα/Igβ heterodimer is an essential molecular complex that initiates signal transduction following cross-linking of the pre-BCR and BCR.[59,60] It is interesting to note that Igα and Igβ are expressed in CD10+/CD19– early B cells prior to the appearance of functional VDJ_H rearrangements.[61] The function of Igα and Igβ in early B cells is unknown. Mice with a targeted disruption of the Igβ gene are blocked at the level of DJ_H rearrangement,[62] suggesting a critical function for the Igβ protein separate from its functional role in the cell surface μ-ψLC pre-BCR. Once pre-B cells successfully rearrange κ or λ light chain genes, they differentiate into immature B cells expressing the BCR. Immature B cells also express high levels of B-cell–restricted cell-surface molecules, including CD20, CD21, CD22, and CD40.

REGULATION OF B-CELL PRECURSOR GROWTH

B-cell development in marrow is regulated by a complex interplay of signals transduced by stromal cells, the extracellular matrix (e.g., fibronectin and type IV collagen), and possibly other lymphohematopoietic cells. The continuous production of B cells throughout life[21] is dependent upon an intact marrow microenvironment.

The interaction or adhesion of human B-cell precursors to the marrow stromal cell microenvironment is mediated through VLA-4 and VLA-5 integrins.[63,64] VLA-4 has two ligands: vascular cell adhesion molecule-1 (VCAM-1) and the CS-1 domain of fibronectin.[65] The ligand for VLA-5 is the central cell-binding domain of fibronectin that contains the amino acid sequence arginine-glycine-aspartic acid, or RGD.[65] Marrow stromal cells constitutively express VCAM-1.[63,64] Functional expression of VCAM-1 can be positively regulated by IL-1β and IL-4 and negatively regulated by TGF-β.[64] VLA-4/VCAM-1 interaction is critical for the adhesion of B-cell precursors to marrow stromal cells, but the function of VLA-4 in B-cell precursors beyond simple adhesion is not well understood.

Human B-cell precursors can be positively or negatively influenced by several different cytokines.[66] IL-7 facilitates the marrow stromal cell–dependent growth of B-cell precursors.[67] The CD19+/CD34+ pro-B cell is the IL-7–responsive population that grows on marrow stromal cells,[68] and IL-7 triggers decreased expression of

RAG-1, RAG-2, and TdT.[68,69] A combination of IL-7, IL-3, and the flt-3 ligand (FL) is the strongest known stimulus for the growth of human pro-B cells.[70] A striking species difference characterizes the requirement for IL-7 signaling in human and murine B-cell development. Murine B-cell development has an absolute requirement for IL-7–IL-7-receptor interaction and subsequent downstream signaling involving the γ_c subunit of the IL-7 receptor and the Jak-3 tyrosine kinase.[71] In contrast, IL-7 is necessary but not sufficient for human B-cell development. X-linked severe combined immunodeficiency patients have mutations in the γ_c cytokine–receptor subunit and exhibit profound thymic hypoplasia, an absence of NK cells, but normal or elevated numbers of B cells.[72] Immunodeficiency patients with mutations in Jak-3[73,74] or the IL-7 receptor[75] also have normal numbers of blood B cells. Furthermore, an in vitro model of human B-cell development is IL-7 independent.[76] These collective results indicate that IL-7 is not essential for at least the numerically normal development of human B cells. The identity of the human marrow stromal cell-derived molecule or molecules that provide the essential proliferative stimulus for human pro-B cells is unknown.

T-CELL DEVELOPMENT

As discussed above, B-cell development can be detected in week 15 human fetal marrow, and the marrow is the primary source of B-cell development throughout life.[21] A fundamental distinction between mammalian B- and T-cell development is that the latter generally consists of an essential progenitor migration step from fetal liver or fetal or postnatal marrow to the thymus. Thus, PSC in fetal liver and marrow or postnatal marrow may differentiate into a progenitor that migrates to the thymus (see Fig. 82-1). The precise phenotype of this migratory progenitor is unknown. Relatively little is known regarding the mechanisms that attract marrow lymphoid precursors to the thymus, but chemotactic factors (e.g., chemokines) produced by thymic stromal cells probably play a role.[77]

ORGANS INVOLVED IN T-CELL DEVELOPMENT

FETAL LIVER AND MARROW

Studies of human T-cell lymphoblastic leukemia revealed the CD7 cell surface molecule as a candidate marker of early T-cell development.[78] In support of this concept, CD7+ lymphoid cells expressing cytoplasmic CD3ε are present in fetal liver at 7 to 8 weeks' gestation.[79,80] Furthermore, CD7+/cytoplasmic CD3ε+ progenitors are present in fetal liver and fetal thorax just prior to colonization of the epithelial thymic rudiment.[79] Rare CD34+/CD7+ lymphoid cells are also present in fetal marrow.[81] One difficulty in interpreting the collective data in these studies is that CD7 is also expressed on NK progenitors and some myeloid cells and is therefore not a T-lineage–specific marker. The developmental relationship between cells that express CD7+ and cytoplasmic CD3ε+ cells versus cells that express CD10 and the IL-7 receptor is unknown (see Fig. 82-1). However, the common lymphoid progenitors contain approximately 10 percent CD7+ cells.[16] Thus, the CD7+/cytoplasmic CD3ε+ cells may be comparable to the common lymphoid progenitors-TRI (see Fig. 82-1). To complicate matters, an alternative pathway of T-cell development that occurs in marrow has been described in the mouse.[82] Whether a T-cell developmental pathway exists in human marrow is unknown. However, extrathymic T-cell maturation may occur in human fetal liver[83] and fetal intestine.[84]

THYMUS

The human thymic microenvironment begins to develop at approximately 4 weeks' gestation[84] and then undergoes at least three developmental phases.[86] The first phase occurs between 4 and 8 weeks' gestation and is characterized by endoderm- and ectoderm-derived thymic epithelial cell proliferation. The second phase occurs between 9 and 15 weeks' gestation and is characterized by the appearance of subcapsular, cortical, and medullary regions. Colonization by fetal liver–derived progenitors begins at about week 9. The third phase occurs from 16 weeks' gestation until 1 to 2 years of age and is characterized by maximal intrathymic T-cell maturation. Historical views have assumed that the thymus only functions in young humans and mice because of its well-known involution during early life.[87] This viewpoint has been seriously challenged by the use of a sophisticated polymerase chain reaction assay that detects extrachromosomal DNA circles called TCR rearrangement excision circles, or TRECs.[88] TRECs are a product of TCR gene rearrangement and represent a molecular marker of thymic function. Using the TREC assay, thymic function was observed to decline by 5-fold at age 35 and 50-fold by age 65, but individuals over 70 years still had TRECs in their blood T cells.[88] The T-cell pool appears to be replenished via a functional thymus (albeit in an age-dependent manner) throughout life.

Thymic T-cell maturation is an extraordinarily complex series of events that results in the development of a functional T-cell repertoire.[89] In addition to the thymocytes, which are at multiple stages of development based on immunologic phenotype (see below), numerous nonlymphoid cells make up the thymic microenvironment.[90] The subcapsular, cortical, and medullary regions of the thymus contain heterogeneous populations of epithelial cells, macrophages, and dendritic/interdigitating cells (see Chap. 5). Current models suggest that positive selection (the process by which T cells recognizing foreign peptides are selected) and negative selection (the process by which T cells recognizing self-peptides are eliminated) occur when developing thymocytes interact with thymic epithelial cells and dendritic/interdigitating cells, respectively. The heterogeneity of the epithelial cell compartment in the thymus is particularly striking,[91,92] and the significance of this heterogeneity in the context of positive selection and other events in thymic T-cell maturation remains to be clarified.

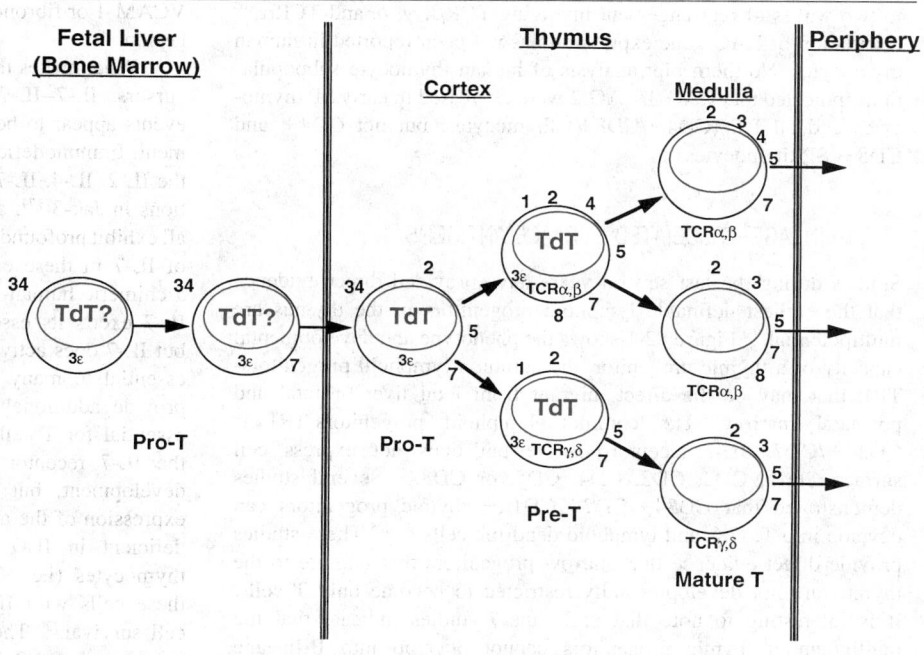

FIGURE 82-3 T-cell development in human thymus. Two potential progenitors of the pro-T cell are shown: T/NK and common lymphoid progenitors-TRI. These two progenitors reflect the two possible pathways shown in Fig. 82-1 wherein either a T/NK or a common lymphoid progenitors-TRI could be the immediate progenitor of the pro-T cell. The TdT and RAG designations indicate nuclear expression of these proteins. The shaded areas indicate active TCR rearrangement at that stage of development. *Thymic stromal cells* is a generic phrase encompassing several different cell types in the thymic microenvironment.

T-CELL RECEPTOR GENE REARRANGEMENT AND EXPRESSION

Like the Ig molecule, the TCR is encoded by distinct gene segments (V, D, J, and C) that rearrange during T-cell development.[93] TCR genes encode polypeptides designated α, β, γ, and δ (see Chap. 84).[93] The α and β proteins pair with one another to form the TCR$\alpha\beta$. The γ and δ proteins pair with one another to form the TCR$\gamma\delta$. The TCR$\alpha\beta$ and TCR$\gamma\delta$ are noncovalently associated with a family of proteins called the CD3 complex. CD3 performs a crucial role in signal transduction following TCR cross-linking, analogous to the role of Igα/Igβ in mediating signal transduction following BCR cross-linking. A more detailed description of TCR genes and proteins is presented in Chap. 84.

Rearrangement of TCRγ and δ genes occurs prior to rearrangement of TCRβ and α genes during human T-cell development.[94,95] The thymocyte compartment containing TCRγ and δ re-

arrangements with most TCRβ genes in germ-line configuration is the pro-T cell (Fig. 82-3). TCRβ rearrangements are initiated in the next stage of T-cell development: the early single-positive (SP) CD4+/CD8− thymocytes. If the TCRβ rearrangement is functional, the encoded TCRβ protein assembles into a complex called the pre-TCR. Cells expressing the pre-TCR are designated early double-positive (DP) thymocytes because they express both CD4 and CD8. If the TCRβ rearrangement is nonfunctional, the early SP thymocytes undergo apoptosis. The elimination of developing T cells by this mechanism mirrors the elimination of pro-B cells that fail to make a functional VDJ$_H$ rearrangement. The pre-TCR consists of TCRβ protein, the CD3 signal transduction protein complex, and an invariant chain designated pTα. The pTα gene was originally cloned in the mouse[96] and subsequently in humans.[97,98] It is interesting to note that the pre-TCR functions as a sensor and facilitates the survival and expansion of pre-TCR+ thymocytes in a process called β selection.[99] Rearrangement of TCRα genes subsequently occurs in intermediate DP thymocytes, eventually culminating in expression of low levels of surface TCR$\alpha\beta$ in late DP thymocytes (see Fig. 82-3).

EXPRESSION OF RECOMBINATION-ASSOCIATED GENES

The role of RAG-1, RAG-2, and TdT in the rearrangement and diversification of the TCR repertoire is very similar to their role in rearrangement and diversification of the BCR repertoire. RAG-1- and RAG-2-deficient mice exhibit profound disruptions in normal thymocyte development due to a failure to initiate TCR rearrangement.[42,43] Likewise, TdT-deficient mice lack N-region insertions and exhibit a restricted diversification of the TCR repertoire.[52,53] RAG gene expression oscillates during murine thymocyte development, corresponding to two waves of rearrangement involving TCRβ, γ, δ, and TCRα.[100] Oscillation of RAG gene expression has not been reported in human thymocytes. Northern blot analysis of human thymocyte subpopulations indicated that RAG-1/RAG-2 were expressed in early SP thymocytes and all DP (CD4+/CD8+) thymocytes, but not CD4+ and CD8+ SP thymocytes.[101]

T-LINEAGE–ASSOCIATED SURFACE ANTIGENS

Studies during the last several years have provided direct evidence that the earliest definable lymphoid progenitors in the thymus are multipotential.[102] Figure 82-1 shows the phenotype and developmental capacity of a thymic progenitor, the common lymphoid progenitors-TRI, that may be the direct migrant from fetal liver or fetal and postnatal marrow. The common lymphoid progenitors-TRI is CD34+/CD7+/IL-7 receptor-positive but does not express cell surface CD1a, CD2, CD3, CD4, CD5, or CD8.[103] Several studies demonstrated that CD34+/CD7+/CD1a− thymic progenitors can develop into T, NK, and lymphoid dendritic cells.[104–106] These studies provide direct evidence that marrow progenitors that migrate to the thymus are not developmentally restricted to become only T cells. It is interesting to note that preliminary studies indicate that the multipotential thymic progenitors cannot develop into B-lineage cells,[102] suggesting that the marrow progenitor designated common lymphoid progenitors-TRI may be the cell that migrates to the thymus (see Fig. 82-1).

As shown in Fig. 82-3, acquisition of cell surface CD1 defines an important checkpoint in T-cell development, and the CD34+/CD1a+ pro-T cell population preferentially develops into the T lineage.[102] The next developmental stage is the early SP thymocyte, which is CD4+/CD8−. Early SP thymocytes are fully committed to the T lineage and can give rise to TCRαβ- or TCRγδ-expressing T cells.[102] Early SP thymocytes differentiate into early DP thymocytes. Early DP thymocytes are easily distinguished from their early SP precursors by the expression of CD8 and the pre-TCR.[101] Figure 83-3 shows three DP stages (early, intermediate, and late) that likely reflect a linear developmental pathway. Early DP thymocytes expressing the pre-TCR undergo substantial expansion in cell numbers. The pre-TCR is lost at the intermediate DP thymocyte stage, coincident with the onset of TCRα rearrangement and subsequent expression of low levels of TCRαβ (the late DP thymocyte). Dstinct subcompartments in the DP thymocyte pool have been identified.[101] Late DP thymocytes differentiate into CD4+/CD8− SP and CD4−/CD8+ SP thymocytes expressing high levels of cell surface TCRαβ. These two populations correspond to helper/inducer and cytotoxic T cells that make up the blood and secondary lymphoid organ T-cell pool. They are discussed in more detail in Chap. 84.

REGULATION OF T-CELL PRECURSOR/THYMOCYTE GROWTH

Growth, differentiation, and apoptosis of thymocytes are regulated by direct physical interaction with thymic stromal cells (i.e., epithelial cells, fibroblasts, and dendritic/interdigitating cells) and cytokines produced by thymic stromal cells. Thymic epithelial cells synthesize and secrete a complex array of cytokines. These include IL-1, IL-3, IL-6, IL-7, stem cell factor, leukemia inhibitory factor, TGF-β, and several colony-stimulating factors.[108–112] Cytokine stimulation probably occurs in the localized microenvironment of a thymic epithelial cell–thymocyte adhesive interaction. This may be accomplished through adhesive interactions mediated by thymocyte CD2 and CD11a interacting with thymic epithelial cell CD58 and CD54.[113,114] Thymocytes also express VLA-4,[81] and it is probable that thymic stromal cell

VCAM-1 or fibronectin serves as the counterreceptor to facilitate adhesion.

What makes thymocytes grow? In contrast to human B-cell precursors, IL-7–IL-7-receptor interaction and downstream signaling events appear to be essential for normal human thymocyte development. Immunodeficiency patients with mutations in the γc subunit of the IL-2, IL-4, IL-7, IL-9, and IL-15 receptors[72]; patients with mutations in Jak-3[73,74]; and patients with mutations in the IL-7 receptor[75] all exhibit profound blocks in thymocyte development. The importance of IL-7 in these experiments of nature has been reproduced using a chimeric human-mouse fetal thymic organ culture.[115] Exactly how IL-7 exerts its essential effect on human thymocytes is unknown, but IL-7 does activate phosphatidylinositol-3 kinase,[116] a lipid kinase essential to many mitogenic pathways. Studies in the mouse may provide additional clues. IL-7 is a nonredundant cytokine that is essential for T-cell development.[117] Mice deficient in expression of the IL-7 receptor α chain exhibit a severe block in thymocyte development, but this deficiency can be overcome by enforced expression of the antiapoptotic protein bcl-2.[118,119] Furthermore, mice deficient in IL-7 show a profound loss of bcl-2 in immature thymocytes (i.e., CD3−/CD4−/CD8−), but short-term culture of these cells with IL-7 increases expression of bcl-2 and promotes cell survival.[120] These collective results indicate that IL-7 functions to enhance bcl-2 levels in early thymocytes, thereby transmitting a survival signal essential for continuing thymocyte development. Whether human thymocyte survival is mediated by a similar IL-7-dependent mechanism is unknown.

NK-CELL DEVELOPMENT

NK cells are large granular lymphocytes that comprise approximately 5 percent of blood and splenic lymphocytes. NK cells play an important role in the innate immune response to infection and some tumors (see Chap. 85). Substantial progress in identifying and characterizing receptors on NK cells that transduce inhibitory signals has been made in the last several years.[1] Due to the lack of NK-specific cell surface markers (see below), a rigorous analysis of NK-cell development has been difficult. However, with the increasing ability to isolate PSC and common lymphoid progenitors by fluorescence-activated cell sorting, coupled with the development of in vitro models for analyzing differentiation into lymphoid lineages, knowledge of NK-cell development has increased.

ORGANS INVOLVED IN NK-CELL DEVELOPMENT

NK-cell development can originate from CD34+ stem cells present in fetal liver, thymus, and marrow. However, it is unclear whether these three tissues generate discrete subsets of NK cells throughout life or whether they reflect a shift in the site of NK-cell development as a function of ontogeny. NK cells can be detected at 6 weeks' gestation in fetal liver,[121] prior to the development of the thymus as a functional organ that supports thymocyte maturation.[85,86] Consistent with this ontogenic observation, fetal liver CD34+ stem cells can differentiate into NK cells in vitro.[122] A close ontogenic relationship exists between NK cells and thymocytes.[102] The development of NK cells from CD34+ thymic progenitors and the supportive capacity of the thymic microenvironment for NK-cell development provide strong evidence for a thymic origin of at least some NK cells.[102,123–125] Thus, a T/NK progenitor is shown as pathway 1 in Fig. 82-1. A second pathway of thymic NK-cell development (see Fig. 82-1) is based on the isolation of a bipotential NK/DC

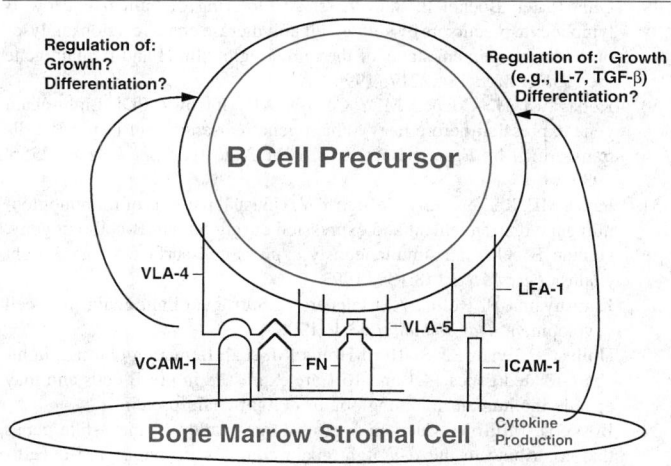

FIGURE 82-4   NK-cell development in human thymus or marrow. Three possible progenitors of the pre-NK cell are shown: common lymphoid progenitors, T/NK, and NK/DC. The common lymphoid progenitors correspond to the common lymphoid progenitors in Fig. 82-1 with multilymphoid lineage developmental potential. The common lymphoid progenitors is a marrow progenitor of the pre-NK cell based on studies by Galy et al.[16] The T/NK is an intrathymic progenitor of the pre-NK cell based on studies summarized by Spits et al.[102] The NK/DC is an intrathymic progenitor of the pre-NK cell based on studies by Márquez et al.[106] Two populations of mature NK cells are shown that circulate in the blood (see the text).

progenitor characterized by high expression of the CD44 cell surface proteoglycan.[126] CD34+ stem cell populations isolated from marrow and cord blood can develop into functional cytolytic NK cells using a variety of in vitro culture systems containing cytokines and stromal cells.[127–133]

NK RECEPTORS AND RECOMBINATION-ASSOCIATED GENES

Unlike T and B cells, NK-cell development does not require a process of receptor gene rearrangement mediated by RAG-1 and RAG-2. Thus, NK-cell development is essentially normal in mice deficient in RAG-1 or RAG-2.[42,43] Human NK-cell recognition of target cells is mediated by two families of so-called inhibitory receptors that recognize polymorphic class I major histocompatibility complex molecules.[1] These receptor families are known as CD94/NKG2 and killer inhibitory receptors (KIR).[1] Following binding to class I, these inhibitory receptors transduce signals that culminate in the inhibition of NK-cell–mediated cytotoxicity and cytokine production. A more detailed discussion of these receptors can be found in Chap. 85.

NK-LINEAGE–ASSOCIATED SURFACE ANTIGENS

Analysis of NK-cell development has been compromised by the absence of NK-lineage–specific cell surface markers. Molecules expressed on the cell surface of NK cells, such as CD16, CD56, CD94, and the inhibitory receptors, are also variably expressed on T-lineage cells.[1,102] Likewise, cell surface molecules commonly found on T cells, such as CD5, CD7, and CD28, are variably expressed on NK cells. The best way to distinguish T-lineage cells from NK cells is to assay for expression of the TCR, a complex found exclusively on T cells. Figure 82-4 shows a tentative scheme of NK-cell development.[102,122,124,127–134] The developmental interface between any multilineage progenitor and the pre-NK cell is very poorly characterized. One of the earliest changes is the appearance of a molecule designated

CD122, the β subunit of the IL-2/IL-15 receptors, on the pre-NK cell.[133] Acquisition of CD56 defines the next stage of development, designated the immature NK cell. The mature NK-cell population (i.e., the population in blood) is composed of two subpopulations. The predominant subpopulation ($\approx$95% of mature NK cells) expresses CD16, low amounts of CD56, and both inhibitory receptor families (CD94 and KIR). The minority subpopulation ($\approx$5% of mature NK cells) expresses high levels of CD56 and CD94 but is KIR$-$ and CD16$-$. There is no evidence that the CD16$-$/KIR$-$ population is a precursor of the CD16+/KIR+ population,[102] and it is also unclear whether the immature NK population can differentiate into the CD16$-$/KIR$-$ population.

REGULATION OF NK-CELL GROWTH

NK cells, like B and T cells, require the complex milieu of the marrow or thymic microenvironment for growth and differentiation. A large number of cytokines have been shown to enhance the development of NK cells from CD34+ stem cells in vitro. These include IL-1α, IL-2, IL-6, IL-7, IL-15, FL, stem cell factor, and granulocyte-macrophage colony stimulating factor.[122,123,126–134] Part of the difficulty in determining which cytokines are important reflects our current inability to distinguish common lymphoid progenitors from the earliest stages of NK development. Figure 82-4 portrays a pre-NK cell, but it is unclear whether a pre-NK cell is committed to the NK lineage. Moreover, the absence of NK-specific antigens has prohibited the use of fluorescence-activated cell sorting to purify NK progenitors. Thus, it is difficult to distinguish the effect of a given cytokine on PSC, common lymphoid progenitors, or an NK progenitor in the context of NK-cell development.

NK-cell development from CD34+ marrow stem cells has been a useful model for evaluating the contribution of marrow stromal cell products to NK-cell development. IL-2 can enhance NK-cell development,[127–130] but IL-2 is only synthesized by antigen-specific T cells and is not produced by marrow stromal cells.[132] IL-15 is a more plausible candidate. IL-15 binds to a receptor complex consisting of a unique α chain, a β chain (CD122) that is used by IL-15 and IL-2, and the common γ chain (γ_c) used by IL-2, IL-4, IL-7, IL-9, and IL-15. Human marrow stromal cells produce IL-15, and IL-15 promotes the development of CD56+ NK cells from CD34+ marrow stem cells.[132] FL also promotes the development of CD56+ NK cells from CD34+ marrow stem cells.[131,133] A recent study suggests a potential hierarchical effect of FL and IL-15 on NK-cell development.[133] FL was found to induce the expression of CD122 and IL-15 receptor α transcripts on CD34+ marrow stem cells. The FL-stimulated CD34+ stem cells could then respond to IL-15 and differentiate into CD56+/KIR+ NK cells with cytolytic activity.[133] In another study, human thymic progenitors cultured in IL-15 gave rise to NK cells.[132] These in vitro studies are consistent with experiments of nature. Severe combined immunodeficiency patients with mutations in the γ_c subunit or Jak-3 tyrosine kinase do not develop NK cells.[72] As mentioned above, these mutations negate the function of IL-2, IL-4, IL-7, IL-9, and IL-15. IL-7 is not likely to be essential for NK-cell development, since patients with mutations in the IL-7 receptor have normal NK-cell development.[75] IL-2 is not likely essential, as discussed above, and there is no known role for IL-4 or IL-9 in NK-cell development. However, IL-15 and IL-15 receptor α chain–deficient mice lack NK cells.[135] These collective data indicate that IL-15 plays a pivotal role in NK-cell development. Definitive evidence for this in humans, however, may require the identification of an immune-deficient patient with a mutation in the IL-15 gene.

REFERENCES

1. Lanier LL: NK cell receptors. *Annu Rev Immunol* 16:359, 1998.

2. Zon LI: Developmental biology of hematopoiesis. *Blood* 86:2876, 1995.

3. Godin IE, Garcia-Porrero JA, Coutinho A, et al: Para-aortic splanchnopleura from early mouse embryos contains B1a cell progenitors. *Nature* 364:67, 1993.

4. Medvinsky AL, Samoylina NL, Muller AM, Dzierzak EA: An early pre-liver intraembryonic source of CFU-S in the developing mouse embryo. *Nature* 364:64, 1993.

5. Cumano A, Dieterlen-Lièvre F, Godin I: Lymphoid potential, probed before circulation in mouse, is restricted to caudal intraembryonic splanchnopleura. *Cell* 86:907, 1996.

6. Kelemen E, Calvo W, Fliedner TM: *Atlas of Human Hemopoietic Development.* Springer-Verlag, Berlin, 1979.

7. Migliaccio G., Migliaccio AR, Petti S, et al: Human embryonic hemopoiesis: Kinetics of progenitors and precursors underlying the yolk sac-→liver transition. *J Clin Invest* 78:51, 1986.

8. Huyhn A, Dommergues M, Izac B, et al: Characterization of hematopoietic progenitors from human yolk sacs and embryos. *Blood* 86:4474, 1995.

9. Tavian M, Coulombel L, Luton D, et al: Aorta-associated CD34+ hematopoietic cells in the early human embryo. *Blood* 87:67, 1996.

10. Labastie M-C, Cortés F, Roméo P-H, et al: Molecular identity of hematopoietic precursor cells emerging in the human embryo. *Blood* 92:3624, 1998.

11. Abramson SR, Miller G, Phillips R: The identification in adult marrow of pluripotent and restricted stem cells of the myeloid and lymphoid systems. *J Exp Med* 146:1567, 1977.

12. Dick J, Magli M, Husser D, et al: Introduction of a selectable gene into primitive stem cells capable of long-term reconstitution of the hematopoietic system of W/WV mice. *Cell* 42:71, 1985.

13. Spangrude GJ, Heimfeld S, Weissman IL: Purification and characterization of mouse hematopoietic stem cells. *Science* 241:58, 1988.

14. Cumano A, Paige CJ, Iscove NN, Brady G: Bipotential precursors of B cells and macrophages in murine fetal liver. *Nature* 356:612, 1992.

15. Hakoda M, Hirai Y, Shimba H, et al: Cloning of phenotypically different human lymphocytes originating from a single stem cell. *J Exp Med* 169:1265, 1989.

16. Galy A, Travis M, Cen Z, Chen B: Human T, B, natural killer and dendritic cells arise from a common marrow progenitor cell subset. *Immunity* 3:459, 1995.

17. Kondo M, Weissman IL, Akashi K: Identification of clonogenic common lymphoid progenitors in mouse marrow. *Cell* 91:661, 1997.

18. Gathings WE, Lawton AR, Cooper MD: Immunofluorescent studies of the development of pre-B-cells, B lymphocytes, and immunoglobulin isotype diversity in humans. *Eur J Immunol* 7:804, 1977.

19. Cooper MD: B lymphocytes, normal development and function. *N Engl J Med* 317:1452, 1987.

20. Solvason N, Kearney JF: The human fetal omentum: A site of B cell generation. *J Exp Med* 175:397, 1992.

21. Nunez C, Nishimoto N, Gartland LG, et al: B cells are generated throughout life in humans. *J Immunol* 156:866, 1996.

22. Brashem CJ, Kersey JH, Bollum FJ, LeBien TW: Ontogenic studies of human lymphoid progenitor cells in human marrow. *Exp Hematol* 10:886, 1982.

23. Alt FW, Oltz EM, Young F, et al: VDJ recombination. *Immunol Today* 13:306, 1992.

24. Matsuda F, Ishii K, Bourvagnet P, et al: The complete nucleotide sequence of the human immunoglobulin heavy chain variable region locus. *J Exp Med* 188:2151, 1999.

25. Nussenzweig MC, Shaw AC, Sinn E, et al: Allelic exclusion in transgenic mice that express the membrane form of immunoglobulin μ. *Science* 236:816, 1987.

26. Ramsden DA, Wu GE: Mouse κ light-chain recombination signal sequences mediate recombination more frequently than those of λ light chain. *Proc Natl Acad Sci USA* 88:10721, 1991.

27. Bertrand FE III, Billips LG, Burrows PD, et al: IgH gene segment transcription and rearrangement prior to surface expression of the pan B-cell marker CD19 in normal human marrow. *Blood* 90:738, 1997.

28. Davi F, Faili A, Gritti C, et al: Early onset of immunoglobulin heavy chain gene rearrangements in normal human marrow CD34+ cells. *Blood* 90:4014, 1997.

29. Ghia P, ten Boekel E, Sanz E, et al: Ordering of human marrow B lymphocyte precursors by single-cell polymerase chain reaction analyses of the rearrangement status of the immunoglobulin H and L chain gene loci. *J Exp Med* 184:2217, 1996.

30. Kubagawa H, Cooper MD, Carroll AJ, Burrows PD: Light-chain gene expression before heavy-chain gene rearrangement in pre-B cells transformed by Epstein-Barr virus. *Proc Natl Acad Sci USA* 86:2356, 1989.

31. Pauza ME, Rehmann JA, LeBien TW: Unusual patterns of immunoglobulin gene rearrangement and expression during human B-cell ontogeny: Human B cells can simultaneously express cell surface κ and λ light chains. *J Exp Med* 178:139, 1993.

32. Karasuyama H, Rolink A, Melchers F: Surrogate light chain in B-cell development. *Adv Immunol* 63:1, 1996.

33. Hollis GF, Evans RJ, Stafford-Hollis JM, et al: Immunoglobulin λ light-chain-related genes 14.1 and 16.1 are expressed in pre-B cells and may encode the human immunoglobulin ω light-chain protein.

34. Bossy D, Milili M, Zucman J, et al: Organization of the λ-like genes that contribute to the μ-ψ light chain complex in human pre-B cells. *Int Immunol* 3:1081, 1991.

35. Wang YH, Nomura J, Faye-Peterson OM, Cooper MD: Surrogate light chain production during B-cell differentiation: Differential intracellular versus cell surface expression. *J Immunol* 161:1132, 1998.

36. Lassoued K, Nunez CA, Billips L, et al: Expression of surrogate light chain receptors is restricted to a late stage in pre-B-cell differentiation. *Cell* 73:73, 1993.

37. Kitamura D, Kudo A, Schaal S, et al: A critical role of λ5 protein in B-cell development. *Cell* 69:823, 1992.

38. Minegishi Y, Coustan-Smith E, Wang YH, et al: Mutations in the human lambda 5/14.1 gene result in B-cell deficiency and agammaglobulinemia. *J Exp Med* 187:71, 1998.

39. Wasserman R, Li YS, Shinton SA, et al: A novel mechanism for B-cell repertoire maturation based on response by B-cell precursors to pre-B receptor assembly. *J Exp Med* 187:259, 1998.

40. ten Boekel E, Melchers F, Rolink AG: Precursor B cells showing H chain allelic inclusion display allelic exclusion at the level of pre-B-cell receptor surface expression. *Immunity* 8:199, 1998.

41. Schatz DG, Oettinger MA, Schlissel MS: V(D)J recombination molecular biology and regulation. *Annu Rev Immunol* 10:359, 1992.

42. Mombaerts P, Iacomini J, Johnson RS, et al: RAG-1-deficient mice have no mature B and T lymphocytes. *Cell* 68:869, 1992.

43. Shinkai Y, Rathbun G, Lam K-P, et al: RAG-2-deficient mice lack mature lymphocytes owing to inability to initiate V(D)J rearrangement. *Cell* 68:855, 1992.

44. Schwarz KG, Gauss GH, Ludwig L, et al: RAG mutations in human B cell-negative SCID. *Science* 274:97, 1996.

45. Oettinger MA: Cutting apart V(D)J recombination. *Curr Opin Genet Dev* 6:141, 1996.

46. Lin WC, Desiderio S: Cell cycle regulation of V(D)J recombination-activating protein RAG-2. *Proc Natl Acad Sci USA* 91:2733, 1994.

47. Fanning L, Bertrand FE, Steinberg C, Wu GE: Molecular mechanisms involved in receptor editing at the heavy chain locus. *Int Immunol* 10:241, 1998.

48. Nussenzweig MC: Immune receptor editing: Revise and select. *Cell* 95:875, 1998.

49. Zarrin AA, Fong I, Malkin L, et al: Cloning and characterization of the human recombination activating gene 1 (RAG1) and RAG2 promoter regions. *J Immunol* 159:4382, 1997.

50. Desiderio SV, Yancopoulos G, Paskind M, et al: Insertion of N regions into heavy-chain genes is correlated with expression of terminal deoxynucleotidyl transferase in B cells. *Nature* 311:752, 1984.

51. Bridges SL, Lee SK, Johnson ML, et al: Somatic mutation and CDR3 lengths of immunoglobulin kappa light chains expressed in patients with rheumatoid arthritis and in normal individuals. *J Clin Invest* 96:831, 1995.

52. Komori T, Okada A, Stewart V, Alt F: Lack of N regions in antigen receptor variable region genes of TdT-deficient lymphocytes. *Science* 261:1171, 1993.

53. Gilfillan S, Dierich A, Lemeur M, et al: Mice lacking TdT: Mature animals with an immature lymphocyte repertoire. *Science* 261:1175, 1993.

54. Gore SD, Kastan MB, Civin CI: Normal human marrow precursors that express terminal deoxynucleotidyl transferase include T-cell precursors and possible lymphoid stem cells. *Blood* 77:1681, 1991.

55. Loken MR, Shah VO, Dattilio KL, Civin CI: Flow cytometric analysis of human marrow: II. Normal B lymphocyte development. *Blood* 70:1316, 1987.

56. LeBien TW, Wörmann B, Villablanca JG, et al: Multiparameter flow cytometric analysis of human fetal marrow B cells. *Leukemia* 4:354, 1990.

57. Barclay AN, Birkeland ML, Brown MH, et al: *The Leukocyte Antigen Handbook.* Academic Press, London, 1993.

58. LeBien TW: B-cell lymphopoiesis in mouse and man. *Curr Opin Immunol* 10:188, 1998.

59. Reth M: Antigen receptors on B lymphocytes. *Annu Rev Immunol* 10:97, 1992.

60. DeFranco AL: The complexity of signaling pathways activated by the BCR. *Curr Opin Immunol* 9:296, 1997.

61. Dworzak MN, Fritsch G, Fröschl G, et al: Four-color flow cytometric investigation of terminal deoxynucleotidyl transferase-positive lymphoid precursors in pediatric marrow: CD79a expression precedes CD19 in early B-cell ontogeny. *Blood* 92:3203, 1998

62. Gong S, Nussenzweig MC: Regulation of an early developmental checkpoint in the B-cell pathway by Ig beta. *Science* 272:411, 1996.

63. Ryan DH, Nuccie BL, Abboud CN, Winslow JM: Vascular cell adhesion molecule-1 and the integrin VLA-4 mediate adhesion of human B-cell precursors to cultured marrow adherent cells. *J Clin Invest* 88:995, 1991.

64. Dittel BN, McCarthy JB, Wayner EA, LeBien TW: Regulation of human B-cell precursor adhesion to marrow stromal cells by cytokines that exert opposing effects on the expression of vascular cell adhesion molecule-1 (VCAM-1). *Blood* 81:2272, 1993.

65. Hynes RO: Integrins, versatility, modulation, and signaling in cell adhesion. *Cell* 69:11, 1992.

66. Jarvis LJ, LeBien TW: Cytokine and stromal influence on early B-cell development, in *Molecular Biology of B-Cell and T-Cell Development,* edited by JG Monroe, EV Rothenberg, p 231. Humana Press, New Jersey, 1998.

67. Wolf ML, Buckley JA, Goldfarb A, et al: Development of a marrow culture for maintenance and growth of normal human B-cell precursors. *J Immunol* 147:3324, 1991.

68. Dittel BN, LeBien TW: The growth response to IL-7 during normal human B-cell ontogeny is restricted to B-lineage cells expressing CD34. *J Immunol* 154:58, 1995.

69. Billips LG, Nunez CA, Bertrand FE III, et al: Immunoglobulin recombinase gene activity is modulated reciprocally by interleukin 7 and CD19 in B-cell progenitors. *J Exp Med* 182:973, 1995.

70. Namikawa R, Muench MO, deVries JE, Roncarolo MG: The FLK2/FLT3 ligand synergizes with interleukin-7 in promoting stromal-cell-independent expansion and differentiation of human fetal pro-B cells in vitro. *Blood* 87:1881, 1996.

71. Candeias S, Muegge K, Durum SK: IL-7 receptor and VDJ recombination: Trophic versus mechanistic actions. *Immunity* 6:501, 1997.

72. Uribe L, Weinberg KI: X-linked SCID and other defects of cytokine pathways. *Semin Hematol* 35:299, 1998.

73. Macchi P, Villa A, Giliani S, et al: Mutations of Jak-3 gene in patients with autosomal severe combined immune deficiency (SCID). *Nature* 377:65, 1995.

74. Russell SM, Tayebi N, Nakajima H, et al: Mutation of Jak3 in a patient with SCID: Essential role of Jak3 in lymphoid development. *Science* 270:797, 1995.

75. Puel A, Ziegler SF, Buckley RH, Leonard WJ: Defective IL7R expression in T(−)B(+)NK(+) severe combined immunodeficiency. *Nat Genet* 20:394, 1998.

76. Pribyl JAR, LeBien TW: IL-7 independent development of human B cells. *Proc Natl Acad Sci USA* 93:10348, 1996.

77. Baggiolini M: Chemokines and leukocyte traffic. *Nature* 392:565, 1998.

78. Vodinelich L, Tax W, Bai Y, et al: A monoclonal antibody (WT1) for detecting leukemias of T cell precursors (T-ALL). *Blood* 62:108, 1983.

79. Haynes BF, Martin ME, Kay HH, Kurtzberg J: Early events in human T cell ontogeny: Phenotypic characterization and immunohistologic lo-

80. Campana D, Janossy G, Constan-Smith E, et al: The expression of T-cell receptor-associated proteins during T-cell ontogeny in man. *J Immunol* 142:57, 1989.

81. Terstappen LWMM, Huang S, Picker LJ: Flow cytometric assessment of human T cell differentiation in thymus and marrow. *Blood* 79:666, 1992.

82. Garcia-Ojeda ME, Dejbakhsh-Jones S, Weissman IL, Strober S: An alternate pathway for T cell development supported by the marrow microenvironment: Recapitulation of thymic maturation. *J Exp Med* 187:1813, 1998.

83. McVay LD, Carding SR: Extrathymic origin of human γδ T cells during fetal development. *J Immunol* 157:2873, 1996.

84. Howie D, Spencer J, DeLord D et al: Extrathymic T cell differentiation in the human intestine early in life. *J Immunol* 161:5862, 1998.

85. Weller GL: Development of the thyroid, parathyroid, and thymus gland in man. *Contrib Embryol Carnegie Inst* 24:95, 1933.

86. Haynes BF: The human thymic microenvironment. *Adv Immunol* 36:87, 1984.

87. Rodewald H-R: The thymus in the age of retirement. *Nature* 396:630, 1998.

88. Douek DC, McFarland RD, Keiser PH, et al: Changes in thymic function with age and during treatment of HIV infection. *Nature* 396:690, 1998.

89. von Boehmer H: Thymic selection: A matter of life and death. *Immunol Today* 13:454, 1992.

90. Boyd RL, Hugo P: Towards an integrated view of thymopoiesis. *Immunol Today* 12:71, 1991.

91. Haynes BF, Scearce RM, Lobach DM, Hensley LL: Phenotypic characterization and ontogeny of mesodermal-derived and endocrine epithelial components of the human thymic microenvironment. *J Exp Med* 159:1149, 1984.

92. Demaagd R, MacKenzie WA, Schuurman H-J, et al: The human thymus microenvironment: Heterogeneity detected by monoclonal anti-epithelial cell antibodies. *Immunology* 54:745, 1984.

93. Moss PAH, Rosenberg WMC, Bell JI: The human T-cell receptor in health and disease. *Annu Rev Immunol* 10:71, 1992.

94. Krangel MS, Yssel H, Brocklehurst C, Spits H: A distinct wave of human T-cell receptor λδ lymphocytes in the early fetal thymus: Evidence for controlled gene rearrangement and cytokine production. *J Exp Med* 172:847, 1990.

95. McVay LD, Cardig SR, Bottomly K, Hayday AC: Regulated expression and structure of T-cell receptor gamma delta transcripts in human thymic ontogeny. *EBMO J* 10:83, 1991.

96. Saint-Ruf C, Ungewiss K, Groettrup M, et al: Analysis and expression of a cloned pre-T cell receptor gene. *Science* 266:1208, 1994.

97. Del Porto P, Bruno L, Mattei MG, et al: Cloning and comparative analysis of the human pre-T-cell receptor alpha-chain gene. *Proc Natl Acad Sci USA* 92:12105, 1995.

98. Ramiro AR, Trigueros C, Márquez C, et al: Regulation of pre-T cell receptor (pTα-TCRβ) gene expression during human thymic development. *J Exp Med* 184:519, 1996.

99. von Boehmer H, Fehling HJ: Structure and function of the pre-T cell receptor. *Annu Rev Immunol* 15:433, 1997.

100. Wilson A, Held W, MacDonald HR: Two waves of recombinase gene expression in developing thymocytes. *J Exp Med* 179:1355, 1994.

101. Trigueros C, Ramiro AR, Carrasco YR, et al: Identification of a late stage of small noncycling pTα− pre-T cells as immediate precursors of T cell receptor α/β+ thymocytes. *J Exp Med* 188:1401, 1998.

102. Spits H, Blom B, Jaleco A-C, et al: Early stages in the development of human T, natural killer and thymic dendritic cells. *Immunol Rev* 165:75, 1998.

103. Galy A, Barcena A, Verma S, Spits H: Precursors of CD3+CD4+CD8+ in the human thymus are defined by expression of CD34: Delineation of early events in human thymic development. *J Exp Med* 178:391, 1993.

104. Sánchez M-J, Muench MO, Roncarolo MG, et al: Identification of a common T/NK cell progenitor in human fetal thymus. *J Exp Med* 180:569, 1994.

105. Res P, Martínez Cáceres E, Jaleco AC, et al: CD34+CD38dim cells in the human thymus can differentiate into T, natural killer and dendritic cells but are distinct from stem cells. *Blood:* 87:5196, 1996.

106. Márquez C, Trigueros C, Franco JM, et al: Identification of a common developmental pathway for thymic natural killer cells and dendritic cells. *Blood* 91:2760, 1998.

107. Reinherz EL, Kung PC, Goldstein G, et al: Discrete stages of human intrathymic differentiation: Analysis of normal thymocytes and leukemic lymphoblasts of T-cell lineage. *Proc Natl Acad Sci USA* 77:1558, 1980.

108. Galy AHM, Spits H: IL-1, IL-4 and IFN-γ differentially regulate cytokine production and cell surface molecule expression in cultured human thymic epithelial cells. *J Immunol* 147:3823, 1991.

109. Le PT, Lazorick S, Whichard LP, et al: Regulation of cytokine production in the human thymus: Epidermal growth factor and transforming growth factor α regulate mRNA levels of IL1α, IL1β and IL6 in human thymic epithelial cells at a post-transcriptional level. *J Exp Med* 174:1147, 1991.

110. Mizutani S, Watt S, Robertson D, et al: Cloning of human thymic subcapsular cortex epithelial cells with T-lymphocyte binding sites and hemopoietic growth factor activity. *Proc Natl Acad Sci USA* 84:4999, 1987.

111. Le PT, Lazorick S, Whichard LP, et al: Human thymic epithelial cells produce IL-6, granulocyte-monocyte CSF and leukemia inhibitory factor. *J Immunol* 145:3310, 1990.

112. Dalloul AH, Arock M, Fourcade C, et al: Human thymic epithelial cells produce interleukin-3. *Blood* 77:69, 1991.

113. Vollger LW, Tuck DT, Springer TA, et al: Thymocyte binding to human thymic epithelial cells is inhibited by monoclonal antibodies to CD2 and LFA3 antigens. *J Immunol* 138:358, 1987.

114. Singer KH, Denning SM, Whichard LP, Haynes BF: Thymocyte LFA-1 and thymic epithelial cell ICAM-1 molecules mediate binding of activated human thymocytes to thymic epithelial cells. *J Immunol* 143:3944, 1989.

115. Plum J, De Smedt M, Leclercq G, et al: Interleukin-7 is a critical growth factor in early human T-cell development. *Blood* 88:4239, 1996.

116. Dadi HK, Roifman CM: Activation of phosphatidylinositol-3 kinase by ligation of the interleukin-7 receptor on human thymocytes. *J Clin Invest* 92:1559, 1993.

117. Akashi K, Kondo M, Weissman IL: Role of interleukin-7 in T-cell development from hematopoietic stem cells. *Immunol Rev* 165:13, 1998.

118. Akashi K, Kondo M, von Freeden-Jeffry U, et al: Bcl-2 rescues T lymphopoiesis in interleukin-7 receptor-deficient mice. *Cell* 89:1033, 1997.

119. Maraskovsky E, O'Reilly LA, Teepe M, et al: Bcl-2 can rescue T lymphocyte development in interleukin-7 receptor-deficient mice but not in mutant rag-1-/-mice. *Cell* 89:1011, 1997.

120. von Freeden-Jeffry U, Solvason N, Howard M, Murray R: The earliest T lineage-committed cells depend on IL-7 for Bcl-2 expression and normal cell cycle progression. *Immunity* 7:147, 1997.

121. Phillips JH, Hori T, Nagler A, et al: Ontogeny of human natural killer (NK) cells: Fetal NK cells mediate cytolytic function and express cytoplasmic CD3 epsilon, delta proteins. *J Exp Med* 175:1055, 1992.

122. Jaleco AC, Blom B, Res P, et al: Fetal liver contains committed NK progenitors, but is not a site for development of CD34+ cells into T cells. *J Immunol* 159:694, 1997.

123. Sanchez MJ, Muench MO, Roncarolo MG, et al: Identification of a common T/natural killer cell progenitor in human fetal thymus. *J Exp Med* 180:569, 1994.

124. Barcena A, Galy AH, Punnonen J, et al: Lymphoid and myeloid differentiation of fetal liver CD34+ lineage-cells in human thymic organ culture. *J Exp Med* 180:123, 1994.

125. Plum J, de Smedt M, Verhasselt B, et al: In vitro intrathymic differentiation kinetics of human fetal liver CD34+CD38− progenitors reveals a phenotypically defined dendritic/T-NK precursor split. *J Immunol* 162:60, 1999.

126. Márquez C, Trigueros C, Franco JM, et al: Identification of a common developmental pathway for thymic natural killer cells and dendritic cells. *Blood* 91:2760, 1998.

127. Miller JS, Verfaillie C, McGlave P: The generation of human natural killer cells from CD34+/DR− primitive progenitors in long-term marrow culture. *Blood* 80:2182, 1992.

128. Lotzova E, Savary CA, Champlin RE: Genesis of human oncolytic natural killer cells from primitive CD34+CD33− marrow progenitors. *J Immunol* 150:5263, 1993.

129. Silva MRG, Hoffman R, Srour EF, Ascensao JL: Generation of human natural killer cells from immature progenitors does not require marrow stromal cells. *Blood* 84:841, 1994.

130. Shibuya A, Nagayoshi K, Nakamura K, Nakauchi H: Lymphokine requirement for the generation of natural killer cells from CD34+ hematopoietic progenitor cells. *Blood* 85:3538, 1995.

131. Miller JS, McCullar V, Punzel M, et al: Single adult human CD34+/Lin−/CD38− progenitors give rise to natural killer cells, B-lineage cells, dendritic cells, and myeloid cells. *Blood* 93:96, 1999.

132. Mrozek E, Anderson P, Caligiuri MA: Role of interleukin-15 in the development of human CD56+ natural killer cells from CD34+ hematopoietic progenitor cells. *Blood* 87:2632, 1996.

133. Yu H, Fehniger TA, Fuchshuber P, et al: Flt3 ligand promotes the generation of a distinct CD34(+) human natural killer cell progenitor that responds to interleukin-15. *Blood* 92:3647, 1998.

134. Leclercq G, Debacker V, De Smedt M, Plum J: Differential effects of interleukin-15 and interleukin-2 on differentiation of bipotential T/natural killer progenitor cells. *J Exp Med* 184:325, 1996.

135. Sevilir Williams N, Klem J, Puzanov IJ, et al: Natural killer cell differentiation: Insights from knockout and transgenic mouse models and in vitro systems. *Immunol Rev* 165:47, 1998.

FUNCTIONS OF B LYMPHOCYTES AND PLASMA CELLS IN IMMUNOGLOBULIN PRODUCTION

THOMAS J. KIPPS

Much of our immune defense against invading organisms is predicated upon the tremendous diversity of immunoglobulin molecules. Immunoglobulins are glycoproteins produced by B lymphocytes and plasma cells. These molecules may be considered receptors, in that the primary function of the immunoglobulin molecule is to bind antigen. A single person can synthesize 10 to 100 million different immunoglobulin molecules, each having a distinct antigen-binding specificity. This great diversity in the so-called humoral immune system allows us to generate antibodies specific for a variety of substances, including synthetic molecules not naturally present in our environment. Despite the diversity in the specificities of antibody molecules, the binding of antibody to antigen initiates a limited series of biologically important effector functions, such as complement activation and/or adherence of the immune complex to receptors on leukocytes. The eventual outcome is the clearance and degradation of the foreign substance. This chapter describes the structure of immunoglobulins and outlines the mechanisms by which B cells can produce molecules of such tremendous diversity with defined effector functions.

IMMUNOGLOBULIN STRUCTURE AND FUNCTION

BASIC IMMUNOGLOBULIN STRUCTURE

All naturally occurring immunoglobulin molecules are composed of one or several basic units consisting of two identical heavy (H) chains and two identical light (L) chains (Fig. 83-1). The four polypeptides are held in a bilaterally symmetrical, Y-shaped structure by disulfide bonds and noncovalent interactions.[1,2] The internal disulfide bonds of the heavy and light chains cause the polypeptides to fold into compact globe-shaped regions, called *domains*, each containing about 110 to 120 amino acid residues.[3] Each domain forms a common fold of a type of protein structure known as *beta-pleated sheets* and is stabilized by a conserved disulfide bond (Fig. 83-1). The light chains have two domains; the heavy chains have four or five domains. The amino-

Acronyms and abbreviations that appear in this chapter include: ADCC, antibody-dependent cell-mediated cytotoxicity; BiP, immunoglobulin "binding protein"; C, constant; CDR, complementarity-determining region; CRIs, cross-reactive idiotypes; D, diversity; FR, framework region; GM-CSF, granulocyte-macrophage colony stimulating factor; H, heavy; INF-γc, interferon gamma; Kde, kappa-deleting element; L, light; NK or K, natural killer cells; RAG-1 or RAG-2, recombination activating genes 1 or 2; RSS, recombination signal sequences; SCID, severe-combined immunodeficient; TdT, terminal deoxynucleotidyl transferase; TNF-α, tumor necrosis factor alpha (or cachectin); V, variable.

terminal domains of the heavy and light chains are designated the variable (V) regions, because their primary structure varies markedly among different immunoglobulin molecules.[4] The carboxy-terminal domains, however, are referred to as constant (C) regions, because their primary structure is the same among immunoglobulins of the same class or subclass. The amino acids in the light- and heavy-chain variable regions interact to form an antigen-binding site.[1,5] Each four-chain immunoglobulin basic unit has two identical binding sites. The constant region domains of the heavy and light chains provide stability for the immunoglobulin molecule. The heavy-chain constant regions also mediate the specific effector functions of the different immunoglobulin classes (Table 83-1).[6]

LIGHT CHAINS

Immunoglobulin light chains have an approximate Mw of 23,000. They are divided into two types, kappa (κ) and lambda (λ), based upon multiple amino acid sequence differences in the single constant region domain.[4] The λ chains are divided further into subclasses. The proportion of κ to λ chains in adult human plasma is about 2 : 1. The immunoglobulin-light chain-constant region has no known effector function. Its main purpose may be to allow for proper assembly and release of an intact immunoglobulin molecule. Soon after synthesis, the antibody light chain constant region associates with the nascent immunoglobulin heavy chain (Fig. 83-1), releasing the latter from the immunoglobulin "binding protein," or BiP. BiP is a heat-shock protein that, in the absence of antibody light chain, binds the first constant region domain of the newly synthesized heavy chain, thereby retaining the heavy chain polypeptide in the cell's endoplasmic reticulum.[7]

HEAVY CHAINS

Immunoglobulin heavy chains have a Mw of 50,000 to 70,000, depending upon the number and length of the constant region domains. The five major isotypes of heavy chains, gamma, alpha, mu, delta, and epsilon, determine the five corresponding classes of immunoglobulin: IgG, IgA, IgM, IgD, and IgE. The individual immunoglobulin molecules of each isotype may contain either κ or λ light chains, but not both. The distinct physical and functional properties of the human immunoglobulin classes are summarized in Tables 83-1 and 83-2.

IgG

Approximately 80 percent of the immunoglobulins in adult plasma are IgG. The IgG molecule is composed of the basic 150,000-dalton immunoglobulin four-chain structure, plus about 3 percent carbohydrate. IgG is the predominant antibody produced during the secondary immune response. IgG molecules effectively penetrate extravascular spaces and readily cross the placental barrier to provide passive immunity to the newborn.

Near the junction of the two arms of the Y-shaped immunoglobulin molecule, the two heavy chains interact to form a flexible "hinge" region (Fig. 83-1). Exposed between constant region globular domains, the hinge region is attacked readily by the proteolytic enzyme papain or pepsin. The cleavage sites are shown in Fig. 83-1. Digestion of IgG with papain yields three fragments. The single Fc piece contains the carboxy-terminal region of both heavy chains. The two identical F(ab) pieces contain the entire light chain and the amino-terminal portion of the heavy chain.

Within the IgG class are four major subclasses, designated IgG$_1$, IgG$_2$, IgG$_3$, IgG$_4$. Each subclass has a distinct heavy-chain constant region and mediates different effector functions (Table 83-3).[6] The average half-life of circulating IgG molecules is approximately 21 days, although the exact value varies among the IgG subclasses (Table 83-3). The most abundant subclass is IgG$_1$, which constitutes 65 percent

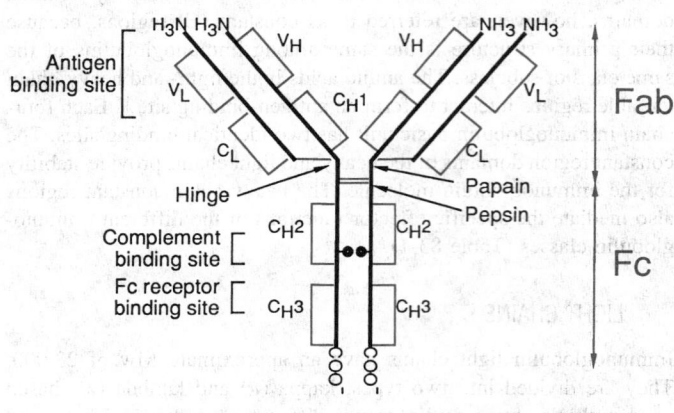

FIGURE 83-1 Schematic model of an IgG molecule of the IgG₁ subclass. The sites of proteolytic cleavage by papain and by pepsin are indicated. The papain-generated fragments Fab and Fc are indicated to the right of the schematic drawing. Thin lines indicate the intrachain disulfide bonds of the variable region domains (V_H and V_L) and constant region domains and the interchain disulfide bonds near the antibody hinge region (labeled *Hinge*). NH₃ or COO− indicate the amino terminus or carboxyl terminus of each polypeptide respectively. Key functional sites of the antibody responsible for antigen binding, complement fixation, or Fc receptor binding are as indicated by the brackets. The glycosylation sites on the constant region carbohydrate groups are indicated by filled circles.

of the total IgG in plasma. Whereas IgG₁ and IgG₃ proteins activate complement via the classical pathway, IgG₂ molecules fix complement poorly and IgG₄ proteins not at all. IgG₃ myeloma protein may aggregate spontaneously to produce a hyperviscosity syndrome.

Either aggregated IgG or antigen-antibody complexes may bind to specific receptors for the Fc fragment, designated FcRI (CD64), FcRII (CD32), and FcRIII (CD16). Of the IgG subclasses, IgG₁ binds best to FcRI (CD64) and FcRII (CD32), with affinities (K_d) of 1×10^{-8} M and 5×10^{-7} M respectively (Table 83-3). IgG₁ and IgG₃ bind equally well to FcRIII (CD16), with an affinity (K_d) of 2×10^{-6} M (Table 83-3). This is the Fc receptor expressed by natural killer cells (NK cells or K cells) that mediate antibody-dependent cell-mediated cytotoxicity (ADCC). Proteins of the IgG₄ or IgG₂ subclass bind poorly to FcRI (CD64) or FcRII (CD32), and to FcRIII (CD16) not at all (Table 83-3).

IgA

IgA comprises about 13 percent of plasma immunoglobulins (Table 83-1). Specific IgA antibodies are synthesized during secondary im-

mune responses. IgA circulates as a monomer, dimer, or higher polymer containing approximately 8 percent carbohydrate. Within the IgA class there are two major subclasses, designated IgA₁ and IgA₂. The most abundant subclass is IgA₁, which constitutes approximately 85 percent of the total IgA in plasma. The half-life of circulating IgA of either subclass is approximately 6 days.

The primary role for IgA is in mucosal immunity.[8,9] A modified form of IgA is the principal antibody in saliva, tears, colostrum, and the fluids of the gastrointestinal, respiratory, and urinary tracts. These secreted immunoglobulins consist of an IgA dimer bound to the J- (or joining) chain polypeptide and a secretory protein of 70,000 daltons. The J chain is required for proper hepatic transport of IgA.[10] The secretory component actually is part of a Fc receptor for dimeric IgA that is not synthesized by B cells but rather by epithelial cells of organs such as the intestine. This protein facilitates the transport of the IgA protein across the epithelial cell and may protect the secreted IgA molecule from proteolytic digestion by enzymes in the intestinal lumen. IgA antibodies do not cross the placenta, fix complement via the classical pathway, or bind efficiently to cell surfaces. Indeed, their main function may be to prevent foreign substances from adhering to mucosal surfaces and entering the blood.

IgM

In a normal adult, approximately 6 percent of the total plasma immunoglobulins belong to the IgM class (Tables 83-1 and 83-2). IgM molecules classically are termed *macroglobulins* because of their large molecular weight. Circulating IgM molecules contain 12 percent carbohydrate and are formed through the linkage of five identical immunoglobulin units by disulfide bonds and by a J chain[10] (Fig. 83-2). IgM represents the predominant immunoglobulin class formed during a primary immune response. IgM macroglobulins do not penetrate easily into extravascular spaces or readily cross the placenta. Compared to monomeric IgG antibodies, pentavalent IgM antibodies fix complement more efficiently. A single IgM molecule on the surface of a red blood cell can initiate complement-mediated hemolysis. IgM is catabolized rapidly, with a plasma half-life of only 6 days. The monomeric form of IgM, with only two heavy and two light chains, is the major immunoglobulin expressed on the B-cell surface (Fig. 83-3).

IgD

Although a trace serum protein that comprises less than 1 percent of plasma immunoglobulins, IgD is expressed on most peripheral B cells along with IgM. The molecule has the basic four-chain constant region and contains 11 percent carbohydrate (Tables 83-1 and 83-2). Sensitive to proteolytic degradation, IgD antibodies do not penetrate extravascular spaces efficiently, cross the placental barrier, or fix complement via the classical pathway. Rather, IgD functions primarily as a B-cell

TABLE 83-1 PHYSICAL PROPERTIES OF HUMAN IMMUNOGLOBULINS

	IgG	IgA	IgM	IgD	IgE
Heavy-chain class	γ	α	μ	δ	ε
Heavy chain subclass	$\gamma1, \gamma2, \gamma3, \gamma4$	$\alpha1, \alpha2$	—	—	—
Number of H chain domains	4	4	5	4	5
Secretory form	Monomer	Monomer, Dimer	Pentamer	Monomer	Monomer
Molecular mass (daltons)	150,000	160,000 (monomer) 400,000 (secretory)	900,000	184,000	188,000
Antigen-binding valency	2	2 (monomer) 4 (secretory)	10	2	2
Serum concentration (mg/ml)	8–16	1.4–4.0	0.5–2.0	0–0.4	17–450 ng/ml
Percent of total immunoglobulin	80	13	6	1	0.002
Electrophoretic mobility	γ	Fast γ to β	Slow γ	Fast γ	Fast γ
Percent carbohydrate	3	8	12	13	12

membrane receptor for antigen that facilitates recruitment of B cells into specific antigen-driven responses.[11]

IgE

Although four human IgE isoforms can be produced by alternative splicing of the epsilon primary transcript,[12] each isoform appears to have similar function. IgE has been called *reaginic* antibody to denote its association with immediate hypersensitivity. It normally constitutes only 0.004 percent of total plasma immunoglobulin (Tables 83-1 and 83-2). In patients with parasitic infestation, and in some children with atopic diseases, plasma IgE levels may rise to 5 to 20 times normal. The IgE molecule consists of a four-chain basic unit, plus 12 percent carbohydrate. Monomeric IgE binds via the Fc region to high-affinity receptors on the surface membranes of basophils and mast cells. When bound to tissue mast cells, IgE has a much longer half-life than in plasma, in which its half-life is only about 2 days (Table 83-2). Cross-linking of cell-bound IgE antibody by antigen induces the release of vasoactive amines, lipid-derived inflammatory mediators, proteases, proteoglycans, and cytokines, such as tumor necrosis factor alpha (TNF-α or cachectin), interferon gamma (INF-γ), granulocyte-macrophage colony stimulating factor (GM-CSF), or interleukins 1, 3, 4, 5, and 6. These substances act on adjacent cells and may regulate the metabolism of the connective tissue extracellular matrix. These lipid mediators and biogenic amines may produce the rapid components of immediate hypersensitivity, such as vascular leakage, vasodilatation, and bronchoconstriction. The released cytokines, on the other hand, are responsible for the late phase of the immediate hypersensitivity response. The physiologic function of this response is not clear. Instead, the immediate hypersensitivity response actually may represent a pathologic systemic exaggeration of a local physiologic process that may potentiate the inflammatory response to invading organisms.

SURFACE IMMUNOGLOBULIN

Any one of the immunoglobulin isotypes may serve as a B-cell membrane receptor for antigen. However, most B cells express surface IgM with or without IgD. Each immunoglobulin is expressed on the surface membrane as a monomer complexed noncovalently with disulfide-linked heterodimeric glycoproteins that, together with surface immunoglobulin, form the B-cell antigen-receptor complex[13] (Fig. 83-3). For surface IgM, each heterodimer is composed of CD79a, an IgM-α chain of 33 kDa, complexed with CD79b, an Ig-β chain of 37 kDa (see Chap. 13). CD79a interacts with the C_H4 domain and the transmembrane domain of the surface IgM molecule (Fig. 83-3). This chain is a product of the human mb-1 gene located at 19q13.2, while CD79b is the product of another gene located on a different chromosome at 17q23.[13] B cells that lack expression of CD79a or CD79b cannot express surface immunoglobulin.

CD79a/CD79b are necessary, not only for transport of the assembled immunoglobulin to the cell surface, but also for signal transduction following surface immunoglobulin-receptor cross-linking by antigen. The cytoplasmic tails of these accessory molecules each contain *immunoreceptor tyrosine activation motifs*, or ITAMs. Such motifs are found in the cytoplasmic domains of several immune system signaling molecules, including those of the T-cell receptor complex (see Chap. 84). Upon surface immunoglobulin cross-linking, the tyrosine residues in these motifs are phosphorylated, allowing cytoplasmic-signaling molecules to recognize and bind to the activated B-cell receptor com-

plex. These signaling molecules in turn activate a variety of other intracellular signaling molecules (see Chap. 15). As such, tyrosine phosphorylation is the first step in the intracellular cascade triggered by antigen binding to specific surface immunoglobulin.[14]

There are three major tyrosine kinases associated with the surface immunoglobulin receptor complex. These tyrosine kinases *Fyn, Blk,* and *Lyn* can phosphorylate tyrosine residues in the ITAMs of CD79a and CD79b. The phosphorylated ITAMs are then recognized and bound by another tyrosine kinase, called *Syk*, that in turns triggers activation of a cascade of intracellular signaling molecules (see Chap. 15).

To mitigate the accidental initiation of signal transduction, the signaling cascade is subject to negative controls.[15,16] One of these acts directly on the receptor-associated kinases that are activated by phosphorylation at one site but are inhibited by phosphorylation at another. Activation of such kinases thus requires dephosphorylation of the inhibitory site and phosphorylation of this activating site. Dephosphorylation of the inhibitory site is mediated by CD45, a membrane phosphatase that also is known as *leukocyte common antigen.* As such, CD45 contributes to the activation of B lymphocytes by removing the inhibitory phosphates from the receptor-associated kinases.[17]

Another protein, called *SH2-domain-containing-phosphotyrosine phosphatase-1* (*SHP-1*) or *protein-tyrosine phosphatase 1c* (*PTP1c*), is responsible for turning off the activated tyrosine kinases, thereby limiting the response of the activated B cell.[17,18] SHP is a cytoplasmic phosphatase that acts by removing the activating phosphate groups from such kinases. The importance of this enzyme is demonstrated in mutant mice that lack this enzyme.[19] The B lymphocytes of such animals are stimulated by much lower concentrations of antigen than the lymphocytes of normal mice. Because of this, these mice have

TABLE 83-2   BIOLOGIC PROPERTIES OF HUMAN IMMUNOGLOBULINS

	IgG	IgA	IgM	IgD	IgE
Percent of body pool in intravascular space	45	42	76	75	51
Percent of intravascular pool catabolized per day	6.7	25	18	37	89
Normal synthetic rate (mg/kg per day)	33	24	6.7	0.4	0.02
Serum half-life (days)	21	5.8	10	2.8	2.3
Placental transfer	Yes	No	No	No	No
Cytophilic for mast cells and basophils	No	No	No	No	Yes
Binding to macrophages and other phagocytes	Yes	No	No	No	Yes
Reactivity with staphylococcal Protein A	Yes	No	No	No	No
Antibody-dependent cell-mediated cytoxicity	Yes	No	No	No	No
Complement fixation:					
Classical pathway	Yes	No	Yes	No	No
Alternate pathway	No	Yes	No	No	No

TABLE 83-3   CHARACTERISTICS OF MAJOR IgG SUBCLASSES

	IgG$_1$	IgG$_2$	IgG$_3$	IgG$_4$
Heavy chain subclass	$\gamma1$	$\gamma2$	$\gamma3$	$\gamma4$
Serum concentration (mg/ml)	9	3	1	0.5
Percent of total IgG	67	22	7	4
Serum half-life (days)	21	20	7	21
Complement fixation:				
Classical Pathway	++	+/−	+++	−
Alternative Pathway	−	−	−	−
FcRI (CD64) binding	++++	+/−	++	+
FcRII (CD32) binding	+++	+/−	+	+
FcRIII (CD16) binding	+	−	+	−
Antibody-dependent cell mediated cytoxicity (ADCC)	+	−	+	−
Heterologous skin sensitization	+	−	+	+

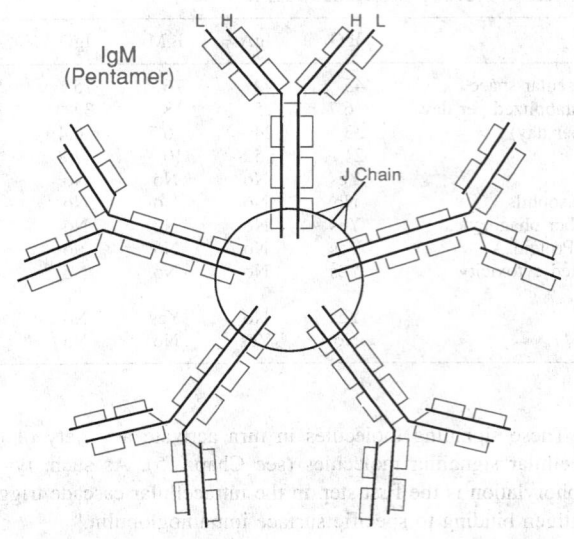

FIGURE 83-2   Schematic model of an IgM pentamer. This diagram shows the positions of the heavy (H) chain, light (L) chains, and the single J chain. Intrachain and interchain disulfide bonds are indicated by the thin lines.

abnormal B-cell proliferation, develop autoimmune disease, and die within a few weeks of birth.

GENETICS OF IMMUNOGLOBULINS

IMMUNOGLOBULIN GENE COMPLEXES

Immunoglobulin genes are inherited in three unlinked gene complexes: one for the heavy-chain classes, one for κ light chains, and one for λ light chains. The immunoglobulin heavy-chain gene complex is located at band q32 of the long arm of chromosome 14. This complex is composed of 51 functional heavy-chain variable region genes (V_H genes), 25 functional 27 diversity (D) segments, 6 functional J_H minigenes, and exons encoding the constant regions for each of the immunoglobulin heavy-chain isotypes (Fig. 83-4).[20–22] The κ light chain gene complex is contained within band p12 on the short arm of chromosome 2. This gene complex consists of approximately 40 functional kappa light-chain variable region genes (V_κ genes), 5 J_κ segments, 1 constant region exon, and 1 kappa-deleting element (Kde) (Fig. 83-5).[23,24] Many of the V_κ genes in the region most proximal to the J_κ segments are in the opposite orientation of the J_κ segments, thus requiring that the V_κ exons in the proximal region undergo inversion during immunoglobulin gene rearrangement (Fig. 83-5). The λ light chain gene complex is located at band q11.12 on the long arm of chromosome 22. This gene complex consists of approximately 39 functional lambda light-chain variable region genes (V_λ genes) along with 4 functional λ constant region genes ($C_\lambda 1$, $C_\lambda 2$, $C_\lambda 3$, and $C_\lambda 7$) and 3 λ constant-region pseudogenes ($C_\lambda 4$, $C_\lambda 5$, and $C_\lambda 6$), each associated with 1 J_λ segment (Fig. 83-5).[25] The constant region elements of the heavy-chain gene complex are proximal to variable region segments on chromosome 14, while the constant region segments of the two light chains are in the opposite orientation, telomeric to the variable region genes.

Each germ line V gene, D element, and J segment is flanked by recognition sequences that are necessary to direct site-specific recombination. Such sequences consist of a highly conserved palindromic heptamer (5′ CACAGTG 3′), a nonconserved spacer of 12 or 23 bp, and a conserved nonamer (5′ ACAAAAACC 3′). Joining

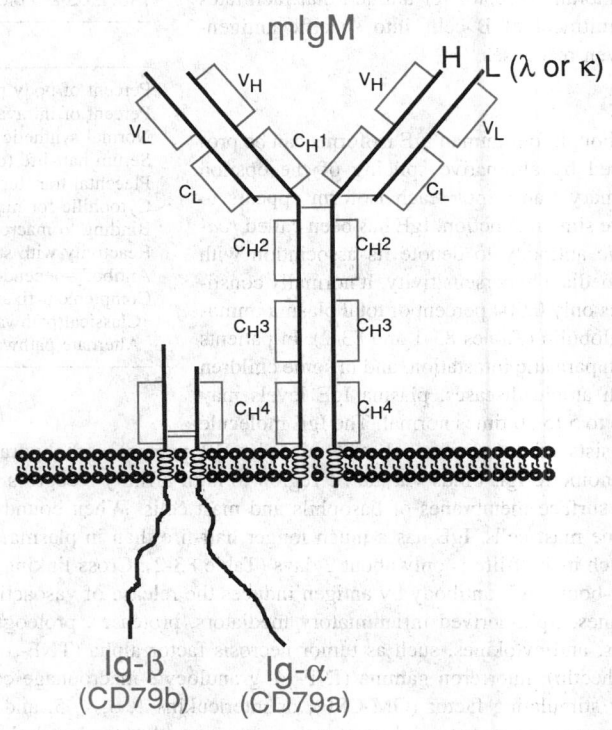

FIGURE 83-3   Schematic of membrane IgM (mIgM) and associated membrane proteins Ig-α and Ig-β or Ig-α and Ig-γ. Intrachain and interchain disulfide bonds are indicated by the thin lines. Filled circles depict the lipid bilayer. The immunoglobulin variable and constant region domains are indicated as in Fig. 83-1.

usually occurs only between segments flanked by recognition sequences with unequal spacers.[26–28] This is referred to as the *12/23 joining rule*. Each spacer varies in sequence, but its length is conserved and corresponds to one or two turns of the DNA double helix. Each spacer serves to bring the heptamer and nonamer sequences to one side of the DNA helix, where they can be bound by the protein complex that catalyzes recombination. Similar recognition sequences flank the elements that rearrange to form the T-cell antigen receptor (see Chap. 84). Such heptamer-spacer-nonamer sequences are targets of lymphocyte-specific recombinases and are often called recombination signal sequences, or RSS.[27,28]

IMMUNOGLOBULIN GENE REARRANGEMENT AND EXPRESSION DURING B-CELL DEVELOPMENT

IMMUNOGLOBULIN GENE REARRANGEMENT

During B-cell ontogeny, the first immunoglobulin gene rearrangements generally occur within the heavy-chain gene complex (Fig. 83-6A).[26] One or more D segments may rearrange and become juxtaposed with a single J_H element, generating a DJ_H complex that then may rearrange with one of the 51 functional V_H genes. Subsequently, gene rearrangements occur in the light-chain loci (Fig. 83-6B). One of the 40 functional V_κ genes can rearrange with any one of five J_κ segments. Should these gene rearrangements fail to generate a functional $V_\kappa J_\kappa$ exon, the kappa-deleting element may rearrange to a site in or immediately downstream of the $V_\kappa J_\kappa$ exon, thus deleting the kappa light-chain constant region exon.[29] Subsequent to kappa light-chain gene rearrangement, one of over 30 functional V_λ exons can rearrange with

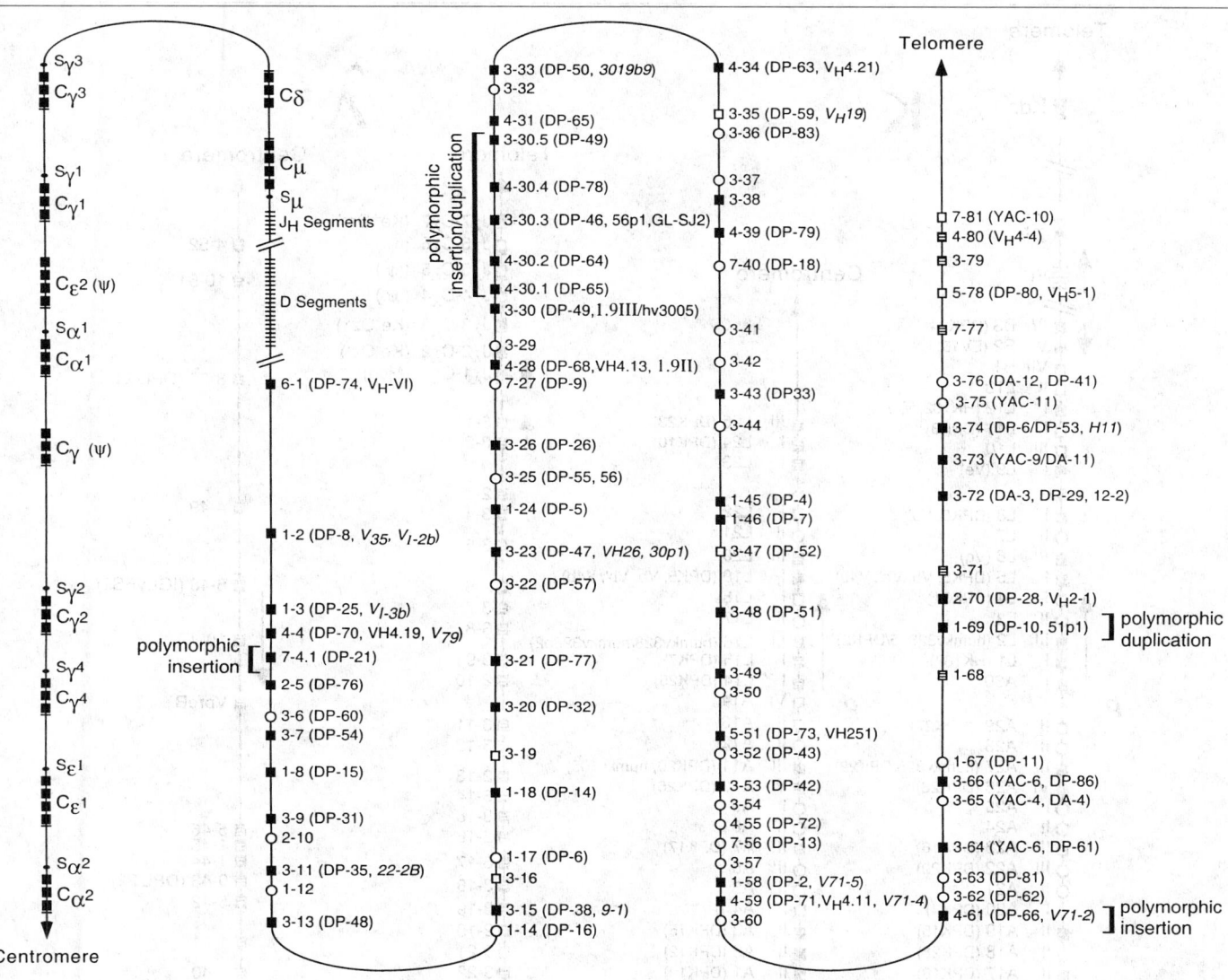

FIGURE 83-4   The human heavy chain immunoglobulin gene complex on chromosome 14q32. The heavy chain exons encoding the constant regions are represented by black boxes, and the associated intronic switch regions (S) are each depicted as a line. These exons are labeled to the right of these symbols. A Ψ next to the heavy chain isotype designation indicates that the gene is a pseudogene. J_H segments and D segments are indicated by lines. Each V_H gene locus is labeled on the right of each symbol. By convention, the loci encoding each of the various V_H genes are assigned a number corresponding to the V_H gene subgroup followed by a hyphen and then the rank order distance from the heavy chain D segments. Listed in parentheses are the alternative names that have been used to designate each locus. Identified polymorphic insertions and/or duplications are indicated with brackets. Black squares represent V_H gene loci that are known to be functional. Open circles represent V_H pseudogenes. The open boxes depict V_H exons that appear functional, but rarely are found to encode a functional heavy chain gene rearrangement. At the end of the line containing the symbols are arrows that indicate the direction to the centromere or the telomere. (For updates see: http://www.mrc-cpe.cam.ac.uk/imt-doc/public/INTRO.html).

any one of the 4 functional J_λ-C_λ exons to generate a gene that can encode a lambda light chain (Fig. 83-6).[25]

The commonest mode of recombination involves the looping-out and deletion of the DNA intervening between two gene segments on the same chromosome. The 12-mer-spaced and 23-mer-spaced recombination signal sequences are brought together by interactions between proteins that specifically recognize the length of spacer between the heptamer and nonamer signals, thus accounting for the 12/23 joining rule.[27,28] The two DNA molecules then are broken and religated.[30] The ends of the heptamer sequences are joined precisely in a head-to-head configuration to form a *signal joint* in a circular piece of DNA that then is lost from the genome when the cell divides. The termini of gene segments that subsequently give

rise to the *coding joint* form short DNA hairpins that subsequently are cleaved at a random site by an endonuclease. Depending on the site of cleavage, the single-stranded DNA may contain nucleotides that originally were complementary in the double-stranded DNA and therefore form short DNA palindromes, also known as *P-nucleotides*. If the cell also expresses the enzyme terminal deoxynucleotidyl transferase (TdT), then nucleotides are added at random to the ends of the single-stranded segments. These nucleotides are called *non-template-encoded nucleotides*, or *N-nucleotides*. The randomness of insertion of P-nucleotides and N-nucleotides at the junction of rearranged gene segments provides an important mechanism with which to generate diversity in the functionally rearranged immunoglobulin genes. A similar process accounts for

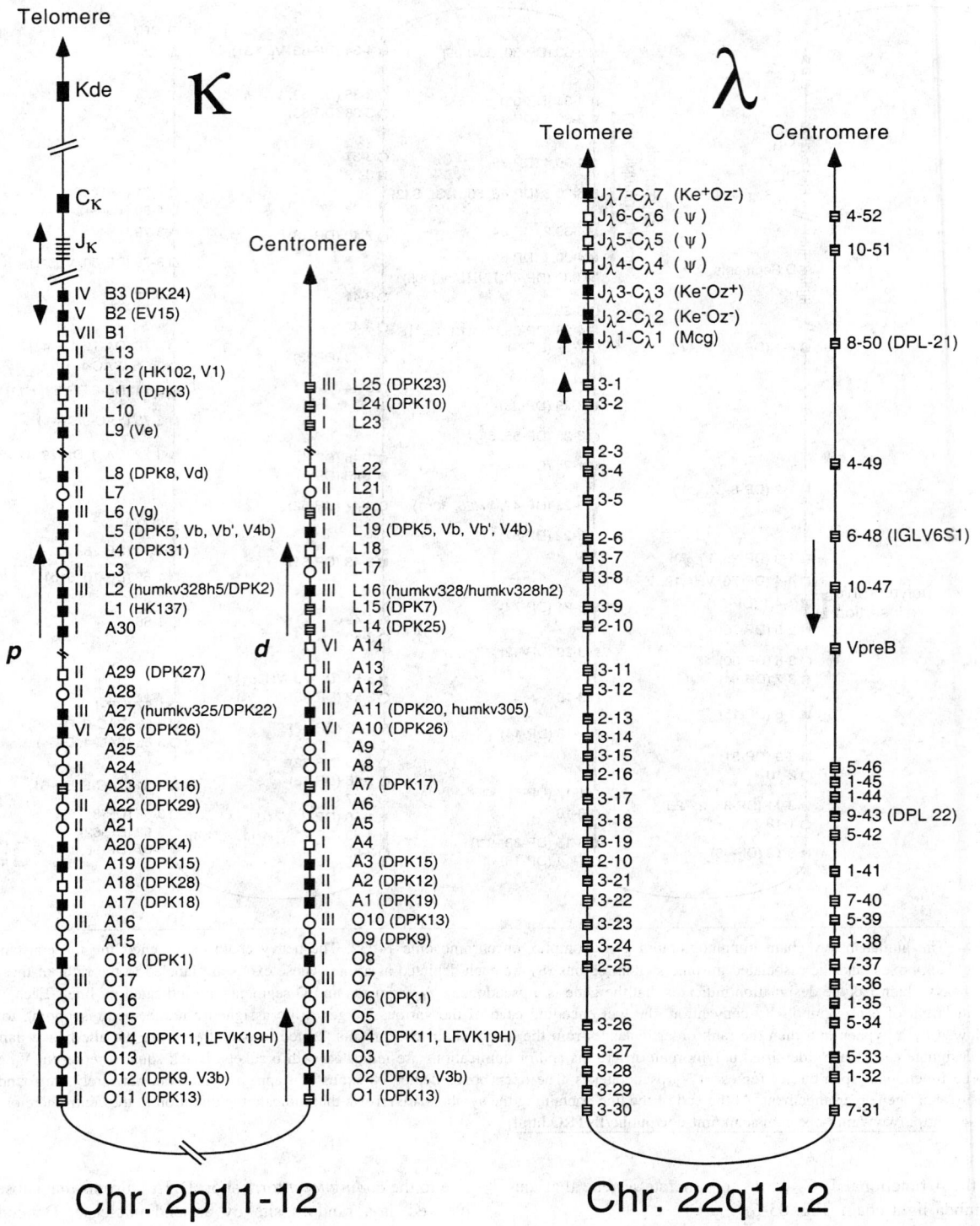

FIGURE 83-5　The immunoglobulin light chain gene complexes. The figure on the left depicts the kappa light-chain gene complex on chromosome 2p11-12. The black boxes in this figure represent the Kde element or the C_κ constant region exon as indicated to the right of each box. Positioned between the C_κ constant region exon and the J_κ segments is the kappa light chain enhancer (E). The J_κ segments are indicated by lines. The V_κ genes are clustered in two regions centromeric to the J_κ and C_κ exons, each region spanning approximately 500 kb. Approximately 800 kb separate the two regions. The region proximal to J_κ and C_κ, designated **p**, contains 40 V_κ genes (B3→B1, L13→L1, A30→A15, and O18→O11), while the distal region (**d** contains 36 gene segments (O1→O10, A1→A14, L14→L25). V_κ genes that can encode functional kappa light chains are represented by black boxes and are labeled to the right of each symbol. Thirty-two of the 76 V_κ genes are pseudogenes (open boxes). The **d** region apparently arose through duplication of a large portion of the **p** region. Consequently, there are 33 pairs of V_κ genes that share 95–100% nucleic acid sequence homology, accounting for 66 of the 76 V_κ genes in the **κ** light chain complex. There V_κ genes can be grouped further into four clusters, A, B,

generation of diversity in the rearrangement of T-cell receptor gene segments (see Chap. 84).

A complex of several enzymes, called *V(D)J recombinase,* acts in concert to mediate somatic V-region gene recombination. This complex mostly is comprised of cleavage and repair enzymes that are present in all cells and that are required for the normal maintenance of genomic DNA integrity. The first cleavage step, however, requires an additional specialized heterodimeric endonuclease encoded by two genes, called *RAG-1* and *RAG-2* for *recombination activating genes 1* and *2.*[31] *RAG-1* and *RAG-2* are adjacent genes located on the short arm of chromosome 11 (11p13-p12)[32] that were isolated based upon their ability to enable fibroblasts to catalyze V(D)J recombination of nonrearranged immunoglobulin genes that were cointroduced via gene transfer. *RAG-1* has sequence similarities to bacterial *topoisomerases* that catalyze the breakage and rejoining of DNA. *RAG-1* and *RAG-2* are coexpressed normally only in developing lymphocytes that are undergoing receptor gene rearrangement. Mice with either RAG gene knocked out cannot undergo immunoglobulin or T-cell receptor gene rearrangements and consequently fail to produce mature B or T lymphocytes.[33] Mutations that impair, but do not completely abolish, the function of *RAG-1* or *RAG-2* in humans result in a form of combined immune deficiency called *Omenn syndrome.*[34]

The other components of the V(D)J recombinase consist of enzymes that normally work to repair double-stranded breaks in genomic DNA. These include an autoantigen, called *Ku,* and DNA-dependent protein kinase. The latter enzyme is required to repair the junctions between the gene segments encoding the coding joints of rearranged gene segments. Consequently, mice that are deficient in this enzyme can make only trivial amounts of immunoglobulin or T-cell receptors and are called *severe-combined immunodeficient* mice, or SCID mice.

SURROGATE LAMBDA LIGHT CHAINS

Precursor B cells that only have rearranged D and J_H elements are referred to as progenitor B cells, or "pro-B cells." The term *pre-B cells* is reserved for precursor B cells that have completed immunoglobulin heavy-chain-gene rearrangement and have a functional $V_H D J_H$ complex. Both pro-B cells and pre-B cells have immunoglobulin light-chain loci in germ line configuration.

Despite this, pre-B cells express some immunoglobulin μ chains in association with "surrogate" λ light chains. One of these proteins, called λ_5, has similarity with known C_λ light-chain domains.[35] Another protein is called *VpreB,* because it resembles a V domain but bears an extra N-terminal protein sequence. Both proteins are encoded by genes located on chromosome 22. The λ_5 gene is situated within a λ-like locus that is telomeric to the true λ light-chain locus. The VpreB

gene is located within the cluster of immunoglobulin V_λ genes (Fig. 83-5), defined by breakpoints of chromosomal translocations found in a few leukemias and lymphomas.[35] Together, VpreB and λ_5 pair with the μ heavy chains to form a primitive immunoglobulin receptor that, together with CD79a and CD79b, may be expressed on the surface membrane of the developing pre-B cell.[36] Monoclonal antibodies that recognize λ_5 or VpreB specifically bind to pre-B cells and can react with B-lineage acute lymphocytic leukemias.[37]

The pre-B cell receptor complex is expressed only transiently, as production of λ_5 ceases as soon as it is formed. Nevertheless, this protein plays an important role in normal B-cell development. In normal mice, the appearance of the pre-B cell receptor coincides with inactivation of the *RAG-2* protein by phosphorylation, and degradation of *RAG-1* and *RAG-2* mRNA, suggesting that this receptor plays a role in suppressing further immunoglobulin gene rearrangement. However, expression of the pre-B cell receptor on the surface membrane is associated with cell activation and proliferation, leading to generation of small, resting pre-B daughter cells that again express *RAG-1* and *RAG-2*. This leads to subsequent light-chain gene rearrangement. As such, expression of the pre-B cell receptor appears to signal that a complete μ heavy-chain gene has been formed, that further rearrangements at this locus should be suppressed, and that development to the next stage can proceed. Therefore, the surrogate light chains play a critical role in normal B-cell development. This is underscored by studies on transgenic mice that lack functional λ_5 genes.[38] In these mice, B-cell development in the marrow is blocked at the pre-B cell stage, thereby markedly reducing in the numbers of functional mature B lymphocytes in the blood and lymphoid tissues.[39] Similarly, humans that have inactivating mutations in the λ_5 genes on both alleles of chromosome 22 have agammaglobulinemia and markedly reduced numbers of B cells.[40]

HEAVY-CHAIN CLASS SWITCHING

During differentiation, a single B lymphocyte can synthesize heavy chains with different constant regions coupled to the same variable region.[41] As pre-B cells develop into mature B cells, intact IgM monomers are inserted into the plasma membrane, followed by IgD molecules with the same antigen-binding specificity. The IgM and IgD constant region genes are closely linked in embryonic DNA (see Fig. 83-4) and may be transcribed together. The differential splicing of the transcript allows the simultaneous synthesis of the two immunoglobulin heavy chains from a single species of messenger RNA.

The secretion of IgM, and the switch from IgM to IgG, IgA, or IgE synthesis, generally requires the prior interaction of lymphocytes with antigen or mitogen. Interleukins provided by antigen-reactive T

L, and O, three of which (A, L, and O) are duplicated and found in both the J_κ-proximal *p* region and the J_κ-distal *d* region. The B cluster, containing V_κ genes B1, B2 (EV15), and B3 (DPK26), is found only in the J_κ-proximal *p* region. Each V_κ gene can be assigned to one of three main subgroups, I-III, and several smaller subgroups (IV, V, VI, and VII) based on nucleotide sequence homology. The largest subgroup is V_κI, with 21 functional genes, depicted as black boxes. The next largest subgroups are V_κ2, with 11 functional genes, and V_κ3, with 7. There are 3 functional genes in the V_κ6 subgroup, and one each for the V_κ4 and V_κ5 subgroups. The V_κ7 subgroup consists of one of the non-functional pseudogene, which are depicted as open squares. Open squares depict V_κ pseudogenes. Black arrows indicate the transcriptional orientation of the V genes in the complex. At the end of the line connecting the symbols are arrows that indicate the direction to the centromere or the telomore.

The figure on the right depicts the lambda-light-chain gene complex on chromosome 22q11.2. The black boxes represent functional J_λ-C_λ exons, whereas open boxes represent J_λ-C_λ pseudogenes. The J_λ-C_λ exon pairs are labeled to the right of each symbol. The figure also depicts as black boxes the 39 functional V_λ genes centromeric to the lambda constant regions. These V_λ genes are arranged into 10 subgroups, each comprised of V_λ genes sharing greater than 75% nucleotide sequence homology. The first number in the labels to the right of each V_λ gene provides the number of the subgroup, followed by a hyphen, and then the relative rank order of the V gene from the constant region exons. Note that the V_λ genes have been mapped into three clusters within 860 kb of the J_λ and C_λ genes that are each separated from one another in the figure by double lines. The cluster most proximal to the J_λ-C_λ exons, designated "A", is comprised of 18 functional V_λ genes mostly belonging to the V_λ2 and V_λ3 gene subgroups. The next cluster, "B", contains 15 functional V_λ genes of the V_λ1, V_λ5, V_λ7, V_λ9 gene subgroups. The third cluster, "C", contains 6 functional V_λ genes of the V_λ4, V_λ6, V_λ8, V_λ10, and V_λ11 gene subgroups along with exon encoding VpreB. Some individuals have an insertion of a functional V_λ gene, 5-39 (5a), marked as "polymorphic insertion". Black arrows indicate the transcriptional orientation of the V genes in the complex.

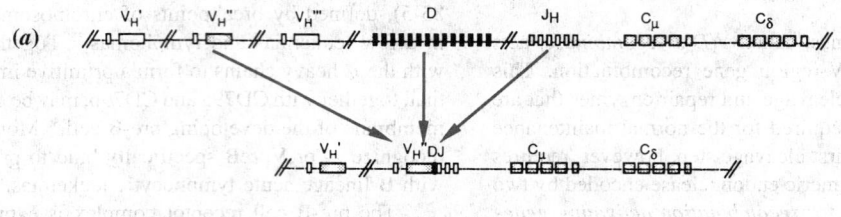

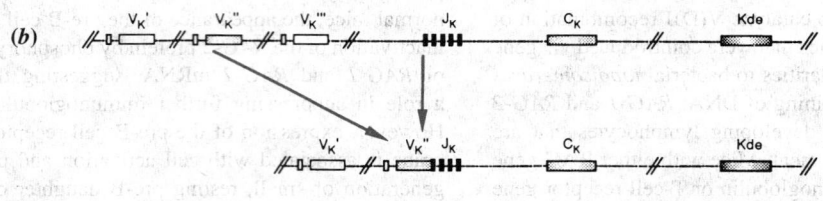

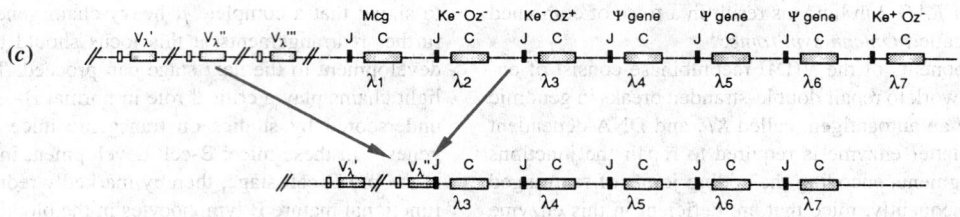

FIGURE 83-6   Immunoglobulin gene complexes and rearrangement. Diagonal double lines indicate that there is a large DNA distance between the flanking genes depicted as rectangular boxes (not drawn to scale). The upper diagram in A, B, or C shows the germ line DNA configuration of the immunoglobulin heavy-chain genes, kappa light-chain genes, or lambda light-chain genes respectively. Depicted on the left side of each immunoglobulin gene complex are exemplary immunoglobulin heavy-chain variable region genes (V_H', V_H'', V_H'''), immunoglobulin kappa light-chain genes (V_κ', V_κ'', V_κ''), or immunoglobulin lambda light-chain variable region genes (V_λ', V_λ'', V_λ''). D denotes the diversity gene segments of the antibody heavy-chain locus. J_H, J_κ, or J_λ indicates the joining gene segments of the antibody heavy chain, κ light chain, or λ light chain respectively. C_μ or C_δ denotes the constant region exons of the μ or δ heavy chain, respectively. Below each is a possible immunoglobulin gene rearrangement comprised of a V_HDJ_H, for the antibody heavy chain, or a $V_\kappa J_\kappa$ or a $V_\lambda J_\lambda$ for the κ or λ light-chain genes respectively. Below the representative λ constant region loci in row C are listed the names of the λ nonallelic genetic markers, Mcg, Ke$^-$ Oz$^-$, Ke$^-$ Oz$^+$, and Ke$^+$ Oz$^-$ on $C_\lambda 1$, $C_\lambda 2$, $C_\lambda 3$, or $C_\lambda 7$ respectively. As indicated, $C_\lambda 4$, $C_\lambda 5$, $C_\lambda 6$ are psuedogenes (Ψ gene) that do not encode protein.

lymphocytes strongly influence (1) which B cells differentiate into IgM-secreting plasma cells and (2) which B cells switch to synthesizing the heavy chain of another immunoglobulin isotype, such as IgG and IgA.[41,42]

Isotype switch recombination occurs in or near the switch region located in the intron between the rearranged VDJ_H sequence and the μ gene and any one of similar regions located upstream of the C genes encoding each of the other heavy-chain isotypes, with the exception of the δ gene (Fig. 83-4). The μ switch region, designated as $S\mu$, consists of approximately 150 repeats of the sequence $(GAGCT)_n(GGGGGT)$, where n is generally three but can be as many as seven. The sequences of the other switch regions (S_λ, S_δ, and S_ε) are similar in that they also contain repeats of the GAGCT and GGGGGT sequences. The switch in heavy-chain classes results from DNA recombination between S_μ and S_λ, S_δ, or S_ε accompanied by the deletion of intervening DNA segments and the apposition of the previously rearranged variable region gene next to the new constant region gene. Switch recombination events produce genes that can encode a functional protein because they involve switch sequences within the introns and therefore cannot cause frame shift mutations in the exons encoding the immunoglobulin molecule.

MECHANISMS FOR GENERATING ANTIBODY DIVERSITY

Several mechanisms contribute to the generation of diversity among immunoglobulin polypeptide variable regions.[26] These are (1) the presence in the germ line of multiple different V, J, and D gene segments; (2) the random joining of these DNA segments to produce a complete variable region exon; (3) uncorrected errors made during the recombination process; (4) the coming together of the heavy- and light-chain polypeptides to produce a complete immunoglobulin monomer capable of binding antigen; and (5) somatic mutations within the rearranged DNA segments themselves. The latter occurs through a process called *somatic hypermutation.*[43]

Somatic hypermutation is not active in all B cells and cannot be triggered merely by mitogen-induced B cell activation. However, during discrete stages of B-cell differentiation, expressed immunoglobulin V genes may incur new mutations at rates as high as 10^{-3} base substitutions per base pair per generation over several cell divisions, particularly during the secondary humoral immune response to antigen. The pattern of somatic mutations in rearranged variable genes differs from that of meiotic mutations, indicating that a different mechanism generates somatic hypermutation than that responsible for spontaneous mutation.[44] Hypermutations begin on the 5' end of rearranged V genes downstream of the transcription initiation site and continue through the V gene and into the 3'-flanking region before tapering off. As such, the mutations are clustered in the region spanning from 300 bp 5' of the rearranged variable region exon to approximately 1 kb 3' of the rearranged mini-gene J segment. Subsequent selection of the immunoglobulin encoded by such mutated immunoglobulin V genes may enhance the frequency of nonconservative base substitutions in the DNA sequences encoding the combining site for antigen.[45]

Under normal conditions, a B lymphocyte or plasma cell synthesizes only one species of light chain and heavy chain, even though the cell has two different sets of each of the immunoglobulin gene complexes that initially undergo seemingly independent immunoglobulin gene rearrangements. Indeed, the specificity of the humoral immune response depends on antigenic selection of unique clones of B cells, each clone expressing a homogeneous set of immunoglobulin receptors. Such restriction is achieved by limiting a given B cell to functional rearrangement and expression of only a single heavy-chain allele and a single light-chain allele. This phenomenon is called *allelic exclusion*. Although occasional neoplastic B cell populations may lack allelic exclusion and express both immunoglobulin alleles, this phenomenon generally is observed with most B-cell tumors.[46]

IMMUNOGLOBULIN VARIABLE REGION STRUCTURE

IMMUNOGLOBULIN VARIABLE REGION SUBGROUPS

Despite the large number of different immunoglobulin variable regions that can be generated through the above mechanisms, each antibody polypeptide may be assigned to one of a relatively small number of variable region subgroups.[4] Comparisons of the amino acid sequences of a large number of different monoclonal immunoglobulin proteins reveal four segments of limited amino acid sequence diversity between different antibody heavy- or light-chain variable regions. These segments are designated the *immunoglobulin variable region frameworks* (FR) (Fig. 83-7). Each immunoglobulin polypeptide may be assigned to one of a relatively small number of variable region subgroups based upon the primary structure of its first three frameworks. Moreover, each subgroup has characteristic framework sequences that serve to distinguish it from other variable region subgroups.

Satisfying expectations that immunoglobulin subgroups defined families of highly related antibody V genes, variable region amino acid subgroup homologies are found to extend to the nucleic acid sequence level.[47–49] Cloned immunoglobulin V genes whose deduced amino acid sequences belong to a given subgroup generally share greater than 80 percent nucleic acid sequence homology. The human heavy-chain variable regions may be grouped into seven subgroups, while kappa or lambda light chains may be divided into 6 or 11 subgroups, respectively.

Crystallographic data of immunoglobulin variable regions indicate that amino acids within the first and third FR regions of either the light or heavy chain form beta bonds on the external surface of the molecule.[5,50] These regions form relatively compact structures on the external solvent-accessible face of the antibody molecule that are not adjacent to the classic antibody combining site for antigen. Accordingly, amino acid differences noted between the different variable region subgroups are amenable to recognition by antisubgroup antibodies.[51]

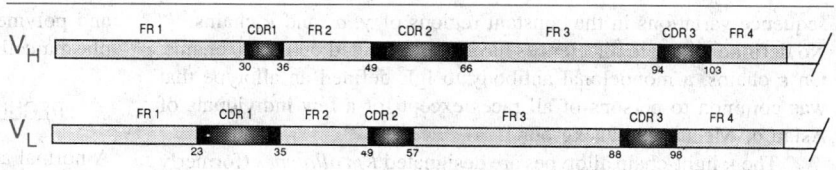

FIGURE 83-7 Schematic diagrams depicting each FR and CDR of the immunoglobulin heavy chain (V_H) or light chain (V_L). The first, second, third, and fourth framework regions are labeled FR1, FR2, FR3, and FR4 respectively. Similarly, the first through third complementarity-determining regions are labeled CDR1, CDR2, and CDR3 respectively. The numbers beneath each diagram indicate the numbers of the amino acid residues that define the borders between these regions according to Kabat.[4]

IMMUNOGLOBULIN IDIOTYPES

Antisubgroup antibodies, however, need to be distinguished from anti-idiotypic antibodies. Positioned between the FR regions are three segments of extreme hypervariability in both light and heavy chain sequences.[4] The third hypervariable region is generated through the recombinatorial process that joins the antibody light-chain V gene with the J segment, in the case of the light chain, or the V_H gene with the somatically generated DJ_H segment of the antibody heavy chain.[52–54] The diversity in first and second hypervariable regions in part reflects germ line DNA-encoded differences between disparate antibody V genes, a diversity often noted even between V genes of the same subgroup.[4,55,56] During an immune response, somatic hypermutation subsequent to V gene rearrangement also may play an important role in increasing the amino acid sequence diversity noted within these regions (discussed above). These hypervariable regions on both chains fold together to form the antigen combining site.[3,50] Hence, each of these regions of hypervariability is designated as being a complementarity-determining region, or CDR (Fig. 83-7).

During secondary immune responses, extensive amino acid substitutions may occur in the complementarity-determining regions. In contrast, amino acid replacement mutations are noted to be much less frequent in the framework regions than would be anticipated if the nucleic acid substitutions were occurring randomly. As a consequence, the subgroup determinants that characterize an entire variable region subgroup may be relatively resilient to the process of somatic hypermutation. On the other hand, the complementarity-determining regions may form determinants of unique specificity that contribute to the epitopes recognized by anti-idiotypic antibodies.

Despite the tremendous potential for diversity in Ig V gene expression and genetic polymorphism, antibodies produced by B-cell malignancies or normal B cells of unrelated persons may share common idiotypic determinants.[57] These common idiotypes, designated cross-reactive idiotypes or CRIs, were defined initially on IgM autoantibodies, such as rheumatoid factors. However, cross-reactive idiotypes may be found on antibodies that do not have anti-self-reactivity. Molecular studies have demonstrated several of these cross-reactive idiotypes to represent serologic markers for expression of conserved immunoglobulin variable region genes with little or no somatic mutation.[58]

GENETIC MARKERS ON IMMUNOGLOBULIN CONSTANT REGIONS

ALLOTYPES

Human immunoglobulins have inherited differences in structure, termed *allotypes*. These genetic markers usually are detected with agglutinating sera from individuals naturally immunized through transfusion or pregnancy. These antibodies recognize minor amino acid sequence variations in the constant regions of γ, α, and κ chains.[59,60] No definite allotypic differences have been detected on μ or δ chains. On ε chains, a monoclonal antibody to IgE defined an allotype that was common to persons of all races except for a few individuals of Asian or Melanesian background.

The κ light-chain allotypes are designated *Km allotypes* (formerly called *inv*). There exist at least three major Km allotypes, designated Km(1), Km(1,2), and Km(3), that may be recognized serologically or, more recently, via the polymerase chain reaction.[61] The α chain allotypes, designated *Am allotypes*, are on the heavy chains of the IgA$_2$ subclass.[60] The γ chain allotypes are on the heavy chains of the IgG$_1$, IgG$_2$, or IgG$_3$ subclasses and are designated *G1m*, *G2m*, and *G3m* respectively. Over 24 Gm allotypic markers have been identified serologically.[60] As discussed earlier, all the heavy-chain constant region genes reside on chromosome 14. Therefore, different combinations of heavy-chain allotype markers are inherited as haplotypic units, in an autosomal codominant manner. The frequency of the various allelic markers differs among ethnic groups.

LAMBDA LIGHT-CHAIN ISOTYPES

The λ light chains have four isotypes, termed Mcg^+, $Ke^- Oz^-$, $Ke^- Oz^+$, and $Ke^+ Oz^-$, that were defined on the basis of their reactivity with the Oz, Kern, and Mcg antisera raised against λ Bence Jones proteins.[62] These isotypes reflect minor nonallelic amino acid differences in the λ light-chain constant regions that are each encoded by one of the multiple constant region genes in the lambda light-chain complex.[25] Mcg^+, $Ke^- Oz^-$, $Ke^- Oz^+$, and $Ke^+ Oz^-$ isotypes are each associated with the $C_\lambda 1$, $C_\lambda 2$, $C_\lambda 3$, or $C_\lambda 7$ λ light-chain constant regions respectively (Fig. 83-6).

IMMUNOGLOBULIN SYNTHESIS AND SECRETION

IMMUNOGLOBULIN SYNTHESIS

The total IgG content of the adult human body is about 75 g, of which 2.2 g is synthesized each day. Most immunoglobulin is produced by mature plasma cells, which have abundant rough endoplasmic reticulum and a well-developed Golgi apparatus.

The final messenger RNA for immunoglobulin light and heavy chains are derived by the processing of large nuclear RNA transcripts. In plasma cells, the rearranged and spliced mRNA molecules for the heavy- and light-chain polypeptides are translated on separate ribosomal complexes. An amino-terminal leader peptide approximately 18 to 30 residues long is cleaved prior to the release of the completed light and heavy chains in the cisternae of the endoplasmic reticulum. There the two polypeptides spontaneously combine to form immunoglobulin half molecules that are stabilized by disulfide bonds. The joining of two identical half molecules by disulfide bonds yields a basic four-chain immunoglobulin unit.

Glycosyltransferase enzymes add a defined sequence of sugars to the assembled immunoglobulin unit to form branched-chain oligosaccharides composed of *N*-acetyl-glucosamine, mannose, galactose, fructose, and sialic acid. The oligosaccharides are attached covalently to the immunoglobulin heavy chain at several sites. The carbohydrate facilitates the transport of the antibody molecule across the plasma membrane and into the extracellular space and increases the solubility of the secreted protein.

Five monomeric units of IgM combine to form a pentameric macroglobulin linked by disulfide bonds and a single J-chain polypeptide. Usually polymerization immediately precedes or occurs simultaneously with IgM secretion. Similarly, IgA molecules form dimers and polymers linked by the J chain just prior to secretion from the plasma cell.

REGULATION OF IMMUNOGLOBULIN SYNTHESIS

A normal adult has preexisting B lymphocytes that can interact with almost any foreign antigen. In the presence of accessory T lymphocytes and macrophages, an antigen-binding clone of B lymphocytes may transform into antibody-secreting plasma cells and memory B cells.[63] Most plasma cells are terminally differentiated and do not divide. Therefore, the continued production of antibody depends upon the rate of plasma cell generation, the functional life span of the plasma cell, and the half-life of the immunoglobulin in the body.[64]

B lymphocytes are produced throughout life by differentiation of hematopoietic cells in the marrow and proliferation of B lymphocytes in secondary lymphoid tissues.[65] Many B lymphocytes survive for but a few weeks without stimulation by antigen and activated accessory T lymphocytes.[66] Without antigen to cross-link their surface immunoglobulin receptors, B lymphocytes that home to the germinal centers of secondary lymphoid tissues will undergo apoptosis, or programmed cell death, within a matter of hours in vitro.[67-69] Not only does this select for B lymphocytes that have surface immunoglobulin with high affinity for antigen,[70] the requirement for antigen-directed surface immunoglobulin cross-linking also allows for secreted specific antibody to regulate its own production. Under normal short-term exposure to antigen, newly formed B lymphocytes must compete with secreted antibody and other antigen-specific B lymphocytes for ever-decreasing amounts of circulating antigen. By preventing the interaction of antigen with immunoglobulin receptors on B lymphocytes, secreted antibody may inhibit the generation of more plasma cells.

REFERENCES

1. Edelman GM: Antibody structure and molecular immunology *Scand J Immunol* 34:1, 1991.
2. Virella G, Wang AC: Immunoglobulin structure. *Immunol Ser* 58:75, 1993.
3. Alzari PM, Lascombe MB, Poljak RJ: Three-dimensional structure of antibodies. *Annu Rev Immunol* 6:555, 1988.
4. Kabat E, Wu TT, Perry HM, et al: *Sequences of Proteins of Immunological Interest*, 5th edition. U.S. Department of Health and Human Services, Bethesda, MD, 1991.
5. Harris LJ, Larson SB, Hasel KW, et al: The three-dimensional structure of an intact monoclonal antibody for canine lymphoma. *Nature* 360:369, 1992.
6. Jefferis R, Lund J, Goodall M: Recognition sites on human IgG for Fc gamma receptors: the role of glycosylation. *Immunol Lett* 44:111, 1995.
7. Lee YK, Brewer JW, Hellman R, Hendershot LM: BiP and immunoglobulin light chain cooperate to control the folding of heavy chains and ensure the fidelity of immunoglobulin assembly. *Mol Biol Cell* 10:2209, 1999.
8. Lamm ME, Nedrud JG, Kaetzel CS, Mazanec MB: IgA and mucosal defense. *Apmis* 103:241, 1995.
9. Corthesy B, Kraehenbuhl JP: Antibody-mediated protection of mucosal surfaces. *Curr Top Microbiol Immunol* 236:93, 1999.
10. Niles MJ, Matsuuchi L, Koshland ME: Polymer IgM assembly and secretion in lymphoid and nonlymphoid cell lines: evidence that J chain is required for pentamer IgM synthesis. *Proc Natl Acad Sci USA* 92:2884, 1995.
11. Roes J, Rajewsky K: Immunoglobulin D (IgD)-deficient mice reveal an auxiliary receptor function for IgD in antigen-mediated recruitment of B cells. *J Exp .Med* 177:45, 1993.
12. Lyczak JB, Zhang K, Saxon A, Morrison SL: Expression of novel secreted isoforms of human immunoglobulin E proteins. *J Biol Chem* 271:3428, 1996.
13. Cambier JC, Campbell KS: Membrane immunoglobulin and its accomplices: new lessons from an old receptor. *FASEB J* 6:3207, 1992.
14. Kurosaki T: Genetic analysis of B cell antigen receptor signaling. *Annu Rev Immunol* 17:555, 1999.

15. Healy JI, Goodnow CC: Positive versus negative signaling by lymphocyte antigen receptors. *Annu Rev Immunol* 16:645, 1998.

16. Cornall RJ, Goodnow CC, Cyster JG: Regulation of B cell antigen receptor signaling by the Lyn/CD22/SHP1 pathway. *Curr Top Micobiol Immunol* 244:57, 1999.

17. Plas DR, Thomas ML: Negative regulation of antigen receptor signaling in lymphocytes. *J Mol Med* 76:589, 1998.

18. Siminovitch KA, Neel BG: Regulation of B cell signal transduction by SH2-containing protein-tyrosine phosphatases. *Semin Immunol* 10:329, 1998.

19. Shultz LD, Rajan TV, Greiner DL: Severe defects in immunity and hematopoiesis caused by SHP-1 protein-tyrosine-phosphatase deficiency. *Trends Biotechnol* 15:302, 1997.

20. Matsuda F, Honjo T: Organization of the human immunoglobulin heavy-chain locus. *Adv Immunol* 62:1, 1996.

21. Tomlinson IM, Cook GP, Walter G, et al: A complete map of the human immunoglobulin VH locus. *Ann NY Acad Sci* 764:43, 1995.

22. Kipps TJ: Human B cell biology. *Int Rev Immunol* 15:243, 1997.

23. Zachau HG: The immunoglobulin kappa locus or what has been learned from looking closely at one-tenth of a percent of the human genome. *Gene* 135:167, 1993.

24. Schäble K, Thiebe R, Flügel A, et al: The human immunoglobulin kappa locus: pseudogenes, unique and repetitive sequences. *Biol Chem Hoppe-Seyler* 375:189, 1994.

25. Pallarès N, Frippiat JP, Giudicelli V, Lefranc MP: The human immunoglobulin lambda variable (IgLV) genes and joining (IgLJ) segments. *Exp Clin Immunogenet* 15:8, 1998.

26. Tonegawa S: The Nobel lectures in immunology. The Nobel Prize for physiology or medicine, 1987. Somatic generation of immune diversity. *Scand J Immunol* 38:303, 1993.

27. Gellert M: Recent advances in understanding V(D)J recombination. *Adv Immunol* 64:39, 1997.

28. Steen SB, Gomelsky L, Speidel SL, Roth DB: Initiation of V(D)J recombination in vivo: role of recombination signal sequences in formation of single and paired double-strand breaks. *EMBO J* 16:2656, 1997.

29. Graninger WB, Goldman PL, Morton CC, et al: The kappa-deleting element. Germline and rearranged, duplicated and dispersed forms. *J Exp Med* 167:488, 1988.

30. Grawunder U, West RB, Lieber MR: Antigen receptor gene rearrangement. *Curr Opin Immunol* 10:172, 1998.

31. Oettinger MA, Schatz DG, Gorka C, Baltimore D: RAG-1 and RAG-2, adjacent genes that synergistically activate V(D)J recombination. *Science* 248:1517, 1990.

32. Oettinger MA, Stanger B, Schatz DG, et al: The recombination activating genes, RAG 1 and RAG 2, are on chromosome 11p in humans and chromosome 2p in mice. *Immunogenetics* 35:97, 1992.

33. Shinkai Y, Rathbun G, Lam KP, et al: RAG-2-deficient mice lack mature lymphocytes owing to inability to initiate V(D)J rearrangement. *Cell* 68:855, 1992.

34. Villa A, Santagata S, Bozzi F, et al: Omenn syndrome: a disorder of Rag1 and Rag2 genes. *J Clin Immunol* 19:87, 1999.

35. Melchers F, Karasuyama H, Haasner D, et al: The surrogate light chain in B-cell development. *Immunol Today* 14:60, 1993.

36. Ten Boekel E, Yamagami T, Andersson J, et al: The formation and selection of cells expressing preB cell receptors and B cell receptors. *Curr Top Micobiol Immunol* 246:3, 1999.

37. Tsuganezawa K, Kiyokawa N, Matsuo Y, et al: Flow cytometric diagnosis of the cell lineage and developmental stage of acute lymphoblastic leukemia by novel monoclonal antibodies specific to human pre-B-cell receptor. *Blood* 92:4317, 1998.

38. Kitamura D, Kudo A, Schaal S, et al: A critical role of lambda 5 protein in B cell development. *Cell* 69:823, 1992.

39. Corcos D, Dunda O, Butor C, et al: Pre-B-cell development in the absence of lambda 5 in transgenic mice expressing a heavy-chain disease protein. *Curr Biol* 5:1140, 1995.

40. Minegishi Y, Coustan-Smith E, Wang YH, et al: Mutations in the human lambda 5/14.1 gene result in B cell deficiency and agammaglobulinemia. *J Exp Med* 187:71, 1998.

41. Stavnezer J: Immunoglobulin class switching. *Curr Opin Immunol* 8:199, 1996.

42. Lorenz MG, Radbruch A: Insights into the control of immunoglobulin class switch recombination from analysis of targeted mice. *Res Immunol* 148:460, 1997.

43. Wabl M, Cascalho M, Steinberg C: Hypermutation in antibody affinity maturation. *Curr Opin Immunol* 11:186, 1999.

44. Winter DB, Gearhart PJ: Dual enigma of somatic hypermutation of immunoglobulin variable genes: targeting and mechanism. *Immunol Rev* 162:89, 1998.

45. Dörner T, Foster SJ, Brezinschek HP, Lipsky PE: Analysis of the targeting of the hypermutational machinery and the impact of subsequent selection on the distribution of nucleotide changes in human VHDJH rearrangements. *Immunol Rev* 162:161, 1998.

46. Rassenti LZ, Kipps TJ: Lack of allelic exclusion in B cell chronic lymphocytic leukemia. *J Exp Med* 185:1435, 1997.

47. Cook GP, Tomlinson IM: The human immunoglobulin VH repertoire. *Immunol Today* 16:237, 1995.

48. Kipps TJ: Human B cell biology. *Int Rev Immunol* 15:243, 1997.

49. Frippiat JP, Williams SC, Tomlinson IM, et al: Organization of the human immunoglobulin lambda light-chain locus on chromosome 22q11.2. *Hum Mol Genet* 4:983, 1995.

50. Poljak RJ: Structure of antibodies and their complexes with antigens. *Mol Immunol* 28:1341, 1991.

51. Jefferis R: Nomenclature of V region markers. *Immunol Today* 16:207, 1995.

52. Tonegawa S: Somatic generation of antibody diversity. *Nature* 302:575, 1983.

53. Sakano H, Kurosawa Y, Weigert M, Tonegawa S: Identification and nucleotide sequence of a diversity DNA segment (D) of immunoglobulin heavy-chain genes. *Nature* 290:562, 1981.

54. Early P, Huang H, Davis M, et al: An immunoglobulin heavy chain variable region gene is generated from three segments of DNA: VH, D and JH. *Cell* 19:981, 1980.

55. Berman JE, Mellis SJ, Pollock R, et al: Content and organization of the human Ig VH locus: definition of three new VH families and linkage to the Ig CH locus. *EMBO J* 7:727, 1988.

56. Zachau HG: The human immunoglobulin kappa locus and some of its acrobatics. *Biol Chem Hoppe-Seyler* 371:1, 1990.

57. Kipps TJ, Carson DA: Autoantibodies in chronic lymphocytic leukemia and related systemic autoimmune diseases. *Blood* 81:2475, 1993.

58. Kipps TJ: Immunologic and therapeutic implications of anti-idiotype antibodies, in *Chronic Lymphocytic Leukemia*, edited by BD Cheson, p 123. Marcel Dekker, New York, 1992.

59. Williams RC Jr, Malone CC, Solomon A: Conformational dependency of human IgG heavy chain-associated Gm allotypes. *Mol Immunol* 30:341, 1993.

60. Schanfield MS, van Loghem E: Human immunoglobulin allotypes, in *Handbook of Experimental Immunology—Genetics and Molecular Immunology*, 4th ed, edited by DM Weir, LA Herzenberg, C Blackwell, L Herzenberg, p 941. Blackwell, Oxford, 1986.

61. Moxley G, Gibbs RS: Polymerase chain reaction-based genotyping for allotypic markers of immunoglobulin kappa shows allelic association of Km with kappa variable segment. *Genomics* 13:104, 1992.

62. Hess M, Hilschmann N, Rivat L, et al: Isotypes in human immunoglobulin lambda-chains. *Nature New Biol* 234:58, 1971.

63. Gray D: Immunologic memory. *Annu Rev Immunol* 11:49, 1993.

64. Virella G, Wang AC: Biosynthesis, metabolism and biological properties of immunoglobulins. *Immunol Ser* 58:91, 1993.

65. Nunez C, Nishimoto N, Gartland GL, et al: B cells are generated throughout life in humans. *J Immunol* 156:866, 1996.

66. Benschop RJ, Cambier JC: B cell development: signal transduction by antigen receptors and their surrogates. *Curr Opin Immunol* 11:143, 1999.

67. Choi YS: Differentiation and apoptosis of human germinal center B-lymphocytes. *Immunol Res* 16:161, 1997.

68. Liu YJ, de Bouteiller O, Fugier-Vivier I: Mechanisms of selection and differentiation in germinal centers. *Curr Opin Immunol* 9:256, 1997.

69. Hollowood K, Goodlad JR: Germinal centre cell kinetics. *J Pathol* 185:229, 1998.

70. Przylepa J, Himes C, Kelsoe G: Lymphocyte development and selection in germinal centers. *Curr Top Micobiol Immunol* 229:85, 1998.

FUNCTIONS OF T LYMPHOCYTES: T-CELL RECEPTORS FOR ANTIGEN

THOMAS J. KIPPS

All T cells express a receptor for antigen that is formed by two polymorphic polypeptides that invariably are associated with a collection of invariant proteins called *CD3*. The latter proteins are necessary for the surface expression and signaling by the T-cell receptor. The two polypeptides that form the T-cell receptor on most T cells are termed α and β; whereas a small subset of T cells have different polypeptides called γ and δ. The polypeptides of the T-cell receptor have a diversity that is comparable to that estimated for immunoglobulin molecules. However, unlike immunoglobulins, the T-cell receptors recognize small fragments of antigen, usually peptides, that are *presented* by major histocompatibility complex (MHC) molecules of another cell. As such, T-cell immune recognition generally requires cognate intercellular interactions between a T cell and another cell, sometimes called the *antigen-presenting cell*. The response of the T cell to antigen depends upon the intensity of the signal generated by ligation of the T-cell receptor. In addition, this signal is modified by the simultaneous ligation of other T-cell receptors for accessory molecules on the plasma membrane of the antigen-presenting cell. Because of this, the outcome of T-cell antigen recognition can range from immune activation and T-cell proliferation to specific T-cell tolerance and/or programmed cell death.

T-LYMPHOCYTE ANTIGEN RECEPTORS

THE T-CELL RECEPTOR FOR ANTIGEN

The receptor proteins of the T-cell antigen receptor are structurally related to immunoglobulin molecules (Fig. 84-1).[1] The receptor for antigen on most T cells is formed by two polypeptides, termed α and β, that are linked to each other via disulfide bonds and associated with a collection of invariant proteins called *CD3* (see Chap. 13).[2-4] Following the rule of allelic exclusion, the T-cell receptor is clonally distributed, each T cell expressing a single α chain and a single β chain. Each chain has a hydrophobic leader sequence of 18 to 29 amino acids and an amino-terminal domain of 102 to 119 amino acids

Acronyms and abbreviations that appear in this chapter include: APC, antigen-presenting cell; CTL, cytolytic T lymphocytes; DTH, delayed-type hypersensitivity; ER, endoplasmic reticulum; GM-CSF, granulocyte-macrophage colony stimulating factor; HIV, human immunodeficiency virus; ICAMs, intercellular adhesion molecules; IL-1, interleukin 1; ITAMs, immunoreceptor tyrosine-based activation motifs; LAG-3, lymphocyte activation gene 3; LFA, lymphocyte-function-associated; MHC, major histocompatibility complex; NK, natural killer; PI 3-kinase, phosphatidylinositol 3-kinase; TCR, T-cell receptor; TNF-β, tumor necrosis factor beta; V-like, variable-region-like; VLA, very late activation.

termed the *variable region*. This designation reflects the variation in the primary structure of these domains among different T-cell receptor polypeptides. Furthermore, each chain has a carboxyl-terminal region segment of 87 to 113 amino acids, termed the *constant region* because this region is invariant among chains of the same class. Owing to their role as surface-membrane receptors, each chain also has a small connecting peptide, a transmembrane region of 20 to 24 amino acids, and a small cytoplasmic region of 5 to 12 residues at the carboxyl terminus.

Like the immunoglobulin domains, the variable and constant regions each contain cysteine residues at positions consistent with the presence of a centrally located disulfide loop of 63 to 69 amino acids. Sequence comparisons indicate that several amino acids that are highly conserved in immunoglobulins, including those involved in domain-domain interactions, also are conserved in the T-cell receptor chains. Furthermore, algorithms that predict a given amino acid primary sequence's hydropathicity, hydrophobicity, and potential for formation of β-pleated sheets and α helices suggest that the T-cell receptor chains fold into very similar tertiary configurations, as do the light and heavy chains of the immunoglobulin molecule. The structural and primary sequence similarities of the T-cell receptor justifiably place the genes encoding these receptor proteins in the so-called immunoglobulin supergene family.[5]

αβ HETERODIMERS

Over 90 percent of mature T cells express an αβ heterodimer, making this the major class of T-cell receptor.[2-4] Each molecule is composed of a single acidic α glycoprotein of 39 to 46 kDa linked to a more basic 40- to 44-kDa β glycoprotein via a disulfide bond between the constant regions of the two chains (Fig. 84-1). Within minutes after being translated into protein, both chains are glycosylated and assembled into a heterodimer for subsequent expression on the cell surface. The α- and β-chain genes each contain at least three sites for N-linked glycosylation. In addition, the β chain contains simple high-mannose glycan side chains. The maximum size of the deglycosylated cell surface forms of the α and β subunits are 27 kDa and 32 kDa respectively.

γδ HETERODIMERS

Less than 10 percent of blood T cells and thymocytes exclusively express a different T-cell receptor heterodimer composed of two glycoproteins designated γ and δ (Fig. 84-1).[6] The development of γδ-expressing T cells appears distinct from that of αβ-expressing T cells.[7,8] In fact, T cells bearing γδ receptors apparently constitute a distinct cell lineage that can undergo relative expansion in response to infection with certain organisms, such as *Listeria monocytogenes*.[9] In secondary lymphoid tissues (see Chap. 5), only about 1 to 5 percent of the CD3-positive cells express γδ receptors. However, in epithelial tissues most T cells express γδ receptors, especially in the epidermis and small intestine of the mouse.

The amino acid sequence of the γ chain is more like that of the T-cell receptor β chain, while the amino acid sequence of the δ chain is more like that of the α chain. Like the αβ heterodimer and immunoglobulins, the γδ heterodimer is clonally distributed. Like the homologous αβ heterodimer, the γδ heterodimer also is associated with the CD3 complex and appears capable of stimulating T-cell activation when bound to specific ligand. Together these two chains have structural and size characteristics similar to those of the αβ heterodimer. However, the tertiary structure of variable regions of γδ T-cell receptors has a closer resemblance to immunoglobulin variable regions than to the variable regions of αβ T-cell receptors.

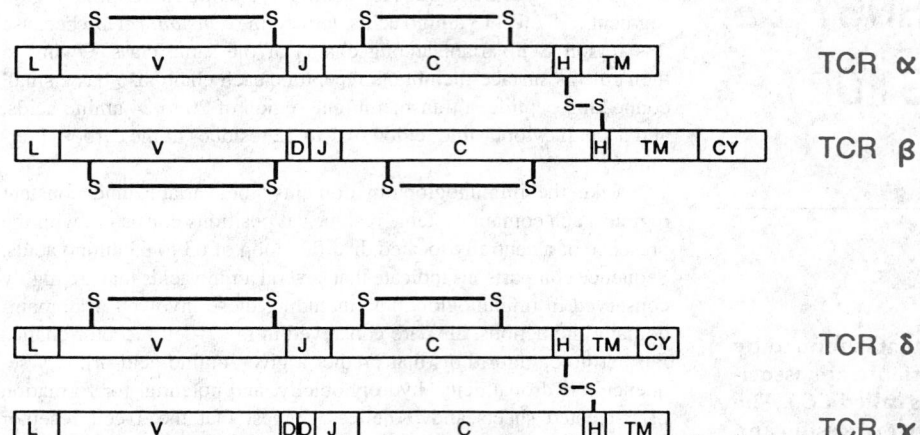

FIGURE 84-1   Schematic diagram of the T-cell receptor (TCR) molecules. Each chain of the TCR is labeled on the far right side of the diagram. TCR-α and TCR-β together form the TCR-αβ heterodimer. Similarly, TCR-δ and TCR-γ form the δγ heterodimer. Lines with S indicate either inter- or intrachain disulfide bridges. Domains of each chain are marked by letters: L, leader peptide; V, variable region; D, diversity segment; J, joining segment; C, constant region; H, hinge region; TM, transmembrane region; CY, cytoplasmic domain.

GENETICS OF THE T-CELL RECEPTOR

Similar to the immunoglobulin genes, each chain of the T-cell receptors is encoded by discrete genetic elements that rearrange during development (Fig. 84-2) (see Chap. 83). Evaluation for T-cell receptor gene rearrangements can distinguish between patients who have clonal T-cell lymphoproliferative diseases from those who have nonneoplastic polyclonal T-cell expansion.[10] Furthermore, molecular analysis for clonal T-cell receptor gene rearrangements can be used to detect minimal residual disease in patients treated for clonal T-cell disorders.[11]

Located at band q35 on the long arm of chromosome 7, the β-chain complex has two closely linked genes, each capable of encoding the β-chain constant region. Each constant region gene is associated with a cluster of functional J_β-gene segments and a single D_β segment. The functional gene encoding the variable region of the β chain is constructed from the rearrangement of any of about 50 variable region gene segments to either one of the two D_β regions and one of 13 J_β regions. The α-chain complex is located at band q11.2 on the long

arm of chromosome 14 and thus is linked to the immunoglobulin heavy-chain complex. The α-chain gene complex consists of one constant region gene and at least 50 different variable region gene segments. The functional gene encoding the α-chain variable region is derived from the juxtaposition of any one of the variable region gene segments with one of the many J_α segments through rearrangement that generally involves the deletion of the intervening DNA.

The organization of the γ and δ genes is similar to that of the α and β genes except for some significant differences. First, the gene complex encoding the δ genes is located entirely within the α-chain gene complex between the V_α and J_α gene segments.[12] Consequently, any rearrangement of the α-chain genes inactivates the genes encoding the δ chain. Second, there are many fewer V gene segments in the γ and δ gene complexes than at either the T-cell receptor α or α gene loci. The γ-gene complex on band p15 on the short arm of chromosome 7, for example, has only about 12 V_γ gene segments, two virtually identical J_γ segments, and two constant region gene segments.[13] Moreover, there are only about four V_δ gene segments, three D_δ gene segments, three J_δ gene segments, and a single constant region gene in the δ gene complex. Consequently, most of the variability in the γ and δ chains is found in the junctional region formed during the process of γδ T-cell receptor gene rearrangement. The amino acids encoded by this region lie at the center of the T-cell receptor binding site.

NATURE OF T-CELL RECEPTOR ANTIGEN RECOGNITION

Although highly similar in structure, there are important differences in the ways that T-cell receptors and immunoglobulins recognize antigen.[1] Whereas immunoglobulins can bind antigens directly, T-cell receptors generally recognize peptide antigens that are bound to a molecule of the MHC on the surface of another cell.

There are two basic classes of MHC molecules. Class I MHC molecules bind peptides that generally are derived from proteins synthesized and degraded in the cytosol. The human histocompatibility antigens HLA-A, -B, or -C are class I molecules. Class II MHC molecules, such as the HLA-D antigens DP, DQ, and DR, generally bind peptides that are derived from exogenous proteins that are degraded in the cellular vesicles. Peptides that bind to MHC class I molecules are usually 8 to 10 amino acids long. The binding of such peptides is stabilized by contacts between atoms in the free amino and carboxyl termini of the peptide and the peptide-binding groove of all MHC class I molecules. Peptides that bind to MHC class II molecules, on the other hand, are at least 13 amino acids long and can be much longer, although they generally are trimmed by peptidases to be 13 to 17 amino acids in most cases. This is because MHC class II molecules do not bind the two ends of the peptide such as the MHC class I molecules.

Nevertheless, for either class I or class II molecules, there exists a discrete binding site for the

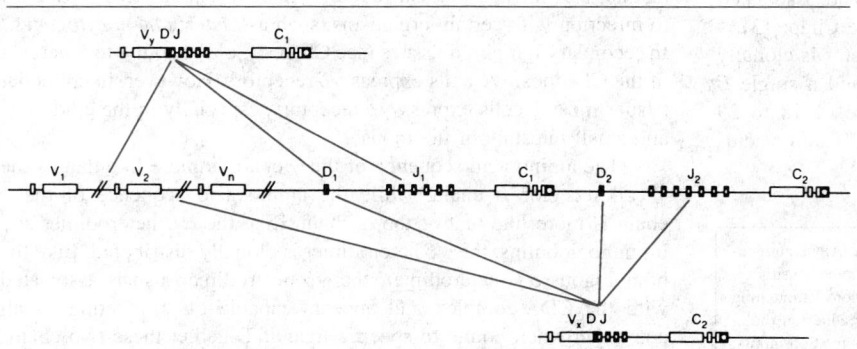

FIGURE 84-2   Schematic diagram of possible rearrangements of the TCR-β-chain genes. The TCR-β-chain genes in the germ-line DNA configuration are depicted in the middle. Possible recombination of either the first constant region (C_1, *above*) or the second constant region (C_2, *below*) with the variable region (V), diversity (D), or joining (J) segments are indicated by the lines.

peptide that lies in a cleft between two α helices of the MHC molecule. Steric factors, hydrogen bonding, and hydrophobic interactions between the peptide and the particular MHC molecule serve to tether the peptide within this cleft, thus generating a tertiary structure that is formed by amino acid residues of both the MHC and the peptide antigen. It is this tertiary structure that is recognized by the T-cell receptor for antigen.

There are several genes for each class of MHC molecule, and each of these is highly polymorphic with many different alleles (see Chap. 138). The particular combination of MHC alleles found on an individual chromosome is known as a *MHC haplotype*. Both maternal and paternal MHC haplotypes are expressed concomitantly. Polymorphism in the MHC molecules primarily affects the amino acids lining the clefts that cradle the peptide antigen.

Each allele encodes a MHC molecule that can bind a restricted set of peptides with a discrete *sequence motif*. Moreover, different alleles of the same MHC molecule will bind peptides with different sequence motifs. This polymorphism combined with biallelic expression of MHC genes and the degeneracy of MHC molecules on any given MHC haplotype ensure that a wide variety of different peptides can be presented to the T cell for immune recognition. However, because T cells actually interact with a tertiary structure that is largely dictated by a particular MHC molecule, T cells manifest MHC-restricted antigen recognition. In other words, a given T cell is specific for one peptide bound to one MHC molecule.

Some T cells, however, do not recognize peptide bound to a given MHC molecule. Such T cells recognize nonpeptide antigens that are presented by MHC class-I-like molecules encoded by genes that map outside the MHC region. One such family of molecules, called *CD1*, first defined as a cell-surface differentiation antigen (see Chap. 13) subsequently was found to present nonpeptide antigens to T cells.[4] For example, in cells infected with mycobacteria, the CD1 molecules are able to bind and present the mycobacterial membrane components such as lipoarabinomannan or mycolic acid. T cells that recognize these complexes play an important role in the immune response to *Mycobacterium tuberculosis*.

Most $\gamma\delta$-expressing T cells may not be restricted by polymorphic self-molecules of the MHC.[15] Furthermore, $\gamma\delta$ receptors bind different ligands than the $\alpha\beta$ T-cell receptors. Some $\gamma\delta$ T cells recognize products of certain *MHC class IB genes*, or variants of the standard MHC class I genes that have little polymorphism (see Chap. 138). Other $\gamma\delta$ receptors apparently recognize antigen directly like immunoglobulin molecules.

GENERATION OF T-CELL RECEPTOR DIVERSITY

Diversity of the T-cell receptor for antigen is achieved by several mechanisms, some of which are the same as those that generate diversity among immunoglobulin molecules[16] (see Chap. 83). The joining of different V, D, and J elements to produce a complete V gene, the presence of uncorrected errors made during the recombination of these genetic elements, and the combinatorial diversity afforded by the random pairing of two chains encoded by separated gene complexes all function to enhance the diversity of the T-cell antigen receptor repertoire.[17,18] An important difference between T cells and B cells in how they may enhance receptor diversity, however, is that B cells are capable of somatic mutation (see Chap. 83). This process apparently occurs uniquely in immunoglobulin genes that have undergone rearrangement and does not operate on the variable region genes of the T-cell receptor.

That T-cell receptor genes do not undergo somatic mutation probably relates to the central role that T cells have in directing host immune defenses. During differentiation, immature precursors to $\alpha\beta$-expressing T cells pass through the thymus, where they are "educated" to distinguish self from nonself vis-à-vis the cell-surface proteins of the major histocompatibility complex (see Chaps. 5 and 82). Because the ligand for the $\alpha\beta$ T-cell receptor is "processed" antigen presented by the proteins of the MHC,[19,20] close interaction with the molecules of the MHC might be lost if the variable region genes of the T-cell receptor were allowed to diverge significantly from the inherited germline repertoire. Furthermore, somatic mutation of expressed T-cell receptor variable region genes may lead to constitutive T-cell activation to processed self-antigen presented by self-MHC molecules, this perhaps leading to autoimmune disease.

THE CD3 COMPLEX

FUNCTION OF THE CD3 COMPLEX

Closely associated with and required for the surface expression of the two polypeptides of the T-cell receptor is the CD3 complex of polypeptides (see Chap. 13). The CD3 polypeptides also are responsible for signal transduction from the T-cell receptor heterodimer to intracellular plasma membrane-associated proteins.[21] Upon binding to specific ligand, the T-cell receptor $\alpha\beta$ (or $\gamma\delta$) heterodimer undergoes steric changes that result in the phosphorylation of the intracellular domains of several polypeptide chains in the CD3 complex. Together, these perturbations of the $\alpha\beta$/CD3 complex result in T-cell activation through a cascade of biochemical events[22] (see Chap. 15). As such, the CD3 surface proteins are integral components of the functional T-cell receptor complex.[23]

The CD3 complex is composed of at least four distinct chains that are designated CD3γ, CD3δ, CD3ϵ, and CD3ζ (see Chap. 13). The CD3γ and CD3δ chains are not to be confused with the γ:δ chains of the T-cell receptor. Rather, the CD3γ, CD3δ, and CD3ϵ chains each form a tight association with the α:β (or γ:δ) receptor heterodimer on the T-cell surface (Fig. 84-3). Each has a negatively charged amino acid in the central portion of the hydrophobic transmembrane region that stabilizes the CD3 complex with the two chains of the T-cell receptor. The CD3ϵ chain couples with either the CD3γ or the CD3δ chain. The CD3ζ chain, on the other hand, forms a disulfide-like homodimer that only weakly associates with the CD3 complex and cannot be coimmunoprecipitated readily with antibodies to the T-cell receptor or other CD3 polypeptides. Very little of the CD3ζ chain is present on the T-cell surface (Fig. 84-3). However, the CD3ζ chain is required for directing the T-cell receptor complex to the cell surface and for receptor-mediated signal transduction,[24] and mice made deficient for expression of the CD3ζ chain have impaired T-cell development.[25] In mice, the CD3ζ chain infrequently may form a disulfide-linked heterodimer with another polypeptide chain, designated CD3η. CD3η actually is generated through alternate RNA splicing of the gene encoding the CD3ζ chain. However, there does not appear to be a CD3η protein in humans.[26]

MOLECULAR FEATURES OF THE CD3 COMPLEX

The genes encoding CD3γ, CD3δ, or CD3ϵ chains are clustered in band q23 on the long arm of chromosome 11. CD3γ has a 16-kDa polypeptide backbone that is heavily glycosylated to assume a final molecular mass of 25 to 28 kDa. CD3δ and CD3ϵ are each 20 kDa in molecular mass. The CD3δ is a glycoprotein consisting of 30 percent carbohydrate. In contrast, CD3ϵ is not glycosylated. CD3δ and CD3γ are highly homologous at both the protein and nucleic acid sequence level. The nucleic acid sequence of each predicts CD3δ and CD3γ to have typical signal peptides, respective hydrophilic extracellular domains of 79 to 89 amino acids, hydrophobic transmembrane regions

Antigen-Presenting Cell

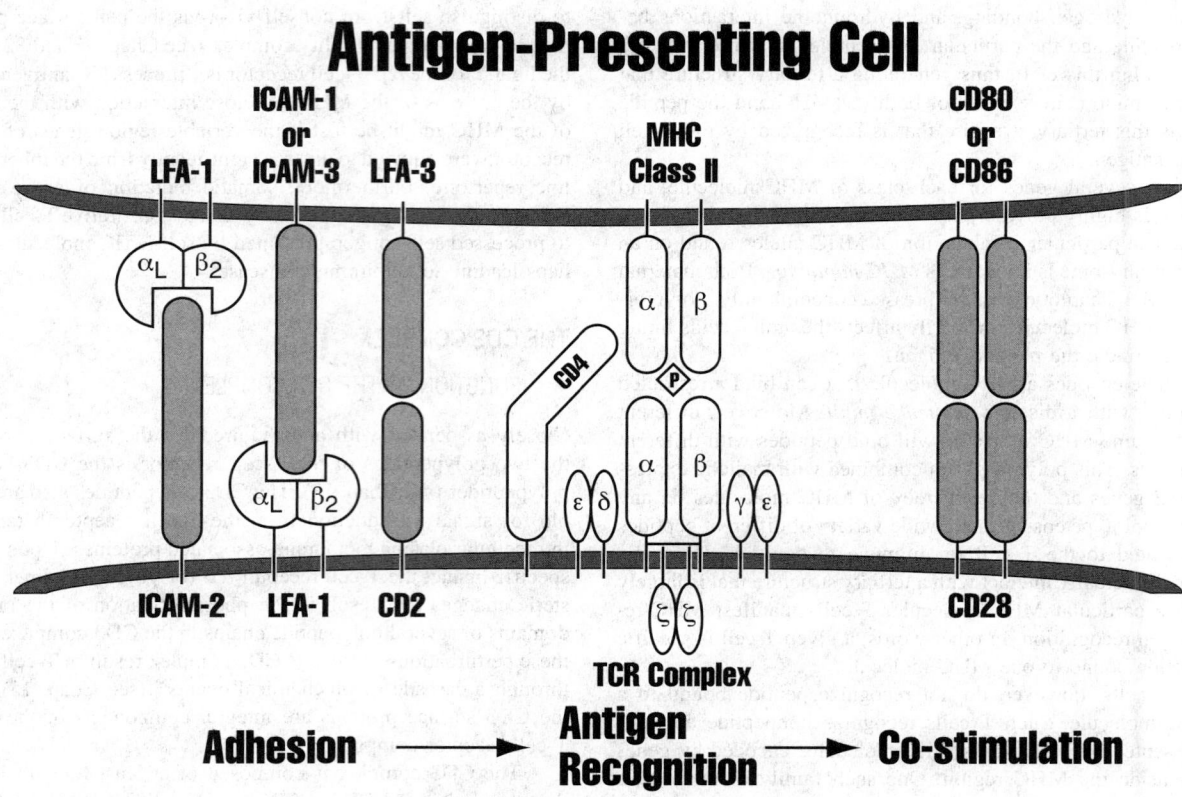

FIGURE 84-3 Schematic diagram of the T-cell interactions with an antigen-presenting cell. The thick gray lines depict the plasma membranes of the interacting cells. The molecules of the antigen-presenting cell, namely LFA-1, ICAM-1 or ICAM-3, LFA-3, MHC class II, and CD80 or CD86, are displayed on top, while the T-cell antigens, ICAM-2, LFA-1, CD2, CD4, the T-cell receptor complex (TCR complex), and CD28, are shown on the bottom of the diagram. Thin lines connecting the stick figures indicate disulfide bridges. The TCR complex consists of the $\alpha\beta$ heterodimer that is noncovalently coupled with the δ, ϵ, γ, and ζ chains of CD3, as indicated. This complex can recognize peptide antigen (designated by the diamond labeled P) that is cradled by the α and β chains of the MHC class II molecule of the antigen-presenting cell. The avidity of this interaction is enhanced by CD4 on the T-cell surface that interacts with nonpolymorphic determinants on the MHC class II molecule. The interaction steps between the T cell and the antigen-presenting cell are listed at the bottom of the figure. T-cell molecules ICAM-2 (CD102), LFA-1 (CD11a/CD18), and CD2 bind to LFA-1, ICAM-1 (CD54) or ICAM-3 (CD50), or LFA-3 (CD58) respectively that are present on the surface of the antigen-presenting cell. These molecules provide for better adhesion between the T cell and the antigen-presenting cell (adhesion), allowing for time for the TCR receptor complex to find the MHC molecule bearing a specific peptide antigen (antigen recognition). Should the antigen-presenting cell express CD80 or CD86, then simultaneous ligation of CD28 will occur (costimulation), leading to activation of the reactive T cell.

of 27 amino acids, and hydrophilic intracellular domains of 44 to 55 amino acids. CD3ϵ is similar, with a 22-residue signal peptide, an extracellular domain of 104 amino acids, a transmembrane domain, and a comparatively long intracellular domain of 81 amino acids. The CD3ζ chain, on the other hand, has no sequence or structural homology to the other three CD3 chains. It is a nonglycosylated protein of 16 kDa in molecular mass that is encoded by a gene found on chromosome 1. The CD3ζ chain has only a very short extracellular domain of 6 to 9 amino acids, a transmembrane domain of 21 amino acids, and a long intracellular domain of 113 amino acids. None of the CD3 polypeptides bear significant homology to immunoglobulins, indicating that the genes encoding the chains of the CD3 complex do not belong to the immunoglobulin supergene family. In addition, there is no variability in the extracellular domains of the CD3 proteins, making it unlikely that these molecules contribute to the specificity of antigen recognition.

Also considered a CD3 polypeptide is CD3ω. This polypeptide is an intracellular protein that transiently associates with the CD3-T-cell receptor complex during its assembly in the endoplasmic reticulum

(ER).[27] However, CD3ω dissociates from the CD3 complex in the ER and does not travel to the plasma membrane. As such, CD3ω plays a role in the intracellular assembly and transport of the intact CD3/T-cell receptor complex.

The cytoplasmic domains of all the CD3 proteins contain sequences called *immunoreceptor tyrosine-based activation motifs* (ITAMs). These sequences allow the CD3 proteins to associate with cytosolic protein tyrosine kinases following receptor ligation, thus transducing a signal to the interior of the T cell (see Chap. 15). The cytoplasmic domains of CD3ϵ and CD3ζ are particularly important in this regard.

CD4 AND CD8

FUNCTION OF CD4 AND CD8

CD4 and CD8 facilitate T-cell antigen recognition by interacting with the glycoproteins of the major histocompatibility complex.[28] Moreover, during antigen recognition, CD4 and CD8 molecules associate on the plasma membrane with components of the T-cell receptor for antigens. For these reasons, these molecules are considered coreceptors of the T-cell receptor for antigen.

The CD8 molecule binds to nonpolymorphic regions of the MHC class I molecule (HLA A, B, or C), and the CD4 molecule binds to nonpolymorphic regions of the MHC class II molecule (HLA-D region–encoded molecules: DP, DQ, and DR). CD8 or CD4 enhance by over 100-fold the adhesion between the T cell's CD3/T-cell receptor complex and the MHC glycoproteins expressed by an antigen-presenting cell (APC) or target cell. These molecules apparently focus MHC molecules of the APC or target cell onto the T-cell surface, allowing for specific recognition of "processed" antigen that is cradled within the MHC glycoproteins. Because CD4 and CD8 differ in their MHC-binding specificities, T cells expressing CD4 or CD8 generally recognize antigens presented by class II or class I MHC glycoproteins respectively.[29] This selectivity is underscored by studies on transgenic mice that lack expression of MHC class II molecules. Such animals fail to develop mature CD4 T cells, owing to their inability to select for such cells in the thymus.[30] In addition, CD4 or CD8 molecules also may enhance antigen responsiveness by transducing a signal either directly or in concert with CD3/T-cell receptor complex.[31]

MOLECULAR FEATURES OF CD4 AND CD8

CD4 and CD8 are glycoproteins that share structural features with other receptor molecules encoded by genes within the immunoglobulin supergene family. CD8 is expressed as a heterodimer of CD8α and CD8β or as a CD8α homodimer. Each chain contains a single immuno-globulin-like domain linked to the membrane by a segment of polypeptide chain that could have an extended conformation. These chains are encoded by genes that are linked closely to the immunoglobulin κ light-chain locus at band p12, on the short arm of chromosome 2. The protein sequence of the amino-terminal domains of each CD8 chain shares greater than 28 percent homology with κ light-chain variable regions. As such, these domains are called the variable-region-like (V-like) domains. Following this V-like domain, the CD8 molecule has a short region rich in prolines, threonines, and serines that resembles the immunoglobulin hinge region. This region also contains sites for O-linked glycosylation. A hydrophobic transmembrane region anchors this hinge-like region. The CD8 molecule has a 28-amino acid cytoplasmic tail consisting of basic residues. Two cysteines within the V-like domain form a disulfide bridge that stabilizes the immuno-globulin-like fold. An additional cysteine residue is located each within the V-like domain, the hinge region, the transmembrane, and cyto-plasmic segments. These cysteines form intermolecular disulfide bridges between two or more CD8 molecules; these bridges stabilizing the CD8 homodimers and multimers that are expressed on the T-cell surface. The cell-surface CD8 homodimer shares the same approximate geometry as heavy- and light-chain immunoglobulin heterodimers.

CD4, on the other hand, does not form such homodimers. It is a 55-kDa monomeric glycoprotein that is encoded by a gene that maps to the short arm of chromosome 12. It consists of five external domains, a stretch of hydrophobic transmembrane residues, and cytoplasmic tail of 40 residues. Similar to CD8, the amino-terminal domain of CD4 also has extensive homology to immunoglobulin light-chain variable regions. However, following this V-like domain is a domain of 270 amino acids that bears little resemblance to other proteins encoded by genes of the immunoglobulin supergene family. Together with this 270-amino acid domain, the V-like domain of the CD4 molecule forms an intramolecular heterodimer on the T-cell surface.

The cytoplasmic regions of CD4 and CD8 are conserved among vertebrates, suggesting that these regions are essential for the function of these molecules. The cytoplasmic region of CD4 contains five

serines and threonines, one or more of which is phosphorylated by protein kinase C upon activation of T cells by phorbol esters or exposure to antigen. Subsequent to phosphorylation, the CD4 glycoprotein is internalized concomitant with T-cell activation. Similarly, the CD8 protein also possesses a highly charged and conserved cytoplasmic domain that may be involved in transmembrane signal transduction. In this light, CD4 and CD8 actually may be integral components of the functional T-cell receptor complex required to trigger T-cell activation and/or function upon exposure to specific antigen.

CD4 also is a coreceptor molecule for the human immunodeficiency virus (HIV).[32,33] Binding of CD4 along with a chemokine receptor facilitates entry of the virus into those T cells that are stimulated specifically in an antigen-driven immune response. Monoclonal antibodies specific for the CD4 glycoprotein can block infection by HIV. Moreover, genetically engineered soluble CD4 can compete with cell-surface CD4 for HIV binding. Finally, disease progression in patients infected with HIV correlates with depletion of blood T cells that express CD4 (see Chap. 89).

DISTRIBUTION OF CD4 AND CD8 ON T-CELL SUBSETS

PRECURSOR THYMOCYTES

CD4 and CD8 are expressed by nearly all T-cell precursors. Only a fraction of thymocytes express neither CD4 nor CD8. These cells are thought to be the marrow-derived precursors to the vast majority of thymocytes that express both CD4 and CD8. More mature thymocytes and all peripheral T cells express either CD4 or CD8, but not both.

HELPER AND SUPPRESSOR (CYTOLYTIC) T CELLS

The mutually exclusive expression of CD4 or CD8 defines two major blood T-cell subsets. Blood T cells that express CD8 are designated *suppressor* T cells. These cells normally constitute 25 to 35 percent of the peripheral T-cell population. Suppressor T cells more appropriately should be designated *cytolytic T lymphocytes* (CTL), in that a main function of these cells is to lyse cells, termed *target cells*, which bear surface antigens for which they are specific. Blood T cells that solely express the CD4 surface antigen are designated *helper* T cells. These cells normally comprise 65 percent of the blood T cells. Generally, helper T cells produce lymphokines upon activation by foreign antigens presented by MHC molecules expressed on the surface of APCs.

CD4+ T-CELL SUBSETS

Mature CD4+ T cells may be divided into at least two subsets, each able to elaborate a distinctive profile of cytokines upon activation.[34,35] The primary differences are that T_H1 cells are the major helper T-cell source of interleukin 2 (IL-2), interferon gamma (IFN-γ), and tumor necrosis factor beta (TNF-β), while T_H2 cells are the predominate producers of IL-4 and IL-5 (Table 84-1). In addition, T_H1 cells may be the major helper T-cell source of tumor necrosis factor alpha (TNF-α) and granulocyte-macrophage colony stimulating factor (GM-CSF), while T_H2 cells apparently are the major T-cell producers of IL-10 and IL-13. A third cell subset, designated T_H0, is comprised of CD4+ helper T cells that may elaborate all of these cytokines and may represent a precursor population to the other two subsets.

These CD4+ T-cell subsets may be distinguished by their differential expression of certain surface molecules. Human T_H1 cells preferentially express CD26, membrane IFN-γ, and the chemokine receptors CCR5 and CXCR3.[36] Moreover, T_H1 cells apparently express higher levels of the *lymphocyte activation gene 3 (LAG-3)*, a ligand for major histocompatibility complex class II antigens that is structurally related to CD4.[37] T_H2 cells, on the other hand, preferentially express CD62L, CD30, and the chemokine receptors CCR3, CCR4, CCR8, and, to

TABLE 84-1　MAJOR CD4+ T-CELL SUBSETS

	CD4+ T-cell Subset	
	T_H1	T_H2
Cytokine production		
IL-2	+	−
IFN-γ	++	−
TNF-β	++	−
IL-4	−	++
IL-5	−	++
TNF-α	++	+
GM-CSF	++	+
IL-10	+/−	++
IL-13	−	++
Functions		
B cell help		
Total Ig	+	+++
IgE	−	++
Mast cell production	−	++
Eosinophil production	−	++
Macrophage activation	++	−
Delayed-type hypersensitivity	++	−

some extent, CXCR4.[36,38,39] Differences in the expression levels of these chemokine receptors may account for the differences in the tissue-specific migration of these helper T-cell subsets.[40]

Each of these two T-cell subsets has a discrete function.[41] T_H1 cells activate the microbicidal properties of macrophages and induce B cells to make IgG antibodies that are very effective at opsonizing extracellular pathogens for uptake by phagocytic cells. In addition, T_H1 cells are the major helper T cells involved in delayed-type hypersensitivity (DTH). The cytokines elaborated by T_H1 cells stimulate macrophage Fc receptor expression, phagocytosis, and antigen presentation, enhancing the capacity of macrophages to kill intracellular pathogens. T_H2 cells, on the other hand, initiate the antibody response to antigen by activating naive antigen-specific B cells to produce IgM antibodies and subsequently stimulate the production of different isotypes, including IgA and IgE and neutralizing and/or weakly opsonizing subtypes of IgG.

Extracellular antigens tend to stimulate the generation of T_H2 cells, whereas pathogens that accumulate in large numbers inside macrophage vesicles tend to stimulate differentiation of T_H1 cells.[42] Immune responses restricted to that of T_H1 cells have been observed in patients with leprosy who have developed cellular immunity to *Mycobacterium leprae*[43] or in patients with arthritis triggered by infection with either *Borrelia burgdorferi* (Lyme disease)[44] or *Yersinia enterocolitica*.[45] The cytokines made by T_H2 cells, on the other hand, facilitate production of IgE antibodies and stimulate mast cells and eosinophils. While these effects may contribute to development of allergy,[46,47] these responses also may be protective in helminth infections.[48,49] Studies demonstrate that eosinophilia and elevated IgE that accompany infection with *Schistosoma mansoni*, for example, are due to the induction of T_H2-type cells in the immune response to parasite ova.[50,51] In addition, because they express IL-4, T_H2 cells appear better suited to induce B-cell responses to antigen.

MEMORY T CELLS

Following a successful immune response to antigen, antigen-specific T lymphocytes may differentiate into memory T cells.[52-54] These cells may have less stringent requirements for activation and an enhanced capacity for lymphokine production upon rechallenge with the same antigen.[55] Alternatively, these cells may develop an impaired responsiveness to antigen when stimulated in the absence of certain costimulatory factors, thus rendering these cells "anergic"[56] (see Chap. 15). In any case, naive and memory CD4+ or CD8+ T lymphocytes apparently differ in surface phenotypes, response to recall antigens, rate of

cycling, and migration.[57,58] These subsets may be distinguished using antibodies specific for isoforms of CD45.[59,60]

CD45, also known as *leukocyte common antigen* or *T200*, consists of a family of membrane glycoproteins, ranging from 180 to 220 kDa, that are expressed on all leukocytes. Each member is the product of a single complex gene on chromosome 1 that contains 34 exons. Exons 3 through 7 may be spliced differently at the RNA transcript level to generate several distinct mRNA and protein products. The deduced amino acid sequences of these protein products have extracellular domains ranging from 391 to 552 amino acids, a transmembrane region, and a highly conserved cytoplasmic domain of 705 amino acids. This large cytoplasmic domain contains an intrinsic tyrosine phosphatase activity that is important in the regulation of various activation pathways involving tyrosine kinase activity, such as those involved in signal transduction via the T-cell receptor for antigen.[61-63] (See Chap. 15)

Differential glycosylation of the CD45 peptide backbone contributes further to the heterogeneity of the members of this family of proteins. Different isoforms of CD45 have distinct patterns of expression during lymphocyte ontogeny and activation.[64] Monoclonal antibodies have been developed that recognize individual members of this family that are expressed on physiologically distinct lymphocyte subsets (see Chap. 13). Isoforms of CD45 that are expressed on such distinct subsets of cells are designated as *CD45R*.

Naive CD4+ T cells express a form of CD45R, called *CD45RA*, whereas memory CD4+ T cells and CD8+ T cells express another isoform of CD45R, designated *CD45RO*. These isoforms can be recognized by monoclonal antibodies 2H4 and UCHL1 respectively.[65] Evaluation for the expression level of another isoform of CD45, designated *CD45RB*, also can be useful for distinguishing memory T cells. Within the CD4+ memory T-cell population, for example, there is an increase of helper activity associated with the shift from a CD45RB^{bright} to a CD45RB^{dim} phenotype.[66] In addition, relative to naive T cells, memory T cells also express lower levels of L-selectin (CD62L) and higher levels of CD29 and CD44[53] (see Chap. 13). It is still uncertain whether the differentiation of CD4+ T cells with the "naive" phenotype (i.e., CD4+CD45RA+CD29^{low}CD44^{low}) to cells having the "memory" phenotype (i.e., CD4+CD45RO+CD29^{high}CD44^{high}) is irreversible,[65] and whether these phenotypic changes are valid for all T_H1- and T_H2-type CD4+ T cells.[67]

ACCESSORY MOLECULES

IMMUNE MODULATORY MOLECULES

CD28

CD28 is a 44-kDa disulfide-linked homodimer that is expressed on most resting T cells and plasma cells.[68,69] Mature thymocytes have higher levels of CD28 than the immature cells. Among peripheral T cells, nearly all CD4+ and approximately 50 percent of CD8 T cells are positive. In general, activation of T cells induces enhanced expression of CD28, but ligation of CD28 leads to its transient downregulation.[69]

CD28 is another member of the immunoglobulin superfamily that is an important receptor for CD80 and CD86. It binds to both CD80 and CD86 using a highly conserved motif (MYPPPY) in a loop that resembles the third complementarity-determining region of immunoglobulin molecules.[70] CD28 binds to CD80 with relatively low affinity ($K_d = 4$ μM) and dissociates very rapidly ($^-K_{off} = 1.6$ s^{-1}).[71] Its binding to CD86 may be even weaker.[72]

CD28 is one of the major costimulatory molecules that is important in T-cell activation.[73] Ligation of CD28 by CD80 or CD86, or by anti-CD28 antibodies, serves as an important cosignal to T-cell receptor cross-linking.[68,74-77] The cytoplasmic domain of CD28 interacts with phosphatidylinositol 3-kinase (PI 3-kinase), the complex between GRB-2 and the guanine nucleotide exchange protein SOS (GRB-2/ SOS), and the tyrosine kinase ITK.[78] The SH2 domains in PI 3-kinase and GRB-2/SOS mediate binding to the CD28 motif YMNMT, after it has been phosphorylated by Lck and Fyn following ligation of CD28.[79,80] (see Chap. 15). Ligation of CD28 thereby activates several signal-transduction pathways.[81] This cosignal enhances the transcription of interleukin-2 and the stability of interleukin-2 transcripts, thereby stimulating the growth of naive T cells.[82] Although mice lacking CD28 can mount effective T-cell responses, they are defective in T-cell-dependent antibody responses, suggesting that CD28 is necessary for T-cell ↔ B-cell interactions and the development of antibody responses to antigen.[83]

The requirement for the same cell to present both the specific antigen and the costimulatory signal plays an important role in preventing destructive autoimmune responses to self-tissues.[84] The initiation of T-cell responses requires simultaneous ligation of the T-cell receptor and CD28. This restricts the initiation of T-cell responses to *antigen-presenting cells* that express both the peptide antigen in the context of self-MHC molecules and the ligands for CD28, namely CD80 and CD86. This is important, as not all self-reactive T cells undergo deletion in the thymus because not all self-peptides are presented in the thymus (see Chap. 5). This is especially true for specialized tissues that express proteins that are never expressed in the thymus. If simultaneous ligation of the T-cell receptor and CD28 was not required, then T cells that recognize the self-peptide expressed by the MHC of such specialized tissues could become activated, leading to autoimmune rejection of the specialized tissue. Instead, ligation of the T-cell receptor in the absence of CD28-ligation leads to a state of anergy, in which the T cell expressing that receptor becomes refractory to activation.[68,85] Anergic T cells are unable to produce interleukin-2 following ligation of their antigen receptors. This prevents these T cells from proliferating and differentiating into effector cells when they encounter antigen. This is an important basis for development of peripheral tolerance for self-antigens that are not expressed in the thymus (see Chaps. 5 and 82).

CTLA-4 (CD152)

CTLA-4 (CD152) is another receptor for CD80 and CD86. It is a 50-kDa disulfide-linked homodimer that shares 31 percent identity with CD28. The gene encoding this receptor is closely linked with that encoding CD28 on the long arm of chromosome 2 at 2q33-q34. However, in contrast to the constitutive expression of CD28, T cells express CD152 only upon activation. Expression of CD152 peaks at approximately 24 h after activation and then subsides by 72 h but is always about 30- to 50-fold lower than that of CD28. Ligation of CD28 is particularly effective in inducing CD152.

CD152 binds to CD80 and CD86 approximately 20 times more avidly than CD28, with K_ds of 0.4 and 2.2 μM respectively.[71,72] Ligation of CD152 transduces a negative signal to the activated T cell, thereby making it less sensitive to stimulation by the antigen-presenting cell.[76,86] Anti-CD152 antibodies can enhance T-cell responses in vitro and in vivo.[87,88] Mice made genetically deficient in CD152 develop a fatal disorder that is characterized by massive lymphocyte proliferation,[89,90] indicating that CD152 serves as an important brake on runaway T-cell activation.

ADHESION MOLECULES

Besides the CD3/T-cell receptor molecules and CD4 or CD8, several other surface proteins are required for efficient T-cell antigen recognition.[91] Some of these surface proteins may be termed *adhesion molecules*, in that they facilitate the adhesion of the T cell to its appropriate antigen-presenting cell or target cell (see Fig. 84-3).[92] By facilitating cell adhesion, these accessory molecules permit the T-cell antigen receptor complex to interact better with the MHC glycoproteins of the other cell, allowing for efficient T-cell antigen recognition and activation. Because each member of this group of accessory molecules has distinctive affinities for the surface molecules expressed by the APC or target cell, differential expression of the accessory molecules may pattern differences in the antigenic specificities and/or cell types with which a given T cell best may interact. As such, the differential expression of these accessory molecules by peripheral T cells may define physiologically distinct T-cell subsets. Other accessory molecules involved in T-cell activation, function, and/or signal transduction are discussed in Chap. 15

LYMPHOCYTE-FUNCTION-ASSOCIATED GLYCOPROTEINS

The lymphocyte-function-associated (LFA) molecules are an important family of glycoproteins that facilitate efficient cell-cell adhesion.[93,94] The molecules were first identified with monoclonal antibodies that could block T-cell function, such as cytotoxic T-cell-mediated killing of target cells. From these early experiments three major surface molecules were identified and designated *LFA-1, LFA-2,* and *LFA-3.* Following international convention, LFA-2 will be referred to as CD2.

LFA-1 belongs to a family of three related glycoproteins: LFA-1, MAC-1, and p150,95 (see Chap. 13). These proteins also are called "integrins" because they are hypothesized to coordinate the binding of cells to other cell types and to extracellular proteins.[95] Each protein consists of a distinct α subunit noncovalently associated with the common β_2 subunit glycoprotein of 95 kDa, designated as *CD18*. Because they share a common β_2 subunit, these molecules also are referred to as the β_2-*integrins*. The α subunit of LFA-1, designated *CD11a*, is a 180-kDa glycoprotein (see Chap. 13). Coupled together with the common β_2 subunit, this 180-kDa molecule is expressed on over one-third of all marrow cells, all T cells, B cells, and natural killer (NK) cells. The α subunit of MAC-1 is a glycoprotein of 170 kDa, designated *CD11b*. MAC-1 is expressed on NK cells, monocytes, macrophages, granulocytes, and small subpopulations of T and B cells. The α subunit of p150,95, designated *CD11c*, is a 150-kDa glycoprotein that is not expressed by T lymphocytes.

The LFA-1 family of glycoproteins is comprised of important adhesion molecules.[93,96] The shared β_2 subunit has extensive sequence homology to the β_3 subunit of the platelet adhesion receptor glycoprotein IIb/IIIa and the β_1 subunit of a family of related adhesion proteins, termed *very late activation* (VLA) antigens. Many of these receptors function in cell-cell interactions and recognize their ligands at sites that contain the amino acid sequence Arg-Gly-Asp. In addition, the α subunit provides some selectivity. LFA-1, because of its α subunit, binds best to cell surface ligands called *intercellular adhesion molecules* (ICAMs), namely ICAM-1 (CD54), ICAM-2 (CD102), and ICAM-3 (CD50) (see Chap. 13). ICAM-1 and ICAM-2 are expressed on endothelial cells as well as antigen-presenting cells. The binding of LFA-1 on lymphocytes to these molecules allows lymphocytes to migrate through blood vessel walls. ICAM-3 is expressed only on leukocytes, including T cells, and is thought to play an important role in the adhesion of T cells with LFA-1 expressed on antigen-presenting cells (Fig. 84-3).

The LFA glycoproteins are required for proper T-cell function and host immunity. Monoclonal antibodies specific for LFA-1 may inhibit T-cell-directed cytolysis of target cells. Furthermore, a few CD8+ or CD4+ cytolytic T-cell clones express MAC-1. Antibodies to CD11b may inhibit conjugate formation between these T-cell clones and their specific target cells and thus block cytotoxic T-lymphocyte-mediated killing. Finally, patients with an inherited deficiency in the ability to produce the common β_2 subunit (CD18) suffer from recurrent life-threatening bacterial and fungal infections and rarely survive beyond childhood.

The LFA molecules are important for initial T-cell interactions with antigen-presenting cells. LFA-1, CD2, and ICAM-3 on the T cell interact with ICAM-1, ICAM-2, LFA-1, and LFA-3 on the antigen-presenting cell (Fig. 84-3). This provides time for the T cell to sample large numbers of MHC molecules on the plasma membrane of the antigen-presenting cell for the presence of specific peptide antigen. When a naive T cell recognizes its specific peptide in the context of the MHC, signaling through the T-cell receptor induces a conformational change in LFA-1 that greatly increases its affinity for ICAM-1 and ICAM-2. This stabilizes the association between the antigen-specific T cell and the antigen-presenting cell. This association can last for several days during which time the naive T cell proliferates, forming daughter cells that also adhere to the antigen-presenting cell and that differentiate into armed effector T cells.

CD2 is a glycoprotein of approximately 50 kDa found on all T lymphocytes, large granular lymphocytes, and thymocytes.[97] CD2 facilitates cell-cell adhesion by binding to LFA-3, a 55- to 70-kDa surface glycoprotein that is expressed on erythrocytes and leukocytes as well as on endothelial, epithelial, and connective tissue cells in most organ studies (Fig. 84-3) (see Chap. 13). Monoclonal antibodies that bind CD2 may inhibit a variety of T-lymphocyte functions, including antigen-specific T-lymphocyte-proliferative responses to lectins, alloantigens, and soluble antigens. Anti-CD2 inhibits cytotoxic T-lymphocyte-mediated cell killing by binding to the T cell rather than to the target, which generally does not express CD2. On the other hand, antibodies directed against LFA-3 inhibit cytotoxic T-lymphocyte-mediated cell killing by binding to LFA-3 on the target cell, thus blocking interaction of CD2 with LFA-3. T cells can be activated by certain monoclonal antibodies to CD2, apparently independent of the CD3/T-cell receptor complex.[98] Thus aside from being a receptor for LFA-3, CD2 also plays a role in transmembrane signal transduction leading to T-cell activation in response to antigen.

REFERENCES

1. Garcia KC, Teyton L, Wilson IA: Structural basis of T cell recognition. *Annu Rev Immunol* 17:369, 1999.
2. Davis MM, Bjorkman PJ: T-cell antigen receptor genes and T-cell recognition [published erratum appears in *Nature* 1988 Oct 20; 335(6192):744]. *Nature* 334:395, 1988.
3. Tonegawa S: Antibody and T-cell receptors. *JAMA* 259:1845, 1988.
4. Marrack P, Kappler JW: The T cell receptors. *Chem Immunol* 49:69, 1990.
5. Barclay AN, Brown MH, Alex Law SK, McKnight AJ, Tomlinson MG, van der Merwe PA: Protein superfamilies and cell surface molecules: *The Leucocyte Antigen Facts Book,* 2nd ed. San Diego, Academic Press, 1997, p 32.
6. Kabelitz D, Wesch D, Hinz T: Gamma delta T cells, their T cell receptor usage and role in human diseases. *Springer Semin Immunopathol* 21:55, 1999.
7. Kang J, Raulet DH: Events that regulate differentiation of alpha beta TCR+ and gamma delta TCR+ T cells from a common precursor. *Semin Immunol* 9:171, 1997.
8. Hayday AC, Barber DF, Douglas N, Hoffman ES: Signals involved in gamma/delta T cell versus alpha/beta T cell lineage commitment. *Semin Immunol* 11:239, 1999.
9. Jouen-Beades F, Paris E, Dieulois C, et al: In vivo and in vitro activation and expansion of gamma delta T cells during *Listeria monocytogenes* infection in humans. *Infect Immun* 65:4267, 1997.
10. Rockman SP: Determination of clonality in patients who present with diagnostic dilemmas: a laboratory experience and review of the literature. *Leukemia* 11:852, 1997.
11. Dibenedetto SP, Lo Nigro L, Di Cataldo A, Schilirò G: Detection of minimal residual disease: methods and relationship to outcome in T-lineage acute lymphoblastic leukemia. *Leuk Lymph* 32:65, 1998.
12. Raulet DH: The structure, function, and molecular genetics of the gamma/delta T cell receptor. *Annu Rev Immunol* 7:175, 1989.
13. Lefranc MP, Rabbitts TH: The human T-cell receptor gamma (TRG) genes. *Trends Biochem Sci* 14:214, 1989.
14. Burdin N, Kronenberg M: CD1-mediated immune responses to glycolipids. *Curr Opin Immunol* 11:326, 1999.
15. Haas W, Pereira P, Tonegawa S: Gamma/delta cells. *Annu Rev Immunol* 11:637, 1993.
16. Krangel MS, Hernandez-Munain C, Lauzurica P, McMurry M, Roberts JL, Zhong XP: Developmental regulation of V(D)J recombination at the TCR alpha/delta locus. *Immunol Rev* 165:131, 1998.
17. Posnett DN: Environmental and genetic factors shape the human T-cell receptor repertoire. *Ann NY Acad Sci* 756:71, 1995.
18. Theofilopoulos AN, Baccalà R, Gonzàlez-Quintial R, et al: T-cell repertoires in health and disease. *Ann NY Acad Sci* 756:53, 1995.
19. Marrack P, Kappler J: The T cell receptor. *Science* 238:1073, 1987.
20. Germain RN, Margulies DH: The biochemistry and cell biology of antigen processing and presentation. *Annu Rev Immunol* 11:403, 1993.
21. Peterson EJ, Koretzky GA: Signal transduction in T lymphocytes. *Clin Exp Rheumatol* 17:107, 1999.
22. Guse AH: Ca²⁺ signaling in T-lymphocytes. *Crit Rev Immunol* 18:419, 1998.
23. Malissen B, Ardouin L, Lin SY, Gillet A, Malissen M: Function of the CD3 subunits of the pre-TCR and TCR complexes during T cell development. *Adv Immunol* 72:103, 1999.
24. Weissman AM, Frank SJ, Orloff DG, Mercep M, Ashwell JD, Klausner RD: Role of the zeta chain in the expression of the T cell antigen receptor: genetic reconstitution studies. *EMBO J* 8:3651, 1989.
25. Tanaka Y, Ardouin L, Gillet A, et al: Early T-cell development in CD3-deficient mice. *Immunol Rev* 148:171, 1995.
26. Clayton LK, Lerner A, Diener AC, Hussey RE, Koyasu S, Reinherz EL: T-cell-receptor isoforms. *Int J Cancer Suppl* 7:1, 1992.
27. Neisig A, Vangsted A, Zeuthen J, Geisler C: Assembly of the T-cell antigen receptor. Paticipation of the CD3ω chain. *J Immunol* 151:870, 1993.
28. Zamoyska R: CD4 and CD8: modulators of T-cell receptor recognition of antigen and of immune responses? *Curr Opin Immunol* 10:82, 1998.
29. Janeway CAJ: The co-receptor function of CD4. *Semin Immunol* 3:153, 1991.
30. Grusby MJ, Johnson RS, Papaioannou VE, Glimcher LH: Depletion of CD4+ T cells in major histocompatibility complex class II-deficient mice. *Science* 253:1417, 1991.
31. Miceli MC, Parnes JR: Role of CD4 and CD8 in T cell activation and differentiation. *Adv Immunol* 53:59, 1993.
32. Virelizier JL: Blocking HIV co-receptors by chemokines. *Dev Biol Stand* 97:105, 1999.
33. Berger EA, Murphy PM, Farber JM: Chemokine receptors as HIV-1 coreceptors: roles in viral entry, tropism, and disease. *Annu Rev Immunol* 17:657, 1999.
34. Romagnani S: Human T_H1 and T_H2 subsets: doubt no more. *Immunol Today* 12:256, 1991.
35. Powrie F, Coffman RL: Cytokine regulation of T-cell function: potential for therapeutic intervention. *Immunol Today* 14:270, 1993.
36. Annunziato F, Galli G, Cosmi L, et al: Molecules associated with human Th1 or Th2 cells. *Eur Cytokine Netw* 9:12, 1998.
37. Huard B, Mastrangeli R, Prigent P, et al: Characterization of the major histocompatibility complex class II binding site on LAG-3 protein. *Proc Natl Acad Sci USA* 94:5744, 1997.
38. Zingoni A, Soto H, Hedrick JA, et al: The chemokine receptor CCR8 is preferentially expressed in T_H2 but not T_H1 cells. *J Immunol* 161:547, 1998.
39. Kim CH, Broxmeyer HE: Chemokines: signal lamps for trafficking of T and B cells for development and effector function. *J Leuk Biol* 65:6, 1999.
40. O'Garra A, McEvoy LM, Zlotnik A: T-cell subsets: chemokine receptors guide the way. *Curr Biol* 8:R646, 1998.
41. Lucey DR: Evolution of the type-1 (T_H1)-type-2 (T_H2) cytokine paradigm. *Infect Dis Clin North Am* 13:1, 1999.
42. Constant SL, Bottomly K: Induction of T_H1 and T_H2 CD4+ T cell responses: the alternative approaches. *Annu Rev Immunol* 15:297, 1997.
43. Haanen JB, de Waal Malefijt R, Res PC, et al: Selection of a human T helper type 1-like T cell subset by mycobacteria. *J Exp Med* 174:583, 1991.
44. Yssel H, Shanafelt MC, Soderberg C, Schneider PV, Anzola J, Peltz

G: *Borrelia burgdorferi* activates a T helper type 1-like T cell subset in Lyme arthritis. *J Exp Med* 174:593, 1991.

45. Lahesmaa R, Yssel H, Batsford S, et al: *Yersinia enterocolitica* activates a T helper type 1-like T cell subset in reactive arthritis. *J Immunol* 148:3079, 1992.

46. Del Prete G: Human Th1 and Th2 lymphocytes: their role in the pathophysiology of atopy. *Allergy* 47:450, 1992.

47. Van Reijsen FC, Bruijnzeel-Koomen CA, Kalthoff FS, et al: Skin-derived aeroallergen-specific T-cell clones of Th2 phenotype in patients with atopic dermatitis. *J Allergy Clin Immunol* 90:184, 1992.

48. Sher A, Coffman RL: Regulation of immunity to parasites by T cells and T cell-derived cytokines. *Annu Rev Immunol* 10:385, 1992.

49. King CL, Nutman TB: Biological role of helper T-cell subsets in helminth infections. *Chem Immunol* 54:136, 1992.

50. Vella AT, Pearce EJ: CD4+ Th2 response induced by *Schistosoma mansoni* eggs develops rapidly through an early, transient, Th0-like stage. *J Immunol* 148:2283, 1992.

51. Contigli C, Silva-Teixeira DN, Del-Prete G, et al: Phenotype and cytokine profile of *Schistosoma mansoni* specific T cell lines and clones derived from schistosomiasis patients with distinct clinical forms. *Clin Immunol* 91:338, 1999.

52. Ahmed R, Gray D: Immunological memory and protective immunity: understanding their relation. *Science* 272:54, 1996.

53. Sprent J, Tough DF, Sun S: Factors controlling the turnover of T memory cells. *Immunol Rev* 156:79, 1997.

54. Tanchot C, Rocha B: The organization of mature T-cell pools. *Immunol Today* 19:575, 1998.

55. Carter LL, Zhang X, Dubey C, Rogers P, Tsui L, Swain SL: Regulation of T cell subsets from naive to memory. *J Immunother* 21:181, 1998.

56. Jenkins MK, Miller RA: Memory and anergy: challenges to traditional models of T lymphocyte differentiation. *FASEB J* 6:2428, 1992.

57. Beverley P: Immunological memory in T cells. *Curr Opin Immunol* 3:355, 1991.

58. McHeyzer-Williams MG, Altman JD, Davis MM: Enumeration and characterization of memory cells in the TH compartment. *Immunol Rev* 150:5, 1996.

59. Plebanski M, Saunders M, Burtles SS, Crowe S, Hooper DC: Primary and secondary human in vitro T-cell responses to soluble antigens are mediated by subsets bearing different CD45 isoforms. *Immunology* 75:86, 1992.

60. Mason D: Subsets of CD4+ T cells defined by their expression of different isoforms of the leucocyte-common antigen, CD45. *Biochem Soc Trans* 20:188, 1992.

61. Janeway CAJ: The T cell receptor as a multicomponent signalling machine: CD4/CD8 coreceptors and CD45 in T cell activation. *Annu Rev Immunol* 10:645, 1992.

62. Turka LA, Kanner SB, Schieven GL, Thompson CB, Ledbetter JA: CD45 modulates T cell receptor/CD3-induced activation of human thymocytes via regulation of tyrosine phosphorylation. *Eur J Immunol* 22:551, 1992.

63. Koretzky GA: Role of the CD45 tyrosine phosphatase in signal transduction in the immune system. *FASEB J* 7:420, 1993.

64. Dianzani U, Redoglia V, Malavasi F, et al: Isoform-specific associations of CD45 with accessory molecules in human T lymphocytes. *Eur J Immunol* 22:365, 1992.

65. Beverley PC: CD45 isoform expression: implications for recirculation of naive and memory cells. *Immunol Res* 10:196, 1991.

66. Tortorella C, Schulze-Koops H, Thomas R, et al: Expression of CD45RB and CD27 identifies subsets of CD4+ memory T cells with different capacities to induce B cell differentiation. *J Immunol* 155:149, 1995.

67. Lee WT, Vitetta ES: Changes in expression of CD45R during the development of Th1 and Th2 cell lines. *Eur J Immunol* 22:1455, 1992.

68. Linsley PS, Ledbetter JA: The role of the CD28 receptor during T cell responses to antigen. *Annu Rev Immunol* 11:191, 1993.

69. Lenschow DJ, Walunas TL, Bluestone JA: CD28/B7 system of T cell costimulation. *Annu Rev Immunol* 14:233, 1996.

70. Peach RJ, Bajorath J, Brady W, et al: Complementarity determining region 1 (CDR1)- and CDR3-analogous regions in CTLA-4 and CD28 determine the binding to B7-1. *J Exp Med* 180:2049, 1994.

71. Van der Merwe PA, Bodian DL, Daenke S, Linsley P, Davis SJ: CD80 (B7-1) binds both CD28 and CTLA-4 with a low affinity and very fast kinetics. *J Exp Med* 185:393, 1997.

72. Greene JL, Leytze GM, Emswiler J, et al: Covalent dimerization of CD28/CTLA-4 and oligomerization of CD80/CD86 regulate T cell costimulatory interactions. *J Biol Chem* 271:26762, 1996.

73. Watts TH, DeBenedette MA: T cell co-stimulatory molecules other than CD28. *Curr Opin Immunol* 11:286, 1999.

74. Boussiotis VA, Freeman GJ, Gribben JG, Nadler LM: The role of B7-1/B7-2:CD28/CLTA-4 pathways in the prevention of anergy, induction of productive immunity and down-regulation of the immune response. *Immunol Rev* 153:5, 1996.

75. Blair PJ, Riley JL, Carroll RG, et al: CD28 co-receptor signal transduction in T-cell activation. *Biochem Soc Trans* 25:651, 1997.

76. Lane P: Regulation of T and B cell responses by modulating interactions between CD28/CTLA4 and their ligands, CD80 and CD86. *Ann NY Acad Sci* 815:392, 1997.

77. Greenfield EA, Nguyen KA, Kuchroo VK: CD28/B7 costimulation: a review. *Crit Rev Immunol* 18:389, 1998.

78. Clements JL, Boerth NJ, Lee JR, Koretzky GA: Integration of T cell receptor-dependent signaling pathways by adapter proteins. *Annu Rev Immunol* 17:89, 1999.

79. June CH, Bluestone JA, Nadler LM, Thompson CB: The B7 and CD28 receptor families. *Immunol Today* 15:321, 1994.

80. Raab M, Cai YC, Bunnell SC, Heyeck SD, Berg LJ, Rudd CE: p56Lck and p59Fyn regulate CD28 binding to phosphatidylinositol 3-kinase, growth factor receptor-bound protein GRB-2, and T cell-specific protein-tyrosine kinase ITK: implications for T-cell costimulation. *Proc Natl Acad Sci USA* 92:8891, 1995.

81. Ward SG: CD28: a signalling perspective. *Biochem J* 318:361, 1996.

82. Powell JD, Ragheb JA, Kitagawa-Sakakida S, Schwartz RH: Molecular regulation of interleukin-2 expression by CD28 co-stimulation and anergy. *Immunol Rev* 165:287, 1998.

83. Shahinian A, Pfeffer K, Lee KP, et al: Differential T cell costimulatory requirements in CD28-deficient mice. *Science* 261:609, 1993.

84. Malvey EN, Telander DG, Vanasek TL, Mueller DL: The role of clonal anergy in the avoidance of autoimmunity: inactivation of autocrine growth without loss of effector function. *Immunol Rev* 165:301, 1998.

85. Sloan-Lancaster J, Allen PM: Signalling events in the anergy induction of T helper 1 cells. *Ciba Found Symp* 195:189, 1995.

86. Chambers CA, Allison JP: Costimulatory regulation of T cell function. *Curr Opin Cell Biol* 11:203, 1999.

87. Kearney ER, Walunas TL, Karr RW, et al: Antigen-dependent clonal expansion of a trace population of antigen-specific CD4+ T cells in vivo is dependent on CD28 costimulation and inhibited by CTLA-4. *J Immunol* 155:1032, 1995.

88. Leach DR, Krummel MF, Allison JP: Enhancement of antitumor immunity by CTLA-4 blockade. *Science* 271:1734, 1996.

89. Tivol EA, Borriello F, Schweitzer AN, Lynch WP, Bluestone JA, Sharpe AH: Loss of CTLA-4 leads to massive lymphoproliferation and fatal multiorgan tissue destruction, revealing a critical negative regulatory role of CTLA-4. *Immunity* 3:541, 1995.

90. Waterhouse P, Penninger JM, Timms E, et al: Lymphoproliferative disorders with early lethality in mice deficient in CTLA-4. *Science* 270:985, 1995.

91. Van Seventer GA, Semnani RT, Palmer EM, McRae BL, van Seventer JM: Integrins and T helper cell activation [see comments]. *Transplant Proc* 30:4270, 1998.

92. Wang J, Springer TA: Structural specializations of immunoglobulin superfamily members for adhesion to integrins and viruses. *Immunol Rev* 163:197, 1998.

93. Springer TA: Adhesion receptors of the immune system. *Nature* 346:425, 1990.

94. De Fougerolles A, Springer TA: Ideas crystallized on immunoglobulin superfamily-integrin interactions. *Chem Biol* 2:639, 1995.

95. Larson RS, Springer TA: Structure and function of leukocyte integrins. *Immunol Rev* 114:181, 1990.

96. Springer TA: Traffic signals for lymphocyte recirculation and leukocyte emigration: the multistep paradigm. *Cell* 76:301, 1994.

97. Davis SJ, Ikemizu S, Wild MK, van der Merwe PA: CD2 and the nature of protein interactions mediating cell-cell recognition. *Immunol Rev* 163:217, 1998.

98. Holter W, Schwarz M, Cerwenka A, Knapp W: The role of CD2 as a regulator of human T-cell cytokine production. *Immunol Rev* 153:107, 1996.

FUNCTIONS OF NATURAL KILLER CELLS

GIORGIO TRINCHIERI
LEWIS L. LANIER

Natural killer (NK) cells, with a predominant morphology of large granular lymphocytes (LGL), represent a third lineage of lymphoid cells with constitutive ability to mediate cytotoxicity of pathologic target cells and to secrete cytokines. Natural killer cells participate in the innate resistance to intracellular pathogens and malignancies and have a modulatory effect on adaptive immunity as well as hematopoiesis. The activity of NK cells is now known to be regulated by the opposite effects of activating and inhibitory receptors. Malignant expansions of NK cells, either acute or chronic, are rare but represent well-identified clinical entities.

IDENTIFICATION AND DEFINITION OF NATURAL KILLER CELLS

DEFINITION

Natural killer cells were originally identified in the peripheral blood and other lymphoid organs of humans and experimental animals as cells capable of killing a variety of cell types, including tumor-derived cell lines, virus-infected cells, and, in some instances, normal cells in the absence of previous deliberate or known sensitization.[1,2] Natural killer cells are currently defined as cytotoxic cells with the predominant morphology of LGL that (1) neither rearrange any of the genes encoding the T-cell receptor (TCR) chains nor express on their surface the CD3 antigen complex or any TCR chain; (2) express on the majority of cells the CD16 (FcγRIIIA) and CD56 (N-CAM) antigens in humans, the NK1.1 antigen in the mouse, and the NKR-PI antigen in the rat; (3) mediate cytolytic reactions even in the absence of MHC class I or class II antigen expression on the target cells. The cytotoxicity mediated by NK cells is clearly distinct from that mediated by cytotoxic T lymphocytes (CTL), which recognize specific antigenic peptides in association with major histocompatibility complex (MHC) class I molecules (see Chap. 84). Cytotoxicity mediated by NK cells is often defined as non-MHC requiring, to distinguish it from the MHC-restricted one mediated by CTL. Certain T lymphocytes that express either an $\alpha\beta$ or a $\gamma\delta$ TCR may exhibit, particularly upon activation, TCR-independent cytolytic activity that resembles that of NK cells. These T lymphocytes are appropriately described as displaying NK-like cytotoxicity or non-MHC-requiring cytotoxicity.

Acronyms and abbreviations that appear in this chapter include: CTL, cytotoxic T lymphocytes; GM-CSF, granulocyte-macrophage colony stimulating factor; IFN, interferon; IL, interleukin; ITIM, immunoreceptor tyrosine-based inhibitory motif; KIR, killer-cell Ig-like receptors; LCMV, lymphocytic choriomeningitis virus; LGL, large granular lymphocytes; M-CSF, macrophage-colony stimulating factor; MHC, major histocompatibility complex; NK, natural killer; TCR, T-cell receptor; TNF, tumor necrosis factor.

MORPHOLOGY

Human LGL are medium- to large-sized lymphocytes with round or indented nuclei, condensed chromatin, and usually prominent nucleoli. The cytoplasm is abundant and contains a variety of organelles. Circular membrane-bound granules (primary lysosomes), which are characteristic of these cells, range in diameter from 50 to 800 nm and contain an electron-dense core (internum) surrounded by a layer of lesser opacity (externum). In addition to lysosomal enzymes, the granules contain phospholipids, proteoglycans, and proteins important for cytotoxic lymphocyte function, such as serine esterases (granzymes) and pore-forming proteins (perforins).[3,4] Although many NK cells have the morphology typical of LGL,[5] a significant proportion of NK cells are indistinguishable from other lymphocytes and may even be agranular.[6]

ORIGIN AND TISSUE DISTRIBUTION

Natural killer cells originate in the marrow. Most are short-lived, with life spans calculated to be from a few days to a few weeks.[7,8] Natural killer cells derive from the common lymphoid progenitor cell that gives rise to T, B, and NK cells. The cytokine IL-15 plays a particularly important role in the differentiation and expansion of NK cells.[9,10] Natural killer cell differentiation does not require the presence of the thymus, although NK cell progenitors can be demonstrated in the thymus, particularly during fetal development.[11] The increased number of NK cells and altered anatomical distribution in response to infection or other stimuli are primarily due to increased NK cell production in the marrow and possibly in part to proliferation of mature peripheral NK cells.[12]

Mature NK cells are mostly present in peripheral blood, where they represent approximately 15 percent of lymphocytes (but with large individual variations), and in the spleen; they are rare or absent in other lymphoid organs.[2,13] Natural killer cells do not normally recirculate through the thoracic duct. In the marrow, they represent less than 1 percent of the cells, indicating that a pool of preformed NK cells is not sequestered in the marrow. Small numbers of NK cells can be identified in the liver (pit cells), lung, and intestinal mucosa.[14,15] Upon activation, as, for example, in response to interferon or viral or bacterial infections, NK cells may accumulate in organs in which they are normally rare, particularly the liver and marrow.[12] Cells with characteristics of activated NK cell (decidual granulocytes) represent the predominant cell type present in the human early pregnancy decidua.[16] The physiologic significance of these cells in the decidua is not clear, but they might have a role in facilitating embryonic implantation, in allowing placenta and embryo growth, or in the modulation of the maternal immune response against embryo antigens.

MECHANISMS OF NATURAL KILLER CELL FUNCTIONS

CELL-MEDIATED CYTOTOXICITY

Cytotoxicity mediated by NK cells depends on binding to the target cells, followed by activation of the lytic mechanism, which usually involves secretion of the granules, including molecules with lytic ability, such as the pore-forming proteins and granzymes.[4] Cytotoxicity is also mediated through the interaction of surface molecules, for example, the interaction of Fas ligand on NK cells with Fas receptor on target cells. Lysis of the target cells is due both to the alteration of membrane permeability and to induction of apoptosis (see Chap. 11).[4] A number of surface molecules have been identified on NK cells that, when stimulated, activate the cytotoxic mechanism.[17] The best characterized of these molecules is the low-affinity receptor for the Fc fragment of IgG (FcγIIIA or CD16) expressed on virtually all human NK cells in association with the signal-transducing CD3ξ or

FcεRIγ chains. When CD16 is cross-linked by IgG antibodies bound to a target cell surface, it triggers antibody-dependent cell-mediated cytotoxicity.[13,18] Other molecules, including receptors able to activate the cytotoxic mechanism and adhesion molecules facilitating the effector–target cell contact, have been shown to be involved in target cell recognition and triggering of the cytotoxic mechanisms. CD16 is not required, in the absence of antibodies, for NK cell cytotoxicity.[17]

Based on the observation that NK cells preferentially kill certain tumor cells lacking expression of MHC class I molecules, Kärre et al[19] proposed that NK cells may detect and eliminate autologous cells lacking MHC class I. This led to the hypothesis that NK cells are regulated by positive signals initiated by activating receptors and negative signals transmitted by putative interactions between inhibitory receptors for MHC class I on the NK cells and autologous MHC class I molecules on potential target cells. A mechanism for immune surveillance against cells that lose expression of MHC class I would be advantageous because, in the absence of class I, these abnormal cells would escape elimination by CTL. Numerous viruses inhibit the synthesis or transport of MHC class I proteins (see Chap. 138), presumably to avoid detection by CTL.[20] In addition, frequent loss of MHC class I expression on tumor cells has been documented.[21]

In humans, two types of NK cell receptors for MHC class I have been identified. The killer-cell Ig-like receptors (KIR) are encoded by about 10 genes present on human chromosome 19q13.4.[22] Certain KIR molecules bind HLA-C ligands, whereas other KIR recognize HLA-B. Another class of NK cell receptors are heterodimeric glycoproteins composed of a CD94 subunit disulfide-bonded to an NKG2 molecule.[22] The *CD94* and *NKG2* genes are on human chromosome 12p12-p13 and are members of the C-type lectin superfamily. The CD94/NKG2 receptor binds to a nonclassical MHC class I molecule, HLA-E, that is unusual in that the peptides present in the HLA-E binding groove are usually leader segments derived from HLA-A, -B, -C, or -G proteins.[23] When synthesis of HLA-A, -B, -C, or -G is disrupted, possibly by viral infection of the host cell, HLA-E cannot be transported to the cell surface for presentation to the CD94/NKG2 receptor. The various KIR and CD94/NKG2 receptors are expressed on overlapping subsets within the NK cell population and also on certain memory T cells. The observation that F1 mice reject marrow grafts from their parents can now be explained by the existence of NK cell subpopulations in the F1 recipient that lack appropriate NK cell receptors for the grafted parental cells.[24] The KIR molecules and the CD94/NKG2A receptor have an immunoreceptor tyrosine-based inhibitory motif (ITIM) sequence in their cytoplasmic domains, which bind to the cytoplasmic tyrosine phosphatase SHP-1, resulting in inhibition of NK cell cytotoxicity and cytokine secretion.[22] Therefore, the functional behavior of NK and T cells expressing KIR or CD94/NKG2 is likely regulated by the balance of positive signals transmitted by a variety of activating receptors and negative signals (resulting in phosphatase recruitment) provided by the inhibitory MHC class I receptors.

Certain receptors of the KIR and CD94/NKG2 families do not possess ITIM sequences and activate, rather than suppress, NK and T cell responses.[22] These receptors noncovalently associate with the homodimeric adapter protein DAP12.[25] Like the CD3ξ and the FcεRI-γ subunits, DAP12 contains an immunoreceptor tyrosine-based activation motif in the cytoplasmic domain. Upon receptor ligation, DAP12 becomes tyrosine phosphorylated, recruits cytoplasmic tyrosine kinases, and induces cellular activation.[25] As yet, the physiologic role of activating NK cell receptors for MHC class I has not been determined, but may have consequences in allogeneic marrow transplantation.

Although resting peripheral blood NK cells are cytotoxic, their activity can be greatly enhanced by both in vivo or in vitro exposure to cytokines such as IFN-α/β, IL-2, IL-12, IL-15, and IL-18.[26–28] Rest-

ing NK cells express intermediate-affinity IL-2 receptors, and IL-2 induces the progression of most NK cells into the cell cycle.[29]

PRODUCTION OF CYTOKINES

Many of the physiologic functions of NK cells are mediated at least in part by their ability to secrete cytokines. Natural killer cells are powerful producers of IFN-γ and granulocyte-macrophage colony stimulating factors (GM-CSF) and have also been shown to be able to produce tumor necrosis factor-α (TNF-α), macrophage-CSF (M-CSF), IL-3, IL-5, IL-8, IL-13, and other cytokines.[2,27,30–32] Stimulation by cytokines such as IL-2, IL-12, IL-18, TNF-α, and IL-1 and triggering of surface receptors, such as CD16 interaction with immune complexes, are among the stimuli that, acting individually or often in synergistic combination, induce NK cells to produce cytokines.[2,33,34]

PHYSIOLOGIC ROLES OF NATURAL KILLER CELLS

NATURAL RESISTANCE

Because of their ability to respond to external stimuli without previous sensitization, NK cells are able to respond rapidly, although nonspecifically, to the presence of infectious microorganisms or, in some cases, neoplastic cells. Together with phagocytic cells, NK cells are effectors of the innate or natural resistance, which represents the first line of defense against infection (Fig. 85-1).

The ability of NK cells to participate in the resistance against infection by certain viruses is well documented in experimental animals[35] and is strongly suggested by the recurrent viral infections in the few patients described to have a selective deficiency of NK cells.[36] In vitro NK cells selectively kill virus-infected cells with a mechanism that is at least in part dependent on the production of IFN-α, a potent stimulator of NK cell activity.[37,38] In vivo virus infection and IFN production are usually accompanied by a rapid activation of and increase in the number of NK cells, both systemic and localized in the infected area.[12] The NK response to virus infection usually peaks at 3 days postinfection and is followed by an antigen-specific T-helper and CTL response, which peaks 7 to 9 days postinfection.[12] The early NK response induces a significant reduction in the titer of certain viruses, including murine cytomegalovirus.[35] Other viruses, such as lymphocytic choriomeningitis virus (LCMV), are resistant to the antiviral effects of NK cells, and NK cell activation induced by these viruses has pathogenic effects.[35]

Natural killer cells have been described to be directly cytotoxic for bacteria and certain parasites.[39] Most important, NK cells enhance the response of phagocytic cells to microorganisms, especially intracellular bacteria and parasites, by producing high levels of the phagocyte-activating cytokines IFN-γ and GM-CSF in response to the microorganisms themselves or to factors such as IL-12 and TNF-α produced by infected phagocytic cells.[40,41]

The observation that NK cells kill in vitro–transformed or tumor-derived cell lines has been used to support the theory that, in immune surveillance, NK cells, rather than T cells, can recognize and kill newly arising malignant tumor cells.[42] In experimental animals, the in vivo activity of NK cells against tumors was investigated by evaluating their effects on long-term growth of tumors, metastasis formation, and short-term elimination of radiolabeled tumor cells.[2] Experiments have clearly shown that NK cells can destroy tumor cells in vivo, and there is some evidence for an effective role of NK cells in resistance to spontaneously arising neoplastic cells. Thus, in human cancer patients, NK cell cytotoxic activity is often decreased, and several studies have suggested that increased NK cell activity tends to correlate with increased survival times and longer intervals before metastasis is observed.[43,44] However, the hypothesis of a role for NK cells in immune surveillance is not yet supported by statistical evidence indicating a correlation between low tumor incidence and high NK cell cytotoxic activity.[45]

REGULATION OF ADAPTIVE IMMUNITY

Natural killer cells, by interacting with infectious agents and antigens early during the immune response, have either stimulatory or inhibitory effects on the function of B and T cells, as well as on antigen-presenting cells.[2] Evidence for an enhancing effect of NK cells on B-cell response has been shown both in vitro and in vivo by studies demonstrating that NK cells in the absence of T cells support antigen-specific B-cell responses, in part by producing IFN-γ.[46,47] In certain bacterial and parasitic infections, NK cells may be necessary for optimal induction of a T-helper type 1 response. Natural killer cells stimulated by microorganisms or by cytokines such as IL-12 and TNF produce large amounts of IFN-γ and other cytokines that facilitate T-helper-cell type 1 development.[48,49]

MODULATION OF HEMATOPOIESIS

Experimental observations in animals, clinical findings in human patients, and in vitro analyses provided strong evidence that NK cells are involved in the regulation of hematopoiesis.[50] The effector role of NK cells in rejection of parental marrow graft in irradiated F1 mice[51] and in suppressing erythropoiesis and phagocytopoiesis in mice infected with LCMV[52] demonstrated that in vivo activated NK cells can affect both allogeneic and syngeneic hematopoietic progenitor cells. Because of the ability of NK cells to kill malignant hematopoietic cells, they have been postulated to play an important role in the graft-versus-leukemia reaction in allogeneic marrow transplantation while playing only a modest, if any, role in graft-versus-host disease (see Chap. 18).[53]

In vivo depletion of NK cells by treatment of mice with anti-NK cell antibodies produces differential effects on various lineages. Natural killer cell depletion in normal mice increases phagocytopoiesis and decreases erythropoiesis and megakaryocytopoiesis.[54,55] Consistent with these results, depletion of NK cells in mice receiving myelosuppressive irradiation results in faster recovery of phagocytopoiesis and slower recovery of megakaryocytopoiesis and erythropoiesis.[56] Clinical evidence for a role of NK cells in the regulation of human hematopoiesis is provided by the demonstration that NK cells are the effector cells mediating suppression of hematopoiesis in some cases of acquired aplastic anemia in both acute and chronic monoclonal NK lymphocytosis and possibly in other clinical conditions.[50] In vitro studies have shown that NK cells have a prevalent inhibitory effect on colony formation from hematopoietic progenitor cells.[57,58] However, NK cells enhance formation of megakaryocytic colonies and, in some experimental conditions, of erythroid and granulocyte-macrophage colonies.[31,59] The effect of NK cells is mostly mediated by secretion of humoral factors and may require the participation of accessory cells.[58] Natural killer cells, constitutively or upon activation, produce several lymphokines, some with mostly inhibitory effects on hematopoiesis, such as TNF and IFN-γ, and some with mostly positive effects, such as GM-CSF, M-CSF, and IL-3.[30,31]

PATHOLOGIC ALTERATIONS IN NATURAL KILLER CELL NUMBER AND FUNCTIONS

Natural killer cell function and, in some, NK cell numbers are often decreased in pathologic conditions, including cancer and AIDS (see

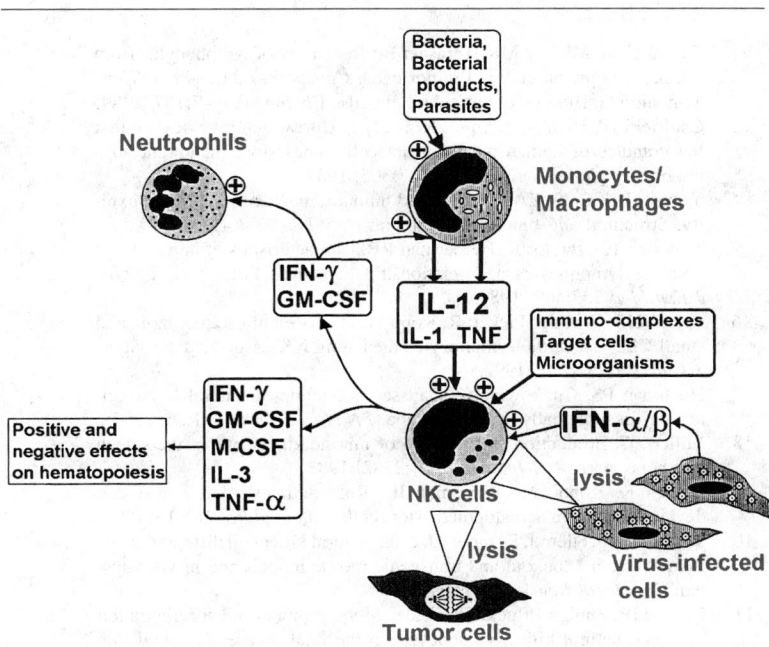

FIGURE 85-1 Schematic depiction of some of the functions and regulatory pathways of NK cells as effector cells of natural resistance. In addition to mediating cytotoxicity, NK cells exert their physiologic roles by releasing several cytokines that affect the functions of other cell types, including hematopoietic cells. Natural-killer-cell activity is also regulated by cytokines. Cytokines IFN-α/β, IL-2, and IL-12 enhance NK-cell-mediated cytotoxicity. IL-2, IL-12, TNF, and IL-1 induce NK-cell lymphokine production. IL-2 and IL-12 induce NK-cell proliferation. The arrows with a + in the figure indicate stimulatory effects resulting in lymphokine secretion, enhancement of NK-cell cytotoxic activity, or activation of phagocytic cells.

Chap. 89).[43,60] The reduced activity or number of NK cells may contribute to the pathology of the disease by decreasing the innate resistance against tumor growth and metastasis in cancer patients or against opportunistic infections in AIDS patients. The complete congenital absence of NK cells is extremely rare and characterized clinically by recurrent, severe viral infections.[36] An NK hyporesponsiveness is observed in patients with Chediak-Higashi syndrome (see Chap 72),[61] a rare autosomal recessive disease associated with cellular dysfunction, including fusion of cytoplasmic granules and defective degranulation of neutrophil lysosomes. Natural killer cells in these patients are in normal numbers but present a single, large granule in the cytoplasm and have a severely reduced ability to mediate cytotoxicity.[61]

Malignant acute expansion of NK cells is rare; it occurs both in the nasopharyngeal region and in nonnasal areas as an NK cell (CD2+, CD3−, CD56+, CD16−, CD57−) leukemia or lymphoma that mostly affects extranodal tissues (see Chaps. 96 and 100). It usually has an extremely aggressive clinical course. It may be associated with Epstein-Barr virus infection.[62-64] More commonly observed is a chronic monoclonal proliferative disorder of large granular lymphocytes with a clinical course that is often relatively benign.[65] Most patients have lymphocytic infiltration of the marrow, and severe neutropenia and anemia are often observed. Associated diseases, most commonly rheumatoid arthritis, hepatitis, or cancer, are present in up to half of the patients.[65] Although cells from all these patients are characterized by an LGL morphology, in approximately two-thirds of the cases they represent a monoclonal expansion of CD8+ T cells, and in only less than one-third do they have the typical phenotype and genotype of CD3−, CD56+, CD57+, and, in some patients, CD16+ NK cells.[65]

REFERENCES

1. Takasugi M, Mickey MR, Terasaki PI: Reactivity of lymphocytes from normal persons on cultured tumor cells. *Cancer Res* 33:2898, 1973.
2. Trinchieri G: Biology of natural killer cells. *Adv Immunol* 47:187, 1989.
3. Caulfield JP, Hein A, Schmidt RE, Ritz J: Ultrastructural evidence that the granules of human natural killer cell clones store membrane in a nonbilayer phase. *Am J Pathol* 127:305, 1987.
4. Young JDE, Cohn ZA: Cellular and humoral mechanisms of cytotoxicity: Structural and functional analogies. *Adv Immunol* 41:269, 1987.
5. Timonen T, Ortaldo JR, Herberman RB: Characteristics of human large granular lymphocytes and relationship to natural killer and K cells. *J Exp Med* 153:569, 1981.
6. Ortaldo JR, Winkler-Pickett R, Kopp W, et al: Relationship of large and small CD3− CD56+ lymphocytes mediating NK-associated activities. *J Leuk Biol* 52:287, 1992.
7. Hochman PS, Cudkowicz G, Dausset J: Decline of natural killer cell activity in sublethally irradiated mice. *J Natl Cancer Inst* 61:265, 1978.
8. Miller SC: Production and renewal of murine killer cells in the spleen and bone marrow. *J Immunol* 129:2282, 1982.
9. Akashi K, Kondo M, Weissman IL: Role of interleukin-7 in T-cell development from hematopoietic stem cells. *Immunol Rev* 165:13, 1998.
10. Williams NS, Klem J, Puzanov IJ, et al: Natural killer cell differentiation: Insights from knockout and transgenic mouse models and in vitro systems. *Immunol Rev* 165:47, 1998.
11. Carlyle JR, Zuniga-Pflucker JC: Lineage commitment and differentiation of T and natural killer lymphocytes in the fetal mouse. *Immunol Rev* 165:63, 1998.
12. Biron CA, Turgiss LR, Welsh RM: Increase in NK cell number and turnover rate during acute viral infection. *J Immunol* 131:1539, 1983.
13. Perussia B, Starr S, Abraham S, et al: Human natural killer cells analyzed by B73.1, a monoclonal antibody blocking Fc receptor functions: I. Characterization of the lymphocyte subset reactive with B73.1. *J Immunol* 130:2133, 1983.
14. Bouwens L, Wisse E: Pit cells in the liver. *Liver* 12:3, 1992.
15. Weissler JC, Nicod LP, Lipscomb MF, Toews GB: Natural killer cell function in human lung is compartmentalized. *Am Rev Respir Dis* 135:941, 1987.
16. Starkey PM, Sargent IL, Redman CWG: Cell populations in human early pregnancy decidua: Characterization and isolation of large granular lymphocytes by flow cytometry. *Immunology* 65:129, 1988.
17. Yokoyama WM: Recognition structures on natural killer cells. *Curr Opin Immunol* 5:67, 1993.
18. Ravetch JV, Perussia B: Alternative membrane forms of FcgRIII(CD16) on human NK cells and neutrophils: Cell-type specific expression of two genes which differ in single nucleotide substitutions. *J Exp Med* 170:481, 1989.
19. Kärre K, Ljunggren HG, Piontek G, Kiessling R: Selective rejection of H-2-deficient lymphoma variants suggests alternative immune defence strategy. *Nature* 319:675, 1986.
20. Ploegh HL: Viral strategies of immune evasion. *Science* 280:248, 1998.
21. Garrido F, Cabrera T, Lopez-Nevot MA, Ruiz-Cabello F: HLA class I antigens in human tumors. *Adv Cancer Res* 67:155, 1995.
22. Long EO: Regulation of immune responses through inhibitory receptors. *Annu Rev Immunol* 17:875, 1999.
23. Braud VM, Allan DS, O'Callaghan CA, et al: HLA-E binds to natural killer cell receptors CD94/NKG2A, B and C. *Nature* 391:795, 1998.
24. Yu YY, George T, Dorfman JR, et al: The role of Ly49A and 5E6 (Ly49C) molecules in hybrid resistance mediated by murine natural killer cells against normal T cell blasts. *Immunity* 4:67, 1996.
25. Lanier LL, Corliss BC, Wu J, et al: Immunoreceptor DAP12 bearing a tyrosine-based activation motif is involved in activating NK cells. *Nature* 391:703, 1998.
26. Trinchieri G, Santoli D: Antiviral activity induced by culturing lymphocytes with tumor-derived or virus-transformed cells: Enhancement of human natural killer cell activity by interferon and antagonistic inhibition of susceptibility of target cells to lysis. *J Exp Med* 147:1314, 1978.
27. Trinchieri G, Matsumoto-Kobayashi M, Clark SC, et al: Response of resting human peripheral blood natural killer cells to interleukin-2. *J Exp Med* 160:1147, 1984.
28. Kobayashi M, Fitz L, Ryan M, et al: Identification and purification of natural killer cell stimulatory factor (NKSF), a cytokine with multiple biologic effects on human lymphocytes. *J Exp Med* 170:827, 1989.
29. London L, Perussia B, Trinchieri G: Induction of proliferation in vitro of resting human natural killer cells: IL-2 induces into cell cycle most peripheral blood NK cells, but only a minor subset of low density T cells. *J Immunol* 137:3845, 1986.
30. Cuturi MC, Anegon I, Sherman F, et al: Production of hematopoietic colony-stimulating factors by human natural killer cells. *J Exp Med* 169:569, 1989.
31. Murphy WJ, Keller JR, Harrison CL, et al: Interleukin-2-activated natural killer cells can support hematopoiesis in vitro and promote marrow engraftment in vivo. *Blood* 80:670, 1992.
32. Peritt D, Robertson S, Gri G, et al: Differentiation of human NK cells into NK1 and NK2 subsets. *J Immunol* 161:5821, 1998.
33. Anegón I, Cuturi MC, Trinchieri G, Perussia B: Interaction of Fcg receptor (CD16) with ligands induces transcription of IL-2 receptor (CD25) and lymphokine genes and expression of their products in human natural killer cells. *J Exp Med* 167:452, 1988.
34. Chan SH, Perussia B, Gupta JW, et al: Induction of IFN-γ production by NK cell stimulatory factor (NKSF): Characterization of the responder cells and synergy with other inducers. *J Exp Med* 173:869, 1991.
35. Welsh RM: Regulation of virus infections by natural killer cells: A review. *Nat Immun Cell Growth Regul* 5:169, 1986.
36. Biron CA, Byron KS, Sullivan JL: Severe herpesvirus infections in an adolescent without natural killer cells. *N Engl J Med* 320:1731, 1989.
37. Santoli D, Trinchieri G, Koproswki H: Cell-mediated cytotoxicity in humans against virus-infected target cells: II. Interferon induction and activation of natural killer cells. *J Immunol* 121:532, 1978.
38. Bandyopadhyay S, Perussia B, Trinchieri G, et al: Requirement for HLA-DR positive accessory cells in natural killing of cytomegalovirus-infected fibroblasts. *J Exp Med* 164:180, 1986.
39. Garcia-Penarrubia P, Koster FT, Kelley RO, et al: Antibacterial activity of human natural killer cells. *J Exp Med* 169:99, 1989.
40. Bancroft GJ, Schreiber RD, Unanue ER: Natural immunity: A T-cell-independent pathway of macrophage activation, defined in the SCID mouse. *Immunol Rev* 124:5, 1991.
41. Gazzinelli RT, Hieny S, Wynn TA, et al: Interleukin 12 is required for the T-lymphocyte-independent induction of interferon gamma by an intracellular parasite and induces resistance in T-cell-deficient hosts. *Proc Natl Acad Sci USA* 90:6115, 1993.
42. Bloom BR: Natural killers to rescue immune surveillance? *Nature* 300:214, 1982.
43. Pross HF: Natural killer cell activity in human malignant disease, in *Natural Immunity Cancer and Biological Response Modification,* edited by E Lotzova and RB Herberman, Karger, Basel, p 196, 1986.
44. Schantz SP, Brown BW, Lira E, et al: Evidence for the role of natural immunity in the control of metastatic spread of head and neck cancer. *Cancer Immunol Immunother* 25:141, 1987.
45. Pross HF, Sterns E, MacGillis DRR: Natural killer activity in women at "high risk" for breast cancer, with and without benign breast syndrome. *Int J Cancer* 34:303, 1984.
46. Mond JJ, Brunswick M: A role for IFN-gamma and NK cells in immune response to T cell-regulated antigens types 1 and 2. *Immunol Rev* 99:105, 1987.
47. Yuan D, Wilder J, Dang T, et al: Activation of B lymphocytes by NK cells. *Int Immunol* 4:1373, 1992.
48. Romagnani S: Induction of TH1 and TH2 responses: A key role for the "natural" immune response? *Immunol Today* 13:379, 1992.
49. Trinchieri G: Interleukin-12 and its role in the generation of Th-1 cells. *Immunol Today* 14:335, 1993.
50. Trinchieri G: Natural killer cells in hematopoiesis, in *The Natural Immune System: Natural Killer Cells,* edited by CE Lewis and J McGee, Oxford University Press, Oxford, England, Vol. 1, p 41, 1992.
51. Cudkowicz G, Hochman PS: Do natural killer cells engage in regulated reaction against self to ensure homeostasis? *Immunol Rev* 44:13, 1979.
52. Randrup-Thomsen A, Pisa P, Bro-Jorgensen K, Kiessling R: Mechanisms of lymphocytic choriomeningitis virus-induced hemopoietic dysfunction. *J Virol* 59:428, 1986.
53. Jiang YZ, Barrett AJ, Goldman JM, Mavroudis DA: Association of natural killer cell immune recovery with a graft-versus-leukemia effect independent of graft-versus-host disease following allogeneic bone marrow transplantation. *Ann Hematol* 74:1, 1997.

54. Hansson M, Petersson M, Koo GC, et al: In vivo function of natural killer cells as regulators of myeloid precursor cells in the spleen. *Eur J Immunol* 18:485, 1988.

55. Pantel K, Nakeff A: Differential effect of natural killer cells on modulating CFU-Meg and BFU-E proliferation in situ. *Exp Hematol* 17:1017, 1989.

56. Pantel K, Boertman J, Nakeff A: Inhibition of hematopoietic recovery from radiation-induced myelosuppression by natural killer cells. *Radiat Res* 122:168, 1990.

57. Hansson M, Beran M, Andersson B, Kiessling R: Inhibition of in vitro granulopoiesis by autologous and allogeneic human NK cells. *J Immunol* 129:126, 1982.

58. Degliantoni G, Murphy M, Kobayashi M, et al: Natural killer (NK) cell-derived hematopoietic colony-inhibiting activity and NK cytotoxic factor: Relationship with tumor necrosis factor and synergism with immune interferon. *J Exp Med* 162:1512, 1985.

59. Gewirtz AM, Xu WY, Mangan KF: Role of natural killer cells, in comparison with T lymphocytes and monocytes, in the regulation of normal human megakaryocytopoiesis in vitro. *J Immunol* 139:2915, 1987.

60. Chehimi J, Starr SE, Frank I, et al: Natural killer (NK) cell stimulatory factor increases the cytotoxic activity of NK cells from both healthy donors and human immunodeficiency virus-infected patients. *J Exp Med* 175:789, 1992.

61. Haliotis T, Roder J, Klein M, et al: Chediak-Higashi gene in humans: I. Impairment of natural-killer function. *J Exp Med* 151:1039, 1980.

62. Kanavaros P, Lescs MC, Briere J, et al: Nasal T-cell lymphoma: A clinicopathologic entity associated with peculiar phenotype and with Epstein-Barr virus. *Blood* 81:2688, 1993.

63. Chan JK, Sin VC, Wong KF, et al: Nonnasal lymphoma expressing the natural killer cell marker CD56: A clinicopathologic study of 49 cases of an uncommon aggressive neoplasm. *Blood* 89:4501, 1997.

64. Jaffe ES: Classification of natural killer (NK) cell and NK-like T-cell malignancies. *Blood* 87:1207, 1996.

65. Reynolds CW, Foon KA: T-gamma-lymphoproliferative disorders in man and experimental animals: A review of the clinical, cellular and functional characteristics. *Blood* 64:1146, 1984.

CLASSIFICATION AND CLINICAL MANIFESTATIONS OF LYMPHOCYTE AND PLASMA CELL DISORDERS

THOMAS J. KIPPS

This chapter outlines the major categories of lymphocyte and plasma cell disorders. Such disorders can be sorted into three main groups. The first is comprised of diseases caused by defects that are intrinsic to lymphoid cells. The second is caused by disorders that result from factors extrinsic to lymphoid cells. The third is comprised of disorders caused by neoplastic or preneoplastic lymphoid cells and is outlined in Chap. 96. While the clinical manifestations of diseases in any one of these three groups may be difficult to distinguish, this grouping can provide a framework with which to proceed in evaluating patients with known or suspected lymphocyte disorders. This chapter introduces this framework and presents a road map to the chapters in the text that discuss each of these disorders in greater detail.

CLASSIFICATION

Lymphocyte and plasma cell disorders can be classified into three major groups. The first group is comprised of lymphocyte disorders that are due to intrinsic defects in lymphoid cells that result in functional abnormalities of marrow-derived (B) lymphocytes, thymic-derived (T) lymphocytes, or both (impaired humoral and cellular immunity) (Table 86-1). These disorders primarily are due to inborn errors in lymphocyte metabolism (see Chaps. 81 and 88) and/or receptor/ligand expression (see Chaps. 15 and 88). These are grouped together as "primary disorders" in Table 86-1. Next are disorders that are caused by factors extrinsic to lymphocytes resulting in immune dysfunction. These conditions most commonly are the result of infection with viruses or other cellular pathogens (see Chaps. 87, 89, and 90) but also may be caused by drugs or systemic disease of nonlymphoid cells. These disorders are listed as "acquired disorders" in Table 86-1. The third group of diseases are comprised of preneoplastic and neoplastic lymphocyte disorders (see Chap. 96).

Different categories of lymphocyte and plasma cell disorders may be difficult to distinguish clinically. For one, lymphocyte disorders can have many clinical manifestations that are not restricted to cells of the immune system. Also, disparate disorders can have similar clinical manifestations, and any one disorder may be associated with a diverse array of clinical pathologies.

In some cases, however, the classification of lymphocyte disorders is influenced by the manifestations of the disease. For example, autoimmune hemolytic disease (see Chaps. 55–57) and autoimmune thrombocytopenia (see Chap. 117) are caused by the inappropriate secretion of autoantibodies by lymphocytes. The blood cell that is coated with autoantibody is presumably normal, yet we classify the disease that can result from hemolytic autoantibodies as an acquired hemolytic anemia. This is because that aspect of the disease is more visible and better understood than is the inappropriate synthesis of antierythrocyte antibody by the disturbed lymphocyte population(s). These disorders are not considered here.

In addition, many diseases, especially infection (e.g., tuberculous adenitis), inflammatory states (e.g., rheumatoid arthritis), autoimmune disease (e.g., systemic lupus erythematosus), or metastatic carcinoma can involve lymph nodes or the spleen as a secondary alteration. These disorders also may be associated with abnormal production of antibodies, such as those resulting in the lupus anticoagulant (see Chap. 128). These disorders also are not considered here because the primary disease is not generally considered a lymphocyte disorder per se.

CLINICAL MANIFESTATIONS

B-LYMPHOCYTE DISORDERS

IMMUNOGLOBULIN DEFICIENCY
The clinical manifestations of B-lymphocyte disorders include the consequences of B-lymphocyte deficiency, dysfunction, or malignant transformation and may consist of a specific deficiency of one of the immunoglobulin isotypes or of several or all normal Ig molecules (panhypogammaglobulinemia) (see Chap. 83). Inability to synthesize or secrete antibodies impairs the clearance of pathogens due to the inability to opsonize microorganisms for phagocytosis, resulting in immune deficiency (see Chap. 88).

ABNORMAL IMMUNOGLOBULIN PRODUCTION
Excess production of immunoglobulin by a clone of B cells can result in essential monoclonal gammopathy (see Chap. 105). This could result from a primary defect in the B-cell clone or expansion of a clone in response to chronic antigen stimulation. Essential monoclonal gammopathy could be a harbinger for development of B-cell neoplastic disease, such as plasma cell myeloma (see Chap. 106) or Waldenström macroglobulinemia (see Chap. 108). Production of abnormal immunoglobulin molecules or immunoglobulin fragments also can be seen associated with chronic infection, leading to development of immunoglobulin heavy-chain disease (see Chap. 109). Deposition of immunoglobulin or immunoglobulin fragments can contribute to formation of amyloid (see Chap. 107). Reactivity of the immunoglobulin with self-antigen(s), such as those found on the red cell membrane (see Chaps. 55 and 56), can result in systemic autoimmune disease.

T-LYMPHOCYTE DISORDERS

IMPAIRED IMMUNOREGULATION
The clinical manifestations of deficiencies or excesses of T lymphocytes depend on the subset of T lymphocytes involved. For example, delayed hypersensitivity normally is mediated by CD4-positive helper T cells (T_H cells) and more specifically T_H1-type cells (see Chap. 84). A deficit or functional disturbance in these T cells can impair the cellular immune response to mycobacteria, listeria, brucella, fungi, or other intracellular organisms associated with the formation of immune granulomas. T_H2-type CD4-positive helper T cells, on the other hand, appear better suited to induce B-cell responses to antigen and direct the immune response against parasitic infestations (see Chap. 84). Depletion of CD4 T cells in patients infected with human immunodeficiency virus accounts in large part to the acquired immune deficiency that develops in patients infected with this virus (see Chap. 89).

T lymphocytes within a marrow allograft are responsible for initiation of the graft-versus-host reaction (see Chap. 18). The acute form of the reaction can lead to severe dermatitis, gastroenteritis,

TABLE 86-1   CLASSIFICATION OF DISORDERS OF LYMPHOCYTES AND PLASMA CELLS

I. Primary disorders
   A. B-lymphocyte deficiency or dysfunction
      1. Agammaglobulinemia (see Chap. 88)
         a. Acquired agammaglobulinemia[1,2]
         b. Associated with plasma cell myeloma[3]
         c. Dysgammaglobulinemia with nodular hyperplasia of intestinal lymphoid areas[4]
         d. Sex-linked agammaglobulinemia of Bruton[5-7]
      2. Selective agammaglobulinemia (see Chap. 88)
         a. IgM deficiency
            i. Bloom syndrome[8,9]
            ii. Isolated [10,11]
            iii. Wiskott-Aldrich syndrome [12,13]
         b. IgA deficiency[2,14]
            i. Isolated asymptomatic[14]
            ii. Steatorrheic[15]
         c. IgA and IgM deficiency (type II dysgammaglobulinemia)[2]
      3. Hyperimmunoglobulin A[16]
      4. Hyperimmunoglobulin D[17,18]
      5. Hyperimmunoglobulin E[19]
      6. Hyperimmunoglobulin E associated with HIV infection[20]
      7. Immunodeficiency with elevated IgM[2,21-24]
      8. X-linked lymphoproliferative disease[2]
   B. T-lymphocyte deficiency or dysfunction (see Chap. 88)[25]
      1. Cartilage-hair hypoplasia[26,27]
      2. Lymphocyte function antigen 1 deficiency[28-30]
      3. Thymic aplasia (DiGeorge syndrome)[2,31-33]
      4. Thymic dysplasia (Nezelof syndrome)[2]
      5. Thymic hypoplasia[34]
      6. Wiskott-Aldrich syndrome[12]
   C. Combined T- and B-cell deficiency or dysfunction (see Chap. 88)[25,33,35]
      1. Ataxia-telangiectasia[2,36-39]
      2. Combined immunodeficiency syndrome (see Chap. 88)
         a. Adenosine deaminase deficiency[40]
         b. Swiss-type autosomal recessive[2]
         c. Thymic alymphoplasia, sex-linked recessive[2]
      3. Defective expression of major histocompatibility antigens[2,41]
      4. IgG and IgA deficiency and impaired cellular immunity (type I dysgammaglobulinemia)[42,43]
      5. Immunodeficiency with thymoma[44,45]
      6. Pyridoxine deficiency[46]
      7. Reticular agenesis (congenital aleukocytosis)[2,47]
      8. ZAP-70 deficiency[48]
II. Acquired disorders
   A. Acquired immunodeficiency syndrome (see Chap. 89)
   B. Reactive lymphocytosis or plasmacytosis (see Chap. 87)[49]
      1. *Bordetella pertussis* lymphocytosis (see Chap. 87)[50]
      2. Cytomegalovirus mononucleosis (see Chap. 90)[49,51]
      3. Drug-induced lymphocytosis[52,53]
      4. Epstein-Barr virus mononucleosis (see Chap. 90)[54]
      5. Inflammatory (secondary) plasmacytosis of marrow
      6. Large granular lymphocytosis[55]
      7. Other viral mononucleosis (see Chaps. 89 and 90)[49,56]
      8. Polyclonal lymphocytosis (see Chap. 87)[57]
      9. Serum sickness[58,59]
      10. T-cell lymphocytosis associated with thymoma[44]
      11. *Toxoplasma gondii* mononucleosis (see Chap. 90)
      12. Viral infectious lymphocytosis[49,60]
   C. T-lymphocyte dysfunction associated with systemic disease
      1. B-cell chronic lymphocytic leukemia (see Chap. 98)
      2. Hodgkin lymphoma (see Chap. 102)
      3. Leprosy[61-63]
      4. Lupus erythematosus[64]
      5. Rheumatoid arthritis[65]
      6. Sarcoidosis[43,66,67]

and hepatitis. The chronic syndrome simulates a collage of vascular diseases, such as scleroderma, xerophthalmia, xerostomia, and pulmonary insufficiency. Eosinophilia, hypergammaglobulinemia, development of autoantibodies, and plasmacytosis also can occur. Infection with classical or opportunistic pathogens is a common complication of both acute and chronic graft-versus-host disease. A similar qualitative reaction, albeit more limited, is seen in mononucleosis that results from Epstein-Barr virus infection (see Chap. 90).

REFERENCES

1. Conley ME, Park CL, Douglas SD: Childhood common variable immunodeficiency with autoimmune disease. *J Pediatr* 108:915, 1986.
2. Buckley RH: Immunodeficiency diseases. *JAMA* 268:2797, 1992.
3. Kyrtsonis MC, Mouzaki A, Maniatis A: Mechanisms of polyclonal hypogammaglobulinaemia in multiple myeloma (MM). *Med Oncol* 16:73, 1999.
4. Hodgson HJ: Immunological aspects of inflammatory bowel diseases of the human gut. *Agents Actions* Spec No: C27, 1992.
5. Smith CI, Bäckesjö CM, Berglöf A, et al: X-linked agammaglobulinemia: lack of mature B lineage cells caused by mutations in the Btk kinase. *Springer Semin Immunopathol* 19:369, 1998.
6. Rawlings DJ: Bruton's tyrosine kinase controls a sustained calcium signal essential for B lineage development and function. *Clin Immunol* 91:243, 1999.
7. Nonoyama S: Recent advances in the diagnosis of X-linked agammaglobulinemia [editorial]. *Intern Med* 38:687, 1999.
8. Auerbach AD, Verlander PC: Disorders of DNA replication and repair. *Curr Opin Pediatr* 9:600, 1997.
9. Chakraverty RK, Hickson ID: Defending genome integrity during DNA replication: a proposed role for RecQ family helicases. *Bioessays* 21:286, 1999.
10. Callard RE, Smith SH, Matthews DJ: Regulation of human B cell growth and differentiation: lessons from the primary immunodeficiencies. *Chem Immunol* 67:114, 1997.
11. Guill MF, Brown DA, Ochs HD, Pyun KH, Moffitt JE: IgM deficiency: clinical spectrum and immunologic assessment. *Ann Allergy* 62:547, 1989.
12. Sullivan KE: Recent advances in our understanding of Wiskott-Aldrich syndrome. *Curr Opin Hematol* 6:8, 1999.
13. Snapper SB, Rosen FS: The Wiskott-Aldrich syndrome protein (WASP): roles in signaling and cytoskeletal organization. *Annu Rev Immunol* 17:905, 1999.
14. Strober W, Sneller MC: IgA deficiency. *Ann Allergy* 66:363, 1991.
15. Collin P, Maki M, Keyrilainen O, Hallstrom O, Reunala T, Pasternack A: Selective IgA deficiency and coeliac disease. *Scand J Gastroenterol* 27:367, 1992.
16. Levenson T, Greenberger PA, Murphy R: Peripheral blood eosinophilia, hyperimmunoglobulinemia A and fatigue: possible complications following rupture of silicone breast implants. *Ann Allergy Asthma Immunol* 77:119, 1996.
17. Livneh A, Drenth JP, Klasen IS, et al: Familial Mediterranean fever and hyperimmunoglobulinemia D syndrome: two diseases with distinct clinical, serologic, and genetic features. *J Rheumatol* 24:1558, 1997.
18. Livneh A, Langevitz P: [Hyperimmunoglobulinemia D—a new periodic syndrome with features simulating familial Mediterranean fever]. *Harefuah* 131:283, 1996.
19. Leung DY, Geha RS: Clinical and immunologic aspects of the hyperimmunoglobulin E syndrome. *Hematol Oncol Clin North Am* 2:81, 1988.
20. Blanche P, Bachmeyer C, Buvry C, Sicard D: Hyperimmunoglobulinemia E syndrome in HIV infection. *J Am Acad Dermatol* 36:106, 1997.
21. Ramesh N, Seki M, Notarangelo LD, Geha RS: The hyper-IgM (HIM) syndrome. *Springer Semin Immunopathol* 19:383, 1998.
22. Notarangelo LD, Duse M, Ugazio AG: Immunodeficiency with hyper-IgM (HIM). *Immunodefic Rev* 3:101, 1992.
23. Fuleihan R, Ramesh N, Loh R, et al: Defective expression of the CD40 ligand in X chromosome-linked immunoglobulin deficiency with normal or elevated IgM. *Proc Natl Acad Sci USA* 90:2170, 1993.
24. Allen RC, Armitage RJ, Conley ME, et al: CD40 ligand gene defects responsible for X-linked hyper-IgM syndrome. *Science* 259:990, 1993.
25. Fischer A, Cavazzana-Calvo M, De Saint Basile G, et al: Naturally

occurring primary deficiencies of the immune system. *Annu Rev Immunol* 15:93, 1997.

26. Makitie O, Kaitila I: Cartilage-hair hypoplasia—clinical manifestations in 108 Finnish patients. *Eur J Pediatr* 152:211, 1993.

27. Makitie O, Rajantie J, Kaitila I: Anaemia and macrocytosis—unrecognized features in cartilage-hair hypoplasia. *Acta Paediatr* 81:1026, 1992.

28. Hogg N, Stewart MP, Scarth SL, et al: A novel leukocyte adhesion deficiency caused by expressed but nonfunctional beta2 integrins Mac-1 and LFA-1. *J Clin Invest* 103:97, 1999.

29. Wright AH, Douglass WA, Taylor GM, et al: Molecular characterization of leukocyte adhesion deficiency in six patients. *Eur J Immunol* 25:717, 1995.

30. Lipnick RN, Iliopoulos A, Salata K, Hershey J, Melnick D, Tsokos GC: Leukocyte adhesion deficiency: report of a case and review of the literature. *Clin Exp Rheumatol* 14:95, 1996.

31. Demczuk S, Aurias A: DiGeorge syndrome and related syndromes associated with 22q11.2 deletions. A review. *Ann Genet* 38:59, 1995.

32. Hong R: The DiGeorge anomaly (CATCH 22, DiGeorge/velocardiofacial syndrome). *Semin Hematol* 35:282, 1998.

33. Harrison LF, Shearer WT: Evaluation and management of B and T cell abnormalities. *Allergy Proc* 12:25, 1991.

34. Frick H, Münger DM, Fauchère JC, Stallmach T: Hypoplastic thymus and T-cell reduction in EECUT syndrome. *Am J Med Genet* 69:65, 1997.

35. Fischer A, Malissen B: Natural and engineered disorders of lymphocyte development. *Science* 280:237, 1998.

36. Meyn MS: Ataxia-telangiectasia, cancer and the pathobiology of the ATM gene. *Clin Genet* 55:289, 1999.

37. Crawford TO: Ataxia telangiectasia. *Semin Pediatr Neurol* 5:287, 1998.

38. Datta U, Sehgal S, Kumar L, et al: Immune status in ataxia telangiectasia. *Indian J Med Res* 94:252, 1991.

39. Taylor AM, Jaspers NG, Gatti RA: Fifth International Workshop on Ataxia-Telangiectasia. *Cancer Res* 53:438, 1993.

40. Hershfield MS: Adenosine deaminase deficiency: clinical expression, molecular basis, and therapy. *Semin Hematol* 35:291, 1998.

41. Griscelli C, Lisowska-Grospierre B, Mach B: Combined immunodeficiency with defective expression in MHC class II genes. *Immunodefic Rev* 1:135, 1989.

42. Standen GR: Wiskott-Aldrich syndrome: a multidisciplinary disease. *J Clin Pathol* 44:979, 1991.

43. Inbal A, Avidor I, Nemesh L, Shaklai M: Persistent lymphocytosis: an unusual feature in sarcoidosis. *Acta Haematol* 74:184, 1985.

44. Barton AD: T-cell lymphocytosis associated with lymphocyte-rich thymoma. *Cancer* 80:1409, 1997.

45. Medeiros LJ, Bhagat SK, Naylor P, Fowler D, Jaffe ES, Stetler-Stevenson M: Malignant thymoma associated with T-cell lymphocytosis. A case report with immunophenotypic and gene rearrangement analysis. *Arch Pathol Lab Med* 117:279, 1993.

46. Trakatellis A, Dimitriadou A, Trakatelli M: Pyridoxine deficiency: new approaches in immunosuppression and chemotherapy. *Postgrad Med J* 73:617, 1997.

47. Gitlin D, Vawter G, Craig JM: Thymic alymphoplasia and congenital aleukocytosis. *Pediatrics* 33:184, 1964.

48. Elder ME: SCID due to ZAP-70 deficiency. *J Pediatr Hematol Oncol* 19:546, 1997.

49. Brown KA: Nonmalignant disorders of lymphocytes. *Clin Lab Sci* 10:329, 1997.

50. Kubic VL, Kubic PT, Brunning RD: The morphologic and immunophenotypic assessment of the lymphocytosis accompanying *Bordetella pertussis* infection. *Am J Clin Pathol* 95:809, 1991.

51. Drew WL, Lalezari JP: Cytomegalovirus: disease syndromes and treatment. *Curr Clin Top Infect Dis* 19:16, 1999.

52. Holcombe RF: Drug-induced granulocytopenia with natural killer lymphocytosis after renal transplantation. *Acta Haematol* 83:96, 1990.

53. Toft P, Tonnesen E, Svendsen P, Rasmussen JW, Christensen NJ: The redistribution of lymphocytes during adrenaline infusion. An in vivo study with radiolabelled cells. *APMIS* 100:593, 1992.

54. Peter J, Ray CG: Infectious mononucleosis. *Pediatr Rev* 19:276, 1998.

55. Zambello R, Semenzato G: Large granular lymphocytosis. *Haematologica* 83:936, 1998.

56. Greenberg MS: Herpesvirus infections. *Dent Clin North Am* 40:359, 1996.

57. Troussard X, Flandrin G: Chronic B-cell lymphocytosis with binucleated lymphocytes (LWBL): a review of 38 cases. *Leuk Lymphoma* 20:275, 1996.

58. Erffmeyer JE: Serum sickness. *Ann Allergy* 56:105, 1986.

59. Virella G: Immune complex diseases. *Immunol Ser* 50:395, 1990.

60. Saulsbury FT: B cell proliferation in acute infectious lymphocytosis. *Pediatr Infect Dis J* 6:1127, 1987.

61. Griffin G, Krishna S: Cytokines in infectious diseases. *J R Coll Physicians Lond* 32:195, 1998.

62. Gulle H, Schoel B, Chiplunkar S, Gangal S, Deo MG, Kaufmann SH: T-cell responses of leprosy patients and healthy contacts toward separated protein antigens of *Mycobacterium leprae*. *Int J Lepr Other Mycobact Dis* 60:44, 1992.

63. Walker KB, Butler R, Colston MJ: Role of Th-1 lymphocytes in the development of protective immunity against *Mycobacterium leprae*. Analysis of lymphocyte function by polymerase chain reaction detection of cytokine messenger RNA. *J Immunol* 148:1885, 1992.

64. Pande I, Sekharan NG, Kailash S, et al: Analysis of clinical and laboratory profile in Indian childhood systemic lupus erythematosus and its comparison with SLE in adults. *Lupus* 2:83, 1993.

65. Masson C, Perroux-Goummy L, Audran M: Felty's syndrome, pseudofelty's syndrome, monoclonal or polyclonal CD3 lymphocytosis of undetermined significance. *Rev Rhum Engl Ed* 63:5, 1996.

66. Moller DR: Cells and cytokines involved in the pathogenesis of sarcoidosis. *Sarcoidosis Vasc Diffuse Lung Dis* 16:24, 1999.

67. Daniele RP, Dauber JH, Rossman MD: Immunologic abnormalities in sarcoidosis. *Ann Intern Med* 92:406, 1980.

LYMPHOCYTOSIS AND LYMPHOCYTOPENIA

THOMAS J. KIPPS

The causes of lymphocytosis or lymphocytopenia are many and varied. This chapter outlines the conditions associated with abnormalities in the numbers of circulating lymphocytes in the blood. It also serves as a useful road map to other chapters in the book that describe in detail those conditions that commonly are associated with abnormalities in the absolute numbers of circulating lymphocytes.

LYMPHOCYTOSIS

DEFINITION

Lymphocytosis is defined as an absolute lymphocyte count exceeding 4×10^9/liter (4000/μl),[1] although somewhat lower threshold values ($>3.1 \times 10^9$/liter ($>3100/\mu$l)) are sometimes used.[2] The normal absolute lymphocyte count is significantly higher in childhood. The methods for determining the absolute lymphocyte count and the normal range for such counts are described in Chap. 2.

The blood film of patients with lymphocytosis should be evaluated for a predominance of reactive lymphocytes associated with infectious mononucleosis (see Chap. 90), large granular lymphocytes associated with large granular lymphocytic leukemia (see Chap. 100), smudge cells associated with chronic lymphocytic leukemia (see Chap. 98), or blasts of acute lymphocytic leukemia (see Chap. 97). A description of normal lymphocyte morphology is provided in Chap. 80.

Characterization of cell surface markers is valuable in distinguishing primary lymphocytosis (leukemic) from secondary lymphocytosis (reactive). New improvements in flow cytometry techniques and reagents have allowed clinical laboratories to perform flow cytometric immunophenotyping to distinguish benign from neoplastic lymphoproliferative disease (see Chap. 13).[3–11] Analysis for immunoglobulin or T-cell receptor gene rearrangement also may provide evidence for monoclonal B-cell or T-cell proliferation, respectively.[12]

PRIMARY LYMPHOCYTOSIS

Primary lymphocytosis defines conditions associated with an increase in the absolute number of lymphocytes secondary to an intrinsic defect in the expanded lymphocyte population (Table 87-1). These conditions also are referred to as lymphoproliferative disorders and most commonly are secondary to the neoplastic accumulation of monoclonal B cells, T cells, natural killer (NK) cells, or less fully differentiated cells of the lymphoid lineage. The chapters describing each of these conditions are indicated in Table 87-1.

Although patients with lymphocytosis secondary to lymphoproli-

ferative disease generally maintain abnormal lymphocyte counts that may rise over time,[13] this is not invariable. Patients with large granular lymphocytic leukemia (see Chap. 100) may have only transient lymphocytosis that is induced by stress or exercise.[14]

MONOCLONAL B-CELL LYMPHOCYTOSIS

The advent of flow cytometric and molecular diagnostic techniques has identified a syndrome in patients who have expanded populations of monoclonal B cells without other associated clinical signs or symptoms.[15–18] This syndrome may resemble that of patients with essential monoclonal gammopathy who otherwise do not have the clinical features of myeloma. Such patients also were identified after improved technology was introduced for evaluating serum immunoglobulins (see Chaps. 104 and 105). Similar to the latter, some patients who have expanded populations of monoclonal B cells may develop progressive neoplastic lymphoproliferative disease.[19]

PERSISTENT POLYCLONAL LYMPHOCYTOSIS OF B LYMPHOCYTES

Lymphocytosis can be secondary to an expansion in the numbers of B cells that are "polyclonal" in their expression of immunoglobulin. Patients with this disorder, termed persistent polyclonal lymphocytosis of B lymphocytes (PPBL), each have increased numbers of kappa and lambda light-expressing B cells that are heterogeneous in their rearrangements of immunoglobulin heavy-chain genes.[20–22] Occasional reports of clonal immunoglobulin rearrangements in this disorder suggest that the polyclonal expansion in some cases may be followed by the emergence of one predominant clone.[23,24]

The cause or causes of PPBL are unknown. Epstein-Barr virus (EBV) genomes have been detected in blood lymphocytes of patients with this disorder.[25–27] One study found a 69 base-pair deletion variant of the gene encoding the EBV latent membrane protein 1 in the lymphocytes of a PPBL patient but not in the lymphocytes of unaffected siblings, suggesting a role for altered LMP1 in the pathogenesis of PPBL.[28] Gender and genotype also may be important in the pathogenesis, since the patients most commonly are young to middle-aged women who often are HLA-DR7 positive.[24] In addition, there are reports of shared cases of PPBL among identical twins,[29] suggesting a possible hereditary or genetic contribution to the pathogenesis. However, the causes of this abnormality may be heterogeneous, as PPBL may not be a single disease entity.

Patients with PPBL can have features that resemble those of patients with various monoclonal B-cell malignancies. In one manifestation of this syndrome, first identified in Japan as hairy B-cell lymphoproliferative disorder,[30] the patients can present with anemia, thrombocytopenia, and splenomegaly, and have an excess of polyclonal B lymphocytes that appear similar in morphology to the neoplastic B cells in hairy-cell leukemia. In another manifestation of this syndrome, the patients have an accumulation of polyclonal B cells that coexpress CD19, CD5, and CD23, thus displaying an immunophenotype similar to that of B-cell chronic lymphocytic leukemia.[31,32]

In perhaps the most common manifestation of PPBL, however, the patients have an accumulation of polyclonal B cells that have an unusual binucleate appearance on the blood film.[21,24,33] These patients often have mild splenomegaly and raised serum IgM levels. This disorder appears more common among cigarette smokers[20,23,34] and most typically is associated the HLA-DR7 haplotype.[24]

Although the lymphocytosis of PPBL generally is not progressive, most patients will have small numbers of blood B cells that have chromosomal abnormalities. These most commonly include an additional isochromosome +i(3q) and premature chromosome condensation,[21,35] although t(14;18) involving the BCL-2 and the immunoglobulin heavy chain loci also have been detected.[22,36,37] In any one patient, these chromosomal abnormalities are restricted to B lymphocytes inde-

---

Acronyms and abbreviations that appear in this chapter include: EBV, Epstein-Barr virus; NK, natural killer; PPBL, persistent polyclonal lymphocytosis of the B lymphocytes; PUVA, psoralen and ultraviolet A irradiation.

TABLE 87-1   CAUSES OF LYMPHOCYTOSIS

I. Primary lymphocytosis
    A. Lymphocytic malignancies
        1. Acute lymphocytic leukemia (Chap. 97)
        2. Chronic lymphocytic leukemia and related disorders (Chap. 98)
        3. Prolymphocytic leukemia
        4. Hairy-cell leukemia (Chap. 99)
        5. Adult T-cell leukemia (Chaps. 98 and 103)
        6. Lymphoma-cell leukemia (Chap. 103)
        7. Large granular lymphocytic leukemia (Chap. 100)
            a. NK-cell leukemia
            b. T gamma lymphocytosis[73,82]
    B. Monoclonal B-cell lymphocytosis of undetermined significance[15-18,83]
    C. Persistent polyclonal B-cell lymphocytosis[31,84]
II. Reactive lymphocytosis
    A. Mononucleosis syndromes (Chap. 90)
        1. Epstein-Barr virus[25]
        2. Cytomegalovirus[43-46]
        3. Toxoplasma gondii[48]
        4. Human immunodeficiency virus[85-92]
        5. Herpes simplex virus type II
        6. Varicella zoster virus
        7. Rubella virus
        8. Adenovirus
        9. Infectious hepatitis virus
    B. Bordetella pertussis[50]
    C. Persistent lymphocytosis (chronic)
        1. Autoimmune disorders[66-69,93]
        2. Cancer[76,77]
        3. Cigarette smoking[20,34,79,94]
        4. Chronic inflammation[77]
        5. Hyposplenism[70,95]
        6. Postsplenectomy[64]
        7. Sarcoidosis[78]
        8. Thymoma[71-75]
        9. Wegener granulomatosis[70]
    D. Stress lymphocytosis (acute)[96]
        1. Cardiovascular collapse[59]
            a. Acute cardiac failure
            b. Myocardial infarction
            c. Septic shock[60]
            d. Drug induced[59,81,97,98]
            e. Hypersensitivity reactions[80]
            f. Major surgery[60,96]
            g. Sickle cell crisis[99]
            h. Status epilepticus[59]
            i. Trauma[2,58,59]

pendent of their expression of immunoglobulin kappa or lambda light chain.[21] For PPBL associated with smoking, these cytogenetic abnormalities apparently persist after the discontinuation of tobacco use.[24] The finding of such chromosome abnormalities is consistent with the notion that PPBL may represent a preneoplastic state. Consistent with this, a small proportion of patients with PPBL ultimately will develop monoclonal B-cell lymphoma or B-cell leukemia.[38,39]

SECONDARY (REACTIVE) LYMPHOCYTOSIS

Secondary lymphocytosis defines conditions associated with an increase in the absolute number of lymphocytes secondary to a physiologic or pathophysiologic response to infection, toxins, cytokines, or unknown factors.[40]

INFECTIOUS MONONUCLEOSIS

The most common reactive lymphocytosis is infectious mononucleosis (see Table 87-1). This syndrome is described in Chap. 90.

ACUTE INFECTION LYMPHOCYTOSIS

A disorder possibly related to infectious mononucleosis is acute infection lymphocytosis, a contagious disease that is characterized by an increase in circulating lymphocytes, often to 20 to 30 $\times$ 10^9/liter (20,000 to 30,000/μl)[41] and occasionally to 100 $\times$ 10^9/liter (100,000/μl).[42] The patients are usually asymptomatic but may have fever, abdominal pain, or diarrhea. Lymph node enlargement and splenomegaly do not occur, and the patient's serum usually is negative for heterophil antibodies. In this regard, the disease resembles infectious mononucleosis caused by viruses other than EBV, such as cytomegalovirus (see Chap. 90).[43-46] In some cases, the lymphocytosis has been found in association with acute infection by coxsackievirus B2.[47] Clinical symptoms last for a few days, but the lymphocytosis may persist for several weeks. Eosinophilia may be present. The marrow has been examined in a few patients and has shown minimal increases in lymphocytes, but marked infiltration with lymphocytes has also been observed.

Toxoplasmosis also can present with reactive lymphocytosis in the absence of lymphadenopathy, especially in the immune-compromised host.[48] Lymphocytosis with atypical lymphocytes also can be part of the early manifestation of acute infection with Falciparum malaria.[49]

BORDETELLA PERTUSSIS

A marked increase in the number of morphologically normal lymphocytes occurs in patients infected with the gram-negative bacterium *Bordetella pertussis*. Absolute lymphocyte counts range from 8 to 70 $\times$ 10^9/liter (8,000 to 70,000/μl), with a mean of approximately 30 $\times$ 10^9/liter (30,000/μl).[50] The lymphocytes are predominantly CD4+ T cells.[51,52]

The lymphocytosis primarily results from the failure of lymphocytes to leave the blood because of a toxin, termed pertussis toxin, released by the bacteria.[53] Pertussis toxin is an ADP-ribosylase that modifies Gi proteins in mammalian lymphocytes and inhibits their capacity to traffic from blood into lymphoid tissues, primarily through the inhibition of chemokine receptors.[54,55] Pertussis toxin also may stimulate egress of maturing T cells from the thymus[52,56] and may bind to neuraminic acid residues of T-cell–surface glycoproteins to induce T-cell activation.[57]

STRESS LYMPHOCYTOSIS

Trauma, surgery, acute cardiac failure, septic shock, myocardial infarction, sickle cell crisis, or status epilepticus may be associated with an elevated lymphocyte count, often above 5 $\times$ 10^9/liter (5000/μl),[58,59] which may revert to normal or below-normal levels within hours.[2] The increased lymphocyte count appears promptly after the event and appears secondary to lymphocyte redistribution.[60] A transient lymphocytosis can be induced by the adrenaline released and/or administered in response to the medical episode.[61-63] Characteristically, two phases are recognized after catecholamine administration: a quick (<30 min) mobilization of lymphocytes, followed by an increase in granulocyte numbers with decreasing lymphocyte numbers.[63]

POSTSPLENECTOMY LYMPHOCYTOSIS

Patients undergoing splenectomy for staging of Hodgkin's disease may develop a chronic postoperative polyclonal lymphocytosis.[64] An absolute lymphocyte count ranging from 4.0 to 8.7 $\times$ 10^9/liter often is noted 4 to 242 (median 70) months after splenectomy and can persist for prolonged periods (e.g., >50 months).[65]

PERSISTENT LYMPHOCYTOSIS

Patients may have subacute or chronic lymphocytosis, termed persistent lymphocytosis, in association with a variety of clinical situations (see Table 87-1).

Autoimmune Disease Patients with rheumatoid arthritis and related disorders may have lymphocytosis secondary to increased numbers of large granular lymphocytes.[66] Occurring in less than 0.6 percent of patients with rheumatoid arthritis, large granular lymphocytic lymphocytosis almost invariably is associated with neutropenia in the absence of splenomegaly and thus may represent a subset disorder of patients with Felty syndrome.[66,67] Patients with autoimmune pure red-cell aplasia or immune thrombocytopenia also may have expanded numbers of polyclonal T cells[68] or NK cells.[69]

Cancer Patients with lymphocytosis may be found to have underlying neoplastic disease.[70] Most notably, patients with malignant thymoma may have a polyclonal T-cell lymphocytosis thought to be secondary to the aberrant release of thymic hormones by the neoplastic thymic epithelium.[71–75] A reactive lymphocytosis or plasmacytosis may be detected in up to 7 percent of patients with acute myeloid leukemia.[76]

Chronic Inflammatory Diseases Persistent lymphocytosis has been reported in patients with systemic diseases associated with inflammation.[70,77] It has been noted in patients with sarcoidosis[78] or Wegener granulomatosis.[70]

Cigarette Smoking Cigarette smokers may have a persistent lymphocytosis secondary to an increase in polyclonal CD4+ T cells and B cells, some of which have an unusual binuclear morphology.[20,34,79]

Hypersensitivity Reactions Delayed hypersensitivity reactions to insect bites may be associated with a large granular lymphocytic lymphocytosis and adenopathy.[80] Idiosyncratic drug reactions also may be associated with subacute lymphocytosis.[81]

LYMPHOCYTOPENIA

DEFINITION

The methods for determining the absolute lymphocyte count and the normal range for such counts are presented in Chap. 2. Lymphocytopenia is defined as a total lymphocyte count of less than 1.0×10^9/liter (1,000/μl),[100] but some consider the lower limit of normal to be 1.5×10^9/liter (1500/μl).[101] Because approximately 80 percent of normal adult blood lymphocytes are T lymphocytes and nearly two-thirds of blood T lymphocytes are CD4+ (helper) T lymphocytes, most patients noted to have lymphocytopenia have reductions in the absolute numbers of T lymphocytes, particularly CD4+ T lymphocytes. The average absolute number of T lymphocytes in normal adult blood is 1.9×10^9/liter (1900/μl), ranging from 1.0 to 2.3×10^9/liter (1000 to 2300/μl).[102] The average absolute number of CD4+ T lymphocytes is 1.1×10^9/liter (1100/μl), ranging from 7.2 to 14×10^8/liter (720 to 1400/μl). The average absolute number of cells of the other major T-cell subgroup, CD8+ T lymphocytes, is 6.5×10^8/liter (650/μl), ranging from 3.8 to 9.7×10^8/liter (380 to 970/μl). Some Asians and blacks may lack or be heterozygous for an epitope on the CD4 molecule that is recognized by the mouse monoclonal antibody OKT4A, thus making these patients appear to have a deficiency in the absolute number of CD4 T cells. The use of other anti-CD4 monoclonal antibodies (e.g., Leu-3a) that bind other epitopes of the CD4 molecule may help rule out factitious CD4+ T-cell depletion.

Table 87-2 summarizes the conditions associated with lymphocytopenia. The mechanism of lymphocytopenia is not established for many of these disorders, and several possible mechanisms exist. Further discussion of lymphocytes and of the diseases associated with lymphocytopenia are presented in the cited reports (see Table 87-2).

The relative incidence of each of these conditions will vary, depending upon the patient population. In one New Zealand survey of patients who had significant lymphocytopenia ($<0.6 \times 10^9$/liter), the patients fell into several categories with some overlap.[103] In order of decreasing frequency, the factors associated with lymphocytopenia

TABLE 87-2   CAUSES OF LYMPHOCYTOPENIA

I. Inherited causes
  A. Congenital immunodeficiency diseases (Chap. 88)
    1. Severe combined immunodeficiency disease[149]
      a. Aplasia of lymphopoietic stem cells
      b. Adenosine deaminase deficiency[150]
      c. Absence of histocompatibility antigens[151]
      d. Absence of CD4+ helper cells[152,153]
      e. Thymic alymphoplasia with aleukocytosis (reticular dysgenesis)[154]
    2. Ataxia-telangiectasia[155]
    3. Wiskott-Aldrich syndrome[156]
    4. Immunodeficiency with short-limbed dwarfism (cartilage-hair hypoplasia)[157,158]
    5. Immunodeficiency with thymoma[159]
    6. Cellular immunodeficiency with immunoglobulins[160]
    7. Purine nucleoside phosphorylase deficiency[160]
    8. Immunodeficiency with veno-occlusive disease of the liver[161]
II. Acquired causes
  A. Aplastic anemia (Chap. 31)[162]
  B. Infectious diseases
    1. Viral diseases (Chap. 89)
      a. Acquired immunodeficiency syndrome[102,105,106]
      b. Hepatitis[102]
      c. Influenza[111]
      d. Herpes virus type 8[163,164]
      e. Other[165]
    2. Bacterial diseases
      a. Tuberculosis[110]
      b. Typhoid fever[166]
      c. Pneumonia[102]
      d. Sepsis[102]
  C. Iatrogenic
    1. Immunosuppressive agents[115]
      a. Anti-lymphocyte globulin therapy[116]
      b. Glucocorticoids[112,118–120]
    2. High-dose PUVA treatment[117]
    3. Neoplastic chemotherapy[114]
    4. Platelet apheresis procedures[125]
    5. Radiation[113]
    6. Major surgery[121–123]
    7. Renal or marrow transplant[167]
    8. Thoracic duct drainage[124]
  D. Systemic disease associated
    1. Autoimmune diseases[126]
      a. Arthritis[168]
      b. Systemic lupus erythematosus[127,128]
      c. Myasthenia gravis[169]
      d. Systemic vasculitis[170]
      e. Behçet's-like syndrome[171]
    2. Hodgkin's disease[101]
    3. Carcinoma[172]
    4. Protein-losing enteropathy[131]
    5. Renal failure[130]
    6. Sarcoidosis[129,141]
    7. Thermal injury[132]
  E. Nutritional and dietary
    1. Ethanol abuse[134]
    2. Zinc deficiency[133]
III. Idiopathic
  A. Idiopathic CD4+ T-lymphocytopenia[135,138,139,148]

were bacterial or fungal sepsis (250 patients), major surgery (228 patients), definite (153 patients) or suspected (53 patients) corticosteroid therapy, malignancy (180 patients), cytotoxic therapy and/or radiotherapy (90 patients), recent trauma or hemorrhage (86 patients), renal allograft (38 patients), marrow allograft (35 patients), "viral infections" other than human immunodeficiency virus (HIV; 26 patients), or infection with HIV (13 patients). Only one patient was suspected of having idiopathic CD4+ T lymphocytopenia.

INHERITED CAUSES

Patients with inherited immunodeficiency diseases may have associated lymphocytopenia (Table 87-2) (see Chap. 88). Inherited immunodeficiency disorders may have a quantitative or qualitative stem cell abnormality, resulting in ineffective lymphopoiesis (see cited references in Table 87-2). Others, such as the Wiskott-Aldrich syndrome, have associated lymphopenia due to premature destruction of T cells secondary to a defect in the lymphocyte cytoskeleton.[104]

ACQUIRED LYMPHOCYTOPENIA

Acquired lymphocytopenia defines syndromes associated with depletion of blood lymphocytes that are not secondary to inherited disease.

INFECTIOUS DISEASES

The most common infectious disease associated with lymphopenia is the acquired immunodeficiency syndrome. The lymphocytopenia is due in part to destruction and/or clearance of CD4+ T cells infected with HIV-1 or HIV-2.[102,105–109] The lymphocytopenia also may reflect impaired lymphocyte production and proliferation secondary to loss of the normal thymic or lymphoid architecture and the high levels of transforming growth factor β that often are noted in patients with this disease (see Chap. 89).

Other viral and bacterial diseases may be associated with lymphocytopenia (see Table 87-2). Patients presenting with active tuberculosis often have lymphocytopenia that usually resolves 2 weeks after initiating appropriate antimicrobial therapy.[110] In acute viral infection, the lymphocytes may be destroyed by the infection, may be trapped in the spleen or nodes, or may migrate to the respiratory tract.[106,111]

IATROGENIC

Radiotherapy, neoplastic chemotherapy, glucocorticoids, and the administration of antilymphocyte globulin all lead to lymphocytopenia by destroying circulating lymphocytes.[103,112–116] Long-term treatment of psoriasis with psoralen and ultraviolet A irradiation (PUVA) may result in T-lymphocyte lymphopenia, possibly through destruction of cells circulating through the cutaneous vasculature.[117] The mechanism by which glucocorticoids cause lymphocytopenia is not clear but may be secondary to a glucocorticoid-induced redistribution of lymphocytes[118,119] in addition to an induced cell destruction.[112,119,120] Redistribution also may be responsible for the lymphocytopenia occurring after surgery.[121–123] In thoracic duct drainage, the lymphocytes are lost from the body.[124] Platelet apheresis similarly lowers the lymphocyte count because of an inadvertent removal of lymphocytes with the platelets.[125]

SYSTEMIC DISEASE ASSOCIATED WITH LYMPHOCYTOPENIA

Patients with systemic autoimmune disease can have lymphocytopenia, either secondary to the underlying disease or to therapy.[126] The lymphocytopenia of patients with systemic lupus erythematosus may be autoantibody mediated.[127,128] The lymphocytopenia of sarcoidosis and renal failure may be due to impaired T-lymphocyte proliferative responses.[129,130] In conditions such as protein-losing enteropathy, lymphocytes may be lost from the body.[131] Severe thermal injury may result in profound T-cell lymphopenia secondary to redistribution of blood T cells to the tissues.[132]

NUTRITIONAL OR DIETARY

Zinc is essential for normal T-cell development and function.[133] Zinc therapy corrects the lymphocytopenia of zinc deficiency, and lymphocytic function also is restored. Excessive intake of ethanol and/or chronic ethanol use may impair lymphocyte proliferative responses. The associated lymphopenia may resolve with abstinence from alcohol.[134]

IDIOPATHIC CD4+ T LYMPHOCYTOPENIA

The advent of immunophenotyping and HIV serologic testing has identified a syndrome of isolated CD4+ T-cell depletion in the absence of evidence for retroviral infection. The syndrome, termed idiopathic CD4+ T lymphocytopenia by the Centers for Disease Control and Prevention in 1993, is defined by a CD4+ T-lymphocyte count of less than 3×10^8/liter (300/μl) on two separate occasions in patients without serologic or virologic evidence of HIV-1 or HIV-2 infection.[135] It is important to exclude congenital immunodeficiency diseases, such as common variable immunodeficiency, that may lead to altered CD4 T-cell counts that are recognized in later life (see Chap. 88).[102,136] The pathogenesis of this disorder is not known, although one study found that the CD4+ T cells from patients with this abnormality were unusually sensitive to programmed cell death induced by T-cell–receptor cross-linking.[137]

Although some patients with idiopathic CD4+ T lymphocytopenia do not have any clinical manifestations,[138–140] over half of all reported cases have had prior opportunistic infections indicative of a cellular immunodeficiency (e.g., recurrent herpes zoster, pulmonary *Mycobacterium avium, Pneumocystis carinii* pneumonia, or cryptococcal osteomyelitis).[141–145] Patients who have such a clinical history are classified by the World Health Organization as having idiopathic CD4+ T lymphocytopenia and severe unexplained HIV-seronegative immune suppression.[102]

The exact proportion of patients with this disorder is unknown, since patients who are not affected clinically by the isolated CD4+ T-cell depletion may not come to medical attention. There are several reports of this abnormality in aged individuals, suggesting that the incidence may be increased in the aged population.[143,146,147] CD4+ T-lymphocytopenic patients with this condition differ from those infected with HIV in that they generally have stable CD4+ counts over time and may manifest reductions in other lymphocyte subgroups.[139,148] Also, patients with this abnormality may have a complete or partial spontaneous reversal in the CD4+ T lymphocytopenia.[139]

REFERENCES

1. Chanarin I, Tidmarsh E, Harrisingh D, Skacel PO: Significance of lymphocytosis in adults. *Lancet* 2:897, 1984.
2. Thommasen HV, Boyko WJ, Montaner JS, Russell JA, Johnson DR, Hogg JC: Absolute lymphocytosis associated with nonsurgical trauma. *Am J Clin Pathol* 86:480, 1986.
3. Francis C, Connelly MC: Rapid single-step method for flow cytometric detection of surface and intracellular antigens using whole blood. *Cytometry* 25:58, 1996.
4. Sun T, Sangaline R, Ryder J, et al: Gating strategy for immunophenotyping of leukemia and lymphoma. *Am J Clin Pathol* 108:152, 1997.
5. Bellido M, Rubiol E, Ubeda J, et al: Rapid and simple immunophenotypic characterization of lymphocytes using a new test. *Haematologica* 83:681, 1998.
6. Crotty PL, Smith BR, Tallini G: Morphologic, immunophenotypic, and molecular evaluation of bone marrow involvement in non-Hodgkin's lymphoma. *Diagn Mol Pathol* 7:90, 1998.
7. Villas BH: Flow cytometry: An overview. *Cell Vision* 5:56, 1998.
8. Schlenke P, Frohn C, Klüter H, et al: Evaluation of a flow cytometric method for simultaneous leukocyte phenotyping and quantification by fluorescent microspheres. *Cytometry* 33:310, 1998.
9. Wells DA, Sale GE, Shulman HM, et al: Multidimensional flow cytometry of marrow can differentiate leukemic from normal lymphoblasts and myeloblasts after chemotherapy and bone marrow transplantation. *Am J Clin Pathol* 110:84, 1998.
10. Kutok JL, Roma AO, Lemire SJ, Dorfman DM: Four-color flow cytometric immunophenotypic determination of peripheral blood CD4+ T-lymphocyte counts: A comparison of validity and cost-effectiveness with a two-color method. *Am J Clin Pathol* 110:465, 1998.
11. Weir EG, Cowan K, LeBeau P, Borowitz MJ: A limited antibody panel

can distinguish B-precursor acute lymphoblastic leukemia from normal B precursors with four color flow cytometry: Implications for residual disease detection. *Leukemia* 13:558, 1999.

12. Rockman SP: Determination of clonality in patients who present with diagnostic dilemmas: A laboratory experience and review of the literature. *Leukemia* 11:852, 1997.

13. Scott CS, Richards SJ, Sivakumaran M, et al: Transient and persistent expansions of large granular lymphocytes (LGL) and NK-associated (NKa) cells: The Yorkshire Leukaemia Group Study. *Br J Haematol* 83:505, 1993.

14. de Pasquale A, Ginaldi L, di Leonardo G, Napoletano C, Quaglino D: Exercise-induced variations of lymphocytosis in the lymphoproliferative disease of large granular lymphocytes [letter]. *Br J Haematol* 82:178, 1992.

15. Kimby E, Mellstedt H, Bjorkholm M, Holm G: Clonal cell surface structures related to differentiation, activation and homing in B-cell chronic lymphocytic leukemia and monoclonal lymphocytosis of undetermined significance. *Eur J Haematol* 43:452, 1989.

16. Garcia C, Rosen A, Kimby E, et al: Higher T-cell imbalance and growth factor receptor expression in B-cell chronic lymphocytic leukemia (B-CLL) as compared to monoclonal B-cell lymphocytosis of undetermined significance (B-MLUS). *Leuk Res* 13:31, 1989.

17. Aman P, Mellstedt H: The leukemic B-cell population of patients with monoclonal lymphocytosis of undetermined significance (MLUS) are functionally distinct from the chronic lymphocytic leukemia (CLL) derived cell population. *Leuk Res* 15:715, 1991.

18. Bassan R, Amaru R, Rambaldi A, Ruggeri M, Borleri GM, Barbui T: The natural history of monoclonal villous lymphocytosis: A chronic lymphoproliferative disorder of CD11c+ B cells. *Leuk Lymph* 21:181, 1996.

19. Ritis K, Tsironidou V, Martinis G, Kartalis G, Sideras P, Bourikas G: Development of CLL in individuals with mild lymphocytosis, without bone marrow infiltration, but with evidence of a monoclonally expanded population in peripheral blood. *Haematologica* 82:184, 1997.

20. Delannoy A, Djian D, Wallef G, et al: Cigarette smoking and chronic polyclonal B-cell lymphocytosis. *Nouv Rev Fr Hematol* 35:141, 1993.

21. Mossafa H, Malaure H, Maynadie M, et al: Persistent polyclonal B lymphocytosis with binucleated lymphocytes: A study of 25 cases. Groupe Français d'Hématologie Cellulaire. *Br J Haematol* 104:486, 1999.

22. Delage R, Roy J, Jacques L, Bernier V, Delâge JM, Darveau A: Multiple bcl-2/Ig gene rearrangements in persistent polyclonal B-cell lymphocytosis. *Br J Haematol* 97:589, 1997.

23. Chan MA, Benedict SH, Carstairs KC, Francombe WH, Gelfand EW: Expansion of B lymphocytes with an unusual immunoglobulin rearrangement associated with atypical lymphocytosis and cigarette smoking. *Am J Respir Cell Mol Biol* 2:549, 1990.

24. Troussard X, Flandrin G: Chronic B-cell lymphocytosis with binucleated lymphocytes (LWBL): A review of 38 cases. *Leuk Lymph* 20:275, 1996.

25. Chow KC, Nacilla JQ, Witzig TE, Li CY: Is persistent polyclonal B lymphocytosis caused by Epstein-Barr virus? A study with polymerase chain reaction and in situ hybridization. *Am J Hematol* 41:270, 1992.

26. Mitterer M, Pescosta N, Fend F, et al: Chronic active Epstein-Barr virus disease in a case of persistent polyclonal B-cell lymphocytosis. *Br J Haematol* 90:526, 1995.

27. Larcher C, Fend F, Mitterer M, Prang N, Schwarzmann F, Huemer HP: Role of Epstein-Barr virus and soluble CD21 in persistent polyclonal B-cell lymphocytosis. *Br J Haematol* 90:532, 1995.

28. Larcher C, McQuain C, Berger C, et al: Epstein-Barr virus–associated persistent polyclonal B-cell lymphocytosis with a distinct 69-base pair deletion in the LMP1 oncogene. *Ann Hematol* 74:23, 1997.

29. Carr R, Fishlock K, Matutes E: Persistent polyclonal B-cell lymphocytosis in identical twins. *Br J Haematol* 96:272, 1997.

30. Machii T, Yamaguchi M, Inoue R, et al: Polyclonal B-cell lymphocytosis with features resembling hairy cell leukemia-Japanese variant. *Blood* 89:2008, 1997.

31. Lush CJ, Vora AJ, Campbell AC, Wood JK: Polyclonal CD5+ B-lymphocytosis resembling chronic lymphocytic leukaemia. *Br J Haematol* 79:119, 1991.

32. Manteiga R, Munoz L, Nomdedéu JF: CD5/CD19/CD23 chronic lymphocytosis [letter]. *Haematologica* 82:510, 1997.

33. Troussard X, Mossafa H, Valensi F, et al: [Polyclonal lymphocytosis with binucleated lymphocytes: Morphological, immunological, cytogenetic and molecular analysis in 15 cases]. *Presse Med* 26:895, 1997.

34. Carstairs KC, Francombe WH, Scott JG, Gelfand EW: Persistent polyclonal lymphocytosis of B lymphocytes, induced by cigarette smoking? [letter]. *Lancet* 1:1094, 1985.

35. Callet-Bauchu E, Renard N, Gazzo S, et al: Distribution of the cytogenetic abnormality +i(3)(q10) in persistent polyclonal B-cell lymphocytosis: A FICTION study in three cases. *Br J Haematol* 99:531, 1997.

36. Granados E, Llamas P, Pinilla I, et al: Persistent polyclonal B lymphocytosis with multiple bcl-2/IgH rearrangements: A benign disorder. *Haematologica* 83:369, 1998.

37. Delage R, Roy J, Jacques L, Darveau A: All patients with persistent polyclonal B cell lymphocytosis present Bcl-2/Ig gene rearrangements. *Leuk Lymph* 31:567, 1998.

38. Roy J, Ryckman C, Bernier V, Whittom R, Delage R: Large cell lymphoma complicating persistent polyclonal B cell lymphocytosis. *Leukemia* 12:1026, 1998.

39. Radossi P, Dazzi F, De Franchis G, et al: Myasthenic syndrome and oligoclonal lymphocytosis: Evolution into chronic lymphocytic leukemia. *Ann Hematol* 76:45, 1998.

40. Brown KA: Nonmalignant disorders of lymphocytes. *Clin Lab Sci* 10:329, 1997.

41. Horwitz MS, Moore GT: Acute infectious lymphocytosis: An etiologic and epidemilogic study of an outbreak. *N Engl J Med* 279:399, 1968.

42. Scalletar HE, Maisel JE, Bramson M: Acute infectious lymphocytosis: Report of an outbreak. *Am J Dis Child* 88:15, 1954.

43. Labalette M, Salez F, Pruvot FR, Noel C, Dessaint JP: CD8 lymphocytosis in primary cytomegalovirus (CMV) infection of allograft recipients: Expansion of an uncommon CD8+ CD57− subset and its progressive replacement by CD8+ CD57+ T cells. *Clin Exp Immunol* 95:465, 1994.

44. Labalette M, Queyrel V, Masy E, Noel C, Pruvot FR, Dessaint JP: Implication of cyclosporine in up-regulation of Bcl-2 expression and maintenance of CD8 lymphocytosis in cytomegalovirus-infected allograft recipients. *Transplantation* 59:1714, 1995.

45. Hertenstein B, Hampl W, Bunjes D, et al: In vivo/ex vivo T cell depletion for GVHD prophylaxis influences onset and course of active cytomegalovirus infection and disease after BMT. *Bone Marrow Transplant* 15:387, 1995.

46. Kunno A, Abe M, Yamada M, Murakami K: Clinical and histological features of cytomegalovirus hepatitis in previously healthy adults. *Liver* 17:129, 1997.

47. Arnez M, Cizman M, Jazbec J, Kotnik A: Acute infectious lymphocytosis caused by coxsackievirus B2. *Pediatr Infect Dis J* 15:1127, 1996.

48. Sijpkens YW, de Knegt RJ, van der Werf SD: Unusual presentation of acquired toxoplasmosis in an immunocompetent adult. *Netherlands J Med* 45:174, 1994.

49. Cunha BA, Bohoan JT, Schlossberg D: Atypical lymphocytes in acute malaria [letter]. *Arch Intern Med* 157:1140, 1997.

50. Kubic VL, Kubic PT, Brunning RD: The morphologic and immunophenotypic assessment of the lymphocytosis accompanying *Bordetella pertussis* infection. *Am J Clin Pathol* 95:809, 1991.

51. De Martino M, Rossi ME, Muccioli AT, Ulivelli A, Vierucci A: Preferential increase of a T-cell subset as a cause of lymphocytosis in children with whooping cough. *Boll Ist Sieroter Milan.* 63:479, 1984.

52. Person PL, Korngold R, Teuscher C: Pertussis toxin-induced lymphocytosis is associated with alterations in thymocyte subpopulations. *J Immunol* 148:1506, 1992.

53. Verschueren H, Dewit J, Van der Wegen A, et al: The lymphocytosis promoting action of pertussis toxin can be mimicked in vitro: Holotoxin but not the B subunit inhibits invasion of human T lymphoma cells through fibroblast monolayers. *J Immunol Methods* 144:231, 1991.

54. Passador L, Iglewski W: ADP-ribosylating toxins. *Methods Enzymol* 235:617, 1994.

55. Burnette WN: AB5 ADP-ribosylating toxins: Comparative anatomy and physiology. *Structure* 2:151, 1994.

56. Suzuki G, Sawa H, Kobayashi Y, et al: Pertussis toxin–sensitive signal controls the trafficking of thymocytes across the corticomedullary junction in the thymus. *J Immunol* 162:5981, 1999.

57. Witvliet MH, Vogel ML, Wiertz EJ, Poolman JT: Interaction of pertussis toxin with human T lymphocytes. *Infect Immun* 60:5085, 1992.

58. Pinkerton PH, McLellan BA, Quantz MC, Robinson JB: Acute lympho-

cytosis after trauma: Early recognition of the high-risk patient? *J Trauma* 29:749, 1989.

59. Teggatz JR, Parkin J, Peterson L: Transient atypical lymphocytosis in patients with emergency medical conditions. *Arch Pathol Lab Med* 111:712, 1987.

60. Toft P, Tonnesen E, Svendsen P, Rasmussen JW, Christensen NJ: The redistribution of lymphocytes during adrenaline infusion: An in vivo study with radiolabelled cells. *APMIS* 100:593, 1992.

61. Tonnesen E, Hohndorf K, Lerbjerg G, Christensen NJ, Huttel MS, Andersen K: Immunological and hormonal responses to lung surgery during one-lung ventilation. *Eur J Anaesthesiol* 10:189, 1993.

62. Mills PJ, Berry CC, Dimsdale JE, Ziegler MG, Nelesen RA, Kennedy BP: Lymphocyte subset redistribution in response to acute experimental stress: Effects of gender, ethnicity, hypertension, and the sympathetic nervous system. *Brain Behav Immun* 9:61, 1995.

63. Benschop RJ, Rodriguez-Feuerhahn M, Schedlowski M: Catecholamine-induced leukocytosis: Early observations, current research, and future directions. *Brain Behav Immun* 10:77, 1996.

64. Juneja S, Januszewicz E, Wolf M, Cooper I: Post-splenectomy lymphocytosis. *Clin Lab Haematol* 17:335, 1995.

65. Domingo P, Fuster M, Muñiz-Diaz E, Ris J, Barrio JL: Spurious postsplenectomy CD4 and CD8 lymphocytosis in HIV-infected patients [letter]. *AIDS* 10:106, 1996.

66. Saway PA, Prasthofer EF, Barton JC: Prevalence of granular lymphocyte proliferation in patients with rheumatoid arthritis and neutropenia. *Am J Med* 86:303, 1989.

67. Stanworth SJ, Green L, Pumphrey RS, Swinson DR, Bhavnani M: An unusual association of Felty syndrome and TCR gamma delta lymphocytosis. *J Clin Pathol* 49:351, 1996.

68. Grossi A, Nozzoli C, Gheri R, et al: Pure red cell aplasia in autoimmune polyglandular syndrome with T lymphocytosis [letter]. *Haematologica* 83:1043, 1998.

69. Garcia-Suarez J, Prieto A, Reyes E, et al: Persistent lymphocytosis of natural killer cells in autoimmune thrombocytopenic purpura (ATP) patients after splenectomy. *Br J Haematol* 89:653, 1995.

70. Tefferi A, Li CY, Phyliky RL: Role of immunotyping in chronic lymphocytosis: Review of the natural history of the condition in 145 adult patients. *Mayo Clin Proc* 63:801, 1988.

71. Medeiros LJ, Bhagat SK, Naylor P, Fowler D, Jaffe ES, Stetler-Stevenson M: Malignant thymoma associated with T-cell lymphocytosis: A case report with immunophenotypic and gene rearrangement analysis. *Arch Pathol Lab Med* 117:279, 1993.

72. Doll DC, Landreneau RJ, List AF: Malignant thymoma associated with peripheral T-cell lymphocytosis. *Med Pediatr Oncol* 19:496, 1991.

73. Lishner M, Ravid M, Shapira J, et al: Delta-T-lymphocytosis in a patient with thymoma. *Cancer* 74:2924, 1994.

74. Smith GP, Perkins SL, Segal GH, Kjeldsberg CR: T-cell lymphocytosis associated with invasive thymomas. *Am J Clin Pathol* 102:447, 1994.

75. Cranney A, Markman S, Lach B, Karsh J: Polymyositis in a patient with thymoma and T cell lymphocytosis. *J Rheumatol* 24:1413, 1997.

76. Rosenthal NS, Farhi DC: Reactive plasmacytosis and lymphocytosis in acute myeloid leukemia. *Hematol Pathol* 8:43, 1994.

77. Quantz MC, Robinson JB, Sachs V, Pinkerton PH: Lymphocyte surface marker studies in the diagnosis of unexplained lymphocytosis. *Can Med Assoc J* 136:835, 1987.

78. Inbal A, Avidor I, Nemesh L, Shaklai M: Persistent lymphocytosis: An unusual feature in sarcoidosis. *Acta Haematol.* 74:184, 1985.

79. Tollerud DJ, Clark JW, Brown LM, et al: The effects of cigarette smoking on T cell subsets: A population-based survey of healthy caucasians. *Am Rev Respir Dis* 139:1446, 1989.

80. Tokura Y, Tamura Y, Takigawa M, et al: Severe hypersensitivity to mosquito bites associated with natural killer cell lymphocytosis. *Arch Dermatol* 126:362, 1990.

81. Sakai C, Takagi T, Oguro M, Tanabe N, Wakatsuki S: Erythroderma and marked atypical lymphocytosis mimicking cutaneous T-cell lymphoma probably caused by phenobarbital. *Intern Med* 32:182, 1993.

82. Berliner N: T gamma lymphocytosis and T cell chronic leukemias. *Hematol Oncol Clin North Am* 4:473, 1990.

83. Kimby E, Mellstedt H, Nilsson B, Bjorkholm M, Holm G: Differences in blood T and NK cell populations between chronic lymphocytic leukemia of B cell type (B-CLL) and monoclonal B-lymphocytosis of undetermined significance (B-MLUS). *Leukemia* 3:501, 1989.

84. Perreault C, Boileau J, Gyger M, et al: Chronic B-cell lymphocytosis. *Eur J Haematol* 42:361, 1989.

85. Itescu S: Diffuse infiltrative lymphocytosis syndrome in children and adults infected with A model of rheumatic illness caused by acquired viral infection. *Am J Reprod Immunol* 28:247, 1992.

86. Itescu S, Brancato LJ, Buxbaum J, et al: A diffuse infiltrative CD8 lymphocytosis syndrome in human immunodeficiency virus (HIV) infection: A host immune response associated with HLA-DR5. *Ann Intern Med* 112:3, 1990.

87. Zambello R, Trentin L, Agostini C, et al: Persistent polyclonal lymphocytosis in human immunodeficiency virus-1-infected patients. *Blood* 81:3015, 1993.

88. Itescu S, Dalton J, Zhang HZ, Winchester R: Tissue infiltration in a CD8 lymphocytosis syndrome associated with human immunodeficiency virus-1 infection has the phenotypic appearance of an antigenically driven response. *J Clin Invest* 91:2216, 1993.

89. Bachmeyer C, Dhôte R, Blanche P, Tulliez M, Sicard D, Christoforov B: Diffuse infiltrative CD8 lymphocytosis syndrome with predominant neurologic manifestations in two HIV-infected patients responding to zidovudine [letter]. *AIDS* 9:1101, 1995.

90. Scharko AM, Graziano FM, Malkovsky M, Pauza CD, Wallace M: Persistent non-B cell lymphocytosis in HIV-infected individuals [letter]. *Immunol Lett* 48:157, 1995.

91. Kazi S, Cohen PR, Williams F, Schempp R, Reveille JD: The diffuse infiltrative lymphocytosis syndrome. Clinical and immunogenetic features in 35 patients. *AIDS* 10:385, 1996.

92. Williams FM, Cohen PR, Jumshyd J, Reveille JD: Prevalence of the diffuse infiltrative lymphocytosis syndrome among human immunodeficiency virus type 1-positive outpatients. *Arthritis Rheum* 41:863, 1998.

93. Smith JG, Smith MA, James I, Blundell E, Maddison PJ: Inhibition of CFU-GM by prostaglandins in a case of chronic T-cell lymphocytosis and neutropenia. *Br J Haematol* 73:148, 1989.

94. Tollerud DJ, Brown LM, Blattner WA, Mann DL, Pankiw-Trost L, Hoover RN: T cell subsets in healthy black smokers and nonsmokers: Evidence for ethnic group as an important response modifier. *Am Rev Respir Dis* 144:612, 1991.

95. Wilkinson LS, Tang A, Gjedsted A: Marked lymphocytosis suggesting chronic lymphocytic leukemia in three patients with hyposplenism. *Am J Med* 75:1053, 1983.

96. Landmann RM, Muller FB, Perini C, Wesp M, Erne P, Buhler FR: Changes of immunoregulatory cells induced by psychological and physical stress: Relationship to plasma catecholamines. *Clin Exp Immunol* 58:127, 1984.

97. Tiberghien P, Racadot E, Deschaseaux ML, et al: Interleukin-2-induced increase of a monoclonal B-cell lymphocytosis: A novel in vivo interleukin-2 effect? *Cancer* 69:2583, 1992.

98. Higa K, Hirata K, Dan K: Mexiletine-induced severe skin eruption, fever, eosinophilia, atypical lymphocytosis, and liver dysfunction. *Pain* 73:97, 1997.

99. Groom DA, Kunkel LA, Brynes RK, Parker JW, Johnson CS, Endres D: Transient stress lymphocytosis during crisis of sickle cell anemia and emergency trauma and medical conditions: An immunophenotyping study. *Arch Pathol Lab Med* 114:570, 1990.

100. Miale JB: *Laboratory Medicine*, vol 15, *Hematology*, 6th ed. Mosby, St Louis, 1982.

101. Hancock BW, Dunsmore IR, Swan HT: Lymphopenia: A bad prognostic factor in Hodgkin's disease. *Scand J Haematol* 29:193, 1982.

102. Laurence J: T-cell subsets in health, infectious disease, and idiopathic CD4+ T lymphocytopenia. *Ann Intern Med* 119:55, 1993.

103. Castelino DJ, McNair P, Kay TW: Lymphocytopenia in a hospital population: What does it signify? *Aust NZ J Med* 27:170, 1997.

104. Molina JM, Kenney DM, Rosen FS, Remold-O'Donnell E: T cell lines characterize events in the pathogenesis of the Wiskott-Aldrich syndrome. *J Exp Med* 176:867, 1992.

105. Phillips AN: CD4 lymphocyte depletion prior to the development of AIDS [editorial]. *AIDS* 6:735, 1992.

106. Maury CP, Lahdevirta J: Correlation of serum cytokine levels with haematological abnormalities in human immunodeficiency virus infection. *J Intern Med* 227:253, 1990.

107. Stricker K, Knipping E, Böhler T, Benner A, Krammer PH, Debatin KM: Anti-CD95 (APO-1/Fas) autoantibodies and T cell depletion in

human immunodeficiency virus type 1 (HIV-1)-infected children. *Cell Death Differ* 5:222, 1998.

108. Jaworowski A, Crowe SM: Does HIV cause depletion of CD4+ T cells in vivo by the induction of apoptosis? *Immunol Cell Biol* 77:90, 1999.

109. Daniel V, Melk A, Süsal C, et al: CD4 depletion in HIV-infected haemophilia patients is associated with rapid clearance of immune complex-coated CD4+ lymphocytes. *Clin Exp Immunol* 115:477, 1999.

110. Pilheu JA, De Salvo MC, Gonzalez J, Rey D, Elias MC, Ruppi MC: CD4+ T-lymphocytopenia in severe pulmonary tuberculosis without evidence of human immunodeficiency virus infection. *Int J Tuberc Lung Dis* 1:422, 1997.

111. Van Campen H, Easterday BC, Hinshaw VS: Destruction of lymphocytes by a virulent avian influenza A virus. *J Gen Virol* 70:467, 1989.

112. Bast RCJ, Reinherz EL, Maver C, Lavin P, Schlossman SF: Contrasting effects of cyclophosphamide and prednisolone on the phenotype of human peripheral blood leukocytes. *Clin Immunol Immunopathol* 28:101, 1983.

113. Petrini B, Wasserman J, Rotstein S, Blomgren H: Radiotherapy and persistent reduction of peripheral T cells. *J Clin Lab Immunol* 11:159, 1983.

114. Calabresi P, Chabner BA: Chemotherapy of neoplastic diseases, in *The Pharmacological Basis of Therapeutics*, 8th ed, edited by AG Gilman, TW Rall, AS Nies, P Taylor, p 1202. Pergamon, New York, 1990.

115. Handschumacher RE: Immunosuppressive agents, in *The Pharmacological Basis of Therapeutics*, 8th ed, edited by AG Gilman, TW Rall, AS Nies, P Taylor, p 1264. Pergamon, New York, 1990.

116. de Planque MM, Brand A, Kluin-Nelemans HC, et al: Haematopoietic and immunologic abnormalities in severe aplastic anaemia patients treated with anti-thymocyte globulin. *Br J Haematol* 71:421, 1989.

117. Borroni G, Zaccone C, Vignati G, et al: Lymphopenia and decrease in the total number of circulating CD3+ and CD4+ T cells during "long-term" PUVA treatment for psoriasis. *Dermatologica* 183:10, 1991.

118. Bloemena E, Weinreich S, Schellekens PT: The influence of prednisolone on the recirculation of peripheral blood lymphocytes in vivo. *Clin Exp Immunol* 80:460, 1990.

119. Bloemena E, Koopmans RP, Weinreich S, Van Boxtel CJ, Schellekens PT: Pharmacodynamic modeling of lymphocytopenia and whole blood lymphocyte cultures in prednisolone-treated individuals. *Clin Immunol Immunopathol* 57:374, 1990.

120. Braat MC, Oosterhuis B, Koopmans RP, Meewis JM, Van Boxtel CJ: Kinetic-dynamic modeling of lymphocytopenia induced by the combined action of dexamethasone and hydrocortisone in humans, after inhalation and intravenous administration of dexamethasone. *J Pharmacol Exp Ther* 262:509, 1992.

121. Jakobsen BW, Pedersen J, Egeberg BB: Postoperative lymphocytopenia and leucocytosis after epidural and general anaesthesia. *Acta Anaesthesiol Scand* 30:668, 1986.

122. Platt MP, Lovat PE, Watson JG, Aynsley-Green A: The effects of anesthesia and surgery on lymphocyte populations and function in infants and children. *J Pediatr Surg* 24:884, 1989.

123. Hauser GJ, Chan MM, Casey WF, Midgley FM, Holbrook PR: Immune dysfunction in children after corrective surgery for congenital heart disease. *Crit Care Med* 19:874, 1991.

124. Ueo T, Tanaka S, Tominaga Y, Ogawa H, Sakurami T: The effect of thoracic duct drainage on lymphocyte dynamics and clinical symptoms in patients with rheumatoid arthritis. *Arthritis Rheum* 22:1405, 1979.

125. Prior CR, Coghlan PJ, Hall JM, Jacobs P: In vitro study of immunologic changes in long-term cytapheresis donors. *J Clin Apheresis* 6:69, 1991.

126. Martin-Suarez I, D'Cruz D, Mansoor M, Fernandes AP, Khamashta MA, Hughes GR: Immunosuppressive treatment in severe connective tissue diseases: effects of low dose intravenous cyclophosphamide. *Ann Rheum Dis* 56:481, 1997.

127. Harley JB, Sestak AL, Willis LG, Fu SM, Hansen JA, Reichlin M: A model for disease heterogeneity in systemic lupus erythematosus: Relationships between histocompatibility antigens, autoantibodies, and lymphopenia or renal disease. *Arthritis Rheum* 32:826, 1989.

128. Noguchi M, Iwamori M, Hirano T, et al: Autoantibodies to T and B cell lines detected in serum samples from patients with systemic lupus erythematosus with lymphopenia and hypocomplementaemia. *Ann Rheum Dis* 51:713, 1992.

129. Daniele RP, Dauber JH, Rossman MD: Immunologic abnormalities in sarcoidosis. *Ann Intern Med* 92:406, 1980.

130. Goldblum SE, Reed WP: Host defenses and immunologic alterations associated with chronic hemodialysis. *Ann Intern Med* 93:597, 1980.

131. Perrick D, Guill MF, Clark J: Chronic abdominal pain, lymphopenia, and hypogammaglobulinemia in a 9-year-old female. *Ann Allergy* 62:287, 1989.

132. Maldonado MD, Venturoli A, Franco A, Nunez-Roldan A: Specific changes in peripheral blood lymphocyte phenotype from burn patients: Probable origin of the thermal injury-related lymphocytopenia. *Burns* 17:188, 1991.

133. Prasad AS: Discovery and importance of zinc in human nutrition. *Fed Proc* 43:2829, 1984.

134. Tonnesen H, Andersen JR, Pedersen AE, Kaiser AH: Lymphopenia in heavy drinkers: Reversibility and relation to the duration of drinking episodes. *Ann Med* 22:229, 1990.

135. Smith DK, Neal JJ, Holmberg SD: Unexplained opportunistic infections and CD4+ T-lymphocytopenia without HIV infection: An investigation of cases in the United States. The Centers for Disease Control Idiopathic CD4+ T-lymphocytopenia Task Force. *N Engl J Med* 328:373, 1993.

136. al-Attas RA, Rahi AH, Ahmed el FE: Common variable immunodeficiency with CD4+ T lymphocytopenia and overproduction of soluble IL-2 receptor associated with Turner's syndrome and dorsal kyphoscoliosis. *J Clin Pathol* 50:876, 1997.

137. Laurence J, Mitra D, Steiner M, Lynch DH, Siegal FP, Staiano-Coico L: Apoptotic depletion of CD4+ T cells in idiopathic CD4+ T lymphocytopenia. *J Clin Invest* 97:672, 1996.

138. Spira TJ, Jones BM, Nicholson JK, et al: Idiopathic CD4+ T-lymphocytopenia: An analysis of five patients with unexplained opportunistic infections. *N Engl J Med* 328:386, 1993.

139. Ho DD, Cao Y, Zhu T, et al: Idiopathic CD4+ T-lymphocytopenia: Immunodeficiency without evidence of HIV infection. *N Engl J Med* 328:380, 1993.

140. Cascio G, Massobrio AM, Cascio B, Anania A: Undefined CD4 lymphocytopenia without clinical complications: A report of two cases. *Panminerva Med* 40:69, 1998.

141. Sinicco A, Maiello A, Raiteri R, et al: *Pneumocystis carinii* in a patient with pulmonary sarcoidosis and idiopathic CD4+ T lymphocytopenia. *Thorax* 51:446, 1996.

142. Manchado Lopez P, Ruiz de Morales JM, Ruiz González I, Rodriguez Prieto MA: Cutaneous infections by papillomavirus, herpes zoster and *Candida albicans* as the only manifestation of idiopathic CD4+ T lymphocytopenia. *Int J Dermatol* 38:119, 1999.

143. Matsuyama W, Tsurukawa T, Iwami F, et al: Two cases of idiopathic CD4+ T-lymphocytopenia in elderly patients. *Intern Med* 37:891, 1998.

144. Ishida T, Hashimoto T, Arita M, Ito I, Osawa M: Pulmonary *Mycobacterium avium* disease in a young patient with idiopathic CD4+ T lymphocytopenia. *Intern Med* 37:622, 1998.

145. Kumlin U, Elmqvist LG, Granlund M, Olsen B, Tärnvik A: CD4 lymphopenia in a patient with cryptococcal osteomyelitis. *Scand J Infect Dis* 29:205, 1997.

146. Belmin J, Ortega MN, Bruhat A, Mercadier A, Valensi P: CD4 lymphopenia in very elderly people [letter]. *Lancet* 347:328, 1996.

147. McBride M: CD4 lymphopenia in elderly patients [letter, comment]. *Lancet* 347:911, 1996.

148. Duncan RA, von Reyn CF, Alliegro GM, Toossi Z, Sugar AM, Levitz SM: Idiopathic CD4+ T-lymphocytopenia: Four patients with opportunistic infections and no evidence of HIV infection. *N Engl J Med* 328:393, 1993.

149. Gelfand EW, Dosch HM: Diagnosis and classification of severe combined immunodeficiency disease. *Birth Defects* 19:65, 1983.

150. Parkman R, Gelfand EW, Rosen FS, Sanderson A, Hirschhorn R: Severe combined immunodeficiency and adenosine deaminase deficiency. *N Engl J Med* 292:714, 1975.

151. Touraine JL, Betuel H, Souillet G, Jeune M: Combined immunodeficiency disease associated with absence of cell-surface HLA-A and -B antigens. *J Pediatr* 93:47, 1978.

152. Edwards KM, Cooper MD, Lawton AR, Sanders DS, Wright PF: Severe combined immunodeficiency associated with absent T4+ helper cells. *J Pediatr* 105:70, 1984.

153. Freier S, Kerem E, Dranitzki Z, et al: Hereditary CD4+ T lymphocytopenia. *Arch Dis Child* 78:371, 1998.

154. Gitlin D, Vawter G, Craig JM: Thymic alymphoplasia and congenital aleukocytosis. *Pediatrics* 33:184, 1964.

155. Datta U, Sehgal S, Kumar L, et al: Immune status in ataxia telangiectasia. *Indian J Med Res* 94:252, 1991.

156. Cooper MD, Chae HP, Lowman JT, Krivit W, Good RA: Wiskott-Aldrich syndrome: An immunologic deficiency disease involving the afferent limb of immunity. *Am J Med* 44:499, 1968.

157. Lux SE, Johnston RBJ, August CS, et al: Chronic neutropenia and abnormal cellular immunity in cartilage-hair hypoplasia. *N Engl J Med* 282:231, 1970.

158. Pierce GF, Polmar SH: Lymphocyte dysfunction in cartilage hair hypoplasia: II. Evidence for a cell cycle specific defect in T cell growth. *Clin Exp Immunol* 50:621, 1982.

159. Korn D, Gelderman A, Cage G, Nathanson D, Strauss AJ: Immune deficiencies, aplastic anemia and abnormalities of lymphoid tissue in thymoma. *N Engl J Med* 276:1333, 1967.

160. Rich KC, Arnold WJ, Palella T, Fox IH: Cellular immune deficiency with autoimmune hemolytic anemia in purine nucleoside phosphorylase deficiency. *Am J Med* 67:172, 1979.

161. Etzioni A, Benderly A, Rosenthal E, et al: Defective humoral and cellular immune functions associated with veno-occlusive disease of the liver. *J Pediatr* 110:549, 1987.

162. Sabbe LJ, Haak HL, Te Velde J, et al: Immunological investigations in aplastic anemia patients. *Acta Haematol* 71:178, 1984.

163. Mazzucchelli I, Vezzoli M, Ottini E, Paulli M, Boveri E, Mazzone A: A complex immunodeficiency: Idiopathic CD4+ T-lymphocytopenia and hypogammaglobulinemia associated with HHV8 infection, Kaposi's sarcoma and gastric cancer [letter]. *Haematologica* 84:378, 1999.

164. García-Silva J, Almagro M, Peña C, et al: CD4+ T-lymphocytopenia, Kaposi's sarcoma, HHV-8 infection, severe seborrheic dermatitis, and onychomycosis in a homosexual man without HIV infection [letter]. *Int J Dermatol* 38:231, 1999.

165. Iwase T, Ojika K, Katada E, et al: An unusual course of progressive multifocal leukoencephalopathy in a patient with idiopathic CD+ T lymphocytopenia. *J Neurol Neurosurg Psychiatry* 64:788, 1998.

166. Abdool Gaffar MS, Seedat YK, Coovadia YM, Khan Q: The white cell count in typhoid fever. *Trop Geogr Med* 44:23, 1992.

167. Ducloux D, Carron PL, Racadot E, et al: CD4 lymphocytopenia in long-term renal transplant recipients. *Transplant Proc* 30:2859, 1998.

168. Symmons DP, Farr M, Salmon M, Bacon PA: Lymphopenia in rheumatoid arthritis. *J R Soc Med* 82:462, 1989.

169. Davis S, Schumacher MJ: Myasthenia gravis and lymphoma: A clinical and immunological association. *JAMA* 242:2096, 1979.

170. Bordin G, Ballaré M, Paglino S, et al: Idiopathic CD4+ lymphocytopenia and systemic vasculitis. *J Intern Med* 240:37, 1996.

171. Venzor J, Hua Q, Bressler RB, Miranda CH, Huston DP: Behçet's-like syndrome associated with idiopathic CD4+ T-lymphocytopenia, opportunistic infections, and a large population of TCR alpha beta+ CD4− CD8− T cells. *Am J Med Sci* 313:236, 1997.

172. Rijnders RJ, van den Ende IE, Huikeshoven FJ: Suspected idiopathic CD4+ T-lymphocytopenia in a young patient with vulvar carcinoma stage IV. *Gynecol Oncol* 61:423, 1996.

IMMUNODEFICIENCY DISEASES

FRED S. ROSEN

The primary immunodeficiency diseases are informative about the normal functioning of the immune system. Defects in B lymphocytes lead to immunoglobulin deficiencies, which render patients susceptible to pyogenic infections. Defects in T lymphocytes lead to deficiencies in cell-mediated immunity, which render patients susceptible to opportunistic infections. Serious T cell deficiencies are life threatening and require bone marrow transplantation as the optimal therapeutic procedure, whereas the consequences of B cell deficiencies can by and large be clinically controlled with intravenous infusions of gamma globulin.

The immunodeficiency diseases are characterized by a decreased capacity to mount an immune defense against foreign antigens. The specific humoral or cellular defects of these diseases are listed in Table 88-1, and the modes of transmission, basic defects, types of infection that occur, and prognoses are summarized in Table 88-2.

X-LINKED AGAMMAGLOBULINEMIA

DEFINITION AND HISTORY

In 1952 Bruton reported the remarkable finding of the absence of γ-globulin from the serum of an 8-year-old boy who had been well up to the age of 4 years, when septic arthritis of the left knee developed. During the next 4 years, the boy had 19 episodes of pneumococcal sepsis, repeated attacks of otitis media, and two bouts of pneumococcal pneumonia. Although these illnesses were successfully treated with antibiotics, immunization with polyvalent pneumococcal vaccines was not protective and did not lead to the appearance of serum antibodies. Further investigation demonstrated that he was unable to produce antibodies after typhoid vaccination, and a Schick test remained positive after attempted diphtheria immunization. Electrophoresis of the serum revealed normal levels of albumin and α- and β-globulins, but no γ-globulin. When given intramuscular injections of γ-globulin, the patient remained well.[1]

ETIOLOGY AND PATHOGENESIS

The study of kindred with multiple occurrences of agammaglobulinemia has shown that it is inherited as an X-linked recessive trait. In most cases no B cells are present in the blood, marrow, or lymph nodes. T-cell function is normal. Blood T lymphocytes of agammaglobulinemic children respond normally to phytohemagglutinin and to antigenic and allogenic stimuli.[2] Homograft rejection is intact in the few agammaglobulinemic patients who have been studied. Normally,

Acronyms and abbreviations that appear in this chapter include: ADA, adenosine deaminase; ATM, ataxia telangiectasia mutated; CVID, common variable, unclassifiable immunodeficiency; DNFB, dinitrofluorobenzene; DPT, diphtheria-pertussis-tetanus; GM-CSF, granulocyte-monocyte colony stimulating factor; MHC, major histocompatibility complex; NP, nucleoside phosphorylase; SCID, severe combined immunodeficiency.

delayed hypersensitivity reactions of both the tuberculin and the skin-contact type can be elicited.

The gene for X-linked agammaglobulinemia has been mapped to Xq21.3-22.[3] In this region a gene encoding a unique tyrosine kinase of the *src* oncogene family, called *btk*, is mutated in affected males. The product of this gene appears to be critical for normal calcium flux in maturing pre-B cells.[4,5]

CLINICAL FEATURES

Male infants with X-linked agammaglobulinemia usually remain well during the first 9 months of life, probably because of the passive protection afforded by maternal γ-globulin. Undue susceptibility to infection gradually develops during the second year of life, but the onset of frequent infections may depend on the environment of the child and the presence of older sibs and social contacts. Almost invariably these children contract infections from the pyogenic organisms, principally staphylococci, pneumococci, streptococci, and *Haemophilus influenzae*. Purulent sinusitis, pneumonia, bacteremia, meningitis, and furunculosis are most common. These types of infection usually can be controlled with antimicrobial chemotherapy, but they recur persistently until proper prophylactic therapy is undertaken.

Agammaglobulinemic children do not have increased susceptibility to the common viral diseases and exanthems of childhood. They usually overcome measles, mumps, varicella, and rubella in an ordinary fashion. When vaccinated with vaccinia virus, they generally exhibit the usual course of a primary take. They have no unusual infections with enterococci or gram-negative bacilli, nor do they have undue susceptibility to mycotic infections.

One-third to one-half of all patients with agammaglobulinemia develop a disease of the large joints that resembles rheumatoid arthritis. The joint disease may develop before susceptibility to infection leads to the establishment of the diagnosis. Joint complications disappear once replacement therapy with γ-globulin is initiated.

Other collagen-vascular diseases have been observed in children with agammaglobulinemia. One of the most distressing (and ultimately fatal) is a syndrome resembling dermatomyositis. Edema, ligneous induration of the muscles, weakness, and rash over the extensor surfaces of the joints are the salient features of this complication. Biopsy and autopsy materials show lymphorrhages around the small blood vessels. Similar involvement of the central nervous system has been observed, producing a progressive and eventually fatal neurologic disease. The disease is fatal despite the use of glucocorticoids and antimetabolite therapy. Echovirus has been persistently cultured from the cerebrospinal fluid of several of these patients.[6] High-dose intravenous γ-globulin has been effective in controlling symptoms and halting progression of this complication.

Hemolytic anemia, drug eruptions, atopic eczema, poison ivy sensitivity, allergic rhinitis, and asthma occur frequently in agammaglobulinemic patients. Wheal-and-flare reactions cannot be elicited.

LABORATORY FEATURES

The serum contains less than 100 mg/dl of IgG. Other serum immunoglobulins, IgA, IgM, IgD, and IgE, are undetectable. Isohemagglutinin is lacking or at a low level. Immunization can be used to demonstrate the basic defect. Stimulation with diphtheria-pertussis-tetanus (DPT) or with any number of other antigens fails to elicit an antibody response. Other serum constituents involved in resistance to infection are normal. Serum complement, lysozyme, and properdin levels; phagocytosis; and interferon synthesis are within normal limits.

The basic deficiency in the disease is an absence of B cells and plasma cells from the lymph nodes, spleen, intestine, blood, and marrow. Moreover, plasma cells do not appear in lymph nodes that

TABLE 88-1   CONCENTRATION OF SERUM IMMUNOGLOBULIN AND BLOOD T AND B LYMPHOCYTES IN THE IMMUNODEFICIENCY DISEASES

	IgG	IgA	IgM	B Cells*	T Cells†
X-linked agammaglobulinemia	Decrease	Decrease	Decrease	Decrease	Normal
Hyper-IgM immunodeficiency	Decrease	Decrease	Increase	Normal	Normal
Selective IgA deficiency	Normal	Decrease	Normal	Normal	Normal
Selective IgG subclass deficiency	Decrease	Normal	Normal	Normal	Normal
Transient hypogammaglobulinemia	Decrease	Decrease	Normal	Normal	Decrease
Common variable agammaglobulinemia	Decrease	Decrease	Decrease	Normal or decrease	Normal or decrease
Severe combined immunodeficiency	Decrease	Decrease	Decrease	Normal or decrease	Decrease
Hereditary ataxia-telangiectasia	Normal	Decrease	Normal	Normal	Decrease
Congenital thymic aplasia	Decrease or normal	Normal	Normal	Normal	Decrease
Wiskott-Aldrich syndrome	Normal	Increase	Decrease	Normal	Decrease
MHC class II deficiency	Decrease	Decrease	Normal	Normal	Normal or Decrease

*As enumerated by surface Ig staining.

†As enumerated by E-rosetting or by mitogenic response to phytohemagglutinin.

NOTE: *Increased*, increased elevated concentration of immunoglobulin or increased number of cells in the blood; *decreased*, decreased concentration of immunoglobulin or decreased number of cells in the blood; *normal*, normal concentration of immunoglobulin or normal number of cells in the blood.

are stimulated with antigen. There are no normal lymph node follicles, but the thymus is normal.

THERAPY, COURSE, AND PROGNOSIS

Periodic intravenous administration of immune serum globulin is effective in preventing the severe recurrent pyogenic infections that affect these males. The optimal therapeutic dose must be determined in each case and usually is at least 400 mg/kg per month. It is best administered at more frequent intervals, divided into weekly or biweekly injections. Appropriate antibiotic therapy should be given for intercurrent infections. With this regimen of therapy the prognosis is excellent.

Inadequate treatment with immune serum globulin (γ-globulin) results in chronic progressive bronchiectasis, as a result of repeated pulmonary infections, and ultimately in death from respiratory failure. The central nervous system infections with echovirus, resulting in the dermatomyositis-like syndrome (see above), also can be controlled with high-dose intravenous γ-globulin. Various products should be screened for relevant antibody to the infecting virus.

THE SELECTIVE IMMUNOGLOBULIN DEFICIENCIES

DEFINITION AND HISTORY

The advent of immunoelectrophoretic techniques led to a more precise definition of immunoglobulin defects that involve deficiencies in only one or two of the immunoglobulin classes. Although there are six possible combinations of deficiencies involving one or more of the three major serum immunoglobulin classes, only two have been reported repeatedly. It has been estimated that about 1 in 200 random hospital admissions has some form of selective immunoglobulin deficiency.[7]

ABSENCE OF IgA AND IgG WITH NORMAL OR ELEVATED IgM

One of the common partial immunoglobulin abnormalities is a deficiency of IgA and IgG with an increased or normal amount of IgM in the serum,[8] commonly called the *hyper-IgM syndrome* or *hyper-IgM immunodeficiency*. IgM levels in this entity range from 150 to 1000 mg/dl, but in spite of the enormous elevation in IgM level, monoclonal components are not present. Also, the distribution of κ and λ light chains in the IgM appears to be normal. Some, but not all, of these patients have an elevated level of serum IgD and IgM subunits. Both hereditary and acquired forms of this defect have been observed. In addition to their undue susceptibility to pyogenic infection, and *Pneumocystis carinii* pneumonia, many of these patients develop thrombocytopenia, neutropenia, renal lesions, and aplastic or hemolytic anemia.[9] Optimal treatment includes immune serum globulin replacement, as in patients with X-linked agammaglobulinemia, and GM-CSF for neutropenia.

The X-linked form of hyper-IgM immunodeficiency is due to a genetic defect in the CD40 ligand,[10–13] a type II membrane glycoprotein expressed on activated T cells. In order for B lymphocytes to undergo

TABLE 88-2   INHERITANCE AND PATHOGENESIS OF PRIMARY IMMUNODEFICIENCIES

SYNDROME	INHERITANCE	BASIC DEFECT	TYPES OF INFECTION	PROGNOSIS
X-linked agammaglobulinemia	X-linked	Mutation of tyrosine kinase (*btk*) at Xq22	Pyogenic	Good
Hyper-IgM immunodeficiency	X-linked (70% of cases); autosomal recessive	Mutation of CD40 ligand unknown	Pyogenic; *Pneumocystis carinii*	Guarded
Selective IgA deficiency	Not known	Not known	Pyogenic	Good
Selective IgG subclass deficiency	Not known	Not known	Pyogenic	Good
Transient hypogammaglobulinemia of infancy	Not known	Not known	Pyogenic	Good
Common variable immunodeficiency	Not known	Not known	Pyogenic	Good
Severe combined immunodeficiency	X-linked or autosomal recessive	Defect in IL-2 receptor γ-chain; deficiency of ADA or PNP or unknown	Opportunistic	Poor
Hereditary ataxia-telangiectasia	Autosomal recessive	Mutation of ATM gene	Pyogenic	Poor
Congenital thymic aplasia	Not hereditary	Not known	Opportunistic	Guarded
Wiskott-Aldrich syndrome	X-linked at Xp11.22	Mutation of WASP gene	Opportunistic and pyogenic	Guarded
MHC class II deficiency	Autosomal recessive	Defect in promoter binding protein	Opportunistic and pyogenic	Poor

isotype switching from IgM and IgD synthesis to IgG, IgA, or IgE synthesis, the B lymphocyte must receive two signals (see Chap. 94). The first signal is a cytokine, such as interleukin-4 for IgE synthesis or interleukin-2 or interleukin-10 for IgG or IgA synthesis. The second signal involves the physical engagement of CD40 on the B cell with the CD40 ligand expressed on activated T cells. The gene for the CD40 ligand maps to Xq26. Several mutations in the CD40 ligand gene have been found in males affected with hyper-IgM syndrome.[10–15]

ABSENCE OF IgA WITH NORMAL IgG AND IgM

The isolated absence of IgA from serum (<5 mg/dl) occurs in a small but significant proportion of the population (1 per 700). This is the most common immunodeficiency in Caucasians.[16] IgA deficiency is encountered only very rarely in other populations. Most IgA-deficient individuals have no symptoms. However, there is a high incidence of lupus erythematosus, rheumatoid arthritis, and other connective tissue diseases in this group of people.[17] They also have a high incidence of allergies and gastrointestinal disease, such as celiac disease and inflammatory bowel disease. About 20 percent of IgA-deficient individuals have concomitant deficiencies of IgG$_2$ and IgG$_4$. These patients are prone to recurrent and progressive respiratory infections and should be treated with intravenous γ-globulin, as outlined above.

Approximately 80 percent of patients with hereditary ataxia-telangiectasia have IgA deficiency. This deficiency also occurs in patients treated with certain drugs, most commonly phenytoin, but also D-penicillamine, gold salts, captopril, antimalarials, and other drugs. A few patients with IgA deficiency may develop IgE antibodies to IgA, which sometimes results in severe anaphylactic reactions during blood or plasma transfusions.[18]

Plasma cells that secrete IgA are absent from patients with IgA deficiency, but they have B lymphocytes with surface IgA. These B cells cannot be induced to secrete IgA in vitro. There is a high familial incidence of IgA deficiency, but the inheritance pattern is complex. This deficiency frequently is associated with a limited number of extended haplotypes of the major histocompatibility complex (MHC), but the significance of this is not yet understood.[19]

SELECTIVE IgG SUBCLASS DEFICIENCY

Patients with recurrent pyogenic infections may have selective deficiency of IgG$_1$, IgG$_2$, IgG$_3$, or IgG$_4$ or of a combination of these subclasses.[20] The basis of IgG subclass deficiency is not understood.[21] As many as 10 percent of the normal population may have gene deletions in the IgG heavy-chain locus. However, this has no apparent clinical consequences for heterozygous individuals who have one normal allele. Rare cases of homozygous deletions in this area of the genome have been described, resulting in immunodeficiency.[22]

TRANSIENT HYPOGAMMAGLOBULINEMIA OF INFANCY

The human fetus is capable of forming antibodies in utero when adequately stimulated after the twentieth week of gestation. Intrauterine infection with syphilis, cytomegalovirus, rubella virus, or *Toxoplasma* results in antibody synthesis. The antibodies synthesized by the human fetus are mainly IgM and at times IgA.

In normal circumstances the full-term newborn infant is provided with maternal IgG, so that umbilical cord serum contains as much IgG as the maternal serum. Infants born of agammaglobulinemic mothers have no detectable immunoglobulin in cord serum. Virtually no maternal IgA and very little maternal IgM traverses the placenta into the fetal circulation. The cord blood contains less than 1 percent of maternal serum levels of IgA, IgD, and IgE and about 10 percent of the maternal IgM level.

The transplacental passage of IgG appears to involve an active transport system that recognizes some specific structural attribute of the Fc fragment. Studies with radioactive iodinated proteins injected into pregnant women near term confirm this conclusion.[23]

Newborns synthesize IgM antibodies, increasing their level of serum IgM to about 75 percent of the adult level by the end of the first year of life. The newborn infant can synthesize IgA by the third week of life. The level of this globulin tends to rise more slowly and approaches 75 percent of the normal adult level by the end of the second year. Thereafter the level rises very slowly throughout childhood. IgA appears in secretions such as tears, however, by the age of 3 weeks. The maternal IgG is slowly catabolized, so that the infant's serum IgG level reaches its low point of approximately 300 mg/ml by the end of the second month of life. With increased synthesis of IgG by the infant, the serum level rises rapidly toward normal adult values by the age of 1 year.

In some infants, the development of immunoglobulin synthesis is abnormally delayed. The nonphysiologic event has been designated *transient hypogammaglobulinemia*. It occurs with equal frequency in males and females. These infants usually develop the ability to synthesize immunoglobulin between 18 and 30 months of age. Before they develop the capacity for normal immunoglobulin synthesis, however, infants with transient hypogammaglobulinemia may have undue susceptibility to infections of the skin, meninges, or respiratory tract, usually due to gram-positive organisms. Recurrent otitis media, bronchitis, and bronchiolitis are the most common types of infection in these infants. Multiple cases in a single family have been observed. Despite the presence of a normal number of B cells in the blood, lymph nodes display small or no germinal centers and few, if any, plasma cells. These infants have a transient deficiency of CD4+ T lymphocytes. As the number of CD4+ T cells returns to normal, the infant usually experiences a spontaneous recovery from the hypogammaglobulinemia.[24] During the period of hypogammaglobulinemia, such infants require immune serum globulin replacement therapy as described above.

COMMON VARIABLE, UNCLASSIFIABLE IMMUNODEFICIENCY

Most patients with immunodeficiency do not fall precisely into any of the aforementioned defined syndromes. Some patients are said to have "acquired" or "late-onset" agammaglobulinemia. Deterioration of T-cell function also may be observed in some instances. The acquisition of agammaglobulinemia has been documented in several cases, but the cause for this depression of immunoglobulin synthesis is unknown.

Primary acquired agammaglobulinemia occurs with equal frequency in males and females. Although there is no defined genetic pattern in its occurrence, multiple cases have occurred in a single kindred. In addition, these patients and their relatives have a high incidence of other immunologic abnormalities, such as lupus erythematosus, immune hemolytic anemia, increased rheumatoid factor titer, and thrombocytopenic purpura.

Undue susceptibility to pyogenic infections, particularly with recurrent sinusitis and pneumonia, is the prominent clinical feature of acquired agammaglobulinemia. Patients with chronic progressive bronchiectasis should, as a routine, be evaluated for this abnormality.

A prominent and frequent complication of acquired agammaglobulinemia, which is rarely seen in the X-linked disease, is a sprue-like syndrome. More than half of all adults with agammaglobulinemia have diarrhea, steatorrhea, protein-losing enteropathy, and a whole range of malabsorption difficulties. Intestinal biopsies usually appear normal, without the characteristic flattening of villi seen in nontropical sprue. Some patients are noted to have nodular lymphoid hyperplasia. *Giardia lamblia* infection is common. Some patients improve on a gluten-free diet, while others benefit from having milk eliminated from their diet. Treatment with metronidazole (Flagyl) is usually helpful.

Another singular feature of the variable form of immunodeficiency is the frequent occurrence of noncaseating granulomas. Most frequently the lungs, spleen, skin, and liver are involved. No microorganisms have been found consistently in these lesions. Steroid therapy has been useful. Several patients have splenomegaly or hepatosplenomegaly and enlarged lymph nodes, and a few patients may develop hypersplenism. Pernicious anemia also has been reported in as many as 50 percent of patients with agammaglobulinemia.[25]

Patients with acquired agammaglobulinemia usually have serum IgG levels that are less than 500 mg/dl but higher than those of patients with X-linked disease. The IgG may not exhibit normal heterogeneity. Both IgA and IgM may be detected in significant quantity in the sera of these patients. Like IgA deficiency, common variable immunodeficiency (CVID) has been associated with extended haplotypes in the MHC.

The lymph nodes of patients with CVID lack plasma cells. However, in contrast to patients with X-linked agammaglobulinemia, these patients may have striking follicular hyperplasia. From in vitro and in vivo studies, it does not appear that an inhibitory factor causes this disease.

B lymphocytes with surface IgM and IgD usually are encountered in normal numbers but they fail to mature into plasma cells. The reasons for this are not understood.[26] Thymomas sometimes are associated with common variable immunodeficiency, and these patients may have refractory anemia and declining T-cell function. Similar to patients with X-linked agammaglobulinemia, patients with CVID should be treated with intravenous immunoglobulin.[27]

SEVERE COMBINED IMMUNODEFICIENCY

DEFINITION AND HISTORY

In 1950, Glanzmann and Riniker described two unrelated infants who succumbed to overwhelming infection during the second year of life after a succession of serious infections, including intractable diarrhea, thrush, and persistent morbilliform rash.[28] They noted persistent and profound lymphopenia in these two infants and designated the disease *essential lymphocytophthisis.* In 1958, Swiss workers pointed out that agammaglobulinemia is a prominent feature of this disease entity.[28] No antibody synthesis can be detected. These infants lack B and T cells and are prey to all kinds of overwhelming infection. The immunodeficiency is uniformly fatal.

ETIOLOGY AND PATHOGENESIS

Initially, it appeared that the disease was transmitted as an autosomal recessive phenomenon, since consanguinity was demonstrated in approximately one-third of the parents of affected children. Further study of these families in America and Europe strongly suggested an additional X-linked transmission of the defect, on the basis of (1) the documentation of affected males in three generations, (2) the appearance of the disease in sons of identical-twin mothers, and (3) the appearance of the disease in sons of the same mother but different fathers. The two different modes of inheritance, autosomal and X-linked recessive, probably account for the 3:1 ratio of males and females observed in the reported cases. The X-linked form of severe combined immunodeficiency (SCID) appears distinctive in that affected males have normal numbers of circulating B cells that do not mature into plasma cells and make antibodies. This is designated T-B+ SCID. X-linked SCID has been found to result from mutations in the gene for the gamma chain of the interleukin-2 receptor.[29] Because this gamma chain of the IL-2 receptor forms part of the IL-4, IL-7, IL-9, and IL-15 receptors, it is designated the gamma common (γ_c) chain. Engagement of the IL-7 receptor is ritual for human T-cell development. When T cells are activated the γ_c chain is phosphorylated by a tyrosine kinase, Jak3. Deficiency of Jak3, which is inherited as an autosomal recessive, also results in T-B+ SCID. In obligate heterozygous women who carry the gene for X-linked SCID, there is nonrandom inactivation of the X chromosome in their peripheral blood T cells. Such nonrandom X inactivation also is found in the B cells of obligate heterozygous women who carry the gene for X-linked agammaglobulinemia. As every female cell randomly inactivates one or the other X chromosome, the finding that T cells (in the case of X-linked SCID) or B cells (in the case of X-linked agammaglobulinemia) only express the normal X chromosome suggests that the defect is restricted to either the T-cell or B-cell lineage, respectively. Susceptible cells that have inactivated the normal X chromosome cannot expand and/or survive with the defective X chromosome.

About half of the infants with the autosomal recessive form have a concomitant deficiency of adenosine deaminase (ADA), the aminohydrolase that converts adenosine to inosine.[30] Prenatal diagnosis is possible by finding this enzyme deficiency in cultured amnion cells.[31] Another cause of defective T-cell immunity is nucleoside phosphorylase (NP) deficiency.[32] In both ADA and NP deficiency the accumulation of toxic metabolites, dATP or dGTP, inhibits normal lymphocyte development[33,34] (see Chap. 90). This is classified as T-B− SCID as affected infants have virtually no T or B cells. T-B− SCID may also result from mutations in the enzymes that cleave double-stranded DNA and initiate VDJ recombination in the genes encoding the T-cell antigen receptor and the immunoglobulins *Rag-1* and *Rag-2.* Missense mutations in these genes may result in a variant of SCID called *Omenn's syndrome,* characterized by marked erythrodermia, hyper IgE, eosinophilia, and oligoclonal expansion of T cells.

CLINICAL FEATURES

There is no discernible difference in the clinical course of the various genetic types. Also, they cannot be separated on the basis of the morbid anatomy of the disease. Infection starts early, between 3 and 6 months of age, and a rapid succession of debilitating infections brings about early demise. Death within the first 2 years of life is the rule. Almost all infants with this disease have chronic watery diarrhea. Stool cultures frequently reveal strains of *Salmonella* or of enteropathic *Escherichia coli.*

In addition, pulmonary infection is almost universal. Lung abscesses that contain *Pseudomonas aeruginosa* are a common cause of death, as is pneumonitis due to *P. carinii*. Extensive moniliasis of the mouth or diaper area that persists beyond the neonatal period is often the first sign of the disease. Usually this is present even before any antibiotic therapy is instituted. These infants, furthermore, are incapable of limiting or overcoming the most benign viral infections. Death has resulted from generalized chickenpox, measles with Hecht's giant cell pneumonia, and, in a few instances, cytomegalovirus and adenovirus infection. Vaccination results in progressive, ultimately fatal vaccinia infection. BCG inoculation also has resulted in progressive BCG infection.

LABORATORY FEATURES

The lymphocyte count is usually less than 2000/μl (2×10^9/liter). The number of lymphocytes may be variable, declining from initially normal neonatal levels [n > 3000/μl (3 × 10^9/liter)] to profound lymphopenia. Accordingly, a single normal lymphocyte count cannot exclude this diagnosis, particularly during its early stages. Neutrophils and platelets are normal. However, leukocytosis may not occur in response to overt infection. Eosinophilia is common, and abnormal granulation of eosinophils has been reported. The number of natural killer cells in the blood may be elevated.

Marrow in normal infants contain up to 20 percent lymphocytic elements, but in SCID the marrow is uniformly deficient in plasma cells, lymphocytes, and lymphoblasts. Lymph node biopsies show complete lack of germinal elements, plasma cells, and lymphocytes. The stroma of the node may contain an occasional mast cell and eosinophils or, rarely, small collections of lymphoid cells without any apparent organization. Lymph node biopsies should not be performed to establish the diagnosis, as the biopsy site usually becomes infected or is a portal of entry for infection. The blood contains virtually no CD3+ cells of the CD4+ or CD8+ subsets. Whatever mature T cells are encountered are usually of maternal origin.[35]

None of the indications of delayed sensitivity can be elicited in these infants. The blood lymphocytes are unresponsive to phytohemagglutinin or allogenic stimulation. Skin grafts are accepted without microscopic or macroscopic signs of rejection. At autopsy, no lymphoid tissue is found in the spleen, tonsils, appendix, or intestinal tract. The thymus has usually failed to descend in the normal manner into the anterior mediastinum and is found with difficulty in the neck. It ordinarily weighs less than 1 g and is composed of primordial spindle-shaped cells, occasionally forming swirls or rosettes. No Hassall's corpuscles and few, if any, lymphocytes are present. The embryonal appearance of the thymus is the uniform characteristic of this entity. The thymus shadow is absent in a chest X-ray antemortem.

THERAPY, COURSE, AND PROGNOSIS

Death within the first 2 years of life, from infection and malnutrition, is almost invariable in this disease. Graft-versus-host disease, however, arising after marrow or whole blood transfusions, has resulted in several fatalities. This complication may result from the persistence of maternal lymphoid cells that are acquired through the placenta. The onset of graft-versus-host disease in any event is marked by the appearance of a characteristic maculopapular rash, starting on the face about 7 days after the injection of immunocompetent incompatible cells. The rash spreads rapidly, ultimately involving all skin surfaces including the palms and soles. Thrombocytopenia, leukopenia, jaundice, and anasarca follow in quick succession. Marrow aplasia leads to death from massive hemorrhage by the twelfth or fourteenth day.[36]

However, transplants of histocompatible marrow, usually from sibling donors but also from unrelated donors, has proved to be lifesaving. It also has been possible to use parental haploidentical marrow from which T cells have been depleted to circumvent graft-versus-host disease.[37] SCID due to ADA deficiency also has been corrected by gene therapy.[38] The ADA gene in a retroviral vector has been inserted into patient lymphocytes in vitro and subsequently reinjected into the patients.

CELLULAR IMMUNE DEFICIENCY SYNDROMES

HEREDITARY ATAXIA-TELANGIECTASIA

Hereditary ataxia-telangiectasia is transmitted as an autosomal recessive disease. Affected persons are first noted to be ataxic and to develop choreoathetoid movements and pseudopalsy of eye movements during infancy.

The telangiectasias appear later, at 5 or 6 years, or occasionally not until adolescence. They invariably involve the conjunctivae and other exposed body areas such as the face, ears, eyelids, and arms. Progressive sinopulmonary infection also appears later in the course. Death from chronic respiratory infection or lymphoreticular malignancy is common in the second or third decade of life.

About 80 percent of patients with ataxia-telangiectasia lack both serum and secretory IgA. Some patients have antibody to IgA, resulting in the rapid catabolism of injected IgA. All patients with ataxia-telangiectasia have a defect in cellular immunity. The thymus gland is dysplastic or hypoplastic, and there is depletion of thymus-dependent areas in the lymph nodes. Delayed hypersensitivity reactions, in vitro response of blood lymphocytes to phytohemagglutinin, and allograft rejection are absent.[39] Immunoglobulin replacement and symptomatic measures have had limited therapeutic success.

It is estimated that 1.4 percent of the population is heterozygous for the hereditary ataxia-telangiectasia gene, and this subpopulation may have a higher incidence of cancer.[40] The ataxia-telangiectasia gene maps to chromosome 11q22-23.[41] It has been cloned and designated ATM (for *ataxia telangiectasia mutated*). The product of this gene is involved in the repair of double-stranded DNA breaks.

WISKOTT-ALDRICH SYNDROME

The Wiskott-Aldrich syndrome is characterized by eczema, thrombocytopenia, and recurrent infections. Inheritance of the syndrome is X-linked. Affected boys rarely survive beyond the first decade of life and succumb to overwhelming infection, hemorrhage, or lymphoreticular malignancy. Both gram-positive and gram-negative bacteria, as well as viruses and fungi, produce severe infections. There appears to be a progressive deterioration of thymus-dependent cellular immunity. In addition, there are concomitant changes in the lymph nodes, resulting in progressive depletion of lymphocytes from the paracortical areas. Serum IgM concentration is usually low, but IgG and IgA levels are normal or elevated. Isohemagglutinins are regularly absent from the serum. This observation suggests a specific inability to respond to polysaccharide antigens. This now has been demonstrated quite conclusively with A and B blood group substances, *Salmonella* Vi lipopolysaccharide, and other similar antigens. The gene for the Wiskott-Aldrich syndrome has been mapped to Xp11.22.[42] The gene has been cloned and designated *WASP*. It encodes a protein comprised of 502 amino acid residues and is involved in cytoskeletal reorganization in a manner that has not yet been completely elucidated. By scanning electron microscopy, the platelets are small and fragmented, and the T cells are bald and lack their usual surface ruffling; these changes are pathognomonic of the disease. Surface sialoglycoproteins, CD43 of the T cells and platelets and gpIb of the platelets, are rapidly degraded on the surface of the cells for unknown reasons.[43]

CONGENITAL THYMIC APLASIA (DIGEORGE'S SYNDROME)

During the sixth week of embryonic life, the thymus primordium arises from the floor of the third pharyngeal pouch and, to a lesser extent, from the fourth pharyngeal pouch. The endodermal epithelial masses rapidly elongate, move down into the neck, and fuse in the midline behind the thyroid primordium in the eighth week of embryonic life. By the twelfth week, the gland comes to occupy its ultimate position in the anterior mediastinum. The epithelial cells form Hassall's corpuscles, and the primordium is invaded by proliferating lymphoblasts.

While the thymus is forming, the parathyroid glands arise simultaneously from the third and fourth pharyngeal pouches and start their downward migration posterior and lateral to the thyroid primordium.

During this same period, the nasomedial processes fuse to form the philtrum of the lip, and the ear tubercles around the hypomandibular cleft form into the external ear.

DiGeorge observed that a congenital anomaly may result from the failure of embryogenesis of the endodermal derivatives of the third and fourth pharyngeal pouches—aplasia of the parathyroid and thymus glands. This abnormality has no increased familial incidence and does not appear to be hereditary. All infants with this syndrome thus far studied have manifested neonatal tetany. The hypocalcemia tends to ameliorate with development during the first year of life. Hypertelorism; a shortened lip philtrum; low-set, notched pinnae; and nasal clefts cause these infants to resemble one another. In addition, anomalies of the great blood vessels are almost always present; tetralogy of Fallot and right-sided aortic arch are the most common defects.[44]

Infants with thymic aplasia who survive the neonatal period exhibit untoward susceptibility to viral, fungal, and bacterial infections that ultimately may be overwhelming. At autopsy, some parathyroid tissue and a miniature thymus gland may be found in an ectopic position by carefully sectioning the neck organs. Nephrocalcinosis has been found in over half the infants examined. The lymphoid tissue, marrow, spleen, and gastrointestinal tract contain a normal number of plasma cells, and the cortical germinal centers of the lymph nodes are normal or hyperplastic. The subcortical ''thymus-dependent region'' shows a moderate to severe depletion of lymphocytes, so that the reticulum cells in this area appear to be unusually prominent. The lymphoid sheaths of the spleen are also depleted of lymphocytes. Blood usually exhibits profound lymphopenia.[45]

Antibody responses to primary stimuli may be normal. Serum concentrations of immunoglobulins are normal. However, patients can neither manifest delayed hypersensitivity to common antigens, such as Candida or streptokinase, nor be sensitized to dinitrofluorobenzene (DNFB). Skin allograft rejection is absent or abnormally delayed. Lymphocyte transfer tests and macrophage-immobilizing factor synthesis are abnormal. The blood lymphocytes respond poorly, if at all, to in vitro stimulation by phytohemagglutinin or allogenic cells.

Transplants of fetal thymic tissue dramatically reverse all these deficits in in vitro and in vivo lymphocyte function into children with this syndrome. Increase in lymphocyte count, population of thymus-dependent areas with lymphocytes, normal skin allograft rejection, and normal responses to intradermal antigens, as well as normalization of phytohemagglutinin response in vitro, have been documented after fetal thymus transplants.[46,47]

COMBINED IMMUNODEFICIENCY WITH DEFECTIVE EXPRESSION IN MHC CLASS II GENES

Several children, principally of North African origin, have been described with severe and repeated opportunistic infections, frequently causing death. These children apparently have normal numbers of T and B cells, but they fail to synthesize and express the MHC class II molecules DP, DQ, and DR. The synthesis of class II molecules cannot be induced with interferon-gamma in affected patients. Because the normal ontogeny of CD4+ T lymphocytes is induced by class II MHC molecules, these children are deficient in CD4+ cells. Consequently they do not have antibody responses and are hypogammaglobulinemic. The in vitro response of their T cells in mixed lymphocyte culture and to mitogens is poor, although they respond normally to anti-CD3 and anti-CD2. Several of these children have been rescued with transplants of bone marrow. The defect does not map to the MHC but rather appears to result from the absence of a promoter binding protein required for coordinate MHC class II synthesis. The four complementation groups of this defect have been identified to result from 4 different promoter proteins.[48]

REFERENCES

1. Bruton OC: Agammaglobulinemia. *Pediatrics* 9:722, 1952.
2. Cooperband SR, Rosen FS, Kibrick S: Studies on the in vitro behavior of agammaglobulinemia lymphocytes. *J Clin Invest* 47:836, 1968.
3. Kwan S-P, Terwilliger J, Parmley R, et al: Identification of a closely linked DNA marker, DXS178, to further refine the X-linked agammaglobulinemia locus. *Genomics* 6:238, 1990.
4. Vetrie D, Vorechovsky I, Sideras P, et al: The gene involved in X-linked agammaglobulinaemia is a member of the *src* family of protein-tyrosine kinases. *Nature* 361:226, 1993.
5. Fruman DA, Snapper SB, Yballe CM, et al: Impaired B cell development and proliferation in absence of phosphoinositide 3-kinase p85alpha. *Science* 283:393, 1999.
6. Wilfert CM, Buckley RH, Mohanakumar T, et al: Persistent and fatal central-nervous-system echovirus infections in patients with agammaglobulinemia. *N Engl J Med* 296:1485, 1977.
7. Hobbs JR: Immune imbalance in dysgammaglobulinemia type IV. *Lancet* 1:110, 1968.
8. Rosen FS, Kevy SV, Merler E, et al: Recurrent bacterial infections and dysgammaglobulinemia: deficiency of 7S gamma globulins in the presence of elevated 19S gamma globulins. *Pediatrics* 28:182, 1961.
9. Hinz CF Jr, Boyer JT: Dysgammaglobulinemia in adults manifested as autoimmune hemolytic anemia. *N Engl J Med* 269:1329, 1963.
10. Allen RC, Armitage RJ, Conley ME, et al: CD40 ligand gene defects responsible for X-linked hyper-IgM syndrome. *Science* 259:990, 1993.
11. DiSanto JP, Bonnefoy JY, Gauchat JF, et al: CD40 ligand mutation in X-linked immunodeficiency with hyper-IgM. *Nature* 361:541, 1993.
12. Aruffo A, Farrington M, Hollenbaugh D, et al: The CD40 ligand, gp39, is defective in activated T cells from patients with X-linked hyper-IgM syndrome. *Cell* 72:291, 1993.
13. Fuleihan R, Ramesh N, Loh R, et al: Defective expression of the CD40 ligand in X chromosome-linked immunoglobulin deficiency with normal or elevated IgM. *Proc Natl Acad Sci USA* 90:2170, 1993.
14. Ramesh N, Fuleihan R, Ramesh V, et al: Deletions in the ligand for CD40 in X-linked immunoglobulin deficiency with normal or elevated IgM (HIGMX-1). *Int Immunol* 5:769, 1993.
15. Korthauer U, Graf D, Mages HW, et al: Defective expression of T-cell CD40 ligand causes X-linked immunodeficiency with hyper-IgM. *Nature* 361:539, 1993.
16. Bachmann R: Studies on the serum gamma A globulin level: III. The frequency of agamma A globulinemia. *Scand J Clin Lab Invest* 17:316, 1965.
17. Ammann AJ, Hong R: Selective IgA deficiency and autoimmunity. *Clin Exp Immunol* 7:343, 1970.
18. Vyas GN, Perkins HA, Fudenerg HH: Anaphylactoid transfusion reactions associated with anti-IgA. *Lancet* 2:312, 1968.
19. Schaffer FM, Monteiro RC, Volanakis JE, et al: IgA deficiency. *Immunodefic Rev* 3:15, 1991.
20. Schur P, Borel H, Gelfand EW, et al: Selective gamma G globulin deficiencies in patients with recurrent pyogenic infection. *N Engl J Med* 283:631, 1970.
21. Preud'Homme J-L, Hanson LA: IgG subclass deficiency. *Immunodefic Rev* 2:129, 1990.
22. Yel L, Minegishi Y, Coustan-Smith E: Mutations in the mu heavy-chain gene in patients with agammaglobulinemia. *N Engl J Med* 335:1486, 1996.
23. Gitlin D, Kumate J, Urrusti J, et al: Selectivity of human placenta in transfer of plasma proteins from mother to fetus. *J Clin Invest* 43:1938, 1964.
24. Siegel RL, Issekutz T, Schwaber J, et al: Deficiency of T helper cells in transient hypogammaglobulinemia of infancy. *N Engl J Med* 305:1307, 1981.
25. Twomey JJ, Jordan PH, Jarrold T, et al: The syndrome of immunoglobulin deficiency and pernicious anemia. *Am J Med* 47:340, 1969.
26. Spickett GP, Webster ADB, Farrant J: Cellular abnormalities in common variable immunodeficiency. *Immunodefic Rev* 2:199, 1990.
27. Eibl M, Wedgwood RJ: Intravenous immunoglobulin: a review. *Immunodefic Rev* 1(suppl):1, 1989.
28. Glanzmann E, Riniker P: Essentielle lymphocytophthise. *Ann Paediatr* 175:1, 1950.
29. Noguchi M, Yi H, Rosenblatt HM, et al: Interleukin-2 receptor gamma

chain mutation results in X-linked severe combined immunodeficiency in humans. *Cell* 73:147, 1993.

30. Giblett ER, Anderson JE, Cohen F, et al: Adenosinedeaminase deficiency in two patients with severely impaired cellular immunity. *Lancet* 2:1067, 1972.

31. Hirschhorn R, Beratis N, Rosen FS, et al: Adenosine deaminase deficiency in a child diagnosed prenatally. *Lancet* 1:73, 1975.

32. Giblett ER, Ammann AJ, Wara DW, et al: Nucleosidephosphorylase deficiency in a child with severely defective T-cell immunity and normal B-cell immunity. *Lancet* 1:1010, 1975.

33. Hirschhorn R: Adenosine deaminase deficiency. *Immunodefic Rev* 2:175, 1990.

34. Markert ML: Purine phosphorylase deficiency. *Immunodefic Rev* 3:45, 1991.

35. Reinherz EL, Cooper MD, Schlossman SF, et al: Abnormalities of T cell maturation and regulation in human beings with immunodeficiency disorders. *J Clin Invest* 68:669, 1981.

36. Kretschmer R, Jeannet M, Mereu TR, et al: Hereditary thymic dysplasia. A graft-versus-host reaction induced by bone marrow cells with a partial 4A series histoincompatibility. *Pediatr Res* 3:34, 1969.

37. O'Reilly RJ, Keever CA, Small TN, et al: The use of HLA-non-identical T-cell-depleted marrow transplants for correction of severe combined immunodeficiency disease. *Immunodefic Rev* 1:273, 1989.

38. Blaese RM, Culver KW: Gene therapy for primary immunodeficiency disease. *Immunodefic Rev* 3:329, 1992.

39. Petersen RDA, Cooper MD, Good RA: Lymphoid tissue abnormalities associated with ataxia telangiectasia. *Am J Med* 41:342, 1966.

40. Swift M: Genetic aspects of ataxia-telangiectasia. *Immunodefic Rev* 2:67, 1990.

41. Gatti RA, Berkel I, Boder E, et al: Localization of the ataxia-telangiectasia gene to chromosome 11q22-23. *Nature* 336:577, 1988.

42. Kwan S-P, Lehner T, Hagemann T, et al: Localization of the gene for the Wiskott-Aldrich syndrome between two flanking markers TIMP and DXS255 on Xp11.22-11.3. *Genomics* 10:29, 1991.

43. Remold-O'Donnell E, Rosen FS: Sialophorin (CD43) and the Wiskott-Aldrich syndrome. *Immunodefic Rev* 2:151, 1990.

44. DiGeorge AM: Congenital absence of thymus and its immunologic consequences: concurrence with congenital hypoparathyroidism, in *Immunologic Diseases in Man*, edited by D. Bergsma. *Birth Defects* 4:116, 1968.

45. Hong R: The DiGeorge anomaly. *Immunodefic Rev* 3:1, 1991.

46. August CS, Rosen FS, Filler RM, et al: Implantation of a foetal thymus, restoring immunological competence in a patient with thymic aplasia (DiGeorge's syndrome). *Lancet* 2:1210, 1968.

47. Cleveland WW, Fogel BJ, Brown WT, et al: Foetal thymic transplant in a case of DiGeorge's syndrome. *Lancet* 2:1211, 1968.

48. Griscelli C, Lisowska-Grospierre B, Mach B: Combined immunodeficiency with defective expression in MHC class II genes. *Immunodefic Rev* 1:135, 1989.

THE ACQUIRED IMMUNODEFICIENCY SYNDROME

HOWARD A. LIEBMAN

TIMOTHY P. COOLEY

ALEXANDRA M. LEVINE

Significant advances have recently been made in the area of HIV and AIDS in terms of the molecular aspects of the virus and immunopathogenesis of the disease. Mechanisms of HIV transmission have been elucidated, with specific means to decrease the transmission to health care workers and to children born to HIV-infected mothers. Detection of specific HIV RNA levels in the blood may both provide prognostic information and help guide treatment decisions. Use of highly active antiretroviral therapy has been associated with a marked decrease in new AIDS-defining illnesses and in mortality from AIDS. HIV may affect virtually all organ systems, with prominent abnormalities related to the marrow and blood. Malignancies associated with HIV include lymphoma, Kaposi sarcoma, and cervical cancer, among others. The pathogenesis of these neoplastic disorders has been elucidated in large part, with new treatment strategies attempting to address the various steps involved in the development of these tumors.

DEFINITION AND HISTORY

DEFINITION

The definition of acquired immunodeficiency syndrome (AIDS) initially was based exclusively upon clinical symptoms and signs.[1] As knowledge of the viral etiopathogenesis evolved, the case definition

Acronyms and abbreviations that appear in this chapter include: AIDS, acquired immunodeficiency syndrome; ANC, absolute neutrophil count; AZT, zidovudine; bDNA, branched-chain DNA; bFGF, basic fibroblast growth factor; CDC, Centers for Disease Control and Prevention; cDNA, copy DNA; CFU-GEMM, colony-forming unit–granulocyte-erythroid-monocyte-macrophage; CNS, central nervous system; d4T, stavudine; DIC, disseminated intravascular coagulation; EBER, Epstein-Barr early region; EBV, Epstein-Barr virus; ELISA, enzyme-linked immunoassay; G-6-PD, glucose-6-phosphate dehydrogenase; G-CSF, granulocyte colony-stimulating factor; GI, gastrointestinal; GM-CSF, granulocyte-monocyte colony-stimulating factor; GP, glycoprotein; HAART, highly active antiretroviral therapy; HHV-8, human herpesvirus 8; HIV, human immunodeficiency virus; ICAM-1, intercellular adhesion molecule-1; Ig, immunoglobulin; IL, interleukin; IM, intramuscular; INF-α, interferon-α ITP, immune thrombocytopenic purpura; IV, intravenous; IVIG, intravenous gamma globulin; MAC, *Mycobacterium avium* complex; m-BACOD, methotrexate, bleomycin, cyclophosphamide, and etoposide combination chemotherapy; M-tropic, macrophage tropic; NK, natural killer; NNRTI, nonnucleoside reverse transcriptase inhibitor; NRTI, nucleoside reverse transcriptase inhibitor; PEL, primary effusion lymphoma; PEP, postexposure prophylaxis; PGL, persistent generalized lymphadenopathy; PI, protease inhibitor; RT-PCR, reverse transcriptase polymerase chain reaction; SAIDS, simian acquired immunodeficiency syndrome; SIC, simian immunodeficiency virus; 3TC, lamivudine; TGF-β, transforming growth factor β, TNF-α, tumor necrosis factor α; TTP, thrombotic thrombocytopenic purpura; VCAM-1, vascular cell adhesion molecule 1; WHO, World Health Organization.

of AIDS underwent multiple revisions by the Centers for Disease Control and Prevention (CDC), with inclusion of additional clinical illnesses and/or a blood CD4 count of less than $200/\mu$l [$0.2(10^9/$liter)] in a patient with serologic evidence of infection with the human immunodeficiency virus (HIV).[2–4]

While this expanded definition is employed in industrialized nations, the World Health Organization (WHO) adopted alternative case-definition systems for diagnosis of AIDS in underdeveloped countries where serologic and immunologic testing is not readily available (Table 89-1).[5,6]

A formal classification system for HIV infection was adopted by the CDC in 1993 that utilized CD4+ cell count and symptoms to better characterize the earlier stages of HIV infection. However, the rapid development of sensitive technologies to quantify HIV in blood and tissues has rapidly supplanted these classification systems as the primary methods of staging and following patients with HIV infection.[7,8]

ORIGINS OF HIV

At approximately the same time that AIDS was first recognized in 1981, reports of a similar immunodeficiency syndrome, characterized by wasting and opportunistic infections, was described in several colonies of macaques housed at primate centers in the United States.[9,10] The illness, known as *simian immunodeficiency syndrome* (SAIDS), was associated with infection by a retrovirus, termed *simian immunodeficiency virus* (SIV).[11] Subsequent testing revealed that over 20 percent of all tested symptomatic African green monkeys or African mangabeys from the wild had serologic evidence of SIV infection.[12–14] The SIV viral strain infecting these monkeys is related to HIV-2, a less virulent strain of human immunodeficiency virus, found primarily in West Africa.[15] An immunodeficiency virus related to HIV-1 and infecting African chimpanzees was also identified.[16] Recent evidence suggests that the subspecies of chimpanzee *Pan troglodyte* may have been the original reservoir of HIV-1.[17]

Based upon these observations, it is postulated that HIV originally may have been transmitted to humans from an African species of ape.[14,17] By the mid- to late 1960s, political and societal circumstances were beginning to change dramatically in ways that were conducive to the rapid spread of this infection in humans. The movement of previously isolated African peoples from rural villages to large urban centers; a change in sexual habits, resulting in widespread exposure to increasing numbers of sexual partners; the worldwide epidemic of parenteral drug abuse; and the advent of commercial air travel all contributed to the current pandemic of HIV infection.

The WHO has estimated that over 30 million people had been infected by HIV worldwide by mid-1998,[18] the majority infected by heterosexual contact, with homosexual contact and injection drug use the predominant modes of transmission in the United States and western Europe. Vertical transmission from infected mother to child is now decreasing in developed countries, although such transmission continues to increase in resource-poor regions of the world.

ETIOLOGY AND PATHOGENESIS

HUMAN IMMUNODEFICIENCY VIRUS-1

HIV-1 is a member of the primate Lentivirinae subfamily of retroviruses,[19,20] RNA viruses that induce a chronic cellular infection by converting their RNA genome into a DNA provirus that is integrated into the genome of the infected cell. Infection by these lentiviruses is characterized by long periods of clinical latency followed by a gradual onset of disease-related symptoms.[21–23]

TABLE 89-1   AIDS-DEFINING CLINICAL CONDITIONS FOR HIV-INFECTED ADOLESCENTS AND ADULTS

Candidiasis of bronchi, trachea, or lungs
Candidiasis, esophageal
Cervical cancer, invasive*
Coccidioidomycosis, disseminated or extrapulmonary
Cryptococcosis, extrapulmonary
Cryptosporidiosis, chronic intestinal (>1 month's duration)
Cytomegalovirus disease (other than liver, spleen, or nodes)
Cytomegalovirus retinitis (with loss of vision)
Encephalopathy, HIV-related
Herpes simplex: chronic ulcer(s) (>1 month's duration) or bronchitis, pneumonitis, or esophagitis
Histoplasmosis, disseminated or extrapulmonary
Isosporiasis, chronic intestinal (>1 month's duration)
Kaposi sarcoma
Lymphoma, Burkitt lymphoma (or equivalent term)
Lymphoma, immunoblastic (or equivalent term)
Lymphoma, primary in brain
Mycobacterium avium complex or *Mycobacterium kansasii*, disseminated or extrapulmonary
Mycobacterium tuberculosis, any site (pulmonary* or extrapulmonary)
Pneumocystis carinii pneumonia
Pneumonia, recurrent*
Progressive multifocal leukoencephalopathy
Salmonella septicemia, recurrent
Toxoplasmosis of brain
Tuberculosis*
Wasting syndrome due to HIV

*Added in the 1993 expansion of the AIDS surveillance case definition.

TRANSMISSION OF HIV

HIV may be transmitted by sexual contact with an infected partner, by parenteral drug use with a contaminated needle, by exposure to infected blood or blood products, and by perinatal exposure from an infected mother to her infant.

General Mechanisms of Sexual Transmission   HIV-1 has been isolated from the semen of HIV-infected men[24] as well as from cell-free seminal fluid[25] and may be detected during the first 3 to 4 weeks after primary infection.[27] Factors associated with increased viral burden in semen include more advanced symptomatic HIV disease, higher levels of HIV-RNA in blood, CD4 cell counts of less than $200/\mu$l, and presence of seminal fluid leukocytosis. HIV infection has been reported after exposure to infected semen during artificial insemination.[27]

HIV has been recovered from cervical and vaginal secretions of HIV-infected women,[28,29] and HIV-infected endothelial cells and macrophages have been detected in cervical biopsies.[30] Factors that influence the levels of HIV-1 in female genital tract secretions include the stage of HIV disease, menstruation status, hormonal parameters, concomitant vaginal infection, age, HIV-1 RNA level in plasma, and antiviral therapy.[31] Although female-to-female transmission of HIV has been reported,[32,33] this appears to be relatively unusual.

HIV transmission may be facilitated by the presence of other sexually transmitted diseases, both with and without ulceration,[34] and HIV has been isolated directly from genital ulcers.[35] Prevention or treatment of sexually transmitted disease has been associated with a decrease in HIV-1 transmission.[36]

Transmission through Parenteral Drug Use   Sharing needles and syringes is an important mode of transmission among parenteral drug users.[37] The use of cocaine has been associated with a particularly high risk of HIV infection,[38] presumably related to its short half-life and the resulting need for greater numbers of injections. Behavioral factors may lead to increased risk of HIV-1 transmission even among nonparenteral illicit drug users.

Transmission through Infected Blood Products   The risk of infection with HIV after receiving 1 unit of infected blood approximates 90 percent.[39] Transfusion of blood products derived from multiple units of pooled blood can also transmit HIV and accounted for the initially high prevalence of HIV infection among patients with hemophilia. Screening of all donated blood, beginning in March 1985, and the subsequent routine heat or solvent detergent treatment of clotting factor concentrates have resulted in a marked decrease in new transfusion-associated HIV infections. Guidelines for proper inactivation of HIV in clotting factor concentrates have been developed.[40,41] Currently, the risk of acquiring HIV through receipt of a unit of blood that tests negative for antibodies to HIV-1 is approximately 1 in 493,000.[42]

Mother-to-Child Transmission   The risk of infection from mother to infant differs in various parts of the world, ranging from approximately 15 percent in Europe to 15–30 percent in the United States and 40–50 percent in Africa.[43–45] HIV-1 may be transmitted in utero,[46,47] intrapartum (at the time of delivery);[48,49] or postpartum, through ingestion of HIV-1 infected mother's milk.[50,51] Several factors predict an increased risk of perinatal transmission. In terms of the mother, more advanced HIV disease,[52,53] higher HIV-1 viral load in the plasma,[54,55] cigarette smoking,[56] and active injection drug use[57] have all been associated with increased risk of transmission. In terms of the details of delivery, premature rupture of the amniotic membranes (over 4 h),[58,59] presence of chorioamnionitis,[57] and vaginal delivery, as opposed to elective cesarean section,[60,61] have each been associated with increased rates of transmission. In terms of the infant, breastfeeding, prematurity, and low gestational age are reported as risk factors.[58,59,62] The CDC has recently made formal recommendations regarding the optimal care for HIV-1 infected pregnant women.[63] These recommendations differ for resource-rich and resource-poor settings. In the United States, the use of antiretroviral agents in pregnancy and delivery, with subsequent administration to the infant for the first 6 weeks of life, has resulted in a dramatic reduction in the rate of transmission, from approximately 25 percent to 8 percent.[64] With the further use of elective cesarean section and avoidance of breast feeding, transmission rates have dropped to approximately 2 percent.[60] The efficacy of shorter courses of zidovudine or neviripine (a non–nucleoside reverse transcriptase inhibitor) have been demonstrated and may be more practically feasible in resource-poor regions of the world.[65,66] The long-term toxicities of in utero exposure to antiretroviral agents are unknown. Nonetheless, their use during pregnancy resulted in a 43 percent decrease in the number of children with perinatally acquired HIV infection in the United States when comparing data from 1992 and 1996.[67]

HIV GENE PRODUCTS

HIV-1 has three structural genes necessary for replication: *GAG*, *POL*, and *ENV*.[19] These viral genes encode proteins that are required for binding to the host cell, intracellular synthesis of provirus by reverse transcription, proviral integration into the host-cell genome, and viral assembly and release. The 9-kb genome of HIV-1 also contains at least six additional genes involved in the regulation of viral gene expression and cellular latency: *VIF, VPU, VPR, TAT, REV,* and *NEF* (Fig. 89-1).[68]

ENV   HIV-1 is an icosahedral virion with a protein-rich envelope in a membrane derived from the host cell[69] (see Fig. 89-1). The surface of the virus particle contains a 120-D glycoprotein (gp120) that is linked noncovalently to a 41-kD transmembrane protein (gp41). Both proteins are derived from a 160-kD precursor protein that is encoded by the *ENV* gene. The intracellular processing of gp160 involves the assembly of oligomeric trimer complexes, which are glycosylated and subsequently cleaved into the respective gp120 and

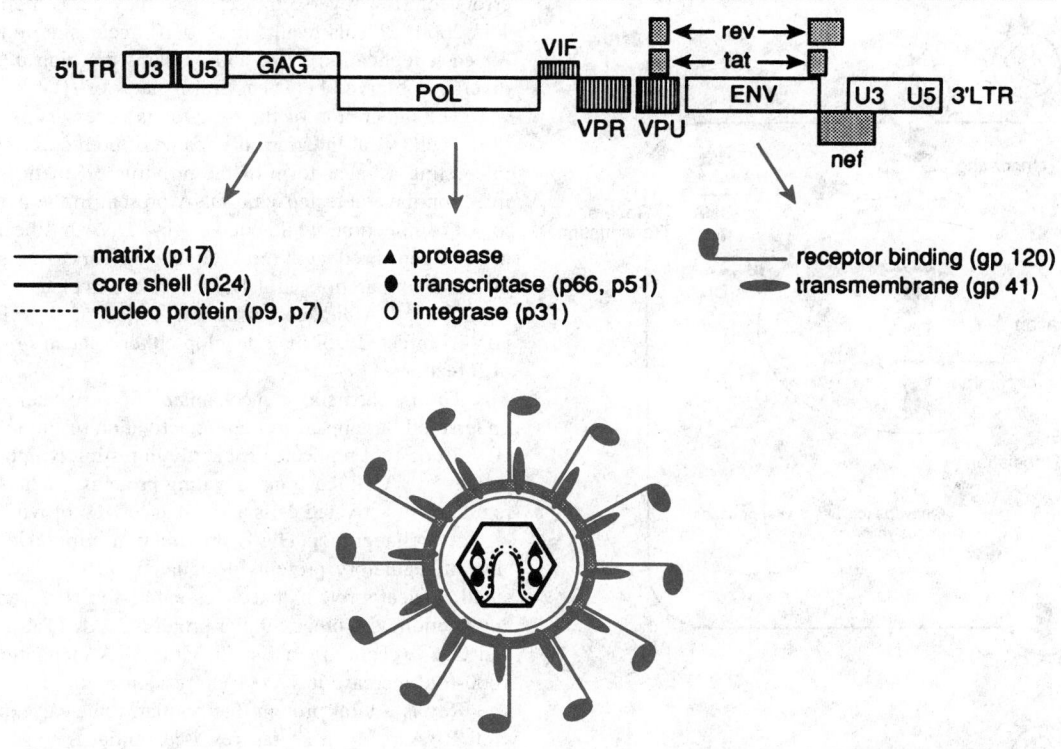

FIGURE 89-1   A schematic representation of the genome and viral structure of HIV-1.

gp41 in the Golgi apparatus of the host cell.[70] HIV gp120 serves as a virion receptor for noninfected cells,[71] first binding to the CD4 antigen and then to one or the other the chemokine receptors CCR5 and CXCR4.[72–74] The CD4-binding domain of gp120 is located on the carboxyl terminal region of the molecule.[75] Within the CD4-binding site of gp120 are a number of regions that display significant genetic variation between different viral isolates without compromising viral binding.[76] The binding of CD4 results in a conformational transition in the V3 variable loop of gp120, exposing the chemokine receptor binding site of the viral molecule and increasing the affinity of gp120 binding to CCR5 by 10- to 100-fold.[70,77] Complexing of gp120 with CD4 and chemokine molecules promotes a second conformational change, which exposes the HIV-1 transmembrane anchoring protein, gp41, ectodomain, which is necessary for fusion of the viral membrane with the membrane of the newly infected cell.[77,78] These viral proteins are immunogenic. Consequently, antibodies against both gp120 and gp41 can be detected in serum of all individuals infected with HIV-1[79] (Fig. 89-2). However, antibodies capable of neutralizing HIV and preventing cellular infection appear to develop only after infection is well established. Further, these antibodies are not capable of efficiently controlling ongoing infection.[70]

GAG   The *GAG* gene encodes a 54-kD precursor protein that is cleaved by a viral protease to form four viral core proteins: p24, p17, p9, and p7 (see Fig. 89-1). The 24-kD protein (p24) forms the shell of the nucleocapsid. The 17-kD myristylated matrix protein (p17) is located between the viral envelope and the nucleocapsid and functions to stabilize the virion and, as part of the p54 *GAG*-precursor protein, to assist in targeting viral assembly at the cell surface. The 7-kD protein (p7) and 9-kD protein (p9) are tightly associated with the viral RNA, stabilizing it in the viral ribonucleoprotein core.[80]

POL   The *POL* gene encodes three critical viral proteins. The first, reverse transcriptase, is a 66-kD protein that generates a copy

DNA (cDNA) from the viral RNA genome. The cDNA then is used as a template, generating a double-stranded DNA provirus, which then integrates into the host cellular genome.[81] The *POL* gene also encodes a 31-kD integrase protein that is required for stable integration of proviral double-stranded DNA into host cellular DNA.[82] The 5′ region of the *POL* gene encodes a viral protease that cleaves the p54 *GAG*

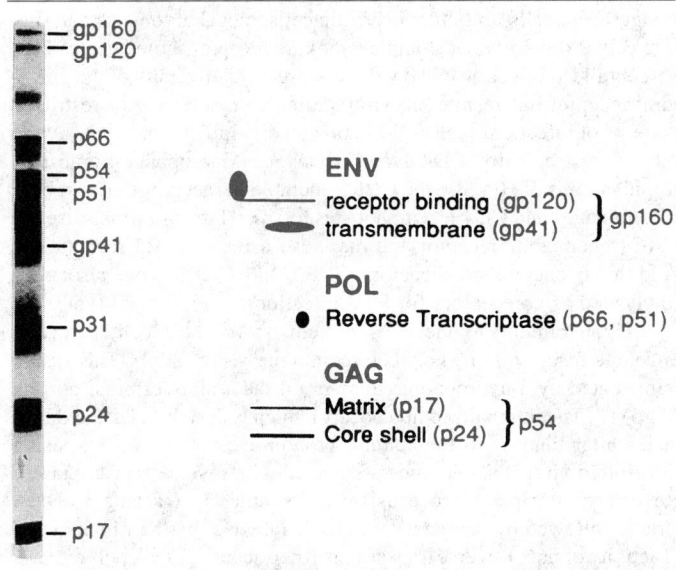

FIGURE 89-2   A Western blot analysis of antibodies against HIV viral proteins from the serum of a patient with AIDS.

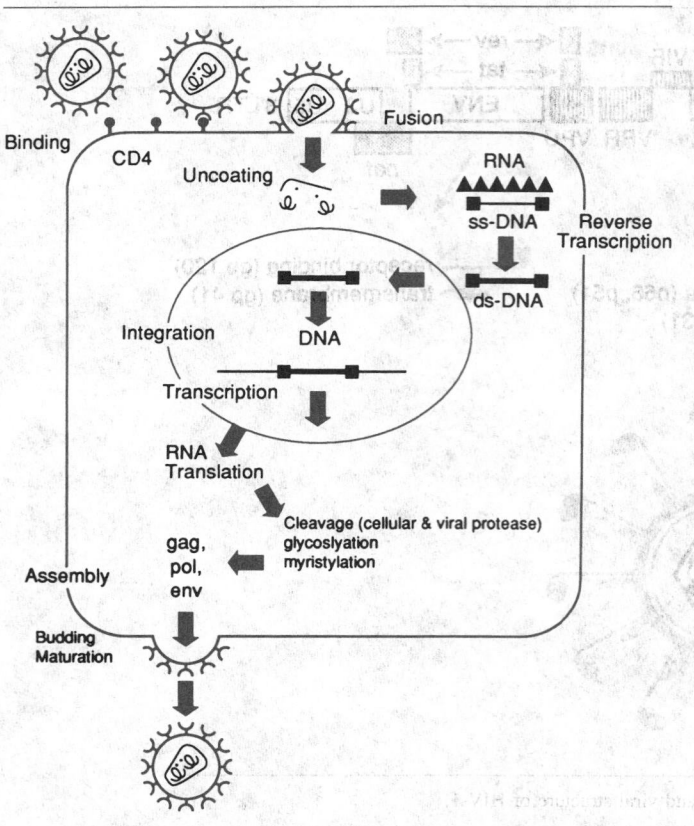

FIGURE 89-3   The life cycle of HIV-1.

precursor protein.[83] A defective protease leads to the production of noninfectious virions.[84]

LIFE CYCLE OF HIV-1

HIV-1 gp120 binds to the CD4 surface membrane protein, resulting in a further high-affinity binding to the chemokine CCR5 receptor.[70,85] Human helper-inducer (CD4) lymphocytes, monocytes-macrophages, Langerhans' cells, follicular dendritic cells, megakaryocytes, and thymic cells express the CD4 and chemokine receptor molecules and are susceptible to infection by HIV-1. The structural diversity of the gp120 viral receptor has resulted in viral strains with selective or restricted patterns of infection, such as those that readily infect monocytes, while others are tropic for CD4 lymphocytes.[76,86] Macrophage-tropic (M-tropic) strains of HIV use the CCR5 chemokine receptor to infect both macrophages and CD4+ lymphocytes.[87,88] The T-tropic strains use the CXC4 chemokine receptor and may also use the CCR5 receptor.[87,88] Additional chemokine receptors CCR2 and CCR3 have also been implicated as coreceptors for HIV infection of certain cell types.[88,89]

Upon binding to the CD4 protein on the host cell, the virus envelope fuses with the host cell membrane[90] (Fig. 89-3). This fusion is mediated by a hydrophobic domain on the amino terminal portion of gp41.[77] The internalized nucleocapsid then is destabilized and dissociates after binding to the cellular protein cyclophilin A,[91] exposing the diploid viral RNA genome associated with reverse transcriptase.[92] Reverse transcription proceeds by the synthesis of a single cDNA strand, followed by degradation of the viral RNA by the ribonuclease H activity of p66. Reverse transcriptase then acts as a DNA polymerase, forming a second DNA strand. This synthesis of the double-stranded DNA provirus must proceed rapidly to prevent the degradation of viral RNA by intracellular enzymes. The estimated rate of base substitution

errors for HIV reverse transcriptase may be as high as 1 in 1700 to 1 in 2000.[93,94] This results in 5 to 10 nucleoside mutations per virus for each replication cycle and explains the high degree of genomic diversity observed between viral isolates of HIV.[95]

The integration of the provirus is necessary for stable infection of the cell. Viral integrase is capable of both cleaving host DNA and integrating a linear form of the provirus.[96] Kinetic studies of HIV-1 infection have detected viral DNA present in the cytoplasm within 2 to 3 h of infection, while nuclear viral DNA has been detected by 24 h.[97] The gene product of the *VPR* gene appears to assist in the transport of the preintegration viral DNA into the nucleus for subsequent integration.[98,99] After successful integration of the viral genome, the HIV-1–infected cell may develop either a latent or a persistent form of infection.

The mechanism or mechanisms of viral latency remain poorly understood but appear to require activation of the infected cell, since HIV-1 does not replicate efficiently in resting lymphocytes or macrophages.[100,101] Cellular transactivating proteins, such as NF-κB, are upregulated in activated cells and enhance HIV proviral transcription.[102]

After integration, HIV-1 proviral transcription leads to the expression of regulatory proteins designated tat, rev, and nef.[97,98] Tat is a small nuclear protein that is essential for HIV replication and, in conjunction with other cellular proteins, TAK (Tat-associated kinase) and CycT (cyclin T), assists in viral RNA elongation, resulting in a 1000-fold increase in HIV-1 expression by the infected cells.[98,103,104]

Rev is a viral protein that regulates nuclear export of unspliced viral RNA.[98,105,106] Like tat, rev is essential for viral replication and must bind to a rev-responsive element located in the *ENV* gene. The other HIV-encoded proteins, designated nef and vpu, have a role in the modulation and down-regulation of the cellular receptor, CD4.[98,107–110]

The structural proteins of the *GAG, POL,* and *ENV* genes are expressed as precursor proteins and subsequently cleaved by viral protease to yield mature viral proteins. Proteolysis of proteins by the viral protease is essential for viral maturation and infectivity. The products of the *ENV* gene, gp120 and gp41, are transported to the cell membrane. The ribonucleoprotein core assembles in the cytoplasm of the host cell and subsequently moves to the membrane surface for budding. The efficient packaging of the viral RNA is dependent upon packaging signals present in the *Gag* region of the viral RNA.[111] The budding of virus appears to be dependent upon the product of the *VPU* gene, which assists in membrane transport of *ENV* gene products.[107,108,112] In addition, viral infectivity appears to require the gene product of the *VIF* gene.[113]

PATHOGENESIS OF HIV INFECTION

HIV infection results in aberrant immune regulation and immunodeficiency. The numerous in vitro and in vivo defects in cellular immune response observed with HIV infection include decreased lymphocyte proliferation to soluble antigens,[114] decreased helper response in immunoglobulin (Ig) synthesis,[115] impaired delayed hypersensitivity,[1,2] decreased interferon-γ production,[116] and decreased T-cell–mediated cytotoxicity of virally infected cells.[117]

DEPLETION OF CD4+ T CELLS

Infection with HIV-1 results in a progressive loss of CD4-positive (CD4+) T lymphocytes, resulting from the direct cytopathic effect of HIV on CD4+ lymphocytes. Formation of syncytial multinucleated giant cells by a mechanism involving fusion of infected cells expressing viral gp120 with noninfected CD4+ T lymphocytes is another mechanism of CD4 depletion.[118] The propensity of certain viral stains to form syncytia appears to be associated with an aggressive clinical course.[117,118] More recent experimental data suggest that an HIV-1 phenotypic switch from an M-tropic (nonsyncytial) to a T-tropic (syncytial) virus may be the central event in acceleration of HIV-induced immunodepletion.[119]

The host immunologic response against HIV-infected lymphocytes also may contribute to the progressive loss of CD4+ lymphocytes by antibody-mediated and cytotoxic T-cell–mediated mechanisms.[120,121] Noninfected lymphocytes may also become ''innocent bystander'' targets for immunologic destruction by binding free gp120 to their surface CD4 protein.

Defective production of immunostimulatory cytokines, such as interleukin-2 (IL-2),[122–124] or exaggerated expression of inhibitors of T-lymphocyte proliferation, such as transforming growth factor-β (TGF-β),[125] can contribute to the progressive decline in CD4 lymphocytes. High-level replication and budding of virus, resulting in membrane injury, has also been proposed as a mechanism for lymphocyte cytotoxicity.

Recent advances in combination antiretroviral therapy have resulted in marked suppression of viral replication, with resulting reductions of blood and tissue viral reservoirs.[126,127] Efficient viral suppression has resulted in significant and prolonged immunologic reconstitution characterized by increased CD4$^+$-lymphocyte numbers, reduced opportunistic infections, and prolonged survival.[128,129] However, significant deficits in the immunologic repertoire persist, and complete immunologic reconstitution has not yet been attained.[130,131]

DEFECTS IN B-CELL IMMUNITY

A number of defects in humoral immunity have been associated with HIV infection. Pronounced polyclonal activation of B lymphocytes is common, resulting in polyclonal hypergammaglobulinemia.[132,133] Spontaneous proliferation of B cells is observed in patients with advanced HIV infection.[134] In contrast, antigen-specific B-cell proliferation and antibody production are decreased in patients with AIDS.[135] This may result from the loss of helper T-lymphocyte activity.

The aberrant B-lymphocyte regulation in HIV infection is associated with a pronounced increase in autoimmune phenomena and an increased risk of B-cell lymphomas.[136] In addition to an increased frequency of positive antiglobulin test results, antibodies against neutrophils,[137,138] lymphocytes,[139] and platelets[140–142] also have been reported.

DEFECTS IN IMMUNE ACCESSORY CELLS
AND NATURAL KILLER CELLS

Monocytes, macrophages, and follicular dendritic cells of the lymph nodes express CD4 antigen and can be infected by HIV.[143,144] Monocytes and macrophages are resistant to HIV-induced cytotoxicity and serve as a chronic reservoir of HIV expression.[143] While functional defects in the chemotaxis of HIV-infected monocytes have been reported,[145] most studies have failed to demonstrate consistent defects.[146,147] The follicular dendritic cells appear to play an important role in HIV clearance in early asymptomatic HIV disease. However, a progressive depletion of these cells is observed over time, resulting in increasing plasma viremia. The loss of follicular dendritic cells results in defective antigen processing in patients with advanced HIV disease.

Natural killer (NK) cell activity is decreased in the blood of HIV-infected individuals.[147,148] In combination with helper T-lymphocyte depletion, decreased NK activity results in defective clearance of virally infected cells. While the number of NK cells is reported to be normal,[147,148] the defect in NK activity appears to result from a deficiency in the signals for cell activation. The addition of exogenous IL-2 can improve NK lymphocyte function.[149]

DIAGNOSIS OF HIV INFECTION

Like the clinical manifestations of acute (primary) HIV infection (''acute retroviral syndrome''), the laboratory markers are nonspecific, with frequent elevation of liver transaminase levels and erythrocyte sedimentation rate. However, HIV viremia is present during the acute illness and can be detected by molecular methods such as reverse transcription polymerase chain reaction (RT-PCR).

The primary diagnostic screening tool is detection of antibody via the enzyme-linked immunoassay (ELISA). However, since a positive ELISA result may not be specific for HIV-1 infection, all positive ELISA screening test results should be verified by immunoblotting HIV-1 antigens (see Fig. 89-2).

By ELISA and immunoblot techniques, the median time from initial infection to first detection of HIV antibody has been estimated to be 2.4 months, while 95 percent of cases are expected to seroconvert within 5.8 months (see Fig. 89-4).[150] HIV infection for longer than 6 months without detectable antibody is extremely uncommon.[151–153]

The presence of the p24 antigen or HIV RNA in serum or plasma may precede seroconversion by several weeks.[154] This initial rise in p24 antigen correlates with the burst of viremia that occurs shortly after primary HIV infection.[155] Despite these observations, p24 antigen screening of donated units of blood appears to provide no benefit over conventional ELISA and immunoblot techniques.[156]

LABORATORY FEATURES OF DISEASE PROGRESSION

With progression from the initial acute infection to the expected asymptomatic period, various laboratory parameters may be used to predict development of more advanced disease.[7,8,157] Quantitation of plasma HIV RNA (viral load) and CD4+ lymphocyte count are the most useful parameters. The CD4+ lymphocyte count falls during the acute retroviral infection and then stabilizes during early asymptomatic infection and may appear relatively normal. The CD4+ count then decreases by approximately 40 to 80 μl/year in the absence of antiretroviral medications,[158] although there is significant variability among patients.[159]

An initial measurement of plasma viral load by RT-PCR or branched-DNA (bDNA) methods provides important prognostic information that can be useful in determining when to start antiretroviral medications.[7,8] The serial assessment of plasma HIV viral load also allows for rapid assessment of efficacy of antiretroviral medications. Changes in viral load usually precede significant alterations in CD4+ lymphocyte counts.[8,128]

Several nonspecific markers of disease progression have been defined, including β_2-microglobulin[160] and neopterin,[161] each of which has independent predictive value in estimating the probability of progression to AIDS. However, each of these surrogate markers has been largely replaced by the more specific molecular assays to quantify plasma HIV viral load.

COURSE AND PROGNOSIS

HIV infection results in a progressive process characterized by gradual depletion of immune function and eventual development of rather nonspecific symptoms, followed by specific infections and/or neoplastic disease. Patients who develop AIDS generally experience relentless deterioration in physical health and ultimately succumb to one or more complications secondary to acquired immunodeficiency, organ dysfunction, and/or malignancy associated with HIV infection.

The recent use of monitoring by means of assessment of the quantity of HIV-1 RNA in the plasma has allowed a more rational basis upon which to predict the course of disease in individual patients.

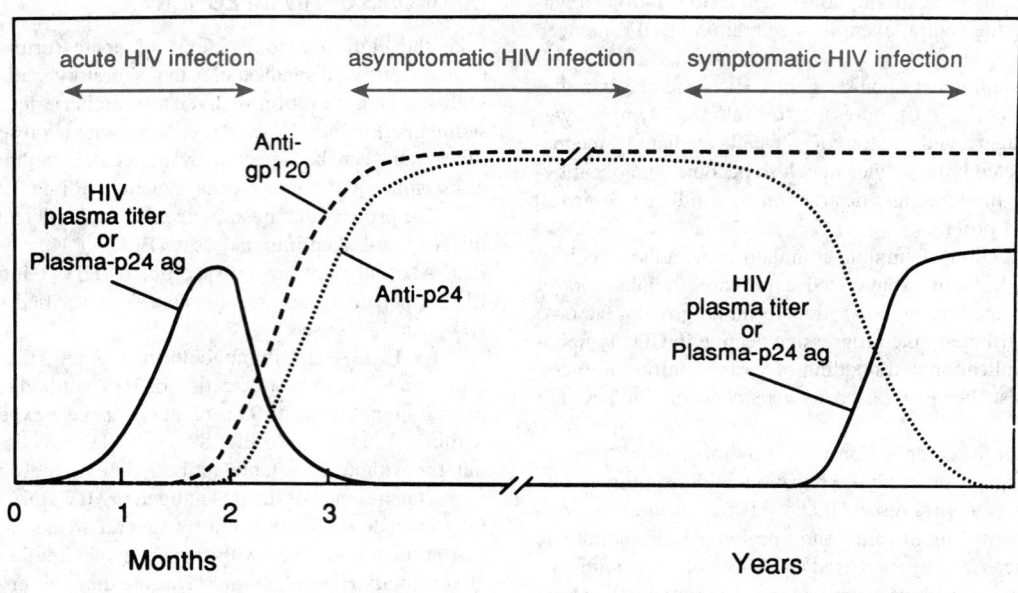

FIGURE 89-4   The virologic, serologic, and clinical course of HIV infection. Antibodies against HIV can first be detected between 2 and 5 months after infection.

In a study performed through the Multicenter AIDS Cohort, a longitudinal cohort study of HIV disease in homosexual and bisexual men, the earliest, baseline level of HIV RNA in plasma was found to correlate significantly with prognosis over time. Thus, a viral load of 5,000 to 10,000 copies/μl was associated with an 8 percent risk of progression to clinical AIDS within the next 5 years, while a viral load in excess of 36,000 copies/μl was associated with a 62 percent 5-year risk of AIDS.[7] In a subsequent study, use of both viral load and CD4[+] cells was found to more accurately predict the prognosis of HIV-infected men.[8]

In addition to the use of viral load monitoring, the development of potent new antiretroviral agents, including the protease inhibitors,[162–164] has recently led to a remarkable improvement in the natural history of HIV infection.[129] The use of combinations of highly active antiretroviral therapies (HAART) was found to be associated with a 73 percent decrease in the incidence of new opportunistic infections and a 49 percent decrease in death due to AIDS when data from 1997–1998 were compared to data from 1994.[129] Remarkable decreases in the incidence of cytomegalovirus disease, atypical *Mycobacterium intracellularis* infections, and other serious opportunistic infections have occurred as a consequence of HAART therapy,[165] and improvement in immune function has also been documented.[166] It may now be possible to discontinue the routine use of prophylaxis against *Pneumocystis carinii* in patients who have been successfully treated with HAART.[167]

ACUTE RETROVIRAL SYNDROME

An acute clinical illness is often associated with initial HIV infection, occurring in approximately 50 to 90 percent of individuals.[155,168,169] This syndrome begins approximately 1 to 3 weeks (range 5 days to 3 months) after primary infection and usually lasts for 1 to 2 weeks. Prominent symptoms include significant fatigue and malaise; fever, which may be as high as 40°C (104°F); headache; photophobia; myalgias; and a morbilliform rash, seen in approximately 40 to 50 percent of patients. Generalized lymphadenopathy may occur toward the end of the acute illness. The symptoms are similar to those of other viral

illnesses, such as infectious mononucleosis (see Chap. 90). All symptoms of this acute retroviral syndrome subside within several weeks. However, headache may persist as an intermittent complaint, as may the generalized lymphadenopathy, termed persistent, generalized lymphadenopathy (PGL), which occurs in approximately 75 percent of patients.[155,169]

EARLY ASYMPTOMATIC HIV DISEASE

After resolution of the acute retroviral syndrome, the patient usually returns to a state of well-being. During this period, the patient harbors HIV in blood and in genital secretions and may transmit the virus to others. This phase of asymptomatic infection persists for approximately a decade or more in the absence of therapy and appears similar in all racial and ethnic groups, all geographic areas, both genders, and all risk groups for HIV infection.[170–173]

ADVANCED SYMPTOMATIC HIV DISEASE

With time, more significant manifestations of disease occur, with more extensive fatigue, fevers, weight loss, night sweats, and the eventual development of opportunistic infections, neurologic symptoms, and/or neoplasms that are considered AIDS-defining conditions (see Table 89-1).

HEMATOLOGIC ABNORMALITIES

ANEMIA IN HIV INFECTION

INCIDENCE OF ANEMIA
Anemia is very common in HIV-infected individuals, occurring in approximately 10 to 20 percent at initial presentation and diagnosed in approximately 70 to 80 percent of patients over the course of disease.[174–176] In an attempt to ascertain the precise incidence of anemia in the setting of HIV infection, Sullivan and colleagues evaluated data derived from the case records of 32,867 HIV-infected persons followed from 1990 through 1996.[176] This cohort, termed the Multistate Adult

and Adolescent Spectrum of HIV Disease Surveillance Project, consists of individuals who receive HIV care in hospitals and HIV clinics in nine U.S. cities. Using a hemoglobin level of less than 10 g/dl to define anemia, the 1-year incidence of anemia was 37 percent among patients with clinical AIDS; 12 percent among patients with immunologic AIDS, as defined by a CD4+ cell count pf less than 200 cells/ml; and 3 percent among HIV-infected individuals with neither clinical nor immunologic AIDS. These data confirm the high incidence of anemia among HIV-infected patients at all stages of disease.

ETIOLOGY OF ANEMIA

Numerous causes for anemia exist in HIV-infected patients (Table 89-2).

ANEMIA DUE TO DECREASED PRODUCTION OF RED BLOOD CELLS

A decrease in production of red blood cells may result from factors suppressing the CFU-GEMM, such as inflammatory cytokines or the HIV virus itself.[174,175] In addition, a blunted production of erythropoietin has been documented in anemic HIV-infected patients, similar to the suppression seen in other states of chronic infection or inflammation.[177] Infiltration of the marrow by tumor, such as lymphoma,[178] or infection, such as *Mycobacterium avium* complex (MAC), may also lead to the decreased production of red cells. In addition, MAC may also be associated with cytokine-induced marrow suppression. Involvement of the gastrointestinal (GI) tract by various infections or tumors may lead to chronic blood loss, with eventual iron deficiency anemia. Another prominent cause of hypoproliferative anemia in patients with

TABLE 89-2   CAUSES AND MECHANISMS OF ANEMIA IN HIV INFECTION

Mechanisms of Anemia	Cause of Anemia
Decreased red cell production	Neoplasm infiltrating the marrow 　Lymphoma 　Kaposi sarcoma 　Others Infection 　Atypical tuberculosis (*Mycobacterium avium intracellularis* or *Mycobacterium avium complex*) 　*Mycobacterium tuberculosis* 　Cytomegalovirus 　B19 parvovirus 　Fungal infection Drugs HIV 　Abnormal growth of burst-forming units–erythroid 　Anemia of chronic disease 　Blunted erythropoietin production or response Iron deficiency anemia secondary to chronic blood loss
Ineffective production	Folic acid deficiency 　Dietary 　Jejunal pathology: malabsorption B_{12} Deficiency 　Malabsorption in ileum 　Gastric pathology with decreased production of intrinsic factor
Increased red cell destruction	Coombs-positive hemolytic anemia Hemophagocytic syndrome Thrombotic thrombocytopenic purpura Disseminated intravascular coagulation Drugs 　Sulfonamides, dapsone 　Oxidant drugs in glucose-6-phosphate dehydrogenase deficiency

HIV infection is the common use of multiple medications, many of which may cause marrow and/or red cell suppression. Zidovudine (AZT), the first licensed antiretroviral agent, is uniformly associated with macrocytosis mean cell volume (MCV >100), which can be used as an objective indication that the patient has been compliant with this medication.[179] It noteworthy that transfusion-dependent anemia (hemoglobin < 8.5 g/dl) has been reported in approximately 30 percent of patients with full-blown AIDS, receiving zidovudine at doses of 600 mg/day. However, the incidence of severe anemia is only 1 percent when the same dose of zidovudine is used in patients with asymptomatic HIV disease.[180]

Infection of the marrow by parvovirus B19 is another cause of hypoproliferative anemia in HIV-infected patients, resulting in specific infection of the pronormoblast.[181,182] Thus, while marrow failure affecting all three lines has been described in association with parvovirus B19 infection, a pure red cell aplasia is the usual consequence. Parvovirus infection is usually acquired during childhood, leading to "fifth disease," one of the common childhood exanthums. Exposure to the virus leads to an antibody response, with subsequent resistance to further infection. Approximately 85 percent of adults have serologic evidence of prior parvovirus infection. However, the seroprevalence of such antibodies among HIV-infected patients is only 64 percent. This would suggest that these individuals may have an ineffective immune response against newly acquired infection. The diagnosis of parvovirus B19 can be made on marrow examination, revealing giant pronormoblasts with clumped basophilic chromatin and clear cytoplasmic vacuoles; diagnosis can be confirmed by in situ hybridization using sequence-specific DNA probes for parvovirus B19. Therapy for parvovirus-induced red cell aplasia consists of infusions of intravenous (IV) gamma globulin that contain antibodies from plasma donors most of whom have been exposed to parvovirus. Relapse of parvovirus B19–induced red cell aplasia may occur, necessitating retreatment in these individuals.[181,182]

ANEMIA DUE TO INCREASED RED CELL DESTRUCTION

Increased red cell destruction may be seen in HIV-infected patients with G-6-PD deficiency who are exposed to oxidant drugs and in HIV-infected patients with disseminated intravascular coagulation (DIC) or thrombotic thrombocytopenic purpura (TTP);[183] presence of fragmented red cells and thrombocytopenia on blood smear will be seen in the latter two conditions, and Heinz bodies will be seen in association with G-6-PD deficiency. Hemophagocytic syndrome has also been described in association with HIV infection. An additional cause of red cell destruction in HIV-infected patients is the development of autoantibodies, with resultant positive Coombs' test result and shortened red cell survival. It is interesting to note that a positive direct Coombs' test result has been reported in as many as 18 to 77 percent of HIV-infected patients, although the incidence of actual hemolysis is quite low. When present, anti-i antibody and antibody against auto-U antigens have been described, occurring in 64 percent and 32 percent of HIV-infected patients, respectively.[184–186] A high incidence of positive direct Coombs' test results has also been detected in patients with other hypergammaglobulinemic states, indicating that the positive Coombs' test results in HIV may simply be secondary to the polyclonal hypergammaglobulinemia that is known to occur in the setting of HIV infection.[187]

ANEMIA DUE TO INEFFECTIVE PRODUCTION OF RED CELLS (B_{12} AND/OR FOLIC ACID DEFICIENCY)

Folic acid is absorbed in the jejunum and is responsible for one carbon transfer required in the synthesis of DNA. A deficiency of folic acid leads to a megaloblastic anemia, with large oval red cells in the blood, hypersegmented neutrophils, and a decrease in all three lines, with resultant anemia, neutropenia, and thrombocytopenia. Since tissue stores of folate are relatively small, a deficiency of folate in the diet lasting as little as 6 to 7 months may lead to anemia. It is thus apparent that HIV-infected patients who are ill and not eating properly, as well as those with underlying disease of the jejunum, may be unable to absorb sufficient folic acid. The classic changes of megaloblastic anemia will be detected upon examination of the bone marrow, while serum and red cell folate levels will be low.

Ineffective production of red cells, with pancytopenia in the blood, elevated indirect bilirubin level, and low reticulocyte count may also be seen in vitamin B_{12} deficiency. The absorption of B_{12} requires initial production of intrinsic factor by parietal cells in the stomach, with subsequent absorption of the complex of B_{12} and intrinsic factor within the ileum. Thus, malabsorption of B_{12} can occur in various disorders of the stomach (achlorhydria), by production of antibodies to intrinsic factor ("pernicious anemia"), or by various disorders of the small bowel and ileum (infection or Crohn's disease). While B_{12} deficiency is highly unlikely on a dietary basis alone, patients with HIV infection appear to be prone to B_{12} malabsorption, presumably due to the myriad infections and other disorders that may occur in the small intestine. Negative vitamin B_{12} balance has been documented in approximately one-third of patients with AIDS, the majority demonstrating defective absorption of the vitamin.[188] Diagnosis of B_{12} deficiency can be made by documenting low serum B_{12} levels, while the earliest indication of negative B_{12} balance is the finding of low B_{12} levels in blood in patients taking transcobalamin II.[189] Monthly administration of parenteral B_{12} will correct the deficiency and the resultant anemia and pancytopenia in the peripheral blood. Since B_{12} deficiency may also cause neurologic dysfunction (subacute combined degeneration of the cord), with motor, sensory, and higher cortical dysfunction, the possibility of vitamin B_{12} deficiency should also be considered in HIV-infected patients with these neurologic symptoms.

CONSEQUENCES OF ANEMIA IN HIV INFECTION

The consequence of anemia in HIV-infected patients was addressed by the Multistate Spectrum of HIV Disease Surveillance Project, in which records from over 32,000 individuals were reviewed. In this study, anemia was defined as a hemoglobin level less than 10 g/dl. It is important to note that anemia was found to be associated with an increased risk of death in this cohort.[176] Thus, the relative risk of death for anemic individuals who began the study with CD4+ counts above 200 cells/ml was 148 percent higher than for individuals at the same CD4+ strata without anemia, while the risk of death was increased by 58 percent for those who entered the study at CD4+ counts less than 200 cells/ml and developed anemia. It is interesting to note that the risk of death decreased in those patients who recovered from anemia, whatever its cause, while the risk of death remained 170 percent higher for patients who did not recover from anemia. A similar relationship between anemia and increased risk of death has also been noted by others.[190]

USE OF ERYTHROPOIETIN IN HIV-INFECTED PATIENTS WITH ANEMIA

A blunted response to erythropoietin is extremely common in the setting of HIV infection;[171,190] it is caused by a posttranscriptional defect, since levels of kidney erythropoietin mRNA are normal. Multiple studies have now confirmed the beneficial effect of erythropoietin in HIV-infected patients with anemia, in whom marrow function has been suppressed as a result of HIV or of other chronic infectious or inflammatory diseases.[190–193] Erythropoietin is also effective in treating the anemia due to zidovudine or other medications, including cancer chemotherapy, which may suppress the marrow.[193] Patients with a baseline endogenous erythropoietin level of less than or equal to 500

IU/liter are expected to respond to erythropoietin therapy, while those with endogenous levels over 500 IU/liter are not. Erythropoietin is administered subcutaneously at a dose of 100 to 200 U/kg body weight three times weekly until normalization of the red cell count is achieved and then given approximately once every week or every other week to maintain the desired hemoglobin concentration. When erythropoietin is prescribed in this manner, statistical increases in the hematocrit are expected, with significant decreases in the number of red cell transfusions required and a significant increase in overall quality of life. Recent data from the Spectrum of Disease Study indicate that correction of anemia is also associated with prolongation of survival.[171,190] Toxicity is uncommon, consisting primarily of local pain at the site of injection, mild fever, or rash. In those patients with endogenous erythropoietin levels less than 500 IU/liter who do not respond to the drug, a search for occult iron deficiency, serum B_{12} or folate deficiency, or other such causes should be made.

NEUTROPENIA

ETIOLOGY OF NEUTROPENIA AND DECREASED GRANULOCYTE FUNCTION IN HIV

Neutropenia is reported in approximately 10 percent of patients with early, asymptomatic HIV infection and in over 50 percent of those individuals with more advanced HIV-related immunodeficiency.[174,175,193] As with other peripheral blood cytopenias in the setting of HIV infection, multiple etiologies may be present, either singly or in combination.[194] Thus, decreased colony growth of the progenitor cell CFU-GM[195] may lead to decreased production of both granulocytes and monocytes. Soluble inhibitory substances produced by HIV-infected cells have been noted to suppress neutrophil production in vitro.[196] Decreased serum levels of G-CSF have been described in HIV-seropositive subjects with afebrile neutropenia (<1000 neutrophils/μl), indicating that a relative deficiency of this specific hematopoeitic growth factor may also contribute to persistent neutropenia.[197] Finally, myelosuppression and neutropenia may result from any one of several medications that are commonly prescribed for HIV-infected patients.

Aside from absolute neutropenia, patients with HIV infection may also experience decreased function of granulocytes and monocytes. Thus, abnormal Fc processing by macrophages has been described, while decreased opsonization and intracellular killing of bacterial or fungal organisms by granulocytes has also been noted.[198]

RISK FACTORS FOR INFECTION IN NEUTROPENIC PATIENTS WITH HIV

In patients with cancer who receive chemotherapy, multiple studies have shown that the risk of bacterial infection rises when the absolute neutrophil count (ANC) falls below 1000 cells/dl and increases again when the ANC falls below 500 cells/μl.[199] Several studies have confirmed the same relationships in patients with HIV infection. Thus, Moore and colleagues found that the risk of bacterial infection increased 2.3-fold for HIV-infected individuals with less than 1000 cells/μl and rose by 7.9-fold in those with ANC levels less than 500 cells/μl.[200] Lower ANC counts are associated with increased risk of hospitalization for serious infection among HIV-infected patients, as shown by a review of 2047 HIV-positive patients. On multivariate analysis, the severity and duration of neutropenia were found to be significant predictors of the incidence of hospitalization for serious bacterial infections.[201]

In a recent study of 62 HIV-infected patients with ANCs less than or equal to 1000 cells/μl, 24 percent developed infectious complications, most commonly within 24 h after the onset of neutropenia.[202] On multivariate analysis, the three factors independently associated with infectious complications included presence of a central venous catheter, neutropenia in the previous 3 months, and a lower nadir of granulocyte count (250 cells/μl in those with infections versus 622 cells/μl in those without). Among patients with medication-associated neutropenia, the most common cause was zidovudine, followed by trimethoprim-sulfamethoxazole, and ganciclovir; neutropenia was less likely to be associated with infection in these patients than in individuals who were neutropenic due to the use of cancer chemotherapy.[202]

USE OF GRANULOCYTE COLONY-STIMULATING FACTOR AND GRANULOCYTE-MACROPHAGE COLONY-STIMULATING FACTOR IN NEUTROPENIC PATIENTS WITH HIV INFECTION

When administered subcutaneously to HIV-infected patients with neutropenia, granulocyte colony-stimulating factor (GM-CSF) results in dose-dependent increases in granulocytes, monocytes, and eosinophils.[203,204]

GM-CSF has been associated with augmentation in the replication of HIV, with increases in viral load, specifically seen in those HIV isolates that are monocyte/macrophage tropic. Thus, use of GM-CSF was associated with a 200-fold increase in HIV p24 levels over baseline when used to prevent neutropenia associated with chemotherapy for AIDS-related lymphoma.[205] However, GM-CSF also increases the uptake and phosphorylation of zidovudine to its active triphosphate form, resulting in a greater antiretroviral effect. It is therefore recommended that antiretroviral therapy be employed in all patients receiving GM-CSF. When used with antiretroviral agents, GM-CSF is not associated with an increased HIV viral load.

Granulocyte colony-stimulating factor (G-CSF) has also been demonstrated to raise granulocyte counts in neutropenic patients with HIV in whom neutropenia has occurred as a consequence of cancer chemotherapy, antiretroviral therapy, and/or antiinfective therapy.[193,206] A retrospective analysis of 152 neutropenic HIV-infected patients, including 71 who received G-CSF and 81 patients who never received G-CSF, was conducted during the years from 1991 to 1994.[207] The two groups had similar baseline characteristics, including median CD4+ count of 37 and 40 cells/μl, respectively. In multivariate analysis, use of G-CSF was associated with a significantly decreased risk of bacteremia ($p = .02$). Further, multivariate analyses revealed a decreased risk of death in patients receiving G-CSF, as well as in those who received antiretroviral agents and/or prophylaxis for *Pneumocystis carinii* pneumonia.[207]

The early recommendations for dosing of G-CSF included an initial induction dose of 5 mg/kg/day given subcutaneously. Recent evidence would suggest, however, that much lower doses of G-CSF may be effective in HIV-infected persons. Thus, an initial dose of 1 mg/kg/day is often initiated and used until the neutrophil count rises to acceptable levels (>1000 cells/μl). This is followed by a titration of dosing, often requiring therapy only once or twice per week, as necessary to maintain the desired response.

G-CSF does not enhance HIV replication in vitro, and its use has not been associated with up-regulation of HIV in vivo. Toxicity of G-CSF has been rather minimal, consisting primarily of bone pain. While patient survival has not increased as a consequence of G-CSF or GM-CSF,[207] these drugs will allow safer administration of other necessary medications.[204,207]

THROMBOCYTOPENIA

Thrombocytopenia is relatively common during the course of HIV infection, occurring in approximately 40 percent of patients and serving as the first symptom or sign of infection in approximately 10 percent.[208,209] Sullivan and colleagues[209] recently evaluated the 1-year incidence of thrombocytopenia (<50,000/μl) in a group of 30,214 HIV-infected patients as part of the retrospective Adult and Adolescent Spectrum of Disease Project. The incidence of thrombocytopenia over 1 year was 8.7 percent in patients with clinical AIDS, 3.1 percent in patients with immunologic AIDS (CD4+ <200 cells/μl), and 1.7 percent in patients with neither. Development of thrombocytopenia was associated with clinical or immunologic AIDS, history of injection drug use, history of anemia or lymphoma, and African American race. After controlling for multiple factors (AIDS, CD4+ count, anemia, neutropenia, antiviral therapy, and receipt of prophylaxis against *P. carinii*), thrombocytopenia was significantly associated with shorter survival (risk ratio = 1.7, 95% confidence interval = 1.6–1.8).[209]

MECHANISMS OF THROMBOCYTOPENIA IN HIV-RELATED THROMBOCYTOPENIC PURPURA

Increased Platelet Destruction   As in "de novo" immune thrombocytopenic purpura (ITP), HIV-infected patients with ITP also demonstrate increased platelet destruction via phagocytosis by macrophages in the spleen.[210] In HIV-related ITP, however, several mechanisms for platelet-associated antibody have been described, often occurring simultaneously in a given patient. Thus, presence of platelet-specific antibodies, immunochemically characterized as anti-glycoprotein (GP)IIb and/or GPIIIa, have been detected in HIV-infected patients with ITP, indicating a mechanism similar to that described in "de novo" disease.[211] However, cross-reactive antibody between HIV GP160/120 and platelet GPIIb/IIIa has also been demonstrated.[212] Thus, Bettaieb and colleagues found that serum antibodies against HIV GP160/120 could be eluted from platelets of patients with HIV-related ITP and that these HIV-specific antibodies shared a common epitope with antibodies against platelet GPIIb/IIIa on the platelet surface. It is thus apparent that molecular mimicry between HIV GP160/120 and platelet GPIIb/IIIa may be operative in the immune destruction of platelets in some cases of HIV-related ITP. A further mechanism of antibody-induced destruction of platelets arises from the absorption of immune complexes against HIV onto the platelet Fc receptor, thus providing a "free" Fc portion for subsequent macrophage binding and phagocytosis.[211]

Decreased Platelet Production   Kinetic studies of platelet production and destruction have been performed in patients with HIV-related ITP, with results compared to a group of normal control subjects and to a group of patients with "de novo" ITP.[210] Mean platelet survival was found to be significantly decreased in patients with HIV ITP, occurring to the same extent in patients receiving zidovudine and in those who were untreated. It is interesting to note that the mean platelet survival was also significantly decreased in HIV-infected patients with normal platelet counts. In addition to this increased destruction of platelets, mean platelet production was found to be significantly decreased in patients with untreated HIV ITP, although those patients receiving zidovudine demonstrated a subsequent increase in platelet production, occurring even in zidovudine-treated HIV-infected individuals without thrombocytopenia. Thus, it is apparent that patients with HIV ITP, while experiencing a moderate increase in platelet destruction, are also faced with significant decreases in platelet production, which occur even in those individuals with normal platelet counts.[210]

Infection of the Megakaryocyte by HIV   The cause for the reduced production of platelets in the setting of HIV infection may be direct infection of the megakaryocyte by HIV. Thus, Kouri and colleagues first demonstrated that human megakaryocytes bear a CD4+ receptor capable of binding HIV-1,[213] while Zucker-Franklin et al. showed that HIV-1 could be internalized by human megakaryocytes.[214] Wang and colleagues demonstrated the presence of the HIV-1 coreceptor, CXCR4, on megakaryocytic progenitors, megakaryocytes, and platelets.[215] Further, employing in situ hybridization techniques and a ^{35}S HIV riboprobe (antisense to an HIV *ENV* sequence), HIV transcripts have been detected in megakaryocytes of 5 of 10 patients with HIV ITP, indicating that the megakaryocyte had been infected by HIV in these cases.[216] Expression of viral RNA was also detected in all 10 patients, using in situ hybridization techniques. Specific ultrastructural damage in the HIV-infected megakaryocytes has also been noted, consisting of blebbing and vacuolization of the surface membrane.[217] The documentation of significant increases in platelet production after receipt of zidovudine[218] would be consistent with the hypothesis that a major mechanism of this disorder is the direct infection of the megakaryocyte by HIV.

Recently, Harker and colleagues described three chimpanzees infected with HIV-1 who developed ITP associated with elevated levels of antibody against platelet GPIIIa. Use of recombinant pegylated human megakaryocyte growth and development factor was associated with a decline in antiplatelet antibodies in serum as well as an increase in peripheral blood platelet counts and an increase in the number of megakaryocytes and megakaryocyte progenitors in the marrow.[219] These changes would imply that the mechanism of ITP in HIV-infected chimps includes insufficient compensatory increases in platelet production.

THERAPY FOR HIV-RELATED ITP

Zidovudine   The Swiss Group for HIV Studies was the first to demonstrate the efficacy of zidovudine therapy in patients with HIV ITP.[218] Ten seropositive patients, with platelet counts ranging from 20,000 to 100,000/μl, received zidovudine at a dose of 2 g/day for 2 weeks, followed by 1 g/day for 6 weeks. This was followed by 8 weeks of placebo. All 10 patients experienced an increase in platelet counts while on zidovudine, with a mean increase of 54,600/μl range (53,200–107,800/μl). In contrast, no patient experienced an increase in platelet count while on placebo. The time to onset of response was approximately 8 days, with full response achieved by day 30. These results were subsequently confirmed by others.[220,221]

The appropriate dose of zidovudine in HIV ITP was studied by Landonio et al., who compared a dose of 500 mg/day in 35 patients with 1000 mg/day in another group of 36 patients.[222] The majority of patients in both groups were injection drug users, with similar mean platelet counts ($\approx$23,000/μl) and mean CD4+ counts ($\approx$400 cells/μl). A response rate of 57 percent was achieved in the low-dose group, with 11 percent experiencing complete response. In contrast, a response rate of 72 percent was achieved in those receiving 1000 mg zidovudine per day, with complete response in 39 percent. At month 6, a significant difference remained between the groups, with a mean platelet count of 56,000/μl in the low-dose group versus 98,200/μl in those receiving high-dose zidovudine. It is apparent from this study that high-dose zidovudine is advantageous in patients with HIV ITP.[222]

Other Antiretroviral Agents   At the present time, very little is known about the efficacy of other reverse transcriptase inhibitors or protease inhibitors in the treatment of HIV ITP. Several case reports would suggest the efficacy of didanosine in both adults and children with HIV ITP, even in one patient who had been refractory to prior zidovudine. However, two additional patients who had been successfully treated with zidovudine subsequently developed relapse of ITP when didanosine was substituted for zidovudine.[223] Recently, increases in platelet counts have been described in 22 patients with advanced HIV disease treated with the protease inhibitor indinavir.[224] It would thus seem appropriate to consider use of other antiretroviral agents in patients with HIV ITP, although full information is still unavailable.[224]

Interferon-α   A prospective, randomized, double-blind, placebo-controlled trial of IFN-α at a dose of 3 million units thrice weekly, given subcutaneously, was conducted in 15 patients with HIV-related ITP.[225] A platelet response was documented in 66 percent, with a mean increase of 60,000/μl. The average time to response was 3 weeks. When interferon therapy was discontinued, platelet counts returned to baseline values within 3 months, indicating the necessity to maintain IFN-α therapy over time. In an attempt to ascertain the mechanisms by which IFN-α exerts its effects, Vianelli et al. demonstrated a prolongation in platelet survival, while no significant increase in platelet production was noted.[226]

High-Dose Intravenous Gamma Globulin   Intravenous gamma globulin (IVIG), at a dose of 1000 to 2000 mg/kg, has been used effectively in pediatric and adult patients with "de novo" ITP, resulting in a significant rise in platelet counts within 24 to 72 h in the majority of individuals.[227] Bussel and Haimi treated 22 patients with HIV-related ITP employing 1 to 2 g/kg during a 2- to 5-day period, depending upon the platelet response.[228] The average platelet count prior to therapy was 22,000/μl, rising to a mean of 182,000/μl (range 10,000–404,000/μl) within 2 to 5 days. Only two patients did not respond, while 77 percent experienced an increase to over100,000/μl, and 86 percent had an increase to over 50,000/μl. However, when IVIG was discontinued, only 25 percent of patients maintained the increased platelet count, while the remainder required repeat infusions approximately every 21 days. The major problem with IVIG appears to be cost, which is quite significant. For this reason, IVIG is often reserved for use in patients who are acutely bleeding or require an immediate increase in platelet count, for example, prior to an invasive procedure.

Anti-Rh Immunoglobulin   The use of anti-Rh IG in nonsplenectomized Rh-positive patients with HIV-related ITP represents another potential mode of therapy.[229] Requirements for effective therapy with anti-Rh (D) include a baseline hemoglobin level adequate to permit a 1- to 2-g decrease, presence of Rh positivity in the patient, and presence of a spleen, the site at which red cells would be preferentially phagocytized. Oksenhendler et al. treated 14 patients with HIV ITP employing 25 mg/kg IV over 30 min on 2 consecutive days.[230] Nine of 11 (83%) Rh-positive patients responded with a platelet count above 50,000/μl, with response first noted at a median of 4 days (range 3–12 days), and median response duration of 13 days (range 0–37 days). Maintenance therapy was administered at a dose of 13 to 25 mg/kg IV every 2 to 4 weeks, resulting in a long-term response (>6 months) in 70 percent of patients. Subclinical hemolysis occurred in all, with a drop of hemoglobin of 0.4 to 2.2 g. Gringeri et al. subsequently confirmed these results and also studied the use of intramuscular (IM) anti-D IG for maintenance treatment after successful induction therapy by the IV route.[229] Patients self-administered the IM anti-Rh at a dose of 6 to 13 mg/kg/week. After induction, 83 percent of patients had achieved a platelet count above 50,000/μl, a response that was maintained in 85 percent over time. It is thus apparent that anti-Rh IG may be used safely and effectively in patients with HIV-related ITP, providing an alternative that in some institutions may be as little as one-tenth the cost of high-dose IVIG.[229,230]

Splenectomy   Splenectomy has been used effectively in patients with "de novo" ITP who are refractory to corticosteroids. At the onset of the AIDS epidemic, several anecdotal case reports described a rapid progression to AIDS postsplenectomy, and the procedure was largely abandoned. More recently, Oksenhendler et al. reported long-term experience with splenectomy in a cohort of 185 patients with HIV ITP.[231] Splenectomy was eventually performed in 68 such patients, at an average of 13 months from initial diagnosis of HIV ITP. The mean platelet count presplenectomy was 18,000/ml, rising to 223,000/ml postoperatively. A response was seen in 92 percent of patients, with complete response (platelet count >100,000/μl) in 85 percent. Maintenance of the elevated platelet count for longer than 6 months was documented in 82 percent. In comparing the survival or rate of progression to AIDS in the 68 splenectomized patients versus the 117 who did not undergo the procedure, no difference was found, indicating that splenectomy was not associated with more rapid progression of HIV disease. Similar conclusions were made by Kemeny et al.[232] It is important to note, however, that 5.8 percent of patients undergoing splenectomy in Oksenhendler's series did experience fulminant infection, consisting of *Streptococcus pneumoniae* meningitis in two and *Haemophilus influenzae* sepsis in one. It is thus apparent that patients must undergo prophylactic vaccination prior to splenectomy and that such surgery may ultimately be safer in those HIV-infected patients who can still achieve an appropriate antibody response to vaccination against *S. pneumoniae* or *H. influenzae*.

Corticosteroids   Corticosteroids remain the initial therapy of choice in patients with "de novo" ITP and at a dose of 1 mg/kg/day are associated with an 80 to 90 percent response rate. Similar results have been documented in patients with HIV-related disease. However, the immunosuppressive effects of high-dose corticosteroids have made such therapy far from optimal in HIV-infected patients. Further, the potential development of fulminant Kaposi sarcoma (KS) in HIV-infected homosexual and bisexual men after use of corticosteroids has further dampened enthusiasm for this therapeutic modality.

SYSTEMIC ORGAN ABNORMALITIES

HIV infection can result in severe organ system dysfunction, involving the brain, peripheral nervous system, heart, lungs, kidneys, and other organs. These disease-related complications can result in significant morbidity and shortened survival but are not within the scope of this chapter.

HIV-ASSOCIATED MALIGNANCIES

Over 40 percent of all HIV-infected patients are eventually diagnosed with cancer.[233] Furthermore, the spectrum of neoplastic disease appears to be wider than initially seen.[233–235] Three cancers are currently considered AIDS-defining in HIV-infected persons: KS, associated with the epidemic from the onset in 1981; intermediate- or high-grade B-cell lymphoma, added to the case definition for AIDS in 1985; and cervical carcinoma, which became an AIDS-defining condition on January 1, 1993. Only AIDS-associated lymphoma and KS are discussed here.

AIDS-RELATED LYMPHOMA

EPIDEMIOLOGY

Patients with AIDS have a risk of developing lymphoma that is nearly 100 times greater than that of the general population.[235–237] The incidence of lymphoma increases with survival and may approach 20 percent for patients with prolonged, far-advanced immunodeficiency.[238,239] The use of HAART has been associated with a significant decrease in the incidence of KS[240] and opportunistic infections[129] in HIV-infected patients. It remains unclear whether the use of HAART will lead to a decreased incidence of AIDS-related lymphoma, although early data have not shown a decreased incidence.[240,241] In the large Swiss HIV Cohort Study, the incidence of new AIDS conditions fell from 157 events per 1000 person years in 1992–1994 to 35 events in 1997–1998, after widespread use of HAART. However, no decrease in the incidence of lymphoma was seen.[242] Lymphoma occurs among all population groups infected with HIV, in all age groups, and in patients from diverse geographic regions.[238,243] The clinical and pathologic characteristics of lymphoma appear similar among all groups.[237,244–246]

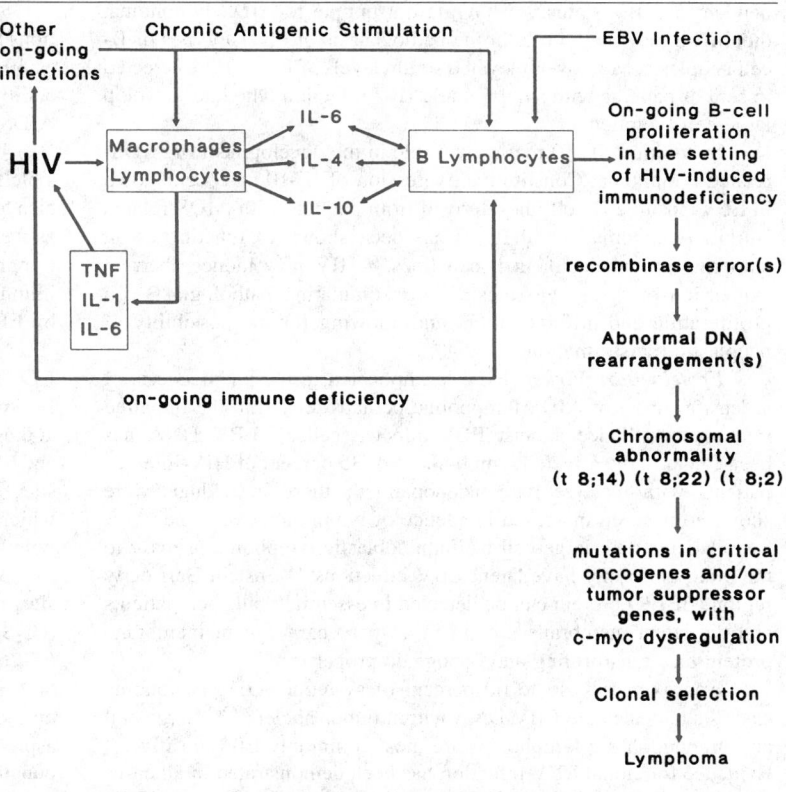

FIGURE 89-5   Schematic representation of the possible sequence of events resulting in the development of lymphoma in HIV disease. (Modified from Martin, et al.[342])

ETIOLOGY AND PATHOGENESIS

The mechanism or mechanisms underlying the development of lymphoma in the setting of HIV are not fully understood. One factor may be immune suppression itself, which is associated with an increased incidence of lymphoma in certain congenital immunodeficiency diseases,[247] autoimmune disorders,[248] or chronic use of immunosuppressive drugs, as in the setting of organ transplantation.[249,250] The lymphomas that develop in these settings are similar to the AIDS lymphomas in terms of the pathologic type, the high frequency of extranodal disease at presentation, and the relatively poor prognosis.

Infection by HIV is associated with myriad immunologic aberrations. These include functional and quantitative defects of CD4+ T cells[125,132,251] and chronic antigenic stimulation of B lymphocytes by antigens, mitogens, or viruses, including Epstein-Barr virus (EBV)[252] and HIV itself.[134,253] Ongoing B-cell expansion and activation result in the development of reactive B-cell hyperplasia in lymphoid tissues, known as PGL,[132,144,147,251] and in polyclonal hypergammaglobulinemia in the serum.[133] Lymphomas may develop after acquisition of genetic errors occurring in the course of polyclonal B-cell proliferation in the setting of underlying immunodeficiency. This has been noted in a primate model, in which high-grade B-cell lymphoma develops between 5 and 15 months after infection with the SIV, coincident with development of severe immunodeficiency.[254]

Cytokine Networks   Dysregulated expression of cytokines may contribute to the chronic B-cell proliferation that characterizes HIV disease. B-cell proliferation and maturation may be induced by several cytokines, including IL-4, IL-6, IL-10, tumor necrosis factor α (TNF-α), and others.[255] B cells from HIV-infected patients with hypergammaglobulinemia constitutively express TNF-α and IL-6.[256] High levels of IL-6 gene expression have been noted in multiple myeloma, chronic lymphocytic leukemia, and both HIV-positive and HIV-negative cases of immunoblastic and large-cell lymphoma, independent of EBV status.[257–259] While not unique to AIDS lymphoma, then, IL-6 may play a role in the pathogenesis of diverse types of B-cell neoplasia. Moreover, elevated serum levels of IL-6 can be detected in sera of patients with symptomatic HIV infection who later develop large-cell lymphoma.[239]

In addition, IL-10 may play a role in the development of AIDS-related lymphoma. Constitutive expression of IL-10 has been shown in EBV-positive B-cell lines derived from patients with AIDS-related Burkitt lymphoma,[260] and IL-10 has been shown to function as an autocrine growth factor in B-cell lines.[261] HIV may induce aberrant expression of these cytokines,[262] thus stimulating pathologic B-cell proliferation and differentiation, and allowing for the possibility of neoplastic transformation.

Epstein-Barr Virus EBV is implicated in the pathogenesis of at least a subset of AIDS lymphoma, perhaps related to the impaired immunosurveillance against EBV-infected cells.[252] EBV DNA has been found in the affected lymph nodes of 35 percent of HIV-infected patients with reactive lymphadenopathy;[263] these individuals were shown to have an increased incidence of lymphoma over time.[263]

Patients with large-cell or immunoblastic lymphoma primary to the brain uniformly have latent EBV infections.[264] Epstein-Barr early region (EBER) protein can be detected in essentially all such patients and the latent membrane protein in 45 percent.[264] Latent membrane protein has transforming and oncogenic properties.[265]

Approximately 40 to 60 percent of systemic AIDS lymphoma cases have detectable EBV DNA within tumor nuclei.[266,267] Large-cell and immunoblastic lymphomas are most commonly EBV positive.[268] Evidence for clonal EBV infection has been demonstrated in all cases examined, indicating that EBV integration occurred before clonal B-cell expansion.[269] This indicates that EBV may play a role in the etiopathogenesis of these lymphomas.

Abnormal DNA Rearrangements During AIDS-related B-cell stimulation induced by HIV, EBV, and/or cytokines, genetic "errors" in Ig gene rearrangement and/or expression may occur, leading to chromosomal translocations involving the Ig heavy- or light-chain genes. There are specific chromosomal translocations that have been described in AIDS-related lymphoma, including t(8;14); t(8;22); or t(8;2).[270–272]

C-MYC Dysregulation Translocations involving chromosome 8 can result in dysregulation of the c-MYC oncogene. Dependent upon the specific breakpoint position on chromosome 8 and the antigen receptor locus on chromosome 14, 2, or 22, different mechanisms for c-MYC dysregulation might apply, as described in the distinct forms of Burkitt lymphoma and in distinct geographic regions of the world.[273,274] However, c-MYC dysregulation is not seen in all cases of AIDS lymphoma. While activation of c-MYC was detected in 100 percent of small, noncleaved lymphomas in one series,[269] such activation was found in only a minority of large-cell or immunoblastic lymphomas.[275] Moreover, the specific mechanisms leading to c-MYC dysregulation appear diverse.[269,276,277] Thus, HIV-1 infection of immortalized B-cell lines in itself can result in upregulation of c-MYC transcripts,[278] while HIV also may affect cellular c-MYC gene expression directly.[277] Whatever the mechanism, dysregulation of c-MYC may contribute to transformation of human B cells in vitro and may cause B-cell lymphoma in transgenic animals carrying Ig-MYC chimeric constructs.[279,280]

BCL-6 Dysregulation and Other Genetic Abnormalities In AIDS-related diffuse large-cell lymphoma, the primary molecular alteration involves mutations of BCL-6.[281,282] While gross rearrangements of BCL-6 are usually absent, small mutations in the 5′ regions of the gene are detectable in as many as 60 percent of cases.[281–283] While the function of these mutations is still unclear, BCL-6 mutations are markers of germinal center derivaton of B cells, indicating that diffuse large-cell lymphomas in AIDS are related to germinal center B cells.[284]

Aside from these genetic abnormalities, other molecular aberrations have been noted, including p53 mutations or deletions in as many as 60 percent of AIDS-related small, noncleaved lymphomas.[275,285] In addition, mutations of RAS have been described in some cases of AIDS-related Burkitt lymphoma.[275]

It is clear that multiple diverse molecular mechanisms are responsible for the various types of AIDS-related lymphomas.[284] Small, noncleaved lymphomas are most often associated with c-MYC aberrations, as well as mutations in p53 and occasionally RAS. Diffuse large-cell lymphomas are associated with mutations in the BCL-6 gene, while immunoblastic and large-cell lymphomas appear to be driven primarily by EBV.

CLINICAL FEATURES

B symptoms, such as fever, night sweats, or weight loss are present at diagnosis in 80 to 90 percent of patients with AIDS lymphoma,[286,287] and 61 to 90 percent have far-advanced disease presenting in extranodal sites.[286,288–293] This is in contrast to non–AIDS-related lymphoma, in which approximately 40 percent of individuals present with extranodal lymphomatous disease.[294]

Virtually any anatomic site may be involved.[286] The more common sites of initial extranodal disease include the central nervous system (CNS; 17–42%), GI tract (4–28%), marrow (21–33%), and liver (9–26%).[286,288–293]

Staging evaluation should include computed tomographic scanning of the chest, abdomen, and pelvis; a gallium-67 scan[295]; marrow aspirate and biopsy; and other studies as clinically indicated. Lumbar puncture should routinely be performed, since approximately 20 percent of patients have leptomeningeal lymphoma, even in the absence of specific symptoms or signs.[296] Intrathecal methotrexate or cytosine arabinoside is often given to prevent isolated CNS relapse.[296]

Primary Central Nervous System Lymphoma Approximately 75 percent of patients with primary CNS lymphoma have far-advanced HIV disease, with median CD4 cell counts less than $50/\mu$l, and a prior history of AIDS.[234,287,297–299] Initial symptoms and signs may be quite variable, with seizures, headache, and/or focal neurologic dysfunction noted in most. However, very subtle changes in behavior may be the only presenting complaint.[297]

Radiographic scanning reveals relatively large mass lesions (2–4 cm), which tend to be few in number (one to three lesions). Ring enhancement may be seen.[300,301] There is no specific radiographic picture. Positron-emission tomography scanning may be useful in differentiating cerebral lymphoma from toxoplasmosis.[302] In addition, thallium-201 single-photon emission computerized tomography scanning may be useful, with median T1 uptake index of greater than 1.5 and a lesion size of greater than 2.5 cm serving as independent predictors of primary CNS lymphoma.[303]

Pathologically, almost all such lymphomas are of diffuse large-cell or immunoblastic subtypes and are uniformly associated with EBV infection within malignant cells.[304] Thus, presence of EBV DNA within spinal fluid may be used as a diagnostic criterion for primary CNS lymphoma.[305]

Optimal therapy for primary CNS lymphoma remains to be defined. Use of cranial radiation is associated with a complete remission rate of only 50 percent and median survival of only 2 or 3 months. While median survival times have not been prolonged with radiation, approximately 75 percent of patients experience an improvement in quality of life.[306] No specific regimen of chemotherapy has yet proven efficacious, perhaps due to the serious level of immunocompromise in affected patients.

Primary Effusion Lymphoma Primary effusion lymphoma (PEL) is uncommon, representing only a small fraction of all AIDS lymphomas. PEL is associated with the newly discovered human herpesvirus, termed KS-associated herpesvirus or human herpesvirus type 8 (HHV-8).[307-309] The disease has been reported in both HIV-positive and HIV-negative patients, although it appears more common in the former. It is interesting to note that PEL has also been diagnosed in a cardiac transplant recipient, whose explanted heart was found, retrospectively, to be infected by HHV-8.[310] Morphologically, the malignant cell is large and appears anaplastic with immunoblastic features. The malignant cell usually lacks B-cell markers but is B lymphoid in origin, based upon presence of Ig gene rearrangement. HHV-8 is present within tumor cells, which often harbor EBV as well. Clinically, patients present with effusions in the pleura, pericardium, or peritoneal cavity. Most patients do not have mass lesions, although such masses have been reported. Despite therapeutic intervention, survival is extremely short, in the range of approximately 2 months.[311]

PATHOLOGY

Eighty to 90 percent of lymphomas associated with AIDS are intermediate- or high-grade B-cell tumors,[312] including immunoblastic or large-cell types, and small noncleaved lymphoma, which may be subclassified as either Burkitt or Burkitt-like. Approximately 80 to 90 percent of patients are diagnosed with one of these pathologic types,[289-293] in sharp contrast to non–HIV-infected patients, in whom high-grade lymphomas are expected in only 10 to 15 percent.[313]

Occasionally, HIV-infected patients with low-grade B-cell lymphomas have been reported,[288,289,293,314] as have relatively young individuals with multiple myeloma or solitary plasmacytoma.[315] The natural history of low-grade lymphoma appears similar in the presence or absence of underlying HIV infection.[314,316] These cases are not considered AIDS defining.

T-cell lymphomas also have been described in HIV-infected individuals.[286] Once again, these cases are not considered AIDS-defining, and their incidence has not increased.

PROGNOSIS AND THERAPY

Prognostic Factors   Poor prognostic indicators for survival include a Karnofsky performance status of less then 70 percent, history of AIDS prior to lymphoma, less than 100 CD4 cells/ml,[287,317] stage III or IV disease, elevated lactate dehydrogenase, history of injection drug use, and age over 35 years.[317]

Patients with primary CNS lymphoma have shorter survival than those with systemic disease.[287] However, in patients with systemic lymphoma who also have leptomeningeal involvement, prognosis is not affected, provided that appropriate therapy to the CNS is given.[287]

Treatment   At the outset of the AIDS epidemic, very dose-intensive regimens were employed. Unfortunately, low complete remission rates (20–33%) were achieved, and there were high rates of complicating opportunistic infections, leading to death in 28 to 78 percent of cases.[298,299,318-320] While occasionally reports noted the efficacy of dose-intensive regimens, these were characterized by the chance inclusion of patients who had presented with good prognostic features.[321]

These observations led to the design and implementation of a low-dose modification of the methotrexate, bleomycin, cyclophosphamide, and etoposide combination chemotherapy (m-BACOD) regimen.[296] A complete response was achieved in 46 percent of patients, with long-term, lymphoma-free survival in 75 percent. The median survival of complete responders was 15 months, while that of all evaluable patients was 6.5 months.[296]

In an attempt to clarify the value of low-dose therapy, the AIDS Clinical Trials Group embarked on a prospective, multicenter trial.[322] Patients were stratified by baseline prognostic indicators and randomized to receive either the low-dose m-BACOD regimen discussed above or standard-dose m-BACOD with hematopoietic growth factor support (GM-CSF). With 192 patients evaluable for response, no statistically significant difference was observed in response rates. While patients with CD4 cell counts below 100/ml did not respond as well as those with higher CD4 cells, the low-dose regimen appeared equivalent to standard-dose m-BACOD in patients with either good risk or poor risk prognostic features. Toxicity was significantly higher in those patients assigned to standard-dose therapy, with grade 3 or 4 toxicity in 70 percent of those assigned to standard dose and 51 percent of those who received low-dose therapy (p < .008). This trial indicates that low-dose m-BACOD is preferable to standard-dose therapy in patients with AIDS lymphoma.[322]

A regimen of continuous infusion chemotherapy, termed CDE, was piloted by Sparano and colleagues.[323] This regimen consists of a 96-h continuous infusion of cyclophosphamide, doxorubicin, and etoposide, which is repeated every 28 days times six. Initial results were excellent, with a complete remission rate of 58 percent and a median overall survival of 18.4 months.[323] When this experience was recently expanded in a multi-institutional trial through the Eastern Cooperative Oncology Group, a complete remission rate of 46 percent was achieved, with median survival of 8.2 months.[324]

Investigators at the National Cancer Institute have recently reported on the EPOCH regimen, employed in 24 patients with newly diagnosed AIDS-lymphoma.[325,326] A 96-h continuous infusion of etoposide, oncovin, and adriamycin was administered, along with a bolus of cyclophosphamide, which was dose adjusted based on patients' CD4 cell count and nadir neutrophil counts. Oral prednisone was also given. A complete remission rate of 79 percent was achieved, and no responding patient has experienced relapse, with a median follow-up of approximately 2 years.

When multiagent chemotherapy is administered together with HAART, pharmacokinetic profiles appear similar to those described in the absence of HAART for adriamycin and indinavir, while the clearance rate for cyclophosphamide appears moderately prolonged. Nonetheless, no increase in clinical or laboratory toxicity was reported. However, the concomitant use of zidovudine with chemotherapy has been associated with significant myelosuppression.

KAPOSI SARCOMA

ETIOLOGY AND PATHOGENESIS

The etiology and pathogenesis of KS is complex, only recently elucidated, and still not fully understood. Underlying immunosuppression clearly increases the risk of KS. Thus, the incidence of KS in organ transplant recipients receiving immunosuppressive therapy is 400- to 500-fold higher than that seen in the general population.[327] Genetic factors may also play a role.[328,329]

In addition to these factors, the epidemiology of AIDS-related KS has always suggested the possibility that another sexually transmitted organism might be involved in the pathogenesis of disease, since the disorder is statistically more likely to occur in homosexual and bisexual men than in other population groups infected by HIV.[330-332] The concept of KS as a sexually transmitted disease independent of HIV infection is also derived from studies of KS in young, sexually active, HIV-negative homosexual men in the United States.[333-335]

The identification of a newly described human herpesvirus, termed KS-associated herpesvirus or HHV-8,[336] provided the anticipated link between KS and a previously unknown sexually transmitted virus. Genomic material from HHV-8 was subsequently found within essentially all KS tissue from virtually all types of KS, including that associated with AIDS, classic Mediterranean KS, endemic KS from Africa, and transplantation-associated KS.[337-340] Subsequent work confirmed that seroconversion to HHV-8 occurred prior to the development of clinical KS[341] and that seropositivity to the virus increased with increasing numbers of sexual contacts.[342] However, the actual means by which HHV-8 is transmitted and the clinical illness associated with initial HHV-8 infection remain speculative at this time.[343]

HHV-8 is a B-lymphotropic γ-DNA herpesvirus with tropism for endothelial cells and keratinocytes.[344] Multiple genes have recently been identified that encode various latent or lytic gene products. Two of these genes, ORF K3 and K5, may decrease major histocompatibility complex expression on the surface of infected cells, thereby enabling escape from immune control.[345] Expression of a viral IL6 homolog (vIL6) has been shown to correlate with development of KS.[346] vIL6 has been shown to induce proliferation of B cells and HIV replication in HIV-infected U1 monocyte cell lines.[347] It is important to note that the lytic gene product, HHV-8 G protein–coupled receptor, which is expressed in the lytic phase of HHV-8, has been shown to transform cells through inflammatory cytokine signaling pathways while also serving as a chemokine homolog and serving to trigger other factors involved in angiogenesis.

In the setting of AIDS-related KS, HHV-8 has been shown to infect endothelial cells, inducing a change in the spindle cell morphology that is characteristic of the disease. These spindle cells then produce numerous autocrine and paracrine growth factors that stimulate both KS and blood vessel proliferation, including basic fibroblast growth factor (bFGF), vascular endothelial growth factor, platelet-derived growth factor, TGF-β, IL-6, IL-8, GM-CSF, and others.[348–352]

HHV-8–encoded gene products thus have the capability of inducing the multiple aberrations that are found within KS tissues. Nonetheless, while the virus appears necessary for development of KS, it is not sufficient in itself. The further addition of immunosuppression and an environment conducive to inflammatory and angiogenic signals is apparently also required.

Aside from inducing the necessary immunosuppression required for development of clinical KS, the HIV TAT gene product is also operative in the pathogenesis of disease. Thus, the Tat protein has been shown to increase the proliferation of KS derived spindle cells.[353,354] Tat also activates the expression of tumor necrosis factor α (TNF-α), IL-6, and various adhesion molecules, such as E-selectin, ICAM-1, and VCAM-1. Tat synergizes with other inflammatory cytokines to stimulate endothelial cells and the invasion of KS spindle cells.

By inducing a mileau of inflammatory cytokines, such as IL-1, TNF-α, IL-6, and others, HIV further indirectly increases the proliferation of the KS lesion, while these inflammatory cytokines also serve to increase the production of various angiogenic factors, such as bFGF.[355–357]

The full pathogenesis of AIDS KS is thus complex, and the very designation of the tumor as a true malignancy is under question. Nonetheless, it is apparent that the full expression of disease requires several components. These include HIV-1 itself, which induces the requisite immunosuppression, as well as the TAT gene product, and a mileau of inflammatory cytokines and angiogenic factors. HHV-8 may induce the initial transforming event as well as myriad gene products that contribute to the cascade of angiogenic and inflammatory cytokines, which induce further growth of the lesion. Conceptually, then, the KS lesion is driven by factors that induce the three components that are integral to the disease: cell proliferation, inflammation, and angiogenesis. These newly recognized concepts will be critical to the development of new methods of treating patients with AIDS KS.

Changing Epidemiology of Kaposi Sarcome in the Era of Highly Active Antiretroviral Therapy

The use of HAART has been associated with a significant decrease in the incidence of KS[240] and opportunistic infections[129] in HIV-infected patients. In the Multicenter AIDS Cohort Study, rates of KS fell by 66 percent between 1989–1994 and 1996–1997,[240] coincident with the widespread use of HAART in the United States.

CLINICAL FEATURES

KS lesions appear as discrete, irregular reddish to violaceous or brown nodules, macules, or plaques and may be symmetrically arranged. They may be several centimeters in circumference or quite small and easy to overlook. Suspicious lesions should undergo biopsy, since many other conditions, such as bacillary angiomatosis, may be confused with KS, even by the experienced observer.

The lesions of KS may occur in any site,[358] although CNS involvement is quite rare. Involvement of the mucous membranes of the mouth is quite common, and, approximately 50 percent of the time, oral KS is associated with KS elsewhere in the GI tract. KS may involve any area of the GI tract. Although usually asymptomatic, GI KS may produce symptoms of retrosternal, epigastric, or rectal pain; blood loss; diarrhea; abdominal cramps; and/or weight loss.[359] Patients suspected of having KS in the GI tract should be evaluated by endoscopy,[360] since barium studies often miss the flat lesions of KS.

Patients with pulmonary KS may have shortness of breath, fever, cough, hemoptysis, and/or chest pain. Occasionally, patients with pulmonary KS are asymptomatic.[361] The radiographic appearance is varied and not specific. Survival in the setting of pulmonary KS is usually short, and systemic therapy is indicated.[361,362]

Patients with KS may present with lymphadenopathy alone, even in the absence of skin or mucous membrane involvement. The diagnosis requires lymph node biopsy.[363] Patients also may present with lymphedema, even in the absence of overlying skin disease. The edema is presumably secondary to capillary leak in the local mileau of inflammatory cytokine and angiogenic factors.

THERAPY, COURSE, AND PROGNOSIS

Antiviral Therapy to Treat KS   With the sharp decline in KS incidence coincident with the widespread use of HAART therapy, the efficacy of HAART as a specific treatment for KS has been discussed. At this time, no prospective trials addressing this issue have been completed. However, anecdotal reports of KS regression while on HAART alone have been published.[364]

Of further interest is the possible use of antiviral agents directed against HHV-8 as a means of treating KS. Studies of in vitro drug sensitivity have shown that HHV-8 is very sensitive to cidofovir, moderately sensitive to ganciclovir and foscarnet, and weakly sensitive to acylovir.[365] A recent prospective randomized trial aimed at determining optimal maintenance therapy for cytomegalovirus (CMV) retinitis in patients with AIDS has also provided information to suggest that treatment of HHV-8 may prevent development of KS.[366] After initial systemic therapy of CMV disease, patients were randomized to receive either a ganciclovir retinal implant alone or the implant with systemic ganciclovir in addition. It is very interesting to note that patients randomized to receive systemic ganciclovir had a statistically decreased risk of progression to KS.[366] The concept that one could treat lytic HHV-8 infection with ganciclovir and in so doing positively affect the development of a tumor is clearly intruiging, and a great deal of further work in this area is expected over the next several years.

Local Therapies   KS is a multicentric disease at presentation and is inherently disseminated. Nevertheless, numerous local therapies have been used efficaciously, including surgical excision, liquid nitrogen cryotherapy, and argon laser therapy.[367–369] Recently, the topical use of cisretinoic acid has proven efficacious in the local therapy of KS and has been licensed in the United States for this purpose.[370,371] Injections of vinblastine, vincristine, or IFN-α directly into the lesion also have been effective.[372–374] These injections may be associated with local pain as the lesion ulcerates and then resolves. Hypo- or hyperpigmented areas may remain. Local radiation therapy also may be effective. Depending upon the indication, complete remission may be achieved in 20 to 70 percent of cases, although postradiation hyperpigmentation has been reported in 20 percent or more, and local relapse may occur.[375,376] Single doses of 800 cGy have been associated with good responses,[377] albeit of short duration in some.[378] Lesions in the oral cavity can be particularly troubling, producing pain or difficulty in eating. Although responses to radiation are expected in the majority, severe confluent mucositis, salivary gland dysfunction with dry mouth, and altered taste for food have been described in patients who were irradiated with as little as 1200 to 1800 cGy to the midline of the oral cavity.[375]

Biologic Response Modifiers Patients with more extensive disease may benefit from therapy with IFN-α, which has been shown to have antiretroviral effects in vitro[379] that correlate with its antitumor efficacy.[380] It is interesting to note that INF-α inhibits angiogenesis, which may be its primary mechanism of activity in KS. Although high doses of IFN-α were initially used to treat AIDS KS, recent studies have confirmed the efficacy of lower doses, from 1 to 10 million units/day, when combined with antiviral therapy.[381-383] Response rates of approximately 40 percent have been reported,[381-383] and maximal response may take up to 3 months.[381,382] Response to IFN-α is associated with enhanced survival.[384]

Systemic Chemotherapy Systemic chemotherapy may be required for patients with rapidly progressive disease, symptomatic visceral disease, pulmonary KS, and/or lymphedema. Multiple single agents have activity in KS, including doxorubicin, vinblastine, vincristine, bleomycin, and etoposide.[385-388] Single-agent use of liposomal daunomycin (DaunoXome) or doxorubicin (Doxil) has been associated with response rates of 40 to 50 percent with acceptable toxicity.[389,390] Taxol, given every 2 or 3 weeks at a dose of 100 to 135 mg/m^2, has also been associated with major response in 55 percent of relapsed or refractory patients.[391]

Combination chemotherapy regimens, such as ABV, consisting of doxorubicin (20 mg/m^2), bleomycin (10 mg/m^2), and vincristine (2 mg),[388] or vincristine and bleomycin (VB) may also be useful.[392] However, discontinuation of chemotherapy eventually results in relapse.

Antiangiogenesis Compounds and Drugs to Decrease the Cascade of Inflammatory Cytokines for Treatment of AIDS KS With the evolving understanding that the KS lesion requires a mileau rich in inflammatory cytokines and angiogenic factors, the possible blockade of these factors has been discussed as a means to treat the disease. In this regard, INF-α has known activity and serves as a potent inhibitor of angiogenic factors.[382,383] A sulfated polysaccharide peptidoglycan (SP-PG) has been shown to inhibit angiogenesis associated with induction of KS-like lesions in vitro.[393] A fumagillin analog with potent antiangiogenesis activity has shown evidence of clinical efficacy in patients with AIDS KS.[394] Multiple additional angiogenesis inhibitors are currently in phase II trial, including IL-12, thalidomide, IM-862, and others. Retinoids have been shown to down-regulate IL-6 and other cytokines that are involved in the pathogenesis of KS, and recent trials have proven some efficacy with the use of oral 9-*cis* retinoic acid.[395] Future directions in the therapy of AIDS KS will clearly involve testing and use of compounds that decrease the cascade of inflammatory cytokines and angiogenic factors that contribute to the pathogenesis of the disease.

ANTIRETROVIRAL THERAPY

Antiretroviral therapy has undergone significant and rapid change over the last several years. In addition to the emergence of an increasing number of effective antiretroviral agents, the development of sensitive assays for the quantitative determination of viral replication and the characterization of mechanisms of viral drug resistance has resulted in more logical and clinically effective therapeutic strategies. However, the rapidity with which HIV therapy has developed and the intensive investigative efforts currently being undertaken suggest that any recommendations made in the context of this chapter will be subject to significant modification, and clinicians should therefore avail themselves of the most current literature regarding HIV antiretroviral therapy.

While controversies exist regarding the optimal time to initiate antiretroviral therapy, current recommendations include treatment of all patients with symptomatic HIV disease or asymptomatic HIV-infected people with CD4 counts lower than 500/μl or plasma HIV RNA greater than 10,000 copies per milliliter by the branched-chain bDNA assay or more than 20,000 copies per milliliter by RT-PCR.[396-398] There are both advantages and disadvantages to initiating early therapy in asymptomatic patients. Early intervention usually results in more effective control of viral replication, with rapid reduction of viral burden and maintenance of near normal immunologic function.[399] An important benefit of rapid and maximal suppression of viral replication is the reduction of viral genomic mutations, which can result in the development of viral drug resistance and the emergence of more aggressive cytopathic viral strains.[400-402] An additional, although theoretical, advantage is that reduced concentrations of virus in body fluids may decrease the risk of viral transmission.

The potential risks of early intervention include reduction in quality of life from drug toxicities, unexpected drug interactions, and an excessive pill burden. In addition, there is growing evidence that some antiretroviral drugs or combinations may have unexpected long-term toxicities, including diabetes, accelerated atherosclerosis, and persistent peripheral neuropathies. Early exposure to antiretroviral medications, especially if associated with poor patient compliance, may lead to early viral drug resistance and a subsequent reduction in therapeutic options due to viral cross-resistance to closely related drugs.[403-409]

The emergence of drug-resistant viral strains has complicated HIV therapy. Well-characterized genomic mutations have been reported in association with viral resistance to certain medications. In addition, some mutations may result in cross-resistance with other antiretroviral agents.[404-406] Transmission of these drug-resistant viral strains has now been reported and therefore may complicate therapy for patients who are apparently therapy naive.[410] Both phenotypic and genotypic assays of drug resistance have been developed.[406,411,412] However, at present these assays are not routinely available.

Viral load should fall at least 1 log in the first 4 weeks after initiation of antiretroviral therapy and should be undetectable by 3 to 6 months.[396-398] Current assays can detect viral RNA to a level of less than 50 copies per milliliter. Data suggest that lowering the viral load to less than 50 copies per milliliter is associated with more complete and durable viral suppression than are levels of 50 to 500 copies per milliliter.[402] Viral load testing should be used to assess the efficacy of treatment and to assist in determining the need modify antiretroviral therapy.

NUCLEOSIDE REVERSE TRANSCRIPTASE INHIBITORS

Nucleoside reverse transcriptase inhibitors (NRTIs) continue to serve as the foundation for most multidrug antiviral regimens. After cellular uptake, NRTIs are converted by cellular kinases to their triphosphate form. The triphosphate form then competes with the natural substrate of HIV reverse transcriptase, which is not present in uninfected human cells. The phosphorylated NRTIs are incorporated into the DNA strand, causing premature termination of the HIV intermediate.[413]

In addition to convenience, the choice of which NRTI combination to use should also be based on efficacy, ability to penetrate the CNS, and effects that one NRTI may have on another. Several studies have found no significant differences among combinations of NRTIs.[414]

Among currently available NRTIs, AZT appears to be the most successful at crossing the blood-brain barrier and has been shown to substantially reduce the risk of developing HIV brain disease.[415,416] Abacavir also effectively crosses the blood-brain barrier and is currently being evaluated as a treatment option for HIV dementia.[417] In the era of triple therapy combinations, including nonnucleoside reverse transcriptase inhibitors (NNRTIs) and protease inhibitors (PIs) that can suppress HIV in the CNS, the absolute need for AZT in an initial regimen may no longer be apparent.

Resistance to lamivudine (3TC) emerges rapidly, especially in patients in whom viral load remains detectable.[417,418] Paradoxically, the mutation that confers 3TC resistance may reverse resistance to AZT by suppressing the effect of AZT mutations at codons 215 and 70.[419] However, this benefit is likely to be transient with the emergence of other mutations that will confer AZT resistance.[420] Response to stavudine (d4T) in people previously treated with AZT may be impaired, sinces chronic AZT therapy may render cells less efficient in phosphorylating other NRTIs.[406]

NONNUCLEOSIDE REVERSE TRANSCRIPTASE INHIBITORS

NNRTIs bind directly and noncompetitively to reverse transcriptase downstream from the active catalytic site to inhibit production of viral DNA, acting at different sites than NRTIs. They do not require phosphorylation for activation.[421] The primary advantages of their use are the ability to delay use of PIs and their relatively easier dosing schedules. NNRTs are not cross-resistant with the NRTIs.[421] However, resistance to this class of drugs can easily develop from a single mutation.[422] In vitro mutations common to all NNRTI-resistant reverse transcriptases include codons 103, 106, 108, 181, and 190.[411,421] Codon 236 mutation appears unique to resistance to delavirdine.[423]

PROTEASE INHIBITORS

PIs represent the most potent antiviral agents available, with the ability to suppress viral replication by 2 logs or more.[396-398,424] PIs prevent HIV from being successfully assembled and released from the infected CD4 cell by inhibiting the viral protease enzyme that cleaves the large viral polyproteins into small functional units.[424] There is clear evidence of durable virologic and immunologic effects with associated improvements in clinical outcome for patients treated with PIs.[424-435] The introduction of PIs into clinical practice in 1996 accounts for the significant improvement in outcome for patients with HIV disease. Despite the potent antiviral effect of PIs, problems with their use include bioavailability, drug interactions, significant toxicity, and the emergence of resistance.[435436-444] Because of concerns for cross-resistance between the drugs in this class, the choice of which drug to use first becomes important because of the potential effect on future treatment options.[396-398,424] Whether these drugs should be used as first-line therapy or reserved for use in people with virologic failure on other regimens is currently under evaluation.

Adverse reactions to PIs have become more apparent with long-term use, and drug-drug interactions are numerous.[398,424,435-444] One newly recognized toxicity of PIs is the "lipodystrophy syndrome," which may occur in 30 to 70 percent of PI-treated patients.[441,442] Clinical features of the lipodystrophy syndrome include increased abdominal girth; loss of subcutaneous fat in the trunk, with increased visceral fat; development of dorsocervical fat pads; and loss of subcutaneous fat pads in the face.[441] Other components of the lipodystrophy syndrome

include the development of pseudo-Cushingoid appearance, hyperglycemia due to development of insulin resistance, and hypercholesterolemia with premature coronary artery disease.[435-444] These toxicities may result from a cross-reaction between the PIs and enzymes for lipid metabolism, including lipoprotein receptor-like protein and cis-retinoic binding protein type1,[441] although the precise mechanism for this toxicity is not yet known.

CLINICAL GUIDELINES

At present, indications for beginning antiretroviral therapy include (1) symptomatic HIV disease, (2) asymptomatic patients with CD4 count less then $500/\mu l$ and viral load greater than 10,000 copies of bDNA per milliliter or greater than 20,000 copies of RNA per milliliter, (3) acute retroviral syndrome or within 6 months of HIV seroconversion, (4) postexposure prophylaxis, and (5) prevention of perinatal transmission.[396-398]

Once a decision has been made to start antiretroviral therapy, the preferred initial regimens at present are a combination of two NRTIs with a PI, NNRTI alone, or two PIs.[396-398]

It is estimated that only 40 to 80 percent of treatment-naive patients will obtain complete virologic suppression with currently available standard regimens.[396-398,445] New studies are attempting to determine whether long-term virologic suppression can be obtained in a higher proportion of patients when they are given a four-drug regimen that incorporates two NRTIs in combination with either two PIs or an NNRTI and a PI.

If therapy is to be discontinued for any reason (e.g., early pregnancy), it is advisable that all drugs be stopped simultaneously to prevent the probable emergence of drug resistance to any one drug when used as monotherapy.[446] Early data from a subgroup of patients in the EARTH study who stopped therapy after 1 year showed a rebound in viral load in all patients. Although all responded to reintroduction of the same regimen used prior to discontinuation, there were declines in CD4 percentages during the period of no treatment.[447] Thus, the concerns with "drug holidays" are related to the potential emergence of viral resistance and also to the adverse effect on immune function.

Indications to change antiretroviral therapy include (1) drug failure, defined as a failure to decrease HIV RNA by more than 0.5 to 0.75 log after 4 weeks of treatment, less than a 1-log reduction by 8 weeks, or a failure to obtain undetectable RNA levels within 4 to 6 months, (2) recurrence of detectable viral RNA from a previously undetectable level, suggesting the development of resistance, (3) significant increase of 0.5 to 0.75 log from nadir viral RNA not attributable to concurrent infection or vaccination, (4) persistently declining CD4 cell counts, (5) clinical deterioration, such as the development of a new major opportunistic infection, (6) toxicity, and (7) nonadherence.[396-398]

It is advisable to base any decision to change therapy on two separate tests of viral load and CD4 counts.[396-398] The decision to change antiretroviral therapy needs to be balanced to include available treatment options, issues of cross-resistance, potential toxicities, and drug interactions. HIV RNA level monitoring should take precedence over CD4 counts in determining the need to switch therapy.

Viral resistance, altered pharmacokinetics, or poor patient adherence may cause failure of a specific regimen. It is essential to differentiate drug failure from drug intolerance, since in the latter situation it may be necessary to change the one offending drug rather than the whole regimen. In contrast, in a failing regimen it is essential to substitute for the old regimen at least two new drugs and preferably an entirely new regimen. For patients with advanced disease and a history of exposure to multiple antiretroviral drugs, it may be necessary to start a regimen that would be deemed suboptimal for initial therapy but that may be a reasonable choice for these patients.

MANAGEMENT OF HIV IN PREGNANCY

Various interventions have recently been explored in an attempt to decrease perinatal HIV-1 transmission. Use of zidovudine in pregnancy, beginning at week 14 and continuing throughout delivery, has been studied by the Pediatric AIDS Clinical Trials Group. A three-part regimen, beginning at week 14 of pregnancy, with IV infusions of zidovudine throughout labor and delivery and subsequent use of oral zidovudine by the infant resulted in a decrease in transmission rate by approximately 70 percent, from 25 percent to 8 percent.[64] More abbreviated courses of zidovudine have also been shown effective, with a 9.3 percent transmission rate in infants who received the drug within 48 h of birth even though their mothers never received it.[65] Short-term toxicity of zidovudine appears acceptable in terms of both mother and infant. However, cancers have developed in offspring of pregnant rodents and monkeys given zidovudine during pregnancy, and much longer follow-up will be required to ascertain the true toxicity of the drug in humans. Preliminary data from Uganda have demonstrated the efficacy of two doses of nevirapine in preventing HIV transmission to the infant. One dose (200 mg) was given orally to the mother at the time of delivery, and the second was given to the newborn within the first 72 h of life.[66] This intervention, if confirmed, would be practically and financially feasible in resource-poor regions of the world. Current recommendations for prevention of perinatal HIV-1 transmission in the United States include use of combination antiretroviral therapy, as would ordinarily be indicated for the mother's own care, with addition of zidovudine.[67] The ultimate decision regarding use of antiretroviral agents in pregnancy must reside with the woman herself, after careful and nonjudgmental discussion with her health care providers. Additional means of decreasing perinatal transmission include avoidance of breast feeding, avoidance of premature rupture of the membranes during delivery, and delivery by elective cesarean section.[51,56,58] Each of these interventions poses particular problems in resource-poor regions of the world.

POSTEXPOSURE PROPHYLAXIS

The guidelines for the management of postexposure prophylaxis (PEP) were outlined in a consensus statement from the CDC in 1998.[448] Recommendations for PEP stem from animal studies and anecdotal human experience, since placebo-controlled clinical trials have not been performed. The risk for acquisition of HIV from a needle-stick exposure from an AIDS patient is 0.4 percent. Risk is increased with a deep injury, presence of visible blood on the device causing the injury, injury with a needle that has been placed in the source patient's artery or vein, terminal illness in the source patient, and lack of use of zidovudine PEP. Based on these risk factors, the recent guidelines have divided PEP regimens into basic and expanded groups. This stratification of risk assessment is fraught with practical problems that are the focus of current debate. Concern for the acquisition of drug-resistant virus has led to the recommendation of the addition of a drug from a class to which the source patient has not been exposed in cases where resistance is known or clinically suspected. In heavily pretreated source patients, this may not be an option. At a minimum, PEP prophylaxis to health care workers should include zidovudine (300 mg orally twice daily) and lamuvidine (150 mg twice a day). These drugs should be started as quickly as possible after the needle stick and should be continued for 4 weeks. If the exposure occurred greater than 72 h from the time of evaluation, antiretroviral drug intervention is not recommended. Attention is currently being focused on the feasibility

of extrapolating these recommendations to cases of sexual exposure and on publishing guidelines for the use of PEP in this setting.

REFERENCES

1. Centers for Disease Control: Case definition of acquired immunodeficiency syndrome. *MMWR* 30:250, 1981.
2. Centers for Disease Control: Revision of the case definition of acquired immunodeficiency syndrome for national reporting. *MMWR* 34:373, 1985.
3. Centers for Disease Control: Revision of the CDC surveillance case definition for acquired immunodeficiency syndrome. *MMWR* 36(1S): 1, 1987.
4. Centers for Disease Control: New case definition of HIV/AIDS. *MMWR* 41:RR17, 1992.
5. Colebunders R, Francis H, Izaley L: Evaluation of a clinical case-definition of acquired immunodeficiency syndrome in Africa. *Lancet* 2:492, 1987.
6. Pan American Health Organization: Working group on AIDS case definition. *Epidemiol Bull PAHO* 10:9, 1990.
7. Mellors JW, Rinaldo CR Jr, Gupta P, White RM, Todd JA, Kingsley LA: Prognosis in HIV-1 infection predicted by the quantity of virus in plasma. *Science* 272:1167, 1996.
8. Mellors JW, Munoz A, Giorgi J, et al: Plasma viral load and CD4+ lymphocytes as prognostic markers of HIV-1 infection. *Ann Intern Med* 126:946, 1997.
9. Letvin NL, Eaton KA, Aldrich WR, et al: Acquired immunodeficiency syndrome in a colony of macaque monkeys. *Proc Natl Acad Sci USA* 80:2718, 1983.
10. Henrickson RV, Maul DH, Osborn KG, et al: Epidemic of acquired immunodeficiency in rhesus monkeys. *Lancet* 1:338, 1983.
11. Kanki PJ, McLane MF, King NW Jr, et al: Serologic identification and characterization of a macaque T-lymphotropic retrovirus closely related to human T-lymphotropic retroviruses (HTLV) type III. *Science* 228:1199, 1985.
12. Kanki PJ, Kurth R, Becker W, et al: Antibodies to simian T-lymphotropic virus type III in African green monkeys and recognition of STLV-III viral proteins by AIDS and related sera. *Lancet* 1:1330, 1985.
13. Kanki PJ, Alroy J, Essex M: Isolation of T-lymphotropic retrovirus related to HTLV-III/LAV from wild-caught African green monkeys. *Science* 230:951, 1985.
14. Essex M: Origin of AIDS, in *AIDS: Etiology, Diagnosis, Treatment and Prevention*, 3rd ed, edited by VT DeVita Jr, S Hellman, SA Rosenberg, p 3. Lippincott, Philadelphia, 1992.
15. Kanki PJ, Barin F, Mboup S, et al: New human T-lymphotropic retrovirus related to simian T-lymphotropic virus type III$_{AGM}$ (STLV-III$_{AGM}$). *Science* 232:238, 1986.
16. Huet T, Cheynier R, Meyerhaus A, et al: Genetic organization of a chimpanzee lentivirus related to HIV-1. *Nature* 345:356, 1990.
17. Gao F, Balles E, Robertson DL, et al: Origin of HIV-1 in chimpanzee *Pan troglodytes troglodytes*. *Nature* 397:436, 1999.
18. Chin J: Present and future dimensions of the HIV/AIDS pandemic. Plenary presentation, 7th International Conference on AIDS, Florence, June 17, 1991.
19. Varmus H: Retroviruses. *Science* 240:1427, 1988.
20. Sharp PM, Robertson F, Gao F, Hahn B: Origins and diversity of human immunodeficiency viruses. *AIDS* 8 (suppl 1):S27, 1994.
21. Gonda MA, Wong-Staal F, Gallo RC, et al: Sequence homology and morphologic similarity of HTLV-III and visna virus, a pathogenic lentivirus. *Science* 227:173, 1985.
22. Daniel MD, Letvin NL, King NW, et al: Isolation of T-cell tropic HTLV-III-like retrovirus from macaques. *Science* 228:1201, 1985.
23. Overbaugh J, Donahue PR, Quackenbush SL, et al: Molecular cloning of a feline leukemia virus that induces fatal immunodeficiency disease in cats. *Science* 239:906, 1988.
24. Ho DD, Schooley RT, Rota TR, et al: HTLV-III in the semen and blood of a healthy homosexual man. *Science* 226:451, 1984.
25. Levy JA: Human immunodeficiency viruses and the pathogenesis of AIDS. *JAMA* 261:2997, 1989.
26. Tindall B, Evans L, Cunningham P, et al: Identification of HIV-1 in semen following primary HIV-1 infection. *AIDS* 6:949, 1992.

27. Chiasson MA, Stoneburner RI, Joseph SC: Human immunodeficiency virus transmission through artificial insemination. *J AIDS* 3:69, 1990.

28. Vogt MW, Witt DJ, Craven DE, et al: Isolation of HTLV-III/LAV from cervical secretions of women at risk for AIDS. *Lancet* 1:525, 1986.

29. Wofsy C, Cohen J, Hauer I, et al: Isolation of AIDS associated retrovirus from genital secretions of women with antibodies to the virus. *Lancet* 1:527, 1986.

30. Pomerants RJ, de la Monte SM, Donegan SP, et al: Human immunodeficiency virus (HIV) infection of the uterine cervix. *Ann Intern Med* 108:321, 1988.

31. Anderson DA, Voeller B: AIDS and contraception, in *Clinical Perspective in Obstetrics and Gynecology*, edited by F Haseltine, D Shoupe, p 192. Springer, New York, 1993.

32. Marmor M, Weiss LR, Lyden M, et al: Possible female to female transmission of human immunodeficiency virus. *Ann Intern Med* 105:969, 1986.

33. Monzon OT, Capellan JM: Female to female transmission of HIV. *Lancet* 2:40, 1987.

34. Stamm WE, Handsfield HH, Rompalo AM, et al: The association between genital ulcer disease and acquisition of HIV infection in homosexual men. *JAMA* 260:1429, 1988.

35. Kreiss JK, Coombs R, Plummer F, et al: Isolation of human immunodeficiency virus from genital ulcers in Nairobi prostitutes. *J Infect Dis* 160:380, 1989.

36. Grosskurth H, Mosha F, Todd J, et al: Impact of improved treatment of sexually transmitted diseases on HIV infection in rural Tanzania: Randomized controlled trial. *Lancet* 356:530, 1995.

37. Sasse H, Salmaso S, Conti S: First Drug User Multicenter Study Group: Risk behaviors for HIV-1 infection in Italian drug users: Report from a multicenter study. *J AIDS* 2:486, 1989.

38. Chaisson RE, Bacchetti P, Osmond D, et al: Cocaine use and HIV infection in intravenous drug users in San Francisco. *JAMA* 261:561, 1989.

39. Donegan E, Stuart M, Niland JC, et al: Infection with human immunodeficiency virus type 1 (HIV-1) among recipients of antibody-positive blood donations. *Ann Intern Med* 113:733, 1990.

40. Centers for Disease Control: Safety of therapeutic products used for hemophilia patients. *MMWR* 37:441, 1988.

41. Pierce GF, Lusher JM, Brownstein AP, et al: The use of purified clotting factor concentrates in hemophilia: Influence of viral safety, cost and supply on therapy. *JAMA* 261:3434, 1989.

42. Schreiber GB, Busch MP, Kleinman SH, Korelitz JJ: The risk of transfusion transmitted viral infections. *N Engl J Med* 334:1685, 1996.

43. Goedert JJ, Mendez H, Drummond JE, et al: Mother to infant transmission of human immunodeficiency virus type 1: Association with prematurity or low anti-gp 120. *Lancet* 2:1351, 1989.

44. Hira SK, Kamanga J, Bhat GJ, et al: Perinatal transmission of HIV-1 in Zambia. *Br Med J* 299:1250, 1989.

45. European Collaborative Study: Risk factors for mother-to-child transmission of HIV-1. *Lancet* 339:1007, 1992.

46. Courgnaud V, Laure F, Brossard A, et al: Frequent and early in utero HIV-1 infection. *AIDS Res Hum Retroviruses* 7:337, 1991.

47. Rouzioux C, Costagliola D, Burgard M, et al: Timing of mother-to-child HIV-1 transmission depends on maternal status: The HIV infection in newborns French Collaborative Study Group. *AIDS* 7(suppl 2):S49, 1993.

48. Burgard M, Mayaux MJ, Blanche S, et al: The use of viral culture and p24 antigen testing to HIV infection in neonates: The HIV infection in newborns French Collaborative Study Group. *N Engl J Med* 327:1192, 1992.

49. Ehrns A, Lindgren S, Dictor M, et al: HIV in pregnant women and their offspring: Evidence for late transmission. *Lancet* 337:203, 1991.

50. van de Perre P, Simonon A, Msellati P, et al: Postnatal transmission of human immunodeficiency virus type 1 from mother to infant: A prospective cohort study in Kigali, Rwanda. *N Engl J Med* 325:593, 1991.

51. Dunn DT, Newell ML, Ades AE, Peckham CS: Risk of human immunodeficiency virus type 1 transmission through breast-feeding. *Lancet* 340:585, 1992.

52. European Collaborative Study: Risk factors for mother-to-child transmission of HIV-1. *Lancet* 339:1007, 1992.

53. Mayzux M-J, Blanche S, Rouzioux C, et al: Maternal factors associated with perinatal HIV-1 transmission: The French cohort study, seven years of follow-up observation. *J AIDS* 8:188, 1995.

54. Fang G, Burger H, Grimson R, et al: Maternal plasma human immunodeficiency virus type 1 RNA level: A determinant and projected threshold for mother-to-child transmission. *Proc Natl Acad Sci USA* 92:12100, 1995.

55. Weiser B, Nachman S, Tropper P, et al: Quantitation of human immunodeficiency virus type 1 during pregnancy: Relationship of viral titer to mother-to-child transmission and stability of viral load. *Proc Natl Acad Sci USA* 91:8031, 1994.

56. Burns DN, Landesman S, Muenz LR, et al: Cigarette smoking, premature rupture of membranes, and vertical transmission of HIV-1 among women with low CD4 levels. *J AIDS* 7:718, 1994.

57. Nair P, Alger L, Hines S, Seiden S, Hebel R, Johnson JP: Maternal and neonatal characteristics associated with HIV infection in infants of seropositive women. *J AIDS* 6:298, 1993.

58. Landesman SH, Kalish LA, Burns DN, et al: Obstetrical factors and the transmission of human immunodeficiency virus type 1 from mother to child. *N Engl J Med* 334:1617, 1996.

59. Simonds RJ, Steketee R, Nesheim S, et al: Impact of zidovudine use on risk and risk factors for perinatal transmission of HIV. *AIDS* 12:301, 1998.

60. The International Perinatal HIV Group: The mode of delivery and the risk of vertical transmission of human immunodeficiency virus type 1: A meta-analysis of 15 prospective cohort studies. *N Engl J Med* 340:977, 1999.

61. European Collaborative Study: Caesarean section and the risk of vertical transmission of HIV-1 infection. *Lancet* 343:1464, 1994.

62. Stratton P, Tuomala RE, Abboud R, et al: Obstetric and newborn outcomes in a cohort of HIV-infected pregnant women: A report of the Women and Infants Transmission Stuidy. *J Acquir Immune Defic Syndr Hum Retroviol* 20:179, 1999.

63. Centers for Disease Control and Prevention: Public Health Service Task Force recommendations for the use of antiretroviral drugs in pregnant women infected with HIV-1 for maternal health and for reducing perinatal HIV-1 transmission in the United States. *MMWR* 47:1, 1998.

64. Connor EM, Sperling RS, Gelver R, et al: Reduction of maternal-infant trnasmission of human immunodeficiency virus type 1 with zidovudine treatment. *N Engl J Med* 331:1173, 1994.

65. Shaffer N, Chauchoowong R, Mock PA, et al: Short-course zidovudine for perinatal HIV-1 transmission in Bangkok, Thailand: A randomized controlled trial. *Lancet* 353:773–780, 1999.

66. Jackson B, Fleming TR: Executive Summary, HIVNET 012. http://www.niaid.nih.gov/newsroom/simple/exec.htm. July 14, 1999.

67. Centers for Disease Control and Prevention: Update: Perinatally acquired HIV/AIDS—United States, 1997. *MMWR* 46:1086, 1997.

68. Gelderblom HR, Hausmann EHS, Ozel M, et al: Fine structure of human immunodeficiency virus (HIV) and immunolocalization of structural proteins. *Virology* 156:171, 1987.

69. Kowalski M, Potz J, Basiripour L, et al: Functional regions of the envelope glycoprotein of human immunodeficiency virus type 1. *Science* 237:1351, 1987.

70. Wyatt R, Sodroski J: The HIV-1 envelope glycoproteins: Fusogens, antigens and immunogens. *Science* 280:1884, 1998.

71. Dalglesh AG, Beverley PCL, Clapham PR, et al: The CD4 (T4) antigen is an essential component of the receptor for the AIDS retrovirus. *Nature* 312:763, 1984.

72. Klatzmann D, Champagne E, Chamaret S, et al: T-lymphocyte T4 molecule behaves as the receptor for human retrovirus LAV. *Nature* 312:767, 1984.

73. Choe H, Farazan M, Sun Y, et al: The beta-chemokine receptors CCR3 and CCR5 facilitate infection by primary HIV isolates. *Cell* 85:1135, 1996.

74. Berberian L, Goodglick L, Kipps TJ, Braun J: Immunoglobulin V_H3 gene products: Natural ligands for HIV gp120. *Science* 261:1588, 1993.

75. Cordonnier A, Montagnier L, Emerman M: Single amino acid changes in HIV envelope affect viral tropisms and receptor binding. *Nature* 340:571, 1989.

76. McKeating JA, Willey RL: Structure and function of the HIV envelope. *AIDS* 3(suppl):S35, 1989.

77. Lapham CK, Ouyang J, Chandrasakhar B, et al: Evidence for cell-

surface association between fusion and CD4-gp120 complex in human cell lines. *Science* 274:602, 1996.

78. Bullough PA, Hughson F, Skehel J, et al: Structure of influenza haemagglutinin at pH of membrane fusion. *Nature* 371:37, 1994.

79. Sarngadharan MG, Popovic M, Bruch L, et al: Antibodies reactive with human T-lymphotropic retroviruses (HTLV-III) in the serum of patients with AIDS. *Science* 224:506, 1984.

80. Mervis RJ, Ahmad N, Lillehoj EP, et al: The gag gene products of human immunodeficiency virus type-1: Alignment with the gag open reading frame, identification of post-translational modifications and evidence for alternative gag precursors. *J Virol* 62:3993, 1988.

81. Mizrahi V: Analysis of the ribonuclease H activity of HIV-1 reverse transcriptase using RNA-DNA hybrid substrates derived from the gag region of HIV-1. *Biochemistry* 28:9088, 1989.

82. Wlodawer A, Miller M, Jaskolski M, et al: Conserved folding in retroviral proteases: Crystal structure of a synthetic HIV-1 protease. *Science* 245:616, 1989.

83. Peng C, Ho BK, Chang TW, Chang NT: Role of human immunodeficiency virus type-1–specific protease in core protein maturation and viral infectivity. *J Virol* 63:2550, 1989.

84. Arthros J, Dean KC, Chalkin MA, et al: Identification of the residues in human CD4 critical for the binding of HIV. *Cell* 57:469, 1989.

85. Fisher AG, Ensoli B, Looney D, et al: Biologically diverse molecular variants within a single HIV-1 isolate. *Nature* 334:444, 1988.

86. Stein BS, Gowda SD, Lifson SD, et al: pH-independent HIV entry into CD4-positive T cells via virus envelope fusion to plasma membrane. *Cell* 49:659, 1987.

87. Berger EA, Doms RW, Fenyo EM, et al: A new classification for HIV-1 [letter]. *Nature* 391:240, 1998.

88. Cairns JS, D'Souza MP: Chemokines and HIV-1 second receptors: The therapeutic connection. *Nature Med* 4:563, 1998.

89. Smith MW, Dean M, Carrington M, et al: Contrasting genetic influence of CCR2 and CCR5 variants on HIV-1 infection and disease progression. *Science* 277:959, 1997.

90. Varmus HE, Swanstrom R: Replication of retroviruses, in *RNA Tumor Viruses*, suppl, edited by R Weiss, N Teich, H Varmus, J Coffin, p 75. Cold Spring Harbor Laboratory, Cold Spring Harbor, NY, 1985.

91. Luban J: Absconding with the chaperone: Essential cyclophin-Gag interaction in HIV-1 viron. *Cell* 87:1157, 1996.

92. Preston BD, Poiesz BJ, Loeb LA: Fidelity of HIV-1 reverse transcriptase. *Science* 242:1108, 1988.

93. Roberts JD, Bebenek K, Kunkel TA: The accuracy of reverse transcriptase of HIV-1. *Science* 242:1171, 1988.

94. Hahn BH, Gonda MA, Shaw GM, et al: Genomic diversity of the acquired immune deficiency syndrome virus HTLV-III: Different viruses exhibit greatest divergence in their envelope genes. *Proc Natl Acad Sci USA* 82:4813, 1985.

95. Ellis J, Bernstein A: Retrovirus vectors containing an internal attachment site: Evidence that circles are not intermediates to murine retrovirus integration. *J Virol* 63:2629, 1989.

96. Kim S, Byrn R, Groopman J, Baltimore D: Temporal aspects of DNA and RNA synthesis during human immunodeficiency virus infection: Evidence for differential gene expression. *J Virol* 63:3708, 1989.

97. Schnittman SM, Psallidopoulos MC, Lane HC, et al: The reservoir for HIV-1 in human peripheral blood is a T cell that maintains expression of CD4. *Science* 245:305, 1989.

98. Emerman M, Malim MH: HIV-1 regulatory/accessory genes: Keys to unraveling viral and host cell biology. *Science* 280:1880, 1998.

99. Popov S, Rexach M, Zybarth G, et al: Viral protein R regulates nuclear import of the HIV-1 pre-integration complex. *EMBO J* 17:909, 1998.

100. Nabel G, Baltimore D: An inducible transcription factor activates expression of human immunodeficiency virus in T cells. *Nature* 326:711, 1987.

101. Kawakami C, Scheidereit C, Roeder RG: Identification and purification of a human immunoglobulin enhancer binding protein NF-κB that activates transcription from a human immunodeficiency virus promoter in vitro. *Proc Natl Acad Sci USA* 85:4700, 1988.

102. Dayton AI, Sodroski JG, Rosen CA, et al: Transactivator gene of the human T cell lymphotropic virus type III is required for replication. *Cell* 44:941, 1986.

103. Laspia M, Rice A, Mathews MB: HIV-1 tat protein increases transcriptional initiation and stabilizes elongation. *Cell* 59:283, 1989.

104. Sodroski J, Goh WC, Rosen C, et al: A second post-transcriptional transactivator gene required for HTLV III replication. *Nature* 321:412, 1986.

105. Malim MH, Bohnlein S, Hauber J, Cullen BR: Functional dissection of the HIV-1 rev transactivation: Derivation of a trans-dominant repressor of rev function. *Cell* 58:205, 1989.

106. Schubert U, Anton LC, Bacik I, et al: CD4-glycoprotein degradation induced by human immunodeficiency virus type 1 Vpu protein requires the function of proteosomes and the ubiquitin conjugating pathway. *J Virol* 72:2280, 1998.

107. Margottin F, Bour SP, Durand H, et al: A novel WD protein, h-beta TrCp, that interacts with HIV-1 Vpu connects CD4 to the ER degradation pathway through F-box motif. *Mol Cell* 1:565, 1998.

108. Greenberg ME, Bronson S, Lock M, et al: Co-localization of the HIV-1 Nef with the AP-2 adaptor protein complex correlates with Nef-induced CD4 down-regulation. *EMBO J* 16: 6964, 1997.

109. Foti M, Mangasarian A, Piguet V, et al: Nef-mediated clathrin-coated pit formation. *J Cell Biol* 139:37, 1997.

110. Jacks T, Power MD, Masiarz FR, et al: Characterization of ribosomal frameshifting in HIV-1 gag-pol expression. *Nature* 331:280, 1987.

111. Klimkait T, Strebel K, Hoggan MD, et al: The human immunodeficiency virus type-1-specific protein vpu is required for efficient virus maturation and release. *J Virol* 64:621, 1990.

112. Strebel K, Daugherty D, Clouse K, et al: The HIV "A" (sor) gene product is essential for virus infectivity. *Nature* 328:728, 1987.

113. Murry HW, Welte K, Jacobs JL, et al: Production of and in vitro response to interleukin 2 in the acquired immunodeficiency syndrome. *J Clin Invest* 76:1959, 1985.

114. Pahwa SG, Quilop MTJ, Lane M, et al: Defective B-lymphocyte function in homosexual men in relation to the acquired immunodeficiency syndrome. *Ann Intern Med* 101:757, 1984.

115. Murry HW, Rubin BY, Masur H, Roberts RB: Impaired production of lymphokines and immune (gamma) interferon in the acquired immunodeficiency syndrome. *N Engl J Med* 310:883, 1984.

116. Rook AH, Masur H, Lane HC, et al: Interleukin-2 enhances the depressed natural killer and cytomegalovirus-specific cytotoxic activities of lymphocytes from patients with the acquired immunodeficiency syndrome. *J Clin Invest* 72:398, 1983.

117. Tersmette M, de Goede REY, Al BJM, et al: Differential syncytium-inducing capacity of human immunodeficiency virus isolates: Frequent detection of syncytium-inducing isolates in patients with acquired immunodeficiency syndrome (AIDS) and AIDS-related complex. *J Virol* 62:2026, 1988.

118. Pantaleo G, Graziosi C, Demarest JF, et al: HIV infection is active and progressive in lymphoid tissue during the clinically latent stage of disease. *Nature* 362:355, 1993.

119. Glushakova S, Grivel J-C, Fitzgerald W, et al: Evidence for the HIV-1 phenotype switch as a causal factor in acquired immunodeficiency. *Nature Med* 4:346, 1998.

120. Walker BD, Chakrabarti S, Moss B, et al: HIV-specific cytotoxic T lymphocytes in seropositive individuals. *Nature* 328:345, 1987.

121. Tsuchiya S, Imaizumi M, Minegishi M, et al: Lack of interleukin-2 production in a patient with OKT4+ T-cell deficiency. *N Engl J Med* 308:1294, 1983.

122. Ebert EC, Stoll DB, Cassens BJ, et al: Diminished interleukin production and receptor generation characterize the acquired immunodeficiency syndrome. *Clin Immunol Immunopathol* 37:283, 1985.

123. Prince HE, Kermani-Arab V, Fahey J: Depressed interleukin-2 receptor expression in acquired immune deficiency and lymphadenopathy syndromes. *J Immunol* 133:1313, 1984.

124. Kekow J, Wachsman W, Gross WL, et al: Transforming growth factor-beta and suppression of humoral immune responses in HIV infection. *J Clin Invest* 87:1010, 1991.

125. Ammann AJ, Abrams D, Conant M, et al: Acquired immune dysfunction in homosexual men: Immunologic profiles. *Clin Immunol Immunopathol* 27:315, 1983.

126. Wong JK, Gunthard HF, Havir DV, et al: Reduction of HIV-1 in blood and lymph nodes following potent antiretroviral therapy of HIV-1 infection. *Proc Natl Acad Sci USA* 94:2574, 1997.

127. Cavert W, Notermans DW, Staskus K, et al: Kinetics of response in lymphoid tissues to antiretroviral therapy of HIV-1 infection. *Science* 276:960, 1997.

128. Hammer SM, Squires KE, Hughes MD, et al: A controlled trial of two

nucleoside analogues plus indinavir in persons with human immunodeficiency virus infection and CD4 cell counts of 200 per cubic millimeter or less. *N Engl J Med* 337:725, 1997.

129. Palella FJ Jr, Delaney KM, Moorman AC et al: Declining morbidity and mortality among patients with advanced human immunodeficiency virus infection. *N Engl J Med* 338:853, 1998.

130. Connors M, Kovacs JA, Krevat S, et al: HIV infection induces changes in CD4+ T-cell phenotype and depletions within the CD4+ T-cell repertroire that are not immediately restored by antiviral or immune-based therapies. *Nature Med* 3:533, 1997.

131. Gorochov G, Neumann AU, Kereveur A, et al: Perturbation of CD4+ and CD8+ T-cell repertoire during progression to AIDS and regulation of the CD4+ repertoire during antiviral therapy. *Nature Med* 4:215, 1998.

132. Chess Q, Daniels J, North E, et al: Serum immunoglobulin elevations in the acquired immunodeficiency syndrome (AIDS): IgG, IgA, IgM, and IgD. *Diagn Immunol* 2:148, 1984.

133. Lane HC, Masur H, Edgar LC, et al: Abnormalities of B-cell activation and immunoregulation in patients with the acquired immunodeficiency syndrome. *N Engl J Med* 309:453, 1983.

134. Pahwa S, Pahwa R, Saxinger C, et al: Influence of the human T-lymphotropic virus/lymphadenopathy–associated virus on functions of human lymphocytes: Evidence for immunosuppressive effects and polyclonal B-cell activation by banded viral preparations. *Proc Natl Acad Sci USA* 82:8198, 1985.

135. Kopelman RG, Zolla-Pazner S: Association of human immunodeficiency virus infection and autoimmune phenomena. *Am J Med* 84:82, 1988.

136. Walsh CM, Nardi MA, Karpatkin S: On the mechanism of thrombocytopenic purpura in sexually active homosexual men. *N Engl J Med* 311:635, 1984.

137. van der Lelie J, Lange JMA, Vos JJE, et al: Autoimmunity against blood cells in human immunodeficiency virus infection. *Br J Haematol* 67:755, 1987.

138. Stricker RB, McHugh TM, Moody D, et al: An AIDS-related cytotoxic autoantibody reacts with a specific antigen on stimulated CD4+ cells. *Nature* 327:170, 1987.

139. Rossi G, Goria R, Stellini R, et al: Prevalence, clinical, and laboratory features of thrombocytopenia in HIV-infected individuals. *AIDS Res Hum Retroviruses* 6:261, 1990.

140. Murphy MF, Metcalfe P, Waters AH, et al: Incidence and mechanism of neutropenia and thrombocytopenia in patients with human immunodeficiency virus infection. *Br J Haematol* 66:337, 1987.

141. Ballem PJ, Belzberg A, Devine DV, et al: Kinetic studies of the mechanism of thrombocytopenia in patients with human immunodeficiency virus infection. *N Engl J Med* 327:1179, 1992.

142. Gartner S, Markovits P, Markovitz DM, et al: The role of mononuclear phagocytes in HTLV-III/LAV infection. *Science* 233:215, 1986.

143. Armstrong GA, Horne R: Follicular dendritic cells and virus-like particles in AIDS-related lymphadenopathy. *Lancet* 2:370, 1984.

144. Poli G, Bottazzi B, Acero R, et al: Monocyte function in intravenous drug abusers with lymphadenopathy syndrome and in patients with the acquired immunodeficiency syndrome: Selective impairment of chemotaxis. *Clin Exp Immunol* 62:136, 1985.

145. Murry HW, Gellene RA, Libby DM, et al: Activation of tissue macrophages from AIDS patients: In vitro response of alveolar macrophages to lymphokines and interferon-gamma. *J Immunol* 135:1501, 1985.

146. Kleinerman ES, Ceccorulli LM, Zwelling LA, et al: Activation of monocyte-mediated tumoricidal activity in patients with acquired immunodeficiency syndrome. *J Clin Oncol* 3:1005, 1985.

147. Creemers PC, Stark DF, Boyko WJ: Evaluation of natural killer cell activity in patients with persistent generalized lymphadenopathy and acquired immunodeficiency syndrome. *Clin Lab Immunol* 14:114, 1984.

148. Klatzman M, Lederman MM: Defective postbinding lysis underlies the impaired natural killer activity in factor VIII–treated human T lymphotropic virus type III seropositive hemophiliacs. *J Clin Invest* 45:406, 1986.

149. Reddy MM, Chinoy P, Grieco MH: Differential effects of interferon alpha and interleukin-2 on natural killer cell activity in patients with the acquired immune deficiency syndrome. *J Biol Res Mod* 3:379, 1984.

150. Horsburgh CR Jr, Ou CY, Jason J, et al: Duration of human immunodeficiency virus infection before detection of antibody. *Lancet* 2:637, 1989.

151. Imagawa DT, Lee MH, Wolinsky SM, et al: HIV-1 infection in homosex-

152. Brettler DB, Somasundaran M, Forsberg AF, et al: Silent human immunodeficiency virus type 1 infection: A rare occurrence in a high-risk heterosexual population. *Blood* 80:2396, 1992.

153. Read S, Cassol S, Coates R, et al: Detection of incident HIV infection by PCR compared to serology. *J AIDS* 5:1075, 1992.

154. Goudsmit J, Lange JM, Krone WJ, et al: Pathogenesis of HIV and its implications for serodiagnosis and monitoring of antiviral therapy. *J Virol Methods* 17:19, 1987.

155. Tindall B, Cooper DA, Donovan B, et al: Primary human immunodeficiency virus infection: Clinical and serologic aspects. *Infect Dis Clin North Am* 2:329, 1988.

156. Alter HJ, Epstein JS, Swensen SG, et al: Prevalence of human immunodeficiency virus type 1 p24 antigen in U.S. blood donors: An assessment of the efficacy of testing in donor screening. *N Engl J Med* 323:1312, 1990.

157. Phillips AN: Studies of prognostic markers in HIV infection: Implications for pathogenesis. *AIDS* 6:1391, 1992.

158. Munoz A, Carey V, Saah AJ, et al: Predictors of decline in CD4 lymphocytes in a cohort of homosexual men infected with human immunodeficiency virus. *J AIDS* 1:396, 1988.

159. Malone JL, Simms TE, Gray GC, et al: Sources of variability in repeated T-helper lymphocyte counts from human immunodeficiency virus type 1 infected patients: Total lymphocyte count fluctuations and diurnal cycle are important. *J AIDS* 3:144, 1990.

160. Anderson RE, Lang W, Shiboski S, et al: Use of beta 2 microglobulin level and CD4 lymphocyte count to predict development of acquired immunodeficiency syndrome in persons with human immunodeficiency virus infection. *Arch Intern Med* 150:73, 1990.

161. Melmed RN, Taylor JMG, Detels R, et al: Serum neopterin changes in HIV infected subjects: Indicator of significant pathology, CD4 T cell changes, and the development of AIDS. *J AIDS* 2:70, 1989.

162. Hammer SM, Squires KE, Hughes MD, et al: A controlled trial of two nucleoside analogues plus indinavir in persons with human immunodeficiency virus infection and CD4 cell counts of 200/mm³ or less. *N Engl J Med* 337:725, 1997.

163. Centers for Disease Control and Prevention: Guidelines for the use of antiretroviral agents in HIV-infected adults and adolescents. *MMWR*, May 5, 1999.

164. Egger M, Hirschel B, Francioli P, et al: Impact of new antiretroviral combination therapies in HIV infected patients in Switzerland: Prospective multicentre study. *BMJ* 315:1194, 1997.

165. Tural C, Romeu J, Sirera G, et al: Long lasting remission of cytomegalovirus retinitis without maintenance therapy in human immunodeficiency virus infected patients. *J Infect Dis* 177:1080, 1998.

166. Li TS, Tubiana R, Katlama C, Calvez V, Mohand A, Autran B: Long-lasting recovery in CD4 T cell function and viral load reduction after highly active antiretroviral therapy in advanced HIV-1 disease. *Lancet* 351:1682, 1998.

167. Furrer H, Egger M, Opravil M, et al: Discontinuation of primary prophylaxis against *Pneumocystis carinii* pneumonia in HIV-1 infected adults treated with combination antiretroviral therapy. *N Engl J Med* 340:1301, 1999.

168. Cooper DA, Maclean P, Finlayson R, et al: Acute AIDS retrovirus infection. *Lancet* 1:537, 1985.

169. Fox R, Eldred LJ, Fuchs EJ, et al: Clinical manifestations of acute infection with human immunodeficiency virus in a cohort of gay men. *AIDS* 1:35, 1987.

170. Lemp GF, Payne SF, Rutherford GW, et al: Projections of AIDS morbidity and mortality in San Francisco. *JAMA* 263:1497, 1990.

171. Moss AR, Bacchetti P: Editorial review: Natural history of HIV infection. *AIDS* 3:55, 1989.

172. Schoenbaum EE, Hartel D, Friedland G: HIV infection and intravenous drug use. *Curr Opin Infect Dis* 3:80, 1990.

173. Volberding P: Clinical spectrum of HIV disease, in *AIDS: Etiology, Diagnosis, Treatment and Prevention*, 3rd ed, edited by VT DeVita Jr, S Hellman, SA Rosenberg, p 123. Lippincott, Philadelphia, 1992.

174. Mitsuyasu R: *AIDS Clin Review 1993/4*. Marcel Dekker, New York, 1993, p189.

175. Zon LI, Arkin C, Groopman JE: Hematologic manifestations of the human immunodeficiency virus (HIV). *Semin Hematol* 25:208, 1988.

176. Sullivan PS, Hanson DL, Chu SY, Jones JL, Ward JW: Epidemiology of anemia in human immunodeficiency virus infected persons: Results from the Multistate Adult and Adolescent Spectrum of HIV Disease Surveillance Project. *Blood* 91:301, 1998.

177. Spivak JL, Barnes DC, Fuchs E, Quinn TC: Serum immunoreactive erythropoietin in HIV infected patients. *JAMA* 261:310, 1989.

178. Seneviratne LS, Tulpule A, Mummaneni M, et al: Clinical, immunological and pathologic correlates of bone marrow involvement in 253 patients with AIDS-related lymphoma. *Blood* 92:244A, 1998.

179. Walker RE, Parker RI, Kovacs JA, et al: Anemia and erythropoiesis in patients with the acquired immunodeficiency syndrome (AIDS) and Kaposi sarcoma treated with zidovudine. *Ann Intern Med* 108:372, 1988.

180. Richman DD, Fischl MA, Grieco MH, et al: The toxicity of azidothymidine (AZT) in the treatment of patients with AIDS and AIDS-related complex: A double-blind, placebo-controlled trial. *N Engl J Med* 317:192, 1987.

181. Anderson LJ: Human parvoviruses. *J Infect Dis* 161:603, 1990.

182. Frickhofen N, Abkowitz JL, Safford M, et al: Persistent B19 parvovirus infection in patients infected with human immunodeficiency virus type 1 (HIV-1): A treatable cause of anemia in AIDS. *Ann Intern Med* 113:926, 1990.

183. Rarick MU, Espina B, Mocharnuk R, Trilling Y, Levine AM: Thrombotic thrombocytopenic purpura in patients with human immunodeficiency virus infection: A report of three cases and review of the literature. *Am J Hematol* 40:103, 1992.

184. Telen MJ, Roberts KB, Bartlett JA: HIV associated autoimmune hemolytic anemia: Report of a case and review of the literature. *AIDS* 3:933, 1990.

185. McGinniss MH, Macher AM, Rook AH, Alter HJ: Red cell autoantibodies in patients with acquired immune deficiency syndrome. *Transfusion* 26:405, 1986.

186. Gupta S, Licorish K: The Coombs' test and the acquired immunodeficiency syndrome. *Ann Intern Med* 100:462, 1984.

187. Toy PTCY, Reid ME, Burns M: Positive direct antiglobulin test associated with hyperglobulinemia in AIDS. *Am J Hematol* 19:145, 1985.

188. Harriman GR, Smith PD, Horne MK, et al: Vitamin B$_{12}$ malabsorption in patients with acquired immunodeficiency syndrome. *Arch Intern Med* 149:2039, 1989.

189. Herbert V, Fong W, Gulle V, Stopler T: Low holotranscobalamin II is the earliest serum marker for subnormal vitamin B$_{12}$ (cobalamin) absorption in patients with AIDS. *Am J Hematol* 34:132, 1990.

190. Moore RD, Keruly JC, Chaisson RE: Anemia and survival in HIV infection *J Acquir Immune Defic Syndr Hum Retrovirol* 19:29, 1998.

191. Henry DH, Beall GN, Benson CA, et al: Recombinant human erythropoietin in the treatment of anemia associated with human immunodeficiency virus (HIV) infection and zidovudine therapy: Overview of four clinical trials. *Ann Intern Med* 117:739, 1992.

192. Demetri G, Wade J, Cella D: Epoetin alfa improves quality of life in cancer patients receiving cytotoxic treatment independent of disease response: Prospective clinical trial results. *Blood* 90:175a, 1997.

193. Miles SA: The use of hematopoietic growth factors in HIV infection and AIDS-related malignancies. *Cancer Invest* 9:229, 1991.

194. Murphy M, Metcalfe P, Waters A: Incidence and mechanism of neutropenia and thrombocytopenia in patients with human immunodeficiency virus infection. *Br J Haematol* 66:337, 1987.

195. Bagnara GP, Zauli G, Giovannini M, Re MC, Furlini G, La Placa M: Early loss of circulating hemopoietic progenitors in HIV-1 infected subjects. *Exp Hematol* 18:426, 1990.

196. Leiderman I, Greenberg M, Adelsberg B, et al: A glycoprotein inhibitor of in vitro granulopoiesis associated with AIDS. *Blood* 70:1267, 1987.

197. Mauss S, Steinmetz HT, Willers R, et al: Induction of granulocyte colony-stimulating factor by acute febrile infection but not by neutropenia in HIV seropositive individuals. *J Acquir Immune Defic Syndr Hum Retrovirol* 14:430, 1997.

198. Elis M, Gupta S, Galant S, et al: Impaired neutrophil function in patients with AIDS or AIDS-related complex: A comprehensive evaluation. *J Infect Dis* 158:1268, 1988.

199. Bodey GP, Buckley M, Sathe US, et al: Qualitative relationships between circulating leukocytes and infection in patients with acute leukemia. *Ann Intern Med* 64:328, 1966.

200. Moore RD, Keruly J, Chaisson RE, et al: Neutropenia and bacterial infection in acquired immunodeficiency syndrome. *Arch Intern Med* 155:1965, 1995.

201. Jacobson MA, Cohen PT, Liu RC, et al: Risk of hospitalization for serious bacterial infection associated with neutropenia severity in patients with HIV [abst 231]. 11th International Conference on AIDS, Vancouver, Canada, 1996.

202. Meynard J-L, Guiguet M, Arsac S, et al: Frequency and risk factors of infectious complications in neutropenic patients infected with HIV. *AIDS* 11:995, 1997.

203. Groopman JE, Feder D: Hematopoietic growth factors in AIDS. *Semin Oncol* 19:408, 1992.

204. Groopman JE, Mitsuyasu RT, DeLeo MJ, et al: Effect of recombinant human granulocyte-macrophage colony stimulating factor on myelopoiesis in the acquired immunodeficiency syndrome. *N Engl J Med* 317:593, 1987.

205. Kaplan L, Kahn J, Crowe S, et al: Clincial and virologic effect of GM-CSF in patients receiving chemotherapy for HIV associated non-Hogkin's lymphoma: Results of a randomized trial. *J Clin Oncol* 9:929, 1991.

206. Kimura S, Matsuda J, Ikematsu S, et al: Efficacy of recombinant human granulocyte colony-stimulating factor on neutropenia in patients with AIDS. *AIDS* 12:1251, 1990.

207. Keiser P, Higgs E, Scanton J: Neutropenia is associated with bacteremia in patients with HIV. *Am J Med Sci* 312:118, 1996.

208. Pechere M, Samii K, Hirschel B: HIV related thrombocytopenia. *N Engl J Med* 328:1785, 1993.

209. Sullivan PS, Hanson DL, Chu SY, Jones JL, Ciesielski CA: Surveillance for thrombocytopenia in persons infected with HIV: Results from the multistate Adult and Adolescent Spectrum of Disease Project. *J Acquir Immune Defic Syndr Hum Retrovirol* 14:374, 1997.

210. Ballem PJ, Belzberg A, Devine DV, et al: Kinetic studies of the mechanism of thrombocytopenia in patients with human immunodeficiency virus infection. *N Engl J Med* 327:1779, 1992.

211. Walsh CM, Nardi MA, Karpatkin S: On the mechanism of thrombocytopenic purpura in sexually active homosexual men. *N Engl J Med* 311:635, 1984.

212. Bettaieb A, Fromont P, Louache F, et al: Presence of cross-reactive antibody between human immunodeficiency virus (HIV) and platelet glycoproteins in HIV related immune thrombocytopenic purpura. *Blood* 80:162, 1992.

213. Kouri Y, Borkowsky W, Nardi M, Karpatkin S, Basch RS: Human megakaryocytes have a CD4+ molecule capable of binding human immunodeficiency virus-1. *Blood* 81:2664, 1993.

214. Zucker-Franklin D, Seremetis S, Heng ZY: Internalization of human immunodeficiency virus type I and other retroviruses by megakaryocytes and platelets. *Blood* 75:1920, 1990.

215. Wang J-F, Liu Z-Y, Groopman JE: The alpha-chemokine receptor CXCR4 is expressed on the megakaryocytic lineage from progenitor to platelets, and modulates migration and adhesion. *Blood* 92:756, 1998.

216. Zucker-Franklin D, Cao Y: Megakaryocytes of human immunodeficiency virus-infected individuals express viral RNA. *Proc Natl Acad Sci USA* 86:5595, 1989.

217. Zucker-Franklin D, Termin CS, Cooper MC: Structural changes in the megakaryocytes of patients infected with the human immunodeficiency virus (HIV-1). *Am J Pathol* 134:1295, 1989.

218. Swiss Group for Clinical Studies on AIDS: Zidovudine for the treatment of thrombocytopenia associated with HIV: A prospective study. *Ann Intern Med* 109:718, 1988.

219. Harker LA, Marzec UM, Novembre F, et al: Treatment of thrombocytopenia in chimpanzees infected with HIV by pegylated recombinant human megakaryocyte growth and development factor. *Blood* 91:4427, 1998.

220. Oksenhendler E, Bierling P, Farcet JP, et al: Response to therapy in 37 patients with HIV related thrombocytopenic purpura. *Br J Haematol* 66:49, 1987.

221. Oksenhendler E, Bierling P, Ferchal F, Clauvel J-P, Seligmann M: Zidovudine for thrombocytopenic purpura related to human immunodeficiency virus (HIV) infection. *Ann Intern Med* 110:365, 1989.

222. Landonio G, Cinque P, Nosari A, et al: Comparison of two dose regimens of zidovudine in an open, randomized, multicenter study for severe HIV related thrombocytpenia. *AIDS* 7:209, 1993.

223. Piketty C, Gilquin J, Kazatchkine MD: Successful treatment of HIV related thrombocytopenia with didanosine (ddI). *J AIDS* 7:521, 1994.

224. Tozzi V, Narcisco P, Sebastiani G, Frigiotti D, D'Amato C: Effects of indinavir treatment on platelet and neutrophil counts in patients with advanced HIV disease. *AIDS* 11:1067, 1997.

225. Marroni M, Gresele P, Landonio G, et al: Interferon-a is effective in the treatment of HIV-1 related, severe, zidovudine-resistant thrombocytopenia: A prospective, placebo-controlled, double-blind trial. *Ann Intern Med* 121:423, 1994.

226. Vianelli N, Catani L, Gugliotta L, et al: Recombinant alpha-interferon 2b in the treatment of HIV related thrombocytopenia. *AIDS* 7:823, 1993.

227. Imbach P, d'Apuzzo V, Hirt A, et al: High dose intravenous gammaglobulin for idiopathic thrombocytopenic purpura in childhood. *Lancet* 1:1228, 1981.

228. Bussel JB, Saimi JS: Isolated thrombocytopenia in patients infected with HIV: Treatment with intravenous gammaglobulin. *Am J Hematol* 28:79, 1998.

229. Gringeri A, Cattaneo M, Santagostino E, Mannucci PM: Intramuscular anti-D immunoglobulins for home treatment of chronic immune thrombocytopenic purpura. *Br J Hematol* 80:337, 1992.

230. Oksenhendler E, Bierling P, Brossard Y, et al: Anti-Rh immunoglobulin therapy for human immunodeficiency virus-related immune thrombocytopenic purpura. *Blood* 71:1499, 1988.

231. Oksenhendler E, Bierling P, Chevret S, et al: Splenectomy is safe and effective in human immunodeficiency virus related immune thrombocytopenia. *Blood* 82:29, 1993.

232. Kemeny MM, Cooke V, Melester TS, et al: Splenectomy in patients with AIDS and AIDS-related complex. *AIDS* 7:1063, 1993.

233. Peters BS, Beck EJ, Coleman DG, et al: Changing disease patterns in patients with AIDS in a referral center in the United Kingdom: The changing face of AIDS. *Br Med J* 302:203, 1991.

234. Pluda JM, Yarchoan R, Jaffe ES, et al: Development of non-Hodgkin's lymphoma in a cohort of patients with severe human immunodeficiency virus (HIV) infection on long-term antiretroviral therapy. *Ann Intern Med* 113:276, 1990.

235. Gail MH, Pluda JM, Rabkin CS, et al: Projections of the incidence of non-Hodgkin's lymphoma related to acquired immunodeficiency syndrome. *J Nat Cancer Inst* 83:695, 1991.

236. Rabkin CS, Biggar RJ, Horm JW: Increasing incidence of cancers associated with the human immunodeficiency virus epidemic. *Int J Cancer* 47:692, 1991.

237. Beral V, Peterman T, Berkelman R, Jaffe H: AIDS-associated non-Hodgkin lymphoma. *Lancet* 337:805, 1991.

238. Biggar RJ, Rabkin CS: The epidemiology of acquired immunodeficiency syndrome-related lymphomas. *Curr Opin Oncol* 4:883, 1992.

239. Pluda JM, Vanzon D, Tosato G, et al: Factors which predict for the development of non-Hodgkin's lymphoma in patients with HIV infection receiving antiretroviral therapy. *Blood* 78:285a, 1991.

240. Jacobson LP: Impact of highly effective anti-retroviral therapy on the incidence of malignancies among HIV infected individuals [abst S5]. *J Acquir Immune Defic Syndr Hum Retrovirol* 17:A39, 1998.

241. Buchsbinder SP, Bittinghoff E, Colfax G, Holmberg S: Declines in AIDS incidence associated with highly active anti-retroviral therapy are not reflected in KS and lymphoma incidence [abst S7]. *J Acquir Immun Defic Syndr Hum Retrovirol* 17:A39, 1998.

242. Ledergerber B, Telenti A, Egger M: Risk of HIV related Kaposi's sarcoma and non-Hodgkin's lymphoma with potent antiretroviral therapy: Prospective cohort study. *BMJ* 319:23, 1999.

243. Roithmann S, Tourani JM, Andrieu JM: AIDS-associated non-Hodgkin's lymphoma. *Lancet* 338:884, 1991.

244. Levine AM, Meyer PR, Begandy MK, et al: Development of B cell lymphoma in homosexual men: Clinical and immunologic findings. *Ann Intern Med* 100:7, 1984.

245. Monfardini S, Vaccher E, Tirelli U: AIDS associated non-Hodgkin's lymphoma in Italy: Intravenous drug users versus homosexual men. *Ann Oncol* 1:208, 1990.

246. Ragni M, Kingsley L, Duzyk A, Obrams I: HIV associated malignancy in hemophiliacs: Preliminary report from the Hemophilia Malignancy Study (HMS). *Blood* 74:38a, 1988.

247. Purtilo DT: Opportunistic non-Hodgkin's lymphoma in X-linked recessive immunodeficiency and lymphoproliferative syndromes. *Semin Oncol* 4:335, 1977.

248. Levine AM, Taylor CR, Schneider DR, et al: Immunoblastic sarcoma of T cell versus B cell origin: I. Clinical features. *Blood* 58:52, 1981.

249. Penn I: Tumors of the immunocompromised patient. *Annu Rev Med* 39:63, 1988.

250. Swinnen LJ, Costanzo-Nordin MR, Fisher SG, et al: Increased incidence of lymphoproliferative disorder after immunosuppression with the monoclonal antibody OKT3 in cardiac transplant recipients. *N Engl J Med* 323:1723, 1990.

251. Pantaleo G, Graziosi C, Fauci AS: Mechanisms of disease: The immunopathogenesis of human immunodeficiency virus infection. *N Engl J Med* 328:327, 1993.

252. Birx DI, Redfield RR, Tosato G: Defective regulation of Epstein-Barr virus infection in patients with acquired immunodeficiency syndrome (AIDS) or AIDS-related disorders. *N Engl J Med* 314:874, 1986.

253. Shear GM, Salahuddin SZ, Markham PD, et al: Prospective study of cytotoxic T lymphocyte responses to influenza virus and antibodies to human T lymphotropic virus-III in homosexual men: Selective loss of influenza-specific human leukocyte antigen-restricted cytotoxic lymphocyte response to human T lymphotropic virus-III positive individuals with symptoms of acquired immunodeficiency syndrome. *J Clin Invest* 76:1699, 1985.

254. Feichtinger H, Rutkonen P, Parravicini C, et al: Malignant lymphomas in *Cynomolgus* monkeys infected with simian immunodeficiency virus. *Am J Pathol* 137:1311, 1990.

255. Jelinek DF, Lipsky PE: Enhancement of human B cell proliferation and differentiation by tumor necrosis factor-alpha and interleukin 1. *J Immunol* 139:2970, 1987.

256. Fauci A, Schnittman SM, Poli G, et al: Immunopathogenetic mechanisms in human immunodeficiency virus (HIV) infection. *Ann Intern Med* 114:678, 1991.

257. Kawano M, Hirano T, Matsuda T, et al: Autocrine generation and requirement of BSF-2/IL-6 for human multiple myelomas. *Nature* 332:83, 1988.

258. Biondi A, Rossi V, Bassan R, et al: Constitutive expression of IL-6 gene in chronic lymphocytic leukemia. *Blood* 73:1279, 1989.

259. Emillie D, Coumbaras J, Raphael M, et al: IL-6 production in high grade B lymphomas: Correlation with presence of malignant immunoblasts in AIDS and in HIV-seronegative patients. *Blood* 80:498, 1992.

260. Benjamin D, Knobloch TJ, Abrams J, Dayton MA: Human B cell IL-10: B cell lines derived from patients with AIDS and Burkitt's lymphoma constitutively secrete large quantities of IL-10. *Blood* 78:384a, 1991.

261. Masood R, Bond M, Scadden D, et al: Interleukin-10: An autocrine B cell growth for human B-cell lymphomas and their progenitors. *Blood* 80:115a, 1992.

262. Poli G, Fauci AS: The effect of cytokines and pharmacologic agents on chronic HIV infection. *AIDS Res Hum Retroviruses* 8:191, 1992.

263. Shibata D, Weiss LM, Nathwani BN, et al: Epstein-Barr virus in benign lymph node biopsies from individuals infected with the human immunodeficiency virus is associated with concurrent or subsequent development of non-Hodgkin's lymphoma. *Blood* 77:1527, 1991.

264. MacMahon EME, Glass JD, Hayward SD, et al: Epstein-Barr virus in AIDS-related primary central nervous system lymphoma. *Lancet* 338:969, 1991.

265. Wang D, Liebowitz D, Kieff E: An EBV membrane protein expressed in immortalized lymphocytes transforms established rodent cells. *Cell* 43:831, 1985.

266. Subar M, Neri A, Inghirami G, et al: Frequent c-myc oncogene activation and infrequent presence of Epstein-Barr virus genome in AIDS-associated lymphoma. *Blood* 72:667, 1988.

267. Shibata D, Weiss LM, Hernandez AM, et al: Epstein-Barr virus–associated non-Hodgkin's lymphoma in patients infected with the human immunodeficiency virus. *Blood* 81:2102, 1993.

268. Hamilton-Dutoit SJ, Raphael M, Audouin M, et al: In situ demonstration of Epstein-Barr virus small RNAs (EBER 1) in AIDS related lymphomas: Correlation with tumor morphology and primary site. *Blood* 82:619, 1993.

269. Neri A, Barriga F, Inghirami G, et al: Epstein-Barr virus infection precedes clonal expansion in Burkitt's and acquired immunodeficiency associated lymphoma. *Blood* 77:1092, 1991.

270. Chaganti RSK, Jhanwar SC, Koziner B, et al: Specific translocations characterize Burkitt's-like lymphoma of homosexual men with the acquired immunodeficiency syndrome. *Blood* 61:1269, 1983.

271. Peterson JM, Tubbs RR, Savage RA, et al: Small noncleaved B cell Burkitt-like lymphoma with chromosome t(8;14) translocation and Epstein-Barr virus nuclear associated antigen in a homosexual man with acquired immunodeficiency syndrome. *Am J Med* 78:141, 1985.

272. Rechavi G, Ben-Bassat M, Berkowicz U, et al: Molecular analysis of Burkitt's leukemia in two hemophilic brothers with AIDS. *Blood* 70:1713, 1987.

273. Pelicci PG, Knowles DM, McGrath IT, Dalla-Favera R: Chromosomal breakpoints and structural alterations of the c-myc locus differ in endemic and sporadic forms of Burkitt lymphoma. *Proc Natl Acad Sci USA* 83:2984, 1986.

274. Shiramizu B, Barriga F, Neequaye J, et al: Patterns of chromosomal breakpoint locations in Burkitt's lymphoma: Relevance to geography and Epstein-Barr virus association. *Blood* 77:1516, 1991.

275. Ballerini P, Gaidano G, Gong JZ, et al: Molecular pathogenesis of HIV-associated lymphomas. *AIDS Res Hum Retroviruses* 8:731, 1992.

276. Pelicci PG, Knowles DM II, Arlin ZA, et al: Multiple monoclonal B cell expansions and c-myc oncogene rearrangements in acquired immune deficiency syndrome-related lymphoproliferative disorders: Implications for lymphomagenesis. *J Exp Med* 164:2049, 1986.

277. Pauza CD, Galindo J, Richman DD: Human immunodeficiency virus infection of monoblastoid cells: Cellular differentiation determines the pattern of virus replication. *J Virol* 62:3558, 1988.

278. Laurence J, Astrin SM: Human immunodeficiency virus induction of malignant transformation in human B lymphocytes. *Proc Natl Acad Sci USA* 88:7635, 1991.

279. Lombardi L, Newcomb EW, Dalla-Favera R: Pathogenesis of Burkitt lymphoma: Expression of an activated c-myc oncogene causes the tumorigenic conversion of EBV infected human B lymphoblasts. *Cell* 46:161, 1987.

280. Adams JM, Harris AW, Pinkert CA, et al: The c-myc oncogene driven by immunoglobulin enhancers induces lymphoid malignancy in transgenic mice. *Nature* 318:553, 1985.

281. Gaidano G, Lo Coco F, Ye BH, et al: Rearrangements of the BCL-6 gene in AIDS associated non-Hodgkin's lymphoma: Association with diffuse large cell subtype. *Blood* 84:397, 1994.

282. Gaidano G, Carbone A, Pastore C, et al: Frequent mutatiuons of the 5′ noncoding region of the BCL-6 gene in acquired immuodeficiency syndrome-related non-Hodgkin's lympomas. *Blood* 89:3755, 1997.

283. Gaidano G, Dalla-Favera R: Biologic aspects of human immunodeficiency virus-related lymphoma. *Curr Opin Oncol* 4:900, 1992.

284. Gaidano G, Carbone A, Dalla-Favera R: Pathogenesis of AIDS-related lymphomas: Molecular and histogenetic heterogeneity. *Am J Pathol* 152:623, 1998.

285. Gaidano G, Ballerini P, Gong JZ, et al: p53 mutations in human lymphoid malignancies: Association with Burkitt lymphoma and chronic lymphocytic luekemia. *Proc Natl Acad Sci USA* 88:5413, 1991.

286. Levine AM: Acquired immunodeficiency syndrome-related lymphoma [review]. *Blood* 80:8, 1992.

287. Levine AM, Sullivan-Halley J, Pike MC, et al: HIV-related lymphoma: Prognostic factors predictive of survival. *Cancer* 68:2466, 1991.

288. Levine AM, Gill PS, Meyer PR, et al: Retrovirus and malignant lymphoma in homosexual men. *JAMA* 254:1921, 1985.

289. Ziegler JL, Beckstead JA, Volberding PA, et al: Non-Hodgkin's lymphoma in 90 homosexual men: Relation to generalized lymphadenopathy and the acquired immunodeficiency syndrome. *N Engl J Med* 311:565, 1984.

290. Kaplan LD, Abrams DI, Feigal E, et al: AIDS-associated non-Hodgkin's lymphoma in San Francisco. *JAMA* 261:719, 1989.

291. Knowles DM, Chamulak GA, Subar M, et al: Lymphoid neoplasia associated with the acquired immunodeficiency syndrome (AIDS): The New York University experience with 105 cases during 1981 through 1986. *Ann Intern Med* 108:744, 1988.

292. Lowenthal DA, Straus DJ, Campbell SW, et al: AIDS-related lymphoid neoplasia: The Memorial Hospital experience. *Cancer* 61:2325, 1988.

293. Ioachim HL, Dorsett B, Cronin W, et al: Acquired immunodeficiency syndrome associated lymphomas: Clinical, pathological, immunologic and viral characteristics of 111 cases. *Hum Pathol* 22:659, 1991.

294. Jones SE, Fuks Z, Bellm M, et al: Non-Hodgkin's lymphoma: IV. Clinicopathologic correlation of 405 cases. *Cancer* 31:806, 1973.

295. Podzamczer D, Ricat I, Bolao F, et al: Gallium-67 scan for distinguishing follicular hyperplasia from other AIDS associated diseases in lymph nodes. *AIDS* 4:683, 1990.

296. Levine AM, Wernz JC, Kaplan L, et al: Low dose chemotherapy with central nervous system prophylaxis and azidothymidine maintenance in AIDS-related lymphoma: A prospective multi-institutional trial. *JAMA* 266:84, 1991.

297. Gill PS, Levine AM, Meyer PR, et al: Primary central nervous system lymphoma in homosexual men: Clinical, immunologic and pathologic features. *Am J Med* 78:742, 1985.

298. Goldstein JD, Dickson DW, Moser FG, et al: Primary central nervous system lymphoma in acquired immunodeficiency syndrome: A clinical and pathologic study with results of treatment with radiation. *Cancer* 67:2756, 1991.

299. Baumgartner JE, Rachlin JR, Beckstead JH, et al: Primary central nervous system lymphomas: Natural history and response to radiation therapy in 55 patients with acquired immunodeficiency syndrome. *J Neurosurg* 73:206, 1990.

300. Gill PS, Graham RA, Boswell W, et al: A comparison of imaging, clinical and pathologic aspects of space occupying lesions within the brain in patients with acquired immunodeficiency syndrome. *Am J Physiol Imaging* 1:134, 1986.

301. Ciricillo SF, Rosenblum ML: Use of CT and MR imaging to distinguish intracranial lesions and to define the need for biopsy in AIDS patients. *J Neurosurg* 73:720, 1990.

302. Hoffman JM, Waskin HA, Schifter T, et al: PDG-PET in differentiating lympoma from nonmalignant central nervous system lesions in patients with AIDS. *J Nucl Med* 34:567, 1993.

303. Alcaide FG, Lomena F, Cruceta A, et al: Predictive value of thallium-201 SPECT in the diagnosis of primary central nervous system lymphoma in AIDS patients [abstr 22291]. 12th World AIDS Conference, Geneva, Switzerland, 1998.

304. MacMahon EME, Glass JD, Hayward SDC, et al: Epstein-Barr virus in AIDS related primary central nervous system lymphoma. *Lancet* 338:969, 1991.

305. Cinque P, Brytting M, Vago L, et al: Epstein-Barr virus DNA in cerebrospinal fluid from patients with AIDS related primary lymphoma of the central nervous system. Lancet 342:398–401, 1993.

306. Baumgartner JE, Rachlin JR, Beckstead JH, et al: Primary central nervous system lymphoma: Natural history and response to radiation therapy in 55 patients with AIDS. *J Neurosurg* 73:206, 1990.

307. Nador RG, Cesarman E, Chadburn A, et al: Primary effusion lymphomas: A distinct clinicopathologic entity associated with the Kaposi's sarcoma-associated herpes virus. *Blood* 88:645, 1996.

308. Chang Y, Cesarman E, Pessin MS, et al: Identification of herpesvirus-like DNA sequences in AIDS associated Kaposi's sarcoma. *Science* 266:1865, 1994.

309. Cesarman E, Chang Y, Moore PS, Said JW, Knowles DM: Kaposi's sarcoma associated herpesvirus like DNA sequences in AIDS-related body cavity based lymphomas. *N Engl J Med* 332:1186, 1995.

310. Jones D, Ballestas ME, Kaye KM, et al: Primary effusion lymphoma and Kaposi's sarcoma in a cardiac transplant recipient. *N Engl J Med* 339:444, 1998.

311. Nador RG, Cesarman E, Chadburn A, et al: Primary effusion lymphoma: A distinct clinicopathologic entity associated with the Kaposi's sarcoma-associated herpes virus. *Blood* 88:645, 1996.

312. Centers for Disease Control: Revision of the case definition of acquired immunodeficiency syndrome for national reporting: United States. *Ann Intern Med* 103:402, 1985.

313. Lukes RJ, Parker JW, Taylor CR, et al: Immunologic approach to non-Hodgkin's lymphomas and related leukemias: Analysis of the results of multiparameter studies of 425 cases. *Semin Hematol* 15:322, 1978.

314. Levine AM, Burkes RL, Walker M, et al: Development of B cell lymphoma in two monogamous homosexual men. *Arch Intern Med* 145:479, 1985.

315. Carbone A, Tirelli U, Vaccher E, et al: A clinicopathologic study of lymphoid neoplasms associated with human immunodeficiency virus infection in Italy. *Cancer* 68:842, 1991.

316. Horning SJ, Rosenberg SA: The natural history of initially untreated low grade non-Hodgkin's lymphomas. *N Engl J Med* 311:1471, 1984.

317. Straus DJ, Huang J, Testa MA, Levine AM, Kaplan LD: Prognostic factors in the treatment of human immunodeficiency virus-associated non-Hodgkin's lymphoma: Analysis of AIDS Clinical Trials Group

protocol 142: Low dose versus standard dose m-BACOD plus granulocyte-macrophage stimulating factor. *J Clin Oncol* 16:3601, 1998.

318. Dugan M, Subar M, Odajnyk C, et al: Intensive multiagent chemotherapy for AIDS related diffuse large cell lymphoma. *Blood* 68:124a, 1986.

319. Odajnyk C, Subar M, Dugan M, et al: Clinical features and correlates with immunopathology and molecular biology of a large group of patients with AIDS associated small non-cleaved lymphoma (SNCL). *Blood* 68:1331a, 1986.

320. Gill PS, Levine AM, Krailo M, et al: AIDS-related malignant lymphoma: Results of prospective treatment trials. *J Clin Oncol* 5:1322, 1987.

321. Bermudez M, Grant KM, Rodvien R, Mendes F: Non-Hodgkin's lymphoma in a population with or at risk for acquired immunodeficiency syndrome: Indications for intensive chemotherapy. *Am J Med* 86:71, 1989.

322. Kaplan LD, Straus DH, Testa MA, et al: Low dose compared with standard dose m-BACOD chemotherapy for non-Hodgkin's lymphoma associated with human immunodeficiency virus infection. *N Engl J Med* 336:1641, 1997.

323. Sparano JA, Wiernik PH, Strack M, Leaf A, Becker N, Valentine ES: Infusional cyclophosphamide, doxorubicin, and etoposide in HIV and HTLV-I related non-Hodgkin's lymphoma: A highly active regimen. *Blood* 81:2810, 1993.

324. Sparano JA, Lee S, Chen M, et al: Phase II trial of infusional cyclophosphamide, doxorubicin and etoposide (CDE) in HIV associated non-Hodgkin's lymphoma: An Eastern Cooperative Oncology Group trial (E1494) [abstr 41]. *Proc ASCO* 18:12a, 1999.

325. Wilson WH, Bryant G, Bates S, et al: EPOCH chemotherapy: Toxicity and efficacy in relapsed and refractory non-Hodgkin's lymphoma. *J Clin Oncol* 11:1573, 1993.

326. Little RF, Pearson D, Steinberg S, et al: Dose adjusted EPOCH chemotherapy in previously untreated HIV associated non-Hodgkin's lymhoma [abstr 33]. *Proc ASCO* 18:10a, 1999.

327. Penn I: The changing pattern of posttransplant malignancies. *Transplant Proc* 23:1101, 1991.

328. Brunson ME, Balakrishnan K, Penn I: HLA and Kaposi's sarcoma in solid organ transplantation. *Hum Immunol* 29:56, 1990.

329. Mann DL, Murray C, O'Donnell M, et al: HLA antigen frequencies in HIV-1 related Kaposi's sarcoma. *J AIDS* 3:51, 1990.

330. Jaffe HW, Choi K, Thomas PA, et al: National case-control study of Kaposi's sarcoma and *Pneumocystis carinii* pneumonia in homosexual men: I. Epidemiologic results. *Ann Intern Med* 99:145, 1983.

331. Beral V, Bull D, Darby S, et al: Risk of Kaposi's sarcoma and sexual practices associated with faecal contact in homosexual or bisexual men with AIDS. *Lancet* 339:632, 1992.

332. Beral V, Peterman TA, Berkelman RL, Jaffe HW: Kaposi's sarcoma among persons with AIDS: A sexually transmitted infection? *Lancet* 335:123, 1990.

333. Afrasiabi R, Mitsuyasu R, Nashanian P: Characterization of a distinct subgroup of high risk persons with Kaposi's sarcoma and good prognosis who present with normal T4 cell number and T4;T8 ratio and negative HTL VIII/LAV serologic test results. *Am J Med* 81:969, 1986.

334. Friedman-Kien AE, Saltzman BR, Cao YZ, et al: Kaposi's sarcoma in HIV-negative homosexual men [letter]. *Lancet* 335:168, 1990.

335. Garcia Muret MP, Pujol RM, Puig I, et al: Disseminated Kaposi's sarcoma not associated with HIV infection in a bisexual man. *J Am Acad Dermatol* 23:1035, 1990.

336. Chang Y, Cesarman E, Pessin ME, et al: Identification of herpes virus-like DNA sequences in AIDS-associated Kaposi's sarcoma. *Science* 266:1865, 1994.

337. Moore PS, Chang Y: Detection of herpesvirus-like DNA sequences in Kaposi's sarcoma in patients with and those without HIV infection. *N Engl J Med* 332:1181, 1995.

338. Huang Y-Q, Li JJ, Kaplan MH, et al: Human herpesvirus-like nucleic acid in various forms of Kaposi's sarcoma. *Lancet* 345:759, 1995.

339. Dupin N, Grandadam MN, Calvez V, et al: Herpesvirus-like DNA sequences in patients with Mediterranean Kaposi's sarcoma. *Lancet* 345:761, 1995.

340. Su I-J, Hsu Y-S, Chang Y-C, Wang I-W: Herpesvirus-like DNA sequences in Kaposi's sarcoma from AIDS and non-AIDS patients in Taiwan. *Lancet* 345:722, 1995.

341. Gao S-J, Kingsley L, Hoover DR, et al: Seroconversion to antibodies against Kaposi's sarcoma-associated herpesvirus-related latent nuclear antigens before the development of Kaposi's sarcoma. *N Engl J Med* 335:233, 1996.

342. Martin JN, Ganem DE, Osmond DH, et al: Sexual transmission and the natural history of human herpesvirus 8 infection. *N Engl J Med* 338:948, 1998.

343. Oksenhendler E, Sazals-Hatem D, Schultz TF, et al: Transient angiolymphoid hyperplasia and Kaposi's sarcoma after primary infection with HHV8 in a patient with HIV infection. *N Engl J Med* 338:1585, 1998.

344. Cerimele E, Cesarman E, Curreli G, et al: In vitro infection of primary human keratinocytes by Kaposi's sarcoma associated herpesvirus [abstr 73]. 3rd National AIDS Malignancy Conference, Bethesda, MD, 1999.

345. Ganem D: KSHV/HHV8 infection and the pathogenesis of AIDS-related neoplasms: An overview [abstr S7]. 3rd National AIDS Malignancy Conference, Bethesda, MD, 1999.

346. Chadburn A, Hyjek E, Ying L, et al: KSHV/HHV8 interluekin 6 (vIL6) expression in HIV related lymphadenopathy correlates with development of Kaposi's sarcoma and survival [abstr 47]. 3rd National AIDS Malignancy Conference, Bethesda, MD, 1999.

347. Breen EC, Gage JR, Magpantay L, et al: Biological effects of the HHV8-encoded IL-6 homologue (v IL6). [abstr 42]. 3rd National AIDS Malignancy Conference, Bethesda, MD, 1999.

348. Ensoli B, Nakamura S, Salahuddin SZ, et al: AIDS-Kaposi's sarcoma derived cells express cytokines with autocrine and paracrine growth effects. *Science* 243:223, 1989.

349. Miles S, Rezai A, Magpantay L, et al: Oncostatin-M is a potent mitogen for AIDS-Kaposi's sarcoma (AIDS-KS) cell lines. *Science* 255:1434, 1991.

350. Brown TJ, Rowe JM, Liu JW, Shoyab M: Regulation of IL-6 expression by oncostatin M. *J Immunol* 147:2175, 1991.

351. Miles SA, Rezai AR, Salazar-Gonzalez JF, et al: AIDS Kaposi's sarcoma derived cells produce and respond to interleukin-6. *Proc Natl Acad Sci USA* 87:4068, 1990.

352. Huang YQ, Li JJ, Nicolaides A, et al: Fibroblast growth factor 6 gene expression in AIDS-associated Kaposi's sarcoma. *Lancet* 339:1110, 1992.

353. Vogel J, Hinrichs SH, Reynolds RK, et al: The HIV tat gene induces dermal lesions resembling Kaposi's sarcoma in transgenic mice. *Nature* 335:606, 1988.

354. Ensoli B, Barillari G, Salahuddin SZ, et al: Tat protein of HIV-1 stimulates growth of cells derived from Kaposi's sarcoma lesions of AIDS patients. *Nature* 345:84, 1990.

355. Albini A, Fontanini G, Masiello L, et al: Angiogenic potential in vivo by KS cell free supernatants and HIV-1 tat product: Inhibition of KS like lesions by tissue inhibitor of metalloproteinase-2. *AIDS* 8:1237, 1994.

356. Breen EC, Rezai AR, Nakajima K, et al: Infection with HIV is associated with elevated IL-6 levels and production. *J Immunol* 144:480, 1990.

357. Molina JM, Scadden DT, Byrn R, et al: Production of tumor necrosis factor alpha and interleukin 1 beta by monocytic cells infected with human immunodeficiency virus. *J Clin Invest* 84:733, 1989.

358. Friedman-Kien AE, Laubenstein LJ, Rubinstein P: Disseminated Kaposi's sarcoma in homosexual men. *Ann Intern Med* 96:693, 1982.

359. Friedman SL, Wright TL, Altman DF: Gastrointestinal Kaposi's sarcoma in patients with acquired immunodeficiency syndrome. *Gastroenterology* 89:102, 1985.

360. Rose HS, Balthazar EJ, Megiobow AJ, et al: Alimentary tract involvement in Kaposi's sarcoma: Radioscopic and endoscopic findings in homosexual men. *Am J Radiol* 13:661, 1982.

361. Gill PS, Akil B, Colletti P, et al: Pulmonary Kaposi's sarcoma: Clinical findings and results of therapy. *Am J Med* 87:57, 1989.

362. Garay SM, Belenko M, Fazzini E, et al: Pulmonary manifestation of Kaposi's sarcoma. *Chest* 91:39, 1987.

363. Levine AM, Meyer PR, Gill PS, et al: Results of diagnostic lymph node biopsy in homosexual men with generalized lymphadenopathy. *J Clin Oncol* 4:165, 1995.

364. Robles R, Lugo D, Gee L, Jacobson MA: Effect of antiviral drugs used to treat cytomegalovirus end-organ disease on subsequent course of previously diagnosed Kaposi's sarcoma in patients with AIDS. *J Acquir Immune Defic Syndr Hum Retrovirol* 20:34, 1999.

365. Medveczky MM, Horvath E, Lund T, Medveczky PG: In vitro antiviral drug sensitivity of the Kaposi's sarcoma-associated herpesvirus. *AIDS* 11:1327, 1997.

366. Martin DF, Kuppermann BD, Wolitz RA, et al: Oral ganciclovir for

patients with cytomegalovirus retinitis treated with a ganciclovir implant. *N Engl J Med* 340:1063, 1999.

367. Serfling U, Hood AF: Local therapies for cutaneous Kaposi's sarcoma in patients with acquired immunodeficiency syndrome. *Arch Dermatol* 127:1479, 1991.

368. Tappero JW, Berger TG, Kaplan LD, et al: Cryotherapy for cutaneous Kaposi's sarcoma (KS) associated with acquired immune deficiency syndromen (AIDS): A phase II trial. *J AIDS* 4:839, 1991.

369. Wheeland RG, Bailin PL: Argon laser photocoagulation therapy of Kaposi's sarcoma: A clinical and histological evaluation. *J Dermatol Surg Oncol* 11:1180, 1985.

370. Bodsworth N: Topical 9-cis retinoic acid gel as treatment of cutaneous AIDS-related Kaposi's sarcoma: Interim results of an international, placebo-controlled trial [abstr 22277]. 12th World AIDS Conference, Geneva, Switzerland, 1998.

371. Friedman-Kien A, Conant M: North American phase III study (protocol L105T-31) of Panretin gel for cutaneous AIDS-related Kaposi's sarcoma [abstr 22283]. 12th World AIDS Conference, Geneva, Switzerland, 1998.

372. Epstein JB, Lozada-Nur F, McLeod A, Spinelli J: Oral Kaposi's sarcoma in the acquired immunodeficiency syndrome: Review of management and report of the efficacy of intra-lesional vinblastine. *Cancer* 64: 2424, 1989.

373. Newman S: Treatment of epidemic Kaposi's sarcoma with intralesional vinblastine injection [abstr]. *Proc Am Soc Clin Oncol* 7:5, 1988.

374. Sulis E, Florio C, Sulis ML, et al: Interferon administered intralesionally in skin and oral cavity lesions in heterosexual drug addicted patients with AIDS-related KS. *Eur J Cancer Clin Oncol* 25:759, 1989.

375. Chak LY, Gill PS, Levine AM, et al: Radiation therapy for acquired immunodeficiency syndrome-related Kaposi's sarcoma. *J Clin Oncol* 6:863, 1988.

376. Cooper JS, Steinfeld AD, Lerch I: Intentions and outcomes in the radiotherapeutic management of epidemic Kaposi's sarcoma. *Int J Radiat Oncol Biol Phys* 20:419, 1991.

377. Berson AM, Quivey JM, Harris JW, Wara WM: Radiation therapy for AIDS-related Kaposi's sarcoma. *Int J Radiat Oncol Biol Phys* 19: 569, 1990.

378. De Wit R, Smith WG, Veenhof KH, et al: Palliative radiation therapy for AIDS associated Kaposi's sarcoma by using a single fraction of 800 cGy. *Radiother Oncol* 19:131, 1990.

379. Stiehm ER, Kronenberg LH, Rosenblatt HM, et al: Interferon: Immunobiology and clinical significance. *Ann Intern Med* 96:80, 1982.

380. Mitsuyasu RT: Interferon alpha in the treatment of AIDS-related Kaposi's sarcoma. *Br J Haematol* 79:69, 1991.

381. Rozenbaum W, Gharakhanian S, Navarette MS, et al: Long-term follow-up of 120 patients with AIDS-related Kaposi's sarcoma treated with interferon alpha-2a. *J Invest Dermatol* 95:161S, 1990.

382. Evans LM, Itri LM, Campion M, et al: Interferon-alpha 2a in the treatment of acquired immunodeficiency syndrome-related Kaposi's sarcoma. *J Immunother* 10:39, 1991.

383. Krown SE, Gold JW, Niedzwiecki D, et al: Interferon-alpha with zidovudine: Safety, tolerance, and clinical and virologic effects in patients with Kaposi's sarcoma associated with the acquired immunodeficiency syndrome. *Ann Intern Med* 112:812, 1990.

384. Krown S, Niedzwiecki D, Bhalla RB, et al: Relationship and prognostic value of endogenous interferon-alpha, β2 microglobulin, and neopterin serum levels in patients with Kaposi's sarcoma and AIDS. *J AIDS* 4:871, 1991.

385. Lassoued K, Clauvel JP, Katlama C, et al: Treatment of the acquired immune deficiency syndrome-related Kaposi's sarcoma with bleomycin as a single agent. *Cancer* 66:1869, 1990.

386. Laubenstein LJ, Krigel RL, Odajnyk CM, et al: Treatment of epidemic Kaposi's sarcoma with etoposide or a combination of doxorubicin, bleomycin, and vinblastine. *J Clin Oncol* 2:1115, 1984.

387. Volberding PA, Abrams DI, Conant M, et al: Vinblastine therapy for Kaposi's sarcoma in the acquired immunodeficiency syndrome. *Ann Intern Med* 103:335, 1985.

388. Gill PS, Rarick MU, McCutchan JA, et al: A systemic treatment of AIDS-related Kaposi's sarcoma: Results of a randomized trial. *Am J Med* 90:427, 1991.

389. Gill PS, Espina B, Cabriales S, et al: Liposomal daunorubicin (Dauno-

390. Northfelt DW, Dezube BJ, Thommes JA, et al: Pegylated-liposomal doxorubicin versus doxorubicin, bleomycin and vincristine in the treatment of AIDS-related Kpaosi's sarcoma: Results of a randomized phase III clinical trial. *J Clin Oncol* 16:2445, 1998.

391. Gill PS, Tulpule A, Espina BM, et al: Taxol for advanced AIDS-related Kaposi's sarcoma. *J Clin Oncol* 17:1876, 1999.

392. Gill PS, Rarick MU, Bernstein-Singer M, et al: Treatment of advanced Kaposi's sarcoma using a combination of bleomycin and vincristine. *Am J Clin Oncol* 13:315, 1990.

393. Nakamura S, Sakurada S, Salahuddin SZ, et al: Inhibition of development of Kaposi's sarcoma-related lesions by a bacterial cell wall complex. *Science* 255:1437, 1992.

394. Dezube BJ, Von Roenn JH, Holden-Wiltse J, et al: Fumagillin analog in the treatment of Kaposi's sarcoma: A phase I CIDS Clinical Trial Group Study. *J Clin Oncol* 16:1444, 1998.

395. Miles S, Dezube B, Lee J, et al: Anti-tumor activity of oral 9-cis retinoic acid in AIDS related Kaposi's sarcoma: AIDS Malignancy Consortium Study 002 [abstr 22276]. 12th World AIDS Conference, Geneva, Switzerland, 1998.

396. Carpenter C, Fischl M, Hammer S, et al: Updated recommendations of the International AIDS Society Panel: USA Panel. *JAMA* 277:1962, 1997.

397. 1998 revision to the British HIV Association guidelines for antiretroviral treatment of HIV seropositive individuals. *Lancet* 352:314, 1998.

398. Department of Health and Human Services: Guidelines for the use of antiretroviral agents in HIV-infected adults and adolescents. www.hivatis.org.

399. Ho D: Time to hit HIV early and hard. *N Engl J Med* 333:450, 1995.

400. O'Brien W, Hartigan P, Daar E, et al: Changes in plasma HIV-1 RNA and CD4 lymphocyte counts predict both response to antiretroviral therapy and therapeutic failure: Veterans Affairs Co-operative Study Group on AIDS. *Ann Intern Med* 126: 933, 1997.

401. Perelson A, Essunger Y, Cao Y, et al: Decay characteristics of HIV-1–infected compartments during combination therapy. *Nature* 387:188, 1997.

402. Raboud J, Montaner J, Conway B, et al: Suppression of plasma viral load below 20 copies/mL is required to achieve a long-term response to therapy. *AIDS* 12:1619, 1998.

403. Wit F, vanLeeuwen R, Weverling G, et al: Outcome and predictors of failure of highly active antiretroviral therapy: One-year follow-up of a cohort of human immunodeficiency virus type 1-infected persons. *J Infect Dis* 179:790, 1999.

404. Mayers D: Prevalence and incidence of resistance to zidovudine and other antiretroviral drugs. *Am J Med* 102:70, 1997.

405. Richman D: Antiretroviral drug resistance: Mechanism, pathogenesis, clinical significance. *Adv Exp Med Biol* 394: 383, 1996.

406. Moyle G: Current knowledge of HIV reverse transcriptase mutations selected during nucleoside analogue therapy: The potential to use resistance data to guide clinical decisions. *J Antimicrob Chemother* 40: 765, 1997.

407. Williams A, Friedland G: Adherence, compliance and HAART. *AIDS Clin Care* 9:51, 1997.

408. Ickovics J, Meisler A: Adherence in AIDS clinical trials: A framework for clinical research and clinical care. *J Clin Epidemiol* 50:385, 1997.

409. Haynes R, McKibbon K, Kanani R: Systematic review of randomised trials of interventions to assist patients to follow prescriptions for medications. *Lancet* 348:383, 1996.

410. Hecht FM, Grant RM, Petropoulos CJ, et al: Sexual transmission of an HIV-1 variant resistant to multiple reverse-transcriptase and protease inhibitors. *N Engl J Med* 339:307, 1998.

411. Hirsh M, Conway B, D'Aquila R, et al: Antiretroviral drug resistance testing in adults with HIV infection: Implications for clinical management. International AIDS Society: USA Panel. *JAMA* 279:1984, 1998.

412. Rodriguez-Rosado R, Briones C, Soriano V: Introduction of HIV drug resistance testing in clinical practice. *AIDS* 12:1007, 1999.

413. Yarchoan R, Mitsuya H, Myers C, et al: Clinical pharmacology of a 3'-azido-2',3'-dideoxythymidine and related didexynucleosides. *N Engl J Med* 321:726, 1989.

414. Molina J-M, Journot V, Ferchal F, et al: ALBI (ANRS 070): A randomized controlled trial to evaluate the efficacy and safety of AZT/3TC vs.

alternating d4T/ddI and AZT/3TC vs. d4T/ddI [abstr 12227]. 12th World AIDS Conference, Geneva, 1998.

415. Yarchoan R, Berg G, Brouwers P, et al: Response of HIV associated neurological disease. *Lancet* 1:132, 1987.

416. Sidtis J, Gatsonis C, Price R, et al: Zidovudine treatment of the AIDS dementia complex: Results of a placebo-controlled trial. *Ann Neurol* 33:343, 1993.

417. Bew B, Brown S, Catalan J, et al: Phase III, randomized, double-blind, placebo controlled, multicentre study to evaluate the safety and efficacy of abacavir (ABC, 1592) in HIV-1 infected subjects with AIDS dementia complex (CNA3001) [abstr 39192]. 12th World AIDS Conference, Geneva, 1998.

418. Van Leeuwen R, Katlama C, Kitchen V, et al: Evaluation and safety of 3TC (lamivudine) with asymptomatic or mildly symptomatic HIV infection: A phase III study. *J Infect Dis* 171:116, 1995.

419. Larder B, Kemp S, Harrigan P: Potential mechanism for sustained antiretroviral efficacy of AZT-3TC combination therapy. *Science* 269:696, 1995.

420. Kemp S, Shi C, Bloor C, et al: A novel polymorphism at codon 333 of HIV type 1 reverse transcriptase can facilitate dual resistance to AZT and 3TC. *J Virol* 72:5093, 1998.

421. DeClercq E: The role of non-nucleoside reverse transcriptase inhibitors (NNRTIs) in the therapy of HIV-1 infection. *Antiviral Res* 153, 1998.

422. Saag M, Emini E, Larkin O, et al: A short-term clinical evaluation of L-697,661, a non-nucleoside inhibitor of HIV-1 reverse transcriptase. *N Engl J Med* 329:1065, 1997.

423. Feimuth WL: Delavirdine mesylate, a potent non-nucleoside HIV-1 reverse transcriptase inhibitor. *Ann Exp Med Biol* 394:279, 1996.

424. Flexner C: Drug therapy: HIV-protease inhibitors. *N Engl J Med* 338:1281, 1998.

425. Collier A, et al: Treatment of human immunodeficiency virus infection with saquinavir, zidovudine, and zalcitabine: AIDS Clinical Trials Group. *N Engl J Med* 334:1011, 1996.

426. Hammer S, Squires K, Hughes M, et al: A controlled trial of two nucleoside analogues plus indinavir in persons with human immunodeficiency virus infection and CD4 counts of 200 per cubic millimeter or less: AIDS Clinical Trials Group 320 Study Section. *N Engl J Med* 337:725, 1997.

427. Gulick R, Mellors J, Havlir D, et al: Treatment with indinavir, zidovudine and lamivudine in adults with human immunodeficiency virus infection and prior antiretroviral therapy. *N Engl J Med* 337:734, 1997.

428. Gulick R, Mellor J, Havlir D: Simultaneous vs. sequential initiation of therapy with indinavir, zidovudine, and lamivudine for HIV-1 infection: 100-week follow-up. *JAMA* 280:35, 1998.

429. Cameron D, Heath-Chiozzi M, Danner S: Randomised placebo-controlled trial of ritonavir in advanced HIV-1 disease: The Advanced HIV Disease Ritonavir Study Group. *Lancet* 351:543, 1998.

430. Hsu A, Granneman F, Bertz R: Ritonavir: Clinical pharmacokinetics and interactions with other anti-HIV drugs. *Clin Pharmacokinet* 35:275, 1998.

431. Cameron D, Japour A, Xu Y: Ritonavir and saquinavir combination therapy for the treatment of HIV infection. *AIDS* 13:213, 1999.

432. Workman C, Musson R, Dyer W, et al: Novel double protease combinations containing indinavir with ritonavir: Results from first study [abstr 22372]. 12th World AIDS Conference, Geneva, 1998.

433. Pedneault L, Fetter A, Hanson C, et al: Amprenavir (141W94, APV): Review of overall safety profile [abstr 386]. 6th Conference on Retroviruses, Chicago, 1999.

434. Haubrich R: Phase 2 study or amprenavir, a novel protease inhibitor, in combination with zidovudine/3TC [abstr 12321]. 12th World AIDS Conference, Geneva, 1998.

435. Eron J, Haubrich R, Richman D: Safety and efficacy of amprenavir in combination with other HIV protease inhibitors [abstr 84]. 4th International Congress on Drug Therapy in HIV Infection, Glasgow, 1998.

436. Reports of diabetes and hyperglycemia in patients receiving protease inhibitors for the treatment of human immunodeficiency virus (HIV): FDA Public Health Advisory. *JAMA* 278:379, 1997.

437. Dube M, Johnson D, Currier J, et al: Protease inhibitor-associated hyperglycemia [letter]. *Lancet* 50:713, 1997.

438. Visnegarwala F, Krause K, Musher D: Severe diabetes associated with protease inhibitor therapy [letter]. *Ann Intern Med* 127:947, 1997.

439. Eastone J, Deckler C: New-onset diabetes mellitus associated with the use of protease inhibitor. *Ann Intern Med* 127:948, 1997.

440. Lo J, Mulligan K, Tai V, et al: Buffalo hump in men with HIV-1 infection. *Lancet* 351:867, 1998.

441. Carr A, Samarras K, Chisholm D, et al: Pathogenesis of HIV-1 protease inhibitor-associated peripheral lipodystrophy, hyperlipidemia and insulin resistance. *Lancet* 351:1881, 1998.

442. Gharakhanian S, Salhi Y, Nguyen H, et al: Frequency of lipodystrophy and factors associated with glucose/lipid abnormalities in a cohort of 650 patients treated by protease inhibitors [abstr 642]. 6th Conference on Retroviruses, Chicago, 1999.

443. Tsiodras S, Mantzoros C, Hammer S, et al: Effects of protease inhibitor use on hyperglycemia and hyperlipidemia: A five year analysis [abstr 643]. 6th Conference on Retroviruses, Chicago, 1999.

444. Henry K, Melroe H, Huebsch J et al: Severe premature coronary artery disease with protease inhibitors [letter]. *Lancet* 351:1328, 1998.

445. Lucas GM, Chaisson RE, Moore RD: Highly active antiretroviral therapy in a large urban clinic: Risk factors for virologic failure and adverse drug reactions. *Ann Intern Med* 131:81, 1999.

446. Wit F, vanLeewen G, Weverling S, et al: Determinants of failure of highly active antiretroviral therapy (HAART) [abstr 12271]. 12th World AIDS Conference, Geneva, 1998.

447. Garcia F, Romeu I, Grau M, et al: An open randomized study comparing the influence of difference therapeutic strategies: No treatment vs. double therapy (ZDV/d4T + 3TC) vs. triple therapy (d4T + 3TC + indinavir) in the progression of chronic HIV-1 infected patients in very early stages (Spanish Early Antiretroviral Therapy in HIV: Spanish EARTH-2 study) [abstr 12238]. 12th World AIDS Conference, Geneva, 1998.

448. Centers for Disease Control and Prevention: Public Health Service recommendations for the management of health-care worker exposures to HIV and recommendations for postexposure prophylaxis. *MMWR* 47(RR-7):1998.

MONONUCLEOSIS SYNDROMES

KUO-LIANG HUANG

ROBERT BETTS

Infectious mononucleosis is an acute illness characterized by lymphocytosis in response to infection. Typically, more than 50 percent of the blood white cells are lymphocytes, of which at least 10 percent are atypical. The most common cause of infectious mononucleosis is Epstein-Barr virus (EBV), followed by cytomegalovirus (CMV), *Toxoplasma gondii*, human immunodeficiency virus type I (HIV-1), and other viruses. Patients with infectious mononucleosis generally present with fever, pharyngitis, lymphadenopathy, and malaise. Depending on the predominant clinical features they may have any one of the three forms: pharyngeal, glandular, or typhoid. About 90 percent of patients with EBV-induced mononucleosis have heterophile antibodies; patients with mononucleosis syndromes caused by other agents that have no heterophile antibodies. Special serologic tests may be needed to determine the specific causative agents. The syndromes generally are self-limited, although complications may occur, especially in immunocompromised patients. Infection occurring during pregnancy may produce congenital anomalies. Treatment of infectious mononucleosis is only symptomatic in most cases. Specific therapy may be indicated in rare cases with serious complications.

DEFINITION AND HISTORY

In 1885 Pfeiffer described a disorder that he designated *Drüsenfieber* (glandular fever).[1] The term *infectious mononucleosis* for what was presumably the same disorder was not introduced until 1920 to describe an acute self-limiting mononuclear leukocytosis seen in patients responding to infection.[2] The sera from such patients were subsequently found by Paul and Bunell to contain antibodies that bound the red cells of other species, such as horse or sheep.[3] Because of this property, the antibodies were called *heterophile* antibodies, and patients having such antibodies are referred to as being *heterophile-positive*. The subsequent development of a differential absorption test greatly improved the specificity of the heterophile antibody titre as a diagnostic measure.[4]

Clinically, infectious mononucleosis is defined as any blood lymphocytosis induced in response to an infectious disease. Usually, over 50 percent of the circulating white cells of patients with mononucleosis are lymphocytes, over 10 percent of which have the morphology of ''atypical'' (reactive) lymphocytes,[5] T lymphocytes undergoing blastogenesis as part of a cellular immune response to infected host cells.

Acronyms and abbreviations found in this chapter include: CMV, cytomegalovirus; EBNA, Epstein-Barr nuclear antigen; EBV, Epstein-Barr virus; ELISA, enzyme-linked immunosorbent assay; PCR, polymerase chain reaction.

ETIOLOGY AND PATHOGENESIS

EPSTEIN-BARR VIRUS

Table 90-1 lists some of the known causes of the infectious mononucleosis syndrome. Most cases of infectious mononucleosis in the United States and other developed countries are caused by EBV,[6,7] a member of the Herpesvirus family. A prolonged period of virus shedding from newly infected cells occurs before establishing latency, and spontaneous reactivation from infected cells may occur frequently during the next 2 years. Immune suppression leads to reactivation of virus from its latent state.[8,9] Previous infection with EBV protects against subsequent EBV-induced mononucleosis.[10]

The patient with infectious mononucleosis often has a history of having entered a close interpersonal relationship with the person who transmits the disease; transmission of EBV requires close mucocutaneous contact between the virus-infected transmitter and the susceptible individual.[4,11] The transmitter usually has no history of recent illness and may not have a history of having had infectious mononucleosis. Because of the social activity that transpires during the teenage years, most persons become infected with EBV in young adulthood. The few that escape infection remain susceptible and usually become infected in later adulthood.[12] Although saliva is believed to be the fluid that most commonly transmits the infection,[13] the detection of the virus in fluid from the uterine cervix has raised the question of sexual transmission as well.[14]

It had been believed that EBV mononucleosis is initiated by entry of EBV into epithelial cells of the oropharynx or B lymphocytes of Waldeyer's ring.[8,15] However, using highly sensitive techniques to detect EBV-DNA and EBV gene products, it has been shown that B lymphocytes are the initial target of EBV during primary infection.[16] EBV enters B cells via the cell surface glycoprotein CD21, the 140-kDa complement receptor type 2, and induces polyclonal B-cell proliferation.[8,17] A neoantigen expressed on infected B cells elicits a polyclonal T-cell immune response.[18] This explains why most of the circulating reactive lymphocytes of patients with infectious mononucleosis are T lymphocytes. Some of these T cells also may be responding nonspecifically.[18] In any case, the cellular immune response to EBV generates cytotoxic T cells that destroy infected tonsillar B lymphocytes, leading to severe pharyngitis. These symptoms subside as the counterresponse to the initial polyclonal B-cell proliferation attenuates.[17,19] Once an individual is infected with EBV, the virus presents throughout the lifetime. However, in the healthy individual only the EBNA-1 antigen is expressed, and this does not elicit a T-cell response because of a glycine-alanine repeat that inhibits its processing.[20]

Besides infectious mononucleosis, EBV has been associated with childhood Burkitt's lymphoma in the malarial belt of Africa,[21] nasopharyngeal carcinoma in adults in the Far East,[22] oral hairy leukoplakia in patients with HIV-1 infection,[23] and with leimyosarcoma or leioma in HIV-1 infected patients and transplant recipients.[24,25]

CYTOMEGALOVIRUS

Like EBV, cytomegalovirus (CMV) is a member of the Herpesvirus family. This virus replicates slowly in cells, causing them to enlarge. It is the second most common cause of infectious mononucleosis.

As with EBV most persons in the developing world are infected with CMV by the age of 5.[26] However, in the United States, childhood infection is less likely to occur. Child-to-child transmission occurs frequently in the child care center, but 60 to 80 percent of 20-year-olds in the United States have never been infected with CMV. For reasons that are not clear, susceptible individuals in their teen years and early twenties are far less likely to become infected with CMV than with EBV. Thus, there is no peak incidence age for CMV mononucleosis.[26] Rather, over the ensuing 50 years of adult life, three-quarters of susceptible persons will become infected with this virus. The patho-

TABLE 90-1   ETIOLOGIC AGENTS ASSOCIATED WITH MONONUCLEOSIS SYNDROME

Epstein-Barr virus
Cytomegalovirus
HIV
Herpes simplex II
Rubella
Toxoplasma gondii
Adenovirus
Hepatitis A or B

TABLE 90-2   CLINICAL MANIFESTATIONS OF MONONUCLEOSIS SYNDROME

	Percent of Subjects		
	EBV	CMV	TOXOPLASMA
Fever	90	90	20
Pharyngitis	80	10	10
Lymphadenopathy	80	10	80
Malaise	70	80	80
Hepatomegaly	50	40	10
Splenomegaly	40	40	10
Palatal petechiae	30	5	
Rash	10	5	20

genesis of CMV infection is less well understood than that of EBV infections. The virus initially may infect neutrophils that subsequently spread the infection to fixed macrophages in the liver, spleen, lung, and possibly other organs.[27] Virus-infected cells that express neoantigens in turn may induce a T-cell immune response, resulting in the generation of reactive lymphocytes and blood lymphocytosis. Circulating monocytes may contain CMV DNA or show signs of being infected, as determined by in vitro assays of monocyte function.[87] Thus, in contrast to EBV, where the B lymphocyte causes the T-cell response, the "reactive lymphocyte" of the CMV-infected patient is a T cell responding to an infected cell of the monocyte/macrophage lineage.

OTHER VIRUSES

Primary infection with HIV-1 may present as a heterophile-negative mononucleosis syndrome.[28,29] The acute syndrome lasts for a few weeks and is usually self-limited. However, severe opportunistic infections have been reported during this acute phase.[28] The pathophysiology of HIV is discussed in Chap. 89. Herpes simplex type II and, less commonly, varicella-zoster virus also may cause a heterophile-negative mononucleosis syndrome. Rubella virus and adenovirus also occasionally may cause such a syndrome. In addition, patients with the clinical picture of acute infectious hepatitis due to hepatitis A or B may have significant lymphocytosis with reactive cells. However, some patients with a heterophile-negative mononucleosis syndrome may not have any evidence for being infected acutely with any of these viruses, suggesting that as yet unidentified agents also may produce this clinical syndrome.

TOXOPLASMA GONDII

The only nonviral agent that commonly is identified as causing a mononucleosis syndrome is *Toxoplasma gondii*. Infection with this organism may produce lymphadenopathy associated with fevers. However, more commonly, infected patients are asymptomatic or have isolated lymphadenopathy without fever.[30,31] Two routes of spread of *T. gondii* are ingestion of cysts in raw meat and ingestion of oocysts in cat feces.[30,32] There is no documented person-to-person transmission.

CLINICAL FEATURES

The incubation periods for CMV and EBV are similar, ranging from 30 to 50 days. However, there are significant differences in the clinical presentation of patients infected with one or another of these two agents. A listing of the symptoms and signs and their frequency in mononucleosis syndrome caused by one of the three common agents is presented in Table 90-2. Clearly the symptoms from different infectious agents overlap, and, although each agent has a typical picture, as discussed below, an etiologic diagnosis cannot be made reliably from the clinical presentation.

Pharyngitis is a prominent part of the presentation of individuals with primary EBV infection. Usually pharyngitis occurs after a week or so of malaise, but it may sometimes be delayed for 2 or 3 weeks. A significant tonsillar exudate is generally present. The pharyngitis

that occasionally occurs with CMV is mild, and exudates are absent. Since mononucleosis caused by EBV has such characteristic exudative tonsillitis and almost always presents with lymphadenopathy, the diagnosis is made easily and quickly.[12] The so-called *typhoidal* form of infectious mononucleosis has a strong component of gastrointestinal symptoms and is much more characteristic of CMV infection, although it may also be caused by EBV.[33] Often unusual diseases are considered and a work-up is well underway before the diagnosis of CMV mononucleosis is appreciated.[26]

Individuals acutely infected with either CMV or EBV may have a fine maculopapular rash as part of their presentation. For both, the frequency of the rash is increased dramatically by administration of ampicillin or amoxicillin. For both infections, palpable hepatomegaly and/or splenomegaly are common. Other manifestations, such as pulmonary or cardiac findings, are uncommon (see Table 90-3). In EBV infection, aplastic anemia or agranulocytosis[34,35] has been noted, as has renal failure.[36] A variety of neurologic syndromes may occur, including encephalopathy/encephalitis, aseptic meningitis, transverse myelitis, psychoses, or cranial nerve palsies.[12,37,26,38,39] The neurologic syndrome most frequently associated with CMV-induced mononucleosis is the Guillain-Barré syndrome. In a case-control study involving 154 Guillain-Barré syndrome patients, CMV was associated with 13 percent of cases.[39] The central nervous system (CNS) syndrome may develop instead of, prior to, or after the development of the mononucleosis syndrome.

Infectious mononucleosis in middle-aged and aged patients usually is due to CMV and not EBV. However, when EBV is the cause, it generally is more severe than in the young.[40]

Infectious mononucleosis caused by agents other than EBV or CMV may have different features. Patients with hepatitis A or B may

TABLE 90-3   COMPLICATIONS OF SUBJECTS WITH EBV OR CMV MONONUCLEOSIS

	EBV	CMV
Hemolytic anemia	++	+
Thrombocytopenia	+	+
Aplastic anemia	+	−
Respiratory obstruction	+	−
Splenic rupture	+	−
Jaundice	+	+
Guillain-Barré*	+	++
Encephalitis*	++	+
Transverse myelitis*	+	+
Renal failure	+	+
Pneumonitis*	+	+
Myocarditis*	+	−
B-cell lymphoma	+	−
Agammaglobulinemia	+	−

*May occur without other signs of mononucleosis. ++, common; +, infrequent; −, not reported.

present with mononucleosis associated with abdominal pain and low-grade fever. These symptoms generally remit prior to the appearance of jaundice. Toxoplasmosis also will produce prominent lymphadenopathy, especially posterior auricular, but it does not produce pharyngitis. Hepatosplenomegaly is less prominent in toxoplasmosis than in either EBV or CMV mononucleosis. A faint rash occasionally occurs. Fever is usually low-grade or absent. Encephalitis or meningitis can occur.[30,31] The other agents that produce mononucleosis syndrome may sometimes produce lymphadenopathy. Rubella usually produces a rash; adenovirus usually causes pharyngitis.

Patients with mononucleosis induced by primary infection with HIV generally present with fever, malaise, sore throat, weight loss, and myalgia. The common physical abnormalities are pharyngits, rash, lymphadenopathy, oral or genital ulceration.[41] Neurologic manifestations such as aseptic meningitis, encephalitis, and polyneuropathy are also frequently reported.[28]

LABORATORY FEATURES

The principal diagnostic feature is the presence of the blood lymphocytosis exceeding 50 percent of the blood white count, with at least 10 percent of blood lymphocytes being reactive. The blood of most cases of infectious mononucleosis are flagged as abnormal by modern hematology analyzers.[42] The one feature that distinguishes EBV from all other infectious causes of mononucleosis is the development of the heterophile antibody. Ninety percent of patients develop detectable antibody after 7 to 21 days of illness. The heterophile antibody is not cross-reactive with EBV itself. Rather, the target antigen is found on the surface of beef, horse, or sheep red blood cells but not guinea pig kidney.[43] The horse erythrocyte has the greatest degree of sensitivity for detecting these antibodies.

A variety of other antibodies are produced, presumably resulting from the polyclonal B-cell activation induced by infection with EBV. Antibodies directed against a variety of self-antigens may be detected. These include platelet glycoproteins, nuclear antigens, and the i antigen of human cord; red blood cells commonly are detected in patients with primary EBV infection. The anti-i autoantibodies usually are cold agglutinins that do not react well with red blood cells at 37°C. However, occasionally patients with acute primary EBV infection may develop severe thrombocytopenia or hemolytic anemia secondary to induced autoantibodies.[44-46] Liver function abnormalities, which are predominantly cholestatic but also hepatocellular in nature, are found regularly, whereas jaundice is decidedly uncommon.[37] With the exception of the heterophile antibody, these laboratory abnormalities also may occur in primary infection with CMV (see Table 90-4). Infectious mononucleosis secondary to acute infection with hepatitis A or B, on the other hand, is associated predominantly with elevation of hepatocellular enzyme levels in the serum and with cholestasis, often culminating in the development of frank jaundice. The typical laboratory findings in

TABLE 90-4   LABORATORY ABNORMALITIES IN MONONUCLEOSIS SYNDROME

	Percent of Subjects	
	EBV	CMV
Heterophile antibody	95	0
Lymphocytosis ≥4500/μl (4.5 × 10^9/liter)]	90	80
>20% reactive lymphocytes	90	70
Abnormal liver function	90	70
Decreased platelet count	50	20
Antinuclear factor	50	20
Cold agglutinins	40	20
Cryoglobulins	40	20

HIV-1-induced mononucleosis include thrombocytopenia, leukopenia, and lymphopenia, followed by CD8 T lymphocytosis and depletion of CD4 cells.[28]

SPECIFIC ANTIBODY TESTS

EPSTEIN-BARR VIRUS

Immunofluorescence techniques to measure specific antiviral antibodies can help establish the diagnosis of primary EBV infection. Even the 10 percent of patients with acute EBV infection who fail to develop a heterophile antibody develop the same antibody response to EBV antigens as do EBV-infected individuals who are heterophile-positive.[47-51] EBV antibodies do not react with CMV or with the heterophile antigen.

Almost all infected patients who are acutely ill already have developed IgG and IgM antibody to the virus capsid antigen when first evaluated. The IgM antibody to virus capsid antigen is a sign of acute infection, persisting for only a few months. The IgG antivirus capsid antigen, on the other hand, persists for life. The heterophile antibody titer rises shortly after the appearance of the antivirus capsid antigen antibodies, peaks 1 to 3 weeks after symptoms develop, and remains high for 1 to 3 months thereafter. Early antigen-specific antibody (i.e., IgG antibody to nuclear antigens that are synthesized by infected B cells before viral-directed DNA synthesis commences) appears slightly later in the illness than IgG anti-Virus capsid antigen and then may persist for years.[47-51] Specific antibody to Epstein-Barr nuclear antigen (EBNA) does not develop until after the acute phase of illness and then persists for life. Complement-fixing antibody and neutralizing antibody also develop. Most laboratories that conduct these studies measure virus capsid antigen and EBNA antibodies. The more difficult tests, for IgM antibody or for antibody to early antigen, are reserved for special cases. A presumptive diagnosis of EBV-induced infectious mononucleosis can be reached if the patient is found to have antivirus capsid antigen antibodies but not anti-EBNA antibodies. Culture techniques can help establish that the patient is infected with EBV and is shedding virus.

CYTOMEGALOVIRUS

Culture techniques can detect CMV, but newer methods such as CMV antigenemia assay and polymerase chain reaction (PCR) for detection of CMV DNA are more sensitive than CMV culture in the diagnosis of CMV infection.[52]

Assaying for antibodies to CMV also may help establish the diagnosis of CMV-induced mononucleosis. Antibodies to CMV antigens are not as well defined as those to EBV. IgM and IgG antibody to antigens in CMV-infected fibroblasts can be demonstrated by immunofluorescence or enzyme-linked immunosorbent assay (ELISA).[53-56] Immunofluorescence techniques, however, may detect IgM antibody to CMV-infected cells in the serum of patients with EBV mononucleosis.[57] An IgM cytolytic antibody to CMV-infected cells, however, is not detected in patients with EBV mononucleosis and may help distinguish patients with primary CMV infection.[58] To determine whether an individual has an acute infection with CMV, it is often necessary to measure changes in the anti-CMV antibody titer. A four-fold rise in complement-fixing anti-CMV antibody titer is considered diagnostic. In most cases, the antibody increase with acute infection is at least 16-fold.

HUMAN IMMUNODEFICIENCY VIRUS

The sera of patients who have a mononucleosis-like illness secondary to primary infection with HIV usually lack specific antibodies to HIV. However, viral p24 antigen or high-titer viral RNA can be detected in the blood of such patients.[41] Between 1 and 2 months after their initial presentation, such patients may develop anti-HIV-1 antibodies.[28]

TOXOPLASMA GONDII

Patients with acute primary toxoplasmosis infection generally have high titers of anti-toxoplasmosis antibodies.[59] Patients with primary infection have particularly high titers of IgM anti-toxoplasmosis antibodies. In contrast, patients with AIDS and CNS toxoplasmosis generally have low titers of anti-toxoplasmosis antibody that almost invariably are of the IgG isotype. Both IgG and IgM anti-toxoplasmosis antibodies may be detected using specific tests, such as the Sabin-Feldman dye test, immunofluorescence assays, or ELISA. These tests are available commercially.

DIFFERENTIAL DIAGNOSIS

MONONUCLEOSIS SYNDROME

EBV mononucleosis presents as a systemic syndrome with severe pharyngitis. The differential diagnosis should include infections by other organisms that may cause pharyngitis, such as β-hemolytic streptococcus, adenovirus, and *Arcanobacter hemolyticum*. Most other viral causes of pharyngitis evolve fairly quickly into typical upper respiratory symptoms. Group A streptococci frequently are isolated from pharyngeal cultures obtained from patients with typical EBV-induced mononucleosis. Although recovery of this organism from the throat cultures of symptomatic patients usually mandates antibiotic therapy, such treatment seldom produces any clinical improvement.

Patients with primary CMV infection present with fever and splenomegaly without other specific findings. Often such patients are suspected to have an underlying lymphoma. Alternatively, the presence of antinuclear antibodies associated with primary CMV infection may suggest that such patients have new-onset systemic lupus erythematosus.

The mononucleosis syndrome of toxoplasmosis has several features that help distinguish it from EBV or CMV mononucleosis (see clinical features). In addition, liver function tests are generally normal. Lymphocytosis occurs in a small percentage of these individuals.[31] Toxoplasma antibody tests can establish the diagnosis.[59] Toxoplasma infection in the CNS of HIV-positive patients generally does not produce a mononucleosis syndrome.

Hepatitis A or B virus also can cause a mononucleosis-like syndrome associated with circulating reactive lymphocytosis and abnormal liver function tests. However, the sera of patients with mononucleosis caused by these viruses generally have marked elevations in serum levels of hepatocellular enzymes. Furthermore, when liver function tests on the sera become abnormal for patients with hepatitis, the fever abates. Symptomatic primary HIV-1 infection has been described in all of the major risk groups. Such a diagnosis should be considered in any patient with an infectious mononucleosis syndrome who is at risk of HIV-1 infection. One of the major manifestations of HIV-1 mononucleosis is aseptic meningitis. Other causes of this process must be considered.

"CHRONIC MONONUCLEOSIS SYNDROME"

A central feature of this syndrome is severe fatigue lasting more than 6 months and reducing activity by 50 percent or more.[60] Initial reports implicated EBV as causing this poorly understood syndrome. However, careful epidemiologic and serologic studies largely have excluded EBV as a major cause for this syndrome.[61] Although antibody titers to EBV antigens may be elevated in some subjects, so are antibody titers to other infectious agents.[62] Since blood mononucleosis is not a component of this syndrome, whereas fatigue is, the descriptor chronic

mononucleosis is a misnomer and should no longer be used. Instead this syndrome has been designated the *chronic fatigue syndrome*.

THERAPY, COURSE, AND PROGNOSIS

Both heterophile-positive and heterophile-negative syndromes are self-limited. Thus, only symptomatic therapy is indicated in most cases. If the spleen is enlarged, patients should temporarily limit their activity because of the small but definite risk of splenic rupture. Although aspirin has been recommended to reduce the fever and pharyngeal inflammation, reports of aspirin producing Reye syndrome in children with EBV[63] make acetaminophen and/or gargling with saline preferable alternatives. Penicillin or erythromycin is indicated if group A streptococcus is isolated from throat cultures of symptomatic patients.

Limited studies suggest that there is very little benefit from glucocorticoid therapy beyond the first 48 to 96 h.[64] There have been reports of encephalitis or myocarditis associated with corticosteroid use in patients with mononucleosis.[65] Most clinicians are reluctant to administer glucocorticoids unless there are severe or life-threatening complications, such as imminent upper airway obstruction, thrombocytopenic purpura, hemolytic anemia, or central nervous system involvement (see Table 90-3).[66] When used, prednisone is given orally at a dose of 40 to 60 mg per day for 4 days. The dosage is slowly reduced over 5 to 7 days and discontinued. Acyclovir alone or in combination with corticosteroid provides no clinical benefit for uncomplicated infectious mononucleosis.[67,68] In an immunocompromised patient with severe, complicated primary EBV infection and infectious mononucleosis, treatment with ganciclovir may produce a favorable outcome.[69] EBV-induced lymphoproliferative disorders are generally not responsive to acyclovir.[70] Various attempts employing interferon-α, interferon-β, interleukin-2, adoptive transfer of EBV-specific T cells, or reducing immunosupressants have been reported to have some beneficial effects in treating these disorders.[71,72] Ganciclovir and foscarnet are effective against cytomegalovirus infection, but their toxicity precludes their use in this self-limited disease except in the immunocompromised host.[73]

Patients with the acute infectious mononucleosis syndrome due to *T. gondii* usually do not require therapy.[30,31,74] If the patient is pregnant, immunocompromised, or has an infection involving vital organs, then pyrimethamine and sulfadiazine should be used.[74] Therapy is initiated with 100 to 200 mg pyrimethamine orally in two divided doses, followed by 1 mg/kg per day in a single dose. In addition, sulfadiazine is given at 75 to 100 mg/kg per day in four divided doses. Treatment is continued for 2 to 4 weeks. Folinic acid (calcium leucovorin) 10 to 20 mg/day may prevent hematologic toxicity.

For patients with acute primary HIV-1 infection, very high titers of HIV are detectable during the acute phase of the illness, i.e., during the mononucleosis-like syndrome. After the resolution of symptoms, the plasma viral RNA level declines rapidly and reaches an inflection point 120 days after infection, then gradually increases. Viral levels 120 to 365 days after acquisition are associated with faster disease progressions.[75] Antiretroviral treatment of primary HIV-1 infection has resulted in clearance of viremia and restoration of CD4 lymphocytes.[41,76] However, the long-term clinical benefit remains to be determined.

MONONUCLEOSIS IN PREGNANCY

Most women of childbearing age are immune to infection with EBV. Hence, congenital infection is rare. This is fortunate, as EBV mononucleosis during gestation may produce severe congenital anomalies, including microcephaly, hepatosplenomegaly, cataracts, mental retardation, and/or death.[37,77] On the other hand, most infants born with congenital CMV are asymptomatic at birth, and 90 percent will develop

TABLE 90-5   SPECIAL PROBLEMS WITH EBV AND CMV INFECTION

	EBV	CMV
In utero infection	+	++
Congenital illness	+	++
Neonatal illness	−	++
Transfusion-associated	+	++
Transplant-associated	+	++
Associated with rheumatoid arthritis	+	−

NOTE: +, reported; ++, recognized with significant frequency; −, not reported.

normally. Such infants generally are born of mothers who were infected many months prior to the onset of pregnancy.[78] However, if a mother develops primary CMV infection, approximately 50 percent of infants will have congenital infection.[79,80] Of these, about one-quarter may be symptomatic. Abortion may be considered for any pregnant woman who develops either CMV or EBV mononucleosis syndrome during pregnancy, especially during the first trimester.

Congenital infection with toxoplasmosis also may produce developmental abnormalities. The mother who already has anti-toxoplasmosis antibody before pregnancy does not transmit the organism to her developing infant. However, if the mother develops a primary infection during her first trimester, there is a risk that the infant may develop congenital abnormalities. Several treatment regimens have been employed to prevent and treat congenital toxoplasmosis. Pyrimethamine, in combination with sulfonamides and/or spiramycin, may eradicate parasites in the placenta and also in the fetus.[32,81] However, multicenter trials testing the safety and efficacy of these regimens are lacking.

HIV-1 can be transmitted from mothers to babies before birth, during labor and delivery, or even after birth (through breast feeding). The maternal plasma HIV-1 RNA level has been demonstrated to be the strongest predictor of the perinatal transmission of HIV-1.[82] With its extremely high level of plasma HI-1 RNA, primary HIV-1 infection during pregnancy may pose a significantly high risk of perinatal HIV-1 transmission. Recent studies have shown that perinatal treatment with zidovudine alone or in combination with elective caesarean section substantially reduces the rate of maternal-infant HIV-1 transmission.[83,84]

THE COMPROMISED HOST

In the compromised host, CMV can cause primary infection if transmitted by blood transfusion or by allografts[85] (Table 90-5). In transplant patients, CMV causes both direct injury involving multiple organs and indirect effects such as allograft rejection and bacterial superinfection.[73] Prevention of CMV infection is of great importance in this population. The use of prophylactic antibiotics has been shown to be safe and effective in reducing CMV disease after organ transplantation.[86]

REFERENCES

1. Pfeiffer E: Drüsenfieber. *Jahrbuch für Kinderheilkunde* 23:257, 1885.
2. Sprunt TP, Evans FA: Mononuclear leukocytosis in reaction to acute infections (''infectious mononucleosis''). *Johns Hopkins Bull* 31:410, 1920.
3. Paul JR, Bunnell WW: The presence of heterophile antibodies in infectious mononucleosis. *Am J Med Sci* 183:91, 1932.
4. Davidsohn I, Walker PH: The nature of the heterophilic antibodies in infectious mononucleosis. *Am J Clin Pathol* 5:455, 1935.
5. Cheeseman SH: Infectious mononucleosis. *Semin Hematol* 25:261, 1988.
6. Evans AS, Niederman JC, McCollum RW: Seroepidemiologic studies of infectious mononucleosis with EB virus. *N Engl J Med* 279:1121, 1978.
7. Klemola E, vonEssen R, Henle G, et al: Infectious mononucleosis-like disease with negative heterophile agglutination test. Clinical features in relation to Epstein-Barr virus and cytomegalovirus antibodies. *J Infect Dis* 121:608, 1970.
8. Thorley-Lawson DA: Basic virological aspects of Epstein-Barr virus infection. *Semin Hematol* 25:247, 1988.
9. Preiksaitis JK, Diaz-Mitoma F, Mirzaryans F, et al: Quantitative oropharyngeal Epstein-Barr virus shedding in renal and cardiac transplant recipients. Relationship to immunosuppressive therapy, serologic responses and the risk of past transplant lymphoproliferative disorder. *J Infect Dis* 166:986, 1992.
10. Sawyer RN, Evans AS, Neiderman JC, McCollum RW: Prospective studies of a group of Yale University freshmen: I. Occurrence of infectious mononucleosis. *J Infect Dis* 123:263, 1971.
11. Chetham MM, Roberts KB: Infectious mononucleosis in adolescents. *Pediatr Ann* 20:206, 1991.
12. Evans AS: Infectious mononucleosis and related syndromes. *Am J Med Sci* 276:325, 1978.
13. Yao QY, Rickinson AB, Epstein MA: A re-examination of the Epstein-Barr virus carrier state in healthy seropositive individuals. *Int J Cancer* 35:35, 1985.
14. Sixbey JW, Lemon SM, Pagano JS: A second site for Epstein-Barr virus shedding: the uterine cervix. *Lancet* 2:1122, 1986.
15. Epstein MA, Adrong BG: Pathogenesis of infectious mononucleosis. *Lancet* 3:1270, 1977.
16. Karajannis MA, Hummel M, Anagnostopoulos I, Stein H: Strict lymphotropism of Epstein-Barr virus during acute infectious mononuleosis in nonimmunocompromised individuals. *Blood* 89:2856, 1997.
17. Yefenef E, Bakas T, Einhorn L, et al: Epstein-Barr virus (EBV) receptors, complement receptors, and EBV infectibility of different lymphocyte fractions of human peripheral blood: I and II. *Cell Immunol* 35:34, 1978.
18. Thorley-Lawson DA: Immunological responses to Epstein-18. Barr virus infection and the pathogenesis of EBV-induced diseases. *Biochim Biophys Acta* 948:263, 1988.
19. Rickinson AB, Moss DJ: Human cytotoxic T lymphocyte responses to Epstein-Barr virus infection. *Annu Rev Immunol* 15:405, 1997.
20. Levitskaya J, Coram M, Levitsky V, et al: Inhibition of antigen processing by the internal repeat region of the Epstein-Barr virus nuclear antigen-1. *Nature* 375:685, 1995.
21. Facer CA, Playfair JHL: Malaria Epstein-Barr virus and the genesis of lymphoma. *Adv Cancer Res* 53:33, 1989.
22. Tam JS, Murray HGS: Nasopharyngeal carcinoma and Epstein-Barr virus-associated serologic markers. *Ear Nose Throat J* 69:261, 1990.
23. Greenspan JS, Greenspan D, Lennette ET: Replication of Epstein-Barr virus within epithelial cells of hairy oral leukoplakia and AIDS associated lesion. *N Engl J Med* 313:1564, 1986.
24. McClain K, Leach CT, Jenson HB, et al: Association of Epstein-Barr virus with leiomyosarcomas in young people with AIDS. *N Engl J Med* 332:12, 1995.
25. Lee ES, Locker J, Nalesnik M, et al: The association of Epstein-Barr virus with smooth muscle tumors occurring after organ transplantation. *N Engl J Med* 332:19, 1995.
26. Betts RF: Syndromes of cytomegalovirus infection. *Adv Intern Med* 26:447, 1980.
27. Zaia JA: Epidemiology and pathogenesis of cytomegalovirus disease. *Semin Hematol* 27(suppl 1):5, 1990.
28. Quinn TC: Grand Rounds at the Johns Hopkins Hospital. Acute primary HIV infection. *JAMA* 278: 58, 1997.
29. Rosenberg ES, Caliendo AM, Walker BD: Acute HIV infection among patients tested for mononucleosis. *N Engl J Med* 340:969, 1999.
30. Krick JA, Remington JS: Current concepts in parasitology: toxoplasmosis in the adult. An overview. *N Engl J Med* 298:500, 1978.
31. Mc Cabe RE, Brooks RG, Dofman RF, Remington JS: Clinical spectrum in 107 cases of toxoplasmic lymphadenopathy. *Rev Infect Dis* 9:754, 1987.
32. Cengir SD, Ortac F, Soylemez F: Treatment and results of chronic toxoplasmosis. Analysis of 33 cases. *Gynecol Obstet Invest* 33:105, 1992.
33. Horwitz CA, Henle W, Henle G, et al: Clinical and laboratory evaluation of cytomegalovirus-induced mononucleosis in previously healthy individuals. *Medicine* 65:124, 1989.

34. Lazarus KH, Braehner RL: Aplastic anemia complicating infectious mononucleosis: a case report and review of the literature. *Pediatrics* 67:907, 1981.

35. Koziner B, Hadler N, Parrillo J, Ellman L: Agranulocytosis following infectious mononucleosis. *JAMA* 225:1235, 1973.

36. Mayer HB, Wanke CA, Williams M, Crosson AW, Federman M, Hammer SM: Epstein-Barr virus-induced infectious mononucleosis complicated by acute renal failure: case report and review. *Clin Infect Dis* 22:1009, 1996.

37. Jones JF: A perspective of Epstein-Barr virus diseases. *Adv Pediatr* 36:307, 1989.

38. Connelly KP, DeWitt LD: Neurologic complications of infectious mononucleosis. *Pediatr Neurol* 10:181, 1994.

39. Jacobs BC, Rothbarth PH, Van der Meche, et al: The spectrum of antecedent infections in Guillain-Barre sydrome. *Neurology* 51:1110, 1998.

40. Auwaerter PG: Infectious mononucleosis in middle age. *JAMA* 281:454, 1999.

41. Kahn J, Walker BD: Acute human immunodeficiency virus type I infection. *N Engl J Med* 339:33, 1998.

42. Brigden ML, Au S, Thompson S, Brigden S, Doyle P, Tsaparas Y: Infectious mononucleosis in an outpatient population. *Arch Pathol Lab Med* 123:875, 1999.

43. Paul JR, Bunnell WW: The presence of heterophile antibodies in infectious mononucleosis. *Am J Med Sci* 183:90, 1932.

44. Matsukawa Y, Okano M, Ishikawa N, Imasi S: Severe thrombocytopenic purpura associated with primary Epstein-Barr virus infection. *J Infect* 29:107, 1994.

45. Whitelaw F, Brook MG, Kennedy N, Weir WR: Haemolytic anaemia complicating Epstein-Barr virus infection. *Br J Clin Pract* 49:212, 1995.

46. Van Spronsen DJ, Breed WP: Cytomegalovirus-induced thrombocytopenia and haemolysis in an immunocompetent adult. *Br J Haematol* 92:218, 1996.

47. Henle W, Henle G, Horwitz CA: Epstein Barr virus. Specific diagnostic tests in infectious mono. *Hum Pathol* 5:551, 1974.

48. Schmitz H, Scherer M: IgM Antibodies to Epstein Barr in infectious mononucleosis. *Arch Gesam Virusforsch* 37:332, 1972.

49. Henle G, Henle W, Haltia K, et al: Antibodies to early antigens induced by Epstein-Barr virus in infectious mononucleosis. *J Infect Dis* 124:58, 1971.

50. Henle G, Henle W, Horwitz CA: Antibodies to Epstein-Barr virus-associated nuclear antigen in infectious mononucleosis. *J Infect Dis* 130:231, 1974.

51. Evans AS, Niederman JC, Cenabre LC, et al: Specificity, sensitivity, and persistence of heterophile and EB-virus specific IgM antibodies in clinical and subclinical infectious mononucleosis. *J Infect Dis* 132:546, 1975.

52. Fischer SH, Masur H: Editorial response: laboratory monitoring of cytomegalovirus disease: is polymerase chain reaction the answer? *Clin Infect Dis* 24:841, 1997.

53. Betts RF, George SD, Rundell BR, et al: Comparative activity of immunofluorescent antibody and complement fixing antibody in cytomegalovirus infection. *J Clin Microbiol* 4:151, 1976.

54. Hanshaw JB, Steinfeld HJ, White CJ: Fluorescent antibody test for cytomegalovirus macroglobulin. *N Engl J Med* 279:566, 1968.

55. Stagno S, Tinker MK, Eliod C, et al: Immunoglobulin M antibodies detected by enzyme-like immunosorbent assay and radioimmunoassay in the diagnosis of cytomegalovirus infection in pregnant women and newborn infants. *J Clin Microbiol* 21:930, 1985.

56. Rasmussen L: Immune response to human cytomegalovirus infection. *Curr Top Microbiol Immunol* 154:222, 1990.

57. Hanshaw JB, Niederman JC, Chessin LN: Cytomegalovirus macroglobulin in cell-associated herpes virus infections. *J Infect Dis* 125:304, 1972.

58. Betts RF, Schmidt SG: Cytolytic IgM antibody to cytomegalovirus in primary cytomegalovirus in humans. *J Infect Dis* 143:821, 1981.

59. Brooks RG, McCabe RE, Remington JS: Role of serology in the diagnosis of toxoplasmic lymphadenopathy. *Rev Infect Dis* 9:775, 1987.

60. Fukuda K, Straus SE, Hickie I, Sharpe MC, Dobbins JG, Komaroff A: The chronic fatigue syndrome: a comprehensive approach to its definition and study. *Ann Intern Med* 121:953, 1994.

61. Hellinger WC, Smith TF, Van Scoy RE, et al: Chronic fatigue syndrome and the diagnostic utility of antibody to Epstein-Barr virus early antigen. *JAMA* 260:971, 1988.

62. Khan AS, Heneine WM, Chapman LE, et al: Assessment of a retrovirus sequence and other possible risk factors for the chronic fatigue syndrome. *Ann Intern Med* 118:241, 1993.

63. Fleisher G, Schwartz J, Lennette ET: Primary Epstein Barr virus in association with Reye's syndrome. *J Pediatr* 97:935, 1980.

64. Brandfonbrener A, Epstein A, Wu S, Phair J: Corticosteroid therapy in Epstein-Barr virus infection. *Arch Intern Med* 146:337, 1986.

65. Straus SE, Cohen JI, Tosato G, Meier J: NIH conference. Epstein-Barr virus infections: biology, pathogenesis, and management. *Ann Intern Med* 118:45, 1993.

66. Peter J, Ray CG: Infectious mononucleosis. *Pediatr Rev* 19:276, 1998.

67. Van der Horst C, Joncas J, Ahronheim G, et al: Lack of effect of peroral acyclovir for the treatment of acute infectious mononucleosis. *J Infect Dis* 164:788, 1991.

68. Tynell E, Aurelius E., Brandell A., et al: Acyclovir and prednisolone treatment of acute infectious mononucleosis: a multicenter, double-blind, placebo-controlled study. *J Infect Dis* 174:324, 1996.

69. Dellemiju PL, Brandenburg A, Niesters HG, Van den Bent MJ, Rothbarth PH, Vlasveld LT: Successful treatment with ganciclovir of presumed Epstein-Barr meningo-encephalitis following bone marrow transplant. *Bone Marrow Transplant* 16:311, 1995.

70. Starzl TE, Nalesnik MA, Porter KA, et al: Reversibility of lymphomas and lymphoproliferative lesions developing under cyclosporin-steroid therapy. *Lancet* 1:583, 1984.

71. Rooney CM, Smith CA, Ng CY, et al: Use of gene-modified virus-specific T lymphocytes to control Epstein-Barr virus related ymphoproliferation. *Lancet* 345:9, 1995.

72. Okano M: Epstein-Barr virus infection and its role in the expanding spectrum of human diseases. *Acta Paediatr* 87:11, 1998.

73. Fishman JA, Rubin RH: Infection in organ-tansplant reciepients. *N Engl J Med* 338:1741, 1998.

74. McCabe RE, Oster S: Current recommendations and future prospects in the treatment of toxoplasmosis. *Drugs* 38:973, 1989.

75. Schacker TW, Hughes JP, Shea T, Coombs RW, Corey L: Biological and virologic characteristics of primary HIV infection. *Ann Intern Med* 128:613, 1998.

76. Zaunders JJ, Cunningham PH, Kelleher AD, et al: Potent antiretroviral therapy of primary human immunodeficiency virus type-1 (HIV-1) infection. Partial normalization of T-lymphocytes subsets and limited reduction of HIV-1 DNA despite clearance of plasma viremia. *J infect Dis* 180:320, 1999.

77. Goldburg GN, Fulginiti VA, Ray G, et al: In utero Epstein-Barr (infectious mononucleosis) infection. *JAMA* 246:1579, 1981.

78. Schopfer K, Lauber E, Krech U: Congenital cytomegalovirus infection in newborn infants of mothers infected before pregnancy. *Arch Dis Child* 53:536, 1978.

79. Stagno S, Pass RF, Dworsky ME, et al: Congenital cytomegalovirus infection: The relative importance of primary or recurrent maternal infection. *N Engl J Med* 306:945, 1982.

80. Boppana SB, Pass RF, Butt WJ: Virus specific antibody responses in mothers and their newborn infants with asymptomatic congenital cytomegalovirus infections. *J Infect Dis* 167:72, 1993.

81. Stray-Pedersen B: Treatment of toxoplasmosis in the pregnant mother and newborn child. *Scand J Infect Dis* 84:23, 1992.

82. Mofenson LM, Lamber JS, Stiehim ER, et al: Risk factors for perinatal transmission of human immunodeficiency virus Type I in women treated with Zidovudine. *N Engl J Med* 341:385, 1999.

83. The international perinatal HIV group: The mode of delivery and the risk of vertical transmission of human immunodeficiency virus Type I—a meta-analysis of 15 prospective cohort studies. *N Engl J Med* 340:977, 1999.

84. Lindegren ML, Byers Jr RH, Thomas P, et al: Trends in perinatal transmission of HIV/AIDs in the United States. *JAMA* 282:531, 1999.

85. Rubin RH: Impact of cytomegalovirus on organ transplant recipients. *Rev Infect Dis* 12:S7, S754, 1990.

86. Lowance D, Neumayer HH, Legendre CM, et al: Valacyclovir for the prevention of cytomegalovirus disease after renal transplantation. *N Engl J Med* 340:1462, 1999.

87. Carney WP, Hirsh MS: Mechanism of immunosuppression in cytomegalovirus mononucleosis. *J Infect Dis* 144:47, 1981.

MALIGNANT DISEASES

CHAPTER 91

CLASSIFICATION AND CLINICAL MANIFESTATIONS OF THE CLONAL MYELOID DISORDERS

MARSHALL A. LICHTMAN

The clonal myeloid disorders result from a mutation of DNA within a pluripotential marrow stem cell or very early progenitor cell. The primary alteration causing the mutation is often evident when cytogenetic analysis is performed. Translocations, inversions, and deletions of chromosomes can result (1) in the expression of fusion genes that encode fusion proteins that are oncogenic or (2) in the over- or underexpression of genes that encode molecules critical to the control of cell growth or programmed cell death.

The different mutations may result in variable phenotypes that range from mild impairment of the steady-state levels of blood cells, insignificant functional impairment of cells, and little consequence on longevity to severe deficiencies in normal blood cell concentration and death in hours to days, if untreated. Although very mild disease expression can be considered a "benign" neoplasm as compared to acute myelogenous leukemia, that term has not been used to classify disorders like idiopathic sideroblastic anemia, because they do have measurable alterations in blood cells and have a propensity to progress to acute myeloid leukemia as compared to age- and gender-matched unaffected persons.

The somatically mutated (neoplastic) stem cell from which the clonal expansion of hematopoietic cells derive retains the ability, albeit imperfectly, to differentiate and mature into each blood cell lineage. The effects of the disorder may alter blood cell numbers, structure, and function and may range from minimal to severe in the various blood cell lineages. The effects occur on one lineage or another in an unpredictable way, even in subjects within the same category of disease. The resulting phenotypes are numerous and varied. In polycythemia vera or thrombocythemia, the maturation of progenitors results in cells nearly normal in appearance and function, although excessive in their level in the blood. Moreover, overlapping features are common, such as thrombocythemia as a feature of polycythemia or chronic myelogenous leukemia. The acquired idiopathic refractory anemias may have insignificant or very consequential neutropenia or thrombocytopenia or sometimes thrombocytosis. This reflects the unpredictable expression

of stem cell capabilities for which the genic explanations are largely unknown. In only a few circumstances are there tight relationships between the cytogenetic alteration and the phenotype and even these are imperfect; for example t(9;22)(q34;q11) with chronic myelogenous leukemia or t(15;17)(q22;q21) with acute promyelocytic leukemia. However, most patients can be grouped into the classical diagnostic designations listed in Table 91-1.

An important feature of the clonal myeloid diseases is that there is potentially reversible suppression of the expression of normal stem cells by the clonally expanded cells. This coexistence and competition forms the basis for the remission-relapse pattern seen in acute myelogenous leukemia after intensive chemotherapy and for the reappearance of polyclonal, normal hematopoiesis in some patients with chronic myelogenous leukemia after interferon-α therapy.

A wide array of clonal (neoplastic) syndromes or diseases can result from a somatic mutation in a stem cell or an early multipotential hematopoietic cell. These several diseases can be grouped, somewhat arbitrarily, by their degree of malignancy, using the classic terminology of experimental carcinogenesis, which logically considers the degree of loss of differentiation potential and the rate of progression of the disease. The term *deviation* relates to the relationship to normal cellular differentiation potential and the regulation of cell population homeostasis (birth and death rates). This terminology has been used to array the well-known diagnostic categories into a framework for the reader.

MINIMAL-DEVIATION MYELOID CLONAL DISORDERS

These neoplasms retain a higher degree of differentiating capability and usually permit life-spans measured in decades without treatment or with minimally toxic treatment approaches,[1] (see Chaps. 61, 92, 118). The use of the term *minimal deviation* should not be construed as indicating that these conditions do not have morbidity, shorten life, and have other consequences to the patient. It is a term that is used relative to acute myelogenous leukemia with an expected life-span if untreated measured in days to weeks.

INEFFECTIVE HEMATOPOIESIS (PRECURSOR APOPTOSIS) PROMINENT

These are a subgroup of clonal hemopoietic stem cell diseases in which cytopenias resulting from ineffective hematopoiesis is the most characteristic feature. A common secondary characteristic is striking dysmorphogenesis of blood cells. These cytologic abnormalities, characteristic of the acquired anemias, bicytopenias, or pancytopenias, include changes in the size (macro- and microcytosis), shape (poikilocytosis), and nuclear or organelle structure (hypo- or hypergranulation, nuclear hypolobulation) of blood cells and their precursors (see Chap. 92). Abnormal maturation of blood cells leads to morphologic, biochemical, and functional alterations of the cells. Ineffective erythropoiesis, the intramedullary death of erythroblasts before they reach full maturation, is a common feature, and ineffective granulopoiesis and thrombopoiesis also can occur. An increase in (leukemic) blast cells is not evident in these syndromes. If they are elevated above the upper limit of 2 percent, they should be considered oligoblastic leukemia (or *refractory anemia with excess blasts*). Because of the variability of marrow differential counts and marrow sampling, such distinctions require several observations.

The term *hematopoietic dysplasia*, later simplified to *myelodysplasia*, has become ensconced as the category into which some of

Acronyms and abbreviations that appear in this chapter include: AML, acute myelogenous leukemia; BFU–E, burst-forming unit–erythroid; CFU–Baso, colony forming unit–basophil; CFU–Eo, colony forming unit–eosinophil; CFU–G, colony-forming unit–granulocyte; CFU–M, colony-forming unit–monocyte-macrophage; CFU–Meg, colony-forming unit–megakaryocyte; 2N, diploid megakaryoblast; CML, chronic myelogenous leukemia.

TABLE 91-1   NEOPLASTIC (CLONAL) MYELOID DISORDERS

Minimal-deviation neoplasms (no leukemic blast cells are evident in marrow)
Underproduction (apoptosis) of mature cells is prominent
Acquired idiopathic sideroblastic anemia (Chap. 92)
Acquired idiopathic nonsideroblastic anemia (Chap. 92)
Pancytopenia with hypercellular marrow (Chap. 92)
Paroxysmal nocturnal hemoglobinuria (Chap. 36)
Overproduction of cells is prominent
Polycythemia vera (Chap. 61)
Primary thrombocythemia (Chap. 118)
Moderate-deviation neoplasms (small proportions of leukemic blast cells usually present in marrow)
Chronic myelogenous leukemia (Chap. 94)
Ph-positive–bcr rearrangement positive CML
Ph-negative–bcr rearrangement positive CML
Idiopathic myelofibrosis (Chap. 95)
Chronic neutrophilic leukemia (Chap. 94)
Moderately severe deviation neoplasms (moderate concentration of leukemic blast cells present in marrow)
Oligoblastic myelogenous leukemia (refractory anemia with excess myeloblasts)
Subacute myelomonocytic leukemia
Severe deviation neoplasms (leukemic blast cells frequent in the marrow)
Acute myelogenous leukemia (Chap. 93)
Myeloblastic (granuloblastic)
Myelomonocytic (granulomonoblastic)
Promyelocytic
Erythroid
Monocytic
Megakaryocytic
Eosinophilic
Basophilic*
Mast cell
Acute biphenotypic (myeloid and lymphoid markers) leukemia†
Acute leukemia with lymphoid markers evolving from a prior clonal hemopathy

---

*Rare cases of basophilic leukemia are Ph-negative and are variants of AML; most cases have the Ph chromosome and evolve from CML.
†About 10 percent of cases of acute myeloblastic leukemia may be biphenotypic (myeloid and lymphoid markers on individual cells) when studied with antimyeloid and antilymphoid monoclonal antibodies (see Chap. 93).

these syndromes, but not others, are grouped. This nomenclature resulted from a meeting in Paris in 1975.[2] In strict pathologic terms, a dysplasia is a nonclonal, nonmalignant change in the cells of a tissue. These myeloid syndromes are clonal, sometimes have aneuploid or pseudodiploid cells in the clone, and can be associated with significant morbidity and premature death and thus fit the features of a neoplasia rather than a dysplasia. They each have a propensity to evolve into acute myelogenous leukemia that far exceeds that of the general population. The term *dysplasia* was used at a time when the prominent dysmorphogenesis was thought to be the singular abnormality. However, the derivation from a single mutant stem cell (monoclonality) mark the syndromes all as neoplasias, and that is the primary feature of these diseases.

OVERPRODUCTION OF CELLS PROMINENT

Polycythemia vera (see Chap. 61), and primary thrombocythemia (see Chap. 118) are clonal hematopoietic stem cell disorders, so named because of the excessive production and overaccumulation of red cells, neutrophils, and platelets in polycythemia and platelets and to a lesser extent neutrophils in thrombocythemia, although each cell lineage is affected in each disorder, reflecting a stem cell origin. The magnitude of the effects is different, however. The effect on red cell production in thrombocythemia is usually slight. Polycythemia vera and primary thrombocythemia do not show morphologic evidence of leukemic hemopoiesis, and differentiation and maturation are maintained. The

proportion of blast cells in the marrow is not increased over normal, and blast cells are not present in the blood. The survival of cohorts of patients with these diseases is slightly less than expected for age- and gender-matched unaffected persons.[1]

MODERATE-DEVIATION CLONAL MYELOID DISORDERS

CML (Chap. 94) and idiopathic myelofibrosis (agnogenic myeloid metaplasia) (Chap. 95) classically share the features of overproduction of granulocytes and platelets and impaired production of red cells. Idiopathic myelofibrosis, however, has the invariable association of marrow fibrosis and striking tear-drop shaped red cells. The cells in the disorder have no specific cytogenetic change. Whereas CML invariably has a rearrangement of BCR on chromosome 22, in about 90 percent of patients this mutation is reflected in t(9;22) at the light microscopic level. Splenomegaly and a gradually progressive course are common to both. Blast cells are very slightly increased in marrow and blood in most patients with these disorders. CML has a very high propensity to transform to acute leukemia. Idiopathic myelofibrosis terminates in acute leukemia in about one out of six patients. Life span in these disorders is usually measured in years but is significantly decreased when compared to age- and gender-matched unaffected cohorts. Therapy is required in virtually all cases of chronic myelogenous leukemia and most cases of idiopathic myelofibrosis at the time of diagnosis. Both diseases can be cured only by stem cell transplantation, although life span has been increased in CML with the use of hydroxyurea and interferon-α therapy.

MODERATELY SEVERE-DEVIATION CLONAL MYELOID DISORDERS

These disorders fall into a group that progresses less rapidly than acute and more rapidly than chronic leukemia. They also have a predisposition to develop with a granulocytic and monocytic phenotype, either morphologically or cytochemically. These diseases also have been called *oligoblastic* or *smoldering leukemia, refractory anemia with excess myeloblasts, subacute myelomonocytic leukemia,* and *atypical myeloproliferative syndromes.* The latter designation is sometimes used for uncommon syndromes that did not fall into easily classifiable designations and usually are seen in patients over 65 years of age. The subacute syndromes produce more morbidity than do the chronic syndromes, and patients have a shorter life expectancy. These are leukemic states that have low or moderate concentrations of leukemic blast cells in marrow and often blood, as well as anemia, thrombocytopenia, and sometimes prominent monocytic maturation of cells (see Chap. 92). The oligoblastic leukemias compose about 80 percent of the cases that have been grouped under the title *myelodysplastic syndromes. Subacute myelomonocytic leukemia* has been withdrawn from the category of myelodysplastic diseases, highlighting the confusion surrounding that term. In all other malignancies, the presence of tumor cells result in the same diagnosis, i.e., carcinoma of the colon or the uterine cervix, whether in situ, invasive, or metastatic. It is illogical to use the percentage of leukemic cells as the basis of a diagnostic distinction. Hence, the preference for oligoblastic leukemia rather than myelodysplasia for patients with increased blast cells, monoclonality, and dysmorphic cell maturation.

SEVERE-DEVIATION CLONAL MYELOID DISORDERS

In 1975, at a conference on the classification of acute leukemia in Paris, Galton and Dacie proposed a classification for the most frequent phenotypic subtypes of AML.[3] They suggested the designation M0 through M6 for seven variants and considered morphology (for example, erythroid, monocytic, granulocytic) and the evidence of maturation in the categorization. Those in attendance at the conference from France (F), America (A), and Britain (B) adopted the proposal and modified it, and it was given the acronym the FAB classification.[4] The latter group used the designations M1 through M7 to indicate the previously recognized, morphologic phenotypes of AML. They later added M0 for another type of undifferentiated myeloblastic leukemia and M7 for megakaryocytic leukemia (see Chap. 93).

Morphologic subclassification of acute myelogenous leukemia is of some importance because it alerts the physician to special epiphenomena (for example, hypofibrinogenic hemorrhage in association with promyelocytic or monocytic leukemia, tissue and central nervous system infiltration in hyperleukocytic monocytic leukemia, etc.). It would be of great significance if it correlated with drug sensitivity. The principal therapy for all morphologic variants of AML is the same. From a clinical standpoint, the most useful classification of acute leukemia would be by drug sensitivity (for example, cytosine arabinoside–sensitive leukemia, glucocorticoid-sensitive leukemia, etc.). There is no set of in vitro tests to accomplish such a prospective classification, but not for lack of trying. Acute promyelocytic leukemia, which uniquely responds to all-*trans*-retinoic acid and arsenic trioxide, is the sole example of the strong correlation of the morphologic subtype of AML with drug sensitivity, and, even in this case, continuous intensive cytotoxic drug use also is required for a sustained effect of therapy (see Chap. 93).

Morphologic and histochemical characteristics of cells on stained films of blood and marrow provide the major basis for the classification of AML. To these two approaches has been added the reactivity pattern of blast cells to monoclonal antibodies with specificity for epitopes on the surface of myeloid or lymphoid cells[5-7] (see Chap. 93). The correlations among observers and between the morphologic method of classification and the monoclonal antibody reactivity–dependent classification of AML is rather imperfect. Cytogenetic characteristics also are used in the classification of some cases of AML (see Chaps. 10 and 93). The importance of these various approaches differs. The morphologic plus cytochemical approach is the most inclusive, since virtually all cases can be placed into a morphologic subtype. Occasionally this requires supplementation by analysis of immunophenotype (the CD representation). Since immunophenotyping has approached the routine in most laboratories in first- and second-world countries, these results are readily available. Classification by cytogenetics is more limited, since many cases have infrequent abnormalities making this approach complex. However, in many cases knowing the cytogenetic alterations is very useful for determining treatment, estimating prognosis, and measuring minimal residual disease by polymerase chain analysis. Thus, combined microscopy, cytochemistry, and immunophenotyping to designate a morphologic classification, supplemented by cytogenetics or molecular diagnostic approaches, is the best approach, currently.

TRANSITIONS AMONG CLONAL MYELOID DISEASES

Patients with minimal, moderate, and moderately severe clonal myeloid disorders have an increased likelihood of progressing to florid AML, with a frequency ranging from about 1 percent of patients with paroxysmal nocturnal hemoglobinuria, 10 percent of patients with acquired refractory sideroblastic anemia, and about 35 percent of patients with pancytopenia with hypercellular marrow. About 15 percent of patients with polycythemia vera evolve to a syndrome indistinguishable from idiopathic myelofibrosis. AML develops as a terminal event in about one percent of patients with polycythemia vera not treated with ^{32}P or alkylating and a larger proportion of those so treated.

About 5 to 15 percent of patients with primary thrombocythemia and idiopathic myelofibrosis and virtually all patients with CML progress to AML. In the case of patients with CML, they may enter a phase that behaves like oligoblastic leukemia before progression to AML.

PATHOGENESIS OF CLONAL MYELOID DISEASES

In AML the mutation in a single stem cell results in a clone that is severely defective and contains precursor cells that are unable to mature. Proliferation of primitive progenitors is excessive when considered in absolute terms, that is, the total number of blast cells proliferating. AML is considered a clinical disease with many forms of morphologic expression. This variation of phenotype is consistent with the behavior of the leukemic stem cell, which is capable of differentiation into all the blood cell lineages (Fig. 91-1). Hence, the asymmetric maturation of leukemic progenitor cells may allow one or another cell type to predominate. There is little difference in the course of these different morphologic variants of AML. There are important epiphenomena related to special features of certain morphologic types of leukemia, such as tissue infiltration (monocyte leukemia), hypofibrinogenemia (promyelocytic leukemia), heart and lung fibrosis (eosinophilic leukemia), marrow fibrosis (megakaryocytic leukemia), and others (see Chap. 93). These morphologic subtypes and epiphenomena are determined by the effect of genic differences. These differences may be evident in gross cytogenic abnormalities that correlate with, and may determine, some phenotypes, for example, t(15;17) with promyelocytic leukemia, t(8;21) with myelomonocytic leukemia, inversion of chromosome 16 with prominent eosinophilic maturation in the marrow (see Chap 93). In CML, the injury to a single cell results in a clone in which there is an enormous expansion of progenitors for granulocytic and, often, megakaryocytic cells. Erythropoiesis is effective but decreased. Unlike AML, maturation of progenitor cells in CML is nearly normal; hence, the predominant leukemic cells in the blood are amitotic, mature, or partially matured cells, such as segmented neutrophils and myelocytes, erythrocytes, and platelets.

Since hemopoiesis is generated by leukemic stem cells, in most patients with AML, CML, and other clonal hemopathies, erythropoiesis and thrombopoiesis as well as granulopoiesis are leukemic, and qualitative abnormalities of structure and function and clonal cytogenic abnormalities affect erythroblasts, megakaryocytes, and granulocyte precursors in most cases of AML (see Chap. 93) and all cases of CML (see Chap. 94).

PHENOTYPE OF MYELOID CLONAL DISEASES AS A RESULT OF THE MATRIX OF DIFFERENTIATION AND MATURATION

The phenotype of the hemopoietic stem cell diseases is a reflection of a neoplastic stem cell's capability to differentiate into committed progenitor cells and the ability of those progenitor cells to mature into identifiable cells of the erythroid, granulocytic (neutrophilic, basophilic, mastocytic, eosinophilic), monocytic, or megakaryocytic lineage[8-13] (Fig. 91-2).

Differentiation represents the changes from the multipotential stem cell to multiple unipotential lineage progenitors. Maturation represents the physical and chemical changes from a unipotential progenitor through a sequence of precursors to the fully mature and functional blood cell, including progression from a BFU-E to proerythroblast to erythrocyte, a CFU-G to myeloblast to segmented neutrophil, a CFU-Eo to a segmented eosinophil, a CFU-Baso to a mature basophil, a colony forming unit–mast cell to a mature mast cell, a CFU-M to promonocyte to monocyte to macrophage, a CFU-Meg to a 2N megakaryoblast to the polyploid megakaryocyte. This matrix, composed of the options of commitment to different lineages and the progressive stages of maturation at which partial or complete arrest can occur, results in the potential for a wide array of morphologic syndromes by which a mutant stem cell can dominate hemopoiesis (see Fig. 91-2).

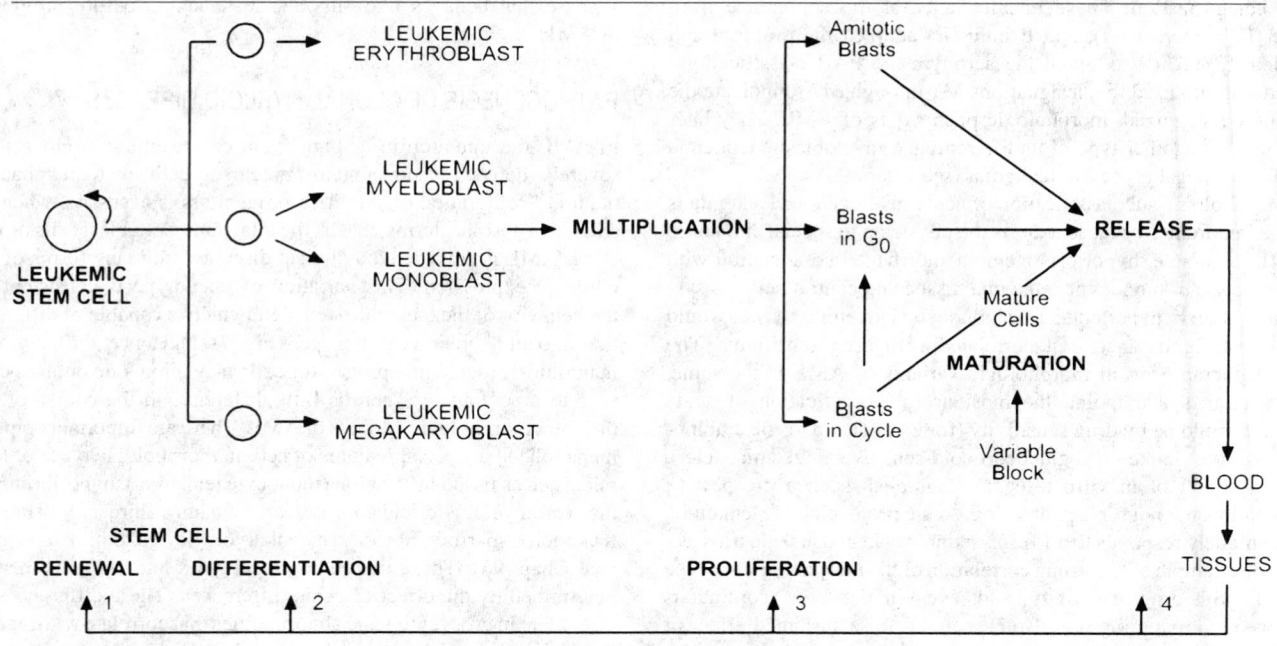

FIGURE 91-1   Hematopoiesis in acute myelogenous leukemia. The malignant process evolves from a single mutant multipotential cell.[45-48] This cell is represented at either level 1 or level 2 in Fig. 91-3. This cell is capable of multivariate commitment to leukemic erythroid, granulocytic, and megakaryocytic progenitors. In most cases, granulocytic commitment predominates, and myeloblasts and monoblasts or their immediate derivatives are the dominant cell types. Leukemic blast cells accumulate in the marrow. The leukemic blast cells may become amitotic (sterile) and undergo programmed cell death, may stop dividing for prolonged periods (blasts in G_0) but have the potential to reenter the mitotic cycle, or may divide and undergo varying degrees of maturation. The maturation may lead to mature cells, such as red cells, segmented neutrophils, monocytes, or platelets. A severe block in maturation is characteristic of AML, whereas a high proportion of leukemic blast cells mature in CML. The disturbance in commitment and maturation in myelogenous leukemia is quantitative, and thus many patterns are possible. At least four major steps in hemopoiesis are regulated: (1) stem cell self-renewal and (2) differentiation into hematopoietic cell lineages (red cells, granulocytes, platelets), (3) proliferation (multiplication) and maturation of progenitor and precursor cells, (4) release of mature cells into the blood. These control points are partially or totally defective in myelogenous leukemia.

In the stem cell diseases in which differentiation and maturation capability is retained, one of the cell lines, for example, erythrocytes, granulocytes, or platelets, tends to accumulate in the blood to a more prominent extent and results in a phenotypic expression of the disease that determines the nosology. In AML, the phenotypic expression may be predominantly myeloblastic (granuloblastic), erythroid, monocytic, megakaryocytic, or combinations thereof. Certain patterns are favored. In AML, myeloblastic leukemia and monocytic leukemia or mixtures of the two are more common than erythroid, megakaryocytic, or eosinophilic leukemia. AML, however, usually has a disturbance in all cell lines. In myeloblastic or myelomonocytic leukemia there may be overt, qualitative abnormalities of erythroblasts and megakaryocytes. The prevalence of the abnormalities in the latter two lineages may not be great enough or evident enough for the observer to designate a case as erythroid or megakaryocytic leukemia.

The continuum of maturation can be completely or partially blocked at various levels, leading to morphologic variants such as acute myeloblastic, promyelocytic, subacute myelogenous, or chronic myelogenous leukemia.

PLURIPOTENTIAL STEM CELL POOL AS SITE OF THE LESION

Evidence points to a lesion in the pluripotential stem cell pool in most of the clonal myeloid diseases, especially in those over age 50, who account for the great proportion of cases. In CML patients, the mutation is in the pluripotential stem cell. In other syndromes, the evidence for involvement of B and T lymphocytes is variable. B lymphocytes are derived from the clone in many cases, whereas evidence for T lymphocyte involvement is less compelling. Evidence that affected T lymphocytes undergo apoptosis before entering the blood in patients with CML may explain their absence in blood lymphocytes in other clonal myeloid disorders.[13]

Thus, the mutation of the cell may be at level 1, between levels 1 and 2, or at level 2 in different patients (see Fig. 91-3).

PROGENITOR CELL LEUKEMIA

An analysis of cases of AML in girls and women who were heterozygous for isotypes A and B of the enzyme glucose-6-phosphate dehydrogenase indicated that the AML clone in the girls was restricted to the granulocyte-monocyte pathway, but in the older women monoclonality was expressed in all cell lines, in keeping with all prior studies of CML and AML by enzymes or chromosome markers.[8,9] These findings support the possibility that a leukemic transformation in some (young) patients can occur in progenitor cells (e.g., CFU-GM) (level 3 in Fig. 91-3) and result in a true acute "granulocytic" leukemia. If progenitor cell leukemia is common in young people, this pattern could explain their better response to treatment. In a subset of patients with acute monocytic leukemia,[31] t(8;21) AML, and t(15;17) AML, their leukemia derives from the neoplastic transformation of a progenitor cell.[10-12]

QUANTITATIVENESS OF CLONAL MYELOID DISEASES

The lesions of the hematopoietic stem cell compartment are qualitative in the sense that there is a distinct alteration from normal in the

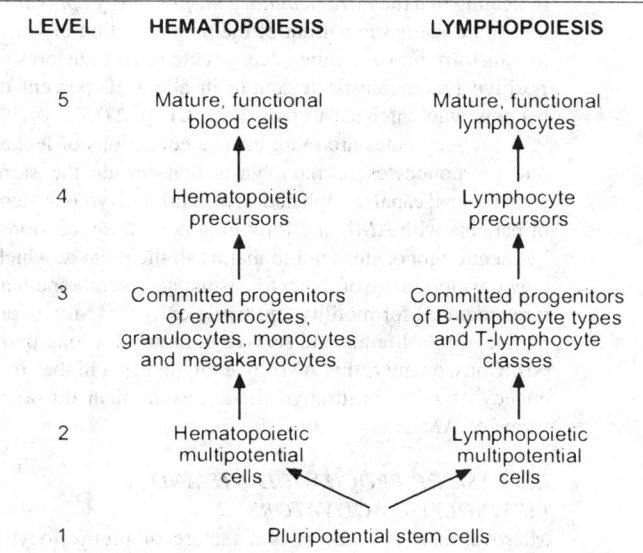

LEVEL	HEMATOPOIESIS	LYMPHOPOIESIS
5	Mature, functional blood cells	Mature, functional lymphocytes
4	Hematopoietic precursors	Lymphocyte precursors
3	Committed progenitors of erythrocytes, granulocytes, monocytes and megakaryocytes	Committed progenitors of B-lymphocyte types and T-lymphocyte classes
2	Hematopoietic multipotential cells	Lymphopoietic multipotential cells
1	Pluripotential stem cells	

FIGURE 91-2   Differentiation and maturation of hematopoietic stem cells. The functioning stem cell pool is thought to be at level 1, the pluripotential cells. In healthy human beings, two multipotential progenitor cell pools may be operative (level 2). The multipotential progenitors differentiate further to unipotential progenitors, which are sensitive to cytokines (level 3). The committed progenitor cells are referred to as colony-forming units (CFU) or colony-forming cells (CFC), since they form colonies of cells in semisolid medium in the presence of the appropriate growth factors. These growth factors are capable of inducing proliferation and maturation of the committed progenitor cells so that they achieve level 4, at which the first morphologically identifiable precursors are present, such as myeloblasts and proerythroblasts, and ultimately level 5, the fully mature, functional blood cells.

function of the cell pool, and this is a reflection of a change in the genome of one hematopoietic stem cell. This qualitative change, however, is such that the stem cell can express all or some of the normal differentiation and maturation options. This expression can mimic the differentiation (commitment) and maturation expected of normal hemopoietic cells such as occurs in CML and polycythemia vera.[15,16]

Most cases tend to conform to readily recognized patterns, but the opportunity for a large number of variations on the most common themes is possible. Thus, some mixed and so-called in-between syndromes occur in which features of ineffective hemopoiesis and myeloproliferation of different cell lineages are present. For example, extreme thrombocytosis, usually confined to primary thrombocythemia, may accompany CML or idiopathic myelofibrosis. Erythrocytosis may accompany CML rarely. Atypical myeloproliferative syndromes or other clonal hemopathies may have mixtures of anemia, granulocytopenia, and thrombocytosis or of anemia, granulocytosis, and thrombocytopenia rather than pancytopenia. Qualitative abnormalities of red cell, granulocyte, or platelet structure or function may be more or less prominent in a given patient. For example, qualitative abnormalities of erythroblast development may result in acquired α thalassemia (hemoglobin H disease) in patients with idiopathic myelofibrosis or other stem cell diseases. In AML, unusual patterns of phenotypic expression occur frequently. For example, one may see patients in whom leukemic erythroblasts and monocytes or eosinophils and monocytes are prominent. Indeed, there is so much opportunity for variation in disease expression among patients with AML that it is unusual to see patients in whom the phenotypes of leukemic cells are identical to those of others. Choice of treatment is little affected by these

variations. The decisions about whether to treat and which drugs to use are greatly influenced by whether a patient has a chronic, subacute, or acute clonal myeloid disease; by the rate of progression of the disease; by the extent of the leukemic blast cell infiltrate; and by the severity of the cytopenias. The diagnostician and therapist usually can identify variants as diseases of a clonal myeloid disorder and can manage them as dictated by their manifestations regardless of precise subclassification.

INTERPLAY OF CLONAL AND POLYCLONAL HEMATOPOIESIS

Although potentially curative chemotherapy of myelogenous leukemia was introduced to kill "the last leukemic cell," two important factors were not explicitly discussed. The first was whether there were residual normal stem cells in marrow to restore polyclonal (normal) hematopoesis if ablation of the leukemia was accomplished. The second was whether, given the early estimates of 1 trillion leukemic cells in a patient, the therapist had to eliminate them all to achieve cure. A corollary of the latter was whether the disease was the result of a mutant stem cell and if so was that the only cell that mattered, ultimately, in the eradication process. We now recognize that remission is the result of sufficient suppression of the leukemic population by intensive chemotherapy to permit restitution of polyclonal hematopoiesis by normal stem cells. Since relapse is the rule, two understudied, nearly ignored, therapeutic approaches should include determining and interfering with the chemicals elaborated by leukemic cells that suppress normal hematopoiesis and assessing whether agents that foster normal stem cell recruitment could tip the balance in favor of those cells. It is unclear also why clonal hematopoiesis is so difficult to subdue, even temporarily, in the chronic myeloid neoplasms (e.g., CML) as compared to the acute myeloid neoplasms (AML). Evidence has accumulated that sustained remission (clinical cure) may occur in some cases with posttherapy minimal residual disease suggesting that a new symbiotic relationship can occur after intensive therapy that suppresses the growth potential of leukemic cells. This phenomenon may be more evident in lymphoid than myeloid neoplasms.

CLINICAL MANIFESTATIONS

DEFICIENCY, EXCESS, OR DYSFUNCTION OF BLOOD CELLS

Alterations in blood cell concentration are the primary manifestations of hematopoietic stem cell disorders. The clinical manifestations of deficiencies or excesses of individual blood cell types are described in the chapters on clinical manifestations of disorders of erythrocytes (see Chap. 30), granulocytes, and monocytes (see Chaps. 70 and 76), and platelets (see Chap. 115).

Several hematopoietic stem cell diseases have as frequent manifestations qualitative abnormalities of blood cells. Abnormal red cell shapes, red cell or granulocyte enzyme deficiencies, abnormal neutrophil granules, bizarre nuclear configurations, disorders of neutrophil chemotaxis, phagocytosis or microbial killing, giant platelets, abnormal platelet granules, and disturbed platelet function can occur in some patients with oligoblastic myelogenous leukemia and idiopathic myelofibrosis. In oligoblastic myelogenous leukemia, the effects of severe cytopenia usually dominate, and the disturbances of cell function are less important. In idiopathic myelofibrosis and primary thrombocythemia, functional platelet abnormalities may contribute to the hemorrhage diathesis, especially if surgery or injury occurs. Paroxysmal nocturnal hemoglobinuria is a hemopoietic stem cell disease in which a highly specific alteration in blood cell membranes renders the cells exquisitely sensitive to complement lysis (see Chap. 36). Patients with CML or polycythemia vera do not usually have clinically

A. DIFFERENTIATION VARIANTS

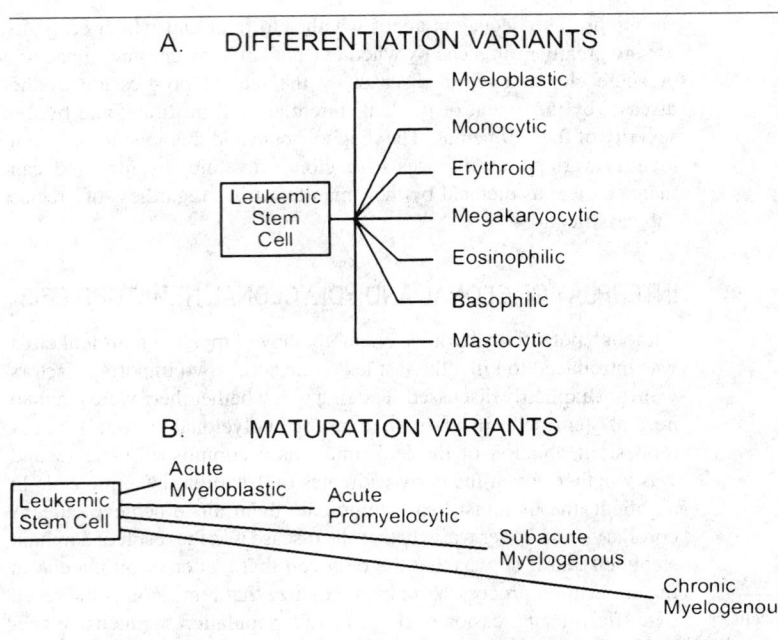

B. MATURATION VARIANTS

FIGURE 91-3 Phenotypic subtypes of acute myelogenous leukemia. Acute myelogenous leukemia has variable morphologic expression and a variable degree of maturation of leukemic cells into recognizable precursors of each blood cell type. This phenotypic variation is a consequence of the fact that the leukemic lesion resides in a cell normally capable of all the different commitment decisions. (*a*) The morphologic variants of AML can be considered differentiation variants in which the cells derived from one of the options of commitment accumulate prominently (e.g., leukemic erythroblasts, leukemic monocytes, leukemic megakaryocytes, etc.). In promyelocytic leukemia and some cases of acute leukemia in younger individuals, the somatic mutation may arise in a somewhat more differentiated progenitor.[8,48] (*b*) Acute myeloblastic leukemia, promyelocytic leukemia, subacute leukemia, and chronic leukemia can be considered maturation variants in which blocks at different levels of maturation are present.

significant functional abnormalities of cells, although in polycythemia vera neutrophils are often activated with heightened metabolic rates and enhanced phagocytosis.

Secondary clinical manifestations occur as a result of the proliferation and accumulation of the malignant (leukemic) cells themselves.

EFFECTS OF LEUKEMIC BLAST CELLS

EXTRAMEDULLARY TUMORS

Granulocytic sarcomas (also called *chloromas* or *myeloblastomas*) are discrete tumors of leukemic myeloblasts and partially matured granulocytes that form in skin and soft tissues, periosteum and bone, lymph nodes, gastrointestical tract, pleura, gonads, urinary tract, central nervous system, and other sites[17] (see Chap. 93). They can develop in patients with AML or the accelerated phase of CML and, rarely, may be the first manifestation of AML, preceding the onset in marrow and blood by months or years.[18] Granulocytic sarcomas can be mistaken for large-cell lymphomas because of the similarity of the histopathology in biopsy specimens from soft tissues. The presence of eosinophils or other granulocytes may arouse suspicion of a granulocytic sarcoma; however, chloracetate esterase, antilysozyme immunoperoxidase stains, or antimyeloblast monoclonal antibodies may be required to establish the granulocytic nature of the process, and these assays should be performed on biopsies of such lesions.[17]

Extramedullary tumors may usher in the accelerated phase of CML. These tumors may be composed of myeloblasts or lymphoblasts, although in each case the Ph chromosome is present in the cells,

indicating that the *extramedullary Ph-positive lymphoblastomas* are the tissue variant of the predisposition of CML to transform into a terminal deoxynucleotidyl transferase–positive lymphoblastic leukemia in about 30 percent of patients who enter blast crisis[19] (see Chap. 27).

Monocytomas are more diffuse collections of leukemic promonocytes or monoblasts that invade the skin, gingiva, anal canal, lymph nodes, or central nervous system of patients with AML and form tumors in those locations. Leukemic monocytes tend to mature to the point at which they develop many of the cytoplasmic and membrane features required for motility and tissue entry.[20–22] Moreover, monocytes proliferate and survive in tissues for long periods. Consequently, this AML phenotype has a higher frequency of overt infiltrative tissue lesions than do other forms of AML.

RELEASE OF PROCOAGULANTS AND FIBRINOLYTIC ACTIVATORS

Microvascular thrombosis is a feature of promyelocytic type of AML, although it can occur in other forms of acute leukemia, especially monocytic leukemia, as well. The leukemic promyelocytes are thought to liberate a procoagulant tissue factor or a plasminogen activator. Each may ultimately contribute to hypofibrinogenemia and hemorrhage. Thrombin generation may mediate the microvascular thrombotic aspect of this process, which can occur in acute promyelocytic, acute monocytic, or acute myelomonocytic leukemia, especially after cytotoxic treatment. A cysteine proteinase procoagulant different from tissue factor may also play a role in thrombosis formation associated with AML. An increase in fibrinolytic activity further complicates the coagulopathy in patients with promyelocytic leukemia[23,24] (see Chap. 93).

HYPERLEUKOCYTIC SYNDROMES

A small proportion of patients with AML (5 percent) and CML (15 percent) manifest extraordinarily high blood leukocyte counts.[25,26] These patients present special problems because of the effects of blast cells in the microcirculation of the lung, brain, eye, ear, and penis and the metabolic effects that result when massive numbers of leukemic cells in blood, marrow, and tissues are simultaneously killed by cytotoxic drugs. Cell concentrations over 75,000/μl (75 $\times$ 10^9/liter) in AML and over 250,000/μl (250 $\times$ 10^9/liter) in CML are usually required to produce such problems. A respiratory distress syndrome attributed to pulmonary leukostasis occurs in some patients with acute promyelocytic leukemia after all-*trans*-retinoic acid therapy. The syndrome is usually but not always associated with neutrophilia. Some cases, however, have been observed in the absence of extreme leukocytosis.[27]

The viscosity of blood is related to the total cytocrit and is usually not increased in hyperleukocytic leukemias because the reduction in hematocrit compensates for the increase in leukocrit. Occasional patients with hyperleukocytic CML who are transfused with red cells may have an increase in blood viscosity above normal.

Leuko-occlusion and vascular invasion in small vessels of the lung, brain, or other sites have been identified in pathologic studies. Since viscosity in the microcirculation is a function of the plasma viscosity and the deformability of individual cells in capillaries, leukocytes should transiently raise the viscosity in such small channels. Flow in microchannels will fall if poorly deformable blast cells enter capillary channels.[28] With high leukocyte counts, chronically reduced flow may reduce oxygen transport to tissues, since the probability of

TABLE 91-2   CLINICAL FEATURES OF THE HYPERLEUKOCYTIC SYNDROME

Pulmonary circulation
   Tachypnea, dyspnea, cyanosis
   Alveolar-capillary block
Pulmonary infiltrates
Postchemotherapy respiratory dysfunction
Central nervous system circulation
   Dizziness, slurred speech, delirium, stupor
   Intracranial (cerebral) hemorrhage
Special sensory organ circulation
Visual blurring
Papilledema
Diplopia
Tinnitus, impaired hearing
Retinal vein distention, retinal hemorrhages
Penile circulation
   Priapism
Spurious laboratory results
   Decreased blood P_{O_2}; increased serum potassium
   Decreased plasma glucose; increased mean corpuscular volume, red cell
      count, hemoglobin, and hematocrit

leukocytes being in microchannels should be increased as a function of white cell count. Moreover, trapped leukemic cells have an oxygen consumption rate that could contribute to deleterious effects in the microcirculation. Leukocyte aggregation, leukocyte microthrombi, release of toxic products from leukocytes, endothelial cell damage, and microvascular invasion can contribute to vascular injury and flow impedance.

High leukemic blast cell counts in acute and chronic myelogenous leukemia may be associated with pulmonary, central nervous system, special sensory, or penile circulatory impairment (Table 91-2). Sudden death can occur in patients with hyperleukocytic acute leukemia as a result of intracranial hemorrhage.[29,30] Hyperleukocytosis should be treated promptly with leukapheresis and with cytotoxic therapy, usually hydroxyurea (see Chaps. 93 and 94). In CML, leukapheresis reverses the hyperleukocytic syndrome, can be used immediately without having to wait for the effect of allopurinol to reduce the risk of uric acid nephropathy, and can reduce the extent of cytolysis-induced hyperuricemia, hyperkalemia, and hyperphosphatemia by reducing the tumor cell mass. The effect of leukapheresis in AML on patient survival appears to be negligible, however.[31]

THROMBOCYTHEMIC SYNDROMES

Hemorrhagic or thrombotic episodes can be the presenting manifestation of thrombocythemia or can develop during the course of primary thrombocythemia.[32,33] Arterial vascular insufficiency and venous thrombosis are the major vascular manifestations of thrombocythemia. Peripheral vascular insufficiency with gangrene and cerebral vascular thrombi can occur. Thrombosis of superficial or deep veins of the extremities occurs frequently. Mesenteric, hepatic, portal, splenic, or penile venous thrombosis can develop. Hemorrhage is a frequent manifestation of thrombocythemia and often occurs concomitantly with thrombotic episodes. Gastrointestinal hemorrhage and cutaneous hemorrhage, the latter especially after trauma, are most frequent, but bleeding from other sites can also occur (see Chap. 118).

Thrombotic complications occur in about one-third of patients with polycythemia vera.[34] Erythrocytosis and thrombocytosis may interact to cause hypercoagulability, especially in the abdominal venous circulation. A syndrome of splanchnic venous thrombosis associated with endogenous erythroid colony growth, the latter characteristic of polycythemia vera, but without blood cell count changes indicative of a myeloproliferative disease, has accounted for a very high proportion of patients with apparent idiopathic hepatic or portal vein thrombosis.[35,36] Thrombosis of the veins of the abdomen, liver, and other organs,

characteristic complications of paroxysmal nocturnal hemoglobinuria, may result from a qualitative abnormality of platelets, which makes them very sensitive to activation of the factor V and X complex because of the absence of cell surface complement inhibitors[37] (see Chap. 36).

SYSTEMIC SYMPTOMS

Fever, weight loss, and malaise occur as an early manifestation of AML. At the time of diagnosis, low-grade fever is present in nearly 50 percent of patients.[37] Although minor infections may be present, systemic infection is relatively uncommon at the time of diagnosis in AML.[37,38] However, fever during cytotoxic therapy, when neutrophil counts are extremely low, is nearly always a sign of infection. Fever also may be a manifestation of the acute leukemic transformation of CML and can occur in some patients with oligoblastic leukemia.

Weight loss occurs in nearly one-fifth of patients with AML.[38] Loss of well-being and intolerance to exertion may be out of proportion to the extent of anemia and may not be corrected by red cell transfusions; the pathogenesis of these effects is still unknown.

METABOLIC SIGNS

Hyperuricemia and hyperuricosuria are very common manifestations of AML and CML. Acute gouty arthritis and hyperuricosuric nephropathy are less common. If therapy is instituted without a reduction in plasma uric acid and without adequate hydration, saturation of the urine with uric acid can lead to precipitation of urate (gravel) and obstructive uropathy. If the uropathy is severe, urine flow can be obliterated, and renal failure ensues. Hyponatremia can occur in AML and in some cases is a result of inappropriate antidiuretic hormone secretion.[39] Hyponatremia can also be a result of an osmotic diuresis of urea, creatinine, urate, and other substances released from blast cells and wasting muscles. Hypokalemia is commonly seen in AML, and it has been thought to be caused by injury to the kidney by increased plasma and urine lysozyme and subsequent kaliuresis. The hypokalemia is related to excessive urinary potassium loss, but the correlation with lysozymuria is imperfect, and other mechanisms are probably responsible in most cases, including osmotic diuresis and tubular dysfunction. Kaliuretic antibiotics, often used in patients with AML, may accentuate the hypokalemia.

Hypercalcemia occurs in about 2 percent of patients with myelogenous leukemia. Several causes have been proposed, including bone resorption as a result of leukemic infiltration. This explanation is in keeping with the normal serum inorganic phosphate in most patients. Occasional patients have had hypercalcemia and hypophosphatemia, and ectopic parathyroid hormone secretion by leukemic blast cells was strongly suggested in one carefully studied case. Lactic acidosis has also been observed in association with myelogenous leukemia, although the mechanism is obscure. Hypoxia can result from the hyperleukocytic syndrome as a consequence of pulmonary vascular leukostasis. Hypophosphatemia can occur because of rapid utilization of plasma inorganic phosphate in some cases of myelogenous leukemia with a high blood blast cell count and a high fraction of proliferative cells.

Increased serum concentrations of lipoprotein A and decreased concentrations both of low- and high-density lipoproteins have been observed in a high proportion of patients with AML.[41] The increase in lipoprotein A, which returns to normal after successful treatment, is correlated with the presence of leukemic blast cells. Serum prolactin is also increased in patients with AML.[41] Leukemic blast cells may be an ectopic source of this hormone.[41]

Colony-stimulating factor 1 is elevated in a variety of lymphoid and hemopoietic malignancies, including AML and CML.[42] It has been proposed that the malignant cells are the source of the excess cytokine.

The plasma levels of protein C antigen, functional protein C, and free protein S are decreased in patients with AML. These changes are not related to liver disease or white cell count.[42]

FACTITIOUS LABORATORY RESULTS

Elevations of serum potassium levels have resulted from the release of potassium from platelets or, less often, leukocytes in patients with myeloproliferative diseases and extreme elevations in those blood cell concentrations.[43] If blood is collected in a tube that contains an anticoagulant and the plasma is removed after high-speed centrifugation, the potassium concentration is normal. Glucose can be falsely decreased, especially since autoanalyzer techniques call for the omission of glycolytic inhibitors such as sodium fluoride in collection tubes. Blood with high leukocyte counts that stands prior to separation of the plasma may have a significant amount of plasma glucose utilized by leukocytes. Factitious hypoglycemia can also occur as a result of red cell utilization of glucose, especially in polycythemic patients. True hypoglycemia has been observed rarely in patients with leukemia. Blood oxygen content also can be lowered spuriously as a result of utilization in vitro by large numbers of leukocytes.

SPECIFIC ORGAN INVOLVEMENT

Myeloproliferative diseases lead to disturbances principally in marrow, blood, and spleen. Although clusters of cells may be found in all organs, major infiltrates and organ dysfunction are unusual. In AML and the acute phase of CML, clinically significant infiltration of the larynx, central nervous system, heart, lungs, bone, joints, gastrointestinal tract, kidney, skin, or virtually any other organ may occur. Splenic enlargement is a feature of the acute and chronic myeloproliferative diseases. In AML, palpable splenomegaly is present in about one-third of cases and is usually slight in extent. In the chronic myeloproliferative diseases, palpable splenomegaly is present in a high proportion of cases (polycythemia vera, 80 percent; CML, 90 percent; idiopathic myelofibrosis, 100 percent). In primary thrombocythemia, splenic enlargement is present in about 60 percent of patients. A predisposition to silent splenic vascular thrombi and splenic atrophy analogous to that which occurs in sickle cell anemia has been postulated for the lower frequency of splenic enlargement. Early satiety, left upper quadrant discomfort, splenic infarctions with painful perisplenitis, diaphragmatic pleuritis, and shoulder pain may occur in patients with splenomegaly, especially in the acute phase of CML and in myeloid metaplasia. In idiopathic myelofibrosis, the spleen can become enormous, occupying the left hemiabdomen. Blood flow through the splenic vein can be so great as to lead to portal hypertension and gastroesophageal varices. Usually, reduced hepatic venous compliance is also present (see Chap. 95). Bleeding and, occasionally, encephalopathy can result from the portosystemic venous shunts.

REFERENCES

1. Rozman CGM, Feliu E, Rubio D, et al: Life expectancy of patients with chronic nonleukemic myeloproliferative disorders. *Cancer* 67:2658, 1991.
2. Bessis M, Bernard J: Hematopoietic dysplasias. *Blood Cells* 2:5, 1976.
3. Galton DAG, Dacie JV: Classification of the acute leukemias. *Blood Cells* 1:17, 1975.
4. Bennett JM, Catovsky D, Daniel MT, et al: Proposals for the classification of the acute leukaemias. *Br J Haematol* 33:451, 1976.
5. Barnard DR, Kalousek DK, Wiersma SR, et al: Morphologic, immuno-

logic, and cytogenetic classification of acute myeloid leukemia and myelodysplastic syndrome in childhood. *Leukemia* 10:5,1996.
6. Bene MC, Castoldi G, Knapp W, et al: Proposals for the immunological classification of acute leukemias. *Leukemia* 9:1783, 1995.
7. Jennings CD, Foon KA: Recent advances in flow cytometry: application to the diagnosis of hematologic malignancy. *Blood* 90:2863, 1997.
8. Fialkow PJ, Singer JW, Adamson JW, et al: Acute nonlymphocytic leukemia: expression in cells restricted to granulocytic and monocytic differentiation. *N Engl J Med* 301:1, 1979.
9. Fialkow PJ, Singer JW, Adamson JW, et al: Acute nonlymphocytic leukemia: heterogeneity of stem cell origin. *Blood* 57:1068, 1981.
10. Ferraris AM, Broccia G, Meloni T, et al: Clonal origin of cells restricted to monocytic differentiation in acute nonlymphocytic leukemia. *Blood* 64:817, 1984.
11. Van Lom K, Hagenmaijer A, Vandekerckhove F, et al: Clonality analysis of hematopoietic cell lineages in acute myeloid leukemia and translocation (8;21): only myeloid cells are part of the malignant clone. *Leukemia* 11:202, 1997.
12. Turhan AG, Lemoine FM, Debert C, et al: Highly purified primitive hematopoietic stem cells are PML-RARa negative and generate non-clonal progenitors in acute promyelocytic leukemia. *Blood* 85:2154, 1995.
13. Takahashi N, Maura I, Saitoh K, Miura AB: Lineage involvement of stem cells bearing the Philadelphia chromosome in chronic myeloid leukemia in the chronic phase as shown by combination of fluorescence-activated cell sorting and fluorescence in situ hybridization. *Blood* 92:4758, 1998.
14. Killman SA: Acute leukemia: development, remission/relapse pattern, relationship between normal and leukaemic haemopoiesis, and the ''sleeper-to-feeder'' stem cell hypothesis. *Baillieres Clin Haematol* 4:577, 1991.
15. Gale RP, Butturini A: Leukemia: stem cells, preleukemia and cure. *Leukemia* 6(suppl 1):80, 1992.
16. Cline MJ: The molecular basis of leukemia. *N Engl J Med* 330:328, 1994.
17. Neiman RS, Barcos M, Berard C, et al: Granulocytic sarcoma: a clinicopathologic study of 61 biopsied cases. *Cancer* 48:1426, 1981.
18. Meis JM, Butler JJ, Osborne BM, Manning JT: Granulocytic sarcoma in non-leukemic patients. *Cancer* 58:2697, 1986.
19. Terjanian T, Kantarjian H, Keating M, et al: Clinical and prognostic features of patients with Philadelphia chromosome-positive chronic myelogenous leukemia and extramedullary disease. *Cancer* 59:297, 1987.
20. Peterson L, Dekner LP, Brunning RD: Extramedullary masses as presenting features of acute monoblastic leukemia. *Am J Clin Pathol* 75:140, 1981.
21. Tobelem G, Jacquillat C, Chastang C, et al: Acute monoblastic leukemia: a clinical and biologic study of 74 cases. *Blood* 55:71, 1980.
22. Lichtman MA, Weed RI: Peripheral cytoplasmic characteristics of leukemia cells in monocytic leukemia: relationship to clinical manifestations. *Blood* 40:52, 1972.
23. Sakata Y, Murakami T, Noro A, et al: The specific activity of plasminogen activator inhibitor-1 in disseminated intravascular coagulation with acute promyelocyte leukemia. *Blood* 77:1949, 1991.
24. Dombret H, Scrobhaci ML, Ghorra P, et al: Coagulation disorders in acute promyelocytic leukemia. *Leukemia* 7:2, 1993.
25. McKee LC, Collins RD: Intravascular leukocyte thrombi and aggregate as a cause of morbidity and mortality in leukemias. *Medicine (Baltimore)* 53:463, 1974.
26. Lichtman MA, Heal J, Rowe JM: Hyperleukocytic leukaemia: rheological and clinical features and management. *Baillieres Clin Haematol* 1:725, 1987.
27. Vosburgh E: Pulmonary leukostasis secondary to all-*trans* retinoic acid in the treatment of acute promyelocytic leukemia in first relapse. *Leukemia* 6:608, 1992.
28. Östergren J, Fagrell B, Björkholm M: Hyperleukocytic effects on skin capillary circulation in patients with leukaemia. *J Intern Med* 231:19, 1992.
29. Dutcher JP, Schiffer CA, Wiernik PH: Hyperleukocytosis in adult acute nonlymphocytic leukemia: impact on remission rate and duration, and survival. *J Clin Oncol* 5:1364, 1987.
30. Wald BR, Heisel MA, Ortega JA: Frequency of early death in children with acute leukemia presenting with hyperleukocytosis. *Cancer* 50:150, 1982.

31. Porcu P, Danielson CF, Orazi A, et al: Therapeutic leukapheresis in hyperleucocytic leukaemias: lack of correlation between degree of cyto-reduction and early mortality rate. *Br J Haematol* 98:433, 1997.

32. Cortelazzo S, Vicero P, Finazzi G, et al: Incidence and risk factors for thrombotic complications in a historical cohort of 100 patients with thrombocythemia. *J Clin Oncol* 8:556, 1990.

33. Landolfi R: Bleeding and thrombosis in myeloproliferative disorders. *Curr Opin Hematol* 5:327, 1998.

34. Anger B, Haugh U, Seidler R, Heimpel H: Polycythemia vera: a clinical study of 141 patients. *Blut* 59:493, 1989.

35. Teofili L, De Stefano V, Leone G, et al: Hematologic causes of venous thrombosis in young people: high incidence of myeloproliferative disor-der as underlying disease in patients with splanchnic venous thrombosis. *Thromb Hemostasis* 67:297, 1992.

36. Vadher BD, Machin SJ, Paterson KG, et al: Life-threatening thrombotic and hemorrhagic problems associated with silent myeloproliferative dis-orders. *Br J Hematol* 85:213, 1993.

37. Wiedmer T, Hall SE, Ortel TL, et al: Complement-induced vesiculation and exposure of membrane prothrombinase sites in platelets of paroxys-mal nocturnal hemoglobinuria. *Blood* 82:1192, 1993.

38. Burke PJ, Braine HG, Rathbun HK, Owens AH Jr: The clinical signifi-cance of fever in acute myelocytic leukemia. *Johns Hopkins Med J* 139:1, 1976.

39. Burns CP, Armitage JO, Frey AL, et al: Analysis of the presenting features of adult acute leukemia. *Cancer* 47:2460, 1981.

40. Mir MA, Delamore JW: Metabolic disorders in acute myeloid leukaemia. *Br J Hematol* 40:79, 1978.

41. Niendorf A, Stang A, Beisiegel U, et al: Elevated lipoprotein (a) levels in patients with acute myeloblastic leukaemia decrease after successful chemotherapeutic treatment. *Clin Invest* 70:683, 1990.

42. Hatfill SJ, Kirby R, Hanley M, et al: Hyperprolactinemia in acute myeloid leukemia and indication of ectopic expression of human prolactin in blast cells of a patient of subtype M4. *Leuk Res* 14:57, 1990.

43. Janowska-Wieczarek A, Belch AR, Jacobs A, et al: Increased circulating colony-stimulating factor-1 in patients with preleukemia, leukemia and lymphoid malignancies. *Blood* 77:1796, 1991.

44. Troy K, Essex D, Rand J, et al: Protein C and S levels in acute leukemia. *Am J Hematol* 37:159, 1991.

45. Westervelt P, Ley TJ: Seed versus soil: the importance of target cell for transgenic models of acute leukemia. *Blood* 93:2143, 1999.

46. Russell NH: Biology of acute leukemia. *Lancet* 349:118, 1997.

47. Ploemacher RE: Characterization and biology of normal human haema-topoietic stem cells. *Haematologica* 84:(EHA-4 educational book)4, 1999.

48. Bonnet D, Dick J: Human acute myeloid leukemia is organized as a hierarchy that originates from a primitive hematopoietic cell. *Nat Med* 3:730, 1997.

MYELODYSPLASTIC DISORDERS (INDOLENT CLONAL MYELOID DISEASES AND OLIGOBLASTIC LEUKEMIA)

MARSHALL A. LICHTMAN

JAMES K. BRENNAN

In contrast to florid acute myelogenous leukemia, there are a group of neoplastic (clonal) myeloid disorders that range from non-progressive to more slowly progressive than AML. The disorders may appear in childhood, but the incidence increases exponentially after age 50 years, and most cases occur between 60 and 90 years of age. These disorders range from acquired idiopathic anemias with or without ringed sideroblasts to oligoblastic myelogenous leukemia. The diseases share a propensity to cytopenias and multilineage dysmorphogenesis of blood cells. Red cells often have striking poikilocytosis, anisocytosis, anisochromia, and stippling. The marrow usually contains increased erythroid precursors with dysmorphic features and nuclear and granular anomalies in neutrophils associated with increased granulocyte precursors. Giant or microcytic platelets, often with abnormal granulation, in the blood are associated with megakaryocytic hyperplasia and atypical lobulation and size of megakaryocytes in the marrow. In the nonprogressive syndromes, anemia is accompanied by only slight variations in neutrophil and platelet levels, and blast cells are not increased in the marrow. Clonal cytogenetic abnormalities occur, however. The syndromes may follow radiation or chemotherapy for another malignancy. In the more progressive syndromes, leukemic blast cells are increased, cytopenias are more severe, and the disease has high morbidity and mortality from infection and bleeding. In each of the syndromes, there is a propensity to evolve into frank AML ranging from about 10 percent in the idiopathic anemias to about 40 percent of patients with trilineage cytopenias and increased marrow blast cells. Mortality from infection also is a high risk in those with severe leukopenia. In the most indolent forms, therapy may not be required. Therapy with cytotoxic drugs, red cell or platelet transfusion, antibiotics, and hematopoietic cytokines may palliate the disease when it is progressive (oligoblastic leukemia).

Acronyms and abbreviations that appear in this chapter include: ALIP, abnormal localized immature precursors; ALL, acute lymphocytic leukemia; AML, acute myelogenous leukemia; ATRA, all-*trans* retinoic acid; CFU-BL, blast cell progenitors; CFU-GM, colony-forming units for granulocytes and monocytes; GM-CSF, granulocyte-macrophage colony-stimulating factor; IRF-1, interferon regulatory factor 1; LE, lupus erythematosus; M-CSF, monocyte colony-stimulating factor; MCV, mean cell volume; NF1, neurofibromatosis; RAEB, refractory anemia with excess blasts; RAEM, refractory anemia with excess myeloblasts; SCF, stem cell factor; WT1, Wilm's tumor.

In young patients allogeneic stem cell transplantation may be very useful.

DEFINITION AND HISTORY

Myelodysplasia is a term used to encompass a spectrum of clonal (neoplastic) myeloid disorders marked by ineffective hematopoiesis, cytopenias, qualitative disorders of blood cells and their precursors, and a variable predilection to undergo clonal evolution to florid AML. The disorders range from relatively indolent idiopathic anemias, with a relatively lower frequency of progression to AML, to more troublesome clonal multilineage cytopenias, to oligoblastic myelogenous leukemias that often progress into overt AML. The somatic mutation that leads to these disorders arises in a multipotential hematopoietic cell. *Dysplasia* is a term that classically implies a polyclonal and, therefore, nonneoplastic process. The choice of the term *myelodysplasia* to denote clonal (neoplastic) disorders is unfortunate because it is hard for students and patients to understand its relationship to other clonal stem cell disorders such as idiopathic myelofibrosis that can have all the features of "myelodysplasia" but are ignored in its classification. Moreover, drawing diagnostic distinctions among 10, 20, and 30 percent leukemic blast cells is inconsistent with the biological behavior of cancer and medicine's classification of cancer. The term myelodysplasia is, however, widely used.[1-3]

The term *indolent clonal myeloid disease*, or *hemopathy*, refers to neoplasias arising in a multipotential hematopoietic marrow cell that result in diseases with no discernible leukemic blast cells in the marrow or blood (e.g., acquired idiopathic anemias) or in oligoblastic leukemia in which an increased number of (leukemic) blast cells is present in the marrow but in which, untreated, the course is smoldering or subacute in contrast to AML.

The boundary between acquired idiopathic anemia and oligoblastic myelogenous leukemia may be indistinct because of the insensitivity of the marrow examination; however, continued observation clarifies the situation. If leukemic blast cells are evident in marrow, the diagnosis of oligoblastic leukemia can be made, maintaining the principle that the histopathologic diagnosis should depend on the presence or absence of tumor cells, not the rate of progression or severity of the manifestations of the malignancy. The proportion of marrow myeloblasts is not increased in reactive states, for example, granulocytic hyperplasia as a result of infection, noninfectious inflammation, solid tumors, and drug-induced granulocytosis (e.g., glucocorticoids, lithium). Indeed, the proportion of blasts usually falls to less than the normal value of 1.0 ± 0.4 SD percent. It is rare to have more than 2.0 percent myeloblasts in a normal marrow in older children and adults, and higher proportions, for example, over 3 percent, are virtually confined to cases of oligoblastic leukemia. The one exception to this rule is that some patients treated with granulocytic growth factors may have a slight increase in blast cells.

The clonal proliferation of multipotential hemopoietic cells is accompanied by variable effects on all blood cell lineages and is usually associated with pathologically enhanced apoptosis of marrow precursor cells such that leukopenia and thrombocytopenia of varying severity often accompany the anemia. Qualitative abnormalities of cell shape, organelle structure, biochemical pathways, and function can occur. The range of clinical expression is broad. Thus, clonal myeloid hemopathies can occur with isolated anemia and a nearly normal-appearing marrow or with severe pancytopenia, profoundly hypercellular marrow, and alterations in blood cell shape, size, and function. The more profound the disorder, the more likely oligoblastic leukemia will be discovered on marrow examination. Since leukemic blast cells may not be evident and some patients with clonal hemopathies do not develop overt leukemia (although their risk is several-thousand-fold that of unaffected individuals), the designation *myelo-dysplasia* has been applied. The choice of the term was intended to highlight the striking dysmorphic appearance of blood and marrow cells neglecting the central alteration, neoplasia. As currently used, *myelodysplasia* encompasses syndromes that are frankly leukemic, such as so-called refractory anemia with excess blasts.[4] Indeed, many of the affected individuals have myelogenous leukemia that is more indolent (smoldering) than overt AML.

HISTORY

At the beginning of the twentieth century, reports of highly morbid cytopenic disorders, refractory to treatment, began to appear in the medical literature.[3] Chevallier and colleagues, in 1942, discussed formally the "odo-leukemia."[5] They chose the Greek word *odo*, meaning threshold, to highlight disorders that are on the threshold of leukemia. Chevallier proposed *leucoses* as the generic term for leukemias so that marked variations in white cell counts and other presenting features would not engender inappropriate terminology. It was a sage but neglected proposal.

In 1949, Hamilton-Paterson used the term *preleukemic anemia* to describe patients with refractory anemia antecedent to the development of AML,[6] and in 1953, Block and coworkers expanded the concept to include cytopenias of all lineages and described cases that closely fit with our current concepts of a clonal myeloid hemopathy prior to the evolution to overt AML.[7] Thus, by midcentury, the relationship of acquired idiopathic cytopenias to the subsequent onset of AML had become broadly appreciated.[8-15] Terms such as *herald state of leukemia, refractory anemia,* sideroachrestic anemia, idiopathic refractory sideroblastic anemia, pancytopenia with hyperplastic marrow, and others were coined to describe the various manifestations of the hematopoietic derangement that preceded the onset of AML.

In 1975, at a conference on unclassifiable leukemias held in Paris, Marcel Bessis, Jean Bernard, and others suggested the term *hemopoietic dysplasia,* later shortened to myelodysplasia for the group of disorders that had a more indolent course than AML.[16,365]

CLASSIFICATION

One classification scheme,[2] which is now undergoing change, separates myelodysplastic syndrome arising *de novo* into several subsets: refractory anemia (with other cytopenias implied), refractory anemia with ringed sideroblasts (with other cytopenias implied), and refractory anemia with excess blasts (smoldering myelogenous leukemia).[2] Chronic myelomonocytic leukemia, although proposed as a myelodysplastic syndrome, can also be included among the chronic myelogenous leukemias[17] (see Chap. 94). The designation *refractory anemia with excess blasts in transformation* has been dropped, since it conveys no additional diagnostic or prognostic information. The myelodysplastic syndromes include entities that have marrow blast percentages ranging from less than 2 percent in refractory anemia to over 20 percent in refractory anemia with excess blasts.[2] This approach is unfortunate, since in no other neoplasms is the designation of the cancer, in this case myelogenous leukemia, called by another name when there is more or less of the tumor cells present. Thus, *myelogenous leukemia,* not refractory anemia, is the name of the tumor whether the marrow has 8 percent or 80 percent blast cells. The arrest in myeloid development is a major component of pathogenesis, not just ineffective hematopoiesis and dysmorphogenesis.

ETIOLOGY AND PATHOGENESIS

ETIOLOGY

There are, not unexpectedly, close similarities to AML in etiologic factors. Benzene,[18-21] chemotherapeutic agents,[363,364] particularly alkyl-ating agents and topoisomerase inhibitors,[21-29] and radiation[30] are exposures that can increase the risk of these indolent clonal hemopathies. These exposures may cause DNA damage, impair DNA repair enzymes, and induce loss of chromosome integrity. Diseases such as Fanconi anemia, known to predispose to the development of AML, occasionally can evolve instead into a clonal myeloid hemopathy.[31,32]

Aging is an important factor in the development of clonal myeloid disorders. They increase exponentially in frequency after the age of 40 years.[33,34]

PATHOGENESIS

These disorders arise from the clonal expansion of a multipotential hematopoietic cell. The clonal origin is supported by studies of women who were heterozygotes for glucose-6-phosphate dehydrogenase isoenzymes A and B and who had such a syndrome. The hematopoietic progenitors[35,36] and in some cases lymphocytes[37,38] of such patients had only one isoenzyme present, supporting the concept of clonal expansion of a neoplastic marrow cell.[39] Clonal studies using X-linked restriction length polymorphisms with probes for hypoxanthine phosphoribosyl transferase or phosphoglycerate kinase also supported the origin of these disorders in a single multipotential stem cell.[40-42]

Fluorescent in situ hybridization of interphase blood cell populations with probes for chromosomes 7 or 8 in patients with monosomy 7 or trisomy 8 indicates that chromosome abnormalities may not be present in lymphoid populations.[42,43] Studies of immunoglobulin heavy-chain gene rearrangement and assay of the human androgen receptor and other genes on the X chromosome have also concluded that lymphocytes are not derived from the neoplastic clone.[44-46] However, pseudodiploidy has been observed in the Epstein-Barr virus-stimulated cell populations of two patients with idiopathic refractory sideroblastic anemia,[47] suggesting that B lymphocytes may be derived from the affected stem cell in some patients.

Molecular genetic studies of patients cells show identifiable gene mutations in about 60 percent. Mutated *RAS* is most common[48-53]; lower frequencies of *FMS* and p53 mutations are present. Codon 12 of *RAS* and codon 969 of *FMS* are the predominant sites of alteration in the respective genes.[54,55] Methylation of p15, an inhibitor of cyclin-dependent kinases 4 and 6, was present in over one-third of patients examined.[56] A variety of other mutations in protooncogenes, or genes encoding proteins involved in the cell cycle, or of transcription factors have been described sporadically.[54,55] Interpretation of these molecular studies is difficult because the mutations are present in advanced disease patients and may be late changes, not seminal in the neoplastic transformation.

The major specific pathophysiologic mechanism in the clonal hemopathies with cytopenias is ineffective hemopoiesis, that is, defective maturation of marrow precursor cells.[57] The specific characteristics of ineffective erythropoiesis and granulopoiesis include a decreased proportion of cells in the DNA synthesis phase of the mitotic cycle and a marked increased in the fraction of late precursor cells undergoing apoptosis.[58-60] Increased levels of apoptotic mediators are present in cells including TNF-α, FAS antigen, and calcium-dependent nuclease activity. Characteristic stepwise degradation of DNA is evident in late precursors.[61-63] The proliferation of progenitor and early precursor cells is usually normal or enhanced, resulting in a hypercellular marrow, but there is a failure to accumulate adequate numbers of mature cells. Mild shortening of cell life-span also contributes to the cytopenias.[9] As the phenotype of the disease evolves toward myelogenous leukemia, proliferative patterns supersede ineffective hematopoeisis as a result of precursor apoptosis.[64] Once the marrow blast percentage is unequivocally above normal (>3 percent) the disease process represents oligoblastic leukemia.

CLINICAL FEATURES

INCIDENCE BY AGE, SEX, AND FAMILIAL OCCURRENCE

The onset of the disease before age 50 years is uncommon except in cases preceded by irradiation or chemotherapy.[33,34,65] Myelodysplasia can occur in children aged 5 months to 15 years at a rate of about 0.5 per million,[66–69,360] and about half of such cases are oligoblastic leukemia. The incidence increases logarithmically after age 40 years to over 20 per 100,000 in septuagenarians.[361] Males are affected about 1.5 to 2.0 times as often as females. Families with an unusually high frequency of clonal myeloid disorders has been described.[70,71,362]

SYMPTOMS AND SIGNS

Patients can be asymptomatic or, if anemia is more severe, can have pallor, weakness, loss of a sense of well-being, and exertional dyspnea.[14,72,73] A small proportion of patients have infections related to granulocytopenia or hemorrhage related to thrombocytopenia at the time of diagnosis, but patients with severe depressions of neutrophil and platelet counts at diagnosis usually have oligoblastic leukemia. Rarely, patients can have fever unrelated to infection.[74] Arthralgias are the initial complaint in some patients.[75] Very rarely, the presentation may mimic a connective tissue disease.[76,77] Hepatomegaly or splenomegaly occurs in about 5 or 10 percent of patients, respectively.

SPECIAL CLINICAL FEATURES

Patients with an indolent phase (smoldering myelogenous leukemia) prior to overt AML may develop diabetes insipidus. Hypothalamic involvement can lead to polyuria, polydipsia, and decreased libido. Hypothalamic-posterior hypophysis insufficiency in clonal myeloid states has been associated with monosomy 7 in hematopoietic cells.[78–80]

Acute neutrophilic dermatosis (Sweet disease) is an acute febrile illness with erythematous patches on arms, face, and legs that progress to painful brown plaques that may ulcerate and produce large necrotizing skin lesions. The histopathology of the skin is that of a dense dermal neutrophilic infiltrate.[81] This syndrome, which occurs principally in middle-aged women, lasts for 6 to 10 weeks, is often associated with blood neutrophilia, and may recur.[82] At least 10 percent of patients with Sweet disease develop AML or another clonal myeloid disease, and occasional cases have been associated with monocytosis or cytogenic abnormalities in marrow cells prior to onset of AML. G-CSF and all-*trans* retinoic acid (ATRA) administration has been followed by Sweet disease in some cases.[83,84] Other dermatopathic conditions also have been associated with clonal myeloid diseases.[85]

A symptom complex that mimics systemic lupus erythematosus (fever, pleurisy, symmetric arthritis, plasma antinuclear antibody, and pancytopenia with a hyperplastic marrow) may precede AML.[76] Several patients with signs of lupus erythematosus (LE) and the LE cell phenomenon have been reported in a review of the clonal hemopathic syndromes.[86] Behcet's disease, glomerulonephritis, seronegative arthritis, and inflammatory bowel disease also have been associated with clonal myeloid disorders.[87–90]

The incidence of other cancers may be increased in subjects with clonal myeloid disorders.[96–99]

LABORATORY FEATURES

BLOOD

RED CELLS

Anemia is present in over 85 percent of patients.[12–15,72] The mean cell volume (MCV) often is increased.[13,14] Red cell shape abnormalities may include oval, elliptical, teardrop, spherical, or fragmented cells.

There is a spectrum of red cell findings. Some patients have only slight anisocytosis. Elliptical red cells sometimes dominate. Basophilic stippling of red cells occurs. Nucleated red cells are seen in the blood film in about 10 percent of cases. Reticulocyte counts are usually low for the degree of anemia. Other abnormalities of red cells also occur, such as an increased proportion of hemoglobin F,[95] decreased red cell enzyme activities, especially acquired pyruvate kinase deficiency.[96] In some cases with pyruvate kinase deficiency, hemolysis has occurred. An enhanced sensitivity of membranes to complement,[97] and modification of red cell blood group antigens may be observed.[98,99] Acquired hemoglobin H disease results in red cell morphology similar to thalassemia (microcytosis, basophilic stippling, target cells, and teardrop cells). Intracellular precipitates of β-chain tetramers (identified by crystal violet stain) reflect an acquired decrease in the rate of α-chain synthesis in erythroblasts.[100,101] The decrease in α-globin chain synthesis is profound, involves each of the four α-chain loci, and results from a transcription abnormality. There are no gross alterations in genes (e.g., insertions, deletions) in these cases.[111]

GRANULOCYTES AND MONOCYTES

Neutropenia is present in about 50 percent of patients at the time of diagnosis.[65] The proportion of monocytes often is increased, and monocytosis per se can be the dominant manifestation of the hematopoietic abnormality for months or years.[102–104] Morphologic abnormalities of neutrophils can occur, sometimes resulting in the acquired Pelger-Huët anomaly. In this condition, the neutrophils have very condensed chromatin and unilobed or bilobed nuclei that often have a pince-nez shape.[105] Ring-shaped nuclei also occur in neutrophils.[106] Neutrophil alkaline phosphatase activity is decreased in some patients.[14] Expression of normal surface antigens on neutrophils and monocytes is decreased, and in some cases abnormal surface antigen expression may occur.[107] Defective primary granules of abnormal size and shape with decreased myeloperoxidase content can be present,[108] and specific neutrophil granules can be decreased in number, producing hypogranular cells.[109] Neutrophil granule membranes frequently are deficient in glycoprotein.[110] Chemotactic, phagocytic, and bactericidal capability may be impaired.[111–113] Formyl-leucyl-methionyl-phenylamine receptor signaling and actin polymerization have been abnormal.[114,115] Muramidase (lysozyme) activity in blood and urine may be increased, a reflection of granulocytic hyperplasia and heightened monocytopoiesis and monocyte turnover.

PLATELETS

About 25 percent of patients may have mild to moderate thrombocytopenia at the time of diagnosis.[14,65] Mild thrombocytosis also can occur.[14,65] Platelets may be abnormally large, have poor granulation, or have large, fused central granules.[116,117] Abnormal platelet function may contribute to a prolonged bleeding time, easy bruising, or exaggerated bleeding. Decreased platelet aggregation in response to collagen or epinephrine is a frequent functional abnormality.[118]

LYMPHOCYTES

Patients with clonal hemopathies may have immunologic deficiencies, such as a decrease in natural killer cells in the blood but no decrease in large granular lymphocytes,[119–122] a decrease in helper T lymphocytes,[120] and a decrease in Epstein-Barr virus receptors on B lymphocytes.[120–123] Antibody-dependent cellular cytotoxicity is normal.[120] Thymidine incorporation after mitogenic stimulation[124,125] and colony growth of T lymphocytes are decreased.[138] Lymphocytes may have an increased sensitivity to irradiation.[124] The defects in lymphoid cells could reflect the site of the somatic mutation in the pluripotential stem cell in some cases[36–38,40,41] (see "Pathogenesis").

PLASMA ABNORMALITIES

Serum iron, transferrin, and ferritin levels may be elevated. Lactic dehydrogenase and uric acid concentrations can be increased as a result of ineffective hemopoiesis and a high death fraction of maturing marrow precursors. Monoclonal gammopathy, polyclonal hypergammaglobulinemia, and hypogammaglobulinemia each occur with an increased frequency.[126,127] The frequency of autoantibodies was increased in one report[127] but not in another.[126]

MARROW

CELLULARITY

Marrow cellularity is usually normal or increased.[128–130] Occasionally, it may be decreased and may simulate hypoplastic anemia or aplastic anemia,[131] although islands of dysmorphic cells are usually present, especially atypical megakaryocytes. An increase in blast cells in this setting suggest hypoplastic myelogenous leukemia (see Chap. 93).

ERYTHROPOIESIS

Erythroid hyperplasia is frequent, and very large or small erythroblasts, nuclear fragmentation, stippled erythroblasts, and poor hemoglobinization may be seen.[13,14,132] Proerythroblasts may be in excess, and the marrow may lack normal clusters or islets of erythroblasts. Erythroblasts may resemble megaloblasts that have nuclear-cytoplasmic maturation asynchrony, nuclear fragmentation, or cytoplasmic nuclear remnants. This pattern is referred to as megaloblastoid erythropoiesis.

Pathologic sideroblasts may be identified when the marrow is treated with Prussian blue stain. These include erythroblasts with an increased number and size of siderosomes (cytoplasmic ferritin–containing vacuoles), referred to as intermediate sideroblasts, or erythroblasts with mitochondrial iron aggregates that take the form of a partial or complete circumnuclear ring of iron globules, referred to as ringed sideroblasts. Macrophage iron often is increased. Some observers believe that ringed sideroblasts are associated with progression to leukemia less often than are sideroblasts with increases in cytoplasmic ferritin.[133,134] Others dispute this conclusion.[135] Ringed sideroblasts, as compared with intermediate sideroblasts, are very uncommon or present only in very low proportions (less than 15 percent) in any clonal myeloid syndrome other than acquired refractory sideroblastic anemia.

GRANULOPOIESIS

Granulocytic hyperplasia is frequent.[13,14,128–130] Marrow monocytes also may be increased in number. Abnormalities of granulocytes include hypogranulation, a monocytoid appearance of neutrophilic granulocytes, and the acquired Pelger-Huët nuclear abnormality of neutrophils. Progranulocytes and myelocytes may be increased. As stated previously, the proportion of blast cells is not increased in clonal hemopathies that are categorized as acquired sideroblastic or nonsideroblastic idiopathic anemia. The latter are syndromes with no increase in blast cells (i.e., less than 2 percent); if the blast percentage is above this level the patient can be considered to have oligoblastic leukemia. Marrow biopsy may show abnormal localized immature precursors (ALIP),[135,136] which are clusters of immature myeloid (? blast) cells located centrally rather than subjacent to the endosteum. These clusters of atypical cells are present in virtually all cases of oligoblastic leukemia where blast cells comprise 3 percent or more of nucleated marrow cells (refractory anemia with excess blasts) and in nearly half the patients with refractory anemia, sideroblastic or nonsideroblastic, suggesting that about half these patients have a disorder closely approaching oligoblastic leukemia. Patients with this abnormality are more prone to develop overt AML.[135] The number of plasma cells may be slightly increased.

THROMBOPOIESIS

Megakaryocytes are present in normal or increased numbers.[13,14,128–130] Micromegakaryocytes (dwarf megakaryocytes) may occur.[128–130,137,138] Megakaryocytes with unilobed or bilobed nuclei may be increased, and hypersegmented and hyposegmented megakaryocytes may be present. Clusters of megakaryocytes may be seen. Megakaryocytes may be distributed laterally from their usual parasinusoidal location.[139]

FIBROSIS

An increase in reticulin and collagen fibers of varying degree is common—especially in oligoblastic leukemias. When fibrosis is prominent, the disorder can resemble primary myelofibrosis, although, in contrast to the latter, splenomegaly is usually not marked. Since idiopathic myelofibrosis is an oligoblastic leukemia with striking dysmorphogenesis of cells, some overlap with other fibrotic clonal myeloid disorders is expected.[140]

The morphologic aberrations (dysmorphogenesis) of blood cells seen in indolent clonal hemopathies can be seen in oligoblastic myelogenous leukemia as well, contributing to the decision to group them together.

CULTURE

The clonal growth of marrow progenitors in soft agar or other viscous culture systems is usually abnormal in patients with clonal hemopathies.[141] Most reports indicate that growth of multipotential (CFU-GEMM) and erythroid progenitors (BFU-E, CFU-E) in the blood or marrow is markedly decreased in subjects with clonal myeloid disorders.[141–144] Biochemical abnormalities of erythroid precursors have been found also. Colony-forming units for granulocytes and monocytes (CFU-GM) are decreased.[140,142] Very small colonies or clusters with impaired maturation often dominate the cultures. Abnormally small and infrequent CFU-GM may be found when blood neutrophil and monocyte counts are nearly normal. Occasionally, overabundant growth is present. Usually, cell culture results become more abnormal as the blood cell abnormalities in the patient worsen.

In overt AML, CFU-GM growth is usually absent. Some studies indicate that very abnormal growth of progenitors in culture (decreased colonies or predominance of small clusters) is a poor prognostic sign and may be a harbinger of overt leukemia.[145,146] Growth that does occur in clonal myeloid hemopathies (and AML) usually remains dependent on growth factors such as erythropoietin and granulocyte-macrophage colony-stimulating factor (GM-CSF).[147,148] Colony growth in children with the monosomy 7 syndrome may occur without added growth factors supporting the view that there is autocrine and paracrine stimulation of progenitor cells.[149–152] Blast cell progenitors (CFU-BL) may be increased in patients with oligoblastic leukemia.[150] The long-term marrow initiating cell is decreased in some patients,[151,152] and the ability of marrow stromal layers to support in vitro hematopoiesis can be impaired.[152]

Circulating M-CSF (CSF-1) has been increased in some patients, as well as in AML and other hematologic malignancies, for no clear reason.[154] Interleukin-1α (IL-1α) and GM-CSF levels have been undetectable in most patients; IL-6, G-CSF, and erythropoietin concentrations have been variable; and tumor necrosis factor has been inversely related to hematocrit.[155] Stem cell factor (SCF), a multilineage hematopoietin, has been decreased in some patients.[156] FLT-3 ligand, another multilineage growth factor, is increased in patients with indolent clonal hemopathies but not oligoblastic leukemia.[157] The inverse relationship between platelet count and thrombopoietin levels is maintained in acquired idiopathic anemia but not oligoblastic leukemia.[158]

CYTOGENETICS

An altered number or form of chromosomes may occur in up to 80 percent of patients with clonal hemopathies, depending on the severity of the syndrome.[159–163] The chromosome abnormalities are nonrandom and often involve chromosomes that are abnormal in patients with AML, although certain chromosomal rearrangements seen in AML such as t(15;17), t(8;21), and inv16 are usually not observed except in oligoblastic leukemias[161–164] (see Chap. 10).

Chromosomal abnormalities involving virtually every chromosome have been noted in marrow cells.[170–178,366,367] Common abnormalities include an extra chromosome 8; loss of the long arm of the chromosome 5, 7, 9, 20, or 21; and monosomy for chromosomes 7 and 9. Losses of part or all of chromosomes 5 and 7 and complex chromosome abberations are particularly common in the oligoblastic myelogenous leukemias (and the overt leukemias) associated with prior treatment with cytotoxic drugs, radiation, or exposure to benzene.[161–167] The Ph chromosome t(9q+;22q) and numerous other occasional chromosome abnormalities have been described in patients with indolent clonal hemopathies.[193,194]

The proportion of cases with chromosome abnormalities is different depending on the severity of the clinical manifestations. Chromosome abnormalities are more frequent in patients with refractory anemia with excess blasts (oligoblastic leukemia) than in those with acquired idiopathic anemia. In general, prevalence of chromosome abnormalities and the likelihood of progression to overt AML are both a function of the number of cell lines involved, the severity of the cytopenias, and the proportion of blast cells present.

THE 5Q-SYNDROME

Patients with the 5q-syndrome have refractory anemia and dysmorphic cells in the marrow containing a deletion in the long arm of chromosome 5 (5q-).[168–171] The refractory anemia, observed most frequently in older women, is associated with marked dyserythropoiesis, erythroid multinuclearity, and hypolobulated and frequently small (''dwarf'') megakaryocytes. The syndrome can occur in children.[171]

The critical regions have been mapped to bands 5q31 to 5q33 with the proximal deletion associated with the spontaneous mutation and the distal region with the posttherapy-related event.[169–171] The genes that encode for the multipotential growth factor IL-3[168]; for the bipotential growth factor for granulocytes and monocytes, GM-CSF[172]; and IL-4, -5, and -9 are located on the portion of chromosome 5 that is deleted in the 5q-syndrome. Gene mapping studies indicate that the IL-3/GM-CSF and IL-4/IL-5 gene clusters are proximal to and excluded from the rearranged region (5q31) associated with myeloid leukemias.[173] The monocyte colony-stimulating factor, M-CSF (CSF-1) gene, previously thought to be on chromosome 5, has been relocated to chromosome 1[174] but the FMS gene, encoding the receptor for M-CSF (CSF-1), is on the long arm of chromosome 5 in the region deleted in the 5q-syndrome.[175,176] The genes for three additional growth factors, IL-1, platelet-derived growth factor, and endothelial cell growth factor, are also on chromosome 5[168] but not on the segment deleted in the 5q-syndrome. The pathogenetic role of the genes deleted in this syndrome is not known, since only a single allele is involved, and unaffected cells (e.g., T lymphocytes, fibroblasts, endothelial cells) also may produce identical growth factors.

A number of other growth-related genes such as the EGR, CDC25C, and interferon regulatory genes also are located on 5q.[168,177–180] A tumor suppressor gene might be located at 5q31, the smallest commonly deleted segment in 5q-syndrome. The interferon regulatory factor-1 (IRF-1) gene, encoding a DNA-binding protein that binds to a promoter element for IFN-α, IFN-β, and other IFN-inducible genes, also has been localized to 5q31. Rearrangements of this gene have been found in some patients with oligoblastic and overt myelogenous leukemia and 5q-.[177–181] The action of IRF-1 is antagonized by IRF-2, and imbalanced expression of IRF-1 relative to that of IRF-2 activity could predispose to neoplastic transformation. The associated proximal break points at 5q12 to 15, sometimes seen in the relatively benign 5q-syndrome, may be associated with preservation of granulocyte and platelet counts and reduced infection and bleeding complications. Patients with this disorder have a risk of developing AML that is similar (about 15 percent) to that of patients with refractory anemia and marrow cells without 5q-.

MONOSOMY 7 SYNDROME

Monosomy 7 is the second most frequent cytogenetic abnormality in the marrow cells of patients with myelodysplasia. It often occurs in marrow cells of subjects exposed to chemicals or radiation and is associated with a poor prognosis and rapid transformation to AML.[184,185] A critical region may reside in bands 7q35–36.[186] Monosomy 7 syndromes, aside from being difficult to classify, usually are not associated with special clinical features in adults, although in children they are characterized by an atypical myeloproliferative disorder or myelomonocytic leukemia with abnormal expression of the neurofibromatosis (NF1) and Wilm's tumor (WT1) genes, unusual susceptibility to infection, and a rapid termination in acute leukemia[66,184–187] (see Chap. 93). Monosomy 7 also occurs in a familial form and during leukemic evolution of Down syndrome and Fanconi anemia.[188,189] A variant of the monosomy 7 syndrome, translocation 1;7, also is seen in adults and children and may be preceded by exposure to cytotoxic treatment.[190,191] The ERB-B gene, which encodes a shortened form of the epidermal growth factor receptor, is amplified in this syndrome.[192]

SPECIFIC CLONAL MYELOID SYNDROMES

These syndromes highlight the variability in expression of the clonal hemopathies (Table 92-1). Most patients have one of the syndromes described below.

ACQUIRED IDIOPATHIC SIDEROBLASTIC ANEMIA

HISTORY

The term *refractory anemia* has been used to define erythropoietic insufficiencies that cannot be assigned to a specific vitamin or mineral deficiency and thus are unresponsive to the known hematinics. In 1956, Bjorkman defined a subset of refractory anemias by the presence of ringed sideroblasts in the marrow.[195] The intramitochondrial location of the iron in the ringed sideroblasts was described a year later.[196]

PATHOGENESIS

The disorder is a multipotential stem cell defect in which ineffective erythropoiesis with normal or slightly shortened red cell survival and only slight impairment of the maturation of other cell lineages occurs.[197–200] The plasma iron turnover is increased, but incorporation of radioactive iron into heme and its delivery to blood as newly synthesized hemoglobin are depressed.[197] Impairment of heme biosynthesis results in mitochondrial iron overload, which may inhibit mitochondrial function and contribute to the premature destruction of marrow

TABLE 92-1 PRODROMAL AND OLIGOBLASTIC (LOW-INFILTRATE) MYELOGENOUS LEUKEMIA

Ineffective hemopoiesis (precursor apoptosis) and dysmorphic cells
    Acquired refractory nonsideroblastic anemia
    Acquired refractory sideroblastic anemia
    Bicytopenia or tricytopenia with hyperplastic marrow
    Oligoblastic leukemia (refractory anemia with excess myeloblasts)

NOTE: Acute and chronic myeloproliferative diseases are listed in Table 91-1.

erythroid precursors.[200] Missense mutations in the gene encoding delta-aminolevulinate synthetase,[201] or in a mitochondrial transfer RNA,[202] and in red cell 5-aminolevulinic acid synthetase (205C) have been described, but a common gene alteration has not been correlated with this disease.

CLINICAL FEATURES

The disease is very uncommon under age 50[33,203–205] except in patients in whom it occurs as a result of radiotherapy or chemotherapy of a malignant tumor.[206] Males and females are affected almost equally. A rare concurrence of familial sideroblastic anemia has been reported.[207] The signs and symptoms are those of anemia: pallor, easy fatigue, weakness, and dyspnea and palpitations on exertion.[199,204] Most patients have the anemia detected as a result of blood cell analysis for other medical reasons. The liver may be slightly enlarged. The spleen is slightly increased in size in about 5 percent of patients. Splenic and hepatic enlargement do not necessarily occur together, and more than slight enlargement is unusual.

LABORATORY FEATURES

Most patients have mild to severe macrocytic anemia.[199,204] The blood film often contains a population of hypochromic cells (dimorphic red cell changes).[198,199,204,205] Red cell anisocytosis, basophilic stippling, and slight poikilocytosis may be present. The total white cell count and platelet count are usually normal, but mild abnormalities may be seen, including a decreased white cell count and an increased or decreased platelet count. Occasionally, the white cell count or platelet count may be increased markedly, or nucleated red cells may be present in the blood film. The reticulocyte percentage is usually between 0.5 and 2.0. Hemoglobin F concentration may be increased slightly.

Marrow cellularity usually is increased as a result of erythroid hyperplasia. Evidence of dyserythropoiesis in the form of vacuolated, small, large, or binucleate erythroblasts may be present. Prussian blue stain of the marrow invariably shows pathological sideroblasts. The latter may have Prussian blue–positive cytoplasmic granules in a partial or complete circumnuclear pattern (ringed sideroblasts) in 15 percent or more of cells or an increased number (more than 5) of Prussian blue–positive granules in their cytoplasm. If the disease progresses to oligoblastic leukemia, sideroblasts may become less prominent.[208] Granulopoiesis and thrombopoiesis are not altered significantly in two-thirds of patients.[205] In the other third, dysgranulopoiesis (hypogranulation, acquired Pelger-Huët anomaly, hypersegmented nuclei, or granule abnormalities) or dysmegakaryocytopoiesis (micromegakaryocytes, large lobulated cells) may be present. Marrow iron stores are increased often.

Cytogenetic abnormalities in marrow cells of patients with acquired refractory sideroblastic anemia provide evidence for the clonal character of the disease. About half of the reported cases with sideroblastic anemia in which cytogenetic studies have been performed have a chromosomal abnormality.[204] Involvement of chromosomes 8, 11, and 20 has been notable[159–162,209–211]; the Philadelphia chromosome has been reported[212]; involvement of chromosome 3 has been associated with thrombocytosis.[213] The absence of the Y chromosome, only in the pathological sideroblasts in one report (45;X/46;XY mosaic), substantiates the dimorphic nature of the erythroid lineage involvement and parallels the hypochromic and normochromic red cell populations.[214] Involvement of the X chromosome (a breakpoint at Xq13) of female patients with sideroblastic anemia[215,216] is of note because a type of hereditary sideroblastic anemia is X chromosome–linked (see Chap. 63).

Serum iron levels and saturation of transferrin are increased. Serum ferritin concentration is increased, reflecting an increase in body iron stores. Bilirubin-proteinate levels (indirect-reacting fraction) may be increased as a result of ineffective erythropoiesis and intramedullary hemolysis.

DIFFERENTIAL DIAGNOSIS

The principal considerations are those anemias with an inadequate reticulocyte response in which erythrocytes are hypochromic. Iron deficiency anemia in contradistinction to sideroblastic anemia is associated with low serum iron levels, saturation of transferrin of less than 16 percent, low serum ferritin concentration, elevated serum transferrin receptors, and absent marrow sideroblasts and macrophage iron. Beta thalassemia minor is characterized by normal to elevated serum iron and ferritin, a low mean red cell volume, elevated hemoglobin A_2 concentration, and evidence of the disease in a parent, siblings, or offsprings. Detection of secondary forms of sideroblastic anemia requires evaluation for exposure to lead or other agents or diseases listed in Chap. 63, as do the hereditary sideroblastic anemias.

THERAPY

Some patients do not require treatment, since the moderate decrease in hemoglobin concentration is tolerated without limitation of usual activities. Occasional patients who have low serum and red cell folate concentrations may have partial improvement in blood hemoglobin concentration after the administration of folic acid (1 mg/day, orally). Rare patients may benefit temporarily from pharmacological doses of pyridoxine (200 mg/day, orally for at least 3 months) or danazol.[217] A therapeutic trial with folic acid and pyridoxine is worthwhile if the anemia is symptomatic, even though only a small percentage of patients are responsive. If anemia is severe or symptoms of heart failure or coronary insufficiency are present, periodic transfusion of red cells is required. Recombinant human erythropoietin generally is not useful unless the pretreatment serum erythropoietin level is below 200 milliunits per ml, an infrequent finding in these patients.[218] The combination of G-CSF with erythropoietin may increase the response rate to over 40 percent.[219] Erythropoietin, 20,000 to 40,000 units subcutaneously, once a week coupled with G-CSF, 300 μg subcutaneously, two or three times per week, is one regimen that can be used if the cytopenias are not tolerated.

COURSE AND PROGNOSIS

In many patients the disorder lasts for years without progression of the anemia or symptoms. A small proportion of patients may have progressive marrow failure, severe cytopenia, and morbidity from infections or hemorrhage. Iron overload is common, and some patients may develop hemochromatosis.[220] The frequency of HLA-A₃ is significantly higher in patients who develop iron overload than in the general population. The frequency is comparable to that found in hereditary hemochromatosis,[221] suggesting that the combination of a genetic predisposition plus sideroblastic anemia facilitates the expression of iron overload in these patients. Evidence in support of this linkage has not been found after search for mutations associated with hemochromatosis.[222] The appearance of hemochromatosis may be accelerated if frequent transfusions have been required for a period of years.[220] Improvement of the anemia and the adverse effects of iron overload in parenchymal tissues can occur following cautious phlebotomy or chelation therapy.[223–225]

Over a 10- to 15-year period about 10 percent of patients with acquired refractory sideroblastic anemia will develop AML.[220,226–229] The progression to leukemia is correlated with the degree of dyshematopoiesis and trilineage abnormalities.[208] Transformation to acute lymphocytic leukemia also has occurred.[230] In one series of 37 patients, 25 had abnormalities confined to the erythroid series, transfusion dependence occurred in 26, and iron overload was common. Five patients progressed to marrow failure and five to AML. Median survival was 72 months.[231] Survival in other series has ranged from 21 to over 60 months.[72] Survival is better in patients without abnormalities in lineages other than erythroid cells and with favorable cytogenetic findings.[232] This also applies to acquired refractory nonsideroblastic anemias and oligoblastic leukemia[233] (see below).

ACQUIRED IDIOPATHIC NONSIDEROBLASTIC ANEMIA

This clonal disorder closely mimics sideroblastic anemia and can occur without prominent sideroblasts in the marrow. The anemia is mild to moderate, with a tendency to macrocytosis. Leukopenia and thrombocytopenia, if present, are usually mild.[205,234] Hyposegmented and hypersegmented neutrophils, giant platelets, and red cell shape, size, and hemoglobinization abnormalities may be present. The marrow is usually cellular, and the precursors may show morphologic evidence of dyshemopoiesis, especially in the erythroid series, but ringed sideroblasts are absent or, in one classification scheme, less than 15 percent of erythroid cells. Since anemia predominates and other cytopenias are slight, the course and management are similar to that of acquired idiopathic sideroblastic anemia with dysmorphogenesis, principally. Patients with low erythropoietin levels may have a significant increase in hemoglobin concentration with weekly injections of the hormone. The proportion of patients transforming into AML and the median survival of patients are similar to patients with acquired idiopathic sideroblastic anemia, particularly cases with accompanying disturbances in granulopoiesis or megakaryopoiesis.[232,235,236] Cytopenias and blood and marrow dysmorphic changes can become more severe, and the course and management in that instance are similar to multilineal cytopenia with hypercellular marrow, discussed below.

MULTILINEAL CYTOPENIA WITH HYPERCELLULAR MARROW

Approximately two-thirds of patients with clonal myeloid hemopathy present with neutropenia and/or thrombocytopenia in addition to anemia.

CLINICAL FINDINGS

These patients present with anemia, neutropenia, and thrombocytopenia; anemia and neutropenia; or anemia and thrombocytopenia. The blood and marrow features are as described above in "Laboratory Features" and lead to a diagnosis, especially in the patient over 50 years of age.[9-16,237,238] The patient usually seeks medical attention for symptoms of anemia: fatigue, dyspnea, and palpitations on exertion, headache, or dizziness. Exaggerated bleeding associated with thrombocytopenia also may be present. Mild hepatomegaly and/or splenomegaly may be present occasionally.

Dysmorphic blood and marrow cell changes are common. Myeloblasts are not increased in the marrow (less than 2 percent) and are absent from the blood. Cytogenetic abnormalities may be present as described under "Cytogenetics." If monocytosis is greater than 1000/μl (1000% 10^6/liter), the disorder merges with chronic myelomonocytic leukemia[149] (see Chap. 94).

DIFFERENTIAL DIAGNOSIS

Mild to moderate bicytopenia (anemia and neutropenia) and sometimes tricytopenia with dysmorphic blood and marrow findings and hypercellular marrow occur in patients with the acquired immune deficiency syndrome[239,240] but have not been associated with progression to acute leukemia. Pancytopenia with hyperplastic marrow has been associated with nonhemopoietic cancers (paraneoplastic syndrome).[241] Megaloblastic anemia can be simulated and can be distinguished by the normal concentration of serum or red cell folate and of serum vitamin B_{12}.

TREATMENT

In patients with pancytopenia and hyperplastic marrow, cytopenias that are not troublesome should not be treated. Transfusion of blood components when necessary is the mainstay of treatment. Regular transfusion of red cells may be used for those who do not adapt to moderate anemia or in whom medical conditions, such as angina pectoris, require a higher packed red cell volume. Erythropoietin with or without G-CSF administration may increase hemoglobin concentration and decrease transfusion frequency. Thrombocytopenia is often not so severe as to require treatment. If thrombocytopenic bleeding occurs, platelet transfusions should be used. Amincaproic acid (Amicar) may be a useful adjunct to platelet transfusion for thrombocytopenic bleeding. Interleukin 11 may increase platelet counts in some patients. Stem cell factor, interleukin 3, or thrombopoietin are not approved for clinical use at this time. Amifostin, an aminothiol agent used for radioprotection, given in doses of 100 to 200 mg/m^2 three times a week may increase blood counts in some patients.[242] Asymptomatic neutropenia should not be treated, but fever should be evaluated promptly and suspected infection treated with broad-spectrum bactericidal antibiotics until the results of cultures are known. In appropriate situations oral antibiotics can be used in patients treated at home.[243,244]

Androgens have not been generally useful. Rare cases may show minor improvement, but the likelihood of substantial or sustained improvement is low. Occasional cases have shown improvement in blood cell counts and, where present, resolution of myelofibrosis following use of glucocorticoids (prednisone, 40 mg/m^2 per day, orally[245] or prednisone, 60 mg qd).[246] Protracted use of glucocorticoids may increase the risk of infection, especially with opportunistic organisms, and has not been shown to increase survival.

For those patients with symptomatic anemia and high transfusion requirements or severe, symptomatic neutropenia, therapeutic trials of erythropoietin[247-250] and/or GM-CSF, G-CSF,[251-255] or IL-3[256] have sometimes been beneficial in increasing counts and improving neutrophil function. Cytokines have not been shown to increase survival and can produce troubling side effects such as local skin reactions, fever, bone pain, and a capillary leak syndrome.[247,257] They also can lead to an increase of immature granulocytes including blasts to increase in marrow and blood.[258]

In uncommon cases with hypoplastic marrows, cyclosporin A and antithymocyte globulin have been used,[259,260] analogous to the responsiveness of some cases of aplastic anemia to such approaches. A variety of chemotherapeutic agents have been used, especially when the disease evolves to oligoblastic or frank AML (see oligoblastic leukemia, "Treatment").

COURSE AND PROGNOSIS

In patients with multicytopenias, morbidity is great; severe infections, exaggerated bleeding, and severe anemia and lassitude may occur. Mortality from infection or hemorrhage occurs in about 25 percent of patients. AML develops in about 50 percent of patients. There is a greater likelihood of transformation to overt AML if the patient has severe cytopenias, more overt qualitative disorders of cells, abnormal localized immature myeloid precursors in marrow, complex chromosome abnormalities, and abnormalities of marrow cell colony growth in culture (excessive growth or decreased growth).[233,261,262] Median survival of patients with clonal hemopathy and multicytopenias is about 20 months.

UNCOMMON PRELEUKEMIC SYNDROMES

ISOLATED THROMBOCYTOPENIA

Amegakaryocytic thrombocytopenia is a very uncommon preleukemic syndrome (less than 1 percent), although bonafide cases have transformed into AML months or years later.[263,264] Among 1220 cases of myelodysplastic syndrome, 11 cases of isolated thrombocytopenia associated with clonal chromosome abnormalities, usually involving chromosomes 3, 5, 8, or 20, were identified. Antiplatelet antibodies were not present, and glucocorticoids were ineffective. Five of the 11 patients progressed to acute myelogenous leukemia.[263] (See Table 92-2.)

ISOLATED NEUTROPENIA

Chronic neutropenic states are rare antecedents of AML.[265] Congenital neutropenia (Kostmann syndrome) has evolved into AML.[265,266] The evolution of Shwachman syndrome (neutropenia and exocrine pancreatic insufficiency) into oligoblastic or overt acute leukemia has been documented.[267] A related disorder, Pearson syndrome (sideroblastic anemia, neutropenia, and exocrine pancreatic insufficiency), is a putative preleukemia disorder in children[268] (see Chap. 31).

MONOCYTOSIS

In a small proportion of patients with preleukemia, monocytosis may be the most striking blood cell abnormality for months or years before the development of acute leukemia.[102–104]

APLASTIC ANEMIA, PAROXYSMAL NOCTURNAL HEMOGLOBINURIA, AND EOSINOPHILIC FASCIITIS

AML occurs in a small fraction of patients (approximately 5 percent) with acquired aplastic anemia.[269,270] Since aplasia itself is a disease with a high early mortality rate, the propensity to leukemia may be greater than is apparent. Patients initially responding to glucocorticoids or antithymocyte globulin have later developed myelodysplastic syndromes.[270]

Paroxysmal nocturnal hemoglobinuria is a hemopoietic stem cell disease that often is associated with marrow hypoplasia (see Chap. 36). AML may ensue in some patients.[97] It is a preleukemic syndrome with a very low incidence of leukemic transformation. There is a propensity for all chronic hemopoietic stem cell disorders (e.g., polycythemia vera, essential thrombocythemia, idiopathic myelofibrosis, chronic myelogenous leukemia) to undergo transformation to AML (see Chap 91). Patients with indolent myeloid clonal disorders may have a PNH-like defect of their blood cell membranes.[27]

Eosinophilic fasciitis mimics the cutaneous manifestations of scleroderma. Symmetrical swelling and induration of arms and legs, sparing the hands and feet, are common.[272,273] Eosinophilia and hypergammaglobulinemia are frequent, and immune cytopenias, aplastic anemia, myelodysplasia, AML, and lymphoma has been associated with the disease.[274] An immune mechanism has been postulated for all the manifestations of the disease. The risk of developing AML is greatly increased compared with healthy individuals.[272–274] Marrow transplantation has been used to treat the aplastic anemia.[275]

OLIGOBLASTIC LEUKEMIAS

DEFINITION AND HISTORY

In 1963, the term *smoldering acute leukemia* was introduced to highlight a subset of patients, usually those over 50 years of age, who had a low proportion of leukemic blast cells in marrow (5 to 30 percent) and blood (0 to 10 percent) and who survived for months or years without specific therapy for leukemia.[276–278] Oligoblastic leukemia has been called refractory anemia with excess myeloblasts, and when the blast count increases further the phrase *in transformation* had been added.[2] The latter distinction has proved of little value and has been abandoned. Chronic myelomonocytic leukemia, previously included under the rubric myelodysplasia, is better linked to the subacute and chronic myelogenous leukemias discussed in Chap. 94. Happily this change further minimizes the oxymoronic classification that considers leukemia a dysplasia.

OLIGOBLASTIC LEUKEMIA (REFRACTORY ANEMIA WITH EXCESS MYELOBLASTS)

This disorder is referred to by the acronym *RAEM* (or RAEB, refractory anemia with excess blasts).[2,279,280] Most patients are over 50 years of age. Males and females are affected about equally. Reticulocytopenic anemia, granulocytopenia, and/or thrombocytopenia are present. Qualitative abnormalities of blood cells may develop as described above under ''Laboratory Features.'' Myeloblasts and progranulocytes constitute from 3 to 30 percent of nucleated marrow cells. Some subclassify this group into RAEB (20 percent or fewer marrow blasts). (*RAEB in transformation* had been used in those cases with 20 to 30 percent marrow blasts but has been dropped.) Auer rods may be present in blast cells. Dysmorphic changes that may occur in marrow precursor cells are described above in ''Laboratory Features.'' This syndrome evolves into overt AML in about 30 to 50 percent of cases.[281] Median survival in RAEB is about 9 months, although there are occasional long-term survivors.

TREATMENT, COURSE, AND PROGNOSIS

The treatment of oligoblastic leukemia should be highly individualized. In some cases no active treatment is required. Periodic evaluation is essential to detect deterioration in well-being or blood cell counts. Most patients will require treatment in weeks to months. The response to cytotoxic therapy is poor, and symptomatic therapy with component transfusion and antibiotics, as required, is the preferable management if that approach can sustain a reasonable functional status. If the disease progresses to frank AML and if the patient is fit, standard therapy as for AML is warranted (see Chap. 93). If the patient is over 70 years, attenuation of doses should be considered. Cytarabine combined with anthracycline antibiotics, etoposide, or topotecan have produced remissions in about half of a group of selected patients.[282–289,370] Recovery may be slow, and remissions tend to be short, however. Patients with a poor performance status, in advanced age, or choosing not to be treated with combined-agent chemotherapy have been treated with low-dose cytarabine, 5-azacytidine or decitabine, etoposide, hydroxyurea, retinoids, butyrates, or interferon coupled with transfusion therapy for palliation of the disease (see below). Although occasional patients have improvement, these approaches have been of limited benefit. Patients under 50 years of age with a histocompatible donor should be considered for stem cell transplantation.[290–292] Other patients

---

TABLE 92-2   HYPOCELLULAR MARROW SYNDROMES THAT OCCASSIONALLY PRECEDE ONSET OF ACUTE MYELOGENOUS LEUKEMIA

Amegakaryocytic thrombocytopenia
Chronic hypoplastic neutropenia
Aplastic anemia with evidence of clonal hematopoiesis
Paroxysmal nocturnal hemoglobinuria–aplastic anemia syndrome

including older individuals who achieve a remission may be considered for intensive therapy and autologous stem cell rescue.[293]

LOW-DOSE CYTARABINE

Chemotherapeutic regimens containing standard doses of cytarabine and daunomycin (see Chap. 93) result in remission in fewer than 20 percent of patients with oligoblastic leukemia. Moreover, a proportion of patients are made worse with intensive chemotherapy. The advanced age and the high frequency of cardiac, renal, immunologic, and other organ system impairment in most patients with oligoblastic leukemia are largely responsible for the poor outcome. Patients who are less than 50 years of age have higher remission rates and should undergo intensive therapy. However, such cases represent only about 10 percent of all patients.

Low-dose cytarabine, 5 to 20 mg/m² per day by subcutaneous injection every 12 h for up to 8 to 16 weeks or by continuous intravenous infusion, has been used in lieu of intensive chemotherapy.[294,295] Although this approach has led to remission in about 20 percent of patients with oligoblastic leukemia, the median duration of remission is only about 10 months, and survival has not been prolonged when compared with supportive care alone. Also, in contrast to AML, survival has not been influenced greatly by induction of a remission. Moreover, low-dose cytosine arabinoside is usually cytotoxic, inducing marrow hypoplasia and worsening cytopenias. Often the patient requires hospitalization and blood cell component transfusion and antibiotic treatment analogous to that used for intensive treatment of AML. In some cases, outpatient therapy is possible with self-administration of subcutaneous cytarabine. Although occasional reports of remission following low-dose cytarabine have been consistent with an effect on leukemia cell maturation, most patients experience suppression of the malignant stem cell clone leading to marrow repopulation with polyclonal hemopoiesis.[289,294,295] Combinations of low-dose cytarabine with growth factors have not shown a clear advantage over chemotherapy alone.[295]

5-AZACYTIDINE

This agent is a pyrimidine analogue that inhibits DNA methyltransferase, reduces cytosine methylation, and induces maturation of some leukemic cell lines. It also is an antiproliferative drug. Administration of the drug and its congener, decitabine, has resulted in improvement of some pateients with oligoblastic leukemia.[287,288] 5-azacytidine in a dose of 75 mg/m² once per day given subcutaneously for 7 consecutive days each month provided significantly more frequent benefit to two-thirds of the patients than did supportive care. Quality of life was enhanced, and disease progression was delayed.[288] The drug is available from the National Cancer Institute on the basis of "compassionate use."

OTHER CYTOTOXIC DRUGS

Agents such as hydroxyurea and low-dose etoposide are useful in controlling leukemic cell proliferation but usually produce only partial responses and do not influence survival duration.[296] Occasional patients have achieved remissions with etoposide (50 mg as a 2-h infusion, two to seven times weekly for 4 weeks; or 100 mg per day, orally, for 3 days and then 50 mg twice weekly).[297] Thalidomide has shown effectiveness in early pilot studies. Further trials alone and in combination with other agents are in progress.[369]

RETINOIDS, VITAMIN D DERIVATIVES, OTHER POTENTIALLY MATURATION-ENHANCING AGENTS

Glucocorticoids, vitamin A analogues (retinoids), vitamin D analogues (dihydroxyvitamin D₃), pyrimidine analogues (cytarabine), hexamethylene bisacetamide, and interferons among other agents can induce in vitro maturation of mouse and human leukemic cells.[298–301] The use of 20 to 100 mg/m² of *cis*-retinoic acid, 25 mg/m² of isotretinoin, or 45 mg/m² of all-*trans* retinoic acid, orally, daily for up to 3 months has produced only slight, transient (few weeks) improvement in a very small proportion of patients with oligoblastic leukemia.[302,303] Adverse effects of these vitamin A derivatives include dry skin, cheilitis, pruritus, lethargy, and arthralgia, which usually disappear after discontinuation of the agent.

A regimen including 2.5 μg per day, orally, of dihydroxyvitamin D₃ for at least 8 weeks has not been beneficial in patients with oligoblastic leukemia.[304,305] Hypercalcemia has been a dose-limiting factor. Analogues with less hypercalcemia-inducing capacity such as alphacalcidol have shown some effect on reducing blasts and promoting monocytoid differentiation, while others have been inactive.[306,307]

A combination of low-dose cytarabine, retinoic acid, and 1,25-dihydroxyvitamin D₃ in 44 patients with oligoblastic leukemias produced 50 percent response rates, with longer survival in responders than in nonresponders.[308] Hexamethylene bisacetamide given in a dosage of 20 to 24 g/m² per day intravenously for 10 days followed by an 18- to 75-day observation period produced increased neutrophil counts and reduced marrow blasts in only 4 of 16 patients with oligoblastic leukemia.[301] In another study no responses were observed.[299] Sodium phenylbutarate is an agent that has shown some activity against oligoblastic leukemia and is in early clinical trials.[300]

Amifostine, pentoxifylline, and dexamethasone has shown effectiveness in prolonging survival of patients. The combination is thought to reverse the exaggerated apoptosis of maturing precursor cells.[368]

INTERFERONS

Interferons also have been used to treat oligoblastic leukemia.[309–312] Doses of IFN-α ranged from 3×10^6 units per day to 1×10^6 units/m² three times a week. Occasional reductions in blast percentages or transfusion requirements have occurred at the price of substantial toxicity. AML occurred in some patients. IFN-γ at 0.01 mg to 0.1 mg/m² three times weekly improved counts and reduced blast percentages in about 40 percent of 30 patients with oligoblastic leukemia in one series. Median survivals were no longer than in untreated historical controls, although they were longer than in untreated concurrent patients. Other reports show little effect from interferon treatment.[313,314]

INTERLEUKIN-2

In one case of therapy-related oligoblastic leukemia developing during a third complete remission of ALL, IL-2 given subcutaneously at 2.5 to 8×10^5 IU twice daily for 30 days enhanced natural killer cell activity and eliminated blasts in the marrow.[315] A phase II clinical trial, however, failed to show improvement in blood counts or decrease in transfusion requirement in patients so treated.[316]

ERYTHROPOIETIN, GM-CSF, G-CSF, IL-3, AND IL-11

Randomized, double-blind studies have not shown that any cytokine prolongs survival or reduces morbidity in oligoblastic leukemia, although the results of early studies suggest that (1) erythropoietin occasionally can reduce transfusion requirement, (2) GM-CSF and G-CSF can increase neutrophil counts and functions, and (3) IL-3 can result in increased white cell count and, less frequently, increased red cell and platelet counts.[248–250,317,318,371] Responses have been seen in oligoblastic leukemias as well as in severe refractory anemias. There is no evidence that cytokines can delay emergence of acute leukemia; rather, they increase blast percentages in a proportion of patients, an event that is not always reversible with cessation of the cytokine.[317,318] In one review, 22 of 83 reported cases of myelodysplasia treated with G-CSF or GM-CSF had an increase in marrow blast percentage, and AML developed in 12 of 69 patients. An increased percentage of abnormal macrophages has also been reported.[319] Use of these agents without chemotherapeutics in oligoblastic leukemias carries a risk of accelerating the leukemia.[320] Combinations of growth factors alone or coupled with maturing agents have not significantly improved response or survival rates.[321,322] IL-11 is being studied as a means of increasing the platelet count in patients with myelodysplasia and symptomatic thrombocytopenia.[373]

STEM CELL TRANSPLANTATION

ALLOGENEIC STEM TRANSPLANTATION

This approach has been used to treat various myelodysplastic syndromes in patients from 1 month to 60 years of age.[323–329,372] Conditioning regimens have been cyclophosphamide plus irradiation or busulfan plus cyclophosphamide. Most patients have received transplants from histocompatible sibling donors, although there is some experience with partially mismatched, related, and unrelated donors. A good representation of the results of this approach using marrow stem cells is the study of 93 patients ranging in age from 1 month to over 60 years (median of 30 years), conditioned with cyclophosphamide and total body irradiation or busulfan and cyclophosphamide, and transplanted with an identical twin donor (3 patients), genotypically HLA-identical sibling (62 patients), HLA-matched family member (2 patients), one to three antigen HLA-mismatched family member (20 patients), or unrelated donor marrow (6 patients). Twenty-nine patients were in the refractory anemia category. Forty-seven recipients were in the oligoblastic leukemia category, and the remainder comprised miscellaneous disorders. Most patients received graft-versus-host disease prophylaxis with methotrexate and cyclosporine, with or without prednisone. The most favorable results were in patients less than age 40 years with shorter duration of disease and without blasts. These patients may have a disease-free survival of 60 percent at 4 years and an overall disease-free survival estimated at 40 percent. Older patients had more peritransplant mortality and higher relapse rates. Actuarial relapse probability at 4 years was 30 percent for the entire group and 50 percent for patients with greater than 5 percent marrow blasts. Cytogenetic abnormalities did not predict outcome in this study, but adverse cytogenetics were an important prognostic factor in other studies. Results with unrelated marrow donors are inferior to those for other donor categories.

AUTOLOGOUS STEM CELL INFUSION

Patients with oligoblastic leukemia have been treated with their own stem cells following intensive chemotherapy therapy.[330] The approach is limited by the contamination of the stem cell product with leukemic cells and the absence of a graft-versus-leukemia effect. The absence of a graft-versus-host reaction makes it more applicable to the age group usually affected. In selected patients, peritransplant mortality with intensive therapy and stem cell rescue has been about 10 percent, and about 50 percent of selected patients have had extended survivals.[331] The more advanced the disease at the time of treatment the worse the outcome.

COURSE AND PROGNOSIS

The median survival in published series of patients with oligoblastic leukemia has varied from 6 to 36 months, with a range of survival of individual patients from 1 to 160 months.[332–336] In a very large single series that included refractory anemia as well, the median survival was 15 months.[278] About half the patients died of infection associated with severe neutropenia or with dysfunctional neutrophils and monocytes, and about 25 percent died of bleeding complications of thrombocytopenia. About 30 percent of cases evolved into AML. The length of survival after diagnosis of patients with oligoblastic leukemia is inversely correlated with the severity of the cytogenetic abnormality, the proportion of blast cells in the marrow, the presence of N-RAS mutations, the presence of adverse cytogenetic patterns, and the severity of the neutropenia and thrombocytopenia.[332–336,374,375]

A rare case of spontaneous disappearance of oligoblastic leukemia has been documented.[337]

PRODROMAL SYNDROMES ANTEDATING LYMPHOCYTIC LEUKEMIA

The indolent clonal disorder usually implies a condition that is an antecedent of myelogenous leukemia. AML often begins with a protracted period (weeks to months) of symptoms or signs preceding clinical diagnosis, and a significant proportion of cases are preceded by a myelodysplastic syndrome. Acute lymphocytic leukemia (ALL) usually begins explosively, and it is rare for symptoms to be present for more than a few weeks prior to diagnosis (see Chap. 97). Intermediate syndromes, for example, smoldering or oligoblastic lymphocytic leukemia or prodromal clonal anemias, are rare, but the latter have been reported, especially in adults.[338–342,376]

Apparent aplastic anemia[343–347] or erythroid hypoplasia[348] has been described as an antecedent to ALL in a few children and a rare adult.[348] The aplasia is promptly improved by glucocorticoids, and ALL ensues quickly, usually within 1 to 8 months. The brief interval between remission of aplastic anemia and the onset of leukemia suggests that the leukemia, although inapparent on marrow biopsy, may in some way initiate the aplasia.[347] Remission of aplasia followed shortly by ALL has occurred in the absence of glucocorticoid or other specific therapy in several cases. The aplastic marrow prodrome of ALL may be distinguishable by its very high prevalence in females (about 90 percent), high prevalence of fibrosis on marrow biopsy (about 90 percent), frequent marrow lymphocytosis (about 60 percent), and spontaneous, temporary recovery (greater than 90 percent).[349]

INDOLENT CLONAL MYELOID DISORDERS OR OLIGOBLASTIC (MYELOGENOUS) LEUKEMIA PRECEDING OR EMERGING IN LYMPHOID MALIGNANCIES OTHER THAN ACUTE LYMPHOCYTIC LEUKEMIA

Sideroblastic anemia sometimes associated with qualitative disorders of other blood cell lines (such as thrombopathy) has developed in patients who have had, or later developed, a lymphoproliferative disease such as hairy-cell leukemia, lymphocytic lymphoma, myeloma, chronic lymphocytic leukemia, or Hodgkin's disease.[350–359] The sideroblastic anemia in these cases was not preceded by cytotoxic therapy. Similar associations have been reported in patients who have received chemotherapy or radiotherapy for a lymphoproliferative disease or a solid tumor, and who later developed a preleukemic syndrome presumed to be the result of the prior treatment. Other types of myelodysplasia also can occur concurrent with B- or T-lymphocyte–derived tumors.[350–359]

REFERENCES

1. Heaney ML, Golde DW: Myelodysplasia. *N Engl J Med* 340:1649, 1999.
2. Bennect JM, Catovsky MT, Daniel, MT et al: Proposals for the classification of the myelodysplastic syndromes. *Br J Haematol* 51:184, 1982.
3. Layton DM, Mufti GJ: Myelodysplastic syndromes: their history, evolution, and relation to acute myeloid leukemia. *Blut* 53:423, 1986.
4. Dreyfus B, Rochant H, Sultan C, et al: Les anémies refractaires avec excès de myeloblastes dans la moelle. Etude de onze observations. *La Presse Med* 78:359, 1970.
5. Chevallier P: Sur la terminologie des leucoses et des affection frontieres. *Le Sang* 15:587, 1942–43.

6. Hamilton-Paterson JL: Preleukaemic anemia. *Acta Haematol* 2:309, 1949.

7. Block M, Jacobson LO, Bethard WJ: Preleukemic acute human leukemia. *JAMA* 152:1018, 1953.

8. Vilter RW, Jarrold T, Will JJ, et al: Refractory anemia with hyperplastic bone marrow. *Blood* 15:1, 1960.

9. Schiller M, Rachmilewitz EA, Izak G: Pancytopenia with hypercellular hemopoietic tissue. *Isr J Med Sci* 5:69, 1969.

10. Saarni MI, Linman JW: Preleukemia. *Am J Med* 55:38, 1973.

11. Linman JW, Saarni MI: The preleukemic syndrome. *Semin Hematol* 11:93, 1974.

12. Pierre RV: Preleukemic states. *Semin Hematol* 11:73, 1974.

13. Dreyfus B: Preleukemic states. *Blood Cells* 2:33, 1976.

14. Linman JW, Bagby GC Jr: The preleukemic syndrome: clinical and laboratory features, natural course and management. *Blood Cells* 2:11, 1976.

15. Linman JW, Bagby GC Jr: The preleukemic syndrome (hemopoietic dysplasia). *Cancer* 42:854, 1978.

16. Bessis M, Bernard J: Hematopoietic dysplasias. *Blood Cells* 2:5, 1976.

17. Bennett JM, Catovsky D, Daniel MT, et al: The chronic myeloid leukaemias: guidelines for distinguishing granulocytic, atypical chronic myeloid, and chronc myelomonocytic leukaemia. *Br J Hematol* 87:746, 1994.

18. Van den Berghe H, Lovwagie A, Broeckart-Van Orshoven A, et al: Chromosome analyses in two unusual malignant blood disorders presumably induced by benzene. *Blood* 53:558, 1979.

19. Askoy M, Erdem S: Follow-up study on the mortality and the development of leukemia in 44 pancytopenic patients with chronic exposure to benzene. *Blood* 52:285, 1978.

20. Smith MT, Zhang L: Biomarkers of leukemic risk: benzene as a model. *Environ Health Perspect* 106(suppl 4):937, 1998.

21. Kitahara M, Cosgriff TM, Eyre HJ: Sideroblastic anemia as a preleukemia event in patients treated for Hodgkin's disease. *Ann Intern Med* 92:625, 1980.

22. Pedersen-Bjergaard J, Ersbøll J, Sørensen HM, et al: Risk of acute nonlymphocytic leukemia and preleukemia in patients treated with cyclophosphamide for non-Hodgkin's lymphomas. *Ann Intern Med* 103:195, 1985.

23. Pedersen-Bjergaard J, Osterlind K, Hansen M, et al: Acute nonlymphocytic leukemia, preleukemia and solid tumors following intensive chemotherapy of small cell carcinoma of the lung. *Blood* 66:1393, 1985.

24. Leone G, Mele L, Pulson A, Equitani F, Pagano L: The incidence of secondary leukemia. *Haematologica* 84:937, 1999.

25. Felix CA: Secondary leukemias induced by topoisomerase-targeted drugs. *Biochim Biophys Acta* 1400:233, 1998.

26. Park DJ, Koeffler HP: Therapy-related myelodysplastic syndromes. *Semin Hematol* 33:256, 1996.

27. Rigolin GM, Cuneo A, Roberti MG, et al: Exposure to myelotoxic agents and myelodysplasia: case-control study and correlation with clinicobiological findings. *Br J Haematol* 103:189, 1998.

28. Sterkers Y, Preudhomme C, Lai JL, et al: Acute myeloid leukemia and myelodysplastic syndromes following essential thrombocythemia treated with hydroxyurea: high proportion of cases with 17p deletion. *Blood* 91:616, 1998.

29. Van Den Neste E, Louviaux I, Michaux JL, et al: Myelodysplastic syndrome with monosomy 5 and/or 7 following therapy with 2-chloro-2′-deoxyadenosine. *Br J Haematol* 105:268, 1999.

30. Nakanishi M, Tanaka K, Shintani T, et al: Chromosomal instability in acute myelocytic leukemia and myelodysplastic syndrome patients among atomic bomb survivors. *J Radiat Res (Toyko)* 40:159, 1999.

31. Nowell P, Bergman G, Besa E, et al: Progressive preleukemia with a chromosomally abnormal clone in a kindred with the Estren-Damashek variant of Fanconi's anemia. *Blood* 64:1135, 1984.

32. Alter BP: Fanconi's anemia and malignancies. *Am J Hematol* 53:99, 1996.

33. McNAlly RJO, Rowland D, Roman E, Cartwright RA: Age and sex distributions of hematological malignancies in the U.K. *Hematol Oncol* 15:173, 1997.

34. Aul C, Gatterman N, Schneider W: Age-related incidence and other epidemiologic aspects of myelodysplastic syndrome. *Br J Haematol* 82:358, 1992.

35. Abkowitz JL, Fialkow PJ, Niebrugge DJ, et al: Pancytopenia as a clonal

36. Rasking WH, Tirumali N, Jacobson R, et al: Evidence for a multistep pathogenesis of a myelodysplastic syndrome. *Blood* 63:1318, 1984.

37. Prchal JT, Throckmorton DW, Caroll AJ, et al: A common progenitor for human myeloid and lymphoid cells. *Nature* 274:590, 1978.

38. Mongkonsritragoon W, Letendre L, Li CY: Multiple lymphoid nodules in bone marrow have the same clonality as underlying myelodysplastic syndrome recognized with fluorescent in situ hybridization technique. *Am J Hematol* 59:252, 1998.

39. Fialkow PJ: Cell lineages in hematopoietic neoplasia studied with glucose-6-phosphate dehydrogenase cell markers. *J Cell Physiol J* 1:37, 1982.

40. Janssen JWG, Buschle M, Layton M, et al: Clonal analysis of myelodysplastic syndromes: evidence of multipotent stem cell origin. *Blood* 73:248, 1989.

41. Tefferi A, Thibodeau SN, Solberg LA Jr: Clonal studies in the myelodysplastic syndrome using X-linked restriction fragment length polymorphisms. *Blood* 75:1770, 1990.

42. Gerritsen WR, Donohue J, Bauman J, et al: Clonal analysis of myelodysplastic syndrome: monosomy 7 is expressed in the myeloid lineage but not in the lymphoid lineage as detected by fluorescent in situ hybridization. *Blood* 80:217, 1992.

43. Anastasi J, Fang J, LeBeau MM, et al: Cytogenetic clonality in myelodysplastic syndromes studied with fluorescence in situ hybridization: lineage, response to growth factor therapy, and clone expansion. *Blood* 81:1580, 1993.

44. Culligan DJ, Cachia P, Whittaker A, et al: Clonal lymphocytes are detectable in only some cases of MDS. *Br J Haematol* 81:346, 1992.

45. Abrahamson G, Boultwod J, Madden J, et al: Clonality of cell population in refractory anaemia using combined approach of gene loss and X-linked restricting fragment length polymorphism–methylation analysis. *Br J Haematol* 79:550, 1991.

46. Delforge M, Demuynck H, Verhoef G, et al: Patients with high-risk myelodysplastic syndrome can have polyclonal or clonal haemopoiesis in complete haematological remission. *Br J Haematol* 102:486, 1998.

47. Lawrence HJ, Broudy VC, Magenis RE, et al: Cytogenetic evidence for involvement of B-lymphocytes in acquired idiopathic sideroblastic anemia. *Blood* 70:1003, 1982.

48. Hirai H, Okada M, Mizoguchi H, et al: Relationship between activated N-ras oncogene and chromosomal abnormality during leukemic progression from myelodysplastic syndrome. *Blood* 71:256, 1988.

49. Nakagawa T, Saitoh S, Imoto S, et al: Multiple point mutation of N-ras and K-ras oncogenes in myelodysplastic syndrome and acute myelogenous leukemia. *Oncology* 49:114, 1992.

50. VanKamp H, dePijper C, Verlaan-de Vries M, et al: Longitudinal analysis of point mutations of the N-ras protooncogene in patients with myelodysplasia using archival blood smears. *Blood* 79:1266, 1992.

51. Paquette RL, Landau EM, Pierre RV, et al: N-ras mutations are associated with poor prognosis and increased risk of leukemia in myelodysplastic syndrome. *Blood* 82:590, 1993.

52. Bartram CR: Molecular genetic aspects of myelodysplastic syndromes. *Semin Hematol* 33:139, 1996.

53. Parker J, Mufti GJ: Ras and myelodysplasia: lessons from the last decade. *Semin Hematol* 33:206, 1996.

54. Padua RA, Guinn BA, Al-Sabah AI, et al: RAS, FMS and p53 mutations and poor clinical outcome in myelodysplasias: a 10-year follow-up. *Leukemia* 12:887, 1998.

55. Plata E, Viniou N, Abazis D, et al: Cytogenetic analysis and RAS mutations in primary myelodysplastic syndromes. *Cancer Genet Cytogenet* 111:124, 1999.

56. Quesnel B, Guillerm G, Vereecque R, et al: Methylation of the p15 (INK4b) gene in myelodysplastic syndromes is frequent and acquired during disease progression. *Blood* 91:2985, 1998.

57. Koeffler HP, Golde DW: Human preleukemia. *Ann Intern Med* 93:347, 1980.

58. Raza A, Gezer S, Mundle S, et al: Apoptosis in bone marrow biopsy samples involving stromal and hematopoietic cells in 50 patients with myelodysplastic syndromes. *Blood* 86:268, 1995.

59. Rajapaksa R, Ginzton N, Rott LS, Greenberg PL: Altered oncoprotein expression and apoptosis in myelodysplastic syndrome marrow cells. *Blood* 88:4275, 1996.

disorder of a multipotent hemopoietic stem cell. *J Clin Invest* 73:258, 1984.

60. Greenberg PL: Apoptosis and its role in the myelodysplastic syndromes: implications for disease natural history and treatment. *Leuk Res* 22:1123, 1998.

61. Raza A, Alvi S, Broady-Robinson L, et al: Cell cycle kinetic studies in 68 patients with myelodysplastic syndromes following intravenous iodo-and/or bromodeoxyuridine. *Exp Hematol* 25:530, 1997.

62. Gersuk GM, Beckham C, Loken MR, et al: A role for tumour necrosis factor-alpha, Fas and Fas-Ligand in marrow failure associated with myelodysplastic syndrome. *Br J Haematol* 103:176, 1998.

63. Mundle SD, Ali A, Cartlidge JD, et al: Evidence for involvement of tumor necrosis factor-alpha in apoptotic death of bone marrow cells in myelodysplastic syndromes. *Am J Hematol* 60:36, 1999.

64. Parker JE, Fishlock KL, Mijovic A, Czepulkowski B, Pagliuca A, Mufti GJ: "Low-risk" myelodysplastic syndrome is associated with excessive apoptosis and an increased ratio of pro- versus anti-apoptotic bcl-2-related proteins. *Br J Haematol* 103:1075, 1998.

65. Groupe Francais de Morphologie Hématologique: French registry of acute leukemia and myelodysplastic syndromes. *Cancer* 60:1385, 1987.

66. Luna-Fineman S, Shannon KM, Atwater SK, et al: Myelodysplastic and myeloproliferative disorders of childhood: a study of 167 patients. *Blood* 93:459, 1999.

67. Hasle H, Jacobsen BB, Pedersen NT: Myelodysplastic syndromes in childhood: a population-based study of nine cases. *Br J Haematol* 81:495, 1992.

68. Gadner H, Haas OA: Experience in pediatric myelodysplastic syndrome. *Hematol Oncol Clin North Am* 6:655, 1992.

69. Martinez-Climent JA, Garcia-Conde J: Chromosomal rearrangements in childhood acute myeloid leukemia and myelodysplastic syndromes. *J Pediatr Hematol Oncol* 2191. 1999

70. Li FP, Marchetto DJ, Vawter FG: Acute leukemia and preleukemia in eight males in a family: an X-linked disorder? *Am J Hematol* 6:61, 1979.

71. Horwitz M, Sabath DE, Smithson WA, Radich J: A family inheriting different subtypes of acute myelogenous leukemia. *Am J Hematol* 52:295, 1996.

72. Noel P, Solberg LA Jr: Myelodysplastic syndromes: pathogenesis, diagnosis and treatment. *Crit Rev Oncol Hematol* 12:193, 1992.

73. Ahmad YH, Kiehl R, Papac RJ: Myelodysplasia. The clinical spectrum of 51 patients. *Cancer* 76:869, 1995.

74. Zanger B, Dorsey HN: Fever—a manifestation of preleukemia. *JAMA* 236:1266, 1976.

75. Varela BL, Chuang C, Woll JE, Bennett JM: Modifications in the classification of primary myelodysplastic syndrome. *Hematol Oncol* 3:55, 1985.

76. Saxne T, Turesson I, Wallheim FA: Preleukemic syndrome simulating SLE. *Acta Med Scand* 212:421, 1982.

77. Hebbar M, Hebbar-Savean K, Fenaux P: Systemic diseases in myelodysplastic syndromes. *Rev Med Intern* 16:897, 1995.

78. Dezza L, Cazzola M, Bergamaschi G, et al: Myelodysplastic syndrome with monosomy 7 in adulthood. *Haematologia* 68:723, 1983.

79. Montecucco C, Cazzola M, Ascari E: Diabetes insipidus in the preleukaemic phase of acute non-lymphocytic leukaemia. *Scand J Haematol* 33:326, 1985.

80. Zijlstra F, Killinger D, Volpe R: Diabetes insipidus associated with dysplastic pancytopenia. *Am J Med* 82:339, 1987.

81. Sweet RD: Acute neutrophilic dermatosis 1978. *Br J Dermatol* 100:93, 1979.

82. Soppi E, Nousiainen T, Seppa A, et al: Acute febrile neutrophilic dermatosis (Sweet's syndrome) in association with myelodysplastic syndromes: a report of three cases and a review of the literature. *Br J Haematol* 73:43, 1989.

83. Arbetter KR, Hubbard KW, Markovic SN, et al: Case of granulocyte colony-stimulating factor-induced Sweet's syndrome. *Am J. Hematol* 61:126, 1999.

84. Arun B, Berberian B, Azumi N, et al: Sweets during treatment with all-trans retinoic acid in a patient with acute promyelocytic leukemia. *Leuk Lymph* 31:613, 1998.

85. Avi I, Rosenbaum H, Levy Y, Rowe J: Myelodysplastic syndrome and associated skin lesions: a review of the literature. *Leuk Res* 23:323, 1999.

86. Weber RFA, Geraedts JPM, Kerkhofs H, Leeksma CHW: The preleukemic syndrome. *Acta Med Scand* 207:391, 1980.

87. Ohno E, Ohtsuka E, Watanabe K, et al: Behcet's disease associated with myelodysplastic syndromes. A case report and a review of the literature. *Cancer* 79:262, 1997.

88. Komatsuda A, Miura I, Ohtani H, et al: Crescentic glomerulonephritis accompanied by myeloperoxidase-antineutrophil cytoplasmic antibodies in a patient having myelodysplastic syndrome with trisomy 7. *Am J Kidney Dis* 31:336, 1998.

89. Saitoh T, Murakami H, Uchiumi H, et al: Myelodysplastic syndromes with nephrotic syndrome. *Am J Hematol* 60:200, 1999.

90. Harewood GC, Loftus EV Jr, Tefferi A, et al: Concurrent inflammatory bowel disease and myelodysplastic syndromes. *Inflamm Bowel Dis* 5:98, 1999.

91. Clark RE, Payne HE, Jacobs A: Primary myelodysplastic syndrome and cancer. *Br Med J* 294:937, 1987.

92. Sans-Sabrafen J, Buxó-Costa J, Woessner S, et al: Myelodysplastic syndromes and malignant solid tumors. *Am J Hematol* 41:1, 1992.

93. Florensa L, Vallespi T, Woessner S, et al: Incidence and characteristics of lymphoid malignancies in untreated myelodysplastic syndromes. *Leuk Lymphoma* 23:609, 1996.

94. Mitterbauer G, Schwarzmeier J, Mitterbauer M, Jaeger U, Fritsch G, Schwarzinger I: Myelodysplastic syndrome/acute myeloid leukemia supervening previously untreated chronic B-lymphocytic leukemia: demonstration of the concomitant presence of two different malignant clones by immunologic and molecular analysis. *Ann Hematol* 74:193, 1997.

95. Craig JE, Sampietro M, Oscier DG, et al: Myelodysplastic syndrome with karyotype abnormality is associated with elevated F-cell production. *Br J Haematol* 93:601, 1996.

96. Kornberg A, Goldfarb A: Preleukemia manifested by hemolytic anemia with pyruvate-kinase deficiency. *Arch Intern Med* 146:785, 1986.

97. Heimstadter V, Arnold H, Blume KG, et al: Acquired pyruvate kinase deficiency with hemolysis in preleukemia. *Acta Haematol* 57:339, 1977.

98. Lopez M, Bonnet-Gajdos M, Reviron M, et al: Acute leukemia augured before clinical signs by blood group antigen abnormalities and low levels of A and H blood group transferase activities in erythrocytes. *Br J Haematol* 63:535, 1986.

99. Harris JW, Koscick R, Lazarus HM, et al: Leukemia arising out of paroxysmal nocturnal hemoglobinuria. *Leuk Lymph* 32:401, 1999.

100. Anagnou NP, Ley TJ, Chesbro B, et al: Acquired α-thalassemia in preleukemia is due to decreased expression of all four α-globin genes. *Proc Natl Acad Sci USA* 80:6051, 1983.

101. Helder J, Deisseroth A: S1 nuclease analysis of α-globin gene expression in preleukemic patients with acquired hemoglobin H disease after transfer to mouse erythroleukemia cells. *Proc Natl Acad Sci USA* 84:2387, 1987.

102. Economopoulos T, Stathakis N, Maragoyannis Z, et al: Myelodysplastic syndrome. Clinical significance of monocyte concentration, degree of blastic infiltration and ring sideroblasts. *Acta Haematol* 65:97, 1981.

103. Jaworkowsky LI, Solovey DY, Rhausova LY, Udris OY: Monocytosis as a sign of subsequent leukemia in patients with cytopenias (preleukemia). *Folia Hematol* 110:395, 1983.

104. Friedland ML, Ward H, Wittels EG, Arlin ZA: A monocytic leukemoid reaction: a manifestation of preleukemia. *Rhode Island Med J* 68:173, 1985.

105. Kuriyama K, Tomonaga M, Matsuo T, et al: Diagnostic significance of pseudo-Pelger-Huët anomalies and micro-megakaryocytes in myelodysplastic syndrome. *Br J Haematol* 63:665, 1986.

106. Langenhuijsen MMAC: Neutrophils with ring-shaped nuclei in myeloproliferative disease. *Br J Haematol* 58:227, 1984.

107. Clark RE, Smith SA, Jacobs A: Myeloid surface antigen abnormalities in myelodysplasia: relation to prognosis and modification by 13-cis retinoic acid. *J Clin Pathol* 40:652, 1987.

108. Cech P, Markert M, Perrin LH: Partial myeloperoxidase deficiency in preleukemia. *Blut* 47:21, 1983.

109. Schofield KP, Stone PCW, Kelsey P, et al: Quantitative cytochemistry of blood neutrophils in myelodysplastic syndromes and chronic granulocytic leukaemia. *Cell Biochem Funct* 1:92, 1983.

110. Elghetany MT, Peterson B, MacCallum J, et al: Deficiency of neutrophilic granule membrane glycoproteins in the myelodysplastic syndromes: a common deficiency in 216 patients studied by the Cancer and Leukemia Group B. *Leuk Res* 21:801, 1997.

111. Ruutu P: Granulocyte function in myelodysplastic syndromes. *Scand J Haematol* 36(suppl 45):66, 1986.

112. Prodan M, Tulissi P, Perticarari S, et al: Flow cytometric assay for the

evaluation of phagocytosis and oxidative burst of polymorphonuclear leukocytes and monocytes in myelodysplastic disorders. *Haematologica* 80:212, 1995.

113. Piva E, De Toni S, Caenazzo A, Pradella M, Pietrogrande F, Plebani M: Neutrophil NADPH oxidase activity in chronic myeloproliferative and myelodysplastic diseases by microscopic and photometric assays. *Acta Haematol* 94:16, 1995.

114. Carulli G, Sbrana S, Minnucci S, et al: Actin polymerization in neutrophils from patients affected by myelodysplastic syndromes—a flow cytometric study. *Leuk Res* 21:513, 1997.

115. Nakaseko C, Asai T, Wakita H, Oh H, Saito Y: Signalling defect in FMLP-induced neutrophil respiratory burst in myelodysplastic syndromes. *Br J Haematol* 95:482, 1996.

116. Pamphilon DH, Aparicio SR, Roberts BE, et al: The myelodysplastic syndromes—a study of haemostatic function and platelet ultrastructure. *Scand J Haematol* 33:486, 1984.

117. Payne CM, Glasser L: An ultrastructural morphometric analysis of platelet grant and fusion granules. *Blood* 67:299, 1986.

118. Rasi V, Lintula R: Platelet-function in the myelodysplastic syndromes. *Scand J Haematol* 36(suppl 45):71, 1986.

119. Hamblin TJ: Immunological abnormalities in myelodysplastic syndromes. *Semin Hematol* 33:150, 1996.

120. Anderson RW, Volsky DJ, Greenberg B, et al: Lymphocyte abnormalities in preleukemia. I. Decreased NK activity, anomalous immunoregulatory cell subsets and deficient EBV receptors. *Leuk Res* 7:389, 1983.

121. Kerndrup G, Meyer K, Ellegaard J, Hokland P: Natural killer (NK)-cell activity and antibody-dependent cellular cytotoxicity (ADCC) in primary preleukemic syndrome. *Leuk Res* 8:239, 1984.

122. Takagi S, Kitagawa S, Takeda A, et al: Natural killer—interferon system in patients with preleukaemic states. *Br J Haematol* 58:71, 1984.

123. Volsky DJ, Anderson RW: Deficiency in Epstein-Barr virus receptors on B lymphocytes of preleukemia patients. *Cancer Res* 43:3923, 1983.

124. Knox SJ, Greenberg BR, Anderson RW, Rosenblatt LS: Studies of T lymphocytes in preleukemic disorders and acute nonlymphocytic leukemia: in vitro radiosensitivity, mitogenic responsiveness, colony formation, and enumeration of lymphocytic subpopulations. *Blood* 61:449, 1983.

125. Baumann MA, Milson TJ, Patrick CW, et al: Immunoregulatory abnormalities in myelodysplastic disorders. *Am J Hematol* 22:17, 1986.

126. Economopoulos T, Economidou J, Giannopoulos G, et al: Immune abnormalities in myelodysplastic syndromes. *J Clin Pathol* 38:908, 1985.

127. Mufti GJ, Figes A, Hamblin TJ, et al: Immunological abnormalities in myelodysplastic syndromes. *Br J Haematol* 63:143, 1986.

128. Tricot G, DeWolf-Peeters C, Vlietinck R, Verwilghen RL: The importance of bone marrow biopsy in myelodysplastic disorders. *Bibl Hematol* 50:31, 1984.

129. Frisch B, Bartol R: Bone marrow histology in myelodysplastic syndromes. *Scand J Haematol* 36(suppl 45):21, 1986.

130. Delacretaz F, Schmidt PM, Piguet D, et al: Histopathology and myelodysplastic syndromes: the FAB classification (proposals) applied to bone marrow biopsy. *Am J Clin Pathol* 87:180, 1987.

131. Fohlmeister I, Fischer R, Modder B, et al: Aplastic anemia and hypocellular myelodysplastic syndrome. *J Clin Pathol* 38:1218, 1985.

132. Reizenstein P, Lagerlof B, Skarberg KO, et al: Alterations in erythropoiesis preceding leukemia. *Acta Haematol* 54:152, 1975.

133. Hast R: Studies on preleukemia. II. Clinical and prognostic significance of sideroblasts in regenerative anaemia with hypercellular bone marrow. *Scand J Haematol* 21:396, 1978.

134. Hast R, Reizenstein P: Sideroblastic anemia and development of leukemia. *Blut* 42:203, 1981.

135. Tricot G, Vlietinck R, Boogaerts MA, et al: Prognostic factors in the myelodysplastic syndromes: importance of initial data on peripheral blood counts, bone marrow cytology, trephine biopsy, and chromosomal analysis. *Br J Haematol* 60:19, 1985.

136. Tricot G, DeWolf-Peeters C, Vlietinck R, Verwilghen RL: Bone marrow histology in myelodysplastic syndromes. II. Prognostic value of ALIP in MDS. *Br J Haematol* 58:217, 1984. 151.

137. Smith WB, Ablin A, Goodman JR, Brecher J: Atypical megakaryocytes in the preleukemic phase of AML. *Blood* 42:535, 1973.

138. Queisser W, Queisser U, Ansmann M, et al: Megakaryocyte polypoloidization in acute leukemia and preleukemia. *Br J Haematol* 28:261, 1974.

139. Bartl R, Frisch B, Baumgart R: Morphologic classification of the myelo-

dysplastic syndromes (MDS): combined utilization of bone marrow aspiratres and trephine biopsies. *Leuk Res* 16:15, 1992.

140. Maschek H, Georgii A, Kaloutsi V, et al: Myelofibrosis in primary myelodysplastic syndromes: a retrospective study of 352 patients. *Eur J Haematol* 148:208, 1992.

141. Greenberg PL: Biologic and clinical implications of marrow culture studies in the myelodysplastic syndromes. *Semin Hematol* 33:163, 1996.

142. Chui DHK, Clarke BJ: Abnormal erythroid progenitor cells in human preleukemia. *Blood* 60:362, 1982.

143. Senn JS, Messner HA, Pinkerton PH, et al: Peripheral blood blast cell progenitors in human preleukemia. *Blood* 59:106, 1982.

144. Juvonen E, Partanen S, Knuutila S, Ruutu T: Megakaryocyte colony formation by bone marrow progenitors in myelodysplastic syndrome. *Br J Haematol* 63:331, 1986.

145. Lidbeck J: In vitro colony and cluster growth haemopoietic dysplasia (the preleukaemic syndrome). I. Clinical correlations. *Scand J Haematol* 24:412, 1980.

146. Raymakers R, DeWitte T, Joziasse J, et al: In vitro growth pattern and differentiation predict for progression of myelodysplastic syndromes to acute nonlymphocytic leukemia. *Br J Haematol* 78:35, 1991.

147. Konwalinka G, Peschel C, Schmalzl F, et al: CFU-GM assay, cytochemical and electron microscopic studies in agar in patients with preleukemia syndrome and aplastic anemia. *Int J Cell Cloning* 3:367, 1985.

148. Koeffler HP, Golde DW: Cellular maturation in human preleukemia. *Blood* 52:355, 1978.

149. Cambier N, Baruchel A, Schlageter MH, et al: Chronic myelomonocytic leukemia: from biology to therapy. *Hematol Cell Ther* 39:41, 1997.

150. Aul C, Gatterman N, Schneider W: Comparison of in vitro growth characteristics of blast cell progenitors (CFU-BL) in patients with myelodysplastic syndromes and acute myeloid leukemia. *Blood* 80:625, 1992.

151. Flores-Figueroa E, Gutierrez-Espindola G, Guerrero-Rivera S, Pizzuto-Chavez J, Mayani H: Hematopoietic progenitor cells from patients with myelodysplastic syndromes: in vitro colony growth and long-term proliferation. *Leuk Res* 23:385, 1999.

152. Sato T, Kim S, Selleri C, Young NS, Maciejewski JP: Measurement of secondary colony formation after 5 weeks in long-term cultures in patients with myelodysplastic syndrome. *Leukemia* 12:1187, 1998.

153. Aizawa S, Nakano M, Iwase O, et al: Bone marrow stroma from refractory anemia of myelodysplastic syndrome is defective in its ability to support normal CD34-positive cell proliferation and differentiation in vitro. *Leuk Res* 23:239, 1999.

154. Janowska-Wieczorek A, Bilch AR, Jacobs A: Increased circulating colony-stimulating factor-1 in patients with preleukemia, leukemia, and lymphoid malignancies. *Blood* 77:1796, 1991.

155. Verhoef GEG, DeSchouder P, Ceuppens JL: Measurement of serum cytokine levels in patients with myelodysplastic syndromes. *Leukemia* 6:1268, 1992.

156. Bowen D, Yancik S, Bennett L, et al: Serum stem cell factor concentration in patients with myelodysplastic syndromes. *Br J Haematol* 85:63, 1993.

157. Zwierzina H, Anderson JE, Rollinger-Holzinger I, Torok-Storb B, Nuessler V, Lyman SD: Endogenous FLT-3 ligand serum levels are associated with disease stage in patients with myelodysplastic syndromes. *Leukemia* 13:553, 1999.

158. Tamura H, Ogata K, Luo S, et al: Plasma thrombopoietin (TPO) levels and expression of TPO receptor on platelets in patients with myelodysplastic syndromes. *Br J Haematol* 103:778, 1998.

159. Parlier V, van Melle G, Beris Ph, et al: Hematologic, clinical, and cytogenetic analysis in 109 patients with primary myelodysplastic syndrome. *Cancer Genet Cytogenet* 78:219, 1994.

160. Jacobs RH, Cornbleet MA, Vordiman JW, et al: Prognostic implications of morphology and karyotype in primary myelodysplastic syndromes. *Blood* 67:1765, 1986.

161. de Greef GE, Hagemeijer A: Molecular and cytogenetic abnormalities in acute myeloid leukemia and myelodysplastic syndromes. *Ballière's Clin Hematol* 9:1, 1996.

162. Fenaux P, Morel P, Lai JL: Cytogenetics of myelodysplastic syndromes. *Semin Hematol* 33:127, 1996.

163. Solé F, Prieto L, Badia L, et al: Cytogenetic studies in 112 cases of untreated myelodysplastic syndromes. *Cancer Genet Cytogenet* 64:12, 1992.

164. Estey E, Trujillo JM, Cork A, et al: AML-associated cytogenetic abnor-

malities (inv 16), del (16), t(8;21) in patients with myelodysplastic syndromes. *Hematol Pathol* 6:43, 1992.

165. Pedersen-Bjergaard J, Pedersen M, Roulston D, Philip P: Different genetic pathways in leukemogenesis for patients presenting with therapy-related myelodysplasia and therapy-related acute myeloid leukemia. *Blood* 86:3542, 1995.

166. Jotterand M, Parlier V: Diagnostic and prognostic significance of cytogenetics in adult primary myelodysplastic syndromes. *Leuk Lymphoma* 23:253, 1996.

167. Zhang L, Rothman N, Wang Y, et al: Increased aneusomy and long arm deletion of chromosomes 5 and 7 in the lymphocytes of chinese workers exposed to benzene. *Carcinogenesis* 19:1955, 1998.

168. Nimer SD, Golde DW: The 5q- abnormality. *Blood* 70:1705, 1987.

169. Boultwood J, Fidler C, Soularue P, et al: Novel genes mapping to the critical region of the 5q-syndrome. *Genomics* 45:88, 1997.

170. Antillon F, Raimondi SC, Fairman J, et al: 5q- in a child with refractory anemia with excess blasts: similarities to 5q-syndrome in adults. *Cancer Genet Cytogenet* 105:119, 1998.

171. Horrigan SK, Westbrook CA, Kim AH, Banerjee M, Stock W, Larson RA: Polymerase chain reaction-based diagnosis of del (5q) in acute myeloid leukemia and myelodysplastic syndrome identifies a minimal deletion interval. *Blood* 88:2665, 1996.

172. Huebner K, Isobe M, Croce CM, et al: The human gene encoding GM-CSF is at 5q21–q32, the chromosome region deleted in the 5q-anomaly. *Science* 230:1281, 1985.

173. LeBeau MM: Deletions of chromosome 5 in malignant myeloid disorders. *Cancer Surv* 15:143, 1992.

174. Morris SW, Valentine MB, Shapiro DN, et al: Reassignment of the human CSF1 gene to chromosome 1p13–p21. *Blood* 78:2013, 1991.

175. Nienhuis AW, Bunn HF, Turner PH, et al: Expression of the human c-fms proto-oncogene in hematopoietic cells and its deletion in the 5q-syndrome. *Cell* 42:421, 1985.

176. LeBeau MM, Westbrook CA, Diaz MO, et al: Evidence for the involvement of GM-CSF and FMS in the deletion (5q) in myeloid disorders. *Science* 231:984, 1986.

177. Willman CL, Sever CE, Pallavicini MG, et al: Deletion of IRF-1, mapping to chromosome 5q31.1, in human leukemia and preleukemic myelodysplasia. *Science* 259:968, 1993.

178. Boultwood J, Fidler C, Lewis S, et al: Allelic loss of IRF1 in myelodysplasia and acute myeloid leukemia: retention of IRF1 on the 5q-chromosome in some patients with the 5q-syndrome. *Blood* 82:2611, 1993.

179. Jaju RJ, Boultwood J, Oliver FJ, et al: Molecular cytogenetic delineation of the critical deleted region in the 5q-syndrome. *Genes Chromosomes Cancer* 22:251, 1998.

180. Boultwood J, Fidler C, Lewis S, et al: Allelic loss of IRF1 in myelodysplasia and acute myeloid leukemia: retention of IRF1 on the 5q-chromosome in some patients with the 5q-syndrome. *Blood* 82:2611, 1993.

181. Harada H, Kitagawa M, Tanaka N, et al: Anti-oncogenic and oncogenic potentials of interferon regulatory factors-1 and -2. *Science* 259:971, 1993.

182. Pedersen B, Jensen IM: Clinical and prognostic implications of chromosome 5q deletions: 96 high-resolution-studied patients. *Leukemia* 5:566, 1991.

183. Mathew P, Tefferi A, Dewald GW, et al: The 5q-syndrome. A single-institution study of 43 consecutive patients. *Blood* 81:1040, 1993.

184. Michiels JJ, Mallios-Zorbala H, Prins MEF, et al: Simple monosomy 7 and myelodysplastic syndrome in thirteen patients without previous cytostatic treatment. *Br J Haematol* 64:425, 1986.

185. Pasquali F, Bernasconi P, Cosalone R, et al: Pathogenetic significance of "pure" monosomy 7 in myeloproliferative disorders. Analysis of 14 cases. *Hum Genet* 62:40, 1982.

186. Dohner K, Brown J, Hehmann U, et al: Molecular cytogenetic characterization of a critical region in bands 7q35-q36 commonly deleted in malignant myeloid disorders. *Blood* 92:4031, 1998.

187. Sessarego M, Fugazza G, Gobbi M, et al: Complex structural involvement of chromosome 7 in primary myelodysplastic syndromes determined by fluorescence in situ hybridization. *Cancer Genet Cytogenet* 106:110, 1998.

188. Hayashi Y, Egushi M, Sugita K, et al: Cytogenetic findings and clinical features in acute leukemia and transient myeloproliferation disorder in Down's syndrome. *Blood* 72:15, 1988.

189. Berger R, LeConiat M, Schaison G: Chromosome abnormalities in bone marrow of Fanconi anemia patients. *Cancer Genet Cytogenet* 65:47, 1993.

190. Bernstein R, Philip P, Ueshima Y: Fourth international workshop on chromosomes in leukemia, 1982. Abnormalities of chromosome 7 resulting in monosomy 7 or in deletion of the long arm (7q-): review of translocations, breakpoints, and associated abnormalities. *Cancer Genet Cytogenet* 11:300, 1984.

191. Smadja N, Krulik M, DeGramont A, et al: Translocation 1;7 in preleukemic states. *Cancer Genet Cytogenet* 18:189, 1985.

192. Woloschak GF, Dewald GW, Gahn RS, et al: Amplification of RNA and DNA specific for erb B in unbalanced 1;7 chromosomal translocation associated with myelodysplastic syndrome. *J Cell Biochem* 32:23, 1986.

193. Canellos GP, Whang-Peng J: Philadelphia-chromosome-positive preleukemic state. *Lancet* 2:1227, 1972.

194. Roth DG, Richman CM, Rowley JD: Chronic myelodysplastic syndrome (preleukemia) with the Philadelphia chromosome. *Blood* 56:262, 1980.

195. Bjorkman SE: Chronic refractory anemia with sideroblastic bone marrow. A study of four cases. *Blood* 11:250, 1956.

196. Caroli J, Bernard J, Bessis M, et al: Hémochromatoses avec anémie hypochrome et absence d'hémoglobine anormale. *Presse Med* 65:1991, 1957.

197. Singh AK, Shinton NK, Williams JDF: Ferrokinetic abnormalities and their significance in patients with sideroblastic anaemia. *Br J Haematol* 18:67, 1970.

198. Barry WE, Day HJ: Refractory sideroblastic anemia: clinical and hematologic study of ten cases. *Ann Intern Med* 61:1029, 1964.

199. Kushner JP, Lee GR, Wintrobe MM, et al: Idiopathic refractory sideroblastic anemia. *Medicine* 50:139, 1971.

200. Geschke W, Beutler E: Refractory sideroblastic and non-sideroblastic anemia. *West J Med* 127:85, 1977.

201. Cotter PD, May A, Fitzsimons EJ, et al: Late-onset X-linked sideroblastic anemia. Missense mutations in the erythroid delta-aminolevulinate synthase (ALAS2) gene in two pyridoxine-responsive patients initially diagnosed with acquired refractory anemia and ringed sideroblasts. *J Clin Invest* 96:2090, 1995.

202. Gattermann N, Retzlaff S, Wang YL, et al: A heteroplasmic point mutation of mitochondrial tRNALeu(CUN) in non-lymphoid haemopoietic cell lineages from a patient with acquired idiopathic sideroblastic anaemia. *Br J Haematol* 93:845, 1996.

203. Bowen DT, Jacobs A: Primary acquired sideroblastic erythropoiesis in non-anaemic and minimally anaemic subjects. *J Clin Pathol* 42:56, 1989.

204. Beris PH, Graf J, Miescher PA: Primary acquired sideroblastic and primary acquired refractory anemia. *Semin Hematol* 20:101, 1983.

205. Garand R, Gardars J, Bizet M, et al: Heterogeneity of acquired idiopathic sideroblastic anema (AISA). *Leuk Res* 16:463, 1992.

206. Kitahara M, Cosgriff TM, Eyre HJ: Sideroblastic anemia as a preleukemic event in patients treated for Hodgkin's disease. *Ann Intern Med* 92:625, 1980.

207. Kardos G, Veerman AJ, de Waal FC, van Oudheusden LJ, Slater R: Familial sideroblastic anemia with emergence of monosomy 5 and myelodysplastic syndrome. *Med Pediatr Oncol* 26:54, 1996.

208. Yoshida Y, Oguma S, Tohyama K, et al: Diagnostic and biological significance of sideroblastic erythropoiesis in the myelodysplastic syndromes. *Int J Hematol* 67:137, 1998.

209. Mecucci C, VanOrshoven A, Vermaelen K, et al: 11 q-chromosome is associated with abnormal iron stores in myelodysplastic syndromes. *Cancer Genet Cytogenet* 27:39, 1987.

210. Schulman P, Kardon N, Weiner R, et al: Acquired idiopathic sideroblastic anemia: a new chromosomal abnormality. *Cancer Genet Cytogenet* 9:341, 1983.

211. Bitran J, Golomb H, Rowley J: Idiopathic refractory sideroblastic anemia: banded chromosome analysis in six patients. *Acta Haematol* 57:15, 1977.

212. Berrebi A, Bruck R, Shtalrid M, Chemke J: Philadelphia chromosome in idiopathic acquired sideroblastic anemia. *Acta Haematol* 72:343, 1984.

213. Carroll AJ, Poon M-C, Robinson NC, Christ WM: Sideroblastic anemia associated with thrombocytosis and a chromosome 3 abnormality. *Cancer Genet Cytogenet* 22:183, 1986.

214. Bennett DD, Stanley WS, Johnson CB: Combined phenotypic and genotypic analysis of ringed sideroblasts in acquired idiopathic sideroblastic anemia. *Acta Haematol* 73:235, 1985.

215. Dewald GW, Pierre RV, Phyliky RL: Three patients with structurally

abnormal X chromosomes, each with X q13 breakpoints and a history of idiopathic acquired sideroblastic anemia. *Blood* 59:100, 1982.

216. DeWald GW, Brecher M, Travis LB, Stupea PJ: Twenty-six patients with hematologic disorders and X-chromosome abnormalities. *Cancer Genet Cytogenet* 42:173, 1989.

217. Chabannori G, Molina L, Pegouri-Bandelier B, et al: A review of 76 patients with myelodysplastic syndromes treated with danazol. *Cancer* 73:3073, 1994.

218. Musto P, Catalano L, Andriani A, et al: Recombinant erythropoietin for refractory anemia with ring sideroblasts. *Hematologia* 77:185, 1992.

219. Hellstrom-Lindberg E, Ahlgren T, Beguin Y, et al: Treatment of anemia in myelodysplastic syndromes with granulocyte colony-stimulating factor plus erythropoietin: results from a randomized phase II study and long-term follow-up of 71 patients. *Blood* 92:68, 1998.

220. Cazzola M, Barosi G, Gobbi PG, et al: Natural history of idiopathic refractory sideroblastic anemia. *Blood* 71:305, 1988.

221. Cartwright GE, Edwards CG, Skolnick MH, Amos BD: Association of HLA-linked hemochromatosis with idiopathic refractory sideroblastic anemia. *J Clin Invest* 65:980, 1980.

222. Beris P, Samii K, Darbellay R, et al: Iron overload in patients with sideroblastic anaemia is not related to the presence of the haemochromatosis Cys282Tyr and His63Asp mutations. *Br J Haematol* 104:97, 1999.

223. Weintraub LR, Conrad ME, Crosby WH: Iron-loading anemia. Treatment with repeated phlebotomy and pyridoxine. *N Engl J Med* 175:169, 1966.

224. French TJ, Jacobs P: Sideroblastic anemia associated with iron overload treated by repeated phlebotomy. *S Afr Med J* 50:594, 1976.

225. Jensen PD, Heickendorff L, Pedersen B, et al: The effect of iron chelation on haemopoiesis in MDS patients with transfusional iron overload. *Br J Haematol* 94:288, 1996.

226. Lewy RI, Kansu E, Gabuzda T: Leukemia in patients with acquired idiopathic sideroblastic anemia. *Am J Hematol* 6:323, 1979.

227. Cheng DS, Kushner JP, Wintrobe MM: Idiopathic refractory sideroblastic anemia. Incidence and risk factors for leukemic transformation. *Cancer* 44:724, 1979.

228. Hast R, Reizenstein P: Sideroblastic anemia and development of leukemia. *Blut* 42:203, 1981.

229. Streeter RR, Presant CA, Reinhard E: Prognostic significance of thrombocytosis in idiopathic sideroblastic anemia. *Blood* 50:427, 1977.

230. Barton JC, Conrad ME, Parmley R: Acute lymphoblastic leukemia in idiopathic refractory sideroblastic anemia. *Am J Hematol* 9:109, 1980.

231. Cazzola M, Barosi G, Gobbi PG: Natural history of idiopathic refractory sideroblastic anemia. *Blood* 71:305, 1988.

232. Gatterman N, Aul C, Schneider W: Two types of acquired idopathic sideroblastic anemia (AISA). *Br J Haematol* 74:45, 1990.

233. Greenberg P, Cox C, LeBeau MM, et al: International scoring system for evaluating prognosis in myelodysplastic syndromes. *Blood* 89:2079, 1997.

234. Feuaux P, Estienne MH, Lepelley P, et al: Refractory anemia according to the FAB classification: a report on 69 cases. *Eur J Haematol* 40:318, 1988.

235. Weisdorf DJ, Oken MM, Johnson LJ, Rydell RE: Chronic myelodysplastic syndrome: short survival with or without evolution to acute leukemia. *Br J Haematol* 55:691, 1983.

236. Vilter RW, Will JJ, Jarrold T: Refractory anemia with hyperplastic bone marrow (regenerative anemia). *Semin Hematol* 4:175, 1967.

237. Rosati S, Mick R, Xu F, et al: Refractory cytopenia with multilineage dysplasia: further characterization of an 'unclassifiable' myelodysplastic syndrome. *Leukemia* 10:20, 1996.

238. Matsuda A, Jinnai I, Yagasaki F, et al: Refractory anemia with severe dysplasia: clinical significance of morphological features in refractory anemia. *Leukemia* 12:482, 1998.

239. Zon LI, Arkin C, Groopman JE: Haematologic manifestations of the human immune deficiency virus (HIV). *Br J Haematol* 66:251, 1987.

240. Thiele J, Zirbas TK, Bertsch HP, et al: AIDS-related bone marrow lesions—myelodysplastic features or predominant inflammatory-reactive changes (HIV-myelopathy)? A comparative morphometric study by immunohistochemistry with special emphasis on apoptosis and PCNA-labeling. *Anal Cell Path* 11:141, 1996.

241. Haznedar R: Pancytopenia with hypercellular bone marrow as a possible paraneoplastic syndrome. *Am J Hematol* 19:205, 1985.

242. List AF, Brasfield F, Heaton R, et al: Stimulation of hematopoiesis by amifostine in patients with myelodysplastic syndrome. *Blood* 90:3364, 1997.

243. Freifeld A, Marchigiani D, Walsh T, et al: A double-blind comparison of empirical oral and intravenous antibiotic therapy for low-risk febrile patients with neutropenia during cancer chemotherapy. *N Engl J Med* 341:305, 1999.

244. Malik IA, Moid I, Aziz Z, Khan S, Suleman M: A randomized comparison of fluconazole with amphotercin B as empiric anti-fungal agents in cancer patients with prolonged fever and neutropenia. *Am J Med* 105:478, 1998.

245. Bagby GC, Gabourel JD, Linman JW: Glucocorticoid therapy in the preleukemic syndrome. *Ann Intern Med* 92:55, 1980.

246. Watts EJ, Majer RV, Grun PJ: Hyperfibrotic myelodysplasia: a report of three cases showing haematologic remission following treatment with prednisone. *Br J Haematol* 78:120, 1991.

247. Schuster MW: Will cytokines alter the treatment of myelodysplastic syndrome? *Am J Med Sci* 305:72, 1993.

248. Schouten HC, Vallenga E, Van Rhinen DJ, et al: Recombinant human erythropoietin in patients with myelodysplastic syndromes. *Leukemia* 5:432, 1991.

249. Stein RS, Abels RI, Krantz SB: Pharmacologic doses of recombinant human erythropoietin in the treatment of myelodysplastic syndromes. *Blood* 78:1658, 1991.

250. Rafanelli D, Grossi A, Longo G, et al: Recombinant human erythropoietin for treatment of myelodysplastic syndromes. *Leukemia* 6:323, 1992.

251. Willemze R, vanderLaly N, Zwierzina H, et al: A randomized phase I/II multicenter study of recombinant human granulocyte-macrophage colony-stimulating factor (GM-CSF) therapy for patients with myelodysplastic syndromes and a relatively low risk of acute leukemia. *Ann Hematol* 64:173, 1992.

252. Gradisher WJ, LeBeau MM, O'Laughlin R, et al: Clinical and cytogenetic responses to granulocyte-macrophage colony-stimulating factor in therapy-related myelodysplasia. *Blood* 80:2463, 1992.

253. Negrin RS, Haeuber DH, Nagler A, et al: Maintenance treatment of patients with myelodysplastic syndromes using recombinant human granulocyte colony-stimulating factor. *Blood* 76:36, 1990.

254. Yoshida Y, Hirashima K, Asano S: A phase II trial of recombinant human granulocyte colony-stimulating factor in the myelodysplastic syndromes. *Br J Haematol* 78:378, 1991.

255. Bessho M, Itho Y, Kataumi S: A hematologic remission by clonal hematopoiesis after treatment with recombinant human granulocyte-macrophage colony-stimulating factor and erythropoietin in a patient with therapy-related myelodysplastic syndrome. *Leuk Res* 16:123, 1992.

256. Ganser A, Seipelt G, Lindemann A, et al: Effects of recombinant human interleukin-3 in patients with myelodysplastic syndromes. *Blood* 76:455, 1990.

257. Ganser A, Hoelzer D: Clinical use of hematopoietic growth factors in the myelodysplastic syndromes. *Semin Hematol* 33:186, 1996.

258. Meyerson HJ, Farhi DC, Rosenthal NS: Transient increase in blasts mimicking acute leukemia and progressing myelodysplasia in patients receiving growth factor [see comments]. *Am J Clin Pathol* 109:675, 1998.

259. Jonasova A, Neuwirtova R, Cermak J, et al: Cyclosporin A therapy in hypoplastic MDS patients and certain refractory anaemias without hypoplastic bone marrow. *Br J Haematol* 100:304, 1998.

260. Molldrem JJ, Jiang YZ, Stetler-Stevenson M, Mavroudis D, Hensel N, Barrett AJ: Haematological response of patients with myelodysplastic syndrome to antithymocyte globulin is associated with a loss of lymphocyte-mediated inhibition of CFU-GM and alterations in T-cell receptor V-beta profiles. *Br J Haematol* 102:1314, 1998.

261. Coiffier B, Adeleine P, Viala JJ, et al: Dysmyelopoietic syndromes: a search for prognostic factors in 193 patients. *Cancer* 52:83, 1983.

262. Garcia S, Sanz MA, Amigo V, et al: Prognostic factors in chronic myelodysplastic syndromes: a multivariate analysis in 107 cases. *Am J Hematol* 27:163, 1988.

263. Minke DM, Colon-Otero G, Cockerill KJ, et al: Refractory thrombocytopenia: a myelodysplastic syndrome that may mimic immune thrombocytopenic purpura. *Am J Clin Pathol* 98:502, 1992.

264. Hoffman R: Acquired pure amegakaryocytic thrombocytopenia purpura. *Semin Hematol* 28:303, 1991.

265. Welte K, Boxer LA: Severe chronic neutropenia: pathophysiology and therapy. *Semin Hematol* 34:267, 1997.

266. Rosen RB, Kang SJ: Congenital agranulocytosis terminating in acute myelomonocytic leukemia. *J Pediatr* 94:406, 1979.

267. Smith OP, Hann IM, Chessells JM, et al: Haematological abnormalities in Shwachman-Diamond syndrome. *Br J Haematol* 94:279, 1996.

268. Pearson HA, Lobel JS, Kocoshis SA, et al: A new syndrome of refractory sideroblastic anemia with vacuolization of marrow precursors and exocrine pancreatic dysfunction. *J Pediatr* 95:976, 1979.

269. Orlandi E, Alessandrino EP, Caldera D, Bernasconi C: Adult leukemia after aplastic anemia: report of 8 cases. *Acta Haematol* 79:174, 1988.

270. DePlanque MM, Bacigalupo A, Wüsch A, et al: Long-term follow up of severe aplastic anemia patients treated with antithymocyte globulin. *Br J Haematol* 73:121, 1989.

271. Dunn DE, Tanawattanacharoen P, Boccuni P, et al: Paroxysmal nocturnal hemoglobinuria cells in patients with bone marrow failure syndromes. *Ann Intern Med* 131:401, 1999.

272. Doyle JA, Ginsburg WW: Eosinophilic fasciitis. *Med Clin North Am* 73:1157, 1989.

273. Lakhanpal S, Ginsburg WW, Michet CJ, et al: Eosinophilic fasciitis: clinical spectrum and therapeutic response in 52 cases. *Semin Arthritis Rheum* 17:221, 1988.

274. Naschitz JE, Boss JH, Misselevich I, et al: The fasciitis-panniculitis syndromes. Clinical and pathologic features. *Medicine* 75:6, 1996.

275. Kim SW, Rice L, Champlin R, Udden MM: Aplastic anemia in eosinophilic fasciitis: response to immunotherapy and marrow transplantation. *Haematologia* 28:131, 1997.

276. Joseph AS, Cinkotal KI, Hunt L, Geary CG: Natural history of smoldering leukemia. *Br J Cancer* 46:160, 1982.

277. Greenberg PL: The smoldering myeloid leukemic states: clinical and biological features. *Blood* 61:1035, 1983.

278. Maddox A-M, Keating MJ, Smith TL, et al: Prognostic factors for survival of 194 patients with low infiltrate leukemia. *Leuk Res* 10:995, 1986.

279. Najean Y, Pecking A: Refractory anemia with excess of myeloblasts in the bone marrow. A clinical trial of androgens in 90 cases. *Br J Haematol* 37:23, 1977.

280. Lavessi AM, Maiolo AT, Chiorboli O, Mozzana R: The bone marrow karyotype in seventeen cases of refractory anemia with excess blasts (RAEB). *Ann Genet* 26:220, 1983.

281. Foucar K, Langdon RM II, Armitage JO, et al: Myelodysplastic syndromes. A clinical and pathologic analysis of 109 cases. *Cancer* 56:553, 1985.

282. Hiddemann W, Jahns-Streubel G, Verbeek W, Wormann B, Haase D, Schoch C: Intensive therapy for high-risk myelodysplastic syndromes and the biological significance of karyotype abnormalities. *Leuk Res* 22 (suppl 1):S23, 1998.

283. Invernizzi R, Pecci A, Rossi G, et al: Idarubicin and cytosine arabinoside in the induction and maintenance therapy of high-risk myelodysplastic syndromes. *Haematologica* 82:660, 1997.

284. Kuriya S, Murai K, Miyairi Y, et al: A combination chemotherapy with low doses of cytarabine and etoposide for high risk myelodysplastic syndromes and their leukemic stage. A pilot study. *Cancer* 78:422, 1996.

285. Estey EH: Incorporating new modalities into guidelines. Topotecan for myelodysplastic syndromes. *Oncology* 12:81, 1998.

286. Estey EH, Thall PF, Pierce S, et al: Randomized phase II study of fludarabine + cytosine arabinoside + idarubicin +/− all-*trans* retinoic acid +/− granulocyte colony-stimulating factor in poor prognosis newly diagnosed acute myeloid leukemia and myelodysplastic syndrome. *Blood* 93:2478, 1999.

287. Silverman LR, Holland JF, Weinberg RS, et al: Effects of treatment with 5-azacytidine on the in vivo and in vitro hematopoiesis in patients with myelodysplastic syndromes. *Leukemia* 7 (suppl 1):21, 1993.

288. Zagonel V, Lo Re G, Marotta G, et al: 5-Aza-2'-deoxycytidine (Decitabine) induces trilineage response in unfavourable myelodysplastic syndromes. *Leukemia* 7 (suppl 1):30, 1993.

289. Cheson BD: Standard and low-dose chemotherapy for the treatment of myelodysplastic syndromes. *Leuk Res* 22 (suppl 1):S17, 1998.

290. Gassmann W, Schmitz N, Loffler H, De Witte T: Intensive chemotherapy and bone marrow transplantation for myelodysplastic syndromes. *Semin Hematol* 33:196, 1996.

291. Appelbaum FR, Anderson J: Allogeneic bone marrow transplantation for myelodysplastic syndrome: outcomes analysis according to IPSS score. *Leukemia* 12 (suppl 1):S25, 1998.

292. Runde V, de Witte T, Arnold R, et al: Bone marrow transplantation from HLA-identical siblings as first-line treatment in patients with myelodysplastic syndromes: early transplantation is associated with improved outcome. Chronic Leukemia Working Party of the European Group for Blood and Marrow Transplantation. *Bone Marrow Transplant* 21:255, 1998.

293. Wattel E, Solary E, Leleu X, et al: A prospective study of autologous bone marrow or peripheral blood stem cell transplantation after intensive chemotherapy in myelodysplastic syndromes. Groupe Francais des Myelodysplasies. Group Ouest-Est d'etude des Leucemies aigues myeloides. *Leukemia* 13:524, 1999.

294. Hellström-Lindberg E, Robért K-H, Gahrton G, et al: A predictive model for the clinical response to low dose ARA-C: a study of 102 patients with myelodysplastic syndromes and acute leukemia. *Br J Haematol* 81:503, 1992.

295. Ganser A, Seipelt G, Eder M, et al: Treatment of myelodysplastic syndromes with cytokines and cytotoxic drugs. *Semin Oncol* 19:95, 1992.

296. Wattel E, Guerci A, Hecquet B, et al: A randomized trial of hydroxyurea versus VP16 in adult chronic myelomonocytic leukemia. Groupe Francais des Myelodysplasies and European CMML Group. *Blood* 88:2480, 1996.

297. Ogata K, Yamada T, Ito T, et al: Low-dose etoposide: a potential therapy for myelodysplastic syndromes. *Br J Haematol* 82:354, 1992.

298. Nagler A, Rikilis I, Tatarsky I, Fabian I: Effect of 1,25-dihydroxyvitamin D_3 and 13-*cis*-retinoic acid on in vitro hematopoiesis in the myelodysplastic syndromes. *J Lab Clin Med* 110:237, 1987.

299. Rowinsky EK, Conley BA, Jones RJ, et al: Hexamethylene bisacetamide in myelodysplastic syndrome: effect of five-day exposure to maximal therapeutic concentrations. *Leukemia* 6:526, 1992.

300. List AF: Hematopoietic stimulation by amifostine and sodium phenylbutyrate: what is the potential in MDS? *Leuk Res* 22 (suppl 1):S7, 1998.

301. Andreeff M, Stone R, Michaeli J, et al: Hexamethylene bisacetamide in myelodysplastic syndrome and acute myelogenous leukemia: a phase II clinical trial with a differentiation-inducing agent. *Blood* 80:2604, 1992.

302. Hast R, Lauren SAL, Reizenstein P: Absent clinical effects of retinoic acid and isotretinoin treatment on the myelodysplastic syndrome. *Hematol Oncol* 7:297, 1989.

303. Ohno R, Naoe T, Hirano M, et al: Treatment of myelodysplastic syndromes with all-trans retinoic acid. *Blood* 81:1152, 1993.

304. Richard C, Mazo E, Cuadrado MA, et al: Treatment of myelodysplastic syndrome with 1,25-dihydroxyvitamin D_3. *Am J Med* 23:175, 1986.

305. Motomura S, Kanamori H, Maruta A, et al: The effect of 1-hydroxyvitamin D_3 for prolongation of leukemic transformation-free survival in myelodysplastic syndromes. *Am J Hematol* 38:67, 1991.

306. Yoshida Y: Japanese experience in the treatment of myelodysplastic syndromes. *Hematol Oncol Clin North Am* 6:673, 1992.

307. Paquette RL, Koeffler HP: Differentiation therapy. *Hematol Oncol Clin North Am* 6:687, 1992.

308. DeRosa L, Montuoro A, DeLaurenzi A: Therapy of "high risk" myelodysplastic syndromes with an association of low-dose ara-c, retinoic acid and 1,25-dihydroxyvitamin D_3. *Biomed Pharmacother* 46:211, 1992.

309. Gisslinger H, Chott H, Linkesch W, et al: Long term α interferon therapy in myelodysplastic syndromes. *Leukemia* 4:91, 1990.

310. Mailo AT, Cortelezzi A, Calori R: Recombinant γ-interferon as first line therapy for high risk myelodysplastic syndromes. *Leukemia* 4:480, 1990.

311. Nand S, Ellis T, Messmore H, et al: Phase II trial of recombinant human interferon-α in myelodysplastic syndromes. *Leukemia* 6:220, 1992.

312. Holcombe RF: Mini-dose interferon-α-2a in the treatment of myelodysplasia. *Leukemia* 7:192, 1993.

313. Maerevoet M, Van Den Neste E, Delannoy A, et al: Limited activity of mini-dose interferon alpha-2a in the treatment of myelodysplastic syndrome. *Leuk Lymphoma* 21:519, 1996.

314. Petti MC, Latagliata R, Avvisati G, et al: Treatment of high-risk myelodysplastic syndromes with lymphoblastoid alpha interferon. *Br J Haematol* 95:364, 1996.

315. Toze CL, Barnett MJ, Klingeman H-G: Response of therapy-related myelodysplasia to low-dose interleukin-2. *Leukemia* 7:463, 1993.

316. Nand S, Stock W, Stiff P, Sosman J, Martone B, Radvany R: A phase

II trial of interleukin-2 in myelodysplastic syndromes. *Br J Haematol* 101:205, 1998.

317. Goy A, Belanger C, Casadevall N, et al: High doses of intravenous recombinant erythropoietin for the treatment of anemia in myelodysplastic syndrome. *Br J Haematol* 84:232, 1993.

318. Vadhan-Raj S, Keating M, LeMaistre A, et al: Effects of recombinant human granulocyte-macrophage colony-stimulating factor in patients with myelodysplastic syndromes. *N Engl J Med* 317:1545, 1987.

319. Verhoef G, VandDenBerghe HV, Boogaerts M: Cytogenetic effects on cells derived from patients with myelodysplastic syndromes during treatment with hemopoietic growth factors. *Leukemia* 6:766, 1992.

320. Tohyama K, Ohmori S, Michishita M: Effects of recombinant G-CSF and GM-CSF on in vitro differentiation of the blast cells of RAEB and RAEB-T. *Eur J Haematol* 42:348, 1989.

321. Ferrero D, Bruno B, Pregno P, et al: Combined differentiating therapy for myelodysplastic syndromes: a phase II study. *Leuk Res* 20:867, 1996.

322. Hofmann WK, Ganser A, Seipelt G, et al: Treatment of patients with low-risk myelodysplastic syndromes using a combination of all-trans retinoic acid, interferon alpha, and granulocyte colony-stimulating factor. *Ann Hematol* 78:125, 1999.

323. Demuynck H, Verhoef GE, Zachee P, et al: Treatment of patients with myelodysplastic syndromes with allogeneic bone marrow transplantation from genotypically HLA-identical sibling and alternative donors. *Bone Marrow Transplant* 17:745, 1996.

324. Anderson JE, Appelbaum FR, Schoch G, et al: Allogeneic marrow transplantation for myelodysplastic syndrome with advanced disease morphology: a phase II study of busulfan, cyclophosphamide, and total-body irradiation and analysis of prognostic factors. *J Clin Oncol* 14:220, 1996.

325. Demuynck H, Delforge M, Verhoef GE, et al: Feasibility of peripheral blood progenitor cell harvest and transplantation in patients with poor-risk myelodysplastic syndromes. *Br J Haematol* 92:351, 1996.

326. De Witte T, Van Biezen A, Hermans J, et al: Autologous bone marrow transplantation for patients with myelodysplastic syndrome (MDS) or acute myeloid leukemia following MDS. Chronic and Acute Leukemia Working Parties of the European Group for Blood and Marrow Transplantation. *Blood* 90:3853, 1997.

327. Woolfrey AE, Gooley TA, Sievers EL, et al: Bone marrow transplantation for children less than 2 years of age with acute myelogenous leukemia or myelodysplastic syndrome. *Blood* 92:3546, 1998.

328. Arnold R, de Witte T, van Biezen A, et al: Unrelated bone marrow transplantation in patients with myelodysplastic syndromes and secondary acute myeloid leukemia: an EBMT survey. European Blood and Marrow Transplantation Group. *Bone Marrow Transplant* 21:1213, 1998.

329. Nevill TJ, Fung HC, Shepherd JD, et al: Cytogenetic abnormalities in primary myelodysplastic syndrome are highly predictive of outcome after allogeneic bone marrow transplantation. *Blood* 92:1910, 1998.

330. Testoni N, Lemoli RM, Martinelli G, et al: Autologous peripheral blood stem cell transplantation in acute myeloblastic leukaemia and myelodysplastic syndrome patients: evaluation of tumour cell contamination of leukaphereses by cytogenetic and molecular methods. *Bone Marrow Transplant* 22:1065, 1998.

331. Wattel E, Solary E, Leleu X, et al: A prospective study of autologous bone marrow or peripheral blood stem cell transplantation after intensive chemotherapy in myelodysplastic syndromes. Groupe Francais des Myelodysplasies. Group Ouest-Est d'etude des Leucemies aigues myeloides. *Leukemia* 13:524, 1999.

332. Sanz GF, Sanz MA, Vallespi T, et al: Two regression models and a scoring system for predicting survival and planning treatment in myelodysplastic syndromes: a multivariate analysis of prognostic factors in 370 patients. *Blood* 74:395, 1989.

333. Ganser A, Hoelzer D: Clinical course of myelodysplastic syndromes. *Hematol Oncol Clin North Am* 6:607, 1992.

334. White AD, Culligan DJ, Hoy TG, Jacobs A: Extended cytogenetic follow-up of patients with myelodysplastic syndrome (MDS). *Br J Haematol* 81:499, 1992.

335. Mufti GJ: A guide to risk assessment in the primary myelodysplastic syndrome. *Hematol Oncol Clin North Am* 6:587, 1992.

336. Pfeilstocker M, Reisner R, Nosslinger T, et al: Cross validation of prognostic scores in myelodysplastic syndromes on 386 patients from a single institution confirms importance of cytogenetics. *Br J Haematol* 106:455, 1999.

337. Brown ER, Heerma NA, Tricot G: Spontaneous remission in myelodysplastic syndrome. *Cancer Genet Cytogenet* 46:125, 1990.

338. Brusamolino E, Isernia P, Alessandrino EP, et al: Terminal deoxynucleotidyl transferase–positive acute leukemias evolving from a myelodysplastic syndrome. *Am J Hematol* 20:187, 1985.

339. Berneman ZN, Van Bockstaele D, DeMeyer P, et al: A myelodysplastic syndrome preceding acute lymphoblastic leukaemia. *Br J Haematol* 60:353, 1985.

340. Ascensao JL, Kay NE, Wright JJ, et al: Lymphoblastic transformation of myelodysplastic syndrome. *Am J Hematol* 22:431, 1986.

341. Bonati A, Delia D, Starich R: Progression of a myelodysplastic syndrome to pre-B-acute lymphoblastic leukaemia with unusual phenotype. *Br J Haematol* 64:487, 1986.

342. Dayton MA, VanBesien K, Tricot G, et al: Preleukemic state preceding adult acute lymphoblastic leukemia. *Am J Med* 89:657, 1990.

343. Saarinen UM, Wegelius R: Preleukemic syndrome in children. Report of four cases and review of literature. *Am J Pediatr Hematol Oncol* 6:137, 1984.

344. Breatnach F, Chessells JM, Greaves MF: The aplastic presentation of childhood leukemia: a feature of common ALL. *Br J Haematol* 49:387, 1981.

345. Klingemann H-G, Storb R, Sanders J, et al: Acute lymphoblastic leukaemia after bone marrow transplantation for aplastic anaemia. *Br J Haematol* 63:47, 1986.

346. Nakamori Y, Takahashi M, Moriyama Y, et al: The aplastic presentation of adult acute lymphoblastic leukaemia. *Br J Haematol* 62:782, 1986.

347. Homans AC, Cohen JL, Barker BE, Marzur EM: Aplastic presentation of acute lymphoblastic leukemia: evidence for cellular inhibition of normal hematopoietic progenitors. *Am J Pediatr Hematol Oncol* 11:456, 1989.

348. DeAlarcon P, Miller M, Stuart MJ: Erythroid hypoplasia: an unusual presentation of childhood leukemia. *Am J Dis Child* 132:763, 1978.

349. Reid MM, Summerfield GP: Distinction between aleukaemic prodrome of childhood acute lymphoblastic leukaemia and aplastic anemia. *J Clin Pathol* 45:697, 1992.

350. MacSween JM, Langley GR: Light-chain disease and sideroblastic anemia–preleukemic chronic granulocytic leukemia. *Can Med Assoc J* 106:995, 1972.

351. Trachida L, Palutke M, Poylik MD, Prasad AS: Primary acquired sideroblastic anemia preceding monoclonal gammopathy and malignant lymphoma. *Am J Med* 55:559, 1973.

352. Papayannis AG, Stathakis NE, Kyrkou K, et al: Primary acquired sideroblastic anemia associated with chronic lymphocytic leukemia. *Br J Haematol* 28:125, 1974.

353. Berkowitz LR, Ross DW, Orringe EP: Hairy cell leukemia with acquired dyserythropoiesis. *JAMA* 140:554, 1980.

354. Catovsky D, Shaw MT, Hoffbrand AV, Dacie JV: Sideroblastic anemia and its association with leukemia and myelomatosis. A report of five cases. *Br J Haematol* 20:385, 1971.

355. Dahlke MA, Nowell PC: Chromosomal abnormalities and dyserythropoiesis in the preleukaemic phase of multiple myeloma. *Br J Haematol* 31:111, 1975.

356. Meckenstock G, Bonatsch CH, Heyll A, et al: T-cell receptor α/δ expressing acute leukemia emerging from sideroblastic anemia: morphologic, immunological, and cytogenetic features. *Leuk Res* 16:379, 1992.

357. Khaleeli M, Keane WM, Lee GR: Sideroblastic anemia in multiple myeloma. A preleukemic change. *Blood* 41:17, 1973.

358. Greenberg BR, Miller C, Cardoff RD, et al: Concurrent development of preleukaemic lymphoproliferative and plasma cell disorders. *Br J Haematol* 53:125, 1983.

359. Copplestone JA, Mufti GJ, Hamblin TJ, Oscier DG: Immunological abnormalities in myelodysplastic syndromes. *Br J Haematol* 63:149, 1986.

360. Nevitzky N, Prindull G: For the European Society of Paediatric Haematology and Immunology: Myelodysplastic syndromes in children. *Am J Hematol* 63:212, 2000.

361. Bauduer F, Ducout L, Dastuque N, et al: Epidemiology of myelodysplastic syndromes in a French general hospital of the Basque country. *Leuk Res* 22:205, 1998.

362. Kumar T, Mandla SG, Greer WL: Familial myelodysplastic syndrome with early age of onset. *Am J Hematol* 64:53, 2000.

363. Krishnan A, Bhatia S, Slovak ML, et al: Predictors of therapy-related leukemia and myelodysplasia following autologous transplantation for lymphoma. *Blood* 95:1588, 2000.

364. Abruzzese E, Radford JE, Miller JS, et al: Detection of abnormal pre-transplant clones in progenitor cells of patients who developed myelodysplasia after autologous transplantation. *Blood* 94:1814, 2000.

365. Vallespi T, Imbert M, Mecucci C, et al: Diagnosis, classification, and cytogenetics of myelodysplastic syndromes. *Haematologica* 83:258, 1998.

366. Mecucci C, La Starza R: Cytogenetics of myelodysplastic syndromes. *Forum* 9:4, 1999.

367. Rossi G, Pelizzari AM, Bellotti D, et al: Cytogenetic analogy between myelodysplastic syndrome and acute myeloid leukemia of elderly patients. *Leukemia* 14:636, 2000.

368. Raza A, Qaui H, Lisak L, et al: Patients with myelodysplastic syndromes benefit from palliative therapy with amifostine, pentoxifylline, and ciprofloxacin with or without dexamethasone. *Blood* 95:1580, 2000.

369. Thomas DA: Pilot studies of thalidomide in acute myelogenous leukemia, myelodysplastic syndromes, and myeloproliferative disorders. *Sem Hematol* 37:26, 2000.

370. Sanz GF, Sanz MA: Progress in intensive chemotherapy for high-risk myelodysplastic syndromes. *Forum* 9:63, 1999.

371. Thompson JA, Gilliland DG, Prchal JT, et al: Effect of recombinant human erythropoietin combined with granulocyte/macrophage colony-stimulating factor in the treatment of patients with myelodysplastic syndrome. *Blood* 95:1175, 2000.

372. Deeg HG, Shulman HM, Anderson JE, et al: Allogeneic and syngeneic marrow transplantation for myelodysplastic syndrome in patients 55 to 66 years of age. *Blood* 95:1188, 2000.

373. Gordon MS: Advances in supportive case of myelodysplastic syndromes. *Sem Hematol* 36:21, 1999.

374. Greenberg PL, Sanz GF, Sanz MA: Prognostic scoring systems for risk assessment in myelodysplastic syndromes. *Forum* 9:17, 1999.

375. Maes B, Meeus P, Michaux L, et al: Application of the International Prognostic Scoring System for myelodysplastic syndromes. *J Oncol* 10:825, 1999.

376. Escudier SM, Albitar M, Robertson LE, et al: Acute lymphoblastic leukemia following preleukemic syndromes in adults. *Leukemia* 10:473, 1996.

CHAPTER 93

ACUTE MYELOGENOUS LEUKEMIA

MARSHALL A. LICHTMAN

JANE L. LIESVELD

Acute myelogenous leukemia (AML) is the result of a somatic mutation in a pluripotential stem cell or a slightly more differentiated progenitor cell. Exposure to very high doses of radiation or chronic exposure to benzene increases the incidence of the disease. A small but increasing proportion of cases develop after the exposure of a patient with lymphoma or a nonhematologic cancer to intensive chemotherapy. The mutant cell gains a growth and/or survival advantage in relationship to the normal pool of stem cells. As the progeny of the mutant cell proliferates to form about ten billion cells or more, normal hematopoiesis is inhibited, and normal red cell, neutrophil, and platelet blood levels fall. The resultant anemia leads to weakness, exertional limitations, and pallor; the thrombocytopenia to spontaneous hemorrhage, usually in the skin; and the neutropenia and monocytopenia to poor wound healing and minor infections. Severe infection usually does not occur at diagnosis but will if the disease progresses for lack of treatment or if chemotherapy-induced impairment of neutrophil and monocyte blood cell levels is superimposed. The diagnosis is made by measurement of the blood cell counts and examination of blood and marrow cells and is based on the identification of blast cells in the marrow and blood. The diagnosis of AML is enhanced in some cases by identification of myeloperoxidase activity in blast cells by cytochemistry or a specific antibody test and by identifying characteristic CD antigens on the blast cells (e.g., CD13, CD33). The leukemic stem cell is capable of imperfect differentiation and maturation, and the clone may contain cells that have the morphologic or immunophenotypic features of erythroblasts, megakaryocytes, monocytes, eosinophils, or rarely basophils in addition to myeloblasts or promyelocytes. When one cell line is sufficiently dominant, the leukemia may be referred to as acute erythroblastic, acute megakaryocytic, acute monocytic, and so on. Certain cytogenetic alterations are very frequent. These include t(8;21), t(15;17), inversion 16, trisomy 8, and deletions of all or part of chromosome 5 or 7; t(15;17) is uniquely associated with acute promyelocytic leukemia. AML usually is treated with cytarabine and an anthracycline antibiotic, although other drugs may be added or substituted in poor-prognosis, refractory, or relapsed patients. High-dose chemotherapy and either autologous stem cell infusion or allogeneic stem cell transplantation may be used in an effort to treat relapse or those at high risk to relapse after chemotherapy alone. The probability of remission ranges from about 75 percent in children to less than 25 percent in octagenarians. The probability for cure decreases from about 35 percent in children to virtually zero in octagenarians.

DEFINITION AND HISTORY

AML is a clonal, malignant disease of hematopoietic tissue that is characterized by (1) the proliferation of abnormal (leukemic) blast cells, principally in the marrow, and (2) impaired production of normal blood cells. Thus, the leukemic cell infiltration in marrow is accompanied, nearly invariably, by anemia and thrombocytopenia. The absolute neutrophil count may be low or normal, depending on the total white cell count.

The first well-documented case of acute leukemia is attributed to Friedreich,[1] but it was Epstein who used the term *acute leukämie* in 1889,[2] and this led to the general appreciation of the clinical distinctions between AML and chronic myelogenous leukemia (CML).[3] In 1878, Neumann, who proposed that marrow was the site of blood cell production, first suggested that leukemia originated in the marrow and used the term *myelogene* (myelogenous) leukemia.[4] The availability of polychromatic stains, as a result of the work of Ehrlich,[5] the description of the myeloblast and myelocyte by Naegeli,[6] and the earliest appreciation of the common origin of red cells and leukocytes by Hirschfield[7] laid the foundation of our current understanding of the disease.

ETIOLOGY AND PATHOGENESIS

ENVIRONMENTAL FACTORS

Table 93-1 lists the major conditions that predispose to subsequent development of AML. Only three well-documented environmental factors are established causal agents: high-dose external low-linear energy transfer radiation exposure,[8,9] chronic benzene exposure,[10–13] and chemotherapeutic agents.[14–19] Most patients have not been exposed to an antecedent causative factor. Exposure to high linear energy transfer radiation from alpha-emitting radioisotopes such as thorium dioxide increases the risk of AML.[20] Case control studies have sometimes found a relationship between AML and organic solvents, petroleum products, radon exposure, pesticides, and herbicides, but these data have not reached the level of the strong association that exists for benzene or high-dose external irradiation or certain chemotherapeutic agents.[21] The aggregate of studies has suggested an association between cigarette smoking and AML.[22,23] Maternal alcohol use has been associated with AML in infancy.[24]

EVOLUTION FROM A CHRONIC CLONAL HEMOPATHY

AML may develop from the progression of other clonal disorders of hematopoietic stem cells including CML, polycythemia vera, idiopathic myelofibrosis, primary thrombocythemia, and certain preleukemic clonal syndromes such as acquired sideroblastic anemias (Table 93-1). This clonal progression can occur spontaneously, although with a different probability of occurrence in each disorder. The frequency of clonal progression to AML is enhanced by radiation or chemotherapy in patients with polycythemia vera (see Chap. 61) or essential thrombocythemia (see Chap. 118).[18,25]

PREDISPOSING DISEASES

Patients who develop AML may have an antecedent predisposing disease, such as aplastic anemia, myeloma,[26] or, rarely, AIDS.[27] A

Acronyms and abbreviations that appear in this chapter include: ACTH, adrenocorticotropic hormone; ALL, acute lymphocytic leukemia; AML, acute myelogenous leukemia; ATRA, all-*trans*-retinoic acid; CML, chronic myelogenous leukemia; FISH, fluorescence in situ hybridization; G-CSF, granulocyte colony stimulating factor; GM-CSF, granulocyte-monocyte colony stimulating factor; PCR, polymerase chain reaction; TAM, transient abnormal myeloproliferation.

TABLE 93-1 CONDITIONS PREDISPOSING TO THE DEVELOPMENT OF ACUTE MYELOGENOUS LEUKEMIA

Environmental factors
    Radiation[8,9,20]
    Benzene[10-13]
    Alkylating agents and other cytotoxic drugs[14-19]
Acquired diseases
  Clonal hematopoietic diseases
    Chronic myelogenous leukemia (Chap. 27)
    Idiopathic myelofibrosis (Chap. 95)
    Primary thrombocythemia (Chap. 118)
    Polycythemia vera (Chap. 30)
    Acquired sideroblastic or nonsideroblastic anemia (Chap. 92)
    Bi- or tricytopenia with hyperplastic marrow (Chap. 92)
    Paroxysmal nocturnal hemoglobinuria (Chap. 92)
  Other hematopoietic disorders
    Aplastic anemia (Chap. 31)
    Eosinophilic fasciitis (Chap. 92)
    Myeloma[26]
Inherited conditions
    Identical sibling with AML[28-30]
    Nonidentical sibling with AML[28-30]
    Down syndrome[31,32]
    Fanconi anemia[33,34]
    Bloom syndrome[35]
    Ataxia-pancytopenia[36]
    Wiskott-Aldrich syndrome[37]
    Dyskeratosis congenita[38]
    Combined immunodeficiency syndrome[37]
    Congenital agranulocytosis[39]
    D-trisomy[40,41]
    Familial AML[42-46]
    Werner syndrome (progeria)[47]
    Neurofibromatosis 1[48]
    Schwachman syndrome[49,788]
    Chromosome 21q disorder[50]

number of inherited conditions, for example, Down syndrome, Fanconi anemia, Bloom syndrome, and others carry an increased risk of AML[28-41] (Table 93-1).

PATHOGENESIS

AML results from a somatic mutation in either a hematopoietic stem cell or a somewhat more differentiated cell.[51] Some cases of monocytic leukemia, of promyelocytic leukemia, and acute myelogenous leukemia in younger individuals are more likely to arise in a progenitor cell with lineage restrictions (progenitor cell leukemia).[51-55] Other morphologic phenotypes and older patients are likely to have the disease originate in a primitive multipotential cell.[51] In the latter case, all blood cell lineages can be derived from the leukemic stem cell, since it retains the ability for some degree of differentiation and maturation.

The somatic mutation results from a chromosomal translocation in nearly 80 percent of patients.[57] The translocations result in rearrangement of a critical region of a protooncogene. The fusion of portions of two genes usually does not prevent the process of transcription, and thus the fusion gene encodes a fusion protein that, because of its abnormal structure, disrupts a normal cell pathway and leads to a malignant transformation of the cell. This protein product is often a transcription factor that disrupts the regulatory sequences that control differentiation, growth rate, or survival of blood cell progenitors.[57-59] Since the mutant stem or early progenitor cell can proliferate and retains the capability to differentiate, a wide variety of phenotypes can emerge from a leukemic transformation. Other genetic changes occur in leukemic cells involving *RAS, FES, MYC, FOS, MPL, KIT*, p53, *RB, WT1*, and other genes.[60-73] In some cases, deletions of all or part of a chromosome, 5- or 7- for example, or additional chromosomes

such as trisomy 4, 8, or 13 are the principal cytogenetic abnormalities (see Chap. 10), although the specific causative "oncogenes" in these latter circumstances have not been defined.

MODE OF INHERITANCE

In most cases there is little evidence for a strong influence of genetic factors. The identical twin of a child with leukemia has a greatly heightened risk (1 in 5) of developing the disease. This risk drops to that of a nonidentical sibling (1 in 800) within about 6 months of age, as compared to a risk of 1 in 3000 in American children of European descent under 15 years of age.[74] This propensity of identical twins to develop leukemia is related to parabiotic metastasis from one twin to another and not an inherent common mutation. This phenomenon explains the rapid attenuation of risk after 6 months of age. Clusters of AML cases in families have been documented, but their frequency is rare.[42-46] Clusters of AML in unrelated persons in a community are very rare and usually appear to be a chance occurrence.

EPIDEMIOLOGY

AML is the predominant form of leukemia during the neonatal period, but it represents a small proportion of cases during childhood and adolescence. The mortality rate from AML is about 0.5 per 100,000 persons under age 10 years and increases progressively until it reaches about 20 per 100,000 persons in the ninth decade of life.[24] AML accounts for 15 to 20 percent of the acute leukemias in children and 80 percent of the acute leukemias in adults.[27,29,70] It is slightly more common in males, and there is little difference in incidence between those of African or European descent at any age. There is an increase in the frequency of AML in Jews, especially of Eastern European descent.

CLASSIFICATION

Variants of AML can be identified by morphologic features of blood films using polychromatic stains and histochemical reactions,[75] monoclonal antibodies against surface markers,[76-80] or by the presence of specific chromosome translocations.[81] There is overlap in the epitopes on the progenitor cells of several phenotypic variants, and several monoclonal antibodies are required to make specific distinctions among cell types (Table 93-2). See also the section "Morphologic Variants of AML" and Table 93-4 later in the chapter. There is a poor correlation between morphologic and immunologic phenotyping of AML as would be expected, since the former method is more subjective, given to observer variation, and is based on qualitative factors, whereas the latter method, which characterizes surface molecular features, is more accurate and reproducible. The correlation is improved only somewhat if morphology and histochemistry are coupled.[82] Chapter 91, "Classification and Clinical Manifestations of Clonal Myeloid Diseases," contains the classification of morphologic variants of AML (Table 91-1 and Fig. 91-2). A need to include functional markers for drug resistance, such as *MDR* expression, has also been proposed to separate more responsive from less responsive AML.[83]

CLINICAL FEATURES

SIGNS AND SYMPTOMS

GENERAL

Signs and symptoms that signal the onset of AML include pallor, fatigue, weakness, palpitations, and dyspnea on exertion. They reflect the development of anemia; however, weakness, loss of sense of well being, and fatigue on exertion can be out of proportion to the severity of anemia.[84-88]

Easy bruising, petechiae, epistaxis, gingival bleeding, conjunctival hemorrhages, and prolonged bleeding from skin injuries reflect thrombocytopenia and are frequent early manifestations of the disease. Very infrequently gastrointestinal, genitourinary, bronchopulmonary, or central nervous system bleeding can occur at the onset of the disease.

Pustules or other minor pyogenic infections of the skin and of minor cuts or wounds are most common. Major infections such as sinusitis, pneumonia, pyelonephritis, and meningitis are uncommon as presenting features of the disease, in part because absolute neutrophil counts under 500/μl (0.5 $\times$ 10^9/liter) are uncommon until chemotherapy is begun. With intensification of neutropenia after chemotherapy, major bacterial, fungal, or viral infections become frequent. Anorexia and weight loss are frequent findings. Fever is present in many patients at the time of diagnosis.[87-91] Palpable splenomegaly or hepatomegaly occurs in about one-third of patients.[84,85,88] Lymphadenopathy is extremely uncommon,[88,92,93] except in the monocytic variant of AML.[94]

SPECIFIC ORGAN SYSTEM INVOLVEMENT

Leukemic blast cells circulate and enter most tissues in small numbers.[95] Occasionally biopsy or autopsy will uncover marked aggregates or infiltrates of leukemic cells, and less frequently collections of such cells may cause functional disturbances. Extramedullary involvement is most common in monocytic or myelomonocytic leukemia.

Skin involvement may be of three types: nonspecific lesions, leukemia cutis, or granulocytic sarcoma of skin and subcutis.[96-101] Nonspecific lesions include macules, papules, vesicles, pyoderma gangrenosum, or vasculitis,[102-104] neutrophilic dermatitis (Sweet's syndrome),[105] cutis vertices gyrata,[106] or erythema multiforme or nodosum.[96,97] Skin involvement preceding marrow and blood involvement is rare.[101,107]

Sensory organ involvement is very unusual, but retinal, choroidal, iridial, and optic nerve infiltration can occur.[108] Otitis externa and interna, inner ear hemorrhage, and mastoid tumors with seventh nerve involvement may be presenting signs.[109-111]

The *gastrointestinal tract* may be involved at any point, but functional disturbances are unusual.[112,113] The mouth, colon, and anal canal are sites of involvement that most commonly lead to symptoms. Oral manifestations may bring the patient to the dentist; gingival or periodontal infiltration and dental abscesses may lead to an extraction followed by prolonged bleeding or an infected tooth socket.[114] Iliotyphlitis (enterocolitis), a necrotizing inflammatory lesion involving the terminal ileum, cecum, and ascending colon, can be a presenting syndrome or occur during treatment.[115-117] Fever, abdominal pain, bloody diarrhea, or ileus may be present and occasionally mimic appendicitis. Intestinal perforation, an inflammatory mass, and associated infection with enteric gram-negative bacilli or clostridial species are often associated with a fatal outcome. Isolated involvement of the gastrointestinal tract is rare.[118,119] Proctitis, especially common in the monocytic variant of AML, can be a presenting sign or a vexing problem during periods of severe granulocytopenia and diarrhea.[112]

The *respiratory tract* can be involved by infiltrates or tumors, leading to laryngeal obstruction, parenchymal infiltrates, alveolar septal infiltration, or pleural seeding. Each of these events can result in severe symptoms and radiologic findings.[120-124]

Cardiac involvement is frequent but rarely causes symptoms. Symptomatic pericardial infiltrates, transmural ventricular infiltrates

TABLE 93-2   IMMUNOLOGIC PHENOTYPES OF AML

	Usually Positive	Usually Negative
Myeloblastic	CD11, CD13, CD15, CD33, CD117, HLA-DR	CD14, CD10 (cALLa), CD20
Myelomonocytic	CD11, CD13, CD14, CD15, CD32, CD33, HLA-DR	CD10, CD20
Erythroblastic	Glycophorin, spectrin, ABH antigens, carbonic anhydrase I, HLA-DR	CD10, CD20
Promyelocytic	CD11, CD13, CD15, CD33	CD14, HLA-DR, CD10, CD20
Monocytic	CD11, CD13, CD14, CD33, HLA-DR	CD10, CD20
Megakaryoblastic	CD34, CD41, CD42, CD61, von Willebrand factor	CD10, CD20

NOTE: The definition of the antigen that represents a cluster of differentiation (CD) may be found in Chap. 13.

with hemorrhage, and endocardial foci with associated intracavitary thrombi can, on occasion, cause heart failure, arrhythmia, and death.[125] Infiltration of the conducting system or valve leaflets or myocardial infarction has occurred.[126]

The *urogenital system* can be affected. The kidneys are infiltrated with leukemic cells in a high proportion of cases, but functional abnormalities are rare. Hemorrhage in the pelvis or collecting system is frequent, however.[127,128] Cases of vulvar, bladder neck, prostatic, or testicular involvement have been described.[129-131]

Osteoarticular symptoms are infrequent. Bone pain, joint pain, and bone necrosis can occur, and rarely arthritis with effusion may be present.[132] Crystal-induced arthritis of either calcium pyrophosphate dihydrate (pseudogout) or monosodium urate (gout) may be responsible for the synovitis in some cases.[133]

Central or peripheral *nervous system* involvement by infiltration of leukemic cells is very uncommon, although in the monocytic type of AML meningeal involvement is an important consideration in treatment.[134,135] There is an association of central nervous system involvement and diabetes insipidus in AML with monosomy 7[136] and inversion of chromosome 16.[137,138]

GRANULOCYTIC SARCOMA

Granulocytic sarcoma is a tumor composed of myeloblasts or monoblasts. It may be found in virtually any location, especially the skin; orbit; paranasal sinuses; bone; chest wall; breast; gastrointestinal, respiratory, or genitourinary tract; central or peripheral nervous system; or lymph nodes.[139,140] These tumors were originally called *chloromas* because of the green color imparted by the high concentration of the enzyme myeloperoxidase present in myelogenous leukemic cells. Chloracetate esterase histochemical stains or antilysozyme immunoperoxidase reaction is positive when biopsy specimens are studied. Granulocytic sarcomas may be the initial manifestation of AML, and the appearance of the disease in the blood and marrow may follow weeks or months later if intensive therapy is not administered.[139,140] AML with the t(8;21) has a propensity to extramedullary leukemia,[141] and patients with granulocytic sarcomas have a poorer outcome with treatment.[142]

LABORATORY FEATURES

BLOOD CELL FINDINGS

Anemia is a constant feature.[84-88] Red cell life span may be mildly shortened, but the principal cause of anemia is inadequate production of red cells. The reticulocyte count is usually between 0.5 and 2.0 percent. Occasionally patients may have rapid destruction of autologous and transfused red cells as a result of an unknown mechanism (milieu hemolysis). The presence of red cell autoantibodies (positive Coombs' test) is very uncommon and may be nonspecific (anti-C_3), perhaps relating to circulating immune complexes or as a result of an anti-I antibody. Red cell morphology is mildly abnormal, with exaggerated variation in cell size and occasional poikilocytes. Nucleated red cells or stippled erythrocytes may be present. Less often, extreme abnormalities of red cell size, shape, and hemoglobin content may occur, but these changes are more often seen in oligoblastic leukemia (see Chap. 92).

Thrombocytopenia is nearly always present at the time of diagnosis. The mechanism of thrombocytopenia is a combination of inadequate production and decreased survival of platelets, and over half the patients have a platelet count less than $50,000/\mu l$ (50×10^9/liter) at the time of diagnosis.[143] Giant platelets and poorly granulated platelets with functional abnormalities can occur.[144] Defects in platelet aggregation and 5-hydroxytryptamine release are frequent.[144]

The total leukocyte count is less than $5000/\mu l$ (5×10^9/liter) in about half the patients at the time of diagnosis.[84,88] The absolute neutrophil count is less than $1000/\mu l$ (1×10^9/liter) in over half the cases at diagnosis.[84,88] Patients with elevated leukocyte counts have a low proportion of mature neutrophils but may have a normal or slightly elevated absolute neutrophil count. Hypersegmented, hyposegmented, and hypogranular mature neutrophils may be present. Cytochemical abnormalities of blood neutrophils include low or absent myeloperoxidase or low alkaline phosphatase activity.[145] Defects in phagocytosis or microbial killing are also common.[146]

Myeloblasts are almost always present in the blood, but in leukopenic patients they may be infrequent. Diligent search may uncover them or examination of a white cell concentrate (buffy coat) may permit their identification. Blood myeloblasts range from 3 to 95 percent of total leukocytes (see Plates XVI and XVII). Classic leukemic blast cells are agranular, but mixtures of immature cells can occur including agranular and slightly granular cells ranging up to overt progranulocytes. Auer rods are elliptical cytoplasmic inclusions about 1.5 μm long and 0.5 μm wide that are derived from azurophilic granules (see Chap. 64). These inclusions are present in the blast cells of about one-quarter of cases, and when present are found in only a small percent of blast cells.[75,147]

MARROW FINDINGS

MORPHOLOGY

The marrow always contains leukemic blast cells. Three to 95 percent of marrow cells are blasts at the time of diagnosis or relapse.[84-88,147] Myeloblasts are distinguished from lymphoblasts by any of three pathognomonic features: reactivity with specific histochemical stains; Auer rods in the cells; or reactivity with specific monoclonal antibodies against epitopes present on myeloblasts (for example, CD11, CD13). Leukemic myeloblasts give positive histochemical reactions for peroxidase, Sudan black B, or naphthyl AS-D-chloroacetate esterase stains. Auer rods can be found in the marrow blast cells in about one-quarter of cases. Blast cells express granulocytic or monocytic surface antigens. They typically do not express either lymphoid surface markers or membrane or cytoplasmic immunoglobulin. No immunoglobulin gene rearrangement or T-lymphocyte receptor gene rearrangement is evident with molecular probes (see also, "Hybrid and Mixed Leukemias"). In a proportion of otherwise typical cases of AML, the cells may contain terminal deoxynucleotidyl transferase.[148,149] Variations in marrow findings are discussed further in "Morphologic Variants of Acute Myelogenous Leukemia," below. Normal erythropoiesis, megakaryocytopoiesis, and granulopoiesis are decreased or absent in the marrow aspirate. The biopsy may contain residual islands of erythroblasts or megakaryocytes. Dyshematopoietic changes, including very small or large erythroblasts with nuclear fragmentation or binucleation or delayed nuclear condensation; small or monolobed megakaryocytes; or hypogranulated, bilobed, or monolobed neutrophils, may occur in 30 percent to 50 percent of patients with de novo AML.[150] Marrow reticulin fibrosis is common but is usually slight to moderate except in cases of megakaryoblastic leukemia, in which intense fibrosis is the rule.[151] Increased blood vessel density (angiogenesis) has been demonstrated in the marrow of patients with AML compared to normal subjects.[56]

MARROW CELL CULTURE

Progenitor cells for granulocytes, for monocytes and macrophages, or for both granulocytes and macrophages form colonies when normal marrow cells are grown in a viscous medium with a source of growth factors. Marrow cells from patients with AML have heterogeneous growth patterns. About 85 percent of patients do not have colony-forming cells in their marrow, but the marrow of 60 percent of patients does have cells capable of forming small clusters in vitro (4 to 40 cells in size). About 15 percent of patients retain colony-forming cells but often in reduced numbers and with abnormal maturation patterns.[152,153] Restoration of colony-forming cells in the marrow of treated patients often precedes morphologic evidence of remission.[154] The correlation of pretreatment marrow colonial growth pattern in vitro with the outcome of intensive chemotherapy is not sufficiently strong to use growth pattern as a prognostic variable.[155]

CYTOGENETIC FEATURES

An abnormal number (aneuploidy) or structure (pseudodiploidy) of chromosomes or both are readily evident in about 75 percent of cases.[156-158] The most prevalent abnormalities are trisomy 8, monosomy 7, monosomy 21, trisomy 21, and loss of an X or Y chromosome, but virtually any chromosome may be rearranged, added, or lost. In cases of AML that occur following chemotherapy or radiotherapy, loss of part or all of chromosome 5 is a common feature,[159-161] as are the cytogenetic findings noted above for AML, occurring de novo. The major abnormalities and translocations seen in AML are presented in Table 93-3 (see Chap. 10). The translocations 8;21, 15;17, and inv 16 confer a more favorable outcome on average; deletion of all or part of chromosomes 5 and 7 or the presence of complex changes confer a less favorable prognosis. Other abnormalities generally confer an intermediate prognosis.[156,157]

PLASMA CHEMICAL FINDINGS

Prior to treatment, mild to moderate increases in serum uric acid and lactic dehydrogenase levels are frequent, and both levels are higher in myelomonocytic and monocytic AML than in other AML phenotypes.[87,88] Occasional patients may have very elevated uric acid levels, but usually this occurs after chemotherapy if proper precautions are not taken (e.g., allopurinol and hydration therapy).[168] Abnormalities of sodium, potassium, calcium, or hydrogen ion concentration are infrequent and usually mild.[169,170] Severe hyponatremia associated with inappropriate antidiuretic hormone secretion has occurred at presentation,[169,170] and severe hypernatremia as a consequence of diabetes insipidus can be an initial event.[171] Hypokalemia is a somewhat more frequent finding at presentation and is related to kaliuresis, although the reason for the proximal renal tubular dysfunction is unclear.[169,170,172] The hypokalemia can be severe, occasionally, and is often worsened by the effects of treatment, especially the use of kaliuretic antibiotics.[172] Factitious elevations in serum potassium levels have been reported in patients with hyperleukocytosis as a result of leakage from white cells in vitro.[173,174] Factitious hypoglycemia and spurious hypoxia from the effects of high blast cell counts also can occur.[173,175]

TABLE 93-3   CLINICAL CORRELATES OF FREQUENT CYTOGENETIC ABNORMALITIES OBSERVED IN AML

Chromosome Abnormality	Genes Affected	Clinical Correlation
Loss or gain of chromosome Deletions of part or all of chromosomes 5 or 7	Not defined	Frequent in patients with acute myelogenous leukemia occurring de novo and in patients with history of chemical, drug, or radiation exposure and/or previous hematologic disease.[156,159,160]
Trisomy 8	Not Defined	Very common abnormality in acute myeloblastic leukemia. Poor prognosis, often a secondary change.[162]
Translocations t(8;21) (q22;q22)	AML1 (CBFα) - ETO	Present in about 12% of patients with AML; associated with loss of Y in males or of X in females in over half the cases. Present in about 40% of myelomonocytic phenotype. High frequency of granulocytic sarcomas.[141,142,255]
t(15;17) (q31; q22)	PML - RARα	Represents about 7% of cases of AML. Translocation involving chromosome 17, t(15;17), t(11;17), or t(5;17) are present in most cases of promyelocytic leukemia.[283,284]
t(9;11); p(22; q23)	ALL1 (MLL) - AF9	Present in about 7% of cases of AML. Associated with monocytic leukemia.[360-362] 11q23 translocations common in infants, carries poor prognosis, rearranges ALL1 (MLL) gene.[163-165] There are many partners (~20) for 11q23 translocation. Present in ~60% of infant AML cases.[325,370]
t(9;22) (q34; q22)	BCR - ABL	Present in about 3% of patients with AML[166,167] (see Chap. 94).
Inversions Inv (16)	CBFB-MYH11	Present in about 12% of cases of AML; associated with increased marrow eosinophils; better response to therapy.[262-265]

Hypercalcemia can occur. The pathogenesis is probably multifactorial,[176] but cases with increased ectopic parathormone-like activity in the plasma have been described.[177] Severe lactic acidosis prior to treatment has been reported.[170,178,179] Hypophosphatemia as a result of phosphate uptake by leukemic cells can occur.[180] Ectopic adrenocorticotropic hormone (ACTH) secretion[181]; circulating immune complexes[182]; and abnormal concentrations of coagulation factors or their inhibitors[183] may be present.

Although prothrombin and partial thromboplastin times are usually normal or near normal, abnormalities in the concentration of coagulation factors are frequent. Elevation of platelet factor 4 and thromboxane-B$_2$ occur often.[184] A decrease in alpha$_2$-antiplasmin, protein C, and antithrombin III levels are also frequent[184] and may be associated with venous thrombosis.[185] Acute promyelocytic and acute monocytic leukemia are associated with hypofibrinogenemia and other indicators of activation of coagulation or fibrinolysis.[186] See ''Morphologic Variants of AML.''

The levels of the shed form of L-selectin[187] and anticardiolipin antibodies[188] are frequently elevated in plasma.

SPECIAL CLINICAL FEATURES

HYPERLEUKOCYTOSIS

About 5 percent of patients with AML develop signs or symptoms attributable to a markedly elevated blood blast cell count, usually in excess of 100,000/μl (100 × 10⁹/liter)[189] (see Chap. 91). The circulation of the central nervous system, lungs, and penis is most sensitive to the effects of leukostasis. Intracerebral hemorrhage from vascular occlusion, invasion, and disruption, and pulmonary insufficiency, sometimes with hemorrhage, are the most virulent manifestations of the syndrome. Dizziness, stupor, dyspnea, and priapism may also occur.[189-192] Diabetes insipidus has been another rare association.[193] A high early mortality in patients with AML is correlated with hyperleukocytosis, greater than 100,000/μl (>100 × 10⁹/liter).[190-192] Chemotherapy in hyperleukocytic patients may also lead to a pulmonary leukostatic syndrome, presumably from the effects of rigid, effete blast cells or the effect of the discharge of large amounts of cell contents and resultant cell aggregation.[194,195] Larger-vessel vascular occlusion as a result of white thrombi or masses of leukemic cells is very rare.[196-199]

HYPOPLASTIC LEUKEMIA

About 10 percent of patients with AML present with a syndrome that includes pancytopenia, often with inapparent blood blast cells, and absence of hepatic, splenic, or lymph nodal enlargement.[200-202] About 75 percent of these patients are men over age 50 years. Marrow biopsy is hypocellular, which is the unusual feature of the syndrome, but leukemic blast cells are evident and in a proportion of 15 to 90 percent of marrow cells. Response to intensive chemotherapeutic treatment has been favorable in some patients.

OLIGOBLASTIC (SMOLDERING) LEUKEMIA

In about 10 percent of cases, usually in patients over age 50, myelogenous leukemia is manifested by anemia and often thrombocytopenia. The leukocyte count may be low, normal, or increased, and a small proportion of blast cells are present in the blood (0 to 15 percent) and marrow (3 to 30 percent). Such cases have been termed oligoblastic leukemia or smoldering leukemia[203-205] or classified as a specific syndrome, especially refractory anemia with excess blasts. The clinical course of the untreated disease can be protracted, but the disease has a high morbidity and mortality from infection and hemorrhage and can evolve into overt (polyblastic) AML. The smoldering or oligoblastic leukemias have historically been grouped with the clonal refractory cytopenias as part of the myelodysplastic syndromes (refractory anemia with excess blasts). For that reason the diagnosis and treatment of these variants are discussed in Chap. 92. Biologically and clinically, this subset of the myelodysplastic syndrome with blast cell proportions in the marrow above normal are leukemias, not dysplasias, but with a slower rate of progression than that of polyblastic myelogenous leukemia. Dysmorphogenesis of red cells, neutrophils, and platelets are more frequent and more striking than in the average case of polyblastic AML (see Chap. 92), but such dysmorphogenesis occurs in polyblastic leukemia as well.[150]

NEONATAL MYELOPROLIFERATION AND LEUKEMIA

Four myeloproliferative syndromes related to AML have been identified in the neonate: transient abnormal myeloproliferation, transient leukemia, congenital leukemia, and neonatal leukemia.

Transient abnormal myeloproliferation (referred to by the acronym TAM) can be present at birth or occur shortly thereafter, principally in infants with Down syndrome.[206–210] The leukocyte count is markedly elevated, blast cells are present in the blood and marrow, and anemia and thrombocytopenia may be present, but the latter are not constant findings. The liver and spleen may be enlarged. Cytogenetic studies and marrow cell culture studies are often normal, except for trisomy 21, characteristic of Down syndrome. The blast cells usually have the phenotype of megakaryocytes. The elevated white cell and blast cell counts disappear over a period of weeks to months. In some cases an additional cytogenetic abnormality is present which disappears after regression of the myeloproliferative syndrome, suggesting a reversible clonal disorder (transient leukemia) that is replaced by normal hematopoiesis. The transient abnormal myeloproliferative syndrome may disappear only to be followed shortly thereafter by acute leukemia. About 25 percent of newborns with Down syndrome and transient leukemia will develop acute megakaryocytic leukemia in the first 4 years of life.[211–213] The response rate of infants with Down syndrome and AML to chemotherapy has been very high over several years of follow-up.[211,214,215] The leukemic blast cells in patients with Down syndrome often have a megakaryoblastic and an erythroid phenotype and may have an interstitial deletion of chromosome 21.[208,209,216,217]

Congenital or neonatal leukemia can occur in apparently normal infants, but this rare syndrome is over 10 times more frequent in newborns with Down syndrome.[215,216] Leukocytosis, blood and marrow blast cells, hepatosplenomegaly, thrombocytopenia, purpura, anemia, and skin infiltrates are usual. Cytogenetic abnormalities can occur and mark the leukemic clone.[217–219] Monocytic leukemia and t(4;11) are the most common phenotype and karyotype.[219,220] A case of vertical (transplacental) transmission of acute monocytic leukemia from mother to son has been reported.[221]

Infants who are normal at birth but develop AML in the first few weeks of life (neonatal leukemia) often display pallor, inadequate food intake, insufficient weight gain, diarrhea, and lethargy. The presence of a cytogenetic abnormality of band q23 on chromosome 11 is a very poor prognostic sign. Infants with congenital or neonatal leukemia rarely survive for more than a few weeks. Since treatment has been largely ineffective, observation to ascertain if a transient myeloproliferative syndrome or a transient leukemia is present has been recommended if the clinical picture is unclear.[222]

HYBRID AND MIXED LEUKEMIAS

Hybrid Leukemias Although coincidental myeloid and lymphoid clonal diseases have been reported for over 30 years, the availability of techniques to identify surface antigens with monoclonal antibodies; immunoglobulin gene and T-lymphocyte receptor gene rearrangements with molecular methods; and chromosome translocations by chromosome banding cytogenetic techniques has led to the appreciation of several types of hybrid acute leukemia.[223–234,237]

Bilineal (interlineal) acute leukemias are cases in which a significant proportion of cells (over 10 percent) have lymphoid and myeloid markers, *interlineal* here referring to lymphocytic and hematopoietic gene expression. Bilineal (biphenotypic) leukemias are heterogeneous in that some cases have cells with both lymphoid and myeloid markers (chimeric) and other cases have cells with either lymphoid or myeloid markers but evidence that all the cells are part of the same malignant clone (mosaic). The bilineal leukemias may be synchronous (that is, lymphoid and myeloid cells are present simultaneously) or asynchronous (in which lymphoid cells are succeeded by myeloid cells or vice versa), but there is evidence for their origin from the same clone.

Cases of biphenotypic leukemia that are morphologically or cytochemically indicative of myelogenous leukemia have been referred to as LY+ AML, and those more indicative of lymphocytic leukemia

MY+ ALL.[225] Interlineal hybrid leukemias, as a group, treated with current regimens, respond to therapy at about the same rate as AML cases without lymphoid markers.[224] Some observers suggest altering drug regimens depending on the balance between lymphoid and myeloid biochemical (drug-response) patterns.[236]

Acute myelogenous leukemias may be intralineal hybrids in that the blast cells have markers for two or more myeloid lineages, for example, erythroid, granulocytic, and megakaryocytic, or in the case of lymphocytic leukemias both immunoglobulin gene rearrangement (B-lymphocyte type) and T-cell receptor gene rearrangement (T-lymphocyte type).

Myeloid–Natural Killer Cell Hybrids and t(8;13) Myeloid-Lymphoid Leukemias Two notable syndromes have been associated with hybrid leukemias: the myeloid leukemia and natural killer cell hybrid[238–240] and the lymphoma, eosinophilia, and myeloid, t(8;13), leukemia hybrid.[241,242] In both syndromes signs of lymphoma such as mediastinal or other lymphadenopathy and extranodal lymphoid tumor are mixed with findings compatible with acute myeloid leukemia. The morphology of the myeloid leukemia simulates acute promyelocytic leukemia.

Hybrid leukemias may result from either lineage infidelity as a result of genetic misprogramming[237] or from promiscuous gene expression, which occurs transiently in the differentiation of normal multipotential hematopoietic stem cells. In the latter case (promiscuity), a persistence of this transient normal event is thought to be present because of the block in differentiation that occurs in these cases.[230] Genetic misprogramming (infidelity) could result from DNA rearrangements of the sequences that control the transcription of genes that designate differentiation antigens.[243]

Mixed Leukemias In these cases lymphoid and myeloid cells are present simultaneously but are derived from separate clones or there is sequential myeloid and lymphoid leukemia but the two lineages are derived from separate clones.

MEDIASTINAL GERM CELL TUMORS AND AML

An unusual but significant concordance has been reported between mediastinal germ cell tumors and AML, especially the megakaryoblastic variant.[244–248] The mediastinal tumors are rare variants of germ cell tumors. The latter ordinarily occur as testicular teratomas and seminomas in men or as ovarian teratomas in women and are thought to be derived from yolk sac cells that failed to migrate.[247,248] AML is a hematopoietic stem cell tumor derived from a cell type that is present in the yolk sac also. Cytogenetic studies are compatible with a clonal relationship (identity) of the mediastinal germ cells and the myelogenous leukemia cells.[244,245] Apparently, hematopoietic lineage genes are predisposed to expression in extragonadal (mediastinal) germ cell tumors.

MORPHOLOGIC VARIANTS OF ACUTE MYELOGENOUS LEUKEMIA

Morphologic variants of AML (Table 93-4) may occur de novo or may be the manifestation of clonal evolution from essential thrombocythemia, idiopathic myelofibrosis, chronic myelogenous leukemia, or other nonacute clonal stem cell disorders. For example, every phenotypic variant of AML can occur as the blast crisis of CML (see Chap. 94).

MYELOBLASTIC LEUKEMIA

The designation *acute myeloblastic leukemia* came into being in the second decade of the twentieth century,[6,7] following the specific description of the myeloblast.[6] About 30 percent of cases of AML have the features of acute myeloblastic leukemia, a variant in which the

TABLE 93-4   MORPHOLOGIC VARIANTS OF AML

Variant	Cytologic Features	Special Clinical Features	Special Laboratory Features
Acute myeloblastic leukemia (M0, M1, M2)	1. Myeloblasts are usually large; nuclear cytoplasmic ratio 1:1. Cytoplasm usually contains granules and occasionally Auer bodies. Nucleus shows fine reticular pattern and distinct nucleoli. 2. Blast cells are Sudanophilic. They are positive for myeloperoxidase and chloroacetate esterase, negative for nonspecific esterase, and negative or diffusely positive for PAS (no clumps or blocks). 3. Electron microscope (EM) shows primary cytoplasmic granules.	1. Most common in adults, and most frequent variety in infants. 2. Three morphologic-cytochemical types (M0, M1, and M2)	1. Chromosomes +8, −5, −7, common. 2. M0 type blast cells positive with antibody to myeloperoxidase and anti-CD34 and CD13 or CD33 coexpression. 3. M1 expresses CD13 and CD33. Positive for myeloperoxidase by cytochemistry. 4. (M2) AML with maturation often associated with t(8;21) karyotype.
Acute promyelocytic leukemia (M3, M3v)	1. Leukemic cells resemble promyelocytes. They have large atypical primary granules and a kidney-shaped nucleus. Branched or adherent Auer rods are common. 2. Peroxidase stain intensely positive. 3. A variant has microgranules (M3v), otherwise the same course and prognosis.	1. Usually in adults. 2. Hypofibrinogenemia and hemorrhage common. 3. Leukemic cells mature in response to all-*trans*-retinoic acid.	1. Cell contains t(15;17) or other alteration in chromosome 17 2. Cells are HLA-DR-negative
Acute myelomonocytic leukemia (M4, M4Eo)	1. Both myeloblastic and monoblastic leukemic cells in blood and marrow. 2. Peroxidase-, Sudan-, chloroacetate esterase-, and nonspecific esterase-positive cells. 3. M4Eo variant has marrow eosinophilia.	1. Similar to myeloblastic leukemia but with more frequent extramedullary disease. 2. Mildly elevated serum and urine lysozyme.	1. Eosinophilic variant has inversion or other abnormalities of chromosome 16.
Acute monocytic leukemia (M5)	1. Leukemia cells are large; nuclear cytoplasmic ratio lower than myeloblast. Cytoplasm contains fine granules. Auer rods are rare. Nucleus is convoluted and may contain large nucleoli. 2. Nonspecific esterase-positive inhibited by NaF; Sudan-, peroxidase-, and chloroacetate esterase-negative. PAS occurs in granules, blocks.	1. Seen in children or young adults. 2. Gum, CNS, lymph node, and extramedullary infiltrations are common. 3. DIC occurs. 4. Plasma and urine lysozyme elevated. 5. Hyperleukocytosis common.	1. t(4;11) common in infants. 2. Rearrangement of q11;q23 very frequent
Acute erythroleukemia (M6)	1. Abnormal erythroblasts are in abundance initially in marrow and often in blood. Later the morphologic findings may be indistinguishable from those of AML.	1. Pancytopenia common at diagnosis.	1. Cells reactive with antihemogloblin antibody. Erythroblasts are usually strongly PAS-positive. 2. Cells reactive with anti Rc-84 (anti-human erythroleukemia cell-line antigen).
Acute megakaryocytic leukemia (M7)	1. Small blasts with pale agranular cytoplasm and cytoplasmic blebs. May mimic lymphoblasts of medium to larger size.	1. Usually presents with pancytopenia. 2. Markedly elevated serum lactic dehydrogenase levels. 3. Marrow aspirates are usually "dry taps" because of the invariable presence of myelofibrosis. 4. Common phenotype in the AML of Down syndrome.	1. Antigens of von Willebrand factor, and glycoprotein Ib (CD42), IIb/IIIa (CD41), IIIa (CD61) on blast cells. 2. Platelet peroxidase-positive.

( ) = FAB designation.

leukemic myeloblast is the predominant cell in the marrow. Acute myeloblastic leukemia has been divided into two forms, designated *M0* and *M1* in the French-American-British (FAB) classification, which converts the descriptive term for a leukemic phenotype into a number. In either type, there is little evidence of maturation of myeloblasts, and the marrow is replaced by a monotonous population of blasts. In the former type, acute myeloblastic leukemia (M0), the patient's age distribution, presenting white cell count, and cytogenetic abnormalities are not distinctive. The blasts are nonreactive when stained for myeloperoxidase activity, and Auer rods are not seen. The blasts do react with antibodies to myeloperoxidase and antibodies to CD13, CD33, and CD34. There is a more frequent presence of abnormal and unfavorable karyotypes (e.g., 5q-,7q-) and higher expression of the multidrug

resistance glycoprotein (p170). This phenotypic variant has a poor prognosis.[249–251] In the other type of myeloblastic leukemia, designated M1, myeloblasts are present in the blood and comprise over 70 percent of the marrow cells. Fewer than 15 percent of marrow cells are promyelocytes and myelocytes. Auer rods may be present in occasional blasts, but azurophilic granules are not evident in the blasts by light microscopy. At least 5 percent, but usually a much higher percentage, of the blast cells have a positive reaction when stained for peroxidase or with Sudan black or react with monoclonal antibodies specific to myeloblasts, such as CD33. This morphologic subtype is denoted as M1 in the FAB classification.

In many cases of myeloblastic leukemia, more prominent granulocytic maturation is evident (FAB type M2). This variant is present in about 25 percent of cases of AML; thus myeloblastic leukemia with or without maturation makes up over 50 percent of cases of AML. Blasts usually constitute at least 30 percent of the marrow cells. Auer rods may be present in blast cells. Promyelocytes, myelocytes, and segmented neutrophils, the latter often with the acquired Pelger-Hüet anomaly, may constitute 30 to 60 percent of marrow granulocytes. The anomaly is reflected in bilobed or monolobed neutrophils. Histochemical and surface markers of blast cells are typical of myeloblastic leukemia, and monocytic markers are absent or infrequent. A translocation between chromosomes 8 and 21 t(8;21)(q22;q22), often concomitant with the loss of the Y chromosome in men or an X chromosome in women, has been associated with this phenotype and occurs in younger patients (average age about 30).[252–254] Patients whose cells contain t(8;21) are prone to granulocytic sarcoma.[141,142]

MYELOMONOCYTIC LEUKEMIA

The ability of AML to express cells of the monocytic and granulocytic lineages was first highlighted in the early 1900s by Naegeli; later, Downey proposed the eponym *Naegeli type* for myelomonocytic leukemia.[256] About 20 percent of patients with AML present with this variant, and they are more likely to have extramedullary infiltrates in gingiva, skin, or central nervous system than those with acute myeloblastic leukemia.[257] A mixture of myeloblasts and monoblasts is found in the blood and marrow. Over 30 percent of marrow cells are myeloblasts, which react with peroxidase or chloracetate esterase, and monoblasts, which react with fluoride-inhibitable nonspecific esterase. Over 20 percent of cells are monoblasts or promonocytes in blood and marrow. In some cases, individual cells react with both monocytic and granulocytic histochemical stains.[258] Serum and urinary lysozyme levels are increased in most cases. This variant of AML is referred to as *M4* in the FAB classification. The proportion of marrow eosinophils[259] or basophils[260] may be increased.

Translocations involving chromosome 3 have been associated with this phenotype.[261] A special variant of myelomonocytic leukemia has increased numbers of marrow eosinophils (10 to 50 percent), Auer rods, and inversion or rearrangement of chromosome 16.[262–265] The eosinophils are abnormally large, and the eosinophilic myelocytes contain large basophilic granules. Macrophages with ingested Charcot-Leyden crystals may be present. This phenotypic variant of AML has been designated *M4Eo* in the FAB classification. A variant of acute myelomonocytic leukemia has an increased number of marrow basophils and a translocation involving chromosomes 6 and 9, t(6;9)(p23;q34).[266] This variant occurs at a younger age, has a poor prognosis, and has a tendency to trilineage dysmorphogenesis and ringed sideroblasts.[267]

ERYTHROLEUKEMIA

Prominence of erythroid cell proliferation in cases of AML was noted by Copelli[268] and DiGuglielmo[269] in the early twentieth century. Erythroleukemia makes up about 5 percent of cases of AML and is referred to as *M6* in the FAB classification. Familial erythroleukemia has been described.[43,44]

Anemia and thrombocytopenia are present in nearly all cases. Some patients may have elevated total leukocyte counts. The red cells show marked anisocytosis, poikilocytosis, anisochromia, and basophilic stippling. Nucleated red cells are present in the blood. The marrow erythroblasts are extremely abnormal, with giant multinucleate forms, nuclear budding, and nuclear fragmentation. Cytogenetic abnormalities are present in about two-thirds of patients. In the earlier stage or less severe form of the disease, so-called erythremic myelosis, granulopoiesis and thrombopoiesis may be only mildly abnormal. This

severe dyserythropoietic phase can be protracted but evolves, sooner or later, into one in which myeloblasts are more prominent; severe neutropenia and thrombocytopenia develop; and the patient progresses to *erythroleukemia*. The disease may evolve further into polyblastic AML.[270–273]

During the erythremic myelosis and erythroleukemia stages, erythropoiesis is markedly ineffective but some normal influences remain, since hypertransfusion decreases both erythropoietin levels and the amount of abnormal erythropoiesis.[274] Spontaneous growth of leukemic erythroid clonogenic cells is a feature of the disease.[275] Periodic acid–Schiff-positive erythroblasts are evident in virutally all cases.[270,273] The frequency of erythroblastic leukemia is increased if methods of detecting erythroid differentiation more sensitive than light microscopy are used. These cell features include glycophorin A, spectrin, carbonic anhydrase I, ABH blood group antigens, or other antigens that occur on early erythroid progenitors.[276–278] Anti-hemoglobin antibody and anti-human erythroleukemic cell-line antibody are often positive.[271]

Erythremic myelosis can have an indolent course and may be managed for a time without intensive chemotherapy. In patients with erythroleukemia, treatment is warranted, and the results are approximately those of other phenotypes in patients of similar age.[273] The more predominant the erythroid component and the less the proportion of myeloblasts, the better the response to therapy.[276]

PROMYELOCYTIC (PROGRANULOCYTIC) LEUKEMIA

The association of an exaggerated hemorrhagic syndrome with certain leukemias was described by French hematologists in 1949,[279] and in 1957 Hillstad bestowed the appellation *promyelocytic leukemia* upon this morphologic-clinical subtype of AML.[280] This variant, which is called *M3* in the FAB classification, occurs at any age and constitutes about 10 percent of cases of AML.[281–284] This subtype of AML occurs with greater frequency than expected among Latinos from Europe and South and Central America[285,286] and among patients with an increased body mass index.[287]

Hemorrhagic manifestations are prominent including hemoptysis, hematuria, vaginal bleeding, melena, hematemesis, and pulmonary and intracranial bleeding, as well as the more typical skin and mucous membrane bleeding. In severely leukopenic patients, blasts may not be evident in the blood. Moderately severe thrombocytopenia [$<50,000/\mu$l ($<50 \times 10^9$/liter)] is present in most cases. The marrow contains few agranular blast cells and some blastlike cells with scant granules. The dominant cells are promyelocytes, which comprise 30 to 90 percent of marrow cells. Auer rods and cells with multiple Auer rods (1 to 10 percent) are present in nearly every case. Promyelocytes with bundles of Auer rods have been referred to as *faggot cells*. Leukemic promyelocytes stain intensely with myeloperoxidase and Sudan black and express CD 9, CD13, and CD33 but not CD34 or HLA-DR.[281–284]

A variant type of promyelocytic leukemia is referred to as *microgranular* (*M3v* in the FAB nomenclature).[288–291] Microgranular cases represent about 20 percent of patients with promyelocytic leukemia. The leukemic cells may mimic promonocytes with convoluted or lobulated nuclei. Auer rods may be present but are less evident. The majority of the leukemic cells contain such small azurophilic granules that they are not visible by light microscopy, but the peroxidase stain is usually strongly positive. Typical hypergranulated promyelocytes are usually present on careful inspection. The total white cell count is often very elevated, and severe coagulopathy is prominent in microgranular cases.[289] Rarely the cells may contain eosinophilic or basophilic granules, but the t(15;17) is present, and the response to all-*trans*-retinoic acid persists.[292–294]

A translocation between chromosome 17 and another chromosome is present in virtually all cases of acute promyelocytic leukemia and in the acute promyelocytic transformation of CML and is not found in other AML variants. The t(15;17) is the most frequent (over 95 percent), but variant translocations between chromosomes 5 or 11 and 17, isochromosome 17, and other less common variants have also been described.[281,283,295,296] In some cases, cytogenetic analysis is inadequate, and Southern blot analysis is required to identify the rearrangement of the RARα gene.

The breakpoint on chromosome 17 is within the gene for the retinoic acid receptor-α, and the breakpoint on chromosome 15 is within the locus of a gene originally referred to as MYL and renamed PML.[297–300] The gene may encode a unique transcription factor. The translocation results in two new chimeric or fusion genes, RARα-PML that is actively transcribed in acute promyelocytic leukemia, and PML-RARα that is also transcribed and may account for the aberrancy in hematopoiesis. The PML-RARα gene has two isoforms that produce a short and a long type fusion mRNA, respectively.[301] Patients with the short isoform may have a worse outcome than those with the longer form. Polymerase chain reaction for the mRNA of the fusion gene can be used to identify residual cells during remission and may predict for relapse. The PML-RARα transgene can reproduce the disease in mice.[302] The specific transforming effects of the protein product are uncertain.[283]

A propensity to hemorrhage is a striking feature of this subtype. The prothrombin and partial thromboplastin times are prolonged and the plasma fibrinogen level decreased in most cases. The disturbance in coagulation was initially thought to be principally the result of intravascular coagulation initiated by procoagulant released from the granules of the leukemic promyelocytes. Elevated thrombin-antithrombin complexes, prothrombin fragment 1+2, and fibrinopeptide A plasma levels support that supposition. Increased levels of fibrinogen-fibrin degradation products, D-dimer, and plasminogen activiation indicate fibrinolysis.[303–305] Decreased levels of plasminogen, increased expression of annexin II on the leukemic cells, and reports of responses to tranexamic acid support an important role for fibrinolysis.[306] Release of nonspecific proteases may further contribute to fibrinogenolysis.

Although acute promyelocytic leukemia responds to chemotherapy regimens for AML, especially those containing an anthracycline antibiotic like daunomycin or rubidazone,[307] the cytologic pattern of response in the marrow was often paradoxical.[308–310] Persistence of leukemic promyelocytes preceded remission in the absence of further therapy, whereas induction of marrow cell hypoplasia was classically considered a requirement for remission in patients with AML. Generally, if leukemic blast cells persist after therapy of AML, relapse ensued unless hypoplasia is induced by more cytotoxic therapy. The unusual pattern of response in acute promyelocytic leukemia was put into context by reports of successful treatment with isomers of retinoic acid, an agent that was known to lead to maturation of leukemic promyelocytes in vitro.[311] In 1988 the success of all-trans-retinoic acid in remission induction was reported[312,313] and confirmed.[283,284] Relapse occurs invariably, however, and thus chemotherapy regimens are required as well. The use of all-trans-retinoic acid has decreased the risk of early hemorrhagic complications and death and enhanced the long-term response to chemotherapy. The approach to therapy and outcome is discussed in the section "Therapy, Course, and Prognosis."

MONOCYTIC LEUKEMIA

Monocytic leukemia was first reported by Reschad and Schilling-Torgau in 1913.[314] About 8 percent of patients with AML present with monocytic leukemia, which is referred to as M5 in the FAB classification. Patients with monocytic leukemia have a higher preva-

lence (50 percent) of extramedullary tumors in the skin, gingiva, eyes, larynx, lung, rectum and anal canal, bladder, lymph nodes, meninges, central nervous system, or other sites than do other phenotypes (<5 percent). Hepatomegaly and splenomegaly also are more frequent in monocytic leukemia.[94,315–317]

The total leukocyte count is higher in a larger proportion of patients, and hyperleukocytosis occurs more frequently (about 35 percent) than in other variants.[318–320] The blood cells may be largely monoblasts or more mature-appearing promonocytes and monocytes. When the blood contains more mature monocytic cells, the marrow contains a lower proportion of blast cells, about 25 to 50 percent, and when the blood monocytes are largely blast cells, the marrow contains about 50 to 90 percent blasts. In nearly all cases 10 to 90 percent of monocytic cells react with nonspecific esterase stains, α-naphthyl acetate esterase, and naphthol AS-D acetate esterase, or with monoclonal antibodies against monocyte surface antigens, especially CD-14. Immunoreactivity of cells for lysozyme is also characteristic. Serum and urine lysozyme levels are elevated in most patients. Serum lactic dehydrogenase and beta-2 microglobulin concentrations are increased in over 80 percent of patients.[321] Plasminogen activator inhibitor-2 is present in the plasma and the cells of a high proportion of patients.[322] Auer rods are absent when monoblasts dominate but are present frequently in cases in which promonocytes and monocytes are prevalent in blood and marrow. Leukemic monocytes have Fc receptors and can ingest and kill microorganisms in some cases.[323,324]

An association between translocations involving chromosome 11, especially region 11q23, and monocytic leukemia is present.[163] In particular, t(9;11) and t(11;17) are found in leukemic monocytes.[317,318,325] In t(9;11) the β₁-interferon gene is translocated to chromosome 11, and the protooncogene ETS-1 is translocated to chromosome 9 adjacent to the α-interferon gene. The latter juxtaposition may be important in the pathogenesis of monocytic leukemia.[164]

The expression of FOS is closely correlated with monocytic maturation of cells in myelomonocytic and monocytic leukemia and in normal monocytopoiesis.[326,327] Absence or markedly decreased expression of the retinoblastoma gene growth suppressor product (p105) is present in about half the patients with monocytic leukemia. These patients express a more dramatic phenotype.[328] A variant of acute monocytic leukemia in which the leukemic cells have monocytoid features and are positive for early and late monocytic lineage antigens and for terminal deoxynucleotidyl transferase activity often occurs after prior radio- or chemotherapy and is relatively resistant to treatment.[329]

The management of monocytic leukemia is complicated by a greater incidence of central nervous system or meningeal disease either at the time of diagnosis or as a form of relapse during remission. Thus, an examination of cerebrospinal fluid should be performed even in the absence of symptoms.[94,317–320] Some therapists recommend prophylactic intrathecal therapy with methotrexate or cytosine arabinoside for patients who enter remission.

Rare cases of dendritic cell or Langerhans' cell phenotype have been described[330,331] (see Chap. 78). Very uncommon cases of histiocytic sarcoma are the tissue or extramedullary variant of monocytic leukemia[332,333] (see Chap. 78).

MEGAKARYOBLASTIC LEUKEMIA

In 1963 Szur and Lewis reported patients with pancytopenia, low percentages of blast cells, and intense myelofibrosis but absence of teardrop red cells, splenomegaly, leukocytosis, and thrombocytosis, the usual features of idiopathic myelofibrosis. They designated the syndrome malignant myelosclerosis.[334] Reports of similar cases ensued, some referring to the syndrome as acute myelofibrosis.[335] The development of methods to phenotype megakaryoblasts indicated that these cases were variants of AML rather than of myelofibrosis and have been designated *acute megakaryocytic* or *acute megakaryoblastic leukemia*.[336,337] This leukemia is referred to as *M7* in the FAB classification. The prevalence of this phenotype is about 5 percent of all cases of AML and is at least twice that frequency in childhood AML.[338] It is an especially prevalent variant of AML that develops in patients with Down syndrome[339,340] or mediastinal germ cell tumors.[244–248]

The leukemic megakaryoblasts and promegakaryocytes can be very difficult to identify by light microscopy using polychrome staining, although with experience heightened suspicion can be engendered by blasts with abundant budding cytoplasm or blasts that have a lymphoid appearance, especially if the marrow cannot be aspirated, because of intense myelofibrosis which is evident on the marrow biopsy. Initially high-resolution histochemistry for platelet peroxidase and identification of the demarcation membrane system using transmission electron microscopy were required for diagnosis. Now antibodies to von Willebrand factor or to glycoprotein Ib (CD42), IIb/IIIa (CD41), or IIIa (CD61) can be used to identify very primitive megakaryocytic cells.[336,337] A small proportion of megakaryoblasts may be present in other cases of AML, but in megakaryocytic leukemia they are prominent (>10 percent) or the dominant leukemic cells; moreover, the other key features of the syndrome are usually present, especially severe myelofibrosis.[338]

Patients usually present with pallor, weakness, excessive bleeding and anemia, and leukopenia. Lymphadenopathy or hepatosplenomegaly is very uncommon at the time of diagnosis. High leukocyte and blood blast cell counts may be present initially or develop later. The platelet count may be normal or elevated in many patients at the time of their presentation. Marrow aspiration is often unsuccessful ("dry tap") because of the extensive marrow fibrosis in most cases. The marrow biopsy contains either small or large blast cells or some combination of both. The former have a high nuclear/cytoplasmic ratio, have dense chromatin with distinct nucleoli, and resemble lymphoblasts. Cases have been mistaken for ALL. The larger blasts may have some features of maturing megakaryocytes with agranular cytoplasm with cytoplasmic protrusions, clusters of plateletlike structures, or shedding of cytoplasmic blebs. The blast cells are peroxidase-negative and tend to aggregate. Confirmation of their megakaryoblastic maturation requires immunocytologic studies of the presence of von Willebrand factor and the immunoreactivity to CD41, CD42, or CD61. The more mature megakaryocytes stain with periodic acid–Schiff reagent, contain sodium fluoride-inhibitable nonspecific esterase, and fail to react for α-naphthylbutyrate esterase.

The serum lactic acid dehydrogenase is frequently strikingly increased and has an isomorphic pattern unlike that seen with other myeloproliferative disorders. An association of megakaryoblastic leukemia in infants with t(1;22)(p13;q13) has been reported.[341] Abnormalities of chromosome 3 have been linked to clonal hemopathies expressing a prominent megakaryocytic phenotype.[342,343] The progression to AML of idiopathic myelofibrosis or essential thrombocythemia may have the phenotype of acute megakaryocytic leukemia.

EOSINOPHILIC LEUKEMIA

Acute eosinophilic leukemia is rare. Increased eosinophils in the marrow but not the blood is seen as a variant of acute myelomonocytic leukemia and inv 16 or other abnormalities of chromosome 16 but is not considered an acute eosinophilic leukemia.[262–265] First described in 1912,[344] acute eosinophilic leukemia is a distinct entity that can arise de novo as AML with 50 to 80 percent of eosinophilic cells in the blood and marrow.[345–347] A specific histochemical reaction, cyanide-resistant peroxidase, permits the identification of leukemic blast cells

with eosinophilic differentiation and the diagnosis of acute eosinoblastic leukemia in some cases of AML with few identifiable eosinophils in blood or marrow.[348] Eosinophilia, not part of the malignant clone, may be a feature of occasional patients with AML. Idiopathic eosinophilia (hypereosinophilic syndrome) is, in some cases, a monoclonal disorder and represents a spectrum of more indolent chronic or subacute eosinophilic leukemia to more progressive acute leukemia[349] (see Chap. 68). Acute eosinophilic leukemia may also evolve in patients who have the chronic form of a hypereosinophilic syndrome. The overexpression of Wilms' tumor gene expression has been proposed as a means of distinguishing acute eosinophilic leukemia from a polyclonal, reactive eosinophilia.[350]

Patients with acute eosinophilic leukemia have a propensity for developing bronchospastic signs and heart failure from endomyocardial fibrosis. Hepatomegaly and splenomegaly are more common than in other variants of AML.

Response to treatment is about the same as in other types of AML.[348]

BASOPHILIC AND MAST CELL LEUKEMIA

First described in 1906,[351] basophilic differentiation as a feature of AML is a very rare event. Most cases of basophilic leukemia evolve from the chronic phase of CML,[352] but de novo acute basophilic leukemia, in which the cells do not contain the Philadelphia chromosome, does occur.[353–356] The cells stain with toluidine blue, and the basophilic granules can be most striking in myelocytes. In some cases of acute myelomonocytic leukemia associated with t(6;9)(p23;q34), basophils may be increased in the marrow but not in the blood. Since CML with t(9;22)(q34;q11) has the same breakpoint (q34) on chromosome 9 as AML with t(6;9) and both diseases are strongly associated with marrow basophilia, a gene or genes at the breakpoint on chromosome 9 may influence basophilopoiesis.[266]

The blood leukocyte count is usually elevated, and proportions of the cells are basophils. The marrow is cellular with a high proportion of blasts and early and late basophilic myelocytes. Special staining with toluidine blue or astra blue is often necessary to distinguish basophilic from neutrophilic promyelocytes and myelocytes. Immunophenotyping may show myeloid markers and CD9 or CD25. Cells may have granules with ultrastructural features of basophils and mast cells.[354] Electron microscopy can be useful in identifying basophilic granules in cases in which none are evident by light microscopy and simulate M0 phenotype. Basophilic leukemia can be confused with promyelocytic leukemia if the basophilic early myelocytes are mistaken for promyelocytes.[357] Prolonged clotting time, intravascular coagulation, and hemorrhage are uncommon presenting features in patients with basophilic leukemia, whereas they are very common in promyelocytic leukemia. Urticaria and elevated blood histamine levels occur in patients with basophilic leukemia. Treatment for acute (Ph-negative) basophilic leukemia is similar to that for other variants of AML.

Mast cell leukemia is a rare manifestation of systemic mast cell disease[358] (see Chap. 69). It can be related to a mutation of the *C-KIT* gene.[359] Extensive, apparently, reactive mast cell tissue infiltrations may be provoked by cytokines during the course of acute myelogenous leukemia.[360]

DIFFERENTIAL DIAGNOSIS

Acute leukemia in infants with Down syndrome should be differentiated from transient myeloproliferative disease (see "Neonatal Myeloproliferation and Leukemia," above). In adults *pseudoleukemia* is the term that has been applied to circumstances that mimic the marrow appearance of promyelocytic leukemia. Recovery from drug-induced or *Pseudomonas aeruginosa*–induced agranulocytosis is characterized by a striking cohort of promyelocytes in the marrow, which on inspection of the marrow aspirate or biopsy mimics promyelocytic leukemia.[361-363]

In pseudoleukemia the platelet count may be normal; the degree of leukopenia is often more profound [<1000/μl (<1.0 × 10^9/liter) than usually seen in AML[361,362]; promyelocytes contain a prominent paranuclear clear (Golgi) zone not covered with granules; and promelocytes do not have Auer rods.[365-368] Similar reactions have been reported after G-CSF administration.[364] In patients suspected of pseudoleukemia, observation for a few days will usually clarify the significance of the marrow appearance, since progressive maturation to segmented neutrophils will normalize the marrow and led to an increasing blood neutrophil count.

In patients with hypoplastic marrows, careful examination of specimens is required to distinguish among aplastic anemia, hypoplastic acute leukemia,[200-202] and hypoplastic oligoblastic leukemia.[69] Leukemic blast cells are evident in the marrow in hypoplastic leukemia, and islands of dysmorphic cells, especially megakaryocytes, are present in hypoplastic oligoblastic leukemia.

Leukemoid reactions and nonleukemic pancytopenias can be distinguished from AML by the absence of leukemic blast cells in the blood or marrow. In older children and adults myeloblasts usually do not constitute more than 2 percent of marrow cells except in patients with leukemia, and the proportion of blast cells usually decreases in the marrow with neutrophilic leukemoid reactions.

THERAPY, COURSE, AND PROGNOSIS

DECISION TO TREAT

Most patients with AML should be advised to undergo treatment promptly after diagnosis. Although remission rates are lower in aged patients, a significant proportion enter remission. Occasionally very elderly patients refuse treatment or are so ill from unrelated illnesses that treatment may be unreasonable. Age per se is not a contraindication to treatment, and septuagenarians and octogenarians can enter sustained remissions. Treatment can be tailored to the decreased tolerance of elderly patients (see ''Treatment of Older Patients,'' below). Associated problems such as hemorrhagic manifestations, severe anemia, or infections should be treated in parallel. Since remission is necessary to eliminate these associated problems, delays in induction chemotherapy treatments are usually detrimental in the long run.

PREPARATION OF THE PATIENT

Orientation of the patient and the family should give them an understanding of the disease, the treatment planned, and the adverse effects of treatment. For example, the likelihood of alopecia and its duration should be discussed and advice about hair pieces provided. While most patients and their families will be focused upon their new diagnosis of leukemia and the induction chemotherapy treatment phase, most will also want information about prognosis and long-term treatment plans. Because most patients will enter a complete remission, and because some patients can expect to have long-term disease-free survival after completion of their treatment regimen, cautious optimism is appropriate.

Pretreatment laboratory examination should include blood cell counts, cytochemistry, immunophenotyping of leukemic cells, and marrow examination, including cytogenetic analysis, blood chemistry studies, chest x-ray films, electrocardiogram, and determination of partial thromboplastin and prothrombin times. More extensive evaluation of coagulation factors should be made if clotting times are abnormal, if bleeding is exaggerated for the level of the platelet count, or if acute promyelocytic or monocytic leukemia is the phenotype. Early HLA typing is useful so that compatible platelet products can be provided if alloimmunization occurs and for patients who will become marrow transplant candidates. It can also be helpful to perform *Herpes simplex* virus and cytomegalovirus serotyping. HIV and hepatitis serology is indicated in certain patients, and patients should have a baseline cardiac scan to determine ejection fraction prior to administration of an anthracycline agent.

A tunneled central venous catheter should be placed (see Chap. 20). This access to the circulation facilitates administration of chemotherapy, blood components, antibiotics, and other intravenous fluids and medications and permits sampling blood for analysis without patient discomfort or concern about venous access.[375] Meticulous skin care at the catheter exit site is required to minimize tunnel infections.[376]

Therapy for hyperuricemia is required if (1) the pretreatment uric acid level is greater than 7.0 mg/dl (0.4 mmol/liter), (2) the marrow is packed with blast cells, or (3) the blood blast cell count is moderately or markedly elevated. Allopurinol, 300 mg/day, orally, should be used. Allopurinol can cause allergic dermatitis, and it should not be used if uric acid is under 7 mg/dl, and the total white cell count is under about 20,000/μl (20 × 10^9/liter), as long as hydration is adequate and urine flow is high (>150 ml/h). The dermatitis appears at a time when antibiotics may be instituted. This concurrence may make it unclear whether the antibiotics can be continued. Thus, allopurinol use should stop after the risk of acute hyperuricosuria or tumor lysis has passed (usually 4 to 7 days).

Attention to decreasing pathogen exposure by assiduous hand washing and meticulous care of catheter and intravenous sites is important, especially when the total neutrophil count is under 500/μl (0.5 × 10^9/liter). Care of the patient in *a single room* is advisable to provide privacy during periods of intensive care and severe discomfort and to help decrease the risk of exogenously acquired infection until recovery of the neutrophil count occurs. Unwashed fruits and vegetables and marijuana are also thought to be sources of pathogenic microorganisms and should be prohibited during the neutropenic period [<500/μl (<0.5 × 10^9/liter)].

REMISSION-INDUCTION THERAPY

PRINCIPLES

The cytotoxic therapy of AML rests on two tenets: (1) two competing populations of cells are present in marrow—a normal, polyclonal and a leukemic, monoclonal population; (2) profound suppression of the leukemic cells to the point that they are inapparent in the marrow aspirate and biopsy is required to permit the restoration of polyclonal hematopoiesis.[377]

Although these two principles hold in most cases, two deviations from these guidelines are the predisposition of patients with acute promyelocytic leukemia to enter remission despite cellular posttherapy marrows[378,379] and the observation that monoclonal hematopoiesis may be present in some cases of AML during remission (see ''Results of Treatment'').

CYTOTOXIC REGIMENS

Current standard induction treatment for AML involves drug regimens with two or more agents,[380,381] which include an anthracycline or anthraquinone and cytarabine.[382-384] The remission rates with such treatment vary from about 50 to 90 percent in adult subjects (Table 93-5) depending on the composition of the population treated. The two most important variables are age of the patients and the proportion of patients with therapy-induced leukemia or an antecedent clonal hemopathy. A

TABLE 93-5   REMISSION INDUCTION FOR AML—COMBINATION OF CYTOSINE ARBINOSIDE AND ANTHRACYCLINE ANTIBIOTIC

DOSE AND SCHEDULE		NO. OF PATIENTS	AGE RANGE (MEDIAN AGE), YEARS	COMPLETE REMISSIONS, %	YEAR OF REPORT	REFERENCE
CYTARABINE	ANTHRACYCLINE ANTIBIOTIC ± ANOTHER AGENT					
3 gm/m² every 12h for 5 days	80 mg/m² (total) mitoxantrone 150 mg/m² etoposide for 3 days	45	<60 (NR)	80	1997	393
3 gm/m², every 12h, days 1, 3, 5, 7	50 mg/m² DNR for 3 days; 75 mg/m² etoposide for 7 days	101	15–60 (45)	71	1996	389
100 mg/m² continuous infusion for 7 days	50 mg/m² DNR for 3 days; 75 mg/m² etoposide for 7 days	102	15–60 (39)	74	1996	389
500 mg/m² by continuous infusion, days 1–3, 8–10	12 mg/m² mitoxantrone for 3 days; 200 mg/m² etoposide IV days 8–10	113	15–70 (43)	60	1995	394
100 mg/m² daily for 7 days	45 mg/m² DNR for 3 days	113	NR (55)	59	1992	382
100 mg/m² daily for 7 days	13 mg/m² IDA for 3 days	101	NR (56)	70	1992	382
200 mg/m² daily for 5 days	50 mg/m² DNR for 3 days	65	19–60 (42)	58	1991	383
200 mg/m² daily for 5 days	12 mg/m² IDA for 3 days	65	17–60 (36)	80	1991	383
3 gm/m² every 12 h for 6 days	45 mg/m² DNR for 3 days	70	17–60 (44)	90	1991	384
100 mg/m² daily for 7 days	50 mg/m² DNR for 3 days	132	15–70 (NR)	56	1990	392
100 mg/m² daily for 7 days	50 mg/m² DNR for 3 days; 75 mg/m² etoposide for 7 days	132	15–70 (NR)	59	1990	392
2 g/m² as a 72-h infusion on days 1 and 10	45 mg/m² DNR for 3 days	75	16–74 (44)	55	1989	391
2 g/m² as a 72-h infusion on day 1	45 mg/m² DNR for 3 days; 200 mg/m² AMSA for 3 days	114	19–79 (55)	54	1989	391

DNR, daunorubicin; IDA, idarubicin; AMSA, amsacrine. The reader is advised to consult the original reports for details of induction and ancillary therapy and consolidation or continuation therapy, which may vary from protocol to protocol. NR = not reported.

combination of an anthracycline and cytarabine has been the standard induction therapy since the 1960s. A current standard induction regimen is daunorubicin at 45 mg/m² for 3 days and cytarabine at 100 mg/m² by continuous infusion for 7 days. Dose or schedule modulation of the anthracycline or cytarabine, addition of other agents such as etoposide, and timed-sequential therapy have represented attempts to improve results above those obtained with standard therapy.[385]

Development of drug resistance is reduced with idarubicin relative to other anthracyclines. Idarubicin does not induce P-glycoprotein expression whereas daunorubicin, doxorubicin, and epirubicin do.[386] Idarubicin 12 mg/m² gives better complete remission rates in younger adults than does daunorubicin 45 mg/m², each given for 3 days. Amsacrine, aclarubicin, and mitoxantrone also give improved results over standard-dose daunorubicin. In older adults, mitoxantrone may reduce cardiotoxicity.[390] Higher doses of daunorubicin may yield higher complete response rates.[387] Dexrazoxane may be given during induction to reduce the risk of cardiotoxicity in patients at higher-than-usual risk because of a history of coronary artery disease or congestive heart failure.[388]

High-dose cytarabine does not increase complete remission rates and increases toxicity when compared to conventional doses, especially in older patients. Patients receiving high-dose cytarabine have more leukopenia, thrombocytopenia, gastrointestinal distress, and eye toxicity. Disease-free survival is better, however, than that achieved with standard therapy, leading some to suggest that high-dose therapy be utilized for induction in patients less than 50 years of age.[389]

Timed, sequential therapy with addition of etoposide may also lead to prolongation of remission duration.[391–394] Timed, sequential chemotherapy combining mitoxantrone on days 1 to 3, etoposide on day 8 to 10, and cytarabine on days 1 to 3 and 8 to 10 resulted in a complete remission in 60 percent, but a toxic death in 9 percent of patients so treated. Median disease-free survival was 9 months.[393] Other studies have not found benefit after addition of high-dose cytarabine to induction regimens. Because many of the studies of various induction regimens differ in age of patients, inclusion criteria, supportive care, and different doses and scheduling of chemotherapy agents, conclusions regarding superiority of any of these regimens compared with standard regimens is difficult. For these reasons, the practice guidelines for AML, other than promyelocytic leukemia, recommend standard-dose cytarabine plus anthracycline treatment.[395] Hematopoietic growth factors used with induction therapy have generally shown no additional benefit.[396]

Patients who have persistent leukemia after the first course of induction chemotherapy are generally given a second similar course. The outcome is worse if two courses of treatment are required even if a complete remission is achieved. About 40 percent of patients with persistent AML after one course of induction therapy have a complete remission after a second course[397] and disease-free survival at 5 years is about 10 percent. The longer the time to remission after the first induction therapy, the shorter the duration of disease-free survival.[235,371] High-risk cytogenetic abnormalities, antecedent hematologic disorders, and other poor prognostic factors can be used to assign nonresponders to a "salvage" chemotherapy regimen rather than repeating induction therapy.

SPECIAL CONSIDERATIONS DURING INDUCTION THERAPY

Hyperleukocytosis   Patients with blast counts greater than 100,000/μl (100 × 10⁹/liter) require prompt treatment to prevent the most serious complication of hyperleukocytosis, intracranial hemorrhage. Cytoreduction therapy can be initiated with hydroxyurea, 1.5

to 2.5 g, orally, every 6 h (total dose of 6 to 10 g/day) for about 36 h. Simultaneous leukapheresis can decrease blast cell concentration within several hours without contributing to the release of uric acid. Each leukapheresis will decrease the blast concentration by about 30 percent.[189] During the first few days of therapy, hydration should be administered to maintain urine flow over 100 ml/h per m². Furosemide administration can be helpful in enhancing urine flow.

Antibiotic Therapy Pancytopenia is worsened or induced shortly after treatment is instituted. Absolute neutrophil counts under 200/μl (0.2 × 10⁹/liter) are to be expected and are a sign of effective drug action. The patient usually becomes febrile [t > 38°C (100.4°F)], often with associated rigors. Cultures of urine, blood, nasopharynx, and if available, sputum should be obtained. Since the inflammatory response is blunted by severe neutropenia and monocytopenia, evidence of exudates on physical examination or in radiographic studies may be minimal or absent. Antibiotics should be started immediately after cultures are obtained.[398] Antibiotic usage in the setting of induction chemotherapy is described in Chap. 17.

Some centers use prophylactic antibacterial, antifungal, and/or antiviral antibiotics whereas others do not. Antifungal prophylaxis can take the form of low-dose amphotericin, fluconazole, or itraconazole.[399,400] Acyclovir prophylaxis during remission-induction therapy of patients with AML does not affect the duration of fever or the need for antibiotics. The incidence of bacteremia is not reduced, but acute oral infections are less severe.[401] Liposomal amphotericin has less infusion-related toxicity and less nephrotoxicity when used in patients with fever and neutropenia[402] but is more expensive to administer than is conventional amphotericin. Some centers are utilizing outpatient supportive therapy immediately after induction therapy in adult AML. Cotrimoxazole, and itraconazole orally until the granulocyte count is over 1,000/μl, and the use of every-other-day platelet transfusions until the count is over 20,000/μl is one approach used.[403]

HEMATOPOIETIC GROWTH FACTORS

Cytokine therapy as an adjunctive treatment for AML remains controversial.[404–406] While accelerating neutrophil recovery, neither GM-CSF nor G-CSF reproducibly decrease major morbidity or mortality,[407] although one study has shown a decrease in mortality from fungal infections in older patients.[408] G-CSF and GM-CSF, when used in untreated leukemia, can increase the percentage of leukemic cells in the DNA synthetic phase resulting in blast population expansion during short-term administration of G-CSF. This can render the cells more sensitive to simultaneous chemotherapy, but clinical benefit from growth factor priming has not been observed[408,409] despite an increase of intracellular cytosine arabinoside triphosphate:deoxycytidine-5'-triphosphate ratios and an enhanced cytarabine incorporation into the DNA of AML blasts.[409]

Use of cytokines during periods of cytopenia following induction therapy is safe, and nearly all trials have shown a modest reduction in the duration of severe neutropenia with a variable effect on the incidence of severe infections, antibiotic usage, and the duration of hospital stays.[405] While no increase in relapse has been noted when growth factors are begun after the completion of chemotherapy, there is no consistent enhancement of remission, event-free survival, or overall survival.[410] The cost-effectiveness of growth factor usage has therefore come into question.[405]

The role of megakaryocyte-stimulating cytokines such as thrombopoietin[411] or interleukin-11[412] is being investigated in AML treatment. Interleukin-11 or keratinocyte growth factor might provide gastrointestinal mucosal protection during AML treatment.[413]

COMPONENT TRANSFUSION THERAPY

Red cell packs should be used to keep the hematocrit above 25 ml/dl, or higher in special cases (e.g., symptomatic coronary artery disease)

(see Chap. 140). Platelet transfusions should be used for hemorrhagic manifestations related to thrombocytopenia and prophylactically if necessary to keep the platelet count between 5000/μl (5 × 10⁹/liter) and 10,000/μl (10 × 10⁹/liter).[414–417] Patients without complicating coagulation abnormalities, anticoagulant use, sepsis, or other complications usually can maintain hemostasis with platelet counts of 5000 to 10,000/μl (5 to 10 × 10⁹/liter). Initially, random donor platelets can be used, although single-donor platelets or HLA-matched platelets are sometimes preferable products and should be tried if random-donor platelets do not raise the platelet count significantly. Platelets from siblings, parents, or offspring can be tried if available but should be avoided if allogeneic marrow transplantation is contemplated (see Chap. 142).

In patients who are platelet-refractory, platelets should be used sparingly unless bleeding occurs. Use of autologous platelet transfusions that are stored in 5% DMSO in liquid nitrogen and transfused during subsequent marrow aplasia can be used in alloimmunized patients, but this approach is obviously not helpful if needed during remission induction regimens.[418] All red cell and platelet products should be depleted of leukocytes, and all products, including granulocytes for transfusions, should be irradiated to prevent transfusion-associated graft-versus-host disease in this immunosuppressed population. This step is particularly important if allogeneic marrow transplantation is to be considered. The benefit of using cytomegalovirus-negative blood products as compared to leukodepletion to prevent virus transmission in patients who are not virus carriers is unsettled.[419]

Granulocyte transfusion should not be used prophylactically for neutropenia but can be used in patients with high fever, rigors, and bacteremia unresponsive to antibiotics, with fungal infections, or with septic shock (see Chap. 141). G-CSF administration to a volunteer donor increases neutrophil yield fourfold and results in posttransfusion blood neutrophil increments for more than 24 h after transfusion.[420] This may be warranted in the treatment of major fungal infections (see Chap. 17).

Jehovah's Witnesses or others who refuse blood product support can survive tailored chemotherapy.[421] In general, phlebotomy is minimized, and antifibrinolytics, hematinics, and growth factors are utilized to support such patients during severe cytopenias.

THERAPY FOR HYPOFIBRINOGENEMIC HEMORRHAGE

Patients with evidence of intravascular coagulation (see Chap. 126) or exaggerated primary fibrinolysis (see Chap. 136) should be considered for platelet and fresh-frozen plasma administration before antileukemic therapy is started, or if the findings are equivocal they should be monitored closely with measurements of fibrinogen levels, fibrin (ogen) degradation products, D-dimer assay, and coagulation times. Intravascular coagulation or primary fibrinolysis may occur in patients with acute promyelocytic leukemia and acute monocytic leukemia but may also occur in occasional patients with acute myeloblastic leukemia with Auer rods.

MANAGEMENT OF CENTRAL NERVOUS SYSTEM DISEASE

Central nervous system disease occurs in about 1 in 50 cases at presentation.[785] Prophylactic therapy is usually not indicated, but examination of the spinal fluid after remission in monocytic subtypes[317–320]; cases with extramedullary disease; the inv 16,[137,138] the t (8;21)[141,142] genotypes, CD7- and CD56-positive (neural cell adhesion molecule) immunophenotypes[786]; or in patients who present with very high blast counts, should be considered. These are situations in which the risk of meningeal leukemia or a brain myeloblastoma is heightened. The treatment of meningeal leukemia can include high-dose cytarabine (which penetrates the blood-brain barrier), intrathecal methotrexate, and cranial radiation in combination.[785] Systemic relapse commonly follows relapse in the meninges, and concurrent systemic treatment is usually indicated. Long-term success is unusual unless allogeneic stem cell transplantation can be used.

REMISSION-MAINTENANCE THERAPY

CYTOTOXIC THERAPY

Some form of postremission therapy is necessary to prolong remission duration and overall survival, but there is no consensus on which is best. Postremission chemotherapy that does not produce profound, prolonged cytopenias, closely simulating intensive induction therapy, has produced on average only slight prolongation of remission or life.[422] Regimens that fall between these intensities have been used with equivocal results. Intensive consolidation therapy after remission results in a somewhat longer remission duration and, more significantly, a subset of patients who have a prolonged remission (more than 3 years).

Whether AML patients in first remission should receive consolidation chemotherapy alone, autologous transplantation, or allogeneic marrow transplantation has now been studied in several randomized trials with no consensus emerging. Allogeneic transplantation was compared to autologous transplantation using unpurged marrow and two courses of intensive chemotherapy in 623 patients who had a complete remission after induction chemotherapy.[423] Disease-free survival was 53 percent at 4 years for those receiving allogeneic marrow; 48 percent for those receiving autologous transplantation; and 30 percent for patients receiving intensive chemotherapy. Overall survival after complete remission was similar in all three groups since patients who relapsed after chemotherapy could be rescued with marrow transplantation. No significant difference in the 4-year disease-free survival between allogeneic marrow transplant (42 percent) and other types of intensive postremission therapy (40 percent) has been found.[424] A reduction of relapse rate in patients receiving autografts was found in another study, but there was no benefit in disease-free or overall survival.[425] In this trial, only 45 percent of patients received the randomly assigned treatments. Thus, in several studies, the early mortality after allogeneic transplantation and the salvageable relapses after autologous marrow transplantation have led to comparable overall survival rates. Autologous transplantation results might be improved by the use of blood stem cells. The mortality after allogeneic transplant in first remission was 43 versus 7 percent for chemotherapy, whereas relapse was less for transplants (24 percent as compared to 63 percent after chemotherapy). Survival was comparable between the groups, but leukemia-free survival was greater after transplantation.[426] When quality of life was measured for patients in complete remission for 1 to 7 years, those treated with chemotherapy had the highest perceived quality and those undergoing allogeneic BMT the lowest.[427]

For patients who do not receive high-dose chemotherapy with autologous or allogeneic transplantation in first remission, consolidation chemotherapy regimens containing high-dose cytarabine provides better results than intermediate-dose cytarabine.[428,429] Long-term disease-free survival at 5 years is generally around 30 percent when two to four such cytarabine-containing regimens are administered.[430–432] Most centers utilize four cycles of 3 g/m^2 twice daily on days 1, 3, and 5, providing 6 total doses per cycle.[432] The optimal number of cycles for this therapy is not known.[433] High-dose cytarabine can be administered at a dose of 3 g/m^2 in a 1-h intravenous infusion every 12 h for periods up to 6 days (12 doses). High-dose cytarabine frequently causes conjunctivitis and photophobia, and glucocorticoid eye drops are usually used every 6 h until 24 h after the last dose of the drug.[434] Cerebellar function abnormalities also may occur, and these require cessation of drug administration. A 1-h duration of infusion of high-dose cytarabine may decrease the likelihood of severe cerebellar

toxicity, as may a reduced dose (e.g., 2 g/m^2).[435] Older patients and patients with renal insufficiency require dose attenuation, e.g., to 2 g/m^2.[436]

Once intensive consolidation chemotherapy has been completed, various forms of less intensive maintenance chemotherapy have been utilized. Many of these regimens consist of monthly chemotherapy; e.g., low-dose 6-thioguanine or cytarabine. While improved disease-free survival is noted in some studies, no improvement in overall survival has been demonstrated in most studies.[437] Other forms of maintenance therapy, such as interleukin-2,[438,439] interleukin-2 plus histamine,[440–442] and induction chemotherapy drugs used at lower doses[443] have also been examined with no definitive benefits on survival reported. Low-dose interleukin-2 alone has not been found beneficial.[444] Leukemic dendritic cells generated ex vivo from myelomonocytic AML cells may have a role in maintenance therapy.[445,446]

The decision to utilize autologous or allogeneic stem cell transplantation or high-dose cytarabine alone for consolidation can be individualized based on patient age and on other prognostic factors such as high-risk cytogenetic findings or antecedent hematologic disease.[395] Patients with good-risk cytogenetics should receive four cycles of high-dose cytarabine. Patients with poor-risk cytogenetics should be considered for allogeneic or autologous stem cell transplantation after 1 or 2 cycles of high-dose cytarabine as discussed below.

CHEMORADIOTHERAPY PLUS AUTOLOGOUS STEM CELL INFUSION

Removal and cryopreservation of postremission marrow or collection of mobilized blood stem cells from patients with AML and reinfusion of these following intensive chemotherapy and/or radiotherapy is a form of postremission therapy[447–450] (see Chap. 18). Autologous marrow rescue can be used in patients with AML who achieve a remission, do not have a compatible stem cell donor, and are up to 70 years of age, potentially tripling the proportion of patients amenable to this from of treatment, as compared to those patients who meet the donor and age requirements for allogeneic marrow transplantation.

Various preparative regimens for autologous transplantation in AML have been utilized[451] such as busulfan/cyclophosphamide, busulfan-etoposide-cytarabine; high-dose cytarabine-mitoxantrone plus total body irradiation; melphalan plus total body irradiation; and cyclophosphamide plus total body irradiation. A disease-free survival rate at 3 years of approximately 40 percent is average after such regimens.[452–455] Long-term disease-free survival can occur in patients who undergo this treatment for AML in second remission.[456] Patients greater than 50 years of age have inferior outcomes, but no strict upper age limit for this procedure has been determined.[457] Administration of two or more courses of consolidation chemotherapy prior to harvest and transplant is associated with decreased relapse rates and improved disease-free survival. A marrow nucleated cell dose greater than 2×10^8/kg improves disease-free survival.[458] Use of marrow grafts purged of residual leukemia cells has not resulted in significantly better results than unpurged marrow in many studies, suggesting that low proportions of leukemic stem cells are extremely difficult to transplant or that they do not survive the freeze-thaw cycle to which autologous marrow is subjected as well as normal stem cells do.[459] The possible benefits of marrow purging thus remain controversial (see Chap. 18). Chemotherapy agents such as 4-hydroperoxycyclophosphamide have been utilized for purging, and various antisense agents have also been reported to diminish leukemic cell contamination.[460]

In long-term cultures from newly diagnosed patients with AML, normal progenitors can be detected and their numbers increased by in vitro culture with cytokines.[461] In oligoblastic leukemia (myelodysplasia), secondary AML, and therapy-related AML, leukapheresis products obtained after chemotherapy and growth factor treatments contain normal progenitors,[462] indicating that mobilized stem cells may be relatively free of leukemic counterparts even in the absence of ex vivo purging.[463] Whether use of mobilized blood versus marrow stem cells will improve long-term outcomes has not been determined.[463]

CHEMORADIOTHERAPY PLUS ALLOGENEIC STEM CELL TRANSPLANTATION

Patients between ages of approximately 1 to 60 years who have AML and are in remission and who have a histocompatible sibling donor are candidates for stem cell transplantation therapy. The patient is prepared with a regimen that includes total-body irradiation and/or high-dose chemotherapy and thereafter is given the donor stem cells by intravenous infusion. Patients given allogeneic blood stem cells have more rapid hematopoietic reconstitution than those given marrow stem cells.[464] Chapter 18 describes the indications, procedure, and preparative regimens for stem cell transplantation.

Disease-free remission after 4 years is about 53 percent.[465] Small series utilizing T-cell depletion have reported 4-year disease-free survival of 65 percent.[466] Leukemia relapses occur in about 20 percent of patients who receive an allogeneic transplant.[465,467] Patients who are alive with good performance status 3 to 4 years after transplant have excellent prospects of long-term survival.[468] In the posttransplant period about one-third of patients die of severe graft-versus-host disease, opportunistic infection, or interstitial pneumonitis. Marrow transplantation therapy is superior to chemotherapy in that the proportion of subjects who have leukemia relapse is lower, but it is uncertain whether marrow transplantation provides an advantage in overall survival at 3 years.[464–471]

About 65 percent of all patients with AML are over 50 years of age, and the current mean family size in the United States is slightly over two children per family. Thus, only about 10 percent of subjects with AML are within the age range and have a sibling donor for marrow transplantation. The ability to extend the proportion of patients who can be transplanted by using histocompatible, unrelated donors or HLA-type-mismatched sibling or parent donors is being studied.[472,473] Molecular matching of class I and class II HLA alleles adds to the clinical success of unrelated donor transplants but makes finding a donor more difficult.[474] Treatment of high-risk acute leukemia with T-cell-depleted stem cells from related donors with one mismatched HLA haplotype with standard conditioning regimens has been successful with an acceptable incidence of graft-versus-host disease. Infectious complications were high, however.[473] HLA-matched or -mismatched cord blood stem cells can be used in adults with acute leukemia, but generally not for those in first remission.[475]

Some form of allograft is usually recommended for patients in early first relapse or second remission, since long-term survival with chemotherapy alone is improbable, whereas histocompatible sibling transplants have a 25 percent survival rate.[476] However, in one study, when transplantation was compared to chemotherapy for AML in second remission, the 3-year probability of event-free survival was 17 percent with chemotherapy and 16 percent with transplant. Patients less than 30 years of age and in remission for at least 1 year fared best.[477] Patients with extramedullary sites of leukemia are more likely to have extramedullary sites of relapse after allogeneic bone marrow transplantation.[478]

In an attempt to decrease the relapse rate after marrow transplantation for advanced acute leukemia, ^{131}I-labeled anti-CD45 antibody to deliver radiation to leukemic cells, followed by a standard transplant preparative regimen, has been utilized. Nine out of 13 patients with AML were disease-free at 8 to 41 months after transplant. With this regimen, more radiation can be delivered to hematopoietic tissues as compared with liver, lung, or kidney, which may improve the efficacy of marrow transplantation.[479]

Patients with AML who relapse after allogeneic marrow transplantation can have a long-term remission if retransplanted.[480–483] The mechanism of benefit of marrow transplantation was thought to be the result of high-dose ablative chemoradiotherapy preparatory to marrow ''rescue.'' The increased relapse rate of AML in patients transplanted with marrow from identical twins, as compared to nonidentical siblings, or transplanted with T-lymphocyte-depleted marrow has indicated that an immunologic effect of donor lymphocytes may determine the results of transplantation. This immunologic reaction, referred to as *graft-versus-leukemia,* may play a role in preventing leukemia relapses.[470,484]

In an attempt to enhance graft-versus-leukemia effects, adoptive immunotherapy with donor mononuclear cell infusions is sometimes utilized to treat relapse of leukemia after allografting.[485] These infusions have been successful in only a minority of patients with AML, but given the high mortality associated with alternative procedures such as second transplants, these infusions are a reasonable approach for relapsed AML after allogeneic transplant. Graft-versus-host disease and marrow aplasia are the major complications of this form of treatment.[486] The graft-versus-leukemia reaction is thought to be directed against minor histocompatibility antigens on the cell surface of hematopoietic cells, but reactions against leukemia-specific antigens are possible. Relapses after donor leukocyte infusions for recurring acute leukemia have a higher probability of being extramedullary.[487] Donor blood stem cells can also be combined with chemotherapy for early relapse of AML after allogeneic stem cell transplantation.[488]

Interleukin-2 has been used to modulate natural killer and T-cell activity after both autologous and allogeneic transplantation. It is too early to determine efficacy of this approach.[489] Minor histocompatibility antigens restricted to hematopoietic cells are an ideal target for antileukemic immune responses. It may be possible to modify leukemic cells to express costimulatory molecules identical to professional antigen-presenting cells to generate cytotoxic T-lymphocyte responses against myeloid leukemia cells.[490] Irradiated B7.1-transduced primary AML cells can be used as therapeutic vaccines in murine AML.[491] B7.1 is the ligand for the T-cell costimulatory molecules CD28 and CTLA-4. Dendritic cells derived in vitro from AML cells may also be utilized to stimulate leukemia-specific cytolytic activity in autologous or allogeneic lymphocytes.[446]

The recurrence of AML in donor cells has been reported in patients who have received marrow transplants from healthy siblings. These recurrences in donor cells occurred in about 1 in 18 relapsed patients who received marrow from a donor of the opposite sex.[491] There is a similar frequency of relapsed AML in recipient cells but with a different clonal cytogenetic abnormality, suggesting a ''new'' leukemia.[491] These frequencies are dependent on the sensitivity and specificity of cytogenetic techniques, which have been challenged.[492] AML developing in a stem cell recipient but of donor cell origin long after transplant has been documented in rare cases.[372]

TREATMENT OF RELAPSED OR REFRACTORY PATIENTS

Patients who relapse after remission-induction and remission-maintenance therapy have a decreased probability of entering a subsequent remission, and the duration of remission is shorter if it occurs. In patients who relapse more than 1 year after the first remission, the original remission-induction regimen can be readministered or a combination salvage chemotherapy regimen can be administered. One regimen includes high-dose cytosine arabinoside without or with another agent such as mitoxantrone,[494] amsacrine,[495] or etoposide.[496] Other salvage chemotherapy regimens are illustrated in Table 93-6.

Refractory disease is defined as that which does not respond to initial induction chemotherapy with cytarabine and an anthracycline

TABLE 93-6 EXAMPLES OF CHEMOTHERAPY USED FOR RELAPSED OR REFRACTORY PATIENTS

REGIMEN	NUMBER OF PATIENTS	COMPLETE REMISSION, %	YEAR	REFERENCE
Mitoxantrone 12 mg/m² days 1 to 5 Etoposide 100 mg/m² days 1 to 5	61	43	1988	497
Mitoxantrone 4 mg/m² days 1 to 3 Etoposide 40 mg/m² days 1 to 3 Cytarabine 1 g/m² days 1 to 3 ± PSC-833	37	32	1999	498
Mitoxantrone 12 mg/m² days 1 to 3 Etoposide 200 mg/m² days 8 to 10 Cytarabine 500 mg/m² days 1 to 3, 8 to 10 GM-CSF 5 μg/kg days 4 to 8	22	30	1993	499
Idarubicin 12 mg/m² days 1, 3, 5 Cytarabine 500 mg/m² every 12 h, days 1 to 7	21	52	1996	500
Fludarabine 30 mg/m² days 1 to 5 Cytarabine 2 g/m² days 1 to 5 ± Idarubicin 12 mg/m² days 1 to 3 G-CSF 400 μg/m² daily until complete remission	85	66	1995	501
Aclarubicin 60 mg/m² days 1 to 5 Etoposide 100 mg/m² days 1 to 5	34	29	1998	502
Idarubicin 12 mg/m² days 1 to 3 Cytarabine 1 g/m² every 12 h, days 1 to 4	23 refractory 38 relapsed	52 68	1997	503
2-Chlorodeoxyadenosine 0.1 mg/kg per day × 7 days continuous infusion ± Daunorubicin 50 mg/m² days 5, 6, 7	19	0*	1998	504
Topotecan 4.75 mg/m² days 1 to 5 Cytarabine 1 g/m² days 1 to 5	53 refractory	4†	1997	505
Carboplatin 300 mg/m² per day × 5 days continuous infusion Cytarabine 500 mg/m² × 3 days	31	29	1999	506
Cyclophosphamide 1g/m² days 1 to 3 Etoposide 200 mg/m² days 1 to 3 Carboplatin 150 mg/m² continuous infusion days 1 to 3 Cytarabine 1 g/m² days 1 to 3	25	12	1998	507

*100% of treated patients had improvement.
†39% of treated patients had improvement.
NOTE: The reader is advised to consult the original reference for details of chemotherapy regimen administration.

antibiotic. Patients with refractory disease are more likely to have disease with adverse cytogenetic findings, a history of antecedent hematologic disturbance, adverse immunophenotypic features, and expression of multidrug resistance.[508,509] Relapsed leukemia is that which recurs following a remission. The duration of remission greatly affects the patient's prognosis and response to additional treatment. The wide range in response rates noted may not only reflect the regimen used but may also reflect variability in patient selection, age, and other prognostic factors.[510–512] Chemotherapy regimens can be divided into cytarabine-based, non-cytarabine-based, and timed, sequential therapy with growth factors and cytotoxic drugs. Despite the response rates shown in Table 93-6, the duration of response is usually only 3 to 6 months. Chemomodulation with drugs designed to overcome multidrug resistance, such as the cyclosporine analog PSC-833, is under study; the use of the latter agent necessitates a two-thirds reduction in mitoxantrone and etoposide doses.[513]

Homoharringtonine, an alkaloid derived from the bark of the Chinese evergreen tree and administered by continuous infusion daily for up to 9 days in a dose of 5 mg/m², has shown effectiveness in de novo, relapsed, or refractory AML.[514,515] Aclacinomycin, an anthracy-

cline antibiotic, has been used successfully in patients with AML[516]; 2-chlorodeoxyadenosine has been found to be active against AML blast cells but is generally not an improvement over existing modalities.[517] Interleukin-2 has been effective in decreasing leukemia cells in the marrow when given in a relatively high dose (e.g., 6 to 8 million units/m² intravenously for 5 days). Occasional complete remissions after IL-2 alone have been observed in refractory patients.[518,519] These successes have occurred in cases of early limited relapsed disease (greater than 5 but less than 30 percent blast cells).[520]

Results from second remission-induction therapy are better in younger patients, those with longer remissions, longer durations since last chemotherapy, and better general health. The probability of a second remission is about 50 percent in younger subjects (15 to 60 years of age) and about 25 percent in older patients (60 to 80 years of age), but the duration of remission is nearly always much shorter than the first remission, and an eventual fatal outcome is nearly certain. Rare patients may have a third (or more) relapse followed by a remission when treated with cytotoxic drugs, but each remission is shorter than the preceding one and is usually measured in weeks.

Marrow transplantation may be the only means to induce a sustained remission in patients with AML who do not enter remission with cytotoxic drug therapy or who relapse after a first remission. About 25 percent of patients with refractory or relapsed AML have a sustained remission of at least 3 years.[521–523] Transplant-related mortality at 3 years is about 50 percent, and relapse rates are higher after sibling than matched unrelated transplantation.[524] If a histocompatible donor is available and the patient is under 50 years of age, marrow transplantation can be as successful if performed at the time of early relapse.[521,522]

NEW TREATMENT MODALITIES

CHEMOTHERAPY
Oral idarubicin can be used in AML when intravenous anthracycline treatment is precluded. Myelosuppression, nausea, vomiting, diarrhea, and mucositis have occurred, but cardiotoxicity has been minimal.[525]

Decitabine, a potent hypomethylating agent, can result in maturation and growth arrest of AML cells. It may have synergism with interferons and retinoids. It has effects as a single salvage agent and has resulted in response rates of 30 to 50 percent in combination with anthracyclines.[526]

GROWTH FACTORS AND RECEPTOR TARGETS
GM-CSF, G-CSF, and IL-3 have been used concurrently with chemotherapy regimens. GM-CSF increases white blood count and blast cell percentage with no constant increase in cells in S-phase. No correlation with in vivo treatment results is usually noted.[527] A ricin fusion toxin attached to human GM-CSF has been found to be selectively toxic to AML cells.[528] A diphtheria toxin and GM-CSF fusion protein is toxic

to AML progenitors.[529] GM-CSF can alter the cellular metabolism of cytarabine and fludarabine in AML patients.[530]

Transforming growth factor beta and dexamethasone enhance c-*JUN* gene expression and inhibit the growth of human monocytic leukemia cells.[531] Recombinant human interferons may induce the differentiation of acute megakaryoblastic leukemia blast cells.[532] Interleukin-1 and its inhibitors have also been found to have anti-leukemic effects.[533] Interleukin-6 can induce improvement in smoldering relapsed AML.[534]

ANTIBODIES TO CD33
Antibodies to the myeloid differentiation antigen, CD33, may have a role in treatment after tumor burden has been reduced by chemotherapy.[535] CD33 antibodies have been conjugated to calicheamicin or have been labeled with [131]I. Humanized CD33 antibodies have been infused in relapsed or refractory AML patients and some antileukemic activity observed, and no immune neutralization of the CD33 antibodies has been observed.[536–538]

MATURATION THERAPIES
A stable benzoic derivative of retinoic acid has been found to induce maturation of promyelocytic leukemic cells. It is 10- to 100-fold more potent than all-*trans*-retinoic acid (ATRA).[539] Several analogs of vitamin D inhibit AML cells by inducing inhibition of cyclin-dependent kinases.[540] *WAF-1* is also induced by vitamin D analogs, and, when combined with retinoids, maturation of leukemic cells is observed.[541] In general, AML cells have not responded to retinoids. Single-strand conformational polymorphism analysis and DNA sequencing of leukemic cells from nonpromyelocytic AML did not find mutations of RARα.[542] Combinations of retinoids, growth factors, and chemotherapeutic agents are being examined for therapeutic potential in AML.[543] Leukemias with 11q, -5, and -7 chromosome abnormalities have high telomerase activity, and this activity can be inhibited by maturation-inducing agents.[544]

OTHER APPROACHES
Phosphorothioate antisense oligonucleotides against multidrug resistance genes[545]; anti-Fas antibodies to mediate apoptosis[546,547]; and 67-gallium[548] inhibit AML cells in vitro. Other antileukemic vaccine strategies have also been proposed.[373,549] In addition, other surface antigen[550] or transcription signal transduction molecules may serve as therapeutic targets.[551–553]

SPECIAL THERAPEUTIC CONSIDERATIONS

ACUTE PROMYELOCYTIC LEUKEMIA
All-trans-Retinoic Acid   ATRA, an analogue of vitamin A, has been used to initiate the therapy of acute promyelocytic leukemia since 1987. The drug is administered in a total dose of 25 mg/m² to 45 mg/m² per day given in two doses orally, with the lower doses equally as effective and less toxic.[554] This drug induces complete remissions in about 80 percent of previously untreated patients.[555–559] In vitro, ATRA is ten times more potent in inducing maturation of leukemic promyelocytes to neutrophils than 13-*cis*-retinoic acid, the other naturally occurring isomer.[560] ATRA induces maturation of the leukemic cells and the suppression of the malignant clone, resulting in a switch in most cases to polyclonal hematopoiesis and a remission.[555,561–563] ATRA may induce synthesis of a protein that selectively degrades PML-RARα, and interferons may regulate PML-RARα expression.[564] Signal transducer and activator of transcription factor STAT-1 is induced and activated by ATRA. As a consequence of elevated amounts of corresponding transcripts, ATRA is capable of modulating the amounts and the state of activation of some of the components of the

IFN intracellular signaling pathways.[563] Promyelocytic leukemia cells with PML-RARα break/fusion sites in PML exon 6 have decreased in vitro responsiveness to ATRA. The t(11;17) variant of APML in which the promyelocytic leukemia zinc finger (*PLZF*) gene is fused to RARα[566] does not respond to ATRA but does mature in the presence of G-CSF.[567] Other types of AML have not been responsive to ATRA therapy.

Toxic Effects of ATRA   ATRA therapy is associated with dryness of the skin and lips, occasionally leading to mild exfoliation, nausea, headache, arthralgias, and bone pain. The white cell count may rise dramatically in the first week or two of therapy. Serum glutamic-pyruvate transaminase and triglyceride concentrations often increase. Leukemic promyelocytes disappear from the blood in 2 to 4 weeks, and a normal marrow aspirate may be obtained in from 4 to 10 weeks. Anemia improves gradually. The majority of patients become PML-RARα negative by PCR after the second consolidation therapy in conjunction with ATRA.[568] ATRA has been used successfully to treat promyelocytic leukemia diagnosed during pregnancy.[569]

A rapid increase in the total blood leukocyte count to as high as 80,000/μl (80 × 10⁹/liter) in the first several weeks of therapy, referred to as the "retinoic acid syndrome," is a potential cause of early death during therapy.[374] Two approaches have been suggested to treat this phenomenon: early use of cytotoxic chemotherapy[570] and glucocorticoid administration.[571] The syndrome consists of fever, weight gain, dependent edema, pleural or pericardial effusion, and bouts of hypotension. Respiratory distress is the key feature, and in fatal cases pulmonary interstitial infiltration with maturing granulocytes is prominent. Once respiratory distress is evident, the patient should receive dexamethasone, 10 mg, intravenously every 12 h for several days.[571] Since the syndrome may occur at relatively low total white cell counts and its onset is unpredictable, high-dose glucocorticoid therapy should be instituted if respiratory symptoms develop even in the absence of pulmonary infiltrates or an elevated white cell count.[572]

Treatment of the Coagulopathy   The risk of early death from hemorrhage as a result of the coagulopathy that accompanies acute promyelocytic leukemia requires use of fresh-frozen plasma and platelet replacement and antifibrinolytic agents.[303,304] Heparin treatment was often utilized during induction chemotherapy in the past to prevent onset of disseminated intravascular coagulopathy during treatments, but this is now rarely used.[573] ATRA may have some corrective effect on coagulation disorders in promyelocytic leukemia. The coagulation abnormalities are due either to release of procoagulant activity, primary fibrinogenolysis, or both mediated by the release of leukocyte proteases. Increased thrombin-antithrombin III complexes, prothrombin fragments 1+2, and D-dimer complexes are seen, but no factor V, AT III, or protein C consumption occurs. With ATRA treatment, more pronounced procoagulant effects versus lytic effects[303,574] may be seen. Abnormally high levels of expression of annexin II on leukemic cells increase the production of plasmin, a fibrinolytic protein. Overexpression of annexin II may be a mechanism for the hemorrhagic complications. Expression of RNA for annexin II disappears after treatment with ATRA.[575] Paradoxcially, hypercoagulable clotting tendency may occur in patients during the first months of ATRA therapy.[561]

Chemotherapy   Induction of remission with ATRA is followed by relapse in weeks to months unless intensive chemotherapy is used.[378,557,558] At relapse, cells show high levels of a cytosolic retinoic-acid-binding protein not detected prior to ATRA therapy.[564] Mechanisms of retinoid resistance in leukemic cells may also involve cytochrome P450 and P glycoprotein due to induction of various P450 enzymes which may alter ATRA metabolism.[576] Chemotherapy with daunorubicin plus cytarabine has produced relatively good results when used as remission-induction therapy. Remission induction with mitoxantrone and high-dose cytarabine or mitoxantrone, etoposide, and high-dose cytarabine may be more effective.[556] Treatment without cytarabine permits administration of more anthracycline antibiotic.[577] Idarubicin, 12 mg/m², for 4 days with 45 mg/m² of ATRA followed by two more courses of idarubicin for 3 days achieved a remission rate of 77 percent, comparable to standard regimens.[577] Patients randomized to receive ATRA alone or conventional daunorubicin and cytarabine as induction therapy followed by two cycles of consolidation chemotherapy with a later randomization either to ATRA maintenance or no further treatment had equivalent results and equivalent treatment mortality rates.[578] ATRA, whether administered as part of induction therapy or as maintenance therapy appeared to confer a disease-free survival advantage; more than 70 percent of patients receiving ATRA at any point were in continuous remission at 2.5 years versus less than 20 percent of patients who never received ATRA.[578] Cure rates have increased from 30 percent to above 50 percent since introduction of the use of ATRA. Acquired in vivo resistance to ATRA requires consolidation of ATRA-induced complete remission with intensive chemotherapy. Maintenance therapy has not been tested in randomized trials.

Age, hemorrhagic diathesis, and initial leukocyte count are prognostic factors for patients treated with ATRA followed by intensive chemotherapy.[581] Secondary cytogenetic changes do not confer a poor prognosis in patients treated with an anthracycline and cytarabine. There is a relationship between PML-RARα S isoform and secondary cytogenetic changes. These secondary chromosome changes have been seen in 30 percent to 85 percent of newly diagnosed patients.[582]

Arsenic Trioxide For patients who relapse, arsenic trioxide (AsO₃) can be useful (see ref. 787). AsO₃ can trigger apoptosis of promyelocytic leukemia cells at high concentrations and maturation at low concentrations. The presence of PML-RARα is important for the response.[579] The apoptosis effect may occur through induction of the expression of proenzymes of caspases 2 and 3 and activation of caspases 1 and 3.[580] AsO₃, 0.06 to 0.12 mg/kg body weight per day until leukemic cells were eliminated in the marrow, induced remission of 12 to 89 days in 11 of 12 patients.[580] Marrow depression did not occur. Rash, lightheadedness, fatigue, and musculoskeletal pain were the main side effects. Conventional chemotherapy is effective after relapse, and patients under age 60 should be considered for allogeneic or autologous transplantation after achieving a second remission or for allogeneic transplantation if a second remission cannot be induced. Transplantation is generally not recommended in first remission for patients with promyelocytic leukemia.

SECONDARY LEUKEMIA

Secondary leukemias arise after a myelodysplastic syndrome or after previous diagnosis and treatment of another malignancy with cytotoxic chemotherapy or radiation. In general, secondary AML has a poorer prognosis than does de novo AML and responds more poorly to chemotherapy and transplantation. Secondary AML accounts for about 15 percent of all AML cases, and this percentage is probably increasing.[583,584] Exposure to topoisomerase II inhibitors can lead to AML with 11q32 rearrangement. Ten of 12 patients with 11q32 rearrangements with secondary leukemia had topoisomerase II exposure, and 9 of those were found to have MLL gene rearrangements on chromosome 11 as seen in de novo AML with 11q32 rearrangements.[585] Patients with secondary leukemia without topoisomerase II inhibitor exposure do not have MLL rearrangements. Inversion 16 is an uncommon aberration in secondary AML and, like balanced translocations of chromosome bands 11q32, 21q22, and t(15;17), is associated with prior chemotherapy with topoisomerase II inhibitors when they are seen in the setting of treatment-induced leukemias. Breakpoints within the MYH11 gene involved in inversion 16 may vary between therapy-induced AML and AML de novo.[586] The latency period with topoisom-

erase II inhibitors is about 2 years. No relationship with higher cumulative dose or a genetic predisposition has been identified.[587] Even the use of low-dose or oral etoposide can be associated with the development of secondary AML.

Alkylating agents cause secondary AML characterized by antecedent myelodysplasia, after a mean latency period of about 6 years and usually with deletion of all or part of chromosome 5 or 7. The risk is related to cumulative alkylating agent dose. Germline aberrancies of NF-1 and p53 may increase the risk. Cisplatin used in the treatment of ovarian cancer also increases the risk of secondary leukemia.[588]

Secondary leukemia is also seen after autologous marrow or blood stem cell transplants which involve high-dose chemotherapy and/or radiotherapy. In a study of 83 patients after autografting, 12 had nonclonal cytogenetic abnormalities and 10 had clonal abnormalities, 5 of whom developed secondary AML. Onset was 12 to 48 months after autografting. The relative contribution of the underlying disease and conditioning therapy is uncertain.[589] Analysis of the human androgen receptor locus in cell samples in patients with lymphoma after autologous transplantation found a clonal marrow cell population 6 months after transplant at a time when there was no morphologic or clinical evidence of AML; AML appeared later in some patients.[590]

Secondary leukemia is generally treated akin to de novo leukemia, but given its lower response rates and remission durations, patients can be treated in clinical trials examining new therapies or treated initially with alternative salvage chemotherapy regimens.[591–594]

TREATMENT OF OLDER PATIENTS

About 60 percent of patients with AML are over 60 years of age at the time of diagnosis.[595] The disease in this age group is less responsive to therapy, and this age group has a higher proportion of patients who have oligoblastic leukemia (myelodysplasia); an antecedent clonal myeloid disease; prior chemotherapy for cancer of the breast, ovary, or another site and comorbid conditions, which decrease the tolerance to intensive chemotherapy programs. The AML cells of elderly patients often have more CD34+ expression, suggesting origin from a more primitive multipotential stem cell. This is thought to contribute to longer duration of postchemotherapy aplasia and to the increased risk of induction deaths in this age group.[596] Patients over 55 years of age also have a high frequency of unfavorable cytogenetic findings (32 percent) and higher MDR1 expression (71 percent) and functional drug efflux (58 percent).[597]

The therapist and patient determine whether a standard regimen, a standard regimen with dose reductions, or a special regimen is used.[598–601] In patients over 60 years of age who are fit and are otherwise considered to be good candidates, standard two-drug therapy can be used. Remission rates of approximately 30 percent can be achieved, whereas in those who are chronically ill or have other reasons for being intolerant to standard therapy, low-dose cytarabine, 10 mg/m², subcutaneously or as a short infusion every 12 h daily for 14 to 28 days, can be used.[602–607] If necessary the cycle can be repeated after about 3 weeks or an attenuated standard regimen can be used. An example of an attenuated regimen is cytarabine, 100 mg/m², subcutaneously every 12 h for 10 doses on days 1 through 5, daunorubicin, 30 mg/m², intravenously on days 1 through 3 of treatment. In previously untreated elderly patients with AML, mitoxantrone induction therapy produces a slightly higher remission rate than does daunorubicin, but it has no significant effect on remission duration and survival.[608,609] In a prospective randomized trial of idarubicin compared to daunorubicin in combination chemotherapy for AML in those 55 to 65, idarubicin resulted in higher remission rates.[610] Oral idarubicin alone has also been used with success.[604]

There is no consensus about the best regimen or the number of treatment cycles for postremission therapy in older adults. Regardless of the consolidation regimen, the duration of the leukemia-free survival is longer with high-dose cytarabine and autologous stem cell transplantation just as it is in other patients,[611] but the percentage of patients able to tolerate this therapy is less. High-dose cytarabine can be used in older adults with AML, but usually at a reduced dose.[612] Older patients treated with attenuated high-dose cytarabine at 750 mg/m² intravenously for 12 doses and then consolidated with 4 to 6 doses had about a 50 percent remission rate with a median duration of remission of 326 days.[613] Fifty-one percent of 110 patients greater than 60 years old had a 9-month median remission duration when consolidated with high-dose cytarabine.[614] The elderly are at higher risk of relapse despite successfully completing intensive consolidation therapy, regardless of whether other adverse prognostic features were present. Others have reported that cytarabine in maintenance therapy may prolong disease-free survival, but it does not improve overall survival.[615]

Patients over 80 years of age do not tolerate treatments well; remission rates are about 30 percent, but the median survival of treated patients is about 1 month. Less than 10 percent survive for 1 year.[616]

Treatment options in the elderly range therefore from no treatment to supportive care to palliative low-dose chemotherapy to attentuated induction chemotherapy designed for older patients to high-dose chemotherapy regimens used in younger patients. AML in the elderly generally has an adverse karyotypic and phenotypic presentation in a patient who has a reduced ability to withstand aggressive chemotherapy regimens. The Medical Research Council of the United Kingdom observed remission rates of 80 percent in children, 70 percent in adults under 50, 68 percent in those 50 to 59, 53 percent in those 60 to 69, 39 percent in those 70 to 75, and 22 percent in those over 75 years old.[617] Remissions, therefore, occur in elderly patients and can occasionally be longer than 12 months. Lower-dose regimens are toxic, also, and can lead to severe cytopenias. The use of colony-stimulating factors permit more elderly patients to tolerate full-dose induction therapy.[408,618,619] In the 15 percent of older patients who remain free of leukemia beyond a year, quality of life is usually good.[620]

TREATMENT OF PREGNANT PATIENTS

Leukemia (AML, ALL, CML) is the second most common malignancy of women in the childbearing age group[621] and can be expected to occur in about 1 in 75,000 pregnancies.[622] There has been no systematic study of the effects of leukemia on pregnancy or delivery, the effects of the leukemia or its treatment on the fetus, or the postnatal development of the offspring exposed in utero to maternal chemotherapy. Folic acid inhibitors, purine analogues, or pyrimidine analogues given during the first trimester of pregnancy will increase the probability of major congenital malformations.[623] Interruption of the pregnancy may be required to provide the patient with intensive therapy. Intensive chemotherapy given to women in the second and third trimesters of pregnancy does not present an inordinate risk to fetal or neonatal development,[624–631] although there is an increase in premature delivery, a higher perinatal mortality, and a lower birth weight for gestational age, especially if the fetus is exposed to chemotherapy. Development of the newborn seems to be normal, however.[628,630] Newborn infants may be cytopenic transiently if the mother is receiving chemotherapy at the time of delivery. Vaginal delivery should be used whenever possible. Although pregnant women with AML who enter remission have little difficulty with childbirth or postparturition, relapse of AML and maternal death are usual. Leukemic infiltrates can be found on the maternal side of the placenta but usually not in the villi.[632] One case of maternal-to-fetal transmission of AML has been documented.[633] Leukapheresis has been employed to treat AML during pregnancy and might be useful in the first trimester,[634] when chemotherapy poses a

high risk to the embryo. ATRA has been used successfully to treat promyelocytic leukemia during pregnancy.[635]

TREATMENT OF CHILDREN

Intensive treatment of patients less than 17 years of age—including remission-induction therapy with cytarabine and daunomycin or doxorubicin, followed by intensive multidrug consolidation and continuation therapy including daunorubicin, cytarabine, 6-thioguanine, etoposide, and intrathecal cytosine arabinoside—has resulted in remission in about 75 percent of children and 3-year relapse-free remissions in about 35 percent of treated children.[636–640] Somewhat better long-term results have also been reported.[641] As in adults, duration of first remission predicts remission rate and long-term survival in children with relapse.[642] Monocytic leukemia and hyperleukocytic [>100,000/μl (>100 × 10⁹/liter)] myelogenous leukemia account for most of the 15 percent of children who either have early deaths from hemorrhage or other causes or present with extramedullary disease and relapse after induction therapy.[636,637,643] Children under the age of 2 years have a poor prognosis when treated with chemotherapy and should be considered for marrow transplantation, if an appropriate donor is available.[644] Relapse rates have been found to be high when children are transplanted at less than 2 years of age. Growth failure and endocrine deficiences are common.[645] Long-term remission in infants can occur after marrow transplantation.[646]

NONHEMATOPOIETIC ADVERSE EFFECTS OF TREATMENT

SKIN RASHES

Over 50 percent of patients with AML develop skin lesions during remission-induction or remission-consolidation therapy. The rash may be on the trunk and extremities and is usually maculopapular initially but can become hemorrhagic in the patient who has thrombocytopenia. Allopurinol, trimethoprim-sulfamethoxazole, and other beta-lactam antibiotics are commonly implicated causes. The use of multiple drugs enhances the reactivity of patients.[647] Cytostatic therapy coupled with the effects of leukemia predisposes patients to an increased frequency of allergic dermatitis.

CARDIAC TOXICITY

Cardiomyopathy occurs in some patients after exposure to the anthracycline antibiotics, daunorubicin, or doxorubicin and is discussed further in Chap. 16. The frequency is a function of the dose used and can reach 10 to 20 percent if between 550 mg/m² and 700 mg/m² of doxorubicin is administered.[648–650] Measurement of the ejection fraction can assist in assessing the risk of proceeding with anthracycline treatment.[650] Since most patients receive total doses of anthracycline below toxic levels, cardiac toxicity has become infrequent. Dexrazoxane may reduce the cardiotoxicity when combined with anthracycline antibiotics.[388]

HEPATITIS

Persistent elevation in serum transaminases occurring after initiation of chemotherapy in patients with AML is usually the result of blood transfusion-transmitted hepatitis C. Hepatitis caused by type A virus is nearly nonexistent early in the course of AML. Cases of type B can occur infrequently. Hepatitis may occur in multiply transfused patients and is usually mild, but persistent hepatitis can develop. Liver biopsy findings do not show fibrosis or bridging necrosis.[651] Screening blood for hepatitis virus C has markedly decreased this risk.

SYSTEMIC CANDIDIASIS SYNDROME

Although microbial sepsis is a common complication of the treatment of AML, the chronic systemic candidiasis syndrome has become of special concern.[652–654] The syndrome is manifested by fever, abdominal pain, and hepatomegaly. Neutrophilia and increased serum alkaline phosphatase activity are often noted. Abdominal computed tomography shows characteristic hepatic lesions: circular areas of decreased attenuation of liver and often spleen, kidney, lung, or paraspinal muscles. Ultrasound reveals multiple hypoechogenic areas with a bull's-eye appearance. Laparoscopic-guided liver biopsy reveals yellow nodules on the liver surface, which on microscopic examination are large granulomas with *Candida* and pseudohyphae. Cure of this infection is possible with long-term (2 to 10 months) amphotericin B, supplemented by fluconazole or itraconazole.[654,655]

NEUTROPENIC TYPHLITIS

Necrotizing inflammation of the cecum with secondary infection can occur in patients with acute leukemia on intensive chemotherapy. The diagnosis can be confirmed by sonography in which a characteristic mucosal thickening and polypoid appearance is evident.[656] Management includes bowel rest, nasogastric suction, parenteral nutrition, and antibiotics. In the absence of resolution, surgical excision should be considered.[657]

THROMBOTIC THROMBOCYTOPENIC PURPURA

This syndrome has been reported in patients with solid tumors treated with cisplatin, bleomycin, vinca alkaloids, or mitomycin C and has been reported in patients in remission of AML during consolidation chemotherapy[658] (see Chap. 51).

FERTILITY AND GONADAL FUNCTION

Women in remission following treatment for AML can be fertile and can become pregnant and deliver healthy infants.[659–661] Histologic studies of the testes show marked suppression of spermatogenesis as a function of duration of treatment for AML and not of the specific agents used or the age of the patient. Residual spermatogenesis in intensively treated patients makes possible the recovery of reproductive function in males.[662] Males receiving intensive daunorubicin, cytosine arabinoside, or 6-thioguanine treatment for AML have conceived children during their therapy.[663] Banking of sperm can be attempted before institution of cytotoxic therapy but is often not logistically possible or successful in males with AML who are often febrile and acutely ill at presentation.

COURSE AND PROGNOSIS

RESULTS OF TREATMENT

Prior to the introduction of chemotherapy for AML 40 years ago, the median survival of patients was about 6 weeks,[664] the 1-year survival was about 3 percent, and longer survival occurred in less than 1 percent of patients. Initial remission rates now approach 90 percent in children, 70 percent in young adults, 50 percent in middle-aged subjects, and 25 percent in the elderly.[665–671] Median survival time has increased to about 12 months, and of those patients who enter remission, about 30 percent are alive at 24 months and about 10 percent 60 months after remission induction.[665–673] Somewhat better survival has been reported for patients who have received allogeneic marrow transplantation in first remission, but the confidence limits for remission duration and survival are widely overlapping for drug-treated and drug- and transplantation-treated groups.[674–678]

CLONAL REMISSIONS

A small proportion of patients who enter remission have their apparently normal hematopoiesis supported by a single clone rather than the expected polyclonal hematopoiesis.[679–684] Evidence points to this clone being a preleukemic cell rather than a normal stem cell.[679–685]

This finding is in keeping with previous hypotheses about the possible patterns of remission and relapse in AML[686–688] and has implications for minimal residual disease detection (see below).

SPONTANEOUS REMISSIONS

Spontaneous disappearance of AML has been reported for over 100 years, although most cases before 1960 had poor documentation of the diagnosis. Bona fide cases of AML that entered complete remission, usually after or concurrent with an infection, do occur but are very rare.[689–691] The occurrence of spontaneous remission with infection is consistent with the observation that the antibody response to *Pseudomonas* vaccine[692] has been correlated with improved probability of chemotherapy-induced remission. Spontaneous remissions are often short-lived but have lasted up to 3 years in adults and over 9 years in children.[693] A particularly notable case of remission of over 60 years has been documented following "treatment" prior to the introduction of chemotherapeutic drugs. The regimen included arsenic.[694]

LONG-TERM SURVIVAL

About 10 percent of adults treated with chemotherapy between the ages of 15 and 60 remain in sustained remission for over 5 years.[692,693] Five-year survival in childhood AML with intensive chemotherapy is projected to be over 60 percent of those treated with intensive chemotherapy and about 70 percent of those who enter remission.[695] Studies of the full age range (0 to over 80 years) have reported about a 20 percent 5-year relapse-free survival.[696]

Relapse (or a new leukemic event) in long-term survivors has been reported as late as 8 years after remission in adults[693,694] and over 16 years in children.[695] Relapse in long-term survivors is nearly always in the marrow in adults and usually in the marrow in children, with occasional childhood cases of central nervous system or gonadal relapses initially, followed by relapse in the marrow.[696] Studies of long-term survivors of AML have shown that most are able to return to work and that at a median follow-up of 9 years, no increased risk of secondary invasive cancer has occurred.[697,698]

FEATURES INFLUENCING OUTCOME OF THERAPY IN ACUTE MYELOGENOUS LEUKEMIA

Numerous features have been found to relate to outcome of treatment in AML.[699] It is often difficult, even with multivariate analysis, to dissect which features are themselves important or are associations that segregate with another prognostic factor (see Table 93-7).

Determining useful prognostic variables in patients with AML is imprecise because negative prognostic factors are being eliminated by better treatment protocols. Moreover, several prognostic factors are significant only when AML is stratified by age or by morphologic phenotype. Conflicting findings are common among studies. In addition, although a prognostic variable may be correlated significantly with a more or less favorable outcome, the lack of a very strong statistical correlation with the outcome of treatment makes its presence or absence of little prognostic value in an individual patient. If a stem cell donor is available, unfavorable prognostic factors could influence the therapist to use allogeneic stem cell transplantation as a means of remission maintenance in patients who enter remission.[753] The impact of prognostic factors may change in relationship to treatment with allogeneic stem cell transplantation.[754,755]

DETECTION OF MINIMAL RESIDUAL DISEASE

General Considerations The tumor cell burden in acute leukemia is about 1 trillion (10^{12}) cells. Apparent marrow aplasia can be induced following chemotherapy with a 2- to 3-log reduction in cell number, which represents a residual tumor cell burden of 1 to 10 billion cells. Intensification therapy is intended to decrease the residual

TABLE 93-7   PROGNOSTIC FACTORS IN ACUTE MYELOGENOUS LEUKEMIA

Better prognosis than average of all patients
  Leukemic cells contain t(8;21), t(15;17), inv(16), trisomy 21[700–702]
  Absence of exaggerated dysmyelopoiesis[699]
  Residual normal metaphases admixed with clonal cytogenetic abnormalities[703]
  High telomerase activity levels[704]
  High levels of caspase 3[705]

Poorer prognosis than average of all patients
  Older age: Age at the time of diagnosis has the greatest impact on the probability of remission and on the duration of survival. Children in the first 15
    years of life, exclusive of the neonatal period, have the highest rate of remission and longest relapse-free remission; patients over 60 years of age have
    only half the chance of a young adult to enter remission and less likelihood of a long relapse-free remission.[665] There is a gradient of poor response to
    treatment through adulthood, with the largest decrease after the sixth decade of life.[617]
  Unfavorable karyotypes: The cytogenetic pattern of leukemic blast cells influences outcome, but the relationship is complex.[706–709] The presence of 5-, 7-,
    5q-, 7q- or of exaggerated hyperdiploidy (<47 chromosomes), trisomy 8, t(6;9), trisomy 11, or multiple chromosomal abnormalities in leukemic cells
    are poor prognostic signs.
  Multidrug resistance phenotype: Leukemic cells expressing P-glycoprotein, a unidirectional drug-efflux pump, encoded by the *MDR1*.[710] Expression of this
    gene product can result in decreased accumulation of anthracyclines, amsacrine, mitoxantrone, and etoposide. Expression of P-glycoprotein does not in-
    fluence outcome of treatment, but if rhodamine 123 efflux also is increased, relapse is more common.[711,712] Frequently, observed in AML cells after re-
    lapse. Associated with CD34 expression and chromosome 7 abnormalities.[713] Alternative non-*MDR1*-mediated drug efflux mechanisms are important
    also.[714–720] *MDR1* expression is low in favorable prognosis subtypes of AML.[721]
  Prior clonal hemopathy: Chemotherapy or radiotherapy remission rates are one-third to one-half that of de novo AML in the same age group and remis-
    sion duration is shorter with remissions over 3 years very uncommon.[722,723] AML developing from the clonal hemopathy may relapse as a smoldering
    leukemia. It then reverts to AML but can be treated with remissions lasting several years.[724–728]
  Higher white cell count: A count greater than 30,000/μl (30 × 10^9/liter) or a blast cell count greater than 15,000/μl (greater than 15 × 10^9/liter).[729,730]
  Very low platelet count [less than 30,000/μl (less than 30 × 10^9/liter)].[709,730]
  High lactic dehydrogenase.[731]
  Another medical disorder. Extreme obesity, diabetes mellitus, chronic renal disease.
  Low serum albumin or prealbumin.
  Need for intubation or ventilator support during induction therapy.[732]
  Autonomous clonal growth of leukemic blast cells.[733]
  High Bcl-2 expression.[734]
  High Mcl-2 expression: Elevated at the time of leukemic relapse. Either suggests prognostic importance or that chemotherapeutic regimen selects for leu-
    kemia cells with elevated levels of apoptosis inhibitors.[735]
  Low expression of retinoblastoma gene.[736]
  High levels of WAF/Cip1 protein: This is a regulator at the G1 checkpoint of cell cycle.[737]
  High CD34 expression: High CD34 antigen expression often in AML subtypes M0, M1, and M4.[738] Remission rate of 61 compared to 88 percent in AML
    not expressing CD34. The correlation is stronger between high-intensity expression of CD34 and lower remission rate.[738,739]
  GATA-1 expression.[740]
  Neural cell adhesion molecule (CD56) expression.[741]
  Elevated soluble L-selectin: seen especially in extramedullary disease.[742]
  Higher expression of interleukin-1β gene.[743]
  Low *FMS* expression[743]
  Expression of the thrombopoietin receptor (c-*MPL*) mRNA.[744]

Factors with no or uncertain prognostic findings
  Morphologic phenotype: The absence of Auer rods has been associated with a poor prognosis.[745–748]
  Myeloid antigens: CD11b expression may be predictive of shorter survival.[749]
  Detection of the WT1 (Wilms tumor) transcript.[750]
  Lung resistance protein: functional test is needed in order to assess activity.[751] Expression may predict poor outcome in de novo AML.[752,789]

cell numbers further. With the advent of specific monoclonal antibodies for leukemic cell antigens and fluorescent in situ hybridization
coupled with flow cytometry and DNA amplification by polymerase
chain reaction, residual cell populations below the 10 billion cells
detectable by light microscopy of stained marrow films can be quantified.[756,757] Sampling remains an important problem, since a marrow
aspiration contains about one ten-thousandth of the marrow cell population, and variation among sites of aspiration is well-documented. In
addition the markers of the leukemic cell used for detection can change
over time during the disease. Persistence of circulating cells containing
t(8;21) in patients with AML in long-term remission, for example,
has been established using PCR.[758]

Routine marrow examinations are not needed in the great majority
of AML patients in first complete remission.[759] Routine cytogenetic
follow-up is also not usually helpful. Emergence of a karyotypically
unrelated clone of de novo AML, especially chromosome 7, can occur.[687] Studies using multiparameter flow cytometry to identify leukemic cells by aberrant antigen expression have a high positive predictive
value with regard to the incidence of relapse.[760] Detection of residual
disease in AML patients by use of double immunologic marker analysis
for terminal deoxynucleotidyl transferase and myeloid markers can be

useful, since expressions of these two markers are expressed on leukemic cells in the majority of patients with AML. These findings are
rare in normal marrow cells.[761,762] In other cases, aberrant combinations
of surface antigens[761,763] or increased expression of various surface
antigens such as CD34 are seen.[764] Other methods to detect minimal
residual disease include: magnetic resonance imaging; fluorescence
DNA in situ hybridization (FISH)[765]; reverse transcriptase PCR to
detect amplification of abnormal fusion genes such as t(15;17), t(8;21),
inv 16, 11q23; and DNA PCR for mutations in the *RAS* coding regions.[757]

Detecting Inversion 16 Minimal residual disease in AML
M4Eo can be detected by nested polymerase chain reaction with allele-
specific amplifications (*CBFB* of 16q and *MYH*11 on 16p).[766–768] This
fusion transcript occurs not only in the majority of cases of AML with
marrow eosinophilia (M4Eo) but also in 10 percent of AML M4
without eosinophilic abnormalities, a much higher incidence than the
sporadic reports of chromosome 16 abnormalities in AML M4 would
suggest. Additional screening by either RT-PCR or FISH should be
performed in patients with AML M4, regardless of morphologic features, to evaluate the prognostic usefulness of this fusion transcript in
minimal disease detection.[769]

Detecting t(8;21)   Transloction 8;21 is one of the most common translocations in AML, occurring in 12 to 15 percent of adult and over one-third of pediatric cases. This fuses the AML1 gene on chromosome 21p to *ETO* on chromosome 8p to produce the fusion gene.[770–773] The fusion has been detected in the majority of patients in remission. One study found its persistence in all patients with t(8;21) after chemotherapy or autologous marrow transplantation.[774–776] By PCR, *AML1-ETO* was found in patients in complete remission for 12 to 150 months but not in those who received allogeneic marrow transplantation. The *PGK* allele, used as a tracking marker, was identical to that detected in the leukemic blasts from the time of initial diagnosis, confirming the persistence and reappearance of leukemic cells from the same clone.[776] This marker may persist after allogeneic marrow transplantation but is compatible with continued remission.[777] Quantitation of the amount of the fusion transcript during remission may be more predictive of cure or relapse than a simple qualitative assessment.[593,778,779] Real-time quantitative RT-PCR can be used for this purpose.[775] A quantitative RT-PCR can predict relapse up to 4 months before the clinical onset.[780] Serial quantification of cases with residual t(8;21) with RT-PCR indicates that at least 0.1 femtograms of *AML1/ETO* competitor-dose is present before cytogenetic relapse occurs.[781] Both *ETO* and *AML*1 are expressed in normal CD34+ progenitors.[782]

Detecting t(15;17)   Unlike the fusion transcript t(8;21), t(15;17) usually disappears after intensive therapy.[568] At least 1 in 100,000 cells with the *PML-RARα* transcript can be detected by RT-PCR.[783] FISH can also be used.[784]

The technology to detect minimal residual disease has increased in sensitivity and availability. In most cases, the use of detection of minimal residual disease to determine a patient's treatment or prognosis remains an evolving area of investigation.

REFERENCES

1. Friedreich N: Ein neuer Fall von Leukämie, *Arch Pathol Anat* 12:37, 1857.
2. Ebstein W: Ueber die acute Leukämie und Pseudoleukämie. *Dtsch Arch Klin Med* 44:343, 1889.
3. Fraenkel A: Ueber acute Leukämie. *Dtsch Med Wochenschr* 21:639,663,676,699,712, 1895.
4. Neumann E: Ueber myelogene leukäemie. *Berl Klin Wochenchr* 15:69, 1878.
5. Ehrlich P: Farbenanolytische Untersuchungen zur Histologie und Klinik des Blutes. Berlin, Hirschwald, 1891.
6. Naegeli O: Ueber rothes Knochenmark und Myeloblasten. *Dtsch Med Wochenschr* 26:287, 1900.
7. Hirschfield H: Zur Kenntnis der Histogenese der granulirten Knochenmarkzellen. *Arch Pathol Anat* 153,335, 1898.
8. Kato H, Schull WJ: Studies on mortality of A-bomb survivors, report 7. Mortality, 1950–78. Part I. Cancer Mortality. *Radiat Res* 90:395, 1982.
9. Moloney WC: Radiogenic leukemia revisited. *Blood* 70:905, 1987.
10. Cronkite EP: Chemical leukemogenesis: benzene as a model. *Semin Hematol* 24:2, 1987.
11. Schattner AR, Nicholich MJ, Bird MG: Determination of leukemogenic benzene exposure concentrations. *Risk Analysis* 16:833, 1996.
12. Smith MT, Zhang L, Wang Y, et al: Increased translocations and aneusomy in chromosomes 8 and 21 among workers exposed to benzene. *Cancer Res* 58:2176, 1998.
13. Smith MT: The mechanism of benzene-induced leukemia. *Environ Health Perspect* 104 (suppl 6):1219, 1966.
14. Levine EG, Bloomfiled CD: Leukemias and myelodysplastic syndromes secondary to drugs, radiation, and environmental exposure. *Semin Oncol* 19:47, 1992.
15. Thirman MJ, Larson RA: Therapy-related myeloid leukemia. *Hematol/Oncol Clin North Am* 10:293, 1996.
16. Pui CH, Relling MV, Behn FG, et al: L-asparaginases may potentiate the leukemogenic effect of the epipodophyllotoxins. *Leukemia* 9:1680, 1995.
17. Travis LB, Holowty EF, Bergfeldt K, et al: Risk of leukemia after platinum-based chemotherapy for ovarian cancer. *N Engl J Med* 340:351, 1999.
18. Sterkers Y, Preudhomme C, Lai J-L, et al: Acute myeloid leukemia and essential thrombocythemia treated with hydroxyurea: high proportion of cases with 17p deletion. *Blood* 91:616, 1998.
19. Van Leeuwen FE: Risk of acute treatment. *Ballière's Clin Haematol* 9:57, 1996.
20. Visfeldt J, Anderson M: Pathoanatomical aspects of malignant haematological disorders among Danish patients exposed to thorium dioxide. *APMIS* 103:29, 1995.
21. Rodella S, Ciccone G, Rege-Cambrin G, et al: Cytogenetics and occupational exposures in acute nonlymphocytic leukemia and myelodysplastic syndrome. *Scand J Work Environ Health* 19:369, 1993.
22. Brownson RC, Novotny TE, Perry MC: Cigarette smoking and adult leukemia: a meta-analysis. *Arch Intern Med* 153:469, 1993.
23. Sandler DP, Shore DL, Anderson JR, et al: Cigarette smoking and risk of acute leukemia: associations with morphology and cytogenetic abnormalities in bone marrow. *J Natl Cancer Inst* 85:1994, 1993.
24. Shu X-O, Ross JA, Pendergrass TW, et al: Parental alcohol consumption, cigarette smoking and risk of infant leukemia. *J Natl Cancer Inst* 88:24, 1996.
25. Najean Y, Rain J-D: Treatment of polycythemia vera. *Blood* 89:2319, 1997.
26. Wiernik P: Leukemias and plasma cell myeloma. *Cancer Chemother Biol Response Modif* 17:390, 1997.
27. Peters BS, Matthews J, Gompels M, et al: Acute myeloblastic leukemia in AIDS. *AIDS* 4:367, 1990.
28. Miller RW: Deaths from childhood leukemia and solid tumors among twins and other sibs in the United States, 1960-67. *J Natl Cancer Inst* 56:203, 1971.
29. Miller RW: Persons with exceptionally high risk of leukemia. *Cancer Res* 27:2420, 1967.
30. Linet MS: *The Leukemias: Epidemiologic Aspects*, chap 3, pp 20–65. Oxford Press, New York, 1985.
31. Zipursky A, Poon A, Doyle J: Leukemia in Down syndrome: a review. *Pediatr Hematol Oncol* 9:139, 1992.
32. Crentzig U, Ritter J, Vormoor J, et al: Myelodyplasia and acute myelogenous leukemia in Down's sndrome. *Leukemia* 10:1677, 1996.
33. Auerbach AD, Allen RG: Leukemia and preleukemia in Fanconi anemia patients. *Cancer Genet Cytogenet* 51:1, 1991.
34. Butturini A, Gale RP, Verlander PC, et al: Hematologic abnormalities in Fanconi anemia: an international Fanconi anemia registry study. *Blood* 84:1650, 1994.
35. German J: Bloom's syndrome: incidence, age of onset, and types of leukemia in the Bloom's syndrome registry, in *Genetics in Hematologic Disorders*, edited by CS Bartsocas, D Loukopoulos, pp 241–258. Hemisphere, Washington, DC, 1992.
36. Daghistani D, Curless R, Toledano SR, Ayyar DR: Ataxia-pancytopenia and monosomy 7. *J Pediatr* 115:108, 1989.
37. Filipovich AH, Heinitz KJ, Robison LL, Frizzera G: The immunodeficiency cancer register. *Am J Pediatr Hematol Oncol* 9:183, 1987.
38. March JCW, Will AJ, Hows JM, et al: "Stem cell" origin of the hemopoietic defect in dyskeratosis congenita. *Blood* 79:3138, 1992.
39. Wong WY, Williams D, Slovak ML, et al: Terminal acute myelogenous leukemia in a patient with congenital agranulocytosis. *Am J Hematol* 43:133, 1993.
40. Zeulzer WW, Thompson RI, Mastrangelo R: Evidence for a genetic factor related to leukemogenesis and congenital anomalies: chromosome abberations in pedigree of an infant with partial D-trisomy and leukemia. *J Pediatr* 72:367, 1968.
41. Fraumeni JF: Constitutional disorders of man predisposing to leukemia and lymphoma. *Monogr Natl Cancer Inst* 32:221, 1969.
42. Horwitz M: The genetics of familial leukemia. *Leukemia* 1:1347, 1997.
43. Novick Y, Marino P, Makower DF, Wiernik PH: Familial erythroleukemia: a distinct clinical and genetic type of familial leukemia. *Leuk Lymph* 80:395, 1998.
44. Lee EJ, Schiffer CA, Misawa S, Testa JR: Clinical and cytogenetic features of familial erythroleukaemia. *Br J Haematol* 65:313, 1987.
45. Horowitz M, Sabath DE, Smithson WA, Radrich J: A family inheriting different subtypes of acute myelogeneous leukemia. *Am J Hematol* 52:295, 1966.
46. Olopade O, Roulston D, Baker T, et al: Familial myeloid leukemia

associated with loss of the long arm of chromosome 5. *Leukemia* 10:669, 1996.

47. Epstein CJ, Martin GM, Schultz AL, Motulsky AG: Werner's syndrome. *Medicine* 45:177, 1996.

48. Lurgaespada DA, Brannan CI, Shaughnessy JD, et al: The neurofibromatosic type 1 (NF1) tumor suppressor gene and myeloid leukemia. *Curr Top Microbiol Immunol* 211:233, 1996.

49. Woods WG, Roloff JS, Lukens JN, Krivit W: The occurrence of leukemia in patients with the Schwachman syndrome. *J Pediatr* 99:425, 1981.

50. Ho CY, Otterud B, Legare RD, et al: Linkage of a familial platelet disorder with a propensity to develop myeloid malignancies to human chromosome 21q22.1 - 22.2. *Blood* 87:5218, 1996.

51. Fialkow PH, Singer JW, Adamson JW, et al: Acute nonlymphocytic leukemia. Heterogeneity of stem cell origin. *Blood* 57:1068, 1991.

52. Ferraris AM, Broccia G, Meloni T, et al: Clonal origin f cells restricted to monocytic differentiation in acute nonlymphocytic leukemia. *Blood* 64:817, 1984.

53. Greaves MF: Stem cell origins of leukaemia and curability. *Br J Cancer* 67:413, 1993.

54. Turhan AG, Lemoire FB, Debert C, et al: Highly purified primitive hematopoietic stem cells are PML-RARA negative and generate nonclonal progenitors in acute promyelocytic leukemia. *Blood* 85:2154, 1995.

55. Van Lom K, Hagenmeijer A, Vandekerckhove F, et al: Clonality analysis of hematopoietic cell lineages in acute myeloid leukemia and translocation (8;21): only myeloid cells are part of malignant clone. *Leukemia* 11:202, 1997.

56. Hussong JW, Rodgers GM, Shami PJ: Evidence of increased angiogensis in patients with acute myeloid leukemia. *Blood* 95:309, 2000.

57. Look AT: Oncogene transcription factors in human acute leukemias. *Science* 278:1097, 1997.

58. Tenen DG, Hromas R, Licht JD, Dong-Er Z: Transcription factors, normal myeloid development, and leukemia. *Blood* 90:489, 1997.

59. Cline MJ: The molecular basis of leukemia. *N Engl J Med* 330:328, 1994.

60. Adams JM, Cosy S: Oncogene cooperation in leukaemogenesis. *Cancer Surv* 15:119, 1992.

61. Farr CJ, Saiki RK, Erlick HA, et al: Analysis of *ras* gene mutations in acute myeloid leukemia by polymerase chain reaction and oligonucleotide probes. *Proc Natl Acad Sci* 85:1629, 1988.

62. Bashey A, Gill R, Levi S, et al: Mutational activation of the N-ras oncogene assessed in primary clonogenic culture of acute myeloid leukemia (AML): implications for the role of N-ras mutation in AML pathogenesis. *Blood* 79:981, 1992.

63. Radich JP, Kopecky KJ, Williams CL, et al: N-ras mutations in adult de novo acute myelogenous leukemia: prevalence and clinical significance. *Blood* 76:801, 1990.

64. Preisler HD, Kinniburgh AJ, Wei-Dong G, Khan S: Expression of the protooncogenes *c-myc, c-fos,* and *c-fms* in acute myelocytic leukemia at diagnosis and in remission. *Cancer Res* 47:874, 1987.

65. Buesco-Ramos DE, Yang Y, de Leon E: The human MDM-2 oncogene is overexposed in leukemia. *Blood* 82:2617, 1993.

66. Mori N, Hidai H, Yokota J, et al: Mutations of the p53 gene in myelodysplastic syndrome and overt leukaemia. *Leuk Res* 19:869, 1995.

67. Slingerland JM, Minden MD, Benchmore S: Mutation of the P53 gene in human acute myelogenous leukemia. *Blood* 77:1500, 1991.

68. Wiede R, Parviz B, Pflüger K-H, et al: The role of decreased retinoblastoma protein expression in acute myelomonocytic and monoblastic leukemias. *Leuk Lymph* 17:135, 1995.

69. Ridge SA, Worwood M, Oscier D, et al: FMS mutations in myelodysplastic, leukemic and normal subjects. *Proc Natl Acad Sci* 87:1377, 1990.

70. Menssen HD, Renki HJ, Rodeck U, et al: Presence of Wilm's tumor gene (wt1) transcripts and the WT1 nuclear protein on the majority of human acute leukemias. *Leukemia* 9:1060, 1995.

71. Ikeda H, Kanakura Y, Tamaki T, et al: Expression and functional role of protooncogene *c-kit* in acute myeloblastic leukemia cells. *Blood* 78:2962, 1991.

72. Wellman CL, Whittaker MH: The molecular biology of acute myeloid leukemia. *Clin Lab Med* 10:769, 1990.

73. Vigon I, Dreyfus F, Melle J, et al: Expression of the c-mpl protooncogene in human hematologic malignancies. *Blood* 82:877, 1993.

74. Groves FD, Linet MS, Devesa SS: Epidemiology of leukemia, in *Leuke-*

mia, 6th ed, edited by ES Henderson, TA Lister, MF Greaves, pp 145–159. Saunders, New York, 1986.

75. Stanley M, McKenna RW, Ellinger G, Brunning RD: Classification of 358 cases of acute myeloid leukemia by FAB criteria: analysis of clinical and morphologic features, in *Chronic and Acute Leukemias in Adults*, edited by CD Bloomfield, pp 147–174. Martinus Nijhoff, Boston, 1985.

76. Scott CS, Den Ottolander GJ, Swirsky D, et al: Recommended procedures for the classification of acute leukaemias. *Leuk Lymph* 11:37, 1993.

77. Jennings CD, Foon KA: Recent advances in flow cytometry: application to the diagnosis of hematologic malignancy. *Blood* 90:2863, 1997.

78. Cassanovas RD, Campos L, Mugneret F, et al: Immunophenotypic patterns and cytogenetic anomalies in acute non-lymphoblastic leukemia subtypes: a prospective study of 432 patients. *Leukemia* 12:34, 1998.

79. Del Vecchio L, Di Noto R, Lo Pardo C, et al: Immunological classification of acute leukemias: comments on the EGIL proposals. *Leukemia* 10:1832, 1996.

80. Paietta E: Classification of acute leukemias: proposals for the immunological classification of acute leukemias. *Leukemia* 9:2147, 1995.

81. De Greef GE, Hagemeiger A: Molecular and cytogenetic abnormalities in acute myeloid leukemia and myelodysplastic syndromes. *Baillière's Clin Haematol* 9:1, 1996.

82. Kheiri SA, MacKerrell T, Bonagura VR, et al: Flow cytometry with or without cytochemistry for the diagnosis of acute leukemias? *Cytometry* 34:82, 1998.

83. Head DR: Revised classification of acute myeloid leukemia. *Leukemia* 10:1826, 1996.

84. Boggs DR, Wintrobe MM, Cartwright GE: The acute leukemias. Analysis of 322 cases and review of the literature. *Medicine* 41:163, 1962.

85. Roath S, Israëls MCG, Wilkinson JF: The acute leukemias: A study of 580 patients. *Q J Med* 33:256, 1964.

86. Choi S-I, Simone JV: Acute non-lymphocytic leukemia in 171 children. *Med Pediatr Oncol* 2:119, 1976.

87. Chessels JM, O'Calloghan U, Hardisty RM: Acute myeloid leukaemia in childhood: clinical features and prognosis. *Br J Haematol* 63:555, 1986.

88. Burns CP, Armitage JO, Frey AL, et al: Analysis of presenting features of adult leukemia. *Cancer* 47:2460, 1981.

89. Goodall PT, Vosti KL: Fever in acute myelogenous leukemia. *Arch Intern Med* 135:1197, 1975.

90. Burke PJ, Braine HG, Rothbun HK, Owens AH: The clinical significance and management of fever in acute myelocytic leukemia. *Johns Hopkins Med J* 139:1, 1976.

91. Chang JC: How to differentiate neoplastic fever from infectious fever in patients with cancer. Usefulness of the naproxen test. *Heart Lung* 16:122, 1987.

92. Gollard RP, Robbins BA, Piro L, Saven A: Acute myelogenous leukemia presenting with bulky lymphadnopathy. *Acta Haematol* 95:129, 1996.

93. Davey DD, Fourcar K, Burns CP, Goekin JA: Acute myelocytic leukemia manifested by prominent generalized lymphadenopathy. *Am J Hematol* 21:89, 1986.

94. Tobelem G, Jacquillat C, Chastang C, et al: Acute monoblastic leukemia: a clinical and biologic study of 74 cases. *Blood* 55:71, 1980.

95. Okano K, Ezumi K, Uda M, et al: Histopathological studies on the mode of leukemic infiltration in various organs. *Med J Osaka Univ* 14:125, 1963.

96. Kaiserling E, Horny H-P, Geerts M-L, Schmid U: Skin involvement in myelogenous leukemia. Morphologic and immunophenotypic heterogeneity of skin infiltrates. *Mod Pathol* 7:771, 1994.

97. Longacre TA, Smoller BR: Leukemia cutis: analysis of 50 biopsy-proven cases with an emphasis on occurrences in myelodysplastic syndromes. *Am J Clin Pathol* 100:276, 1993.

98. Shaikh BS, Frantz E, Lookingbill DP: Histologically proven leukemia cutis carries a poor prognosis in acute nonlymphocytic leukemia. *Cutis* 39:57, 1987.

99. Sipp N, Radaszkiemicz T, Meijer CJLM, et al: Specific skin manifestations in acute leukemia with monocytic differentiation. *Cancer* 71:124, 1993.

100. Baer MR, Barcos M, Farrell H, et al: Acute myelogenous leukemia in leukemia cutis. *Cancer* 63:2192, 1989.

101. Long JC, Mihm MC: Multiple granulocytic tumors of the skin: Report of six cases of myelogenous leukemia with initial manifestations in the skin. *Cancer* 39:2004, 1977.

102. Bourantas K, Malamou-Mitsi V, Christou L, et al: Cutaneous vasculitis

as the initial manifestation in acute myelomonocytic leukemia. *Ann Intern Med* 121:942, 1994.

103. Sheps M, Shapero H, Ramsay C: Bullous pyoderma gangrenosum and acute leukemia. *Arch Dermatol* 114:1842, 1978.

104. Lewis SJ, Poh-Fitzpatrick MB, Walther RR: A typical pyoderma gangrenosum with leukemia. *JAMA* 239:935, 1978.

105. Cho K-H, Han K-H, Sim S-W, et al: Neutophilic dermatoses associated with myeloid malignancy. *Clin Exp Dermatol* 22:269, 1997.

106. Cheson BD, Christensen RM: Cutis verticis gyrata: Unusual chloromatous disease in acute myelogenous leukemia. *Am J Hematol* 8:415, 1980.

107. Muller CP, Ziegler A, Steinke B, et al: Myelosarcomatosis of the skin preceding leukemic generalization of acute myelomonocytic leukemia. *Blut* 58:165, 1987.

108. Kincaid MC, Green WR: Ocular and orbital involvement in leukemia. *Surv Ophthalmol* 27:211, 1983.

109. Paparella MM, Berlinger NT, Oda M: Otological manifestations of leukemia. *Laryngoscope* 83:1510, 1973.

110. Bertrand Y, Lefrère J-J, L'Evergren G, et al: Acute myeloblastic leukemia presenting as apparent acute otitis media. *Am J Hematol* 27:136, 1988.

111. Shiknecht HF, Igarashi M, Chasin WD: Inner ear hemorrhage in leukemia. *Laryngoscope* 75:662, 1965.

112. Dewar GJ, Lim C-NH, Michalyshyn B, Akabutu J: Gastrointestinal complications in patients with acute and chronic leukemia. *Can J Surg* 24:67, 1981.

113. Hunter TB, Bjelland JC: Gastrointestinal complications of leukemia and its treatment. *Am J Roentgenol* 142:513, 1984.

114. Duffy JH, Driscoll EJ: Oral manifestations of leukemia. *Oral Surg* 11:484, 1958.

115. Ahsan N, Schen-Chih, JS, John DD: Acute iliotyphlitis as presenting manifestation of acute myelogenous leukemia. *Am J Clin Pathol* 89:407, 1988.

116. Rodgers B, Seibert JJ: Unusual combination of an appendicolith in a leukemic patient with typhlitis-ultrasound diagnosis. *J Clin Ultrasound* 18:141, 1990.

117. Abramson SJ, Berdon WE, Baker DH: Childhood typhlitis: Its increasing association with acute myelogenous leukemia. *Radiology* 146:61, 1983.

118. Roy J, Vercellotti G, Fenderson M, et al: Isolated relapse of acute myelogenous leukemia presenting as a gastric ulcer. *Am J Hematol* 37:270, 1991.

119. Thompson BC, Feczko PJ, Mezwa DG: Dysphagia caused by acute leukemia infiltration of the esophagus. *Am J Radiol* 155:654, 1990.

120. Ti M, Villafuerte R, Chase PH, Dosik H: Acute leukemia presenting as laryngeal obstruction. *Cancer* 34:427, 1974.

121. Bodey GP, Powell RD, Hersh EM, et al: Pulmonary complications of acute leukemia. *Cancer* 19:781, 1966.

122. Maile CW, Moore AV, Ulreich S, Putnam CE: Chest radiographic-pathologic correlation in adult leukemia patients. *Invest Radiol* 18:495, 1983.

123. Armstrong P, Dyer R, Alford BA, O'Hara M: Leukemic pulmonary infiltrates. Rapid development mimicking pulmonary edema. *Am J Roentgenol* 135:373, 1980.

124. Wu KK, Burns CP: Leukemic pleural infiltrates during bone marrow remission of acute myelocytic leukemia. *Cancer* 33:1179, 1974.

125. Roberts WC, Bodey GP, Wertlake PT: The heart in acute leukemia. A study of 420 autopsy cases. *Am J Cardiol* 21:388, 1968.

126. Lisker SA, Finkelstein D, Brody JI, Beizer LH: Myocardial infarction in acute leukemia. *Arch Intern Med* 119:332, 1967.

127. Norris NH, Weiner J: The renal lesions in leukemia. *Am J Med Sci* 241:512, 1961.

128. Uno Y: Histopathological study of leukemic cell infiltration in the kidney. *Med J Osaka Univ* 18:185, 1967.

129. Russo A, Basquez E, Russo G, Schilvio G: Testicular relapse in acute myelogenous leukemia after 3 1/2 years of complete remission. *Acta Haematol* 65:131, 1981.

130. Quien ET, Wallach B, Sandhaus L, et al: Primary extramedullary leukemia of the prostate. *Am J Hematol* 53:267, 1996.

131. Vanden Broecke R, Van Droogenbroek J, Dhont M: Vulvovaginal manifestations of acute myeloblastic leukemia. *Obstet Gynecol* 88:735, 1996.

132. Marsh WL, Byland DJ, Heath VC, Anderson MJ: Osteoarticular and pulmonary manifestations of acute leukemia. *Cancer* 57:385, 1986.

133. Weinberger A, Schumacher R, Schimmer BM, et al: Arthritis in acute leukemia. *Arch Intern Med* 141:1183, 1981.

134. Pavlovsky S, Eppinger-Helft M, Murill FS: Factors that influence the appearance of central nervous system leukemia. *Blood* 42:935, 1973.

135. Meyer RJ, Ferreira PP, Cuttner J, et al: Central nervous system involvement at presentation in acute granulocytic leukemia. *Am J Med* 68:691, 1980.

136. Castagnola C, Morra E, Bernasconi P, et al: Acute myeloid leukemia and diabetes insipidus: results in five patients. *Acta Haematol* 93:1, 1995.

137. Holmes R, Keating MJ, Cork A, et al: A unique pattern of central nervous system leukemia in acute myelomonocytic leukemia associated with inv (16) (p13;q32). *Blood* 65:1071, 1985.

138. Glass JP, VanTassel P, Keating MJ, et al: Central nervous system complications of a newly recognized subtype of leukemia: AMML with a pencentric inversion of chromosome 16. *Neurology* 38:639, 1987.

139. Byrd JC, Edenfield WJ, Shields DJ, Dawson NA: Extramedullary myeloid cell tumors in acute nonlymphocytic leukemia. A clinical review. *J Clin Oncol* 13:1800, 1995.

140. Neiman RS, Barcos M, Berard C, et al: Granulocytic sarcoma: A clinicopathologic study of 61 biopsied cases. *Cancer* 48:426, 1981.

141. Tallman MS, Hakerman D, Shaw JM, et al: Granulocytic sarcoma is associated with the 8;21 translocation in acute myeloid leukemia. *J Clin Oncol* 11:690, 1993.

142. Byrd JC, Weiss RB, Arthur DC, et al: Extramedullary leukemia adversely affects hematologic complete remission rate and overall survival in patients with t(8;21) (q22;q22): results from Cancer and Leukemia Group B 8461. *J Clin Oncol* 15:466, 1997.

143. Rowe JM: Clinical and laboratory features of the myeloid and lymphoid leukemias. *Am J Med Technol* 49:103, 1983.

144. Woodcock BE, Cooper PC, Brown PR, et al: The platelet defect in acute myeloid leukemia. *J Clin Pathol* 37:1339, 1984.

145. Hofmann W-K, Stauch M, Höffken K: Impaired granulocytic function in patients with acute leukaemia: only partial normalization after successful remission-inducing treatment. *Clin Res Clin Oncol* 124:113, 1998.

146. Suda T, Onai T, Maekawa T: Studies on abnormal polymorphonuclear neutrophils in acute myelogenous leukemia. *Am J Hematol* 15:45, 1983.

147. Glick AD, Paniker K, Flexner JM, et al: Acute leukemia of adults: ultrastructural, cytochemical, and histological observations in 100 cases. *Am J Pathol* 73:459, 1980.

148. San Miguel JF, Conzalez M, Canizo MC, et al: TdT activity in acute myeloid leukemias defined by monoclonal antibodies. *Am J Hematol* 23:9, 1986.

149. Kaplan SS, Penchansky L, Krause JR, et al: Simultaneous evaluation of terminal deoxynucleotidyl transferase and myeloperoxidase in acute leukemias using an immunocytochemical method. *Am J Clin Pathol* 87:732, 1987.

150. Kahl, C, Florschütz A, Müller G, et al: Prognostic significance of dysplastic features of hematopoiesis in patients with de novo acute myelogenous leukemia. *Ann Hematol* 75:91, 1997.

151. Manoharan A, Horsley R, Pitney WR: The reticulin content of bone marrow in acute leukemia in adults. *Br J Haematol* 43:185, 1979.

152. Moore MAS, Spitzer G, Williams N, et al: Agar culture studies in 127 cases of untreated acute leukemia: the prognostic value of reclassification of leukemia according to in vitro growth characteristics. *Blood* 44:1, 1974.

153. Knudtzon S: In vitro culture of leukaemic cells from 81 patients with acute leukemia. *Scand J Haematol* 18:377, 1977.

154. Spitzer G, Dicke KA, McCredre KB, Barlogie B: The early detection of remission in acute myelogenous leukaemia by in vitro cultures. *Br J Haematol* 35:411, 1977.

155. Goldberg J, Tice D, Nelson DA, Gottliev AJ: Predictive value of in vitro colony and cluster formation in acute nonlymphocytic leukemia. *Am J Med Sci* 277:81, 1979.

156. Mrózek K, Heinonen K, de la Chapelle A, Bloomfield C: Clinical significance of cytogenetics in acute myeloid leukemia. *Semin Oncol* 24:17, 1997.

157. Stasi R, Del Poeta G, Masi M, et al: Incidence of chromosome abnormalities and clinical significance of karyotype in de novo acute myeloid leukemia. *Cancer Genet Cytogenet* 66:28, 1993.

158. Martinez-Climent JA, Lane NJ, Rubin CM, et al: Clinical and prognostic significance of chromosomal abnormalities in childhood acute myeloid leukemia de novo. *Leukemia* 9:95, 1995.

159. Pedersen-Bjergaard J, Philip P: Chromosome characteristics of therapy-related acute nonlymphocytic leukemia and preleukemia: possible implications for pathogenesis of the disease. *Leuk Res* 11:315, 1987.

160. Zaccarea A, Alimena G, Baccarani M, et al: Cytogenetic analyses in 89 patients with secondary hematologic disorders: Results of a cooperative study. *Cancer Genet Cytogenet* 26:65, 1987.

161. Bitter MA, LeBeau MM, Rowley JD, et al: Association between morphology, karyotype, and clinical features in myeloid leukemias. *Human Pathol* 18:211, 1987.

162. Byrd JC, Lawrence D, Arthur DC, et al: Patients with isolated trisomy 8 in acute myeloid leukemia are not cured with cytarabine-based chemotherapy: results from Cancer and Leukemia Group B 8461. *Clin Cancer Res* 4:1235, 1998.

163. Mrózek K, Heinonen K, Lawrence D, et al: Adult patients with de novo acute myeloid leukemia and t(9;11) (p22;q23) have a superior outcome to patients with other translocations involving band 11q23: a Cancer and Leukemia Group B study. *Blood* 90:4532, 1997.

164. Diaz MO, LeBeau MM, Pitha P, Rowley JD: Interferon and *c-est*-1 genes in the translocation (9;11)(p22;q23) in human acute monocytic leukemia. *Science* 231:265, 1986.

165. Ziemin vander Poel S, McCabe NR, Gill HJ, et al: Identification of a gene, *MLL*, that spans the breakpoint in 11q23 translocations associated with human leukemias. *Proc Natl Acad Sci USA* 89:4220, 1992.

166. Kurzock R, Shtalrid M, Talpaz M, et al: Expression of c-abl in Philadelphia-positive acute myelogenous leukemia. *Blood* 70:1584, 1987.

167. Tien H-F, Wang C-W, Chuang S-M, et al: Characterization of Philadelphia-chromosome-positive acute leukemia by clinical, cytochemical, and gene analysis. *Leukemia* 6:907, 1992.

168. Kjellstrand CM, Campbell DC, von Hartitzsch B, Buselmeier TJ: Hyperuricemic acute renal failure. *Arch Intern Med* 133:349, 1974.

169. O'Regan S, Carson S, Chesney RW, Drummond KN: Electrolyte and acid-base disturbances in the management of leukemia. *Blood* 49:345, 1977.

170. Mir MA, Delamore IW: Metabolic disorders in acute myeloid leukaemia. *Br J Haematol* 40:79, 1978.

171. Bergman GE, Baluarte HJ, Naiman JL: Diabetes insipidus as a presenting manifestation of acute myelogenous leukemia. *J Pediatr* 88:355, 1976.

172. Mir MA, Brabin B, Tang OT, et al: Hypokalemia in acute myeloid leukaemia. *Ann Intern Med* 82:54, 1975.

173. Salomon J: Spurious hypoglycemia and hyperkalemia in myelomonocytic leukemia. *Am J Med Sci* 267:359, 1974.

174. Bellevue R, Disik H, Speigel G, Gussoff BD: Pseudohyperkalemia and extreme leukocytosis. *J Lab Clin Med* 85:660, 1975.

175. Fox MJ, Brody JS, Weintraub LR, et al: Leukocyte larceny: a cause of spurious hypoxia. *Am J Med* 67:742, 1979.

176. Palva IP, Salokannel SJ: Hypercalcemia in acute leukemia. *Blut* 24:209, 1972.

177. Zidar BL, Shadduck RK, Winkelstein A, et al: Acute myeloblastic leukemia and hypercalcemia. *N Engl J Med* 295:692, 1976.

178. Roth GJ, Poite D: Chronic lactic acidosis and acute leukemia. *Arch Intern Med* 125:317, 1970.

179. Wainer RA, Wiernik PH, Thompson WL: Metabolic and therapeutic studies of a patient with acute leukemia and severe lactic acidosis of prolonged duration. *Am J Med* 55:255, 1973.

180. Zamkoff KW, Kirshner JJ: Marked hypophosphatemia associated with acute myelomonocytic leukemia. *Arch Intern Med* 140:1523, 1980.

181. Pflüger K-H, Gramse M, Gropp C, Havemann K: Ectopic ACTH production with autoantibody formation in a patient with acute myeloblastic leukemia. *N Engl J Med* 305:1632, 1981.

182. Carpenter NA, Fiere DM, Schuh D, et al: Circulating immune complexes and the prognosis of acute myeloid leukemia. *N Engl J Med* 307:1174, 1982.

183. Bratt G, Bromback M, Paul C, et al: Factors and inhibitors of blood coagulation and fibrinolysis in acute nonlymphoblastic leukaemia. *Scand J Haematol* 34:332, 1985.

184. Reddy VB, Kowal-Vern A, Hoppensteadt DA, et al: Global and molecular hemostatic markers in acute myeloid leukemia. *Am J Clin Pathol* 94:397, 1990.

185. Tsumita Y, Matsushima T, Uchiumi H, et al: Acute myeloid leukemia accompanied by multiple thrombophlebitis. *Intern Med* 36:595, 1997.

186. Weltermann A, Pabinger I, Geiseler K, et al: Hypofibrinogenemia in non-M3 acute myeloid leukemia. Incidence, clinical and laboratory characteristics and prognosis. *Leukemia* 12:1182, 1998.

187. Spertini O, Callegari P, Cordey A-S, et al: High levels of the shed form of L-selectin are present in patients with acute leukemia and inhibit blast cell adhesion to activated endothelium. *Blood* 84:1249, 1994.

188. Lossos IS, Bogomolski-Yahalom V, Matzner Y: Anticardiolipin antibodies in acute myeloid leukemia: prevalence and significance. *Am J Hematol* 57:139, 1998.

189. Lichtman MA, Heal J, Rowe JM: Hyperleukocytic leukaemia: rheological and clinical features and management. *Ballière's Clin Hematol* 1:725, 1987.

190. Ventura GJ, Hester JP, Smith TL, Keating MJ: Acute myeloblastic leukemia with hyperleukocytosis: risk factors for early mortality in induction. *Am J Hematol* 27:34, 1988.

191. Dutcher J, Schiffer CA, Wiernik PH: Hyperleukocytosis in adult acute nonlymphocytic leukemia: impact on remission rate, duration and survival. *J Clin Oncol* 5:1364, 1987.

192. VanBuchem MA, Te Velde J, Willemze R, Spaander PJ: Leucostasis, an underestimated cause of death in leukaemia. *Blut* 56:39, 1988.

193. Dilek I, Uysal A, Demirer T, et al: Acute myeloblastic leukemia associated with hyperleukocytosis and diabetes insipidus. *Leuk Lymph* 30:657, 1998.

194. Nagler A, Brenner B, Zuckerman E, et al: Acute respiratory failure in hyperleukocytic acute myeloid leukemia. *Am J Hematol* 27:65, 1988.

195. Von Eyben FE, Siddiqui MZ, Spanosi G: High-voltage irradiation and hydroxyurea for pulmonary leukostasis in acute myelomonocytic leukemia. *Acta Haematol* 77:180, 1987.

196. Koote AMM, Thompson J, Bruijn JA: Acute myelocytic leukemia with acute aortic occlusion as presenting symptoms. *Acta Hematol* 75:120, 1986.

197. Foss R, Haddad M, Zaizov R, et al: Recurrent peripheral arterial occlusion by leukemic cells sedimentation in acute promyelocytic leukemia. *J Pediatr Surg* 27:665, 1992.

198. Mataix R, Gómez-Casares MT, Campo C, et al: Acute leg ischaemia as a presentation of hyperleukocytosis syndrome in acute myeloid leukaemia. *Am J Hematol* 51:250, 1996.

199. Murray JC, Dorfman SR, Brandt ML, Dreyer ZE: Renal venous thrombosis complicating acute myeloid leukemia in the hyperleukocytosis. *J Pediatr Hematol Oncol* 18:327, 1996.

200. Berdeaux DH, Glosser L, Serokmann R: Hypoplastic acute leukemia. Review of 70 cases with multivariate regression analysis. *Hematol Oncol* 4:291, 1986.

201. Tuzuner N, Cox C, Rowe JM, Bennett JM: Hypocellular acute leukemia. *Hematol Pathol* 9:195, 1995.

202. Nagai K, Kohno T, Chen Y-X, et al: Diagnostic criteria for hypocelluar acute leukemia. *Leuk Res* 7:563, 1996.

203. Barlogie B, Johnston DA, Keating M, et al: Evolution of oligoleukemia. *Cancer* 53:2115, 1984.

204. Maddox A-M, Keating MJ, Smith TL, et al: Prognostic factors for survival of 194 patients with low infiltrate leukemia. *Leuk Res* 10:995, 1986.

205. Niissler V, Sauer H, Pelka-Fleischer R, et al: Clinical, biochemical and cytokinetic parameters for distinguishing smouldering and rapidly proliferating variants of acute leukemia. *Eur J Haematol* 45:19, 1990.

206. Yumura-Yagi K, Hara J, Talva A, Kawa-Ha K: Phenotypic characteristics of acute megakaryocytic leukemia and transient myelopoiesis. *Leuk Lymph* 13:393, 1994.

207. Bhatt S, Schreck R, Graham JM, et al: Transient leukemia with trisomy 21. *Am J Med Genet* 58:310, 1995.

208. Litz CE, Davies S, Brunning RD, et al: Acute leukemia and the transient myeloproliferative disorder associated with Down syndrome: morphologic immunophenotypic and cytogenetic manifestations. *Leukemia* 9:1432, 1999.

209. Ito E, Kasai M, Hayashi Y, et al: Expression of erythroid-specific genes in acute megakaryoblastic leukaemia and transient myeloproliferative disorder in Down syndrome. *Br J Haematol* 90:607, 1995.

210. Kurukashi H, Junichi H, Keiko Y, et al: Monoclonal nature of transient abnormal myelopoiesis in Down's syndrome. *Blood* 77:1161, 1991.

211. Zipursky A, Poon A, Doyle J: Leukemia in Down syndrome: a review. *Pediatr Hematol Oncol* 9:139, 1992.

212. Creutzig U, Ritter J, Vormoor J, et al: Myelodysplasia and acute myelogenous leukemia in Down's syndrome. *Leukemia* 10:1677, 1996.

213. Avet-Loiseau H, Mechinaud F, Harousseau J-L: Clonal hematologic disorders in Down syndrome. *J Pediatr Hematol Oncol* 17:19, 1995.

214. Ravindranath Y, Abella E, Kruscher JP, et al: Acute myeloid leukemia (AML) in Down's syndrome is highly responsive to chemotherapy: experience on Pediatric Oncology Group AML Study 8498. *Blood* 80:2210, 1992.

215. Pui C-H, Kane JR, Crist WM: Biology and treatment of infant leukemias. *Leukemia* 9:762, 1995.

216. McCoy JP Jr, Overton WR: Immunophenotyping of congenital leukemia. *Cytometry* 22:85, 1995.

217. Kempski HM, Chessells JM, Reeves BR: Deletions of chromosome 21 restricted to the leukemia cells of children with Down syndrome and leukemia. *Leukemia* 11:1973, 1997.

218. Lampert F, Harbott J, Ritterbach J: Cytogenetic findings in acute leukaemias of infants. *Br J Cancer* 66(Suppl XVII):S20, 1992.

219. Nagasaka M, Maeda S, Maeda H, et al: Four cases of t(4;11) acute leukemia and its myelomonocytic nature in infants. *Blood* 61:1174, 1983.

220. Hunger SP, Cleary ML: What significance should we attribute to the detection of MLL fusion transcripts? *Blood* 92:709, 1998.

221. Osada S, Horibe K, Oiwa K, et al: A case of infantile acute monocytic leukemia caused by vertical transmission of the mother's leukemic cells. *Cancer* 65:1146, 1990.

222. Lampkin BC, Peipon JJ, Price JK, et al: Spontaneous remission of presumed congenital acute nonlymphoblastic leukemia (ANLL) in a karyotypically normal neonate. *Am J Pediatr Hematol Oncol* 7:346, 1985.

223. Gale RP, Ben Bassat I: Hybrid acute leukaemia. *Br J Haematol* 65:261, 1987.

224. Lauria F, Raspadori D, Ventura MA, et al: The presence of lymphoid-associated antigens in adult acute myeloid leukemia is devoid of prognostic relevance. *Stem Cells* 13:428, 1995.

225. Pui C-H, Raimondi SC, Head DR, et al: Characterization of childhood acute leukemia with multiple myeloid and lymphoid markers at diagnosis and at relapse. *Blood* 78:1327, 1991.

226. Carbonell F, Swansbury J, Min T, et al: Cytogenetic findings in acute biphenotypic leukaemia. *Leukemia* 10:1283, 1996.

227. Gagnon GA, Childs CC, LeMaistre A, et al: Molecular heterogeneity in acute leukemia lineage switch. *Blood* 74:2088, 1989.

228. Greaves MF, Chan LC: Mixed lineage leukemia: the implication for hemopoietic differentiation. *Blood* 68:598, 1986 (letter).

229. Piu C-H, Raimondi SC, Behm FG, et al: Shifts in blast cell phenotype and karyotype at relapse of childhood lymphoblastic leukemia. *Blood* 68:1306, 1986.

230. Greaves MF, Chan LC, Furley AJW, et al: Lineage promiscuity in hemopoietic differentiation and leukemia. *Blood* 67:1, 1986.

231. Neame PB, Soamboonsrup P, Browman G, et al: Simultaneous or sequential expression of lymphoid and myeloid phenotypes in acute leukemia. *Blood* 65:142, 1985.

232. Stass S, Mirro J, Melvin S, et al: Lineage switch in acute leukemia. *Blood* 64:701, 1984.

233. Scott CS, Vulliamy T, Catovsky D, et al: DNA genotypic conservation during phenotypic switch from T-cell acute lymphoblastic leukaemia to acute myeloblastic leukaemia. *Leuk Lymph* 1:21, 1989.

234. Jensen AW, Hokland M, Jorgensen H, et al: Solitary expression of CD 7 among T-cell antigens in acute myeloid leukemia. *Blood* 78:1291, 1991.

235. Estey EH, Shen Yu, Thall PF: Effect of time to complete remission on subsequent survival and disease-free survival time in AML, RAEB-t, and RAEB. *Blood* 95:72, 2000.

236. Ferra F, DelVecchio L: Clinical relevance of acute mixed-lineage leukemia. *Blood* 79:2799, 1992.

237. Miwa H, Nakase K, Kita K: Biological characteristics of CD7(+) acute leukemia. *Leuk Lymph* 21:239, 1996.

238. Suzuki R, Yamamoto K, Seto M, et al: CD7$^+$ and CD56$^+$ myeloid/natural killer cell precursor acute leukemia: a distinct hematolymphoid disease entity. *Blood* 90:2417, 1997.

239. Scott AA, Head DR, Kropecky KJ, et al: HLA-DR$^-$, CD33$^+$, CD56$^+$, CD16$^-$ myeloid/natural killer cell acute leukemia. *Blood* 84:244, 1994.

240. Paietta E, Gallagher RE, Wiernik PH: Myeloid/natural killer cell acute leukemia. *Blood* 84:2824, 1994.

241. Inhorn RC, Aster JC, Roach SA, et al: A syndrome of lymphoblastic lymphoma, eosinophilia, and myeloid hyperplasia malignancy associated with t(8;13) (p11;q11): description of a distinctive clinical entity. *Blood* 85:1881, 1995.

242. Still IH, Chernova O, Hurd D, et al: Molecular characterization of the t(8;13) (p11;q12) translocation associated with an atypical myeloproliferative disorder: Evidence for three discrete loci involved in myeloid leukemias on 8 p11. *Blood* 90:3136, 1997.

243. Mirro J, Kitchingman GR, Williams DL, Murphy SB: Mixed lineage leukemia: the implication for hemopoietic differentiation. *Blood* 68:597, 1986 (letter).

244. Ladanyi M, Samaniego F, Reuter VE, et al: Cytogenetic and immunohistochemical evidence for the germ cell origin of a subset of acute leukemias associated with mediastinal germ cell tumors. *J Natl Cancer Inst* 82:221, 1990.

245. DeMent, CR, Roth BJ, Heerema N, et al: Hematologic neoplasia associated with primary mediastinal germ-cell tumors. *Human Pathol* 21:699, 1990.

246. Nichols CR, Roth BJ, Heerema N, et al: Hematologic neoplasia associated with primary mediastinal germ-cell tumors. *N Engl J Med* 322:1425, 1990.

247. Kiffer JD, Sandeman TF: Primary malignant mediastinal germ cell tumors: a study of eleven cases and a review of the literature. *Int J Radiat Oncol Biol Phys* 17:835, 1990.

248. Nichols CR: Mediastinal germ cell tumors: Clinical features and biologic correlates. *Chest* 99:472, 1991.

249. Cuneo A, Ferrant A, Michaux JL, et al: Cytogenetic profile of minimally differentiated (FAB M0) acute myeloid leukemia: correlation with clinicobiologic findings. *Blood* 85:3688, 1995.

250. Venditti A, Del Poeta G, Buccisano F, et al: Minimally differentiated acute myeloid leukemia (AML M0): comparison of 25 cases with other French-American-British subtypes. *Blood* 89:621, 1997.

251. Villamor N, Zarco M-A, Rozman M, et al: Acute myeloblastic leukemia with minimal myeloid differentiation: phenotypical and ultrastructural characteristics. *Leukemia* 12:1071, 1998.

252. Maruyami F, Stass SA, Estey EH, et al: Detection of AML1/ETO fusion transcript as a tool for diagnosing t(8;21) positive acute myelogenous leukemia. *Leukemia* 8:40, 1994.

253. Schoch C, Haase D, Haferlach T, et al: Fifty-one patients with acute myeloid leukemia and translocation t(8;21) (q22; q22): an additional deletion in 9q is an adverse prognostic factor. *Leukemia* 10:1288, 1996.

254. Wang J, Wang M, Liu JM: Transformation properties of the ETO gene, fusion partner in t(8;21) leukemias. *Cancer Res* 57:2951, 1997.

255. Andrieu V, Radford-Weill I, Troussand X, et al: Molecular detection of t(8;21)/AML1-ETO in AML M1/M2: correlation with cytogenetics, morphology and immunophenotype. *Br J Haematol* 92:855, 1996.

256. Watkins CH, Hall BE: Monocytic leukemia of the Naegeli and Schilling types. *Am J Clin Pathol* 10:387, 1940.

257. Huhn D, Twardzik L: Acute myelomonocytic leukemia and the French-American-British classification. *Acta Haematol* 69:36, 1983.

258. Scott CS, Morgan M, Limbert HJ, et al: Cytochemical, immunological and ANAE-isoenzyme studies in acute myelomonocytic leukaemia: a study of 39 cases. *Scand J Haematol* 35:284, 1985.

259. Creictzig U, Niederbiermann G, Kitter J, et al: Prognostic significance of eosinophilia in acute myelomonocytic leukemia in relation to induction treatment. *Haematol Blood Transf* 33:226, 1990.

260. Hoyle CF, Sherrington PD, Fischer P, Hayhoe FGT: Basophils in acute leukemia. *J Clin Pathol* 42:785, 1989.

261. Bloomfield CD, Garson OM, Knuutila S, de la Chapelle A: t(1;3)(p36;q21) in acute nonlymphocytic leukemia: a new cytogeneticclinicopathologic association. *Blood* 66:1409, 1985.

262. Plantier I, Lai JL, Wattel E, et al: Inv (16) may be one of the many ''favorable'' factors in acute myeloid leukemia. *Leuk Res* 18:885, 1994.

263. Haferlach T, Gassman W, Löffler H, et al: Clinical aspects of acute myeloid leukemias of the FAB types M3 and M4Es. *Ann Hematol* 66:165, 1993.

264. Poirel H, Radford-Weiss I, Rack K, et al: Detection of the chromosome 16 CBFβ - MYH11 fusion transcript in myelomonocytic leukemias. *Blood* 85:1313, 1995.

265. Haferlach T, Winkemann M, Löffler H, et al: The abnormal eosinophils are part of the leukemic cell population in acute myelomonocytic leukemia with abnormal eosinophils (AML M4 Eo) and carry pericentric inversion 16: a combination of May-Grünwald-Giemsa a staining and fluorescence in situ hypbridization. *Blood* 87:2459, 1996.

266. Pearson MG, Vardiman JW, LeBeau MM, et al: Increased numbers of marrow basophils may be associated with t(6;9) in ANLL. *Am J Hematol* 18:393, 1985.

267. Alsabeh R, Byrnes RK, Slovak ML, Arber DA: Acute myeloid leukemia with t(6;9) (p23;q34): association with myelodysplasia, basophilia, and initial CD34 negative phenotype. *Am J Clin Pathol* 107:430, 1997.

268. Copelli M: Di una emopatia sistemizzata rappresentata da una iperplasia eritroblastica (eritromatosis). *Path Riv Quindicin* 4:460, 1912.

269. DiGuglielmo G: Richerche di hematologia: I. Una casa di eritroleucemia. *Folia Med* 13:386, 1917.

270. Cuneo A, VanOrshoven A, Michaux JL, et al: Morphologic, immunologic and cytogenetic studies in erythroleukemia: evidence for multilineage involvement and identification of two distinct cytogenetic-clinico-pathologic types. *Br J Haematol* 75:346, 1990.

271. Goldberg SL, Noel P, Klumpp TR, Dewald GW: The erythroid leukemias. *Am J Clin Oncol* 21:42, 1998.

272. Olopade OI, Thangavelu M, Larson RA, et al: Clinical, morphologic, and cytogenetic characteristics of 26 patients with acute erythroblastic leukemia. *Blood* 80:2873, 1992.

273. Davey FR, Abraham N Jr, Bronetto VL, et al: Morphologic characteristics of erythroleukemia (Acute myeloid leukemia; FAB-M6): a CALGB study. *Am J Hematol* 49:29, 1995.

274. Adamson JW, Finch CA: Erythropoietin and the regulation of erythropoiesis in diGuglielmo's syndrome. *Blood* 36:590, 1970.

275. Mitjavila MT, Villeval JL, Cramer P, et al: Effects of granulocyte-macrophage colony-stimulating factor and erythropoietin on leukemic erythroid colony formation in human early erythroblastic leukemias. *Blood* 70:965, 1987.

276. Mazella FM, Kowel-Vern A, Shrit MA, et al: Acute erythroleukemia evaluation of 48 cases with reference to classification, cell proliferation, cytogenetics, and prognosis. *Am J Clin Pathol* 110:590, 1998.

277. Breton-Gorius J: Phenotypes of blasts in acute erythroblastic and megakaryoblastic leukemia—a review. *Keio J Med* 36:23, 1987.

278. Peterson BA, Levine EG: Uncommon subtypes of acute nonlymphocytic leukemia: clinical features and management of FAB M5, M6 and M7. *Semin Oncol* 14:425, 1987.

279. Croizat P, Favre-Gilly J: Les aspects du syndrome hémorrhagiue des leucémies. *Sang* 20:417, 1949.

280. Hillstad LK: Acute promyleocytic leukemia. *Acta Med Scand* 159:189, 1957.

281. LoCoco F, Nervi C, Avvisati G, Mandelli F: Acute promyelocytic leukemia: a curable disease. *Leukemia* 12:1866, 1998.

282. Warrell RP Jr, deThé H, Wang Z-Y, Degos L: Acute promyelocytic leukemia. *N Engl J Med* 329:177, 1993.

283. Grignani F, Fagioli M, Alcalay M, et al: Acute promyelocytic leukemia from genetics to treatment. *Blood* 83:10, 1994.

284. LoCoco F, Diverio D, Falini B, et al: Genetic diagnosis and molecular monitoring in the management of acute promyelocytic leukemia. *Blood* 94:12, 1999.

285. Dover BD, Preston-Martin S, Chang E, et al: High frequency of acute promyelocytic leukemia among Latinos with acute myeloid leukemia. *Blood* 87:308, 1996.

286. Otero JC, Santillana S, Fereyros G: High frequency of acute promyelocytic leukemia among Latinos with acute myeloid leukemias. *Blood* 88:377, 1996.

287. Estey E, Thall P, Kantarjian H, et al: Association between increased body mass index and a diagnosis of acute promyelocytic leukemia in patients with acute myeloid leukemia. *Leukemia* 11:1661, 1997.

288. Golomb HM, Rowley JD, Vardiman J, et al: "Microgranular" acute promyelocytic leukemia: a distinct clinical, ultrastructural, and cytogenetic entity. *Blood* 55:253, 1980.

289. McKenna RW, Parkin J, Bloomfield C, et al: Acute promyelocytic leukaemia: a study of 39 cases with identification of a hyperbasophilic microgranular variant. *Br J Haematol* 50:201, 1982.

290. Rovelli A, Biondi A, Rajnoldi AC, et al: Microgranular variant of acute promyelocytic leukemia in children. *J Clin Oncol* 10:1413, 1992.

291. Castoldi GL, Liso V, Speechia G, Thomasi P: Acute promyelocytic leukemia: morphological aspects. *Leukemia* 8 (suppl 2):S27, 1994.

292. Umeda M, Nojima Z, Yamaguchi R, et al: Two cases of acute promyelocytic leukemia with marked basophilia—a variant type of APL with the capability of differentiating into basophilis. *Rinsho Ketsveki* 28:2004, 1987.

293. Gotoh H, Murakani S, Oku N, et al: Translocation t(15;17) and t(9;14) (q34;q22) in a case of acute promyelocytic leukemia with increased number of basophils. *Cancer Genet Cytogenet* 36:103, 1988.

294. Yu R-Q, Huang W, Chen S-J, et al: A case of acute eosinophilic granulocytic leukemia with PML-RAR alpha fusion gene expression and response to all-*trans*-retinoic acid. *Leukemia* 11:609, 1997.

295. Rowley JD, Golomb HM, Dogherty C: 15/17 translocation, a consistent chromosomal change in acute promyelocytic leukaemia. *Lancet* 1:549, 1977.

296. Lavau C, Dejean A: The t(15;17) translocation in acute promyelocytic leukemia. *Leukemia* 8:1615, 1994.

297. DeThé H, Chomienne C, Lanotte M, et al: The t(15;17) translocation of acute promyelocytic leukaemia fuses the retinoic acid receptor α-gene to a novel transcribed locus. *Nature* 347:558, 1990.

298. Borrow J, Goddard AD, Sheer D, Soloman E: Molecular analysis of acute promyelocytic breakpoint cluster region in chromosome 17. *Science* 249:1577, 1990.

299. Alcalay N, Zangrilli D, Pandolfi PP, et al: Translocation breakpoint of acute promyelocytic leukemia lies within the retinoic acid receptor a locus. *Proc Natl Acad Sci* 88:1977, 1991.

300. Kakizuka A, Miller WH Jr, Umesono K, et al: Chromosomal translocation t(15;17) in human acute promyelocytic leukaemia fuses RAR α with a novel putative transcription factor γ PML. *Cell* 66:663, 1991.

301. Huang W, Sun G-L, Li X-S, et al: Acute promyelocytic leukemia: clinical relevance of two major PML-RARα isoforms and detection of minimal residual disease by retrotranscriptase/polymerase chain reaction to predict relapse. *Blood* 82:1264, 1993.

302. Brown D, Kogan S, Lagasse E, et al: A PML-RARα transgene initiates murine acute promyelocytic leukemia. *Proc Natl Acad Sci USA* 94:2251, 1997.

303. Dombret H, Scrobohaci ML, Ghorra P, et al: Coagulation disorder associated with acute promyelocytic leukemia: correct effect of all-*trans* retinoic acid. *Leukemia* 7:2, 1993.

304. Tallman MS, Kwaan HC: Reassessing the hemostatic disorder associated with acute promyelocytic leukemia. *Blood* 79:543, 1992.

305. Barbui T, Finazzi G, Falanga A: The impact of all-*trans* retinoic acid on the coagulopathy of acute promyelocytic leukemia. *Blood* 91:3093, 1998.

306. Avvisati G, ten Cate JW, Büller H, Mandelli F: Tranexamic acid for control of haemorrhage in patients with acute promyelocyte leukaemia. *Lancet* ii:122, 1989.

307. Fenaux P, Tertian G, Castaigne S, et al: A randomized trial of amsacrine and rubidasone on 39 patients with acute promyelocytic leukemia. *J Clin Oncol* 9:1556, 1991.

308. Craddock CG, Crandall BF, Como R: Restoration of effective hemopoiesis preceding suppression of leukemia clone in myeloblastic leukemia. *Am J Med* 59:737, 1975.

309. Amato R, Kantarjian H, Walter R, Keating M: Rebound peripheral blastosis with subsequent remission during induction in a patient with acute promyelocytic leukemia. *Cancer* 61:650, 1988.

310. Stone RM, Maguire M, Goldberg MA, et al: Complete remission in acute promyelocytic leukemia despite persistence of abnormal marrow promyelocytes during induction therapy: experience in 34 patients. *Blood* 71:690, 1988.

311. Breitman TR, Collins SJ, Keene BR: Terminal differentiation of human promyelocytic leukemic cells in primary culture in response to retinoic acid. *Blood* 57:1000, 1981.

312. Huang ME, Ye YC, Chen SR, et al: Use of all-*trans* retinoic acid in the treatment of acute promyelocytic leukemia. *Blood* 72:567, 1988.

313. Wu X, Wang X, Qen X, et al: Four years experience with treatment of all-*trans* retinoic acid in acute promyelocytic leukemia. *Am J Hematol* 43:183, 1993.

314. Reschad H, Schilling-Torgau V: Ueber eine neue Leukämie durch echte Uebergangsformen (Splenozyten-leukämie) und ihre Bedeutung für die Selbstständigkeit dieser Zellen. *Münch Med Wochenschr* 60:1981, 1913.

315. Straus DJ, Mertelsmann R, Koziner B, et al: The acute monocytic leukemias. *Medicine* 59:409, 1980.

316. Janvier M, Tobelem G, Daniel MT, et al: Acute monoblastic leukaemia. Clinical, biological data and survival in 45 cases. *Scand J Haematol* 32:385, 1984.

317. Finaux P, Vanhaesbroucke C, Estienne MH, et al: Acute monocytic leukaemia in adults: Treatment and prognosis in 99 cases. *Br J Haematol* 75:41, 1990.

318. Fung H, Shepard JD, Naiman SC, et al: Acute monocytic leukemia: a single institution experience. *Leuk Lymph* 19:259, 1995.

319. Cuttner J, Conjalka MS, Reilly M, et al: Association of monocyte leukemia in patients with extreme leukocytosis. *Am J Med* 69:555, 1980.

320. Jourdan E, Dombret H, Glaisner S, et al: Unexpected high incidence of intracranial subdural haematoma during intensive chemotherapy for acute myeloid leukaemia with a monoblastic component. *Br J Haematol* 89:527, 1995.

321. Scott CS, Stark AN, Limbert HJ, et al: Diagnostic and prognostic factors in acute monocytic leukemia: an analysis of 51 cases. *Br J Haematol* 69:247, 1988.

322. Scherrer A, Kruithof EKO, Grob J-P: Plasminogen activator inhibitor-2 in patients with monocytic leukemia. *Leukemia* 5:479, 1991.

323. Van Furth R, van Zwet TL: Cytochemical, functional, and proliferative characteristics of promonocytes and monocytes from patients with monocytic leukemia. *Blood* 62:298, 1983.

324. Van Furth R, Leijh PCJ, van Zwet TL, van den Barselaar MT: Phagocytic and intracellular killing by peripheral blood monocytes of patients with monocytic leukemia. *Blood* 59:1234, 1982.

325. Swansbury GJ, Slater R, Bain BJ, et al: Hematologic malignancies with t(9;11) (p21-22; q23)—a laboratory and clinical study of 125 cases. *Leukemia* 12:792, 1998.

326. Mavilo F, Testa U, Sposi NM, et al: Selective expression of *fos* protooncogene in human acute myelomonocytic and monocytic leukemias: a molecular marker of terminal differentiation. *Blood* 69:160, 1987.

327. Pinto A, Colletta G, deVecchio L, et al: *c-fos* oncogene expression in human hemopoietic malignancies is restricted to acute leukemias with monocytic phenotype and to subsets of B cell leukemias. *Blood* 70:1450, 1987.

328. Weide R, Parviz B, Pflüger K-H, Haveman K: Altered expression of the human retinoblastoma gene in monocytic leukaemias. *Br J Haematol* 83:428, 1993.

329. Cuttner J, Seremetis S, Najfield V, et al: TdT-positive acute leukemia with monocytoid characteristics: clinical, cytochemical, cytogenetic, and immunologic findings. *Blood* 64:237, 1984.

330. Santiago-Schwarz F, Coppock DL, Hindenburg A, Kern J: Identification of a malignant counterpart of the monocytic-dendritic cell progenitor in acute myeloid leukemia. *Blood* 84:3054, 1994.

331. Srivastava BIS, Srivastava A, Srivastava MD: Phenotype, genotype and cytokine production in acute leukemia involving progenitors of dendritic Langerhans' cells. *Leuk Res* 18:499, 1994.

332. Elghetany MT: True histiocytic lymphoma: is it an entity? *Leukemia* 11:762, 1997.

333. Esteve J, Rozman M, Campo E, et al: Leukemia after true histiocytic lymphoma: another type of acute monocytic leukemia with histiocytic differentiation (AML-M5c). *Leukemia* 9:1389, 1995.

334. Lewis SM, Szur L: Malignant myelosclerosis. *Br Med J* 2:472, 1963.

335. Bergsman KL, VanSlyck EJ: Acute myelofibrosis. *Ann Intern Med* 74:232, 1971.

336. Huang MJ, Li CY, Nichols WL, et al: Acute leukemia with megakaryocytic differentiation. A study of twelve cases identified immunocytochemically. *Blood* 64:427, 1984.

337. Gassman W, Löffler H: Acute megakaryoblastic leukemia. *Leuk Lymph* 18:69, 1995.

338. Cripe LD, Hromas R: Malignant disorders of megakaryocytes. *Semin Hematol* 35:200, 1998.

339. Lange BJ, Kobrinsky N, Barnard DR, et al: Distinctive demography, biology, and outcome of acute myeloid leukemia and myelodysplatic syndrome in children with Down syndrome: Childrens Cancer Group Studies 2861 and 2891. *Blood* 91:608, 1998.

340. Zipursky A, Brown E, Christensen H, et al: Leukemia and/or myeloproliferative syndrome in neonates with Down syndrome. *Semin Perinatol* 21:97, 1997.

341. Carroll A, Civin C, Schneider N, et al: The t(1;22)(p13;q13) is nonrandom and restricted to infants with acute megakaryoblastic leukemia: a pediatric oncology group study. *Blood* 78:748, 1991.

342. Cuneo A, Mecucci C, Kerim S, et al: Multipotent stem cell involvement in megakaryoblastic leukemia: cytologic and cytogenetic evidence in 15 patients. *Blood* 74:1781, 1989.

343. Dhyashiki K, Ohyashiki JH, Hojo H, et al: Cytogenetic findings in adult acute leukemia in myeloproliferative disorders with an involvement of megakaryocytic lineage. *Cancer* 65:940, 1990.

344. Stillman RG: A case of myeloid leukemia with predominance of eosinophilic cells. *Med Rec* 81:594, 1912.

345. Harrington DS, Peterson C, Ness M, et al: Acute myelogenous leukemia with eosinophilic differentiation. *Am J Clin Pathol* 90:464, 1988.

346. Kueck BD, Smith RE, Parkin J, et al: Eosinophilic leukemia: A myeloproliferative disorder distinct from the hypereosinophilic syndrome. *Hematol Pathol* 5:195, 1991.

347. Sanada I, Asou N, Kajima S, et al: Acute myelogenous leukemia (FAB M1) associated with t(5;16) and eosinophilia. *Cancer Genet Cytogenet* 43:139, 1989.

348. Gabbas AG, Li CF: Acute non-lymphocytic leukemia with eosinophilic differentiation. *Am J Hematol* 21:29, 1986.

349. Brito-Babapulle F: Clonal eosinophilic disorders and the hypereosinophilic syndrome. *Blood Rev* 11:129, 1997.

350. Menssen HD, Renkl H-J, Rieder H, et al: Distinction of eosinophilic leukaemia from idiopathic hypereosinophilic syndrome by analysis of Wilms tumor gene expression. *Br J Haematol* 101:325, 1998.

351. Joachim G: Über mastzellenleukämien. *Dtsch Arch Klin Med* 87:437, 1906.

352. Goh KO, Anderson FW: Cytogenetic studies in basophilic chronic myelocytic leukemia. *Arch Pathol Lab Med* 193:288, 1979.

353. Kubota M, Akiyama Y, Tabata Y, et al: Acute nonlymphocytic leukemia with basophilic differentiation and t(9;11)(p22;q23) in a child. *Am J Hematol* 31:133, 1989.

354. Mezger J, Permanetter W, Gerhartz H, et al: Philadelphia chromosome-negative acute hematopoietic malignancy: Ultrastructural, cytochemical, and immunocytochemical evidence of mast cell and basophil differentiation. *Leukemia Res* 14:169, 1990.

355. Duchayne E, Demur C, Rubie H, et al: Diagnosis of acute basophilic leukemia. *Leuk Lymph* 32:269, 1999.

356. Petersen LC, Parken JL, Arthur DC, Brunning RD: Acute basophilic leukemia. *Hematopathology* 96:160, 1991.

357. Kubonishi I, Fijishita M, Niiya K, et al: Basophilic differentiation in acute promyelocytic leukaemia. *Acta Haematol Jpn* 48:1390, 1985.

358. Travis WD, Li C-Y, Hoaglan HC, et al: Mast cell leukemia. Report of a case and review of the literature. *Mayo Clin Proc* 61:957, 1986.

359. Beghini A, Cairoli R, Morra E, Larizza L: In vivo differentiation of mast cells from acute myeloid leukemia blasts carrying a novel activating ligand-independent c-Kit mutation. *BCMD* 24:262, 1998.

360. Fukuda T, Kakihara T, Kamishima T, et al: Leukemic cell membrane from acute myelogenous leukemias with massive mast cell infiltration has a mast cell differentiation activity under culture condition containing interleukin 3. *Leuk Res* 18:749, 1994.

361. Levine PH, Weintraub LR: Pseudoleukemia during recovery from dapsone-induced agranulocytosis. *Ann Intern Med* 68:1060, 1968.

362. Sanal SM, Campbell EW, Bowdler AJ, Brat PJ: Pseudoleukemia. *Postgrad Med* 65:143, 1979.

363. Dreskin SC, Iberti TJ, Watson-Williams EJ: Pseudoleukemia due to infection. *J Med* 14:147, 1983.

364. Reykdal S, Sham R, Phatak P, Kouides P: Pseudoleukemia following the use of G-CSF. *Am J Hematol* 49:258, 1995.

365. Lanham GR, Dahl GV, Billings FT, Stass SA: *Pseudomonas aeruginosa* infection with marrow suppression simulating acute promyelocytic leukemia. *Am J Clin Pathol* 80:404, 1983.

366. Orchard PJ, Moffet HL, Hafez R, Sondel PM: Pseudomonas sepsis simulating acute promyelocytic leukemia. *Pediatr Infect Dis J* 7:66, 1988.

367. Innes DJ, Hess CE, Bertholf MF, Wade P: Promyelocyte morphology: differentiation of acute promyelocytic leukemia from benign myeloid proliferations. *Am J Clin Pathol* 88:725, 1987.

368. Ahmed MAM: Promyelocytic leukaemoid reaction: an atypical presentation of mycobacterial infection. *Acta Haematol* 85:143, 1991.

369. Fohlmeister F, Fischer R, Modder B, et al: Aplastic anemia and the hypocellular myelodysplastic syndrome. *J Clin Pathol* 38:1218, 1985.

370. Poirel H, Rack K, Dalbesse E, et al: Incidence and characterization of MLL gene (11q23) rearrangements in acute myeloid leukemia M1 and M5. *Blood* 87:2496, 1996.

371. Kern W, Scoch C, Haferlach T, et al: Multivariate analysis of prognostic factors in patients with refractory and relapsed acute myeloid leukemia. *Leukemia* 14:226, 2000.

372. Cooley LD, Sears DA, Udden MN, et al: Donor cell leukemia: Report

of a case occurring 11 years after allogeneic bone marrow transplantation and review of the literature. *Am J Hematol* 63:46, 2000.

373. Dunussi-Joannopoulos K, Runyon K, Erickson J, et al: Vaccines with interleuken-12-transduced acute myeloid leukemia elicit very potent therapeutic and long-lasting protective immunity. *Blood* 94:4263, 1999.

374. Tallman MS, Andersen JW, Schiffer CA, et al: Clinical description of 44 patients with acute promyelocytic leukemia who developed the retinoic acid syndrome. *Blood* 95:90, 2000.

375. Wade JC, Newman KA, Schimpff SC, et al: Two methods for improved venous access in acute leukemia patients. *JAMA* 246:140, 1981.

376. Corona ML, Peters SG, Narr BJ, et al: Infections related to central venous catheters. *Mayo Clin Proc* 65:979, 1990.

377. LoCoco F, Pelicci PG, D'Adamo F, et al: Polyclonal hematopoietic reconstitution in leukemia patients in remission after suppression of specific gene rearrangements. *Blood* 82:606, 1993.

378. Petti MC, Avvisati G, Amadori S, et al: Acute promyelocytic leukaemia: Clinical aspects and results of treatment in 62 patients. *Haematologica* 72:151, 1987.

379. Sanz MA, Jarque I, Martin G, et al: Acute promyelocytic leukemia. *Cancer* 6:7, 1988.

380. Marie J-P, ZiHoun R: Chemotherapy of acute myelogenous leukaemia. *Clin Haematol* 4:97, 1991.

381. Foon KA, Gale RP: Therapy of acute myelogenous leukaemia. *Blood Rev* 6:15, 1992.

382. Wiernik PH, Banks PLC, Case DC Jr, et al: Cytarabine plus idarubicin or daunorubicin as induction and consolidation therapy for previously untreated adult patients with acute myeloid leukemia. *Blood* 79:313, 1992.

383. Berman E, Heller G, Santorsa J, et al: Results of a randomized trial comparing idarubicin and cytosine arabinoside with daunorubicin and cytosine arabinoside in adult patients in the newly diagnosed acute myelogenous leukemia. *Blood* 77:1666, 1991.

384. Phillips GL, Reece DE, Shepard JD, et al: High-dose cytarabine and daunorubicin induction and postremission chemotherapy for the treatment of acute myelogenous leukemia in adults. *Blood* 77:1429, 1991.

385. Rowe JM: What is the best induction regimen for acute myelogenous leukemia? *Leukemia* 12 (suppl 1):516, 1998.

386. Hargrave RM, Davey MW, Davey RA, Kidman AD: Development of drug resistance in reduced idarubicin relative to other anthracyclines. *Anticancer Drugs* 6:432, 1995.

387. Usui N, Dobashi N, Kobayashi T, et al: Role of daunorubicin in the induction therapy for adult acute myeloid leukemia. *J Clin Oncol* 16:2086, 1998.

388. Woodlock TJ, Lifton R, DiSalle M: Coincident acute myelogenous leukemia and ischemic heart disease: use of the cardioprotectant dexrazoxane during induction chemotherapy. *Am J Hematol* 59:246, 1998.

389. Bishop JF, Matthews JP, Young GA, et al: A randomized study of high-dose cytarabine in induction in acute myeloid leukemia. *Blood* 87:1710, 1996.

390. Feldman EJ: High-dose mitoxantrone in acute leukaemia: New York Medical College experience. *Eur J Cancer Care* 6:27, 1997.

391. Bishop JF, Lowenthal RM, Joshua D, et al: Etoposide in acute non-lymphocytic leukemia. *Blood* 75:27, 1990.

392. Geller RB, Burke PJ, Karp JE, et al: A two-step timed sequential treatment for acute myelocytic leukemia. *Blood* 74:1499, 1989.

393. Archimbaud E, Thomas X, Leblond V, et al: Timed sequential chemotherapy for previously treated patients with acute myeloid leukemia: long-term follow-up of the etoposide, mitoxantrone, and cytarabine-86 trial. *J Clin Oncol* 13:11, 1995.

394. Archimbaud E, Leblond V, Fenaux P, et al: Timed sequential chemotherapy for advanced acute myeloid leukemia. *Hematol Cell Ther* 38:161, 1996.

395. O'Donnel MR, Appelbaum F, Bishop M, et al: NCCN Acute Leukemia Practic Guidelines. The National Comprehensive Cancer Network. *Oncology* 10:205, 1996.

396. Zittoun R, Suciu S, Mandelli F, et al: Granulocyte-macrophage colony-stimulating factor associated with induction treatment of acute myelogenous leukemia: a randomized trial by the European Organization for Research and Treatment of Cancer Leukemia Cooperative Group. *J Clin Oncol* 14:2150, 1996.

397. Anderlini P, Ghaddar HM, Smith TL, et al: Factors predicting complete remission and subsequent disease-free survival after a second course of

induction therapy in patients with acute myelogenous leukemia resistant to the first. *Leukemia* 10:964, 1996.

398. Hughes WT, Armstrong D, Bodey GP, et al: 1997 guidelines for the use of antimicrobial agents in neutropenic patients with unexplained fever. Infectious Diseases Society of America. *Clin Infect Dis* 25:551, 1997.

399. Uzun O, Anaissie EJ: Antifungal prophylaxis in patients with hematologic malignancies: a reappraisal. *Blood* 86:2063, 1995.

400. Glasmacher A, Molitor E, Hahn C, et al: Antifungal prophylaxis with itraconazole in neutropenic patients with acute leukaemia. *Leukemia* 12:1338, 1998.

401. Bergmann OJ, Mogensen SC, Ellermann-Eriksen S, Ellegaard J: Acyclovir prophylaxis and fever during remission-induction therapy of patients with acute myeloid leukemia: a randomized, double-blind, placebo-controlled trial. *J Clin Oncol* 15:2269, 1997.

402. Walsh TJ, Finberg RW, Arndt C, et al: Liposomal amphotericin B for empirical therapy in patients with persistent fever and neutropenia. National Institute of Allergy and Infectious Disease Mycoses Study Group. *N Engl J Med* 340:764, 1999.

403. Ruiz-Arguelles GJ, Apreza-Molina MG, Aleman-Hoey DD, et al: Outpatient supportive therapy after induction to remission therapy in adult acute myelogenous leukaemia (AML) is feasible: a multicentre study. *Eur J Haematol* 54:18, 1995.

404. Estey E: Hematopoietic growth factors in the treatment of acute leukemia. *Curr Opin Oncol* 10:23, 1998.

405. Jakubowski A, Gordon M, Tafuri A, et al: A pilot study of the biologic and therapeutic effects of granulocyte colony-stimulating factor (Filgrastim) in patients with acute myelogenous leukemia. *Leukemia* 9:1799, 1995.

406. Schiffer CA: Hematopoietic growth factors as adjuncts to the treatment of acute myeloid leukemia. *Blood* 88:3675, 1996.

407. Stone RM, Berg DT, George SL, et al: Granulocyte-macrophage colony-stimulating factor after initial chemotherapy for elderly patients with primary acute myelogenous leukemia. Cancer and Leukemia Group B. *N Engl J Med* 332:1671, 1995.

408. Rowe JM, Anderson JW, Mazza JJ, et al: A randomized placebo-controlled phase III study of granulocyte-macrophage colony-stimulating factor in adult patients (>55 to 70 years of age) with acute myelogenous leukemia: a study of the Eastern Cooperative Oncology Group (E1490). *Blood* 86:457, 1995.

409. Ganser A, Heil G: Use of hematopoeitic growth factors in the treatment of acute myelogenous leukemia. *Curr Opin Hematol* 4:191, 1997.

410. Hoelzer D, Seipelt G: Granulocyte colony-stimulating factor and granulocyte-macrophage colony-stimulating factor in the treatment of myeloid leukemia. *Curr Opin Hematol* 2:196, 1995.

411. Kasper C, Schwarzer A, De Wynter EA, et al: Recombinant human megakaryocyte growth and development factor (MGDF) increases the numbers of megakaryocyte progenitor cells to normal values in long-term bone marrow cultures of patients with AML in first remission. *Leukemia* 12:907, 1998.

412. Sonis S, Edwards L, Lucey C: The biological basis for the attenuation of mucositis: the example of interleukin-11. *Leukemia* 13:831, 1999.

413. Farrell CL, Bready JV, Rex KL, et al: Keratinocyte growth factor protects mice from chemotherapy and radiation-induced gastrointestinal injury and mortality. *Cancer Res* 58:933, 1998.

414. Schlichter SJ, Harker LA: Thrombocytopenia: Mechanisms and management. *Clin Haematol* 7:523, 1978.

415. Gmür J, Burger J, Schanz U, et al: Safety of stringent prophylactic platelet transfusion policy for patients with acute leukemia. *Lancet* 338:1223, 1991.

416. Solomon J, Bofenkamp T, Fahey JL, et al: Platelet prophylaxis in acute non-lymphoblastic leukemia. *Lancet* 1:267, 1978.

417. Beutler E: Platelet transfusions: the 20,000/μl trigger. *Blood* 81:1441, 1993.

418. Funke I, Wiesneth M, Koerner K, et al: Autologous platelet transfusion in alloimmunized patients with acute leukemia. *Ann Hematol* 71:169, 1995.

419. Luban NL: An update on transfusion-transmitted viruses. *Curr Opin Pediatr* 10:53, 1998.

420. Schiffer CA: Granulocyte transfusion therapy. *Curr Opin Hematol* 6:3, 1999.

421. Cullis JO, Duncombe AS, Dudley JM, et al: Acute leukaemia in Jehovah's Witnesses. *Br J Haematol* 100:664, 1998.

422. Cassileth PA, Harrington DP, Hines, JD, et al: Maintenance chemotherapy prolongs remission duration in adult non-lymphocytic leukemia. *J Clin Oncol* 6:583, 1988.

423. Zittoun RA, Madelli F, Willemze R, et al: Autologous or allogeneic bone marrow transplantation compared with intensive chemotherapy in acute myelogenous leukemia. European Organization for Research and Treatment of Cancer (EORTC) and the Gruppo Italiano Malattie Ematologiche Maligne dell-Adulto (GIMEMA) Leukemia Cooperative Groups. *N Engl J Med* 332:217, 1995.

424. Harousseau JL, Cahn JY, Pignon B, et al: Comparison of autologous bone marrow transplantation and intensive chemotherapy as postremission therapy in adult acute myeloid leukemia The Group Ouest Est Leucemies Aigues Myeloblastiques (GOELAM). *Blood* 90:2978, 1997.

425. Cassileth PA, Harrington DP, Appelbaum FR, et al: Chemotherapy compared with autologous or allogeneic bone marrow transplantation in the mangement of acute myeloid leukemia in first remission. *N Engl J Med* 339:1649, 1998.

426. Gale RP, Buchner T, Zhang MF, et al: HLA-identical sibling bone marrow transplants vs chemotherapy for acute myelogenous leukemia in first remission. *Leukemia* 10:1687, 1996.

427. Zittoun R, Suciu S, Watson M, et al: Quality of life in patients with acute myelogenous leukemia in prolonged first complete remission after bone marrow transplantation (allogeneic or autologous) or chemotherapy: a cross-sectional study of the EORTC-GIMEMA AML 8A trial. *Bone Marrow Transplant* 20:307, 1997.

428. Shpilberg O, Haddad N, Sofer O, et al: Postremission therapy with two different dose regimens of cytarabine in adults with acute myelogenous leukemia. *Leuk Res* 19:893, 1995.

429. Heil G, Mitrou PS, Hoeizer D, et al: High-dose cytosine arabinoside and daunorubicin postremission therapy in adults with de novo acute myeloid leukemia. Long-term follow-up of a prospective multicenter trial. *Ann Hematol* 71:219, 1995,

430. Schiller G, Gajewski J, Territo M, et al: Long-term outcome of high-dose cytarabine-based consolidation chemotherapy for adults with acute myelogenous leukemia. *Blood* 80:2977, 1992.

431. Schiller G: Dose-intensive treatment of acute myelogenous leukemia: improved survival? [Letter; comment]. *J Clin Oncol* 13:1828, 1995.

432. Mayer RJ, Davis RB, Schiffer CA, et al: Intensive postremission chemotherapy in adults with acute myeloid leukemia. Cancer and Leukemia Group B. *N Engl J Med* 331:896, 1994.

433. Elonen E, Almqvist A, Hanninen A, et al: Comparison between four and eight cycles of intensive chemotherapy in adult acute myeloid leukemia: a randomized trial of the Finnish Leukemia Group. *Leukemia* 12:1041, 1998.

434. Graves T, Hooks MA: Drug-induced toxicities associated with high-dose cytosine arabinoside infusions. *Pharmacotherapy* 9:23, 1989.

435. Lazarus HM, Herzig RH, Herzig GP, et al: Central nervous system toxicity of high dose systemic cytosine arabinoside. *Cancer* 48:2577, 1981.

436. Smith GA, Damon LE, Rugo HS, et: High-dose cytarabine dose modification reduces the incidence of neurotoxicity in patients with renal insufficiency. *J Clin Oncol* 15:833, 1997.

437. Hewlett J, Kopecky KJ, Head D, et al: A prospective evaluation of the roles of allogeneic marrow transplantation and low-dose monthly maintenance chemotherapy in the treatment of adult acute myelogenous leukemia (AML): a Southwest Oncology Group study. *Leukemia* 9:562, 1995.

438. Bergmann L, Heil G, Kolbe K, et al: Interleukin-2 bolus infusion as late consolidation therapy in 2nd remission of acute myeloblastic leukemia. *Leuk Lymph* 16:271, 1995.

439. Cortes JE, Kantarjian HM, O'Brien S, et al: A pilot study of interleukin-2 for adult patients with acute myelogenous leukemia in first complete remission. *Cancer* 85:1506, 1999.

440. Hellstrand K, Mellqvist UH, Wallhult E, et al: Histamine and interleukin-2 in acute myelogenous leukemia. *Leuk Lymph* 27:429, 1997.

441. Brune M, Hellstrand K: Remission maintenance therapy with histamine and interleukin-2 in acute myelogenous leukaemia. *Br J Haematol* 92:620, 1996.

442. Brune M, Hansson M, Mellqvist UH, et al: NK cell-mediated killing of AML blasts: role of histamine, monocytes and reactive oxygen metabolites. *Eur J Haematol* 57:312, 1996.

443. Volger WR, Weiner RS, Moore JO: Long-term follow-up of a randomized post-induction therapy trial in acute myelogenous leukemia (a Southeastern Cancer Study Group trial). *Leukemia* 9:1456, 1995.

444. Spiekermann K, O'Brien S, Estey E: Relapse of acute myelogenous leukemia during low dose interleukin-2 (IL-2) therapy. Phenotypic evolution associated with strong expression of the IL-2 receptor alpha chain. *Cancer* 75:1594, 1995.

445. Choudhury BA, Liang JC, Thomas EK, et al: Dendritic cells derived in vitro from acute myelogenous leukemia cells stimulate autologous, antileukemic T-cell responses. *Blood* 93:780, 1999.

446. Choudhury A, Toubert A, Sutaria S, et al: Human leukemia-derived dendritic cells: ex-vivo development of specific antileukemic cytotoxicity. *Crit Rev Immunol* 18:121, 1998.

447. Beelen DW, Quabeck K, Graeven U, et al: Acute toxicity and first clinical results of intensive post induction therapy using a modified busulfan and cyclophosphamide regimen in the autologous bone marrow rescue in first remission of acute myeloid leukemia. *Blood* 74:1507, 1989.

448. Gorin NC, Aegerter P, Auvert B, et al: Autologous bone marrow transplantation for acute myelocytic leukemia in first remission: a European survey of the role of marrow purging. *Blood* 75:1606, 1990.

449. Ball ED, Mills LE, Cornwell GG III, et al: Autologous bone marrow transplantation for acute myeloid leukemia using monoclonal antibody-purged bone marrow. *Blood* 76:1199, 1990.

450. Chao NJ, Stein AS, Long GD, et al: Busulfan/etoposide-initial experience with a new preparatory regimen for autologous bone marrow transplantation in patients with acute non-lymphocytic leukemia. *Blood* 81:319, 1993.

451. Gorin NC: Autologous stem cell transplantation in acute myelocytic leukemia. *Blood* 92:1073, 1998.

452. Schiller G, Lee M, Miller T, et al: Transplantation of autologous peripheral blood progenitor cells procured after high-dose cytarabine-based consolidation chemotherapy for adults with acute myelogenous leukemia in first remission. *Leukemia* 11:1533, 1997.

453. Gondo H, Harada M, Miyamoto T, et al: Autologous peripheral blood stem cell transplantation for acute myelogenous leukemia. *Bone Marrow Transplant* 20:821, 1997.

454. Stein AS, O'Donnell MR, Chai A, et al: In vivo purging with high-dose cytarabine followed by high-dose chemoradiotherapy and reinfusion of unpurged bone marrow for adult acute myelogenous leukemia in first complete remission. *J Clin Oncol* 14:2206, 1996.

455. Miggiano MC, Gherlinzoni F, Rosti G, et al: Autologous bone marrow transplantation in late first complete remission improves outcome in acute myelogenous leukemia. *Leukemia* 10:402, 1996.

456. Meloni G, Vignetti M, Avvisati G, et al: BAVC regimen and autograft for acute myelogenous leukemia in second complete remission. *Bone Marrow Transplant* 18:693, 1996.

457. Kusnierz-Glaz CR, Schlegel PG, Wong RM, et al: Influence of age on the outcome of 500 autologous bone marrow transplant procedures for hematologic malignancies. *J Clin Oncol* 15:18, 1997.

458. Mehta J, Powles R, Singhal S, et al: Autologous bone marrow transplantation for acute myeloid leukemia in first remission: identification of modifiable prognostic factors. *Bone Marrow Transplant* 16:499, 1995.

459. To LB, Haylock DN, Thorp D, et al: The optimization of collection of peripheral blood stem cells for autotransplantation in acute myeloid leukaemia. *Bone Marrow Transplant* 4:41, 1989.

460. Bishop MR, Jackson JD, Tarantolo SR, et al: Ex vivo treatment of bone marrow with phosphorothioate oligonucleotide OL(l) p53 for autologous transplantation in acute myelogenous leukemia and myelodysplastic syndrome. *J Hematother* 6:441, 1997.

461. Hogge DE, Ailles LE, Gerhard B: Cytokine responsiveness of primitive progenitors in acute myelogenous leukemia. *Leukemia* 11:2220, 1997.

462. Carella AM, Dejana A, Lerma E, et al: In vivo mobilization of karyotypically normal peripheral blood progenitor cells in high-risk MDS, secondary or therapy-related acute myelogenous leukaemia. *Br J Haematol* 95:127, 1996.

463. Mehta J, Powles R, Horton C et al: Factors affecting engraftment and hematopoietic recovery after unpurged autografting in acute leukemia. *Bone Marrow Transplant* 18:319, 1996.

464. Lemoli RM, Bandini G, Leopardi G, et al: Allogeneic peripheral blood stem cell transplantation in patients with early-phase hematologic malignancy: a retrospective comparison of short-term outcome with bone marrow transplantation. *Haematologica* 83:48, 1998.

465. Santos GW: Marrow transplantation in acute nonlymphocytic leukemia. *Blood* 74:901, 1989.

466. Soiffer RJ, Fairclough D, Robertson M, et al: CD6-depleted allogeneic bone marrow transplantation for acute leukemia in first complete remission. *Blood* 89:3039, 1997.

467. Champlin R, Gale RP: Bone marrow transplantation for acute leukemia: Recent advances and comparison with alternative therapies. *Semin Hematol* 24:55, 1987.

468. Mehta J, Powles R, Treleaven J, et al: Long-term follow-up of patients undergoing allogeneic bone marrow transplantation for acute myeloid leukemia in first complete remission after cyclophosphamide-total body irradiation and cyclosporine. *Bone Marrow Transplant* 18:741, 1996.

469. Fefer A: Allogeneic marrow transplantation for acute nonlymphoblastic leukemia. *J Natl Cancer Inst* 76:1275, 1986.

470. Sullivan KM, Werden PL, Storb RP, et al: Influence of acute and chronic graft-versus-host disease in relapse and survival after bone marrow transplantation from HLA-identical siblings as treatment of acute and chronic leukemia. *Blood* 73:1720, 1989.

471. Conde E, Iriondo A, Richard C, et al: Allogeneic bone marrow transplantation versus intensification chemotherapy for acute myelogenous leukaemia in first remission: a prospective controlled trial. *Br J Haematol* 68:219, 1988.

472. Petersdorf EW, Gooley TA, Anasefti C, et al: Optimizing outcome after unrelated marrow transplantation by comprehensive matching of HLA class I and II alleles in the donor and recipient. *Blood* 92:3515, 1998.

473. Aversa F, Tabilio A, Velardi A, et al: Treatment of high-risk acute leukemia with T-cell-depleted stem cells from related donors with one fully mismatched HLA haplotype. *N Engl J Med* 339:1186, 1998.

474. Sasazuki T, Juji T, Morishima Y, et al: Effect of matching of class I HLA alleles on clinical outcome after transplantation of hematopoietic stem cells from an unrelated donor. Japan Marrow Donor Program. *N Engl J Med* 339:1177, 1998.

475. Gian VG, Moreb JS, Abdef-Mageed A, et al: Successful salvage using mismatched umbilical cord blood transplant in an adult with recurrent acute myelogenous leukemia failing autologous peripheral blood progenitor cell transplant: a case history and review. *Bone Marrow Transplant* 21:1197, 1998.

476. Clift RA, Buckner CD, Thomas ED, et al: The treatment of acute nonlymphoblastic leukemia by allogeneic marrow transplantation. *Bone Marrow Transplant* 2:243, 1987.

477. Gale RP, Horowitz MM, Rees JK, et al: Chemotherapy versus transplants for acute myelogenous leukemia in second remission. *Leukemia* 10:13, 1996.

478. Michel G, Boulad F, Small TN, et al: Risk of extramedullary relapse following allogeneic bone marrow transplantation for acute myelogenous leukemia with leukemia cutis. *Bone Marrow Transplant* 20:107, 1997.

479. Matthews DC, Appelbaum FR, Eary JF, et al: Development of a marrow transplant regimen for acute leukemia using targeted hematopoietic irradiation delivered by ^{131}I-labeled anti-CD45 antibody, combined with cyclophosphamide and total body irradiation. *Blood* 85:1122, 1995.

480. Wagner JE, Santos GW, Burns WH, Sacal R: Second bone marrow transplantation after leukemia relapse in 11 patients. *Bone Marrow Transplant* 4:115, 1989.

481. Saunders JE, Buckner RA, Clift A, et al: Second marrow transplants in patients with leukemia who relapse after allogeneic marrow transplantation. *Bone Marrow Transplant* 3:11, 1989.

482. Blume KG, Forman SJ: High dose busulfan/etoposide as a preparatory regimen for second bone marrow transplants in hematologic malignancies. *Blut* 55:49, 1987.

483. Atkinson K, Biggs J, Concannon A, et al: Second marrow transplants for recurrence of haematologic malignancy. *Bone Marrow Transplant* 1:159, 1986.

484. Shlomchik WD, Emerson SG: The immunobiology of T cell therapies for leukemias. *Acta Haematol* 96:189, 1996.

485. Porter DL, Roth MS, Lee SJ, et al: Adoptive immunotherapy with donor mononuclear cell infusions to treat relapse of acute leukemia or myelodysplasia after allogeneic bone marrow transplantation. *Bone Marrow Transplant* 18:975, 1996.

486. Van Rhee F, Kolb HJ: Donor leukocyte transfusions for leukemic relapse. *Curr Opin Hematol* 2:423, 1995.

487. Berthou C, Leglise MC, Herry A, et al: Extramedullary relapse after favorable molecular response to donor leukocyte infusions for recurring acute leukemia. *Leukemia* 12:1676, 1998.

488. Trenschel R, Bernier M, Stryckmans P, et al: Complete remission following donor PBSC after low-dose cytarabine chemotherapy for early relapse of acute myelogenous leukemia after allogeneic stem cell transplantation. *Bone Marrow Transplant* 19:381, 1997.

489. Goodman M, Cabral L, Cassileth P: Interleukin-2 and leukemia. *Leukemia* 12:1671, 1998.

490. Falkenburg JH, Smit WM, Willemze R: Cytotoxic T-lymphocyte (CTL) responses against acute or chronic myeloid leukemia. *Immunol Rev* 157:223, 1997.

491. Dunussi-Joannopoulos K, Krenger W, Weinstein HJ, Ferrara JL, Croop JM: CD8+ T cells activated during the course of murine acute myelogenous leukemia elicit therapeutic responses to late B7 vaccines after cytoreductive treatment. *Blood* 89:2915, 1997.

492. Boyd CN, Ramberg RC, Thomas ED: The incidence of recurrence of leukemia in donor cells after allogeneic bone marrow transplantation. *Leuk Res* 6:833, 1982.

493. Minden MD, Messner HA, Blech A: Origin of leukemic relapse after bone marrow transplantation detected by restriction fragment length polymorphism. *J Clin Invest* 75:91, 1985.

494. Hiddeman W, Krentzmann H, Straif K, et al: High-dose cytosine arabinoside in combination with mitoxantrone: a highly effective regimen in refractory acute myeloid leukemia. *Blood* 69:744, 1987.

495. Arlin ZA, Ahmed T, Mittleman A, et al: A new regimen of amsacrine with high dose cytarabine is safe and effective therapy for acute leukemia. *J Clin Oncol* 5:371, 1987.

496. Parikh P, Powles R, Treleaven J, et al: High-dose cytosine arabinoside plus etoposide as initial treatment for acute myeloid leukaemia. *Br J Cancer* 62:830, 1990.

497. Ho AD, Lipp T, Ehninger G, et al: Combination of mitoxantrone and etoposide in refractory acute myelogenous leukemia—an active and well-tolerated regimen. *J Clin Oncol* 6:213, 1988.

498. Advani R, Saba HI, Tallman MS, et al: Treatment of refractory and relapsed acute myelogenous leukemia with combination chemotherapy plus the multidrug resistance modulator PSC 833 (Valspodar). *Blood* 93:787, 1999.

499. Archimbaud E, Fenaux P, Reiffers J, et al: Granulocyte-macrophage colony-stimulating factor in association to timed-sequential chemotherapy with mitoxantrone, etoposide, and cytarabine for refractory acute myelogenous leukemia. *Leukemia* 7:372, 1993.

500. De Witte T, Suciu S, Selleslag D, et al: Salvage treatment for primary resistant acute myelogenous leukemia consisting of intermediate-dose cytosine arabinoside and interspaced continuous infusions of idarubicin: a phase-11 study (no. 06901) of the EORTC Leukemia Cooperative Group. *Ann Hematol* 72:119, 1996.

501. Estey EH, Kantarjian HM, O'Brien, et al: High remission rate, short remission duration in patients with refractory anemia with excess blasts (RAEB) in transformaiton (RAEB-t) given acute myelogenous leukemia (AML)-type chemotherapy in combination with granulocyte-CSF (G-CSF). *Cytokines Mol Ther* 1:21, 1995.

502. Kern W, Braess J, Grote-Metke A, et al: Combination of aclarubicin and etoposide for the treatment of advanced acute myeloid leukemia: results of a prospective multicenter phase 11 trial. German AML Cooperative Group. *Leukemia* 12:1522, 1998.

503. De La Serna J, Francisco Tomas J, Solano C, et al: Idarubicin and intermediate dose ARA-C followed by consolidation chemotherapy or bone marrow transplantation in relapsed or refractory acute myeloid leukemia. *Leuk Lymph* 25:365, 1997.

504. Van Den Neste E, Martiat P, Mineur P, et al: 2-Chlorodeoxyadenosine with or without daunorubicin in relapsed or refractory acute myeloid leukemia. *Ann Hematol* 76:19, 1998.

505. Seiter K, Feldman EJ, Halicka HD, et al: Phase I clinical and laboratory evaluation of topotecan and cytarabine in patients with acute leukemia. *J Clin Oncol* 15:44, 1997.

506. Larrea L, Martinez JA, Sanz GF, et al: Carboplatin plus cytarabine in the treatment of high-risk acute myeloblastic leukemia. *Leukemia* 13:161, 1999.

507. Kornblau SM, Kantarjian H, O'Brien S, et al: CECA-cyclophosphamide, etoposide, carboplatin and cytosine arabinoside—a new salvage regimen for relapsed or refractory acute myelogenous leukemia. *Leuk Lymph* 28:371, 1998.

508. Schiller G, Emmanoulides C, Lastrebner MC, et al: High-dose cytarabine and recombinant human granulocyte colony-stimulating factor for the treatment of resistant acute myelogenous leukemia. *Leuk Lymph* 20:427, 1996.

509. Schiller GJ: Treatment of resistant disease. *Leukemia* 12 (suppl) I:S20, 1998.

510. Estey E: Treatment of refractory AML. *Leukemia* 10:932, 1996.

511. Estey E, Kornblau S, Pierce S, et al: A stratification system for evaluating and selecting therapies in patients with relapsed or primary refractory acute myelogenous leukemia. *Blood* 88:756, 1996.

512. Estey E, Thall P, David C: Design and analysis of trials of salvage therapy in acute myelogenous leukemia. *Cancer Chemother Pharmacol* 40:S9, 1997.

513. Kornblau SM, Estey E, Madden T, et al: Phase I study of mitoxantrone plus etoposide with multidrug blockade by SDZ PSC-833 in relapsed or refractory acute myelogenous leukemia. *J Clin Oncol* 15:1796, 1997.

514. Warrell RP Jr, Coonley CJ, Gee TS: Homoharringtonine: an effective new drug for remission induction in refractory non-lymphoblastic leukemia. *J Clin Oncol* 3:617, 1985.

515. Feldman E, Arlin Z, Ahmed T, et al: Homoharringtonine in combination with cytarabine for patients with acute myelogenous leukemia. *Leukemia* 6:1189, 1992.

516. Rowe JM, Chang AYC, Bennett JM: Aclacinomycin A and etoposide (VP-16-213): an effective regimen in previously treated patients with refractory acute myelogenous leukemia. *Blood* 74:992, 1988.

517. Kornblau SM, Gandhi V, Andreeff HM, et al: Clinical and laboratory studies of 2-chlorodeoxyadenosine ±cytosine arabinoside for relapsed or refractory acute myelogenous leukemia in adults. *Leukemia* 10:1563, 1996.

518. Foa R, Fierro MT, Tosti S, et al: Induction and persistence of complete remission in a resistant acute myeloid leukemia patient with recombinant interleukin-2. *Leuk Lymph* 1:113, 1990.

519. Mandelli F, Vignetti M, Tosti S, et al: Interleukin-2 treatment in acute myelogenous leukemia. *Stem Cells* 11:263, 1993.

520. Meloni G, Vignetti M, Andrizzi C, et al: Interlekin-2 for the treatment of advanced acute myelogenous leukemia patients with limited disease: updated experience with 20 cases. *Leuk Lymph* 21:429, 1996.

521. Applebaum FR: Marrow transplantation for hematologic malignancies: a brief review of current status and future prospects. *Semin Hematol* 25:16, 1988.

522. Biggs JC, Horowitz MM, Gale RP, et al: Bone marrow transplants may cure patients with acute leukemia never achieving remission with chemotherapy. *Blood* 80:1090, 1992.

523. Greinix HT, Keil F, Brugger SA, et al: Long-term leukemia-free survival after allogeneic marrow transplantation in patients with acute myelogenous leukemia. *Ann Hematol* 72:53, 1996.

524. Greinix HT, Reiter E, Keil F, et al: Leukemia-free survival and mortality in patients with refractory or relapsed acute leukemia given marrow transplants from sibling and unrelated donors. *Bone Marrow Transplant* 21:673, 1998.

525. Buckley MM, Lamb HM: Oral idarubicin. A review of its pharmacological properties and clinical efficacy in the treatment of haematological malignancies and advanced breast cancer. *Drugs Aging* 11:61, 1997.

526. Kantarjian HM, O'Brien SM, Estey E, et al: Decitabine studies in chronic and acute myelogenous leukemia. *Leukemia* 11(suppl 1):S35, 1997.

527. Lacombe F, Puntous M, Dumain P, et al: Influence of rhGM-CSF on Ara-C sensitivity of patients with acute myeloid leukemia in relapse: a flow cytometry study. *Leuk Res* 20:481, 1996.

528. Burbage C, Tagge EP, Harris B, et al: Ricin fusion toxin targeted to the human granulocyte-macrophage colony stimulating factor receptor is selectively toxic to acute myeloid leukemia cells. *Leuk Res* 21:681, 1997.

529. Hogge DE, Willman CL, Kreitman RJ, et al: Malignant progenitors from patients with acute myelogenous leukemia are sensitive to a diphtheria toxin-granulocyte-macrophage colony-stimulating factor fusion protein. *Blood* 92:589, 1998.

530. Gandhi V, Estey E, Du M, et al: Modulation of the cellular metabolism of cytarabine and fludarabine by granulocyte-colony-stimulating factor during therapy of acute myelogenous leukemia. *Clin Cancer Res* 1:169, 1995.

531. Kanatani Y, Kasukabe T, Okabe-Kado J, et al: Transforming growth factor beta and dexamethasone cooperatively enhance c-jun gene expression and inhibit the growth of human monocytoid leukemia cells. *Cell Growth Differ* 7:187, 1996.

532. Hassan HT, Grell S, Borrmann-Danso U, Freund M: Effect of recombinant human interferons in inducing differentiation of acute megakaryoblastic leukaemia blast cells. *Leuk Lymph* 16:329, 1995.

533. Kurzrock R, Wetzler M, Estrov Z, Talpaz M: Interleukin-1 and its inhibitors: a biologic and therapeutic model for the role of growth regulatory factors in leukemias. *Cytokines Mol Ther* 1:177, 1995.

534. Estey E, Andreeff M: Phase 11 study of interleukin-6 in patients with smoldering relapse of acute myelogenous leukemia. *Leukemia* 9:1440, 1995.

535. Appelbaum FR: Antibody-targeted therapy for myeloid leukemia. *Sem Hematol* 36:2, 1999.

536. Caron PC, Dumont L, Scheinberg DA: Supersaturating infusional humanized anti-CD33 monoclonal antibody HuM1 95 in myelogenous leukemia. *Clin Cancer Res* 4:1421, 1998.

537. Jurcic JG, Caron PC, Nikula TK, et al: Radiolabeled anti-CD33 monoclonal antibody M1 95 for myeloid leukemias. *Cancer Res* 55:5908s, 1995.

538. Pagliaro LC, Liu B, Munker R, et al: Humanized M1 95 monoclonal antibody conjugated to recombinant gelonin: an anti-CD33 immunotoxin with antileukemic activity. *Clin Cancer Res* 4:1971, 1998.

539. Gianni M, Li Calzi M, Terao M, et al: AM580, a stable benzoic derivative of retinoic acid, has powerful and selective cyto-differentiating effects on acute promyelocytic leukemia cells. *Blood* 87:1520, 1996.

540. Munker R, Kobayashi T, Eistner E, et al: A new series of vitamin D analogs is highly active for clonal inhibition, differentiation, and induction of WAF1 in myeloid leukemia. *Blood* 88:2201, 1996.

541. Munker R, Zhang W, Elstner E, Koeffler HP: Vitamin D analogs, leukemia and WAF1. *Leuk Lymph* 31:279, 1998.

542. Morosetti R, Grignani F, Liberatore C, et al: Infrequent alterations of the RAR alpha gene in acute myelogenous leukemias, retinoic acid–resistant acute promyelocytic leukemias, myelodysplastic syndromes, and cell lines. *Blood* 87:4399, 1996.

543. Usuki K, Kitazume K, Endo M, et al: Combination therapy with granulocyte colony-stimulating factor, all-*trans* retinoic acid, and low-dose cytotoxic drugs for acute myelogenous leukemia. *Intern Med* 34:1186, 1995.

544. Zhang W, Piatyszek MA, Kobayashi T, et al: Telomerase activity in human acute myelogenous leukemia: inhibition of telomerase activity by differentiation-inducing agents. *Clin Cancer Res* 2:799, 1996.

545. Motomura S, Motoji T, Takanashi M, et al: Inhibition of P-glycoprotein and recovery of drug sensitivity of human acute leukemic blast cells by multidrug resistance gene (mdrl) antisense oligonucleotides. *Blood* 91:3163, 1998.

546. Komada Y, Zhou YW, Zhang XL, et al: Fas receptor (CD95)-mediated apoptosis is induced in leukemic cells entering G 1 B compartment of the cell cycle. *Blood* 86:3848, 1995.

547. Munker R, Andreeff M: Induction of death (CD95/FAS), activation and adhesion (CD54) molecules on blast cells of acute myelogenous leukemias by TNF-alpha and IFN-gamma. *Cytokines Mol Ther* 2:147, 1996.

548. Jonkhoff AR, Huijgens PC, Versteegh RT, et al: Radiotoxicity of 67-gallium on myeloid leukemic blasts. *Leuk Res* 19:169, 1995.

549. Arceci RJ: The potential for antitumor vaccination in acute myelogenous leukemia. *J Mol Med* 76:80, 1998.

550. Wang JC, Beauregard P, Soamboonsrup P, Neame PB: Monoclonal antibodies in the management of acute leukemia. *Am J Hematol* 50:188, 1995.

551. Karp JE: Molecular pathogenesis and targets for therapy in myelodysplastic syndrome (MDS) and MDS-related leukemias. *Curr Opin Oncol* 10:3, 1998.

552. Nichols J, Nimer SD: Transcription factors, translocations, and leukemia. *Blood* 80:2953, 1992.

553. MacKenzie KL, Dolnikov A, Millington M, et al: Mutant N-ras induces myeloproliferative disorders and apoptosis in bone marrow repopulated mice. *Blood* 93:2043, 1999.

554. Castaigne S, Lefebvre P, Chomienne C, et al: Effectiveness and pharmacokinetics of low-dose all-*trans* retinoic acid (25 mg/m^2) in acute promyelocytic leukemia. *Blood* 82:3560, 1993.

555. Castaigne S, Chomienne C, Daniel MT, et al: All-*trans* retinoic acid as

differentiating therapy for acute promyelocytic leukemia: I. Clinical results. *Blood* 76:1704, 1990.

556. Tallman MS: Differentiating therapy with all-*trans* retinoic acid in acute myeloid leukemia. *Leukemia* 10(suppl 1):S12, 1996.

557. Warrell RP Jr, Frankel SR, Miller WH Jr, et al: Differentiation therapy of acute promyelocytic leukemia with tretinoin (all-*trans*-retinoic acid). *N Engl J Med* 324:1385, 1991.

558. Fenaux P, Chastang C, Cherret S, et al: A randomized comparison of all-*trans* retinoic acid followed by chemotherapy and ATRA plus chemotherapy and the role of maintenance therapy in newly diagnosed acute promyelocytic leukemia. *Blood* 94:1192, 1999.

559. White KL, Wiley JS, Frost T, et al: All-*trans* retinoic acid in the treatment of acute promyelocytic leukemia. *Aust NZ J Med* 22:449, 1992.

560. Chomienne C, Ballerini P, Balitrans N, et al: All-*trans* retinoic acid in acute promyelocytic leukemia: II. In vitro studies: structure-function relationship. *Blood* 76:1710, 1990.

561. Degos L: Is acute promyelocytic leukemia a curable disease? Treatment strategy for a long-term survival. *Leukemia* 8:911, 1994.

562. Head D, Kopecky KJ, Weick J, et al: Effect of aggressive daunomycin therapy on survival in acute promyelocytic leukemia. *Blood* 86:1717, 1995.

563. Gianni M, Terao M, Fortino L, et al: Stat 1 is induced and activated by all-*trans* retinoic acid in acute promyelocytic leukemia cells. *Blood* 89:1001, 1997.

564. Degos L, Dombret H, Chomienne C, et al: All-*trans*-retinoic acid as a differentiating agent in the treatment of acute promyelocytic leukemia. *Blood* 85:2643, 1995.

565. Gallagher RE, Li YP, Rao S, et al: Characterization of acute promyelocytic leukemia cases with PML-RAR alpha break/fusion sites in PML exon 6: identification of a subgroup with decreased in vitro responsiveness to all-*trans* retinoic acid. *Blood* 86:1540, 1995.

566. Licht JD, Chomienne C, Goy A, et al: Clinical and molecular characterization of a rare syndrome of acute promyelocytic leukemia associated with translocation (11;17). *Blood* 85:1083, 1995.

567. Jansen JH, de Ridder MC, Geertsma WM, et al: Complete remission of t(11;17) positive acute promyelocytic leukemia induced by all-*trans* retinoic acid and granulocyte colony-stimulating factor. *Blood* 94:39, 1999.

568. Martinelli G, Ottaviani E, Testoni N, et al: Disappearance of PML/RAR alpha acute promyelocytic leukemia associated transcript during consolidation chemotherapy. *Haematologica* 83:985, 1998.

569. Incerpi MH, Miller DA, Posen R, Byrne JD: All-*trans* retinoic acid for the treatment of acute promyelocytic leukemia in pregnancy. *Obstet Gynecol* 89:826, 1997.

570. Frankel SR, Eardley A, Lauwers G, et al: The ''retinoic acid syndrome'' in acute promyelocytic leukemia. *Ann Intern Med* 117:292, 1992.

571. Azlin ZA, Ahmed T: Cure in acute promyelocytic leukemia—now more readily achievable with less toxic therapy. *Blood* 79:2492, 1992.

572. De Botton S, Dombret H, Sanz M, et al: Incidence, clinical features, and outcome of all *trans*-retinoic acid syndrome in 413 cases of newly diagnosed acute promyelocytic leukemia. The European APL Group. *Blood* 92:2712, 1998.

573. Goldberg MA, Ginsburg D, Mayer RJ, et al: Is heparin administration necessary during induction chemotherapy for patients with acute promyelocytic leukemia? *Blood* 69:187, 1987.

574. Zhu J, Guo WM, Yao YY, et al: Tissue factors on acute promyelocytic leukemia and endothelial cells are differently regulated by retinoic acid, arsenic trioxide and chemotherapeutic agents. *Leukemia* 13:1062, 1999.

575. Menell JS, Cesarman GM, Jacovina AT et al: Annexin II and bleeding in acute promyelocytic leukemia. *N Engl J Med* 340:994, 1999.

576. Kizaki M, Ueno H, Yamazoe Y, et al: Mechanisms of retinoid resistance in leukemic cells: possible role of cytochrome P450 and P-glycoprotein. *Blood* 87:725, 1996.

577. Estey E, Thall PF, Pierce S, et al: Treatment of newly diagnosed acute promyelocytic leukemia without cytarabine. *J Clin Oncol* 15:483, 1997.

578. Tallman MS, Andersen JW, Schiffer CA, et al: All-*trans*-retinoic acid in acute promyelocytic leukemia. *N Engl J Med* 337:1021, 1997.

579. Chen GQ, Shi XG, Tang W, et al: Use of arsenic trioxide (As$_2$O$_3$) in the treatment of acute promyelocytic leukemia (APL): 1. As$_2$O$_3$ exerts dose-dependent dual effects on APL cells. *Blood* 89:3345, 1997.

580. Soignet SL, Maslak P, Wang ZG, et al: Complete remission after treatment of acute promyelocytic leukemia with arsenic trioxide. *N Engl J Med* 339:1341, 1998.

581. Asou N, Adachi K, Tamura J, et al: Analysis of prognostic factors in newly diagnosed acute promyelocytic leukemia treated with all-*trans* retinoic acid and chemotherapy. Japan Adult Leukemia Study Group. *J Clin Oncol* 16:78, 1998.

582. Slack JL, Arthur DC, Lawrence D, et al: Secondary cytogenetic changes in acute promyelocytic leukemia-prognostic importance in patients treated with chemotherapy alone and association with the intron 3 breakpoint of the PML gene: a Cancer and Leukemia Group B study. *J Clin Oncol* 15:1786, 1997.

583. Smith MA, McCaffrey RP, Karp JE: The secondary leukemias: challenges and research directions. *J Natl Cancer Inst* 88:407, 1996.

584. Smith MA, Rubinstein L, Anderson JR, et al: Secondary leukemia or myelodysplastic syndrome after treatment with epipodophyllotoxins. *J Clin Oncol* 17:569, 1999.

585. Super HJ, McCabe NR, Thirman MJ, et al: Rearrangements of the MLL gene in therapy-related acute myeloid leukemia in patients previously treated with agents targeting DNA-topoisomerase 11. *Blood* 82:3705, 1993.

586. Dissing M, Le Beau MM, Pedersen-Bjergaard J: Inversion of chromosome 16 and uncommon rearrangements of the CBFB and MYHI1 genes in therapy-related acute myeloid leukemia: rare events related to DNA-topoisomerase II inhibitors? *J Clin Oncol* 16:1890, 1998.

587. Felix CA: Secondary leukemias induced by topoisomerase-targeted drugs. *Biochim Biophys Acta* 1400:233, 1998.

588. Pogliani EM, Pioltelli P, Russini F, et al: Acute leukemia following cisplatin for ovarian cancer. *Hematologica* [Letter] 72:184, 1987.

589. Lambertenghi Deliliers G, Annaloro C, Pozzoli E, et al: Cytogenetic and myelodysplastic alterations after autologous hemopoietic stem cell transplantation. *Leuk Res* 23:291, 1999.

590. Legare RD, Gribben JG, Maragh M, et al: Prediction of therapy-related acute myelogenous leukemia (AML) and myelodysplastic syndrome (MDS) after autologous bone marrow transplant (ABMT) for lymphoma. *Am J Hematol* 56:45, 1997.

591. Amadori S, Picardi A, Fazi P, et al: A phase 11 study of VP-16, intermediate-dose Ara-C and carboplatin (VAC) in advanced acute myelogenous leukemia and blastic chronic myelogenous leukemia. *Leukemia* 10:766, 1996.

592. De Witte T, Suciu S, Peetermans M, et al: Intensive chemotherapy for poor prognosis myelodysplasia (MDS) and secondary acute myeloid leukemia (SAML) following MDS of more than 6 months duration. A pilot study by the Leukemia Cooperative Group of the European Organisation for Research and Treatment in Cancer (EORTC-LCG). *Leukemia* 9:1805, 1995.

593. Tobal K, Newton J, Macheta M, et al: Molecular quantitation of minimal residual disease in acute myeloid leukemia with t(8;21) can identify patients in durable remission and predict relapse. *Blood* 95:815, 2000.

594. Estey EH: Treatment of acute myelogenous leukemia and myelodysplastic syndromes. *Semin Hematol* 32:132, 1995.

595. Brincker H: Estimate of overall treatment results in acute nonlymphocytic leukemia based on age-specific rates of incidence and complete remission. *Cancer Treat Rep* 69:5, 1985.

596. Pinto A, Zulian GB, Archimbaud E: Acute myelogenous leukaemia. *Crit Rev Oncol Hematol* 27:161, 1998.

597. Leith CP, Kopecky KJ, Godwin J, et al: Acute myeloid leukemia in the elderly: assessment of multidrug resistance (MDR1) and cytogenetics distinguishes biologic subgroups with remarkably distinct responses to standard chemotherapy. A Southwest Oncology Group study. *Blood* 89:3323, 1997.

598. Champlin RE, Gajewski TL, Golde DW: Treatment of acute myelogenous leukemia in the elderly. *Semin Oncol* 16:51, 1989.

599. Ballester O, Moscinski LC, Morris D, Balducci L: Acute myelogenous leukemia in the elderly. *J Am Geriatr Soc* 40:277, 1992.

600. Copplestone JA, Prentice AG: Acute myeloblastic leukaemia in the elderly. *Leukemia Res* 12:617, 1988.

601. Stein RS, Volger WR, Winton EF, et al: Therapy of acute myelogenous leukemia in patients over age 50: A randomized Southeastern Cancer Study Group Trial. *Leukemia Res* 14:895, 1990.

602. Powell BL, Capizzi RL, Muss HB, et al: Low-dose Ara-c therapy for acute myelogenous leukemia in elderly patients. *Leukemia* 3:23, 1989.

603. Tucker J, Thomas AE, Gregoy WM, et al: Acute myeloid leukemia in elderly adults. *Hematol Oncol* 8:13, 1990.

604. Harousseau JF, Rigal-Huguet F, Hurteloup P, et al: Treatment of acute myeloid leukemia in elderly patients with oral idarubicin as a single agent. *Eur J Haematol* 42:182, 1989.

605. Smith AG, Whitehouse JM, Roath OS, et al: Acute leukaemia in the elderly, remission induction versus palliative therapy. *Haematol Blood Transf* 30:330, 1987.

606. Walters RS, Kantarjian HM, Keating MJ, et al: Intensive treatment of acute leukemia in adults 70 years of age and older. *Cancer* 60:149, 1987.

607. Worsley A, Mufti GJ, Copplestone JA, et al: Very-low-dose cytarabine for myelodysplastic syndromes and acute myeloid leukemia in the elderly. *Lancet* 1:966, 1986.

608. Lowenberg B, Suciu S, Archimbaud E, et al: Mitoxantrone versus daunorubicin in induction-consolidation chemotherapy—the value of low-dose cytarabine for maintenance of remission, and an assessment of prognostic factors in acute myeloid leukemia in the elderly: final report. European Organization for the Research and Treatment of Cancer and the Dutch-Belgian Hemato-Oncology Cooperative Hovon Group. *J Clin Oncol* 16:872, 1998.

609. Lowenberg B, Suciu S, Archimbaud E, et al: Use of recombinant GM-CSF during and after remission induction chemotherapy in patients aged 61 years and older with acute myeloid leukemia: final report of AML-11, a phase III randomized study of the Leukemia Cooperative Group of European Organisation for the Research and Treatment of Cancer and the Dutch Belgian Hemato-Oncology Cooperative Group. *Blood* 90:2952, 1997.

610. Reiffers J, Huguet F, Stoppa AM, et al: A prospective randomized trial of idarubicin vs daunorubicin in combination chemotherapy for acute myelogenous leukemia of the age group 55 to 75. *Leukemia* 10:389, 1996.

611. Schiller GJ: Postremission therapy of acute myeloid leukemia in older adults. *Leukemia* 10(suppl 1):S18, 1996.

612. Herzig RH: High-dose ara-C in older adults with acute leukemia. *Leukemia* 10 (suppl 1):S10, 1996.

613. Letendre L, Noel P, Litzow MR, et al: Treatment of acute myelogenous leukemia in the older patient with attenuated high-dose ara-C. *Am J Clin Oncol* 21:142, 1998.

614. Schiller G, Lee M: Long-term outcome of high-dose cytarabine-based consolidation chemotherapy for older patients with acute myelogenous leukemia. *Leuk Lymph* 25:111, 1997.

615. Lowenberg B: Post-remission treatment of acute myelogenous leukemia. *N Engl J Med* 332:260, 1995.

616. DeLima M, Ghaddar H, Pierce S, Estey E: Treatment of newly-diagnosed acute myelogenous leukaemia in patients aged 80 years and above. *Br J Haematol* 93:89, 1996.

617. Johnson PR, Yin JA: Prognostic factors in elderly patients with acute myeloid leukaemia. *Leuk Lymph* 16:51, 1994.

618. Volm MD, Tallman MS: Developments in the treatment of acute leukemia in adults. *Curr Opin Oncol* 7:28, 1995.

619. Dombret H, Chastang C, Fenaux P, et al: A controlled study of recombinant human granulocyte colony stimulating factor in elderly patients after treatment for acute myelogenous leukemia. AML Cooperative Study Group. *N Engl J Med* 332:1678, 1995.

620. Maslak PG, Weiss MA, Berman E, et al: Granulocyte colony-stimulating factor following chemotherapy in elderly patients with newly diagnosed acute myelogenous leukemia. *Leukemia* 10:32, 1996.

621. McLain CR: Leukemia in pregnancy. *Clin Obstet Gynecol* 17:185, 1974.

622. Yahia C, Hyman GA, Phillips JL: Acute leukemia and pregnancy. *Obstet Gynecol Surv* 13:1, 1958.

623. Doll DC, Rigenberg QS, Yarbro JW: Management of cancer during pregnancy. *Arch Intern Med* 148:2058, 1988.

624. Catanzarite VA, Ferguson JE: Acute leukemia and pregnancy: a review of outcome and management, 1972-1982. *Obstet Gynecol Surv* 39:663, 1984.

625. Fassas A, Kartabs G, Klearchou N, et al: Chemotherapy for acute leukemia during pregnancy. Five case reports. *Nouv Rev Fr Hematol* 26:19, 1984.

626. D'Emilio A, Dragone P, DeNegri G, et al: Acute myelogenous leukemia in pregnancy. *Haematologica* (Pavia) 74:601, 1989.

627. Aviles A, Diaz-Magusco JC, Talavera A, et al: Growth and development of children of mothers treated with chemotherapy during pregnancy: Current status of 43 children. *Am J Hematol* 36:243, 1991.

628. Caligiuri MA, Mayer RJ: Pregnancy and leukemia. *Semin Oncol* 16:388, 1989.

629. Volkenandt M, Buchner T, Hiddemann W, VandeLoo J: Acute leukaemia during pregnancy. *Lancet* 2:1521, 1987.

630. Renosos EE, Shepard FA, Messner HA, et al: Acute leukemia during pregnancy: The Toronto Leukemia Study Group Experience with long-term follow-up of children exposed in utero to chemotherapeutic agents. *J Clin Oncol* 5:1098, 1987.

631. Juarez S, Cuadrado-Pastor JM, Feliu J, et al: Association of leukemia and pregnancy: Clinical and obstetric aspects. *Am J Clin Oncol* 11:159, 1988.

632. Gonbunova ZB, Streneva TN: On the transplacental transmission of acute leukemia. *Probl Gematol Perel Krovi* 12:36, 1964.

633. Osada S, Horibe K, Oiwa K, et al: A case of infantile acute monocytic leukemia caused by vertical transmission of the mother's leukemic cells. *Cancer* 65:1146, 1990.

634. Meyer R, Cuttner J, Truog P, et al: Therapeutic leukapheresis of acute myelomonocytic leukemia in pregnancy. *Med Pediatr Oncol* 4:77, 1978.

635. Lipovsky MM, Biesma DH, Christiaens GC, Petersen EJ: Successful treatment of acute promyelocytic leukaemia with all-*trans* retinoic acid during late pregnancy. *Br J Haematol* 94:669, 1996.

636. Amadori S, Ceci A, Comelli A, et al: Treatment of acute myelogenous leukemia in children: Results of the Italian cooperative study AIEOP/LAM 8204. *J Clin Oncol* 5:1356, 1987.

637. Boulad F, Kernan NA: Treatment of childhood acute nonlymphoblastic leukemia: a review. *Cancer Invest* 11:534, 1993.

638. Steinhorn SC, Ries LG: Improved survival among children with acute leukemia in the United States. *Biomed Pharmacother* 42:675, 1988.

639. Zittoun R: Chemotherapy of acute myelogenous leukemia: a review. *Leukemia* 6(suppl 2):36, 1992.

640. Hurwitz CA, Krance R, Schell MJ, et al: Current strategies for treatment of acute myeloid leukemia at St. Jude Children's Research Hospital. *Leukemia* 6(suppl 2):39, 1992.

641. Nygaard R, Moe PJ: Outcome after cessation of therapy in childhood leukemia. *Acta Paediatrica Scand Suppl* 354:4, 1989.

642. Stahnke K, Boos J, Bender-Gotze C, et al: Duration of first remission predicts remission rates and long-term survival in children with relapsed acute myelogenous leukemia. *Leukemia* 12:1534, 1998.

643. Creutzig U, Stahnke K, Pollman H, et al: The problem of early death in childhood AML. *Haematol Blood Transf* 30:524, 1987.

644. Johnson FL, Sanders JE, Ruggiero M, et al: Bone marrow transplantation for treatment in acute nonlymphocytic leukemia in children aged less than 2 years. *Blood* 71:1277, 1988.

645. Woolfrey AE, Gooley TA, Sievers EL, et al: Bone marrow transplantation for children less than 2 years of age with acute myelogenous leukemia or myelodysplastic syndrome. *Blood* 92:3546, 1998.

646. Vormoor J, Boos J, Stahnke K, et al: Therapy of childhood acute myelogenous leukemias. *Ann Hematol* 73:11, 1996.

647. Verhagen C, Stalpers LJA, dePauw BE, Haanen C: Drug-induced skin reactions in patients with acute non-lymphocytic leukaemia. *Eur J Haematol* 38:225, 1987.

648. Young RC, Ozols RF, Myers CE: The anthracycline antineoplastic drugs. *N Engl J Med* 305:139, 1981.

649. Couch RD, Loh KK, Sugino J: Sudden cardiac death following adriamycin therapy. *Cancer* 48:38, 1981.

650. Nitchi JL, Senger JW, Thorning D, et al: Anthracycline cardiotoxicity: clinical and pathological outcomes assessed by radionuclide ejection fractions. *Cancer* 46:1109, 1980.

651. Wade JC, Gaffey M, Wiernik PH, et al: Hepatitis in patients with acute non-lymphocytic leukemia. *Am J Med* 75:413, 1983.

652. Thaler M, Pastakia B, Shawker TA, et al: Hepatic candidiasis in cancer patients: the evolving picture of the syndrome. *Ann Intern Med* 108:88, 1988.

653. VonEiff M, Essink M, Roos N, et al: Hepatosplenic candidiasis, a late manifestation of candida septicemia in neutropenic patients with haematologic malignancies. *Blut* 60:242, 1990.

654. Blade J, Lopez-Guillermo A, Rozman C, et al: Chronic systemic candidiasis in acute leukemia. *Ann Hematol* 64:240, 1992.

655. Walsh TJ, Pizzo A: Treatment of systemic fungal infections: recent progress and current problems. *Eur J Clin Microbiol Infect Dis* 7:460, 1988.

656. Alexander JE, Williamson SL, Seibert JJ, et al: The ultrasonographic diagnosis of typhlitis (neutropenic colitis). *Pediatr Radiol* 18:200, 1988.

657. Moir CR, Scudamore CH, Benny WB: Typhlitis: selective surgical management. *Am J Surg* 151:1563, 1986.

658. Byrnes JJ, Baqueriro H, Gonzalez M, Henseley GT: Thrombotic thrombocytopenic purpura subsequent to acute myelogenous leukemia chemotherapy. *Am J Hematol* 21:299, 1986.

659. Milliken S, Poweles R, Parikh P, et al: Successful pregnancy following bone marrow transplantation for leukemia. *Bone Marrow Transplant* 5:135, 1990.

660. Hinterberger-Fischer M, Kier P, Kalhs P, et al: Fertility, pregnancies and offspring complications after bone marrow transplantation. *Bone Marrow Transplant* 7:5, 1991.

661. Giri N, Vowels MR, Barr AL, Mameghan H: Successful pregnancy after total body irradiation and bone marrow transplantation for acute leukaemia. *Bone Marrow Transplant* 10:93, 1992.

662. Maguire LC, Dick FR, Sherman BM: The effects of anti-leukemic therapy on gonadal histology in adult males. *Cancer* 48:1967, 1981.

663. Matthews JH, Wood JK: Male fertility during chemotherapy for acute leukemia. *N Engl J Med* 303:1235, 1980.

664. MacMahon B, Forman D: Variations in the duration of survival of patients with acute leukemia. *Blood* 12:683, 1957.

665. Copplestone JA, Smith AG, Oscier DG, Hamblin TJ: True outlook in acute myeloblastic leukaemia. *Lancet* 1:1104, 1986.

666. Beguin Y, Sautois B, Forget P: Long-term follow-up of patients with acute myelogenous leukemia who received the daunorubicin, vincristine, and cytosine arabinoside regimen. *Cancer* 79:1351, 1997.

667. Berman E: Recent advances in the treatment of acute leukemia. *Curr Opin Hematol* 4:256, 1997.

668. Bigelow CL, Kopecky K, Files JC, et al: Treatment of acute myelogenous leukemia in patients over 50 years of age with V-TAD: a Southwest Oncology Group study. *Am J Hematol* 48:228, 1995.

669. Feldman EJ: Acute myelogenous leukemia in the older patient. *Semin Oncol* 22:21, 1995.

670. Harousseau JL, Pignon B, Witz F, et al: Treatment of acute myeloblastic leukemia in adults. The GOELAM experience. *Hematol Cell Ther* 38:381, 1996.

671. Zittoun R: The EORTC trials for acute myelogenous leukemia. EORTC Leukemia Cooperative Group. European Organisation of Research and Treatment of Cancer. *Hematol Cell Ther* 38:247, 1996.

672. Bennett JM, Andersen JW, Cassileth PA: Long-term survival in acute myeloid leukemia: The Eastern Cooperative Oncology Group (ECOG) experience. *Leukemia Res* 15:223, 1991.

673. Vignefti M, Orsini E, Petti MC, et al: Probability of long-term disease-free survival for acute myeloid leukemia patients after first relapse: a single-centre experience. *Ann Oncol* 7:933, 1996.

674. Berman E: Chemotherapy in acute myelogenous leukemia: high dose, higher expectations? *J Clin Oncol* 13:1, 1995.

675. Burnett AK: Transplantation in first remission of acute myeloid leukemia. *N Engl J Med* 339:1698, 1998.

676. Burnett AK, Goldstone AH, Stevens RM, et al: Randomised comparison of addition of autologous bone-marrow transplantation to intensive chemotherapy for acute myeloid leukaemia in first remission: results of MRC AML 10 trial. UK Medical Research Council Adult and Children's Leukaemia Working Parties. *Lancet* 351:700, 1998.

677. Clift RA, Buckner CD: Marrow transplantation for acute myeloid leukemia. *Cancer Invest* 16:53, 1998.

678. Gale RP, Butturini A: Transplants for acute myelogenous leukemia. *Cancer Invest* 16:66, 1998.

679. Jacobson RJ, Temple MJ, Singer JW, et al: A clonal complete remission in a patient with acute nonlymphocytic leukemia originating in a multipatient stem cell. *N Engl J Med* 710:1513, 1984.

680. Tilly H, Bostard C, Bizet M, et al: Low-dose cytarabine: persistence of a clonal abnormality during complete remission of acute nonlymphocytic leukemia. *N Engl J Med* 314:246, 1986.

681. Fialkow PJ, Singer JW, Roskind WH, et al: Clonal development, stem cell differentiation and the nature of clinical remissions in acute non-lymphocytic leukemia: studies of patients heterozygous for glucose-6-phosphate dehydrogenase. *N Engl J Med* 317:468, 1987.

682. Bartram CR, Ludwig W-D, Hiddemann W, et al: Acute myeloid leukemia: analysis of *ras* gene mutations and clonality defined by polymorphic X-linked loci. *Leukemia* 3:247, 1989.

683. Fialkow PJ, Janssen JWG, Bartram CR: Clonal remissions in acute nonlymphocytic leukemia: evidence for a multistep pathogenesis of the malignancy. *Blood* 77:1415, 1991.

684. Busque L, Gilliland DG: Clonal evolution in acute myeloid leukemia. *Blood* 82:337, 1993.

685. Gale RE, Wheadon H, Goldstone AH, et al: Frequency of clonal remission in acute myeloid leukaemia. *Lancet* 341:138, 1993.

686. Killman S-A: Acute leukemia: development, remission/relapse pattern, relationship between normal and leukaemic haemopoiesis, and the "sleeper-to-feeder" stem cell hypothesis. *Ballière's Clin Haematol* 4:577, 1991.

687. Kudoh S, Asou H, Kyo T, et al: Emergence of karyotypically unrelated clone in remission of de novo acute myeloblastic leukaemias. *Br J Haematol* 89:531, 1995.

688. Jinnai 1, Nagai K, Yoshida S, et al: Incidence and characteristics of clonal hematopoiesis in remission of acute myeloid leukemia in relation to morphological dysplasia. *Leukemia* 9:1756, 1995.

689. Robert EE: Spontaneous complete remission in acute promyelocytic leukemia. *N Y State J Med* 86:662, 1985.

690. Takue Y, Culbert SJ, van Eys J, et al: Spontaneous cure of end-stage acute nonlymphocytic leukemia complicated with chloroma (granulocytic sarcoma). *Cancer* 58:1101, 1986.

691. Jehn UW, Mempel MA: Spontaneous remission of acute myeloid leukemia. *Blut* 52:165, 1986.

692. Passe S, Miké V, Mertelsmann R, et al: Acute nonlymphoblastic leukemia: prognostic factors in adults with long-term follow-up. *Cancer* 50:1462, 1982.

693. Evansen SA, Stavem P: Long-term survival in acute leukemia. *Acta Med Scand* 219:79, 1986.

694. Grunwald HW: The cure of acute myeloblastic leukemia in adults. *JAMA* 247:1698, 1982.

695. Lie S, Slørdahl SH: Long-term relapse-free survival in childhood acute non-lymphocytic leukemia. *Semin Oncol* 14(suppl 1):7, 1987.

696. Kawashima K, Nagura E-L, Yamaoa K, et al: Leukemia relapse in long-term survivors of acute leukemia. *Cancer* 56-88, 1985.

697. De Lima M, Strom SS, Keating M, et al: Implications of potential cure in acute myelogenous leukemia: development of subsequent cancer and return to work. *Blood* 90:4719, 1997.

698. Greenberg DB, Kornblith AB, Herndon JE, et al: Quality of life for adult leukemia survivors treated on clinical trials of Cancer and Leukemia Group B during the period 1971–1988: predictors for later psychologic distress. *Cancer* 80:1936, 1997.

699. Buchner T, Heinecke A: The role of prognostic factors in acute myeloid leukemia. *Leukemia* 10(suppl) 1:S28, 1996.

700. Billström R, Nilsson PG, Mitelman F: Chromosomes, Auer rods and prognosis in acute myeloid leukaemia. *Eur J Haematol* 40:273, 1988.

701. Berger R, Bernheim A, Ochva-Noguera ME, et al: Prognostic significance of chromosomal abnormalities in acute nonlymphocytic leukemia. A study of 343 patients. *Cancer Genet Cytogenet* 28:293, 1987.

702. Cortes JE, Kantarjian H, O'Brien S, et al: Clinical and prognostic significance of trisomy 21 in adult patients with acute myelogenous leukemia and myelodysplastic syndromes. *Leukemia* 9:115, 1995.

703. Ghaddar HM, Pierce S, Reed P, Estey EH: Prognostic value of residual normal metaphases in acute myelogenous leukemia patients presenting with abnormal karyotype. *Leukemia* 9:779, 1995.

704. Seol JG, Kim ES, Park WH, et al: Telomerase activity in acute myelogenous leukaemia: clinical and biological implications. *Br J Haematol* 100:156, 1998.

705. Estrov Z, Thall PF, Talpaz M, et al: Caspase 2 and caspase 3 protein levels as predictors of survival in acute myelogenous leukemia. *Blood* 92:3090, 1998.

706. Weh HJ, Kuse R, Hoffman R, et al: Prognostic significance of chromosome analysis in de novo acute myeloid leukemia (AML). *Blut* 56:19, 1988.

707. Arthur DC, Berger R, Golomb HM, et al: The clinical significance of karyotype in acute myelogenous leukemia. *Cancer Genet Cytogenet* 40:203, 1989.

708. Garsm OM, Hagemeijer A, Sakurai M, et al: Cytogenetic studies of 103 patients with acute myelogenous leukemia in relapse. *Cancer Genet Cytogenet* 40:187, 1989.

709. Pedersen-Bjergaard J, Philip P, Larsen SO, et al: Chromosome aberrations and prognostic factors in therapy-related myelodysplasia and acute nonlymphocytic leukemia. *Blood* 76:1083, 1990.

710. Paietta E: Classical multidrug resistance in acute myeloid leukaemia. *Med Oncol* 14:53, 1997.

711. Ino T, Miyazaki H, Isogai M, et al: Expression of P-glycoprotein in de novo acute myelogenous leukemia at initial diagnosis: results of molecular and functional assays and correlation with treatment outcome. *Leukemia* 8:1492, 1994.

712. Hart SM, Ganeshaguru K, Hoffbrand AV: Expression of the multidrug resistance-associated protein (MRP) in acute leukaemia. *Leukemia* 8:2163, 1994.

713. Guerci A, Merlin JL, Missoum N, et al: Predictive value for treatment outcome in acute myeloid leukemia of cellular daunorubicin accumulation and P-glycoprotein expression simultaneously determined by flow cytometry. *Blood* 85:2147, 1995.

714. Leith CP, Chen IM, Kopecky KJ, et al: Correlation of multidrug resistance (MDR1) protein expression with functional dye/drug efflux in acute myeloid leukemia by multiparameter flow cytometry: identification of discordant MDR/efflux+ and MDR1+/efflux- cases. *Blood* 86:2329, 1995.

715. Kohler T, Eller J, Leiblein S, et al: Mechanisms responsible for therapy resistance of acute myelogenous leukemia (AML). *Int J Clin Pharmacol Ther* 36:97, 1998.

716. Longo R, Bensi L, Vecchi A, et al: P-glycoprotein expression in acute myeloblastic leukemia analyzed by immunocytochemistry and flow cytometry. *Leuk Lymph* 17:121, 1995.

717. Haber DA: Multidrug resistance (MDR) in leukemia: is it time to test? *Blood* 79:295, 1992.

718. Michieli M, Damiani D, Michelutti A, et al: Overexpression of multidrug resistance-associated p170-glycoprotein in acute non-lymphocytic leukemia. *Eur J Haematol* 48:87, 1992.

719. Marie JP, Zittoun R, Sikic BI: Multidrug resistance (mdr 1) gene expression in adult acute leukemias: correlation with treatment outcome and in vitro drug sensitivity. *Blood* 78:586, 1991.

720. Massaad-Massade L, Ribrag V, Marie JP, et al: Glutathione system, topoisomerase II level and multidrug resistance phenotype in acute myelogenous leukemia before treatment and at relapse. *Anticancer Res* 17:4647, 1997.

721. Drach D, Zhao S, Drach J, Andreeff M: Low incidence of MDR1 expression in acute promyelocytic leukaemia. *Br J Haematol* 90:369, 1995.

722. Hoyle CF, deBastos M, Wheatley K, et al: AML associated with previous cytotoxic therapy, MDS or myeloproliferative disorders: results from the MRC's 9th AML trial. *Br J Haematol* 72:45, 1989.

723. DeWitte T, Muus P, DePauw B, Haanen C: Intensive antileukemic treatment of patients younger than 65 years with myelodysplastic syndromes and secondary acute myelogenous leukemia. *Cancer* 66:831, 1990.

724. Brito-Babapulle F, Catovsky D, Galton DAG: Clinical and laboratory features of de novo acute myeloid leukaemia with trilineage myelodysplasia. *Br J Haematol* 66:445, 1987.

725. Brito-Babapulle F, Catovsky D, Galton DAG: Myelodysplastic relapse of de novo acute myeloid leukaemia with trilineage myelodysplasia. *Br J Haematol* 68:411, 1988.

726. Rosenthal NS, Farhi DC: Dysmegakaryopoiesis resembling acute megakaryoblastic leukemia in treated acute myeloid leukemia. *Am J Clin Pathol* 95:556, 1991.

727. Layton DM, Ireland RM, Mufti GJ, Bellingham AJ: Myelodysplastic relapse of de novo AML: a heterogenous entity. *Leukemia Res* 11:1055, 1987.

728. Jowitt SN, Yin JAL, Saunders MJ: Relapsed myelodysplastic clone differs from acute onset clone as shown by X-linked DNA polymorphism patterns in a patient with acute myeloid leukemia. *Blood* 82:613, 1993.

729. O'Brien S, Kantarjian HM, Keating M, et al: Association of granulocytosis with poor prognosis in patients with acute myelogenous leukemia and translocation of chromosomes 8 and 21. *J Clin Oncol* 7:1081, 1989.

730. Krykowski E, Polkowska-Kulesza E, Robak T, et al: Analysis of prognostic factors in acute leukemias in adults. *Haematol Blood Transf* 30:369, 1987.

731. Bernard P, Reiffers J, LaComb F, et al: A stage classification for prognosis in adult acute myelogenous leukaemia based upon patient's age, bone marrow karyotype, and clinical features. *Scand J Haematol* 32:429, 1984.

732. Tremblay LN, Hyland RH, Schouten BD, Hanly PJ: Survival of acute myelogenous leukemia patients requiring intubation/ventilatory support. *Clin Invest Med* 18:19, 1995.

733. Hunter AE, Rogers SY, Roberts IAG, et al: Autonomous growth of blast cells is associated with reduced survival in acute myeloblastic leukemia. *Blood* 82:399, 1993.

734. Campos L, Rouault JP, Sabido O, et al: High expression of bcl-2 protein in acute myeloid leukemia cells is associated with poor response to chemotherapy. *Blood* 81:3091, 1993.

735. Kaufmann SH, Karp JE, Svingen PA, et al: Elevated expression of the apoptotic regulator Mcl-1 at the time of leukemic relapse. *Blood* 91:991, 1998

736. Zhang W, Kornblau SM, Kobayashi T, et al: High levels of constitutive WAFl/Cipl protein are associated with chemoresistance in acute myelogenous leukemia. *Clin Cancer Res* 1:1051, 1995.

737. Zhang W, Xu HJ, Kornblau SM, et al: Growth-factor stimulation reveals two mechanisms of retinoblastoma gene inactivation in human myelogenous leukemia cells. *Leuk Lymph* 16:191, 1995.

738. Raspadori D, Lauria F, Ventura MA, et al: Incidence and prognostic relevance of CD34 expression in acute myeloblastic leukemia: analysis of 141 cases. *Leuk Res* 21:603, 1997.

739. Dalal Bi, Wu V, Barnett MJ, et al: Induction failure in de novo acute myelogenous leukemia is associated with expression of high levels of CD34 antigen by the leukemic blasts. *Leuk Lymph* 26:299, 1997.

740. Shimamoto T, Ohyashiki K, Ohyashiki JH, et al: The expression pattern of erythrocyte/megakaryocyte-related transcription factors GATA-1 and the stem cell leukemia gene correlates with hematopoietic differentiation and is associated with outcome of acute myeloid leukemia. *Blood* 86:3173, 1995.

741. Baer MR, Stewart CC, Lawrence D, et al: Expression of the neural cell adhesion molecule CD56 is associated with short remission duration and survival in acute myeloid leukemia with t(8;21)(q22;q22). *Blood* 90:1643, 1997.

742. Extermann M, Bacchi M, Monai N, et al: Relationship between cleaved L-selectin levels and the outcome of acute myeloid leukemia. *Blood* 92:3115, 1998.

743. Raza A, Preisler HD, Li YQ, et al: Biologic characteristics of newly diagnosed poor prognosis acute myelogenous leukemia. *Am J Hematol* 42:359, 1993.

744. Wetzler M, Baer MR, Bernstein SH, et al: Expression of c-mpl MRNA, the receptor for thrombopoietin, in acute myeloid leukemia blasts identifies a group of patients with poor response to intensive chemotherapy. *J Clin Oncol* 15:2262, 1997.

745. Griffin JD, Davis R, Nelson DA, et al: Use of surface marker analysis to predict outcome of adult acute myeloblastic leukemia. *Blood* 68:1232, 1986.

746. San Miguel JF, Ojeda E, Gonzalez M, et al: Prognostic value of immunologic markers in acute myeloblastic leukemia. *Leukemia* 3:108, 1989.

747. Mertelsmann R, Thaler HT, To L, et al: Morphologic classification, response to therapy, and survival in 263 adult patients with acute non-lymphoblastic leukemia. *Blood* 56:773, 1980.

748. Swirsky DM, deBastos M, Parish SE, et al: Features affecting outcome during remission induction of acute myeloid leukaemia in 619 adult patients. *Br J Haematol* 64:435, 1986.

749. Bradstock K, Matthews J, Benson E, et al: Prognostic value of immunophenotyping in acute myeloid leukemia. Australian Leukaemia Study Group. *Blood* 84:1220, 1994.

750. Gaiger A, Schmid D, Heinze G, et al: Detection of the WT1 transcript by RT-PCR in complete remission has no prognostic relevance in de novo acute myeloid leukemia. *Leukemia* 12:1886, 1998.

751. Legrand O, Simonin G, Zittoun R, Marie JP: Lung resistance protein (LRP) gene expression in adult acute myeloid leukemia: a critical evaluation by three techniques. *Leukemia* 12:1367, 1998.

752. Filipits M, Pohl G, Stranzl T, et al: Expression of the lung resistance protein predicts poor outcome in de novo acute myeloid leukemia. *Blood* 91:1508, 1998.

753. Keating MJ, Smith TL, Gehan EA, et al: A prognostic factor analysis for use in the development of predictive models for response of adult acute leukemia. *Cancer* 50:457, 1988.

754. Gale RP, Horowitz MM, Weiner RS, et al: Impact of cytogenetic abnormalities on outcome of bone marrow transplants in acute myelogenous leukemia in first remission. *Bone Marrow Transplant* 16:203, 1995.

755. Zapatero A, Martin de Vidales C, Pinar B, et al: Prognostic factors

affecting leukemia relapse after allogeneic BMT conditioned with cyclo-phosphamide and fractionated TBI. *Bone Marrow Transplant* 18:591, 1996.

756. Hagenbeek A: Minimal residual disease in leukemia: state of the art 1991. *Leukemia* 6 (suppl 2):12, 1992.

757. Sievers EL, Loken MR: Detection of minimal residual disease in acute myelogenous leukemia. *J Pediatr Hematol Oncol* 17:123, 1995.

758. Nucifora G, Larson RA, Rowley JD: Persistence of the 8;21 translocation in patients with acute myeloid leukemia type M2 in long-term remission. *Blood* 82:712, 1993.

759. Estey E, Pierce S: Routine bone marrow exam during first remission of acute myeloid leukemia. *Blood* 87:3899, 1996.

760. Ball ED: Immunophenotyping of acute myeloid leukemia cells. *Clin Lab Med* 10:721, 1990.

761. Adriaansen HJ, Jacobs BC, Kappers-Klunne MC, et al: Detection of residual disease in AML patients by use of double immunological marker analysis for terminal deoxynucleotidyl transferase and myeloid markers. *Leukemia* 7:472, 1993.

762. Reading CL, Estey EH, Huh YO, et al: Expression of unusual immuno-phenotype combinations in acute myelogenous leukemia. *Blood* 81:3083, 1993.

763. Kita K, Miwa H, Nakase K, et al: Clinical importance of CD7 expression in acute myelocytic leukemia. The Japan Cooperative Group of Leuke-mia/Lymphoma. *Blood* 81:2399, 1993.

764. Porwit-MacDonald A, Janossy G, Ivory K, et al: Leukemia-associated changes identified by quantitative flow cytometry: IV. CD34 overexpres-sion in acute myelogenous leukemia M2 with t(8;21). *Blood* 87:1162, 1996.

765. Arkesteijn GJ, Erpelinck SL, Martens AC, et al: The use of FISH with chromosome specific repetitive DNA probes for the follow-up of leukemia patients. Correlations and discrepancies with bone marrow cytology. *Cancer Genet Cytogenet* 88:69. 1996.

766. Hebert J, Cayuela JM, Daniel MT, et al: Detection of minimal residual disease in acute myelomonocytic leukemia with abnormal marrow eosin-ophils by nested polymerase chain reaction with allele specific amplifica-tion. *Blood* 84:2291, 1994.

767. Laczika K, Novak M, Hilgarth B, et al: Competitive CBFbeta/MYHl1 reverse-transcriptase polymerase chain reaction for quantitative assess-ment of minimal residual disease during postremission therapy in acute myeloid leukemia with inversion(16): a pilot study. *J Clin Oncol* 16:1519, 1998.

768. Costello R, Sainty D, Blaise D, et al: Prognosis value of residual disease monitoring by polymerase chain reaction in patients with CBF beta/MYH11-positive acute myeloblastic leukemia. *Blood* 89:2222, 1997.

769. Poirel H, Radford-Weiss 1, Rack K, et al: Detection of the chromosome 16 CBF beta-MYH11 fusion transcript in myelomonocytic leukemias. *Blood* 85:1313, 1995.

770. Erickson P, Gao J, Chank K-S, et al: Identification of breakpoints in t(8;21) acute myelogenous leukemia and isolation of a fusion transcript, AML 1/ETO with similarity to *Drosophila* segmentation gene, runt. *Blood* 80:1825, 1992.

771. Nucifora G, Birn DJ, Erickson P, et al: Detection of DNA rearrangements in the AML1 and ETO loci and of an AML 1/ETO fusion mRNA in patients with t(8;21) acute myeloid leukemia. *Blood* 81:1573, 1993.

772. Maseki N, Miyoshi H, Shimuzu K, et al: The 8;21 chromosome transloca-tion in acute myeloid leukemia is always detectable by molecular analysis using AML 1. *Blood* 81:1573, 1993.

773. Inokuchi K, Iwakiri R, Futaki M, et al: Minimal residual disease in acute myelogenous leukemia with PML/RAR alpha or AMLl/ETO mRNA and phenotypic analysis of possible T and natural killer cells in bone marrow. *Leuk Lymph* 29:553, 1998.

774. Kusec R, Laczika K, Knobl P, et al: AMLl/ETO fusion mRNA can be detected in remission blood samples of all patients with t(8;21) acute myeloid leukemia after chemotherapy or autologous bone marrow trans-plantation. *Leukemia* 8:735, 1994.

775. Marcucci G, Livak KJ, Bi W, et al: Detection of minimal residual disease in patients with AMLl/ETO-associated acute myeloid leukemia using a novel quantitative reverse transcription polymerase chain reaction assay. *Leukemia* 12:1482, 1998.

776. Miyamoto T, Nagafuji K, Akashi K, et al: Persistence of multipotent progenitors expressing AMLl/ETO transcripts in long-term remission patients with t(8;21) acute myelogenous leukemia. *Blood* 87:4789, 1996.

777. Jurlander J, Caligiuri MA, Ruutu T, et al: Persistence of the AMLl/ETO fusion transcript in patients treated with allogeneic bone marrow transplantation for t(8;21) leukemia. *Blood* 88:2183, 1996.

778. Miyamoto T, Nagafuji K, Harada M, et al: Quantitative analysis of AMLl/ETO transcripts in peripheral blood stem cell harvests from pa-tients with t(8;21) acute myelogenous leukaemia. *Br J Haematol* 91:132, 1995.

779. Miyamoto T, Nagafuji K, Harada M, Niho Y: Significance of quantitative analysis of AMLl/ETO transcripts in peripheral blood stem cells from t(8;21) acute myelogenous leukemia. *Leuk Lymph* 25:69, 1997.

780. Tobal K, Liu Yin JA: Molecular monitoring of minimal residual disease in acute myeloblastic leukemia with t(8;21) by RT-PCR. *Leuk Lymph* 31:115, 1998.

781. Muto A, Mori S, Matsushita H, et al: Serial quantification of minimal residual disease of t(8;21) acute myelogenous leukaemia with RT-com-petitive PCR assay. *Br J Haematol* 95:85, 1996.

782. Erickson PF, Dessev G, Lasher RS, et al: ETO and AML1 phosphopro-teins are expressed in CD34+ hematopoietic progenitors: implications for t(8;21) leukemogenesis and monitoring residual disease. *Blood* 88:1813, 1996.

783. Takatsuki H, Umemura T, Sadamura S, et al: Detection of minimal residual disease by reverse transcriptase polymerase chain reaction for the PML/RAR alpha fusion MRNA: a study in patients with acute promyelocytic leukemia following peripheral stem cell transplantation. *Leukemia* 9:889, 1995.

784. Zhao L, Chang KS, Estey EH, et al: Detection of residual leukemic cells in patients with acute promyelocytic leukemia by the fluorescence in situ hybridization method: potential for predicting relapse. *Blood* 85:495, 1995.

785. Castagnola C, Nozza A, Corso A, Bernasconi C: The value of combina-tion therapy in adult acute myeloid leukemia with central nervous system involvement. *Haematologia* 82:577, 1997.

786. Hatano Y, Miura I, Horiuchi T, et al: Cerebellar myeloblastoma forma-tion in CD7-positive, neural cell adhesion molecule (CD56)-positive acute myelogenous leukemia (M1). *Ann Hematol* 75:125, 1997.

787. Niu C, Yan H, Yu T, et al: Studies on treatment of acute promyelocytic leukemia with arsenic trioxide. *Blood* 94:3315, 1999.

788. Dror Y, Freedman MH: Schwachmann-Diamond syndrome. *Blood* 94:3048, 1999.

789. Filipits M, Stranzl T, Pohl G, et al: Drug resistance factors in acute myeloid leukemia. *Leukemia* 14:68, 2000.

CHRONIC MYELOGENOUS LEUKEMIA AND RELATED DISORDERS

MARSHALL A. LICHTMAN

JANE L. LIESVELD

The chronic myelogenous leukemias include classical chronic myelogenous leukemia, chronic myelomonocytic leukemia, juvenile myelomonocytic leukemia, and chronic neutrophilic leukemia. The term *chronic*, as a contrast to *acute*, once had prognostic implications, but, although the terms remain useful for nosology, they no longer reflect an invariable difference in prognosis. For example, acute myelogenous leukemia in children and young adults has a higher remission and cure rate than chronic or juvenile myelomonocytic leukemia in children or adults.

Classical chronic myelogenous leukemia presents with anemia, exaggerated granulocytosis, a large proportion of mature neutrophils, absolute basophilia, normal or elevated platelet counts, and frequently, splenomegaly. The marrow is very hypercellular, and cytogenetic analysis will show a Ph chromosome in 90 percent of cases, and molecular diagnostic analysis will reveal a rearrangement of the BCR gene on chromosome 22 in 99 percent of cases. The disease is usually responsive to hydroxyurea, interferon-α, and cytarabine, and median survival has been extended to about 6 years. Inevitably, an accelerated phase ensues that often terminates in acute leukemia, at which point therapy is usually unsuccessful and survival is measured in weeks or months. Allogeneic stem cell transplantation can cure the disease, especially if applied early in the chronic phase. A group of acute leukemias have a translocation between chromosomes 9 and 22, a molecular alteration similar to classic chronic myelogenous leukemia. The translocation results in the fusion gene encoding an oncoprotein that may be similar in size to that in classical chronic myelogenous leukemia, 210 kDa, whereas in some cases it is smaller, 185 kDa. These acute leukemias may in some cases reflect the presentation of the disease in acute blastic transformation without a preceding chronic phase and in other cases a different phenotype resulting from a similar geno-

type. The associated genetic alterations that determine these variations are not clear.

Chronic myelomonocytic leukemia has variable presenting features. Anemia may be accompanied by mildly or moderately elevated leukocyte counts and an elevated total monocyte count; a low, normal, or elevated platelet count; splenomegaly sometimes; and, although cytogenetic abnormalities may be present, there is no specific genetic marker of the disease. Juvenile myelomonocytic leukemia occurs in infancy or very early childhood. Anemia, thrombocytopenia, and leukocytosis with monocytosis is usual. The disease is very refractory to treatment, and, even with current maximal therapy and stem cell rescue, cures are very rare.

Chronic neutrophilic leukemia presents with mild anemia and exaggerated neutrophilia with very few immature cells in the blood. Splenomegaly is common. The disease usually occurs after age 60 years and is usually refractory to current treatment approaches. Chronic and juvenile myelomonocytic leukemia and chronic neutrophilic leukemia have a propensity to transition to acute leukemia. Prior to that time morbidity and mortality is related to infection, hemorrhage, or complicating medical conditions.

DEFINITION AND HISTORY

Chronic myelogenous leukemia (CML) is a pluripotential stem cell disease that is characterized by anemia, extreme blood granulocytosis and granulocytic immaturity, basophilia, often thrombocytosis, and splenomegaly. The hematopoietic cells contain a reciprocal translocation between chromosome numbers 9 and 22 in over 90 percent of patients, which leads to an overtly foreshortened long arm of one of the chromosome pair number 22 (i.e., 22, 22q-) referred to as the *Philadelphia (Ph) chromosome*. A rearrangement of the breakpoint cluster region, a segment of the long arm of chromosome 22, is probably present in all subjects with CML, even the 10 percent without an overt 22q- abnormality. The disease has a very high propensity to evolve into an accelerated, rapidly fatal phase resembling acute leukemia.

In 1845, Bennett in Scotland[1] and Virchow in Germany[2] published descriptions of patients with splenic enlargement, severe anemia, and enormous concentrations of granulocytes in their blood at autopsy. Bennett initially favored an extreme pyemia as the explanation, but Virchow argued against suppuration as a cause. Additional cases were reported by Craige[3] and others, and in 1847 Virchow introduced the designation *weisses Blut* and *leukämie* (leukemia).[4] In 1878 Neumann proposed that the marrow not only was the site of normal blood cell production but was the site from which leukemia originated and used the term *myelogene* (myelogenous) leukemia.[5] Subsequent observations amplified the clinical and laboratory features of the disease, but few fundamental insights were gained until the discovery by Nowell and Hungerford, reported in 1960, that two patients with the disease had an apparent loss of the long arm of chromosome number 21 or 22,[6] an abnormality that was quickly confirmed[7-9] and designated the Philadelphia chromosome.[7] This observation led to a new approach to diagnosis, a marker to study the pathogenesis of the disease, and a focus for future studies of the molecular pathology of the disease. The availability of more sensitive banding techniques to define the structure of chromosomes[10,11] led to the discovery, by Rowley, that the apparent lost chromosomal material on chromosome 22 was part of a reciprocal translocation between chromosomes 9 and 22.[12] The discovery that the cellular oncogene, *ABL*, on chromosome number 9 and a segment of chromosome 22, the breakpoint cluster region,

Acronyms and abbreviations that appear in this chapter include: ALL, acute lymphocytic leukemia; BCR, breakpoint cluster region; CFU-GM, colony forming unit–granulocyte-monocyte; CLL, chronic lymphocytic leukemia; CML, chronic myelogenous leukemia; CMML, chronic myelomonocytic leukemia; FISH, fluorescence in situ hybridization; G, Giemsa; GM-CSF, granulocyte-monocyte colony stimulating factor; GVH, graft-versus-host; HPRT, hypoxanthine phosphoribosyltransferase; IFN-α, interferon α; IRF, interferon regulatory factor; LTC-IC, long-term culture initiating cells; MCP-1, monocyte chemotactic protein-1; MIP-1α, macrophage inflammatory protein-1 alpha; PCR, polymerase chain reaction; Ph, Philadelphia chromosome; Q, quinacrine; Rb, retinoblastoma; RT-PCR, reverse transcriptase–polymerase chain reaction; SCID, severe combined immunodeficiency; TdT, terminal deoxynucleotidyl transferase; TGF-β, transforming growth factor beta; WT, Wilms' tumor.

BCR, fuse as a result of the translocation has provided a basis for the study of the molecular cause of the disease[13,14] (see "Pathogenesis," below).

ETIOLOGY

Exposure to very high doses of ionizing radiation can increase the occurrence of CML above the expected frequency in comparable populations. Three major populations, the Japanese exposed to the radiation released by the atomic bomb detonations at Nagasaki and Hiroshima[15]; British patients with ankylosing spondylitis treated with spine irradiation[16,17]; and women with uterine cervical carcinoma who required radiation therapy[18] had a frequency of CML (as well as acute leukemia) significantly above that expected in comparable unexposed groups. The median latent period was about 4 years in irradiated spondylitics, among whom about 20 percent of the leukemia cases were CML; 9 years in the uterine cervical cancer patients, of whom about 30 percent had CML; and 11 years in the Japanese survivors of the atomic bombs, of whom about 30 percent of the leukemia patients had CML.[19] Chemical leukemogens such as benzene and alkylating agents have not been identified as causative agents of CML, although they are well established to produce a dose-dependent increase in acute myelogenous leukemia. DNA topoisomerase II inhibitors may be an exception, since they have been found to have a propensity to induce t(9;22)-positive leukemia.[20]

Subjects with CML have an increased frequency of HLA antigens CW3 and CW4, suggesting that these may be markers for susceptibility genes for this leukemia.[21] Multiple occurrence of CML in families is very infrequent, however. One exception to the absence of a familial pattern has been reported,[22] but overall the evidence for inheritance being a causative factor is very weak compared, for example, to chronic lymphocytic leukemia.[23]

PATHOGENESIS

ORIGIN FROM A STEM CELL CLONE

Chronic myelogenous leukemia results from the malignant transformation of a single stem cell. The disease is acquired (somatic mutation), since the identical twin of patients with CML and the offspring of mothers with the disease neither carry the Ph chromosome nor develop the disease.[24] The origin of CML from a single hematopoietic stem cell is supported by the following lines of evidence:

1. The involvement of erythropoiesis, neutrophilopoiesis, eosinophilopoiesis, basophilopoiesis, monocytopoiesis, and thrombopoiesis in chronic phase CML[25]
2. The presence of the Ph chromosome (22q-) in erythroblasts; neutrophilic, eosinophilic, and basophilic granulocytes; macrophages; and megakaryocytes[26]
3. The presence of a single glucose-6-phosphate dehydrogenase isoenzyme in red cells, neutrophils, eosinophils, basophils, monocytes, and platelets, but not in fibroblasts or other somatic cells in women with CML who are heterozygotes for isoenzymes A and B[27-29]
4. The presence of the Ph translocation only on a structurally anomalous chromosome 9 or 22 of each chromosome pair in every cell analyzed in occasional patients with a structurally dissimilar 9 or 22 chromosome within the pair[30-32]
5. The presence of the Ph chromosome in one but not the other cell lineage of patients who are a mosaic for sex chromosomes, as in Turner syndrome (45X/46XX)[33] and Klinefelter syndrome (46XY/47XXY)[34]
6. Molecular studies that show variation in the breakpoint of chromosome 22 among different patients with CML but precisely the same breakpoint among cells within a single patient with CML[35,36]
7. A combined DNA hybridization-methylation analysis of women who have restriction fragment length polymorphisms at the X-linked locus for hypoxanthine phosphoribosyltransferase (HPRT) which enables distinction of the two alleles of the HPRT gene in heterozygous females coupled with methylation-sensitive restriction enzyme cleavage patterns, which permits delineation of whether cells contain either the maternally derived or the paternally derived copy of the gene[37]

The foregoing observations placed the parent cell of the clone at least at the level of the hematopoietic stem cell.

PLURIPOTENTIAL VERSUS HEMATOPOIETIC STEM CELL LESION

Some patients in chronic phase CML have lymphocytes that are derived from the primordial malignant cell. Evidence for this includes: a single isoenzyme for glucose-6-phosphate dehydrogenase has been found in some T and B lymphocytes in women with chronic myelogenous leukemia who are heterozygous for isoenzymes A and B[38]; blood cells from patients with CML induced to proliferate with Epstein-Barr virus (presumptive B lymphocytes) are of the same glucose-6-phosphate dehydrogenase isoenzyme type, have cytoplasmic immunoglobulin heavy and light chains, and contain the Ph chromosome[39]; blood lymphocytes stimulated with B-lymphocyte mitogens contain the Ph chromosome[40,41]; purified B lymphocytes from the blood in chronic phase CML contain an abnormal, elongated phosphoprotein coded for by the chimeric gene resulting from the t(9;22)[42]; fluorescence in situ hybridization has detected the BCR-ABL fusion gene in about 25 percent of B lymphocytes in patients in chronic phase[43] in some but not all patients.[44] These findings suggest that B lymphocytes are derived from the malignant clone, placing the lesion closer to, if not in, the pluripotential stem cell.[38-42] Virtually all studies find that the B-lymphocyte pool is a mosaic, containing both Ph chromosome and BCR-ABL-positive and Ph chromosome or BCR-ABL-negative cells. The studies examining the derivation of T lymphocytes from the malignant clone are more ambiguous but indicate that T lymphocytes are derived from the malignant clone in some but not most patients.[38,40,45-54,832] Natural killer cells isolated from patients with chronic phase CML do not contain the BCR-ABL.[55] It is possible that myelopoiesis is invariably clonal and lymphopoiesis is an unpredictable mosaic derived largely from normal residual stem cells. This conclusion is supported by the finding that progenitors of T, B, and NK lymphocytes contain the Ph chromosome and BCR-ABL, but most B-cell and all T-cell progenitors derived from the leukemic clone undergo apoptosis, leaving unaffected cells in the blood.[56,831,833]

ETIOLOGIC ROLE OF THE Ph CHROMOSOME

Early studies indicated that the Ph chromosome may appear after the initial leukemogenic event.[57-60] Patients with CML have developed the Ph chromosome during the course of the disease, have had periods of the disease when the Ph chromosome disappeared,[61] or have had Ph-chromosome-positive and Ph-chromosome-negative cells concurrently.[62-66]

Nearly all, if not all, patients with CML have an abnormality of chromosome 22 at a molecular level (BCR rearrangement). Thus, earlier studies indicating an absence of a Ph chromosome were not a valid measure of the normality of chromosome 22. The molecular abnormality in CML involving the *ABL* gene on chromosome 9 and the *BCR* gene on chromosome 22 have been established as being the proximate cause of the chronic phase of the disease (see "Molecular Pathology," below).

COEXISTENCE OF NORMAL STEM CELLS

Most, if not all, patients with CML have hematopoietic stem cells which, after treatment[67–69] or culture in vitro[70–72]; use of special cell isolation techniques[73,74]; or use of cell transfer to NOD/SCID mice,[75] do not have the Ph chromosome[76,77] or the *BCR-ABL* fusion gene.[78–81] The switch to Ph-chromosome-negative cells in vitro is associated with a loss of monoclonal glucose-6-phosphate dehydrogenase isoenzyme patterns, indicating the persistence and reemergence of normal polyclonal hematopoiesis rather than reversion to a Ph-chromosome-negative clone.[82] Very primitive hematopoietic cells, the so-called long-term culture initiating cells (LTC-IC), are present in Ph-chromosome-negative cytapheresis samples collected during early recovery after chemotherapy for CML.[83] These are most commonly present when cells are collected within 3 months of diagnosis.[84] Variable levels of *BCR-ABL*-negative progenitors are found in the CD34+DR− population, but low levels are found in the CD34+CD38− population.[85] Preprogenitors for the CD34+DR− cells are predominantly *BCR-ABL*-negative in both marrow and blood at diagnosis.[86] Some cells with surface marker characteristics of very primitive normal hematopoietic cells do express the *BCR-ABL* gene, however.[87] Both normal and leukemic SCID-repopulation cells coexist in the marrow and blood from CML patients in chronic phase, whereas only leukemic SCID repopulating cells are detected in blast crisis.[88,89]

PROGENITOR CELL CHARACTERISTICS IN CML

PROGENITOR CELL DYSFUNCTION

The leukemic transformation resulting from the *BCR-ABL* fusion oncogene leads to a marked expansion of erythroid, granulocytic, and megakaryocytic progenitor populations and to a decreased sensitivity of progenitors to regulation.[90–92] This expansion is especially dramatic in the more mature progenitor cell compartment and less so in the primitive progenitor compartments.[90,93] The proliferative capacity of individual granulocytic progenitors is decreased compared to normal cells. Thus, the progenitor cell population in marrow and blood expands proportionately more than the increase in granulopoiesis.[94,95] Moreover, the progenitors have buoyant density that is lighter than their normal counterparts but similar to hepatic fetal granulopoietic progenitors, suggesting an oncofetal pattern.[94] Sensitivity to growth factors and maturation of granulocyte progenitors in culture is similar to normal, however. The marked expansion of the total blood granulocyte pool is the result of a total expansion of granulopoiesis,[93,96] with a minor contribution from prolonged intravascular circulation time.[97]

Erythroid progenitors are expanded, erythroid precursor maturation is blocked at the basophilic erythroblast stage, and the extent of the impairment of erythropoiesis is inversely proportional to the total white cell count.[98]

PROGENITOR CELL CHARACTERIZATION

Phenotypic differences of stem and progenitor cells in CML patients as compared to normals have been identified.[99] For example, a greater proportion of the circulating leukemic CFU-GM express high levels of the adhesion receptor CD44[100] and low levels of L-selectin[101] in contrast to normal cells. Leukemic CD34+ cells overexpress the P-glycoprotein which determines the multidrug resistance phenotype.[102]

BCR-ABL-positive progenitors survive less well in long-term culture than do their normal counterparts. Leukemic CFU-GM colonies, unlike normal colonies, decrease in long-term cultures that are deficient in *kit* ligand,[103] whereas their proliferation is favored in the presence of *kit* ligand.[104] Macrophage inflammatory protein-1 alpha (MIP-1α) does not inhibit growth factor-mediated proliferation of CD34+ cells from CML patients as it does CD34+ cells from normal subjects, even though the MIP-1α receptor is expressed.[105] Another chemokine, monocyte chemotactic protein-1 (MCP-1), unlike MIP-1α, is an endogenous chemokine that has been found to cooperate with transforming growth factor beta (TGF-β) to inhibit the cycling of primitive normal but not CML progenitors in long-term human marrow cultures.[106] Leukemic progenitors are less sensitive than normal progenitors to the antiproliferative effects of TGF-β.[107]

EFFECTS OF *BCR-ABL* ON CELL ADHESION

Primitive progenitors and blast colony-forming cells from patients with CML have decreased adherence to marrow stromal cells.[108,109] This defect is normalized if stromal cells are treated with interferon α (IFN-α).[109,110] As a result, *BCR-ABL*-negative progenitors are enriched in the adherent fraction of circulating CD34+ cells in chronic phase CML patients. The most primitive *BCR-ABL*-positive cells in the blood of patients with CML differ from their normal counterparts. They are increased in frequency and are activated, such that signals that block cell mitosis are bypassed.[111]

Ph-chromosome-positive colony-forming cells adhere less to fibronectin (as well as to marrow stroma) than do their normal counterparts. Adhesion is fostered as a result of restoration of cooperation between activated β_1 integrins and the altered epitopes of CD44.[112–114] CML granulocytes have reduced and altered binding to P-selectin due to modification in the CD15 antigens.[115] *BCR-ABL*-induced defects in integrin function may underlie the abnormal circulation and proliferation of progenitors,[116] since growth signaling can occur through the fibronectin receptor.[117] IFN-α restores normal integrin-mediated inhibition of hematopoietic progenitor proliferation by the marrow microenvironment.[118]

BCR-ABL-encoded fusion protein p210[bcr–abl] binds to actin, and several cytoskeletal proteins are thereby phosphorylated. The p210[bcr–abl] interacts with actin filaments through an actin-binding domain. *BCR-ABL* transfection is associated with an increase in spontaneous motility, membrane ruffling, formation of long actin extensions (filopodia), and accelerated rate of protrusion and retraction of pseudopodia on fibronectin-coated surfaces. Alpha-interferon treatment slowly converts the abnormal motility phenotype of *BCR-ABL*-transformed cells toward normal.[119] Integrins regulate the c-*ABL*-encoded tyrosine kinase activity and its cytoplasmic-nuclear transport.[120] The p210[bcr–abl] abrogates the anchorage requirement but not the growth factor requirement for proliferation.[121]

In normal cells exposed to IL-3, paxillin tyrosine residues are phosphorylated. In cells transformed by p210[bcr–abl], the tyrosines of paxillin, vinculin, p125FAK, talin, and tensin are constitutively phosphorylated. Pseudopodia enriched in focal adhesion proteins[122] are present in cells expressing p210[bcr–abl].

MOLECULAR PATHOLOGY

THE Ph CHROMOSOME

The genic disturbance became evident with the knowledge that CML was derived from a primitive cell that contains a 22q-abnormality.[6,11] The abnormal chromosome contained only 60 percent of the DNA in other G-group chromosomes.[123] Cytogenetic analysis indicated the G-group chromosome involved was different from the extra G-group chromosome in Down syndrome, which had been assigned number 21, and thus the former was assigned number 22—even though it proved to be slightly longer than the chromosome involved in Down syndrome.[11,124] The Paris Conference on Nomenclature decided not to undo the concept that Down syndrome is trisomy 21, and assigned the Ph chromosome and its normal counterpart, 22.[125] Rowley, by using quinacrine (Q) and Giemsa (G) banding, reported in 1973 that the material missing from chromosome 22 was not lost (deleted) from the cell but was translocated to the distal portion of the long arm of chromosome 9.[12] The amount of material translocated to chromosome 9 was approximately equivalent to that lost from 22, and it was predicted that the translocation was balanced.[12] Moreover the breaks were localized to band 34 on the long arm of 9 and band 11 on the long arm of 22. The classical Ph chromosome is, therefore, t(9;22)(q34;q11), abbreviated t(Ph) (Fig. 94-1). The Ph chromosome can develop on either the maternal or the paternal member of the pair.[126]

MUTATION OF ABL AND BCR GENES

The mutations of the *ABL* gene on chromosome 9 and the *BCR* gene on chromosome 22 are central to the development of CML (Fig. 94-2).[127-129]

In 1982 the human cellular homolog, *ABL,* of the transforming sequence of the Ableson murine leukemia virus, was localized to human chromosome number 9.[130] In 1983 *ABL* was shown to be on the segment of chromosome 9 that is translocated to chromosome 22[131] by showing reaction to hybridization probes for *ABL* only in somatic cell hybrids of human CML cells containing 22q- but not those containing 9q+. *ABL* is closely homologous to the viral oncogene *v-abl,* which is the cell-transforming portion of the gene. This gene can induce malignant transformation of cells in culture and can induce leukemia in susceptible mice.[132]

The *ABL* gene is rearranged and amplified in cell lines from patients with CML.[133] Cell lines and fresh isolates of CML cells contain an abnormal, elongated 8-kb RNA transcript,[134-137] which is transcribed

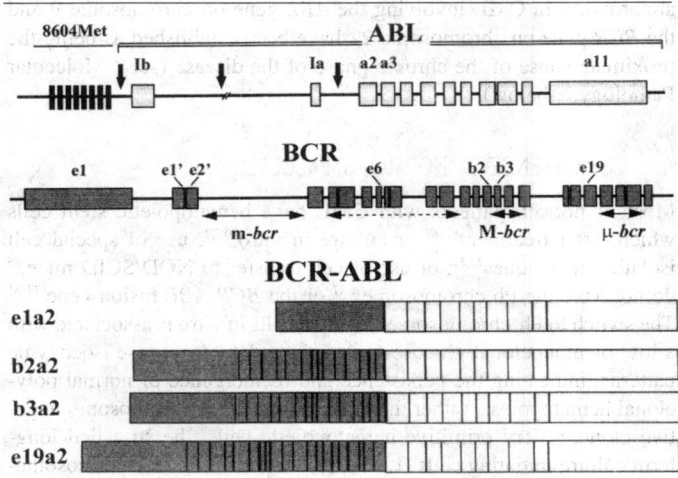

FIGURE 94-2 Schematic representation of the normal *ABL* and *BCR* genes and of the *BCR-ABL* fusion transcripts. In the upper portion of the diagram, the possible breakpoint positions in *ABL* are illustrated by vertical arrows. Note the position immediately upstream of the *ABL* locus of the *8604Met* gene, for which the function is unknown. The *BCR* gene contains 25 exons, including first (e1′) and second (e2′) exons. The position of the three breakpoint cluster regions, m-bcr, M-bcr, and μ-bcr, is shown. The lower portion of the figure shows the structure of the *BCR-ABL* messenger RNA fusion transcripts. Breakpoints in μ-bcr result in *BCR-ABL* transcripts with an e19a2 junction. *b* or *e* represents the breakpoint in *ABL*. The associated number designates the exon (location) at which the break occurs in each gene. (Reprinted with permssion from *Blood* 88:2376, 1966.)

from the new chimeric gene produced by the fusion of the 5′ portion of the *BCR* gene left on chromosome 22 with the 3′ portion of the *ABL* gene translocated from chromosome 9[131] (Fig. 94-3). The fusion mRNA leads to the translation of a unique tyrosine phosphoprotein kinase of 210 kDa (p210[bcr–abl]), which can phosphorylate tyrosine residues on cellular proteins similar to the action of the v-abl protein product.[138-142] The anomalous tyrosine kinase is difficult to identify in chronic phase cells because of inhibitors in granulocytes[142]; molecular variants reflect variations in the breakpoint on chromosome 22.[143]

The *ABL* locus contains at least two alleles, one having a 500-bp deletion.[144] In normal cells, the *ABL* protooncogene codes for a tyrosine kinase of molecular weight 145,000, which only is translated in trace quantities and lacks any in vitro kinase activity.[139] It is hypothesized that the fusion product expressed by the *BCR-ABL* gene leads to malignant transformation because of the abnormally regulated phosphorylating activity of the chimeric tyrosine protein kinase.[140,141,145,146] Construction of *BCR-ABL* fusion genes indicated that *BCR* sequences could also activate a microfilament-binding function, but the tyrosine-kinase and microfilament-binding functions were not linked. Nevertheless, the tyrosine kinase modification of actin filament function has been proposed as a step in leukemogenesis.[147]

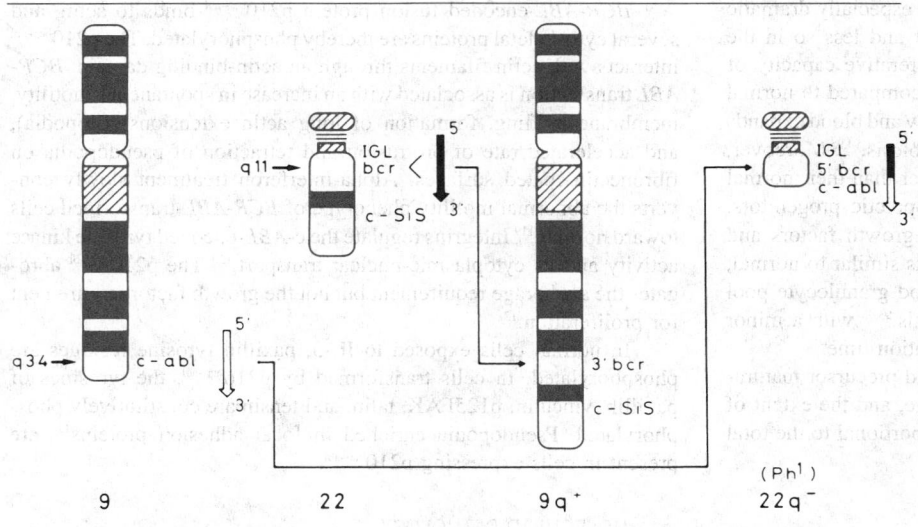

FIGURE 94-1 Schematic diagram of normal chromosome 9 showing the *ABL* gene between band q34 and qter of chromosome 22, which has the *BCR* and *SIS* genes between band q11 and qter. The t(9;22) is shown on the right. The *ABL* from chromosome 9 is transposed to the chromosome 22 M-bcr sequences, and the terminal portion of chromosome 22 is transposed to the long arm of chromosome 9. The 22q- is the Ph chromosome. bcr, breakpoint cluster region; c-sis, cellular homolog of the viral simian sarcoma virus-transforming gene; IgL, gene for immunoglobulin light chains. (Reprinted with permission from *Mutation Res* 186:161, 1987.)

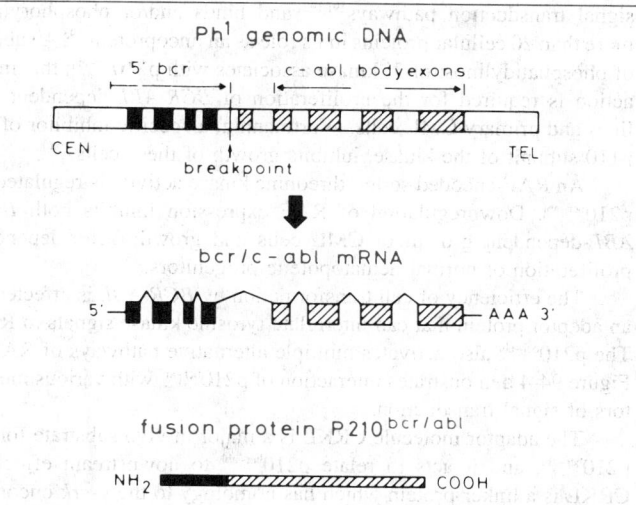

FIGURE 94-3 The molecular effects of the Ph chromosome translocation t(9;22)(q34;q11). The upper representation is of the physically joined 5' *BCR* and the 3' *ABL* regions on chromosome 22. The exons are solid (from chromosome 22, *BCR*) and hatched (from chromosome 9, *ABL*). The middle representation depicts transcription of chimeric messenger RNA, and the lower representation is the translated fusion protein with the amino terminus derived from the *BCR* of 22 and the carboxy terminus from the *ABL* of 9. (Reprinted with permission from *Mutation Res* 186:161, 1987.)

THE p210 FUSION PROTEIN

The breakpoints on chromosome 9 are not narrowly clustered, ranging from about 15 to over 40 kb upstream from the most proximate region (first exon) of the *ABL* gene.[130,131,148] The breakpoints on chromosome 22 occur over a very short, approximately 5- to 6-kb, stretch of DNA referred to as the breakpoint cluster region (M-*bcr*),[149,150] which is part of a much longer breakpoint cluster region gene, *BCR*[151,152] (Fig. 94-3). Three main breakpoint cluster regions have been characterized on chromosome 22: major (M-*bcr*), minor (m-*bcr*), and micro (μ-*bcr*). They encode a p210, p190, and p230 fusion proteins, respectively (Fig. 94-2). The overwhelming majority of CML patients have a *BCR-ABL* fusion gene that encodes a fusion protein of 210 kDa (p210[bcr-abl]) and for which mRNA transcripts have a b3a2 or a b2a2 fusion junction[153] (Fig. 94-2). A *BCR-ABL* with an e1a2 type of junction has been identified in approximately 50 percent of the Ph-chromosome-positive acute lymphoblastic leukemia cases (see "Ph-Chromosome-Positive Acute Leukemia") and results in the production of a *BCR-ABL* protein of 190 kDa (p190[bcr-abl]). Virtually all CML cases at diagnosis that encode a p210[bcr-abl] also express *BCR-ABL* transcripts for p190.[154] The biological or clinical significance of these dual transcripts is not known. Transgenic mice expressing p210[bcr-abl] develop acute lymphoblastic leukemia in the founder mice, but all transgenic progeny have a myeloproliferative disorder resembling CML.[155]

The *BCR* gene encodes a 160-kDa serine-threonine kinase, which, when it oligomerizes, autophosphorylates and transphosphorylates several protein substrates.[156] Aberrant methylation of the M-*bcr* in CML occurs.[153] The first exon sequences of the *BCR* gene potentiate the tyrosine kinase of *ABL* when they fuse as a result of the translocation.[157] The central portion of *BCR* has homology to *DBL*, a gene involved in the control of cell division after S-phase of the cell cycle. The C-terminus of *BCR* has a GTPase-activating protein for p21[rac], a member of the *RAS* family of GTP-binding proteins.[158] A reciprocal hybrid gene *ABL-BCR* is formed on chromosome 9q+, when *BCR-ABL* fuses on chromosome 22. The *ABL-BCR* fusion gene actively transcribes in most patients with CML.[159]

Variations in breakpoints involving smaller stretches of chromosome 9 and rearrangements outside the M-*bcr* of chromosome 22 can occur.[36] In a few cases of CML in which there has been no evident elongation of chromosome 9, molecular probes have shown that *ABL* is still translocated to chromosome 22.[160] In occasional patients with Ph-chromosome-positive CML, the break in chromosome 22 is outside the M-*bcr*, and there is a failure to transcribe a fusion RNA of the usual type or a fusion RNA is transcribed that does not hybridize with the classical M-*bcr* cDNA probe.[161]

In cases in which the Ph chromosome is not found, *BCR-ABL* may still be located on chromosome 9 (a masked Ph chromosome).[162] The *BCR* gene can recombine with genomically distinct sites on band 11q13 in complex translocations in a region rich in Alu repeat elements.[163] ETV6/ABL fusion genes have also been found in *BCR-ABL*-negative CML.[164]

The *BCR* breakpoint site has been examined as a factor in disease prognosis. Some studies have shown no correlation between CML chronicity and breakpoint site, although thrombocytosis may be more common with 3' breakpoint sites and basophilia with 5' breakpoint sites.[165] No difference in response to IFN-α therapy was noted, and survival was not significantly different, although patients with 3' deletions tended to have shorter survival.[166] A better response to IFN-α in patients with a 3' rearrangement has been observed by others.[167]

CML patients with m-*bcr* breakpoints develop a blast crisis with monocytosis and an absence of splenomegaly and basophilia.[168] The p230 encoded by μ-*bcr* is rarely expressed but has been associated with neutrophilic-CML or thrombocytosis (see "Special Clinical Features"). Other rare breakpoints have been described.[169] For example, a case with a 12-bp insert between BCR1 and ABL1 resulted in a *BCR-ABL*-negative (false negative), Ph-chromosome-positive CML with thrombocythemia.[170] Another novel *BCR-ABL* fusion gene (e6a2) in a patient with Ph-chromosome-negative CML encoded an oncoprotein of 185 kDa.[171] Typical CML has also been associated with an e19a2 junction *BCR-ABL* transcript.[172]

Experimental support for the hypothesis that p210[bcr-abl] tyrosine phosphoprotein kinase is transforming is provided by a retroviral gene transfer system that permits expression of the protein. Mouse marrow cells transfected with *BCR-ABL* develop clonal outgrowths of immature cells expressing the p210[bcr-abl] tyrosine kinase. Some clones progress to a malignant phenotype, can be transplanted, and can induce tumors in syngeneic mice.[173] Similar studies suggest the p210[bcr-abl] can transform 3T3 murine fibroblasts if the *gag* gene sequence from a helper virus cooperates.[174] The *BCR-ABL* gene from a retroviral vector has been expressed in an interleukin-3 (IL-3)-dependent cell line. Clones derived from the infected line transform over months to IL-3 independency; are capable of increased proliferation; and develop chromosomal abnormalities.[175]

A series of mouse models in which the *BCR-ABL* was used to induce leukemogenesis have been described.[176–184] Lethally irradiated mice have been reconstituted with marrow enriched for cycling stem cells infected with a *BCR-ABL*-bearing retrovirus. Fatal diseases with abnormal accumulations of macrophagic, erythroid, mast, and lymphoid cells develop.[175] Classical CML did not occur, and complete transformation was not documented. The cell lines from spleen and marrow from mice with a *BCR-ABL* retrovirus infection were predominantly mast cells; however, these cell lines were shown to spontaneously switch in some cases to either erythroid and megakaryocytic, erythroid, or granulocytic lineages displaying maturation. They were transplantable (transformed) and contained the same proviral inserts as the original mast cell line.[185] Murine marrow also has been infected with a retrovirus encoding p210[bcr-abl] and transplanted into irradiated syngeneic recipients.[176] Although several types of hematologic malignancies developed, a syndrome mimicking human CML occurred, also. Mice transgenic for a p190[bcr–abl] develop an acute lymphocytic leukemia-lymphoma syndrome,[177] resembling human Ph-chromosome-positive ALL. When a p210[bcr–abl] transcript is introduced into a mouse germ line (one-cell fertilized eggs), the p210 founder and progeny transgenic animals developed leukemia of B or T lymphoid or of myeloid origin after a relatively long latency period. In contrast, p190-transgenic mice exclusively developed leukemia of B-cell origin, with a relatively short period of latency. This was felt to be consistent with the apparent indolence of human CML during the chronic phase.[178] When transgenic mice express p210[bcr–abl], the transgenes develop ALL, whereas the progeny develop a myeloproliferative disorder.[179]

BCR-ABL *IN HEALTHY SUBJECTS*

BCR-ABL fusion genes can be found in the leukocytes of some normal individuals using a two-step reverse transcriptase polymerase chain reaction assay. Thus, while *BCR-ABL* may be expressed relatively frequently in hematopoietic cells, only infrequently do the cells acquire the additional changes necessary to produce leukemia.[186,187]

BCR-ABL *AND SIGNAL TRANSDUCTION*

The tyrosine phosphoprotein kinase activity of the p210[bcr–abl] has been causally linked to the development of Ph-chromosome-positive leukemia in man.[188–199] The p210[bcr–abl] interacts with several components of

signal transduction pathways[191,192] and binds and/or phosphorylates more than 20 cellular proteins in its role as an oncoprotein.[193] A subunit of phosphatidylinositol-3' kinase associates with p210[bcr–abl]; this interaction is required for the proliferation of *BCR-ABL*-dependent cell lines and primary CML cells. Wortmannin, a specific inhibitor of the p110 subunit of the kinase, inhibits growth of these cells.[194]

An RAF-encoded serine-threonine kinase activity is regulated by p210[bcr–abl]. Downregulation of RAF expression inhibits both *BCR-ABL*-dependent growth of CML cells and growth-factor-dependent proliferation of normal hematopoietic progenitors.[195]

The efficiency of cell transformation by *BCR-ABL* is affected by an adaptor protein that can interrelate tyrosine kinase signals to RAS. The p210[bcr–abl] also activates multiple alternative pathways of RAS.[196] Figure 94-4 demonstrates interaction of p210[bcr–abl] with various mediators of signal transduction.

The adaptor molecule CRKL is a major in vivo substrate for the p210[bcr–abl], and it acts to relate p210[bcr–abl] to downstream effectors. CRKL is a linker-protein which has homology to the v-*crk* oncogene product. Antibodies to CRKL immunoprecipate paxillin, a focal adhesion protein[197] which is phosphorylated by p210[bcr–abl]. The p210[bcr–abl] may be physically linked to paxillin by CRKL. CRKL binds to CBL, an oncogene product that induces B-cell and myeloid leukemias in mice.[198] The Src homology 3 domains of CRKL do not bind to CBL, but they do bind *BCR-ABL*. CRKL therefore mediates the oncogenic signal of *BCR-ABL* to CBL. The p120[CBL] and the adaptor proteins CRKL and c-CRK also link c-abl, p190[bcr–abl], and p210[bcr–abl] to the phosphatidylinositol-3' kinase (PI3K) pathway.[199] The p120[CBL] also coprecipitates with the p85 subunit of P13K, CRKL, and c-CRK. The p210[bcr–abl] may, therefore, induce the formation of multimeric complexes of signaling proteins.[200] These complexes contain paxillin and talin and may explain some of the adhesive defects of CML cells.[201]

Hef2 also binds to CRKL in leukemic tissues of p190[bcr–abl] transgenic mice. Hef2 is involved in the integrin signaling pathway[202] and encodes a protein that accelerates GTP hydrolysis of RAS-encoded proteins and neurofibromin. The latter negatively regulates GM-CSF signaling through RAS in hematopoietic cells.[203] P62dok, a constitutively tyrosine-phosphorylated, p120[ras] GAP-associated protein, which is rapidly tyrosine-phosphorylated upon activation of the c-kit receptor,[204] is also associated with ABL.[205]

NF kappa B activation is also required for p210[bcr–abl]-mediated transformation.[206] The expression of p210[bcr–abl] leads to activation of NF kappa B-dependent transcription via nuclear translocation.[207]

Cell lines that express p210[bcr–abl] also demonstrate constitutive activation of JAKs and STATs, usually STAT5.[208] STAT5 is also activated in primary mouse bone marrow cells acutely transformed by the *BCR-ABL*[209]; p210[bcr–abl] coimmunoprecipitates with and constitutively phosphorylates the common beta subunit of the IL-3 and GM-CSF receptors and JAK 2.[210] Both *ABL* and *BCR* are also multifunctional regulators of a GTP-binding protein family, Rho,[211,212] and a growth-factor-binding

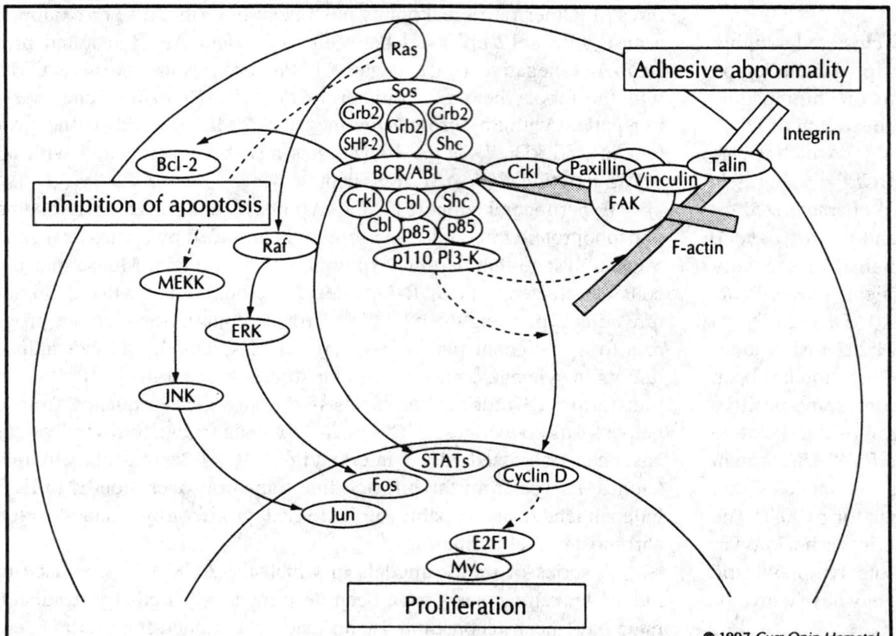

FIGURE 94-4   Major intracellular signaling events associated with *BCR/ABL*. Constitutive activation of ABL protein tyrosine kinase (PTK) induces phosphorylation of the tyrosine moiety of various substrates including autophosphorylation of *BCR/ABL* and complex formation of *BCR/ABL* with adaptor proteins. This subsequently activates multiple intracellular signaling pathways including *RAS* activation and phosphatidylinositol-3' kinase (P1-3-K) activation pathways. *BCR/ABL* also activates the c-MYC pathway, which involves *ABL*-SH2 domain. *BCR/ABL* inhibits apoptosis possibly, in part, through upregulation of Bcl-2, and alters cellular adhesive properties, possibly by interacting with focal adhesion proteins and the actin cytomatrix. *Broken lines* indicate hypothetical pathways. ERK, extracellular signal-regulated kinase; MEKK, MEK kinase; JNK, Jun N-terminal kinase; FAK, focal adhesion kinase; Sos, Son-of-sevenless; STAT, signal transducer and activator of transcription. (Reprinted with permission from *Curr Opin Hematol* 4:3, 1997.)

protein (Grb2), which links tyrosine kinases to RAS and forms a complex with *BCR-ABL* and the nucleotide exchange factor Sos that leads to activation of *RAS*.[213]

The p210[bcr-abl] also activates Jun kinase and requires Jun for transformation.[214] In some CML cells lines, p210[bcr-abl] is associated with the retinoblastoma (Rb) protein.[215] Loss of the neurofibromatosis (NF1) tumor suppressor gene, a RAS GTPase activating protein, is also sufficient to produce a myeloproliferative syndrome in mice akin to human CML due to RAS-mediated hypersensitivity to GM-CSF.[216]

EFFECTS OF BCR-ABL ON APOPTOSIS

Whether p210[bcr-abl] influences the expansion of the malignant clone in CML by inhibition of apoptosis is uncertain. In one study, the survival of normal and CML progenitors was the same after in vitro incubation in serum-deprived conditions and after treatment with x-irradiation or glucocorticoids.[217] P210[bcr-abl] has been found to inhibit apoptosis by delaying the G_2/M transition of the cell cycle after DNA damage.[218] The p210[bcr-abl] may also exert an antiapoptotic effect in factor-dependent hematopoietic cells.[219,220]

P210[bcr-abl] does not prevent apoptotic death induced by human natural killer or lymphokine-activated killer cells directed against CML or normal cells.[221] In accelerated and blast phases, rates of apoptosis were lower in CML neutrophils. G-CSF and GM-CSF considerably decreased the rate of apoptosis in CML neutrophils.[222]

THE SIS GENE

SIS, the human homolog of the transforming gene of the simian sarcoma virus,[223] is found on chromosome 22[224] and is translocated to chromosome 9 in the t(9;22)(q34;q11).[225] *SIS,* like v-*sis,*[226] encodes for a protein which is identical to platelet-derived growth factor.[227] The *SIS* gene, which is distant from the breakpoint on chromosome 22, is not expressed in chronic phase cells but can be expressed in the accelerated phase of the disease, although the transcript when expressed is normal in size (4.0 kb).[228] Activation of *SIS* is not thought to be related to the transforming events leading to the chronic phase of CML.

TELOMERASE

Some patients with CML present with normal telomere length at diagnosis, and this may be associated with response to interferon-α therapy.[229] A significant increase in telomerase activity has been noted in blast phase of CML as compared to chronic phase.[230]

CLINICAL FEATURES

EPIDEMIOLOGY

CML accounts for about 15 percent of all cases of leukemia, and the death rate from it is about 0.9 per 100,000 population per year in the United States. The disease occurs slightly more often in men than women but has similar manifestations and a similar course in both sexes. The age-specific mortality rate for CML increases with age from less than 0.1 per 100,000 population between ages 0 to 14 years to about 1 per 100,000 in the mid-40s, to over 8 per 100,000 in octogenarians.[231] Although CML occurs in children and adolescents, only about 10 percent of all cases occur in subjects between 5 and 20 years of age. CML represents about 3 percent of all childhood leukemias. There is no concordance of the disease between identical twins.

SIGNS AND SYMPTOMS

In the 70 percent of patients who are symptomatic at diagnosis, the most frequent complaints include easy fatigability, loss of sense of

well-being, decreased tolerance to exertion, anorexia, abdominal discomfort, and early satiety (related to splenic enlargement), weight loss, and excessive sweating.[232-234] The symptoms are vague, nonspecific, and gradual in onset (weeks to months). A physical examination may detect pallor and splenomegaly. The latter was present in about 90 percent of patients at diagnosis, but with medical care being sought earlier, the presence of splenomegaly is decreasing in frequency at the time of diagnosis.[233] Sternal tenderness, especially the lower portion, is common; occasionally, patients will notice it themselves.

Uncommon presenting symptoms include those of dramatic hypermetabolism (night sweats, heat intolerance, weight loss) simulating thyrotoxicosis; acute gouty arthritis, presumably related in part to hyperuricemia; priapism, tinnitus, or stupor from the leukostasis associated with greatly exaggerated blood leukocyte count elevations[235-237]; left upper quadrant and left shoulder pain as a consequence of splenic infarction and perisplenitis; vasopressin-responsive diabetes insipidus[238,239]; and acne urticata associated with hyperhistaminemia.[240] Acute febrile neutrophilic dermatosis (Sweet's syndrome), a perivascular infiltrate of neutrophils in the dermis, can occur. Fever accompanied by painful maculonodular violaceous lesions on trunk, arms, leg, and face are characteristic.[241,242] Spontaneous rupture of the spleen is a rare event.[243,244] Digital necrosis has been reported as a rare paraneoplastic event.[245,246]

In an increasing proportion of patients, the disease is discovered, coincidentally, when blood cell counts are measured at a ''routine'' medical examination.

LABORATORY FINDINGS

BLOOD

The presumptive diagnosis of CML can be made from the results of the blood cell counts and examination of the blood film.[25,232,233] The hematocrit is decreased in most patients at the time of diagnosis. Red cells are usually only slightly altered, with an increase in variation from small to large size and only occasional misshapen (elliptical or irregular) erythrocytes. Small numbers of nucleated red cells are commonly present. The reticulocyte count is normal or slightly elevated, but clinically significant hemolysis is rare.[232,247] A positive direct antiglobulin test may develop in patients during interferon therapy.[248] Rare cases of mild erythrocytosis[249,250] or erythroid aplasia[251,252] have been documented.

The total leukocyte count is always elevated at the time of diagnosis and is nearly always over 25,000/μl (25 × 10⁹/liter); half the patients have total white counts over 100,000/μl (100 × 10⁹/liter)[25,232,233] (Fig. 94-5). The total leukocyte count rises progressively in untreated patients. Rare patients may have dramatic cyclic variations in white cell counts of as much as an order of magnitude with cycle intervals of about 60 days.[253,254] Granulocytes at all stages of development are present in the blood and are generally normal in appearance. The mean blast cell prevalence is about 3 percent but can range from 0 to 10 percent; progranulocyte prevalence is about 4 percent; myelocytes, metamyelocytes, and bands account for about 40 percent; and segmented neutrophils about 35 percent of total leukocytes (Table 94-1). Hypersegmented neutrophils are commonly present (Plate XIX).

Neutrophil alkaline phosphatase activity is low or absent in over 90 percent of patients with CML.[255-257] The mRNA for alkaline phosphatase is undetectable in neutrophils of patients with CML.[258] The activity increases toward or to normal in the presence of intense inflammation or infection and when the total leukocytic count is decreased to or near normal with treatment.[257,259] CML neutrophils regain alkaline phosphatase activity after infusion into leukopenic recipients, suggesting the effect of regulators or factors extrinsic

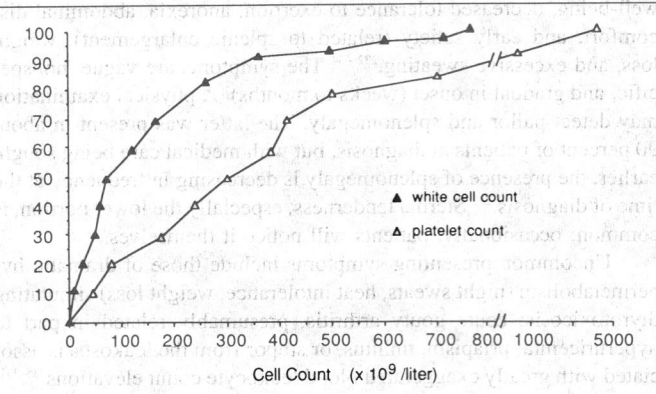

FIGURE 94-5   The total white cell count and platelet count of 90 patients with CML at the time of diagnosis. The cumulative percent of patients is on the ordinate, and the cell count is on the abscissa. Fifty percent of patients had a white cell count over 100×10^9/liter and a platelet count over about 300×10^9/liter at the time of diagnosis.

to the neutrophils.[260] In vitro, a monocyte-derived soluble mediator is capable of inducing increased alkaline phosphatase activity in neutrophils from CML patients.[261] Neutrophil alkaline phosphate is decreased sporadically in a variety of disorders and conditions[262] but is decreased markedly and consistently in paroxysmal nocturnal hemoglobinuria,[262] hypophosphatasia,[263] in about a quarter of patients with idiopathic myelofibrosis, and in patients using androgens. Neutrophil alkaline phosphatase is increased in polycythemia vera, in 25 percent of patients with idiopathic myelofibrosis, in pregnant women, and in subjects with inflammatory disorders or infections.

The proportion of eosinophils is usually not increased, but the absolute eosinophil count is nearly always increased. Rarely, eosinophils may be so prominent as to dominate the granulocytic cells and lead to the designation *Ph-positive eosinophilic CML*.[264–267] An absolute increase in the basophil concentration is present in virtually every patient, and this finding can be useful in preliminary consideration of differential diagnosis.[25,268] Basophilic progentior cells are increased in the blood.[269] The proportion of basophils is usually not above 10 to 15 percent during chronic phase but may, in rare patients,

TABLE 94-1   BLOOD WHITE CELL DIFFERENTIAL COUNT AT THE TIME OF DIAGNOSIS IN 90 CASES OF CHRONIC MYELOGENOUS LEUKEMIA

	PERCENT OF TOTAL LEUKOCYTES (MEAN VALUES)
Myeloblasts	3
Promyelocytes	4
Myelocytes	12
Metamyelocytes	7
Band forms	14
Segmented forms	38
Basophils	3
Eosinophils	2
Nucleated red cells	0.5
Monocytes	8
Lymphocytes	8

SOURCE: University of Rochester Medical Center.
NOTE: In these 90 patients, the mean hematocrit was 31 ml/dl, mean total white cell count was 160×10^9/liter, and the mean platelet count was 442×10^9/liter at the time of diagnosis.

represent 30 to 80 percent of the total leukocyte count during chronic phase and lead to the designation of Ph-chromosome-positive basophilic CML.[270] Unlike mastocytosis, hyperhistaminemia usually is not associated with elevated basophil counts. Cases of exaggerated basophilia and disabling pruritus, urticaria, and gastric hyperacidity have occurred, associated with enormous increases (several hundredfold) of blood histamine concentration.[271,272] Granulocytes containing both eosinophilic and basophilic granules are commonly present.[273]

The total absolute lymphocyte count is increased (mean about 15×10^9/liter) in patients with CML at the time of diagnosis[274] as a result of the balanced increase in T-helper and T-suppressor cells.[275] B lymphocytes are not increased.[275] T lymphocytes also are increased in the spleen.[276] Natural killer cell activity is defective in CML patients as a result of decreased maturation of these cells in vivo.[277,278] The absolute number of circulating NK cells is decreased in patients with CML. The CD56 bright subset is particularly decreased. These cells are reduced more as CML progresses, and they respond less to stimuli that recruit clonogenic natural killer cells as compared to NK cells from normal subjects.[279]

The platelet count is elevated in about 50 percent of patients at the time of diagnosis and is normal in most of the rest.[280] The platelet count may increase during the course of the chronic phase; platelet counts over 1,000,000/μl (1000×10^9/liter) are not unusual, and platelet counts as high as 5,000,000 to 7,000,000/μl (5000 to 7000×10^9/liter) have occurred. Thrombohemorrhagic complications of thrombocytosis are infrequent. Occasionally, the platelet count may be below normal at the time of diagnosis, but this usually signals an impending progression to the accelerated phase of the disease (see "Accelerated Phase of CML").

Functional abnormalities of neutrophils (adhesion, emigration, phagocytosis) are mild; are compensated for by high neutrophil concentrations; and do not predispose patients in chronic phase to infections by either usual or opportunistic organisms.[281–283] Platelet dysfunction can occur but is not associated with spontaneous or exaggerated bleeding. A decrease in the second wave of epinephrine-induced platelet aggregation is the most common abnormality and is associated with a deficiency of adenine nucleotides in the storage pool.[284,285]

MARROW

Morphology   The marrow is markedly hypercellular, and hematopoietic tissue takes up 75 to 90 percent of the marrow volume, fat being reduced markedly.[286,287] Granulopoiesis is dominant, with a granulocytic/erythroid ratio of between 10 and 30:1 rather than the normal 2 to 4:1. Erythropoiesis is usually decreased, and megakaryocytes are normal or increased in number. Eosinophils and basophils may be increased, usually in proportion to their increase in the blood. Mitotic figures are increased in number. Macrophages that mimic Gaucher cells in appearance are sometimes seen. This finding is a result of the inability of normal cellular glucocerebrosidase activity to degrade the increased glucocerebroside load associated with markedly increased cell turnover.[288] Macrophages also can become engorged with lipids, which, when oxidized and polymerized, yield ceroid pigment. This pigment imparts a granular and bluish cast to the cells after polychrome staining; such cells have been referred to as *sea-blue histiocytes*[288] (Plate IX).

Collagen type III, which takes the silver impregnation stain, is commonly increased at the time of diagnosis (reticulin fibrosis) and is strikingly increased in nearly half the patients[289] and is correlated with the proportion of megakaryocytes in the marrow.[290,291] Increased fibrosis is correlated also with larger spleen size, more severe anemia, and a higher proportion of marrow and blood blast cells.

Progenitor Cell Growth   Cells that form colonies of neutrophils and macrophages or eosinophils (CFUs) are increased in the marrow and blood. The increase in CFUs in marrow is about 20-fold normal and in blood about 500-fold normal. The CFUs are of lighter buoyant density than those in normal marrow.[94] More primitive progenitors that can initiate long-term cultures of hematopoiesis are also markedly increased.[292] Spontaneous blood-derived granulocyte-macrophage colony growth is common, although CFUs also respond to growth factor stimulation.[95]

Cytogenetics   The marrow and nucleated blood cells of over 90 percent of patients with clinical and laboratory signs that fall within the criteria for the diagnosis of CML contain the Ph chromosome, t(9;22)(q34;q11). The chromosome is present in all blood cell lineages (erythroblasts, granulocytes, monocytes, megakaryocytes, T- and B-cell progenitors) but is not present in the majority of blood B or in most T lymphocytes.[45,47] About 70 percent of patients in chronic phase have the classic Ph chromosome in their cells.[293] The remaining 20 percent have, in addition, a missing Y chromosome, t(Ph),-Y; an additional C-group chromosome, usually number 8, that is t(Ph),+8; an additional chromosome 22q-, but without the 9q+, that is t(Ph), 22q-, or t(Ph) plus either another stable translocation or another minor clone.[74] These variations have not been shown to affect the duration of the chronic phase. Deletion of the Y chromosome occurs in about 10 percent of healthy men over age 60 years.[294,295]

Variant Ph chromosome translocations occur in about 5 percent of subjects with CML and involve complex rearrangements (three chromosomes), and every chromosome except the Y chromosome can be involved.[296–300] The Ph chromosome, that is, 22q-, is present, but the gross exchange of chromosomal material involves a chromosome other than 9 (simple variant) or involves exchange of material among chromosomes 9,22, and a third or more chromosomes (complex variant) (Fig. 94-6). High-resolution techniques have indicated that 9q34-qter is transposed to 22q11 in simple as well as complex translocations.[301,302] Thus, the fusion of 9q34 with 22q11 seems to occur in the cells of most patients with CML.[303] Complex translocations involving chromosome 3 have been notable.[303–305] In rare cases, a reciprocal translocation with a chromosome other than 9 to chromosome 22 is larger than usual, and the posttranslocation shortening of the long arms of 22 is not apparent. This circumstance has been referred to as a *masked Ph chromosome* or *masked translocation,* since the 22q- is not evident by microscopic examination,[306,307] although t(9;22) may occur as judged by banding techniques or molecular probes.[308]

Molecular Probes   In a small proportion of patients with a clinical disease analogous to CML, cytogenetic studies do not disclose a classical, variant, or masked Ph chromosome. In these cases, use of a panel of restriction enzymes and Southern blotting analyses with a molecular probe for the breakpoint cluster region on chromosome 22 nearly always detects rearrangement of fragments. This finding has led to the conclusion that virtually all cases of CML have an abnormality of the long arm of chromosome number 22 (*BCR*-rearrangement).[309–313] Ph-chromosome-negative CML cells with *BCR* rearrangement can express the p210[bcr–abl], and such patients have a clinical course similar to Ph-chromosome-positive CML.[309,312–317]

The ability to identify the molecular consequences of the t(9;22), that is, *BCR* rearrangement, mRNA transcripts of the mutant fusion gene, and the p210[bcr–abl], has resulted in diagnostic tests supplementary to cytogenetic analysis.[303] These tests include Southern blot analysis

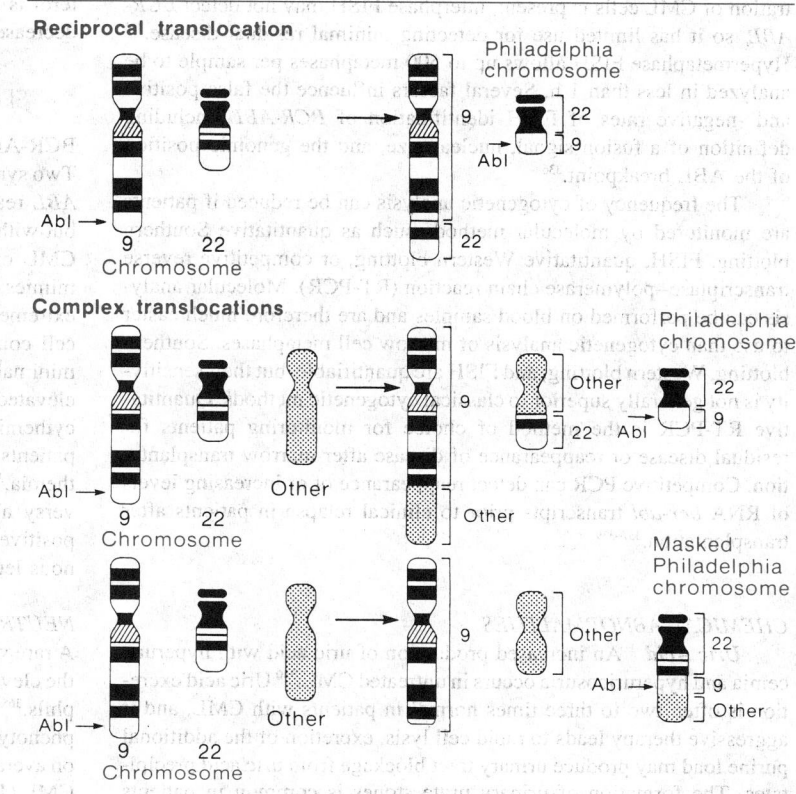

FIGURE 94-6   Translocations involved in chronic myelogenous leukemia. The positions of the *ABL* gene in each of the chromosomes before and after the translocation is noted. The origin of the chromosomal segments in each of the translocated chromosomes is indicated by a bracket on the side of the chromosome. (Reprinted with permission from Rosson D, Reddy EP: Activation of the abl oncogene and its involvement in chromosomal translocations in human leukemia. *Mutation Res* 195:231, 1988.)

of *BCR* rearrangement,[315–319] polymerase chain reaction (PCR) amplification of the abnormal mRNA,[320] and a less complex variation on the latter, a hybridization protection assay.[321]

Southern blot of the DNA extracted from samples of blood cells should be correlated with marrow cytogenetic analysis; some occasional discordant cases in which Southern blot analysis does not detect *BCR* gene rearrangement but the marrow cells have Ph-chromosome-positive metaphases can occur. Thus, marrow cytogenetic analysis should be performed if patients achieve a complete disappearance of *BCR*-rearranged cells by Southern blot to avoid overestimating the degree of response.[322]

The PCR can achieve a sensitivity of 1 positive cell in about 500,000 to 1 million cells. This extreme sensitivity requires special care in analysis and the inclusion of negative controls.[323–326]

Immunodiagnosis of CML by identification of the p210[bcr–abl] is possible, also. This tumor-specific protein for CML is unique, based on the amino acids at the junction between the *ABL* and *BCR* sequences. Oligopeptides corresponding to the junctional amino acids have been synthesized and used as antigens[327–330] to develop specific antibodies to the p210[bcr–abl]. A multicolor fluorescence in situ hybridization (FISH) method to detect the *BCR-ABL* fusion in patients with CML is a rapid and sensitive alternative to Southern blot and PCR-dependent methods.[331] For diagnostic purposes, FISH appears to be simple, accurate, and sensitive and can detect the various molecular fusions (e.g., b2a2, b3a2, e1a2).[332–334,834] Interphase FISH is faster and more sensitive than cytogenetics to identify the Ph chromosome. If a very low concentration of CML cells is present, interphase FISH may not detect *BCR-ABL*, so it has limited use for detecting minimal residual disease.[335] Hypermetaphase FISH allows up to 500 metaphases per sample to be analyzed in less than 1 h. Several factors influence the false-positive and -negative rates of FISH identification of *BCR-ABL*, including definition of a fusion signal, nuclear size, and the genomic position of the ABL breakpoint.[336]

The frequency of cytogenetic analysis can be reduced if patients are monitored by molecular methods such as quantitative Southern blotting, FISH, quantitative Western blotting, or competitive reverse transcriptase–polymerase chain reaction (RT-PCR). Molecular analysis can be performed on blood samples and are therefore much easier to use than cytogenetic analysis of marrow cell metaphases. Southern blotting, Western blotting, and FISH are quantifiable, but their sensitivity is not generally superior to classical cytogenetic methods. Quantitative RT-PCR is the method of choice for monitoring patients for residual disease or reappearance of disease after marrow transplantation. Competitive PCR can detect reappearance of or increasing levels of RNA *bcr-abl* transcripts prior to clinical relapse in patients after transplantation.[337-339]

CHEMICAL ABNORMALITIES

Uric Acid An increased production of uric acid with hyperuricemia and hyperuricosuria occurs in untreated CML.[340] Uric acid excretion is often two to three times normal in patients with CML, and if aggressive therapy leads to rapid cell lysis, excretion of the additional purine load may produce urinary tract blockage from uric acid precipitates. The formation of urinary urate stones is common in patients with CML, and some with latent gout may develop acute gouty arthritis or uric acid nephropathy.[341] The likelihood of complications from urate overproduction is greatly increased by starvation, acidosis, renal disease, or diuretic drug therapy.

Serum Vitamin B₁₂-Binding Proteins and Vitamin B₁₂ Neutrophils contain vitamin B_{12}-binding proteins, including transcobalamin I and III (syn: R-type B_{12}-binding protein or cobalophilin).[342-345] Patients with myeloproliferative diseases have an increased serum level of B_{12}-binding capacity, and the source of the protein is principally mature neutrophilic granulocytes.[342,343] The increase in transcobalamin level and the resultant increase in vitamin B_{12} concentration are particularly notable in CML, although any increase in the number of neutrophilic granulocytes such as in leukemoid reactions can be accompanied by an increase in serum B_{12}-binding protein levels and vitamin B_{12} concentration.[345] The serum B_{12} level in CML patients is increased on the average to over 10 times normal.[346] The increase is proportional to the total leukocyte count in untreated patients and falls toward normal levels with treatment, although increased B_{12} levels commonly persist even after the white cell count is lowered to near normal with therapy.

Rarely pernicious anemia and CML may coexist. In this situation the tissues are vitamin B_{12} deficient, but the serum vitamin B_{12} level may be normal because of the elevation in the level of transcobalamin I, a binder with a very high affinity for vitamin B_{12}.[346]

Serum Lactic Dehydrogenase, Potassium, Calcium, Cholesterol The level of serum lactic dehydrogenase (LDH) is elevated in CML.[347] Pseudohyperkalemia due to the release of potassium from white cells during clotting[348] and spurious hypoxemia or pseudohypoglycemia from in vitro utilization of oxygen or glucose by granulocytes can occur. Hypercalcemia[349] or hypokalemia[350] has occurred during the chronic phase of the disease, but such complications are very rare until the disorder transforms to acute leukemia. Elevations in serum and urinary lysozyme levels are features of leukemia with greater monocytic components and are not features of CML.[351] Serum cholesterol is decreased in patients with CML,[352,353] and the severity of the decrease is correlated with shortened duration of patient survival.[353]

SPECIAL CLINICAL FEATURES

BCR-ABL *POSITIVE THROMBOCYTHEMIA*

Two syndromes, thrombocythemia with the Ph chromosome and *BCR-ABL* rearrangement or thrombocythemia without a Ph chromosome but with the *BCR-ABL* rearrangement may precede the overt signs of CML or its accelerated phase.[354-360] In general, the disease closely mimics classical thrombocythemia initially; marked platelet elevation, extreme megakaryocytic hyperplasia, normal or mildly elevated white cell count, no or very slight myeloid immaturity in the blood, and minimal anemia. In some cases, the absolute basophil count is mildly elevated. About 5 percent of patients with apparent essential thrombocythemia have a Ph chromosome,[356] and about 5 to 7 percent of CML patients present with a classical picture of essential thrombocythemia.[357,358] Evolution to blast crisis may occur.[355,361,362] There is controversy about the frequency of Ph-chromosome-negative, *BCR-ABL*-positive thrombocythemia and its relationship to chronic myelogenous leukemia.[363,364]

NEUTROPHILIC-CHRONIC MYELOGENOUS LEUKEMIA

A rare variant of *BCR-ABL*-positive CML has been described in which the elevated white cell count is composed principally of mature neutrophils.[365,366] Too few cases have been described to be certain of its other phenotypic distinctions, but the white cell count appears to be lower on average (30 to 50,000/μl) at the time of diagnosis than with classical CML (100 to 200,000/μl). Moreover, patients with neutrophilic CML usually do not have basophilia, notable myeloid immaturity in the blood, prominent splenomegaly, or low leukocyte alkaline phosphatase scores. These patients' cells have the Ph chromosome but have an unusual *BCR-ABL* fusion gene in that the breakpoint in the *BCR* gene is between exons 19 and 20 resulting in most of the *BCR* gene fusing with *ABL*, which results in a larger fusion protein (230 kDa) as compared to the fusion protein in classical CML (210 kDa) (Fig. 94-2). This correlation between genotype and phenotype was not observed in all cases.[367]

MINOR-BCR-BREAKPOINT-POSITIVE CML

A very small number of patients with Ph-chromosome-positive myeloproliferative disease have had the breakpoint on the *BCR* gene in the first intron (m-*bcr*) resulting in a 190-kDa fusion protein instead of the classical 210-kDa protein observed in patients with CML (Fig. 94-2). The m-*bcr* molecular lesion is similar to that observed in about 60 percent of patients with *BCR* rearrangement-positive ALL. In patients with m-*bcr* CML, monocytes are more prominent, the white cell count lower on average, and basophilia and splenomegaly less prominent than in disease with classical *BCR* breakpoint (M-*bcr*). The few cases reported have had a short interval before either myeloid or lymphoid blast transformation has developed.[368]

HYPERLEUKOCYTOSIS

About 15 percent of patients present with symptoms or signs referable to leukostasis as a result of the intravascular flow-impeding effects of white cell counts over 300,000/μl (300 × 10⁹/liter).[235] Hyperleukocytosis is more prevalent in children with Ph-chromosome-positive CML.[236] The effects of total leukocyte counts from 300,000 to 800,000/μl (300 to 800 × 10⁹/liter) include impairment of the circulation of the lung, central nervous system, special sensory organs, and penis, resulting in some combination of tachypnea, dyspnea, cyanosis, dizziness, slurred speech, delirium, stupor, visual blurring, diplopia, retinal vein distention, retinal hemorrhages, papilledema, tinnitus, impaired hearing, or priapism.[237] Such symptoms or signs usually respond to the rapid decrease in white cell count by a combination of leukapheresis and hydroxyurea therapy.

CONCURRENCE OF LYMPHOID MALIGNANCIES

CML has an association with lymphoproliferation that can take four principal forms: (1) Patients may develop CML years after irradiation treatment of lymphoma or Hodgkin disease; (2) about one-third of CML patients enter the accelerated phase of the disease by evolution and dedifferentiation of the CML clone into one that supports lymphoblastic proliferation (acute lymphoblastic transformation); (3) patients may have concurrent lymphoproliferative or plasmacytic malignancies and CML. Lymphoma or lymphoblastic leukemia,[369–373] essential monoclonal gammopathy,[374,375] myeloma,[376,377,838] or Waldenström macroglobulinemia[378] have occurred in association with CML. Several cases have been reported of CML emerging in patients with established chronic lymphocytic leukemia (CLL).[379,380] A few patients have presented with both diseases occurring simultaneously.[365,366] A single case has been reported of lymphocytic leukemoid reaction simulating CLL which regressed as CML emerged.[367] In some cases, the CLL lymphocytes have not contained the Ph chromosome, whereas the CML cells did, suggesting the presence of two independent clonal disorders,[379–381] and in other cases the Ph chromosome was present in the myeloid and lymphoid cells indicating a common origin.[382] (4) Patients may present with Ph-chromosome-positive acute lymphoblastic leukemia and, following chemotherapy-induced remission, develop the features of typical CML.[383]

DIFFERENTIAL DIAGNOSIS

DISEASES MIMICKING CML

The diagnosis of CML is made on the basis of the characteristic granulocytosis, white cell differential count, increased absolute basophil count, and splenomegaly coupled with the presence of the Ph chromosome or its variants (greater than 95 percent of patients) or a BCR rearrangement on chromosome 22 (greater than 99 percent of patients).

Patients with other chronic hematopoietic stem cell diseases such as polycythemia vera, primary thrombocythemia, or idiopathic myelofibrosis only occasionally have closely overlapping features. For example, the total white cell count is above 30×10^9/liter in over 90 percent of patients with CML and increases inexorably over weeks or months of observation, whereas it is below 30×10^9/liter in over 90 percent of patients with the three other classical chronic hematopoietic stem cell diseases and usually does not change significantly over months to years. Polycythemia vera is associated with an increase in red cell mass and hematocrit and displays clinical signs of plethora; CML does not have these features. Patients with idiopathic myelofibrosis invariably have marked teardrop poikilocytes and other severe red cell shape, size, and chromicity changes and prominent nucleated red cells in the blood; CML rarely has these features. Patients with primary thrombocythemia have a platelet count over $750,000/\mu l$ (750×10^9/liter) and usually only mild neutrophilia, the latter white cell findings distinguishing it from the small proportion (10 percent) of CML patients with platelet counts over $750,000/\mu l$ (750×10^9/liter) at the time of diagnosis. In addition, patients with the clinical features of polycythemia vera or idiopathic myelofibrosis do not have the Ph chromosome or BCR rearrangement in their blood and marrow cells, except in extremely rare cases. The case of essential thrombocythemia is more complex (see previous section). Increasing awareness of the features of related disorders such as chronic myelomonocytic leukemia and an appreciation that elderly patients are prone to atypical stem

cell diseases have minimized the inappropriate diagnosis of Ph-chromosome-negative CML, which should be avoided unless the clinical features are characteristic of classical CML and a masked Ph chromosome or BCR rearrangement is found. If neutrophil alkaline phosphatase reactivity is normal or elevated and the clinical features are atypical, the diagnosis of CML is unlikely; however, the test is too insensitive and nonspecific to be the deciding factor in the diagnosis.

Reactive leukocytosis can occur with absolute neutrophil counts of 30 to $100,000/\mu l$ (30 to 100×10^9/liter). Usually these leukemoid reactions occur in the setting of an overt inflammatory disease, cancer, or infection. If the incitant is not apparent, the absence of granulocytic immaturity, basophilia, splenomegaly, and decreased neutrophil alkaline phosphatase activity would argue against CML. The absence of a cytogenetic or molecular abnormality in chromosome 22 would virtually eliminate classical CML as a consideration.

The precise diagnosis of CML is of help in estimating prognosis for the patient, the choice of drugs for treatment, and the timing of special therapies, such as stem cell transplantation.

PH-CHROMOSOME-POSITIVE CHRONIC HEMATOPOIETIC STEM CELL DISEASES

The Ph chromosome has been found rarely in patients with apparent polycythemia vera,[26,384] polycythemia vera that later evolves into Ph-chromosome-positive CML,[385–387] idiopathic myelofibrosis,[265,388,389] or a myelodysplastic syndrome.[390,391] Molecular studies to determine the presence of the BCR-ABL were not performed in cases reported before 1985. Primary (essential) thrombocythemia with a Ph chromosome and/or BCR-ABL rearrangement is discussed above in "Special Clinical Features."

THERAPY

GENERAL CONSIDERATIONS

Hyperuricemia and hyperuricosuria are frequent features of CML at diagnosis or in relapse.[392] Treatment of hyperuricemia is a function of the elevation of the pretreatment serum uric acid concentration, the blood white cell concentration, spleen size, and the dose of chemotherapy planned. If these variables suggest a high risk for a significant amount of cell lysis. Allopurinol, 300 mg per day, orally, and adequate hydration to maintain a good urine flow should be instituted prior to chemotherapy. If hyperuricemia is extreme, alkalinization of urine can be achieved with sodium bicarbonate . Allopurinol is associated with a high frequency of allergic skin reactions and should be discontinued after the blood leukocyte count and spleen size are decreased and the risk of exaggerated cell lysis has passed.

Treatment of chronic myelogenous leukemia is evolving as new drugs and drug combinations are being applied in clinical trials.[393] A current approach for patients under age 60 years is shown in Fig. 94-7. While progress has been made in the treatment of CML, even in the era of IFN-α and new transplantation strategies, most people die of the disease. Only a small fraction of patients are suitable for allogeneic stem cell transplantation, and only a small fraction have a complete cytogenetic response with IFN-α.

INITIAL CYTOREDUCTION THERAPY

IFN-α is utilized in virtually all patients less than 60 years of age, most patients between 60 and 70, and some patients in older age groups, even in circumstances in which minimal white cell elevation is present. In cases in which the white cell count is markedly elevated, hydroxyurea is used prior to IFN-α. If rapid cytoreduction is required

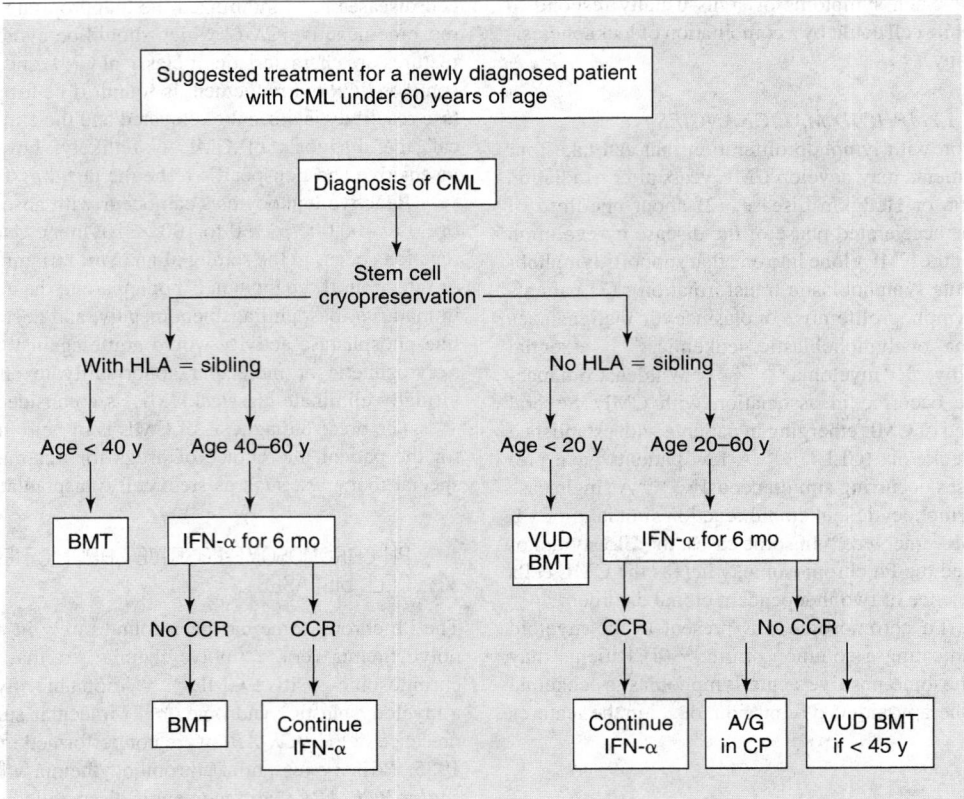

FIGURE 94-7   Treatment for a newly diagnosed patient with CML under 60 years of age. It is suggested that patients under 40 years of age with HLA-identical siblings should be treated by allografting soon after diagnosis; those aged 40 to 60 years should receive a trial of IFN-α, and stem cell transplantation should be delayed if they achieve a complete cytogenetic response (CCR). All patients with an HLA-identical sibling should receive a trial of IFN-α. Complete responders should continue on IFN-α. Those who fail to achieve CCR should be considered for treatment by allografting with an alternative donor, usually a volunteer unrelated donor (VUD), or by autografting (A/G) while still in chronic phase (CP). Some centers delay stem cell cryopreservation for those patients already treated with IFN-α rather than preserving stem cells at diagnosis. These guidelines cannot be applied without individual consideration of each patient's circumstances. (Reprinted with permission from *Clin Haematol* 10:405, 1997.)

because of signs of the hyperleukocytic syndrome, leukapheresis and hydroxyurea are often combined.

LEUKAPHERESIS

Leukapheresis can control CML only temporarily. For this reason, it is useful in two types of patient: the hyperleukocytic patient in whom rapid cytoreduction can reverse symptoms and signs of leukostasis (e.g., stupor, tinnitus, papilledema, priapism)[236,237] and the pregnant patient with CML who can be controlled by leukapheresis treatment without chemotherapy either during the early months of pregnancy when chemotherapy poses a higher risk to the fetus or, in some cases, throughout the pregnancy.[394,395] Because of the large body burden of leukocytes in marrow, blood, and spleen, and the high proliferative rate in CML, the leukocyte reduction by apheresis is less efficient than in other types of leukemias.[237] Leukapheresis reduces the burden of tumor cells subject to chemotherapeutically induced cytolysis and thus the production and the excretion of uric acid. In hyperleukocytic nonpregnant patients, leukapheresis is best used in conjunction with hydroxyurea to ensure rapid and optimal reduction in white cell count.

HYDROXYUREA

Hydroxyurea now is preferred to busulfan for the control of white cell elevation. It is less toxic, may sustain the chronic phase of CML

for a longer time, and may permit greater success with stem cell transplantation. Hydroxyurea 1 to 6 g per day, orally, depending on the height of the white cell count, can be used to initiate elective therapy.[396] Urgent treatment of extraordinary total white cell counts may require higher doses. The dose of hydroxyurea should be decreased as the total white cell count decreases and is usually given at 1 to 2 g per day when the total white cell count reaches 20,000/μl (20 × 10⁹/liter). Thereafter, dosing should be adjusted individually to keep the white count between 5000 to 15,000/μl (5–15 × 10⁹/liter). Initially, blood cell counts should be obtained 2 to 3 times per week, decreased to every 2 to 6 weeks depending on their stability, but eventually, if stable, may only be required every 2 or 3 months. Patients require chronic administration of hydroxyurea to control the chronic phase of CML usually at a dose of about 0.5 to 2.0 g per day, orally. The drug should be temporarily discontinued if the white cell count drops below 5000/μl (5 × 10⁹/liter). If hydroxyurea is being used in combination with IFN-α, it is usually tapered and discontinued once a hematologic response to IFN-α is observed.

The major side effect of hydroxyurea is an extension of its pharmacological effect, that is, reversible suppression of hematopoiesis, often with megaloblastic erythropoiesis. The median survival of patients with CML treated with hydroxyurea alone is about 5 years (Table 94-2). Studies with high-dose hydroxyurea indicate that marrow

TABLE 94-2 SURVIVAL OF PATIENTS WITH CHRONIC MYELOGENOUS LEUKEMIA

	No. of Patients		Significant Cytogenic Response, %		Median Survival, months		5-Year Survival, %	
	IFN	Chemo	IFN	Chemo	IFN	Chemo	IFN	Chemo
Germany, 1993[440]*		187(a)	—	—	—	58	—	48
		184(b)				45		28
United States, 1995[398]†	274	—	38	—	89	—	63	—
Germany, 1997[436]	133	194	10	2	66	56	59	44
United Kingdom, 1995[401]	293	294	11	3	63	43	52	34
Japan, 1998[402]‡	80	79	16	5	71	55	58	32
Benelux, 1998[435]	100	95	16	2	64	68	55	55
Italy, 1998[403]¶	218	104	28	0	104	64	56	43

Significant cytogenetic response is 66 to 100 percent Ph-chromosome-negative metaphases.
*A prospective, randomized trial of hydroxyurea (a) compared to busulfan (b).
†The results of treatment of patients with interferon-α.
‡Seven-year survival was 36 percent for IFN-α and 23 percent for chemotherapy treatment.
¶Ten-year survival was 47 percent for IFN-α and 30 percent for chemotherapy treatment.

metaphase cells in some patients lose the Ph chromosome either partially or completely after such therapy.[397] The drug may be very useful in patients at advanced ages, with comorbid conditions, or other factors that limit their tolerance to IFN therapy.

INTERFERON

Treatment with IFN-α offers a survival advantage as compared to treatment with hydroxyurea or busulfan alone[398–403] (Table 94-2). IFN-α has a very slowly progressive effect, and patients may require hydroxyurea and/or leukapheresis therapy during the first week or two of IFN-α therapy.

Initiation of Treatment Several guidelines for the use of IFN-α in CML have been published.[393,404] While some study groups have reported that doses of 3×10^6 units/m^2 injected subcutaneously per day are as effective as higher doses (e.g., 5×10^6 units/m^2 per day),[399–405] some groups have found that patients receiving 5×10^6 units/m^2 per day have the greatest incidence of cytogenetic remission.[406] A hematologic response has been observed in up to 80 percent of patients, partial disappearance of Ph-chromosome-positive cells (<35 percent of cells) in 50 percent of patients, and nearly complete cytogenetic responses (<5 percent of cells) in 15 percent of patients, regardless of the patient's age.[407]

IFN-α can be started at a dose of 3 million units/day subcutaneously in the evening on a Monday, Wednesday, Friday schedule and then escalated after 1 week to 5 million units/day, three times per week. If symptoms allow, the dose can then be increased to 5 million units/m^2, three times per week, for 1 week and then to 5×10^6 units/m^2 per day. Doses can be adjusted based on white cell and platelet counts. Hydroxyurea may be used to control the white cell count during any phase of interferon therapy. Hydroxyurea should be adjusted to maintain a white cell count of 5000 to 10,000/μl and generally is discontinued when the white cell count is less than 5000/μl. Greater leukopenia requires reduction or cessation of the interferon dose. Platelet count depressions below 50,000/μl require a decrease in the dose or the frequency of dosing, or even temporary discontinuation of interferon.

Maintenance Therapy IFN-α is usually required continuously, although many patients can be maintained in a hematologic remission with one to two doses of 3 to 5×10^6 units/m^2 per week. A complete hematologic response within 3 months of initiation of IFN-α is associated with the highest likelihood of a complete cytogenetic response.[408] Polyclonal hematopoiesis has been demonstrated after IFN-α induced cytogenetic remission.[409] The greater the decrease in Ph-chromosome-positive cells, the greater the duration of survival, but long-term control

of disease by IFN-α occurs only in a minority of patients.[410] Rare sustained remissions in which the blood cells do not have *BCR* rearrangment after cessation of treatment do occur.[411] After 6 months of therapy, patients with a partial hematologic response or resistant disease are very unlikely (<10 percent) to achieve a later major cytogenetic response.[405] Two studies have shown no advantage of IFN-α use compared to hydroxyurea in survival from diagnosis,[435,436] but the dose intensity of either IFN-α or hydroxyurea as well as the difference in the compositions of patient populations may contribute to these different results. Meta-analysis of randomized trials comparing IFN-α to other therapies, however, have shown a survival advantage for those treated with IFN-α[400] (Table 94-2). However, the most efficacious dose of IFN-α; the benefit, if any, of continuing it in patients who have no cytogenetic response; the timing of its use in relationship to allogeneic stem cell transplantation; and its use in combination with other agents all remain to be determined.[393]

Mechanism of Action IFN-α's beneficial effect in CML may relate to a direct inhibition of DNA polymerase activity.[412] Expression of interferon regulatory factor (IRF) genes, specifically a high ratio of IRF-1 to IRF-2, may be associated with a good cytogenetic and molecular response.[413] IFN-α has also been found to affect Fas-mediated apoptosis in CML.[414] The response to IFN-α is correlated with transcript numbers of *BCR-ABL*.[415,840] In CML patients who demonstrate a long-term response to IFN-α, a specific immune response directed against p210$^{bcr-abl}$ occurs.[416] The progressive methylation of the *ABL* promoter correlates inversely with a response to IFN-α.[417] The site of M-*bcr* rearrangement has been reported to be predictive for the response to IFN-α with 5′ breakpoints responding more favorably,[418] but others have not found a significant difference in the breakpoint locus and the time to transformation.[419]

Monitoring Response Hypermetaphase FISH on blood films to detect the frequency of Ph-chromosome-positive cells during IFN-α treatment permits assessment of the response.[420,421] Patients with IFN-α who maintain long-term complete cytogenetic responses may remain positive by RT-PCR for mRNA$^{bcr-abl}$, indicating that the disease is not eradicated.[422] The number of mRNA$^{bcr-abl}$ transcripts that persist in patients treated with IFN-α who achieve a complete cytogenetic remission (no Ph-chromosome-positive cells) has been found to vary by as much as four orders of magnitude.[423] When quantitative PCR has been used to monitor residual disease in CML during treatment with IFN-α, detection of elevated transcripts may precede signs of hematologic or cytogenetic disease progression by up to 8 months.[424] The *BCR-ABL* can persist as judged by FISH despite negative or very weakly positive levels measured by quantitative RT-PCR. This discordance may be explained by persistence of nonproliferating affected cells that do not express the transcripts.[842]

Toxic Effects   IFN-α requires subcutaneous administration. Its early side effects may include fever, fatigue, sweating, anorexia, headache, muscle pain, nausea, and bone pain. These occur in about 50 percent of patients. Later effects include apathy; agitation; insomnia; depression; bone pain; muscle pain; hepatic, renal, or cardiac dysfunction; immune-hemolytic anemia; thrombocytopenia; and hypothyroidism.[425] Elevation of liver enzymes is frequent, and hypertriglyceridemia is nearly universal. Toxicities may necessitate dose reduction or discontinuation of IFN-α. The acute side effects, however, can be minimized by evening doses and premedication with acetaminophen and/or diphenhydramine.

IFN-γ is less active than IFN-α in CML,[426] but combinations of the interferons may decrease the total dose required and increase the response rate.[427] Patients who do not respond to IFN-α may respond to hydroxyurea or busulfan. Development of neutralizing anti-interferon antibodies can occur during treatment.[428] Some patients with antibodies who are resistant to recombinant IFN-α respond to lymphoblastoid IFN-α.[429]

The effect of IFN-α use in patients with marrow fibrosis is controversial. Some reports indicate that it may prevent fibrosis in those responding to treatment,[430] whereas others have found that it may speed progression of marrow fibrosis.[431]

Prolonged administration of IFN-α may adversely affect allogeneic stem cell transplantation outcomes.[432] Higher rates of graft failure and posttransplant infections were found in patients pretreated with IFN-α, although there was no influence on GVH disease or relapse rate. Prolonged IFN-α treatment may also adversely affect matched, unrelated donor transplant outcomes.[433] IFN-α can induce cytogenetic remission in patients with cytogenetic relapse following stem cell transplantation.[434]

USE OF OTHER CHEMOTHERAPEUTIC AGENTS IN CHRONIC PHASE

Cytarabine   Daily infusion of low-dose cytarabine (15–30 mg/m^2 per day) to outpatients by a portable pump has resulted in control of the disease and a partial decrease or complete absence of metaphase cells containing the Ph chromosome.[437] Combinations of hydroxyurea, interferon-α, and cytarabine also are being studied.[438] For example, IFN-α2b combined with cytarabine (20mg/m^2 for 10 days each month) in chronic phase was associated with a greater proportion of major cytogenetic response at 12 months after randomization and with greater survival prolongation than was IFN-α alone.[439]

Busulfan   Once the mainstay of treatment for the chronic phase, use of busulfan largely has been replaced by IFN-α and/or hydroxyurea.[440] It is used primarily as part of the preparative regimen for allografting or autografting. Busulfan in doses of 4 to 6 mg per day orally can be used until the white cell count falls to about 30,000/μl (30 $\times$ 10^9/liter). After stopping the drug, the effect persists for days to weeks, and a further decrease usually occurs toward or to normal levels. Some patients may get a sustained effect and not require further treatment immediately. After reaching its nadir, the total leukocyte count will increase in most patients and require maintenance therapy, which can be as little as 2 mg twice a week, orally. The drug leads to a decrease in the white cell count, decrease in spleen size, increase in the hematocrit, and a restoration of a sense of well-being in about 95 percent of patients treated in the chronic phase. Periodic blood cell counts should be obtained to follow the response of the patient to the drug, and intervals between counts should not extend beyond 4 to 6 weeks in apparently stabilized patients and should be more frequent in unstable patients.

Control of the disease with busulfan does not usually induce disappearance of the Ph chromosome. The intensity of therapy is not sufficient to cause suppression of the abnormal clone. The objective of busulfan therapy has been to control the chronic phase of the disease and eliminate or minimize its morbidity.[440]

The chronic use of the drug has been associated with a syndrome that simulates adrenal insufficiency manifested by skin pigmentation, weakness, fever, and diarrhea[441,442] or with pulmonary fibrosis.[443] Prolonged aplasia of the marrow can occur with busulfan[444] and in one large series was a cause of death in patients. In some patients who survive aplasia induced by busulfan, prolonged remissions may occur along with disappearance of the Ph chromosome.[445]

Homoharringtonine   Homoharringtonine, a plant alkaloid, has been reported to induce responses, including cytogenetic responses, in patients in late chronic phase.[446] Homoharringtonine has also been utilized in combination with IFN-α and cytosine arabinoside.[447]

Other Cytotoxic Agents   The nucleoside analogs, deoxycoformycin and fludarabine do not have a significant effect in chronic phase CML.[448]

Several other chemotherapeutic agents can control the chronic phase of the disease, notably dibromomannitol.[449] Although a wide variety of other agents have been used including melphalan, cyclophosphamide, 6-mercaptopurine, 6-thioguanine, demecolcine, and uracil mustard, they are largely inferior to hydroxyurea in the proportion of patients who respond well to them.[450]

Intensive multidrug regimens have been used to study whether such an approach can eradicate the Ph-chromosome-positive clone and lead to prolongation of remission or cure of the disease. This approach has not significantly increased survival.[451]

Vitamin A has been reported to have benefit when used in conjunction with busulfan.[452] All *trans*-retinoic acid and 13 *cis*-retinoic acid may also play a role in management.[453–455]

Anagrelide   Anagrelide has been utilized to treat markedly elevated platelet counts in CML, especially where thrombosis or bleeding is present. This agent acts directly to decrease megakaryocyte mass, and it can lead to a precipitous fall in platelet counts.[456]

ANTISENSE OLIGODEOXYNUCLEOTIDES

Gene target-selective destruction of cells containing the *BCR-ABL* fusion gene is a theoretical possibility and has been studied in vitro. This approach to therapy is highly specific, but several important issues remain to be resolved regarding delivery of these agents in vivo.[457,821,836,837]

ANTI–TYROSINE KINASE DRUGS

The p210 product of the *BCR-ABL* oncogene is a protein phosphokinase and is the principal oncogenic factor in the onset of CML. Drugs that act to prevent the action of this protein kinase are under study and have reached the stage of clinical trials. The experimental agent, referred to as *STI 571* is administered daily by mouth. If its therapeutic effects are sufficiently dramatic and sustained and are not countered by exaggerated toxicity, it looms as a new primary mode of therapy for patients in the chronic phase.[820,821,835] The drug or its congeners could interrupt the leukemic process and result in reestablishment of polyclonal, normal hematopoiesis.

RADIOTHERAPY

Splenic irradiation may be useful occasionally in subjects who have entered accelerated or advanced chronic phase and are troubled with extreme splenomegaly with splenic pain, perisplenitis, and encroachment of the spleen on the gastrointestinal tract.[458] The result of splenic irradiation is usually short-lived.

Radiotherapy may be useful for extramedullary tumors, which may occur occasionally in bone or soft tissue during the chronic phase.

SPLENECTOMY

Splenectomy does not prolong the chronic phase of CML, delay the onset of the accelerated phase, enhance sensitivity to standard or intensive chemotherapy, or prolong survival of patients.[459] In carefully selected patients with symptomatic thrombocytopenia unresponsive to chemotherapy and a greatly enlarged spleen, splenectomy may be useful. Postoperative morbidity from infection, thrombosis, or hemorrhage has been high. Splenectomy does not decrease recurrence of disease after therapy. Splenectomy has not been found to influence the severity of GVH disease or survival after allogeneic stem cell transplantation.[460]

HIGH-DOSE CHEMOTHERAPY WITH AUTOLOGOUS STEM CELL INFUSION

Ph-chromosome-negative stem cells are present in most patients with CML at the time of diagnosis. Techniques to use these cells to reconstitute hematopoiesis after high-dose therapy have been developed.[461] Ph-chromosome-negative progenitors can be mobilized with G-CSF and collected from the blood in patients who have responded to prior treatment with IFN-α.[462] Such cells can also be collected after recovery from chemotherapy regimens, such as after idarubicin and cytarabine, followed by G-CSF stimulation.[461,463] BCR-ABL-negative primitive myeloid cells can be selected for autografting early in chronic phase.[464] Patients autografted with Ph-chromosome-negative progenitors after myeloablative conditioning regimens may have long-term remissions in some cases.[465,466] There is as yet no evidence that this approach prolongs survival.[467]

In addition to positive selection of Ph-chromosome-negative progenitors, based on their lack of HLA-DR expression,[463] negative selection by purging of BCR-ABL-positive progenitors in vitro can be used. These approaches have included treatment of cell suspensions with either IFN-α, specific T-cell subsets, natural killer cells,[468,469] antisense oligonucleotides,[470] ribozymes,[471] various inhibitors of signal transduction pathways, such as genistein,[472] or an inhibitor of the ABL tyrosine kinase.[473] In vitro culture of CML marrow favors outgrowth of normal progenitors and offers a means of depleting leukemic progenitors.[474] When such techniques have been used to select cells for autografting, most patients have relapsed.[475] No randomized trials have been conducted to demonstrate that marrow purged of BCR-ABL-positive progenitors improves remission rates or duration of survival. Thus, although autografting in CML may have therapeutic benefit in select patients, it remains an investigational approach.

Dendritic cells possessing the Ph chromosome that induce CD8+ cytotoxic T cells specific for leukemia cells can be isolated from CML patients.[476] The ability to identify CML-specific T cells after transplant has not been uniform, however.[477] Such cells could be utilized in a state of minimal disease after autologous stem cell transplantation to achieve a specific anti-CML effect.

ALLOGENEIC AND SYNGENEIC STEM CELL TRANSPLANTATION

Patients in the chronic phase of CML who are less than 65 years of age and who have an identical twin[478] or a histocompatible sibling[479-481] or who are less than 55 with access to a histocompatible, unrelated donor[482] can be transplanted after intensive therapy, usually cyclophosphamide and fractionated total-body irradiation or a combination of busulfan and cyclophosphamide.

ALLOGRAFTING

Stem cell transplantation from HLA-compatible siblings results in engraftment and an actual or projected long-term survival in 45 to 70 percent of recipients.[483] There is about a 20 percent risk of relapse of CML. Transplanted T lymphocytes, especially if activated by a (mild) GVH reaction, may be an important factor in preventing leukemic relapse. This phenomenon, referred to as graft-versus-leukemia reaction, is thought to suppress the leukemic process through T-cell-mediated cytotoxicity.[481] The beneficial effect of graft-versus-leukemia phenomena may be present in blast crisis[484] and in chronic phase.[485,486] Graft failure is rare in properly conditioned patients in chronic phase. The 5-year probability of survival is about 60 percent for chronic phase patients and about 20 percent for accelerated phase patients.[487] The majority of survivors have no evidence of residual leukemia cells.[488]

The best outcomes are seen in younger patients when the transplant is performed within 1 year of diagnosis.[489,490] Choice of pretransplant conditioning does not appear to have an impact on outcome, but previous exposure to busulfan has a negative impact.[491] IFN-α does not increase the probability of treatment failure.[492] In the first 18 months after the diagnosis of CML, mortality is higher in the patients who have received a stem cell transplant than in the cohort treated without transplants; between 18 to 56 months, mortality is similar in the two groups; and after 56 months, the mortality is lower in the patients who were transplanted.[493] Survival after 7 years was 48 percent with transplant and 32 percent with hydroxyurea or IFN-α treatment.[493] The relative benefit of marrow as compared to mobilized blood stem cells as the source of the allograft has not been established.[494]

For younger patients who do not have a histocompatible sibling, utilization of unrelated donor or a mismatched family member as a source of stem cells is feasible. The toxicity of this procedure is greater than that of an HLA-identical sibling donor transplant. Five-year disease-free survival is about 40 percent.[495] Younger patients with cytomegalovirus-seronegative donors who are matched at the HLA-DRB1 allele by molecular methods fare better.[496] When class I HLA genes are typed with molecular methods, one may expect an improvement in matching and better outcomes using unrelated donors. Cord blood stem cell transplantation from an unrelated donor has also been used in adults with CML.[497]

The major causes of failure of a stem cell allograft in CML include conditioning regimen-related toxicity, GVH disease, and relapse of leukemia. Prophylaxis of GVH disease may include various methods of T-cell depletion in vitro or in vivo and prevention of the reaction with cyclosporine and methotrexate. Glucocorticoids are the mainstay of treatment for established GVH disease. The risk of leukemia relapse is higher if the allograft is depleted of T cells in vitro. Using non-T-cell-depleted grafts, the 5-year relapse rate is about 20 percent and in unrelated donor transplants, 3 percent.[498] The use of unrelated stem cell allografts compensates for the reduced graft-versus-leukemia activity associated with T-cell depletion in patients transplanted in chronic phase.[499] Disease status after the allograft can be monitored with cytogenetic studies, PCR, or FISH analysis. A positive PCR assay at 3 months after allogeneic BMT has not been found to correlate with an increased risk of relapse compared with PCR-negative patients. A positive assay 6 months and beyond is associated with subsequent relapse. In one series, 42 percent of patients with a positive PCR assay at 6 to 12 months relapsed versus 3 percent with a negative assay.[500]

Patients who remain *BCR-ABL*-positive more than 36 months after a transplant have little propensity for relapse.[500] Graft-versus-leukemia may act to suppress minimal residual disease after allogeneic marrow transplantation.[501]

Infection with cytomegalovirus, fungi, herpes simplex or herpes zoster virus can cause severe morbidity and early posttransplantation mortality, but these causes of death have decreased in frequency significantly. Poorly controlled GVH disease is the major cause of early posttransplantation mortality. The early posttransplantation mortality of about 25 percent has stimulated studies that define the optimal time of transplantation in chronic phase by considering variables such as age, percent blood blasts, spleen size, the likelihood of remaining in chronic phase for a prolonged period, and the probability of successful marrow transplantation in the accelerated phase.[502]

Marrow transplantation can eradicate the Ph-chromosome-carrying clone and has led to apparent cure of some patients.[503] Some believe that marrow transplantation should be undertaken during the first year of chronic phase, if a histocompatible sibling or identical twin donor is available.[504] The improvement in survival with hydroxyurea and interferon-α therapy and the exploration of new drug combinations for therapy may influence these recommendations.[505] Figure 94-7 outlines possible treatment options. Individual patient preferences enter into the decision.

IMMUNOTHERAPY: ADOPTIVE CELL THERAPY FOR POSTTRANSPLANT RELAPSE

There is substantial evidence that the effectiveness of allografting in CML is not due solely to the eradication of the leukemic clone with the high-dose chemoradiotherapy conditioning regimens but also to adoptive immunotherapy provided by lymphocytes in the allograft, the graft-versus-leukemia effect.[484] This phenomenon has been recreated to produce a therapeutic response by infusion of stem-cell-donor lymphocytes after relapse following allogeneic stem cell transplantation.[506,839] Ten million mononuclear cells per kilogram body weight may be enough to achieve a graft-versus-leukemic effect in the absence of GVH disease.[507] The overall response rate to such treatment is about 75 percent. The response rate is higher when this approach is employed early after detecting a relapse by PCR.[508] This approach may avoid the need for high-dose cytotoxic chemotherapy that would accompany a second transplant procedure.[509]

The main toxicities of donor-lymphocyte infusion have been induction of GVH disease and myelosuppression. Attempts to diminish these toxicities have included the use of CD8-depleted donor leukocyte infusions and the infusion of smaller numbers of T cells.[510,511] Donor lymphocytes can also be transfected with vectors containing the herpes simplex virus genome in a replication defective form. If GVH disease occurs, the lymphocytes can be eradicated with systemic ganciclovir treatment. The ultimate utility of such approaches is still unmeasured.[512]

Ways to administer more specific immune effector cells have been sought. *BCR-ABL*-specific T cells with marked cytotoxic activity against CML cells can be generated and amplified from the blood of a normal donor.[513,514] HLA-DR1-restricted *BRC-ABL* (b3a2)-specific, CD4-positive T lymphocytes respond to dendritic cells pulsed with b3a2-peptide and antigen-presenting cells exposed to b3a2-containing cell lysates.[515] Peptides derived from the whole sequence of *BCR-ABL* bind to several class I molecules, allowing specific induction of human cytotoxic T lymphocytes.[516] Such *BCR-ABL* junction peptides, when bound to HLA class I molecules, allow specific induction of human cytotoxic T lymphocytes.[517] Whether such cells utilized in adoptive immunotherapy will be more effective than donor leukocytes in preventing or treating relapse is not known.

COURSE AND PROGNOSIS

Several large studies of treatment during the 1970s and early 1980s reported a similar survival of patients with CML treated with standard chemotherapy, that is, busulfan or hydroxyurea, during the chronic phase.[518–526] Median survival ranged from 39 to 47 months, the 5-year survival was about 25 to 35 percent of patients, and the 8-year survival 8 to 17 percent of patients. A large randomized study comparing hydroxyurea to busulfan has shown a significant prolongation of chronic phase with hydroxyurea[440] and a further prolongation with IFN-α therapy (Table 94-2). Occasional patients have remained in chronic phase from 10 to 25 years.[527–534]

At the time of diagnosis the variables most closely associated with duration of chronic phase, and thus survival, are percent blasts in the blood, liver and spleen size, and total basophil plus eosinophil count. Using these variables in large numbers of patients, the population segregates into three risk groups: better risk, with a median of survival of about 5.0 years; intermediate risk, with a median survival of 3.5 years; and poor risk, with a median survival of 2.5 years.[535–537] In the better-risk group, 40 percent are alive at 7 years, and in the poor-risk group, 10 percent or fewer are alive at 7 years. These figures are based on large numbers of patients treated principally with busulfan. If prolongation of chronic phase by hydroxyurea and interferon treatment is validated, the median survival in each group may be extended by several years. Prognostic indices, therefore, may be important in interpreting the results of chemical therapies and may have a major role in deciding the timing of stem cell transplantation because of the relatively high peritransplant mortality.[502,538] The indices may not have sufficient specificity and sensitivity to be applied to a single patient, however. Studies that link the precise (3-prime) location of the breakpoint in the *BCR* gene with shortened duration of chronic phase[539] have not been confirmed.[540] Most patients die as a result of conversion from the chronic to the accelerated phase of the disease even in the era of IFN-α treatment and increased transplant donor availability.[541] Spontaneous remissions of CML have been reported,[542,543] but the disease may recur.[544]

DETECTION OF MINIMAL RESIDUAL DISEASE

The detection of minimal residual disease by molecular probes makes it possible to identify about one cell in a million that is derived from the CML clone.[545] Such studies have detected CML cells in patients who appeared to be free of Ph-chromosome-positive cells by cytogenetic analysis following allogeneic stem cell transplantation.[546–549] PCR permits observation of the regression of subclinical disease following therapy, the persistence of subclinical disease following therapy, or the progression of subclinical disease prior to its becoming overt. The stable persistence of subclinical disease does not invariably predict early relapse.[546,549] There is an increased risk of misinterpreting negative results of RT-PCR when very small numbers of transcripts are present.[325] The dilution threshold for reproducible amplification is 250,000 cells. mRNA$^{bcr-abl}$ can also be detected in single progenitor colonies after culture.[550] A good correlation has been found between the proportion of Ph-chromosome-positive metaphase cells and levels of mRNA$^{bcr-abl}$, and no difference in levels of the fusion mRNA was found between Ph-chromosome-positive and Ph-chromosome-negative, *BCR-ABL*-positive patients.[551] Through utilization of quantitative PCR, an increase of mRNA$^{bcr-abl}$ expression has been found to precede disease progression. This increase was detected up to 16 months before laboratory or clinical parameters showed phenotypic transformation of the malignant clone.[552] The technique of detecting minimal residual disease is very sensitive but is subject to false-positive reactions.

RELATED DISEASES WITHOUT THE PH CHROMOSOME

CHRONIC NEUTROPHILIC LEUKEMIA

HISTORY AND PATHOGENESIS

Tuohey in 1920 described the first recorded case of an unusual sustained neutrophilia with splenomegaly without fever, inflammation, cancer, or another cause of a leukemoid reaction.[553] Since that time, about 80 cases have been reported.[554–577] The disease is a clonal hemopathy and a rare form of a clonal myeloproliferative disorder. Some cases may arise in the hematopoietic stem cell, others in a later progenitor cell[578] (see Chap 92).

CLINICAL FEATURES

Symptoms and Signs   About 90 percent of patients have been over 60 years of age.[561–564] Younger patients have been described, however.[565] Somewhat more men than women have been reported. Patients may complain of weakness, anorexia, weight loss, abdominal pain, and easy bruising. Symptoms and signs of gouty arthritis occur in about one-third of the cases. The spleen has been enlarged in all cases, and the liver is frequently enlarged. Lymphadenopathy is very infrequent.[578] A hemorrhagic tendency is present in some patients.[561,564,569,576,579]

Laboratory Findings   Although some patients may have a normal hemoglobin concentration, most have anemia on presentation. The reticulocytic count is usually between 0.5 and 3.0 percent. The platelet count is rarely below 125,000/μl (125 × 10⁹/liter) and usually is normal. Coagulation times are normal. The total leukocyte count is between 25,000 and 50,000/μl (25 and 50 × 10⁹/liter) in most cases and only rarely exceeds 100,000/μl (100 × 10⁹/liter). Neutrophils make up 90 to 95 percent of the white cells and, although segmented cells usually dominate, occasional cases have 20 to 50 percent band forms. Very infrequent metamyelocytes, myelocytes, and nucleated red cells may be present in occasional patients. Blasts are usually not present in the blood. Neutrophil alkaline phosphatase activity is increased in virtually all cases.

The marrow invariably shows granulocytic hyperplasia with M:E ratios as high as 10:1. Myeloblasts are not overtly increased in number (0.5 to 3.0 percent). Megakaryocytes are either normal or increased in number. Erythropoiesis is usually mildly decreased. Unlike CML, reticulin fibrosis is very unusual. A few cases have been reported with dysplastic features in the marrow (acquired Pelger-Hüet anomaly, erythroid, dysplasia and micromegakaryocytes).[580] The Ph chromosome, *BCR* gene rearrangements, and *BCR-ABL* transcripts have been absent in the cases that have had such studies.[577,581–586] Occasional, nonrandom abnormalities of chromosomes have been reported.[554,561,564,574,583,587,588] Most patients have normal karyotypes. Use of X-chromosome-linked polymorphic genes in blood cells and fluorescence in situ hybridization of chromosome abnormalities have been indicative of a clonal disorder.[581,584,585]

Serum vitamin-B₁₂-binding protein and vitamin B₁₂ levels are both markedly increased above normal. Serum uric acid concentration is increased, and serum lactic dehydrogenase activity may be increased.

Virtually every case examined postmortem has had liver and splenic enlargement.[561,564] Portal hepatic and splenic red pulp infiltrates of neutrophils or islands of extramedullary hematopoiesis with immature myeloid cells and megakaryocytes are characteristic.

DIFFERENTIAL DIAGNOSIS

Most leukemoid reactions will be associated with an obvious underlying cause such as pancreatitis, carcinoma of the lung, or bacterial infection. Molecular studies to identify *BCR* gene rearrangement or the presence of *BCR-ABL* transcripts should distinguish chronic neutrophilic leukemia from neutrophilic-chronic myelogenous leukemia (see "Special Clinical Features").

TREATMENT

There are no systematic studies of treatment. Although busulfan or hydroxyurea may decrease the white count and spleen size transiently,[568,571] the disease generally has been difficult to control.

COURSE AND PROGNOSIS

The disease is fatal, with a median survival of about 2 to 3 years and a range of 0.5 to 6 years.[561,562,564,569,572] A case of spontaneous remission has been reported.[573] The prognosis is considerably worse than CML despite the prevalence of mature neutrophils and the paucity of blasts in most cases. Severe hemorrhage, despite normal platelet counts and coagulation times, has been the cause of death in several patients. Severe infection has occurred in a few patients. Acute myelogenous leukemia has been the terminal event in several cases.[559,561,580,583] A remarkable frequency of concordant essential monoclonal gammopathy or myeloma has been described.[558,560,563,571,573,575,585,589–591] In two cases, the extreme neutrophilia proved to be a polyclonal response to plasma cell disorder.[585,592] Chronic neutrophilic leukemia has evolved from polycythemia vera or oligoblastic leukemia,[593,594] supporting its relationship to the clonal hemopathies.[585,595,596] The disease usually afflicts elderly subjects, and cardiac, pulmonary, and vascular diseases contribute to a fatal outcome in most cases.

CHRONIC MONOCYTIC LEUKEMIA

HISTORY

In 1937, Osgood reviewed his experience with monocytic leukemia and included a case which probably represented the rare disorder chronic monocytic leukemia.[597] In 1981, about 28 bona fide cases had been reported, 5 cases were added, and the characteristics were reviewed.[598]

CLINICAL FINDINGS

Patients range from 30 to 80 years of age. Males are affected more frequently than females. Fever, fatigue, and left upper quadrant pain are the most common complaints. Splenomegaly and hepatomegaly are nearly constant findings.[598–600]

LABORATORY FINDINGS

Anemia is mild. Anisocytosis and poikilocytosis are usually present. The leukocyte count is usually normal or low but can be elevated in a minority of patients. The percent of monocytes is increased, but the absolute monocyte count is often normal in the range of 300 to 1500/μl (0.3 to 1.5 × 10⁹/liter) or mildly elevated. Occasional patients may have more striking monocyte counts. The platelet count may be normal or decreased. Rare nucleated red cells may be present in the blood. The monocytes in the blood contain alpha-naphthol acetate esterase, tartrate-sensitive acid phosphatase, fluoride-sensitive naphthol AS-D acetate esterase, and peroxidase as judged by histochemical tests. The marrow is cellular, often without an increase in monocytes. The Ph chromosome is absent. The leukemic cells are similar to mature monocytes with abundant cytoplasm. Erythrophagocytosis or thrombocytophagocytosis by monocytes may be seen.

The disease is often not recognized, since the total white cell count, the monocyte count, and the number of marrow monocytes may not be elevated until the spleen is removed, usually for diagnostic purposes.[598] Following splenectomy, a gradual leukocytosis may develop 3000 to 100,000/μl (3 to 100 × 10⁹/liter).[598] The absolute monocyte count increases dramatically, often from under 1000/μl (1 × 10⁹/

liter) to as high as 75,000/µl (75 × 10^9/liter). The marrow may contain more than 50 percent mature monocytes following splenectomy.

The spleen is enlarged (300 to 2500 g). The red pulp is infiltrated with mononuclear cells, often obliterating sinus lumens. Erythrophagocytosis by the mononuclear cells is frequently evident. Liver biopsy may show a mononuclear infiltrate in the sinusoids. Although clinical lymph node enlargement is rare, lymph node biopsies show striking infiltration by leukemic monocytes.

COURSE, PROGNOSIS, AND TREATMENT

Median survival is about 25 months, and patients often die of septicemia[598–600] or acute monocytic leukemia.[601,602] Therapy has not been studied systematically, but neither intensive combination chemotherapy nor glucocorticoids have changed the course of the disease.[421]

JUVENILE MYELOMONOCYTIC LEUKEMIA

DEFINITION

Ph-chromosome-positive, adult-type CML occurring below the age of 15 years makes up about 3 percent of childhood leukemias and about 10 percent of all cases of CML.[236,603] Although CML occurs in children of all ages, it is rare under age 5. With the exception of a propensity to present with higher total leukocyte counts and with leukostatic signs or symptoms,[236] CML in children has the typical manifestations and course of the disorder as seen in adults.

A disorder different from adult-type CML, which has been designated *juvenile myelomonocytic leukemia* (juvenile CML), represents about 1.5 percent of childhood leukemias. It occurs most often in infants and children under 4 years of age and is similar in some respects to adult subacute or chronic myelomonocytic leukemia (see Chap. 92).[604–606]

PATHOGENESIS

This disorder is a clonal hemopathy that originates in an early hematopoietic progenitor cell.[607] *RAS* mutations in hematopoietic cells are present in about 20 percent of patients.[608] About 1 of 10 patients with juvenile myelomonocytic leukemia have mutations of *NF*1 and manifest type 1 neurofibromatosis. This frequency is about 400 times the expected occurrence.[609–611] The linkage between neurofibromin, the protein encoded by the *NF*1 gene; guanosine triphosphatase-activity proteins; and the activation state of *RAS*-encoded proteins have led to a postulated sequence of events that may be triggered by the extraordinarily heightened sensitivity of the colony-forming cells in the marrow and blood of infants with the disease to the proliferative effects of granulocytic-monocytic colony stimulating factor. The latter initiates signal transduction from the cell membrane to the nucleus via *RAS* protein activation.[606,612]

CLINICAL FINDINGS

Symptoms and Signs   Infants present with failure to thrive, and children present with malaise, fever, persistent infections, and exaggerated skin, oral, or nasal bleeding. Hepatomegaly can occur. Splenomegaly, sometimes massive, is present in virtually every case. Lymphadenopathy is frequent.[604,605] Over half the patients have eczematoid or maculopapular skin lesions[613] and xanthomatous lesions, and multiple café au lait spots (neurofibromatosis) may occur also.[605] The xanthomas may be the earliest signs of neurofibromatosis.[604,605]

Laboratory Findings   Anemia, thrombocytopenia, and moderate leukocytosis are common. The blood has an increased concentration of monocytes 1000 to 100,000/µl (1 to 100 × 10^9/liter), immature granulocytes including blast cells, and nucleated red cells. Fetal hemoglobin concentration is increased in about two-thirds of the patients. The marrow aspirate is hypercellular as a result of granulocytic hyperplasia; the number of erythroblasts and of megakaryocytes usually are decreased. Monocytic cells are increased. Leukemic blast cells are present in modest proportions.

Cell culture of blood and marrow shows a striking preponderance of monocytic progenitors, even in the absence of overt monocytosis in the marrow.[614,615] Granulocyte-monocyte colony forming cells show a marked tendency to spontaneous growth if adherent (monocytic) cells are not depleted from culture.[615] The effect is mediated by a release of large quantities of granulocyte-monocyte colony stimulating factor by monocytes in culture.[616]

Although clonal chromosome abnormalities have been found in some cases, there is no consistent pattern to the cytogenetic abnormalities, and over half the patients have normal karyotypes. The Ph chromosome is not present.[617,618] The phenotype of monosomy 7 syndrome overlaps with juvenile myelomonocytic leukemia, and this cytogenetic abnormality is present in about 15 percent of patients.[604]

COURSE, PROGNOSIS, AND TREATMENT

The median survival of patients with juvenile CML is less than 2 years.[604,605] The disease has been refractory to chemotherapy. Although improvement in survival after stem cell transplantation from a histocompatible sibling occurs,[619] cure is uncommon. A minority of patients will have a smoldering course for 1 to 3 years but, thereafter, rapidly progress and succumb to infection or hemorrhage. Some children convert to a full-blown acute myelogenous leukemia with a rapidly fatal outcome. Occasional patients have a very long survival (over 10 years) despite persistence of abnormal blood counts and splenomegaly, independent of the type or intensity of therapy. Younger children (less than 2 years) are more likely to have a protracted course.[605] In a study of nine patients, four treated with five or six drug-intensive regimens had a remission of 11 to 27+ months, compared with untreated or lightly treated patients, four of whom died in 7 months.[620] Even in the treated patients, complete suppression of the disease did not occur, and treatment protocols to induce and sustain remissions are lacking.[615] Future studies of isotretinoin, interleukin-10, interleukin-1 receptor antagonist, GM-CSF antagonist (E21R), and blockers of RAS protein farnesylation hold promise for ameliorating the disease.[604]

CHRONIC MYELOMONOCYTIC LEUKEMIA

This leukemia is part of the spectrum of clonal myeloid diseases that may have findings that simulate CML. In the past, when rigorous criteria for the diagnosis of CML were not applied, chronic myelomonocytic leukemia was among a heterogenous group of related diseases that were sometimes referred to as *Ph-chromosome-negative CML.*[621]

Most patients with chronic myelomonocytic leukemia (CMML) are over 50 years of age, and about 75 percent of cases are over 60 years of age at the time of diagnosis. Cases also have been reported in children and as a complication of polycythemia vera. The onset is usually insidious, and weakness, infection, or exaggerated bleeding may bring patients to medical attention.[823–828] Hepatomegaly and splenomegaly occur in about 40 percent of patients.

The disease is characterized by anemia and blood monocytosis usually in excess of 1,000/µl (1 × 10^9/liter). The white cell count may be slightly decreased, normal, or moderately elevated. Immature granulocytes may be present in the blood. Blood myeloblasts may be absent or, when present, do not exceed 10 percent of total white cells. Most patients have thrombocytopenia, but normal or elevated platelet counts may occur. The marrow is hypercellular as a result of granulomonocytic hyperplasia; the dominant cells are early myelocytes. The proportions of myeloblasts and progranulocytes are increased but do not exceed 20 percent of marrow cells. Promonocytes also are increased in number. Distinction between poorly granulated myelocytes and promonocytes with primary granules can be difficult. Macronormoblasts and hyper- or hyposegmented (Pelger-Huët) neutrophils are frequent. Despite thrombocytopenia, megakaryocytes are usually present in the marrow. Plasma and urine lysozyme concentrations are nearly always elevated. Eosinophilia may be so prominent in occasional cases that the designation chronic eosinophilic leukemia may be appropriate.[264,267,843,844] CMML also is characterized by frequent *RAS* gene mutations. In some cases, there is homozygous deletion of the genes encoding the macrophage CSF-1 receptor and, also, in "spontaneous" cluster/colony growth in vitro. The latter may be due to autocrine or paracrine production of growth factors such as GM-CSF and IL-3. Chronic myelomonocytic leukemia is closely related clinically to chronic monocytic leukemia and to so-called Philadelphia-chromosome-negative, breakpoint-cluster-region-negative chronic myelogenous leukemia. Translocation between chromosomes 5 and 12, which juxtaposes the gene encoding platelet-derived growth factor beta receptor with the *TEL* gene, is present in cases of CMML.[829] This fusion gene encodes a transforming protein that activates beta R kinase signaling pathways. The *RAS* gene may also be involved in the transforming events.[830]

Treatment has been unsatisfactory, and remissions of any duration are rare. The age and performance status of the patient is considered in determining the intensity of treatment. Cytarabine, either standard or low-dose, etoposide, hydroxyurea, and other approaches used for the oligoblastic myelogenous leukemias have been tried with little success (see Chap. 92). Median survival in CMML is about 20 months, with a range from about 10 to over 60 months.

PH-CHROMOSOME-NEGATIVE OR *BCR*-REARRANGEMENT-NEGATIVE CML

An ever-diminishing proportion of patients with clinical manifestations within the limits usually applied to the diagnosis of CML have neither a Ph chromosome (classical, variant, or masked) nor evidence of rearrangement within the M-*bcr* on chromosome 22.[622,623] This circumstance represents true Ph-chromosome-negative CML, perhaps better referred to as *BCR*-rearrangement-negative CML. The literature describing Ph-chromosome-negative CML prior to 1987 is difficult to evaluate because many cases were not studied carefully for masked or variant translocations and for *BCR* gene rearrangement. Ph-chromosome-negative CML is a clonal disease[624] which has the propensity for lymphoid as well as myeloid transformation.[625-627] Although most cases of *BCR*-rearrangement-negative CML cases are closer in manifestations to chronic myelomonocytic leukemia,[622,623,628-631] a few residual cases are difficult to distinguish from classical CML.[632-634] In the latter group, absence of acute blast transformation as a terminal event has been observed. As the disease progresses, the patient develops severe cytopenias.[633] Some patients have been shown to have transposition of *ABL* to chromosome 22 but not the classical translocation.[635,636] Some cases of hypereosinophilia have been shown to be clonal (neoplastic) myeloproliferative disorders and may have blood and marrow findings similar to CML with eosinophilic dominance[637] (see Chap. 68). The hematopoietic cells in these cases do not contain the Ph chromosome or *BCR* gene rearrangement and have been dubbed *chronic eosinophil leukemia*.[638,639]

PH-CHROMOSME-POSITIVE ACUTE LEUKEMIA

MYELOGENOUS

About 2 percent of cases of acute myelogenous leukemias have the Ph chromosome t(9;22)(q34;q11) in a significant proportion (10 to 100 percent) of leukemic blast cells.[640-643] The blast cells have surface antigens characteristic of myeloid leukemias.[644] One interpretation of this concurrence is that it represents CML presenting in myeloid blast crisis.[645-649] The arguments in favor of this proposal are (1) that blast crisis may occur within days after diagnosis of Ph-chromosome-positive CML, (2) that several of the cases presented with additional cytogenetic changes comparable to CML in blast crisis,[650] (3) that marked hepatosplenomegaly is present,[645,649,650] (4) that platelet counts are normal and basophils exhibit intermittent increases,[645,648,649] (5) that a long prodromal period of weakness and weight loss and the appearance of some features of CML, such as granulocytosis, follow treatment with chemotherapy,[640,647,651] (6) that Ph-chromosome-positive AML has a very poor prognosis like myeloid blast crisis, (7) that the breakpoint on chromosome 22 in the M-*bcr* is typical of CML and the product of the fusion *BCR-ABL* gene is a p210 tyrosine kinase identical to that in classical CML,[649-654] and (8) that some patients enter a remission by converting to a phenotype analogous to chronic phase CML.[451] An alternative view has been promulgated because (1) most cases of Ph-chromosome-positive AML are a mosaic (normal karyotypes as well as abnormal), (2) the Ph chromosome may appear later in the course of the disease,[655] (3) additional chromosomal abnormalities are often different from those seen in the myeloblastic crisis of CML,[656,657] and (4) the Ph chromosome in these cases is not associated with breaks in the M-*bcr* on chromosome 22,[652,654,657-659] the latter being characteristic of CML. Moreover, Ph-chromosome-positive AML has developed following Ph-chromosome-negative oligoblastic leukemia.[660] Some cases of Ph-chromosome-positive acute leukemia are myeloid-lymphoid hybrids.[661] It appears that Ph-chromosome-positive AML comes in two varieties: one with a break in M-*bcr* of chromosome 22 with a p210 product, which could be considered analogous to acute blast crisis of CML, and one with a molecular pathology such that the oncogene product is a p190 protein. These distinctions may be important if future therapy is keyed to the specific fusion oncogene product.

LYMPHOCYTIC

About 3 percent of cases of childhood acute lymphocytic leukemia (ALL)[662-668] and 20 percent of cases of adult ALL[662,666,669] cells contain the Ph chromosome. In children the clinical and laboratory findings in the disease are similar whether the lymphoblasts contain the Ph chromosome or not, but the prognosis is worse for those with the Ph chromosome; lower frequencies of remission, much shorter remission duration, and less chance of cure with chemotherapy.[665,667,669] Remission rates and median survivals are also significantly lower in adults with ALL and the Ph chromosome (see Chap. 97). Marrow transplantation may hold hope for successful treatment of this variant of ALL in some patients with a histocompatible donor.[668,669]

Molecular studies of the chromosomes and cells of patients with ALL indicate the disease is heterogeneous. Some adults and few, if any, children with ALL have the t(9;22)(q34;q11) with a *BCR-ABL* fusion gene that codes for and expresses the p210[bcr-abl] tyrosine kinase.[651-653,670-685] The leukemic cells of some adults with ALL and virtually all children with the disease have the Ph chromosome, but their cells have a rearrangement of the *BCR* gene that involves sequences outside the 5.8-kb M-*bcr*. In these cases, a 7.0-kb chimeric RNA is transcribed that directs the translation of a p190[bcr-abl] product and that also has tyrosine kinase activity.[671,686] The Ph-chromosome-positive, 5.8-kb *BCR*-rearrangement-positive ALL patients may revert to CML after intensive chemotherapy, whereas the Ph-chromosome-positive, *BCR*-rearrangement-negative ALL patients who enter remission have reappearance of normal hematopoiesis. The former group of Ph-chromosome-positive, *BCR*-rearrangement-positive ALL is thought to represent presentation of CML in lymphocytic blast crisis; the Ph-chromosome-positive, *BCR*-rearrangement-negative ALL represents *de novo* ALL.[687,688] The somatic mutation, however, appears to involve a cell that can differentiate into all hematopoietic lineages.[689] A subgroup of the latter with concomitant monosomy 7 has been described, also.[690] Patients with ALL with the BCR rearrangement restricted to lymphoid cells have a more favorable prognosis than those with BCR rearrangement present in myeloid and lymphoid cells.[691,692]

Phenotyping of blast cells with panels of antibodies to surface antigens, histochemical reactions, and gene rearrangement probes indicates that Ph-chromosome-positive leukemias also may be biphenotypic (lymphoid and myeloid lineage) and be heterogenous in the site in the BCR gene in which rearrangements occur.[662,692]

ACCELERATED PHASE OF CHRONIC MYELOGENOUS LEUKEMIA

DEFINITION

In most cases of CML, the patient's disease eventually changes to a more aggressive, more symptomatic and troublesome phase, which is poorly responsive to therapy that formerly controlled the chronic phase. The failure of IFN-α, hydroxyurea, or another previously successful modality simultaneously to restore near-normal red cell and white cell counts, decrease spleen size, and maintain a feeling of well-being is the most consistent clinical hallmark of the metamorphosis of the chronic to the accelerated phase of CML.

The terminology used has included *acute phase, acute transformation,* or *blast crisis,* but the metamorphosis, which can be acute or blastic, is often more gradual and manifested by severe dyspoiesis, refractory splenomegaly, and extramedullary tumor masses; hence the preference for *transformation* or *accelerated phase* to describe this transition from a controllable to an uncontrollable malignancy. Blast crisis is the most severe manifestation of the accelerated phase.

PATHOGENESIS

Cytogenetic evidence indicates that the accelerated phase of the disease results from a progressive change in the clone that supported the chronic phase. Often chromosomal abnormalities occur in addition to the Ph chromosome, but the Ph chromosome persists.[693–697] Progression of the clone to a more malignant one is reflected also in a more disordered growth and maturation pattern of progenitor cells in culture, ultimately mimicking the growth failure of acute leukemia,[695] and in increased morphologic and functional abnormalities of blood cells,[698–700] eventuating in a total block in maturation and replacement of blood and marrow by blast cells.

FISH has been used to determine which cells have secondary cytogenetic abnormalities, and these cells often are not the blast cells. This finding suggests that some chromosomal abnormalities merely denote genomic instability.[701] About 65 percent of patients have cytogenetic abnormalities in addition to the Ph chromosome. A double Ph chromosome, trisomy 8, and isochromosome 17p are the secondary changes most commonly seen.[702] Clonal instability has also been found in cases of lymphoid blast crisis. Clones distinct from those identified later may be detected before overt lymphoid transformation. The identification of these abortive clones suggests clonal instability before the onset of transformation, which might have prognostic value.[703]

The abnormal mRNA and protein product p210[bcr–abl] are present in the marrow and blood cells of patients who have transformed to acute leukemia.[704–706] Although the breakpoint site on M-bcr was thought to be correlated with the time of the onset of the accelerated phase,[706] subsequent studies have not indicated a correlation between length of chronic phase and the specific site of the BCR-ABL fusion.[707] Rare cases have had deletion of the BCR-ABL fusion gene, loss of transcription of the message, and loss of expression of the p210 tyrosine kinase after transformation, the latter finding suggesting the abnormal protein kinase may not play a unique role in sustaining the acute state.[708]

Numerous molecular changes have been identified in the cells of patients with acute transformation that might contribute to the increased malignant behavior of the CML clone: activation of the N-RAS gene,[709,710] rearrangement of the p53 gene,[710–713] and hypermethylation of the calcitonin gene[714] have been described. One series found p53 mutations in 17 percent of blast crisis patients. An association between a failure of CML cells to express the retinoblastoma gene product and acute blast crisis with a megakaryoblastic phenotype has also been reported.[715]

Homozygous deletions of the p16 tumor suppressor gene have been associated with lymphoid transformation of CML,[716] but such deletions have not been seen in chronic phase and in myeloid blast crisis. P16 is also known as the *cyclin-dependent kinase 4 inhibitor gene* and is located on chromosome 9p21.[717] This gene inhibits a kinase, CDK-4, that regulates a cell cycle checkpoint prior to commitment to DNA synthesis. The Wilms' tumor (*WT*) gene on chromosome 11p13 encodes a zinc-finger-motif-containing transcription factor found in CML patients only after progression to blast crisis.[718] Overexpression of the *EVI*-1 gene has also been found in CML blast crisis.[719,720] Microsatellite instability has not been found to be involved with progression to blast crisis.[721] Roles for *BCL-2, c-MYC,* and various other genes have also been implicated in the evolution of CML.[722–725]

CLINICAL FEATURES

The features that signal the conversion of the chronic to the accelerated phase include unexplained fever, bone pain, weakness, night sweats, weight loss, loss of sense of well-being, arthralgias, or left upper quadrant pain. These may occur weeks in advance of laboratory evidence of the accelerated phase. Localized or diffuse lymphadenopathy or enlarging masses in extralymphatic sites containing myeloblasts or Ph-chromosome-positive lymphoblasts may develop. An increase of the basophil count (>10 percent); a decrease of the platelet count to less than $100,000/\mu l$ ($<100 \times 10^9$/liter); an increase in the proportion of blood (>5 percent) or marrow (>10 percent) blasts; new cytogenetic abnormalities; decreased progenitor cell growth in culture; or poor response in blood cell counts and splenic size to therapy for the chronic phase may be evident.[726–728] Splenic enlargement, unresponsive to previously successful cytotoxic therapy, may occur. Symptoms due to histamine excess in basophilic crisis can be present.[729]

Several of these changes may occur in series or in parallel. The time of onset of transformation and the final appearance of the blastic phase and its clinical expression is unpredictable.

LABORATORY FEATURES

BLOOD FINDINGS[726–728]

Anemia may worsen and be associated with increasing poikilocytosis, anisocytosis, and anisochromia. Nucleated red cells may increase in number. These red cell changes may be accentuated further if advancing marrow fibrosis is a feature of the disease, also.

The total leukocyte count may fall without treatment. The proportion of blasts may increase in blood and marrow and may represent 50 to 90 percent of the cells at the time of blastic crisis. Myelocytes decrease in number. Hyposegmented neutrophils (Pelger-Huët cells) may become evident. Basophils may increase and occasionally reach levels of 30 to 80 percent of the total blood leukocytes.

Thrombocytopenia may develop. Giant platelets, micromegakaryocytes, and megakaryocyte fragments may enter the blood.

MARROW FINDINGS[726–728]

The marrow findings are widely variable. Marked dysplastic changes in one, two, or three of the major cell lineages; marrow morphology simulating subacute myelomonocytic leukemia; or, in the extreme, florid blastic transformation can occur. Reticulin fibers may increase, and occasionally severe reticulin and collagen fibrosis can develop.

EXTRAMEDULLARY BLAST CRISIS

A variety of symptoms or signs may occur as a result of the specific effects of new extramedullary blastic tumors, referred to as *extramedullary blast crisis*.[730–733] Extramedullary blast crisis is the first manifestation of accelerated phase in about 10 percent of patients with CML. Lymph nodes,[731,733,734] serosal surfaces,[734–738] skin and soft tissue,[730–733] breast,[733,739] gastrointestinal or genitourinary tract,[731,733,740] bone,[731,733,741–744] and central nervous system[733,745–748] are among the principal areas involved. Isolated or diffuse lymphadenopathy may occur. Bone involvement may lead to severe pain, tenderness, and x-ray changes. The central nervous system involvement is usually meningeal and may be preceded by headache, vomiting, stupor, cranial nerve palsies, and papilledema and is associated with an increase in cells, protein, and the presence of blasts in the spinal fluid.[733,746–748]

Appropriate histochemical and immunological tests are required to determine if the extramedullary disease is composed of phenotypic myeloblasts or lymphoblasts. Since the tumor cells may have features of lymphoma cells, the terms *granulocytic sarcoma, chloroma,* and *myeloblastoma* can be misnomers, and the term *extramedullary blast crisis* is used for this circumstance in CML.[747,749–752] The lymphoblasts, like the myeloblasts, are Ph-chromosome-positive. A combination of morphology, histochemistry (e.g., peroxidase, lysozyme), terminal transferase assay, and monoclonal antibodies specific for lymphoid or myeloid cells can be used to classify the extramedullary blast cells. It is probable that older reports (1930s to 1960s) of concurrent lymphoma and CML were, in many cases, examples of extramedullary lymphoblast crisis in lymph nodes or other sites.

MARROW BLAST CRISIS

Most patients with CML enter the accelerated phase by developing acute leukemia. The onset of blast crisis can develop from days[753] to decades after diagnosis of CML. The signs and symptoms may include fever, hemorrhage, bone pain, and lymphadenopathy.[754–757] The morphology of the acute leukemia is usually myeloblastic or myelomonocytic.[755–757] A substantial proportion of myeloid leukemia in this setting may not have myeloperoxidese demonstrable by cytochemistry.[758] The proportion of cases classified as erythroblastic leukemia is about 10 percent based on morphologic features[759] but may be as high as 20 percent if the expression of glycophorin-A is used as the determinant.[760] Occasional cases have megakaryoblastic transformation.[715,761–763] These cases may be difficult to identify by light microscopy because the megakaryoblasts may be mistaken for lymphoid cells or undifferentiated blasts. Myelofibrosis is a feature of this variant. Antiplatelet glycoprotein antibodies and other monoclonal antiplatelet antibodies are now available as reagents to identify megakaryoblasts without the need for ultrastructural studies.[763] Promyelocytic[764–766] and eosinophilic[767] blast crises also can occur. Basophilic leukemia is known to be a variant of CML.[768] Patients with promyelocytic crisis often have t(15;17) in addition to the Ph chromosome, and some have presented with disseminated intravascular coagulation.[769]

CML may transform into acute lymphoblastic leukemia in nearly one-third of CML patients in blastic crisis.[748,770–774] The lymphoid cells generally express terminal deoxynucleotidyl transferase (TdT),[770,771] and are of the B-cell lineage,[774–776] as judged by anti-immunoglobulin staining. TdT is a DNA polymerase that adds deoxynucleoside monophosphates from triphosphate substrates to single-stranded DNA by end addition, differing in the latter respect from replicative polymerases.[777] The enzyme is present in normal immature thymocytes and the blast cells of nearly all patients with acute lymphoblastic leukemia.[778] Rare patients have blasts with a T-lymphocyte phenotype.[779–781] Some cases are biphenotypic, the blasts having both lymphoid and myeloid markers.[757,782–784] Some of these may have myeloperoxidase and express CD33 or CD13. Myeloid to lymphoid clonal succession following autologous transplantation in second chronic phase has been described.[785] Patients with lymphoid blast crisis seldom have an intermediate accelerated phase, have less splenomegaly and basophilia, and usually have a higher degree of marrow blast infiltration. Survival is usually somewhat longer in cases of lymphoid as compared to myeloid blast crisis.[786]

CYTOGENETIC STUDIES

Most large studies have shown four principal changes in patients' cells prior to, or during, the accelerated phase: additional 22q-, isochromosome 17, trisomy 8, and trisomy 19.[787–789] In addition, a large number of other chromosome abnormalities have been described.[790–796] In one study, 63 percent of 73 blast crisis patients had secondary cytogenetic abnormalities, and these were more common in myeloid blast crisis and associated with shorter remission.[702] These changes may be features of myeloid blast crisis as compared to lymphoid crisis.[788,793] Some abnormalities such as inv 16 have been associated with early transformation to AML.[789]

In cases where the blastic transformation is in extramedullary sites, like lymph nodes or spleen, the additional cytogenetic abnormalities may be in the cells at those sites, but not in cells in the blood or marrow.[797]

TREATMENT

The treatment approach is predicated on the phenotype of the blast cells in CML patients with blast crisis.

In patients with myeloid phenotypes the approach has been similar to that used for acute myelogenous leukemia: combinations of an anthracycline antibiotic, such as idarubicin or daunorubicin, with intermediate-dose cytosine arabinoside and etoposide. Because this approach produces few remissions and they are of short duration, a variety of other drug combinations incorporating high-dose cytosine arabinoside, methotrexate, busulfan, mitoxantrone, 5-azacytidine, etoposide, hydroxyurea, plicamycin, and others have been used with as yet little significant benefit[798–801]; 2-chlorodeoxyadenosine has also been used in myeloid blast crisis.[802] Tiazofurin, a selective blocker of inosine 5'-phosphate dehydrogenase activity may become useful in treating myeloid blast crisis.[803]

In patients with lymphoid phenotypes, vincristine sulfate, 1.4 mg/m^2 (not to exceed 2 mg/dose) intravenously once per week, and prednisone, 60 mg/m^2 orally per day, are the mainstay of treatment.[804–806] A minimum of two cycles of treatment (2 weeks) should be given to judge responsivity. About one-third of patients with lymphoid blast transformation will reenter chronic phase after such treatment, but, since only about a third of patients have lymphoid blasts, this represents a remission rate of only about 10 percent of patients who enter blast crisis. Some relapsed patients become TdT-negative (myeloblastic relapse). However, even if relapsed patients remain TdT-positive, they are not likely to respond to a second treatment. Some therapists argue for a more intensive induction regimen for the patient with lymphoblastic crisis, akin to regimens for de novo adult ALL or high-risk childhood ALL, and report somewhat better results: higher remission rates and longer remissions.[807,808] The experience is not yet sufficient to judge the net benefit of such an intensive approach, since remission durations have been modest. TdT-positive, CD10 (CALLA)-positive lymphoblasts may be the lymphoblast phenotype most responsive to vincristine and prednisone.[773,808]

Stem cell transplantation from a histocompatible twin or sibling has been used in some patients after entry into the blastic phase. Occasional patients have had long-term survival. The 3-year survival is about 15 to 20 percent,[809–811] unlike transplantation in the chronic phase in which the 3-year survival is 50 to 60 percent.[483] However, for patients who present in blast crisis, who develop it in the first year of the chronic phase, or who delay transplantation for other reasons, transplantation remains the best hope for long-term survival if a histocompatible donor is available.[809,810] Relapse of accelerated phase after allogeneic stem cell transplantation has responded to infusion of donor, in-vitro-selected, cytotoxic T lymphocytes.[822]

Autografting in accelerated phase or blast crisis, either with stem cells collected during chronic phase[812] or with mobilized Ph-chromosome-negative progenitor cells collected upon cell rebound after intensive chemotherapy[813] has resulted in apparent prolonged remission in some patients.[814–817]

Splenectomy may be performed for palliation of painful splenic infarctions or hemorrhage, but complication rates are high.[818]

COURSE AND PROGNOSIS

The accelerated phase of CML, generally, is a treatment-refractory and morbid state that is fatal in weeks to months in all but a very few patients who have a successful stem cell transplant from a histocompatible donor. Patients with myeloid blast crisis have a median survival of about 5 months,[785] while those with lymphoid blast crisis have a median survival of about 12 months. The median survival after evidence of clonal evolution in patients in chronic phase is about 19 months. Poorer survival was seen with abnormalities of chromosome 17, other superimposed translocations, or a high percentage of abnormal metaphases.[819] Severe cytopenias from repeated courses of cytotoxic therapy contribute to infections, hemorrhage, and organ dysfunction, especially liver and kidney dysfunction. Opportunistic infections with herpes viruses, cytomegalovirus, or fungi often supervene.

REFERENCES

1. Bennett JH: Case of hypertrophy of the spleen and liver, in which death took place from suppuration of the blood. *Edinburgh Med Surg J* 64:313, 1845.
2. Virchow R: Weisses blut. *Froiep's Notizen* 36:151, 1845.
3. Craige D: Case of disease of the spleen in which death took place in consequence of the presence of purulent matter in the blood. *Edinburgh Med Surg J* 64:400, 1845.
4. Virchow R: *Die leukaemie in gesammelte abhandlungen zur wissenschaftlichen medizin*, p. 190. Frankfort, Meidinger, 1865.
5. Neumann E: Ueber myelogene leukämie. *Berl Klin Wochenschr* 15:69, 1878.
6. Nowell PC, Hungerford DA: A minute chromosome in human chronic granulocytic leukemia. *J Natl Cancer Inst* 25:85, 1960.
7. Baike AG, Court Brown WM, Buckton KE, et al: A possible specific chromosome abnormality in human chronic myeloid leukemia. *Nature* 188:1165, 1960.
8. Nowell PC, Hungerford DA: Chromosome studies in human leukemia: II. Chronic granulocytic leukemia. *J Natl Cancer Inst* 27:1013, 1961.
9. Tough IM, Court Brown WM, Buckton KE, et al: Cytogenetic studies in chronic leukemia and acute leukemia associated with mongolism. *Lancet* 1:411, 1961.
10. Caspersson T, Zech L, Johansson C, Modest EJ: Identification of human chromosomes by DNA binding fluorescent agents. *Chromosoma* 30:215, 1970.
11. Caspersson T, Gahrton G, Lindsten J, Zech L: Identification of the Philadelphia chromosome as a number 22 by quinicrine mustard fluorescence analysis. *Exp Cell Res* 63:238, 1970.
12. Rowley JD: A new consistent abnormality in chronic myelogenous leukemia identified by quinacrine fluorescence and Giemsa staining. *Nature* 243:290, 1973.
13. DeKlein A, VanKessel AG, Grosveld G, et al: A cellular oncogene is translocated to the Philadelphia chromosome in chronic myelocytic leukemia. *Nature* 300:765, 1982.
14. Bartram CR, deKlein A, Hagameijer A, et al: Translocation of c-abl oncogene correlates with the presence of a Philadelphia chromosome in chronic myelocytic leukemia. *Nature* 306:277, 1983.
15. Ichimaru M, Ichimaru T, Belsky JL: Incidence of leukemia in atomic bomb survivors belonging to a fixed cohort in Hiroshima and Nagasaki, 1950–1971. *J Radiat Res* 19:262, 1978.
16. Court Brown WM, Doll R: Adult leukemia: trends in mortality in relation to etiology. *Br Med J* 1:1063, 1959.
17. Court Brown WM, Doll R: Adult leukemia. *Br Med J* 1:1753, 1960.
18. Boice JD Jr, Day NE, Anderson A, et al: Second cancers following radiation treatment for cervical cancer. *J Natl Cancer Inst* 74:955, 1985.
19. Maloney WC: Radiation leukemia revisited. *Blood* 70:905, 1987.
20. Pederson-Bjergaard J, Bondum-Nielsen K, Karle H, Johansson B: Chemotherapy-related and late-occuring Philadelphia chromosome in AML, ALL and CML. Similar events related to treatment with DNA topoisomerase II inhibitors? *Leukemia* 11:1571, 1997.
21. Bortin MM, D'Amaro J, Bach FH, et al: HLA association with leukemia. *Blood* 70:227, 1987.
22. Tokuhata GK, Neely CL, Williams DL: Chronic myelocytic leukemia in identical twins and a sibling. *Blood* 31:216, 1968.
23. Leukemia, Lymphoma, Myeloma 1999 Facts. Leukemia Society of America. www.leukemia.org.
24. Whang-Peng J, Knutsen T: Chromosomal abnormalities, in *Chronic Granulocytic Leukaemia, edited by MT Shaw, pp 49–92. Praeger, East Sussex, UK, 1982*.
25. Spiers ASD, Bain BJ, Turner JE: The peripheral blood in chronic granulocytic leukemia: a study of 50 untreated Philadelphia positive cases. *Scand J Haematol* 18:25, 1977.
26. Sandberg AA: The leukemias: the Philadelphia chromosome, in *The Chromosomes in Human Cancer and Leukemia*, 2nd ed, pp 183–261. Elsevier, New York, 1990.
27. Fialkow PJ, Garther SM, Yoshida A: Clonal origin of chronic myelocytic leukemia in men. *Proc Natl Acad Sci USA* 58:1468, 1967.
28. Fialkow PJ, Jacobsen RJ, Papayannopoulou T: Chronic myelocytic leukemia: clonal origin in a stem cell common to granulocyte, erythrocyte, platelet and monocyte/macrophage. *Am J Med* 63:125, 1977.
29. Koeffler HP, Levine AM, Sparkes LM, Sparkes RS: Chronic myelocytic leukemia: eosinophils involved in the malignant clone. *Blood* 55:1063, 1980.
30. Hayata I, Kakati S, Sandberg AA: On the monoclonal origin of chronic myelocytic leukemia. *Proc Jpn Acad* 30:351, 1974.
31. Lawler SD, O'Malley F, Lobb DS: Chromosome banding studies in Philadelphia chromosome positive myeloid leukemia. *Scand J Haematol* 17:17, 1976.
32. Harrison CJ, Chang J, Johnson D, et al: Chromosomal evidence of a common stem cell in acute lymphoblastic leukemia and chronic granulocytic leukemia. *Cancer Genet Cytogenet* 13:331, 1984.
33. Chaganti RSK, Bailey RB, Jhanwar SC, et al: Chronic myelogenous leukemia in the monosomic cell line of a fertile Turner syndrome mosaic (45,X/46,XX). *Cancer Genet Cytogenet* 5:215, 1982.
34. Fitzgerald PH, Pickering AF, Eiby JR: Clonal origin of the Philadelphia chromosome and chronic leukemia. *Br J Haematol* 21:473, 1971.
35. Groffen J, Stephenson JR, Heisterkamp N, et al: Philadelphia chromosomal breakpoints are clustered within a limited region, bcr, on chromosome 22. *Cell* 36:93, 1984.
36. Leibowitz D, Schaefer-Rego K, Popenoe DW, et al: Variable breakpoints on the Philadelphia chromosome in chronic myelogenous leukemia. *Blood* 66:243, 1985.
37. Yoffe G, Chinault AG, Talpaz M, et al: Clonal nature of Philadelphia chromosome positive and negative chronic myelogenous leukemia by DNA hybridization analysis. *Exp Hematol* 15:725, 1987.
38. Fialkow PJ, Denman AM, Jacobsen RJ, Lowenthal MN: Chronic myelo-

cytic leukemia. Origin of some lymphocytes from leukemic stem cells. *J Clin Invest* 62:815, 1978.

39. Martin PJ, Najfeld V, Hansen JA, et al: Involvement of the B-lymphoid system in chronic myelogenous leukaemia. *Nature* 287:49, 1980.

40. Boggs DR: Hematopoietic stem cell theory in relation to possible lymphoblastic conversion in chronic myeloid leukemia. *Blood* 44:449, 1974.

41. Bernheim A, Berger R, Preud'homme JL, et al: Philadelphia chromosome positive blood B lymphocytes in chronic myelocytic leukemia. *Leuk Res* 5:331, 1981.

42. Collins S, Coleman H, Groudine M: Expression of bcr and bcr-abl fusion transcripts in normal and leukemic cells. *Mol Cell Biol* 7:2870, 1987.

43. Al-Amin A, Lennartz K, Runde V, et al: Frequency of clonal B lymphocytes in chronic myelogenous leukemia evaluated by fluorescence in situ hybridization. *Cancer Genet Cytogenet* 104: 45, 1998.

44. Torlakovic E, Litz CE, McClure JS, Brunning RD: Direct detection of the Philadelphia chromosome in CD20-positive lymphocytes in chronic myelogenous leukemia by tri-color immunophenotyping/FISH. *Leukemia* 8:1940, 1994.

45. Kearney L, Orchard KH, Hibbin JA, Goldman JM: T-cell cytogenetics in chronic granulocytic leukaemia. *Lancet* 1:858, 1981.

46. Nogueira-Costa R, Spitzer G, Cock A, Trijillo JM: E rosette-positive agar colonies containing the Philadelphia chromosome in chronic myeloid leukemia. *Scand J Haematol* 34:184, 1985.

47. Bartram CR, Raghavachar A, Anger B, et al: T lymphocytes lack rearrangement of the bcr gene in Philadelphia chromosome-positive chronic myelogenous leukemia. *Blood* 69:1682, 1985.

48. Fauser AA, Kanz L, Bross KJ, et al: T cells and probably B cells arise from the malignant clone in chronic myelogenous leukemia. *J Clin Invest* 75:1080, 1985.

49. Nitta M, Kato Y, Strife A, et al: Incidence of the B and T lymphocyte lineages in chronic myelogenous leukemia. *Blood* 66:1053, 1985.

50. Nogueira-Costa R, Spitzer G, Khorana S, et al: T-cell involvement in benign phase chronic myelogenous leukemia. *Leuk Res* 10:1433, 1986.

51. Ariad S, Dajee D, Willem P, Bezwoda WR: Lack of involvement of T-lymphocytes in the leukaemic population during prolonged chronic phase of Philadelphia chromosome positive chronic myeloid leukaemia. *Leuk Lymphoma* 10:217, 1993.

52. Tsukamoto N, Karasawa M, Maehara T, et al: The majority of T lymphocytes are polyclonal during the chronic phase of chronic myelogenous leukemia. *Ann Hematol* 72:61, 1996.

53. Garicochea B, Chase A, Lazaridou A, Goldman JM: T lymphocytes in chronic myelogenous leukaemia (CML). *Leukemia* 8:1197, 1994.

54. Jonas D, Lubbert M, Kawasaki ES, et al: Clonal analysis of bcr-abl rearrangement in T lymphocytes from patients in the chronic myelogenous leukemia. *Blood* 79:1017, 1992.

55. Verfaillie C, Miller W, Kay N, McClave P: Adherent lymphokine-activated killer cells in chronic myelogenous leukemia: a benign cell population with potent cytotoxic activity. *Blood* 74:793, 1989.

56. Takahashi N, Miura I, Saitoh K, Miura AB: Lineage involvement of stem cells bearing the Philadelphia chromosome in chronic myeloid leukemia in the chronic phase as shown by a combination of fluorescence-activated cell sorting and fluorescence in situ hybridization. *Blood* 92:4758, 1998.

57. Fialkow PJ, Martin PJ, Najfeld V, et al: Evidence for a multistep pathogenesis of chronic myelogenous leukemia. *Blood* 58:158, 1981.

58. Lisker R, Casas L, Mutchinick O, et al: Late-appearing Philadelphia chromosome in two patients with chronic myelogenous leukemia. *Blood* 56:812, 1980.

59. Kamada N, Uchino H: Chronologic sequence in appearance of clinical and laboratory findings characteristic of chronic myelogenous leukemia. *Blood* 51:843, 1978.

60. Smadja N, Krulik M, DeGramont A, et al: Acquisition of a Philadelphia chromosome concomitant with transformation of a refractory anemia into an acute leukemia. *Cancer* 55:1477, 1985.

61. Fegan C, Morgan G, Whittaker JA: Spontaneous remission in a patient with chronic myeloid leukaemia. *Br J Haematol* 72:594, 1989.

62. Brandt L, Mitelman F, Panani A, Lenner HC: Extremely long duration of chronic myeloid leukaemia with Ph[1] negative and Ph[1] positive bone marrow cells. *Scand J Haematol* 16:321, 1976.

63. Hagemeijer A, Smith EME, Lowenberg B, Abels J: Chronic myeloid leukemia with permanent disappearance of the Ph[1] chromosome and development of new clonal subpopulations. *Blood* 53:1, 1979.

64. Singer JN, Arlin ZA, Najfeld V, et al: Restoration of nonclonal hematopoiesis in chronic myelogenous leukemia (CML) following a chemotherapy induced loss of the Ph[1] chromosome. *Blood* 56:356, 1980.

65. Sokal JE: Significance of Ph[1]-negative marrow cells in Ph[1] positive chronic granulocytic leukemia. *Blood* 56:1072, 1980.

66. Smadja N, Krulik M, Audebert AA, et al: Spontaneous regression of cytogenetic and haematologic anomalies in Ph[1]-positive chronic myelogenous leukaemia. *Br J Haematol* 63:257, 1986.

67. Goldman JM, Kearney L, Pittman S, et al: Hemopoietic stem cell grafting for chronic granulocytic leukaemia. *Exp Hematol* 10:76, 1982.

68. Reiffers J, Vezon G, David B, et al: Philadelphia negative cells in a patient treated with autografting for Ph[1] positive chronic granulocytic leukaemia in transformation. *Br J Haematol* 55:382, 1983.

69. Reiffers J, Broustet A, Goldman JM: Philadelphia chromosome-negative progenitors in chronic granulocytic leukaemia. *N Engl J Med* 309: 1460, 1983.

70. Coulombel L, Kalousek DK, Eaves CJ, et al: Long-term marrow culture reveals chromosomally normal hemopoietic progenitor cells in patients with Philadelphia chromosome-positive chronic myelogenous leukemia. *N Engl J Med* 308:1493, 1983.

71. Degliantoni G, Mangori L, Rizzoli V: In vitro restoration of polyclonal hematopoiesis in a chronic myelogenous leukemia after in vitro treatment with 4-hydroperoxy-cyclophosphamide. *Blood* 65:753, 1985.

72. Barnett MJ, Eaves CJ, Phillips GL, et al: Successful autografting in chronic myeloid leukemia after maintenance of marrow in culture. *Bone Marrow Transplant* 4:345, 1989.

73. Verfaillie CM, Miller WJ, Boylan K, McGlave PB: Selection of benign primitive hematopoietic progenitors in chronic myelogenous leukemia on the basis of HLA-DR antigen expression. *Blood* 79:1003, 1992.

74. Leemhuis T, Leibowitz D, Cox G, et al: Identification of BCR/ABL-negative primitive hematopoietic progenitor cells within chronic myeloid leukemia marrow. *Blood* 81:801, 1993.

75. Wang JCY, Lapidot T, Cashman JD, et al: High level engraftment of NOD/SCID mice by primitive normal and leukemic hemopoietic cells from patients with chronic myeloid leukemia in chronic phase. *Blood* 91:2406, 1998.

76. Dunbar CE, Stewart FM: Separating the wheat from the chaff: selection of benign hematopoietic cells in chronic myeloid leukemia. *Blood* 79:1107, 1992.

77. Strife A, Clarkson B: Biology of chronic myelogenous leukemia: is discordant maturation the primary defect? *Semin Hematol* 25:1, 1988.

78. Heinzinger M, Waller CF, Rosentiel A, et al: Quality of IL-3 and G-CSF-mobilized peripheral blood stem cells in patients with early chronic phase CML. *Leukemia* 12:333, 1998.

79. Verfaillie CM, Bhatia R, Miller W, et al: BCR/ABL-negative primitive progenitors suitable for transplantation can be selected from the marrow of most early-chronic phase but not accelerated-phase chronic myelogenous leukemia patients. *Blood* 87:4770, 1996.

80. Grand FH, Marley SB, Chase A, et al: BCR/ABL-negative progenitors are enriched in the adherent fraction of CD34+ cells circulating in the blood of chronic phase chronic myeloid leukemia patients. *Leukemia* 11:1486, 1997.

81. Carella AM, Podesta M, Frassoni R, et al: Collection of "normal" blood repopulating cells during early hemopoietic recovery after intensive conventional chemotherapy in chronic myelogenous leukemia. *Bone Marrow Transplant* 12:267, 1993.

82. Hogge DE, Coulumbel L, Kalousek D, et al: Nonclonal hemopoietic progenitors in a G6PD heterozygote with chronic myelogenous leukemia revealed after long-term marrow culture. *Am J Hematol* 24:389, 1987.

83. Van den Berg D, Wessman M, Murray L, et al: Leukemic burden in subpopulations of CD34+ cells isolated from the mobilized peripheral blood of alpha-interferon-resistant or -intolerant patients with chronic myeloid leukemia. *Blood* 87:4348, 1996.

84. Podesta M, Piaggio G, Frassoni F, et al: Very primitive hemopoietic cells (LTC-IC) are present in Philadelphia negative cytaphereses collected during early recovery after chemotherapy for chronic myeloid leukemia (CML). *Bone Marrow Transplant* 16:549, 1995.

85. Kirk JA, Reems JA, Roecklein BA, et al: Benign marrow progenitors are enriched in the CD34+/HLA-DRlo population but not in the CD34+/CD38lo population in chronic myeloid leukemia: an analysis using interphase fluorescence in situ hybridizaiton. *Blood* 86:737, 1995.

86. Lewis ID, Haylock DN, Moore S, et al: Peripheral blood is a source

of BCR-ABL-negative pre-progenitors in early chronic phase chronic myeloid leukemia. *Leukemia* 11:581, 1997.

87. Maguer-Satta V, Petzer AL, Eaves AC, Eaves CJ: BCR-ABL expression in different subpopulations of functionally characterized Ph+ CD34+ cells from patients with chronic myeloid leukemia. *Blood* 88:1796, 1996.

88. Sirard C, Lapidot T, Vormoor J, et al: Normal and leukemia SCID-repopulating cells (SRC) coexist in the bone marrow and peripheral blood from CML patients in chronic phase, whereas leukemic SRC are detected in blast crisis. *Blood* 87:1539, 1996.

89. Dazzi F, Capelli D, Hasserjian R, et al: The kinetics and extent of engraftment of chronic myelogenous leukemia cells in non-obese diabetic/severe combined immunodeficiency mice reflect the phase of the donor's disease: an in vivo model for chronic myelogenous leukemia biology. *Blood* 92:1390, 1998.

90. Strife A, Lambek C, Wisniewski D, et al: Discordant maturation as the primary biological defect in chronic myelogenous leukemia. *Cancer Res* 48:1035, 1988.

91. Eaves C, Cashman J, Eaves A: Defective regulation of leukemic hematopoiesis in chronic myeloid leukemia. *Leuk Res* 22:1085, 1998.

92. Clarkson BD, Strife A, Wisniewski D, et al: New understanding of the pathogenesis of CML: a prototype of early neoplasia. *Leukemia* 11:1404, 1997.

93. Bedi A, Zehnbauer BA, Collector MI, et al: BCR-ABL gene rearrangement and expression of primitive hematopoietic progenitors in chronic myeloid leukemia. *Blood* 81:2898, 1993.

94. Moore MAS: In vitro culture studies in chronic granulocytic leukaemia. *Clin Haematol* 6:97, 1977.

95. Siitonen T, Zheng A, Savolainen E-R, Koistinen P: Spontaneous granulocyte-macrophage colony growth by peripheral blood mononuclear cells in myeloproliferative disorders. *Leukemia Res* 20:187, 1996.

96. Eaves CJ, Eaves AC: Cell culture studies in CML. *Baillieres Clinical Haematol* 1:931, 1987.

97. Galbraith PR, Abu-Zahra HT: Granulopoiesis in chronic granulocytic leukemia. *Br J Haematol* 22:135, 1972.

98. Sjögren U, Brandt L: Composition and mitotic activity of the erythropoietic part of the bone marrow in chronic myeloid leukaemia. *Scand J Haematol* 12:18, 1974.

99. Verfaillie CM: Stem cells in chronic myelogenous leukemia. *Hematol-Oncol Clin North Am* 11:1079, 1997.

100. Ghaffari S, Dougherty GJ, Lansdorp PM, et al: Differentiation-associated changes in CD44 isoform expression during normal hematopoiesis and their alteration in chronic myeloid leukemia. *Blood* 86:2976, 1995.

101. Kawaishi K, Kimura A, Katch O, et al: Decreased L-selectin expression in CD34-positive cells from patients with chronic myelocytic leukaemia. *Br J Haematol* 93:367, 1996.

102. Turkina AG, Baryshnikov AY, Sedyakhina NP, et al: Studies of P-glycoprotein in chronic myelogenous leukaemia patients: expression, activity and correlations with CD34 antigen. *Br J Haematol* 92:88, 1996.

103. Agarwal R, Doren S, Hicks B, Dunbar CE: Long-term culture of chronic myelogenous leukemia marrow cells on stem cell factor-deficient stroma favors benign progenitors. *Blood* 85:1306, 1995.

104. Moore S, Haylock DN, Levesque J-P, et al: Stem cell factor as a single agent induces selective proliferation of the Philadelphia chromosome positive fraction of chronic myeloid leukemia CD34+ cells. *Blood* 92:2461, 1998.

105. Chasty RC, Lucas GS, Owen-Lynch PJ, et al: Macrophage inflammatory protein-1 alpha receptors are present on cells enriched for CD34 expression from patients with chronic myeloid leukemia. *Blood* 86:4270, 1995.

106. Cashman JD, Eaves CJ, Sarris AH, Eaves AC: MCP-1, not MIP-1α is the endogenous chemokine that cooperates with TGF-β to inhibit the cycling of primitive normal but not leukemic (CML) progenitors in long-term human marrow cultures. *Blood* 92:2338, 1998.

107. Murohashi I, Endho K, Nishida S, et al: Differential effects of TGF-beta 1 on normal and leukemic human hematopoietic cell proliferation. *Exp Hematol* 23:970, 1995.

108. Gordon MY, Dowding C, Riley G, et al: Altered adhesive interactions with marrow stroma of haematopoietic progenitor cells in chronic myeloid leukaemia. *Nature* 328:342, 1987.

109. Dowding C, Guo A-P, Osterholz J, et al: Interferon-α overrides the deficient adhesion of chronic myeloid leukemia primitive progenitor cells to bone marrow stromal cells. *Blood* 78:499, 1991.

110. Bhatia R, Wayner EA, McGlave PB, Verfaillie CM: Interferon-α restores normal adhesion of chronic myelogenous leukemia hematopoietic progenitors to bone marrow stroma by correcting impaired β1 integrin receptor function. *J Clin Invest* 94:384, 1994.

111. Verfaillie CM: Stem cells in chronic myelogenous leukemia. *Hematol Oncol Clin North Am* 11:1079, 1997.

112. Bhatia R, Munthe HA, Verfaillie CM: Tyrphostin AG957, a tyrosine kinase inhibitor with anti-BCR/ABL tyrosine activity restores β1 integrin-mediated adhesion and inhibiting signaling in chronic myelogenous leukemia hematopoietic progenitors. *Leukemia* 12:1708, 1998.

113. Lundell BI, McCarthy JB, Kovach NL, Verfaillie CM: Activation of beta1 integrins on CML progenitors reveals cooperation between beta1 integrins and CD44 in the regulation of adhesion and proliferation. *Leukemia* 11:822, 1997.

114. Ghaffari S, Dougherty GJ, Eaves AC, Eaves CJ: Altered patterns of CD44 epitope expression in human chronic and acute myeloid leukemia. *Leukemia* 10:1773, 1996.

115. Vijayan KV, Advani SH, Zingde SM: Chronic myeloid leukemic granulocytes exhibit reduced and altered binding to P-selectin; modification in the CD15 antigens and sialyation. *Leuk Res* 21:59–65, 1997.

116. Verfaillie CM, Hurley R, Lundell BI, et al: Integrin-mediated regulation of hematopoiesis: do BCR/ABL-induced defects in integrin function underlie the abnormal circulation and proliferation of CML progenitors? *Acta Haematol* 29:40, 1997.

117. Symington BE: Growth signalling through the alpha 5 beta 1 fibronectin receptor. *Biochem Biophys Res Commun* 208:126, 1995.

118. Bhatia R, McCarthy JB, Verfaillie CM: Interferon-alpha restores normal beta 1 integrin-mediated inhibition of hematopoietic progenitor proliferation by the marrow microenvironment in chronic myelogenous leukemia. *Blood* 87:3883, 1996.

119. Salgia R, Li JL, Ewaniuk DS, et al: BCR/ABL induces multiple abnormalities of cytoskeletal function. *J Clin Invest* 100:46, 1997.

120. Lewis JM, Baskaran R, Taagepera S, et al: Integrin regulation of c-ABL tyrosine kinase activity and cytoplasmic-nuclear transport. *Proc Natl Acad Sci* 93:15174, 1996.

121. Renshaw MW, McWhirter JR, Wang JY. The human leukemia oncogene bcr-abl abrogates the anchorage requirement but not the growth factor requirement for proliferation. *Mol Cell Biol* 15:1286, 1995.

122. Salgia R, Brunkhorst B, Pisick E, et al: Increased tyrosine phosphorylation of focal adhesion proteins in myeloid cell lines expressing p210BCR/ABL. *Oncogene* 11:1149, 1995.

123. Rudkin GT, Hungerford DA, Nowell PC: DNA content of chromosome Ph¹ and chromosome 21 in human chronic granulocytic leukemia. *Science* 144:1229, 1964.

124. O'Riordan ML, Robinson JA, Buckton KE, Evans HJ: Distinguishing between the chromosome involved in Down's syndrome (trisomy 21) and chronic myeloid leukaemia (Ph¹) by fluorescence. *Nature* 230:167, 1971.

125. Lawler SD: The cytogenetics of chronic granulocytic leukemia. *Clin Haematol* 6:55, 1977.

126. Melo JV, Yan XH, Diamond J, Goldman JM: Balanced parental contribution to the ABL component of the BCR-ABL gene in chronic myeloid leukemia. *Leukemia* 9:734, 1995.

127. Chissoe SL, Bodenteich A, Wang YF, et al: Sequence and analysis of the human ABL gene, the BCR gene, and regions involved in the Philadelphia chromosomal translocation. *Genomics* 27:67, 1995.

128. Melo JV: The molecular biology of chronic myeloid leukaemia. *Leukemia* 10:751, 1996.

129. Daley GQ, Beu Neriah Y: Implicating the bcr/abl gene in the pathogenesis of Philadelphia chromosome-positive human leukemia. *Adv Cancer Res* 57:151, 1991.

130. Heisterkamp N, Groffen J, Stephenson JR, et al: Chromosomal localization of human cellular homologues of two viral oncogenes. *Nature* 299:747, 1982.

131. Heisterkamp N, Stephenson JR, Groffen J, et al: Localization of the c-abl oncogene adjacent to a translocation breakpoint in chronic myelocytic leukemia. *Nature* 306:239, 1983.

132. Konopka JB, Witte ON: Activation of the abl oncogene in murine and human leukemias. *Biochem Biophys Acta* 823:1, 1985.

133. Collins SJ, Groudine MT: Rearrangements and amplification of c-abl sequences in the human chronic myelogenous leukemia cell line K562. *Proc Natl Acad Sci USA* 80:4813, 1983.

134. Canaani E, Gale RP, Steiner-Seltz D, et al: Altered transcription of an oncogene in chronic myelocytic leukemia. *Lancet* 1:593, 1984.

135. Gale RP, Canaani E: An 8 kilobase abl RNA transcript in chronic myelogenous leukemia. *Proc Natl Acad Sci USA* 81:5648, 1984.

136. Collins SJ, Kubonishi I, Miyoshi I, Groudine MT: Altered transcription of the c-abl oncogene in K562 and other chronic myelogenous leukemia cells. *Science* 225:72, 1984.

137. Leibowitz D, Cubbon RM, Bank A: Increased expression of a novel c-abl related RNA in K562 cells. *Blood* 65:526, 1985.

138. Konopka JB, Watanabe SM, Witte ON: An alteration of the human c-abl protein in K562 leukemia cells unmasks associated tyrosine kinase activity. *Cell* 37:1035, 1984.

139. Konopka JB, Watanabe SM, Singer JW, et al: Cell lines and clinical isolates derived from Ph^1-positive chronic myelogenous leukemia patients express c-abl proteins with a common structural alteration. *Proc Natl Acad Sci USA* 82:1810, 1985.

140. Stam K, Heisterkamp N, Grosveld G, et al: Evidence of a new chimeric bcr/c-abl mRNA in patients with chronic myelocytic leukemia and the Philadelphia chromosome. *N Engl J Med* 313:1429, 1985.

141. Ben-Neriah Y, Daley GQ, Mes-Masson A-M, et al: The chronic myelogenous leukemia-specific P210 protein is the product of the bcr/abl hybrid gene. *Science* 233:212, 1985.

142. Maxwell SA, Kurzrock R, Parson SJ, et al: Analysis of P210$^{bcr/abl}$ tyrosine protein kinase activity in various subtypes of Philadelphia chromosome-positive cells from chronic myelogenous leukemia patients. *Cancer Res* 47:1731, 1987.

143. Kurzrock R, Kloetzer WS, Talpaz M, et al: Identification of molecular variants of P210$^{bcr-abl}$ in chronic myelogenous leukemia. *Blood* 70:233, 1987.

144. Xu DQ, Galibert F: Restriction fragment length polymorphism caused by a deletion within the human c-abl gene (ABL). *Proc Natl Acad Sci USA* 83:3447, 1986.

145. Popenoe DW, Schaefer-Rego K, Mears JC, et al: Frequent and extensive deletion during the 9,22 translocation in CML. *Blood* 68:1123, 1986.

146. Shtivelman E, Gale RP, Dreazen O, et al: bcr-abl RNA in patients with chronic granulocytic leukemia. *Blood* 69:971, 1987.

147. McWhirter JR, Wang JJ: Activation of tyrosine kinase and microfilament-binding functions of c-abl by bcr sequences in bcr/abl fusion proteins. *Mol Cell Biol* 11:1553, 1991.

148. Bernards A, Rubin CM, Westbrook CA, et al: The first intron in the human c-abl gene is at least 200 kilobases long and is the target for translocations in chronic myelogenous leukemia. *Mol Cell Biol* 7:3231, 1987.

149. Eisenberg A, Silver R, Soper L, et al: The location of breakpoints within the breakpoint cluster region (bcr) of chromosome 22 in chronic myeloid leukemia. *Leukemia* 2:642, 1988.

150. Collins SJ: Breakpoints on chromosome 9 and 22 in Philadelphia chromosome-positive chronic myelogenous leukemia. *J Clin Invest* 78:1392, 1986.

151. Heisterkamp N, Stam K, Groffen J, et al: Structural organization of the bcr gene and its role in the Ph^1 translocation. *Nature* 315:758, 1985.

152. Gao L-M, Goldman J: Long-range mapping of the normal BCR gene. *Leukemia* 5:555, 1991.

153. Melo JV: BCR-ABL gene variants. *Baillieres Clin Haematol* 10:203, 1997.

154. Saglio G, Pane F, Gottardi E, et al: Consistent amounts of acute leukemia-associated P190BCR/ABL transcripts are expressed by chronic myelogenous leukemia patients at diagnosis. *Blood* 87:1075, 1996.

155. Honda H, Oda H, Suzuki T, et al: Development of acute lymphoblastic leukemia and myeloproliferative disorder in transgenic mice expressing p210bcr/abl: a novel transgenic model for human Ph1-positive leukemias. *Blood* 91:2067, 1998.

156. Maru Y, Witte ON: The BCR gene encodes a novel serine/threonine kinase activity within a single exon. *Cell* 67:459, 1991.

157. Muller AJ, Young JC, Pendergast A-M, et al: BCR first exon sequences specifically activate the BCR/ABL tyrosine kinase oncogene of Philadelphia chromosome-positive human leukemia. *Mol Cell Biol* 11:1785, 1991.

158. Diekmann D, Brill S, Garrett MD, et al: BCR encodes a GTPase-activating protein for p21^{rac}. *Nature* 351:400, 1991.

159. Melo JV, Gordon DE, Goldman JM: The ABL-BCR fusion gene is expressed in chronic myeloid leukemia. *Blood* 81:158, 1993.

160. Bartram CR, deKlein A, Hagemeijer A, et al: Translocation of the human c-abl oncogene correlates with the presence of a Philadelphia chromosome in chronic myelocytic leukaemia. *Nature* 306:277, 1983.

161. Selleri L, Narni F, Emilia G, et al: Philadelphia-positive chronic myeloid leukemia with a chromosome 22 breakpoint outside the breakpoint cluster region. *Blood* 70:1659, 1987.

162. Mohamed AN, Koppitch F, Varterasian M, et al: BCR/ABL fusion located on chromosome 9 in chronic myeloid leukemia with a masked Ph chromosome. *Genes Chromosom Cancer* 13:133, 1995.

163. Morris C, Jeffs A, Smith T, et al: BCR gene recombines with genomically distinct sites on band 11Q13 in complex BCR-ABL translocations of chronic myeloid leukemia. *Oncogene* 12:677, 1996.

164. Andreasson P Johansson B, Carlsson M, et al: BCR/ABL-negative chronic myeloid leukemia with ETV6/ABL fusion. *Genes Chromosom Cancer* 20:299, 1997.

165. Rozman C, Urbano-Ispizua A, Cervantes F, et al: Analysis of the clinical relevance of the breakpoint location within M-BCR and the type of chimeric mRNA in chronic myelogenous leukemia. *Leukemia* 9:1104, 1995.

166. Verschraegen CF, Kantarjian HM, Hirsch-Ginsberg C, et al: The breakpoint cluster region site in patients with Philadelphia chromosome-positive chronic myelogenous leukemia. Clincial, laboratory, and prognostic correlations. *Cancer* 76:992, 1995.

167. Zaccaria A, Martinelli G, Testoni N, et al: Does the type of BCR/ABL junction predict the survival of patients with Ph1-positive chronic myeloid leukemia? *Leuk Lymph* 16:231, 1995.

168. Ohno T, Hada S, Sugiyama T, et al: Chronic myeloid leukemia with minor bcr breakpoint developed hybrid type of blast crisis. *Am J Hematol* 57:320, 1998.

169. Melo JV: The diversity of BCR-ABL fusion proteins and their relationship to leukemia phenotype. *Blood* 88:2375, 1996.

170. Rubinstein R, Purves LR: A novel BCR-ABL rearrangement in a Philadelphia chromosome-positive chronic myelogenous leukaemia variant with thrombocythaemia. *Leukemia* 12:230, 1998.

171. Hochhaus A, Reither A, Skladny H, et al: A novel BCR-ABL fusion gene (e6a2) in a patient with Philadelphia chromosome-negative chronic myelogenous leukemia. *Blood* 88:2236, 1996.

172. Briz M, Vilches C, Cabrera R, et al: Typical chronic myelogenous leukemia with e19a2 junction BCR/ABL transcript. *Blood* 90:5024, 1997.

173. McLaughlin J, Chianese E, Witte ON: In vitro transformation of immature hemopoietic cells by P210 bcr/abl oncogene product of the Philadelphia chromosome. *Proc Natl Acad Sci USA* 84:6558, 1987.

174. Daley GQ, McLaughlin J, Witte ON, Baltimore D: The CML-specific P210 bcr/abl protein, unlike v-abl, does not transform NIH/3T3 fibroblasts. *Science* 237:532, 1987.

175. Elefanty AG, Hariharan IK, Cory S: bcr-abl, the hallmark of chronic myeloid leukaemia in man, induces multiple haemopoietic neoplasms in mice. *EMBO* 9:1069, 1990.

176. Daley GQ, VanEtten RA, Baltimore D: Induction of chronic myelogenous leukemia in mice by the p210$^{bcr/abl}$ gene of the Philadelphia chromosome. *Science* 247:824, 1990.

177. Voncken JW, Morris C, Pattengale P, et al: Clonal development and karyotype evolution during leukemogenesis of BCR/ABL transgenic mice. *Blood* 79:1029, 1992.

178. Gishizky ML, Johnson-White J, Witte O: Efficient transplantation of BCR-ABL-induced chronic myelogenous leukemia-like syndrome in mice. *Proc Natl Acad Sci USA* 90:3755, 1993.

179. Daley GQ: Animal models of BCR/ABL-induced leukemias. *Leuk Lymphoma* 11:57, 1993.

180. Voncken JW, Kaartinen V, Pattengale PK, et al: BCR/ABL P210 and P190 cause distinct leukemia in transgeneic mice. *Blood* 86:4603, 1995.

181. Honda H, Oda H, Suzuki T, et al: Development of acute lymphoblastic leukemia and myeloproliferative disorder in transgenic mice expressing p210bcr/abl: a novel transgenic model for human Ph1-positive leukemias. *Blood* 91:2067, 1998.

182. Pear WS, Miller JP, Xu L, et al: Efficient and rapid induction of a chronic myelogenous leukemia-like myeloproliferative disease in mice receiving P210 bcr/abl-transduced bone marrow. *Blood* 92:3780, 1998.

183. Honda M, Ohno S, Takahashi T, et al: Establishment, characterization, and chromosomal analysis of new leukemic cell lines derived from MT/p210/bcr/abl transgenic mice. *Exp Hematol* 26:188, 1998.

184. Zhang X, Ren R: Bcr-Abl efficiency induces in a myeloproliferative

disease and production of excess interleuken-3 and granulocyte-macrophage colony-stimulating factor in mice: a novel model for chronic myelogenous leukemia. *Blood* 92:3829, 1998.

185. Elefanty AG, Corsy S: *bcr-abl*-induced cell lines can switch from mast cell to erythroid or myeloid differentiation in vitro. *Blood* 79:1271, 1992.

186. Bose S, Deininger M, Goora-Tybor J, et al: The presence of typical and atypical BCR-ABL fusion genes in leukocytes of normal individuals: biological significance and implications for the assessment of minimal residual disease. *Blood* 92:3362, 1998.

187. Biernaux C, Loss M, Sels A, et al: Detection of major bcr-abl gene expression at a very low level in blood of some healthy individuals. *Blood* 86:3118, 1995.

188. Hirai HS, Tanaka M, Azuma Y, et al: Transforming genes in human leukemia cells. *Blood* 66:1371, 1985.

189. Clarkson BD, Strife A, Wisniewski D, et al: New understanding of the pathogenesis of CML: A prototype of early neoplasia. *Leukemia* 11:1404, 1997.

190. Verfaillie CM: Chronic myelogenous leukemia: from pathogenesis to therapy. *J Hemotherap* 8:3, 1999.

191. Pasternak G, Hochhaus A, Schultheis B, Hehlmann R: Chronic myelogenous leukemia: molecular and cellular aspects. *J Cancer Res Clin Oncol* 124:643, 1998.

192. Gotoh A, Broxmeyer HE: The function of BCR/ABL and related proto-oncogenes. *Curr Opin Hematol* 4:3, 1997.

193. Sattler M, Salgi AR: Activation of hematopoietic growth factor signal transduction pathways by the human oncogene BCR/ABL. *Cytokine Growth Factor Rev* 8:63, 1997.

194. Skorski T, Kanakaraj P, Nieborowska-Skorska M, et al: Phosphatidylinositol-3 kinase activity is regulated by BCR/ABL and is required for the growth of Philadelphia chromosome-positive cells. *Blood* 86:726, 1995.

195. Skorski T, Nieborowska--Skorska M, Szczylik C, et al: C-RAF-1 serine/threonine kinase is required in BCR/ABL-dependent and normal hematopoiesis. *Cancer Research* 55:2275, 1995.

196. Goga A, McLaughlin J, Afar DE, et al: Alternative signals to RAS for hematopoietic transformation by the BCR-ABL oncogene. *Cell* 82:981, 1995.

197. Salgia R, Uemura N, Okuda K, et al: CRKL links p210BCR/ABL with paxillin in chronic myelogenous leukemia cells. *J Biol Chem* 270:29145, 1995.

198. De Jong R, ten Hoeve J, Heisterkamp N, Groffen J: Crkl is complexed with tyrosine-phosphorylated Cbl in Ph-positive leukemia. *J Biol Chem* 270:21468, 1995.

199. Salgia R, Pisick E, Sattler M, et al: P130CAS forms a sginalling complex with the adapter protein CRKL in hematopoietic cells transformed by the BCR/ABL oncogene. *J Biol Chem* 271:25198, 1996.

200. Sattler M, Salgia R, Okuda K, et al: The proto-oncogene product p120^CBL and the adaptor proteins CRKL and c-CR link c-ABL, p190BCR/ABL and p210BCR/ABL to the phosphatidylinositol-3; kinase pathway. *Oncogene* 12:832, 1996.

201. Salgia R, Sattler M, Pisick E, et al: P210BCR/ABL induces formation of complexes containing focal adhesion proteins and the protooncogene product p120c-CBL. *Exp Hematol* 24:310, 1996.

202. De Jong R, van Wijk A, Haataja L, et al: BCR/ABL-induced leukemogenesis causes phosphorylation of Hef2 and its association with Crkl. *J Biol Chem* 272:32649, 1997.

203. Bollag G, Clapp DW, Shih S, et al: Loss of NF1 results in activation of the Ras signaling pathway and leads to aberrant growth in haematopoietic cells. *Nature Genet* 12:144, 1996.

204. Carpino N, Wisniewski D, Strife A, et al: p62dok: a constitutively tyrosine-phosphorylated, GAP-associated protein in chronic myelogneous leukemia progenitor cells. *Cell* 88:197, 1997.

205. Yamanashi Y, Baltimore D: Identification of the Abl-and ras GAP-associated 62 kDa protein as a docking protein, Dok. *Cell* 88:205, 1997.

206. Reuther JY, Reuther GW, Cortez D, et al: A requirement for NF-kappaB activation in BCR/ABL-mediated transformation. *Genes Dev* 1:12:968, 1998.

207. LaMontagne KR, Flint AJ, Franza BR, et al: Protein tyrosine phosphatase 1B antagonizes signalling by oncoprotein tyrosine kinase p210 bcr/abl in vivo. *Mol Cell Biol* 18:2965, 1998.

208. Chai SK, Nichols GL, Rothman P: Constitutive activation of JAKs and STATs in BCR-abl-expressing cell lines and peripheral blood cells derived from leukemic patients. *J Immunol* 159:4720, 1997.

209. Shuai K, Halpern J, ten Hoeve J, et al: Constitutive activation of STAT5 by the BCR-ABL oncogene in chronic myelogenous leukemia. *Oncogene* 13:247, 1996.

210. Wilson-Rawls J, Xie S, Liu J, et al: P210 Bcr-Abl interacts with the interleukin 3 receptor beta (c) subunit and constitutively induces its tyrosine phosphorylation. *Cancer Res* 56:3426, 1996.

211. Chuang TH, Xu X, Kaartinen V, et al: Abl and Bcr are multifunctional regulators of the Rho GTP-bindng protein family. *Proc Natl Acad Sci* 92:10282, 1995.

212. Afar DE, Witte O: Characterization of breakpoint cluster region kinase and SH2-binding activites. *Methods Enzymol* 256:125, 1995.

213. Gishizky ML, Cortez D, Pendergast AM: Mutant forms of growth factor-binding protein-2 reverse BCR-ABL-induced transformation. *Proc Natl Acad Sci USA* 92:10889, 1995.

214. Raitano AB, Halpern JR, Hambuch TM, Sawyers CL: The Bcr-Abl leukemia oncogene activates Jun kinase and requires Jun for transformation. *Proc Natl Acad Sci* 92:11746, 1995.

215. Miyamura T, Nishimuar J, Yufu Y, Nawata H: Interaction of Bcr-Abl with the retinoblastoma protein in Philadelphia chromosome-positive cell lines. *Int J Hematol* 67:115, 1997.

216. Largaespada DA, Brannan CI, Jenkins NA, Copeland NG: NF1 deficiency causes Ras-mediated granulocyte/macrophage colony stimulating factor hypersensitivity and chronic myeloid leukaemia. *Nature Genet* 12:137, 1996.

217. Amos TA, Lewis JL, Grand FH, et al: Apoptosis in chronic myeloid leukaemia: normal responses by progenitor cells to growth factor deprivation, X-irradiation and glucocorticoids. *Br J Haematol* 91:387, 1995.

218. Bedi A, Barber JP, Bedi GC, et al: BCR-ABL-mediated inhibition of apoptosis with delay of G2/M transition after DNA damage: a mechanism of resistance to multiple anticancer agents. *Blood* 86:1148, 1995.

219. Amarante-Mendes GP, Naekyung KC, Liu L, et al: Bcr-Abl exerts its antiapoptotic effect against diverse apoptotic stimuli through blockage of mitochondrial release of cytochrome C and activation of caspase-3. *Blood* 92:1700, 1998.

220. Maguer-Satta V, Burl S, Liu L, et al: C. BCR-ABL accelerates C2-ceramide-induced apoptosis. *Oncogene* 16:237, 1998.

221. Pierson BA, Miller JS: CD56+bright and CD56+dim natural killer cells in patients with chronic myelogenous leukemia progressively decrease in number, respond less to stimuli that recruit clonogenic natural killer cells, and exhibit decreased proliferation on a per cell basis. *Blood* 88:2279, 1996.

222. Gissinger H, Kurzrock R, Wetzler M, et al: Apoptosis in chronic myelogenous leukemia: studies of stage-specific differences. *Leuk Lymphoma* 25:121, 1997.

223. Doolittle RF, Hienkapiller MW, Hood LE, et al: Simian sarcoma virus oncogene, v-sis, is derived from the gene (or genes) encoding a platelet-derived growth factor. *Science* 221:275, 1983.

224. Dalla-Favera R, Gallo RC, Giallongo A, Croce C: Chromosomal localization of the human homolog (c-sis) of the simian sarcoma virus onc gene. *Science* 218:686, 1982.

225. Bartram CR, deKlein A, Hagemeijer A, et al: Localization of the c-sis oncogene in Ph¹ positive and Ph¹ negative chronic myelogenous leukemia by in situ hybridization. *Blood* 63:223, 1984.

226. Waterfield MD, Scarce GT, Whittle N, et al: Platelet derived growth factor is structurally related to the putative transforming protein P28sis of simian sarcoma virus. *Nature* 304:35, 1983.

227. Joseph SF, Ratner L, Clark MF, et al: Transforming potential of human c-sis nucleotide sequences encoding platelet derived growth factor. *Science* 225:636, 1984.

228. Romero P, Blick M, Talpaz M, et al: C-sis and c-abl expression in chronic myelogenous leukemia and other hematologic malignancies. *Blood* 67:839, 1986.

229. Iwama H, Ohyashiki K, Ohyashiki JH, et al: The relationship between telomere length and therapy-associated cytogenetic resposnes in patients with chronic myeloid leukemia. *Cancer* 79:1552, 1997.

230. Ohyashiki K, Ohyashiki JH, Iwama H, et al: Telomerase activity and cytogenetic changes in chronic myeloid leukemia with disease progression. *Leukemia* 11:190, 1997.

231. Selvin S, Levin LI, Merrill DW, Winkelstein W Jr: Selected epidemiologic observations of cell-specific leukemia mortality in the United States, 1969–1977. *Am J Epidemiol* 117:140, 1983.

232. Thompson RB, Stainsby D: The clinical and haematological features of chronic granulocytic leukaemia in the chronic phase, in *Chronic Granulocytic Leukaemia,* edited by MT Shaw, pp 137–167. Praeger, East Sussex, UK, 1982.

233. Cortes JE, Talpaz M, Kantarkian H: Chronic myelogenous leukemia: a review. *Am J Med* 100:555, 1996.

234. Goldman JM: Chronic myeloid leukemia. *Curr Opin Hematol* 4:277, 1997.

235. Lichtman MA, Rowe JM: Hyperleukocytic leukemias: rheological, clinical and therapeutic considerations. *Blood* 60:279, 1982.

236. Rowe JM, Lichtman MA: Hyperleukocytosis and leukostasis: common features of childhood chronic myelogenous leukemia. *Blood* 63:1230, 1984.

237. Lichtman MA, Heal J, Rowe JM: Hyperleukocytic leukaemia. *Baillieres Clin Haematol* 1:725, 1987.

238. Ungaro PC, Gonzalez JJ, Werk EE, MacKay JC: Chronic myelogenous leukemia presenting clinically as diabetes insipidus. *N C Med J* 45:640, 1984.

239. Juan D, Hsu S-D, Hunter J: Case report of vasopressin-responsive diabetes insipidus associated with chronic myelogenous leukemia. *Cancer* 56:1468, 1985.

240. Brydon J, Lucky PA, Duffy T: Acne urticaria associated with chronic myelogenous leukemia. *Cancer* 56:2083, 1985.

241. Cohen PR, Talpaz M, Kurzrock R: Malignancy-associated Sweet's syndrome: a review of the world's literature. *J Clin Oncol* 6:1887, 1988.

242. López JLB, Fonseca E, Mauso F: Sweet's syndrome during the chronic phase of chronic myeloid leukemia. *Acta Haematol* 84:207, 1990.

243. Nestok BR, Goldstein JD, Lipkovic P: Splenic rupture as a cause of sudden death in undiagnosed chronic myelogenous leukemia. *Am J Forensic Med Pathol* 9:241, 1988.

244. Giagounidis AAN, Burk M, Meckenstock G, et al: Pathological rupture of the spleen in hematologic malignancies. *Ann Hematol* 73:297, 1996.

245. Hild DH, Myers TJ: Hyperviscosity in chronic granulocytic leukemia. *Cancer* 46:1418, 1980.

246. D'Hondt L, Guillaume TH, Hemblit Y, Symann M: Digital necrosis associated with chronic myeloid leukemia. *Acta Clin Belgica* 52:49, 1997.

247. Arbaje YM, Betran G: Chronic myelogenous leukemia complicated by autoimmune hemolytic anemia. *Am J Med* 88:197, 1990.

248. Steegman JL, Pinilla I, Requena MJ, et al: The direct antiglobulin test is frequently positive in chronic myeloid leukemia patients treated with interferon-α. *Transfusion* 37:446, 1997.

249. Hoppin EC, Lewis JP: Polycythemia rubra vera progressing to Ph¹-positive chronic myelogenous leukemia. *Ann Intern Med* 83:820, 1975.

250. Shenkenberg TD, Waddell CC, Rice L: Erythrocytosis and marked leukocytosis in overlapping myeloproliferative diseases. *South Med J* 75:868, 1982.

251. Haas O, Hinterberger W, Morz R: Pure red cell aplasia as possible early manifestation of chronic myeloid leukemia. *Am J Hematol* 27:20, 1986.

252. Mijovic A, Rolovic Z, Novak A, et al: Chronic myeloid leukemia associated with pure red cell aplasia and terminating in promyelocytic transformation. *Am J Hematol* 31:128, 1989.

253. Inbal A, Aktein E, Barak I, Meytes D: Cyclic leukocytosis and long survival in chronic myeloid leukemia. *Acta Haematol* 69:353, 1983.

254. Umemura T, Hirata J, Kaneko S, et al: Periodic appearance of erythropoietin-independent erythropoiesis in chronic myelogenous leukemia with cyclic oscillation. *Acta Haematol* 76:230, 1986.

255. Mitus WJ, Kiossoglou KA: Leukocyte alkaline phosphatase in myeloproliferative syndrome. *Ann NY Acad Sci* 155:976, 1968.

256. DePalma L, Delgado P, Werner M: Diagnostic discrimination and cost-effective assay strategy for leukocyte alkaline phosphate. *Clin Chim Acta* 6:83, 1996.

257. Pedersen F: Functional and biochemical phenotype in relation to cellular age of differentiated neutrophils in chronic myeloid leukemia. *Br J Haematol* 51:339, 1982.

258. Rambaldi A, Terao M, Bettoni S, et al: Differences in the expression of alkaline phosphatase in mRNA in chronic myelogenous leukemia and paroxysmal nocturnal hemoglobinuria polymorphonuclear leukocytes. *Blood* 73:1113, 1989.

259. Perillie PE: Studies of the changes in leukocyte alkaline phosphatase following pyrogen stimulation in chronic granulocytic leukemia. *Blood* 29:401, 1967.

260. Rustin GJS, Goldman JM, McCarthy D, et al: An extracellular factor controls neutrophil alkaline phosphatase in chronic granulocytic leukemia. *Br J Haematol* 45:381, 1980.

261. Matsuo T: In vitro modulation of alkaline phosphatase activity in neutrophils from patients with chronic myelogenous leukemia by monocyte-derived activity. *Blood* 67:492, 1986.

262. Tanaka KR, Valentine WN, Fredricks RE: Diseases or clinical conditions associated with low leukocyte alkaline phosphatase. *N Engl J Med* 262:912, 1960.

263. Stinson RA, McPhee J, Lewanczk R, Dinwoodie A: Neutrophil alkaline phosphatase in hypophosphatasia. *N Engl J Med* 312:1642, 1985.

264. Gruenwald H, Kiossoglou KA, Mitus WJ, Dameshek W: Philadelphia chromosome in eosinophilic leukemia. *Am J Med* 39:1003, 1965.

265. Kiossoglou KA, Mitus WJ, Dameshek W: Cytogenetic studies in the chronic myeloproliferative syndrome. *Blood* 28:241, 1966.

266. Elves MW, Israels MCG: Cytogenetic studies in unusual forms of chronic myeloid leukemia. *Acta Haematol* 38:129, 1967.

267. Chusid MJ, Dale DC, West BC, Wolff SM: The hypereosinophilic syndrome: analysis of fourteen cases with review of the literature. *Medicine* 54:1, 1975.

268. Kamada N, Uchino H: Chronologic sequence in appearance of clinical and laboratory findings characteristic of chronic myelocytic leukemia. *Blood* 51:843, 1978.

269. Denberg JA, Wilson WEC, Goodacre R, Brenenstock J: Chronic myeloid leukemia—evidence for basophil differentiation and histamine synthesis from cultured peripheral blood cells. *Br J Haematol* 45:13, 1980.

270. Goh K-O, Anderson FW: Cytogenetic studies in basophilic chronic myelocytic leukemia. *Arch Pathol Lab Med* 103:288, 1979.

271. Youman JD, Taddeini L, Cooper T: Histamine excess symptoms in basophilic chronic granulocytic leukemia. *Arch Intern Med* 131:560, 1973.

272. Rosenthal S, Schwartz JH, Canellos GP: Basophilic chronic granulocytic leukemia with hyperhistaminemia. *Br J Haematol* 36:367, 1977.

273. Weil SC, Hrisinko MA: A hybrid eosinophilic-basophilic granulocyte in chronic granulocytic leukemia. *Am J Clin Pathol* 87:66, 1987.

274. Velardi A, Rambotti P, Cernetti C, et al: Monoclonal antibody defined T-cell phenotypes and phytohemagglutinin reactivity of E-rosette forming circulating lymphocytes from untreated chronic myelocyte leukemia patients. *Cancer* 53:913, 1984.

275. Dowding C, Th'ng KH, Goldman JM, Galton DAG: Increased T-lymphocyte numbers in chronic granulocytic leukemia before treatment. *Exp Hematol* 12:811, 1984.

276. Kaur J, Catovsky D, Spiers ASD, Galton DAG: Increase of T-lymphocytes in the spleen in chronic granulocytic leukaemia. *Lancet* 1:834, 1974.

277. Fujimiya Y, Bakke A, Chang WC, et al: Natural killer-cell immunodeficiency in patients with chronic myelogenous leukemia. *Int J Cancer* 37:639, 1986.

278. Fujimiya Y, Chang WC, Bakke A, et al: Natural killer cell immunodeficiency in patients with chronic myelogenous leukemia. *Cancer Immunol Immunother* 24:213, 1987.

279. Pierson BA, Miller JS: The role of autologous natural killer cells in chronic myelogenous leukemia. *Leukemia* 11:1404, 1997.

280. Mason JE, DeVita VT, Canellos GP: Thrombocytosis in chronic granulocytic leukemia: incidence and clinical significance. *Blood* 44:483, 1974.

281. Pederson B: Kinetics and cell function, in *Chronic Granulocytic Leukaemia,* edited by MT Shaw, pp 93–135. Praeger, East Sussex, UK, 1982.

282. Radhika V, Thennarasu S, Naik NR, et al: Granulocytes from chronic myeloid leukemia (CML) patients show differential response to different chemoattractments. *Am J Hematol* 52:155, 1996.

283. Kasimir-Bauer S, Ottinger H, Brittinger G, König W: Philadelphia chromosome-positive chronic myelogenous leukemia: functional defects in circulating mature neutrophils of untreated and interferon-α-treated patients. *Exp Hematol* 22:426, 1994.

284. Adams T, Schultz L, Goldberg L: Platelet function abnormalities in the myeloproliferative disorders. *Scand J Haematol* 13:215, 1974.

285. Gerrard JM, Stoddard SF, Shapiro RS, et al: Platelet storage pool deficiency and prostaglandin synthesis in chronic granulocytic leukaemia. *Br J Haematol* 40:597, 1978.

286. Knox WF, Bhavani M, Davson J, Geary CG: Histological classification of chronic granulocytic leukaemia. *Clin Lab Haematol* 6:171, 1984.

287. Lorand-Metze I, Vassalo J, Souza CA: Histological and cytological heterogeneity of bone marrow in Philadelphia-positive chronic myelogenous leukaemia at diagnosis. *Br J Haematol* 67:45, 1987.

288. Kelsey PR, Geary CG: Sea-blue histiocytes and Gaucher's cells in bone marrow of patients with chronic myeloid leukaemia. *J Clin Path* 41:960, 1988.

289. Dezmezian R, Kantarjian HM, Keating MJ, et al: The relevance of reticulin stain-measured fibrosis at diagnosis in chronic myelogenous leukemia. *Cancer* 59:1739, 1987.

290. Ghosh K, Varma N, Varma S, Dash S: Cellular composition and reticulin fibrosis in chronic myeloid leukaemia. *Indian J Cancer* 25:128, 1988.

291. Buhr T, Choritz H, Georgü A: The impact of megakaryocyte proliferation for the evolution of myelofibrosis. *Virchows Archiv A Pathol Anat* 420:473, 1992.

292. Udomsakdi C, Eaves CJ, Lansdorp PM, Eaves AC: Phenotypic heterogeneity of primitive leukemic hematopoietic cells in patients with chronic myeloid leukemia. *Blood* 80:2522, 1992.

293. Huret JL: Complex translocations, simple variant translocation and Ph-negative cases in chronic myelogenous leukaemia. *Hum Genet* 85:565, 1990.

294. Sakurai M, Sandberg AA: The chromosomes and causation of human cancer and leukemia: XVIII. The missing Y in acute myeloblastic leukemia (AML) and Ph¹-positive chronic myelocytic leukemia. *Cancer* 38:762, 1976.

295. Berger R, Bernheim A: Y chromosome loss in leukemias. *Cancer Genet Cytogenet* 1:1, 1979.

296. Ishihara T, Sasaki M, Oshimura M, et al: A summary of cytogenetic studies on 534 cases of chronic myelogenous leukemia in Japan. *Cancer Genet Cytogenet* 9:81, 1983.

297. Mitelman F: Catalogue of chromosomal aberrations in cancer. *Cytogenet Cell Genet* 36:9, 1983.

298. Heim S, Billstrom R, Kristoffersson U, et al: Variant Ph translocations in chronic myeloid leukemia. *Cancer Genet Cytogenet* 18:215, 1985.

299. Bartram CR, Anger B, Carbonell F, Kleihauer E: Involvement of chromosome 9 in variant Ph¹ translocation. *Leuk Res* 9:1133, 1985.

300. Morris CM, Rosman I, Archer SA, et al: A cytogenetic and molecular analysis of five variant Philadelphia translocations in chronic myeloid leukemia. *Cancer Genet Cytogenet* 35:179, 1988.

301. Teyssier JR, Bartram CR, DeVille J, et al: c-abl oncogene and chromosome 22 "bcr" juxtaposition in chronic myelogenous leukemia. *N Engl J Med* 312:1393, 1985.

302. Hagemeijer A, Bartram CR, Smith EME, et al: Is the chromosomal region 9q34 always involved in variants of the Ph¹ translocation? *Cancer Genet Cytogenet* 13:1, 1984.

303. DeBraikeleer M, Chiu H-K, Fiser J, Gardner HA: A further case of Philadelphia chromosome-positive chronic myeloid leukemia with t(3;9;22). *Cancer Genet Cytogenet* 35:279, 1988.

304. Latoge-Pochitaloff-Huvalé M, Sainty D, Adriaansen HJ, et al: Translocation (3;21) in Philadelphia positive chronic myeloid leukemia. *Leukemia* 3:554, 1989.

305. Thompson PW, Whittaker JA: Translocation 3;21 in Philadelphia chromosome positive chronic myeloid leukemia at diagnosis. *Cancer* 39:143, 1989.

306. Engel E, McGee BJ, Flexner JM, et al: Philadelphia chromosome (Ph¹) translocation in an apparently Ph¹ negative, minus G22, case of chronic myeloid leukemia. *N Engl J Med* 291:154, 1974.

307. Verma RS, Dosik H: "Masked" Ph¹ chromosome in chronic myelogenous leukaemia (CML). *Blut* 50:129, 1985.

308. Hagemeijer A, deKlein A, Godde-Saltz E, et al: Translocation of c-abl to "masked" Ph in chronic myeloid leukemia. *Cancer Genet Cytogenet* 18:95, 1985.

309. Melo JV: The diversity of BCR-ABL fusion proteins and their relationship to leukemic phenotype. *Blood* 88:2375, 1996.

310. O'Brien S, Thall PR, Siciliano MJ: Cytogenetics of chronic myeloid leukemia. *Baillieres Clin Haematol* 10:259, 1997.

311. Bartram CR, Carbonell F: bcr rearrangement in Ph-negative CML. *Cancer Genet Cytogenet* 21:183, 1986.

312. Bartram CR: Rearrangement of bcr and c-abl sequences in Ph-positive acute leukemias and Ph-negative CML—an update. *Hematol Blood Transfus* 31:160, 1987.

313. Ganesan TS, Rassool F, Guo A-P, et al: Rearrangement of the bcr gene in Philadelphia-chromosome negative chronic myeloid leukemia. *Hematol Blood Transfus* 31:153, 1987.

314. Wiedemann LM, Karhi K, Chan LC: Similar molecular alterations occur in related leukemias with and without the Philadelphia chromosome. *Hematol Blood Transfus* 31:149, 1987.

315. Benn P, Loper L, Eisenberg A, et al: Utility of molecular genetic analysis of bcr rearrangement in the diagnosis of chronic myeloid leukemia. *Cancer Genet Cytogenet* 29:1, 1987.

316. Epner DE, Koeffler AP: Molecular genetic advances in chronic myelogenous leukemia. *Ann Intern Med* 113:3, 1990.

317. Dubé I, Dixon J, Beckett T, et al: Location of breakpoints within the major breakpoint cluster region (bcr) in 33 patients with bcr rearrangement-positive chronic myeloid leukemia with complex or absent Philadelphia chromosomes. *Genes Chromosom Cancer* 1:106, 1989.

318. Morris C, Heisterkamp N, Kennedy MA, et al: Ph-negative chronic myeloid leukemia: molecular analysis of ABL insertion into M-BCR on chromosome 22. *Blood* 76:1812, 1990.

319. Blennerhassett GT, Furth ME, Anderson A, et al: Clinical evaluation of DNA probe assay for the Philadelphia (Ph¹) translocation in chronic myelogenous leukemia. *Leukemia* 2:648, 1988.

320. Lange W, Snyder DS, Castro R, et al: Detection by enzymatic amplification of bcr-abl mRNA in peripheral blood and bone marrow cells of patients with chronic myelogenous leukemia. *Blood* 73:1735, 1989.

321. Dhingra K, Talpaz M, Riggs MC, et al: Hybridization protection assay: A rapid, sensitive, and specific method for detection of Philadelphia chromosome-positive leukemias. *Blood* 77:238, 1991.

322. Gaiger A, Henn T, Horth E, et al: Increase of bcr-abl chimeric mRNA expression in tumor cells of patients with chronic myeloid leukemia precedes disease progression. *Blood* 86:2371, 1995.

323. Stock W, Westbrook CA, Peterson B, et al: Value of molcular monitoring during the treatment of chronic myeloid leukemia: a Cancer and Leukemia Group B study. *J Clin Oncol* 15:26, 1997.

324. Frenoy N, Chabli A, Sol D, et al: Application of a new protocol for nested PCR to the detection of minimal residual bcr/abl transcripts. *Leukemia* 8:1411, 1994.

325. Melo JV, Yan XH, Diamond J, et al: Reverse transcription/polymerase chain reaction (RT/PCR) amplification of very small numbers of transcripts: the risk in misinterpreting negative results. *Leukemia* 10:1217, 1996.

326. Lin F, Chase A, Bunget J, et al: Correlation between the proportion of Philadelphia chromosome-positive metaphase cells and levels of BCR-ABL mRNA in chronic myeloid leukaemia. *Genes Chromosom Cancer* 13:110, 1995.

327. VanDenderen J, Hermans A, Meeuwsen T, et al: Antibody recognition of the tumor-specific bcr-abl joining region in chronic myeloid leukemia. *J Exp Med* 169:87, 1989.

328. Hagemeyer A, vanderPlas DC, Solkarman D, et al: The Philadelphia translocation in CML and ALL: Recent investigations, new detection methods. *Nouv Rev Fr Hematol* 32:83, 1990.

329. Maxwell SA, Kurzrock R, Parsons SJ, et al: Analysis of p210 bcr-abl tyrosine protein kinase activity in various subtypes of Philadelphia chromosome-positive cells from chronic myelogenous leukemia patients. *Cancer Res* 47:1731, 1987.

330. Guo JQ, Lian JY, Xian YM, et al: BCR-ABL protein expression in peripheral blood cells of chronic myelogenous leukemia patients undergoing therapy. *Blood* 83: 3629, 1994.

331. Dewald GW, Schad CR, Christensen ER, et al: The application of in situ flourescent hybridization to detect M bcr/abl fusion in variant Ph chromosomes in CML and ALL. *Cancer Genet Cytogenet* 71:7, 1993.

332. Cox MC, Maffei L, Buffolino S, et al: A comparative analysis of FISH, RT-PCR, and cytogenetics for the diagnosis of bcr-abl-positive leukemias. *Am J Clin Pathol* 109:24, 1998.

333. Sinclair PB, Green AR, Grace C, Nacheva EP: Improved sensitivity of BCR-ABL detection: a triple-probe three-color fluorescence in situ hybridization system. *Blood* 90:1395, 1997.

334. Acar H, Stewart J, Boyd E, Connor MJ: Identification of variant translocations in chronic myeloid leukemia by fluorescence in situ hybridization. *Cancer Genet Cytogenet* 93:115, 1997.

335. Werner M, Ewig M, Nasarek A, et al: Value of fluorescence in situ hyridization for detecting the bcr/abl gene fusion in interphase cells of routine bone marrow specimens. *Diagn Mol Pathol* 6:282, 1997.

336. Chase A, Grand F, Zhang JG, et al: Factors influencing the false positive

and negative rates of BCR-ABL fluorescence in situ hybridizaiton. *Genes Chromosom Cancer* 18:246, 1997.

337. Hochhaus A, Reiter A, Skladny H, et al: Molecular monitoring of residual disease in chronic myelogenous leukemia patients after therapy. *Recent Results Cancer Res* 144:36, 1998.

338. Wells SJ, Phillips CN, Winton EF, Farhi DC: Reverse transcriptase-polymerase chain reaction for bcr-abl fusion in chronic myelogenous leukemia. *Am J Clin Pathol* 105:756, 1996.

339. Cox MC, Maffei L, Buffolino S, et al: A comparative analysis of FISH, RT-PCR, and cytogenetics for the diagnosis of bcr-abl-positive leukemias. *Am J Clin Pathol* 109:24, 1998.

340. Krackoff IH: Studies of uric acid biosynthesis in the chronic leukemias. *Arthritis Rheum* 8:772, 1965.

341. Vogler WR, Bain JA, Huguley CM Jr, et al: Metabolic and therapeutic effects of allopurinol in patients with leukemia and gout. *Am J Med* 40:548, 1966.

342. Zittoun J, Marquet J, Zittoun R: The intracellular content of the three cobalamins at various stages of normal and leukaemic myeloid cell development. *Br J Haematol* 31:299, 1975.

343. Zittoun J, Zittoun R, Marquet J, Sultan C: The three transcobalamins in myeloproliferative disorders and acute leukemia. *Br J Haematol* 31:287, 1975.

344. Rosner F, Schreiber ZA: Serum vitamin B_{12} and vitamin B_{12} binding capacity in chronic myelogenous leukemia and other disorders. *Am J Med Sci* 263:473, 1972.

345. Sternman U-H: Intrinsic factor and the B_{12} binding proteins. *Clin Haematol* 5:473, 1976.

346. Corcino JJ, Zalusky R, Greenberg M, Herbert V: Coexistence of pernicious anaemia and chronic myeloid leukaemia: an experiment of nature involving vitamin B_{12} metabolism. *Br J Haematol* 20:511, 1971.

347. Gomez GA, Sokal JE, Walsh D: Prognostic features at diagnosis of chronic myelocytic leukemia. *Cancer* 47:2470, 1981.

348. Bellevue R, Dosik H, Spergel G, Gussoff BD: Pseudohyperkalemia and extreme leukocytosis. *J Lab Clin Med* 85:660, 1975.

349. Ballard HS, Marcus AJ: Hypercalcemia in chronic myelogenous leukemia. *N Engl J Med* 282:663, 1970.

350. Evans JJ, Bozdech MJ: Hypokalemia in nonblastic chronic myelogenous leukemia. *Arch Intern Med* 141:786, 1981.

351. Perillie PE, Finch SC: Muramidase studies in Philadelphia-chromosome-positive and chromosome-negative chronic granulocytic leukemia. *N Engl J Med* 283:456, 1970.

352. Gilbert HS, Ginsberg H: Hypocholesterolemia as a manifestation of disease activity in chronic myeloid leukemia. *Cancer* 51:1428, 1983.

353. Muller CP, Wagner AN, Maucher C, Steinke B: Hypocholesterolemia, an unfavorable feature of prognostic value in chronic myeloid leukemia. *Eur J Haematol* 43:235, 1989.

354. Morris CM, Fitzgerald PH, Hollings PE, et al: Essential thrombocythemia and the Philadelphia chromosome. *Br J Haematol* 70:13, 1988.

355. Stoll DB, Peterson P, Exten R, et al: Clinical presentation and natural history of patients with essential thrombocythemia and the Philadelphia chromosome. *Am J Hematol* 27:77, 1988.

356. Sessarego M, Defferrari R, Dejana AM, et al: Cytogenetic analysis in essential thrombocythemia at diagnosis and at transformation. *Cancer Genet Cytogenet* 43:57, 1989.

357. Cervantes F, Colomer D, Vives-Corrows JL, et al: Chronic myeloid leukemia of thrombocythemic onset: a CML subtype with distinct hematological and molecular features. *Leukemia* 11:617, 1997.

358. Blickstein D, Aviram A, Luboshitz J, et al: BCR-ABL transcripts in bone marrow aspirates of Philadelphia-negative essential thrombocythemia patients: clinical presentation. *Blood* 90:2768, 1997.

359. Cerventes F, Colomer D, Vives-Corrons JL, et al: Chronic myeloid leukemia of thrombocythemic onset: a CML subtype with distinct hematological and molecular features. *Leukemia* 10:1241, 1996.

360. Martiat P, Ifrah N, Rassool F, et al: Molecular analysis of Philadelphia positive essential thrombocythemia. *Leukemia* 3:563, 1989.

361. Paietta E, Rosen N, Roberts M, et al: Philadelphia chromosome positive essential thrombocythemia evolving into lymphoid blast crisis. *Cancer Genet Cytogenet* 25:227, 1987.

362. Michiels JJ, Prins ME, Hagermeijer A, et al: Philadelphia chromosome-positive thrombocythemia and megakaryoblast leukemia. *Am J Clin Pathol* 88:645, 1987.

363. Kwong YL, Chiu EK, Liang RH, Chan V, Chan TK: Esential thrombocy-

themia with BCR/ABL rearrangement. *Cancer Genet Cytogenet* 89:74, 1996.

364. Marasca R, Luppi M, Zucchini P, et al: Might essential thrombocythemia carry Ph anomaly? *Blood* 91:3084, 1998.

365. Sanadi I, Yamamoto S, Ogata M, et al: Detection of the Philadelphia chromosome in chronic neutrophilic leukemia. *Jpn J Clin Oncol* 15:553, 1985.

366. Christopoulus C, Kottoris K, Mikraki V, Anevlavis E: Presence of bcr/abl rearrangement in a patient with chronic neutrophilic leukaemia. *J Clin Pathol* 49:1013, 1996.

367. Pane F, Frigeri F, Sindina M, et al: Neutrophilic-chronic myeloid leukemia: a distinct disease with a specific molecular marker (BCR/ABL with C3/A2 junction). *Blood* 88:2410, 1996.

368. Saglio G, Guerrasio A, Rosso C, et al: New type of BCR/ABL junction in Philadelphia chromosome-positive chronic myelogenous leukemia. *Blood* 87:1075, 1996.

369. Knowles DM: Thymoma and chronic myelogenous leukemia. *Cancer* 38:414, 1976.

370. Vannier JP, Bizet M, Bastard C, et al: Simultaneous occurrence of a T-cell lymphoma and a chronic myelogenous leukemia with an unusual karyotype. *Leuk Res* 8:647, 1984.

371. Djulbegovi B, Hadley T, Yen F: Occurrence of high-grade T-cell lymphoma in a patient with Philadelphia chromosome-negative chronic myelogenous leukemia with breakpoint cluster region rearrangement. *Am J Hematol* 36:63, 1991.

372. Tittley P, Trempe JM, vanderJagt R, et al: Occurrence of T-cell lymphoma in a patient with Philadelphia chromosome-positive chronic myelogenous leukemia with rearrangements of BCR and TCR-β genes in the lymph nodes. *Am J Hematol* 42:229, 1993.

373. Hornstein P, Nordenson I, Wahlin A: Philadelphia chromosome negative acute lymphoblastic leukemia preceding Philadelphia positive chronic myelogenous leukemia. *Cancer Genet Cytogenet* 39:147, 1989.

374. Naparstek Y, Zlotnick A, Polliack A: Coexistent chronic myeloid leukemia and IgA monoclonal gammopathy: report of a case and review of the literature. *Am J Med Sci* 292:111, 1980.

375. Shoenfeld Y, Berliner S, Ayalone A, et al: Monoclonal gammopathy in patients with chronic and acute myeloid leukemia. *Cancer* 54:280, 1984.

376. Tanaka M, Kimura R, Matsutani A, et al: Coexistence of chronic myelogenous leukemia and multiple myeloma. *Acta Haematol* 99:221, 1998.

377. Guglielmi P, Davi F, Brouet JC: Prevalence of monoclonal Ig with λ light chains in chronic myelocytic leukemia. *Br J Haematol* 73:331, 1989.

378. Vitali C, Bombardieri S, Spremolla G: Chronic myeloid leukemia in Waldenström's macroglobulinemia. *Arch Intern Med* 141:1349, 1981.

379. Whang-Peng J, Gralnick HR, Johnson RE, et al: Chronic granulocytic leukemia (CGL) during the course of chronic lymphocytic leukemia (CLL): correlation of blood, marrow, and spleen morphology and cytogenetics. *Blood* 43:333, 1974.

380. Schrieber ZA, Axelrod MR, Abebe LS: Coexistence of chronic myelogenous leukemia and chronic lymphocytic leukemia. *Cancer* 54:697, 1984.

381. Esteve J, Cervantes F, Rives S, et al: Simultaneous occcurrence of B-cell chronic lymphocytic leukemia and chronic meyloid leukemia with further evolution to lymphoic blast status. *Haematologica* 82:596, 1997.

382. Leoni F, Ferrini PR, Castoldi GL, et al: Simultaneous occurrence of chronic granulocytic leukemia and chronic lymphoid leukemia. *Haematologia* 72:253, 1987.

383. Faguet GB, Little T, Agee JF, Garver FA: Chronic lymphatic leukemia evolving into chronic myelocytic leukemia. *Cancer* 52:1647, 1983.

384. Jantunen E, Nousiainen T: Ph-positive chronic myelogenous leukemia evolving after polycythemia vera. *Am J Hematol* 37:212, 1991.

385. Hoppen EC, Lewis JP: Polycythemia rubra vera progressing to Ph-positive chronic myelogenous leukemia. *Ann Intern Med* 83:820, 1975.

386. Haq AU: Transformation of polycythemia vera to Ph-positive chronic myelogenous leukemia. *Am J Hematol* 356:110, 1990.

387. Roth AD, Oral A, Przepiorka D, et al: Chronic myelogenous leukemia and acute lymphoblastic leukemia occurring in the course of polycythemia vera. *Am J Hematol* 43:123, 1993.

388. Foviester RH, Louro JM: Philadelphia chromosome abnormality in agnogenic myeloid metaplasia. *Ann Intern Med* 64:622, 1966.

389. Nowell PC, Kant JA, Finan JB, et al: Marrow fibrosis associated with a Philadelphia chromosome. *Cancer Genet Cytogenet* 59:89, 1992.

390. Roth DG, Richman CM, Rowley JD: Chronic myelodysplastic syndrome (preleukemia) with the Philadelphia chromosome. *Blood* 56:262, 1980.

391. Berrebi A, Bruck R, Shtalrid M, Chemke J: Philadelphia chromosome in idiopathic acquired sideroblastic anemia. *Acta Haematol* 72:343, 1984.

392. Hande K: Hyperuricemia, uric acid nephropathy and the tumor lysis syndrome, in *Renal Complications of Neoplasia*, edited by TD McKinney, pp 134–156. Praeger, New York, 1986.

393. Goldman JM: Treatment of chronic myeloid leukaemia: some topical questions. *Baillieres Clin Haematol* 10:405, 1997.

394. Fitzgerald D, Rowe JM, Heal J: Leukapheresis for control of chronic myelogenous leukemia during pregnancy. *Am J Hematol* 22:213, 1986.

395. Bazarbashi MS, Smith MR, Karanes C, et al: Successful management of Ph chromosome chronic myelogenous leukemia with leukapheresis during pregnancy. *Am J Hematol* 38:235, 1991.

396. Kennedy BJ: The evolution of hydroxyurea therapy in chronic myelogenous leukemia. *Sem Oncol* 19(Suppl 9):21, 1992.

397. Kolitz JE, Kempin SF, Schluger A, et al: A phase II trial of high-dose hydroxyurea in chronic myelogenous leukemia. *Semin Oncol* 19(Suppl 9):27, 1992.

398. Kantarjian HM, Smith TL, O'Brien S, et al: Prolonged survival in chronic myelogenous leukemia after cytogenetic response to interferon-alpha therapy. *Ann Intern Med* 122:254, 1995.

399. Wetzler M, Kantarjian H, Kurzrock R, Talpaz M: Interferon-alpha therapy for chronic myelogenous leukemia. *Am J Med* 99:402, 1995.

400. Chronic Myeloid Leukemia Trialist's Collaborative Group. Interferon alfa versus chemotherapy for chronic myeloid leukemia: a meta-analysis of seven randomized trials. *J Natl Cancer Inst* 89:1616, 1997.

401. Allan NC, Richards SM, Shepherd PCA, et al: UK Medical Research Council randomized, multicentric trial of interferon-α for chronic myeloid leukemia: improved survival irrespective of cytogenetic response. *Lancet* 345:1392, 1995.

402. Ohnishi K, Tomonagu M, Kamada N, et al: A long-term follow-up of a randomized trial comparing interferon-α with busulfan for chronic myelogenous leukemia. *Leuk Res* 22:779, 1998.

403. The Italian Cooperative Study Group on Chronic Myeloid Leukemia: Long-term follow-up of the Italian trial of interferon-α vs. conventional chemotherapy in chronic myeloid leukemia. *Blood* 92:1541, 1998.

404. O'Brien S, Kantarjian H, Talpaz M. Practical guidelines for the management of chronic myelogenous leukemia with interferon alpha. *Leuk Lymphoma* 23:247, 1996.

405. Sacchi S, Kantarjian HM, Smith TL, et al: Early treatment decisions with interferon-alfa therapy in early chronic phase chronic myelogenous leukemia. *J Clin Oncol* 16:882, 1998.

406. Schofield JR, Robinson WA, Murphy JR, Rovira DK: Low doses of interferon-α are as effective as higher doses in inducing remission and prolonging survival in chronic myeloid leukemia. *Ann Intern Med* 121:736, 1944.

407. Cortes J, Kantarjian H, O'Brien S, et al: Result of interferon-alpha therapy in patients with chronic myelogenous leukemia 60 years of age and older. *Am J Med* 100:452, 1996.

408. Montastruc M, Mahon FX, Faberes C, et al: Response to recombinant interferon alpha in patients with chronic myelogenous leukemia in a single center: results and analysis of predictive factors. *Leukemia* 9:1997, 1995.

409. Claxton D, Deisseroth A, Talpaz M, et al: Polyclonal hematopoiesis in interferon-induced cytogenetic remissions of chronic myelogenous leukemia. *Blood* 79:997, 1992.

410. Kloke O, Niederle N, Opaika B, et al: Prognostic impact of interferon-alpha-induced cytogenetic remission in chronic myelogenous leukaemia: long-term follow-up. *Eur J Haematol* 56:78, 1996.

411. Rio B, Ramond S, Lacorte JM, et al: Unmaintained cytogenetic and molecular remission in chronic myelogenous leukaemia following treatment by interferon. *Br J Haematol* 92:504, 1996.

412. Nicolson NL, Talpaz M, Nicolson GL: Interferon-alpha directly inhibits DNA polymerase activity in isolated chromatin nucleoprotein complexes: correlation with IFN-alpha treatment outcome in patients with chronic myelogenous leukemia. *Gene* 159:105, 1995.

413. Hochhaus A, Yan XH, Willer A, et al: Expression of interferon regulatory factor (IRF) genes and response to interferon-alpha in chronic myeloid leukaemia. *Leukaemia* 11:933, 1997.

414. Sellieri C, Sato T, DelVecchio L, et al: Involvement of Fas-mediated apoptosis in the inhibitory effects of interferon-alpha in chronic myelogenous leukemia. *Blood* 89:957, 1997.

415. Hochhaus A, Lin F, Reiter A, et al: Quantification of residual disease in chronic myelogenous leukemia patients on interferon-alpha therapy by competitive polymerase chain reaction. *Blood* 87:1549, 1996.

416. Oka T, Sastry KJ, Nehete P, et al: Evidence for specific immune response against p210 BCR-ABL in long-term remission CML patients treated with interferon. *Leukemia* 12:1550, 1998.

417. Ben-Yehuda D, Krichevsky S, Rachmilewitz EA, et al: Molecular follow-up of disease progression and interferon therapy in chronic myelocytic leukemia. *Blood* 90:4918, 1997.

418. Elliott SL, Taylor KM, Taylor DL, et al: Cytogenetic response to alpha-interferon is predicted in early chronic phase chronic myeloid leukemia by M-bcr breakpoint location. *Leukemia* 9:946, 1995.

419. The Italian Cooperative Study Group on Chronic Myeloid Leukemia: Chronic myeloid leukemia, BCR/ABL transcript, response to alph-interferon and survival. *Leukemia* 9:1648, 1995.

420. Seong DC, Kantarjian HM, Ro JY, et al: Hypermetaphase fluorescence in situ hybridization for quantitative monitoring of Philadelphia chromosome-positive cells in patients with chronic myelogenous leukemia during treatment. *Blood* 86:2343, 1995.

421. Muhlmann J, Thaler J, Hilbe W, et al: Fluorescence in situ hybridization (FISH) on peripheral blood smears for monitoring Philadelphia chromosome-positive chronic myeloid leukemia (CML) during interferon treatment: a new strategy for remission assessment. *Genes Chromosom Cancer* 21:90, 1998.

422. Bihou-Nabera C, Marit G, Gharbi MJ, et al: Chronic myelocytic leukemia patients achieving complete cytogenetic conversion under interferon alpha therapy: minimal residual disease follow-up. *Leukemia* 9:2067, 1995.

423. Hochhaus A, Lin F, Reiter A, et al: Variable number of BCR-ABL transcripts persist in CML patients who achieve complete cytogenetic remission with interferon-alpha. *Br J Haematol* 91:126, 1995.

424. Lion T, Gaiger A, Henn T, et al: Use of quantitative polymerase chain reaction to monitor residual disease in chronic myelogenous leukemia during treatment with interferon. *Leukemia* 9:1353, 1995.

425. Talpaz M, Kantarjian HM, McCredie KB, et al: Clinical investigations of human alpha interferon in chronic myelogenous leukemia. *Blood* 69:1280, 1987.

426. Kurzrock R, Talpaz M, Kantarjian H, et al: Therapy of chronic myelogenous leukemia with recombinant interferon. *Blood* 70:943, 1987.

427. Kloke O, May D, Wandl U, et al: Treatment of chronic myelogenous leukemia with interferon alpha and gamma. *Blut* 61:45, 1990.

428. Freund M, VonWussow P, Diedrich H, et al: Recombinant human interferon alpha-2b in chronic myelogenous leukemia: dose dependency of response and frequency of neutralizing anti-interferon antibodies. *Br J Haematol* 72:350, 1989.

429. Russo D, Candoni A, Zuffa E, et al: Neutralizing anti-interferon-alpha antibodies and response to treatment in patients with Ph+ chronic myeloid leukaemia sequentially treated with recombinant and lymphoblastoid interferon-alpha. *Br J Haematol* 94:300, 1996.

430. Wilhelm M, Bueso-Ramos C, O'Brien S, et al: Effect of interferon-alpha therapy on bone marrow fibrosis in chronic myelogenous leukemia. *Leukemia* 12:65, 1998.

431. Thiele J, Kvasnicka HM, Niederle N, et al: The impact of interferon versus busulfan therapy on the reticulin stain-measured fibrosis in CML—a comparative morphometric study on sequential trephine biopsies. *Ann Hematol* 70:121, 1995.

432. Beelen DW, Graeven U, Elmaagacli AH, et al: Prolonged administration of interferon-alpha in patients with chronic-phase Philadelphia chromosome-positive chronic myelogenous leukemia before allogeneic bone marrow transplantation may adversely affect transplant outcome. *Blood* 85:2981, 1995.

433. Marten AJ, Gooley T, Hansen JA, et al: Association between pretransplant interferon-α and outcome after unrelated donor marrow transplantation for chronic myelogenous leukemia. *Blood* 92:394, 1998.

434. Higano CS, Chielens D, Rashkind W, et al: Use of alpha-2a-interferon to treat cytogenetic relapse of chronic myeloid leukemia after marrow transplantation. *Blood* 90:2549, 1997.

435. The Benelux CML Study Group: Randomized study on hydroxyurea alone versus hydroxyurea combined with low-dose interferon-alpha 2b from chronic myeloid leukemia.. *Blood* 91:2713, 1998.

436. Hehlmann R, Willer A, Heimpel H, et al: Randomized studies with interferon in chronic myelogenous leukemia (CML) and comparative molecular aspects. *Leukemia* 3:506, 1997.

437. Robertson MJ, Tantravaki R, Griffin JD, et al: Hematologic remission and cytogenetic improvement after treatment of stable phase chronic myelogenous leukemia with continuous infusion low-dose cytosine arabinoside. *Am J Hematol* 43:95, 1993.

438. Giulhot F, Dreyfus B, Brizard A, et al: Cytogenetic remission in chronic myelogenous leukemia using interferon alpha-2a and hydroxyurea with or without low-dose cytosine arabinoside. *Leuk Lymphoma* 4:49, 1991.

439. Guilhot F, Chastang C, Michallet M, et al: Interferon alfa-2b combined with cytarabine versus interferon alone in chronic myelogenous leukemia. *N Engl J Med* 337:223, 1997.

440. Hehlmann R, Heimpel H, Hasford J, et al: Randomized comparison of busulfan and hydroxyurea in chronic myelogenous leukemia: prolongation of survival by hydroxyurea. *Blood* 82:398, 1993.

441. Harrold BP: Syndrome resembling Addison's disease following prolonged treatment with busulfan. *Br Med J* 1:463, 1966.

442. Feingold ML, Koss LG: Effects of long-term administration of busulfan. *Arch Intern Med* 124:66, 1969.

443. Kirshner RH, Esterly JR: Pulmonary lesions associated with busulfan therapy of chronic myelogenous leukemia. *Cancer* 27:1074, 1971.

444. Wetherall DJ, Galton DA, Kay HE: Busulfan and bone marrow depression. *Br Med J* 1:638, 1969.

445. Finney R, McDonald GA, Baikie AG, Douglas AS: Chronic granulocytic leukemia with Ph1- negative cells in bone marrow and a ten year remission after busulfan hypoplasia. *Br J Haematol* 23:283, 1972.

446. O'Brien S, Kantarjian H, Keating M, et al: Homoharringtonine therapy induces responses in patients with chronic myelogenous leukemia in late chronic phase. *Blood* 86:3322, 1995.

447. Visani G, Russo D, Ottaviani E, et al: Effects of homoharringtonine alone and in combination with alpha interferon and cytosine arabinoside on ''in vitro'' growth and induction of apoptosis in chronic myeloid leukemia and normal hematopoietic progenitors. *Leukemia* 11:624, 1997.

448. Cortes J, Kantarjian H, Talpaz M, et al: Treatment of chronic myelogneous leukemia with nucleoside analogs deoxycoformycin and fludarabine. *Leukemia* 11:788, 1997.

449. Dibromomannitol Cooperative Study Group: Survival of chronic myeloid leukemia patients treated by dibromomannitol. *Eur J Cancer* 9:583, 1973.

450. Talpaz M, Kantarjian HM, Kurzrock R, Gutterman J: The therapy of chronic myelogenous leukemia: Chemotherapy and interferons. *Semin Hematol* 25:62, 1988.

451. Clarkson B: Chronic myelogenous leukemia: Is aggressive treatment indicated? *J Clin Oncol* 3:135, 1985.

452. Meyskens FL, Kopecky KJ, Appelbaum FR, et al: Effects of vitamin A on survivial in patients with chronic myelogenous leukemia: SWOG randomized trial. *Leuk Res* 19:605, 1995.

453. Cortes J, Kantarjian H, O'Brien S, et al: A pilot study of all-trans retinoic acid in patients with Philadelphia chromosome-positive chronic myelogenous leukemia. *Leukemia* 11:929, 1997.

454. Handa H, Hegde UP, Kotelnikov VM, et al: The effects of 13-*cis* retinoic acid and interferon-alpha in chronic myelogenous leukemia cells in vivo in pati*ent*s. Leuk Res *21:1087, 1997.*

455. Zheng A, Savolainen ER, Koistinen P: All-*trans* retinoic acid combined with interferon-alpha effectively inhibits granulocyte-macrophage colony formation in chronic myeloid leukemia. *Leuk Res* 20:243, 1996.

456. Petitt R, Silverstein MN, Petrone ME: Anagrelide for control of thrombocythemia in polycythemia and other myeloproliferative disorders. *Semin Hematol* 34:51, 1997.

457. Gewirtz AM: Antisense oligonucleotide therapeutics for human leukemia. *Crit Rev Oncol* 8:93, 1997.

458. Wagner H, McKeough PG, Desforges J, Madoc-Jones H: Splenic irradiation in the treatment of patients with chronic myelogenous leukemia or myelofibrosis and myeloid metaplasia. *Cancer* 58:1204, 1986.

459. The Italian Cooperative Study Group on Chronic Myeloid Leukemia. Results of a prospective randomized trial of early splenectomy in chronic myeloid leukemia. *Cancer* 54:333, 1984.

460. Kalhs P, Schwarzinger I, Anderson G, et al: A retrospective analysis of the long-term effect of splenectomy on late infections, graft-versus-host disease, relapse, and survival after allogeneic marrow transplantation for chronic myelogenous leukemia. *Blood* 86:2028, 1995.

461. Goldman J: Autologous stem-cell transplantation for chronic myelogenous leukemia. *Semin Hematol* 30:53, 1993.

462. Talpaz M, Kantarjian H, Liang J, et al: Percentage of Philadelphia chromosome (Ph)-negative and Ph-positive cells found after autologous transplantation for chronic myelogenous leukemia depends on percentage of diploid cells induced by conventional dose chemotherapy before collection of autologous cells. *Blood* 85:3257, 1995.

463. Verfaillie CM, Bhatia R, Steinbuch M, et al: Comparative analysis of autografting in chronic myelogenous leukemia: effects of priming regimen and marrow or blood origin of stem cells. *Blood* 92:1820, 1998.

464. Bhatia R, Verfaillie CM: Autografting for chronic myelogenous leukemia. *Curr Opin Hematol* 2:436, 1995.

465. Kantarjian HM, Talpaz M, Hester J, et al: Collection of peripheral-blood diploid cells from chronic myelogenous leukemia patients early in the recovery phase from myelosuppression induced by intensive-dose chemotherapy. *J Clin Oncol* 18:553, 1995.

466. Carella AJ, Cunningham I, Benvenuto E, et al: Mobilization and transplantation of Philadelphia-negative peripheral blood progenitor cells early in chronic myelogenous leukemia. *J Clin Oncol* 15:1575, 1997.

467. Reiffers J, Mahon FX, Boiron JM, et al: Autografting in chronic myeloid leukemia: an overview. *Leukemia* 10:385, 1996.

468. Choudhury A, Gajewski JL, Liang JF, et al: Use of leukemic dendritic cells for the generation of antileukemic cellular cytotoxicity against Philadelphia chromosome-positive chronic myelogenous leukemia. *Blood* 89:1133, 1997.

469. Scheffold C, Brandt K, Johnston V, et al: Potential of autologous immunologic effector cells for bone marrow purging in patients with chronic myeloid leukemia. *Bone Marrow Transplant* 15:33, 1995.

470. De Fabritiis P, Petti MC, Montefusco E, et al: BCR-ABL antisense oligodeoxynucleotide in vitro purging and autologous bone marrow transplantation for patients with chronic myelogenous leukemia in advanced phase. *Blood* 91:3156, 1998.

471. Wright LA, Milliken S, Biggs JC, Kearney P: Ex vivo effects associated with the expression of a bcr-abl-specific ribozyme in a CML cell line. *Antisense Nucleic Acid Drug Dev* 8:15, 1998.

472. Carlo-Stella C, Dotti G, Manguni L, et al: Selection of myeloid progenitors lacking BCR/ABL in chronic myelogenous leukemia patients after in vitro treatments with the tyrosine kinase inhibitor, genistein. *Blood* 88:3091, 1996.

473. Druker BH, Tamura S, Buchdunger E, et al: Effects of a selective inhibitor of the Abl tyrosine kinase on the growth of Bcr-Abl positive cells. *Nat Med* 2:561, 1996.

474. Fogli M, Amabile M, Martinelli G, et al: Selective expansion of normal haemopoietic progenitors from chronic myelogenous leukemia marrow. *Br J Haematol* 101:119, 1998.

475. Coutinho LH, Chang J, Brereta ML, et al: Autografting in Philadelphia (Ph)+ chronic myeloid leukemia using cultured marrow: an update of a pilot study. *Bone Marrow Transplant* 19:969, 1997.

476. Eibl B, Ebner S, Duba C, et al: Dendritic cells generated from blood precursors of chronic myelogenous leukemia patients carry the Philadelphia translocation and can induce a CML-specific primary cytotoxic T-cell response. *Genes Chromosom Cancer* 20:215, 1997.

477. Lewalle P, Hensel N, Guimaeraes A, et al: Helper and cytotoxic lymphocyte responses to chronic myeloid leukemia: implications for adoptive immunotherapy with T cells. *Br J Haematol* 92:587, 1996.

478. Thomas ED, Clift RA, Fefer A, et al: Marrow transplantation for the treatment of chronic myelogenous leukemia. *Ann Intern Med* 104:155, 1986.

479. Apperley JF: Hematopoietic stem cell transplantation in chronic myeloid leukemia. *Curr Opin Hematol* 5:445, 1998.

480. Cooperative Study Group on Chromosomes in Transplanted Patients. Cytogenetic follow-up of 100 patients submitted to bone marrow transplantation for Philadelphia chromosome-positive chronic myeloid leukemia. *Eur J Haematol* 40:50, 1988.

481. Trint RL, Ash RC: Manipulation of T-cell content in transplanted human bone marrow: Effect on GVH and GVL reactions, in *Cellular Immunotherapy of Cancer*, edited by RL Truitt, RP Gale, MM Bortin, p 409. Liss, New York, 1987.

482. McGlave P, Bartoch G, Anasetti C, et al: Unrelated donor marrow transplantation therapy for chronic myelogenous leukemia. *Blood* 81:543, 1993.

483. Clift RA, Anasetti C: Allografting for chronic myeloid leukaemia. *Baillieres Clin Haematol* 10:319, 1997.

484. Sullivan KM: Marrow transplantation for disorders of hematopoieis. *Leukemia* 7:1098, 1993.

485. Horowitz MM, Gale RP, Sondell PM, et al: Graft-versus-leukemia reaction after bone marrow transplantation. *Blood* 75:555, 1990.

486. Antin JH: Graft-versus-leukemia: no longer an epiphenomenon. *Blood* 82:2273, 1993.

487. Savage DG, Szydlo RM, Chase A, et al: Bone marrow transplantation for chronic myeloid leukaemia: the effects of differing criteria for defining chronic phase on probabilities of survival and relapse. *Br J Haematol* 99:30, 1997.

488. Van Rhee F, Szydlo RM, Hermans J, et al: Long-term results after allogeneic bone marrow transplantation for chronic myelogenous leukemia in chronic phase: a report from the Chronic Leukemia Working Party of the European Groups for Blood and Marrow Transplantation. *Bone Marrow Transplant* 20:553, 1997.

489. Lee SJ, Kuntz KM, Horowitz MM, et al: Unrelated donor bone marrow transplantation for chronic myelogenous leukemia; a decision analysis. *Ann Intern Med* 127:1080, 1997.

490. Enright H, Daniels K, Arthur DC, et al: Related donor marrow transplant for chronic myeloid leukemia: patients' characteristics predictive of outcome. *Bone Marrow Transplant* 17:537, 1996.

491. Goldman JM, Szydlo R, Horowitz MM, et al: Choice of pretransplant treatment and timing of transplants for chronic myelogenous leukemia in chronic phase. *Blood* 82:2235, 1993.

492. Tomas JF, Lopez-Lorenzo JL, Requena MJ, et al: Absence of influence of prior treatments with interferon on the outcome of allogeneic bone marrow transplantation for chronic myeloid leukemia. *Bone Marrow Transplant* 22:47, 1998.

493. Gale RP, Hehlmann R, Zhang MJ, et al: Survival with bone marrow transplantation versus hydroxyurea or interferon for chronic myelogenous leukemia. *Blood* 91:1810, 1998.

494. Byrne JL, Stainer C, Hyde H, et al: Low incidence of acute graft-versus-host disease and recurrent leukaemia in patients undergoing allogeneic haemopoietic stem cell transplantation from sibling donors with methotrexate and dose-monitored cyclosporin A prophylaxis. *Bone Marrow Transplant* 22:541, 1988.

495. Szydlo R, Goldman JM, Klein JP, et al: Results of allogeneic bone marrow transplants using donors other than HLA-identical siblings. *J Clin Oncol* 15:1767, 1997.

496. Petersdorf EW, Longton GM, Anasetti C, et al: The significance of HLA-DRB1 matching on clinical outcome after HLA-A, B and DR identical unrelated donor transplantation. *Blood* 86:1606, 1995.

497. Laporte JP, Gorin NC, Rubinstein P, et al: Cord-blood transplantation from an unrelated donor in an adult with chronic myelogenous leukemia. *N Engl J Med* 335:167, 1997.

498. Enright H, Davies SM, DeFor T, et al: Relapse after non-T cell depleted allogeneic bone marrow transplantation for chronic myelogenous leukemia: early transplant, use of an unrelated donor and chronic graft-versus-host disease are protective. *Blood* 88:714, 1996.

499. Hessner MJ, Endean DJ, Casper JT, et al: Use of unrelated marrow grafts compensate for reduced graft-versus-leukemia reactivity after T-cell-depleted allogeneic marrow transplantation for chronic myelogenous leukemia. *Blood* 86:3987, 1995.

500. Radich JP, Gehly G, Gooley T, et al: Polymerase chain reaction detection of the BCR-ABL fusion transcript after allogeneic marrow transplantation for chronic myeloid leukemia: results and implications in 346 patients. *Blood* 85:2632, 1995.

501. Okamoto R, Harano H, Matsuzaki M, et al: Predicting relapse of chronic myelogenous leukemia after allogeneic bone marrow transplantation by BCR/ABL mRNA and DNA fingerprinting. *Am J Clin Pathol* 104:510, 1995.

502. Segel GB, Simon W, Lichtman MA: Variables influencing the timing of marrow transplantation in patients with chronic myelogenous leukemia. *Blood* 68:1055, 1986.

503. Champlin RE, Goldman JM, Gale RP: Bone marrow transplantation in chronic myelogenous leukemia. *Semin Hematol* 25:74, 1988.

504. Thomas ED, Clift RA: Indications for marrow transplantation in chronic myelogenous leukemia. *Blood* 73:861, 1989.

505. Goldman JM: Chronic myeloid leukemia. *Curr Opin Hematol* 4:277, 1997.

506. Kolb HJ, Mittermuller J, Clemm CH, et al: Donor leukocyte transfusions for treatment of recurrent chronic myelogenous leukemia in marrow transplant patients. *Blood* 76:2462, 1990.

507. Mackinnon S, Papadopoulos EB, Carabasi MH, et al: Adoptive immunotherapy evaluating escalating doses of donor leukocytes for relapse of chronic myeloid leukemia after bone marrow transplantation: separation of graft-versus-leukemia responses from graft-versus-host disease. *Blood* 86:1261, 1995.

508. Van Rhee F, Lin F, Cullis JO, et al: Relapse of chronic myeloid leukemia after allogeneic bone marrow transplant: the case of giving donor leukocyte transfusions before the onset of hematologic relapse. *Blood* 83:3377, 1994.

509. Soiffer RJ, Alyea EP, Ritz J: Immunomodulatory effects of donor lymphocyte infusions following allogeneic bone marrow transplantation. *J Clin Apheresis* 10:139, 1995.

510. Mackinnon S: Donor leukocyte infusions. *Baillieres Clin Haematol* 10:357, 1997.

511. Giralt S, Hester J, Huh T, et al: CD8-depleted donor lymphocyte infusion as treatment for relapsed chronic myelogenous leukemia after allogeneic bone marrow transplantation. *Blood* 86:4337, 1995.

512. Verzeletti S, Bonini C, Marktel S, et al: Herpes simplex virus thymidine kinase gene transfer for controlled graft-versus-host disease and graft-versus-leukemia: clinical follow-up and improved new vectors. *Hum Gene Ther* 9:2243, 1998.

513. Nieda M, Nicol A, Kikuchi A, et al: Dendritic cells stimulate the expansion of BCR-ABL-specific CD8+ T cells with cytotoxic activity against leukemic cells from patients with chronic myeloid leukemia. *Blood* 92:977, 1998.

514. Smit WM, Rijnbeek M, van Bergen CA, et al: Generation of dendritic cells expressing BCR-ABL from CD34-positive chronic myeloid leukemia precursor cells. *Hum Immunol* 53:216, 1997.

515. Mannering SI, McKenzie JL, Fearnley DB, Hart DN: HLA-DR1-restricted BCR-ABL (b3a2)-specific CD4+ T lymphocytes respond to dendritic cells pulsed with b3a2 peptide and antigen-presenting cells exposed to b3a2 containing cell lysates. *Blood* 90:290, 1997.

516. ten Bosch GJA, Kessler JH, Joosten AM, et al: A BCR-ABL oncoprotein p210b2a2 fusion region sequence is recognized by HLA-DR2a restricted cytotoxic T lymphocytes and presented by HLA-DR matched cells transfected with an Ii(b2a2) construct. *Blood* 94:1038, 1999.

517. Greco G, Fruci D, Accapezzato D, et al: Two bcr-abl junction peptides bind HLA-A3 molecules and allow specific induction of human cytotoxic T lymphocytes. *Leukemia* 10:693, 1996.

518. Kardinal CG, Bateman JR, Weiner J: Chronic myeloid leukemia. Review of 356 cases. *Arch Intern Med* 136:305, 1976.

519. Tura S, Baccarini M, Corbelli G: Staging of chronic myeloid leukemia. *Br J Haematol* 47:105, 1981.

520. Gomez GA, Sokal JE, Walsh D: Prognostic features at diagnosis of chronic myelogenous leukemia. *Cancer* 47:2470, 1981.

521. Cervantes F, Rozman C: A multivariate analysis of prognostic factors in chronic myeloid leukemia. *Blood* 60:1298, 1982.

522. Sokal JE, Cox EB, Baccarani M, et al: Prognostic discrimination in "good-risk" chronic granulocytic leukemia. *Blood* 63:789, 1984.

523. Sokal JE, Baccarini M, Tura S, et al: Prognostic discrimination among younger patients with chronic granulocytic leukemia: relevance to bone marrow transplantation. *Blood* 66:1352, 1985.

524. Kantarjian HM, Keating MJ, Walters RS, et al: Clinical and prognostic features of Philadelphia chromosome-negative chronic myelogenous leukemia. *Cancer* 58:2023, 1986.

525. Sokal JE, Baccarini M, Russo D, Tura S: Staging and prognosis in chronic myelogenous leukemia. *Semin Hematol* 25:49, 1988.

526. Kantarjian HM, Keating MK, Smith TL, et al: Proposal for a single synthesis prognostic staging system in chronic myelogenous leukemia. *Am J Med* 88:1, 1990.

527. Dreazen I, Berman M, Gaoe RP: Molecular abnormalities of bcr and c-abl in chronic myelogenous leukemia associated with a long chronic phase. *Blood* 71:797, 1988.

528. Nowell PC, Jackson L, Weiss A, Kurzrock P: Historical communication: Philadelphia positive chronic myelogenous leukemia followed for 27 years. *Cancer Genet Cytogenet* 34:57, 1988.

529. Selleir L, Emilia G, Temperani P, et al: Philadelphia-positivie chronic myelogenous leukemia with typical *bcr/abl* molecular features and aytpical, prolonged survival. *Leukemia* 3:538, 1989.

530. Birnie GD, MacKenzie Ed, Goyns MH, Pollock A: Sequestration of Philadelphia chromosome-positive cells in the bone marrow of a chronic myeloid leukemia patient in very prolonged remission. *Leukemia* 4:452, 1990.

531. Larry TH, Dauriac C, PePrise PY: Long-term survival in chronic granulocytic leukaemia. *Br J Haematol* 73:279, 1989.

532. Johansson B, Martens F, Fioretos T, et al: Remarkably long survival of a patient with Ph1-positive chronic myeloid leukemia and 5/bcr rearrangement. *Leukemia* 4:448, 1990.

533. Singer CRJ, McDonald GA, Douglas AS: Twenty-five year survival of chronic granulocytic leukemia with spontaneous karyotype conversion. *Br J Haematol* 57:309, 1984.

534. Wodzinski MA, Potter AM, Lawrence ACK: Prolonged survival in chronic granulocytic leukemia associated with loss of the Philadelphia chromosome. *Br J Haematol* 71:296, 1989.

535. Kantarjian HM, Smith TL, McCredie KB, et al: Chronic myelogenous leukemia: a multivariate analysis of the associations of patient characteristics and therapy with survival. *Blood* 66:1326, 1985.

536. Kantarjian HM, Talpaz M: Treatment of chronic myelogenous leukemia. *Hematology* 14:105, 1991.

537. Baccarini M, Russo D, Zuffa E, et al: The prognosis of chronic myeloid leukemia. *Bone Marrow Transplant* 1(suppl 4):126, 1989.

538. Simon W, Segel GB, Lightman, MA: Upper and lower time limits in the decision to recommend marrow transplantation for patients with chronic myelogenous leukemia. *Br J Haematol* 70:31, 1988.

539. Grossman A, Silver RT, Arlin Z, et al: Fine mapping of chromosome 22 breakpoints within the breakpoint cluster region (bcr) implies a role for bcr exon 3 in determining disease duration in chronic myeloid leukemia. *Am J Hum Genet* 45:729, 1989.

540. Morris SW, Daniel L, Ahmed CMI, et al: Relationship of bcr breakpoint to chronic phase duration, survival, and blast crisis lineage in chronic myelogenous leukemia patients presenting in early chronic phase. *Blood* 75:2035, 1990.

541. Giralt S, Kantarjian H, Talpaz M: The natural history of chronic myelogenous leukemia in the interferon era. *Semin Hematol* 32:152, 1995.

542. Smadja N, Krulik M, Audebert AA, et al: Spontaneous regression of cytogenetic and hematologic anomalies in Ph1-positive chronic myelogenous leukemia. *Br J Haematol* 63:257, 1986.

543. Musashi M, Abe S, Yamada T, et al: Spontaneous remission in a patient with chronic myelogenous leukemia. *N Engl J Med* 336:337, 1997.

544. Provan AB, Smith AG: Re-emergence of Philadelphia chromosome positive clone on a patient with previous spontaneous remission of chronic myeloid leukemia. *Leukemia* 9:1600, 1995.

545. Yee K, Anglin P, Keating A: Molecular approaches to the detection and monitoring of chronic myeloid leukemia: theory and practice. *Blood Reviews* 13:105, 1999.

546. Negrin RS, Blume KG: The use of the polymerase chain reaction for the detection of minimal residual malignant disease. *Blood* 78:255, 1991.

547. Delage R, Soiffer RJ, Dean K, Ritz J: Clinical significance of bcr-abl gene rearrangement detected by polymerase chain reaction after allogeneic bone marrow transplantation in chronic myelogenous leukemia. *Blood* 78:2759, 1991.

548. Thompson JD, Brodsky I, Yunis JJ: Molecular quantification of residual disease in chronic myelogenous leukemia after bone marrow transplantation. *Blood* 79:1629, 1992.

549. Lee M-S, Kantarjian H, Talpaz M, et al: Detection of minimal residual disease by polymerase chain reaction in Philadelphia chromosome-positive chronic myelogenous leukemia following interferon therapy. *Blood* 79:1920, 1992.

550. Schulze E, Krahl R, Thalmeier K, Helbig W: Detection of bcr-abl mRNA in single progenitor colonies from patients with chronic myeloid leukemia by PCR: comparison with cytogenetics and PCR from uncultured cells. *Exp Hematol* 23:1649, 1995.

551. Lin F, Chase A, Bungey J, et al: Correlation between the proportion of Philadelphia chromosome-positive metaphase cells and levels of BCR-ABL mRNA in chronic myeloid leukaemia. *Genes Chromosom Cancer* 13:110, 1995.

552. Gaiger A, Henn T, Horth E, et al: Increase of bcr-abl chimeric mRNA expression in tumor cells of patients with chronic myeloid leukemia precedes disease progression. *Blood* 86:2371, 1995.

553. Tuohey EL: A case of splenomegaly with polymorphonuclear neutrophil hyperleukocytosis. *Am J Med Sci* 160:18, 1920.

554. Tanzer J, Harel P, Borron M, Bernard J: Cytochemical and cytogenetic findings in a case of chronic neutrophilic leukaemia of mature cell type. *Lancet* 1:387, 1964.

555. Jackson IMD, Clark RM: A case of neutrophilic leukemia. *Am J Med Sci* 249:72, 1965.

556. Rubin H: Chronic neutrophilic leukemia. *Ann Intern Med* 65:93, 1966.

557. Silberstein EB, Kellner DC Shivakumar BN, Burgen LA: Neutrophilic leukemia. *Ann Intern Med* 80:110, 1974.

558. Turz T, Flandrin G, Brouet JC, et al: Coexistence d'un myélome et d'une leucémie granuleuse en l'absence de tout traitement. Etude de quatre observations. *Nouv Rev Fr Hématol* 14:693, 1974.

559. Shindo T, Sakai C, Shibata A: Neutrophilic leukemia and blastic crisis. *Ann Intern Med* 87:66, 1977.

560. Vorobiof DA, Benjamin A, Kaplan H, Dvilansky A: Chronic granulocytic leukemia, neutrophilic type with paraproteinemia (IgA type K). *Acta Haematol* 60:316, 1978.

561. You W, Weisbrot IM: Chronic neutrophilic leukemia: report of two cases and review of the literature. *Am J Clin Pathol* 72:223, 1979.

562. Sanz MA: Long-term survival in chronic neutrophilic leukemia. *Am J Clin Pathol* 74:717, 1980.

563. Carcassonne Y, Gastaut JA, Sebahoun G, Gratecos N: Découverte simultanée chez un même malade d'un myélome, d'une leucémie granuleuse (à polynucléaires neutrophils) et d'une maladie de Paget. *Nouv Rev Fr Hématol* 18:240, 1977.

564. Bareford D, Jacobs P: Chronic neutrophilic leukemia. *Am J Clin Pathol* 73:837, 1980.

565. Hasle H, Olesen G, Kerndrup G, et al: Chronic neutrophilic leukaemia in adolescence and young adulthood. *Br J Haematol* 94:628, 1996.

566. Pérez-Simon JA, Hernandez-Rivas JM, Flores T: Lymph node myeloid metaplasia associated with chronic neutrophilic leukaemia. *Haematologica* 82:126, 1997.

567. Dotten DA, Pruzanski W, Wong D: Functional characterization of the cells in chronic neutrophilic leukaemia. *Am J Hematol* 12:157, 1982.

568. Yam LT: Neutrophilic leukemia. *South Med J* 75:870, 1982.

569. Yamaya T, Kamata Y, Nassi K, Sawada Y: An autopsy case of chronic neutrophilic leukemia and the review of Japanese literature. *Rinsho Ketsueki* 23:1808, 1982.

570. Watanabe, A, Yoshida Y, Yamamoto H, et al: A case of chronic neutrophilic leukemia with paraproteinemia (IgG type lambda and IgA type K). *Jpn J Med* 23:39, 1984.

571. Franchi F, Seminara P, Gruinchi G: Chronic neutrophilic leukemia and myeloma. Report on long survival. *Tumori* 70:105, 1984.

572. Mehrotra PK, Winfield DA, Fergusson LH: Cellular abnormalities and reduced colony-forming cells in chronic neutrophilic leukaemia. *Acta Haematol* 73:47, 1985.

573. Ito T, Kojima H, Otani K, et al: Chronic neutrophilic leukemia associated with monoclonal gammopathy of undetermined significance. *Acta Haematol* 95:140, 1996.

574. DiDonato D, Croci G, Lazzari S, et al: Chronic neutrophilic leukemia: Description of a new case with karyotypic abnormalities. *Am J Clin Pathol* 85:369, 1986.

575. Lewis MJ, Oelbaum MH, Coleman M, Allen S: An association between chronic neutrophilic leukaemia and multiple myeloma with a study of cobalamin-binding proteins. *Br J Haematol* 63:173, 1986.

576. Hossfeld DK, Lokhorst HW, Garbrecht M: Neutrophilic leukemia accompanied by hemorrhagic diathesis: report of two cases. *Blut* 54:109, 1987.

577. Zitton R, Rèa D, Huang L, Ramond S: Chronic neutrophilic leukemia: a study of four cases. *Ann Hematol* 68:55, 1994.

578. Yanagisawa K, Ohminami H, Sato M, et al: Neoplastic involvement of granulocytic lineage, not granulocytic-monocytic, monocytic or erythrocytic lineage in a patient with chronic neutrophilic leukemia. *Am J Hematol* 57:221, 1998.

579. Sponoza E, Virgolini L, Tosato F, Paladini G: Chronic neutrophilic leukemia: report of a case. *Haematologica* 71:143, 1986.

580. Zorembos NC, Symeonidis A, Kourakli-Symeonidas A: Chronic neutrophilic leukemia with dysplastic features. *Acta Haematol* 82:156, 1989.

581. Froberg MK, Brunning RD, Dorion P, et al: Demonstration of clonality in neutrophils using FISH in a case of chronic neutrophilic leukemia. *Leukemia* 12:623, 1998.

582. Storek J: Chronic neutrophilic leukemia. *Am J Hematol* 41:304, 1992.

583. Matano S, Nakamura S, Kobayashi K, et al: Deletion of the long arm of chromosome 20 in a patient with chronic neutrophilic leukemia: cytogenetic findings. *Am J Hematol* 54:72, 1997.

584. Kwong YL, Cheng G: Clonal nature of chronic neutrophilic leukemia. *Blood* 82:1035, 1993.

585. Standen GR, Steers FJ, Jones L: Clonality in chronic neutrophilic leukemia associated with myeloma: analysis using the X-linked probe M27β. *J Clin Pathol* 46:297, 1993.

586. Foa P, Iurlo A, Saglio G, et al: Chronic neutrophilic leukemia associated with polycythemia vera. *Br J Haematol* 78:286, 1991.

587. Lorente JA, Peña JM, Ferro T, et al: A case of chronic neutrophilic leukemia with original chromosomal abnormalities. *Eur J Haematol* 41:285, 1988.

588. Orazi A, Cattoretti G, Sozzi G: A case of chronic neutrophilic leukemia in the trisomy 8. *Acta Haematol* 81:148, 1989.

589. Rovira M, Cervantes F, Namdedeu B, Rozman C: Chronic neutrophlic leukaemia preceding for seven years the development of multiple myeloma. *Acta Haematol* 3:94, 1990.

590. Standen GR, Jasani B, Wagstaff M, Wardrop CAJ: Chronic neutrophilic leukemia and multiple myeloma. *Cancer* 66:162, 1990.

591. Nagai M, Oda S, Iwamoto M, et al: Granulocyte-colony stimulating factor concentrates in a patient with plasma cell dyscrasia and clinical features of chronic neutrophilic leukemia. *J Clin Pathol* 49:858, 1996.

592. Masini L, Salvarani C, Macchioni P, et al: Chronic neutrophilic leukemia (CNL) with karyotype abnormalities associated with plasma cell dyscrasia. *Haematologica* 77:277, 1992.

593. Pascucci M, Dorion P, Makary A, Froberg MK: Chronic neutrophilic leukemia evolving from the myelodysplastic syndrome. *Acta Haematol* 98:163, 1997.

594. Takamatsu Y, Kondo S, Inoue M, Tamura K: Chronic neutrophilic leukemia with dysplastic features mimicking myelodysplastic syndrome. *Int J Hematol* 63:65, 1996.

595. Higuchi T, Oba R, Endo M, et al: Transition of polycythemia vera to chronic neutrophilic leukemia. *Leuk Lymphoma* 33:203, 1999.

596. Iurlo A, Foa P, Mailo AT, et al: Polycythemia vera terminating in chronic neutrophilic leukemia. *Am J Hematol* 35:139, 1990.

597. Osgood EE: Monocytic leukemia. Report of six cases and review of one hundred and twenty-seven cases. *Arch Intern Med* 59:931, 1937.

598. Bearman RM, Kjeldsberg CR, Pangalis GA, et al: Chronic monocytic leukemia in adults. *Cancer* 48:2239, 1981.

599. Beattie JW, Seal RME, Crowther KV: Chronic monocytic leukemia. *Q J Med* 20:131, 1951.

600. Sinn CW, Dick FW: Monocytic leukemia. *Am J Med* 20:588, 1956.

601. Rodgers GM, Carrera CJ, Ries CA, Bainton DF: Blastic transformation of a well differentiated monocytic leukemia. Changes in cytochemical and cell surface markers. *Leuk Res* 6:613, 1982.

602. Wahlin A, Nordenson I, Roos G: Chronic monocytic leukemia terminating in blastic transformation. *Blut* 53:405, 1986.

603. Castro-Malaspina H, Schaison G, Brier J, et al: Philadelphia chromosome positive chronic myelocytic leukemia in children: Survival and prognostic factors. *Cancer* 51:721, 1983.

604. Arico M, Biondi A, Pui C-H: Juvenile myelomonocytic leukemia. *Blood* 90:479, 1997.

605. Neimeye CM, Arico M, Basso A, et al: Chronic myelomonocytic leukemia in childhood. *Blood* 89:3535, 1997.

606. Emanual PD, Shannon KM, Castleberry RP: Juvenile myelomonocytic leukemia: molecular understanding and prospects for therapy. *Mol Med Today* 468, 1996.

607. Busque L, Gilliland DG, Prchal JT, et al: Clonality in juvenile chronic myelogenous leukemia. *Blood* 85:21, 1995.

608. Miyauchi J, Asada M, Sasaki M, et al: Mutations of the N-*ras* gene in juvenile chronic myelogenous leukemia. *Blood* 83:2248, 1994.

609. Bader JL, Miller RW: Neurofibromatosis and childhood leukemia. *J Pediatr* 92:925, 1978.

610. Brodeur GM: The NF1 gene in myelopoiesis and childhood myelodysplastic syndrome. *N Engl J Med* 330: 637, 1994.

611. Shannon KM: Loss of normal NF1 allele from the bone marrow of children with type 1 neurofibromatosis and malignant myeloid disorders. *N Engl J Med* 330:597, 1994.

612. Bollag G: Loss of NF1 results in activation of RAS signaling pathway and leads to aberrant growth in haematopoietic cells. *Nat Genet* 12:137, 1996.

613. Owen G, Lewis IJ, Morgan M, et al: Prognostic factors in juvenile chronic granulocytic leukaemia. *Br J Cancer* 66(suppl XVIII):S68, 1992.

614. Estrov Z, Grunberger T, Chan HSL, Freedman MH: Juvenile chronic myelogenous leukemia. Characterization of the disease using cell cultures. *Blood* 67:1382, 1986.

615. Estrov Z, Dube ID, Chan HSL, Freedman MH: Residual juvenile chronic myelogenous leukemia cells detected in peripheral blood during clinical remission. *Blood* 70:1466, 1987.

616. Emanuel PD, Bates LJ, Zhu S-W, et al: The role of monocyte-derived hemopoietic growth factors in the regulation of myeloproliferation in juvenile chronic myelogenous leukemia. *Exp Hematol* 19:1017, 1991.

617. Inoue S, Ravindranath Y, Thompson RI, et al: Cytogenetics of juvenile type chronic granulocytic leukemia. *Cancer* 39:2017, 1977.

618. Brodeur GM, Dow LW, Williams DL: Cytogenetic features of juvenile chronic myelogenous leukemia. *Blood* 53:812, 1979.

619. Locatelli F, Niemeyer C, Angelucci E, et al: Allogeneic bone marrow transplantation for chronic myelomonocytic leukemia in childhood. *J Clin Oncol* 15:556, 1997.

620. Chan HSL, Estrov Z, Weitzman SS, Freedman MH: The value of intensive combination chemotherapy for juvenile chronic myelogenous leukemia. *J Clin Oncol* 5:1960, 1987.

621. Kantarjian HM, Kurzrock R, Talpaz M: Philadelphia chromosome-negative chronic myelogenous leukemia and chronic myelomonocytic leukemia. *Hematol Oncol Clin North Am* 4:389, 1990.

622. Morris CM, Reeve AE, Fitzgerald PH, et al: Genomic diversity correlates with clinical variation in Ph¹-negative chronic myeloid leukemia. *Nature* 320:281, 1986.

623. Fitzgerald PH, Beard MEJ, Heaton DC, Reeve AE: Ph-negative chronic myeloid leukemia. *Br J Haematol* 66:311, 1987.

624. Fialkow PJ, Jacobsen RJ, Singer JW, et al: Philadelphia chromosome (Ph¹)-negative chronic myelogenous leukemia (CML): a clonal disease with origin in a multipotent stem cell. *Blood* 56:70, 1980.

625. Hughes A, McVerry BA, Walker H, et al: Heterogeneity of blast crises in Philadelphia negative chronic granulocytic leukaemia. *Br J Haematol* 47:563, 1981.

626. Soda H, Kuriyama K, Tomonaga M, et al: Lymphoid crisis with T-cell phenotypes in a patients with Philadelphia chromosome negative chronic myeloid leukemia. *Br J Haematol* 59:671, 1985.

627. Kessler JF, Grogan TM, Greenberg BR: Philadelphia-chromosome-negative chronic myelogenous leukemia with lymphoid stem cell blastic transformation. *Am J Hematol* 18:201, 1985.

628. Dobrovic A, Morley AA, Seshadri R, Januszewicz EH: Molecular diagnosis of Philadelphia negative CML using the polymerase chain reaction and DNA analysis: clinical features and course of M-bcr negative and M-bcr positive CML. *Leukemia* 5:187, 1990.

629. Martiat P, Michaux JL, Rohain J, et al: Philadelphia-negative (Ph⁻) chronic myeloid leukemia (CML): comparison with Ph⁺ CML and chronic myelomonocytic leukemia. *Blood* 78:205, 1991.

630. VanderPlas DC, Grosveld G, Hagemeijer A: Review of clinical, cytogenetic, and molecular aspects of Ph-negative CML. *Cancer Genet Cytogenet* 52:143, 1991.

631. Galton DA: Haematological differences between chronic granulocytic leukemia, atypical chronic myeloid leukaemia and chronic myelomonocytic leukaemia. *Leuk Lymphoma* 7:343, 1992.

632. Kato Y, Sawada H, Tashima M et al: Heterogeneous features of Ph-negative CML—possible existence of Ph-negative, bcr-rearrangement-negative CML. *Acta Haematol JPN* 52:1004, 1989.

633. Kurzrock R, Kantarjian HM, Shtalrid M, et al: Philadelphia chromosome-negative chronic myelogenous leukemia without breakpoint cluster region rearrangement: a chronic myeloid leukemia with a distinct clinical course. *Blood* 75:445, 1990.

634. Costello R, Sainty D, LaFage-Pochitaloff M, Gabert J: Clinical and biological aspects of Philadelphia-negative/BCR-negative chronic myeloid leukemia. *Leuk Lymphoma* 25:225, 1997.

635. Selleri L, Emilia G, Luppi M, et al: Chronic myelogenous leukemia with typical clinical and morphological features can be Philadelphia chromosome negative and "bcr negative." *Hematol Pathol* 4:67, 1990.

636. Stopera SA, Davie JR, Ray M: Transposition of the abl protooncogene in Philadelphia-negative chronic myeloid leukemia and acute lymphocytic leukemia. *Cytobios* 61:161, 1990.

637. Malbrain MLNG, Van den Bergh, H, Zachée P: Futher evidence for the clonal nature of the idiopathic hypereosinophilic syndrome: complete

haematological and cytogenetic remission induced by interferon-alpha in a case with a unique chromosomal abnormality. *Br J Haematol* 92:176, 1996.

638. Duell T, Mittermüller J, Schmetzer HM, et al: Chronic myeloid leukemia-associated hypereosinophilic syndrome with a clonal t(4;7) (q11;132). *Cancer Genet Cytogenet* 94:91, 1997.

639. Juneja S, Stewart J, McKenzie A, et al: Hypereosinophilic syndrome or chronic eosinophilic leukemia: report of a case with a lytic bone lesion. *Leukemia* 11:765, 1997.

640. Whang-Peng J, Henderson ES, Knutsen T, et al: Cytogenetic studies in acute myelocytic leukemia with special emphasis on the occurrence of Ph[1] chromosome. *Blood* 36:448, 1970.

641. Sandberg AA: Ph[1]-positive acute myeloblastic leukemia, in *The Chromosomes in Human Cancers and Leukemias*, pp 270–275. Elsevier, New York, 1980.

642. Bloomfield CD, Lindquist LL, Brunning RD, et al: The Philadelphia chromosome in acute leukemia. *Virchow Arch [Cell Pathol]* 29:81, 1978.

643. Woods WG, Nesbit ME, Buckley J, et al: Correlation of chromosome abnormalities with patient characteristics, histologic subtype, and induction success in children with acute non-lymphocytic leukemia. *J Clin Oncol* 3:3, 1985.

644. Neuman MP, deSolas I, Parkin JL, et al: Monoclonal antibody study of Philadelphia chromosome-positive blastic leukemias using the alkaline phosphatase anti-alkaline phosphatase (APAAP) technique. *Am J Clin Pathol* 85:564, 1986.

645. Hammonda F: Chromosome abnormalities in acute leukemia. *Lancet* 2:410, 1963.

646. Kiossoglou KA, Mitus WJ, Dameshek W: Two Ph[1] chromosomes in acute granulocytic leukemia. A study of two cases. *Lancet* 2:665, 1965.

647. Mastrangelo R, Zuelzer WW, Thompson RI: The significance of the Ph[1] chromosome in acute myeloblastic leukemia: serial cytogenetic studies in a critical case. *Pediatrics* 40:834, 1967.

648. Bornstein RS, Nesbit M, Kennedy BJ: Chronic myelogenous leukemia presenting in blast crisis. *Cancer* 30:939, 1972.

649. Peterson LC, Bloomfield CD, Brunning RD: Blast crisis as an initial or terminal manifestation of chronic myeloid leukemia. *Am J Med* 60:209, 1976.

650. Worm A-M, Pedersen-Bjergaard J: Chronic myelocytic leukemia presenting in blast transformation. *Scand J Haematol* 18:288, 1977.

651. Kantarjian HM, Talpaz M, Chingra K, et al: Significance of the p210 versus p190 molecular abnormalities in adults with Philadelphia chromosome-positive acute leukemia. *Blood* 78:2411, 1991.

652. Chen SJ, Flandrin G, Daniel M-T, et al: Philadelphia-positive acute leukemia: Lineage promiscuity and inconsistently rearranged breakpoint cluster region. *Leukemia* 2:261, 1988.

653. Price CM, Rasool F, Shirji MKK, et al: Rearrangement of the breakpoint cluster region and expression of p210 BCR-ABL in a "masked" Philadelphia chromosome-positive acute myeloid leukemia. *Blood* 72:1829, 1988.

654. Westbrook CA, Hooberman AL, Spino C, et al: Clinical significance of the BCR-ABL fusion gene in adult acute lymphoblastic leukemia: a Cancer and Leukemia Group B study. *Blood* 80:2983, 1992.

655. Vandenberge E, Martiat P, Baens M, et al: Megakaryoblastic leukemia with an N-ras mutation and late acquisition of a Philadelphia chromosome. *Blood* 5:683, 1991.

656. Helenglass G, Testa JR, Schiffer CA: Philadelphia chromosome-positive acute leukemia. *Am J Hematol* 25:311, 1987.

657. Mecucci C, Noens L, Aventin A, et al: Philadelphia-positive acute myelomonocytic leukemia with inversion of chromosome 16 and eosinobasophils. *Am J Hematol* 27:69, 1988.

658. Chen SJ, Chen Z, Font M-P, et al: Structural alterations in the BCR and ABL genes in Ph1 positive acute leukemias with rearrangements in the BCR gene first intron: Further evidence implicating Alu sequences in the chromosome translocation. *Nucleic Acid Res* 17:7631, 1989.

659. Kurzrock R, Shtalrid M, Talpaz M, et al: Expression of c-abl in Philadelphia-positive acute myelogenous leukemia. *Blood* 70:1584, 1987.

660. Smadja N, Krulik M, DeGramont A, et al: Acquisition of Philadelphia chromosome concomitant with transformation of a refractory anemia into acute leukemia. *Cancer* 55:1477, 1985.

661. LoCoco F, Basso G, DiCello PF, et al: Molecular characterization of Ph[1]+ hybrid acute leukemia. *Leukemia* Res 13:1061, 1989.

662. Catovsky D: Ph[1]-positive acute leukaemia and chronic granulocytic leukaemia: one or two diseases. *Br J Haematol* 42:493, 1979.

663. Ribeiro RC, Abromowitch M, Raimondi SC, et al: Clinical and biologic hallmarks of the Philadelphia chromosome in childhood acute lymphoblastic leukemia. *Blood* 70:948, 1987.

664. Christ N, Carroll A, Shuster J, et al: Philadelphia chromosome positive childhood acute lymphoblastic leukemia: clinical and cytogenetic characteristics and treatment outcome. *Blood* 76:489, 1990.

665. Pui C-H, Crist WM, Look AT: Biology and clinical significance of cytogenetic abnormalities in childhood acute lymphoblastic leukemia. *Blood* 76:1449, 1990.

666. Bloomfield CD, Peterson LC, Yunis JJ, et al: The Philadelphia chromosome (Ph[1]) in adults presenting with acute leukaemia: a comparison of Ph[1]+ and Ph[1]- patients. *Br J Haematol* 36:347, 1977.

667. Priest JR, Robison LL, McKenna RW: Philadelphia chromosome positive childhood acute lymphoblastic leukemia. *Blood* 56:15, 1980.

668. Reece DE, Buskard NA, Hill RS, et al: Allogeneic bone marrow transplantation for Philadelphia-chromosome positive acute lymphoblastic leukemia. *Leuk Res* 10:457, 1986.

669. Forman SJ, O'Donnell MR, Nademanee DS, et al: Bone marrow transplantation for patients with Philadelphia chromosome-positive acute lymphoblastic leukemia. *Blood* 70:587, 1987.

670. Erikson J, Griffin CA, Ar-Rushdi A, et al: Heterogeneity of chromosome 22 breakpoint in Philadelphia positive acute lymphoblastic leukemia. *Proc Natl Acad Sci USA* 83:1807, 1986.

671. Chan LC, Karhi KK, Rayter SI, et al: A novel abl protein expressed in Philadelphia chromosome positive acute lymphoblastic leukaemia. *Nature* 325:635, 1987.

672. Kurzrock R, Shtalrid M, Romero P, et al: A novel c-abl protein product in Philadelphia-positive acute lymphoblastic leukemia. *Nature* 325:631, 1987.

673. Dreazen O, Klisak I, Jones G, et al: Multiple molecular abnormalities in Ph[1] chromosome positive acute lymphoblastic leukaemia. *Br J Haematol* 67:319, 1987.

674. Clark SS, Crist WM, Witte ON: Molecular pathogenesis of Ph-positive leukemias. *Ann Rev Med* 40:113, 1989.

675. Schaefer-Rego K, Arlin Z, Shapiro LG, et al: Molecular heterogeneity of adult Philadelphia chromosome-positive ALL. *Cancer Res* 48:866, 1988.

676. Hermans A, Heisterkamp N, vonLindern M, et al: Unique fusion of bcr and c-abl genes in Philadelphia chromosome positive acute lymphoblastic leukemia. *Cell* 51:33, 1987.

677. Clark SS, McLaughlin J, Crist WM, et al: Unique forms of the abl tyrosine kinase distinguish Ph[1]-positive ALL. *Science* 235:85, 1987.

678. Chen SJ, Chen Z, Hillion J, et al: Ph1-positive, bcr-negative acute leukemias: clustering of breakpoints on chromosome 22 in the 3/end of the BCR gene first intron. *Blood* 73:1312, 1989.

679. Rubin CM, Carrino JJ, Dickler MN, et al: Heterogeneity of genomic fusion of *BCR* and *ABL* in Philadelphia chromosome-positive acute lymphoblastic leukemia. *Proc Natl Acad Sci USA* 85:2795, 1988.

680. Hooberman AL, Rubin CM, Barton KP, Westerbrook CA: Detection of the Philadelphia chromosome in acute lymphoblastic leukemia by pulsed-field gel electrophoresis. *Blood* 74:1101, 1989.

681. Dow LW, Tachibana N, Raimondi SC, et al: Comparative biochemical and cytogenetic studies of childhood acute lymphoblastic leukemia with the Philadelphia chromosome and other 22q11 variants. *Blood* 73:1291, 1989.

682. Seckler-Walker LM, Cooke HMG, Browett PJ, et al: Variable Philadelphia breakpoints and potential lineage restriction of bcr rearrangements in acute lymphoblastic leukemia. *Blood* 72:784, 1988.

683. Hermans A, Gow J, Selleri L, et al: bcr-abl oncogene activation in Philadelphia chromosome-positive acute lymphoblastic leukemia. *Leukemia* 2:628, 1988.

684. Melo JV, Gordon DE, Tuszynski A, et al: Expression of the ABL-BCR fusion gene in Philadelphia-positive acute lymphoblastic leukemia. *Blood* 81:2488, 1993.

685. Suryanarayan K, Hunger SP, Kohler S, et al: Consistent involvement of the BCR gene by 9;22 breakpoints in pediatric acute leukemias. *Blood* 77:324, 1991.

686. Clark SS, McLaughlin J, Timmons M, et al: Expression of a distinctive BCR-ABL oncogene in Ph[1]-positive acute lymphocytic leukemia (ALL). *Science* 239:775, 1988.

687. DeKlein A, Hagemeijer A, Bartram CR, et al: bcr rearrangement and translocation of the c-abl oncogene in Philadelphia positive acute lymphoblastic leukemia. *Blood* 68:1369, 1986.

688. Anastasi J, Feng J, Dickstein JI, et al: Lineage involvement by BCR/ABL in Ph+ lymphoblastic leukemias: chronic myelogenous leukemia presenting in lymphoid blast phase vs Ph+ acute lymphoblastc leukemia. *Leukemia* 10:795, 1996.

689. Schenk TM, Keyhani A, Bottcher S, et al: Multilineage involvement of Philadelphia chromosome postivie acute lymphoblastic leukemia. *Leukemia* 12:666, 1998.

690. Russo C, Carroll A, Kohler S, et al: Philadelphia chromosome and monosomy 7 in childhood acute lymphoblastic leukemia. *Blood* 77:1050, 1991.

691. Secker-Walker LM, Craig JM: Prognostic implications of breakpoint and lineage heterogeneity in Philadelphia-positive acute lymphoblastic leukemia: a review. *Leukemia* 7:147, 1993.

692. Hirsch-Ginsberg C, Childs C, Chang K-S, et al: Phenotypic and molecular heterogeneity in Philadelphia chromosome-positive acute leukemia. *Blood* 71:186, 1988.

693. DeGrouchy J, DeNava C, Cantu J-M, et al: Models of clonal evolutions: a study of chronic myelogenous leukemia. *Am J Hum Genet* 18:485, 1966.

694. Carbonell F, Benitez J, Prieto F, et al: Chromosome banding patterns in patients with chronic myelocytic leukemia. *Cancer Genet Cytogenet* 7:287, 1982.

695. Lowenberg B, Hagemeijer A, Swart K, Abels J: Serial follow-up of patients with chronic myeloid leukemia (CML) with combined cytogenetic and colony culture methods. *Exp Hematol* 10:123, 1982.

696. Haas OA, Schwarzmeier JD, Nachera E, et al: Investigations on karyotype evolution in patients with chronic myeloid leukemia (CML). *Blut* 48:33, 1984.

697. Swolin B, Weinfeld A, Westin J, et al: Karyotypic evolution in Ph-positive chronic myeloid leukemia in relation to management and disease progression. *Cancer Genet Cytogenet* 18:65, 1985.

698. Pederson B: Pathogenesis and blastic transformation of chronic myeloid leukemia as consequences of Ph-positive stem cell hyperplasia: a unifying concept. *Blood Cells* 3:535, 1977.

699. Coiffier B, Byron PA, Flere D, et al: Chronic granulocytic leukemia: early detection of metamorphosis with ''in vitro'' culture of granulocytic progenitors. *Biomedicine* 33:96, 1980.

700. Todd MB, Waldron JA, Jennings TA, et al: Loss of myeloid differentiation antigens precedes blastic transformation in chronic myelogenous leukemia. *Blood* 70:122, 1987.

701. Anastasi J, Feng J, LeBeau MM, et al: The relationship between secondary chromosomal abnormalities and blast transformation in chronic myelogenous leukemia. *Leukemia* 9:628, 1995.

702. Gnesshammer M, Heinze B, Bangerter M, et al: Karyotype abormalities and their clinical significance in blast crisis at chronic myeloid leukemia. *J Mol Med* 75:8836, 1997.

703. Spencer A, Vulliamy T, Kaeda J, et al: Clonal instability preceding lymphoid blastic transformation of chronic myeloid leukemia. *Leukemia* 11:195, 1997.

704. Bartram CR, DeKlein A, Hagemeijer A, et al: Additional C-abl/bcr rearrangements in a CML patient exhibiting two Ph¹ chromosomes during blast crisis. *Leuk Res* 10:221, 1986.

705. Collins SJ, Grudine MT: Chronic myelogenous leukemia: amplification of a rearranged c-abl oncogene in both chronic phase and blast crisis. *Blood* 69:893, 1987.

706. Schaefer-Rego K, Dudik H, Popenoe D, et al: CML patients in blast crisis have breakpoints localized to a specific region of the bcr. *Blood* 70:448, 1987.

707. Mills KI, Benn P, Birnie GD: Does the breakpoint within the major breakpoint region (M-bcr) influence the duration of the chronic phase in chronic myeloid leukemia? An analytical comparison of current literature. *Blood* 78:1155, 1991.

708. Bartram CR, Janssen JWG, Becher R, et al: Persistence of chronic myelocytic leukemia despite deletion of rearranged bcr/c-abl sequences in blast crisis. *J Exp Med* 164:1389, 1986.

709. Okabe M, Matsushima S: Philadelphia chromosome-positive leukemia: molecular analysis of bcr and abl genes and transforming genes. *Acta Haematol Jpn* 51:1471, 1988.

710. Ahuja H, Bar-Eli M, Arlin Z, et al: The spectrum of molecular alterations in the evolution of chronic myelocytic leukemia. *J Clin Invest* 87:2042, 1991.

711. Kelman Z, Prokocimer M, Peller S, et al: Rearrangements in the p53 gene in Philadelphia chromosome positive chronic myelogenous leukemia. *Blood* 74:2318, 1989.

712. Mashal R, Shtalrid M, Talpaz M, et al: Rearrangement and expression of p53 in the chronic phase and blast crisis of chronic myelocytic leukemia. *Blood* 75:180, 1990.

713. Guinn BA, Mello KI: p53 mutations, methylation and genomic instability in the progression of chronic myeloid leukemia. *Leuk Lymphoma* 26:241, 1997.

714. Malinen T, Palotie A, Pakkala S, et al: Acceleration of chronic myeloid leukemia correlates with calcitonin gene methylation. *Blood* 77:2435, 1991.

715. Towatari M, Adachi K, Kato H, Saito H: Absence of the human retinoblastoma gene product in the megakaryoblastic crisis of chronic myelogenous leukemia. *Blood* 78:2178, 1991.

716. Sill H, Goldman JM, Cross NC: Homozygous deletions of the p16 tumor-suppressor gene are associated with lymphoid transformation of chronic myeloid leukemia. *Blood* 85:2013, 1995.

717. Serra A, Gottardi E, Della Ragione F, et al: Involvement at the cyclin-dependent kinase-4 inhibitor (CDKN2) gene in the pathogenesis of lymphoid blast crisis of chronic myelogenous leukaemia. *Br J Haematol* 91:625, 1995.

718. Menssen HD, Renki JMJ, Rodeck U, et al: Presence of Wilms' tumor gene (wt1) transcripts and the WT1 nuclear protein in the majority of human acute leukemias. *Leukemia* 9:1060, 1995.

719. Mitarri K, Ogawa S, Tanaka T, et al: Generation of the AML1-EVI-1 fusion gene in the t(3;21) (q26;q22) causes blastic crisis in chronic myelocytic leukemia. *EMBO* 13:504, 1994.

720. Carapeti M, Goldman JM, Cross NC: Overexpression of EV-l in blast crisis of chronic myeloid leukemia. *Leukemia* 10:1561, 1996.

721. Mori N, Takeuchi S, Tasaka T, et al: Absence of microsatellite instability during the progression of chronic myelocytic leukemia. *Leukemia* 11:151, 1997.

722. Handa H, Hegde UP, Kuteninikov VM, et al: Bcl-2 and c-myc expressions, cell cycle kinetics and apoptosis during the progression of chronic myelogenous leukemia from diagnosis to blastic phase. *Leuk Res* 21:479, 1997.

723. Daheron L, Salmeron S, Patri S, et al: Identification of several genes differentially expressed during progression of chronic myelogenous leukemia. *Leukemia* 12:326, 1998.

724. Foti A, Ahuja HG, Allen SL, et al: Correlation between molecular and clinical events in the evolution of chronic myelocytic leukemia to blast crisis. *Blood* 77:2441, 1991.

725. Mori N, Morosetti R, Loe S, et al: Allelotype analysis in the evolution of chronic myelocytic leukemia. *Blood* 90:2010, 1997.

726. Spiers ASD: Metamorphosis of chronic granulocytic leukemia: diagnosis, classification and management. *Br J Haematol* 49:1, 1979.

727. Grignani F: Chronic myelogenous leukemia. CRC Critical Review. *Oncol Hematol* 4:31, 1985.

728. Matsuo T, Tomonaga M, Kuriyama K, et al: Prognostic significance of the morphological dysplastic changes in chronic myelogenous leukemia. *Leuk Res* 10:331, 1986.

729. Ishii N, Murakami H, Matsushima T, et al: Histamine excess symptoms in basophilic crisis of chronic myelogenous leukemia. *J Med* 26:235, 1995.

730. Specchia G, Palumbo G, Pastore D, et al: Extramedullary blast crisis in chronic myeloid leukemia. *Leuk Res* 20:905, 1996.

731. Inveradi D, Lazzarino M, Morra E, et al: Extramedullary disease in Ph-positive chronic myelogenous leukemia: frequency, clinical features, prognostic signifance. *Haematologica* 75:146, 1990.

732. Jacknow J, Fizzera G, Gajl-Peczalska K, et al: Extramedullary presentation of the blast crisis of chronic myelogenous leukemia. *Br J Haematol* 61:225, 1985.

733. Terjanian T, Kantarjian H, Keating M, et al: Clinical and prognostic features of patients with Philadelphia chromosome-positive chronic myelogenous leukemia and extramedullary disease. *Cancer* 59:297, 1987.

734. Woodson DL, Bennett DE, Sears DA: Extramedullary myeloblastic transformation of chronic myelocytic leukemia. *Arch Intern Med* 134:523, 1974.

735. Miksanek T, Reyes CV, Semkuo Z, Molnar ZJ: Granulocytic sarcoma of the peritoneum. *CA* 33:40, 1983.

736. Lancon JP, Charve P, Favre JP, Caillaux D: Pleural myeloid metaplasia revealing chronic myelogenous leukemia. *Crit Care Med* 14:834, 1986.

737. Jones TI: Pleural blast crisis in chronic myelogenous leukemia. *Am J Hematol* 44:75, 1993.

738. Sacchi S, Temperani P, Selleri L, et al: Extramedullary pleural blast crisis in chronic myelogenous leukemia. *Acta Hematologica* 83:198, 1990.

739. Pascoe HR: Tumors composed of immature granulocytes occurring in the breast in chronic granulocytic leukemia. *Cancer* 25:697, 1970.

740. Kwan Y-L, Singh S, Vincent PC, Gunz FW: Metamorphosis of chronic granulocytic leukemia arising in an extramedullary site. *Leuk Res* 1:301, 1977.

741. Chabner BA, Haskell CM, Canellos GP: Destructive bone lesions in chronic granulocytic leukemia. *Medicine* 48:401, 1969.

742. Licht A, Many N, Rachmilewitz EA: Myelofibrosis, osteolytic bone lesions and hypercalcemia in chronic myeloid leukemia. *Acta Haematol* 49:182, 1973.

743. Lee CH, Morris TCM: Bone marrow necrosis and extramedullary myeloid tumor necrosis in aggressive chronic myeloid leukemia. *Pathology* 11:551, 1979.

744. Asarro S, Sato N, Ueshima Y, et al: Localized blastoma preceding blastic transformation in Ph¹-positive chronic myelogenous leukemia. *Scand J Haematol* 25:251, 1980.

745. Ohyashiki K, Ito H: Characterization of extramedullary tumors in a case of Ph-positive chronic myelogenous leukemia. *Cancer Genet Cytogenet* 15:119, 1985.

746. Schwartz JH, Canellos GP, Young RC, DeVita VT: Meningeal leukemia in the blastic phase of chronic granulocytic leukemia. *Am J Med* 59:819, 1975.

747. Sun T, Susin M, Koduru P, et al: Extramedullary blast crisis in chronic myelogenous leukemia. *Cancer* 68:605, 1991.

748. Saikia TK, Dhabhar B, Iyer RS, et al: High incidence of meningeal leukemia in lymphoid blast crisis of chronic myelogenous leukemia. *Am J Hematol* 43:10, 1993.

749. Ohyashiki K, Oshimura M, Uchida H, et al: Characterization of extramedullary tumors in a case of Ph-positive chronic myelogenous leukemia: Possible involvement of immature T-lymphocytes. *Cancer Genet Cytogenet* 15:119, 1985.

750. Falini B, Tabilio A, Pelicci PG, et al: T-cell receptor B-chain gene rearrangement in a case of Ph¹-positive chronic myeloid leukaemia blast crisis. *Br J Haematol* 62:776, 1986.

751. Giannone L, Whitlock JA, Kinney MC, et al: Use of the BCR probe to demonstrate extramedullary recurrence of CML with a T cell lymphoid phenotype following bone marrow transplantation. *Bone Marrow Transplant* 3:631, 1988.

752. Ohyashiki J, Ohyashiki K, Shimizu H, et al: Testicular tumor as the first manifestation of B-lymphoid blastic crisis in a case of Ph-positive chronic myelogenous leukemia. *Am J Hematol* 29:164, 1988.

753. Neirhout RC: Chronic granulocytic leukemia. Early blast crisis simulating acute leukemia. *Am J Dis Child* 115:66, 1968.

754. Rosenthal S, Canellos GP, DeVita VT, Gralnick HR: Characteristics of blast crisis in chronic granulocytic leukemia. *Blood* 49:705, 1977.

755. Barton JC, Conrad ME: Current status of blastic transformation in chronic myelogenous leukemia. *Am J Hematol* 4:281, 1978.

756. Peterson LC, Bloomfield CD, Brunning RD: Blast crisis as an initial or terminal manifestation of chronic myeloid leukemia. *Am J Med* 60:209, 1976.

757. Bettelheim P, Lutz D, Majdic O, et al: Cell lineage heterogeneity in blast crisis of chronic myeloid leukaemia. *Br J Haematol* 59:395, 1985.

758. Nair C, Chopra M, Shinde S, et al: Immunophenotype and ultrastructural studies in blast crisis of chronic myeloid leukemia. *Leuk Lymphoma* 19:309, 1995.

759. Rosenthal S, Canellos GP, Gralnick HR: Erythroblastic transformation of chronic granulocytic leukemia. *Am J Med* 63:116, 1977.

760. Ekhlom M, Borgstrom G, vonWillebrand E, et al: Erythroid blast crisis in chronic myelogenous leukemia. *Blood* 62:591, 1983.

761. Udomratn T, Steinberg MH, Dreiling BJ, Lockhard V: Circulating micro-megakaryocytes signaling blast transformation of chronic myeloid leukaemia. *Scand J Haematol* 16:394, 1976.

762. Bain B, Catovsky C, O'Brien M, et al: Megakaryoblastic transformation of chronic granulocytic leukemia. *J Clin Pathol* 30:235, 1977.

763. Lingg G, Schmalzl F, Breton-Gorius J, et al: Megakaryoblastic micro-megakaryocytic crisis in chronic myeloid leukemia. *Blut* 51:275, 1985.

764. Castaigne S, Berger R, Jolly V, et al: Promyelocytic blast crisis of chronic myelocytic leukemia with both t(9;22) and t(15;17) in M3 cells. *Cancer* 54:2409, 1984.

765. Berger R, Bernheim A, Daniel MT, Flandrin G: t(15;17) in a promyelocytic form of chronic myeloid leukemia blastic crisis. *Cancer Genet Cytogenet* 8:149, 1983.

766. Misawa S, Lee E, Schiffer CA, et al: Association of translocation (15;17) with malignant proliferation of promyelocytes in acute leukemia and chronic myelogenous leukemia in blast crisis. *Blood* 67:270, 1986.

767. Marinone G, Rossi G, Verzura P: Eosinophilic blast crisis in a case of chronic myeloid leukaemia. *Br J Haematol* 55:251, 1983.

768. Goh K-O, Anderson FW: Cytogenetic studies in basophilic chronic myelocytic leukemia. *Arch Pathol Lab Med* 103:288, 1979.

769. Rosenthal NS, Knapp D, Farhi DC: Promyelocytic blast crisis of chronic myelogenous leukemia. A rare subtype associated with disseminated intravascular coagulation. *Am J Clin Path* 103:185, 1995.

770. Lemes A, Gomez Casares MT, de la Iglesia S, Matutes E, Molero MT: p190 BCR-ABL rearrangement in chronic myeloid leukemia and acute lymphoblastic leukemia. *Cancer Genet Cytogenet* 113:100, 1999.

771. Bertazzoni U, Brusamolino E, Isernia P, et al: Diagnostic significance of terminal transferase and adenosine deaminase in acute and chronic myeloid leukemia. *Blood* 60:685, 1982.

772. Schuh AC, Sutherland DR, Horsfall W, et al: Chronic myeloid leukemia arising in a progenitor common to T cells and myeloid cells. *Leukemia* 4:631, 1990.

773. Uike N, Takeichi N, Kimura N, et al: Dual arrangement of immunoglobulin and T-cell receptor genes in blast crisis of CML. *Eur J Haematol* 42:460, 1989.

774. Greaves MF, Verbi W, Reeves, BR, et al: "Pre-B" phenotypes in blast crisis of Ph¹ positive CML: evidence for a pluripotential stem cell "target." *Leuk Res* 3:181, 1979.

775. Bakhshi A, Minowada J, Arnold A, et al: Lymphoid blast crisis of chronic myelogenous leukemia represents stages in the development of B-cell precursors. *N Engl J Med* 309:826, 1983.

776. Griffin JD, Todd RF, Ritz J, et al: Differentiation patterns in the blastic phase of chronic myeloid leukemia. *Blood* 61:85, 1983.

777. Bollum FJ: Terminal deoxynucleotidyl transferase, in *The Enzymes*, edited by RD Boyer, pp 145–171. Academic, New York, 1974.

778. McCaffrey R, Lilliquist A, Sallan S, et al: Clinical utility of leukemia cell terminal transferase measurements. *Cancer Res* 41:4814, 1981.

779. Dorfman DM, Longtine JA, Fox EA, et al: T-cell blast crisis in chronic myelogenous leukemia. *Am J Clin Path* 107:168, 1997.

780. Allouche M, Bourinbaiar A, Georgoulias V, et al: T-cell lineage involvement in lymphoid blast crisis of chronic myeloid leukemia. *Blood* 66:1155, 1985.

781. Gramatzki M, Bartram CR, Muller D, et al: Early T-cell differentiated chronic myeloid leukemia blast crisis with rearrangement of the breakpoint cluster region but not of the T-cell receptor Beta chain genes. *Blood* 69:1082, 1987.

782. Dastugue N, Kuhlein E, Duchayne E, et al: t(14;14)(q11;q32) in biphenotypic blastic phase of chronic myeloid leukemia. *Blood* 68:949, 1986.

783. Kuriyama K, Tomonaga M, Yao E, et al: Dual expression of lymphoid/basophil markers on single blast cells transformed from chronic myeloid leukemia. *Leuk Res* 10:1015, 1986.

784. Yasukawa M, Iwamasa K, Kawamura S, et al: Phenotypic and genotypic analysis of chronic myelogenous leukaemia with T lymphoblastic and megakaryoblastic mixed crisis. *Br J Haematol* 66:331, 1987.

785. Spencer A, Vulliamy T, Chase A, et al: Myeloid to lymphoid clonal suppression following autologous transplantation in second chronic phase of chronic myeloid leukemia. *Leukemia* 9:2138, 1995.

786. Cervantes F, Villamor N, Esteve J, et al: "Lymphoid" blast crisis of chronic myeloid leukaemia is associated with distinct clinicohaematological features. *Br J Haematol* 100:123, 1998.

787. Stoll C, Oberline F: Non-random clonal evolution in 45 cases of chronic myeloid leukemia. *Leuk Res* 46:61, 1980.

788. Sandberg AA: The cytogenetics of chronic myelocytic leukemia (CML): chronic phase and blastic crisis. *Cancer Genet Cytogenet* 1:217, 1980.

789. Myint H, Ross FM, Hall JL, et al: Early transformation to acute myeloblastic leukaemia with the acquisition of inv(16) in Ph positive chronic granulocytic leukaemia. *Leuk Res* 21:473, 1997.

790. Sandberg AA: Chronic myelocytic leukemia, in *The Chromosomes in Human Cancer and Leukemia*, 2nd ed, pp 465–477. Elsevier North Holland, New York, 1990.

791. O'Malley FM, Garson OM: Chronic granulocytic leukemia: correlation of blastic transformation with karyotypic evolution. *Am J Hematol* 20:313, 1985.

792. Singh S, Wass J, Vincent PC, et al: Significance of secondary cytogenetic changes in patients with Ph-positive chronic granulocytic leukemia in the acute phase. *Cancer Genet Cytogenet* 21:209, 1986.

793. Diez-Martin JL, DeWald GW, Pierre RV: Possible cytogenetic distinction between lymphoid and myeloid blast crisis in chronic granulocytic leukemia. *Am J Hematol* 27:194, 1988.

794. Mitani K, Miyazono K, Urabe A, Takaku F: Karyotypic changes during the course of blastic crisis of chronic myelogenous leukemia. *Cancer Genet Cytogenet* 39:299, 1989.

795. Heim S, Christensen EB, Fioretos T, et al: Acute myelomonocytic leukemia with inv(16) (p13q22) complicating Philadelphia chromosome positive chronic myeloid leukemia. *Cancer Genet Cytogenet* 59:35, 1992.

796. Feinstein E, Cimino G, Gale RP, Canaani E: Initiation and progression of chronic myelogenous leukemia. *Leukemia* 6(suppl 1): 37, 1992.

797. Hogge DE, Misawa S, Testa JR, et al: Unusual karyotypic changes and B-cell involvement in a case of lymph node blast crisis of chronic myelogenous leukemia. *Blood* 64:123, 1984.

798. Wiernik P: The current status of therapy for the prevention of blast crisis of chronic myelocytic leukemia. *J Clin Oncol* 2:329, 1984.

799. Koller CA, Miller DM: Preliminary observations on the therapy of the myeloid blast phase of chronic granulocytic leukemia with plicamycin and hydroxyurea. *N Engl J Med* 315:1433, 1986.

800. Rosenthal S, Canellos G, Whang-Peng J, Gradwick A: Blast crisis of chronic granulocytic leukemia. *Am J Med* 63:542, 1977.

801. Kouides PA, Rowe JM: A dose intensive regime of cytosine arabinoside and daunorubicin for chronic myelogenous leukemia in blast crisis. *Leuk Res* 19:763, 1995.

802. Gollard R, Miller WE, Piro LD, Saven A: 2-chlorodeoxyadenosine administration to patients with the myeloid blast phase of chronic myelogenous leukemia. *Leuk Lymphoma* 28:183, 1997.

803. Tricot G, Weber G: Biochemically targeted therapy of refractory leukemia and myeloid blast crisis of chronic granulocytic leukemia with Tiazofurin, a selective blocker of inosine 5'-phosphate dehydrogenase activity. *Anticancer Res* 16:334, 1996.

804. Marks SM, Baltimore D, McCaffrey R: Terminal transferase as a predictor of initial responsiveness to vincristine and prednisone in blastic chronic myelogenous leukemia. *N Engl J Med* 298:812, 1978.

805. Janossy G, Woodruff RK, Pippard MJ, et al: Relation of lymphoid phenotype and response to chemotherapy incorporating vincristine-prednisone in the acute phase of Ph[1] positive leukemia. *Cancer* 43:426, 1979.

806. Tanaka M, Kaneda T, Hirota Y, et al: Terminal deoxynucleotidyl transferase in the blastic phase of chronic myelogenous leukemia. An indicator of response to vincristine and prednisone. *Am J Hematol* 9:287, 1980.

807. deWitte T, dePauw B, Haanen C: Remission-induction of acute lymphoblastic transformation of chronic myeloid leukemia, followed by long-term maintenance therapy. *Blut* 52:231, 1986.

808. Jain K, Arlin Z, Mertelsmann R, et al: Philadelphia chromosome and terminal transferase-positive acute leukemia: Similarity of terminal phase of chronic myelogenous leukemia and de novo acute presentation. *J Clin Oncol* 1:669, 1983.

809. Champlain R, Ho W, Arenson E, Gale RP: Allogeneic bone marrow transplantation for chronic myelogenous leukemia in chronic or accelerated phase. *Blood* 60:1038, 1982.

810. McGlave PB, Kim TH, Hard DD, et al: Successful allogeneic bone-marrow transplantation for patients in the accelerated phase of chronic granulocytic leukaemia. *Lancet* 2:625, 1982.

811. Martin PJ, Clift RA, Fisher LD, et al: HLA-identical marrow transplantation during accelerated-phase chronic myelogenous leukemia: analysis of survival and remission duration. *Blood* 77:1978, 1988.

812. Buckner CD, Stewart P, Clift RA, et al: Treatment of blastic transformation of chronic granulocytic leukemia by chemotherapy, total body irradiation and infusion of cryopreserved autologous marrow. *Exp Hematol* 6:96, 1978.

813. Goldman JM, Johnson SA, Islam A, et al: Haematological reconstitution after autografting for chronic granulocytic leukemia in transformation: the influence of previous splenectomy. *Br J Haematol* 45:223, 1980.

814. Haines ME, Goldman JM, Worsley AM, et al: Chemotherapy and autografting for chronic granulocytic leukaemia in transformation. Probably prolongation of survival for some patients. *Br J Haematol* 58:711, 1984.

815. DeWitte T, Raymakers R, dePauw B, Haanen C: Repetitive cycles of cytoreductive therapy followed by stem cell autografting for non-lymphoblastic transformation of chronic granulocytic leukaemia. *Scand J Haematol* 35:421, 1985.

816. Reiffers J, Gorin NC, Michallet M, et al: Autografting for chronic granulocytic leukemia in transformation. *J Natl Cancer Inst* 76:1307, 1986.

817. Carella AM, Gaozza E, Raffo MR, et al: Therapy of acute phase chronic myelogenous leukemia with intensive chemotherapy, blood cell autotransplant and cyclosporin A. *Leukemia* 5:517, 1991.

818. Bouvet M., Babiera GV, Termuhlen PM, et al: Splenectomy in the accelerated or blastic phase of chronic myelogenous leukemia: a single-institution, 25-year experience. *Surgery* 122:20, 1997.

819. Majiis A, Smith TL, Talpaz M, et al: Signficance of cytogenetic clonal evolution in chronic myelogenous leukemia. *J Clin Oncol* 14:196, 1996.

820. Sawyers CL, Druker B: Tyrosine kinase inhibitors in chronic myeloid leukemia. *Cancer* 5:63, 1999.

821. Warmuth M, Danhauser-Reidel S, Hallek M: Molecular pathogenesis of chronic myeloid leukemia: implications for new therapeutic strategies. *Ann Hematol* 78:49, 1999.

822. Falkenberg JHF, Wafelman AR, Joosten P, et al: Complete remission of accelerated phase chronic myeloid leukemia by treatment with leukemia-reactive cytotoxic T lymphocytes. *Blood* 94:1201, 1999

823. Sexauer J, Kass L, Schnitzer B: Subacute myelomonocytic leukaemia: a distinct haematological entity. *Am J Med* 57:853, 1974.

824. Zittoun R: Subacute and chronic myelomonocytic leukaemia: a distinct haematological entity. *Br J Haematol* 32:1, 1976.

825. Stark AN, Thorogood J, Head C, et al: Prognostic factors and survival in chronic myelomonocytic leukaemia (CMML). *Br J Cancer* 56:59, 1987.

826. Fenaux P, Jouet JP, Zandecki M, et al: Chronic and subacute myelomonocytic leukaemia in the adult. *Br J Haematol* 65:101, 1987

827. Bennett JM, Catavosky D, Daniel MT, et al: The chronic myeloid leukemias: guidelines for distinguishing chronic granulocytic, atypical chronic myeloid, and chronic myelomonocytic leukaemia. *Br J Haematol* 87:746, 1994.

828. Cambier N, Baruchel A, Schlageter MH, et al: Chronic myelomonocytic leukemia: from biology to therapy. *Hematol Cell Ther* 39:41, 1997.

829. Wessels JW, Fibbe WE, van der Keur D, et al: t(5;12)(q31;p12): a clinical entity with features of both myeloid leukemia and chronic myelomonocytic leukemia. *Cancer Genet Cytogenet* 65:7, 1993.

830. Maher J, Colonna F, Baker D, et al: Retroviral-mediated gene transfer of a mutant H-ras gene into a normal human bone marrow alters myeloid cell proliferation and differentiation. *Exp Hematol* 22:8,1994.

831. Miura A: Progress in laboratory medicine in chronic myeloid leukemia. *Jap J Clin Pathol* 46:1226, 1998.

832. Haferlach T, Winkemann M, Nickening C, et al: Which components are involved in Philadelphia-chromosome-positive chronic leukemia? *Br J Haematol* 97:99, 1997.

833. Muñoz L, Bellido M, Sierra J, Nomdedéu JF: Flow cytometric detection of B cell abnormal maturation in chronic myeloid leukemia. *Leukemia* 14:339, 1999.

834. Yanagi M, Shinjo K, Takeshita A, et al: Simple and reliably sensitive diagnosis and monitoring of Philadelphia chromosome-positive cells in chronic myeloid leukemia by interphase fluorescence *in situ* hybridization of peripheral blood cells. *Leukemia* 13:542, 1999.

835. Druker BJ, Lydon NB: Lessons learned fvrom the development of an Abl tyrosine kinase inhibitor for chronic myelogenous leukemia. *J Clin Invest* 105:3, 2000.

836. James HA: The potential application of ribozymes for the treatment of hematologic disorders. *J Leuk Biol* 66:361, 1999.

837. Verfaillie CM, McIvor RS, Zhao CH: Gene therapy for chronic myelogenous leukemia. *Mol Med Today* 5:359, 1999.

838. Nitta M, Tsuboi K, Yamashita S, et al: Multiple myeloma preceding development of chronic myelogenous leukemia. *Int J Hematol* 69:170, 1999.

839. Dazzi F, Szydlo RM, Goldman JM: Donor lymphocyte infusion for

relapse of chronic myeloid leukemia after allogeneic stem cell transplant: where we now stand. *Exp Hematol* 27:1477, 1999.

840. Pane F, Mostarda I, Sellari C: BCR/ABL mRNA and the P210 BCR/ABL protein are downmodulated by Interferon-α in chronic myeloid leukemia patients. *Blood* 94:2200, 1999.

841. Hochhaus A, Reiter A, Saubele S, et al: Molecular heterogeneity in complete cytogenetic responders after interferon-α therapy for chronic myelogenous leukemia. *Blood* 95:62, 2000.

842. Chomel J-C, Brizard F, Veinstein A, et al: Persistence of BCR-ABL genomic rearrangement in chronic myeloid leukemia patients in complete sustained cytogenetic remission after interferon-α therapy or allogeneic bone marrow transplantation. *Blood* 95:404, 2000.

843. Golub TR, Barker GF, Love HM, Gilliland DG: Fusion of PDGF receptor β to a novel *ets*-like gen, *tel*, in chronic myelomonocytic leukemia with t(5;12) chromosomal translocation. *Cell* 77:307, 1994.

844. Bain BJ: Hypereosinophilia. *Curr Opin Hematol* 7:21, 2000.

IDIOPATHIC MYELOFIBROSIS (AGNOGENIC MYELOID METAPLASIA)

MARSHALL A. LICHTMAN

Idiopathic myelofibrosis is one of several disorders in the spectrum of clonal hemopathies, malignant diseases that originate in the clonal expansion of a single neoplastic hematopoietic stem cell. It is characterized by anemia, mild neutrophilia, thrombocytosis, and splenomegaly. Immature myeloid and erythroid precursors, teardrop-shaped erythrocytes, and large platelets are constant features of the blood film. The marrow has increased reticulin fibers, and this reactive fibroplasia is the result of cytokines released locally by the numerous abnormal megakaryocytes. The disease may be complicated by portal hypertension, as a result of a very large splenic blood flow and the loss of compliance of hepatic vessels, and by fibrohematopoietic tumors that can develop in any tissue and lead to symptoms by compression of vital structures. Treatment may include hydroxyurea for thrombocytosis and massive splenomegaly, red cell transfusions for severe anemia, local irradiation of fibrohematopoietic tumors or of the spleen, and splenectomy. Portosystemic shunt surgery may be required for gastroesophageal variceal bleeding. The disease may remain indolent for years or may progress rapidly by further deterioration in hematopoiesis, by massive splenic enlargement and its sequelae, or by transformation to acute myelogenous leukemia. Overall median survival is about five years.

DEFINITION AND HISTORY

Idiopathic myelofibrosis is a chronic myeloproliferative disorder characterized by (1) anemia, (2) splenomegaly, (3) immature granulocytes, erythroblasts, and teardrop-shaped red cells in the blood, and (4) marrow fibrosis. The disorder was originally described by Heuck in 1879 under the title ''Two Cases of Leukemia and Peculiar Blood and Bone Marrow Findings.''[1] Silverstein, in his monograph, traces the history of the concepts set forth during the first half of the twentieth century to explain the pathogenesis of this disease, including its origin in the marrow, the appearance of extramedullary hemopoiesis, and the relationship of fibrosis to hematopoietic changes.[2] Over 30 designations for the disease have been proposed or used, and different ones are preferred in different countries.[3] *Agnogenic myeloid metaplasia* and, more recently, *idiopathic myelofibrosis* are the two most frequently used terms for the disease. Neither designation accommodates the three key phenomena of a clonal hematopoietic stem cell abnormal-

ity, a propensity to extramedullary fibrohematopoietic tumors, and the secondary intense marrow fibrosis.[302]

ETIOLOGY AND PATHOGENESIS

Marrow fibrosis associated with compromise of intramedullary hematopoiesis and development of ectopic foci of hemopoiesis have been induced in animals by chemicals such as lead acetate and saponin, after infection with the Rauscher rat leukemia and S37 sarcoma viruses, by high doses of estrogens, and by overexpression of thrombopoietin.[2,4] These models do not replicate the pathogenesis of human disease, which is the result of a somatic mutation in an hematopoietic stem cell.

Animals injected with marrow extracts, antimarrow serum, or egg albumin have developed marrow fibrosis and splenic hematopoiesis.[2] These observations, along with reports of myelofibrosis in patients with lupus erythematosus, have suggested the possibility of immunologic-mediated hyperplasia of marrow connective tissue.[2] This form of myelofibrosis is different from the monoclonal stem cell disease being considered in this chapter.

Exposure to benzene[5-7] or very high dose ionizing radiation[8,9] has preceded the development of idiopathic myelofibrosis in a small proportion of patients with the disease. These two incitants are well-established environmental causes of clonal myeloid disorders.

CLONAL HEMOPATHY

The disease arises from the neoplastic transformation of a single hemopoietic stem cell, a conclusion derived from studies in women with idiopathic myelofibrosis who were also heterozygous for isotypes A and B of G-6-PD.[10,11] Although the nonhemopoietic tissues of these patients expressed both isotypes, each patient had blood cells with only one G-6-PD isotype. These findings strongly imply that the blood cells of each patient arose from only one transformed stem cell. Further, chromosome studies of colonies of hemopoietic progenitor cells in idiopathic myelofibrosis have established that a clonal cytogenetic abnormality is present in erythroblasts, neutrophils, macrophages, basophils, and megakaryocytes.[12] These studies have been confirmed by (1) examining X-linked restriction fragment length polymorphisms in women with idiopathic myelofibrosis with heterozygosity for the X chromosome-linked genes[13,14] and (2) verifying the presence of a mutation of codon 12 of the N-*RAS* gene in five blood cell lineages of a patient with the disease.[15,16]

Myeloproliferation is usually the dominant abnormality in the granulocytic and megakaryocytic marrow lineages resulting in blood granulocytosis and thrombocytosis. Ineffective or hypoplastic hemopoiesis can be present initially or emerge as the dominant pathogenetic process later, leading to granulocytopenia and/or thrombocytopenia. Anemia is a frequent finding as a result of a combination of hypoplastic erythropoiesis, shortened red cell survival, and the effects of massive splenomegaly on the distribution of red cells in the circulation. Hemolysis can be a prominent factor in some cases.

FIBROPLASIA

Four of the five major types of collagen[17] are present in normal marrow: type I found in bone, type III found in blood vessels, and types IV and V found in basement membranes. The fine reticulin fibers that are visible after silver impregnation of normal marrow are principally type III collagen. They do not stain with trichrome dyes. The thicker collagen fibers are principally type I collagen and stain with trichrome dyes but do not impregnate with silver. The fine fibrous network in normal marrow that is stained by silver impregnation techniques[18] is increased in amount in the marrow of virtually all patients with idio-

Acronyms and abbreviations that appear in this chapter include: G-6-PD, glucose-6-phosphate dehydrogenase; IL, interleukin.

TABLE 95-1   FIBROPLASIA IN IDIOPATHIC MYELOFIBROSIS

Marrow Stroma

Increased Amount of
Total collagen (hydroxyproline)[20,24]
Type I collagen[20–22,25]
Type III collagen[20–22,25]
Type III procollage[21–26]
Type IV collagen[21,27,28]
Laminin[21,27,29]
Fibronectin[30,31]
Tenascin[32]
Vitronectin[33]

Plasma

Increased Concentration of
Prolylhydroxylase[34]
C-terminal peptide of procollagen type I[23]
N-terminal peptide of procollagen type III[22,35,36]
Type IV collagen[22,29]
Laminin[22,29]
Fibronectin[31]
Hyaluronan[37]

pathic myelofibrosis[19] (Table 95-1). The fibrous network contains collagen and can progress occasionally to include thick collagen bands that are evident with trichrome stains. Collagen types I, III, IV, and V are increased in myelofibrosis, but type III collagen is increased uniformly and preferentially.[20–23] The latter occurrence accounts also for the increase in the plasma concentration of procollagen III amino terminal peptide, a component of collagen type III, which is cleaved during the biosynthesis of collagen.[22,24] Serum prolylhydroxylase and marrow and plasma fibronectin are also increased in patients with idiopathic myelofibrosis or myelofibrosis from other causes.[14,21,22]

Marrow fibrosis in idiopathic myelofibrosis is most closely correlated with an increase of dysmorphic megakaryocytes in the marrow, and even densely fibrotic marrow with little residual granulopoiesis or erythropoiesis usually has numerous megakaryocytes scattered throughout the fibrotic areas.[19,38]

The enhanced collagen types I and III content of marrow is the result of release of fibroblast growth factors. These include platelet-derived growth factor,[39,40] epidermal growth factor,[41] endothelial cell growth factor,[41] transforming growth factor-β[42,43] and basic fibroblast growth factor,[44] each of which is present in megakaryocyte α granules. Other factors, such as tumor necrosis factor-α and IL-1 α and β, which can be released from marrow cells, also can stimulate fibroblasts.[45,46] Platelet factor 4, also derived from megakaryocytes, inhibits collagenase and could contribute to collagen accumulation,[38] although studies showing a poor correlation between plasma platelet factor 4 concentration and marrow fibrosis have dampened enthusiasm for the role of this factor.[47] The high urinary excretion of platelet-derived calmodulin, a putative fibroblast growth factor, in patients with myelofibrosis has added this compound to the array of factors that may contribute to the fibroplasia.[45] The pathogenetic role of released growth factors in fibroplasia is incompletely understood. Generalizations from in vitro experiments or correlation between two variables provide only a limited perspective. For example, transforming growth factor-β can stimulate or inhibit fibroblast growth, depending on the repertoire of other growth factors in the environment.[42,43]

The fibroplasia in idiopathic myelofibrosis is associated with an increase in the number and size of marrow sinuses,[19,48] the number of endothelial cells,[49] an increase in vascular volume in the marrow,[50] and an increase in blood flow through the marrow.[27,51] These processes are responsible for the increase in marrow collagen types IV and V

and laminin synthesized by endothelial cells in the marrow of patients with myelofibrosis.[41]

The fibroblastic proliferation in marrow is not an intrinsic part of the abnormal clonal expansion of hemopoiesis.[52] In cases of idiopathic myelofibrosis in which G-6-PD isoenzyme studies or chromosome karyotyping establish monoclonal growth of hemopoietic cells, marrow fibroblasts contain both G-6-PD isoenzymes and do not share the clonal chromosome abnormality.[53] These findings strongly imply that the fibroblasts differentiate from a primordial cell different from the hemopoietic stem cell and that their proliferation and enhanced collagen synthesis is a secondary result of the abnormal hemopoiesis.

EXTRAMEDULLARY HEMATOPOIESIS

Extramedullary hemopoiesis is consistently present in liver and spleen,[54–56] where it contributes to organ enlargement. Escape of progenitor cells from marrow and their lodgment in other organs may contribute to extramedullary blood formation. Reversion of the liver and spleen to their fetal hemopoietic functions is not held to be a major factor in the extramedullary hemopoiesis, and quantitatively significant, effective hemopoiesis does not occur outside of the marrow.

CLINICAL FEATURES

AGE AND SEX

Idiopathic myelofibrosis characteristically occurs after age 50.[2,54–61] The median age at diagnosis is about 65 years,[57–59] but the disease can occur from the neonatal period to the ninth decade.[57,58,62,63] Its occurrence in children is usually in the first 3 years of life.[63–65] In adults the disease occurs with about equal frequency in men and women,[57–61] whereas in young children girls are afflicted with the disease twice as frequently as boys.[63] The disease, rarely, can be familial.[67,68]

PRESENTING SYMPTOMS

About one-quarter of patients are asymptomatic at the time of diagnosis, being detected by medical examination for an unrelated reason. In symptomatic patients, fatigue, weakness, shortness of breath, and palpitations are nonspecific but frequent complaints.[54–56] Weight loss is common, but anorexia is less so and night sweats occur very infrequently. A dragging sensation in the left upper abdomen caused by an enlarged spleen or early satiety from encroachment of the spleen on the stomach may occur. Severe left upper quadrant or left shoulder pain can occur from splenic infarction and perisplenitis. Patients may also report unexpected bleeding. Rarely, bone pain may be prominent, especially in the lower extremities.

PRESENTING SIGNS

Hepatomegaly is detectable in two-thirds of patients, and splenomegaly is present in virtually every patient at the time of diagnosis.[2,54–61] The spleen is mildly enlarged in one-third and massively enlarged in one-third. Muscle wasting, peripheral edema, and purpura are present infrequently. Bone tenderness may be present.

Neutrophilic dermatosis, a syndrome that closely mimics the raised and tender plaques of Sweet syndrome may develop.[69–71] It can be the presenting or a significant complicating feature of myelofibrosis and can progress to bullae or pyoderma gangrenosum.[69,72] The dermatopathology of neutrophilic dermatosis is different from leukemia cutis and is unrelated to infection or vasculitis. The predominant lesion is an intense polymorphonuclear neutrophilic infiltrate.

Skin infiltrates related to hematopoietic cells (leukemia cutis) are very uncommon.[73]

SPECIAL CLINICAL FEATURES

FIBROHEMOPOIETIC EXTRAMEDULLARY TUMORS

Foci of hemopoiesis are often present in adrenals, kidneys, and lymph nodes and may become clinically apparent as fibrohemopoietic tumors in the adrenal glands,[74] subcapsular renal space,[75] and lymph nodes.[76,77] Tumors composed of hemopoietic tissue, sometimes with intense fibrosis, can develop in the bowel,[78–81] breast,[82–84] lungs,[85,86] mediastinum,[85] mesentery,[85] skin,[87,88] synovium,[89] thymus,[85] thyroid,[90] prostate,[91] or the kidney and urinary tract.[92–96]

Extramedullary hemopoiesis in the intracranial or intraspinal epidural space can lead to serious neurologic complications, including subdural hemorrhage,[97] delirium,[98,99] increased intracranial pressure,[99] papilledema,[100] coma,[101] motor and sensory impairment,[102–105] spinal cord compression,[103] and limb paralysis.[102,103] Intraspinal myelography,[103,104] computed axial tomography,[97,99,101,106] positron emission tomography after [52]Fe infusion,[98] and magnetic resonance imaging[107,108] each have been used to define the location and nature of the masses.

Hemopoietic foci on serosal surfaces can produce effusions, sometimes massive, in the thorax,[109] abdomen,[110,111] and pericardial space.[112–115] The effusion fluid often contains megakaryocytes, immature granulocytes, and occasionally erythroblasts.[116–118] Splenectomy is sometimes followed by extramedullary hemopoietic tumors in soft tissues,[119] in body cavities, or on serosal surfaces,[115] perhaps as a result of an increase in circulating hematopoietic progenitors[120] and the loss of the filtration function of the spleen. In rare cases, extramedullary soft tissue megakaryoblastic tumors simulate the granulocytic sarcomas of other types of myelogenous leukemia.[121,122]

PORTAL HYPERTENSION AND VARICES

In patients with idiopathic myelofibrosis there can be a massive increase in splenoportal blood flow and a decrease in hepatic vascular compliance or the presence of hepatic vein thrombosis, either of which can result in severe portal hypertension, ascites, esophageal and gastric varices, intraluminal gastrointestinal bleeding, and hepatic encephalopathy.[123–125] Perisinusoidal fibrosis,[126–128] collagen bundles in the spaces of Disse,[127] perisinusoidal fibroplasia,[126–129] and foci of hemopoietic cells[127] each appear to contribute to the decreased sinusoidal compliance.

Portal vein thrombosis is a complication of idiopathic myelofibrosis and can occasionally precede the onset of the disease.[130]

IMMUNE MANIFESTATIONS

Abnormalities of humoral immune mechanisms have been observed in up to one-half of patients with idiopathic myelofibrosis.[131–136] The array of immune products and events reported includes anti-red-cell antibodies,[135,137] antiplatelet antibodies,[138,139] antinuclear antibodies,[131,132,136] elevated plasma soluble IL-2 receptor,[140] anti-Gal (galactosidic determinants) antibodies,[141] anti-gamma-globulins,[131,132,136] antiphospholipid antibodies,[136,142] antitissue or organ-specific antibodies,[132,135] and circulating immune complexes,[136,143–145] as well as complement activation,[136,146] immune complex deposition,[133] interstitial immunoglobulin deposition,[133] increased numbers of marrow plasmacytoid lymphocytes,[133,143] and the development of amyloidosis.[144,147] Occasional reports of myelofibrosis associated with lupus erythematosus,[148–152] vasculitis,[153] polyarteritis nodosa,[136,154] scleroderma,[155] and acute reversible myelofibrosis responsive to glucocorticoids[156] have raised the possibility that immune mechanisms may play a role in the development of marrow fibrosis in some circumstances.

BONE CHANGES

A large proportion of patients develop osteosclerosis,[57,157] reflected by increased bone density on radiographic studies and also evident on marrow biopsy.[158] The proximal femur and humerus, pelvis, vertebrae, ribs, and skull may be involved. The x-ray picture may mimic the bone reaction to metastatic carcinoma. Osteolytic lesions are rare[159] and may reflect a granulocytic sarcoma.[160] Periostitis can lead to debilitating bone pain.[54–56,161]

LABORATORY FEATURES

BLOOD CELL COUNTS AND MORPHOLOGY

The range of values for blood cell counts at the time of diagnosis is very broad. Normocytic-normochromic anemia is present in most, but not all, patients.[2,54–60,162–165] The mean hemoglobin concentration at diagnosis was 9.5 to 11.6 g/dl, with a range of 4 to 20 g/dl among a total of 539 patients in four studies.[56,60,163,164] Anisocytosis and poikilocytosis are a constant finding, and teardrop-shaped red cells (dacrocytes) are present in all cases in sufficient number to be found in every oil-immersion field (Fig. 95-1). Nucleated red cells are present in the blood film of most patients and average 2 percent of nucleated cells, with a range of 0 to 30 percent. The percentage of reticulocytes is mildly increased but may vary widely in a given case. Anemia may be worsened by an expansion of plasma volume and a higher-than-normal proportion of the red cell volume in an enlarged spleen. Ineffective erythropoiesis can result in a decrease in red cell mass,[162] and erythroid hypoplasia is present in many patients.[166,167] In some patients hemolysis may be prominent, and polychromatophilia and very elevated reticulocyte counts can occur.[56,60,163,164] The antiglobulin (Coombs') test is usually negative, but red cell autoantibodies can develop and lead to immune-mediated hemolysis.[56,136,137,168] Occasional patients have a positive acid hemolysis and sucrose hemolysis test, reflecting concurrent paroxysmal nocturnal hemoglobinuria.[169] Acquired hemoglobin H disease, coincident with typical white cells and platelet changes of myelofibrosis, can occur[170] and results in hemolysis, hypochromic-microcytic red cells, marked poikilocytosis, and hemoglobin H inclusions that stain with brilliant cresyl blue. Red cell aplasia, in association with myelofibrosis, has also been observed.[165,171]

The total white cell count in patients with idiopathic myelofibrosis is usually elevated mildly as a result of granulocytosis.[2,54–61] The mean total white cell count was 10 to 14 $\times10^9$/l in four large studies. The range of white cell counts was 0.4 to 237 $\times 10^9$/l at the time of diagnosis.[56,60,163,164] Myelocytes and promyelocytes are present in small proportions in most patients, and a low proportion of blast cells (1–2%) may be found in the blood film in many patients. The range of blood blast cells is zero to 20 percent at the time of diagnosis. Hypersegmentation, hyposegmentation (acquired Pelger-Huët anomaly), and abnormal granulation of neutrophils may be present.[2,54–56] Neutrophil alkaline phosphatase scores may be elevated (25 percent of patients) or decreased (25 percent of patients).[2,172] The percent of basophils may be slightly increased.[164] Neutropenia is present in about 20 percent of patients at the time of diagnosis.[58]

The mean platelet count has ranged from 175 to 580 $\times 10^9$/l, and the range of individual counts was from 15 to 3215 $\times 10^9$/l.[6,60,163,164] The platelet count is elevated in about 40 percent of patients.[58,164] Mild to moderate thrombocytopenia is present in about one-third of patients at the time of diagnosis. Giant platelets and abnormal platelet granulation are characteristic features of this disease.

About 10 percent of patients may present with pancytopenia because of severe impairment of hematopoiesis affecting each cell lineage, coupled with sequestration in a massively enlarged spleen.[2,54,55] Pancytopenia is usually associated with intense marrow fibrosis.

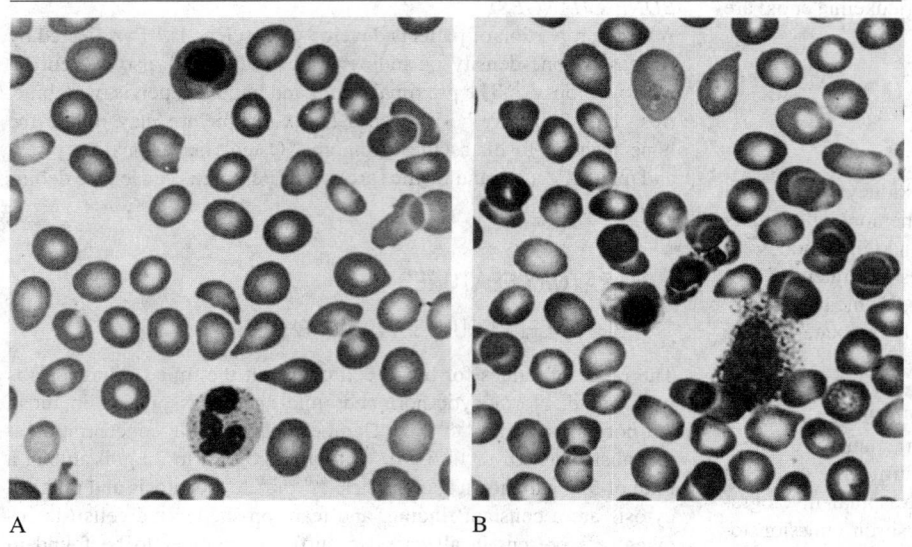

FIGURE 95-1 Blood films from two patients with idiopathic myelofibrosis. (*a*) Characteristic teardrop poikilocytes, a nucleated red cell, and a segmented neutrophil are evident. (*b*) Teardrop red cells, a nucleated red cell, and a promyelocyte are present.

Increased concentrations of pluripotential,[173] granulocytic,[174,175] monocytic,[176,177] and erythroid[178] progenitor cells are present in the blood of patients as measured by clonogenic assays of blood cells in semisolid cultures. Megakaryocytes are also present in the systemic venous blood.[177]

FUNCTIONAL ABNORMALITIES OF BLOOD CELLS

The neutrophils of some patients have impaired phagocytosis, oxygen consumption, nitroblue tetrazolium reduction, and hydrogen peroxide generation, as well as decreased myeloperoxidase[178,179] and glutathione reductase activities.[179] Bleeding time can be prolonged out of proportion to the platelet count.[180,181] Abnormalities of platelets in patients with idiopathic myelofibrosis include impaired aggregation in response to epinephrine, depletion of dense granule adenosine diphosphate content,[182] decreased platelet lipoxygenase pathway activity,[183] and others.[184,185] The correlation of bleeding or thrombosis with platelet functional abnormalities is weak, however.[184,185] The lupus anticoagulant has been present, but only rarely.[141]

MARROW EXAMINATION

MORPHOLOGY

Marrow aspiration is often unsuccessful because of the fibrosis.[18,54,60] The marrow biopsy is often cellular and shows granulocytic and megakaryocytic hyperplasia.[19,164] Erythroid cells may be decreased, normal, or increased in number. Hematoxylin and eosin stains of the biopsy may show slight collagen fibrosis, but this may be extreme on occasion. In some subjects, osteosclerosis is found.[19,60,164] Silver stain shows an increase in reticulin fibers, and in half the patients a striking increase in reticulin fibers is present.[60,164] In intensely fibrotic marrows cellularity may be decreased, but megakaryocytes usually remain evident.[60,164] Giant megakaryocytes and micromegakaryocytes, abnormal nuclear lobulation, and naked megakaryocyte nuclei may be present.[60,186] Granulocytes may show hyperlobulation and hypolobulation of the nucleus, acquired Pelger-Huët anomaly, nuclear blebs, and

nuclear-cytoplasmic maturation asynchrony.[187] Dilated marrow sinusoids are common. Intrasinusoidal, immature hemopoietic cells, and megakaryocytes are present.[19,48]

CYTOGENETIC FINDINGS

Chromosome abnormalities of hemopoietic cells are evident in about forty percent of the patients at the time of diagnosis.[188–191] The most frequent findings are partial trisomy 1q, interstitial deletion of a segment of the long arm of chromosome 13, del 13 (q13q21), which bears the retinoblastoma gene,[16,189–191] and del 20q. Involvement of chromosomes 5, 7, 9, 13, 20, or 21 occurs with heightened frequency. Aneuploidy, as a result of monosomy or trisomy, is common. Pseudodiploidy, manifested by partial deletions and translocations, occurs also. Patients with typical idiopathic myelofibrosis have had the Ph chromosome in their marrow cell.[192] This association is rare, however. Clonal chromosomal abnormalities found in hemopoietic cells have not been found in fibroblasts.[53]

MAGNETIC RESONANCE IMAGING

Fibrosis in the marrow alters the hyperintensity of T1-weighted images that normally result from the marrow fat. As fibrosis progresses, hypointensity of T1- and T2-weighted images develops. These abnormalities are similar to those that occur with marrow hemosiderosis. Histologic confirmation by marrow biopsy of MR images is important for verification. MR imaging cannot distinguish between idiopathic myelofibrosis and secondary causes of fibrosis.[193,194]

PLASMA AND URINE CHEMICAL CHANGES

The serum levels of uric acid, lactic dehydrogenase, bilirubin, alkaline phosphatase, and high-density lipoprotein are frequently elevated,[54,58] and those of albumin and cholesterol are frequently decreased.[58,195] Hypocalcemia[196] or hypercalcemia[197] may occur. Plasma levels of thrombopoietin and IL-6 are elevated but do not correlate with either platelet or megakaryocyte mass.[198] Urinary excretion of calmodulin is about three times normal.[45]

DIFFERENTIAL DIAGNOSIS

Chronic myelogenous leukemia (see Chap. 94) should be considered in the differential diagnosis of idiopathic myelofibrosis. In chronic myelogenous leukemia the white cell count is over $30 \times 10^9/l$ (30,000/μl) in virtually all patients and over 100×10^9/liter (100,000/μl) in half the patients, but in myelofibrosis it is usually less than $30 \times 10^9/l$ (30,000/μl) at the time of diagnosis. In chronic myelogenous leukemia red cell shape is usually normal or slightly perturbed, whereas in myelofibrosis teardrop poikilocytes are present in every oil-immersion field and exaggerated anisocytosis and anisochromia are often prominent. The marrow in chronic myelogenous leukemia shows intense granulocytic hyperplasia with virtually 100 percent cellularity and usually no or very slight fibrosis.[199] In myelofibrosis, the marrow has mildly increased cellularity or is hypocellular, with moderate to marked fibrosis. The Ph chromosome or the *BCR-ABL* fusion gene is present in chronic myelogenous leukemia and absent in idiopathic myelofibrosis. Rarely, patients with chronic myelogenous leukemia may develop intense marrow fibrosis and dysmorphic blood cell changes that make distinction between the two diseases difficult.[199] Most cases are readily separable on the basis of the aforementioned distinctions.

Patients with idiopathic myelofibrosis may have pancytopenia or bicytopenia and in that respect mimic patients with oligoblastic leukemia (myelodysplasia) (see Chap. 92). Contrariwise, patients with oligoblastic leukemia may rarely have intense fibrosis. Prominent splenomegaly is expected in patients with idiopathic myelofibrosis but not in patients with oligoblastic leukemia, which also helps to distinguish the former from the latter patients. The absence of a high frequency of teardrop shaped red cells, nucleated red cells, and striking aniso-poikilocytosis would mitigate against idiopathic myelofibrosis.

Since some patients with idiopathic myelofibrosis have platelet counts over $600,000 \times 10^9$/l, the diagnosis of primary thrombocythemia may be considered. The aniso-poikilocytosis, nucleated red cells, and myeloid immaturity in the blood film characteristic of myelofibrosis is not present in patients with thrombocythemia. Marrow fibrosis is usually insignificant in thrombocythemia, and splenic enlargement is often absent or slight. There is for these reasons usually a clear distinction between the two disorders.[164,200]

Hairy cell leukemia (see Chap. 99), when it is associated with shape abnormalities of red cells, pancytopenia, splenomegaly, and fibrotic marrow, can mimic idiopathic myelofibrosis closely. Usually, careful scrutiny of the blood and marrow by microscopy, histochemistry, and cell immunophenotype will show evidence of the abnormal mononuclear (hairy) cells that characterizes the disease.

Metastatic carcinoma, especially derived from carcinoma of the breast or prostate tumors[201–206] or from disseminated mycobacterial infection, can induce reactive marrow fibrosis[207] and occasionally simulate idiopathic myelofibrosis. The demonstration of metastatic carcinoma cells or mycobacteria in the marrow indicates the etiology. Other disorders reported with secondary myelofibrosis include mastocytosis,[208,209] angioimmunoblastic lymphadenopathy,[210] lymphoma,[211] multiple myeloma,[212–217] renal osteodystrophy,[218] hypertrophic osteoarthropathy,[219] gray platelet syndrome,[220] systemic lupus erythematosus,[148–151] polyarteritis nodosa,[153] hypereosinophilic syndrome,[221] tretinoin administration,[222] neuroblastoma,[223] giant lymph node hyperplasia,[224] vitamin D deficiency rickets,[225,226] Langerhans cell histiocytosis,[227] and malignant histiocytosis.[228] Correction or amelioration of the primary disorder can lead to disappearance of the marrow fibrosis.

Lymphoma,[229,230] chronic lymphocytic leukemia,[231] hairy cell leukemia,[232] macroglobulinemia,[233] amyloidosis,[144,147] myeloma,[234,235] malignant teratoma,[236] and essential monoclonal gammopathy[237] have been reported to coincide with idiopathic myelofibrosis.

TRANSITIONS TO AND FROM MYELOFIBROSIS AMONG CLONAL HEMOPATHIES

All clonal hematopoietic diseases may have increased marrow reticulin fibers but only infrequently have collagen fibrosis.[238] Acute megakaryoblastic leukemia is accompanied by intense marrow fibrosis (see Chap. 93). At least 25 percent of patients with polycythemia vera, whether treated by phlebotomy, alkylating agents, or ^{32}P, develop a clinical state indistinguishable from idiopathic myelofibrosis during twenty years of observation[239–241] (see Chap. 61).

Sideroblastic anemia has also been observed to progress to idiopathic myelofibrosis.[242] Rarely, idiopathic myelofibrosis reverts to polycythemia vera, with disappearance of the marrow fibrosis.[243–245]

THERAPY

THE DECISION TO TREAT

A very large proportion of asymptomatic patients will remain stable for years, not requiring specific treatment.[2,54–61]

ANDROGENS AND GLUCOCORTICOIDS

Severe anemia may improve with androgen therapy in some patients.[246–249] Testosterone, oxymethalone, and fluoxymesterone have been used but have virilizing effects, in addition to the potential for hepatic injury and other side effects. Danazol, 600 mg orally per day for weeks to months can be used. Patients on androgen therapy should have periodic assessment of liver size by physical examination, measurement of liver function tests, and if appropriate, ultrasound imaging to detect liver injury (e.g., peliosis) or tumors.[250] Patients with significant hemolytic anemia may benefit from glucocorticoid therapy. A trial of prednisone, 25 mg/m^2 per day, orally, can be tried. If tolerated, this dose can be continued for one to two months and thereafter tapered gradually. In children, high-dose glucocorticoid therapy has been reported to ameliorate marrow fibrosis and improve hematopoiesis.[251,252]

RECOMBINANT HUMAN ERYTHROPOIETIN

Serum erythropoietin levels are appropriate to the severity of anemia in patients with myelofibrosis.[253] Use of erythropoietin to treat anemia has been largely unsuccessful.[254,255]

CHEMOTHERAPY

A variety of cytotoxic drugs have been used in the treatment of massive splenomegaly, thrombocytosis or constitutional symptoms. Hydroxyurea has become the most commonly used and preferred agent.[256–258] Hydroxyurea can decrease the size of the spleen and liver; decrease or eliminate constitutional symptoms of night sweats or weight loss; and lead to an increase in hemoglobin concentration, a decrease of elevated platelet counts, and occasionally a decrease in the degree of marrow fibrosis. Patients with myelofibrosis often do not have the marrow tolerance to chemotherapy of patients with other chronic myeloproliferative diseases. Hydroxyurea can be administered in doses of 0.5 to 1.0 g per day or 1.0 to 2.0 g two to three times per week, orally, depending on the level of the pretreatment blood cell counts. Patients should be evaluated for dose adjustment at least every week for a month and, if appropriate, extended to every two weeks for two months. Thereafter, monthly evaluation of dose may be appropriate. Although alkylating agents, especially busulfan and other cytotoxic agents, have been used successfully they have largely been replaced by hydroxyurea.[259]

Ascites resulting from peritoneal hemopoietic implants has been treated by intraperitoneal cytarabine.[260]

INTERFERONS

Interferon alpha and interferon gamma act synergistically to inhibit myeloproliferation[261] and are effective antiproliferative agents in chronic myelogenous leukemia (see Chap. 94). Although it has not been used extensively in idiopathic myelofibrosis, interferon alpha has been useful in treating splenic enlargement, bone pain, and thrombocytosis in selected patients.[262] Trials comparing interferon therapy with chemotherapy have not been reported. Hydroxyurea is easier to use and has less frequent side effects than interferon.

BISPHOSPHONATES

Debilitating bone pain can be a vexing problem in some patients with osteosclerosis and periostitis. A report of dramatic improvement in bone pain and hematopoiesis after etidronate, 6 mg/kg, on alternate months may indicate the potential usefulness of this family of drugs.[264]

RADIOTHERAPY

There are five situations in which radiotherapy can be useful for patients with idiopathic myelofibrosis: In the presence of (1) severe splenic pain (splenic infarctions) or (2) massive splenic enlargement with a contraindication to splenectomy (e.g., thrombocytosis),[264–266] doses of 50 to 200 rad (0.5 to 2 Gy) to the spleen can produce an amelioration of pain. The other situations in which radiation may be useful are (3) ascites resulting from myeloid metaplasia of the peritoneum;[267] (4) focal areas of severe bone pain (periostitis or the osteolysis of a granulocytic sarcoma);[161,268] and (5) extramedullary fibrohemopoietic tumors,[76] especially of the epidural space.[104]

SPLENECTOMY

Splenectomy is important in the management of idiopathic myelofibrosis.[269–272,303] The major indications for splenectomy include (1) painful enlarged spleen, (2) excessive transfusion requirements or refractory hemolytic anemia, (3) severe thrombocytopenia, and (4) portal hypertension.

Patients who have a prolonged bleeding time or coagulation times are at serious risk of hemorrhage with surgery and should not have the procedure unless these abnormalities can be corrected by platelet transfusion or factor replacement therapy. Evidence of low-grade intravascular coagulation, such as elevated D-dimer levels, may require prophylactic heparin therapy and platelet transfusion should there be excessive bleeding. In one series 50 patients had splenectomy: 26 of 27 patients splenectomized for pain, 5 of 9 patients splenectomized for refractory hemolysis, 4 of 10 patients splenectomized for refractory thrombocytopenia, and 4 of 4 patients splenectomized for portal hypertension had improvement.[271]

Removal of the spleen in patients with idiopathic myelofibrosis may be difficult. The spleen is usually adherent to neighboring serosal surfaces and structures and has numerous collateral vessels and very dilated splenoportal arteries and veins. Immediate postoperative mortality is a function of surgical experience and skill and of the rapidity of recognition of postoperative complications. In experienced hands, perioperative mortality should be less than 10 percent. Postoperative morbidity from hemorrhage, subphrenic hematoma, subphrenic abscess, injury to the tail of the pancreas, pancreatic fistulas, or portal vein stump thrombosis occurs in about 30 percent of patients. Later, postoperative changes include liver enlargement,[273] extramedullary hemopoietic tumors,[115,119] and a decrease in teardrop-shaped red cells.[274] Postoperative liver enlargement and thrombocytosis have responded to treatment with cladribine.[275] Anagrelide may also be useful for exaggerated thrombocytosis (see Chap. 118). The morbidity and mortality from splenectomy and the modest extension of life on the average has led to increasing conservatism in its use.[276] Splenectomy, however, can improve the state of patients who are selected carefully and in a timely fashion.

Five patients with idiopathic myelofibrosis were among 91 patients who had subtotal splenectomy, preserving the upper pole of the spleen and its blood supply. No surgical mortality occurred, but details of outcome were not reported.[277]

PORTAL-SYSTEMIC VASCULAR SHUNT SURGERY

Patients who are operated on for portal hypertension and bleeding varices or refractory ascites should have circulatory dynamic studies performed at the time of surgery. In patients in whom the hepatic wedge-pressure elevations are a result of the markedly increased blood flow from the spleen to the liver, the preferred treatment procedure for portal hypertension is splenectomy. In those patients who have portal hypertension as a result of intrahepatic block or hepatic vein thrombosis, a splenorenal shunt is usually performed.[278]

MARROW CURETTAGE, COLLAGEN SYNTHESIS INHIBITORS, VITAMIN D CONGENERS, IMMUNOGLOBULINS, AND CYCLOSPORINES

Several experimental forms of therapy have been used in a small number of patients. Hematologic remission has been described in one case of myelofibrosis treated by bilateral iliac-crest marrow curettage.[279]

Investigative approaches to the disease include the use of agents that prevent collagen formation, such as monoamine oxidase inhibitors and lysylaldehyde chelators such as dehydroproline.[280]

1,25-Dihydroxyvitamin D therapy was associated with improvement of patients with myelofibrosis, although hypercalcemia and hypophosphatemia may prevent continued use.[281] The mechanism of action could relate to a profound antiproliferative effect of 1,25-dihydroxyvitamin D on megakaryocytes, which are the putative source of most of the fibroblast activation factors. In two other reports no benefit was found from administration of this vitamin D analog.[282,283] 1,25-Dihydroxycholecalciferol has also been reported to ameliorate myelofibrosis.[284] Single cases of improvement in hematopoiesis and decrease in osteosclerosis after intravenous immune globulin[285] and sustained improvement in anemia after cyclosporine[286] have been reported.

MARROW TRANSPLANTATION

Marrow transplantation therapy, which is efficacious in acute megakaryocytic leukemia with intense myelofibrosis, could be used in appropriate candidates who are under the age of 40 and have a histocompatible sibling.[287–289] Patients engraft at a rate similar to patients with hematologic diseases without marrow fibrosis[289] (see Chap. 18).

COURSE AND PROGNOSIS

The rate of progression of the disease has been associated with at least ten variables measured at the time of diagnosis. Shorter survival has been associated with older age, severity of anemia, severity of thrombocytopenia, exaggerated leukocytosis or leukopenia, the proportion of blast cells in the blood, degree of liver enlargement, extent of marrow fibrosis, abnormal clonal cytogenetic abnormalities, and constitutional symptoms of fever, sweating, or weight loss at the time of diagnosis. Each retrospective study has found a different subset of these factors to be significant prognostic factors. The most consistent predictive variables appear to be advanced age, severity of anemia, and clonal cytogenetic abnormality at the time of diagnosis, each of which represents a poor prognostic indicator.[57–60,163,164,191,290]

The median survival of all patients with idiopathic myelofibrosis is approximately 5 years from the time of diagnosis.[57–60] The 5-year survival is about forty percent of that expected for healthy age- and sex-matched controls.[2,55,291] Retrospective analysis of prognostic variables permits stratification of patients into slowly progressive and rapidly progressive cohorts.[55,57–59,163,167,291]

The major causes of death are infection, hemorrhage, postsplenectomy mortality, and acute leukemic transformation).[2,54-56,292-294,301] Acute leukemia occasionally may be preceded by the development of granulocytic sarcomas.[160,269,295] Evolution of the disease to acute lymphocytic leukemia or lymphoma also may occur.[296,297] An increased risk of progression to leukemia has been reported in splenectomized patients.[298] Rare spontaneous remissions of apparent idiopathic myelofibrosis have been documented.[299,300]

REFERENCES

1. Heuck G: Zwei Fälle von Leukämie mit eigenthümlichem Blut-resp Knochenmarksbefund. *Virchows Arch (Pathol Anat)* 78:475, 1879.

2. Silverstein MN: *Agnogenic Myeloid Metaplasia.* Publishing Science, Boston, 1975.

3. Heller EL, Lewisohn MG, Palin WE: Aleukemic myelosis, chronic nonleukemic myelosis, agnogenic myeloid metaplasia, osteosclerosis, leukoerythroblastic anemia, and synonymous designations. *Am J Pathol* 23:327, 1947.

4. Yan X-Q, Lacey D, Hill D, et al: A model of myelofibrosis and osteosclerosis in mice induced by overexpressing thrombopoietin (mpl ligand). *Blood* 88:402, 1996.

5. Aksoy M, Erdem S, Dincol G: Two rare complications of chronic benzene poisoning: myeloid metaplasia and paroxysmal nocturnal hemoglobinuria. *Blut* 30:255, 1975.

6. Hu H: Benzene-associated myelofibrosis. *Ann Intern Med* 106:171, 1987.

7. Tondel M, Perrson B, Carstensen J: Myelofibrosis and benzene exposure. *Occup Med* 45:31, 1995.

8. Anderson RE, Hoshino T, Yamamoto T: Myelofibrosis with myeloid metaplasia in survivors of the atomic bomb in Hiroshima. *Ann Intern Med* 60:1, 1964.

9. Dungworth DL, Goldman M, Switzer JW, et al: Development of a myeloproliferative disorder in beagles continuously exposed to ^{90}Sr. *Blood* 34:610, 1969.

10. Jacobson RS, Salo A, Fialkow PS: Agnogenic myeloid metaplasia: A clonal proliferation of hematopoietic stem cells with secondary myelofibrosis. *Blood* 51:189, 1978.

11. Kahn A, Bernard JF, Cottreau D, et al: A deficient G-6-PD variant with hemizygous expression in blood cells of a woman with primary myelofibrosis. *Humangenetick* 30:41, 1975.

12. Sato Y, Suda T, Suda J, et al: Multilineage expression of haemopoietic precursors with an abnormal clone in idiopathic myelofibrosis. *Br J Haematol* 64:657, 1986.

13. Kreipe H, Jaquet K, Falgner J, et al: Clonal granulocytes and bone marrow cells in the cellular phase of agnogenic myeloid metaplasia. *Blood* 78:1814, 1991.

14. Tsukamoto N, Morita K, Maehara T, et al: Clonality in chronic myeloproliferative disorders defined by X-chromosome linked probes. *Br J Haematol* 86:253, 1994.

15. Buschle M, Janssen JWG, Drexler H, et al: Evidence for pluripotent stem cell origin of idiopathic myelofibrosis: Clonal analysis of a case characterized by a N-*ras* gene mutation. *Leukaemia* 2:658, 1988.

16. Lebowitz P, Papac R, Ghosh PK: Impaired retinoblastoma susceptibility (Rb) gene expression in agnogenic myeloid metaplasia. *Blood* 76(suppl 1):236A, 1990.

17. Prockop DJ, Kivirikko KI, Tuderman L, et al: The biosynthesis of collagen and its disorders. *N Engl J Med* 301:13, 1979.

18. Bauermeister DE: Quantitation of bone marrow reticulin: A normal range. *Am J Clin Pathol* 56:24, 1971.

19. Ivànyi JL, Mahunka M, Papp A, Telek B: Prognostic significance of bone marrow reticulum fibers in idiopathic myelofibrosis: evolution of clinicopathological parameters in a scoring system. *Hematologia* 26:75, 1994.

20. McCarthy DM: Annotation: Fibrosis of the bone marrow: Content and causes. *Br J Haematol* 59:1, 1985.

21. Apaja-Sarkkinen M, Autio-Harmainen H, Alavaikko M, et al: Immunohistochemical study of basement membrane proteins and type III procollagen in myelofibrosis. *Br J Haematol* 63:571, 1986.

22. Hasselbalch H, Junker P, Lisse I, et al: Serum markers for type IV collagen and type III procollagen in the myelofibrosis-osteomyelo-

sclerosis syndrome and other chronic myeloproliferative disorders. *Am J Hematol* 23:101, 1986.

23. Reilly JT: Pathogenesis of idiopathic myelofibrosis: Role of growth factors. *J Clin Pathol* 45:461, 1992.

24. Charron D, Robert L, Couty MC, Binet JL: Biochemical and histological analysis of bone marrow collagen in myelofibrosis. *Br J Haematol* 41:151, 1979.

25. Gay S, Gay RE, Prohal JT: Immunohistological studies of bone marrow collagen, in *Myelofibrosis and the Biology of Connective Tissue,* edited by P Berk, H Castro-Malaspina, LR Wasserman, pp 291–306. Liss, New York, 1984.

26. Hasselbalch H, Junker P, Horslev-Patersen K, et al: Procollagen type III amino-terminal peptide in serum in idiopathic myelofibrosis and allied conditions. *Am J Hematol* 33:18, 1990.

27. Reilly JT, Nash JRG, Mackie MJ, McVerry BA: Endothelial cell proliferation in myelofibrosis. *Br J Haematol* 60:625, 1985.

28. Baglin TP, Crocker MA, Timmins A, et al: Bone marrow hypervascularity in patients with myelofibrosis identified by infrared thermography. *Clin Lab Haematol* 13:341, 1991.

29. Dolan G, Forrest P, Eastham J, et al: Serum laminin, procollagen terminal peptide III and thrombocyte platelet derived growth factor concentrations in idiopathic myelofibrosis. *Br J Haematol* 77(suppl 1):73, 1991.

30. Reilly JT, Nash JRG, Mackie MJ, McVerry BA: Immunoenzymatic detection of fibronectin in normal and pathological haemopoietic tissue. *Br J Haematol* 59:497, 1985.

31. Hasselbalch H, Clemmensen I: Plasma fibronectin in idiopathic myelofibrosis and related chronic myeloproliferative disorders. *Scand J Clin Lab Invest* 47:429, 1987.

32. Soini Y, Kamel D, Apaja-Sarkkinen M, et al: Tenascin immunoreactivity in normal and pathological bone marrow. *J Clin Pathol* 46:218, 1993.

33. Reilly JT, Nash JRG: Vitronectin (serum spreading factor): Its localization in normal and fibrotic tissue. *J Clin Pathol* 41:1269, 1988.

34. Wang JC, Wong C, Kao WW: Immunoreactive prolylhydroxylase in patients with primary and secondary myelofibrosis. *Br J Haematol* 65:171, 1987.

35. Barosi G, Costa A, Liberato LN, et al: Serum procollagen III peptide level correlates with disease activity in myelofibrosis with myeloid metaplasia. *Br J Haematol* 72:16, 1989.

36. Hochweiss S, Fruchtman S, Hahn EG, et al: Increased serum procollagen III amino-terminal peptide in myelofibrosis. *Am J Hematol* 15:343, 1983.

37. Hasselbalch H, Junker P, Lisse I, et al: Circulating hyaluronan in the myelofibrosis/osteomyelosclerosis syndrome and other myeloproliferative disorders. *Am J Hematol* 36:1, 1991.

38. Thiele J, Kvasnicka HM, Fischer R, Diehl V: Clinicopathological impact of the interactivity between megakaryocytes and myeloid stroma in chronic myeloproliferative disorders: a concise update. *Leuk Lymph* 24:463, 1997.

39. Rosenfeld M, Keating A, Bowen-Pope BF, et al: Responsiveness of the in vitro hematopoietic microenvironment to platelet-derived growth factor. *Leuk Res* 9:427, 1985.

40. Bernabei PA, Arcangeli A, Casini M, et al: Platelet-derived growth factor(s) mitogenic activity in patients with myeloproliferative disease. *Br J Haematol* 63:353, 1986.

41. Thiele J, Rompick V, Wagner S, Fischer R: Vascular architecture and collagen type IV in primary myelofibrosis and polycythemia vera. *Br J Haematol* 80:227, 1992.

42. Johnston JB, Dalal BI, Israels SJ, et al: Deposition of transforming growth factor-β in the marrow in myelofibrosis, and the intracellular localization and secretion of TGF-β by leukemic cells. *Am J Clin Pathol* 103:574, 1995.

43. Martré M-C: TGF-β and megakaryocytes in the pathogenesis of myelofibrosis in myeloproliferative disorders. *Leuk Lymph* 20:39, 1995.

44. Martré M-C, LeBousse-Kerdiles M-C, Romquin N, et al: Elevated levels of basic fibroblast growth factor in megakaryocytes and platelets from patients with idiopathic myelofibrosis. *Br J Haematol* 97:441, 1997.

45. Dalley A, Smith JM, Reilly JT, MacNeil S: Investigation of calmodulin and basic fibroblast growth factor (bFGF) in idiopathic myelofibrosis: evidence for a role of extracellular calmodulin in fibroblast proliferation. *Br J Haematol* 93:856, 1996.

46. Nathan C: Secretory products of macrophages. *J Clin Invest* 79:319, 1987.

47. Burstein SA, Malpass TW, Yee E, et al: Platelet factor-4 excretion in

myeloproliferative disease: Implication for the aetiology of myelofibrosis. *Br J Haematol* 57:383, 1984.

48. Kvasnica HM, Thiele J, Amend T, Fischer R: Three-dimensional reconstruction of histiologic structures in human bone marrow from serial sections of trephine biopsies. *Anal Quant Cytol Hist* 16:159, 1994.

49. Reilly JT, Nash JR, Mackie MJ, et al: Endothelial cell proliferation in myelofibrosis. *Br J Haematol* 60:625, 1985.

50. Charbord P: Increased vascularity of bone marrow in myelofibrosis. *Br J Haematol* 62:595, 1986.

51. VanDyke D, Anger HO, Parker H, et al: Markedly increased bone blood flow in myelofibrosis. *J Nucl Med* 12:506, 1971.

52. Hotta T, Utsumi M, Katoh T, et al: Granulocytic and stromal progenitors in the bone marrow of patient with primary myelofibrosis. *Scand J Haematol* 34:251, 1985.

53. Greenberg BR, Woo L, Veomett JC, et al: Cytogenetics of bone marrow fibroblastic cells in idiopathic chronic myelofibrosis. *Br J Haematol* 66:487, 1987.

54. Ward HP, Block MH: The natural history of agnogenic myeloid metaplasia (AMM) and a critical evaluation of its relationship with myeloproliferative syndrome. *Medicine* 50:357, 1971.

55. Varki A, Lottenberg R, Griffith R, et al: The syndrome of idiopathic myelofibrosis. *Medicine* 62:353, 1983.

56. Hasselbalch H: Idiopathic myelofibrosis. *Am J Hematol* 34:291, 1990.

57. Kvasnicka H-M, Thiele J, Werden C, et al: Prognostic factors in idiopathic (primary) osteo-myelofibrosis. *Cancer* 80:708, 1997.

58. Cervantes F, Pereira A, Esteve J, et al: Identification of ''short-lived'' and ''long-lived'' patients at presentation of idiopathic myelofibrosis. *Br J Haematol* 97:635, 1997.

59. Dupriez B, Morel P, Demory JL, et al: Prognostic factors in agnogenic myeloid metaplasia: a report on 195 cases with a new scoring system. *Blood* 88:1013, 1996.

60. Rupoli S, DaLio L, Sisti S, et al: Primary myelofibrosis: a detailed analysis of the clinicopathologic variables influencing survival. *Ann Hematol* 68:205, 1994.

61. Ozen S, Ferhanoglu B, Senocak M, Tüzüner N: Idiopathic myelofibrosis (agnogenic myeloid metaplasia). *Leuk Res* 21:125, 1997.

62. Shalev O, Goldfarb A, Ariel I, et al: Myelofibrosis in young adults. *Acta Haematol* 70:396, 1983.

63. Selehar M, Prentice HG, Poyat U, et al: Idiopathic myelofibrosis in children. *Br J Haematol* 93:394, 1996.

64. Sekhar M, Prentice HG, Popat U, et al: Idiopathic myelofibrosis in children. *Br J Haematol* 93:394, 1996.

65. Cohn SL, Cohn RA, Chou P, et al: Infantile myelofibrosis with nephromegaly secondary to myeloid metaplasia. *Clin Pediatrics* 30:59, 1991.

66. Mallouh AA, Sa'di AR: Agnogenic myeloid metaplasia in children. *Am J Dis Child* 146:965, 1992.

67. Kaufman S, Briere J, Bernard J: Familial myeloproliferative syndromes: Study of 6 families and review of literature. *Nouv Rev Fr Hematol* 20:1, 1978.

68. Péres-Encinas M, Bello JL, Perez-Crespo S, et al: Familial myeloproliferative syndrome. *Am J Hematol* 46:225, 1994.

69. Caughman W, Stern R, Haynes H: Neutrophilic dermatosis of myeloproliferative disorders: Atypical forms of pyoderma gangrenosum and Sweet's syndrome associated with myeloproliferative disorders. *J Am Acad Dermatol* 9:751, 1983.

70. Gibson LE, Dicken CH, Flach DB: Neutrophilic dermatoses and myeloproliferative disease: Report of two cases. *Mayo Clin Proc* 60:735, 1985.

71. Su WPD, Alegre VA, White WL: Myelofibrosis discovered after diagnosis of Sweet's syndrome. *Int J Dermatol* 29:201, 1990.

72. Kanel KT, Kroboth FJ, Swartz WM: Pyoderma gangrenosum with myelofibrosis. *Am J Med* 82:1031, 1987.

73. Loewy G, Matthew A, Distenfeld A: Skin manifestations of agnogenic myeloid metaplasia. *Am J Hematol* 45:167, 1994.

74. King BF, Kopecky KK, Baker MK, et al: Extramedullary hematopoiesis in the adrenal glands: CT characteristics. *J Comput Assist Tomogr* 11:342, 1987.

75. Redlin L, Francis RS, Orlando MM: Renal abnormalities in agnogenic myeloid metaplasia. *Radiology* 121:605, 1976.

76. Shaver RW, Close FC: Extramedullary hemopoiesis in myeloid metaplasia. *Am J Radiol* 137:874, 1981.

77. Williams ME, Innes DJ, Hutchison WT, et al: Extramedullary hemato-

78. Sharma BK, Pounder RE, Cruse JP, et al: Extramedullary haemopoiesis in the small bowel. *Gut* 27:873, 1986.

79. MacKinnon S, McNicol AM, Lee FD, et al: Myelofibrosis complicated by intestinal extramedullary haemopoiesis and acute small bowel obstruction. *J Clin Pathol* 39:677, 1986.

80. Soloman D, Goodman H, Jacobs P: Rectal stenosis due to extramedullary hematopoiesis. *Clin Radiol* 49:726, 1994.

81. Sunderland K, Barratt J, Pidcock M: Extramedullary hemopoiesis arising in the gut mimicking carcinoma of the cecum. *Pathol* 26:62, 1994.

82. Brooks JJ, Krugman DT, Danjanor I: Myeloid metaplasia presenting as a breast mass. *Am J Surg Pathol* 4:281, 1980.

83. Martinelli G, Santini D, Bazzocchi F, et al: Myeloid metaplasia of the breast: A lesion which clinically mimics carcinoma. *Virchows Arch* 401:203, 1983.

84. Zonderland HM, Michiels JJ, ten Kate FJW: Mammographic and sonographic demonstration of extramedullary hematopoiesis of the breast. *Clin Radiol* 44:64, 1991.

85. Yusen RD, Kollef MH: Acute respiratory failure due to extramedullary hematopoiesis. *Chest* 108:1170, 1995.

86. Asakura S, Colby T: Agnogenic myeloid metaplasia with extramedullary hemopoiesis and fibrosis in the lung. *Chest* 105:1866, 1994.

87. Pierard GE: Cutaneous hematopoiesis and myelofibrosis. *Ann Pathol* 7:73, 1987.

88. Mizoguchi M, Kawa Y, Minami T, et al: Cutaneous extramedullary hematopoiesis in myelofibrosis. *J Am Acad Dermatol* 22:351, 1990.

89. Heinicke MH, Zarrabi MH, Gorevic PD: Arthritis due to synovial involvement by extramedullary haematopoiesis in myelofibrosis with myeloid metaplasia. *Ann Rheum Dis* 42:196, 1983.

90. Leoni F, Fabbri R, Pascarella A, et al: Extramedullary hematopoiesis in thyroid multinodular goiter preceding clinical evidence of agnogenic myeloid metaplasia. *Histopathology* 28:559, 1996.

91. Humphrey PA, Vollmer RT: Extramedullary hematopoiesis in the prostate. *Am J Surg Pathol* 15:486, 1991.

92. Balogh K, O'Hara CJ: Myeloid metaplasia masquerading as a urethral caruncle. *J Urol* 135:789, 1986.

93. Oesterling JE, Keating JP, Leroy AJ, et al: Idiopathic myelofibrosis with myeloid metaplasia involving the renal pelvis, ureters and bladder. *J Urol* 147:1360, 1992.

94. Gryspeerdt S, Oyen R, Van Hoe L, et al: Extramedullary hematopoiesis encasing the pelvicalyceal system. *Ann Hematol* 71:53, 1995.

95. Perazella MA, Buller GK: Nephrotic syndrome associated with agnogenic myeloid metaplasia. *Am J Nephrol* 14:223, 1994.

96. Holt SG, Field P, Carmichael P, et al: Extramedullary haemopoiesis in the renal parenchyma as a cause of acute renal failure in myelofibrosis. *Nephrol Dial Transplant* 10:1438, 1995.

97. Brown JA, Gomez-Leon G: Subdural hemorrhage secondary to extramedullary hematopoiesis in postpolycythemic myeloid metaplasia. *Neurosurg* 14:588, 1984.

98. Cornfield DB, Shipkin P, Alluvia A, et al: Intracranial myeloid metaplasia: Diagnosis by CT and Fe52 scans and treatment by cranial irradiation. *Am J Hematol* 15:273, 1983.

99. Lundh B, Brandt L, Cronqvist S, et al: Intracranial myeloid metaplasia in myelofibrosis. *Scand J Haematol* 28:91, 1982.

100. Cameron WR, Ronnert M, Brun A: Extramedullary hematopoiesis of CNS in postpolycythemic myeloid metaplasia. *N Engl J Med* 305:765, 1981.

101. Ligumski M, Polliack A, Benbassat J: Metaplasia of the central nervous system in patients with myelofibrosis and agnogenic myeloid metaplasia. *Am J Med Sci* 275:99, 1979.

102. Stahl SM, Ellinger G, Baringer JR: Progressive myelopathy due to extramedullary hematopoiesis. *Ann Neurol* 5:485, 1979.

103. Cook G, Sharp RA: Spinal cord compression due to extramedullary haemopoiesis in myelofibrosis. *J Clin Pathol* 47:464, 1994.

104. Price F, Bell H: Spinal cord compression due to extramedullary hematopoiesis: Successful treatment in a patient with long-standing myelofibrosis. *JAMA* 253:2876, 1985.

105. Ohtsubo M, Hayaski K, Fukushima T, et al: Intracranial extramedullary haematopoiesis in postpolycythemia myelofibrosis. *Br J Radiol* 67:299, 1994.

106. Urman M, O'Sullivan RA, Nugent RA, Lentle BC: Intracranial extramedullary hematopoiesis. *Clin Nucl Med* 16:431, 1991.

107. Lanir A, Aghai E, Simon JS, et al: MR imaging in myelofibrosis. *J Comput Assist Tomogr* 10:634, 1986.

108. Koch BL, Bisset GS, Bisset RR, Zimmer MB: Intracranial extramedullary hematopoiesis: MR findings with pathologic correlation. *Am J Roentgenol* 162:1419, 1994.

109. Bartlett RP, Greipp PR, Tefferi A, et al: Extramedullary hematopoiesis manifesting as a symptomatic pleural effusion. *Mayo Clin Proc* 70:1165, 1995.

110. Knobel B, Melamud E, Virage I, Meytes D: Ectopic medullary hematopoiesis as a cause of ascites in agnogenic myeloid metaplasia. *Acta Haematol* 89:104, 1993.

111. Lioté F, Yeni P, Teillet-Thiebaud F, et al: Ascites revealing peritoneal and hepatic extramedullary hematopoiesis with peliosis in agnogenic myeloid metaplasia. *Am J Med* 90:111, 1991.

112. Vilaseca J, Arnau JM, Tallada N, et al: Agnogenic myeloid metaplasia presenting as massive pericardial effusion due to extramedullary hematopoiesis. *Acta Haematol (Basel)* 73:239, 1985.

113. Haedersdal C, Hasselbalch H, Devantier A, et al: Pericardial haematopoiesis with tamponade in myelofibrosis. *Scand J Haematol* 34:270, 1985.

114. Imam TH, Doll DC: Acute cardiac tamponade associated with pericardial extramedullary hematopoieses in agnogenic myeloid metaplasia. *Acta Haematol* 98:42, 1997.

115. Nagler A, Brenner B, Argov S, et al: Postsplenectomy pericardial effusion in two patients with myeloid metaplasia. *Arch Intern Med* 146:600, 1986.

116. Pedio G, Krause M, Jansova I: Megakaryocytes in ascitic fluid in a case of agnogenic myeloid metaplasia (letter). *Acta Cytol* 29:89, 1985.

117. Silverman JF: Extramedullary hematopoietic ascitic fluid cytology in myelofibrosis. *Am J Clin Pathol* 84:125, 1985.

118. Stephenson RW, Britt DA, Schumann GB: Primary cytodiagnosis of peritoneal extramedullary hematopoiesis. *Diag Cytopathol* 2:241, 1986.

119. Hocking WG, Lazar GS, Lipsett JA, et al: Cutaneous extramedullary hematopoiesis following splenectomy for idiopathic myelofibrosis. *Am J Med* 76:956, 1984.

120. Partanen S, Ruutu T, Jubonen E, et al: Effect of splenectomy on circulating haematopoietic progenitors in myelofibrosis. *Scand J Haematol* 37:87, 1986.

121. Chubachi A, Wakui H, Miura I, et al: Extramedullary megakaryoblastic tumors following an indolent phase of myelofibrosis *Leuk Lymph* 17:351, 1995.

122. Chan ACL, Kwong Y-L, Lam CCK: Granulocytic sarcoma megakaryoblastic differentiation complicating chronic idiopathic myelofibrosis. *Hum Pathol* 27:417, 1996.

123. Oishi N, Swisher SN, Stormont JM, et al: Portal hypertension in myeloid metaplasia. *Arch Surg* 81:80, 1960.

124. Rosenbaum DL, Murphy GW, Swisher SN: Hemodynamic studies of the portal circulation in myeloid metaplasia. *Am J Med* 41:360, 1966.

125. Jacobs P, Maze S, Tayob F, et al: Myelofibrosis, splenomegaly, and portal hypertension. *Acta Haematol* 74:45, 1985.

126. Degott C, Carpon JP, Bettan L, et al: Myeloid metaplasia, perisinusoidal fibrosis, and nodular regenerative hyperplasia of the liver. *Liver* 5:276, 1985.

127. Bioulac-Sage P, Roux D, Quinton A, et al: Ultrastructure of sinusoids in patients with agnogenic myeloid metaplasia. *J Submicrosc Cytol* 18:815, 1986.

128. Roux D, Merlio JP, Quinton A, et al: Agnogenic myeloid metaplasia, portal hypertension and sinusoidal abnormalities. *Gastroenterology* 92:1067, 1987.

129. Tsao MS: Hepatic sinusoidal fibrosis in agnogenic myeloid metaplasia. *Am J Clin Pathol* 91:302, 1989.

130. Valla d, Casadevall N, Huisse MG, et al: Etiology of portal vein thrombosis in adults. *Gastroenterology* 94:1063, 1988.

131. Boivin P, Bernard JF, Hakim J, et al: Anomalies immunitaires au cours de splenomegalies myeloides myelosclerose. *Acta Haematol (Basel)* 51:91, 1974.

132. Lang JM, Oberling F, Mayer S, et al: Autoimmunity in primary myelofibrosis. *Biomedicine* 25:39, 1976.

133. Barge J, Slabodshy-Brousse N, Bernard JF: Histoimmunology of myelofibrosis: A study of 100 cases. *Biomedicine* 29:73, 1978.

134. Vellenga E, Mulder N, The T, et al: A study of the cellular and humoral immune response in patients with myelofibrosis. *Clin Lab Haematol* 4:239, 1982.

135. Rondeau E, Solal-Celigny P, Dhermy D, et al: Immune disorders in agnogenic myeloid metaplasia: Relations to myelofibrosis. *Br J Haematol* 53:467, 1983.

136. Gordon B: Immunological abnormalities in myelofibrosis. *Prog Clin Biol Res* 154:455, 1984.

137. Khumbanonda M, Horowitz HI, Eyster ME: Coombs' positive hemolytic anemia in myelofibrosis with myeloid metaplasia. *Am J Med Sci* 258:89, 1969.

138. Schreiber ZA: Immune thrombocytopenia in postpolythemic myelofibrosis. *Am J Hematol* 54:146, 1997.

139. Seelen MAJ, de Meijer PHEM, Posthuma EF, Meinders AE: Myelofibrosis and thrombocytopenic purpura. *Ann Hematol* 75:129, 1997.

140. Wang JC, Wang A: Plasma soluble interleukin-2 receptor in patients with primary myelofibrosis. *Br J Haematol* 86:380, 1994.

141. Leoni P, Rupoli S, Salvi A, et al: Antibodies against terminal galactosyl alpha(1–3) galactose epitopes in patients with idiopathic myelofibrosis. *Br J Haematol* 85:313, 1993.

142. Bernhardt B, Valleta M: Lupus anticoagulant in myelofibrosis. *Am J Med Sci* 272:229, 1976.

143. Cappio FC, Vigliani R, Novarino A, et al: Idiopathic myelofibrosis: A possible role for immune-complexes in the pathogenesis of bone marrow fibrosis. *Br J Haematol* 49:17, 1981.

144. Akikusa B, Komatsu T, Kondo Y, et al: Amyloidosis complicating idiopathic myelofibrosis. *Arch Pathol Lab Med* 111:525, 1987.

145. Hasselbalch H, Nielsen H, Berild D, et al: Circulating immune complexes in myelofibrosis. *Scand J Haematol* 34:177, 1985.

146. Gordon BR, Coleman M, Kohen P, et al: Immunologic abnormalities in myelofibrosis with activation of the complement system. *Blood* 58:904, 1981.

147. Ferhanoglu B, Erzin Y, Baslar Z, Tüzüner HAN: Secondary amyloidosis in the course of idiopathic myelofibrosis. *Leuk Res* 21:897, 1997.

148. El Mouzan MI, Ahmed MAM, Saleh MAF, et al: Myelofibrosis and pancytopenia in systemic lupus erythematosus. *Am J Med* 81:935, 1986.

149. Matsouka CH, Lioouris J, Andrianokis A: Systemic lupus erythematosus and myelofibrosis. *Clin Rheumatol* 8:402, 1989.

150. Paquette RL, Meshkinpour A, Rosen PJ: Autoimmune myelofibrosis. A steroid-responsive cause of bone marrow fibrosis associated with systemic lupus erythematosus. *Medicine* 73:145, 1994.

151. Ramakrishna R, Kyle PW, Day PJ, Mansharan A: Evan's syndrome, myelofibrosis and systemic lupus erythematosus: role of procollagens in myelofibrosis. *Pathol* 27:255, 1995.

152. Aharon A, Levy Y, Bar-Dayan Y, et al: Successful treatment of early secondary myelofibrosis in SLE with IVIG. *Lupus* 6:408, 1997.

153. Von Knorring J, Selroos OW, Wegelius O: Myeloid metaplasia in disseminated vascular disease. *Acta Med Scand* 195:137, 1974.

154. Connelly TJ, Abruzzo JL, Schwab RH: Agnogenic myeloid metaplasia with polyarteritis. *J Rheumatol* 9:954, 1982.

155. Ben-Chetrit E, Gross DJ, Ikon E, et al: The association between autoimmunity and agnogenic myeloid metaplasia. *Scand J Haematol* 31:410, 1983.

156. Hasselbalch H, Jans H, Nielsen PL: A distinct subtype of idiopathic myelofibrosis with bone marrow features mimicking hairy cell leukemia: Evidence of an autoimmune pathogenesis. *Am J Hematol* 25:225, 1987.

157. Thiele J, Chen Y-S, Kvasnicka H-M, et al: Evolution of fibro-osteosclerotic bone marrow lesions in primary (idiopathic) osteomyelofibrosis—a histomorphometric study on sequential trephine biopsies. *Leuk Lymph* 14:163, 1994.

158. Coindre JM, Reiffers J, Goussot JF, et al: Histomorphometric analysis of sclerotic bone from idiopathic myeloid metaplasia. *J Pathol* 144:163, 1984.

159. Cassi E, DePaoli A, Tosi A, et al: Pure osteolytic lesions in myelofibrosis: Report of 2 cases. *Haematologica* 70:178, 1985.

160. Fayemi AO, Gerber MA, Cohen I, et al: Myeloid sarcoma. *Cancer* 32:253, 1973.

161. Yu JS, Greenway G, Resnick D: Myelofibrosis associated with prominent periosteal bone apposition. *Clin Imaging* 18:89, 1994.

162. Barosi G, Cazzoli M, Frassoni F: Erythropoiesis in myelofibrosis with myeloid metaplasia: Recognition of different classes of patients by erythrokinetics. *Br J Haematol* 48:263, 1981.

163. Barosi G, Berzuinic C, Liberato LN, et al: A prognostic classification of myelofibrosis with myeloid metaplasia. *Br J Haematol* 70:397, 1988.

164. Thiele J, Kvasnicka H-M, Werden C, et al: Idiopathic primary osteomyelofibrosis. *Leuk Lymph* 22:303, 1996.

165. Njoku OS, Lewis SM, Catovsky D, et al: Anaemia in myelofibrosis: Its value in prognosis. *Br J Haematol* 54:79, 1983.

166. Howarth JE, Waters HM, Hyde K, Geary CG: Detection of erythroid hypoplasia in myelofibrosis using erythrokinetic studies. *J Clin Path* 42:1250, 1989.

167. Thiele J, Windecker R, Kvasnicka HM, et al: Erythropoiesis in primary (idiopathic) osteomyelofibrosis. *Am J Hematol* 46:36, 1994.

168. Bird GW, Wingham J, Richardson SG: Myelofibrosis, autoimmune haemolytic anaemia and Tn-polyagglutinability. *Haematologia* 18:99, 1985.

169. Kuo CY, VanVoolen GA, Morrison AN: Primary and secondary myelofibrosis: Its relationship to the PNH-like defect. *Blood* 40:875, 1972.

170. Veer A, Kosciolek BA, Bauman AW, et al: Acquired hemoglobin H disease in idiopathic myelofibrosis. *Am J Hematol* 6:199, 1979.

171. Barosi G, Baraldi A, Cassola M, et al: Red cell aplasia in myelofibrosis with myeloid metaplasia. *Cancer* 52:1290, 1983.

172. Silverstein MN, Elveback LR: Leukocyte alkaline phosphatase in agnogenic myeloid metaplasia. *Am J Clin Pathol* 61:307, 1974.

173. Douer D, Fabian I, Cline MJ: Circulation pluripotent haemopoietic cells in patients with myeloproliferative disorders. *Br J Haematol* 54:373, 1983.

174. Partanen S, Ruutu T, Vuopio P: Circulating haematopoietic progenitors in myelofibrosis. *Scand J Haematol* 29:325, 1982.

175. Wang JC, Cheung CP, Ahmed F, et al: Circulating granulocyte and macrophage progenitor cells in primary and secondary myelofibrosis. *Br J Haematol* 54:301, 1983.

176. Kornberg A, Fibach E, Treves A, et al: Circulating erythroid progenitors in patients with ''spent'' polycythaemia vera and myelofibrosis with myeloid metaplasia. *Br J Haematol* 52:573, 1982.

177. Tinggaard-Pedersen N, Laursen B: Megakaryocytes in cubital venous blood in patients with chronic myeloproliferative diseases. *Scand J Haematol* 30:50, 1983.

178. Marquetty C, Labro-Bryskier MT, Perianin A, et al: Impaired metabolic activity of phagocytosis neutrophils in agnogenic osteomyelofibrosis with splenomegaly. *Am J Med* 16:243, 1984.

179. Perianin A, Labro-Bryskier MT, Marquetty C, et al: Glutathione reductase and nitroblue tetrazolium reduction deficiencies in neutrophils of patients with primary idiopathic myelofibrosis. *Clin Exp Immunol* 57:244, 1984.

180. Murphy S, Davis JL, Walsh PN, et al: Template bleeding time and clinical hemorrhage in myeloproliferative disease. *Arch Intern Med* 138:1251, 1978.

181. Malpass TW, Savage B, Hanson SR, et al: Correlation between bleeding time and depletion of platelet dense granule ADP in patients with myelodysplastic and myeloproliferative disorders. *J Lab Clin Med* 103:894, 1984.

182. Cunietti E, Gandini R, Marcaro G, et al: Defective platelet aggregation and increased platelet turnover in patients with myelofibrosis and other myeloproliferative diseases. *Scand J Haematol* 26:339, 1981.

183. Schafer AL: Deficiency of platelet lipoxygenase activity in myeloproliferative disorders. *N Engl J Med* 306:381, 1982.

184. Shafer AL: Bleeding and thrombosis in the myeloproliferative disorders. *Blood* 64:1, 1984.

185. Barbui T, Cortelazzo S, Viero P, et al: Thrombohaemorrhagic complications in 101 cases of myeloproliferative disorders: Relationship to platelet number and function. *Eur J Cancer Clin Oncol* 19:1593, 1983.

186. Thiele J, Lorenzen J, Manich B, et al: Apoptosis (programmed cell death) in idiopathic (primary) osteo-/myelofibrosis. *Acta Haematol* 97:137, 1997.

187. Thiele J, Holgado S, Choritz H, et al: Chronic megakaryocyte-granulocytic myelosis—an electron microscope study including freeze-fracture. *Virchows Arch[A]* 375:129, 1977.

188. Miller JB, Testa JR, Lindgren V, et al: The patterns and clinical significance of karyotypic abnormalities in patients with idiopathic polycythemic myelofibrosis. *Cancer* 55:582, 1985.

189. Damor JL, Dupriez B, Fenaux P, et al: Cytogenetic studies and their prognostic significance in agnogenic myeloid metaplasia. *Blood* 72:855, 1988.

190. Nakamura H, Sadamori N, Mine M, et al: Effects of short-term liquid culture of peripheral blood mononuclear cells with recombinant human granulocyte or granulocyte-macrophage colony-stimulating factor in cytogenetic studies of myelofibrosis with myeloid metaplasia. *Leukemia* 6:853, 1992.

191. Reilly JT, Snowden JA, Spearing RL, et al: Cytogenetic abnormalities and their prognostic significance in idiopathic myelofibrosis. *Br J Haematol* 98:96, 1997.

192. Forrester RH, Louro JM: Philadelphia chromosome abnormality in agnogenic myeloid metaplasia. *Ann Intern Med* 64:622, 1966.

193. Weda F, Takashima T, Suzuki M, Kadoya M: MR diagnosis of myelofibrosis *Radiat Med* 12:135, 1994.

194. Amano Y, Onda M, Amano M, Kumazaki T: Magnetic resonance imaging of myelofibrosis. STIR and gadolinium-enhanced MR images. *Clin Imaging* 21:264, 1997.

195. Gilbert HS, Ginsberg H, Fagerstrom R, Brown WV: Characterization of hypocholesterolemia in myeloproliferative diseases. *Am J Med* 71:595, 1981.

196. Naggar L, Jaeger P, Burckhardt P, et al: Hypocalcemia and myelofibrosis: An unrecognized association. *Schweiz Med Wochenschr* 116:1771, 1986.

197. Voss A, Schmidt K, Hasselbalch H, Junker P: Hypercalcemia in idiopathic myelofibrosis. *Am J Hematol* 39:231, 1992.

198. Wang JC, Chen C, Lou L-H, Mora M: Blood thrombopoietin, IL-6 and IL-11 levels in patients with agnogenic myeloid metaplasia. *Leukemia* 11:1827, 1997.

199. Dekmezian R, Kantarjian HM, Heating MJ, et al: The relevance of reticulin stain-measured fibrosis at diagnosis in chronic myelogenous leukemia. *Cancer* 59:1739, 1987.

200. Thiele J, Zankovich R, Steinberg T, et al: Primary (essential) thrombocythemia versus initial hyperplastic stages of agnogenic myeloid metaplasia with thrombocytosis. *Acta Haematol* 81:192, 1989.

201. Fortunato A, Mazzone A, Ricevuti G: Myelofibrosis caused by cancer: Presentation of a clinical case with a very difficult diagnosis. *Minerva Med* 76:1051, 1985.

202. Yablonski-Peretz T, Sulkes A, Polliack A, et al: Secondary myelofibrosis with metastatic breast cancer simulating agnogenic myeloid metaplasia: Report of a case and review of the literature. *Med Pediatr Oncol* 13:92, 1985.

203. Ishimura J, Fukushi M: Scintigraphic evaluation of secondary myelofibrosis associated with prostatic cancer before hormonal therapy. *Clin Nucl Med* 15:330, 1990.

204. Smart HE, Canney PA, Kerr DJ: Myelofibrosis associated with metastatic seminoma. *Clin Oncol* 4:132, 1992.

205. Takahashi T, Akihama T, Yamaguchi A, et al: Lysozyme secreting tumor: A case of gastric cancer associated with myelofibrosis due to disseminated bone marrow metastasis. *Jpn J Med* 26:58, 1987.

206. Rubins JM: The role of myelofibrosis in malignant leukoerythroblastosis. *Cancer* 51:308, 1983.

207. Hashim MSK, Kordofani AYA, El Dabi MA: Tuberculosis and myelofibrosis in children. *Ann Trop Paediatrics* 17:61, 1997.

208. Sawers AH, Davson J, Braganza J, et al: Systemic mastocytosis, myelofibrosis and portal hypertension. *J Clin Pathol* 35:617, 1982.

209. Reisberg IR, Oyakawa S: Mastocytosis with malabsorption, myelofibrosis, and massive ascites. *Am J Gastroenterol* 82:54, 1987.

210. Brenner B, Green J, Rosenbaum H, et al: Severe pancytopenia due to marked marrow fibrosis associated with angioimmunoblastic lymphadenopathy. *Acta Haematol* 74:43, 1985.

211. Meckenstock G, Wehmeier A, Schaefer HE, et al: Lymphoid myelofibrosis associated with high grade B cell lymphoma of the liver. *Leuk Lymph* 26:197, 1997.

212. Vandermolen L, Rice L, Lynch EL: Plasma cell dyscrasia with marrow fibrosis. *Am J Med* 79:297, 1985.

213. Humphrey CA, Morris TCM: The intimate relationship of myelofibrosis and myeloma: Effect of therapy. *Br J Haematol* 73:269, 1989.

214. Patterson KG, Treleavan JG, Zuiable A: Marrow fibrosis in myeloma: Improvement by alkylating agent therapy. *Clin Lab Haematol* 18:221, 1988.

215. Murayama T, Matsui T, Hayaski Y, et al: Plasma cell leukemia with myelofibrosis. *Ann Hematol* 69:151, 1994.

216. Schmidt U, Ruwe M, Leder LD: Multiple myeloma with bone marrow

biopsy features simulating concomitant chronic idiopathic myelofibrosis. *Nouv Rev Franc d'Hematol* 37:159, 1995.

217. Abildgaard N, Bendix-Hanse K, Kristensen JE, et al: Bone marrow fibrosis and disease activity in multiple myeloma monitored by the autoterminal propeptide of procollagen III in serum. *Br J Haematol* 99:641, 1997.

218. Nomura S, Ogawa Y, Osawa G, et al: Myelofibrosis secondary to renal osteodystrophy. *Nephron* 72:683, 1996.

219. Fontenay-Roupie M, Dupuy E, Berrou E, et al: Increased proliferation of bone-marrow-derived fibroblasts in primary hypertropic osteoarthropy with severe myleofibrosis. *Blood* 85:3229, 1995.

220. Jantunen E, Hänninen A, Naukkarinen A, et al: Gray platelet syndrome with splenomegaly and signs of extramedullary hematopoiesis. *Am J Hematol* 46:218, 1994.

221. Sadoun A, Lacotte L, Delwail V, et al: Allogeneic bone marrow transplantation for hypereosinophilic syndrome with advanced myelofibrosis. *Bone Marrow Transplant* 19:741, 1997.

222. Hatake K, Ohtsuki T, Uwai M, et al: Tretinoin induces bone marrow collagenous fibrosis in acute promyelocytic leukemia. *Br J Haematol* 93:646, 1996.

223. Labotka RJ, Morgan RR: Myelofibrosis with neuroblastoma. *Med Pediatr Oncol* 10:21, 1982.

224. Karcher DS, Pearson CE, Butler WM, et al: Giant lymph node hyperplasia involving the thymus with associated nephrotic syndrome and myelofibrosis. *Am J Clin Pathol* 77:100, 1982.

225. Walka MM, Daümling S, Hadorn HB, et al: Vitamin D dependent rickets type II with myelofibrosis and immune dysfunction. *Eur J Pediatr* 114:213, 1989.

226. Al-Eissa YA, Al-Mashhadami SA: Myelofibrosis in severe combined immunodeficiency due to vitamin D deficiency rickets. *Acta Haematol* 92:160, 1994.

227. Sartoris DJ, Resnick D: Myelofibrosis arising in treated histiocytosis X. *Eur Pediatr* 144:200, 1985.

228. Shah-Reddy I, Subramanian L, Narang S: Myelofibrosis and true histiocytic lymphoma. *Tumor* 71:509, 1985.

229. Jennings WH, Li CY, Kiely JM: Concomitant myelofibrosis with agnogenic myeloid metaplasia and malignant lymphoma. *Mayo Clin Proc* 58:617, 1983.

230. Epstein RJ, Joshua DE, Kronenberg H: Idiopathic myelofibrosis complicated by lymphoma: Report of two cases. *Acta Haematol* 73:40, 1985.

231. Kaufman S, Iuclea S, Reif R: Idiopathic myelofibrosis complicated by chronic lymphatic leukaemia. *Clin Lab Haematol* 9:81, 1987.

232. Subramanian VP, Gomez GA, Han T, et al: Coexistence of myeloid metaplasia with myelofibrosis and hairy-cell leukemia. *Arch Intern Med* 145:164, 1985.

233. Ji SQ, Zhu M, Wang YZ: Primary macroglobulinemia with myelofibrosis: Report of a case. *Chin Med J* 100:83, 1987.

234. Humphrey CA, Morris TCM: The intimate relationship of myelofibrosis and myeloma. *Br J Haematol* 73:269, 1989.

235. Meerkin D, Ashkenazi Y, Gottschalk-Sabag S, Hershko C: Plasma cell dyscrasia with myelofibrosis. *Cancer* 73:625, 1994.

236. Kakkar N, Vashishta RK, Banerjee AK, et al: Primary pulmonary malignant teratoma with yolk sac element associated with hematologic neoplasia. *Respiration* 63:52, 1996.

237. Berner Y, Berrebi A: Myeloproliferative disorders and nonmyelomatous paraprotein: A study of five patients and review of the literature. *Isr J Med Sci* 22:109, 1986.

238. Ellis JT, Peterson P: Myelofibrosis in the myeloproliferative disorders. *Prog Clin Biol Res* 154:19, 1984.

239. Najean Y, Rain JD, Dresch C, et al: Risk of leukaemia, carcinoma and myelofibrosis in ³²P- or chemotherapy-treated patients with polycythaemia vera. *Leuk Lymph* 22(suppl 1):111, 1996.

240. Najean Y, Rain JD: Treatment of polycythemia vera: use of ³²P- alone or in combination with maintenance therapy using hydroxyurea in 461 patients greater than 65 years of age. *Blood* 89:2319, 1997.

241. Randi ML, Barbone E, Fabris F, et al: Post-polycythemia myeloid metaplasia. *J Med* 25:363, 1994.

242. Lukowicz DF, Myers TJ, Grasso JA, et al: Sideroblastic anemia terminating in myelofibrosis. *Am J Hematol* 13:253, 1982.

243. Hasselbalch H, Berild D: Transition of myelofibrosis to polycythaemia vera. *Scand J Haematol* 30:161, 1983.

244. Talarico L, Wolf BC, Kumar A, Weintraub LR: Reversal of bone marrow

fibrosis and subsequent development of polycythemia vera in patients with myeloproliferative disorders. *Am J Hematol* 30:248, 1989.

245. Palphilon DH, Creamer P, Keeling DH, et al: Restoration of active haemopoiesis in a patient with myelofibrosis and subsequent termination in acute myeloblastic leukaemia: Case report and review of the literature. *Eur J Haematol* 38:279, 1987.

246. Besa EC, Nowell PC, Geller NI, Gardner F: Analysis of androgen response of 23 patients with agnogenic myeloid metaplasia. *Cancer* 49:308, 1982.

247. Silverstein MN: Treatment of myelofibrosis, in *Myelofibrosis: Pathophysiology and Clinical Management,* edited by SM Lewis, pp 195–202. Marcel Dekker, New York, 1985.

248. Chabannon C, Pegourie B, Sotto JJ, Hallard D: Clinical and hematological improvement in a patient receiving danazol therapy for myelofibrosis with myeloid metaplasia. *Nouv Rev Fr Hematol* 32:165, 1990.

249. Lévy V, Bourgarit A, Delmer A, et al: Treatment of agnogenic myeloid metaplasia with danazol. *Am J Hematol* 53:239, 1996.

250. Makdisi WJ, Cherian R, Vanveldhuizen PJ, et al: Fatal peliosis of the liver and spleen in a patient with agnogenic myeloid metaplasia treated with danazol. *Am J Gastroenterol* 90:317, 1995.

251. Ozsoylu S, Ruacan S: High-dose intravenous corticosteroid treatment in childhood idiopathic myelofibrosis. *Acta Haematol* 75:49, 1986.

252. Cetingül N, Yener E, Oztop S, et al: Agnogenic myeloid metaplasia in childhood: A report of two cases and efficiency of intravenous high dose methylprednisolone treatment. *Acta Pediatr Jpn* 36:697, 1994.

253. Barois G, Liberato LN, Guarnone R: Serum erythropoietin in patients with myeloid metaplasia. *Br J Haematol* 83:365, 1993.

254. Rodrigues JN, Martino ML, Muniz R, Prados D: Recombinant human erythropoietin for the treatment of anemia in myelofibrosis with myeloid metaplasia. *Am J Hematol* 39:435, 1994.

255. Tefferi A, Silverstein MN: Recombinant human erythropoietin therapy in patients with myelofibrosis with myeloid metaplasia. *Br J Haematol* 86:893, 1994.

256. Lofvenberg E, Wahlin A: Management of polycythaemia vera, essential thrombocythaemia and myelofibrosis with hydroxyurea. *Eur J Haematol* 41:375, 1988.

257. Lofvenberg E, Wahlin A, Roos G, Ost A: Reversal of myelofibrosis by hydroxyurea. *Eur J Haematol* 44:33, 1990.

258. Manoharan A: Management of myelofibrosis with intermittent hydroxyurea. *Br J Haematol* 71:252, 1991.

259. Manoharan A, Pitney WR: Chemotherapy resolves symptoms and reverses marrow fibrosis in myelofibrosis. *Scand J Haematol* 33:453 1984.

260. Stahl RL, Hoppstein L, Davidson TG: Intraperitoneal chemotherapy with cytosine arabinoside in agnogenic myelofibrosis with myeloid metaplasia and ascites due to peritoneal extramedullary hematopoiesis. *Am J Hematol* 43:156, 1993.

261. Carlo-Stella C, Cazzola M, Gasner A, et al: Effects of recombinant alpha and gamma interferons on the in vitro growth of circulating hematopoietic progenitors from patients with myelofibrosis and myeloid metaplasia. *Blood* 70:1014, 1987.

262. Sacchi S: The role of α-interferon in essential thrombocythaemia, polycythaema vera and myelofibrosis with myeloid metaplasia (MMM): a concise update. *Leuk Lymph* 19:13, 1995.

263. Sivera P, Cesano L, Guerrasio A, et al: Clinical and hematological improvement in a patient with idiopathic myelofibrosis and osteosclerosis. *Br J Haematol* 86:397, 1994.

264. Greenberger JS, Chaffey JT, Rosenthal DS, et al: Irradiation for control of hypersplenism and painful splenomegaly in myeloid metaplasia. *Int J Radiat Oncol Biol Phys* 2:1083, 1977.

265. Parmentier C, Charbord P, Tibi M, et al: Splenic irradiation in myelofibrosis, clinical findings and ferrokinetics. *Int J Radiat Oncol Biol Phys* 2:1075, 1977.

266. Wagner H Jr, McKeough PG, Desforges J, et al: Splenic irradiation in the treatment of patients with chronic myelogenous leukemia or myelofibrosis with myeloid metaplasia. *Cancer* 58:1204, 1986.

267. Jacobs P, Wood L, Robson S: Refractory ascites in the chronic myeloproliferative syndrome. *Am J Hematol* 37:128, 1991.

268. Jacobs P, Sellars S: Granulocytic sarcoma preceding leukaemic transformation in myelofibrosis. *Postgrad Med J* 61:1069, 1985.

269. Benbassat J, Penchas S, Ligumski M: Splenectomy in patients with agnogenic myeloid metaplasia: An analysis of 321 published cases. *Br J Haematol* 42:207, 1979.

270. Brenner B, Nagler A, Tatarsky I, Häsmonai M: Splenectomy in agnogenic myeloid metaplasia and post-polycythemic myeloid metaplasia. *Arch Intern Med* 148:2501, 1988.

271. Barosi G, Ambrosetti A, Buratti A, et al: Splenectomy for patients with myelo-fibrosis with myeloid metaplasia. *Leukemia* 7:200, 1993.

272. Lafaye F, Rain JD, Clot P, Najean Y: Risks and benefits of splenectomy in myelofibrosis: analysis of 39 cases. *Nouv Rev Franc d'Hematol* 36:359, 1994.

273. Towell BL, Levine SP: Massive hepatomegaly following splenectomy for myeloid metaplasia: Case report and review of the literature. *Am J Med* 82:371, 1987.

274. DiBella NJ, Silverstein MN, Hoagland HC: Effect of splenectomy on teardrop-shaped erythrocytes in agnogenic myeloid metaplasia. *Arch Intern Med* 137:380, 1977.

275. Tefferi A, Silverstein MN, Li CY: 2-chlorodeoxyadenosine treatment after splenectomy in patients who have myelofibrosis with myeloid metaplasia. *Br J Haematol* 99:352, 1997.

276. Benbassat J, Gilon D, Penchas S: The choice between splenectomy and medical treatment in patients with advanced agnogenic myeloid metaplasia. *Am J Hematol* 33:128, 1990.

277. Petroianu A, Da Silva RG, Simal CJ, et al: Late postoperative follow-up of patients submitted to subtotal splenectomy. *Am Surg* 63:735, 1997.

278. Tefferi A, Barrett SM, Silverstein NM, Nagorney DM: Outcome of portal-systemic shunt surgery for portal hypertension associated with intrahepatic obstruction in patients with agnogenic myeloid metaplasia. *Am J Hematol* 46:325, 1994.

279. Matzner Y, Polliack A: Bone marrow curettage in myelodysplastic disorders: A stimulus for regeneration in disturbed hematopoiesis. *JAMA* 246:1926, 1981.

280. Fruchtman SM: Therapeutic implications of collagen metabolism in myelofibrosis. *Prog Clin Biol Res* 154:467, 1984.

281. Petrini M, Cecconi N, Azzara A, et al: 1,25-dihydroxy-vitamin D on the treatment of idiopathic myelofibrosis. *Br J Haematol* 62:399, 1986.

282. Richard C, Mazzora F, Iriondo A, et al: The usefulness of 1,25-dihydroxy-vitamin in the treatment of idiopathic myelofibrosis. *Br J Haematol* 62:399, 1986.

283. Eugster C, Brun-del-Re GP, Bucher U: The role of 1,25-dihydroxy-vitamin D$_3$ (1,25(OH)2D3) in the treatment of idiopathic myelofibrosis (letter). *Br J Haematol* 65:381, 1987.

284. Arlet P, Nicodeme R, Adoue D, et al: Clinical evidence for 1-dihydroxy-cholecalciferol action in myelofibrosis (letter). *Lancet* 1:1013 1984.

285. Rewald E. de las Mercedes Francischetti: Combining interferon-alpha2b (IFN) and intravenous immunoglobulins IgG, IgM and IgA (IVIG) in rapid progressive myelofibrosis (MF) with Trisomy 1 (letter). *Am J Hematol* 54:340, 1997.

286. Pietrasanta D, Clavio M, Vallebella E, et al: Long-lasting effect of cyclosporin-A on anemia associated with idiopathic myelofibrosis. *Haematologica* 82:458, 1997.

287. Singhal S, Powles R, Treleaven J, et al: Allogeneic bone marrow transplantation for primary myelofibrosis. *Bone Marrow Transplant* 16:743, 1995.

288. Guardiola P, Anderson JE, Bandini G, et al: Allogeneic bone marrow transplantation for agnogeneic myeloid metaplasia. *Blood* 93:2831, 1999.

289. Przepiorka D, Giralt S, Khour I, et al: Allogeneic marrow transplantation for myeloproliferative disorders other than chronic myelogenous leukemia: review of forty cases. *Am J Hematol* 7:24, 1998.

290. Visini G, Finelli C, Castelli U, et al: Myelofibrosis with myeloid metaplasia: Clinical and haematological parameters predicting survival in a series of 133 patients. *Br J Haematol* 75:4, 1990.

291. Rozman C, Giralt M, Feliu E, et al: Life expectancy of patients with chronic non-leukemic myeloproliferative disorders. *Cancer* 67:2658, 1991.

292. Silverstein MN, Brown AL, Linman JW: Idiopathic myeloid metaplasia, its evolution into acute leukemia. *Arch Intern Med* 132:709, 1973.

293. Marcus RE, Hibbin JA, Matutes E, et al: Megakaryoblastic transformation of myelofibrosis with expression of the c-*sis* oncogene. *Am J Haematol* 36:186, 1986.

294. Hernandez JM, SanMiguel JF, Gonzalez M, et al: Development of acute leukaemia after idiopathic myelofibrosis. *J Clin Pathol* 45:427, 1992.

295. Chan ACL, Kwong Y-L, Lam CCK: Granulocytic sarcoma of megakaryoblastic differentiation complicating chronic idiopathic myelofibrosis. *Hem Pathol* 27:417, 1996.

296. Polliack A, Prokocimer M, Matzner Y, et al: Lymphoblastic leukemic transformation (lymphoblastic crisis) in myelofibrosis and myeloid metaplasia. *Am J Hematol* 9:211, 1980.

297. Yinon A, Kopolovic J, Dollberg L, Hershko C: Evolution of malignant lymphoma in agnogenic myeloid metaplasia. *Oncology* 45:373, 1988.

298. Barosi G, Ambrosetti A, Centra A: Splenectomy and risk of blast transformation in myelofibrosis with myeloid metaplasia. *Blood* 91:3630, 1998.

299. Shreiner DP: Spontaneous hematologic remission in agnogenic myeloid metaplasia. *Am J Med* 60:1014, 1976.

300. Rani MV, Shreiner DP: Spontaneous "remission" of agnogenic myeloid metaplasia and termination in acute myeloid leukemia. *Arch Intern Med* 141:1481, 1981.

301. Mesa R, Silverstein MN, Jacobsen SJ, et al: Population-based incidence and survival figures in essential thrombocythemia and agnogenic myeloid metaplasia: an Olmstead County Study, 1976–1995. *Am J Hematol* 61:10, 1999.

302. Tefferi A: Myelofibrosis with myeloid metaplasia. *New Eng J Med* 342:1255, 2000.

303. Tefferi A, Mesa RA, Nagorney DM, et al: Splenectomy in myelofibrosis with myeloid metaplasia. *Blood* 95:2226, 2000.

CLASSIFICATION OF MALIGNANT LYMPHOID DISORDERS

THOMAS J. KIPPS

> This chapter outlines the category of neoplastic or pre-neoplastic lymphocyte and plasma cell disorders. It introduces a framework for evaluating neoplastic lymphocyte and plasma cell disorders, outlines clinical syndromes associated with such disorders, and presents a road-map to the chapters in the text that discuss each of these disorders in greater detail. The diseases caused by non-neoplastic disorders of lymphocytes and plasma cells are outlined in Chap. 86.

CLASSIFICATION

Lymphocyte malignancies comprise a wide spectrum of different morphologic and clinical syndromes (Table 96-1). Lymphocyte neoplasms can originate from cells that are at a stage prior to T- and B-lymphocyte differentiation from a primitive stem cell or from cells at stages of maturation after stem cell differentiation. Thus, acute lymphocytic leukemias arise from a primitive lymphoid stem cell that may give rise to cells with either B- or T-cell phenotypes (see Chap. 97). On the other hand, chronic lymphocytic leukemia arises from a more differentiated B-lymphocyte progenitor (see Chap. 98), and multiple myeloma from progenitors at even later stages of B-lymphocyte maturation (see Chap. 106). Variability in expression of a lymphopoietic stem cell disorder may result in the spectrum of lymphocytic diseases, such as a B-lymphocyte or T-lymphocyte lymphoma (see Chap. 103), and different types of diseases, such as hairy-cell leukemia (see Chap. 99), prolymphocytic leukemia (see Chap. 98), natural killer cell large granular lymphocytic leukemia (see Chap. 100), or plasmacytoma (see Chap. 106).

To provide a unified international basis for clinical and investigative work in this field, the International Lymphoma Study Group proposed a new classification termed revised European-American lymphoma (REAL) classification (see Chap. 101).[1] This classification scheme makes use of the pathologic, immunophenotypic, genetic, and clinical features of a given lymphocyte tumor to delineate them into separate disease entities (see Table 96-1).[2] Studies have verified the clinical utility of this classification scheme.[3,4]

ASSOCIATED CLINICAL SYNDROMES

ABNORMAL PRODUCTION OF IMMUNOGLOBULIN

When B lymphocytes undergo neoplastic transformation and clonal proliferation, they can secrete monoclonal proteins inappropriately (see Chap. 104). If the monoclonal protein is IgM, IgA, or a member of certain subclasses of IgG (e.g., namely IgG_3), this may increase the viscosity of the blood, impairing blood flow through the microcirculation (see Chaps. 106 and 108). This may be impeded further by the associated erythrocyte-erythrocyte aggregation (pathologic rouleaux) that often occurs in blood with a high concentration of immunoglobulin protein. Collectively this may result in the hyperviscosity syndrome, manifested clinically by headache, dizziness, diplopia, stupor, retinal venous engorgement, or frank coma (see Chap. 108).[5,6]

Monoclonal immunoglobulin proteins also can interact with cell surfaces and impair granulocyte or platelet function, or interact with coagulation proteins to impair their function in hemostasis. Excessive excretion of immunoglobulin light chains can lead to several types of renal tubular dysfunction and renal insufficiency (see Chap. 106). IgM deposited in glomerular tufts also can lead to renal disease (see Chap. 108). Cryoglobulins [or immunoglobulins that precipitate at temperatures below 37°C (98.6°F)] can result in Raynaud syndrome, skin ulcerations, purpura, and digital infarction and gangrene (see Chap. 56). These manifestations are the result of immune complex formation and complement activation as well as precipitation of cryoglobulins in cutaneous blood vessels. Finally, excessive production of monoclonal immunoglobulin or immunoglobulin fragments in plasma cell myeloma (see Chap. 106) of heavy-chain disease (see Chap. 109) may lead to formation of amyloid, resulting in primary amyloidosis (see Chap. 107).

Production of autoreactive antibodies spontaneously or in relationship to a B-lymphocyte neoplasia may lead to autoimmune hemolytic anemia (see Chap. 55), autoimmune thrombocytopenia (see Chap. 117), or, rarely, autoimmune neutropenia (see Chap. 71). Autoantibodies directed against tissues are implicated in the etiopathogenesis of such diseases as autoimmune thyroiditis, adrenalitis, encephalitis, or other organ involvement. Peripheral neuropathies, as a result of demyelinization, can occur in patients with monoclonal immunoglobulin (see Chaps. 106 and 108). The neural injury is often related to antibody activity against myelin-associated glycoproteins or absorption by nerve tissue. Rarely, the polyneuropathy is associated with organomegaly, endocrinopathy, a monoclonal protein, and skin chains, or POEMS syndrome (see Chap. 106).

MARROW AND OTHER TISSUE INFILTRATION

Well-differentiated malignant B-lymphocytes, such as those found in early stages of chronic lymphocytic leukemia or macroglobulinemia, may infiltrate the marrow extensively, causing minimal impairment of hemopoiesis. Eventually, however, further infiltration of marrow by malignant B lymphocytes can suppress normal hemopoiesis, resulting in varying combinations of anemia, granulocytopenia, and/or thrombocytopenia (see Chap. 98). Malignant B-lymphocyte proliferation or infiltration may result in any combination of splenomegaly and lymphadenopathy of either superficial or deep lymph nodes. Many B-cell lymphomas tend to involve isolated lymph node groups (see Chaps. 102 and 103), whereas B-cell chronic lymphocytic leukemia and most low-grade lymphomas tend to involve many superficial and deep lymph node-bearing areas and the spleen (see Chaps. 98 and 103). Prolymphocytic leukemia and hairy-cell leukemia, two uncommon B-lymphocyte malignancies, are prone to infiltrate the marrow and spleen, sometimes causing massive enlargement of the latter (see Chaps. 98 and 99).

LYMPHOKINE-INDUCED DISORDERS

In addition to the consequences of monoclonal immunoglobulin and tumor proliferation noted above, some lymphocyte malignancies may elaborate cytokines that contribute to the disease morbidity. Patients with cutaneous T-cell lymphomas have been found to have elevated plasma levels of T_H2-type associated cytokines (see Chap. 84), which

Acronyms and abbreviations that appear in this chapter include: IL-1, interleukin-1.

TABLE 96-1

Lymphocyte Neoplasm	Morphology	Phenotype	Genotype
B-Cell Neoplasms			
Precursor B-cell Neoplasms			
Lymphoblastic leukemia (see Chap. 97)	Medium to large cells with finely stippled chromatin and scant cytoplasm	TdT$^+$, sIg$^-$, CD10, CD13$^{+/-}$, CD19, CD34$^{+/-}$, CD33$^{+/-}$, CD79a	t(1;19), t(9;22), and 11q13-defects associated with poor prognosis
Lymphoblastic lymphoma (see Chap. 103)	Large cells with high nuclear:cytoplasmic ratio	see above	see above
Mature B-cell Neoplasms			
Leukemias			
Chronic lymphocytic leukemia (see Chap. 98)	Small cells with round, dense nuclei	Dull sIg, CD5, CD10$^-$, CD19, dull CD20, CD23, CD38$^{+/-}$	IgR, trisomy 12 (~30%), del at 13q14 (~50%), 11q-
Prolymphocytic leukemia (see Chap. 98)	≥55% prolymphocytes	Bright sIg, CD5$^{+/-}$, CD19, CD22	IgR, trisomy 12 (~30%)
Hairy cell leukemia (see Chap. 99)	Small cells with cytoplasmic projections	Dull sIg, CD5$^{+/-}$, CD10$^-$, CD19, CD20, CD103	IgR
Lymphomas (see Chap. 103)			
Small lymphocytic lymphoma	Small round cells	Dull sIg, CD5, CD19, dull CD20, CD23	IgR, trisomy 12 (~30%), del at 13q14 (~40%), 11q$^-$
Lymphoplasmacytoid lymphoma	Small cells with plasmacytoid features	Dull cIg, CD5$^-$, CD10$^-$, CD19, CD20$^{+/-}$	IgR, t(9;14) (~50%) involving PAX-5
Mantle cell lymphoma	Small- to medium-sized cells	sIgM/IgD, CD5, CD10$^-$, CD19, CD20, CD23$^-$	IgR, t(11;14) (~70%) involving BCL1
Follicular lymphoma (follicle center lymphoma)	Small, medium, or large cells with cleaved nuclei	sIg, CD5$^-$, CD10, CD19, bright CD20, CD23$^{+/-}$	IgR, t(14;18) (~85%) involving BCL2
Marginal zone B-cell lymphoma	Small or large monocytoid cells	sIgM$^+$, sIgD$^-$, cIg (~50%), CD5$^-$, CD11c$^{+/-}$, CD19, CD20, CD23$^-$, CD43$^{+/-}$	IgR, commonly with trisomy 3 and/or t(11;18)
Mucosa-associated lymphoid tissue (''MALT'') type	see above	see above	see above
Nodal type	see above	see above	see above
Splenic marginal zone B-cell lymphoma	Small to large monocytoid and/or villous lymphocytes	sIgM$^+$, sIgD$^-$, CD5$^-$, CD19, CD20, CD23$^-$	IgR
Diffuse large B-cell lymphoma	Large, irregular cells that can resemble centroblasts, immunoblasts, multilobate cells, or even RS-like cells	sIgM$^+$, sIgD$^{+/-}$, CD5$^{+/-}$, CD10$^{+/-}$, CD19, CD20	IgR, 3q27 abnormalities involving BCL6 (~40%) or t(14,18) (~25%) involving BCL-2
Primary mediastinal large B-cell lymphoma	same as above	sIg$^-$, CD5$^-$, CD19, CD20, CD22	same as above
Burkitt lymphoma	Medium-sized, round cells with abundant cytoplasm	sIgM$^+$, CD5$^-$, CD10, CD19, CD20, CD23$^-$	t(8;14), t(2;8), or t(8;22) involving C-MYC
Burkitt-like lymphoma	Medium-sized, round cells with abundant cytoplasm	same as above except sIg$^-$, cIg$^{+/-}$, and CD10$^-$	same as above except ~30% have BCL-2 rearrangements
Plasma Cell Neoplasms			
Plasma cell myeloma (see Chap. 106)	Plasma cells with occasional plasmablasts	cIg, CD5$^-$, CD19, CD20$^-$, CD22, CD38, CD56	IgR, complex karyotypes common
Plasma cell leukemia	Plasmablastic cells with prominent nucleoli	same as above	same as above
Plasma cell lymphoma	Plasma cells	same as above	same as above
Waldenström macroglobulinemia (see Chap. 108)	Plasmacytoid cells	CD5$^{+/-}$, CD10$^{+/-}$, CD19, CD20, CD22, CD38$^{+/-}$	IgR, complex karyotypes common
Hodgkin Disease (see Chap. 104)			
T-Cell Neoplasms			
Precursor T-cell Neoplasms			
Acute lymphoblastic leukemia (see Chap. 97)	Medium to large cells with finely stippled chromatin and scant cytoplasm	CD2$^{+/-}$, cytoplasmic CD3, CD5$^{+/-}$, CD7, CD10$^{+/-}$, CD4$^+$/CD8$^+$ or CD4$^-$/CD8$^-$	Abnormalities in TCR loci at 14q11 (TCR-α), 7q34 (TCR-β), or 7p15 (TCR-γ), and t(9;17)(q34;q23)
Lymphoblastic lymphoma (see Chap. 103)	same as above	same as above	same as above
Mature T-cell Neoplasms			
Leukemias			
T-cell prolymphocytic leukemia	Small cells with prominent nucleoli and abundant cytoplasm	TdT$^-$, CD2, CD3, CD5, CD7, CD4$^+$/CD8$^-$ is more common than CD4$^-$/CD8$^+$	α/β TCR rearrangement, inv14(q11;q32) (~75%)
Large granular lymphocytic leukemia (see Chap. 100)	abundant cytoplasm and azurophilic granules	TdT$^-$, CD2, CD3, CD8, CD16$^{+/-}$, CD56$^-$, CD57$^{+/-}$	α/β TCR rearrangement

TABLE 96-1 (*CONTINUED*)

LYMPHOCYTE NEOPLASM	MORPHOLOGY	PHENOTYPE	GENOTYPE
Lymphomas (see Chap. 103)			
T-cell lymphoma, nasal and nasal-type ("angiocentric lymphoma")	Angiocentric and angiodestructive growth	CD2, CD3$^{+/-}$, CD5$^{+/-}$, CD56, cytoplasmic CD3	TCR rearrangements variable, EBV present
Cutaneous T-cell lymphoma	Small to large cells with cerebriform nuclei	TdT$^-$, CD2, CD3, CD4, CD5, CD7$^{+/-}$, CD25$^-$	α/β TCR rearrangement
Mycosis fungoides	same as above	same as above	same as above
Sézary syndrome	same as above	same as above	same as above
Angioimmunoblastic T-cell lymphoma	Small immunoblasts with pale-staining or clear cells		α/β TCR rearrangement with rare incomplete IgR, trisomy 3 or 5 noted
Peripheral T-cell lymphoma (unspecified)	highly variable	CD2, CD3, CD5, CD7$^-$, CD4 > CD8 > CD4/CD8	α/β TCR rearrangement often with incomplete IgR
Subcutaneous panniculitic T-cell lymphoma	Medium-sized atypical cells with irregular nuclei and hyperchromasia	CD2, CD3, CD5, CD7$^-$, CD4 or CD8	α/β TCR rearrangement
Intestinal T-cell lymphoma	Small to large atypical lymphocytes	CD2, CD3, CD5, CD7$^-$, CD4$^-$/CD8$^-$ or CD4$^-$/CD8$^+$, CD103	β TCR rearrangement
Hepatosplenic γ:δ T-cell lymphoma	small to medium-size cells with condensed chromatin and round nuclei	CD2, CD3, CD4$^-$, CD5, CD7$^-$, CD8$^{+/-}$	γ/δ TCR rearrangement, isochromosome 7q
Adult T-cell lymphoma	Highly variable with multilobed nuclei	CD2, CD3, CD5, CD7$^-$, CD25, CD4 >> CD8	α/β TCR rearrangement and integrated HTLV-1
Anaplastic large-cell lymphoma	Large blastic pleomorphic cells with "horseshoe"-shaped nuclei, prominent nucleoli, and abundant basophilic cytoplasm	TdT$^-$, CD2, CD3, CD5, CD7$^{+/-}$, CD25$^{+/-}$, CD30, CD45$^{+/-}$	TCR rearrangement, t(2;5)(p23;q35) resulting in nucleophosmin - anaplastic lymphoma kinase fusion protein
Primary cutaneous CD30-positive lymphoma	Anaplastic large cells as above in cutaneous nodules	TdT$^-$, CD2, CD3, CD5, CD7$^{+/-}$, CD25$^{+/-}$, CD30	TCR rearrangement, without t(2;5)(p23;q35)
Natural Killer Cell Neoplasms			
Large granular lymphocytic leukemia (see Chap. 100)	abundant cytoplasm and azurophilic granules	TdT$^-$, CD2, CD3$^-$, CD8$^{+/-}$, CD16, CD56, CD57$^{+/-}$	No TCR rearrangement
Aggressive natural killer cell leukemia	same as above	same as above	No TCR rearrangement, EBV present
Natural killer-cell lymphoma, nasal and nasal-type ("angiocentric lymphoma")	Angiocentric and angiodestructive growth	CD2, CD5$^{+/-}$, CD56, cytoplasmic CD3	No TCR rearrangment, EBV present

*The immunohistochemical and surface-antigen phenotypes that typically are found for neoplastic cells of a given disorder are listed. If a CD antigen is indicated (see Chap. 13), then most of the neoplastic cells express that particular surface protein that are expressed by most tumor cells. CD antigens that have a minus sign "−" suffix are characteristically not expressed by the neoplastic cells of that disease entity. CD antigens that have a ± sign suffix are not expressed by the neoplastic cells of all patients with that entity or are expressed at low or variable levels on the tumor cells.

†The common genetic features associated with a given type of neoplasm are indicated. The numbers in parentheses provide the approximate proportion of cases that have the defined phenotype or genetic abnormality.

ABBREVIATIONS: α/β TCR, = T-cell receptor genes encoding the α and β chains of the T-cell receptor (see Chap. 84); cIg, = cytoplasmic immunoglobulin; EBV, = Epstein-Barr virus; γ δ TCR, = T-cell receptor genes encoding the γ and δ chains of the T-cell receptor (see Chap. 84); IgR, = immunoglobulin gene rearrangement; sIg, = surface immunoglobulin (see Chap. 83); sIgM, = surface IgM; sIgD, = surface IgD; RS-like cells, = Reed-Sternberg–like cells.

may account for the relatively high incidence of eosinophilia and eosinophilic pneumonia observed in patients with this disease.[7] In addition, the neoplastic plasma cells in multiple myeloma may secrete interleukin-1 (IL-1), a cytokine that can stimulate osteoclast proliferation and activity leading to extensive osteolysis, severe bone pain, and pathologic fractures (see Chap. 106).[8] In addition, IL-1 may stimulate production of antidiuretic hormone and contribute to a syndrome of inappropriate secretion of antidiuretic hormone.[9] Dysregulated extrarenal production of calcitriol, the active metabolite of vitamin D, appears to underlie the hypercalcemia associated with Hodgkin lymphoma and other lymphomas (see Chaps. 102 and 103).[10]

SYSTEMIC SYMPTOMS

Large-cell lymphoma, poorly differentiated lymphoma, and Hodgkin lymphoma frequently are associated with fever, night sweats, weight loss, and anorexia (see Chaps. 102 and 103). Patients with lymphomas or Hodgkin lymphoma have an increased incidence of localized or disseminated herpes zoster, and 10 percent or more of these patients may be affected sometime during the course of their illness. Pruritus

is common in Hodgkin lymphoma, and its severity parallels disease activity. Systemic symptoms may be present in Hodgkin lymphoma in the absence of obvious, bulky lymph node or splenic tumors, whereas, in well-differentiated small-cell lymphomas, such as chronic lymphocytic leukemia and Waldenström macroglobulinemia, fever, night sweats, and significant weight loss are uncommon, despite generalized lymphadenopathy and splenomegaly. Rather, fever in patients with chronic lymphocytic leukemia or macroglobulinemia usually is secondary to infectious disease.

METABOLIC SIGNS

Lymphocytic malignancies are associated with the most dramatic metabolic disturbances associated with cancers (see Chap. 103). Some lymphomas and lymphocytic leukemias may have an extremely high proliferative rate, a high death fraction of cells, and, therefore, an enormous turnover of nucleoproteins, sometimes causing hyperuricemia and extreme hyperuricosuria. Burkitt lymphoma or acute lymphocytic leukemia is particularly likely to cause an extreme degree of hyperuricemia, sometimes leading to renal failure prior to cytotoxic therapy. Also, because these and other lymphocytic malignancies are sensitive to cytotoxic drugs and glucocorticoids, cytotoxic therapy may cause extreme hyperuricemia, hyperuricosuria, hyperkalemia, and hyperphosphatemia.[11] This has been called the tumor lysis syndrome. Precipitation of uric acid in the renal tubules and collecting system can lead to acute obstructive nephropathy and renal failure unless precautions are taken, such as pre-treatment with allopurinol, hydration, and alkalization of the urine.

Hypercalcemia and calciuria are common complications of multiple myeloma because of osteolysis. Hypercalcemia also may occur during the course of lymphomas (see Chap. 103) or plasma cell myeloma (see Chap. 106). This may be caused by several mechanisms, including tumor- cell- production of IL-1, ectopic parathyroid hormone elaboration, excessive bone resorption, and impaired bone formation.[8]

ORGAN INFILTRATION (EXTRANODAL INVOLVEMENT)

T-cell leukemias and lymphomas, in addition to causing lymph node and spleen enlargement, also may involve the skin, mediastinum, or central nervous system. As the name implies, cutaneous T-cell lymphomas have malignant cells that home to the skin, sometimes producing a severe desquamating erythroderma in Sézary syndrome, small (<2 cm) subcutaneous nodules in primary cutaneous CD30-positive lymphoma, or a variety of nodular infiltrative lesions in mycosis fungoides (see Chap. 103). T-cell acute lymphocytic leukemia and lymphoblastic lymphoma frequently cause mediastinal enlargement (see Chap. 103). These diseases frequently involve the leptomeniges and other structures that are transverse to the subarachnoid space, such as the cranial and peripheral nerves.

B-cell lymphomas frequently may involve the salivary glands, endocrine glands, joints, heart, lung, kidney, bowel, bone, and, less frequently, other extra-nodal sites. These diseases may begin as an extranodal tumor, or the tumor may develop during the course of

the disease. Marginal zone B-cell lymphoma of mucosa-associated lymphoid tissue (MALT) type frequently involves the stomach and salivary glands, although the disease may be encountered in any extranodal site distinguished by the presence of a columnar or cuboidal epithelium.

REFERENCES

1. Harris NL, Jaffe ES, Stein H, et al: A revised European-American classification of lymphoid neoplasms: A proposal from the International Lymphoma Study Group. *Blood* 84:1361, 1994.
2. Segal GH, Kjeldsberg CR: Practical lymphoma diagnosis: An approach to using the information organized in the REAL proposal. Revised European-American Lymphoid Neoplasm. *Anat Pathol* 3:147, 1998.
3. A clinical evaluation of the International Lymphoma Study Group classification of non-Hodgkin's lymphoma: The Non-Hodgkin's Lymphoma Classification Project. *Blood* 89:3909, 1997.
4. Fisher RI, Miller TP, Grogan TM: New REAL clinical entities. *Cancer J Sci Am* 4(suppl) 2:S5, 1998.
5. Kwaan HC, Bongu A: The hyperviscosity syndromes. *Semin Thromb Hemost* 25:199, 1999.
6. Kyle RA: Sequence of testing for monoclonal gammopathies. *Arch Pathol Lab Med* 123:114, 1999.
7. Hirshberg B, Kramer MR, Lotem M, et al: Chronic eosinophilic pneumonia associated with cutaneous T-cell lymphoma. *Am J Hematol* 60:143, 1999.
8. Roodman GD: Mechanisms of bone lesions in multiple myeloma and lymphoma. *Cancer* 80:1557, 1997.
9. Chubachi A, Miura I, Hatano Y, et al: Syndrome of inappropriate secretion of antidiuretic hormone in patients with lymphoma-associated hemophagocytic syndrome. *Ann Hematol* 70:53, 1995.
10. Seymour JF, Gagel RF: Calcitrol: The major humoral mediator of hypercalcemia in Hodgkin's disease and non-Hodgkin's lymphomas. *Blood* 82:1383, 1993.
11. Lorigan PC, Woodings PL, Morgenstern GR, Scarffe JH. Tumour lysis syndrome, case report and review of the literature. *Ann Oncol* 7:631, 1996.

C H A P T E R   9 7

ACUTE LYMPHOBLASTIC LEUKEMIA

CHING-HON PUI

Acute lymphoblastic leukemia (ALL) is a malignant disorder that originates in a single B- or T-lymphocyte progenitor. The proliferation and accumulation of blast cells in the marrow results in suppression of hematopoiesis and, thereafter, anemia, thrombocytopenia, and neutropenia. Extramedullary accumulations of lymphoblasts may occur in various sites, especially the meninges, gonads, thymus, liver, spleen, or lymph nodes. The disease is most common in children but can occur at any age. ALL has many subtypes and can be classified using morphologic, immunologic, cytogenetic, and molecular genetic methods. These approaches can identify biologic subtypes that require different treatment approaches. These differences include the specific drug combination, drug dosages, and duration of treatment required to achieve optimal results. For example, childhood ALL with a hyperdiploid karyotype responds well to extended treatment with methotrexate and 6-mercaptopurine, while cases with adverse genetic changes, such as _MLL-AF4_ fusion, require intensive treatment with genotoxic agents. The relative lack of therapeutic success in adult ALL corresponds to a high frequency of cases with unfavorable genetic lesions, such as the _BCR-ABL_ oncogene resulting from the rearrangement of chromosomes 9 and 22. This poor outlook in adults is improving, however, as a result of better drug combinations and the use of allogeneic stem cell transplantation. Currently, 80 percent of children and 35 percent of adults can expect long-term leukemia-free survival, and probable cure, following intensive therapy on contemporary protocols. As cure rates increase, new approaches are required to prevent second malignancies, cardiotoxicity, growth stunting, and other severe side effects that may accompany long-term survivors.

DEFINITION AND HISTORY

Acute lymphoblastic leukemia is a neoplastic disease that results from somatic mutation in a single lymphoid progenitor cell at one of several discrete stages of development. The immunophenotype of the leukemic cells at diagnosis reflects the level of differentiation achieved by the dominant clone. The clonal origin of ALL has been established by cytogenetic analysis and analysis of restriction fragments in females who are heterozygotes for polymorphic X chromosome-linked genes (Chap. 8). These female patients have both alleles expressed in normal

tissue cells but only a single active parental allele is expressed in leukemic lymphoblasts. Also, analysis of T-cell receptor gene or immunoglobulin gene rearrangements has documented the monoclonal nature of the disease.[1] The leukemic cells divide more slowly and take a longer time to synthesize DNA than do their normal hematopoietic counterparts,[2] but they accumulate relentlessly, competing successfully with normal hematopoietic cells and resulting in anemia, thrombocytopenia, and neutropenia. At diagnosis, the leukemic cells not only have replaced normal marrow cells but have disseminated to various extramedullary sites. Studies suggest that the activation of telomerase in leukemic cells contribute their growth advantage and to disease progression.[3,4]

The earliest report of leukemia is generally credited to Velpeau, writing in 1827,[5] although it was not until 1845 that Virchow,[6] Bennett,[7] and Craigie,[8] in separate reports, recognized this condition as a distinct entity. In 1847, Virchow coined the term _leukemia_, applying it to two distinct types of the disease, splenic and lymphatic, that could be distinguished from each other on the basis of splenomegaly and enlarged lymph nodes, as well as the morphologic similarities of the leukemic cells to those normally residing in the spleen and lymph glands.[9] Ehrlich's introduction of staining methods in 1891 allowed further distinction of leukemia subtypes.[10] Splenic and myelogenous leukemias were soon recognized as the same disease. By 1913, leukemia could be classified as acute or chronic, and as lymphatic or myelogenous.[11] The increased prevalence of acute leukemia in children, especially those between 1 and 5 years, was recognized in 1917.[12]

Shortly after the recognition of leukemia as a discrete disease entity, physicians began to use chemicals as palliative therapy for this disorder. The first advance came with the use of a 4-amino antimetabolite of folic acid (aminopterin), prompted by Farber's observation that folic acid might have accelerated the proliferation of leukemic cells. The results were striking! For the first time, children achieved complete clinical and hematologic remissions that lasted for several months.[13] A year after the report of aminopterin-induced clinical remissions, a 1949 conference revealed that a newly isolated adrenocorticotrophic hormone (ACTH) also could induce prompt though brief remissions in patients with leukemia.[14] Almost concurrently, Hitchings and Elion[15] synthesized antimetabolites that interfere with purine and pyrimidine synthesis, leading to the introduction of 6-mercaptopurine, 6-thioguanine, and allopurinol into clinical use. The decade from 1950 to 1960 witnessed the introduction of many new antileukemic agents and occasional cures. A "total therapy" approached devised by Pinkel at St. Jude Children's Research Hospital in 1962 consisted of four treatment phases: remission induction, intensification or consolidation, therapy for subclinical central nervous system leukemia (or preventive meningeal treatment), and prolonged continuation therapy. By the early 1970s, it was clear that as many as 50 percent of children could be cured with this innovative strategy.[16,17] During the same period, a better understanding of the genetics of human histocompatibility and wider use of HLA typing culminated in the successful use of bone marrow transplantation to treat children with relapsed leukemia.[18] It was eventually recognized that ALL is a broad term encompassing a heterogeneous group of diseases—clinically, immunologically, and genetically[19,20]—setting the stage for risk-directed therapy.

Progress in the treatment of ALL has been incremental, beginning with the development of effective therapy for central nervous system disease, followed by intensification of early treatment, especially for patients at high risk of relapse. The current cure rates of nearly 80 percent in children (Fig. 97-1) and 30 to 40 percent in adults attest to the steady progress that has been made in treating this disease.[21] The development of genetic probes to the genotype as well as the phenotype of leukemic lymphoblasts has improved the selection of therapy and the estimation of individual disease.

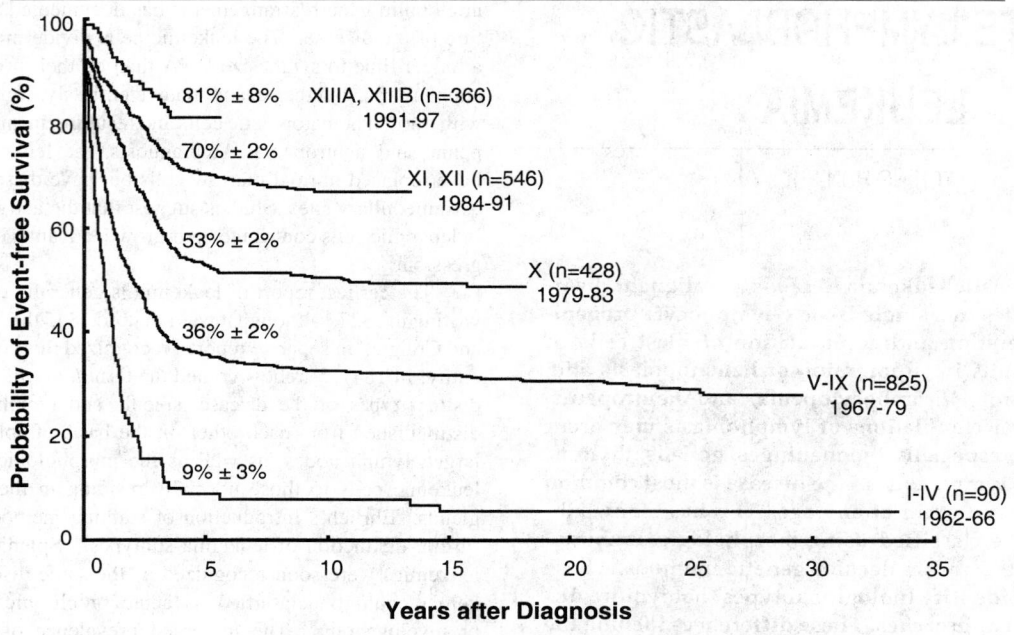

FIGURE 97-1 Kaplan-Meier analysis of event-free survival in 2255 children with ALL treated in 13 consecutive Total Therapy studies at St. Jude Children's Research Hospital. Early intensification of systemic as well as intrathecal chemotherapy in the 1990s has boosted the event-free survival estimate to 81 plus or minus 8 (SE) %. (From Pui and Evans.[21])

ETIOLOGY AND PATHOGENESIS

The initiation and progression of ALL is driven by successive mutations that differ according to the developmental stages of the affected blast cells. Thus, specific subtypes of ALL appear to have genetically distinct origins linked to different causative mechanisms. Environmental agents, such as ionizing radiation and chemical mutagens, have been implicated in the induction of ALL in some patients. However, the vast majority of cases lack discernible etiologic factors. The favored concept is that leukemogenesis reflects the interaction between multiple genetic and environmental factors, a model that needs to be confirmed in well-designed population and molecular epidemiologic studies.

INCIDENCE

ALL represents about 12 percent of all leukemias diagnosed in the United States, and 60 percent of all cases occur in persons younger than 20 years.[22] ALL is the most common malignancy diagnosed in patients under the age of 15 years, accounting for one-fourth of all cancers and 76 percent of all leukemias in this age group.[23] Age-specific incidence patterns are characterized by a peak between the ages of 2 and 5 years, followed by falling rates during later childhood, adolescence, and young adulthood (Fig. 97-2).[22] The incidence rates rise again, beginning in the sixth decade and reaching a second, smaller peak in the elderly. The sharp incidence peak of ALL during childhood has only been observed since the 1930s in the United Kingdom and the United States.[24] In the United States, the peak first appeared in children of European descent and was subsequently observed in children of African descent in the 1960s. The age peak is absent in many developing or underdeveloped countries, suggesting a leukemogenic contribution from factors associated with industrialization. With the exception of a slight female predominance in infancy,[25] males of European descent are affected by ALL more often than females in all

age groups; a similar frequency distribution has been noted among those of African descent.[22] In most age groups, the incidence of ALL is higher in those of European descent than in those of African descent, especially among children from 2 to 5 years of age.

There are substantial geographic differences in the incidence of ALL. Higher rates are evident among populations in Northern and Western Europe, North America, and Oceania, with lower rates apparent in Asian and African populations.[26] In Europe, the highest rates of ALL among males are found in Spain and the highest rates among females in Denmark. In the United States, the highest rates for both genders are among Latinos in Los Angeles. A survey by the Surveillance, Epidemiology, and End Results Program indicated that during the period 1973 to 1995, the age-adjusted incidence of childhood ALL in the United States increased from 2.7 to 3.3 cases per 100,000 children aged 0 to 14 years.[22] However, changes in diagnostic specificity from the mid-1970s to later eras, resulting in the recognition of not-otherwise-specified forms of lymphoid leukemia as ALL, could account for this apparent increase in incidence.[27] Indeed, a recent survey showed a plateau of the incidence curve.[22]

RISK FACTORS

Despite the paucity of knowledge of factors that increase the risk of ALL, a minority (5 percent) of cases are associated with inherited, predisposing genetic syndromes, often involving genes whose encoded proteins affect genomic stability and DNA repair.[28] A variety of normal inherited genetic polymorphisms may also contribute indirectly to the risk of leukemia, for example, those involving enzymes important in carcinogen metabolism and detoxification and those affecting the regulation of immune responses.[29]

GENETIC SYNDROMES

Children with Down syndrome have a 10- to 30-fold increased risk of leukemia. Acute megakaryoblastic leukemia predominates in patients

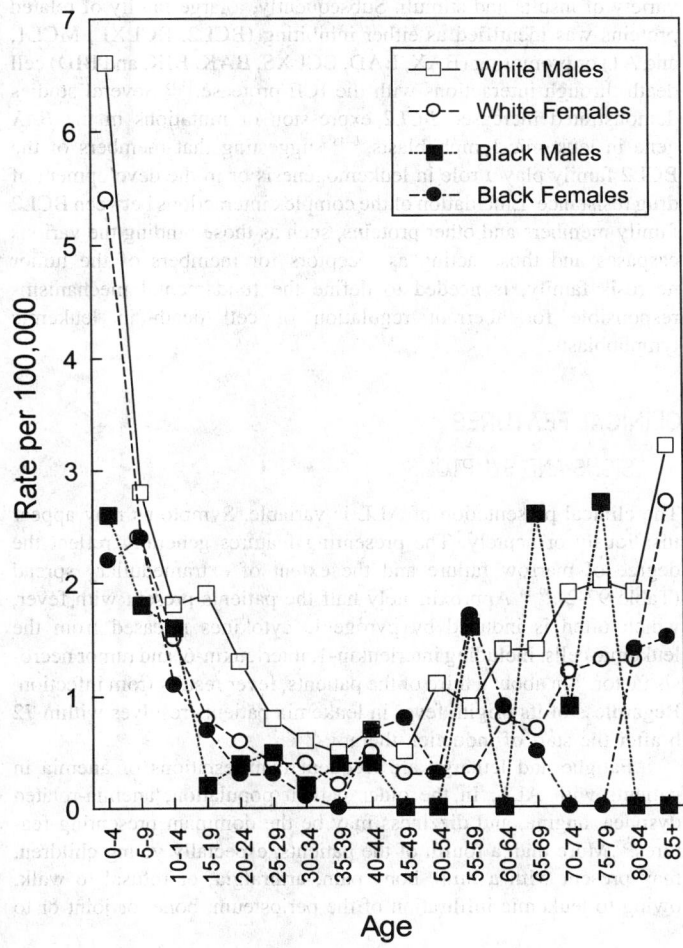

FIGURE 97-2   Age-specific incidence rates for ALL by race and sex. (From SEER data, 1991 to 1995.[22])

FAMILIAL LEUKEMIA

Reports of two or more leukemia cases in the same family are rare, reinforcing the notion that heredity plays only a minor role in the causation of this disease. Even so, fraternal twins and siblings of affected children have a twofold to fourfold greater risk of developing leukemia than do unrelated children during the first decade of life. When leukemia occurs in one identical twin, the other twin has a 20 percent chance of developing the disease. If leukemia develops in the index twin before the age of 1 year, the other twin almost invariably will develop leukemia, typically within a few months. Molecular studies have demonstrated that intrauterine metastasis from one twin to the other via their shared placental circulation is responsible for the concordant leukemia.[33,34] The same route of transmission appears to operate in older twins, emphasizing the long latent period of ALL in some patients.[35] This finding also supports speculation that many cases of ALL arise in utero, with the most aggressive forms presenting in infants and the remainder appearing in later childhood.[27]

ENVIRONMENTAL FACTORS

In utero (but not postnatal) exposure to diagnostic X-rays confers a slightly increased risk for the development of ALL, which correlates positively with the number of exposures.[36] The evidence for an association between the development of ALL and nuclear fallout; occupational, natural terrestrial, or cosmic ionizing radiation exposure; or paternal preconception radiation exposure is weak.[28] Nonionizing radiation in the form of low-energy electromagnetic fields produced by residential power supply and appliances is not a factor in the development of childhood ALL according to a recent comprehensive study.[37] Pesticide exposure (occupational or home use) and parental cigarette smoking before or during pregnancy have been suggested as causes of childhood ALL. Other proposed causes of childhood ALL include neonatal administration of vitamin K, maternal alcohol consumption during pregnancy, and increased consumption of dietary nitrites. However, each of these associations is controversial, and most have been refuted after careful, controlled investigation. An increased incidence of ALL has also been reported among women whose drinking water was contaminated with trichloroethylene and among smokers older than 60 years.[24] Both of these findings require confirmation.

HYPOTHESES

Despite numerous provocative clues, the instigating factors in most cases of ALL remain a mystery. Some researchers now believe that many childhood cases, especially those diagnosed between 2 and 5 years of age, result from rare abnormal responses to common infections occurring at a later time than was typical in the past.[28,38] Such "delayed" exposures at a time when there is increased lymphoid cell proliferation would be expected to increase the chance of unfavorable genetic mutations and hence the development of leukemia. This theory is supported by the higher frequency of childhood ALL in industrialized as opposed to developing countries and in locations where large numbers of infected and uninfected persons come into contact with each other (e.g., new towns). Two large-scale epidemiologic studies now under way in the United States and the United Kingdom are designed to test this theory.

ACQUIRED GENETIC CHANGES

The lymphoblasts from virtually all cases of ALL have acquired genetic changes, at least two-thirds of which are nonrandom and, in all likelihood, contribute in major ways to the generation and expansion of leukemic clones.[39] Such lesions include changes in both the number (ploidy) and structure of chromosomes. The latter comprise translocations (the most frequent abnormality), inversions, deletions, point mu-

younger than 3 years and ALL in older age groups. Down syndrome cases are more likely to have B-cell precursor ALL, and their leukemic cells lack adverse genetic abnormalities.[30] Autosomal recessive genetic diseases associated with increased chromosomal fragility and a predisposition to ALL include ataxia-telangiectasia, Nijmegen breakage syndrome, and Bloom syndrome.[31] The lymphocytes and leukemic cells of patients with ataxia-telangiectasia frequently have chromosomal rearrangements involving bands 7p13-p14, 7q32-q35, and 14q11 (sites of the T-cell receptor gamma, beta, and alpha/delta genes respectively), as well as band 14q32 (site of the immunoglobulin heavy-chain gene). The mutation of ataxia-telangiectasia patients may allow a large increase in production of translocations at the time of V(D)J recombination, leading to an increased predisposition to ALL.[31] Patients with other constitutional or acquired immunodeficiency diseases, such as congenital X-linked agammaglobulinemia, immunoglobulin A deficiency, and variable immunodeficiency, are also at increased risk for this disease.[32] Although impaired immune surveillance contributes to the increased risk of Epstein-Barr-virus-related malignancies in patients with acquired immunodeficiencies, there is no compelling evidence that defective immunity contributes to the predisposition to ALL in patients with ataxia-telangiectasia or other congenital immunodeficiency syndromes.

tations, and amplifications (see Chap. 10). These rearrangements affect gene expression in ways that subvert normal programs of cell differentiation, proliferation, and survival, and these factors likely act in concert with each other in multistep pathways leading to leukemic transformation.

There are two general mechanisms of leukemia induction. One depends on the activation of a proto-oncogene or the creation of a fusion gene with oncogenic properties. In both cases, genes that encode transcription factors are the most frequent mutational targets, reflecting the pivotal roles of these regulatory proteins in cell function.[39] Transcription factors are usually classified by their shared structural motifs, denoting participation in similar regulatory processes (Table 97-1).

The second mechanism involves the loss or inactivation of one or more tumor suppressor genes (e.g., *p53* and *INK4a,* encoding p16 and p19^{ARF}). Wild-type p53 function can be inhibited by overexpression of the MDM-2 oncoprotein, a protein capable of complexing with p53.[40] These tumor suppressors act at specific points in the cell cycle: p53 expression is increased by DNA damage, blocks cell division at G1 in the cell cycle to allow DNA repair, and is capable of stimulating apoptosis of cells that have irreparable DNA damage[41]; p16 and p19^{ARF} negatively regulate the cell cycle by inhibiting cyclin-dependent kinase phosphorylation of retinoblastoma protein, decreasing the proportion of cells entering S-phase.[42] Hence, the loss of tumor suppressor function either endows the leukemic cell with a proliferative advantage or prevents its normal programmed cell death. While *p53* mutation occurs rarely in ALL, homozygous deletions of p15 and *p16* have been detected in 20 percent to 30 percent of B-cell precursor ALL and 60 percent to 80 percent of T-cell ALL. Studies have shown that homozygous p15/p16 deletions are frequently acquired at relapse, suggesting that loss of function of the proteins encoded by these genes plays an important role in disease progression.[43]

The first mammalian antiapoptotic gene identified was *BCL2,* whose overexpression can render cells relatively resistant to a wide variety of insults and stimuli. Subsequently, a large family of related proteins was identified as either inhibiting (BCL2, BCLXL, MCL1, and A1) or promoting (BAX, BAD, BCLXS, BAK, BIK, and BID) cell death through interactions with the ICE protease.[44,45] Several studies demonstrated increased *BCL2* expression or mutations in the *BAX* gene in leukemic lymphoblasts,[46–48] suggesting that members of the BCL2 family play a role in leukemogenesis or in the development of drug resistance. Elucidation of the complex interactions between BCL2 family members and other proteins, such as those binding the various caspases and those acting as receptors for members of the tumor necrosis family, is needed to define the fundamental mechanisms responsible for aberrant regulation of cell death in leukemic lymphoblasts.

CLINICAL FEATURES

SIGNS AND SYMPTOMS

The clinical presentation of ALL is variable. Symptoms may appear insidiously or acutely. The presenting features generally reflect the degree of marrow failure and the extent of extramedullary spread (Table 97-2).[49–54] Approximately half the patients present with fever, which often is induced by pyrogenic cytokines released from the leukemic cells, including interleukin-1, interleukin-6, and tumor necrosis factor.[55] In about a third of the patients, fever results from infection. Regardless of its origin, fever in leukemia patients resolves within 72 h after the start of induction therapy.[49]

Fatigue and lethargy are frequent manifestations of anemia in patients with ALL. In the older patient population, anemia-related dyspnea, angina, and dizziness may be the dominant presenting features.[53] More than a fourth of the patients, especially young children, may present with a limp, bone pain, arthralgia, or refusal to walk, owing to leukemic infiltration of the periosteum, bone, or joint or to

TABLE 97-1 GENES AFFECTED BY CHROMOSOMAL TRANSLOCATIONS

PROTEIN FAMILY	FUNCTION OF PROTEIN PRODUCT	TRANSLOCATION	INVOLVED GENES	PHENOTYPE	FREQUENCY, % CHILDREN	FREQUENCY, % ADULTS
Basic helix-loop-helix (bHLH proteins)	Transcription factor	t(8;14)(q24.1;q32)	MYC/IGH	B-cell	2–3	3–4
		t(2;8)(p12;q24.1)	IGK/MYC	B-cell	<1	<1
		t(8;22)(q24.1;q11)	MYC/IGL	B-cell	<1	<1
		t(8;14)(q24.1;q11.2)	MYC/TCRA	T-cell	<1	<1
		t(7;19)(q35;p13)	TCRB/LYL1	T-cell	<1	<1
		t(1;7)(p32;q35)	TAL1/TCRB	T-cell	<1	<1
		t(1;14)(p32;q11.2)	TAL1/TCRD	T-cell	0.5	~20
		t(7;9)(q35;q32)	TCRB/TAL2	T-cell	<1	<1
Cysteine-rich (LIM) proteins	Transcription factor	t(11;14)(p15;q11.2)	RHOM1/TCRD	T-cell	<1	<1
		t(11;14)(p13;q11.2)	RHOM2/TCRD	T-cell	1	5–7
		t(7;11)(q35;p13)	TCRB/RHOM2	T-cell	<1	<1
Homeodomain (HOX) proteins	Transcription factor	t(10;14)(q24;q11.2)	HOX11/TCRD	T-cell	<1	3–7
		t(7;10)(q35;q24)	TCRB/HOX11	T-cell	<1	<1
		t(1;19)(q23;p13.3)	E2A-PBX1	Pre-B	5–6	3
Basic region/leucine-zipper (bZIP) proteins	Transcription factor	t(17;19)(q22;p13.3)	E2A-HLF	Early pre-B	<1	<1
Trithorax homology	Probably involved in transcription regulation	t(4;11)(q21;q23)	MLL-AF4	Early pre-B	2	3–5
		t(11;19)(q23;p13.3)	MLL-ENL	Early pre-B	1	<1
ETS-like (*TEL*)	Transcription factor	t(12;21)(p13;q22)	TEL-AML1	Early pre-B	20–25	<1
Runt homology (*AML1*)	Transcription factor	t(12;21)(p13;q22)	TEL-AML1	Early pre-B	20–25	<1
Tyrosine kinase	Signal transduction	t(9;22)(q34;q11.2)	BCR-ABL	Early pre-B	3–4	20–30
		t(1;7)(p34;q35)	LCK/TCRB	T-cell	<1	<1
Growth factor	Cytokine	t(5;14)(q31;q32)	IL3/IGH	Early pre-B	<1	<1
Notch receptor	Signal transduction	t(7;9)(q34;q34)	TCRB/TAN1	T-cell	<1	<1

TABLE 97-2   PRESENTING CLINICAL FEATURES IN CHILDREN AND ADULTS

	PERCENT OF TOTAL	
FEATURE	CHILDREN	ADULTS
Age (yr)		
<1	3	—
1–9	77	—
10–19	20	—
20–39	—	55
40–59	—	36
≥60	—	9
Male	55	62
Symptoms		
Fever	57	33–56
Fatigue	50	?
Bleeding	43	33
Bone or joint pain	25	25
Lymphadenopathy		
None	30	51
Marked (>3 cm)	15	11
Hepatomegaly		
None	34	65
Marked (below umbilicus)	17	?
Splenomegaly		
None	41	56
Marked (below umbilicus)	17	?
Mediastinal mass	8	15
Central nervous system leukemia	3	8
Testicular leukemia	1	0.3

SOURCE: Data presented in Pui and Crist,[49] McKenna and Baehner,[50] Reiter et al.,[51] and Chessells et al.,[52] for childhood ALL; and in Chessells et al.,[52] Hoelzer,[53] and Larson et al.,[54] for adult ALL.

expansion of the marrow cavity by leukemic cells. Children with prominent bone pain frequently have nearly normal blood counts, which can contribute to a delay in diagnosis.[56] In a small proportion of patients, marrow necrosis can result in severe bone pain and tenderness, fever, and a very high serum lactate dehydrogenase level.[57] Arthralgia and bone pain are less severe in adult patients. Less common signs and symptoms include headache, vomiting, alteration of mental function, oliguria, and anuria. Occasional patients present with a life-threatening infection or bleeding (e.g., intracranial hematoma). Very rarely, ALL does not produce any signs or symptoms and is detected during routine examination.

PHYSICAL FINDINGS

Pallor, petechiae, and ecchymosis in the skin and mucous membranes and bone tenderness due to leukemic infiltration or hemorrhage that stretches the periosteum frequently are evident. Liver, spleen, and lymph nodes are the most common sites of extramedullary involvement, and the degree of organomegaly is more pronounced in children than in adults. An anterior mediastinal (thymic) mass is present in 7 to 10 percent of childhood cases and 15 percent of adult cases (Fig. 97-3). A bulky anterior mediastinal mass can compress the great vessels and trachea and possibly lead to the superior vena cava syndrome or the superior mediastinal syndrome.[58] Patients with this syndrome present with cough, dyspnea, orthopnea, dysphagia, stridor, cyanosis, facial edema, increased intracranial pressure, and sometimes syncope. Such patients tolerate anesthesia poorly.

Painless enlargement of the scrotum can be a sign of a testicular leukemia or hydrocele, the latter resulting from lymphatic obstruction. Both conditions can be readily diagnosed by ultrasonography. Overt testicular disease is relatively rare and generally occurs in infants or patients with T-cell leukemia with hyperleukocytosis.[59] Other uncom-

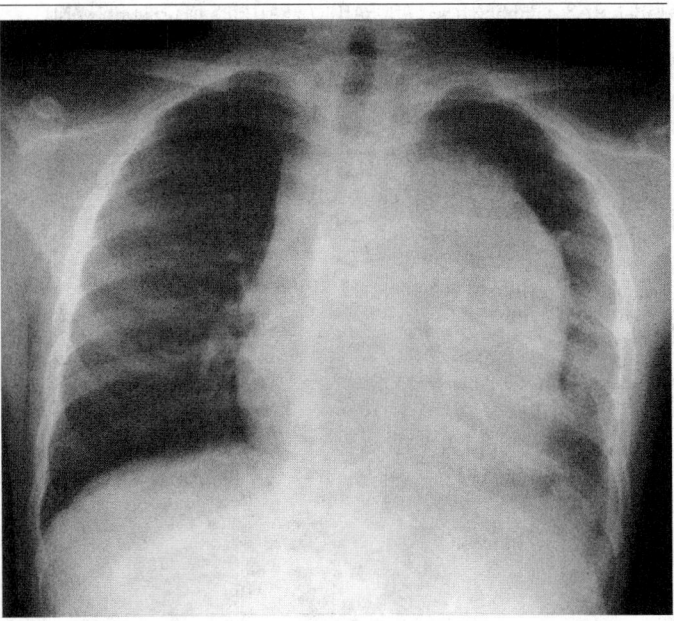

FIGURE 97-3   Chest x-ray of a 12-year-old black boy with T-cell ALL and an anterior mediastinal mass.

mon presenting features include ocular involvement (leukemic infiltration of the orbit, optic nerve, retina, iris, cornea, or conjunctiva), subcutaneous nodules (leukemia cutis), enlarged salivary glands (Mikulicz's syndrome), cranial nerve palsy, and priapism (due to leukostasis of the corpora cavernosa and dorsal veins or sacral nerve involvement). Epidural spinal cord compression is a rare but serious presenting finding that requires immediate treatment to prevent permanent paraparesis or paraplegia. In some pediatric patients, infiltration of tonsils, adenoids, appendix, or mesenteric lymph nodes leads to surgical intervention before leukemia is diagnosed.

LABORATORY FEATURES

Anemia, neutropenia, and thrombocytopenia are common findings in patients with newly diagnosed ALL, and their severity reflects the degree of marrow replacement by leukemic lymphoblasts (Table 97-3).[49–54] Presenting leukocyte counts range widely, from 0.1 to 1500×10^9/liter (median, 10 to 12×10^9/liter), with hyperleukocytosis ($>100 \times 10^9$/liter) occurring in 10 percent to 16 percent of patients. Profound neutropenia ($<0.5 \times 10^9$/liter) is found in 20 percent to 40 percent of patients, rendering them at high risk for infection. Most patients have circulating leukemic blast cells. Hypereosinophilia, generally reactive, may precede the diagnosis of ALL by several months.[60] Some patients, principally males, have ALL with the t(5;14)(q31;q32) chromosomal abnormality and a hypereosinophilia syndrome (pulmonary infiltration, cardiomegaly, and congestive heart failure). Activation of the interleukin-3 gene on chromosome 5 by the enhancer element of the immunoglobulin heavy-chain gene on chromosome 14 is thought to play a central role in leukemogenesis and the associated eosinophilia in these cases.[61] In patients with anemia, there is a strong inverse relationship between the hemoglobin level and age at diagnosis.[52] Occasionally, a child can present with a hemoglobin level as low as 1 g/dl.

Decreased platelet counts often are present at diagnosis (median, $48–52 \times 10^9$/liter). This finding differs from immune thrombocytopenia, since it is almost always accompanied by anemia and or leuko-

TABLE 97-3   PRESENTING LABORATORY FEATURES IN CHILDREN AND ADULTS

FEATURE	PERCENT OF TOTAL	
	CHILDREN	ADULTS
Leukocyte count ($\times 10^9$/liter)		
<10	50	41
10–49	31	31
50–99	9	12
>100	10	16
Hemoglobin (g/dl)		
<8	52	28
8–10	28	26
>10	20	46
Platelet count ($\times 10^9$/liter)		
<50	48	52
50–100	20	22
>100	32	26
Leukemic blasts in bone marrow, %		
<90	19	29
>90	81	71
Leukemic blasts in blood		
Present	84	92
Absent	16	8

SOURCE: Data presented in Pui and Crist,[49] McKenna and Baehner,[50] Reiter et al.,[51] and Chessells et al.,[52] for childhood ALL; and in Chessells et al.,[52] Hoelzer,[53] and Larson et al.,[54] for adult ALL.

cyte abnormalities.[62] Severe bleeding is uncommon, even when platelet counts are as low as 20×10^9/liter, provided that infection and fever are absent.[63] Occasionally patients, principally males, present with thrombocytosis (>400×10^9/liter).[64] Pancytopenia followed by a period of spontaneous hematopoietic recovery may precede the diagnosis of ALL in rare cases (see Chap. 92).[65] Coagulopathy, usually mild, can occur in 3 percent to 5 percent of patients, most of whom have T-cell ALL, and is only rarely associated with clinical bleeding.[53,66] The serum lactate dehydrogenase level is elevated in most patients with ALL and correlates well with the size of the leukemic infiltrate and prognosis.[67] Increased serum uric acid levels are common in patients with a large leukemic cell burden, reflecting an increased rate of purine catabolism. Patients with massive renal involvement can have increased levels of creatinine, urea nitrogen, uric acid, and phosphorus. Occasionally, patients with T-cell ALL present with acute renal failure, despite a relatively small leukemic infiltrate.[68] Rarely, patients present with hypercalcemia due to the release of parathyroid hormonelike protein from lymphoblasts and leukemic infiltration of bone.[69] Liver dysfunction due to leukemic infiltration occurs in 10 percent to 20 percent of patients, is usually mild, and has no important clinical or prognostic consequences.[49] Serum immunoglobulin levels (mostly IgA and IgM classes) are modestly decreased in approximately a third of children with ALL, reflecting the decreased number and impaired function of normal lymphocytes.[70] Urinalysis may disclose microscopic hematuria and the presence of uric acid crystals.

A chest radiograph is needed to detect enlargement of the thymus or mediastinal nodes, with or without pleural effusion (Fig. 97-3). Although bony abnormalities, such as metaphyseal banding, periosteal reactions, osteolysis, osteosclerosis, or osteopenia, can be found in half of the patients, especially children with low presenting leukocyte counts,[71] skeletal roentgenograms are not necessary for patient management. Spinal roentgenography is useful in patients suspected of having vertebral collapse.

Examination of the cerebrospinal fluid (CSF) is an essential diagnostic procedure. Leukemic blasts can be identified in as many as a third of childhood ALL patients at diagnosis, the majority of whom will lack neurologic symptoms.[72] Traditionally, central nervous system

(CNS) leukemia is defined by the presence of at least five leukocytes per microliter of CSF (with leukemic blast cells apparent in a cytocentrifuged sample) or by the presence of cranial nerve palsies. There are conflicting conclusions regarding the clinical importance of blast cells in diagnostic CSF samples containing fewer than five leukocytes per microliter.[73–76] Some studies have shown that the presence of any leukemic blast cells in the CSF is an indication to intensify CNS-directed therapy to prevent subsequent CNS relapse.[73,74] There are also different opinions on when the first lumbar puncture should be performed. Many leukemia therapists perform the procedure at diagnosis but do not instill intrathecal chemotherapy in the event a second diagnostic test is needed to verify the presence of leukemic cells. Others delay the examination because of concern that circulating leukemic cells from the peripheral blood will "seed" the CNS. A recent study has shown that contamination of the CSF by leukemic cells, due to a traumatic lumbar puncture at diagnosis, was associated with an inferior treatment outcome.[77] However, this potential hazard must be weighed against the benefit associated with early intensification of intrathecal therapy.[72] Thus, we perform lumbar puncture at diagnosis in all of our patients under deep sedation or general anesthesia and administer intrathecal therapy immediately after a CSF sample is obtained for examination.

DIAGNOSIS AND CELL CLASSIFICATION

Careful examination of marrow cells is essential to establishing the diagnosis of ALL because as many as 16 percent of patients lack blasts in the blood film at the time of diagnosis. Also, the morphology of leukemic cells in blood may differ from that in marrow. Fibrosis or tightly packed marrow can lead to difficulties with marrow aspiration, necessitating biopsy. A touch preparation of the biopsied tissue can be used for cytological diagnosis. Multiple marrow aspirations are sometimes needed to obtain diagnostic tissue from patients with marrow necrosis.

MORPHOLOGIC AND CYTOCHEMICAL ANALYSIS

The diagnosis of ALL begins with morphologic analysis of Romanowsky-stained (Wright-Giemsa or May-Grünwald-Giemsa) bone marrow smears. Lymphoblasts tend to be relatively small (ranging from the same size to twice the size of small lymphocytes) with scanty, often light-blue cytoplasm; a round, clefted or slightly indented nucleus; fine to slightly coarse and clumped chromatin; and inconspicuous nucleoli (Fig. 97-4). In some cases, the lymphoblasts are large with

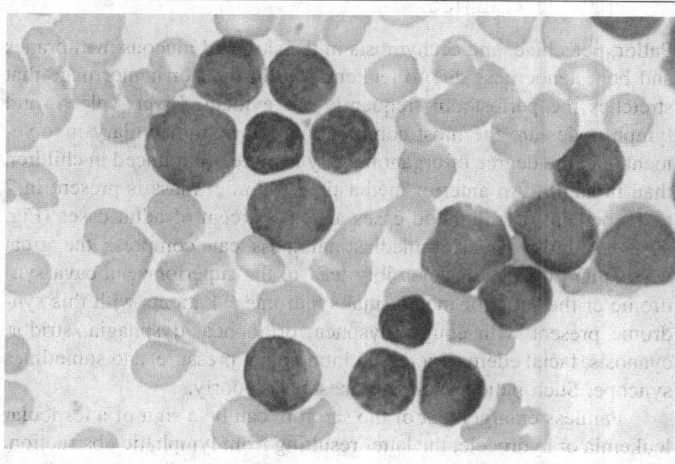

FIGURE 97-4   Typical lymphoblasts with scanty cytoplasm, regular nuclear shape, fine chromatin, and indistinct nucleoli (Wright-Giemsa, ×1000).

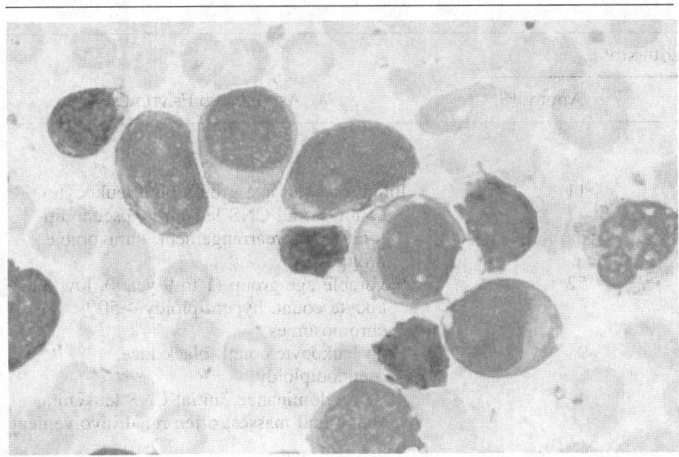

FIGURE 97-5   ALL with large blasts showing prominent nucleoli and moderate amounts of cytoplasm, with an admixture of smaller blasts (Wright-Giemsa, ×1000).

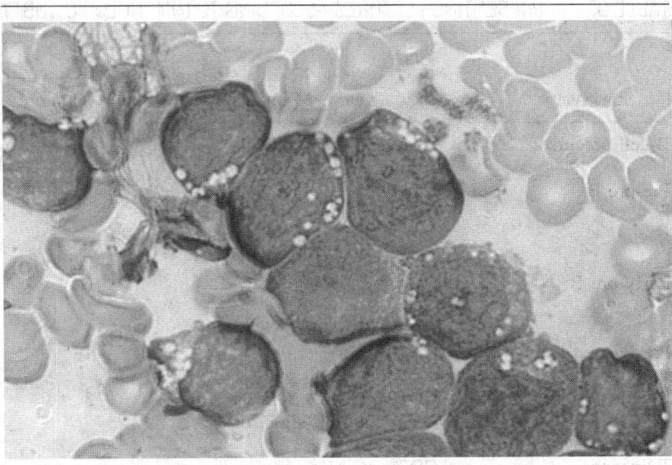

FIGURE 97-7   B-lineage lymphoblasts. The blasts are characterized by intensely basophilic cytoplasm, regular cellular features, and cytoplasmic vacuolation (Wright-Giemsa, ×1000).

prominent nucleoli and moderate amounts of cytoplasms, with an admixture of smaller blasts (Fig. 97-5). Cytoplasmic granules are found in the lymphoblasts of some cases of ALL (Fig. 97-6); such granules are usually amphophilic (fuchsia) and readily distinguishable from the primary myeloid granules (deep purple). B-cell ALL blasts are characterized by intensely basophilic cytoplasm, regular cellular features, prominent nucleoli, and cytoplasmic vacuolation (Fig. 97-7).

Analysis of only a Romanowsky-stained smear is not sufficient for a certain distinction between ALL and AML. The cytochemical stains needed to discriminate between the two leukemias are myeloperoxidase, Sudan black, and nonspecific esterases, including alpha naphthyl butyrate and alpha naphthyl acetate esterase. These stains do not react with leukemic lymphoblasts. By contrast, staining with periodic acid–Schiff reagent is positive in over 70 percent of ALL cases, while acid phosphatase reactivity can be demonstrated in about 70 percent of cases with a T-cell immunophenotype. However, neither stain reacts exclusively with leukemic lymphoid cells.

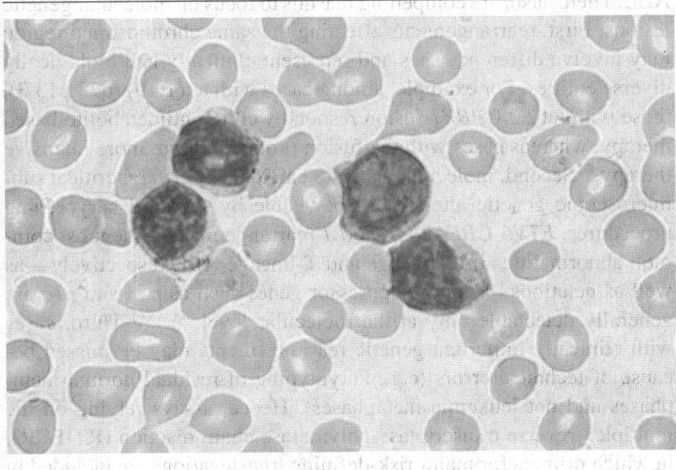

FIGURE 97-6   ALL with cytoplasmic granules. Fuchsia-colored granules are present in the cytoplasm of many blasts. Such granules may lead to a misdiagnosis of acute myeloid leukemia; however, the granules are negative for myeloperoxidase and myeloid-pattern Sudan black B (Wright-Giemsa, ×1000).

IMMUNOLOGIC CLASSIFICATION

Because leukemic lymphoblasts lack specific morphologic and cytochemical features, immunophenotyping is an essential part of the diagnostic evaluation. The antibodies that distinguished clusters of differentiation (CD) groups recognize the same cellular antigen but not necessarily the same epitope. Most leukocyte antigens lack specificity; hence, a panel of antibodies is needed to establish the diagnosis and to distinguish among the different immunologic subclasses of leukemic cells. The panel used at St. Jude Children's Research Hospital includes at least one highly sensitive marker (CD19 for B-lineage cells, CD7 for T-lineage cells, and CD13 or CD33 for myeloid cells) and one marker that is highly specific (cytoplasmic CD79a for B-lineage cells, cytoplasmic CD3 for T-lineage cells, and cytoplasmic myeloperoxidase for myeloid cells).[21] By using this method of analysis, one can make a firm diagnosis in 99 percent of cases.

Although cases can be further subclassified according to the recognized steps of normal maturation within the B-lineage (early pre-B, pre-B, transitional pre-B, and mature B) and T-lineage (early, mid-, and late thymocyte) pathways,[78,79] the only distinctions of therapeutic importance are those between T-cell, mature B, and other B-lineage (B-cell precursor) immunophenotypes.[21] Pre-B ALL (with the presence of cytoplasmic immunoglobulin), which occurs in 20 percent of childhood and 10 percent of adult cases, was once considered to be a specific phenotypic subgroup. However, the high-risk features formerly ascribed to this subgroup were found to be more closely associated with the presence of the t(1;19) and the *E2A-PBX1* fusion gene (discussed later).[80] Transitional pre-B ALL is characterized by the expression of cytoplasmic and surface immunoglobulin mu heavy chains without kappa or lambda light chains. Transitional pre-B ALL is found in approximately 3 percent of childhood ALL cases and is associated with a low presenting leukocyte count, hyperdiploidy, and a favorable prognosis,[78] but this ALL phenotype has not been studied in the adult population. In some studies, cases of B-cell-precursor ALL are subdivided into CD10-postive (so-called common ALL) and CD10-negative (pre-pre-B or CD10-negative B-cell-precursor) leukemias, while cases of T-lineage ALL are further classified as pre-T (or pro-T) and mature T-cell leukemias.[79–82] Despite their prognostic implications, these refined categories of ALL have not been used in treatment assignments. Table 97-4 summarizes the salient presenting features of six recognized immunologic subtypes of ALL.

TABLE 97-4 PRESENTING FEATURES ACCORDING TO IMMUNOLOGIC SUBTYPE

| SUBTYPE | TYPICAL MARKERS | FREQUENCY | | ASSOCIATED FEATURES |
		CHILDHOOD, %	ADULT, %	
B-cell precursor	CD19$^+$, CD22$^+$, CD79a$^+$, cIg$^\pm$, sIgμ^-, HLA-DR$^+$			
Pre-pre-B	CD10$^-$	5	11	Infant or adult age group, high leukocyte count, initial CNS leukemia, pseudodiploidy, *MLL* rearrangement, unfavorable prognosis
Early pre-B	CD10$^+$	63	52	Favorable age group (1 to 9 years), low leukocyte count, hyperdiploidy >50 chromosomes
Pre-B	CD10$^\pm$, cIg$^+$	16	9	High leukocyte count, black race, pseudodiploidy
B-cell	CD19$^+$, CD22$^+$, CD79a$^+$, cIg$^+$, sIgμ^+, sIgκ^+ or sIgλ^+	3	4	Male predominance, initial CNS leukemia, abdominal masses, often renal involvement
T-lineage	CD7$^+$, cCD3$^+$			
T-cell	CD2$^+$, CD1$^\pm$, CD4$^\pm$, CD8$^\pm$, HLA-DR$^-$, TdT$^\pm$	12	18	Male predominance, hyperleukocytosis, extramedullary disease
Pre-T	CD2$^-$, CD1$^-$, CD4$^-$, CD8$^-$, HLA-DR$^\pm$, TdT$^+$	1	6	Male predominance, hyperleukocytosis, extramedullary disease, unfavorable prognosis

ABBREVIATIONS: cCD3, cytoplasmic CD3; cIg, cytoplasmic immunoglobulin; sIg, surface immunoglobulin; TdT, terminal deoxynucleotidyl transferase.

Expression of myeloid-associated antigens may occur on otherwise typical lymphoblasts. Because of differences in the monoclonal antibodies and immunophenotyping techniques, the frequencies of myeloid-associated antigen expression have ranged from 5 percent to 30 percent in childhood cases and 10 percent to 50 percent in adult cases.[54,83,84] The pattern of myeloid-associated antigen expression correlates with certain blast cell genetic features—CD15, CD33, and CD65 in cases with a rearranged *MLL* gene, and CD13 and CD33 in those with *ETV6-CBFA2* (*TEL-AML1*) fusion.[83,84] The presence of myeloid antigens lacks significance in contemporary treatment programs,[54,83,84] but it can be useful in immunologic monitoring of patients for minimal residual leukemia (as discussed later).[85]

GENETIC CLASSIFICATION

Acute lymphoblastic leukemia arises from a lymphopoietic progenitor cell that has sustained specific genetic damage leading to malignant transformation and proliferation. Thus, genetic classification of blast cells could be expected to yield more relevant biologic information than could be obtained by other means. Approximately 60 percent of adult cases and 70 percent of childhood cases can be readily classified into therapeutically relevant subgroups based on the modal chromosome number (or DNA content estimated by flow cytometry), specific chromosomal rearrangements, and molecular genetic changes.[21,86–89] Table 97-5 summarizes the prominent clinical and biologic features of cases with the most common genetic abnormalities.

Two ploidy groups (hyperdiploidy >50 chromosomes and hypodiploidy <45 chromosomes) have clinical relevance. Hyperdiploidy, which occurs in approximately 25 percent of childhood cases and 6 to 7 percent of adult cases, confers a favorable prognosis that may reflect an increased cellular accumulation of methotrexate and its polyglutamates, an increased sensitivity to therapeutic antimetabolites, and a marked propensity of these cells to undergo apoptosis.[90–92] By contrast, hypodiploidy is associated with an exceptionally poor prognosis.[86,88,93] Flow cytometric determination of cellular DNA content is a useful adjunct to cytogenetic analysis because it is automated, rapid, and inexpensive, and its measurements are not affected by the mitotic index of the cell population; results can be obtained in virtually all cases. Flow cytometric studies can sometimes identify a small but drug-resistant subpopulation of near-haploid or tetraploid cells that may have been missed by standard cytogenetic analysis.[93,94]

Phenotype-specific reciprocal translocations are the most biologically and clinically significant karyotypic changes in ALL. Many translocations identified in cases of B-cell and T-cell ALL arise from mistakes in the normal recombination mechanisms that generate antigen receptor genes (Table 97-1). Such rearrangements can mobilize the promotor/enhancer element of the immunoglobulin heavy- or light-chain gene or the T-cell antigen receptor (TCR) beta or alpha/delta gene to sites adjacent to a variety of transcription factors. More often, in cases of B-cell precursor ALL, the rearrangements create fusion genes with transforming properties. The major translocations in ALL affect proteins that have critical functions in cell proliferation, differentiation, or survival.[39]

The correlations of specific cytogenetic findings with presenting clinical features and blast cell phenotypes (Table 97-5) indicate the prognostic significance of chromosomal abnormalities in patients with ALL. There, also, are compelling reasons to focus on molecular genetic lesions. First, rearrangements affecting the same chromosomal region may involve different genes and represent clinically and biologically diverse entities. For example, among cases with a t(1;19) (q23;p13.3), those without *E2A-PBX1* fusion respond well to antimetabolite-based therapy, whereas cases with the fusion product require more intensive therapy.[80] Second, molecular analyses can identify several critical submicroscopic genetic alterations not visible by standard karyotyping procedures. *ETV6-CBFA2* and *TAL1* rearrangements—the most common abnormalities in B-lineage and T-lineage ALL respectively—as well as deletions of tumor suppressor genes such as *p53* and *p16* are generally detectable only at the molecular level.[40,43,95,96] Third, cases with clinically important genetic rearrangements may be missed because of technical errors (e.g., karyotyping of residual normal metaphases and not leukemic metaphases). Hence, assays relying on the multiplex reverse transcriptase-polymerase chain reaction (RT-PCR), in which primers for major risk-defining translocations are included in a single PCR reaction tube, have been developed to facilitate molecular diagnosis.[97] By combining such assays with rapid, semiautomated, and nonradioactive detection systems, one can identify translocations in a single PCR reaction mixture within 24 to 36 h.

TABLE 97-5   CLINICAL AND BIOLOGIC FEATURES ASSOCIATED WITH THE MORE COMMON GENETIC SUBTYPES

SUBTYPE	ASSOCIATED FEATURES	ESTIMATED EVENT-FREE SURVIVAL, %	
		CHILDREN	ADULTS
Hyperdiploidy >50 chromosomes	Predominant B-cell-precursor phenotype; low leukocyte count; favorable age group (1-9 yr) and prognosis in children	80–90 at 5 yr	30–50 at 5 yr
Hypodiploidy <45 chromosomes	Predominant B-cell-precursor phenotype; increased leukocyte count; poor prognosis	30 at 3 yr	10–20 at 3 yr
ETV6-CBFA2 fusion	CD13$^\pm$/CD33$^\pm$ B-cell-precursor phenotype; pseudodiploidy; age 1-9 yr; favorable prognosis	85–90 at 5 yr	Unknown
t(1;19)(q23; p13.3) with *E2A-PBX1* fusion	CD10$^+$/CD20$^\pm$/CD34$^-$ pre-B phenotype; pseudodiploidy; increased leukocyte count; black race; CNS leukemia; intermediate prognosis	70–80 at 5 yr	20–40 at 3 yr
t(9;22)(q34;q11)	Predominant B-cell precursor phenotype; older age; increased leukocyte count; dismal outcome in adults and in children with poor early responses to induction or leukocyte counts >25 × 10^9/liter	20–40 at 5 yr	<10 at 3 yr
t(4;11)(q21;q23)	CD10$^-$/CD15$^\pm$/CD33$^\pm$/CD65$^\pm$ B-cell precursor phenotype; infant and older adult age groups; hyperleukocytosis; CNS leukemia; dismal outcome	10–35 at 5 yr	10–20 at 3 yr
t(8;14)(q24; q32.3)	B-cell phenotype; L3 morphology; male predominance; bulky extramedullary disease; favorable prognosis with short-term intensive chemotherapy including high-dose methotrexate, cytarabine, and cyclophosphamide	75–85 at 5 yr	50–55 at 4 yr
t(1;14)(p34;q11)	CD10$^-$ T-cell phenotype; male predominance; hyperleukocytosis; intermediate prognosis	65–75 at 5 yr	50 at 3 yr
dic(9;12)(p11-12; ?p12)	CD10$^+$ B-cell precursor phenotype; male predominance; young age (<25 yr); low leukocyte count; excellent prognosis	80–90 at 5 yr	Unknown

SOURCE: Data presented in Pui and Evans,[21] Secker-Walker et al.,[86] Faderl et al.,[87] Groupe Français de Cytogénétique Hématologique,[88] Martinez-Clement.[89]

DIFFERENTIAL DIAGNOSIS

The initial manifestations of ALL may mimic a variety of disorders. The acute onset of petechiae, ecchymoses, and bleeding may suggest idiopathic thrombocytopenic purpura. The latter disorder is often associated with a recent viral infection, large platelets in blood smears, and normal hemoglobin concentration and no leukocyte abnormalities in blood or marrow. Both ALL and aplastic anemia may present with pancytopenia and complications associated with marrow failure, but in aplastic anemia, hepatosplenomegaly and lymphadenopathy are rare, and the skeletal changes associated with leukemia are absent. The results of bone marrow aspiration or biopsy usually distinguish these two diseases, although the diagnosis may be difficult in a patient presenting with a hypocellular marrow later replaced by lymphoblasts. In one study, transient pancytopenia preceded ALL in 2 percent of all cases of childhood ALL.[98] PCR analysis disclosed monoclonality during the preleukemic phase in these patients, suggesting that hypoplasia was due to the inhibition of normal hematopoiesis by leukemic cells.[99] ALL should be considered in the differential diagnosis of patients with hypereosinophilia, which may be a presenting feature of leukemia or precede its diagnosis by several months.[60]

Infectious mononucleosis and other viral infections, especially those associated with thrombocytopenia or hemolytic anemia, can be confused with leukemia. Detection of atypical lymphocytes or serologic evidence of Epstein-Barr virus infection helps to establish the diagnosis. Patients with pertussis or parapertussis may have marked lymphocytosis; however, even in cases with leukocyte counts as high as 50 × 10^9/liter, the affected cells are mature lymphocytes rather than lymphoblasts. Bone pain, arthralgia, and occasionally arthritis may mimic juvenile rheumatoid arthritis, rheumatic fever, other collagen diseases, or osteomyelitis. Hence, the marrow should be examined if one plans to initiate glucocorticoid treatment for presumed rheumatic diseases.

Childhood ALL should also be distinguished from pediatric small round cell tumors that involve the bone marrow, including neuroblastoma, rhabdomyosarcoma, and retinoblastoma. Generally, in patients with solid tumors, a primary lesion may be found by standard diagnostic studies; disseminated tumor cells often present in characteristic aggregate, and immunophenotypic characteristics of lymphocytes are absent.

THERAPY

SUPPORTIVE CARE

Optimal management of patients with ALL requires careful attention to several facets of supportive care, including the immediate treatment or prevention of metabolic and infectious complications, as well as the rational use of blood products. Other important supportive care measures, such as the use of indwelling catheters (see Chap. 19), amelioration of nausea and vomiting, pain control (see Chap. 20), and continuous psychosocial support for the patient and family are essential.

METABOLIC COMPLICATIONS

Hyperuricemia and hyperphosphatemia with secondary hypocalcemia are frequently encountered at diagnosis, even before chemotherapy is initiated, especially in patients with B-cell or T-cell ALL or B-cell-precursor leukemia with high leukemic cell burden. These patients should be given intravenous hydration, sodium bicarbonate to alkalinize the urine, allopurinol to treat hyperuricemia, and a phosphate binder to treat hyperphosphatemia, such as aluminum hydroxide, calcium carbonate or acetate (if the serum calcium concentration is low), or sevelamer. Allopurinol, by inhibiting de novo purine synthesis in leukemic blast cells, may reduce the peripheral blast cell count before chemotherapy.[100] Allopurinol may decrease both the anabolism and catabolism of 6-mercaptopurine by depleting intracellular phosphoribosyl pyrophosphate and inhibiting xanthine oxidase.[101] If oral 6-mercaptopurine and allopurinol are given together, the dosage of

6-mercaptopurine generally needs to be reduced. Allopurinol can cause skin rashes but seldom produces severe allergic reactions.

Nonrecombinant urate oxidase, available in France and Italy, converts uric acid to allantoin, a readily excreted metabolite that is 5 to 10 times more soluble than uric acid and decreases the serum uric acid concentration more rapidly than does allopurinol.[102] However, this agent can cause acute hypersensitivity reactions and, in patients with glucose-6-dehydrogenase deficiency, can cause methemoglobulinemia or hemolytic anemia. A recombinant form of urate oxidase has proved to be a safe, highly effective, and rapidly acting uricolytic agent.[103]

HYPERLEUKOCYTOSIS

For patients with extreme leukocytosis (leukocyte count $>200 \times 10^9$/liter), either leukapheresis or exchange transfusion (in small children) can be used to reduce the burden of leukemic cells.[104,105] In theory, either treatment should reduce the metabolic complications associated with leukostasis; however, the short- and long-term benefits of these procedures remain in question.[106,107] Emergency cranial irradiation, once advocated by some leukemia therapists, probably has no role in these patients.[104–106] Preinduction therapy with low-dose glucocorticoids, adding vincristine and cyclophosphamide in cases of B-cell ALL, is a favored means of ameliorating hyperleukocytosis. Pioneered by French investigators, this method when used in conjunction with urate oxidase has largely eliminated the tumor lysis syndrome and the need for hemodialysis in patients with B-cell ALL.[108]

INFECTION CONTROL

Infections are common in febrile patients with newly diagnosed ALL. Thus, any patient presenting with fever, especially those with neutropenia, should be given broad-spectrum antibiotics until infection is excluded. Remission induction therapy can increase susceptibility to infection by exacerbating myelosuppression and mucosal breakdown. Indeed, at least 50 percent of patients undergoing induction therapy will experience infections. Special precautions should be taken to reduce the risk of infection during this critical phase of treatment, including reverse protective isolation and air filtration; elimination of contact with people with infectious or potentially contaminated food products, such as raw cheese, uncooked vegetables, or unpeeled fruits; and antiseptic mouthwash or sitz baths, especially in patients with mucositis. Administration of granulocyte colony-stimulating factor may hasten the recovery from neutropenia and reduce the complications of intensive chemotherapy, but it does not improve the event-free survival rate in either children or adults.[109–111] The diagnosis and treatment of fungal or viral infections are addressed in Chap. 16.

At most medical centers, all patients with ALL are given trimethoprim-sulfamethoxazole, 3 days per week, as prophylactic therapy for Pneumocystis carinii pneumonia.[112] Alternative treatments for patients who cannot tolerate trimethoprim-sulfamethoxazole include aerosolized pentamidine, dapsone, and atovaquone.[113–115] Live virus vaccine should not be administered during immunosuppressive therapy. Siblings and other children who have frequent contact with patients should be given inactivated poliomyelitis vaccine but can be immunized against measles, mumps, and rubella. Susceptible patients exposed to varicella should receive zoster immunoglobulin within 96 h of exposure, which usually prevents or modifies the clinical manifestations of varicella. Patients exposed to active cases of influenza A virus infection should be given rimantadine or amantadine prophylactically.

HEMATOLOGIC SUPPORT

ALL or its treatment can lead to thrombocytopenia. Hemorrhagic manifestations are common but are usually limited to the skin and mucous membranes. Although rare, bleeding in the CNS, lungs, or gastrointestinal tract can be life-threatening. Patients with extremely high leukocyte counts at diagnosis are more likely to develop such complications. Coagulopathy attributable to disseminated intravascular coagulation, hepatic dysfunction, or chemotherapy is usually mild.[53,66] Patients receiving induction treatment, including L-asparaginase and a glucocorticoid, are generally in a hypercoagulable state.[116,117] Platelet transfusions should be given therapeutically for overt bleeding and may be indicated when platelet counts are less than 10×10^9/liter.[118] Children generally do not have active bleeding during remission induction therapy with prednisone, vincristine, and L-asparaginase even when platelet counts are less than 10×10^9/liter. A higher threshold for prophylactic platelet transfusions should be considered for active toddlers and patients with fever or infection. Recombinant thrombopoietin accelerates platelet recovery in solid tumor patients undergoing chemotherapy or marrow transplantation, and it improves the yield of platelet apheresis in normal donors, resulting in higher increments of platelet recovery in the recipients. Additional clinical trials are needed to establish the role of this procedure in patients with ALL.[119] Transfusion of packed red cells is indicated in patients with anemia and marrow suppression. Granulocyte transfusions are needed only rarely in patients with absolute neutropenia and documented gram-negative septicemia or disseminated fungal infection who have responded poorly to antimicrobial treatment. All blood products should be irradiated to prevent graft-versus-host disease.

ANTILEUKEMIC THERAPY

ALL is a heterogeneous disease with many distinct subtypes; a uniform approach to therapy is no longer appropriate. A stringent assessment of the relapse hazard is necessary in order to avert undertreatment or overtreatment. There is disagreement over the risk criteria and the terminology for defining prognostic subgroups. Usually, childhood ALL cases are divided into low-, standard- (intermediate- or average-), and high-risk groups, while adult cases are considered to have either standard- or high-risk features. The only exception is B-cell ALL, which requires a unique treatment approach. At many medical centers, infants with ALL are considered to be a special subgroup and are treated differently from other children.

B-CELL ALL

The most effective contemporary treatment regimens for B-cell ALL are drug combinations that include cyclophosphamide given over a relatively short time (3 to 6 months). The first major breakthrough in this disease was reported by French investigators, who achieved a 68 percent event-free survival rate in their LMB 84 study that featured high-dose cyclophosphamide, high-dose methotrexate, vincristine, doxorubicin, and conventional doses of cytarabine.[108] More recently, in the LMB 89 study, the same group reported a cure rate of 80 percent, obtained with increased doses of both methotrexate (to 8 g/m² per dose) and cytarabine (2 g/m² per dose) and the addition of etoposide (for patients with a large leukemic cell burden).[120] This achievement established a standard against which other trials are now measured. Successful treatments have also been developed by the Berlin-Frankfurt-Münster (BFM) consortium, using a multiagent regimen that incorporated fractionated cyclophosphamide, high-dose methotrexate (5 g/m²), etoposide, ifosfamide, and cytarabine (2 g/m² per dose);[121] and by the Pediatric Oncology Group study, using fractionated cyclophosphamide, vincristine, and doxorubicin, alternating with high-dose methotrexate and cytarabine.[122] Whether etoposide or ifosfamide contributed to the improved results will require further study.

Effective CNS therapy is an essential component of successful high-dose regimens for B-cell ALL, and generally consists of methotrexate and cytarabine administered both systemically and intrathecally. Whether or not cranial irradiation should be used in therapy for CNS leukemia is controversial. Although it was a component of a very successful French regimen,[120] cranial irradiation was not included in other successful protocols, and the French group has excluded it from their current trial. B-cell ALL rarely, if ever, recurs after the first year, so that prolonged continuation therapy is not a requirement in this disease.

The same treatment approach has also been taken in adults with B-cell ALL, yielding promising results in several trials.[123,124] A cure rate of approximately 50 percent can now be achieved in adult patients, including those with initial CNS leukemia. Some investigators recommend reduced doses of methotrexate and cytarabine for adults over 60 years of age in order to reduce toxicity.[124]

B-CELL-PRECURSOR AND T-CELL ALL

Treatment for leukemias affecting the B-cell-precursor and T-cell lineages consists of three standard phases: remission induction, intensification (consolidation), and prolonged continuation therapy. CNS-directed therapy, which overlaps with other treatments, is begun early and is given for different lengths of time, depending on the patient's risk of relapse and the intensity of the primary systemic regimen.

Remission Induction   The first goal of therapy for patients with leukemia is to induce a complete remission with restoration of normal hematopoiesis. The induction regimen invariably includes a glucocorticoid (prednisone, prednisolone, or dexamethasone) and vincristine, as well as L-asparaginase for children or an anthracycline for adults.[21,125–127] With improvements in chemotherapy and supportive care, the rate of complete remission now ranges from 97 to 99 percent in children and from 70 to 90 percent in adults. At the time a complete clinical remission is induced, patients have various degrees of residual leukemia, and some may still have as many as 10 billion leukemic cells.[128] Since the extent of residual disease correlates well with long-term outcome,[85,129–131] the concept of a "molecular" or "immunologic" remission, defined as leukemic involvement of less than 0.01 percent of nucleated marrow cells,[21] is beginning to supplant the traditional perception of remission, which is based solely on blast cell morphologic criteria.

Intensive induction therapy with four or more drugs has been credited with improving long-term clinical outcomes in several pediatric trials.[51,132–134] This approach is driven by the premise that more rapid and complete reduction of the leukemic cell burden will forestall the development of drug resistance. Similar approaches in adults have been limited by a low tolerance to drug toxicities.[125–127] However, use of a five-drug induction regimen (cyclophosphamide, daunorubicin, vincristine, prednisone, and L-asparaginase) in two consecutive CALGB studies produced a complete remission rate of 85 percent,[54,111] while 2 weeks of L-asparaginase added to standard induction therapy with prednisone, vincristine, and daunorubicin yielded a remission rate of 88 percent in 109 adults with ALL.[135] Similarly, a combination of prednisone, vincristine, L-asparaginase, and high-dose daunorubicin (270 mg/m²) resulted in a remission rate of 93 percent in 60 adults.[136] Fifty-eight of 66 adults (88%) attained remission when given a "preinduction" course of etoposide and cytarabine, followed by prednisone, vincristine, and doxorubicin.[137]

Perhaps because of its increased penetration into cerebrospinal fluid and its longer half-life,[138] dexamethasone, when used in induction and continuation therapy, provides better control of systemic and CNS disease than does prednisone in children with ALL.[139,140] Three forms of L-asparaginase, each with a different pharmacokinetic profile, are available—one derived from *Erwinia carotovora*, another prepared from *Escherichia coli*, and a third made of a polyethylene glycol (PEG) form of the *E. coli* product.[141] The dosages of these three products are based on their half-lives. PEG L-asparaginase, which has the longest half-life, is usually administered at 2500 IU/m² every other week for two doses in cases of newly diagnosed ALL. By contrast, the *Erwinia* product, with the shortest half-life, is generally given at 10,000 IU/m² three times per week for 6 to 12 doses. The dosages of *E. coli* L-asparaginase range from 6000 to 10,000 IU/m², administered two to three times per week for 6 to 12 doses. In one randomized trial, the clinical outcome in patients treated with L-asparaginase derived from *E. coli* was better than that in patients treated with *Erwinia carotovora*, given at the same dosage.[142] Different *E. coli* preparations have different pharmacologic and pharmacokinetic properties,[143] mandating dosage adjustment to avoid excessive toxicities.[144,145] Among the various anthracyclines (daunorubicin, doxorubicin, and mitoxantrone) given to adults with ALL, one has not proved superior to another[146,147]; however, daunorubicin is used most commonly.

Intensification (Consolidation) Therapy   With restoration of normal hematopoiesis, patients in remission become candidates for intensification therapy. Such treatment, administered shortly after remission induction, refers to high doses of multiple agents not used during the induction phase or to readministration of the induction regimen. More commonly used regimens in childhood cases include high-dose methotrexate with or without 6-mercaptopurine[51,132,148,149]; high-dose L-asparaginase given for an extended period[133,150]; an epipodophyllotoxin plus cytarabine[132,151]; or a combination of dexamethasone, vincristine, L-asparaginase, doxorubicin, and thioguanine, with or without cyclophosphamide.[51,134] This phase of therapy has improved outcome, even in patients with low-risk ALL.[151] A very high dose of methotrexate (5 g/m²) appears to improve the outcome of treatment in patients with T-cell ALL.[51] This finding is consistent with data indicating that T-lineage blast cells accumulate methotrexate polyglutamates (active metabolites of the parent compound) less avidly than do B-cell precursors,[152] so that higher serum levels of the drug are needed for an adequate therapeutic effect.[153] In fact, the conventional dose of methotrexate (1 g/m²) may be too low for many patients with B-cell-precursor ALL.[154,155]

The value of intensification treatment is less certain in adults with ALL. In two randomized trials, high doses of cytarabine and daunorubicin, which had been effective against acute myelogenous leukemia, failed to improve the clinical outcome over results achieved without these agents.[156,157] In another randomized trial, prolonged (4-month) consolidation therapy with methotrexate, cytarabine, thioguanine, cyclophosphamide, and L-asparaginase yielded essentially the same leukemia-free survival rate as did short (1-month) consolidation therapy with cyclophosphamide and L-asparaginase.[158] These results notwithstanding, the outcomes of several nonrandomized studies strongly suggest a benefit from intensive consolidation therapy, especially in young adults. In cases of T-cell ALL, the benefit derives from both cyclophosphamide and cytarabine; while in other standard-risk and high-risk ALL, it derives from high-dose cytarabine.[54,125,159,160] More striking perhaps is the markedly improved results in two German multicenter trials with high-dose cytarabine and mitoxantrone in cases bearing the t(4;11), which generally confers a dismal outcome.[161]

Continuation Therapy   Excluding cases of mature B-cell leukemia, children with ALL require prolonged continuation therapy for reasons that are still poorly understood. Perhaps, long-term drug exposure or the host immune system is needed to kill residual, slowly dividing leukemic cells or to suppress their growth, allowing programmed cell death to occur. In one study, attempts to shorten the duration of moderately intensive chemotherapy to 18 months or less resulted in a high rate of relapse after cessation of therapy.[162] In a meta-analysis of 42 trials, a third year of continuation therapy reduced the likelihood of relapse during the third year, but there was no advantage to prolonging treatment beyond 3 years.[163] Several studies have demonstrated that the third year of continuation therapy benefits boys but not girls.[164–166] Hence, the general rule is to discontinue all therapy in girls who remain in remission for 2 to 2 1/2 years and in boys whose remissions have continued for 3 years. It remains unclear whether the duration of therapy can be shortened for patients who have received contemporary forms of intensive therapy. It is also uncertain whether adults with ALL require prolonged continuation therapy. In two trials of postremission treatment given for 5 to 10 months, the median durations of remission ranged from 9 to 12 months.[146,157] These poor results may reflect inadequate treatment for remission induction or inadequate consolidation therapy. In most adult trials, continuation therapy is given for 2 years.

A combination of methotrexate administered weekly and mercaptopurine administered daily constitutes the usual continuation regimen for children with ALL. Accumulation of higher intracellular concentrations of the active metabolites of methotrexate and administration of this combination to the limits of tolerance (as indicated by low leukocyte counts) have been associated with an improved clinical outcome.[167–170] One recent study showed that the dose intensity of 6-mercaptopurine was the most important pharmacologic factor influencing treatment outcome.[171] The effect of 6-mercaptopurine is better when the drug is given to patients in the evening.[172] It should not be given with milk or milk products, as both decrease its bioavailability.[173] Although the merits of oral versus parenteral administration of methotrexate continue to be debated, the latter route affords a way to circumvent problems of decreased bioavailability and poor compliance, especially in adolescents.[174] Prolonged oral administration of methotrexate in divided doses has proved inferior to intermittent intravenous infusions of the drug at higher doses.[175] By contrast, 6-mercaptopurine is best given orally on a daily basis. Its intravenous administration does not improve outcome and may produce an inferior result.[175] Antimetabolite treatment should not be withheld because of isolated elevations of liver enzymes, since such abnormalities in liver function are tolerable and reversible.[176]

A few patients (1 in 300) have an inherited deficiency of thiopurine S-methyltransferase, the enzyme that catalyzes the S-methylation (inactivation) of 6-mercaptopurine. In these patients standard doses of 6-mercaptopurine have potentially fatal hematologic side effects. The drug should be given in much smaller doses (e.g., 10-fold reduction).[177] Further, about 10 percent of the affected patients are heterozygous for this enzyme deficiency and thus have intermediate levels of the methyltransferase.[178] This subgroup can be treated safely with only moderate reductions in 6-mercaptopurine dosage and appears to have better clinical outcome than patients with homozygous wild-type phenotype. The genetic basis of this autosomal codominant trait was recently identified, opening the way for molecular diagnosis of these cases.[179] To this end, emphasis has been placed on the study of inherited differences in the metabolism and disposition of various chemotherapeutic drugs, due to genetic polymorphisms in drug-metabolizing enzymes, drug transporters, receptors, and targets.[29] Ultimately, therapy can be designed according to the hosts' and leukemic cells' genetic constitution.

Intermittent pulses of vincristine and a glucocorticoid improve the efficacy of antimetabolite-based continuation regimens[163] and therefore have been widely adopted in the treatment of childhood ALL. Another integral component of many protocols is reinduction therapy introduced relatively soon after patients have attained their first remission. This treatment, which relies on the same drugs that were used during the initial phase of induction therapy, has improved outcomes in both children and adults with ALL.[51,159,163] Prolonged intensification including a second reinduction phase or rotational administration of noncross-resistant drug pairs during continuation treatment may further improve outcome in patients with standard- or high-risk ALL.[180–182]

Therapy of the Central Nervous System The CNS is a frequent sanctuary site for leukemic cells requiring presymptomatic therapy for CNS involvement in patients with ALL. Cranial irradiation (2400 cGy) plus intrathecal methotrexate, administered after the induction of complete remission, became the cornerstone of ALL therapy in the 1970s.[183] Concern that cranial irradiation may cause late neurologic sequelae and occasional brain tumors stimulated efforts to replace this modality with intensive intrathecal and systemic chemotherapy administered early in the clinical course to patients with a low risk of CNS relapse. This approach has lowered rates of CNS relapse to 2 percent or less in several studies.[72,149,180,184–186]

Whether certain groups of patients at high risk of relapse should be treated with cranial irradiation is unclear. In one retrospective study, children with T-cell ALL and leukocyte counts less than 100×10^9/liter had similar outcomes whether or not they received cranial irradiation. However, among those with higher leukocyte counts, the irradiated group had significantly better long-term responses than did patients given intrathecal therapy exclusively.[186] These results are not conclusive because systemic chemotherapy differed between the two groups and may have been more effective in the irradiated patients. Nonetheless, in the context of effective systemic chemotherapy, a radiation dose as low as 1200 cGy appears to provide adequate protection against CNS relapse, even in high-risk patients (e.g., those with T-cell ALL and leukocyte counts $> 100 \times 10^9$/liter).[186]

Allogeneic Stem Cell Transplantation Hematopoietic stem cell transplantation during first remission remains controversial. In adult ALL, long-term event-free survival rates range from 30 to 40 percent with chemotherapy alone and from 40 to 60 percent with allogeneic transplantation.[187–189] However, it is difficult to interpret these results because the proportions of patients in similar risk groups differed from study to study, as did the criteria for patient selection. Even so, the results of both the adult and pediatric studies suggested that allogeneic transplantation may be of benefit in some high-risk cases.[189,190] Thus, because of their unfavorable prognosis, patients with the Ph chromosome, the t(4;11), or poor initial response to induction therapy commonly receive allogeneic stem cell transplantation during the first remission.[126,189–192] Exceptions to this general rule include children with Ph-chromosome-positive ALL and low presenting leukocyte counts ($<25 \times 10^9$/liter) or good initial responses to prednisone, as well as children 1 to 9 years of age with the t(4;11) translocation—all of whom are potentially curable with intensive chemotherapy.[193–196] Even adults with the t(4;11) can expect a 50 percent prospect of long-term event-free survival when treated with high-dose cytarabine and mitoxantrone.[161] Hence, the indications for transplantation in first remission are variable and should be reevaluated as chemotherapy continues to improve. Currently, allogeneic stem cell transplantation is the treatment of choice for adults and most children with Ph-chromosome-positive ALL and those who require extended induction therapy to attain complete remission.

COURSE AND PROGNOSIS

RELAPSE

Relapse is defined as the reappearance of leukemic cells at any site in the body. Most relapses occur during treatment or within the first 2 years after its completion, although in some instances initial relapses have been observed 10 years or more after diagnosis.[197] The marrow remains the most common site of relapse in ALL. Anemia, leukocytosis, leukopenia, thrombocytopenia, enlargement of the liver or spleen, bone pain, fever, or a sudden decrease in tolerance to chemotherapy may signal the onset of marrow relapse. In other sites, such as the CNS and testes, the frequency of relapse has decreased, and in contemporary programs of childhood ALL treatment, the rates of CNS and testicular relapse are generally less than 2 percent.[198] Leukemic relapse occasionally occurs at other extramedullary sites, including the eye, ear, ovary, uterus, bone, muscle, tonsil, kidney, mediastinum, pleura, and paranasal sinus.[199]

Marrow relapse, with or without extramedullary involvement, portends a poor outcome for most patients. Factors indicating an especially poor prognosis in previously treated patients include relapse on therapy or after a short initial remission, after intensive primary therapy, a T-cell immunophenotype, the Ph chromosome, the presence of circulating blasts, or a high leukocyte count at relapse.[200–206] Prolonged second remissions (>3 years) may be obtained with chemotherapy in as many as one-half of patients with late relapses (i.e., >6 months after cessation of therapy) but in only approximately 10 percent of those with early relapse.[200,201,205] In patients who develop hematologic relapse on therapy or shortly thereafter, allogeneic hematopoietic stem cell transplantation is the treatment of choice.[207–213] Autologous transplantation offers no substantial advantage over chemotherapy as post-induction treatment.[214–216] For patients without histocompatible related donors, transplantation of stem cells from matched unrelated donors has yielded encouraging results.[217,218] Umbilical cord blood offers a second transplant option that does not require the same degree of histocompatibility as procedures relying on marrow stem cells from children or adults.[219–221] Whether the lower risk of graft-versus-host disease associated with cord blood transplants will lead to an increased risk of relapse due to a reduced graft-versus-leukemia effect is uncertain. Transplantation with large doses of T-cell-depleted hematopoietic stem cells from haploid-identical donors, following enhanced myeloablation and immunosuppression, has produced a disease-free survival rate that compares favorably with results in patients receiving transplants from matched unrelated donors.[222] For patients who relapse after allogeneic transplantation, a second transplant or donor T-lymphocyte infusion may occasionally result in sustained remission.[223,224] For patients who receive only chemotherapy therapy, a second course of CNS-directed treatment is needed to prevent subsequent CNS relapse.[225]

Although extramedullary relapse frequently presents as an isolated finding, most, if not all, occurrences are associated with minimal residual disease in the marrow.[226,227] Hence, these patients require intensive systemic treatment to prevent subsequent hematologic relapse. The efficacy of retrieval therapy for patients with an isolated CNS relapse depends largely on whether they have received prior CNS irradiation. Intensive chemotherapy and craniospinal irradiation can be expected to secure long-term second remissions in at least half of the previously unirradiated group.[205,228,229] For patients with earlier prophylactic irradiation, this rate generally does not exceed 30 percent; hence, some investigators have selected hematopoietic stem cell transplantation as a treatment option for this small subgroup.[216,230] There is no firm evidence indicating an advantage of either autologous or allogeneic transplantation over intensive chemotherapy.

One-third of patients with early testicular relapse and two-thirds with late recurrences in this site became long-term survivors after salvage chemotherapy and bilateral testicular irradiation.[231–235] Whether this experience can be extrapolated to patients who have received contemporary intensive treatment is uncertain. One study showed that some patients with late isolated testicular relapses can be successfully treated with chemotherapy, including very high dose methotrexate, without the addition of radiotherapy.[236] The optimal treatment and prognosis for patients who relapse at unusual extramedullary sites are also unclear. However, the same principles that apply to the clinical management of CNS or testicular relapse would likely hold for this subgroup.

TREATMENT SEQUELAE

Despite the increasing intensity of curative treatment for childhood ALL, judicious use of supportive care has reduced the rate of early death from 8 percent in the early 1970s to less than 2 percent in the 1990s.[21] However, the death rate among older patients receiving remission induction therapy can be as high as 30 percent, owing to increased hematologic and nonhematologic toxicities (e.g., hepatotoxicity and cardiotoxicity).[53] This poor tolerance of chemotherapy and consequent reduction of dose intensity largely account for the generally poor clinical outcome in elderly patients.

Table 97-6 summarizes the more common side effects associated with antileukemic therapy. Hyperglycemia develops in 10 percent of children during induction therapy with prednisone, vincristine, and L-asparaginase and may require short-term insulin treatment. An adolescent age, obesity, a positive family history for diabetes mellitus, and Down syndrome are associated with an increased susceptibility to this complication.[237] This induction regimen can also cause a hypercoagulable state,[238] leading to cerebral thromboses, peripheral vein thromboses, or both in up to 2 percent of patients. Cerebral thrombosis should be distinguished from transient ischemic lesions, which are associated with acute hypertension and severe constipation. These lesions are located at the watershed areas between the major cerebral arteries and are generally reversible.[239] Sagittal sinus thrombosis, on the other hand, can be diagnosed by magnetic resonance imaging or computed tomography (Fig. 97-8).

Emphasis on intensive use of methotrexate and glucocorticoids has led to an increased frequency of neurotoxicity[240–242] and aseptic necrosis of bone,[243–246] respectively, underscoring the need for judicious use of even seemingly benign agents. For example, methotrexate given in divided doses of 25 mg/m^2 every 6 h four times daily in four weekly courses can result in acute neurologic toxicity if subsequent leucovorin treatment is inadequate.[240] Many of the long-term survivors of childhood ALL have developed severe osteoporosis,[247,248] focusing attention on the need for early identification of bone lesions and the introduction of therapy to prevent fractures.

Treatment with anthracyclines can produce severe cardiomyopathy, especially when these agents are given to young girls in high cumulative and peak doses.[249,250] Whether there is a safe cumulative dose of anthracycline is controversial.[251,252] Several ongoing trials will evaluate whether dexrazoxane can prevent anthracycline-induced cardiotoxicity without interfering with antileukemic activity.[253] Cranial irradiation has been implicated as the cause of numerous late sequelae in children, including neuropsychologic deficits and endocrine abnormalities leading to obesity, short stature, precocious puberty, and osteoporosis.[21] In general, these complications are seen in girls more often than in boys and in young children more often than in older ones. Many children with profound deficiencies of growth hormone are receiving hormone replacement therapy, which permits acceptable final heights to be attained without an increase in the relapse hazard.[21] The current practice of limiting both the use and dose of cranial irradiation promises to lower the frequency of many treatment sequelae.

The most devastating complication is the development of a second cancer, especially brain tumors and acute myelogenous leukemia. Children who received cranial irradiation at 6 years of age or younger and those with ETV6-CBFA2 fusion in their leukemic lymphoblasts are most susceptible to the development of brain tumors.[254,255] The intensive use of antimetabolites before and during cranial irradiation also increases the risk for brain tumor development.[255] The median latency period for high-grade brain tumor is 9 years but almost 20 years for low-grade tumors (e.g., meningioma).[254] Patients with low-grade brain tumors have an excellent prognosis, while the outcome for those with

TABLE 97-6   SIDE EFFECTS ASSOCIATED WITH ANTILEUKEMIC THERAPY

TREATMENT	ACUTE COMPLICATIONS	DELAYED COMPLICATIONS
Prednisone (or prednisolone)	Hyperglycemia, hypertension, changes in mood or behavior, acne, increased appetite, weight gain, peptic ulcer, hepatomegaly, myopathy	Avascular necrosis of bone, osteoporosis, growth retardation
Dexamethasone	Same as prednisone, with the exception of increased changes in mood or behavior but less salt retention.	Same as prednisone
Vincristine	Peripheral neuropathy, constipation, chemical cellulitis, seizures, hair loss	None
Daunorubicin, idarubicin, doxorubicin, or epirubicin	Nausea and vomiting, hair loss, mucositis, bone marrow suppression, chemical cellulitis, increased skin pigmentation, hair loss	Cardiomyopathy (from high cumulative dose)
L-asparaginase	Nausea and vomiting, allergic reactions (manifested as rashes, bronchospasm, severe pain at intramuscular injection site), hyperglycemia, pancreatitis, liver dysfunction, thrombosis, encephalopathy	None
6-Mercaptopurine	Nausea and vomiting, mucositis, bone marrow suppression, solar dermatitis, liver dysfunction. Increased hematologic toxicity in individuals who lack thiopurine S-methyltransferase	Osteoporosis (long-term use)
Methotrexate	Nausea and vomiting, liver dysfunction, bone marrow suppression, mucositis (from high-dose treatment), solar dermatitis	Leukoencephalopathy, osteoporosis (long-term use)
Etoposide, teniposide	Nausea and vomiting, hair loss, mucositis, bone marrow suppression, allergic reactions (bronchospasm, urticaria, angioedema, hypotension)	Acute myeloid leukemia (schedule- and dose-dependent)
Cytarabine	Nausea and vomiting, fever, skin rashes, mucositis, bone marrow suppression, liver dysfunction, conjunctivitis (from high-dose treatment)	Decreased fertility (from high cumulative dose)
Cyclophosphamide	Nausea and vomiting, hemorrhagic cystitis, bone marrow suppression, syndrome of inappropriate ADH secretion, hair loss	Bladder cancer or acute myeloid leukemia (rare), decreased fertility (from high cumulative dose)
Intrathecal methotrexate	Headache, fever, seizure, bone marrow suppression, mucositis (in patients with renal dysfunction)	? Encephalopathy or myelopathy (from high cumulative dose)
Brain irradiation	Hair loss, postirradiation somnolence syndrome (6 to 10 weeks following treatment)	Seizure, mineralizing microangiopathy, growth hormone deficiency, thyroid dysfunction, obesity, osteoporosis, brain tumors (rare), hair loss, cataract (rare), dental abnormalities

high-grade tumors is very poor. Acute myelogenous leukemia has been linked to intensive treatment with the epipodophyllotoxins (teniposide and etoposide), with the risk of disease development apparently depending on treatment schedule and the concomitant use of other agents (e.g., L-asparaginase, alkylating agents, and perhaps antimetabolites).[256,257] The long-term survival rate for patients with this complication is very low, even when they undergo allogeneic stem cell trans-

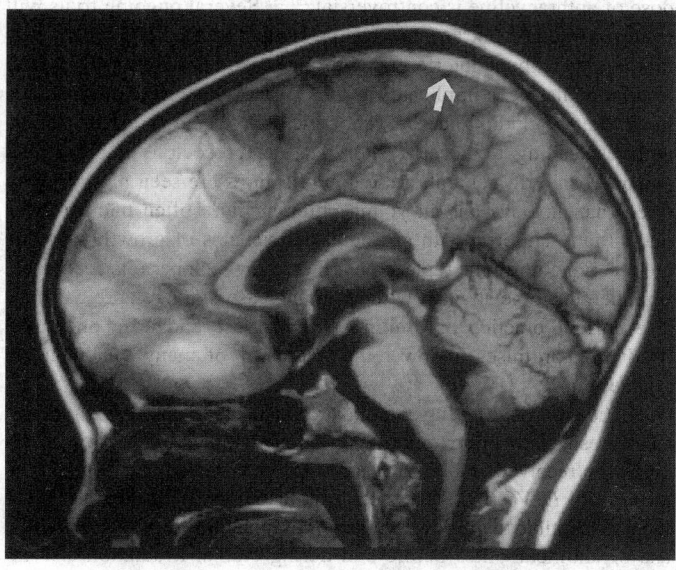

FIGURE 97-8   This T1-weighted magnetic resonance image without contrast demonstrates a clot in the superior sagittal sinus (*arrow*) and several frontal lobe hematomas.

plantation.[257] There has been no indication that the incidence of cancer or birth defects has increased among the offspring of adult survivors of childhood ALL.[258–260]

PROGNOSTIC FACTORS

The cornerstone of the modern therapeutic approach to childhood ALL has been careful assessment of the risk of relapse, so that only standard- or high-risk cases are treated with intensive therapy, with less toxic treatments, usually antimetabolites, reserved for low-risk cases. By contrast, virtually all adult patients are candidates for intensive therapy. Of the many variables that influence prognosis, treatment is the most important.[261] Some of the factors that have emerged as useful prognostic indicators disappeared as treatment improved; others have shown predictive strength in one or several trials but not in others. For example, T-cell and B-cell ALL, once associated with a very bad prognosis, now have long-term response rates of 70 percent to 80 percent in children[51,108,120–122] and 50 percent to 60 percent in adults[53,123,124] as a result of effective intensive chemotherapy.

Age and leukocyte count continue to be used for risk classification in virtually every pediatric clinical trial involving B-cell-precursor ALL. In a workshop sponsored by the U.S. National Cancer Institute, participants agreed on a presenting age between 1 and 9 years and a leukocyte count of less than 50×10^9/liter as the minimal criteria for low-risk ALL.[262] This criterion probably applies only to B-cell precursor ALL and not to T-cell ALL. Among adults, the outcome of therapy worsens with increasing age and leukocyte count.[52–54,125–127,263–265] However, there are no clear guidelines for assigning prognostic value to particular increments of age or leukocyte numbers. In general, an age of less than 60 years is considered to be a practical guide for selecting candidates who might benefit from intensive therapy, including allogeneic transplantation. Any decision to begin aggressive treatment in

TABLE 97-7   RISK CLASSIFICATION SYSTEM IN ST. JUDE TOTAL THERAPY STUDY XIV

RISK GROUP	FEATURE
Low	B-cell-precursor phenotype with age 1–9 years and presenting leukocyte count less than 50×10^9/liter, ETV6-CBFA2 fusion, or hyperdiploidy more than 50 chromosomes (DNA index greater than 1.16)
	Must not have CNS leukemia (CNS-3 status), testicular leukemia, t(9;22), t(1;19), rearranged MLL or hypodiploidy or poor early response
Standard	T-cell ALL and all cases of B-cell precursor ALL not meeting the criteria for low- or high-risk ALL
High	t(9;22)(BCL-ABL) with leukocyte $>25 \times 10^9$/liter or poor early response, rearranged MLL gene with age more than 12 months, or induction failure

patients older than 60 years must be weighed against the risk of increased morbidity and mortality.

Gender has long been recognized as a significant prognostic factor in childhood ALL. Despite the consistency of this finding, gender differences have attracted only scant attention from leukemia therapists, until recently.[198,266,267] Although both boys and girls have benefited from recent improvement in therapy, boys continue to fare worse than girls, a result only partially explained by the higher frequency of T-cell ALL in boys.[198] Gender has less influence in adult ALL; however, when a sex difference in survival was observed, males had the inferior outcome.[53] The historically poor prognosis for children of African ancestry with ALL has largely been abolished by more effective treatment.[268]

Age and certain genetic subtypes of ALL are strongly correlated with prognosis. For example, 70 percent to 80 percent of infants (<1 year old) have rearrangements of the MLL gene and a very poor survival rate.[269] Adolescent and adult patients have relatively high frequencies of MLL rearrangements and the Ph chromosome, together with low rates of long-term survival.[52,88,270] By contrast, two favorable genetic abnormalities—hyperdiploidy (>50 chromosomes per cell) and ETV6-CBFA2 fusion—occur mainly in children 1 to 9 years of age.[21,95,96] Despite their close relation to the biologic properties of leukemic blast cells, genetic abnormalities do not offer a precise guide to clinical outcome. For example, as many as 20 percent of children with hyperdiploid- or ETV6-CBFA2-positive ALL eventually have a relapse.[21] On the other hand, there are subgroups of patients with MLL rearrangements and a favorable age[195,196,271,272] or BCR-ABL with low initial leukocyte counts or a good response to early treatment[193,194,273] who fare well on contemporary protocols.

A useful adjunct in risk assessment is the response to early treatment, as measured by the rate of clearance of leukemic cells from the blood or marrow[274–276] or by the level of minimal residual disease after the induction of a clinical remission.[85,129–131,277,278] We have now included this factor in our risk classification system (Table 97-7). Whether the alteration of treatment intensity according to the level of minimal residual disease will improve long-term outcome in patients with ALL remains to be determined.

REFERENCES

1. Gale RE, Wainscoat JS: Clonal analysis using X-linked DNA polymorphisms. Br J Hematol 85:2, 1993.
2. Saunders EF, Lampkin BC, Mauer AM: Variation of proliferative activity in leukemic cell populations of patients with acute leukemia. J Clin Invest 46:1356, 1967.
3. Shay JW, Werbin H, Wright WE: Telomeres and telomerase in human leukemias. Leukemia 10:1225, 1996.
4. Ohyashiki JH, Ohyashiki K, Iwama H, Hayashi S, Toyama K, Shay JW: Clinical implications of telomerase activity levels in acute leukemia. Clin Cancer Res 3:619, 1997.
5. Velpeau A: Sur la resorption du pus et sur l'alteration du sang dans les maladies, Clinique de persection nenemant. Premier observation. Rev Med 26:216, 1827.
6. Virchow R: Weisses blut. Notiz Geg Natur Heilk 36:152, 1845.
7. Bennett JH: Case of hypertrophy of the spleen and liver in which death took place from suppuration of the blood. Edinburgh Med Surg J 64:413, 1845.
8. Craigie D: Case of disease of the spleen, in which death took place in consequence of the presence of purulent matter in the blood. Edinburgh Med Surg J 64:400, 1845.
9. Virchow R: Weisses Blut und Milztumoren. Part II. Med Z, 1847, 16, 9; and Virchow's Arch Path Anat Physiol 1:565, 1847.
10. Ehrlich P: Farbenanalytische untersuchungen zur histologie und klinick des blutes. Berlin Hirschwald, p 137, 1891.
11. Reschad H, Schilling-Torgau V: Ueber eine neue Leukämie durch echte Uebergangsformen (Splenozytenleuämie) und ihre bedeutung für dies, selbständigkeit dieser Zellen. Munchener Med Wochenschr 60:1981, 1913.
12. Ward G: The infective theory of acute leukemia. Br J Child Dis 14:10, 1917.
13. Farber S, Diamond LK, Mercer, RD, et al: Temporary remissions in acute leukemia in children produced by folic acid antagonist, 4-aminopteroyl-glumatic acid (aminopterin). N Engl J Med 238:787, 1948.
14. Farber S: The effect of ACTH in acute leukemia in childhood, in Proceedings of the First Clinical Conference on the Use of ACTH, edited by JR Mote, p 325. Blakiston, Philadelphia, 1950.
15. Elion GB, Hitchings GH, Vanderwerff H: Antagonists of nucleic acid derivatives; purines. J Biol Chem 192:505, 1951.
16. Pinkel D, Hernandez K, Borella L, et al: Drug dosage and remission duration in childhood lymphocytic leukemia. Cancer 27:247, 1971.
17. Aur RJA, Simone JV, Hustu HO, Verzosa MS: A comparative study of central nervous system irradiation and intensive chemotherapy early in remission of childhood acute lymphocytic leukemia. Cancer 29:381, 1972.
18. Thomas ED, Buckner CD, Rudolph RH, et al: Allogeneic marrow grafting for hematological malignancy using HLA-matched donor-recipient pairs. Blood 38:267, 1971.
19. Sen L, Borella L: Clinical importance of lymphoblasts with T markers in childhood acute leukemia. N Engl J Med 292:828, 1975.
20. Williams DL, Look AT, Melvin SL, et al: New chromosomal translocations correlate with specific immunophenotypes of childhood acute lymphoblastic leukemia. Cell 36:101, 1984.
21. Pui CH, Evans WE: Acute lymphoblastic leukemia. N Engl J Med 339:605, 1998.
22. SEER Cancer Statistics Review, 1973-1995, National Cancer Institute, 1998.
23. Gurney JG, Davis S, Severson RK, et al: Trends in cancer incidence among children in the U.S. Cancer 78:532, 1996.
24. Sandler DP, Ross JA: Epidemiology of acute leukemia in children and adults. Semin Oncol 24:3, 1997.
25. Reaman GH, Sposto R, Sensel MG, et al: Treatment outcome and prognostic factors for infants with acute lymphoblastic leukemia treated on two consecutive trials of the Children's Cancer Group. J Clin Oncol 17:445, 1999.
26. Parkin DM, Muir CS, Whelan SL, et al: Cancer incidence in five continents. IARC Scientific Publication. Vol 6. No 120, Lyon, 1992.
27. Pui C-H: Acute leukemia in children. Curr Opin Hematol 3:249, 1996.
28. Greaves MF: Aetiology of acute leukaemia. Lancet 349:344, 1997.
29. Evans WE, Relling MV: Pharmacogenomics: translating functional genomics into rational therapeutics. Science 286:487, 1999.
30. Pui C-H, Raimondi SC, Borowitz MJ, et al: Immunophenotypes and karyotypes of leukemic cells in children with Down syndrome and acute lymphoblastic leukemia. J Clin Oncol 11:1361, 1993.
31. Vanasse GJ, Concannon P, Willerford DM: Regulated genomic instability and neoplasia in the lymphoid lineage. Blood 94:3997, 1999.
32. Filipovich AH, Mathur A, Kamat D, et al: Lymphoproliferative disorders and other tumors complicating immunodeficiencies. Immunodeficiency 5:91, 1994.

33. Ford AM, Ridge SA, Cabrera ME, et al: In utero rearrangements in the trithorax-related oncogene in infant leukaemias. *Nature* 363:358, 1993.

34. Wiemels JL, Cazzaniga G, Daniotti M, et al: Prenatal origin of acute lymphoblastic leukaemia in children. *Lancet* 354:1499, 1999.

35. Ford AM, Pombo-de-Oliveira MS, McCarthy KP, et al: Monoclonal origin of concordant T-cell malignancy in identical twins. *Blood* 89:281, 1997.

36. Doll R, Wakeford R: Risk of childhood cancer from fetal irradiation. *Br J Radiol* 70:130,1997.

37. Linet MS, Hatch EE, Kleinerman RA, et al: Residential exposure to magnetic fields and acute lymphoblastic leukemia in children. *N Engl J Med.* 337:1, 1997.

38. Kinlen LJ: High-contact paternal occupations, infection and childhood leukaemia: five studies of unusual population mixing of adults. *Br J Cancer* 76:1539,1997

39. Look AT: Oncogenic transcription factors in the human acute leukemias. *Science* 278:1059, 1997.

40. Zhou M, Gu L, Abshire TC, et al: Incidence and prognostic significance of MDM2 oncoprotein overexpression is relapsed childhood acute lymphoblastic leukemia. *Leukemia* 14:61, 2000.

41. Kirsch DG, Kastan MB: Tumor-suppressor p53: implications for tumor development and prognosis. *J Clin Oncol* 16:3158, 1998.

42. Kamijo T, Zindy F, Roussel MF, et al: Tumor suppression at the mouse *INK4a* locus mediated by the alternative reading frame product p19*ARF*. *Cell* 91:649, 1997.

43. Maloney KW, McGavran L, Odon LF, Hunger SP: Acquisition of *P16INK4A* and *P15INK4B* gene abnormalities between initial diagnosis and relapse in children with acute lymphoblastic leukemia. *Blood* 93:2380, 1999.

44. Knudson CM, Korsmeyer SJ: *BCL-2* and *Bax* function independently to regulate cell death. *Nat Genet* 16:358, 1997.

45. Reed JC: Dysregulation of apoptosis in cancer. *J Clin Oncol* 17:2941, 1999

46. Coustan-Smith E, Kitanaka A, Pui CH, et al: Clinical relevance of *BCL-2* overexpression in childhood acute lymphoblastic leukemia. *Blood* 87:1140, 1996.

47. Findley HW, Gu L, Yeager AM, Zhou M: Expression and regulation of Bcl-2, Bcl-xl, and Bax correlate with p53 status and sensitivity to apoptosis in childhood acute lymphoblastic leukemia. *Blood* 89:2986, 1997.

48. Meijerink JPP, Mensink EJBM, Wang K, et al: Hematopoietic malignancies demonstrate loss-of-function mutations of *BAX*. *Blood* 91:2991, 1998.

49. Pui C-H, Crist WM: Acute lymphoblastic leukemia, in *Childhood Leukemia*, edited by C-H Pui, p 288. Cambridge University Press, New York, 1999.

50. McKenna SM, Baehner RL: Diagnosis and treatment of childhood acute lymphoblastic leukemia, in *Neoplastic Diseases of the Blood,* 3rd ed, edited by PH Wiernik, GP Canellos, JP Dutcher, RA Kyle, p 271. Churchill Livingstone, New York, 1996.

51. Reiter A, Schrappe M, Ludwig WD, et al: Chemotherapy in 998 unselected childhood acute lymphoblastic leukemia patients. Results and conclusions of the multicenter trial ALL-BFM 86. *Blood* 84:3122, 1994.

52. Chessells JM, Hall E, Prentice HG, et al: The impact of age on outcome in lymphoblastic leukemia; MRC UKALL X and XA compared: a report from the MRC Paediatric and Adult Working Parties. *Leukemia* 12:463, 1998.

53. Hoelzer DF: Diagnosis and treatment of adult acute lymphoblastic leukemia, in *Neoplastic Diseases of the Blood,* 3rd ed, edited by PH Wiernik, GP Canellos, JP Dutcher, RA Kyle, p 295. Churchill Livingstone, New York, 1996.

54. Larson LA, Dodge RK, Burns CP, et al: A five-drug remission induction regimen with intensive consolidation for adults with acute lymphoblastic leukemia: Cancer and Leukemia Group B study 8811. *Blood* 85:2025, 1995.

55. Dinarello CA, Bunn PA Jr: Fever. *Semin Oncol* 24:288, 1997.

56. Jonsson OG, Sartain P, Ducore JM, Buchanan GR: Bone pain as an initial symptom of childhood acute lymphoblastic leukemia: association with nearly normal hematologic indexes. *J Pediatr* 117:233, 1990.

57. Pui C-H, Stass S, Green A: Bone marrow necrosis in children with malignant disease. *Cancer* 56:1522, 1985.

58. Ingram L, Rivera GK, Shapiro DN: Superior vena cava syndrome associ-

ated with childhood malignancy: analysis of 24 cases. *Med Pediatr Oncol* 18:476, 1990.

59. Gajjar A, Ribeiro RC, Mahmoud HH, et al: Overt testicular disease at diagnosis is associated with high risk features and a poor prognosis in patients with childhood acute lymphoblastic leukemia. *Cancer* 78:2437, 1996.

60. Bain BJ: Eosinophilic leukaemias and the idiopathic hypereosinophilic syndrome. *Br J Haematol* 95:2, 1996.

61. Meeker TC, Hardy D, Willman C, et al: Activation of the interleukin-3 gene by chromosome translocation in acute lymphocytic leukemia with eosinophilia. *Blood* 76:285, 1990.

62. Dubansky AS, Boyett JM, Falletta J, et al: Isolated thrombocytopenia in children with acute lymphoblastic leukemia: a rare event in a Pediatric Oncology Group study. *Pediatr* 84:1068, 1989.

63. Beutler E: Platelet transfusions: the 20,000/μL trigger. *Blood* 81:1411, 1993.

64. Blatt J, Penchansky L, Horn M: Thrombocytosis as a presenting feature of acute lymphoblastic leukemia in childhood. *Am J Hematol* 31:46, 1989.

65. Hasle H, Heim S, Schroeder H, et al: Transient pancytopenia preceding acute lymphoblastic leukemia (pre-ALL). *Leukemia* 9:605, 1995.

66. Ribeiro RC, Pui CH: The clinical and biological correlates of coagulopathy in children with acute leukemia. *J Clin Oncol* 4:1212, 1986.

67. Pui C-H, Dodge RK, Dahl GV, et al: Serum lactic dehydrogenase level has prognostic value in childhood acute lymphoblastic leukemia. *Blood* 66:778, 1985.

68. Jones DP, Stapleton FB, Kalwinsky D, et al: Renal dysfunction and hyperuricemia at presentation and relapse of acute lymphoblastic leukemia. *Med Pediatr Oncol* 18:283, 1990.

69. McKay C, Furman WL: Hypercalcemia complicating childhood malignancies. *Cancer* 72:256, 1993.

70. Welch JC, Lilleyman JS: Immunoglobulin concentrations in untreated lymphoblastic leukaemia. *Pediatr Hematol Oncol* 12:545, 1995.

71. Müller HL, Horwitz AE, Kühl J: Acute lymphoblastic leukemia with severe skeletal involvement: a subset of childhood leukemia with a good prognosis. *Pediatr Hematol Oncol* 15:121, 1998.

72. Pui CH, Mahmoud HH, Rivera GK, et al: Early intensification of intrathecal chemotherapy virtually eliminates central nervous system relapse in children with acute lymphoblastic leukemia. *Blood* 92:411, 1998.

73. Mahmoud HH, Rivera GK, Hancock ML, et al: Low leukocyte counts with blast cells in cerebrospinal fluid of children with newly diagnosed acute lymphoblastic leukemia. *N Engl J Med* 329:314, 1993.

74. Lauer S, Shuster J, Kirchner P, et al: Prognostic significance of cerebrospinal fluid (CSF) lymphoblasts (LB) at diagnosis (dx) in children with acute lymphoblastic leukemia (ALL). *Proc ASCO* 13:317, 1994.

75. Gilchrist GS, Tubergen DG, Sather HN, et al: Low numbers of CSF blasts at diagnosis do not predict for the development of CNS leukemia in children with intermediate-risk acute lymphoblastic leukemia: a Childrens Cancer Group report. *J Clin Oncol* 12:2594, 1994.

76. Van den Berg H, Vet R, den Ouden E, Behrendt H: Significance of lymphoblasts in cerebrospinal fluid in newly diagnosed pediatric acute lymphoblastic malignancies with bone marrow involvement: possible benefit of dexamethasone. *Med Pediatr Oncol* 25:22, 1995.

77. Gajjar A, Harrison PL, Sandlund JT, et al: Traumatic lumbar puncture at diagnosis adversely affects outcome in childhood acute lymphoblastic leukemia (ALL). *Blood* 92(suppl 1):512a, 1998.

78. Pui CH, Behm FG, Crist WM: Clinical and biologic relevance of immunologic marker studies in childhood acute lymphoblastic leukemia. *Blood* 82:343, 1993.

79. Béné MC, Bernier M, Castoldi G, et al: Impact of immunophenotyping on management of acute leukemias. *Haematologica* 84:1024, 1999.

80. Pui CH, Raimondi SC, Hancock ML, et al: Immunologic, cytogenetic, and clinical characterization of childhood acute lymphoblastic leukemia with the t(1;19) (q23;p13) or its derivative. *J Clin Oncol* 12:2601, 1994.

81. Pui CH, Rivera GK, Hancock ML, et al: Clinical significance of CD10 expression in childhood acute lymphoblastic leukemia. *Leukemia* 7:35, 1993.

82. Ludwig WD, Reiter A, Löffler H, et al: Immunophenotypic features of childhood and adult acute lymphoblastic leukemia (ALL): experience of the German multicentre trials ALL-BFM and GMALL. *Leuk Lymphoma* 13:71, 1994.

83. Putti MC, Rondelli R, Cocito MG, et al: Expression of myeloid markers

lacks prognostic impact in children treated for acute lymphoblastic leukemia: Italian experience in AIEOP-ALL 88-91 studies. *Blood* 92:795, 1998.

84. Pui CH, Rubnitz JE, Hancock ML, et al: Reappraisal of the clinical and biologic significance of myeloid-associated antigen expression in childhood acute lymphoblastic leukemia. *J Clin Oncol* 16:3768, 1998.

85. Coustan-Smith E, Behm FG, Sanchez J, et al: Immunological detection of minimal residual disease in children with acute lymphoblastic leukaemia. *Lancet* 351:550, 1998.

86. Secker-Walker LM, Prentice HG, Durrant J, et al: Cytogenetics adds independent prognostic information in adults with acute lymphoblastic leukaemia on MRC trial UKALL XA. *Br J Hematol* 96:601, 1997.

87. Faderl S, Kantarjian HM, Talpaz M, Estrov Z: Clinical significance of cytogenetic abnormalities in adult acute lymphoblastic leukemia. *Blood* 91:3995, 1998.

88. Group Français de Cytogénétique Hématologique: Cytogenetic abnormalities in adult acute lymphoblastic leukemia: correlations with hematologic findings and outcome. A collaborative study of the Groupe Français de Cytogénétique Hématologique. *Blood* 87:3135, 1996.

89. Martinez-Clement JA: Molecular cytogenetics of childhood hematological malignancies. *Leukemia* 11:1999,1997.

90. Synold TW, Relling MV, Boyett JM, et al: Blast cell methotrexate-polyglutamate accumulation in vivo differs by lineage, ploidy, and methotrexate dose in acute lymphoblastic leukemia. *J Clin Invest* 94:1996, 1994.

91. Kaspers GJL, Smets LA, Pieters R, et al: Favorable prognosis of hyperdiploid common acute lymphoblastic leukemia may be explained by sensitivity to antimetabolites and other drugs: results of an in vitro study. *Blood* 85:751, 1995.

92. Ito C, Kumagai M, Manabe A, et al: Hyperdiploid acute lymphoblastic leukemia with 51 to 65 chromosomes: a distinct biological entity with a marked propensity to undego apoptosis. *Blood* 93:315, 1999.

93. Pui CH, Carroll AJ, Raimondi SC, et al: Clinical presentation, karyotypic characterization, and treatment outcome of childhood acute lymphoblastic leukemia with a near-haploid or hypodiploid <45 line. *Blood* 75:1170, 1990.

94. Pui CH, Carroll AJ, Head D, et al: Near-triploid and near-tetraploid acute lymphoblastic leukemia of childhood. *Blood* 76:590, 1990.

95. Romana SP, Poirel H, Leconiat M, et al: High frequency of t(12;21) in childhood B-lineage acute lymphoblastic leukemia. *Blood* 86:4263, 1995.

96. Rubnitz JE, Pui CH, Downing JR: The role of *TEL* fusion genes in pediatric leukemias. *Leukemia* 13:6, 1999.

97. Scurto P, Hsu Rocha M, Kane JR, et al. A multiplex RT-PCR assay for the detection of chimeric transcripts encoded by the risk-stratifying translocations of pediatric acute lymphoblastic leukemia. *Leukemia* 12:1994, 1998.

98. Hasle H, Heim S, Schroeder H, et al: Transient pancytopenia preceding acute lymphoblastic leukemia (pre-ALL). *Leukemia* 9:605, 1995.

99. Morely AA, Brisco MJ, Rice M, et al: Leukaemia presenting as marrow hypoplasia: molecular detection of the leukaemic clone at the time of initial presentation. *Br J Haematol* 98:940, 1997.

100. Masson E, Synold TW, Relling MV, et al: Allopurinol inhibits de novo purine synthesis in lymphoblasts of children with acute lymphoblastic leukemia. *Leukemia* 10:56, 1996.

101. Keuzenkamp-Jansen CW, De Abrue RA, Bökkerink JPM, et al: Metabolism of intravenously administered high-dose 6-mercaptopurine with and without allopurinol treatment in patients with non-Hodgkin lymphoma. *J Pediatr Hematol/Oncol* 18:145, 1996.

102. Pui CH, Relling MN, Lascombes F, et al: Urate oxidase in prevention and treatment of hyperuricemia associated with lymphoid malignancies. *Leukemia* 11:1813, 1997.

103. Pui CH, Wiley JM, Woods GM, et al: Recombinant urate oxidase corrects hyperuricemia in patients treated for leukemia or lymphoma. *Blood* 92(suppl 1):482a, 1998.

104. Bunin NJ, Pui CH: Differing complications of hyperleukocytosis in children with acute lymphoblastic or acute nonlymphoblastic leukemia. *J Clin Oncol* 3:1590, 1985.

105. Maurer HS, Steinherz PG, Gaynon PS, et al: The effect of initial management of hyperleukocytosis on early complications and outcome of children with acute lymphoblastic leukemia. *J Clin Oncol* 6:1425, 1988.

106. Nelson SC, Bruggers CS, Kurtzberg J, Friedman HS: Management of leukemic hyperleukocytosis with hydration, urinary alkalinization, allopurinol. Are cranial irradiation and invasive cytoreduction necessary? *Am J Pediatr Hematol/Oncol* 15:351, 1993.

107. Basade M, Dhar AK, Kulkarni SS, et al: Rapid cytoreduction in childhood leukemic hyperleukocytosis by conservative therapy. *Med Pediatr Oncol* 25:204, 1995.

108. Patte C, Philip T, Rodary C, et al: High survival rate in advanced-stage B-cell lymphomas and leukemias without CNS involvement with a short intensive polychemotherapy: results from the French Pediatric Oncology Society of a randomized trial of 216 children. *J Clin Oncol* 9:123, 1991.

109. Pui CH, Boyett JM, Hughes WT, et al: Human granulocyte colony-stimulating factor after induction chemotherapy in children with acute lymphoblastic leukemia. *N Engl J Med* 336:1781, 1997.

110. Geissler K, Koller E, Hubmann E, et al: Granulocyte colony-stimulating factor as an adjunct to induction chemotherapy for adult acute lymphoblastic leukemia—a randomized phase-III study. *Blood* 90:590, 1997.

111. Larson RA, Dodge RK, Linker CA, et al: A randomized controlled trial of filgrastim during remission induction and consolidation chemotherapy for adults with acute lymphobastic leukemia: CALGB study 9111. *Blood* 92:1556, 1998.

112. Hughes WT, Rivera GK, Schell MJ, et al: Successful intermittent chemoprophylaxis for *Pneumocystis carinii* pneumonitis. *N Engl J Med* 316:1627, 1987.

113. Weinthal J, Frost JD, Briones G, Cairo MS: Successful *Pneumocystis carinii* pneumonia prophylaxis using aerosolized pentamidine in children with acute leukemia. *J Clin Oncol* 12:136, 1994.

114. Pui CH, Hughes WT, Evans WE, Crist WM: Prevention of *Pneumocystis carinii* pneumonia in children with cancer. *J Clin Oncol* 12:1522, 1994.

115. Hughes W, Leoung G, Kramer F, et al: Comparison of atovaquone (566C80) with trimethoprim-sulfamethoxazole to treat *Pneumocystis carinii* pneumonia in patients with AIDS. *N Engl J Med* 328:1521, 1993.

116. Pui CH, Jackson CW, Chesney C, et al: Sequential changes in platelet function and coagulation in leukemic children treated with L-asparaginase, prednisone, vincristine. *J Clin Oncol* 1:380, 1983.

117. Mitchell L, Hoogendoorn H, Giles AR, et al: Increased endogenous thrombin generation in children with acute lymphoblastic leukemia: risk of thrombotic complications in L-asparaginase-induced antithrombin III deficiency. *Blood* 83:386, 1994.

118. Heckman KD, Weiner GJ, Davis CS, et al: Randomized study of prophylactic platelet transfusion threshold during induction therapy for adult acute leukemia: 10,000/μL versus 20,000/μL. *J Clin Oncol* 15:1143, 1997.

119. Kaushansky K: Thrombopoietin. *N Engl J Med* 339:746, 1998.

120. Patte C: Pediatric update: non-Hodgkin's lymphoma. *Eur J Cancer* 34:359, 1998.

121. Reiter A, Schrappe M, Tiemann M, et al: Improved treatment results in childhood B-cell neoplasms with tailored intensification of therapy: a report of the Berlin-Frankfurt-Münster group trial NHL-BFM90. *Blood* 94:3294, 1999.

122. Bowman W, Shuster JJ, Cook B, et al: Improved survival for children with B-cell acute lymphoblastic leukemia and stage IV small noncleaved-cell lymphoma: a pediatric oncology group study. *J Clin Oncol* 14:1252, 1996.

123. Hoelzer D, Ludwig WD, Thiel E, et al: Improved outcome in adult B-cell acute lymphoblastic leukemia. *Blood* 87:495, 1996.

124. Soussain C, Patte C, Ostronoff M, et al: Small noncleaved cell lymphoma and leukemia in adults: a retrospective study of 65 adults treated with the LMB pediatric protocols. *Blood* 85:664, 1995.

125. Cortes JE, Kantarjian HM: Acute lymphoblastic leukemia: a comprehensive review with emphasis on biology and therapy. *Cancer* 76:2393, 1995.

126. Copelan EA, McGuire EA: The biology and treatment of acute lymphoblastic leukemia in adults. *Blood* 85:1151, 1995.

127. Laport GF, Larson RA: Treatment of adult acute lymphoblastic leukemia. *Semin Oncol* 24:70, 1997.

128. Campana D, Pui CH: Detection of minimal residual disease in acute leukemia: methodologic advances and clinical significance. *Blood* 85:1416, 1995.

129. Jacquy C, Delepaut B, VanDaele S, et al: A prospective study of minimal residual disease in childhood B-lineage acute lymphoblastic leukaemia: MRD level at the end of induction is a strong predictive factor of relapse. *Br J Haemat* 98:140, 1997.

130. Cave H, Bosch JV, Suciu S, et al: Clinical significance of minimal residual disease in childhood acute lymphoblastic leukemia. *N Engl J Med* 339:591, 1998.

131. Van Dongen JJM, Seriu T, Panzer-Grümayer ER, et al: Prognostic value of minimal residual disease in acute lymphoblastic leukemia in childhood. *Lancet* 352:1731, 1998.

132. Rivera GK, Raimondi SC, Hancock ML, et al: Improved outcome in childhood acute lymphoblastic leukaemia with reinforced early treatment and rotational combination chemotherapy. *Lancet* 337:61, 1991.

133. Neimeyer CM, Gelber RD, Tarbell NJ, et al: Low-dose versus high-dose methotrexate during remission induction in childhood acute lymphoblastic leukemia (protocol 81-01 update). *Blood* 78:2514, 1991.

134. Gaynon PS, Steinherz PG, Bleyer WA, et al: Improved therapy for children with acute lymphoblastic leukemia and unfavorable presenting features: a follow-up report of the Children's Cancer Group study CCG-106. *J Clin Oncol* 11:2234, 1993.

135. Linker CA, Levitt LJ, O'Donnell M, et al: Treatment of adult acute lymphoblastic leukemia with intensive cyclical chemotherapy: a follow-up report. *Blood* 78:2814, 1991.

136. Todeschini G, Tecchio C, Meneghini V, et al: Estimated 6-year event-free survival of 55% in 60 consecutive adult acute lymphoblastic leukemia patients treated with an intensive phase II protocol based on high induction dose of daunorubicin. *Leukemia* 12: 144, 1998.

137. Daenen S, Van Imhoff GW, Van Den Berg E, et al: Improved outcome of adult acute lymphoblastic leukaemia by moderately intensified chemotherapy which includes a "pre-induction" course for rapid tumour reduction: preliminary results on 66 patients. *Br J Haematol* 100:273, 1998.

138. Balis FM, Lester CM, Chrousos GP, et al: Differences in cerebrospinal fluid penetration of corticosteriods: possible relationship to the prevention of meningeal leukemia. *J Clin Oncol* 5:202, 1987.

139. Jones B, Freeman AI, Shuster JJ, et al: Lower incidence of meningeal leukemia when prednisone is replaced by dexamethasone in the treatment of acute lymphocytic leukemia. *Med Pediatr Oncol* 19:269, 1991.

140. Bostrom B, Gaynon PS, Sather H, et al: Dexamethasone (DEX) decreases central nervous system (CNS) relapse and improves event-free survival (EFS) in lower risk acute lymphoblastic leukemia (ALL). *Proc Am Soc Clin Oncol* 17:527, 1998.

141. Asselin BL, Whitin JC, Coppola DJ, et al: Comparative pharmacokinetic studies of three asparaginase preparations. *J Clin Oncol* 11:1780, 1993.

142. Otten J, Suciu S, Luz P, et al: The importance of L-asparaginase (A'ase) in the treatment of acute lymphoblastic leukemia (ALL) in children: results of the EORTC 58881 randomized phase III trial showing greater efficiency of *Escherichia coli (E. coli)* as compared to *Erwinia (Erw)* A'ase. *Blood* 88(suppl 1):669, 1996.

143. Boos J, Werber G, Ahlke E, et al: Monitoring of asparaginase activity and asparagine levels in children on different asparaginase preparations. *Eur J Cancer* 32a:1544, 1996.

144. Ahlke E, Nowak-Göttl U, Schulze-Westhoff P, et al: Dose reduction of asparaginase under pharmacokinetic and pharmacodynamic control during induction therapy in children with acute lymphoblastic leukaemia. *Br J Haematol* 96:675, 1997.

145. Liang DC, Hung IJ, Yang CP, et al: Unexpected mortality from the use of *E. coli* L-asparaginase during remission induction therapy for childhood acute lymphoblastic leukemia: a report from the Taiwan Pediatric Oncology Group. *Leukemia* 13:155, 1999.

146. Cuttner J, Mick R, Budman DR, et al: Phase III trial of brief intensive treatment of adult acute lymphocytic leukemia comparing daunorubicin and mitoxantrone: a CALGB study. *Leukemia* 5:425, 1991.

147. Fiére D, Lepage E, Sebban C, et al: Adult acute lymphoblastic leukemia: a multicentric randomized trial testing bone marrow transplantation as postremission therapy. *J Clin Oncol* 11:1990, 1993.

148. Mahoney DH, Shuster J, Nitschke R, et al: Intermediate-dose intravenous methotrexate with intravenous mercaptopurine is superior to repetitive low-dose oral methotrexate with intravenous mercaptopurine for children with lower-risk B-lineage acute lymphoblastic leukemia: a Pediatric Oncology Group Phase III trial. *J Clin Oncol* 16:246, 1998.

149. Veerman AJP, Hählen K, Kamps WA, et al: High cure rate with a moderately intensive treatment regimen in non-high-risk childhood acute lymphoblastic leukemia: results of protocol ALL VI from the Dutch Childhood Leukemia Study group. *J Clin Oncol* 14:991, 1996.

150. Schorin MA, Blattner S, Gelber RD, et al: Treatment of childhood acute lymphoblastic leukemia: results of Dana-Farber Cancer Institute/ Children's Hospital Acute Lymphoblastic Leukemia Consortium Protocol 85-01. *J Clin Oncol* 12:740, 1994.

151. Chessells JM, Bailey C, Richards SM: Intensification of treatment and survival in all children with lymphoblastic leukaemia: results of UK Medical Research Council Trial UKALL X. *Lancet* 345:143, 1995.

152. Synold TW, Relling MV, Boyett JM, et al: Blast cell methotrexate-polyglutamate accumulation in vivo differs by lineage, ploidy, and methotrexate dose in acute lymphoblastic leukemia. *J Clin Invest* 94:1996, 1994.

153. Galpin AJ, Schuetz JD, Masson E, et al: Differences in folylpolyglutamate synthetase and dihydrofolate reductase expression in human B-lineage versus T-lineage leukemic lymphoblast: mechanisms for lineage differences in methotrexate polyglutamylation and cytotoxicity. *Mol Pharm* 52:155, 1997.

154. Evans WE, Crom WR, Abromowitch M, et al: Clinical pharmocodynamics of high-dose methotrexate in acute lymphocytic leukemia. Identification of a relation between concentration and effect. *N Engl J Med* 314:471, 1986.

155. Evans WE, Relling MV, Rodman JH, et al: Conventional compared with individualized chemotherapy for childhood acute lymphoblastic leukemia. *N Engl J Med* 338:499, 1998.

156. Ellison RR, Mick R, Cuttner J, et al: The effects of postinduction intensification treatment with cytarabine and daunorubicin in adult acute lymphocytic leukemia: a prospective randomized clinical trial by Cancer and Leukemia Group B. *J Clin Oncol* 9:2002, 1991.

157. Cassileth PA, Anderson JW, Bennett JM, et al: Adult acute lymphocytic leukemia: the Eastern Cooperative Oncology Group experience. *Leukemia* 6(suppl 2):178, 1992.

158. Stryckmans P, DeWitte TH, Marie JP, et al: Therapy of adult ALL: overview of 2 successive EORTC studies: (ALL-2 & ALL-3). *Leukemia* 6(suppl 2):199, 1992.

159. Hoelzer D, Thiel E, Ludwig WD, et al: The German multicentre trials for treatment of acute lymphoblastic leukemia in adults. *Leukemia* 6(suppl 2):175, 1992.

160. Rohatiner AZS, Bassan R, Battista R, et al: High dose cytosine arabinoside in the initial treatment of adults with acute lymphoblastic leukaemia. *Br J Cancer* 62:454, 1990.

161. Ludwig WD, Rieder H, Bartram CR, et al: Immunophenotypic and genotypic features, clinical characteristics, and treatment outcome of adult pro-B acute lymphoblastic leukemia: results of the German multicenter trials GMALL 03/87 and 04/89. *Blood* 92:1898, 1998.

162. Riehm H, Gadner H, Henze G, et al: Results and significance of six randomized trials in four consecutive ALL-BFM studies. *Haem Blood Trans* 33:439, 1990.

163. Childhood ALL Collaborative Group: Duration and intensity of maintenance chemotherapy in acute lymphoblastic leukaemia: overview of 42 trials involving 12,000 randomised children. *Lancet* 347:1783, 1996.

164. Sather H, Miller D, Nesbit M, et al: Differences in prognosis for boys and girls with acute lymphoblastic leukaemia. *Lancet* i:741, 1981.

165. The Medical Research Council's Working Party on Leukaemia in Childhood: Duration of chemotherapy-in-childhood acute lymphoblastic leukaemia. *Med Pediatr Oncol* 10:511, 1982.

166. Trigg ME, Sather H, Coccia P, et al: Duration of maintenance therapy for childhood acute lymphoblastic leukemia. *Proc ASCO* 12:324a, 1993.

167. Lennard L, Lilleyman JS, Loon JV, Weinshilboum RM: Genetic variation in response to 6-mercaptopurine for childhood acute lymphoblastic leukaemia. *Lancet* 336:225, 1990.

168. Whitehead VM, Vuchich MJ, Lauer SJ, et al: Accumulation of high levels of methotrexate polyglutamates in lymphoblasts from children with hyperdiploid (>50 chromosomes) B-lineage acute lymphoblastic leukemia: a Pediatric Oncology Group Study. *Blood* 80:1316, 1992.

169. Schmiegelow K, Schrøder H, Gustafsson G, et al: Risk of relapse in childhood acute lymphoblastic leukemia is related to RBC methotrexate and mercaptopurine metabolites during maintenance chemotherapy. *J Clin Oncol* 13:345, 1995.

170. Chessells JM, Harrison G, Lilleyman JS, et al: Continuing (maintenance) therapy in lymphoblastic leukaemia: lessons from MRC UKALL X. *Br J Haematol* 98:945, 1997.

171. Relling MV, Hancock ML, Boyett JM, et al: Prognostic importance of 6-mercaptopurine dose intensity in acute lymphoblastic leukemia. *Blood* 93:2817, 1999.

172. Schmiegelow K, Glomstein A, Kristinsson J, et al: Impact of morning

versus evening schedule for oral methotrexate and 6-mercaptopurine on relapse risk for children with acute lymphoblastic leukemia. *J Pediatr Hematol/Oncol* 19:102, 1997.

173. Rivard GE, Lin KT, Leclerc JM, David M: Milk could decrease the bioavailability of 6-mercaptopurine. *Am J Pediatr Hematol/Oncol* 11:402, 1989.

174. Lancaster D, Lennard L, Lilleyman JS: Profile of non-compliance in lymphoblastic leukaemia. *Arch Dis Child* 76:365, 1997.

175. Mahoney DH, Shuster J, Nitschke R, et al: Intermediate-dose intravenous methotrexate with intravenous mercaptopurine is superior to repetitive low-dose oral methotrexate with intravenous mercaptopurine for children with lower-risk B-lineage acute lymphoblastic leukemia: a Pediatric Oncology Group Phase III trial. *J Clin Oncol* 16:246, 1998.

176. Farrow AC, Buchanan GR, Zwiener RJ, et al: Serum aminotransferase elevation during and following treatment of childhood acute lymphoblastic leukemia. *J Clin Oncol* 15:1560, 1997.

177. Evans WE, Horner M, Chu YQ, et al: Altered mercaptopurine metabolism, toxic effects, and dosage requirement in a thiopurine methyltransferase-deficient child with acute lymphocytic leukemia. *J Pediatr* 119:985, 1991.

178. Relling MV, Hancock ML, Rivera GK, et al: Mercaptopurine therapy intolerance and heterozygosity at the thiopurine *S*-methyltransferase gene locus. *J Natl Cancer Inst* 91:2001, 1999.

179. Yates CR, Krynetski EY, :pemmecjem T, et al: Molecular diagnosis of thiopurine *S*-methyltransferase deficiency: genetic basis for azathioprine and mercaptopurine intolerance. *Ann Intern Med* 126:608, 1997.

180. Nachman J, Sather HN, Gaynon PS, et al: Augmented Berlin-Frankfurt-Munster therapy abrogates the adverse prognostic significance of slow early response to induction chemotherapy for children and adolescents with acute lymphoblastic leukemia and unfavorable presenting features: a report from the Children's Cancer Group. *J Clin Oncol* 15:2222, 1997.

181. Nachman JB, Sather HN, Sensel M, et al: Augmented post-induction therapy for children with high-risk acute lymphoblastic leukemia and a slow response to initial therapy. *N Engl J Med* 338:1663, 1998.

182. Sackmann-Muriel F, Pavlovsky S, Lastiri F, et al: Latin American trials in childhood acute lymphoblastic leukemia. GATLA/GLATHEM report of results from 1967 through 1994. *Int J Pediatr Hematol/Oncol* 5:177, 1998.

183. Pinkel D, Woo S: Prevention and treatment of meningeal leukemia in children. *Blood* 84:355, 1994.

184. Kantarjian HM, O'Brien S, Smith TL, et al: Results of treatment with Hyper-CVAD, a dose-intensive regimen, in adult acute lymphocytic leukemia. *J Clin Oncol* 18:547, 2000.

185. Conter V, Aricò M, Valsecchi MG, et al: Extended intrathecal methotrexate may replace cranial irradiation for prevention of CNS relapse in children with intermediate-risk acute lymphoblastic leukemia treated with Berlin-Frankfurt-Münster-based intensive chemotherapy. *J Clin Oncol* 13:2497, 1995.

186. Conter V, Schrappe M, Aricò M, et al: Role of cranial radiotherapy for childhood T-cell acute lymphoblastic leukemia with high WBC count and good response to prednisone. *J Clin Oncol* 15:2786, 1997.

187. Chao NJ, Forman SJ, Schmidt GM, et al: Allogeneic bone marrow transplantation for high-risk acute lymphoblastic leukemia during first complete remission. *Blood* 78:1923, 1991.

188. De Witte T, Awwad B, Boezeman J, et al: Role of allogeneic bone marrow transplantation in adolescent or adult patients with acute lymphoblastic leukaemia or lymphoblastic lymphoma in first remission. *Bone Marrow Transplant* 14:767, 1994.

189. Sebban C, Lepage E, Vernant JP, et al: Allogeneic bone marrow transplantation in adult acute lymphoblastic leukemia in first complete remission: a comparative study. *J Clin Oncol* 12:2580, 1994.

190. Chessells JM, Bailey C, Wheeler K, Richards SM: Bone marrow transplantation for high-risk childhood lymphoblastic leukaemia in first remission: experience in MRC UKALL X. *Lancet* 340:565, 1992.

191. Appelbaum FR: Allogeneic hematopoietic stem cell transplantation for acute leukemia. *Semin Oncol* 24:114, 1997.

192. Marks DI, Bird JM, Cornish JM, et al: Unrelated donor bone marrow transplantation for children and adolescents with Philadelphia-positive acute lymphoblastic leukemia. *J Clin Oncol* 16:931, 1998.

193. Ribeiro RC, Broniscer A, Rivera GK, et al: Philadelphia chromosome-positive acute lymphoblastic leukemia in children: durable responses to chemotherapy associated with low initial white blood cell counts. *Leukemia* 11:1493, 1997.

194. Schrappe M, Aricò M, Harbott J, et al: Philadelphia chromosome-positive (Ph+) childhood acute lymphoblastic leukemia: good initial steroid response allows early prediction of a favorable treatment outcome. *Blood* 92:2730, 1998.

195. Pui CH, Frankel LS, Carroll AJ, et al: Clinical characteristics and treatment outcome of childhood acute lymphoblastic leukemia with the t(4;11) (q21;q23): a collaborative study of 40 cases. *Blood* 77:440, 1991.

196. Johansson B, Moorman AV, Haas OA, et al: Hematologic malignancies with t(4;11) (q21;q23)—a cytogenetic, morphologic, immunopheno-typic and clinical study of 183 cases. *Leukemia* 12:779, 1998.

197. Vora A, Frost L, Goodeve A, et al: Late relapsing childhood lymphoblastic leukemia. *Blood* 92:2334, 1998.

198. Pui CH, Boyett JM, Relling MV, et al: Sex differences in prognosis for children with acute lymphoblastic leukemia. *J Clin Oncol* 17:818, 1999.

199. Bunin NJ, Pui CH, Hustu HO, Rivera GK: Unusual extramedullary relapses in children with acute lymphoblastic leukemia. *J Pediatr* 109:665, 1986.

200. Henze G, Fengler R, Hartmann R, et al: Six-year experience with a comprehensive approach to the treatment of recurrent childhood acute lymphoblastic leukemia (All-REZ BFM 85). A relapse study of the BFM group. *Blood* 78:1166, 1991.

201. Sadowitz PD, Smith SD, Shuster J, et al: Treatment of late bone marrow relapse in children with acute lymphoblastic leukemia: A Pediatric Oncology Group study. *Blood* 81:602, 1993.

202. Schroeder H, Garwicz S, Kristinsson J, et al: Outcome after first relapse in children with acute lymphoblastic leukemia: a population-based study of 315 patients from the Nordic Society of Pediatric Hematology and Oncology (NOPHO). *Med Pediatr Oncol* 25:372, 1995.

203. Bührer C, Hartmann R, Fengler R, et al: Peripheral blast counts at diagnosis of late isolated bone marrow relapse of childhood acute lymphoblastic leukemia predict response to salvage chemotherapy and outcome. *J Clin Oncol* 14:2812, 1996.

204. Beyermann B, Adams HP, Henze G: Philadelphia chromosome in relapsed childhood acute lymphoblastic leukemia; a matched-pair analysis. *J Clin Oncol* 15:2231, 1997.

205. Gaynon PS, Qu RP, Chappell RJ, et al: Survival after relapse in childhood acute lymphoblastic leukemia. Impact of site and time to first relapse—the Children's Cancer Group experience. *Cancer* 82:1387, 1998.

206. Guglielmi C, Cordone I, Boecklin F, et al: Immunophenotype of adult and childhood acute lymphoblastic leukemia: changes at first relapse and clinico-prognostic implications. *Leukemia* 11:1501, 1997.

207. Barrett AJ, Horowitz MM, Pollock BH, et al: Bone marrow transplants form HLA-identical siblings as compared with chemotherapy for children with acute lymphoblastic leukemia in a second remission. *N Engl J Med* 331:1253, 1994.

208. Uderzo C, Valsecchi MG, Bacigalupo A, et al: Treatment of childhood acute lymphoblastic leukemia in second remission with allogenic bone marrow transplantation and chemotherapy: ten-year experience of the Italian Bone Marrow Transplantation Group and the Italian Pediatric Hematology Oncology Association. *J Clin Oncol* 13:352, 1995.

209. Feig SA, Harris RE, Sather HN: Bone marrow transplantation versus chemotherapy for maintenance of second remission of childhood acute lymphoblastic leukemia: a study of the Children's Cancer Group (CCG-1884). *Med Pediatr Oncol* 29:534, 1997.

210. Bordigoni P, Esperou H, Souillet G, et al: Total body irradiation-high-dose cytosine arabinoside and melphalan followed by allogeneic bone marrow transplantation from HLA-identical siblings in the treatment of children with acute lymphoblastic leukaemia after relapse while receiving chemotherapy: a Société Française de Greffe de Moelle study. *Br J Haematol* 102:656, 1998.

211. Martino R, Bellido M, Brunet S, et al: Allogeneic or autologous stem cell transplantation following salvage chemotherapy for adults with refractory or relapsed acute lymphoblastic leukemia. *Bone Marrow Transplant* 21:1023, 1998.

212. Boulad F, Steinherz P, Reyes, B, et al. Allogeneic bone marrow transplantation versus chemotherapy for the treatment of childhood acute lymphoblastic leukemia in second remission: a single-institution study. *J Clin Oncol* 17:197, 1999.

213. Zecca M, Pession A, Messina C, et al: Total body irradiation, thiotepa, and cyclophosphamide as a conditioning regimen for children with acute

lymphoblastic leukemia in first or second remission undergoing bone marrow transplantation with HLA-identical siblings. *J Clin Oncol* 17:1838, 1999.

214. Borgmann A, Schmid H, Hartmann R, et al: Autologous bone-marrow transplants compared with chemotherapy for children with acute lymphoblastic leukaemia in a second remission: a matched-pair analysis. *Lancet* 346:873, 1995.

215. Weisdorf DJ, Billett AL, Hannan P, et al: Autologous versus unrelated donor allogeneic marrow transplantation for acute lymphoblastic leukemia. *Blood* 90:2962, 1997.

216. Wheeler K, Richards S, Bailey C, Chessells J: Comparison of bone marrow transplant and chemotherapy for relapsed childhood acute lymphoblastic leukaemia: the MRC UKALL X experience. *Br J Haematol* 101:94, 1998.

217. Davies SM, Wagner JE, Shu XO, et al: Unrelated donor bone marrow transplantation for children with acute leukemia. *J Clin Oncol* 15:557, 1997.

218. Hongeng S, Krance RA, Bowman LC, et al: Outcomes of transplantation with matched-sibling and unrelated-donor bone marrow in children with leukaemia. *Lancet* 350:767, 1997.

219. Kurtzberg J, Laughlin M, Graham ML, et al: Placental blood as a source of hematopoietic stem cells for transplantation into unrelated recipients. *N Engl J Med* 335:157, 1996.

220. Gluckman E, Rocha V, Boyer-Chammard A, et al: Outcome of cord blood transplantation from related and unrelated donors. *N Engl J Med* 337:373, 1997.

221. Rubinstein P, Carrier C, Scaradavou A, et al: Outcomes among 562 recipients of placental-blood transplants from unrelated donors. *N Engl J Med* 339:1565, 1998.

222. Aversa F, Tabilio A, Veldardi A, et al: Treatment of high-risk acute leukemia with T-cell depleted stem cells from related donors with one fully mismatched HLA haplotype. *N Engl J Med* 339:1186, 1998.

223. Bosi A, Bacci S, Miniero R, et al: Second allogeneic bone marrow transplantation in acute leukemia: a multicenter study from the Gruppo Italiano Trapianto Di Midollo Osseo (GITMO). *Leukemia* 11:420, 1997.

224. Atra A, Millar B, Shepherd V, et al: Donor lymphocyte infusion for childhood acute lymphoblastic leukaemia relapsing after bone marrow transplantation. *Br J Haematol* 97:165, 1997.

225. Bührer C, Hartmann R, Fengler R, et al: Importance of effective central nervous system therapy in isolated bone marrow relapse of childhood acute lymphoblastic leukemia. *Blood* 83:3468, 1994.

226. Neale GAM, Pui CH, Mahmoud HH, et al: Molecular evidence for minimal residual bone marrow disease in children with "isolated" extramedullary relapse of T-cell acute lymphoblastic leukemia. *Leukemia* 8:768, 1994.

227. Lal A, Kwan E, Al Mahr M, et al: Molecular detection of acute lymphoblastic leukemia in boys with testicular relapse. *J Clin Pathol: Mol Pathol* 51:277, 1998.

228. Ribeiro RC, Rivera GK, Hudson M, et al: An intensive re-treatment protocol for children with an isolated CNS relapse of acute lymphoblastic leukemia. *J Clin Oncol* 13:333, 1995.

229. Ritchey AK, Pollock BH, Lauer SJ, et al: Improved survival of children with isolated CNS relapse of acute lymphoblastic leukemia: a Pediatric Oncology Group study. *J Clin Oncol* 17:3745, 1999.

230. Messina C, Valsecchi MG, Aricò M, et al: Autologous bone marrow transplantation for treatment of isolated central nervous system relapse of childhood acute lymphoblastic leukemia. *Bone Marrow Transplant* 21:9, 1998.

231. Uderzo C, Zurlo MG, Adamoli L, et al: Treatment of isolated testicular relapse in childhood acute lymphoblastic leukemia: an Italian multicenter study. *J Clin Oncol* 8:672, 1990.

232. Buchanan GR, Boyett JM, Pollock BH, et al: Improved treatment results in boys with overt testicular relapse during or shortly after initial therapy for acute lymphoblastic leukemia: a Pediatric Oncology Group study. *Cancer* 68:48, 1991.

233. Wofford MM, Smith SD, Shuster JJ, et al: Treatment of occult or late overt testicular relapse in children with acute lymphoblastic leukemia: a Pediatric Oncology Group study. *J Clin Oncol* 10:624, 1992.

234. Finklestein JZ, Miller DR, Feusner J, et al: Treatment of overt isolated testicular relapse in children on therapy for acute lymphoblastic leukemia. A report from the Children's Cancer Group. *Cancer* 73:219, 1994.

235. Grundy RG, Leiper AD, Stanhope R, Chessells JM: Survival and endo-
crine outome after testicular relapse in acute lymphoblastic leukaemia. *Arch Dis Child* 76:190, 1997.

236. Van den Berg H, Langeveld NE, Veenhof CHN, Behrendt H: Treatment of isolated testicular recurrence of acute lymphoblastic leukemia without radiotherapy. Report from the Dutch Late Effects Study Group. *Cancer* 79:2257, 1997.

237. Pui CH, Burghen GA, Bowman WP, Aur RJA: Risk factors for hyperglycemia in children with leukemia receiving L-asparaginase and prednisone. *J Pediatr* 99:46, 1981.

238. Pui CH, Chesney CM, Weed J, Jackson CW: Altered von Willebrand factor molecule in children with thrombosis following asparaginase-prednisone-vincristine therapy for leukemia. *J Clin Oncol* 3:1266, 1985.

239. Pihko H, Tyni T, Virkola K, et al: Transient ischemic cerebral lesions during induction chemotherapy for acute lymphoblastic leukemia. *J Pediatr* 123:718, 1993.

240. Winick NJ, Bowman WP, Kamen BA, et al: Unexpected acute neurologic toxicity in the treatment of children with acute lymphoblastic leukemia. *J Natl Cancer Inst* 84:252, 1992.

241. Mahoney DH, Shuster JJ, Nitschke R, et al: Acute neurotoxicity in children with B-precursor acute lymphoid leukemia: an association with intermediate-dose intravenous methotrexate and intrathecal triple therapy—a Pediatric Oncology Group study. *J Clin Oncol* 16:1712, 1998.

242. Rubnitz JE, Relling MV, Harrison PL, et al: Transient encephalopathy following high-dose methotrexate treatment in childhood acute lymphoblastic leukemia. *Leukemia* 12:1176, 1998.

243. Chan-Lam D, Prentice AG, Copplestone JA, et al: Avascular necrosis of bone following intensified steroid therapy for acute lymphoblastic leukaemia and high-grade malignant lymphoma. *Br J Haematol* 86:227, 1994.

244. Ojala AE, Lanning FP, Pääkkö E, Lanning BM: Osteonecrosis in children treated for acute lymphoblastic leukemia: a magnetic resonance imaging study after treatment. *Med Pediatr Oncol* 29:260, 1997.

245. Ojala AE, Pääkkö E, Lanning FP, Lanning M: Osteonecrosis during the treatment of childhood acute lymphoblastic leukemia: a prospective MRI study. *Med Pediatr Oncol* 32:11, 1999.

246. Körholz D, Bruder M, Engelbrecht V, et al: Aseptic osteonecrosis in children with acute lymphoblastic leukemia. *Pediatr Hematol/Oncol* 15:307, 1998.

247. Nysom K, Holm K, Michaelsen KF, et al: Bone mass after treatment for acute lymphoblastic leukemia in childhood. *J Clin Oncol* 16:3752, 1998.

248. Boot AM, van den Heuvel-Eibrink MM, Hählen K, et al: Bone mineral density in children with acute lymphoblastic leukemia. *Ear J Cancer* 35:1693, 1999.

249. Lipshultz SE, Lipsitz SR, Mone SM, et al: Female sex and higher drug dose as risk factors for late cardiotoxic effects of doxorubicin therapy for childhood cancer. *N Engl J Med* 332:1738, 1995.

250. Grenier MA, Lipshultz SE: Epidemiology of anthracycline cardiotoxicity in children and adults. *Semin Oncol* 25:72, 1998.

251. Sorensen K, Levitt G, Bull C, et al: Anthracycline dose in childhood acute lymphoblastic leukemia: issues of early survival versus late cardiotoxicity. *J Clin Oncol* 15:61, 1997.

252. Nysom K, Holm K, Lipsitz SR, et al: Relationship between cumulative anthracycline dose and late cardiotoxicity in childhood acute lymphoblastic leukemia. *J Clin Oncol* 16:545, 1998.

253. Wexler LH: Ameliorating anthracycline cardiotoxicity in children with cancer: clinical trials with dexrazoxane. *Semin Oncol* 25:86, 1998.

254. Walter AW, Hancock ML, Pui CH, et al: Secondary brain tumors in children treated for acute lymphoblastic leukemia at St. Jude Children's Research Hospital. *J Clin Oncol* 16:3761, 1998.

255. Relling MV, Rubnitz JE, Rivera GK, et al: High incidence of secondary brain tumors after radiotherapy and antimetabolites. *Lancet* 354:34, 1999.

256. Pui CH, Ribeiro RC, Hancock ML, et al: Acute myeloid leukemia in children treated with epipodophyllotoxins for acute lymphoblastic leukemia. *N Engl J Med* 325:1682, 1991.

257. Pui C-P, Relling MV: Topoisomerase II inhibitor–related acute myeloid leukemia. *Br J Haematol* (in press).

258. Hawkins MM, Draper GJ, Winter DL: Cancer in the offspring of survivors of childhood leukaemia and non-Hodgkin lymphomas. *Br J Cancer* 71:1335, 1995.

259. Kenney LB, Nicholson HS, Brasseux C, et al: Birth defects in offspring of adult survivors of childhood acute lymphoblastic leukemia. A Children's

Cancer Group/National Institutes of Health Report. *Cancer* 78:169, 1996.

260. Sankila R, Olsen JH, Anderson H, et al: Risk of cancer among offspring of childhood-cancer survivors. *N Engl J Med* 338:1339, 1998.

261. Pui C-H, Crist WM: Biology and treatment of acute lymphoblastic leukemia. *J Pediatr* 124:491, 1994.

262. Smith M, Arthur D, Camitta B, et al: Uniform approach to risk classification and treatment assignment for children with acute lymphoblastic leukemia. *J Clin Oncol* 14:18, 1996.

263. Ellison RR, Mick R, Cuttner J, et al: The effects of postinduction intensification treatment with cytarabine and daunorubicin in adult acute lymphocytic leukemia: a prospective randomized clinical trial by Cancer and Leukemia Group B. *J Clin Oncol* 9:2002, 1991.

264. Taylor PRA, Reid MM, Bown N, et al: Acute lymphoblastic leukemia in patients aged 60 years and over: a population-based study of incidence and outcome. *Blood* 80:1813, 1992.

265. Boucheix C, David B, Sebban C, et al: Immunophenotype of adult acute lymphoblastic leukemia, clinical parameters, and outcome: an analysis of a prospective trial including 562 tested patients (LALA87). *Blood* 84:1603, 1994.

266. Chessells JM, Richards SM, Bailey CC, et al: Gender and treatment outcome in childhood lymphoblastic leukaemia: report from the MRC UKALL trials.*Br J Haematol* 89:364, 1995.

267. Shuster JJ, Wacker P, Pullen J, et al: Prognostic significance of sex in childhood B-precursor acute lymphoblastic leukemia: a Pediatric Oncology Group Study. *J Clin Oncol* 16:2854, 1998.

268. Pui C-H, Boyett JM, Hancock ML, et al: Outcome of treatment for childhood cancer in black as compared with white children. The St. Jude Children's Research Hospital experience, 1962 through 1992. *JAMA* 273:633, 1995.

269. Pui C-H, Kane JR, Crist WM: Biology and treatment of infant leukemias. *Leukemia* 9:762, 1995.

270. Behm FG, Raimondi SC, Frestedt JL, et al: Rearrangement of the *MLL* gene confers a poor prognosis in childhood acute lymphoblastic leukemia, regardless of presenting age. *Blood* 87:2870, 1996.

271. Rubnitz JE, Camitta BM, Mahmoud H, et al: Childhood acute lymphoblastic leukemia with the *MLL-ENL* fusion and t(11;19)(q23;p13.3) translocation. *J Clin Oncol* 17:191, 1999.

272. Dordelmann M, Reiter A, Borkhardt A, et al: Prednisone response is the strongest predictor of treatment outcome in infant acute lymphoblastic leukemia. *Blood* 94:1209, 1999.

273. Aricò M, Valsecchi MG, Camitta B, et al: Treatment of Philadelphia-chromosome positive acute lymphoblastic leukemia in 326 children. *N Engl J Med* (in press).

274. Gajjar A, Ribeiro R, Hancock ML, et al: Persistence of circulating blasts after 1 week of multiagent chemotherapy confers a poor prognosis in childhood acute lymphoblastic leukemia. *Blood* 86:1292, 1995.

275. Lilleyman JS, Gibson BES, Stevens RF, et al: Clearance of marrow infiltration after 1 week of therapy for childhood lymphoblastic leukaemia: clinical importance and the effect of daunorubicin. *Br J Haematol* 97:603, 1997.

276. Gaynon PS, Desai AA, Bostrom BC, et al: Early response to therapy and outcome in childhood acute lymphoblastic leukemia. A review. *Cancer* 80:1717, 1997.

277. Panzer-Grümayer ER, Schneider M, Panzer S, et al: Rapid molecular response during early induction chemotherapy predicts a good outcome in childhood acute lymphoblastic leukemia. *Blood* 95:790, 2000.

278. Pui C-H, Campana D: New definition of remission in childhood acute lymphoblastic leukemia. *Leukemia* (in press).

CHRONIC LYMPHOCYTIC LEUKEMIA AND RELATED DISEASES

THOMAS J. KIPPS

Chronic lymphocytic leukemia (CLL) is a neoplastic disease characterized by the accumulation of small mature-appearing CD5+ B lymphocytes in the blood, marrow, and lymphoid tissues. The causes of this disease are unknown, although it appears likely that genetic factors contribute to its development. The leukemic cells from nearly 50 percent of CLL patients can be found to have clonal chromosomal abnormalities, of which del 13q14-23.1 is the most common chromosomal abnormality in CLL, followed in order by trisomy 12, del 11q22.3-q23.1, del 6q21-q23, and 14q abnormalities. Mutations of the P53 tumor suppressor gene at 17q13 are uncommon except in advanced disease. Assessing for clinical stage and various prognostic markers can be useful in deciding when to initiate therapy. Treatment with chlorambucil, with or without prednisone, has been the mainstay of initial treatment, although recent studies confirm the high activity of deoxyadenosine analogs such as fludarabine in this disease. Combination drug therapy has not been shown to be more effective as frontline therapy. However, new drug combinations, autologous and allogeneic stem cell transplantation, monoclonal antibodies, and gene therapy are being evaluated, as there are no established cures or demonstrated survival benefit from current treatments. This chapter also discusses prolymphocytic leukemia, which can be of B- or T-cell origin. The latter includes cases that formerly were designated T-cell CLL. Although B-cell prolymphocytic leukemia can evolve from preexisting cases of CLL, it has many distinctive features including a more adverse clinical outcome. Treatments for B-cell prolymphocytic leukemia are similar to those used in CLL, but the response rates are lower and of shorter duration. Similarly, T-cell prolymphocytic leukemia is more aggressive than CLL. Rearrangements and mutations in the ataxia-telangiectasia mutated gene and in T-cell leukemia 1 (TCL-1) and related genes apparently contribute to the pathogenesis of T-cell prolymphocytic leukemia. About a third of patients will have cutaneous involvement causing erythroderma. Treatment with deoxyadenosine analogs appears effective in a subset of patients with this disease. Investigation into the use of new agents, stem cell transplantation, and/or monoclonal antibodies, such as CAMPATH-1H, is ongoing, as there are no established cures.

CHRONIC LYMPHOCYTIC LEUKEMIA

DEFINITION AND HISTORY

Chronic lymphocytic leukemia is a neoplastic disease characterized by the accumulation of small mature-appearing lymphocytes in the blood, marrow, and lymphoid tissues. CLL has an average incidence of 2.7 persons per 100,000 in the United States. The risk of developing CLL increases progressively with age and is 2.8 times higher for older men than for older women.[1] Because of its relative indolence, this disease accounts for approximately 0.8 percent of all cancers and nearly 30 percent of all leukemias at any point in time. It is the most common adult leukemia in Western societies. Generally, the neoplastic lymphocytes are of the B-cell lineage. In less than 2 percent of cases, however, the neoplastic cells are of T-cell origin and are considered under the heading T-cell prolymphocytic leukemia.

The first descriptions of patients with CLL were published in the early nineteenth century.[2-4] In the 1840s, Virchow described two forms of chronic leukemia, these probably corresponding to CLL and chronic myelogenous leukemia.[4-6] Patients with the former were noted to have mild-to-moderate splenic enlargement, lymphadenopathy, and large numbers of small agranular cells in the blood that resembled those found in enlarged lymph nodes.[5] Virchow considered this type of leukemia to be principally related to disease of the lymph nodes rather than of the spleen. In 1893, Kundrat introduced the term lymphosarcoma to describe an indolent disease that affected lymph nodes.[7] Histochemical staining techniques introduced by Ehrlich at the turn of the century[8] made it possible for pathologists to distinguish between myeloid and lymphocytic leukemias. These methods enabled Türk in 1903 to establish a relationship of the leukemic cells in CLL to those in lymphosarcoma.[9] He proposed the term lymphomatoses to describe several lymphoproliferative disorders including CLL. Owing to its indolent nature, CLL was considered a "benign" lymphomatosis.

In 1924, Minot and Isaacs described the natural history of 98 patients with CLL,[10] challenging the notion that CLL was a "benign" process. These investigators noted that although gamma radiation could reduce lymph node enlargement or splenomegaly, it apparently did not prolong survival. Radioactive phosphorus later was found effective in reducing lymph node swelling.[11] However, this also was noted to be of limited therapeutic value because of its marrow toxicity and its inability to reverse disease-related cytopenias or to improve survival.[11] In 1954, Tivey published the survival data of 685 patients with CLL, observing that the median survival time was approximately 3 years from the onset of symptoms related to CLL.[12] Soon thereafter,

Acronyms and abbreviations that appear in this chapter include: ACE, cytosine arabinoside, cisplatin, and etoposide; ADCC, antibody-dependent cellular cytotoxicity; A-T, ataxia-telangiectasia; ATM gene, ataxia-telangiectasia mutated gene; BCL-1, B-cell leukemia 1; CAP, cyclophosphamide, doxorubicin, and prednisone without vincristine; CCP, cladribine in combination with cyclophosphamide and prednisone; CHOP, cyclophosphamide, doxorubicin, vincristine, and prednisone; CLL, chronic lymphocytic leukemia; CTL, cytotoxic T lymphocytes; CVP, cyclophosphamide, vincristine, and prednisone; DBM, disrupted in B-cell malignancies; DiSC, differential staining cytotoxicity; EBV, Epstein-Barr virus; FAB Cooperative Group, French-American-British Cooperative Group; FC, fludarabine/cyclophosphamide; FISH, fluorescence-in-situ hybridization; GM-CSF, granulocyte-macrophage colony-stimulating factor; G6PD, glucose-6-phosphate dehydrogenase; GVHD, graft-versus-host disease; HCV, type C hepatitis virus; HTLV-I, human T lymphotropic virus type I; HTLV-1+, human T lymphotropic virus type I-positive adult T-cell leukemia/lymphoma; ICAM, intercellular adhesion molecule; IL-6, interleukin 6; LDH, lactate dehydrogenase; LT-α, lymphotoxin alpha; MDR-1, multidrug resistance 1 gene; MEN-1, multiple endocrine neoplasia syndrome type 1; NF-2, neurofibromatosis type 2 tumor suppressor gene; Pgp, P-glycoprotein; PLL, prolymphocytic leukemia; RDX, radixin; Rh-IL-6, recombinant human interleukin 6; SCL, Sézary-cell leukemia; SCT, stem cell transplantation; SS, Sézary syndrome; sVCAM-1, soluble vascular cell adhesion molecule 1; TCL-1, T-cell leukemia 1; TdT, terminal deoxynucleotidyl transferase; TGF-β, transforming growth factor beta; TK, thymidine kinase; TNF-α, tumor necrosis factor alpha; TRAP, tartrate-resistant isozyme 5 of acid phosphatase; TSEB, total skin electron beam; VAD, vincristine, doxorubicin, and dexamethasone; VCAM-1, vascular cellular adhesion molecule 1; YAC, yeast artificial chromosome.

alkylating agents,[13] and later glucocorticoids,[14] were found to be effective therapy for CLL. These agents became the mainstays of treatment.

In 1967, Dameshek hypothesized that CLL was an accumulative disease of immunologically incompetent lymphocytes.[15] In the early 1970s, the leukemic cells from most cases of CLL were found to express surface immunoglobulin, indicating that the neoplastic cells were of B-cell origin.[16] Subsequent studies demonstrated that the CLL cells of female patients who were heterozygous for glucose-6-phosphate dehydrogenase (G6PD) expressed only one G6PD allele,[17] indicating that the leukemia cells arose from a single B-cell clone. Consistent with this notion, the CLL cells from any one patient were found to express only one type of immunoglobulin light chain[18] and idiotype,[19–21] indicating their uniformity in the expression of immunoglobulin.

A clinical staging system for patients with CLL was introduced in 1975 by Rai and colleagues,[22] delineating the adverse implication of anemia or thrombocytopenia on patient survival. In the late 1980s, purine analogs, such as fludarabine or 2′-chlorodeoxyadenosine (cladribine), were found to be effective in the treatment of CLL. Other treatment modalities are being examined, including passive or active immunotherapy or ablative chemotherapy with marrow transplantation, as the disease still is not considered curable.

ETIOLOGY AND PATHOGENESIS

ENVIRONMENTAL FACTORS

Environmental factors do not appear to play a role in the pathogenesis of B-cell CLL. Although one study noted an increase in CLL in a rural farming community,[23] the incidence of CLL was not associated with exposure to pesticides, sunlight, ionizing radiation, or known carcinogens.[24–29] A few epidemiologic studies have noted an increase in CLL among persons chronically exposed to electromagnetic fields.[30–32] However, it is not determined whether this association reflects a causal relationship.

Antibodies specific for type C hepatitis virus (HCV) and/or viral DNA have been identified in some patients, suggesting a pathogenic role.[33] However, more recent studies have failed to verify an association between the development of CLL and infection with hepatitis C virus.[34,35] CLL cells are resistant to infection with Epstein-Barr virus (EBV), except in unusual cases,[36] making it unlikely that EBV plays a pathogenic role.

The incidence of CLL in men is twice that of women. One retrospective study of women noted a nonsignificant trend toward reduced risk of CLL with increasing parity, prompting speculation that pregnancy lowers the risk for CLL.[37] However, hormones have not been demonstrated to play any role in the development of CLL.

HEREDITARY FACTORS

Genetic factors apparently contribute to the development of CLL. Although B-cell CLL is the most common adult leukemia in Western societies, it is relatively rare in Asia. In the United States, the annual incidence of CLL is 3.9 or 2.0 per 100,000 males or females, respectively. However, in Korea, the estimated incidence of this disease is only 1.5 percent of this rate.[38] Similarly, B-cell CLL is relatively uncommon in China and rare in Japan.[39–41] A very low incidence of B-cell CLL is noted even among Japanese immigrants to the United States.[39,42] Likewise, the incidence of B-cell CLL in Israel is significantly higher among European immigrants than among those from Africa or Asia.[43]

Although most cases of CLL are sporadic, multiple cases of CLL may be found within a single family. There are numerous reports of families with multiple members having B-cell CLL.[44–49] First-degree relatives of patients with CLL are more than three times at risk for having this disorder or other lymphoid neoplasms than is the general population.[47] Afflicted individuals within such families often present at a younger age than most patients with CLL, suggesting that genetic factors in familial CLL may contribute to early leukemogenesis.

The genetic factors that contribute to the increased incidence of CLL in certain families are unknown. There is no apparent association between HLA haplotype and disease susceptibility.[50] One study noted that the leukemic cells of affected family members sometimes might express the same immunoglobulin heavy-chain variable region gene.[51] However, each patient's leukemia cells have distinct immunoglobulin gene rearrangements,[48,51] even those of monozygous twins,[52] indicating that they originate from distinct somatic events.

GENETICS

Detection of chromosomal abnormalities initially was hampered by the inability to induce leukemic cell proliferation. These cells generally do not grow spontaneously in cell culture and are much more refractory to activation by mitogens or to transformation by Epstein-Barr virus than normal B cells.[15,53] As such, the normal karyotypes noted in some samples could reflect an outgrowth of normal bystander lymphocytes.

Using Q-banding and/or G-banding techniques (see Chap. 10), and improved methods for inducing leukemia-cell proliferation in vitro,[54,55] the leukemic cells from nearly 50 percent of CLL patients are noted to have clonal chromosomal abnormalities.[56–59] Interphase cytogenetics using fluorescence-in-situ hybridization (also referred to as FISH) has increased the sensitivity for detecting translocations, deletions, or chromosome trisomy. Using these techniques, it appears that del 13q14-23.1 is the most common chromosomal abnormality in CLL, followed in order by trisomy 12, del 11q22.3-q23.1, del 6q21-q23, 14q abnormalities, and deletions/mutations of the P53 tumor suppressor gene at 17q13.[60] Deletions or duplications account for most of the observed genetic defects, as chromosomal translocations are relatively rare in CLL.

Chromosome 13 Anomalies Deletions on the long arm of chromosome 13 are the most common genetic abnormality in CLL. These deletions generally occur in the absence of chromosome translocation. Nevertheless, those CLL cells with translocations often are noted to have ones involving the long arm of chromosome 13 with any one of several different chromosomes.[61] Because these translocations generally result in deletions at 13q14, deletions at 13q14 may be the contributing genetic lesion, rather than translocation per se.

Deletions in the long arm of chromosome 13 can be detected in approximately half of the cases of CLL. One group noted deletions at 13q12.3, in and around the breast cancer susceptibility gene, BRCA2, in the leukemia cells of 80 percent of 35 CLL patients.[62] Subsequent studies by other investigators, however, failed to confirm this.[63] Instead, these and several other groups have identified deletions at 13q14.3, particularly in a region that is telomeric to the retinoblastoma gene RB-1 and centromeric to and including the D13S25 marker.[64–68] A tumor suppressor gene is hypothesized to reside in this region, referred to as *DBM* (for disrupted in B-cell malignancies). Candidate tumor suppressor genes that map to this region include LEU1 and LEU2.[69] However, CLL cells do not appear to have mutations in both alleles of these genes, making it less likely that they are the actual tumor suppressor genes involved in CLL. Another candidate tumor suppressor gene is LEU5. This gene encodes a zinc-finger domain of the RING type and shares homology with genes involved in tumorigenesis, including the RET finger protein and BRCA1.[70]

Chromosome 12 Anomalies Trisomy 12 is found in the leukemia cells of 10 to 30 percent of all patients with CLL.[71,72] However, studies using molecular techniques, such as fluorescence-in-situ hybridization, have noted a higher proportion of cases with trisomy 12, as well as other chromosomal abnormalities.[58,73–75] Studies using restriction fragment length polymorphism analysis revealed that the leukemia cells with trisomy 12 have one duplicated chromosome 12, while retaining the other homologue.[76,77] As such, it appears that this genetic lesion is not recessive, as would be the case for the loss of a tumor suppressor gene, but rather provides for a gene dosage effect. More recent studies on partial trisomy 12 are consistent with this notion, suggesting that trisomy 12 reflects a gene dosage effect of some genes located between 12q13 and 12q22.[71]

Trisomy 12 may be a secondary event that occurs within an established leukemic clone, or preleukemic B cell.[78] Leukemia cells with trisomy 12 often have complex karyotypic abnormalities[79] and atypical and/or prolymphocytic morphology.[65,71,80–82] One study using fluorescence-in-situ hybridization found that nearly half of the cases with 13q14 deletions also had trisomy 12.[83] Trisomy 12 may not be detectable at diagnosis but is more commonly seen in the leukemia cells of patients with advanced disease or who develop Richter transformation.[79,84,85] Furthermore, this abnormality often may be detected in only a subset of the leukemia cells from any one patient.[86,87] Finally, studies suggest that the leukemia-cell subset with trisomy 12 may expand during disease progression.[64] Collectively, these studies suggest that trisomy 12 is acquired during the evolution of the disease, rather than being a defining genetic event in the etiopathogenesis of CLL.

Chromosome 11 Anomalies Approximately 10 to 20 percent of patients may have leukemia cells with deletions in the long arm of chromosome 11, termed *11q−*.[88–90] These patients tend to be younger in age (less than 55 years) and to have more aggressive disease than those without such genetic changes.[89] Furthermore, the leukemia cells of such patients may express lower levels of surface CD11a/CD18, CD11c/CD18, CD31, CD48, and CD58 than CLL cells from patients without 11q−, arguing that such cells may have a distinctive biology.[91]

CLL B cells can have translocations or deletions involving 11q13, a region that contains the tumor suppressor gene associated with multiple endocrine neoplasia syndrome type I (MEN-1).[92] However, deletions on chromosome 11 more commonly cluster between 11q14-24, particularly at 11q22.3-q23.1, in a region defined by yeast artificial chromosome (YAC) clones 801e11, 975h6, and 755b11.[88,89] Potential tumor suppressor genes within this region include ATM and RDX. RDX, or radixin, has homology with the neurofibromatosis type 2 tumor suppressor gene (NF-2). ATM, on the other hand, is the gene mutated in ataxia-telangiectasia. Upon DNA damage, the normal gene plays an important role in the activation of the tumor suppressor gene-product P53, leading to cell-cycle arrest and DNA repair.[93] The ATM gene has been noted to be lost through deletion or mutation in leukemia cells of patients with relatively aggressive disease.[88,89,94–96] Some CLL patients carry one defective copy of this gene in the germ-line DNA, suggesting that mutations in ATM may be involved in the pathogenesis of aggressive B-CLL.[95,97]

Chromosome 6 Anomalies Another recurring chromosome abnormality involves the short arm of chromosome 6, but the genes altered have not been identified.[65] The most frequent abnormalities on chromosome 6 involve breaks between 6q23 and 6q24, frequently resulting in deletions at 6q25-27, 6q21, and particularly 6q23.[98–101] Patients with abnormalities between 6q21 and 6q24 generally have higher proportions of blood prolymphocytes and more aggressive disease.

One study described an association between CLL and particular alleles of the gene encoding tumor necrosis factor alpha (TNF-α),[102] designated *TNF-1* and located on 6q, 220 kb centromeric of the major histocompatibility complex. In addition, patients with aggressive disease had a particular allele of a contiguous gene encoding lymphotoxin alpha (LT-α), designated *TNFB*2, more often than control subjects. These alleles are associated with functional differences in the levels of inducible TNF-α or LT-α. Prospective studies are required to determine whether such alleles are genetic risk factors for CLL.

Chromosome 14 Anomalies Located on chromosome 14, at band 14q32, are the genes encoding the immunoglobulin heavy chain (see Chap. 83). This band frequently is the site of translocations in B-cell malignancies, with breakpoints often occurring within or near the immunoglobulin heavy-chain J segment minigenes or the immunoglobulin heavy-chain isotype switch regions.[103] Band q11.2 of chromosome 14 also contains genes encoding the α chain and the δ chain of the human T-cell receptor (see Chap. 84). Leukemic cells with inversions of chromosome 14, inv(14) (q11q32), most often are derived from the T-cell lineage and express T-cell differentiation antigens.[104–106] These lesions are common in T-cell prolymphocytic leukemia. Translocations at either of these loci are postulated to reflect an aberrant immunoglobulin or T-cell receptor gene rearrangement that in turn activates a proto-oncogene located on the other chromosome involved in the translocation.

t(11;14)(q13;q32) A small minority of patients with B-cell CLL may have leukemia cells with translocations involving chromosome 14, at band 14q32, and chromosome 11, at band 11q13, or t(11;14)(q13;q32).[59,107–109] The translocation juxtaposes the heavy-chain immunoglobulin genes with a proto-oncogene, designated *BCL-1*, for B-cell leukemia 1,[107,110] that subsequently was identified as PRAD1, a gene encoding cyclin D1.[111,112] Overexpression of PRAD1 can contribute to cell transformation[113] and may play a role in the development of some cases of B-cell CLL.[113] However, among lymphoid malignancies, the highest incidence of t(11;14) and/or PRAD1 overexpression is noted in mantle zone cell lymphoma.[114–118] Because the neoplastic B cells of this intermediate-grade lymphoma can share many phenotypic features with the leukemic B cells in CLL (see Chaps. 96 and 103), cases of CLL that previously were thought to have t(11;14)(q13;q32) instead may have represented the leukemic phase of mantle cell lymphoma.[116,117,119–121]

t(14;18) Rarely, the leukemic cells in B-cell CLL can have t(14;18) translocations that more commonly are found in low-grade nodular B-cell lymphomas (see Chap. 103).[122,123] This translocation juxtaposes the immunoglobulin heavy chain genes with the BCL-2 oncogene.

t(14;19)(q32;q13.1) Although an initial report of t(14;19) translocations in CLL found this translocation in 3 of 30 cases,[124] cytogenetic analyses of 4487 patients with indolent lymphoproliferative diseases, including those with CLL, revealed only six cases to have t(14;19).[125] Only 23 CLL cases have been reported to have t(14;19) to date. Such translocations generally involve the isotype switch regions of IgA on chromosome 14 and result in increased transcription of BCL3, a gene near the breakpoint on chromosome 19 that encodes a protein of the IκB family of transcription factors.[125,126] There is a striking association of t(14;19) with trisomy 12. The presence of this and other CLL-associated features argues that patients with t(14;19) do not have a lymphoproliferative disease distinct from that of CLL. Rather, t(14;19) may be an acquired cytogenetic abnormality that occurs during the evolution of preexisting CLL.

ABNORMALITIES IN SPECIFIC GENES

P53 The P53 gene, located on the short arm of chromosome 17 at 17p13.1, encodes a 53-kDa nuclear phosphoprotein.[127] Upon damage to the cell's DNA, P53 plays an important role in inducing p21/WAF1, leading to inhibition of cyclin-dependent kinase activity; failure to phosphorylate key substrates, such as the retinoblastoma protein; and consequent cell-cycle arrest. Mutations or defects in this gene probably play a pathogenic role in nearly half of all human cancers[128,129] (see Chap. 10).

However, deletions in the short arm of chromosome 17, in and around P53, have been noted in leukemia cells from only about 10 to 15 percent of patients.[82] A similar proportion of patients are noted to have leukemic cells with mutations in the P53 gene.[130,131–133] These mutations commonly occur in the highly conserved exons 4 through 8 of the P53 gene and often are associated with loss of heterozygosity for chromosome 17p.[132]

Patients who have CLL cells with P53 mutations generally have more advanced disease, a higher leukemia-cell proliferative rate, a shorter survival, and greater resistance to first-line therapy.[133–136] Moreover, the neoplastic cells from nearly half of the patients with Richter transformation or B-cell prolymphocytic leukemia have been noted to have P53 mutations.[130] As such, it appears that P53 gene mutations are acquired in some B-cell CLL, resulting in leukemic cells that have a selective growth advantage and a more aggressive clinical behavior.

Multidrug-Resistance (MDR) Gene   The leukemic cells from approximately 40 percent of CLL patients express elevated levels of the multidrug resistance 1 gene, designated *MDR-1*, especially in response to chemotherapy.[137–142] MDR-1, located on the long arm of chromosome 7 at 7q21.1, encodes a 170-kDa transmembrane P-glycoprotein (Pgp) that can function as an energy-dependent, efflux pump for a wide variety of cytotoxic drugs, thus lowering their intracellular concentration to sublethal levels.[143] Elevated expression of this gene appears to be peculiar to the CLL B cell, as it is not noted in normal B cells.[139] However, because MDR-1 can be induced by treatment or by changes in a preexistent leukemia clone, aberrant MDR gene expression more likely plays a role in disease progression of some B-cell CLL rather than in primary pathogenesis.

BCL-2   Approximately 5 percent of CLL patients may have leukemic cells that have aberrant immunoglobulin gene rearrangements with the BCL-2 proto-oncogene located on the long arm of chromosome 18, at 18q21.[122,123,144] In contrast to BCL-2 gene rearrangements in nodular B-cell lymphomas, the rearrangements in B-cell CLL generally occur at breakpoints in the 5′-end of the BCL-2 gene and involve the κ or λ immunoglobulin light-chain genes on chromosomes 2 or 22, respectively.[144] Independent of BCL-2 gene rearrangement, however, the leukemic cells from nearly all patients with B-cell CLL express high levels of the bcl-2 protein that are comparable to that noted for lymphoma cells carrying the t(14;18)(q32;q21) translocation.[145,146] This is associated with hypomethylation of the BCL-2 locus.[147] Using pulse-field gel electrophoresis to examine for BCL-2 gene rearrangements in DNA fragments of 50,000 to 10,000 kilobases, one study found that each of nine CLL cases had somatic rearrangements that would not have been detected by conventional techniques.[148] This suggests that there may be previously undetected genetic abnormalities in CLL involving chromosome 18 that may be responsible for the high-level expression of the BCL-2.

IMMUNOGLOBULIN GENES

Immunoglobulin Characteristics   The leukemic cells from over 90 percent of patients express low levels of monoclonal surface immunoglobulin with either κ or λ light chains. Sixty percent of cases express κ light chains, while the other 40 percent express λ light chains.[149–151] Of the heavy-chain isotypes, over half of all cases have surface IgM and IgD (55 percent), a quarter have IgM exclusive of IgD, and approximately 7 percent have immunoglobulin isotypes other than IgM or IgD (usually IgG or IgA). Less than 5 percent of cases express IgD without detectable IgM. Both IgM and IgM/IgD expressing CLL frequently express cross-reactive idiotypes (see Chap. 83) that commonly are found on IgM autoantibodies.[152]

The immunoglobulins expressed in B-cell CLL often have reactivity for self-antigens, most notably for the constant region of human IgG (reviewed in Caligaris-Cappio[153]). An important feature of these autoantibodies is their "polyreactivity," or binding activity for two or more seemingly disparate self-antigens. Such polyreactivity is a characteristic of some antibodies produced during early B-cell development, even in animals raised in apparent germ-free environments.[154,155] Because of this, several investigators have used the term natural autoantibodies to describe these autoantibodies.

Immunoglobulin Variable Region Genes   CLL B cells can be segregated into at least two groups that differ in the extent to which their expressed immunoglobulin variable region genes (V genes) have undergone somatic mutation.[156] About half of all cases have leukemia cells that express nonmutated V genes, whereas the rest express V genes with levels of base substitutions that distinguish them from their germ-line counterparts. As such, the later resemble more the cases of CLL that express IgA or IgG.[157–160] The extent to which V genes are mutated does not vary within any one leukemia cell population,[161] even when examined over a period of years.[162]

The leukemia cells from approximately 5 percent of CLL patients, however, may lack immunoglobulin heavy-chain allelic exclusion[163] (see Chap. 83). Leukemia cells lacking allelic exclusion express at least two different immunoglobulin heavy chains encoded by each allele. Some leukemia cells have been found to express both mutated and nonmutated immunoglobulin V genes simultaneously.[163] This may complicate the use of somatic mutation as a means to segregate distinct leukemia subtypes.

Nevertheless, CLL B cells that express nonmutated immunoglobulin V genes may constitute a distinct subset of CLL. Leukemia cells that express nonmutated immunoglobulin V genes may have trisomy 12 and atypical morphology more often than those that expressed mutated immunoglobulin V genes, which in turn more frequently tend to have abnormalities involving 13q14.[164] Furthermore, patients with leukemia cells that express mutated immunoglobulin V genes may have a more indolent clinical course than patients with leukemia cells that express nonmutated immunoglobulin V genes.[165,166]

Certain immunoglobulin V genes expressed by CLL B cells may play a role in leukemogenesis. Some V genes, such as the 51p1 allele of V_H1-69, are expressed at high frequency and without mutation in CLL.[167] Moreover, CLL B cells that express the 51p1 have restricted use of certain amino acid sequences within the third complementarity determining region[156,168] (see Chap. 83). This restriction is not a feature of "polyreactive antibodies" per se or of antibodies expressed by B cells during fetal development.[169,170] Rather, it appears that the antibodies used in CLL may be selected because of some undefined binding specificity and/or play a role in leukemogenesis.

CYTOGENESIS

Immunophenotype   The leukemic cells of most patients express pan-B-cell surface antigens, such as CD19 and CD20 (see Chap. 13), indicating that they are derived from the B-lymphocyte lineage. The level at which the CD20 antigen is expressed, however, is substantially lower than that found on normal circulating B cells.[171–173]

Some of the patterns of lymphoid infiltration in CLL reflect expression of certain integrins.[174,175] CLL B cells generally express the β_1 (CD29) and β_2 (CD18) integrins with varying amounts of α_3 (CD49c), α_4 (CD49d), or α_5 (CD49e). The α chains that normally are associated with β_1, such as α_2 (CD49b), α_6 (CD49f), or α_V (CD51), generally are not expressed in CLL. Also, expression of the β_2 integrins, such as leukocyte function antigen-1 (LFA-1), is variable. In one study,[175] low-level expression of β_2 integrins was associated with a diffuse marrow infiltrate and aggressive disease.

The leukemia cells from most patients also express ligands for LFA-1, namely intercellular adhesion molecule (ICAM)-1 (CD54), ICAM-2 (CD102), and ICAM-3 (CD50).[176] CLL cells can bind weakly to nonstimulated endothelium via such ICAMs. Stimulation of endothelium to express the vascular cellular adhesion molecule 1 (VCAM-1) allows for enhanced binding of CLL cells that express the

VCAM-1 ligand, $\alpha_4\beta_1$.[174] Expression of $\alpha_4\beta_1$ also may allow the CLL cells to localize at major sites of VCAM-1 expression, e.g., marrow, liver, and spleen.

CD5 B Cells (B1 B Cells)   The leukemic cells of more than 95 percent of patients express CD5 (Leu 1, OKT1). Most cases of CLL with monoclonal leukemia B cells that do not express CD5 actually may be found to represent lymphoproliferative diseases other than CLL upon more rigorous phenotypic and pathologic analyses.[177]

The physiologic counterpart to such cells is the CD5 B cell.[178] These cells constitute a small subpopulation of human B lymphocytes in the lymphoid organs and peripheral blood of normal adults and most B cells in fetal spleen. Human B cells in lymphoid tissue that express CD5 reside primarily in the mantle zones surrounding the germinal centers of secondary B-cell follicles.[179] These cells are enriched for B cells that spontaneously may produce polyreactive IgM autoantibodies[180,181] and frequently express autoantibody-associated cross-reactive idiotypes.[179,182] Although they share many characteristics, these cells may not be phenotypically identical with CLL B cell.[183]

Because detectable levels of the CD5 antigen (1) are not noted on all B cells that otherwise satisfy other criteria for "CD5 B cells,"[184] (2) may be induced on non-"CD5 B cells,"[185,186] and (3) can be reduced on "CD5 B cells" by treatment with various cytokines,[187] the term CD5 B cell was not considered adequate. For these reasons, long-lived, recirculating, and/or self-replenishing B cells that are enriched for cells expressing "natural" IgM autoantibodies are referred to by many investigators as B-1 B cells.[188] Short-lived B cells that are generated continuously in the adult marrow are referred to as conventional, or B-2 B, cells.

LEUKEMIA CELL ACCUMULATION

Growth Kinetics   There is a small pool of proliferating cells. In the spleen, proliferation of CLL cells occurs preferentially in the white pulp zones, even in cases in which both the white and red pulp are extensively infiltrated.[189] However, CLL cells in the blood incorporate extremely low amounts of ^{3}H-thymidine in vitro[190] and are mainly in the G_0 stage of the cell cycle, as assessed by flow cytometry.[191] Because most CLL cells are not proliferating, the life span of CLL lymphocytes appears long. Consistent with this, human CLL B cells can survive for many weeks after transfer into mice with severe combined immune deficiency.[192]

Resistance to Apoptosis   CLL cells accumulate, as they are resistant to programmed cell death, or apoptosis (see Chap. 11). CLL B cells express high-levels of the anti-apoptotic protein bcl-2.[147,193–200] In addition, the neoplastic B cells of patients with CLL also characteristically express high levels of other anti-apoptotic proteins, such as bcl-x_L, mcl-1, and bag-1,[201] and low levels of the pro-apoptotic protein bax or bcl-x_s.[195] Bcl-2 and bax proteins form homodimers and heterodimers that influence the susceptibility to apoptosis.[202,203] Moreover, it appears that the relative ratio of bcl-2 and/or bcl-x_L to bax in leukemia cells is related to their resistance to drugs in vitro[194,196,199,204] and possibly also in vivo.

Drugs that are active in the treatment of CLL can alter the relative ratio of bcl-2 to bax. Increasing the relative concentration of bcl-2 decreases the relative sensitivity to apoptosis, whereas increasing the relative concentration of bax increases contributes to cell death (reviewed in Yang and Korsmeyer[205]). In vitro, fludarabine (9-β D-arabinofuranosyl-2-fluoradenine, F-ara-A) can down-regulate expression of BCL-2 mRNA and bcl-2 protein by some leukemia cells in vitro. Furthermore, the sensitivity of leukemia cell samples to fludarabine-induced down-regulation of BCL-2 correlated loosely with the therapeutic response to this drug in vivo.[206] It remains to be established whether the modulation in the relative levels of bcl-2 to bax by such drugs in vitro can predict the clinical response to such drugs in vivo.

In any case, the sensitivity of CLL cells to undergoing spontaneous- or drug-induced apoptosis may be influenced by the leukemia-cell microenvironment. Glucocorticoids, for example, also may induce a decrease in the relative concentration of bcl-2 to bax in CLL B cells, thereby enhancing leukemia-cell susceptibility to apoptosis.[207] However, this effect can be mitigated by contact with cells bearing receptors for certain proteins expressed on the leukemia cell surface, such as CD6.[208,209] In addition, CLL B cells can survive for long periods ex vivo when cultured with marrow stromal cells.[210,211] The ability of stromal cells to inhibit spontaneous apoptosis in vitro is not mediated by soluble factors, but apparently is dependent upon direct cell-cell contact involving the β_1 and β_2 integrins.

IMMUNOLOGIC DEFECTS

Most patients with CLL have an acquired immune deficiency.[212] CLL patients have an increased risk for herpes zoster infection.[213] Also, patients with CLL have a higher risk for skin cancers, including basal cell carcinoma, than age-matched controls.[214]

Patients with CLL have a greater susceptibility to infection due to numerous factors, including hypogammaglobulinemia, low complement levels,[215] functional defects in bystander T cells,[216] altered leukemia-cell expression of major histocompatibility complex class II antigens,[217] and impaired granulocytic function.[218]

The leukemia cells themselves can contribute to the immunodeficiency noted in patients with this disease. Leukemia B cells elaborate immune suppressive cytokines, such as transforming growth factor beta (TGF-β),[219,220] and release soluble surface molecules, such as CD27,[183,221,222] that can interfere with cognate intercellular interactions that are required for immune activation. High levels of TGF-β also may account for the reversal in the ratio of CD4 to CD8 T cells that often is noted in the patients with CLL.[223] CLL B cells have little stimulatory activity in autologous or even allogeneic mixed lymphocyte culture.[224,225] Aside from TGF-β, this in part is related to the surface phenotype of the leukemic B cells. Important accessory molecules required for cognate B-cell↔T-cell interactions, such as CD80 (see Chaps. 15 and 84), are absent or present at low levels on the leukemic cell surface. This makes leukemic cells poor antigen-presenting cells but possible effective inducers of T-cell anergy (see Chap. 84).

CLL B cells also are effective in down-modulating expression of the CD40-ligand (CD154), a surface glycoprotein that ordinarily is expressed on CD4+ T cells following immune activation.[226,227] Because CD154 plays a critical role in the development of an immune response (reviewed in Grewal and Flavell[228]), such down-modulation may be responsible for the immune deficiency that is acquired in CLL. Given the role of CD154 in T-cell induction of immunoglobulin class switching, this acquired functional defect in CD154 may account for the acquired deficiency of CLL patients to produce IgG of each of the various subclasses.[229] Indeed, the acquired immune deficiency of patients with CLL has features in common with that of persons with inherited functional defects in the gene encoding CD154 (see Chaps. 15 and 88).

These shared features include the frequent development of intermittent and intercurrent systemic autoimmunity despite profound immune deficiency. Patients with congenital lack of CD154 commonly develop autoimmune hemolytic anemia (see Chap. 55) and immune thrombocytopenic purpura (see Chap. 117).[230] These also are the most common autoimmune diseases that develop in patients with CLL.[15,231,232] Much less frequently, patients with CLL may develop pure red blood cell aplasia[233] or neutropenia[231] secondary to the development of autoantibodies against marrow hematopoietic progenitor cells. Although patients with rheumatoid arthritis have been reported to have an increased prevalence of CLL compared to that of the general population,[234] CLL patients in general do not appear to have an increased incidence of pathologic autoimmunity other than that directed against hematopoietic cells.[231,232] The pathogenic autoantibodies generally do not appear to be produced by the malignant B-cell clone.[152]

CLINICAL FEATURES

PATIENT POPULATION

At diagnosis, most patients are over 60 years of age, and 90 percent are over age 50. The disease is extremely rare in persons under 25 years of age. There is a 2:1 male to female incidence and prevalence of CLL.

GENERAL SYMPTOMS

Over 25 percent of patients are asymptomatic at diagnosis. Such patients generally are detected because of the discovery of nontender lymphadenopathy or an unexplained absolute lymphocytosis. Otherwise, patients may have only mild symptoms of reduced exercise tolerance, fatigue, or malaise. Patients may experience such symptoms even when they apparently lack major organ involvement or anemia. Because of the advanced age of the affected population, patients sometimes present with an exacerbation of another underlying medical condition, such as pulmonary, cerebrovascular, or coronary artery disease.

Some cases may present with chronic rhinitis secondary to nasal involvement of CLL cells.[235] In rare cases, patients may present with a sensorimotor polyneuropathy associated with IgM antibody to various gangliosides.[55] For unknown reasons, patients may note exaggerated responses to insect bites, particularly to those of mosquitoes.[236,237]

Patients who present with more advanced disease may experience weight loss, recurrent infections, bleeding secondary to thrombocytopenia, and/or symptomatic anemia. However, night sweats and fevers (the so-called B symptoms) are uncommon and should prompt evaluation for complicating infectious disease. Indeed, patients with CLL are more prone to viral or bacterial infections secondary to impaired T-cell immunity or hypogammaglobulinemia, respectively.

LYMPHADENOPATHY

Nearly 80 percent of all CLL patients have nontender lymphadenopathy at diagnosis, most commonly involving the cervical, supraclavicular, or axillary lymph nodes. Lymph node enlargement ranges from minimal to massive, the latter potentially causing local disfiguration or organ dysfunction. Some patients may develop symptoms of upper airway obstruction due to oral-pharyngeal lymphadenopathy. However, it is unusual for the lymphadenopathy in CLL to cause obstruction of vascular or lymphatic channels. Lymphedema of the extremities is rare, even in the setting of massive axillary and cervical adenopathy, and superior vena cava obstruction is so uncommon that it should alert the clinician to the possibility of a secondary pulmonary neoplasm. Computerized axial tomography of the abdomen can detect intraabdominal lymph node enlargement in a large number of patients. However, such information has yet to be incorporated into clinical staging schemes. Large retroperitoneal adenopathy can result in ureteral obstruction and hydronephrosis. Rarely, patients may develop periportal lymph node enlargement that results in biliary tract obstruction. Occasional patients may experience acute, painful swelling in previously nontender, chronically enlarged lymph nodes secondary to acute lymphadenitis resulting from infection with herpes simplex virus.[238,239]

SPLENOMEGALY AND HEPATOMEGALY

Approximately half of all CLL patients present with mild to moderate splenomegaly. Occasionally, this may cause symptoms of early satiety and/or abdominal fullness. Sometimes, splenic enlargement may result in hypersplenism, contributing to anemia and thrombocytopenia. However, in CLL such cytopenias are more commonly secondary to extensive marrow involvement with CLL and/or intermittent expression of autoantibodies.[231,240-243] Less frequently, patients develop hepatomegaly secondary to leukemic cell infiltration of the liver. Derangement of hepatic function secondary to visceral involvement is usually mild, and cholestatic jaundice is unusual in the absence of nodal disease causing biliary tract obstruction.

EXTRANODAL INVOLVEMENT

Organ infiltration with leukemic cells is frequently detected at autopsy but is not commonly symptomatic. For example, leukemic cell infiltration of the renal parenchyma can be detected in over half of all patients examined postmortem. However, CLL only rarely is associated with impaired renal function. Leukemic cell infiltration, however, may become symptomatic when it develops in certain locations, such as in the retro-orbit, where it can produce proptosis. Lymph tissue also may develop in the scalp, subconjunctivae, prostate, gonads, or pharynx, the latter sometimes causing symptoms of upper airway obstruction. Infiltration of the pericardium by leukemia cells can produce a constrictive pericarditis[244] or result in cardiac tamponade.[245]

Occasionally, the leukemic cells infiltrate the lung parenchyma, producing nodular or miliary pulmonary infiltrates that can be detected on chest x-ray. This may be associated with pulmonary function test abnormalities. The respiratory tract mucosa also may be involved. Leukemic infiltration of the pleura may result in hemorrhagic or chylous pleural effusions.[246-248]

The gastrointestinal tract also may be infiltrated with leukemic cells, causing abnormal mucosal thickening. This may result in ulceration, gastrointestinal bleeding, or malabsorption. The latter may cause dietary deficiencies of essential nutrients, such as folate. Finding iron deficiency should alert the physician to evaluate for gastrointestinal bleeding that may be due to mucosal ulcerations or to a secondary gastrointestinal malignancy.

Leukemic cell infiltration of the central nervous system is unusual but may produce headache, meningitis, cranial nerve palsy, obtundation, or coma.[249] The development of neurologic changes in CLL, however, also may be caused by infections with unusual organisms, including fungi, *Cryptococcus neoformans*, *Listeria monocytogenes*, or other pathogens that generally only afflict an immune compromised host.

LABORATORY FEATURES

BLOOD FINDINGS

The diagnosis of CLL requires a sustained monoclonal lymphocytosis greater than $5000/\mu l$ (5×10^9/liter). At diagnosis, the absolute lymphocyte count generally exceeds $10,000/\mu l$ (10×10^9/liter) and is sometimes greater than $100,000/\mu l$ (100×10^9/liter). Morphologically, the leukemic cells generally appear similar to normal resting lymphocytes. Typically these cells have scanty, bluish cytoplasm upon Wright-Giemsa staining, moderately condensed and mature-appearing nuclei, and an MCV of 170 fl (see Plate XX-4). A few cells can have prominent nucleoli. During the preparation of the blood film, many CLL lymphocytes apparently are disrupted and appear as smudge cells. Leukemic leukocytosis in excess of $800,000/\mu l$ (800×10^9/liter) may produce blood hyperviscosity.

The red cells typically are normocytic and normochromic. About 15 percent of patients present with normocytic anemia. In the setting of extreme lymphocytosis, the packed red cell volume may be overestimated unless care is taken to exclude from the measurement the expanded buffy coat containing the leukemic cells. About 20 percent of all CLL patients have a positive Coombs' test at some time during their disease due to the production of IgG anti-red cell autoantibodies by bystander nonleukemic B cells. Autoimmune hemolytic anemia, however, develops in only about 8 percent of CLL patients.

During the most advanced disease stage, patients have thrombocytopenia due to marrow replacement and hypersplenism. At any stage, however, patients can develop immune thrombocytopenia due to antiplatelet antibodies. Generally, the platelet morphology is not remarkable.

MARROW FINDINGS

The marrow invariably is infiltrated with leukemic cells. There are four patterns of marrow involvement.[250–252] (Fig. 98-1). In approximately one-third of patients, the marrow has an interstitial, or lacy, pattern that is associated with a better prognosis and/or early-stage disease. About 10 percent of patients present with a nodular pattern of marrow involvement, and approximately 25 percent have a mixed nodular-interstitial pattern. These patterns also are associated with a better prognosis. A quarter of the patients present with extensive marrow replacement, producing a diffuse pattern that is associated with advanced clinical stage and/or more aggressive disease.[252,253]

LYMPH NODE FINDINGS

The lymph node architecture typically is effaced by a diffuse infiltration of small lymphocytes that have the same morphology as that of the circulating leukemic cells. The node histology is identical to that of low-grade small lymphocytic lymphoma. As the disease progresses, the nodes may coalesce and form large fixed masses. In rare cases, the lymph node can contain a few scattered cells that have the morphology and phenotype of Reed-Sternberg cells typically seen in Hodgkin disease (see Chap. 102).[254]

IMMUNOLOGIC STUDIES

Several tests are recommended as part of the laboratory evaluation of patients with CLL. Lymphocyte surface immunologic markers can determine monoclonality and the presence of CLL-type lymphocytes. The direct Coombs' test can uncover those patients who have or are at risk for an immune hemolytic anemia. Measurement of serum immunoglobulin quantifies the depression of IgG, IgA, and IgM that predisposes to infection. Skin test with PPD and other recall antigens can detect anergy. The frequency of the concomitant T-cell functional defect increases in advanced stages of CLL.

IMMUNOPHENOTYPING

Flow cytometric analyses can evaluate leukemic cells for expression of B-cell or T-cell differentiation antigens, surface immunoglobulin, and κ or λ light chains. Such studies can distinguish B-cell CLL from not only T-cell leukemias but also other B-cell leukemias that can otherwise mimic B-cell CLL (Table 98-1). Useful markers for this are CD5, CD10, CD11c, CD19, CD20, CD22, CD23, CD25, CD38, and CD103 (see Chap. 13).[151,255–258] The differential expression of these antigens helps to distinguish between the various B-cell leukemias (see Table 98-1). Analyses for other cell surface markers also may be clinically useful.

Cytoplasmic immunoglobulin can be detected in CLL B cells and may be a valuable adjunct in B-cell phenotyping.[259] Compared to normal cells, CLL B cells have a lower density of surface but a higher content of cytoplasmic immunoglobulin. Rarely, intracytoplasmic inclusions of crystalloid immunoglobulin have been seen. Over three-fourths of patients with CLL may have excess light chains in the Golgi complex and the cisternae of the rough endoplasmic reticulum.[260–262]

PROTEIN ELECTROPHORESIS

The most common finding on serum protein electrophoreses is hypogammaglobulinemia. Nearly three-fourths of all B-cell CLL patients develop severe hypogammaglobulinemia during the course of their disease. Reduction in the serum levels of IgM precedes that of IgG and IgA. The degree of hypogammaglobulinemia correlates loosely with clinical stage, and virtually all patients with advanced disease have decreased concentrations of serum immunoglobulin.

However, 5 percent of patients have a serum monoclonal immunoglobulin paraprotein. The serum paraprotein generally is the same type as that present on the leukemic cell surface. When the concentration of IgM paraprotein is high, hyperviscosity may ensue, and the clinical picture can be confused with that of Waldenström macroglobulinemia (see Chap. 108). In some cases, there is defective and/or unbalanced immunoglobulin chain synthesis by the leukemic B-cell clone, resulting in mu heavy-chain disease and/or immunoglobulin light-chain proteinuria (see Chap. 109). The latter can be detected on urine immunoelectrophoresis (see Chap. 104).

When high-resolution agarose gel electrophoresis is combined with immunofixation, small paraprotein spikes can be identified in the sera or urine samples of nearly two-thirds of all patients.[18,263–265] These paraprotein spikes generally have immunoglobulin heavy chains that belong to isotypes other than those expressed by the leukemic B-cell clone.[18]

DIFFERENTIAL DIAGNOSIS

The differential diagnosis of lymphocytosis is discussed in Chap. 87. Lymphocytosis can occur in persons infected with various viruses, *Bordetella pertussis*, or *Toxoplasma gondii* (see Chap. 87). However, the patients who usually encounter such illness generally are much younger than patients with CLL. Also, in contrast to the reactive lymphocytosis that occurs in response to these infections, the lymphocytosis of patients with CLL is persistent and monoclonal. The latter characteristic is important in distinguishing CLL from unusual cases of persistent polyclonal lymphocytosis of B cells that sometimes can masquerade as B-cell CLL.[266,267] Flow cytometric analyses of blood mononuclear cells generally can differentiate between reactive lymphocytosis, polyclonal B-cell lymphocytosis, and monoclonal lymphocytosis secondary to lymphoproliferative disease.[268]

PROLYMPHOCYTIC LEUKEMIA

Prolymphocytic leukemia is a subacute variant of CLL in which over half of the blood leukemic cells are large lymphocytes, termed prolymphocytes. These cells can be distinguished from the leukemic cells in CLL by size and morphology.[269] Prolymphocytes measure 10 to 15 μm in diameter, whereas CLL cells generally have the size of small resting lymphocytes (7–10 μm in diameter). Also, prolymphocytes in the blood or marrow have round or indented nuclei, each possessing a single prominent thick-rimmed nucleolus and chromatin that is more dense than that of a lymphoblast but less dense than that of a typical mature lymphocyte or a CLL B cell (see Plate XX-5). The cytoplasm generally is pale blue and agranular, except for occasional intracytoplasmic inclusions that are visible by electron, and sometimes light,

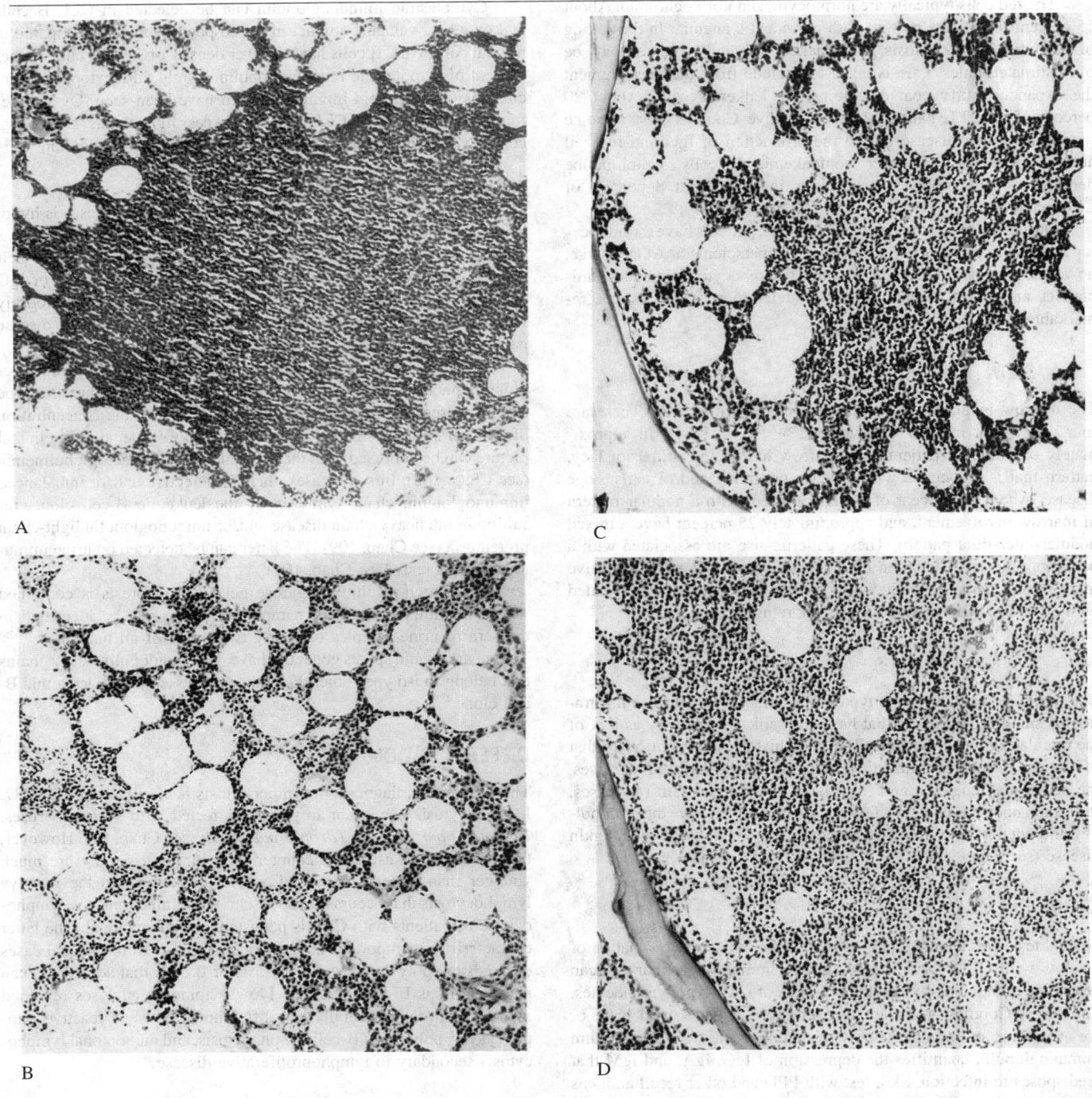

FIGURE 98-1   Photomicrographs of marrow sections demonstrating (a) nodular, (b) interstitial, (c) mixed nodular and interstitial, and (d) diffuse patterns of infiltration. (Reproduced with permission from Pangalis GA, Roussou PA, Kittas C, et al.[251])

microscopy.[270] By scanning electron microscopy, these prolympho-cytes often have more surface microvilli than do leukemic cells from patients with B-cell CLL. They may involve lymph nodes, generally producing a pseudonodular pattern of infiltration that is distinct from that of the diffuse pattern typical of CLL.[271] In contrast to the leukemic B cells in CLL, prolymphocytes typically express high levels of surface immunoglobulin and stain brightly with SN8, a mAb specific for CD79b (see Chaps. 13 and 83).[272,273] These and other features that distinguish CLL from prolymphocytic leukemia are presented in Table

98-1. Other features of this disease are discussed in the section on prolymphocytic leukemia at the end of this chapter.

HAIRY CELL LEUKEMIA

The clinical and laboratory features that assist in distinguishing CLL from hairy cell leukemia and its variants, hairy cell leukemia variant, and splenic lymphoma with villous lymphocytes,[274] are presented in Table 98-1. These diseases are discussed in Chap. 99.

TABLE 98-1   IMMUNOPHENOTYPE OF CHRONIC B-CELL LEUKEMIAS/LYMPHOMAS

DISEASE ENTITY	sIg	CD5	CD10	CD11c	CD19	CD20	CD22	CD23	CD25	CD103
Chronic lymphocytic leukemia	+/−	++	−	−/+	+	+/−	−/+	++	−/+	−
Prolymphocytic leukemia	++	+	−	−/+	+	+/−	+	+/−	−	−
Hairy cell leukemia	+/−	−/+	−	++	+	+	++	−/+	+	++
Mantle cell lymphoma	+	++	−	−	+	+	+	−/+	−	−
Splenic marginal zone lymphoma	+	−/+	−/+	+	+	+	+/−	−/+	−	−
Lymphoplasmacytoid lymphoma	+/−	−/+	−	−	+	+/−	+/−	−/+	+/−	−
Follicular center lymphoma	+	−	+	−	+	++	+	−/+	−	−

− Leukemia cells do not express the surface antigen; + leukemia cells from most cases express the surface antigen; +/−, low-level expression; −/+, most cases either do not express the antigen or express it at very low levels; ++, high-level expression of the surface antigen in nearly all cases.

The neoplastic B cells in hairy cell leukemia are larger than CLL cells (MCV 400 fl) and have more abundant cytoplasm, often with fine filamentous "hairy" projections (see Plate XX-7). These cells are strongly positive for tartrate-resistant isozyme 5 of acid phosphatase (TRAP) activity. Finally, in contrast to CLL B cells, the neoplastic cells in hairy cell leukemia express high levels of CD11c, the α^X chain of the β_2 integrins, and CD103, the α^E subunit of the β_7 integrins (see Chap. 99).

LYMPHOMAS

Lymphomas can have circulating neoplastic cells, sometimes producing a blood lymphocytosis that may be mistaken for CLL. The lymphomas are discussed in Chap. 103. Those lymphomas that most closely can resemble B-cell CLL are listed below.

SMALL LYMPHOCYTIC LYMPHOMA
Low-grade small lymphocytic B-cell lymphoma is closely related to B-cell CLL in its biology and clinical features. The neoplastic cells in small lymphocytic lymphoma with blood involvement are the same morphologically as the leukemic cells in CLL. Moreover, the histology of the involved lymph nodes in CLL and small lymphocytic lymphoma are indistinguishable.[275] Similar to the B cells in CLL, the neoplastic B cells in small lymphocytic lymphoma frequently express immunoglobulins that bear autoantibody-associated cross-reactive idiotypes and that are encoded by nonmutated immunoglobulin genes.[149,276] Finally, the neoplastic B cells in both diseases express many of the same surface antigens, including CD5.[277] For these reasons, the distinction between these diseases is primarily clinical, in that CLL invariably is associated with a blood lymphocytosis (greater than 4000 lymphocytes/μl), whereas small lymphocytic lymphoma invariably is associated with lymph node involvement. Also, although patients with CLL invariably have marrow lymphocytosis, the marrow in small lymphocytic lymphoma need not be involved. When the marrow is involved, the pattern in small lymphocytic lymphoma typically is nodular, rather than interstitial or diffuse.[252] This disorder is discussed further in Chap. 103.

MANTLE CELL LYMPHOMA
Mantle cell lymphoma (previously called centrocytic lymphoma, mantle zone lymphoma, or intermediate lymphoma) in the Working Formulation is an intermediate-grade B-cell lymphoma (see Chaps. 96, 101, and 103). In contrast to the diffuse lymph node involvement typical in CLL, the histology of lymph nodes in mantle cell lymphoma typically is one of reactive germinal centers surrounded by well-defined, expanded mantle zones of monoclonal B cells.[278] However, heavily involved lymph nodes may lose this architecture and appear diffusely infiltrated, assuming histology similar to that of lymph nodes involved in CLL.

The neoplastic B cells in mantle cell lymphoma express many of the same surface antigens as do CLL B cells, including CD5 (Table 98-1). However, in contrast to CLL B cells, mantle cell lymphoma cells generally do not express CD23. Mantle cell lymphoma cells also tend to express higher levels of CD79a than do CLL cells.[279]

LYMPHOMAS OF FOLLICULAR CENTER CELL ORIGIN
Low-grade lymphomas of follicular center cell origin also can involve the blood. There is often marked adenopathy and occasionally massive splenomegaly. The leukemic cells are small and typically have cleaved nuclei with well-delineated nucleoli. Follicular center small cleaved cell lymphomas frequently express the CD10 (CALLA) antigen. In contrast to CLL, these cells often express high levels of surface immunoglobulin and generally express neither mouse rosette receptors nor the CD5 antigen (Table 98-1). The cells are FMC7-positive. Biopsy of a lymph node will confirm nodular or diffuse small cleaved cell (poorly differentiated lymphocytic) lymphoma. These diseases are discussed in Chap. 103.

LYMPHOPLASMACYTIC LEUKEMIAS

Plasmacytoid lymphocytes can be seen on the blood films and are always present in the marrow of patients with Waldenström macroglobulinemia (see Chap. 108). These cells have abundant, often basophilic, cytoplasm with mature lymphoid nuclei. By flow cytometric analysis (see Chap. 81), these cells express pan-B lymphocyte surface antigens CD19, CD20, and CD24 (see Chap. 13) and are monoclonal as defined by immunoglobulin light-chain expression. Similar to CLL B cells, these cells often express CD5 and CD11b. However, they can be distinguished from CLL cells by their expression of the CD10 (CALLA) and/or CD9 antigens and by their lymphoplasmacytic morphology (see Chaps. 96 and 101).

Patients with plasma cell myeloma may develop plasma cell leukemia. The leukemic cells can be distinguished from those in B-cell CLL by their plasmacytic morphology, their expression of CD38, PCA-1, CD56, and CD85, and their low-level or lack of expression of CD19, CD20, CD24, CD72, and HLA-DR (Table 98-1). Plasma cell myeloma is discussed in Chap. 106.

T-CELL CHRONIC LYMPHOPROLIFERATIVE DISORDERS

T-cell variants of CLL constitute a heterogeneous group of disorders that must be distinguished from B-cell CLL. T-cell chronic lymphoproliferative diseases are much less common. Several have counterparts in the various B-cell leukemias and are discussed in other chapters, including T-cell prolymphocytic leukemia (discussed in the section on prolymphocytic leukemia at the end of this chapter) and T-cell lymphoma (see Chap. 103). A subset of large granular lymphocytic leukemias represents another T-cell chronic leukemia that is discussed in Chap. 100.

TABLE 98-2   RAI CLINICAL STAGING SYSTEM

Stage	Clinical Features at Diagnosis	Median Survival, Months
0	Blood and marrow lymphocytosis	>150
I	Lymphocytosis and enlarged lymph nodes	101
II	Lymphocytosis and enlarged spleen and/or liver	>71
III	Lymphocytosis and anemia (hemoglobin below 11 g/dl)	19
IV	Lymphocytosis and thrombocytopenia (platelets below 100,000/μl)	19

These diseases can be distinguished from lymphoproliferative disorders of B cells or natural killer cells by immunophenotype. The leukemic cells from all T-cell malignancies lack expression of monoclonal surface immunoglobulin or B-cell restricted surface differentiation antigens, such as CD19 or CD20 (see Chap. 13), and generally lack immunoglobulin light-chain gene rearrangements (see Chap. 83). Characteristically, chronic T-cell leukemias have rearrangement and expression of the genes encoding the T-cell receptor for antigen (see Chap. 84) and express the CD3 surface antigens (see Chaps. 13 and 84). The latter is a property exclusive to lymphocytes of the T-cell lineage and can be used to distinguish large granular lymphocytic leukemia of T-cell versus natural killer cell origin (see Chap. 100).

THERAPY, COURSE, AND PROGNOSIS

CLINICAL STAGING

Wide variability exists in the rate of disease progression and the incidence of disease-related complications among patients with CLL. Because of this, the life expectancies of patients with newly diagnosed CLL can vary tremendously. Staging helps to define prognosis and to decide when to initiate therapy.

Two major staging systems have been developed, each having established value in helping to predict survival.[280] The first widely used system was introduced by Rai and colleagues in 1975.[22] This staging system designated five clinical stages using Roman numerals 0 through IV. Patients in stages 0 and I have a favorable prognosis, while patients in stages III and IV have a relatively short survival (Table 98-2). The prognosis of patients in stage II is intermediate. Although confirmed to have useful predictive value,[281] the number of stages was considered excessive by some investigators. Accordingly, in 1981, Binet and colleagues proposed a three-stage classification system that considered the total lymphoid mass.[282] The most advanced stage, stage C, describes all patients who have anemia and/or thrombocytopenia due to impaired marrow function (Table 98-3). The remaining patients are divided into stages A or B, based upon the number of enlarged lymphoid areas (of which there are five: cervical, axillary, or inguinofemoral lymph nodes, and liver or spleen). Patients in groups A or B have less than three or greater than or equal to three areas of lymphoid enlargement respectively (Table 98-3). Most physicians use either the Binet or the Rai staging system. Generally, disease progression follows a stepwise pattern from earlier to later stages.

In 1987, Rai reorganized his original staging system into three categories: low-risk (stage 0), intermediate-risk (stages I and II), and high-risk (stages III and IV) patients.[283] Low-risk patients have a projected median survival of greater than 150 months (Table 98-2). In contrast, intermediate- and high-risk patients have median survivals of approximately 90 months and 19 months respectively. Both the Binet classification and modified Rai classification have proven utility in helping to access disease outcome.[283]

OTHER PROGNOSTIC INDICATORS

In addition to the widely accepted staging systems of Rai and Binet, there are additional indicators that can help identify high-risk patients who may benefit from closer follow-up and/or early therapy. These variables could be considered when deciding whether to initiate therapy.

LEUKEMIC CELL DOUBLING TIME
CLL B cells generally do not have a high mitotic index and express low levels of the cyclin-dependent kinase inhibitor $p27^{kip1}$ (p27), a protein that ordinarily increases as a cell progresses into S phase. However, some patients have leukemia cells that have high-level expression of p27.[284] Such patients may have shorter blood lymphocyte doubling times and survival than average patients with CLL.

Patients whose lymphocyte counts double within 1 year have progressive disease, whereas those with stable counts represent a good-risk population. Independent of stage, the median survival for patients with a doubling time less than 12 months was 5 years, whereas it was greater than 12 years if the doubling time was greater than 12 months.[285]

MARROW HISTOLOGY
Biopsy can reveal characteristic patterns of marrow infiltration, defined as nodular, interstitial, mixed, or diffuse.[286,287] (See Fig. 98-1). A diffuse replacement of the marrow is associated with a worse prognosis than a nodular or interstitial pattern.[250–252,288] The marrow biopsy is more reliable than the aspirate is distinguishing patients with favorable disease (nodular and/or interstitial) versus nonfavorable disease (diffuse) independent of clinical stage.[286] However, both the aspirate and biopsy appear to have independent prognostic value.[286,289] As such, evaluation of the marrow is considered desirable, especially for patients prior to therapy.[290]

LEUKEMIA CELL PHENOTYPE
Atypical lymphocyte morphology is associated with a more adverse clinical course.[291] If more than 50 percent of the leukemia cells have a prolymphocytic morphology, then the patient's disease may have evolved to prolymphocytic leukemia.

A more adverse clinical course has been associated with leukemic cells that express CD38[166] or that express only surface IgM rather than both IgM and IgD.[292,293] Another study noted that advanced-stage disease was associ-

TABLE 98-3   BINET CLINICAL STAGING SYSTEM

Stage	Clinical Features at Diagnosis	Median Survival, Years
A	Blood and marrow lymphocytosis and less than 3 areas* of palpable lymphoid-tissue enlargement	>7
B	Blood and marrow lymphocytosis and 3 or more areas of palpable lymphoid-tissue enlargement	<5
C	Same as B with anemia (hemoglobin below 11 g/dl in men or 10 g/dl in women) or thrombocytopenia (platelets less than 100,000/μl)	<2

*An area is defined as the cervical, axillary, or inguinofemoral lymph nodes, or the liver and spleen. The liver and spleen together count as one area, as do the right and left cervical lymph nodes. However, bilateral enlargement of the axillary lymph nodes or the inguinofemoral lymph nodes each count as two areas. Thus, the number of enlarged lymphoid areas can range from one to five.

ated with low to nondetectable expression levels of CD11a and CD18 but had no significant relation to the relative expression of CD11c.[175]

KARYOTYPE

Survival of patients with abnormal karyotypes is significantly shorter than that of comparably staged patients with normal karyotypes.[294,295] Multiple abnormalities in association with trisomy 12 carry a worse prognosis than trisomy 12 alone.[56,294,296,297] However, patients who have trisomy 12 as the only cytogenetic abnormality fare worse than those with a normal karyotype or those with isolated abnormalities involving 13q14.[298,299] Patients who have structural abnormalities of chromosomes 14, 6, or 11q− also generally have a more adverse clinical course than those with a normal karyotype.[89,300] The prognostic effect of 11q deletion on survival is most apparent for patients younger than 55 years of age.

SERUM FACTORS

Provided the patient has normal renal function, there are several serum proteins that become elevated in patients with aggressive disease. Moreover, the relative level of each of these proteins has been found to correlate with the kinetics of tumor progression and/or tumor burden. For this reason, potential prognostic value can be obtained by measuring the relative serum levels of: beta-2 microglobulin (β_2M),[288,301,302] thymidine kinase (TK),[303] soluble CD23,[288,304,305] soluble vascular cell adhesion molecule-1 (sVCAM-1),[306] or soluble CD27.[183,307] Lactate dehydrogenase (LDH) also is generally elevated in patients with aggressive disease and in nearly all patients with Richter transformation.[308,309] On the other hand, progressive disease more typically is associated with a greater suppression of T-cell function and a more marked decline in serum IgA.[310] Hypercalcemia is rare in patients with CLL[311] and may indicate Richter transformation[312] (see below).

However, it should be recognized that certain treatments, diseases, or renal dysfunction could affect the relative level of each of these factors, mitigating their potential to have predictive value. This is evident, for example, in patients treated with granulocyte-macrophage colony-stimulating factor (GM-CSF).[313] GM-CSF can induce substantial increases in the serum levels of β_2M and TK that do not appear related to disease progression or impaired renal function.[314]

TELOMERASE ACTIVITY

Progressive shortening of chromosome telomeres occurs with repeated cell division and may result in cell senescence. Erosion of chromosome telomeres is prevented by telomerase, a ribonucleoprotein enzyme that synthesizes TTAGGG repeats on the ends of chromosomes using its RNA component as a template.[315,316] Mean telomere lengths and telomerase activity have been correlated with survival in B-CLL.[317] Mean telomere length is inversely correlated with telomerase activity. Leukemia cells with telomere lengths of less than 6.0 kb had high telomerase activity, whereas leukemia cells with telomere lengths of greater than 6.0 kb had low telomerase activity. Patients with leukemia cells that had high telomerase activity had a significantly shorter median survival than patients whose leukemia cells had low telomerase activity.

INDICATIONS FOR THERAPY

There are no proven cures for CLL. Moreover, treatment of early-stage patients with chemotherapy does not appear to offer any survival advantage over that achieved with conservative management.[318] However, for certain patients therapy can reduce morbidity and/or improve survival significantly.

TABLE 98-4 INDICATIONS FOR THERAPY IN B-CELL CLL

Anemia
Thrombocytopenia
Disease-related symptoms
Markedly enlarged or painful spleen
Symptomatic lymphadenopathy
Blood lymphocyte count doubling time < 6 months
Prolymphocytic transformation
Richter transformation

A number of criteria are useful for deciding when to initiate therapy (Table 98-4). Generally, an elevated blood lymphocyte count by itself is not an indication for therapy. Complications from extreme lymphocytosis, such as leukostasis, are rare in patients with nonprolymphocytic CLL who have blood lymphocyte counts below 800,000/μl.[319] Also, minor or moderate lymphadenopathy in the absence of other indications is usually not treated. Lymphadenopathy that causes functional disturbances should be treated. Such disturbances include pain due to nerve impingement from nodal encroachment; obstruction of the small bowel, ureter, or upper airway; or extreme adenopathy causing cosmetic disfigurement.

Newly diagnosed patients without the criteria listed in Table 98-4 should be followed monthly for the next several months. During follow-up exams, the hemogram should be monitored to access the rate of increase in the lymphocyte count and to evaluate for anemia or thrombocytopenia. Thereafter, patients with early-stage disease and good prognostic features should be followed at 2- to 6-month intervals without chemotherapy.

When the decision is made to initiate treatment, the objectives for therapy should be defined. Once the reasons for initiating chemotherapy are resolved, then treatment should be stopped, as there is no evidence that continued maintenance therapy improves survival.

Independent of the criteria listed in Table 98-4, patients who develop autoimmune hemolytic anemia (see Chap. 55), immune thrombocytopenia (see Chap. 117), or other pathologic autoimmune process warrant therapy appropriate for the autoimmune disease.

RESPONSE CRITERIA

In 1996, a National Cancer Institute–sponsored Working Group recommended criteria with which to describe the response to therapy in CLL.[290] The definition of a complete response is largely clinical rather than biological. A patient has a complete response when he/she becomes free of clinical disease for at least 2 months. The patient must maintain a normal complete blood, with at least 1500 neutrophils, 100,000 platelets, and fewer than 4000 lymphocytes per μl of blood. The hemoglobin must be greater than 11 g/dl without requiring red cell transfusion. In addition, the patient must lack constitutional symptoms, hepatosplenomegaly, or detectable adenopathy. Finally, the marrow must contain fewer than 30 percent lymphocytes and lack lymphocyte nodules.

To classify as having a partial response, the patient must experience at least a 50 percent reduction in the number of blood lymphocytes and have at least a 50 percent reduction in lymphadenopathy or hepatosplenomegaly. In addition, one or more of the following criteria must be achieved and maintained for at least 2 months: platelets are greater than 100,000/μl, hemoglobin is greater than 11 g/dl, or a 50 percent improvement in platelet or red cell counts over pretreatment values without transfusions. Treated patients who fulfill all the criteria for a complete response but have persistent lymphocyte nodules in the marrow are classified as having had a nodular partial response.[290]

Progressive disease is defined by at least one of the following: increase greater than or equal to 50 percent in the absolute lymphocyte count or a transformation to a more aggressive histology; increase greater than or equal to 50 percent in the size of the liver and/or spleen or the new appearance of palpable hepatomegaly or splenomegaly; increase greater than 50 percent in the sum of the products of at least two lymph nodes (one of which must be greater than 2 cm) on two consecutive physical examinations performed 2 weeks apart; or the appearance of new palpable lymphadenopathy. Patients who do not achieve a complete or partial remission and who do not have progressive disease are defined as having stable disease.

SINGLE-AGENT CHEMOTHERAPY

GLUCOCORTICOIDS

Glucocorticoids are effective as single agents in CLL, especially for patients with autoimmune hemolytic anemia or immune thrombocytopenia (see Chaps. 55 and 117). Even for nonautoimmune manifestations, prednisone, as a single agent, can control the disease temporarily in approximately 10 percent of patients.[320] Generally, prednisone is given orally at a dose of 40 to 60 mg/day for 1 week and then tapered and stopped after another week. Thereafter, prednisone is given every month for 5 days at 60 mg/day.

Partial responses may be achieved by treatment with intravenous methylprednisolone at 1 g/m^2/day for 5 days at monthly intervals for 7 months.[321,322] Concomitant therapy with H2 antagonists and prophylactic antibiotics can reduce the rate of treatment-related complications, which also include fluid retention and hyperglycemia.

ALKYLATING AGENTS

Chlorambucil Since its introduction in 1952, chlorambucil (Leukoran) has been the main alkylating agent used for CLL. Although chlorambucil is useful in the palliative therapy of patients with advanced-stage disease, it does not appear to improve survival and should not be used for asymptomatic patients with early-stage disease.[323]

Given orally, it generally is well tolerated, without the side effects that sometimes may be seen with other alkylating agents, such as cystitis, alopecia, or gastrointestinal distress. There seems to be some sparing of the myeloid and megakaryocytic series. Generally patients are started on a daily oral dose of 2 to 4 mg. This can be advanced to 6 to 8 mg per day if the patient does not experience intolerable hematologic toxicity. Alternatively, patients can be treated intermittently with a total oral dose of approximately 0.4 to 0.7 mg/kg. This dose can be given on day 1 or divided into four equal daily doses and given on days 1 through 4. The cycle is repeated every 2 to 4 weeks, depending on the time to marrow recovery. Pulse chlorambucil is as effective as continuous administration and is less myelotoxic.[320] Complete response rates of 15 percent and partial response rates of 65 percent are common.[324]

The effectiveness of chlorambucil for inducing apoptosis of leukemia cells in vitro can augmented by theophylline,[325–327] a phosphodiesterase inhibitor that commonly is used to treat adult asthma. This suggests that there may be therapeutic advantage to administering both drugs simultaneously to patients with CLL. In a nonrandomized trial involving 12 patients with progressive disease, responses were noted in 11 cases at doses of chlorambucil that were 3- to 38-fold lower than that used in previous cycles.[328]

High-dose chlorambucil has been studied for patients with advanced-stage CLL.[329] Chlorambucil was given for less than 6 months at a fixed dose of 15 mg per day until the patient achieved a complete response, or grade 3 toxicity. This treatment was noted in one single-institution study to effect a higher complete and partial response rate (89.5 percent) than that achieved with cyclophosphamide, doxorubicin,

vincristine, and prednisone (CHOP) (e.g., six monthly cycles of doxorubicin at 25 mg/m^2 on day 1, vincristine 1 mg/m^2 on day 1, cyclophosphamide 30 mg/m^2 per day, and prednisone 40 mg/m^2 per day on days 1 to 5). However, significant myelotoxicity was observed.

Cyclophosphamide Cyclophosphamide is as active as chlorambucil in CLL.[330] Patients can be started on daily oral doses of 50 to 100 mg. Alternatively, patients can be treated intermittently with 500 to 750 mg/m^2 given intravenously or orally every 3 to 4 weeks, depending on the time to marrow recovery. Because intermittent or daily oral cyclophosphamide predisposes to hemorrhagic cystitis, it should be taken as a single dose in the morning rather than at bedtime. Patients should be encouraged to drink at least 2 to 3 liters of fluid per day.

DEOXYADENOSINE ANALOGS

Fludarabine Fludarabine (9-β-D-arabinofuranosyl-2-fluoradenine, F-ara-A) is a fluorinated monophosphate derivative of an adenosine analog that has significant activity in the treatment of CLL.[331] Given as a 30-min intravenous infusion at a dose of 25 mg/m^2 daily for 5 days at 4-week intervals, this drug can induce hematologic complete and partial responses in a high percentage of patients.[332–337] An oral form of fludarabine has been developed that has good bioavailability and low intra-individual variation in its pharmacodynamics[338] making it feasible to consider alternative dosing regimens.

Multicenter trials typically have observed overall response rates to parenteral fludarabine of approximately 45 percent, including 10 percent with complete responses, in previously treated patients. Furthermore, overall response rates of approximately 70 percent, including 38 percent with complete responses, are achieved when fludarabine is given as front-line therapy.[339–342] Fludarabine, as a single agent, appears more effective in CLL than some combination chemotherapy regimens, such as CAP (cyclophosphamide 750 mg/m^2 and doxorubicin 50 mg/m^2 on day 1, and prednisone 50 mg/m^2 per day on days 1 to 5).[343,344] Moreover, remission duration appears significantly longer in patients achieving a response with fludarabine than in those who respond to such combination regimens.

Long-term follow-up studies indicate that even those patients who achieved complete response to fludarabine ultimately will have recurrent disease.[342,345] The median time to progression of responders was 33 months for those who had not received prior chemotherapy, and 21 months for those who had. The median times to progression were 27 months for patients with a partial response and 30 to 37 months for those achieving a complete response.[342] Although multicenter clinical trials have confirmed the activity of single-agent fludarabine in CLL,[339–341] treatment of patients with this drug has not been shown to improve overall survival.

About one-third of patients who have not received prior therapy and nearly half of those who are refractory to treatment with chlorambucil will not achieve even a partial response to treatment with fludarabine. Logistic regression analysis in one study indentified four factors that were associated with poorer response to fludarabine: Rai stage III-IV disease, prior therapy, older age, and low albumin levels.[346] In vitro drug-sensitivity testing using a differential staining cytotoxicity (DiSC) assay may have predictive value in identifying patients with fludarabine-response disease.[347,348] In addition, patients who do not show evidence for a response to the first two cycles of therapy are unlikely to achieve a partial or complete response to subsequent cycles of treatment. For this reason, patients who fail to show any clinical benefit from two cycles of treatment should be considered for alternative types of therapy to minimize toxicity.

The major toxicities are hematologic and immunologic. Neutropenia is noted in approximately two-thirds of treated patients with advanced disease,[335] although this usually is not dose-limiting. Patients also may experience reversible neurologic toxicity, even after receiving the standard dose of fludarabine.[349] Highly responsive patients may experience the tumor-lysis syndrome.[336,350,351]

The major morbidity associated with fludarabine is immune suppression. Fludarabine produces a pronounced decrease in the number of blood T cells, especially CD4+ T cells, that often persists for more than a year after therapy.[352,353] Treated patients apparently have an increased incidence of infection with opportunistic organisms, including herpes simplex, herpes zoster, *Listeria monocytogenes*, and *Pneumocystis carinii*.[336,346,353]

Patients treated with fludarabine have been noted to have an increased incidence of new-onset autoimmune diseases, such as autoimmune hemolytic anemia, immune thrombocytopenia, or pure red cell aplasia.[344,354,355] However, it is controversial whether this defines a causal relationship. Tumor lysis syndrome can be another therapy-related complication.[356,357] Finally, CLL patients treated with fludarabine also may develop transfusion-associated graft-versus-host disease,[358,359] possibly reflecting the overall impairment to the host immune system that is induced by this drug. Despite the associated immune suppression, treatment with fludarabine does not appear to increase the risk for secondary malignancies in patients with CLL.[360]

2'-Chlorodeoxyadenosine (Cladribine) 2'-Chlorodeoxyadenosine (cladribine) is another deoxyadenosine analog that has activity in CLL[361] (see Chap. 81). Different dosage schedules or administrations routes have proved effective, although the response rates do not appear to be better than those achieved with fludarabine. Monthly courses of cladribine given via intravenous infusion over 2 h at 0.12 mg/kg, daily for 5 consecutive days, has resulted in overall response rates of approximately 40 percent to 60 percent in patients who were previously treated with alkylating agents.[362–364] Higher overall response rates are observed in previously nontreated patients. Although one study found that patients refractory to fludarabine still could respond to cladribine,[365] a subsequent and larger study found that patients with advanced CLL refractory to fludarabine therapy were not likely to benefit from treatment with cladribine.[366]

Cladribine also appears effective when administered orally.[367] Overall response rates of 75 percent were noted in previously nontreated CLL patients given cladribine at 10 mg/m² per day orally for 5 consecutive days.[368]

Treatment with cladribine has not been shown to prolong survival. The median duration of partial remissions is approximately 9 months, and nonresponding patients have a relatively short median survival of approximately 4 months. DiSC assays[347] have been reported to have predictive value in assessing a given patient's potential response to therapy.[369] However, the most evident predictor of a good response was a rapid decrease of blood lymphocyte counts following the first course of therapy. As with fludarabine, patients who fail to show any clinical benefit from two cycles of cladribine should be considered for alternative types of therapy to minimize toxicity.

The toxicities of treatment with cladribine are similar to those with fludarabine. Thrombocytopenia is a common dose-limiting toxicity, as is general myelosuppression. As with fludarabine, treated patients experience long-lasting reductions in the levels of blood T cells and have impaired cellular immunity to viral infections. Systemic fungal infections and opportunistic infections are a common cause of morbidity and mortality. There is one case report of a patient with refractory CLL who experienced the tumor-lysis syndrome following therapy with cladribine,[370] although the incidence of this appears to be very low.

2'-Deoxycoformycin (Pentostatin) Deoxycoformycin (pentostatin) is a purine analog synthesized by *Streptomyces antibioticus* that structurally is related to adenosine.[371] This drug inhibits adenosine deaminase, an enzyme important in lymphocyte purine metabolism (see Chap. 81). Pentostatin generally is administered intravenously at a dosage of 4 mg/m² weekly for 3 weeks, then 4 mg/m² every other week for 6 weeks and once a month for 6 months.[371,372] This drug appears less effective in CLL than fludarabine or cladribine, effecting complete or partial responses in approximately 25 percent of patients.[372] Since the toxicity of pentostatin is comparable to those noted for fludarabine or cladribine, it appears to offer no unique advantage for the treatment of CLL.

OTHER AGENTS

Cytosine Arabinoside High-dose cytosine arabinoside has modest activity in advanced-stage CLL.[373] It is administered intravenously at a dosage of 3 g/m² delivered over 2 h. This may be repeated one to three times every 12 h to complete one cycle.

Etoposide Patients who failed alkylator-based chemotherapy have been noted to achieve partial responses with oral etoposide, lasting 2 to 18 months.[374] Etoposide was administered as a single drug at a dosage of 50 mg/m² per day for 21 days in a 28-day cycle. Myelosuppression was the most common and serious dose-limiting effect.

Melarsoprol Melarsoprol, an organic arsenical compound used for treatment of trypanosomiasis, was noted to effect down-modulation of BCL-2 and induce apoptosis of CLL cells in vitro.[375] Because of this, a clinical trial was conducted in which patients received escalating intravenous doses daily for 3 days, repeated weekly for 3 weeks, with doses of 1 mg/kg on day 1, 2 mg/kg on day 2, and 3.6 mg/kg on day 3 and on all days thereafter, up to a maximum daily dose of 200 mg.[376] However, treatment was associated with significant central nervous system toxicity and limited clinical benefit.

COMBINATION CHEMOTHERAPY

CHLORAMBUCIL AND PREDNISONE

The standard regimen for treating patients who warrant the initiation of chemotherapy has been the combination of oral chlorambucil and prednisone. Each cycle consists of chlorambucil at 0.4 to 0.7 mg/kg on day 1, with prednisone at 80 mg per day on days 1 through 5. This course is repeated every 2 to 4 weeks, depending on the time to marrow recovery. The dosage of chlorambucil may be divided and given over 2 days. It is raised or lowered based upon the response and the degree of myelosuppression. When the white cell count declines below 10,000/μl the dose of chlorambucil should be reduced to maintain the white cell count between 5000/μl and 10,000/μl. The addition of prednisone to chlorambucil may provide a therapeutic advantage over chlorambucil alone.[324] However, more recent studies have challenged this notion.[377,378] Nevertheless, responses to the combination of chlorambucil and prednisone occur in about 80 percent (complete remissions in 15 percent plus partial remissions in 65 percent) of patients.[320,379–381]

FLUDARABINE-CONTAINING REGIMENS

Fludarabine/Cyclophosphamide (FC) Combinations of fludarabine, at 20 to 30 mg/m² daily for 3 days, and cyclophosphamide, at 200 to 300 mg/m² daily for 3 days, given every 28 days can result in favorable clinical responses in extensively pretreated patients.[382] However, this combination does not appear to offer a significant response or survival advantage over single-agent fludarabine in previously nontreated patients. As such, this combination should only be considered as salvage therapy. Use of this combination is associated with a relatively high rate of nausea and vomiting (20 percent and 10 percent respectively) and skin rash. Myelosuppression can be severe and is a major dose-limiting toxicity.

Fludarabine/Mitoxantrone Treatment with fludarabine, given at 30 mg/m² on days 1 through 3 of a 28-day cycle, along with mitoxantrone, given at 10 mg/m² on the first day of each cycle, has achieved overall response rates of 80 percent in previously nontreated patients and 60 percent in patients who were refractory to therapy with alkylating agents.[382] As such, this treatment may not provide for a significant advantage over that using single-agent fludarabine in previously nontreated patients. Its utility as salvage therapy is under investigation. Myelosuppression is the major dose-limiting toxicity.

Fludarabine/Cisplatin Cisplatin, administered at 100 mg/m² via continuous intravenous infusion over 4 days, has been used in combination with fludarabine given at 30 mg/m² via bolus intravenous infusion on days 3 and 4 of a 28-day cycle.[383] These two drugs, alone or in combination with cytosine arabinoside at 500 mg/m² on day 4 of the cycle, did not appear to offer significant benefit over that of single-agent fludarabine for the treatment of patients refractory to alkylating agents. Its use as a salvage regimen is under investigation. Myelosuppression is the major dose-limiting toxicity.

Fludarabine/Prednisone Concomitant use of prednisone with fludarabine does not improve the response rate but rather increases the risk for opportunistic infection, resulting in poorer outcome than use of fludarabine alone.[342,346] Because of this, fludarabine/prednisone combinations are not recommended for patients with CLL.

Fludarabine/Chlorambucil Fludarabine has been used in combination with chlorambucil.[350] Chlorambucil was given orally on day 1 at 15 or 20 mg/m², and fludarabine was administered intravenously on days 1 to 5 at 10, 15, or 20 mg/m², every 28 days. With chlorambucil at 15 mg/m² given on day 1, the maximum tolerated dose for fludarabine was 20 mg/m². Although responses were observed, treatment with this combination has not been shown to be significantly better than that with fludarabine alone.[350]

CLADRIBINE-CONTAINING REGIMENS
The response to cladribine in combination with cyclophosphamide and prednisone (CCP) has been evaluated in patients with CLL.[384] Patients received cladribine at 0.1 mg/kg per day as a subcutaneous bolus injection on days 1 to 3 with intravenous cyclophosphamide 500 mg/m² on day 1 and oral prednisone 40 mg/m² on days 1 to 5 of a 28-day cycle for a maximum of six cycles. Overall response rates of 88 percent were observed, with 4 patients achieving a complete clinical and hematologic response and 12 achieving a partial response.

CYCLOPHOSPHAMIDE, VINCRISTINE, AND PREDNISONE
The combination of cyclophosphamide, vincristine, and prednisone (CVP) is effective in previously untreated patients and in some patients with refractory CLL.[385] The dosages are cyclophosphamide 300 to 400 mg/m², orally, daily for 5 days, vincristine 1 to 2 mg intravenously on day 1, and prednisone 40 mg/m² orally per day for 5 days. The cycle is repeated every 3 to 4 weeks. About 25 percent of patients achieve a complete remission, and approximately 50 percent obtain a partial remission when treated with this regimen.[385] No differences were noted in response rates or survival of CLL patients treated in randomized trials with either CVP versus chlorambucil and prednisone[381] or chlorambucil alone.[386]

Patients previously treated with chlorambucil and prednisone may respond to CVP. Prolonged therapy over a 12- to 18-month period may prolong survival.[379] In one series, Rai stages III and IV patients had a median survival of 4.2 years following 18 months of therapy, with the median survival of complete responders over 60 months. This may be compared historically with the 19-month median survival reported for stages III and IV patients in the mid-1970s.[22] Therapy with cyclophosphamide, vincristine, and prednisone is associated with significant neurotoxicity and with more severe marrow toxicity than is therapy with chlorambucil and prednisone.

CYCLOPHOSPHAMIDE, DOXORUBICIN, VINCRISTINE, AND PREDNISONE
The addition of doxorubicin to CVP chemotherapy (CHOP) has been evaluated in patients with advanced CLL.[387] These patients were treated with CVP, and half also received doxorubicin 25 mg/m² on day 1. Adding doxorubicin to the chemotherapeutic regimen increased the median survival from less than 2 years to more than 4 years in one study. However, the mean survival of patients treated with CHOP was similar to that of patients who received CVP over an 18-month period. Vincristine does not appear to add substantially to the CHOP regimen. In a randomized multicenter clinical trial, patients with stage B or stage C CLL were treated with CHOP or with cyclophosphamide, doxorubicin, and prednisone without vincristine (CAP). The rates of partial response and overall response were, respectively, 64 percent and 75 percent for the CHOP-treated patients, and 65 percent and 72 percent for the CAP-treated patients.[388] However, these response rates compare unfavorably with that of a third group of comparably staged CLL who were treated only with fludarabine, this group achieving partial or overall response rates in this same study of 75 percent and 94 percent respectively. This is consistent with other studies that show that fludarabine appears more effective as a single agent in CLL than these combination regimens.[343]

VINCRISTINE, DOXORUBICIN, AND DEXAMETHASONE
The regimen consisting of vincristine, doxorubicin, and dexamethasone (VAD) appears to have limited activity in CLL. In one study, patients received a 96-h infusion of 1.6 mg vincristine and 36 mg/m² of doxorubicin and took 40 mg of dexamethasone orally each day for 4 days. This cycle was repeated every 3 weeks, inducing a 21 percent partial response rate and no complete responses.[343]

CYTOSINE ARABINOSIDE, CISPLATIN, AND ETOPOSIDE (ACE)
Combination therapy with cytosine arabinoside (4 doses at 2 g/m² every 12 h), cisplatin (2 doses of 35 mg/m² every 24 h), and etoposide (2 doses at 100 mg/m²) has induced partial responses and occasional complete responses in advanced-stage patients with refractory disease, sometimes inducing an acute tumor-lysis syndrome.[389]

SPLENECTOMY

Splenectomy may ameliorate the cytopenias associated with advanced-stage CLL, particularly thrombocytopenia.[390,391] In one study, patients who underwent splenectomy for thrombocytopenia and/or anemia had a trend toward improved 3-year actuarial survival (31 percent ± 9 percent) over matched subjects who did not undergo splenectomy (12 percent ± 7 percent).[391] Preoperative performance status appeared to be the best predictor of perioperative and postoperative survival.

RADIATION THERAPY

Systemic irradiation was the first therapeutic modality used in CLL that was found to effect some degree of patient improvement.[10] However, it soon was recognized that the therapeutic benefit was short-lived and often resulted in severe marrow suppression.[392]

Irradiation remains a useful technique for localized treatment to ameliorate symptoms due to nerve impingement, vital organ compromise, painful bone lesions, or bulky disfigurement. Delivery of 200 Gy can result in rapid shrinkage of lymph nodes or masses.

Splenic irradiation is useful in patients with painful splenomegaly,[393] especially in patients considered poor candidates for surgical splenectomy.[394] Patients may experience systemic improvement after splenic irradiation, possibly due to irradiation of leukemic cells circulating through the spleen. However, the low rate of response and the short remission duration argue that splenic irradiation should be combined with other therapeutic approaches.[395]

Endolymphatic radiotherapy[396] and extracorporeal irradiation of blood[397] appear to provide limited improvement in lymphocyte counts but do not appear to improve patient survival. Extracorporeal photochemotherapy also has been tried in B-cell CLL but was found ineffective.[398]

LEUKAPHERESIS

Intensive leukapheresis may reduce organomegaly and improve hemoglobin and platelet levels.[399] The measure has been advocated for patients with marrow failure who are refractory to standard therapy.[400] This treatment has not been shown to improve patient survival.

INVESTIGATIONAL THERAPIES

MARROW OR BLOOD STEM CELL TRANSPLANTATION

Autologous Stem Cell Transplantation   Several studies have examined the benefit of high-dose chemotherapy with stem cell rescue in patients with CLL (see Chap. 18). Complicating autologous stem cell transplantation (SCT) is the high probability that stem cell collections are contaminated with CLL cells, even in patients who have been treated to minimal residual disease.[401–403] This has prompted investigation into more effective purging techniques to remove unwanted leukemia cells prior to transplantation. Nevertheless, a few studies with small numbers of patients have shown that complete clinical responses can be achieved in CLL.[404–406] However, it is not yet known whether patients who have achieved complete responses in the setting of SCT have been cured of their disease.

Of some concern, however, are studies that identified trisomy 12 or 13q deletions in the CD34+ progenitor cells of the marrow or blood in a subset of patients with CLL.[402,403] This suggests that patients with CLL might have CD34+ progenitor cells that harbor cytogenetic lesions that contribute to leukemia development. As such, eradication of the B cells that have differentiated from an aberrant pluripotent clone may not completely eliminate the risk for recurrent neoplastic transformation. Consistent with this are cases of recurrent CLL following high-dose therapy and autologous stem cell transplantation that have immunoglobulin gene rearrangements that were distinct from those of the original CLL clone.[407]

Allogeneic Stem Cell Transplantation   Transplantation with allogeneic stem cells is being evaluated for younger patients with poor-prognosis CLL.[408–413] Treatment-related morbidity rates in some series have been high, occurring in approximately half the treated patients.[410] Autologous transplantation requires elimination of leukemia cells that invariably are found in the marrow following conventional treatments. Aggressive treatment may eradicate the leukemia cells to the levels that cannot be detected using sensitive PCR techniques to detect clonal immunoglobulin gene rearrangements.[408] Patients who relapse following allogeneic marrow transplantation may respond to infusions of donor leukocytes, demonstrating the effectiveness of a graft-versus-leukemia effect.[412,413] Collectively, these studies provide encouraging evidence that transplantation may be curative in a subset of patients with CLL.

''Mini'' Allogeneic Stem Cell Transplantation   Because patients who receive allogeneic cells appear to benefit from a graft-versus-leukemia response, some groups have treated CLL patients with nonmyeloablative doses of chemotherapy prior to allogeneic SCT. Khouri and colleagues[414] treated 15 patients (median age 55; range 45 to 71 years) in this fashion, using a pretransplant regimen consisting of fludarabine and cyclophosphamide. Two to three months after transplant, the patients were infused with donor lymphocytes if

they did not have graft-versus-host disease (GVHD) (see Chap. 18). Eleven patients had engraftment of donor cells, eight of which achieved a complete response. However, only 7 of the 15 treated patients (47 percent) were alive after a median follow-up of 180 days (range, 90 to 767 days), indicating that this approach is associated with a high mortality.

Another study examined allogeneic marrow transplantation for 15 CLL patients who were refractory to fludarabine.[415] Three patients received a one- or two-antigen-mismatched graft, and the remainder received HLA-identical sibling donor grafts. Fourteen patients engrafted, and thirteen (87 percent) achieved a complete remission with a median follow-up of 3 to 60 months. These results are comparable to those observed after allogeneic marrow transplantation for CLL patients who had never been treated with fludarabine.

IMMUNOTHERAPY AND BIOLOGIC RESPONSE MODIFIERS

Cytokines   Recombinant interferon-α has been reported effective in patients with early-stage disease,[416] inducing partial responses in about two-thirds of treated patients.[417] This agent lowers the lymphocyte count with minimal side effects.[418] In contrast, patients with advanced CLL may experience an acceleration of their disease when treated with higher doses of interferon.[419]

A clinical trial examined whether treatment of patients with human interleukin-6 (h-IL-6) for 5 days prior to CHOP chemotherapy could enhance leukemia-cell proliferation and response to chemotherapy. Of note, leukemia-cell expression of CD20 increased during the period of treatment with Rh-IL-6, raising the prospect of using Rh-IL-6 in combination with anti-CD20 monoclonal antibodies. However, Rh-IL-6 did not appear to enhance the proportion of leukemia cells in S phase, as assessed by labeling studies with bromodeoxyuridine or the observed response to CHOP chemotherapy.

Passive Immunotherapy   Passive immunotherapy with monoclonal antibodies targeted to immunoglobulin idiotypes expressed by CLL cells have not resulted in significant therapeutic benefit.[420] Infusion with anti-T101 (CD5), a murine monoclonal antibody, has shown transient beneficial effects, but modulation of the surface antigen by the target cells and allergic reactions to the murine antibody limited the usefulness of this approach.[421,422] Phase I trials have been performed testing the safety of treating CLL with toxin-conjugated antibodies specific for CD19 (B4)[423] or the CD25 (Tac)[424] antigen.

Rituximab, IDEC-C₂B₈.   Rituximab is humanized monoclonal antibody specific for human CD20.[425] Infusion of this mAb at 375 mg/m² per day for 4 days per cycle can induce responses in nearly half of patients treated with relapsed follicular lymphoma,[426,427] possibly by directing antibody-dependent cellular cytotoxicity (ADCC) against CD20-bearing lymphoma B cells. However, CLL B cells express nearly tenfold lower levels of CD20 than most lymphoma cells and appear less sensitive to treatment with rituximab. Several clinical trials testing rituximab in CLL are ongoing. Nevertheless, some patients have experienced tumor-lysis syndrome following treatment with rituximab.[428] Moreover, patients with leukemia cell counts exceeding 50×10^9/liter at the time of treatment have been noted to experience a severe cytokine-release syndrome secondary to release of tumor necrosis factor alpha (TNF-α) and interleukin-6 (IL-6).[429] Elevated cytokine levels during treatment were associated with clinical symptoms, including fever, chills, nausea, vomiting, hypotension, and dyspnea. Lymphocyte and platelet counts dropped to 50 to 75 percent of baseline values within 12 h after the onset of the infusion. Simultaneously, there was a 5-fold to 10-fold increase of liver enzymes, D-dimers, and lactate dehydrogenase, as well as a prolongation of the prothrombin time. This complication may be mitigated by use of a fractionated dosing schedule with infusion of 50 mg rituximab on the first day, 150 mg on day 2, and the rest of the 375-mg/m² dose on day 3.[429]

CAMPATH-1H. CAMPATH-1H is humanized monoclonal antibody-specific human CD52.[430–432] This antibody binds to a surface antigen present on most lymphocytes, including CLL B cells, and can induce complement-mediated and antibody-dependent T-cell cytotoxicity. In one study, patients who were refractory to chemotherapy were given intravenous infusions of 30 mg CAMPATH-1H three times a week for 12 weeks.[433] Of the 29 patients to receive such therapy, 38 percent experienced a partial remission, and 4 percent achieved a complete remission with median response duration of 12 months. CAMPATH-1H does not appear to have a significant impact on lymphadenopathy.

To minimize the "first-dose" reactions to intravenous CAMPATH-1H, such as fever, chills, and/or rash, CAMPATH-1H also has been administered subcutaneously at 30 mg three times per week for at least 6 weeks.[431] Although partial remissions also were achieved, the duration of the response to CAMPATH-1H by either route is relatively short. Also, CAMPATH-1H treated patients appear to have an increased susceptibility to opportunistic infections (especially cytomegalovirus), possibly secondary to a further depletion of normal T-cells following treatment with this mAb.[431,433] Moreover, responses appear to be short-lived and associated with an increased incidence of opportunistic infections. Nevertheless, CAMPATH-1H may be of value in eradicating residual disease prior to autologous transplantation for patients who have persistent disease after treatment with chemotherapy.[433,434]

Lym-1. Lym-1 is an IgG$_{2a}$ mouse mAb specific for human B cells that has been used in the radioimmune therapy of CLL.[435,436] Conjugated with ¹³¹I, this mAb has been used in phase I/II trials in which patients received ¹³¹I-Lym-1 in escalating amounts from 1480 Mbq/m² to 3700 Mbq/m² (40 to 100 mCi/m²).[437,438] For patients with splenomegaly, most of the administered radiolabeled antibody localized to the spleen and did not distribute uniformly through other lymphoid tissue. Nevertheless, the treatment was well tolerated and associated with reductions in spleen size and/or lymphocytosis. Although argued to possibly increase survival, the numbers of treated patients and duration of follow-up preclude definitive conclusions at this time.

GENE THERAPY

Infection of leukemia B cells with a replication-defective adenovirus vector encoding recombinant CD154 (Ad-CD154) induces expression of a variety of coreceptors, including CD54, CD58, CD80 (B7-1), CD86 (B7-2), and CD70, on both infected and bystander leukemia B cells, rendering such cells more proficient in presenting antigens to autologous T cells.[222] Furthermore, Ad-CD154-infected CLL B cells can induce autologous T cells to generate cytotoxic T lymphocytes (CTL) in vitro specific for noninfected leukemia cells. This formed the basis for a clinical trial of gene therapy for CLL whereby leukemia B cell are transduced with Ad-CD154 ex vivo and then infused back into the same patient to induce host anti-leukemia-cell immune rejection.[439]

DISEASE COMPLICATIONS

INFECTION

Infection is major cause of morbidity and mortality in CLL.[440] Patients often have an impaired antibody response to microbes and hypogammaglobulinemia, making them highly susceptible to recurrent infection. *Streptococcus pneumoniae, Staphylococcus aureus, Streptococcus pyogenes, Escherichia coli,* and the herpes zoster-varicella virus account for most infections, and the lungs, skin, and

urinary tract are the sites most frequently affected.[440] Fungal, mycobacterial, and cryptococcal infections are uncommon. However, as noted above, patients treated with purine analogs, such as fludarabine, apparently have an increased incidence of infection with other opportunistic organisms, including herpes simplex, cytomegalovirus, herpes zoster, *Listeria monocytogenes, Pneumocystis carinii,* and mycobacteria.[336,346,353,441]

Infections usually respond well to antibiotics in CLL patients with early-stage disease. However, at later stages, the response is less satisfactory and more often associated with systemic complications. For such patients it often is necessary to administer antibiotics for prolonged periods to eradicate soft-tissue or urinary tract infection. Patients may be immunized with nonviable vaccines, such as those used to immunize patients against influenza or *S. pneumoniae.* However, the response to immunization is often poor. The use of live vaccines is contraindicated due to the risk of the attenuated agent being virulent in the immunocompromised host.

Patients with advanced-stage disease, hypogammaglobulinemia, and low levels of specific antibodies to pneumococcal capsular polysaccharide appear to be at greatest risk for severe or multiple infections.[442,443] Immunoglobulin deficiency is the factor that correlates best with the frequency, severity, and pattern of infection.[440] For this reason, investigators have examined the utility of administering intravenous gammaglobulin at 400 mg/kg every 3 weeks to patients with severe hypogammaglobulinemia associated with recurrent infections. While such therapy may decrease the frequency of bacterial infections,[444] it may not improve survival.[445]

SYSTEMIC AUTOIMMUNE DISEASE

CLL patients have an increased risk of autoimmune disease. Prednisone at a dosage of 1 mg/kg per day is used to treat autoimmune hemolytic anemia or immune thrombocytopenia and can be tapered slowly to the minimum dosage necessary. These diseases, and various treatment regimens for refractory disease, are discussed in Chaps. 55 and 117.

For CLL patients who develop pure red cell aplasia presumed secondary to pathogenic autoantibodies, the combination of cyclosporine and prednisone appears superior to prednisone alone.[446]

SECOND MALIGNANCIES

Patients with CLL have an increased risk of second malignancies.[440,447,448] The most frequent second tumors are melanoma, soft-tissue sarcoma, and colorectal and lung carcinoma. Multiple myeloma occurs at 10 times the expected rate in patients with CLL[449] but evidently does not arise from the same malignant B-cell clone.[450–452] Both untreated and treated CLL patients can develop acute myelogenous leukemia or myelodysplastic syndrome.[453,454] The concurrence of AML or MDS and untreated CLL may represent two separate disease processes. Nucleoside analogs do not appear to enhance the risk for secondary malignancies.[360] However, for some patients, alkylating agents may contribute to the development of second malignancy. In one large multicenter trial, patients with stage A CLL who were treated with intermittent chlorambucil had a poorer survival than that of a matched control group of untreated CLL patients, in part because they experienced a higher incidence of epithelial neoplasms.[455]

LEUKEMIA CELL TRANSFORMATION

CLL can undergo transformation into either of three disease entities, each of which has an adverse prognostic implication.

RICHTER TRANSFORMATION

In 1928, Maurice N. Richter described an aggressive lymphoma that developed in a patient with CLL.[456] Now described as Richter transformation, this transition from an indolent leukemia to an aggressive, large B-cell, high-grade lymphoma can occur at any time in the course of CLL, occurring in approximately 3 percent of all patients at median interval of 2 years following the initial diagnosis of CLL.[309,457]

It is debated whether these lymphomas arise from the original CLL clone or from a de novo lymphoproliferation in the setting of CLL.[458] However, nucleic acid sequence analyses of the immunoglobulin genes expressed by the original leukemic cells and the high-grade lymphoma of a patient with Richter transformation have provided irrefutable evidence that such lymphomas can arise from the original CLL clone.[459] Some cases, however, may represent a genetically unrelated, independent second cancer. As noted, CLL patients with Richter transformation have a higher incidence of P53 mutations than do CLL patients with indolent disease,[130] suggesting that cytogenetic abnormalities acquired in the course of CLL may generate a neoplasm with more aggressive growth properties.

The most common clinical and laboratory features associated with Richter transformation (with their respective incidence indicated in parentheses) include: (1) elevation of serum lactate dehydrogenase (82 percent); (2) rapid lymph node enlargement (64 percent); (3) systemic symptoms of fever and/or weight loss (59 percent); (4) a monoclonal gammopathy on serum protein electrophoresis (44 percent); and (5) extranodal disease (41 percent).[309] Patients also may have abdominal symptoms due to increasing hepatosplenomegaly or neurologic symptoms secondary to central nervous system involvement.[460–462] Occasional patients may present with an extranodal mass lesion.[463] Patients with Richter transformation often have bulky retroperitoneal adenopathy and massive splenomegaly.

The diagnosis of Richter transformation requires lymph node biopsy. Involved lymph nodes are effaced by large immunoblastic cells with abundant basophilic cytoplasm and irregular nuclei with prominent nucleoli.[275] The marrow may be infiltrated with these immature cells, sometimes resulting in osteolytic lesions. Descriptions of the lymphoma cells in tissue vary from what the Working Formulation currently describes as either small noncleaved cell lymphoma, large-cell lymphoma (cleaved or noncleaved), or large-cell lymphoma with tumor giant cells.[457,460,461,464] All these types are considered high-grade lymphomas in both the Working Formulation and the Kiel classification (see Chap. 101) and are distinguished readily from the small lymphocytic lymphoma that typifies the tissue phase of CLL.[275]

The treatment for patients with Richter transformation is similar to that used for patients with high-grade lymphoma (see Chap. 103). Although occasional patients have achieved long-term remissions following intensive multiagent chemotherapy,[462] most patients at best achieve only a partial remission and have a very poor prognosis. Overall, patients with Richter transformation have median survival of 5 months from diagnosis.[309]

CLL/PLL AND PROLYMPHOCYTIC TRANSFORMATION

In nearly 15 percent of B-cell CLL patients, the population of leukemic cells consists of a mixture of small lymphocytes and prolymphocytes, the latter cell type accounting for between 10 to 50 percent of the lymphoid cells.[465,466] These patients have been termed to have CLL/PLL, although this term is not in frequent use. These patients have a degree of lymphadenopathy and age distribution similar to that of patients with CLL but more pronounced splenomegaly. In 80 percent of CLL/PLL cases, the proportion of prolymphocytes remains stable, and survival does not differ from that of CLL patients with comparable clinical-stage disease.[467] Such patients generally do not have blood prolymphocyte counts above 15,000/μl or massive splenomegaly.

The remaining patients with CLL/PLL will undergo a prolymphocytic transformation. This is characterized by a decrease in the proportion of leukemic cells able to form rosettes with mouse erythrocytes,

increases in the proportions of blood lymphocytes with prolymphocyte morphology and immunophenotype, and progressive splenomegaly. One study noted the leukemic cells in transformation apparently acquired the t(6;12) translocation that commonly is associated with prolymphocytic leukemia.[468] Patients with this transformation respond poorly to chemotherapy, and survival is limited. In one study, the mean survival of patients after transformation to prolymphocytic leukemia was 9 months.[469]

ACUTE LYMPHOBLASTIC LEUKEMIA

Very rarely, patients with B-cell CLL may develop acute lymphoblastic leukemia.[470] Studies of a few of the dozen cases reported indicate that the acute leukemia can arise from the same B-cell clone as that of the CLL cells.[471–474] Blastic transformation has been associated with a seven- to eightfold increase in the expression of *C-MYC* and immunoglobulin genes.[474] Leukemic blast cells generally express terminal deoxynucleotidyl transferase (TdT) and high levels of surface immunoglobulin and HLA-DR.

PROGNOSIS

There are no established cures for CLL, and spontaneous remissions are extremely rare.[475,476] Nevertheless, the prognosis can vary substantially between different patients, depending upon clinical stage and the presence or absence of disease features that have been associated with disease progression and/or a more adverse clinical outcome (see section on clinical staging).

Patient age had been argued to be an independent prognostic factor.[298,308,477,478] However, a large study from the U.S. National Cancer Data Base revealed that the 5-year relative survival was 69.5 percent, 72.2 percent, 63.1 percent, and 41.7 percent for age groups under 40, 40 to 59, 60 to 79, and 80+ years respectively, indicating that the 5-year survival does not vary significantly between these different age groups.[1] As such, it appears that CLL, and not comorbid disease, caused the greatest percentage of deaths, even among the aged.

Another study also found that younger and older patients have a similar overall median survival probability but had different distributions of causes of deaths.[479] CLL-unrelated deaths and secondary malignancies predominated in the older age group, whereas the direct effects of leukemia were prevalent in the younger age group. At diagnosis, younger and older patients displayed a similar distribution of clinical features, except for a significantly higher male/female ratio in younger patients (2.85 versus 1.29; p less than 0.0001). Both groups had an elevated rate of second malignancies (8.3 percent versus 10.7 percent), whereas the occurrence of Richter syndrome was significantly higher in younger patients (5.9 percent versus 1.2 percent; p less than 0.00001). Two subsets of young CLL patients with a different prognostic outcome could be identified. One group, comprising 40 percent of the patients under age 55, had long-lasting stable disease without treatment and an actuarial survival probability of 94 percent at 12 years from diagnosis. The remaining patients had progressive disease and a median survival probability of 5 years after therapy.[479] A key feature of patients with the more adverse prognosis is evidence for disease progression.[480]

B-CELL PROLYMPHOCYTIC LEUKEMIA

HISTORY AND DEFINITION

B-cell prolymphocytic leukemia (PLL) is a clinical and morphologic variant of CLL that first was described as a distinct entity in 1973.[481] It is a subacute lymphoid leukemia with an incidence that is about 10 percent that of CLL. The diagnosis of prolymphocytic leukemia requires that at least 55 percent of the circulating leukemic lymphocytes have a prolymphocytic morphology.[465] Such cells are larger than resting lymphocytes and have a high nucleocytoplasmic ratio, a basophilic cytoplasm devoid of granules, moderately condensed chromatin, and a single prominent nucleolus. In 80 percent of such cases, the prolymphocytes are neoplastic B cells,[482] whereas the remaining cases are derived from mature T cells.

ETIOLOGY AND PATHOGENESIS

The etiology is unknown. There is a 4:1 male to female predominance, suggesting that males are much more susceptible to developing this disease. Also, B-cell prolymphocytic leukemia can evolve from B-cell CLL.[466] As such, factors that contribute to the pathogenesis or progression of CLL may operate in B-cell prolymphocytic leukemia.

CYTOGENETICS

The karyotype of the leukemia cells from many patients displays the $14q^+$ abnormality.[483] Trisomy 12 is another recurrent abnormality.[484,485] Deletions of the long arm of chromosome 6 ($6q^-$) and rearrangement affecting chromosomes 1 and 12 are occasionally observed. One study observed a t(6;12)(q15;p13) chromosomal anomaly in several independent cases, leading the investigators to postulate that this anomaly is distinctive for a subset of patients with prolymphocytic leukemia.[468] The (2;13)(q35;q14) translocation that commonly is associated with pediatric rhabdomyosarcoma also has been identified.[486]

Loss of heterozygosity at 17p13.3 associated with inactivating mutations in the P53 gene is observed in as many as three-quarters of the cases examined.[487,488] The high frequency of P53 mutations in B-cell prolymphocytic leukemia is in marked contrast to what is observed in B-cell CLL and may explain the relative resistance of this disease to therapy. In addition, some cases of B-cell prolymphocytic leukemia have t(2;8) translocations involving the C-MYC gene that are similar to those observed in Burkitt lymphoma (see Chap. 103).[489] Such mutations may account for the aggressive clinical course of prolymphocytic leukemia relative to that of B-cell CLL.

CYTOGENESIS

B-cell prolymphocytic leukemia is derived from mature B cells that have undergone immunoglobulin gene rearrangement (see Chap. 83). These cells invariably have monoclonal immunoglobulin gene rearrangements and express many of the same B-cell surface antigens as do leukemic cells in CLL. In many cases, the disease may evolve from preexistent CLL. The immunoglobulins expressed by prolymphocytic leukemia cells frequently bear autoantibody-associated cross-reactive idiotypes, suggesting a biased use of immunoglobulin variable region genes similar to that of leukemic cells in B-cell CLL.[490] However, sequence analyses indicate the prolymphocytic leukemia cells from at least half of the patients express nonmutated variable region genes, whereas the remaining cases express mutated variable region genes.[491] The presence of such somatic mutations suggests that the B-cell PLL cells from at least some individuals may be derived from a postgerminal center B cell (see Chaps. 5 and 83).

CLINICAL FEATURES

Over 50 percent of the patients are over 70 years of age at diagnosis. Presenting symptoms include fatigue, weakness, weight loss, an acquired bleeding tendency, or early satiety with abdominal discomfort due to splenomegaly. Splenomegaly is massive in nearly two-thirds of the patients. The liver also may be enlarged. Nevertheless, patients typically have minimal palpable lymphadenopathy.

In rare cases, patients may present with leukemic meningitis,[492,493] leukemic pleural effusion,[494] or malignant ascites.[495] A few patients develop cardiopulmonary complications due to leukostasis associated with extreme leukocytosis.[496]

LABORATORY FEATURES

Over three-fourths of the patients have blood lymphocyte counts greater than $100,000/\mu l$.[271,277] The marrow commonly is infiltrated diffusely with neoplastic prolymphocytes. At autopsy, these cells can be found to have infiltrated most other organs.[484] At presentation, patients commonly have a normochromic and normocytic anemia, with blood hemoglobin less than 11 g/dl and/or blood platelet counts below $100,000/\mu l$. As in CLL, patients commonly have hypogammaglobulinemia.[497] However, many patients have a monoclonal gammopathy on serum protein electrophoresis.

Prolymphocytic leukemia B cells express B-cell differentiation antigens similar to those of B-cell CLL. However, expression of CD5 is variable.[465] Even in cases that have evolved from CD5+ CLL B cells, the leukemia cells have low to negligible expression of CD5 (see Table 98-1). Also, in contrast to CLL B cells, prolymphocytic leukemia cells generally express very high levels of surface immunoglobulin, usually IgM with or without IgD[498] and react strongly with the antibody FMC7. In addition, prolymphocytic leukemia cells generally express high levels of CD22 and often are negative for CD23. Finally, in contrast to CLL B cells, prolymphocytic leukemia B cells generally stain brightly with SN8, a mAb specific for CD79b (see Chaps. 13 and 83).[272,273]

THERAPY, COURSE, AND PROGNOSIS

At presentation, patients commonly have advanced-stage disease that requires treatment. Most patients present with prominent splenomegaly and hyperleukocytosis and have rapid progression soon after diagnosis. Nevertheless, some patients may have a more indolent course.[499] As such, the indications for therapy are similar to those used for patients with CLL. These include disease-related symptoms, symptomatic splenomegaly, progressive marrow failure, or a blood prolymphocyte count of more that $200,000/\mu l$.

Treatments for patients with prolymphocytic leukemia are similar to those described for patients with CLL. Alkylating agents similar to those used in CLL are commonly used. However, chlorambucil or cyclophosphamide, in combination with prednisone and/or vincristine, typically yield response rates of less than 20 percent.[465] Treatment with high-dose glucocorticoids appears less effective for patients with prolymphocytic leukemia than for those with CLL.[322] Partial and complete responses have been observed in approximately half the patients treated with intensive combination chemotherapy regimens similar to those used to treat high-grade lymphomas (see Chap. 103), such as CHOP. Unfortunately, responses are relatively short-lasting. Although occasional patients may respond to salvage regimens,[500,501] the long-term survival is generally poor.

The deoxyadenosine analogs are active in this disease. Cladribine given at 0.1 mg/kg per day for 7 days by continuous infusion every 28 to 35 days has been noted to induce complete and partial remission in approximately half of the patients with de novo B-cell prolymphocytic leukemia.[502–504] Similarly, fludarabine at a dose of 30 mg/m^2 over 30 min daily for 5 days every 4 weeks produced complete and partial remissions in nearly 40 percent of the patients treated.[505] In another study, the response rates to fludarabine were similar to that noted for B-cell CLL.[351] Rapid response to fludarabine may be complicated by the tumor-lysis syndrome.[506,507]

Pentostatin also appears effective, although less so than fludarabine. Twenty patients with prolymphocytic leukemia were treated with pentostatin (2'-deoxycoformycin) at a dosage of 4 mg/m^2 intravenously once a week for 3 weeks, then every other week for three doses. The major hematologic toxicity of this regimen was thrombocytopenia. Although 45 percent achieved a partial remission, no patients achieved a complete response. The median duration of the remission was 9 months. Patients with B-cell prolymphocytic leukemia had a higher rate of response and duration of remission (12 months) than those with disease of T-cell origin.[508] However, pentostatin also has some activity in T-cell prolymphocytic leukemia.[509]

Splenectomy may ameliorate symptoms, but only transiently.[390] Splenic irradiation, with 1000 to 1600 Gy delivered to the splenic bed, has been advocated as a primary therapy for this disease.[510,511] especially for symptomatic patients who are considered poor candidates for chemotherapy and/or splenectomy.[512]

Case reports indicate that interferon-α can be effective in inducing cytoreduction in prolymphocytic leukemia.[513-515] There is one report of a patient who achieved a 5-year survival following a complete response to interferon-α following splenic irradiation.[516] However, generally interferon-α appears less effective than chemotherapy.

Spontaneous remissions are extremely rare.[517]

T-CELL PROLYMPHOCYTIC LEUKEMIA

DEFINITION AND HISTORY

In 1989, the French-American-British (FAB) Cooperative Group distinguished five subgroups of T-cell leukemia, namely T-cell CLL; T-cell prolymphocytic leukemia; human T lymphotropic virus type I-positive (HTLV-I⁺) adult T-cell leukemia/lymphoma; and Sézary syndrome.[518] When a new entity called large granular lymphocytic leukemia was defined (see Chap. 100), the existence of T-cell CLL as a distinct entity became a topic of debate.[519-522] Because of this the World Health Organization commissioned a panel of experts to draft a new classification of the hematologic neoplasms.[523] At a meeting in November 1997, this panel proposed a categorization of peripheral T-cell neoplasms that largely was based on the Revised European-American Lymphoma classification, or REAL classification[524] (see Chap. 101). However, because of its aggressive clinical behavior, T-cell CLL was reclassified under the heading of T-cell prolymphocytic leukemia, without regard to subtle differences in morphology.[525] Even together they account for less than 5 percent of all chronic lymphoid leukemias.

ETIOLOGY AND PATHOGENESIS

The etiology is unknown. There is a 3:2 male to female predominance, suggesting that males are more susceptible to developing this disease.

Infection with human T lymphotropic virus type I (HTLV-I) has been speculated to play a role in the development of at least some cases of T-cell prolymphocytic leukemia. Evidence for HTLV-I can be found in the leukemia cells of patients with T-cell prolymphocytic leukemia, suggesting a causal relationship.[526] However, another study involving 36 patients with T-cell prolymphocytic leukemia from an area that was nonendemic for HTLV-I failed to reveal any evidence for HTLV-I or human T lymphotropic virus type II (HTLV-II) DNA or transcripts in the leukemia cells.[527] As such, the association of HTLV-I and T-cell prolymphocytic leukemia cells may be coincidental in areas with high rates of HTLV-I infection. Alternatively, there may be multiple mechanisms involved in leukemogenesis, some involving HTLV-I in endemic areas.[528]

Consistent with this hypothesis, the cytogenetic features of T-cell prolymphocytic leukemia appear to vary depending upon the patient population studied. In the United States and Europe, inv(14q), del(11q), translocations involving 11q23, i(8q), trisomy 8q, and rearranged Xq28 are the commonest nonrandom chromosomal abnor-

malities in T-prolymphocytic leukemia.[529] Moreover, abnormalities of the short arm of chromosome 12 are often observed.[530] In contrast, chromosome 14 and 8 abnormalities are infrequently noted in the T-cell prolymphocytic leukemia cells of Japanese patients,[531] suggesting that T-cell prolymphocytic leukemia is a heterogeneous disorder.

ATAXIA-TELANGIECTASIA MUTATED GENE

Patients with ataxia-telangiectasia have a high risk of developing T-cell prolymphocytic leukemia. Ataxia-telangiectasia is an autosomal recessive disorder characterized by cerebellar ataxia, oculocutaneous telangiectasia, immune deficiency, genome instability, and predisposition to malignancies, particularly T-cell neoplasms. The responsible gene, called ataxia-telangiectasia mutated (ATM), maps to chromosomal region 11q22.3-23.1, is 150 kb in length, consists of 66 exons, and encodes a nuclear phosphoprotein of approximately 350 kDa.[93] Patients with ataxia-telangiectasia (A-T) frequently develop clonal expansions of T-cells that often progress to T-cell prolymphocytic leukemia, suggesting that ATM is a predisposing factor. Furthermore, inactivating mutations in ATM frequently are observed in both alleles of T-prolymphocytic leukemia cells from patients who do not have ataxia-telangiectasia.[532-534] Moreover, ATM mutations appear associated with T-cell prolymphocytic leukemia and are infrequent in other T-cell malignancies, such as T-cell ALL.[535] These findings suggest that ATM functions as a tumor-suppressor gene in T-cell prolymphocytic leukemia.

T-CELL LEUKEMIA 1 AND RELATED GENES

Studies of t(X;14)(q28;q11) chromosomal rearrangements in T-cell prolymphocytic leukemia have implicated two additional genes, designated MTCP1 or TCL1, in the pathogenesis of this disease.[529,536,538] These genes encode two homologous proteins, designated p13(MTCP1) and p14(TCL1), with highly similar tertiary structure[539] that often are dysregulated in T-cell prolymphocytic leukemia. In addition, clonal T-cell expansions similar to that of T-cell prolymphocytic leukemia that develop in patients with ataxia-telangiectasia also frequently have aberrant expression of these genes and/or harbor translocations involving the 14q32.1 or Xq28 regions, where the TCL1 and MTCP1 are located.[537] Finally, mice transgenic for MTCP1 under the control of CD2 regulatory elements spontaneously develop T-cell leukemias that share many features in common with T-cell prolymphocytic leukemia.[540] As such, the proteins encoded by these genes may play an important role in the pathogenesis of this disease.

CLINICAL FEATURES

Presenting symptoms include fatigue, weakness, weight loss, and early satiety with abdominal discomfort due to splenomegaly.[519,522,541] On presentation, patients generally have blood lymphocyte counts in excess of $10 \times 10^3/\mu l$, marrow infiltration, and splenomegaly. In contrast to B-cell prolymphocytic leukemia, lymphadenopathy is a common finding in T-cell prolymphocytic leukemia.

About a third of patients have cutaneous involvement on the torso, arms, and face, which generally is present at the time of diagnosis.[542] Skin manifestations include a diffuse infiltrated erythema; infiltration localized to the face and ears; nodules; and erythroderma, producing a nonscaling, papular, nonpruritic rash. Some cases present with a cutaneous infiltration mimicking a cellulitis that is resistant to antibiotic therapy.[543]

LABORATORY FEATURES

Biopsy of erythematous skin lesions generally shows a perivascular or periappendageal dermal infiltrate of lymphoid cells with a prolymphocytic morphology.[542]

Neoplastic T cells invariably can be found infiltrating the marrow, often in an interstitial pattern, with varying degrees of involvement.

The leukemia cells express the T-cell differentiation antigens CD2, CD3, CD5, and CD7, but not CD1, HLA-DR, or terminal transferase, reflecting a mature T-cell phenotype (see Chaps. 13 and 84). In over 75 percent of cases the leukemia cells have a helper T-cell phenotype as they express CD4 but not CD8.[544] About 15 percent of cases have leukemia cells that express CD8 but not CD4.[519,525,545] In less than 10 percent of the cases, the leukemic T cells express both CD4 and CD8,[546] a less mature phenotype implying derivation from a more primitive T cell (see Chaps. 5 and 82). Monoclonal gene rearrangements in the genes encoding the α and β chains of the T-cell receptor can be detected in the leukemia-cell genomic DNA (see Chap. 84).

DIFFERENTIAL DIAGNOSIS

The lymphocytosis of T-cell prolymphocytic leukemia can be distinguished readily from that of B-cell leukemias by immunophenotypic analyses (see section on differential diagnosis for CLL).

POLYCLONAL T-CELL LYMPHOCYTOSIS
T-cell prolymphocytic leukemia should be distinguished from other lymphoproliferative processes that can present with T-cell lymphocytosis (see Chap. 87), such as the reactive T-cell lymphocytosis that can occur in infectious mononucleosis (see Chap. 90). Lymphocytosis due to polyclonal T-cell expansion generally consists of both CD4+/CD8− and CD4−/CD8+ T cells and lacks clonal T-cell receptor gene rearrangements (see Chap. 84). Southern analyses for T-cell receptor gene rearrangements or evaluation for expression of T-cell receptor variable region genes can help distinguish T-cell prolymphocytic leukemia from this entity.

LARGE GRANULAR LYMPHOCYTIC LEUKEMIA
The leukemic cells in this disorder have the distinctive morphology of large granular lymphocytes (see Chaps. 96 and 100). These cells have abundant cytoplasm that contains many azurophilic granules. Two major subtypes are defined. In the more common type, the leukemic cells are derived from the T-cell lineage and generally express the CD3 surface antigen. This disorder formerly was called Tγ-CLL. In the other subtype, the leukemic cells are derived from natural killer cells and lack expression of CD3. These diseases are discussed in Chap. 100.

ADULT T-CELL LEUKEMIA/LYMPHOMA
Adult T-cell leukemia/lymphoma is endemic to the southwest of Japan and the Caribbean region. Most patients have lymphadenopathy, hypercalcemia, and high white blood cell counts. Skin involvement, lytic bone lesions, and hepatomegaly are common. The leukemic cells have polylobed or convoluted nuclei. The diagnosis can be confirmed by demonstration of antibodies to HTLV-I. It is an aggressive disorder with short survival and is discussed in Chap. 103.

MYCOSIS FUNGOIDES AND SÉZARY SYNDROME
Cutaneous T-cell lymphomas (Sézary syndrome and mycosis fungoides) have a helper CD4+ T-cell phenotype and often have blood involvement. This disease is discussed in Chap. 103.

Sézary-cell leukemia (SCL) is a mature T-cell leukemia with characteristic cerebriform nuclei, whereas Sézary syndrome (SS) involves a mature T-cell lymphoma with a similar nuclear morphology. However, the distinction between T-cell prolymphocytic leukemia and Sézary-cell leukemia is not straightforward. The leukemia cells in either disease can have similar immune phenotypes and cytogenetic

abnormalities.[547] Moreover, clinical manifestations are similar, as is the overall clinical course. This has led some investigators to consider Sézary-cell leukemia as a variant form of T-cell prolymphocytic leukemia.[547,548]

T-CELL CLL
The major feature distinguishing T-cell CLL from T-cell prolymphocytic leukemia was the morphology of the leukemia cells.[522] However, because T-cell CLL and T-cell prolymphocytic leukemia share so many other clinical and laboratory features, the distinction of T-cell CLL as a separate entity is currently not considered to have clinical utility. Instead, more attention should be given to distinguishing T-cell prolymphocytic leukemia with the usual CD4+/CD8− phenotype from exceptional cases of T-cell prolymphocytic leukemia/T-cell CLL that have a CD4−/CD8+ phenotype, generally lack prolymphocytic morphology, and have an even more aggressive clinical course than typical T-cell prolymphocytic leukemia.[525,545]

THERAPY, COURSE, AND PROGNOSIS

The disease is aggressive and generally refractory to conventional alkylator-based chemotherapy, with a median survival of about 7.5 months.[549]

Treatment with deoxyadenosine analogs yields higher response rates, although it has not been determined whether these drugs provide a survival benefit. Two articles describe treatment of T-cell PLL with cladribine.[550,551] Pentostatin given intravenously at 4 mg/m^2 weekly for the first 4 weeks and then every 2 weeks until maximal responses is effective in inducing complete or partial responses in about half of patients with T-cell prolymphocytic leukemia.[509]

Patients with extensive cutaneous involvement may benefit from treatments that commonly are used for mycosis fungoides, such as topical corticosteroids, mechlorethamine, carmustine, ultraviolet light B, PUVA, or total skin electron beam (TSEB) therapy.[552] These treatments are discussed in Chap. 103. However, systemic therapy is warranted for patients with T-cell prolymphocytic leukemia, and this generally obviates local therapy.

The humanized monoclonal antibody specific for CD52, CAMPATH-1H, causes significant T-cell depletion when used to treat patients with B-cell CLL. Because of this, it is being evaluated for use in patients with T-cell prolymphocytic leukemia. In one study of 15 patients, 11 (73 percent) treated with CAMPATH-1H had major responses, compared with 40 percent with pentostatin. Complete remissions were documented in nine (60 percent) of the CAMPATH-1H-treated cases, and only three (12 percent) were obtained with pentostatin.[553] Treatment with CAMPATH-1H can result in complete remissions, even in patients with large tumor burdens and high blood leukemia cell counts.[554]

Treatment of patients with T-cell prolymphocytic leukemia with high-dose chemoradiotherapy and allogeneic stem cell transplantation from HLA-matched sibling donors has resulted in anecdotal success.[555]

COURSE AND PROGNOSIS
In one large study, median survival was 3 years for patients with prolymphocytic leukemia and 8 years for those with CLL.[467] Patients with T-cell prolymphocytic leukemia, however, may have an even poorer prognosis than those with B-cell prolymphocytic leukemia and have a median survival of only approximately 7 months.[556-558] However, some patients may experience an initial indolent clinical course with stable moderate leukocytosis.[559] Also, it is not certain how these survival times may improve with the advent of monoclonal antibody therapy and other new modalities of treatment for this disease.

REFERENCES

1. Diehl LF, Karnell LH, Menck HR: The American College of Surgeons Commission on Cancer and the American Cancer Society. The National Cancer Date Base report on age, gender, treatment, and outcomes of patients with chronic lymphocytic leukemia. *Cancer* 86:2684, 1999.

2. Velpeau A: Sur la resorption du pusuaet sur l'alteration du sang dans les maladies clinique de persection nenemant. Premier observation. *Rev Med* 2:216, 1827.

3. Fuller H: Particulars of a case in which enormous enlargement of the spleen and liver, together with dilation of all the blood vessels of the body, were found coincident with a peculiarly altered condition of the blood. *Lancet* 2:43, 1846.

4. Virchow R: Weisses Blut. Froriep's *Notizen* 36:151, 1845.

5. Virchow R: Weisses Blut und Milztumoren. I. *Med Z* 15:157, 1846.

6. Virchow R: Weisses Blut und Milztumoren. II. *Med Z* 16:9, 1847.

7. Kundrat H: Über Lympho-Sarkomatosis. *Wien Med Wochenschr* 6:211, 1893.

8. Ehrlich P: *Farbenanalytische Untersuchungen zur Histologie und Klinik des Blutes*. Hirschwald, Berlin, 1891.

9. Türk W: Ein System der Lymphomatosen. *Wien Kinische Wochenschriften* 16:1073, 1903.

10. Minot GR, Isaacs R: Lymphatic leukemia; age incidence, duration and benefit derived from irradiation. *Boston Med Surg* 191:1, 1924.

11. Reinhard EH, Neely CL, Samples DM: Radioactive phosphorus in the treatment of chronic leukemias: long term results over a period of 15 years. *Ann Intern Med* 50:942, 1959.

12. Tivey H: The prognosis for survival in chronic granulocytic and lymphocytic leukemia. *Am J Roentgenol* 72:68, 1954.

13. Galton DAG, Isreals LG, Nabarro JDN, et al: Clinical trials of p(di-2-chloroethylamino)-phenybutyric acid (CD 1348) in malignant lymphoma. *Br Med J* 2:1172, 1955.

14. Shaw RK, Boggs DR, Silberman HR, et al: A study of prednisone therapy in chronic lymphocytic leukemia. *Blood* 17:182, 1961.

15. Dameshek W: Chronic lymphocytic leukemia—an accumulative disease of immunologically incompetent lymphocytes. *Blood* 29(suppl):566, 1967.

16. Rubin AD, Schultz E: Surface immunoglobulins on lymphocytes in leukemia. *N Engl J Med* 287:989, 1972.

17. Fialkow PJ, Najfeld V, Reddy AL, Singer J, Steinmann L: Chronic lymphocytic leukaemia: clonal origin in a committed B-lymphocyte progenitor. *Lancet* 2:444, 1978.

18. Preud'homme JL, Seligmann M: Surface bound immunoglobulins as a cell marker in human lymphoproliferative diseases. *Blood* 40:777, 1972.

19. Salsano F, Froland SS, Natvig JB, Michaelsen TE: Same idiotype of B-lymphocyte membrane IgD and IgM. Formal evidence for monoclonality of chronic lymphocytic leukemia cells. *Scand J Immunol* 3:841, 1974.

20. Fu SM, Winchester RJ, Feizi T, Walzer PD, Kunkel HG: Idiotypic specificity of surface immunoglobulin and the maturation of leukemic bone-marrow-derived lymphocytes. *Proc Natl Acad Sci USA* 71:4487, 1974.

21. Schroer KR, Briles DE, Van Boxel JA, Davie JM: Idiotypic uniformity of cell surface immunoglobulin in chronic lymphocytic leukemia. Evidence for monoclonal proliferation. *J Exp Med* 140:1416, 1974.

22. Rai KR, Sawitsky A, Cronkite EP, Chanana AD, Levy RN, Pasternack BS: Clinical staging of chronic lymphocytic leukemia. *Blood* 46:219, 1975.

23. Waterhouse D, Carman WJ, Schottenfeld D, Gridley G, McLean S: Cancer incidence in the rural community of Tecumseh, Michigan: a pattern of increased lymphopoietic neoplasms. *Cancer* 77:763, 1996.

24. Cronkite EP: An historical account of clinical investigations on chronic lymphocytic leukemia in the Medical Research Center, Brookhaven National Laboratory. *Blood Cells* 12:285, 1987.

25. Zahm SH, Weisenburger DD, Babbitt PA, Saal RC, Vaught JB, Blair A: Use of hair coloring products and the risk of lymphoma, multiple myeloma, and chronic lymphocytic leukemia. *Am J Pub Health* 82:990, 1992.

26. Inskip PD, Kleinerman RA, Stovall M, et al: Leukemia, lymphoma, and multiple myeloma after pelvic radiotherapy for benign disease. *Radiat Res* 135:108, 1993.

27. Neugut AI, Ahsan H, Robinson E, Ennis RD: Bladder carcinoma and other second malignancies after radiotherapy for prostate carcinoma. *Cancer* 79:1600, 1997.

28. Rushton L, Romaniuk H: A case-control study to investigate the risk of leukaemia associated with exposure to benzene in petroleum marketing and distribution workers in the United Kingdom. *Occup Environ Med* 54:152, 1997.

29. Adami J, Gridley G, Nyren O, et al: Sunlight and non-Hodgkin's lymphoma: a population-based cohort study in Sweden. *Int J Cancer* 80:641, 1999.

30. Floderus B, Persson T, Stenlund C, Wennberg A, Ost A, Knave B: Occupational exposure to electromagnetic fields in relation to leukemia and brain tumors: a case-control study in Sweden. *Cancer Causes Control* 4:465, 1993.

31. Stone R: Polarized debate: EMFs and cancer [news]. *Science* 258:1724, 1992.

32. Feychting M, Forssen U, Floderus B: Occupational and residential magnetic field exposure and leukemia and central nervous system tumors. *Epidemiology* 8:384, 1997.

33. La Civita L, Zignego AL, Monti M, et al: Type C hepatitis and chronic lymphocytic leukaemia [letter]. *Eur J Cancer* 32A:1819, 1996.

34. Luppi M, Grazia Ferrari M, Bonaccorsi G, et al: Hepatitis C virus infection in subsets of neoplastic lymphoproliferations not associated with cryoglobulinemia. *Leukemia* 10:351, 1996.

35. McColl MD, Singer IO, Tait RC, McNeil IR, Cumming RL, Hogg RB: The role of hepatitis C virus in the aetiology of non-Hodgkins lymphoma a regional association? *Leuk Lymphoma* 26:127, 1997.

36. Avila-Carino J, Lewin N, Tomita Y, et al: B-CLL cells with unusual properties. *Int J Cancer* 70:1, 1997.

37. Adami HO, Tsaih S, Lambe M, et al: Pregnancy and risk of non-Hodgkin's lymphoma: a prospective study. *Int J Cancer* 70:155, 1997.

38. Ahn YO, Koo HH, Park BJ, Yoo KY, Lee MS: Incidence estimation of leukemia among Koreans. *J Korean Med Sci* 6:299, 1991.

39. Haenszel W, Kurihara M: Studies of Japanese migrants: I. Mortality from cancer and other diseases among Japanese in the United States. *J Natl Cancer Inst* 40:43, 1968.

40. Nishiyama H, Mokuno J, Inoue T, Relative frequency and mortality rate of various types of leukemia in Japan. *Gann* 60:71, 1969.

41. Zheng W, Linet MS, Shu XO, Pan RP, Gao YT, Fraumeni JFJ: Prior medical conditions and the risk of adult leukemia in Shanghai, People's Republic of China. *Cancer Causes Control* 4:361, 1993.

42. Yanagihara ET, Blaisdell RK, Hayashi T, Lukes RJ: Malignant lymphoma in Hawaii-Japanese: a retrospective morphologic survey. *Hematol Oncol* 7:219, 1989.

43. Bartal A, Bentwich Z, Manny N, Izak G: Ethical and clinical aspects of chronic lymphocytic leukemia in Israel: a survey on 288 patients. *Acta Haematol* 60:161, 1978.

44. Gunz FW: The epidemiology and genetics of the chronic leukaemias. *Clin Haematol* 6:3, 1977.

45. Conley CL, Misiti J, Laster AJ: Genetic factors predisposing to chronic lymphocytic leukemia and to autoimmune disease. *Medicine* (Baltimore) 59:323, 1980.

46. Linet MS, Van Natta ML, Brookmeyer R, et al: Familial cancer history and chronic lymphocytic leukemia. A case-control study. *Am J Epidemiol* 130:655, 1989.

47. Cuttner J: Increased incidence of hematologic malignancies in first-degree relatives of patients with chronic lymphocytic leukemia. *Cancer Invest* 10:103, 1992.

48. Shah AR, Maeda K, Deegan MJ, Roth MS, Schnitzer B: A clinicopathologic study of familial chronic lymphocytic leukemia. *Am J Clin Pathol* 97:184, 1992.

49. Yuille MR, Houlston RS, Catovsky D: Anticipation in familial chronic lymphocytic leukemia. *Leukemia* 12:1696, 1998.

50. Jones HP, Whittaker JA: Chronic lymphatic leukaemia: an investigation of HLA antigen frequencies and white cell differential counts in patients, relatives and controls. *Leuk Res* 15:543, 1991.

51. Shen A, Humphries C, Tucker P, Blattner F: Human heavy-chain variable region gene family nonrandomly rearranged in familial chronic lymphocytic leukemia. *Proc Natl Acad Sci USA* 84:8563, 1987.

52. Brok-Simoni F, Rechavi G, Katzir N, Ben Bassat I: Chronic lymphocytic leukaemia in twin sisters: monozygous but not identical [letter]. *Lancet* 1:329, 1987.

53. Rickinson AB, Finerty S, Epstein MA: Interaction of Epstein-Barr virus

with leukaemic B cells in vitro: I. Abortive infection and rare cell line establishment from chronic lymphocytic leukaemic cells. *Clin Exp Immunol* 50:347, 1982.

54. Solé F, Woessner S, Pérez-Losada A, et al: Cytogenetic studies in seventy-six cases of B-chronic lymphoproliferative disorders. *Cancer Genet Cytogenet* 93:160, 1997.

55. Hilgenfeld E, Padilla-Nash H, Schrock E, Ried T: Analysis of B-cell neoplasias by spectral karyotyping (SKY). *Curr Topics Microbio Immunol* 246:169, 1999.

56. Han T, Ozer H, Sadamori N, et al: Prognostic importance of cytogenetic abnormalities in patients with chronic lymphocytic leukemia. *N Engl J Med* 310:288, 1984.

57. Juliusson G, Gahrton G, Oscier D, et al: Cytogenetic findings and survival in B-cell chronic lymphocytic leukemia. Second IWCCLL compilation of data on 662 patients. *Leuk Lymphoma* 5S:21, 1991.

58. Losada AP, Wessman M, Tiainen M, et al: Trisomy 12 in chronic lymphocytic leukemia: an interphase cytogenetic study. *Blood* 78:775, 1991.

59. Crossen PE: Cytogenetic and molecular changes in chronic B-cell leukemia. *Cancer Genet Cytogenet* 43:143, 1989.

60. Döhner H, Stilgenbauer S, Dohner K, Bentz M, Lichter P: Chromosome aberrations in B-cell chronic lymphocytic leukemia: reassessment based on molecular cytogenetic analysis. *J Mol Med* 77:266, 1999.

61. Gardiner AC, Corcoran MM, Oscier DG: Cytogenetic, fluorescence in situ hybridisation, and clinical evaluation of translocations with concomitant deletion at 13q14 in chronic lymphocytic leukaemia. *Genes Chromosomes Cancer* 20:73, 1997.

62. Garcia-Marco JA, Caldas C, Price CM, Wiedemann LM, Ashworth A, Catovsky D: Frequent somatic deletion of the 13q12.3 locus encompassing BRCA2 in chronic lymphocytic leukemia. *Blood* 88:1568, 1996.

63. Panayiotidis P, Ganeshaguru K, Rowntree C, Jabbar SA, Hoffbrand VA, Foroni L: Lack of clonal BCRA2 gene deletion on chromosome 13 in chronic lymphocytic leukemia. *Br J Haematol* 97:844, 1997.

64. Garcia-Marco JA, Price CM, Catovsky D: Interphase cytogenetics in chronic lymphocytic leukemia. *Cancer Genet Cytogenet* 94:52, 1997.

65. Crossen PE: Genes and chromosomes in chronic B-cell leukemia. *Cancer Genet Cytogenet* 94:44, 1997.

66. Bouyge-Moreau I, Rondeau G, Avet-Loiseau H, et al: Construction of a 780-kb PAC, BAC, and cosmid contig encompassing the minimal critical deletion involved in B cell chronic lymphocytic leukemia at 13q14.3 *Genomics* 46:183, 1997.

67. Corcoran MM, Rasool O, Liu Y, et al: Detailed molecular delineation of 13q14.3 loss in B-cell chronic lymphocytic leukemia. *Blood* 91:1382, 1998.

68. Stilgenbauer S, Nickolenko J, Wilhelm J, et al: Expressed sequences as candidates for a novel tumor suppressor gene at band 13q14 in B-cell chronic lymphocytic leukemia and mantle cell lymphoma. *Oncogene* 16:1891, 1998.

69. Liu Y, Corcoran M, Rasool O, et al: Cloning of two candidate tumor suppressor genes within a 10 kb region on chromosome 13q14, frequently deleted in chronic lymphocytic leukemia. *Oncogene* 15:2463, 1997.

70. Kapanadze B, Kashuba V, Baranova A, et al: A cosmid and cDNA fine physical map of a human chromosome 13q14 region frequently lost in B-cell chronic lymphocytic leukemia and identification of a new putative tumor suppressor gene, Leu5. *FEBS Letters* 426:266, 1998.

71. Dierlamm J, Michaux L, Criel A, Wlodarska I, Van den Berghe H, Hossfeld DK: Genetic abnormalities in chronic lymphocytic leukemia and their clinical and prognostic implications. *Cancer Genet Cytogenet* 94:27, 1997.

72. Hjalmar V, Kimby E, Matutes E, et al: Trisomy 12 and lymphoplasmacytoid lymphocytes in chronic leukemic B-cell disorders. *Haematologica* 83:602, 1998.

73. Anastasi J, Le Beau MM, Vardiman JW, Fernald AA, Larson RA, Rowley JD: Detection of trisomy 12 in chronic lymphocytic leukemia by fluorescence in situ hybridization to interphase cells: a simple and sensitive method. *Blood* 79:1796, 1992.

74. Que TH, Marco JG, Ellis J, et al: Trisomy 12 in chronic lymphocytic leukemia detected by fluorescence in situ hybridization: analysis by stage, immunophenotype, and morphology. *Blood* 82:571, 1993.

75. Acar H, Connor MJ: Detection of trisomy 12 and centromeric alterations in CLL by interphase and metaphase-FISH. *Cancer Genet Cytogenet* 100:148, 1998.

76. Einhorn S, Burvall K, Juliusson G, Gahrton G, Meeker T: Molecular analyses of chromosome 12 in chronic lymphocytic leukemia. *Leukemia* 3:871, 1989.

77. Crossen PE, Horn HL: Origin of trisomy 12 in B-cell chronic lymphocytic leukemia [letter]. *Cancer Genet Cytogenet* 28:185, 1987.

78. Matutes E: Trisomy 12 in chronic lymphocytic leukaemia. *Leuk Res* 20:375, 1996.

79. Sole F, Woessner S, Perez-Losada A, et al: Cytogenetic studies in seventy-six cases of B-chronic lymphoproliferative disorders. *Cancer Genet Cytogenet* 93:160, 1997.

80. Woessner S, Sole F, Perez-Losada A, Florensa L, Vila RM: Trisomy 12 is a rare cytogenetic finding in typical chronic lymphocytic leukemia. *Leuk Res* 20:369, 1996.

81. Matutes E, Oscier D, Garcia-Marco J, et al: Trisomy 12 defines a group of CLL with atypical morphology: correlation between cytogenetic, clinical and laboratory features in 544 patients. *Br J Haematol* 92:382, 1996.

82. Amiel A, Arbov L, Manor Y, et al: Monoallelic p53 deletion in chronic lymphocytic leukemia detected by interphase cytogenetics. *Cancer Genet Cytogenet* 97:97, 1997.

83. Navarro B, Garcia-Marco JA, Jones D, Price CM, Catovsky D: Association and clonal distribution of trisomy 12 and 13q14 deletions in chronic lymphocytic leukaemia. *Br J Haematol* 102:1330, 1998.

84. Brynes RK, McCourty A, Sun NC, Koo CH: Trisomy 12 in Richter's transformation of chronic lymphocytic leukemia. *Am J Clin Pathol* 104:199, 1995.

85. Shahidi H, Leslie WT, Wool NL, Gregory SA: Transformation of chronic lymphocytic leukemia to immunoblastic lymphoma (Richter's syndrome) [clinical conference]. *Med Pediatr Oncol* 29:146, 1997.

86. Garcia-Marco J, Matutes E, Morilla R, et al: Trisomy 12 in B-cell chronic lymphocytic leukaemia: assessment of lineage restriction by simultaneous analysis of immunophenotype and genotype in interphase cells by fluorescence in situ hybridization. *Br J Haematol* 87:44, 1994.

87. Mould S, Gardiner A, Corcoran M, Oscier DG: Trisomy 12 and structural abnormalities of 13q14 occurring in the same clone in chronic lymphocytic leukaemia. *Br J Haematol* 92:389, 1996.

88. Stilgenbauer S, Liebisch P, James MR, et al: Molecular cytogenetic delineation of a novel critical genomic region in chromosome bands 11q22.3-q23.1 in lymphoproliferative disorders. *Proc Natl Acad Sci USA* 93:11837, 1996.

89. Döhner H, Stilgenbauer S, James MR, et al: 11q deletions identify a new subset of B-cell chronic lymphocytic leukemia characterized by extensive nodal involvement and inferior prognosis. *Blood* 89:2516, 1997.

90. Karhu R, Knuutila S, Kallioniemi OP, et al: Frequent loss of the 11q14–24 region in chronic lymphocytic leukemia: a study by comparative genomic hybridization. Tampere CLL Group. *Genes Chromosomes Cancer* 19:286, 1997.

91. Sembries S, Pahl H, Stilgenbauer S, Döhner H, Schriever F: Reduced expression of adhesion molecules and cell signaling receptors by chronic lymphocytic leukemia cells with 11q deletion. *Blood* 93:624, 1999.

92. Thieblemont C, Pack S, Sakai A, et al: Allelic loss of 11q13 as detected by MEN1-FISH is not associated with mutation of the MEN1 gene in lymphoid neoplasms. *Leukemia* 13:85, 1999.

93. Lavin MF, Khanna KK: ATM: the protein encoded by the gene mutated in the radiosensitive syndrome ataxia-telangiectasia. *Int J Radiat Biol* 75:1201, 1999.

94. Starostik P, Manshouri T, O'Brien S, et al: Deficiency of the ATM protein expression defines an aggressive subgroup of B-cell chronic lymphocytic leukemia. *Cancer Res* 58:4552, 1998.

95. Bullrich F, Rasio D, Kitada S, et al: ATM mutations in B-cell chronic lymphocytic leukemia. *Cancer Res* 59:24, 1999.

96. Bevan S, Yuille MR, Marossy A, Catovsky D, Houlston RS: Ataxia telangiectasia gene mutations and chronic lymphocytic leukaemia [letter]. *Lancet* 353:753, 1999.

97. Stankovic T, Weber P, Stewart G, et al: Inactivation of ataxia telangiectasia mutated gene in B-cell chronic lymphocytic leukaemia. *Lancet* 353:26, 1999.

98. Offit K, Louie DC, Parsa NZ, et al: Clinical and morphologic features of B-cell small lymphocytic lymphoma with del(6)(q21q23). *Blood* 83:2611, 1994.

99. Glassman AB, Harper-Allen EA, Hayes KJ, Hopwood VL, Gutterman

EE, Zagryn SP: Chromosome 6 abnormalities associated with pro-lymphocytic acceleration in chronic lymphocytic leukemia. *Ann Clin Lab Sci* 28:24, 1998.

100. Finn WG, Kay NE, Kroft SH, Church S, Peterson LC: Secondary abnormalities of chromosome 6q in B-cell chronic lymphocytic leukemia: a sequential study of karyotypic instability in 51 patients. *Am J Hematol* 59:223, 1998.

101. Amiel A, Mulchanov I, Elis A, et al: Deletion of 6q27 in chronic lymphocytic leukemia and multiple myeloma detected by fluorescence in situ hybridization. *Cancer Genet Cytogenet* 112:53, 1999.

102. Demeter J, Porzsolt F, Ramisch S, Schmidt D, Schmid M, Messer G: Polymorphism of the tumour necrosis factor-alpha and lymphotoxin-alpha genes in chronic lymphocytic leukaemia. *Br J Haematol* 97:107, 1997.

103. Croce CM: Molecular biology of lymphomas. *Semin Oncol* 20:31, 1993.

104. Zech L, Gahrton G, Hammarstrom L, et al: Inversion of chromosome 14 marks human T-cell chronic lymphocytic leukaemia. *Nature* 308:858, 1984.

105. Hecht F, Morgan R, Hecht BK, Smith SD: Common region on chromosome 14 in T-cell leukemia and lymphoma. *Science* 226:1445, 1984.

106. Larramendy ML, Peltomaki P, Salonen E, Knuutila S: Chromosomal abnormality limited to T4 lymphocytes in a patient with T-cell chronic lymphocytic leukaemia. *Eur J Haematol* 45:52, 1990.

107. Erikson J, Finan J, Tsujimoto Y, Nowell PC, Croce CM: The chromosome 14 breakpoint in neoplastic B cells with the t(11;14) translocation involves the immunoglobulin heavy chain locus. *Proc Natl Acad Sci USA* 81:4144, 1984.

108. Pittman S, Catovsky D: Prognostic significance of chromosome abnormalities in chronic lymphocytic leukaemia. *Br J Haematol* 58:649, 1984.

109. Meeker TC, Grimaldi JC, O'Rourke R, Louie E, Juliusson G, Einhorn S: An additional breakpoint region in the BCL-1 locus associated with the t(11;14)(q13;q32) translocation of B-lymphocytic malignancy. *Blood* 74:1801, 1989.

110. Davey MP, Bertness V, Nakahara K, et al: Juxtaposition of the T-cell receptor alpha-chain locus (14q11) and a region (14q32) of potential importance in leukemogenesis by a 14;14 translocation in a patient with T-cell chronic lymphocytic leukemia and ataxia-telangiectasia. *Proc Natl Acad Sci USA* 85:9287, 1988.

111. Motokura T, Bloom T, Kim HG, et al: A novel cyclin encoded by a bcl1-linked candidate oncogene. *Nature* 350:512, 1991.

112. Seto M, Yamamoto K, Iida S, et al: Gene rearrangement and overexpression of PRAD1 in lymphoid malignancy with t(11;14)(q13;q32) translocation. *Oncogene* 7:1401, 1992.

113. Hinds PW, Dowdy SF, Eaton EN, Arnold A, Weinberg RA: Function of a human cyclin gene as an oncogene. *Proc Natl Acad Sci USA* 91:709, 1994.

114. Rimokh R, Berger F, Cornillet P, et al: Break in the BCL1 locus is closely associated with intermediate lymphocytic lymphoma subtype. *Genes Chromosomes Cancer* 2:223, 1990.

115. Ambinder RF, Griffin CA: Biology of the lymphomas: cytogenetics, molecular biology, and virology. *Curr Opin Oncol* 3:806, 1991.

116. Brito-Babapulle V, Ellis J, Matutes E, et al: Translocation t(11;14)(q13;q32) in chronic lymphoid disorders. *Genes Chromosomes Cancer* 5:158, 1992.

117. Williams ME, Swerdlow SH, Rosenberg CL, Arnold A: Characterization of chromosome 11 translocation breakpoints at the bcl-1 and PRAD1 loci in centrocytic lymphoma. *Cancer Res* 52:5541s, 1992.

118. Swerdlow SH, Saboorian MH, Pelstring RJ, Williams ME: Centrocytic lymphoma: a morphometric study with comparison to other small cleaved follicular center cell lymphomas and genotypic correlates. *Am J Pathol* 142:329, 1993.

119. Einhorn S, Meeker T, Juliusson G, Burvall K, Gahrton G: No evidence of trisomy 12 or t(11;14) by molecular genetic techniques in chronic lymphocytic leukemia cells with a normal karyotype. *Cancer Genet Cytogenet* 48:183, 1990.

120. Rechavi G, Katzir N, Brok-Simoni F, et al: A search for bcl1, bcl2, and c-myc oncogene rearrangements in chronic lymphocytic leukemia. *Leukemia* 3:57, 1989.

121. Newman RA, Peterson B, Davey FR, et al: Phenotypic markers and BCL-1 gene rearrangements in B-cell chronic lymphocytic leukemia: a Cancer and Leukemia Group B study. *Blood* 82:1239, 1993.

122. Jonveaux P, Hillion J, Bennaceur AL, et al: t(14;18) and bcl-2 gene rearrangement in a B-chronic lymphocytic leukaemia. *Br J Haematol* 81:620, 1992.

123. Raghoebier S, van Krieken JH, Kluin-Nelemans JC, et al: Oncogene rearrangements in chronic B-cell leukemia. *Blood* 77:1560, 1991.

124. Ueshima Y, Bird ML, Vardiman JW, Rowley JD: A 14;19 translocation in B-cell chronic lymphocytic leukemia: a new recurring chromosome aberration. *Int J Cancer* 36:287, 1985.

125. Michaux L, Mecucci C, Stul M, et al: BCL3 rearrangement and t(14;19)(q32;q13) in lymphoproliferative disorders. *Genes Chromosomes Cancer* 15:38, 1996.

126. McKeithan TW, Takimoto GS, Ohno H, et al: BCL3 rearrangements and t(14;19) in chronic lymphocytic leukemia and other B-cell malignancies: a molecular and cytogenetic study. *Genes Chromosomes Cancer* 20:64, 1997.

127. Zambetti GP, Levine AJ: A comparison of the biological activities of wild-type and mutant p53. *FASEB J* 7:855, 1993.

128. Marshall CJ: Tumor suppressor genes. *Cell* 64:313, 1991.

129. Harris CC: p53: at the crossroads of molecular carcinogenesis and risk assessment. *Science* 262:1980, 1993.

130. Gaidano G, Ballerini P, Gong JZ, et al: p53 mutations in human lymphoid malignancies: association with Burkitt lymphoma and chronic lymphocytic leukemia. *Proc Natl Acad Sci USA* 88:5413, 1991.

131. Fenaux P, Preudhomme C, Lai JL, et al: Mutations of the p53 gene in B-cell chronic lymphocytic leukemia: a report on 39 cases with cytogenetic analysis. *Leukemia* 6:246, 1992.

132. el Rouby S, Bayona W, Pisharody SM, Newcomb EW: p53 mutations in B-cell chronic lymphocytic leukemia. *Curr Top Microbiol Immunol* 182:313, 1992.

133. el Rouby S, Thomas A, Costin D, et al: p53 gene mutation in B-cell chronic lymphocytic leukemia is associated with drug resistance and is independent of MDR1/MDR3 gene expression. *Blood* 82:3452, 1993.

134. Lens D, De Schouwer PJ, Hamoudi RA, et al: p53 abnormalities in B-cell prolymphocytic leukemia. *Blood* 89:2015, 1997.

135. Cordone I, Masi S, Mauro FR, et al: p53 expression in B-cell chronic lymphocytic leukemia: a marker of disease progression and poor prognosis. *Blood* 91:4342, 1998.

136. Callet-Bauchu E, Salles G, Gazzo S, et al: Translocations involving the short arm of chromosome 17 in chronic B-lymphoid disorders: frequent occurrence of dicentric rearrangements and possible association with adverse outcome. *Leukemia* 13:460, 1999.

137. Holmes J, Wareing C, Jacobs A, Hayes JD, Padua RA, Wolf CR: Glutathione-s-transferase pi expression in leukaemia: a comparative analysis with mdr-1 data. *Br J Cancer* 62:209, 1990.

138. Michieli M, Raspadori D, Damiani D, et al: The expression of the multidrug resistance-associated glycoprotein in B-cell chronic lymphocytic leukaemia. *Br J Haematol* 77:460, 1991.

139. Sparrow RL, Hall FJ, Siregar H, Van der Weyden MB: Common expression of the multidrug resistance marker P-glycoprotein in B-cell chronic lymphocytic leukaemia and correlation with in vitro drug resistance. *Leuk Res* 17:941, 1993.

140. Sonneveld P, Nooter K, Burghouts JT, Herweijer H, Adriaansen HJ, van Dongen JJ: High expression of the mdr3 multidrug-resistance gene in advanced-stage chronic lymphocytic leukemia. *Blood* 79:1496, 1992.

141. Warr JR, Levie SE, Perkins LJ, et al: Levels of expression of mdr-3 and glutathione-S-transferase genes in chronic lymphocytic leukemia lymphocytes [letter]. *Blood* 82:1937, 1993.

142. Friedenberg WR, Spencer SK, Musser C, et al: Multi-drug resistance in chronic lymphocytic leukemia. *Leuk Lymphoma* 34:171, 1999.

143. Ueda K, Cardarelli C, Gottesman MM, Pastan I: Expression of a full-length cDNA for the human "MDR1" gene confers resistance to colchicine, doxorubicin, and vinblastine. *Proc Natl Acad Sci USA* 84:3004, 1987.

144. Adachi M, Tefferi A, Greipp PR, Kipps TJ, Tsujimoto Y: Preferential linkage of bcl-2 to immunoglobulin light chain gene in chronic lymphocytic leukemia. *J Exp Med* 171:559, 1990.

145. Pezzella F, Tse AG, Cordell JL, Pulford KA, Gatter KC, Mason DY: Expression of the bcl-2 oncogene protein is not specific for the 14;18 chromosomal translocation. *Am J Pathol* 137:225, 1990.

146. Schena M, Larsson LG, Gottardi D, et al: Growth- and differentiation-associated expression of bcl-2 in B-chronic lymphocytic leukemia cells. *Blood* 79:2981, 1992.

147. Hanada M, Delia D, Aiello A, Stadtmauer E, Reed JC: bcl-2 gene

hypomethylation and high-level expression in B-cell chronic lympho-cytic leukemia. *Blood* 82:1820, 1993.

148. Laytragoon-Lewin N, Kashuba V, Mellstedt H, Klein G: bcl-2 re-arrangement detected by pulsed-field gel electrophoresis (PFGE) in B-chronic lymphocytic leukemia (CLL) cells. *Int J Cancer* 76:909, 1998.

149. Kipps TJ, Robbins BA, Tefferi A, Meisenholder G, Banks PM, Carson DA: CD5-positive B-cell malignancies frequently express cross-reactive idiotypes associated with IgM autoantibodies. *Am J Pathol* 136:809, 1990.

150. Geisler CH, Larsen JK, Hansen NE, et al: Prognostic importance of flow cytometric immunophenotyping of 540 consecutive patients with B-cell chronic lymphocytic leukemia. *Blood* 78:1795, 1991.

151. Legac E, Chastang C, Binet JL, Michel A, Debre P, Merle-Beral H: Proposals for a phenotypic classification of B-chronic lymphocytic leu-kemia, relationship with prognostic factors. *Leuk Lymphoma* 5S:53, 1991.

152. Kipps TJ, Carson DA: Autoantibodies in chronic lymphocytic leukemia and related systemic autoimmune diseases. *Blood* 81:2475, 1993.

153. Caligaris-Cappio F: B-chronic lymphocytic leukemia: a malignancy of anti-self B cells. *Blood* 87:2615, 1996.

154. Guigou V, Guilbert B, Moinier D, et al: Ig repertoire of human polyspe-cific antibodies and B cell ontogeny. *J Immunol* 146:1368, 1991.

155. Lydyard PM, Quartey-Papafio R, Broker B, et al: The antibody repertoire of early human B cells: I. High frequency of autoreactivity and polyreac-tivity. *Scand J Immunol* 31:33, 1990.

156. Fais F, Ghiotto F, Hashimoto S, et al: Chronic lymphocytic leukemia B cells express restricted sets of mutated and unmutated antigen receptors. *J Clin Invest* 102:1515, 1998.

157. Friedman DF, Moore JS, Erikson J, et al: Variable region gene analysis of an isotype-switched (IgA) variant of chronic lymphocytic leukemia. *Blood* 80:2287, 1992.

158. Ebeling SB, Schutte ME, Logtenberg T: Molecular analysis of VH and VL regions expressed in IgG-bearing chronic lymphocytic leukemia (CLL): further evidence that CLL is a heterogeneous group of tumors. *Blood* 82:1626, 1993.

159. Hashimoto S, Dono M, Wakai M, et al: Somatic diversification and selection of immunoglobulin heavy and light chain variable region genes in IgG+ CD5+ chronic lymphocytic leukemia B cells. *J Exp Med* 181:1507, 1995.

160. Matolcsy A, Casali P, Nador RG, Liu YF, Knowles DM: Molecular characterization of IgA- and/or IgG-switched chronic lymphocytic leu-kemia B cells. *Blood* 89:1732, 1997.

161. Kipps TJ, Tomhave E, Chen PP, Carson DA: Autoantibody-associated kappa light chain variable region gene expressed in chronic lymphocytic leukemia with little or no somatic mutation. Implications for etiology and immunotherapy. *J Exp Med* 167:840, 1988.

162. Schettino EW, Cerutti A, Chiorazzi N, Casali P: Lack of intraclonal diversification in Ig heavy and light chain V region genes expressed by CD5+ IgM+ chronic lymphocytic leukemia B cells: a multiple time point analysis. *J Immunol* 160:820, 1998.

163. Rassenti LZ, Kipps TJ: Lack of allelic exclusion in B cell chronic lymphocytic leukemia. *J Exp Med* 185:1435, 1997.

164. Oscier DG, Thompsett A, Zhu D, Stevenson FK: Differential rates of somatic hypermutation in V(H) genes among subsets of chronic lymphocytic leukemia defined by chromosomal abnormalities. *Blood* 89:4153, 1997.

165. Hamblin TJ, Davis Z, Gardiner A, Oscier DG, Stevenson FK: Unmutated Ig V(H) genes are associated with a more aggressive form of chronic lymphocytic leukemia. *Blood* 94:1848, 1999.

166. Damle RN, Wasil T, Fais F, et al: Ig V gene mutation status and CD38 expression as novel prognostic indicators in chronic lymphocytic leukemia. *Blood* 94:1840, 1999.

167. Kipps TJ, Tomhave E, Pratt LF, Duffy S, Chen PP, Carson DA: Develop-mentally restricted VH gene expressed at high frequency in chronic lymphocytic leukemia. *Proc Natl Acad Sci USA* 86:5913, 1989.

168. Johnson TA, Rassenti LZ, Kipps TJ: Ig VH1 genes expressed in B-cell chronic lymphocytic leukemia exhibit distinctive molecular features. *J Immunol* 158:235, 1997.

169. Martin T, Crouzier R, Weber JC, Kipps TJ, Pasquali JL: Structure-function studies on a polyreactive (natural) autoantibody. Polyreactivity

is dependent on somatically generated sequences in the third complemen-tarity-determining region of the antibody heavy chain. *J Immunol* 152:5988, 1994.

170. Schroeder HWJ, Mortari F, Shiokawa S, Kirkham PM, Elgavish RA, Bertrand FE: Developmental regulation of the human antibody reper-toire. *Ann NY Acad Sci* 764:242, 1995.

171. Marti GE, Zenger V, Caproaso NE, et al: Antigenic expression of B-cell chronic lymphocytic leukemic lymphocytes. *Anal Quant Cytol Histol* 11:315, 1989.

172. Marti GE, Faguet G, Bertin P, et al: CD20 and CD5 expression in B-chronic lymphocytic leukemia. *Ann NY Acad Sci* 651:480, 1992.

173. Almasri NM, Duque RE, Iturraspe J, Everett E, Braylan RC: Reduced expression of CD20 antigen as a characteristic marker for chronic lymphocytic leukemia. *Am J Hemat* 40:259, 1992.

174. Vincent AM, Cawley JC, Burthem J: Integrin function in chronic lymphocytic leukemia. *Blood* 87:4780, 1996.

175. Domingo A, Gonzalez-Barca E, Castellsague X, et al: Expression of adhesion molecules in 113 patients with B-cell chronic lymphocytic leukemia: relationship with clinico-prognostic features. *Leuk Res* 21:67, 1997.

176. Molica S, Dattilo A, Mannella A, Levato D: Intercellular adhesion molecules (ICAMs) 2 and 3 are frequently expressed in B cell chronic lymphocytic leukemia. *Leukemia* 10:907, 1996.

177. Huang JC, Finn WG, Goolsby CL, Variakojis D, Peterson LC: CD5-small B-cell leukemias are rarely classifiable as chronic lymphocytic leukemia. *Am J Clin Pathol* 111:123, 1999.

178. Kipps TJ: The CD5 B Cell. *Adv Immunol* 47:117, 1989.

179. Kipps TJ, Duffy SF: Relationship of the CD5 B cell to human tonsillar lymphocytes that express autoantibody-associated cross reactive idio-types. *J Clin Invest* 87:2087, 1991.

180. Burastero SE, Casali P: Characterization of human CD5 (Leu-1, OKT1)+ B lymphocytes and the antibodies they produce. *Contrib Mi-crobiol Immunol* 11:231, 1989.

181. Hardy RR, Hayakawa K, Shimizu M, Yamasaki K, Kishimoto T: Rheu-matoid factor secretion from human Leu-1+ B cells. *Science* 236:81, 1987.

182. Axelrod O, Silverman GJ, Dev V, Kyle R, Carson DA, Kipps TJ: Idiotypic cross-reactivity of immunoglobulins expressed in Walden-strom's macroglobulinemia, chronic lymphocytic leukemia, and mantle zone lymphocytes of secondary B-cell follicles. *Blood* 77:1484, 1991.

183. Van Oers MH, Pals ST, Evers LM, et al: Expression and release of CD27 in human B-cell malignancies. *Blood* 82:3430, 1993.

184. Herzenberg LA, Herzenberg LA: Toward a layered immune system. *Cell* 59:953, 1989.

185. Miller RA, Gralow J: The induction of Leu-1 antigen expression in human malignant and normal B cells by phorbol myristic acetate (PMA). *J Immunol* 133:3408, 1984.

186. Freedman AS, Freeman G, Whitman J, Segil J, Daley J, Nadler LM: Studies of in vitro activated CD5+ B cells. *Blood* 73:202, 1989.

187. Caligaris-Cappio F, Riva M, Tesio L, Schena M, Gaidano G, Bergui L: Human normal CD5+ B lymphocytes can be induced to differentiate to CD5- B lymphocytes with germinal center cell features. *Blood* 73:1259, 1989.

188. Allison A, Alt F, Arnold L, et al: A new nomenclature for B cells. *Immunol Today* 12:383, 1991.

189. Lampert IA, Wotherspoon A, Van Noorden S, Hasserjian RP: High expression of CD23 in the proliferation centers of chronic lymphocytic leukemia in lymph nodes and spleen. *Hum Pathol* 30:648, 1999.

190. Zimmerman TS, Godwin HA, Perry S: Studies of leukocyte kinetics in chronic lymphocytic leukemia. *Blood* 31:277, 1968.

191. Andreeff M, Darzynkiewicz Z, Sharpless TK, Clarkson BD, Melamed MR: Discrimination of human leukemia subtypes by flow cytometric analysis of cellular DNA and RNA. *Blood* 55:282, 1980.

192. Kobayashi R, Picchio G, Kirven M, et al: Transfer of human chronic lymphocytic leukemia to mice with severe combined immune deficiency. *Leuk Res* 16:1013, 1992.

193. Robertson LE, Plunkett W, McConnell K, Keating MJ, McDonnell TJ: Bcl-2 expression in chronic lymphocytic leukemia and its correlation with the induction of apoptosis and clinical outcome. *Leukemia* 10:456, 1996.

194. McConkey DJ, Chandra J, Wright S, et al: Apoptosis sensitivity in

chronic lymphocytic leukemia is determined by endogenous endonuclease content and relative expression of BCL-2 and BAX. *J Immunol* 156:2624, 1996.

195. Gottardi D, Alfarno A, De Leo AM, et al: In leukaemic CD5+ B cells the expression of BCL-2 gene family is shifted toward protection from apoptosis. *Br J Haematol* 94:612, 1996.

196. Pepper C, Bentley P, Hoy T: Regulation of clinical chemoresistance by bcl-2 and bax oncoproteins in B-cell chronic lymphocytic leukaemia. *Br J Haematol* 95:513, 1996.

197. Petersen AJ, Brown RD, Gibson J, et al: Nucleoside transporters, bcl-2 and apoptosis in CLL cells exposed to nucleoside analogues in vitro. *Eur J Haematol* 56:213, 1996.

198. Tangye SG, Raison RL: Leukaemic CD5+ B-cell apoptosis: co-incidence of cell death and DNA fragmentation with reduced bcl-2 expression. *Br J Haematol* 92:950, 1996.

199. Agular-Santelises M, Rottenberg ME, Lewin N, Mellstedt H, Jondal M: Bcl-2, Bax and p53 expression in B-CLL in relation to in vitro survival and clinical progression. *Int J Cancer* 69:114, 1996.

200. Smets LA, van den Berg JD: Bcl-2 expression and glucocorticoid-induced apoptosis of leukemic and lymphoma cells. *Leuk Lymphoma* 20:199, 1996.

201. Kitada S, Andersen J, Akar S, et al: Expression of apoptosis-regulating proteins in chronic lymphocytic leukemia: correlations with in vitro and in vivo chemoresponses. *Blood* 91:3379, 1998.

202. Korsmeyer SJ: Bcl-2 initiates a new category of oncogenes: regulators of cell death. Blood 80:879, 1992.

203. Coulie PG: Human tumour antigens recognized by T-cells: new perspectives for anti-cancer vaccines? *Mol Med Today* 3:261, 1997.

204. Thomas A, el Rouby S, Reed JC, et al: Drug-induced apoptosis in B-cell chronic lymphocytic leukemia: relationship between p53 gene mutation and bcl-2/bax proteins in drug resistance. *Oncogene* 12:1055, 1996.

205. Yang E, Korsmeyer SJ: Molecular thanatopsis: a discourse on the BCL2 family and cell death. *Blood* 88:386, 1996.

206. Gottardi D, De Leo AM, Alfarano A, et al: Fludarabine ability to down-regulate Bcl-2 gene product in CD5+ leukaemic B cells: in vitro/in vivo correlations. *Br J Haematol* 99:147, 1997.

207. McConkey DJ, Aguilar-Santelises M, Hartzell P, et al: Induction of DNA fragmentation in chronic B-lymphocytic leukemia cells. *J Immunol* 146:1072, 1991.

208. Osorio LM, De Santiago A, Aguilar-Santelises M, Mellstedt H, Jondal M: CD6 ligation modulates the Bcl-2/Bax ratio and protects chronic lymphocytic leukemia B cells from apoptosis induced by anti-IgM. *Blood* 89:2833, 1997.

209. Aruffo A, Bowen MA, Patel DD, et al: CD6-ligand interactions: a paradigm for SRCR domain function? *Immunol Today* 18:498, 1997.

210. Panayiotidis P, Jones D, Ganeshaguru K, Foroni L, Hoffbrand AV: Human bone marrow stromal cells prevent apoptosis and support the survival of chronic lymphocytic leukaemia cells in vitro. *Br J Haematol* 92:97, 1996.

211. Lagneaux L, Delforge A, Bron D, De Bruyn C, Stryckmans P: Chronic lymphocytic leukemic B cells but not normal B cells are rescued from apoptosis by contact with normal bone marrow stromal cells. *Blood* 91:2387, 1998.

212. Winkelstein A, Jordan PS: Immune deficiencies in chronic lymphocytic leukemia and multiple myeloma. *Clin Rev Allergy* 10:39, 1992.

213. Bower JH, Hammack JE, McDonnell SK, Tefferi A: The neurologic complications of B-cell chronic lymphocytic leukemia. *Neurology* 48:407, 1997.

214. Levi F, Randimbison L, Te VC, La Vecchia C: Non-Hodgkin's lymphomas, chronic lymphocytic leukaemias and skin cancers. *Br J Cancer* 74:1847, 1996.

215. Schlesinger M, Broman I, Lugassy G: The complement system is defective in chronic lymphatic leukemia patients and in their healthy relatives. *Leukemia* 10:1509, 1996.

216. Rossi E, Matutes E, Morilla R, Owusu-Ankomah K, Heffernan AM, Catovsky D: Zeta chain and CD28 are poorly expressed on T lymphocytes from chronic lymphocytic leukemia. *Leukemia* 10:494, 1996.

217. Veenstra H, Jacobs P, Dowdle EB: Abnormal association between invariant chain and HLA class II alpha and beta chains in chronic lymphocytic leukemia. *Cell Immunol* 171:68, 1996.

218. Itala M, Vainio O, Remes K: Functional abnormalities in granulocytes

219. Lotz M, Ranheim E, Kipps TJ: Transforming growth factor beta as endogenous growth inhibitor of chronic lymphocytic leukemia B cells. *J Exp Med* 179:999, 1994.

220. Lagneaux L, Delforge A, Bron D, Massy M, Bernier M, Stryckmans P: Heterogenous response of B lymphocytes to transforming growth factor-beta in B-cell chronic lymphocytic leukaemia: correlation with the expression of TGF-beta receptors. *Br J Haematol* 97:612, 1997.

221. Ranheim EA, Cantwell MJ, Kipps TJ: Expression of CD27 and its ligand, CD70, on chronic lymphocytic leukemia B cells. *Blood* 85:3556, 1995.

222. Kato K, Cantwell MJ, Sharma S, Kipps TJ: Gene transfer of CD40-ligand induces autologous immune recognition of chronic lymphocytic leukemia B cells. *J Clin Invest* 101:1133, 1998.

223. Matutes E, Wechsler A, Gomez R, Cherchi M, Catovsky D: Unusual T-cell phenotype in advanced B-chronic lymphocytic leukaemia. *Br J Haematol* 49:635, 1981.

224. Fu SM, Chiorazzi N, Kunkel HG: Differentiation capacity and other properties of the leukemic cells of chronic lymphocytic leukemia. *Immunol Rev* 48:23, 1979.

225. Ranheim EA, Kipps TJ: Activated T-cells induce expression of B7/BB1 on normal or leukemic B cells through a CD40-dependent signal. *J Exp Med* 177:925, 1993.

226. Cantwell MJ, Hua T, Pappas J, Kipps TJ: Acquired CD40-ligand deficiency in chronic lymphocytic leukemia. *Nat Med* 3:984, 1997.

227. Kneitz C, Goller M, Wilhelm M, et al: Inhibition of T-cell/B-cell interaction by B-CLL cells. *Leukemia* 13:98, 1999.

228. Grewal IS, Flavell RA: The CD40 ligand. At the center of the immune universe? *Immunol Res* 16:59, 1997.

229. Lacombe C, Gombert J, Dreyfus B, Brizard A, Preud'Homme JL: Heterogeneity of serum IgG subclass deficiencies in B chronic lymphocytic leukemia. *Clin Immunol* 90:128, 1999.

230. Rosen FS: Autoimmunity and immunodeficiency disease. *Ciba Found Symp* 129:135, 1987.

231. Hamblin TJ, Oscier DG, Young BJ: Autoimmunity in chronic lymphocytic leukaemia. *J Clin Pathol* 39:713, 1986.

232. Duhrsen U, Augener W, Zwingers T, Brittinger G: Spectrum and frequency of autoimmune derangements in lymphoproliferative disorders: analysis of 637 cases and comparison with myeloproliferative diseases. *Br J Haematol* 67:235, 1987.

233. Bhavnani M: Cyclosporin A treatment of pure red cell aplasia associated with B-CLL. *Br J Haematol* 79:137, 1991.

234. Taylor HG, Nixon N, Sheeran TP, Dawes PT: Rheumatoid arthritis and chronic lymphatic leukaemia. *Clin Exp Rheumatol* 7:529, 1989.

235. Amir R, Dowdy YG, Goldberg AN: Chronic rhinitis: a manifestation of chronic lymphocytic leukemia. *Am J Otolaryngol* 20:328, 1999.

236. Weed RI: Exaggerated delayed hypersensitivity to mosquito bites in chronic lymphocytic leukemia. *Blood* 26:257, 1965.

237. Barzilai A, Shpiro D, Goldberg I, et al: Insect bite-like reaction in patients with hematologic malignant neoplasms. *Arch Dermatol* 135:1503, 1999.

238. Higgins JP, Warnke RA: Herpes lymphadenitis in association with chronic lymphocytic leukemia. *Cancer* 86:1210, 1999.

239. Mariette X, Molina JM, Asli B, Brouet JC: A patient with chronic lymphoid leukemia and recurrent necrotic herpetic lymphadenitis [letter]. *Am J Med* 107:403, 1999.

240. Rustagi PK, Han T, Ziolkowski L, Farolino DL, Currie MS, Logue GL: Granulocyte antibodies in leukaemic chronic lymphoproliferative disorders. *Br J Haematol* 66:461, 1987.

241. Lischner M, Prokocimer M, Zolberg A, Shaklai M: Autoimmunity in chronic lymphocytic leukaemia. *Postgrad Med J* 64:590, 1988.

242. Chablani AT, Badakere SS, Bhatia HM: Incidence of antibodies to nuclear antigens, platelets and circulating immune complexes in leukaemias. *Indian J Med Res* 88:348, 1988.

243. Koerner TA, Weinfeld HM, Bullard LS, Williams LC: Antibodies against platelet glycosphingolipids: detection in serum by quantitative HPTLC-autoradiography and association with autoimmune and alloimmune processes. *Blood* 74:274, 1989.

244. Habboush HW, Dhundee J, Okati DA, Davies AG: Constrictive pericarditis in B cell chronic lymphatic leukaemia. *Clin Lab Haematol* 18:117, 1996.

245. Giannini O, Schönenberger-Berzins R: Fulminant cardiac tamponade in chronic lymphocytic leukemia [letter]. *Ann Oncol* 8:1168, 1997.

246. Sivakumaran M, Qureshi H, Chapman CS: Chylous effusions in CLL [letter; comment]. *Leuk Lymphoma* 18:365, 1995.

247. Zeidman A, Yarmolovsky A, Djaldetti M, Mittelman M: Hemorrhagic pleural effusion as a complication of chronic lymphocytic leukemia. *Haematologia (Budap)* 26:173, 1995.

248. Miyahara M, Shimamoto Y, Sano M, Nakano H, Shibata K, Matsuzaki M: Immunoglobulin gene rearrangement in T-cell-rich reactive pleural effusion of a patient with B-cell chronic lymphocytic leukemia. *Acta Haematol* 96:41, 1996.

249. Elliott MA, Letendre L, Li CY, Hoyer JD, Hammack JE: Chronic lymphocytic leukaemia with symptomatic diffuse central nervous system infiltration responding to therapy with systemic fludarabine. *Br J Haematol* 104:689, 1999.

250. Montserrat E, Marques-Pereira JP, Gallart MT, Rozman C: Bone marrow histopathologic patterns and immunologic findings in B-chronic lymphocytic leukemia. *Cancer* 54:447, 1984.

251. Pangalis GA, Roussou PA, Kittas C, et al: Patterns of bone marrow involvement in chronic lymphocytic leukemia and small lymphocytic (well differentiated) non-Hodgkin's lymphoma. Its clinical significance in relation to their differential diagnosis and prognosis. *Cancer* 54:702, 1984.

252. Pangalis GA, Boussiotis VA, Kittas C: Malignant disorders of small lymphocytes. Small lymphocytic lymphoma, lymphoplasmacytic lymphoma, and chronic lymphocytic leukemia: their clinical and laboratory relationship. *Am J Clin Pathol* 99:402, 1993.

253. Pangalis GA, Roussou PA, Kittas C, Kokkinou S, Fessas P: B-chronic lymphocytic leukemia. Prognostic implication of bone marrow histology in 120 patients experience from a single hematology unit. *Cancer* 59:767, 1987.

254. Kanzler H, Küppers R, Helmes S, et al: Hodgkin and Reed-Sternberg-like cells in B-cell chronic lymphocytic leukemia represent the outgrowth of single germinal-center B-cell-derived clones: potential precursors of Hodgkin and Reed-Sternberg cells in Hodgkin's disease. *Blood* 95:1023, 2000.

255. Baldini L, Cro L, Cortelezzi A, et al: Immunophenotypes in "classical" B-cell chronic lymphocytic leukemia. Correlation with normal cellular counterpart and clinical findings. *Cancer* 66:1738, 1990.

256. Sarfati M, Fournier S, Christoffersen M, Biron G: Expression of CD23 antigen and its regulation by IL-4 in chronic lymphocytic leukemia. *Leuk Res* 14:47, 1990.

257. Batata A, Shen B: Immunophenotyping of subtypes of B-chronic (mature) lymphoid leukemia. A study of 242 cases. *Cancer* 70:2436, 1992.

258. De Rossi G, Zarcone D, Mauro F, et al: Adhesion molecule expression on B-cell chronic lymphocytic leukemia cells: malignant T-cell phenotypes define distinct disease subsets. *Blood* 81:2679, 1993.

259. Pianezze G, Gentilini I, Casini M, Fabris P, Coser P: Cytoplasmic immunoglobulins in chronic lymphocytic leukemia B cells. *Blood* 69:1011, 1987.

260. Yasuda N, Kanoh T, Shirakawa S, Uchino H: Intracellular immunoglobulin in lymphocytes from patients with chronic lymphocytic leukemia: an immunoelectron microscopic study. *Leuk Res* 6:659, 1982.

261. Newell DG, Hannam-Harris A, Karpas A, Smith JL: The differential ultrastructural localization of immunoglobulin heavy and light chains in human haematopoietic cell lines. *Br J Haematol* 50:445, 1982.

262. Newell DG, Harris AH, Smith JL: The ultrastructural localization of immunoglobulin in chronic lymphocytic lymphoma cells: changes in light and heavy chain distribution induced by mitogen stimulation. *Blood* 61:511, 1983.

263. Deegan MJ, Abraham JP, Sawdyk M, Van Slyck EJ: High incidence of monoclonal proteins in the serum and urine of chronic lymphocytic leukemia patients. *Blood* 64:1207, 1984.

264. Sinclair D, Dagg JH, Dewar AE, et al: The incidence, clonal origin and secretory nature of serum paraproteins in chronic lymphocytic leukaemia. *Br J Haematol* 64:725, 1986.

265. Pangalis GA, Moutsopoulos HM, Papadopoulos NM, Costello R, Kokkinou S, Fessas P: Monoclonal and oligoclonal immunoglobulins in the serum of patients with B-chronic lymphocytic leukemia. *Acta Haematol* 80:23, 1988.

266. Gordon DS, Jones BM, Browning SW, Spira TJ, Lawrence DN: Persistent polyclonal lymphocytosis of B lymphocytes. *N Engl J Med* 307:232, 1982.

267. Wilkinson LS, Tang A, Gjedsted A: Marked lymphocytosis suggesting chronic lymphocytic leukemia in three patients with hyposplenism. *Am J Med* 75:1053, 1983.

268. Batata A, Shen B: Diagnostic value of clonality of surface immunoglobulin light and heavy chains in malignant lymphoproliferative disorders. *Am J Hematol* 43:265, 1993.

269. Melo JV, Wardle J, Chetty M, et al: The relationship between chronic lymphocytic leukaemia and prolymphocytic leukaemia: III. Evaluation of cell size by morphology and volume measurements. *Br J Haematol* 64:469, 1986.

270. Robinson DS, Melo JV, Andrews C, Schey SA, Catovsky D: Intracytoplasmic inclusions in B prolymphocytic leukaemia: ultrastructural, cytochemical, and immunological studies. *J Clin Pathol* 38:897, 1985.

271. Bearman RM, Pangalis GA, Rappaport H: Prolymphocytic leukemia: clinical, histopathological, and cytochemical observations. *Cancer* 42:2360, 1978.

272. Moreau EJ, Matutes E, A'Hern RP, et al: Improvement of the chronic lymphocytic leukemia scoring system with the monoclonal antibody SN8 (CD79b). *Am J Clin Pathol* 108:378, 1997.

273. Zomas AP, Matutes E, Morilla R, Owusu-Ankomah K, Seon BK, Catovsky D: Expression of the immunoglobulin-associated protein B29 in B cell disorders with the monoclonal antibody SN8 (CD79b). *Leukemia* 10:1966, 1996.

274. Matutes E, Morilla R, Owusu-Ankomah K, Houlihan A, Catovsky D: The immunophenotype of splenic lymphoma with villous lymphocytes and its relevance to the differential diagnosis with other B-cell disorders. *Blood* 83:1558, 1994.

275. Dick FR, Maca RD: The lymph node in chronic lymphocytic leukemia. *Cancer* 41:283, 1978.

276. Pratt LF, Rassenti L, Larrick J, Robbins B, Banks P, Kipps TJ: Immunoglobulin gene expression in small lymphocytic lymphoma with little or no somatic hypermutation. *J Immunol* 143:699, 1989.

277. Medeiros LJ, Strickler JG, Picker LJ, Gelb AB, Weiss LM, Warnke RA: "Well-differentiated" lymphocytic neoplasms. Immunologic findings correlated with clinical presentation and morphologic features. *Am J Pathol* 129:523, 1987.

278. Ellison DJ, Turner RR, van Antwerp R, Martin WE, Nathwani BN: High-grade mantle zone lymphoma. *Cancer* 60:2717, 1987.

279. Bell PB, Rooney N, Bosanquet AG: CD79a detected by ZL7.4 separates chronic lymphocytic leukemia from mantle cell lymphoma in the leukemic phase. *Cytometry* 38:102, 1999.

280. Skinnider LF, Tan L, Schmidt J, Armitage G: Chronic lymphocytic leukemia. A review of 745 cases and assessment of clinical staging. *Cancer* 50:2951, 1982.

281. Phillips EA, Kempin S, Passe S, Mike V, Clarkson B: Prognostic factors in chronic lymphocytic leukaemia and their implications for therapy. *Clin Haematol* 6:203, 1977.

282. Binet JL, Auquier A, Dighiero G, et al: A new prognostic classification of chronic lymphocytic leukemia derived from a multivariate survival analysis. *Cancer* 48:198, 1981.

283. Rai KR: A critical analysis of staging in CLL, in *Chronic Lymphocytic Leukemia: Recent Progress and Future Directions,* edited by Gale RP, Rai KR, p. 253. Alan R. Liss, New York, 1987.

284. Vrhovac R, Delmer A, Tang R, Marie JP, Zittoun R, Ajchenbaum-Cymbalista F: Prognostic significance of the cell cycle inhibitor p27Kip1 in chronic B-cell lymphocytic leukemia. *Blood* 91:4694, 1998.

285. Montserrat E, Sanchez-Bisono J, Vinolas N, Rozman C: Lymphocyte doubling time in chronic lymphocytic leukaemia: analysis of its prognostic significance. *Br J Haematol* 62:567, 1986.

286. Montserrat E, Villamor N, Reverter JC, et al: Bone marrow assessment in B-cell chronic lymphocytic leukaemia: aspirate or biopsy? A comparative study in 258 patients. *Br J Haematol* 93:111, 1996.

287. Geisler CH, Hou-Jensen K, Jensen OM, et al: The bone-marrow infiltration pattern in B-cell chronic lymphocytic leukemia is not an important prognostic factor. Danish CLL Study Group. *Eur J Haematol* 57:292, 1996.

288. Molica S, Levato D, Cascavilla N, Levato L, Musto P: Clinico-prognostic implications of simultaneous increased serum levels of soluble CD23 and beta2-microglobulin in B-cell chronic lymphocytic leukemia. *Eur J Haematol* 62:117, 1999.

289. Jarque I, Larrea L, Gomis F, et al: Bone marrow assessment in B-cell chronic lymphocytic leukaemia: aspirate or biopsy? [letter]. *Br J Haematol* 95:754, 1996.

290. Cheson BD, Bennett JM, Grever M, et al: National Cancer Institute-sponsored Working Group guidelines for chronic lymphocytic leukemia: revised guidelines for diagnosis and treatment. *Blood* 87:4990, 1996.

291. Oscier DG, Matutes E, Copplestone A, et al: Atypical lymphocyte morphology: an adverse prognostic factor for disease progression in stage A CLL independent of trisomy 12. *Br J Haematol* 98:934, 1997.

292. Baldini L, Mozzana R, Cortelezzi A, et al: Prognostic significance of immunoglobulin phenotype in B cell chronic lymphocytic leukemia. *Blood* 65:340, 1985.

293. Oscier DG, Stevens J, Hamblin TJ, Pickering RM, Fitchett M: Prognostic factors in stage A0 B-cell chronic lymphocytic leukaemia. *Br J Haematol* 76:348, 1990.

294. Han T, Henderson ES, Emrich LJ, Sandberg AA: Prognostic significance of karyotypic abnormalities in B cell chronic lymphocytic leukemia: an update. *Semin Hematol* 24:257, 1987.

295. Escudier SM, Pereira-Leahy JM, Drach JW, et al: Fluorescent in situ hybridization and cytogenetic studies of trisomy 12 in chronic lymphocytic leukemia. *Blood* 81:2702, 1993.

296. Juliusson G, Robert KH, Ost A, et al: Prognostic information from cytogenetic analysis in chronic B-lymphocytic leukemia and leukemic immunocytoma. *Blood* 65:134, 1985.

297. Tefferi A, Bartholmai BJ, Witzig TE, et al: Clinical correlations of immunophenotypic variations and the presence of trisomy 12 in B-cell chronic lymphocytic leukemia. *Cancer Genet Cytogenet* 95:173, 1997.

298. Juliusson G, Oscier DG, Fitchett M, et al: Prognostic subgroups in B-cell chronic lymphocytic leukemia defined by specific chromosomal abnormalities. *N Engl J Med* 323:720, 1990.

299. Montserrat E, Bosch F, Rozman C: B-cell chronic lymphocytic leukemia: recent progress in biology, diagnosis, and therapy. *Ann Oncol* 8(Suppl 1):93, 1997.

300. Oscier DG, Stevens J, Hamblin TJ, Pickering RM, Lambert R, Fitchett M: Correlation of chromosome abnormalities with laboratory features and clinical course in B-cell chronic lymphocytic leukaemia. *Br J Haematol* 76:352, 1990.

301. Spati B, Child JA, Kerruish SM, Cooper EH: Behaviour of serum beta 2-microglobulin and acute phase reactant proteins in chronic lymphocytic leukaemia. A multicentre study. *Acta Haematol* 64:79, 1980.

302. Hallek M, Wanders L, Ostwald M, et al: Serum beta(2)-microglobulin and serum thymidine kinase are independent predictors of progression-free survival in chronic lymphocytic leukaemia and immunocytoma. *Leuk Lymphoma* 22:439, 1996.

303. Hallek M, Langenmayer I, Nerl C, et al: Elevated serum thymidine kinase levels identify a subgroup at high risk of disease progression in early, nonsmoldering chronic lymphocytic leukemia. *Blood* 93:1732, 1999.

304. Sarfati M, Chevret S, Chastang C, et al: Prognostic importance of serum soluble CD23 level in chronic lymphocytic leukemia. *Blood* 88:4259, 1996.

305. Knauf WU, Ehlers B, Mohr B, et al: Prognostic impact of the serum levels of soluble CD23 in B-cell chronic lymphocytic leukemia [letter]. *Blood* 89:4241, 1997.

306. Christiansen I, Sundstrom C, Totterman TH: Elevated serum levels of soluble vascular cell adhesion molecule-1 (sVCAM-1) closely reflect tumour burden in chronic B-lymphocytic leukaemia. *Br J Haematol* 103:1129, 1998.

307. Molica S, Vitelli G, Levato D, et al: CD27 in B-cell chronic lymphocytic leukemia. Cellular expression, serum release and correlation with other soluble molecules belonging to nerve growth factor receptors (NGFr) superfamily. *Haematologica* 83:398, 1998.

308. Lee JS, Dixon DO, Kantarjian HM, Keating MJ, Talpaz M: Prognosis of chronic lymphocytic leukemia: a multivariate regression analysis of 325 untreated patients. *Blood* 69:929, 1987.

309. Robertson LE, Pugh W, O'Brien S, et al: Richter's syndrome: a report on 39 patients. *J Clin Oncol* 11:1985, 1993.

310. Everaus H, Luik E, Lehtmaa J: Active and indolent chronic lymphocytic leukaemia—immune and hormonal peculiarities. *Cancer Immunol Immunother* 45:109, 1997.

311. Vlasveld LT, Pauwels P, Ermens AA, Aarnoudse WH, Ooms HW, Haak HR: Parathyroid hormone-related protein (PTH-rP)-associated hypercalcemia in a patient with an atypical chronic lymphocytic leukemia. *Neth J Med* 54:21, 1999.

312. Beaudreuil J, Lortholary O, Martin A, et al: Hypercalcemia may indicate

313. de Nully Brown P, Hansen MM: GM-CSF treatment in patients with B-chronic lymphocytic leukemia. *Leuk Lymphoma* 32:365, 1999.

314. Itala M, Pelliniemi TT, Remes K: GM-CSF raises serum levels of beta 2-microglobulin and thymidine kinase in patients with chronic lymphocytic leukaemia. *Br J Haematol* 94:129, 1996.

315. Lundblad V, Wright WE: Telomeres and telomerase: a simple picture becomes complex. *Cell* 87:369, 1996.

316. Ohyashiki K, Ohyashiki JH: Telomere dynamics and cytogenetic changes in human hematologic neoplasias: a working hypothesis. *Cancer Genet Cytogenet* 94:67, 1997.

317. Bechter OE, Eisterer W, Pall G, Hilbe W, Kuhr T, Thaler J: Telomere length and telomerase activity predict survival in patients with B cell chronic lymphocytic leukemia. *Cancer Res* 58:4918, 1998.

318. CLL Trialists' Collaborative Group: Chemotherapeutic options in chronic lymphocytic leukemia: a meta-analysis of the randomized trials. *J Natl Cancer Inst* 91:861, 1999.

319. Lichtman MA, Rowe JM: Hyperleukocytic leukemias: rheological, clinical, and therapeutic considerations. *Blood* 60:279, 1982.

320. Sawitsky A, Rai KR, Glidewell O, Silver RT: Comparison of daily versus intermittent chlorambucil and prednisone therapy in the treatment of patients with chronic lymphocytic leukemia. *Blood* 50:1049, 1977.

321. Patel PM, Selby PJ, Graham MA, Viner C, Newell DR, McElwain TJ: Pharmacokinetics of high dose methylprednisolone and use in hematological malignancies. *Hematol Oncol* 11:89, 1993.

322. Thornton PD, Hamblin M, Treleaven JG, Matutes E, Lakhani AK, Catovsky D: High dose methyl prednisolone in refractory chronic lymphocytic leukaemia. *Leuk Lymphoma* 34:167, 1999.

323. Dighiero G, Maloum K, Desablens B, et al: Chlorambucil in indolent chronic lymphocytic leukemia. French Cooperative Group on Chronic Lymphocytic Leukemia. *N Engl J Med* 338:1506, 1998.

324. Han T, Ezdinli EZ, Shimaoka K, Desai DV, Chlorambucil vs. combined chlorambucil-corticosteroid therapy in chronic lymphocytic leukemia. *Cancer* 31:502, 1973.

325. Mentz F, Mossalayi MD, Ouaaz F, et al: Theophylline synergizes with chlorambucil in inducing apoptosis of B-chronic lymphocytic leukemia cells. *Blood* 88:2172, 1996.

326. Mentz F, Merle-Beral H, Dalloul AH: Theophylline-induced B-CLL apoptosis is partly dependent on cyclic AMP production but independent of CD38 expression and endogenous IL-10 production. *Leukemia* 13:78, 1999.

327. Makower D, Malik U, Novik Y, Wiernik PH: Therapeutic efficacy of theophylline in chronic lymphocytic leukemia. *Med Oncol* 16:69, 1999.

328. Binet JL, Mentz F, Leblond V, Merle-Beral H: Synergistic action of alkylating agents and methylxanthine derivatives in the treatment of chronic lymphocytic leukemia [letter]. *Leukemia* 9:2159, 1995.

329. Jaksic B, Brugiatelli M, Krc I, et al: High dose chlorambucil versus Binet's modified cyclophosphamide, doxorubicin, vincristine, and prednisone regimen in the treatment of patients with advanced B-cell chronic lymphocytic leukemia. Results of an international multicenter randomized trial. International Society for Chemo-Immunotherapy, Vienna. *Cancer* 79:2107, 1997.

330. Huguley CMJ: Treatment of chronic lymphocytic leukemia. *Cancer Treat Rev* 4:261, 1977.

331. Keating MJ, O'Brien S, Plunkett W, et al: Fludarabine phosphate: a new active agent in hematologic malignancies. *Semin Hematol* 31:28, 1994.

332. Keating MJ: Fludarabine phosphate in the treatment of chronic lymphocytic leukemia. *Semin Oncol* 17:49, 1990.

333. Feldman EJ, Keating MJ: Fludarabine in the treatment of lymphoproliferative malignancies. *Cancer Invest* 11:314, 1993.

334. De Rossi G, Mauro FR, Caruso R, Monarca B, Mandelli F: Fludarabine and prednisone in pretreated and refractory B-chronic lymphocytic leukemia (B-CLL) in advanced stages. *Haematologica* 78:167, 1993.

335. Zinzani PL, Lauria F, Rondelli D, et al: Fludarabine in patients with advanced and/or resistant B-chronic lymphocytic leukemia. *Eur J Haematol* 51:93, 1993.

336. Bergmann L, Fenchel K, Jahn B, Mitrou PS, Hoelzer D: Immunosuppressive effects and clinical response of fludarabine in refractory chronic lymphocytic leukemia. *Ann Oncol* 4:371, 1993.

337. Hiddemann W, Rottmann R, Wormann B, et al: Treatment of advanced

Richter's syndrome: report of four cases and review. *Cancer* 79:1211, 1997.

chronic lymphocytic leukemia by fludarabine. Results of a clinical phase-II study. *Ann Hematol* 63:1, 1991.

338. Foran JM, Oscier D, Orchard J, et al: Pharmacokinetic study of single doses of oral fludarabine phosphate in patients with "low-grade" non-Hodgkin's lymphoma and B-cell chronic lymphocytic leukemia. *J Clin Oncol* 17:1574, 1999.

339. Gjedde SB, Hansen MM: Salvage therapy with fludarabine in patients with progressive B-chronic lymphocytic leukemia. *Leuk Lymphoma* 21:317, 1996.

340. Angelopoulou MA, Poziopoulos C, Boussiotis VA, Kontopidou F, Pangalis GA: Fludarabine monophosphate in refractory B-chronic lymphocytic leukemia: maintenance may be significant to sustain response. *Leuk Lymphoma* 21:321, 1996.

341. Sorensen JM, Vena DA, Fallavollita A, Chun HG, Cheson BD: Treatment of refractory chronic lymphocytic leukemia with fludarabine phosphate via the group C protocol mechanism of the National Cancer Institute: five-year follow-up report. *J Clin Oncol* 15:458, 1997.

342. Keating MJ, O'Brien S, Lerner S, et al: Long-term follow-up of patients with chronic lymphocytic leukemia (CLL) receiving fludarabine regimens as initial therapy. *Blood* 92:1165, 1998.

343. Friedenberg WR, Anderson J, Wolf BC, Cassileth PA, Oken MM: Modified vincristine, doxorubicin, and dexamethasone regimen in the treatment of resistant or relapsed chronic lymphocytic leukemia. An Eastern Cooperative Oncology Group study. *Cancer* 71:2983, 1993.

344. Johnson S, Smith AG, Loffler H, et al: Multicentre prospective randomised trial of fludarabine versus cyclophosphamide, doxorubicin, and prednisone (CAP) for treatment of advanced-stage chronic lymphocytic leukaemia. The French Cooperative Group on CLL. *Lancet* 347:1432, 1996.

345. Keating MJ, O'Brien S, Kantarjian H, et al: Long-term follow-up of patients with chronic lymphocytic leukemia treated with fludarabine as a single agent. *Blood* 81:2878, 1993.

346. O'Brien S, Kantarjian H, Beran M, et al: Results of fludarabine and prednisone therapy in 264 patients with chronic lymphocytic leukemia with multivariate analysis-derived prognostic model for response to treatment. *Blood* 82:1695, 1993.

347. Mason JM, Drummond MF, Bosanquet AG, Sheldon TA: The DiSC assay. A cost-effective guide to treatment for chronic lymphocytic leukemia? *Int J Technol Assess Health Care* 15:173, 1999.

348. Bosanquet AG, Johnson SA, Richards SM: Prognosis for fludarabine therapy of chronic lymphocytic leukaemia based on ex vivo drug response by DiSC assay. *Br J Haematol* 106:71, 1999.

349. Cohen RB, Abdallah JM, Gray JR, Foss F: Reversible neurologic toxicity in patients treated with standard-dose fludarabine phosphate for mycosis fungoides and chronic lymphocytic leukemia. *Ann Intern Med* 118:114, 1993.

350. Elias L, Stock-Novack D, Head DR, et al: A phase I trial of combination fludarabine monophosphate and chlorambucil in chronic lymphocytic leukemia: a Southwest Oncology Group study. *Leukemia* 7:361, 1993.

351. List AF, Kummet TD, Adams JD, Chun HG: Tumor lysis syndrome complicating treatment of chronic lymphocytic leukemia with fludarabine phosphate. *Am J Med* 89:388, 1990.

352. Wijermans PW, Gerrits WB, Haak HL: Severe immunodeficiency in patients treated with fludarabine monophosphate. *Eur J Haematol* 50:292, 1993.

353. Anaissie E, Kontoyiannis DP, Kantarjian H, Elting L, Robertson LE, Keating M: Listeriosis in patients with chronic lymphocytic leukemia who were treated with fludarabine and prednisone. *Ann Intern Med* 117:466, 1992.

354. Myint H, Copplestone JA, Orchard J, et al: Fludarabine-related autoimmune haemolytic anaemia in patients with chronic lymphocytic leukaemia. *Br J Haematol* 91:341, 1995.

355. Maclean R, Meiklejohn D, Soutar R: Fludarabine-related autoimmune haemolytic anaemia in patients with chronic lymphocytic leukaemia. *Br J Haematol* 92:768, 1996.

356. Nakhoul F, Green J, Abassi ZA, Carter A: Tumor lysis syndrome induced by fludarabine monophosphate: a case report [letter]. *Eur J Haematol* 56:254, 1996.

357. Cheson BD, Frame JN, Vena D, Quashu N, Sorensen JM: Tumor lysis syndrome: an uncommon complication of fludarabine therapy of chronic lymphocytic leukemia. *J Clin Oncol* 16:2313, 1998.

358. Briz M, Cabrera R, Sanjuan I, et al: Diagnosis of transfusion-associated

359. graft-versus-host disease by polymerase chain reaction in fludarabine-treated B-chronic lymphocytic leukaemia. *Br J Haematol* 91:409, 1995.

359. Briones J, Pereira A, Alcorta I: Transfusion-associated graft-versus-host disease (TA-GVHD) in fludarabine-treated patients: is it time to irradiate blood component? [letter]. *Br J Haematol* 93:739, 1996.

360. Cheson BD, Vena DA, Barrett J, Freidlin B: Second malignancies as a consequence of nucleoside analog therapy for chronic lymphoid leukemias. *J Clin Oncol* 17:2454, 1999.

361. Beutler E: New chemotherapeutic agent: 2-chlorodeoxyadenosine. *Semin Hematol* 31:40, 1994.

362. Piro LD, Carrera CJ, Beutler E, Carson DA: 2-Chlorodeoxyadenosine: an effective new agent for the treatment of chronic lymphocytic leukemia. *Blood* 72:1069, 1988.

363. Juliusson G, Liliemark J: High complete remission rate from 2-chloro-2'-deoxyadenosine in previously treated patients with B-cell chronic lymphocytic leukemia: response predicted by rapid decrease of blood lymphocyte count. *J Clin Oncol* 11:679, 1993.

364. Robak T, Blasinka-Morawiec M, Krykowski E, et al: Intermittent 2-hour intravenous infusions of 2-chlorodeoxyadenosine in the treatment of 110 patients with refractory or previously untreated B-cell chronic lymphocytic leukemia. *Leuk Lymphoma* 22:509, 1996.

365. Juliusson G, Elmhorn-Rosenborg A, Liliemark J: Response to 2-chlorodeoxyadenosine in patients with B-cell chronic lymphocytic leukemia resistant to fludarabine. *N Engl J Med* 327:1056, 1992.

366. O'Brien S, Kantarjian H, Estey E, et al: Lack of effect of 2-chlorodeoxyadenosine therapy in patients with chronic lymphocytic leukemia refractory to fludarabine therapy. *N Engl J Med* 330:319, 1994.

367. Juliusson G, Liliemark J: Complete remission of B-cell chronic lymphocytic leukaemia after oral cladribine [letter]. *Lancet* 341:54, 1993.

368. Juliusson G, Christiansen I, Hansen MM, et al: Oral cladribine as primary therapy for patients with B-cell chronic lymphocytic leukemia. *J Clin Oncol* 14:2160, 1996.

369. Bosanquet AG, Copplestone JA, Johnson SA, et al: Response to cladribine in previously treated patients with chronic lymphocytic leukaemia identified by ex vivo assessment of drug sensitivity by DiSC assay. *Brit J Haematol* 106:474, 1999.

370. Dann EJ, Gillis S, Polliack A, Okon E, Rund D, Rachmilewitz EA: Brief report: tumor lysis syndrome following treatment with 2-chlorodeoxyadenosine for refractory chronic lymphocytic leukemia. *N Engl J Med* 329:1547, 1993.

371. Dillman RO: A new chemotherapeutic agent: deoxycoformycin (pentostatin). *Semin Hematol* 31:16, 1994.

372. Ho AD, Thaler J, Stryckmans P, et al: Pentostatin in refractory chronic lymphocytic leukemia: a phase II trial of the European Organization for Research and Treatment of Cancer. *J Natl Cancer Inst* 82:1416, 1990.

373. Robertson LE, Hall R, Keating MJ, et al: High-dose cytosine arabinoside in chronic lymphocytic leukemia: a clinical and pharmacologic analysis. *Leuk Lymphoma* 10:43, 1993.

374. Shaklai S, Bairey O, Blickstein D, et al: Severe myelotoxicity of oral etoposide in heavily pretreated patients with non-Hodgkin's lymphoma or chronic lymphatic leukemia. *Cancer* 77:2313, 1996.

375. Konig A, Wrazel L, Warrell RPJ, et al: Comparative activity of melarsoprol and arsenic trioxide in chronic B-cell leukemia lines. *Blood* 90:562, 1997.

376. Soignet SL, Tong WP, Hirschfeld S, Warrell RP Jr: Clinical study of an organic arsenical, melarsoprol, in patients with advanced leukemia. *Cancer Chemother Pharmacol* 44:417, 1999.

377. Catovsky D, Richards S, Fooks J, Hamblin TJ: CLL Trials in the United Kingdom. *Leuk Lymphoma* 5(suppl):105, 1991.

378. Montserrat E, Fontanilles M, Estapé J: Treatment of chronic lymphocytic leukemia: a preliminary report of Spanish (Pethema) trials. *Leuk Lymphoma* 5(supp):89, 1991.

379. Keller JW, Knospe WH, Raney M, et al: Treatment of chronic lymphocytic leukemia using chlorambucil and prednisone with or without cycle-active consolidation chemotherapy. A Southeastern Cancer Study Group Trial. *Cancer* 58:1185, 1986.

380. Montserrat E, Alcala A, Alonso C, et al: A randomized trial comparing chlorambucil plus prednisone vs cyclophosphamide, melphalan, and prednisone in the treatment of chronic lymphocytic leukemia stages B and C. *Nouv Rev Fr Hematol* 30:429, 1988.

381. Raphael B, Andersen JW, Silber R, et al: Comparison of chlorambucil

and prednisone versus cyclophosphamide, vincristine, and prednisone as initial treatment for chronic lymphocytic leukemia: long-term follow-up of an Eastern Cooperative Oncology Group randomized clinical trial. *J Clin Oncol* 9:770, 1991.

382. O'Brien S, Kantarjian H, Beran M, et al: Fludarabine and granulocyte colony-stimulating factor (G-CSF) in patients with chronic lymphocytic leukemia. *Leukemia* 11:1631, 1997.

383. Giles FJ, O'Brien SM, Santini V, et al: Sequential cisplatin and fludarabine with or without arabinosyl cytosine in patients failing prior fludarabine therapy for chronic lymphocytic leukemia: a phase II study. *Leuk Lymphoma* 36:57, 1999.

384. Laurencet FM, Zulian GB, Guetty-Alberto M, Iten PA, Betticher DC, Alberto P: Cladribine with cyclophosphamide and prednisone in the management of low-grade lymphoproliferative malignancies. *Br J Cancer* 79:1215, 1999.

385. Oken MM, Kaplan ME: Combination chemotherapy with cyclophosphamide, vincristine, and prednisone in the treatment of refractory chronic lymphocytic leukemia. *Cancer Treat Rep* 63:441, 1979.

386. French Cooperative Group: A randomized clinical trial of chlorambucil versus COP in stage B chronic lymphocytic leukemia. The French Cooperative Group on Chronic Lymphocytic Leukemia. *Blood* 75:1422, 1990.

387. French Cooperative Group: Prognostic and therapeutic advances in CLL management: the experience of the French Cooperative Group. French Cooperative Group on Chronic Lymphocytic Leukemia. *Semin Hematol* 24:275, 1987.

388. French Cooperative Group: Comparison of fludarabine, cyclophosphamide/doxorubicin/prednisone, and cyclophosphamide/doxorubicin/vincristine/prednisone in advanced forms of chronic lymphocytic leukemia: preliminary results of a controlled clinical trial. The French Cooperative Group on Chronic Lymphocytic Leukemia. *Semin Oncol* 20:21, 1993.

389. McCroskey RD, Mosher DF, Spencer CD, Prendergast E, Longo WL: Acute tumor lysis syndrome and treatment response in patients treated for refractory chronic lymphocytic leukemia with short-course, high-dose cytosine arabinoside, cisplatin, and etoposide. *Cancer* 66:246, 1990.

390. Coad JE, Matutes E, Catovsky D: Splenectomy in lymphoproliferative disorders: a report on 70 cases and review of the literature. *Leuk Lymphoma* 10:245, 1993.

391. Seymour JF, Cusack JD, Lerner SA, Pollock RE, Keating MJ: Case/control study of the role of splenectomy in chronic lymphocytic leukemia. *J Clin Oncol* 15:52, 1997.

392. Rubin P, Bennett JM, Begg C, Bozdech MJ, Silber R: The comparison of total body irradiation vs chlorambucil and prednisone for remission induction of active chronic lymphocytic leukemia: an ECOG study. Part I: total body irradiation-response and toxicity. *Int J Radiat Oncol Biol Phys* 7:1623, 1981.

393. Byhardt RW, Brace KC, Wiernik PH: The role of splenic irradiation in chronic lymphocytic leukemia. *Cancer* 35:1621, 1975.

394. Aabo K, Walbom-Jorgensen S: Spleen irradiation in chronic lymphocytic leukemia (CLL): palliation in patients unfit for splenectomy. *Am J Hematol* 19:177, 1985.

395. Chisesi T, Capnist G, Dal Fior S: Splenic irradiation in chronic lymphocytic leukemia. *Eur J Haematol* 46:202, 1991.

396. Chiappa S, Bonadonna G, Uslenghi C, Marano P, Molinari R: The role of endolymphatic radiotherapy in the treatment of chronic lymphatic leukaemia. *Br J Cancer* 20:480, 1966.

397. Chanana AD, Cronkite EP, Rai KR: The role of extracorporeal irradiation of blood in treatment of leukemia. *Int J Radiat Oncol Biol Phys* 1:539, 1976.

398. Wieselthier JS, Rothstein TL, Yu TL, Anderson T, Japowicz MC, Koh HK: Inefficacy of extracorporeal photochemotherapy in the treatment of B-cell chronic lymphocytic leukemia: preliminary results. *Am J Hematol* 41:123, 1992.

399. Marti GE, Folks T, Longo DL, Klein H: Therapeutic cytapheresis in chronic lymphocytic leukemia. *J Clin Apheresis* 1:243, 1983.

400. Cooper IA, Ding JC, Adams PB, Quinn MA, Brettell M: Intensive leukapheresis in the management of cytopenias in patients with chronic lymphocytic leukaemia (CLL) and lymphocytic lymphoma. *Am J Hematol* 6:387, 1979.

401. Gribben JG, Neuberg D, Barber M, et al: Detection of residual lymphoma cells by polymerase chain reaction in peripheral blood is significantly less predictive for relapse than detection in bone marrow. *Blood* 83:3800, 1994.

402. Gahn B, Schafer C, Neef J, et al: Detection of trisomy 12 and Rb-deletion in CD34+ cells of patients with B-cell chronic lymphocytic leukemia. *Blood* 89:4275, 1997.

403. Gahn B, Schafer C, Neef J, et al: Detection of trisomy 12 in CD34+ progenitor cells in a patient with B-cell chronic lymphocytic leukemia by fluorescence in situ hybridization. *Ann Oncol* 8(suppl 2):55, 1997.

404. Dreger P, von Neuhoff N, Kuse R, et al: Early stem cell transplantation for chronic lymphocytic leukaemia: a chance for cure? *Br J Cancer* 77:2291, 1998.

405. Pavletic ZS, Bierman PJ, Vose JM, et al: High incidence of relapse after autologous stem-cell transplantation for B-cell chronic lymphocytic leukemia or small lymphocytic lymphoma. *Ann Oncol* 9:1023, 1998.

406. Sutton L, Maloum K, Gonzalez H, et al: Autologous hematopoietic stem cell transplantation as salvage treatment for advanced B cell chronic lymphocytic leukemia. *Leukemia* 12:1699, 1998.

407. Gribben JG: Bone marrow transplantation for low-grade B-cell malignancies. *Curr Opin Oncol* 9:117, 1997.

408. Provan D, Bartlett-Pandite L, Zwicky C, et al: Eradication of polymerase chain reaction-detectable chronic lymphocytic leukemia cells is associated with improved outcome after bone marrow transplantation. *Blood* 88:2228, 1996.

409. Khouri I, Champlin R: Allogenic bone marrow transplantation in chronic lymphocytic leukemia [letter]. *Ann Intern Med* 125:780, 1996.

410. Michallet M, Archimbaud E, Bandini G, et al: HLA-identical sibling bone marrow transplantation in younger patients with chronic lymphocytic leukemia. European Group for Blood and Marrow Transplantation and the International Bone Marrow Transplant Registry. *Ann Intern Med* 124:311, 1996.

411. Mehta J, Powles R, Singhal S, et al: T-cell-depleted allogeneic bone marrow transplantation from a partially HLA-mismatched unrelated donor for progressive chronic lymphocytic leukemia and fludarabine-induced bone marrow failure. *Bone Marrow Transplant* 17:881, 1996.

412. Mehta J, Powles R, Singhal S, Iveson T, Treleaven J, Catovsky D: Clinical and hematologic response of chronic lymphocytic and pro-lymphocytic leukemia persisting after allogeneic bone marrow transplantation with the onset of acute graft-versus-host disease: possible role of graft-versus-leukemia. *Bone Marrow Transplant* 17:371, 1996.

413. Rondon G, Giralt S, Huh Y, et al: Graft-versus-leukemia effect after allogeneic bone marrow transplantation for chronic lymphocytic leukemia. *Bone Marrow Transplant* 18:669, 1996.

414. Khouri IF, Keating M, Korbling M, et al: Transplant-lite: induction of graft-versus-malignancy using fludarabine-based nonablative chemotherapy and allogeneic blood progenitor-cell transplantation as treatment for lymphoid malignancies. *J Clin Oncol* 16:2817, 1998.

415. Khouri IF, Przepiorka D, van Besien K, et al: Allogeneic blood or marrow transplantation for chronic lymphocytic leukaemia: timing of transplantation and potential effect of fludarabine on acute graft-versus-host disease. *Br J Haematol* 97:466, 1997.

416. Rozman C, Montserrat E, Vinolas N, et al: Recombinant alpha 2-interferon in the treatment of B chronic lymphocytic leukemia in early stages. *Blood* 71:1295, 1988.

417. Morabito F, Callea V, Oliva B, et al: Alpha 2-interferon in B-cell chronic lymphocytic leukemia: clinical response, serum cytokine levels, and immunophenotype modulation. *Leukemia* 7:366, 1993.

418. Pozzato G, Franzin F, Moretti M, et al: Low-dose "natural" alpha-interferon in B-cell derived chronic lymphocytic leukemia. *Haematologica* 77:413, 1992.

419. Foon KA, Bottino GC, Abrams PG, et al: Phase II trial of recombinant leukocyte alpha interferon in patients with advanced chronic lymphocytic leukemia. *Am J Med* 78:216, 1985.

420. Allebes WA, Knops R, Bontrop RE, et al: Phenotypic and functional changes of tumour cells from patients treated with monoclonal anti-idiotypic antibodies. *Scand J Immunol* 32:441, 1990.

421. Foon KA, Schroff RW, Bunn PA, et al: Effects of monoclonal antibody therapy in patients with chronic lymphocytic leukemia. *Blood* 64:1085, 1984.

422. Dillman RO, Shawler DL, Sobol RE, et al: Murine monoclonal antibody therapy in two patients with chronic lymphocytic leukemia. *Blood* 59:1036, 1982.

423. Grossbard ML, Lambert JM, Goldmacher VS, et al: Anti-B4-blocked

ricin: a phase I trial of 7-day continuous infusion in patients with B-cell neoplasms. *J Clin Oncol* 11:726, 1993.

424. Kreitman RJ, Chaudhary VK, Kozak RW, FitzGerald DJ, Waldman TA, Pastan I: Recombinant toxins containing the variable domains of the anti-Tac monoclonal antibody to the interleukin-2 receptor kill malignant cells from patients with chronic lymphocytic leukemia. *Blood* 80:2344, 1992.

425. Reff ME, Carner K, Chambers KS, et al: Depletion of B cells in vivo by a chimeric mouse human monoclonal antibody to CD20. *Blood* 83:435, 1994.

426. Maloney DG, Grillo-López AJ, White CA, et al: IDEC-C2B8 (Rituximab) anti-CD20 monoclonal antibody therapy in patients with relapsed low-grade non-Hodgkin's lymphoma. *Blood* 90:2188, 1997.

427. McLaughlin P, Grillo-López AJ, Link BK, et al: Rituximab chimeric anti-CD20 monoclonal antibody therapy for relapsed indolent lymphoma: half of patients respond to a four-dose treatment program. *J Clin Oncol* 16:2825, 1998.

428. Yang HH, Rosove MH, Figlin RA: Tumor lysis syndrome occurring after the administration of rituximab in lymphoproliferative disorders: high-grade non-Hodgkin's lymphoma and chronic lymphocytic leukemia. *Am J Hematol* 62:247, 1999.

429. Winkler U, Jensen M, Manzke O, Schulz H, Diehl V, Engert A: Cytokine-release syndrome in patients with B-cell chronic lymphocytic leukemia and high lymphocyte counts after treatment with an Anti-CD20 monoclonal antibody (Rituximab, IDEC-C2B8). *Blood* 94:2217, 1999.

430. Hale G, Dyer MJ, Clark MR, et al: Remission induction in non-Hodgkin lymphoma with reshaped monoclonal antibody CAMPATH-1H. *Lancet* 2:1394, 1988.

431. Bowen AL, Zomas A, Emmett E, Matutes E, Dyer MJ, Catovsky D: Subcutaneous CAMPATH-1H in fludarabine-resistant/relapsed chronic lymphocytic and B-prolymphocytic leukaemia. *Br J Haematol* 96:617, 1997.

432. Osterborg A, Fassas AS, Anagnostopoulos A, Dyer MJ, Catovsky D, Mellstedt H: Humanized CD52 monoclonal antibody CAMPATH-1H as first-line treatment in chronic lymphocytic leukaemia. *Br J Haematol* 93:151, 1996.

433. Osterborg A, Dyer MJ, Bunjes D, et al: Phase II multicenter study of human CD52 antibody in previously treated chronic lymphocytic leukemia. European Study Group of CAMPATH-1H Treatment in Chronic Lymphocytic Leukemia. *J Clin Oncol* 15:1567, 1997.

434. Dyer MJ, Kelsey SM, Mackay HJ, et al: In vivo 'purging' of residual disease in CLL with CAMPATH-1H. *Br J Haematol* 97:669, 1997.

435. Shen S, DeNardo GL, O'Donnell RT, Yuan A, DeNardo DA, DeNardo SJ: Impact of splenomegaly on therapeutic response and ^{131}I-LYM-1 dosimetry in patients with B-lymphocytic malignancies. *Cancer* 80:2553, 1997.

436. DeNardo GL, Lamborn KR, Goldstein DS, Kroger LA, DeNardo SJ: Increased survival associated with radiolabeled Lym-1 therapy for non-Hodgkin's lymphoma and chronic lymphocytic leukemia. *Cancer* 80:2706, 1997.

437. DeNardo GL, DeNardo SJ, Shen S, et al: Factors affecting ^{131}I-Lym-1 pharmacokinetics and radiation dosimetry in patients with non-Hodgkin's lymphoma and chronic lymphocytic leukemia. *J Nucl Med* 40:1317, 1999.

438. DeNardo GL, O'Donnell RT, Rose LM, Mirick GR, Kroger LA, DeNardo SJ: Milestones in the development of Lym-1 therapy. *Hybridoma* 18:1, 1999.

439. Kipps TJ, Cantwell MJ, Sharma S, Kato K: Gene therapy of chronic lymphocytic leukemia. *Cancer Res Ther Control* 7:37, 1998.

440. Robertson TI: Complications and causes of death in B cell chronic lymphocytic leukaemia: a long term study of 105 patients. *Aust NZ J Med* 20:44, 1990.

441. Morra E, Nosari A, Montillo M: Infectious complications in chronic lymphocytic leukaemia. *Hematol Cell Ther* 41:145, 1999.

442. Griffiths H, Lea J, Bunch C, Lee M, Chapel H: Predictors of infection in chronic lymphocytic leukaemia (CLL). *Clin Exp Immunol* 89:374, 1992.

443. Itala M, Helenius H, Nikoskelainen J, Remes K: Infections and serum IgG levels in patients with chronic lymphocytic leukaemia. *Eur J Haematol* 48:266, 1992.

444. Cooperative Group for the Study of Immunoglobulin in Chronic Lymphocytic Leukemia: Intravenous immunoglobulin for the prevention of infection in chronic lymphocytic leukemia. A randomized, controlled clinical trial. *N Engl J Med* 319:902, 1988.

445. Stiehm ER: New uses for intravenous immune globulin [editorial; comment]. *N Engl J Med* 325:123, 1991.

446. Chikkappa G, Pasquale D, Zarrabi MH, Weiler RJ, Divakara M, Tsan MF: Cyclosporine and prednisone therapy for pure red cell aplasia in patients with chronic lymphocytic leukemia. *Am J Hematol* 41:5, 1992.

447. Greene MH, Hoover RN, Fraumeni JFJ: Subsequent cancer in patients with chronic lymphocytic leukemia–a possible immunologic mechanism. *J Natl Cancer Inst* 61:337, 1978.

448. Quaglino D, Lusvarghi E, Piccinini L, di Prisco AU, Guerzoni O, Mauri C: The association between chronic lymphocytic leukaemia and a solid tumor: a survey study of 258 cases of chronic lymphocytic leukaemia covering an eleven year period. *Haematologica* 61:456, 1976.

449. Quaglino D, Paterlini P, De Pasquale A, Cretara G, Venturoni L: Association of chronic lymphocytic leukaemia and multiple myeloma: report of a case and review of the literature. *Haematologica* 67:576, 1982.

450. Hoffman KD, Rudders RA: Multiple myeloma and chronic lymphocytic leukemia in a single individual. *Arch Intern Med* 137:232, 1977.

451. Jeha MT, Hamblin TJ, Smith JL: Coincident chronic lymphocytic leukemia and osteosclerotic multiple myeloma. *Blood* 57:617, 1981.

452. Pedersen-Bjergaard J, Petersen HD, Thomsen M, Wiik A, Wolff-Jensen J: Chronic lymphocytic leukaemia with subsequent development of multiple myeloma. Evidence of two B-lymphocyte clones and of myeloma-induced suppression of secretion of an M-component and of normal immunoglobulins. *Scand J Haematol* 21:256, 1978.

453. Lai R, Arber DA, Brynes RK, Chan O, Chang KL: Untreated chronic lymphocytic leukemia concurrent with or followed by acute myelogenous leukemia or myelodysplastic syndrome. A report of five cases and review of the literature. *Amer J Clin Pathol* 111:373, 1999.

454. Coso D, Costello R, Cohen-Valensi R, et al: Acute myeloid leukemia and myelodysplasia in patients with chronic lymphocytic leukemia receiving fludarabine as initial therapy [letter]. *Ann Oncol* 10:362, 1999.

455. French Cooperative Group: Effects of chlorambucil and therapeutic decision in initial forms of chronic lymphocytic leukemia (stage A): results of a randomized clinical trial on 612 patients. The French Cooperative Group on Chronic Lymphocytic Leukemia. *Blood* 75:1414, 1990.

456. Richter MN: Generalized reticular cell sarcoma of lymph nodes associated with lymphatic leukemia. *Am J Pathol* 4:285, 1928.

457. Long JC, Aisenberg AC: Richter's syndrome. A terminal complication of chronic lymphocytic leukemia with distinct clinicopathologic features. *Am J Clin Pathol* 63:786, 1975.

458. Foon KA, Thiruvengadam R, Saven A, Bernstein ZP, Gale RP: Genetic relatedness of lymphoid malignancies. Transformation of chronic lymphocytic leukemia as a model. *Ann Intern Med* 119:63, 1993.

459. Cherepakhin V, Baird SM, Meisenholder GW, Kipps TJ: Common clonal origin of chronic lymphocytic leukemia and high-grade lymphoma of Richter's syndrome. *Blood* 82:3141, 1993.

460. Foucar K, Rydell RE: Richter's syndrome in chronic lymphocytic leukemia. *Cancer* 46:118, 1980.

461. Trump DL, Mann RB, Phelps R, Roberts H, Conley CL: Richter's syndrome: diffuse histiocytic lymphoma in patients with chronic lymphocytic leukemia. A report of five cases and review of the literature. *Am J Med* 68:539, 1980.

462. Harousseau JL, Flandrin G, Tricot G, Brouet JC, Seligmann M, Bernard J: Malignant lymphoma supervening in chronic lymphocytic leukemia and related disorders. Richter's syndrome: a study of 25 cases. *Cancer* 48:1302, 1981.

463. Milkowski DA, Worley BD, Morris MJ: Richter's transformation presenting as an obstructing endobronchial lesion. *Chest* 116:832, 1999.

464. Fitzgerald PH, McEwan CM, Hamer JW, Beard ME: Richter's syndrome with identification of marker chromosomes. *Cancer* 46:135, 1980.

465. Melo JV, Catovsky D, Galton DA: The relationship between chronic lymphocytic leukaemia and prolymphocytic leukaemia: I. Clinical and laboratory features of 300 patients and characterization of an intermediate group. *Br J Haematol* 63:377, 1986.

466. Melo JV, Catovsky D, Galton DA: The relationship between chronic lymphocytic leukaemia and prolymphocytic leukaemia: II. Patterns of evolution of 'prolymphocytoid' transformation. *Br J Haematol* 64:77, 1986.

467. Melo JV, Catovsky D, Gregory WM, Galton DA: The relationship between chronic lymphocytic leukaemia and prolymphocytic leukaemia:

IV. Analysis of survival and prognostic features. *Br J Haematol* 65:23, 1987.

468. Sadamori N, Han T, Minowada J, Bloom ML, Henderson ES, Sandberg AA: Possible specific chromosome change in prolymphocytic leukemia. *Blood* 62:729, 1983.

469. Ghani AM, Krause JR, Brody JP: Prolymphocytic transformation of chronic lymphocytic leukemia. A report of three cases and review of the literature. *Cancer* 57:75, 1986.

470. Zarrabi MH, Grunwald HW, Rosner F: Chronic lymphocytic leukemia terminating in acute leukemia. *Arch Intern Med* 137:1059, 1977.

471. Brouet JC, Preud'homme JL, Seligmann M, Bernard J: Blast cells with monoclonal surface immunoglobulin in two cases of acute blast crisis supervening on chronic lymphocytic leukaemia. *Br Med J* 4:23, 1973.

472. McPhedran P, Heath CWJ: Acute leukemia occurring during chronic lymphocytic leukemia. *Blood* 35:7, 1970.

473. Frenkel EP, Ligler FS, Graham MS, Hernandez JA, Kettman JRJ, Smith RG: Acute lymphocytic leukemic transformation of chronic lymphocytic leukemia: substantiation by flow cytometry. *Am J Hematol* 10:391, 1981.

474. Torelli UL, Torelli GM, Emilia G, et al: Simultaneously increased expression of the c-myc and mu chain genes in the acute blastic transformation of a chronic lymphocytic leukaemia. *Br J Haematol* 65:165, 1987.

475. Büchi G, Termine G, Zappalà C, Girotto M, Grosso E, Autino R: Spontaneous complete remission of CLL. Report of a case studied with monoclonal antibodies. *Acta Haematol* 70:198, 1983.

476. Bernard M, Drenou B, Pangault C, et al: Spontaneous phenotypic and molecular blood remission in a case of chronic lymphocytic leukaemia [letter]. *Br J Haematol* 107:213, 1999.

477. Mandelli F, De Rossi G, Mancini P, et al: Prognosis in chronic lymphocytic leukemia: a retrospective multicentric study from the GIMEMA group. *J Clin Oncol* 5:398, 1987.

478. Jaksic B, Vitale B, Hauptmann E, Planinc-Peraica A, Ostojic S, Kusec R: The roles of age and sex in the prognosis of chronic leukaemias. A study of 373 cases. *Br J Cancer* 64:345, 1991.

479. Mauro FR, Foa R, Giannarelli D, et al: Clinical characteristics and outcome of young chronic lymphocytic leukemia patients: a single institution study of 204 cases. *Blood* 94:448, 1999.

480. Molica S, Levato D, Dattilo A: Natural history of early chronic lymphocytic leukemia. A single institution study with emphasis on the impact of disease progression on overall survival. *Haematologica* 84:1094, 1999.

481. Catovsky D, Galetto J, Okos A, Galton DA, Wiltshaw E, Stathopoulos G: Prolymphocytic leukaemia of B and T-cell type. *Lancet* 2:232, 1973.

482. Katayama I, Aiba M, Pechet L, Sullivan JL, Roberts P, Humphreys RE: B-lineage prolymphocytic leukemia as a distinct clinicopathologic entity. *Am J Pathol* 99:399, 1980.

483. Pittman S, Catovsky D: Chromosome abnormalities in B-cell prolymphocytic leukemia: a study of nine cases. *Cancer Genet Cytogenet* 9:355, 1983.

484. Stone RM: Prolymphocytic leukemia. *Hematol Oncol Clin North Am* 4:457, 1990.

485. Solé F, Woessner S, Espinet B, et al: Cytogenetic abnormalities in three patients with B-cell prolymphocytic leukemia. *Cancer Genet Cytogenet* 103:43, 1998.

486. Adami F, Sancetta R, Trentin L, et al: The pediatric rhabdomyosarcoma translocation (2;13)(q35;q14) in B-prolymphocytic leukemia [letter]. *Leukemia* 7:1676, 1993.

487. Lens D, De Schouwer PJ, Hamoudi RA, et al: p53 abnormalities in B-cell prolymphocytic leukemia. *Blood* 89:2015, 1997.

488. De Angeli C, Cuneo A, Aguiari G, et al: 5' region and exon 7 mutations of the TP53 gene in two cases of B-cell prolymphocytic leukemia. *Cancer Genet Cytogenet* 107:137, 1998.

489. Lens D, Coignet LJ, Brito-Babapulle V, et al: B cell prolymphocytic leukaemia (B-PLL) with complex karyotype and concurrent abnormalities of the p53 and c-MYC gene. *Leukemia* 13:873, 1999.

490. Shokri F, Mageed RA, Richardson P, Jefferis R: Immunophenotypic and idiotypic characterisation of the leukaemic B-cells from patients with prolymphocytic leukaemia: evidence for a selective expression of immunoglobulin variable region (IgV) gene products. *Leuk Res* 17:669, 1993.

491. Davi F, Maloum K, Michel A, et al: High frequency of somatic mutations in the V$_H$ genes expressed in prolymphocytic leukemia. *Blood* 88:3953, 1996.

492. Hoffman MA, Valderrama E, Fuchs A, Friedman M, Rai K: Leukemic meningitis in B-cell prolymphocytic leukemia. A clinical, pathologic, and ultrastructural case study and a review of the literature. *Cancer* 75:1100, 1995.

493. Pastor E, Grau E, Real E: Leukemic meningitis in a patient with B-cell prolymphocytic leukemia [letter]. *Haematologica* 82:511, 1997.

494. Andrieu V, Encaoua R, Carbon C, Couvelard A, Grange MJ: Leukemic pleural effusion in B-cell prolymphocytic leukemia. *Hematol Cell Ther* 40:275, 1998.

495. Shimoni A, Shvidel L, Shtalrid M, Klepfish A, Berrebi A: Prolymphocytic transformation of B-chronic lymphocytic leukemia presenting as malignant ascites and pleural effusion [letter]. *Am J Hematol* 59:316, 1998.

496. Dietrich PY, Pedraza E, Casiraghi O, Bayle C, Hayat M, Pico JL: Cardiac arrest due to leucostasis in a case of prolymphocytic leukaemia. *Br J Haematol* 78:122, 1991.

497. Takenaka T, Nakamine H, Nishihara T, Tsuda T, Tsujimoto M, Maeda J: Prolymphocytic leukemia with IgM hypogammaglobulinemia. *Am J Clin Pathol* 80:237, 1983.

498. Caligaris-Cappio F, Janossy G: Surface markers in chronic lymphoid leukemias of B cell type. *Semin Hematol* 22:1, 1985.

499. Shividel L, Shtalrid M, Bassous L, Klepfish A, Vorst E, Berrebi A: B-cell prolymphocytic leukemia: a survey of 35 patients emphasizing heterogeneity, prognostic factors and evidence for a group with an indolent course. *Leuk Lymphoma* 33:169, 1999.

500. Lambertenghi-Deliliers G, Maiolo AT, Annaloro C, Pogliani E, Baldini L, Polli E: Complete remission in prolymphocytic leukemia with 4-demethoxydaunorubicin and arabinosyl cytosine. *Cancer* 54:199, 1984.

501. Swift JF, Wold HG, Gandara DR, Redmond J, George CB: Prolymphocytic leukemia. Serial responses to therapy. *Cancer* 54:978, 1984.

502. Barton K, Larson RA, O'Brien S, Ratain MJ: Rapid response of B-cell prolymphocytic leukemia to 2-chlorodeoxyadenosine [letter]. *J Clin Oncol* 10:1821, 1992.

503. Saven A, Lee T, Schlutz M, et al: Major activity of cladribine in patients with de novo B-cell prolymphocytic leukemia. *J Clin Oncol* 15:37, 1997.

504. Lorand-Metze I, Oliveira GB, Aranha FJ: Treatment of prolymphocytic leukemia with cladribine. *Ann Hematol* 76:85, 1998.

505. Kantarjian HM, Childs C, O'Brien S, et al: Efficacy of fludarabine, a new adenine nucleoside analogue, in patients with prolymphocytic leukemia and the prolymphocytoid variant of chronic lymphocytic leukemia. *Am J Med* 90:223, 1991.

506. Smith RE, Stoiber TR: Acute tumor lysis syndrome in prolymphocytic leukemia. *Am J Med* 88:547, 1990.

507. Cannon LM, Spilove L, Rhodes R, Garfinkel H, Pezzimenti J: Acute tumor lysis syndrome complicating fludarabine treatment of prolymphocytic leukemia. *Conn Med* 57:651, 1993.

508. Döhner H, Ho AD, Thaler J, et al: Pentostatin in prolymphocytic leukemia: phase II trial of the European Organization for Research and Treatment of Cancer Leukemia Cooperative Study Group. *J Natl Cancer Inst* 85:658, 1993.

509. Dearden C, Matutes E, Catovsky D: Deoxycoformycin in the treatment of mature T-cell leukaemias. *Br J Cancer* 64:903, 1991.

510. Muncunill J, Villa S, Domingo A, Domenech P, Arnaiz MD, Callis M: Splenic irradiation as primary therapy for prolymphocytic leukaemia. *Br J Haematol* 76:305, 1990.

511. Yamamoto K, Hamaguchi H, Nagata K, Shibuya H, Takeuchi H: Splenic irradiation for prolymphocytic leukemia: is it preferable as an initial treatment or not? *Jpn J Clin Oncol* 28:267, 1998.

512. Singh AK, Bates T, Wetherley-Mein G: A preliminary study of low-dose splenic irradiation for the treatment of chronic lymphocytic and prolymphocytic leukaemias. *Scand J Haematol* 37:50, 1986.

513. Terashima T, Ohtake K, Ogawa T: Prolymphocytic leukemia treated with natural and recombinant alpha-interferon. *Am J Hematol* 35:56, 1990.

514. Delannoy A, Balligand JL, Ledant T: Interferon and B-cell prolymphocytic leukaemia [letter]. *Br J Haematol* 66:579, 1987.

515. Jacobs P, le Roux I, Wood L, Bolding E: Interferon response in B-cell prolymphocytic leukemia [letter]. *Br J Haematol* 65:375, 1987.

516. Vivaldi P, Garuti R, Rubertelli M, Mazzon C: Prolymphocytic leukemia: a very satisfactory response to treatment with recombinant interferon alpha. *Haematologica* 77:169, 1992.

517. Blecher TE: ''Spontaneous'' complete remission in a case of prolymphocytic leukemia [letter]. *Br J Haematol* 63:395, 1986.

518. Bennett JM, Catovsky D, Daniel MT, et al: Proposals for the classsifica-

tion of chronic (mature) B and T lymphoid leukaemias. French-American-British (FAB) Cooperative Group. *J Clin Pathol* 42:567, 1989.

519. Matutes E, Brito-Babapulle V, Swansbury J, et al: Clinical and laboratory features of 78 cases of T-prolymphocytic leukemia. *Blood* 78:3269, 1991.

520. Matutes E, Catovsky D: CLL should be used only for the disease with B-cell phenotype [letter]. *Leukemia* 7:917, 1993.

521. Foon KA, Gale RP: Is there a T-cell form of chronic lymphocytic leukemia? [editorial]. *Leukemia* 6:867, 1992.

522. Hoyer JD, Ross CW, Li CY, et al: True T-cell chronic lymphocytic leukemia: a morphologic and immunophenotypic study of 25 cases. *Blood* 86:1163, 1995.

523. Pileri SA, Milani M, Fraternali-Orcioni G, Sabattini E: From the R.E.A.L. Classification to the upcoming WHO scheme: a step toward universal categorization of lymphoma entities? *Ann Oncol* 9:607, 1998.

524. Harris NL, Jaffe ES, Stein H, et al: A revised European-American classification of lymphoid neoplasms: a proposal from the International Lymphoma Study Group [see comments]. *Blood* 84:1361, 1994.

525. Ascani S, Leoni P, Fraternali Orcioni G, et al: T-cell prolymphocytic leukaemia: does the expression of CD8+ phenotype justify the identification of a new subtype? Description of two cases and review of the literature. *Ann Oncol* 10:649, 1999.

526. Kojima K, Sawada T, Yasukawa M, et al: Deleted HTLV provirus in peripheral blood cells of a patient with T-cell prolymphocytic leukaemia. *Br J Haematol* 100:567, 1998.

527. Pawson R, Schulz TF, Matutes E, Catovsky D: The human T-cell lymphotropic viruses types I/II are not involved in T prolymphocytic leukemia and large granular lymphocytic leukemia. *Leukemia* 11:1305, 1997.

528. Kojima K, Sawada T, Ikezoe T, et al: Defective human T-lymphotrophic virus type I provirus in T-cell prolymphocytic leukemia. *Br J Haematol* 105:376, 1999.

529. Maljaei SH, Brito-Babapulle V, Hiorns LR, Catovsky D: Abnormalities of chromosomes 8, 11, 14, and X in T-prolymphocytic leukemia studied by fluorescence in situ hybridization. *Cancer Genet Cytogenet* 103:110, 1998.

530. Salomon-Nguyen F, Brizard F, Le Coniat M, Radford I, Berger R, Brizard A: Abnormalities of the short arm of chromosome 12 in T-cell prolymphocytic leukemia. *Leukemia* 12:972, 1998.

531. Kojima K, Kobayashi H, Imoto S, et al: 14q11 abnormality and trisomy 8q are not common in Japanese T-cell prolymphocytic leukemia. *Int J Hematol* 68:291, 1998.

532. Stilgenbauer S, Schaffner C, Litterst A, et al: Biallelic mutations in the ATM gene in T-prolymphocytic leukemia. *Nat Med* 3:1155, 1997.

533. Yuille MA, Coignet LJ, Abraham SM, et al: ATM is usually rearranged in T-cell prolymphocytic leukaemia [published erratum appears in *Oncogene* 1998 Jun 4;16:2955]. *Oncogene* 16:789, 1998.

534. Stoppa-Lyonnet D, Soulier J, Laugé A, et al: Inactivation of the ATM gene in T-cell prolymphocytic leukemias. *Blood* 91:3920, 1998.

535. Luo L, Lu FM, Hart S, et al: Ataxia-telangiectasia and T-cell leukemias: no evidence for somatic ATM mutation in sporadic T-ALL or for hypermethylation of the ATM-NPAT/E14 bidirectional promoter in T-PLL [published erratum appears in *Cancer Res* 1998 Aug 1;58:3488]. *Cancer Res* 58:2293, 1998.

536. Madani A, Choukroun V, Soulier J, et al: Expression of p13MTCP1 is restricted to mature T-cell proliferations with t(X;14) translocations. *Blood* 87:1923, 1996.

537. Thick J, Metcalfe JA, Mak YF, et al: Expression of either the TCL1 oncogene, or transcripts from its homologue MTCP1/c6.1B, in leukaemic and non-leukaemic T-cells from ataxia telangiectasia patients. *Oncogene* 12:379, 1996.

538. Gritti C, Choukroun V, Soulier J, et al: Alternative origin of p13MTCP1-encoding transcripts in mature T-cell proliferations with t(X;14) translocations. *Oncogene* 15:1329, 1997.

539. Hoh F, Yang YS, Guignard L, et al: Crystal structure of p14TCL1, an oncogene product involved in T-cell prolymphocytic leukemia, reveals a novel beta-barrel topology. *Structure* 6:147, 1998.

540. Gritti C, Dastot H, Soulier J, et al: Transgenic mice for MTCP1 develop T-cell prolymphocytic leukemia. *Blood* 92:368, 1998.

541. Matutes E, Catovsky D: Similarities between T-cell chronic lymphocytic leukemia and the small-cell variant of T-prolymphocytic leukemia [letter]. *Blood* 87:3520, 1996.

542. Mallett RB, Matutes E, Catovsky D, Maclennan K, Mortimer PS, Holden CA: Cutaneous infiltration in T-cell proplymphocytic leukaemia. *Br J Dermatol* 132:263, 1995.

543. Serra A, Estrach MT, Martí R, Villamor N, Rafel M, Montserrat E: Cutaneous involvement as the first manifestation in a case of T-cell prolymphocytic leukaemia. *Acta Derm Venereol* 78:198, 1998.

544. Catovsky D, Wechsler A, Matutes E, et al: The membrane phenotype of T-prolymphocytic leukaemia. *Scand J Haematol* 29:398, 1982.

545. Hui PK, Feller AC, Pileri S, Gobbi M, Lennert K: New aggressive variant of suppressor/cytotoxic T-CLL. Am *J Clin Pathol* 87:55, 1987.

546. Kluin-Nelemans HC, Gmelig-Meyling FH, Kootte AM, et al: T-cell prolymphocytic leukemia with an unusual phenotype CD4+ CD8+. *Cancer* 60:794, 1987.

547. Brito-Babapulle V, Maljaie SH, Matutes E, Hedges M, Yuille M, Catovsky D: Relationship of T leukaemias with cerebriform nuclei to T-prolymphocytic leukaemia: a cytogenetic analysis with in situ hybridization. *Br J Haematol* 96:724, 1997.

548. Pawson R, Matutes E, Brito-Babapulle V, et al: Sezary cell leukaemia: a distinct T-cell disorder or a variant form of T prolymphocytic leukaemia? *Leukemia* 11:1009, 1997.

549. Matutes E, Brito-Babapulle V, Swansbury J, et al: Clinical and laboratory features of 78 cases of T-prolymphocytic leukaemia. *Blood* 78:3269, 1991.

550. Palomera L, Domingo JM, Agulló JA, Soledad Romero M: Complete remission in T-cell prolymphocytic leukemia with 2-chlorodeoxyadenosine [letter]. *J Clin Oncol* 13:1284, 1995.

551. Uike N, Choi I, Tokoro A, et al: Adult T-cell leukemia-lymphoma successfully treated with 2-chlorodeoxyadenosine. *Intern Med* 37:411, 1998.

552. Zackheim HS: Cutaneous T-cell lymphoma: update of treatment. *Dermatology* 199:102, 1999.

553. Pawson R, Dyer MJ, Barge R, et al: Treatment of T-cell prolymphocytic leukemia with human CD52 antibody. *J Clin Oncol* 15:2667, 1997.

554. Dyer MJ: The role of CAMPATH-1 antibodies in the treatment of lymphoid malignancies. *Semin Oncol* 26:52, 1999.

555. Collins RH, Piñeiro LA, Agura ED, Fay JW: Treatment of T prolymphocytic leukemia with allogeneic bone marrow transplantation. *Bone Marrow Transplant* 21:627, 1998.

556. Tsai LM, Tsai CC, Hyde TP, Thomas LA, Broun GOJ: T-cell prolymphocytic leukemia with helper-cell phenotype and a review of the literature. *Cancer* 54:463, 1984.

557. Pawson R, Richardson DS, Pagliuca A, et al: Adult T-cell leukemia/lymphoma in London: clinical experience of 21 cases. *Leuk Lymphoma* 31:177, 1998.

558. López-Guillermo A, Cid J, Salar A, et al: Peripheral T-cell lymphomas: initial features, natural history, and prognostic factors in a series of 174 patients diagnosed according to the R.E.A.L. Classification. *Ann Oncol* 9:849, 1998.

559. Garand R, Goasguen J, Brizard A, et al: Indolent course as a relatively frequent presentation in T-prolymphocytic leukaemia. Groupe Français d'Hématologie Cellulaire. *Br J Haematol* 103:488, 1998.

HAIRY-CELL LEUKEMIA

ALAN SAVEN

Hairy-cell leukemia is a rare chronic lymphoproliferative disorder of B-lymphocytes that display prominent cytoplasmic projections and that infiltrate the marrow and spleen in a characteristic way. Afflicted individuals are often middle-aged males who present with pancytopenia, splenomegaly, or recurrent serious infections. Treatment with cladribine has greatly improved the prognosis for patients with this disorder.

DEFINITION AND HISTORY

Hairy-cell leukemia is a B-lymphocyte neoplasm that principally involves the marrow and spleen. Reactive marrow fibrosis and blood cytopenias are frequent features. It was first recognized in 1923 by Ewald, who described the condition as *leukämische reticuloendotheliose*.[1] In 1958, Bouroncle recognized the disorder to be a distinct clinicopathologic entity and referred to it as leukemic reticuloendotheliosis.[2] The descriptive term *hairy-cell leukemia* was coined by Schrek and Donnelly in 1966 to emphasize the irregular cytoplasmic projections of the abnormal mononuclear cells seen in the blood or marrow.[3] Until the mid-1980s, the principal treatment modality for this disease was splenectomy, which resulted in transiently improved blood counts. During the past decade, the successful introduction of three effective systemic therapies—interferon-α, pentostatin (2'-deoxycoformycin), and cladribine (2-chlorodeoxyadenosine—has dramatically improved the prognosis of patients with this disease.

ETIOLOGY AND PATHOGENESIS

With 600 new patients being diagnosed annually, the disease hairy-cell leukemia accounts for approximately 2 percent of all adult leukemias in the United States. The disease is very rare in persons of African or Asian descent. It is predominantly a disease of middle-aged males, with a median age at presentation of 52 years. The disease has not been described in children or teenagers. There is a 4:1 male predominance, with Ashkenazi Jewish males being more frequently affected. Familial cases have been described.[4,5] The possible association of human T-cell leukemia virus II (HTLV-II) infection with a rare T-cell hairy-cell leukemia variant has been disputed by some investigators.[6] Prior exposure to radiation and organic solvents is more frequent among hairy-cell leukemia patients than among healthy persons.[7,8] A possible etiologic role of the Epstein-Barr virus has been suggested in the development of the disease hairy-cell leukemia,[9] but this has been disputed by other investigators.[10] When cytogenetic analyses were performed in 30 patients with hairy-cell leukemia, chromosome 5 was involved in clonal aberrations in 12 (40 percent) patients, most

commonly as trisomy 5 or pericentric inversions and interstitial deletions involving band 5q13.[11]

The normal function and precise site of origin in lymphocytic ontogeny of the hairy cell remains elusive, although it is generally accepted that hairy cells represent clonal expansions of mature B cells with phenotypic features of activation.[12] Hairy cells have clonal immunoglobulin gene rearrangements[13] and express the pan B-cell surface differentiation antigens CD19, CD20, and CD22, as well as monoclonal surface immunoglobulin.[14] These immunologic markers of B-cell differentiation indicate an intermediate level of maturity of the hairy cell. Thus, cell surface markers normally lost in the terminal stages of B-cell maturation and CD20 are present on hairy cells, while early cell surface markers, such as CD10, are absent. Hairy cells express the early plasma cell marker PCA-1, consistent with the notion that they represent a cell at a stage of B-cell development analagous to a pre-plasma cell.[15]

Hairy cells secrete cytokines, such as tumor necrosis factor α. The cytokines produced by hairy cells may contribute to the impaired hematopoiesis seen in this disease by reducing the number of erythroid colony-forming units (CFU-E).[16] Macrophage colony-stimulating factor (M-CSF) induces hairy-cell motility,[17] and specific integrin receptors, $\alpha v_{\beta 3}$, have been identified that are responsible for their motile behavior.[18]

CLINICAL FEATURES

Patients with hairy-cell leukemia generally have the diagnostic triad of pancytopenia, splenomegaly, and circulating hairy cells. Pancytopenia occurs in 50 percent of the patients, and the remaining half usually have a combination of cytopenias. In a series of 102 patients with hairy-cell leukemia, 86 had anemia, 84 thrombocytopenia, and 78 neutropenia at the time of diagnosis.[19] On initial presentation, one-quarter of patients present with fatigue and weakness, and another quarter with easy bruising from thrombocytopenia or with opportunistic infections from leukopenia. An additional 25 percent have early satiety or abdominal fullness from splenomegaly. The remaining patients present with an incidental finding of splenomegaly or abnormal blood counts on examination for an unrelated condition.[20,21]

Splenomegaly, which may be massive, is found in 90 percent of patients.[22,23] Hepatomegaly is rarely a significant finding. Palpable lymphadenopathy is distinctly uncommon and when found is usually localized. However, with the advent of computed tomography scans, significant internal adenopathy can be demonstrated in up to one-third of patients with hairy-cell leukemia.[24,25] In 3 percent of patients, the disease manifests itself as painful bony lesions, most commonly involving the proximal femur. Patients with skeletal complications tend to have higher tumor burdens, with their marrow being more diffusely infiltrated by hairy-cell leukemia. Diffuse osteoporosis, as well as focal or diffuse osteosclerosis, may occur. Lytic lesions, primarily involving the skeleton, have been reported.[26]

At diagnosis, up to 30 percent of hairy-cell leukemia patients will have an absolute blood neutrophil count of less than 0.5×10^9/liter. Most patients will demonstrate monocytopenia.[27] These cytopenias predispose patients to infection from a wide variety of typical and opportunistic organisms. Impaired interferon production by blood mononuclear cells in hairy-cell leukemia also may enchance the risk for intracellular infections.[28] Organisms encountered in febrile hairy-cell leukemia patients include *Mycobacterium kansasii* (accounting for 5–10 percent of mycobacterial disease in this population), *Pneumocystis carinii*, aspergillus, histoplasma, cryptococcus, and *Toxoplasma gondii*.[29] During the follow-up of 137 patients with hairy-cell leukemia, 47 had culture-proved infections, 48 had clinically significant infectious episodes without positive cultures, and 48 had no infectious complications.[30] Other laboratory abnormalities include liver function

Acronyms and abbreviations that appear in this chapter include: CFU-E, erythroid colony-forming units; G-CSF, granulocyte colony-stimulating factor; IL-2, interleukin-2; HML-1, human mucosal lymphocyte 1; HTLV-II, human T-cell leukemia virus II; M-CSF, macrophage colony-stimulating; TRAP, tartrate-resistant acid phosphatase.

test abnormalities in 19 percent, azotemia in 27 percent, and hyperglobulinemia in 18 percent, which may be monoclonal.[31] Hypogammaglobulinemia, unlike chronic lymphocytic leukemia, is rare. These paraproteinemias may, in part, contribute to some of the unusual manifestations experienced by some patients with hairy-cell leukemia, including cutaneous vasculitis, leukocytoclastic angiitis, erythema nodosum, and Raynaud's phenomenon.[31] Hypocholesterolemia, mainly due to a low concentration of low-density lipoprotein cholesterol, is a frequent finding in advanced hairy-cell leukemia but is resolved after successful treatment.[32,33]

In a series of 116 patients with hairy-cell leukemia followed for over two decades, several unusual presentations and complications were encountered, including spontaneous rupture of the spleen; massive splenomegaly from hairy-cell infiltration, with normal blood counts; spinal cord compression with paralysis; protein-losing enteropathy from infiltration of the bowel by hairy cells; and esophageal perforation with a fistulous tract.[34] In rare cases, hairy-cell leukemia patients may have serous or chylous ascites, or pleural or pericardial effusions.[35] The disease can involve soft tissues and has been implicated as a cause of uveitis in one case report.[36]

LABORATORY FEATURES

BLOOD

Hairy cells are mononuclear cells with eccentric or central nuclei.[37] Nuclear morphology is variable, being round, ovoid, reniform, or convoluted. Nuclear forms tend to have a reticular chromatin pattern. Hairy cells have variable amounts of cytoplasm. This typically is blue-gray in appearance, exhibiting thin cytoplasmic projections (Fig. 99-1). Rarely, granules or broad-shaped inclusions can be seen in the cytoplasm, which correspond to the ribosomal lamellar complex seen on electron microscopy.[38] More than 80 percent of patients have absolute neutropenia and monocytopenia.[37,39-41]

MARROW

The hairy cells in the marrow aspirate tend to have a slightly coarser reticular chromatin-staining pattern than those found in the blood. The marrow usually contains hairy-cell infiltrates, which in some patients may be patchy or difficult to discern. Marrow involvement may be diffuse or focal. The marrow may be hypocellular, with scant infiltra

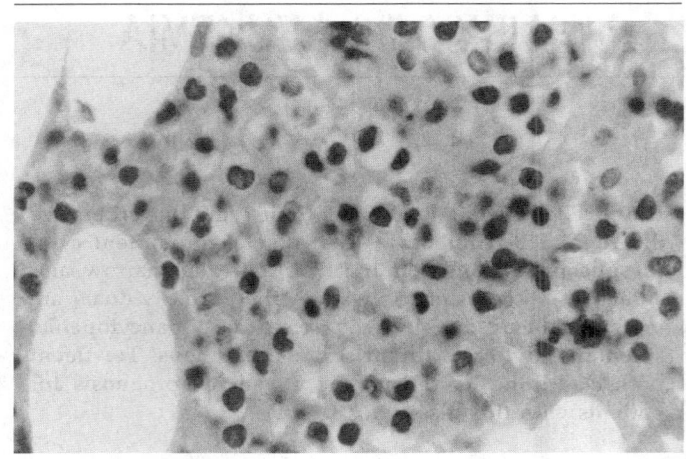

FIGURE 99-2   Marrow biopsy. Diffuse infiltration by hairy cells with wide spaces between nuclei, a pattern often called "fried-egg" appearance (×2000).

tion by hairy cells admixed with residual hematopoietic tissue.[37,39] Hairy cells have monotonous round, oval, or spindle-spaced nuclei that are separated by abundant quantities of pale-staining cytoplasm in a fine fibrillar network. This separation of individual hairy-cell nuclei is characteristic and referred to as the ''fried-egg'' appearance (Fig. 99-2). Because of marked marrow reticulin fibrosis, the marrow is frequently difficult or impossible to aspirate (Fig. 99-3). Fibroblast infiltration and overt collagen fibrosis are generally absent. It has been shown that hairy cells can synthesize and assemble a fibronectin matrix that likely is responsible for the marrow fibrosis characteristic of the disease.[42] The pale and delicate network of fibrils is usually recognizable but is often better appreciated with the periodic acid-Schiff stain. Occasionally, the marrow has dilated sinuses with extravasated erythrocytes, similar to the red blood cell lakes that are seen in the spleen.

SPLEEN AND OTHER SITES

The spleen is usually enlarged, with a median weight of 1300 g.[43] On section, the spleen has a dark-red, smooth surface. On light microscopy, the hairy cells involve the splenic red pulp. Later, the white pulp atrophies and is replaced. Red cell lakes are characteristic; these lakes

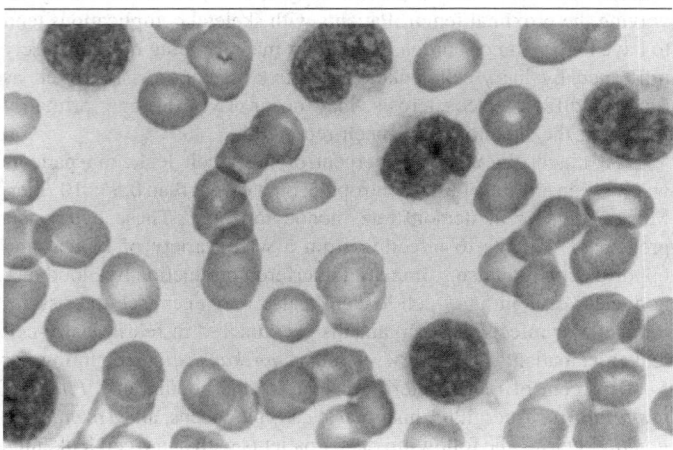

FIGURE 99-1   Blood fetus. The hairy cells are small to medium in size, have ovoid or reniform nuclei with finely clumped chromatin, and demonstrate abundant, frayed cytoplasm (×1500).

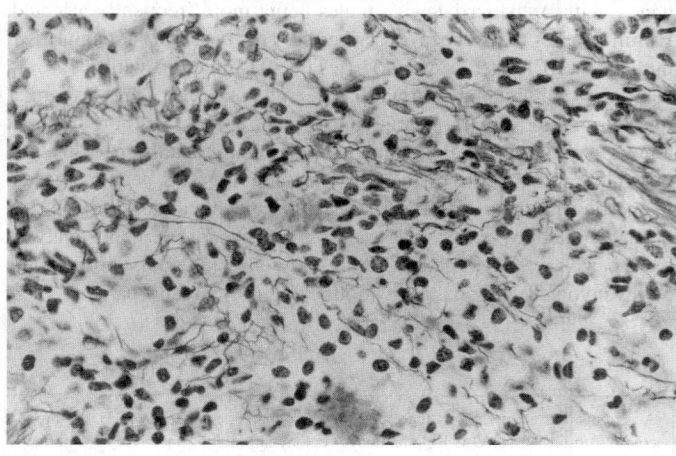

FIGURE 99-3   Marrow biopsy showing marked increase in reticulin fibrils in patients with hairy-cell leukemia (×2500).

are blood-filled spaces lined by hairy cells that have disrupted the normal sinus architecture.[44] These blood-filled spaces are sometimes referred to as pseudosinuses.

Hepatic infiltration is both sinusoidal and portal.[44] Lymph node involvement is marked by both sinusoidal and interstitial involvement.[45] Bony infiltration can progress from the medullary cavity to the cortex, resulting in osteolytic lesions.[46]

CYTOCHEMISTRY

The hairy-cell cytoplasm usually stains strongly for tartrate-resistant acid phosphatase (TRAP). Isoenzyme 5 acid phosphatase, present in the hairy-cell cytoplasm, resists decolorization by tartrate.[47,48] A TRAP stain that involves at least two cells with more than 40 granules or with numerous granules obscuring the nucleus is usually diagnostic. TRAP staining of the fetus of the buffy coat is positive in 90 percent of cases.[47] Normal neutrophils and platelets also contain acid phosphatases but are not resistant to decolorization by tartrate. Weak to moderate TRAP staining may occur in other diseases, including prolymphocytic leukemia and lymphoma.[49]

ELECTRON MICROSCOPY

Hairy cells in hairy-cell leukemia have circumferential cytoplasmic projections. Hairy cells have a few blunt microvilli. The cells of patients with splenic lymphoma with circulating B lymphocytes have more numerous and finer projections that are polarized at one end of the cell (Fig. 99-4).[50–52] Ribosomal lamella complexes can be found in the cytoplasm of hairy cells by transmission electron microscopy in 50 percent of patients.[47] This cytoplasmic inclusion is a cylindrical structure composed of a central hollow space and an outer sheath of multiple parallel lamellae, with ribosomal-like granules in the interlamellar space.[53] These complexes also have been described in other lymphoproliferative disorders.[54]

IMMUNOPHENOTYPE

Hairy cells express the pan B-cell antigens CD19, CD20, and CD22 but not CD21.[13,55,56] Hairy cells have a pattern of surface marker expression that distinguishes them from the neoplastic cells of other lymphoproliferative disorders.[57] Most distinctively, hairy cells express high levels of the CD11c, CD22, CD25, and CD103 surface antigens.[58] The CD11c antigen, the 150-kD α chain of the 150/95 β_2-integrin that ordinarily is expressed on monocytes and neutrophils,[58,59] is expressed at levels 30-fold higher than those in chronic lymphocytic leukemia.[60]

Hairy-cell leukemia was the first B-cell lymphoproliferative disorder identified that expressed CD25, the α chain of the interleukin-2 (IL-2) receptor.[61] Serum levels of soluble IL-2 receptor are elevated in hairy-cell leukemia patients and correlate with disease activity following treatment.[62] CD103 (Bly-7) has the greatest sensitivity and specificity for hairy-cell leukemia.[62] CD103 is the α^E subunit of the $\alpha^E\beta_7$-integrin, known as the human mucosal lymphocyte 1 (HML-1) antigen because HML-1 is primarily expressed by intraepithelial T lymphocytes. This integin is thought to be involved with the process of lymphocyte homing and adhesion.[63–65]

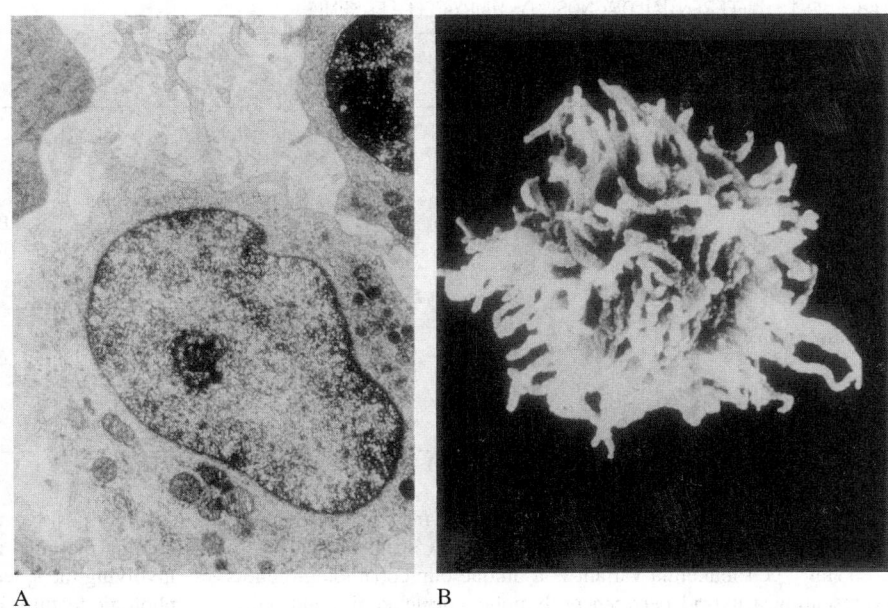

A   B

FIGURE 99-4   (A) Scanning and (B) transmission electron micrographs of blood hairy cells showing the characteristic circumferential, villiform cytoplasmic projections ($\times 7000$).

CD22 also is expressed more intensely on hairy cells than in other B-cell chronic lymphoproliferative disorders. For example, hairy cells express CD22 at 50-fold higher levels than in chronic lymphocytic leukemia.[57] In 26 percent of cases there is weak expression of CD10 (the CALLA antigen), and in 5 percent of cases there is weak expression of CD5.

Multiparameter immunofluorescence analysis is especially useful in identifying hairy cells because it permits identification of cells coexpressing CD11c, CD25, or CD103 antigens, together with a pan B-cell antigen, such as CD19, CD20, or CD22. Using peripheral blood flow cytometry, 92 percent of 161 patients with hairy-cell leukemia had identifiable circulating hairy cells, in some patients representing less than 1 percent of lymphocytes.[57] In contrast, a thorough morphologic evaluation of the blood from these same patients revealed hairy cells in only 80 percent.

IMMUNOHISTOCHEMISTRY

Immunohistochemistry performed on marrow biopsy samples can aid in the diagnosis of hairy-cell leukemia and is useful for the detection of minimal residual disease following systemic therapies. Most monoclonal antibodies used to detect circulating hairy cells in the blood, including anti-CD103 antibodies, require that the marrow be processed by frozen section, since these antigens are destroyed by fixation and standard processing.[67] In contrast, the CD20 antibody (L26) and another monoclonal antibody (DBA.44) can be used to stain hairy cells in routinely processed paraffin sections of the marrow.[68–70] L26 staining is membranous and accentuates the ruffled, abundant cytoplasm of hairy cells, while DBA.44, an undefined antigen, stains in both a cytoplasmic granular and membranous pattern. DBA.44 is not specific for hairy-cell leukemia, since 30 percent of low-grade lymphomas also stain positively with this antibody.

DIFFERENTIAL DIAGNOSIS

The development of highly effective systemic therapy for hairy-cell leukemia makes distinguishing it from other lymphoproliferative disorders imperative (Table 99-1).

TABLE 99-1　DIFFERENTIAL DIAGNOSIS OF HAIRY-CELL LEUKEMIA

MARGINAL PARAMETERS	HAIRY-CELL LEUKEMIA VARIANT	VILLOUS LYMPHOCYTES	SPLENIC lYMPHOMA WITH ZONE LYMPHOMA	MONOCYTOID B-CELL LYMPHOMA/
Peripheral blood				
Morphology				
Nuclear shape	Ovoid, reniform	Round	Round	Irregular
Chromatin	Reticular ± nucleolus	Coarse with central nucleolus	Coarse ± nucleolus	Coarse
Cytoplasm	Blue-gray, abundant	Blue-gray, abundant	Basophilic, scant to moderate	Pale, abundant
Monocytopenia	+	−	−	−
TRAP stain	+++	±	±	±
Aspirable bone marrow	−	+	+	+
Splenic involvement	Red pulp	Red pulp	White pulp	White pulp
Flow cytometry				
CD22	+++	++	++	++
CD11c	+++	++	+	±
CD25	++	−	±	±
CD103	++	±	−	−

Myelofibrosis usually can be distinguished from hairy-cell leukemia by careful review of the blood and marrow specimens.

Hairy-cell leukemia variant is a unique clinicopathologic entity representing a hybrid between prolymphocytic leukemia and hairy-cell leukemia; the nucleus most closely resembles a prolymphocyte and the cytoplasm a hairy cell.[71] Hairy-cell variant cells generally have higher nuclear-to-cytoplasmic ratios, more highly condensed chromatin, and more conspicuous central nucleoli than do the neoplastic cells of patients with classic hairy-cell leukemia.[72] Afflicted individuals present with massive splenomegaly and are frequently in a leukemia phase. TRAP staining of hairy-cell variant cells is either negative or only weakly positive. Unlike classical hairy cells, the cells in the variant disease are usually CD25- and CD103-negative. Distinction of hairy-cell leukemia is based on nuclear morphology, the leukemia presentation, the lack of monocytopenia, the aspirable marrow, and the morphologic appearance of the cells seen in the marrow biopsy. Also, on electron microscopy, hairy-cell leukemia variant cells mostly lack ribosomal-lamellar complexes. There is also a blastic variant of hairy-cell leukemia, in which the patients have massive splenomegaly, peripheral adenopathy, and cytopenias.[73] These cells stain positively with TRAP and do not express myeloperoxidase. More recently, a new entity, called hairy B-cell lymphoproliferative disorder, has been described in Japan.[74] Patients with this disease have splenomegaly without lymphadenopathy and have a persistent lymphocytosis consisting of abnormal lymphocytes with long microvilli. The circulating lymphocytes are polyclonal B cells that are CD25-negative and only weakly TRAP positive.

Splenic lymphoma with circulating villous lymphocytes is a closely related disorder that can be difficult to distinguish from hairy-cell leukemia. Patients with splenic lymphoma with circulating villous lymphocytes also can have massive splenomegaly without lymphadenopathy. However, unlike hairy-cell leukemia, lymphocytosis is common.[75] In this disorder, the lymphocytes have more basophilic cytoplasm, and the cytoplasmic projections tend to be polar and more subtle.[76] Circulating plasmacytoid cells are frequently noted.[51] TRAP staining is either negative or very weakly positive.[47,77] The cells express high levels of CD11c but are frequently CD103 negative. Peripheral monocytopenia is usually absent. Sections of spleen show predominantly white pulp involvement resembling that of low-grade lymphoma.[75]

B-cell prolymphocytic leukemia is often confused with the prolymphocytic variant of hairy cell leukemia. Both disorders generally occur in elderly men with prominent splenomegaly. B-cell prolymphocytic leukemia lymphocytes are only focally TRAP-positive, whereas hairy cell leukemia classic and variant hairy cells are diffusely and strongly positive with TRAP staining. Other splenic lymphomas, including marginal zone lymphoma and monocytoid B-cell lymphoma involving the spleen, also need to be excluded.[79,80] Although the morphologic features of these two disorders may approximate hairy cells, they are generally TRAP stain negative.[81,82]

Hairy-cell leukemia also should be differentiated from mast cell disease, especially when the infiltrates are composed of spindle-shaped cells. Mast cells are shown to contain metachromatic granules on Giemsa staining. The granules also test positive for chloroacetate esterase.[83] On immunohistochemical analysis, the cells react with KPI (CDBP), a macrophage marker, but not L26 (CD20). Aged blood samples from patients with B-cell chronic lymphocytic leukemia may demonstrate artifactual cytoplasmic projections due to cytoplasmic distortion, but, unlike hairy cells, they are CD5 positive.[84] Leukocytosis in chronic lymphocytic leukemia is more pronounced, and monocytopenia is usually absent.

THERAPY, COURSE, AND PROGNOSIS

THERAPY

INDICATIONS FOR THERAPY
Ninety percent of patients with hairy-cell leukemia require treatment at presentation or sometime during the course of their disease. Standard hematologic parameters for initiating therapy include anemia (hemoglobin < 9 g/dl), thrombocytopenia (platelet count < 50–100 × 10^9/liter), or neutropenia (absolute neutrophil count < 0.5–1.0 × 10^9/liter), especially if associated with recurrent, serious infections. Other, less common indications for initiating treatment are symptomatic splenomegaly, leukocytosis with a high proportion of hairy cells (white blood cell count > 20 × 10^9/liter), bulky or painful lymphadenopathy, vasculitis, and bony involvement.

TREATMENTS OF HISTORICAL INTEREST
Splenectomy　Splenectomy was the first standard treatment modality employed in hairy-cell leukemia, since it rapidly reverses peripheral cytopenias. Ninety percent of patients will have improvement in at least one hematologic parameter, and 40 to 60 percent will have normalization of blood counts.[85,86] The present indications for splenectomy are active or uncontrolled infections, thrombocytopenic bleeding, massive painful and/or ruptured splenomegaly, and failure to respond to chemotherapy including a purine analog.

Chlorambucil　Chlorambucil at 2 to 4 mg orally daily for 6 to 9 months induces a consistent number of hematologic responses. The absolute neutrophil count, however, rarely improves with chlorambucil.[89] There are brief reports of the salutory effects of protracted androgen[90] and lithium administration in hairy-cell leukemia.[91] These treatments are rarely used today, given availability of more effective systemic treatments.

Irradiation   Lytic bone lesions, especially in the proximal femur, may be managed with low-dose irradiation, 1500 to 3000 Gy.[46,92]

Interferon   The standard dose recommendation for interferon-α_{2b} is 2 million units/m^2 administered subcutaneously three times per week for 12 months, and for interferon-α_{2a} is 3 million units/m^2 subcutaneously given daily for 6 months and then decreased to three times per week for an additional 6 months.

The commonest side effect of interferon is a flulike syndrome consisting of fever, myalgias, and malaise. Acetaminophen often ameliorates these symptoms, and tachyphylaxis frequently develops over time. There is an unexpectedly high incidence of second neoplasms in patients after treatment of hairy-cell leukemia with interferon-α_{2b}.[99] Of 69 patients followed for a median of 91 months, 13 patients (19 percent) developed a second neoplasm; 6 were of hematopoietic origin, and 7 were adenocarcinomas. The median survival after diagnosis of the second neoplasm was only 9 months.

While interferon-α is an active agent in hairy-cell leukemia, it does not induce the same high complete response rates seen with the purine nucleoside analogs. Accordingly, it is likely that the use of interferon-α in the treatment of hairy-cell leukemia will be reserved for those patients with active infections and therefore unable to undergo purine nucleoside analog therapy, given their associated T-cell immunosuppression.[29,107] It also may be useful in patients who have failed prior systemic therapy with a purine nucleoside analog.[108]

PENTOSTATIN (2'-DEOXYCOFORMYCIN)

The response rates of several pentostatin clinical trials are summarized in Table 99-2. The standard dose of pentostatin for patients with hairy-cell leukemia is 4 mg/m^2 every other week for 3 to 6 months until maximum response is achieved.

Pentostatin-induced toxicities include fever, nausea, vomiting, photosensitivity, and keratoconjunctivitis.[118,119] Severe myelosuppression may occur soon after the initiation of pentostatin therapy, especially in those patients with preexisting marrow compromise.[114,120] Severe infections, including the disseminated herpes zoster, *Escherichia coli, Haemophilus influenzae* and pneumococcal and fungal infections were observed soon on after the initiation of pentostatin.[119] Pentostatin is best avoided in those patients with active and uncontrolled infections, a poor performance status, or impaired renal function.[113] Pentostatin is strongly immunosuppressive.[121] During pentostatin therapy and for at least 1 year thereafter, CD4 and CD8 lymphocytes may decrease to levels below 200 cells/μl. Low doses of pentostatin are also potently immunosuppressive.[29]

CLADRIBINE (2-CHLORODEOXYADENOSINE)

Cladribine is the treatment of choice for hairy-cell leukemia. In one large series, 91 percent of 349 patients achieved an initial complete response and 7 percent a partial response, with an overall median duration of response follow-up at 52 months. Response rates to cladribine were independent of prior therapy, including pentostatin. Twenty-six percent of the patients relapsed at a median of 29 months, and, of 53 patients treated with a second course of cladribine at first relapse, 62 percent achieved a complete response. In one study, there was a slight excess of second neoplasms in cladribine-treated patients; in another study there was no such excess.

Fever is the principal toxic effect of cladribine therapy in hairy-cell leukemia, occurring in 42 percent of patients treated. The fever is related to the disappearance of hairy cells and appears most marked in those patients with the greatest pretreatment hairy-cell leukemia

burden, manifested principally as splenomegaly. Documented infections unrelated to a peripherally inserted central catheter device used to deliver the cladribine are uncommon. Dermatomal herpes zoster is the most frequent late infection reported.[125] Like pentostatin, 2-chlorodeoxyadenosine (cladribine) is also immunosuppressive.[107] In one study, there was a tendency toward restoration of CD4 cells at 6 and 12 months,[130] while other studies have shown more profound and long-lasting CD4 lymphocytopenia.[131]

Although in the Scripps Clinic study the time–to–treatment failure rate for complete responders was 16.3 percent at 4 years, there was no obvious plateau on the time–to–treatment failure curve.[125] Thus, it is unclear what proportion of patients, if any, will be cured. Twenty-five to fifty percent of patients in morphologic complete remission after cladribine have minimal residual disease detected by immunohistochemical stains of marrow biopsies.[132,133] Using the polymerase chain reaction and clonogenic probes derived from the immunoglobulin heavy-chain genes, all seven patients in apparent complete remission following cladribine showed detectable minimal residual disease.[134]

Cladribine can induce long-lasting complete responses in the vast majority of patients following only a single 7-day infusion. The response rates to cladribine have been shown in several published chemical trials. Relapse rates for complete responders are low, and patients who relapse can be successfully retreated with cladribine. The recommended dose of cladribine is 0.1 mg/kg per day by continuous intravenous infusion for 7 days. The optimum route and method of administration for cladribine remain under investigation. The successful administration of subcutaneous cladribine has been reported,[135] as well as a weekly intravenous administration schema.[136] These methods of drug delivery remain to be tested in large numbers of patients, and longer follow-up is needed to determine whether these methods of drug administration are equivalent to the continuous intravenous infusion method.

FLUDARABINE

Fludarabine, although rigorously evaluated in patients with chronic lymphocytic leukemia,[137,138] has only been evaluated in small numbers of patients with hairy-cell leukemia (see Table 99-2). Although results have been less than dramatic than with other purine nucleoside analogs, some patients with a hariy-cell variant disease did achieve partial responses.[139–141]

SUPPORTIVE THERAPY

Granulocyte Colony-Stimulating Factor   G-CSF abrogates the early myelosuppressive effects of interferon[142] and reverses neutropenia in some hairy-cell leukemia patients. The role of G-CSF in the management of hairy-cell leukemia will likely be principally adjunctive to systemic therapy. It does have a role in the initial treatment of actively infected hairy-cell leukemia patients. Of four patients with hairy-cell leukemia treated with G-CSF at 1 to 6 μg/kg per day for 6 weeks, 3 patients had normalization of their absolute neutrophil count in 1 to 2 weeks.[142] A single patient with hairy-cell leukemia and a history of cutaneous vasculitis developed acute neutrophilic dermatosis (Sweet syndrome) following the administration of G-CSF.

COURSE AND PROGNOSIS

Ten percent of patients, usually elderly males with smaller-sized spleens, normal blood counts, and a lower hairy-cell burden, may be observed for protracted intervals, since they generally do not require treatment.[143] Prior to the successful application of interferon and purine nucleoside analogs in the treatment of hairy-cell leukemia, patients with hairy-cell leukemia had a median survival time of only 53 months.[143] Now, with purine nucleoside analog therapy, overall survival rates in excess of 95 percent at 4 years have been reported.[125] Regardless of the curative potential of purine nucleoside analog therapy, patients with hairy-cell leukemia can now anticipate long survival.

REFERENCES

1. Ewald O: Die leukämische reticuloendotheliose. *Dtsch Arch Klin Med* 142:222, 1923.
2. Bouroncle BA, Wiseman BK, Doan CA: Leukemic reticuloendotheliosis. *Blood* 13:609, 1958.
3. Schrek R, Donnelly J: Hairy cells in blood lymphoreticular neoplastic disease and "flagellated" cells of normal lymph nodes. *Blood* 27:199, 1966.
4. Wylis RF, Greene MH, Palretke M, et al: Hairy cell leukemia in three siblings: An apparent HLA-linked disease. *Cancer* 49:538, 1982.
5. Egli FL, Koller B, Furrer J: Hairy cell leukemia and glucose-6-phosphatase dehydrogenase deficiency in two brothers [letter]. *N Engl J Med* 322:1159, 1990.
6. Wachsman W, Golde DW, Chen IS: Hairy cell leukemia and human T cell leukemia virus. *Semin Oncol* 11:446, 1984.
7. Oleske D, Golomb HM, Farber MD, et al: A case-control inquiry into the etiology of hairy cell leukemia. *Am J Epidemiol* 121:675, 1985.
8. Stewart DJ, Keating MJ: Radiation exposure as a possible etiologic factor in hairy cell leukemia. *Cancer* 46:1577, 1980.
9. Wolf BC, Martin AW, Heiman RS, et al: The detection of Epstein-Barr virus in hairy cell leukemia cells by *in situ* hybridization. *Am J Pathol* 136:717, 1990.
10. Chang KL, Chen YY, Weiss LM: Lack of evidence of Epstein-Barr virus in hairy cell leukemia and monocytoid B-cell lymphoma. *Hum Pathol* 24:58, 1993.
11. Haglund U, Juliusson G, Stellan B, et al: Hairy cell leukemia is characterized by clonal chromosome abnormalities clustered to specific regions. *Blood* 83:2637, 1994.
12. Burthem J, Zuzel M, Cawley JC: What is the nature of the hairy cell and why should we be interested? [annotation]. *Br J Haematol* 97:511, 1997.
13. Korsmeyer SJ, Greene WC, Cossman J, et al: Rearrangement and expression of immunoglobulin genes and expression of Tac antigen in hairy cell leukemia. *Proc Natl Acad Sci USA* 80:4522, 1983.
14. Golomb HM, Davis S, Wilson C, et al: Surface immunoglobulins on hairy cells of 55 patients with hairy cell leukemia. *Am J Hematol* 12:397, 1982.
15. Anderson KC, Boyd AW, Fisher DC, et al: Hairy cell leukemia: A tumor of pre-plasma cells. *Blood* 65:620, 1985.
16. Lindemann A, Ludwig WD, Oster W, et al: High-level secretion of tumor necrosis factor-alpha contributes to hematopoietic failure in hairy cell leukemia. *Blood* 73:880, 1989.
17. Burthem J, Baker PK, Hunt JA, et al: The function of c-fms in hairy-cell leukemia: Macrophage colony-stimulating factor stimulates hairy-cell movement. *Blood* 83:1381, 1994.
18. Burthem J, Baker PK, Cawley JC: Hairy cell interactions with extracellular matrix: Expression of specific integrin receptors and their role in the cell's response to specific adhesive proteins. *Blood* 84:873, 1994.
19. Turner A, Kjeldsberg CR: Hairy cell leukemia: A review. *Medicine (Baltimore)* 57:477, 1978.
20. Flandrin G, Sigaux F, Sebahoun G, et al: Hairy cell leukemia: Clinical presentation and follow-up of 211 patients. *Semin Oncol* 11:458, 1984.
21. Catovsky D: Hairy cell leukemia and prolymphocytic leukemia. *Clin Haematol* 6:245, 1977.
22. Katayama I, Finkel HE: Leukemic reticuloendotheliosis: A clinicopathologic study with review of the literature. *Am J Med* 57:115, 1974.
23. Golomb HM: Hairy cell leukemia, an unusual lymphoproliferative disease: A study of 24 patients. *Cancer* 42:946, 1978.
24. Hakimian D, Tallman MS, Hogan DK, et al: Prospective evaluation of internal adenopathy in a cohort of 43 patients with hairy cell leukemia. *J Clin Oncol* 12:268, 1994.
25. Mercieca J, Matutes E, Moskovic E, et al: Massive abdominal lymphadenopathy in hairy cell leukaemia: A report of 12 cases. *Br J Haematol* 82:547, 1992.
26. Quesada JR, Keating MJ, Libshitz HI, et al: Bone involvement in hairy cell leukemia. *Am J Med* 74:228, 1983.
27. Goyette RE: Hairy cell leukemia, in *Hematology: A Comprehensive Guide to the Diagnosis and Treatment of Blood Disorders*, edited by RE Goyette, p 576. PMIC, Los Angeles, 1997.
28. Siegal FP, Shodell M, Shah K, et al: Impaired interferon alpha response in hairy cell leukemia is corrected by therapy with 2-chloro-2'-deoxyadenosine: Implications for susceptibility to opportunistic infections. *Leukemia* 8:1474, 1994.
29. Kraut EH, Neff JC, Bouroncle BA, et al: Immunosuppressive effects of pentostatin. *J Clin Oncol* 8:848, 1990.
30. Golomb HM, Hadad LJ: Infectious complications in 127 patients with hairy cell leukemia. *Am J Hematol* 16:393, 1984.
31. Dorsey JK, Penick GD: The association of hairy cell leukemia with unusual immunologic disorders. *Arch Intern Med* 142:902, 1982.
32. Juliusson G, Vitols S, Liliemark J: Mechanisms behind hypocholesterolaemia in hairy cell leukaemia. *BMJ* 310:27, 1995.
33. Juliusson G, Vitols S, Liliemark J: Disease-related hypocholesterolemia in patients with hairy cell leukemia. *Cancer* 76:423, 1995.
34. Bouroncle BA: Unusual presentations and complications of hairy cell leukemia. *Leukemia* 1:288, 1987.
35. Davies GE, Wiernik PH: Hairy cell leukemia with chylous ascites. *JAMA* 238:1541, 1977.
36. Robinson A, Eting E, Zeidman A, et al: Ocular manifestation of hairy cell leukemia with dramatic response to 2-chloro-deoxy-adensosine. *Am J Ophthalmol* 121:7, 1997.
37. Bartl R, Frisch B, Hill W, et al: Bone marrow histology in hairy cell leukemia. *Am J Clin Pathol* 79:531, 1983.
38. Katayama I: Bone marrow in hairy cell leukemia. *Hematol Oncol Clin North Am* 2:585, 1988.
39. Burke JS: The value of the bone-marrow biopsy in the diagnosis of hairy cell leukemia. *Am J Clin Pathol* 70:876, 1978.
40. Naeim F, Jacobs AD: Bone marrow changes in patients with hairy cell leukemia treated by recombinant alpha-2 interferon. *Hum Pathol* 16:1200, 1985.
41. Ratain MJ, Golomb HM, Bardawil RG, et al: Durability of responses to interferon alfa-2b in advanced hairy cell leukemia. *Blood* 69:872, 1987.
42. Burthem J, Cawley JC: The bone marrow fibrosis of hairy-cell leukemia is caused by the synthesis and assembly of a fibronectin matrix by the hairy cells. *Blood* 83:497, 1994.
43. Golomb HM, Vardiman JW: Response to splenectomy in 65 patients with hairy cell leukemia: An evaluation of spleen weight and bone marrow involvement. *Blood* 61:349, 1983.
44. Nanba K, Soban EJ, Bowling MC, et al: Splenic pseudosinuses and hepatic angiomatous lesions: Distinctive features of hairy cell leukemia. *Am J Clin Pathol* 67:415, 1977.
45. Vardiman JW, Golomb HM: Autopsy findings in hairy cell leukemia. *Semin Oncol* 11:370, 1984.
46. Lembersky BC, Ratain MJ, Golomb HM: Skeletal complications in hairy cell leukemia: Diagnosis and therapy. *J Clin Oncol* 6:1280, 1988.
47. Yam LT, Janckila AJ, Li C-Y, et al: Cytochemistry of tartrate-resistant acid phosphatase: Fifteen years' experience. *Leukemia* 1:285, 1987.
48. Li CY, Yam LT, Lam KW: Studies of acid phosphatase isoenzymes in human leukocytes: Demonstration of isoenzyme specificity. *J Histochem Cytochem* 18:901, 1970.
49. Drexler HG, Gaedicke G, Minowade J: Isoenzyme studies in human leukemia-lymphoma cell lines: II. Acid phosphatase. *Leuk Res* 9:537, 1985.
50. Katayama I, Li CY, Yam LT: Ultrastructural characteristics of the "hairy cells" of leukemic reticuloendotheliosis. *Am J Pathol* 361:370, 1972.
51. Melo JV, Robinson DS, Gregory C, et al: Splenic B cell lymphoma with "villous" lymphocytes in the peripheral blood: A disorder distinct from hairy cell leukemia. *Leukemia* 1:294, 1987.
52. Catovsky D, O'Brien M, Melo JV, et al: Hairy cell leukemia variant: An intermediate disease between hairy cell leukemia and B prolymphocytic leukemia. *Semin Oncol* 11:362, 1984.
53. Rosner MC, Golomb HM: Ribosome-lamella complex in hairy cell leukemia: Ultrastructure and distribution. *Lab Invest* 42:236, 1980.
54. Brunning RD, Parkin J: Ribosome-lamella complexes in neoplastic hematopoietic cells. *Am J Pathol* 79:565, 1975.
55. Hsu S, Yang K, Jaffe ES: Hairy cell leukemia: A B-cell neoplasm with a unique antigenic phenotype. *Am J Clin Pathol* 80:421, 1983.
56. Falini B, Schwarting R, Erber W, et al: The differential diagnosis of hairy cell leukemia with a panel of monoclonal antibodies. *Am J Clin Pathol* 83:289, 1985.

57. Robbins BA, Ellison DJ, Spinosa JC, et al: Diagnostic application of two-color flow cytometry in 161 cases of hairy cell leukemia. *Blood* 82:1277, 1993.

58. Visser L, Shaw A, Slupsky J, et al: Monoclonal antibodies reactive with hairy cell leukemia. *Blood* 74:320, 1989.

59. Schwarting R, Stein H, Wang CY: The monoclonal antibodies alpha S-hairy cell leukemia 1 (alpha Leu-14) and alpha S-hairy cell leukemia 3 (alpha Leu-M5) allow the diagnosis of hairy cell leukemia. *Blood* 65:974, 1985.

60. Hanson CA, Gribbin TE, Schnitzer B, et al: CD11c (Leu-M5) expression characterizes a B-cell chronic lymphoproliferative disorder with features of both chronic lymphocytic leukemia and hairy cell leukemia. *Blood* 76:2360, 1990.

61. de Totero D, Tazzari PL, Lauria F, et al: Phenotypic analysis of hairy cell leukemia: "Variant" cases express the interleukin-2 receptor beta chain, but not the alpha chain (CD25). *Blood* 82:528, 1993.

62. Steis RG, Marcon L, Clark J, et al: Serum soluble IL-2 receptor as a tumor marker in patients with hairy cell leukemia. *Blood* 77:1304, 1988.

63. Micklem KJ, Dong Y, Willis A, et al: HML-1 antigen on mucosa-associated T cells, activated cells, and hairy leukemic cells is a new integrin containing the $\beta 7$ subunit. *Am J Pathol* 139:1297, 1991.

64. Flenghi L, Spinozzi F, Stein H, et al: LF61: A new monoclonal antibody directed against a trimeric molecule (150 kDa, 125 kDa, 105 kDa) associated with hairy cell leukemia. *Br J Haematol* 76:451, 1990.

65. Cepek KL, Parker CM, Madara JL, et al: Integrin alpha E beta F mediates adhesion of T lymphocytes to epithelial cell. *J Immunol* 150:3459, 1993.

66. Linde GA, Hammarstrom L, Persson MAA, et al: Virus-specific antibody activity of different subclasses of immunoglobulins G and A in cytomegalovirus infections. *Infect Immun* 42:237, 1983.

67. Thaler J, Denz H, Dietze O, et al: Immunohistological assessment of bone marrow biopsies from patients with hairy cell leukemia: Changes following treatment with alpha-2-interferon and deoxycoformycin. *Leuk Res* 13:377, 1989.

68. Stroup R, Sheibani K: Antigenic phenotypes of hairy cell leukemia and monocytoid B-cell lymphoma: An immunohistochemical evaluation of 66 cases. *Hum Pathol* 23:172, 1992.

69. al Saati T, Caspar S, Brousset P, et al: Production of anti-B monoclonal antibodies (DBB.42, DBA.44, DNA.7, and DND.53) reactive on paraffin-embedded tissues with a new B-lymphoma cell line grafted into athymic nude mice. *Blood* 74:2476, 1989.

70. Hounieu H, Chittal SM, al Saati T, et al: Hairy cell leukemia: Diagnosis of bone marrow involvement in paraffin-embedded sections with monoclonal antibody DBA.44. *Am J Clin Pathol* 98:26, 1992.

71. Sainati L, Matutes E, Mulligan S, et al: A variant form of hairy cell leukemia resistant to alpha-interferon: Clinical and phenotypic characteristics of 17 patients. *Blood* 76:157, 1990.

72. Cawley JC, Burns GF, Hayhoe RGH: A chronic lymphoproliferative disorder with distinctive features: A distinct variant of hairy cell leukemia. *Leuk Res* 4:547, 1980.

73. Diez-Martin JL, Li CY, Banks PM: Blastic variant of hairy cell leukemia. *Am J Clin Pathol* 87:576, 1987.

74. Machii T, Yamaguchi M, Inoue R, et al: Polyclonal B-cell lymphocytosis with features resembling hairy cell leukemia-Japanese variant. *Blood* 89:2008, 1997.

75. Sun T, Susin M, Brody J, et al: Splenic lymphoma with circulating villous lymphocytes: Report of seven cases and review of the literature. *Am J Hematol* 45:39, 1994.

76. Hanson CA, Ward PC, Schnitzer B: A multilobular variant of hairy cell leukemia with morphologic similarities to T-cell lymphoma. *Am J Surg Pathol* 13:671, 1989.

77. Yam LT, Li CY, Lam KW: Tartrate-resistant acid phosphatase isoenzyme in the reticulum cells of leukemic reticuloendotheliosis. *N Engl J Med* 284:357, 1971.

78. Slovak ML, Weiss LM, Nathwan BN, et al: Cytogenetic studies of composite lymphomas: Monocytoid B-cell lymphoma and other B-cell non-Hodgkin's lymphomas. *Hum Pathol* 24:1086, 1993.

79. Sheibani K, Burke JS, Swartz WG, et al: Monocytoid B-cell lymphoma: Clinicopathologic study of 21 cases of a unique type of low-grade lymphoma. *Cancer* 62:1531, 1988.

80. Shin SS, Sahibani K: Monocytoid B-cell lymphoma. *Am J Clin Pathol* 99:421, 1973.

81. Saven A, Piro LD: Hairy cell leukemia, in *Hematology: Basic Principles and Practice*, edited by Hoffman R, Benz EJ, Shattil SJ, Furie B, et al, p 1322. Churchill Livingstone, New York, 1995.

82. Traweek ST, Sheiban K: Monocytoid B-cell lymphoma: The biologic and clinical implications of peripheral blood involvement. *Am J Clin Pathol* 97:591, 1992.

83. Burke JS, Rappaport H: The differential diagnosis of hairy cell leukemia in bone marrow and spleen. *Semin Oncol* 11:334, 1984.

84. Keating MJ: Chronic lymphoproliferative disorders: Chronic lymphocytic leukemia and hairy cell leukemia. *Curr Opin Oncol* 5:35, 1993.

85. Mintz U, Golomb HM: Splenectomy as initial therapy in twenty-six patients with leukemic reticuloendotheliosis (hairy cell leukemia). *Cancer Res* 39:2366, 1979.

86. Jansen J, Hermans J: Splenectomy in hairy cell leukemia: A retrospective multicenter analysis. *Cancer* 47:2066, 1981.

87. Lewis SM, Catovsky D, Hows JM, et al: Splenic red cell pooling in hairy cell leukemia. *Br J Haematol* 35:351, 1977.

88. Golde DW: Therapy of hairy-cell leukemia. *N Engl J Med* 307:495, 1982.

89. Golomb HM: Progress report on chlorambucil therapy in postsplenectomy patients with progressive hairy cell leukemia. *Blood* 57:464, 1981.

90. Lusch CJ, Ramsey HE, Katayama I: Leukemic reticuloendotheliosis: Report of a case with peripheral blood remission on androgen therapy. *Cancer* 41:1964, 1978.

91. Blum SF: Lithium in hairy cell leukemia. *N Engl J Med* 303:464, 1983.

92. Arkel YS, Lake-Lewin D, Sarapoulous AA, et al: Bone lesions in hairy cell leukemia. *Cancer* 53:2401, 1984.

93. Quesada JR, Reuben J, Manning JT, et al: Alpha-interferon for induction of remission in hairy cell leukemia. *N Engl J Med* 310:15, 1984.

94. Golomb HM, Jacobs A, Fefer A, et al: Alpha-2 interferon therapy of hairy cell leukemia: A multicenter study of 64 patients. *J Clin Oncol* 4:900, 1986.

95. Golomb HM, Ratain MJ, Fefer A, et al: Randomized study of the duration of treatment with interferon alfa-2b in patients with hairy cell leukemia. *J Natl Cancer Inst* 80:369, 1988.

96. Berman E, Heller G, Kempin S, et al: Incidence of response and long-term follow-up in patients with hairy cell leukemia with recombinant alpha-2a. *Blood* 75:839, 1990.

97. Quesada JR, Hersh EM, Manning J, et al: Treatment of hairy cell leukemia with recombinant alpha-interferon. *Blood* 68:493, 1986.

98. Von Wussow P, Pralle H, Hochkeppel H, et al: Effective natural interferon-α therapy in recombinant interferon-α-resistant patients with hairy cell leukemia. *Blood* 78:38, 1991.

99. Ratain MJ, Golomb HM, Vardiman JW, et al: Relapse after interferon alpha-2b therapy for hairy-cell leukemia: Analysis of diagnostic variables. *J Clin Oncol* 6:1714, 1988.

100. Ratain MJ, Golomb HM, Vardiman JW, et al: Interferon alpha-2b therapy for hairy cell leukemia in 69 patients: A 6-year update [abstr]. *Blood* 74:76, 1989.

101. Kampmeier P, Spielberger R, Dickstein J, et al: Increased incidence of second neoplasms in patients treated with interferon α-2b for hairy cell leukemia: A clinicopathologic assessment. *Blood* 83:2931, 1994.

102. Ruco LP, Procapio A, Maccallini V, et al: Severe deficiency of natural killer activity in the peripheral blood of patients with hairy cell leukemia. *Blood* 61:1132, 1983.

103. Lee SH, Kelley S, Chin H, et al: Stimulation of natural killer cell activity and inhibition of proliferation of various leukemic cells by purified human leukocyte interferon subtypes. *Cancer Res* 42:1312, 1982.

104. Lieberman D, Voloch Z, Aviv H, et al: Effects of interferon on hemoglobin synthesis and leukemia virus production in Friend cells. *Mol Biol Rep* 1:447, 1974.

105. Taylor-Papadimitriou J: Effects of interferons on cell growth and function, in *Interferon 1980*, vol 2, edited by I Gresser, p 13. Academic Press, New York, 1980.

106. Jansen JH, Van der Harst D, Wientjens G-JHM, et al: Induction of CD11a/leukocyte function antigen-1 and CD54/intercellular adhesion molecule-1 on hairy cell leukemia cells is accompanied by enhanced susceptibility to T-cell but not lymphokine-activated killer cell cytotoxicity. *Blood* 80:478, 1992.

107. Juliusson G, Lenkei R, Liliemark J: Flow cytometry of blood and bone marrow cells from patients with hairy cell leukemia: Phenotype of hairy cells and lymphocyte subsets after treatment with 2-chlorodeoxyadenosine. *Blood* 83:3672, 1994.

108. Seymour JF, Estey EH, Keating MJ, et al: Response to interferon-α in patients with hairy cell leukemia relapsing after treatment with 2-chlorodeoxyadenosine. *Leukemia* 9:929, 1995.

109. Giblett ER, Anderson JE, Cohen F, et al: Adenosine deaminase deficiency in two patients with severely impaired cellular immunity. *Lancet* 2:1067, 1972.

110. Cohen A, Hirshhorn R, Horowitz SD, et al: Deoxyadenosine triphosphate as a potentially toxic metabolite in adenosine deaminase deficiency. *Proc Natl Acad Sci USA* 75:472, 1978.

111. Carson DA, Wasson DB, Kaye J, et al: Deoxycytidine kinase-mediated toxicity of deoxyadenosine analogs toward malignant human lymphoblasts *in vitro* and toward murine L1210 leukemia *in vivo*. *Proc Natl Acad Sci USA* 77:6865, 1980.

112. Spiers ASD, Parekh SJ: Pentostatin (2′-deoxycoformycin, DCF) is active in hairy cell leukemia (hairy cell leukemia) [abstr]. *Blood* 62:208, 1983.

113. Spiers ASD, Moore D, Cassileth PA, et al: Remissions in hairy cell leukemia with pentostatin (2′-deoxycoformycin). *N Engl J Med* 316:825, 1987.

114. Cassileth PA, Cheuvant B, Spiers ASD, et al: Pentostatin induces durable remissions in hairy cell leukemia. *J Clin Oncol* 9:243, 1991.

115. Ho AD, Thaler J, Stryckmans P, et al: Pentostatin in resistant chronic lymphocytic leukemia: A phase II trial of the European organization for research and treatment of cancer. *Proc Am Soc Clin Oncol* 9:206, 1990.

116. Grever M, Kopecky K, Foucar K, et al: Randomized comparison of pentostatin versus interferon alfa-2a in previously untreated patients with hairy cell leukemia: An Iintergroup study. *J Clin Oncol* 13:974, 1995.

117. Kraut EH, Grever MR, Bouroncle BA: Long-term follow-up of patients with hairy cell leukemia after treatment with 2′-deoxycoformycin. *Blood* 84:4061, 1994.

118. Spiers ASD, Parekh SJ, Bishop MB: Hairy-cell leukemia: Induction of complete remission with pentostatin (2′-deoxycoformycin). *J Clin Oncol* 2:1336, 1984.

119. Johnston JB, Glazer RI, Pugh L, et al: The treatment of hairy-cell leukemia with 2′-deoxycoformycin. *Br J Haematol* 63:525, 1986.

120. Ho AD, Thaler J, Stryckmans P, et al: Pentostatin in refractory chronic lymphocytic leukemia: A phase II trial of the European Organization for Research and Treatment of Cancer. *J Natl Cancer Inst* 82:1416, 1990.

121. Urba WJ, Baseler MW, Kopp WC, et al: Deoxycoformycin-induced immunosuppression in patients with hairy cell leukemia. *Blood* 73:38, 1989.

122. Piro LD, Carrera CJ, Carson DA, et al: Lasting remissions in hairy cell leukemia induced by a single infusion of 2-chlorodeoxyadenosine. *N Engl J Med* 322:1117, 1990.

123. Juliusson G, Liliemark J: Rapid recovery from cytopenia in hairy cell leukemia after treatment with 2-chloro-2′-deoxyadenosine (CdA): Relation to opportunistic infections. *Blood* 79:888, 1992.

124. Estey EM, Kurzrock R, Kantarjian HM, et al: Treatment of hairy cell leukemia with 2-chlorodeoxyadenosine (2-CdA). *Blood* 79:882, 1992.

125. Saven A, Burian C, Koziol JA, et al: Long-term follow-up of patients with hairy cell leukemia following cladribine treatment. *Blood* 92:1918, 1998.

126. Saven A, Piro LD: Complete remissions in hairy cell leukemia with 2-chlorodeoxyadenosine after failure with 2′-deoxycoformycin. *Ann Intern Med* 119:278, 1993.

127. Kurzrock R, Strom SS, Estey E, et al: Second cancer risk in hairy cell leukemia: Analysis of 350 patients. *J Clin Oncol* 15:1803, 1997.

128. Tallman MS, Hakimian D, Rademaker AW, et al: Relapse of hairy cell leukemia after 2-chlorodeoxyadenosine: Long-term follow-up of the Northwestern University experience. *Blood* 88:1954, 1996.

129. Hoffman MA, Janson D, Rose E, et al: Treatment of hairy cell leukemia with cladribine: Response, toxicity and long-term follow-up. *J Clin Oncol* 15:1138, 1997.

130. Carrera CJ, Piro LD, Saven A, et al: Restoration of lymphocyte subsets following 2-chlorodeoxyadenosine remission induction in hairy cell leukemia [abstr]. *Blood* 76(suppl 1):260a, 1990.

131. Seymour J, Kurzrock R, Freireich EJ, et al: 2-Chlorodeoxyadenosine induces durable remissions and prolonged suppression of CD4+ lymphocyte counts in patients with hairy cell leukemia. *Blood* 83:2906, 1994.

132. Hakimian D, Tallman MS, Kiley C, et al: Detection of minimal residual disease by immunostaining of bone marrow biopsies after 2-chlorodeoxyadenosine for hairy cell leukemia. *Blood* 82:1798, 1993.

133. Ellison DJ, Sharpe RW, Robbins BA, et al: Immunomorphologic analysis of bone marrow biopsies after treatment with 2-chlorodeoxyadenosine for hairy cell leukemia. *Blood* 84:4310, 1994.

134. Filleul B, Delannoy A, Ferrant A, et al: A single course of 2-chlorodeoxyadenosine does not eradicate leukemic cells in hairy cell patients in complete remission. *Leukemia* 8:1153, 1994.

135. Juliusson G, Heldal D, Hippe E, et al: Subcutaneous injections of 2-chlorodeoxyadenosine for symptomatic hairy cell leukemia. *J Clin Oncol* 13:989, 1995.

136. Lauria F, Bocchia M, Marotta G, et al: Weekly administration of 2-chlorodeoxyadenosine in patients with hairy cell leukemia: A new treatment schedule effective and safer in preventing infectious complications [letter]. *Blood* 89:1838, 1998.

137. Keating MJ, Kantarjian H, Talpaz M, et al: Fludarabine: A new agent with major activity against chronic lymphocytic leukemia. *Blood* 74:19, 1989.

138. Keating MJ, Kantarjian H, O'Brien S, et al: Fludarabine: A new agent with marked cytoreductive activity in untreated chronic lymphocytic leukemia. *J Clin Oncol* 9:44, 1991.

139. Kantarjian HM, Redman J, Keating MJ: Fludarabine phosphate therapy in other lymphoid malignancies. *Semin Oncol* 17(suppl 8):66, 1990.

140. Kantarjian HM, Schachner J, Keating MJ: Fludarabine therapy in hairy cell leukemia. *Cancer* 67:1291, 1991.

141. Kraut E, Chun H: Fludarabine phosphate in refractory hairy cell leukemia. *Am J Hematol* 37:59, 1991.

142. Glaspy JA, Baldwin GC, Robertson PA, et al: Therapy for neutropenia in hairy cell leukemia with recombinant human granulocyte colony-stimulating factor. *Ann Intern Med* 109:789, 1988.

143. Golomb HM, Catovsky D, Golde DW: Hairy cell leukemia: A clinical review of 71 cases. *Ann Intern Med* 89:677, 1978.

144. Quesada JR, Gutterman J, Hersh EM: Treatment of hairy cell leukemia with alpha interferons. *Cancer* 57:1678, 1986.

145. Foon KA, Maluish AE, Abrams PG, et al: Recombinant leukocyte A interferon therapy for advanced hairy cell leukemia: Therapeutic and immunologic results. *Am J Med* 80:351, 1986.

146. Rai K, Mick R, Ozer H, et al: Alpha-interferon therapy in untreated active hairy cell leukemia: A Cancer and Leukemia Group B (CALGB) study [abstr]. *Proc Am Soc Clin Oncol* 6:159, 1987.

147. Golomb H, Fefer A, Golde D, et al: Update of a multi-institutional study of 195 patients (pts) with hairy cell leukemia treated with interferon alfa-2b (IFN) [abstr]. *Proc Am Soc Clin Oncol* 6:215, 1990.

148. Grever M, Kopecky K, Foucar MK, et al: Randomized comparison of pentostatin versus interferon alfa-2a in previously untreated patients with hairy cell leukemia: An Intergroup study. *J Clin Oncol* 13:974, 1995.

149. Kraut EH, Bouroncle BA, Grever MR: Pentostatin in the treatment of advanced hairy cell leukemia. *J Clin Oncol* 7:168, 1989.

150. Grem J, King S, Cheson B, et al: Pentostatin in hairy cell leukemia: Treatment by the special exception mechanism. *J Natl Cancer Inst* 81:448, 1989.

LARGE GRANULAR LYMPHOCYTIC LEUKEMIA

THOMAS P. LOUGHRAN

MARSHALL E. KADIN

Clonal diseases of larger granular lymphocytes (LGL) can arise from either T cells or natural killer (NK) cells. Although T-LGL and NK-LGL cells have a similar morphology, they have distinctive surface antigen phenotypes and represent two discrete diseases with different clinical features and clinical outcomes. Current treatment for either disease is not considered curative. This chapter describes these two disease entities and outlines current therapeutic approaches.

DEFINITION AND HISTORY

A clinical syndrome of chronic neutropenia associated with increased numbers of circulating LGL was described in 1977.[1] Clonal cytogenetic abnormalities established its neoplastic nature, and the term *LGL leukemia* was introduced.[2] Other terms used include *Tγ-lymphoproliferative disease*[3] and *lymphoproliferative disease of granular lymphocytes*.[4]

LGL comprise 10 to 15 percent of normal blood mononuclear cells and may be of either CD3− (NK cell) or CD3+ (T cell) lineage. LGL leukemia is classified into *T-LGL leukemia* and *NK-LGL leukemia,* reflecting different cellular origins.[5,6] T-LGL leukemia is defined as a clonal proliferation of CD3+ LGL; NK-LGL leukemia as a clonal proliferation of CD3− LGL. T-cell receptor gene rearrangement studies are useful for confirming the clonality of T-LGL leukemia.[7] NK-cell leukemia also is a clonal disease, as demonstrated by cytogenetics.[8] However, NK cells, and NK-cell leukemia, lack convenient clonal markers, such as antigen receptor gene rearrangements.

ETIOLOGY AND PATHOGENESIS

The etiology of T-LGL leukemia is unknown. Infection with HTLV-II has been detected in two patients. However, most patients are not infected with either HTLV-I or HTLV-II.[9] Nevertheless, serologic findings show frequent reactivity to the BA-21 epitope of the p21e *env* protein of HTLV-I, suggesting that a cellular or retroviral protein with homology to BA-21 may be important in pathogenesis.[9] Epstein-Barr virus infection has been implicated in the pathogenesis of NK-LGL leukemia.[10]

Leukemic LGL show many characteristics of antigen-activated cytotoxic T cells (CTL), suggesting that an initial step in LGL expansion is an antigen-driven mechanism. Normal CTL are regulated through apoptosis. Dysregulated apoptosis is a characteristic finding in LGL leukemia and is thought to underlie the pathogenesis of the disease. Leukemic LGL constitutively express high levels of Fas, yet are resistant to Fas-mediated death.[11] Defective apoptosis, therefore,

Acronyms and abbreviations that appear in this chapter include: CTL, cytotoxic T cells; LGL, large granular lymphocytes; NK, natural killer.

may contribute to extended cell survival of leukemic LGL. Leukemic LGL also constitutively express Fas ligand, and patient sera contain high levels of this protein.[12,13] It is conceivable that disease manifestations such as neutropenia and rheumatoid arthritis are related to circulating Fas ligand in these patients.

CLINICAL FEATURES

Clinical features of T-LGL leukemia are summarized in Table 100-1. Rheumatoid arthritis may be a prominent feature of LGL leukemia, sometimes resulting in a clinical picture resembling that of Felty syndrome.[14] The clinical presentation of NK-LGL leukemia is different from that of T-LGL leukemia. Patients with NK-LGL leukemia usually are younger, more often have systemic B symptoms, and typically have more massive hepatosplenomegaly. Lymphadenopathy and gastrointestinal tract involvement are common.[8]

LABORATORY FEATURES

HEMATOLOGIC FINDINGS

Examination of the blood film is important to diagnose T-LGL leukemia, since approximately 25 percent of patients do not have an increased total lymphocyte count.[6] LGL can be identified by morphology, although immunophenotyping is necessary to distinguish whether the LGL are of T-cell or NK-cell lineage (see below). The median LGL count of patients with T-LGL leukemia, however, is 4200/μl (4.2 × 10^9/liter). Patients with NK-LGL leukemia generally have much higher LGL counts, sometimes exceeding 50,000/μl (5.0 × 10^{10}/liter).

Most patients (84 percent) with T-LGL leukemia have chronic neutropenia, and about half (48 percent) have neutrophil counts less than 500/μl (5 × 10^8/liter).[6] In contrast, less than one-fifth (18 percent) of patients with NK-LGL have severe neutropenia.[6] Anemia is observed in 50 percent and 100 percent of cases of T- and NK-LGL leukemia respectively. Pure red cell aplasia and Coombs' positive hemolytic anemia are seen with T-LGL leukemia.[2,6] Indeed, LGL leukemia is the most commonly associated disease in patients with pure red cell aplasia.[15] Thrombocytopenia and coagulopathy are features of NK-LGL leukemia.[6] Moderate thrombocytopenia occurring with T-LGL leukemia can resemble idiopathic thrombocytopenic purpura.[2]

IMMUNOPHENOTYPING

Immunophenotyping can distinguish T-LGL leukemia from NK-LGL leukemia. T-leukemic LGL usually are CD3+, CD4−, CD8+, CD16+, CD56−, CD57+, and often HLA-DR+. Cases of LGL leukemia expressing CD3 and CD56 may have a more aggressive clinical course.[16] Leukemic T-LGL usually are T-cell receptor (TCR) $\alpha\beta$+, although TCR $\gamma\delta$+ cases with similar clinical features have been described.[17] NK-leukemic LGL are usually CD3−, CD4−, CD8−, CD16+, CD56+, and CD57−.[8]

IMMUNE ABNORMALITIES

Patients with T-LGL leukemia frequently have humoral immune abnormalities, including positive tests for rheumatoid factor or antinuclear antibodies, polyclonal hypergammaglobulinemia, circulating immune complexes, and antineutrophil antibodies (Table 100-2). These patients also may have defects in cellular immunity, such as diminished NK activity.[2] Immune function has not been evaluated in most patients with NK-LGL leukemia.

HISTOPATHOLOGIC FEATURES

T-LGL leukemia invariably affects the spleen, where the major findings are leukemic infiltration of the red pulp cords and sinuses, plasma

TABLE 100-1   CLINICAL FEATURES OF CD3+ LGL LEUKEMIA*

Feature	Cases, %
Recurrent infections	20–40
B symptoms	20–30
Splenomegaly	20–50
Hepatomegaly	1–23
Lymphadenopathy	1–3

*Data on two series of 128 and 68 patients.[5,26]
SOURCE: Reprinted with permission from Lamy T, Loughran TP Jr: Large granular lympho-cyte leukemia. *Cancer Control* 5:25, 1998.

cell hyperplasia, and prominent germinal centers.[2,18] Liver sinusoids and portal areas are infiltrated by LGL. The marrow biopsy may contain nodules of B lymphocytes and scattered LGL, which are better seen in the aspirate. Granulocyte maturation arrest and pure red cell aplasia have been observed. Lymph nodes usually are not involved but can have expanded paracortical areas containing plasma cells and LGL.

DIFFERENTIAL DIAGNOSIS

The diagnosis of T-LGL leukemia should be considered in patients with chronic or cyclic neutropenia[19] or in patients with pure red cell aplasia or rheumatoid arthritis who have increased concentrations of LGL cells. Cytomegalovirus or HIV infection can lead to a mild increase in the concentration of LGL cells. However, the LGL are not monoclonal.[20] Some patients may have elevated numbers of CD3– LGL but lack the clinical features of NK-LGL leukemia and have a chronic clinical course.[21] Molecular studies using X-linked probes indicate that these patients have polyclonal expansion of LGL.[22] Of interest, sera from these patients with chronic NK lymphocytosis also have frequent reactivity to BA-21.[23]

THERAPY, COURSE, AND PROGNOSIS

Morbidity and mortality usually result as consequences of neutro-penia.[6] Optimum treatment for correction of neutropenia is not defined. Treatment with oral low-dose methotrexate, cyclosporine, or oral cy-clophosphamide has been efficacious in small series.[24–26] Clinical im-provement may be associated with reductions in levels of circulating Fas ligand. Treatment with glucocorticoids has ameliorated the neutro-penia of some patients. However, neutropenia generally recurs as the medication is tapered. Splenectomy is also of limited benefit. Experience with recombinant growth factors is limited.[27,28] Single-agent chemotherapy with prednisone, cyclophosphamide, or chloram-bucil is effective in correcting pure red cell aplasia associated with T-LGL leukemia.[6] In contrast to the chronic course of T-LGL leukemia, NK-LGL leukemia has an acute presentation and poor clinical out-

TABLE 100-2   SEROLOGIC FINDINGS IN CD3+ LGL LEUKEMIA*

Feature	Cases, %
Rheumatoid factor	60
Antinuclear antibody	40
Polyclonal hypergammaglobulinemia	10–40
Monoclonal gammopathy	8
Circulating immune complexes	55
Antineutrophil antibody	40
Positive Coombs' test	15

*Data from two series of 128 and 68 patients.[5,26]
SOURCE: Reprinted with permission from Lamy T, Loughran TP Jr: Large granular lympho-cyte leukemia. *Cancer Control* 5:25, 1998.

come. Most patients die within 2 months of diagnosis from dissemi-nated disease with multiorgan failure, despite aggressive combination chemotherapy.[8] Patients with chronic NK lymphocytosis do not usually require treatment.

To better define the natural history of LGL leukemia, a registry has been formed. Clinical trials are also being administered through the registry. For more information, the registry can be contacted at *www.moffitt.usf.edu/lgl-leukemia*, which can be accessed through the Williams Hematology, 6th edition, web page.

REFERENCES

1. McKenna RW, Parkin J, Kersey JH, et al: Chronic lymphoproliferative disorder with unusual clinical, morphologic, ultrastructural and mem-brane surface marker characteristics. *Am J Med* 62:588, 1977.
2. Loughran TP Jr, Kadin ME, Starkebaum G, et al: Leukemia of large granular lymphocytes: association with clonal chromosomal abnormali-ties and auto-immune neutropenia, thrombocytopenia and hemolytic anemia. *Ann Intern Med* 102:169, 1985.
3. Reynolds CW, Foon KA: Tγ Lymphoproliferative disease and related disorders in humans and experimental animals. A review of the clinical, cellular, and functional characteristics. *Blood* 64:1146, 1984.
4. Semenzato G, Pandolfi F, Chisesi T, et al: The lymphoproliferative disease of granular lymphocytes. A heterogeneous disorder ranging from indolent to aggressive conditions. *Cancer* 60:2971, 1987.
5. Loughran TP Jr: Clonal diseases of large granular lymphocytes. *Blood* 82:1, 1993.
6. Lamy T, Loughran TP Jr: Large granular lymphocyte leukemia. *Cancer Control* 5:25, 1998.
7. Rambaldi A, Pelicci P-G, Allavena P, et al: T cell receptor β chain gene rearrangements in lymphoproliferative disorders of large granular lymphocytes/natural killer cells. *J Exp Med* 162:2156, 1985.
8. Taniwaki M, Tagawa S, Nishigaki H, et al: Chromosomal abnormalities define clonal proliferation in CD3- large granular lymphocyte leukemia. *Am J Hematol* 33:32, 1990.
9. Loughran TP Jr, Hadlock KG, Perzova R, et al: Epitope mapping of HTLV envelope seroreactivity in LGL leukemia. *Br J Haematol* 101:318, 1998.
10. Kawa-Ha K, Ishihara S, Ninomiya T, et al: CD3-negative lymphopro-liferative disease of granular lymphocytes containing Epstein-Barr viral DNA. *J Clin Invest* 84:51, 1989.
11. Lamy T, Liu JH, Landowski TH, et al: Dysregulation of CD95/CD95 ligand-apoptotic pathway in CD95+ LGL leukemia. *Blood* (in press).
12. Tanaka M, Suda T, Haze K, et al: Fas ligand in human serum. *Nat Med* 2:317, 1996.
13. Perzova R, Loughran TP Jr: Constitutive expression of Fas ligand in LGL leukemia. *Br J Haematol* 97:123, 1997.
14. Loughran TP Jr, Starkebaum G, Kidd P, Neiman P: Clonal proliferation of large granular lymphocytes in rheumatoid arthritis. *Arthritis Rheum* 31:31, 1988.
15. Lacy MQ, Kurtin PJ, Tefferi A, et al: Pure red cell aplasia: association with large granular lymphocyte leukemia and the prognostic value of cytogenetic abnormalities. *Blood* 87:3000, 1996.
16. Gentile TC, Uner AH, Hutchison RE, et al: CD3+, CD56+ aggressive variant of large granular lymphocyte leukemia. *Blood* 84:2315, 1994.
17. Foroni L, Matutes E, Foldi J, et al: T-cell leukemias with rearrangement of the γ but not β T-cell receptor genes. *Blood* 71:356, 1988.
18. Agnarsson BA, Loughran TP Jr, Starkebaum G, Kadin ME: The pa-thology of large granular lymphocyte leukemia. *Hum Pathol* 20:643, 1989.
19. Loughran TP Jr, Hammond WP: Adult onset cyclic neutropenia is a "benign" neoplasm associated with clonal proliferation of large granular lymphocytes. *J Exp Med* 164:2089, 1986.
20. Zambello R, Trentin L, Agostini C, et al: Persistent polyclonal lymphocy-tosis in HIV-1 infected patients. *Blood* 81:3015, 1993.
21. Tefferi A, Li CY, Witzig TE, et al: Chronic natural killer cell lymphocy-tosis: a descriptive clinical study. *Blood* 84:2721, 1994.
22. Nash R, McSweeney P, Zambello R, et al: Clonal studies of CD3-negative lymphoproliferative disease of granular lymphocytes. *Blood* 81:2363, 1993.
23. Loughran TP Jr, Hadlock KG, Yang Q, et al: Seroreactivity to an

envelope protein of human T-cell leukemia/lymphoma virus in patients with CD3-(NK) lymphoproliferative disease of granular lymphocytes. *Blood* 90:1977, 1997.

24. Loughran TP Jr, Kidd PG, Starkebaum G: Treatment of large granular lymphocyte leukemia with oral low-dose methotrexate. *Blood* 84:2164, 1994.

25. Sood R, Stewart CC, Aplan PD, et al: Neutropenia associated with T-cell large granular lymphocyte leukemia: long-term response to cyclosporine therapy despite persistence of abnormal cells. *Blood* 91:3372, 1998.

26. Dhodapkar MU, Li CY, Lust JA, et al: Clinical spectrum of clonal proliferations of T-large granular lymphocytes: a T-cell clonopathy of undetermined significance? *Blood* 84:1620, 1994.

27. Thomssen C, Nissen C, Gratwohl A, et al: Agranulocytosis associated with T-gamma-lymphocytosis: no improvement of peripheral blood granulocyte count with human-recombinant granulocyte-macrophage colony-stimulating factor (GM-CSF). *Br J Haematol* 71:157, 1989.

28. Kaneko T, Ogawa Y, Hirata Y, et al: Agranulocytosis associated with granular lymphocyte leukaemia: improvement of peripheral blood granulocyte count with human recombinant granulocyte colony-stimulating factor (G-CSF). *Br J Haematol* 74:121, 1990.

PATHOLOGY OF MALIGNANT LYMPHOMAS

PETER M. BANKS

Clonal diseases of larger granular lymphocytes (LGL) can arise from either T cells or natural killer (NK) cells. Although T-LGL and NK-LGL cells have a similar morphology, they have distinctive surface antigen phenotypes and represent two discrete diseases with different clinical features and clinical outcomes. Current treatment for either disease is not considered curative. This chapter describes these two disease entities and outlines current therapeutic approaches.

DEFINITION AND HISTORY

In 1832 Thomas Hodgkin published the first treatise on primary lymphatic malignancy: *"On Some Morbid Appearances of the Absorbent Glands and Spleen."* His work derived from clinical and gross autopsy findings in seven cases.[5] Subsequently, Virchow distinguished lymphoma from leukemia in 1846[6] and coined the terms *lymphoma*[7] and *lymphosarcoma*.[8] Billroth, in 1871, was the first to use the term *malignant lymphoma*.[9]

The category of follicular lymphomas initially was recognized in 1916 by Ghon and Roman, who related such neoplasms to normal lymphoid follicles.[13] Brill and others, in 1925,[14] and Symmers, in 1927,[15] failed to appreciate the neoplastic nature among many of their cases of "giant follicular hyperplasia"; however, this oversight was corrected in 1938 with information gained through long-term follow-up.[16] Thus, the neoplastic, albeit indolent, nature of this category of lymphomas became recognized.

In addition to perceiving the aggressive nature of lymphomas composed of large cells, Roulet, in 1930, proposed that the origin of such neoplasms was the sinus lining, and he compared their morphology with that of the normal reticulum, or syncytial network of nodal sinuses.[17] His term *Retothelsarkom* was subsequently popularized but mistranslated as reticulum *cell* sarcoma, and the term *reticulum cell* was applied in varying ways in diverse disorders.[18]

By the middle of the twentieth century, clinically useful systems of classification were formulated. For Hodgkin lymphoma, the Jackson and Parker system (1947) separated the unfavorable sarcoma and favorable, but rare, paragranuloma from the large intermediate grouping of granuloma.[20] In 1966, Lukes, Butler, and Hicks, incorporating others' observations, proposed a six-part pathologic subclassification of Hodgkin lymphoma that correlated closely with clinical survival.[21]

For the lymphomas two fundamental features were correlated with differences in survival, namely the identification of certain cell types and growth patterns. Neoplasms composed of small, nonreplicating lymphocytes (lymphocytic, well-differentiated lymphocytic) were recognized as a favorable group. Those featuring atypical, mitotically active lymphocytes (lymphoblastic, poorly differentiated lymphocytic) were less favorable. Those made up of large cells were erroneously, in retrospect, considered as nonlymphoid (stem cells, clasmatocytic, undifferentiated, or histiocytic) in derivation. The presence of a follicular or nodular growth pattern was an important, favorable predictive feature.[22] Based upon these simple principles, with ever-increasing detail and precision, sequential classification systems were developed: those of Gall and Mallory (1942), Gall and Rappaport (1958), and Rappaport (1966).[23–25] During the 1970s, great strides were achieved in the therapy of lymphomas, as the predictive accuracy of the Rappaport system was demonstrated in selecting those aggressive histologic types for which intensive intervention was required (see Chap. 103).[26] The Working Formulation for Clinical Usage represented a simple, morphologically based system for stratification of lymphomas into major predictive groups[27] (see Table 101-1). Even as this system gained widespread popularity, its scientific validity came into question in the face of data from newly applied methods.

CONTRIBUTION OF IMMUNOLOGY TO LYMPHOMA CLASSIFICATION

Advances in immunology and immunogenetics have provided new insights into the cytogenesis of lymphomas, allowing for a newer classification system.[4] For example, immunophenotyping of large cell lymphomas dispelled the previously popular "reticulum cell" or histiocytic theories of this lymphoma's cytogenesis.[28] Analyzing immunoglobulins from whole-tumor homogenates, a monoclonal B-cell composition in most lymphomas was demonstrated, including the large cell types—reticulum cell or histiocytic.[29] Subsequent studies using immunophenotyping and molecular techniques have characterized these large cell lymphomas as being either B-cell or, less commonly, T-cell proliferations.[30] Only rarely are cases found to be of true histiocytic origin.[31]

Lymphomas with a nodular or follicular growth pattern are neoplastic counterparts of germinal centers. Desmosomal dendritic reticulum cells are present in both benign and neoplastic follicles.[32] Immunologic analyses show that they have common functional properties.[33]

Burkitt and "Burkitt-like" lymphoma variants, designated as undifferentiated in the Rappaport system, are B-cell neoplasms.[30]

Lymphoblastic lymphoma is an important clinicopathologic entity. It is distinct from other lymphomas with which it had been included as "poorly differentiated lymphocytic" in the original Rappaport system. Immunologic, enzymatic, and cytochemical evidence revealed this neoplasm to be of embryonic precursor cell type, more often having a pre-T cell rather than a pre-B cell phenotype.[34] Such neoplasms uniformly possess nuclear terminal deoxynucleotidyl transferase activity and often progress to an unfavorable form of acute lymphoblastic leukemia (see Chap. 101). This entity corresponds to Sternberg's mediastinal "leukosarcoma,"[35] thus explaining Cooke's clinical observations made four decades previously (see "History").

Within the Working Formulation type of diffuse, small cleaved cell lymphoma is an entity newly recognized in relation to both clinical and molecular genetic characteristics—mantle cell lymphoma.[36] These neoplasms are composed of small cleaved B lymphocytes with a diffuse or faintly follicular growth pattern. Unlike neoplasms of germinal center differentiation, i.e., follicular lymphomas, these B-cell tumors coexpress the T cell-related antigen CD5. In addition, these tumors frequently have genetic translocations that involve *BCL-1*, a proto-oncogene that encodes a protein cyclin D1 involved in regulation of cell proliferation.[37] Clinically this is an unfavorable disease of older males, usually with disseminated lymph node involvement or, less commonly, leukemia.[38] A spectacular clinical variant presentation of this process is so-called lymphomatous polyposis of the gastrointestinal tract.[39]

Another distinctive entity deriving largely from the Working Formulation diffuse, small cleaved cell grouping is B-marginal zone lymphoma. Although there is little specific to the B-cell immunophenotype of these tumors, microscopically they are characterized by a subtle mixture of small round lymphocytes, small cleaved cells with

TABLE 101-1   ALPHABETIC DESIGNATIONS FOR CATEGORIES OF NON-HODGKIN LYMPHOMAS OF WORKING FORMULATION* ALLOW COMPARISON WITH REVISED EUROPEAN-AMERICAN LYMPHOMA ("REAL") CLASSIFICATION OF 1994† (MODIFIED 1999)‡

WORKING FORMULATION 1982	"REAL" CLASSIFICATION 1994† (MODIFIED 1999)‡	
Low Grade	**B-cell neoplasms**	**T-cell neoplasms**
A Small lymphocytic, with or without plasmacytoid differentiation	I Precursor B-cell lymphoblastic lymphoma/leukemia	I Precursor T-cell lymphoblastic lymphoma/leukemia
B Follicular, small cleaved	**Mature B-cell neoplasms**	**Mature T-cell & Natural Killer Cell Neoplasms**
C Follicular, mixed small cleaved and large cell	A B-cell small lymphocytic lymphoma/chronic lymphocytic leukemia	A T-cell prolymphocytic leukemia
Intermediate-grade	A B-cell prolymphocytic leukemia	A T-cell large granular lymphocytic leukemia
D Follicular, large cell	A Lymphoplasmacytic (lymphoplasmacytoid) lymphoma	K Aggressive natural killer cell leukemia
E Diffuse, small cleaved	B,E Mantle cell lymphoma	E,F T/NK-cell lymphoma, nasal and nasal-type ("angiocentric lymphoma")
F Diffuse, mixed, small and large cell	B,C,D Follicular lymphoma (follicle center lymphoma)	A,E,K Mycosis fungoides
G Diffuse, large cell	B,C,D Cutaneous follicle center lymphoma	A Sezary syndrome
High-grade	B,C,E,F Marginal zone B-cell lymphoma of mucosa-associated lymphoid tissue ("MALT") type	F,H Angioimmunoblastic T-cell lymphoma
H Large cell, immunoblastic	B,C,E,F Nodal marginal zone lymphoma	E,F,G,H Peripheral T-cell lymphoma (unspecified)
I Lymphoblastic (convoluted or nonconvoluted)	B,C,E,F Splenic marginal zone B-cell lymphoma	K Adult T-cell lymphoma/leukemia
J Small noncleaved cell	K Hairy cell leukemia	H Anaplastic large-cell lymphoma
Others	G,H Diffuse large B-cell lymphoma	E,F,G,H Peripheral T-cell lymphoma (unspecified)
K Hairy cell, cutaneous T-cell, histiocytic neoplasia, plasmacytic, etc.	Mediastinal (thymic)	K Adult T-cell lymphoma/leukemia
	Intravascular	H Anaplastic large-cell lymphoma (T-and null-cell types)
	Primary effusion lymphoma	H Primary cutaneous CD30-positive T-cell lymphoproliferative disorders
	J Burkitt lymphoma	F,K Subcutaneous panniculitic T-cell lymphoma
	K Plasmacytoma	F,H Enteropathy-type intestinal T-cell lymphoma
	K Plasma cell lymphoma	E,F,K Hepatosplenic gamma/delta T-cell lymphoma

*Cancer 1982; 49:2121[27]
†Blood 1994; 84:1362[4]
‡With permission, Jaffe ES, Modern Pathology, 1999; 12:113[52]

clear cytoplasm (monocytoid B-cells), and plasmacytic or plasmacytoid forms. Interestingly, clinical behavior depends largely on distribution. Tumors localized to extranodal parenchymal tissues (stomach, salivary gland, lung, skin, etc.) tend to remain restricted to these sites with potential for cure, in striking contrast to most low-grade lymphomas. This phenomenon corresponds to the mucosa associated lymphoid tissue (MALT) lymphoma concept pioneered by Isaacson.[40] Early gastric MALT type lymphomas often regress with antimicrobial therapy for Helicobacter pylori.[41] Trisomy 3 is the cytogenetic abnormality most closely associated with MALT type lymphomas.[42] B-marginal zone lymphomas of lymph nodes behave clinically in a manner similar to other low-grade lymphoma, i.e. with systemic distribution and a protracted course.[36] Those presenting with splenic enlargement, so-called "splenic lymphoma with villous lymphocytes" show cellular, immunophenotypic and clinical overlap with hairy cell disease[43] (see Chapter 99).

Although relatively uncommon, anaplastic large cell lymphoma affords conceptual insights into the relationship between Hodgkin and non-Hodgkin lymphoma.[44,45] The process was first described in 1982 as "regressing atypical histiocytosis" of the skin.[46] Histologically, tumor cells show extreme nuclear anaplasia and abundant cytoplasm with a cohesive growth pattern suggestive of metastatic carcinoma or histiocytic malignancy. The surprisingly favorable clinical behavior seen in some cases seems to correlate with its propensity to afflict young patients and to be limited to the skin.[47] Another independent favorable prognostic factor is the expression of the p80 or ALK-1 protein, based on a t(2;5) translocation.[48] The immunophenotype is that of activated lymphocytes. Most notably these tumors express the activation antigen CD30 (Ki-1) and an incomplete constellation of lymphoid markers, usually those associated with the cytotoxic T-cell subset. Unlike the tumor cells of Hodgkin lymphoma, those of anaplastic large cell lymphoma usually do express both CD45 (leuko-

cyte common antigen) and epithelial membrane antigen (see Fig. 101-2).

A predominance of T-cell lymphoma was observed in the southern islands of Japan.[49] This observation led to the discovery of the association between the human T-lymphotropic virus, (HTLV-1) and adult T-cell leukemia-lymphoma. Sporadic HTLV-1-positive cases were subsequently observed among native Caribbean and American southern blacks.[50]

THE REVISED EUROPEAN-AMERICAN LYMPHOMA (REAL) CLASSIFICATION

Although the Working Formulation for Clinical Usage served as a practical system for classifying lymphomas into major predictive groupings, by the late 1980s it was becoming clear that it was imprecise in not specifically recognizing these newly identifiable types of lymphoma.[51] Furthermore, there was divergence in the practice of lymphoma classification, as most Europeans used the Kiel classification with its inclusion of immunologic criteria,[1] and some in North America preferred the Lukes-Collins system[2] for similar reasons. In 1993 the International Lymphoma Study Group began a year-long effort to establish a new classification which would acknowledge recent advances in discernment of distinct types of lymphoma, based on combined clinical, microscopic, immunologic, and, in some cases, genetic data. This system was entitled the "REAL" classification, an acronym for Revised European-American Lymphoma; the term also signified the basis for distinguishing the respective lymphoma types as real, i.e., actual, bioglogically distinct entities.[4] Emphasized in this classification are the immune cell types to which the various neoplasms correspond. Thus, the major division of lymphomas is between B-cell and T-cell (see Table 101-1). Explicit in the REAL Classification's exposition is the mutability of any such system in deference to clinical

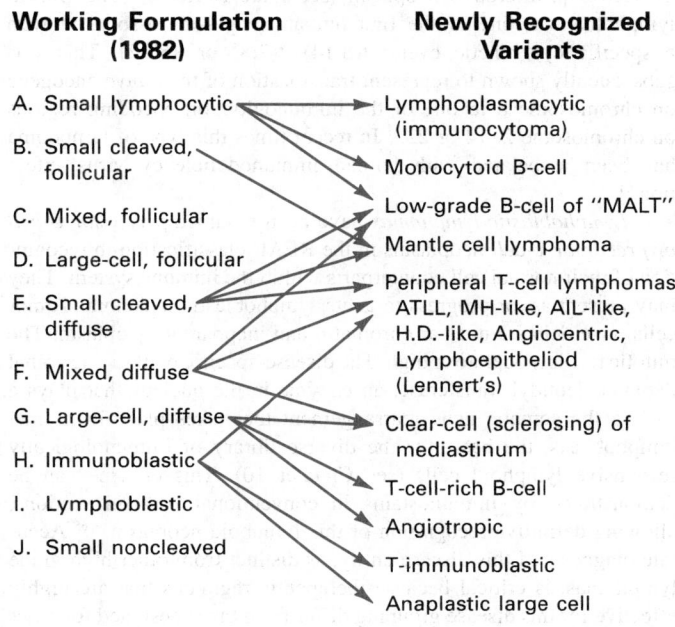

Working Formulation (1982)	Newly Recognized Variants
A. Small lymphocytic	Lymphoplasmacytic (immunocytoma)
B. Small cleaved, follicular	Monocytoid B-cell
C. Mixed, follicular	Low-grade B-cell of "MALT"
D. Large-cell, follicular	Mantle cell lymphoma
E. Small cleaved, diffuse	Peripheral T-cell lymphomas: ATLL, MH-like, AIL-like, H.D.-like, Angiocentric, Lymphoepitheliod (Lennert's)
F. Mixed, diffuse	
G. Large-cell, diffuse	Clear-cell (sclerosing) of mediastinum
H. Immunoblastic	T-cell-rich B-cell
I. Lymphoblastic	Angiotropic
J. Small noncleaved	T-immunoblastic
	Anaplastic large cell

FIGURE 101-1   Newly recognized distinct variants of certain lymphomas (right column) are related to types in the Working Formulation (left column). The following abbreviations are used: AIL, angioimmunoblastic lymphoma; ATLL, adult T-cell leukemia/lymphoma; H.D.-like, Hodgkin disease-like; and MH, malignant histiocytosis. (From Banks,[45] with permission.)

and scientific advances. Members of the original International Lymphoma Study Group collaborated with an assembly of other specialists, both clinicians and pathologists, to develop a modified, updated REAL Classification[52] (see Table 101-1). In the summary presentation which follows, emphasis is placed on major groupings of

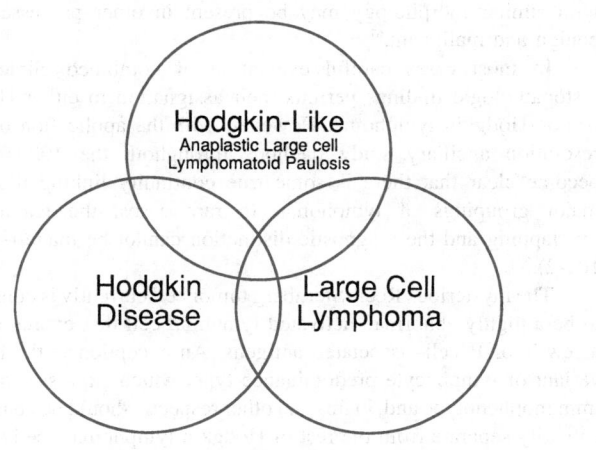

FIGURE 101-2   Simplified conceptual schema representing the interrelationship of Hodgkin lymphoma with other lymphomas. In general, lymphomas are composed of neoplastic cells that have immunophenotypes very similar to that of their normal cell counterparts, whereas Hodgkin lymphoma tumor cells are activated, very abnormal cells that express very few lymphocyte-associated antigens. The Hodgkin-like grouping is intermediate with respect to these two extremes. Note that there is a partial overlap of these groupings, representing cases that are difficult to assign to one or the other group.

lymphomas according to aggressiveness on natural, untreated tumor behavior.

MAJOR PREDICTIVE GROUPINGS OF NON-HODGKIN LYMPHOMA LOW-GRADE

Almost all favorable lymphomas are of B-cell immunophenotype, the prototype being *follicle center lymphomas* (types "B" and "C," follicular small cleaved and follicular mixed types of the Working Formulation (see Table 101-1). These neoplasms correspond to germinal centers, and can be confidently recognized as B-cell tumors by virtue of their follicular growth pattern which, as in benign follicles, is imparted by associated dendritic cells (see Plate XXII-7). There is always some mixture of small cleaved lymphocytes and larger, proliferative "centroblasts." There is a predominance of small cells in the small cleaved cell type (grade I of the REAL classification) (see Plate XXII-8). The distinction from follicular mixed type (grade II of the REAL classification) is often somewhat subjective, and so has been described as an exercise in grading rather than classification in the REAL system.[4] These lymphomas are usually disseminated and, with conventional therapy, effectively incurable, however, patients survive with this disease for prolonged periods (see Chapter 103).[53] These neoplasms appear to represent neoplastic immortalization of germinal center cell lines by bcl-2 (or bcl-6) translocation.[54]

Another major type of low-grade lymphoma is *small lymphocytic* type, which shows a strong tendency to circulate as *chronic lymphocytic leukemia*. Microscopically, this is a diffuse lymphoma, but faint nodules are usually discernible, so-called proliferation centers, representing concentrations of prolymphocytes (see Plate XXII-5). This pattern is useful in recognition of this process, both in relation to accurate classification and in distinguishing this process from benign lymphocytic infiltrates.[55] The neoplastic cells are indistinguishable from benign inactive lymphocytes, featuring clumped heterochromatin and inapparent cytoplasm (see Plate XXII-6). Mitotic figures are infrequent. Immunologically, this is a homogeneous entity, with tumor cells positive for B-cell CD markers such as CD19 and CD20 and with coexpression of CD5. Surface immunoglobulin is expressed faintly. Cases with *plasmacytoid* or *plasmacytic* features correspond clinically and serologically to immunosecretory disorders such as Waldenström macroglobulinemia (see Chapter 108). Rare cases with similar microscropic features are of T-cell phenotype. These most often exhibit subtle pleomorphism with a dispersion of prolymphocytes and abundant mitotic figures, and are of helper subset T-cell phenotype. *Prolymphocytic* variants, whether B-cell or T-cell, pursue an aggressive clinical course.[56] The only T-cell neoplasms that behave as low-grade disease are the *large granular (CD8) lymphocytosis* (see Chapter 100)[57] and early (patch stage) *cutaneous T-cell lymphomas*.[58]

Newly recognized by the REAL classification is the low-grade grouping of *B-marginal zone lymphomas*, characterized microscopically by a heterogenous mixture of small round and cleaved lymphocytes, often with some plasmacytic differentiation and a component of monocytoid B-cells. Immunologically, these are B-cell neoplasms expressing heavy chain other than IgD, usually without CD5 coexpression. They can be usefully subdivided into three types clinically. Nodal marginal zone lymphomas behave as classic low-grade lymphoma,[36] splenic marginal zone lymphomas show some overlap with hairy cell disease[43] (see Chapter 99) and extranodal marginal zone (MALT) lymphomas behave unlike typical low-grade disease, remaining long localized to primary parenchymal sites for a long period of time.[40,41]

INTERMEDIATE GRADE

This grouping is extremely diverse, including lymphomas of different immunophenotype and pathobiology. Two of the Working Formulation types, diffuse small cleaved and diffuse mixed, have disappeared entirely in the REAL classification, having been distributed into various more precisely defined entities. Most lymphomas originally classified as diffuse small cleaved cell type are recognizable today as either low-grade B-marginal zone lymphomas or as intermediate grade *mantle cell lymphomas*. The latter is composed of relatively uniform small cleaved cells, coexpresses CD5 and is positive for cyclin D1 by virtue of the bcl-1 t(11;4) translocation.[36,37] Blastic variants of mantle cell lymphoma are extremely aggressive, truly high-grade neoplasms.[38]

Diffuse mixed lymphoma is only a starting point, a simple microscopic description of lymphomas, which tells the managing physician little about predicted clinical behavior.[59] Neoplasms now separately recognizable within this crude grouping include low-grade pleomorphic variants of small lymphocytic lymphoma and B-marginal zone lymphoma, intermediate grade diffuse counterparts of follicle center neoplasms, and high-grade T-cell lymphomas and so-called T-cell-rich B-cell lymphomas.[60]

Although most T-cell lymphomas are heterogenous in cellular composition, often including a rich interspersion of benign inflammatory elements recruited by T-cell lymphokines, several clinically distinctive entities have been identified in the updated REAL system.[52] These include nasal NK/T-cell (''angiocentric'') type, associated with Epstein-Barr virus (''destructive midline granuloma''); angioimmunoblastic T-cell lymphoma, usually presenting as a systemic syndrome; subcutaneous panniculitic T-cell lymphoma, with a stuttering progression of widespread skin lesions and often eventuating in a hemophagocytic syndrome; and enteropathy-type intestinal T-cell lymphoma, an extremely aggressive neoplasm often derived from preexistent gluten enteropathy.[61]

There is a continuum of clinical aggressiveness among both B-cell and T-cell lymphomas with ''diffuse mixed'' microscopic appearance, ranging from intermediate- to high-grade.[53,59] In general, a high proliferative rate, as gauged by the pathologist on the basis of frequency of mitotic figures, is a useful predictor for more aggressive behavior.[62] Large B-cell lymphomas likely to follow an intermediate grade course are those with preserved (even focally) follicular growth pattern, the more delicate cellular microscopic features of large follicle center cells (see Plate XXII-10) rather than immunoblastic features, and a relatively low mitotic rate.

HIGH-GRADE

Lymphomas with a high mitotic rate have an aggressive natural course, representing a therapeutic emergency (see Chapter 103). Since these tumors may present at early stage, prognosis is highly influenced by such evaluation.

Large B-cell lymphomas with immunoblastic features or with a high mitotic rate should be considered high-grade. Some such tumors show microscopic, immunophenotypic, genetic, and clinical features overlapping those of Burkitt lymphoma, and have been described as ''Burkitt-like.'' Large-cell lymphomas of T-cell immunophenotype usually display pleomorphic immunoblastic features. It is important to distinguish the subgrouping of *anaplastic large-cell lymphomas*, since these often behave in a more favorable way, particularly if the translocation protein product p80 or ALK-1 is expressed.[47,48] Immunostaining for CD30 reveals uniformly strong reactivity among the neoplastic cells of anaplastic large-cell lymphoma.

Burkitt lymphomas show an extremely high mitotic rate and are composed of medium sized cells with one to four prominent nucleoli and deeply basophilic cytoplasm (see Plate XXII-17). The characteristic ''starry sky'' low magnification appearance is imparted by interspersed macrophages, reflecting the high cellular turnover

of such a proliferative neoplasm (see Plate XXII-16). The Burkitt lymphoma was one of the first human neoplasms associated with a specific cytogenetic event: t(8;14), t(2;8) or t(8;22). This was subsequently shown to represent translocation of the *c-myc* oncogene on chromosome 8 to one of the immunoglobulin encoding regions on chromosome 2, 14 or 22.[63] In recent times this type of lymphoma has been associated with human immunodeficiency virus infection.[64]

Lymphoblastic lymphomas have been renamed *precursor B-cell or precursor T-cell* neoplasms in the REAL classification in recognition of their normal cell counterparts within the immune system. They may present as, or progress to acute lymphoblastic leukemia. Tumor cells have delicate nuclear chromatin and inapparent cytoplasm. The mitotic rate is moderate or high. The disease-specific marker is terminal deoxynucleotidyl transferase, an enzyme in the nucleus that plays a role in the somatic gene rearrangement that takes place in normal lymphoblasts, the basis for the diverse library of immunologically responsive lymphoid cells (see Chapter 10). This enzyme can be demonstrated by immunostains in conventional paraffin sections, allowing definitive recognition of this lymphoid neoplasm.[34,65] Accurate diagnosis of this disease entity, as distinct from other high-grade lymphomas, is critical because therapeutic regimens that are highly effective for this disease grouping differ from those designed for other aggressive lymphoma types.[66]

HODGKIN LYMPHOMA

The histologic hallmark of Hodgkin lymphoma that sets it apart from other lymphomas is the mixture of benign, reactive cells with neoplastic cells. Efforts to isolate and characterize the tumor cells have been impeded by the intimate association of these cells with reactive host inflammatory cells. The diagnosis of Hodgkin lymphoma should not be made unless bizarre, giant (Reed-Sternberg) tumor cells are present (see Plate XXII-13). To qualify, a cell must be large and have two or more nuclei (or nuclear lobes), each containing a large amphophilic or eosinophilic inclusion-like nucleolus. The presence of Reed-Sternberg cells, however, is not diagnostic of Hodgkin lymphoma, since cells with similar morphology may be present in other processes, both benign and malignant.[67]

In most cases careful evaluation of combined clinical and histopathologic findings permits their assignation to either Hodgkin or non-Hodgkin lymphoma. However, with the application of high-resolution ancillary study methods throughout the 1980s it has become clear that there is some true continuity linking these two major groupings of lymphoma. In rare cases, the features are overlapping and the diagnostic distinction cannot be made (see Fig. 101-2).[68]

The mysterious Reed-Sternberg tumor cell currently is considered to be a highly abnormal, activated lymphoid cell that expresses only a few T or B cell–associated antigens. An exception is the nodular variant of lymphocyte predominance type, which expresses a B-cell immunophenotype and, in this and other respects, should be considered an entity separate from the rest of Hodgkin lymphoma (see below)[69]. Typically, however, the Reed-Sternberg cells, and the mononuclear variant forms (''Hodgkin cells''), express CD30 (Ki-1) and CD15 (Leu-M1) antigens but not CD45 (leukocyte common) antigen.[44] These Hodgkin cells express other ''activation'' markers, including interleukin-2 receptors, transferrin receptors, and DR antigens. Recent highly sensitive molecular probe studies of single, isolated Reed-Sternberg cells indicate them to be abnormal ''crippled'' immunoblasts which are incapable of successfully producing immunoglobulin.[70,71]

TABLE 101-2   PATHOLOGIC CLASSIFICATION OF HODGKIN LYMPHOMA BASED ON THE "REAL" CLASSIFICATION OF 1994† (MODIFIED 1999)‡

NODULAR LYMPHOCYTE-PREDOMINANT HODGKIN LYMPHOMA

Classical Hodgkin Lymphoma
  Nodular sclerosis (grades I and II)
  Lymphocyte-rich
  Mixed cellularity
  Lymphocyte-depleted (includes most cases of "Hodgkin-like anaplastic
     large-cell lymphoma")

†*Blood* 1994; 84:1362[4]
‡With permission, Jaffe ES, *Modern pathology*, 1999; 12:113[52]

The original six-part classification of Lukes, Butler, and Hicks[21] has been modified in the REAL classification into a five-part system (see Table 101-2).

NODULAR LYMPHOCYTE-PREDOMINANCE HODGKIN LYMPHOMA

Lymphocyte predominance Hodgkin lymphoma, clinically the most favorable type, exhibits a very low ratio of neoplastic cells to reactive cells, and very few Reed-Sternberg cells. Variant forms of atypical cells, so-called "L and H" cells, predominate (see Plate XXII-12). These have sparse cytoplasm and delicate, mutilobed nuclei with small nucleoli. Reactive cells consist of any combination of small lymphocytes, benign epithelioid histiocytes, and occasional plasma cells. Neutrophils and eosinophils usually are not present, and necrosis is not associated with this type of disease (see Plate XXII-11). Two forms of this type are recognized in the original six-part system: the nodular and the diffuse.[21] In the diffuse type, although neoplastic cells may show some clustering, the background cellularity has a diffuse pattern, resembling a diffuse lymphoma at low magnification. Using immunostain for B-cells, some nodularity can be perceived even in these cases which initially appear diffuse in conventional stains. In the nodular type, the reactive cells of the background are massed into nodules, and the neoplastic cells are centrally located within these nodules. At low magnification, this process resembles follicular lymphoma. Indeed, large peculiar follicles, so-called progressively transformed germinal centers, often are associated with this process, and the large L and H variant cells express B-cell phenotype. These have been demonstrated to be clonal post-follicular B-cells.[70,71] The nodular variant is the most indolent of all the Hodgkin lymphoma types but has a predilection for late relapse and also for eventual development into high-grade lymphoma.[72,73]

CLASSICAL HODGKIN LYMPHOMA

In the REAL classification most types of Hodgkin lymphoma are considered "classical", in that these show many overlapping clinical, microscopic, and immunophenotypic features. Tumor cells (Reed-Sternberg and Hodgkin cells) are largely negative by immunostaining for B-cell and T-cell lymphoid markers, positive for CD30 (Ki-1) and often but not invariably positive for CD15(Leu-M1).

LYMPHOCYTE-RICH TYPE

A newly apearing term, lymphocyte-rich type connotes classical Hodgkin lymphoma in which tumor giant cells are relatively sparse in an inflammatory background which is predominately lymphocytic.[74] The distinction from nodular lymphocyte predominance Hodgkin lymphoma on the basis of conventional microscopy can be difficult

or impossible.[75] Immunostains are necessary to ascertain the nature of the tumor cells, i.e., whether B-cell or as in classical Hodgkin lymphoma.

MIXED CELLULARITY TYPE

Mixed cellularity type Hodgkin lymphoma contains an intermediate ratio of neoplastic cells to reactive cells. Usually, though not always, Reed-Sternberg cells are identified readily, and mononuclear variant forms of Reed-Sternberg cells are abundant (see Plate XXII-13). Reactive cells consist of any combination of lymphocytes, histiocytes, plasma cells, neutrophils, or eosinophils. A mixed background of reactive cells need not be present. There may be suppuration and necrosis. Recent studies suggest a strong association between mixed cellularity type and Epstein-Barr virus.[76]

LYMPHOCYTE DEPLETION TYPE

Lymphocytic depletion Hodgkin lymphoma is the least favorable type clinically. The more common reticular form has a high ratio of neoplastic cells to reactive cells, and extremely large, bizarre, malignant giant cells are often present. With the advent of specific cell lineage markers, many cases previously considered reticular lymphocytic depletion Hodgkin lymphoma actually have proved to be anaplastic large-cell lymphomas. The diagnosis is very uncommon and is effectively one of exclusion. The distinction of reticular variant lymphocyte depletion Hodgkin lymphoma from anaplastic large cell lymphoma is, at most, a very subtle one.[78] The diffuse fibrosis variant is rare but diagnostically less controversial than the reticular variant. A hypocellular process replaces involved tissues with nonbirefrigent precollagen matrix, scant inflammatory cells, and rare diagnostic Reed-Sternberg cells.

NODULAR SCLEROSIS TYPE

Nodular sclerosis Hodgkin lymphoma is distinctive clinically and pathologically. Young adult females are most commonly affected and there is strong predilection for disease involving the anterior mediastinum (see Chap. 102). Part of the reactive background includes fibrosis emanating from the capsule and connective tissue trabecula. This response begins with the formation of granulation tissue and progresses to the formation of dense bands of hyaline fibrosis that encircle nodules of cells (see Plate XXII-14). Within these nodules is a mixture of reactive and neoplastic cells, and the proportion may range from "lymphocyte predominance" to "lymphocyte depletion," a finding that apparently does have slight predictive value.[79] Reed-Sternberg cells may be present, but more often only lacunar cell variants are evident on which to base the diagnosis. Lacunar cells contain abundant clear cytoplasm that retracts from the surrounding lymphocytes upon fixation with formalin, producing a space, or lacuna. These bizarre cells contain many nuclear lobes, sometimes in a circular or semicircular array at the cell margin and sometimes clustered centrally, each containing a small nucleolus (see Plate XXII-15). Lymph nodes with very early involvement by nodular sclerosing disease do not exhibit capsular or trabecular fibrosis but rather show only nodules with central clusters of lacunar cells. Such a pattern has been described as a "cellular" or "presclerotic" phase of the disease.

PRACTICAL CONSIDERATIONS FOR DIAGNOSIS

Pathologists should interpret a lymph node biopsy in a way that provides answers to the following questions: Is the process an orderly immune response? Are there features that suggest a specific cause, for example, an infection? Is there evidence of neoplasia, and, if

TABLE 101-3 ANCILLARY SPECIAL STUDIES FOR LYMPH NODE INTERPRETATION

METHOD	APPLICATIONS	PRACTICALITY
Paraffin immunostains[65,81]	Exclusion of other malignancies stimulating lymphoma, clonality of Ig light chains in some (plasmacytic) processes	Most practical, conventional processing only, fast convenient, (fixation critical)
Frozen section immunostains[82]	Definitive phenotyping, even surface Ig detected, all antigens preserved	Fast, convenient, but frozen tissue must be allocated
Air-dried imprint immunostains[65]	Cytomorphology ideal with individual cell localization of antigens	No tissue consumed, fast, inexpensive; however, obscured by plasma proteins
Genetic probe analysis[83]	Highly sensitive, for clonality (T- and B-cell), for DNA, RNA markers of oncogenes, virsus, etc.	Tissue requirements simple, frozen tissue in small amounts, time-consuming, expensive
Automated cytometry[84,85]	Quantitative analysis of cell populations, Ig light-chain comparison, phenotyping, DNA histograms	Very rapid for phenotyping, fresh tissue expended, inferential, only cells attaining suspension studied
Cytogenetics[86]	Clonality, marker chromosomal abnormalities for evidence of neoplasia, in some instances useful for classification	Fastidious, fresh (sterile) tissue needed, time-consuming, expensive
Kinetics[62]	Proliferative activity of (neoplastic) processess	Diversity of methods, most requiring very fresh tissue, clinical utility unproved except in plasma cell disease

so, is it lymphoid in origin?[80] And what are the implications for the therapist?

Effective study of lymph node biopsy specimens requires careful tissue sampling and processing. In consultation with the hematologist and pathologist, the surgeon should biopsy the largest and most pathologically involved lymph nodes. The pathologist should monitor the laboratory's methods to assure that good-quality conventional slides are made and that adequate tissue samples are allocated for special studies (Table 101-3).[65,81]

Reactive hyperplastic lymph nodes may contain clues to the pathogenesis of the lymphadenopathy.[87] Certain infectious agents, such as *Toxoplasma gondii* and the cat-scratch bacillus, elicit specific cellular responses. Other clinicopathologic entities, such as angiofollicular lymph node hyperplasia (Castleman disease) and sinus histiocytosis with massive lymphadenopathy (Rosai-Dorfman disease), can be identified but are of unknown etiology.[88,89]

The most important task for the pathologist is to distinguish benign from malignant proliferations.[80] Hyperplasia can exhibit features that suggest neoplasia, e.g., extreme cellular pleomorphism, abundant mitotic activity, and cellular atypia. On the other hand, lymphoid neoplasia can be difficult to recognize when there is only early, partial involvement of a lymph node or when the neoplasm is composed of small, mitotically inactive cells. The diagnosis of malignancy can be made confidently if the normal functional components of a lymph node are totally replaced by a process of uniform cellular composition (see Plate XXII-5) or if cytomorphologic study reveals features of atypia beyond the limits of reactive lymphoid or histiocytic response.

In some instances ancillary studies must be applied to achieve a definitive diagnosis. Frozen section immunostaining for immunoglobulin light chains is a practical and decisive means of distinguishing low-grade B-cell lymphoma (follicular or small lymphocytic) from hyperplasia.[82] In cases of T-cell proliferation, even detailed immunophenotyping often fails to provide direct evidence of malignancy, and cytogenetics or gene probe studies may be necessary to prove the presence of a monoclonal (neoplastic) process (see Table 101-3).[83]

Even with sophisticated methodology, the pathologist should be circumspect, since in exceptional situations monoclonality is not equivalent to clinical malignancy, for example, the salivary gland lesions in Sjogren syndrome[90] or the bizarre cellular infiltrate in lymphomatoid papulosis.[91]

Exceptionally strong immune stimuli, especially in patients with primary or induced immunodeficiency, can elicit cellular responses in nodal or tonsillar tissues so atypical in appearance as to simulate neoplasm.[80,92] In some cases, such processes may progress eventually to actual lymphoma.[93]

Even when a lymph node obviously is effaced by malignancy, there is potential for diagnostic error. Anaplastic malignancies converge in histomorphologic appearance, so that high-grade lymphomas, in particular, are closely simulated by other neoplasms, such as granulocytic sarcoma (myeloblastoma) and anaplastic carcinoma. Special methods, including immunophenotyping, histochemistry (chloroacetate esterase for granulocytic differentiation), electron microscopy (for subtle features of epithelial differentiation), and immunostaining, may be required to determine cellular origin.[65,80] Since these distinctions are crucial for clinical management, sometimes rebiopsy specifically for ancillary studies is necessary.

REFERENCES

1. Lennert K: *Histopathology of Non-Hodgkin's Lymphomas (Based on the Kiel Classification)*. Springer, New York, 1981.
2. Lukes RJ: The immunologic approach to the pathology of malignant lymphomas. *Am J Clin Pathol* 72:657, 1979.
3. Aster J, Kumar V: White cells, lymph nodes, spleen, and thymus, in *Pathologic Basis of Disease*, Sixth Edition, edited by RS Cotran, V Kumar, T Collins, pp. 651-675. Saunders, Philadelphia, 1999.
4. Harris NL, Jaffe ES, Stein H, Banks PM, Chan KC, et al. A revised European-American classification of lymphoid neoplasms: A proposal from the International Lymphoma Study Group. *Blood* 84:1361,1994.
5. Hodgkin T: On some morbid appearances of the absorbent glands and spleen. *Trans Med Chir Soc Lond* 17:68, 1832.
6. Virchow R: Weisses Blut and Milztumoren. *Med Zgt Berlin* 15:157, 1846.
7. Virchow R: *Die Cellularpathologie in ihrer Begrundung auf Physiologische und Pathologische Gewebelehr*. Hirschwald, Berlin, 1858.
8. Virchow R: *Die Krankhaften Geschwulste*. Hirschwald, Berlin, 1863.
9. Billroth T: Multiple Lymphome: Erfolgreiche Behandlung mit Arsenik. *Wien Med Wochenschr* 21:1066, 1871.
10. Wilks S: Cases of enlargement of the lymphatic glands and spleen (or Hodgkin's disease). *Guys Hosp Rep* 11:56, 1865.
11. Sternberg C: Über eine Eigenartige unter dem Bilde der Pseudoleukämie verlaufende Tuberculose des lymphatischen Apparates. *Z Heilk* 19:21, 1898.
12. Reed DM: On the pathologic changes in Hodgkin's disease, with especial reference to its relation to tuberculosis. *Johns Hopkins Hosp Rep* 10:133, 1902.
13. Ghon A, Roman B: Über das Lymphosarkom. *Frankfurt Z Pathol* 19:1, 1916.
14. Brill NE, Baehr G, Rosenthal N: Generalized giant lymph follicle hyperplasia of lymph nodes and spleen: A hitherto undescribed type. *JAMA* 84:668, 1925.
15. Symmers D: Follicular lymphadenopathy with splenomegaly: A newly recognized disease of the lymphatic system. *Arch Pathol* 3:816, 1927.
16. Symmers D: Giant follicular lymphadenopathy with or without splenomegaly: Its transformation into polymorphous cell sarcoma of the lymph

follicles and its association with Hodgkin's disease, lymphatic leukemia and an apparently unique disease of the lymph nodes and spleen—a disease entity believed heretofore undescribed. *Arch Pathol* 26:603, 1938.

17. Roulet F: Das primäre Retothelsarkom der Lymphknoten. *Virchows Arch (Pathol Anat)* 227:15, 1930.

18. Gall EA: Enigmas in lymphoma: Reticulum cell sarcoma and mycosis fungoides. *Minn Med* 38:674, 1955.

19. Cooke JV: Mediastinal tumor in acute leukemia: A clinical and roentgenologic study. *Am J Dis Child* 44:1153, 1932.

20. Jackson H Jr, Parker F Jr: *Hodgkin's Disease and Allied Disorders*, p 17. Oxford, New York, 1947.

21. Lukes RJ, Butler JJ, Hicks EB: Natural history of Hodgkin's disease as related to its pathologic picture. *Cancer* 19:317, 1966.

22. Rappaport H, Winter WJ, Hicks EB: Follicular lymphoma: A reevaluation of its position in the scheme of malignant lymphoma, based on a survey of 253 cases. *Cancer* 9:792, 1956.

23. Gall EA, Mallory TB: Malignant lymphoma: A clinicopathologic survey of 618 cases. *Am J Pathol* 18:381, 1942.

24. Gall EA, Rappaport H: Seminar on diseases of lymph nodes and spleen, in *Proceedings of the 23rd Seminar of the American Society of Clinical Pathologists*, edited by JR McDonald. American Society of Clinical Pathologists, Chicago, 1958.

25. Rappaport H: Tumors of the hematopoietic system, in *Atlas of Tumor Pathology, sec* III, fasc 8. Armed Forces Institute of Pathology, Washington, DC, 1966.

26. Rosenberg SA: Non-Hodgkin's lymphoma—selection of treatment on the basis of histologic type. *N Engl J Med* 301:924, 1979.

27. The Non-Hodgkin's Lymphoma Pathologic Classification Group: NCI-sponsored study of classifications of non-Hodgkin's lymphomas: Summary and description of a working formulation for clinical usage. *Cancer* 49:2112, 1982.

28. Lennert K: Classification of malignant lymphomas (European concept), in *Progress in Lymphology*, edited by A Ruttimann, p 103. Thieme, Stuttgart, 1967.

29. Stein H, Lennert K, Parwaresch MR: Malignant lymphomas of B-cell type. *Lancet* 2:855, 1972.

30. Foon KA, Todd RF III: Immunologic classifications of leukemia and lymphoma. *Blood* 68:1, 1986.

31. Wilson MS, Weiss LM, Gatter KC, et al: Malignant histiocytosis: A reassessment of cases previously reported in 1975 based on paraffin section immunophenotyping studies. *Cancer* 66:530, 1990.

32. Lennert K, Niedorf HR: Nachweis von desmosomal verknupften Reticulumzellen in follikularen Lymphoma (Brill Symmers). *Virchows Arch (Cell Pathol)* 4:148, 1969.

33. Jaffe ES, Shevach EM, Frank MM, et al: Nodular lymphoma—evidence for origin from follicular B lymphocytes. *N Engl J Med* 290:813, 1974.

34. Cossman J, Chused TM, Fisher RI, et al: Diversity of immunological phenotypes of lymphoblastic lymphoma. *Cancer Res* 43:4486, 1983.

35. Smith JL, Clein GP, Barker CR, Collins RD: Characterization of malignant mediastinal lymphoid neoplasm (Sternberg sarcoma) as thymic in origin. *Lancet* 1:74, 1973.

36. Fisher RI, Dahlberg S, Nathwani BN, Banks PM, Miller TP, and Grogan TM: A clinical analysis of two indolent lyphoma entities: Mantle cell lymphoma and marginal zone lymphoma (including the mucosa-associated lymphoid tissue and monocytoid B-cell subcategories): A Southwest Oncology Group Study. *Blood* Vol 85(4):1075-1082, 1995.

37. Weisenburger DD, Armitage JO: Mantle cell lymphoma—An entity comes of age. *Blood* 87:4483, 1996.

38. Argatoff LH, Connors JM, Klasa RJ, Horsman DE, and Gascoyne RD: Mantle cell lymphoma: A clinicopathologic study of 80 cases. *Blood* 89:2067, 1997.

39. Triozzi PL, Borowitz MJ, Gockerman JP: Gastro-intestinal involvement and multiple lymphomatous polyposis in mantle zone lymphoma. *J Clin Oncol* 4:866, 1986.

40. Pelstring RJ, Essell JH, Kurtin PJ, et al: Diversity of organ site involvement among malignant lymphomas of mucosa-associated tissues. *Am J Clin Pathol* 96:738, 1991.

41. Banks PM, Isaacson PG: MALT lymphomas in 1997—Where do we stand? *Am J Clin Pathol* Vol 111(Suppl 1):S75, 1999.

42. Blanco R, Lyda M, Davis B, Kraus M, and Fenoglio-Preiser C: Trisomy 3 in gastric lymphomas of extranodal marginal zone B-cell (mucosa-

associated lymphoid tissue)–Origin demonstrated by FISH in intact paraffin sections. *Hum Pathol* 30:706, 1999.

43. Matutes E, Morilla R, Owusu-Ankomah K, Houliham A, Meeus P and Catovsky D: The immunophenotype of hairy cell leukemia (HCL). Proposal for a scoring system to distinguish HCL from B-cell disorders with hairy or villous lymphocytes. *Leuk Lymphoma* 14:57, 1994.

44. Banks PM: The pathology of Hodgkin's disease. *Semin Oncol* 4:866, 1990.

45. Banks PM: Newly recognized variant forms of non-Hodgkin's lymphomas. *Hematol Oncol Clin North Am* 5:935, 1991.

46. Flynn KJ, Dehner LP, Gajl-Peczalska KJ, et al: Regressing atypical histiocytosis: A cutaneous proliferation of atypical neoplastic histiocytes with unexpectedly indolent biologic behavior. *Cancer* 49:959, 1982.

47. Gascoyne RD, Aoun PA, Wu D, Chhanabhai M, Skinnider BF, et al. Prognostic significance of anaplastic lymphoma kinase (ALK) protein expression in adults with anaplastic large cell lymphoma. *Blood* 93:3913,1999.

48. Benharroch D, Meguerian-Bedoyan Z, Lamant L, Amin C, Brugleres, et al. ALK-Positive lymphoma: A single disease with a broad spectrum of morphology. *Blood* 91:2076, 1998.

49. Blattner WA, Blayney DW, Robert-Guroff M, et al: Epidemiology of human T-cell leukemia/lymphoma virus (HTLV). *J Infect Dis* 147:406, 1983.

50. Bunn PA, Schechter GP, Jaffe ES, et al: Retrovirus-associated adult T-cell lymphoma in the United States: Staging, evaluation, and management. *N Engl J Med* 309:257, 1983.

51. Banks PM: Changes in diagnosis of non-Hodgkin's lymphomas over time. *Cancer Res (suppl)* 52:5453s, 1992.

52. Jaffe ES. Hematopathology—Integration of morphologic features and biologic markers for diagnosis. *Mod Pathol* 12:109, 1999.

53. A Clinical Evaluation of the International Lymphoma Study Group Classification of Non-Hodgkin's Lymphoma. By the Non-Hodgkin's Lymphoma Classification Project. *Blood* 89:3909, 1997.

54. Gribben JG, Freedman AS, Woo SD, et al: All advanced stage non-Hodgkin's lymphomas with a polymerase chain reaction amplifiable breakpoint of *bcl-2* have residual cells containing the *bcl-2* rearrangement at evaluation and after treatment. *Blood* 78:3275, 1991.

55. Ellison DJ, Nathwani BN, Cho SY, Martin SE: Interfollicular small lymphocytic lymphoma: The diagnostic significance of pseudofollicles. *Hum Pathol* 20:1108, 1989.

56. Witzig TE, Phyliky RL, Li C-Y, Homburger HA: T-cell chronic lymphocytic leukemia with a helper/inducer membrane phenotype: A distinct clinicopathologic entity with a poor prognosis. *Am J Hematol* 21:139, 1988.

57. Aisenberg AC, Krontiris TG, Mak TW, Wilkes BM: Rearrangement of the gene for the beta chain of the T-cell receptor in T-cell chronic lymphocytic leukemia and related disorders. *N Engl J Med* 313:529, 1985.

58. Diamandidou E, Cohen PR, and Kurzrock R. Mycosis fungoides and sezary syndrome. *Blood* 88:2385, 1996.

59. Foucar K, Armitage JO, and Dick FR. Malignant lymphoma, diffuse mixed small and large cell—A clinicopathologic study of 47 cases. *Cancer* 51:2090, 1983.

60. Krishman J, Wallberg K, and Frizzera G. T-Cell rich large B-cell lymphoma—A study of 30 cases, supporting its histologic heterogeneity and lack of clinical distinctiveness. *Am J Surg Pathol* 18:455, 1994.

61. Badgi E, Diss TC, Munson P, and Isaacson PG. Mucosal intra-epithelial lymphocytes in enteropathy-associated T-cell lymphoma, ulcerative jejunitis, and refractory celiac disease constitute a neoplastic population. *Blood* 94:260, 1999.

62. Miller TP, Grogan TM, Dahlberg S, Spier CM, Braziel RM, Banks PM et al. Prognostic significance of the Ki-67-associated proliferative antigen in aggressive non-Hodgkin's lymphomas—A prospective Southwest Oncology Group trial. *Blood* 83:1460, 1994.

63. Yano T, van Krieken HJM, Magrath IT, et al: Histogenetic correlations between subcategories of small non-cleaved cell lymphomas. *Blood* 79:1282, 1992.

64. Levine AM: Acquired immunodeficiency syndrome-related lymphoma. *Blood* 80:8, 1992.

65. Banks PM: Technical factors in the preparation and evaluation of lymph node biopsies, in *Neoplastic Hematopathology*, edited by DM Knowles, p 367. Williams & Wilkins, Baltimore, 1992.

66. Wilson JF, Jenkin RDT, Anderson JR, et al: Studies on the pathology of non-Hodgkin's lymphoma of childhood. *Cancer* 53:1695, 1984.

67. Strum SB, Park JK, Rappaport H: Observation of cells resembling Sternberg-Reed cells in conditions other than Hodgkin's disease. *Cancer* 26:176, 1970.

68. Banks PM: The distinction of Hodgkin's disease from T cell lymphoma. *Semin Diagn Pathol* 9:279, 1992.

69. Mason DY, Banks PM, Chan J, et al: Nodular lymphocyte predominance Hodgkin's disease: A distinct clinicopathological entity. *Am J Surg Pathol* 18:526, 1994.

70. Kanzler H, Küppers R, Hansmann ML, and Rajewsky K. Hodgkin and Reed-Sternberg cells in Hodgkin's disease represent the outgrowth of a dominant tumor clone derived from (crippled) germinal center B cells. *J Exp Med* 184:1, 1996.

71. Bräuninger A, Hansmann ML, Strickler JG, Dummer R, Burg G, Jajewsky K, and Küppers R. Identification of common germinal-center B-cell precursors in two patients with both Hodgkin's disease and non-Hodgkin's lymphoma. *N Eng J Med* 340:1239, 1999.

72. Regula DP Jr, Hoppe RT, Weiss LM: Nodular and diffuse types of lymphocyte predominance Hodgkin's disease. *N Engl J Med* 318:214, 1988.

73. Sundeen JT, Cossman J, Jaffe ES: Lymphocyte predominant Hodgkin's disease nodular subtype with coexistent ''large cell lymphoma'': Histological progression or composite malignancy? *Am J Surg Pathol* 12:599, 1988.

74. Harris NL. Hodgkin's disease: Classification and differential diagnosis. *Mod Pathol* 12:159, 1999.

75. Diehl V, Stein H, Sextro M, et al. Lymphocyte-predominant Hodgkin's disease: A European Task Force on Lymphoma project [abstract]. *Blood* 88:294a, 1996.

76. Delsol G, Brousset P, Chittal S, Rigal-Huguet F: Correlation of the expression of Epstein-Barr virus latent membrane protein and in situ hybridization with biotinylated BamH1-W probes in Hodgkin's disease. *Am J Pathol* 140:247, 1992.

77. Weiss LM, Lopategui JR, Sun LH, Kamel OW, Koo CH, and Glackin C. Absence of the t(2;5) in Hodgkin's disease. *Blood* 85:2845, 1995.

78. Zellers RA, Thibodeau SN, Banks PM: Primary splenic lymphocyte-depletion Hodgkin's disease. *Am J Clin Pathol* 94:453, 1990.

79. Ferry J, Linggood R, Convery K, Efrid J, Eliseo R, Harris N. Hodgkin's disease, nodular sclerosis type: Implications of histologic subclassification. *Cancer* 71:457, 1993.

80. Banks PM. Microscopic mimicry of lymphomas: Diagnostic pitfalls. *Mod Pathol* 12:116, 1999.

81. Collins RD: Lymph node examination: What is an adequate workup? *Arch Pathol Lab Med* 109:797, 1985.

82. Harris NL, Data RE: The distribution of neoplastic and normal B-lymphoid cells in nodular lymphomas. *Hum Pathol* 13:610, 1982.

83. Gill JI, and Gulley ML. Immunoglobulin and T-cell receptor gene rearrangement. *Hematol Oncol Clin N Am* 8:751, 1994.

84. Witzig TE, Banks PM, Stenson MJ, Griepp PR, Katzmann JA, Habermann TM, et al. Rapid immunophenotyping of B-cell non-Hodgkin's lymphomas by flow cytometry—A comparison with the standard frozen section method. *Am J Clin Pathol* 94:280, 1990.

85. Jennings CD and Foon KA. Recent advances in flow cytometry: Application to the diagnosis of hematologic malignancy. *Blood* 90:2863, 1997.

86. Inwards DJ, Habermann TM, Banks PM, et al: Cytogenetic findings in 21 cases of peripheral T-cell lymphoma. *Am J Hematol* 35:88, 1990.

87. Chan JKC, Tsang WYW. Reactive lymphadenopathies in Pathology of Lymph Nodes. Edited by LM Weiss, pp. 81-168, Churchill Livingstone, New York, 1996.

88. Menke DM, Camoriano JK, Banks PM: Angiofollicular lymph node hyperplasia: A comparison of unicentric, multicentric, hyaline vascular, and plasma cell types of disease by morphometric and clinical analysis. *Mod Pathol* 5:525, 1992.

89. Rosai J, Dorfman RF: Sinus histiocytosis with massive lymphadenopathy: A newly recognized benign clinicopathological entity. *Arch Pathol* 87:63, 1969.

90. Collins RD. Is clonality equivalent to malignancy: Specifically, is immunoglobulin gene rearrangement diagnostic of malignant lymphoma? *Hum Pathol* 28:757, 1997.

91. Weiss LM, Wood GS, Trela M, et al: Clonal T-cell populations in lymphomatoid papulosis. *N Engl J Med* 315:475, 1986.

92. Craig F, Gulley M, Banks PM: Post-transplantation lymphoproliferative disorders. *Am J Clin Pathol* 99:265, 1993.

93. Knowles DM. Immunodeficiency-associated lymphoproliferative disorders. *Mod Pathol* 12:200, 1999.

HODGKIN LYMPHOMA

SANDRA J. HORNING

Hodgkin lymphoma is a neoplasm of lymphoid tissue defined by the presence of the malignant Reed-Sternberg and Hodgkin cells (RS-H) with an appropriate cellular background. Four histologic types (lymphocyte predominance, nodular sclerosis, mixed cellularity, and lymphocyte depletion) are distinguished on the basis of the appearance and relative proportions of RS-H cells, lymphocytes, and fibrosis. The anatomic extent of disease and, to a lesser degree, the histologic subtype are the primary factors determining the presenting features, prognosis, and optimal therapy of Hodgkin lymphoma.

The goal of treatment is to cure the greatest number of patients with minimal complications. Outstanding results have been achieved by combining radiotherapy and chemotherapy, each of which are independently effective in Hodgkin lymphoma, with ongoing efforts to minimize cumulative exposure to each modality. This chapter discusses both modalities and their application to presentations of Hodgkin lymphoma at diagnosis and upon relapse, as well as the complications of treatment.

DEFINITION AND HISTORY

In his historic 1832 paper entitled "On Some Morbid Appearances of the Absorbent Glands and Spleen," Thomas Hodgkin described the clinical histories and gross postmortem findings of seven cases of the disease that was later to bear his name.[1] In 1856 Samuel Wilks independently described 10 cases of "a peculiar enlargement of the lymphatic glands frequently associated with disease of the spleen," including four of Hodgkin's original cases.[2] Upon discovering Hodgkin's original report, he used the appellation "Hodgkin's Disease" in a subsequent series of 15 cases published in 1865.[3]

Thirteen years after Hodgkin's original paper, Craigie,[4] Bennett,[5] and Virchow[6] described the first cases of leukemia. Cases in which the neoplastic cells remained confined to the lymphatic system were described by Dreschfield (1892)[7] and Kundrat (1893)[8]; the latter gave the name *lymphosarcoma* to these cases. The description of additional members of the lymphoma-leukemia complex has continued throughout the twentieth century up to the present time.

Carl Sternberg (1898)[9] and Dorothy Reed (1902)[10] are credited with the first definitive and thorough descriptions of Hodgkin lymphoma, although a number of investigators from England, Germany, and France had previously recognized the characteristic multinucleated giant cells. In 1926 Fox examined microscopic sections from the gross specimens preserved in the Gordon Museum of Guy's Hospital in London of three of Hodgkin's original cases.[11] It is remarkable that the preserved microanatomy allowed him to confirm the histopathologic diagnosis in two of these cases. Jackson and Parker made the first serious effort at histopathologic classification, correlating their findings with prognosis.[12] A second advance was made in 1966 when Lukes, Butler, and Hicks proposed a classification that related well to clinical presentation and course.[13] Their proposal was slightly modified into the Rye classification, in which four histopathologic subtypes were described: lymphocyte predominance, nodular sclerosis, mixed cellularity, and lymphocyte depletion. The new proposed World Health Organization classification of lymphoid neoplasms (1999) specifically recognizes Hodgkin lymphoma as a lymphoma and clearly delineates the nodular lymphocyte predominance subtype from classical Hodgkin lymphoma. A new category of "lymphocyte-rich" classical Hodgkin lymphoma is introduced (Table 102-1).

Peters described a clinical staging system in 1950, emphasizing the diagnostic evaluation of the anatomic extent of disease.[14,15] In 1952 Kinmouth introduced lower-extremity lymphangiography, which allowed roentgenologic visualization of the pelvic and retroperitoneal lymph nodes and was found to be far more sensitive than palpation or other radiographic methods.[16] The frequency of unsuspected splenic involvement was revealed in a group of 65 patients subjected to laparotomy and splenectomy with biopsy of splenic hilar, para-aortic and mesenteric nodes, and liver at Stanford University.[17] These diagnostic procedures led to improved understanding of the mode of dissemination of disease and correlated well with prognosis, culminating in the modern concepts of staging codified at the Rye, New York conference in 1965[18] and further refined at the workshop on the staging of Hodgkin disease in Ann Arbor, Michigan, in 1971.[19]

Pusey (1902)[20] and Senn (1903)[21] were the first to report dramatic regressions of lymphadenopathy with the x-rays newly discovered by Roentgen in 1896. Based upon the nearly inevitable appearance of recurrences in untreated areas, Gilbert proposed the systematic treatment of both involved and uninvolved areas in 1939.[22] Peters (1950) is given credit for the first demonstration of the curative potential of radiotherapy in her classic paper.[14] The development of megavoltage radiotherapy (doses >4000 cGy), as reported by Kaplan in 1962,[23] permitted the delivery of tumoricidal doses to virtually all lymphoid regions in the body within acceptable limits of normal tissue tolerance.

The chemotherapy of Hodgkin lymphoma originated as a by-product of the wartime work on the mustard gases.[24,25] Following the initial work with the nitrogen mustards, antimetabolites were synthesized, and a number of alkaloids and antibiotics extracted from various plant, fungus, and microbial sources became available for clinical use. DeVita and colleagues introduced the first highly effective combination chemotherapy, "MOPP" (nitrogen mustard, vincristine, procarbazine, prednisone), based on experimental studies indicating the desirability of combining agents with nonoverlapping toxicities.[26] Combination chemotherapy extended the curative potential to advanced disease.

ETIOLOGY AND PATHOGENESIS

Difficulty in the characterization of the neoplastic cells, which account for only about 1 to 2 percent of the cellular composition, led to controversy regarding the etiology and pathogenesis of Hodgkin

TABLE 102-1   WORLD HEALTH ORGANIZATION CLASSIFICATION OF
HODGKIN LYMPHOMA

Nodular lymphocyte predominant Hodgkin lymphoma
Classic Hodgkin lymphoma
    Lymphocyte-rich
    Nodular sclerosis (grades I and II)
    Mixed cellularity
    Lymphocyte depletion

lymphoma for more than 150 years. New techniques affording molecular analyses of single cells have facilitated the study.

ORIGIN OF THE REED-STERNBERG CELL

The histologic diagnosis is based on the recognition of the Reed-Sternberg cell in an appropriate cellular background. The classic Reed-Sternberg cell has a bilobed nucleus with prominent eosinophilic nucleoli separated by a clear space from the thickened nuclear membrane (Fig. 102-1). Mononuclear variants (Hodgkin cells) have similar

nuclear characteristics and may represent Reed-Sternberg cells cut in a plane that shows only one lobe of the nucleus. Reed-Sternberg cells are not pathognomonic for Hodgkin lymphoma; they may be seen in reactive and other neoplastic conditions. Study of the Reed-Sternberg cell has been complicated by the fact that the neoplastic cells are sparsely interspersed among a reactive mixed cell population of lymphocytes, eosinophils, histiocytes, plasma cells, and neutrophils.

IMMUNOHISTOCHEMISTRY

Reed-Sternberg cells and their mononuclear variants (RS-H) demonstrate inconsistent lineage-specific antigen expression. Approximately 85 percent of cases of nodular sclerosis and mixed cellularity express the CD30 antigen (Ki-1), which was identified by Stein and colleagues.[27] This antigen is a marker of lymphocyte activation and is expressed by both reactive and neoplastic lymphoid cells, including a number of non-Hodgkin lymphomas.[28,29] The majority of RS-H cells in classic Hodgkin lymphoma express the CD15 antigen, which is characteristically expressed in the late stages of granulopoiesis.[30,31] However, CD15 expression is not limited to granulocytes and monocytes; it has been identified in activated T cells and cytomegalovirus-

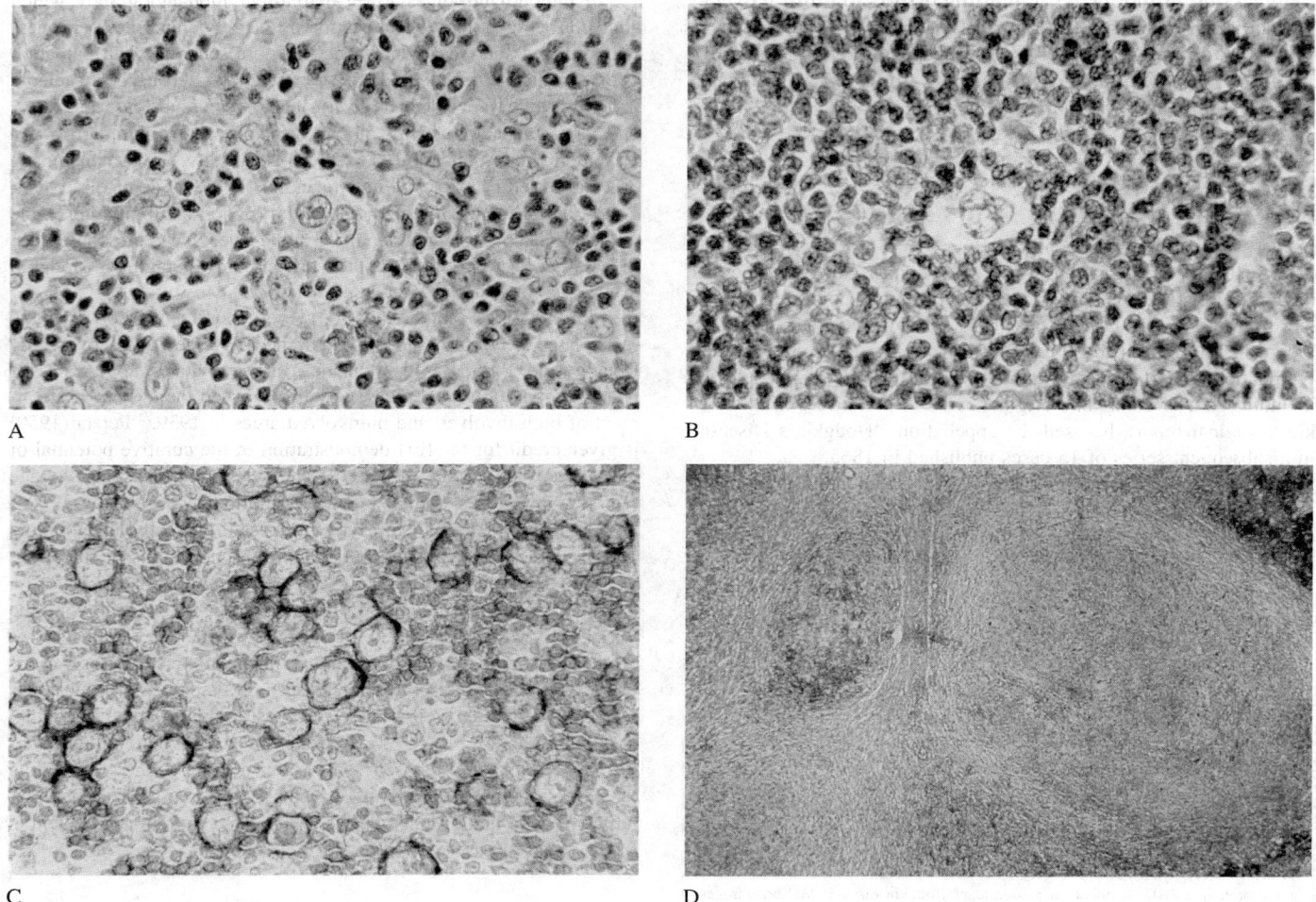

FIGURE 102-1   (*a*) Characteristic Reed-Sternberg cell of Hodgkin disease and surrounding mononuclear variants. (*b*) Lymphocyte and histiocyte (L&H) variant of the nodular form of lymphocyte predominance. (The ''histiocyte'' may actually be a lymphocyte.) Note the multilobulated ''popcorn'' nucleus and surrounding small lymphocytes. (*c*) Immunoperoxidase staining of the L & H variant of the nodular form of lymphocyte predominance with the L26 antibody directed against a pan-B-cell antigen (CD20) outlines the large atypical cells. (*d*) Low-power view of nodular sclerosis, demonstrating broad bands of collagen partitioning the lymph node into nodules.

infected cells as well as nonlymphoid cells.[32–34] Most RS-H cells express the interleukin 2 receptor, (CD25 or Tac), characteristic of activated T cells.[35] The B-cell antigens CD19 and CD20 are expressed by RS-H cells in about 35 to 40 percent of nodular sclerosis and mixed cellularity cases.[36–39]

Immunohistochemical analysis of Hodgkin lymphoma provides evidence that nodular lymphocyte predominance (LPHD) is a distinctive subtype. The RS-H cells in this subtype, known as *lymphocyte and histiocyte* (L&H) variants, have a unique polylobated, "popcorn" appearance, and they consistently express B-cell markers such as CD20 and CD45 (leukocyte common antigen)[40] (Figure 102-1B). They lack expression of CD15 and have variable expression of CD30.[41] The synthesis of cytoplasmic J chain and immunoglobulin also indicates the B-cell origin of this subtype.[42] Although most investigators describe polyclonal staining for light chains, others have reported light-chain restriction.[43,44]

The new category of lymphocyte-rich Hodgkin lymphoma requires immunohistochemistry for diagnosis. As in nodular lymphocyte predominance, the majority of cells are small B lymphocytes, and a nodular or follicular pattern may be seen. The RS-H cells express CD15 and CD30, lack CD45, and may or may not express CD20. Thus, although the morphologic features of the lymphocyte-rich subtype may be confused with lymphocyte predominance, the immunophenotype of the RS-H cells is that of classical Hodgkin lymphoma.

Historically, a macrophage origin of RS-H cells was postulated by the presence of polyclonal immunoglobulins in the cytoplasm, the expression of HLA-DR (Ia), and the presence of natural sugar receptors detected by lectins such as peanut agglutinin (PNA-binding).[45,46] The interdigitating reticulum cell or T-zone macrophage was proposed as the cell of origin because, like RS-H cells, this cell expresses CD15, HLA-DR, the transferrin receptor, intercellular adhesion molecule-1 (ICAM-1), or CD54, and forms spontaneous T-cell rosettes.[47,48] Molecular analyses of single cells indicate that RS-H cells largely represent clonal populations, as discussed below.

LYMPHOCYTE ANTIGEN RECEPTOR GENE STUDIES

Because the configuration of antigen receptor genes is a reliable clonal marker of the B-cell lymphomas, these genes were studied for clues to the etiology of Hodgkin lymphoma. However, it was more challenging to detect clonal populations in Hodgkin lymphoma, since RS-H cells comprise less than 1 to 2 percent of the total cell population, the limit of detection for the DNA hybridization methods used in most studies. The majority of studies in unselected cases demonstrated a germline configuration of antigen receptor genes.[49–53] Clonal immunoglobulin heavy-chain and light-chain rearrangements were reported in cases selected for a larger proportion of RS-H cells or enrichment for these cells in vitro, but *clonality* was not confirmed by others.[51,53,54]

In 1994, RS-H cells were isolated by micromanipulation of histologic sections of three cases of Hodgkin lymphoma and individual cells analyzed for immunoglobulin variable gene rearrangements by polymerase chain reaction (PCR).[55] In each case a single variable gene rearrangement was amplified, indicative of a single clone. In 1997 evidence was found for clonal gene rearrangements in 13 of 14 cases.[56] The rearranged V_H genes carried extensive somatic mutations, indicating a germinal center origin. The presence of stop codons in some RS-H cells has led to the hypothesis that these cells have acquired crippling mutations that prevent antigen selection but escape apoptosis through some transforming event.[57] Of considerable interest with regard to possible mechanisms of escape, constitutive expression of the nuclear transcription factor NFκB has been found in R-SH cells, and inactivation of NFκB in cell lines restored sensitivity to apoptosis.[58] The lost capacity to express functional antigen receptor may be due

to mutations in the untranslated regions as well as the coding region of the immunoglobulin gene.[59]

Single-cell analyses in lymphocyte predominant Hodgkin lymphoma demonstrated identical rearranged variable genes, but sequencing studies demonstrated that they were highly mutated.[60–62] The monoclonal expansion of cells with intraclonal diversity suggests that the L&H cells are of germinal center origin.

Immunoglobulin variable gene rearrangements have also served as clonal markers when multiple sites were examined and at primary diagnosis and upon relapse.[63,64] This observation of an identical clone at diagnosis and upon relapse after intensive treatment defines the malignant nature of RS-H cells. A common B-cell precursor has also been reported for two cases of classic Hodgkin lymphoma and non-Hodgkin lymphoma.[65]

In sum, the RS-H cell in most cases of Hodgkin lymphoma represent monoclonal outgrowths of germinal center B cells that have lost the ability to express antigen receptor through crippling mutations, which in turn, escape apoptosis through mechanisms such as viruses or regulator genes.[66]

ONCOGENES

The demonstration that transforming proteins related to Epstein-Barr virus (EBV) are capable of upregulating *BCL-2* in cultured cells created further interest in a relationship between *BCL-2* expression and Hodgkin lymphoma. However, correlation between *BCL-2* expression, seen in about 35 to 40 percent of cases, and EBV detection or expression of EBV-related transforming protein has not been found.[37,67,68] Whereas *BCL-2* expression does not appear to correlate with EBV-infection or the t(14;18) translocation, several reports suggest that *BCL-2* expression may be related to prognosis, as has been established in the non-Hodgkin lymphomas.[69,70]

The tumor suppressor gene p53 has been found in most cases of classical Hodgkin lymphoma with nuclear accumulation.[71–73] The significance of this finding remains uncertain as mutations in the p53 gene have been rarely detected.[72,74] Overexpression of MDM2 gene product, an antagonist of p53, has been described in RS-H cells.[75] Preservation of p53 function is suggested by expression of p21 in a proportion of RS-H cells.[76] To date, no characteristic patterns of genomic alteration or deregulated expression of oncogenes have been detected but clinical correlative data are just emerging.

CYTOGENETIC STUDIES

Karyotypes are usually hyperdiploid with structural abnormalities but without pathognomonic chromosomal aberration or specific defects. Relatively few cases have been well documented by banding techniques due to the paucity of RS-H cells and the difficulty of growing the cells in culture. However, clonal populations with numeric or structural chromosome abnormalities have been demonstrated by cytogenetic studies in over half of the cases that have been well-studied.[77–79]

In one large series, the most common breakpoints identified (11q23, 14q32, 6q11–21, and 8q22–24) are shared with the non-Hodgkin lymphomas, and this has been used as further support of a lymphoid origin.[77] Deletions or translocation of the short arm of chromosomes 12 and 13 have also been described.[77] The most commonly observed aberrations in a genetic analysis of sorted RS-H cells using comparative genomic hybridization were a loss on 16q11–21, a gain on 1p13, and a gain on 7q35–36.[80] The large number of chromosomal alterations, gains, and losses in each studied case, suggests that genetic stability plays a role in the etiology of Hodgkin lymphoma.

The t(14;18) (q32,q21) translocation in which *BCL-2* on chromosome 18 is juxtaposed to the joining region of the immunoglobulin heavy-chain gene has been the subject of several investigations in Hodgkin tissues. Although rearranged *BCL-2* was found in about a third of the cases in one report, using PCR technique, subsequent studies failed to confirm this finding.[81-83] Using micromanipulation, it has been established that the translocation is found in bystander B cells.[84] However, identical clonal rearrangements were identified in a composite follicular and Hodgkin lymphoma.[65]

ASSOCIATION WITH EBV

Although long suspected on the basis of epidemiological and serologic data, the presence of EBV genomes in Hodgkin lymphoma was not confirmed until 1987.[85] With highly sensitive in situ hybridization methods, there is agreement that about 50 percent of Hodgkin cases are EBV-associated and associated with a monoclonal population of cells. An active role for EBV in pathogenesis is further supported by the demonstration that EBV-positive malignant cells express the viral latent-membrane protein (LMP).[86,87] This protein has transforming potential in transfection assays and upregulates a number of cellular genes. However, EBV cannot be implicated as the transforming factor in all cases because it is detectable in only half the cases. As discussed below, detection of EBV genomes is positively associated with mixed cellularity histology, very young and old age, low socioeconomic status, and human immunodeficiency virus (HIV) infection.

ASSOCIATION WITH THE NON-HODGKIN LYMPHOMAS

There are numerous reports of the coexistence of Hodgkin lymphoma with a non-Hodgkin lymphoma, either occurring as sequential events or in the same site, where they are referred to as *composite*. The most common association is between lymphocyte predominance and large cell lymphoma.[86,88,89] The association of other subtypes of Hodgkin lymphoma is common with follicular lymphoma.[90] In a series of cases with coexisting CLL and RS-H cells, several patients subsequently developed disseminated Hodgkin lymphoma.[91,92] While these findings are consistent with a B-lineage origin of RS-H cells, rare association with mycosis fungoides, a T-lineage neoplasm, has been reported.[93,94]

With microdissection techniques, the clonal relationship between the non-Hodgkin lymphomas/leukemia and Hodgkin lymphoma can be addressed. Such studies confirmed a clonal relationship in Hodgkin lymphoma and CLL.[95] Amplification and sequencing of genomic DNA from the rearranged immunoglobulin variable chain genes from two patients with both Hodgkin lymphoma and non-Hodgkin lymphoma (one follicular and one T-cell rich) demonstrated clonal identity.[65] In contrast, a small non-cleaved-cell lymphoma was found to be derived from the same clone of B cells as that accounting for a preceding Hodgkin lymphoma.[96]

CYTOKINES

The relative amounts of collagen sclerosis and inflammatory cells, and the cytology of the malignant RS-H cells, define the histologic subtypes of Hodgkin lymphoma. It is hypothesized that these subtypes result from the cytokines elaborated by RS-H cells or the "bystander" cells. The autocrine or paracrine interactions between RS-H and bystander cells are complex. Observations have been made on primary tissues and several well-characterized Hodgkin-lymphoma cell lines. CD40 ligand (CD154), IL-4, IL-6, and IL-9 appear to stimulate the growth of RS-H cells.[97-102] RS-H cells secrete a variety of cytokines that may be responsible for the presence and characteristics of the nonmalignant cells surrounding them. In turn, these reactive cells produce cytokines that can affect RS-H cells and further influence the surrounding cellular milieu. For example, secretion of IL-5 by RS-H

cells attracts eosinophils, which then express CD30-ligand (CD30L) and transforming growth factor beta (TGF-β). Another example is IL-8 release by RS-H cells which attracts neutrophils that express CD30L. Cytokines can also influence the expression of RS-H cell surface adhesion molecules such as CD54 (ICAM-1), LDFA-3, CD40, and the integrin family including CD15 and others. RS-H cells have receptors for interleukin-2, CD30L, and CD154.[103] Human IL-10 expression has been associated with EBV infection in Hodgkin lymphoma. Because of its potential inhibitory effects on cell-mediated immunity, expression of IL-10 may inhibit development of cytotoxic responses directed at this antigen.[104] An IL-9-mediated autocrine loop has been suggested for Hodgkin lymphoma; of interest, in vivo overexpression of IL-9 results in the development of thymic lymphomas.[105] Elevated levels of IL-13 were identified in RS-H cells by gene expression pattern analyses.[106] Treatment of a Hodgkin lymphoma-derived cell line with a neutralizing antibody resulted in inhibition, suggesting that modulation of the IL-13 signaling pathway might be a target for future therapeutic strategies. The expression of selected cytokines and factors—IL-2 receptor (IL-2R), IL-6, IL-10, and CD30—in tissues and secretion into the serum have been found to correlate with constitutional symptoms and advanced disease.[107-111]

The different types of Hodgkin lymphoma have different quantities of cytokines, and these appear to relate to the distinctive histopathologic features. Adhesion molecules, modulated by cytokines, affect the interaction of RS-H cells with surrounding T cells and probably affect the spread of disease.

IMMUNOLOGIC DYSFUNCTION

Hodgkin lymphoma is associated with abnormal cellular immunity. Abnormalities include impaired delayed cutaneous hypersensitivity, decreased natural killer cytotoxicity, enhanced suppressor T-cell and suppressor monocyte activity, high levels of circulating immune complexes with increased immunoglobulin production, production of anti-lymphocyte and anti-Ia antibodies, and an impaired proliferative response to T-cell mitogen stimulation and lymphokine production.[112-115] Some of these defects persist for several years following successful treatment. Patients observed to be free of disease for several years continued to have suppressed hypersensitivity to neoantigens, although anergy to recall antigens was reversible.[116-118] Responses to concanavalin-A and phytohemagglutinin were significantly less than in normal controls.[119] Lymphopenia is common in advanced Hodgkin lymphoma and is also seen as a consequence of radiotherapy. This treatment primarily decreases the CD4+ T-cell population that slowly regenerates after treatment is completed.[120] Profound defects in naive CD4 and CD8 T cells persist up to 30 years in patients treated with mediastinal irradiation.[121]

The immunophenotype and cytokine production of the T cells surrounding RS-H cells are consistent with a Th2-type response, which is characterized by IL-4 and interferon gamma (IFN-γ) production, but not IL-2. Absence of IL-2 production is also characteristic of anergic cells. The cytokine TGF-β produced by RS-H cells has potent immunosuppressive effects. The immune response may also be modulated toward a Th2 type by IL-10. Production of the chemokine TARC by RS-H cells provides a possible explanation for the attraction of a Th2-subset in Hodgkin lymphoma.[122] The expression of cytokines described above on RS-H cells and their natural ligands by surrounding lymphocytes may also play a role. For instance, expression of the FAS ligand (CD95L) may induce apoptosis of activated, FAS-expressing, CD8+ T cells and NK cells. A range of factors appears to contribute to the apparent paradox of a rich inflammatory infiltrate, ineffective host response, and generalized immune deficiency.

EPIDEMIOLOGY

DESCRIPTIVE EPIDEMIOLOGY

The incidence of Hodgkin lymphoma in the United States has been stable over the past several decades with an incidence of 3.2 per 100,000 population.[123] It is higher among men than women and higher among Americans of European than of African descent.

Unlike most malignancies, Hodgkin lymphoma has a bimodal age-incidence curve: rates rise through early life, peaking in the third decade and declining until age 45, after which the incidence increases steadily.[124-126] The clinical presentation tends to be different in childhood (ages 0 to 14), young adult (15 to 34 years), and older adults. The nodular sclerosis subtype predominates in young adults while the mixed cellularity subtype is more common in the pediatric population and at older ages. There is a male predominance at all ages, but this is most marked in childhood cases (85 percent).

An increased risk of Hodgkin lymphoma in the young adult population has been associated with high socioeconomic status in multiple studies.[124,127,128] High intelligence, small family size, single-family dwelling, and high educational attainment of patients and their immediate families have all been associated with increased risk.

The geographic patterns vary for the three major age groups: the incidence of Hodgkin lymphoma is greater in childhood, and there is a predominance of mixed cellularity histology in less developed countries, while the incidence peaks in young adulthood and is associated with more favorable histologic subtypes in developed countries.[129] An intermediate picture may be seen in rural areas of developing countries. Together these data suggest a remarkable association between socioeconomic and environmental factors in the incidence of Hodgkin lymphoma.

POSSIBLE INFECTIOUS ETIOLOGY

The demographic features have long supported the concept that one or more subtypes of Hodgkin lymphoma have an infectious etiology. In 1966 MacMahon proposed that the first age peak in young adults was infectious in nature while that seen in the second peak resulted from causes similar to other lymphomas.[124]

Several reports of clustering of Hodgkin lymphoma at the time of diagnosis suggested the possibility of infectious transmission.[130,131] The weaknesses of the retrospective methodology in these studies have been critically assessed, and further statistical analyses indicate that these likely occurred by chance alone.[129] Some population-based studies have found significant case aggregation (shared exposure) in schools, but these results have been seriously questioned on the basis of the methods used.[132-135]

Several large studies have demonstrated that a prior history of serologically confirmed infectious mononucleosis confers about a threefold increased risk of young adult Hodgkin lymphoma.[136-138] Elevations in titers of EBV, the etiologic agent of infectious mononucleosis, have been reported in people diagnosed with Hodgkin lymphoma. A large population study showed that people who developed Hodgkin lymphoma had abnormally high titers of some anti-EBV antibodies in prediagnostic sera.[139] The demonstration of EBV viral genomes in RS-H cells discussed above further supports a relationship between EBV and Hodgkin lymphoma.

The epidemiological features of Hodgkin lymphoma appear to fit a polio model where delayed age at infection leads to an increased risk of young adult disease. In less developed countries where early infection is probable, childhood Hodgkin lymphoma is more common than young adult disease while the reverse is true in developed countries. A similar pattern of geographic occurrence and age at initial infection also occurs for EBV infection. However, the presence of EBV in tumor tissue presents some unexpected results.

Whereas it is the young-adult, nodular sclerosis type that is associated with the epidemiological factors that suggest an association with EBV, the highest proportion of EBV-positive cases are in the mixed cellularity category.[140,141] Several studies report a high incidence of EBV association, 85 to 100 percent in pediatric Hodgkin lymphoma.[142-145] Geographic, ethnic, and racial factors have been implicated in the association of EBV with pediatric Hodgkin lymphoma.[143] A high frequency of EBV within RS-H cells is reported in HIV-infected individuals with Hodgkin lymphoma.[146]

GENETIC BASIS

Evidence that supports a genetic basis for increased susceptibility to Hodgkin lymphoma includes the increased risk among siblings and close relatives and an association with other tumor types in a familial setting. Hodgkin-lymphoma-prone families, with or without other forms of cancer, have been described.[147-150] Hodgkin lymphoma has also been described in monozygotic twins.[151-153] Examples of consanguinity have been reported as well.[127,154] The fact that the time interval between diagnoses in affected siblings is shorter than their age differences supports an environmental influence in Hodgkin-lymphoma-prone families.[155] The increased incidence in same sex siblings (ninefold) versus opposite sex siblings (fivefold) also supports an environmental influence.[156] However, connubial occurrence in Hodgkin lymphoma is rare.[157] Lack of concordance of EBV association in tissues and serology does not indicate a viral role in the pathogenesis in familial Hodgkin lymphoma.[158]

In addition to the presentation of both Hodgkin lymphoma and a non-Hodgkin lymphoma in the same individual, both diagnoses have been noted in lymphoma-prone families, favoring a common mechanism of lymphomagenesis.[149,159,160]

Immunoregulatory genes within or near the major histocompatibility complex that may govern susceptibility to viral infections have been postulated to influence susceptibility to Hodgkin lymphoma.[161] This hypothesis is supported by the data that demonstrate that patients have lifelong, depressed cellular immunity that also has been noted in their healthy relatives.[162] Studies have implicated specific human lymphocyte antigen (HLA) regions in the etiology of Hodgkin lymphoma, and there is increased HLA haplotype sharing among relatives in multiple-case families.[161,163,164] Epidemiological and prognostic associations between HLA-DP alleles and Hodgkin lymphoma have been made in several studies using molecular techniques.[165-167]

CLINICAL FEATURES

PRESENTING MANIFESTATIONS

HISTORY AND PHYSICAL EXAMINATION

Constitutional symptoms, some of which confer a less favorable prognosis, may accompany the diagnosis. Patients with fever in excess of 38°C, drenching night sweats, and weight loss exceeding 10 percent of baseline body weight during the 6 months preceding diagnosis are designated as having "B" disease. Fevers, present in 27 percent of patients at diagnosis, are usually of low grade and irregular.[168] Rarely, a cyclic pattern of high fevers for 1 to 2 weeks alternating with afebrile periods of similar duration is present at diagnosis. This classic Pel-Ebstein fever is virtually diagnostic.[169,170] Generalized pruritus, often accompanied by marked excoriation, may be present at diagnosis, but is not of prognostic significance.[171] Pain in involved lymph nodes immediately after the ingestion of alcohol is a curious complaint that is nearly specific to Hodgkin lymphoma. It occurs in fewer than 10 percent of patients and has no prognostic significance.[172] The etiology of these symptoms has been the subject of speculation but remains unexplained. Patients with extensive intrathoracic disease may present with cough, chest pain, dyspnea, and, rarely, hemoptysis. Infrequently, patients present with bone pain, including the constellation of back pain accompanied by signs and symptoms of spinal cord compression.

Detection of an unusual mass or swelling in the superficial lymph nodes is the most common presentation. Lymphadenopathy is usually nontender and has a rubbery consistency. A diffuse, puffy swelling rather than a discrete mass may be apparent in the supraclavicular, infraclavicular, or anterior chest wall regions. Infrequently, compression of the superior vena cava will result in facial swelling and engorgement of the veins in the neck and upper chest. Auscultation of the chest may reveal a pleural effusion. Palpation is an insensitive method for the detection of intraabdominal adenopathy or organ enlargement, but examination should be oriented toward the liver, spleen, and upper retroperitoneal area. While parenchymal or meningeal involvement of the central nervous system is rare, paraneoplastic syndromes of several varieties have been described. Patients have presented with signs of progressive multifocal leukoencephalopathy,[173] subacute cerebellar degeneration,[174,175] necrotizing myelopathy,[176] subacute sensory or motor neuropathy,[177] episodic neurologic dysfunction,[178] memory loss,[179] the Guillain-Barré syndrome,[180] and granulomatous angiitis of the central nervous system.[181]

RADIOGRAPHIC FEATURES

Intrathoracic disease is present at diagnosis in two-thirds of patients. Mediastinal adenopathy is common, particularly in young women with nodular sclerosis.[182] Hilar adenopathy, pulmonary parenchymal involvement, pleural effusions, pericardial effusions, and chest wall masses may be appreciated by computed tomography of the chest; these are more common in the presence of extensive mediastinal disease.

Bipedal lymphography is accomplished by cannulation of the lymphatics on the dorsum of each foot, followed by the injection of a radiopaque contrast material. When the lymphangiographic interpretation was correlated with histologic findings in surgically removed lymph nodes in 197 consecutive patients, the overall predictive accuracy was 92 percent, with no false negatives and a 25 percent false positive rate.[183] Extensive experience with lymphography has demonstrated that about 30 to 60 percent of patients with clinical disease limited to the supradiaphragmatic regions had involvement of the abdominal or pelvic lymph nodes.[184] A significant advantage of this technique is that contrast material may remain for months to years and can be used to assess the response to treatment and in follow-up.

Computerized tomography (CT) of the chest, abdomen, and pelvis is routinely employed in diagnostic evaluation. Although technologic advances have greatly increased the resolution of this technique, the correlation with histologic involvement of the spleen has been disappointing. CT has been valuable in detecting lymph nodes such as celiac, portal, splenic hilar, and mesenteric which are not appreciated by lymphography. Although lymphography is more sensitive than CT because it can detect filling defects in normal-size lymph nodes, it is becoming less and less available except at specialized treatment centers.[185-187]

Gallium-67 scintigraphy is useful in evaluating the mediastinum or areas that appear abnormal on bone scan and in the evaluation of residual masses following treatment. Single photon-emitted computed tomography (SPECT) increases the accuracy of the gallium scan. Whole-body positron emission tomography (PET) correlates well with CT evaluation and may demonstrate additional areas of disease, although this information results in few changes in stage or therapy.[188,189] Magnetic resonance imaging has been disappointing in the evaluation of abdominal disease or residual mediastinal masses in treated patients.[190,191]

CLINICAL AND PATHOLOGIC CORRELATION

There is a strong correlation among age at onset, the anatomic extent of disease, and histologic subtype of Hodgkin lymphoma (see Table 102-1). About 10 percent of patients present with nodular lymphocyte predominance (NLPHD) which, as stated above, is considered to be a special subtype. Progressive transformation of germinal centers may precede or follow NLPHD in other sites.[44,192] The cellular composition is predominantly benign B lymphocytes, with or without histiocytes. Patients most commonly present with stage I disease (70 percent), particularly in the axillae, and there is a 4:1 male predominance.[193] This subtype has been associated with large-cell non-Hodgkin lymphoma as a composite tumor, or the large cell lymphoma may occur at a later date.[88,89]

Nodular sclerosis is noted for its distinctive histologic features and frequent involvement of the lower cervical, supraclavicular, and mediastinal lymph nodes in adolescents and young adults, particularly females. About 70 percent of patients present with limited-stage disease. Nodular sclerosis constitutes the majority of cases, ranging from 40 to 70 percent. One of the distinguishing histologic features is the lacunar cell, an RS variant that results from retraction of the cytoplasm of RS cells during formalin fixation. Another feature is the thickened capsule and fibrous bands which divide the lymphoid tissue into cellular nodules (Fig. 102-1C). Nodular sclerosis has been subclassified as type I or II based on the frequency of malignant cells and normal lymphocytes. The malignant cells are numerous in the lymphocyte-depleted type (II), also referred to as the *syncytial variant*. The clinical and prognostic significance of nodular sclerosis subtypes is controversial.[194,195]

Mixed cellularity Hodgkin lymphoma involves both pediatric and older age groups and is more commonly associated with advanced-stage disease, constitutional symptoms, and immunodeficiency. About 30 to 50 percent of patients have this histology. Classic RS-H cells are easily found amid a cellular background composed of lymphocytes, eosinophils, plasma cells, and histiocytes (Fig. 102-1d). A worse prognosis has been characteristic of this subtype in the historical literature, but these differences have been largely blurred by modern therapy.

The incidence of lymphocyte-depletion Hodgkin lymphoma is much lower than originally reported, as many cases have been reclassified as non-Hodgkin lymphoma.[196] Two subtypes have been described: reticular and diffuse fibrosis. The reticular variant contains abundant pleomorphic neoplastic cells. The more common diffuse fibrosis variant, as the name implies, has a prominent fibroblastic proliferation with few normal lymphocytes. RS-H cells are sparse. The disease presents in the older age group with symptomatic, extensive disease. Peripheral and mediastinal adenopathy is much less common than in other cases of Hodgkin lymphoma.[197] Presentation with fever of unknown origin, jaundice, hepatosplenomegaly, or pancytopenia is not uncommon. This subtype is also associated with the acquired immunodeficiency syndrome.

The 1999 World Health Organization classification of lymphoma introduces a new subtype for the first time in 25 years. *Lymphocyte-rich Hodgkin lymphoma* was discovered during an expert pathology review of cases of lymphocyte predominance.[198] As noted above, the two subtypes differ subtly on morphologic grounds, but the major difference is that the RS-H cells in lymphocyte-rich have a classic immunophenotype. The presenting features are very similar, although patients with the lymphocyte-rich subtype tend to be older.

ANATOMIC DISTRIBUTION OF DISEASE

About 60 to 80 percent of clinical presentations are in the cervical nodes, 6 to 20 percent are in axillary nodes and 6 to 12 percent in the inguinal nodes.[168] A minority of patients presents with exclusive subdiaphragmatic disease. Figure 102-2 illustrates the anatomic distri-

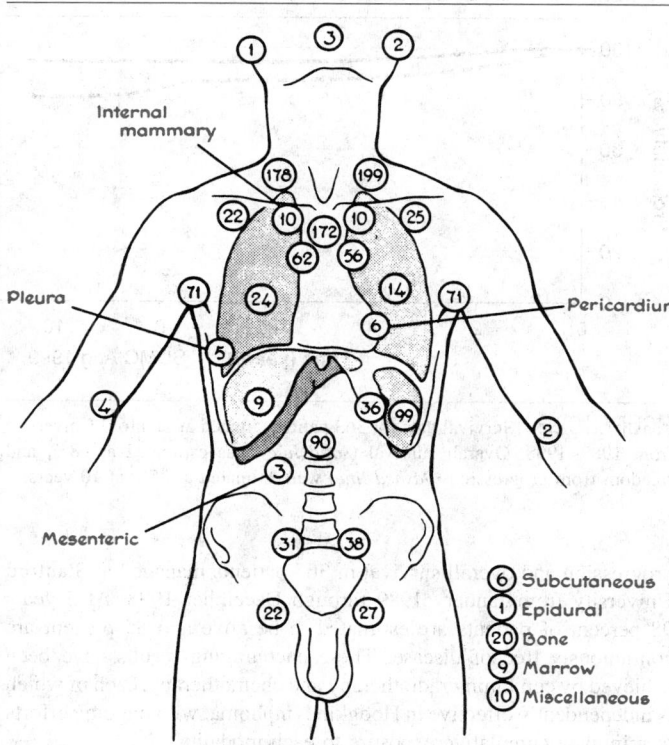

FIGURE 102-2   Anatomical distribution of sites of involvement in 285 consecutive, previously untreated patients with Hodgkin disease, 272 of whom were submitted to staging laparotomy with splenectomy. (Reprinted with permission from Kaplan et al.[206])

bution of sites of involvement in 285 consecutive, unselected, and untreated patients. Involvement of abdominal lymph nodes and spleen was documented in 272 of these patients at staging laparotomy, a surgical diagnostic procedure in which the intraabdominal and pelvic lymph nodes are sampled, the spleen is removed and examined pathologically in thin slices, the liver is biopsied by needle and wedge technique, and the bone marrow is biopsied. The frequency of splenic involvement at laparotomy in untreated patients averages 37 percent in 17 published series.[168] Involvement is strongly dependent on histologic subtype; it is present in 60 percent of mixed cellularity and lymphocyte depletion cases compared with 34 percent of lymphocyte predominance or nodular sclerosis. Hepatic and marrow diseases are invariably associated with splenic involvement.

Two different theories, the *contiguity* theory of Kaplan and Rosenberg[199] and the *susceptibility* theory of Smithers,[200] have been proposed to account for the mode of spread of Hodgkin lymphoma. In support of the former, most cases of Hodgkin lymphoma appear to spread via lymphatic channels to contiguous lymphatic structures in a predictable, nonrandom pattern. Controversy has surrounded the mode of spread to the spleen, which lacks afferent lymphatics. When four or more lymph node regions are involved, the possibility of spread by hematogenous distribution appears more likely.[201] Disseminated disease is more common in mixed cellularity and lymphocyte depletion, consistent with the presence of vascular invasion reported in these subtypes.[201] While vascular invasion is controversial, it has been reported to be more common in the spleen compared to lymph nodes and to connote a poor prognosis.[202,203] Even when involvement beyond the lymphatic system occurs, patterns of association are evident as described by Kaplan and Rosenberg.

TABLE 102-2   ANN ARBOR STAGING CLASSIFICATION*

STAGE	DEFINITION
I	Involvement of a single lymph node region (I) or of a single extralymphatic organ or site (I_E)
II	Involvement of two or more lymph node regions on the same side of the diaphragm (II) or localized involvement of an extralymphatic organ or site and of one or more lymph node regions on the same side of the diaphragm (II_E)
III	Involvement of lymph node regions on both sides of the diaphragm (III), which may also be accompanied by involvement of the spleen (III_S) or by localized involvement of an extralymphatic organ or site (III_E) or both (III_{SE})
IV	Diffuse or disseminated involvement of one or more extralymphatic organs or tissues, with or without associated lymph node involvement

The absence or presence of fever, night sweats, and/or unexplained loss of 10 percent or more of body weight in the 6 months preceding diagnosis are to be denoted in all cases by the suffix letters A or B, respectively.

*Adopted at the Workshop on the Staging of Hodgkin Disease held at Ann Arbor, Michigan, in April 1971.

STAGING

The extent of Hodgkin lymphoma is classified using the four-stage Ann Arbor classification, as indicated in Table 102-2.[19] *Clinical stage* refers to the results of physical, radiographic, and laboratory examination, while *pathologic stage* refers to the use of additional biopsy procedures. The presence or absence of constitutional symptoms further characterizes the classification. Extranodal disease, representing extracapsular extension of lymph node disease that can be treated with a curative dose of radiotherapy, is distinguished from disseminated, stage IV disease. The correlation of this staging classification system with prognosis has been extensively verified. Prognostic information such as mediastinal bulk, other bulky nodal masses, and the extent of subdiaphragmatic nodal disease is included in a modification of the Ann Arbor system, known as the *Cotswold* classification.[204]

Recommended staging procedures for untreated patients have evolved with changes in therapy. Exploratory laparotomy and splenectomy are reserved for a small subset of patients who are candidates for management with limited radiotherapy only. Historically, staging laparotomy advanced about one-third of clinical stage I and II patients to pathologic stage III and IV while reducing fewer than one-fourth of clinical stage III patients to pathologic stage I or II.[205–208] Prognostic indicators of laparotomy findings have been described.[209,210] For instance, clinical stage I women, patients with intrathoracic-only disease or high neck disease of favorable histology, and men with lymphocyte predominance have less than a 5 to 10 percent risk of subdiaphragmatic disease. In Europe and Canada, where most patients were clinically staged without laparotomy, a number of prognostic factors for the risk of relapse were identified as discussed below.

Marrow involvement occurs in 5 to 20 percent of new patients and is more common in patients of older age, advanced stage, less favorable histology, or those with constitutional symptoms or immunodeficiency. Because the marrow is almost never involved in young, asymptomatic patients with favorable clinical stage I or II presentations, marrow biopsy may be omitted in their staging. Bone scans are indicated in patients with bone pain; skeletal x-rays may demonstrate osteolytic, osteoblastic, or mixed lesions.[215]

LABORATORY FEATURES

There are no diagnostic laboratory features of Hodgkin lymphoma. A complete blood count may reveal granulocytosis,[211] eosinophilia,[212] lymphocytopenia,[213] thrombocytosis,[214] or anemia.[215] The anemia is usually due to chronic disease but rarely may be due to hemolysis secondary to high fever[216] or associated with a positive direct antiglobulin test (Coombs' test).[217] Thrombocytopenia may occur as a result of marrow involvement, hypersplenism, or an autoimmune mechanism.[218-220] Autoimmune neutropenia has been reported.[221] Cytopenias are particularly common in advanced-stage disease and lymphocyte depletion histology. Elevation of the erythrocyte sedimentation rate is most common in advanced disease and correlates with constitutional symptoms.[222,223] The degree of elevation has been correlated with prognosis, particularly in limited-stage disease.[224] Although nonspecific, it may be useful in follow-up, heralding recurrent disease. Serum lactate dehydrogenase levels are elevated in 30 to 40 percent of patients at diagnosis.[225,226] The alkaline phosphatase may be elevated, nonspecifically in limited disease or in association with involvement of liver, bone, or bone marrow in advanced disease.[227] Hypercalcemia is unusual but when it occurs may be secondary to synthesis of increased levels of 1,25-dihydroxyvitamin D by Hodgkin lymphoma tissue.[228] A variety of other abnormalities have been reported, including hypoglycemia[229,230] due to an autoantibody to insulin receptors and inappropriate secretion of antidiuretic hormone.[231]

Anemia, granulocytosis, lymphopenia, and low serum albumin constitute four of seven adverse prognostic factors identified in advanced Hodgkin lymphoma by an international consortium.[232] As in the non-Hodgkin lymphomas, serum beta 2 microglobulin levels correlate with tumor burden and prognosis.[233] Serum levels of cytokines including soluble CD30, IL-6, IL-10, and the IL-2 receptor have been reported to correlate with constitutional symptoms and advanced disease.[107-111]

Examination of pleural fluid may reveal transudative, exudative, or chylous properties. Because cytology rarely yields diagnostic RS-H cells, the etiology is most often considered to be one of central lymphatic obstruction. Laboratory abnormalities may be prominent in rare presentations of Hodgkin lymphoma. These include abnormal liver function tests associated with marked enlargement of porta hepatis nodes and biliary obstruction or intrahepatic cholestasis.[234] The nephrotic syndrome is a rare presentation.[235,236]

DIFFERENTIAL DIAGNOSIS

Clinically enlarged lymph nodes may be associated with a variety of infectious, inflammatory, autoimmune, or neoplastic disorders. Biopsies of suspicious adenopathy should be reviewed by a competent hematopathologist. The differential diagnosis is usually between Hodgkin lymphoma and a non-Hodgkin lymphoma. The syncytial variant of nodular sclerosis may be particularly troublesome. Mixed cellularity Hodgkin lymphoma may demonstrate a spectrum of pattern and cellular and stromal composition and should be distinguished from peripheral T-cell lymphoma and T-cell-rich, B-cell lymphoma. In these cases and those of lymphocyte depletion histology, immune markers as described above have proved invaluable. Nonneoplastic conditions that may simulate Hodgkin lymphoma include viral infections, particularly infectious mononucleosis. Depleted nodes of any histology may resemble the diffuse fibrosis variant of lymphocyte depletion, including the depleted phase of lymph nodes from HIV-infected patients. The diagnosis in an extranodal site depends upon the organ involved and whether there is a known diagnosis of Hodgkin lymphoma. Diagnostic RS cells are not required in liver and bone marrow because the foci of involvement are so small. Of course, the rare presentations of Hodgkin lymphoma, such as those in the CNS, liver, or as a fever of unknown origin, may have an extensive differential diagnosis.

THERAPY, COURSE, AND PROGNOSIS

The goal of treatment is to cure the greatest number of patients with minimal complications. Figure 102-3 illustrates the freedom from

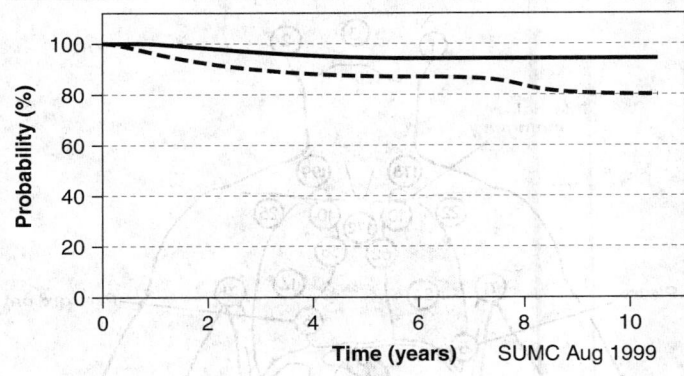

FIGURE 102-3   Survival data for 363 patients treated at Stanford University from 1989–1998. Overall survival (*solid line*) was estimated at 98%, and freedom from progression (*dashed line*) was estimated at 85% at 10 years.

progression and overall survival in 363 patients managed at Stanford University from January 1989 through December 1998. At 5 years 98 percent of patients are estimated to be alive and 85 percent are continuously free of disease. These encouraging results have been achieved by combining radiotherapy and chemotherapy, each of which is independently effective in Hodgkin lymphoma, with ongoing efforts to minimize cumulative exposure to each modality.

TREATMENT MODALITIES

RADIOTHERAPY

The pioneering work of Vera Peters in Toronto[14,15] and of Henry S. Kaplan and his colleagues at Stanford University provided the basis for modern radiotherapy. Hodgkin lymphoma first became a curable neoplasm through the systematic study of the spread of the disease and the use of supervoltage radiotherapy techniques.

Kaplan and others[237,238] provided evidence for a tumoricidal dose level. This important concept led to the incorporation of high doses that could permanently ablate Hodgkin lymphoma. Modern supervoltage techniques allow high doses of radiation to be given in large volumes with acceptable normal tissue tolerance. This method has the advantage of increased depth of dose that spares the skin and sharp beam edges that reduce scatter. The modern linear accelerator provides x-rays in the 4- to 8-MeV range. When radiotherapy is used alone, involved fields usually receive doses of 3500 to 4400 cGy with prophylactic doses of 3000 to 3500 cGy to uninvolved tissues, but 3000 cGy may be adequate.[239] Tumor doses of 150 to 200 cGy are given daily five times per week.

The classic regions of radiotherapy employed in Hodgkin lymphoma include the mantle, paraaortic region, and pelvis. The mantle region encompassed the cervical, supraclavicular, infraclavicular, axillary, mediastinal, and hilar nodes. The paraaortic region included the splenic pedicle or the spleen, if still intact. Together, these regions were referred to as *subtotal lymphoid irradiation*. The combination of the paraaortic region and the pelvic region was called an *inverted Y*, and *total lymphoid irradiation* referred to the combined mantle and inverted Y regions. In the current management of Hodgkin lymphoma, wide-field irradiation is infrequently used. When used, match lines between fields must not overlap to ensure that the spinal cord does not receive excessive radiation that can result in myelopathy. Pelvic irradiation requires careful shielding of the testes in men and consideration for oophoropexy plus shielding in premenopausal women.[240,241]

In the setting of combined chemotherapy and radiotherapy treatment, modifications of the mantle field have been made to address

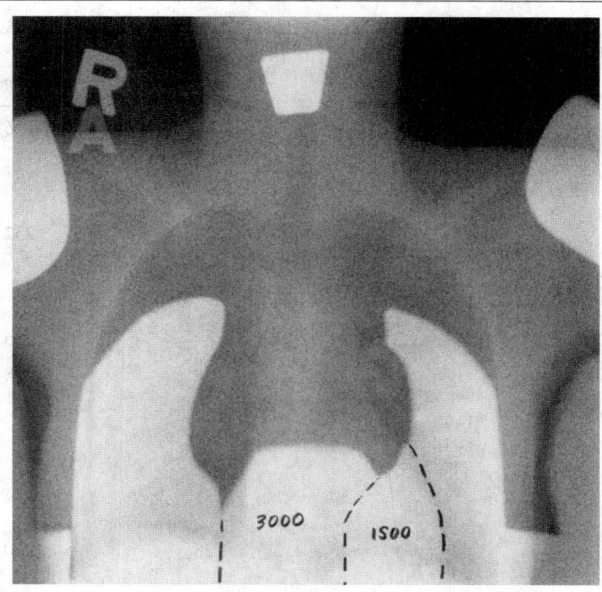

FIGURE 102-4 Simulated film for radiation treatment of mediastinal Hodgkin disease. The contours of the lung-shielding blocks are outlined. Note that a small portion of the left lung block is cut separately and omitted when mediastinal adenopathy is present. In this case, a dose of 1,500 cGy is given to the heart, and then the block is inserted for the remaining treatment. The subcarinal block is placed after a dose of 3,000 cGy is delivered.

adverse consequences of treatment. Figure 102-4 illustrates a typical simulated chest film for a modified mantle. The axillae and the upper neck are not included in the field. Lung blocks are shaped to ensure adequate irradiation of the tumor volume. The whole heart is not treated unless there is evidence of pericardial involvement. A pericardial block is placed at 1500 cGy, and a subcarinal block is placed at 3000 cGy. The technical aspects of radiotherapy are extremely important. These include use of simulators, individually constructed blocks, detailed patient positioning, careful beam definition, and verification of dose with dosimetry.

CHEMOTHERAPY

From 1942 through 1963 a number of chemotherapy drugs became available for clinical use.[24,25] Nitrogen mustard, other alkylating agents, the antifols, corticosteroids, the vinca alkaloids, and a new agent with exciting activity in Hodgkin lymphoma, procarbazine, were all studied as single agents in advanced disease. While responses were observed, there was no evidence of cure. The first modern combination chemotherapy program was devised by DeVita and colleagues.[26] The MOPP program differed from previous attempts in its curative intent, longer (6-month) treatment program, and the introduction of a sliding scale for dose adjustment based upon hematologic toxicity. The national mortality figures for Hodgkin lymphoma decreased by more than 60 percent in the decade that followed the introduction of MOPP chemotherapy.[242] In the 20-year follow-up of the original series of 188 advanced-stage patients treated with MOPP, 54 percent were continuously free of disease.[243]

A number of modifications were made to the original MOPP regimen by others with the intent to reduce acute toxicity, particularly the neuropathy and nausea and vomiting.[244] Of the MOPP-like regimens, the MVPP regimen that substitutes vinblastine for vincristine, and the ChlVPP regimen, which substitutes chlorambucil for nitrogen mustard and vinblastine for vincristine, had comparable efficacy with somewhat improved tolerance.[245–248] Neither the use of maintenance

therapy nor the addition of bleomycin resulted in improved outcome when compared with the original MOPP program administered in full doses.[244,249–251]

An important alternative regimen, ABVD (adriamycin, bleomycin, vinblastine, and dacarbazine) was effective in the treatment of patients who had failed MOPP.[252,253] In addition, as discussed below, this regimen has a different toxicity profile than MOPP. ABVD was subsequently employed alone, in combination with radiotherapy, and used together with MOPP in alternating or "hybrid" programs.[254–260]

Multiple alternative chemotherapy regimens have been introduced for the treatment of Hodgkin lymphoma. An abbreviated 12-week combination, Stanford V (doxorubicin, vinblastine, vincristine, bleomycin, nitrogen mustard, etoposide, prednisone), has been developed.[263,264] Table 102-3 describes the drugs, doses, and schedules of combination chemotherapy programs effective in the management of Hodgkin lymphoma.

DISEASE STAGE

FAVORABLE, LIMITED-STAGE DISEASE

Favorable, limited-stage disease may be defined as asymptomatic stage I or II supradiaphragmatic disease with no bulky sites and no or only one extranodal site. As defined above, staging may or may not include exploratory laparotomy. Extended field (subtotal lymphoid) radiotherapy, usually administered after staging laparotomy, was the treatment of choice for these patients in the United States for many years. This treatment was based on a pivotal clinical trial in which patients with stage I-IIA disease were randomized to involved field or extended field radiotherapy.[265] With more than 15 years follow-up, extended field radiotherapy yielded a highly significant advantage in freedom from relapse, 80 percent, compared with 32 percent for involved field. The overall survival was no different in the two groups due to effective treatment at relapse. Subsequent reports from multiple institutions have confirmed the high rate of cures in stage I and II with extended field radiotherapy. A metaanalysis concluded that more extensive radiotherapy increased the chance of cure by more than 30 percent, although no survival benefit was seen at 10 years.[266]

A very favorable group of patients (40 years old or younger with nodular sclerosis or lymphocyte predominance, laparotomy-stage I and IIA with mediastinal disease, and ESR less than 70) was studied to determine the role of prophylactic abdominal radiotherapy.[267,268] A 1997 update of this randomized trial showed no difference between mantle radiotherapy or subtotal lymphoid radiotherapy either for treatment failure or overall survival.[269] These results with mantle irradiation alone in selected laparotomy-stage (PS) patients have been corroborated in other retrospective studies.[270–272]

The description of prognostic factors for the probability of occult disease, improvements in radiographic imaging, and the desire to eliminate staging laparotomy have resulted in the more routine use of clinical staging for favorable, limited Hodgkin lymphoma. However, mantle radiotherapy alone is not sufficient for clinical stage patients, even those selected for very favorable prognostic features. Mature follow-up of a clinical trial resulted in a 6-year event-free survival of 66 percent, an unacceptably high rate of relapse among this very favorable group of clinical stage IA women aged 40 or younger with lymphocyte predominance or nodular sclerosis histology.[273]

The treatment of early-stage disease has become so successful that at 15 to 20 years, the overall mortality rate from other causes exceeds deaths due to Hodgkin lymphoma.[274] As detailed below, the largest cause of mortality is second cancers, and these seem to be related to the extent of radiotherapy treatment. Thus, there is interest in reducing the volume and dose of radiotherapy in limited Hodgkin lymphoma without compromising the therapeutic results.

TABLE 102-3   COMBINATION CHEMOTHERAPY REGIMENS FOR HODGKIN LYMPHOMA

Acronym	Drugs	Dose	Route	Schedule, Days	Interval Between Cycles, Days	Reference
MOPP	Nitrogen mustard	6 mg/m²	IV	1, 8	28	26
	Vincristine*	1.4 mg/m²	IV	1, 8		
	Procarbazine	100 mg/m²	PO	1–14		
	Prednisone	40 mg/m²	PO	1–14**		
ABVD	Adriamycin	25 mg/m²	IV	1, 15	28	252
	Bleomycin	10 u/m²	IV	1, 15		
	Vinblastine	6 mg/m²	IV	1, 15		
	Dacarbazine	375 mg/m²	IV	1, 15		
MOPP/ABVD	Alternate cycles of MOPP and ABVD					255
MOPP/ABV hybrid (Canada)	Nitrogen mustard	6 mg/m²	IV	1	28	258
	Vincristine*	1.4 mg/m²	IV	1		
	Procarbazine	100 mg/m²	PO	1–7		
	Prednisone	40 mg/m²	PO	1–14		
	Adriamycin	35 mg/m²	IV	8		
	Bleomycin	10 u/m²	IV	8		
	Vinblastine	6 mg/m²	IV	8		
MOPP/ABVD hybrid (Milan)	Nitrogen mustard	6 mg/m²	IV	1	28	260
	Vincristine*	1.4 mg/m²	IV	1		
	Procarbazine	100 mg/m²	PO	1–7		
	Prednisone	40 mg/m²	PO	1–7		
	Adriamycin	25 mg/m²	IV	15		
	Bleomycin	10 u/m²	IV	15		
	Vinblastine	6 mg/m²	IV	15		
	Dacarbazine	375 mg/m²	IV	15		
BEACOPP (Escalated BEACOPP)	Bleomycin	10 u/m²	IV	8	21	262
	Etoposide	100 (200) mg/m²	IV	1–3		
	Adriamycin	25 (35) mg/m²	IV	1		
	Cyclophosphamide	650 (1250) mg/m²	IV	1		
	Vincristine*	1.4 mg/m²	IV	8		
	Procarbazine	100 mg/m²	PO	1–7		
	Prednisone	40 mg/m²	PO	1–14		
	G-CSF	– (5) μg/kg	SQ	8+		
Stanford V	Vinblastine	6 mg/m²	IV	weeks 1, 3, 5, 7, 9, 11		264
	Adriamycin	25 mg/m²	IV	weeks 1, 3, 5, 7, 9, 11		
	Vincristine*	1.4 mg/m²	IV	weeks 2, 4, 6, 8, 10		
	Bleomycin	5 u/m²	IV	weeks 2, 4, 6, 8, 10		
	Nitrogen mustard	6 mg/m²	IV	weeks 1, 5, 9		
	Etoposide	60 x 2 mg/m²	IV	weeks 3, 7, 11		
	Prednisone	40 mg/m²	PO	weeks 1–10, taper		
	G-CSF	5 μg/kg	SQ	upon first delay/reduction		

*Vincristine dose may be capped at 2 mg.
**Prednisone given on cycles 1 and 4 in original report.

Stanford University first demonstrated that chemotherapy could substitute for extended field radiotherapy in stage I and II patients. In sequential clinical trials, MOPP and VBM (vinblastine, bleomycin, and methotrexate) were given as adjuvants to involved field radiotherapy with equivalent or superior results.[265,275] In a subsequent trial, clinical stage I and II patients were randomized to subtotal lymphoid radiotherapy or a combination of limited radiotherapy and VBM, with excellent results in both treatment arms.[276] Six cycles of EBVP (epirubicin, bleomycin, vinblastine, and prednisone) plus involved field radiotherapy or subtotal radiotherapy were randomly assigned selected clinical stage I-IIA patients with favorable prognostic features. At 6 years, the event-free survival on the combined modality arm was 90 percent, significantly higher than radiotherapy alone.[273]

In recent years, clinical trials have been designed to test the optimal number of cycles of chemotherapy and the volume and dose of radiotherapy when both modalities are used in limited Hodgkin lymphoma. Greater than 95 percent disease control was achieved with four cycles of ABVD and radiotherapy. No advantage of extended field over involved field treatment was found.[277] Preliminary data in favorable I-II patients indicate that two cycles of ABVD followed by subtotal radiotherapy are superior to subtotal radiotherapy alone.[278] Excellent preliminary results, 91 percent progression-free survival at 3 years, have also been published with just 4 weeks of VAPEC-B (vinblastine, doxorubicin, prednisone, etoposide, cyclophosphamide, and bleomycin) chemotherapy and limited radiotherapy.[279] An 8-week course of Stanford V and limited field and dose radiotherapy appear to yield comparable results in favorable CS I-IIA patients as 95 percent event-free survival at 3 years has been reported.[280] Although these outstanding results with modest therapy are encouraging, the strategy of short-course chemotherapy and involved field radiotherapy allows omission of mediastinal radiotherapy, a source of considerable morbidity, in just 20 percent of patients. Thus there is considerable interest in chemotherapy alone in limited-stage Hodgkin lymphoma.

MOPP and ChlVPP have been studied in pediatric Hodgkin lymphoma.[281,282] Excellent results have been achieved with both, with cures above 75 to 80 percent. Similarly, an excellent outcome for chemotherapy alone was reported for CVPP (cyclophosphamide substituted for mustard) alone compared with combined chemotherapy and radiotherapy.[283] MOPP chemotherapy alone and subtotal lymphoid irradiation have been compared in pathologically staged patients in two prospective randomized trials. In a study of stage I-IIA or B and selected IIIA patients,[284] freedom from progression at 10 years significantly favored chemotherapy; however, when the subset of patients with massive mediastinal or stage III disease was excluded, the difference was no longer significant. In a study of similar design,[285] no difference was seen in relapse-free survival among stage I and IIA patients, but the overall survival significantly favored the radiotherapy group (93 percent versus 56 percent at 8 years) due to the limited ability to cure patients who failed MOPP. It was speculated that the chemotherapy arm might induce chemoresistant clones. Because MOPP chemotherapy has an undesirable toxicity profile, clinical trials in Europe and North America are exploring the use of ABVD in limited Hodgkin lymphoma. Ongoing studies in North America and Europe test the efficacy of ABVD alone, the number of cycles of chemotherapy (two versus four) and the optimal dose of radiotherapy (2000 cGy versus 3000 cGy).

Several subsets of limited patients deserve further mention. CS I patients presenting with inguinofemoral disease may be treated with inverted Y (paraaortic and pelvic) radiation only. Other subdiaphragmatic presentations of Hodgkin lymphoma are best managed with combined modality therapy or chemotherapy alone. A number of reports indicate that patients with extensive mediastinal disease have a much less favorable outcome with radiotherapy alone.[286,287] About half of patients with masses greater than one-third of the chest diameter relapsed. Although selected patients have been managed with radiation therapy incorporating careful CT planning, most are managed with combined treatment as in the following section.[288] Similarly, IIB patients are generally managed with chemotherapy or combined modality. Although a series of PS IIB patients with extended field radiotherapy enjoyed an excellent outcome, the requirement for laparotomy and the development of less toxic chemotherapy led to abandoning this approach for most IIB patients.[289]

LOCALLY EXTENSIVE, LIMITED-STAGE HODGKIN LYMPHOMA

Extensive mediastinal Hodgkin lymphoma is frequently accompanied by extranodal extension to lung, pericardium, and chest wall. Pleural effusions may also be seen. The use of combined chemotherapy and radiation (combined modality therapy) results in freedom from relapse in 80 percent or more of such patients compared with only 40 to 55 percent following radiation alone.[287] Significant numbers of patients can be effectively treated with chemotherapy after radiation failure, and their ultimate survival is similar to patients treated with combined modality. However, in addition to the psychological trauma of recurrent disease, patients managed with radiotherapy alone are subject to the potential morbidity of extensive radiation to normal heart and lung tissue. In question are the optimal chemotherapy regimen and its duration, the radiation dose, and the sequence of therapy for combined treatment. Two hundred thirty-two patients were randomized to six courses of MOPP or ABVD combined with subtotal lymphoid irradiation.[256,290] Many of these patients had extensive mediastinal disease. The ABVD/RT combination was significantly superior to MOPP/RT as measured by both freedom from progression and survival. The major concerns in choice of chemotherapy relate to late effects, specifically the concern for sterility and acute leukemia ascribed to alkylating agents and the potential for enhanced cardiopulmonary toxicity with ABVD, especially when combined with radiotherapy. Subsequently, the efficacy of four cycles of ABVD and involved field radiotherapy in stage I-II patients, many of whom had massive mediastinal disease, was reported.[277] The 12-week Stanford V program together with modified mantle radiotherapy was very effective in these patients also.[263]

As described below, an Intergroup randomized clinical trial testing ABVD with radiotherapy versus Stanford V with radiotherapy is in progress. There are relatively few data regarding the use of chemotherapy alone for bulky mediastinal Hodgkin lymphoma. A retrospective report of the results with MOPP alone or MOPP with adjuvant radiotherapy in this subset described cure of less than half of these patients with MOPP alone, leading to the recommendation of combined treatment for massive mediastinal Hodgkin lymphoma.[291]

ADVANCED DISEASE

Historically, there was controversy regarding the treatment of stage IIIA Hodgkin lymphoma. Because the most favorable presentations (involvement of the spleen, celiac, splenic hilar, or porta hepatis nodes only) required total nodal irradiation, there is general agreement that IIIA patients should be managed with chemotherapy alone or with combined modality treatment if bulky mediastinal or other sites are observed. Patients with IIIA disease fared superbly in the original NCI MOPP trial, and multiple studies have corroborated a 90 percent disease-free survival in this group.

As noted above, 20-year follow-up of the original MOPP series demonstrated that the actuarial freedom from progression was 54 percent, and 48 percent were alive.[243] Constitutional symptoms, male sex, advanced-stage disease, and administration of vincristine lower than the projected rate were prognostic for complete response. Bonadonna and colleagues tested a program of MOPP alternating with ABVD for 12 monthly cycles in a randomized trial in stage IV patients.[255] The control arm received 12 courses of MOPP. The 8-year freedom-from-progression rates were significantly different: 65 percent versus 36 percent for the MOPP/ABVD and MOPP groups respectively. Although overall survival rates were superior for MOPP/ABVD (84 percent) compared with MOPP (64 percent), these differences did not achieve statistical significance because of the relatively small number of patients in the trial. A large multi-institutional comparison of MOPP for 8 cycles, ABVD for 8 cycles, or MOPP alternating with ABVD for 12 monthly cycles was undertaken in patients with stages IIIA, IIIB, and IV disease.[257] The ABVD and MOPP/ABVD results were superior to MOPP as described in Table 102-4. The failure-free survival rates were similar for ABVD (61 percent) and MOPP/ABVD (65 percent), and both were significantly better than those achieved with MOPP (50 percent). Two groups combined MOPP and ABVD in a slightly different hybrid regimen as detailed in Table 102-3.[259,260] Both of these hybrid strategies have been compared with MOPP alternating with ABVD in randomized trials. In one study equivalent outcome for the two study arms was seen, but the hybrid regimen was more toxic, particularly in older patients.[259] Similarly, freedom from progression and overall survival were not different in the alternating and hybrid arms in the other study.[260]

In a subsequent study patients were randomized to ABVD alone versus a hybrid regimen. The study was stopped early due to excess deaths and second cancers in the hybrid arm. At the time the study was reported, there were no differences in efficacy with 65 percent of ABVD patients and 67 percent of hybrid patients failure-free.[292] These results were achieved with 8 to 10 monthly cycles of chemotherapy. In aggregate the constellation of clinical trials indicate that 60 to 70 percent of patients with advanced Hodgkin lymphoma are cured with ABVD, hybrid, or alternating combinations. ABVD alone has emerged as the preferred treatment because it has a more favorable toxicity profile.

In an attempt to further improve outcomes in advanced Hodgkin lymphoma, the BEACOPP regimen was developed.[261,262] This treatment program is delivered every 3 weeks and features relatively dose-intense etoposide and cyclophosphamide. An escalated version incorporates very high doses of these drugs facilitated by granulocyte col-

TABLE 102-4   RESULTS OF COMBINATION CHEMOTHERAPY FOR ADVANCED HODGKIN LYMPHOMA

GROUP	ACRONYM	No.	% FAILURE-FREE SURVIVAL	% OVERALL SURVIVAL	FOLLOW-UP YEARS	REFERENCE
NCI	MOPP	188	54*	48	20	243
CALGB	MOPP vs	123	50	66	5	257
	ABVD vs	115	61	73		
	MOPP/ABVD	123	65	75		
Milan	MOPP/ABVD vs	150	67*	74	5	260
	MOPP-ABVD hybrid	150	65*	72		
Canada	MOPP/ABVD vs	141	67	83	5	259
	MOPP/ABV hybrid	146	71	81		
CALGB	MOPP/ABV hybrid vs	428	67	85	3	292
	ABVD	428	65	87		
GHSG	COPP/ABVD* vs	182	75	88	2	261
	BEACOPP (standard and escalated)	323	84	92		

*Freedom from progression.

ony-stimulating factor. Patients with initial tumor bulk or residual radiographic disease received radiotherapy after chemotherapy. Several interim analyses showed superior outcomes for BEACOPP compared with the standard alternating chemotherapy arm. The results achieved, cure rates in excess of 80 percent, are the best recorded for a large phase III trial in advanced Hodgkin lymphoma. Multiple second cancers were reported in these early reports, and long-term follow-up is required to determine the combined efficacy and toxicity of this approach. Investigators tested an alternate approach to locally extensive and advanced Hodgkin lymphoma, abbreviating the duration of therapy and reduction of the cumulative drug doses. The Stanford V regimen was administered over 12 weeks and given in combination with radiotherapy for patients with bulky (5 cm or larger) nodal or macroscopic splenic disease. Freedom from progression in excess of 85 percent and overall survival in excess of 95 percent were reported with this approach in single-arm studies.[263,264,293] ABVD versus Stanford V is being tested in locally extensive and advanced Hodgkin lymphoma with zero to two adverse international prognostic factors as defined below (Table 102-5).[232]

Low-dose irradiation as a consolidation to combination chemotherapy was reported as a successful strategy in adults and children in single-arm experiences.[294,295] However, when compared with chemotherapy alone in randomized trials, low-dose consolidative radiotherapy provided no significant advantage.[296-299]

PROGNOSTIC FACTORS

A number of complex prognostic factor schemes have been developed for limited Hodgkin lymphoma treated with radiotherapy alone. Massive mediastinal disease and constitutional symptoms were consistently identified as independent predictors of relapse, whereas only older age was predictive of inferior survival. Investigators incorporated gender, age, ESR, number of Ann Arbor disease sites, stage, and histology into stratifications for favorable, very favorable, and unfavorable disease categories.[268,302] The significance of these factors when newer combined modality treatments are used for limited disease is unknown, but it is important to be aware of the variable eligibility criteria when interpreting the literature. An international consortium pooled patient data and identified a prognostic score for advanced Hodgkin lymphoma based on seven factors (Table 102-5).[232] These include male sex, age greater than or equal to 45 years, stage IV, white blood count greater than or equal to 15,000/μl, lymphocyte count less than 6 percent or less than 800/μl, hemoglobin less than 10.5 g/dl, and albumin less than 4 g/dl. The presence of each factor reduced the freedom from progression by about 7 percent. Only 7 percent of patients were in the worst prognostic group (five to seven factors), and the freedom from progression in this subset was 42 percent at 5 years. Consensus with regard to prognostic factors promotes uniformity in clinical trial design and provides a rationale for new approaches such as dose intensification and autologous bone marrow transplantation in high-risk subsets.[303] As noted, the influence of age in Hodgkin lymphoma is consistent regardless of tumor burden. Reports in the older age groups indicate that dose reductions may explain inferior results in a subset of patients, but results in older patients are worse, even when therapy is controlled.[304,305]

These clinical prognostic factors are surrogates for the underlying biology of Hodgkin lymphoma. Prognostic significance has been ascribed to a variety of biologic parameters including histopathologic grading of nodular sclerosis, immunophenotype, oncogene expression, and characteristics of the T-cell infiltrate.[38,70,194,306] As noted earlier, serum levels of cytokines including soluble CD30, Il-6, IL-10, and the IL-2 receptor have been reported to correlate with constitutional symptoms and advanced disease.[107-111]

TABLE 102-5   INTERNATIONAL PROGNOSTIC FACTORS FOR ADVANCED HODGKIN LYMPHOMA

Stage IV
Male sex
Age $\geq$ 45 years
Hemoglobin < 10.5 g/dl
WBC $\geq$ 15,000/μl
Lymphocyte count < 800/μl or < 6%
Albumin < 4 g/dl

No. of FACTORS	POPULATION (%)	ESTIMATED % FREEDOM FROM PROGRESSION AT 5 YEARS
0	7	84
1	22	77
2	29	67
3	23	60
4	12	51
5–7	7	42

TREATMENT OF RECURRENT DISEASE

Patients who relapse after radiotherapy alone have an excellent rate of cure with chemotherapy.[307,308] Most of the accumulated experience is with MOPP. Patients with extensive disease at recurrence and those with constitutional symptoms have a less favorable prognosis.[309] The outlook is significantly less favorable for patients who relapse after chemotherapy alone or chemotherapy given in combination with radiotherapy. The length of prior remission, greater or less than 1 year, has a significant effect on the ability of patients to respond to subsequent treatment and maintain their response.[310] The relapse-free survival for long initial remissions was 24 percent at 11 years compared with 11 percent for those with short initial remissions in the updated MOPP experience.[311] About half of the deaths in the group with longer remissions were due to second cancers and other treatment complications, indicative of the cumulative effects of cancer treatment. The importance of initial remission duration following primary chemotherapy has been confirmed.[312,313] Among those with long initial remissions, treatment results were quite good with 45 percent free of disease at 5 years. The results were equivalent whether the same regimen, a non-cross-resistant regimen, or an alternating approach was used.[313]

The availability of chemotherapy and autologous stem cell transplantation has markedly increased the options for treatment of recurrent Hodgkin lymphoma because these approaches allow dose intensification of drugs with dose-limiting myelotoxicity, such as cyclophosphamide, carmustine, etoposide, cytosine arabinoside, or melphalan. Initially, these strategies were tested in unfavorable patients resistant to standard chemotherapy; despite this, complete responses were seen in up to half. In the last several years high-dose therapy and stem cell rescue has been offered to patients in first relapse with encouraging results.[314-317] Disease-free survival rates of 50 to 60 percent are reported at 4 to 5 years, and, in addition, transplant-related mortality has reduced from 10 to 25 percent to less than 5 percent. Although these data reflect selection bias, two randomized clinical trials provide compelling evidence for the superiority of transplantation in relapsed Hodgkin lymphoma. Patients were randomized to conventional or high-dose BEAM (carmustine, etoposide, cytosine arabinoside, melphalan), the latter with autologous stem cell transplantation.[318] This study was stopped because the 3-year event-free survival was markedly superior in the high-dose arm compared with standard BEAM, 53 percent versus 10 percent, respectively. The largest multicenter trial was conducted in Europe, where patients with relapsed Hodgkin lymphoma were randomly assigned to four cycles of dexa-BEAM (dexamethasone and BEAM) or two cycles of dexa-BEAM followed by autologous stem cell transplantation.[319] Interim analysis of this trial demonstrated superior freedom from treatment failure in the transplant group, 53 percent, versus 39 percent for patients receiving dexa-BEAM alone, $P = 0.025$. No survival advantage was seen. Similarly, no survival advantage was seen in retrospective analysis of patients treated with conventional or high-dose therapy.[320] Seven to eight years of follow-up are required for the survival curve to plateau, and early and late treatment-related mortality must be considered in the final analysis.

Prognostic factors for the success of autologous transplantation have been described by several groups.[316,321,322] Among patients transplanted earlier in their disease course, sensitivity to chemotherapy, disease in extranodal sites at relapse, and constitutional symptoms at relapse have emerged as consistent prognostic features. Primary treatment induction failures present a special challenge to clinicians. Single-institution and registry data indicate that a subset of refractory patients, as many as 38 to 49 percent, were alive and disease-free after high-dose therapy and transplantation with follow-up of 3 to 4 years.[323-325] These results have encouraged investigators to consider treatment of adverse-risk patients with high-dose therapy and trans-

plantation in the primary management; randomized clinical trials utilizing this strategy are in progress.

COMPLICATIONS OF TREATMENT

The treatment of Hodgkin lymphoma is associated with a wide array of acute and chronic side effects. While the acute complications of chemotherapy and radiotherapy may be troublesome, they are relatively easily managed. Late treatment effects in the form of sterility, cardiopulmonary disease, and second malignancy are more serious.

SECOND CANCERS

Acute leukemia and myelodysplasia were the initial second malignancies to be observed after successful treatment for Hodgkin lymphoma with MOPP chemotherapy.[326-328] The risk was proportional to the cumulative dose of alkylating agents, which in some cases included maintenance therapy, prolonged treatment, or salvage therapy.[329,330] Actuarial risks of 1 to 10 percent with relative risks in excess of 100 have been reported over a 7- to 10-year period. It is unclear if the risk plateaus at 10 years or this finding is an artifact of inadequate follow-up.[331,332] In a multi-institutional, case-control study of 29,552 Hodgkin lymphoma patients, the relative risk of acute leukemia was increased in patients receiving more than six cycles of MOPP chemotherapy, but no increased risk was found with combined radiation and chemotherapy.[329] Several studies have suggested that prior splenectomy increases the risk about twofold.[329,333] The risk of acute leukemia is significantly less after ABVD chemotherapy, although it is not zero.

There is an increased relative risk of non-Hodgkin lymphomas after treatment for Hodgkin lymphoma.[332,333] These are diffuse, aggressive B-cell lymphomas that may occur early or late after treatment. There is no clear relationship to the type of primary treatment. Some have considered the non-Hodgkin lymphomas to be a result of the ongoing immunodeficiency while others have suggested a common cell of origin.

An increased risk of solid cancers after treatment for Hodgkin lymphoma has been identified by several authors.[332,334,335] The risk is related to radiotherapy exposure, with tumors occurring infield or at the edges of the radiotherapy field. The overall actuarial risk of second solid cancer malignancy at 15 years was about 18 percent in the Stanford series.[332] Cancers of the lung, stomach, bone, and soft tissue were observed in a temporal pattern consistent with radiation-induced neoplasms. The latency for developing second cancers is an important consideration. For instance, an increased risk of breast cancer and thyroid cancer was only appreciated when mean follow-up was 10 or more years.[336-338] Breast cancer is increased in women treated before age 30 and is markedly increased in children and adolescents.[336,338,339]

CARDIOPULMONARY EFFECTS

Mediastinal radiotherapy is associated with an increased risk of cardiac disease. An increased risk of death from coronary artery disease and acute myocardial infarction has been identified in adults and children.[274,340,341] Other types of cardiac disease following chest radiotherapy include valvular disease, constrictive pericarditis, and cardiomyopathy. The risks of radiation-related heart disease do not appear to be influenced significantly by the addition of chemotherapy. The onset of increased risk is within 5 to 10 years. The incidence of radiation pneumonitis depends on the volume of lung irradiated and the total dose. Symptoms include cough, dyspnea, and fever. Although prospective assessment of pulmonary function demonstrates reduction of lung volumes following mantle radiotherapy, recovery is seen in 12 to 24 months, and symptomatic radiation pneumonitis is unusual.[349,350]

REPRODUCTIVE EFFECT

About 90 percent of males are permanently sterilized by six cycles of MOPP chemotherapy.[342] The risk is related to the cumulative dose of alkylating agents such that two to three cycles of MOPP result in azoospermia in about 50 percent of patients.[343] Female fertility after MOPP is related to age at treatment as well as cumulative alkylating agent dose.[344,345] Women over 25 at treatment have an 80 percent probability of sterility following six courses of MOPP. The ABVD combination is associated with temporary amenorrhea or azoospermia with full recovery noted in 50 to 90 percent of patients.[346,347] Pregnancy has been a possible outcome following treatment for Hodgkin lymphoma. No increases in birth defects or complications of pregnancy have been seen.[345]

OTHER COMPLICATIONS

Lhermitte's sign, or the induction of a sharp or lancinating sensation or pain down the spine produced by flexion, is a common complication of mantle radiotherapy.[348] An elevated thyroid-stimulating hormone level, with or without a low T3 or T4, is seen in about 30 percent of patients following mantle radiotherapy.[337] Rarely, hyperthyroidism, Grave's ophthalmopathy, or thyroid neoplasms occur after neck radiotherapy.[337]

Full-dose radiation therapy interferes with normal growth and development in children. Current therapy programs use low-dose or no radiotherapy for all stages of disease. Overwhelming sepsis is a rare event in patients who have had their spleen removed and been treated for Hodgkin lymphoma and occurs particularly in children.[351,352] Vaccination against encapsulated organisms 10 to 14 days prior to the onset of treatment is advised. However, neither vaccines nor antibiotic prophylaxis can provide certain protection.

Psychosocial sequelae of treatment for Hodgkin lymphoma deserve further study.[353] With the high rates of cure currently attained in the management of Hodgkin lymphoma (see Fig. 102-3), reduction in late effects and quality of life assume even greater importance.

REFERENCES

1. Hodgkin T: On some morbid appearances of the absorbent glands and spleen. *Med Chir Trans* 17:68, 1832.
2. Wilks S: Cases of lardaceous disease and some allied affections, with remarks. *Guys Hosp Rep* 17:103, 1856.
3. Wilks S: Cases of enlargement of the lymphatic glands and spleen, or Hodgkin's disease, with remarks. *Guys Hosp Rep* 11:56, 1865.
4. Craigie D: Case of disease of the spleen, in which death took place in consequence of the presence of purulent matter in the blood. *Edinburgh Med Surg J* 64:400, 1845.
5. Bennett J: Case of hypertrophy of the spleen and liver, in which death took place from suppuration of the blood. *Edinburgh Med Surg J* 64:413, 1845.
6. Virchow R: Weisses Blut. *Neue Notizen Geb Natur-Heilkunde.* 36:151, 1845.
7. Dreschfield J: Clinical lecture on acute Hodgkin's (or pseudoleucocythemia). *Brit Med J* 1:893, 1892.
8. Kundrat H: Uber Lympho-sarkomatosis. *Wien Wochnschr* 6:211, 1893.
9. Sternberg C: Uber eine eigenartige unter dem Bilde der Pseudoleukamie verlaufende Tuberculose des lymphatischen Appartes. *Z Heilk* 19:21, 1898.
10. Reed D: On the pathological changes in Hodgkin's disease, with especial reference to its relation to tuberculosis. *Johns Hopkins Hosp Rep* 10:133, 1902.
11. Fox H: Remarks on the presentation of microscopial preparations made from some of the original tissue described by Thomas Hodgkin. *Ann Med History* 8:370, 1926.
12. Jackson H, Parker F: *Hodgkin's Disease and Allied Disorders.* Oxford University Press, New York, 1947.
13. Lukes RJ, Butler JJ, Hicks EB: Natural history of Hodgkin's disease as related to its pathologic picture. *Cancer* 19:317, 1966.
14. Peters M: A study of survivals in Hodgkin's disease treated radiologically. *Am J Roentgenol* 63:299, 1950.
15. Peters M: A study of Hodgkin's disease treated by irradiation. *Am J Roentgenol* 79:114, 1958.
16. Kinmouth J: Lymphangiography in man: method of outlining lymphatic trunks and operation. *Clin Sci* 11:13, 1952.
17. Glatstein E, Guerney J, Rosenberg S, Kaplan H: The value of laparotomy and splenectomy in the staging of Hodgkin's disease. *Cancer* 24:709, 1969.
18. Rosenberg S: Report of the committee on the staging of Hodgkin's disease. *Cancer Res* 26:1310, 1966.
19. Carbone P, Kaplan H, Musshoff K: Report of the committee on the Hodgkin's disease staging. *Cancer Res* 31:1860, 1971.
20. Pusey W: Cases of sarcoma and of Hodgkin's disease treated by exposures to x-rays: a preliminary report. *JAMA* 38:166, 1902.
21. Senn N: Therapeutical value of roentgen ray in treatment of pseudoleukemia. *NY Med J* 77:665, 1903.
22. Gilbert R: Radiotherapy in Hodgkin's disease (malignant granulomatosis): anatomic and clinical foundations, governing principles, results. *Am J Roentgenol* 41:198, 1939.
23. Kaplan H: The radical radiotherapy of regionally localized Hodgkin's disease. *Radiology* 78:553, 1962.
24. Goodman L, Wingtrobe M, Dameshek W, Goodman MJ, Gilman A, McLennan MT: Nitrogen mustard therapy: use of methyl-bis(β-chloroethyl)amine hydrochloride and tris(β-chloroethyl)amine hydrochloride for Hodgkin's disease, lymphosarcoma, leukemia, and certain allied and miscellaneous disorders. *JAMA* 251:2255, 1984.
25. Jacobson L, Spurr C, Baron EG: Nitrogen mustard therapy: use of methyl-bis(β-chloroethyl)amine hydrochloride on neoplastic disorders of the hematopietic system. *JAMA* 132:263, 1946.
26. DeVita V, Serpick A, Carbone P: Combination chemotherapy in the treatment of advanced Hodgkin's disease. *Ann Intern Med* 73:881, 1970.
27. Stein H, Mason DY, Gerdes J, et al: The expression of the Hodgkin's disease associated antigen Ki-1 in reactive and neoplastic lymphoid tissue: evidence that Reed-Sternberg cells and histiocytic malignancies are derived from activated lymphoid cells. *Blood* 66:848, 1985.
28. Miettinen M: CD30 distribution. Immunohistochemical study on formaldehyde-fixed, paraffin-embedded Hodgkin's and non-Hodgkin's lymphomas. *Arch Pathol Lab Med* 116:1197, 1992.
29. Penny RJ, Blaustein JC, Longtine JA, Pinkus GS: Ki-1-positive large cell lymphomas, a heterogenous group of neoplasms. Morphologic, immunophenotypic, genotypic, and clinical features of 24 cases. *Cancer* 68:362, 1991.
30. Schienle HW, Stein N, Muller RW: Neutrophil granulocytic cell antigen defined by a monoclonal antibody—its distribution within normal haemic and non-haemic tissue. *J Clin Pathol* 35:959, 1982.
31. Stein H, Uchánska-Ziegler B, Gerdes J, Ziegler A, Wernet P: Hodgkin and Sternberg-Reed cells contain antigens specific to late cells of granulopoiesis. *Int J Cancer* 29:283, 1982.
32. Pinkus GS, Said JW: Leu-M1 immunoreactivity in nonhematopoietic neoplasms and myeloproliferative disorders. An immunoperoxidase study of paraffin sections. *Am J Clin Pathol* 85:278, 1986.
33. Rushin JM, Riordan GP, Heaton RB, Sharpe RW, Cotelingam JD, Jaffe ES: Cytomegalovirus-infected cells express Leu-M1 antigen. A potential source of diagnostic error. *Am J Pathol* 136:989, 1990.
34. Swerdlow SH, Wright SA: The spectrum of Leu-M1 staining in lymphoid and hematopoietic proliferations. *Am J Clin Pathol* 85:283, 1986.
35. Hsu SM, Tseng CK, Hsu PL: Expression of p55 (Tac) interleukin-2 receptor (IL-2R), but not p75 IL-2R, in cultured H-RS cells and H-RS cells in tissues. *Am J Pathol* 136:735, 1990.
36. Schmid C, Pan L, Diss T, Isaacson PG: Expression of B-cell antigens by Hodgkin's and Reed-Sternberg cells. *Am J Pathol* 139:701, 1991.
37. Lauritzen AF, Moller PH, Nedergaard T, Guldberg P, Hou-Jensen K, Ralfkiaer E: Apoptosis-related genes and proteins in Hodgkin's disease. *APMIS* 107:636, 1999.
38. Von Wasielewski R, Mengel M, Fischer R, et al: Classical Hodgkin's disease. Clinical impact of the immunophenotype. *Am J Pathol* 151:1123, 1997.
39. Papadimitriou CS, Bai MK, Kotsianti AJ, Costopoulos JS, Hytiroglou P: Phenotype of Hodgkin and Sternberg-Reed cells and expression of CD57 (LEU7) antigen. *Leuk Lymphoma* 20:125, 1995.

40. Pinkus GS, Said JW: Hodgkin's disease, lymphocyte predominance type, nodular—further evidence for a B cell derivation. L & H variants of Reed-Sternberg cells express L26, a pan B cell marker. *Am J Pathol* 133:211, 1988.

41. Pinkus GS, Said JW: Hodgkin's disease, lymphocyte predominance type, nodular—a distinct entity? Unique staining profile for L&H variants of Reed-Sternberg cells defined by monoclonal antibodies to leukocyte common antigen, granulocyte-specific antigen, and B-cell-specific antigen. *Am J Pathol* 118:1, 1985.

42. Stein H, Hansmann ML, Lennert K, Brandtzaeg P, Gatter KC, Mason DY: Reed-Sternberg and Hodgkin cells in lymphocyte-predominant Hodgkin's disease of nodular subtype contain J chain. *Am J Clin Pathol* 86:292, 1986.

43. Schmid C, Sargent C, Isaacson PG: L and H cells of nodular lymphocyte predominant Hodgkin's disease show immunoglobulin light-chain restriction. *Am J Pathol* 139:1281, 1991.

44. Poppema S, Kaiserling E, Lennert K: Nodular paragranuloma and progressively transformed germinal centers. Ultrastructural and immunohistologic findings. *Virchows Arch B Cell Pathol* 31:211, 1979.

45. Kadin ME, Stites DP, Levy R, Warnke R: Exogenous immunoglobulin and the macrophage origin of Reed-Sternberg cells in Hodgkin's disease. *N Engl J Med* 299:1208, 1978.

46. Ree HJ, Kadin ME: Macrophage-histiocytes in Hodgkin's disease. The relation of peanut-agglutinin-binding macrophage-histiocytes to clinicopathologic presentation and course of disease. *Cancer* 56:333, 1985.

47. Mori N, Oka K, Sakuma H, Tsunoda R, Kojima M: Immunoelectron microscopic study of Hodgkin's disease. *Cancer* 56:2605, 1985.

48. Hsu SM, Yang K, Jaffe ES: Phenotypic expression of Hodgkin's and Reed-Sternberg cells in Hodgkin's disease. *Am J Pathol* 118:209, 1985.

49. Knowles D, Neri A, Pelicci PG, et al: Immunoglobulin and T-cell receptor beta-chain gene rearrangement analysis of Hodgkin's disease: implications for lineage determination and differential diagnosis. *Proc Natl Acad Sci USA* 83:7942, 1986.

50. Brinker MG, Poppema S, Buys CH, Timens W, Osinga J, Visser L: Clonal immunoglobulin gene rearrangements in tissues involved by Hodgkin's disease. *Blood* 70:186, 1987.

51. Weiss LM, Warnke RA, Sklar J: Clonal antigen receptor gene rearrangements and Epstein-Barr viral DNA in tissues of Hodgkin's disease. *Hematol Oncol* 6:233, 1988.

52. Roth MS, Schnitzer B, Bingham EL, Harnden CE, Hyder DM, Ginsburg D: Rearrangement of immunoglobulin and T-cell receptor genes in Hodgkin's disease. *Am J Pathol* 131:331, 1988.

53. Raghavachar A, Binder T, Bartram CR: Immunoglobulin and T-cell receptor gene rearrangements in Hodgkin's disease. *Cancer Res* 48:3591, 1988.

54. Sundeen J, Lipford E, Uppenkamp M, et al: Rearranged antigen receptor genes in Hodgkin's disease. *Blood* 70:96, 1987.

55. Küppers R, Rajewsky K, Zhao M, et al: Hodgkin disease: Hodgkin and Reed-Sternberg cells picked from histological sections show clonal immunoglobulin gene rearrangements and appear to be derived from B cells at various stages of development. *Proc Natl Acad Sci USA* 91:10962, 1994.

56. Küppers R, Roers A, Kanzler H: Molecular single cell studies of normal and transformed lymphocytes. *Cancer Surv* 30:45, 1997.

57. Kanzler H, Küppers R, Hansmann ML, Rajewsky K: Hodgkin and Reed-Sternberg cells in Hodgkin's disease represent the outgrowth of a dominant tumor clone derived from (crippled) germinal center B cells. *J Exp Med* 184:1495, 1996.

58. Bargou RC, Emmerich F, Krappmann D, et al: Constitutive nuclear factor-kappaB-RelA activation is required for proliferation and survival of Hodgkin's disease tumor cells. *J Clin Invest* 100:2961, 1997.

59. Jox A, Zander T, Küppers R, et al: Somatic mutations within the untranslated regions of rearranged Ig genes in a case of classical Hodgkin's disease as a potential cause for the absence of Ig in the lymphoma cells. *Blood* 93:3964, 1999.

60. Braeuninger A, Küppers R, Strickler JG, Wacker HH, Rajewsky K, Hansmann ML: Hodgkin and Reed-Sternberg cells in lymphocyte predominant Hodgkin disease represent clonal populations of germinal center-derived tumor B cells. *Proc Natl Acad Sci USA* 94:9337, 1997.

61. Ohno T, Stribley JA, Wu G, Hinrichs SH, Weisenburger DD, Chan WC: Clonality in nodular lymphocyte-predominant Hodgkin's disease. *N Engl J Med* 337:459, 1997.

62. Marafioti T, Hummel M, Anagnostopoulos I, et al: Origin of nodular lymphocyte-predominant Hodgkin's disease from a clonal expansion of highly mutated germinal-center B cells. *N Engl J Med* 337:453, 1997.

63. Vockerodt M, Soares M, Kanzler H, et al: Detection of clonal Hodgkin and Reed-Sternberg cells with identical somatically mutated and rearranged VH genes in different biopsies in relapsed Hodgkin's disease. *Blood* 92:2899, 1998.

64. Jox A, Zander T, Kornacker M, et al: Detection of identical Hodgkin-Reed Sternberg cell specific immunoglobulin gene rearrangements in a patient with Hodgkin's disease of mixed cellularity subtype at primary diagnosis and in relapse two and a half years later. *Ann Oncol* 9:283, 1998.

65. Bräuninger A, Hansmann ML, Strickler JG, et al: Identification of common germinal-center B-cell precursors in two patients with both Hodgkin's disease and non-Hodgkin's lymphoma. *N Engl J Med* 340:1239, 1999.

66. Stein H, Hummel M, Marafioti T, Anagnostopoulos I, Foss HD: Molecular biology of Hodgkin's disease. *Cancer Surv* 30:107, 1997.

67. Bhagat SK, Medeiros LJ, Weiss LM, Wang J, Raffeld M, Stetler SM: bcl-2 expression in Hodgkin's disease. Correlation with the t(14;18) translocation and Epstein-Barr virus. *Am J Clin Pathol* 99:604, 1993.

68. Jiwa NM, Oudejans JJ, Bai MC, et al: Expression of bcl-2 protein and transcription of the Epstein-Barr virus bcl-2 homologue BHRF-1 in Hodgkin's disease: implications for different pathogenic mechanisms. *Histopathology* 26:547, 1995.

69. Smolewski P, Niewiadomska H, B*o*nski JZ, Robak T, Krykowski E: Expression of proliferating cell nuclear antigen (PCNA) and p53, bcl-2 or C-erb B-2 proteins on Reed-Sternberg cells: prognostic significance in Hodgkin's disease. *Neoplasma* 45:140, 1998.

70. Brink AA, Oudejans JJ, van den Brule AJ, et al: Low p53 and high bcl-2 expression in Reed-Sternberg cells predicts poor clinical outcome for Hodgkin's disease: involvement of apoptosis resistance? *Mod Pathol* 11:376, 1998.

71. Doglioni C, Pelosio P, Mombello A, Scarpa A, Chilosi M: Immunohistochemical evidence of abnormal expression of the antioncogene-encoded p53 phosphoprotein in Hodgkin's disease and CD30+ anaplastic lymphomas. *Hematol Pathol* 5:67, 1991.

72. Gupta RK, Patel K, Bodmer WF, Bodmer JG: Mutation of p53 in primary biopsy material and cell lines from Hodgkin disease. *Proc Natl Acad Sci USA* 90:2817, 1993.

73. Niedobitek G, Agathanggelou A, Barber P, Smallman LA, Jones EL, Young LS: P53 overexpression and Epstein-Barr virus infection in undifferentiated and squamous cell nasopharyngeal carcinomas. *J Pathol* 170:457, 1993.

74. Chen WG, Chen YY, Kamel OW, Koo CH, Weiss LM: p53 mutations in Hodgkin's disease. *Lab Invest* 75:519, 1996.

75. Chilosi M, Doglioni C, Menestrina F, et al: Abnormal expression of the p53-binding protein MDM2 in Hodgkin's disease. *Blood* 84:4295, 1994.

76. Sánchez-Beato M, Piris MA, Martinez-Montero JC, et al: MDM2 and p21WAF1/CIP1, wild-type p53-induced proteins, are regularly expressed by Sternberg-Reed cells in Hodgkin's disease. *J Path* 180:58, 1996.

77. Cabanillas F, Pathak S, Trujillo J, et al: Cytogenetic features of Hodgkin's disease suggest possible origin from a lymphocyte. *Blood* 71:1615, 1988.

78. Schouten HC, Sanger WG, Duggan M, Weisenburger DD, MacLennan KA, Armitage JO: Chromosomal abnormalities in Hodgkin's disease. *Blood* 73:2149, 1989.

79. Tilly H, Bastard C, Delastre T, et al: Cytogenetic studies in untreated Hodgkin's disease. *Blood* 77:1298, 1991.

80. Oshima K, Ishiguro M, Ohgami A, et al: Genetic analysis of sorted Hodgkin and Reed-Sternberg cells using comparative genomic hybridization. *Int J Cancer* 82:250, 1999.

81. Stetler SM, Crush SS, Cossman J: Involvement of the bcl-2 gene in Hodgkin's disease. *J Natl Cancer Inst* 82:855, 1990.

82. Louie DC, Kant JA, Brooks JJ, Reed JC: Absence of t(14;18) major and minor breakpoints and of Bcl-2 protein overproduction in Reed-Sternberg cells of Hodgkin's disease. *Am J Pathol* 139:1231, 1991.

83. Athan E, Chadburn A, Knowles DM: The bcl-2 gene translocation is undetectable in Hodgkin's disease by Southern blot hybridization and polymerase chain reaction. *Am J Pathol* 141:193, 1992.

84. Gravel S, Delsol G, Al Saati T: Single-cell analysis of the

t(14;18)(q32;q21) chromosomal translocation in Hodgkin's disease demonstrates the absence of this translocation in neoplastic Hodgkin and Reed-Sternberg cells. *Blood* 91:2866, 1998.

85. Weiss LM, Strickler JG, Warnke RA, Purtilo DT, Sklar J: Epstein-Barr viral DNA in tissues of Hodgkin's disease. *Am J Pathol* 129:86, 1987.

86. Herbst H, Dallenbach F, Hummel M, et al: Epstein-Barr virus latent membrane protein expression in Hodgkin and Reed-Sternberg cells. *Proc Natl Acad Sci USA* 88:4766, 1991.

87. Pallesen G, Hamilton DS, Rowe M, Young LS: Expression of Epstein-Barr virus latent gene products in tumour cells of Hodgkin's disease. *Lancet* 337:320, 1991.

88. Miettinen M, Franssila KO, Saxen E: Hodgkin's disease, lymphocytic predominance nodular. Increased risk for subsequent non-Hodgkin's lymphomas. *Cancer* 51:2293, 1983.

89. Sundeen JT, Cossman J, Jaffe ES: Lymphocyte predominant Hodgkin's disease nodular subtype with coexistent "large cell lymphoma." Histological progression or composite malignancy? *Am J Surg Pathol* 12:599, 1988.

90. Gonzalez CL, Medeiros LJ, Jaffe ES: Composite lymphoma. A clinico-pathologic analysis of nine patients with Hodgkin's disease and B-cell non-Hodgkin's lymphoma. *Am J Clin Pathol* 96:81, 1991.

91. Williams J, Schned A, Cotelingam JD, Jaffe ES: Chronic lymphocytic leukemia with coexistent Hodgkin's disease. Implications for the origin of the Reed-Sternberg cell. *Am J Surg Pathol* 15:33, 1991.

92. Momose H, Jaffe ES, Shin SS, Chen YY, Weiss LM: Chronic lymphocytic leukemia/small lymphocytic lymphoma with Reed-Sternberg-like cells and possible transformation to Hodgkin's disease. Mediation by Epstein-Barr virus. *Am J Surg Pathol* 16:859, 1992.

93. Lipa M, Kunynetz R, Pawlowski D, Kerbel G, Haberman H: The occurrence of mycosis fungoides in two patients with preexisting Hodgkin's disease. *Arch Dermatol* 118:563, 1982.

94. Caya JG, Choi H, Tieu TM, Wollenberg NJ, Almagro UA: Hodgkin's disease followed by mycosis fungoides in the same patient. Case report and literature review. *Cancer* 53:463, 1984.

95. Ohno T, Smir BN, Weisenburger DD, Gascoyne RD, Hinrichs SD, Chan WC: Origin of the Hodgkin/Reed-Sternberg cells in chronic lymphocytic leukemia with "Hodgkin's transformation." *Blood* 91:1757, 1998.

96. Ohno T, Trenn G, Wu G, Abou-Elella A, Reis HE, Chan WC: The clonal relationship between nodular sclerosis Hodgkin's disease with a clonal Reed-Sternberg cell population and a subsequent B-cell small noncleaved cell lymphoma. *Mod Pathol* 11:485, 1998.

97. Carbone A, Gloghini A, Gattei V, et al: Expression of functional CD40 antigen on Reed-Sternberg cells and Hodgkin's disease cell lines. *Blood* 85:780, 1995.

98. Newcom SR, Ansari AA, Gu L: Interleukin-4 is an autocrine growth factor secreted by the L-428 Reed-Sternberg cell. *Blood* 79:191, 1992.

99. Jücker M, Abts H, Li W, et al: Expression of interleukin-6 and interleukin-6 receptor in Hodgkin's disease. *Blood* 77:2413, 1991.

100. Tesch H, Jücker M, Klein S, et al: Hodgkin and Reed-Sternberg cells express interleukin 6 and interleukin 6 receptors. *Leuk Lymphoma* 7:297, 1992.

101. Foss HD, Herbst H, Oelmann E, et al: Lymphotoxin, tumour necrosis factor and interleukin-6 gene transcripts are present in Hodgkin and Reed-Sternberg cells of most Hodgkin's disease cases. *Br J Haematol* 84:627, 1993.

102. Merz H, Houssiau FA, Orscheschek K, et al: Interleukin-9 expression in human malignant lymphomas: unique association with Hodgkin's disease and large cell anaplastic lymphoma. *Blood* 78:1311, 1991.

103. Springer TA: Traffic signals for lymphocyte recirculation and leukocyte emigration: the multistep paradigm. *Cell* 76:301, 1994.

104. Herbst H, Foss HD, Samol J, et al: Frequent expression of interleukin-10 by Epstein-Barr virus-harboring tumor cells of Hodgkin's disease. *Blood* 87:2918, 1996.

105. Demoulin JB, Renauld JC: Interleukin 9 and its receptor: an overview of structure and function. *Int Rev Immunol* 16:345, 1998.

106. Kapp U, Yeh WC, Patterson B, et al: Interleukin 13 is secreted by and stimulates the growth of Hodgkin and Reed-Sternberg cells. *J Exp Med* 189:1939, 1999.

107. Pizzolo G, Vinante F, Chilosi M, et al: Serum levels of soluble CD30 molecule (Ki-1 antigen) in Hodgkin's disease: relationship with disease activity and clinical stage. *Br J Haematol* 75:282, 1990.

108. Nadali G, Vinante F, Ambrosetti A, et al: Serum levels of soluble CD30

are elevated in the majority of untreated patients with Hodgkin's disease and correlate with clinical features and prognosis. *J Clin Oncol* 12:793, 1994.

109. Kurzrock R, Redman J, Cabanillas F, Jones D, Rothberg J, Talpaz M: Serum interleukin 6 levels are elevated in lymphoma patients and correlate with survival in advanced Hodgkin's disease and with B symptoms. *Cancer Res* 53:2118, 1993.

110. Pizzolo G, Chilosi M, Vinante F, et al: Soluble interleukin-2 receptors in the serum of patients with Hodgkin's disease. *Br J Cancer* 55:427, 1987.

111. Sarris AH, Kliche KO, Pethambaram P, et al: Interleukin-10 levels are often elevated in serum of adults with Hodgkin's disease and are associated with inferior failure-free survival. *Ann Oncol* 10:433, 1999.

112. Slivnick DJ, Ellis TM, Nawrocki JF, Fisher RI: The impact of Hodgkin's disease on the immune system. *Semin Oncol* 17:673, 1990.

113. Levy R, Kaplan HS: Impaired lymphocyte function in untreated Hodgkin's disease. *N Engl J Med* 290:181, 1974.

114. Corder MP, Young RC, Brown RS, DeVita VT: Phytohemagglutinin-induced lymphocyte transformation: the relationship to prognosis of Hodgkin's disease. *Blood* 39:595, 1972.

115. Romagnani S, Ferrini PL, Ricci M: The immune derangement in Hodgkin's disease. *Semin Hematol* 22:41, 1985.

116. Bjorkholm M, Holm G, Mellstedt H: Immunologic profile of patients with cured Hodgkin's disease. *Scand J Haematol* 18:361, 1977.

117. Young RC, Corder MP, Haynes HA, DeVita VT: Delayed hypersensitivity in Hodgkin's disease. A study of 103 untreated patients. *Am J Med* 52:63, 1972.

118. King GW, Yanes B, Hurtubise PE, Balcerzak SP, LoBuglio AF: Immune function of successfully treated lymphoma patients. *J Clin Invest* 57:1451, 1976.

119. Fisher RI, DeVita VJ, Bostick F, et al: Persistent immunologic abnormalities in long-term survivors of advanced Hodgkin's disease. *Ann Intern Med* 92:595, 1980.

120. Fisher RI: Implications of persistent T cell abnormalities for the etiology of Hodgkin's disease. *Cancer Treat Rep* 66:681, 1982.

121. Watanabe N, De Rosa SC, Cmelak A, Hoppe R, Herzenberg LA, Roederer M: Long-term depletion of naive T cells in patients treated for Hodgkin's disease. *Blood* 90:3662, 1997.

122. Van den Berg A, Visser L, Poppema S: High expression of the CC chemokine TARC in Reed-Sternberg cells. A possible explanation for the characteristic T-cell infiltrate in Hodgkin's lymphoma. *Am J Pathol* 154:1685, 1999.

123. Landis SH, Murray T, Bolden S, Wingo PA: Cancer statistics, 1999. *CA Cancer J Clin* 49:8, 1999.

124. MacMahon B: Epidemiology of Hodgkin's disease. *Cancer Res* 26:1189, 1966.

125. Grufferman S, Duong T, Cole P: Occupation and Hodgkin's disease. *J Natl Cancer Inst* 57:1193, 1976.

126. Young JJ, Percy CL, Asire AJ, et al: Cancer incidence and mortality in the United States, 1973–77. *Natl Cancer Inst Monogr* 1, 1981.

127. Abramson JH, Pridan H, Sacks MI, Avitzour M, Peritz E: A case-control study of Hodgkin's disease in Israel. *J Natl Cancer Inst* 61:307, 1978.

128. Gutensohn N, Cole P: Childhood social environment and Hodgkin's disease. *N Engl J Med* 304:135, 1981.

129. Grufferman S, Delzell E: Epidemiology of Hodgkin's disease. *Epidemiol Rev* 6:76, 1984.

130. Vianna NJ, Greenwald P, Davies JN: Extended epidemic of Hodgkin's disease in high-school students. *Lancet* 1:1209, 1971.

131. Klinger RJ, Minton JP: Case clustering of Hodgkin's disease in a small rural community, with associations among cases. *Lancet* 1:168, 1973.

132. Vianna NJ, Greenwald P, Davies JNP: Epidemiologic evidence for transmission of Hodgkin's disease: the lymphoid tissue barrier. *N Engl J Med* 10:499, 1974.

133. Cuneo JM: Infectious aspects of Hodgkin's disease. *N Engl J Med* 290:345, 1974.

134. Pike MC, Henderson BE, Casagrande J: Infectious aspects of Hodgkin's disease. *N Engl J Med* 290:341, 1974.

135. Grufferman S, Cole P, Levitan TR: Evidence against transmission of Hodgkin's disease in high schools. *N Engl J Med* 300:1006, 1979.

136. Rosdahl N, Larsen SO, Clemmesen J: Hodgkin's disease in patients with previous infectious mononucleosis: 30 years' experience. *Br Med J* 2:253, 1974.

137. Munoz N, Davidson RLJ, Witthoff B: Infectious mononucleosis and Hodgkin's disease. *Int J Cancer* 22:10, 1978.

138. Kvale G, Hoiby EA, Pedersen E: Hodgkin's disease in patients with previous infectious mononucleosis. *Int J Cancer* 23:593, 1979.

139. Mueller N, Evans A, Harris N: Altered antibody titers to Epstein-Barr virus before the diagnosis of Hodgkin's disease. *N Engl J Med* 320:689, 1989.

140. Boiocchi M, De RV, Dolcetti R, Carbone A, Scarpa A, Menestrina F: Association of Epstein-Barr virus genome with mixed cellularity and cellular phase nodular sclerosis Hodgkin's disease subtypes. *Ann Oncol* 3:307, 1992.

141. Herbst H, Pallesen G, Weiss LM, et al: Hodgkin's disease and Epstein-Barr virus. *Ann Oncol* 4:27, 1992.

142. Armstrong AA, Alexander FE, Paes RP, et al: Association of Epstein-Barr virus with pediatric Hodgkin's disease. *Am J Pathol* 142:1683, 1993.

143. Ambinder RF, Browning PJ, Lorenzana I, et al: Epstein-Barr virus and childhood Hodgkin's disease in Honduras and the United States. *Blood* 81:462, 1993.

144. Chang KL, Albújar PF, Chen YY, Johnson RM, Weiss LM: High prevalence of Epstein-Barr virus in the Reed-Sternberg cells of Hodgkin's disease occurring in Peru. *Blood* 81:496, 1993.

145. Weinreb M, Day PJ, Murray PG, et al: Epstein-Barr virus (EBV) and Hodgkin's disease in children: incidence of EBV latent membrane protein in malignant cells. *J Pathol* 168:365, 1992.

146. Herndier BG, Sanchez HC, Chang KL, Chen YY, Weiss LM: High prevalence of Epstein-Barr virus in the Reed-Sternberg cells of HIV-associated Hodgkin's disease. *Am J Pathol* 142:1073, 1993.

147. Lynch HT, Saldivar VA, Guirgis HA, et al: Familial Hodgkin's disease and associated cancer. A clinical-pathologic study. *Cancer* 38:2033, 1976.

148. Creagan ET, Fraumeni JJ: Familial Hodgkin's disease. *Lancet* 2:547, 1972.

149. Buehler SK, Firme F, Fodor G, Fraser GR, Marshall WH, Vaze P: Common variable immunodeficiency, Hodgkin's disease, and other malignancies in a Newfoundland family. *Lancet* 1:195, 1975.

150. Manigand G, Macrez C, Chome J: Maladie de Hodgkin's familial. *Presse Med* 72:1871, 1964.

151. Bohunicky L, Poliakova L, Krizan Z, Cerny V, Hal'ko J: The incidence of lymphogranulomatosis in single-ovum twins. *Neoplasma* 18:283, 1971.

152. Gracz K, Kofman S, Economou SG: Hodgkin disease in monozygotic twins: a case report. *J Surg Oncol* 12:221, 1979.

153. Razis DV, diamond HD, Craver LF: Familial Hodgkin's disease—its significance and implications. *Ann Intern Med* 51:933, 1953.

154. Haim N, Cohen Y, Robinson E: Malignant lymphoma in first-degree blood relatives. *Cancer* 49:197, 1982.

155. Vianna NJ, Davies JN, Polan AK, Wolfgang P: Familial Hodgkin's disease: an environmental and genetic disorder. *Lancet* 2:854, 1974.

156. Grufferman S, Cole P, Smith PG, Lukes RJ: Hodgkin's disease in siblings. *N Engl J Med* 296:248, 1977.

157. Vianna NJ: *Lymphoreticular Malignancies, Epidemiologic and Related Aspects.* University Park Press, Baltimore, 1975.

158. Lin AY, Kingma DW, Lennette ET, et al: Epstein-Barr virus and familial Hodgkin's disease. *Blood* 88:3160, 1996.

159. Bjerrum OW, Hasselbalch HC, Drivsholm A, Nissen NI: Non-Hodgkin malignant lymphomas and Hodgkin's disease in first-degree relatives. Evidence for a mutual genetic predisposition? *Scand J Haematol* 36:398, 1986.

160. Fraumeni JF, Wertelecki W, Blattner WA, Jensen RD, Leventhal BG: Varied manifestations of a familial lymphoproliferative disorder. *Am J Med* 59:145, 1975.

161. Hors J, Dausset J: HLA and susceptibility to Hodgkin's disease. *Immunol Rev* 70:167, 1983.

162. Cimino G, Lo CF, Cartoni C, et al: Immune-deficiency in Hodgkin's disease (HD): a study of patients and healthy relatives in families with multiple cases. *Eur J Cancer Clin Oncol* 24:1595, 1988.

163. Bodmer JG, Tonks S, Oza AM, Lister TA, Bodmer WF: HLA-DP based resistance to Hodgkin's disease. *Lancet* 1:1455, 1989.

164. Berberich FR, Berberich MS, King MC, Engleman EG, Grumet FC: Hodgkin's disease susceptibility: linkage to the HLA locus demonstrated by a new concordance method. *Hum Immunol* 6:207, 1983.

165. Oza AM, Tonks S, Lim J, Fleetwood MA, Lister TA, Bodmer JG: A clinical and epidemiological study of human leukocyte antigen-DPB alleles in Hodgkin's disease. *Cancer Res* 54:5101, 1994.

166. Tonks S, Oza AM, Lister TA, Bodmer JG: Association of HLA-DPB with Hodgkin's disease. *Lancet* 340:968, 1992.

167. Klitz W, Aldrich CL, Fildes N, Horning SJ, Begovich AB: Localization of predisposition to Hodgkin disease in the HLA class II region. *Am J Human Genet* 54:497, 1994.

168. Kaplan HS: *Hodgkin's Disease.* Harvard University Press, Cambridge, MA, 1980.

169. Pel PK: Zur symptomatolgie der sogennanten pseudoleukamie. II. Pseudokeukamie oder chronisches Ruckfallsfieber? *Berlin Klin Wochenschr* 24:844, 1887.

170. Ebstein WV: Das chronische Ruckfallsfieber, eine neu infectionskrankheit. *Berlin Klin Wochenshr* 24:565, 1887.

171. Tubiana M, Attie E, Flamant R, Gerard MR, Hayat M: Prognostic factors in 454 cases of Hodgkin's disease. *Cancer Res* 31:1801, 1971.

172. Atkinson K, Austin DE, McElwain TJ, Peckham MJ: Alcohol pain in Hodgkin's disease. *Cancer* 37:895, 1976.

173. Bjerrum OW, Hansen OE: Progressive multifocal leucoencephalopathy in Hodgkin's disease. *Scand J Haematol* 34:442, 1985.

174. Trotter JL, Hendin BA, Osterland CK: Cerebellar degeneration with Hodgkin disease. An immunological study. *Arch Neurol* 33:660, 1976.

175. Greenberg HS: Paraneoplastic cerebellar degeneration. A clinical and CT study. *J Neurooncol* 2:377, 1984.

176. Dansey RD, Hammond TG, Lai K, Bezwoda WR: Subacute myelopathy: an unusual paraneoplastic complication of Hodgkin's disease. *Med Pediatr Oncol* 16:284, 1988.

177. Sagar HJ, Read DJ: Subacute sensory neuropathy with remission: an association with lymphoma. *J Neurol Neurosurg Psychiatry* 45:83, 1982.

178. Feldmann E, Posner JB: Episodic neurologic dysfunction in patients with Hodgkin's disease. *Arch Neurol* 43:1227, 1986.

179. Carr I: The Ophelia syndrome: memory loss in Hodgkin's disease. *Lancet* 1:844, 1982.

180. Julien J, Vital C, Aupy G, Lagueny A, Darriet D, Brechenmacher C: Guillain-Barré syndrome and Hodgkin's disease—ultrastructural study of a peripheral nerve. *J Neurol Sci* 45:23, 1980.

181. Rewcastle NB, Tom MI: Non-infectious granulomatis angiitis of the nervous system associated with Hodgkin's disease. *J Neurol Neurosurg Psychiatry* 25:51, 1962.

182. Filly R, Bland N, Castellino RA: Radiographic distribution of intrathoracic disease in previously untreated patients with Hodgkin's disease and non-Hodgkin's lymphoma. *Radiology* 120:277, 1976.

183. Castellino RA, Billingham M, Dorfman RF: Lymphographic accuracy in Hodgkin's disease and malignant lymphoma with a note on the "reactive" lymph node as a cause of most false-positive lymphograms. *Invest Radiol* 9:155, 1974.

184. Kaplan HS: Survival and relapse rates in Hodgkin's disease: Stanford experience 1961–1971. *Natl Cancer Inst Monogr* 36:489, 1973.

185. Mansfield CM, Fabian C, Jones S, et al: Comparison of lymphangiography and computed tomography scanning in evaluating abdominal disease in stages III and IV Hodgkin's disease. A Southwest Oncology Group study. *Cancer* 66:2295, 1990.

186. Castellino RA, Hoppe RT, Blank N, et al: Computed tomography, lymphography, and staging laparotomy: correlations in initial staging of Hodgkin disease. *Am J Roentgenol* 143:37, 1984.

187. Castellino RA: Imaging techniques for staging abdominal Hodgkin's disease. *Cancer Treat Rep* 66:697, 1982.

188. Jerusalem G, Warland V, Najjar F, et al: Whole-body 18F-FDG PET for the evaluation of patients with Hodgkin's disease and non-Hodgkin's lymphoma. *Nucl Med Comm* 20:13, 1999.

189. Bangerter M, Moog F, Buchmann I, et al: Whole-body 2-[18F]-fluoro-2-deoxy-D-glucose positron emission tomography (FDG-PET) for accurate staging of Hodgkin's disease. *Ann Oncol* 9:1117, 1998.

190. Skillings JR, Bramwell V, Nicholson RL, Prato FS, Wells G: A prospective study of magnetic resonance imaging in lymphoma staging. *Cancer* 67:1838, 1991.

191. Gasparini MD, Balzarini L, Castellani MR, et al: Current role of gallium scan and magnetic resonance imaging in the management of mediastinal Hodgkin lymphoma. *Cancer* 72:577, 1993.

192. Burns BF, Colby TV, Dorfman RF: Differential diagnostic features of nodular L & H Hodgkin's disease, including progressive transformation of germinal centers. *Am J Surg Pathol* 8:253, 1984.

193. Hansmann ML, Zwingers T, Boske A, Loffler H, Lennert K: Clinical features of nodular paragranuloma (Hodgkin's disease, lymphocyte predominance type, nodular). *J Cancer Res Clin Oncol* 108:321, 1984.

194. MacLennan KA, Bennett MH, Tu A, et al: Relationship of histopathologic features to survival and relapse in nodular sclerosing Hodgkin's disease. A study of 1659 patients. *Cancer* 64:1686, 1989.

195. Masih AS, Weisenburger DD, Vose JM, Bast MA, Armitage JO: Histologic grade does not predict prognosis in optimally treated, advanced-stage nodular sclerosing Hodgkin's disease. *Cancer* 69:228, 1992.

196. Kant JA, Hubbard SM, Longo DL, Simon RM, DeVita VJ, Jaffe ES: The pathologic and clinical heterogeneity of lymphocyte-depleted Hodgkin's disease. *J Clin Oncol* 4:284, 1986.

197. Neiman RS, Rosen PJ, Lukes RJ: Lymphocyte-depletion Hodgkin's disease. A clinicopathological entity. *N Engl J Med* 288:751, 1973.

198. Diehl V, Sextro M, Franklin J, et al: Clinical presentation, course, and prognostic factors in lymphocyte-predominant Hodgkin's disease and lymphocyte-rich classical Hodgkin's disease: report from the European Task Force on Lymphoma Project on Lymphocyte-Predominant Hodgkin's Disease. *J Clin Oncol* 17:776, 1999.

199. Rosenberg SA, Kaplan HS: Evidence for an orderly progression in the spread of Hodgkin's disease. *Cancer Res* 26:1225, 1966.

200. Smithers DW: Spread of Hodgkin's disease. *Lancet* 1:1262, 1970.

201. Hutchison GB: Anatomic patterns by histologic type of localized Hodgkin's disease of the upper torso. *Lymphology* 5:1, 1972.

202. Kirschner RH, Abt AB, O'Connell MJ, Sklansky BD, Greene WH, Wiernik PH: Vascular invasion and hematogenous dissemination of Hodgkin's disease. *Cancer* 34:1159, 1974.

203. Naeim F, Waisman J, Coulson WF: Hodgkin's disease: the significance of vascular invasion. *Cancer* 34:655, 1974.

204. Lister TA, Crowther D, Sutcliffe SB, et al: Report of a committee convened to discuss the evaluation and staging of patients with Hodgkin's disease: Cotswold meeting. *J Clin Oncol* 7:1630, 1989.

205. Piro AJ, Hellman S: Invited discussion: Laparotomy alters treatment in Hodgkin's disease. *Natl Cancer Inst Monogr* 36:307, 1973.

206. Kaplan HS, Dorfman RF, Nelsen TS, Rosenberg SA: Staging laparotomy and splenectomy in Hodgkin's disease: analysis of indications and patterns of involvement in 285 consecutive, unselected patients. *Natl Cancer Inst Monogr* 36:291, 1973.

207. Desser RK, Golomb HM, Ultmann JE, et al: Prognostic classification of Hodgkin disease in pathologic stage III, based on anatomic considerations. *Blood* 49:883, 1977.

208. Stein RS, Golomb HM, Diggs CH, et al: Anatomic substages of stage III-A Hodgkin's disease. A collaborative study. *Ann Intern Med*: 159, 1980.

209. Leibenhaut MH, Hoppe RT, Efron B, Halpern J, Nelsen T, Rosenberg SA: Prognostic indicators of laparotomy findings in clinical stage I-II supradiaphragmatic Hodgkin's disease. *J Clin Oncol* 7:81, 1989.

210. Mauch P, Larson D, Osteen R, et al: Prognostic factors for positive surgical staging in patients with Hodgkin's disease. *J Clin Oncol* 8:257, 1990.

211. Simmons AV, Spiers AS, Fayers PM: Haematological and clinical parameters in assessing activity in Hodgkin's disease and other malignant lymphomas. *Q J Med* 42:111, 1973.

212. Tauro GP: Hodgkin's disease associated with raised eosinophil counts. *Med J Aust* 2:604, 1966.

213. MacLennan KA, Hudson BV, Jelliffe AM, Haybittle JL, Hudson GV: The pretreatment peripheral blood lymphocyte count in 1100 patients with Hodgkin's disease: the prognostic significance and the relationship to the presence of systemic symptoms. *Clin Oncol* 7:333, 1981.

214. Ultmann JE, Cunningham JK, Gellhorn A: The clinical picture of Hodgkin's disease. *Cancer Res* 26:1047, 1966.

215. MacLennan KA, Vaughan HB, Easterling MJ, Jelliffe AM, Vaughan HG, Haybittle JL: The presentation haemoglobin level in 1103 patients with Hodgkin's disease (BNLI report no. 21). *Clin Radiol* 34:491, 1983.

216. Storgaard L, Karle H: Fever and haemolysis in Hodgkin's diseases. *Acta Med Scand* 197:311, 1975.

217. Jones SE: Autoimmune disorders and malignant lymphoma. *Cancer* 31:1092, 1973.

218. Sonnenblick M, Kramer R, Hershko C: Corticosteroid responsive immune thrombocytopenia in Hodgkin's disease. *Oncology* 43:349, 1986.

219. Cohen JR: Idiopathic thrombocytopenic purpura in Hodgkin's disease: a rare occurrence of no prognostic significance. *Cancer* 41:743, 1978.

220. Kedar A, Khan AB, Mattern JQ, Fisher J, Thomas PR, Freeman AI: Autoimmune disorders complicating adolescent Hodgkin's disease. *Cancer* 44:112, 1979.

221. Hunter JD, Logue GL, Joyner JT: Autoimmune neutropenia in Hodgkin's disease. *Arch Intern Med* 142:386, 1982.

222. Le Bourgeois J, Tubiana M: The erythrocyte sedimentation rate as a monitor for relapse in patients with previously treated Hodgkin's disease. *Int J Radiat Oncol Biol Phys* 2:241, 1977.

223. Haybittle JL, Hayhoe FG, Easterling MJ, et al: Review of British National Lymphoma Investigation studies of Hodgkin's disease and development of prognostic index. *Lancet* 1:967, 1985.

224. Tubiana M, Henry AM, van dW, et al: A multivariate analysis of prognostic factors in early stage Hodgkin's disease. *Int J Radiat Oncol Biol Phys* 11:23, 1985.

225. Schilling RF, McKnight B, Crowley JJ: Prognostic value of serum lactic dehydrogenase level in Hodgkin's disease. *J Lab Clin Med* 99:382, 1982.

226. Friedenberg WR, Gatlin PF, Mazza JJ, et al: Prognostic value of serum lactic dehydrogenase level in Hodgkin's disease. *J Lab Clin Med* 103:489, 1984.

227. Aisenberg AC, Kaplan MM, Rieder SV: Serum alkaline phosphatase at the onset of Hodgkin's disease. *Cancer* 26:318, 1970.

228. Mercier RJ, Thompson JM, Harman GS, Messerschmidt GL: Recurrent hypercalcemia and elevated 1,25-dihydroxyvitamin D levels in Hodgkin's disease. *Am J Med* 84:165, 1988.

229. Braund WJ, Naylor BA, Williamson DH, et al: Autoimmunity to insulin receptor and hypoglycaemia in patient with Hodgkin's disease. *Lancet* 1:237, 1987.

230. Walters EG, Tavare JM, Denton RM, Walters G: Hypoglycaemia due to an insulin-receptor antibody in Hodgkin's disease. *Lancet* 1:241, 1987.

231. Eliakim R, Vertman E, Shinhar E: Syndrome of inappropriate secretion of antidiuretic hormone in Hodgkin's disease. *Am J Med Sci* 291:126, 1986.

232. Hasenclever D, Diehl V: A prognostic score for advanced Hodgkin's disease. International Prognostic Factors Project on Advanced Hodgkin's Disease. *N Engl J Med* 339:1506, 1998.

233. Dimopoulos MA, Cabanillas F, Lee JJ, et al: Prognostic role of serum beta 2-microglobulin in Hodgkin's disease. *J Clin Oncol* 11:1108, 1993.

234. Lieberman DA: Intrahepatic cholestasis due to Hodgkin's disease. An elusive diagnosis. *J Clin Gastroenterol* :304, 1986.

235. Moorthy AV, Zimmerman SW, Burkholder PM: Nephrotic syndrome in Hodgkin's disease. Evidence for pathogenesis alternative to immune complex deposition. *Am J Med* 61:471, 1976.

236. Routledge RC, Hann IM, Jones PH: Hodgkin's disease complicated by the nephrotic syndrome. *Cancer* 38:1735, 1976.

237. Kaplan HS: Evidence for a tumoricidal dose level in the radiotherapy of Hodgkin's disease. *Cancer Res* 26:1221, 1966.

238. Vijayakumar S, Myrianthopoulos LC: An updated dose-response analysis in Hodgkin's disease. *Radiother Oncol* 24:1, 1992.

239. Hanks GE, Kinzie JJ, Herring DF, Kramer S: Patterns of care outcome studies in Hodgkin's disease: results of the national practice and implications for management. *Cancer Treat Rep* 66:805, 1982.

240. Trueblood HW, Enright LP, Ray GR, Kaplan HS, Nelsen TS: Preservation of ovarian function in pelvic radiation for Hodgkin's disease. *Arch Surg* 100:236, 1970.

241. Pedrick TJ, Hoppe RT: Recovery of spermatogenesis following pelvic irradiation for Hodgkin's disease. *Int J Radiat Oncol Biol Phys* 12:117, 1986.

242. Feuer EJ, Kessler LG, Baker SG, Triolo HE, Green DT: The impact of breakthrough clinical trials on survival in population based tumor registries. *J Clin Epidemiol* 44:141, 1991.

243. Longo DL, Young RC, Wesley M, et al: Twenty years of MOPP therapy for Hodgkin's disease. *J Clin Oncol* 4:1295, 1986.

244. De Vita VT Jr, Hubbard SM, Longo DL: The chemotherapy of lymphomas: looking back, moving forward—the Richard and Hinda Rosenthal Foundation award lecture. *Cancer Res* 47:5810, 1987.

245. Nicholson WM, Beard ME, Crowther D, et al: Combination chemotherapy in generalized Hodgkin's disease. *Br Med J* 3:7, 1970.

246. Sutcliffe SB, Wrigley PF, Peto J, et al: MVPP chemotherapy regimen for advanced Hodgkin's disease. *Br Med J* 1:679, 1978.

247. McElwain TJ, Toy J, Smith E, Peckham MJ, Austin DE: A combination of chlorambucil, vinblastine, procarbazine and prednisolone for treatment of Hodgkin's disease. *Br J Cancer* 36:276, 1977.

248. Selby P, Patel P, Milan S, et al: ChlVPP combination chemotherapy for Hodgkin's disease: long-term results. *Br J Cancer* 62:279, 1990.

249. Frei E, Luce JK, Gamble JF, et al: Combination chemotherapy in advanced Hodgkin's disease. Induction and maintenance of remission. *Ann Intern Med* 79:376, 1973.

250. Cadman E, Bloom AF, Prosnitz L, et al: The effective use of combined modality therapy for the treatment of patients with Hodgkin's disease who relapsed following radiotherapy. *Am J Clin Oncol* 6:313, 1983.

251. Coltman CA, Jr: Chemotherapy of advanced Hodgkin's disease. *Semin Oncol* 7:155, 1980.

252. Santoro A, Bonadonna G: Prolonged disease-free survival in MOPP-resistant Hodgkin's disease after treatment with adriamycin, bleomycin, vinblastine and dacarbazine (ABVD). *Cancer Chemother Pharmacol* 2:101, 1979.

253. Santoro A, Bonfante V, Bonadonna G: Salvage chemotherapy with ABVD in MOPP-resistant Hodgkin's disease. *Ann Intern Med* 96:139, 1982.

254. Santoro A, Bonadonna G, Bonfante V, Valagussa P: Alternating drug combinations in the treatment of advanced Hodgkin's disease. *N Engl J Med* 306:770, 1982.

255. Bonadonna G, Valagussa P, Santoro A: Alternating non-cross-resistant combination chemotherapy or MOPP in stage IV Hodgkin's disease. A report of 8-year results. *Ann Intern Med* 104:739, 1986.

256. Santoro A, Bonadonna G, Valagussa P, et al: Long-term results of combined chemotherapy-radiotherapy approach in Hodgkin's disease: superiority of ABVD plus radiotherapy versus MOPP plus radiotherapy. *J Clin Oncol* 5:27, 1987.

257. Canellos GP, Anderson JR, Propert KJ, et al: Chemotherapy of advanced Hodgkin's disease with MOPP, ABVD, or MOPP alternating with ABVD. *N Engl J Med* 327:1478, 1992.

258. Klimo P, Connors JM: MOPP/ABV hybrid program: combination chemotherapy based on early introduction of seven effective drugs for advanced Hodgkin's disease. *J Clin Oncol* 3:1174, 1985.

259. Connors JM, Klimo P, Adams G, et al: Treatment of advanced Hodgkin's disease with chemotherapy—comparison of MOPP/ABV hybrid regimen with alternating courses of MOPP and ABVD: a report from the National Cancer Institute of Canada clinical trials group. *J Clin Oncol* 15:1638, 1997.

260. Viviani S, Bonadonna G, Santoro A, et al: Alternating versus hybrid MOPP and ABVD combinations in advanced Hodgkin's disease: ten-year results. *J Clin Oncol* 14:1421, 1996.

261. Diehl V, Franklin J, Hasenclever D, et al: BEACOPP, a new dose-escalated and accelerated regimen, is at least as effective as COPP/ABVD in patients with advanced-stage Hodgkin's lymphoma: interim report from a trial of the German Hodgkin's Lymphoma Study Group. *J Clin Oncol* 16:3810, 1998.

262. Diehl V, Sieber M, Rüffer U, et al: BEACOPP: an intensified chemotherapy regimen in advanced Hodgkin's disease. The German Hodgkin's Lymphoma Study Group. *Ann Oncol* 8:143, 1997.

263. Horning SJ, Rosenberg SA, Hoppe RT: Brief chemotherapy (Stanford V) and adjuvant radiotherapy for bulky or advanced Hodgkin's disease: an update. *Ann Oncol* 7 (Suppl) 4:105, 1996.

264. Bartlett NL, Rosenberg SA, Hoppe RT, Hancock SL, Horning SJ: Brief chemotherapy, Stanford V, and adjuvant radiotherapy for bulky or advanced-stage Hodgkin's disease: a preliminary report. *J Clin Oncol* 13:1080, 1995.

265. Rosenberg SA, Kaplan HS: The evolution and summary results of the Stanford randomized clinical trials of the management of Hodgkin's disease: 1962–1984. *Int J Radiat Oncol Biol Phys* 11:5, 1985.

266. Specht L, Gray RG, Clarke MJ, Peto R: Influence of more extensive radiotherapy and adjuvant chemotherapy on long-term outcome of early-stage Hodgkin's disease: a meta-analysis of 23 randomized trials involving 3,888 patients. International Hodgkin's Disease Collaborative Group. *J Clin Oncol* 16:830, 1998.

267. Carde P, Burgers JM, Henry AM, et al: Clinical stages I and II Hodgkin's disease: a specifically tailored therapy according to prognostic factors. *J Clin Oncol* 6:239, 1988.

268. Tubiana M, Henry AM, Carde P, et al: Toward comprehensive management tailored to prognostic factors of patients with clinical stages I and II in Hodgkin's disease. The EORTC Lymphoma Group controlled clinical trials: 1964–1987. *Blood* 73:47, 1989.

269. Wirth A, Byram D, Chao M, Corry J, Davis S: Long term results of mantle irradiation alone in 261 patients with clinical stage I-II supradiaphragmatic Hodgkin's disease. *Int J Radiat Oncol Biol Phys* (Abstract) 78:174, 1997.

270. Mandelli F, Anselmo AP, Cartoni C, Cimino G, Maurizi Enrici R, Biagini C: Evaluation of therapeutic modalities in the control of Hodgkin's disease. *Int J Radiat Oncol Biol Phys* 12:1617, 1986.

271. Ganesan TS, Wrigley PF, Murray PA, et al: Radiotherapy for stage I Hodgkin's disease: 20 years experience at St Bartholomew's Hospital. *Br J Cancer* 62:314, 1990.

272. Mauch PM, Canellos GP, Shulman LN, et al: Mantle irradiation alone for selected patients with laparotomy-staged IA to IIA Hodgkin's disease: preliminary results of a prospective trial. *J Clin Oncol* 13:947, 1995.

273. Noordijk EM, Carde P, Hagenbeek A, Mandard A-M, Kluin-Nelemans JC: Combination of radiotherapy and chemotherapy is advisable in all patients with clinical stage I-II Hodgkin's disease. Six year results of the EORTC-GPMC controlled clinical trials 'H7-VF', 'H7-F', and 'H7-UF'. *Int J Radiat Oncol Biol Phys* (Abstract) 77:173, 1997.

274. Hancock SL, Hoppe RT, Horning SJ, Rosenberg SA: Intercurrent death after Hodgkin disease therapy in radiotherapy and adjuvant MOPP trials. *Ann Intern Med* 109:183, 1988.

275. Horning SJ, Hoppe RT, Hancock SL, Rosenberg SA: Vinblastine, bleomycin, and methotrexate: an effective adjuvant in favorable Hodgkin's disease. *J Clin Oncol* 6:1822, 1988.

276. Horning SJ, Hoppe RT, Mason J, et al: Stanford-Kaiser Permanente G1 study for clinical stage I to IIA Hodgkin's disease: subtotal lymphoid irradiation versus vinblastine, methotrexate, and bleomycin chemotherapy and regional irradiation. *J Clin Oncol* 15:1736, 1997.

277. Bonfante V, Santoro A, Vivani S, Devizzi L: ABVD plus radiotherapy (subtotal nodal vs involved field) in early-stage Hodgkin's disease (HD). *Proc Am Soc Clin Oncol* (Abstract) 1262:373, 1994.

278. Tesch H, Sieber M, Ruffer JU, Franklin J: 2 cycles ABVD plus radiotherapy is more effective than radiotherapy alone in early stage HD—interim analysis of the HD7 trial of the GHSG. *Proc Am Soc Hematol* (Abstract) 2001, 1998.

279. Radford JA, Cowan RA, Ryder WDJ, Deakin DP, James RD: Four weeks of neo-adjuvant chemotherapy significantly reduces the progression rate in patients treated with limited field radiotherapy for clinical stage IA/IIA Hodgkin's disease. Results of a randomized trial. *Ann Oncol* (Abstract) 066:21, 1996.

280. Horning SJ, Hoppe RT, Breslin S, Baer DM, Mason J, Rosenberg SA: Very brief (8 week) chemotherapy and low dose (30 Gy) radiotherapy for limited stage Hodgkin's disease: Preliminary results of the Stanford-Kaiser G4 study of Stanford V + RT. *Proc Am Soc Hematol*, 1999.

281. Olweny CL, Katongole ME, Kiire C, Lwanga SK, Magrath I, Ziegler JL: Childhood Hodgkin's disease in Uganda: a ten year experience. *Cancer* 42:787, 1978.

282. Ekert H, Waters KD, Smith PJ, Toogood I, Mauger D: Treatment with MOPP or ChlVPP chemotherapy only for all stages of childhood Hodgkin's disease. *J Clin Oncol* 6:1845, 1988.

283. Pavlovsky S, Maschio M, Santarelli MT, et al: Randomized trial of chemotherapy versus chemotherapy plus radiotherapy for stage I-II Hodgkin's disease. *J Natl Cancer Inst* 80:1466, 1988.

284. Longo DL, Glatstein E, Duffey PL, et al: Radiation therapy versus combination chemotherapy in the treatment of early-stage Hodgkin's disease: seven-year results of a prospective randomized trial [see comments]. *J Clin Oncol* 9:906, 1991.

285. Biti GP, Cimino G, Cartoni C, et al: Extended-field radiotherapy is superior to MOPP chemotherapy for the treatment of pathologic stage I-IIA Hodgkin's disease: eight-year update of an Italian prospective randomized study. *J Clin Oncol* 10:378, 1992.

286. Mauch P, Gorshein D, Cunningham J, Hellman S: Influence of mediastinal adenopathy on site and frequency of relapse in patients with Hodgkin's disease. *Cancer Treat Rep* 66:809, 1982.

287. Hoppe RT, Coleman CN, Cox RS, Rosenberg SA, Kaplan HS: The management of stage I-II Hodgkin's disease with irradiation alone or combined modality therapy: the Stanford experience. *Blood* 59:455, 1982.

288. Hoppe RT: The management of stage II Hodgkin's disease with a large mediastinal mass: a prospective program emphasizing irradiation. *Int J Radiat Oncol Biol Phys* 11:349, 1985.

289. Crnkovich MJ, Leopold K, Hoppe RT, Mauch PM: Stage I to IIB

Hodgkin's disease: the combined experience at Stanford University and the Joint Center for Radiation Therapy. *J Clin Oncol* 5:1041, 1987.

290. Bonfante V, Santoro A, Viviani S, Valagussa P, Bonadonna G: ABVD in the treatment of Hodgkin's disease. *Semin Oncol* 19:38, 1992.

291. Longo DL, Russo A, Duffey PL, et al: Treatment of advanced-stage massive mediastinal Hodgkin's disease: the case for combined modality treatment. *J Clin Oncol* 9:227, 1991.

292. Duggan D, Petroni G, Johnson J: MOPP/ABV vs ABVD for advanced Hodgkin's disease: a preliminary report of CALGB 8952. *Proc Am Soc Clin Oncol* (Abstract) 12a:41, 1997.

293. Horning SJ, Williams J, Bartlett NL, et al: E1492: Assessment of the Stanford V regimen and consolidative radiotherapy for bulky and advanced Hodgkin's disease. *J Clin Oncol* 1999.

294. Prosnitz LR, Farber LR, Kapp DS, et al: Combined modality therapy for advanced Hodgkin's disease: 15-year follow-up data. *J Clin Oncol* 6:603, 1988.

295. Donaldson SS, Link MP: Combined modality treatment with low-dose radiation and MOPP chemotherapy for children with Hodgkin's disease. *J Clin Oncol* 5:742, 1987.

296. Meerwaldt JH, Coleman CN, Fischer RI, Lister TA, Diehl V: Role of additional radiotherapy in advanced stages of Hodgkin's disease. *Ann Oncol* 4:83, 1992.

297. Fabian CJ, Mansfield CM, Dahlberg S, et al: Low-dose involved field radiation after chemotherapy in advanced Hodgkin disease. A Southwest Oncology Group randomized study. *Ann Intern Med* 120:903, 1994.

298. Diehl V, Loeffler M, Pfreundschuh M, et al: Further chemotherapy versus low-dose involved-field radiotherapy as consolidation of complete remission after six cycles of alternating chemotherapy in patients with advance Hodgkin's disease. German Hodgkins' Study Group (GHSG). *Ann Oncol* 6:901, 1995.

299. Weiner MA, Leventhal B, Brecher ML, et al: Randomized study of intensive MOPP-ABVD with or without low-dose total-nodal radiation therapy in the treatment of stages IIB, IIIA2, IIIB, and IV Hodgkin's disease in pediatric patients: a Pediatric Oncology Group study. *J Clin Oncol* 15:2769, 1997.

300. Specht L, Nordentoft AM, Cold S, Clausen NT, Nissen NI: Tumor burden as the most important prognostic factor in early stage Hodgkin's disease. Relations to other prognostic factors and implications for choice of treatment. *Cancer* 61:1719, 1988.

301. Mauch PM: Controversies in the management of early stage Hodgkin's disease. *Blood* 83:318, 1994.

302. Gospodarowicz MK, Sutcliffe SB, Clark RM, et al: Analysis of supradiaphragmatic clinical stage I and II Hodgkin's disease treated with radiation alone. *Int J Radiat Oncol Biol Phys* 22:859, 1992.

303. Carella AM, Carlier P, Congiu A, et al: Autologous bone marrow transplantation as adjuvant treatment for high-risk Hodgkin's disease in first complete remission after MOPP/ABVD protocol. *Bone Marrow Transplant* 8:99, 1991.

304. Kennedy BJ, Loeb VJ, Peterson V, Donegan W, Natarajan N, Mettlin C: Survival in Hodgkin's disease by stage and age. *Med Pediatr Oncol* 20:100, 1992.

305. Enblad G, Glimelius B, Sundstrom C: Treatment outcome in Hodgkin's disease in patients above the age of 60: a population-based study. *Ann Oncol* 2:297, 1991.

306. Oudejans JJ, Jiwa NM, Kummer JA, et al: Activated cytotoxic T cells as prognostic marker in Hodgkin's disease. *Blood* 89:1376, 1997.

307. Portlock CS, Rosenberg SA, Glatstein E, Kaplan HS: Impact of salvage treatment on initial relapses in patients with Hodgkin disease, stages I-III. *Blood* 51:825, 1978.

308. Timothy AR, Sutcliffe SB, Wrigley PF, Jones AE: Hodgkin's disease: combination chemotherapy for relapse following radical radiotherapy. *Int J Radiat Oncol Biol Phys* 5:165, 1979.

309. Roach Md, Brophy N, Cox R, Varghese A, Hoppe RT: Prognostic factors for patients relapsing after radiotherapy for early-stage Hodgkin's disease. *J Clin Oncol* 8:623, 1990.

310. Fisher RI, DeVita VT, Hubbard SP, Simon R, Young RC: Prolonged disease-free survival in Hodgkin's disease with MOPP reinduction after first relapse. *Ann Intern Med* 90:761, 1979.

311. Longo DL, Duffey PL, Young RC, et al: Conventional-dose salvage combination chemotherapy in patients relapsing with Hodgkin's disease after combination chemotherapy: the low probability for cure. *J Clin Oncol* 10:210, 1992.

312. Viviani S, Santoro A, Negretti E, Bonfante V, Valagussa P, Bonadonna G: Salvage chemotherapy in Hodgkin's disease. Results in patients relapsing more than twelve months after first complete remission. *Ann Oncol* 1:123, 1990.

313. Bonadonna G, Santoro A, Gianni AM, et al: Primary and salvage chemotherapy in advanced Hodgkin's disease: the Milan Cancer Institute experience. *Ann Oncol* 1:9, 1991.

314. Chopra R, McMillan AK, Linch DC, et al: The place of high-dose BEAM therapy and autologous bone marrow transplantation in poor-risk Hodgkin's disease. A single-center eight-year study of 155 patients. *Blood* 81:1137, 1993.

315. Bierman PJ, Anderson JR, Freeman MB, et al: High-dose chemotherapy followed by autologous hematopoietic rescue for Hodgkin's disease patients following first relapse after chemotherapy. *Ann Oncol* 7:151, 1996.

316. Horning SJ, Chao NJ, Negrin RS, et al: High-dose therapy and autologous hematopoietic progenitor cell transplantation for recurrent or refractory Hodgkin's disease: analysis of the Stanford University results and prognostic indices. *Blood* 89:801, 1997.

317. Reece DE, Connors JM, Spinelli JJ, et al: Intensive therapy with cyclophosphamide, carmustine, etoposide +/− cisplatin, and autologous bone marrow transplantation for Hodgkin's disease in first relapse after combination chemotherapy. *Blood* 83:1193, 1994.

318. Linch DC, Winfield D, Goldstone AH, et al: Dose intensification with autologous bone-marrow transplantation in relapsed and resistant Hodgkin's disease: results of a BNLI randomised trial. *Lancet* 341:1051, 1993.

319. Schmitz N, Sextro M, Pfistner B, Hasenclever D, Tesch H: High dose therapy followed by hematopoietic stem cell transplantation for relapsed chemosensitive Hodgkin's disease: Final results of a randomized GHSG and EBMT trial (HDR-1). *Proc Am Soc Clin Oncol* (Abstract) 5:2a, 1999.

320. Yuen AR, Rosenberg SA, Hoppe RT, Halpern JD, Horning SJ: Comparison between conventional salvage therapy and high-dose therapy with autografting for recurrent or refractory Hodgkin's disease. *Blood* 89:814, 1997.

321. Nademanee A, O'Donnell MR, Snyder DS, et al: High-dose chemotherapy with or without total body irradiation followed by autologous bone marrow and/or peripheral blood stem cell transplantation for patients with relapsed and refractory Hodgkin's disease: results in 85 patients with analysis of prognostic factors. *Blood* 85:1381, 1995.

322. Lohri A, Barnett M, Fairey RN, et al: Outcome of treatment of first relapse of Hodgkin's disease after primary chemotherapy: identification of risk factors from the British Columbia experience 1970 to 1988. *Blood* 77:2292, 1991.

323. Lazarus HM, Rowlings PA, Zhang MJ, et al: Autotransplants for Hodgkin's disease in patients never achieving remission: a report from the Autologous Blood and Marrow Transplant Registry. *J Clin Oncol* 17:534, 1999.

324. Horning SJ: Primary refractory Hodgkin's disease. *Ann Oncol* 9 Suppl 5:S97, 1998.

325. Reece DE, Barnett MJ, Shepherd JD, et al: High-dose cyclophosphamide, carmustine (BCNU), and etoposide (VP16–213) with or without cisplatin (CBV +/− P) and autologous transplantation for patients with Hodgkin's disease who fail to enter a complete remission after combination chemotherapy. *Blood* 86:451, 1995.

326. Arseneau JC, Sponzo RW, Levin DL, et al: Nonlymphomatous malignant tumors complicating Hodgkin's disease. Possible association with intensive therapy. *N Engl J Med* 287:1119, 1972.

327. Canellos GP, Arseneau JC, DeVita VT, Whang PJ, Johnson RE: Second malignancies complicating Hodgkin's disease in remission. *Lancet* 1:947, 1975.

328. Coleman CN, Williams CJ, Flint A, Glatstein EJ, Rosenberg SA, Kaplan HS: Hematologic neoplasia in patients treated for Hodgkin's disease. *N Engl J Med* 297:1249, 1977.

329. Kaldor JM, Day NE, Clarke EA, et al: Leukemia following Hodgkin's disease. *N Engl J Med* 322:7, 1990.

330. Levine EG, Bloomfield CD: Leukemias and myelodysplastic syndromes secondary to drug, radiation, and environmental exposure. *Semin Oncol* 19:47, 1992.

331. Blayney DW, Longo DL, Young RC, et al: Decreasing risk of leukemia with prolonged follow-up after chemotherapy and radiotherapy for Hodgkin's disease. *N Engl J Med* 316:710, 1987.

332. Tucker MA, Coleman CN, Cox RS, Varghese A, Rosenberg SA: Risk of second cancers after treatment for Hodgkin's disease. *N Engl J Med* 318:76, 1988.

333. Van LF, Somers R, Taal BG, et al: Increased risk of lung cancer, non-Hodgkin's lymphoma, and leukemia following Hodgkin's disease. *J Clin Oncol* 7:1046, 1989.

334. Boivin JF, Hutchison GB, Lyden M, Godbold J, Chorosh J, Schottenfeld D: Second primary cancers following treatment of Hodgkin's disease. *J Natl Cancer Inst* 72:233, 1984.

335. Henry AM: Second cancers after radiotherapy and chemotherapy for early stages of Hodgkin's disease. *J Natl Cancer Inst* 71:911, 1983.

336. Hancock SL, Tucker MA, Hoppe RT: Breast cancer after treatment of Hodgkin's disease. *J Natl Cancer Inst* 85:25, 1993.

337. Hancock SL, Cox RS, McDougall IR: Thyroid diseases after treatment of Hodgkin's disease. *N Engl J Med* 325:599, 1991.

338. Shapiro CL, Mauch PM: Radiation-associated breast cancer after Hodgkin's disease: risks and screening in perspective. *J Clin Oncol* 10:1662, 1992.

339. Bhatia S, Robison LL, Oberlin O, et al: Breast cancer and other second neoplasms after childhood Hodgkin's disease. *N Engl J Med* 334:745, 1996.

340. Hancock SL, Donaldson SS, Hoppe RT: Cardiac disease following treatment of Hodgkin's disease in children and adolescents. *J Clin Oncol* 11:1208, 1993.

341. Boivin JF, Hutchison GB, Lubin JH, Mauch P: Coronary artery disease mortality in patients treated for Hodgkin's disease. *Cancer* 69:1241, 1992.

342. Chapman RM, Sutcliffe SB, Rees LH, Edwards CR, Malpas JS: Cyclical combination chemotherapy and gonadal function. Retrospective study in males. *Lancet* 1:285, 1979.

343. Da CM, Meistrich ML, Fuller LM, et al: Recovery of spermatogenesis after treatment for Hodgkin's disease: limiting dose of MOPP chemotherapy. *J Clin Oncol* 2:571, 1984.

344. Chapman RM, Sutcliffe SB, Malpas JS: Cytotoxic-induced ovarian failure in women with Hodgkin's disease: I. Hormone function. *JAMA* 242:1877, 1979.

345. Horning SJ, Hoppe RT, Kaplan HS, Rosenberg SA: Female reproductive potential after treatment for Hodgkin's disease. *N Engl J Med* 304:1377, 1981.

346. Anselmo AP, Cartoni C, Bellantuono P, Maurizi ER, Aboulkair N, Ermini M: Risk of infertility in patients with Hodgkin's disease treated with ABVD vs MOPP vs ABVD/MOPP. *Haematologica* 75:155, 1990.

347. Viviani S, Santoro A, Ragni G, Bonfante V, Bestetti O, Bonadonna G: Gonadal toxicity after combination chemotherapy for Hodgkin's disease. Comparative results of MOPP vs ABVD. *Eur J Cancer Clin Oncol* 21:601, 1985.

348. Carmel RJ, Kaplan HS: Mantle irradiation in Hodgkin's disease. An analysis of technique, tumor eradication, and complications. *Cancer* 37:2813, 1976.

349. Smith LM, Mendenhall NP, Cicale MJ, Block ER, Carter RL, Million RR: Results of a prospective study evaluating the effects of mantle irradiation on pulmonary function. *Int J Radiat Oncol Biol Phys* 16:79, 1989.

350. Horning SJ, Adhikari A, Rizk N, Hoppe RT, Olshen RA: Effect of treatment for Hodgkin's disease on pulmonary function: results of a prospective study. *J Clin Oncol* 12:297, 1994.

351. Donaldson SS, Kaplan HS: Complications of treatment of Hodgkin's disease in children. *Cancer Treat Rep* 66:977, 1982.

352. Rosner F, Zarrabi MH: Late infections following splenectomy in Hodgkin's disease. *Cancer Invest* 1:57, 1983.

353. Bloom JR, Fobair P, Gritz E, et al: Psychosocial outcomes of cancer: a comparative analysis of Hodgkin's disease and testicular cancer. *J Clin Oncol* 11:979, 1993.

LYMPHOMAS

KENNETH A. FOON
RICHARD I. FISHER

The lymphomas are a heterogenous group of clonal (neo-plastic) diseases that share the single characteristic of arising as the result of a somatic mutation(s) in a lymphocyte progenitor. The progeny of the affected cell usually carry the phenotype of a B, T, or NK cell as judged by immunophenotyping or gene rearrangement studies. Any site of the lymphatic system may be the primary site of origin of the disorder including lymph nodes, gut-associated lymphatic tissue, skin, or spleen. Any organ, e.g., thyroid, lung, bone, brain, gonads, etc. may be involved either by spread from lymphatic sites or as a manifestation of primary extranodal disease. The classification of the subtypes of disease has been difficult but newer systems couple immunologic phenotype with histopathologic and cytologic features to arrive at definition of subtypes. By historical convention, lymphocytic malignancies originating in the marrow are referred to as lymphocytic leukemia, whereas those originating in any other lymphoid site are referred to as lymphoma. In the former case, lymphoid sites may be involved and in the latter case the marrow may be involved. Diagnosis is usually made by histological examination of a biopsy specimen, supplemented by immunophenotyping and molecular analysis for clonal origin. Patients are often put through staging procedures that may involve imaging studies, other biopsies, and blood chemical studies. Treatment depends on the type of lymphoma and the distribution of clinically evident disease. Combinations of drugs are often required. Radiotherapy may be useful for localized disease. Perhaps the most exciting progress in the treatment of lymphomas has been for the follicular B cell lymphomas. Combinations of chemotherapies including fludarabine and mitoxantrone or cyclophosphamide have demonstrated responses in 75 to 95 percent of patients. The majority of these responses are complete responses, and many of them appear to be quite durable. Newer agents such as Rituximab, which is a human mouse chimeric monoclonal antibody that binds to the CD20 antigen, demonstrate responses in over 50 percent of patients. [131]I- and ^{90}Y-labeled anti-CD20 antibodies have also demonstrated outstanding responses in previously treated patients. The role of autologous and allogeneic bone marrow transplant is well established for intermediate-risk and high-risk lymphomas and is being better defined for patients with low-risk lymphoma. Better therapies clearly need to be defined for mantle zone cell lymphoma and adult T-cell leukemia lymphoma, neither of which consistently respond to any current therapeutic regimens.

DEFINITION AND HISTORY

Lymphomas are a heterogeneous group of malignancies of B cells or T cells that usually originate in the lymph nodes but may originate in any organ of the body. Lymphoma previously was referred to as *reticulum cell sarcoma, lymphosarcoma,* or *giant follicular lymphoma.*[1-5] In 1966, Rappaport published a classification system based on the patterns of lymphoma cell growth, size, and shape that attempted to correlate morphology with clinical outcome.[6] The classification proved to have some inaccuracies, such as the term *histiocytic* to describe tumors of large transformed lymphocytes that were not derived from the macrophage lineage (see Chap. 101). Nonetheless, the Rappaport classification was an important milestone and became the most widely used classification in the United States. In 1974, Lukes and Collins proposed another classification system that incorporated morphology with immunologic subtype, which was endorsed by the Committee on Nomenclature.[7] Another scheme, the Kiel classification, has been more popular in Europe.[8] In 1982, a Working Formulation sponsored by the National Cancer Institute attempted to reconcile the large number of competing classifications then in use.[9] The Working Formulation was very useful clinically and gained wide popularity. However, with advances in our understanding of the immune system, particularly the use of monoclonal antibodies to subdivide lymphoid cells, and increasing molecular and genetic advances, a new classification schema became necessary. In 1994, a revised European-American classification of lymphoid neoplasm (REAL) was proposed by the International Lymphoma Study Group[10] and is presented in Chap. 101. This group distinguished three major categories of lymphoid malignancies which included B-cell, T-cell, and Hodgkin disease. Lymphomas were defined by current morphologic, immunologic, and genetic techniques. Many of the lymphomas were associated with distinct clinical presentations, and cases that did not fit into defined entities were left unclassified. Further subclassification[11] divided each of the B- and T-cell lineages into: (1) indolent lymphomas (low risk), (2) aggressive lymphomas (intermediate risk), and (3) very aggressive lymphomas (high risk) (Table 103-1). Diseases presented in Table 103-1 that are not presented in this chapter are shown in brackets.

ETIOLOGY AND PATHOGENESIS

INCIDENCE AND EPIDEMIOLOGY

In 1998, the new cases of lymphoma in the United States are estimated to be 55,000 with 25,000 estimated deaths.[12] This represents 4 percent of cancer incidence and 4 percent of all cancer-related deaths. The incidence of lymphoma has increased dramatically in the last half of the twentieth century. This increase has affected men and women, all age groups, and most histologic types and has been documented in industrialized countries in Europe as well as in the United States. The increase preceded the appearance of AIDS, but the latter has added to the effect somewhat. The increase in incidence, which was about 4 percent per year, slowed to about 1 percent in the 1990s, but the mortality rate continues to increase significantly. Case control studies have suggested that chemical lymphomagens in herbicides and pesti-

Acronyms and abbreviations that appear in this chapter include: ACLC, anaplastic large-cell lymphoma; ALL, acute lymphoblastic leukemia; ALT, adult T-cell leukemia/lymphoma; CALGB, Cancer and Acute Leukemia Group B; CLL, chronic lymphocytic leukemia; CNS, central nervous system; CT scan, computed tomographic scan; DFS, disease-free survival; EBV, Epstein-Barr virus; EFS, event-free survival; FAB, French-American British; GELA, Groupe d'Etudes des Lymphomes des l'Adulte; HTLV-I, human T-cell leukemia-lymphoma virus I; IL-2, interleukin 2; IPI, International Lymphoma Prognostic Factor Index; KLH, keyhole limpet hemocyanin; LAK, lymphokine-activated killer; LDH, lactic dehydrogenase; MALT, mucosa-associated lymphoid tissue; MRI, magnetic resonance imaging; PCR, polymerase chain reaction; PFS, progression-free survival; PUVA, psoralen and ultraviolet A light; REAL, revised European-American classification of lymphoid neoplasm; SLVL, splenic lymphoma with villus lymphocytes; SWOG, Southwest Oncology Group; TdT, terminal deoxynucleotidyl transferase.

TABLE 103-1   REVISED EUROPEAN-AMERICAN CLASSIFICATION OF LYMPHOID NEOPLASMS

B-Cell Lineage	T-Cell Lineage

I. Indolent lymphomas (low-risk)
  Chronic lymphocytic leukemia/small lympho-
    cytic lymphoma*
  [Lymphoplasmacytic lymphoma/immunocy-
    toma†/Waldenström macroglobulinemia]‡
  [Hairy cell leukemia]
  Splenic marginal zone lymphoma
  Marginal zone B-cell lymphoma
    Extranodal (MALT-B-cell lymphoma)
    Nodal (monocytoid)
  Follicle center lymphoma/follicular (small
    cell)—grade I
  Follicle center lymphoma/follicular (mixed
    small and large cell)—grade II
	I. Indolent lymphomas (low-risk)
	  [Large granular lymphocytic leukemia; T- and
	    NK-cell types]_
	  Mycosis fungoides/Sézary syndrome
	  Smoldering and chronic adult T-cell leukemia
	    leukemia/lymphoma (HTLV1⁺)_

II. Aggressive lymphomas (intermediate-risk)
  [Prolymphocytic leukemias]_
  [Plasmacytoma/multiple myeloma]
  Mantle cell lymphoma
  Follicle center lymphoma/follicular (large
    cell)—grade III
  Diffuse large B-cell lymphoma (includes im-
    munoblastic and diffuse large and
    centroblastic lymphoma)
  Primary mediastinal (thymic) large B-cell
    lymphoma
High-grade B-cell lymphoma, Burkitt-like_
	II. Aggressive lymphomas (intermediate-risk)
	  [Prolymphocytic leukemia]_
	  Peripheral T-cell lymphoma, unspecified_
	  Angioimmunoblastic lymphoma_
	  Angiocentric lymphoma
	  Intestinal T-cell lymphoma_
	  Anaplastic large cell lymphoma (T- and null-
	    cell type)

III. Very aggressive lymphomas (high-risk)
  [Precursor B-lymphoblastic lymphoma/leuke-
    mia]
  Burkitt lymphoma/B-cell acute leukemia
  [Plasma cell leukemia]
IV. [Hodgkin's disease]
	III. Very aggressive lymphomas (high-risk)
	  Precursor T-lymphoblastic lymphoma/leuke-
	    mia
	  Adult T-cell lymphoma/leukemia

cides may account for some of the increase. Large-scale studies are underway at the National Cancer Institute to examine possible environmental causal relationships. Variations in racial incidence, histology, and immunologic subtypes are found throughout the world. Lymphoma is more common in males than females and in whites than blacks. There exists a lower incidence of follicular lymphomas in China and Japan.[13] The United States has a higher total incidence of lymphoma than does Japan, while the incidence of extranodal disease is higher in Japan.[14] While there is a preadolescent peak in incidence, there is generally a logarithmic increase with age.[15] Burkitt lymphoma occurs most frequently in tropical Africa, while T-cell leukemia lymphoma is most common in southwest Japan and the Caribbean basin.[16] Cutaneous T-cell lymphoma is an uncommon malignancy in the United States, with about 1000 new cases reported per year.[281] The average annual adjusted mortality rate is about 400 to 500 deaths per year.

EPIDEMIOLOGY AND ETIOLOGY

ENVIRONMENTAL FACTORS

An increased incidence of lymphoma has been reported among chemists, farmers, and individuals involved in rubber production and asbestos and arsenic processing.[17-26] This increased incidence is attributed to exposure to a variety of agents, including benzene and herbicides. Studies regarding agent orange, a herbicide that was used as a defoliant during the Vietnam war, have been inconclusive.[27] Small but significant increases in lymphoma have been associated with radiation exposure.[28] Increased lymphomas were reported in survivors of the atomic bomb in Hiroshima who were exposed to 10 Gy or more.[29,30] An increased incidence of lymphomas also has been reported for individuals radiated for ankylosing spondylitis.[31] It is also well known that patients with

Hodgkin disease who were patients with radiation therapy and chemotherapy have an increased incidence of lymphoma.

INFECTIOUS AGENTS

The most compelling evidence for a viral etiology of lymphoma is adult T-cell leukemia/lymphoma (ATL). A C-type RNA tumor virus was isolated from patients that was designated *human T-cell leukemia-lymphoma virus I* (HTLV-I).[49] HTLV-I is an acquired retrovirus that is not related to other known animal retroviruses. HTLV-I was demonstrated to immortalize lymphoid cells in culture and induce malignancy in an infected human host. Incidence of infection with HTLV-I in endemic areas is very high, yet few of these patients develop ATL. HTLV-I also leads to a neurologic disorder called *tropical spastic paraparesis*.[50] There appear to be host factors that affect transformation of lymphocytes by HTLV-I, and evidence suggests that there may be host-related genetic factors.[51] Development of adult T-cell leukemia/lymphoma is associated with infection by the human T-cell leukemia virus I.[390-393] Serum specimens from Japanese patients with adult T-cell leukemia/lymphoma were found to be positive for HTLV-I, as were serum samples from adult T-cell leukemia/lymphoma patients in the Caribbean, where adult T-cell leukemia/lymphoma was endemic.[394,395] Moreover, the highest prevalence of adult T-cell leukemia/lymphoma in Japan is in the southern island of Kyushi, where 10 to 15 percent of the population have antibody to HTLV-I.[395,396] On Japanese islands where adult T-cell leukemia/lymphoma is rare, the rate is less than 1 percent. It is apparent from these and additional data from the Caribbean, the southeastern United States, South America, and Africa that adult T-cell leukemia/lymphoma clusters in regions where HTLV-I is prevalent.[395-397] It is not known how these regions are linked. One hypothesis is that HTLV-I was brought to the Americas from Africa by the slave trade, and then to the southern islands of Japan by trade with Japan and Africa.[395]

Several studies suggest that host susceptibility or a shared environmental exposure or both contribute to HTLV-I infection. The prevalence of HTLV-I antibodies in close family members is three to four times higher than in the corresponding normal population.[398] In some instances, cell cultures of antibody-positive, clinically normal patients yielded HTLV-I isolates.[399] Blood donors are routinely screened for antibodies to HTLV-I to prevent transmission by this route.

Some B-cell lymphomas may be caused by Epstein-Barr virus (EBV). EBV is a DNA virus in the herpes virus family that first was described in cultured lymphoblasts from patients with African Burkitt lymphoma.[32] EBV binds to the CD21 antigen (also the receptor for the C3d component of complement) on B lymphocytes.[33] It is capable of transforming B lymphocytes into lymphoblastoid cells that may proliferate perpetually in cell culture.[34] EBV is present in over 95 percent of cases of endemic Burkitt lymphoma and in approximately 20 percent of cases of nonendemic Burkitt lymphoma.[35,36] Malaria is holoendemic in the regions where endemic Burkitt lymphoma exists.[37] A three-step process in the development of this lymphoma has been proposed.[38,39] (1) EBV initiates a polyclonal proliferation of B cells; (2) malaria stimulates further the proliferating B cells; and (3) the transforming B cells incur specific reciprocal translations of chromosome 8, with either chromosomes 2, 14, or 22.

H. pylori can cause MALT lymphomas of the stomach and is probably the cause of some of the higher grade lymphomas, either from transformation of a MALT or de novo large cell lymphoma.[151–153] This spiral gram-negative bacillus is the first bacterium demonstrated to cause a human neoplasm.

IMMUNOSUPPRESSION

There exist a variety of examples of immunosuppressed individuals who develop lymphoma. AIDS-related lymphoma is discussed in Chap. 89. Individuals who are immunosuppressed by drugs following organ transplantation have a range of abnormalities from benign proliferations of EBV-infected polyclonal B cells to aggressive malignant lymphoma.[40,41] Extranodal involvement is extremely common in post-transplant lymphomas. The incidence and rapidity of lymphomas has increased with the introduction of immunosuppressive agents such as cyclosporine and OKT3 (murine monoclonal anti-CD3).[42,43] There has also been an increased incidence of lymphomas in recipients of mismatched T-cell-depleted marrow grafts. Individuals with inherited or acquired immunodeficiency also have B-cell lymphomas that are caused by EBV. The X-linked lymphoproliferative syndrome is an example of a genetic defect in immunoregulation that leads to an inability to generate an active anti-EBV immune response.[44–48]

CHROMOSOMAL ABNORMALITIES

Chromosomal abnormalities are common in lymphomas (see Chap. 10). For example, approximately 85 percent of follicle center lymphomas carry the chromosomal translocation t(14;18)(q32;q21) in which the BCL-2 oncogene on chromosome 18q21 is brought in continuity with the Ig heavy-chain loci on 14q32.[156,157] The expression of the BCL-2 protein is increased.[158,159] The accumulation of the BCL-2 protein permits accumulation of long-lived centrocytes, as BCL-2 protein inhibits programmed cell depth (apoptosis), leading to a longer cell life (see Chap. 11).[160,161] The BCL-2 rearrangement may be detected by both Southern blot hybridization and the polymerase chain reaction. In Burkitt lymphoma the common genetic abnormality is the translocation of the C-MYC oncogene from chromosome 8 to either the immunoglobulin heavy-chain region on chromosome 14, t(8;14)(q24;q32) or, less commonly, the κ region on chromosome 2 t(2;8)(p13;q24) or the λ region on chromosome 22, t(8;22)(q24;q11). In the African endemic cases, the breakpoint on chromosome 14 includes the heavy-chain joining region, suggesting translocation occurs before complete immunoglobulin gene rearrangement in an early B cell. In nonendemic cases, the translocation involves the immunoglobulin heavy-chain switch region, suggesting the translocation occurs at a later stage of B-cell development.[272,273] Epstein-Barr virus genomes are demonstrated in the tumor cells in most of the African cases, in approximately one-third of the cases associated with AIDS[274–276] but less frequently in non-African, non-immune-deficient cases. The translocation t(2;5)(p23;q35) of anaplastic large cell lymphoma involves the NPM gene at 5p35 and the ALK gene at 2p23,[375] leading to expression of a novel fusion protein p80.[376] This translocation has been identified in approximately 50 percent of systemic cases and may be higher in children with ALCL.[377,378] The t(2;5) is not common in primary cutaneous anaplastic large-cell lymphoma (ALCL).[379] Several cytogenetic abnormalities have been reported in adult T-cell leukemia/lymphoma cells. The most common abnormalities are trisomy, or partial trisomy, of 3q, 6q, 14q, and inv.[14] Less common cytogenetic abnormalities include loss of the X chromosome, 7(9;21), 5p, 2q+, 17q+, and trisomy 18.[406–412] In some studies, survival correlates with karyotype abnormalities.

T-CELL LYMPHOMAS

The cause of cutaneous T-cell lymphoma is not known. Environmental, infectious, and genetic influences may be important.[283–285] Exposure to toxic chemicals and physical agents, and employment in manufacturing, particularly textiles, petrochemicals, and machinery, is associated with an increased incidence of cutaneous T-cell lymphoma, but this remains controversial.[283–285] HTLV-I originally was isolated in the United States from patients thought to have cutaneous T-cell lymphoma.[286] Seroepidemiologic studies, however, suggest that HTLV-I is associated with adult T-cell leukemia/lymphoma.[287] Fewer than 1 percent of patients with cutaneous T-cell lymphoma in the United States have serologic evidence for prior infection with HTLV-I. In a series of CD25-negative cutaneous T-cell lymphoma patients from Italy, a new retrovirus, called HTLV-V, was isolated. The significance of this finding is not clear.[288] Evidence for genetic factors in the cause of cutaneous T-cell lymphoma is less impressive. Cutaneous T-cell lymphoma is less common in African-Americans. Also, first-degree relatives of patients with cutaneous T-cell lymphoma may have an increased incidence of lymphoma or leukemia.[289] Data conflict regarding whether there is an increased incidence of cutaneous T-cell lymphoma among family members.

CLINICAL FEATURES

HISTORY AND PHYSICAL EXAMINATION

It is important to ascertain whether the patient has night sweats, fever, or metabolic wasting resulting in loss of more than 10 percent of body weight within the preceding 6 months. The presence of such "B" symptoms has unfavorable prognostic significance.

An examination should be made of all lymph node areas. Involved nodes are typically nontender, firm, and rubbery. The throat should be examined for involvement of the oropharyngeal lymphoid tissue (Waldeyer ring). The aggressive lymphomas are more likely to involve extranodal sites such as the skin and the central nervous system (see "Extranodal Lymphoma").

STAGING

The staging procedures that may be used are shown in Table 103-2. Generally, staging laparotomy is not indicated. Surgery may be indicated to definitively treat low-grade lymphomas of the gastrointestinal tract and for the diagnosis of extranodal or nodal disease confined to

TABLE 103-2   STAGING PROCEDURES FOR LYMPHOMA

Initial studies
  History and physical examination
  Pathologic diagnosis from biopsy specimen
  Laboratory studies
    Blood chemistries and complete blood counts
    Bilateral posterior iliac crest marrow biopsies
  Chest roentgenogram (CT scan if x-ray is suspicious)
  CT scans of abdomen and pelvis
Subsequent studies
  Ultrasonography and MRI to clarify abnormalities
  Gallium scan (particularly useful to follow large masses)
  Lumbar puncture if neurologic signs or symptoms of aggressive lymphoma
    with marrow involvement
  Gastrointestinal studies if Waldeyer ring involvement
  CT scan or MRI of brain if neurologic signs or symptoms
  Immunoglobulin and T-cell receptor gene rearrangement studies
  Polymerase chain reaction for BCL-1 and BCL-2
  Flow cytometry
  Immunohistochemistry
  Cytogenetics

TABLE 103-3   ANN ARBOR STAGING SYSTEM

Stage I*	Restricted to one lymph node-bearing area
Stage II*	Two or more areas of nodal involvement on one side of the diaphragm
Stage III*	Lymphatic involvement on both sides of the diaphragm
Stage IV	Liver, marrow, or other extensive extranodal disease
Symptom status A	Absence of fevers, sweats, or weight loss
Symptom status B	Unexplained fevers higher than 38°C, drenching night sweats, weight loss of more than 10% of body weight in the preceding 6 months
Clinical stage	The assigned stage based only on history, physical findings, and laboratory and radiologic studies
Pathologic stage	The assigned stage based only on areas of biopsy-proven involvement
Substage E	Localized, extranodal disease

*The spleen is considered nodal.

the abdomen. The role of surgery for large intraabdominal masses (larger than 10 cm) is controversial and is not routinely recommended.

The Ann Arbor staging classification (Table 103-3) is not optimal for staging lymphoma[52] but is still considered the gold standard and impacts patient survival. The staging system was created for Hodgkin disease, which spreads by contiguity from lymph node areas, rather than hematogenously as does lymphoma. For this reason, more than 80 percent of patients with low-grade lymphoma and more than 50 percent of patients with intermediate- or high-grade lymphoma present with stage III or stage IV disease. However, staging is critically important for patients that are truly stages I and II who are treated by potentially curative radiation therapy if they have low-risk follicle center lymphomas or a combination of radiation therapy and limited cycles of chemotherapy if they have an intermediate- or high-risk lymphoma.

EXTRANODAL LYMPHOMA

Lymphomas involving extranodal sites most commonly occur simultaneously with nodal involvement, either at the time of diagnosis or sometime during the course of disease. Where extranodal involvement occurs as the only evidence of lymphoma, it is referred to as *primary extranodal lymphoma*.

CENTRAL NERVOUS SYSTEM

Between 5 and 10 percent of patients with nodal presentation of lymphoma may develop CNS involvement. These patients have a high incidence of marrow involvement and typically have aggressive histology.[70–72] Epidural, testes,[73,74] and paranasal sinus[75] involvement commonly are associated with CNS disease. CNS presentation may include spinal cord compression, leptomeningeal spread, and/or intracerebral mass lesions. Spinal cord compression typically presents with back pain followed by extremity weakness, paresis, and paralysis. Leptomeningeal spread may present with cranial nerve palsies and signs of meningeal irritation. Intracerebral mass lesions may present with headaches, lethargy, papilledema, focal neurologic signs, or seizures.

Primary lymphomas originating and confined to the brain[76,77] or spinal cord[78] are rare. They almost always have an aggressive histology. Intracerebral tumors have increased dramatically in recent years because of the association with AIDS-related aggressive lymphomas (Chap. 89). Progressive multifocal leukoencephalopathy occurs as a result of polyoma virus infection in the brain and is characterized by demyelination; it is typically fatal.[79] Paraneoplastic neurologic syndromes such as myasthenia gravis, cerebellar degeneration, peripheral neuropathies, and transverse myelopathy also may be associated with lymphomas.[80]

EYE

The most common presentation of ocular lesions is the periorbital soft tissues, in particular the conjunctival mucosal surfaces and the area surrounding the lacrimal gland.[81] These lesions are typically low-risk and commonly have the histology of a mucosa-associated lymphoid tissue (MALT) or follicle center lymphoma. The preferred therapy is radiation in the range of 25 to 30 Gy, which is curative in the majority of patients.[82] Bilateral involvement, particularly with MALT lymphomas, may be seen. In the rare situation where large-cell lymphoma involves the periorbital soft tissue, treatment follows the overall clinical picture.

Intraocular lymphomas are a rare presentation of lymphoma of the eye.[83] Most cases are B-cell large-cell lymphomas, but they often have a unique indolent pattern. The diagnosis is established by a vitrectomy. There is approximately a 50 percent chance that the disease will be bilateral. Also, it is frequently associated with brain or leptomeningeal involvement. The mainstay of therapy is radiation, but most patients relapse within the eye or brain. Chemotherapeutic agents do not typically penetrate the eye or brain. Most patients are offered palliation with radiation and steroids, but recurrence is typical. These tumors behave much like large B-cell lymphomas of the brain, and consideration of more aggressive therapy would be reasonable.

PARANASAL SINUSES

Lymphomas may involve the frontal, maxillary, ethmoid, and sphenoid sinuses. These lymphomas typically involve bone and present with pain, upper airway obstruction, rhinorrhea, facial swelling, or epistaxis. Periorbital tumors may present with proptosis, visual loss, or dyplopia. These lymphomas are typically large-cell lymphomas.[84] Following staging, treatment is planned in three phases that include systemic, local, and prophylaxis therapy to prevent spread to the CNS.[81] With localized disease, three cycles of chemotherapy are recommended followed by involved field radiation. For more advanced disease, six to eight cycles of chemotherapy are recommended. Following standard therapy, six doses of intrathecal chemotherapy over 3 weeks are recommended because of the high incidence of CNS disease. Using this three-step approach to management, the majority of patients will be cured.[81]

SKIN

Cutaneous T-cell lymphoma and adult T-cell leukemia/lymphoma typically involve the skin. Anaplastic large-cell lymphoma also commonly involves the skin. However, any lymphoma may secondarily infiltrate the skin. The lesions are typically reddish-purplish[85] nodules and are more common with aggressive lymphomas, but low-grade lymphoma may also infiltrate the skin. Primary extranodal involvement of the skin is rarely seen in B-cell lymphomas and may have a more favorable prognosis.[86]

LUNG

Pulmonary involvement is not common at diagnosis but may be seen with progressive disease.[87] This typically is associated with lymphatic spread of tumor from hilar and mediastinal nodes. It may be seen in approximately 20 percent of cases at presentation. Primary lymphomas of the lung are rare and typically have a low-grade histology.[88] Pleural effusions are quite common, occurring in approximately 25 percent of patients secondary to either central lymphatic obstruction or pleural seeding.

GASTROINTESTINAL TRACT

Approximately 15 percent of patients with nodal disease also have gastrointestinal involvement, and nearly half of patients have disease at autopsy.[89] Patients may present with anorexia, nausea, vomiting, abdominal mass, or pain. Adjacent mesenteric nodes may be involved and may contribute to the symptoms.[90] Intestinal involvement may be multifocal and may be associated with Waldeyer ring disease. The histologic pattern is usually that of an aggressive lymphoma.[91] Ascites typically develops only late in the disease and is most commonly secondary. Primary involvement of the gastrointestinal tract is seen in approximately 5 percent of cases. The most frequent site of primary gastrointestinal lymphoma is the stomach, followed by the small intestine, rectum, and colon.[92,93] Lymphoma of the stomach typically causes dyspeptic symptoms and sometimes anorexia or early satiety. Hemorrhaging is unusual but suggests a high-grade lymphoma. Diagnosis is typically made by gastroscopic biopsy. At gastroscopy, mild to severe gastritis is common. Adequate biopsies are critical at multiple sites so there is adequate material to determine the presence of *H. pylori*. MALT lymphoma is very common, but diffuse large B-cell lymphoma also may arise de novo or be found in the background of a MALT lymphoma. If both histologies are present, the treatment should be directed at the large-cell lymphoma.[94-97]

TESTICULAR LYMPHOMA

Lymphoma of the testis typically presents as a painless enlargement of the testis in an older man.[98-100] It is typically a diffuse large B-cell lymphoma. At presentation, two-thirds of cases are localized to the testicle alone or the testicle and pelvic or abdominal lymph nodes. In the remaining cases, the testicle is one site of metastatic involvement in patients with widespread disease. After the orchiectomy has established the diagnosis, patients are staged with a special focus on the remaining testicle. If the sonography of the remaining testicle demonstrates a solid mass, it should be assumed to be lymphoma.

LIVER

Hepatic involvement secondary to infiltration of the portal tract is more common in patients with low-risk lymphoma,[101,102] whereas hepatic mass lesions are more commonly seen in patients with aggressive lymphomas.[103] Liver involvement may not be associated with spleen involvement, as is typically seen in Hodgkin disease.[104] Hepatomegaly and jaundice occur in about one-third of patients during the course of their disease. Primary lymphomas of the liver are quite rare and usually are associated with aggressive lymphomas.[105]

SPLEEN

Splenic involvement is found in nearly half of patients with lymphoma.[101,102] Primary involvement of the spleen is quite rare and may occur in all subtypes of lymphoma.[106,107]

BONE

Bone involvement in patients with nodal presentation is rare, as is primary bone involvement.[104] Typically, this is restricted to aggressive lymphoma, and the lesions are usually lytic.[108]

MARROW

Marrow involvement is very common in low-grade follicle center lymphomas and small lymphocytic lymphoma. Aggressive lymphomas that commonly are associated with marrow involvement include lymphoblastic lymphoma and small-noncleaved-cell lymphoma. Diffuse large-cell lymphoma involves the marrow in 10 percent of cases. Rarely, the marrow is the primary site of lymphoma involvement.[109-112]

GENITOURINARY

Retroperitoneal urethral obstruction by lymph nodes is the most common urinary tract finding.[113] This may be observed at diagnosis but more commonly is seen later in the course of the disease. While kidney involvement is common at autopsy, it rarely causes clinical overt disease. An unusual clinical manifestation is enlarged kidneys grossly involved with lymphoma; this rarely occurs at presentation. The nephritic syndrome is also unusual and may be due to renal vein occlusion, glomerulonephritis, or minimal change glomerulopathy. Glomerulopathy is more commonly associated with Hodgkin disease. Lymphomas involving the prostate,[114] testes,[73,74] or ovary[115] are uncommon and typically have aggressive histology and clinical behavior.

OTHER SITES

Clinical disease related to cardiac involvement by lymphoma is very unusual. However, cardiac involvement may be found at autopsy in 20 percent of cases.[103,116] Other uncommon sites include the salivary glands,[117] adrenals,[118] and thyroid.[119] Thyroid lymphoma is usually associated with Hashimoto thyroiditis.

B-CELL LINEAGE INDOLENT LYMPHOMAS (LOW RISK)

SMALL LYMPHOCYTIC LYMPHOMA

Small lymphocytic, or small lymphocytic lymphoma constitutes approximately 5 to 10 percent of all lymphomas.[120-122] This lymphoma has a histologic appearance that is analogous to that of involved lymph nodes of patients with chronic lymphocytic leukemia (CLL).[123] These neoplastic cells share the same morphologic and immunologic features, including low-intensity monoclonal surface immunoglobulin, gene rearrangement of heavy and light immunoglobulin chains, pan B-cell surface antigens (e.g., CD19 or CD20), and CD5[124,125] (see Chap. 13). Similar to patients with CLL, the median age of patients with small lymphocytic lymphoma is 60 years. The disease tends to be indolent, with painless lymphadenopathy and eventual marrow involvement. Some patients with small lymphocytic lymphoma develop CLL. Staging is the same as that used in CLL and should include chest x-ray and a CT scan of the abdomen to determine if there are any lymph nodes compromising vital organs. Examination of the marrow should be performed to determine if there is tumor involvement and, if present, its histologic pattern (i.e., nodular versus diffuse) (see Chap. 98).

Fewer than 1 percent of patients with small lymphocytic lymphoma have lymphoma composed of neoplastic T cells rather than B lymphocytes.[126,127] This represents an entirely different disease than that of B-cell small lymphocytic lymphoma and is often more aggressive. The cytogenetic abnormality inv (14)(q11;q32) has been observed in some cases, suggesting that at least some of these cases are the lymph node counterpart of T-prolymphocytic leukemia.[128-131]

MARGINAL ZONE B-CELL LYMPHOMA

Marginal zone B-cell lymphomas have cellular heterogeneity, including marginal zone cells, monocytoid B-cells, small lymphocytes, and plasma cells. The immunophenotype is that of mature B cells, with surface membrane immunoglobulin, IgM greater than IgG, and B-cell-associated antigens including CD19, CD20, CD22 without CD5, CD10, CD23, or CD11C.[125] This is a tumor of adults with a slight female predominance.

EXTRANODAL MARGINAL ZONE LYMPHOMA OR LOW-GRADE B-CELL LYMPHOMA OF MUCOSA-ASSOCIATED LYMPHOID TISSUE (MALT)

A history of autoimmune disease such as Sjögren syndrome or Hashimoto thyroiditis is common. Most patients present with stage I or II extranodal disease of epithelial tissue, most frequently the stomach. Less common sites are small intestine, lung, salivary gland, thyroid, skin, and other soft tissues.[132-135] Dissemination occurs in one-third of the cases, often in other extranodal sites with long disease-free intervals. It has been hypothesized that this disease may be multifocal. Abnormal karyotypes are observed commonly, often with rearrangements of chromosome 1p and numerical abnormalities of chromosomes 3 and 7.[136] A t(11;18)(q21lq21) translocation was reported in a high frequency of patients with indolent MALT lymphoma.[137] Staging studies are usually negative. Transformation to diffuse large B-cell lymphoma may occur.

NODAL MARGINAL ZONE MONOCYTOID B-CELL LYMPHOMA

The morphologic and immunophenotypic features of nodal marginal zone lymphoma is the same as MALT lymphoma. Most patients with nodal marginal zone monocytoid B-cell lymphoma have localized disease, commonly head and neck lymph nodes, and may have parotid gland involvement.[138–140]

Approximately 15 percent of such patients have Sjögren syndrome.[141,142] Similar to patients with low-grade B-cell lymphomas of MALT, most patients with this lymphoma respond to local therapy. This is likely the nodal equivalent of MALT lymphoma or a closely related condition. Transformation to large cell lymphoma may occur.

SPLENIC MARGINAL ZONE LYMPHOMA WITH OR WITHOUT VILLOUS LYMPHOCYTES

Splenic marginal zone lymphoma appears to be morphologically and clinically distinct from extranodal MALT lymphomas and nodal marginal zone B-cell lymphomas.[143,144] There is overlap between this entity and splenic lymphoma with villous lymphocytes (SLVL).[145] The spleen pathology appears to be identical between these identities with involvement of both mantle and marginal zones of the splenic white pulp usually with a central residual germinal center and involvement of red pulp. The malignant cells range from small lymphocytes in the mantle zone to larger cells with irregular nuclei and pale cytoplasm in the marginal zones. The immunophenotype is identical to MALT and nodal marginal zone lymphomas. At presentation, the patients typically have marrow and blood involvement, usually without peripheral lymphadenopathy. A small M component may be present. These patients typically have a very indolent course.

FOLLICLE CENTER LYMPHOMA, FOLLICULAR

Follicle center lymphoma, follicular are tumors composed of follicle center cells, usually a mixture of cleaved follicle center cells (centrocytes) and large noncleaved follicle center cells (centroblasts). Diffuse areas may be present and, in fact, may even predominate, but follicles exist. Sclerosis also may be seen in diffuse areas. The REAL classification proposes that the term *follicle center lymphoma, follicular* encompasses most of the tumors that were previously classified by pattern as follicular center lymphomas in the Working Formulation and, by cytology, follicular center cell lymphoma in the Lukes and Collins classification, or centroblastic/centrocytic in the Kiel classification. Follicle center lymphoma, follicular show a wide variation in the number of large cells, and it is difficult to sharply divide the distinct subtypes. The REAL classification proposes the term *follicle center lymphoma, follicular grade I, grade II,* or *grade III* to distinguish predominantly small-cell, mixed small and large cell, and large-cell respectively. Grade I or II are treated similarly, while grade III disease is treated the same as diffuse large B-cell lymphoma.

The disease is typically widespread at diagnosis and has an indolent course. Clinical involvement tends to be systemic with lymph nodes, marrow, liver, and spleen involvement. Progression to large-cell lymphoma is common. Tumor cells typically express surface immunoglobulin and CD10, but not CD5, CD23, CD43, and CD11c.[125]

INTERMEDIATE-GRADE LYMPHOMAS

LARGE B-CELL LYMPHOMA SUBTYPE: PRIMARY MEDIASTINAL (THYMIC) LARGE B-CELL LYMPHOMA

This tumor typically involves the thymus at presentation and is composed of large cells resembling centroblasts, large centrocytes, or multilobated cells.[230,231] In some cases the predominant cells are immunoblast, and Reed-Sternberg-like cells may also be present. Sclerosis is a common feature. The cells typically do not express surface immunoglobulin but have the typical B-cell-associated antigens, including CD19, CD20, and CD22, and may have weak expression of CD30.[232,233] They have no specific genetic abnormality. This disease is predominantly found in women with a median age at presentation of 40 years.[234,235] These patients typically present with a locally invasive anterior mediastinal mass originating from the thymus. Patients may have airway compromise or superior vena cava syndrome. Upon relapse, patients tend to have extranodal disease. While the disease is aggressive, it responds well to therapy with a similar outcome as diffuse large B-cell lymphoma.

MANTLE ZONE CELL LYMPHOMA

This tumor is defined in the Kiel classification as centrocytic lymphoma. The tumor is typically composed of small to medium lymphocytes with irregular or "cleaved" nuclei.[255] A small proportion of cases have larger nuclei with more dispersed chromatin, referred to as the *blastic* variant. The pattern of mantle zone cell lymphoma is usually diffuse or vaguely nodular. Some cases involve the mantle zone of reactive follicles, but rarely does a purely mantle zone pattern occur. The immunophenotype has some similarities to CLL/SLL in that the lymphoma cells express surface IgM and IgD and the B-cell-associated antigens CD19 and CD20 along with CD5.[256,257] However, in contrast to CLL/SLL, mantle zone cell lymphoma express CD22 but not CD23 or CD11c. The chromosomal translocation of t(11;14)(q13;q32) involving the *BCL-1* locus at chromosome 11 and the immunoglobulin heavy-chain locus on chromosome 14 occurs in about 50 percent of cases.[258–264] This results in overexpression of the gene known as *PRAD1*, which encodes cyclin D1, a cell cycle protein that is not normally expressed in lymphoid cells. Patients with mantle cell lymphoma are predominantly males and have a median age of 60 years.[265–269] The disease is typically widespread at diagnosis involving lymph nodes, spleen, Waldeyer ring, marrow, blood, and extranodal sites, especially the gastrointestinal tract (lymphomatous polyposis).

FOLLICLE CENTER LYMPHOMA/DIFFUSE SMALL CELL (PROVISIONAL)

These cases are rare lymphomas composed of cells that resemble centrocytes, with minor components with centroblasts, but are entirely diffuse. They represent the diffuse counterpart of the follicle center lymphoma.[10] In some cases, this may be a sampling problem as additional biopsies may show follicular elements. These cases have been called *diffuse small-cleaved-cell lymphoma* by the Working Formulation. The immunophenotype is identical to other follicle center lymphomas. A large retrospective study[270] demonstrated that the vast majority of cases previously referred to as *diffuse small-cleaved-cell lymphoma* when reevaluated were predominantly marginal cell lymphomas and mantle cell lymphomas (SWOG).

PROVISIONAL ENTITY: HIGH-GRADE B-CELL LYMPHOMA, BURKITT-LIKE

In the Working Formulation, this disease entity was called *small noncleaved cell, non-Burkitt.* The International Lymphoma Study Group noted that often these cases were confused with large-cell lymphomas and suggested that many of the cases had been designated undifferentiated, non-Burkitt in the Rappaport classification, and small noncleaved cell, non-Burkitt-type in the Working Formulation.[10] Some cases classified as *small noncleaved non-Burkitt type*, lacked the C-MYC rearrangement but often had the BCL-2 rearrangement, suggesting that they were not Burkitt lymphoma. This classification, therefore, represents cases in which the cell size and nuclear morphology are intermediate between Burkitt lymphoma and typical large-cell lymphoma, in which there is a high proliferative index with or without a starry-sky pattern. The Study Group emphasizes that this is not a reproducible category and likely does not represent a single-disease entity. The tumors typically expressed surface immunoglobulin-positive and B-cell-associated antigens, but not CD5 or CD10. The C-MYC rearrangement is rare, and one-third of cases have the BCL-2 rearrangement. This disease occurs mostly in adults and may or may not be associated with immunosuppression. Involvement of lymph nodes is more common than extranodal sites. In children, the disease appears to behave very much as classic Burkitt lymphoma. In adults, it appears to be a highly aggressive disease.

B-CELL LINEAGE VERY AGGRESSIVE LYMPHOMA (HIGH RISK)-BURKITT LYMPHOMA

Under the Working Formulation, Burkitt lymphoma is small non-cleaved cell, Burkitt's type. The cells are monomorphic, with round nucleoli, and are intermediate in size between small-cell lymphomas and large-cell lymphomas. When these cells are present in the blood, the patient may be classified as having L3 acute lymphoblastic leukemia (ALL) by the French-American-British (FAB) criteria (see Chap. 97). Cytoplasmic lipid vacuoles are typically present. This tumor has an extremely high proliferative index and high rate of spontaneous cell death. The classic starry-sky pattern is secondary to macrophages that have ingested remnants of the tumor cells. Immunophenotypically, the cells express surface IgM and B-cell-associated antigens CD19, CD20, CD22, and CD10 but not CD5 or CD23.[271]

Burkitt lymphoma is commonly a disease of children, but the adult cases are predominantly in the AIDS population. The male:female ratio is approximately 2:1. In the endemic cases, facial bones and, most particularly, the jaws are involved, while in the nonendemic cases, the jaw tumors are less common, and the majority of cases present with disease in the abdomen, most commonly in the distal ileum cecum, and/or mesentery, or other abdominal organs.[277]

T-CELL LINEAGE INDOLENT LYMPHOMAS (LOW RISK)

MYCOSIS FUNGOIDS/SÉZARY SYNDROME

Cutaneous T-cell lymphoma consists of mycosis fungoides and the Sézary syndrome. These disorders are malignant proliferations of T lymphocytes of the helper phenotype. In 1938, Sézary and Bouvrain described a syndrome of pruritus, generalized exfoliative erythroderma, and abnormal hyperconvoluted lymphoid cells in the blood.[282] Today this is referred to as *Sézary syndrome*, a syndrome seen in a subset of patients with mycosis fungoides. Sézary syndrome has biological features similar to the other forms of mycosis fungoides. Most patients with generalized erythroderma have varying numbers of circulating Sézary cells. One-fourth of those with plaque or tumor stage also have circulating Sézary cells.

The initial clinical manifestation of cutaneous T-cell lymphoma occurs more commonly in males, with a 2:1 ratio. The median age at diagnosis is 55 years. Initial skin lesions are clinically and histologically nonspecific, and it may take many years before the diagnosis is confirmed.

The initial clinical manifestation of cutaneous T-cell lymphoma is cutaneous infiltration, and the diagnosis is usually established by skin biopsy. Early lesions may show polymorphic infiltrations compatible with several benign diseases as well as cutaneous T-cell lymphoma. Characteristically, the malignant infiltrate in early cutaneous T-cell lymphoma is epidermotrophic, with exocytosis of single or clusters of convoluted cutaneous T-cell lymphoma cells. Epidermal clusters of these cells are termed *Pautrier microabscesses*. The epidermis also may show parakeratosis and acanthosis. A bandlike infiltrate in the upper dermis is composed of lymphocytes, neutrophils, eosinophils, plasma cells, and histiocytes in early lesions. The atypical, convoluted lymphocytes are present in clusters. In more advanced stages, the infiltrate is less polymorphic with a predominance of atypical cells extending deeper into the dermis; epidermotrophism may be lost. Lymph nodes that drain affected areas may show partial or complete effacement of normal architecture with a monomorphic infiltrate of cutaneous T-cell lymphoma cells. In most lymph nodes, the architecture is not effaced, and dermatopathic changes with varying numbers of atypical lymphocytes in the T-cell paracortical areas of the node are present. The cytologic appearance of the malignant cells in visceral organs is similar to that in the skin.[290]

Most cases of cutaneous T-cell lymphoma progress through distinct stages of skin involvement. These stages begin with a premycotic, erythematous, or eczematoid stage, progress to an infiltrative plaque stage, and eventuate in the tumor stage.[291] Progression is variable but commonly occurs over several years.[292] The premycotic or erythematous stage of cutaneous T-cell lymphoma is nonspecific; it is characterized by localized or widespread areas of erythema or dry eczema.[291] Lesions may be associated with pruritus. Histologic features also are nonspecific, and a definitive diagnosis is often not possible. This stage may last for months to years before progression. The plaque stage is distinguished by palpable, pruritic, indurated lesions. The tumor stage is characterized by large lesions; these may develop in previously normal skin or in premycotic lesions or plaques. The lesions occur most often on the face and in body folds, often in a "bathing trunk" distribution. Tumors are often generalized, and ulceration is common. Pruritus is absent.

The erythrodermic form of cutaneous T-cell lymphoma is manifested by generalized erythroderma and may precede the appearance of other cutaneous T-cell lymphoma lesions by many years. It also may be preceded by premycotic lesions or may appear simultaneously with plaques or tumors. Two common types of erythroderma are exfoliative erythroderma, characterized by intense scaling, and "I'homme rouge" or "red-man" syndrome, in which redness rather than scaling predominates. Transition between forms is common. Lymphadenopathy and alopecia are frequent manifestations.

Cutaneous lesions are classified by using the T staging system. *T1* (limited plaque stage) consists of erythematous patches and plaques covering less than 10 percent of the body. Plaques covering 10 percent of the skin surface are designated *T2*. Cutaneous tumors are designated *T3*, and generalized erythroderma, *T4*. Patients with limited plaque disease have an intermediate prognosis; those with tumor or erythroderma have the worst prognosis.[293]

Lymphadenopathy is present in about half of patients and increases with progressive cutaneous involvement.[294] Lymphangiograms were formerly used to assess pretreatment involvement of intraabdominal lymph nodes. CT scans are less invasive, however, and reveal similar information.[281,295,296] In most cases the cells express CD3, CD5, and CD4, a phenotype associated with mature helper-inducer T lymphocytes[297–299] (see Chap. 13). These cells function as helper T lymphocytes in in vitro assays.[300] The CD7 antigen, expressed by more than 85 percent of normal circulating T lymphocytes, also is present on mycosis fungoides cells in the skin but not on circulating Sézary cells.[301] The cells are generally negative for markers of T-cell activation, such as HLA-DR or CD25 (IL-2 receptor). Like most malignant T cells, the cutaneous T-cell lymphoma cells stain for acid phosphatase, alpha-naphthyl acetate esterase, and beta glucoronidase. They are generally negative for peroxidase, alkaline phosphatase, and esterase. PAS-positive granules are present in some cases. Rearrangement of the T-cell receptor beta gene can be identified.

A wide range of chromosomal abnormalities are described in cutaneous T-cell lymphoma[302] (see Chap. 10). Chromosomes 1 and 6 are frequently involved in structural abnormalities, whereas chromosomes 7, 11, 21, and 22 frequently are involved in numeric abnormalities. Rearrangement of chromosome 10 was common in one study.[303] Chromosomal abnormalities often correlate with extent of disease and survival.

Circulating Sézary cells have been thought to increase with advancing disease. These cells are particularly prominent in patients with generalized erythroderma. Malignant cells also can be detected using sensitive techniques such as cytogenetics or T-cell receptor gene-rearrangement studies.[304-308] Patients with blood involvement have a higher likelihood of lymphadenopathy, visceral involvement, and shorter survival. Marrow infiltration is infrequently detected by biopsy despite circulating malignant cells; it is identified at autopsy in 30 to 40 percent of cases. Using a highly sensitive PCR technique, one group reported a high frequency of clonal T cells in the blood of early mycosis fungoides, suggesting that early systemic disease is quite common.[309]

Smoldering adult T-cell leukemia/lymphoma has a number of clinical features similar to cutaneous T-cell lymphoma, but it usually can be distinguished by the presence of antibodies to HTLV-1 and by its regional occurrence. Pagetoid reticulosis is a rare skin disorder consisting of solitary or localized cutaneous plaques. The involved areas show a prominent atypical mononuclear cell infiltrate with hyperplastic epidermis.[310]

Although this disease is usually indolent and localized, some patients present with a disseminated form referred to as the *Ketron-Goodman variant*.[311] Studies have demonstrated that this is a disease of an activated T lymphocyte that only occasionally expresses the helper T-cell CD4 antigen.[312] Like cutaneous T-cell lymphoma, the neoplastic cells have T-cell receptor gene rearrangements.

T-CELL LINEAGE AGGRESSIVE LYMPHOMAS (INTERMEDIATE RISK)

PERIPHERAL T-CELL LYMPHOMAS, UNSPECIFIED (PROVISIONAL CYTOLOGIC CATEGORIES; MEDIUM-CELL, MIXED MEDIUM- AND LARGE-CELL, LARGE-CELL)

Many of the large T-cell lymphomas cannot be specifically diagnosed and, therefore, are grouped under this heading.[10] These peripheral T-cell lymphomas typically are made up of a mixture of small and large atypical lymphocytes. In the Working Formulation, they have been identified as either diffuse mixed small- and large-cell type or the large-cell immunoblastic. They are extremely heterogeneous and uncommon in the Western world. The International Lymphoma Study Group suggested that, until they can further subclassify this entity, they will be under this current heading.[10] Immunophenotypically, they have T-cell-associated antigens, but many of these antigens may be absent. The cases are predominantly CD4-positive but may be CD8-positive or may be CD4/CD8-negative. The cells lack B-cell antigens. T-cell receptor genes are usually rearranged. Clinically, the cases represent approximately 10 percent of the cases in the United States but appear to be more common in other parts of the world. It is typically a disease of adults who present with systemic disease occasionally with eosinophilia, pruritus, or a hemophagocytic syndrome. Clinical course is typically aggressive, although potentially curable, but relapses are more common than are seen in large B-cell lymphomas. The treatment is identical for large B-cell lymphomas.

LENNERT LYMPHOMA (MALIGNANT LYMPHOMA WITH HIGH CONTENT OF EPITHELIOID HISTIOCYTES)

Lymphoepithelioid lymphoma was first described by Lennert[346] and later by Lennert and Mestdagh[347] and was believed to be a variant of Hodgkin disease. It is now believed that Lennert lymphoma is a distinct lymphoma with a multifocal epithelioid histiocytic reaction.[348] The neoplasms are composed of small and large atypical lymphoid cells, some resembling Reed-Sternberg cells, reactive lymphocytes, or epithelioid histiocytes. They are typically mature T-cells with a helper T-cell immunophenotype and T-cell receptor chain gene rearrangement.[349,350] Cytogenetic studies show a variety of chromosome abnormalities, especially involving chromosome 3[351,352] (see Chap. 10). Lennert lymphoma is most often placed in the diffuse, mixed small- and large-cell category of the Working Formulation. However, patients tend to be older and to have disseminated disease that commonly involves the lung, spleen, lymph nodes, and marrow.[348] Lymphoma involvement of Waldeyer ring is common, as are B symptoms. The clinical course is variable, some patients having a rapidly progressive course. The more aggressive form of the disease is treated with combination chemotherapy, while the indolent form is treated similar to low-grade lymphomas.

ANGIOCENTRIC IMMUNOPROLIFERATIVE LESIONS

Angiocentric immunoproliferative lesions previously were termed *polymorphic reticulosis* and *lymphomatoid granulomatosis*.[353,354] They are composed of atypical lymphoid cells mixed with histiocytes and plasma cells that invade and destroy blood vessels. The atypical lymphoid cells express T-cell antigens but usually do not have T-cell receptor gene rearrangements.[355-357] Angiocentric immunoproliferative lesions are classified into three groups based on the degree of cytologic atypia and number of large lymphoid cells. Grade I lesions have the least atypia and fewest large cells, while grade III have the most and are termed *angiocentric lymphoma*. Grade II is intermediate. The lower-grade lesions often progress to frank lymphoma. Association of EBV within the tumor cells of grade III lesions suggests a role for EBV in the pathogenesis of this disease.[355,356,358] Grade III patients often respond with durable complete responses to chemotherapy with CHOP, while grades I and II patients who progress to grade III generally do not.[357]

ANGIOIMMUNOBLASTIC LYMPHADENOPATHY-LIKE LYMPHOMA

Angioimmunoblastic lymphadenopathy is a rare disease predominantly seen in elderly patients who typically have fever, chills, night sweats, and malaise, generalized lymphadenopathy, hepatospenomegaly, pruritic skin rash, polyclonal hypergammaglobulinemia, anemia (often with a positive Coombs' test), and eosinophilia.[359] Histologically there is loss of lymphoid architecture with a polymorphous infiltrate, including medium-size lymphocytes, plasma cells, esoinophils, and immunoblasts. A hallmark of the disease is arborizing proliferation of small blood vessels and absence of lymphoid follicles.

Approximately 30 percent of patients with angioimmunoblastic lymphadenopathy develop angioimmunoblastic lymphadenopathy-like lymphoma. The neoplasms are either diffuse mixed or large-cell immunoblastic. The tumors of most patients have T-cell surface antigens, as well as T-cell receptor β gene rearrangement[360-362] and nonrandom chromosomal abnormalities.[363,364] Some angioimmunoblastic lymphadenopathy-like lymphoma patients develop B-cell lymphomas that may be related to EBV.[365] Many consider angioimmunoblastic lymphadenopathy-like lymphoma to be a preneoplastic disorder causing abnormalities of the immune system and predisposing to either B- or T-cell malignancies.

INTESTINAL T-CELL LYMPHOMA

This disease is a T-cell lymphoma of the intestines and typically presents with jejunal ulcers which may be multiple and may have perforations.[10,368] The tumors contain an admixture of small, medium, large, or anaplastic lymphocytes.[10] Immunophenotypically, the cells are CD3-positive, CD7-positive, sometimes CD8-positive, CD4-negative, and CD103-positive. The TCR beta chain genes are rearranged. This is a disease of adults who often have a history of gluten-sensitive enteropathy. They may have as the initial event typical histologic features of sprue in the resected intestine. This is a very uncommon disease in the United States and Europe but is seen in areas where gluten-sensitive enteropathies are common. The typical presentation is abdominal pain, often associated with jejunal perforation. Other areas of the gastrointestinal tract are less commonly involved. The course is aggressive, and death usually occurs from intestinal perforation.

ANAPLASTIC LARGE-CELL LYMPHOMA

Anaplastic large-cell lymphoma, formally referred to as *Ki-1 lymphoma*, is now a world-recognized pathologic entity that accounts for 2 to 8 percent of all lymphomas. It was first noted that the cells from large-cell lymphomas reacted with the anti-Ki-1 antibody, a monoclonal antibody raised against the Reed-Sternberg cells of Hodgkin disease patients.[369–371] Pathologically, the lymph nodes are partially involved and the B-cell follicles are spared, but the sinuses are infiltrated by tumor cells.[10] There exists a proliferation of pleomorphic large neoplastic lymphoid cells usually growing in a cohesive pattern and peripherally spreading in the lymph node sinuses. The majority of ALCL cases express antigens of the T-cell lineage; however, many cases may lack lymphoid antigens and others may express B-cell antigens.[10,372–374] The REAL classification includes the B-cell type of ALCL among the morphologic variants of diffuse large B-cell lymphoma, limiting ALCL to T-cell and null-cell types.[10]

The two distinct clinical forms of primary ALCL are cutaneous and systemic. The primary cutaneous form of ALCL is uncommon before age 20, may undergo spontaneous regression, and has a favorable prognosis. The systemic form is common in children and adolescents, has a bimodal age distribution, and has an aggressive clinical course, frequently presenting with systemic symptoms, advanced disease, and extranodal localization of disease. While response to treatment and overall survival of systemic ALCL in children is good, prognosis in adults is controversial. In one study[373] comparing 146 adult patients with primary systemic ALCL to 1695 cases of nonanaplastic diffuse large-cell lymphoma, a number of conclusions were drawn. Patients with ALCL were more likely to be male, were younger, and had more frequent B-cell symptoms. Skin and lung involvement was more frequent in ALCL, while bone marrow involvement was identical. The immunophenotype was rather equally divided between B-cell, T-cell, and null-cell phenotypes. Response to chemotherapy, event-free survival, and overall survival were superior for ALCL.

MALIGNANT LYMPHOMA, LYMPHOBLASTIC

Clinically, lymphoblastic lymphoma is very similar to acute lymphoblastic leukemia. It is an aggressive lymphoma that frequently spreads to the CNS. The published experience in adult patients is relatively limited.

PRECURSOR T-CELL-LYMPHOBLASTIC LYMPHOMA/LEUKEMIA

This is a disease caused by lymphoblasts with round or convoluted nuclei, fine chromatin, scant cytoplasm, and an inconspicuous nucleoli.[10] These cells have an identical morphology to that of precursor B lymphoblastic neoplasms. However, the cells have a distinguishing immunophenotype in that they typically express CD7 and CD3. Cytoplasmic CD3 is typically present even if surface membrane CD3 is absent. The expression of other T-cell-associated antigens is variable, and the expression of CD4 and CD8 is quite variable with double positives, double negatives, or either CD4 or CD8 alone.[125,380–382] TdT

is positive, and B-cell-associated antigens are negative. The rearrangement of the T-cell receptor gene is variable, depending on the maturity of the cells.[383]

Patients are typically young adult males. This disease constitutes 40 percent of childhood lymphomas and 15 percent of acute lymphoblastic leukemias.[384] The typical presentation is a rapidly enlarging thymic mass and/or peripheral adenopathy. It is a rapidly fatal disease if untreated and usually terminates in acute leukemia with central nervous system involvement.

ADULT T-CELL LEUKEMIA/LYMPHOMA

Adult T-cell leukemia/lymphoma is a T-cell lymphoproliferative syndrome first described in Japan in 1977 and later identified in the United States, the Caribbean, and other countries.[385–389] Adult T-cell leukemia/lymphoma is characterized by pleomorphic neoplastic cells with membrane features of mature helper T lymphocytes. Presenting features include lymphadenopathy, hepatomegaly, splenomegaly, cutaneous infiltration, hypercalcemia (with or without lytic bone lesions), and interstitial pulmonary infiltrate.

Patients with adult T-cell leukemia/lymphoma have varied clinical presentations, including an aggressive acute syndrome with leukemia, a lymphoma without lymphocytosis, a chronic process with a modest leukemia phase, and a smoldering condition.[400] The median age of patients with the aggressive acute type of adult T-cell leukemia/lymphoma is 40 years. Typical presentation includes an elevated leukocyte count, ranging from 5000 to 100,000/μl (5 to 100 $\times$ 10^9/liter) with circulating malignant lymphocytes.[385,386] Anemia and thrombocytopenia are uncommon at presentation. Onset of symptoms is typically acute, with rapidly developing cutaneous lesions, hypercalcemia, or both. The appearance of skin lesions is variable. Some patients have discrete tumors, and others have confluent smaller nodules. Some patients present with plaques, papules, nonspecific erythematous patches, or erythroderma. Patients with hypercalcemia typically have weakness, lethargy, confusion, polyuria, and polydipsia.

Lymph node enlargement occurs in all patients, although the nodes are initially small in some. Many have generalized lymphadenopathy, and most have retroperitoneal adenopathy. Hilar adenopathy is common, but a mediastinal mass is rare. The patient's marrow may be infiltrated with leukemia cells. Additional sites of disease include the lung, liver, skin, gastrointestinal tract, and central nervous system. In addition, adult T-cell leukemia/lymphoma is associated with lymphomas of several histologic subtypes, including diffuse, poorly differentiated small-cell; mixed large- and small-cell; and large-cell immunoblastic. No apparent correlation exists between clinical course and lymph node morphology. Opportunistic infections are common in patients with adult T-cell leukemia/lymphoma. *Pneumocystis carinii* infection is common, as is cryptococcal meningitis. Bacterial and fungal infections are also common.

Cutaneous involvement occurs in about two-thirds of patients with adult T-cell leukemia/lymphoma. Focal epidermal infiltration with adult T-cell leukemia/lymphoma cells, or Pautrier microabscesses, is seen in most patients with cutaneous involvement. Pautrier microabscesses were thought to be pathognomonic of cutaneous T-cell lymphoma, but they also can also be found in some patients with adult T-cell leukemia/lymphoma. The absence of a chronic premycotic phase in most patients with adult T-cell leukemia/lymphoma distinguishes it from typical cutaneous T-cell lymphoma. Furthermore, serologic studies in cases of cutaneous T-cell lymphoma show no association with HTLV-I infection, although rare patients with cutaneous T-cell lymphoma are HTLV-I positive.

An important pathologic feature of adult T-cell leukemia/lymphoma is the presence of pleomorphic lymphoid cells in the blood.

Not all patients have blood involvement at diagnosis, even though circulating leukemia cells are identified in most cases eventually. Adult T-cell leukemia/lymphoma cells have moderately condensed nuclear chromatin, inconspicuous nucleoli, and a markedly irregular nuclear contour that divides the nucleus into several lobes. These cells are characteristic of HTLV-I-associated disease and can be distinguished from Sézary cells and cells of other mature and immature T-cell malignancies. In about 20 percent of the cases, nuclear irregularities are less extreme, and the cells may be difficult to distinguish from Sézary cells.

The malignant cells from patients with adult T-cell leukemia/lymphoma typically have the phenotype of mature helper T cells[401] and express the CD2, CD3, and CD4 antigens (see Chap. 13). They also express CD25, the p55 subunit of the IL-2 receptor. Clonal rearrangements of the T-cell receptor β chain are present.[402–405] Leukemia cells have been reported to suppress B-cell immunoglobulin secretion by a complex mechanism involving induction of suppressor cells after activation of normal suppressor cell precursors.[401]

Radionuclide bone scans of patients with the acute adult T-cell leukemia/lymphoma syndrome typically show a diffuse increased uptake throughout the skeleton, most prominent in the joints and skull. These scans are referred to as "super" scans and are unusual in other patients with malignant lymphomas. Isolated lytic bone lesions also may occur. Typically, the serum alkaline phosphatase level is elevated.

LABORATORY FEATURES

BLOOD

Laboratory tests include standard chemistry and hematology studies. The indolent lymphomas are more likely to involve the blood. If anemia or reticulocytosis is present at diagnosis, a Coombs' test should be obtained to determine whether autoimmune hemolytic anemia is present. Thrombocytopenia may be related to marrow replacement, hypersplenism, or autoimmune destruction. Marrow involvement, as well as autoimmune complications, is more common with low-grade lymphomas. Elevation of serum lactic dehydrogenase (LDH) is common and suggests a poorer prognosis.

LYMPH NODE BIOPSY

A biopsy is essential to establish the diagnosis of lymphoma. This usually involves excisional biopsy of an affected lymph node. If the disease is extranodal, then a surgical biopsy of the site of involvement is necessary. A needle aspiration biopsy is not adequate for the initial diagnosis, except in unusual circumstances.

A portion of the biopsy specimen should be placed in formalin for histology, and another portion frozen for immunologic and molecular studies that may be necessary. Special studies such as immunoglobulin and T-cell receptor gene rearrangement studies, polymerase chain reaction (PCR) for the BCL-1 or BCL-2 oncogene rearrangements, cytogenetics, flow cytometry, and immunohistochemistry may be critical for diagnosis in a minority of cases or may support the diagnosis in other cases.

MARROW EXAMINATION

Evaluation of the marrow of patients with suspected or newly diagnosed lymphoma may assist in establishing the diagnosis or in staging the extent of disease respectively. Because the marrow involvement by most lymphomas is spotty, patients generally should undergo bilateral posterior iliac crest biopsies. Except in Burkitt lymphoma and lymphoblastic lymphoma, the incidence of marrow involvement is higher in indolent lymphomas (20 to 95 percent) than in the more aggressive lymphomas (10 percent). Lymphoma involvement of the marrow can be detected by morphologic evaluation if there is 5 percent or greater infiltration by malignant cells. Additional techniques, such as flow cytometry, Southern Blot analysis, or evaluation for clonal excess, may detect lymphoma cells in the marrow when they constitute a smaller proportion of marrow cells, e.g., greater than 1 percent. The polymerase chain reaction can be used to detect abnormalities, such as the t(14;18) translocation involving BCL-2, in the range of one lymphoma cell in 10^5 to 10^6 normal cells. PCR is not entirely reliable, as 10 to 20 percent of patients with follicular lymphomas do not have a PCR-amplified breakpoint. PCR also may have a role in detecting minimal residual disease following therapy. However, PCR cannot be considered a standard tool unless the results of the PCR changes our approach to therapy. Patients who have intermediate- or high-grade lymphoma in the marrow have a higher likelihood of central nervous system disease and should undergo a spinal tap.

RADIOGRAPHIC STUDIES

Chest roentgenograms should be performed in all patients found to have lymphoma. A computed tomographic (CT) scan of the chest is indicated if the chest roentgenogram is abnormal or questionable. A CT scan of the abdomen and pelvis should be performed to evaluate for abdominal or pelvic nodes and masses. Lymphangiography has been abandoned for this purpose. Gallium scan may be very useful in the setting of large masses to follow responses to therapy and to evaluate residual tumor in a large mass that has responded to treatment. Ultrasonography and magnetic resonance imaging (MRI) may clarify abnormalities found on other studies. Lymphoma involvement of Waldeyer ring is commonly associated with lymphoma in the gastrointestinal tract, and vice versa. Therefore, patients who have Waldeyer ring involvement should be evaluated with an upper gastrointestinal series that includes a small-bowel follow-through and a barium enema. Such barium contrast studies also should be performed if any abnormality involving the gastrointestinal tract is suspected from the history or physical examination.

THERAPY, COURSE, AND PROGNOSIS

GENERAL PROGNOSTIC FACTORS

One important prognostic factor is the histologic subtype. This is described in detail below and divides the lymphomas into different risk groups. Low-risk lymphomas may transform over a number of years to intermediate- or high-risk lymphomas that typically have a more aggressive clinical course than de novo intermediate- or high-risk disease. Advanced stage is associated with poorer survival. Systemic B symptoms generally are considered adverse,[53] although some studies have not confirmed this finding.[54] Age is considered a prognostic factor. Patients over 60 years of age have a poorer survival,[55,56] although this is disputed by some investigators.[57] This may be related to the lower tolerance of the elderly for chemotherapeutic drugs.[58] Extranodal disease is considered an adverse prognostic factor, particularly in CNS disease. Primary CNS disease usually is associated with more aggressive histologies and has a high incidence in individuals with AIDS. The testes are another extranodal site, and radiation of the uninvolved testis generally is recommended because of the high incidence of recurrent disease. As described above, patients with Waldeyer ring involvement have an increased risk of gastrointestinal lymphoma.

Tumor bulk and growth rate also have been associated with prognosis. Tumor masses larger than 10 cm generally have been considered a poor prognostic factor.[59–61] Elevated serum LDH is an unfavorable prognostic factor as it reflects increased tumor burden.[62] Some studies have reported that a T-cell phenotype in advanced aggressive disease is an adverse prognostic factor,[63,64] although this remains controversial.[65] A high proliferative index as measured by the Ki-67 antigen was associated with a poor prognosis in one study.[66] Nonrandom chromosomal abnormalities also have been associated with a poorer prognosis.[67]

The International Lymphoma Prognostic Factor Index (IPI) is a predictive model for aggressive lymphoma.[68] The project was undertaken to develop a model for predicting outcome in patients with aggressive lymphoma on the basis of patients' clinical characteristics before treatment, because the Ann Arbor classification was inconsistent in distinguishing between patients. Five risk factors were identified as poor prognostic factors (Table 103-4). These included age greater than 60 years, elevated serum LDH concentration, poor performance status, stage III or IV disease, and more than one extranodal disease site. Based on these factors, four risk groups were identified with 5-year survival rates of 73 percent, 51 percent, 43 percent, and 26 percent (Table 103-5).

While the original classification was identified for patients with aggressive lymphoma, it was later demonstrated that the same model could predict prognosis for a variety of histologic types of lymphoma.[69] Interestingly, the histologic diagnosis of anaplastic large-cell lymphoma was associated with good survival even with a high prognostic index.

LOW-GRADE LYMPHOMAS

SMALL LYMPHOCYTIC LYMPHOMA

Treatment of small lymphocytic lymphoma is similar to that for CLL and is presented in Chap. 98. Systemic therapy is initiated with single agent chlorambucil, fludarabine, or cladrabine but is not curative.[123] Some investigators consider fludarabine the treatment of choice for previously untreated patients.[131]

The rare T-cell variant of small lymphocytic leukemia may be more aggressive and require therapeutic intervention earlier. Doxorubicin-based regimens often are initiated, although pentostatin (deoxycoformycin) might be a reasonable alternative.[129] There exists no standard therapy for the T-cell variant.

MALT LYMPHOMA AND MONCYTOID B-CELL LYMPHOMA

MALT lymphoma and monocytoid B-cell lymphoma often are localized and may be cured by surgery or local radiation, depending on the site of disease.[146–148] Single-agent chemotherapy also has been recommended.[149] Unless there is residual disease, there are no data to

TABLE 103-5   OUTCOME ACCORDING TO RISK GROUP DEFINED BY THE INTERNATIONAL INDEX*

INTERNATIONAL INDEX	NO. OF RISK FACTORS	COMPLETE RESPONSE RATE (%)	RELAPSE-FREE SURVIVAL 2-YR	RELAPSE-FREE SURVIVAL 5-YR	SURVIVAL 2-YR	SURVIVAL 5-YR
Low	0 or 1	87	79	70	84	73
Low-intermediate	2	67	66	50	66	51
High-intermediate	3	55	59	49	54	43
High	4 or 5	44	58	40	34	26

*Adapted from reference 68.

support the use of postoperative radiation therapy. It has been suggested that the lymphoma may be multifocal and that patients should have frequent follow-up with endoscopy and biopsy of suspicious lesions. Disseminated disease may be followed without therapy until necessary to relieve symptoms. When therapy is indicated, it usually is initiated with an alkylating agent or multiagents including an anthracycline.[149,150]

Successful treatment of the *H. pylori* frequently leads to complete regression of the MALT lymphoma.[154,155] The diagnosis of *H. pylori*-associated MALT lymphoma requires biopsy proof of both the lymphoma and the presence of *H. pylori*. The patient is then treated with antibiotics effective against *H. pylori*. If the *H. pylori* is not eradicated, which appears in approximately 10 percent of the cases, a second course of antibiotics is indicated. Even if the *H. pylori* is eliminated, the MALT lymphoma may persist. This should be followed with serial endoscopies as there may be a gradual regression of the MALT lymphoma. If the MALT lymphoma does not continue to decrease in size or persists beyond 6 months, further antilymphoma therapy should be initiated with either single-agent chlorambucil or cyclophosphamide or upper abdominal radiation. Biopsies should rule out coexistant large-cell lymphoma.

FOLLICLE CENTER LYMPHOMA

Follicle center lymphomas grade III are more aggressive than the small cleaved or mixed small cleaved and large cell lymphomas and represents 10 percent of the total cases. The cells may be cleaved or noncleaved. They more commonly present with localized tumors, as compared to grade I and grade II tumors. However, despite the early clinical stage at diagnosis, they have the least favorable prognosis of the follicle center lymphomas, with frequent recurrences and progression to diffuse large-cell lymphoma. The number of centroblasts and the size of the centrocytes appear to correlate with the prognosis.[162,163] Controversy exists over whether cases classified as follicular mixed cell type may be curable with aggressive therapy, while the small cleaved cell variant is not considered curable with therapy. The proportion of the tumor that has a follicular pattern also is correlated with prognosis.[164,165] The rare purely diffuse cases appear to have the worse prognosis.[166] Progression to diffuse large B-cell lymphoma may occur.

Over time the follicular pattern tends to progress to a diffuse pattern, and the fraction of tumor cells that are large cleaved or noncleaved increases. The growth fraction increases with the number of large cells in the tumor, and the number of cytogenetic abnormalities increases with acceleration of the disease. The ability to obtain durable responses to initial therapy, however, also increases as a function of the number of large cells in the tumor.

Patients with follicle center lymphoma grades I and II are treated in a similar fashion. There are data to suggest that patients with grade II disease may have a more durable response to therapy. However,

TABLE 103-4   THE INTERNATIONAL NON-HODGKIN'S LYMPHOMA PROGNOSTIC FACTOR INDEX*

RISK FACTORS
Age (≤60 vs. >60)
Serum LDH (≤1 × normal vs. >1 × normal)
Performance status (0 or 1 vs. 2–4)
Stage I or II vs. III or IV
Extranodal involvement (≤1 site vs. >1 site)

*Adapted from reference 68.
ABBREVIATION: LDH, lactic dehydrogenase.

the approach to therapy is the same. However, patients with grade III disease are treated similarly to patients with diffuse large B-cell lymphoma and are not included in this section.

Patients who have stage I or stage II disease represent fewer than 20 percent of all cases. These patients often are treated with involved-field radiation therapy alone. Between 50 and 75 percent of such patients are cured. There is no evidence that adjuvant chemotherapy in this setting improves survival or diminishes the risk for recurrent disease. A retrospective review of 177 patients with stage I and stage II disease with either follicle center lymphomas grade I or grade II demonstrated a median survival of 14 years following radiation therapy as a single modality.[167] Most of these patients received either involved- or extended-field radiation therapy ranging from 35 to 50 Gy. Approximately 50 percent of the patients were relapse-free at 5 to 10 years, but only 5 of 47 patients who reached 10 years without relapse subsequently developed recurrence.

The concept of ''watch and wait'' for patients with stage III or IV disease proposes that patients are followed without therapy until they develop progressive disease or systemic symptoms. Some untreated patients have spontaneous remissions and are spared chemotherapy. The median survival of patients so managed was reported to be over 7 years in one study[168] and 4 years in another.[169] In another trial, patients were randomized to a watch-and-wait protocol or to a protocol of combined therapy with prednisone, methotrexate, doxorubicin, cyclophosphamide, and etoposide, then mechlorethamine, vincristine, procarbazine, and prednisone (ProMACE/MOPP) followed by total nodal irradiation.[170] The overall survival rates for the two groups were similar. However, the number of complete remissions and the disease-free survival rates were longer in the patients treated with combined modality therapy. Responses to single-agent therapy such as chlorambucil or a nucleoside (Table 103-6) range from 75 to 90 percent of patients.[171–177] All patients eventually relapse. In randomized trials, single-agent alkylating therapy was compared to CVP. Patients treated with CVP had more complete responses and shorter median time to complete response than patients treated with single-agent therapy but did not have significantly longer overall survival rates.[171,173,174,178–181] Similarly, intensive combination regimens including doxorubicin also have demonstrated excellent responses for patients with follicle center lymphoma, but there is no evidence that such treatment prolongs survival.[182–185]

Approximately 90 percent of relapsed follicle center lymphoma patients responded to fludarabine, mitoxantrone, and dexamethasone with 50 percent complete responses.[186] Twenty-seven of 27 previously untreated follicle center lymphoma patients responded to a combination of cyclophosphamide and fludarabine with over 90 percent complete responses.[187] Similar responses were reported with three courses of full-dose fludarabine followed by six to eight courses of cyclophosphamide, mitoxantrone, vincristine, and prednisone with 96 percent responses, and 65 percent complete responses.[188]

Rituximab, an anti-CD20 human-mouse chimeric monoclonal antibody, has been approved by the U.S. Food and Drug Administration for the treatment of follicle center lymphoma.[189,190] Response rates of 50 percent are reported following a dose of 375mg/m^2 given weekly for four doses to previously treated patients. The majority of responses were partial responses but tended to be very durable with a median time to progression of 13 months. ^{131}I- and ^{90}Y-labeled murine monoclonal anti-CD20 antibody trials have demonstrated excellent responses in previously treated patients treated with either a one-time low-dose of ^{131}I- or ^{90}Y-labeled antibody[191,192] or a marrow ablative dose of ^{131}I-labeled antibody.[193,194] Previously untreated patients with follicle center lymphomas were treated with 75 cGy delivered on 35mg of anti-CD20 murine monoclonal antibody with 100 percent response rates and predominantly complete responses.[195] The major toxicity was moderate reversible myelosuppression.

Autologous and allogeneic stem cell transplantation is an additional therapeutic approach for patients with follicle center lymphoma (see Chap 18). In most studies, patients were treated for recurrent disease. Similar survival outcomes are reported for autologous and allogeneic transplantation, although allogeneic transplant has a much higher incidence of treatment-

TABLE 103-6   SINGLE AND COMBINATION AGENTS USED TO TREAT FOLLICLE CENTER LYMPHOMA, FOLLICULAR GRADES I AND II

AGENT(S)	DOSE	ROUTE	DAYS(S) OF TREATMENT	REPEAT CYCLED, DAYS
SINGLE AGENTS				
Chlorambucil	0.08–0.12 mg/kg	PO	Daily	
	or 0.4–1.0 mg/kg	PO	1	28
Cyclophosphamide	50–100 mg/m^2	PO	Daily	
	or 300 mg/m^2	PO	1–5	28
Fludarabine	25 mg/m^2/day	IV	1–5	28
Pentostatin	4 mg/m^2	IV	1	14
Cladribine	0.1 mg/kg/day	IV (continuous)	1–7	28
	or 0.14 mg/kg/day	IV (2 h)	1–5	28
Rituximab	375 mg/m^2/day	IV	1, 8, 15, 22	
COMBINATION THERAPIES				
CVP				
Cylophosphamide	400 mg/m^2	PO	1–5	21
Vincristine	1.4 mg/m^2 (maximum 2 mg)	IV	1	
Prednisone	100 mg/m^2	PO	1–5	
COPP				
Cyclophosphamide	400–650 mg/m^2	IV	1 and 8	28
Vincristine	1.4 mg/m^2 (maximum 2 mg)	IV	1 and 8	
Procarbazine	100 mg/m^2	PO	1–14	
Prednisone	40 mg/m^2	PO	1–14	
CHOP				
Cyclophosphamide	750 mg/m^2	IV	1	21
Doxorubicin	50 mg/m^2	IV	1	
Vincristine	1.4 mg/m^2	IV	1	
Prednisone	100 mg	PO	1–5	
FND				
Fludarabine	25 mg/m^2	IV	1–3	28
Mitoxantrone	10 mg/m^2	IV	1	
Dexamethasone	20 mg	IV or PO	1–5	
CF				
Cyclophosphamide	600–1000 mg/m^2	IV	1	
Fludarabine	20 mg/m^2	IV	1–5	21–28
F-CNOP				
Fludarabine	25 mg/m^2	IV	1–5	28
Cyclophosphamide	750 mg/m^2	IV	1	
Mitoxantrone	12 mg/m^2	IV	1	
Vincristine	1.4 mg/m^2 (maximum 2 mg)	IV	1	
Prednisone	100 mg	PO	1	

related death, while autologous transplants have a higher incidence of disease recurrence. In one large retrospective study of 113 follicle center lymphoma patients that received allografts, the 3-year probability of disease-free survival was 49 percent.[196] Allografts should likely be considered for younger patients with follicle center lymphoma who do not have an initial conventional chemotherapy-induced remission.

Autografts are more popular than allografts because of age and donor limitations. Some investigators have used monoclonal antibodies specific for B-cell surface antigens for ex vivo "purging" of tumor cells from autologous marrow. In one study, detection of residual lymphoma by PCR for the *BCL-2* oncogene rearrangement in the purged marrow proved to be the most important predictor of early relapse following transplantation.[197] Several investigators have failed to show benefit from purging in low-grade lymphoma; however, large randomized studies have not been reported.[198–200] Unfortunately, while high-dose therapy may prolong disease-free survival, there is no definitive evidence to date that it prolongs overall survival compared with conventional approaches. Furthermore, there is no evidence that blood stem cells are superior to marrow, stem cells, that regimens which include total body irradiation are superior to drug-only regimens, or that outcome of patients with follicle center lymphoma, grade II (mixed cellularity) is superior to that of patients with grade I (small cleaved cell) disease.[198]

An aggressive approach to follicle center lymphoma is autologous marrow transplantation in first remission. In one study, 83 patients with previously untreated follicle center lymphoma were treated with anthracycline-based chemotherapy and 77 were eligible for stem cell transplantation.[201] Forty-three patients entered complete remissions at a median follow-up of 45 months. The 3-year estimated disease-free survival was 63 percent, and the overall survival at 3 years was 89 percent. A patient whose marrow was PCR-negative after purging had a significantly longer freedom from recurrence than patients who were PCR-positive.

High-dose interferon-α is active in heavily pretreated patients with follicle center lymphoma.[202,203] Based on these results, studies were designed to determine the role of interferon-α both in the induction phase of treatment as well as in maintenance therapy. A number of phase III trials were designed to address these issues. Two of four trials included doxorubicin-based regimens, one included cyclophosphamide, vincristine, and prednisone, and one had cyclophosphamide as a single agent.[204–208] These studies included relatively low doses of interferon given intermittently, ranging from 2 to 6 million U/m². In one of the studies, disease-free survival and overall survival were improved.[204] In two studies, there was increased remission duration without an improvement in overall survival.[205–207] A fourth study demonstrated interferon to have no impact on remission or survival.[208] Five large randomized trials evaluated interferon-α as postinduction therapy.[205,209–212] Patients were randomized to relatively low-doses of interferon-α three times per week following chemotherapy (2 to 5 million U/m²). The duration of remission was improved in three of the five trials, but it is not clear that there was an impact on overall survival. These studies demonstrate activity for interferon-α in follicle center lymphoma. However, it is not clear that there is a survival benefit.

Interleukin-2 (IL-2) has been used to treat patients with low-grade lymphoma. In one study, IL-2 and exogenous lymphokine-activated killer (LAK) cells had no activity in patients with advanced low-grade or intermediate-grade lymphoma.[213] In another study IL-2, alone or in combination with interferon-α, also demonstrated no activity in patients with lymphoma.[214] A subsequent study, using higher doses of IL-2 with exogenous LAK cells, observed objective responses in 3 of 6 patients with low-grade lymphoma.[215] However, considering the toxicity and modest activity of this regimen, it is difficult to envision a major role for IL-2 in the treatment of this disease.

B-cell malignancies are clonal; All cells within the tumor express immunoglobulin with the same variable region structure that can be recognized uniquely by anti-idiotype antibodies. Therefore, an anti-idiotype antibody raised against patients' tumor cells may recognize a "tumor-specific" antigen. Infusion with murine monoclonal anti-idiotype antibodies, either combined with interferon-α, chlorambucil, or antibody alone have demonstrated approximately 50 percent response rates in patients with advanced follicle center lymphoma.[216–218] Several problems have been identified with the anti-idiotype antibody therapy, including the high cost of generating custom-made antibodies for each patient's tumor and the fact that idiotype variants within the tumor may be selected during treatment that are nonresponsive to subsequent therapy with the original anti-idiotype antibodies.[219] Current studies are focused on idiotype vaccines. Isolating the idiotypic protein and coupling it to keyhole limpet hemocyanin (KLH) combined with an immunologic adjuvant generates specific immune responses in approximately 50 percent of patients treated.[220] There appeared to be an improved clinical outcome for those patients who generated a specific immune response against the idiotype.[221,222] In more recent studies, autologous dendritic cells were pulsed ex vivo with tumor-specific idiotype protein, and 4 of 4 patients with follicle center lymphoma developed measurable antitumor cellular immune responses measured by T-cell proliferation, and 3 of these 4 patients demonstrated clinical responses.[223]

Monoclonal antibody specific for tumor-associated antigens may be conjugated to toxins producing immunotoxins. Such immunotoxins may directly deliver toxin to tumor cells. The most common toxin used in clinical studies is ricin. Ricin is a heterodimeric protein that inhibits protein synthesis with the action of its cytotoxic A chain. The A chain is linked covalently to a B chain that binds galactose, a sugar found in glycoproteins of virtually all mammalian cells. By removing or chemically blocking the B chain, the cell-binding activity of ricin is eliminated. Conjugating this modified ricin to monoclonal antibody allows for specific delivery of the toxic A chain to cells recognized by the monoclonal antibody. Clinical trials with antibody conjugated to either ricin A chain or using the whole ricin with the B chain chemically blocked have demonstrated modest responses.[224–226]

B-CELL LINEAGE AGGRESSIVE LYMPHOMAS (INTERMEDIATE RISK)

GENERAL PRINCIPLES

Early-Stage Disease Clinical data from the 1960s and 1970s indicated that about half of all patients with localized diffuse large-cell lymphoma could be cured with involved- or extended-field radiation therapy. The patients who relapsed had undetected microscopic disease at distinct sites. Early phase II pilot studies demonstrated that higher cure rates were noted for patients treated with combination chemotherapy, with or without involved-field radiation.[238] Such systemic therapy also obviated staging laparotomy, thereby reducing the morbidity and mortality of the initial patient evaluation. National cooperative group studies have evaluated the optimal number of cycles of chemotherapy for such patients and whether local radiation therapy is necessary. Investigators demonstrated that nonbulky patients with stage I or II disease had a superior overall survival when treated with three cycles of CHOP (cyclophosphamide, doxorubicin, vincristine and prednisone) chemotherapy plus involved field radiation therapy compared to eight cycles of CHOP chemotherapy alone.[239] The 5-year estimates of overall survival for patients receiving CHOP plus radiation therapy was 82 percent. Patients with localized disease who have larger tumor bulks have also been studied in a prospective randomized trial.[240] They demonstrated that patients treated with eight cycles of CHOP plus low-dose radiation had a superior result compared to those patients receiving eight cycles of CHOP alone. Six-year overall survival was approximately 64 percent. Therefore, it appears from these two large, prospective randomized clinical trials, that combined modality treatment with CHOP plus radiotherapy is superior to CHOP chemotherapy alone for patients with localized diffuse large B-cell lymphoma. The number of cycles of chemotherapy should be determined by the stage of disease (I versus II) and the tumor bulk.

Advanced-Stage Disease Combination chemotherapy may be curative for patients with advanced-stage high-grade lymphomas. The most active chemotherapeutic agents for treating the aggressive lymphomas are cyclophosphamide and doxorubicin. Initial studies using the "first-generation" chemotherapeutic regimens, such as C-MOPP (cyclophosphamide, vincristine, procarbazine and prednisone) or CHOP, produced complete response rates of 40 to 55 percent, with 30 to 35 percent long-term survivors (Table 103-7).[236] A 10- to 15-year follow-up revealed that only a few successfully treated patients experienced a late-disease relapse. Assuming that higher cure rates could be achieved using a larger number of chemotherapeutic agents, several complex treatment regimens were developed. These regimens

often included drugs that, by themselves, had little activity in patients with such lymphomas. The most commonly used regimens included m-BACOD (methotrexate with leucovorin rescue, bleomycin, doxorubicin, cyclophosphamide, vincristine, and dexamethasone),[241] ProMACE/CytaBOM (prednisone, doxorubicin, cyclophosphamide, and etoposide followed by cytarabine, bleomycin, vincristine, and methotrexate with leucovorin rescue),[242] and MACOP-B (methotrexate with leucovorin rescue, doxorubicin, cyclophosphamide, vincristine, prednisone and bleomycin).[243] Single-institution pilot studies reported that 55 to 65 percent of the patients treated with any one of these complex regimens achieved a complete remission. However, longer follow-up of these patients and multicenter clinical trials failed to substantiate that these complex and costly regimens yielded a significant improvement in survival over that achieved by CHOP.[244] Thus the ultimate conclusions concerning the efficacy of these new regimens awaited the results of prospective randomized trials. The Southwest Oncology Group (SWOG) conducted a randomized trial comparing standard therapy, CHOP, to the third generation chemotherapy regimens, m-BACOD, ProMACE-CytaBOM, or MACOP-B.[245] Fatal toxicity was 1 percent for CHOP, 3 percent for ProMACE/CytaBOM, 5 percent for m-BACOD, and 6 percent for MACOP-B. After over 6 years, there is still no difference in response rate, time to treatment failure, or overall survival between CHOP and the third-generation regimens. Other randomized trials comparing CHOP with each of the previously mentioned third-generation chemotherapy regimens gave similar results.[246] Thus CHOP remains the best available standard of care; the recognition of this fact has resulted in significant cost savings and the avoidance of unnecessary toxicity. However, based on the fact that fewer than 50 percent of all patients are cured and, as noted subsequently, that we can now identify subsets of patients with even lower cure rates, it is absolutely essential that oncologists develop new and improved therapeutic approaches for patients with advanced stage, aggressive histology lymphoma. The IPI described above[68] reported that patients in the high-risk IPI group had a CR rate of 44 percent and a 5-year survival rate of only 26 percent as compared to a CR rate of 87 percent and a 5-year survival of 73 percent in patients in the low-risk IPI group. Therefore, those patients with a low IPI, whose outcome is predicted to be favorable with conventional therapy, should be spared the added toxicity that often is associated with more aggressive experimental therapy. On the other hand, those with a high-intermediate or high-risk IPI, in whom a CR is unlikely with conventional therapy, should be identified as candidates for more aggressive treatment. When patients on the National High Priority Lymphoma Study are divided into these four risk groups and each risk group is analyzed for time to treatment failure and overall survival, there is no significant difference between the curves for any of the combination chemotherapy regimens in any of the risk groups.

Seventy-five patients with poor risk aggressive lymphoma were randomized to treatment with MACOP-B or with a novel high-

TABLE 103-7 COMBINATION CHEMOTHERAPY FOR INTERMEDIATE- AND HIGH-GRADE LYMPHOMA

CHOP—See Table 6

COP-BLAM

Cylophosphamide	400 mg/m²	IV	1	21
Doxorubicin	40 mg/m²	IV	1	
Vincristine	1 mg/m²	IV	1	
Procarbazine	100 mg/m²	PO	1–10	
Prednisone	40 mg/m²	PO	1–10	
Bleomycin	15 mg/m²	IV	14	

ProMACE/CytaBOM

Cyclophosphamide	650 mg/m²	IV	1	21
Doxorubicin	25 mg/m²	IV	1	
Etoposide	120 mg/m²	IV	1	
Cytarabine	300 mg/m²	IV	8	
Bleomycin	5 mg/m²	IV	8	
Vincristine	1.4 mg/m²	IV	8	
Methotrexate	120 mg/m²	IV	8	
Leucovorin	25 mg/m²	PO	9 (q 6 h × 4)	
Prednisone	60 mg/m	PO	1–14	
Cotrimoxazole	2 PO bid			

MACOP-B

Methotrexate	400 mg/m²	IV	8, 36, 64	one-12 week cycle
Leucovorin	15 mg/m²	PO (q 6 h × 6)	9, 37, 65	
Doxorubicin	50 mg/m²	IV	1, 15, 29, 43, 57, 71	
Vincristine	1.4 mg/m²	IV	8, 22, 36, 50, 64, 78	
Bleomycin	10 mg/m²	IV	22, 50, 78	
Prednisone	75 mg/m²	PO	1–84 (tapered over days 70–84)	
Cotrimoxazole	2 PO bid			

m-BACOB

Methotrexate	200 mg/m²	IV	8, 15	21
Leucovorin	10 mg/m²	PO (q 6 h × 6)	9, 16	
Bleomycin	4 mg/m²	IV	1	
Doxorubicin	45 mg/m²	IV	1	
Cyclophosphamide	600 mg/m²	IV	1	
Vincristine	1 mg/m²	IV	1	
Dexamethasone	6 mg/m²	PO	1–5	

ESHAP (for relapsed lymphoma)

Etoposide	40 mg/m²	IV/2 h	1–4	21
Methylprednisone	500 mg/m²	IV	1–4	
Cytarabine	2 mg/m²	IV/3 h	5	
Cisplatin	25 mg/m²	CIV	1–4	

DHAP (for relapsed lymphoma)

Dexamethasone	40 mg/m²	PO or IV	1–4	21
Cisplatin	100 mg/m²	CIV	1	
Cytarabine	2 mg/m²	IV/q 12 h × 2	2	

dose chemotherapy regimen requiring hematopoietic progenitor cell autotransplantation.[247] The toxic death rate on the high-dose arm of the study was initially high (16 percent) but has decreased with modification of the treatment regimen. Thirty-eight patients were randomized to the high-dose therapy, and 37 patients were randomized to MACOP-B. After a median follow-up of 43 months there is a statistically significant improvement in relapse-free survival (93 percent versus 68 percent, $P = 0.05$) and freedom from progression (88 percent versus 41 percent, $P = 0.0001$) in favor of the high-dose therapy arm. Overall survival was not statistically improved, however, with 73 percent on the high-dose arm versus 62 percent on the MACOP-B arm.

The Groupe d'Etudes des Lymphomes des l'Adulte (GELA) randomized 464 patients who were induced with anthracycline-containing regimens to autotransplant versus sequential chemotherapy. With a median follow-up of 28 months, the 3-year disease-free survival rate was 52 percent in the autotransplant arm ($P = 0.46$). The 3-year survival did not differ between the two arms. This trial was instituted before the publication of the IPI. Therefore, patients were not stratified by IPI as important prognostic factors. A subsequent retrospective analysis did reveal a relapse-free and overall survival benefit for the patients who were reclassified as having the high-intermediate and high-risk characteristics according to the IPI.[249] Prospective randomized trials will be required to determine whether this subset of patients truly benefits from high-dose therapy.

Support for the concept that high-dose therapy after standard induction chemotherapy may be beneficial only for the high-intermediate and high-risk IPI groups has been provided.[250] Patients were randomized to receive either standard VACOP-B chemotherapy or VACOP-B followed by autologous marrow transplantation. While there was no difference in the disease-free survival (DFS) or progression-free survival (PFS) for the entire group of 124 patients, there was a statistical improvement in DFS ($P = 0.008$) and a favorable trend in PFS ($P = 0.08$) for the high-intermediate and high-risk IPI groups assigned to high-dose therapy.

Based on the previously described data, the lymphoma committees and the marrow transplant committees of SWOG, ECOG, and CALGB (Cancer and Acute Leukemia Group B) have agreed to jointly conduct a randomized clinical trial of early versus delayed high-dose therapy for patients with high-intermediate and high-risk large-cell lymphoma. Patients under the age of 65 years will each receive five cycles of CHOP; responding patients will then be randomized to receive either three more cycles of CHOP, or one additional cycle of CHOP followed by high-dose therapy with autologous stem-cell rescue. Patients on the standard CHOP treatment who relapse will then receive the same high-dose therapy. If this study confirms the benefit of high-dose therapy in this patient group, subsequent trials will attempt to increase the number of responding patients who become eligible for high-dose therapy.

Relapsed or Refractory Aggressive Lymphomas   Patients who develop progressive disease during initial therapy or who relapse following the completion of therapy have historically had a very poor prognosis. Retreatment with any of the front-line chemotherapy programs is not associated with a long-term benefit. Salvage regimens such as ESHAP (etoposide, methylprednisolone, cytarabine, cisplatin), DHAP (dexamethasone, high-dose cytarabine and cisplatin), and MIME (methyl-GAG, ifosfamide, methotrexate and etoposide) may provide long-term disease-free survival in approximately 20 to 40 percent of patients who are eligible for transplantation.[251,252] The role of high-dose therapy with stem-cell rescue has been provided by the results of the Parma trial.[253] Relapsed patients under the age of 60 years were first treated with two courses of conventional salvage chemotherapy; patients responding with a CR or PR were considered to be chemosensitive and were then randomized to receive involved-field radiotherapy and high-dose BEAC chemotherapy versus DHAP chemotherapy for 6 additional months followed by involved-field radiotherapy. The event-free survival (EFS) of patients randomized to high-dose therapy was 46 percent compared to 12 percent for patients continuing to receive salvage chemotherapy ($P = 0.001$) OS also was superior in the high-dose therapy group ($P = 0.038$). Thus all relapsed patients with aggressive lymphoma should be evaluated for eligibility for high-dose therapy. Patients not eligible because of age or medical factors should receive one of the previously described salvage regimens.

Treatment of the Elderly Patient   As noted, age is an important prognostic factor. The poorer survival of aged patients is secondary, in part, to their increased tendency to experience treatment-related toxicity. Efforts to reduce the amount of chemotherapy given to elderly patients to avoid such toxicities have resulted in fewer initial responses and poorer survival. Because of this, treatment regimens designed specifically for the elderly have been developed. In any case, the ability of elderly patients to tolerate combination chemotherapy is based on their physiologic and not chronologic age.[254] Palliative therapy should be considered for appropriate patients who cannot tolerate combination drug chemotherapy.

DIFFUSE LARGE B-CELL LYMPHOMA

Under the Working Formulation this was diffuse large cell cleaved, noncleaved, immunoblastic, or diffuse mixed small and large cell. The predominant cell represents either a large noncleaved cell or an immunoblast, or a mixture of both cell types.[10] Other cell types include large cleaved or multilobated cells and anaplastic large cells. In some cases there may be a predominance of small T lymphocytes or histiocytes resembling either a T-cell lymphoma or Hodgkin disease of the lymphocyte predominant variety.[10,227–229] The REAL classification suggests that with current technology, this tumor should not be subclassified but rather designated *large B-cell lymphoma*, and future studies should focus on identifying clinically relevant subtypes.[10] All cases express classic B-cell-associated antigens CD19, CD20, and CD22, with or without surface immunoglobulin, and typically do not express CD5 or CD10. *BCL-2* is rearranged in approximately 30 percent of cases, and C-MYC is rearranged in a minority of cases.

Large B-cell lymphomas represent approximately 40 percent of adult lymphomas with a median age of 60 years. Patients typically present with an enlarging mass at a single nodal or extranodal site, and 40 percent of the cases present with extranodal involvement. It is a very aggressive disease, but is potentially curable with anthracycline-based therapy. Chemotherapeutic regimens routinely used for diffuse large-cell lymphoma are not adequate. Effective regimens include prophylactic therapy of the CNS and are similar to those developed to treat patients with acute lymphoblastic leukemia.

LARGE B-CELL LYMPHOMA SUBTYPE: PRIMARY MEDIASTINAL (THYMIC) LARGE B-CELL LYMPHOMA

The treatment goal for all patients with diffuse large B-cell lymphoma is cure, which can be accomplished for approximately half of all patients. While it was previously thought that the complete remission rate would invariably reflect the number of cured patients, recent studies in advanced stage patients have demonstrated that this is not universally correct.[236,237] Thus failure-free survival and overall survival have become the most meaningful endpoints in determining the results of new therapies. The selection of a patient's therapy should be based primarily on the clinical stage, rather than the histologic subtype. As described later, patients with early-stage disease, defined as stage I or II (nonbulky), have a much better prognosis than patients with advanced-stage disease, defined as stage II (bulky), stage III, or stage IV. These conclusions are based on studies of patients with the most common high-grade lymphoma, namely diffuse large-cell lymphoma (malignant lymphoma, diffuse, large-cell, or immunoblastic in the Working Formulation). Since the clinical behavior of most other intermediate- and high-grade lymphomas appears similar to that of diffuse large-cell lymphoma and since these histologic subtypes are difficult to categorize reproducibly, most studies have treated all patients with intermediate- or high-grade lymphomas in a similar manner.

Diffuse large-cell lymphomas have been referred to as the *aggressive* lymphomas to distinguish them from the indolent or low-grade histologies. The new REAL classification, in fact, groups all of these B-cell aggressive lymphomas into one category, termed *diffuse large B-cell lymphoma*.[10] Patients with lymphoblastic lymphoma or Burkitt lymphoma are exceptions to this and will be discussed separately.

MANTLE ZONE CELL LYMPHOMA

The disease course is aggressive and there is no known curative therapies. Median survival is 3 to 5 years. The blastoid variant is more aggressive. The overall response rate of 524 patients with mantle zone cell lymphoma treated on 12 trials with conventional chemotherapy was 84 percent, with 46 percent achieving objective complete responses.[269] The median progression-free survival was 20 months in these patients, and the median overall survival was 36 months. There has been no convincing evidence from any of these studies to suggest that any conventional chemotherapy regimen is curative. Hence, consideration of innovative treatment protocols appear warranted. Since prospective, randomized clinical trials will be necessary to define optimal treatment strategies for mantle zone cell lymphoma, patients should be encouraged to participate in cooperative group protocols whenever possible. Off protocol, it seems reasonable to individualize therapy. Patients presenting with slowly progressive disease (especially those with the mantle zone variant) might be managed using oral chlorambucil, cyclophosphamide, or CVP. Patients who are markedly symptomatic or who have rapidly progressive disease are probably best treated with CHOP, if they are not eligible for cooperative group protocols.

B-CELL LINEAGE VERY AGGRESSIVE LYMPHOMA (HIGH RISK)

The small noncleaved cell malignant lymphomas include Burkitt and non-Burkitt lymphoma. Even though these two entities cannot be easily separated by expert hematopathologists, patients with non-Burkitt lymphomas traditionally have been treated with chemotherapy similar to that used for patients with the diffuse large-cell lymphomas. Burkitt lymphoma is an aggressive, rapidly dividing malignant lymphoma, most commonly seen in children. The tumor is highly aggressive but potentially curable. Prognosis, particularly in children, correlates inversely with bulky disease at the time of diagnosis.[278] The staging evaluation should be considered a medical emergency, and the patient should receive chemotherapy within 48 to 72 h after establishing the diagnosis. These lymphomas are exquisitely sensitive to chemotherapy.[279,280] Therefore, treated patients are at high risk for developing the rapid-tumor-lysis syndrome unless they are concomitantly treated with allopurinol and forced alkaline diuresis. Frequent monitoring of electrolytes and renal function are recommended during therapy. Successful treatment regimens use high dose of cyclophosphamide, moderate to high doses of methotrexate, and CNS prophylaxis.

T-CELL LINEAGE INDOLENT LYMPHOMAS (LOW RISK)

MYCOSIS FUNGOIDS/SÉZARY SYNDROME

Four therapeutic modalities produce remissions in most patients with cutaneous T-cell lymphoma: topical nitrogen mustard, photochemotherapy with psoralen and ultraviolet A light (PUVA), systemic chemotherapy, and radiation therapy (particularly total-body electron beam therapy). Each induces remission, but cure is uncommon and possible only in early disease.

Topical Nitrogen Mustard Topical nitrogen mustard is used predominantly in patients with early cutaneous stages of disease. In more advanced stages, this approach is used to supplement other therapies. The major advantage of topical therapy is that it is relatively nontoxic. Disadvantages include the inconvenience of daily application to large areas of skin, the allergic reactions in up to half of cases,[313] the potential for development of skin cancer,[314] and the inability to cure the disease. Nitrogen mustard (10 mg diluted to 60 ml of tap water or 60 g of a water-miscible cream or an anhydrous ointment, which may have less allergic sensitization) is administered daily using a cotton swab or small pain brush. Therapy is continued for up to 12 months in responders. Frequency is then reduced to every other day for an additional 1 to 2 years. Therapy is discontinued after 3 years or when cutaneous lesions disappear completely.

Psoralen Psoralen is a phototoxic furocoumarin activated by ultraviolet A light. In its active form, it bonds covalently and irreversibly to DNA. Ultraviolet A light penetrates only the upper part of the dermis. Therefore, psoralen activated by ultraviolet A light affects cells primarily in the epidermis and papillary dermis. A 60 percent complete remission rate has been reported with psoralen; patients with generalized erythroderma and tumors have lower response rates than those with plagues.[315–317] Psoralen is usually given at a dose of 0.6 mg/kg orally, 2 h before the ultraviolet A light therapy. Treatments are initially given three times weekly. Maintenance therapy may be given every 2 to 4 weeks indefinitely. Adverse effects of PUVA therapy include mild nausea, pruritus, and sunburnlike changes with atrophy and dry skin. PUVA is not cross-resistant with other treatment modalities. Disadvantages of this therapy are its inability to cure and its expense. Long-term side effects are not yet reported.

Chemotherapy The largest experience with single-agent chemotherapy is with alkylating agents, including nitrogen mustard, 0.4 mg/kg intravenously every 4 to 6 weeks; cyclophosphamide; and chlorambucil. Response rates of 60 percent, with 15 percent complete remissions, have been reported.[292,321–324] Similar results occur with methotrexate, 2.5 to 10 mg/day by mouth; bleomycin, 7.5 to 15 mg intramuscularly twice weekly; and doxorubicin, 60 mg/m^2 once monthly.[292,325–331] Single-agent therapy does not cure cutaneous T-cell lymphoma. Combination therapy with these and other drugs produces objective responses in more than 80 percent of patients and complete responses in about one-fourth of cases.[292,332,333] Duration of remission varies, with a median of about 1 year; no long-term disease-free survival has been reported.

Electron Beam Therapy Electron beam therapy penetrates only into the upper dermis, and there are minimal systemic effects and an 80 percent complete remission rate.[318–320] Twenty percent of patients remain relapse-free at 3 years. Typically, treatment is 4 Gy per week to a total dose of 36 Gy in 8 to 9 weeks. The advantage of electron beam therapy is a high frequency of durable complete responses without systemic toxicity. Disadvantages are alopecia, atrophy, edema, dermatitis, and high cost.

Combined Modality Therapy Randomized trials with wholebody electron beam therapy as a single modality compared with electron beam therapy followed by topical nitrogen mustard suggest a benefit of combined therapy.[334] Studies of electron beam therapy combined with chemotherapy suggest no advantage over either alone,[335] although combined modality therapy produced disease-free survival in some patients with early-stage disease; those with advanced disease failed to benefit. A report on patients randomized either to early intensive therapy with cyclophosphamide, doxorubicin, vincristine, and etoposide combined with either topical nitrogen mustard or 30

Gy of electron beam radiation therapy or to topical or radiation therapy only showed no difference.[336]

Investigational Therapy   Many therapeutic approaches to cutaneous T-cell lymphoma are being evaluated. One study reported a 50 percent response with high-dose interferon-α.[337] In another study, three of four patients receiving 13 cis-retinoic acid improved.[338] Some investigators claimed success using leukapheresis to treat patients with cutaneous T-cell lymphoma.[339] In other studies,[340] subjects received oral psoralen followed by leukapheresis. The lymphocyte-enriched blood fraction was exposed to ultraviolet A light and returned. This approach decreased lymphocyte viability by 90 percent. Twenty-seven of 37 patients with otherwise resistant cutaneous T-cell lymphoma responded to the treatment. Treatment of four patients with advanced cutaneous T-cell lymphoma with pentostatin resulted in two complete and two partial responses.[341] A response rate of 30 percent has been reported for cladrabine.[342,343] Finally, therapy with monoclonal antibodies was also studied. Unlabeled monoclonal antibodies had only a minimal transient effect,[344] while ^{131}I-labeled monoclonal antibody produced more prolonged and consistent responses.[345]

Prognosis   Median survival after histologic diagnosis of cutaneous T-cell lymphoma is about 10 years. However, lymph node involvement is associated with a poorer prognosis than disease limited to the skin.[292,293] Patients with cutaneous T-cell lymphoma with visceral involvement that includes liver, spleen, pleura, and lung have the poorest prognosis. Such patients have a median survival of less than 1 year.

Fifty percent of deaths of patients with cutaneous T-cell lymphoma result from infections. These are usually staphylococcus- and pseudomonas-related and develop from cutaneous lesions.[292] Septicemia and bacterial pneumonia are common. Herpes infections occur in up to 10 percent of patients with advanced cutaneous T-cell lymphoma. Visceral involvement does not appear until late in the course of the disease. Progressive cutaneous T-cell lymphoma with widespread visceral involvement is the next most common cause of death.

T-CELL LINEAGE AGGRESSIVE LYMPHOMAS (INTERMEDIATE RISK)

Patients with adult T-cell leukemia/lymphoma treated with combination chemotherapy are usually treated using a regimen that includes doxorubicin, such as CHOP. Complete and partial responses are attained in most patients. However, most patients relapse within 6 to 12 months, and cures are not reported. Encouraging responses have been observed in patients who received passive immunotherapy or radioimmunotherapy using monoclonal antibodies specific for antigens expressed by the neoplastic T cells, such as CD25.[413,414] Other biological agents, such as interferon-α, have had modest effects.[415,416] Therapy with the nucleoside pentostatin may benefit some patients with this disease.[417] Responses to combination therapy with interferon-α and zidovudine have been reported.[418,419]

Patients with the smoldering type of adult T-cell leukemia/lymphoma have an indolent course, if they do not succumb to opportunistic infections.[385,420] They typically have a long survival without therapy and without hypercalcemia. Skin lesions are characteristic and occur as erythema, papules, or nodules. The proportion of adult T-cell leukemia/lymphoma cells in the blood is low (less than 5 percent), with minimal lymphadenopathy, hepatosplenomegaly, and marrow infiltration. One patient developed aggressive adult T-cell leukemia/lymphoma after more than 5 years of illness and another after 13 years. Patients with smoldering adult T-cell leukemia/lymphoma are more likely to have a normal karyotype.

In one study, 28 patients with angioimmunoblastic lymphadenopathy-like lymphoma were treated with either prednisone or prednisone with combination chemotherapy including cyclophosphamide, doxorubicin, bleomycin, vincristine, procarbazine, ifosfamide, methotrexate, etoposide, and mesna.[366] Complete remissions were more common in the chemotherapy arm of the protocol, but there was no significant difference in survival. Others have reported responses and long complete remissions in patients treated with combination chemotherapy.[367] Based on these results, combination chemotherapy with a CHOP-like regimen would be a reasonable first choice for therapy for patients with angioimmunoblastic lymphadenopathy-like lymphoma. Prednisone may be considered for elderly patients with a more indolent disease. Mean survival is 30 months; infection is the most common cause of death.

EXTRANODAL DISEASE

GASTRIC LYMPHOMA

There may be a role for surgery in patients with gastric lymphoma.[94–97] Patients who present with a major hemorrhage or perforation will require partial gastrectomy in addition to chemotherapy and radiation therapy. Patients with stage I and II diffuse B-cell large-cell lymphoma can be treated with upper abdominal radiation after three cycles of chemotherapy. Those with B symptoms, bulky disease, or stage III or IV disease will require a full course of chemotherapy with radiation reserved for residual disease following chemotherapy.

TESTICULAR LYMPHOMA

Definitive therapy of testicular lymphoma depends on the stage of disease. If the patient receives systemic chemotherapy, the risk of relapse in the opposite testicle is 25 percent.[98–100] The addition of 25 Gy of radiation eliminates this risk.[84] CNS involvement is unusual as an isolated site of relapse for patients who present with primary disease of the testicle. However, for patients with systemic lymphoma, with the testicle as a site of disease, prophylactic CNS intrathecal chemotherapy is recommended.

REFERENCES

1. Oberling C: Les Reticulosarcomes et les reticuloendotheliosarcomes de la moelle ossue se (sarcomes d'Ewing). *Bull Assoc Fr Etude Cancer* 17:259, 1928.
2. Roulet F: Das primare Retothelsarkom der Lymphknoten. *Virchows Arch (Pathol Anat)* 277:15, 1930.
3. Ewing J: Endothlioma of lymph nodes. *J Med Res* 28:1, 1913.
4. Brill NE, Baehr G, Rosenthal N: Generalized giant lymph follicle hyperplasia of lymph nodes and spleen: a hitherto undescribed type. *JAMA* 84:668, 1925.
5. Symmers D: Follicular lymphadenopathy with splenomegaly: a newly recognized disease of the lymphatic system. *Arch Pathol Lab Med* 3:816, 1927.
6. Rappaport H: Tumors of the hematopoietic system, in *Atlas of Tumor Pathology*, sec 3, fasc 8, Washington, DC, 1966, US Armed Forces Institute of Pathology.
7. Lukes RJ, Craver LF, Hall TC, Rappaport H, Ruben P: Report of the nomenclature committee. *Cancer Res* 26:1311, 1966.
8. Lennert K, Mohri N, Stein H, Kaiserling E: The histopathology of malignant lymphoma. *Br J Haematol* 31(suppl): 193, 1975.
9. The Non-Hodgkin's Lymphoma Pathologic Classification Project: National Cancer Institute sponsored study of classifications of non-Hodgkin's lymphomas: summary and description of a Working Formulation for clinical usage. *Cancer* 49:2112, 1982.
10. Harris NL, Jaffe ES, Stein H, et al: A revised European-American classification of lymphoid neoplasms: a proposal from the International Lymphoma Study Group. *Blood* 84:1361, 1994.
11. Hiddemann W, Longo DL, Coiffier B, et al: Lymphoma classification—the gap between biology and clinical management is closing. *Blood* 88:4085, 1996.

12. Landis SH, Murray T, Bolden S, Wingo PA: Cancer Statistics, 1998. *Cancer* 48:6, 1998.

13. Ng CS, Chan JKC, Lo STH, et al: Immunophenotypic analysis of Hodgkin's lymphomas in Chinese. A study of 75 cases in Hong Kong. *Pathology* 18:419, 1986.

14. Kadin ME, Bernard CW, Nanba K, Wakasa H: Lymphoproliferative diseases in Japan and Western countries: proceedings of United States-Japan seminar. *Hum Pathol* 14:745, 1983.

15. Cutler SJ, Young JL: Third national cancer survey: incidence data. *Natl Cancer Inst Monogr* 40(6):1, 1975.

16. Shih L-Y, Liang D-C: Non-Hodgkin's lymphoma in Asia. *Hematol Oncol Clin North Am* 5:983, 1991.

17. Olin GR: The hazards of chemical laboratory environment: a study of the mortality in two cohorts of Swedish chemists. *Am Ind Hyg Assoc J* 39:557, 1978.

18. Wong O: An industry wide mortality study of chemical workers occupationally exposed to benzene: II. Dose response analyses. *Br J Indust Med* 44:382, 1987.

19. Woods JS, Polissar L, Severson RK, et al: Soft tissue sarcoma and non-Hodgkin's lymphoma in relation to phenoxyherbicide and chlorinated phenol exposure in Western Washington. *J Natl Cancer Inst* 78:899, 1987.

20. Pearce NE, Sheppard RA, Smith AH, et al: Non-Hodgkin's lymphoma and farming: An expanded case-control study. *Int J Cancer* 39:155, 1987.

21. Morrison HI, Wilkins K, Semenel WR, et al: Herbicides and cancer. *J Natl Cancer Inst* 84:1866, 1992.

22. Levin PH, Hoover RN: The emerging epidemic of non-Hodgkin's lymphoma: current knowledge regarding etiologic factors. *Cancer Res* 52:54325, 1992.

23. Li FP, Fraumeni JR Jr, Mantel N, et al: Cancer mortality among chemists. *JNCI* 43:1159, 1969.

24. Axelson O, Dahlgren E, Jansson CD, et al: Arsenic exposure and mortality: a case-referent study from a Swedish copper smelter. *Br J Ind Med* 35:8, 1978.

25. Ross R, Dworsky R, Nichols P, et al: Asbestos exposure and lymphomas of the gastrointestinal tract and oral cavity. *Lancet* 2:1118, 1982.

26. Cantor KP: Farming and mortality from non-Hodgkin's lymphoma: a case-control study. *Int J Cancer* 29:239, 1982.

27. Dalager NA, Kang HK, Burt VL, Weatherbee L: Non-Hodgkin's lymphomas among Vietnam veterans. *J Occup Med* 33:774, 1991.

28. Beebe GW, Kato H, Land C: Studies of the mortality of A-bomb survivors. Mortality and radiation dose. 1950–1974. *Radiat Res* 75:138, 1978.

29. Anderson RE, Nishiyama H, Yohei I, et al: Pathogenesis of radiation related leukemia and lymphoma. Speculations based primarily on experience of Hiroshima and Nagasaki. *Lancet* 1:1060, 1972.

30. Miller RW: Delayed radiation effects in atomic bomb survivors. *Science* 166:569, 1969.

31. Court-Brown WM, Doll R: Leukemia and aplastic anemia in patients irradiated for ankylosing spondylitis. Medical Research Council Special Report Series, No. 295 London: Her Majesty's Stationery Office, 1957.

32. Epstein MA, Achang BG, Barr YH: Virus particles in cultured lymphoblasts from Burkitt's lymphoma. *Lancet* 1:702, 1964.

33. Nemerow GR, Wolfert R, McNaughton ME, Cooper NR: Identification and characterization of the Epstein-Barr virus receptor on human B-lymphocytes and its relation to the C3d complement receptor (CR2). *J Virol* 55:347, 1985.

34. Henle W, Diehl V, Kohn G, et al: Herpes-type virus and chromosome marker in normal leucocytes after growth with irradiated Burkitt cells. *Science* 157:1064, 1967.

35. Anderson M, Klein G, Ziegler J, Henle W: Association of Epstein-Barr viral genomes with American Burkitt lymphoma. *Nature* 260:357, 1976.

36. Potter M, Mushinski JF: Oncogenes in B neoplasia. *Cancer Invest* 2:285, 1984.

37. Morrow RH Jr: Epidemiological evidence for the role of falciparum malaria in the pathogenesis of Burkitt's lymphoma, in *Burkitt's Lymphoma: A Human Cancer Model*, edited by Lenoir G, O'Conor T, Olweny CLM, p 177. ARC Scientific, Lyon, France, 1985.

38. Klein G: Lymphoma development in mice and humans: diversity of initiation is followed by convergent cytogenetic evolution. *Proc Natl Acad Sci USA* 76:2442, 1979.

39. Klein G: Specific chromosomal translocations and the genesis of B-cell-derived tumors in mice and men. *Cell* 19:311, 1983.

40. Penn I: The incidence of malignancies in transplant recipients. *Transplant Proc* 7:323, 1975.

41. Matas AJ, Hertel BJ, Rosai J, et al: Post-transplant malignant lymphoma. Distinctive morphologic features related to its pathogenesis. *Am J Med* 61:716, 1976.

42. Penn I: Cancers complicating organ transplantation. *N Engl J Med* 23:1767, 1990.

43. Swinnen IJ, Costanzo-Nordin MR, Fisher SG, et al: Increased incidence of lymphoproliferative disorder after immunosuppression with the monoclonal antibody OKT3 in cardiac-transplant receipts. *N Engl J Med* 323:1723, 1990.

44. Robinson JE, Brown N, Andiman W: Diffuse polyclonal B-cell lymphoma during primary infection with Epstein-Barr virus. *N Engl J Med* 302:1293, 1980.

45. Purtilo DT, Klein G: Introduction to Epstein-Barr virus and lymphoproliferative diseases in immunodeficient individuals. *Cancer Res* 41:4209, 1981.

46. Sullivan JL: Epstein-Barr virus and lymphoproliferative disorders. *Semin Hematol* 25:269, 1988.

47. Purtilo DT, Cassel CK, Yang JPS, Harper R: X-linked recessive progressive combined variable immunodeficiency (Duncan's disease). *Lancet* 1:935, 1975.

48. Fudenberg HH: Are autoimmune diseases immunologic deficiency states? *Hosp Pract* 3:43, 1968.

49. Polesz BJ, Ruscetti FW, Gazdar AF, et al: Detection and isolation of type C retrovirus particles from fresh and cultured lymphocytes of a patient with cutaneous T-cell lymphoma. *Proc Natl Acad Sci USA* 77:7415, 1980.

50. Jacobson S, Raine CS, Mingioli ES, et al: Isolation of an HTLV-V-I-like retrovirus from patients with tropical spastic paraparesis. *Nature* 331:540, 1988.

51. Snoda S: Relationship of HTLV-I-related adult T-cell leukemia and HTLV-I-associated myelopathy to distinct HLA haplotypes. *Jikken Igaku* 5:769, 1987.

52. Carbone PP: Report on the committee on Hodgkin's Disease Staging Classification. *Cancer Res* 31:1860, 1971.

53. Cabanillas F, Burke JS, Smith TL, et al: Factors predicting for response and survival in adults with advanced non-Hodgkin's lymphoma. *Arch Intern Med* 138:413, 1978.

54. Jones SE, Fuks Z, Bull M, et al: Non-Hodgkin's lymphomas: IV. Clinicopathologic correlation in 405 cases. *Cancer* 31:806, 1973.

55. Dixon DO, Neilan B, Jones JE, et al: Effect of age on therapeutic outcome in advanced diffuse histiocytic lymphoma: the Southwest Oncology Group experience. *J Clin Oncol* 4:295, 1986.

56. Todd MB, Portlock CS, Farber LR, et al: Prognostic indicators in diffuse large cell (histiocytic) lymphoma. *J Radiat Oncol Biol Phys* 12:593, 1986.

57. Vose JM, Armitage JO, Weisenberger DD, et al: The importance of age in survival of patients treated with chemotherapy for aggressive non-Hodgkin's lymphoma. *J Clin Oncol* 6:1838, 1988.

58. Armitage JO, Potter JF: Aggressive chemotherapy for diffuse histiocytic lymphoma in the elderly: increased complications with advancing age. *J Am Geriatr Soc* 32:269, 1984.

59. Jagannath S, Velasquez WS, Tucker SL, et al: Tumor burden assessment and its implication for a prognostic model in advanced diffuse large cell lymphoma. *J Clin Oncol* 4:859, 1986.

60. Shipp MA, Harrington DP, Klatt MM, et al: Identification of major prognostic subgroups of patients with large cell lymphoma treated with m-BACOD or M-BACOD. *Ann Intern Med* 104:757, 1986.

61. Fisher RI, DeVita VT, Johnson BL, et al: Prognostic factors for advanced diffuse histiocytic lymphoma following treatment with combination chemotherapy. *Am J Med* 63:177, 1977.

62. Ferraris AA, Giuntini P, Gaetani GF: Serum lactic dehydrogenase as a prognostic tool for non-Hodgkin's lymphomas. *Blood* 54:928, 1979.

63. Coiffier B, Berger F, Bryon PA, et al: T-cell lymphoma, immunologic, histologic, clinical and therapeutic analysis of 63 cases. *J Clin Oncol* 6:1584, 1988.

64. Armitage JO, Vose JM, Linder J, et al: Clinical significance of immunophenotyping in diffuse aggressive non-Hodgkin's lymphoma. *J Clin Oncol* 7:1783, 1989.

65. Horning SJ, Weiss CM, Crabtree CG, Warnke RA: Clinical and phenotypic diversity of T-cell lymphomas. *Blood* 67:1578, 1986.

66. Grogan TM, Lippman SM, Spier CM, et al: Independent prognostic significance of a nuclear proliferation antigen in diffuse large cell lymphomas as determined by the monoclonal antibody Ki-67. *Blood* 71:1157, 1988.

67. Levine EG, Arthur DC, Frizzera G, et al: Cytogenetic abnormalities predict clinical outcome in non-Hodgkin's lymphoma. *Ann Intern Med* 108:14, 1988.

68. The International non-Hodgkin's Lymphoma Prognostic Factors Project: A predictive model for aggressive non-Hodgkin's lymphoma. *N Engl J Med* 329:987, 1993.

69. A clinical evaluation of the International lymphoma study group classification of non-Hodgkin's lymphoma. The non-Hodgkin's lymphoma classification project. *Blood* 11:3909, 1997.

70. Herman TS, Hammond N, Jones SE, et al: Involvement of the central nervous system by non-Hodgkin's lymphoma: The Southwest Oncology Group experience. *Cancer* 43:390, 1979.

71. Recht L, Straus DJ, Cirrincione C, et al: Central nervous system metastases from non-Hodgkin's lymphoma: treatment and prophylaxis. *Am J Med* 84:425, 1988.

72. Mackintosh FR, Colby TV, Podosky WJ, et al: Central nervous system involvement in non-Hodgkin's lymphoma: an analysis of 105 cases. *Cancer* 49:586, 1982.

73. Woolley PV, Osborne CK, Levi JA, et al: Extranodal presentation of non-Hodgkin's lymphomas in the testis. *Cancer* 38:1026, 1976.

74. Martenson JA Jr, Buskirk SJ, Illstrup DM, et al: Patterns of failure in primary testicular non-Hodgkin's lymphoma. *J Clin Oncol* 6:297, 1988.

75. Frierson HF, Mills SE, Innes DJ: Non-Hodgkin's lymphomas of the sinonasal region: Histologic subtypes and their clinicopatholic features. *Am J Clin Pathol* 81:721, 1984.

76. Bonnie JM, Garcia JH: Primary malignant non-Hodgkin's lymphoma of the central nervous system. *Pathol Ann* 22:353, 1987.

77. Pollack IF, Lunsford LD, Flickinger JC, et al: Prognostic factors in the diagnosis and treatment of primary central nervous system lymphomas. *Cancer* 63:939, 1989.

78. Epelbaum R, Haim N, Ben-Shahar M, et al: Non-Hodgkin's lymphoma presenting with spinal epidural involvement. *Cancer* 58:2120, 1986.

79. Richardson EP Jr: Progressive multifocal leukoencephalopathy 30 years later. *N Engl J Med* 318:315, 1988.

80. Henson RA, Urich H: *Cancer and the Nervous System.* Blackwell, Oxford, 1982.

81. Conners JM. Problems in lymphoma management: special sites of presentation. *Oncology* 12:188, 1998.

82. Esik O, Ikeda H, Mukai K, Kaneko A: A retrospective analysis of different modalities for treatment of primary orbital non-Hodgkin's lymphomas. *Radiother Oncol* 38:13, 1996.

83. Whitecup SM, de Smet MD, Rubin BI, et al: Intraocular lymphoma: clinical and histopathologic diagnosis. *Ophthalmology* 100:1399, 1993.

84. Abbondanzo SL, Wenig BM: Non-Hodgkin's lymphoma of the sinonasal tract: a clinicopathologic and immunophenotypic study of 120 cases. *Cancer* 75:1281, 1995.

85. Wood GS, Burke JS, Horning S, Doggett RS, Levy R, Warnke RA: The immunologic and clincopathologic heterogeneity of cutaneous lymphomas other than mycosis fungoides. *Blood* 62:464, 1983.

86. Willemze R, Meijer CJLM, Scheffer E, et al: Diffuse large cell lymphomas of follicular center cell origin presenting in the skin: a clinicopathologic and immunologic study of 16 patients. *Am J Pathol* 126:325, 1987.

87. Manoharan A, Pitney WR, Schonnel ME, Bader LV: Intrathoracic manifestations in non-Hodgkin's lymphoma. *Thorax* 34:29, 1979.

88. Kennedy JL, Nasthwani BN, Burke JS, Hill LR, Rappaport H: Pulmonary lymphomas and other pulmonary lymphoid lesions: a clincopathologic and immunologic study of 64 patients. *Cancer* 56:539, 1985.

89. Solidoro A, Salazar F, Flor J, Sanchez J, Otero J: Endoscopic tissue diagnosis of gastric involvement in the staging of non-Hodgkin's lymphoma. *Cancer* 48:1053, 1981.

90. Kim H, Dorfman RF: Morphological studies of 84 untreated patients subjected to laparotomy for the staging of non-Hodgkin's lymphomas. *Cancer* 33:657, 1974.

91. List AF, Greer JP, Cousar JC, et al: Non-Hodgkin's lymphomas of the gastrointestinal tract: an analysis of clinical and pathologic features affecting outcome. *J Clin Oncol* 6:1125, 1988.

92. Haber DA, Mayer RJ: Primary gastrointestinal lymphoma. *Semin Oncol* 15:154, 1988.

93. Lewin KJ, Ranchod M, Dorfman RF: Lymphomas of the gastrointestinal tract. *Cancer* 42:693, 1978.

94. Shchepotin IB, Evans SR, Shabahang M, et al: Primary non-Hodgkin's lymphoma of the stomach: three radical modalities of treatment in 75 patients. *Ann Surg Oncol* 3:277, 1996.

95. Rabbi C, Aitini E, Cavazzini G, et al: Stomach preservation in low-and high-grade primary gastric lymphomas: preliminary results. *Haematologica* 81:15, 1996.

96. Ernst M, Stein H, Ludwig D, Boese-Landgraf J, Ritz J, Haring R: Surgical therapy of gastrointestinal non-Hodgkin's lymphomas. *Eur J Surg Oncol* 22:177, 1996.

97. Haim N, Leviov M, Ben-Arieh Y, et al: Intermediate and high-grade gastric non-Hodgkin's lymphoma: a prospective study of non-surgical treatment with primary chemotherapy, with or without radiotherapy. *Leuk Lymphoma* 17:321, 1995.

98. Connors JM, Klimo P, Voss N, Fairey RN, Jackson S: Testicular lymphoma: improved outcome with early brief chemotherapy. *J Clin Oncol* 6:776, 1988.

99. Doll DC, Weiss RB: Malignant lymphoma of the testis. *Am J Med* 81:515, 1986.

100. Touroutoglou N, Dimopoulos MA, Younes A, et al: Testicular lymphoma: late relapses and poor outcome despite doxorubicin-based therapy. *J Clin Oncol* 13:1361, 1995.

101. Goffinet DR, Castellino RA, Kim H: Staging laparotomies in unselected previously untreated patients with non-Hodgkin's lymphomas. *Cancer* 32:672, 1973.

102. Moran EM, Ultmann JE, Ferguson DJ, Hoffer PB, Ranniger K, Rappaport H: Staging laparotomy in non-Hodgkin's lymphoma. *Br J Cancer* 31(suppl II):228, 1975.

103. Risdall R, Hoppe RT, Warnke R: Non-Hodgkin's lymphoma: a study of the evolution of the disease based upon 92 autopsied cases. *Cancer* 44:529, 1979.

104. Rosenberg SA, Diamond HD, Jaslowitz B, et al: Lymphosarcoma: a review of 1269 cases. *Medicine* 40:31, 1961.

105. DeMent SH, Mann RB, Staal SP, Kuhajda FP, Boitnott JK: Primary lymphomas of the liver: report of six cases and review of the literature. *Am J Clin Pathol* 88:255, 1987.

106. Kehoe J, Straus DJ: Primary lymphoma of the spleen: clinical features and outcome after splenectomy. *Cancer* 62:1433, 1988.

107. Narang S, Wolf BC, Neiman RS: Malignant lymphoma presenting with prominent splenomegaly: a clinicopathologic study with special reference to intermediate cell lymphoma. *Cancer* 55:1948, 1985.

108. Clayton F, Butler JJ, Ayala AG, Ro JY, Zornoza J: Non-Hodgkin's lymphoma in bone: pathologic and radiologic features with clinical correlates. *Cancer* 60:2494, 1987.

109. Rosenburg SA: Bone marrow involvement in the non-Hodgkin's lymphomata. *Br J Cancer* 31(suppl II):261, 1975.

110. Stein RS, Ultmann JE, Byrne GE Jr, Moran EM, Golomb HM, Oetzel N: Bone marrow involvement in non-Hodgkin's lymphoma. *Cancer* 37:629, 1976.

111. Bitran JD, Golomb HM, Ultmann JE: Non-Hodgkin's lymphoma, poorly differentiated lymphocytic and mixed cell types: results of sequential staging procedures, response to therapy and survival of 100 patients. *Cancer* 42:88, 1978.

112. Chabner BA, Johnson RE, Young RC, et al: Sequential nonsurgical and surgical staging of non-Hodgkin's lymphoma. *Ann Intern Med* 85:149, 1976.

113. Coggins CH: Renal failure in lymphoma. *Kidney Int* 17:847, 1980.

114. Bostwick DG, Mann RB: Malignant lymphomas involving the prostate; a study of 13 cases. *Cancer* 56:2932, 1985.

115. Paladugu RR, Bearman RM, Rappaport H: Malignant lymphoma with primary manifestation in the gonad. *Cancer* 45:561, 1980.

116. Levitt LJ, Ault KA, Pinkus GS, Sloss LJ, McManus BM: Pericarditis and early cardiac tamponade as a primary manifestation of lymphosarcoma cell leukemia. *Am J Med* 67:719, 1979.

117. Colby TV, Dorfman RF: Malignant lymphomas involving the salivary glands. *Pathol Ann* 14(part 2):307, 1979.

118. Harris GJ, Tio FO, Von Hoff DD: Primary adrenal lymphoma. *Cancer* 63:799, 1989.

119. Hamburger JI, Miller JM, Kini SR: Lymphoma of the thyroid. *Ann Int Med* 99:685, 1983.

120. Jones SE, Fuks Z, Bull M: Non-Hodgkin's lymphomas: IV. Clinicopathologic correlation in 405 cases. *Cancer* 31:806, 1973.

121. Anderson T, Chabner BA, Young RC, et al: Malignant lymphoma: I. The histology and staging of 473 patients at the National Cancer Institute. *Cancer* 50:2699, 1982.

122. Ben-Ezra J, Burke JS, Swartz WG, et al: Small lymphocytic lymphomas: clinicopathologic analysis of 268 cases. *Blood* 73:579, 1989.

123. Foon KA, Rai KR, Gale RP: Chronic lymphocytic leukemia: new insights into biology and therapy. *Ann Intern Med* 113:525, 1990.

124. Foon KA, Todd RF III: Immunologic classification of leukemia and lymphoma. *Blood* 68:1, 1986.

125. Jennings CD, Foon KA. Recent advances in flow cytometry: application to the diagnosis of hematologic malignancy. *Blood* 90:2863, 1997.

126. Tubbs RR, Fishleder A, Weiss RA, et al: Immunohistologic cellular phenotypes of lymphoproliferative disorders. *Am J Pathol* 113:207, 1983.

127. Picker LJ, Weiss LM, Medeiros LJ, Wood GS, Warnke RA: Immunophenotypic criteria for the diagnosis of non-Hodgkin's lymphoma. *Am J Pathol* 128:181, 1987.

128. Medeiros LJ, Bagg A, Crossman J: Application of molecular genetics to the diagnosis of hematopoietic neoplasms, in *Neoplastic Hematopathology*, edited by DM Knowles, pp 263–298. Williams and Wilkins, Baltimore, 1992.

129. Matutes E, Brito-Babapulle V, Swansbury J, et al: Clinical and laboratory features of 78 cases of T-prolymphocytic leukemia. *Blood* 78:3269, 1991.

130. Gonzalez CL, Medeiros LJ: Non-Hodgkin's lymphomas and the working formulation: Part 1 *Contemporary Oncol* 3:34, 1993.

131. Rai KR, Peterson B, Elias L, et al: A randomized comparison of fludarabine and chlorambucil for patients with previously untreated chronic lymphocytic leukemia. A CALGB, SWOG, CTG/NCI-C, and ECOG inter-group study. *Blood* 88:552a, 1996.

132. Isaacson PG, Spencer J: Malignant lymphoma of mucosa-associated lymphoid tissue. *Histopathology* 11:445, 1987.

133. Pelstring RJ, Essell JH, Kurtin PJ, Cohen AR, Banks PM: Diversity of organ site involvement among malignant lymphomas of mucosa-associated tissues. *Am J Clin Pathol* 96:738, 1991.

134. Wotherspoon AC, Doglioni C, Isaacson PG: Low-grade gastric B-cell lymphoma of mucosa-associated lymphoid tissue (MALT): a multifocal disease. *Histopathology* 20:29, 1992.

135. Thieblemont C, Bastion Y, Berger F, et al: Mucosa-associated lymphoid tissue gastrointestinal and nongastrointestinal lymphoma behavior: analysis of 108 patients. *J Clin Oncol* 15:1624, 1997.

136. Wotherspoon AC, Pan LX, Diss TC, Isaacson PG: Cytogenetic study of B-cell lymphoma of mucosa-associated lymphoid tissue. *Cancer Genet Cytogenet* 58:35, 1992.

137. Ott G, Katzenberger T, Greiner A, et al: The t(11;18)(q21;q21) chromosome transolocation is a frequent and specific aberration in low-grade but not high-grade malignant non-Hodgkin's lymphomas of the mucosa-associated lymphoid tissue (MALT) type. *Cancer Res* 57:3944, 1997.

138. Sheibani K, Burke JS, Swartz WG, Nademanee A, Winberg CD: Monocytoid B-cell lymphoma: clinicopathologic study of 21 cases of a unique type of low-grade lymphoma. *Cancer* 62:1531, 1988.

139. Nizze H, Cogliatti SB, von Schilling C, Feller AC, Lennert K: Monocytoid B-cell lymphoma: morphological variants and relationship to low-grade B-cell lymphoma of the mucosa-associated lymphoid tissue. *Histopathology* 18:403, 1991.

140. Piris M, Rivas C, Morente M, Cruz M, Rubio C, Oliva H: Monocytoid B-cell lymphoma, a tumour related to the marginal zone. *Histopathology* 12:383, 1998.

141. Ngan B-Y, Warnke R, Wilson M, Takagi K, Cleary M, Dorfman R. Monocytoid B-cell lymphoma: a study of 36 cases. *Hum Pathol* 22:409, 1991.

142. Shin S, Sheibani K, Fishleder A, et al: Monocytoid B-cell lymphoma in patients with Sjogren's syndrome: a clinicopathologic study of 13 patients. *Hum Pathol* 22:422, 1991.

143. Schmid C, Kirkham N, Diss T, Isaacson P: Splenic marginal zone cell lymphoma. *Am J Surg Pathol* 16:455, 1992.

144. Hollema H, Visser L, Poppema S: Small lymphocytic lymphomas with predominant splenomegaly: a comparison of immunophenotypes with cases of predominant lymphadenopathy. *Mod Pathol* 4:712, 1991.

145. Melo J, Hegde U, Parreira A, Thompson I, Lampert I, Catovsky D: Splenic B-cell lymphoma with circulating villous lymphocytes: differential diagnosis of B-cell leukaemias with large spleens. *J Clin Pathol* 40:642, 1987.

146. Bartlett DL, Karpeh MS Jr, Filippa DA, Brennan MF: Long-term follow-up after curative surgery for early gastric lymphoma. *Ann Surg* 223:53, 1996.

147. Roukos DH, Hottenrott C, Encke A, Baltogiannis G, Casioumis D: Primary gastric lymphomas: a clinicopathologic study with literature review. *Surg Oncol* 3:115, 1994.

148. Schechter NR, Portlock CS, Yahalom J: Treatment of mucosa-associated lymphoid tissue lymphoma of the stomach with radiation alone. *J Clin Oncol* 16:1916, 1998.

149. Hammel P, Haioun C, Chaumette MT, et al: Efficacy of single-agent chemotherapy in low-grade B-cell mucosa lymphoid tissue lymphoma with prominent gastric expression. *J Clin Oncol* 13:2524, 1995.

150. Nakamura S, Akazawa K, Yao T, Tsuneyoshi M: A clinicopathologic study of 233 cases with special reference to evaluation with the MIB-1 index. *Cancer* 76:1313, 1995.

151. Isaacson PG, Spencer J: Gastric lymphoma and *Helicobacter pylori*. *Important Adv Oncol* 111, 1996.

152. Nakamura S, Yao T, Aoyagi K, Iida M, Fujishima M, Tsuneyoshi M: *Helicobacter pylori* and primary gastric lymphoma: a histopathologic and immunohistochemical analysis of 237 patients. *Cancer* 79:3, 1997.

153. Savio A, Franzin G, Wotherspoon AC, et al: Diagnosis and posttreatment follow-up of *Helicobacter pylori*-positive gastric lymphoma of mucosa-associated lymphoid tissue: Histology, polymerase chain reaction, or both? *Blood* 87:1255, 1996.

154. Roggero E, Zucca E, Pinotti G, et al: Eradication of *Helicobacter pylori* infection in primary low-grade gastric lymphoma of mucosa-associated lymphoid tissue. *Ann Intern Med* 122:767, 1995.

155. Wotherspoon AC, Doglioni C, Diss TC, et al: Regression of primary low-grade B-cell gastric lymphoma of mucosa-associated lymphoid tissue type after eradication of *Helicobacter pylori*. *Lancet* 342:575, 1993.

156. Rowley JD: Chromosome studies in the non-Hodgkin's lymphomas: the role of the 14;18 translocation. *J Clin Oncol* 6:919, 1988.

157. Yunis JJ, Frizzera G, Oken MM, McKenna J, Theologides A, Arnesen M: Multiple recurrent genomic defects in follicular lymphoma. A possible model for cancer. *N Engl J Med* 316:79, 1987.

158. Ngan B-Y, Chen-Levy Z, Weiss LM, Warnke RA, Cleary ML: Expression in non-Hodgkin's lymphoma of the bcl-2 protein associated with the t(14;18) chromosomal translocation. *N Engl J Med* 318:1638, 1988.

159. Korsmeyer SJ: Bcl-2 initiates a new category of oncogenes: regulators of cell death. *Blood* 80:879, 1992.

160. Hockenbery D, Zutter M, Hickey W, Nahm M, Korsmeyer S: BCL2 protein is topographically restricted in tissues characterized by apoptotic cell death. *Proc Natl Acad Sci USA* 88:6961, 1991.

161. McDonnell T, Deane N, Platt F, Nunez G, Jaeger U, McKearn J, Korsmeyer S: BCL-2-immunoglobulin transgenic mice demonstrate extended B-cell survival and follicular lymphoproliferation. *Cell* 57:79, 1989.

162. Mann R, Berard C. Criteria for the cytologic subclassification of follicular lymphomas: a proposed alternative method. *Hematol Oncol* 1:187, 1982.

163. Nathwani B, Metter G, Miller T, et al: What should be the morphologic criteria for the subdivision of follicular lymphomas? *Blood* 68:837, 1986.

164. Warnke R, Kim H, Fuks Z, Dorfman R: The co-existence of nodular and diffuse patterns in nodular non-Hodgkin's lymphomas. *Cancer* 40:1229, 1977.

165. Ezdinli E, Costello W, Kucuk O, Berard C: Effect of the degree of nodularity on the survival of patients with nodular lymphomas. *J Clin Oncol* 5:413, 1987.

166. Brittinger G, Bartels H, Common H, et al: Clinical and prognostic relevance of the Kiel classification of non-Hodgkin lymphomas: results of a prospective multicenter study by the Kiel lymphoma study group. *Hematol Oncol* 2:269, 1984.

167. Manus MPM, Hoppe RT: Is radiotherapy curative for stage I and II low-grade follicular lymphoma? Results of a long-term follow-up study of patients treated at Stanford University. *J Clin Oncol* 14:1282–1290, 1996.

168. Portlock CS, Rosenberg SA: No initial therapy for stage III and IV non-Hodgkin's lymphoma of favorable histologic types. *Ann Intern Med* 90:10, 1979.

169. Straus DJ, Gaynor JJ, Leiberman PH, Filippa DA, Koziner B, Clarkson

BD: Non-Hodgkin's lymphomas: characteristics of long-term survivors following conservative treatment. *Am J Med* 82:247, 1986.

170. Young RC, Longo DL, Glatstein E, Ihde DC, Jaffe ES, Devita VT Jr: The treatment of indolent lymphomas: watchful waiting v aggressive combined modality treatment. *Semin Hematol* 25:11, 1988.

171. Kennedy BJ, Bloomfield CD, Kiang DT, Vosika G, Peterson BA, Theologides A: Combination versus successive single agent chemotherapy in lymphocytic lymphoma. *Cancer* 41:23, 1978.

172. Jones SE, Rosenberg SA, Kaplan HS, Kadin ME, Dorfman RF: Non-Hodgkin's lymphomas: II. Single agent chemotherapy. *Cancer* 30:31, 1972.

173. Portlock CS, Rosenberg SA, Glatstein E, Kaplan HS: Treatment of advanced non-Hodgkin's lymphomas with favorable histologies: preliminary results of a prospective trial. *Blood* 47:747, 1976.

174. Hoppe RT, Kushlan P, Kaplan HS, Rosenberg SA, Brown BW: The treatment of advanced stage favorable histology non-Hodgkin's lymphoma: a preliminary report of randomized trial comparing single agent chemotherapy, combination chemotherapy, and whole body irradiation. *Blood* 58:592, 1981.

175. Hochster HS, Kim K, Green MD, et al: Activity of fludarabine in previously treated non-Hodgkin's low-grade lymphoma: results of an Eastern Cooperative Oncology Group Study. *J Clin Oncol* 10:28, 1992.

176. Kay AC, Saven A, Carrera CJ, et al: 2-Chlorodeoxyadenosine treatment of low-grade lymphomas. *J Clin Oncol* 10:371, 1992.

177. Duggan DB, Anderson JR, Dillman R, Case D, Glttlieb AJ: 2'Deoxycoformycin (pentostatin) for refractory non-Hodgkin's lymphoma: a CALGB phase II study. *Med Pediatr Oncol* 18:203, 1990.

178. Lister TA, Cullen MH, Beard MEJ, et al: Comparison of combined and single-agent chemotherapy in non-Hodgkin's lymphoma of favorable histological type. *BMJ* 1:533, 1978.

179. Luce JK, Gamble JF, Wilson HE, et al: Combined cyclophosphamide, vincristine and prednisone therapy of malignant lymphoma. *Cancer* 28:306, 1971.

180. Bagley Jr CM, DeVita VT Jr, Berard CW, Canellos GP: Advanced lymphosarcoma: Intensive cyclical combination chemotherapy with cyclophosphamide, vincristine and prednisone. *Ann Intern Med* 76:227, 1972.

181. Schein PS, Chabner BA, Cannellos GP, Young RC, Berard C, DeVita VT: Potential for prolonged disease-free survival following combination chemotherapy of non-Hodgkin's lymphoma. *Blood* 43:181, 1974.

182. Peterson BA, Anderson JR, Fizzera G, Bloomfield CD, Gottlieb AJ, Holland JF: Nodular mixed lymphoma (NML): a comparative trial of cyclophosphamide (CTX) and cyclophosphamide, adriamycin, vincristine, prednisone and bleomycin (CAVPB). *Blood* 66:216, 1985.

183. Jones SE, Grozea PN, Metz EN, et al: Improved complete remission rates and survival for patients with large cell lymphoma treated with chemoimmunotherapy. *Cancer* 51:1083, 1983.

184. McLaughlin P, Fuller LM, Velasquez WS, et al: Stage III follicular lymphoma: Durable remissions with a combined chemotherapy-radiotherapy regimen. *J Clin Oncol* 5:867, 1987.

185. Dana BW, Dahlberg S, Nathwani BN, et al: Long-term follow-up of patients with low-grade malignant lymphomas treated with Doxorubicin-based chemotherapy of chemoimmunotherapy. *J Clin Oncol* 11:644, 1993.

186. McLaughlin P, Hagemeister FB, Romoguera JE, et al: Fludarabine, Mitoxantrone, and Dexamethasone: an effective new regimen for indolent lymphoma. *J Clin Oncol* 14:1262, 1996.

187. Hochster H, Oken M, Winter J, et al: Prolonged time to progression (TTP) in patients with low grade lymphoma (LGL) treated with cyclophosphamide and fludarabine [ECOG 1491]. *ASCO* 16:66a, 1998.

188. Foon KA, Hicks L, Gohmann J, Doukas M, Garrison J, Larocca R: Excellent responses to sequential fludarabine followed by cyclophosphamide, mitoxantrone, vincristine, and prednisone (cnop) in previously untreated patients with follicle center lymphoma, grade I and II. *Blood* 1998.

189. Maloney DG, Grillo-López AJ, Bodkin DJ, et al: IDEC-C2B8: results of a phase I multi-dose trial in patients with relapsed non-Hodgkin's lymphoma. *J Clin Oncol* 15:3266, 1997.

190. McLaughlin P, Grillo-Lépez A, Link BK, et al: Rituximab chimeric anti-CD20 monoclonal antibody therapy for relapsed indolent lymphoma: half of patients respond to a four-dose treatment program. *J Clin Oncol* 16:2825, 1998.

191. Kaminski MS, Zasadny KR, Francis IR, et al: Radioimmunotherapy of B-cell lymphoma with ^{131}I anti-B1 (Anti-CD20) antibody. *N Engl J Med* 329:459, 1993.

192. Knox SJ, Goris ML, Trisler K, et al: Yttrium-90-labeled anti-CD20 monoclonal antibody therapy of recurrent B-cell lymphoma. *Clin Cancer Res* 2:457, 1996.

193. Press OW, Eary JF, Appelbaum FR, et al: Radiolabeled-antibody therapy of B-cell lymphoma with autologous bone marrow support. *N Engl J Med* 329:1219, 1993.

194. Liu SY, Eary JF, Petersdorf SH, et al: Follow-up of relapsed B-cell lymphoma patients treated with Iodine-131-labeled anti-CD20 antibody and autologous stem cell rescue. *J Clin Oncol* 16:3270, 1998.

195. Kaminski MS, Gribbin T, Estes J, et al: I-131 anti-B1 antibody for previously untreated follicular lymphoma (FL): clinical and molecular remissions. *ASCO* 17:6a, 1998.

196. Van Biesen K, Sobocinski KA, Rowlings PA, et al: Allogeneic bone marrow transplantation for low grade lymphoma. *Blood* 92:1832,1998.

197. Gribben JG, Freedman AS, Neuberg D, et al: Immunologic purging of marrow assessed by PCR before autologous bone marrow transplantation for B-cell lymphoma. *N Engl J Med* 325:1525, 1991.

198. Bierman PJ, Vose JM, Anderson JR, Bishop MR, Kessinger A, Armitage JO: High-dose therapy with autologous hematopoietic rescue for follicular low-grade non-Hodgkin's lymphoma. *J Clin Oncol* 15:445, 1997.

199. Colombat P, Donadio D, Fouillard L, et al: Value of autologous bone marrow transplantation in follicular lymphoma: a France autogreffe retrospective study of 42 patients. *Bone Marrow Transplant* 13:157, 1994.

200. Cervantes F, Shu XO, McGlave PB, et al: Autologous bone marrow transplantation for non-transformed low-grade non-Hodgkin's lymphoma. *Bone Marrow Transplant* 16:387, 1995.

201. Freedman AS, Gribben JG, Neuberg D, et al: High-dose therapy and autologous bone marrow transplantation in patients with follicular lymphoma during first remission. *Blood* 88:2780, 1996.

202. Foon KA, Sherwin SA, Abrams PG, et al: Treatment of advanced non-Hodgkin's lymphoma with recombinant leukocyte A interferon. *N Engl J Med* 311:1148, 1984.

203. Horning SJ, Merigan TC, Krown SE, et al: Human interferon alpha in malignant lymphoma and Hodgkin's disease. Results of the American Cancer Society trial. *Cancer* 56:1305, 1985.

204. Solal-Céligny P, Lepage E, Brousse N, et al: Doxorubicin-containing regimen with or without interferon alfa-2b for advanced follicular lymphomas: final analysis of survival and toxicity in the groupe d'Etude des lymphomes folliculaires 86 trial. *J Clin Oncol* 16:2332, 1998.

205. Arranz R, Garcia-Alfonso P, Sobrino P, et al: Role of interferon alfa-2b in the induction and maintenance treatment of low-grade non-Hodgkin's lymphoma: results from a prospective, multicenter trial with double randomization. *J Clin Oncol* 16:1538, 1998.

206. Smalley RV, Andersen JW, Hawkins MJ, et al: Interferon alfa combined with cytotoxic chemotherapy for patients with non-Hodgkin's lymphoma. *N Engl J Med* 327:1336, 1992.

207. Andersen JW, Smalley RV: Interferon alfa plus chemotherapy for non-Hodgkin's lymphoma: five-year follow-up [letter]. *N Engl J Med* 329:1821, 1993.

208. Peterson BA, Petroni GR, Oken MM, et al: Cyclophosphamide versus cyclophosphamide plus interferon alpha-2b in follicular low-grade lymphomas: an intergroup phase III trial (CALGB 8691 and EST 7486). *Proc Am Soc Clin Oncol* 16:48a, 1997.

209. Hagenbeek A, Carde P, Meerwaldt JH, et al: Maintenance of remission with human recombinant interferon alfa-2a in patients with stages III and IV low-grade malignant non-Hodgkin's lymphoma. European Organization for Research and Treatment of Cancer Lymphoma Cooperative Group. *J Clin Oncol* 16:41, 1998.

210. Price CG, Rohatiner AZ, Steward W, et al: Interferon alfa-2b in addition to chlorambucil in the treatment of follicular lymphoma: preliminary results of a randomized trial in progress. *Eur J Cancer* 27(suppl 4):S34, 1991.

211. Unterhalt M, Herman R, Koch P, et al: Long term interferon alpha maintenance prolongs remission duration in advanced low-grade lymphomas and is related to the efficacy of the initial cytoreductive chemotherapy. *Blood* 88(suppl 1):1801a, 1996.

212. Dana BW, Unger J, Fisher RI: A randomized study of alpha-interferon

consolidation in patients with low-grade lymphoma who have responded to PRO-MACE-MOPP (Day 1–8). *Proc ASCO* 17:3a, 1998.

213. Bernstein ZP, Vaickus L, Friedman N, et al: Interleukin-2 lymphokine-activated killer cell therapy of non-Hodgkin's lymphoma and Hodgkin's disease. *J Immunother* 10:141, 1991.

214. Duggan DB, Santarelli MT, Zamkoff K, et al: A phase II study of recombinant interleukin-2 with or without recombinant interferon-β in non-Hodgkin's lymphoma. A study of the cancer and leukemia group B. *J Immunother* 12:115, 1992.

215. Weber JS, Yang JC, Topalian SL, Schwartzentruber DJ, White DE, Rosenberg SA: The use of interleukin-2 and lymphokine-activated killer cells for the treatment of patients with non-Hodgkin's lymphoma. *J Clin Oncol* 10(1):33, 1992.

216. Meeker TC, Lowder J, Maloney DG, et al: A clinical trial of anti-idiotype therapy of B-cell malignancy. *Blood* 65:1349, 1985.

217. Brown SL, Miller RA, Horning SJ, et al: Treatment of B-cell lymphoma with anti-idiotypic antobidies alone and in combination with alpha interferon. *Blood* 73:651, 1989.

218. Maloney DG, Brown S, Czerwinski DK, et al: Monoclonal anti-idiotype antibody therapy of B-cell lymphoma: the addition of a short course of chemotherapy does not interfere with the antitumor effect nor prevent the emergence of idiotype-negative variant cells. *Blood* 80:1502, 1992.

219. Cleary ML, Meeker TL, Levy S, et al: Clustering of extensive somatic mutations in the variable region of an immunoglobulin heavy chain gene from a human B-cell lymphoma. *Cell* 44:97, 1986.

220. Kwak LW, Campbell MJ, Czerwinski DK, Hart S, Miller RA, Levy R: Induction of immune responses in patients with B-cell lymphoma against the surface-immunoglobulin idiotype expressed by their tumors. *N Engl J Med* 327:1209, 1992.

221. Nelson EL, Li X, Hsu FJ, et al: Tumor-specific, cytotoxic T-lymphocyte response after idiotype vaccination for B-cell, non-Hodgkin's lymphoma. *Blood* 88:580, 1996.

222. Hsu FJ, Caspar CB, Czerwinski D, et al: Tumor-specific idiotype vaccines in the treatment of patients with B-cell lymphoma-long-term results of a clinical trial. *Blood* 89:3129, 1997.

223. Hsu F, Benike C, Fagnoni F, et al: Vaccination of patients with B cell lymphoma using autologous antigen pulsed dendritic cells. *Nat Med* 2:1038, 1996.

224. Stone MJ, Sausville EA, Fay JW, et al: A phase I study of bolus versus continuous infusion of the anti-CD19 immunotoxin, IgG-HD37-dgA, in patients with B-cell lymphoma. *Blood* 88:1188, 1996.

225. Grossbard ML, Freeman AS, Ritz J, et al: Serotherapy of B-cell neoplasms with anti-B4 blocked ricin: a phase I trial of daily bolus infusion. *Blood* 79:576, 1992.

226. Conry RM, Khazaeli MB, Saleh MN, et al: Phase I trial of an anti-CD19 Deglycosylated Ricin A chain immunoto xin in non-Hodgkin's lymphoma: effect of an intensive schedule of administration. *J Immunol* 18:231, 1996.

227. Ramsay A, Smith W, Isaacson P: T-cell-rich B-cell lymphoma. *Am J Surg Pathol* 12:433, 1988.

228. Chittal S, Brousset P, Voight J, Delsol G: Large B-cell lymphoma rich in T-cells and simulating Hodgkin's disease. *Histopathology* 19:211, 1991.

229. Delabie J, Vandenberghe E, Kennes C, et al: Histiocyte-rich B cell lymphoma. Adistinct clinicopathologic entity possibly related to lymphocyte predominant Hodgkin's disease, paragranuloma subtype. *Am J Surg Pathol* 1637, 1992.

230. Addis B, Isaacson P: Large cell lymphoma of the mediastinum: a B-cell tumor of probable thymic origin. *Histopathology* 10:379, 1986.

231. Lamarre L, Jacobson J, Aisenberg A, Harris N: Primary large cell lymphoma of the mediastinum. *Am J Surg Pathol* 13:730, 1989.

232. Yousem S, Weiss L, Warnke R: Primary mediastinal non-Hodgkin's lymphomas: A morphologic and immunologic study of 19 cases. *Am J Clin Pathol* 83:676, 1985.

233. Moller P, Moldenhauer G, Momburg F, Lammler B, Eberlein-gonska M, Kiesel S, Dorken B: Mediastinal lymphoma of clear cell type is a tumor corresponding to terminal steps of B cell differentiation. *Blood* 69;1087, 1987.

234. Levitt l, Aisenberg A, Harris N, Linggood R, Poppema S: Primary non-Hodgkin's lymphoma of the mediastinum. *Cancer* 50:2486, 1982.

235. Jacobson J, Aisenberg A, Lamarre L, et al: Mediastinal large cell lymphoma: an uncommon subset of adult lymphoma curable with combined modality therapy. *Cancer* 62:1893, 1988.

236. Fisher RI, Hubbard SM, DeVita VT, et al: Factors predicting long-term survival in diffuse mixed, histiocytic, or undifferentiated lymphoma. *Blood*. 58:45, 1981.

237. Fisher RI, DeVita VT Jr, Hubbard SM, et al: Diffuse aggressive lymphomas: increased survival after alternating flexible sequences of proMACE and MOPP chemotherapy. *Ann Intern Med*. 98:304, 1983.

238. Miller TP, Jones SE: Initial chemotherapy for clinically localized lymphomas of unfavorable histology. *Blood*. 62:413, 1983.

239. Miller TP, Dahlberg S, Cassady JR, et al: Chemotherapy alone compared with chemotherapy plus radiotherapy for localized intermediate- and high-grade non-Hodgkin's lymphoma. *N Engl J Med*. 339:21, 1998.

240. Glick JH, Kim K, Earle J, O'Connell MJ: An ECOG randomized phase III trial of CHOP versus CHOP plus radiotherapy for intermediate grade early stage non-Hodgin's lymphoma. *Proc Am Soc Clin Oncol* 14:391, 1995.

241. Shipp MA, Yeap BY, Harrington DP, et al: The m-BACOD combination chemotherapy regimen in large-cell lymphoma: analysis of the completed trial and comparison with the M-BACOD regimen. *J Clin Oncol*. 8:84, 1990.

242. Longo DL, DeVita VT, Duffey PL, et al: Superiority of ProMACE-CytaBOM over ProMACE-MOPP in the treatment of advanced diffuse aggressive lymphoma: results of a prospective randomized trial. *J Clin Oncol*. 9:25, 1991.

243. Connors JM, Klimo P: MACOP-B Chemotherapy for malignant lymphomas and related conditions: 1987 update and additional observations. *Semin Hematol*. 25:41, 1988.

244. Miller TP, Dahlberg S, Weick JK, et al: Unfavorable Histologies of Non-Hodgkin's Lymphoma Treated with ProMACE-CytaBOM: a Groupwide Southwest Oncology Group Study. *J Clin Oncol*. 8:1951, 1990.

245. Fisher RI, Gaynor ER, Dahlberg S, et al: Comparison of a standard regimen (CHOP) with three intensive chemotherapy regimens for advanced non-Hodgkin's lymphoma. *N Engl J Med*. 328:1002, 1993.

246. Gordon LI, Harrington D, Andersen J, et al: Comparison of a second-generation combination chemotherapeutic regimen (m-BACOD) with a standard regimen (CHOP) for advanced diffuse non-Hodgkin's lymphoma. *N Engl J Med*. 327:1342, 1992.

247. Gianni AM, Bregni M, Siena S, et al: 5-year update of the Milan Cancer Institute randomized trial of high-dose squential (HDS) vs MACOP-B therapy for diffuse large-cell lymphomas. *Proc Am Soc Clin Oncol* 13:373a, 1994.

248. Haioun C, Lepage E, Gisselbrecht C, et al: Comparison of autologous bone marrow transplantation with sequential chemotherapy for intermediate and high-grade non-Hodgkin's lymphoma in first complete remission: a study of 464 patients. Groupe d'Etude des Lymphomes de l'Adulte. *J Clin Oncol* 12:2543, 1994.

249. Haioun C, Lepage E, Gisselbrecht C, et al: Benefit of autologous bone marrow transplantation over sequential chemotherapy in poor-risk aggressive non-Hodgkin's lymphoma: updated results of the prospective study LNH87–2. Groupe d'Etude des Lymphomes de l'Adulte *J Clin Oncol*. 15:1131, 1997.

250. Santini G, Salvagno L, Leoni P, et al: VACOP-B versus VACOP-B plus autologous bone marrow transplantation for advanced diffuse non-Hodgkin's lymphoma: results of a prospective randomized trial by the non-Hodgkin's lymphoma cooperative study group. *J Clin Oncol*. 16:2796, 1998.

251. Cabanillas F, Hagemeister FB, Bodey GP, Freireich EJ: IMVP-16: An effective regimen for patients with lymphoma who have relapsed after initial combination chemotherapy. *Blood*. 60:693, 1982.

252. Cabanillas F, Hagemeister FB, McLaughlin P, et al: Results of MIME salvage regimen for recurrent or refractory lymphoma. *J Clin Oncol*. 5:407, 1987.

253. Philip T, Guglielmi C, Hagenbeek A, et al: Autologous bone marrow transplantation as compared with salvage chemotherapy in relapses of chemotherapy-sensitive non-Hodgkin's lymphoma. *N Engl J Med*. 333:1540, 1995.

254. O'Reilly SE, Klimo P, Connors JM: Low dose ACOP-B and VABE: weekly chemotherapy for elderly patients with advanced-stage diffuse large-cell lymphoma. *J Clin Oncol*. 9:741, 1991.

255. Weisenburger DD, Armitage JO: Mantle cell lymphoma—an entity comes of age. *J Am Soc Hematol* 87:4483, 1996.

256. Swerdlow SH, Habeshaw JA, Murray LJ, Dhaliwal HS, Lister TA, Stansfeld AG. Centrocytic lymphoma. A distinct clinicopathologic and

immunologic entity. A multiparameter study of 18 cases at diagnosis and relapse. *Am J Pathol* 113:181, 1983.

257. Lardelli P, Bookman MA, Sundeen J, Longo DL, Jaffe ES: Lymphocytic lymphoma of intermediate differentiation. Morphologic and immunophenotypic spectrum and clinical correlations. *Am J Surg Pathol* 14: 752, 1990.

258. Segal GH, Masih AS, Fox AC, Jorgensen T, Scott M, Braylan RC: CD5-expressing B-cell non-Hodgkin's lymphomas with bcl-1 gene rearrangement have a relatively homogeneous immunophenotype and are associated with an overall poor prognosis. *Blood* 85:1570, 1995.

259. Medeiros L, van Krieken J, Jaffe E, Raffeld M: Association of bcl-1 rearrangements with lymphocytic lymphoma if intermediate differentiation. *Blood* 76:2086, 1990.

260. Rimokh R, Berger F, Cornillet P, et al: Break in the BCL1 locus is closely associated with intermediate lymphocytic lymphoma subtype. *Genes Chrom Cancer* 2:223, 1990.

261. Williams ME, Westermann CD, Swerdlow SH: Genotypic characterization of centrocytic lymphoma: frequent rearrangment of the chromosome 11 bcl-1 locus. *Blood* 76:1387, 1990.

262. Vandenberghe E, De Wolf-Peeters C, Van den Oord J, et al: Translocation (11;14): a cytogenetic anomaly associated with B-cell lymphomas of non-follicle center cell lineage. *J Pathol* 163:13, 1991.

263. Rosenberg C, Wong E, Petty E, Bale A, Tsujimoto Y, Harris N, Arnold A: Overexpression of PRAD1, a candidate BCL1 breakpoint region oncogene, in centrocytic lymphomas. *Proc Natl Acad Sci USA* 88:9638, 1991.

264. Williams M, Swerdlow S, Rosenberg C, Arnold A: Characterization of chromosome 11 tranlocation breakpoints at the bcl-1 and PRAD 1 loci in centrocytic lymphoma. *Cancer Res* 52:5541, 1992.

265. Hiddemann W, Unterhalt M, Herrmann R, et al: Mantle-cell lymphoma have more widespread disease and a slower response to chemotherapy compared with follicle-center lymphomas: results of a prospective comparative analysis of the German low-grade lymphoma study group. *J Clin Oncol* 16:1922, 1998.

266. Velders GA, Kluin-Nelemans JC, De Boer CJ, et al: Mantle-cell lymphoma: a population-based clinical study. *J Clin Oncol* 14:1269, 1996.

267. Argatoff LH, Connors JM, Klasa RJ, Horsman DE, Gascoyne RD: Mantle cell lymphoma: a clinicopathologic study of 80 cases. *Blood* 89:2067, 1997.

268. Majlis A, Pugh WC, Rodriguez MA, Benedict WF, Cabanillas F: Mantle cell lymphoma: correlation of clinical outcome and biologic features with three histologic variants. *J Clin Oncol* 15:1664, 1997.

269. Press OW, Grogan TM, Fisher RI: Evaluation and management of mantle cell lymphoma. *Adv Leuk Lymphoma* 6:3, 1996.

270. Fisher RI, Dahlberg S, Nathwani BN, Banks PM, Miller TP, Grogan TM: A clinical analysis of two indolent lymphoma entities: mantle cell lymphoma and marginal zone lymphoma (including the mucosa-associated lymphoid tissue and monocytoid B-cell subcategories): a Southwest Oncology Group study. *Blood* 85:1075, 1995.

271. Garcia C, Weiss L, Warnke R: Small noncleaved cell lymphoma: an immunophenotypic study of 18 cases and comparison with large cell lymphoma. *Hum Pathol* 17:454, 1986.

272. Pelicci P, Knowles D, Mcgrath IU, Dalla-Favera R: Chromosomal breakpoints and structural alterations of the c-myc locus differ in endemic and sporadic forms of Burkitt lymphoma. *Proc Natl Acad Sci USA* 83:2984, 1986.

273. Neri A, Barriga F, Knowles D, Magrath I, Dalla-Favera R: Different regions of the immunoglobulin heavy-chain locus are involved in chromosomal translocations in distinct pathogenetic forms of Burkitt lymphoma. *Proc Natl Acad Sci USA* 85:2748, 1988.

274. Hamilton-Dutoit S, Pallesen G, Franzmann M, et al: AIDS-related lymphoma. Histopathology, immunophenotype, and association with Epstein-Barr virus as demonstrated by in situ nucleic acid hybridization. *Am J Pathol* 138:149, 1991.

275. Meeker T, Shiramizu B, Kaplan L, et al: Evidence for molecular subtypes of HIV-associated lymphoma: division into peripheral monoclonal, polyclonal and central nervous system lymphoma. *AIDS* 5:669, 1991.

276. Ballerini P, Gaidano G, Gong J, et al: Multiple genetic lesions in AIDS-related non-Hodgkin's lymphoma. *Blood* 81:166, 1993.

277. Magrath I, Shiramizu B: Biology and treatment of small non-cleaved cell lymphoma. *Oncology* 3:41, 1989.

278. Hutchinson R, Murphy S, Fairclough D, et al: Diffuse small noncleaved cell lymphoma in children, Burkitt's versus non-Burkitt's types. *Cancer* 64:23, 1989.

279. Magrath IT, James C, Edwards BK, et al: An effective therapy for both undifferentiated (including Burkitt's) lymphomas and lymphoblastic lymphomas in children and young adults. *Blood* 5:1102, 1984.

280. Longo DL, Duffey PL, Jaffe ES, et al: Diffuse small noncleaved-cell, non-Burkitt's lymphoma in adults: a high-grade lymphoma responsive to ProMACE-based combination chemotherapy. *J Clin Oncol* 12:2153, 1994.

281. Lorincz AL: Cutaneous T-cell lymphoma (mycosis fungoides). *Lancet* 347:871, 1996.

282. Sézary A, Bouvrain Y: Erythrodermie avec présence de cellules monstrueses dans le derme et dans lang circulant. *Bull Soc Fr Dermatol Syph* 45:254, 1938.

283. Fischman AB, Bunn PA, Guccion JG, et al: Exposure to chemicals, physical agents and biologic agents in mycosis fungoides and Sezary syndrome. *Cancer Treat Rep* 63:591, 1979.

284. Cohen SR: Mycosis fungoides: clinicopathologic relationships, survival and therapy in 59 patients with observations on occupation as a new prognostic factor. *Cancer* 46:2654, 1980.

285. Whittemore AS, Holly EA, Lee IM, et al: Mycosis fungoides in relation to environmental exposures and immune response: a case-control study. *J Natl Cancer Inst Cancer* 81:1560, 1989.

286. Poiesz BJ, Ruscetti FW, Gazdar AF, et al: Detection and isolation of type-C retrovirus particles from fresh and cultured lymphocytes of a patient with cutaneous T-cell lymphoma. *Proc Natl Acad Sci USA* 77:7415, 1980.

287. Gallo RC, Kalyanaraman VS, Sarngadharan MG, et al: Association of the human type C retrovirus with a subset of adult T-cell cancers. *Cancer Res* 43:3892, 1983.

288. Manzari V, Gismondi A, Barillari G, et al: HTLV-V: a new human retrovirus isolated in a tac-negative T-cell lymphoma/leukemia. *Science* 238(4833):1581, 1987.

289. Greene MH, Pinto HA, Kant JA, et al: Lymphomas and leukemias in the relatives of patients with mycosis fungoides. *Cancer* 49:737, 1982.

290. Long JC, Mihm MC: Mycosis fungoides with extracutaneous dissemination: a distinct clinicopathologic entity. *Cancer* 34:1745, 1974.

291. Winkler CF, Bunn PA: Cutaneous T-cell lymphoma: a review. *CRC Crit Rev Oncol Hematol* 1:49, 1983.

292. Epstein EH Jr, Levin DL, Croft JD Jr, et al: Mycosis fungoides: survival, prognostic features, response to therapy, and autopsy findings. *Medicine* 51:61, 1972.

293. Bunn PA, Humberman MS, Whang-Peng J, et al: Prospective staging evaluation of patients with cutaneous T-cell lymphomas: demonstration of high frequency of extra-cutaneous dissemination. *Ann Intern Med* 93:223, 1980.

294. Green SB, Byar DP, Lamberg SI: Prognostic variables in mycosis fungoides. *Cancer* 47:2671, 1981.

295. Castellino RA, Hoppe RT, Blank N, Young SW, Fuks Z: Experience with lymphography in patients with mycosis fungoides. *Cancer Treat Rep* 63:581, 1979.

296. Hamminga L, Mulder JD, Evans C, et al: Staging lymphography with respect to lymph node histology, treatment, and follow-up in patients with mycosis fungoides. *Cancer* 47:692, 1981.

297. Haynes BF, Metzgar RS, Minna JD, Bunn PA: Phenotypic characterization of cutaneous T-cell lymphoma. *N Engl J Med* 304:1319, 1981.

298. Kung PC, Berger CL, Goldstein G, LoGerfo P, Edelson RL: Cutaneous T-cell lymphoma: characterization by monoclonal antibodies. *Blood* 57:261, 1981.

299. Schroff RW, Foon KA, Billing RJ, Fahey JL: Immunologic classification of lymphocytic leukemias based on monoclonal antibody-defined cell surface antigens. *Blood* 59:207, 1982.

300. Broder S, Edelson RL, Lutzner M, et al: The Sezary syndrome: a malignant proliferation of helper T-cells. *J Clin Invest* 58:1297, 1976.

301. Haynes BF, Hensley LL, Jegasothy BV: Phenotypic characterization of skin-infiltrating T-cells in cutaneous T-cell lymphoma: comparison with benign cutaneous T-cell infiltrates. *Blood* 60:463, 1982.

302. Whang-Peng J, Bunn PA, Knutsen T, Matthews MJ, Schechter G, Minna JD: Clinical implications of cytogenetic studies in cutaneous T-cell lymphoma (CTCL). *Cancer* 50:1139, 1982.

303. Shapiro PE, Warburton D, Berger CL, Edelson RL: Clonal chromosomal

abnormalities in cutaneous T-cell lymphoma. *Cancer Genet Cytogenet* 28:267, 1987.

304. Weiss LM, Wood GS, Hu E, Abel EA, Hope RT, Sklar J: Detection of clonal T-cell receptor gene rearrangements in the peripheral blood of patients with mycosis fungoides/Sezary syndrome. *J Invest Dermatol* 92:601, 1989.

305. Weiss LM, Hu E, Wood GS, et al: Clonal rearrangements of T-cell receptor genes in mycosis fungoides and dermatopathic lymphadenopathy. *N Engl J Med* 313:539, 1985.

306. Whittaker SJ, Smith NP, Jones RR, Luzzatto L: Analysis of beta, gamma, and delta T-cell receptor genes in mycosis fungoides and Sezary syndrome. *Cancer* 68;1572, 1991.

307. Bakels V, Van Oostveen JW, Gordijn RL, Walboomers JM, Meijer CJ, Willemze R: Frequency and prognostic significance of clonal T-cell receptor B-gene rearrangements in the peripheral blood of patients with mycosis fungoides. *Arch Dermatol* 128:1602, 1992.

308. Dommann SNW, Dommann-Scherrer CC, Dours-Zimmermann MT, Zimmermann DR, Kural-Serbes B, Burg G: Clonal disease in extracutaneous compartments in cutaneous T-cell lymphomas. A comparative study between cutaneous T-cell lymphomas and pseudolymphomas. *Arch Dermatol Res* 288:163, 1996.

309. Muche Marcus J, Lukowsky A, Asadullah K, Gellrich S, Sterry W: Demonstration of frequent occurrence of clonal T cells in the peripheral blood of patients with primary cutaneous T-cell lymphoma. *Blood* 90:1636, 1997.

310. Deneau DG, Wood GS, Beckstead J, Hoppe RT, Price N: Woringer-Kolopp disease (Pagetoid reticulosis): four cases with histopathologic ultrastructural, and immunohistologic observations. *Arch Dermatol* 120:1045, 1984.

311. Ketron LW, Goodman MH: Multiple lesions of skin apparently of epithelial origin resembling clinically mycosis fungoides: report of a case. *Arch Dermatol Syph* 24:758, 1931.

312. Wood GS, Weiss LM, Hu C-H, et al: T-cell antigen deficiencies and clonal rearrangements of T-cell receptor genes in pagetoid reticulosis (Woringer-Kolopp disease). *N Engl J Med* 318:164, 1988.

313. Vonderheid EC, Van Scott EJ, Johnson WC, Grekin DA, Asbell SO: Topical chemotherapy and immunotherapy of mycosis fungoides: intermediate term results. *Arch Dermatol* 113:454, 1977.

314. Deviver A, Vonderheid EC, Can Scott EJ, Urbach F: Mycosis fungoides, nitrogen mustard and skin cancer. *Br J Dermatol* 99:61, 1978.

315. Gilchrest BA: Methoxsalen photochemotherapy for mycosis fungoides. *Cancer Treat Rep* 63:633, 1979.

316. Roenigk HH: Photochemotherapy of mycosis fungoides: long-term follow-up study. *Cancer Treat Rep* 63:699, 1979.

317. Briffa DV, Warin AP, Harrington CI, Bleehen SJ: Photochemotherapy in mycosis fungoides: a study of 73 patients. *Lancet* 2:49, 1980.

318. Lo TC, Salzman FA, Moschella SL, Tolman EL, Wright KA: Whole body surface electron irradiation in the treatment of mycosis fungoides: an evaluation of 200 patients. *Radiology* 130:453, 1979.

319. Vonderheid EC, Van Scott EJ, Wallner PE, Johnson WC: A 10 year experience with patients treated by total-skin electron beam radiation therapy. *Cancer Treat Rep* 63:681, 1979.

320. Hoppe RT, Cox RS, Fuks Z, Price NM, Bagshaw MA, Farber EM: Electron-beam therapy for mycosis fungoides: the Stanford University experience. *Cancer Treat Rep* 63:691, 1979.

321. Kierland RR, Watkins CH, Shullenberger CC: The use of nitrogen mustard in the treatment of mycosis fungoides. *J Invest Dermatol* 940:195, 1947.

322. Van Scott EJ, Grekin DA, Kalmanson JD, Vonderheid EC, Barry WE: Frequent low doese of intravenous mechlorethamine for late-stage mycosis fungoides lymphoma. *Cancer* 36:1613, 1975.

323. Van Scott EJ, Auerbach R, Clendenning WE: Treatment of mycosis fungoides with cyclophosphamide. *Arch Dermatol* 85:107, 1962.

324. Wright JC, Lyons MM, Walker DB, et al: Observations on the use of cancer chemotherapeutic agents in patients with mycosis fungoides. *Cancer* 17:1045, 1964.

325. Haynes HA, Van Scott EJ: Therapy of mycosis fungoides. *Prog Dermatol* 3:1, 1968.

326. Wright JC, Gumport SL, Golomb FM: Remissions produced with the use of methotrexate in patients with mycosis fungoides. *Cancer Chemother Rep* 9:11, 1960.

327. McDonald CJ, Bertino JR: Treatment of mycosis fungoides lymphomas: effectiveness of infusions of methotrexate followed by oral citovorum factor. *Cancer Treat Rep* 62:1009, 1979.

328. Takeda K, Sagawa T, Arakawa T: Therapeutic effect of bleomycin for skin tumors. *Cancer* 61:207, 1970.

329. Spigel SC, Coltman CA Jr: Therapy of mycosis fungoides with bleomycin. *Cancer* 32:767, 1975.

330. Yagoda A, Mukherji B, Young C, et al: Bleomycin, an anti-tumor antibiotic. *Ann Intern Med* 77:861, 1972.

331. Levi JA, Diggs CH, Wiernik PH: Adriamycin therapy in advanced mycosis fungoides. *Cancer* 39:1967, 1977.

332. Grozea PN, Jones SE, McKelvey EM, Coltman CA Jr, Fisher R, Haskins CL: Combination chemotherapy for mycosis fungoides: a Southwest Oncology Group Study. *Cancer Treat Rep* 63:647, 1979.

333. Leavell UW Jr, DeSimone P: Combined chemotherapy (COP), in treatment of mycosis fungoides: report of four cases. *South Med J* 69:915, 1976.

334. Price NM, Hoppe RT, Constantine VS, Fuks ZY, Farber EM: The treatment of mycosis fungoides: adjuvant topical mechlorethamine after electron beam therapy. *Cancer* 40:2851, 1977.

335. Winkler CF, Sausville EA, Ihde DC, et al: Combined modality treatment of cutaneous T-cell lymphoma: results of a 6 year follow-up. *J Clin Oncol* 4:1094, 1986.

336. Kaye F, Eddy J, Ohde DC, et al: Conservative vs aggressive therapy in mycosis fungoides. *Proc ASCO* 8:257, 1989.

337. Bunn PA Jr, Ihde DC, Foon KA: The role recombinant leukocyte A interferon in the therapy of cutaneous T-cell lymphomas. *Cancer* 57:1315, 1986.

338. Kessler JF, Meyskens FL Jr, Levine N, Lynch PJ, Jones SE: Treatment of cutaneous T-cell lymphoma (mycosis fungoides) with 13-cis-retinoic acid. *Lancet* 1:1345, 1983.

339. Edelson R, Facktor M, Andrews A, Lutzner M, Schein P: Successful management of the Sezary syndrome: mobilization and removal of extravascular neoplastic T-cells by leukapheresis. *N Engl J Med* 291:293, 1974.

340. Edelson R, Berger C, Gasparro F, et al: Treatment of cutaneous T-cell lymphoma by extracorporeal photochemotherapy: preliminary results. *N Engl J Med* 316:297, 1987.

341. Bisccia ER, Grever MR, Scarborough DA, et al: 2-deoxycoformycin (CDF) induced remission in advanced cutaneous T-cell lymphomas (CTCL). *Proc Am Soc Clin Oncol* (abstract) 18:158, 1982.

342. Saven A, Carrera CJ, Beutler E, Piro LD: 2-Chlorodeoxyadenosine: an active agent in the treatment of cutaneous T-cell lymphoma. *Blood* 80:587, 1992.

343. Kuzel TM, Hurria A, Samuelson E, et al: Phase II trial of 2-chlorodeoxyadenosine for the treatment of cutaneous T-cell lymphoma. *Blood* 87:906, 1996.

344. Miller RA, Oseroff AR, Stratte PT, Levy R: Monoclonal antibody therapeutic trials in seven patients with T-cell lymphoma. *Blood* 62:988, 1983.

345. Rosen S, Zimmer AM, Goldman-Neiken R, et al: Radioimmunodetection and radioimmunotherapy antibody; an Illinois Cancer Council Study. *J Clin Oncol* 5:562, 1987.

346. Lennert K: *Zur Histologischen Diagnose der Lymphogranulomatose.* Frankfurt, FRG, Habil-Schrift, 1952.

347. Lennert K, Mestdeagh J: Hodgkin's disease with constantly high content of epithelioid cells. *Virchows Arch* (B) 344:1, 1968.

348. Kim H, Jacobs C, Warnke RA, Dorfman RF: Malignant lymphoma with a high content of epithelioid histiocytes: a distinct clinicopathologic entity and a form of so-called Lennert's lymphoma. *Cancer* 41:620, 1978.

349. Feller AC, Griesser GH, Mak TW, Lennert K: Lymphoepithelioid lymphoma (Lennert's lymphoma) is a monoclonal proliferation of helper/inducer T cells. *Blood* 68:663, 1986.

350. Stonesifer KJ, Benson NA, Ryden SE, Pawliger DF, Braylan RC: The malignant cells in a Lennert's lymphoma are T lymphocytes with a mature helper surface phenotype. A multiparameter flow cytometric analysis. *Blood* 68:426, 1986.

351. Godde-Salz E: Aberrations of chromosome 3, a marker of T-cell lymphomas? *J Genet Hum* 31:39, 1983.

352. Godde-Salz E, Feller AC, Lennert K: Cytogenetic and immunohistochemical analysis of lympho-epitheloid cell lymphoma (Lennert's lymphoma): Further substantiation of its T-cell nature. *Leuk Res* 10:313, 1985.

353. Liebow AA, Carrington CB, Friedman RJ: Lymphomatoid granulomatosis. *Hum Pathol* 3:457, 1972.

354. Eichel BS, Harrison EG Jr, Devine KD, Scanlon PW, Brown HA: Primary lymphoma of the nose including a relationship to lethal midline granuloma. *Am J Surg* 112:597, 1966.

355. Medeiros LJ, Jaffe ES, Chen Y-Y, Weiss LM: Localization of Epstein-Barr viral genomes in angiocentric immunoproliferative lesions. *Am J Surg Pathol* 16:439, 1992.

356. Medeiros LJ, Peiper SC, Elwood L, Yano T, Raffeld M, Jaffe ES: Angiocentric immunoproliferative lesions: a molecular analysis of eight cases. *Hum Pathol* 22:1150, 1991.

357. Lipford EH, Margolick JB, Longo DL, Fauci AS, Jaffe ES: Angiocentric immunoproliferative lesions: a clinicopathologic spectrum of post-thymic T-cell proliferations. *Blood* 72:1674, 1988.

358. Tsai T-F, Su I-J, Lu Y-C, et al: Cutaneous angiocentric T-cell lymphoma associated with Epstein-Barr virus. *J Am Acad Dermatol* 26:31, 1992.

359. Frizzera G, Kaneko Y, Saturai M: Angioimmunoblastic lymphadenopathy and related disorders: a retrospective look in search of definitions. *Leukemia* 3:1, 1989.

360. Weiss LM, Strickler JG, Dorfman RF, Horning SJ, Warnke RA, Sklar J: Clonal T cell populations in angioimmunoblastic lymphadenopathy and angioimmunoblastic lymphadenopathy-like lymphoma. *Am J Pathol* 122:392, 1986.

361. Griesser H, Feller AC, Lennert K, Minden M, Mak TW: Rearrangement of the beta-chain of the T cell antigen receptor and immunoglobulin genes in lymphoproliferative disorders. *J Clin Invest* 78:1179, 1986.

362. Tobiani K, Minato K, Ohtsu T, et al: Clinicopathologic, immunophenotypic and immunogenotypic analyses of immunoblastic lymphadenopathy-like T-cell lymphoma. *Blood* 72:1000, 1988.

363. Kaneko Y, Maseki N, Sakurai M, et al: Characteristic karyotypic pattern in T-cell lymphoproliferative disorders with reactive "angioimmunoblastic lymphadenopathy with dysproteinemia-type" features. *Blood* 72:413–421, 1988.

364. Schlegelberger B, Feller A, Godde-Satz E, Grote W, Lennert K: Stepwise development of chromosomal abnormalities in angioimmunoblastic lymphadenopathy (AILD). *Cancer Genet Cytogenet* 50:15, 1990.

365. Weiss LM, Jaffe ES, Liu X-F, Chen YY, Shibata D, Medeiros LJ: Detection and localization of Epstein-Barr viral genomes in angioimmunoblastic lymphadenopathy and angioimmunoblastic lymphadenopathy-like lymphoma. *Blood* 79:1789, 1992.

366. Siegert W, Agthe A, Griesser H, et al: Treatment of angioimmunoblastic lymphadenopathy (AILD)-type T-cell lymphoma using prednisone with or without the COPBLAM/IMVP-16 regimen. *Ann Intern Med* 117:364, 1992.

367. Pangalis GA, Moran EM, Nathwani BN, Zelman RJ, Kim H, Rappaport H: Angioimmunoblastic lymphoadenopathy, long-term follow-up study. *Cancer* 52:318, 1983.

368. Isaacson P, Spencer J, Connolly C, et al: Malignant histiocytosis of the intestine: a T-cell lymphoma. *Lancet* 2:688, 1985.

369. Stein H, Mason DY, Gerdes J, et al: The expression of the Hodgkin's disease associated antigen Ki-1 in reactive and neoplastic lymphoid tissue: evidence that Reed-Sternberg cells and histiocytic malignancies are derived from activated lymphoid cells. *Blood* 66:848, 1985.

370. Agnarsson BA, Kadin ME: Ki-1 positive large cell lymphoma. A morphologic and immunologic study of 19 cases. *Am J Surg Pathol* 12:264, 1988.

371. Delsol G, Al Saati T, Gatter K, et al: Coexpression of epithelial membrane antigen (EMA), Ki-1, and interleukin-2 receptor by anaplastic large cell lymphomas: diagnostic value in so-called malignant histiocytosis. *Am J Pathol* 130:59, 1988.

372. Zinzani PL, Bendandi M, Martelli M, et al: Anaplastic large-cell lymphoma: clinical and prognostic evaluation of 90 adult patients. *J Clin Oncol* 14:955, 1996.

373. Tilly H, Gaulard P, Lepage E, et al: Primary anaplastic large-cell lymphoma in adults: clinical presentation, immunophenotype, and outcome. *Blood* 90:3727, 1997.

374. Filippa DA, Ladanyi M, Wollner N, et al: CD30 (Ki-1)-positive malignant lymphomas: clinical, immunophenotypic, histologic and genetic characteristics and differences with Hodgkin's disease. *Blood* 87:2905, 1996.

375. Morris SW, Kirstein MN, Valentine MB, et al: Fusion of a kinase gene

376. Morris S, Kirstein M, Valentine M, et al: Fusion of a kinase gene, ALK, to a nucleolar protein gene, NPM, in non-Hodgkin's lymphoma. *Science* 263:1282, 1994.

377. Lopategui JR, Sun L-H, Chan JKC, et al: Low frequency association of the t(2;5)(p23;q35) chromosomal translocation with CD30+ lymphomas from American and Asian patients. *Am J Pathol* 146:323, 1995.

378. Downing JR, Shurtleff SA, Zielenska M, et al: Molecular detection of the (2;5) translocation of non-Hodgkin's lymphoma by reverse transcriptase polymerase chain reaction. *Blood* 85:3416, 1995.

379. DeCoteau JF, Butmarc JR, Kinney MC, Kadin ME: The t(2;5) chromosomal translocation is not a common feature of primary cutaneous CD30+ lymphoproliferative disorders: comparison with anaplastic large-cell lymphoma of nodal origin. *Blood* 87:3437, 1996.

380. Bernard A, Boumsell L, Reinherz L, et al: Cell surface characterization of malignant T-cells from lymphoblastic lymphoma using monoclonal antibodies: evidence for phenotypic differences between malignant T-cells from patients with acute lymphoblastic leukemia and lymphoblastic lymphoma. *Blood* 57:1105, 1981.

381. Weiss L, Bindl J, Picozzi V, Link M, Warnke R: Lymphoblastic lymphoma: an immunophenotype study of 26 cases with comparison to T-cell acute lymphoblastic leukemia. *Blood* 67:474, 1986.

382. Sheibani K, Nathwani B, Winberg C: Antigenically defined subgroups of lymphoblastic lymphoma: relationship to clinical presentation and biological behavior. *Cancer* 60:183, 1987.

383. Falini B, Flenghi L, Fagioli M, et al: T-lymphoblastic lymphomas expressing the non-disulfide-linked form of the T-cell receptors. *Blood* 74:2501, 1989.

384. Nathwani B, Diamond L, Winberg C, et al: Lymphoblastic lymphoma: a clinicopathologic study of 95 patients. *Cancer* 48:2347, 1981.

385. Uchiyama T, Yodoi J, Sagawa K, Takatsuki K, Uchino H: Adult T-cell leukemia: clinical and hematologic features of 16 cases. *Blood* 50:481, 1977.

386. Bunn PA, Schechter GP, Jaffe E, et al: Clinical course of retrovirus associated adult T-cell lymphoma in the United States: staging, evaluation and management. *N Engl J Med* 309:257, 1983.

387. Catovsky D, Greaves MF, Rose M, et al: Adult T-cell lymphoma/leukemia in blacks from the West Indies. *Lancet* 1:639, 1982.

388. Bunn PA: Clinical features, in T-cell lymphoproliferative syndrome associated with human T-cell leukemia/lymphoma virus. *Ann Intern Med* 100:543, 1984.

389. Blattner WA, Kalyanaraman VS, Robert-Guroff M, et al: The human type-C retrovirus HTLV, in blacks from the Caribbean region, and relationship to adult T-cell leukemia/lymphoma. *Int J Cancer Cancer* 30:257, 1982.

390. Popovic M, Sarin PS, Robert-Guroff M, et al: Isolation and transmission of human retrovirus (human T-cell leukemia virus). *Science* 219:856, 1983.

391. Kinoshita K, Amagasaki P, Ikedas S, et al: Preleukemic state of adult T-cell leukemia: abnormal T-lymphocytosis induced by human T-cell leukemia-lymphoma virus. *Blood* 66:120, 1985.

392. Posner LE, Robert-Guroff M, Kalyanaraman VS, et al: Natural antibodies to the human T-cell lymphoma virus in patients with T-cell lymphomas. *J Exp Med* 154:333, 1981.

393. Kalyanaraman VS, Sarngadharan MG, Bunn PA, Minna JD, Gallo RC: Antibodies in human sera reactive against an internal structural protein of human T-cell lymphoma virus. *Nature* 294:271, 1981.

394. Greenberg SJ, Tendler CL, Manns A, et al: Altered cellular gene expression in human retroviral-associated leukemogenesis. *Hum Retrovirol* (in press).

395. Wong-Staal F, Gallo RC: The family of human T-lymphotropic leukemia viruses: HTLV-I as the cause of adult T cell leukemia and HTLV-III as the cause of acquired immunodeficiency syndrome. *Blood* 65:253–263,1985.

396. Blattner WA, Clark JW, Gibbs WN, et al: Human T cell leukemia/lymphoma virus: epidemiology and relationship to human malignancy, in *Human T-Cell Leukemia/Lymphoma Virus*, edited by RC Gallo, M Essex, L Gros, p 267. Cold Spring Harbor Laboratory, Cold Spring Harbor, New York, 1984.

397. Saxinger W, Blattner WA, Levine PH, et al: Human T-cell leukemia virus (HTLV-I) antibodies in Africa. *Science* 225:1473, 1984.

398. Robert-Guroff M, Kalyanaraman VS, Blattner WA, et al: Evidence for human T-cell lymphoma-leukemia virus infection of family members of human T cell lymphoma-leukemia virus positive T-cell leukemia-lymphoma patients. *J Exp Med* 157:248, 1983.

399. Sarin PS, Aoki T, Shibata A, et al: High incidence of human type-C retrovirus (HTLV) in family members of a HTLV-positive Japanese T-cell leukemia patient. *Proc Natl Acad Sci USA* 80:2370, 1983.

400. Shimoyama M: Diagnostic criteria and classification of clinical subtypes of adult T-cell leukemia-lymphoma: a report from the Lymphoma Study Group [1984–87]. *Br J Haematol* 79:428, 1991.

401. Waldmann TA, Greene WC, Sarin PS, et al: Functional and phenotypic comparison of human T-cell leukemia/lymphoma virus positive adult T-cell leukemia with human T-cell leukemia/lymphoma virus negative Sezary leukemia, and their distinction using anti-tac. *J Clin Invest* 73:1711, 1984.

402. Flug F, Pelicci PG, Bonetti F, Knowles DM II, Dalla-Favera R: T-cell receptor gene rearrangements as markers of lineage and clonality in T-cell neoplasms. *Proc Natl Acad Sci* 82:3460, 1984.

403. Waldmann TA, David MM, Bongiovanni KF, Korsmeyer SJ: Re-arrangements of genes for the antigen receptor on T-cells as markers of lineage and clonality in human lymphoid neoplasms. *N Engl J Med* 313:776, 1985.

404. Bertness V, Lirsch I, Hollis G, Johnson B, Bunn PA Jr: T-cell receptor gene arrangements as clinical markers of human T-cell lymphomas. *N Engl J Med* 313:534, 1985.

405. Aisenberg AC, Krontiris TG, Mak TW, Wilkes BM: Rearrangement of the gene for the beta-chain of the T-cell receptor in T-cell chronic lymphocytic leukemia and related disorders. *N Engl J Med* 313:530, 1985.

406. Sanada I, Tanaka R, Kumagai E, et al: Chromosomal aberrations in adult T-cell leukemia:relationship to the clinical severity. *Blood* 65:649, 1985.

407. Verma RS, Macera MJ, Krishnamurthy M, Abramson J, Kapelner S, Dosik H: Chromosomal abnormalities in adult T-cell leukemia/lymphoma (ATL). *J Cancer Res Clin Oncol* 113:892, 1985.

408. Miyamoto K, Tomita N, Ishii A, et al: Specific abnormalities of chromosome 14 in patients with acute type of adult T-cell leukemia/lymphoma. *Int J Cancer Cancer* 40:461, 1987.

409. Shiraishi Y, Taguchi T, Kubonishi I, Taguchi H, Miyoshi I: Chromosome abnormalities, sister chromatid exchanges, and cell cycle analysis in phytohemagglutinin-stimulated adult T cell leukemia lymphocytes. *Cancer Genet Cytogenet* 15:65, 1985.

410. Whang-Peng J, Bunn PA, Knutsen T, et al: Cytogenetic studies in human T-cell lymphoma virus (HTLV)-positive leukemia-lymphoma in the United States. *J Natl Cancer Inst* 74:357, 1985.

411. Shimoyama M, Abe T, Miyamoto K, et al: Chromosome aberrations and clinical features of adult T-cell leukemia-lymphoma not associated with human T-cell leukemia virus type I. *Blood* 69:984, 1987.

412. Brito-Babpulle V, Matutes E, Parreira L, Catovsky D: Abnormalities of chromosome 7q and Tac expression in T-cell leukemia. *Blood* 67:516, 1986.

413. Waldmann TA, Goldman CK, Bongiovanni KF, et al: Therapy of patients with human T-cell lymphotrophic virus I-induced adult T-cell leukemia with anti-Tac, a monoclonal antibody to the receptor for interleukin-2. *Blood* 72:1805, 1988.

414. Waldmann TA, White JD, Carrasquillo JA, et al: Radioimmunotherapy of interleukin-2R α-expressing adult T-cell leukemia with Yttrium-90-labeled Anti-Tac. *Blood* 86:4063, 1995.

415. Tamura K, Makino S, Araki Y, Imamura T, Seita M: Recombinant interferon beta and gamma in the treatment of adult T-cell leukemia. *Cancer* 59:1069, 1987.

416. Saigo K, Shiozawa S, Shiozawa K, et al: Alpha-interferon treatment for adult T-cell leukemia: low levels of circulating alpha-interferon and its clinical effectiveness. *Blut* 56:83, 1988.

417. Daenen R, Rojer A, Smit JW, Halie MR, Nieweg HO: Successful chemotherapy with deoxycoformycin in adult T-cell lymphoma-leukaemia. *Br J Haematol* 58:7237, 1984.

418. Gill PS, Harrington W Jr, Kaplan MH, et al: Treatment of adult T-cell leukemia-lymphoma with a combination of interferon alfa and zidovudine. *N Engl J Med* 332:1744, 1995.

419. Hermine O, Bouscary D, Gessain A, et al: Brief report: treatment of adult T-cell leukemia-lymphoma with zidovudine and interferon alfa. *N Engl J Med* 332:1749, 1995.

420. Yamaguchi K, Nishimura H, Kohrogi H, Jono M, Miyamoto Y, Takatsuki K: A proposal for smoldering adult T-cell leukemia: a clinicopathologic study of five cases. *Blood* 62:758, 1983.

PLASMA CELL NEOPLASMS: GENERAL CONSIDERATIONS

STEPHEN M. BAIRD

Plasma cell neoplasms are monoclonal tumors of plasma cells and their precursors. It is important to distinguish these conditions from conditions that are considered benign and that do not require specific therapy. Although monoclonal immunoglobulin protein generally is detected in plasma cell myeloma, other conditions also may result in the production of a relative excess of monoclonal immunoglobulin. This chapter summarizes the laboratory studies that are used to evaluate for monoclonal proteinemia or monoclonal immunoglobulin gene rearrangements. This chapter also delineates laboratory features that can be used to distinguish plasma cell myeloma from related conditions that may give rise to a relative excess of monoclonal immunoglobulin. This chapter provides references to relevant chapters in the textbook that focus on a particular plasma cell or B-cell disorder.

DEFINITION AND HISTORY

PLASMA CELL NEOPLASMS

Plasma cell neoplasms are monoclonal tumors comprised of plasma cells and their precursors. All the differentiated cells within such a neoplasm produce the same whole immunoglobulin chain or chain fragment. In a given neoplasm the monoclonal proteins generally have the same heavy-chain class (γ, α, μ, δ, or ε), same light-chain (κ or λ), and same idiotypes (or antigenic determinants of the immunoglobulin variable regions, see Chap. 83).[1] The neoplastic plasma cells and their precursor small lymphocytes have the same immunoglobulin gene rearrangements and chromosomal anomalies, if any are present.[2–5] Since Henry Bence Jones first discovered what turned out to be monoclonal light chains in the urine of multiple myeloma patients 150 years ago,[6] the monoclonal immunoglobulin molecules (or their constituent chains) produced by plasma cell neoplasms have remained the best examples of tumor-specific antigens in the entire field of oncology. These proteins are usually called *M* proteins, which at various times in history has stood for *malignant, myeloma,* and now, *monoclonal* proteins. The diseases associated with M proteins are listed in Table 104-1. Some are benign and nonprogressive, while some are frankly malignant.

ESSENTIAL MONOCLONAL GAMMOPATHY

The term *benign* must be used with caution when describing monoclonal gammopathies in patients who do not have overt malignant

plasmacytoma or multiple myeloma. Clinical and laboratory features consistent with essential monoclonal gammopathy are an M protein level less than 2.5 g/dl, few or no monoclonal light chains in the urine, and no anemia or change in serum calcium (Table 104-2). There are no bony lesions on skeletal surveys, and the plasmacytosis in the marrow, if present, is less than 30 percent.[12,13] The concept that this condition is benign is based on its generally indolent biologic behavior. However, a low but significant percentage of patients with monoclonal gammopathy develop frank B-cell malignancies each year.[7–11] For this reason, the term *benign monoclonal gammopathy* largely has been replaced by the term *essential monoclonal gammopathy* (see Chap. 105).

CHRONIC COLD AGGLUTININ SYNDROME

Chronic cold agglutinin syndrome is a disease in which elderly patients produce a monoclonal IgM molecule that binds red blood cells and causes their agglutination at temperatures significantly below 37°C (98.6°F) (see Chap. 56). It may be seen in patients without other apparent evidence of malignant disease, in patients with lymphoma (see Chap. 103), or in patients with Waldenström macroglobulinemia (see Chap. 108). The apparently benign form of the disease also may progress to malignancy.[19,20] This disorder bears no relationship to acute, postinfectious cold agglutinin syndrome, in which the offending immunoglobulins are polyclonal and disappear after the inciting infectious agent is eradicated.

CRYOGLOBULINS

Cryoglobulins are complexes of immunoglobulins that precipitate on exposure to cold (see Chap. 108).[21] Three classes of cryoglobulins have been recognized for convenience of description. *Type 1 cryoglobulins* are monoclonal IgM, IgG, or IgA molecules. *Type 2 cryoglobulins* are monoclonal immunoglobulins, usually of the IgM class, with antibody activity against other immunoglobulins, usually IgG. An association of type 2 cryoglobulins with hepatitis B and C infection has been reported.[21–23] *Type 3 cryoglobulins* are composed of polyclonal immunoglobulins with anti-immunoglobulin activity. Cryoglobulins may cause a variety of pathologic conditions, all related to the formation of immune complexes and the attendant inflammation and coagulation disorders. They are detected by allowing serum to stand and precipitate at 4°C (39.2°F) for 24 to 72 h.

TRANSIENT M PROTEINS

Transient M proteins occasionally may be associated with inflammation (see Chap. 105).[24–26] Molecules also have been described in hyperimmunized laboratory animals. They do not progress to malignant disease and are not always high-affinity antibodies to the presumed cause of inflammation or experimental immunogen.

Patients with any of a variety of congenital immunodeficiencies in which the T-cell arm of immunity is more affected than the B-cell arm may develop transient, low-level monoclonal gammopathies, typically of the IgM class (see Chap. 105). These have become apparent as more-sensitive techniques for their detection have been developed. Immunodeficient patients receiving marrow transplants also frequently exhibit a transient monoclonal gammopathy early in their posttransplant course.[27,28] If the patient or donor is infected with Epstein-Barr virus (EBV), the gammopathy may be oligoclonal and herald the development of an EBV-driven lymphoproliferative disorder that may be fatal.

The incidence of multiple myeloma in individuals over 25 years of age is about 30 per 100,000. The incidence of monoclonal gammopathy is about 100 times as high, and the transient monoclonal gammopa-

TABLE 104-1   DISEASES ASSOCIATED WITH M PROTEINS

DISEASE	REFERENCE
Benign	
Essential monoclonal gammopathy	Chapter 105
Chronic cold agglutinin syndrome	Chapter 56
Transient (after inflammation)	Chapter 105
Transient (after marrow transplant)	Chapter 18
Immunodeficiency (see particularly T cell)	Chapter 89
Neoplastic	
Plasma cell myeloma	Chapter 106
Neoplasms producing γ, α, μ, δ, or ε heavy chains and either κ or λ light chains	
Neoplasms producing only κ or λ light chains	
Neoplasms that do not make detectable immunoglobulin	
Neoplasms causing amyloidosis or light-chain deposition in tissues	Chapter 107
Neoplasms causing dermatologic lesions	
Waldenström macroglobulinemia	Chapter 108
Heavy-chain disease: α, γ, μ, or rarely δ, but no light chains	Chapter 109
Chronic lymphocytic leukemia and related lymphomas	Chapter 98

thies associated with all the various forms of inflammation and immunodeficiency are about 400 times more frequent.[15] All rise dramatically with age. The monoclonal gammopathies in immunodeficient hosts occur at a much younger age than multiple myeloma or monoclonal gammopathy.

ETIOLOGY AND PATHOGENESIS

GENETIC BACKGROUND

In the mouse, the genetic background of the animal is an important risk factor for developing monoclonal gammopathy or plasmacytomas. About 60 percent of C57BL/Ka mice develop M proteins of the IgM class by 21 months of age. Also, about 40 percent of C3H and NZB mice develop M proteins of the IgM class. However, BALB/c and CBA/Kij strains have a very low incidence of spontaneous plasma cell neoplasm.[14] Surprisingly, mice of the BALB/c strain are most susceptible to developing plasmacytomas following repeated intraperitoneal injections of mineral oil. NZB mice also are fairly susceptible to the induction of plasmacytomas by this method. However, C57BL/Ka mice are resistant.[29]

Human families with a high incidence of plasma cell neoplasms also have been reported.[30,31] No consistent genetic aberrations have been described in these families. Multiple myeloma also occurs more frequently in relatives of patients with the disease than in the general population.[32,33] In the United States, African Americans have a higher incidence of multiple myeloma than Caucasians.[34] All these observa-

tions indicate that the genetic background of the host is an important risk factor for the development of plasma cell neoplasms in mammals.

There have been numerous attempts to induce plasmacytomas that secrete antibodies to specific antigens in BALB/c mice. Such animals were hyperimmunized with any one of a variety of antigens in mineral oil. Although plasmacytomas arose, they virtually never made antibodies reactive with the injected antigen.[35] Thus, there is no apparent relationship between chronic antigenic stimulation and the development of plasma cell neoplasms in these animals. However, this is not the case with Aleutian minks infected with the Aleutian disease virus.[36] Many of these animals develop M proteins consisting of antibodies that bind specifically to the infecting virus. In humans, there is no consistent relationship between prior inflammatory disease and subsequent development of a plasma cell neoplasm. However, monoclonal gammopathies have been described to occur at increased frequency in patients with inflammatory and autoimmune diseases.[24,25,37–39]

CHROMOSOMAL ANOMALIES

About 90 percent of mouse plasmacytomas induced by mineral oil in mice show consistent chromosomal anomalies.[40] In these the c-myc gene on mouse chromosome 15 is fused with either the immunoglobulin heavy-chain locus on mouse chromosome 12 or the immunoglobulin κ light-chain locus on mouse chromosome 6.[40,41] The fusion of c-myc with an immunoglobulin heavy- or light-chain locus resembles the typical chromosomal anomalies seen in human Burkitt lymphoma.[42] However, the biologic behaviors of murine plasmacytomas and human Burkitt lymphoma are radically different, and no virus (such as EBV) has been associated with murine or human plasmacytomas.

Certain chromosomal abnormalities in neoplastic cells may be seen repeatedly in patients with multiple myeloma or plasma cell leukemia (a late, preterminal stage of multiple myeloma) (see Chap. 106).[43] Additions to the long arm of chromosome 14 ($14q^+$) have been described in 30 to 50 percent of multiple myeloma patients. Often the donated material is from chromosome 11, generating a t(11;14) (q13;q32).[44] Multiple myeloma and plasma cell leukemia cells also may have abnormalities of chromosome 1 in about 50 to 70 percent of the cases. These anomalies are highly variable, though, and no consistent deletions, additions, or translocations have been found. Finally, rare patients have deletions of chromosome 22 in the region of the immunoglobulin λ light-chain locus. Interestingly, chromosomal anomalies associated with the immunoglobulin κ light-chain region on chromosome 2 have not been described in humans, even though about two-thirds of M proteins express κ light chains.

Patients with trisomies of chromosomes 6, 9, and 17 tend to have prolonged survival while patients with monosomy 13 (loss of Rb) have shortened survival[66] (see Chap. 106). However, cytogenetic studies are not normally performed on multiple myeloma patients. Because neoplastic plasma cells or their precursors often divide relatively slowly, the inability to find an abnormal karyotype in some biopsy specimens merely may reflect the fact that only normal hematopoietic cells were induced into metaphase. Therefore, negative results may be false negatives.

CYTOKINES

Interleukin-6 (IL-6) is a potent stimulator of plasmacytoma growth.[45–49] In cultures of freshly isolated marrow cells from patients with multiple myeloma, IL-6 is produced predomi-

TABLE 104-2   SOME BIOLOGICAL FEATURES OF MONOCLONAL GAMMOPATHY

	MULTIPLE MYELOMA	MONOCLONAL GAMMOPATHY	IMMUNODEFICIENCY
Clonal size	Large	Medium	Small
Immunoglobulin production	>25 mg/ml	<25 mg/ml	<2.5 mg/ml
Proliferation	Progressive	Persistent	Transient
Abnormal immunoglobulin structure	Frequent	Rare	Never
Bone destruction	Frequent	Never	Never
Mouse models:			
Transformed clone	+	+	−
Transplantable generations	<4	−	
Autonomous growth	+	+?	
Immortality	+	−	−

SOURCE: Modified from Radl.[15]

nantly by monocytoid cells and fibroblasts. With time in culture, the myeloma cells themselves may produce IL-6, which in turn may stimulate plasma cell growth in vitro. IL-6 may play such a role in patients with multiple myeloma. In one study, injected monoclonal antibodies to IL-6 significantly inhibited tumor cell growth in vivo.[48] In addition, other cytokines, such as granulocyte-monocyte colony stimulating factor (GM-CSF), IL-3, IL-1, or low-dose interferon alpha (IFN-α), may synergize with IL-6 to stimulate the growth of plasmacytomas. Kaposi's sarcoma-associated herpesvirus (KSHV) has been found in bone marrow dendritic cells of patients with multiple myeloma and occasionally in patients with MGUS. KSHV-encoded IL-6 was shown to be transcribed in these bone marrow dendritic cells.[67] Malignant precursors of myeloma cells appear to adhere to these dendritic cells.[68] Finally, rearrangements of the IL-6 receptor gene in myeloma cells also have been described, in at least one case. As the tumor progresses, malignant cells may escape from their dependency on IL-6. None of these studies has related the effects of cytokines to the observed chromosomal anomalies prevalent in multiple myeloma. The gene for IL-1 is on chromosome 2q; IL-3 and GM-CSF are on 5q; IFN-α is on 9p; IFN-γ is on 12q; and IL-6 is on 7p.[44]

The malignant cells of multiple myeloma also produce other cytokines that contribute to the noted pathophysiology of this disease. *Multiple myeloma* means multiple tumors in the marrow. This term was adopted because patients with this disease often develop numerous tumors in the bone that can be detected radiographically as osteolytic lesions. These osteolytic lesions result in the weakening of the bone matrix and may lead to pathologic fractures. These lesions are produced by osteoclasts that are activated by cytokines released by the malignant plasma cells themselves. Formerly called *osteoclast activating factor* (OAF), it is now thought that the factor involved actually may be a combination of different cytokines, including IL-1, tumor necrosis factor-alpha (TNF-α), IL-5, TNF-β, and/or IL-6.[18,50,51]

LABORATORY FEATURES

SURFACE MARKERS

Cell marker studies have shown a great deal of lineage infidelity in multiple myeloma. Malignant B cells may express both early and late B-cell antigens along with antigens characteristic of granulocytes, monocytes, or megakaryocytes.[52–54] This has led some investigators to suggest that the transformed cell of multiple myeloma is really the marrow stem cell. However, lineage infidelity commonly is seen in marker studies of a variety of neoplasms. Such lineage infidelity may be reflective of dysregulation in the expression of cellular differentiation antigens secondary to malignant transformation. Nonetheless, it is probable that multiple myeloma is not a disease in which the transforming event occurs in mature plasma cells.

Cells resembling small lymphocytes may have the same immunoglobulin gene rearrangements, immunoglobulin idiotypes, and surface antigens as all malignant plasma cells.[52] As such, these neoplasms may be composed of transformed B cells that have retained their ability to mature into plasma cells. Thus myeloma contrasts with lymphocytic lymphomas which usually do not produce significant numbers of plasma cells. This may be analogous to the difference between chronic myelogenous leukemia, in which malignant cells may mature into segmented neutrophils, and acute myelogenous leukemia, in which very few do (see Chaps. 93 and 94). Indeed, in the spectrum of M-protein-producing disorders, we find tumors of small lymphocytes, such as CLL and small lymphocytic lymphoma, and tumors of plasmacytoid lymphocytes, such as Waldenström macroglobulinemia. These types of tumor usually produce IgM, whereas plasmacytomas usually produce IgG or IgA.

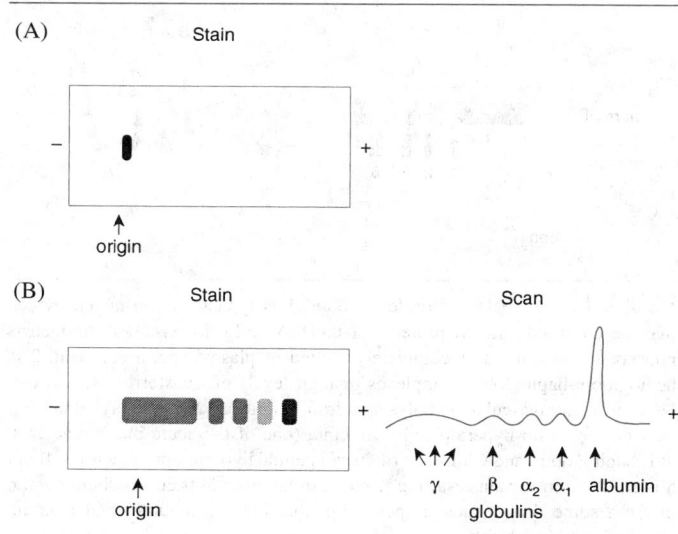

FIGURE 104-1   Normal serum electrophoresis. (*A*) Apply serum to support medium; (*B*) electrophoretically separate proteins, stain, observe, scan.

In the case of multiple myeloma, cells from a single transformed clone can have the morphology of a small lymphocyte, a lymphoblast, or a plasma cell. Although it is conventional to assume that a fully mature plasma cell cannot reenter the cycle of cell division, this has not been demonstrated rigorously in plasma cell neoplasms. In fact, on histologic sections of marrow from multiple myeloma patients, many plasma cells have nuclei with an immature chromatin pattern, rather than the highly condensed pattern of normal plasma cells. There also is an increased frequency of bi- or multinucleate cells. The ability to divide or incorporate tritiated thymidine into DNA are criteria that are quite useful in distinguishing "malignant" plasma cell neoplasms from "benign."[12,51] These criteria are not routinely used in the clinical laboratory because other, less expensive tests yield similar information.

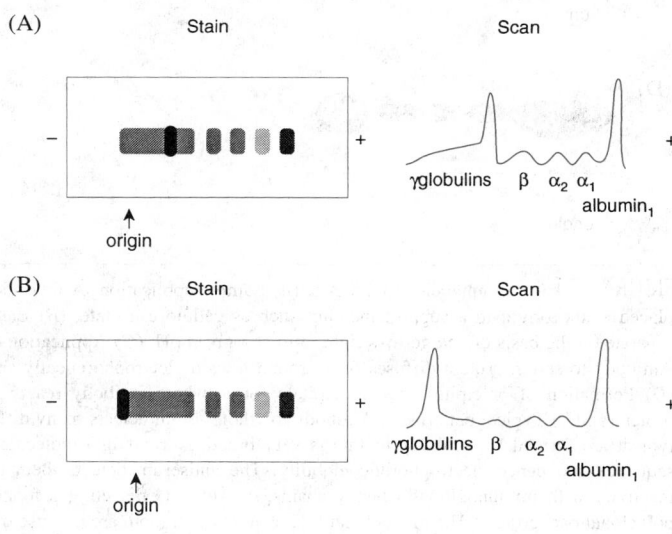

FIGURE 104-2   M protein electrophoresis. (*A*) Fast-moving M protein spike; (*B*) slow-moving M protein spike.

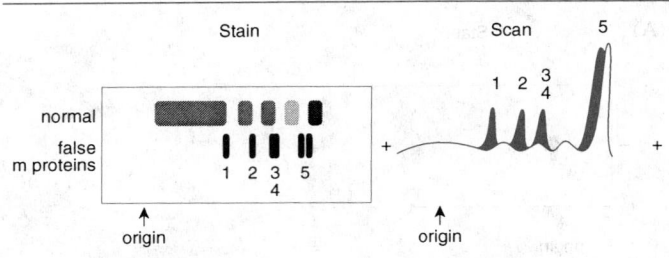

FIGURE 104-3 False M proteins. Band 1 is typical of fibrinogen, which may be confused with M proteins of the IgA or IgM class. If fibrinogen is present, the serum was incompletely clotted or plasma was used. Band 2 is hemoglobin-haptoglobin complexes or high levels of transferrin, which may be seen in intravascular hemolysis or iron deficiency respectively. Band 3/4 may be seen with hyperalphaglobulinemia (one of the acute phase reactants, as is haptoglobin) and with some of the congenital hyperlipoproteinemias. Band 5 is an albumin variant resulting from a rare autosomal trait, bisalbuminemia, or from some drugs, such as penicillin, that bind to albumin and alter its electrophoretic mobility.

ZONAL ELECTROPHORESIS

SERUM

The most common screening test for an M protein is serum electrophoresis. In this test, a few microliters of serum are spotted onto a support medium, such as cellulose acetate, that has been equilibrated at a basic pH. When an electric current is applied across the support medium, the proteins in the serum migrate toward the anode with a velocity proportional to the ratio of their negative charge to molecular weight. After a period of migration of about half an hour, depending on the precise conditions, the cellulose acetate is taken up, dried, immersed in a stain that detects proteins, such as Ponceau SX or Coomassie Blue, and examined by eye or densitometry. The procedure and typical results are illustrated in Fig. 104-1.

The most abundant protein in normal serum is albumin. This protein migrates as a sharp peak because, except in rare cases, all albumin molecules have exactly the same amino acid sequence and hence the same electrophoretic mobility. In contrast, the gamma globulins comprise immunoglobulins that have millions of different amino acid sequences and varying carbohydrate side chains. Consequently these proteins migrate in a very broad band that typically contains IgA and IgM in the front (toward the β globulins) and IgG spread through the entire range of globulins. IgD and IgE are normally secreted at such low levels that they are not detectable by this method. When a plasma cell neoplasm produces an M protein, the electrophoretic pattern is altered, as shown in Fig. 104-2.

A monoclonal immunoglobulin protein may migrate anywhere in the globulin region. IgM and IgA M proteins tend to migrate faster than most IgG molecules. Accordingly, the M protein in example 1 of Fig. 104-2 probably is an IgA or IgM, while the spike in example 2 probably is an IgG molecule. To distinguish these immunoglobulin classes with certainty requires either immunoelectrophoresis or immunofixation electrophoresis, which will be described later. False monoclonal proteins are illustrated in Fig. 104-3.

SPINAL FLUID AND URINE

Electrophoresis also can be performed on concentrated specimens of cerebrospinal fluid (CSF) or urine. Evaluation of the cerebrospinal fluid allows for detection of an M-protein-secreting plasmacytoma in the central nervous system. Evaluation of the urine is useful for detecting excessive and unbalanced synthesis of immunoglobulin molecules. Because the proteins larger than albumin (or 67 kDa) normally do not pass through the glomeruli, whole immunoglobulins ordinarily do not pass into the urine. However, free immunoglobulin light chains are only approximately 25 kDa and hence pass freely through the glomerulus. Patients with a circulating M protein who pass whole immunoglobulins in their urine generally have severe renal dysfunction, often due to renal amyloidosis secondary to deposition of immunoglobulin chains in the renal parenchyma.

When free light chains appear in the urine, they can be detected by sulfosalicylic acid precipitation, electrophoresis of concentrated urine, immunoelectrophoresis, or immunofixation electro-

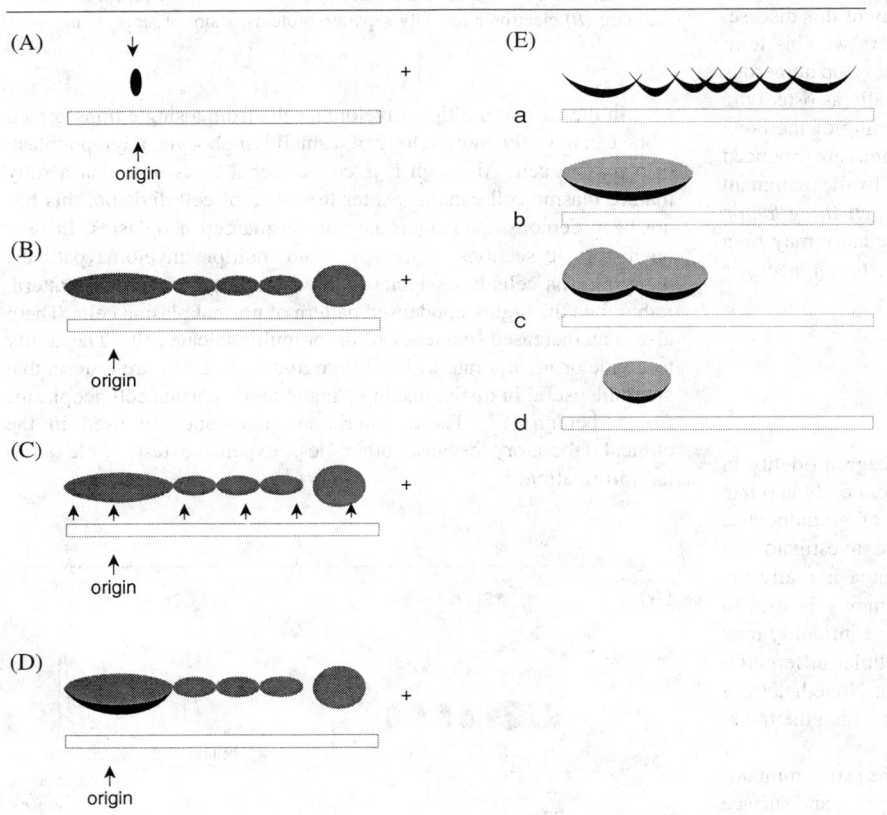

FIGURE 104-4 Immunoelectrophoresis. (A) Sample application. A few microliters of serum are placed at the origin in a support medium such as cellulose acetate. (B) Electrophoresis. Proteins separate on the basis of charge-to-weight ratio at a given pH. (C) Application of antibody in trough. Antibody to serum protein diffuses from trough toward electrophoretically size-separated proteins. (D) Formation of precipitin arcs. Precipitate forms where antibody reacts with antigenic serum protein(s). (E) Typical patterns: a, Antibody to whole serum detects many different proteins. b, The typical arc formed by antibody to IgG is very broad. Normal IgG molecules vary in amino acid sequence and hence electrophoretic mobility. The antiserum detects them all, due mostly to its reactivity with immunoglobulin heavy chains. c, Anti-IgG detecting a monoclonal IgG within a polyclonal background. The monoclonal IgG distorts the smooth arc because of its increased amount relative to that of other IgG species and its unique electrophoretic mobility. d, A monoclonal immunoglobulin heavy or light chain with no polyclonal background. The arc is narrower than the polyclonal pattern because of the unique electrophoretic mobility of the monoclonal proteins.

phoresis. These last two techniques also are useful for evaluation of whether the immunoglobulin light chains are only κ, λ, or both. The common urine dipstick relies on bromphenol blue, a dye that binds rather specifically to albumin.[55] Thus, dipsticks are not reliable screening tools for Bence Jones protein, and sulfosalicylic acid should be used.

Urine electrophoresis is one of the most important tools for the diagnosis and follow-up of patients with plasma cell neoplasms. The neoplastic B cells of many myeloma patients produce excess immunoglobulin light chain or light chain alone. When the amount of immunoglobulin light chain filtered through the glomeruli exceeds the resorption capacity of the proximal tubules, free light chains are excreted into the urine. The amount of light chain excreted in a fixed amount of time often is proportional to the amount of light chain produced, which in turn is proportional to the number of neoplastic plasma cells. Thus, serial measurements of the amount of immunoglobulin light chain excreted over time are a convenient way to follow tumor mass and the effects of therapy.

Measurements of immunoglobulin light chains in urine, however, do not always correlate with the rate of immunoglobulin light-chain production. Immunoglobulin light chains normally are reabsorbed and metabolized in the proximal tubules of the kidney. As renal damage progresses, the amount of light chains excreted in the urine increases, in part due to deteriorating renal function. For this reason, the best estimate of tumor cell mass in a patient with multiple myeloma is through the measurement of the M protein in the serum. However, mutations of tumor cells causing them to secrete less immunoglobulin, hydration of the patient, and renal disease also may influence the amount of serum M protein independent of tumor cell burden.

IMMUNOELECTROPHORESIS AND IMMUNOFIXATION ELECTROPHORESIS

The principles of immunoelectrophoresis and immunofixation electrophoresis are illustrated in Figs. 104-4 and 104-5 respectively. These techniques are useful for identifying the immunoglobulin heavy-chain class and light-chain type in putative M proteins.

Table 104-3 lists several clinical conditions that generally are associated with a serum protein abnormality that could be detected by electrophoresis, immunoelectrophoresis, or immunofixation electrophoresis. Note that these techniques are useful for detecting a variety of serum protein abnormalities other than M proteins.

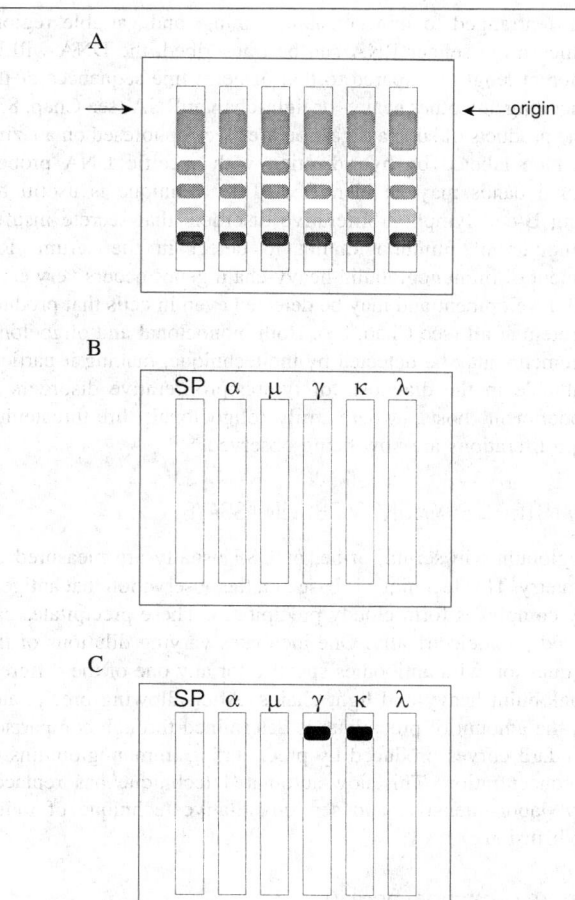

FIGURE 104-5   Immunofixation electrophoresis. (*a*) Serum samples are placed in each of several lanes of an agarose gel support medium for protein electrophoresis. (*b*) Overlay each lane with antiserum to a specific immunoglobulin heavy or light chain, typically anti-α, -μ, -γ, -κ, or -λ. Allow precipitation to occur. (*c*) Wash and stain. Only immunoprecipitates remain in the gel. Nonprecipitated proteins wash out. Results show an IgG$_\kappa$ M protein.

IMMUNOGLOBULIN GENE REARRANGEMENTS

The most specific means to determine whether a lymphoproliferative disorder is monoclonal is through analysis for immunoglobulin gene rearrangement. In the laboratory the most *common* technique is flow cytometry, looking for light-chain (κ or λ) restriction on tumor cells. Because B cells rearrange both immunoglobulin heavy- and light-chain genes to produce unique immunoglobulin genes, the detection of non-germ-line DNA immunoglobulin gene fragments following digestion with restriction endonucleases has become a common research technique (see Chap. 83). Genomic DNA isolated from a suspected B-cell neoplasm is digested with one or more restriction endonucleases that each cut DNA at specific recognition sequences. If the DNA between these target

TABLE 104-3   CLINICAL INDICATIONS FOR ELECTROPHORESIS OF SERUM AND URINE PROTEINS

CLINICAL INDICATIONS	ABNORMALITY AND INTERPRETATION
Unexplained edema or ascites	Hypoalbuminemia
Suspected liver disease	Hypoalbuminemia frequent; hyperglobulinemia suggests cirrhosis or chronic active hepatitis
Collagen diseases, sarcoidosis	Polyclonal hyperglobulinemia
Collagen diseases, sarcoidosis	Hypo- or agammaglobulinemia
CLL, malignant lymphoma	Hypogammaglobulinemia or, rarely, IgG or IgM M proteins
Unexplained proteinuria	Albumin or a mixture of all serum proteins found with urinary tract infections or the nephrotic syndrome; homogeneous urine proteins that migrate in the globulin region usually indicative of plasma cell neoplasms secreting free light or heavy chains
Evidence of plasma cell myeloma	Serum or urinary monoclonal neoplasms, e.g., bone pain, protein, with reduced normal immunoglobulins, frequent infections, elevated immunoglobulins and sedimentation rate, rouleaux, hypoalbuminemia, proteinuria, hyperviscosity, or osteolytic skeletal lesions
Amyloidosis	Monoclonal serum or urinary proteins frequent
Acquired clotting disorders	M proteins or amyloid bind to some clotting factors such as I, II, VIII, IX, X, and XI.
Acquired neuropathy	M proteins infiltrate peripheral nerves

sites has rearranged to join constant, joining, and variable regions from which a messenger RNA can be transcribed, the DNA will be of a different length compared to that of germ line sequences or the DNA encoding any other heavy- or light-chain mRNA (see Chap. 83). When the products of such a digestion are electrophoresed on a sizing gel and then labeled by hybridization with specific DNA probes, monoclonal bands may be identified. This technique is useful for evaluating B-cell lymphoproliferative disorders that secrete insufficient amounts of immunoglobulin to detect in the serum. Rearrangement of immunoglobulin heavy-chain genes occurs very early in B-cell development and may be detected even in cells that produce no M protein at all (see Chap. 83). Both monoclonal and oligoclonal rearrangements may be detected by the technique, making it particularly valuable in the diagnosis of lymphoproliferative disorders in immunodeficient hosts, where truly oligoclonal, life-threatening lymphoproliferations are now being observed.[56-58]

QUANTITATIVE IMMUNOGLOBULIN ASSAYS

Immunoglobulins in serum, urine, or CSF usually are measured by nephelometry. This technique is based on the observation that antigen-antibody complexes form cloudy precipitates. These precipitates can be detected photoelectrically. One incubates varying dilutions of the fluid in question with antibodies specific for any one of the different immunoglobulin heavy and light chains. After allowing precipitates to form, the amount of precipitate is determined through comparison with standard curves produced by precipitating immunoglobulins of known concentration. This now-automated technique has replaced the slow, labor-intensive, and semiquantitative technique of radial immunodiffusion.

SERUM β2-MICROGLOBULIN

β_2-Microglobulin is the light chain of class I molecules of the major histocompatibility complex (MHC). Class I molecules are present on essentially all nucleated cells, including lymphocytes and plasma cells. In rapidly dividing cell populations, membrane turnover leads to shedding of many molecules, including class I MHC. Because β_2-microglobulin is not covalently linked to its heavy chain, it is released into the extracellular fluid and the blood. Because its molecular weight is less than 12,000, it is filtered through the normal glomerulus. However, β_2-microglobulin is reabsorbed by normal proximal renal tubules and does not appear in significant quantities in the urine. In patients with plasma cell neoplasms, however, β_2-microglobulin increases in the serum due to increased neoplastic cell turnover. Also, as myeloma-protein-induced renal damage occurs, reduced glomerular filtration will increase serum β_2-microglobulin levels. Renal tubular dysfunction increases serum levels even further. Serum β_2-microglobulin therefore provides another parameter with which to monitor for neoplastic cell mass, cell turnover, effect on renal function, and response to treatment.[59-62]

SERUM VISCOSITY

Large molecules such as IgM pentamers or IgA dimers can increase serum viscosity significantly. Some IgG molecules, particularly those of the IgG3 subclass, also tend to aggregate and increase serum viscosity.[63] In vivo this can cause sludging of capillary flow and disturbances of vision, other central nervous system abnormalities, and some clotting disorders (see "Waldenstrom Macroglobulinemia," Chap. 108). In the laboratory, serum viscosity is measured as resistance to flow through standardized glass tubing compared to distilled water. The test is usually performed at room temperature, which is highly variable.

If a patient has cryoglobulins, which aggregate increasingly at temperatures below 37°C (98.6°F), then serum viscosity measurements should be performed at 37°C (98.6°F) to obtain clinically relevant information. The relative viscosity of normal serum ranges up to 1.8 times that of water. Patients usually do not experience clinical symptoms with serum viscosities of 4 or less.

AMYLOIDOSIS

The type of amyloidosis associated with plasma cell neoplasms is caused by the deposition of light chains or light-chain fragments in tissues (see Chap. 107). The name *amyloid,* meaning "starchlike," comes from the polysaccharide groups attached to immunoglobulin light- (and heavy-) chain molecules. Amyloid can deposit in any tissue and often has a predilection for packing in and around the walls of small blood vessels. Amyloid is best detected by tissue biopsy, often of the kidney, liver, rectum, oral cavity, heart, or skin. Tissue light-chain deposition has a regular order and binds dyes such as Congo red or Thioflavin B.[64] Under polarized light, or with a fluorescent microscope, these lesions have a characteristic appearance that permits one to establish the diagnosis. Amyloidosis may severely impair organ function and is a potentially serious complication of plasma cell neoplasms. One should also keep in mind that tissue amyloid deposits may interfere with hemostasis and complicate needle biopsies of internal organs.[65]

REFERENCES

1. Kubagawa H, Vogler LB, Capra JD, et al: Studies on the clonal origin of multiple myeloma: Use of individually specific (idiotype) antibodies to trace the oncogenic event to its earliest point of expression in B-cell differentiation. *J Exp Med* 150:792, 1979.
2. Berenson J, Wong R, Kim K, et al: Evidence of peripheral blood B lymphocyte but not T lymphocyte involvement in multiple myeloma. *Blood* 70:1550, 1987.
3. Lindstrom FD, Hardy WR, Eberle BJ, et al: Multiple myeloma and benign monoclonal gammopathy: Differentiation by immunofluorescence of lymphocytes. *Ann Intern Med* 78:837, 1973.
4. Ueshima Y, Rowley JD: Chromosome studies in patients with multiple myeloma and related paraproteinemias, in *Neoplastic Diseases of the Blood,* edited by PH Wiernick, GP Canellos, RA Kyle, et al, vol 1, pp 499–512. Churchill Livingstone, New York, 1985.
5. Lewis JP, MacKenzie MR: Non-random chromosome aberrations associated with multiple myeloma. *Hematol Oncol* 2:307, 1984.
6. Bence Jones H: Papers on Chemical Pathology, Lecture 3. *Lancet* 2:269, 1847.
7. Axelsson U, Backmann R, Hallen J: Frequency of pathological proteins (M-components) in 6995 sera from an adult population. *Acta Med Scand* 179:235, 1966.
8. Axelsson U: An eleven-year follow-up on 64 subjects with M-components. *Acta Med Scand* 201:173, 1977.
9. Kyle RA, Greipp PR: Monoclonal gammopathies of undetermined origin, in *Neoplastic Diseases of the Blood,* edited by PH Wiernick, GP Canellos, RA Kyle, et al, vol 2, pp 653–676. Churchill Livingstone, New York, 1985.
10. Hallen J: Frequency of "abnormal" serum globulins (M-components) in the aged. *Acta Med Scand* 173:737, 1963.
11. Englisova M, Englis M, Kyral V, et al: Changes of immunoglobulin synthesis in old people. *Exp Gerontol* 3:125, 1968.
12. Boccadoro M, Gavarotti P, Fossati G, et al: Low plasma cell ^{3}H-thymidine incorporation in monoclonal gammopathy of undetermined significance (MGUS), smouldering myeloma and remission phase myeloma: A reliable indicator of patients not requiring therapy. *Br J Haematol* 58:689, 1984.
13. Kyle RA: "Benign" monoclonal gammopathy: a misnomer? *JAMA* 251:1849, 1984.
14. Radl J, Hollander CF, Van Den Berg P, et al: Idiopathic paraproteinemia: I. Studies in an animal model—the aging C57BL/KaLwRij mouse. *Clin Exp Immunol* 33:395, 1978.

15. Radl J: Age-related monoclonal gammopathies: clinical lessions from the aging C57BL mouse. *Immunol Today* 11:234, 1990.

16. Dimopoulos MA, Goldstein J, Fuller L, et al: Curability of solitary bone plasmacytomas. *J Clin Oncol* 10:587, 1992.

17. Moulopoulos LA, Dimopoulos MA, Weber D, et al: Magnetic resonance imaging in the staging of solitary plasmacytoma of bone. *J Clin Oncol* 11:1311, 1993.

18. Barlogie B, Epstein J, Selvanayagam P, et al: Plasma cell myeloma: new biological insights and advances in therapy. *Blood* 73:865, 1989.

19. Frank M, Atkinson JP, Gadek J: Cold agglutinins and cold agglutinin disease. *Annu Rev Med* 28:291, 1977.

20. Crisp D, Pruzanski W: B cell neoplasms with homogeneous cold-reacting antibodies (cold agglutinins). *Am J Med* 72:915, 1982.

21. Brouet J, Clouvel JP, Danon F, et al: Biologic and clinical significance of cryoglobulins: A report of 86 cases. *Am J Med* 57:775, 1974.

22. De Bandt M, Ribard P, Meyer O, et al: Type II IgM monoclonal cryo-globulinemia and hepatitis C virus infection (letter). *Clin Exp Rheumatol* 9:659, 1991.

23. Gorevic PD, Kassab HJ, Levo Y, et al: Mixed cryoglobulinemia: clinical aspects and long-term follow-up of 40 patients. *Am J Med* 69:287, 1980.

24. Penny R, Hughes S: Repeated stimulation of the reticuloendothelial system and the development of plasma cell dyscrasias. *Lancet* 1:77, 1970.

25. Rosenblatt J, Hall CA: Plasma-cell dyscrasia followed prolonged stimulation of reticuloendothelial system. *Lancet* 1:301, 1970.

26. Turesson I, Rausing A: Gaucher's disease and benign monoclonal gammopathy. *Acta Med Scand* 197:507, 1975.

27. Fischer AM, Simon F, Le Deist F, et al: Prospective study of the occurrence of monoclonal gammopathies following bone marrow transplantation in young children. *Transplantation* 49:731, 1990.

28. Mitus AJ, Stein R, Rappeport JM, et al: Monoclonal and oligoclonal gammopathy after bone marrow transplantation. *Blood* 74:2764, 1989.

29. Potter M, Pumphrey JG, Bailey DW: Genetics of susceptibility of plasmacytoma induction: I. BALB/c AnN(C), C57BL/6N(B6), C57BL/Ka(BK), (CxB6)F₁, (CxBK)F₁ and CxB recombinant inbred strains. *J Natl Cancer Inst* 54:1413, 1976.

30. Blattner WA: Multiple myeloma and macroglobulinemia, in *Cancer, Epidemiology and Prevention,* edited by D Schottenfeld, JF Fraumeni Jr, p 795. Saunders, Philadelphia, 1982.

31. Meijers KAE, Leeuw B, Voormolen-Kalova M: The multiple occurrence of myeloma and asymptomatic paraproteinemia within one family. *Clin Exp Immunol* 12:185, 1972.

32. Williams RC, Erickson JL, Polesky HF, et al: Studies on monoclonal immunoglobulins (M-components) in various kindreds. *Ann Intern Med* 67:309, 1967.

33. Kalff MW, Higmans W: Immunoglobulin analysis in families of macroglobulinemia patients. *Clin Exp Immunol* 5:479, 1969.

34. Potter LM, Blattner WA: Etiology an epidemiology of multiple myeloma and related disorders, in *Neoplastic Diseases of the Blood,* edited by PH Wiernick, GP Canellos, RA Kyle, et al, vol 1, pp 413–429. Churchill Livingstone, New York, 1985.

35. Cohn M, Notani G, Rice SA: Characterization of the antibody to the C carbohydrate produced by a transplantable mouse plasmacytoma. *Immunochemistry* 6:111, 1969.

36. Porter DD, Larsen AE, Porter HG: Aleutian disease of mink. *Adv Immunol* 29:261, 1980.

37. Goldenberg GJ, Paraskevas F, Israels LG: The association of rheumatoid arthritis with plasma cell and lymphocytic neoplasms. *Arthritis Rheum* 12:569, 1969.

38. Wegelius O, Skrifvars B: Rheumatoid arthritis terminating in plasmacytoma. *Acta Med Scand* 187:133, 1970.

39. Isomaki HA, Hakulmen T, Joutsenlahti U: Excess risk of lymphomas, leukemias and myelomas in patients with rheumatoid arthritis. *J Chronic Dis* 31:691, 1978.

40. Potter M: Concepts of pathogenesis and experimental models of immunoglobulin-secreting tumors in animals, in *Neoplastic Diseases of the Blood,* edited by PH Wiernick, GP Canellos, RA Kyle, et al, vol 1, pp 393–412. Churchill Livingstone, New York, 1985.

41. Mushinski JF, Bauer SR, Potter M, et al: Increased expression of myc and related oncogene RNA characterizes most BALB/c plasmacytomas induced by pristane or Abelson virus. *Proc Natl Acad Sci USA* 80:1073, 1983.

42. Rowley JD: Human oncogene locations and chromosome aberrations. *Nature* 301:290, 1983.

43. Heim S, Mitelman F: Chronic lymphoproliferative disorders, in *Cancer Cytogenetics,* pp 175–199. Liss, New York, 1987.

44. Cavanaugh M, Chan HS, Cohen IH, et al: Regional localization of genes and DNA segments on human chromosomes: Number 5, HGM10. Howard Hughes Medical Institute and Yale University, pp 26–29, 1989.

45. Klein B, Zhang XG, Jourdan M, et al: Interleukin 6 is the central tumor growth factor in vitro and in vivo in multiple myeloma. *Eur Cytokine Netw* 1:193, 1990.

46. Hirano T: Interleukin 6 (IL-6) and its receptor: their role in plasma cell neoplasias. *Int J Cell Cloning* 9:166, 1991.

47. Nilsson K, Jernberg H, Pettersson M: IL-6 as a growth factor for human multiple myeloma cells—a short overview. *Curr Top Microbiol Immunol* 166:3, 1990.

48. Klein B, Zhang X-G, Jourdan M, et al: Interleukin-6 is a major myeloma cell growth factor in vitro and in vivo especially in patients with terminal disease. *Curr Top Microbiol Immunol* 166:23, 1990.

49. Suematsu S, Hibi M, Sugita T, et al: Interleukin 6 (IL-6) and its receptor (IL-6R) in myeloma/plasmacytoma. *Curr Top Microbiol Immunol* 166:13, 1990.

50. Lichtenstein A, Berenson J, Norma D, et al: Production of cytokines by bone marrow cells obtained from patients with multiple myeloma. *Blood* 74:1206, 1989.

51. Bataille R, Jourdan M, Zhang X-G, et al: Serum levels of interleukin 6, a potent myeloma cell growth factor, as a reflection of disease severity in plasma cell dyscrasias. *J Clin Invest* 84:2008, 1989.

52. Bergsagel DE: Plasma cell myeloma: biology and treatment. *Annu Rev Med* 42:167, 1991.

53. Grogan TM, Durie B, Spier CM, et al: Myelomonocytic antigen positive myeloma. *Blood* 73:763, 1989.

54. Epstein J, Xiao H, He X: Markers of multiple hematopoietic lineages in multiple myeloma. *N Engl J Med* 322:664, 1990.

55. Smith JK: The significance of the "protein error" of indicators in the diagnosis of Bence Jones proteinuria. *Acta Haematol* 530:144, 1963.

56. Harnly ME, Swan SH, Holly EA, et al: Temporal trends in the incidence of non-Hodgkin's lymphoma and selected malignancies in a population with a high incidence of acquired immunodeficiency syndrome (AIDS). *Am J Epidemiol* 128:261, 1988.

57. Cleary ML, Dorfman RF, Sklar J: Failure in immunological control of the virus infection: Post-transplant lymphomas, in *The Epstein-Barr Virus: Recent Advances,* edited by MA Epstein, BG Achong, pp 163–182. Heinemann Medical, London, 1986.

58. Beral V, Peterman T, Berkelman R, et al: AIDS-associated non-Hodgkin lymphoma. *Lancet* 337:805, 1991.

59. Child AJ, Kushwaha MRS: Serum beta 2-microglobulin in lymphoproliferative and myeloproliferative diseases. *Hematol Oncol* 2:391, 1984.

60. Bataille R, Grenier J, Sany J, et al: Beta-2-microglobulin: optimal use for staging, prognosis and treatment—a prospective study of 160 patients. *Blood* 63:468, 1984.

61. Bataille R, Durie BGM, Grenier J, et al: Prognostic factors and staging in multiple myeloma: a reappraisal. *J Clin Oncol* 4:80, 1986.

62. Cuzik J, Cooper EH, MacLennan ICM: The prognostic value of serum β2 microglobulin compared with other presentation features in myelomatosis. *Br J Cancer* 52:1, 1985.

63. Capra JD, Kunkel HG: Aggregation of γ3 proteins: Relevance to the hyperviscosity syndrome. *J Clin Invest* 49:610, 1970.

64. Franklin EC: Immunopathology of the amyloid diseases. *Hosp Pract* 15:70, 1980.

65. Kyle RA, Greipp PR: Amyloidosis (AL): clinical and laboratory features in 229 cases. *Mayo Clin Proc* 58:665, 1983.

66. Perez-Simon JA, Garcia-Sanz R, Taberno MD, et al: Prognostic value of numerical chromosome aberrations in multiple myeloma: a FISH analysis of 15 different chromosomes. *Blood* 91:3366, 1998.

67. Retteg MB, Ma HJ, Vescio RA, et al: Kaposi's sarcoma-associated herpesvirus infection of bone marrow-dendritic cells from multiple myeloma patients. *Science* 276:1851, 1997.

68. Vidriales MB, Anderson KC: Adhesion of multiple myeloma cells to the bone marrow microenvironment: implications for future therapeutic strategies. *Mol Med Today* 2:425, 1996.

ESSENTIAL MONOCLONAL GAMMOPATHY

MARSHALL A. LICHTMAN

Essential monoclonal gammopathy is defined by two key features: the presence of a monoclonal immunoglobulin G, A, or M in the serum or of monoclonal light chains in the urine and the absence of evidence for an overt or progressive malignancy of B lymphocytes or plasma cells (e.g., lymphoma, myeloma, or amyloidosis). Since the latter diseases may be about to emerge at the time the monoclonal immunoglobulin is first detected, follow-up of the patient over several months is required to ascertain if essential monoclonal gammopathy is the appropriate diagnosis. Long-term follow-up at appropriate intervals is prudent to detect conversion from a stable, benign condition to a progressive lymphoma or myeloma, which occurs in about 1 percent of cases per year. Essential monoclonal gammopathy increases in prevalence from about 1 percent in 30-year-old individuals to 10 percent in those 80 years of age or older. The condition has been reported in association with a large variety of disorders, especially nonlymphocytic cancers, but these coincidences are thought to be the chance concurrence of conditions that have a high prevalence in older populations. Some cases of essential monoclonal gammopathy are symptomatic because the immunoglobulin can interact with plasma proteins or neural tissue and cause serious dysfunction. In such cases, disability may be so great that attempts to remove the immunoglobulin by apheresis and to suppress its production using cytotoxic therapy can be warranted. In the absence of such findings, careful periodic follow-up is all that is required.

DEFINITION AND HISTORY

The syndrome of essential monoclonal gammopathy has two important characteristics. The first characteristic is a plasma immunoglobulin or urinary immunoglobulin light chain that has the molecular features of the product of a single clone of B lymphocytes or plasma cells: homogeneous electrophoretic migration and a single light-chain type. The second feature is the absence of evidence of an overt neoplastic disorder of B lymphocytes or plasma cells, such as lymphoma or multiple myeloma.

The observations that Bence Jones proteinuria can precede by many years the clinical signs of multiple myeloma[1] and that hyperglobulinemia without evidence of multiple myeloma can occur in some patients[2] antedated the concept of monoclonal gammopathy as a syndrome. With the more frequent clinical application of zonal electrophoresis of plasma proteins during the 1950s and 1960s, patients were discovered who had a monoclonal immunoglobulin either without an associated disease or with diseases such as nonlymphoid cancers, infections, and inflammatory disorders, which are not typically associated with a monoclonal proliferation of B lymphocytes.[3–10] The presence of a monoclonal protein in plasma or urine is referred to as *essential monoclonal gammopathy* if it is not associated with a disease. Over 30 synonyms for the syndrome have been used, particularly *essential monoclonal gammopathy* and *benign monoclonal gammopathy.*[6] *Monoclonal gammopathy of unknown significance* (MGUS) has been proposed as a designation preferable to *benign monoclonal gammopathy* because about one-third of patients were noted to progress to myeloma, macroglobulinemia, amyloidosis, or a B-cell lymphoma in over 25 years of observation.[10] The term *essential monoclonal gammopathy* seems best, since it neither highlights a benign process nor indicates that the risks of subsequent lymphoma or myeloma are unknown. A classification of monoclonal gammopathies is presented in Table 105-1.

OCCURRENCE

Monoclonal gammopathy can occur at any age, but it is unusual before puberty, and its frequency increases with age.[11] The frequency of a serum paraprotein using zonal electrophoresis is about 1 percent in persons over age 25 years,[4] about 3 percent in those over age 70 years,[4,9] and about 10 percent in those over age 80 years.[3] A much higher prevalence of monoclonal gammopathy has been reported using more sensitive screening methods, such as isoelectric focusing or immunoblotting.[12,13] The prevalence rate among Americans of African descent is significantly greater than among those of European descent in each age group over 50 years.[14,15] Familial occurrence also has been described.[16,17] An increased incidence of monoclonal gammopathy has been associated with several occupation groups, including farmers and industrial workers.[18]

ETIOLOGY AND PATHOGENESIS

Monoclonal gammopathy can be compared with any benign tumor, such as a colonic polyp, that can stay the same size indefinitely or undergo malignant transformation at an unpredictable future time.

Monoclonal gammopathy is caused by the proliferation of a single B lymphocyte, a plasma cell progenitor, leading to a clonal population that reaches a steady state at or below about 1×10^{11} cells. At this cell population density, marrow plasma cell prevalence is indistinguishable from that of normal marrow. The expanded clone secretes monoclonal immunoglobulin at a rate per cell sufficient to be detected by standard tests. The clonal expansion, however, does not cause osteolysis, inhibit hematopoietic proliferation and maturation, or impair differentiation of polyclonal B lymphocytes to plasma cells. As such, immunoglobulin synthesis is normal, and patients do not necessarily incur an increased risk of infection. The cells in the benign clone do not accumulate further and do not elaborate significant amounts of osteoclast-activating factors [i.e., interleukin (IL)-1 β, IL-6, soluble IL-6 receptor α, and macrophage colony stimulating factor (M-CSF)] that are responsible for bone destruction. Remarkably, despite these significant differences from myeloma in the behavior of the neoplastic B cells, cytogenetic abnormalities akin to those seen in myeloma involving chromosomes 3, 7, 11, and 18 are present in plasma cells derived from the clone.[19–21]

The C57BL mouse provides a model of benign monoclonal gammopathy. The frequency of monoclonal gammopathy increases with mouse age.[22] The disease can be transferred to either irradiated or nonirradiated mice by marrow or spleen cells.[23] The transfer can only be accomplished during the first four consecutive transplantations, and there is no effect on the survival of the recipient compared with that of appropriate control subjects. In contrast, if mouse B-cell

TABLE 105-1   TYPES OF MONOCLONAL IMMUNOGLOBULIN SYNTHESIZED
BY ABNORMAL CELL CLONE

IgG, IgA, IgM,[6-10] IgE,[27] or IgD[28,29]
IgG + IgA, IgG + IgM, IgG + IgA +IgM[30-33]
Monoclonal κ or λ light chain (Bence Jones proteinuria)[10,34]

---

lymphoma or myeloma cells are transplanted into normal mice, the engraftment frequency is higher than that of B cells from mice with benign gammapathy, and passage from the original recipient to a new recipient is unlimited; progressive disease develops, and survival of recipients is decreased. Thus, there is an intrinsic difference in the growth potential (degree of malignancy) of these two B-cell clones.[23] The frequency of monoclonal gammapathy increases with age, but the progression to multiple myeloma in the C57BL mouse is a rare event.[24] Studies in transgenic mice and their litter mates replicate the increased incidence of B-cell clones and gammapathy with aging.[25]

Occasionally, monoclonal gammapathy may occur from the exaggerated production of natural antibody by a B-lymphocyte clone.[26] For example, patients with cold agglutinins may have monoclonal IgM for years. A few monoclonal IgMs act as rheumatoid factors and may form cryoglobulins through complex formation with IgG molecules.

CLINICAL FEATURES

Characteristically, individuals are detected by the unexpected identification of a monoclonal protein in plasma or urine in the absence of symptoms or signs caused by diseases associated with monoclonal proteins (e.g., anemia, marrow plasmacytosis, lymph node enlargement, plasmacytoma, bone lesions, or amyloid deposits).[6-10,26-34]

Some patients may have monoclonal proteins with antibody specificity directed against plasma or cell proteins, resulting in symptomatic pathophysiologic effects, such as immune hemolytic anemia,[35] acquired von Willebrand disease,[36,37] immune neutropenia,[38] or other functional manifestations listed in Table 105-2.

Rare patients with essential urinary light-chain excretion and renal disease have been described.[43-45]

There is a significant association between the occurrence of neuropathies and essential monoclonal gammapathy.[46-56] About 10 percent of patients with idiopathic neuropathy have a monoclonal immunoglobulin, a frequency about eight times that of healthy comparison groups.[46,47,50] Monoclonal antibodies can react with peripheral nerve myelin, specifically with myelin-associated glycoprotein, glycolipids, or sulfitides.[48,52,56-59] Neuropathy in the absence of such reactivity implies that other mechanisms also may operate to cause nerve damage.[49,52]

Patients with essential IgM gammapathy and neuropathy can have dysesthesia of the hands and feet, loss of vibration and position sense, atrophy of distal muscles, ataxia, and intention tremor.[56-60] In contrast, patients with essential IgG or IgA gammapathy usually have a chronic axonal sensorimotor neuropathy, sometimes with limb paral-

TABLE 105-2   FUNCTIONAL ABNORMALITIES ASSOCIATED WITH
ESSENTIAL MONOCLONAL GAMMOPATHY

Plasma protein disturbances
    Antierythrocyte antibodies,[35] acquired von Willebrand disease,[36,37] immune neutropenia,[38] cryoglobulinemia,[10] cryofibrinogenemia,[10] acquired C1 esterase inhibitor deficiency (angioedema),[10] acquired antithrombin,[39] insulin antibodies,[40,41] antiacetylcholine receptor antibodies,[42] "antiphospolipid" antibodies[176]
Renal disease[43-45]
Neuropathies[46-73]

---

ysis and occasionally with a remitting-relapsing course.[61-64] Essential IgA gammapathy has been associated with dysautonomia.[49] The presence or absence of antibody to myelin-associated glycoprotein may have an effect on the specific nature of the neuropathic manifestations.[52,56-60]

Demyelinization is reflected in a marked decrease in conduction velocity. Axonal loss is reflected in decreased sensory potentials.[50,52,55,56,61-64] Electromyography shows denervation of muscles.[50,52,65-67] Immunofluorescence studies of sural nerve or of skin biopsies may uncover immunoglobulin binding to nerve.[52,56,58]

Four treatment approaches may result in improvement in the neuropathies: (1) intravenous gamma globulin administration, (2) immunoadsorption of perfused blood with staphylococcal protein A, (3) plasmapheresis, or (4) immunosuppressive chemotherapy, such as cyclophosphamide or chlorambucil with or without glucocorticoids.[52,55,59,60,65-70] In some cases use of plasmapheresis has been followed by cytotoxic therapy in an effort to produce a sustained effect. Response rates to each form of therapy are low and duration of response is variable,[52,60,65-70] but some patients appear to obtain significant improvement for prolonged periods.

Monoclonal gammapathy unrelated to a clinically evident proliferation of B lymphocytes or plasma cells has been observed in association with a wide variety of conditions, shown in Table 105-3.[71-101] Although they are grouped under the designation *monoclonal gammopathy with an associated disease,* few such reports have examined whether the coincidence is greater than would be expected in a control group matched for age and ethnicity, the two variables that have the greatest impact on incidence of monoclonal gammapathy. Non-B-cell malignancies, including solid tumors,[3,5,6,102-104] myeloproliferative disorders,[105-111] and non-B-cell lymphomas,[112-115] have been associated with paraproteinemia. These relationships could be the result of (1) patients with an M component having an increased risk of developing cancer, (2) the M component being an antibody against some antigen associated with the cancer, (3) the globulin being the product of

TABLE 105-3   DISORDERS REPORTED IN COINCIDENCE WITH
MONOCLONAL GAMMOPATHY

Connective tissue diseases and autoimmune diseases: e.g., Crohn disease, Hashimoto thyroiditis, lupus erythematosus, myasthenia gravis, pernicious anemia, polymyalgia rheumatica, psoriatic arthritis, rheumatoid arthritis, scleroderma, Sjögren disease[71-79]
Corneal diseases: pseudo-Kayser-Fleischer ring,[80] corneal gammapathy[81]
Cutaneous diseases: e.g., hyperkeratotic spicules, pyoderma gangrenosum (neutrophilic dermatoses), psoriasis, scleromyxedema, Schnitzler syndrome,[85,178] urticaria[82-84,86,87]
Endocrine diseases: e.g., hyperparathyroidism[88,89]
Gaucher disease[90,91]
Hepatic disease: e.g., hepatitis,[179] cirrhosis[79]
Hereditary spherocytosis[92]
Infectious diseases: e.g., bacterial endocarditis, *Corynebacterium* species, cytomegalovirus, human immunodeficiency virus, *Mycobacterium tuberculosis,* purpura fulminans[79,93-97]
Metabolic disease: hyperlipidemia[98]
Pregnancy[177]
Pseudomyeloma (severe osteoporosis)[99,100]
Silicone breast implants[101,102]
Non-B-cell or plasma cell neoplasms
Carcinomas: e.g., colon, lung, prostate, others[3,5,6,103-105]
Myeloproliferative diseases: e.g., acute and chronic myelogenous leukemia, polycythemia vera[106-111]
T-cell lymphomas: e.g., Sézary syndrome[112-115]
After chemotherapy, radiotherapy, or marrow, kidney, or liver transplantation[116-121]
Miscellaneous diseases[122-124]
Transient, monoclonal, or oligoclonal gammapathies[125-127]
Factitious hyperferremia[128]

cancer cells, or (4) coincidence. The last possibility is favored by one epidemiologic study that found the same frequency of monoclonal gammopathy in a matched control group as in cancer patients.[9] Furthermore, where the monoclonal immunoglobulin is associated with a cancer, it usually persists after surgical excision of the tumor.

Chemotherapy, radiotherapy, and organ or marrow transplantation have been associated with a transient or persistent monoclonal immunoglobulin,[116-121] as have other miscellaneous disorders (Table 105-3).[5,7,10,15,16,78,79]

The high prevalence of monoclonal proteins and associated diseases, especially after age 50 years, indicates that some of these associations may be coincidental. Thus, although surgical correction of hyperparathyroidism has been associated with disappearance of the plasma monoclonal protein,[88] statistical studies of this disorder suggest a coincidental relationship in most patients.[89] In hematopoietic stem cell diseases, some observers have proposed that the paraprotein reflects subtle B-cell lineage involvement. In inflammatory, autoimmune, and infectious diseases, the association has been viewed as an unusual expansion of a restricted population of B lymphocytes. Following marrow transplantation, the presence of oligoclonal blood B-lymphocyte populations may reflect the effect of a reconstitution of the B-cell population.

LABORATORY FEATURES

PLASMA AND URINARY IMMUNOGLOBULINS

The monoclonal protein is usually IgG; however, IgM, IgA, IgD, and IgE urinary light chains, double gammopathy involving IgA and IgG or IgM and IgA, and triple gammopathy can occur (Table 105-1).[103-107,129] By definition, no findings other than a plasma or urinary M component are present that would permit a diagnosis of a B-lymphocyte or plasma cell malignancy.

In monoclonal gammopathy of the IgG type, the concentration of monoclonal immunoglobulin is usually less than 3.0 g/dl, and in the IgA or IgM type, it is usually below 2.5 g/dl.[10,129] However, there are dramatic exceptions to this rule, with occasional patients with essential monoclonal gammopathy having concentrations as high as 6.0 g/dl. Some patients have Bence Jones proteinuria as the sole manifestation of monoclonal gammopathy.[1,10] The amount of urinary light chains excreted may occasionally be large (>1.0 g/day), and renal dysfunction can develop.[43]

Most patients with myeloma or macroglobulinemia have a significant depression in the nonmonoclonal immunoglobulin levels. For example, patients with IgG myeloma usually have very low IgA and IgM concentrations as well as a reduction in polyclonal IgG level. Patients with monoclonal gammopathy usually have normal polyclonal immunoglobulin levels, and depression of their polyclonal immunoglobulin levels, when it occurs, is usually not as severe as in myeloma.[10,129,130]

OLIGOCLONAL AND MONOCLONAL IMMUNOGLOBULINS

Oligoclonal or monoclonal serum immunoglobulins have been detected with high-resolution agarose gel electrophoresis in hospitalized patients with acute phase reactions or polyclonal hyperglobulinemia.[127] Oligoclonal immunoglobulin bands are frequently seen in the cerebrospinal fluid and serum of patients with a variety of neurological conditions, especially in patients with multiple sclerosis when the fluids are analyzed by isoelectric focusing.[131] Patients with acquired immunodeficiency syndrome (AIDS) have B-cell activation and aberrancies of B-cell regulation. High-resolution electrophoresis has indicated that most AIDS patients with advanced disease have monoclonal or oli-

goclonal serum immunoglobulin bands. Subjects with AIDS, lymphadenopathy syndrome, or antibody to the human immunodeficiency virus also have oligoclonal or monoclonal immunoglobulin bands by standard zonal electrophoresis.[94,96] These monoclonal proteins are IgG.

LYMPHOCYTE AND PLASMA CELL PHENOTYPES

The concentration of plasma cells in the marrow is less than 5 percent, and the incorporation of tritiated thymidine into marrow plasma cells is negligible (<1 percent) in essential monoclonal gammopathy. Blood T-lymphocyte subset levels are normal in monoclonal gammopathy, whereas CD4+ T cell levels are lower and CD8+ T cell levels higher in myeloma and macroglobulinemia.[132-135] Blood B-cell concentration is normal in monoclonal gammopathy but is often decreased in myeloma patients. Clonally restricted, idiotype-positive blood B cells are characteristic of myeloma but not of monoclonal gammopathy.[136]

β_2 microglobulin is the light chain of cell surface HLA molecules, and normally it is present at low concentrations in serum. Its concentration in serum frequently is elevated in myeloma, and the magnitude of the elevation is positively correlated with tumor mass. β_2 microglobulin concentration is not elevated in essential monoclonal gammopathy.[137,138]

The distinction between stable essential monoclonal gammopathy and emerging (so-called larval myeloma) with a very low tumor burden is blurred at the margins. This has not kept investigators from looking for a distinguishing test. Over 20 variables have been studied as an index for discriminating benignity from malignancy (Table 105-4).

TABLE 105-4   VARIABLES THAT HAVE BEEN USED IN AN ATTEMPT TO DISTINGUISH ESSENTIAL MONOCLONAL GAMMOPATHY FROM MYELOMA

LYMPHOCYTES AND IMMUNOGLOBULINS

M protein serum concentration[129,130,139,141]
Ig κ light chain[141]
Light chains in urine[141]
Polyclonal Ig serum concentration[141]
β_2-microglobulin or C-reactive protein serum concentration[137,138,140-142]
Ig-secreting cells in blood[143]
Idiotype-reactive blood T lymphocytes[144,145]
CD4-to-CD8 lymphocyte ratio in blood or marrow[134,146-148]
Clonally restricted B lymphocytes[136,149,150]
Natural killer cell frequency[151]

PLASMA CELLS

Frequency[6,7,9,10,141]
Morphology[132,152,153]
MB2 antibody reactivity[154]
Proliferative index[132,133,142,152]
DNA content or interphase fluorescent in situ hybridization[19-21,152]
Blood or marrow concentration[10,132,133,141,149]
J chains[155]
Acid phosphatase[156]
Multidrug resistance expression[157]
CD19 expression[158]
5′ nucleotidase[159]

BONE INTEGRITY

Magnetic resonance imaging[160,161]
Dual-energy x-ray absorptiometry[162]
Histomorphometry[163]
Urinary pyridinium-collagen complexes[164]

MISCELLANEOUS

Neural cell adhesion molecules[165]
Serum IL-6, IL-10, soluble CD16, soluble IL-6 receptor, IL-1β[166-169,174,175]
Hemoglobin concentration

No single test is sufficiently sensitive and specific to be useful in an individual patient. Periodic examination of the patient is the best method of detecting the emergence of myeloma or a related disease. Measurement of the concentration of the serum monoclonal protein, urinary light chains, serum β_2-microglobulin, and hemoglobin concentration at appropriate intervals is required. Practical methods of measuring serum IL-6 and bone density may become additional useful measures of stability or progression.

COURSE, PROGNOSIS, AND THERAPY

Longitudinal studies have reported three major patterns of outcome for patients with essential monoclonal gammopathy.[10,129,130,139,170–172] About 25 percent of patients do not progress. In this group, occasional patients may experience increases in monoclonal protein concentration of up to 50 percent of their initial diagnostic value. However, these patients restabilize and do not develop signs of myeloma, macroglobulinemia, amyloidosis, or lymphoproliferative disease. About one-half of patients die of an unrelated cause. The remaining one-quarter of the patients develop myeloma, amyloidosis, macroglobulinemia, or lymphoma over two decades of observation. The latter group of patients continues to increase slowly without reaching a plateau, and evolution to myeloma has been observed more than 20 years after the diagnosis of monoclonal gammopathy. The actuarial risk of progressing to lymphoma or myeloma is about 1 percent per year.[139,141,170–173] In rare patients, the monoclonal protein may appear transiently in relation to a disease (e.g., infection)[125–127] or may disappear spontaneously even when not associated with a disease.[3]

Generally, the diagnosis of essential monoclonal gammopathy cannot be made with certainty at the time of the initial evaluation. Periodic reexamination is required to document a stable clinical course. Therapy usually is not required unless there is a confirmed diagnosis of myeloma, macroglobulinemia, amyloidosis, or lymphoma with evidence of progressive disease. Therapy may also be indicated in the uncommon circumstance that the monoclonal protein interferes with the vital function of a normal plasma or tissue constituent.

REFERENCES

1. Prentiss RG Jr: Multiple myeloma with diffuse skeletal involvement: case report. *Mil Surg* 80:294, 1937.
2. Waldenstrom JG: Incipient myelomatosis or essential hyperglobulinemia with fibrinogenopenia: a new syndrome? *Acta Med Scand* 117:216, 1944.
3. Hallen J: Frequency of "abnormal serum globulins" (M-components) in the aged. *Acta Med Scand* 173:737, 1963.
4. Axelsson U, Bachmann R, Hallen J: Frequency of pathological proteins (M-components) in 6995 sera from an adult population. *Acta Med Scand* 179:235, 1966.
5. Migliore PJ, Alexanian R: Monoclonal gammopathy in human neoplasia. *Cancer* 21:1127, 1968.
6. Ritzmann SE, Loukes D, Sakai H, et al: Idiopathic (asymptomatic) monoclonal gammopathies. *Arch Intern Med* 135:95, 1975.
7. Amies A, Ko HS, Pruzanski W: M-components: a review of 1242 cases. *Can Med Assoc J* 114:889, 1976.
8. Lindstrom FD, Dahlstrom V: Multiple myeloma or benign monoclonal gammopathy? A study of differential diagnostic criteria in 44 cases. *Clin Immunol Immunopathol* 10:168, 1978.
9. Salerin JP, Vicariot M, Deroff P, et al: Monoclonal gammopathies in the adult population of Finistère, France. *J Clin Pathol* 35:63, 1982.
10. Kyle RA: Monoclonal gammopathy of undetermined significance and solitary myeloma. *Hematol Oncol Clin North Am* 11:71, 1997.
11. Ligthart GL, Radl J, Corberand JX, et al: Monoclonal gammopathies in human aging: increased occurrence with age and correlation with health status. *Mech Ageing Dev* 52:235, 1990.
12. Sinclair D, Sheehan T, Parrott DMV, Stott DI: The incidence of monoclonal gammopathy in a population over 45 years old determined by isoelectric focusing. *Br J Haematol* 67:745, 1986.
13. Radl J, Wels J, Hoogeven CM: Immunoblotting with (sub)class specific antibodies reveals a high frequency of monoclonal antibodies in persons thought to be immunodeficient. *Clin Chem* 34:1839, 1988.
14. Schecter GP, Shoff N, Chan C, et al: The frequency of monoclonal gammopathy in black and white veterans in a hospital population, in Obrams GI, Potter M (eds): *Epidemiology and Biology of Multiple Myeloma.* New York, Springer-Verlag, pp 83–85.
15. Singh J, Dudley AW, Kulig KA: Increased incidence of monoclonal gammopathy of undetermined significance in blacks and its age-related differences with whites on the basis of a study of 397 men and one woman in a hospital setting. *J Lab Clin Med* 116:785, 1990.
16. Bizzaro N, Pasini P: Familial occurrence of multiple myeloma and monoclonal gammopathy of undetermined significance in siblings. *Haematologica* 75:58, 1990.
17. Jensen TS, Schroeder HD, Jonsson V, et al: IgM monoclonal gammopathy and neuropathy in two siblings. *J Neurol Neurosurg Psychiatry* 51:1308, 1988.
18. Pasqualetti P, Collacciani A, Casole R: Risk of monoclonal gammopathy of undetermined significance. *Am J Hematol* 52:217, 1996.
19. Drach J, Angerler J, Schuster J, et al: Interphase fluorescence in situ hybridization identifies chromosomal abnormalities in plasma cells from patients with monoclonal gammopathy of undetermined significance. *Blood* 86:3915, 1995.
20. Zandecki M, Lai JL, Genevieve F, et al: Several cytogenetic subclones may be identified within plasma cells from patients with monoclonal gammopathy of undetermined significance both at diagnosis and during the indolent course of the disease. *Blood* 90:3682, 1997.
21. Zandecki M, Obein V, Bernardi F, et al: Monoclonal gammopathy of undetermined significance: chromosome changes as a common finding within bone marrow plasma cells. *Br J Haematol* 90:693, 1995.
22. Radl J, Hollander CF: Homogeneous immunoglobulins in sera of mice during aging. *J Immunol* 112:2271, 1974.
23. Radl J, DeGlopper E, Schuit HRE, Zurcher C: Idiopathic paraproteinemia: II. Transplantation of the paraprotein-producing clone from old to young 57B1/KaLwRij mice. *J Immunol* 122:609, 1979.
24. Radl J: Age-related monoclonal gammopathies: clinical lessons from the aging C57BL mouse. *Immunol Today* 11:234, 1990.
25. van Arkel C, Hopstaken CM, Zurcher C, et al: Monoclonal gammopathies in aging m,x-transgenic mice: involvement of the B-1 cell lineage. *Eur J Immunol* 27:2436, 1997.
26. George G, Gilburd B, Schoenfeld Y: The emerging concept of pathogenic natural antibodies. *Hum Antibod* 8:70, 1997.
27. Ludwig H, Vormittag W: "Benign" monoclonal Ig E gammopathy. *Br Med J* 281:539, 1980.
28. O'Connor ML, Rice DT, Buss DH, Muss HB: Immunoglobulin D benign monoclonal gammopathy. *Cancer* 68:611, 1991.
29. Kinoshita K, Nagai H, Murate T, et al: Ig D monoclonal gammopathy of undetermined significance. *Int J Hematol* 65:169, 1997.
30. Imhof JW, Balliux RE, Mul NAJ, Poen H: Monoclonal and diclonal gammopathies. *Acta Med Scand* 179(suppl 455):102, 1966.
31. Jensen K, Jensen B, Olesen H: Three M-components in serum from an apparently healthy person. *Scand J Haematol* 4:485, 1967.
32. Kyle RA, Robinson RA, Katzmann JA: The clinical aspects of biclonal gammopathies: review of 57 cases. *Am J Med* 71:999, 1981.
33. Riddell S, Traczyk Z, Paraskevas F, Israels LG: The double gammopathies: clinical and immunological studies. *Medicine (Baltimore)* 65:135, 1986.
34. Kyle RA, Greipp PR: "Idiopathic" Bence-Jones proteinuria. *N Engl J Med* 306:564, 1982.
35. Kay NE, Gordon LI, Douglas SD: Autoimmune hemolytic anemia in association with monoclonal IgM(k) with anti-i-activity. *Am J Med* 64:845, 1978.
36. Federici AB, Stabile F, Castaman G, et al: Treatment of acquired von Willebrand syndrome in patients with monoclonal gammopathy of uncertain significance: comparison of three different therapeutic approaches. *Blood* 92:2707, 1998.
37. Lopez-Fernandez MF, Lopez-Berges C, Martin R, et al: Unique multimeric pattern of von Willebrand factor in a patient with a benign monoclonal gammopathy. *Scand J Haematol* 36:302, 1986.
38. Carrington PA, Walsh SE, Houghton JB: Benign paraproteinemia and immune neutropenia. *Clin Lab Haematol* 2:407, 1989.

39. Gabriel DA, Carr ME, Cook L, Roberts HR: Spontaneous antithrombin in a patient with benign paraprotein. *Am J Hematol* 25:85, 1987.

40. Sluiter WJ, Marrink J, Houwen B: Monoclonal gammopathy with an insulin binding IgG(K) M-component, associated with severe hypoglycaemia. *Br J Haematol* 62:679, 1986.

41. Wasada T, Egueli Y, Takayama S, Yoo K, et al: Insulin autoimmune syndrome associated with benign monoclonal gammopathy. *Diabetes Care* 12:147, 1989.

42. Ahlberg RE, Lefvert AK: Monoclonal gammopathy and antibody activity against the acetylcholine receptor. *Am J Hematol* 29:49, 1988.

43. Maldonado JE, Velosa JA, Kyle RA, et al: Fanconi syndrome in adults: a manifestation of a latent form of myeloma. *Am J Med* 58:354, 1975.

44. Gavarotti P, Fortina F, Costa D, et al: Benign monoclonal gammopathy presenting with severe renal failure. *Scand J Haematol* 36:115, 1986.

45. Kebler R, Kithier K, McDonald FD, Cadnapaphornchai P: Rapidly progressive glomerulonephritis and monoclonal gammopathy. *Am J Med* 78:133, 1985.

46. Kahn SN, Riches PG, Kohn J: Paraproteinemia in neurologic disease: incidence, associations, and classification of monoclonal immunoglobulins. *J Clin Pathol* 33:617, 1980.

47. Kelly JJ Jr, Kyle RA, O'Brien PC, Dyck PJ: Prevalence of monoclonal protein in peripheral neuropathy. *Neurology* 31:1480, 1981.

48. Lee KW, Inghirami G, Spatz L, et al: The B-cells that express anti-MAG antibodies in neuropathy and non-malignant IgM monoclonal gammopathy belong to the CD5 subpopulation. *J Neuroimmunol* 31:83, 1991.

49. Bailey RO, Ritaccio AL, Bishop MB, Wu AY: Benign monoclonal IgAk gammopathy associated with polyneuropathy and dysautonomia. *Acta Neurol Scand* 73:574, 1986.

50. Simmons Z, Albers JW, Bromberg MB, Feldman EL: Presentation and initial clinical course in patients with chronic inflammatory demyelinating polyradiculoneuropathy: comparison of patients without and with monoclonal gammopathy. *Neurology* 43:2202, 1993.

51. Vallatt JM, Jauberteau MO, Bordessoule D, et al: Link between peripheral neuropathy and monoclonal dysglobulinemia: a study of 66 cases. *J Neurol Sci* 137:124, 1996.

52. Ropper AH, Gorsin KC: Neuropathies associated with paraproteinemia. *N Engl J Med* 338:1601, 1998.

53. Kissel JT, Mendell JR: Neuropathies associated with monoclonal gammopathies. *Neuromuscular Disord* 6:3, 1996.

54. Lavrnic D, Vidakovic A, Miletic V, et al: Motor neuron disease and monoclonal gammopathy. *Eur Neurol* 35:104, 1995.

55. Gorsin KC, Allan G, Ropper AH: Chronic inflammatory demyelinating polyneuropathy: clinical features and response to treatment in 67 consecutive patients with and without a monoclonal gammopathy. *Neurology* 48:321, 1997.

56. Chassande B, Léger J-M, Younes-Chennoufi AB, et al: Peripheral neuropathy associated with IgM monoclonal gammopathy: correlation between M-protein antibody activity and clinical/electrophysicological features in 40 cases. *Muscle Nerve* 21:55, 1998.

57. Pestronk A, Li F, Bieser BS, et al: Anti-MAG antibodies. *Neurology* 44:1131, 1994.

58. Johnsson V, Jensen TS, Früs ML, et al: Immunoglobulin deposits in peripheral nerve endings detected by skin biopsy in patients with IgM M proteins and neuropathy. *Neurology* 37:303, 1987.

59. Ellie E, Vital A, Steck A, et al: Neuropathy associated with ''benign'' anti-myelin-associated glycoprotein IgM gammopathy: clinical, immunological, neurophysiological pathological findings and response to treatment in 33 cases. *J Neurol* 243:34, 1996.

60. Notermans NC: Monoclonal gammopathy and neuropathy. *Curr Opin Neurol* 9:334, 1996.

61. Barbieri S, Sandroni P, Orazio-Noble E, et al: Small fiber involvement in neuropathy associated with IgG, IgA and IgM monoclonal gammopathy. *Electromyogr Clin Neurophysiol* 35:39, 1995.

62. Notermans NC, Wokke JHJ, vanden Berg LH, et al: Chronic idiopathic axonal polyneuropathy. *Brain* 119:421, 1996.

63. Jonsson V, Schroder HD, Trojaborg W, et al: Autoimmune reactions in patients with M-component and peripheral neuropathy. *J Intern Med* 232:185, 1992.

64. Gorsin KC, Ropper AH: Axonal neuropathy associated with monoclonal gammopathy of undertermined significance. *J Neurol Neurosurg Psychiatry* 63:163, 1997.

65. Latov N: Pathogensis and therapy of neuropathies associated with monoclonal gammopathies. *Ann Neruol* 37(suppl 1):532, 1995.

66. Frayne J, Stark RJ: Peripheral neuropathy with gammopathy responding to plasmapheresis. *Clin Exp Neurol* 21:195, 1985.

67. Kiprov DD, Miller RG: Paraproteinemia associated with demyelinating polyneuropathy or myositis: treatment with plasmapheresis and immunosuppressive drugs. *Artif Organs* 9:47, 1985.

68. Dyck PJ, Low PA, Windeback AJ, et al: Plasma exchange in polyneuropathy associated with monoclonal gammopathy in undetermined significance. *N Engl J Med* 325:1482, 1991.

69. Blume G, Pestronk A, Goodnough LT: Anti-MAG antibody-associated polyneuropathies: improvement following immunotherapy with monthly plasma exchange and IV cyclophosphamide. *Neurology* 45:1577, 1995.

70. Oksenhendler E, Chevret S, Léger JM, et al: Plasma exchange and chlorambucil in polyneuropathy associated with monoclonal IgM gammopathy. *J Neurol Neurosurg Psychiatry* 59:243, 1995.

71. Burner E, Swahlen A, Cruchaud A: Nonmalignant monoclonal immunoglobulinemia, pernicious anemia, and gastric carcinoma: a model of immunologic dysfunction. *Am J Med* 60:1019, 1976.

72. Rowland LP, Osserman EF, Scharfman WB, et al: Myasthenia gravis with a myeloma-type gamma-G (IgG) immunoglobulin abnormality. *Am J Med* 46:599, 1969.

73. Ilfeld D, Barzilay J, Vana D, et al: IgG monoclonal gammopathy in four patients with polymyalgia rheumatica (letter). *Ann Rheum Dis* 44:501, 1985.

74. Nanji AA: Monoclonal gammopathy associated with Crohn's disease during treatment with total parenteral nutrition. *J Parenteral Nutr* 9:621, 1985.

75. Wallach D, Carado Y, Foldes C, Cottennot F: Dermatomyositis and monoclonal gammopathy. *Ann Dermatol Venereol* 112:783, 1985.

76. McFadden N, Ree K, Syland E, Larse TE: Scleredema adultorum associated with a monoclonal gammopathy and generalized hyperpigmentation. *Arch Dermatol* 123:629, 1987.

77. Oikarinen A, Ala-Kokko L, Palatsi R, et al: Scleroderma and paraproteinemia. *Arch Dermatol* 123:226, 1987.

78. Johnsson V, Svendsen B, Vostrup S, et al: Multiple autoimmune manifestations in monoclonal gammopathy of undetermined significance and chronic lymphocytic leukemia. *Leukemia* 10:327, 1996.

79. Kyle RA: Monoclonal gammopathy of unknown significance (MGUS). *Ballière's Clin Haematol* 8:761, 1995.

80. Probst LE, Hoffman E, Cherian MG, et al: Ocular copper deposition associated with benign monoclonal gammopathy and hypercupremia. *Cornea* 15: 94, 1996.

81. Secundo W, Seifert P: Monoclonal corneal gammopathy: topographic considerations. *Ger J Ophthalmol* 5:262, 1996.

82. Doutre MS, Beylot C, Bioluac P, Bezian JH: Monoclonal IgM and chronic urticaria: two cases. *Ann Allergy* 58:413, 1987.

83. Samochocki Z, Szudzinski A: Gangrenous pyoderma in monoclonal IgA gammopathy and functional disorders of T lymphocytes. *Przegl Dermatol* 73:409, 1986.

84. Abraham Z, Feuerman EJ: IgA benign monoclonal gammopathy with recurrent self-healing skin tumors. *J Am Acad Dermatol* 21:1303, 1989.

85. Puddu P, Cianchini G, Giardelli CR, et al: Schnitzler's syndrome: report of a new case and review of the literature. *Clin Exper Rheumatol* 15:91, 1997.

86. Wayte JA, Rogers S, Powell FC: Pyoderma gangrenosum, erythema elevatum diutinum and Ig A monoclonal gammopathy. *Australas J Dermatol* 36:21, 1995.

87. Paul C, Fermaud J-P, Flageul B, et al: Hyperkeratotic spicules and monoclonal gammopathy. *J Am Acad Dermatol* 33:346, 1995.

88. Schnur MJ, Appel GB, Bilezikian JP: Primary hyperparathyroidism and benign monoclonal gammopathy. *Arch Intern Med* 137:1201, 1977.

89. Rao DS, Antonelli R, Kane KR, et al: Primary hyperparathyroidism and monoclonal gammopathy. *Henry Ford Hosp Med J* 39:41, 1991.

90. Schoenfeld Y, Berliner S, Pinkhas J, Beutler E: The association of Gaucher's disease and dysproteinemias. *Acta Haematol (Basel)* 64:241, 1980.

91. Brady K, Corash L, Bhargava E: Multiple myeloma arising from monoclonal gammopathy of unknown significance in a patient with Gaucher's disease. *Arch Pathol Lab Med* 121:1108, 1997.

92. Schafer AL, Miller JB, Lester EP, et al: Monoclonal gammopathy in

hereditary spherocytosis: a possible pathogenetic relation. *Ann Intern Med* 88:45, 1978.

93. Danon F, Bussel A, Perol Y: Immunoglobulines monoclonales infections a cytomegalovirus et hémopathies malignes. *Ann Immunol* 128A:83, 1977.

94. Papadopoulos NM, Lane HC, Costello R, et al: Oligoclonal immunoglobulins in patients with the acquired immunodeficiency syndrome. *Clin Immunol Immunopathol* 35:43, 1985.

95. Heriot K, Hallquist AE, Tomar RH: Paraproteinemia in patients with acquired immunodeficiency syndrome (AIDS) or lymphadenopathy syndrome (LAS). *Clin Chem* 31:1224, 1985.

96. Kouns DM, Marty AM, Sharpe RW: Oligoclonal bands in serum protein electrophoretograms of individuals with human immunodeficiency virus antibodies. *JAMA* 256:2343, 1986.

97. Ong F, Hermans J, Noordik EM, et al: A population-based registry on paraproteinaemia in the Netherlands. *Br J Haematol* 99:914, 1997.

98. Johnston JD, Lumb PJ, Wierzbicki AS: Hyperlipidaemia in association with benign paraproteinemia. *Ann Clin Bichem* 34:697, 1997.

99. Buonocore E, Solmon A, Kerley HE: Pseudomyeloma. *Radiology* 95:41, 1970.

100. Maldonado JE, Riggs L, Bayrd ED: Pseudomyeloma. *Arch Intern Med* 135:267, 1975.

101. Silverman S, Vescio R, Silver D, et al: Silicone gel implants and monoclonal gammopathies. *Curr Top Microbiol Immunol* 210:367, 1996.

102. Kyle RA: Monoclonal gammopathy of unknown significance. *Curr Top Microbiol Immunol* 210:375, 1996.

103. Solomon A: Homogeneous (monoclonal) immunoglobulins in cancer. *Am J Med* 63:169, 1977.

104. Colls BM, Lorier MA: Immunocytoma, cancer, and other associations of monoclonal gammopathy: a review of 224 cases. *N Z Med J* 82:121, 1975.

105. Abdul M, Hassein NM: Gammopathy associated with advanced prostate cancer. *Urol Res* 23:185, 1995.

106. Thys LG, Hijmans W, Leene W, et al: Blast cell leukemia associated with IgA paraproteinemia and Bence-Jones protein. *Br J Haematol* 19:485, 1970.

107. Shoenfeld Y, Berliner S, Ayalone A, et al: Monoclonal gammopathy in patients with chronic and acute myeloid leukemia. *Cancer* 54:280, 1984.

108. Berner Y, Berrebi A: Myeloproliferative disorders and nonmyelomatous paraprotein. *Isr J Med Sci* 22:109, 1986.

109. Tosato F, Fossaluzza V, Rossi P, et al: Monoclonal gammopathy of undetermined significance in a case of primary thrombocythemia. *Haematologica (Pavia)* 71:417, 1986.

110. Economopoulos T, Economidou J, Papageorgiou E, et al: Monoclonal gammopathy in chronic myeloproliferative disorders. *Blut* 58:7, 1989.

111. Ito T, Kojima H, Otani K, et al: Chronic neutrophilic leukemia associated with monoclonal gammopathy of unknown significance. *Acta Haematol* 95:140, 1996.

112. Offit K, Macris NT, Hellman G, Rotterdam, HZ: Consecutive lymphoma with monoclonal gammopathy in a married couple. *Cancer* 57:277, 1986.

113. Venencie PY, Winkelmann RK, Puissant A, Kyle RA: Monoclonal gammopathy in Sézary syndrome: report of three cases and review of the literature. *Arch Dermatol* 120:605, 1984.

114. Kamihira S, Taguchi H, Kinoshita K, Ichimaru M: Monoclonal gammopathy in adult T-cell leukemia/lymphoma: a report of three cases. *Jpn J Clin Oncol* 14:699, 1984.

115. Chisesi I, Capnist G, Barbui T: Two serum IgG M-components of differing light chain types in a case of Hodgkin's disease. *Acta Haematol (Basel)* 55:250, 1976.

116. VanCamp B, Reynaerts PH, Naets JP, Radl J: Transient IgA$_1$-λ paraproteinemia during treatment of acute myeloblastic leukemia. *Blood* 55:21, 1980.

117. Hammarstrom L, Smith CIE: Frequent occurrence of monoclonal gammopathies with an imbalanced light-chain ratio following bone marrow transplantation. *Transplantation* 43:447, 1987.

118. Mitus AJ, Stein R, Rappeport JM, et al: Monoclonal and oligoclonal gammopathy after bone marrow transplantation. *Blood* 74:2764, 1989.

119. Passweg J, Thiel G, Bock HA: Monoclonal gammopathy after intense induction immunosuppression in renal transplant patients. *Nephrol Dial Transplant* 11:2461, 1996.

120. Badley AD, Portela DF, Patel R, et al: Development of monoclonal gammopathy precedes the development of Epstein-Barr virus-induced posttransplant lymphoproliferatve disorder. *Liver Transplantl Surg* 2:375, 1996.

121. Touchard G, Pasdeloup T, Parpeix J, et al: High prevalence and usual persistence of serum monoclonal immunoglobulins evidenced by sensitive methods in renal transplant recipients. *Nephrol Dial Transplant* 12:1199, 1997.

122. Ho JL, Polde PA, McEniry D, et al: Acquired immunodeficiency syndrome with progressive multifocal leukoencephalopathy and monoclonal B-cell proliferation. *Ann Intern Med* 100:693, 1984.

123. Nagler A, Ben-Arieh Y, Brenner B, et al: Eosinophilic fibrohistiocytic lesion of bone marrow associated with monoclonal gammopathy and osteolytic lesions. *Am J Hematol* 23:277, 1986.

124. Hineman VL, Phyliky RL, Banks PM: Angiofollicular lymph node hyperplasia and peripheral neuropathy: association with monoclonal gammopathy. *Mayo Clin Proc* 57:379, 1982.

125. Radl J, VandenBerg A: Transitory appearance of homogeneous immunoglobulins—paraproteins—in children with severe combined immunodeficiency before and after transplantation, in Peeters H (ed): *Protides of Biological Fluids,* vol 20. Oxford, Pergamon, 1973, p 203–211.

126. DelCarpio J, Espinoza LR, Lauater S, Osterland CK: Transient monoclonal proteins in drug hypersensitivity reactions. *Am J Med* 66:1051, 1979.

127. Keshgegian AA: Prevalence of small monoclonal proteins in the serum of hospitalized patients. *Am Soc Clin Pathol* 77:436, 1982.

128. Bakker AJ, Kothman-Tijkotte MJ: Artifactually high concentration of iron determined in serum from a patient with a monoclonal immunoglobulin. *Clin Chem* 36:1517, 1990.

129. Malacrida V, De-Francesco D, Banfi G, et al: Laboratory investigation of monoclonal gammopathy during 10 years of screening in a general hospital. *J Clin Pathol* 40:793, 1987.

130. Moller-Petersen J, Schmidt EB: Diagnostic value of the concentration of M-component in initial classification of monoclonal gammopathy. *Scand J Haematol* 26:295, 1986.

131. Link H, Kostulas V: Utility of isoelectric focusing of cerebrospinal fluid and serum of agarose evaluated for neurological patients. *Clin Chem* 29:810, 1983.

132. Greipp PR, Kyle RA: Clinical, morphological and cell kinetic differences among multiple myeloma, monoclonal gammopathy of undetermined significance and smoldering myeloma. *Blood* 62:166, 1983.

133. Boccadoro M, Gavarotti P, Fossati G: Low plasma cell 3(H)-thymidine incorporation in MGUS, smoldering myeloma and remission phase myeloma: reliable identification of patients not requiring therapy. *Br J Haematol* 58:689, 1984.

134. San Miguel JF, Caballero MD, Gonzalez M: T-cell subpopulations in patients with monoclonal gammopathies: essential monoclonal gammopathy, multiple myeloma and Waldenstrom macroglobulinemia. *Am J Hematol* 20:267, 1985.

135. Lindstrom FD, Hardy WR, Eberle BJ, Williams RC Jr: Multiple myeloma and benign monoclonal gammopathy: differentiation by immunofluorescence of lymphocytes. *Ann Intern Med* 78:837, 1973.

136. Billadeau D, Greipp P, Ahmann G, et al: Detection of B-cells clonally related to the tumor population in multiple myeloma and MGUS. *Curr Top Microbiol Immunol* 194:9, 1995.

137. Morrell A, Riesen W: Serum B$_2$-macroglobulin, serum creatinine and bone marrow plasma cells in benign and malignant monoclonal gammopathy. *Acta Haematol (Basel)* 64:87, 1980.

138. Fine JM, Lambin P, Desjobert H: Serum neopterin and B$_2$-microglobulin concentrations in monoclonal gammopathies. *Acta Med Scand* 224:179, 1988.

139. Vuckovic J, Ilic A, Knezevic N, et al: Progress in monoclonal gammopathy of undetermined significance. *Br J Haematol* 97:649, 1997.

140. Bataille R: New insights in the clinical biology of multiple myeloma. *Sem Hematol* 34:23, 1997.

141. Baldini L, Guffanti A, Cesana BM, et al: Role of different hematologic variables in defining the risk of malignant transformation in monoclonal gammopathy. *Blood* 87:92, 1996.

142. French M, Fench P, Remy F, et al: Plasma cell proliferation in monoclonal gammopathy: relations with other biologic variables—diagnostic and prognostic significance. *Am J Med* 98:60, 1995.

143. Witzig TE, Gonchoroff NJ, Katzmann JA, et al: Peripheral blood B cell labeling indices are a measure of disease activity in patients with monoclonal gammopathies. *J Clin Oncol* 6:1041, 1988.

144. Yi Q, Eriksson I, He W, et al: Idiotype-specific T lymphocytes in monoclonal gammopathies: evidence for the presence of CD4+ and CD8+ subsets. *Br J Haematol* 96:338, 1997.

145. Yi Q, Osterborg A, Bergenbrant S, et al: Idiotype-reactive T-cell subsets and tumor load in monoclonal gammopathies. *Blood* 86:3043, 1995.

146. Halapi E, Werner A, Wahlstrom J, et al: T cell repertoire in patients with multiple myeloma and monoclonal gammopathy of undetermined significance: clonal CD8+ T cell expansions are found preferentially in patients with a low tumor burden. *Eur J Immunol* 27:2245, 1997.

147. Corso A, Castelli G, Pagnucco G, et al: Bone marrow T-cell subsets in patients with monoclonal gammopathies: correlation with clinical stage and disease. *Haematologia* 82:43, 1997.

148. Miguel-Garcia A, Matutes E, Tarin F, et al: Circulating Ki 67 positive lymphocytes in multiple myeloma and benign monoclonal gammopathy. *J Clin Pathol* 48:835, 1995.

149. Billadeau D, Van Ness B, Kimlinger T, et al: Clonal circulation cells are common in plasma cell proliferative disorders: a comparison of monoclonal gammopathy, smoldering myeloma, and active myeloma. *Blood* 88:289, 1996.

150. Isaksson E, Bjockholm M, Holm G, et al: Blood clonal B-cell excess in patients with monoclonal gammopathy of undetermined significance (MGUS): association with malignant transformation. *Br J Haematol* 92:71, 1996.

151. Sawanoborj M, Suzuki K, Nakagawa Y, et al: Natural killer cell frequency and serum cytokine levels in monoclonal gammopathies: correlation of bone marrow granular lymphocytes to prognosis. *Acta Haematol* 98:150, 1997.

152. Leo E, Kropff M, Lindemann A, et al: DNA aneuploidy, increased proliferation and nuclear area of plasma cells in monoclonal gammopathy of undetermined significance and multiple myeloma. *Anal Quant Cytol Histol* 17:113, 1995.

153. Turesson I: Nucleolar size in benign and malignant plasma cell proliferation. *Acta Med Scand* 197:7, 1975.

154. Dehou MF, Schots R, Lacor P, Arras N, et al: Diagnostic and prognostic value of the MB2 monoclonal antibody in paraffin-embedded bone marrow sections of patients with multiple myeloma and monoclonal gammopathy of undetermined significance. *J Clin Pathol* 94:287, 1990.

155. Yasuda N, Kanoh T, Uchino H: J chain synthesis in human myeloma cells: light and electron microscopic studies. *Clin Exp Immunol* 40:573, 1980.

156. Cassuto JP, Hammore JC, Pastorelli E, et al: Plasma cell acid phosphatase, a discriminative test for benign and malignant monoclonal gammopathies. *Biomed* 27:97, 1977.

157. Sonneveld P, Durie BGM, Lokhorst HM, et al: Analysis of multidrug-resistance (MDR-1) glycoprotein and CD56 expression to separate monoclonal gammopathy from multiple myeloma. *Br J Haematol* 83:63, 1993.

158. Zandecki N, Facon T, Bernard F, et al: CD19 and immunophenotype of bone marrow plasma cells in monoclonal gammopathy of undetermined significance. *J Clin Pathol* 48:548, 1995.

159. Majumdar G, Heard SE, Singh AK: Use of cytoplasmic 5-prime nucleotidase for differentiating malignant from benign monoclonal gammopathies. *J Clin Pathol* 43:891, 1990.

160. Van de Berg BC, Michaux L, Lecouvet FE, et al: Nonmyelomatous monoclonal gammopathy: correlation of bone marrow MR images with laboratory findings and spontaneous clinical outcome. *Radiology* 202:249, 1997.

161. Bellaiche L, Laredo J-D, Lioté F, et al: Magnetic resonance appearance of monoclonal gammopathies of unknown significance and mutiple myeloma. *Spine* 22:2551, 1997.

162. Laroche M, Attal M, Pouilles JM, et al: Dual-energy x-ray absorption in patients with multiple myeloma and benign gammopathies. *Clin Exp Rheumatol* 14:108, 1996.

163. Bataille R, Chappard D, Basle M: Quantifiable excess of bone resorption in monoclonal gammopathy is an early symptom of malignancy: a prospective study of 87 bone biopsies. *Blood* 87:4762, 1996.

164. Pecherstorfer M, Seibel MJ, Woitge HW, et al: Bone resorption in multiple myeloma and in monoclonal gammopathy of undetermined significance: quantification by urinary pyridinium cross-links of collagen. *Blood* 90:3743, 1997.

165. Ong F, Kaiser U, Seelen PJ, et al: Serum neural cell adhesion molecule differentiates multiple myeloma from paraproteinemias due to other causes. *Blood* 87:712, 1996.

166. Greco C, Ameglio F, Alvino S, et al: Selection of patients with monoclonal gammopathy of undetermined significance is mandatory for a reliable use of interleukin-6 and other nonspecific multiple myeloma serum markers. *Acta Haematol* 92:1, 1994.

167. Mathiot C, Mary JY, Tartour E, et al: Soluble CD16 (sCD16), a marker of malignancy in individuals with monoclonal gammopathy of undetermined significance (MGUS). *Br J Haematol* 95:660, 1996.

168. Gaillard JP, Bataille R, Brailly H, et al: Increased and highly stable levels of functional soluble interleukin-6 receptor levels in sera of patients with monoclonal gammopathy. *Eur J Immunol* 23:820, 1993.

169. DuVillard L, Guiguet M, Casasnovas R-O, et al: Diagnostic value of serum IL-6 level in monoclonal gammopathies. *Br J Haematol* 89:243, 1995.

170. Pasqualetti P, Festucci V, Collacciani A, Casale R: The natural history of monoclonal gammopathy of undetermined significance. *Acta Haematol* 97:174, 1997.

171. Van de Poel MHW, Coebergh JWW, Hillen HFP: Malignant transformation of monoclonal gammopathy of undetermined significance among out-patients of a community hospital in southeastern Netherlands. *Br J Haematol* 91:121, 1995.

172. Kyle RA: Monoclonal gammopathy of undetermined significance. *Blood Review* 8:135, 1994.

173. Pasqualetti P, Casale R: Risk of malignant transformation in patients with monoclonal gammopathy of undetermined significance. *Biomed Pharmacother* 51:74, 1997.

174. Cozzolino F, Torcia M, Aldinucci D, et al: Production of interleukin-1 by bone marrow myeloma cells. *Blood* 74:380, 1989.

175. Donovan KA, Lacy MQ, Kline MP, et al: Contrast in cytokine expression between patients with monoclonal gammopathy of undetermined significance or multiple myeloma. *Leukemia* 12:593, 1998.

176. Disdier P, Swiader L, Aillaud M-F, et al: Ig M monoclonal gammopathy, lymphoid proliferations and lupus anticoagulant. *Am J Med* 102:319, 1997.

177. Chryssikkopoulos A, Dalamaga AL, Hassiakos D: Monoclonal gammopathy of unknown significance in pregnancy. *Clin Exp Obstet Gynecol* 24:31, 1997.

178. deKleijn EM, Telgt D, Laan R: Schnitzler's syndrome presenting as fever of unknown origin (FUO): the role of cytokines in its systemic features. *Neth J Med* 51:140, 1997.

179. Andreone P, Zignego AL, Cursaro C, et al: Prevalence of monoclonal gammopathies in patients with hepatitis C virus infection. *Ann Intern Med* 129:294, 1998.

PLASMA CELL MYELOMA

BART BARLOGIE

JOHN SHAUGHNESSY

NIKHIL MUNSHI

JOSHUA EPSTEIN

Multiple myeloma is a B-cell malignancy of neoplastic plasma cells that generally produce a monoclonal immunoglobulin protein. It remains controversial whether all cases of myeloma evolve from an essential monoclonal gammopathy or MGUS condition (monoclonal gammopathy of undetermined significance). Through intricate interactions with the marrow microenvironment, myeloma plasma cells receive critical survival signals, which may explain the relative resistance of this generally hypoproliferative tumor to chemotherapy. This disease causes clinical symptoms by way of tumor mass effects (pain), cytokine production (anemia), and protein deposition in organs (kidney, heart). Clinical manifestations of myeloma vary as a result of the heterogeneous biology and span the entire spectrum from indolent disease to highly aggressive myeloma presenting with extramedullary features. Magnetic resonance imaging (MRI) has become an important staging tool to distinguish truly solitary plasmacytoma of bone from multiple myeloma and, within the latter category, to document the extent and pattern of marrow involvement that can be diffuse or distinctly macrofocal. Prognosis is best correlated with serum levels of beta-2-microglobulin and C-reactive protein but also with the plasma cell labeling index. Recent studies indicate that cytogenetics may help delineate a subgroup of patients who have neoplastic cells with deletions in chromosome 13 and a more adverse prognosis. Standard therapy with melphalan-prednisone or similar agents has been palliative. High-dose melphalan requiring hemopoietic stem cell support has increased the incidence of true complete remission from 5 percent to approximately 50 percent. Additional therapeutic developments include thalidomide that is active in one-third of patients relapsing after high-dose therapy, consolidation chemotherapy following high-dose stem-cell-supported therapy, and immune therapy. Bisphosphonates and recombinant erythropoietin represent two important adjuncts alleviating myeloma-associated bone disease and anemia, respectively.

DEFINITION

Multiple myeloma (MM) accounts for approximately 1 percent of all malignancies and 10 percent of hematological tumors and represents the second most frequently occurring hematological malignancy in the United States. At any one time, 40,000 people suffer from MM, and approximately 13,000 are diagnosed each year. The median age is approximately 65 years, although occasionally MM occurs in the second decade of life. Myeloma is a disease of neoplastic plasma cells that synthesize abnormal amounts of immunoglobulin or immunoglobulin fragments. Clinical manifestations are heterogeneous but include the formation of tumor, monoclonal immunoglobulin production, decreased immunoglobulin secretion by normal plasma cells leading to hypogammaglobulinemia, impaired hematopoiesis, osteolytic bone disease, hypercalcemia, and renal dysfunction. Symptoms are caused by tumor mass effects, cytokines released directly by tumor cells or indirectly by host cells (marrow stroma and bone cells) in response to adhesion of tumor cells, and, finally, by the abnormal MM protein leading to deposition diseases (AL amyloidosis and light-chain deposition) or autoimmune disorders (e.g., coagulopathies).

This disease belongs to a spectrum of disorders referred to as *plasma cell dyscrasias*. These include clinically benign conditions, such as essential monoclonal gammopathy (see Chap. 105, "Essential Monoclonal Gammopathy"); rare and biologically intriguing disorders, such as Castleman disease and alpha-heavy-chain disease (see Chap. 109, "Heavy-chain disease"); macroglobulinemia (see Chap. 108, "Macroglobulinemia"); solitary plasmacytoma with a high potential for cure when arising in soft tissue; and the most common malignant entity, plasma cell myeloma, a disseminated B-cell malignancy, not curable with standard dose-chemotherapy. All disorders share plasma-cell morphologic features, and most are associated with the production of immunoglobulin molecules (see Chap. 107, "Functions of B lymphocytes and plasma cells"). While most plasma cell dyscrasias result from the expansion of a single clone of cells, with resultant monoclonal protein secretion, oligoclonal and polyclonal protein abnormalities accompany some conditions, such as Castleman disease or angioimmunoblastic lymphoproliferative disease, now recognized as a T-cell lymphoma (see Chap. 103, "Lymphomas").

ETIOLOGY AND PATHOGENESIS

ANIMAL MODELS

Plasmacytoma or myeloma can be induced in BALB/c mice by pristane oil or can develop spontaneously in some mouse strains.[1,2] In the former, pristane oil induces an oil granuloma characterized by lymphoplasmacytic reaction to the chemical. This progresses to an autonomously growing plasmacytoma with uncontrolled expression of *c-MYC* due to its gene rearrangement. Generally, these plasmacytomas secrete monoclonal immunoglobulin of the IgA isotype. Essential monoclonal gammopathies and a malignancy resembling human plasma cell myeloma may arise spontaneously in inbred mice.[3,4]

Human myeloma cell lines can survive and disseminate in mice with severe combined immunodeficiency (SCID).[5,6] Fetal bone implants (SCID-hu) can sustain survival and expansion of primary human myeloma cells from untreated patients with a high success rate.[7] Thus, at last, the SCID-hu model provides a suitable in vivo read out system to study human myeloma biology. Tumor self-renewal capacity can be examined in relation to maturation stage and the contributions of host accessory cells and cytokines to disease manifestation and progression elucidated. It is anticipated that new treatment principles aimed, for example, at inactivating the marrow microenvironment (e.g., bisphosphonates[8,9]) and targeting neoangiogenesis (e.g., Thalidomide[10,11]) can be evaluated.

ENVIRONMENTAL EXPOSURE

Environmental exposure to radiation and chemicals has been associated with an increased incidence of myeloma.[12] Studies of atomic bomb survivors observed an increased incidence of plasma cell myeloma 15 to 20 years after radiation exposure.[13] On the other hand, epidemiological studies attempting to establish associations between myeloma and certain infections or autoimmune diseases have remained inconclusive.[14]

Human herpes virus, (HHV-8) (also called Kaposi-sarcoma herpes virus [KSHV]), already shown to be involved in the pathogenesis of Castleman disease,[15] pleural cavity lymphoma[16] and Kaposi sarcoma,[17] has recently been shown to be present in marrow dendritic cells of the majority of patients with myeloma.[18,19] Although confirmed by some groups,[20,21] others failed to identify HHV-8 in dendritic cells generated from mobilized peripheral blood stem cells.[22,23] Additionally, serologic evidence of HHV-8 infection has not been demonstrated.[24] Using nested PCR, 60 percent of 30 myeloma samples were positive, but ORF 26 sequence was also amplified in 44 percent of 25 normal controls; other viral genome regions (ORF 72 and 75) were uniformly negative in all myeloma and control samples.[24] The proposed pathogenic mechanism for HHV-8 in myeloma is unique in that tumorigenesis would involve the infection of a normal cell lineage (dendritic cells) exerting tumor cell-survival- and growth-promoting signals.

PATHOGENESIS AND GENETIC ALTERATIONS

A multistep process is probably involved in the malignant transformation leading to myeloma[25-27] (Table 106-1, Figs. 106-1 and 106-2). Early mutations may be cryptic and involve virgin and memory B cells that, in the process of recycling through lymphoid follicles and antigen-triggered replication, accumulate genetic damage. Such "migrant plasmablasts" may be involved in the pathogenesis of solitary plasmacytoma, essential monoclonal gammopathy, and the progression to plasma cell myeloma[27,28] (see Fig. 106-1). Although the tissue site of malignant transformation and incipient tumor growth in human myeloma is unknown, myeloma cell expansion occurs in the marrow in close interaction with normal stromal cell compartments. The presence of clonotypic cells in the blood even at diagnosis underscores the importance of hematogenous spread for disease dissemination and homing to the marrow, which may be distinctly macrofocal as recognized clinically on magnetic resonance imaging.[29-39]

The tremendous karyotypic complexity, with an average of 11 abnormalities per karyotype and lack of obvious recurrent chromosomal changes in myeloma has precluded a focused search for specific molecular lesions.[40-43] Screening for abnormalities of oncogenes and tumor suppressor genes involved in B-cell lymphomas and leukemias has revealed infrequent rearrangements of BCL-1, BCL-2, and C-MYC genes.[44] Abnormal size C-MYC transcripts as well as high-level expression of c-MYC RNA and protein have been reported in the majority of patients studied.[45] Mutations of N-RAS occur in up to 50 percent of patients.[46-50] BCL2 protein is abundant in both normal and malignant plasma cells.[51,52] Using fluorescence in situ hybridization (FISH), investigators have found RB1 or P53 mutations and deletions in malig-

TABLE 106-1　PLASMA CELL MYELOMA: BIOLOGY AND THERAPY

FEATURES	NOTES
Symptoms	
Anemia	Secondary to marrow replacement with neoplastic plasma cells and secretion of IL-6, IL-1, TNF-α, and/or TNF-β
Bone lesions	Secondary to secretion of IL-1-β, TNF-β, and/or IL-6
Renal failure	Secondary to light chain casts (Bence Jones proteinuria), hypercalcemia with interstitial nephritis, AL or LCDD
Infections	B-cell and T-cell immunodeficiency (secondary to TGF-β, FAS ligand production by MM cells)
Hypoalbuminemia	Secondary to IL-6
Cytogenetics	DNA hyperdiploidy noted in 80% of cases
Complex "myeloma signature"	Trisomy or monosomy common; 14q32 translocations involving many translocation partners; monosomy 13 or del 13q present in 15%–20% mostly involving 13q14
Oncogenes and cell proliferation genes	RAS mutations in 30%; MYC RNA over-expressed in 25%, excess myc protein noted in > 80%; BCL-1 (cyclin D 1) over-expressed in cell lines, rarely in patient samples; FGFR3 and MMSET on 4p16 in cell lines and some patient samples?
Anti-apoptosis and cell cycle regulatory genes	BCL-2 expressed in normal and malignant plasma cells; p53 and Rb deletions/mutations; MDM2 (murine double minute 2 gene) products inhibit p53 function; NF-κB central modulator of apoptosis
Phenotype	Monoclonal cytoplasmic immunoglobulin; pre-B-cell, T-cell, myeloid, erythroid, megakaryocyte, and NK cell markers; preplasmacyte compartment also in blood (CD11b$^+$, CD19$^+$, CD45$^+$); syndecan-1 expression used to purify MM cells (BB-4 antibody) although syndecan-1-negative cells exist
Growth factors and receptors	IL-6 receptors on most myeloma cells; IL-6 effects on tumor cell proliferation, differentiation, and survival (anti-apoptotic signal); in vitro proliferative effects of IL-1, IL-3, GM-CSF, HGF; inhibition of proliferation and induction of apoptosis by soluble syndecan-1
Staging	Serum β_2-microglobulin, C-reactive protein, Durie-Salmon system, plasma cell labeling index, lactic dehydrogenase, chromosome 13 deletion, Rb deletion
Treatment	Glucocorticoids highly effective; melphalan and prednisone, VAD (Vincristine, Adriamycin, Dexamethasone) for standard therapy; high-dose melphalan +/− TBI and autologous or allogeneic stem cell transplantation; high-dose prednisone or IFN for maintenance
Outcome with standard therapy (melphalan and prednisone)	50% improved; complete remissions in less than 5% of treated patients; median survival of 3 years
Outcome with high-dose therapy (tandem transplants with melphalan 200 mg/m^2)	40%–50% CR; 60% in continuous CR at 7 years when B2M < 4 mg/L and del 13 absent; median durations of event-free survival and overall survival of 3.3 and 5.7 years respectively
Secondary problems	High-grade transformation; plasma cell leukemia; organ failure due to AL or LCDD; AML in less than 5%; myelodysplasia in 5–15% by cytogenetics, depending on prior therapy

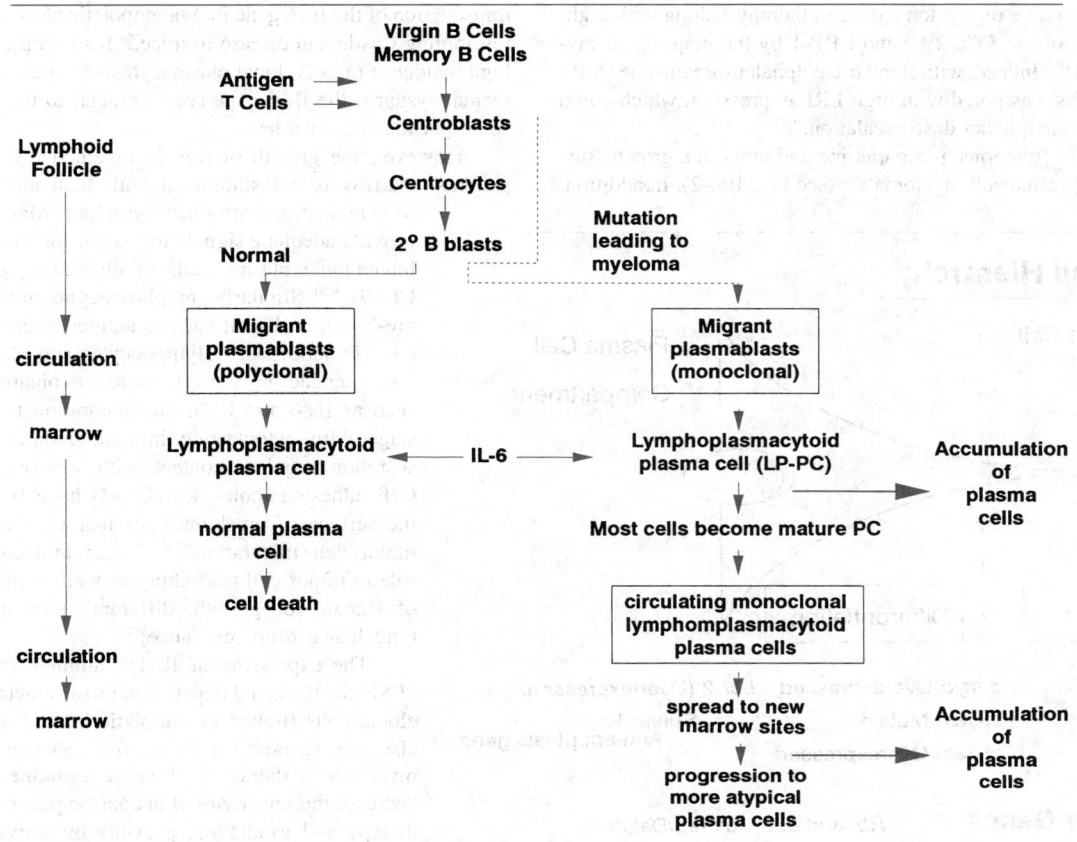

FIGURE 106-1 The origin of multiple myeloma in terms of site of transformation has not yet been elucidated. A putative model assumes a mutation to occur at the level of memory B cells undergoing antigen or T-cell stimulation to centroblasts/centrocytes and secondary B blasts, resulting in monoclonal migrant plasmablasts that circulate in the blood and eventually home to the marrow, where differentiation to mature plasma cells occurs. Thus, the pathogenesis of myeloma may occur in lymphoid follicles with subsequent blood circulation and spread to marrow sites. The sustained life span of malignant B cells with lymphoplasmacytoid/plasmacytic characteristics may be related to an imbalance of cytokine expression, especially IL-6. (Reproduced from Potter,[11] with permission.)

nant plasma cells of up to 50 percent of the patients studied.[49,53–55] P53 can be inactivated by MDM 2, which is overexpressed in myeloma cell lines but rarely in clinical specimens [56]

Unlike CLL, considered a pregerminal center B-cell malignancy with limited Ig gene hypermutations (see Chap. 98, "Chronic Lymphocytic Leukemia"), myeloma has all the hallmarks of a germinal center-derived tumor with a post-switch B-cell phenotype (IgM myeloma is exceedingly rare) and is characterized by extensive Ig gene hypermutation, reflecting antigenic stimulation.[57–61] Given the recent findings that somatic mutation of other loci besides the immunoglobulin genes occurs in B cells, e.g., *BCL6*,[62] it is possible to envision that oncogenes and/or tumor suppressor genes could also be affected by a somatic hypermutation mechanisms in myeloma.

Translocations involving 14q32, the site of the immunoglobulin heavy-chain (IgH) locus, occur in 20 to 40 percent of cases with abnormal karyotypes.[27,41,42] In approximately 30 percent of the cases, the translocation affects the *BCL1* (cyclin D) locus on 11q13.[27] In most cases the partner loci are not identified and the chromosome is designated as an add 14q32. G-banded and spectral karyotyping of patient samples has demonstrated that the add 14q32 chromosome is frequently a t(14;16)(q32;q22~23).[63] Molecular analysis of this translocation has shown that it results in a fusion of IgH switch region with the sequences near the *c-MAF* oncogene.[64] Additional recurrent 14q32 translocations cloned from myeloma cell lines involve 4p16 (FGFR3

and MMSET[65,66] and 6p25 (MUM1/IRF4).[67] The promiscuous array of exchange partners involved in the 14q32 translocations makes it unclear as to their importance in myelomagenesis as the clinical implications of these translocations have not been reported.

Recent studies have demonstrated that partial or complete deletion of chromosome 13 represents an important negative prognostic variable and represents the first chromosomal abnormality linked to clinical outcome. While initially observed in the context of high-dose therapy,[68,69] the high-risk implications of chromosome 13 deletion have recently been confirmed in the context of standard therapy using either G-banding or FISH using the *RB1* gene.[70,71] Further scrutiny of the entire length of chromosome 13 by molecular cytogenetic analysis in interphase cells has revealed deletions in nearly 90 percent of patients.[72] Critical regions of the chromosome appear to lie in the 13q12, 13q14, and 13q21-22 bands. It is anticipated that myeloma-specific tumor suppressor genes will soon be identified on 13q.

PHENOTYPE AND CYTOKINES

The expression of the multidrug resistance gene (*MDR*) is observed in myeloma cells, even prior to therapy.[73] This may explain the resistance to chemotherapeutic agents whose cellular efflux is mediated by the *MDR* pump.[74–78] *De novo MDR* expression, albeit by only a small fraction of tumor cells,[74] suggests that *MDR* may facilitate the survival and resistance of myeloma cells to therapy[79] along with high-level expression of the *BCL-2*[51,52] and LRP-1 by the majority of myeloma plasma cells. Indeed, with standard melphalan-prednisone (MP), inferior prognosis was noted with high LRP expression, which could be overcome by melphalan dose escalation.[80,81]

Interleukin-6 functions as a paracrine and autocrine growth/survival factor for plasma cell myeloma[82–85] (see Fig. 106-2). In addition,

transduction of the IL-6 gene into hemopoietic cells leads to a disorder resembling Castleman disease in mice.[86] IL-6 transgenic mice have a high incidence of polyclonal plasmacytosis.[87] Thus, at least in experimental systems, the IL-6 gene seems crucial to the manifestation of some plasma cell disorders.

However, the growth of freshly obtained myeloma cells from patients' marrow is not stimulated with IL-6 alone, or with IL-6 in combination with other cytokines. Marrow stromal cells provide adequate signals for expansion and maturation into monoclonal plasma cells of circulating B cells (CD11b, CD19).[89,90] Similarly, preplasmacytic myeloma cells with pre-B-cell or B-cell surface antigen expression (see Chap. 83, "Functions of B lymphocytes and plasma cells") can be expanded in vitro with a combination of cytokines such as IL-6 and IL-3, but maturation to the plasma cell stage with cytoplasmic immunoglobulin expression and secretion requires contact with marrow stromal cells.[90] Cell adhesion molecules (CAM) have been identified on the surface of myeloma cells that vary with the stage of tumor cell maturation.[91–95] These molecules may play a role in tumor cell trafficking as well as in the transduction of signals for growth, differentiation, and cell survival (and hence drug resistance).[96]

The expression of IL-1β, tumor necrosis factor beta (TNF-β), IL-6, and hepatocyte growth factor (HGF) by myeloma cells (linked to osteolytic bone disease, see below) also may account for the relative resistance of plasma cell myeloma to therapy.[97–103] These cytokines apparently can decrease the sensitivity of neoplastic plasma cells to chemotherapy and irradiation, possibly by activation of NF-κB, which is a central modulator of myeloma cell apoptosis.[104,105]

Syndecan-1, a heparin proteoglycan present in pre-B cells, is reexpressed at the plasma cell differentiation stage, including the neoplastic myeloma plasma cell.[106,107] The molecule is shed so that, similar to beta-2-microglobulin, its serum concentration reflects tumor burden.[108] In vitro and in vivo experimental studies have documented a role of syndecan-1 in cell-cell and cell-matrix adhesion, delaying cell cycle progression and inducing myeloma cell apoptosis suggestive of a potentially important autoregulatory loop.[109] Syndecan-1 may also serve to trap growth-regulatory molecules such as insulin growth factor (IGF) and fibroblast growth factor (FGF).[110] Moreover, syndecan-1 promotes osteoblast activation and inhibits osteoclast differentiation, thereby exerting a potentially beneficial effect on bone.[109]

The feasibility of in vivo propagation of human myeloma cell lines (SCID mice)[5,6] and of primary human tumor cells also from previously untreated patients (SCID-hu system)[7,110] has opened up entirely new research avenues to identify in vivo the critical growth-promoting and growth-inhibitory cytokines and their host cell sources and to elucidate the mechanisms involved. Furthermore, the recapitulation of human disease in the SCID-hu system with anemia, bone destruction, wasting, and renal failure should serve as a powerful tool to identify therapies directed not only at myeloma growth control but at palliation of symptoms. Administration of bisphosphonates not only halts bone destruction, it also inhibits myeloma growth in this system, presumably by interfering with the interactions between the human marrow microenvironment and the myeloma cells, thus opening a novel avenue of myeloma growth control aimed at inactivating the "soil" on which the "seed" of tumor cells survive and expand.

Tumor Cell Hierarchy

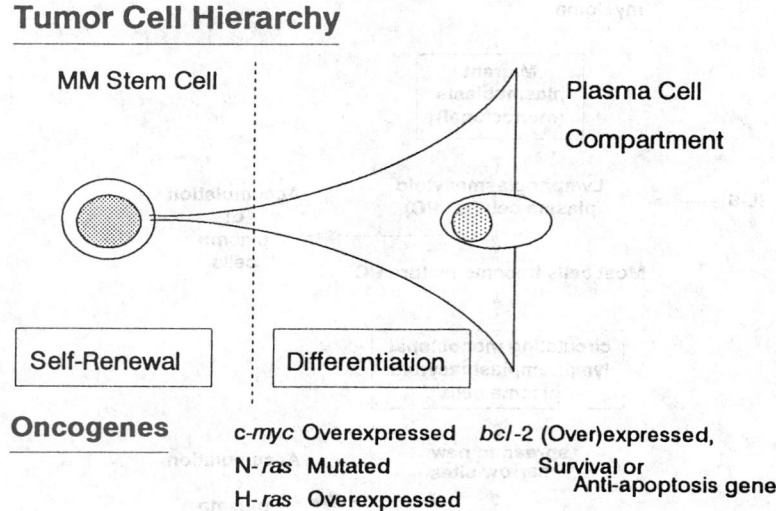

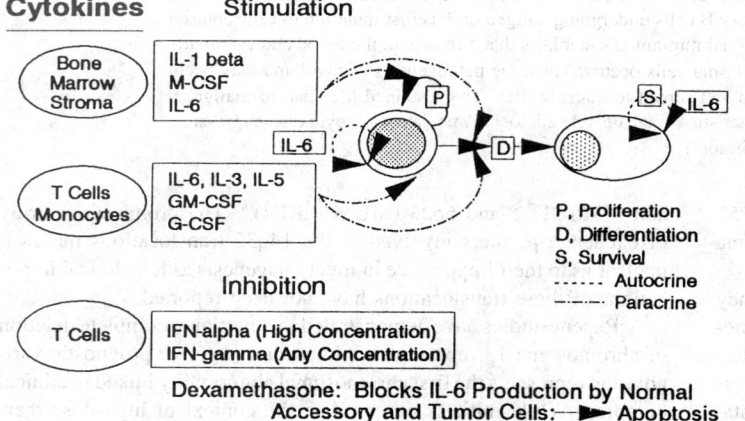

FIGURE 106-2   Biology of multiple myeloma. *Tumor cell hierarchy:* The predominant tumor cell population in the marrow consists of mature plasma cells, and the tumor stem cell compartment with unlimited self-renewal capacity remains elusive. It appears that tumor progenitor cells are relatively infrequent and maintain, through a variety of cytokines, a systemic malignancy with a predominantly terminal B-cell phenotype. *Oncogenes:* As in the mouse model, c-*MYC* is overexpressed at the RNA and protein level in more than 80 percent of patients; *MYC* rearrangement is infrequent, however, but abnormal *MYC* RNA transcripts are commonly observed. N-*RAS* is mutated in about one-third of cases, H-ras protein is overexpressed in approximately 80 percent, and high *BCL-2* expression is noted in both myeloma and normal plasma cells. *Suppressor genes:* Mutations and deletions of both *RB* and *p53* have been reported. *Cytokines:* The cytokine network in myelomatosis is exceedingly complex, involving many of the cytokines also important in regulation of normal hemopoiesis. IL-6 induces tumor cells to proliferate, to differentiate, or to resist undergoing apoptosis at various stages of tumor cell differentiation. Inhibitory molecules include IFN-α (at high concentrations) and IFN-γ (also at lower concentrations). Glucocorticoids block IL-6 production by tumor and normal accessory cells and thus induce apoptosis, which can be counteracted by exogenous IL-6.

MYELOMA BIOLOGY

Consistent with results seen in other germinal center cell-derived B-cell malignancies, such as follicular and diffuse large-cell lymphomas, plasma cell myelomas express immunoglobulin genes that have undergone somatic mutation. In addition, the BCL-6 in myeloma also can harbor mutations in the 5′ autoregulatory site. Conceivably, other tumor suppressor genes may be affected by the natural, but potentially pathogenic, process of immunoglobulin somatic mutation.''

A key candidate site for such mutations is located on chromosome 13, which, when morphologically deleted, is associated with rapid disease progression and grave prognosis. Molecular genetic studies employing FISH of interphase cells have recently demonstrated that nearly 90 percent of both newly diagnosed and previously treated patients harbor chromosome 13 deletions. The presence of biallelic deletions at specific loci at 13q12, q14, and q21 and the seemingly progressive acquisition of additional deletions on chromosome 13 are consistent with tumor suppressor gene activity in this region conferring survival or proliferation advantage. The clinically more benign numeric aberrations, mainly involving gains in the number of chromosomes, may result from centrosome disorganization.[111]

Myeloma cells are endowed with receptors for a multiplicity of potentially growth-promoting cytokines IL-6, IL-11, oncostatin-M, leukemia inhibitory factor (LIF), granulocyte colony stimulating factor (G-CSF), stem cell factor (SCF), interferon alpha (INF-α and IL-10), tumor necrosis factor (TNF-α), insulin growth factor (IGF-I and IGF-II).[26,27] Antibodies to IL-6, as well as high concentrations of IFN-α, INFγ, and soluble syndecan-1 inhibit cell growth. Most of these results have been observed in established myeloma cell lines, so that their relevance for clinical disease sustenance and progression remains to be elucidated. This is now possible with the availability of the SCID-hu host system for myeloma. The expression of multiple cell adhesion molecules such as CD44, CD49d (VLA-4), CD54 (ICAM-1), CD56 (NCAM), and CD138 (syndecan-1) is important for mediating adherence of myeloma cells to the marrow stroma, triggering the secretion of IL-6 and other cytokines in stromal cells that, in the case of IL-6, involves NF-κB activation of the IL-6 promoter, which may be mediated by RANKL.[112]

A role for tumor angiogenesis also has been demonstrated for myeloma where high microvessel density was associated with markedly inferior prognosis.[113] Angiogenic factors such as vascular endothelial growth factor 1 (VEGF-1) are expressed by myeloma cells, and VEGF receptors (Flt-1) are present on endothelial cells.[114] The recently observed clinical antitumor activity of thalidomide in about one-third of patients with far advanced disease may involve an antiangiogenic mechanism, possibly involving the down-regulation of VEGF.[115,11]

The progression of myeloma is intimately linked to the marrow microenvironment. Circulating clonotypic B cells, present even in the earliest stages of the disease, including solitary plasmacytoma, adhere to marrow stoma through unique adhesion molecule combinations. The survival of these cells is enhanced by growth signals elaborated by the various components of the marrow microenvironment. The genomic complexity, unique among B-cell malignancies, confers an unusual degree of resistance of typically hypoproliferative myeloma cells to both endogenous and exogenous (i.e., therapeutic) apoptosis-inducing signals. In the terminal disease phase, hyperproliferative features are acquired either due to mutations of cell cycle repressor genes or by way of translocations involving cell cycle activators such as cyclin D1. Thus, the B-cell maturation stage-dependent susceptibility to Ig gene mutations probably extends to critical cell cycle repressor genes and master switch genes such as BCL-6 that collectively lead to expression of genes that facilitate marrow adhesion and clinical disease development. Marrow stromal cell activation may be conferred by additional exogenous stimuli, such as viruses or other carcinogens.

CLINICAL FEATURES

Patients may present with symptoms of anemia, bone pain, pathologic fractures, a bleeding tendency, and/or peripheral neuropathies. These signs and symptoms generally result from tumor mass effects or from the proteins or cytokines secreted by tumor cells or normal accessory cells under the influence of tumor cell products (see Table 106-1 and Fig. 106-2).

PAIN

Pain suffered by subjects with myeloma results most frequently from vertebral compression fractures at sites of osteopenia or, more typically, lytic bone lesions. These are due to excessive osteoclast activating factor (OAF) activity exerted by IL-1-β,[97] TNF-β,[98] and/or IL-6.[116] These factors apparently also inhibit compensatory osteoblastic activity.[117] Localized pain can also be induced by regional tumor growth toward the spinal cord and nerve roots. Painful mass effects also can be provoked by amyloid deposition (see Chap. 107, ''Amyloidosis'') in various anatomic sites, e.g., the median nerve sheath, as in amyloid-associated carpal tunnel syndrome.[118]

INFECTIONS

Deficiencies in cellular immune function account for the recurrent infections commonly seen in myeloma.[119–121] The mechanisms underlying this immunodeficiency remain obscure, although transforming growth factor beta (TGF-β)[122] and FAS-ligand have been incriminated.[123] In addition, patients are impaired in their ability to mount a humoral immune response to antigen and, except for the myeloma protein, have low levels of other serum immunoglobulins. As a result, myeloma patients are more susceptible to serious infections with bacteria that ordinarily may be opsonized by specific antibody, such as Streptococcus pneumoniae.

NEPHROPATHY

Abnormalities of renal function occur when the tubular absorptive capacity of light chains is exhausted, resulting in interstitial nephritis with light-chain casts.[124,125] The second most common cause of nephropathy is hypercalcemia with hypercalciuria, leading to volume depletion and prerenal azotemia. In addition, hypercalcemia is conducive to calcium deposits in the renal tubules, also producing interstitial nephritis.[126,127] AL amyloidosis associated with light-chain proteinuria usually presents as nephrotic syndrome but can lead, over time, to renal failure[128–130] (see Chap. 107, ''Amyloidosis''). AL amyloidosis is more common in patients with λ light-chain myeloma proteins than in patients with κ light-chain myeloma, especially those with λ light-chain proteins that have immunoglobulin variable regions belonging to the VI λ light-chain subgroup. Probably underestimated, however, is the frequency of immunoglobulin light-chain deposition disease, a disease more commonly associated with κ light-chain myeloma proteins. This also leads to impaired glomerular filtration.[130,131]

Tumor cell involvement of the kidneys is uncommon but should be suspected in patients with renal enlargement, which, however, is more often due to AL amyloid[129] (see Chap. 107, ''Amyloidosis''). Complicating factors in the pathogenesis of renal failure in myeloma include the frequent use of nonsteroidal anti-inflammatory drugs for pain control.[132] Recent studies using IL-6 transgenic mice that express an IL-6 transgene under the control of the metallothionin-1 promoter indicate that constitutive high-level expression of IL-6 in the liver can induce dysproteinemia and a protracted acute-phase response leading to renal pathology with features remarkably similar to those in human myeloma kidney.[133]

EXTRAMEDULLARY DISEASE

Although uncommon at diagnosis, extramedullary disease manifestations are observed with increasing frequency as the duration of disease control can be extended by high-dose therapy. Liver, lymph nodes, spleen, kidneys, various subcutaneous and cutaneous sites, as well as meninges and brain-parenchyma, can be involved, sometimes accompanying secondary plasma cell leukemia.[134–136] Such visceral organ involvement is typically associated with immunoblastic morphology, high LDH serum levels, high tumor-cell-labeling index, and complex karyotypes.

NEUROPATHIES

Neurologic abnormalities generally are caused by regional tumor growth compressing the spinal cord or cranial nerves. Polyneuropathies are observed with perineuronal or perivascular (*vasa nervorum*) amyloid deposition[118] but also can be seen with osteosclerotic myeloma, sometimes as part of the complete POEMS syndrome (*p*olyneuropathy, *o*rganomegaly, *e*ndocrinopathy, *m*onoclonal gammopathy, and *s*kin changes).[137,138] The humoral and cellular mechanisms mediating this peculiar syndrome are unknown.

HYPERVISCOSITY

Hyperviscosity occurs in fewer than 10 percent of patients with myeloma.[139,140–142] Although noted in a higher proportion of patients with Waldenström macroglobulinemia (see Chap. 108, "Macroglobulinemia"),[143] hyperviscosity actually may be seen more commonly in association with myeloma because of its 10-fold higher incidence.[144] Symptoms of hyperviscosity result from circulatory problems, leading to cerebral, pulmonary, renal, and other organ dysfunction (see "Hyperviscosity Syndrome," Chap. 108, "Macroglobulinemia"). Hyperviscosity often is associated with bleeding.

While there is a general correlation between clinical symptoms and relative serum viscosity, the relationship between serum immunoglobulin levels and symptoms is not consistent from one patient to the next. This may be related to the different physicochemical properties of each of the classes and subclasses of immunoglobulin molecules (see Chap. 83, "Function of B cells and plasma cells"). Because of a greater tendency for IgA to form polymers, patients with IgA myeloma more often have hyperviscosity than patients with IgG myeloma, and almost one-quarter of IgA myeloma patients may have features of the hyperviscosity syndrome.[141] Among patients with IgG myeloma, those with tumors expressing immunoglobulins of the IgG$_3$ subclass are the most susceptible to developing this syndrome.[145]

BLEEDING AND THROMBOSIS

Bleeding has been reported in 15 percent of patients with IgG myeloma and in over 30 percent of patients with IgA myeloma.[146,147] This may be due to anoxia and thrombosis in capillary circulation, to perivascular amyloid, and/or to an acquired coagulopathy.[144] Thrombocytopenia, however, even with extensive marrow involvement, is rare in early phases of myeloma.[148]

Some patients present with thromboembolic disease. These patients may have a hypercoagulable state secondary to acquired deficiencies in protein C or to a lupus anticoagulant (see Chap. 128, "Lupus anticoagulants and related disorders").

LABORATORY FEATURES

The diagnosis even of symptomatic plasma cell myeloma is often delayed by months. Patients may have complaints of persistent back pain following minor trauma or of recurrent infections. Such complaints in the setting of unexplained hyperproteinemia or proteinuria, anemia, renal insufficiency, hypoalbuminemia, dysproteinemia, or marked elevation of the erythrocyte sedimentation rate should prompt laboratory evaluation for plasma cell myeloma.

INITIAL EVALUATION

Minimal requirements include evaluation of the hemogram, inspection of the blood film for the presence of rouleaux, radiographic examination of axial skeleton (skull, entire spine, and pelvis) (Fig. 106-3), serum protein electrophoresis (see Chap. 106, "Plasma Cell Neoplasms: General Considerations"), measurement of urinary protein excretion, and marrow aspiration and biopsy.

HEMATOLOGIC ABNORMALITIES

Neoplastic myeloma cells may replace the normal hemopoietic tissue in the marrow. These cells consist predominantly of plasma cells exhibiting varying degrees of maturity. A larger cell with prominent nucleoli and scant cytoplasm is usually present in small numbers. Such plasmablasts tend to increase with disease progression and may represent the dominant tumor cell population during the terminal disease phase.[149,150] Tumor involvement of the marrow typically causes anemia, the degree of which appears related to tumor mass (see below).

Serum erythropoietin levels are relatively low for the degree of anemia present.[151] This blunted erythropoietin response to anemia may be due to abundant production of cytokines such as IL-1 and TNF-β.[152] This also has been attributed to increased serum viscosity levels.[153] Overproduction of IL-6 by marrow stroma, normal accessory cells, and/or tumor cells may contribute to the anemia of myeloma. However, possibly because of the thrombopoietic activity of this cytokine, myeloma patients typically do not manifest significant thrombocytopenia, in the absence of other factors.

However, thrombocytopenia may develop subsequent to therapy or from autoimmune mechanisms, such as those accounting for anemia or factor VIII deficiency.[154–156] The antibody portion (Fab) of the myeloma protein may bind to fibrin during clotting and prevent fibrin aggregation. This probably represents the most common coagulopathy in patients with myeloma.[157] Factor X deficiency associated with systemic AL amyloidosis apparently cannot be traced to an inhibitor in vitro[158] (see Chap. 107, "Amyloidosis").

Some patients present with thrombocytosis secondary to hyposplenism because of AL amyloid. In addition, hypercoagulable states may result from protein C deficiency, perhaps as a consequence of monoclonal immunoglobulins exhibiting anti-protein-C activity. Lupus anticoagulants also have been reported in association with myeloma. However, these have not been traced to be a direct action of the monoclonal immunoglobulin.[159]

DETECTION OF MONOCLONAL IMMUNOGLOBULIN

Most patients with myeloma secrete a monoclonal immunoglobulin that may be detected by immunoelectrophoresis or, more sensitively, by immunofixation analysis (see Chap. 106, "Plasma Cell Neoplasms: General Considerations"). Of the patients with plasma cell myeloma, approximately 60 percent have detectable monoclonal IgG (usually greater than 3.5 g/dl), 20 percent have monoclonal IgA (typically greater than 2 g/dl), and 20 percent only have monoclonal immunoglobulin light chains. A small proportion of patients have "*nonsecretory myeloma,*" in which the neoplastic plasma cells do not produce significant amounts of monoclonal immunoglobulin. Myelomas pro-

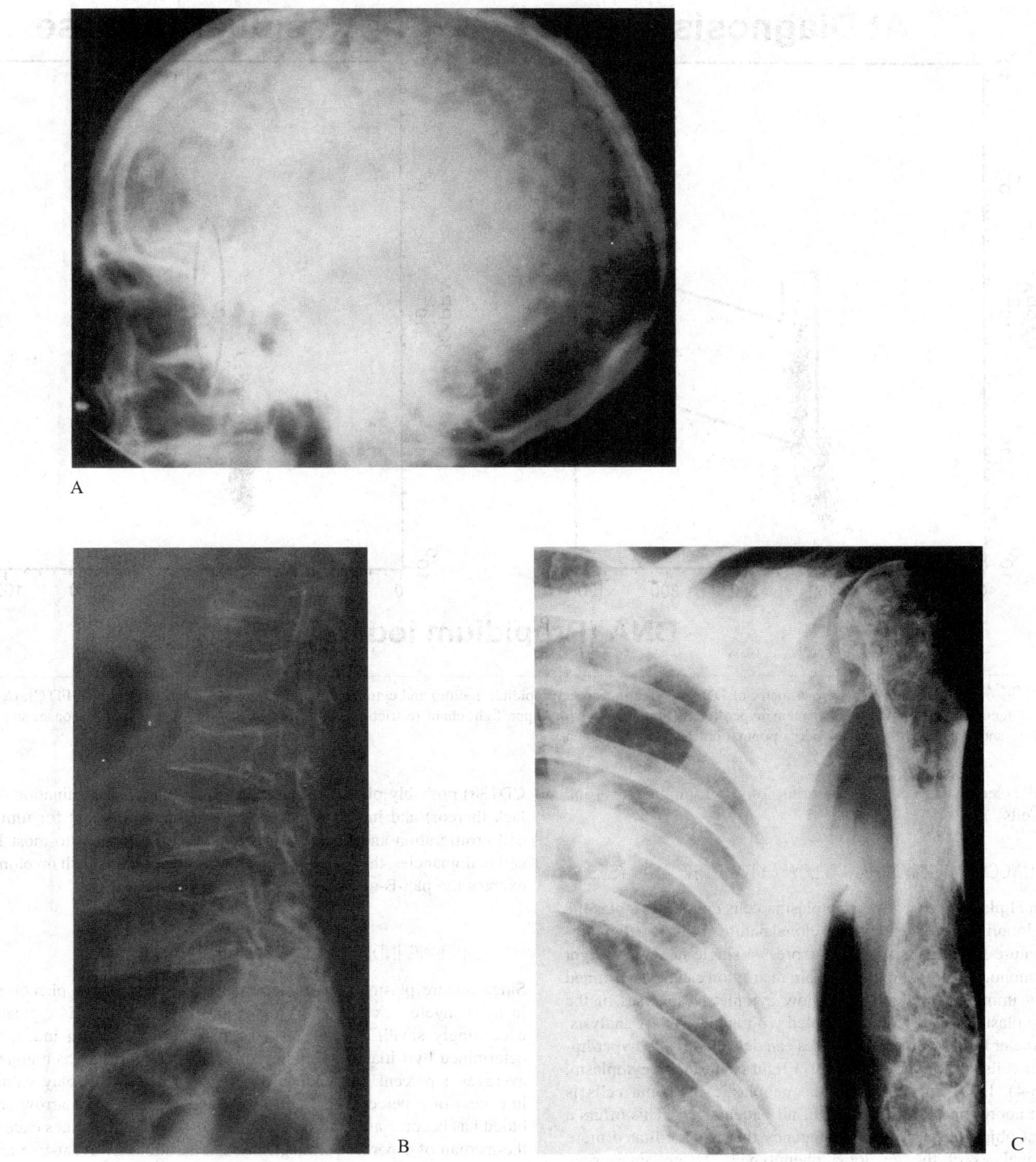

FIGURE 106-3   Typical skeletal changes on roentgenogram. (*a*) Example of "punched-out" lytic lesions in skull. (*b*) Diffuse osteopenia with compression fractures of spine. (*c*) Lytic lesions in the left humerus. (Courtesy of Edgardo J. Angtuaco.)

ducing monoclonal IgD, IgE, IgM, or more than one immunoglobulin class are rare.

Suppression of uninvolved immunoglobulin classes is typical for symptomatic myeloma. Even patients with light-chain myeloma, nonsecretory myeloma, or IgD or IgE myeloma, often have depressed levels of serum IgG, IgA, and IgM. Unlike other myeloma isotypes, IgD myelomas make immunoglobulins that more commonly have λ,

rather than κ, light chains. Patients with plasma cell myeloma often have Bence Jones proteinuria due to the excretion of κ or λ immunoglobulin light chains, often in excess of 1g per 24-h period.

The monoclonal nature of tumor cells can be verified by analyses of immunoglobulin gene rearrangements in the DNA isolated from neoplastic plasma cells.[160,161] In addition, the immunoglobulins produced by the tumor cells can be found to have unique immunoglobulin

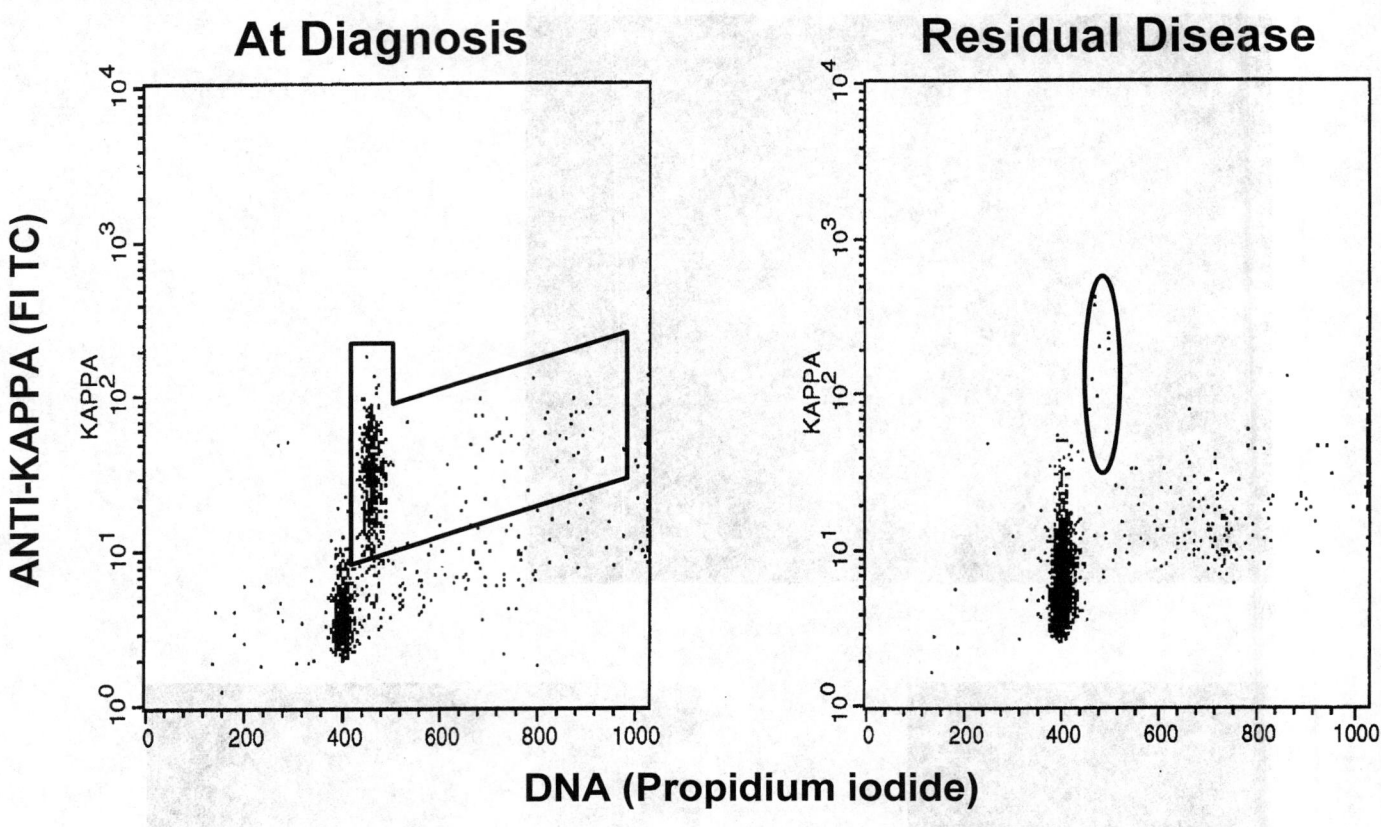

FIGURE 106-4   Two parameter flow cytometry of DNA content (abscissa, propidium iodide) and cytoplasmic immunoglobulin (ordinate, anti-κ FITC); *(left panel)* at diagnosis: approximately 30 percent hyperdiploid tumor cells with kappa light-chain restriction; *(right panel)* at time of maximal response: small hyperdiploid and kappa light-chain-restricted population (less than 1 percent).

idiotypes[32] (see Chap. 83, "Functions of B Lymphocytes and Plasma Cells").

IMMUNOCYTOCHEMICAL AND FLOW CYTOMETRIC ANALYSES

Like normal plasma cells, myeloma plasma cells contain cytoplasmic immunoglobulin. Consistent with the clonal nature of this B-cell malignancy, mature tumor cells typically express a single heavy and light chain. Immunoglobulin κ or λ light-chain restriction can be determined readily by immunocytochemical or flow cytometric analyses of the neoplastic plasma cells.[162] When coupled with nuclear DNA analysis, two-parameter flow cytometric analyses can detect typically hyperdiploid tumor cells with monoclonal κ or λ light chain in the cytoplasm. (Fig. 106-4). DNA aneuploidy in the neoplastic myeloma cells is present in approximately 80 percent of all patients.[163,164] This offers a convenient objective marker of malignancy that has facilitated more detailed analysis of the myeloma phenotype.[165] Using appropriate monoclonal antibodies, myeloma cells have been found to express a wide array of early and late differentiation markers pertaining to myeloid, monocytic, erythroid, megakaryocytic, B-cell, T-cell, and/or natural killer cell lineages.[91,165–169] Some of these markers are coexpressed with cytoplasmic immunoglobulin, an infrequent phenotype in normal B-cell development.[165] Other DNA aneuploid and diploid cells express B and pre-B features (CD10, CD11b, CD19, and CD20) without cytoplasmic immunoglobulin.[33,165] Such cells, present in both marrow and blood, are capable, under suitable in vitro conditions, of differentiating into monoclonal plasma cells.[88,170] The expression of maturation-dependent cell adhesion molecules (e.g., CD56, CD54, or

CD138) probably plays an important role in tumor dissemination (or lack thereof) and in the transduction of signals important for tumor cell proliferation and/or differentiation.[91,106,167] In contrast to most B-cell malignancies, the neoplastic plasma cells of patients with myeloma express the pan-B-cell antigen, CD20, in less than 20%.

LABELING INDEX

Since mature plasma cells represent the dominant tumor phenotype in most myeloma cases, the proportion of cycling cells is typically exceedingly small.[163,171–174] Thus, the plasma cell labeling index, as determined by tritiated thymidine or bromodeoxyuridine techniques, averages 1 percent. Fewer than 5 percent of patients display values in excess of 5 percent.[173,175] The BrdU labeling index of marrow and blood has become an important prognostic variable. As values exceed the median of 1 percent at diagnosis, the durations of event-free and overall survival are progressively shortened.[176]

CYTOGENETICS

It is the low proliferative activity of most morphologically recognizable tumor cells that accounts for the great difficulty in obtaining cytogenetic data, requiring dividing cells to be arrested in metaphase.[40–42,177] Contrasting with DNA aneuploidy in the majority of patients, abnormal karyotypes are observed in only 30 percent of untreated myeloma patients, suggesting that the normal diploid karyotype in the remaining cases originates in normal hemopoietic cells.[164]

Myeloma karyotypes have some of the most complex chromosomal aberrations observed in human malignancies. Marked numeric and structural changes involve virtually all chromosomes (Fig. 106-5). Although these anomalies do not appear random, unique myeloma-specific alterations have not been identified. Translocations common in other B-cell tumors, such as t(8;14), t(11;14), and t(14;18),[27] also are observed in about 5 to 30 percent of patients with myeloma, although with different molecular breakpoints (see below).[44,178-180] Most translocations involving 14q32 are unbalanced and involve IgH switch regions with a multiplicity of translocation partners.[181,182] Whereas historical studies in individual patients failed to demonstrate further genetic evolution during the course of the disease,[183] recent longitudinal investigations have clearly demonstrated clonal evolution including the fascinating observation that myelodysplasia-type anomalies can be acquired not only by normal hemopoietic cells but by myeloma cells as well.[184,185] The acquisition of such "leukemic signature" in addition to the original myeloma karyotypic abnormalities conferred poor prognosis.[184]

The application of FISH using appropriate marker probes has made possible the detection of mainly numeric chromosomal aberrations in interphase cells so that the incidence of genetic abnormalities has been raised beyond 90 percent in some studies.[186] This represents an important advance since chromosome 13 deletion abnormalities have been recognized as the dominant adverse pretreatment laboratory feature with both standard[71] and high-dose therapy,[68] recognized however on standard Giemsa-banded metaphase spreads in only 15 to 20 percent of cases. Rb-1 deletion, on the other hand, can be detected by FISH in interphase cells in approximately 40 percent[55] and seems to distinguish a prognostically unfavorable group of patients receiving standard therapy.[70,187] The application of a chromosome 13 cocktail covering the entire length of 13q has yielded molecular deletions in up to 90 percent of cases, although implications for therapy have yet to be defined.[72] Other chromosomal abnormalities have failed to impart similar prognostic implications when controlled for chromosome 13 deletions.[69] Recent studies with FISH, however, have demonstrated favorable effects of chromosomal gains resulting in trisomy of certain chromosomes,[70] suggesting clinically relevant suppressor gene activity. Translocation (11;14), frequently associated with primary plasma cell leukemia,[183] does not per se confer inferior outcome. Hypodiploidy recognized by DNA flow cytometry was associated with primary drug resistance,[188] and deletion 6q was associated with more extensive bone disease.[189]

DIFFERENTIAL DIAGNOSIS

In most patients, the diagnosis of plasma cell myeloma is readily established.[210,211] Major criteria include the demonstration of marked

TABLE 106-2   CRITERIA FOR DIAGNOSIS OF PLASMA CELL MYELOMA*

Major criteria
Plasmacytomas on tissue biopsy
  Marrow plasmacytosis with >30% plasma cells
  Monoclonal globulin spike on serum electrophoresis >3.5 g/dl for IgG or >2.0 g/dl for IgA; 1.0 g/24 h of κ or λ light-chain excretion on urine electrophoresis in the absence of amyloidosis
Minor criteria
  Marrow plasmacytosis 10–30%
  Monoclonal globulin spike present, but less than the levels defined above
  Lytic bone lesions
  Normal IgM < 0.05 g/dl, IgA < 0.1 g/dl, or IgG < 0.6 g/dl

*The diagnosis of plasma cell myeloma is confirmed when at least one major and one minor criterion or at least *three minor criteria* are documented in *symptomatic* patients with *progressive* disease. The presence of features not specific for the disease supports the diagnosis, particularly if of recent onset: anemia, hypercalcemia, azotemia, bone demineralization, or hypoalbuminemia.

TABLE 106-3   CRITERIA FOR DIAGNOSIS OF ESSENTIAL MONOCLONAL GAMMOPATHY

Monoclonal immunoglobulin in serum
M-component level
  IgG < 3.5 g/dl
  IgA < 2.0 g/dl
  Bence Jones proteinuria < 1.0 g/24 h
Marrow plasma cells < 10%
No bone lesions
No bone marrow lesions on MRI
No symptoms

marrow plasmacytosis, lytic bone lesions, and monoclonal protein in serum and/or urine (Table 106-2). In the absence of lytic bone lesions or diffuse osteopenia, other criteria should feature more prominently, especially anemia, levels of monoclonal protein, marrow plasmacytosis, and/or renal insufficiency. MRI abnormalities are especially useful in assessing for nonsecretory myeloma.

It is important to distinguish plasma cell myeloma from essential monoclonal gammopathy[212,213] (Table 106-3). This condition is associated with lower serum levels of monoclonal protein, less Bence Jones proteinuria, and less detectable monoclonal plasmacytosis in the marrow (see Chap. 108, "Plasma Cell Neoplasms: General Considerations"). Patients with essential monoclonal gammopathy do not have associated anemia, bone lesions, or MRI abnormalities. The monoclonal plasma cells of essential monoclonal gammopathy may be aneuploid.[29] However, these plasma cells have a lower labeling index than that of plasma cell myeloma so that the presence of abnormal metaphases on cytogenetic examination is incompatible with benign gammopathy.[214]

SOLITARY PLASMACYTOMA
Solitary plasmacytoma of bone[204,215,216] *or soft tissue*[217,218] requires the absence of indicators of systemic disease, such as marrow plasmacytosis, anemia, or other lytic or soft tissue lesions. Computed axial tomography (CT) is recommended for more-detailed evaluation of early bone disease not recognized on standard roentgenographic examination.[219] MRI is a powerful tool for detecting plasma cell myeloma involving the marrow in a macrofocal fashion (see Fig. 106-6a) or solitary plasmacytoma (see Fig. 106-6b).[204-209] The detection of a solitary MRI lesion (cytologically proven) in the setting of an otherwise benign gammopathy changes the diagnosis to solitary plasmacytoma. In contrast to most patients with plasma cell myeloma, patients with solitary plasmacytoma or essential monoclonal gammopathy have normal serum immunoglobulin levels.

AMYLOIDOSIS
Additional diagnostic procedures are indicated for patients with lymphadenopathy or hepatosplenomegaly to evaluate for extramedullary disease or protein deposition disease. The diagnosis of AL amyloid (see Chap. 107, "Amyloidosis") often can be made by fine-needle aspiration of subcutaneous fat or by biopsy of the rectal mucosa.[220] Staining the tissue with Congo red may reveal perivascular amyloid with its classical apple-green birefringence when viewed under polarized light.[221] AL amyloid also may be detectable on marrow biopsy.[130] Amyloidosis should be suspected in patients with macroglossia, "racoon's eyes" (resulting from periorbital subcutaneous hemorrhages due to vascular fragility), carpal tunnel syndrome, nephrosis, or cardiomegaly associated with arrhythmias or low-voltage and conduction defects on electrocardiogram.[222] Patients suspected of having isolated cardiac amyloid with myeloma should be evaluated via echocardiography.[223] Endomyocardial biopsy may establish the diagnosis. Orthostatic hypotension also should alert to the possibility of systemic amyloidosis

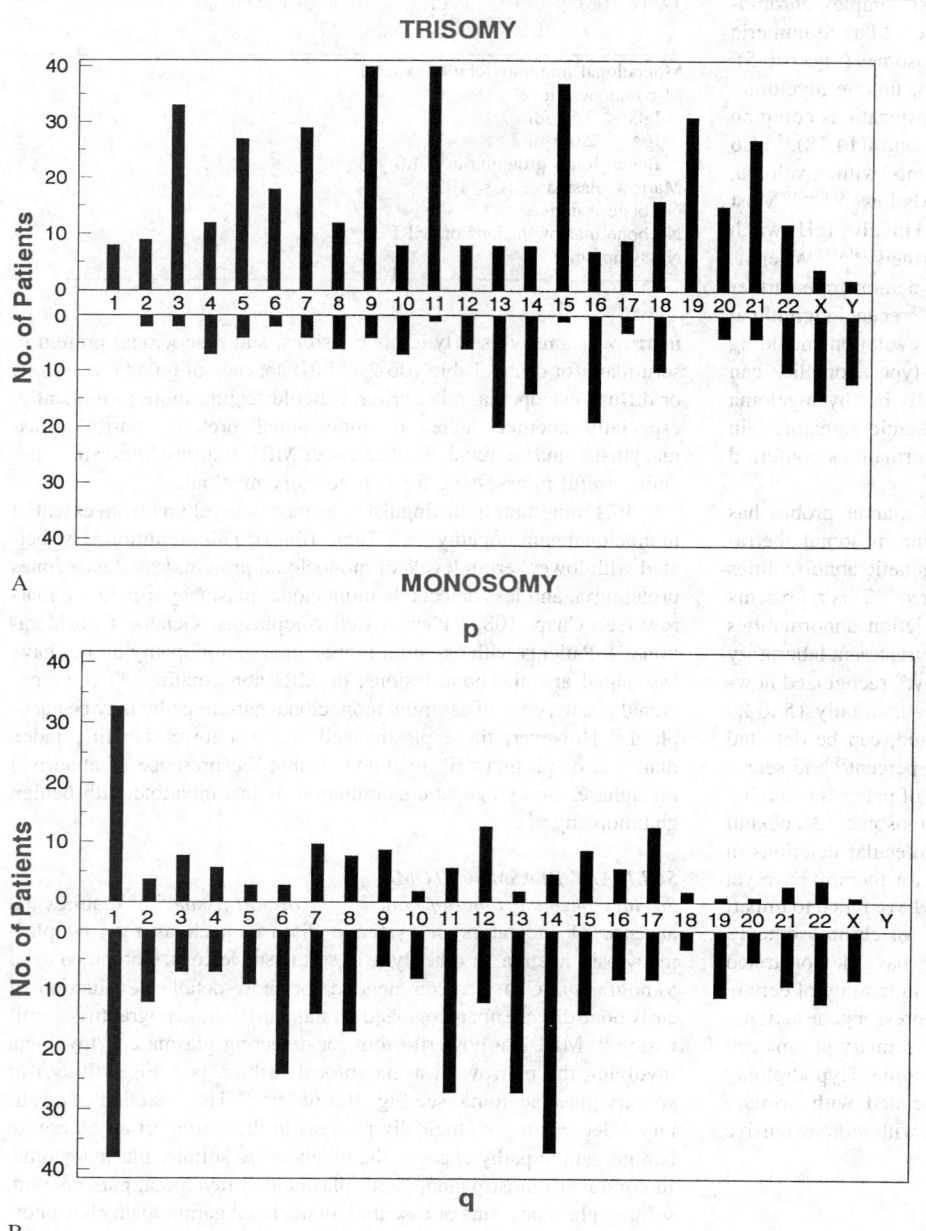

FIGURE 106-5   Cytogenetics in multiple myeloma. (a) Summary of numeric abnormalities ovbserved among 100 abnormal karyoptyes, portraying the incidence of trisomies (*top*) and monosomies (*bottom*). The most common trisomies include those of chromosomes 3, 5, 7, 9, 11, 15, 19, and 21; monosmoies most commonly involve chromsomes 13 and 16. (b) Summary of chromosomal breakpoints involving the short arm (p, *top*) or the long arm (q, *bottom*) of each chromosome that were observed among 100 abnormal karyotypes. Translocations, deletions, and breakpoints most commonly involve both short and long arms of chromosome 1 as well as the long arm of chromosomes 6, 11, 13, and 14 (see part c). (c) Ideogram of 100 abnormal karyotypes, with 459 chromosomal breakpoints delineated by dots. Breakpoints involve areas of known oncogenes such as L-MYC (1p32), N-MYC (2p24), c-MYC (8q24), BCL-1 (11q13), BCL-2 (18q22), N-RAS (1p22), and H-RAS (11p15). Deletions in breakpoints are also seen at sites of suppressor genes (Rb, 13q14; p53, 17q13.) (Courtesy of Jeffery R. Sawyer)

as a result of amyloid deposition in *vasa nervorum* of the autonomic nervous system or in adrenal glands resulting in hypo-adrenalism. It can be difficult to recognize amyloidosis as a major cause of morbidity and mortality in patients with myeloma. Since immunoglobulin and mainly light-chain deposition disease (LCDD) can mimic many mani-

festations of AL but requires immunofluores-cence analysis of unfixed tissue, formalin fix-ation should be avoided whenever protein deposition disease is suspected.

THERAPY, COURSE, AND PROGNOSIS

STAGING

Once the diagnosis of plasma cell myeloma has been established (Table 106-2), tumor staging should be performed[190] (Table 106-4). Studies measuring in vitro immunoglobulin production by patients' myeloma cells have led to a clinically applicable method to esti-mate tumor mass.[191] A tumor-staging system has been derived using standard laboratory measurements, including hemoglobin concen-tration, protein levels in serum and urine, pres-ence of hypercalcemia, and extent of bone disease.[190] The Durie-Salmon staging system has remained in use for more than 20 years and has permitted better interpretation of therapeutic trials according to comparably staged patients.

However, due to the variable interpreta-tion especially of lytic bone lesions, other variables have been used for tumor staging which are more quantitative and discrimina-tory as far as risk assessment is concerned. Among a long list of individually relevant measurements, the serum concentration of β_2-microglobulin currently provides the most re-liable and quantitative prognosticator for sur-vival in plasma cell myeloma.[192-194] Additional independent factors include the plasma cell labeling index[163,176] and C-reactive protein levels, reflecting in vivo IL-6 activity.[196] Increased IL-6 activity mediates many of the abnormalities encountered in myeloma, including hypoalbuminemia, anemia, and lytic bone disease.[197-199] The degree of mar-row plasmacytosis, as assessed by flow cy-tometry of DNA and cytoplasmic immuno-globulin, obviously reflects tumor burden and hence has prognostic utility.[162,200] How-ever, this evaluation is compromised by the patchy marrow involvement often observed in this malignancy. Hypodiploidy identifies marked resistance to standard drug regimens and, as a result, is associated with inferior survival.[188]

Cytologically plasmablastic myeloma, present in 8 percent of newly diagnosed pa-tients, is an adverse parameter frequently as-sociated with high labeling index[149,150] (see Plate XVI-7), higher incidence of extramedul-lary disease, elevated serum LDH levels,[135,201] and a high incidence of karyotypic anomalies, all recognized to confer poor prognosis independently. In the setting of high-dose therapy, histological evaluation of marrow biopsy sections identified short event-free and overall survival in the 20 percent of patients presenting with immature morphology (Bartl grade greater than 1) and increased mitotic activity (greater than or equal to 1 per high-power field), regardless of beta-2-microglobulin, CRP, or cytogenetics (Fig. 106-7).[202,203] Recently, marrow microvessel density (MVD) has been associated with prognosis. High MVD, possibly reflecting VEGF expression by most myeloma cells,[114] conferred short event-free and overall survival.[113]

MAGNETIC RESONANCE IMAGING (MRI) MRI-STIR images of the axial skeleton (skull, spine, and pelvis) are very useful not only for the delineation of truly solitary plasmacytoma of bone[204] but for the assessment of tumor burden and the recognition of macrofocal disease where random marrow sampling from the iliac crest may not yield diagnostic information.[204-208] In such circumstances, CT-guided fine-needle aspiration can render a cytological diagnosis and provide important prognostic information in terms of labeling index and karyotypic analysis.[209] Virtually all patients with myeloma have abnormal MR images at diagnosis, presenting either as hyperintense diffuse, heterogeneous or as focal patterns (Fig. 106-6). As high-dose therapy approaches aim at cure, residual MRI abnormalities remaining in otherwise stringently defined complete remission (CR, see below) need to be recognized.

C

FIGURE 106-5   (*continued*)

RISK ASSESSMENT

Given the multiplicity of prognostically relevant staging parameters, it is recommended that all patients with myeloma should have analysis performed of beta-2-microglobulin (B2M), C-reactive protein (CRP), LDH, and cytogenetics, as well as marrow biopsy evaluation to evaluate for key features with dominant adverse implications.

On the basis of the above considerations, high-risk myeloma can be identified on the basis of one of the following: cytogenetics revealing chromosome 13 deletion, plasma cell labeling index greater than 2 percent, LDH greater than 2 times normal unexplained by liver function abnormalities or hemolytic anemia, hemoglobin less than 8 percent in association with extensive marrow plasmacytosis greater than 50 percent, B2M and CRP elevations greater than 4 mg/liter, hypercalcemia or excess paraprotein production with IgG greater than 7 g/dl, IgA greater than 5g/dl, Bence Jones protein excretion greater than 10 g/liter. Low-risk disease requires the absence of unfavorable cytogenetics, labeling index not exceeding 1 percent, LDH within institutional normal range, hemoglobin greater than 12 percent, B2M and CRP less than 2.5 mg/liter, marrow plasmacytosis not exceeding 20 percent, normocalcemia, normal albumin. All others have an intermediate risk.

THERAPY FOR SOLITARY PLASMACYTOMA

The recommended therapy for solitary plasmacytoma lesions of soft tissue or bone is radiotherapy at potentially curative doses of 40 to 50 Gy. Using this approach, approximately 70 percent of patients with soft-tissue plasmacytoma can be cured,[218,224-226] contrasting with less than 30 percent of those with solitary bone lesions.[227] This discrepancy is probably due to the relative insensitivity of standard staging procedures for marrow and bone disease. Higher cure rates are anticipated when solitary plasmacytoma lesions are defined with more-sensitive techniques, such as CT scans[219] or MRI.[206,228]

THERAPY FOR INDOLENT MYELOMA

Patients who have systemic but asymptomatic myeloma may have a low tumor mass and slow disease progression[229,230] (see Table 106-5).

TABLE 106-4   ASSESSMENT OF TUMOR MASS (DURIE-SALMON)

1. High tumor mass (stage III) ($> 1.2 \times 10^{12}/m^2$)*
   One of the following abnormalities must be present:
   a. Hemoglobin < 8.5 g/dl, hematocrit $< 25\%$
   b. Serum calcium >12 mg/dl
   c. Very high serum or urine myeloma protein production rates:
      (1) IgG peak > 7 g/dl
      (2) IgA peak > 5 g/dl
      (3) Bence Jones protein > 12 g/24 h
   d. > 3 lytic bone lesions on bone survey (bone scan not acceptable)
2. Low tumor mass (stage I) ($< 0.6 \times 10^{12}/m^2$)*
   All of the following must be present:
   a. Hemoglobin > 10.5 g/dl or hematocrit $> 32\%$
   b. Serum calcium normal
   c. Low serum myeloma protein production rates:
      (1) IgG peak < 5 g/dl
      (2) IgA peak < 3 g/dl
      (3) Bence Jones protein < 4 g/24 h
   d. No bone lesions or osteoporosis
3. Intermediate tumor mass (stage II) ($0.6-1.2 \times 10^{12}/m^2$)*
All patients who do not qualify for high or low tumor mass categories are considered to have intermediate tumor mass.
   a. No renal failure (creatinine ≤ 2mg/dl)
   b. Renal failure (creatinine > 2 mg/dl)

*Estimated number of neoplastic plasma cells.

Panel A

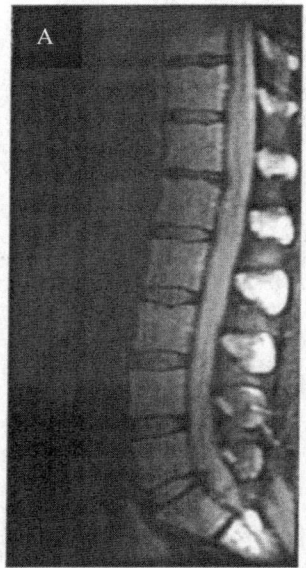 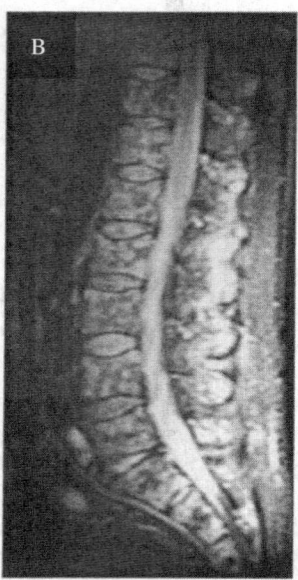 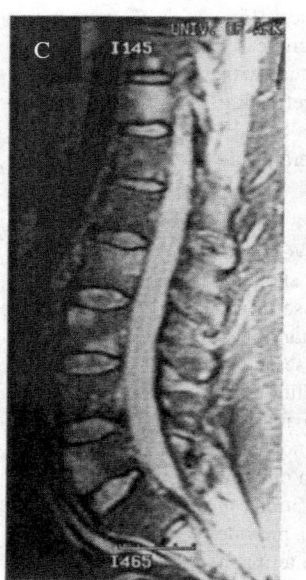 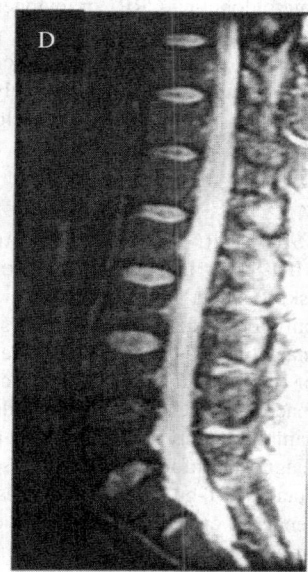

Diffuse
33%

Heterogeneous
33%

Focal
33%

Normal
<5%

Panel B

Normal pelvis
L4 focal lesion

T 2 focal
lesion

CT FNA of L4

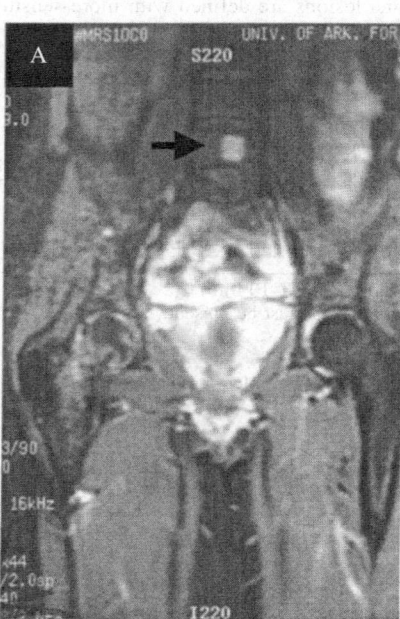 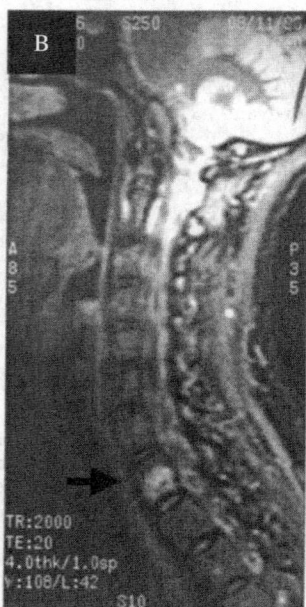 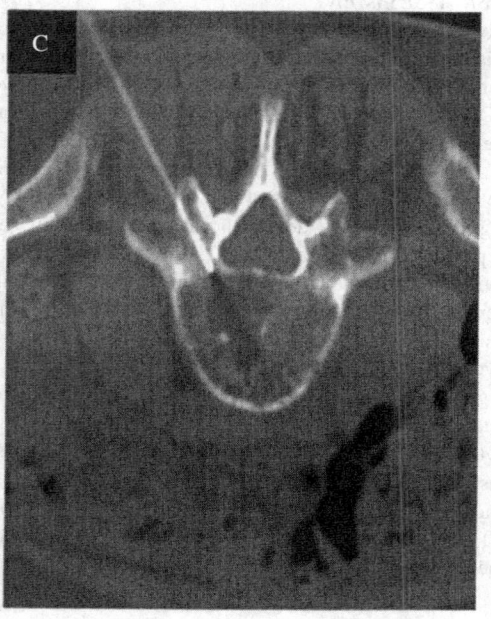

FIGURE 106-6   Magnetic resonance imaging (MRI) pattern in multiple myeloma at diagnosis: (a) STIR (short inversion-time inversion recovery) imaging shows approximately one-third each presenting with diffuse homogeneous pattern (*panel A*), heterogeneous pattern (*panel B*), and focal plasmacytoma lesions (*panel C*). Few patients have a hypo-intense and homogenous pattern seen also in normal individuals (*panel D*). (b) Some patients present with macrofocal disease. *Panel A:* normal pelvis and isolated L-4 lesion, *panel B:* T(2) focal lesion; *panel C:* computed-tomography-guided fine needle aspiration of L-4 lesion. Examination in 72 patients with MRI-focal disease showed tumor in 92 percent, indicating that MR focal lesions in myeloma represent tumor.

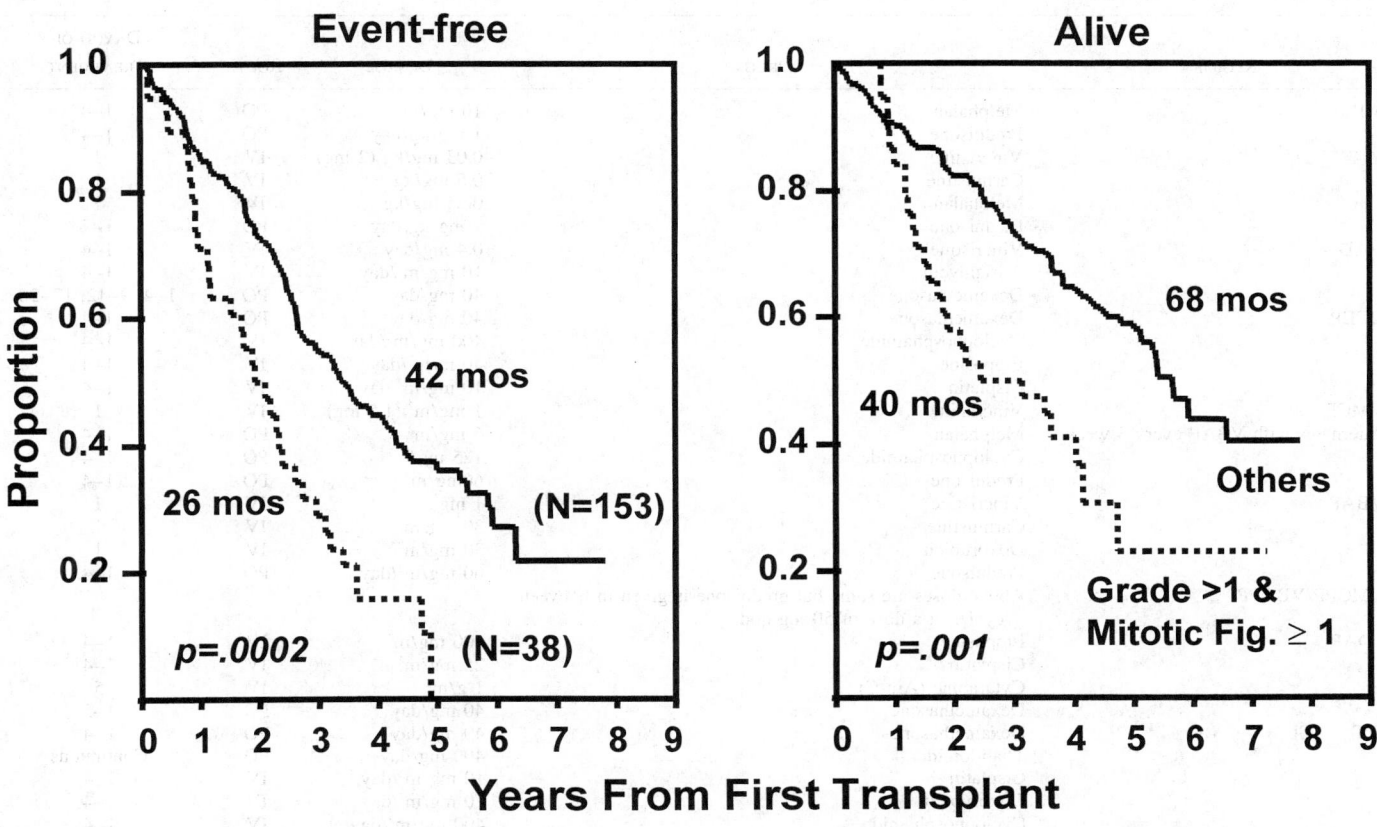

FIGURE 106-7   Bone marrow histology and prognosis with high-dose therapy (total therapy[262]). In the presence of Bartl grade greater than 1 and more than one mitotic figure per high-power field (38 pts), event-free (*left panel*) and overall survival (*right panel*) were significantly shorter in patients lacking these features (153 pts).

Such patients generally do not have a marrow plasmacytosis that exceeds 30 percent of the marrow cells. Also, the monoclonal serum immunoglobulin levels, while exceeding those found in patients with essential monoclonal gammopathy, typically range from 3.5 g/dl to 7 g/dl for indolent IgG myeloma, or 2 g/dl to 5 g/dl for indolent IgA myeloma. Also, Bence Jones proteinuria generally does not exceed 10 g per day in indolent myeloma. Bone lesions typically are small and few in number. Severe anemia (hemoglobin less than 10 g/dl), renal failure (creatinine greater than 2 mg/dl), recurrent infections, and hypercalcemia are typically absent. The plasma cell labeling index is usually less than 1 percent[124] (hypoproliferative myeloma). Such patients can be recognized only retrospectively, although reports sug-

gest earlier progression to symptomatic myeloma in the presence of lytic bone lesions or serum myeloma protein levels in excess of 3 g/dl and Bence Jones proteinuria.[231] Focal MRI abnormalities and hyperintense background signal on STIR images by MRI have also been associated with earlier disease progression. Treatment, previously withheld until the onset of symptoms or until disease progression, has recently been performed with pamidronate to delay the onset of bone disease and possibly progression of the disease process.

THERAPY FOR SYMPTOMATIC MULTIPLE MYELOMA

"STANDARD THERAPY"

Therapeutic progress has been slow in myeloma. Oral melphalan and prednisone, introduced over 30 years ago, have remained standard therapy (Table 106-6), providing control of symptoms and/or tumor mass reduction by no more than 50 percent in one-half of patients treated.[232,233] Various combination drug regimens have been tested that include nitrosoureas, doxorubicin, vinca alkaloids, and cyclophosphamide, in addition to melphalan and prednisone.[234–236] Most studies, however, have failed to show that such regimens improve patient survival (Fig. 106-8). This is not surprising, considering that the overall cytotoxic dose intensity was low to avoid marked myelosuppression. Given the low incidence of stringently defined complete remissions (5 percent), the degree of tumor cytoreduction from standard therapy has typically not affected prognosis.[237] However, patients achieving "plateau phase" fared significantly better than those with disease

TABLE 106-5   CRITERIA FOR DIAGNOSIS OF INDOLENT MYELOMA*

Few bone lesions (if any, < 4) and no compression fractures
M-component levels
   IgG < 7 g/dl
   IgA < 5 g/dl
No symptoms or associated disease features:
   Performance status > 50%
   Hemoglobin >10 g/dl
   Normal serum calcium levels
   Serum creatinine ≤ 2.0 mg/dl
   No infections

*The criteria for diagnosis of plasma cell myeloma presented in Table 106-2 must be satisfied. However, patients with indolent myeloma have all of the features listed in this table.

TABLE 106-6　CHEMOTHERAPY REGIMENS IN MYELOMA

REGIMEN	DRUG	DOSAGE	ROUTE	DAY(S) OF TREATMENT
MP	Melphalan	10 mg/m²	PO	1–4
	Prednisone	1 mg/kg/day	PO	1–4
M-2	Vincristine	0.03 mg/kg (2 mg)	IV	1
	Carmustine	0.5 mg/kg	IV	1
	Melphalan	0.25 mg/kg	IV	1
	Prednisone	1 mg/kg/day	PO	1–7
VAD	Vincristine	0.4 mg/day	IV	1–4
	Adriamycin	10 mg/m²/day	IV	1–4
	Dexamethasone	40 mg/day	PO	1–4, 9–12, 17–20
DCEP	Dexamethasone	40 mg/day	PO	1–4
	Cyclophosphamide	400 mg/m²/day	IV	1–4
	Etoposide	40 m/m²/day	IV	1–4
	Cisplatin	10 mg/m²/day	IV	1–4
VMCP	Vincristine	1 mg/m² (1.5 mg)	IV	1
Alternates with VBAP every 3 weeks	Melphalan	6 mg/m²	PO	1–4
	Cyclophosphamide	125 mg/m²	PO	1–4
	Prednisone	60mg/m²	PO	1–4
VBAP	Vincristine	1 mg	IV	1
	Carmustine	30 mg/m²	IV	1
	Doxorubicin	30 mg/m²	IV	1
	Prednisone	60 mg/m²/day	PO	1–4
VMCPP/VBAPP	Above doses are same but prednisone is given in between cycles at a dose of 50 mg qod			
EDAP	Etoposide	100 mg/m²	IV	1–4
	Cisplatin	25 mg/m²	IV	1–4
	Cytarabine (Ara-C)	1 g/m²	IV	5
	Dexamethasone	40 mg/day	PO	1–5
D.T. PACE	Dexamethasone	40 mg/day	PO	1–4
	Thalidomide	400 mg/day	PO	Continuous
	Cisplatin	10 mg/m²/day	IV	1–4
	Doxorubicin	10 mg/m²/day	IV	1–4
	Cyclophosphamide	400 mg/m²/day	IV	1–4
	Etoposide	40 mg/m²/day	IV	1–4

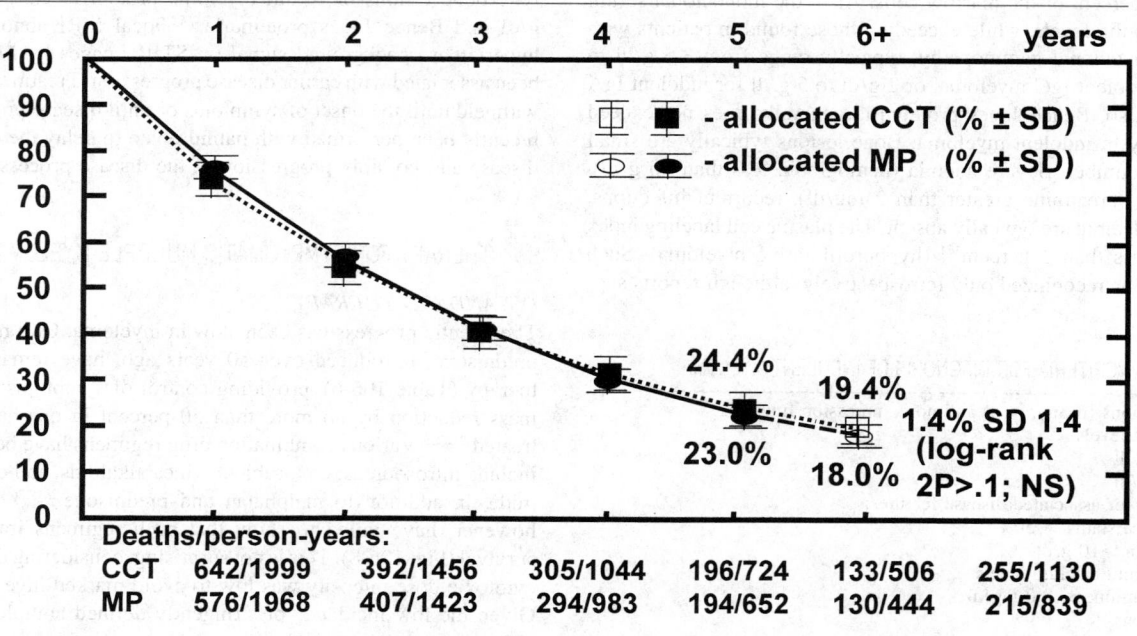

FIGURE 106-8　Survival with combination chemotherapy (CCT) versus standard melphalan and prednisone (MP). Results of a meta-analysis of randomized trials revealed no difference in almost 2000 patients enrolled in CCT versus MP trials.

progression[238] Although previous randomized trials showed no benefit due to maintenance therapy with cytotoxic agents,[239,240] including interferon immunotherapy,[241-243] significant extension of event-free and overall survival has recently been observed with high-dose prednisone.[244]

As a consequence of prolonged administration of alkylating agents targeting hemopoietic progenitor cells, myelotoxicity accumulates, potentially leading to myelodysplasia (MDS) or acute myeloid leukemia (AML)[245] (see Chap. 93, "Acute Myelogenous Leukemia"). Myeloma and MDS/AML may share MDS cytogenetic features ("leukemic signature," see above) without indicating, however, a common ancestral origin.

INTENSIVE GLUCOCORTICOID THERAPY AND VAD

Therapeutic benefit from high doses of glucocorticoids had been reported in occasional myeloma patients.[246] However, serious investigations into the role of high-dose glucocorticoid therapy were conducted first as part of the VAD regimen, combining continuous infusions of vincristine, Adriamycin (doxorubicin), and 4-day pulses of high-dose dexamethasone at 40 mg daily[247] (Table 106-6). In myeloma refractory to myelosuppressive doses of standard alkylating agent regimens, VAD produced rapid and marked cytoreduction of over 75 percent in more than 50 percent of treated patients, especially in those with relapsing disease (i.e., with prior response). Subsequent studies with high-dose dexamethasone alone revealed response rates comparable to VAD among subjects who had primary drug resistance.[248] Responders to VAD or dexamethasone had not only protein reduction but also marrow remission (fewer than 5 percent tumor cells). These results represented a major advance, since there previously had not been effective salvage therapy for plasma cell myeloma resistant to alkylating agents.

Therapy with VAD, or modifications thereof, produced responses in about 65 percent of previously untreated myeloma patients, with a short median tumor halving time of about 21 days compared to 6 to 8 weeks with standard melphalan-prednisone.[249,250] Signs and symptoms of disease resolved more quickly than with standard therapy with alkylating agents and prednisone. The faster tumor cytoreduction with high-dose glucocorticoid-containing regimens may result from down-regulation of various cytokines possibly involved in the pathogenesis of myeloma. Down-regulation of IL-6 induced by glucocorticoids, for example, is accompanied by rapid apoptosis of cultured human myeloma cells, explaining the absence of a tumor lysis syndrome clinically despite often dramatically rapid responses. Apoptosis can be prevented by coincubation of myeloma cells with recombinant IL-6[100] or by stromal cell exposure.[103]

Despite its more profound and rapid cytoreduction, the VAD regimen failed to markedly extend the survival of newly diagnosed patients in comparison with standard alkylating drug-containing regimens.[249-252] This may be due to the primordial tumor cells preferentially producing IL-6,[253] which confers resistance to dexamethasone,[100] and expressing MDR,[77-80] which confers resistance to vincristine and doxorubicin. However, with VAD or dexamethasone alone, hemopoietic function was preserved. The 4-day continuous infusion regimen of doxorubicin is virtually devoid of cardiomyopathy, even after extended application, probably because of the lower drug serum levels that are used. Myelosuppression is uncommon with VAD, and dexamethasone accounts for most of the toxicity observed.

Recent randomized trials comparing VAD with standard VMCP-VBAP or VMCPP-VBAPP (Table 106-6) with more extensive prednisone revealed superior outcome with the more dose intensive glucocorticoid regimens,[251] in line with subsequent observations that higher doses of prednisone are also beneficial in the setting of maintenance.[244]

BISPHOSPHONATES

An important adjunct is the administration of *pamidronate*, a newer-generation bisphosphonate, which has been shown to delay the onset of myeloma-related skeletal events and to prolong survival.[268,269] Pamidronate inhibits osteoclast activity and seems to mediate antitumor activity through down-regulation of myeloma-survival signals elaborated by the marrow microenvironment.[8,9,270] Pamidronate has been shown, in randomized trials, not only to delay the onset of *myeloma-related skeletal events*[268] but also to extend overall survival.[269] The survival extension may be due to direct or indirect antitumor effects, possibly involving the inhibition of cytokines sustaining myeloma growth and survival. Bone mineral density measured by DEXA (dual energy x-ray absorptiometry) has also been shown to increase substantially after monthly administrations of pamidronate at 90 to 180 mg.[289] Observations of antitumor activity with pamidronate in smoldering myeloma form the basis for its current investigation along with glucocorticoids for patients over age 70 who may not be candidates for high-dose therapy.[270]

INTERFERON ALPHA

The role of interferon alpha (IFN-α) in the setting of standard therapy remains controversial. Meta-analyses evaluating the role of during induction or maintenance have, on the whole, shown more positive than negative results.[242] Growth-inhibiting effects of IFM-α may be either direct or mediated by modulation of the immune response or through antiangiogenesis mechanisms.

HIGH-DOSE THERAPY WITH AUTOLOGOUS HEMOPOIETIC STEM CELL SUPPORT

Recent results of randomized and historically controlled clinical trials have demonstrated that, as a result of mainly melphalan-based high-dose therapy, the incidence of complete remission can be raised from 5 percent up to 50 percent, and event-free and overall survival durations have been extended from 1.5 to well over 3 years and from 3 to 5 to 6 years respectively.[256,257] The use of peripheral blood stem cells, mobilized with stem cell-sparing cyclophosphamide alone, in combination with hemopoietic growth factor, such as G-CSF or GM-CSF, as well as G-CSF alone, have accelerated both neutrophil and platelet recovery so that the duration of marrow aplasia typically does not exceed 5 days and critical levels of granulocytes greater than $500/\mu l$ and platelets greater than $50,000/\mu l$ are typically attained within 2 weeks from autograft administration.[258] Such results are superior to earlier studies utilizing autologous marrow as a source of hemopoietic stem cells. Melphalan at 200 mg/m² as preparative regimen is well tolerated even by patients up to age 70.[259] This regimen can be given in the setting of renal failure although it is associated with a higher incidence and greater degree of extramedullary toxicities.[260] There is no indication that the addition of total body irradiation to chemotherapy with melphalan is beneficial.[261] If the promise holds, also in myelomatosis, that CR is a necessary but possibly not sufficient first step toward prolonged disease control and eventual cure, high-dose therapy should be conducted early during the disease when CR can be attained most readily.[262] Indeed, in the case of 2 cycles of high-dose therapy with melphalan 200 mg/m² ("total therapy"), CR can be obtained in almost 50 percent of patients. Median CR duration exceeds 4 years with 60 percent projected in continuous complete remission at 6 years in those lacking chromosome 13 deletion and presenting with low B2M. The median event-free and overall survival durations were 3.3 and 5.7 months with 25 percent remaining relapse-free and 45 percent alive at 8 years (Fig. 106-9). Treatment-related mortality within the first year of total therapy was 7 percent.[262] Issues currently under investigation

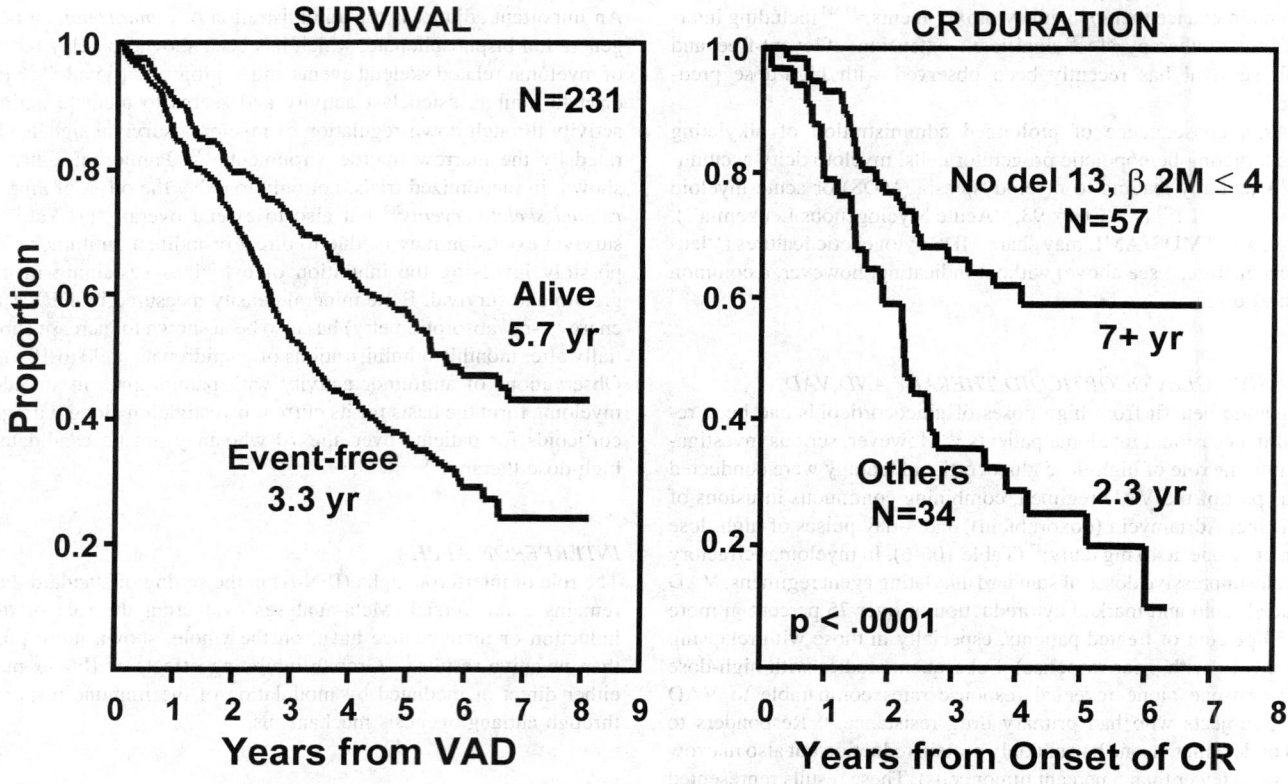

FIGURE 106-9   Event-free and overall survival (*left panel*) as well as CR duration (*right panel*) following total therapy[262] for newly diagnosed patients. Total therapy consisted of remission induction with non-cross-resistant regimens followed by two cycles of high-dose therapy with melphalan 200 mg/m^2 and interferon-α_2 maintenance. In the absence of chromosome 13 deletion and with B$_2$M levels $\leq$ 4 mg/L (present in 57 of 91 CR patients), CR duration was markedly extended with about 60 percent remaining in continuous complete remission at 6 years compared to less than 10 percent among the remaining subjects.

include the role of multiple cycles of high-dose therapy,[263] tumor cell removal by selection of CD34 hemopoietic progenitor cells,[263,264] and post-high-dose therapy maintenance strategies.

To date, *CD34 selection* has not resulted in superior event-free survival or overall survival when compared in randomized trials with nonselected autografts in support of BUCY[263] or MEL 140 + TBI,[262] indicating that residual disease remaining after high-dose therapy dominantly affects prognosis. Even when very early hemopoietic stem cells devoid of clonal B cells (CD34$^+$, Thy-1$^+$, Lin$^-$) were employed, relapses especially of deletion 13 disease were common.[264] Importantly, compared to nonselected cells, hemopoietic and immune reconstitution were significantly delayed resulting in considerable morbidity and mortality.

CONSOLIDATION CHEMOTHERAPY

Consolidation chemotherapy with DCEP (dexamethasone 40mg on days 1–4; continuous infusions of cyclophosphamide 400mg/m^2, etoposide 40mg/m^2, and cisplatin 10mg/m^2; all daily for 4 days) after tandem transplant (Table 106-6), effective for posttransplant relapses,[265] not only delayed relapses but also converted PR to CR in almost 30 percent of 50 patients treated.[266] Maintenance immunotherapy with IFN-α is currently being tested in a U.S. Intergroup trial of early versus late myeloablative therapy for patients achieving at least partial remission. *Idiotype vaccination* strategies have been promising in low-grade lymphoma and currently are being evaluated for their

ability to generate tumor-specific anti-idiotype T- and B-cell responses in patients with myeloma, as well.[267]

ALLOGENEIC STEM CELL TRANSPLANTATION

In the case of HLA-identical twins, *syngeneic transplants* should be offered in support of maximally cytoreductive therapy such as with melphalan 200 mg/m^2 or TBI-containing regimens. Data from the European Bone Marrow Registry involving 16 subjects indicate a complete remission rate of 50 percent, and median durations of event-free and overall survival were 32 and 60 months, respectively.[271]

RELATED HLA-MATCHED ALLOGENEIC TRANSPLANTS

HLA-matched sibling donor transplant data in myeloma from EBMT and several individual institutions indicate a high transplant-related mortality of typically 50 percent within the first year, usually as a result of pneumonia, sepsis, or graft-vs-host disease. Event-free survival at 6 years for those achieving CR was 34 percent.[272,273] At 7 years, 28 percent of all patients survived. Results were superior when prior therapy was limited to one regimen and when CR was attained. In comparing results of patients undergoing allogeneic transplantation with matched patients undergoing autograft-supported high-dose therapy, an obvious survival advantage was observed with autologous transplant due to high treatment-related mortality (41 percent versus 13 percent); however, in patients surviving more than 1 year after a transplant, there was a significantly better progression-free survival

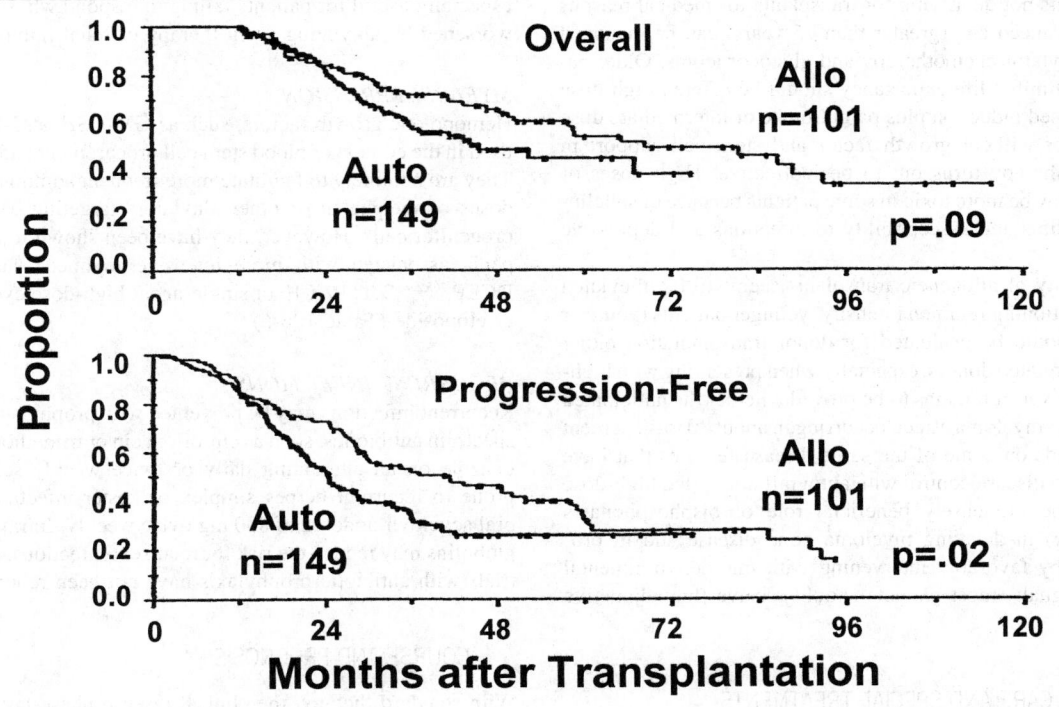

FIGURE 106-10   Improved progression-free and overall survival following allogeneic transplantation compared to autologous transplantation in patients alive at 1 year.

(p = 0.02) and a trend toward better long-term survival (p = 0.07) after allotransplants (Fig. 106-10).[274] Additional advances can be expected from careful selection of patients early after diagnosis whose prognosis, due to disease-intrinsic features, has been poor with autograft-supported high dose therapy (e.g., chromosome 13 deletion myeloma) and from graft manipulation to take advantage of a graft-vs.-myeloma effect[275] while reducing the grave toxicities of graft-vs.-host disease. Similar considerations apply to matched unrelated donor transplants. Current efforts focus, like in other hemopoietic malignancies, on reducing the conditioning regimen intensity ("mini-allotransplants")[276] and hastening hemopoietic reconstitution by administering high doses of donor peripheral blood stem cells mobilized with G-CSF. Results indicate that morbidity and mortality can be decreased markedly even in older patients.

SALVAGE THERAPIES
Such strategies must take into consideration the type and duration of prior therapy, disease responsiveness, and patient tolerance. High-dose dexamethasone alone, at 40 mg/day PO on days 1 to 4 each week, or combined with vincristine and doxorubicin (VAD regimen) represents a key element of therapy for myeloma unresponsive to or relapsing from remission induced with standard alkylating agent therapy.[247] Such remissions can be further consolidated with autograft-supported high-dose melphalan when adequate quantities of hemopoietic stem cells can be procured. This is more likely when the patient has a normal platelet count over $150,000/\mu$ liter and expected when CD34 quantities exceed 2×10^6/kg with up to 24 months of therapy and greater than 5×10^6/kg with more extended duration of treatment.[257]

In the case of high-risk disease with high LDH, labeling index greater than 2 percent and especially cytogenetic abnormalities involving chromosome 13 or other translocations, DCEP combination chemotherapy (Table 106-6) has proved effective in reestablishing disease

control (approximately 75 percent tumor mass reduction) in up to 40 percent of cases, including true CR in 15 percent.[265]

Exciting results have been reported with thalidomide. This drug presumably works through an antiangiogenesis mechanism. It can produce both paraprotein and marrow responses in about one-third of cases treated mainly for posttransplant relapse often with high-risk cytogenetic features.[11] Current trials are evaluating D.T. PACE (dexamethasone 40 mg daily × 4, thalidomide 400 mg daily continuously and 4-day continuous infusions of daily doses of cisplatin 10 mg/m², doxorubicin 10 mg/m², cyclophosphamide 400 mg/m² and etoposide 40 mg/m²) followed by G-CSF administered subcutaneously until hemopoietic recovery.[277]

PRIMARY TREATMENT STRATEGY

Upon confirmation of a diagnosis of multiple myeloma, either symptomatic or progressive, a long-term strategy should be developed that considers, in addition to host features, the key myeloma prognosticators including B2M, CRP, labeling index, and, most important, cytogenetics or FISH to detect deletion 13 myeloma. These prognostic variables pertain to both standard and high-dose therapies. Given the rapid progress in myeloma biology and therapy during the past decade, practicing physicians and hematologists/oncologists should be aware of the latest developments offered as part of clinical research trials aimed at increasing the chance of durable complete remissions. Remission induction should avoid stem-cell-toxic therapy so that all patients can benefit potentially from dose-intensive regimens with autograft support. Available data clearly indicate that, although high-dose therapy induces CR with similar frequencies in good and high-risk myeloma, patients in the latter category require additional treatment to prevent relapse.

Those patients not qualifying for transplants for medical reasons or because of advanced age (greater than 75 years) can be managed with standard alkylator chemotherapy and glucocorticoids. Older patients with more limited life expectancy should be offered high-dose glucocorticoid-based induction plus pamidronate or intermediate dose melphalan with or without growth factor and stem cell support in case the former therapy turns out to be ineffective. High doses of glucocorticoids may be more toxic in some patients because of subclinical diabetes mellitus and susceptibility to infections and depressive disorders.

As the toxicity of allogeneic transplants seems to be alleviated by reducing conditioning regimen intensity, younger patients (younger than 60 years) should be evaluated for donor transplantation either from sibling or unrelated donors, especially when presenting with high-risk disease. However, it remains to be proved whether the anticipated beneficial graft-vs.-myeloma effect, occurring in about 30 to 40 percent of patients, depends on some of the same disease features that have been an obstacle to disease control with autograft-supported high-dose therapy. Given the immensely beneficial role of bisphosphonates (e.g., pamidronate) in delaying myeloma bone disease and in prolonging survival by favorably intervening with microenvironmental tumor survival signals, most patients should receive this adjunctive therapy.[268,269]

SUPPORTIVE CARE AND SPECIAL TREATMENTS

HYPERCALCEMIA AND RENAL FAILURE

Hypercalcemia and renal failure are best managed with high doses of dexamethasone alone or with the full VAD regimen. Occasionally, especially in refractory myeloma, calcitonin or pamidronate may be required. Hemodialysis should be used as clinically indicated for the management of acute or chronic renal failure.

In refractory conditions of persistent disease with recent onset of renal failure, high-dose therapy with melphalan and peripheral blood stem cell support should be considered in order to achieve maximum antitumor effect that, not infrequently, is associated with improvement or even normalization of renal function.

SPINAL CORD COMPRESSION

Spinal cord compression has traditionally been treated with local radiotherapy and/or decompressive laminectomy. While local radiotherapy has curative potential for the management of truly solitary plasmacytoma as demonstrated on MR imaging of axial marrow, its role in palliation has to be assessed in the context of long-term management and in light of the underlying cause. In more recently treated patients suffering from systemic disease, chemotherapy that includes high-dose dexamethasone pulsing with VAD or DCEP has been shown to provide remarkable activity. In the absence of symptom relief with tumor volume reduction on MRI within 1 week, local radiation and/or decompressive laminectomy should be added.

In case of cord compression as a result of vertebral collapse without readily identifiable plasmacytoma on MRI, radiation may not be beneficial, and decompressive laminectomy should be the treatment of choice. The local doses of radiotherapy to the spinal cord should not exceed 30 Gy, and liberal use of local radiation for the management of rib fractures is discouraged.

SYMPTOMATIC ANEMIA

Symptomatic anemia usually improves with therapy, especially with high doses of dexamethasone. Responses can be hastened by subcutaneous administration of recombinant erythropoietin at doses of 10,000 units thrice weekly or 40,000 once weekly.[285,286] Such treatment is especially useful for patients failing to respond whose anemia is often worsened by alkylating agent therapy or renal failure.

MYELOSUPPRESSION

Hemopoietic growth factors, such as GM-CSF or G-CSF, are mainly used in the context of blood stem cell procurement and after transplant. They are not likely to facilitate more frequent administration of higher doses of melphalan or other alkylators targeting early hemopoietic progenitor cells. However, they have been shown to alleviate neutropenia associated with more intensive regimens such as EDAP,[287] DCEP,[265,266] D.T. PACE, or single-agent high-dose cyclophosphamide or etoposide (Table 106-6).[288]

RECURRENT INFECTIONS

Recurrent infections may be prevented with prophylactic use of broad-spectrum antibiotics, such as ciprofloxacin or trimethoprim-sulfamethoxazole on an alternating daily or twice weekly schedule. Patients prone to recurrent herpes simplex or zoster infections benefit from oral acyclovir at doses of 800 mg twice weekly. Intravenous immunoglobulins may reduce the risk for recurrent infections, but comparative trials with antibiotic prophylaxis have not been reported.

COURSE AND PROGNOSIS

With standard therapy, the clinical disease phase lasts an average of only 3 years, as a result of only temporary growth control with alkylating agents and glucocorticoids. Patients then succumb either to the consequences of rapid tumor cell expansion, akin to blast crisis of chronic myelogenous leukemia or transformation from an indolent to an aggressive malignant lymphoma,[135] or to the consequences of marrow failure from chronic alkylating agent therapy, sometimes associated with the development of a myelodysplastic syndrome or frank acute myelogenous leukemia.[245]

Successful remissions induced by initial standard chemotherapy usually do not exceed a median of 18 months, and median survival of all patients averages 30 to 36 months. Few patients obtain true complete responses (as defined by absence of monoclonal protein production on immunofixation analysis and normal marrow aspirate and biopsy), typically on the order of 5 percent. Similarly, about 5 percent survive 10 to 15 years, usually when presenting with low tumor mass and responding to standard-dose regimens.[254,255] However, virtually all patients with plasma cell myeloma receiving standard therapy succumb to their malignancy.

SECONDARY HEMOPOIETIC MALIGNANCIES

Due to their often advanced age, patients also may have a co-existing myelodysplastic syndrome. This can be recognized prior to the development of morphologic changes and cytopenia using cytogenetic analysis and, more recently, FISH using suitable probes to detect deletions of chromocome 5, 7, and 20, as well as trisomy 8. As in Hodgkin disease and malignant lymphoma, where autograft-supported high-dose therapy has been used extensively for salvage or for consolidation of high-risk disease, an accentuated frequency of myelodysplasia has been observed beginning about 2 years after autotransplants for myeloma.[184,290] At 5 to 7 years, the incidence of MDS cytogenetic lesions did not exceed 1 to 2 percent in patients whose age did not exceed 50 years and when standard alkylating agent therapy was limited to 12 months. Otherwise, the frequency of cytogenetically recognized MDS reached 7 to 10 percent, especially when CD34 mobilization was impaired (Fig. 106-11). Thus, with a background of alkylating agent-induced DNA damage, hemopoietic stem cell replication stress after high-dose therapy may be associated with telomere shortening

Panel A

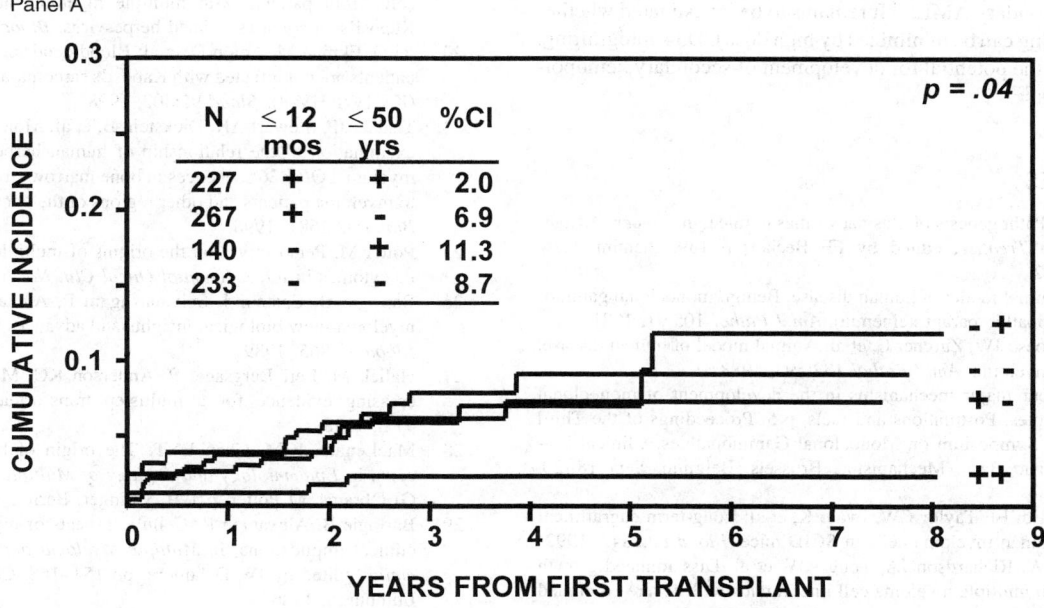

Panel B

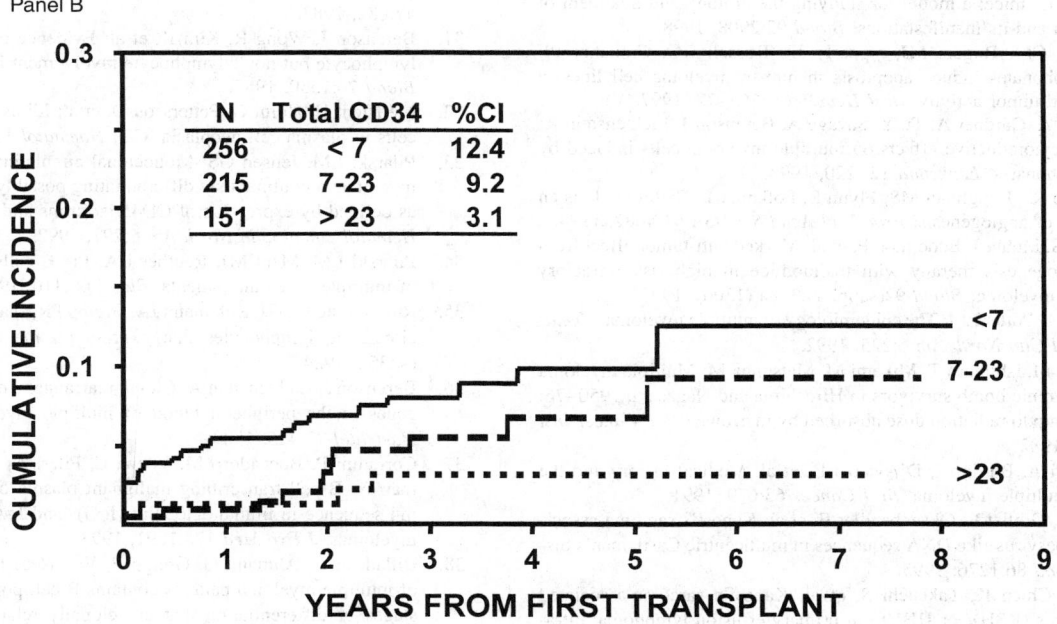

FIGURE 106-11 Development of myelodysplasia using cytogenetic criteria (5 or del 5q, 7 or del 7q, trisomy 8, del 20q11) following autologous hematopoietic stem cell-supported high-dose therapy with melphalan 200 mg/m² (one or two cycles). *Panel A*: cumulative incidence of cytogenetic MDS in relationship to months of prior therapy (less than 12 versus greater than 12 months) and age (less than 50 versus greater than 50 years). Patients with no more than 12 months of prior therapy and aged 50 years or younger had the lowest risk of MDS compared to the three other groups. *Panel B*: examination of CD34 stem cell mobilization (CD34 × 10⁶/kg) on MDS development among the 622 patients with either more than 12 months of prior therapy or more than 50 years of age. Note: MDS was least common in the subgroup with high CD34 yield (>23 × 10⁶/kg).

causing genomic instability and increasing the chance for clonal myelo-dysplasia and secondary AML.[291] It remains to be investigated whether telomere shortening can be minimized by high dose CD34 autografting. This may reduce the potential for development of secondary hemopoietic malignancies.[292]

REFERENCES

1. Potter M: Pathogenesis of plasmacytomas in mice, in *Cancer: A Comprehensive Treatise*, edited by FF Becker, p 139. Plenum, New York, 1982.
2. Radl J: Animal model of human disease. Benign monoclonal gammopathy (idiopathic paraproteinemia). *Am J Pathol* 105:91, 1981.
3. Radl J, Croese JW, Zurcher C, et al: Animal model of human disease. Multiple myeloma. *Am J Pathol* 132:593, 1988.
4. Radl J: Four major mechanisms in the development of monoclonal gammapathies. Postulations and facts, p 5. Proceedings of the Third EURAGE Symposium on Monoclonal Gammopathies: Clinical Significance and Basic Mechanisms, Brussels, Belgium, Sept 18–20, 1991.
5. Feo-Zuppardi FJ, Taylor CW, Iwato K, et al: Long-term engraftment of fresh human myeloma cells in SCID mice. *Blood* 80:2843, 1992.
6. Huang Y-W, Richardson JA, Tong AW, et al: Disseminated growth of a human multiple myeloma cell line in mice with severe combined immunodeficiency disease. *Cancer Res* 53:1392, 1993.
7. Yaccoby S, Barlogie B, Epstein J: Primary myeloma cells growing in SCID-hu mice: a model for studying the biology and treatment of myeloma and its manifestations. *Blood* 92:2908, 1998.
8. Shipman CM, Rogers MJ, Apperly JF, Russell RG, Croucher PI: Bisphosphonates induce apoptosis in human myeloma cell lines: a novel anti-tumor activity. *Br J Hem* 98(3):665–72, 1997.
9. Aparicio A, Gardner A, Tu Y, Savage A, Berenson J, Lichtenstein A: In vitro cytoreductive effects on multiple myeloma cells induced by bisphosphonates. *Leukemia* 12: 220, 1998.
10. D'Amato RJ, Loughnan MS, Flynn E, Folkman J: Thalidomide is an inhibitor of angiogenesis. *Proc Natl Acad Sci USA* 91:4082, 1994.
11. Singhal S, Mehta J, Eddelmon P, et al: Marked anti-tumor effect from anti-angiogenesis therapy with thalidomide in high risk refractory multiple myeloma. *Blood* 92(suppl 1):318a (1306), 1998.
12. Riedel DA, Potter LM: The epidemiology of multiple myeloma. *Hematol Oncol Clin North Am* 6:225, 1992.
13. Ichimaru M, Ishimaru T, Mikami M, Matsunga M: Multiple myeloma among atomic bomb survivors in Hiroshima and Nagasaki, 1950–76: relationship to radiation dose absorbed by marrow. *J Natl Cancer Inst* 69:323, 1982.
14. Gramenzi A, Buttino I, D'Avanzo B, et al: Medical history and the risk of multiple myeloma. *Br J Cancer* 63:679, 1991.
15. Soulier J, Grollet L, Oksenhendler E, et al: Kaposi's sarcoma-associated herpesvirus-like DNA sequences in multicentric Castleman's disease. *Blood* 86:1276, 1995.
16. Said W, Chien K, Takeuchi S, et al: Kaposi's sarcoma-associated herpesvirus (KSHV or HHV8) in primary effusion lymphoma: ultrastructural demonstration of herpesvirus in lymphoma cells. *Blood* 87:4937, 1996.
17. Schalling M, Ekman M, Kaaya EE, Linde A, Biberfeld P: A role for a new herpes virus (KSHV) in different forms of Kaposi's sarcoma. *Nat Med* 1:707, 1995.
18. Rettig MB, Ma HJ, Vescio RA, et al: Kaposi's sarcoma-associated herpesvirus infection of bone marrow dendritic cells from multiple myeloma patients. *Science* 276:1851, 1997.
19. Said JW, Rettig MR, Heppner K, et al: Localization of Kaposi's sarcoma-associated herpesvirus in bone marrow biopsy samples from patients with multiple myeloma. *Blood* 90:4278, 1997.
20. Chauhan D, Bharti A, Raje N, et al: Detection of Kaposi's sarcoma herpesvirus DNA sequences in multiple myeloma bone marrow stromal cells. *Blood* 93:1482, 1999.
21. Raje N, Gong J, Chauhan D, et al: Bone marrow and peripheral blood dendritic cells from patients with multiple myeloma are phenotypically and functionally normal despite the detection of Kaposi's sarcoma herpesvirus gene sequences. *Blood*. 93:1487, 1999.
22. Tarte K, Olsen SJ, Yang LZ, et al: Clinical-grade functional dendritic cells from patients with multiple myeloma are not infected with Kaposi's sarcoma-associated herpesvirus. *Blood* 91:1852, 1998.
23. Yi Q, Ekman M, Anton D, et al: Blood dendritic cells from myeloma patients are not infected with Kaposi's sarcoma-associated herpesvirus (KSHV/HHV-8). *Blood* 92:402, 1998.
24. Tisdale JF, Stewart AK, Dickstein B, et al: Molecular and serological examination of the relationship of human herpesvirus 8 to multiple myeloma: ORF 26 sequences in bone marrow stroma are not restricted to myeloma patients and other regions of the genome are not detected. *Blood* 92:2681, 1998.
25. Potter M: Perspectives on the origins of multiple myeloma and plasmacytomas in mice. *Hematol Oncol Clin North Am* 6:211, 1992.
26. Barlogie B, Epstein J, Selvanayagam P, Alexanian R: Plasma cell myeloma–new biological insights and advances in therapy. [Review]. *Blood* 73:865, 1989.
27. Hallek M, Leif Bergsagel P, Anderson KC: Multiple myeloma: increasing evidence for a multistep transformation process. *Blood* 91:3, 1998.
28. MacLennan ICM, Chan EYT: The origin of bone marrow plasma cells, in *Epidemiology and Biology of Multiple Myeloma,* edited by GI Obrams, M Potter, p 129. Springer, Berlin, 1991.
29. Barlogie B, Alexanian R: Cellular aspects of myeloma: biologic and clinical implications, in *Multiple Myeloma and Other Paraproteinemias,* edited by IW Delamore, pp 154–168. Churchill Livingstone, Edinburgh, 1986.
30. Bast E, van Camp B, Reynaert P, et al: Idiotypic peripheral blood lymphocytes in monoclonal gammopathy. *Clin Exp Immunol* 47:682, 1982.
31. Berenson J, Wong R, Kim K, et al: Evidence of peripheral blood B lymphocyte but not T lymphocyte involvement in multiple myeloma. *Blood* 70:1550, 1987.
32. Mellstedt H, Holm G, Pettersson D, et al: Idiotype-bearing lymphoid cells in plasma cell neoplasia. *Clin Haematol* 11:65, 1982.
33. Pilarski LM, Jensen GS: Monoclonal circulating B cells in multiple myeloma: a continuously differentiating possibly invasive population as defined by expression of CD45 isoforms and adhesion molecules. *Hematol/Oncol Clin North Am* 6:297, 1992.
34. Pilarski LM, Mant MJ, Reuther BA: Pre-B cells in peripheral blood of multiple myeloma patients. *Blood* 66:416, 1985.
35. Ruiz-Arguelles GJ, Katzmann JA, Greipp PR, et al: Multiple myeloma: circulating lymphocytes that express plasma cell antigens. *Blood* 64:352, 1984.
36. Berenson J, Lichtenstein A: Clonal rearrangement of immunoglobulin genes in the peripheral blood of multiple myeloma patients. *Br J Haematol* 73;425, 1989.
37. Corradini P, Boccadoro M, Voena C, Pileri A: Evidence for a bone marrow B cell transcribing malignant plasma cell VDJ joined to C mu sequence in immunoglobulin (IgG)- and IgA- secreting multiple myelomas. *J Exp Med* 178:1091, 1993.
38. Billadeau D, Ahmann G, Greipp P, Van Ness B: The bone marrow of multiple myeloma patients contains B cell populations at different stages of differentiation that are clonally related to the malignant plasma cell. *J Exp Med* 178:1023, 1993.
39. Chen BJ, Epstein J: Circulating clonal lymphocytes in myeloma constitute a minor subpopulation of B cells. *Blood* 87:1972, 1996.
40. Gould J, Alexanian R, Goodacre A, et al: Plasma cell karyotype in multiple myeloma. *Blood* 71:453, 1988.
41. Dewald GW, Kyle RA, Hicks GA, Greipp PR: The clinical significance of cytogenetic studies in 100 patients with multiple myeloma, plasma cell leukemia, or amyloidosis. *Blood* 66(2):380, 1985.
42. Sawyer JR, Waldron JA, Jagannath S, Barlogie B: Cytogenetic findings in 200 patients with multiple myeloma. *Cancer Genet Cytogenet* 82(1):41, 1995.
43. Feinman R, Sawyer, J, Hardin J, Tricot G: Cytogenetics and molecular genetics in multiple myeloma. *Hematol/Oncol Clin North Am* 11:1, 1997.
44. Selvanayagam P, Blick M, Narni F, et al: Alteration and abnormal expression of the c-*MYC* oncogene in human multiple myeloma. *Blood* 71:30, 1988.
45. Greil R, Fasching B, Loidl P, Huber H: Expression of the c-*MYC* proto-

oncogene in multiple myeloma and chronic lymphocytic leukemia: an in situ analysis. *Blood* 78:180, 1991.

46. Neri A, Murphy JP, Cro L, et al: *RAS* oncogene mutation in multiple myeloma. *J Exp Med* 170:1715, 1989.

47. Ernst TJ, Gazdar A, Ritz J, Shipp MA: Identification of a second transforming gene, RASN, in a human multiple myeloma line with a rearranged c-*MYC* allele. *Blood* 72:1163, 1989.

48. Paquette RL, Berenson J, Lichtenstein A, et al: Oncogenes in multiple myeloma: point mutation of N-*RAS*. *Oncogene* 5:1659, 1990.

49. Portier M, Moles J-P, Mazars G-R, et al: *p53* and *RAS* gene mutations in multiple myeloma. *Oncogene* 7:2539, 1992.

50. Liu P, Leong T, Quam L, et al: Activating mutations of N- and K-ras in multiple myeloma show different clinical associations: analysis of the Eastern Cooperative Oncology Group phase III trial. *Blood* 88: 2699, 1996.

51. Hamilton MS, Barker HF, Ball J, et al: Normal and neoplastic human plasma cells express *BCL-2* antigen. *Leukemia* 5:768, 1991.

52. Pettersson M, Jernberg-Wiklund H, Larson LG, et al: Expression of the *BCL-2* gene in human multiple myeloma cell lines and normal plasma cells. *Blood* 79:495, 1992.

53. Neri A, Baldini L, Trecca D, et al: *p53* gene mutations in multiple myeloma are associated with advanced forms of malignancy. *Blood* 81:128, 1993.

54. Drach J, Ackermann J, Fritz E, et al: Presence of a p53 gene deletion in patients with multiple myeloma predicts for short survival after conventional-dose chemotherapy. *Blood* 92:802, 1998.

55. Dao DD, Sawyer JR, Epstein J, Hoover RG, Barlogie B, Tricot G: Deletion of the retinoblastoma gene in multiple myeloma. *Leukemia* 8:1280, 1994.

56. Teoh G, Urashima M, Ogata A, et al: MDM2 protein overexpression promotes proliferation and survival of multiple myeloma cells. *Blood* 90:1982, 1997.

57. Korganow AS, Martin T, Weber JC, et al: Molecular analysis of rearranged VH genes during B cell chronic lymphocytic leukemia: intraclonal stability is frequent but not constant. *Leuk Lymphoma* 14:55, 1994.

58. Oscier DG, Thompsett A, Zhu D, Stevenson FK: Differential rates of somatic hypermutation in V(H) genes among subsets of chronic lymphocytic leukemia defined by chromosomal abnormalities. *Blood* 89:4153, 1997.

59. Fais F, Ghiotto F, Hashimoto S, et al: Chronic lymphocytic leukemia B cells express restricted sets of mutated and unmutated antigen receptors. *J. Clin. Invest.* 102:1515, 1998.

60. Bakkus MH, Heirman C, Van RietI, Van Camp B, Thielemans K: Evidence that multiple myeloma Ig heavy chain VDJ genes contain somatic mutations but show no intraclonal variation. *Blood* 80:2326, 1992.

61. Vescio RA, Cao J, Hong CH, et al: Myeloma Ig heavy chain V region sequences reveal prior antigenic selection and marked somatic mutation but no intraclonal diversity. *J Immunol* 155:2487, 1995.

62. Shen HM, Peters A, Baron B, Zhu X, Storb U: Mutation of BCL-6 gene in normal B cells by the process of somatic hypermutation of Ig genes. *Science.* 280:1750, 1998.

63. Sawyer JR, Lukacs J, Munshi N, et al: Identification of new nonrandom translocations in multiple myeloma with multicolor spectral karyotyping. *Blood* 92:4269, 1998.

64. Chesi M, Bergsagel PL, Shonukan OO, et al: Frequent dysregulation of the c-maf proto-oncogene at 16q23 by translocation to an Ig locus in multiple myeloma. *Blood* 91:4457, 1998.

65. Chesi M, Nardini E, Brents LA, et al: Frequent translocation t(4;14)(p16.3;q32.3) in multiple myeloma is associated with increased expression and activating mutations of fibroblast growth factor receptor 3. *Nat Genet* 16:260, 1997.

66. Chesi M, Nardini E, Lim RS, Smith KD, Kuehl WM, Bergsagel PL: The t(4;14) translocation in myeloma dysregulates both FGFR3 and a novel gene, MMSET, resulting in IgH/MMSET hybrid transcripts. *Blood* 92:3025, 1998.

67. Iida S, Rao PH, Butler M, et al: Deregulation of MUM1/IRF4 by chromosomal translocation in multiple myeloma. *Nat Genet* 17:226, 1997.

68. Tricot G, Barlogie B, Jagannath S, et al: Poor prognosis in multiple myeloma is associated only with partial or complete deletions of

chromosome 13 or abnormalities involving 11q and not with other karyotypes abnormalities. *Blood* 86:4250, 1995.

69. Barlogie B, Sawyer J, Ayers D, et al: Chromosome 13 myeloma is a distinct entity with poor prognosis despite tandem autotransplants. *Blood* 92(suppl 1):258a(#1059).

70. Perez-Simon JA, Garcia-Sanz R, Tabernero MD, et al: Prognostic value of numerical chromosome aberrations in multiple myeloma: a FISH analysis of 15 different chromosomes. *Blood* 91: 3366, 1998.

71. Seong C, Delasalle K, Hayes K, et al: Prognostic value of cytogenetics in multiple myeloma. *Br J Haematol* 101:189, 1998.

72. Shaughnessy J, Tian E, Bell T, et al: Molecular cytogenetic analysis of chromosome 13q14, site of a putative tumor suppressor gene in multiple myeloma. *Blood* 92(suppl 1):259a, 1998.

73. Epstein J, Barlogie B: Tumor resistance to chemotherapy associated with expression of the multidrug resistance phenotype. *Cancer Bull* 41:41, 1989.

74. Epstein J, Xiao H, Oba BK: P-glycoprotein expression in plasma cell myeloma is associated with resistance to VAD. *Blood* 74:913, 1989.

75. Dalton WS, Durie BGM, Alberts DS, et al: Characterization of a new drug resistant human myeloma cell line which expresses P-glycoprotein. *Cancer Res* 46:5125, 1986.

76. Dalton WS, Grogan TM, Durie BGM, et al: Drug-resistance in multiple myeloma and non-Hodgkin's lymphoma: detection of P-glycoprotein and potential circumvention by addition of verapamil to chemotherapy. *J Clin Oncol* 7:415, 1989.

77. Dalton WS, Grogan TM, Rybski JA, et al: Immunohistochemical detection and quantitation of P-glycoprotein in multiple drug-resistant human myeloma cells: association with level of drug resistance and drug accumulation. *Blood* 73;747, 1989.

78. Dalton WS: Detection of multidrug resistance gene expression in multiple myeloma. [Review]. *Leukemia* 11:1166, 1997.

79. Chaudhary PM, Roninson IB: Expression and activity of p-glycoprotein, a multidrug efflux pump, in human hematopoietic stem cells. *Cell* 66:85, 1991.

80. Sonneveld P, Lokhorst HM, Vossebeld P: Drug resistance in multiple myeloma. [Review] *Semin Hematol* 34:34, 1997.

81. Raaijmakers HG, Izquierdo MA, Lokhorst HM, et al: Lung-resistance-related protein expression is a negative predictive factor for response to conventional low but not to intensified dose alkylating chemotherapy in multiple myeloma. *Blood* 91:1029, 1998.

82. Kawano M, Hirano T, Matsuda T, et al: Autocrine generation and requirement of BSF-2/IL-6 for human multiple myelomas. *Nature* 332:83, 1988.

83. Klein B, Zhang XG, Jourdan M, et al: Paracrine rather than autocrine regulation of myeloma-cell growth and differentiation by interleukin-6. *Blood* 73:517, 1989.

84. Caligaris-Cappio F, Bergui L, Gaidano GL, et al: In vitro studies provide evidence that multiple paracrine loops may be operating in multiple myeloma, in *Epidemiology and Biology of Multiple Myeloma*, edited by GI Obrams, M Potter, p 123. Springer, Berlin, 1991.

85. Hata H, Xiao H, Petrucci MT, Woodliff J, Chang R, Epstein J: Interleukin-6 gene expression in multiple myeloma: a characteristic of immature tumor cells. *Blood* 81:3357, 1993.

86. Brandt S, Bodine D, Dunbar C, Nienhuis A: Dysregulated interleukin-6 expression produces a syndrome resembling Castleman's disease in mice. *J Clin Invest* 86:592, 1990.

87. Suematsu S, Matsusaka T, Matsuda T, et al: Generation of plasmacytomas with the chromosomal translocation t(12;15) in interleukin 6 transgenic mice. *Proc Natl Acad Sci USA* 89(1):232, 1992.

88. Caligaris-Cappio F, Bergui L, Gregoretti MG, et al: Role of bone marrow stromal cells in the growth of human multiple myeloma. *Blood* 77:2688, 1991.

89. Thomas X, Xiao HQ, Chang R, Epstein J: Circulating B lymphocytes in multiple myeloma patients contain an autocrine IL-6 driven pre-myeloma cell population. *Curr Top Microbiol Immunol* 182:201, 1992.

90. Epstein J: Myeloma phenotype: clues to disease origin and manifestation. *Hematol Oncol Clin North Am* 6:249, 1992.

91. Van Camp B, Durie BGM, Spier C, et al: Plasma cells in multiple myeloma express a natural killer cell-associated antigen: CD56 (NKH-1; Leu-19). *Blood* 75:377, 1990.

92. Kawano MM, Huang N, Harada H, et al: Identification of immature

and mature myeloma cells in the bone marrow of human myelomas. *Blood* 82:564, 1993.

93. Omede P, Boccadoro M, Fusaro A, Gallone G, Pileri A: Multiple myeloma: ''early'' plasma cell phenotype identifies patients with aggressive biological and clinical characteristics. *Br J Haematol* 85:504, 1993.

94. Huang N, Kawano MM, Harada H, et al: Heterogeneous expression of a novel MPC-1 antigen on myeloma cells: possible involvement of MPC-1 antigen in the adhesion of mature myeloma cells to bone marrow stromal cells. *Blood* 82:3721, 1993.

95. Stauder R, Van Driel M, Schwarzler C, et al: Different CD44 splicing patterns define prognostic subgroups in multiple myeloma. *Blood* 88:3101, 1996.

96. Damiano JS, Cress AE, Hazlehurst LA, Shtil AA, Dalton WS: Cell adhesion mediated drug resistance (CAM-DR): role of integrins and resistance to apoptosis in human myeloma cell lines. *Blood* 93:1658, 1999.

97. Cozzolino F, Torcia M, Adinucci D, et al: Production of interleukin-1 by bone marrow myeloma cells. *Blood* 74:380, 1989.

98. Garrett IR, Durie BGM, Nedwin GE, et al: Production of lymphotoxin, a bone resorbing cytokine, by cultured human myeloma cells. *N Engl J Med* 317:526, 1989.

99. Mundy GR, Raisz LG, Cooper RA, et al: Evidence for the secretion of an osteoclast-stimulating factor in myeloma. *N Engl J Med* 291:1041, 1974.

100. Hardin J, MacLeod S, Grigorieva I, et al: Interleukin-6 prevents dexamethasone-induced myeloma cell death. *Blood* 84:3063, 1994.

101. Xu F, Gardner A, Tu Y, Michl P, Prager D, Lichtenstein A: Multiple myeloma cells are protected against dexamethasone-induced apoptosis by insulin-like growth factors. *Br J Haematol* 97:429, 1997.

102. Borset M, Hjorth-Hansen H, Seidel C, Sundan A, Waage A: Hepatocyte growth factor and its receptor c-met in multiple myeloma. *Blood* 88:3998, 1996.

103. Grigorieva I, Thomas X, Epstein J: The bone marrow stromal environment is a major factor in myeloma cell resistance to dexamethasone. *Exp Hematol* 26:597, 1998.

104. Eastgate J, Moreb J, Nick HS, et al: A role for manganese superoxide dismutase in radioprotection of hematopoietic stem cells by interleukin-1. *Blood* 81:639, 1993.

105. Feinman R, Koury J, Thames M, Barlogie B, Epstein J, Siegel DS: Role of NF-κB in the rescue of multiple myeloma cells from glucocorticoid-induced apoptosis by bcl-2. *Blood* (in press) 1999.

106. Ridley RC, Xiao H, Hata H, Woodliff J, Epstein J, Sanderson RD: Expression of syndecan regulates human myeloma plasma cell adhesion to type I collagen. *Blood* 81:767, 1993.

107. Wijdenes J, Vooijs WC, Clement C, et al: A plasmocyte selective monoclonal antibody (BB4) recognizes syndecan-1. *Br J Haematol* 94:318, 1996.

108. Dhodapkar MV, Kelly T, Theus A, Athota AB, Barlogie B, Sanderson RD: Elevated levels of shed syndecan-1 correlate with tumour mass and decreased matrix metalloproteinase-9 activity in the serum of patients with multiple myeloma. *Br J Haematol* 99:368, 1997.

109. Dhodapkar M, Abe E, Theus A, et al: Syndecan-1 is a multifunctional regulator of myeloma pathobiology: control of tumor cell survival, growth and bone cell differentiation. *Blood* 91:2679, 1998.

110. Kleeff J, Ishiwata T, Kumbasar A, et al: The cell-surface heparan sulfate proteoglycan glypican-1 regulates growth factor action in pancreatic carcinoma cells and is overexpressed in human pancreatic cancer. *J Clin Invest* 102:1662, 1998.

111. Pihan GA, Purohit A, Wallace J, et al: Centrosome defects and genetic instability in malignant tumors. *Cancer Res* 58:3974, 1998.

112. Hofbauer LC, Heufelder AE: Osteoprotegerin and its cognate ligand: a new paradigm of osteoclastogenesis. *Eur J Endocrinol* 139:152, 1998.

113. Munshi N, Wilson CS, Penn J, et al: Angiogenesis in newly diagnosed multiple myeloma: poor prognosis with increased microvessel density (MVD) in bone marrow biopsies *Blood* 92(suppl 1):97a, 1998.

114. Bellamy WT, Richter L, Frutiger Y, Grogan TM: Expression of vascular endothelial growth factor and its receptors in hematopoietic malignancies. *Cancer Res* 59:728, 1999.

115. Kruse FE, Joussen AM, Rohrschneider K, Becker MD, Volcker HE: Thalidomide inhibits corneal angiogenesis induced by vascular endo-

116. Bataille R, Klein B: The bone resorbing activity of interleukin-6. *J Bone Min Res* 9:1144, 1991.

117. Bataille R, Chappard D, Marcelli C, et al: Mechanism of bone destruction in multiple myeloma. The importance of an unbalanced process in determining the severity of lytic bone disease. *J Clin Oncol* 7:1909, 1989.

118. Hind CRK, Baltz ML, Pepys MB: Amyloidosis, in *Multiple Myeloma and Other Paraproteinaemias*, edited by IW Delamore, p 234. Churchill Livingstone, Edinburgh, 1986.

119. Ullrich S, Zolla-Pazner S: Immunoregulatory circuits in myeloma. *Clin Hematol* 11:87, 1982.

120. Jacobson DR, Zolla-Pazner S: Immunosuppression and infection in multiple myeloma. *Semin Oncol* 2:282, 1986.

121. Broder S, Humphrey R, Durm M, et al: Impaired synthesis of (non-paraprotein) immunoglobulins by circulating lymphocytes from patients with multiple myeloma. *N Engl J Med* 293:887, 1975.

122. Lynch RG: A role for TGF-beta in the immunodeficiency of malignant plasma cell tumors, abstract. Proceedings of the Third EURAGE Symposium, Brussels, Belgium, Sept 18–20, 1991.

123. Villunger A, Egle A, Marschitz I, et al: Constitutive expression of Fas (Apo-1/CD95) ligand on multiple myeloma cells: a potential mechanism of tumor-induced suppression of immune surveillance. *Blood* 90:12, 1997.

124. Solomon A, Weiss DT: A perspective of plasma cell dyscrasias: clinical implications of monoclonal light chains in renal disease, in *The Kidney in Plasma Cell Dyscrasias*, edited by L Minetti, G D'Amico, C Ponticelli, p 3. Kluwer, Dordrecht, Netherlands, 1988.

125. Solomon A, Weiss DT, Kattine AA: Nephrotoxic potential of Bence Jones proteins. *N Engl J Med* 324:1845, 1991.

126. Alexanian R, Barlogie B, Dixon D: Renal failure in multiple myeloma: pathogenesis and prognostic implications. *Arch Intern Med* 150:1693, 1990.

127. Alexanian R, Barlogie B: Implications of renal failure in multiple myeloma, in *The Kidney in Plasma Cell Dyscrasias*, edited by L Minetti, G D'Amico, C Ponticelli, p 260. Kluwer, Dordrecht, Netherlands, 1988.

128. Zucker-Franklin D: Renal amyloidosis: new perspectives, in *The Kidney in Plasma Cell Dyscrasias*, edited by L Minetti, G D'Amico, C Ponticelli, p 45. Kluwer, Dordrecht, Netherlands, 1988.

129. Kyle RA, Greipp PR: Amyloidosis (AL): clinical and laboratory features in 229 cases. *Mayo Clinic Proc* 58:665, 1983.

130. Buxbaum J: Mechanisms of disease: monoclonal immunoglobulin deposition. *Hematol Oncol Clin North Am* 6:323, 1992.

131. Gallo G, Buxbaum J: Monoclonal immunoglobulin deposition disease: immunopathologic aspects of renal involvement, in *The Kidney in Plasma Cell Dyscrasias*, edited by L Minetti, G D'Amico, C Ponticelli, p 171. Kluwer, Dordrecht, Netherlands, 1988.

132. Reeves WB, Foley RJ, Weinman EJ: Nephrotoxicity from nonsteroidal anti-inflammatory drugs. *South Med J* 78:318, 1985.

133. Fattori E, Della Rocca C, Costa P, et al: Development of progressive kidney damage and myeloma kidney in interleukin-6 transgenic mice. *Blood* 83:2570, 1994.

134. Spiers ASD, Halpern R, Ross SC, et al: Meningeal myelomatosis. *Arch Intern Med* 140:256, 1980.

135. Barlogie B, Smallwood L, Smith T, Alexanian R: High serum levels of lactic dehydrogenase identify a high-grade lymphoma-like myeloma. *Ann Intern Med* 110:521, 1989.

136. Bichel J, Efferse P, Gormsen H, Harboe N: Leukemic myelomatosis (plasma cell leukemia). A review with report of four cases. *Acta Radiol* 37:196, 1952.

137. Waldenström JG, Adner A, Gydell K, Zettervall O: Osteosclerotic ''plasmacytoma'' with polyneuropathy, hypertrichosis and diabetes. *Acta Med Scand* 203:297, 1978.

138. Miralles GD, O'Fallon JR, Talley NJ: Plasma-cell dyscrasia with polyneuropathy—the spectrum of POEMS syndrome. *N Engl J Med* 327:1919, 1992.

139. Pruzanski W, Watt JG: Serum viscosity and hyperviscosity syndrome in IgG multiple myeloma. *Ann Intern Med* 77:853, 1972.

140. Preston FE, Cooke KB, Foster ME, et al: Myelomatosis and the hyperviscosity syndrome. *Br J Haematol* 38:517, 1978.

thelial growth factor. *Graefes Arch Clin Exp Ophthalmol* 236:461, 1998.

141. Chandy KG, Stockley RG, Leonard RCF, et al: Relationships between serum viscosity and intravascular IgA polymer concentration in IgA myeloma. *Clin Exp Immunol* 46:653, 1981.

142. Somer T: Hyperviscosity syndrome in plasma cell dyscrasias. *Adv Microcirculation* 6:1, 1975.

143. Waldenström JG: Incipient myelomatosis or "essential" hyperglobulinaemia with fibrinogenopenia—a new syndrome. *Acta Med Scand* 117:216, 1944.

144. Kelsey PR, Delamore IW: Clinical features of multiple myeloma, in *Multiple Myeloma and Other Paraproteinaemias*, edited by IW Delamore, p 117. Churchill Livingstone, Edinburgh, 1986.

145. Capra JD, Kunkel HG: Aggregation of IgG3 proteins. Relevance to the hyperviscosity syndrome. *J Clin Invest* 49:610, 1970.

146. Perkins HA, MacKenzie MR, Fudenberg HH: Haemostatic defects in dysproteinaemias. *Blood* 35:695, 1970.

147. Lackner H: Haemostatic abnormalities associated with dysproteinaemias. *Semin Haematol* 10:125, 1973.

148. Barlogie B, Gale RP: Multiple myeloma and chronic lymphocytic leukemia: parallels and contrasts. *Am J Med* 93:443, 1992.

149. Greipp R, Raymond NM, Kyle RA, O'Fallon WM: Multiple myeloma: significance of plasmablastic subtype in morphological classification. *Blood* 65:305, 1985.

150. Greipp PR, Leong T, Bennett JM, et al: Plasmablastic morphology—an independent prognostic factor with clinical and laboratory correlates: Eastern Cooperative Oncology Group (ECOG) myeloma trial E9486 report by the ECOG Myeloma Laboratory Group. *Blood* 91:2501, 1998.

151. Ludwig H, Pecherstorfer M, Leitgeb C, Fritz E: Recombinant human erythropoietin for the treatment of chronic anemia in multiple myeloma and squamous cell carcinoma *Stem Cells* (Dayt) 11:348, 1993.

152. Faquin WC, Schneider TJ, Goldberg MA: Effect of inflammatory cytokines on hypoxia-induced erythropoietin production. *Blood* 79:1987, 1992.

153. Singh A, Eckardt KU, Zimmermann A, et al: Increased plasma viscosity as a reason for inappropriate erythropoietin formation. *J Clin Invest* 91:251, 1993.

154. Gleuck HI, Hong RA: Circulating anticoagulant in multiple myeloma: its modification by penicillin. *J Clin Invest* 44:1866, 1965.

155. Wenz B, Freidman G: Acquired factor VIII inhibitor in a patient with malignant lymphoma. *Am J Med* Sci 268:295, 1974.

156. Kelsey PR, Leyland MJ: Acquired inhibitor to human factor VIII associated with paraproteinaemia and subsequent development of chronic lymphatic leukaemia. *Br Med J* 285:174, 1982.

157. Coleman M, Vigliano EM, Weksler ME, Nachman RL: Inhibition of fibrin monomer polymerization by lambda myeloma globulin. *Blood* 39:210, 1972.

158. Furie B, Greene E, Furie BC: Syndrome of acquired factor X deficiency and systemic amyloidosis. In vivo studies of the metabolic fate of factor X. *N Engl J Med* 297:81, 1977.

159. Kunkel LA: Acquired circulating anticoagulants in malignancy. *Semin Thromb Hemost* 18:416, 1992.

160. Billadeau D, Quam L, Thomas W, et al: Detection and quantitation of malignant cells in the peripheral blood of multiple myeloma patients. *Blood* 80:1818, 1992.

161. Aubin J, Davi F, Nguyen-Salomon F, et al: Description of a novel FR1 IgH PCR strategy and its comparison with three other strategies for the detection of clonality in B cell malignancies. *Leukemia* 9:471, 1995.

162. Barlogie B, Alexanian R, Pershouse M, et al: Cytoplasmic immunoglobulin content in multiple myeloma. *J Clin Invest* 76:765, 1985.

163. Latreille J, Barlogie B, Johnston D, Drewinko B, Alexanian R: Ploidy and proliferative characteristics in monoclonal gammopathies. *Blood* 59:43, 1982.

164. Latreille J, Barlogie B, Dosik G, Johnston DA, Drewinko B, Alexanian R: Cellular DNA content as a marker of human multiple myeloma. *Blood* 55:403, 1980.

165. Epstein J, Barlogie B, Alexanian R: Phenotypic heterogeneity in aneuploid multiple myeloma indicates pre-B cell involvement. *Blood* 71:861, 1988.

166. Grogan TM, Durie BG, Lomen C, et al: Delineation of a novel pre-B cell compartment in plasma cell myeloma: immunochemical, immunophenotypic, genotypic, cytologic, cell culture and kinetic features. *Blood* 70:832, 1987.

167. Grogan TM, Durie BGM, Spier CM, et al: Myelomonocytic antigen positive multiple myeloma. *Blood* 73:763, 1989.

168. Epstein J, Xiao H-Q, He X-Y: Markers of multiple hematopoietic-cell lineages in multiple myeloma. *N Engl J Med* 322:664, 1990.

169. Durie BGM, Grogan TM: cALLa-positive myeloma: an aggressive subtype with poor survival. *Blood* 66:229, 1985.

170. Caligaris-Cappio F, Bergui L, Tesio L, et al: Identification of malignant plasma cell precursors in the bone marrow of multiple myeloma. *J Clin Invest* 76:1243, 1985.

171. Drewinko B, Alexanian R, Boyer H, et al: The growth fraction of human myeloma cells. *Blood* 57:333, 1981.

172. Durie BGM, Salmon SE, Moon TE: Pretreatment tumor mass, cell kinetics, and prognosis in multiple myeloma. *Blood* 55:364, 1980.

173. Greipp PR, Witzig TE, Gonchoroff NJ, et al: Immunofluorescence labeling indices in myeloma and related monoclonal gammopathies. *Mayo Clin Proc* 62:969, 1987.

174. Boccadoro M, Massaia M, Dianzani U, et al: Multiple myeloma: biological and clinical significance of bone marrow plasma cell labelling index. *Haematologica* 72:171, 1987.

175. Witzig TE, Gonchoroff NJ, Katzmann JA, et al: Peripheral blood B cell labeling indices are a measure of disease activity in patients with monoclonal gammopathies. *J Clin Oncol* 6:1041, 1988.

176. Greipp PR, Lust JA, O'Fallon WM, Katzmann JA, Witzig TE, Kyle RA: Plasma cell labeling index and beta 2-microglobulin predict survival independent of thymidine kinase and C-reactive protein in multiple myeloma. *Blood* 81:3382, 1993.

177. Van Den Berghe H: Chromosomes in plasma-cell malignancies. *Eur J Haematol* 43(suppl 51):47, 1989.

178. Meeus P, Stul MS, Mecucci C, Cassiman JJ, Van den Berghe H: Molecular breakpoints of t (11;14)(q13;q32) in multiple myeloma. *Cancer Genet Cytogenet* 83:25, 1995.

179. Ladanyi M, Wang S, Niesvizky R, Feiner H, Michaeli J: Proto-oncogene analysis in multiple myeloma *Am Pathol* 141:949, 1992.

180. Avet-Loiseau H, Li JY, Facon T, et al: High incidence of translocations t(11;14)(q13;q32) and t(4;14)(p16;q32) in patients with plasma cell malignancies. *Cancer Res* 58:5640, 1998.

181. Nishida K, Tamura A, Nakazawa N, et al: The Ig heavy chain gene is frequently involved in chromosomal translocations in multiple myeloma and plasma cell leukemia as detected by in situ hybridization. *Blood* 90(2):526, 1997.

182. Bergsagel PL, Chesi M, Nardini E, Brents LA, Kirby SL, Kuehl WM: Promiscuous translocations into immunoglobulin heavy chain switch regions in multiple myeloma. *Proc Natl Acad Sci USA* 93:13931, 1996.

183. Durie BGM: Cellular and molecular genetic features of myeloma and related disorders. *Hematol Oncol Clin North Am* 6:463, 1992.

184. Drach J, Ayers D, Govindarajan R, Sawyer J, et al: MDS-associated cytogenetic abnormalities (CG?) in both hematopoietic and neoplastic cells after autotransplants (AT) in 868 patients with multiple myeloma (MM). Blood 92(suppl 1):97a(#398).

185. Pedersen-Bjergaard J, Timshel S, Andersen MK, Andersen AS, Philip P: Cytogenetically unrelated clones in therapy-related myelodysplasia and acute myeloid leukemia: experience from the Copenhagen series updated to 180 consecutive cases. *Genes Chromosomes Cancer* 23:337, 1998.

186. Shaughnessy J, Barlogie B: Chromosome 13 deletion in myeloma. *Curr Top Microbiol Immunol* 246:199, 1999.

187. Dallinger S, Kaufmann H, Ackermann J, et al: Interphase fluorescence in situ hybridization (FISH) confirms the poor prognosis of patients with multiple myeloma (mm) and deletion of 13q. *Blood* 92(suppl 1):97a, 1998.

188. Smith L, Barlogie B, Alexanian R: Biclonal and hypodiploid multiple myeloma. *Am J Med* 80:841, 1986.

189. Durie BGM, Baum VE, Vela EE, Mundy GR: Abnormalities of chromosome 6q and osteoclast activating factor (LAF: TNF-β) production in multiple myeloma. *Blood* 68:208a, 1986.

190. Durie B, Salmon S: A clinical staging system for multiple myeloma. *Cancer* 36:842, 1975.

191. Salmon SE, Smith BA: Immunoglobulin synthesis and total body tumor cell number in IgG multiple myeloma. *J Clin Invest* 49:114, 1970.

192. Child JA, Norfolk DR, Cooper EH: Serum beta-2-microglobulin in myelomatosis: potential value in stratification and monitoring. *Br J Haematol* 63:406, 1986.

193. Garewal H, Durie BGM, Kyle RA, et al: Serum beta-2-microglobulin in the initial staging and subsequent monitoring of monoclonal plasma cell disorders. *J Clin Oncol* 2:51, 1984.

194. Alexanian R, Barlogie B, Fritsche H: Beta 2 microglobulin myeloma: optimal use for staging, prognosis and treatment—a prospective study of 160 patients. *Blood* 63:468, 1984.

195. Durie BGM, Young LA, Salmon SE: Human myeloma in vitro colony growth: interrelationship between drug sensitivity, cell kinetics and patient survival duration. *Blood* 61:929, 1983.

196. Bataille R, Boccadoro M, Klein B, et al: C-reactive protein and beta-2-microglobulin produce a simple and powerful myeloma staging system. *Blood* 80:733, 1992.

197. Klein B, Bataille R: Cytokine network in human multiple myeloma. *Hematol Oncol Clin North Am* 6:273, 1992.

198. Bataille R, Chappard D, Klein B: Mechanisms of bone lesions in multiple myeloma. *Hematol Oncol Clin North Am* 6:285, 1992.

199. Bataille R, Harousseau JL: Multiple myeloma. *N Engl J Med* 336(23): 1657, 1997.

200. Cherng NC, Asal NR, Kuebler JP, Lee ET, Solanki D: Prognostic factors in multiple myeloma. *Cancer* 67:3150, 1991.

201. Dimopoulos MA, Alexanian R, Barlogie B: High serum lactic dehydrogenase as a marker of drug resistance in multiple myeloma. *Ann Intern Med* 115:931, 1991.

202. Bartl R, Frisch B, Fateh-Moghadam A, Kettner G, Jaeger K, Sommerfeld W: Histologic classification and staging of multiple myeloma. A retrospective and prospective study of 674 cases. *Am J Clin Pathol* 87:342, 1987.

203. Waldron J, Jazieh R, Jagannath S, et al: Bone marrow morphology (BMM) adds critical prognostic information to other standard parameters (SP) including cytogenetics among newly diagnosed multiple myeloma (MM) patients (PTS) receiving total therapy (TT). *Blood* 90:90a, 1997.

204. Dimopoulos MA, Moulopoulos A, Delasalle K, Alexanian R: Solitary plasmacytoma of bone and asymptomatic multiple myeloma. *Hematol Oncol Clin North Am* 6:359, 1992.

205. Daffner RH, Lupetin AR, Dash N, et al: MRI in the detection of malignant infiltration of bone marrow. *Am J Roentgenol* 146:353, 1986.

206. Moulopoulos L, Dimopoulos M, Weber D, et al: Magnetic resonance imaging in the staging of solitary plasmacytoma of bone. *J Clin Oncol* 11:1311, 1993.

207. Dohner H, Guckel F, Knowf W, et al: Magnetic resonance imaging of bone marrow in lymphoproliferative disorders: correlation with bone marrow biopsy. *Br J Haematol* 73:12, 1989.

208. Moulopoulos LA, Dimopoulos MA, Weber D, Fuller L, Libshitz HI, Alexanian R: Magnetic resonance imaging in the staging of solitary plasmacytoma of bone. *J Clin Oncol* 11:1311, 1993.

209. Angtuaco E, Jazieh A, Ferris E, et al: Complete remission by MRI (MR-CR) after tandem autotransplants associated with superior survival blood. 92(Suppl1):97a(#4117).

210. Kyle RA: Diagnostic criteria of multiple myeloma. *Hematol Oncol Clin North Am* 6:347, 1992.

211. Alexanian R: Diagnosis and management of multiple myeloma, in *Neoplastic Diseases of the Blood*, 2d ed, edited by PH Weirnile, GP Canellos, RA Kyle, CA Schiffer, pp 453–465. Churchill Livingstone, New York, 1991.

212. Waldenström JG: Benign monoclonal gammopathy. *Acta Med Scand* 216:435, 1984.

213. Kyle RA: Monoclonal gammopathy of determined significance: natural history in 241 cases. *Am J Med* 64:814, 1978.

214. Greipp PR, Kyle RA: Clinical morphological and cell kinetic differences among multiple myeloma, monoclonal gammopathy of undetermined significance, and smoldering multiple myeloma. *Blood* 62: 166, 1983.

215. Bataille R, Sany J: Solitary myeloma: clinical and prognostic features of a review of 114 cases. *Cancer* 48:845, 1981.

216. Corwin J, Lindberg RD: Solitary plasmacytoma of bones versus extra-medullary plasmacytomas and their relationship to multiple myeloma. *Cancer* 43:1007, 1979.

217. Knowling MA, Harwood AR, Bergsagel DF: Comparison of extramedullary plasmacytomas with solitary and multiple plasma cell tumors of bone. *J Clin Oncol* 1:255, 1983.

218. Whittaker JA: Solitary plasmacytoma, in *Multiple Myeloma and Other Paraproteinaemias*, edited by IW Delamore, p 193. Churchill Livingstone, New York, 1986.

219. Kyle R, Schreiman J, McLeod R, et al: Computed tomography in diagnosis of multiple myeloma and its variants. *Arch Intern Med* 145:1451, 1985.

220. Libbey CA, Skinner M, Cohen AS: Use of abdominal fat tissue aspirate in the diagnosis of systemic amyloidosis. *Arch Intern Med* 143:1549, 1983.

221. Cooper JH: A histochemical construct of the amyloid fibril, in *Amyloidosis E.A.R.S.*, edited by CR Tribe, PA Bacon, pp 31–34. Wright, Bristol, 1983.

222. Ridolfi RL, Bulkley BH, Hutchins GM: The conduction system in cardiac amyloidosis. *Am J Med* 62:677, 1977.

223. Hind CRK, Gibson DG, Lavender JP, Pepys MB: Non-invasive demonstration of cardiac involvement in acquired forms of systemic amyloidosis. *Lancet* 1:1417, 1984.

224. Woodruff RK, Whittle JM, Malpas JS: Solitary plasmacytoma. I: Extramedullary soft tissue plasmacytoma. *Cancer* 43:2340, 1979.

225. Mill WB, Griffith R: The role of radiation therapy in the management of plasma cell tumors. *Cancer* 45:647, 1980.

226. Liebross RH, Ha CS, Cox JD, Weber D, Delasalle K, Alexanian R: Solitary bone plasmacytoma: outcome and prognostic factors following radiotherapy. *Int J Radiat Oncol Biol Phys* 41:1063, 1998.

227. Woodruff RK, Malpas JS, White FE: Solitary plasmacytoma. II: Solitary plasmacytoma of bone. *Cancer* 43:2344, 1979.

228. Fruehwald FXJ, Tscholakoff D, Schwaighoffer B, et al: Magnetic resonance imaging of the lower vertebral column in patients with multiple myeloma. *Radiology* 23:193, 1988.

229. Alexanian R: Localized and indolent myeloma. *Blood* 56:521, 1980.

230. Kyle RA, Greipp R: Smoldering multiple myeloma. *N Engl J Med* 302:1347, 1980.

231. Dimopoulos M, Moulopoulos A, Smith T, et al: Risk of disease progression in asymptomatic multiple myeloma. *Am J Med* 94:57, 1993.

232. Bergsagel DE, Sprague CC, Austin C, Griffith KM: Evaluation of new chemotherapeutic agents in the treatment of multiple myeloma IV: l-phenylalanine mustard. *Cancer Chemother Rep* 21:87, 1962.

233. Alexanian R, Haut A, Khan AU, et al: Treatment of multiple myeloma: combination chemotherapy with different melphalan dose regimens. *JAMA* 208:1680, 1969.

234. Boccadoro M, Marmont F, Tribalto M, et al: Multiple myeloma: VMCP/VBAP alternating combination chemotherapy is not superior to melphalan and prednisone even in high-risk patients. *J Clin Oncol* 9:444, 1991.

235. Gregory WM, Richards MA, Malpas JS: Combination chemotherapy versus melphalan and prednisolone in the treatment of multiple myeloma: an overview of published trials. *J Clin Oncol* 10:334, 1992.

236. Combination chemotherapy versus melphalan plus prednisone as treatment for multiple myeloma: an overview of 6,633 patients from 27 randomized trials. Myeloma Trialists' Collaborative Group. *J Clin Oncol* 16:3832, 1998.

237. Palmer M, Belch A, Hanson J, et al: Reassessment of the relationship between M-protein decrement and survival in multiple myeloma. *Br J Cancer* 59:110, 1989.

238. Durie BGM, Russel DH, Salmon SE: Reappraisal of plateau phase in myeloma. *Lancet* 1:65, 1980.

239. Alexanian R, Gehan E, Haut A, et al: Unmaintained remission in multiple myeloma. *Blood* 51:1005, 1978.

240. Belch A, Shelley W, Bergsagel D, et al: A randomized trial of maintenance versus no maintenance melphalan and prednisone in responding multiple myeloma patients. *Br J Cancer* 57:94, 1988.

241. Mandelli F, Avvisati G, Amadori S, et al: Maintenance treatment with recombinant interferon alfa-2b in patients with multiple myeloma responding to conventional induction chemotherapy. *N Engl J Med* 20:1430, 1990.

242. Ludwig H, Cohen AM, Polliack A, et al: Interferon-alpha for induction and maintenance in multiple myeloma: results of two multicenter randomized trials and summary of other studies. *Ann Oncol* 6:467, 1995.

243. Salmon SE, Crowley JJ, Balcerzak SP, et al: Interferon versus interferon plus prednisone remission maintenance therapy for multiple myeloma: a Southwest Oncology Group Study. *J Clin Oncol* 16:890, 1998.

244. Berenson J, Crowley J, Barlogie B, Salmon S: Alternate day oral prednisone maintenance therapy improves progression-free and overall survival in multiple myeloma patients *Blood* 92(suppl1):97a, 1998.

245. Bergsagel DE, Bailey AJ, Langley GR, et al: The chemotherapy of plasma cell myeloma and the incidence of acute leukemia. *N Engl J Med* 301:743, 1979.

246. Salmon SE, Shadduck RK, Schilling A: Intermittent high dose prednisone therapy for multiple myeloma. *Cancer Chemother Rep* 51:179, 1967.

247. Barlogie B, Smith L, Alexanian R: Effective treatment of advanced multiple myeloma refractory to alkylating agents. *N Engl J Med* 310:1353, 1984.

248. Alexanian R, Barlogie B, Dixon D: High dose glucocorticoid treatment for resistant multiple myeloma. *Ann Intern Med* 105:8, 1986.

249. Alexanian R, Barlogie B, Tucker S: VAD-based regimens as primary treatment for multiple myeloma. *Am J Hematol* 33:86, 1990.

250. Samson D, Gaminara E, Newland A, et al: Infusion of vincristine and doxorubicin with oral dexamethasone as first-line therapy for multiple myeloma. *Lancet* 2:882, 1989.

251. Salmon SE, Crowley JJ, Grogan TM, Finley P, Pugh RP, Barlogie B: Combination chemotherapy glucocorticoids, and interferon alfa in the treatment of multiple myeloma: a Southwest Oncology Group study. *J Clin Oncol* 12:2405, 1994.

252. Alexanian R, Dimopoulos MA, Delasalle K, Barlogie B: Primary dexamethasone treatment of multiple myeloma. *Blood* 80:887, 1992.

253. Hata H, Xiao H, Petrucci MT, Woodliff J, Chang R, Epstein J: Interleukin-6 gene expression in multiple myeloma: a characteristic of immature tumor cells. *Blood* 81:3357, 1993.

254. Kyle RA: Long-term survival in multiple myeloma. *N Engl J Med* 308:314, 1983.

255. Alexanian R: Ten year survival in multiple myeloma. *Arch Intern Med* 145:2073, 1985.

256. Attal M, Harousseau JL, Stoppa AM, et al: A prospective, randomized trial of autologous bone marrow transplantation and chemotherapy in multiple myeloma. Intergroupe Francais du Myelome. *N Engl J Med* 335:91, 1996.

257. Barlogie B, Jagannath S, Vesole D, et al: Superiority of tandem autologous transplantation over standard therapy for previously untreated multiple myeloma. *Blood*, 89:789, 1997.

258. Tricot G, Jagannath S, Vesole DH, et al: Peripheral blood stem cell transplants for multiple myeloma identification of favorable variables for rapid engraftment in 225 patients. *Blood* 85:588, 1995.

259. Siegel DS, Desikan KR, Mehta J, et al: Age is not a prognostic variable with autotransplants for multiple myeloma. *Blood* 93:51, 1999.

260. Mehta J, Tricot G, Jagannath S, et al: High-dose chemotherapy with carboplatin, cyclophosphamide and etoposide and autologous transplantation for multiple myeloma relapsing after a previous transplant. *Bone Marrow Transplant* 20:113, 1997.

261. Desikan KR, Fassas A, Siegel D, et al: Superior outcome with melphalan 200 mg/m^2 (MEL 200) for scheduled second autotransplant compared MEL+TBI or CTX for myeloma (MM) in pre-Tx-2 PR. *Blood* 90:231a, 1997.

262. Barlogie B, Jagannath S, Desikan KR, et al: Total therapy with tandem transplants for newly diagnosed multiple myeloma *Blood* 93:55, 1999.

263. Vescio R, Schiller G, Stewart AK, et al: Multicenter phase III trial to evaluate CD34(+) selected versus unselected autologous peripheral blood progenitor cell transplantation in multiple myeloma. *Blood* 93:1858, 1999.

264. Tricot G, Gazitt Y, Leemhuis T, et al: Collection, tumor contamination and engraftment kinetics of highly purified hematopoietic prognitor cells to support high dosetherapy in multiple myeloma. *Blood* 91:4489, 1998.

265. Munshi NC, Desikan KR, Jagannath S, et al: Dexamethasone, cyclophosphamide, etoposide and cis-platinum (DCEP) an effective regimen for relapse after high-dose chemotherapy and autologous transplantation (AT). *Blood* 88:586a, 1996.

266. Desikan R, Siegel D, Fassas A, et al: DCEP consolidation after tandem autotransplants (AT) in high risk multiple myeloma (MM)—improved prognosis compared to matched historical controls. *Blood* 92(suppl 1):97a, 1998.

267. Kwak LW, Taub DD, Duffey PL, et al: Transfer of myeloma idiotype-specific immunity from an actively immunised marrow donor. *Lancet* 345:1016, 1995.

268. Berenson JR, Lichtenstein A, Porter L, et al: Efficacy of pamidronate in reducing skeletal events in patients with advanced multiple myeloma. Myeloma Aredia Study Group. *N Engl J Med* 334:488, 1996.

269. Berenson JR, Lichtenstein A, Porter L, et al: Long-term pamidronate treatment of advanced multiple myeloma patients reduces skeletal events. Myeloma Aredia Study Group. *J Clin Oncol* 16:593, 1998.

270. Dhodapkar MV, Singh J, Mehta J, et al: Anti-myeloma activity of pamidronate in vivo. *Br J Haematol* 103:530, 1998.

271. Gahrton G, Svensson H, Bjorkstrand B, et al: Syngeneic bone marrow transplantation in multiple myeloma. *BMT* 19:S88, 1997.

272. Gahrton G, Tura S, Ljungman P: Allogeneic bone marrow transplantation in multiple myeloma. *N Engl J Med* 325:1267, 1991.

273. Bensinger WI, Gahrthon G: Allogeneic hematopoietic cell transplantation for multiple myeloma, in *Hematopoietic Cell Transplantation*, 2nd ed, edited by S Forman, K Blume, E Thomas.: Blackwell Science, Oxford, UK 1999.

274. Bjorkstrand BB, Ljungman P, Svensson H, et al: Allogeneic bone marrow transplantation versus autologous stem cell transplantation in multiple myeloma: a retrospective case-matched study from the European Group for Blood and Marrow Transplantation. *Blood* 88:4711, 1996.

275. Tricot G, Vesole DH, Jagannath S, Hilton J, Munshi NC, Barlogie B: Graft vs myeloma effect: proof of principle. *Blood* 87:1196, 1996.

276. Khouri IF, Keating M, Korbling M, et al: Transplant-lite: induction of graft-versus-malignancy using fludarabine-based nonablative chemotherapy and allogeneic blood progenitor-cell transplantation as treatment for lymphoid malignancies. *J Clin Oncol* 16:2817, 1998.

277. Barlogie B, Desikan R, Munshi N, et al: Single course D.T. PACE anti-angiochemotherapy effects CR in plasma cell leukemia and fulminant multiple myeloma (MM). 92(suppl 1):97a, 1998.

278. Cunningham D, Paz-Ares L, Gore ME, et al: High-dose melphalan for multiple myeloma: long-term follow-up data. *J Clin Oncol* 12:764, 1994.

279. Cunningham D, Paz-Ares L, Milan S, et al: High-dose melphalan and autologous bone marrow transplantation as consolidation in previously untreated myeloma. *J Clin Oncol* 12:759, 1994.

280. Anderson KC, Andersen J, Soiffer R, et al: Monoclonal antibody-purged bone marrow transplantation therapy for multiple myeloma. *Blood* 82:2568, 1993.

281. Bensinger WI, Rowley SD, Demirer T, et al: High-dose therapy followed by autologous hematopoietic stem cellfusion for patients with multiple myeloma. *J Clin Oncol* 14:1447, 1996.

282. Bjorkstrand B, Ljungman P, Bird JM, et al: Autologous stem cell transplantation in multiple myeloma: results of the European Group for Bone Marrow Transplantation. *Stem Cells* (Dayt) 13(suppl 2):140, 1995.

283. Fermand JP, Chevret S, Ravaud P, Divine M, Leblond V, Dreyfus F, Mariette X, Brouet JC High-dose chemoradiotherapy and autologous blood stem cell transplantation in multiple myeloma: results of a phase II trial involving 63 patients. *Blood* 82:2005, 1993.

284. Harousseau JL, Attal M, Divine M, Marit G, Leblond V, Stoppa AM, Bourhis JH, Caillot D, Boasson M, Abgrall JF, et al: Autologous stem cell transplantation after first remission induction treatment in multiple myeloma: a report of the French Registry on autologous transplantation in multiple myeloma. *Blood* 85:3077, 1995.

285. Ludwig H, Fritz E, Kotzmann H, et al: Erythropoietin treatment of anemia associated with multiple myeloma. *N Engl J Med* 322:1693, 1990.

286. Barlogie B, Beck T: Recombinant human erythropoietin and the anemia of multiple myeloma. *Stem Cell* 11:88, 1993.

287. Barlogie B, Alexanian R, Cabanillas F: Etoposide, dexamethasone, cytarabine, and cisplatin in vincristine, doxorubicin, and dexamethasone-refractory myeloma. *J Clin Oncol* 7:1514, 1989.

288. Dimopoulos MA, Delasalle KB, Champlin R, Alexanian R: Cyclophosphamide and etoposide therapy with GM-CSF for VAD-resistant multiple myeloma. *Br J Haematol* 83:240, 1993.

289. Dhodapkar MV, Weinstein R, Tricot G, et al: Biologic and therapeutic determinants of bone mineral density in multiple myeloma. *Leuk Lymphoma* 32:121, 1998.

290. Govindarajan R, Jagannath S, Flick J, et al: Preceeding standard therapy is the likely cause of MDS after autotransplants for multiple myeloma. *Br J Haematol* 95:349, 1996.

291. Counter CM, Gupta J, Harley CB, Leber B, Bacchetti S: Telomerase activity in normal leukocytes and in hematologic malignancies. *Blood* 85:2315, 1995.

292. Engelhardt M, Kumar R, Albanell J, Pettengell R, Han W, Moore MA: Telomerase regulation, cell cycle, and telomere stability in primitive hematopoietic cells. *Blood* 90:182, 1997.

THE AMYLOIDOSES

JOEL N. BUXBAUM

DANIEL R. JACOBSON

The amyloidoses are disorders of secondary structure, in which a protein, synthesized and secreted from the cell as a soluble molecule, forms insoluble, fibrillar tissue deposits, leading to organ dysfunction. The site and rate of deposition determine the clinical presentation. All amyloid deposits contain a single major fibrillar component and minor nonfibrillar components. To date, 19 fibril proteins have been isolated from different forms of human amyloidosis; one of these is immunoglobulin light chain. Light-chain amyloidosis (AL) is a monoclonal plasma cell disease in which the secreted immunoglobulin, because of its amino acid sequence, is predisposed to fibrillogenesis under physiologic conditions. AL is characterized by fatigue, weight loss, purpura, heart failure, proteinuria, renal failure, gastrointestinal dysfunction, neuropathy, and various other symptoms, depending upon the organ involved. Diagnosis is made by biopsy of an affected organ or subcutaneous fat aspiration followed by Congo red staining and immunohistochemistry of the specimen, to determine the type of amyloid. In the face of similar clinical features, immunohistochemistry distinguishes AL tissue deposition from that of other systemic amyloidoses in which AL-specific treatment would be inappropriate. Chemotherapy with melphalan and prednisone reduces the size of the plasma cell clone producing the amyloidogenic light chain and prolongs survival.

DEFINITION AND HISTORY

The amyloidoses are characterized by the extracellular accumulation of insoluble protein fibrils. Deposits were first identified in autopsy specimens by their homogeneous, eosinophilic appearance in conventional histologic sections stained with hematoxylin and eosin. Subsequently they were shown to bind metachromatic dyes and to possess the property of *Congophilia*, i.e., binding the dye Congo red, with a characteristic apple-green-appearing birefringence when the stained tissues were examined under polarized light. Electron microscopy and x-ray diffraction revealed a fibrillar ultrastructure, with extensive β-pleated sheet secondary structure. All the amyloidoses, regardless of the clinical setting or chemical composition, possess these staining and ultrastructural properties.

Historically, the amyloidoses were classified according to the clinical or pathologic features of the associated diseases. Secondary

amyloidosis accompanied chronic inflammatory processes. Familial amyloidosis was recognized by distinctive clinical manifestations within a kindred. All other types, except that occurring with myeloma, were termed *primary*, in the sense of idiopathic, although some investigators had drawn attention to similarities between primary amyloidosis and the myeloma-related form. The development of methods for dissolving and fractionating amyloid fibrils extracted from tissues permitted the identification of nineteen different proteins as amyloid precursors to date (Table 107-1). Classification is now based on the chemical nature of the fibrillar component of the deposits. Terms such as *primary* and *secondary* amyloidosis, and descriptive clinical diagnoses, such as *senile, dialysis-associated,* and *myeloma-associated,* have been abandoned in favor of the etiologically based, chemical terminology.[1]

All amyloid deposits contain a major (85 to 95 percent) fibrillar component, which is soluble in water and buffers of low ionic strength, and nonfibrillar components that are extractable with conventional ionic strength buffers. The nonfibrillar components include P (pentagonal) component, apolipoprotein E, and heparan sulfate proteoglycans, which are found in all types of amyloid. Complement components, proteases, and membrane constituents have been demonstrated in some, but not all, tissue deposits. P component comprises 5 to 10 percent of the total deposited protein. It is derived from circulating serum amyloid P (SAP) component, which behaves as a typical acute phase reactant in the mouse, but not in humans. P component has structural homology to C-reactive protein and belongs to the pentraxin group of proteins.[2]

ETIOLOGY AND PATHOGENESIS

MECHANISMS OF AMYLOID FORMATION

The amyloid precursor proteins are relatively small, with molecular weights between 4000 and 25,000. They do not share any detectable amino acid sequence homology, although the secondary structures of most have substantial β-pleated sheet structure. The known exceptions are serum amyloid A-related protein (SAA) and Prp^c, which contain little or no β-folding in the precursor despite extensive β-sheet in the deposited fibrils. The clinical amyloidoses are in vivo disorders of secondary protein structure in which the precursor proteins are secreted from the cell in a soluble form, only to become insoluble at some tissue site, ultimately compromising organ function. They represent an extracellular subset of a spectrum of disorders of secondary protein structure. The protein aggregates in the intracellular forms, Parkinson's disease (cytoplasmic) and Huntington's disease (intranuclear), lack the amyloid-defining properties.[3,4]

In some cases, the aberrant secondary structure seen in amyloid formation reflects a hereditary alteration in sequence that predisposes to fibril formation, e.g., transthyretin (TTR), lysozyme, fibrinogen, cystatin c, gelsolin, AβPP, ApoA1. In other cases wild-type molecules are the fibril precursor (TTR, AβPP, β_2M, ApoA1). The deposits are primarily extracellular, but there have been reports of fibrillar structures within lysosomes of macrophages and the cisternae of plasma cells in AL marrow.[5] In the localized forms of amyloidosis, the deposits are found close to the site of synthesis of the precursor, while in the systemic amyloidoses the deposits may form either locally or at a distance from the precursor-producing cells. AL is usually a systemic disorder, but localized AL may occur in the setting of an apparently confined plasma cell proliferation.

The role of P component and that of the other accessory molecules in amyloid deposition is not clear. While they do not appear to be an absolute requirement for fibril formation, they may stabilize the fibril, protecting it from proteolysis once it is formed, or enhance the transition from prefibril to fibril. In experimental systems, the rate of amyloid deposition is slower in the absence of P component.[6] Intravenously

TABLE 107-1   THE MODERN (CHEMICAL) CLASSIFICATION OF HUMAN AMYLOIDOSIS

AMYLOID PROTEIN	PRECURSOR PROTEIN	CLINICAL SYNDROME(S)	REFERENCES
AL	Immunoglobulin light chains or light-chain fragments	Plasma-cell disorders	This chapter
AH	Immunoglobulin heavy chain	Systemic amyloidosis	25
ATTR	Transthyretin (TTR)	Familial amyloidotic polyneuropathy, familial amyloid cardiomyopathy, senile systemic amyloidosis, isolated vitreous amyloidosis	103, 104
AA	Apo-SAA	Familial Mediterranean fever, inflammation-associated, Muckle Wells syndrome	119, 124, 130
$A\beta_2M$	β_2 microglobulin	Dialysis-associated amyloid	131
AApoAI	Apolipoprotein AI	Familial amyloidosis involving various organs	138, 139
AFib	Fibrinogen α chain	Familial renal amyloidosis	141
ALys	Lysozyme	Familial systemic amyloidosis	142
ACys	Cystatin C	Hereditary cerebral hemorrhage with amyloidosis-Icelandic type	143
$A\beta$	β-protein precursor	Alzheimer disease, Down syndrome, hereditary cerebral hemorrhage with amyloidosis, Dutch type	144, 145
APrP	Prion protein	Creutzfeldt-Jakob & Gerstmann-Sträussler-Scheinker diseases	146
AGel	Gelsolin	Hereditary corneal amyloidosis	148
AKE	Kerato-epithelin	Hereditary corneal amyloidosis	149
ALac	Lactoferrin	Hereditary corneal amyloidosis	150
ACal	Calcitonin	Medullary carcinoma of the thyroid (in multiple endocrine neoplasia)	152
AIAPP	Amylin (Islet amyloid polypeptide)	Insulinoma, type II diabetes mellitus	153
AANF	Atrial natriuretic factor	Isolated atrial amyloidosis	151
APro	Prolactin	Pituitary amyloid	154
AKer	Keratin	Cutaneous amyloidosis	155, 156

injected purified P component will preferentially bind to amyloid deposits; this property has been exploited clinically, using radiolabeled P component, to localize and quantify the total body burden of amyloid.[7]

Apolipoprotein E has been found in all types of amyloid deposits.[8] One Apo E allele (Apo E4) is strongly associated with Alzheimer's disease. Apo E4 also may be a genetic risk factor for other forms of amyloidosis; however, its association with other amyloidoses is less well supported by the epidemiological evidence.[9–13] The mechanism of Apo E involvement is not known.

Heparan sulfate proteoglycans are basement membrane components that are intimately associated with all types of tissue amyloid deposits.[14] As with P component and Apo E, their role in amyloidogenesis remains undefined. Compounds known to bind to heparan sulfate proteoglycans, such as anionic sulphonates, have been shown to decrease fibril deposition in murine models of acquired amyloid (AA) disease and have been suggested as potential therapeutic agents.[15]

In some instances (e.g., uniformly in AA, frequently in AL, and inconsistently, perhaps in a tissue-related manner, in TTR) the amyloid precursors undergo proteolysis which may enhance the kinetics of folding into a profibrillar structural intermediate. It is also possible that in some of the amyloidoses (e.g., Aβ or AA), a normal proteolytic process is disturbed, yielding a higher than normal concentration of a profibrillar molecule. Whether tissue deposition is purely physicochemical, or depends upon an interaction equivalent to that between ligand and receptor in which some component of tissue ground substance is the binding target, is unknown. In cases in which proteolysis is seen, it is unclear when cleavage takes place relative to deposition. In AL, Aβ, and A-TTR, there is both clinicopathological and experimental evidence for deposition of nonfibrillar, non–Congo-red–binding forms of the same molecules as found in the fibrils.[16–18] Nonfibrillar deposits probably represent a processing or deposition intermediate but may represent an alternative form of deposition.

STRUCTURE OF IMMUNOGLOBULIN-RELATED AMYLOID FIBRILS

When examined by immunofluorescent and immunohistologic techniques or immunogold electron microscopy, tissue AL amyloid deposits show binding of antibodies to a single Ig polypeptide chain class. In nearly all cases, the deposits consist of monoclonal L-chains and/or their derived peptides.[19] Rarely, the deposits contained only H-chain determinants and were classified as AH rather than AL.[20]

Extraction of L-chain–related amyloid deposits using either distilled water or low ionic strength buffers has yielded fibril subunits comprised of L-chain fragments, whole chains, or both. The fragments include the amino terminus of the chain and extend into the constant region. They are usually about 16,000 Da in molecular mass but may be as small as 5000 Da.[19] In 90 percent of patients the deposited peptides include constant region sequence, accounting for the property of staining with commercially available anti–L-chain sera which are specific for constant region determinants. These observations are consistent with the failure, even in experienced laboratories, of 10 percent of deposits to bind either anti-κ or anti-λ antisera. In most cases, the deposits contain complete L-chains and L-chain fragments. In a minority of cases only complete chains are deposited. Molecules larger than conventionally sized L-chains, representing enzymatically glycosylated L-chains, have also been found.

The prominence of fragments in the deposits has suggested a proteolytic origin of the fibril precursor from an intact amyloidogenic L-chain; however, direct in vivo evidence for this hypothesis is lacking. Occasional ultrastructural demonstration of L-chain fibrils within the cisternae of malignant plasma cells or within macrophages have been used to support the role of lysosomal digestion of the precursor to yield fibril.[5] It has been argued, however, that such findings could also be explained by phagocytic ingestion of preformed fibrils. A single cell culture experiment suggested plasma cell-macrophage interaction in the production of AL fibrils.[21] In vitro experiments have shown that lysosomal enzymes can digest L-chains to molecules that form fibrils in the test tube.[22] In other studies, the propensity of a light chain to form amyloid fibrils in vitro following protease digestion did not correlate with in vivo amyloid formation.[23] Marrow cells, obtained from all patients with well-documented tissue AL deposition, synthesize excess L-chains, regardless of whether free L-chains are detected in the patients' serum or urine. In some instances the cells contained L-chain fragments, but the synthetic or degradative origin of the fragments was not definitively established.[24]

In addition to the chemical analysis of deposited AL fibrils, considerable information has been obtained from the study of light chains isolated from the serum and/or urine of patients with AL. In some instances, the fibrils were also available, but in others the L-chains were assumed, but not proved, to be identical with the deposited proteins based on the immunohistochemistry. The most common AL precursor proteins are L-chains of the λ class: λ AL is about twice as prevalent as κ AL.[19] In contrast, in nonamyloid monoclonal immunoglobulin deposition disease (MIDD), κ chains are the predominant precursor. In the instances in which H-chains were the major amyloid component, chemical analysis revealed that the precursor H-chain displayed domain deletions resulting in polypeptides the size of L-chains.[20] In studies of nonamyloid MIDD containing both H- and L-chain deposition, the heavy chains are also smaller than normal.[25]

Within L-chain classes, not all variable regions have the same fibrillogenic potential. L-chains of the $V_{\lambda vi}$ class appear to be the most amyloidogenic: Clonal plasma cell proliferative diseases in which the $V_{\lambda vi}$ gene is expressed are always associated with amyloid deposition.[26,27] Recent data, using molecular probes specific for germline V-region genes, have suggested that monoclonal Igs of the $V_{\lambda vi}$ class are more likely to be associated with renal disease than with other organ involvement and are less likely to be associated with myeloma. To date no such pattern has been demonstrated for other germline V-genes expressed in amyloid proteins. Among κ V-genes, the $V_{\kappa I}$ subgroup is overrepresented among amyloid forming L-chains, while some other subclasses appear underrepresented in amyloidosis in comparison to plasma cell disorders without amyloidosis.[28]

Within the V-region families certain amino acid residues occurring at particular positions in the L-chain sequence seem to render those chains more amyloidogenic. When a combination of such residues is present the chances of a L-chain being associated with tissue amyloid deposition is increased.[29] Other substitutions seem more likely to be associated with the nonfibrillar deposits of MIDD.[30] Another structural feature that appears to predispose to AL deposition is enzymatic glycosylation of the L-chain. While approximately 15 percent of human L-chains bear sugar residues, almost one-third of amyloidogenic L-chains are glycosylated.[31] The nature of the contribution of glycosylation to the process is unknown.

CLINICAL FEATURES

GENERAL FEATURES

AL is the most common form of systemic amyloidosis in the United States. In Olmstead County, Minnesota, AL prevalence is about 1 case per 100,000 people.[32] It is not clear if the estimate, obtained in a relatively homogeneous northern European–derived population, would apply in an ethnically diverse setting.

The clinical picture of patients with AL varies widely. The median age at diagnosis in one large series of AL patients was 64 years. The most common presenting symptoms are weakness and weight loss, followed by purpura, particularly in loose facial tissue. Prognosis depends upon the pattern of tissue deposition. The kidneys are the most frequent sites of AL deposits; the heart, peripheral nerves, gastrointestinal tract, and liver are also affected. Any organ can be involved, with symptoms and physical findings reflecting the extent of anatomic compromise. Patients with clinical cardiac involvement have the worst prognosis, while patients with signs and symptoms limited to peripheral nerves have the longest survival.[33] Other favorable prognostic features include a small number of clonal plasma cells in the marrow and normal renal function.[34,35]

Initial physical findings include peripheral edema, hepatomegaly, purpura, orthostatic hypotension, peripheral neuropathy, carpal tunnel syndrome, and macroglossia.[32,36,37] Peripheral edema and hypotension may be related to congestive heart failure and/or the nephrotic syndrome. Purpura results from vascular fragility produced by amyloid deposition in the subendothelium of the small blood vessels. It may be very prominent in patients with coagulopathy.[38,39] In recent series, macroglossia has been less common at the time of initial presentation than in older studies, perhaps because of earlier diagnosis. When it does occur, it is highly suggestive that the amyloid is of the AL type, as it has only been seen in AL and occasionally in β_2M amyloid.[40]

It is not known what leads to the pattern of tissue deposition in a given patient. Amyloid in a particular organ leads to similar clinical consequences regardless of the chemical type. For example, cardiac AL and cardiac TTR amyloidosis produce similar symptoms and findings on electrocardiography and echocardiography, although AL cardiomyopathy typically runs a more rapid clinical course.[41,42] In recent analyses, the median survival following diagnosis of AL was slightly longer than 1 year, with fewer than 10 percent surviving 5 years.[32] Patients with cardiac presentation had a median survival of about 6 months.[33] Renal and cardiac involvement were the most common causes of death before aggressive dialysis was used in patients with renal amyloid; more recently, cardiac deaths predominate.

RENAL INVOLVEMENT

The most common renal manifestation of AL disease is proteinuria; 30 percent to 50 percent of AL patients excrete at least a gram of predominantly non–L-chain protein per day in the urine.[43–45] AL can also cause hematuria. Azotemia is a late manifestation of renal AL, but dialysis can stabilize the course of patients with extensive kidney involvement and is an option in patients developing renal failure.[46] Renal biopsy reveals deposits in the glomerular mesangium and, later, along the basement membrane. Nonamyloid immunoglobulin deposits will also be detected by immunohistochemical staining.[47]

CARDIOVASCULAR INVOLVEMENT

AL deposits in the heart occur in the ventricular interstitium and along the conduction system.[48,49] The amyloid causes diastolic dysfunction, congestive heart failure, and arrhythmias, including heart block, premature ventricular contractions, and various tachyarrhythmias.[50] Deposits in the coronary arteries, usually the smaller intracardiac arterioles, may cause a clinical picture similar to atherosclerotic coronary artery disease.[51] The interstitial deposition leads to thickening of the ventricular walls without the increase in chamber volume that occurs in heart failure arising from long-standing hypertension. Late in the course, the stiff myocardium can yield cardiac catheterization data similar to constrictive pericarditis. Cardiac involvement eventually occurs in over 75 percent of patients with AL.[32,52] Death is due to cardiac deposition with congestive heart failure or arrhythmias in about half of AL patients. The actual number may be higher because some patients have undiagnosed terminal arrhythmias.

No noninvasive test is sufficiently sensitive or specific for diagnosing cardiac amyloidosis. Electrocardiography often shows a low voltage QRS complex in the limb leads.[53] In some cases, loss of anterior forces suggests anteroseptal infarction that is not confirmed at autopsy.[54] The most useful diagnostic test for cardiac amyloidosis, apart from endomyocardial biopsy, is echocardiography, which reveals increased ventricular wall thickness, increased septal thickness, and the appearance of granular "sparkling." The latter finding is neither sensitive nor specific enough to be diagnostic but is suggestive when present. Evaluation of diastolic function by Doppler echocardiography shows impaired ventricular relaxation early with shortened deceleration times later, ultimately showing a pattern much like that of constrictive pericarditis. The ejection fraction is preserved until late in disease. Other echocardiographic findings include valvular thickening and insufficiency, atrial enlargement, and rare atrial thrombosis.[55–57] Scanning with radiolabeled P component (available only in Europe as of 1999) is a sensitive noninvasive means of detecting and monitoring the amount of amyloid in many organs.[6] It is not useful for diagnosing cardiac amyloid because the myocardial signal does not stand out from the background created by the label in the intracardiac blood. The combined use of electrocardiography plus echocardiography appears to have the most diagnostic value.[53,58]

AL (and other systemic amyloidoses) can lead to severe orthostatic hypotension with restriction of normal activity and syncope.[32] Poor cardiac contractility resulting from myocardial deposition, autonomic neuropathy secondary to amyloid deposits in the peripheral nerves, and impaired arteriolar responsiveness resulting from endothelial deposition all may contribute. Diuretic treatment of heart failure or the nephrotic syndrome with reduction of intravascular volume also predisposes to symptomatic hypotension.

NEUROLOGIC INVOLVEMENT

Sensorimotor neuropathy, consequent to deposition in peripheral nerves with axonal degeneration of the small nerve fibers, occurs in about 20 percent of AL cases. The symmetric sensory impairment and weakness, sometimes accompanied by painless ulcers, is similar to that of diabetic neuropathy.[32] The lower extremities are usually affected more severely than the upper. Diagnosis can be made by sural nerve biopsy, although the actual deposits may be proximal to the sural nerve and not in the biopsy specimen.[60] Cranial neuropathy is occasionally seen.[61] Autonomic neuropathy, leading to orthostatic hypotension, diarrhea, or impotence, may be incapacitating.[62] The combination of severe peripheral and autonomic neuropathy is also a common presentation of familial transthyretin-amyloidosis, but the patient's age, absence of other organ involvement, and family history should be discriminated.

CARPAL TUNNEL SYNDROME

Carpal tunnel syndrome was the initial presenting finding in one-fifth of AL patients evaluated in a large referral center.[32] Involvement of the carpal ligament is also seen in β_2M amyloid in patients undergoing dialysis, and in TTR amyloidosis, with or without a TTR variant.[63] Treatment is surgical. At the time of carpal tunnel release, the tissue specimen can be stained with Congo red and immunohistochemistry performed if a definitive diagnosis has not been previously established. Amyloidosis is responsible for only a small fraction of symptomatic individuals undergoing surgery for relief of median nerve compression.

GASTROINTESTINAL INVOLVEMENT

All forms of systemic amyloidosis involve the gastrointestinal tract. Most patients with AL have histologic evidence of infiltration of the gut, particularly in the blood vessels, but the deposition is symptomatic in only a minority.[32,64] Macroglossia can become severe enough to interfere with swallowing and breathing. Gastric AL can cause hematemesis, nausea, and vomiting.[65] Intestinal AL can impair motility and cause hemorrhage, obstruction, constipation, and diarrhea, or alternating constipation and diarrhea.[66–70] Malabsorption from AL is rare. AL autonomic neuropathy also contributes to impaired gastrointestinal motility.

Hepatic AL, causing hepatomegaly, is common, although liver function abnormalities are rare even in cases with massive deposition.[39,71] Splenomegaly may also develop and is usually asymptomatic, but functional asplenism may produce Howell-Jolly bodies in the peripheral blood. Spontaneous rupture of a massively infiltrated liver or spleen is a surgical emergency.[72]

RESPIRATORY TRACT INVOLVEMENT

Systemic AL commonly deposits in the respiratory tract, in a nodular or diffuse pattern. Any part of the respiratory tree, from nasopharynx to pulmonary alveoli, may be involved. Involvement is often asymptomatic, although alveolar or diffuse interstitial involvement can cause dyspnea. Chest radiography reveals a reticular nodular pattern or interstitial infiltration.[73–75]

MUSCULOSKELETAL SYSTEM

AL deposits in the joints may resemble seronegative rheumatoid arthritis.[76] Deposits in the glenohumeral articulation may cause localized pain and swelling, the "shoulder pad sign,"[77] while deposits in skeletal muscle may produce pseudohypertrophy.[78,79] Congophilic fibrils may be seen in the synovial fluid.

LOCALIZED AL

Localized amyloid deposits, including amyloid masses termed *amyloidomas*, may be found in various sites even in the absence of systemic disease. In some cases, plasma cells have been demonstrated histologically surrounding the deposits; in one case DNA sequencing revealed that the local plasma cells were producing the deposited L-chains.[80] For unknown reasons, the respiratory tract is the most common site of localized AL. It often remains confined, without progression to systemic disease.[81,82] Similar AL deposits involving the lower urinary tract, the mediastinum, retroperitoneum and skin, as either plaques or nodules, have been described.[83,84]

BLEEDING

Bleeding may be a severe manifestation of AL, or indeed of any of the systemic amyloidoses. Subendothelial deposition results in capillary fragility and mucocutaneous hemorrhage.[85] A deficiency in coagulation factor X, secondary to its binding to AL amyloid fibrils, can produce life-threatening bleeding.[38] Less often, extensive liver involvement can lead to decreased levels of other vitamin K–depending clotting factors.[39]

CLINICAL FINDINGS IN MIDD

Patients with MIDD, without myeloma, usually present with proteinuria or the full nephrotic syndrome with nodular glomerulosclerosis and slowly developing renal failure. When MIDD accompanies myeloma the histology is characterized by tubular deposits and Bence-Jones cast nephropathy with rapidly developing renal failure.[47] As in AL, cardiac involvement can occur in either group. Despite the differences in the intramyocardial distribution of amyloid and MIDD deposits, the physiologic consequences of alterations in relaxation and compliance, distortions in the voltage/mass relationship, diastolic dysfunction, arrhythmias, and congestive heart failure are similar.[86]

LABORATORY FEATURES

Amyloidosis is diagnosed by demonstration of Congo red–binding material with the characteristic apple-green fluorescence under polarized light in a biopsy specimen. Sampling of relatively accessible tissues under direct vision provides a reliable means for determining the presence of amyloid deposition. For many years, rectal biopsy was

TABLE 107-2   BIOPSY DIAGNOSIS OF AMYLOIDOSIS

Site	Sensitivity	Advantages	Disadvantages
Subcutaneous fat	80–90%	No mortality, little morbidity[88]	Insensitive in β_2M and AA amyloid associated with FMF
Rectal mucosa	75–85%	Routine processing	Occasional complication (bleeding); must include vessels
Marrow	30–40% in AL	Can be assessed at same time as presence of myeloma[89]	Not reliable in other than AL amyloid
Gingiva	15–20%	Easily accessible	Insensitive
Stomach	75–85%	High sensitivity in single center[91]	Requires endoscopy; sensitivity needs confirmation in other centers
Salivary gland	75%	High sensitivity in single center[90]	Needs confirmation in other centers and in broader spectrum of amyloidoses
Involved organ (liver, kidney, lung, heart)	90–100%	High sensitivity, high specificity: allows definitive attribution of clinical features to amyloid deposition	Occasional serious complication

the procedure of choice. Currently subcutaneous fat aspiration is the first approach to obtaining material for Congo red and immunohistochemical staining.[87,88] The combination of fat aspiration and rectal biopsy will identify 80 to 90 percent of patients later found to have amyloid elsewhere. Other sampling sites include salivary glands, stomach, and marrow (Table 107-2). Biopsy of an organ with impaired function, such as kidney or heart, is a high-yield procedure that definitively establishes the relationship between organ dysfunction and amyloid deposition.

Because different types of amyloidosis require different approaches to treatment, it is no longer adequate to determine only that a patient has amyloidosis. Although the clinical situation may suggest the type of amyloidosis, the diagnosis must be established by immunohistochemistry of a biopsy specimen using antibodies against the major amyloid fibril precursors. AL, TTR, and β_2M amyloidoses can all present as carpal tunnel syndrome or gastrointestinal amyloidosis, but each has a different etiology, requiring different approaches to treatment. Distinguishing between AL and TTR cardiac amyloidosis on clinical grounds alone is particularly difficult, as the age of the patient, the patterns of organ involvement, and the clinical consequences of deposition are often similar. For instance, in individuals over age 70, a group in which serum M-proteins are common, the most prevalent form of cardiac amyloidosis is TTR-derived.[41,92] When cardiac amyloidosis is suspected because of the results of noninvasive cardiac testing, the definitive distinction between AL and A-TTR can be made by endomyocardial biopsy, with Congo red and immunohistochemical staining of the tissue sample. In a patient with congestive heart failure and noninvasive testing suggestive of amyloidosis, subcutaneous fat aspiration can provide material for definitive diagnosis, avoiding the more invasive endomyocardial biopsy. Without immunohistologic identification of the deposited protein, an incorrect presumptive diagnosis of AL could lead to ineffective and perhaps harmful treatment.

MONOCLONAL IMMUNOGLOBULINS

The cardinal laboratory finding in AL and MIDD, a monoclonal immunoglobulin light chain, is detected on clinical laboratory testing in the serum or concentrated urine of 80 to 90 percent of patients.[19,32,36] It is likely that a monoclonal protein would be detected in all patients with systemic deposition disease if a sufficiently sensitive assay were available.[93] The concentration of normal immunoglobulins is often decreased, as in myeloma.[36,94] The combination of hypogammaglobulinemia and proteinuria should suggest a diagnosis of AL or MIDD. In contrast, systemic AA is usually associated with polyclonal hyperglobulinemia related to the persistent inflammation and increase in cytokine (Il-6) production.

About 40 percent of patients have more than 10 percent plasma cells in the marrow.[32,89] Light-chain immunophenotyping of the marrow, even in the absence of increased numbers of plasma cells, will usually reveal the distortion in the κ/λ ratio reflecting the L-chain type of the amyloid precursor.

COAGULATION SYSTEM ABNORMALITIES

Many clotting system abnormalities have been described in AL. Factor X may bind to amyloid fibrils, leading to its rapid clearance from the blood, with consequent prolongation of the prothrombin and partial thromboplastin times.[38] Elevation in tissue and urine plasminogen activators and decrease in tissue plasminogen activator inhibitor, leading to hyperfibrinolytic states, have also been reported.[97]

DIFFERENTIAL DIAGNOSIS

The differential diagnosis of AL includes MIDD, or, if a diagnosis of amyloidosis has already been made, nonimmunoglobulin forms of systemic amyloidosis. Diagnostic confusion in the evaluation of biopsies can be created by the binding of Congo red to collagen. The nonspecific nature of the binding can usually be clarified by immunohistochemical analysis and electron microscopy.

TRANSTHYRETIN (TTR) AMYLOIDOSIS

Transthyretin (formerly known as *thyroxine binding prealbumin*) is a normal serum protein that transports thyroxine and retinol binding protein. It is synthesized in the liver, choroid plexus, and retina being regulated independently in the liver and choroid.[98] Hepatic, but not choroid plexus, synthesis is decreased during inflammation and malnutrition. The protein consists of 4 identical subunits of 127 amino acids, and contains considerable β-pleated sheet structure.

TTR amyloidosis resembles AL in affecting the peripheral and autonomic nervous systems, heart, and gastrointestinal tract. It differs in that renal disease is rarely a dominant manifestation. TTR amyloid occurs in two molecular contexts. Normal-sequence TTR commonly forms amyloid deposits in the cardiac ventricles, gastrointestinal tract, carpal ligament, and other organs of elderly people.[41,54,63,99–101] It may be confused with AL, since monoclonal serum or urine proteins may occur coincidentally in such patients. The variant forms of TTR, containing point mutations, form systemic deposits, usually involving the heart and/or peripheral nerves, but usually at an earlier age.[102]

In clinical practice normal TTR was utilized as an indicator of malnutrition.[103] It was first noted to be involved in disease pathogenesis when a mutant molecule (TTR Met$_{30}$) was found to be the fibril precursor of the amyloid found in the systemic and peripheral nerve deposits in Portuguese patients with familial amyloidotic polyneuropathy (FAP). FAP is characterized by predominant peripheral and autonomic neuropathy, as well as involvement of the heart, gastrointestinal tract, and vitreous.[104] The pattern of organ involvement varies among kindreds. The age of onset varies from the teens to beyond age 60. In the advanced stage of disease, proteinuria, renal failure, lower cranial nerve involvement, decreased salivation, macroglossia, goiter, and neuropathic knee or ankle damage may occur. It is in the latter stages when, in the absence of a positive family history, the disorder is most apt to be confused with AL, but the long clinical course distinguishes TTR amyloid from AL.

Other familial amyloid syndromes with different clinical patterns of involvement (predominant upper or lower extremity neuropathy, varying involvement of the heart, kidneys, GI tract, and eye) have been reported. Often the clinical phenotype is specific for a particular TTR mutation, but even with the same mutation phenotypic variation is seen.[105,108] When TTR primarily affects the heart, without significant neuropathy, and a TTR mutation is present, the disease is termed *familial amyloidotic cardiomyopathy* (FAC). As of June 1999, 71 different amyloid-associated amino acid substitutions had been discovered at 55 of the 127 positions in the TTR molecule.[106] TTR Met_{30} FAP has been treated with liver transplantation to replace the gene encoding the variant TTR with a wild type gene. This form of gene therapy has resulted in some clinical improvement, particularly in autonomic neuropathy. It is not clear if it is effective in patients with other mutations, especially those with predominant cardiac involvement.[104,107]

Isolated ventricular amyloid in elderly people, generally without a family history of amyloidosis, was originally called *senile cardiac amyloid* (SCA). While the deposition was originally thought to be incidental, it now appears that in half the cases the deposits are the cause of death.[101,108] Detailed autopsy studies indicated that many patients with SCA also had deposits in the lungs and blood vessels, and the alternative name *senile systemic amyloidosis* (SSA) was proposed. Ventricular TTR deposition has been found at autopsy in 10 to 25 percent of people over age 80. Functional abnormalities, including atrial fibrillation and congestive heart failure, occur in the absence of any anatomically definable cardiac disease other than the amyloid deposits. In several patients the TTR deposits in SCA/SSA have been shown to be of wild-type sequence.[109]

Occasional patients present in the sixth to eighth decades with severe cardiac TTR-amyloidosis and no known family history. Despite the negative family history, some have been found to have a TTR mutation; thus, they have FAC, not SCA/SSA.[110-112] The most common mutation in this age group is a substitution of Ile for Val at position 122, which is carried by 3 to 4 percent of African Americans.[113] Thus, there are 1.3 million gene carriers in the United States, with approximately 150,000 over the age of 60 at risk for cardiac deposition.[110] None of the patients with TTR Ile_{122} cardiomyopathy has been noted to be associated with neuropathy. Patients presenting in this manner might be incorrectly assumed to have AL with predominant cardiac manifestations.

AA AMYLOID

Worldwide, AA amyloid is the most common of the systemic amyloidoses.[114] The AA protein comprises the fibril in the amyloid deposition accompanying chronic inflammatory diseases of either infectious (e.g., leprosy, osteomyelitis, tuberculosis) or noninfectious (e.g., rheumatoid arthritis, familial mediterranean fever, or FMF,) etiologies. In emerging nations, AA is more likely to occur subsequent to untreated or long-standing infections. In contrast, most patients in the United States and Western Europe with AA have an underlying rheumatic

disorder such as long-standing rheumatoid arthritis. Even in association with noninfectious inflammatory disease, the incidence of AA varies considerably among countries with apparently similar levels of economic development, suggesting that factors other than the degree of industrialization play a significant role.

About 70 percent of patients with AA have renal disease (tubular disorders, nephrotic syndrome, and/or renal insufficiency) at the time of diagnosis.[37,115] Renal vein thrombosis may occur, although it is not clear if it is more frequent in amyloidosis than it is in nephrotic syndrome from other causes.[116] Gastrointestinal involvement, hepatomegaly, and splenomegaly are common. Adrenal deposits can be seen, but clinical adrenal insufficiency is rare. Peripheral neuropathy and clinically significant cardiac involvement are rare. For unclear reasons, subcutaneous fat aspiration is not usually useful in patients with AA associated with FMF.[117]

The precursor molecule apo-SAA circulates in the serum bound to high-density lipoprotein and behaves as an acute phase reactant. The concentration of SAA in normal serum is barely detectable, but with inflammation it may increase by 2 to 3 orders of magnitude. SAA is involved in the intracellular metabolism of cholesterol by inflammatory cells; the production of apo-SAA, but not its tissue deposition, is part of the normal inflammatory response.[118] Three SAA genes, two of which have multiple alleles, encode the expressed isoforms of the protein; there is also an SAA pseudogene.[119] SAA1 is the predominantly deposited protein in human AA disease. SAA1 allele frequencies vary in different ethnic groups. The differences may be responsible for the variation in the incidence of AA in the course of inflammatory diseases, some populations having alleles of greater amyloidogenicity.[120]

Renal AA has also been found in association with some tumors, most commonly renal cell carcinoma, Hodgkin's lymphoma, and rarely atrial myxomas.[121,122] The relationship may be secondary to cytokine production by the tumor or by inflammatory cells responding to the tumor.

Differences in the frequency of AA disease have been seen in different ethnic groups with the autosomal recessive disease familial Mediterranean fever, a periodic febrile disorder with serositis, arthritis, and skin rashes, associated with high levels of SAA production.[123] The febrile disease is associated with mutations in the pyrin/marenostrin gene, which is expressed in granulocytes. The normal function of the pyrin/marenostrin protein may be to inhibit, or turn off, the inflammatory response. In Armenian kindreds the frequency of renal amyloidosis is quite low, while in Sephardic Jews renal involvement, ultimately fatal, is common by age 30.[124] It has been suggested that the ethnic discrepancy may be related to differences in the spectrum of mutations in each group, variation in other genes controlling the process of amyloidogenesis, or differences in environmental influences in the different populations.[125]

In AA associated with FMF, colchicine prophylaxis reduces the frequency and severity of the febrile episodes.[126] It is likely that the elimination of renal amyloidosis in patients who adhere to the thrice-daily regimen results from a reduction in inflammation, rather than an amyloid-specific effect. Colchicine has also been reported to inhibit experimental AA formation in murine inflammatory models.[127] Because of these two sets of observations, colchicine has also been used empirically in patients with AA unrelated to FMF. The evidence for its benefit in these is largely anecdotal.[128]

Other hereditary periodic febrile disorders have been described in association with AA. In the Muckle-Wells syndrome, AA deposition accompanies deafness, urticaria, and febrile episodes. It appears to display autosomal dominant inheritance. The responsible gene is unknown, although a candidate region for the gene has recently been localized to chromosome 1q44.[129]

β2 MICROGLOBULIN AMYLOID

Patients undergoing long-term hemodialysis develop carpal tunnel amyloid consisting of β_2 microglobulin (β_2M)–derived fibrils. This type of amyloid primarily involves synovial membranes, causing trigger finger, bone cysts, and destructive spondyloarthropathy. The heart, GI tract, liver lung, prostate, adrenals, and tongue may also be involved.[130,131] β_2M amyloidosis increases with the duration of hemodialysis: It first appears after about 5 years and increases to 20 percent at 10 years, 30 to 50 percent at 15 years, and 80 to 100 percent at 20 years.[132] Deposits also occur in patients treated with continuous ambulatory peritoneal dialysis and have been reported in patients with renal failure who have not undergone dialysis.[133,134] Diagnosis is made in the clinical setting of long-standing renal failure treated by dialysis, the characteristic x-ray lesions, which resemble the punched-out lytic bone lesions of myeloma, and biopsy demonstration of amyloid staining with anti-β_2M antiserum. Subcutaneous fat aspiration is not usually helpful.[135] The long history of renal failure and dialysis in a patient with carpal tunnel syndrome should allow the distinction between AL and β_2M amyloid to be made easily on clinical grounds and confirmed by biopsy. Kidney transplantation may arrest amyloid progression in these patients.

β_2M, the light-chain component of the major histocompatibility complex, is both excreted and catabolized in the kidney. In renal failure, it accumulates in the serum. Because of its size β_2M is not removed by conventional dialysis membranes and serum levels may reach 30 to 60 times normal in dialysis patients. Originally it was believed that the mass-action effect was responsible for this form of amyloid deposition, so more permeable dialysis membranes with larger pore sizes were developed to reduce this debilitating complication of dialysis. Current data suggest that the pathogenesis is more complicated, involving macrophage activation by dialysis membranes with increased β_2M production, nonenzymatic glycation of the protein and additional activation via the receptor for advanced glycation end-products.[136]

OTHER FORMS OF AMYLOIDOSIS

HEREDITARY RENAL AMYLOIDOSES

Each of the hereditary amyloidoses (AApoAI, Afib, Alys) should be considered when a renal biopsy is reported to show amyloid deposition.[137–141] The clinical differentiation between the hereditary renal amyloidoses and AL with a dominant renal presentation should be easily established on the basis of family history and immunoglobulin studies. The definitive diagnosis is made by immunohistologic staining of the biopsy material with antibodies specific for the candidate amyloid precursor proteins.

AMYLOIDOSES LOCALIZED TO THE CENTRAL NERVOUS SYSTEM

There should be little clinical confusion between AL disease and any of the primarily CNS amyloidoses, as AL deposits are rarely found in the central nervous system, though they may be found in the cerebral vessels. The authors have seen one case of a cerebral AL amyloidoma in a patient with a circulating monoclonal IgM protein. The primary CNS amyloidoses include Acys, hereditary cerebral hemorrhage with amyloidosis-Icelandic type, in which the precursor is the protease inhibitor cystatin c[142]; the Aβ amyloidoses, including Dutch-type hereditary cerebral hemorrhage with amyloidosis, Alzheimer's disease, and Down's syndrome[143,144]; APrp, the prionoses including Creutzfeldt-Jakob disease (CJD), Gerstmann-Sträussler-Scheinker (GSS) disease, fatal familial insomnia (FFI), bovine spongiform encephalopathy, kuru, and scrapie in goats and sheep.[145,146]

CORNEAL AMYLOIDOSES

Three proteins, gelsolin (Agel),[147] kerato-epithelin (AKE),[148] and lactoferrin (Alac),[149] have been found in fibrils from patients with autosomal dominant corneal amyloidosis. Whether there is a pathophysiologic relationship among these disorders is not yet clear.

OTHER LOCALIZED AMYLOIDOSES

Four polypeptide hormones have been defined as the fibril precursors in tissue-specific localized amyloidoses: AANF in isolated atrial amyloid[150]; Acal in medullary carcinoma of the thyroid[151]; AIAPP seen in the pancreatic islets of the elderly, putatively involved in the pathogenesis of type II diabetes mellitus[152]; APro from pituitary adenomas[153]; and Aker localized to the skin.[154,155]

THERAPY, COURSE, AND PROGNOSIS

Potential treatments of any of the amyloidoses can be directed at interfering with any or all of several pathogenetic processes. Production of the precursor can be reduced or its catabolism enhanced; generation of the profibrillar intermediate can be blocked; interactions between profibrillar molecules to yield the fibril can be inhibited; deposition can be slowed; or deposits can be actively mobilized. At present, standard treatment for AL involves only one of these strategies, i.e., that of reducing production of the monoclonal immunoglobulin precursor via chemotherapy, or occasionally via radiotherapy or surgery of a localized amyloidogenic plasmacytoma. Equally important are supportive measures that maintain organ function in the absence of specific treatment or while specific therapy is being administered.

CHEMOTHERAPY

The rationale for chemotherapy assumes that AL, like myeloma, is caused by proliferation of a plasma cell clone; therefore, drugs likely to benefit AL patients are the same as those that are useful for myeloma. It is more difficult to assess the response to therapy in AL than in myeloma, since it requires indirect measurements of end-organ damage, serial biopsies, or serial P-component scans where available. In addition, studies of AL therapy require that all cases have a tissue diagnosis of the type of amyloid (e.g., AL versus ATTR). The recognition that there are different amyloid precursor proteins, which can be distinguished using readily available antisera, has made histologic diagnosis unequivocal.

The first effective regimen for myeloma was melphalan and prednisone. After the combination was shown to be of use in myeloma, it was tried in AL, with several case reports suggesting occasional benefit. In the initial randomized studies of melphalan and prednisone versus placebo or colchicine, several patients demonstrated objective responses to chemotherapy. In one study, a trend toward improved survival was seen with chemotherapy; however, statistical significance was not attained.[156,157] In a subsequent trial,[158] patients were randomized to one of three arms: (1) melphalan and prednisone; (2) melphalan, prednisone, and colchicine; or (3) colchicine alone. Median survival was greater in the melphalan-prednisone-colchicine and melphalan-prednisone arms (18 and 17 months, respectively) than in the colchicine alone arm (8.5 months). In a second trial, 100 patients were randomized to receive oral melphalan, prednisone, and colchicine, or colchicine alone.[159] Overall survival in the melphalan-prednisone-colchicine group was 12.2 months, as compared with 6.7 months in the colchicine alone group. The difference did not reach statistical significance ($P = .087$), because of the small sample size and early deaths of patients with severe cardiac or renal disease in both treatment arms. Taken together, these studies demonstrate a survival benefit of melphalan and prednisone, as compared with placebo, in AL. Patients most likely to respond to chemotherapy with objective improvement in end-organ damage are those with the renal involvement and the nephrotic syndrome. Approximately a quarter of this group will have at least a 50 percent decrease in proteinuria, with most showing its complete disappearance. Functional improvement can occur in nearly any affected organ but is least common in neuropathy.[33,59]

Other regimens used for myeloma have also been explored in AL. In one study, patients were randomized to either melphalan and prednisone or a 5-drug regimen, i.e., vincristine, carmustine, melphalan, cyclophosphamide, and prednisone; response rates and survival were not different between the two groups.[160] In a phase II trial, high-dose dexamethasone also produced responses in some AL patients, but survival was not superior to what would have been expected from melphalan and prednisone based on historic controls.[161] High-dose dexamethasone also gave objective organ responses in 3 of 19 patients who had previously received chemotherapy.[162] Melphalan plus prednisone can now be considered standard therapy for AL, with any other regimen shown to be effective in myeloma being a reasonable second choice.

For patients who respond to chemotherapy, there are no data defining the optimal duration of treatment. In those with objective improvement in organ function who do not develop toxicity, some investigators have continued chemotherapy for 1 or 2 years. When disease initially responds and then progresses off treatment, chemotherapy—the same or a different regimen—can be resumed. There is little information whether any maintenance therapy such as α interferon is of use, mirroring the situation in myeloma.

Melphalan has considerable leukemogenic potential: The actuarial risk for acute myelogenous leukemia (AML) in one study of patients with myeloma treated with melphalan was 17 percent at 50 months.[163] In two other studies 5 percent of patients developed myelodysplasia (including several with chromosomal abnormalities and/or progression to AML) in 3 years of follow-up.

In order to obtain better survival in myeloma, protocols using "high-dose" chemotherapy, followed by autologous marrow or peripheral blood stem cell rescue, have been instituted. Several phase II trials of high-dose therapy in selected patients have demonstrated favorable response and survival rates as compared with historical controls.[164] A panel of myeloma experts, reviewing the data available in 1998, concluded that high-dose therapy was appropriate in myeloma patients under age 55 with stage 3 disease and a complete or partial response or stable disease after initial chemotherapy. It is possible that further trials will justify extension of the procedure to other groups.[165]

Following the myeloma model, several centers have reported phase II trials of high-dose chemotherapy followed by rescue with autologous marrow or peripheral blood stem cells in AL.[166,167] In one highly selected group of patients (median age 48, exclusion of patients with severely impaired cardiac, pulmonary, or renal function), a response, as assessed by objective improvement in end-organ function, was reported in 11 of 17 patients (65 percent). Based on these data, some centers now employ high-dose chemotherapy regimens for all patients able to tolerate the conditioning regimen. In the initial studies of high-dose therapy with peripheral blood stem cell rescue, patients with severe cardiac involvement experienced very high early mortality.[168] The risk has been attributed to intolerance of the fluid shifts that accompany peripheral blood stem cell harvesting. Patients with severe cardiac involvement, i.e., those with the worst prognosis of any AL subgroup, have been excluded from high-dose therapy trials. Another concern with high-dose therapy followed by stem cell rescue is that autologous stem cells collected for reinfusion will generally contain clonal cells producing the amyloidogenic light chain.[169]

Until the results of phase III randomized trials comparing standard to high-dose chemotherapy are available, the choice in individual patients will remain difficult and will require discussion of the risks and possible benefits with the patient.[170] In view of the limited numbers of patients diagnosed with AL and the large numbers of patients required to perform such studies in a timely manner, referral of patients to specialized centers performing such randomized phase III trials is essential.

THERAPY OF LOCALIZED AL

The treatment of localized AL (most often in the pulmonary tract) has not been systematically studied. Since progression to systemic disease does not occur often, chemotherapy may not be indicated. Localized radiotherapy, aimed at destroying the local collection of plasma cells producing the AL precursor, is a reasonable therapeutic approach.[171] In patients with massive macroglossia, conventional surgical resection has not been effective. Relief can sometimes be achieved with laser techniques, although formal studies of efficacy have not been reported.

PHARMACOLOGIC AGENTS DESIGNED TO BREAK DOWN AMYLOID FIBRILS

The antiamyloid activity of 4-iododoxorubicin (Idox), an anthracycline analogue of doxorubicin was discovered serendipitously when it was being studied as a cytotoxic chemotherapeutic agent for myeloma. One patient with myeloma and AL began excreting a large amount of light chains into the urine, and dramatically improved clinically within days.[172] Subsequently, five of eight patients treated in a pilot trial responded with clinical improvement, which appeared unrelated to any cytotoxic effect on the plasma cell clone. From 1995 to 1997 Idox was given to a further 14 patients in a single-institution study and to 28 patients at other institutions on a compassionate basis. Of these 42 patients, 13 had disease responses, and 15 showed stabilized disease. Responses were transient, however, and disease typically progressed after a period of months. In mid-1999, a phase II trial of Idox for AL was begun at two centers in the United States.

Laboratory studies demonstrated that Idox binds to various types of amyloid. It is possible that its most effective use may be in combination with cytotoxic chemotherapy, in an effort to simultaneously decrease clonal light-chain production and enhance mobilization of deposited light chains. Other small molecules that may bind to amyloid fibrils, of the AL and other types, are under investigation.

TREATMENT OF NONAMYLOID MIDD

As in AL, once a diagnosis of MIDD is established, it should be determined whether the patient has myeloma (e.g., serum and urine evaluation for monoclonal protein, marrow aspiration and biopsy, skeletal survey). Regimens effective in myeloma and AL should be utilized to reduce end organ damage, as MIDD is a similar monoclonal plasma cell disorder. However, no published studies have addressed chemotherapeutic treatment of nonamyloid MIDD in a systematic fashion.

SUPPORTIVE MEASURES FOR AL

CARDIAC INVOLVEMENT

Diuretics and angiotensin-converting inhibitors are the mainstay of therapy for congestive heart failure resulting from amyloidosis. Hypotension, resulting from a low ejection fraction and/or autonomic neuropathy, may limit diuretic use. On the other hand, if edema is troubling and hypotension is asymptomatic, diuretics can be increased. The use of digoxin and calcium channel blockers must be avoided in both

AL and TTR cardiac amyloidosis because these compounds bind to amyloid fibrils and have been reported to increase congestive heart failure and produce arrhythmias.[173-175] Pacemakers are of use in some patients with symptomatic bradycardia.[176,177] Cardiac transplants have been performed in a small number of AL patients. This therapy may be lifesaving for patients with severe disease, but in the absence of effective systemic therapy to eliminate production of the amyloidogenic light chain, amyloid recurs in the transplanted organ.[178,179] For young patients with severe cardiac involvement, cardiac transplantation followed by high-dose therapy and autologous stem cell reinfusion has been utilized, but its efficacy has not been established.

RENAL INVOLVEMENT

Hemodialysis and peritoneal dialysis are indicated in patients with AL and renal failure.[46] Renal transplantation has been utilized in patients with amyloidosis, but most have not been of the AL type. Since AL is a systemic disease and hemodialysis is generally effective, renal transplantation is rarely indicated, except perhaps in occasional patients who have had particularly good responses to chemotherapy, where long survival may be expected. In the absence of effective chemotherapy, reaccumulation of amyloid in the transplanted kidney has been reported.

REFERENCES

1. International Nomenclature Committee on Amyloidosis: Part 1. Nomenclature of amyloid fibril proteins. *Amyloid: Int J Exp Clin Invest* 6:63, 1999.
2. Emsley J, White HE, O'Hara BP, et al: Structure of pentameric human serum amyloid P component. *Nature* 367:338, 1994.
3. Conway KA, Harper JD, Lansbury PT: Accelerated *in vitro* fibril formation by a mutant alpha synuclein linked to early-onset Parkinson's Disease. *Nat Med* 4:1318, 1998.
4. Karpuj MV, Garren H, Slunt H, et al: Transglutaminase aggregates huntingtin into nonamyloidogenic polymers, and its enzymatic activity increases in Huntington's disease brain nuclei. *Proc Natl Acad Sci USA* 96:7388, 1999.
5. Ishihara T, Takahashi M, Koga M, Yakota T, Yamashita Y, Uchino F: Amyloid fibril formation in the rough endoplasmic reticulum of plasma cells from a patient with localized Alambda amyloidosis. *Lab Invest* 64:265, 1991.
6. Botto M, Hawkins PN, Bickerstaff MC, et al: Amyloid deposition is delayed in mice with targeted deletion of the serum amyloid P component gene. *Nat Med* 3:855, 1997.
7. Hawkins PN, Aprile C, Capri G, et al: Scintigraphic imaging and turnover studies with iodine-131 labelled serum amyloid P component in systemic amyloidosis. *Eur J Nucl Med* 25:701, 1998.
8. Gallo G, Wisniewski T, Choi-Miura N-H, Ghiso J, Frangione B: Potential role of apolipoprotein-E in fibrillogenesis. *Am J Pathol* 145:526, 1994.
9. Gejyo F, Suzuki S, Kimura H, et al: Increased risk of dialysis-related amyloidosis in patients with the apolipoprotein E4 allele. *Amyloid: Int J Exp Clin Invest* 4:13, 1997.
10. Hasegawa H, Nishi SI, Ito S, et al: High prevalence of serum apolipoprotein E4 isoprotein in rheumatoid arthritis patients with amyloidosis. *Arth Rheum* 39:1728, 1996.
11. Kindy MS, deBeer FC, Markesbery WR, et al: Apolipoprotein E genotypes in AA and AL amyloidoses. *Amyloid: Int J Exp Clin Invest* 2:159, 1995.
12. Lovat LB, Booth SE, Booth DR, et al: Apolipoprotein E4 genotype is not a risk factor for systemic AA amyloidosis or familial amyloid polyneuropathy. *Amyloid: Int J Exp Clin Invest* 2:163, 1995.
13. Korpela MM, Lehtimaki T, Mustonen JT, Pasternack A: Prevalence of serum apolipoprotein E4 isoprotein is not increased in rheumatoid arthritis patients with amyloidosis: comment on article by Hasegawa et al. *Arth Rheum* 41:1328, 1998.
14. Kisilevsky R, Fraser P: Proteoglycans and amyloid fibrillogenesis, in *The Nature and Origin of Amyloid Fibrils*, p 58. Wiley, New York, 1996.
15. Kisilevsky R, Lemieux LJ, Fraser PE, Kong X, Hultin PG, Szarek WA:

Arresting amyloidosis in vivo using small molecule anionic sulphonates or sulphates: implications for Alzheimer's disease. *Nat Med* 1:143, 1995.
16. Teng M, Yin J, Vidal R, et al: Gender dependent amyloid deposition in aging mice transgenic for human transthyretin, in *Amyloid and Amyloidosis 1998*, p 224. Parthenon, New York, 1999.
17. Gallo G, Picken M, Buxbaum J: Deposits in monoclonal immunoglobulin deposition disease lack amyloid P-component. *Mod Pathol* 1:453, 1988.
18. Tagliavini F, Ghiso J, Timmers W, Giaccone G, Bugiani O, Frangione B: Coexistence of Alzheimer's amyloid precursor protein and amyloid protein in cerebral vessel walls. *Lab Invest* 62:761, 1990.
19. Buxbaum J: Mechanisms of disease: monoclonal immunoglobulin deposition. Amyloidosis, light chain deposition disease, and light and heavy chain deposition disease. *Hematol Oncol Clin North Am* 6:323, 1992.
20. Solomon A, Weiss DT, Murphy C: Primary amyloidosis associated with a novel heavy-chain fragment (AH amyloidosis). *Am J Hematol* 45:171, 1994.
21. Durie B, Persky B, Soehnlen BJ, Grogan TM, Salmon SE: Amyloid production in human myeloma stem-cell culture with morphologic evidence of amyloid secretion by associated macrophages. *N Engl J Med* 307:1689, 1982.
22. Epstein WV, Tan M, Wood IS: Formation of "amyloid" fibrils in vitro by action of human kidney lysomal enzymes on Bence Jones proteins. *J Lab Clin Med* 84:107, 1974.
23. Linke RP, Zucker-Franklin D, Franklin EC: Morphologic, chemical and immunologic studies of amyloid-like fibrils formed from Bence Jones proteins by proteolysis. *J Immunol* 111:10, 1973.
24. Buxbaum J: Aberrant immunoglobulin synthesis in light chain amyloidosis. Free light chain and light chain fragment production by human bone marrow cells in short-term tissue culture. *J Clin Invest* 78:798, 1986.
25. Moulin B, Deret S, Mariette X, et al: Nodular glomerulosclerosis with deposition of monoclonal immunoglobulin heavy chains lacking CH1. *J Am Soc Nephrol* 10:519, 1998.
26. Comenzo RL, Wally J, Kica G, et al: Clonal immunoglobulin light chain variable region germline gene use in AL amyloidosis: association with dominant amyloid-related organ involvement and survival after stem cell transplantation. *Br J Haematol* 106:744, 1999.
27. Solomon A, Frangione B, Franklin EC: Bence Jones proteins and light chains of immunoglobulins. Preferential association of the V lambda VI subgroup of human light chains with amyloidosis AL (lambda). *J Clin Invest* 70:453, 1982.
28. Raffen R, Dieckman LJ, Szpunar M, et al: Physicochemical consequences of amino acid variations that contribute to fibril formation by immunoglobulin light chains. *Protein Sci* 8:509, 1999.
29. Hurle MR, Helms LR, Li L, Chan W, Wetzel R: A role for destabilizing amino acid replacements in light chain amyloidosis. *Proc Natl Acad Sci USA* 91:5446, 1994.
30. Gallo G, Goni F, Boctor F, et al: Light chain cardiomyopathy: structural analysis of the light chain tissue deposits. *Am J Pathol* 148:1397, 1996.
31. Stevens FJ, Kisilevsky R: Immunoglobulin light chains, glycosaminoglycans and amyloid. *Cell Mol Life Sci* 57:441, 2000.
32. Kyle RA, Gertz MA: Primary systemic amyloidosis: clinical and laboratory features in 474 cases. *Semin Hematol* 32:45, 1995.
33. Gertz MA, Kyle RA, Greipp PR: Response rates and survival in primary systemic amyloidosis. *Blood* 77:257, 1991.
34. Perfetti V, Colli Vignarelli M, Anesi E, et al: The degrees of plasma cell clonality and marrow infiltration adversely influence the prognosis of AL amyloidosis patients. *Haematologica* 84:218, 1999.
35. Kyle RA, Gertz MA, Greipp PR, et al: Long-term survival (10 years or more) in 30 patients with primary amyloidosis. *Blood* 93:1062, 1999.
36. Pruzanski W, Katz A: Clinical and laboratory findings in primary generalized and multiple-myeloma-related amyloidosis. *Can Med Assoc J* 114:906, 1976.
37. Browning MJ, Banks RA, Tribe CR, et al: Ten years' experience of an amyloid clinic—a clinicopathological survey. *Q J Med* 54:213, 1985.
38. Lucas FV, Fishleder AJ, Becker RC, Cavalier DS, Tubbs RR: Acquired factor X deficiency in systemic amyloidosis. *Cleve Clin J Med* 54:399, 1987.
39. Gertz MA, Kyle RA: Hepatic amyloidosis (primary [AL], immunoglobulin light chain): the natural history in 80 patients. *Am J Med* 85:73, 1988.
40. Matsuo K, Nakamoto M, Yasunaga C, Goya T, Sugimachi K: Dialysis-

related amyloidosis of the tongue in long-term hemodialysis patients. *Kidney Int* 52:832, 1997.

41. Olson LJ, Gertz MA, Edwards WD, et al: Senile cardiac amyloidosis with myocardial dysfunction. Diagnosis by endomyocardial biopsy and immunohistochemistry. *N Engl J Med* 317:738, 1987.

42. Moyssakis I, Triposkiadis F, Rallidis L, Hawkins P, Kyriakidis M, Nihoyannopoulos P: Echocardiographic features of primary, secondary and familial amyloidosis. *Eur J Clin Invest* 29:484, 1999.

43. Desikan KR, Dhodapkar MV, Hough A, et al: Incidence and impact of light chain associated (AL) amyloidosis on the prognosis of patients with multiple myeloma treated with autologous transplantation. *Leuk Lymphoma* 27:315, 1997.

44. Schena FP, Pannarale G, Carbonara MC: Clinical and therapeutic aspects of renal amyloidosis. *Nephrol Dial Transplant* 11(suppl 9):63, 1996.

45. Montseny JJ, Kleinknecht D, Meyrier A, et al: Long-term outcomes according to renal histological lesions in 118 patients with monoclonal gammopathies. *Nephrol Dial Transplant* 13:1438, 1998.

46. Gertz MA, Kyle RA, O'Fallon WM: Dialysis support of patients with primary systemic amyloidosis. *Arch Intern Med* 152:2245, 1992.

47. Buxbaum J, Gallo G: Non-amyloidotic monoclonal immunogloblin deposition disease. *Hematol Oncol Clin North Am* 13:14–1, 1999.

48. Ridolfi RL, Bulkley BH, Hutchins GM: The conduction system in cardiac amyloidosis: clinical and pathologic features of 23 patients. *Am J Med* 62:677, 1977.

49. Arbustini E, Merlini G, Gavazzi A, et al: Cardiac immunocyte-derived (AL) amyloidosis: an endomyocardial biopsy study in 11 patients. *Am Heart J* 130:528, 1995.

50. Falk RH, Rubinow A, Cohen AS: Cardiac arrhythmias in systemic amyloidosis: correlation with echocardiographic abnormalities. *J Am Coll Cardiol* 3:107, 1984.

51. Smith RRL: Ischemic heart disease secondary to amyloidosis of intramyocardial arteries. *Am J Cardiol* 44:413, 1979.

52. Hamer JPM, Janssen S, van Rijswijk MH, Lie KI: Amyloid cardiomyopathy in systemic non-hereditary amyloidosis. Clinical, echocardiographic and electrocardiographic findings in 30 patients with AA and 24 patients with AL amyloidosis. *Eur Heart J* 13:623, 1992.

53. Carroll JD, Gaasch WH, McAdam KPWJ: Amyloid cardiomyopathy: characterization by a distinctive voltage/mass relationship. *Am J Cardiol* 49:9, 1982.

54. Smith TJ, Kyle RA, Lie JT: Clinical significance of histopathologic patterns of cardiac amyloidosis. *Mayo Clin Proc* 59:547, 1984.

55. Klein AL, Hatle LK, Taliercio CP, et al: Prognostic significance of Doppler measures of diastolic function in cardiac amyloidosis: a Doppler echocardiography study. *Circulation* 83:808, 1991.

56. Cueto-Garcia L, Tajik J, Kyle RA, et al: Serial echocardiographic observations in patients with primary systemic amyloidosis: an introduction to the concept of early (asymptomatic) amyloid infiltration of the heart. *Mayo Clin Proc* 59:589, 1984.

57. Tei C, Dujardin KS, Hodge DO, Kyle RA, Tajik J, Seward JB: Doppler index combining systolic and diastolic myocardial performance: clinical value in cardiac amyloidosis. *J Am Coll Cardiol* 28:658, 1996.

58. Simons M, Isner JM: Assessment of relative sensitivities of noninvasive tests for cardiac amyloidosis in documented cardiac amyloidosis. *Am J Cardiol* 68:425, 1992.

59. Glenner GG, Murphy MA: Amyloidosis of the nervous system. *J Neurol Sci* 94:1, 1989.

60. Simmons Z, Blaivas M, Aguilera AJ, Feldman EL, Bromber MB, Towfighi J: Low diagnostic yield of sural nerve biopsy in patients with peripheral neuropathy and primary amyloidosis. *J Neurol Sci* 120:60, 1993.

61. Traynor AE, Gertz MA, Kyle RA: Cranial neuropathy associated with primary amyloidosis. *Ann Neurol* 29:451, 1991.

62. Nordborg C, Kristensson K, Olsson Y, Sourander P: Involvement of the autonomic nervous system in primary and secondary amyloidosis. *Acta Neurol Scand* 49:31, 1973.

63. Kyle RA, Gertz MA, Linke RP: Amyloid localized to tenosynovium at carpal tunnel release: immunohistochemical identification of amyloid type. *Am J Clin Pathol* 97:250, 1992.

64. Reinish EI, Raviv M, Srolovitz H, Gornitsky M: Tongue, primary amyloidosis, and multiple myeloma. *Oral Surg Oral Med Oral Pathol* 77:121, 1994.

65. Menke DM, Kyle RA, Fleming CR, Wolfe JT3, Kurtin PJ, Oldenburg

66. WA: Symptomatic gastric amyloidosis in patients with primary systemic amyloidosis. *Mayo Clin Proc* 68:763, 1993.

66. Brandt K, Cathcart ES, Cohen AS: A clinical analysis of the course and prognosis of forty-two patients with amyloidosis. *Am J Med* 44:955, 1968.

67. Battle WM, Rubin MR, Cohen S, Snape WJ Jr: Gastrointestinal motility dysfunction in amyloidosis. *N Engl J Med* 301:24, 1979.

68. Jarnum S: Gastrointestinal hemorrhage and protein loss in primary amyloidosis. *Gut* 6:14, 1965.

69. Brandt K, Cathcart ES, Streiff R, Cohen AS: Amyloidosis of the stomach associated with impaired gastric secretion of intrinsic factor and the development of vitamin B12 deficiency. *Isr J Med Sci* 4:1005, 1968.

70. Carlson HC, Breen JF: Amyloidosis and plasma cell dyscrasias: gastrointestinal involvement. *Semin Roentgenol* 21:128, 1986.

71. Gertz MA, Kyle RA: Hepatic amyloidosis: clinical appraisal in 77 patients. *Hepatology* 25:118, 1997.

72. Gastineau DA, Gertz MA, Rosen CB, Kyle RA: Computed tomography for diagnosis of hepatic rupture in primary systemic amyloidosis. *Am J Hematol* 37:194, 1991.

73. Attwood HD, Price CG, Riddell RJ: Primary diffuse tracheobronchial amyloidosis. *Thorax* 27:620, 1972.

74. Talbot AR: Laryngeal amyloidosis. *J Laryngol Otol* 104:147, 1990.

75. Hui AN, Koss MN, Hochholzer L, Wehunt WD: Amyloidosis presenting in the lower respiratory tract. Clinicopathologic, radiologic, immunohistochemical, and histochemical studies on 48 cases. *Arch Pathol Lab Med* 110:212, 1986.

76. Wiernik PH: Amyloid joint disease. *Medicine (Baltimore)* 51:465, 1972.

77. Katz GA, Peter JB, Pearson CM, Adams WS: The shoulder-pad sign—a diagnostic feature of amyloid arthropathy. *N Engl J Med* 288:354, 1973.

78. Yamada M, Tsukagoshi H, Hatakeyama S: Skeletal muscle amyloid deposition in AL-(primary or myeloma-associated), AA-(secondary), and prealbumin-type amyloidosis. *J Neurol Sci* 85:223, 1988.

79. Santiago RM, Scharnhorst D, Ratkin G, Crouch EC: Respiratory muscle weakness and ventilatory failure in AL amyloidosis with muscular pseudohypertrophy. *Am J Med* 83:175, 1987.

80. Hamidi Asl K, Liepnicks JJ, Nakamura M, Benson MD: Organ-specific (localized) synthesis of Ig light chain amyloid. *J Immunol* 162:5556, 1999.

81. Michaels L, Hyams VJ: Amyloid in localised deposits and plasmacytomas of the respiratory tract. *J Pathol* 128:29, 1979.

82. Lim JS, Lebowitz RA, Jacobs JB: Primary amyloidosis presenting as a nasopharyngeal mass. *Am J Rhinol* 13:209, 1999.

83. Krishnan J, Chu WS, Elrod JP, Frizzera G: Tumoral presentation of amyloidosis (amyloidomas) in soft tissues. A report of 14 cases. *Am J Clin Pathol* 100:135, 1993.

84. Piette WW: Myeloma, paraproteinemias, and the skin. *Med Clin North Am* 70:155, 1986.

85. Rapoport M, Yona R, Kaufman S, Segal M, Kornberg A: Unusual bleeding manifestations of amyloidosis in patients with multiple myeloma. *Clin Lab Haematol* 16:349, 1994.

86. Buxbaum J, Genega E, Kronzon I, Tunick P, Gallo G: Non-amyloid infiltrative cardiomyopathy in plasma cell dyscrasias: an underappreciated feature of systemic light chain deposition. *JACC* 31(suppl A):67A, 1998.

87. Gertz MA, Lacy MQ, Dispenzieri A: Amyloidosis: recognition, confirmation, prognosis, and therapy. *Mayo Clin Proc* 74:490, 1999.

88. Kaplan B, Vidal R, Kumar A, Ghiso J, Gallo G: Immunochemical microanalysis of amyloid proteins in fine-needle aspirates of abdominal fat. *Am J Clin Pathol* 112:403, 1999.

89. Wolf BC, Kumar A, Vera JC, Neiman RS: Bone marrow morphology and immunology in systemic amyloidosis. *Am J Clin Pathol* 86:84, 1986.

90. Yamada M, Hatakeyama S, Tsukagoshi H: Gastrointestinal amyloid deposition in AL (primary or myeloma associated) and AA (secondary) amyloidosis. Diagnostic value of gastric biopsy. *Hum Pathol* 16:1206, 1985.

91. Dupond J, de Wazieres B, Saile R, et al: Systemic amyloidosis in the elderly: diagnostic value of the test of subcutaneous abdominal fat and the labial salivary glands. Prospective study in 100 aged patients. *Rev Med Interne* 16:314, 1995.

92. Kyle RA, Lust JA: Monoclonal gammopathies of undetermined significance, in *Neoplastic Diseases of the Blood,* 2nd ed, p 571. Churchill Livingstone, New York, 1991.

93. Perfetti V, Garini P, Vignarelli MC, Marinone MG, Zorzoli I, Merlini G: Diagnostic approach to and follow-up of difficult cases of AL amyloidosis. *Haematologica* 80:409, 1995.

94. Cathcart ES, Ritchie RF, Cohen AS, Brandt K: Immunoglobulins and amyloidosis. An immunologic study of sixty-two patients with biopsy-proved disease. *Am J Med* 52:93, 1972.

97. Sane DC, Pizzo SV, Greenberg CS: Elevated urokinase-type plasminogen activator level and bleeding in amyloidosis: case report and literature review. *Am J Hematol* 31:53, 1989.

98. Herbert J, Wilcox JN, Pham KC, et al: Transthyretin: a choroid plexus-specific transport protein in human brain. *Neurol* 36:900, 1986.

99. Rocken C, Saeger W, Linke RP: Gastrointestinal amyloid deposits in old age. *Path Res Pract* 190:641, 1994.

100. Pitkänen P, Westermark P, Cornwell GG III: Senile systemic amyloidosis. *Am J Pathol* 117:391, 1984.

101. Hodkinson HM, Pomerance A: The clinical significance of senile cardiac amyloidosis: a prospective clinico-pathological study. *Q J Med* XLVI:381, 1977.

102. Saraiva MJM: Transthyretin mutations in health and disease. *Hum Mutation* 5:191, 1995.

103. Smith FR, Suskind R, Thanangkul O, Leitzmann C, Goodman DS, Olson RE: Plasma vitamin A, retinol-binding protein and prealbumin concentrations in protein-calorie malnutrition. III. Response to varying dietary treatments. *Am J Clin Nutr* 28:732, 1975.

104. Coelho T: Familial amyloid polyneuropathy: new developments in genetics and treatment. *Curr Opin Neurol* 9:355, 1996.

105. Plante-Bordeneuve V, Lalu T, Misrahi M, et al: Genotypic-phenotypic variations in a series of 65 patients with familial amyloid polyneuropathy. *Neurol* 51:708, 1998.

106. Buxbaum JN, Tagoe CE: The genetics of the amyloidoses. *Annu Rev Med* 51:543, 2000.

107. Dubrey SW, Davidoff R, Skinner M, Bergethon P, Lewis D, Falk RH: Progression of ventricular wall thickening after liver transplantation for familial amyloidosis. *Transplantation* 64:74, 1997.

108. Lie JT, Hammond H: Pathology of the senescent heart: anatomic observations on 237 autopsy studies of patients 90 to 105 years old. *Mayo Clin Proc* 63:552, 1988.

109. Gustavsson Å, Jahr H, Tobiassen R, Jacobson DR, Sletten K, Westermark P: Amyloid fibril composition and transthyretin gene structure in senile systemic amyloidosis. *Lab Invest* 73:703, 1995.

110. Jacobson DR, Pastore RD, Yaghoubian R, et al: Variant-sequence transthyretin (isoleucine 122) in late-onset cardiac amyloidosis in black Americans. *N Engl J Med* 336:466, 1997.

111. Jacobson DR, Pan T, Kyle RA, Buxbaum JN: Transthyretin Ile20, a new variant associated with late-onset cardiac amyloidosis. *Hum Mutation* 9:83, 1997.

112. Dupuy O, Blétry O, Blanc AS, et al: A novel variant of transthyretin (Glu42Asp) associated with sporadic late-onset cardiac amyloidosis. *Amyloid: Int J Exp Clin Invest* 5:285, 1998.

113. Jacobson DR, Pastore R, Pool S, et al: Revised transthyretin Ile 122 allele prevalence in African-Americans. *Hum Genet* 98:236, 1996.

114. Buxbaum J: The amyloidoses, in *Textbook of Rheumatology,* 2nd ed, p 8.27.1. Mosby, London, 1998.

115. Helin HJ, Korpela MM, Mustonen JT, Pasternack AI: Renal biopsy findings and clinicopathologic correlations in rheumatoid arthritis. *Arth Rheum* 38:242, 1995.

116. Ekelund L: Radiologic findings in renal amyloidosis. *Am J Roentgen* 129:851, 1977.

117. Tishler M, Pras M, Yaron M: Abdominal fat tissue aspirate in amyloidosis of familial Mediterranean fever. *Clin Exp Rheumatol* 6:395, 1988.

118. Marhaug G, Dowton SB: Serum amyloid A: an acute phase apolipoprotein and precursor of AA amyloid. *Ballière's Clin Rheumatol* 8:553, 1994.

119. International Nomenclature Committee on Amyloidosis: Part 2. Revised nomenclature for serum amyloid A (SAA). *Amyloid: Int J Exp Clin Invest* 6:67, 1999.

120. Booth DR, Booth SE, Gillmore JD: SAA1 Alleles as risk factors in reactive systemic AA amyloidosis. *Amyloid: Int J Exp Clin Invest* 5:262, 1998.

121. Champion M, Richards R: Amyloidosis in Hodgkin's disease: a Scottish survey. *Scot Med J* 24:9, 1979.

122. Dictor M, Hasserius R: Systemic amyloidosis and non-hematologic malignancy in a large autopsy series. *Acta Path Microbiol Scand* sect A 89:411, 1981.

123. Samuels J, Aksentijevich I, Torosyan Y, et al: Familial Mediterranean fever at the millennium; clinical spectrum, ancient mutations and a survey of 100 American referrals to the National Institutes of Health. *Medicine* 77:268, 1998.

124. Pras M, Bronshpigel N, Zemer D, Gafni J: Variable incidence of amyloidosis in familial Mediterranean fever among different ethnic groups. *Johns Hopkins Med J* 150:22, 1982.

125. Livneh A, Langevitz P, Shinar Y, et al: MEFV mutation analysis in patients suffering from amyloidosis of familial mediterranean fever. *Amyloid: Int J Exp Clin Invest* 6:1, 1999.

126. Zemer D, Pras M, Sohar E, Modan M, Cabili S, Gafni J: Colchicine in the prevention and treatment of the amyloidosis of familial mediterranean fever. *N Engl J Med* 314:1001, 1986.

127. Shirahama T, Cohen A: Blockage of amyloid induction by colchicine in an animal model. *J Exp Med* 140:1102, 1999.

128. Kagan A, Husar M, Frumkin A, Rapoport J: Reversal of nephrotic syndrome due to AA amyloidosis in psoriatic patients on long-term colchicine treatment. Case report and review of the literature. *Nephron* 82:348, 1999.

129. Cuisset L, Drenth JP, Berthelot JM, et al: Genetic linkage of the Muckle-Wells syndrome to chromosome 1q44. *Am J Hum Genet* 65:1054, 1999.

130. Kay J: β_2-microglobulin amyloidosis. *Amyloid: Int J Exp Clin Invest* 4:187, 1997.

131. Zingraff JJ, Noel LH, Bardin T, et al: Beta 2 microglobulin amyloidosis in chronic renal failure. *N Engl J Med* 323:1070, 1990.

132. Jimenez RE, Price DA, Pinkus GS, et al: Development of gastrointestinal beta2-microglobulin amyloidosis correlates with time on dialysis. *Am J Surg Pathol* 22:729, 1998.

133. Tan SY, Baillod R, Brown E, et al: Clinical, radiological and serum amyloid P component scintigraphic features of beta2-microglobulin amyloidosis associated with continuous ambulatory peritoneal dialysis. *Nephrol Dial Transplant* 14:1467, 1999.

134. Jadoul M, Garbar C, Vanholder R, et al: Prevalence of histological beta2-microglobulin amyloidosis in CAPD patients compared with hemodialysis patients. *Kidney Int* 54:956, 1998.

135. Varga J, Idelson BA, Felson D, Skinner M, Cohen AS: Lack of amyloid in abdominal fat aspirates from patients undergoing longterm hemodialysis. *Arch Intern Med* 147:1455, 1987.

136. Miyata T, Inagi R, Lida Y, et al: Involvement of Beta$_2$ microglobulin with advanced glycation end products in the pathogenesis of hemodialysis-associated amyloidosis. *J Clin Inv* 93:521, 1994.

137. Van Allen MW, Frohlich JA, Davis JR: Inherited predisposition to generalised amyloidosis. Clinical and pathological study of a family with neuropathy, nephropathy and peptic ulcer. *Neurology* 19:10, 1969.

138. Genschel J, Haas R, Propsting MJ, Schmidt HH: Apolipoprotein A-I induced amyloidosis. *FEBS Lett* 430:145, 1998.

139. Westermark P, Mucchiano G, Marthin T, Johnson KH, Sletten K: Apolipoprotein A1-derived amyloid in human aortic atherosclerotic plaques. *Am J Pathol* 147:1186, 1995.

140. Benson MD, Liepnieks J, Uemichi T, Wheeler G, Correa R: Hereditary renal amyloidosis associated with a mutant fibrinogen α-chain. *Nat Genet* 3:252, 1993.

141. Pepys MB, Hawkins PN, Booth DR, et al: Human lysozyme gene mutations cause hereditary systemic amyloidosis. *Nature* 362:553, 1993.

142. Olafsson I, Thorsteinsson L, Jensson O: The molecular pathology of hereditary cystatin C amyloid angiopathy causing brain hemorrhage. *Brain Pathol* 6:121, 1996.

143. Bornebroek M, Haan J, Maat-Schieman ML, Van Duinen SG, Roos RA: Hereditary cerebral hemorrhage with amyloidosis-Dutch type (HCHWA-D): I. A review of clinical, radiologic and genetic aspects. *Brain Pathol* 6:111, 1996.

144. Mann DM, Esiri MM: The pattern of acquisition of plaques and tangles in the brains of patients under 50 years of age with Down's syndrome. *Neurol Sci* 89:169, 1989.

145. Wisniewski T, Aucouturier P, Soto C, Frangione B: The prionoses and other conformational disorders. *Amyloid: Int J Exp Clin Invest* 5:212, 1998.

146. Price DL, Sisodia SS, Borchelt DR: Genetic neurodegenerative diseases: the human illness and transgenic models. *Science* 282:1079, 1998.

147. Kiuru S: Gelsolin-related familial amyloidosis, Finnish type (FAF), and its variants found worldwide. *Amyloid: Int J Exp Clin Invest* 5:55, 1998.

148. Korvatska E, Munier FL, Chaubert P, et al: On the role of kerato-epithelin in the pathogenesis of 5q31-linked corneal dystrophies. *Invest Ophthalmol Vis Sci* 40:2213, 1999.

149. Klintworth GK, Valnickova Z, Kielar R, Baratz KH, Campbell RJ, Enghild JJ: Familial subepithelial corneal amyloidosis—a lactoferrin-related amyloidosis. *Invest Ophthalmol Vis Sci* 38:2756, 1997.

150. Looi LM: Isolated atrial amyloidosis: a clinicopathologic study indicating increased prevalence in chronic heart disease. *Hum Pathol* 24:602, 1993.

151. Saad MF, Ordonez NG, Rashid RK, et al: Medullary carcinoma of the thyroid: a study of the clinical features and prognostic factors in 161 patients. *Medicine* 63:319, 1984.

152. Kahn SE, Andrikopoulos S, Verchere CB: Islet amyloid: a long-recognized but underappreciated pathological feature of type 2 diabetes. *Diabetes* 48:241, 1999.

153. Westermark P, Eriksson L, Engstrom U, Enestrom S, Sletten K: Prolactin-derived amyloid in the aging pituitary gland. *Am J Pathol* 150:67, 1997.

154. Norén P, Westermark P, Cornwell GG, Murdoch W: Immunofluorescence and histochemical studies of localized cutaneous amyloidosis. *Br J Dermatol* 108:277, 1983.

155. Huilgol SC, Ramnarain N, Carrington P, Leigh IM, Black MM: Cytokeratins in primary cutaneous amyloidosis. *Australas J Dermatol* 39:81, 1998.

156. Kyle RA, Greipp PR: Primary systemic amyloidosis: Comparison of melphalan/prednisone versus placebo. *Blood* 52:818, 1978.

157. Kyle RA, Greipp PR, Garton JP, Gertz MA: Primary systemic amyloidosis. Comparison of melphalan/prednisone versus colchicine. *Am J Med* 79:708, 1985.

158. Kyle RA, Gertz MA, Greipp PR, et al: A trial of three regimens for primary amyloidosis: colchicine alone, melphalan and prednisone, and melphalan, prednisone, and colchicine. *N Engl J Med* 336:1202, 1997.

159. Skinner M, Anderson JJ, Simms R, et al: Treatment of 100 patients with primary amyloidosis: a randomized trial of melphalan, prednisone, and colchicine versus colchicine only. *Am J Med* 100:290, 1996.

160. Gertz MA, Lacy MQ, Lust JA, Greipp PR, Witzig TE, Kyle RA: Prospective randomized trial of melphalan and prednisone versus vincristine, carmustine, melphalan, cyclophosphamide, and prednisone in the treatment of primary systemic amyloidosis. *J Clin Oncol* 17:262, 1999.

161. Gertz MA, Lacy MQ, Lust JA, Greipp PR, Witzig TE, Kyle RA: Phase II trial of high-dose dexamethasone for untreated patients with primary systemic amyloidosis. *Med Oncol* 16:104, 1999.

162. Gertz MA, Lacy MQ, Lust JA, Greipp PR, Witzig TE, Kyle RA: Phase II trial of high-dose dexamethasone for previously treated immunoglobulin light-chain amyloidosis. *Am J Hematol* 61:115, 1999.

163. Bergsagel DE, Bailey AJ, Langley GR, MacDonald RN, White DF, Miller AB: The chemotherapy of plasma-cell myeloma and the incidence of acute leukemia. *N Engl J Med* 301:743, 1979.

164. Attal M, Harousseau JL, Stoppa AM, et al: A prospective, randomized trial of autologous bone marrow transplantation and chemotherapy in multiple myeloma. Intergroupe Francais du Myelome [see comments]. *N Engl J Med* 335:91, 1996.

165. Gale RP, Park RE, Dubois RW, et al: Delphi-panel analysis of appropriateness of high-dose therapy and bone marrow autotransplants in newly diagnosed multiple myeloma. *Leuk Lymphoma* 33:511, 1999.

166. Comenzo RL, Vosburgh E, Falk RH, et al: Dose-intensive melphalan with blood stem-cell support for the treatment of AL (amyloid light-chain) amyloidosis: survival and responses in 25 patients. *Blood* 91:3662, 1998.

167. Moreau P, Leblond V, Bourquelot P, et al: Prognostic factors for survival and response after high-dose therapy and autologous stem cell transplantation in systemic AL amyloidosis: a report on 21 patients. *Br J Haematol* 101:766, 1998.

168. Falk RH, Reisinger J, Dubrey SW, et al: The effect of cardiac involvement on the outcome of intravenous melphalan therapy and autologous stem cell rescue for AL amyloidosis, in *Amyloid and Amyloidosis 1998: The Proceedings of the VIIIth International Symposium on Amyloidosis*, p 111. Parthenon, New York, 1999.

169. Perfetti V, Ubbiali P, Magni M, et al: Cells with clonal light chains are present in peripheral blood at diagnosis and in apheretic stem cell harvests of primary amyloidosis. *Bone Marrow Transplant* 23:323, 1999.

170. Kyle RA: High-dose therapy in multiple myeloma and primary amyloidosis: an overview. *Semin Oncol* 26:74, 1999.

171. Kurrus JA, Hayes JK, Hoidal JR, Menendez MM, Elstad MR: Radiation therapy for tracheobronchial amyloidosis. *Chest* 114:1489, 1998.

172. Merlini G, Anesi E, Garini P, et al: Treatment of AL amyloidosis with 4′-lodo-4′-deoxydoxorubicin: an update. *Blood* 93:1112, 1999.

173. Gertz MA, Skinner M, Connors LG, Falk RH, Cohen AS, Kyle RA: Selective binding of nifedipine to amyloid fibrils. *Am J Cardiol* 55:1646, 1985.

174. Gertz MA, Falk RH, Skinner M, Cohen AS, Kyle RA: Worsening of congestive heart failure in amyloid heart disease treated by calcium channel-blocking agents. *Am J Cardiol* 55:1845, 1985.

175. Rubinow A, Skinner M, Cohen AS: Digoxin sensitivity in amyloid cardiomyopathy. *Circulation* 63:1285, 1981.

176. Mathew V, Olson LJ, Gertz MA, Hayes DL: Symptomatic conduction system disease in cardiac amyloidosis. *Am J Cardiol* 80:1491, 1997.

177. Mathew V, Chaliki H, Nishimura RA: Atrioventricular sequential pacing in cardiac amyloidosis: an acute Doppler echocardiographic and catheterization hemodynamic study. *Clin Cardiol* 20:723, 1997.

178. Hosenpud JD, DeMarco T, Frazier OH, et al: Progression of systemic disease and reduced long-term survival in patients with cardiac amyloidosis undergoing heart transplantation: follow-up results of a multicenter survey. *Circulation* 84(suppl 3):III338, 1991.

179. Dubrey S, Simms RW, Skinner M, Falk RH: Recurrence of primary (AL) amyloidosis in a transplanted heart with four-year survival. *Am J Cardiol* 76:739, 1995.

WALDENSTRÖM MACROGLOBULINEMIA

THOMAS J. KIPPS

This chapter focuses on Waldenström macroglobulinemia, a B-cell malignancy in which there is abnormal production of a monoclonal IgM protein. It is important to distinguish this disorder from other causes of macroglobulinemia that also are described in this chapter. Recent observations are reviewed that provide insight into the potential etiology and pathogenesis of Waldenström macroglobulinemia. This chapter also discusses the clinical manifestations of this disease and outlines current approaches to therapy, including the use of purine analogues.

DEFINITION AND HISTORY

The term *macroglobulinemia* describes an increase in the blood concentration of IgM. Although this term commonly connotes Waldenström macroglobulinemia, several other disorders also may be associated with a monoclonal macroglobulinemia.[1,2] In addition, some conditions may be associated with an increase in polyclonal serum IgM protein.[3]

The types of disorders associated with a monoclonal macroglobulinemia vary with the study population. Physicians in specialized centers may see macroglobulinemia primarily associated with lymphoplasmacytic and B-lymphocyte neoplasms. On the other hand, physicians at primary treatment centers that use serum electrophoresis as a screening test more commonly may see patients with essential macroglobulinemia, or macroglobulinemia that is not associated with overt lymphoproliferative disease. Of 430 patients with monoclonal IgM investigated at the Mayo Clinic, 242 (56 percent) were classified as having essential monoclonal macroglobulinemia.[4] Seventeen percent of these patients developed Waldenström macroglobulinemia, chronic lymphocytic leukemia, lymphoma, or amyloidosis, and an additional 8 percent had progressive increases in serum IgM to 5 g/liter or more.

LYMPHOPLASMACYTIC NEOPLASMS

WALDENSTRÖM MACROGLOBULINEMIA

In 1944, Jan Waldenström described two male patients who had fatigue, a tendency to bleed from the gums and nasal mucosa, lymphadenopathy, worsening normochromic anemia, a low serum fibrinogen despite an "excessive sedimentation of the erythrocytes," and an extremely high serum viscosity secondary to a pathologic serum "euglobulin" (macroglobulin) of approximately 1,000,000 kDa.[5,6] These patients lacked any lytic bone lesions on X-ray and did not have any typical signs of myeloma, even on postmortem examination. Now known as Waldenström macroglobulinemia, this syndrome is the manifestation of a neoplastic disease in a clone of IgM-producing B cells. This chapter focuses primarily on this disorder.

Compared to myeloma, Waldenström macroglobulinemia is relatively less common. In the United States, the age-adjusted incidence rate per 1 million person-years at risk is 3.4 for men and 1.7 for women.[7] These rates increase sharply with age, from 0.1 for those who are less than 45 to 36.3 and 16.4 for men and women, respectively, who are 75 or older.

IgM MYELOMA AND EXTRAMEDULLARY PLASMACYTOMA

Patients with monoclonal macroglobulinemia associated with lytic bone lesions or hypercalcemia may be diagnosed as having IgM myeloma. The neoplastic plasma cells have a surface phenotype with characteristics that overlap with those of Waldenström macroglobulinemia and plasma cell myeloma. Plasma cells of IgM myeloma have high-level expression of CD38 but weak or negligible expression of CD5, CD10, CD20, CD22, CD23, CD45, HLA-DR, FMC7, and surface immunoglobulin.[8] Extramedullary plasmacytomas also may produce an excess in monoclonal IgM protein and have features in common with plasma cell myeloma. These conditions are discussed in Chap. 106.

B-LYMPHOCYTIC NEOPLASMS

Patients with low-grade B-cell lymphomas or B-cell chronic lymphocytic leukemia may have a monoclonal macroglobulinemia due to the IgM produced by the neoplastic B-cell clone. These diseases are discussed in Chaps. 103 and 98, respectively.

ESSENTIAL MONOCLONAL MACROGLOBULINEMIA

Patients may have monoclonal macroglobulinemia without associated anemia, lymphadenopathy, hepatosplenomegaly, bone lesions, or evidence of disease progression. Such patients are classified as having essential monoclonal macroglobulinemia, a subtype of essential monoclonal gammopathy. Patients with essential monoclonal gammopathy are at increased risk for developing plasma cell myeloma or Waldenström macroglobulinemia.[9] This condition is discussed in Chap. 105. Should the excess monoclonal IgM protein have binding activity for the "i" or "I" carbohydrate determinant found predominately on neonatal and adult erythrocytes, respectively, the macroglobulin may agglutinate red cells in the cold. Patients who have hemolytic anemia secondary to the continuous production of such autoantibodies have the cold agglutinin syndrome. This condition is discussed in Chap. 56.

ETIOLOGY AND PATHOGENESIS

ETIOLOGY

The etiology of Waldenström macroglobulinemia is unknown. Although there are a few reports of patients developing Waldenström macroglobulinemia years after radiation therapy,[10] a significant increase in incidence of this disease has not been noted in persons previously exposed to ionizing radiation or other environmental toxins.[11]

Hepatitis C infection has been associated with development of Waldenström macroglobulinemia.[12] An association between macroglobulinemia and hepatitis C infection was noted in a study of B-cell malignancies in Japan that included four patients with Waldenström macroglobulinemia.[13] Another report noted the unusual development of Waldenström macroglobulinemia in five young Americans of African descent with a median age of 38 that was associated with hepatitis C infection and a history of intravenous heroin and cocaine use.[14] The finding that patients with hepatitis C may have an associated macro-

Acronyms and abbreviations that appear in this chapter include: CLL, chronic lymphocytic anemia; IgM, immunoglobulin M.

globulinemia that can resolve after treatment with interferon alpha[15] suggests a possible relationship between uncontrolled hepatitis C infection and the development of Waldenström macroglobulinemia. However, it is controversial whether hepatitis C is involved in all or most of cases of macroglobulinemia.[16]

Some investigators have speculated that infection of marrow stromal dendritic cells by human herpesvirus type 8 (HHV-8), also known as Kaposi's sarcoma–associated herpesvirus, might be a key factor in the etiology and pathogenesis of monoclonal gammopathies, including Waldenström macroglobulinemia.[17,18] However, in one survey of 20 patients, only one was found to have evidence of HHV-8 in the marrow.[19]

Although an uncommon disease, Waldenström macroglobulinemia has been noted in the kindred of certain families[16,20–22] and in monozygotic twins.[23] Moreover, occasionally "unaffected" family members may have macroglobulinemia or other serum immunoglobulin abnormalities.[20,24] This has led some investigators to speculate that genetic factors contribute to the etiopathogenesis of this disease.

Various chromosomal abnormalities have been described in neoplastic cells of patients with Waldenström macroglobulinemia.[25–31] In one study of 19 patients, 89 percent were found to have chromosome abnormalities, most commonly involving chromosomes 9, 10, 11, and 12.[25] However, no one particular chromosomal abnormality is identified in the majority of patients with this disease. In this study, monosomy of chromosome 9 was associated with disease progression. In another study, a significant proportion of cases were found to carry the translocation t(9;14)(p13;q32) involving the PAX-5 gene.[32] Yet another study using nonstimulated short-term marrow cell cultures identified chromosomal abnormalities in only 15 percent of the patients with Waldenström macroglobulinemia.[31] Rearrangements in the long arm of chromosome 14, at band 32, also have been identified.[26,31,33] Abnormalities of chromosome 6, particularly partial deletions affecting 6q, have been detected using sensitive G-banding techniques (see Chap. 10).[28] Finally, the neoplastic cells of a few patients may be found to have mutations in the p53 tumor-suppressor gene that may be acquired during the evolution of the disease.[34]

PATHOGENESIS

Much of the morbidity associated with Waldenström macroglobulinemia is caused by the IgM produced by the neoplastic B cells. The blood viscosity increases when the concentration of IgM in the blood rises. High blood viscosity affects platelet function[35] and impairs capillary blood flow, reducing oxygen delivery through the microcirculation.[36] This may result in the patient developing the hyperviscosity syndrome, described below. High blood viscosity also has been associated with viscous pancreatic secretions, increasing the risk for developing pancreatitis.[37] In addition, high serum levels of macroglobulins may cause abnormal cerebrovascular permeability, either by a direct toxic effect or by way of viscosity-related ischemia. This may lead to infiltration of the cerebral parenchyma by IgM and lymphoplasmacytic cells, and, ultimately, focal degeneration of the white matter, resulting in leukoencephalopathy.[38]

Occasionally, the monoclonal IgM protein may react with self-antigens to cause disease.[39–41] For example, the monoclonal IgM may have rheumatoid factor activity or binding activity for the constant region of human IgG.[42] IgM rheumatoid factors may form immune complexes with IgG, especially at low temperatures, leading to complement activation and tissue destruction secondary to immune complex deposition.[43,44] Some patients can develop myopathy associated with monoclonal IgM proteins that react with muscle self-antigens.[45] More often, the IgM protein reacts with red blood cells, particularly at low temperatures, sometimes causing autoimmune hemolytic anemia (see

Chap. 56).[46] On rare occasions, the monoclonal IgM may react with platelets, causing immune thrombocytopenic purpura.[47]

Although in most cases the monoclonal IgM protein does not react with any specific antigen,[48] in some patients it reacts with the myelin-associated glycoprotein or other components of peripheral nerve sharing a common carbohydrate determinant with myelin-associated glycoprotein.[49–52] Other patients may have an IgM that reacts with chrondroitin sulfate C,[53] myelin basic protein,[54] or nerve glycolipids, such as GM1 ganglioside.[55–57] Patients with an IgM reactive with myelin-associated glycoprotein often develop a sensory demyelinating peripheral neuropathy, whereas elevated titers of anti-GM1 ganglioside antibodies are associated with lower motor neuron syndromes with multifocal motor conduction block.[57] The severity of neuropathy may be related to the level of monoclonal IgM autoantibody.

If the monoclonal IgM protein precipitates from the serum on cooling, it is called a cryoglobulin. Cryoglobulins in general may be classified as type I (monoclonal), type II (mixed), or type III (polyclonal). Monoclonal IgM of patients with Waldenström macroglobulinemia may be either type I or type II according to whether they form cryoprecipitates, respectively, by themselves or as an immune complex, usually with polyclonal IgG. Patients with cryoglobulinemia may develop cold hypersensitivity, particularly if the cryoglobulin precipitates at temperatures above 22°C (71.6°F) and is present at blood concentrations greater than 20 g/liter.[58]

In some patients, the abnormal monoclonal IgM protein interferes with hemostasis.[59,60] Coating of platelets by the monoclonal IgM protein may produce defects in platelet aggregation secondary to impaired release of platelet factor 3.[61] Also, some monoclonal IgM proteins bind coagulation factors and inhibit coagulation.[59] For example, some IgM proteins bind to fibrin and inhibit fibrin monomer aggregation, resulting in a bulky, gelatinous, transparent clot with impaired clot retraction.[43] When combined with impaired platelet function, this may produce a bleeding diathesis. Also, monoclonal IgM proteins have been noted to inhibit factor VIII, factor V, or factor VII.[59] Such IgM proteins also may lead to depletion of one or more coagulation factors in vivo. Finally, the plasma of Waldenström macroglobulinemia patients may have strong lupus anticoagulant activity if the monoclonal IgM has binding activity for the phosphatidylserine or phosphatidylethanolamine of cephalin.[62]

CLINICAL FEATURES

Generally, patients with Waldenström macroglobulinemia are in their sixth or seventh decade of life. The median age at diagnosis is 63 years.[4] Although occasionally young adults can develop Waldenström macroglobulinemia,[14] less than 3 percent of patients are under age 40. The disease is more common in men.

The patients most commonly present with complaints of fatigue, weakness, and weight loss. They also often note episodic bleeding, particularly from the gums and nasal mucosa. Patients also may present with symptoms and signs of the hyperviscosity syndrome.

The most common physical findings are lymphadenopathy and hepatosplenomegaly. It is common to find dependent purpura and evidence of bleeding from the mucosal surfaces of the gastrointestinal tract. Secondary to serum hyperviscosity, Waldenström macroglobulinemia patients often have dilated and tortuous retinal veins.

The physical properties of the IgM paraprotein may produce symptoms. Patients with cryoglobulinemia may complain of cold hypersensitivity, noting that exposure to low temperatures precipitates urticaria, purpura, acral cyanosis, or Raynaud phenomenon. Some patients may have multiple flesh-colored, sometimes pruritic papules on extensor skin surfaces secondary to skin deposition of monoclonal

IgM. In some cases, the IgM protein has been found to react with epidermal basement membrane antigens.[41,63]

Various skin lesions are associated with Waldenström macroglobulinemia. Patients can have purpura, ulcers, or urticarial lesions caused by hyperviscosity of the blood, immune complex-mediated vascular damage, paraprotein deposition, or amyloid deposition.[64] In addition, some patients have translucent, flesh-colored papules, resulting from monoclonal IgM deposits. When such deposits occur in the tarsal conjunctiva and tarsus, the patient can develop eyelid thickening and ptosis.[65] Some patients may develop a bullous dermatosis associated with the monoclonal IgM protein.[66,67] In such cases, deposits of the macroglobulin often can be found lining the subepidermis at the point of separation in the upper dermis, suggesting that the monoclonal IgM has an unusual reactivity for skin-associated antigens. Finally, a few patients may develop violaceous skin lesions composed of lymphoplasmacytic infiltrates. The latter cutaneous manifestations may be a harbinger that the disease is undergoing transformation into high-grade lymphoma.

Not infrequently, patients may develop a peripheral neuropathy. Most commonly, this produces symptoms of a slowly progressive, symmetric, and predominantly sensory peripheral neuropathy that affects the legs more severely than the arms.[68] These symptoms may antedate the diagnosis of Waldenström macroglobulinemia by several years and sometimes bear no defined relationship to the duration or severity of the macroglobulinemia, particularly if the monoclonal IgM protein does not react with nerve-associated antigens. Often one can detect high serum titers of antibodies to such antigens as myelin-associated glycoprotein.[68] However, nearly half of the macroglobulinemia patients with neuropathy have monoclonal IgM proteins that have no detectable reactivity with such nerve components, implying that the pathogenesis of macroglobulinemia-associated neuropathy is heterogeneous.

Occasionally, organ-system disease may develop from direct involvement by the neoplastic B cells. Some patients may have involvement of the gastrointestinal tract with B-cell lymphoma.[69–72] Furthermore, a few patients can have endobronchial lesions with direct infiltration of the pulmonary parenchyma by lymphocytes, plasma cells, and amyloid as the primary clinical manifestation of their disease.[73,74] Hilar and mediastinal lymphadenopathy is not uncommon in such settings.

A few patients with Waldenström macroglobulinemia may develop features of POEMS syndrome (polyneuropathy, organomegaly, endocrinopathy, monoclonal gammopathy, and skin changes),[75] a syndrome that more commonly is noted for patients with plasma cell myeloma (see Chap. 106).

THE HYPERVISCOSITY SYNDROME

Waldenström macroglobulinemia patients may develop a hyperviscosity syndrome. Although usually associated with severe macroglobulinemia, this syndrome also may be noted occasionally in patients with IgG or IgA myeloma (see Chap. 106).

Symptoms generally do not develop unless the serum viscosity is more than four times that of water.[36] However, plasma viscosity is not a perfect indicator of blood viscosity in macroglobulinemia, since red cell concentration also is an important determinant of blood viscosity.[76] Possibly secondary to an expanded plasma volume and increased intracranial pressure, headache is a common early symptom. Patients also may complain of visual blurring. Occasionally, these patients may have mental status changes, ranging from impaired mentation to frank dementia. Ataxia, nystagmus, vertigo, confusion, disturbances of consciousness progressing to coma, and a diffuse brain syndrome, sometimes designated coma paraproteinaemicum, also may develop

in patients with marked hyperviscosity. Patients with hyperviscosity-induced stroke[77] and dementia[78] who improve following plasmapheresis have been described. Secondary to anemia, an increased blood viscosity, and an expanded plasma volume, these patients also may develop symptoms and signs of congestive heart failure.

Funduscopic evaluation may reveal dilatation and segmentation of retinal and conjunctival vessels.[79] This may give the retinal veins a "link-sausage" appearance. In addition, these patients often are noted to have retinal hemorrhages and sometimes frank papilledema. Less commonly, patients may develop central retinal vein occlusion.[80]

LABORATORY FINDINGS

SERUM IMMUNOGLOBULIN AND BLOOD VISCOSITY

By definition, the serum IgM level is elevated in macroglobulinemia. The blood levels of the other immunoglobulin classes usually are normal or depressed. On serum protein electrophoresis, the serum IgM usually produces a tall, narrow peak or a dense band that migrates to the γ region of the serum electrophoresis pattern (see Chap. 104). Patients with macroglobulinemia who develop symptoms generally have serum IgM concentrations greater than 30 g/liter.

The IgM is usually a pentamer with a molecular weight of approximately 900,000 (see Chap. 83). Some patients also have a monomeric serum IgM protein of 165,000 molecular weight that diffuses more rapidly in a gel. This may create a double ring when the IgM is measured by immunodiffusion (see Chap. 104), causing some laboratories to overestimate of the amount of serum IgM.

The immunoglobulins expressed in Waldenström macroglobulinemia apparently constitute a skewed repertoire. The light chain of the monoclonal IgM is κ in 75 percent of patients.[4] In addition, these immunoglobulins often bear cross-reactive idiotypes that frequently are found on immunoglobulins expressed in chronic lymphocytic leukemia and by mantle zone B cells (see Chap. 98).[81]

The serum viscosity is elevated in most patients, but only 20 percent have symptoms related to hyperviscosity. Patients with a serum viscosity greater than four times that of water may develop the hyperviscosity syndrome. However, higher plasma viscosity can be offset by the anemia that commonly is associated with this disease. For this reason, blood rheology performed on whole blood at +32°C (+89.6°F) to +37°C (+98.6°F) at low shear rates may be the best indicator of the actual blood viscosity.[76]

BLOOD AND MARROW CELLS

Nearly four-fifths of the patients with Waldenström macroglobulinemia present with a hemoglobin concentration less than 120 g/liter.[4] Leukopenia also may be present at diagnosis. The platelet count may be depressed[47] but is usually in the normal range.

The anemia usually results from a mild decrease in red cell survival time and impaired erythropoiesis. The erythrocytes usually are normocytic and normochromic. However, the electronically measured mean corpuscular volume may be elevated spuriously due to erythrocyte aggregation. Also, the severity of the anemia often is exaggerated artificially due to an expanded plasma volume. This results from the increased oncotic pressure of plasma that contains an elevated concentration of IgM protein.[82]

The blood may contain a population of monoclonal B lymphocytes, even in asymptomatic patients.[83–85] By flow cytometric analysis, these cells express pan–B-lymphocyte surface antigens CD19, CD20, and CD24 (see Chap. 13) and are monoclonal, as defined by immunoglobulin light-chain expression, idiotype expression, or Southern blot analysis of the rearranged immunoglobulin genes. Unlike normal circulating B cells, the monoclonal B cells often express CD5, CD10 (CALLA), CD11b, and CD9 and are heterogeneous in their expression of CD45 isoforms that are found on B cells at various stages of differentiation.[85,86] The latter observation has been interpreted to indicate ongoing differentiation within the monoclonal B-cell population. The size of the circulating monoclonal B-lymphocyte population correlates with the clinical course of the disease, increasing in those who fail to respond or who progress.

The marrow aspirate often is hypocellular. However, marrow biopsy specimens generally are hypercellular and diffusely infiltrated with lymphocytes, plasmacytoid lymphocytes, and some plasma cells.[87] Similar to the marrow in chronic lymphocytic leukemia (see Chap. 98), different patterns of marrow infiltration can be delineated. In a retrospective survey of patient marrow specimens, the patterns of lymphocyte infiltration were diffuse (seen in 45%), nodular-interstitial (22%), mixed paratrabecular-nodular (20%), and paratrabecular (13%).[88] Mast cells also are often increased in number. The lymphocytes tend to be small, basophilic, and well-differentiated cells, often resembling plasma cells. Periodic acid–Schiff-positive material (Dutcher bodies) may be seen occasionally in lymphoid cells, in the interstitium, and in blood vessel walls. The lymphocytes, plasmacytoid lymphocytes, and plasma cells are monoclonal by an analysis of surface membrane and cytoplasmic immunoglobulins, using antisera that react specifically with the idiotype of the patient's IgM.[89] The monoclonal cells, however, are of different levels of maturity, consisting of small lymphocytes carrying surface IgM/IgD, or IgM plasmacytoid cells and mature plasma cells with only cytoplasmic IgM.

DISORDERS OF HEMOSTASIS

The clotting abnormality detected most frequently is prolongation of the thrombin time.[43] Less frequently, a patient's plasma may have an elevated prothrombin time or activated partial thromboplastin time secondary to depletion of a coagulation factor or factors or presence of lupus anticoagulant.[59,62]

Platelet function often is impaired, resulting in a prolonged bleeding time, impaired clot retraction, defective prothrombin consumption, poor thromboplastin generation with the patient's platelets, defective platelet aggregation in vivo, and defective platelet adhesion in vitro.[35,61,90]

RENAL ABNORMALITIES

Renal insufficiency is less frequent in patients with Waldenström macroglobulinemia than in patients with plasma cell myeloma,[91] although the blood urea nitrogen is elevated above 8 mmol/liter (25 mg/dl) in about one-third of patients.[92,93] The urine of nearly 80 percent of patients has detectable immunoglobulin light chains that apparently are produced by the population of monoclonal B cells.[4,94] However, since the amount of light chain excreted rarely exceeds 2.0 g/24 h,[93] its detection generally requires that the urine sample be concentrated prior to zonal electrophoresis or immunoelectrophoresis.

Glomerular lesions are more frequent in patients with Waldenström macroglobulinemia than in those with myeloma. IgM may precipitate on the endothelial side of the glomerular basement membrane, forming deposits that are so large that they occlude the glomerular capillaries. In the renal parenchyma of a minority of patients there may exist amyloid deposits and interstitial infiltrates of lymphocytes and plasma cells similar to those found in the marrow.[93]

Some patients may develop an immunologically mediated glomerulonephritis associated with the nephrotic syndrome. One patient was noted to have monoclonal granular deposits of IgM, IgG, and the third component of complement along the glomerular basement membrane that was associated with a low serum complement level.[95] Another was found to have a monoclonal IgM that reacted with glomerular antigens, resulting in the deposition of IgM in glomerular and interstitial capillaries.[96]

DIFFERENTIAL DIAGNOSIS

It is important to distinguish patients with essential monoclonal macroglobulinemia from those with Waldenström macroglobulinemia or IgM myeloma.[97] The clinical and laboratory findings presented in Table 108-1 are helpful in making this distinction. In addition to being symptomatic, patients with IgM-producing lymphoplasmacytic neoplasms usually have anemia, a monoclonal IgM protein level greater than 30 g/liter, increased serum viscosity, and symptoms and signs that progress over time. For this reason, patients deemed to have essential monoclonal macroglobulinemia should receive follow-up evaluation for evidence of disease progression.

Monoclonal macroglobulinemia can develop in patients with a variety of lymphoid neoplasms. Patients with chronic lymphocytic leukemia generally have a monoclonal B-cell lymphocytosis of more than $5000/\mu l$ (5×10^9/liter). In contrast to the abnormal blood B cells of patients with Waldenström macroglobulinemia, the leukemic B cells of patients with CLL do not express CD10 (CALLA) and do not have lymphoplasmacytic features by morphology (see Chap. 98). Patients with lymphoma may be diagnosed by biopsy of a lymph node or other tissue (see Chap. 103). Lytic skeletal lesions and hypercalcemia indicate that the monoclonal macroglobulinemia is secondary to IgM myeloma (see Chap. 106).

THERAPY, COURSE, AND PROGNOSIS

THERAPY

Waldenström macroglobulinemia is an incurable disease. Therefore, therapy is directed toward prevention and/or palliation of the associated clinical sequelae of macroglobulinemia.

Asymptomatic patients may be followed without specific therapy. These patients should be evaluated periodically, however, for reduction in hemoglobin, rise in serum IgM, deterioration in renal function, or other clinical manifestations of the disease, such as hyperviscosity, lymphadenopathy, hepatosplenomegaly, bleeding tendencies, or neurologic changes. Symptomatic patients should receive chemotherapy.[97]

ALKYLATOR THERAPY

Chlorambucil is an effective agent. Patients may receive an initial daily dose of 2 to 8 mg orally. Alternatively, patients may receive oral high-dose intermittent chlorambucil of 0.7 mg/kg on day 1, or 0.2 to 0.3 mg/kg on days 1 through 4. This often is administered with 40 to 60 mg prednisone on days 1 through 4. This cycle may be repeated every 21 to 28 days. Hematologic monitoring is essential. The initial dose often needs to be altered, depending on the platelet and leukocyte count and the therapeutic response. Unfortunately, no randomized trials comparing the effectiveness of treatment for symptomatic macroglobulinemia have been reported.

The M-2 protocol (carmustine, cyclophosphamide, vincristine, melphalan, and prednisone) also may be effective for patients with this disease. In one institution, 33 patients with symptomatic Waldenström macroglobulinemia received therapy every 5 weeks for 2 years and every 10 weeks for an additional 1 to 3 years.[98] Responses were observed in 27 patients (81%), of whom 21 (63%) had partial responses. Survival ranged from 1 to 120+ months, with 58 percent of patients projected to be alive at 10 years.

In another institution, 34 patients with Waldenström macroglobulinemia received 7 days of oral melphalan (6 mg/m^2), cyclophosphamide (125 mg/m^2), and prednisone (40 mg/m^2).[99] Courses were repeated every 4 to 6 weeks for a total of 12 courses. Responding patients subsequently received continuous treatment with chlorambucil and prednisone until relapse. Following the induction, 23 of 31 evaluated patients (74%) responded to induction therapy, and 8 (26% of the 31 evaluated patients) achieved a complete remission.

TABLE 108-1   DISTINCTIONS BETWEEN ESSENTIAL VERSUS WALDENSTRÖM MACROGLOBULINEMIA

	ESSENTIAL MACROGLOBULINEMIA	WALDENSTRÖM MACROGLOBULINEMIA
Symptoms	Usually none, but may have peripheral neuropathy or cold sensitivity	Fatigue, weight loss, headache, epistaxis, neurologic symptoms, or cold hypersensitivity
Physical findings	Usually none	Hepatosplenomegaly, purpura, lymphadenopathy, Raynaud, neurologic signs, retinopathy
Laboratory findings		
IgM protein (g/liter)	Usually <30 and stable	Often >30 and increasing
Hemoglobin (g/liter)	Usually >120	<120 in 80% of patients
Serum viscosity	Normal	Increased

NUCLEOSIDE ANALOGUES

2-Chlorodeoxyadenosine (Cladribine)

The adenine nucleoside analogue 2-chlorodeoxyadenosine (cladribine) is an effective agent in the treatment of patients with newly diagnosed or refractory Waldenström macroglobulinemia. This drug usually is administered as a continuous intravenous infusion at a dose of 0.1 mg/kg body weight per day for 7 days. This is often repeated 1 month later. In some cases, repeated treatments are given at monthly intervals to patients who fail to respond adequately to the first two courses.

Using this regimen, over 40 percent of the patients who are refractory to an alkylating agent therapy can experience reduction in IgM macroglobulinemia and resolution of symptoms.[100] In one study, 46 alkylator-refractory patients received two courses of cladribine. Twenty of the patients (43%) had an objective response, with a median progression-free survival of 12 months. A higher response frequency was noted in patients with disease relapsing off therapy (78%) or with primary resistant disease within the first year (57%) than in those with later phases of disease (22%). The median survival after treatment was 28 months and the median progression-free survival of responding patients was 12 months.[101]

Patients who had not received any prior chemotherapy had even higher response rates. Twenty-six previously untreated but symptomatic patients with Waldenström macroglobulinemia each received two courses of cladribine, and responding patients were followed up without further therapy until relapse. Twenty-two of 26 patients responded (85%; 95% confidence interval, 65–96%), including 3 patients who achieved a complete response and 19 patients who had a partial response. A similar high response rate was noted in a study of 10 previously nontreated patients with Waldenström macroglobulinemia.[102] The response rates are higher than that achieved using chlorambucil and prednisone or other nucleoside analogues. Nevertheless, patients who are refractory to fludarabine generally do not respond to cladribine and vice versa.[103]

Alternative methods for administering cladribine to patients with Waldenström macroglobulinemia have been examined. In one study 20 patients, including 7 who were not treated previously, each were given 2 h of intravenous infusion of cladribine at 0.12 mg/kg each day for 5 consecutive days. Three cycles were given to all patients at monthly intervals. Responding patients received an additional fourth cycle.[104] One patient achieved a complete response (5%) and 10 achieved a partial response (50%). Overall, 4 of 7 (57%) untreated and 7 of 13 (54%) previously treated patients responded. The median duration of response follow-up was 28 months (range, 1–37 months). In another study, cladribine was given as subcutaneous bolus injections. In this phase II multi-institutional study, 25 patients received cycles of 0.5 mg/kg of cladribine administered in 5 equal daily subcutaneous bolus injections.[105] All but one patient had been treated previously with more than one regimen (median 2, range 0–10). Ten patients (40%) achieved a partial remission. Maximum responses were reached no later than the third cycle. Median time to treatment failure

and remission duration were 4.4 (range, 0.5–33) and 8 months (range, 5–29), respectively. These response rates are similar to those of patients who received the drug via continuous intravenous infusion through an indwelling central catheter. However, another study suggests that such alternative modes of drug delivery may be associated with higher rates of significant myelosuppression and less efficacy in the treatment of Waldenström macroglobulinemia than in continuous intravenous infusion.[106]

Cladribine has been used in combination with cyclophosphamide and prednisone in the treatment of macroglobulinemia. In one study of indolent lymphoproliferative disease in 19 patients that included 3 with macroglobulinemia, the subjects received cladribine at a dose of 0.1 mg/kg per day as a subcutaneous bolus injection on days 1 through 3.[107] In addition, they were given intravenous cyclophosphamide at a dose of 500 mg/m^2 on day 1 and oral prednisone 40 mg/m^2 on days 1 through 5. This course was repeated every 4 weeks up to a maximum of six courses. The overall response rate was 88 percent, with only four (21%) achieving a complete clinical remission. Two patients developed grade 4 neutropenia, and one had grade 3 infection. During the follow-up, five patients had greater than grade 3 hematologic toxicity, and another five had grade 3 nonhematologic toxicity.

The major toxicity of cladribine is acute myelosuppression and chronic immune suppression secondary to depletion of CD4+ T cells. This results in a higher risk of both common and opportunistic infections in patients after treatment with this drug.[108] One case report described a patient who, following treatment with cladribine, developed Epstein-Barr-virus–associated lymphoproliferative disease and lymphoma similar to that seen in posttransplant patients receiving systemic immunosuppressive therapy.[109]

Fludarabine

The adenine nucleoside analogue fludarabine also is effective in the treatment of Waldenström macroglobulinemia. This drug generally is given as a daily intravenous dose of 25 mg/m^2 for 5 days every 4 weeks. Many patients receive up to six courses of treatment, although fewer courses also may be effective.

Fludarabine is effective in treating patients who are refractory to alkylating agent therapy. Twenty-six patients with Waldenström macroglobulinemia who were resistant to therapy with chlorambucil received fludarabine.[110] Of these, 31 percent responded, achieving a nonmaintained remission that lasted for a median of 38 months. In another institution, fludarabine was given to 11 patients, 10 of whom had failed prior standard chemotherapy.[111] Five patients (45%) responded with more than a 50 percent reduction of IgM tumor mass for a projected median duration of longer than 1 year. This response rate is similar to that noted in another study of 12 alkylator-refractory patients (5 of 12 responders, or 41%).[112] Finally, in a more recent study of 71 patients who were resistant to alkylator therapy, 21 (30%) achieved a partial response and 50 (70%) were considered treatment failures after a median of six courses of fludarabine.[113] The overall median survival time of all treated patients was 23 months, and the time to treatment failure was 32 months. The only factor that favorably influenced the response to fludarabine was a longer interval between the first treatment and the start of fludarabine. Pretreatment factors associated with shorter survival in the entire population were hemoglobin level less than 95 g/liter ($P = .02$) and platelet count less than 75×10^9/liter ($P = .02$). These studies indicate that fludarabine is an effective agent for patients with Waldenström macroglobulinemia, with response rates in alkylator-resistant patients that are similar to those of cladribine.[112,114]

Higher response rates to fludarabine are noted in previously non-treated patients.[110] In a phase II multicenter trial, newly diagnosed and nontreated patients were given single-agent intravenous fludarabine until they achieved a maximum response, plus two further cycles as consolidation.[115] Myelosuppression was relatively common, and the treatment-related mortality rate was 5 percent, mostly associated with pancytopenia and infection. This regimen yielded an overall response rate of 63 percent in patients with macroglobulinemia (and a 15% complete response rate), with a median duration of response of approximately 2.5 years.[115]

After treatment with fludarabine, patients may be at increased risk for developing opportunistic infections.[116] One case report described a patient who, following treatment with fludarabine, developed watery diarrhea, nausea, and vomiting secondary to uncontrolled infection with astrovirus that was successfully treated with intravenous immuno-globulin infusions.[117]

MARROW TRANSPLANTATION

Marrow transplantation has been tried in only a few patients, with anecdotal success. Two patients with aggressive Waldenström macroglobulinemia who progressed in spite of multiagent chemotherapy and autologous stem cell transplantation underwent allogeneic stem cell transplantation using stem cells from HLA-matched donors.[118] The patients were reported to be alive with event-free survivals of 3 and 9 years, respectively.

PLASMAPHERESIS

Patients with symptomatic hyperviscosity should be treated with plasmapheresis. In some cases, plasmapheresis can be used to alleviate the autoimmune pathology resulting from a self-reactive monoclonal IgM protein.[119] Conventional plasma exchange is superior to cascade filtration, in which proteins are removed as a function of their size.[120] Daily plasma exchanges of 3000 to 4000 ml with albumin, rather than plasma, are particularly effective in reducing the serum IgM level and serum viscosity.[36,121] This often is initiated concomitantly with chemotherapy to reduce the production of the abnormal monoclonal IgM protein.

RED CELL TRANSFUSIONS

Patients with Waldenström macroglobulinemia may require periodic transfusions of packed red cells because of symptomatic anemia. However, it should be recognized that these patients often have artificially low hemoglobin and hematocrit levels due to an expanded plasma volume. Consequently, these patients should not receive red cell transfusions simply on the basis of low hemoglobin. Moreover, because of the increased serum viscosity of macroglobulinemia, these patients actually may have reduced capillary blood flow following transfusions of packed red cells due to increased blood viscosity. For this reason, patients with symptomatic hyperviscosity should not be transfused unless therapy is implemented to reduce the serum IgM level. In addition, patients should be monitored for signs of fluid overload or congestive heart failure prior to and during red cell transfusion. Packed red cells should be administered slowly, at a rate not to exceed 1 unit per 2-h period.

COURSE AND PROGNOSIS

Waldenström macroglobulinemia is an indolent disease that generally progresses over a period of years. The median survival from diagnosis is approximately 5 years.[4] However, the clinical course is variable. Features that are associated with poorer prognosis are hemoglobin levels below 9 g/dl, age of greater than 70 years, weight loss, and cryoglobulinemia.[122] Patients with the worse prognosis have at diagnosis two or more of these features or any one associated with low platelet count, splenomegaly, lymphadenopathy, and/or high levels of serum macroglobulin.[88] Elevated serum beta-2-microglobulin also may be associated with a poorer prognosis. However, marrow histology or plasma cell expression of proliferating cell nuclear antigen does not have an apparent relationship to survival.[88]

Hyperviscosity, anemia, hemorrhage, thrombosis, or infections often are contributory causes of death. Neoplastic lymphocytes may infiltrate the liver, spleen, marrow, lymph nodes, lung, skin, and/or gastrointestinal mucosa. In some patients, the concentration of IgM paraprotein may fall as the tumor burden increases. Further dedifferentiation of the neoplastic cells and loss of their ability to produce IgM protein may explain this effect. This suggests that the neoplastic cells may dedifferentiate and lose their ability to produce IgM protein. This often is associated with an accelerated deterioration in the clinical course. In some cases, the disease evolves into a high-grade lymphoma with characteristics similar to those of Richter transformation in chronic lymphocytic leukemia.[123,124] In such cases, the patient may develop hypercalcemia or infiltrative skin lesions as an early manifestation of the transformation to high-grade lymphoma.[64,124] Some patients develop acute myelogenous leukemia,[125–127] immunoblastic sarcoma,[128–130] or chronic myelogenous leukemia[131] as a preterminal event. Most of these cases have occurred after treatment with alkylating agents.

REFERENCES

1. Baldini L, Guffanti A, Cesana BM, et al: Role of different hematologic variables in defining the risk of malignant transformation in monoclonal gammopathy. *Blood* 87:912, 1996.
2. Herrinton LJ: The epidemiology of monoclonal gammopathy of unknown significance: A review. *Curr Top Microbiol Immunol* 210:389, 1996.
3. Fuleihan RL: The X-linked hyperimmunoglobulin M syndrome. *Semin Hematol* 35:321, 1998.
4. Kyle RA, Garton JP: The spectrum of IgM monoclonal gammopathy in 430 cases. *Mayo Clin Proc* 62:719, 1987.
5. Waldenström J: Incipient myelomatosis or "essential" hyperglobulinemia with fibrinogenopenia: A new syndrome? *Acta Med Scand* 117:216, 1944.
6. Kyle RA, Anderson KC: A tribute to Jan Gosta Waldenström [editorial]. *Blood* 89:4245, 1997.
7. Groves FD, Travis LB, Devesa SS, et al: Waldenström's macroglobulinemia: Incidence patterns in the United States, 1988–1994. *Cancer* 82:1078, 1998.
8. Haghighi B, Yanagihara R, Cornbleet PJ: IgM myeloma: Case report with immunophenotypic profile. *Am J Hematol* 59:302, 1998.
9. Isaksson E, Björkholm M, Holm G, et al: Blood clonal B-cell excess in patients with monoclonal gammopathy of undetermined significance (MGUS): Association with malignant transformation. *Br J Haematol* 92:71, 1996.
10. Epenetos AA, Rohatiner A, Slevin M, Woothipoom W: Ankylosing spondylitis and Waldenström's macroglobulinaemia: A case report. *Clin Oncol* 6:83, 1980.
11. Tepper A, Moss CE: Waldenström's macroglobulinemia: Search for occupational exposure. *J Occup Med* 36:133, 1994.

12. Silvestri F, Barillari G, Fanin R, et al: Risk of hepatitis C virus infection, Waldenström's macroglobulinemia, and monoclonal gammopathies. *Blood* 88:1125, 1996.

13. Izumi T, Sasaki R, Tsunoda S, et al: B cell malignancy and hepatitis C virus infection. *Leukemia* 11(suppl)3:516, 1997.

14. Ahmed S, Shurafa MS, Bishop CR, Varterasian M: Waldenström's macroglobulinemia in young African-American adults. *Am J Hematol* 60:229, 1999.

15. Schott P, Pott C, Ramadori G, Hartmann H: Hepatitis C virus infection-associated noncryoglobulinaemic monoclonal IgM-kappa gammopathy responsive to interferon-alpha treatment. *J Hepatol* 29:310, 1998.

16. Custodi P, Cerutti A, Cassani P, et al: Familial occurrence of IgMκ gammopathy: No involvement of HCV infection [letter]. *Haematologica* 80:484, 1995.

17. Agbalika F, Mariette X, Marolleau JP, et al: Detection of human herpesvirus-8 DNA in bone marrow biopsies from patients with multiple myeloma and Waldenström's macroglobulinemia [letter]. *Blood* 91:4393, 1998.

18. Mikala G, Xie J, Berencsi G, et al: Human herpesvirus 8 in hematologic diseases. *Pathol Oncol Res* 5:73, 1999.

19. Brousset P, Theriault C, Roda D, et al: Kaposi's sarcoma-associated herpesvirus (KSHV) in bone marrow biopsies of patients with Waldenström's macroglobulinaemia. *Br J Haematol* 102:795, 1998.

20. Blattner WA, Garber JE, Mann DL, et al: Waldenström's macroglobulinemia and autoimmune disease in a family. *Ann Intern Med* 93:830, 1980.

21. Renier G, Ifrah N, Chevailler A, et al: Four brothers with Waldenström's macroglobulinemia. *Cancer* 64:1554, 1989.

22. Ogmundsdóttir HM, Jóhannesson GM, Sveinsdóttir S, et al: Familial macroglobulinaemia: Hyperactive B-cells but normal natural killer function [published errata appear in Scand J Immunol 41:650, 1995]. *Scand J Immunol* 40:195, 1994.

23. Fine JM, Muller JY, Rochu D, et al: Waldenström's macroglobulinemia in monozygotic twins. *Acta Med Scand.* 220:369, 1986.

24. Taleb N, Tohme A, Abi Jirgiss D, et al: Familial macroglobulinemia in a Lebanese family with two sisters presenting with Waldenström's disease. *Acta Oncol* 30:703, 1991.

25. Palka G, Spadano A, Geraci L, et al: Chromosome changes in 19 patients with Waldenström's macroglobulinemia. *Cancer Genet Cytogenet* 29:261, 1987.

26. Nishida K, Taniwaki M, Misawa S, Abe T: Nonrandom rearrangement of chromosome 14 at band q32.33 in human lymphoid malignancies with mature B-cell phenotype. *Cancer Res* 49:1275, 1989.

27. Carbone P, Caradonna F, Granata G, et al: Chromosomal abnormalities in Waldenström's macroglobulinemia. *Cancer Genet Cytogenet* 61:147, 1992.

28. White AD, Clark RE, Jacobs A: Isochromosome (6p) in Waldenström's macroglobulinemia. *Cancer Genet Cytogenet* 58:89, 1992.

29. Johansson B, Waldenström J, Hasselblom S, Mitelman F: Waldenström's macroglobulinemia with the AML/MDS-associated t(1;3)(p36;q21). *Leukemia* 9:1136, 1995.

30. Panayiotidis P, Kotsi P: Genetics of small lymphocyte disorders. *Semin Hematol* 36:171, 1999.

31. Calasanz MJ, Cigudosa JC, Odero MD, et al: Cytogenetic analysis of 280 patients with multiple myeloma and related disorders: Primary breakpoints and clinical correlations. *Genes Chromosomes Cancer* 18:84, 1997.

32. Pangalis GA, Angelopoulou MK, Vassilakopoulos TP, et al: B-chronic lymphocytic leukemia, small lymphocytic lymphoma, and lymphoplasmacytic lymphoma, including Waldenström's macroglobulinemia: A clinical, morphologic, and biologic spectrum of similar disorders. *Semin Hematol* 36:104, 1999.

33. Chong YY, Lau LC, Lui WO, et al: A case of t(8;14) with total and partial trisomy 3 in Waldenström macroglobulinemia. *Cancer Genet Cytogenet* 103:65, 1998.

34. Sugimoto K, Toyoshima H, Sakai R, et al: Mutations of the p53 gene in lymphoid leukemia. *Blood* 77:1153, 1991.

35. van Breugel HF, de Groot PG, Heethaar RM, Sixma JJ: Role of plasma viscosity in platelet adhesion. *Blood* 80:953, 1992.

36. Reinhart WH, Lutolf O, Nydegger UR, et al: Plasmapheresis for hyperviscosity syndrome in macroglobulinemia Waldenström and multiple myeloma: Influence on blood rheology and the microcirculation. *J Lab Clin Med* 119:69, 1992.

37. Hertan HI, Pitchumoni CS: Chronic calcific pancreatitis in a patient with Waldenström's macroglobulinemia. *Am J Gastroenterol* 86:633, 1991.

38. Scheithauer BW, Rubinstein LJ, Herman MM: Leukoencephalopathy in Waldenström's macroglobulinemia: Immunohistochemical and electron microscopic observations. *J Neuropathol Exp Neurol* 43:408, 1984.

39. Waldenström JG: Antibody activity of monoclonal immunoglobulins in myeloma, macroglobulinemia and benign gammopathy. *Med Oncol Tumor Pharmacother* 3:135, 1986.

40. Merlini G, Farhangi M, Osserman EF: Monoclonal immunoglobulins with antibody activity in myeloma, macroglobulinemia and related plasma cell dyscrasias. *Semin Oncol* 13:350, 1986.

41. Cobb MW, Domloge-Hultsch N, Frame JN, Yancey KB: Waldenström macroglobulinemia with an IgM-kappa antiepidermal basement membrane zone antibody. *Arch Dermatol* 128:372, 1992.

42. Artandi SE, Canfield SM, Tao MH, et al: Molecular analysis of IgM rheumatoid factor binding to chimeric IgG. *J Immunol* 146:603, 1991.

43. Coleman M, Vigliano EM, Weksler ME, Nachman RL: Inhibition of fibrin monomer polymerization by lambda myeloma globulins. *Blood* 39:210, 1972.

44. Vital A, Vital C: Immunoelectron identification of endoneurial IgM deposits in four patients with Waldenström's macroglobulinemia: A specific ultrastructural pattern related to the presence of cryoglobulin in one case. *Clin Neuropathol* 12:49, 1993.

45. al-Lozi MT, Pestronk A, Yee WC, Flaris N: Myopathy and paraproteinemia with serum IgM binding to a high-molecular-weight muscle fiber surface protein. *Ann Neurol* 37:41, 1995.

46. Gologan R, Dima I, Butoianu E, et al: Autoimmune hemolytic anemia with warm antibodies complicated with an intercurrent attack of hemolysis with cold agglutinins in a case of Waldenström disease. *Rom J Intern Med* 34:149, 1996.

47. Varticovski L, Pick AI, Schattner A, Shoenfeld Y: Anti-platelet and anti-DNA IgM in Waldenström macroglobulinemia and ITP. *Am J Hematol* 24:351, 1987.

48. Lacroix-Desmazes S, Mouthon L, Pashov A, et al: Analysis of antibody reactivities toward self-antigens of IgM of patients with Waldenström's macroglobulinemia. *Int Immunol* 9:1175, 1997.

49. Nobile-Orazio E, Francomano E, Daverio R, et al: Anti-myelin-associated glycoprotein IgM antibody titers in neuropathy associated with macroglobulinemia. *Ann Neurol* 26:543, 1989.

50. Vrethem M, Cruz M, Wen-Xin H, et al: Clinical, neurophysiological and immunological evidence of polyneuropathy in patients with monoclonal gammopathies. *J Neurol Sci* 114:193, 1993.

51. Vital C, Vital A, Deminiere C, et al: Myelin modifications in 8 cases of peripheral neuropathy with Waldenström's macroglobulinemia and anti-MAG activity. *Ultrastructural Pathol* 21:509, 1997.

52. Steck A: Neurological manifestations of malignant and non-malignant dysglobulinaemias. *J Neurol* 245:634, 1998.

53. Sherman WH, Latov N, Hays AP, et al: Monoclonal IgM kappa antibody precipitating with chondroitin sulfate C from patients with axonal polyneuropathy and epidermolysis. *Neurology* 33:192, 1983.

54. Kira J, Inuzuka T, Hozumi I, et al: A novel monoclonal antibody which reacts with a high molecular weight neuronal cytoplasmic protein and myelin basic protein (MBP) in a patient with macroglobulinemia. *J Neurol Sci* 148:47, 1997.

55. Ilyas AA, Quarles RH, Dalakas MC, Brady RO: Polyneuropathy with monoclonal gammopathy: Glycolipids are frequently antigens for IgM paraproteins. *Proc Natl Acad Sci USA* 82:6697, 1985.

56. Lieberman F, Marton LS, Stefansson K: Pattern of reactivity of IgM from the sera of eight patients with IgM monoclonal gammopathy and neuropathy with components of neural tissues: Evidence for interaction with more than one epitope. *Acta Neuropathol (Berlin)* 68:6, 1985.

57. Bosch EP, Smith BE: Peripheral neuropathies associated with monoclonal proteins. *Med Clin North Am* 77:125, 1993.

58. Letendre L, Kyle RA: Monoclonal cryoglobulinemia with high thermal insolubility. *Mayo Clin Proc* 57:629, 1982.

59. Lackner H: Hemostatic abnormalities associated with dysproteinemias. *Semin Hematol* 10:125, 1973.

60. Harbord M, Ivanova S, Akhtar N, Gupta Y: Waldenström macroglobulinaemia presenting as bleeding diathesis with paradoxical coagulation of blood samples. *J Accid Emerg Med* 15:331, 1998.

61. Penny R, Castaldi PA, Whitsed HM: Inflammation and haemostasis in paraproteinaemias. *Br J Haematol* 20:35, 1971.

62. Wisloff F, Michaelsen TE, Godal HC: Monoclonal IgM with lupus anticoagulant activity in a case of Waldenström's macroglobulinaemia. *Eur J Haematol* 38:456, 1987.

63. Lowe L, Fitzpatrick JE, Huff JC, et al: Cutaneous macroglobulinosis: A case report with unique ultrastructural findings. *Arch Dermatol* 128:377, 1992.

64. Appenzeller P, Leith CP, Foucar K, et al: Cutaneous Waldenström macroglobulinemia in transformation. *Am J Dermatopathol* 21:151, 1999.

65. Klapper SR, Jordan DR, Pelletier C, et al: Ptosis in Waldenström's macroglobulinemia. *Am J Ophthalmol* 126:315, 1998.

66. Whittaker SJ, Bhogal BS, Black MM: Acquired immunobullous disease: A cutaneous manifestation of IgM macroglobulinaemia. *Br J Dermatol* 135:283, 1996.

67. West NY, Fitzpatrick JE, David-Bajar KM, Bennion SD: Waldenström macroglobulinemia-induced bullous dermatosis. *Arch Dermatol* 134:1127, 1998.

68. Rudnicki SA, Harik SI, Dhodapkar M, et al: Nervous system dysfunction in Waldenström's macroglobulinemia: Response to treatment. *Neurology* 51:1210, 1998.

69. Rosenthal JA, Curran WJ Jr, Schuster SJ: Waldenström's macroglobulinemia resulting from localized gastric lymphoplasmacytoid lymphoma. *Am J Hematol* 58:244, 1998.

70. Qutub HM, Wilbur AC, Dada S: Gastric involvement in Waldenström macroglobulinemia: CT findings. *Abdom Imaging* 22:461, 1997.

71. Yasui O, Tukamoto F, Sasaki N, et al: Malignant lymphoma of the transverse colon associated with macroglobulinemia. *Am J Gastroenterol* 92:2299, 1997.

72. Kaila VL, el-Newihi HM, Dreiling BJ, et al: Waldenström's macroglobulinemia of the stomach presenting with upper gastrointestinal hemorrhage. *Gastrointest Endosc* 44:73, 1996.

73. Fadil A, Taylor DE: The lung and Waldenström's macroglobulinemia. *South Med J* 91:681, 1998.

74. Zatloukal P, Bezdícek P, Schimonová M, et al: Waldenström's macroglobulinemia with pulmonary amyloidosis. *Respiration* 65:414, 1998.

75. Pavord SR, Murphy PT, Mitchell VE: POEMS syndrome and Waldenström's macroglobulinaemia. *J Clin Pathol* 49:181, 1996.

76. Persson SU, Larsson H, Odeberg H: How should blood rheology be measured in macroglobulinaemia? *Scand J Clin Lab Invest* 58:669, 1998.

77. Pavy MD, Murphy PL, Virella G: Paraprotein-induced hyperviscosity: A reversible cause of stroke. *Postgrad Med* 68:109, 1980.

78. Mueller J, Hotson JR, Langston JW: Hyperviscosity-induced dementia. *Neurology* 33:101, 1983.

79. Lekhra OP, Sawhney IM, Gupta A, et al: Venous stasis retinopathy in Waldenström's macroglobulinemia. *J Assoc Physicians India* 44:61, 1996.

80. Avashia JH, Fath DF: Bilateral central retinal vein occlusion in Waldenström's macroglobulinemia. *J Am Optom Assoc* 60:657, 1989.

81. Axelrod O, Silverman GJ, Dev V, et al: Idiotypic cross-reactivity of immunoglobulins expressed in Waldenström's macroglobulinemia, chronic lymphocytic leukemia, and mantle zone lymphocytes of secondary B-cell follicles. *Blood* 77:1484, 1991.

82. MacKenzie MR, Fudenberg HH: Macroglobulinemia: An analysis for forty patients. *Blood* 39:874, 1972.

83. Smith BR, Robert NJ, Ault KA: In Waldenström's macroglobulinemia the quantity of detectable circulating monoclonal B lymphocytes correlates with clinical course. *Blood* 61:911, 1983.

84. Pilarski LM, Andrews EJ, Serra HM, et al: Abnormalities in lymphocyte profile and specificity repertoire of patients with Waldenström's macroglobulinemia, multiple myeloma, and IgM monoclonal gammopathy of undetermined significance. *Am J Hematol* 30:53, 1989.

85. Jensen GS, Andrews EJ, Mant MJ, et al: Transitions in CD45 isoform expression indicate continuous differentiation of a monoclonal CD5+ CD11b+ B lineage in Waldenström's macroglobulinemia. *Am J Hematol* 37:20, 1991.

86. Jensen GS, Poppema S, Mant MJ, Pilarski LM: Transition in CD45 isoform expression during differentiation of normal and abnormal B cells. *Int Immunol* 1:229, 1989.

87. Rywlin AM, Civantos F, Ortega RS, Dominguez CJ: Bone marrow histology in monoclonal macroglobulinemia. *Am J Clin Pathol* 63:769, 1975.

88. Andriko JA, Aguilera NS, Chu WS, et al: Waldenström's macroglobulinemia: A clinicopathologic study of 22 cases. *Cancer* 80:1926, 1997.

89. Pettersson D, Mellstedt H, Holm G: Characterization of the monoclonal blood and bone marrow B lymphocytes in Waldenström's macroglobulinaemia. *Scand J Immunol* 11:593, 1980.

90. Doumenc J, Prost RJ, Samama M, Bousser J: [Anomalies of platelet aggregation during Waldenström's disease (apropos of 3 cases).] Anomalie de l'agregation plaquettaire au cours de la maladie de Waldenström (à-propos de 3 cas). *Nouv Rev Fr Hematol* 6:734, 1966.

91. Kyle RA: Monoclonal gammopathies and the kidney. *Annu Rev Med* 40:53, 1989.

92. Krajny M, Pruzanski W: Waldenström's macroglobulinemia: Review of 45 cases. *Can Med Assoc J* 114:899, 1976.

93. Morel-Maroger L, Basch A, Danon F, et al: Pathology of the kidney in Waldenström's macroglobulinemia: Study of sixteen cases. *N Engl J Med* 283:123, 1970.

94. Solomon A, Weiss DT, Macy SD, Antonucci RA: Immunocytochemical detection of kappa and lambda light chain V region subgroups in human B-cell malignancies. *Am J Pathol* 137:855, 1990.

95. Martelo OJ, Schultz DR, Pardo V, Perez-Stable E: Immunologically mediated renal disease in Waldenström's macroglobulinemia. *Am J Med* 58:567, 1975.

96. Lindstrom FD, Hed J, Enestrom S: Renal pathology of Waldenström's macroglobulinaemia with monoclonal antiglomerular antibodies and nephrotic syndrome. *Clin Exp Immunol* 41:196, 1980.

97. Quaglino D, Di Leonardo G, Pasqualoni E, et al: Therapeutic management of hematological malignancies in elderly patients: Biological and clinical considerations: IV. Multiple myeloma and Waldenström's macroglobulinemia. *Aging* 10:5, 1998.

98. Case DCJ, Ervin TJ, Boyd MA, Redfield DL: Waldenström's macroglobulinemia: Long-term results with the M-2 protocol. *Cancer Invest* 9:1, 1991.

99. Petrucci MT, Avvisati G, Tribalto M, et al: Waldenström's macroglobulinaemia: Results of a combined oral treatment in 34 newly diagnosed patients. *J Intern Med* 226:443, 1989.

100. Dimopoulos MA, Kantarjian H, Estey E, et al: Treatment of Waldenström macroglobulinaemia with 2-chlorodeoxyadenosine. *Ann Intern Med* 118:195, 1993.

101. Dimopoulos MA, Weber D, Delasalle KB, et al: Treatment of Waldenström's macroglobulinemia resistant to standard therapy with 2-chlorodeoxyadenosine: Identification of prognostic factors. *Ann Oncol* 6:49, 1995.

102. Fridrik MA, Jäger G, Baldinger C, et al: First-line treatment of Waldenström's disease with cladribine. Arbeitsgemeinschaft Medikamentöse Tumortherapie. *Ann Hematol* 74:7, 1997.

103. Dimopoulos MA, Weber DM, Kantarjian H, et al: 2-Chlorodeoxyadenosine therapy of patients with Waldenström macroglobulinaemia previously treated with fludarabine. *Ann Oncol* 5:288, 1994.

104. Liu ES, Burian C, Miller WE, Saven A: Bolus administration of cladribine in the treatment of Waldenström macroglobulinaemia. *Br J Haematol* 103:690, 1998.

105. Betticher DC, Hsu Schmitz SF, Ratschiller D, et al: Cladribine (2-CDA) given as subcutaneous bolus injections is active in pretreated Waldenström's macroglobulinaemia. Swiss Group for Clinical Cancer Research (SAKK). *Br J Haematol* 99:358, 1997.

106. Delannoy A, Ferrant A, Martiat P, et al: 2-Chlorodeoxyadenosine therapy in Waldenström's macroglobulinaemia. *Nouv Rev Fr Hematol* 36:317, 1994.

107. Laurencet FM, Zulian GB, Guetty-Alberto M, et al: Cladribine with cyclophosphamide and prednisone in the management of low-grade lymphoproliferative malignancies. *Br J Cancer* 79:1215, 1999.

108. Van Den Neste E, Delannoy A, Vandercam B, et al: Infectious complications after 2-chlorodeoxyadenosine therapy. *Eur J Haematol* 56:235, 1996.

109. Niesvizky R, Zhu AX, Louie D, Michaeli J: Epstein-Barr virus-associated lymphoma after treatment of macroglobulinaemia with cladribine [letter]. *N Engl J Med* 341:55, 1999.

110. Dimopoulos MA, O'Brien S, Kantarjian H, et al: Fludarabine therapy in Waldenström's macroglobulinaemia. *Am J Med* 95:49, 1993.

111. Kantarjian HM, Alexanian R, Koller CA, et al: Fludarabine therapy in macroglobulinaemic lymphoma. *Blood* 75:1928, 1990.

112. Zinzani PL, Gherlinzoni F, Bendandi M, et al: Fludarabine treatment in resistant Waldenström's macroglobulinaemia. *Eur J Haematol* 54: 120, 1995.

113. Leblond V, Ben-Othman T, Deconinck E, et al: Activity of fludarabine in previously treated Waldenström's macroglobulinaemia: A report of 71 cases. Groupe Coopératif Macroglobulinémie. *J Clin Oncol* 16: 2060, 1998.

114. O'Brien , Kantarjian H, Keating MJ: Purine analogs in chronic lymphocytic leukemia and Waldenström's macroglobulinaemia. *Ann Oncol* 7(suppl 6):S27, 1996.

115. Foran JM, Rohatiner AZ, Coiffier B, et al: Multicenter phase II study of fludarabine phosphate for patients with newly diagnosed lymphoplasmacytoid lymphoma, Waldenström's macroglobulinaemia, and mantle-cell lymphoma. *J Clin Oncol* 17:546, 1999.

116. Costa P, Luzzati R, Nicolato A, et al: Cryptococcal meningitis and intracranial tuberculoma in a patient with Waldenström's macroglobulinaemia treated with fludarabine. *Leuk Lymphoma* 28:617, 1998.

117. Björkholm M, Celsing F, Runarsson G, Waldenström J: Successful intravenous immunoglobulin therapy for severe and persistent astrovirus gastroenteritis after fludarabine treatment in a patient with Waldenström's macroglobulinaemia. *Int J Hematol* 62:117, 1995.

118. Martino R, Shah A, Romero P, et al: Allogeneic bone marrow transplantation for advanced Waldenström's macroglobulinaemia. *Bone Marrow Transplant* 23:747, 1999.

119. Patel TC, Moore SB, Pineda AA, Witzig TE: Role of plasmapheresis in thrombocytopenic purpura associated with Waldenström's macroglobulinaemia. *Mayo Clin Proc* 71:597, 1996.

120. Höffkes HG, Heemann UW, Teschendorf C, et al: Hyperviscosity syndrome: Efficacy and comparison of plasma exchange by plasma separation and cascade filtration in patients with immunocytoma of Waldenström's type. *Clin Nephrol* 43:335, 1995.

121. Siami GA, Siami FS: Plasmapheresis and paraproteinemia: Cryoprotein-induced diseases, monoclonal gammopathy, Waldenström's macroglobulinaemia, hyperviscosity syndrome, multiple myeloma, light chain disease, and amyloidosis. *Ther Apher* 3:8, 1999.

122. Gobbi PG, Bettini R, Montecucco C, et al: Study of prognosis in Waldenström's macroglobulinaemia: A proposal for a simple binary classification with clinical and investigational utility. *Blood* 83:2939, 1994.

123. Marinella MA, Kim MH, Anderson MM: Waldenström's macroglobulinaemia transformed into immunoblastic lymphoma presenting with malignant ascites [letter]. *Am J Hematol* 51:249, 1996.

124. Beaudreuil J, Lortholary O, Martin A, et al: Hypercalcemia may indicate Richter's syndrome: Report of four cases and review. *Cancer* 79: 1211, 1997.

125. Salberg D, Kurtides S, McKeever WP: Monomyelocytic leukemia in an untreated case of Waldenström macroglobulinaemia. *Arch Intern Med* 137:514, 1977.

126. Horsman DE, Card RT, Skinnider LF: Waldenström macroglobulinaemia terminating in acute leukemia: A report of three cases. *Am J Hematol* 15:97, 1983.

127. Rodríguez JN, Fernández-Jurado A, Martino ML, Prados D: Waldenström's macroglobulinaemia complicated with acute myeloid leukemia: Report of a case and review of the literature [letter]. *Haematologica* 83:91, 1998.

128. Leonhard SA, Muhleman AF, Hurtubise PE, Martelo OJ: Emergence of immunoblastic sarcoma in Waldenström's macroglobulinaemia. *Cancer* 45:3102, 1980.

129. Abe M, Takahashi K, Mori N, Kojima M: "Waldenström's macroglobulinaemia" terminating in immunoblastic sarcoma: A case report. *Cancer* 49:2580, 1982.

130. Emmerich B, Pemsl M, Wust I, et al: Conversion of an IgM secreting immunocytoma in a high grade malignant lymphoma of immunoblastic type. *Blut* 46:81, 1983.

131. Vitali C, Bombardieri S, Spremolla G: Chronic myeloid leukemia in Waldenström's macroglobulinaemia. *Arch Intern Med* 141:1349, 1981.

HEAVY-CHAIN DISEASES

JOEL N. BUXBAUM

ALICE ALEXANDER

The heavy-chain diseases are rare B-cell proliferative disorders of varying degrees of malignancy. Their characteristic feature is the production of a monoclonal immunoglobulin molecule in which the heavy chain is truncated and there is no covalent attachment of light chains, either because of absent L-chain production or failure of formation of H-L disulfide bonds. The analysis of the domain structure of the heavy-chain disease proteins provided one of the early clues to the exon-intron structure of immunoglobulin genes. Immunoelectrophoresis or immunofixation of serum, urine, or secretory fluids or immunohistologic analysis of the proliferating cells establishes the diagnosis. The diseases behave clinically as B-cell lymphomas with the class of their monoclonal protein generally reflective of the major site of involvement. Gamma heavy-chain disease (γ-heavy-chain disease) behaves as a systemic lymphoma, alpha heavy-chain disease (α-heavy-chain disease) as a predominantly gut-associated lymphoproliferative disorder, and mu heavy-chain disease (μ-heavy-chain disease) as a systemic lymphoma with some patients presenting features of chronic lymphocytic leukemia. Prognosis is variable and definitive effective treatment regimens have not yet been established, except perhaps in the case of α-heavy-chain disease occurring in nonindustrialized environments.

DEFINITION AND HISTORY

The heavy-chain diseases are proliferative disorders of B cells that synthesize and secrete incomplete immunoglobulin (Ig) heavy chains. These initially were recognized as gammopathies by the presence of monoclonal proteins in the patients' serum or urine. The disorders were defined in terms of the production of structurally aberrant immunoglobulin molecules. Since the neoplastic cells displayed plasmacytic features, they were viewed as myeloma variants and studied for the insights they could provide to immunoglobulin structure. The immunochemical description of the first heavy-chain disease protein suggested that the gamma chain was divided into domains. Moreover, it suggested the possibility that the domains were encoded by separate genes (or gene segments).[1]

The original definition, which remains valid for clinical diagnostic purposes, demanded that patients' serum or urine contain a deleted Ig H-chain without a bound L-chain.[2,3] Later work demonstrated that heavy-chain molecules with similar structures could be identified within neoplastic cells of some cases of so-called nonsecretory myeloma or lymphoma. Also, in some instances defective immunoglobulin light chains could be identified.[4] In μ-heavy-chain disease, despite the absence of immunoglobulin light chains in the serum protein, L-chain production by the μ-fragment-synthesizing cells is seen in the majority of cases. Even in the first case of μ-heavy-chain disease, intact immunoglobulin light chains were identified in the proliferating cells, but they were not linked to the μ fragment via a covalent bond in either the cells or the serum.[5,6] While the identification of heavy-chain disease proteins is still largely consistent with the original criteria, variations on the theme, detectable by more precise molecular techniques, have allowed an expanded view of the circumstances leading to the production of the benchmark proteins.

ETIOLOGY AND PATHOGENESIS

The etiology of heavy-chain disease is not known. Some of the factors responsible for this disease may be similar to those involved in the etiology and pathogenesis of plasma cell myeloma or chronic lymphocytic leukemia. The etiology of plasmacytic and lymphocytic disorders is discussed in Chap. 106 and Chap. 98.

The observations that none of the heavy-chain disease disorders resembled plasma cell myeloma or Waldenström macroglobulinemia stimulated investigations into the nature of the heavy-chain disease cell and attempts to place it somewhere in the relatively orderly scheme of B-cell differentiation (see Chap. 82). While the infiltrates contain plasma cells, the predominant cell is a lymphocyte, perhaps more precisely reflecting the nature of the tumor stem cell that retains some capacity to mature.

CHRONIC ANTIGENIC STIMULATION

Infection is thought to play a role, at least for some types of heavy-chain disease, particularly α-heavy-chain disease. The latter is more frequently observed in nonindustrialized societies in which gastrointestinal infections are common. A causal relationship between infection and pathogenesis is supported by the observation that early stages of this disease can be treated successfully with antibiotics alone (see discussion below).

There is a high frequency of autoimmune disorders preceding or concurrent with the diagnosis of heavy chain disease, particularly γ-heavy-chain disease. This may be related to disease pathogenesis of γ-heavy-chain disease in the same fashion as the exposure to gastrointestinal organisms is to the pathogenesis of α-heavy-chain disease.

DEFECTIVE IMMUNOGLOBULIN MOLECULES

STRUCTURAL ANALYSES

Defective Gamma Heavy Chains Structural analysis of the defective monoclonal gamma heavy chains of 23 patients with γ-heavy-chain disease reveals several characteristic features (Fig. 109-1A). In two cases of γ-heavy-chain disease, OMM[7] and RIV,[8] cDNA and genomic sequence data are available (Fig. 109-2). The proteins usually initiate with a normal variable region amino acid sequence. In most cases, this sequence is short and abruptly interrupted by a large deletion encompassing the remainder of the V region, although four of the proteins shown in Fig. 109-1A appear to have retained most or all of their V, D, and J sequences.[9–12] In all γ-heavy-chain disease proteins, the entire CH1 domain is also deleted, with normal sequence reinitiating at the hinge (or occasionally the CH2 domain). No light chains are associated with the defective heavy chains, which usually exist in the serum as disulfide-linked dimers.

Defective Alpha Heavy Chains As a group, the alpha heavy chains of patients with α-heavy-chain disease have several general features in common with those of the defective gamma heavy chains of patients with γ-heavy-chain disease. These include deleted V regions, missing CH1 domains, and the absence of associated light chains. In

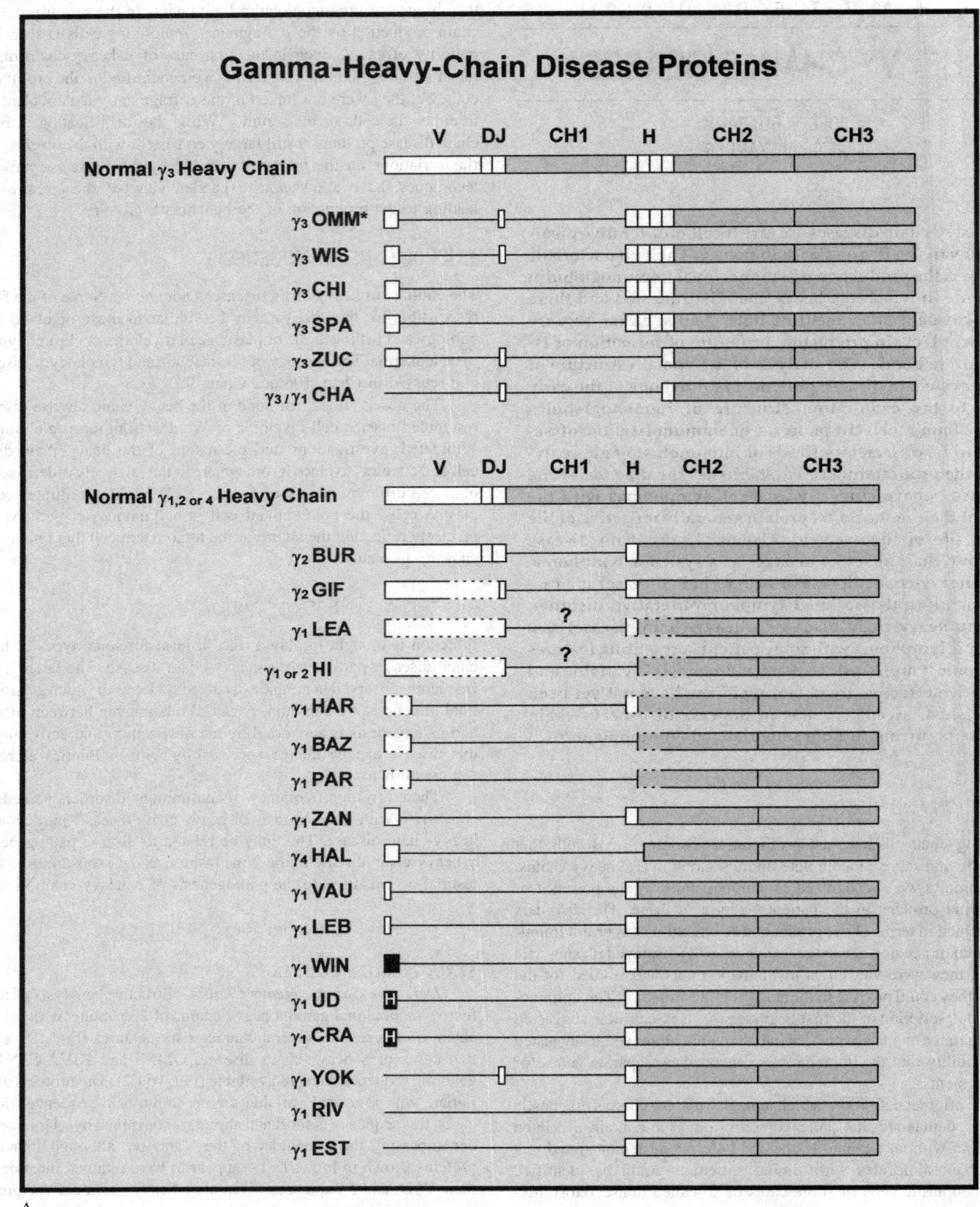

FIGURE 109-1 A and B

*Structures shown are primary synthetic protein products synthesized by the heavy chain disease cells. Serum proteins were modified after synthesis and did not contain any amino acids before the hinge.

**Structures shown are deduced amino acid sequences determined by cDNA sequencing.

H Indicates unusual and heterogeneous amino acid sequences.

■ Indicates unusual amino acid sequences.

Boxes indicate coding regions.

Lines indicate deletions.

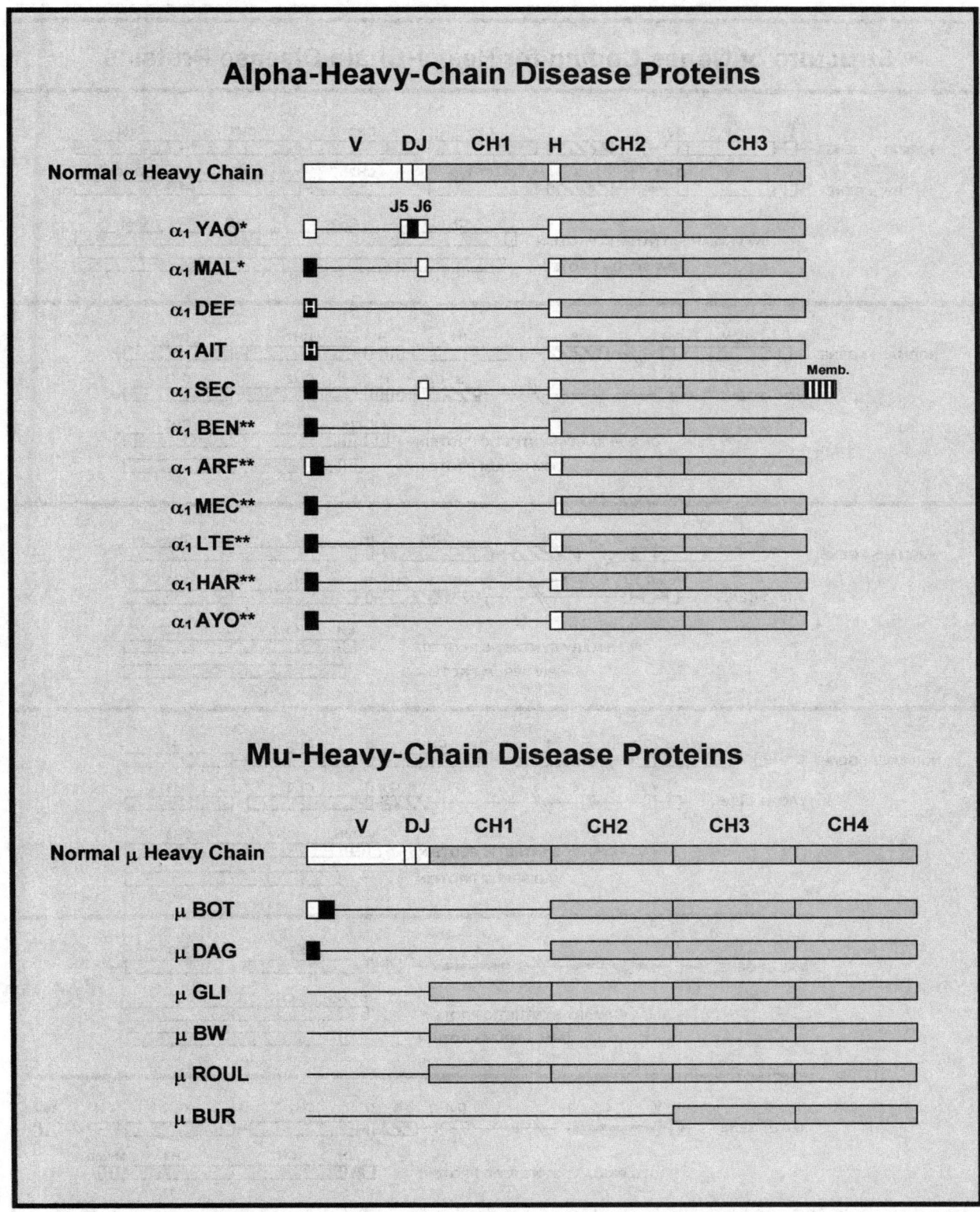

FIGURE 109-1 (*Continued*)

Dashed lines indicate likely structures for which sequence data are missing.

? indicates probable missing domain based on molecular weight and partial protein structure analysis.

V = variable region, D = diversity segment, J = joining region, H = hinge region, CH1, CH2, CH3, CH4 = constant regions of heavy chains, Memb. = membrane exon OMM,[7] WIS,[50] CHI,[51] SPA,[52] ZUC,[53] CHA,[54] γBUR,[9] GIF,[10] LEA,[11] HI,[12] HAR,[11] BAZ,[55] PAR,[56] ZAN,[57] HAL,[58] VAU, LEB,[59] WIN,[17] UD,[57] CRA,[61] YOK,[62] RIV,[8] EST,[63] YAO,[4] MAL,[18] DEF,[65] AIT,[66] SEC,[3] BEN, ARF, MEC, LTE, HAR, AYO,[41] BOT,[67] DAG,[68] GLI,[69] BW,[14] ROUL,[16] μBUR.[70]

Structure of Genes Coding for Heavy-Chain Disease Proteins

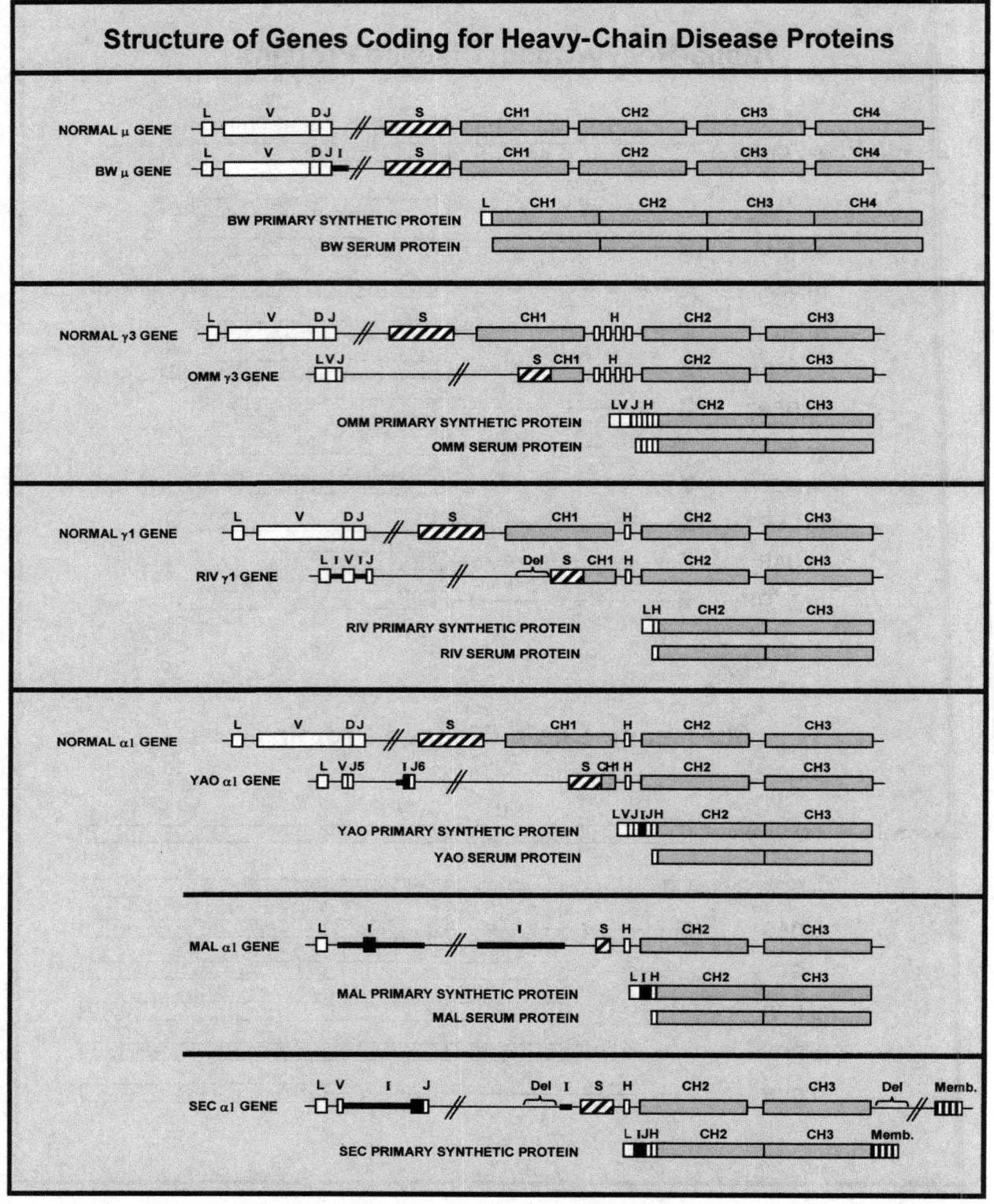

FIGURE 109-2   Boxes indicate coding regions.

◻ Indicates switch region.

■ Indicates inserted coding sequence.

■ Indicates inserted non-coding sequence.

Lines indicate intervening (non-coding) sequences.

L = leader region, V = variable region, D = diversity segment, J = joining region, I = inserted sequence, Del = deleted sequence, S = switch region, H = hinge region, CH1, CH2, CH3, CH4 = constant regions of heavy chains, Memb. = membrane exon.

BW,[14] OMM,[7] RIV, [8] YAO,[64] MAL,[18] SEC.[13]

the cases where amino acid or nucleotide-sequence data are available (Fig. 109-1B), most α-heavy-chain disease proteins were shown to contain short unusual sequences of unknown origin at the amino-terminus.

The complete sequences of the genes encoding three α-heavy-chain disease proteins are shown in Fig. 109-2. As in the γ-heavy-chain disease genes, OMM and RIV, strikingly similar noncontiguous deletions are present in the V/J and switch/CH1 regions of the α-heavy-chain disease genes. The genomic structures show that the unusual coding regions are actually part of larger regions containing unusual sequences of varying length, which include noncoding as well as coding nucleotides. These inserted regions show no homology to any known sequences, and their mechanism of origin is unclear.

Defective Mu Heavy Chains   In common with the defective heavy chains of patients with other types of heavy-chain disease, the defective mu heavy chains of patients with μ-heavy-chain disease contain large variable region deletions (Fig. 109-1B). In contrast to the other classes, the μ proteins often contain normal constant regions, including CH1 domains.

There is sequence for only one gene coding for a μ-heavy-chain disease protein (Fig. 109-2). This gene encodes a normal μ constant region containing CH1. The VDJ region is present but was shown to contain a single base deletion generating three stop-codons.[14] An inserted stretch of nucleotides immediately 3' to J destroyed the J donor splice site, causing the cell to splice the 3' donor site of the leader directly to the CH1 domain, eliminating variable region sequences from the mature mRNA.

Immunoglobulin Light Chains   Many patients with μ-heavy-chain disease also synthesize monoclonal light chains detectable as Bence Jones proteins in serum and/or urine. In some cases, immunofluorescence studies showed that the same cells produced both the light and heavy chains.[15,16] The light chains can associate in the serum with the short μ heavy chains but do not form covalent bridges even in cases where the CH1 domain, containing the H—L interchain disulfide bond, was shown to be present.[16] Monoclonal immunoglobulin light-chain production is rare in patients with γ- or α-heavy-chain disease but synthesis of truncated fragments has been noted.[4,17-20]

GENETIC BASIS FOR DEFECTIVE IMMUNOGLOBULINS

The structural features of the heavy-chain disease proteins can be interpreted in terms of the current knowledge of immunoglobulin gene structure. As expected for secretory proteins, heavy-chain disease genes encode a leader peptide, which is cleaved from the molecule before secretion (see Chaps. 9 and 83). If the heavy-chain disease gene contains intact V and J splice sites, those regions will be present in the mature mRNA and primary synthetic product, even if they contain extensive deletions, insertions, or other in-frame mutations. If there are no intact V or J splice sequences, the donor splice site of the leader peptide will be spliced to the next available acceptor site (Fig. 109-2).

The presence of large deletions in the switch/CH1 regions of the five γ- and α-heavy-chain disease genes sequenced so far explain why their corresponding heavy-chain disease proteins lack CH1. Since the normal CH1 acceptor splice site is deleted in these genes, the donor splice site of the leader or J region is alternatively spliced directly to the next available site at the hinge or CH2 domain. It would be expected that other heavy-chain disease proteins with missing CH1 domains contain similar switch/CH1 deletions in their genes. Thus, deletions and mutations of coding regions and splice sites explain why entire domains can be missing from the cytoplasmic mRNA and protein.

Any explanation for the origin of heavy-chain disease proteins must account for the three main defects in heavy-chain disease cells:

the two noncontiguous deletions in the V/J and switch/CH1 regions of the heavy-chain genes and the absence of associated light chains.

If the heavy-chain disease abnormalities occurred at random, it should be possible to isolate molecules from serum, which contain any combination of the three defects. Normal heavy chains unassociated with light chains have never been isolated from serum. Biosynthetic studies of immunoglobulin secreting cells have shown that in the absence of light chains, the CH1 domain of heavy chains will bind to the heavy-chain binding protein (BIP) inside the cell or undergo degradation rather than secretion.[21] If light chains are present, they will bind to the CH1 domain of the heavy chains and prevent the attachment to BIP. Four γ-heavy-chain disease proteins have been described which contain CH1 deletions and appear to have intact VDJ regions.[9-12] In these cells, the absence of light chains does not prevent secretion of the aberrant heavy chains, because they are missing CH1 domains and cannot bind BIP; γ- and α-heavy-chain disease serum proteins containing only the V/J deletion and intact CH1 domains have not been described. Such structures might be synthesized but would not be secreted from the cell in the absence of light chains due to intracellular binding of BIP at the CH1 domain. This was demonstrated in a study of a nonsecreting myeloma, which produced no light chains but synthesized deleted heavy chains that contained CH1 domains and missing VDJ regions.[22] The abnormal H chains were shown to undergo intracellular degradation rather than secretion. Thus, ascertainment bias may partly explain the observed association of the three defects in heavy-chain disease.

It is unclear whether the V/J or switch/CH1 deletion occurs first in heavy-chain disease cells, and it is not known whether the first deletion influences the second. Abnormal VDJ recombination, as an initial event, is suggested by the finding of a significant fraction of cells with aberrant joins when normal human peripheral mononuclear cells are exposed to Epstein-Barr virus (EBV).[23] If the cells persist after EBV infection or are generated at some rate throughout life, they could represent potential tumor stem cells. However, deletion of the V region during VDJ joining would render the early B cell unable to synthesize membrane immunoglobulin containing a normal antigen-combining site, and such cells could no longer be stimulated by the antigen cognate for the original antibody. Since switching is generally considered an antigen-dependent event, and most heavy-chain disease cells have switched from μ to γ or α, the occurrence of a V region deletion before switching would require the isotype change to be driven by an antigen-independent mechanism such as cytokine stimulation or a proliferative oncogenic event. In only one instance has an activating oncogene (N-ras) mutation been identified in a patient with heavy-chain disease.[24]

The switch region deletion as the initial abnormality is suggested by the existence of four γ-heavy-chain disease proteins (Fig. 109-1A) that appear to contain intact variable regions and switch/CH1 deletions.[9-12] Alternatively, these molecules may represent a category of heavy-chain disease proteins arising by a different, independent mechanism, either related to or a result of oncogenic transformation.

The variable region deletions and insertions in heavy-chain disease may be a consequence of the hypermutation process. During affinity maturation of normal B cells, the visible consequences of hypermutation are single base substitutions rather than deletions or insertions. However, a study involving single-cell PCR analysis of normal human lymphocytes showed that deletions and insertions were also common in germinal-center–derived B cells undergoing hypermutation but were rare in naive pregerminal center B cells.[25,26] The role of this mechanism in the generation of V region deletions in heavy-chain disease would be strengthened if the cells synthesizing the abnormal proteins were shown to carry germinal center markers.

Heavy-chain disease proteins of the γ-3 and α-1 classes are overrepresented relative to their frequency among intact human IgG proteins. The reason for this is not known. However, it is noteworthy that the Ig H-chain genes encoding these two heavy chains are arranged in two closely linked clusters in the germ line DNA (see Chap. 83). The first cluster contains the μ/δ pair followed sequentially by the gene encoding the γ_3, γ_1, and α_1 genes, while the second cluster, located 3' to the first, contains γ_2, γ_4, and α_2. The preference for isotypes of the first cluster in heavy-chain disease may be a function of their proximity to μ. Switching from μ to an isotype in the second cluster would require the switching mechanism to operate over greater distances, possibly decreasing the likelihood of forming a functional gene. Alternatively, the switch/CH1 deletion in heavy-chain disease proteins may prematurely terminate a sequential switching process, in which cells switch initially from μ to another isotype in the first cluster and then switch again to a gene from the second cluster. Support for this concept comes from studies in which cells were shown to undergo sequential switching, selecting constant region genes in a 5' to 3' direction.[27]

CLINICAL FEATURES

At first it appeared as if each class of heavy-chain disease had a characteristic clinical phenotype. Patients with γ-heavy-chain disease typically present with a systemic lymphoma particularly involving lymphoid structures in the head and neck.[28] Alpha-heavy-chain disease (α-HCD) is primarily a gut-associated lymphoproliferative state sometimes responding to antibiotics, while μ-heavy-chain disease is an apparent aberrant form of chronic lymphocytic leukemia.[29,30] Although the original associations were correct, time has revealed that the deleted proteins are associated with a broader spectrum of clinical syndromes.

GAMMA-HEAVY-CHAIN DISEASE

From the initial report in 1964 to 1989 almost one hundred cases of γ-heavy-chain disease were reported.[31,32] Since 1989 only 6 new instances have been recorded, suggesting that knowledge concerning the clinical aspects of the disorder has been incorporated into the body of medical practice; γ-heavy-chain disease appears to have the broadest range of clinical presentations among the heavy-chain diseases. As in μ-heavy-chain disease, the most common initial symptom complex is systemic with anemia, weight loss, and occasionally fever. In a significant fraction of patients the detection of lymphadenopathy or splenomegaly is the event that triggers further diagnostic investigation. Some form of lymphoproliferative disease is the final diagnosis in approximately three-quarters of the patients.

The waxing and waning lymphadenopathy and palatal and uvular swelling on the basis of involvement of Waldeyer's ring, described in the early cases of the disease, are not as frequent as originally believed. While it is characteristic when it occurs, it is found in fewer than 20 percent of γ-heavy-chain disease patients.

There has been a striking association of the occurrence of γ-heavy-chain disease in patients with preexisting or concurrent autoimmune disease.[33] Fully one-third of the reported patients have had some form of immunologically based inflammatory disease, most commonly rheumatoid arthritis. Autoimmune hemolytic anemia, systemic and discoid lupus erythematosus, and Sjögrens syndrome also have been seen associated with this disease

The clinical features of γ-heavy-chain disease differ from multiple myeloma (Table 109-1), as those of μ-heavy-chain disease differ from those of Waldenström's disease (Table 109-2). Renal disease and osteolytic lesions are far less common in γ-heavy-chain disease. Renal failure secondary to Bence-Jones proteinuria or AL amyloid is rare,

TABLE 109-1   CLINICAL FEATURES OF MULTIPLE MYELOMA AND GAMMA-HEAVY-CHAIN DISEASE

FEATURE	MULTIPLE MYELOMA	γ-HEAVY-CHAIN DISEASE
Anemia	Common	Common
Fever	Occasional	Occasional
Frequent infections	Yes	Yes
Lymphadenopathy	No	Yes
Hepatomegaly	Rare	Common
Splenomegaly	Rare	Common
Osteolytic lesions	Common	Very rare
Renal failure (cast nephropathy)	Common	Not reported
Renal amyloidosis	Occasional	Rare

owing to the lack of production or secretion of immunoglobulin light chains.

Lymphadenopathy is present in approximately half the cases; splenomegaly is detectable in between half and three-quarters; hepatomegaly occurs in about one-third. Extralymphoid presentations have been seen in 10 to 15 percent, with cutaneous or thyroid infiltrates specifically reported. In contrast to μ-heavy-chain disease, only two individuals with γ-heavy-chain disease proteins have been noted to have chronic lymphocytic leukemia (CLL).

ALPHA-HEAVY-CHAIN DISEASE

Unlike the other heavy-chain diseases, most cases of α-HCD arise in a characteristic environmental setting. The patients are usually young, in their teens and twenties, and live in nonindustrialized locales with relatively poor sanitation. The disease has been described as ''little more than an academic curiosity'' in industrialized nations, but it is a widely prevalent, debilitating illness in developing countries.[34] Thus significant clinical series and systematic approaches to therapy have been reported from Tunisia, Iran, Pakistan, India, Thailand, South Africa, and Mexico. The index case and the cases in which the structural features of the proteins have been best characterized have been from North Africa.

The most common clinical presentation is that of recurrent or chronic diarrhea with abdominal pain and weight loss due to malabsorption. Fever is common. For a period of time there was confusion over whether Mediterranean lymphoma with malabsorption and α-heavy-chain disease were different conditions, primarily because the heavy-chain disease protein could not be demonstrated in many cases of the lymphoma. It is now clear that most patients with the clinical picture of Mediterranean lymphoma produce the defective IgA proteins

TABLE 109-2   CLINICAL FEATURES OF WALDENSTRÖM'S MACROGLOBULINEMIA AND MU-HEAVY-CHAIN DISEASE

FEATURE	WALDENSTRÖM MACROGLOBULINEMIA	μ-HEAVY-CHAIN DISEASE
Anemia	Common	Common
Fever	Occasional	Occasional
Frequent infections	Yes	Yes
Lymphadenopathy	Yes	Yes
Hepatomegaly	Yes	Yes
Splenomegaly	Yes	Yes
Hyperviscosity	Common	Never
Osteolytic lesions	Rare	20%
Renal failure (cast nephropathy)	Occasional	Rare
Renal amyloidosis	Occasional	Occasional
Peripheral neuropathy	Common	Not reported

at some time in their course. In many cases the protein can only be found in the intestinal secretions, and in others it can only be found within the cytoplasm of the infiltrating plasma cells. All of these patients are now classified as having immunoproliferative small intestinal disease (IPSID).[35,36]

In addition to the diarrhea, malabsorption, and weight loss, growth retardation is common, and digital clubbing is found in 33 to 66 percent of patients. Mesenteric lymphadenopathy is frequently manifested as an intestinal mass, but extraabdominal lymphadenopathy is rare. Splenic involvement is also uncommon. Moderate hepatomegaly occurs in 20 to 25 percent of the patients. Ascites is sometimes seen, as is peripheral edema, both on the basis of hypoalbuminemia.

MU-HEAVY-CHAIN DISEASE

Of the major Ig classes, μ-heavy-chain disease is the least common. Approximately 30 cases have been documented in the literature since its original description.[5,37] It is likely that more cases have been identified but not reported, particularly in the last 10 years. Alternatively, since it is now apparent that the clinical picture is not specific, it is possible that many additional cases have been diagnosed as CLL- or B-cell lymphoma, and the protein abnormality was not recognized. Initially the reported cases all had a clinical picture consistent with CLL; however, with better diagnostic procedures and a higher index of suspicion the defining protein abnormality has been noted in a broader range of clinical settings. Currently, it appears that only about one-third of the patients with μ-heavy-chain disease have CLL. Thorough investigation of serum proteins in over 150 consecutive patients with CLL failed to identify a single instance of μ-heavy-chain disease, suggesting that fewer than 1 percent of cases of CLL actually are associated with production of an abnormal μ fragment.[38] Other clinical presentations varied from essential monoclonal gammopathy with little or no clinical symptoms of B-cell lymphoma (20 percent). Ten percent of the cases were associated with the simultaneous detection of an intact IgM protein in the serum, and another 10 percent with clinical multiple myeloma or extramedullary plasmacytoma.

The presentation is usually that of a systemic disease with weight loss, sometimes fever, anemia, and recurrent infections. Splenomegaly is found in almost all cases, hepatomegaly in three-quarters, and peripheral lymphadenopathy in approximately 40 percent of patients with μ-heavy-chain disease.

DELTA- AND EPSILON-HEAVY-CHAIN DISEASE

No cases have been reported in which an incomplete epsilon chain has been identified. A single case of delta-heavy-chain disease has been described. The patient presented with the clinical features of multiple myeloma with osteolytic lesions of the skull, marrow plasmacytosis, and the rapid development of renal failure and death. While the immunochemical analysis of the patient's serum was consistent with the presence of a polymerized δ fragment, no definitive sequence data were obtained.[39]

LABORATORY FEATURES

DETECTION OF ABNORMAL IMMUNOGLOBULIN PROTEIN

As a rule the neoplastic cells do not produce large amounts of immunoglobulin. This makes it sometimes difficult to detect the abnormal immunoglobulin produced in heavy-chain disease. Nevertheless, a combination of electrophoretic, immunoelectrophoretic, and immunofixation techniques[40] can establish the diagnosis. In a minority of cases the proteins can be initially identified as a discrete homogeneous band of β mobility on serum or urine electrophoresis. The immunoelectro-

phoretic pattern, when developed with specific anti-heavy- and anti-light-chain antisera, reveals an H-chain specific arc not reacting with either the anti-κ or anti-λ antisera. This is most readily apparent in proteins of the γ class, since occasionally intact monoclonal IgA or IgM M-proteins will not react with some anti-L-chain sera. This is more common with immunoelectrophoresis than with immunofixation techniques. In those cases it may be necessary to separate the monoclonal proteins from the sera, treat them with reducing agents to cleave the disulfide bonds, and subject them to gel electrophoresis to determine the size of the immunoglobulin heavy chain polypeptide.

More commonly the proteins are present in smaller amounts and give heterogeneous patterns on electrophoresis, either because of N-terminal proteolysis or partial digestion of the glycosyl-chains attached to the heavy chains. Again, immunoelectrophoresis or immunofixation with development of the patterns with a panel of anti-H and anti-L antibodies can strongly suggest the diagnosis. More detailed, structural analysis can be performed on the isolated, reduced, and alkylated H-chain monomer and confirm the presence or absence of immunoglobulin light chains in specialized laboratories.

GAMMA-HEAVY-CHAIN DISEASE

As in patients without μ-heavy-chain disease, marrow aspirates or biopsies often show a pleiomorphic histologic picture with lymphocytes, plasma cells, and cells called *lymphocytoid plasma cells*, or *plasmacytoid lymphocytes*, making up a significant proportion of the infiltrate. In 25 to 30 percent of cases the marrow is nondiagnostic or normal. Immunophenotyping of the marrow aspirate has been performed in a minority of patients. In experienced laboratories such studies have usually revealed a lymphoid population staining only for the gamma H-chain with no staining for immunoglobulin light chains. In some cases in which the heavy-chain disease protein could not be detected in the serum or urine, or in which the concentration of heavy-chain disease protein was too low or heterogeneous by electrophoresis, these studies provided the definitive diagnostic test. In a few the analyses revealed the presence of more than a single proliferating clone, and in at least three instances demonstrated a major population of proliferating T cells and a quantitatively minor B-cell clone producing the γ-heavy-chain disease protein.

ALPHA-HEAVY-CHAIN DISEASE

Occasionally, most commonly in α-heavy-chain disease, the protein cannot be seen in the serum, urine, or even the gastrointestinal secretion. Instead a population of plasmacytoid cells may be found in the intestinal epithelium, lymph nodes, or the marrow that stain for only H-chain determinants. In these cases the typical molecular abnormality of heavy-chain disease (see below) can be identified by analysis of cDNA derived from the heavy-chain disease positive cells.[41]

Serial small-bowel biopsies have shown that the early phases of the disease are characterized by dense mucosal and lamina propria infiltration mature plasma cells producing a monoclonal alpha-chain-fragment.[42] The jejunum is the usual site of involvement with the duodenum and ileum involved less often. Involvement may be patchy, and different areas may be in different stages of the disease at the same time, requiring biopsies from multiple sites for accurate staging. As the disease progresses, fewer plasma cells are seen and the dominant cells, still derived from the same clone, are more blastic with little or no production of the alpha fragment. At this point the cells have infiltrated beyond the lamina propria into the muscularis layer. In the latter stage there is extensive infiltration of regional nodes with similar cells and final pathologic diagnoses have included lymphoma of the low, intermediate, or high-grade immunoblastic type, mantle zone lymphoma, or parafollicular B-cell lymphoma. Rarely the tumor cells may be seen in the marrow, although the frequency of marrow involvement has not been precisely determined.

As expected with this sequence of involvement, early imaging of the small bowel reveals a pseudopolypoid appearance. When the muscularis is penetrated a more cobblestone-like picture is found. In the late stages tumor masses are defined, and surface ulceration is detectable. The diagnosis requires small-bowel biopsies from more than one site along the jejunum, and the presence of the alpha fragment in the serum, the intestinal secretions, or in the cells infiltrating the gastric mucosa. If there is demonstrable nodal involvement, mesenteric lymph node biopsy may yield the same findings. The differential diagnosis includes celiac disease, diffuse intestinal giardiasis, Western type intestinal lymphoma (which is not associated with α-fragment production), bacterial overgrowth syndrome, and Whipple disease. Interestingly, many of these patients may have concomitant parasitic infestation or chronic infection with bacteria, such as *Helicobacter pylori*. The relevance of these infections to pathogenesis is unclear, although they certainly contribute to the symptoms and must be treated.

Instances of patients producing α-heavy-chain disease proteins have been found in other clinical contexts in more industrialized parts of the world. A single three-year-old with frequent infections, hypogammaglobulinemia, and leukopenia was found to have a defective alpha chain,[43] but no detailed structural studies were reported. Rare patients in the United States and Japan, with Western type lymphomas involving only the gut or with more widespread disease, have been noted to have a similar circulating protein.[44] Single patients with goiter or skin lesions and no detectable systemic disease also have been described. These may represent a different mode of pathogenesis.

MU-HEAVY-CHAIN DISEASE

Marrow involvement is characterized by infiltration with lymphocytes and plasma cells. Cells that often are described as lymphocytic plasmacytes or plasmacytoid lymphocytes are prominent. Although the marrow of almost all patients contains the multivacuolated plasma cells described in the index case, the vacuoles are not universally apparent.[15] Their identification has sometimes been the clinical feature that has suggested the diagnosis, subsequently confirmed by the appropriate electrophoretic and immunoelectrophoretic studies.

The presence or absence of osteolytic lesions or pathologic fractures only has been noted in half the reported patients, with bone involvement occurring in 40 percent of those. It is likely that the true incidence is lower but still approaches the frequency seen in multiple myeloma, rather than that in Waldenström's macroglobulinemia, where it is quite rare.

Urinary excretion of the μ fragment was noted in only two patients, presumably because in most patients the polymers of the carboxy-terminal μ fragment were too large to be filtered by intact renal glomeruli. Monoclonal light chains have been found in the urine in two-thirds of cases. Nonetheless, renal complications have been infrequent. Cast nephropathy, with renal failure, has been reported in one case, and two patients, including the first reported case, had AL amyloidosis.[45] Immunoglobulin light chains capable of producing amyloid are found in approximately 12 percent of cases, an incidence that is not significantly different from that found in patients with multiple myeloma.

THERAPY, COURSE, AND PROGNOSIS

GAMMA-HEAVY-CHAIN DISEASE

The clinical course has been extremely variable. Survival, ranging from one month to 20 years from the finding of the protein abnormality, has reflected the nature of the associated disease. Patients with a lymphoma on presentation have a more aggressive course than do the patients with little clinical evidence of lymphoproliferative disease.

The lymphomas have been treated with a variety of regimens including splenic or other local irradiation and combinations of chemotherapy, usually including cyclophosphamide, or vincristine and prednisone, although other agents have been used in some patients. A single case has been reported in which there was a complete response to fludarabine after a partial remission with epirubicin, chlorambucil, and prednisone.[46] Patients with predominant autoimmune disease have been treated with prednisone, and some patients have received no treatment. Disappearance of the γ-heavy-chain disease protein in response to treatment has not always been predictive of a good overall therapeutic response.

ALPHA-HEAVY-CHAIN DISEASE

Since 1965 ten series with more than 10 patients each have assessed the impact of therapy on the course of disease and survival. The total number of patients included is 206. The utility of clinical staging was not recognized until the late 1970s, hence details of responsiveness prior to that time are difficult to interpret. However it appeared from those data that mean overall survival was approximately 8 months in the absence of a therapeutic response and that fewer than half the patients responded to any treatment. Since the early studies, most series have classified patients into those with only mucosal infiltration with plasma cells (stage A) and the remainder with deeper infiltration or nodal spread (stages B and C).[47-49] When stage A patients are treated with antibiotics (usually tetracycline at 1 to 2 g/d for 6 to 8 months), response rates range from 25 percent to 72 percent. The cumulative response rate to antibiotic therapy is 53 percent, with overall survival between 29 percent and 75 percent at 5 years and disease-free survival in one series of 43 percent at 5 years. An occasional stage A patient also received abdominal irradiation. Stage B and C patients were sometimes treated with similar antibiotic regimens and a variety of chemotherapy regimens, usually including cyclophosphamide and prednisone (such as COPP or CHOP, sometimes followed by BACOP, see Chap. 103).

MU-HEAVY-CHAIN DISEASE

The course is variable in duration with survival ranging from 1 to 11 months after the appearance of symptoms. Because of its rarity no large series of patients treated in a systematic way in a single center has been reported. A variety of drug protocols have been used with most including alkylating agents (chlorambucil, melphalan, and cyclophosphamide) with inconsistent responses. It is possible that more aggressive regimens will be more effective, but to date there is no reported experience bearing on that question.

REFERENCES

1. Kataoka T, Yamawaki-Kataoka Y, Yamagishi H, Honjo T: Cloning immunoglobulin gamma2b chain gene of mouse: characterization and partial sequence determination. *Proc Natl Acad Sci USA* 76:4240, 1979.
2. Franklin EC, Lowenstein J, Bigelow B, Meltzer M: Heavy chain disease—a new disorder of serum gamma-globulins. *Am J Med* 37:332, 1964.
3. Osserman EF, Takatsuki K: Clinical and immunochemical studies of four cases of heavy (H gamma) chain disease. *Am J Med* 37:351, 1964.
4. Matuchansky C, Cogne M, Lemaire M, et al: Nonsecretory alpha chain disease with immunoproliferative small intestinal disease. *N Engl J Med* 320:1534, 1989.
5. Ballard HS, Hamilton LM, Marcus AJ, Illes CH: A new variant of heavy chain disease (mu chain disease). *N Engl J Med* 282:1060, 1970.
6. Buxbaum J, Franklin EC, Scharff MD: Immunoglobulin M heavy chain disease: intracellular origin of the mu chain fragment. *Science* 169:770, 1970.

7. Alexander A, Anicito I, Buxbaum J: Gamma heavy chain disease in man: genomic sequence reveals two noncontiguous deletions in a single gene. *J Clin Invest* 82:1244, 1988.

8. Guglielmi P, Bakhshi A, Cogne M, Seligmann M, Korsmeyer SJ: Multiple genomic defects result in an alternative RNA splice creating a human gamma H chain disease protein. *J Immunol* 141:1762, 1988.

9. Prelli F, Frangione B: Franklin's disease: Ig gamma2 H chain mutant BUR. *J Immunol* 148:949, 1992.

10. Cooper SM, Franklin EC, Frangione B: Molecular defect in a gamma2 heavy chain. *Science* 176:187, 1972.

11. Frangione B, Franklin EC, Smithies O: Unusual genes at the aminoterminus of human immunoglobulin variants. *Nature* 273:400, 1978.

12. Terry WD, Ohms J: Implications of heavy chain disease protein sequences for multiple gene theories of immunoglobulin synthesis. *Proc Natl Acad Sci USA* 66:558, 1970.

13. Cogne M, Preud'homme J: Gene deletions force nonsecretory alpha-chain disease plasma cells to produce membrane-form alpha-chain only. *J Immunol* 145:2455, 1990.

14. Bakhshi A, Guglielmi P, Siebenlist U, Ravetch J, Jensen JP, Korsmeyer SJ: A DNA insertion/deletion necessitates an aberrant RNA splice accounting for a mu heavy chain disease protein. *Proc Natl Acad Sci USA* 83:2689, 1986.

15. Zucker-Franklin D, Franklin EC: Ultrastructural and immunofluorescence studies of the cells associated with mu-chain disease. *Blood* 37:257, 1971.

16. Cogne M, Aucouturier P, Brizard A, Dreyfus B, Duarte F, Preud'homme J: Complete variable region deletion in a mu heavy chain disease protein (ROUL). Correlation with light chain secretion. *Leukemia Res* 17:527, 1993.

17. Adlersberg JB, Grann V, Zucker-Franklin D, Frangione B, Franklin EC: An unusual case of a plasma cell neoplasm with an IgG3-lambda myeloma and a gamma3 heavy chain disease protein. *Blood* 51:85, 1978.

18. Tsapis A, Bentaboulet M, Pellet P, et al: The productive gene for alpha-H chain disease protein MAL is highly modified by insertion-deletion processes. *J Immunol* 143:3821, 1989.

19. Cogne M, Bakhshi A, Korsmeyer SJ, Guglielmi P: Gene mutations and alternate RNA splicing result in truncated Ig L chains in human gamma H chain disease. *J Immunol* 141:1738, 1988.

20. Hauke G, Schiltz E, Bross KJ, Hollmann A, Peter HH, Krawinkel U: Unusual sequence of immunoglobulin L-chain rearrangements in a gamma heavy chain disease patient. *Scand J Immunol* 36:463, 1992.

21. Hendershot L, Bole D, Kohler G, Kearney JF: Assembly and secretion of heavy chains that do not associate posttranslationally with immunoglobulin heavy chain-binding protein. *J Cell Biol* 104:761, 1987.

22. Cogne M, Guglielmi P: Exon skipping without splice site mutation accounting for abnormal immunoglobulin chains in nonsecreting human myeloma. *Eur J Immunol* 23:1289, 1993.

23. Brokaw JL, Wetzel SM, Pollok BA: Conserved patterns of somatic mutation and secondary VH gene rearrangement create aberrant Ig-encoding genes in Epstein-Barr Virus-transformed and normal human B lymphocytes. *Int Immunol* 4:197, 1992.

24. Moskovits T, Jacobson DR, Buxbaum JN: N-*ras* oncogene activation in a patient with gamma heavy chain disease. *Am J Hematol* 41:302, 1992.

25. Goossens T, Klein U, Kuppers R: Frequent occurrence of deletions and duplications during somatic hypermutation: implications for oncogene translocations and heavy chain disease. *Proc Natl Acad Sci USA* 95:2463, 1998.

26. Klein U, Goossens T, Fischer M, et al: Somatic hypermutation in normal and transformed human B cells. *Immunol Rev* 162:261, 1998.

27. Petrini J, Shell B, Hummel M, Dunnick W: The immunoglobulin heavy chain switch: structural features of gamma1 recombinant switch regions. *J Immunol* 138:1940, 1987.

28. Buxbaum J: Heavy chain diseases in man. *La Ricerca in Clinica e in Laboratorio* 6:301, 1976.

29. Rambaud JC, Bognel C, Prost A, et al: Clinico-pathological study of a patient with "Mediterranean" type of abdominal lymphoma and a new type of IgA abnormality ("Alpha Chain Disease"). *Digestion* 1:321, 1968.

30. Franklin EC: μ-chain disease. *Arch Intern Med* 135:71, 1975.

31. Fermand J, Brouet J, Danon F, Seligmann M: Gamma heavy chain "disease": heterogeneity of the clinicopathologic features. Report of 16 cases and review of the literature. *Medicine* 68:321, 1989.

32. Kyle RA, Greipp PR, Banks PM: The diverse picture of gamma heavy chain disease. Report of seven cases and review of literature. *Mayo Clin Proc* 56:439, 1981.

33. Husby G, Blichfeldt P, Brinch L, et al: Chronic arthritis and gamma heavy chain disease: coincidence or pathogenic link? *Scand J Rheumatol* 27:257, 1998.

34. Ryan JC: Premalignant conditions of the small intestine. *Semin Gastrointestinal Dis* 7:88, 1996.

35. Rambaud JC, Halphen M, Galian A, Tsapis A: Immunoproliferative small intestinal disease (IPSID): relationships with alpha chain disease and "Mediterranean" lymphomas. *Springer Semin Immunopathol* 12:239, 1990.

36. Martin IG, Aldoori MI: Immunoproliferative small intestinal disease: Mediterranean lymphoma and alpha heavy chain disease. *Br J Surg* 1:20, 1994.

37. Wahner-Roedler DL, Kyle RA: Mu-heavy chain disease: presentation as a benign monoclonal gammopathy. *Am J Hematol* 40:56, 1992.

38. Bonhomme J, Seligmann M, Mihaesco C, et al: Mu-chain disease in an African patient. *Blood* 43:485, 1974.

39. Vilpo JA, Irjala K, Viljanen MK, Klemi P, Kouvonen I, Ronnemaa T: Delta-heavy chain disease. A study of a case. *Clin Immunol Immunopathol* 17:584, 1980.

40. Franklin EC: The heavy chain diseases. *The Harvey Lectures* 78:1, 1984.

41. Fakhfakh F, Dellagi K, Ayadi H, et al: Alpha heavy chain disease alpha mRNA contain nucleotide sequences of unknown origins. *Eur J Immunol* 22:3037, 1992.

42. Galian A, Lecestre M, Scotto J, Bognel C, Matuchansky C, Rambaud J: Pathological study of alpha-chain disease, with special emphasis on evolution. *Cancer* 39:2081, 1977.

43. Faux JA, Crain JD, Rosen FS, Merler E: An alpha heavy chain abnormality in a child with hypogammaglobulinemia. *Clin Immunol Immunopathol* 1:282, 1973.

44. Cohen HJ, Gonzalvo A, Krook J, Thompson TT, Kremer WB: New presentation of alpha heavy chain disease: North American polypoid gastrointestinal lymphoma. Clinical and cellular studies. *Cancer* 41:1161, 1978.

45. Preud'homme J, Bauwens M, Dumont G, Goujon JM, Dreyfus B, Touchard G: Cast nephropathy in mu heavy chain disease. *Clin Nephrol* 48:118, 1997.

46. Agrawal S, Abboudi Z, Matutes E, Catovsky D: First report of fludarabine in gamma-heavy chain disease. *Br J Haematol* 88:653, 1994.

47. Akbulut H, Soykan I, Yakaryilmaz F, et al: Five-year results of the treatment of 23 patients with immunoproliferative small intestinal disease. A Turkish experience. *Cancer* 80:8, 1997.

48. Ben-Ayed F, Halphen M, Najjar T, et al: Treatment of alpha chain disease. Results of a prospective study in 21 Tunisian patients by the Tunisian-French intestinal lymphoma study group. *Cancer* 63:1251, 1989.

49. Salimi M, Spinelli JJ: Chemotherapy of Mediterranean abdominal lymphoma. Retrospective comparison of chemotherapy protocols in Iranian patients. *Am J Clin Oncol* 19:18, 1996.

50. Frangione B, Rosenwasser E, Prelli F, Franklin EC: Primary structure of human gamma3 immunoglobulin deletion mutant: gamma3 heavy-chain disease protein Wis. *Biochem* 19:4304, 1980.

51. Frangione B: A new immunoglobulin variant: gamma3 heavy chain disease protein CHI. *Proc Natl Acad Sci USA* 73:1552, 1976.

52. Frangione B, Franklin EC: Correlation between fragmented immunoglobulin genes and heavy chain deletion mutants. *Nature* 281:600, 1979.

53. Wolfenstein-Todel C, Frangione B, Prelli F, Franklin EC: The amino acid sequence of "heavy chain disease" protein ZUC. Structure of the Fc fragment of immunoglobulin G3. *Biochem Biophys Res Commun* 71:907, 1976.

54. Arnaud P, Wang A, Gianazza E, et al: Gamma heavy chain disease protein CHA: immunological and structural studies. *Mol Immunol* 18:379, 1981.

55. Smith LL, Barton BP, Garver FA, et al: Physicochemical and immunochemical properties of gamma1 heavy chain disease protein BAZ. *Immunochemistry* 15:323, 1978.

56. Rabin BS, Moon J: Clinical findings in a case of newly defined gamma heavy chain disease protein. *Clin Exp Immunol* 14:563, 1973.

57. Franklin EC, Prelli F, Frangione B: Human heavy chain disease protein

WIS: implications for the organization of immunoglobulin genes. *Proc Natl Acad Sci USA* 76:452, 1979.

58. Frangione B, Lee L, Haber E, Bloch KJ: Protein Hal: partial deletion of a "gamma" immunoglobulin gene(s) and apparent reinitiation at an internal AUG codon. *Proc Natl Acad Sci USA* 70:1073, 1973.

59. Franklin EC, Kyle R, Seligmann M, Frangione B: Correlation of protein structure and immunoglobulin gene organization in the light of two new deleted heavy chain disease proteins. *Mol Immunol* 16:919, 1979.

60. Sala P, Tonutti E, Pizzolitto S, et al: Immunochemical and structural characterization of an IgG1 heavy chain disease. *Res Clin Lab* 19:59, 1989.

61. Franklin EC, Frangione B: The molecular defect in a protein (CRA) found in gamma1 heavy chain disease, and its genetic implications. *Proc Natl Acad Sci USA* 68:187, 1971.

62. Nabeshima Y, Ikenaka T, Arima T: N- and C-terminal amino acid sequences of a gamma heavy chain disease protein YOK. *Immunochemistry* 13:245, 1976.

63. Biewenga J, Frangione B, Franklin EC, Van Loghem E: A gamma1 heavy-chain disease protein (EST) lacking the entire VH and CH1 domains. *Scand J Immunol* 11:601, 1980.

64. Bentaboulet M, Mihaesco E, Gendron M, Brouet J, Tsapis A: Genomic alterations in a case of alpha heavy chain disease leading to the generation of composite exons from the JH region. *Eur J Immunol* 19:2093, 1989.

65. Wolfenstein-Todel C, Mihaesco E, Frangione B: "Alpha chain disease" protein DEF: Internal deletion of a human immunoglobulin A1 heavy chain. *Proc Natl Acad Sci USA* 71:974, 1974.

66. Wolfenstein-Todel C, Mihaesco E, Frangione B: Variant of a human immunoglobulin: "alpha chain disease" protein AIT. *Biochem Biophys Res Commun* 65:47, 1975.

67. Barnikol-Watanabe S, Mihaesco E, Mihaesco C, Barnikol HU, Hilschmann N: The primary structure of mu-chain-disease protein BOT. *Hoppe-Seyler's Z Physiol Chem* 365:105, 1984.

68. Mihaesco C, Ferrara P, Guillemot JC, et al: A new extra sequence at the amino terminal of a mu heavy chain disease protein (DAG). *Mol Immunl* 27:771, 1990.

69. Franklin EC, Frangione B, Prelli F: The defect in mu heavy chain disease protein GLI. *J Immunol* 116:1194, 1976.

70. Lebreton JP, Ropartz C, Rousseaux J, Roussel P, Dautrevaux M, Biserte G: Immunochemical and biochemical study of a human Fc mu-like fragment (mu-chain disease). *Eur J Immunol* 5:179, 1975.

PART X

HEMOSTASIS
AND
THROMBOSIS

MEGAKARYOPOIESIS AND THROMBOPOIESIS

DAVID J. KUTER

Large, polyploid, bone marrow megakaryocytes shed enucleate platelets into the circulation. Most of the proteins and granules that determine the characteristics of these platelets are made in the megakaryocytes. In response to an increased need for platelets, megakaryocytes increase their number, size, and ploidy; the opposite effects occur when the demand decreases. The growth of megakaryocytes and the production of platelets are regulated almost entirely by the amount of thrombopoietin in the circulation. Upon binding to the thrombopoietin receptor, c-Mpl, thrombopoietin increases the growth of early marrow precursors of all lineages but only stimulates the maturation of late precursors of the megakaryocyte lineage and thereby increases only platelet production. Thrombopoietin is produced at a constant rate in the liver, and its level is determined primarily by the rate of clearance by c-Mpl receptors on platelets and possibly megakaryocytes. Characteristic changes in megakaryocytes occur in a wide variety of disorders of abnormal platelet production. Recombinant thrombopoietins as well as other hematopoietic growth factors such as interleukin-11 can increase platelet production and may become clinically useful.

The derivation of blood platelets from megakaryocytes has been known since 1906,[1] but the process of platelet production (termed *thrombopoiesis* or *thrombocytopoiesis*) remains enigmatic. Megakaryocytes are very large, polyploid bone marrow cells whose low prevalence has made their investigation difficult. During the past two decades, in vitro cloning of megakaryocytic progenitors, production of monoclonal antibodies that specifically identify megakaryocytes and their constituents, and new molecular techniques have advanced our knowledge of megakaryocyte biology (called *megakaryopoiesis* or *megakaryocytopoiesis*). With the purification of *thrombopoietin*[2-7] great strides have been made in understanding the physiology of platelet production from megakaryocytes.

ANATOMY OF MEGAKARYOCYTES

In lower vertebrate species such as fish and birds, all the circulating blood cells, including the erythrocytes and the platelets (called *thrombocytes*), are nucleated and are produced by diploid bone marrow

Acronyms and abbreviations that appear in this chapter include: 5–FU, 5–fluorouracil; CHO, Chinese hamster ovary; GEMM-CFC, or mix-CFC, granulocyte-erythroid-macrophage-megakaryocyte colony-forming cells; HIV, human immunodeficiency virus; ITP, idiopathic thrombocytopenic purpura; MGDF, megakaryocyte growth and development factor; meg-BFC, megakaryocytic burst-forming cell; meg-CFC, megakaryocyte colony-forming cell; MPV, mean platelet volume; PEG-rHuMGDF, pegylated, recombinant megakaryocyte growth and development factor; PF4, platelet factor 4; rHuTPO, recombinant human thrombopoietin; vWf, von Willebrand factor.

precursor cells.[8] However, in higher vertebrates platelets are produced by a different mechanism whose evolutionary advantage is unclear. Anucleate platelets[9] are generated from unusual bone marrow cells, the megakaryocytes. Megakaryocytes normally account for approximately 0.05 to 0.1 percent of all nucleated human bone marrow cells, but their number increases as the demand for platelets rises. In contrast to the erythrocyte with a diameter of $5\mu m$ and a volume of 85 to 100 fl, megakaryocytes have average diameters of 20 to 25 μm and volumes of 4700 ± 100 fl.[10] Some of the largest megakaryocytes may have diameters of 50 to 60 μm and volumes of 65,000 to 100,000 fl. These unique cells are polyploid and contain platelet-specific granules and proteins.

POLYPLOIDY

Mature megakaryocytes are invariably polyploid and contain from two (4N) to 32 (64N) times the normal diploid amount of DNA.[11,12] Human megakaryocytes have a mean ploidy of 16N. Unlike the small percentage of hepatocytes and macrophages that have two- to four-fold the normal diploid content of DNA and whose DNA is contained in multiple separate nuclei, all of the DNA in megakaryocytes is contained within one highly lobulated nuclear envelope where each nuclear lobule represents one diploid amount (2N) of DNA. In general there is a relationship between increased ploidy and increased megakaryocyte size, but given the time needed for the cytoplasm of megakaryocytes to mature, not all small megakaryocytes are of low ploidy. In fetal life megakaryocytes are less polyploid; cultured mature megakaryocytes from fetal liver at 8 to 10 weeks of gestation are only 2N and 4N, while 8N megakaryocytes are detected at 20 weeks of gestation.[13]

At some ill-defined point in the megakaryocytic differentiation pathway, mitosis ceases and the unusual process of *endomitosis* (also called *polyploidization* or *endoreduplication*) commences.[14] Endomitosis is a process in which DNA replication occurs but neither the nucleus nor the cell undergoes division (*cytokinesis*). Morphologically, endomitosis is associated with the dissolution of the nuclear membrane and the formation of a multipolar mitotic spindle.[15] While initially it was assumed that endomitosis was simply the absence of mitosis after each round of DNA replication, studies in mice[16] showed that megakaryocytes indeed enter mitosis and progress through normal prophase, prometaphase, metaphase, and up to anaphase A, but not to anaphase B, telophase, or cytokinesis. After anaphase, the nuclear membrane is reassembled about the sister chromatids as a single nucleus skipping telophase and cytokinesis, and the cells enter the next round of DNA replication.

Cessation of mitosis in the diploid megakaryocyte progenitors is apparently directly coupled to the start of endoreduplication, and it is generally assumed that most cells greater than 4N in ploidy are committed to endomitosis and rarely divide mitotically. The probability of entering the endomitotic pathway is hierarchically dependent upon the state of differentiation of the progenitor.[17] Thus, the more primitive the progenitor is, the more likely it is to remain a mitotic cell. Genes with known roles in regulating the cell cycle such as the cyclin-dependent kinases and the cyclins have been studied. Although results are incomplete, during endomitosis cyclin D3 is increased,[18] and the levels of cyclin B1 and cyclin B1-dependent Cdc2 kinase are reduced.[19] These events may allow the megakaryocyte to abort some aspects of mitosis and reenter a phase of DNA replication without cytokinesis.[20]

MEGAKARYOCYTE GRANULES

Since platelets can produce only very small amounts of protein, their cytoplasmic characteristics are mostly determined by the megakaryocytes from which they come. Four distinct categories of granules differing in their internal constituents are produced by maturing megakaryocytes: alpha (α), dense, lysosomal, and microperoxisomal (Fig. 110-1*a*–*e*).

α GRANULES

The α granules (which are azurophilic on stained smears) are the most numerous granules seen with the electron microscope.[21] The granule body itself is made early in megakaryocyte development before the demarcation membrane system and first appears in the Golgi apparatus of megakaryoblasts (stage I megakaryocytes).[22] Several platelet proteins, including von Willebrand factor (vWf), platelet factor 4 (PF4), and thrombospondin have been detected in early megakaryocyte progenitors prior to the appearance of α granules.[23] Figure 110-1*b* shows that α granules exhibit distinct zones: a diffuse granular matrix, a dense nucleoid, and a third electron-lucent compartment containing from one to six tubular structures close to the membrane.[24] Immunoelectron microscopy has shown that several of the α granule proteins are compartmentalized; for example, vWf is associated with tubular structures similar to those of the vWf storage organelles of the vascular endothelium (Weibel-Palade bodies). Thrombospondin and fibrinogen are localized in the matrix,[25–27] and β-thromboglobulin (β-TG) and PF4, together with mucopolysaccharides, are present in the dense nucleoid.[28–30]

Although some of the α granule proteins such as platelet-derived growth factor, transforming growth factor-β, PF4, and vWf are synthesized in the megakaryocyte and transported to the α granules,[31] other proteins such as fibrinogen undergo GPIIb/IIIa receptor-mediated endocytosis from the plasma into the α granules of both megakaryocytes and platelets.[32–35] Still others, such as albumin and IgG are pinocytosed from the plasma into the α granules of megakaryocytes and platelets.[36] The location of megakaryocytes in close proximity to vascular sinuses may facilitate uptake of these circulating proteins.[37]

Several proteins have been detected on the membrane of α granules: GPIIb/IIIa,[38] P-selectin (CD62P; GMP-140 or PADGEM),[39] GMP-33,[40] and platelet osteonectin.[41]

DENSE GRANULES

Dense granules constitute a class of granules distinguishable from α granules by their morphology (Fig. 110-1*c*) and their content: a nonmetabolic pool of adenine nucleotides synthesized by megakaryocytes, and calcium and serotonin.[42] Dense granules of platelets are physically dense, and because of their content of serotonin and calcium, they are also electron-dense when viewed with the transmission electron microscope. The dense granule membrane bodies are made in megakaryocytes but do not acquire their content of serotonin and calcium until platelets are released into the circulation and then uptake calcium and most of the body's circulating serotonin.[43,44] This ability to accumulate and store serotonin constitutes an early marker of megakaryocytes, since even the earliest megakaryocyte progenitors are able to incorporate exogenous serotonin.[44,45] The membrane of dense bodies expresses granulophysin[46] and P-selectin.[47]

LYSOSOMAL GRANULES

Lysosomal granules are a unique class of granules as judged by ultrastructural cytochemical localization of arylsulfatase and acid phosphatase (Fig. 110-1*d*), the immunolocalization of cathepsin D, and the identification of lysosome-associated membrane protein.[48–50] They are formed very early during maturation, prior to the appearance of α granules.

MICROPEROXISOME GRANULES

Small granules (90 nm) that arise prior to α granule formation have been shown to contain catalase.[51] These granules appear similar to the microperoxisomes of other cells (Fig. 110-1*e*).

MEGAKARYOCYTE SURFACE MEMBRANE

DEMARCATION MEMBRANE SYSTEM

The surface membrane of the mature megakaryocyte is deeply invaginated and highly redundant (Fig. 110-1*a*). It divides the cytoplasm into platelet-sized "territories" and has thus been termed the *demarcation membrane system*.[52,53] Since the lumen of the demarcation membrane system stains with extracellular tracers (Fig. 110-1*f*), it is continuous with the extracellular medium.[52,54] The total area of the surface and demarcation membranes may increase by 26-fold during a 72-h maturation period.[52] This enormous amplification of the surface membrane is required to form platelets.[52,55,56]

PLATELET GLYCOPROTEINS

Both the megakaryocyte cell membrane and the demarcation membrane system express GPIIb/IIIa and GPIb/IX complexes; however, these platelet glycoproteins appear first on the plasma membrane prior to the formation of the demarcation membrane system.[57] One of the first signs of differentiation along the megakaryocyte lineage is the appearance on the surface of CD34+ progenitors of the platelet GPIIb/IIIa receptor,[58] and its expression increases in parallel with the decline of CD34 expression during maturation.[59] GPIIb has been considered to be specific for the megakaryocyte-platelet lineage.[60] This is later followed by the appearance of the GPIb/IX complex[57] and the collagen receptors. Expression of GPIb/IX, a receptor for vWf,[61] correlates with the onset of ploidization.[59] This complex has been thought to be platelet-specific, although cytokine-activated endothelial cells may also express a form of GPIb.[62–64]

LIGHT MICROSCOPIC APPEARANCE OF MEGAKARYOCYTES

The large, mature, polyploid megakaryocytes are readily identified by light microscopy (see Plate XXX) and are often located adjacent to bone marrow sinusoids.[37] Occasionally they may actually be seen to be shedding platelets.[1,65] In addition to the mature megakaryocytes, several other earlier maturational stages of megakaryocytes may be identified[66] using a classification scheme based on the nuclear/cytoplasmic ratio, nuclear shape, basophilia, and granularity (Table 110-1).[67] These early megakaryocytes are often distant from the sinusoid.

Also present in the bone marrow are small, diploid megakaryocyte progenitor cells called *promegakaryoblasts* that are transitional cells committed to the process of endomitosis but not yet polyploid.[68–72] In humans these cells have the size and morphology of lymphocytes and express GPIIb on their membrane and vWf or PF4 in their cytoplasm.[23,73,74] This population is equivalent to the small acetylcholinesterase-positive marrow cells in rodents.[69] (In rodents and cats, acetylcholinesterase is a specific marker for platelets and megakaryocytes[69]; in humans acetylcholinesterase appears to be present in immature, but not mature megakaryocytes.[75]) Some of these cells may retain proliferative capacity,[72] but the majority of these transitional cells do not form colonies in culture. They are, however, capable of maturing into typical polyploid megakaryocytes[71,76] and constitute 4 percent of all megakaryocytes.[77–79] Ultrastructurally, human promegakaryoblasts are recognizable by the cytochemical demonstration of *platelet peroxidase*, which is present exclusively in the endoplasmic reticulum (Fig. 110-2).[54] This enzyme, which is present throughout megakaryocytic maturation and is detectable in platelets, is involved in prostaglandin synthesis.[80] Although several other types of marrow cells capable of transient prostaglandin synthesis exhibit a similar peroxidase activity, nonmegakaryocytes possess characteristics that distinguish them from promegakaryoblasts.[81,82] Simultaneous analysis of membrane GPIIb

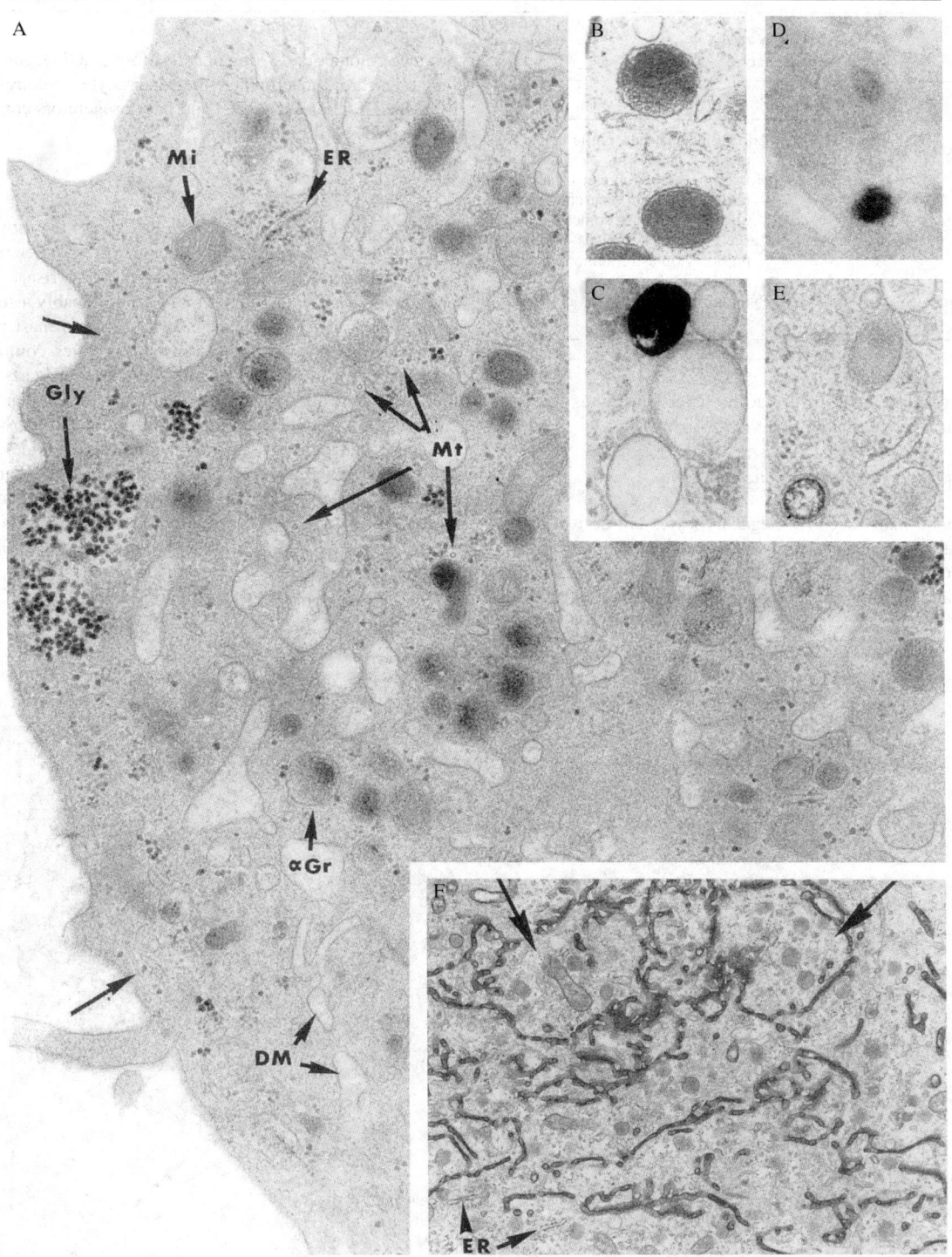

FIGURE 110-1 *(a)* Ultrastructure of the cytoplasm of a mature megakaryocyte. The majority of the granules are α granules (α-Gr) exhibiting dense nucleoid. Demarcation membranes (DM) are slightly dilated. Transverse sections of microtubules (Mt) are dispersed; at the periphery, a longitudinal microtubule runs under the cell membrane *(arrows)*. Dense aggregates of glycogen (Gly), small cisternae of endoplasmic reticulum (ER), and free ribosomes can be recognized. ×30,320. *(b)* Morphology of an α granule. Dense nucleoid is located at the top; in a clear zone at the opposite pole, four transverse sections of tubular structures are seen adjacent to the granule membrane. ×37,200. *(c)* A dense body can be distinguished from an α granule by the black deposit when calcium is added to the fixative. ×37,200. *(d)* Cytochemical detection of acid phosphatase using β-glycophosphate as substrate and cerium as a trapping agent. Dense cerium-phosphate precipitates are present in lysosomal granules while α granules are unreactive. ×37,200. *(e)* Microperoxisome visualized using alkaline diaminobenzidine. Note the small size of a reactive granule compared to an α granule. ×37,200. *(f)* Distribution of a dense tracer filling the lumen of the demarcation membrane system in a maturing megakaryocyte. This system appears to outline some platelet territories *(arrows)*. In contrast to the demarcation membrane system, which is open to the extracellular space, the endoplasmic reticulum (ER) is not labeled. ×9700. (Courtesy of Dr. Janine Breton-Gorius.)

TABLE 110-1 MATURATION STAGES OF MEGAKARYOCYTES

TERM	SIZE, μM	MORPHOLOGY
Megakaryoblast (stage I)	>15	Lobed nucleus, basophilic cytoplasm
Basophil megakaryocyte (stage II)	>20	Horseshoe-shaped nucleus, basophilic cytoplasm, azurophil granules around centrosome
Granular megakaryocyte (stage III)	>25–50	Large multilobed nucleus, acidophilic cytoplasm, numerous azurophil granules
Mature megakaryocyte (stage IV)	>25–50	Pyknotic nucleus, groups of 10–12 azurophil granules

and platelet peroxidase has shown that the latter constitutes the first marker of megakaryocyte maturation.[83]

THE ORIGIN OF MEGAKARYOCYTES

Like all other bone marrow cells, megakaryocytes are derived from the pluripotential stem cell (Fig. 110-3). The cellular steps by which the stem cell becomes a megakaryocyte have been defined by in vitro colony studies and include early progenitors having the capacity to produce colonies consisting of cells of several lineages [such as granulocyte-erythroid-macrophage-megakaryocyte colony-forming cells (GEMM-CFC) or Mix-CFC] and later progenitors committed only to megakaryocyte differentiation.[84,85]

EARLY MEGAKARYOCYTE PROGENITORS

Although most CD34+/CD38− cells express the thrombopoietin receptor, c-Mpl, on their surface,[86] few express other megakaryocyte-specific antigens. These cells ultimately give rise to multipotential progenitors such as the GEMM-CFC and probably also to progenitors committed to erythrocyte, megakaryocyte, and mast cell differentiation. There is no specific assay for this latter common progenitor cell, but there is a close relationship between early erythroid and megakaryocyte differentiation at the molecular, cellular, and pathological levels. For example, common transcription factors exist in these two lineages,[87] and their regulatory hematopoietic cytokines, erythropoietin and thrombopoietin, are 50 percent similar.[3] Both share the common *cis*-acting sequence, GATA-1,[88,89] which is present in the promoter regions of many genes. In addition, in mice in which the thymidine kinase gene was expressed under the control of the GPIIb promoter, administration of gancyclovir resulted in eradication of both megakaryocyte and erythroid progenitors,[90] suggesting that the GPIIb promoter

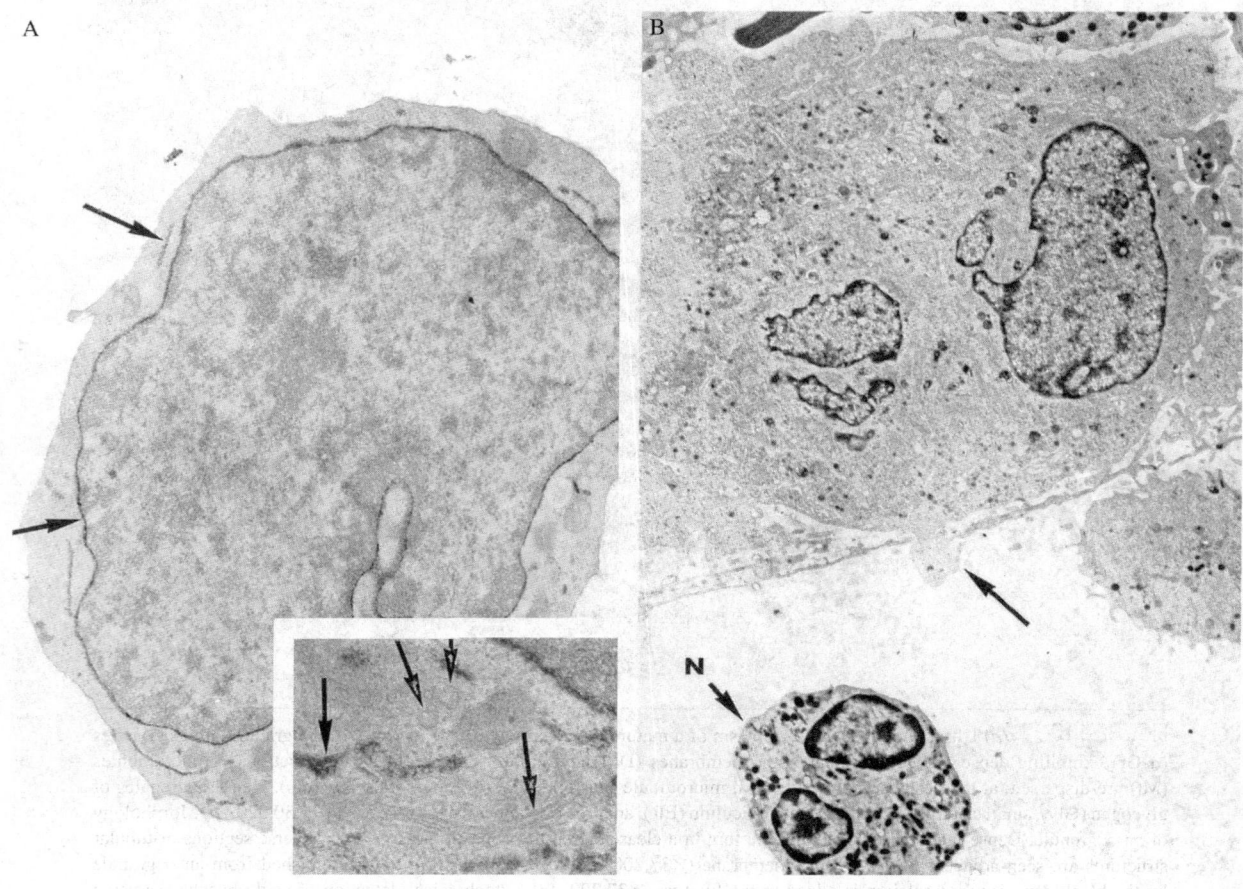

FIGURE 110-2 (a) Electron micrograph of a normal human marrow promegakaryocyte treated for the detection of platelet peroxidase. This small cell (<9 μm) exhibits a dense reaction product, demonstrating the presence of platelet peroxidase in the perinuclear space and in the endoplasmic reticulum (*arrows*). ×12,150. (Inset) Enlargement of the Golgi zone. The Golgi saccules and vesicles are devoid of platelet peroxidase (*open arrows*), while the endoplasmic reticulum contains platelet peroxidase activity (*closed arrow*). ×25,000. (b) Maturing megakaryocyte in the marrow. The large megakaryocyte is located close to the sinus endothelium, and a small cytoplasmic bleb (*arrow*) is in direct contact with the blood. A neutrophil (N) is seen in the sinus. ×3600. (Courtesy of Dr. Janine Breton-Gorius.)

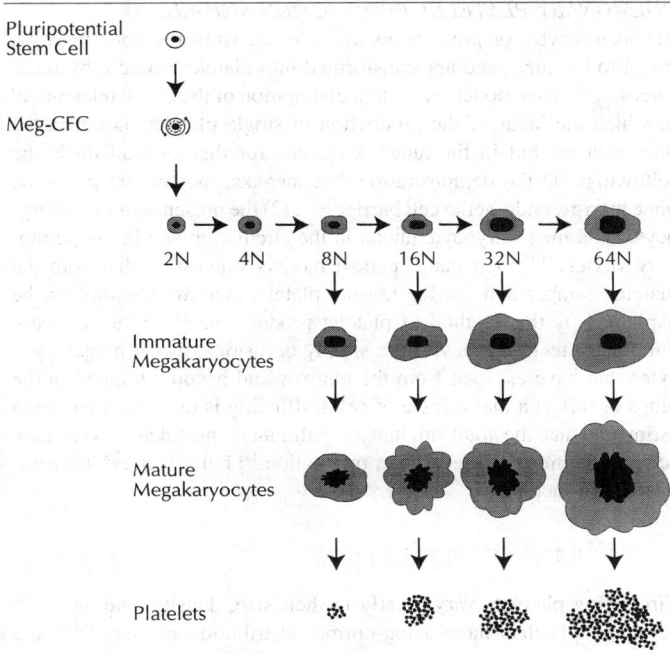

FIGURE 110-3 The origin and development of megakaryocytes. The pluripotential stem cell produces a progenitor cell committed to megakaryocyte differentiation (meg-CFC) which can undergo mitosis. Eventually the meg-CFC stops mitosis and enters endomitosis during which neither cytoplasm nor nucleus divides but DNA replication proceeds and gives rise to polyploid immature precursor cells. Upon completion of endomitosis, the immature progenitor cells become large, morphologically identifiable, mature megakaryocytes that shed platelets.

was transcriptionally active in a bipotential progenitor cell[91] and possibly in a totipotent progenitor cell.[92]

LATE MEGAKARYOCYTE PROGENITORS

At some point, the differentiation process produces precursor cells committed only to megakaryocyte differentiation. The transition between multipotent progenitors and megakaryocyte-restricted progenitors may involve the *c-mpl* oncogene, which is highly expressed in megakaryocyte cell lines and progenitor cells.[93] Inhibition of *c-mpl* function in vitro has been reported to decrease megakaryocyte differentiation of primitive progenitors.[94] A hierarchical classification system of megakaryocytic progenitors has been devised based on proliferative characteristics in culture, membrane antigen expression, and physical properties.[95–98] The more immature progenitors have the greatest capacity for proliferation, a capacity that declines as the progenitor differentiates.[99] The earliest definable committed progenitor, the *megakaryocytic burst-forming cell* (meg-BFC),[95] gives rise to clusters of megakaryocytes (100 cells or more), is fully expressed at 21 days following initiation of culture, is resistant to 5-fluorouracil (5-FU) treatment, expresses the hematopoietic stem cell marker CD34, and is HLA-DR-negative.[96,99]

A later progenitor, the *megakaryocyte colony-forming cell* (meg-CFC),[100,101] gives rise to colonies composed of smaller numbers of megakaryocytes, is expressed at 12 days of culture, is sensitive to 5-FU, expresses membrane GPIIb/IIIa[102,103] and HLA-DR antigens,[99] and undergoes mitosis.[104] The CD34 antigen declines progressively with increasing maturity of the progenitors and is lost in the polyploid immature megakaryocyte.[59]

Eventually the meg-CFC stops mitosis and enters endomitosis in which polyploid precursors with scant cytoplasm are produced (Fig. 110-3). Upon the completion of endomitosis, immature megakaryocytes develop a mature cytoplasm, become morphologically identifiable, and eventually release platelets. Overall, it takes approximately 5 to 7 days to progress from the meg-CFC to the platelet. Morphologically identifiable megakaryocytes rarely divide.

EFFECTS OF THROMBOPOIETIC GROWTH FACTORS

The primary regulator of platelet production, thrombopoietin, has a major effect on almost all steps of megakaryocyte differentiation and maturation. It promotes the growth of meg-CFC, dramatically increases the rate of endomitosis, and stimulates megakaryocyte maturation.[105,106] Increased megakaryocyte ploidy is seen at even very low concentrations of thrombopoietin and is the most sensitive indicator of the effect of thrombopoietin. However, the final stage of platelet release is not dependent on thrombopoietin and actually may be inhibited by large amounts of thrombopoietin.[107] Other cytokines such as IL-3,[108–111] IL-6,[112–120] and IL-11[121–124] can also promote meg-CFC growth and megakaryocyte maturation but lack much effect on endomitosis; they can all increase platelet production in vivo. Transforming growth factor β inhibits megakaryocyte growth and platelet production in vitro and in vivo.[125–127] Interferon alpha and beta inhibit the growth of meg-CFC,[128–133] but interferon gamma stimulates meg-CFC growth.[134] Interferon alpha has been used clinically to reduce the platelet count in patients with essential thrombocythemia and other myeloproliferative disorders[129,135,136]; in patients with chronic hepatitis, interferon alpha produces a rapid decrease in the platelet count.[137]

PLATELET PRODUCTION AND RELEASE

THE FORMATION OF PLATELETS FROM MEGAKARYOCYTES

Although historically one of the first observations was the apparent shedding of platelets by megakaryocytes,[1,65] the exact mechanism by which platelets are produced remains unclear. Incomplete data suggest that platelets are not shed from megakaryocytes with ploidy less than 8N and that larger megakaryocytes make more platelets than smaller ones. Each megakaryocyte produces an average of 1000 to 3000 platelets, and it has been estimated that 35,000 to 45,000 platelets per microliter of blood are produced per day.[10,138,139] During times of marked platelet demand, normal production may increase sixfold.[10] Three different mechanisms of platelet production from megakaryocytes have been proposed.

PLATELET TERRITORIES MODEL

The megakaryocyte cytoplasm is divided by the demarcation membrane system into future platelet "territories" (Fig. 110-1*f*), and the megakaryocyte then simply fractures into separate platelets.[140] The platelets would be released into the marrow and then somehow pass into the sinusoids, leaving behind the bare megakaryocyte nucleus. Support for this mechanism comes primarily from electron microscopic data showing these platelet territories in megakaryocytes but not the more dynamic process of them fracturing into platelets. However, few bare megakaryocyte nuclei are seen in the bone marrow, and there is no evidence that platelets pass through the endothelial cells lining the sinusoids.

PROPLATELET MODEL

Megakaryocytes use the highly redundant demarcation membrane system to send pseudopodia out into the bone marrow sinusoids,[52,55,141–143] and platelets and proplatelets bud off. *Proplatelets* are elongated

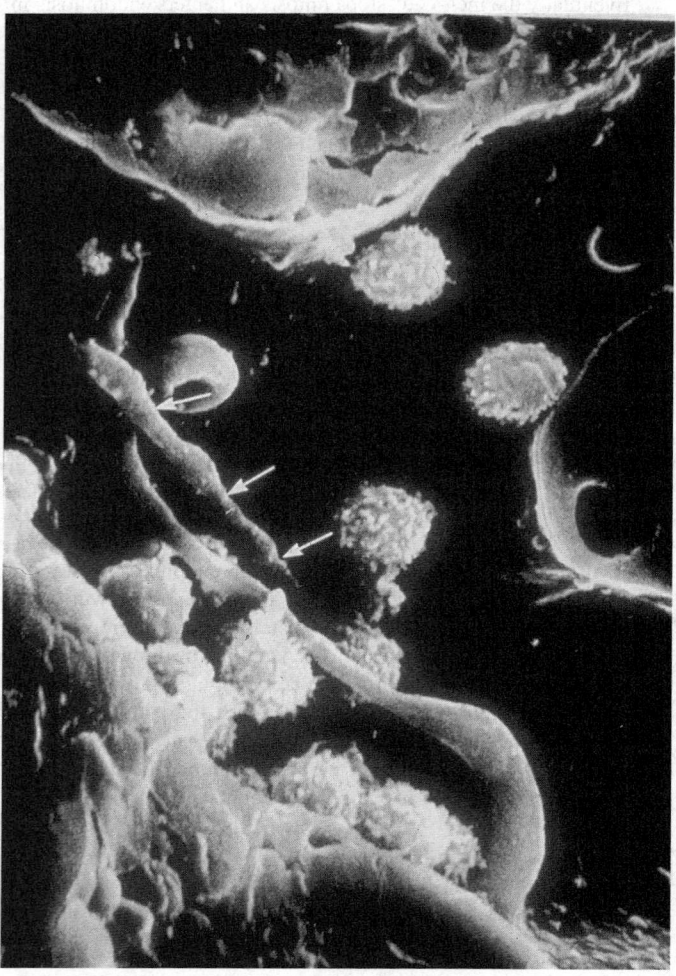

FIGURE 110-4　Megakaryocyte proplatelet processes in the bone marrow sinusoid. This scanning electron micrograph shows the luminal view of the confluence of two bone marrow sinusoids with two proplatelet processes protruding through the lining endothelial cells. One of the processes has intermittent constrictions (*arrows*) indicating potential sites for platelet formation. Other cells depicted include lymphocytes and erythrocytes (×3000). Reproduced by permission from reference 141.

strands of megakaryocyte cytoplasm (Fig. 110-4) that are larger than normal platelets[141,144] and later fragment into a number of platelets. The bone marrow sinusoids are lined by very thin endothelial cells that are tightly bound to each other and may even overlap.[141] The megakaryocyte pseudopodia actually pass through, not between, the endothelial cells, which may in turn play some role in regulating the process.[141] This is the method initially suggested in 1906,[1,65] and most subsequent data confirm many elements of this model. For example, the culture of mature megakaryocytes on basement membrane matrix leads to increased proplatelet formation.[145–147] Platelets may then be liberated from these elongated processes by rupture of the links. In mice recovering from severe thrombocytopenia there are increased numbers of proplatelet processes in the sinusoids.[90] Also in mice lacking the transcription factor NF-E2, the severe thrombocytopenia that is present is probably related to the inability of the megakaryocytes to form proplatelet processes.[148,149] A similar defect occurs in mice with selective loss of the transcription factor GATA-1.[150]

PULMONARY PLATELET PRODUCTION MODEL

Megakaryocytes or proplatelets are released from the bone marrow, travel to the lung, and are transformed into platelets therein by shear forces.[151–153] This model is a further elaboration of the proplatelet model in which the locus of the production of single platelets is not in the bone marrow but in the lungs. Evidence for this mechanism is the following: (1) the demonstration that megakaryocytes can cross the bone marrow endothelial cell barrier[90,154]; (2) the presence of megakaryocytes and megakaryocyte nuclei in the circulation and in the pulmonary vessels[151,153]; (3) mathematical models suggesting that both the platelet number and the log-normal platelet size distribution can be explained by this method of platelet production.[152,155] Whether these pulmonary megakaryocytes are simply occasional errant megakaryocytes that have escaped from the marrow and become trapped in the lungs or reflect a major route of cell trafficking is unclear. It has been estimated that the total amount of pulmonary megakaryocytes may account for most of the platelet production,[156] but direct evidence for this is still lacking.

REGULATION OF PLATELET SIZE

Circulating platelets vary greatly in their size, density, and age.[157,158] Although platelets have a log-normal distribution of sizes,[152,155] the cellular mechanisms accounting for the size of platelets is poorly understood. It is unclear whether large platelets come from large, high-ploidy megakaryocytes or small, low-ploidy megakaryocytes; evidence for either exists.[158–160] In general, the mean platelet volume (MPV) increases as the platelet count decreases[160,161] and the larger platelets are assumed to be younger[162–166] and more reactive.[167] This effect is seen clinically in patients with chronic idiopathic thrombocytopenic purpura (ITP) in whom the MPV is increased due to an increased number of large platelets, called *megathrombocytes;* the presence of megathrombocytes is useful in distinguishing ITP from some of the other thrombocytopenic disorders.[163–166] In reactive thrombocytosis the MPV is not increased.

The effect of thrombopoietin on platelet size is variable. In mice, administration of low doses of thrombopoietin decreased the MPV, intermediate doses produced an initial increase followed by a later decrease, and high doses gave an initial increase followed by a normalization of the MPV.[168,169] In humans administered a recombinant form of thrombopoietin, the MPV usually decreased in a manner inversely proportional to the platelet count.[170]

THE MOLECULAR BIOLOGY OF MEGAKARYOCYTE DIFFERENTIATION

The molecular mechanisms by which cells become committed to the megakaryocyte lineage are just starting to be unraveled. Unlike hematopoietic growth factors such as thrombopoietin, which appear to prevent apoptosis and stimulate growth of cells already committed to megakaryocyte differentiation, *intrinsic lineage-specific transcription factors* become expressed in uncommitted precursor cells and then establish cell-specific phenotypes. The transcription factors *GATA-1* and *NF-E2* have been shown to be important in megakaryocyte development. The lineage-specific genes that are, in turn, controlled by these factors remain unknown.

GATA-1

This zinc-finger transcription factor is expressed in erythroid cells, megakaryocytes, eosinophils, and mast cells. Elimination of the entire GATA-1 gene results in embryonic death due to severe anemia.[171] Since GATA-1 is found in megakaryocytes, and GATA-1 binding sites are found in many genes specific for megakaryocytes and platelets, it was anticipated that GATA-1 played a role in megakaryocyte development. When a unique portion of the GATA-1 promoter was disrupted, GATA-1 expression was eliminated in megakaryocytes but not in erythrocytes. Animals with this disrupted GATA-1 promoter were not anemic, but they had platelet counts 15 percent of normal and an increased number of small, abnormal megakaryocytes with multilobulated nuclei.[150] The megakaryocytes had scant cytoplasm, few demarcation membranes, no platelet "territories," and few platelet granules; they rarely formed proplatelets, suggesting an early defect in cytoplasmic maturation and consequently diminished platelet production. In addition these megakaryocytes had an increased proliferative capacity in vitro.[87]

NF-E2

This heterodimeric basic leucine zipper transcription factor is composed of a widely expressed p18 subunit and a p45 subunit present only in erythroid cells, megakaryocytes, and mast cells. When NF-E2 was disrupted, mice developed a mild anemia and a profound thrombocytopenia associated with a high rate of early hemorrhagic death.[172,173] These mice had adequate numbers of large, abnormal megakaryocytes with hyperlobulated nuclei, rare granules, and adequate amounts of demarcation membranes, but no platelet "territories." The mice never appear to form proplatelets.[149] NF-E2 appears to affect megakaryocyte cytoplasmic differentiation and platelet production at a somewhat later step than GATA-1.[174]

THE REGULATION OF MEGAKARYOCYTOPOIESIS AND THROMBOPOIESIS

PHYSIOLOGICAL PRINCIPLES

Over the past 50 years a number of principles of the regulation of platelet production have emerged from clinical studies[175]:

1. The platelet count in any individual remains constant throughout life unless perturbed by physiological (e.g., pregnancy) or pathological (e.g., myelodysplasia) processes.[176]
2. Among normal individuals there is a large variation in platelet counts, ranging from $150-450 \times 10^9$/liter.[162] This is unlike the erythrocyte count, which is much less variable between individuals.
3. There is an inverse relationship between the normal platelet count and the normal mean platelet volume (MPV),[177] and this produces a roughly constant circulating platelet mass.[158,178] This inverse relationship extends to other species; for example, mice have a normal platelet count of 1200×10^9/liter and an MPV of 4.7 fl whereas porcupines have a normal platelet count of 30×10^9/liter and an MPV of 105 fl.[179]
4. The body "defends" the total *mass of platelets,* not the platelet count. Normally approximately one-third of the total platelet mass is sequestered in an exchangeable splenic pool.[180] In animals[181,182] or humans with enlarged spleens,[180] the platelet count decreases proportionally to the increase in the size of the spleen, but the total body mass of platelets remains normal and unchanged.
5. The bone marrow megakaryocytes respond to changes in the demand for platelets by altering their number, size, and ploidy. In animals[12,183,184] made thrombocytopenic by the injection of antibody to platelets, bone marrow megakaryocytes increase their number, size, and ploidy. In animals made thrombocytotic by

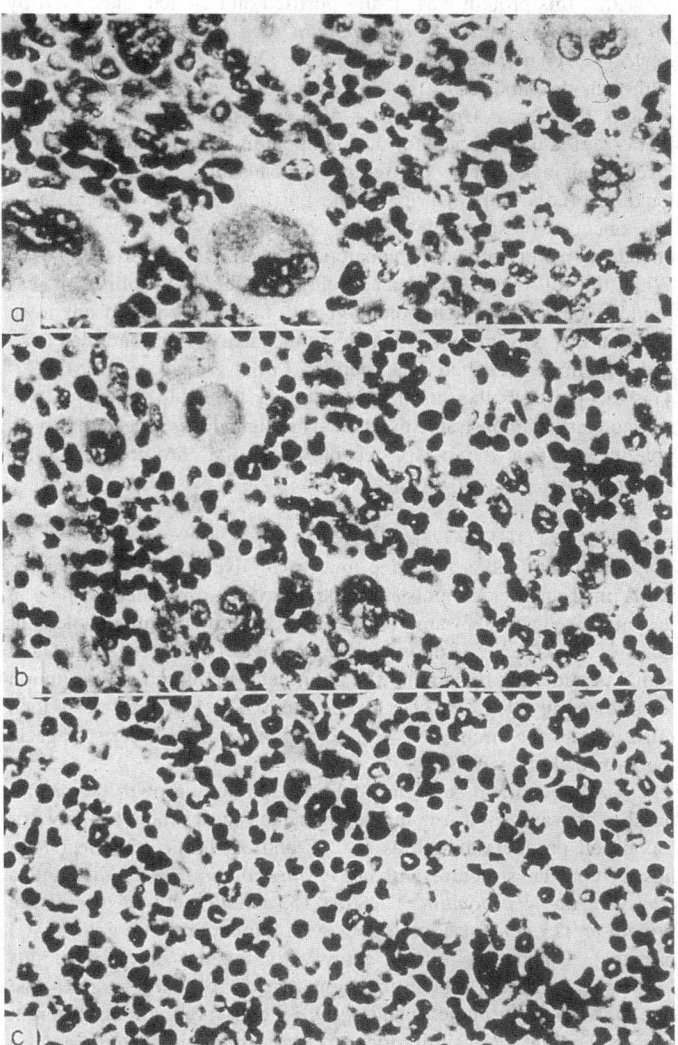

FIGURE 110-5   The physiological response of bone marrow megakaryocytes to changes in the platelet count. Mice were made acutely thrombocytopenic by the injection of antiplatelet antibody *(a)* or made thrombocytotic by the transfusion of platelets *(c)* and compared with untreated mice *(b).* The number, size, and nuclear lobulation of bone marrow megakaryocytes increased during thrombocytopenia and decreased during thrombocytosis when compared with normal animals ($\times 16$). Reproduced by permission.[184]

platelet transfusion, the opposite changes in megakaryocytes occur (Fig. 110-5).
6. Meg-CFC do not respond acutely to the stimulus of thrombocytopenia[185,186]; rather, increased meg-CFC are observed subsequent to the alterations that are noted in the more differentiated megakaryocytes.[185] Similarly, thrombocytosis does not result in a compensatory decrease in meg-CFC.[185] These in vivo observations imply that the initial response to platelet demand is focused on the more mature nonmitotic megakaryocytes.

THROMBOPOIETIN

For almost 50 years it had been assumed that a *thrombopoietin* existed that regulated platelet production just as erythropoietin controlled the production of erythrocytes.[187] Despite heroic efforts, it was not until

1994 that this protein was finally purified and cloned and called by several different names: *thrombopoietin*,[5,188] *c-Mpl ligand*,[3] *megakaryocyte growth and differentiation factor* (MGDF),[6] or *megapoietin*.[2] Although thrombopoietin is the historically accepted name for this protein, the term *c-Mpl ligand* is also appropriate given the finding that c-Mpl is the receptor for thrombopoietin. This receptor had been discovered in a murine retrovirus that caused a myeloproliferative leukemia (i.e., "mpl") prior to the purification of thrombopoietin. The oncogene responsible for that syndrome, *v-mpl*, was found to encode a novel truncated hematopoietic growth factor receptor.[189] When the full-length cellular homologue, *c-mpl*, was cloned, it was found to be a new hematopoietic growth factor receptor of unknown function that was present primarily on megakaryocytes and platelets[93] and if inhibited resulted in a decrease in the growth of meg-CFC.[94] This receptor was then used to help purify the c-Mpl ligand. It was subsequently demonstrated that the c-Mpl ligand was indeed thrombopoietin and that the c-Mpl receptor was the thrombopoietin receptor.[190–193]

STRUCTURE OF THROMBOPOIETIN

Thrombopoietin is produced primarily in liver parenchymal cells, while much smaller amounts are made in the kidney.[194] Thrombopoietin is synthesized as a 353–amino acid precursor protein with a molecular mass of 36 kDa.[3,6,195] Following the removal of the 21–amino acid signal peptide, the remaining 332 amino acids undergo glycosylation to produce an 80- to 90-kDa glycoprotein. The glycoprotein is then released into the circulation with no apparent intracellular storage in the liver or kidney.

Thrombopoietin is an unusual hematopoietic growth factor in a number of ways. First it is much larger than most other regulators of blood cell production such as G-CSF and erythropoietin. Second it has an unusual structure with an *erythropoietin-like domain* and a *carbohydrate-rich domain*. The first 153 amino acids of the mature protein are 23 percent homologous with human erythropoietin[196] and probably 50 percent similar if conservative amino acid substitutions are considered. This region also contains four cysteine residues just like those in erythropoietin and is highly conserved among different species. Despite these similarities with erythropoietin, thrombopoietin does not bind to the erythropoietin receptor and erythropoietin does not bind to the thrombopoietin receptor.

Amino acids 154 to 332 comprise a novel sequence that contains six N-linked glycosylation sites; this region is less well conserved among different species. Structure-function studies have demonstrated that while the first 153 amino acids of the c-Mpl ligand are all that are required for its thrombopoietic effect in vitro,[3,6,197] this truncated molecule has a markedly decreased circulatory half-life compared to the 20- to 40-h half-life of the native protein.[198] Presumably, the carbohydrate-rich half of the molecule confers stability and prolongs the circulatory half-life. Similar carbohydrate sequences regulate the stability of erythropoietin.[199] In addition, this part of the molecule assists in the secretion of the intact molecule from the hepatocytes by serving as a molecular chaperone or guide in protein folding; truncated muteins of this portion of the molecule have diminished secretion.[200]

There is a single copy of the gene for thrombopoietin on human chromosome 3q27-28.[195,196,201] The gene spans approximately 7 kb with seven exons, the first two of which are noncoding. The third exon contains part of the 5'-untranslated mRNA sequence and part of the signal peptide. The erythropoietin-like region is coded for by exons 4 to 7, and all of the carbohydrate domain is encoded by exon 7. Comparison with the erythropoietin gene shows conservation of the boundaries of the coding exons except for the addition of the carbohydrate domain sequence in the final exon of the thrombopoietin gene. In addition to the functional mRNA encoded (TPO-1), two other nonfunctional m-RNA sequences (TPO-2 and TPO-3) are present due to alternative splicing.[195,196]

THE THROMBOPOIETIN RECEPTOR

It is now known that the *thrombopoietin receptor* (c-Mpl) is present on platelets and megakaryocytes, and at lesser density on most other hematopoietic precursor cells. Upon binding to thrombopoietin, the receptor undergoes dimerization, resulting in a number of signal transduction events that improve cell viability, promote growth, and possibly increase differentiation.[202] In addition, receptor binding provides the major mechanism by which thrombopoietin is removed from the circulation by platelets and possibly megakaryocytes.[2,203–205] Upon binding thrombopoietin, the receptor-ligand complex undergoes internalization, and the bound thrombopoietin is degraded.[206] The receptor is not reexpressed on the surface.[207]

THE EFFECTS OF THROMBOPOIETIN IN VITRO

Binding of thrombopoietin to its receptor prevents apoptosis of megakaryocytes[208] and increases their number, size, and ploidy. The rate of cellular maturation is probably also increased. These events are mediated via signal transduction pathways involving JAK, STAT, and other intracellular mediators.[209–217] Addition of thrombopoietin to CD34+ cells can actually result in the majority of cells becoming megakaryocytes and then shedding platelets.[218]

Although thrombopoietin stimulates early precursor cells of all lineages as well as pluripotential stem cells,[219] it stimulates late maturation only in megakaryocytes.

THE EFFECTS OF THROMBOPOIETIN IN VIVO

When administered to normal animals, thrombopoietin stimulates an increase in bone marrow and peripheral blood meg-CFC, an increase in bone marrow megakaryocytes, and a rise in the platelet count.[220–222] Interestingly, both erythroid and multipotential precursor cells are also increased in the bone marrow and peripheral blood, but without affecting the erythrocyte or neutrophil count.

Following the daily administration of a recombinant form of thrombopoietin to normal baboons, a predictable response occurs.[221,222] During the first 4 days of administration, bone marrow megakaryocyte ploidy rises to a maximum, but there is no change in the platelet count. On day 5 the platelet count begins to rise and does so at a dose-dependent rate. With continued administration of thrombopoietin, a dose-dependent plateau platelet count is attained on days 8 to 12. There is a log-linear relationship between the thrombopoietin dose and the plateau platelet count, with a maximum sixfold increase in the rate of platelet production. Upon stopping the growth factor, the platelet count returns to its baseline over 10 days without a rebound thrombocytopenia. In humans a similar time course and platelet response have been demonstrated with no acute toxicity[220] but with subsequent studies indicating the potential of individuals to make antibodies to at least one of the thrombopoietin preparations under development (see Recombinant Thrombopoietic Growth Factors and Their Clinical Uses, below).

In addition to increasing the number of megakaryocytes and platelets, thrombopoietin can also affect the function of platelets. When thrombopoietin binds to its platelet receptor, it induces phosphorylation of the c-Mpl receptor and a number of other molecules in several different signal transduction pathways[223–225] but does not directly cause platelet activation. However, such thrombopoietin treatment reduces by 50 percent the threshold for activation by other platelet agonists like ADP and collagen. It is unclear if this is a clinically relevant effect.

THE ROLE OF THROMBOPOIETIN IN NORMAL PHYSIOLOGY

THROMBOPOIETIN IS THE ONLY PHYSIOLOGICALLY RELEVANT REGULATOR OF PLATELET PRODUCTION

Thrombopoietin serves to ''amplify'' the basal production rate of megakaryocytes and platelets. When thrombopoietin or its receptor has been ''knocked out'' by homologous recombination in mice,[226–228] the megakaryocyte and platelet mass are reduced to about 10 percent of normal, but the animals are healthy and do not spontaneously bleed. The neutrophil and erythrocyte counts are normal. In animals in which only one of the thrombopoietin genes has been deleted, the platelet count is reduced to about 65 percent of normal. However, such thrombopoietin-deficient mice can increase their platelet count if treated with other thrombopoietic growth factors such as IL-6, IL-11, or stem cell factor.[229]

THROMBOPOIETIN AFFECTS BONE MARROW PRECURSOR CELLS OF ALL LINEAGES

In the animals made deficient in thrombopoietin or c-Mpl, the megakaryocyte precursor cells (meg-CFC) are reduced by 90 to 95 percent, as expected. However, the myeloid and erythroid precursor cells are also reduced by 60 to 80 percent.[226,229] Presumably the normal neutrophil and erythrocyte counts in these animals are maintained by the intact feedback mechanisms mediated by G-CSF and erythropoietin.

THERE IS NO ''SENSOR'' OF THE PLATELET MASS

Hepatic thrombopoietin production is constitutive, and the circulating levels are determined by the circulating platelet mass (Fig. 110-6). While the production of red blood cells is regulated by a cytochrome P-450 system that senses changes in oxygen delivery to tissues and alters the rate of transcription of the erythropoietin gene, thrombopoietin mRNA is produced at the same rate in normal and thrombocytopenic individuals.[2,203–205,230,231] No drug or clinical condition has yet been shown to increase hepatic thrombopoietin production. Platelets and megakaryocytes contain high-affinity thrombopoietin receptors (c-Mpl) that bind and clear thrombopoietin from the circulation and thereby directly determine the circulating thrombopoietin level. When platelet production is decreased, clearance of thrombopoietin is reduced and levels rise. This type of feedback system is not unusual in hematology. Indeed, both M-CSF and G-CSF are normally regulated primarily by the amount of circulating monocytes and neutrophils, respectively.[232,233] It appears that only for erythropoietin is there a true sensor of the circulating blood cell mass that in turn alters production of this hematopoietic growth factor.

MEGAKARYOCYTES IN DISEASE

As initially described in 1910,[65] characteristic changes in megakaryocytes are associated with several disease processes. Most of these clinical conditions have been extensively studied with bone marrow and platelet kinetic studies[10] and thrombopoietin levels.[234]

MEGAKARYOCYTE HYPOPLASIA SECONDARY TO CHEMOTHERAPY

The thrombocytopenia that follows chemotherapy is due to a decreased number of megakaryocytes. This results in elevated levels of thrombopoietin[235] that increase the average ploidy of the remaining megakaryocytes in an effort to increase platelet production. Platelet kinetic studies

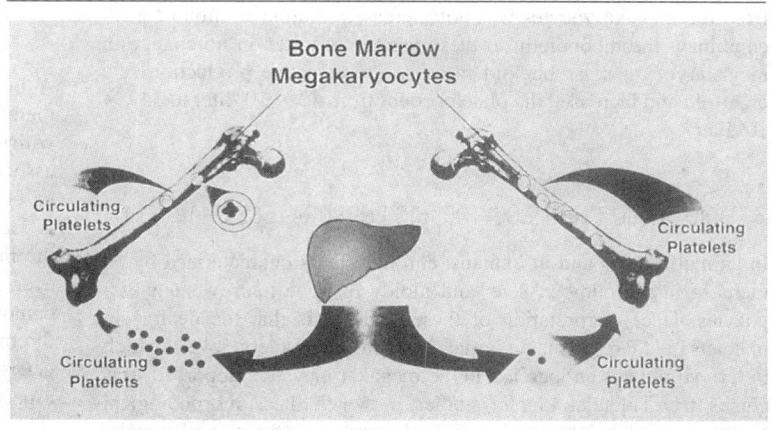

FIGURE 110-6   The mechanism by which thrombopoietin (TPO) regulates platelet production from megakaryocytes. TPO (width of arrows indicates relative concentration) is produced at a constant rate by the liver and enters the circulation. *Left side*: When the platelet count is normal, high-affinity TPO receptors on the platelet clear most of the TPO and produce a normal plasma TPO concentration, thereby providing basal stimulation of bone marrow megakaryocytes and a normal rate of platelet production. *Right side*: When platelet production and the platelet count are low, the overall clearance of TPO is reduced, subsequently increasing the plasma TPO concentration and megakaryocyte and platelet production. Modified from reference 2.

have also demonstrated some element of ineffective platelet production (*ineffective thrombopoiesis*) in this setting.[10]

PERNICIOUS ANEMIA (SEE CHAP. 37)

In severe pernicious anemia the low platelet count is associated with a marked increase in the number of megakaryocytes but diminished ploidy resulting in an expanded megakaryocyte mass but reduced platelet production per megakaryocyte.[10] This *ineffective platelet production* from the megakaryocytes is comparable to the ineffective erythrocyte production also seen in this disorder.

CONGESTIVE SPLENOMEGALY (SEE CHAP. 59)

As suggested above, the thrombocytopenia seen in splenomegaly secondary to liver disease has long been felt to be due to a redistribution of the normal circulating mass of platelets from the circulation to the spleen.[180,236] Platelet kinetic studies have analyzed this situation further and demonstrated that the modest thrombocytopenia is not accompanied by a decrease in platelet survival but does give rise to a small increase in the number and ploidy of megakaryocytes and a small overall increase in platelet production.[10] These results are at odds with data showing a reduced level of thrombopoietin and a reduction in platelet production rates in patients with cirrhosis.[237]

THROMBOCYTOPENIA ASSOCIATED WITH HUMAN IMMUNODEFICIENCY VIRUS (HIV) (SEE CHAP. 114)

Thrombocytopenia is commonly seen in both early and late HIV infection and has been considered due to immune complex binding to platelet Fc receptors and consequent platelet removal by the spleen.[238] Antiretroviral treatment is often associated with improvement. However, platelet kinetic studies suggest that platelet survival is only slightly reduced, and there is marked ineffective production of platelets from megakaryocytes.[139,239] In the thrombocytopenic HIV-infected patients studied,[239] megakaryocyte mass and megakaryocyte size were increased two- to threefold, but the total effective platelet production from the megakaryocytes was not increased. Administration of a recombinant thrombopoietin to these patients resulted in no change in megakaryocyte mass but did increase the effective production rate eightfold and increased the platelet count from 42×10^9/liter to 349×10^9/liter.

IDIOPATHIC THROMBOCYTOPENIC PURPURA (SEE CHAP. 114)

In animal models and in humans, chronic ITP is characterized by an increase in the number, size, and ploidy of bone marrow megakaryocytes. One interpretation of these findings is that the decline in platelets in ITP results in an initial rise in thrombopoietin levels, which in turn stimulates an increase in the megakaryocytes. Support for this comes from platelet kinetic studies in which these morphological findings are associated with a sixfold increase in the rate of platelet production[10,240,241] and a shortened platelet survival time. However, subsequent platelet kinetic studies[242] have failed to demonstrate an increase in platelet production in ITP and suggest that the morphological findings might be related to ineffective platelet production akin to that described for HIV infection. The observation that thrombopoietin levels are normal in this patient group is consistent with either hypothesis.[234,243]

REACTIVE THROMBOCYTOSIS (SEE CHAP. 115)

Reactive thrombocytosis occurs in association with iron deficiency, malignancy, and inflammatory states. It is associated with an increased number of megakaryocytes but with ploidy less than normal, an increased megakaryocyte mass, and an increased rate of platelet production. The increased platelet count is probably secondary to the expansion of the megakaryocyte number due to inflammatory cytokines such as IL-6,[244] and ploidy is reduced due to a decreased level of thrombopoietin secondary to increased thrombopoietin clearance by the expanded platelet mass.

ESSENTIAL THROMBOCYTHEMIA (SEE CHAP. 115)

Although the clonal nature of essential thrombocythemia has been challenged,[245] in essential thrombocythemia and the related myeloproliferative disorders such as chronic myeloid leukemia and polycythemia vera, there is a proliferation of megakaryocytes that are of high ploidy and actively produce platelets. Whether the normal regulatory mechanism via thrombopoietin and its receptor is functioning is unclear. Platelet kinetic data suggest the proliferation is autonomous of thrombopoietin in that at increased platelet mass there is a greatly increased megakaryocyte ploidy despite a normal thrombopoietin level.[234,246] Evidence suggests that platelet and possibly megakaryocyte thrombopoietin receptors are decreased tenfold in essential thrombocythemia.[246]

MYELODYSPLASTIC SYNDROMES (SEE CHAP. 90)

Thrombocytopenia as well as thrombocytosis are found in myelodysplastic syndromes and attributed to abnormal megakaryocytes. The morphological picture is that of an increased number of small megakaryocytes of low ploidy, occasionally displaying a characteristic "pawn ball" nucleus with three lobes.[247] Platelet kinetic studies[10] have demonstrated a greatly expanded megakaryocyte mass (increased number of megakaryocytes of low ploidy) and ineffective platelet production from the megakaryocytes.

HEMATOPOIETIC DISORDERS ASSOCIATED WITH ABNORMAL CHROMOSOME 3Q

A number of hematopoietic disorders associated with thrombocythemia or abnormal megakaryocyte formation have been associated with defects involving chromosome 3q,[248] and some myeloid leukemias associated with thrombocytosis have a characteristic rearrangement of chromosome 3q21 and 3q26.[201] Since the thrombopoietin gene is located on chromosome 3q27-28, it has been suggested that the thrombopoietin gene might be mediating these effects.[195,196,201] However, analysis of the chromosome regions in these patients has not demonstrated involvement of the thrombopoietin gene, and blood thrombopoietin levels are normal.[201,249] These results suggest that other genes close to the thrombopoietin gene may be responsible for other aspects of megakaryocyte differentiation and growth.

AGNOGENIC MYELOFIBROSIS WITH MYELOID METAPLASIA (SEE CHAP. 93)

The typical finding in this myeloproliferative disorder is an increase in bone marrow megakaryocytes without dysplasia as well as a large amount of fibrosis. The fibrotic response is a polyclonal proliferation of fibroblasts which has been attributed to the release of mesenchymal growth factors such as *platelet-derived growth factor* or *transforming growth factor–β* from the abnormal megakaryocytes. Subsequent data suggest that this may not be the entire mechanism.[250] Overexpression of the thrombopoietin gene using adenovectors in immunodeficient SCID mice results in thrombocytosis, increased marrow megakaryocytes, fibrosis, and extramedullary hematopoiesis that mimics the clinical disorder. However, similar overexpression of thrombopoietin in NOD-SCID mice (which have reduced monocyte and macrophage function in addition to the lymphocyte deficiency in SCID mice) produced similar thrombocytosis and megakaryocytosis but no fibrosis. These results imply that other monocyte/macrophage mediators may be involved in causing the fibrosis.

DISORDERS OF THROMBOPOIETIN PRODUCTION

The thrombopoietin physiology described above suggests possible mechanisms for clinical disorders associated with abnormalities in platelet count.[231] A few of these postulated disorders have been identified.

INHERITED THROMBOCYTHEMIA

A few families have been described that have a disorder that is clinically like the more common, sporadic cases of essential thrombocythemia.[251,252] Analysis of one of these families[252] identified a single point mutation in the splice donor site of intron 3 of the thrombopoietin gene that produced a new thrombopoietin mRNA with a normal protein coding region but with a shortened 5′ untranslated region that was more efficiently translated than the normal thrombopoietin transcripts. The 5′ untranslated region of thrombopoietin mRNA is unusual in that it contains numerous translation initiation sites, only one of which produces the active protein. A reduction in the number of these alternative translation initiation sites yields thrombopoietin mRNA that is more efficiently translated.[253] In the families with inherited thrombocythemia, loss of these sites by mutation results in more thrombopoietin protein synthesis, higher plasma thrombopoietin levels, and chronically elevated platelet counts. In individuals with the more common, sporadic cases of essential thrombocythemia none of these mutations have been found.

LIVER DISEASE

Since the liver is the primary site of thrombopoietin production,[254] and the thrombopoietin gene is apparently not inducible, thrombopoietin deficiency may be potentially responsible (along with splenic sequestration) for the thrombocytopenia in patients with liver failure. In animals, partial resection of the liver results in a proportional decrease in the platelet count.[255] In patients with liver failure, thrombopoietin levels appear to be inappropriately low,[237] leading to the suggestion that recombinant forms of thrombopoietin may be an effective therapy.

RECOMBINANT THROMBOPOIETIC GROWTH FACTORS AND THEIR CLINICAL USES

THROMBOPOIETIN

Two recombinant thrombopoietins have been extensively studied and demonstrate some clinical effect. One is a glycosylated molecule produced in Chinese hamster ovary (CHO) cells consisting of the full-length, native human amino acid sequence (*recombinant thrombopoietin, rHuTPO*) which has a circulatory half-life of 20 to 40 h.[256-258] The other is a nonglycosylated, truncated molecule produced in *E. coli* composed of the first 163 amino acids of the native molecule and chemically coupled on the amino terminus to polyethylene glycol (*pegylated, recombinant megakaryocyte growth and development factor, PEG-rHuMGDF*).[220,259,260] The half of the native thrombopoietin molecule contained in the latter drug is 50 percent similar to erythropoietin and contains all of the receptor-binding domain of thrombopoietin; it has a very short circulatory half-life and thus little biological activity in vivo. The addition of the polyethylene glycol moiety serves to stabilize the molecule in the circulation and replaces the domain that normally confers longer intravascular survival. The polyethylene glycol-thrombopoietin conjugate has a half-life of 30 to 40 h. Neither recombinant thrombopoietin product has received approval for clinical use. Some patients given PEG-rHuMGDF subcutaneously have developed antibodies to the molecule that cross-react to the endogenous thrombopoietin and cause thrombocytopenia. Intravenous administration of PEG-rHuMGDF has not been associated with antibody formation, and development of PEG-rHuMGDF by this route continues.

These recombinant thrombopoietins have demonstrated some benefit in the primary prophylaxis of thrombocytopenia associated with chemotherapy by reducing the duration, and often the depth, of the thrombocytopenia.[257,259,260] In addition, they may decrease the need for platelet transfusions.[257] However, when used in myeloablative chemotherapy settings such as AML[261] or stem cell transplantation,[262-264] neither has shown significant benefit. Both are potent mobilizers of peripheral blood progenitor cells[260] and can expand cord blood progenitor cells ex vivo.[265] Both can stimulate an increase in platelet count in normal platelet donors and increase the yield of plateletpheresis.[266,267] Platelet counts in thrombocytopenic HIV-infected patients can also be increased.[239,268]

INTERLEUKIN-11

IL-3, IL-6, and IL-11 produce significant stimulation of platelet production. IL-3 and IL-6 are probably too toxic for most clinical uses, but recombinant IL-11 has modest side effects and has been approved by the FDA for use in the prevention of chemotherapy-induced thrombocytopenia.[269] Recombinant human IL-11 (Neumega) stimulates megakaryocyte growth and increases platelet production with a time course similar to that of thrombopoietin. Its thrombopoietic action is not mediated through thrombopoietin release or synergism and is independent of the thrombopoietin receptor.[123] Surprisingly, when the gene for the IL-11 receptor was eliminated in mice, there was no effect on

the production of platelets or any other blood cell, suggesting that IL-11 is not important for normal hematopoiesis.[270,271] However, in clinical studies IL-11 reduced the extent of chemotherapy-induced thrombocytopenia[123,269] and in one study actually reduced the need for platelet transfusions by 27 percent.[124] Its major side effects are dilutional anemia, pleural effusions, and atrial arrhythmias.

OTHER THROMBOPOIETIC GROWTH FACTORS

There is also a growing number of other molecularly designed platelet growth factors based on the structure of thrombopoietin or its receptor that are just entering preclinical testing. One of these, *promegapoietin*,[272] is a molecular modification of thrombopoietin in which the receptor-binding region is coupled to the hematopoietic growth factor IL-3. This molecule can bind to and activate both the thrombopoietin and IL-3 receptor. Another is a thrombopoietin peptide mimetic (*TPO peptide mimetic*) that consists of a dimer of two identical 14–amino acid peptides with no sequence homology to thrombopoietin and that avidly binds to and activates the thrombopoietin receptor, c-Mpl.[273] Neither of these molecules has entered clinical testing. These molecules define a new and growing family of molecules called the *Mpl ligand family*[274] based on their common ability to bind and activate the receptor for thrombopoietin, c-Mpl.

Novel molecularly designed proteins[275] currently under development include *myelopoietin* (an IL-3 receptor agonist) and *progenipoietin-G* (a fusion protein of flt-3 ligand and G-CSF)[276]; they both stimulate platelet production as well as cells of other lineages and give the promise of being "panpoietins."

REFERENCES

1. Wright JH: The origin and nature of blood plates. *Boston Med Surg J* 154:643, 1906.
2. Kuter DJ, Beeler DL, Rosenberg RD: The purification of megapoietin: a physiological regulator of megakaryocyte growth and platelet production. *Proc Natl Acad Sci USA* 91:11104, 1994.
3. De Sauvage FJ, Hass PE, Spencer SD, et al: Stimulation of megakaryocytopoiesis and thrombopoiesis by the c-Mpl ligand. *Nature* 369:533, 1994.
4. Kato T, Ogami K, Shimada Y, et al: Purification and characterization of thrombopoietin. *J Biochem* 118:229, 1995.
5. Lok S, Kaushansky K, Holly RD, et al: Cloning and expression of murine thrombopoietin cDNA and stimulation of platelet production in vivo. *Nature* 369:565, 1994.
6. Bartley TD, Bogenberger J, Hunt P, et al: Identification and cloning of a megakaryocyte growth and development factor that is a ligand for the cytokine receptor Mpl. *Cell* 77:1117, 1994.
7. Kaushansky K: Thrombopoietin: the primary regulator of megakaryocyte and platelet production. *Thromb Haemost* 74:521, 1995.
8. Levin J: The evolution of mammalian platelets, in *Thrombopoiesis and Thrombopoietins: Molecular, Cellular, Preclinical, and Clinical Biology*, edited by DJ Kuter, P Hunt, W Sheridan, D Zucker-Franklin, p 63. Humana Press, Ottowa, 1997.
9. Wright JH: A rapid method for the differential staining of blood films and malarial parasites. *J Med Res* 7:138, 1902.
10. Harker LA, Finch CA: Thrombokinetics in man. *J Clin Invest* 48:963, 1969.
11. Kuter DJ, Greenberg SM, Rosenberg RD: Analysis of megakaryocyte ploidy in rat bone marrow cultures. *Blood* 74:1952, 1989.
12. Jackson CW, Brown LK, Somerville BC, et al: Two-color flow cytometric measurement of DNA distributions of rat megakaryocytes in unfixed, unfractionated marrow cell suspensions. *Blood* 63:768, 1984.
13. Hegyi E, Nakazawa M, Debili N, et al: Developmental changes in human megakaryocyte ploidy. *Exp Hematol* 19:87, 1991.
14. Jackson CW: Megakaryocyte endomitosis: a review. *Int J Cell Cloning* 8:224, 1990.
15. Radley J, Green S: Ultrastructure of endomitosis in megakaryocytes. *Nouv Rev Fr Hematol* 31:232a, 1989.
16. Nagata Y, Muro Y, Todokoro K: Thrombopoietin-induced polyploidiza-

tion of bone marrow megakaryocytes is due to a unique regulatory mechanism in late mitosis. *J Cell Biol* 139:449, 1997.

17. Paulus JM, Prenant M, Deschamps JF, Henry-Amar M: Polyploid megakaryocytes develop randomly from a multicompartmental system of committed progenitors. *Proc Nat Acad Sci USA* 79:4410, 1982.

18. Zimmet JM, Ladd D, Jackson CW, et al: A role for cyclin D3 in the endomitotic cell cycle. *Mol Cell Biol* 17:7248, 1997.

19. Zhang Y, Wang Z, Liu DX, et al: Ubiquitin-dependent degradation of cyclin B is accelerated in polyploid megakaryocytes. *J Biol Chem* 273:1387, 1998.

20. Zimmet JM, Toselli P, Ravid K: Cyclin D3 and megakaryocyte development: exploration of a transgenic phenotype. *Stem Cells* 16(Suppl 2): 97, 1998.

21. Jones O: Origin of megakaryocyte granules from Golgi vesicles. *Anat Rec* 138:105, 1960.

22. Behnke O, Pedersen NT: Ultrastructural aspects of megakaryocyte maturation and platelet release, in *Platelets: Production, Function, Transfusion, and Storage*, edited by MG Baldini, S Ebbe, p 21. Grune & Stratton, New York, 1974.

23. Vinci G, Tabilio A, Deschamps JF, et al: Immunological study of in vitro maturation of human megakaryocytes. *Br J Haematol* 56:589, 1984.

24. White JG: Tubular elements in platelet granules. *Blood* 32:148, 1968.

25. Cramer EM, Meyer D, le Menn R, Breton-Gorius J: Eccentric localization of von Willebrand factor in an internal structure of platelet alpha-granule resembling that of Weibel-Palade bodies. *Blood* 66:710, 1985.

26. Wencel-Drake JD, Painter RG, Zimmerman TS, Ginsberg MH: Ultrastructural localization of human platelet thrombospondin, fibrinogen, fibronectin, and von Willebrand factor in frozen thin section. *Blood* 65:929, 1985.

27. Suzuki H, Katagirl Y, Tsukita S, et al: Location of adhesive proteins in two newly subdivided zones in electron-lucent matrix of human α-granules. *Histochemistry* 94:337, 1990.

28. Sander HJ, Slot JW, Bouma BN, et al: Immunocytochemical localization of fibrinogen, platelet factor 4, and beta thromboglobulin in thin frozen sections of human blood platelets. *J Clin Invest* 72:1277, 1983.

29. Hegyi E, Nakeff A: Ultrastructural localization of platelet factor 4 in rat megakaryocytes and platelets by gold-labeled antibody detection. *Exp Hematol* 17:223, 1989.

30. Harrison P, Savidge GF, Cramer EM: The origin and physiological relevance of alpha-granule adhesive proteins. *Br J Haematol* 74:125, 1990.

31. Greenberg SM, Kuter DJ, Rosenberg RD: In vitro stimulation of megakaryocyte maturation by megakaryocyte stimulatory factor. *J Biol Chem* 262:3269, 1987.

32. Handagama PJ, Shuman MA, Bainton DF: The origin of platelet α-granule protein, in *Molecular Biology and Differentiation of Megakaryocytes*, edited by J Breton-Gorius, J Levin, AT Nurden, N Williams, p 119. Wiley-Liss, New York, 1990.

33. Handagama PJ, Bainton DF, Jacques Y, et al: Kistrin, an integrin antagonist, blocks endocytosis of fibrinogen into guinea pig megakaryocyte and platelet α-granules. *J Clin Invest* 91:193, 1993.

34. Handagama PJ, Amrani DL, Shuman MA: Endocytosis of fibrinogen into hamster megakaryocyte α-granules is dependent on dimeric gamma A configuration. *Blood* 85:1790, 1995.

35. Harrison P, Wilbourn B, Debili N, et al: Uptake of plasma fibrinogen into alpha granules of human megakaryocytes and platelets. *J Clin Invest* 84:1320, 1989.

36. Handagama PJ, Shuman MA, Bainton DF: Incorporation of intravenously injected albumin, immunoglobulin G, and fibrinogen in guinea pig megakaryocyte granules. *J Clin Invest* 84:73, 1989.

37. Lichtman MA, Chamberlain JK, Simon W, Santillo PA: Parasinusoidal location of megakaryocytes in marrow: a determinant of platelet release. *Am J Hematol* 4:303, 1978.

38. Cramer EM, Savidge GF, Vainchenker W, et al: Alpha-granule pool of glycoprotein IIb-IIIa in normal and pathologic platelets and megakaryocytes. *Blood* 75:1220, 1990.

39. Stenberg PE, McEver RP, Shuman MA, et al: A platelet alpha-granule membrane protein (GMP-140) is expressed on the plasma membrane after activation. *J Cell Biol* 101:880, 1985.

40. Metzelaar MJ, Heijnen HF, Sixma JJ, Nieuwenhuis HK: Identification of a 33-kd protein associated with the alpha-granule membrane (GMP-

33) that is expressed on the surface of activated platelets. *Blood* 79:372, 1992.

41. Breton-Gorius J, Clezardin P, Guichard J, et al: Localization of platelet osteonectin at the internal face of the alpha-granule membranes in platelets and megakaryocytes. *Blood* 79:936, 1992.

42. Da Prada M, Richard SJG, Kettler R: Amine storage organelles in platelets, in *Platelets in Biology and Pathology*, edited by AS Gordon, p 107. Elsevier/North Holland, Amsterdam, 1981.

43. White JG: Serotonin storage organelles in human megakaryocytes. *Am J Pathology* 63:403, 1971.

44. Schick PK, Weinstein M: A marker for megakaryocytes: serotonin accumulation in guinea pig megakaryocytes. *J Lab Clin Med* 98:607, 1981.

45. Bricker LJ, Zuckerman KS: Serotonin uptake by progeny of murine megakaryocyte precursors (CFU-M) in vitro. *Exp Hematol* 12:672, 1984.

46. Gerrard JM, Lint D, Sims PJ, et al: Identification of a platelet dense granule membrane protein that is deficient in a patient with the Hermansky-Pudlak syndrome. *Blood* 77:101, 1991.

47. Israels SJ, Gerrard JM, Jacques YV, et al: Platelet dense granule membranes contain both granulophysin and P-selectin (GMP-140). *Blood* 80:143, 1992.

48. Bentfeld-Barker ME, Bainton DF: Identification of primary lysosomes in human megakaryocytes and platelets. *Blood* 59:472, 1982.

49. Sixma JJ, van den Berg A, Hasilik A, et al: Immuno-electron microscopical demonstration of lysosomes in human blood platelets and megakaryocytes using anti-cathepsin D. *Blood* 65:1287, 1985.

50. Metzelaar MJ, Clevers HC: Lysosomal membrane glycoproteins in platelets. *Thromb Haemost* 68:378, 1992.

51. Breton-Gorius J, Guichard J: Two different types of granules in megakaryocytes and platelets as revealed by the diaminobenzidine method. *J Microsc Biol Cell* 23:197, 1975.

52. Behnke O: An electron microscope study of the megakaryocyte of the rat bone marrow: I. The development of the demarcation membrane system and the platelet surface coat. *J Ultrastruct Res* 24:412, 1968.

53. MacPherson GG: Origin and development of the demarcation system in megakaryocytes of rat bone marrow. *J Ultrastruct Res* 40:167, 1972.

54. Breton-Gorius J, Reyes F: Ultrastructure of human bone marrow cell maturation. *Int Rev Cytol* 46:251, 1976.

55. Radley, JM, Haller CJ: The demarcation membrane system of the megakaryocyte: a misnomer. *Blood* 60:213, 1982.

56. MacPherson GG: Changes in megakaryocyte development following thrombocytopenia. *Br J Haematol* 26:105, 1974.

57. Debili N, Kieffer N, Nakazawa M, et al: Expression and isolation of a platelet GPIb-like protein in human umbilical vein endothelial cells and bovine aortic smooth muscle cells. *Blood* 76:368, 1990.

58. Berridge MV, Ralph SJ, Tan AS: Cell-lineage antigens of the stem cell-megakaryocyte-platelet lineage are associated with the platelet IIb/IIIa glycoprotein complex. *Blood* 66:76, 1985.

59. Debili N, Issaad C, Masse JM, et al: Expression of CD34 and platelet glycoproteins during human megakaryocytic differentiation. *Blood* 80:3022, 1992.

60. Uzan G, Prenant M, Prandini MH, et al: Tissue-specific expression of the platelet GPIIb gene. *J Biol Chem* 266:8932, 1991.

61. Roth GJ: Developing relationships: arterial platelet adhesion, glycoprotein Ib, and leucine-rich glycoproteins. *Blood* 77:5, 1991.

62. Asch AS, Adelman B, Fujimoto M, Nachman RL: Identification and isolation of a platelet GPIb-like protein in human umbilical vein endothelial cells and bovine aortic smooth muscle cells. *J Clin Invest* 81:1600, 1988.

63. Wu G, Essex DW, Meloni FJ, et al: Human endothelial cells in culture and in vivo express on their surface all four components of the glycoprotein Ib/IX/V complex. *Blood* 90:2660, 1997.

64. Kelly MD, Essex DW, Shapiro SS, et al: Complementary DNA cloning of the alternatively expressed endothelial cell glycoprotein Ib beta (GPIb beta) and localization of the GPIb beta gene to chromosome 22. *J Clin Invest* 93:2417, 1994.

65. Wright JH: The histogenesis of the blood platelets. *J Morph* 21:263, 1910.

66. Odell TT, Jackson CW: Polyploidy and maturation of rat megakaryocytes. *Blood* 32:102, 1968.

67. Williams N, Levine RF: The origin, development and regulation of megakaryocytes. *Br J Haematol* 52:173, 1982.

68. Mazur EM, Hoffman R, Chasis J, et al: Immunofluorescent identification

of human megakaryocyte colonies using an antiplatelet glycoprotein antiserum. *Blood* 57:277, 1981.

69. Jackson CW: Cholinesterase as a possible marker for early cells of the megakaryocytic series. *Blood* 42:413, 1973.

70. Long MW, Williams N, McDonald TP: Immature megakaryocytes in the mouse: in vitro relationship to megakaryocyte progenitor cells and mature megakaryocytes. *J Cell Physiol* 112:339, 1982.

71. Long MW, Williams N, Ebbe S: Immature megakaryocytes in the mouse: physical characteristics, cell cycle status, and in vitro responsiveness to thrombopoietic stimulatory factor. *Blood* 59:569, 1982.

72. Young KM, Weiss L: Megakaryocytopoiesis: incorporation of tritiated thymidine by small acetylcholinesterase-positive cells in murine bone marrow during antibody-induced thrombocytopenia. *Blood* 69:290, 1987.

73. Rabellino EM, Nachman RL, Williams N, et al: Human megakaryocytes: I. Characterization of the membrane and cytoplasmic components of isolated marrow megakaryocytes. *J Exp Med* 149:1273, 1979.

74. Vainchenker W, Deschamps JF, Bastin JM, et al: Two monoclonal antiplatelet antibodies as markers of human megakaryocyte maturation: immunofluorescent staining and platelet peroxidase detection in megakaryocyte colonies and in in vivo cells from normal and leukemic patients. *Blood* 59:514, 1982.

75. Lev-Lehman E, Deutsch V, Eldor A, Soreq H: Immature human megakaryocytes produce nuclear-associated acetylcholinesterase. *Blood* 89:3644, 1997.

76. Kavnoudias H, Jackson H, Ettlinger K, et al: Interleukin 3 directly stimulates both megakaryocyte progenitor cells and immature megakaryocytes. *Exp Hematol* 20:43, 1992.

77. Breton-Gorius J, Gordin M, Reyes F: Ultrastructure of the leukemic cell, in *The Leukemic Cell*, edited by D Catovsky, p 87. Churchill Livingston, London, 1981.

78. Long MW, Henry RL: Thrombocytosis-induced suppression of small acetylcholinesterase-positive cells in bone marrow of rats. *Blood* 54:1338, 1979.

79. Rabellino EM, Levine RB, Leung LL, Nachman RL: Human megakaryocytes: II. Expression of platelet proteins in early marrow megakaryocytes. *J Exp Med* 154:88, 1981.

80. Gerrard JM, White JG, Rao GH, Townsend D: Localization of platelet prostaglandin production in the platelet dense tubular system. *Am J Path* 83:283, 1976.

81. Breton-Gorius J, Vainchenker W: Expression of platelet proteins during the in vitro and in vivo differentiation of megakaryocytes and morphological aspects of their maturation. *Semin Hematol* 23:43, 1986.

82. Breton-Gorius J, Villeval JL, Mitjavila MT, et al: Ultrastructural and cytochemical characterization of blasts from early erythroblastic leukemias. *Leukemia* 1:173, 1987.

83. Breton-Gorius J: Megakaryocyte maturation and platelet release in normal pathologic conditions, in *Blood Cell Biochemistry*, edited by JR Harris, p 1. Plenum, New York, 1991.

84. Nakahata T, Ogawa M: Identification in culture of a class of hemopoietic colony-forming units with extensive capability to self-renew and generate multipotential hemopoietic colonies. *Proc Natl Acad Sci USA* 79:3843, 1982.

85. Fauser AA, Messner HA: Identification of megakaryocytes, macrophages, and eosinophils in colonies of human bone marrow containing neutrophilic granulocytes and erythroblasts. *Blood* 53:1023, 1979.

86. Solar GP, Kerr WG, Zeigler FC, et al: Role of c-mpl in early hematopoiesis. *Blood* 92:4, 1998.

87. Orkin SH, Shivdasani RA, Fujiwara Y, McDevitt MA: Transcription factor GATA-1 in megakaryocyte development. *Stem Cells* 16(Suppl 2):79, 1998.

88. Martin DI, Zon LI, Mutter G, Orkin SH: Expression of an erythroid transcription factor in megakaryocytic and mast cell lineages. *Nature* 344:444, 1990.

89. Orkin SH: GATA-binding transcription factors in hematopoietic cells. *Blood* 80:575, 1992.

90. Poujol C, Tronik-Le Roux D, Tropel P, et al: Ultrastructural analysis of bone marrow hematopoiesis in mice transgenic for the thymidine kinase gene driven by the a$_{IIb}$ promoter. *Blood* 92:2012, 1998.

91. Tronik-Le Roux D, Roullot V, Schweitzer A, et al: Suppression of erythro-megakaryocytopoiesis and the induction of reversible thrombo-cytopenia in mice transgenic for the thymidine kinase gene targeted by the platelet glycoportein a$_{IIb}$ promoter. *J Exp Med* 181:2141, 1995.

92. Tropel P, Roullot V, Vernet M, et al: A 2.7-kb portion of the 5' flanking region of the murine glycoprotein a$_{IIb}$ is transcriptionally active in primitive hematopoietic progenitor cells. *Blood* 90:2995, 1997.

93. Vigon I, Mornon J-P, Cocault L, et al: Molecular cloning and characterization of MPL, the human homolog of the v-mpl oncogene: Identification of a member of the hematopoietic growth factor receptor superfamily. *Proc Natl Acad Sci USA* 89:5640, 1992.

94. Methia N, Louache F, Vainchenker W, Wendling F: Oligodeoxynucleotides antisense to the proto-oncogene c-mpl specifically inhibit in vitro megakaryocytopoiesis. *Blood* 82:1395, 1993.

95. Long MW, Gragowski LL, Heffner CH, Boxer LA: Phorbol diesters stimulate the development of an early murine progenitor cell. The burst-forming unit-megakaryocyte. *J Clin Invest* 76:431, 1985.

96. Briddell RA, Brandt JE, Straneva JE, et al: Characterization of the human burst-forming unit-megakaryocyte. *Blood* 74:145, 1989.

97. Gewirtz AM, Hoffman R: Human megakaryocyte production: cell biology and clinical considerations. *Hematol Oncol Clin North Am* 4:43, 1990.

98. Briddell RA, Hoffman R: Cytokine regulation of the human burst-forming unit-megakaryocyte. *Blood* 76:516, 1990.

99. Hoffman R: Regulation of megakaryocytopoiesis. *Blood* 74:1196, 1989.

100. Metcalf D, MacDonald HR, Odartchenko N, Sordat B: Growth of mouse megakaryocyte colonies in vitro. *Proc Natl Acad Sci USA* 72:1744, 1975.

101. Vainchenker W, Bouguet J, Guichard J, Breton-Gorius J: Megakaryocyte colony formation from human bone marrow precursors. *Blood* 54:940, 1979.

102. Miyazaki H, Inoue H, Yanagida M, et al: Purification of rat megakaryocyte colony-forming cells using a monoclonal antibody against rat platelet glycoprotein IIb/IIIa. *Exp Hematol* 20:855, 1992.

103. Levine RB, Lamaziere J, Broxmeyer HE, et al: Human megakaryocytes: V. Changes in the phenotypic profile of differentiating megakaryocytes. *J Exp Med* 161:457, 1985.

104. Nakeff A: Colony-forming unit, megakaryocyte (CFU-m): its use in elucidating the kinetics and humoral control of the megakaryocytic committed progenitor cell compartment, in *Experimental Hematology Today*, edited by SJ Baum, DG Ledney, p 111. Springer, New York, 1977.

105. Broudy VC, Lin NL, Fox N, et al: Thrombopoietin stimulates colony-forming unit-megakaryocyte proliferation and megakaryocyte maturation independently of cytokines that signal through the gp130 receptor subunit. *Blood* 88:2026, 1996.

106. Dolzhanskiy A, Basch RS, Karpatkin S: The development of human megakaryocytes: III. Development of mature megakaryocytes from highly purified committed progenitors in synthetic culture media and inhibition of thrombopoietin-induced polyploidization by interleukin-3. *Blood* 89:426, 1997.

107. Choi ES, Hokom MM, Chen JL, et al: The role of megakaryocyte growth and development factor in terminal stages of thrombopoiesis. *Br J Haematol* 95:227, 1996.

108. Carrington PA, Hill RJ, Stenberg PE, et al: Multiple in vivo effects of interleukin-3 and interleukin-6 on murine megakaryocytopoiesis. *Blood* 77:34, 1991.

109. Stahl CP, Winton EF, Monroe MC, et al: Differential effects of sequential, simultaneous, and single agent interleukin-3 and granulocyte-macrophage colony-stimulating factor on megakaryocyte maturation and platelet response in primates. *Blood* 80:2479, 1992.

110. Ganser A, Lindemann A, Seipelt G, et al: Effects of recombinant human interleukin-3 in patients with normal hematopoiesis and in patients with bone marrow failure. *Blood* 76:666, 1990.

111. Kurzrock R, Talpaz M, Estrov Z, et al: Phase I study of recombinant human interleukin-3 in patients with bone marrow failure. *J Clin Oncol* 9:1241, 1991.

112. Ishibashi T, Kimura H, Shikama Y, et al: Interleukin-6 is a potent thrombopoietic factor in vivo in mice. *Blood* 74:1241, 1989.

113. Ishibashi T, Kimura H, Uchida T, et al: Human interleukin-6 is a direct promoter of maturation of megakaryocytes in vitro. *Proc Natl Acad Sci USA* 86:5953, 1989.

114. Kishimoto T: The biology of interleukin-6. *Blood* 74:1, 1989.

115. Imai T, Koike K, Kubo T, et al: Interleukin-6 supports human megakaryocytic proliferation and differentiation in vitro. *Blood* 78:1969, 1991.

116. Kimura H, Ishibashi T, Uchida T, et al: Interleukin-6 is a differentiation factor for human megakaryocytes in vitro. *Eur J Immunol* 20:1927, 1990.

117. Hill RJ, Warren MK, Levin J: Stimulation of thrombopoiesis in mice by human recombinant interleukin-6. *J Clin Invest* 85:1242, 1990.

118. Asano S, Okano A, Ozawa K, et al: In vivo effects of recombinant human interleukin-6 in primates: stimulated production of platelets. *Blood* 75:1602, 1990.

119. Mayer P, Geissler K, Valent P, et al: Recombinant human interleukin-6 is a potent inducer of the acute phase response and elevates the blood platelets in nonhuman primates. *Exp Hematol* 19:688, 1991.

120. Stahl CP, Zucker-Franklin D, Evatt BL, Winton EF: Effects of human interleukin-6 on megakaryocyte development and thrombocytopoiesis in primates. *Blood* 78:1467, 1991.

121. Teramura M, Kobayashi S, Hoshino S, et al: Interleukin-11 enhances human megakaryocytopoiesis in vitro. *Blood* 79:327, 1992.

122. Teramura M, Kobayashi S, Yoshinaga K, et al: Effect of interleukin-11 on normal and pathological thrombopoiesis. *Cancer Chemother Pharmacol* 38(suppl):S99, 1996.

123. Du X, Williams DA: Interleukin-11: Review of molecular, cell biology, and clinical use. *Blood* 89:3897, 1997.

124. Tepler I, Elias L, Smith JW, et al: A randomized placebo-controlled trial of recombinant human interleukin-11 in cancer patients with severe thrombocytopenia due to chemotherapy. *Blood* 87:3607, 1996.

125. Carlino JA, Higley HR, Creson JR, et al: Transforming growth factor beta 1 systemically modulates granuloid, erythroid, lymphoid, and thrombocytic cells in mice. *Exp Hematol* 20:943, 1992.

126. Ishibashi T, Miller SL, Burstein SA: Type beta transforming growth factor is a potent inhibitor of murine megakaryocytopoiesis in vitro. *Blood* 69:1737, 1987.

127. Kuter DJ, Gminski DM, Rosenberg RD: Transforming growth factor β inhibits megakaryocyte growth and endomitosis. *Blood* 79:619, 1992.

128. Bellucci S, Han ZC, Caen JP: Positive and negative regulation of megakaryocytopoiesis. *C R Seances Soc Biol Fil* 190:515, 1996.

129. Gugliotta L, Bagnara GP, Catani L, et al: In vivo and in vitro inhibitory effect of alpha-interferon on megakaryocyte colony growth in essential thrombocythaemia. *Br J Haematol* 71:177, 1989.

130. Han ZC, Bellucci S, Caen JP: Regulation of human megakaryocytopoiesis. *Nouv Rev Fr Hematol* 32:395, 1990.

131. Han ZC, Bellucci S, Caen JP: Megakaryocytopoiesis: characterization and regulation in normal and pathologic states. *Int J Hematol* 54:3, 1991.

132. Hassan HT, Freund M: Characteristic biological features of human megakaryoblastic leukaemia cell lines. *Leuk Res* 19:589, 1995.

133. Hassan HT, Drexler HG: Interleukins and colony stimulating factors in human myeloid leukemia cell lines. *Leuk Lymphoma* 20:1, 1995.

134. Muraoka K, Tsuji K, Yoshida M, et al: Thrombopoietin-independent effect of interferon-gamma on the proliferation of human megakaryocyte progenitors. *Br J Haematol* 98:265, 1997.

135. Gisslinger H, Chott A, Scheithauer W, et al: Interferon in essential thrombocythaemia. *Br J Haematol* 79 (Suppl) 1:42, 1991.

136. Murphy S, Peterson P, Iland H, Laszlo J: Experience of the Polycythemia Vera Study Group with essential thrombocythemia: a final report on diagnostic criteria, survival, and leukemic transition by treatment. *Semin Hematol* 34:29, 1997.

137. Shiota G, Okubo M, Kawasaki H, Tahara T: Interferon increases serum thrombopoietin in patients with chronic hepatitis C. *Br J Haematol* 97:340, 1997.

138. Chernoff A, Levine RF, Goodman DS: Origin of platelet-derived growth factor in megakaryocytes in guinea pigs. *J Clin Invest* 65:926, 1980.

139. Ballem PJ, Belzberg A, Devine DV, et al: Kinetic studies of the mechanism of thrombocytopenia in patients with human immunodeficiency virus infection. *N Engl J Med* 327:1779, 1992.

140. Yamada F: The fine structure of the megakaryocyte in the mouse spleen. *Acta Anat* 29:267, 1957.

141. Becker RP, De Bruyn PPH: The transmural passage of blood cells into myeloid sinusoids and the entry of platelets into the sinusoidal circulation; a scanning electron microscopic investigation. *Am J Anat* 145:183, 1975.

142. Behnke O: An electron microscope study of the rat megacaryocyte: II. Some aspects of platelet release and microtubules. *J Ultrastruct Res* 26:111, 1969.

143. Radley JM, Scurfield G: The mechanism of platelet release. *Blood* 56:996, 1980.

144. Tong M, Seth P, Penington DG: Proplatelets and stress platelets. *Blood* 69:522, 1987.

145. Topp KS, Tablin F, Levin J: Culture of isolated bovine megakaryocytes on reconstituted basement membrane matrix leads to proplatelet process formation. *Blood* 76:912, 1990.

146. Leven RM, Tablin F: Extracellular matrix stimulation of guinea pig megakaryocyte proplatelet formation in vitro is mediated through the vitronectin receptor. *Exp Hematol* 20:1316, 1992.

147. Hunt P, Hokom MM, Wiemann B, et al: Megakaryocyte proplatelet-like process formation in vitro is inhibited by serum prothrombin, a process which is blocked by matrix-bound glycosaminoglycans. *Exp Hematol* 21:372, 1993.

148. Lecine P, Blank V, Shivdasani R: Characterization of the hematopoietic transcription factor NF-E2 in primary murine megakaryocytes. *J Biol Chem* 273:7572, 1998.

149. Lecine P, Villeval J, Vyas P, et al: Mice lacking transcription factor NF-E2 provide in vivo validation of the proplatelet model of thrombocytopoiesis and show a platelet production defect that is intrinsic to megakaryocytes. *Blood* 92:1608, 1998.

150. Shivdasani RA, Fujiwara Y, McDevitt MA, Orkin SH: A lineage-specific knockout establishes the critical role of transcription factor GATA-1 in megakaryocyte growth and platelet development. *EMBO J* 16:3965, 1997.

151. Kaufman RM, Airo R, Pollack S, Crosby WH: Circulating megakaryocytes and platelet release in the lung. *Blood* 26:720, 1965.

152. Trowbridge EA, Martin JF, Slater DN: Evidence for a theory of physical fragmentation of megakaryocytes, implying that all platelets are produced in the pulmonary circulation. *Thromb Res* 28:461, 1982.

153. Pedersen NT: Occurrence of megakaryocytes in various vessels and their retention in the pulmonary capillaries in man. *Scand J Haematol* 21:369, 1978.

154. Tavassoli M, Aoki M: Migration of entire megakaryocytes through the marrow-blood barrier. *Br J Haematol* 48:25, 1981.

155. Martin JF, Slater DN, Trowbridge EA: Evidence that platelets are produced in the pulmonary circulation by a physical process. *Prog Clin Biol Res* 215:405, 1986.

156. Levine RF, Eldor A, Shoff PK, et al: Circulating megakaryocytes: delivery of large numbers of intact, mature megakaryocytes to the lungs. *Eur J Haematol* 51:233, 1993.

157. Corash L, Mok Y, Levin J, Baker G: Regulation of platelet heterogeneity: effects of thrombocytopenia on platelet volume and density. *Exp Hematol* 18:205, 1990.

158. Frojmovic MM, Milton JG: Human platelet size, shape, and related functions in health and disease. *Physiol Reviews* 62:185, 1982.

159. Garg SK, Amorosi EL, Karpatkin S: Use of the megathrombocyte as an index of megakaryocyte number. *N Engl J Med* 284:11, 1971.

160. Corash L, Chen HY, Levin J, et al: Regulation of thrombopoiesis: effects of the degree of thrombocytopenia on megakaryocyte ploidy and platelet volume. *Blood* 70:177, 1987.

161. Cole JL, Marzec UM, Gunthel CJ, et al: Ineffective platelet production in thrombocytopenic human immunodeficiency virus-infected patients. *Blood* 91:3239, 1998.

162. Giles C: The platelet count and mean platelet volume. *Br J Haematol* 48:31, 1981.

163. Garg SK, Lackner H, Karpatkin S: The increased percentage of megathrombocytes in various clinical disorders. *Ann Intern Med* 77:361, 1972.

164. Karpatkin S: Biochemical and clinical aspects of megathrombocytes. *Ann N Y Acad Sci* 201:262, 1972.

165. Karpatkin S, Garg SK: The megathrombocyte as an index of platelet production. *Br J Haematol* 26:307, 1974.

166. Chatterji AK, Lynch EC, Garg SK, et al: Circulating large platelets. *N Engl J Med* 284:1440, 1971.

167. van der Loo B, Martin JF: Megakaryocytes and platelets in vascular disease. *Baillieres Clin Haematol* 10:109, 1997.

168. Ulich TR, del Castillo J, Senaldi G, et al: Systemic hematologic effects of PEG-rHuMGDF-induced megakaryocyte hyperplasia in mice. *Blood* 87:5006, 1996.

169. Daw NC, Arnold JT, Abushullaih BA, et al: A single intravenous dose of murine megakaryocyte growth and development factor potently stimulates platelet production, challenging the necessity for daily administration. *Blood* 91:466, 1998.

170. O'Malley CJ, Rasko JE, Basser RL, et al: Administration of pegylated recombinant human megakaryocyte growth and development factor to humans stimulates the production of functional platelets that show no evidence of in vivo activation. *Blood* 88:3288, 1996.

171. Fujiwara Y, Browne CP, Cunniff KC, et al: Arrested development of embryonic red cell precursors in mouse embryos lacking transcription factor GATA-1. *Proc Natl Acad Sci USA* 93:12355, 1996.

172. Shivdasani RA, Rosenblatt MF, Zucker-Franklin D, et al: Transcription factor NF-E2 is required for platelet formation independent of the actions of thrombopoietin/MGDF in megakaryocyte development. *Cell* 81:695, 1995.

173. Shivdasani RA, Orkin SH: Erythropoiesis and globin gene expression in mice lacking the transcription factor NF-E2. *Proc Natl Acad Sci USA* 92:8690, 1995.

174. Lecine P, Shivdasani RA: Cellular and molecular biology of megakaryocyte differentiation in the absence of lineage-restricted transcription factors. *Stem Cells* 16(Suppl 2):91, 1998.

175. Kuter DJ: The physiology of platelet production. *Stem Cells* 14(Suppl 1): 88, 1996.

176. Brecher G, Cronkite E: Morphology and enumeration of human blood platelets. *J Appl Physiol* 3:365, 1950.

177. Bessman JD, Williams LJ, Gilmer PR: The inverse relation of platelet size and count in normal subjects and an artifact of other particles. *Am J Clin Pathol* 76:289, 1981.

178. Thompson CB: From precursor to product; how do megakaryocytes produce platelets, in *Megakaryocyte Development and Function*, edited by RF Levine, N Williams, J Levin, B Evatt, p 361. Liss, New York, 1986.

179. Von Behrens WE: Evidence of phylogenetic canalization of the circulating platelet mass in man. *Thromb Diath Haemorrh* 27(suppl):159, 1972.

180. Aster RH: Pooling of platelets in the spleen: role in the pathogenesis of "hypersplenic" thrombocytopenia. *J Clin Invest* 45:645, 1966.

181. De Gabriele G, Penington DG: Regulation of platelet production: "hypersplenism" in the experimental animal. *Br J Haematol* 13:383, 1967.

182. Aster RH: Studies of the mechanism of "hypersplenic" thrombocytopenia in rats. *J Lab Clin Med* 70:736, 1967.

183. Kuter DJ, Rosenberg RD: Regulation of megakaryocyte ploidy in vivo in the rat. *Blood* 75:74, 1990.

184. Penington DG, Olsen TE: Megakaryocytes in states of altered platelet production: cell numbers, size and DNA content. *Br J Haematol* 18:447, 1970.

185. Burstein SA, Adamson JW, Erb SK, Harker LA: Megakaryocytopoiesis in the mouse: response to varying platelet demand. *J Cell Physiol* 109:333, 1981.

186. Levin J, Levin FC, Metcalf D: The effects of acute thrombocytopenia on megakaryocyte-CFC and granulocyte-macrophage-CFC in mice: studies of bone marrow and spleen. *Blood* 56:274, 1980.

187. Kelemen E, Cserhati I, Tanos B: Demonstration and some properties of human thrombopoietin in thrombocythaemic sera. *Acta Haematol* 20:350, 1958.

188. Kato T, Ogami K, Shimada Y, et al: Purification and characterization of thrombopoietin. *J Biochem* 119:229, 1995.

189. Souryi M, Vigon I, Penciolelli J-F, et al: A putative truncated cytokine receptor gene transduced by the myeloproliferative leukemia virus immortalizes hematopoietic progenitors. *Cell* 63:1137, 1990.

190. Wendling F, Maraskovsky E, Debili N, et al: c-Mpl ligand is a humoral regulator of megakaryocytopoiesis. *Nature* 369:571, 1994.

191. Methia N, Debili N, Titeux M, et al: From the v-mpl oncogene to thrombopoietin. *C R Acad Sci III* 318:479, 1995.

192. Vainchenker W, Methia N, Debili N, et al: c-mpl, the thrombopoietin receptor. *Thromb Haemost* 74:526, 1995.

193. Wendling F, Vainchenker W: Thrombopoietin and its receptor, the proto-oncogene c-mpl. *Curr Opin Hematol* 2:331, 1995.

194. Nomura S, Ogami K, Kawamura K, et al: Cellular localization of thrombopoietin mRNA in the liver by in situ hybridization. *Exp Hematol* 25:565, 1997.

195. Foster DC, Sprecher CA, Grant FJ, et al: Human thrombopoietin: gene structure, cDNA sequence, expression, and chromosomal localization. *Proc Natl Acad Sci USA* 91:13023, 1994.

196. Gurney AL, Kuang WJ, Xie MH, et al: Genomic structure, chromosomal localization, and conserved alternative splice forms of thrombopoietin. *Blood* 85:981, 1995.

197. Foster D, Hunt P: The biological significance of truncated and full-length forms of Mpl ligand, in *Thrombopoiesis and Thrombopoietins: Molecular, Cellular, Preclinical, and Clinical Biology*, edited by DJ Kuter, P Hunt, W Sheridan, D Zucker-Franklin, p 203. Humana Press, Ottowa, 1997.

198. Hokom MM, Lacey D, Kinstler OB, et al: Pegylated megakaryocyte growth and development factor abrogates the lethal thrombocytopenia associated with carboplatin and irradiation in mice. 86:4486, 1995.

199. Spivack JL, Hogans BB: The in vivo metabolism of recombinant human erythropoietin in the rat. *Blood* 73:90, 1989.

200. Foster D, Lok S: Biological roles for the second domain of thrombopoietin. *Stem Cells* 14(Suppl 1):102, 1996.

201. Schnittger S, de Sauvage FJ, Le Paslier D, Fonatsch C: Refined chromosomal localization of the human thrombopoietin gene to 3q27-q28 and exclusion as the responsible gene for thrombocytosis in patients with rearrangements of 3q21 and 3q26. *Leukemia* 10:1891, 1996.

202. Kaushansky K: Thrombopoietin: the primary regulator of platelet production. *Blood* 86:419, 1995.

203. Kuter DJ: Thrombopoietin: biology and clinical applications. *Oncologist* 1:98, 1996.

204. Kuter DJ: Thrombopoietin: biology, clinical applications, role in the donor setting. *J Clin Apheresis* 11:149, 1996.

205. Kuter DJ, Rosenberg RD: The reciprocal relationship of thrombopoietin (c-Mpl ligand) to changes in the platelet mass during busulfan-induced thrombocytopenia in the rabbit. *Blood* 85:2720, 1995.

206. Fielder PJ, Hass P, Nagel M, et al: Human platelets as a model for the binding and degradation of thrombopoietin. *Blood* 89:2782, 1997.

207. Li J, Xia Y, Romo J, Kuter DJ: C-mpl-mediated thrombopoietin internalization in human platelets. *Blood* 90(Suppl 1):55a, 1997.

208. Zauli G, Vitale M, Falcieri E, et al: In vitro senescence and apoptotic cell death of human megakaryocytes. *Blood* 90:2234, 1997.

209. Bacon CM, Tortolani PJ, Shimosaka A, et al: Thrombopoietin (TPO) induces tyrosine phosphorylation and activation of STAT5 and STAT3. *FEBS Lett* 370:63, 1995.

210. Dorsch M, Fan PD, Bogenberger J, Goff SP: TPO and IL-3 induce overlapping but distinct protein tyrosine phosphorylation in a myeloid precursor cell line. *Biochem Biophys Res Commun* 214:424, 1995.

211. Drachman JG, Kaushansky K: Dissecting the thrombopoietin receptor: functional elements of the Mpl cytoplasmic domain. *Proc Natl Acad Sci USA* 94:2350, 1997.

212. Ezumi Y, Takayama H, Okuma M: Thrombopoietin, c-Mpl ligand, induces tyrosine phosphorylation of Tyk2, JAK2, and STAT3, and enhances agonist-induced aggregation in platelets in vitro. *FEBS Lett* 374:48, 1995.

213. Gurney AL, Wong SC, Henzel WJ, de Sauvage FJ: Distinct regions of c-Mpl cytoplasmic domain are coupled to the JAK-STAT signal transduction pathway and Shc phosphorylation. *Proc Natl Acad Sci USA* 92:5292, 1995.

214. Miyakawa Y, Oda A, Druker BJ, et al: Thrombopoietin induces tyrosine phosphorylation of Stat3 and Stat5 in human blood platelets. *Blood* 87:439, 1996.

215. Morella KK, Bruno E, Kumaki S, et al: Signal transduction by the receptors for thrombopoietin (c-mpL) and interleukin-3 in hematopoietic and nonhematopoietic cells. *Blood* 86:557, 1995.

216. Morita H, Tahara T, Matsumoto A, et al: Functional analysis of the cytoplasmic domain of the human Mpl receptor for tyrosine-phosphorylation of the signaling molecules, proliferation and differentiation. *FEBS Lett* 395:228, 1996.

217. Pallard C, Gouilleux F, Benit L, et al: Thrombopoietin activates a STAT5-like factor in hematopoietic cells. *Embo J* 14:2847, 1995.

218. Choi ES, Nichol JL, Hokom MM, et al: Platelets generated in vitro from proplatelet-displaying human megakaryocytes are functional. *Blood* 85:402, 1995.

219. Kaushansky K, Lin N, Grossmann A, et al: Thrombopoietin expands erythroid, granulocyte-macrophage, and megakaryocytic progenitor cells in normal and myelosuppressed mice. *Exp Hematol* 24:265, 1996.

220. Basser RL, Rasko JE, Clarke K, et al: Thrombopoietic effects of pegylated recombinant human megakaryocyte growth and development factor (PEG-rHuMGDF) in patients with advanced cancer. *Lancet* 348:1279, 1996.

221. Harker LA, Marzec UM, Hunt P, et al: Dose-response effects of pegy-

lated human megakaryocyte growth and development factor on platelet production and function in nonhuman primates. *Blood* 88:511, 1996.

222. Harker LA, Hunt P, Marzec UM, et al: Regulation of platelet production and function by megakaryocyte growth and development factor in nonhuman primates. *Blood* 87:1833, 1996.

223. Chen J, Herceg-Harjacek L, Groopman JE, Grabarek J: Regulation of platelet activation in vitro by the c-Mpl ligand, thrombopoietin. *Blood* 86:4054, 1995.

224. Kubota Y, Arai T, Tanaka T, et al: Thrombopoietin modulates platelet activation in vitro through protein-tyrosine phosphorylation. *Stem Cells* 14:439, 1996.

225. Montrucchio G, Brizzi MF, Calosso G, et al: Effects of recombinant human megakaryocyte growth and development factor on platelet activation. *Blood* 87:2762, 1996.

226. Alexander WS, Roberts AW, Nicola NA, et al: Deficiencies in progenitor cells of multiple hematopoietic lineages and defective megakaryocytopoiesis in mice lacking the thrombopoietic receptor c-Mpl. *Blood* 87:2162, 1996.

227. Gurney AL, Carver-Moore K, de Sauvage FJ, Moore MW: Thrombocytopenia in c-mpl-deficient mice. *Science* 265:1445, 1994.

228. De Sauvage FJ, Carver-Moore K, Luoh SM, et al: Physiological regulation of early and late stages of megakaryocytopoiesis by thrombopoietin. *J Exp Med* 183:651, 1996.

229. Carver-Moore K, Broxmeyer HE, Luoh SM, et al: Low levels of erythroid and myeloid progenitors in thrombopoietin-and c-mpl-deficient mice. *Blood* 88:803, 1996.

230. Stoffel R, Wiestner A, Skoda RC: Thrombopoietin in thrombocytopenic mice: evidence against regulation at the mRNA level and for a direct regulatory role of platelets. *Blood* 87:567, 1996.

231. Kuter DJ: The regulation of platelet production, in *Thrombopoiesis and Thrombopoietins: Molecular, Cellular, Preclinical and Clinical Biology*, edited by DJ Kuter, P Hunt, W Sheridan, D Zucker-Franklin, p 377. Humana, Ottowa, 1997.

232. Bartocci A, Mastrogiannis DS, Migliorati G, et al: Macrophages specifically regulate the concentration of their own growth factor in the circulation. *Proc Natl Acad Sci USA* 84:6178, 1987.

233. Layton JE, Hockman H, Sheridan WP, Morstyn G: Evidence for a novel in vivo control mechanism of granulopoiesis: mature cell-related control of a regulatory growth factor. *Blood* 74:1303, 1989.

234. Nichol JL: Thrombopoietin levels after chemotherapy and in naturally occurring human diseases. *Curr Opin Hematol* 5:203, 1998.

235. Nichol JL, Hokom MM, Hornkohl A, et al: Megakaryocyte growth and development factor. Analyses of in vitro effects on human megakaryopoiesis and endogenous serum levels during chemotherapy-induced thrombocytopenia. *J Clin Invest* 95:2973, 1995.

236. Penington DG: Studies of platelet production and sequestration in the experimental animal. *Proc R Soc Med* 61:601, 1968.

237. Peck-Radosavljevic M, Zacherl J, Meng YG, et al: Is inadequate thrombopoietin production a major cause of thrombocytopenia in cirrhosis of the liver? *J Hepatol* 27:127, 1997.

238. Karpatkin S: HIV-1-related thrombocytopenia. *Hematol Oncol Clin North Am* 4:193, 1990.

239. Harker LA, Carter RA, Marzec UM, et al: Correction of thrombocytopenia and ineffective platelet production in patients infected with human immunodeficiency virus (HIV) by PEG-rHuMGDF therapy. *Blood* 92(Suppl 1):707a, 1998.

240. Harker LA: Kinetics of thrombopoiesis. *J Clin Invest* 47:458, 1968.

241. Harker LA: Regulation of thrombopoiesis. *Am J Physiol* 218:1376, 1970.

242. Ballem PJ, Segal GM, Stratton JR, et al: Mechanisms of thrombocytopenia in chronic autoimmune thrombocytopenic purpura. *J Clin Invest* 80:33, 1987.

243. Emmons RV, Reid DM, Cohen RL, et al: Human thrombopoietin levels are high when thrombocytopenia is due to megakaryocyte deficiency and low when due to increased platelet destruction. *Blood* 87:4068, 1996.

244. Beck JT, Hsu SM, Wijdenes J, et al: Brief report: alleviation of systemic manifestation of Castleman's disease by monoclonal anti-interleukin-6 antibody. *New Engl J Med* 330:602, 1994.

245. Harrison CN, Gale RE, Machin SJ, Linch DC: A large proportion of patients with a diagnosis of essential thrombocythemia do not have a clonal disorder and may be at lower risk of thrombotic complications. *Blood* 93:417, 1999.

246. Li J, Xia Y, Kuter DJ: Analysis of the thrombopoietin receptor (MPL) on platelets from normal and essential thrombocythemic (ET) patients. *Blood* 88:545a, 1996.

247. Rosenthal DS, Moloney WS: Refractory dysmyelopoietic anemia and acute leukemia. *Blood* 63:314, 1984.

248. Pinto MR, King MA, Goss GD, et al: Acute megakaryoblastic leukaemia with 3q inversion and elevated thrombopoietin (TSF): an autocrine role for TSF? *Br J Haematol* 61:687, 1985.

249. Bouscary D, Fontenay-Roupie M, Chretien S, et al: Thrombopoietin is not responsible for the thrombocytosis observed in patients with acute myeloid leukemias and the 3q21q26 syndrome. *Br J Haematol* 91:425, 1995.

250. Frey BM, Rafii S, Teterson M, et al: Adenovector-mediated expression of human thrombopoietin cDNA in immune-compromised mice: insights into the pathophysiology of osteomyelofibrosis. *J Immunol* 160:691, 1998.

251. Kondo T, Okabe M, Sanada M, et al: Familial essential thrombocythemia associated with one-base deletion in the 5′-untranslated region of the thrombopoietin gene. *Blood* 92:1091, 1998.

252. Wiestner A, Schlemper RJ, van der Maas AP, Skoda RC: An activating splice donor mutation in the thrombopoietin gene causes hereditary thrombocythaemia. *Nat Genet* 18:49, 1998.

253. Ghilardi N, Wiestner A, Skoda RC: Thrombopoietin production is inhibited by a translational mechanism. *Blood* 92:4023, 1998.

254. Quin S, Fu F, Li W, et al: Primary role of the liver in thrombopoietin production shown by tissue-specific knockout. *Blood* 92:2189, 1998.

255. Siemensma NP, Bathal PS, Penington DG: The effect of massive liver resection on platelet kinetics in the rat. *J Lab Clin Med* 86:817, 1975.

256. Vadhan-Raj S, Murray LJ, Bueso-Ramos C, et al: Stimulation of megakaryocyte and platelet production by a single dose of recombinant human thrombopoietin in patients with cancer. *Ann Int Med* 126:673, 1997.

257. Vadhan-Raj S, Verschraegen C, McGarry L, et al: Recombinant human thrombopoietin (rhTPO) attenuates high-dose carboplatin (C)-induced thrombocytopenia in patients with gynecological malignancy. *Blood* 90:580a, 1997.

258. Vadhan-Raj S: Recombinant human thrombopoietin: clinical experience and in vivo biology. *Semin Hematol* 35:261, 1998.

259. Fanucchi M, Glaspy J, Crawford J, et al: Effects of polyethylene glycol-conjugated recombinant human megakaryocyte growth and development factor on platelet counts after chemotherapy for lung cancer. *N Engl J Med* 336:404, 1997.

260. Basser RL, Rasko JE, Clarke K, et al: Randomized, blinded, placebo-controlled phase I trial of pegylated recombinant human megakaryocyte growth and development factor with filgrastim after dose-intensive chemotherapy in patients with advanced cancer. *Blood* 89:3118, 1997.

261. Archimbaud E, Ottmann O, Lin J, et al: A randomized, double-blind, placebo-controlled study using PEG-rHuMGDF as an adjunct to chemotherapy for adults with de-novo acute myeloid leukemia (AML): Early results. *Blood* 99:447a, 1996.

262. Nash R, Kurzrock R, DiPersio J, et al: Safety and activity of recombinant human thrombopoietin (rhTPO) in patients (pts) with delayed platelet recovery (DPR). *Blood* 90:262a, 1997.

263. Bolwell B, Vredenburgh J, Overmoyer B, et al: Safety and biological effect of pegylated recombinant megakaryocyte growth and development factor (PEG-rHuMGDF) in breast cancer patients following autologous peripheral blood progenitor cell transplantation (PBPC). *Blood* 90:171a, 1997.

264. Glaspy J, Vredenburgh J, Demetri GD, et al: Effects of pegylated recombinant human megakaryocyte growth and development factor (PEG-rHuMGDF) before high dose chemotherapy (HDC) with peripheral blood progenitor cell (PBPC) support. *Blood* 90:580a, 1997.

265. Piacibello W, Sanavio F, Garetto L, et al: Extensive amplification and self-renewal of human primitive hematopoietic stem cells from cord blood. *Blood* 89:2644, 1997.

266. Kuter DJ: The use of PEG-rHuMGDF in platelet apheresis. *Stem Cells* 16(Suppl 2):231, 1998.

267. Goodnough LT, DiPersio J, McCullough J, et al: Pegylated recombinant human megakaryocyte growth and development factor (PEG-rHuMGDF) increases platelet (PLT) count (CT) and apheresis yields of normal PLT donors: initial results. *Transfusion* 37:266S, 1997.

268. Harker LA, Marzec UM, Novembre F, et al: Treatment of thrombocytopenia in chimpanzees infected with human immunodeficiency virus by

pegylated recombinant human megakaryocyte growth and development factor. *Blood* 91:4427, 1998.

269. Kaye JA: FDA Licensure of NEUMEGA to prevent severe chemotherapy-induced thrombocytopenia, in *Thrombopoietin: From Molecule to Medicine*, edited by MJ Murphy, DJ Kuter, p 207. AlphaMed Press, Miamisburg, 1998.

270. Robb L, Li R, Hartley L, et al: Infertility in female mice lacking the receptor for interleukin-11 is due to a defective uterine response to implantation. *Nat Med* 4:303, 1998.

271. Nandurkar HH, Robb L, Tarlinton D, et al: Adult mice with targeted mutation of the interleukin-11 receptor (IL11Ra) display normal hematopoiesis. *Blood* 90:2148, 1997.

272. Giri JG, Smith WG, Kahn LE, et al: Promegapoietin, a chimeric growth factor for megakaryocyte and platelet restoration. *Blood* 90:580a, 1997.

273. Cwirla SE, Balasubramanian P, Duffin DJ, et al: Peptide agonist of the thrombopoietin receptor as potent as the natural cytokine. *Science* 276:1696, 1997.

274. Sheridan WP, Kuter DJ: Mechanism of action and clinical trials of Mpl ligand. *Curr Opin Hematol* 4:312, 1997.

275. Kuter D: Thrombopoietins and thrombopoiesis: a clinical perspective. *Vox Sang* 74:75, 1998.

276. MacVittie TJ, Farese AM, Lind LB, et al: Progenipoietin-G stimulates hematopoietic recovery following myelosuppression. *Blood* 90:581a, 1997.

PLATELET MORPHOLOGY, BIOCHEMISTRY, AND FUNCTION

LESLIE V. PARISE
SUSAN S. SMYTH
BARRY S. COLLER

Platelets are small anucleate cell fragments adapted to adhere to damaged blood vessels, aggregate one with another, and facilitate the generation of thrombin. These actions contribute to hemostasis by forming a platelet plug and then reinforcing the plug by the action of thrombin converting fibrinogen to fibrin strands. To accomplish these tasks, platelets have surface receptors that can bind adhesive glycoproteins (GP); these include the GPIb/IX/V complex, which supports platelet adhesion by binding von Willebrand factor even under conditions of high shear, and the GPIIb/IIIa receptor, which is platelet-specific and mediates platelet aggregation by binding fibrinogen and/or von Willebrand factor. Other receptors for adhesive glycoproteins [GPIa/IIa ($\alpha 2\beta 1$), GPVI, and GP65 for collagen; GPIc*/IIa ($\alpha 5\beta 1$) for fibronectin; and GPIc/IIa ($\alpha 6\beta 1$) for laminin] also contribute to platelet adhesion, but their precise contributions are less well defined. Activated platelets express surface P-selectin, which mediates interactions with leukocytes. Platelet coagulant activity results from the exposure of negatively charged phospholipids on the surface of platelets and platelet microparticles, along with release and activation of platelet factor V and perhaps exposure of specific receptors for activated coagulation factors. Platelets change shape with activation as a result of complex changes in the platelet membrane skeleton and cytoskeleton. With activation, platelets undergo release of α granule, dense body, and lysosomal contents. The activation process involves a number of receptors for agonists such as ADP, epinephrine, thrombin, collagen, thrombox-

ane A_2, and platelet-activating factor, as well as several signal transduction pathways, including phosphoinositide metabolism, arachidonic acid release and conversion into thromboxane A_2, and phosphorylation of a number of different target proteins. Increases in intracellular calcium result from, and further contribute to, platelet activation. Platelet activation results in a change in the conformation of the GPIIb/IIIa receptor, leading to high-affinity ligand binding and platelet aggregation.

Platelets also act as storehouses for a variety of molecules that affect platelet function, inflammation, vascular tone, fibrinolysis, and wound healing; these agents are actively released upon platelet activation. Other vasoactive and platelet activating substances are newly synthesized when platelets are activated. Through cooperative biochemical interactions, platelets can communicate with, and are affected by, other blood cells and endothelial cells.

Quantitative and qualitative disorders of platelets result in hemorrhagic diatheses (see Chaps. 117, 119, 120). In pathologic states, uncontrolled platelet thrombus formation can lead to vasoocclusion and ischemic necrosis, as, for example, in myocardial infarction and stroke (see Chaps. 130 and 131). Platelets may also facilitate tumor metastasis.

PLATELET MORPHOLOGY AND BIOCHEMISTRY

LIGHT MICROSCOPIC APPEARANCE

On films made from blood anticoagulated with the strong calcium chelating agent ethylenediaminetetraacetic acid (EDTA) and stained with Wright stain, platelets appear as small bluish-gray, oval-to-round bodies with several purple-red granules (Plate XIV) (see Chap. 2). The mean diameter of platelets varies in different individuals, ranging from about 1.5 to 3.0 μm, approximately one-third to one-fourth that of erythrocytes. There is also considerable variability in the size of platelets in a single individual, with occasional platelets in normal blood samples having diameters greater than half the diameter of erythrocytes. Overall, platelet size appears to follow a log normal distribution. When unanticoagulated blood is used to prepare blood films, platelets undergo variable activation and spreading, and thus platelet aggregates are commonly seen; platelets from such specimens may demonstrate three or four very long and thin processes extending out from the body of the platelet (filopodia), and some platelets may be devoid of granules.

ELECTRON MICROSCOPIC APPEARANCE AND BIOCHEMISTRY

Electron microscopy reveals a fuzzy coat (glycocalix) extending 14 to 20 nm from the platelet surface, which is thought to be composed of membrane glycoproteins, glycolipids, mucopolysaccharides, and adsorbed plasma proteins (Fig. 111-1).[1] Platelets move in an electric field as if they have a net negative surface charge; sialic acid residues attached to proteins and lipids are major contributors to this negative charge.[2] The electrostatic repulsion created by the negative surface charge may help prevent resting platelets from attaching to each other or to negatively charged endothelial cells.

The surface of the platelet has a number of indentations that are thought to be the openings of the open canalicular system, which is an elaborate channel system composed of invaginations of the plasma membrane that extend throughout the platelet (see Fig. 111-1 and "Membrane Systems" below). The contents of platelet granules can gain access to the outside when the granules fuse with either the plasma

Acronyms and abbreviations that appear in this chapter include: ADP, adenosine 5'-diphosphate; ATP, adenosine 5'-triphosphate; BTK, Bruton's tyrosine kinase; cAMP, cyclic AMP; COX, cyclooxygenase; CTAP-III, connective-tissue-activating peptide III; DAG, diacylglycerol; DTS, dense tubular system; Edg, endothelial differentiation gene; EDTA, ethylenediaminetetraacetic acid; ERK2, extracellular-signal-regulated kinase 2; FcRγ, Fc receptor γ; GP, glycoproteins; HPS, Hermansky-Pudlak syndrome; IAP, integrin-associated protein; IP$_3$, inositol 1,4,5-trisphosphate; ITAMs, immuno-receptor tyrosine-containing activation motifs; JNK, Jun N-terminal kinase; LAT, linker-for-activator T cells; LIBS, ligand-induced binding sites; LPA, lysophosphatidic acid; MIDAS, metal-ion-dependent adhesion site; mRNA, messenger RNA; NAP1, neutrophil-activating peptide 1; NO, nitric oxide; PAF, platelet-activating factor; PAI-1, plasminogen activator inhibitor 1; PAR-1, protease-activated receptor 1; PC, phosphatidylcholine; PCR, polymerase chain reaction; PDE, phosphodiesterase; PDGF, platelet-derived growth factor; PE, phosphatidylethanolamine; PECAM-1, platelet-endothelial cell adhesion molecule 1; PF4, platelet factor 4; PG, prostaglandin; PH, pleckstrin homology; PIP$_2$, phosphatidylinositol 4,5-bisphosphate; PKC, protein kinase C; PLA$_2$, phospholipase A$_2$; PLC, phospholipase C; PSGL-1, P-selectin glycoprotein ligand 1; RIBS, receptor-induced binding sites; SH2, Src homology 2; sPLA$_2$, secretory PLA$_2$; TGF-β, transforming growth factor beta; TSP, thrombospondin; uPAR, urokinase receptor; VEGF, vascular endothelial growth factor; vWF, von Willebrand factor;

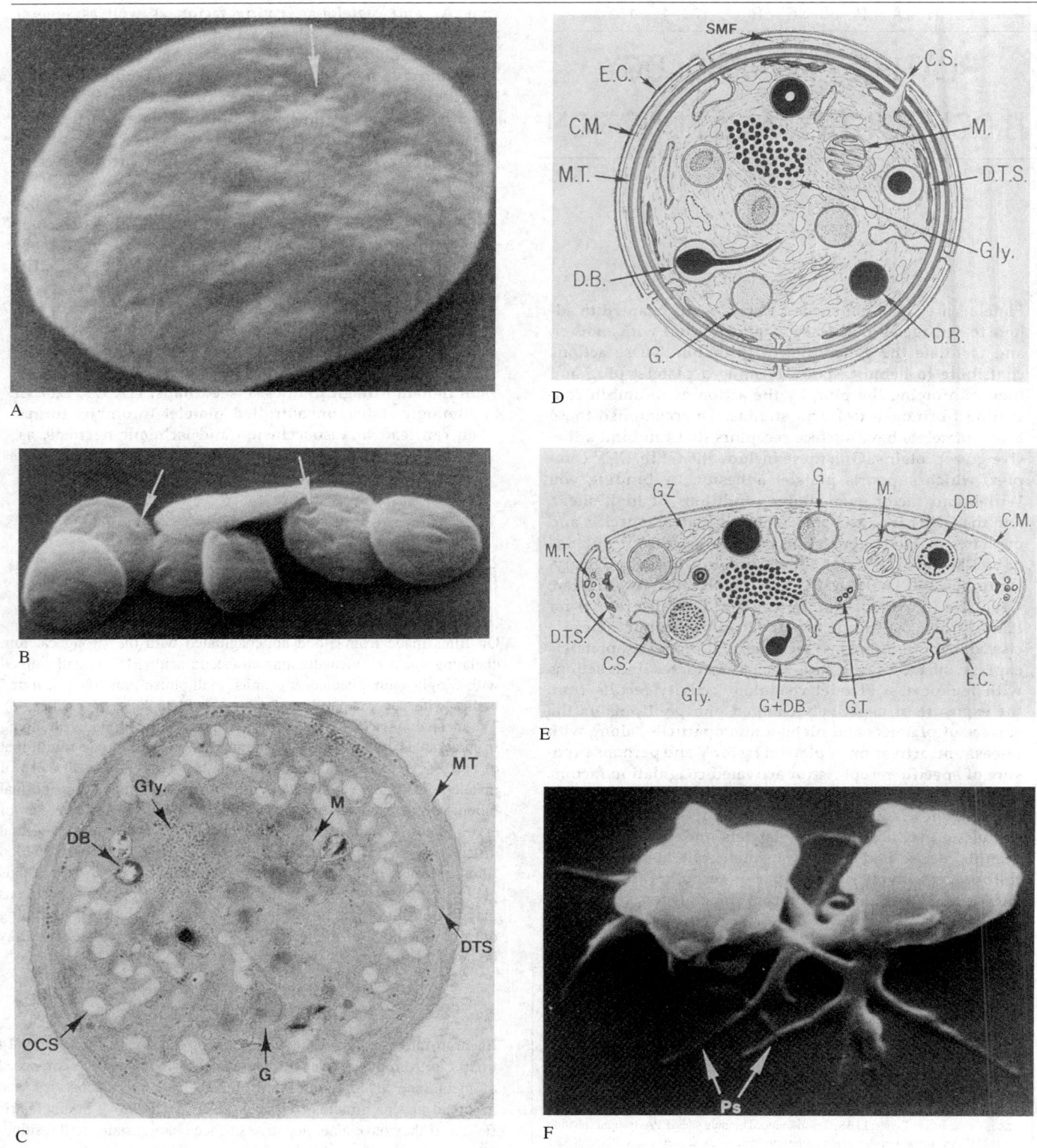

FIGURE 111-1 (A) and (B). Discoid platelets. The lentiform shape of blood platelets is well preserved in samples fixed in glutaraldehyde and critical-point-dried for study in the scanning electron microscope. The indentations apparent on the otherwise smooth surfaces of the platelets (*arrows*) indicate sites where channels of the open canalicular system (OCS) communicate with the cell exterior. (A × 13,200; B × 35,000.) (C), (D), and (E). Ultrastructural features observed in thin sections of discoid platelets cut in the equatorial plane (C and D) or cross-section (E). Components include the exterior coat (EC), trilaminar unit membrane (CM), and submembrane area containing the specialized filaments (SMF) of the membrane skeleton. The plasma membrane indentations form the walls of the channels of the surface-connected canalicular system (CS and OCS). The circumferential band of microtubules (MT) is seen as a continuous band beneath the plasma membrane on the equatorial section and as small open cylinders at the ends of the platelet on the cross-section. Glycogen granules (Gly) are prominent punctate structures in the cytoplasm, and residual Golgi zones (GZ) can also be identified. Organelles include mitochondria (M), dense bodies (DB), and α granules (G), many of which have regions of electron density (nucleoids). The dense tubular system (DTS), the platelet equivalent of the

1358

TABLE 111-1   PLATELET LIPIDS

I   17% dry weight, primarily in membranes
II   Membranes
   A   Protein 57%
   B   Lipid 35%
   C   Carbohydrate 8%
III   Membrane lipids
   A   Phospholipid 75%
   B   Neutral lipid 20%
   C   Glycolipid 5%
IV   Phospholipids
   A   Phosphatidylcholine (PC) 38%
   B   Phosphatidylethanolamine (PE) 27%
   C   Sphingomyelin (SPH) 17%
   D   Phosphatidylserine (PS) 10%
   E   Phosphatidylinositol (PI) 5%
V   Membrane phospholipid asymmetry (percentage of each phospholipid in the exterior leaflet)
   A   Uncharged phospholipids
      1   PC 45%
      2   SPH 93%
   B   Negatively charged phospholipids
      1   PE 20%
      2   PI 16%
      3   PS 9%
VI   Neutral lipids
   A   Cholesterol 95%
   B   Cholesterol: phospholipid = 0.5 on molar basis
VII   Glycolipids
   A   Gangliosides [0.5% of total lipids; 6% of total sialic acid; primarily hematoside (GM3)]
   B   Neutral glycolipids (64% lactosyl ceramide)
   C   Ceramides (A and B)
VIII   Arachidonic acid (29;4)
   1   42% of fatty acids in PI
   2   32% of fatty acids in PE
   3   23% of fatty acids in PS

SOURCE: Adapted from Coller,[788] with permission.

THE PLASMA MEMBRANE

membrane or any region of the open canalicular system. Similarly, glycoproteins contained within granule membranes can join the plasma membrane after granule fusion with either the plasma membrane or the open canalicular system.

The plasma membrane is a trilaminar unit composed of a bilayer of phospholipids in which cholesterol, glycolipids, and glycoproteins are embedded.[1] Platelets prepared by the freeze-fracture technique demonstrate more intramembranous particles embedded in the outer platelet membrane leaflet than in the inner leaflet, which is the reverse of findings in erythrocytes; this observation presumably reflects the many external receptors that mediate platelet interactions. The plasma membrane is thought to contain the sodium- and calcium-ATPase pumps that control the intracellular ionic environment of the platelet. Approximately 57 percent of platelet phospholipids are contained in the plasma membrane (Table 111-1). The phospholipids are asymmetrically organized in the plasma membrane; the negatively charged phospholipids are almost exclusively present in the inner leaflet, whereas the others are more evenly distributed.[3] The negatively charged phospholipids, especially phosphatidylserine, are able to accelerate several steps in the coagulation sequence and so their presence in the inner leaflet of resting platelets, separated from the plasma

coagulation factors, is thought to be a control mechanism for preventing inappropriate coagulation.[4] During platelet activation induced by select agonists, the aminophospholipids may become exposed on the platelet surface or on the surface of platelet microparticles (see ''Platelet Coagulant Activity'' below).[4–6]

The phospholipid asymmetry in resting platelets may be maintained by an ATP-dependent aminophospholipid translocase that actively pumps phosphatidylserine and phosphatidylethanolamine from the outer to the inner leaflet.[4,7] Interactions of negatively charged phospholipids with cytoskeletal or other cytoplasmic elements may also contribute to the asymmetry.[8,9]

The lipid composition of platelet membranes is outlined in Table 111-1. The enrichment of selected phospholipids with arachidonic acid is quite striking, furnishing a store of arachidonic acid for release and conversion into thromboxane A_2 (TXA_2) (see ''Signaling Pathways in Platelet Activation and Aggregation'' below).

The glycoproteins in the plasma membrane are discussed below.

CYTOSKELETAL ELEMENTS

Membrane Cytoskeleton   A planar network of thin, elongated spectrin tetramers interconnected by the ends of actin filaments is present immediately below the plasma membrane and the membranes of the open canalicular system.[10] Actin-binding protein (filamin-1) is able to interact with both the transmembrane glycoprotein GPIbα and the actin immediately below the membrane, thus connecting these components to the spectrin network and forming a membrane cytoskeleton that probably stabilizes the membrane's discoid shape. In addition, the association of GPIbα with the membrane skeleton restricts the expansion of the spectrin network and probably helps to organize receptors into linear arrays on the platelet surface, thus enhancing receptor cooperation.[11,12] Other proteins that have been found in the membrane skeleton include talin, vinculin, dystrophin-related protein, molecules implicated in signal transduction, and several isoenzymes of protein kinase C (see below).[11] The protein vimentin (M_r 58,000), which is an important component of intermediate filaments, is present in platelets and may contribute to the membrane cytoskeleton. With platelet activation, GPIIb/IIIa and α2β1 may also join the cytoskeleton. Thus, interactions with the cytoskeleton determine whether receptors are free to move in the plane of the membrane; they may also have a role in moving certain receptors from the surface to the interior of platelets and vice versa via the open canalicular system.[11–13] The membrane skeleton may also be important in platelet spreading after adhesion.

Microtubules   The circumferential band of microtubules present below the plasma membrane probably contributes to the platelet's discoid shape,[1] but it may also be involved in platelet formation from megakaryocytes.[14] On cross-section, approximately 8 to 12 separate coils are observed at the tapered ends of the platelet, but this probably represents a single coil of about 100 μm wound multiple times. Microtubules are 25-nm hollow polymers composed of 13 protofilaments made up of polymers of M_r 110,000 subunits, each composed of two proteins of M_r 55,000 (α- and β-tubulin) that associate with several high-molecular-weight proteins (microtubule-associated proteins).[15–17] Approximately 60 percent of the platelet tubulin is in microtubules, and there is a dynamic equilibrium between the polymerized and free tubulin subunits.[18] Motor proteins of the dynein and kinesin families are also associated with microtubules.[19]

sarcoplasmic reticulum sequesters calcium. (C × 30,000.) (F). Platelet shape change. Platelets exposed to ADP and then fixed and examined by scanning electron microscopy. The platelets lose their discoid shape and become spiny spheres with long extensions, variably referred to as *filopodia* or *pseudopodia* (Ps). (×17,000.) (From White,[786] with permission.)

Microfilaments   The platelet is rich in actin, a protein that can polymerize into microfilamentous bundles (see below).[10,11,20] In resting platelets, microfilaments are not prominent, but when platelets change shape, the filopodia they form contain bundles of microfilaments made up of actin and associated proteins.[1,16]

ORGANELLES

Peroxisomes   Peroxisomes are very small organelles present in platelets. They are thought to contribute to lipid metabolism, especially plasmalogen synthesis, and may participate in the synthesis of platelet-activating factor (PAF).[21] They contain acyl-CoA:dihydroxyacetone phosphate acyltransferase, which catalyzes the first step in the synthesis of ether phospholipids. Deficiencies of this enzymatic activity in platelets have been identified in the cerebro-renal Zellweger syndrome.[22,23]

Mitochondria   Platelets contain, on average, approximately seven mitochondria of relatively small size that are involved in oxidative energy metabolism (see "Energy Metabolism" below).[24] Abnormalities of mitochondrial enzymes, including NADH coenyzme Q reductase (complex I), have been implicated in the pathophysiology of aging and several neurodegenerative disorders, including some patients with Parkinson disease. Assays of platelet mitochondrial enzyme levels have been used in these studies.[25,26]

Lysosomes   Platelets have lysosomal granules that contain acid hydrolases typical of these organelles. Among the enzymes thought to originate from platelet lysosomes are β-glucuronidase, cathepsins, aryl sulfatase, β-hexosaminidase, β-galactosidase, endoglucosidase (heparitinase), β-glycerophosphatase, elastase, and collagenase.[24] When platelets undergo secretion, lysosomal contents are more slowly and incompletely released than are the contents of α granules and dense bodies.[27,28] Moreover, stronger inducers of activation are required to induce release of lysosomal contents. Proteins present in lysosomal membranes (e.g., CD63) have been identified, and their appearance on the plasma membrane serves as a marker of the platelet release reaction.[29,30] The elastase and collagenase activities may contribute to vascular damage at sites of platelet thrombus formation. The heparitinase may be able to cleave heparin-like molecules from the surface of endothelial cells, and the resulting soluble molecules appear to inhibit growth of smooth muscle cells.[31]

Dense Bodies   Platelets contain, on average, approximately three to eight electron-dense organelles, 20 to 30 nm in diameter (see Fig. 111-1).[1,32] The intrinsic electron density of dense bodies when viewed as unstained whole mounts derives from their high content of calcium (see Table 111-2)[1,24]; the granules are also dense when viewed by transmission electron microscopy because they are highly osmophilic.[32] Dense granules contain high concentrations of serotonin, which is taken up from plasma by a plasma membrane carrier and then trapped in the dense bodies.[32] Trapping of serotonin may occur as a result of the lower pH ($\sim$6.1) maintained in dense granules due to the action of an H+ pumping ATPase on the dense body membrane.[32] Adenosine 5'-diphosphate (ADP) and adenosine 5'-triphosphate (ATP) are also highly concentrated in dense bodies.[24] There is more ADP than ATP in the dense bodies (ATP:ADP = 2:3), which is the reverse of their relative concentrations in the cytoplasm (ATP:ADP = 8:1). Since there is very little connection between the pools of adenine nucleotides in the cytoplasm and the dense bodies, they have been respectively designated as the *metabolic* and *storage pools* of adenine nucleotides.[24] Storage of adenine nucleotides at such a high concentration in dense bodies appears to be achieved by stacking the ATP and ADP purine rings vertically in aggregates that are stabilized by the interactions of calcium ions with the polyphosphate groups.[33,34] The planar hydroxyindole rings of serotonin may also enter these stacks, helping to account for the trapping mechanism. Trapping of serotonin

TABLE 111-2   PLATELET GRANULE AND CYTOPLASMIC CONTENTS

Dense bodies[789]	
ADP	653 m*M*
ATP	436 m*M*
Calcium	2181 m*M*
Serotonin	65 m*M*
Pyrophosphate	326 m*M*

α Granules[43,46,48]
  Platelet-specific proteins:
    Platelet factor 4 (PF4)
    β-Thromboglobulin (β-TG) family (platelet basic protein, low-affinity platelet factor 4, β-thromboglobulin, and β-thromboglobulin-F)
  Multimerin
  Adhesive glycoproteins:
    Fibrinogen
    Von Willebrand factor (vWF)
    Fibronectin
    Thrombospondin
    Vitronectin
  Coagulation factors:
    Factor V
    Protein S
    Factor XI
  Mitogenic factors:
    Platelet-derived growth factor (PDGF)
    Transforming growth factor-β (TGF-β)
    Endothelial cell growth factor
    Epidermal growth factor (EGF)
  Angiogenic factors:
    Vascular endothelial growth factor
    Platelet factor 4 (inhibitor)
  Fibrinolytic inhibitors:
    α_2-Plasmin inhibitor (α_2-PI)
    Plasminogen activator inhibitor 1 (PAI-1)
  Albumin
  Immunoglobulins
  Granule membrane-specific proteins:
    P-selectin (CD62P)
    CD63
    GMP 33
Other secreted or released proteins[43,48]
  Protease nexin I
  Peptidase
  Amyloid β-protein precursor (protease nexin II)
  Tissue factor pathway inhibitor (TFPI)
  Factor XIII
α_1-Protease inhibitor
  Cl-inhibitor
  High-molecular-weight kininogen
  α_2-Macroglobulin
  Vascular permeability factor
  Interleukin-Iβ

must differ from that of adenine nucleotides, however, since dense granule serotonin exchanges readily with external serotonin.[24]

The membrane of dense granules contains glycoproteins that are also found on the plasma membrane and the membranes of α granules and lysosomes, including CD36, LAMP-2, P-selectin, GPIIb/IIIa, and GPIb/IX. Since patients with Hermansky-Pudlak syndrome (HPS) (see Chap. 119) have abnormal dense bodies, it is likely that the HPS gene product, which contains two transmembrane domains, is also associated with dense granules.[35] Similarly, the product of the Chediak-Higashi syndrome gene, although lacking a transmembrane domain, has been proposed to associate with the dense granule membrane.[36]

Release of dense granule contents from activated platelets constitutes an important positive feedback mechanism for platelet aggregation, since ADP is a potent platelet agonist and serotonin is a weak agonist (see below). ATP is a partial antagonist of ADP-induced activation, but since ATP is rapidly catabolized to ADP in plasma ($T_{1/2}$ = 1.5 min), and ADP is rapidly catabolized to AMP ($T_{1/2}$ = 4 min) and then to adenosine,[24] a platelet inhibitor,[37] it is difficult to predict the overall effect of ATP release. Adding to the complexity in vivo is the presence of an ecto-ATP diphosphohydrolase (ATPDase) (CD39; ecto-ADPase) present on endothelial and lymphoid cells, which can metabolize ATP and ADP to AMP and thus probably limits the amount of ADP present.[38] ATP released from platelets may also serve as a high-energy phosphate source for platelet ecto-protein kinases, which can phosphorylate several proteins, including GPIV.[39–42]

α Granules   α granules are the most abundant granules in platelets, numbering about 50 to 80 per platelet.[43] They are about 200 nm in diameter on cross-section and demonstrate internal variation in electron density, often with an eccentric area of accentuated electron density, termed a *nucleoid*, in which β-thromboglobulin, platelet factor 4, and proteoglycans are concentrated (Fig. 111-1).[1] The more electron-lucent areas contain tubular elements in which von Willebrand factor (vWF), multimerin, and factor V are preferentially localized.[44] Some of the most important proteins present in α granules are listed in Table 111-2. It appears that small amounts of virtually all plasma proteins are nonspecifically taken up into α granules, and thus the plasma levels of these proteins determines their platelet levels.[45,46] For example, since the α-granule pool of immunoglobulins represents the vast majority of platelet immunoglobulin, total platelet immunoglobulin is much more affected by plasma immunoglobulin levels than by changes in surface immunoglobulin[45,46] (see Chap. 117).

The platelet-specific proteins (platelet factor 4 and the β-thromboglobulin family) are present in α granules at concentrations that are about 20,000 times higher than their plasma concentrations (when each is expressed as a fraction of total protein in platelets or plasma respectively) (Table 111-2).[47,48] These M_r 7000 to 11,000 proteins all bind to heparin, but with varying affinities. They also share amino acid sequence homology with each other and with other members of the "intercrine-cytokine" family of molecules, such as interleukin-8 (neutrophil-activating peptide 1, NAP1), which are active in inflammation, cell growth, and malignant transformation (Fig. 111-2).[49–51]

Platelet factor 4 (PF4) is a chemokine in the CXC family that does not contain the Glu-Leu-Arg (ELR) conserved sequence.[52] PF4 binds to heparin with high affinity and can neutralize heparin's anticoagulant activity.[47,53–55] It is thought to exist as a PF4 tetramer complexed to a proteoglycan carrier.[56,57] Specific lysine residues (amino acids 61, 62, 65, and 66) have been implicated in its binding to heparin. X-ray crystallography indicates that these lysines are on the surface of the PF4 tetramer and that heparin winds around this core.[58,59]

After PF4 is released from platelets, it binds to heparin-like molecules on the surface of endothelial cells.[59] Heparin administration can mobilize this endothelial-bound pool of PF4 into the circulation.[59] PF4-heparin complexes and PF4-heparin-like molecule complexes on endothelial cells have been implicated as the target antigens in heparin-induced thrombocytopenia with thrombosis.[60] PF4 also binds to hepatocytes, which take it up and catabolize it.[61] PF4 is a weak neutrophil and fibroblast attractant.[52,62] It inhibits angiogenesis, perhaps through inhibition of endothelial cell proliferation.[63] A large number of other activities have been ascribed to PF4, including histamine release from basophils[64]; inhibition of tumor growth[65] and megakaryocyte maturation[66,67]; reversal of immunosuppression[62,68]; enhancement of fibroblast attachment to substrata[69]; potentiation of platelet aggregation[70]; inhibition of contact activation,[71] and enhancement of polymorphonuclear leukocyte responsiveness to the activating peptide f-Met-Leu-Phe and monocyte responsiveness to lipopolysaccharide.[72,73]

The β-thromboglobulin family of proteins are CXC chemokines that contain the conserved Glu-Leu-Arg (ELR) sequence.[52] They include platelet basic protein, low-affinity platelet factor 4 (connective-tissue-activating peptide III; CTAP-III), β-thromboglobulin, and β-thromboglobulin-F (NAP2) (see Table 111-2 and Fig. 111-2).[48,74–76] All of these proteins share the same carboxy terminus but differ in the length of their amino termini, presumably due to proteolytic digestion of the parent molecule, platelet basic protein (Fig. 111-2). These proteins bind to heparin but with lower affinity than PF4, and thus they neutralize heparin less well. Unlike PF4, they are cleared from the circulation by the kidney rather than the liver.[77] CTAP-III is a weak fibroblast mitogen, and β-thromboglobulin is chemoattractant for fibroblasts.[52] β-thromboglobulin-F (NAP2) is chemotactic for granulocytes and activates them to undergo endocytosis.[52,76]

The biochemistry of the adhesive glycoproteins contained in α granules and others variably present in plasma and extracellular matrix is described in Table 111-3 and in other chapters (Chap. 112 for fibrinogen and Chap. 135 for vWF). Their relative concentrations in α granules varies significantly. Presumably they are localized in platelets so that when platelets undergo the release reaction they will be present at high concentrations at the site of vascular injury.

Multimerin comprises a family of disulfide-linked homo-multimers, ranging from M_r 450,000 to many millions of daltons in size.[78] The M_r 450,000 multimer is thought to be a trimer of a single subunit of either M_r 167,000[79] or M_r 155,000[78] that is synthesized in megakaryocytes and endothelial cells and stored in the electron-lucent region of α granules in platelets and dense-core granules in endothelial cells.[80] It colocalizes with vWF in platelets but not in endothelial cells. Although multimerin's multimeric structure is similar to that of vWF, the deduced amino acid sequence of its subunit is not homologous to that of vWF.[78] The prepromultimerin subunit contains 1228 amino acids. It undergoes glycosylation and proteolysis during synthesis. It is composed of a number of domains, including an amino-terminal region that includes an RGD sequence, coiled coil sequences, epider-

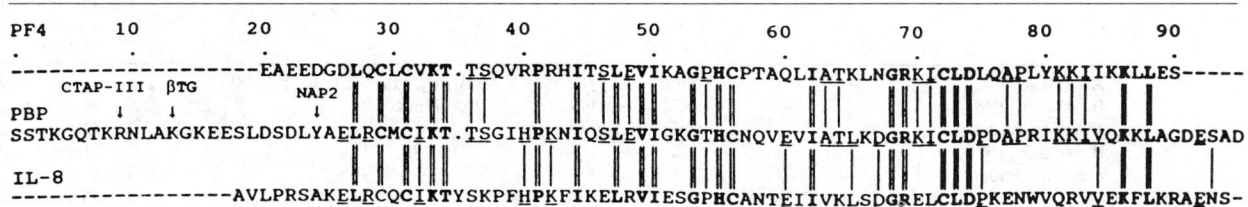

FIGURE 111-2   Comparison of the amino acid sequences of platelet factor 4 (PF4), platelet basic protein (PBP), and interleukin-8/NAP1 (IL-8). Double vertical lines indicate identical amino acids (underlined) in two of the three proteins. Dots (.) denote artificial breaks inserted to improve alignment. Note that the PBP and IL-8 share the ELR sequence (amino acids 26–28 in PBP) conserved in a number of CXC chemokines, but PF4 does not contain this sequence. Cleavage of peptide bond between R9 and N10 of PBP yields low-affinity platelet factor 4 (LA-PF4/CTAP-III); cleavage of peptide bond between K13 and G14 yields β-thromboglobulin (βTG); cleavage of peptide bond between Y24 and A25 yields β-thromboglobulin fragment (βTG-F/NAP2). Cleavage points follow the amino acid indicated by the arrows. (Adapted from Niewiarowski,[47] with permission.)

TABLE 111-3   ADHESIVE GLYCOPROTEINS

Protein	Subunit, kDa	Unusual 1° Structural Features & Modifications	Domain Homologies & Binding Regions	Mature Protein Composition	Mature Protein M_r	Known Interactions
Collagens	95–180	Gly-Pro-X repeating sequence Hydroxylysine Hydroxyproline	RGD Right-handed triple helix	Tropocollagen = 3 chains		Variable
Type I	$\alpha1(I)$ $\alpha2(I)$			$[\alpha1(I)]_2\alpha2(I)$ $[\alpha1(I)]_3$ (minor component)		Thrombospondin Fibronectin von Willebrand factor ?Fibrinogen
Type III	$\alpha1(III)$			$[\alpha1(III)]_3$		
Type IV	$\alpha1(IV)$ $\alpha2(IV)$			$[\alpha1(IV)]_2\alpha2(IV)$, $[\alpha1(IV)]_3$ and $[\alpha2(IV)]_3$		
Type V	$\alpha1(V)$ $\alpha2(V)$ $\alpha3(V)$			$[\alpha1(V)]_2\alpha2(V)$ $\alpha1(V)\alpha2(V)\alpha3(V)$		
Type VI	$\alpha1(VI)$ $\alpha2(VI)$ $\alpha3(VI)$			$\alpha1(VI)\alpha2(VI)$ $\alpha3(VI)$?		
Von Willebrand factor	220 (2,050 amino acids)	Large propeptide (741 amino acids); A, B, C, D, E repeats	GPIIb/IIIa—RGD 1,789–1,791 GPIb—I Domain 230–310	Dimer = protomer Multimers of protomers from 2 to ~40 via disulfide bonds	880,000– ~20,000,000	Collagen Heparin Factor VIII Fibrin
Fibrinogen	$A\alpha$ = 63 (625 amino acids) $B\beta$ = 56 (427 amino acids) γ = 47 (411 amino acids)	Alternately spliced γ chains Phosphorylation of $A\alpha$	2 RGDs in $A\alpha$ (95–97 and 572–574) $\alpha V\beta3$—RGD 572–574 GPIIb/IIIa-C-terminal γ-chain dodecamer (400–411)	2 $A\alpha$, 2 $B\beta$, 2 γ via disulfide bonds	340,000	Thrombospondin ?Collagen Staphylococci
Vitronectin	1 chain = 75 (458 amino acids) 2 chain = 65+10 via disulfide bonds	Met→Thr polymorphism	RGD Somatomedin B Hemopexin	Same as subunits	75,000 and 65,000 + 10,000	Glass Plastic Heparin Serine protease: serpin complexes PAI-1 uPAR
Fibronectin	220 (2355 amino acids)	Type I, II, and III repeats Alternately spliced forms	RGD (1493–1495)	Dimer via disulfide bonds	440,000	Fibrin Heparin Collagen DNA Staphylococci
Thrombospondin	180 (1150 amino acids)		RGD (?functional) $\alpha1(I)$ Collagen Epidermal growth factor Malaria antigen	Trimer via disulfide bonds	450,000	Calcium Plasminogen Collagen Fibrinogen Histidine-rich glycoprotein Fibronectin Laminin Heparin
Laminin	A = 400 B_1 = 215 (1765 amino acids) B_2 = 205 (1576 amino acids)		YIGSR RGD (?functional) Epidermal growth factor	A, B_1, B_2, via disulfide bonds	850,000	Collagen type IV Nidogen/entactin Osteonectin Heparin sulfate C1q Plasminogen Plasmin
Multimerin	155 or 167	Large prepropeptide (1228 amino acids)	RGD in N-terminal region EGF		450,000– ~5,000,000	Factor V

* Assumes, 10^{11} platelets per ml of packed platelets.
RDG, arginine-glycine-aspartic acid sequence; YIGSR, amino acid sequence involved in laminin function; PAI-1, plasminogen activator

(table continued on opposite page)

Known Platelet Receptors	Electron Microscopy Structure	Plasma Concentration, μg/ml	Platelet Concentration,* μg/ml	Ratio Platelet/ Plasma	Sites of Synthesis
GPIa/IIa ($\alpha2\beta1$; CD49b/CD29; VLA-2) GPIV (CD36) GPVI	Tropocollagen = rodlike coil, 15 × 3,000 Å; other forms have variable degrees of fibril formation	—	—	—	Fibroblasts
GPIb (CD42b, c) GPIIb/IIIa (αIIbβ3; CD41/CD61)	Elliptical, nodular coil, length 5,000, but with some 11,000 Å	10	34	3.4	Endothelial cells Megakaryocytes
GPIIb/IIIa (αIIbβ3; CD41/CD61) αVβ3 (CD51/CD61)	Trinodular, asymmetrical; 475 Å diameter	3,000	7,300	2.4	Hepatocytes
GPIIb/IIIa (αIIbβ3; CD41/CD61) αVβ3 (CD51/CD61)		350	800	2.3	?Hepatocytes
GPIc*/IIa ($\alpha5\beta1$; CD49e/CD29; VLA-5) GPIIb/IIIa (αIIbβ3; CD41/CD61)	Extended antiparallel dimeric structure	300	315	1.1	Hepatocytes Fibroblasts ?Endothelial cells Megakaryocytes Monocytes, etc.
GPIV (CD36) ?GPIIb/IIIa (αIIbβ3; CD41/CD61) Integrin Associated Protein (CD47)	3 Asymmetrical dumbbells, joined near smaller globular domains	0.16	4,900	30,625	Megakaryocytes Many cultured cells
GPIc/IIa ($\alpha6\beta1$; CD49f/CD29; VLA-6)	Cross-like structure	—	—	—	Fibroblasts Many other cell types
Unknown	Unknown	—	—	—	Megakaryocytes Endothelial cells

mal growth factor-like domains, and a carboxy-terminal globular head similar to that found in the complement protein C1q. Multimerin binds both factor V and factor Va, and all of the biologically active factor V in platelets is bound to multimerin.[44] With thrombin activation of platelets, factor V separates from multimerin, and is released from platelets (see below); the higher M_r multimerin multimers bind to the platelet membrane. Multimerin does not circulate in plasma at an appreciable concentration, but it may act as an adhesive extracellular matrix protein.

Fibrinogen is concentrated in α granules, as judged by the ratio of platelet/plasma fibrinogen. Megakaryocytes do not appear to synthesize fibrinogen; instead, it is taken up from plasma by a process that involves the GPIIb/IIIa receptor.[81] Since fibrinogen molecules that contain altered sequences in the γ chain are not stored in α granules, even when the molecules are heterodimeric (i.e., contain one normal and one abnormal γ chain), it is possible that uptake requires simultaneous binding of a fibrinogen molecule to two different GPIIb/IIIa receptors via the γ-chain carboxy-terminal sequence[81,82] (see GPIIb/IIIa below and Chap. 119).

The vWF stored in platelet α granules appears to contribute to hemostasis because in certain pathologic states it correlates better with bleeding symptoms than does plasma vWF (see Chap. 135). vWF is made in megakaryocytes and endothelial cells (see Chaps. 114 and 135). The multimeric structure of platelet vWF is thought to reflect endothelial vWF more nearly than plasma vWF, since higher M_r multimers are present (see Chap. 135).

Fibronectin is present in α granules, and, although it interacts with a number of adhesive glycoproteins and can bind to thrombin-stimulated platelets under certain circumstances, no precise role in platelet function has been identified for this adhesive protein.

Vitronectin, a molecule that binds readily to glass, also binds to plasminogen activator inhibitor 1 (PAI-1), the urokinase receptor (uPAR), collagen, and heparin and forms ternary complexes with serine proteases and serpins in the coagulation and complement systems. It is present in platelets at levels that suggest it is concentrated,[83] but it does not appear to be synthesized in megakaryocytes. Mice deficient in vitronectin develop normally but demonstrate a predisposition to develop thrombosis when challenged, suggesting that vitronectin serves an antithrombotic function.[84]

Thrombospondin-1 is unique among the adhesive glycoproteins in blood in that it is present almost exclusively inside the platelet.[85,86] It constitutes about 20 percent of the released platelet proteins. Thrombospondin-1 is synthesized by megakaryocytes, cultured endothelial cells, and other cultured cells.[87,88] Although GPIIb/IIIa, $\alpha V\beta 3$, proteoglycans, integrin-associated protein, and GPIV (CD36) have all been implicated as receptors for thrombospondin, controversy remains as to its mechanism of binding to platelets.[89–94] The phosphorylation state of GPIV (CD36) may affect its ability to bind thrombospondin.[91] Thrombospondin contains an Arg-Gly-Asp (RGD) sequence, which may contribute to its binding to platelets, but other regions are probably also involved.[86] The conformation of thrombospondin varies with the calcium concentration of the surrounding environment. Thrombospondin can interact with many other adhesive glycoproteins, including fibronectin and fibrinogen,[95,96] and it is a component of the extracellular matrix.[97] Thrombospondin appears to stabilize platelet aggregates that are formed[98]; it may also modulate fibrinolysis and activate latent transforming growth factor beta (TGF-β) (see below).[99,100] Thrombospondin and a peptide derived from its cell-binding domain can activate platelets via binding to integrin-associated protein, a membrane protein that is a member of the immunoglobulin superfamily and is associated with both GPIIb/IIIa and $\alpha 2\beta 1$ (see ''Signaling Pathways in Platelet Activation and Aggregation'' below).[93,94,101,102]

Platelets contribute about 20 percent of the factor V present in whole blood, with nearly all of it in α granules.[103,104] Megakaryocytes probably synthesize factor V,[105,106] and it associates with multimerin when stored in α granules. During platelet activation and release, platelet-derived factor V appears to undergo proteolytic activation by at least two separate enzymes.[4,107,108] Evidence from patients with inhibitors and deficiencies of plasma and platelet factor V indicate that platelet-derived factor V has an important role in hemostasis.[109,110] Platelets undergo microvesiculation when activated, and the microvesicles, which are rich in factor V, are potent promoters of coagulation.[111]

Protein S (see Chap. 113), PAI-1 (see Chap. 116), and α_2-plasmin inhibitor (see Chap. 116) are also contained in α granules and can be released from platelets. Similarly, tissue factor pathway inhibitor (see Chap. 113), α_1-protease inhibitor, and C-1 inhibitor (see Chap. 113) have also been identified in platelets.

Platelet-derived growth factor (PDGF) is a disulfide-linked dimeric molecule of M_r 30,000 that is mitogenic for smooth-muscle cells.[112] Platelet α granules contain a mixture of the homodimer PDGF B-B (30 percent) and the heterodimer PDGF A-B (70 percent); the different forms appear to have different functional activities.[113] PDGF may play a role in normal cell proliferation, as well as in the development of atherosclerosis, tumor growth, wound repair, and fibroproliferative responses.[114–116] After it was discovered in platelets and named *platelet-derived growth factor*, other cells were found to produce the same factor; thus the name *PDGF* is misleading. PDGF is structurally related to the putative transforming protein p28^{sis} of simian sarcoma virus,[117,118] and its receptor is in the tyrosine kinase family.[119]

Platelet-derived endothelial cell growth factor is a protein of M_r 45,000 that stimulates endothelial cell proliferation and angiogenesis.[120] This protein is thought to be present in the cytoplasm of platelets and thus is only released at the time of platelet disintegration.

Platelets contain high concentrations of vascular endothelial growth factor (VEGF), an important stimulator of angiogenesis, and can release VEGF after stimulation in vitro and during the hemostatic response to a bleeding time wound.[121–123] Megakaryocytes express mRNA of the three VEGF isoforms (121, 165, and 189 amino acids),[124] and by immunoblot VEGF protein bands of M_r 34,000 and 44,000 are identifiable in platelets.[125] Platelets and megakaryocytes also express the gene transcript for a VEGF receptor termed *KDR*.[126] Another endothelial growth factor structurally related to VEGF, VEGF-C, has also been identified in platelets.[127] Platelet levels of VEGF have been reported to be increased in malignancies,[128] and platelet VEGF has been postulated to play a role in tumor growth[129] and proliferative retinopathy in sickle cell disease.[130,131]

Epidermal growth factor has also been identified in platelets, but the kinetics of its release upon thrombin or collagen stimulation differs from that of other granule proteins.[132]

An amyloid β-protein precursor protein (protease nexin II) (M_r about 115,000) is present in high concentrations in platelets and can be released with platelet activation.[133,134] Unique proteolysis products of this protein are found in cerebral amyloid deposits in patients with Alzheimer's disease, and such patients may have altered proteolysis of their platelet protease nexin II as well.[135] This protein also inhibits factors IX and XI, and heparin accelerates the inhibition.[136–138]

Factor XIII is present in platelets but differs from plasma factor XIII in having only the ''a'' subunits (see Chap. 112).[139,140] Platelet factor XIII accounts for about 50 percent of total blood factor XIII.[139,140]

Transforming growth factor beta (TGF-β) is an M_r 25,000 homodimeric protein that promotes the growth of certain cells and inhibits the growth of others.[141] It also induces synthesis of extracellular matrix proteins, PAI-1, and metalloproteinases. Migration of endothelial cells is inhibited by TGF-β, but it acts as a chemoattractant for monocytes and fibroblasts. TGF-β has a wide tissue distribution and is concentrated in platelet α granules, from which it can be released with platelet activation.[142] TGF-β released from platelets is inactive (latent) because it is complexed with a portion of its precursor protein, and the latter is covalently coupled to another protein, the latent TGF-β-binding protein. Activation of latent TGF-β is a complex process that appears to require the cooperation of two different cell types and involves proteolytic digestion, perhaps by plasmin, abetted by transglutaminase.[141] Complex formation between latent TGF-β and thrombospondin may also activate TGF-β.[100] Active TGF-β can bind to three different cell surface proteins, a proteoglycan (beta glycan) and two serine/threonine kinases.[143,144] TGF-β can increase thrombopoietin production by bone marrow stromal cells, and in turn, thrombopoietin induces megakaryocyte expression of TGF-β receptors I and II, allowing TGF-β to arrest the maturation of megakaryocyte colony-forming units.[145] TGF-β can also stimulate smooth muscle cells to express and release VEGF, thus perhaps supporting reendothlialization after vascular injury.[146]

Platelets may also release proteins that affect the uptake of oxidized low-density lipoproteins by macrophages, furnishing another potential link between platelet activation and atherosclerosis.[147]

Ribosomes and Messenger RNA Platelets contain only a relatively small number of ribosomes, have only remnants of a Golgi apparatus (Fig. 111-1), and have only a small amount of messenger RNA (mRNA)[148,149] Since they lack nuclei, they cannot synthesize mRNA. The application of the polymerase chain reaction (PCR) to platelet mRNA has permitted the molecular biologic analysis of platelet membrane glycoproteins and select plasma proteins that are synthesized in platelets, such as von Willebrand factor.[150,151] Regulated synthesis of new proteins by platelets has been reported after thrombin activation, and it appears that signaling produced by ligand engagement of GPIIb/IIIa is required to initiate the process.[152,153] Signaling through GPIa/IIa ($\alpha 2\beta 1$) also can initiate platelet protein synthesis.[153]

MEMBRANE SYSTEMS

Open Canalicular System The surface-connected open canalicular system is an elaborate series of conduits that begin as indentations of the plasma membrane and course throughout the interior of the platelet.[1,154] Tracer studies demonstrate that the open canalicular system is contiguous with the exterior of the platelet, even though elements of the open canalicular system may appear as closed vesicles or vacuoles by electron microscopy of sectioned platelets.[1,154,155]

The open canalicular system may serve several functions. It provides a mechanism for entry of external elements into the interior of the platelet. It also provides a potential route for the release of granule contents to the outside, eliminating the need for granule fusion with the plasma membrane itself.[155] This latter function is especially important because, under most circumstances, platelet granules appear to move to the center of the platelet upon platelet activation rather than to the periphery.[1,156] Controversy remains, however, regarding the relative frequency with which secretion occurs via the open canalicular system versus direct fusion with the plasma membrane.[1,157]

The open canalicular system also represents an extensive internal store of membrane. Both filopodia formation and platelet spreading after adhesion result in a dramatic increase in surface plasma membrane compared to the plasma membrane of resting platelets, and it is not possible for new membrane to be synthesized during the short timecourse of these phenomena. Thus, the membrane of the open canalicular system most likely contributes to the increase in plasma membrane under these conditions; the membranes of α granules, dense bodies, and, to a lesser extent, lysosomes may also contribute, but only if the stimulus is sufficient to induce the fusion of these organelles with the plasma membrane (release reaction). Finally, the membrane of the open canalicular system may serve as a storage site for plasma membrane glycoproteins. For example, under certain conditions, platelet activa-

tion by thrombin leads to a consistent, selective loss of GPIb/IX from the platelet surface; electron microscopy indicates that the GPIb/IX becomes sequestered in the open canalicular system.[13,158,159] Plasmin may produce a similar phenomenon.[13,160] Platelet activation leads to an increase in surface GPIIb/IIIa, and, although much of this is thought to derive from α-granule membranes, at least some may come from GPIIb/IIIa receptors in the membranes of dense bodies and the open canalicular system.[13,161]

Dense Tubular System The dense tubular system is a closed-channel network of residual endoplasmic reticulum characterized histocytochemically by the presence of peroxidase activity.[1,162,163] The channels of the dense tubular system are less extensive than those of the open canalicular system and tend to cluster in regions in close approximation to the open canalicular system.[1] The dense tubular system has been likened to the sarcoplasmic reticulum of muscle because it can sequester ionized calcium and release it when platelets are activated.[164,165] Calreticulin, a calcium-binding protein found in the dense tubular system, probably helps to sequester calcium.[17,166] Release of calcium from the dense tubular system involves the binding of inositol 1,4,5 trisphosphate (IP$_3$), a messenger molecule formed during signal transduction, to receptors on the dense tubular system membrane. Cyclic AMP (cAMP) inhibits calcium release from the dense tubular system, either by enhancing the calcium pumping mechanism[167] or by inhibiting release induced by IP$_3$.[168]

The dense tubular system membrane is also probably a major site of prostaglandin and thromboxane synthesis[165,169]; in fact, the peroxidase activity used to identify the dense tubular system is an enzymatic component of prostaglandin synthesis.[169,170]

PLATELET PHYSIOLOGY AND BIOCHEMISTRY

OVERVIEW OF PLATELET ADHESION, AGGREGATION, AND PLATELET THROMBUS FORMATION

The hemostatic system is under elaborate control mechanisms lest the response either be inadequate to meet the hemorrhagic challenge or result in inappropriate thrombosis in response to trivial provocation. Evolutionary pressures have probably favored a highly active hemostatic system, since individuals with more active hemostatic systems were more likely to avoid death from hemorrhage prior to attaining sexual maturity or during childbirth. Our active hemostatic system appears to be less well adapted to our modern age, which is characterized by long life-spans and progressive vascular disease, since the deposition of a platelet-fibrin thrombus on a damaged atherosclerotic plaque can lead to myocardial infarction or stroke.

The platelet's major function is to seal openings in the vascular tree. It is appropriate, therefore, that the initiation signal for platelet deposition and activation is exposure of underlying portions of the blood vessel wall that are normally concealed from circulating platelets by an intact endothelial lining (Fig. 111-3 and Table 111-4). Additional parameters that probably control the platelet response are: (1) the depth of injury, with deeper damage exposing more platelet-reactive materials and tissue factor[171-174] (see Chap. 113); (2) the vascular bed, with the blood vessels serving mucocutaneous tissues especially dependent on platelets for hemostasis, in contrast to the vascular beds in muscles and joints, which rely more on the coagulation mechanism; (3) the age of the individual, since the composition of the blood vessel wall probably changes with age; (4) the hematocrit, since increased numbers of erythrocytes enhance platelet interactions with the blood vessel wall by forcing platelets to the periphery of the bloodstream (as the erythrocytes disproportionately occupy the axial region) and by imparting radially directed energy to platelets as the erythrocytes engage in flip-flop motions[175]; and (5) the speed of blood flow and

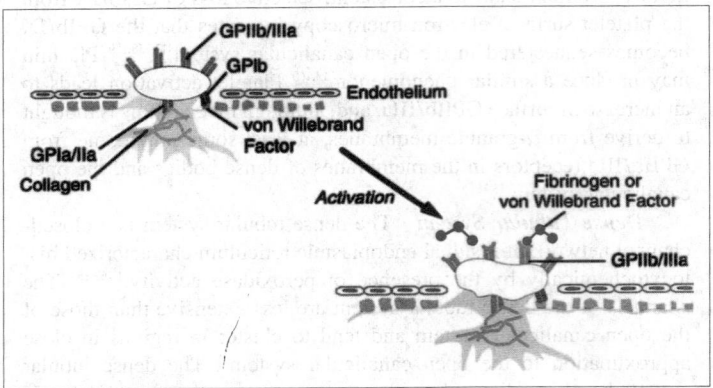

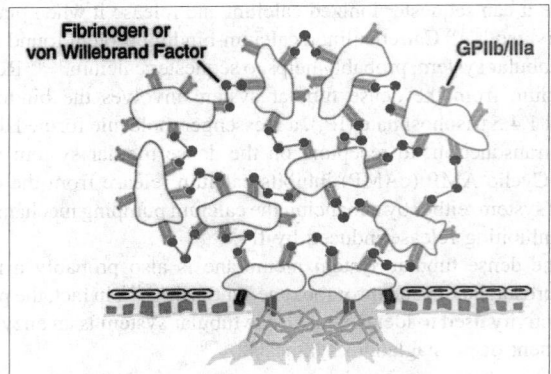

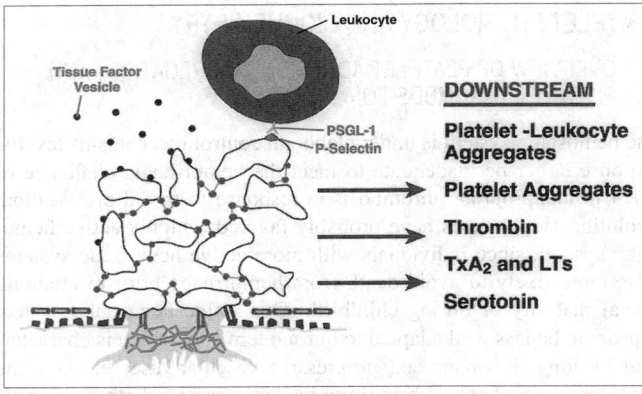

FIGURE 111-3   Platelet adhesion, activation, aggregation, and platelet-leukocyte interactions. A. Platelet adhesion is initiated by loss of endothelial cells (or in the case of an atherosclerotic lesion, rupture or erosion of the plaque), which exposes adhesive glycoproteins such as collagen and von Willebrand factor in the subendothelium. Other adhesive glycoproteins are also probably exposed, and these are listed in Table 111-3. In addition, von Willebrand factor and perhaps other adhesive glycoproteins in the plasma deposit on the damaged area. Platelets adhere to the subendothelium via receptors that bind to the adhesive glycoproteins. GPIb binding to von Willebrand factor plays a prominent role, but GPIa/IIa ($\alpha2\beta1$) binding to collagen and other platelet receptors listed in Table 111-5 probably also play a role. After platelets adhere they undergo an activation process that leads to a conformational change in GPIIb/IIIa receptors, resulting in their ability to bind multivalent adhesive proteins including fibrinogen and von Willebrand factor, with high affinity. B. Platelet aggregation occurs when the multivalent adhesive glycoproteins bind simultaneously to GPIIb/IIIa receptors on two different platelets, resulting in receptor clustering and cross-linking. C. After platelets adhere and aggregate, they bind tissue-factor-containing vesicles circulating in the plasma, expose negatively charged phospholipids on their surface (not shown), release platelet factor V (not shown) and release procoagulant microparticles (not shown). In addition,

TABLE 111-4   COMPONENTS OF THE BLOOD VESSEL WALL THAT ARE HEMOSTATICALLY ACTIVE

I	Subendothelium
	Von Willebrand factor
	Collagen (types IV, V, and VI)
	Fibronectin
	Thrombospondin
	Laminin
	Vitronectin
	Fibrinogen (fibrin)
	Tissue factor (trace amounts)
II	Media
	Collagen (types I and III)
IV	Adventitia
	Collagen (types I and III)
	Tissue factor

SOURCE: From Coller,[172] with permission.

the size of the blood vessel, which will determine the number of platelets passing by in a given time, the amount of time a platelet has to interact with the blood vessel wall or other platelets, the rate of dilution of platelet activating agents, and the forces tending to pull a platelet from the vessel wall or another platelet (shear rate).[172,175] The vasospastic response that accompanies vascular injury, to which platelets contribute by release of thromboxane A_2 and serotonin, probably plays a key role in decreasing hemorrhage and facilitating platelet and fibrin deposition via its effect on blood flow. Finally, platelet thrombi appear to be able to rapidly recruit tissue factor from the blood; the tissue factor is associated with small lipid-containing vesicle and may derive from leukocyte membranes.[176]

The shear rate differentially affects platelet adhesion to surfaces; vWF-dependent adhesion is most important at higher shear rates, probably because high shear rates cause conformational changes in vWF and/or platelet GPIb.[177–180] Very high shear rates can cause platelets to aggregate via a mechanism that involves vWF binding to GPIb/IX followed by activation of GPIIb/IIIa.[181–183] Platelets contribute more significantly to arterial thrombi than to venous thrombi, perhaps as a result of differences in the shear rates in the different beds.[172]

The subendothelial layer immediately subjacent to the endothelium contains a large number of adhesive proteins (Table 111-4),[172,178] and the platelet has receptors for many of these (Tables 111-3 and 111-5). GPIb/IX is a receptor complex that is particularly important in mediating adhesion to vWF immobilized in the subendothelium, and this receptor appears to dominate the adhesion process at high shear[184] (see Chap. 135). Three different sources of vWF may contribute to the subendothelial vWF; synthesis by endothelial cells, deposition from plasma, or release from platelet α granules.[178,184] Subendothelial vWF appears to associate with type VI collagen,[185] but it can bind to multiple collagen types. The interaction between GPIbα and vWF does not itself cause firm adhesion; rather, it results in tethering and slow translocation, probably because the bonds between vWF and GPIbα not only form rapidly but also dissociate rapidly.[179] Adhesion

activated platelets express P-selectin on their surface, which leads to leukocyte adhesion via P-selectin glycoprotein ligand-1 expressed on the surface of leukocytes. Other interactions between platelets and leukocytes are detailed in Fig. 111-13. Thrombus formation is a dynamic cyclical process, with platelets repeatedly adhering, aggregating, and then breaking off and going downstream. Platelet-leukocyte aggregates, thrombin, thromboxane A_2 (TxA$_2$), leukotrienes (LTs), and serotonin probably also go downstream and affect the microvasculature. Ultimately the vessel either becomes fully occluded or it loses its thrombogenic reactivity, that is, it becomes passivated. (From Coller, ref. 786a with permission.)

initiated by GPIbα-vWF interactions are stabilized by interactions between vWF and GPIIb/IIIa.[186]

The biologic contributions of the interactions between the GPIc/IIa ($\alpha6\beta1$) receptor and laminin, the GPIc*/IIa ($\alpha5\beta1$) receptor and fibronectin, and the $\alpha V\beta3$ receptor and vitronectin or other ligands in initiating platelet adhesion remain unknown. GPIIb/IIIa may function as an adhesion receptor for immobilized fibrinogen even in the absence of platelet activation,[187,188] but platelet activation is required for GPIIb/IIIa-mediated adhesion to vWF and fibronectin.[188] Platelets may interact directly with exposed collagen via GPIa/IIa ($\alpha2\beta1$) or perhaps other receptors implicated in platelet-collagen interactions (GPIV, GPVI, p65).[189] In addition,[189-197] fibrinogen, fibronectin, and vWF, whether released from platelets or circulating in plasma, may also bind to collagen. In turn, these proteins may then interact with platelet GPIIb/IIIa, GPIc*/IIa ($\alpha5\beta1$), and/or GPIb/IX, completing a sandwich mechanism initiated by collagen exposure.[193]

Depending on the vascular bed, available adhesive glycoproteins, and shear conditions, it is likely that various combinations of platelet receptors, including GPIbα, GPIa/IIa ($\alpha2\beta1$), GPVI, p65, and GPIIb/IIIa act in concert to transform the tethering and slow translocation of platelets initiated by GPIbα interacting with vWF into stable platelet adhesion.[179,196,198,199]

For platelet plug formation to occur, platelets must undergo activation as well as adhesion. Figure 111-4 lists physiologic and pathologic platelet agonists that can initiate platelet activation, along with some of the signal transduction pathways that lead to activation of platelet GPIIb/IIIa receptors and their clustering. Agonists can be subclassified as either strong (e.g., high-dose thrombin and collagen) and weak (e.g., epinephrine, ADP, serotonin) based on their ability to initiate the platelet release reaction without the added stimulation that comes with platelet aggregation. Most of these activators are released or synthesized at the site of vascular injury, resulting in a local response. In addition, cooperative biochemical interactions between erythrocytes and platelets may enhance platelet activation.[200]

It has been speculated that vascular injury results in release of ADP from erythrocytes, thus leading to platelet activation. Adhesion of platelets to subendothelial structures may itself lead to platelet activation, including generation of TXA$_2$, release of ADP and serotonin, and activation of the GPIIb/IIIa receptors on the luminal side of the platelet to their high-affinity ligand-binding states.[201] These positive feedback mechanisms ensure an adequate hemostatic response. Depending on the nature of the surface to which they adhere, platelets also undergo variable spreading reactions and become anchored by a process that at least partially involves GPIIb/IIIa ligation and clustering, cytoskeletal reorganization, and tyrosine phosphorylation; these reactions also contribute to initiating the release reaction.[202-204]

The activated luminal GPIIb/IIIa receptors on adherent platelets may then bind vWF and/or fibrinogen and await the interaction with another platelet, which itself may have undergone activation of its GPIIb/IIIa receptors as a result of exposure to released ADP and TXA$_2$. Alternatively, a platelet may become activated and bind vWF or fibrinogen while still circulating, in which case the platelet-ligand complex may bind directly to an activated GPIIb/IIIa receptor on the luminal surface. This process of the binding of adhesive ligands to platelet receptors repeats itself, resulting in the recruitment of additional layers of platelets, and ultimately the formation of a hemostatic plug. Intravital videomicroscopy of the mesenteric circulation of mice after endothelial cell damage demonstrates that, at least in this vascular bed, platelet thrombus formation is initially a very dynamic process, with many platelets depositing but then breaking off and moving downstream. The thrombus grows relatively slowly compared to what its growth would be if all of the platelets that deposited remained attached to the surface.[205]

The aggregated platelets can facilitate thrombin generation by one or more different mechanisms, including formation of microvesicles, exposure of activated factor V, exposure of negatively charged phospholipids, and perhaps activation of the contact system (see below). The thrombin thus generated further activates platelets, leading to more extensive degranulation; thrombin also further activates coagulation and initiates the deposition of fibrin strands that reinforce the platelet plug as well as serve as sites for more vWF deposition.[206] Thrombin may also help to consolidate the plug by initiating platelet-mediated clot retraction (see below). Finally, thrombin affects the surface membrane receptors, downregulating GPIb/IX and upregulating GPIIb/IIIa, perhaps facilitating the transition from platelet adhesion to platelet aggregation.[13,158,159,207]

Release of vasoactive and mitogenic agents from platelets no doubt contributes to the inflammatory response, as does the appearance of P-selectin on the surface of platelets and endothelial cells, which is likely to localize neutrophils to the damaged region (see "Platelet-Leukocyte Interactions" below).[208,209] Platelets themselves will roll on endothelial cells that have been activated to expose P-selectin on their surface,[210] and at least one of the counterreceptors for endothelial cell P-selectin is platelet GPIbα.[180] Platelets also express CD40 ligand on their surface after activation,[211] which can interact with CD40 on lymphocytes, monocytes, and endothelial cells, leading to cell activation and an enhanced inflammatory response. Finally, the platelet-fibrin thrombi resolve, most likely by a combination of embolization, fibrinolysis, and macrophage removal of debris.

Several inhibitory factors serve to balance platelet activation and prevent excessive platelet deposition (Table 111-6). The dilutional effects of flowing blood are probably most important; thus, alterations in the surface of the blood vessel that produce local areas of stasis in which platelets and coagulation factors may concentrate increase the likelihood of thrombosis.[172,175] Endothelial cells can synthesize two potent inhibitors of platelet activation, prostacyclin and nitric oxide (see below and Chap. 114). Basal synthesis of prostacyclin probably is too low to influence formation of platelet aggregates, but activated endothelial cells produce more prostacyclin. Activated platelets can also facilitate prostacyclin synthesis via production and release of endoperoxide intermediates and compounds that can activate endothelial prostacyclin production via receptor-mediated mechanisms. In addition, activated platelets can release microparticles that can transfer arachidonic acid to endothelial cells.[212] Thus, prostacyclin may contribute significantly to platelet inhibition at sites of injury.[213] Nitric oxide, which is synthesized by endothelial cells, is a potent inhibitor of ex vivo platelet adhesion and aggregation. It is not clear, however, whether the normal basal level of nitric oxide affects platelets. Nitric oxide synthesis is probably enhanced at sites of injury, and so it may well contribute to platelet inhibition, especially since it apparently synergizes with prostacyclin.[213] Endothelial cells also have CD39, an ecto-ATP diphosphohydrolase (ecto-ADPase) that can digest ATP and ADP to AMP, and thus limit the effects of released ADP.[38,42] Under certain conditions, leukocytes appear to interact biochemically with platelets to limit platelet activation,[214] but cathepsin G released from activated leukocytes can activate platelets.[215,216]

Since thrombin is such a potent activator of platelets, the control mechanisms that limit thrombin production also can be considered control mechanisms for platelet aggregation (see Chap. 113). Platelets can also become desensitized to stimulation by some agonists if they have previously been exposed to low concentrations of that agonist (homologous desensitization). It is possible that in the penumbra of released platelet agonists some platelets become inhibited by this mechanism.[217-219]

Since the GPIIb/IIIa receptor occupies a central role in determining the extent of platelet aggregation, it is notable that this receptor

TABLE 111-5 PLATELET SURFACE PROTEIN

Gene Family	Common Name	Platelet Chain Designation	Integrin Designation	VLA† Designation	CD+ Designation		M_r Nonreduced		M_r Reduced
Integrin	Fibrinogen receptor	GPIIb/IIIa	αIIbβ3		IIb/IIIa-CD41a				
					IIb-CD4lb	GPIIb	145,000	GPIIbα	125,000
								GPIIbβ	23,000
					IIIa-CD61	GPIIIa	90,000		114,000
	Collagen receptor	GPIa/IIa	α2β1	VLA-2	Ia-CD49b	GPIa	150,000		
					IIa-CD29	GPIIa	138,000		148,000
	Fibronectin receptor	GPIc*/IIa	α5β1	VLA-5	Ic*-CD49e	GPIc*	140,000		
					IIa-CD29	GPIIa	138,000		148,000
	Laminin receptor	GPIc/IIa	α6β1	VLA-6	Ic-CD49f	GPIc	140,000		
					IIa-CD29	GPIIa	138,000		148,000
	Vitronectin receptor	αV/GPIIIa	αVβ3		αV-CD51	αV	150,000	αVα	125,000
								αVβ	25,000
					IIIa-CD61	GPIIIa	90,000		114,000
Leucine-rich glyco-proteins	von Willebrand factor receptor	GPIb/IX			Ib/IX-CD42	GPIb	170,000	GPIbα	145,000
					Ibα-CD42b			GPIbβ	22,000
					Ibβ-CD42c				
					IX-CD42a	GPIX	17,000		17,000
		GPV				GPV	82,000		82,000
Immunoglobulin cell adhesion molecules	PECAM-I				CD31		130,000		
	Fcγ-RII				CD32		40,000		
	HLA-Class 1								
	ICAM-2				CD102				59,000
	GPVI						62,000		65,000
	IAP				CD47		50,000		
Selectins	P-Selectin (GMP 140; PADGEM)				CD62P		140,000		
Tetraspanins	p24				CD9		24,000		
	PETA-3				CD151		27,000		
	Lamp 3 (granulo-physin)				CD63		53,000		
Miscellaneous	GPIV				CD36		88,000		
	Lamp 1				CD107a		110,000		
	Lamp 2				CD107b		120,000		
	67 kD Laminin receptor						67,000		
	ADP PX1 Receptor						70,000		
	Leukosialin, sialophorin				CD43		90,000		
Seven transmembrane domain (G protein-linked)	PAR-1						70,000		
	PAR-4								
	Thromboxane A$_2$ receptor								55,000
	α_2-Adrenergic receptor								64,000
	Vasopressin receptor						125,000		
	ADP P2Y1 Receptor								

ABBREVIATIONS: Fib, fibrinogen; vWf, von Willebrand factor; Fn, fibronectin; Vn, vitronectin; TSP, thrombospondin; PSGL-1, P-selectin glycoprotein ligand-1; IAP, integrin-associated protein; Osp, ospeontin; TxA$_2$, thromboxane A$_2$
* Number of leucine-rich repeats.
†VLA, very late antigen; CD, cluster of differentiation, see Chap. 13

(table continued on opposite page)

Amino Acids	Carbohydrate	Lipid	Phosphorylated	Chromosome	Ligands	Platelet Specific	Function	Molecules on Platelet Surface (S) or Internal (I)
GPIIb 1039	+	−	−	17	Fib, vWf, Fn, Vn, ?TSP	+	Adhesion, aggregation, protein trafficking	(S) 80,000
GPIIIa 762	+	−	+	17		+		(I) 40,000
GPIa 1152				5	Collagen	−	Adhesion	(S) 1,000
GPIIa 778				10		−		
GPIc* 1008				12	Fn	−	Adhesion	(S) 1,000
GPIIa 778				10				
GPIc				2	Laminin	−	Adhesion	(S) 1,000
GPIIa 778				10				
α_v 1048				2	Vn, Fib, vWf, Fn, ?TSP, Osp	−	?Adhesion, ?protein trafficking	(S) 100
GPIIIa 762	+	−		17				
GPIbα 610(7)*	+	−		1	vWf, Thrombin	+?	Adhesion (high shear), ?thrombin binding	(S) 25,000
GPIbβ 181(1)*	+	+	−	22		+?		(S) 25,000
GPIX 160(1)*	+	+	+	3		+?		(S) 25,000
GPV 544(15)*	+	+	+	3		+?		(S) 12,500
PECAM-1 738	+	?	+	17	Heparin, PECAM-1	−	?Adhesion	(S) 8,000
Fcγ-RII 324	+		+	1	Immune complexes	−	Immune complex binding	(S) ~1,000
HLA	+			6	−		Histocompatibility	(S)
ICAM-2 274				17	LFA-1	−	Platelet-leukocyte adhesion	(S) 2,600
GPVI 316	+	−		?	Collagen	+	Activation	(S) ~2,000
IAP 287	+			3	TSP	−	Activation	
P-Selectin 830	+	+	+	1	Sialyl-Le^x, PSGL-1	−	Platelet-leukocyte adhesion	(I) 20,000
CD9 228	+				?	−	Activation	(S) 40,000
CD151 253	+	−	−	11	?	−	Activation	(I) ~2,000
Lamp 3 238	+							(I) 10,000
GPIV 471	+		+	7	Collagen, TSP	−	Adhesion, fatty acid transport	(S) 20,000
Lamp 1 389	+			13	?	−	?	(I) 1,200
Lamp 2 381	+			X	?			
67kD ?295				X	Laminin	−	Adhesion	
PX1 399	+			17	ADP	−	Activation	(S) 13–130
CD43 400	+		+	16	ICAM-1	−	Adhesion	
PAR-1 425				5	Thrombin	−	Activation	(S) ~1,800
PAR-4 385	+		+	19	Thrombin	−	Activation	
TxA$_2$ 343				19	PGH$_2$/thromboxane A$_2$	−	Activation	~200
α_2-Adrenergic 450				10	Epinephrine	−	Activation	~250
Vasopressin 418				?X	Vasopressin	−	Activation	~75
P2Y1 373	+			3	ADP	−	Activation	

Platelet activation and aggregation

Agonists	Transducing mechanisms	Effectors
1. **Adhesion**	1. **Arachidonic acid**	1. **GPIIb/IIIa activation**
2. **Thrombin**	2. **Protein kinase C**	2. **GPIIb/IIIa clustering**
3. **Thromboxane A$_2$**	3. **Tyrosine kinases**	
4. **ADP**	4. **Phosphatases**	
5. **Epinephrine**	5. **Calcium**	
6. **Serotonin**	6. **?**	
7. **Vasopressin**		
8. **Thrombospondin**		
9. **Von Willebrand factor**		
10. **Fibrinogen**		
11. **PAF**		
12. **Immune complexes**		
13. **Plasmin**		
14. **t-PA/SK**		
15. **Shear**		

FIGURE 111-4   Platelet activation. Many different agents and phenomena can initiate platelet activation, and these are listed as agonists. Virtually all of these are released, synthesized, or occur at sites of vascular injury, resulting in both geographical and temporal restriction of the response. These agonists can initiate aggregation either alone or in combination with one or more other agonists. A number of different signal transduction mechanisms have been defined that convert the agonist signal into a change in the conformation of the GPIIb/IIIa receptor and cytoskeletal changes that result in ligand binding, receptor clustering, and platelet aggregation. (Adapted, with permission, from the Annual Review of Medicine, Volume 43, © 1992, by Annual Reviews www.AnnualReviews.org.)

is present at extraordinarily high density on the platelet surface (receptors are probably less than 20 nm apart).[220–222] This permits the receptor to rapidly initiate platelet aggregation. On the other hand, the receptor is not in its high-affinity ligand-binding state on resting platelets but rather needs to be activated by agonists, including ADP, serotonin, thrombin, collagen, and TXA$_2$, that are localized to sites of vascular injury.[204,221,222] As a result, platelets can circulate in plasma containing high concentrations of the GPIIb/IIIa ligands fibrinogen and vWF without ongoing platelet thrombus formation.

Thus, platelet adhesion is controlled by the exposure of the subendothelium, with the platelet GPIb/IX receptor for immobilized vWF and the GPIIb/IIIa receptor for immobilized fibrinogen always competent to interact with these adhesive ligands.[178,187,188] In contrast, the ability of GPIIb/IIIa to mediate platelet aggregation by binding fluid-phase vWF[223] or fibrinogen[221,222,224] is under the control of an elaborate activation mechanism that limits the response to sites of vascular injury.

The agonists that activate the GPIIb/IIIa receptor are likely to work in combination in vivo. In fact, the mixture of agonists present in a thrombus is likely to change as the process unfolds, with perhaps

TABLE 111-6   PHYSIOLOGIC INHIBITORY ELEMENTS THAT OPPOSE PLATELET ACTIVATION

Flowing blood
Prostacyclin (PGI$_2$)
Nitric oxide, also known as endothelial-derived relaxation factor (EDRF)
Endothelial cell CD39 (ATP diphosphohydrolase; ecto-ADPase)
Platelet refractoriness
Leukocyte-platelet interactions
Inhibitors of thrombin generation and thrombin action

SOURCE: Adapted from Coller,[172] with permission.

collagen more important at the beginning, thrombin more important later on, and with the other agonists in varying mixtures throughout. Platelet activation induced by multiple agonists simultaneously is not simply additive; synergistic interactions are well documented (see below).[225,226] Epinephrine, although a relatively weak platelet agonist itself, probably plays an important role by enhancing the platelet's response to other agonists, including the ability to overcome aspirin-induced inhibition of platelet thrombus formation.[227] Changes in epinephrine levels that can accompany cigarette smoking or vascular collapse, as during myocardial infarction, may therefore have significant effects on platelet thrombus formation.[227–229] Finally, platelets can also be activated by shear stresses ex vivo; while the in vivo significance of this phenomenon remains unknown, it offers another potential link between the blood vessel narrowing produced by atherosclerotic vascular disease and platelet activation.[182,183,230]

PLATELET ENERGY METABOLISM

Platelets have sizable stores of glycogen that can often be seen on electron microscopy (Fig. 111-1). Glycogen can be broken down into glucose 1-phosphate, and platelets can also take up glucose from their surrounding medium. Both sources of glucose can be converted to glucose 6-phosphate, which can then enter glycolysis or the hexose monophosphate shunt. Platelet glycolysis rates significantly exceed those of erythrocytes and skeletal muscle.[231] Oxidative metabolism probably contributes to energy production in resting platelets, but it has been estimated that less than 1 percent of the pyruvic acid produced by glycolysis actually enters the citric acid cycle, the remainder terminating in lactate or pyruvate, which leave the platelet.[232] Platelet mitochondria are capable of β oxidation of fatty acids, but it is not clear how much this contributes to energy production.[233–235] Platelets can actively metabolize acetate, and this ability has been exploited to improve platelet storage conditions.[236] Amino acids may also act as energy sources and feed into the citric acid cycle, but the contribution of this process to platelet energy metabolism is uncertain.

As in all cells, ATP consumption by platelets is partially devoted to maintaining ionic and osmotic homeostasis.[237,238] In addition, the continuous polymerization and depolymerization of actin involves conversion of ATP to ADP, and this may account for as much as 40 percent of the ATP consumption in resting platelets.[239] The inositol phosphates, which are important in signal transduction, undergo continual dephosphorylation and rephosphorylation; these reactions have been estimated to consume as much as 7 percent of the total ATP produced.[240] Protein phosphorylation also occurs as an ongoing event, but its fractional use of ATP is not clear.

Depleting platelets of the metabolic pool of ATP and ADP decreases their ability to respond to stimuli, but the effect is not uniform: thus, shape change is only minimally affected, whereas there is an increasingly significant effect on platelet aggregation, α-granule and dense granule secretion, arachidonic acid liberation, and lysosome secretion.[28,241]

Platelet stimulation is accompanied by a marked increase in both glycolytic activity and oxidative ATP production, perhaps due to the abrupt decrease in ATP that occurs with platelet activation or the increase in cytoplasmic pH.[234] The increased ATP appears to be utilized, at least in part, in phosphoinositide phosphorylation and protein phosphorylation.

PLATELET CONTRACTILE ELEMENTS AND PLATELET SHAPE CHANGE, SECRETION, AND CLOT RETRACTION

The major components of the platelet contractile system are listed in Table 111-7. These elements are thought to contribute to platelet shape change, secretion, and clot retraction after platelet activation.

THE PLATELET CYTOSKELETON

The platelet cytoskeleton, namely, those elements that contribute to the maintenance and change of its shape, is operationally defined as proteins that are insoluble in the presence of the nonionic detergent Triton X-100 under defined ionic conditions (see also "Membrane Cytoskeleton").[11,242,243] The cytoskeleton of resting platelets consists of the membrane skeleton described above, which lies just beneath the membrane, and a lacy cytoplasmic actin filament network, which also contains, α-actin, tropomyosin, vinculin, and caldesmon.[242,244,245]

With platelet activation, phosphorylated myosin joins the cytoskeleton, as does talin, and the cytoskeleton becomes an electron-dense mass of bundled filaments.[242,246,247] Platelet membrane glycoproteins GPIIb/IIIa and GPIa/IIa ($\alpha 2\beta 1$) also join the cytoskeleton of activated platelets, probably via some interaction between actin, vinculin, talin, and the cytoplasmic domains of the membrane glycoproteins.[11,248] The tyrosine kinase pp125[Fak] may also play a role in the process,[202,249] as may the tyrosine kinase pp60[src], which is very abundant in platelets[249]; cortactin, an 85-kD protein that is phosphorylated on tyrosine; and small GTP-binding proteins such as Rho, Rac, and Cdc 42.[10,11,250]

Platelets contain calpains, which are calcium-dependent, sulfhydryl, neutral proteases composed of two subunits that preferentially cleave cytoskeletal proteins, in particular actin-binding protein (filamin-1) and talin,[250,251] but have also been reported to cleave the cytoplasmic domain of GPIIIa, and a number of molecules involved in signaling, including kinases and phosphatases [see "Calcium-Dependent Proteases (Calpains)" below]. It has been proposed that calpains are involved in cytoskeletal reorganization upon platelet activation and perhaps binding of ligand to GPIIb/IIIa.[252,253] Calpains have also been implicated in platelet spreading, microparticle formation, and the generation of platelet coagulant activity.[250,254,255]

TABLE 111-7   PLATELET CYTOSKELETAL PROTEINS*

PROTEIN	PROPERTIES	PROTEIN	PROPERTIES
Actin[790]	$M_r = 42,000$ 20–30% of total platelet protein (0.55 M) β and γ forms present at a ratio of 5:1 Monomeric actin (G-actin) bound to calcium-ATP (or ADP) Polymerization requires energy (ATP→ADP) and produces F-actin F-actin filaments: two strands of intertwined helices with polarity based on ability to interact with myosin fragment ("pointed" and "barbed" ends) Steady-state polymerization: monomers lost from pointed end while others join barbed end ("treadmilling")	Talin[798]	$M_r = 235,000$ 3% of platelet protein Binds to vinculin, α-actinin, and perhaps integrin receptors and actin α
		α-Actinin[791]	$M_r = 100,000$ and 102,000; dimer Binds actin at 1:10 stoichiometry; binds Ca^{2+} Forms gel with F-actin; cooperates with actin-binding protein; promotes actin polymerization
		Vinculin[799,800]	$M_r = 130,000$ Binds to talin; may link actin to membrane proteins at adhesion sites
		Myosin II[801,802]	$M_r = 480,000$ ($2 \times 200,000$; $2 \times 20,000$; $2 \times 16,000$) 2–5% of platelet protein; 325×111-nm filaments Myosin light chain ($M_r = 20,000$); phosphorylated; required for ATPase activity
Profilin[791]	$M_r = 15,200$ Forms 1:1 reversible complex with actin monomer Prevents actin polymerization May help "recharge" actin monomers with ATP	Myosin light-chain kinase[803]	$M_r = 105,000$ Phosphorylates myosin light chain and activates actomyosin ATPase leading to contraction
Gelsolin[792]	$M_r = 91,000$ Binds to barbed end of F-actin filaments Severs actin filaments Facilitates nucleation Produces shorter filaments with gel→sol transformation	Calmodulin[804]	$M_r = 17,000$ Binds four calciums and activates myosin light-chain kinase
		CapZ[10]	$M_r = 36,000$ and 32,000 Heterodimer Binds barbed ends of actin filaments
Thymosin β_4[793]	$M_r = 5,000$ Binds actin monomer Inhibits actin polymerization	Cofilin[10]	$M_r = 20,000$ Accelerates depolymerization of actin filaments
Tropomyosin[794]	$M_r = 28,000$; rod-shaped dimer of 35-nm length Binds to groove on actin filaments (six actins: one tropomyosin) Not all actin filaments have bound tropomyosin	Fimbrin (L-plastin)[10]	$M_r = 68,000$ Bundles actin filaments Found in microvilli
Caldesmon[795]	$M_r = 80,000$; asymmetric Binds to actin, tropomyosin, myosin, and calmodulin May control actin filament bundling and actomyosin ATPase	VASP[10]	$M_r = 50,000$ Tetrameric Binds profilin, vinculin, zyxin
		GTPases[250]	Cdc42—filopodia Rho—stress fibers Rac—lamellipods and ruffles Rap1b—GPIIb/IIIa control
Actin-binding protein[10,11,796,797] (Filamin 1)	$M_r = 260,000$ subunit; tail-to-tail dimer; elongated 162-nm flexible rod; phosphorylated 2–3% of platelet protein Binds actin with 1 actin binding protein molecule per 14 actin molecules Binds GPIbα cytoplasmic domain and links GPIb/IX to actin Cross-links actin filaments to form a gel Dephosphorylation leads to loss of activity	Tyrosine kinases	pp60[src] pp125[Fak]–GPIIb/IIIa signaling pp72[syk]–GPVI signaling
		Adaptor proteins	14-3-3ζ—binds to GPIbα Pleckstrin—phosphorylated on activation
		PI kinases	PI-3 kinase PI$_4$P-5 kinase

* See Fox,[11] Daniel,[20] Furman et al,[242] and Hartwig[10,805]

PLATELET SHAPE CHANGE

Platelet shape change occurs in response to many different agonists. It involves loss of the platelet's normal discoid shape (about 1.5 to 2.5 μm diameter and about 0.5 to 0.9 μm width) and transformation to a spiny sphere with long, thin filopodia extending several μm out from the platelet and ending in points that are as small as 0.1 μm in diameter (Fig. 111-1).[1,256] Although the reason platelets undergo shape change is unclear, one possibility is that it reduces electrostatic repulsion even without reducing surface charge density; thus, the tip of a platelet can approach and make contact with a surface or a cell, with the great bulk of the repulsive surface charge now at a distance.[2]

Actin fibril formation, which is an important component in shape change, is a complex, energy-requiring process that depends on nucleation, polymerization, helix winding, and filament bundling.[242] The proteins listed in Table 111-7 either facilitate or inhibit these processes. In resting platelets, actin monomers and small, thin actin filaments predominate (60 percent), but with activation, actin polymerization occurs and monomeric actin decreases to 20 to 40 percent of total actin.[20,242] Actin filaments in resting platelets are relatively stable because their barbed ends (the ends from which they can grow by adding additional actin monomers) are capped with the protein CapZ (Fig. 111-5).[10]

The initial step in shape change is the activation of gelsolin, which then both severs existing actin filaments and caps the newly created barbed ends. This increases the number of actin filaments by an estimated tenfold and substitutes gelsolin for CapZ as the capping protein.[10] Severing of actin filaments that interact with the planar lattice of actin-binding protein (filamin-1), GPIb, and spectrin in the membrane cytoskeleton releases the constraints on the spectrin network. This allows the membrane skeleton to swell (but not produce filopodia) (Fig. 111-6) by incorporating into the plasma membrane the membranes from the open canalicular system, and later the membranes from the granules that release their contents.

The protrusive force for filopodia development comes from subsequent actin polymerization on the newly severed actin filaments, including those attached to the plasma membrane. Uncapping of the actin filaments appears to be accomplished by the inactivation of gelsolin by phosphoinositides (ppIs) that are produced during platelet activation, including phosphatidylinositol 3,4 bisphosphate ($PI_{3,4}P_2$), $PI_{4,5}P_2$, and $PI_{3,4,5}P_3$.[10] The uncapped actin filaments act as nuclei onto which actin monomers (which are maintained in an available pool by association with thymosin-β4) can assemble. Profilin accelerates actin polymerization by facilitating the transfer of actin from the actin-thymosin-β4 complex to the barbed ends of the actin filaments. Other proteins that have been implicated in organizing the tips of the filopodia where the actin bundles attach to the plasma membrane are the small GTPase Cdc 42, the exchange protein WASP (which is abnormal in Wiskott-Aldrich syndrome) (see Chap. 119), vinculin, VASP, zyxin, and profilin.[17] As the filopodia form, the platelet's granules and organelles move to the center, surrounded by the microtubule coil, resulting in an increase in electron density. Activation of myosin via phosphorylation of myosin light-chain kinase, contributes to the inward contractile force by its interaction with the actin fibers.

PLATELET SPREADING AND SURFACE-INDUCED ACTIVATION

After platelets adhere to surfaces, they undergo variable degrees of spreading and activation. The patterns of spreading and activation depend primarily on the protein surface on which they spread, with collagen consistently inducing the most activation.[195,257] Activation can result in release of granule contents and exposure of activated GPIIb/IIIa receptors on the luminal surface of the platelets, where it is strategically located to bind adhesive glycoprotein ligands that can

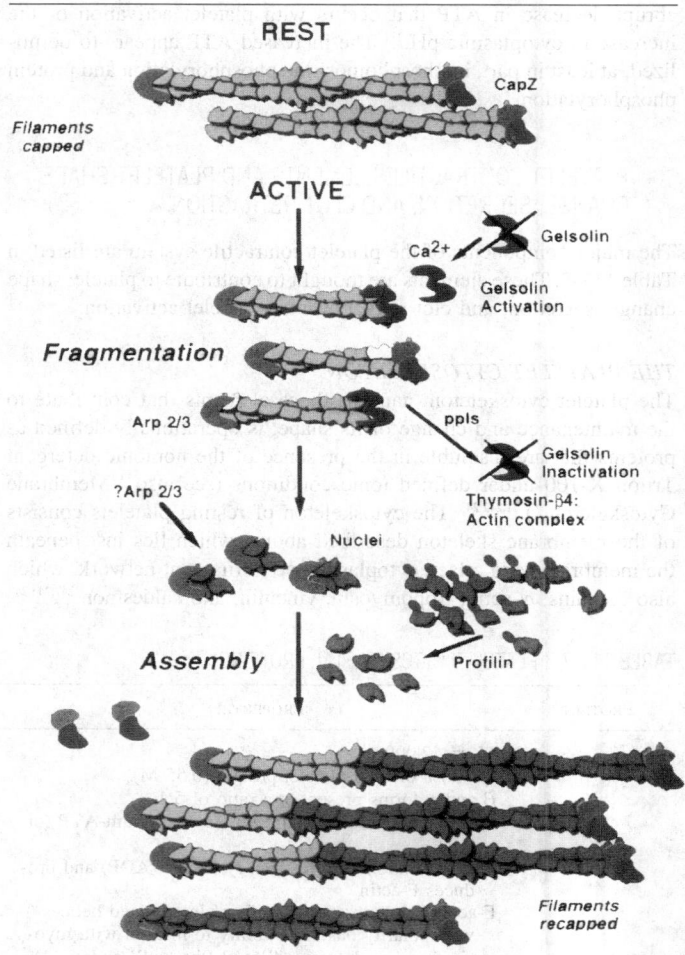

FIGURE 111-5 Control of platelet actin assembly. Rest: Forty percent of the actin in the resting cell is filamentous. The rest of the actin is soluble (60 percent) and is in a 1:1 complex with β_4-thymosin. Filaments are stable because they are capped on their barbed ends by capZ. Active: Shape change begins when calcium rises into the micromolar level and gelsolin becomes active. Gelsolin binds to actin filaments, interdigitates, and causes filaments to fragment. After fragmentation gelsolin remains bound to the barbed filament end. Assembly of actin begins when capping proteins are dissociated from the barbed ends of the filament fragments formed in the rounding step by polyphosphoinositides (ppIs) and when the actin-related protein (ARP) 2/3 complex in platelets is activated to nucleate de novo filaments. Actin monomers, stored in complex with β_4-thymosin, are the source of the actin for this polymerization event. Transfer of actin from β_4-thymosin to the barbed ends of actin filaments is facilitated by profilin. Once assembly is complete, capZ recaps the barbed filament ends. (From Hartwig,[10] with permission.)

recruit additional platelets.[201] If the surface density of platelets is sufficient, the platelets can also enter into lateral associations, which appear to depend on GPIIb/IIIa, leading to syncytial development. In general, platelet spreading results in the development of broad lamellipodia rather than spikelike filopodia.[10,250] The different morphologies of platelet spreading reflect differences in the organization of the orthogonal network of actin filaments. In turn, these differences reflect the different signals initiated by the adhesion process, and both ppIs and the small GTPase molecules Rac and Rho appear to be particularly important in this process.[17] Pleckstrin, a platelet protein that is phosphorylated during platelet activation, appears to participate in this process by binding to ppIs and affecting Rac via an exchange

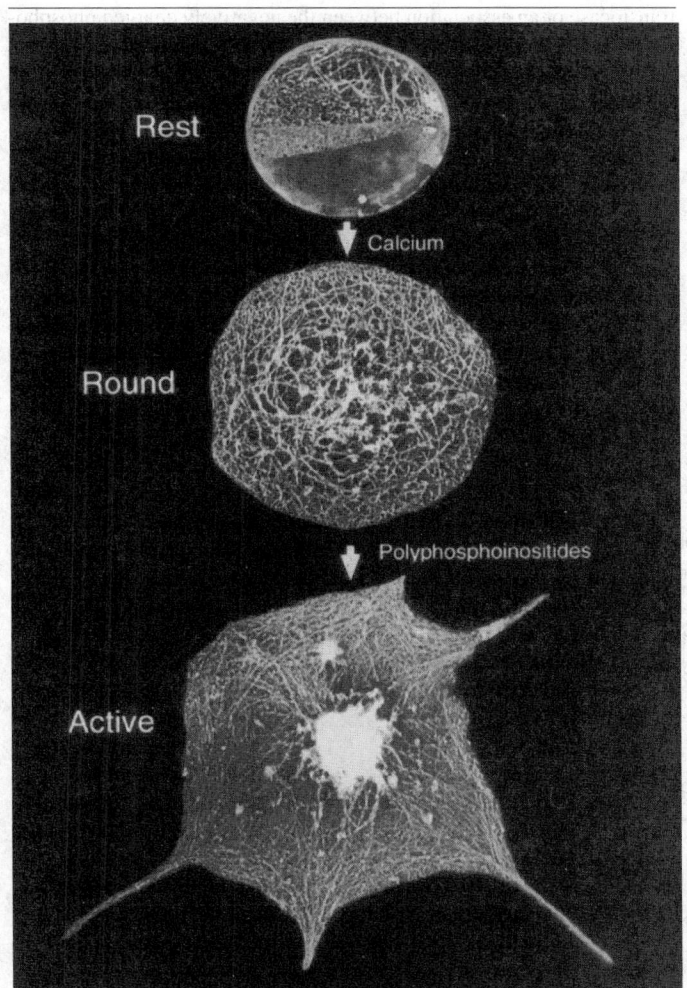

FIGURE 111-6   Control of platelet shape change. Resting platelets are small discs. Platelets convert from discs in two steps. In the first, a calcium transient activates platelet gelsolin. Gelsolin binds, severs, and caps actin filaments. The fragmentation of endogenous filaments causes the cell to become spherical. In the second step, spherical cells protrude lamellae and filopods. Actin filament assembly drives the protrusion of cellular processes. (From Hartwig,[10] with permission.)

factor.[258] Signaling after adhesion results from the assembly of protein complexes on the cytoplasmic surfaces of the receptor(s) involved in the adhesion process. These complexes then initiate local cytoskeletal rearrangements as well as the generation of signaling molecules that probably act throughout the platelet.[153,204]

Membrane glycoproteins are affected by cytoskeletal rearrangements associated with platelet shape change and spreading. Activation of platelets in suspension under certain conditions results in movement of GPIb/IX receptors from the surface of platelets to the open cannalicular system.[158,159] With adherent platelets, the GPIb/IX internalization is much slower.[17] The initial effect of activation on GPIIb/IIIa is an increase in receptors on the plasma membranes as the GPIIb/IIIa receptors in α granules, and perhaps dense bodies and the open cannalicular system, join the plasma membrane. After activation, more GPIIb/IIIa molecules become associated with the cytoskeleton, and this presumably reflects ligand-induced GPIIb/IIIa clustering, resulting in the development of protein complexes, including cytoskeletal proteins, on the cytoplasmic surface of the receptor.[204]

When platelets are adherent, and ligand-coated beads bind to GPIIb/IIIa receptors, the beads are transported to the center of the platelets, indicating that the cytoskeleton can move GPIIb/IIIa receptors that have ligand attached to them.[259,260] Finally, it has been suggested that the GPIIb/IIIa activation process itself, in which GPIIb/IIIa adopts a high-affinity binding state, is due to the loss of the basal constraints imposed on GPIIb/IIIa by the cytoskeleton.[261]

PLATELET SECRETION

The contractile mechanism involving actin and myosin is thought to mediate granule secretion and clot retraction, but the details remain obscure.[32,242] After the initial platelet shape change, actin becomes organized centrally into thick filamentous masses, where it probably associates with myosin filaments.[242] The contractile response is thought to be initiated by an increase in cytosolic calcium, which results in the formation of a calcium-calmodulin complex that then activates myosin light-chain kinase; phosphatases and cAMP-dependent kinase A can modulate the response (see below). The centralization of organelles in a contractile ring correlates well with secretion.[1] There is controversy, however, as to whether platelets secrete the contents of their granules by fusion with the open canalicular system in the center of the platelet or by direct fusion with the plasma membrane.[1,157]

A two-step model for granule secretion has been proposed in which the first step is docking of granules to the inner leaflet of the plasma membrane and the second step is the fusion of the lipid bilayers.[32,262] The docking process is thought to involve small GTPases, notably rab 3, which is phosphorylated when platelets are activated.[263] The rab 3 is thought to form complexes with SNARE proteins present on both the granule and plasma membrane, including syntaxins 2 and 4, leading to the development of a 7S docking complex.[262] The docking reaction does not require ATP, but the subsequent priming reaction, which prepares the complexes for membrane fusion, is energy dependent.[264] The 7S docking complex interacts with other proteins, including N-ethylmaleimide-sensitive factor (NSF) and both α- and γ-synaptosomal-associated proteins (SNAPs), forming a large 20S fusion complex. Phosphoinositides and cytoskeletal proteins, including myosin light-chain kinase, also participate in the priming reactions.[265] In the fusion step, it has been proposed that SNAP interactions with NSF activates the NSF ATPase activity, resulting in release of SNAREs from the 20S complex. Calcium plays an important role, probably acting in concert with a homologue of synaptotagamin, in creating fusion pores between the membranes, and the process is aided by synaptophysin and synaptogyrin (or their homologues).[266]

CLOT RETRACTION

When blood initially clots in the test tube, the fibrin mesh extends throughout, trapping virtually all of the serum in a gel-like state. If platelets are present, within minutes to hours, the clot retracts, extruding a very large fraction of the serum.[267] This process is thought to mimic in vivo phenomena that result in consolidation of thrombi and perhaps enhancement of wound healing. Clot retraction has also been implicated in decreasing the efficiency of thrombolysis, which may partially account for the resistance of platelet-rich thrombi to fibrinolytic agents.[268] Although the platelet requirement for clot retraction is indisputable, and temporal studies strongly incriminate an actinomyosin contractile mechanism,[269,270] no model describing the details of the process has gained acceptance.[271] Proposed mechanisms include movement of platelet filopodia along fibrin strands, tugging of fibrin strands by filopodia, and internalization of fibrin by the action of the membrane skeleton.[269–273] Platelet GPIIb/IIIa is required for clot retraction, as demonstrated by studies of patients with Glanzmann thrombasthenia (see Chap. 119) and studies of normal platelets in the presence of agents that block the GPIIb/IIIa receptor.[272,274,275] Results with these agents demonstrate, however, differences in their ability to inhibit clot retraction that do not correlate with their ability to block fibrinogen binding to platelets. Moreover, fibrinogen lacking the γ-chain sequence that mediates binding to platelet GPIIb/IIIa is still capable of supporting clot retraction.[276,277] Thus, while GPIIb/IIIa is required for clot retraction, the process is not a simple reflection of fibrinogen binding to GPIIb/IIIa.

PLATELET COAGULANT ACTIVITY

In resting platelets, the negatively charged phospholipids, including phosphatidyl serine, are almost exclusively present in the inner leaflet. The mechanisms responsible for this assymetry are not clear but may involve unidirectional enzymatic movement by an aminophospholipid

translocase or an association between the negatively charged phospholipids and elements in the cytoplasm, including cytoskeletal elements and their accompanying proteins.[4,7,9,278,279] The mechanisms responsible for the redistribution of negatively charged phospholipids to the platelet surface are also not fully understood but probably involve a calcium-activated plasma membrane enzyme of M_r 37,000 that counters the assymetric distribution ("scrambalase") (Fig. 111-7).[279–281] Since platelet activation with certain agonists results in the formation microparticles, which are particularly rich in surface-exposed negatively charged phospholipids, it is possible that the molecular reorganization of the membrane that produces microparticles also results in surface exposure of negatively charged phospholipids on both the microparticles and the residual platelet membrane. Microparticles also are rich in factor Va and thus actively support thrombin generation.[5,212,282]

Microparticle formation can be induced in vitro by activation of platelets with ionophore A23187, complement C5b-9, or the combina-

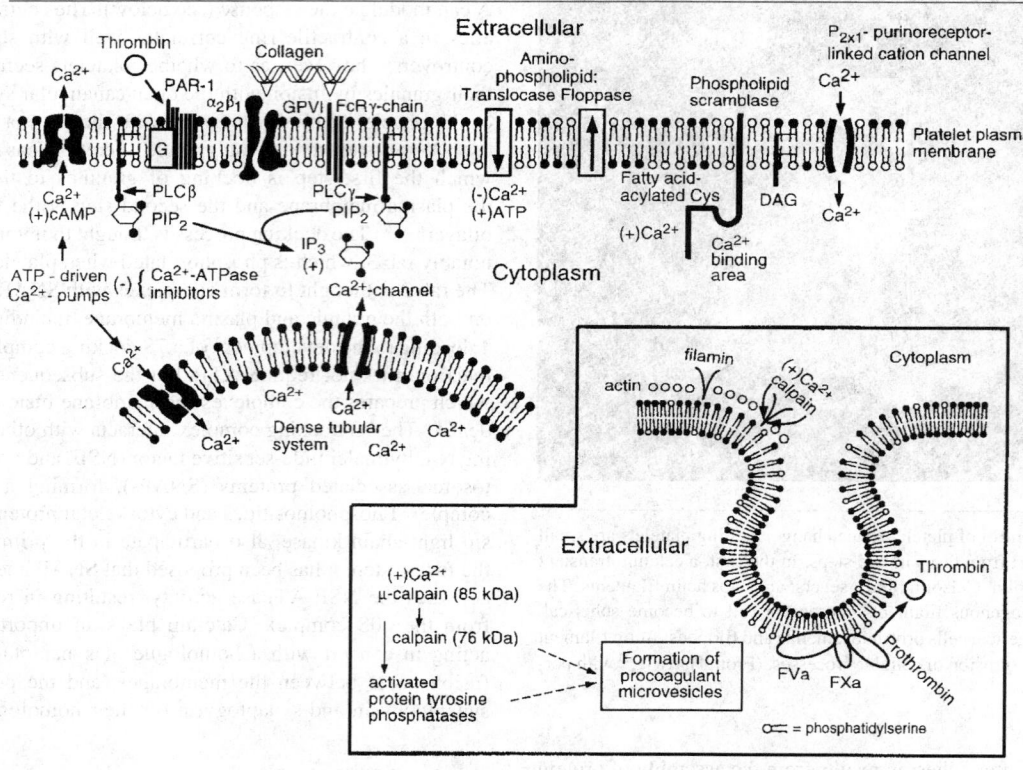

FIGURE 111-7 Schematic representation of platelet calcium homeostasis and the reactions leading to procoagulant expression. Thrombin activates protease-activated receptor 1 (PAR-1), which interacts with G proteins and stimulates phospholipase Cβ (PLCβ) to split phosphatidylinositol-4,5-bisphosphate (PIP₂) into 1,2-diacylglycerol (DAG) and inositol-1,4,5-triphosphate (IP₃). Collagen binds to the integrin receptor GPIa/IIa (α2β1) and activates platelets through tyrosine phosphorylation of the Fc receptor γ chain (FcRγ-chain), which is associated with the membrane glycoprotein GPVI. This leads to tyrosine phosphorylation and activation of PLCγ2, which, like PLCβ, splits PIP₂ and produces IP₃. The IP₃ opens Ca²⁺ channels in the intracellular membrane system called the *dense tubular system*, which serves as an intracellular Ca²⁺ store. ATP-driven Ca²⁺ pumps, both in dense tubular system membranes and in the plasma membrane, carry Ca²⁺ out of cytosol by active transport. This can be inhibited by specific Ca²⁺-ATPase inhibitors. Further platelet activation via diacylglycerol (DAG) and protein kinase C and activation of phospholipase A₂ with formation of thromboxane A₂ are not shown. Activation of the phospholipid scramblase by Ca²⁺ ions and a concomitant Ca²⁺-mediated inhibition of ATP-dependent aminophospholipid translocase that serves to maintain the normal phospholipid asymmetry lead to translocation of negatively charged phosphatidylserine to the outer membrane bilayer. This is a prerequisite for formation of the complexes of coagulation factors on the platelet surface. A Ca²⁺-induced activation of the proteolytic enzyme calpain is important for the formation of microvesicles. Protein tyrosine phosphatase activities are associated with calpain activation and microvesiculation in an as-yet-unknown manner. The microvesicles express a procoagulant surface. Substances that activate or inhibit the various processes are labeled with + or − respectively. FVa and FXa indicate factors Va and Xa, respectively. (Reproduced from Solum[278] with permission.)

tion of thrombin and collagen; by adding tissue factor to recalcified platelet-rich plasma; or by high shear stress.[212,283,284] Incubation of platelets with sera from patients with heparin-induced thrombocytopenia can also produce microparticles,[285] perhaps accounting, in part, for the thrombosis that is sometimes associated with this disorder. Elevations of cytosolic Ca^{++}, calpain activation, cytoskeletal reorganization, protein phosphorylation, and phospholipid translocation have all been implicated in microparticle formation. Inhibiting GPIIb/IIIa, and perhaps $\alpha V \beta 3$, decreases tissue-factor-induced platelet coagulant activity and microparticle formation in the presence or absence of fibrin,[283] whereas inhibiting GPIb inhibits tissue factor-induced microparticle formation only in the presence of fibrin.[286]

The biologic relevance of microparticles is supported by the finding of increased circulating levels of platelet microparticles in patients with activated coagulation and fibrinolysis, diabetes mellitus, sickle cell anemia, human immunodeficiency virus infection, unstable angina, and patients with respiratory distress syndrome.[212,287] Microparticles can bind to fibrin thrombi via one or more of the receptors present on their surface [GPIIb/IIIa, GPIb/IX, GPIa/IIIa ($\alpha 2 \beta 1$), and P-selectin].[288]

Microparticles bind factor VIII, factor Va, and factor Xa, allowing them to form both the tenase and prothrombinase complexes on their surface.[212] They can also bind protein S, which could serve an anticoagulant function. In addition, microparticles can activate platelets by supplying arachidonic acid. In a similar manner, they can activate endothelial cells and monocytes, resulting in enhanced monocyte attachment to endothelial cells, a potential contributor to atherosclerosis.[212]

Platelet activation leading to increased platelet coagulant activity shares several features with cell apoptosis, including surface exposure of negatively charged phospholipids and membrane blebbing leading to microparticle formation. Platelets contain the apoptosis-related proteins procaspase-3 and procaspase-9, as well as the caspase activators APAF-1 and cytochrome c.[289,290] There are conflicting data, however, regarding the relative roles of caspases and calpains in the development of platelet coagulant activity.[289,290]

There is incontrovertible evidence that platelets accelerate thrombin formation, but the precise mechanisms involved remain controversial.[4,292–296] The effect of platelets on activation of factor X by factors IXa and VIIIa and the activation of prothrombin by factors Xa and Va have been extensively studied.[4,292,296] Both reactions are accelerated by platelets, most dramatically when the platelets have been activated by thrombin or other agonists (see Chap. 112). Platelets also are able to accelerate factor VIII activation by thrombin.[297] It is likely that factor VIIIa on platelets acts as a binding site for factor IXa and that factor Va on platelets acts as a binding site for factor Xa.[298] A separate receptor for factor IXa may also exist. What remains unclear is whether factors VIIIa and Va bind to specific receptors on platelets or whether they bind nonspecifically to negatively charged phospholipids, most particularly phosphatidylserine, that join the outer leaflet of the platelet plasma membrane bilayer when platelets are activated.[279,293,294,298] The assembly of the factor IXa/factor VIIIa/platelet complex increases the catalytic efficiency of factor X activation (k_{cat}/K_m) by a factor of 2.4 × 10^6.[4] In addition, the binding of activated coagulation factors to the surface of platelets appears to protect them from inactivation by inhibitors in plasma and platelets.[4] The relatively large platelet pool of factor V,[103,105] which appears to be complexed to multimerin,[78] and the ability of platelet proteases to activate it[108,299] also probably contribute to platelet coagulant activity. The importance of platelet factor V in normal hemostasis can be inferred from the presence of a bleeding diatheses in patients with Quebec platelet syndrome (related to proteolysis of platelet α-granule proteins, including factor V) (see Chap. 119), as well as in a patient with abnormal platelet factor V.[296]

The physiologic importance of microparticle formation is supported by observations on patients with significant bleeding diatheses and defects in platelet microparticle formation (see Chap. 119).[294,296,300] Platelets from the most intensively studied patient had impaired ability to accelerate both factor X and prothrombin activation, did not bind factor Va normally, and did not expose negatively charged phospholipids normally. In flow chamber studies, the patient's platelets did not support normal fibrin deposition. The defect in microparticle formation appears to be the primary abnormality, since the patient's erythrocytes also failed to undergo normal vesiculation in response to the calcium ionophore A23187.[294,301]

In addition to the platelet's role in accelerating the activation of factor X and prothrombin, there are other connections between platelets and the coagulation system. These include: (1) the presence of fibrinogen in α granules and perhaps on the surface of platelets, where it is strategically located for interactions with locally generated thrombin[4,81]; (2) the presence of intracellular vWF and the binding of extracellular vWF to platelets, with the potential colocalization of factor VIII attached to the vWF (see Chap. 135); (3) the presence of factor XI or a factor XI-like protein associated with platelet membranes[4,302,303]; (4) the presence of cytoplasmic factor XIII (see Chap. 112); (5) the presence in platelets of inhibitors of coagulation (α_1-protease inhibitor, C-1 inhibitor, tissue factor pathway inhibitor, the thrombin inhibitor protease nexin I, and the factors IXa and XIa inhibitor protease nexin II or β-amyloid precursor protein)[4,136]; and (6) the ability of activated platelets to facilitate factor XI activation and prevent its inactivation by α_1-protease inhibitor.[4]

PLATELET MEMBRANE GLYCOPROTEINS, PLATELET ADHESION, AND PLATELET AGGREGATION

Platelet membrane glycoproteins mediate the interactions between the platelet and its external environment. Receptors can receive signals from outside the platelet and send signals inside. In addition, receptors can receive signals from inside the platelet that affect their external domains. Platelet glycoprotein receptors are derived from several different receptor families (integrins, leucine-rich glycoproteins, immunoglobulin cell adhesion molecules, selectins, tetraspanins, and seven transmembrane domain receptors) (see Table 111-5). One member of the integrin family, GPIIb/IIIa, is unique to platelets; the leucine-rich glycoproteins GPIb/IX and GPV appear to have highly restricted expression, including primarily platelets and cytokine activated endothelial cells.[304–306]

INTEGRINS

Integrin receptors are heterodimeric complexes composed of an α subunit containing three or four divalent cation-binding domains and a β subunit rich in disulfide bonds. Both subunits are transmembrane glycoproteins and are encoded by different genes. There are at least 14 α subunits and 7 β subunits.[220,307–309] Three major families of integrin receptors are recognized based on the β subunit: β_1, β_2, and β_3. Integrins are widely distributed on different cell types, and each integrin demonstrates unique ligand-binding properties. Integrin receptors mediate interactions between cells and between proteins and cells; they are also involved in protein trafficking in cells. Integrin receptors can also transduce messages from outside the cell to inside the cell, and from inside the cell to outside the cell.

GPIIb/IIIa (Fibrinogen Receptor; $\alpha IIb \beta 3$; CD41/CD61) The GPIIb/IIIa complex, a member of the β_3-integrin receptor family, is the dominant platelet receptor, with 80,000 to 100,000 receptors present on the surface of a resting platelet.[220,221,309,310] Another 20,000 to 40,000 receptors are present inside platelets, primarily in α-granule membranes, but also in dense bodies and the membranes lining the open canalicular system; these receptors are able to join the plasma membrane when platelets are activated and undergo the release reaction.[311-313] On average, GPIIb/IIIa receptors are less than 20 nm apart on the platelet surface and thus are among the most densely expressed adhesion/aggregation receptors present on any cell type. By electron microscopy, the receptors appear to have a globular head of 8×12 nm, composed of the amino termini of both subunits, and two 18-nm tails representing the carboxy-terminal regions of each subunit, including their transmembrane and intracytoplasmatic domains.[314] Biochemical studies of GPIIb/IIIa proteolytic digestion fragments, however, are not entirely consistent with this structural model.[315]

GPIIb/IIIa shares the same basic structural features of all integrin receptors (Table 117-5). GPIIb, the α subunit, is a transmembrane protein with four calmodulin-like domains that are able to bind divalent cations (see Fig. 119-5). The mature protein contains 1008 amino acids and consists of a heavy (α) chain which is extracytoplasmic, and a light (β) chain that contains the transmembrane and intracytoplasmatic domains.[220,309,316] GPIIIa, the β subunit, contains 762 amino acids and has a characteristic cysteine-rich region near its transmembrane domain.[220,309,317] The genes coding for GPIIb and GPIIIa are very close to each other on chromosome 17 at q21.32 but are not so close as to share common regulatory domains.[318,319] Both proteins are made in megakaryocytes and join to form a calcium-dependent, noncovalent complex in the rough endoplasmic reticulum (see Fig. 119-2).[309,320] They subsequently undergo further processing in the Golgi apparatus, where the carbohydrate structures undergo maturation and the pro-GPIIb molecule is cleaved into its heavy and light chains.[309,321,322] Approximately 15 percent of the mass of both GPIIb and GPIIIa is composed of carbohydrate.[323] The mature GPIIb/IIIa complex is then transported to the plasma membrane or the membranes of α granules or dense bodies. If GPIIb and GPIIIa do not form a proper complex, either because of a structural abnormality or the failure to synthesize one of the subunits, the glycoproteins that are synthesized are rapidly degraded and so are not expressed on the membrane surface (see Chap. 119).[219,220]

The GPIIb/IIIa receptors in α granules appear to cycle to and from the plasma membrane.[324] This recycling helps to explain the ability of GPIIb/IIIa to take up fibrinogen from plasma and transport it to α granules, where it is concentrated.[81,83]

On resting platelets, GPIIb/IIIa will support adhesion of platelets to immobilized fibrinogen, but it has low affinity for fibrinogen in solution; when platelets are activated with ADP, epinephrine, thrombin, or other agonists, however, GPIIb/IIIa binds fibrinogen relatively strongly.[221,222,224] The signal-transduction mechanisms that mediate activation are discussed below. Activation induces changes in the GPIIb/IIIa receptor itself that are responsible for the change in fibrinogen-binding affinity,[325,326] but changes in the microenvironment surrounding GPIIb/IIIa may also be involved. The cytoplasmic domains of GPIIb and GPIIIa have been implicated in controlling the activation process.[204,327,328]

The precise areas of GPIIb/IIIa that are involved in binding fibrinogen are not known with certainty, but data from ligand cross-linking studies and peptide inhibition studies, and deductions from patients with mutations in GPIIb/IIIa that affect fibrinogen binding (see Chap. 119), suggest that the regions in GPIIIa between amino acids 109 to 171 and 211 to 222 are important (see Fig. 119-4).[329-332] These regions of GPIIIa contain sequences that are similar to those of the metal-ion-dependent adhesion site (MIDAS) present in the I domain of some integrin α subunits, including a DxSxS motif (Asp 119, Ser 121, Ser 123), lending support to the importance of this region in cation and ligand binding.[333,334] Based on studies of other integrin α subunits, a β propeller model structure with 7 blades has been proposed for this family of subunits; the fundamental features

of this structure may be applicable to GPIIb.[335] Each blade of the propeller radiates out from the center and is composed of a repeat sequence that includes four beta strands that are linked by loops that either extend above (between strands 2 and 3 of the same blade, and between strand 4 and strand 1 of the next blade) or below (between strands 1 and 2, and between strands 3 and 4) the plane of the propeller (Fig. 119-5). A 3 dimensional version of this image is available from the Williams Hematology website (http//www.williamshematology.com). The loops that extend below the propeller contain the E-F hand-like calcium-binding sequences, which appear to be important in receptor biosynthesis, whereas the loops that extend above the propeller appear to be involved in ligand binding. Data from patients with Glanzmann thrombasthenia appear to be in accord with this model (see Chap. 119). Divalent cations are required for the binding of all ligands, but there are differences in the optimal cation (calcium, magnesium, manganese) and its concentration, depending on the ligand.[222,224,336]

Data from other integrin receptors identified a cell recognition sequence composed of Arg-Gly-Asp (RGD) in the ligand fibronectin.[337,338] Fibrinogen contains one RGD sequence near the carboxy terminus of each of the two Aα chains (amino acids 572 to 574) and another at amino acids 95 to 97.[339] In addition, the carboxy-terminal 12 amino acids of each of the two γ chains (amino acids 400 to 411) contains a sequence that includes Lys-Gln-Ala-Gly-Asp-Val, and it appears that the Lys and Gly-Asp form a molecular mimic of the RGD sequence.[340] The γ-chain sequence appears to be the most important in the binding of fibrinogen to platelets, but the RGD sequences may also participate.[188,341-343] Small, synthetic peptides containing the RGD or γ-chain sequence inhibit the binding of fibrinogen to platelets, and these observations have been exploited to produce therapeutic agents to inhibit platelet thrombus formation (see Chap. 131).[344] Similarly, monoclonal antibodies that inhibit binding of ligands to GPIIb/IIIa have been developed and a murine/human chimeric Fab fragment of one of them has been shown to be effective as an antiplatelet agent (see Chap. 131).[344]

The binding of fibrinogen to GPIIb/IIIa appears to be a multistep process[221]: (1) the initial interaction is divalent cation-dependent and most likely involves the γ-chain carboxy-terminal regions[188,342,343]; (2) subsequent interactions, which may include internalization of the fibrinogen,[345] render the binding irreversible, even when divalent cations are removed[346]; (3) binding of fibrinogen induces changes in the receptor that can be recognized by antibodies (ligand-induced binding sites; LIBS)[241]; and (4) binding of fibrinogen to GPIIb/IIIa induces changes in fibrinogen that can be recognized by antibodies (receptor-induced binding sites, RIBS) and may involve exposure of the Aα chain Arg-Gly-Asp-Phe (RGDF) sequence at amino acids 95 to 98.[347,348]

Binding of fibrinogen to platelet GPIIb/IIIa leads to platelet aggregation, presumably via cross-linking of GPIIb/IIIa molecules on two different platelets by fibrinogen.[349,350] The dimeric and relatively rigid structure of fibrinogen, and the location of the binding sites at the extremes of the γ chains, are all consistent with such a model since the two binding sites on a single fibrinogen molecule are probably more than 45 nm apart. Soon after fibrinogen binds, it can be dissociated from the platelet by chelating the divalent cations, but the binding becomes irreversible within an hour.[346] Fibrinogen binding alone is not sufficient for platelet aggregation, but the events necessary after fibrinogen binding, which probably include ligand- and/or cytoskeletal-mediated receptor clustering, are not well understood.[1,346,349,351] After ligands bind to GPIIb/IIIa, "outside-in" signaling through GPIIb/IIIa can occur, resulting in a number of phosphorylation events, changes in the platelet cytoskeleton, and even initiation of protein translation.[153,204]

In addition to fibrinogen, several other adhesive glycoproteins that contain RGD sequences can bind to GPIIb/IIIa on activated platelets, including vWF, fibronectin, vitronectin, and thrombospondin.[89,352] There are subtle differences in the binding of each of these ligands with regard to divalent cation preference and competent activating agents.[325] The binding of all of these other ligands can also be inhibited by RGD-containing peptides, indicating a common requirement for the interaction between the RGD sequence in the protein and the RGD-binding site in GPIIb/IIIa.[353,354]

Platelet aggregation measured in an aggregometer ex vivo depends upon fibrinogen binding to GPIIb/IIIa. It is less clear whether fibrinogen is the most important ligand supporting platelet aggregation in vivo, since studies performed in model systems under flowing conditions indicate that vWF is the major ligand at higher shear rates.[223] Even in the aggregometer, vWF can partially substitute for fibrinogen if the fibrinogen concentration is very low.[355]

In contrast to the requirement for platelet activation in order for platelets to bind soluble fibrinogen (or other adhesive glycoproteins), unactivated platelets will adhere to fibrinogen immobilized on a surface.[187,188,356] This activation-independent adhesion may be due to alterations in the structure of fibrinogen when it is immobilized on a surface.[348,357] Alternatively, it may result from there always being a few GPIIb/IIIa receptors that are transiently in the proper conformation to bind fibrinogen, and the favorable kinetics achieved as a result of the high local density of fibrinogen that accompanies immobilization on a surface.

Fibrinogen and/or fibrin have been identified on the surface of damaged blood vessels; thus it is possible that GPIIb/IIIa mediates platelet adhesion under those circumstances.[358] In contrast, GPIIb/IIIa on unactivated platelets does not appear to be able to mediate adhesion to vWF or fibronectin[188]; if platelets are activated, however, GPIIb/IIIa can support adhesion to these glycoproteins.[353] In models of platelet accumulation under flowing conditions, GPIIb/IIIa acts in synergy with GPIb/IX, von Willebrand factor, and fibrinogen at the apex of thrombi, where shear forces are greatest.[186,198,199] GPIIb/IIIa has also been implicated in platelet spreading after adhesion,[201,203] and it is necessary for clot retraction (see above) and the accumulation of platelet α-granule fibrinogen.[81,83]

Less well defined roles for GPIIb/IIIa have been suggested in the binding of plasminogen[359] and factor XIIIa[360] to platelets; calcium transport across the platelet membrane (see below)[361-363]; IgE binding to platelets leading to parasite cytotoxicity[364]; and interaction with the Borellia species spirochetes that cause Lyme disease.[365]

GPIa/IIa (Collagen Receptor; VLA-2; α2β1; CD49b/CD29)
The GPI/IIa (α2β1) receptor, a member of the β1 integrin family, is widely distributed on different cell types and can mediate adhesion to collagen.[189,192-194,366-369] The GPIa (α2) subunit contains a region of 191 amino acids inserted in the amino-terminal region (I domain) that is homologous to similar regions in other proteins that are known to interact with collagen, including vWF and cartilage matrix protein.[370] This region has a metal-ion-dependent adhesion site (MIDAS domain) and probably mediates the interactions with collagen.

Platelet adhesion to collagen mediated by GPIa/IIa (α2β1) is enhanced in the presence of magnesium or manganese and is inhibited by calcium, and thus the conditions in human blood, where calcium is abundant and magnesium is only present at low levels, do not

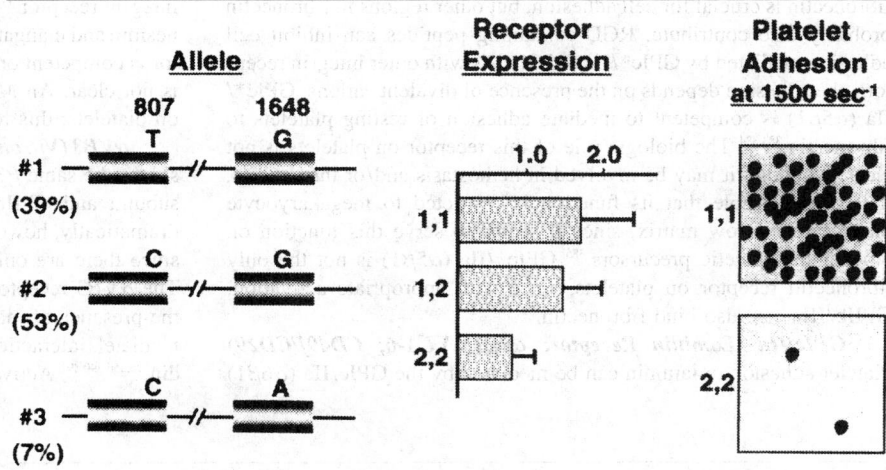

FIGURE 111-8 Polymorphisms of integrin α₂. The left panel shows a cartoon of the three alleles and their frequency. The nucleotide position in the cDNA is shown above. The 807 T/C substitution is silent, not altering an amino acid; the 1648 G/A substitution causes an amino acid alteration (glutamic acid to lysine) and is responsible for the Br^b and Br^a alloantigens respectively. The middle panel indicates the association of the different genotypes containing alleles 1 and 2 (807 T and 807 C respectively) with platelet receptor density, shown as arbitrary units on the horizontal axis. The right panel is a schematic drawing indicating platelet deposition to immobilized collagen under shear stress according to the α₂ genotypes 1,1 and 2,2. (From Bray,[377] with permission.)

provide optimal cation concentrations for GPI/IIa function.[189,193] GPIa/IIa (α2β1) can, however, mediate platelet adhesion to collagen in heparinized blood.[193,194] Regions of collagen type I have been implicated as potential binding sites for GPIa/IIa (α2β1)[371]; the peptide sequences 502–516 of collagen type I alpha 1 chain, containing a Gly-Glu-Arg sequence, may be of particular importance,[372] but other interactions may also be important.[373] In type III collagen, amino acids 522–528 of fragment alpha 1 (III) CB4 contains a binding region for GPIa/IIa (α2β1).[374] Evidence from patients with diminished platelet GPIa/IIa (α2β1) supports a role for this receptor in hemostasis (see Chap. 119).[369,375]

There are at least three alleles for α2 that differ at nucleotides 807 (T or C) and 1648 (G or A) (Fig. 111-5). The 807 substitution does not affect the amino acid sequence, but the 1648 substitution causes a change from Glu to Lys, resulting in the Br^b and Br^a alloantigens. Allele 1 (T-G) is present in 39 percent of individuals, allele 2 (C-G) in 53 percent, and allele 3 (C-A) in 7 percent (Fig. 111-8).[376,377] Individuals with allele 1 have higher GPIb/IIa (α2β1) platelet density than individuals with allele 2, and individuals with allele 3 have the lowest density. The density of GPIb/IIa (α2β1) receptors correlates with platelet deposition on collagen under flow. Individuals with allele 1 have been reported to be at increased risk of developing myocardial infarction[378,379] and stroke.[380]

GPIa/IIa (α2β1) is probably linked to the membrane skeleton and is competent to mediate adhesion on resting platelets.[12] Its ligand specificity appears to be determined by the cell on which it is expressed, since on platelets it appears to function only as a collagen receptor, whereas on endothelial cells it functions as a laminin receptor as well as a collagen receptor.[381,382] Engagement of GPIa/IIa (α2β1) is capable of initiating platelet protein synthesis.[153]

GPIc*/IIa (Fibronectin Receptor; α5β1; VLA-5; CD49e/CD29)
GPIc*/IIa (α5β1) is a β1-integrin receptor that is expressed on a wide variety of different cells and mediates adhesion to fibronectin.[337,338] It is important in interactions with extracellular matrix, and data from cells other than platelets indicate a role for this receptor in developmental biology and tumor metastasis. The RGD sequence in

fibronectin is crucial for cell adhesion, but other regions in fibronectin probably also contribute. RGD-containing peptides can inhibit cell adhesion mediated by GPIc*/IIa ($\alpha5\beta1$). As with other integrin receptors, the adhesion depends on the presence of divalent cations. GPIc*/IIa ($\alpha5\beta1$) is competent to mediate adhesion of resting platelets to fibronectin.[383,384] The biologic role of this receptor on platelets is not clear. Although it may be involved in hemostasis and/or thrombosis, it is also possible that its function is restricted to megakaryocyte binding to marrow matrix, since it seems to serve this function on other hematopoietic precursors.[385] GPIc*/IIa ($\alpha5\beta1$) is not the only fibronectin receptor on platelets, since with appropriate activation, GPIIb/IIIa can also bind fibronectin.[89]

GPIc/IIa (Laminin Receptor; $\alpha6\beta1$; VLA-6; CD49f/CD29)
Platelet adhesion to laminin can be mediated by the GPIc/IIa ($\alpha6\beta1$)

integrin receptor.[178,386,387] The adhesion is best demonstrated with magnesium and manganese; calcium does not support adhesion. This receptor is competent on resting platelets, but its role in platelet physiology is not clear. An M_r 67,000 laminin receptor has also been identified on platelets; this receptor is present on other cells as well.[388]

$\alpha V\beta3$ (Vitronectin Receptor; CD51/CD61)   The $\alpha V\beta3$ receptor shares the same $\beta3$ subunit as GPIIb/IIIa (see Fig. 119-3).[317] The αV subunit and GPIIb have 36 percent sequence identity.[389] It differs dramatically, however, from GPIIb/IIIa in its platelet surface density, since there are only about 50 to 100 $\alpha V\beta3$ receptors per platelet.[336] The $\alpha V\beta3$ receptor can mediate adhesion to vitronectin, but only in the presence of magnesium or manganese, not calcium.[336] It also can mediate interactions with fibrinogen, vWF, and thrombospondin.[90,356,390,391] Activated $\alpha V\beta3$ may also uniquely mediate adhesion to osteopontin, a protein found in high concentrations in atherosclerotic plaques.[392] Its role in platelet physiology is not defined, but it may contribute to the development of platelet coagulant activity.[283]

The $\alpha V\beta3$ receptor is also present on endothelial cells,[341,391] osteoclasts,[393] and other cells; it has been implicated in bone resorption,[394] endothelial-matrix interactions,[341] lymphoid cell apoptosis,[395] neovascularization,[396] tumor angiogenesis,[397] and both smooth-muscle cell migration and intimal hyperplasia after vascular injury.[398] Binding of adhesive proteins to $\alpha V\beta3$ can be inhibited by RGD-containing peptides.

The presence or absence of $\alpha V\beta3$ on the platelets of patients with Glanzmann thrombasthenia can help localize the abnormality to either GPIIb (if $\alpha V\beta3$ is present in normal or increased amounts) or GPIIIa (if $\alpha V\beta3$ is reduced or absent) (see Chap. 119).

LEUCINE-RICH REPEAT GLYCOPROTEIN RECEPTORS
GPIb/GPIX (CD42)   GPIb is composed of GPIbα (CD42b) (610 amino acids) disulfide-bonded to GPIbβ (CD42c) (122 amino acids) (Fig. 111-9).[177,304,399,400] The GPIbα gene is on the short arm of chromosome 17, and the GPIbβ gene is on the long arm of chromosome 22. A genetic polymorphism in GPIbα affects the number of repeating 13-amino-acid units (1, 2, 3, or 4) and produces changes in the M_r of GPIbα.[401] The two-repeat variant is most common, but there is considerable ethnic variation in the frequency of the different numbers of repeats. This M_r polymorphism has been linked to the Sib and Ko alloantigens, which have been localized to a Thr→Met variation at amino acid 145 of GPIbα, with Met associated with either three or four repeats and Thr associated with either one or two repeats (Fig. 111-10 and see Chap. 138).[377] Two reports suggest an association between the alleles with the larger number of repeats and coronary artery disease,[402,403] but inconsistent results have been reported on the impact of these polymorphisms on the risk of cerebrovascular disease.[403,404] Two other GPIbα polymorphisms have been de-

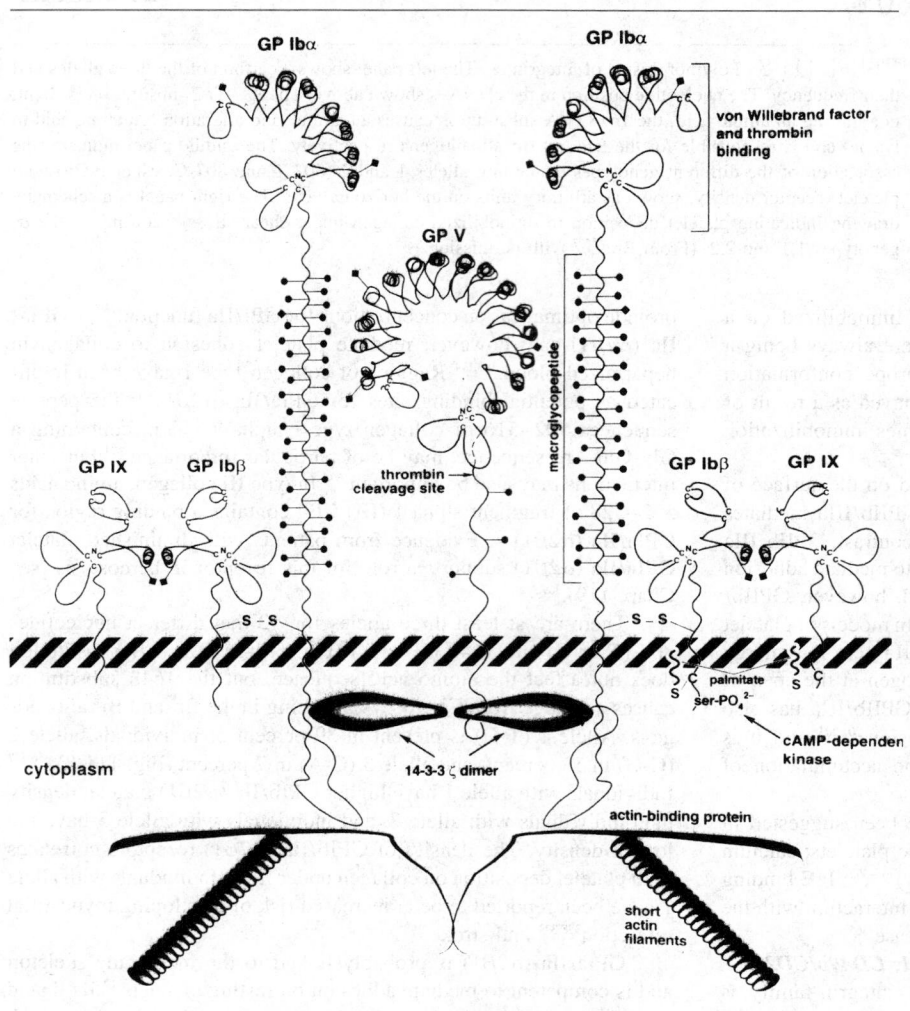

FIGURE 111-9   Schematic view of the platelet GPIb-IX-V complex. Key structural features of the complex are shown. The leucine-rich repeats of the four polypeptides are drawn based on the structure determined for the porcine ribonuclease inhibitor, a protein made up entirely of leucine-rich repeats. The depicted polypeptide arrangement is based on the published stoichiometry determined by monoclonal antibody binding and on the associations determined for the polypeptides. A caveat about this depiction: the quantity of GPV on the platelet surface has only been determined using 2 GPV monoclonal antibodies, which could lead to overestimates or underestimates of true polypeptide number. In addition, no quantitation has ever been performed to indicate that every GPV molecule on the platelet surface is associated with the complex. Complexes of greater complexity having the same stoichiometry are also possible. Diamonds on stalks represent N-linked carbohydrates and circles on stalks represent O-linked carbohydrate. (From Lopez et al,[400] with permission.)

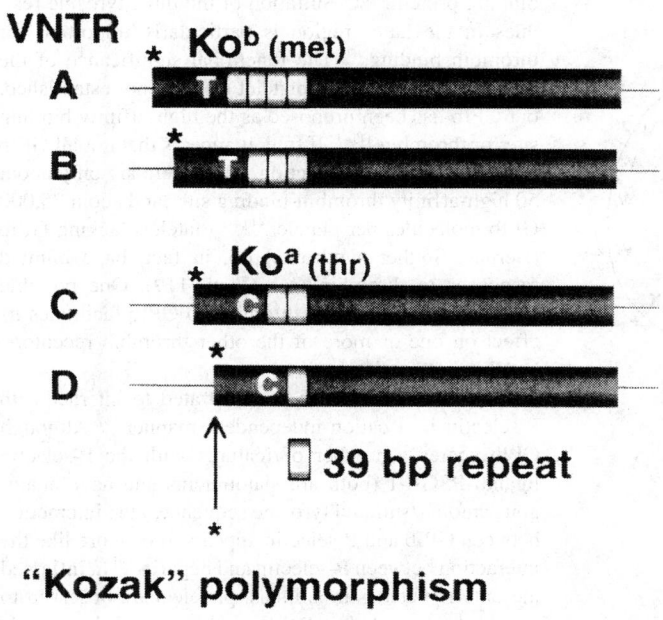

"Kozak" polymorphism

FIGURE 111-10   Polymorphisms of platelet GPIbα. The four alleles of GPIbα that have been defined by the VNTR, Ko, and Kozak polymorphisms. The 4 variable number of tandem repeat (VNTR) polymorphisms are defined as A–D, according to the number of 39 base pair repeats: A has four repeats, B has three repeats, C has two repeats, and D has one repeat. The Ko polymorphism results from a T to C nucleotide substitution that alters the amino acid from methionine (met) to threonine (thr). The "*" indicates the location of the nucleotide substitution, which generates a sequence that better conforms to the consensus Kozak sequence. (From Bray,[377] with permission.)

scribed: (1) C or T at position 5 from the ATG start codon (RS system), and (2) a nucleotide dimorphism at the third bases of the codon for Arg 358.[400,405,406] A C at position 5 is present in only 8 to 17 percent of individuals and more closely resembles the sequence surrounding the ATG start codon (Kozak sequence) considered optimal for translation. In fact, this polymorphism is associated with higher levels of platelet surface GPIb and may be a risk for early myocardial infarction.[407] GPIb has been implicated as a target antigen in autoimmune thrombocytopenia and in quinine and quinidine-induced thrombocytopenia (see Chap. 117).

GPIbα has a large number of O-linked carbohydrate chains terminating in sialic acid residues,[408] and the latter contribute significantly to the negative charge of the platelet membrane.[2] Electron micrographic analysis indicates that GPIb exists as a long flexible rod (60 nm) with two globular domains of about 9 and 16 nm.[409] Thus, GPIb probably extends much further out from the platelet's surface than does GPIIb/IIIa, which may account for its primacy in platelet adhesion, as well as the increased risk of cardiovascular disease in individuals with longer GPIb molecules due to an increased number of 13-amino-acid repeats. The long extension may also make it susceptible to conformational changes induced by shear forces.[304] The extracellular region of GPIbα is readily cleaved by a variety of proteases, including platelet calpains,[410] yielding a soluble fragment named *glycocalicin* that circulates in normal plasma at 1 to 3 μg/ml.[411] Levels of plasma glycocalicin correlate with platelet production and thus can be used to differentiate thrombocytopenia due to decreased platelet production from thrombocytopenia due to increased platelet destruction.[412,413]

GPIbβ has a free sulfhydryl group in its cytoplasmic domain.[414] In addition, its cytoplasmic domain can undergo phosphorylation of

serine 166 by cAMP-dependent kinase, which may affect actin polymerization and GPIb function.[304,415] The cytoplasmic domain of GPIbα connects GPIb to actin-binding protein, thus connecting GPIb to the platelet cytoskeleton.[12,180,416] Alterations in the cytoskeleton can affect GPIb functional activity.[417–419] The cytoplasmic domain is probably also a site of palmitic acid attachment, which may enhance attachment to the lipid bilayer.[420] The GPIbα cytoplasmic domain also has a site that binds protein 14-3-3ζ, which has been implicated in GPIb-mediated intracellular signaling that results in GPIIb/IIIa activation.[180] GPIb also appears to be in close proximity to FcγRIIA and the Fc receptor γ chain, two receptors that can initiate signaling.[421,422]

GPIb appears to exist on the surface of platelets in a one-to-one complex with GPIX (160 amino acids).[423–425] The function of GPIX is unknown, but it is probably required for efficient surface expression of GPIb.[426] GPIbα has seven leucine-rich repeats in the amino-terminal region of its extracellular domain, whereas GPIbβ and GPIX have one each.[177,399,425] These repeats are consensus sequences of 24 amino acids with seven regularly spaced leucines; well-defined disulfide loop sequences flank the repeats.[304] Similar leucine-rich repeats are present in a variety of other proteins; crystallographic studies of one of these proteins (porcine ribonuclease inhibitor) identified a unique β sheet-α helix recurring structure for each of the leucine-rich repeats.[427] Immediately C-terminal to the leucine-rich repeat flanking sequence in GPIbα is a 19-amino-acid sequence rich in negatively charged amino acids that contains three sulfated tyrosines.[180,400]

GPIb mediates platelet interaction with vWF, with the binding site in the vWF AI domain (residues 480–718).[400] Both Asp 514 to Glu 542 and the region encompassing Glu 596 and Lys 599 have been proposed as recognition sites.[180,400] This region is distinct from the RGD-containing region of vWF that mediates binding to GPIIb/IIIa (see Chap. 135).

The vWF-binding domain on GPIbα has been localized to the first 300 amino acids, and three different regions appear to contribute: the anionic, sulfated-tyrosine sequence; a portion of the carboxy-terminal leucine-rich repeat flanking sequence; and the leucine-rich repeats themselves (Figs. 111-6 and 111-8).[400,428–431] Support for the importance of the carboxy-terminal repeat region in vWF binding also comes from the observation that patients with pseudo (platelet-type) von Willebrand disease, whose platelet GPIb/IX complex has enhanced affinity for vWF, have mutations within this region (Fig. 111-11 and see Chap. 119). Plasma vWF will not bind to GPIb under static conditions unless the antibiotic ristocetin or the snake venom botrocetin is added. The mechanism by which ristocetin induces vWF binding to GPIb is unclear but appears to involve changes in platelet surface charge, and requires dimerization of ristocetin molecules.[184,304,432] Botrocetin binds to vWF, exposing the site that binds to GPIb.[433] Peptide studies implicate the anionic, sulfated tyrosine region of GPIb as the binding site for botrocetin-treated vWF.[304]

Unlike GPIIb/IIIa, which requires intact, activated platelets to bind to vWF, GPIb-mediated vWF binding does not require platelet activation or even platelet metabolic integrity, since formaldehyde-fixed platelets are readily agglutinated in the presence of vWF and either ristocetin or botrocetin.[184] This observation forms the basis of the assay of plasma vWF activity (see Chap. 135).

Platelets will adhere to vWF when the latter is immobilized on a surface, even in the absence of ristocetin or botrocetin.[178,184,434] Under these circumstances, the vWF may undergo a conformational change that allows for direct interactions. It may not, however, be necessary to propose a change in vWF conformation, since the interaction between vWF and GPIb appears to have both high association and dissociation rates, permitting tethering and translocation on a surface coated with vWF but minimal interaction in fluid phase.[179] Similarly,

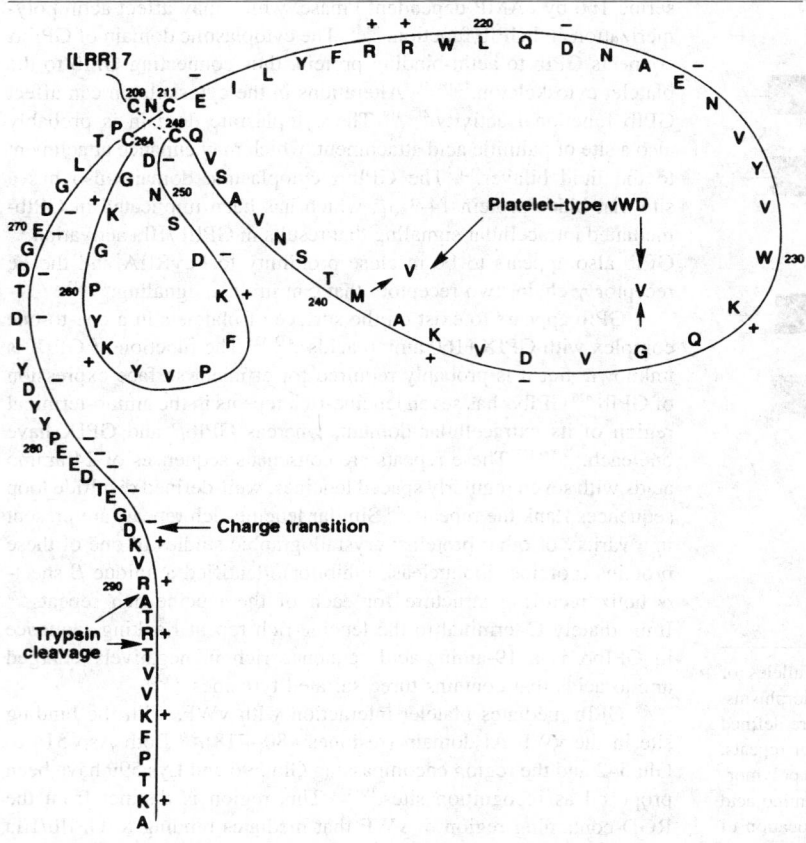

FIGURE 111-11   The region in GPIbα from amino acids 209–302. Disulfide bonds between Cys209 and Cys248 and between Cys211 and Cys264 create two loops. Mutations in the loop between Cys209 and Cys248 result in enhanced interaction between von Willebrand factor and GPIb, producing platelet-type von Willebrand disease (see Chap. 119). This loop has also been implicated in regulating von Willebrand factor binding to GPIb. The region between amino acids 235–279 has been implicated in ristocetin-induced binding of von Willebrand factor, whereas the region between amino acids 271–285 has been implicated in botrocetin-induced von Willebrand factor binding. The region between amino acids 269 and 287 bears resemblance to the thrombin-binding peptide hirudin, and so it has been postulated to be part of the thrombin-binding region. (From Lopez,[304] with permission.)

vWF associated with fibrin can interact with platelet GPIb without ristocetin or botrocetin.[206,435]

Shear stress is an important factor in GPIb-mediated adhesion of platelets to immobilized vWF and subendothelial surfaces.[177,178,434,436,437] Platelets deficient in GPIb or platelets in which GPIb has been blocked with monoclonal antibodies[178,436] adhere poorly to subendothelial surfaces at all shear rates, but the defect in blood from patients with von Willebrand disease is manifest primarily at higher shear rates.[178] In what may be a related phenomenon, subjecting platelets to high shear stresses can induce platelet aggregation, which is mediated by vWF binding to GPIb, followed by platelet activation and GPIIb/IIIa-dependent platelet aggregation.[181,183,438] Whether the shear rates generated in vivo in stenotic blood vessels are of sufficient magnitude and duration to produce a similar degree of platelet activation is unknown. It is also uncertain as to whether the effect of shear is acting on GPIb, on vWF, or on both[177,179,183,304] but shear-induced changes in the structure of vWF, leading to a more extended conformation, have been defined.[439]

GPIbα also functions as a binding site for thrombin.[304,440,441] The region between amino acids 216 and 240 has been proposed as the binding site, but the region between amino acids 269 and 287 has also been suggested because of its similarity to hirudin, a thrombin-

binding protein.[304,429] Sulfation of the three tyrosine residues in the latter region is particularly important for thrombin binding.[180] The functional significance of the binding of thrombin to platelet GPIb is not established, but GPIb has been proposed as the high-affinity binding site for thrombin.[440,442] If true, it appears that not all GPIb molecules serve this function, since there are only about 50 high-affinity thrombin-binding sites and about 25,000 GPIb molecules per platelet.[440,441] Platelets lacking GPIb (Bernard-Soulier syndrome) do, in fact, have blunted responses to thrombin (see Chap. 119). One possible model is that binding of thrombin to GPIb facilitates its effect on one or more of the other thrombin receptors, but this is speculation.

GPIb has also been demonstrated to interact with P-selectin in a cation-independent manner.[180] Although GPIb shares a number of features with the P-selectin ligand, PSGL-1 (both are sialomucins and have analogous anionic/sulfated tyrosine sequences) the interaction between GPIb and P-selectin appears to be more like the interaction between P-selectin and heparin.[180] In inflamed mesenteric venules in animals, platelets are observed to roll on the activated endothelium,[443] and so it is possible that platelet GPIb interacts with endothelial P-selectin in this interaction.[180]

GPV   Glycoprotein V is an M_r 82,000 protein composed of 544 amino acids that contains 15 leucine-rich repeats.[444–447] GPV appears to form a noncovalent complex with GPIb/IX, but since the number of GPV molecules on the surface of platelets is approximately 50 percent of the number of GPIb and GPIX molecules,[448] it has been suggested that the basic unit consists of two GPIb molecules, two GPIX molecules, and one GPV molecule.[304,400] GPV is deficient in platelets from patients with Bernard-Soulier syndrome (see Chap. 119), who have defects in GPIb or GPIX, but GPV is not required for surface expression of the GPIb/IX complex.[449] A soluble fragment of M_r 69,000 is cleaved from GPV by thrombin, but cleavage does not correlate with thrombin-induced platelet activation.[450] Platelets from mice lacking GPV appear to respond more actively to thrombin and ADP than wild-type mice, raising the possibility that GPV inhibits platelet activation.[451] The platelets from these mice also adhere to immobilized vWF and can bind vWF in the presence of botrocetin, indicating that GPV is not required for the interaction between vWF and the GPIb/IX/V complex.[451]

IMMUNOGLOBULIN FAMILY OF CELL SURFACE ADHESION RECEPTORS

PECAM-1 (CD31)   Platelet-endothelial cell adhesion molecule 1 (PECAM-1) is an M_r 130,000 transmembrane glycoprotein of the immunoglobulin gene family with six immunoglobulin-like domains of the C2 group.[452] In addition to platelets and endothelial cells, it is expressed on monocytes, myeloid cells, and some lymphocyte subsets (see Chap. 13). There are approximately 8000 PECAM-1 molecules on the surface of platelets.[453]

Crosslinking of PECAM-1 molecules on the platelet surface enhances platelet adhesion and aggregate formation under low shear conditions and enhances ADP- and PAF-induced platelet aggregation.[454] These effects correlate with tyrosine phosphorylation of PECAM-1 and suggest that PECAM-1 is a costimulatory agonist, working in concert with platelet GPIIb/IIIa.[454] Phosphorylated PECAM-1 can recruit a protein tyrosine phosphatase (SHP-2), which may participate in the enhanced platelet function found when PECAM-1 is activated.[455]

In endothelial cells, PECAM-1 is localized to the contact areas between endothelial cells, where it is likely to be involved in controlling transmigration of leukocytes.[456] It appears to be capable of both homotypic and heterotypic adhesive interactions, with the latter perhaps mediated by glycosaminoglycan interactions with a region in the second immunoglobulin domain.[457] An antibody to PECAM-1 decreases neutrophil accumulation and myocardial infarct size in a rat model of ischemia-reperfusion injury.[458]

FcγRIIA (CD32)   The FcγRIIA is a low-affinity immunoglobulin receptor of M_r 40,000 that is widely distributed on hematopoietic cells (see Chap. 13). Three different mRNA transcripts (A, B, and C) make similar FcγRIIA receptors,[459] and these are preferentially expressed on different cells. In addition, a polymorphism within FcγRIIA, H131R, affects the binding of different IgG subclasses.[460]

The FcγRIIA on platelets may bind immune complexes generated in certain diseases.[461,462] It may also provide a second binding site for antibodies that bind to platelets via their antibody-binding site (see "CD9" below). This second interaction can potentially lead to bridging between platelets, with the antibody binding to an antigen on one platelet and an FcγRIIA receptor on another platelet.[463] It is also possible that antibodies can bind to both an antigen and FcγRIIA receptor on a single platelet. These interactions can lead to platelet activation, because crosslinking of FcγRIIA can initiate tyrosine phosphorylation, phosphoinositol metabolism, activation of phospholipase Cγ2, calcium signaling, and cytoskeletal rearrangements.[464,465] FcγRIIA expression on platelets shows considerable variation among individuals (about 600 to 1500 molecules per platelet), and this variation correlates with FcγRIIA-mediated function.[462] This variation in receptor density may explain individual differences in immune-mediated disorders such as heparin-induced thrombocytopenia with thrombosis.[466] The H131R polymorphism may also have clinical significance, since the homozygous H/H genotype is overrepresented in patients with heparin-induced thrombocytopenia,[467] but the R/R 131 genotype may confer a higher risk of developing thrombosis in patients with heparin-induced thrombocytopenia.[468] The R/R genotype may also be associated with the likelihood of requiring splenectomy in patients with immune thrombocytopenia.[469] FcγRIIA has also been suggested to be in close proximity to the GPIb/IX/V complex,[304] and it appears that the signal transduction that accompanies vWF binding to GPIb may be mediated through FcγRIIA.[470] Cooperation between FcγRIIA and C1q receptor has also been reported.[471]

Fc Receptor γ-chain   Platelets contain the Fc receptor γ (FcRγ) chain,[472] although they lack the Fc receptors for FcεR1, FcγRI, and FcγRIII that normally form signaling complexes with FcRγ chain in other cell types. In platelets, the FcRγ chain exists as an M_r 20,000 homodimer believed to be involved in signal transduction. The FcRγ chain, along with FcγRIIA, are the only known platelet proteins with immune-receptor tyrosine-containing activation motifs (ITAMs). Much of the understanding of the role of proteins with ITAM-containing domains comes from studies in cells other than platelets, where phosphorylation of the ITAM domain serves to recruit proteins with Src homology 2 (SH2) domains,[473,474] many of which are involved in signal transduction. FcRγ-chain is associated with GPVI[475] and GPIbα[422] and may activate intracellular signaling pathways in response to platelet adhesion to collagen and vWF respectively. Phosphorylation

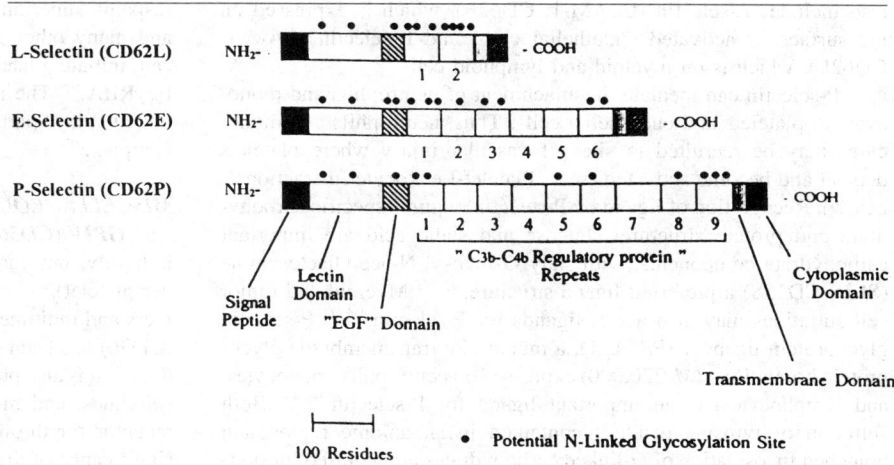

FIGURE 111-12   Structures of the selectins, L-selectin (CD62L), E-selectin (CD62E), and P-selectin (CD62P). (Modified from McEver,[787] with permission.)

of the ITAM sequence of FcRγ-chain recruits syk,[476] activates PI-3 kinase,[477] and appears to be involved in activation of PLCγ[478] and polyphosphoiniositide hydrolysis (see "Signaling Pathways in Platelet Activation and Aggregation" below).

ICAM-2 (CD102)   Intracellular adhesion molecule 2 (ICAM-2), a member of the immunoglobulin family of receptors that is also present on endothelial cells, is a ligand for the β_2-integrin $\alpha L\beta 2$ (LFA-1) on lymphocytes and myeloid cells.[479] Approximately 2600 ICAM-2 molecules are present on platelets, distributed on the membrane surface and open canalicular system.[479] Platelet ICAM-2 may contribute to platelet-leukocyte interactions (see "Platelet-Leukocyte Interactions" below).

GPVI   GPVI is an M_r 62,000 transmembrane glycoprotein of 316 amino acids.[191] Its extracellular region contains two immunoglobulin C2-like domains, and its transmembrane domain contains an Arg residue that may make a salt bridge with the FcRγ-chain. For a discussion of the role of GPVI as a receptor for collagen, see "Collagen Signaling" below.

Human Leukocyte Antigens (HLA)   HLA class I molecules are expressed on the surface of platelets. They are discussed in Chap. 138.

SELECTINS

P-selectin (GMP140, PADGEM, CD62P)   P-selectin is an M_r 140,000 glycoprotein that is present in the membrane of α granules in resting platelets and joins the plasma membrane when platelets are activated.[208,209,480] Approximately 13,000 molecules are detected by antibodies on the surface of activated platelets. The expression of P-selectin on circulating platelets has, therefore, been used as an indicator of in vivo activation of platelets.[30,325] It is also present in the Weibel-Palade body membranes of endothelial cells; as in platelets, it joins the plasma membrane when endothelial cells are activated.[208,480]

P-selectin has a modular structure in which the amino-terminal region has a calcium-dependent lectin domain that binds carbohydrates. Adjacent to the lectin domain is an epidermal growth factor domain, followed by nine repeats that are homologous to complement regulatory proteins ("sushi" domains), a transmembrane domain, and a cytoplasmic domain (Fig. 111-12).[209,480] The cytoplasmic domain contains serine, threonine, tyrosine, and histidine residues that can be phosphorylated. In addition, a cysteine residue becomes acylated with stearic or palmitic acid. Alternatively spliced forms of P-selectin may be produced in which sushi domains are omitted. The selectin family also includes E-selectin (ELAM-1; CD62E), which is expressed on the surface of activated endothelial cells, and L-selectin (LAM-1; CD62L), which is on myeloid and lymphoid cells.[481]

P-selectin can mediate the attachment of neutrophils and monocytes to platelets and endothelial cells. Thus, neutrophils and monocytes may be recruited to sites of vascular injury where platelets deposit and become activated (see "Platelet-Leukocyte Interactions" below). Recognition of ligand by P-selectin requires specific carbohydrate and protein structures. Fucose and sialic acid are important carbohydrate components, with sialyl-3-fucosyl-N-acetyllactosamine (SLe^x; CD15S) a preferred ligand structure.[482–485] Myeloid and tumor cell sulfatides may also act as ligands for P-selectin.[486,487] P-selectin glycoprotein ligand 1 (PSGL-1), a mucin-like transmembrane glycoprotein homodimer (M_r 220,000) expressed on neutrophils, monocytes, and lymphocytes, is an important ligand for P-selectin.[488–490] Both sulfation of tyrosine residues contained in an anionic region and branched fucosylation of O-linked carbohydrates are required for optimal binding to P-selectin. Binding of P-selectin to PSGL-1 on monocytes can trigger tissue factor synthesis.[491]

In intact blood vessels, the rapid on and off rates of the interactions between PSGL-1 on neutrophils and P-selectin on endothelial cells allows leukocytes to roll on the endothelium, the first step in leukocyte transmigration (see Chap. 67).[492] The rapid upregulation of surface P-selectin after endothelial cell activation allows for a quick response. Platelets have been reported to roll on activated endothelium, and this appears to result from an interaction between endothelial P-selectin and perhaps platelet GPIbα.[180,443] An antibody to P-selectin can image thrombi, and an antibody that blocks P-selectin binding can inhibit fibrin deposition in experimental systems.[493]

A cDNA encoding a soluble form of P-selectin, lacking the transmembrane domain, has been identified, and an increase in plasma levels of soluble P-selectin has been reported in thrombotic and inflammatory disorders.[494]

TETRASPANINS

CD9   CD9 is a protein of 228 amino acids that contains four putative transmembrane domains, making it a member of the tetraspanin superfamily.[495,496] CD9 is also present on endothelial cells, smooth muscle cells, cultured fibroblasts, some lymphoblasts, eosinophils, basophils, and other cells. CD9 is present at high density on the platelet surface (about 40,000/platelet).[497] It colocalizes with GPIIb/IIIa on the inner surface of α granules in resting platelets and on pseudopods of activated platelets.[498] Binding of monoclonal antibodies specific for CD9 to platelets results in platelet aggregation by triggering phosphatidylinositol metabolism via a mechanism that also requires binding to the platelet FcγRII receptor.[499–501] The platelet activation induced by the binding of such antibodies requires external calcium and results in an association between CD9 and GPIIb/IIIa.[502]

CD63 (Granulophysin, LAMP-3)   CD63, an M_r 53,000 protein member of the tetraspanin superfamily, appears to be present in both lysosomal and dense granule membranes in platelets.[29,503] CD63 is also present in Weibel-Palade bodies in endothelial cells, the lysosomal membranes of a variety of other cells, as well as the membranes of melanosomes. It joins the surface membrane when platelets are activated, making it a useful marker for platelet activation.[29,30] CD63 appears to be markedly reduced or absent from the dense bodies of patients with Hermansky-Pudlak syndrome,[503] who have oculocutaneous albinism and a defect in platelet dense bodies (see Chap. 119). The amino acid sequence of CD63 has been deduced from cDNA cloning.[504]

Platelet-Endothelial Cell Tetra-Span Antigen (PETA-3; CD151)   PETA-3 is an M_r 27,000 glycoprotein member of the tetraspanin superfamily.[505,506] It is present on platelets, endothelial cells, and many other cells.[507] Antibodies to PETA-3, like those to CD9, can initiate platelet aggregation by binding to both PETA-3 and FcγRIIA.[505] The role of PETA-3 in platelet physiology is uncertain, but it may participate with FcγRIIA as a signal transduction complex.[505]

MISCELLANEOUS

GPIV (CD36)   GPIV (CD36) is an M_r 88,000 glycoprotein that is highly, but variably, expressed on platelets (about 20,000 copies per platelet).[92,308,508–510] Biochemical data suggest that it may form dimers and multimers.[511] Increased platelet surface expression of GPIV (CD36) has been described in patients with myeloproliferative disorders.[512] It is also present on monocytes, endothelial cells, hematopoietic cell lines, and melanoma cells. It has been proposed as a platelet receptor for thrombospondin[513] and collagen,[514,515] but the functional significance of these interactions remains unclear because individuals with inherited deficiencies of GPIV (CD36) (Nak^a-negative) do not have a bleeding disorder (see Chap. 119).[516] GPIV (CD36) may play a role in the thrombospondin-mediated interaction reported between platelets and sickle erythrocytes[517] and in the binding of *Plasmodium falciparum*-infected erythrocytes to endothelial cells and monocytes.[518] It has also been implicated in monocyte binding of oxidized LDL and myocardial uptake of long-chain fatty acids.[519]

The nucleotide sequence of GPIV cDNA encodes a protein of 471 residues with an M_r of 53,000 and ten potential N-linked glycosylation sites.[518] It is unusual in having two putative transmembrane domains and two short cytoplasmic tails. The cytoplasmic regions may associate with intracellular tyrosine kinases of the src family and undergo phosphorylation.[520] Moreover, the phosphorylation status of the extracellular region of the protein may control its ligand-binding properties,[91] offering a potential explanation for some of the variable results obtained under different conditions.[91,92,521]

LAMP-1 and LAMP-2 (CD107a, CD107b)   LAMP-1 and LAMP-2 are lysosome-associated membrane proteins that are about 30 percent homologous. They are integral membrane glycoproteins of 110 and 120 kDa respectively that are contained within lysosomal membranes.[522] When platelets undergo the release reaction, they join the plasma membrane. Each protein has two extracellular disulfide-bonded loops containing 36 to 38 amino acids. The loops are separated by a region rich in proline and serine that shares homology with the hinge region of IgA. There are multiple N-linked glycosylation sites on each glycoprotein, and they contain more than 60 percent carbohydrate. Among the carbohydrate residues are polylactosaminoglycans that may possess sialylated Lewis^x structures, which are thought to interact with selectins (see above).

C1q Receptors   Platelets have several receptors for C1q, an M_r 460,000 glycoprotein composed of six globular domains attached to a short collagen-like triple helix.[523,524] One is for the collagen-like domain (cC1qR, M_r 60,000 to 67,000 nonreduced and 72,000 to 75,000 reduced), and another is for the globular domain (gC1qR, M_r 28,000 to 33,000).[525,526] A third receptor of M_r 126,000 enhances phagocytosis.[527] C1q circulates with C1r and C1s as a calcium-dependent complex, but interaction with immune complexes leads ultimately to dissociation of the complex and release of free C1q, with its collagen-like domain exposed. cC1qR has sequence homology to calreticulin and can modulate platelet-collagen interactions at low collagen concentrations. It may also localize immune complexes, and when cross-linked by aggregated C1q, it can initiate platelet activation, aggregation, secretion, and expression of platelet coagulant activity.[528] Thus, the binding of C1q monomers to platelets inhibits collagen-induced platelet aggregation but has little effect on platelet adhesion to collagen.[529] C1q multimers support platelet adhesion and can induce aggregation via activation of GPIIb/IIIa.[528] C1q can also augment platelet aggregation induced by aggregated IgG.[471] The gC1qR is present on platelets and other cells, including endothelial cells, where it functions as a receptor for high-molecular-weight kininogen.[526] It may, therefore, participate in contact activation.

67-kD Laminin Receptor   An M_r 67,000 protein identified as a laminin receptor on several different cells has also been detected on platelets. It can mediate platelet adhesion to laminin under certain conditions.[388] The relative roles of this receptor and the integrin receptor GPIc/IIa ($\alpha 6\beta 1$), which also mediates the interaction between platelets and laminin, are unknown.

GMP-33   An M_r 33,000, predominantly α-granule membrane protein has been identified that joins the plasma membrane when platelets undergo the release reaction. Approximately 4000 antibody molecules directed against GMP-33 bind to unactivated platelets, and 19,000 bind to activated platelets.[530] The function of GMP-33 is unknown.

Leukosialin, Sialophorin (CD43)   Leukosialin, a glycoprotein of M_r 90,000, may act as a ligand for ICAM-1.[531] It is expressed on myeloid and some lymphoid cells. Abnormalities in leukosialin have been described in Wiskott-Aldrich syndrome (see Chap. 119).

PLATELETS AND THROMBOLYSIS

The interactions between platelets and the fibrinolytic system are complex, and Table 111-8 contains a partial listing.[532-534] Both profi-

TABLE 111-8   PLATELETS AND THROMBOLYSIS

Profibrinolytic effects of platelets
  Tissue plasminogen activator (t-PA) and single-chain urokinase-type t-PA identified on or in platelets.
  Unactivated platelets bind plasminogen, and binding is enhanced by thrombin.
  Thrombospondin, a plasminogen-binding protein, is expressed on the surface of platelets after activation.
  Activation of plasminogen by t-PA is enhanced by platelets.
  Clot lysis is enhanced by platelets in some model systems.
Antifibrinolytic effects of platelets
  Plasminogen activator inhibitor-1 and α_2-antiplasmin are present in platelet granules.
  Platelets release a protein that stimulates cells to release a fibrinolysis inhibitor.
  Platelets contain factor XIII, which can cross-link fibrin, making it resist fibrinolysis, and can cross-link α_2-antiplasmin to fibrin, enhancing its antifibrinolytic effects.
  Platelet GPIIb/IIIa can bind plasma factor XIIIa, localizing it to the site of thrombus formation.
  Platelets facilitate clot retraction, which diminishes the efficiency of fibrinolysis.
Platelet-activating effects of thrombolytic agents
  Streptokinase and t-PA activate platelets in vivo and in vitro.
  Plasmin, at high doses, can aggregate platelets.
  Thrombolytic agents may generate the potent platelet agonist thrombin or release it from thrombi.
  Thrombolytic agents may blunt the prostacyclin increase that accompanies acute thrombosis.
Platelet-inhibiting effects of thrombolytic agents
  Plasmin, at low doses, can inhibit platelet activation and aggregation.
  Platelets can be disaggregated by t-PA by selective lysis of platelet-bound fibrinogen.
  Plasmin can cause redistribution and/or cleavage of platelet glycoprotein Ib.
  Inhibition of platelet aggregation by the depletion of plasma fibrinogen, if severe, and generation of fibrin(ogen) degradation products.
  Proteolysis of plasma von Willebrand factor.
  Prolongation of the bleeding time.

SOURCE: Adapted from Coller,[172] with permission.

brinolytic[99,359,535-540] and antifibrinolytic[268,360,541-546] effects of platelets have been described, and so it is difficult to predict the net effect. Since platelet-rich thrombi are known to resist thrombolysis in animal models, the antifibrinolytic effects of platelets appear to predominate in vivo.[547]

The effects of fibrinolytic agents on platelets are also complex, with considerable evidence that fibrinolytic agents can activate platelets soon after administration,[548-554] via either a direct effect of plasmin[555,556] or an indirect effect through the paradoxical generation of thrombin.[534,557-560] A direct effect of tissue plasminogen activator on fibrinopeptide release from fibrinogen has also been described.[561]

Stimulation of platelets by thrombolytic agents may prolong the time required for reperfusion and may contribute to reocclusion after successful reperfusion.[172,532] In animal models and in humans, potent antiplatelet agents can, in fact, speed reperfusion, abolish reocclusion, and diminish the size of myocardial infarcts.[562-565]

With prolonged use of thrombolytic agents, however, there may be inhibition of platelet function via a variety of mechanisms,[160,551,554,566-576] which might contribute to some of the hemorrhagic phenomena and the prolonged bleeding times observed with this therapy. The inhibition may be caused by the thrombolytic agents making the platelets refractory to further stimulation.

PLATELET-LEUKOCYTE INTERACTIONS, PLATELET-TISSUE FACTOR INTERACTIONS, AND THE ROLE OF PLATELETS IN INFLAMMATION

Leukocytes can bind to activated platelets and in model systems transmigrate through a platelet monolayer (reviewed in Coller[577]). These interactions may be important at sites of vascular injury where leukocytes have been shown to deposit on adherent and aggregated platelets. Many mechanisms of platelet-leukocyte interactions have been defined, but the initial interaction appears to be mediated primarily by the interaction between P-selectin (CD62P) expressed on the surface of activated platelets and P-selectin glycoprotein ligand-1 (PSGL-1) on the surface of neutrophils and monocytes (Fig. 111-13).[480,482,578-582] Activated $\alpha M\beta 2$ on leukocytes can interact with fibrinogen via a region on the γ chain (amino acids 190–202,[583] perhaps with the cooperation of amino acids 377–395[584]), and thus fibrinogen bound to platelet GPIIb/IIIa and/or $\alpha V\beta 3$ may also support leukocyte binding to platelets. Platelets can synthesize and release PAF, which can activate leukocyte $\alpha M\beta 2$, as can the CXC chemokines released by activated platelets (ENA-78, GRO-α) and produced by the action of leukocyte cathepsin G on β-thromboglobulin secreted by platelets (neutrophil-activating peptide-2, NAP-2) (reviewed in Weber and Springer[585]). Thrombospondin may also serve as a bridging molecule between CD36 receptors, which are expressed on both platelets and mononuclear cells.[586] Platelets also have ICAM-2 on their surface, which is a ligand for the leukocyte integrin receptor $\alpha L\beta 2$[479]; although this ligand-receptor interaction appears to have only a minor role in platelet-leukocyte adhesion, it may be more important in leukocyte tethering.[585]

Animal models and studies of human tissue demonstrate that within hours after vascular injury, leukocytes became enmeshed in platelet thrombi and/or transiently form a monolayer on top of adherent or aggregated platelets.[587,588] The initial surface association of leukocytes with platelets is usually transient, lasting less than a day. Since leukocytes, and in particular, monocytes, contain and can produce tissue factor, especially when P-selectin binds to PSGL-1, the platelet-leukocyte interaction may be important in initiating coagulation.

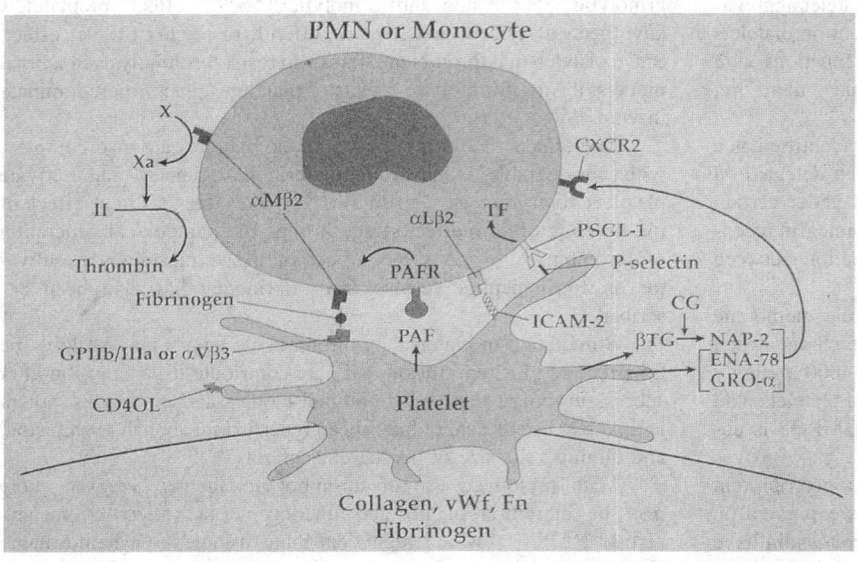

FIGURE 111-13   Platelet-leukocyte interactions. A number of interactions can occur between platelets and leukocytes, including polymorphonuclear leukocytes (PMN) and monocytes. The interaction between platelet P-selectin and leukocyte P-selectin glycoprotein ligand-1 (PSGL-1) is probably the most important interaction [and can lead to tissue factor (TF) synthesis by monocytes], but fibrinogen binding simultaneously to activated $\alpha M\beta 2$ on leukocytes and either GPIIb/IIIa or $\alpha V\beta 3$ on platelets may play a role under certain circumstances. Platelets can release platelet activation factor (PAF), which can interact with a PAF receptor (PAFR) on leukocytes, leading to $\alpha M\beta 2$ activation and binding of fibrinogen and factor X. Platelets also can release CXC chemokines (ENA-78 and GRO-α), and β-thromboglobulin (βTG) released by platelets can be converted by leukocyte cathepsin G (CG) into the potent chemotatic CXC chemokine, NAP-2. The chemokines, in turn, activate leukocytes by binding to the chemokine receptor CXCR2. Platelets also contain the potent immune-stimulating molecule, CD40 ligand (CD40L), and both express it on the platelet surface and release it into the circulation upon platelet activation. Not shown is the interaction between thrombospondin and CD36 molecules on both platelets and some leukocytes, or the interaction between GPIb and $\alpha M\beta 2$.

Platelet aggregates that form in animal models of vascular injury and in vitro systems stain positively for tissue factor antigen even when the perfusion is as brief as 5 min.[176] Since this is too short a time for significant protein synthesis to occur, the tissue factor appears to be derived from circulating microvesicular structures.

Several clinical observations support a potential role for platelet-leukocyte interactions in vascular disease, including the presence of circulating platelet-leukocyte aggregates in patients with unstable angina[589] and after coronary artery angioplasty[590]; in the latter situation, the presence of such aggregates appears to confer a worse prognosis for ischemic vascular complications.[590]

Transcellular metabolism of eicosanoids can result in production of unique products (see Chap. 114) and leukocytes can modify platelet activation.[591] In a complemetary fashion the intimate relationship between leukocytes and platelets allows the latter to contribute to the inflammatory response, including the release of chemokines that can activate leukocytes; platelet-derived growth factor, which can affect fibroblast and smooth-muscle cells; transforming growth factor beta (TGF-β), which both stimulates and inhibits cellular growth; and PF-4, which can prime neutrophils and has antiangiogenic activity. Platelets also contain FcγIIA receptors that can localize IgG and immune complexes, resulting in complement activation. Finally, platelets express CD40 ligand on their surface after activation, and this molecule can interact with CD40, a member of the tumor necrosis factor receptor family, on leukocytes and endothelial cells, leading to their activation and their elaboration of a number of proinflammatory molecules.[211,592,593]

SIGNALING PATHWAYS IN PLATELET ACTIVATION AND AGGREGATION

OVERVIEW

Platelets generally circulate in a quiescent state but are poised to be activated in response to a variety of agonists that become available at sites of vascular injury or ruptured atherosclerotic plaques. A number of different phenomena occur with platelet activation, and these are listed in Table 111-9. Agonists differ in their intrinsic ability to produce these phenomena, and added complexity derives from differences in dose responses to each agonist and the synergistic effects of agonists used in combination. Agonists are diverse (Fig. 111-4) and include small and large soluble molecules, enzymes, and immobilized adhesive glycoproteins. They can be classified as either ''strong'' or ''weak,'' depending on whether full activation, including the release reaction, can be initiated without the augmenting effect of platelet aggregation itself (Fig. 111-4). Low doses of strong agonists behave like weak agonists. Most agonists are released, synthesized, or formed at the site of vascular injury and this undoubtedly serves to localize the response.

Agonists bind to receptors of two general categories: seven-transmembrane, G-protein-coupled receptors and receptors that can initiate phosphorylation of target proteins (Fig. 111-14). In both cases, a sequence of signaling events ultimately leads to platelet activation. Physiologic responses of platelets to agonists are listed in Table 111-9, with all of them leading to activation of the GPIIb/IIIa receptor to a high-affinity ligand binding state leading to subsequent platelet aggregation. Moreover, binding of ligands to platelets and platelet aggregation itself further propagates signals that are required for stabilization of the platelet aggregates and clot retraction. In this section, the major agonists, receptors, and signaling pathways involved in early stages of platelet activation that lead to shape change, granule secretion, and platelet aggregation, as well as post-aggregation signaling events are described.

PLATELET ACTIVATION, ACTIVATORS, AND ACTIVATOR RECEPTORS

Many, but not all, platelet agonists initiate platelet activation by binding to seven transmembrane heterotrimeric, G-protein-coupled receptors. When such receptors are activated, the Gα subunit exchanges GDP for GTP and dissociates from the $\beta\gamma$ complex. The free Gα subunit, and in some cases, the $\beta\gamma$ complex can activate some relatively common

TABLE 111-9   PHENOMENA ASSOCIATED WITH PLATELET ACTIVATION

Increased platelet cytosolic calcium
Shape change
Change in GPIIb/IIIa to high-affinity binding state
Generation of arachidonic acid metabolites (e.g., thromboxane A_2)
Phosphorylation of select platelet proteins
Platelet aggregation
Induction of platelet coagulant activity
Release of α-granule contents
Release of dense granule contents
Release of lysosomal contents
Surface expression of proteins contained in lysosomal membranes
Surface expression of proteins contained in α-granule membranes

downstream pathways and initiate positive feedback loops (Figs. 111-7 and 111-14). Activation of these pathways is usually intertwined. One common pathway involves the activation of one or more isozymes of phospholipase C (PLC), leading to phosphoinositide hydrolysis. Three classes of PLC (β,γ, and δ), have been described, and multiple isozymes exist within each class.[594] The best-studied PLCs in platelets include PLCβ and PLCγ2. PLCβ is often activated downstream of the seven transmembrane, G-protein-coupled, receptor family, whereas PLCγ2 can be activated by phosphorylation on tyrosine, which is a downstream signal from other types of agonist receptors (Fig. 111-14). PLC of either type hydrolyzes phospholipids between the glycerol backbone and the phosphate moiety; both PLCβ and PLCγ2 are inositol-lipid specific. The hydrolysis of one particular phosphoinositide, phosphatidylinositol 4,5-bisphosphate (PIP$_2$), by either class of PLC is critical in platelet function, since it results in the formation of two important products, inositol 1,4,5-trisphosphate (IP$_3$) and diacylglycerol (DAG). IP$_3$ binds to specific receptors on the dense tubular system, causing release of Ca^{2+} into the intracellular space. Increases in intracellular Ca^{2+} are important for activation of a number of signalling enzymes and proteins involved in cytoskeletal reorganization (see below). Increases in calcium are also important in granule fusion and the release reaction. DAG binds to protein kinase C (PKC) and participates in its conversion to an active enzyme. For many agonists, activation of one or more of the multiple isozymes of PKC is an obligatory step in the conversion of GPIIb/IIIa to a high-affinity fibrinogen receptor and subsequent platelet aggregation.[595-597] The precise mechanism by which PKC causes GPIIb/IIIa activation, however, remains unclear. One consequence of protein kinase C activation is to cause the release of ADP from dense granules to the extracellular space. Released ADP then acts on its own seven transmembrane G-protein coupled receptor and/or a ligand-gated calcium channel to potentiate the action of numerous agonists.

Activation of a number of receptors also leads to the activation of phospholipase A$_2$ (PLA$_2$), which releases arachidonic acid from membrane lipid stores. Arachidonic acid is then rapidly converted in the dense tubular system to the prostaglandin products, PGH$_2$ and TXA$_2$, which are themselves potent activators of platelet aggregation (see below).

ADP ADP is present in platelet dense granules and is secreted when platelets are activated by adequate concentrations of most, if not all, agonists. Another source of ADP is the red blood cell; damaged red blood cells or those subjected to high shear stress may release ADP and increase the local ADP concentration. ADP is an important physiological agonist not only because it can induce platelet aggregation independent of other agonists but because secreted ADP contributes significantly to the full aggregation response induced by many other agonists. This has been convincingly demonstrated in experimental systems in which secreted ADP is rapidly degraded or inhibited. Moreover, submaximal concentrations of ADP synergize with other agonists, and this has been most studied with epinephrine (see below). ADP also induces or contributes to a variety of responses in platelets: shape change, granule release, TXA$_2$ production, activation of GPIIb/IIIa, and platelet aggregation.[598] Recent pharmacologic and cloning and sequencing studies suggest that ADP exerts its full effect on platelets through at least three receptors (reviewed in Kunapuli[598]) (Fig. 111-15). Two of these receptors, P2Y1 and P2TAC, are G-protein-coupled and are responsible for most of the physiologic effects of ADP, and the third, P2X1, is a ligand gated ion channel.

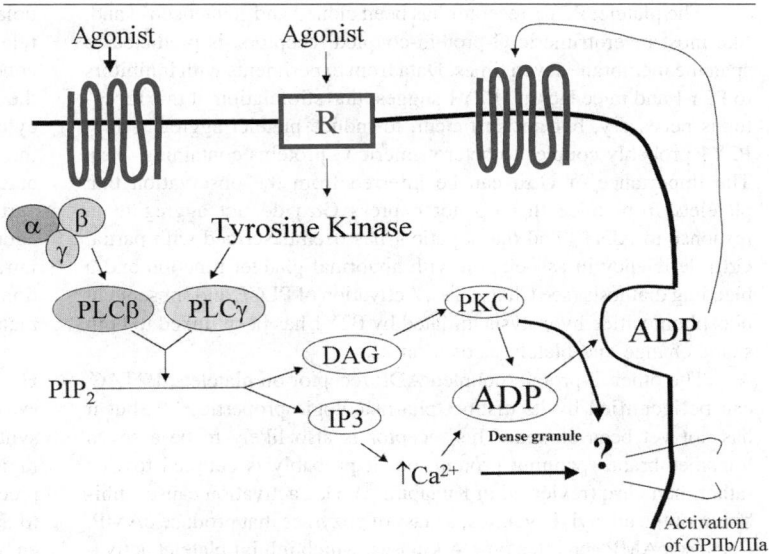

FIGURE 111-14   General scheme of agonist activation of platelets. Agonists stimulate specific platelet receptors such as seven-transmembrane G-protein-coupled receptors (GPCR) (left) or receptors coupled to tyrosine kinases (right). GPCRs activate a heterotrimeric G-protein by converting the α subunit to a GTP-bound state. The α subunit, after separating from the $\beta\gamma$ subunit, binds and activates phospholipase Cβ (PLCβ). Similarly, some tyrosine kinases (e.g., Syk) that are activated by other receptors activate PLCγ. PLCβ or PLCγ catalyze the hydrolysis of phosphatidylinositol bisphosphate (PIP$_2$), which generates diacylglycerol (DAG) and inositol trisphosphate (IP$_3$). IP$_3$ acts on specific receptors to increase intracellular Ca^{2+}, whereas DAG facilitates the activation of protein kinase C (PKC). These events promote dense granule fusion with the plasma membrane and release of ADP and other bioactive molecules and the activation of the major platelet integrin, GPIIb/IIIa. The exact signaling pathways leading to granule release and integrin activation are not well defined.

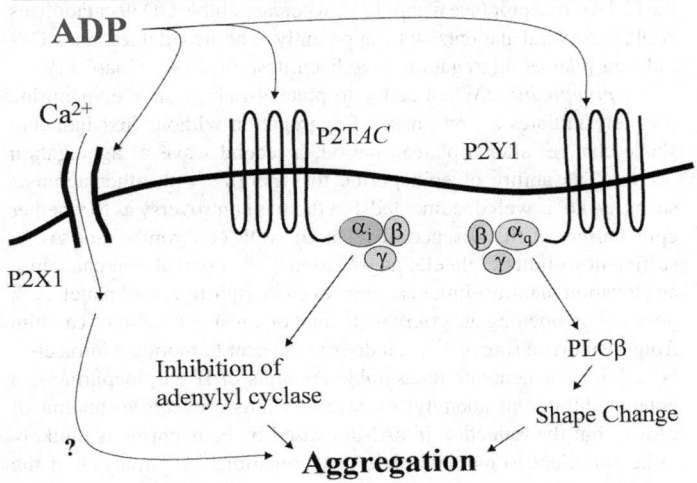

FIGURE 111-15   ADP activation of platelets. ADP potentially activates three separate receptors on platelets, a ligand-gated Ca^{2+} channel called *P2X1*, and 2 seven-transmembrane G-protein-coupled receptors, P2Y1, and a postulated receptor termed P2TAC. P2Y1 activates Gαq, which then activates PLCβ, whereas P2TAC is believed to activate Gαi, which inhibits adenylyl cyclase. Current evidence suggests that activation of both P2Y1 and P2TAC are required for maximal aggregation by ADP. Preliminary data suggest that P2X1 may also be important.

The platelet P2Y1 receptor has been cloned and sequenced[599] and, like most heterotrimeric G-protein-coupled receptors, is predicted to span the membrane seven times. Data from experiments with inhibitors to P2Y1 and mice lacking P2Y1 suggest that stimulation of this receptor is necessary, but not sufficient, to induce platelet aggregation.[600] P2Y1 probably couples to heterotrimeric G-proteins containing $G\alpha q$. The importance of $G\alpha q$ can be inferred from the observation that platelets from mice that do not express $G\alpha q$ do not aggregate in response to ADP[601] and that a patient has been described with partial $G\alpha q$ deficiency in association with abnormal platelet function and a bleeding diathesis (see Chap. 119). Activation of $PLC\beta$ and subsequent phosphoinositide hydrolysis initiated by P2Y1 has been linked to both shape change and platelet activation.

The other G-protein-coupled ADP receptor on platelets, P2TAC, can be identified by its distinct pharmacologic properties[602,603] but it has not yet been cloned. This receptor is also likely to be a seven transmembrane spanning protein, but it probably is coupled to $G\alpha i$ rather than $G\alpha q$ (reviewed in Kunapuli[598]). $G\alpha i$ activation causes inhibition of the adenylyl cyclases, a class of enzymes that produce cAMP. Because cAMP activates type A kinases, which inhibit platelet activation by a variety of effects, it is an attractive notion that inhibition of cAMP production promotes platelet aggregation. However, a decrease in cAMP levels alone is insufficient to activate platelets.[604,605] Synergistic effects between the signaling pathways of the P2Y1 and P2AC receptors (and perhaps the P2X1 receptor discussed below) appear to be sufficient to induce platelet aggregation.

Platelets contain mRNA for a third ADP receptor, P2X1. Receptors of the P2X family are ligand-gated ion channels rather than G-protein-coupled receptors.[606] The amino acid sequence of P2X1 suggests that it spans the plasma membrane twice and is largely extracellular.[607] ADP binding to this receptor is proposed to cause a rapid Ca^{2+} influx. However, Ca^{2+} influx induced by stimulation of this receptor appears to be insufficient in and of itself to induce platelet shape change or aggregation.[604] It may, however, cooperate in a positive manner with the other platelet ADP receptors.

Several antiplatelet agents inhibit ADP-induced platelet activation. Thus, metabolites of ticlopidine and clopidogrel appear to inhibit the P2TAC receptor (see Chap. 131), whereas soluble CD39 catabolizes ADP.[608] Several patients with apparently inherited defects in ADP-induced platelet aggregation have been described (see Chap. 119).

Epinephrine   When added to platelet-rich plasma, epinephrine uniquely initiates a first phase of aggregation without first inducing shape change; after a plateau period, a second wave of aggregation occurs. The ability of epinephrine to synergize with other agonists such as ADP is well documented, but there is controversy as to whether epinephrine, in the absence of released ADP or thromboxane A_2, is sufficient to initiate platelet aggregation.[609-611] Epinephrine can cause an elevation in intracellular calcium, even in aspirin-treated platelets,[612] possibly by opening an external channel or causing release of calcium from membrane sources[613,614]; it does not appear to mobilize intracellular calcium or generate measurable amounts of IP_3. Epinephrine is a potent inhibitor of adenylyl cyclase and thus prevents formation of cAMP, but the reduction in cAMP caused by epinephrine is unlikely to be sufficient to mediate platelet aggregation.[615-617] Analysis of the purified epinephrine receptor and its nucleotide sequence identify it as a seven-transmembrane, G-protein-coupled, $\alpha 2$ adrenergic receptor of M_r 64,000.[618,619]

Prostaglandin H_2/Thromboxane A_2 (TXA_2)   The metabolism of arachidonic acid to TXA_2 is a fundamental pathway contributing to agonist-induced platelet activation and aggregation. TXA_2 is a potent platelet agonist that stimulates its own seven-transmembrane-spanning G-protein-coupled receptor. Many agonists stimulate the release of arachidonic acid from phosphatidylcholine (PC) and phosphatidyletha-

nolamine (PE) in the plasma membrane.[620] Most arachidonic acid is released by the action of PLA_2, but some is also released by: (1) the concerted actions of PLC and DAG kinase, followed by PLA_2, or (2) the action of PLC followed by the action of DAG lipase. PLA_2 is a cytosolic enzyme, with multiple isoforms in platelets.[621] PLA_2 acts on the C2 position of triacylglycerols such as PC and PE to form free arachidonic acid and the resulting lysophospholipid. PLA_2 also converts phosphatidic acid into lysophosphatidic acid, a potent platelet agonist. Some PLA_2 isozymes are activated by the rise in platelet intracellular Ca^{2+} that occurs during agonist-stimulated activation, whereas other isozymes are activated in a Ca^{2+}-independent manner.

Arachidonic acid is subsequently metabolized by prostaglandin H_2 synthase 1 (cyclooxygenase-1 or COX-1) in the dense tubular system, to prostaglandin (PG)G_2, and then to PGH_2.[622] Thromboxane synthase next converts PGH_2 to TXA_2, which is spontaneously and rapidly converted to the inactive metabolite, TXB_2.[623] TXA_2 and its precursor, PGH_2, can both stimulate platelet thromboxane receptors to induce platelet aggregation.[623,624] An inducible cyclooxygenzase enzyme (COX-2) is present in many cells involved in mediating the inflammatory response, but only trace amounts are present in platelets.[625] Cyclooxygenase (COX) inhibitors such as aspirin inhibit platelet function by inhibiting COX-1 and decreasing TXA_2 production.[626,627]

Pharmacologic studies have suggested the existence of two distinct TXA_2 receptor subtypes based on differing affinities for agonist ligands. It appears that the low-affinity binding sites mediate platelet aggregation and granule secretion, whereas the high-affinity sites are associated with platelet shape change.[628] Only one thromboxane A_2 receptor, however, has been cloned to date.[628a] Two alternatively spliced forms of the receptor have been reported,[628a] $TXR\alpha$ cloned from placenta, and $TXR\beta$ cloned from the endothelium, which differ only at the carboxy terminus.[628a] The alternative splicing significantly affects the function of these two receptors, as $TXR\beta$ but not α undergoes agonist-induced internalization.[629] Although both $TXR\alpha$ and $TXR\beta$ mRNA can be detected in platelet lysates, it appears that $TXR\alpha$ is the dominant form.[630] The TXA_2 receptor has been localized to the platelet plasma membrane,[631] and on SDS-polyacrylamide gel electrophoresis it migrates as a broad band of M_r 55,000 to 57,000,[632,633] due to variability in glycosylation.[630] The thromboxane receptor is coupled to $G\alpha q$ and $G\alpha 13$[634,635] and possibly $G\alpha 11$,[636] $G\alpha 12$,[636a] and $G\alpha i2$.[637] Studies of TXA_2 receptor-deficient mice demonstrate that this one gene locus is responsible for most, if not all, biological effects attributed to TXA_2 receptor subtypes.[638] Bleeding times in these mice are prolonged, confirming the importance of this pathway in normal hemostasis. Moreover, platelet aggregation in response to collagen but not ADP is delayed, demonstrating the importance of TXA_2 production in collagen-induced platelet aggregation.

A significant portion of PGH_2/TXA_2-induced platelet aggregation is actually mediated by secreted ADP, since ADP scavenger systems reportedly block aggregation induced by a stable PGH_2/TXA_2 analogue either partially (30 percent)[639] or totally.[640]

Thrombin   Thrombin is derived from the inactive zymogen, prothrombin, which circulates in plasma. When acted upon by the prothrombinase complex (factor Xa, factor Va, Ca^{2+}), assembled on activated platelets and other cells, prothrombin is cleaved into thrombin[641] (see Chap. 112), one of the most potent platelet agonists. The proteolytic activity of thrombin is required for its role as a platelet agonist.[642] Thrombin activates the protease-activated receptor 1 (PAR-1), a seven-transmembrane G-protein-coupled receptor on platelets and other cells,[643,644] by cleaving an extracellular 41 amino acid peptide from the N-terminus of the receptor (Fig. 111-16). Removal of this peptide results in a new amino-terminus, which acts as a "tethered ligand" by binding to another region of PAR-1 to activate the receptor and initiate signal transduction. The 41 amino acid cleavage product of PAR-1 can also induce platelet aggregation by a poorly defined mechanism.[645]

Surprisingly, platelets from PAR-1 knockout mice respond almost normally to thrombin. These unexpected results led to the search for, and discovery of other members of the PAR family, including PAR-3[646] and PAR-4.[647] A full response of platelets to thrombin appears to require at least two thrombin receptors, PAR-1 and PAR-4 on human platelets,[647,648] and PAR-3 and PAR-4 on mouse platelets.[647,649]

When platelets are exposed to subaggregating concentrations of thrombin, they become relatively insensitive to the addition of an aggregating concentration of thrombin, a process termed *homologous desensitization*. Part of this mechanism involves rapid PAR-1 internalization, but other biochemical changes probably are also involved.[650] Trafficking of the thrombin receptor to lysosomes is dictated by sequence in the cytoplasmic tail of PAR.[651]

Thrombin can bind to GPIbα, and platelets from patients lacking the GPIb/IX complex (Bernard-Soulier syndrome) have decreased thrombin-induced platelet aggregation (see Chap. 119). A region on GPIbα with three sulfated tyrosines and a large number of anionic amino acids (with homology to the high-affinity thrombin inhibitor hirudin) contains the thrombin binding site. Despite these data, it is not clear that the binding of thrombin to GPIbα initiates a signal or is of physiologic significance.

Platelet Activating Factor Platelet-activating factor (a mixture of 1-O-hexadecyl-2-acetyl-sn-glycero-3-phosphocholine and 1-O-octadecyl-2-acetyl-sn-glycero-3-phosphocholine[652]) is a phospholipid ether produced by platelets, leukocytes, and other cells. PAF is a potent platelet agonist and proinflammatory mediator.[653] Cellular responses to PAF are mediated by a specific seven-transmembrane, G-protein-coupled receptor.[654,655] PAF induces G-protein-dependent inhibition of adenylyl cyclase and activation of PLC,[656] which causes phosphoinositide turnover, leading to the activation of PKC and an increase in intracellular Ca^{2+}.[655] PAF also indirectly activates PLA_2, which causes release of arachidonic acid from the platelet membrane.[657] All of these effects contribute to the overall platelet response to PAF.

Serotonin Platelets serve as the major storage site in the circulation for serotonin because they have an extensive capacity to take it up actively into dense granules. The release of serotonin from the dense granules during platelet activation may amplify platelet aggregation and granule release. The receptor that mediates serotonin's effects on platelet function has been classified pharmacologically as a 5HT2 receptor,[658] and the 5HT2-receptor-blocking compound ketanserin antagonizes serotonin's stimulatory effects on platelets.[659] The receptor has been cloned from platelets and shown to be essentially identical to the seven-transmembrane, G-protein-coupled, 5-HT2A receptor present in the brain frontal cortex.[660,661] Two naturally occurring amino acid substitutions have been identified in the receptor.[662] Platelets from

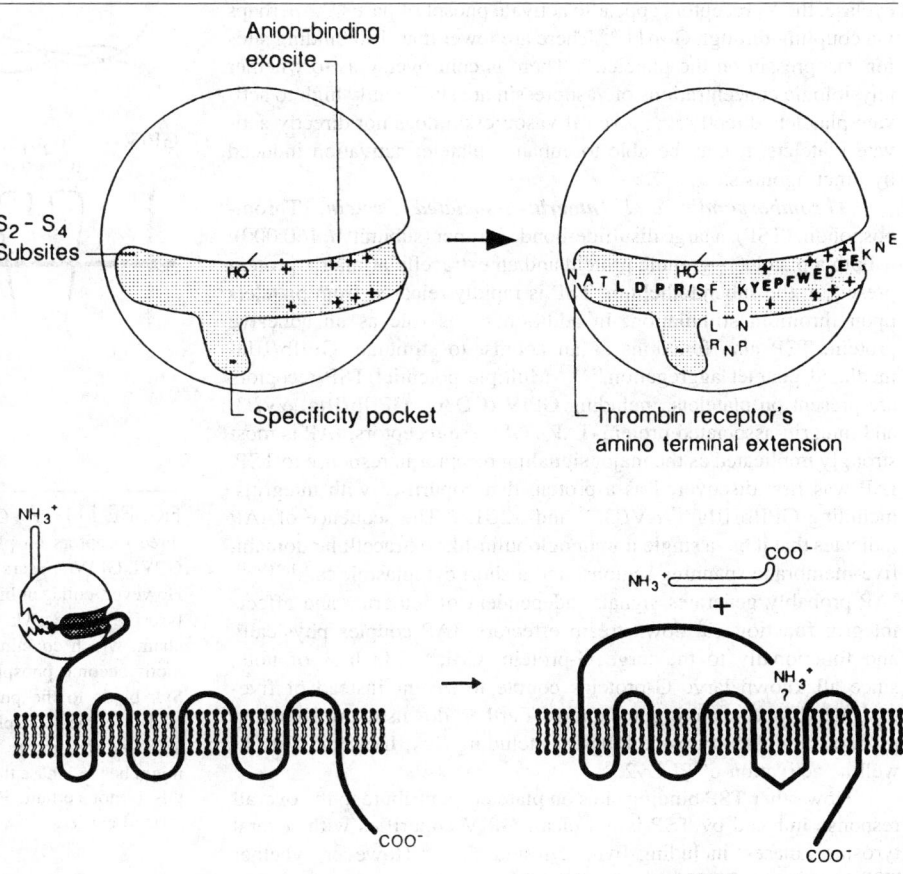

FIGURE 111-16   *Above.* Model for thrombin-protease activated receptor 1 (PAR-1). The receptor's LDPR sequence interacts with thrombin's subsites, and the receptor's YEPFWEDEE sequence binds to thrombin's anion-binding exosite. Thrombin cleaves the receptor between R41 and S42. *Below.* After cleavage, the new amino terminus acts as a tethered ligand and inserts into the membrane, initiating activation. (From Vu et al.[787a] Reprinted by permission from *Nature* (353:674–677). Copyright 1991 Macmillan Magazines Limited.)

patients heterozygous for the H452Y polymorphism have a blunted calcium response when stimulated with serotonin compared to platelets from patients homozygous for H452.[662] Many studies have been performed correlating platelet serotonin transporter activity and 5-HT2A receptors with a number of neuropsychiatric disorders.[663–667] There is some concern, however, about the correlation between 5-HT2A receptors on platelets and those in the brain.[668]

Addition of serotonin in micromolar concentrations to platelets in vitro causes elevation of intracellular calcium, PLC activation, protein phosphorylation, and mild aggregation.[669,670] In whole blood, serotonin does not itself cause platelet aggregation, but it does enhance aggregation induced by ADP and thrombin.[671] Serotonin released from platelets can cause vasoconstriction of blood vessels that have suffered endothelial damage,[672] further promoting thrombus formation. Inhibition of serotonin's action has a favorable effect in animal models of thrombosis and vascular damage, but it is not clear whether the benefit derives from effects on platelet aggregation or vasoconstriction.[673]

Vasopressin Vasopressin interacts with platelets to induce shape change, aggregation, and dense granule release.[674] These events follow an induced rise in intracellular calcium and PLC activation.[675] The platelet binding site is classified pharmacologically as a V_1-type receptor,[676] and radiolabeled vasopressin binds to it with a K_D of 1 to 10 nM.[677] Unlike the case with V_2 receptors that activate adenylate cyclase, the V_1 receptors appear to activate phospholipase C,[678] perhaps via coupling through Gαq11.[679] There are fewer than 100 binding sites for vasopressin on the platelet.[680] There is controversy as to whether physiologic concentrations of vasopressin are sufficiently high to activate platelets directly[681,682]; even if vasopressin does not directly activate platelets, it may be able to enhance platelet activation induced by other agonists.

Thrombospondin and Integrin-Associated Protein Thrombospondin (TSP), a large disulfide-bonded trimer (subunit M_r 160,000), is both a platelet α-granule protein and an extracellular matrix protein present in the subendothelium. TSP is rapidly released from platelets upon thrombin stimulation. In addition to its role as an adhesive protein, TSP also functions as an agonist to stimulate GPIIb/IIIa-mediated platelet aggregation.[683,684] Multiple potential TSP receptors are present on platelets, including GPIV (CD36), GPIIb/IIIa, αVβ3, and integrin-associated protein (IAP). Of these receptors, IAP is most strongly implicated as the major signaling receptor in response to TSP. IAP was first discovered as a protein that copurifies with integrins, including GPIIb/IIIa,[683] αVβ3,[685] and α2β1.[686] The sequence of IAP indicates that it has a single immunoglobulin-like extracellular domain, five-membrane spanning regions, and a short cytoplasmic tail.[102,684,685] IAP probably generates signals independent of integrins and affects integrin function via downstream effectors. IAP couples physically and functionally to the large G-protein, Gαi,[687] which is of note, since all known large G-proteins couple to seven- instead of five-transmembrane spanning receptors. Further downstream signaling probably involves tyrosine kinases, including Syk, Lyn, and Fak, as well as activation of PLCγ2.[683]

How other TSP binding sites on platelets contribute to the overall response induced by TSP is not clear. GPIV copurifies with several tyrosine kinases, including Fyn, Lyn and Yes.[688] However, whether TSP binding to GPIV activates these kinases and whether they then contribute to the observed platelet response is unknown.

Collagen Upon vascular injury, collagens in the subendothelium become exposed to flowing blood and promote both platelet attachment and activation, thereby contributing to normal hemostasis. Collagen is also thought to be one of the most thrombogenic substances in atherosclerotic plaques, and upon plaque rupture is believed to contribute to platelet aggregation and thrombus formation, leading to ischemic damage.[689] The types of collagen present in the subendothelium include: I, III, IV, V, VI, VIII, and XIII,[690] the most abundant being types I and III (more than 95 percent). Under conditions that mimic physiologic blood flow, platelets adhere tightly to collagen types I, III, and IV, weakly to types VI, VII, and VIII, and not at all to type V. However, under static conditions, platelets can adhere to types II and V collagens as well as to the other collagens listed above.[691]

Collagen-induced platelet activation probably involves multiple receptors (Figs. 111-7 and 111-17). The best characterized collagen receptor on platelets is the GPIa/IIa (α2β1) integrin (see "GPIa/IIa" above). The I, or inserted, domain in the Ia (α2) subunit is homologous to a number of collagen-binding domains in other proteins and probably mediates adhesion of the receptor to collagen. Another platelet collagen receptor, which appears to be important in collagen-induced signaling, is GPVI. This M_r 62,000 glycoprotein from the immunoglobulin superfamily[191,692–694] functions in concert with the Fc receptor γ chain (FcRγ), with the latter initiating intracellular signaling.[695] Other collagen receptors on platelets include GPIV (CD36)[510] and an M_r 65,000 protein (GP65).[696] The potential interrelation of all these collagen receptors is unknown, but there is considerable evidence that they probably work in concert, perhaps by assembling intracellular proteins into complexes, since interactions of collagen with both GPIa/IIa (α2β1) and GPVI are required for a full platelet response.[375,697,698]

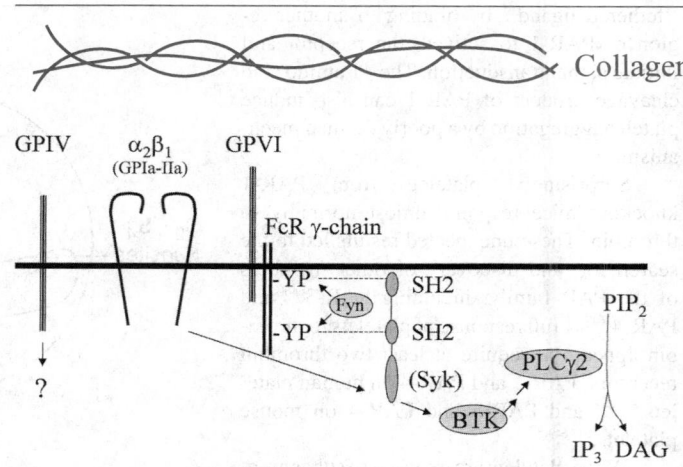

FIGURE 111-17 Collagen activation of platelets. Collagen binds to at least three receptors on platelets, glycoprotein IV (GPIV), GPIa/IIa (α2β1), and GPVI. GPIV appears to play little or no role in collagen activation of platelets. However, collagen binding to both α2β1 and GPVI is required to activate the tyrosine kinase, Syk. GPVI is physically and functionally coupled to the FcRγ chain, which contains an ITAM motif. The tyrosines (Y) within the ITAM motif become phosphorylated (P), most likely by Fyn. The tyrosine kinase Syk binds to the phosphorylated ITAM motif through SH2 domains. Syk itself becomes phosphorylated (probably by Fyn or Lyn tyrosine kinases) and activated, leading to the activation of Bruton's tyrosine kinase (BTK). BTK might be the kinase that directly phosphorylates and activates PLCγ2, although this is not certain. PLCγ2 hydrolyzes PIP$_2$, forming IP3 and DAG as described earlier.

Glycoprotein VI exists in a stable physical complex with the FcRγ chain. In GPVI-deficient platelets, the FcRγ chain is also absent.[475] The addition of either collagen or an antibody that can cross-link GPVI induces tyrosine phosphorylation of the FcRγ chain.[475] The kinases contributing to this event are likely to be the nonreceptor kinases Fyn and/or Lyn.[699] Tyrosine phosphorylation of the immune-receptor tyrosine-based activation motif (ITAM) on the FcRγ chain increases the affinity of the ITAM for SH2 domains, resulting in the recruitment of proteins with SH2 domains to the FcRγ chain. The nonreceptor tyrosine kinase Syk contains two adjacent SH2 domains and a tyrosine kinase domain. In platelets from normal mice, Syk physically associates with the FcRγ chain and becomes phosphorylated and activated after collagen stimulation,[475] whereas in platelets from mice lacking FcRγ chain, collagen is unable to induce Syk phosphorylation and activation.[695] Similarly, in platelets lacking GPVI or in platelets in which the GPIa/IIa (α2β1) integrin is blocked, collagen-induced Syk phosphorylation is also inhibited, demonstrating that GPVI, GPIa/IIa (α2β1), and Syk all participate in the platelet response to collagen. The β subunit of the GPIa/IIa (α2β1) receptor also has tyrosines spaced in a manner reminiscent of an ITAM motif, and thus it is possible that Syk might also associate with this collagen receptor. In addition to Syk,[700] Src[701] also becomes tyrosine phosphorylated in response to collagen. Although Src is an abundant kinase in platelets, its role in platelet signaling is unclear, since mice lacking Src do not suffer from any obvious bleeding disorder.[702] Syk, on the other hand, appears to play a critical role in collagen activation of platelets, since platelets from mice lacking Syk do not aggregate or undergo secretion in response to collagen.[695]

Collagen stimulation of platelets also results in tyrosine phosphorylation and activation of PLCγ2,[703] and, as discussed above, activation of this enzyme causes phosphoinositide hydrolysis, leading to GPIIb/

IIIa activation. PLCγ2 activation occurs downstream of Syk, as evidenced by the findings that collagen is unable to activate PLCγ2 in platelets pretreated with a Syk-selective inhibitor[697] or in platelets from Syk knock-out mice.[695] It is unknown whether Syk activates PLCγ2 directly, but Bruton's tyrosine kinase (BTK) might be positioned between Syk and PLCγ2 because patients lacking BTK not only exhibit the B-cell deficiency X-linked agammaglobulinaemia but also show reduced platelet responsiveness to collagen and diminished phosphorylation of PLCγ2.[704]

GPIV (CD36) can also bind collagen and antibodies to GPIV partially inhibit platelet adhesion to collagen.[704a] There is currently no evidence that GPIV contributes to collagen-induced signaling in platelets, since platelets from patients lacking GPIV respond normally to collagen.[704b]

Platelets stimulated with collagen exhibit several distinct responses. While elevated cAMP levels normally inhibit platelet aggregation, collagen-stimulated platelets are relatively resistant to inhibition by cAMP.[705] This may be related to the fact that collagen stimulates the PLCγ isotype, which is insensitive to cAMP-mediated inhibition, whereas other agonists such as thrombin stimulate PLCβ, which is inhibited by cAMP. Another difference has been noted with the phosphatase inhibitor, phenylarsine oxide, which inhibits collagen, but not thrombin or ADP-induced platelet aggregation.[706] This suggests that one or more phosphatases are critical in collagen-induced platelet aggregation.

Von Willebrand Factor—GPIb/IX/V   The GPIb/IX/V complex functions as a signaling receptor upon vWF binding, resulting in platelet activation and GPIIb/IIIa-mediated aggregation. Thus, ristocetin-mediated interaction of vWF with platelets results in PIP_2 metabolism, activation of PKC, and an increase in intracellular Ca^{2+}. Shear forces can also initiate signaling through the binding of vWF to GPIb/IX/V.[707] GPIb/IX/V signaling causes arachidonic acid to be released and metabolized to form TXA_2. These proaggregatory events are specifically inhibited by monoclonal antibodies that recognize GPIb, but not antibodies to GPIIb/IIIa.[708] This signaling appears to be mediated in part by an M_r 29,000 protein termed 14-3-3ζ that binds directly to the cytoplasmic domains of both GPIbα and GPIbβ and may have PLA_2-related properties[709,710] (Fig. 111-9). The binding site for 14-3-3ζ on GPIbα has been mapped to the last 15 residues of the C-terminus of the cytoplasmic domain, with the last 5 residues being especially important.[711] Protein 14-3-3ζ exists as a dimer, allowing it to link GPIb molecules.[712] The helix I region of 14-3-3ζ (residues 202–231) is required for binding to GPIbα, and another region binds the serine/threonine kinase c-RAF,[712] suggesting a direct link to the Raf/MEK/MAPK signaling pathway.

The GPIb/IX/V complex also appears to be involved in transmitting at least one cAMP-dependent inhibitory signal. Thus, elevated cAMP, which activates protein kinase A, induces phosphorylation of GPIbβ on serine 166.[713] Elevated cAMP also normally inhibits agonist-induced platelet actin polymerization. However, in platelets from patients with Bernard-Soulier syndrome, which lack GPIb/IX/V, actin polymerization proceeds normally after collagen stimulation, even when cAMP is elevated, suggesting that cAMP-mediated phosphorylation of GPIbβ may be required for the cAMP-mediated inhibition.[714]

Lysolipid Phosphate Activators: Lysophosphatidic Acid and Sphingosine-1-Phosphate   Platelets possess cell surface receptors for the lysolipid phosphates, lysophosphatidic acid (LPA)[715] and sphingosine-1-phosphate,[716] which stimulate platelet aggregation. The receptor(s) for these lipids are believed to be members of the endothelial differentiation gene (Edg) family of G-protein-coupled receptors; they can activate PLC and initiate tyrosine kinase phosphorylation.[715,717] Lysolipid phosphates are synthesized by both *de novo* and agonist-stimulated pathways.[718] Platelets accumulate sphingosine-1-phosphate

due to a lack of sphingosine-1-phosphate lyase activity and high levels of sphingosine-1-phosphate kinase activity. One pathway for LPA formation involves agonist-stimulated production of phosphatidic acid, either by PLD or the sequential actions of PLC and DAG kinase. Phosphatidic acid in the outer portion of the plasma membrane or in platelet-derived microvesicles is hydrolyzed by secretory PLA_2 ($sPLA_2$) to LPA,[719,720] which then can act on its extracellular receptors to induce platelet aggregation. Mild oxidation of LDL generates LPA, and the LPA component of oxidized LDL in the lipid-rich thrombogenic core of atherosclerotic lesions exposed during plaque rupture may be a potent stimulus for platelet activation.[721] LPA levels in plasma are approximately $0.2\ \mu M$, whereas they are $10\ \mu M$ in serum, reflecting mainly the secretion of LPA-precursors by activated platelets.[712] Phosphatidic acid in platelet-derived microparticles is believed to be a substrate for $sPLA_2$ and the principle source for plasma LPA. Plasma LPA circulates bound to albumin, activates endothelial cells, stimulates fibroblast proliferation and smooth-muscle cell contraction, and is a monocyte chemoattractant. LPA is degraded by cell-associated phosphatases located on platelets and other cells. Thus, LPA activates platelets and activated platelets at sites of vascular injury may provide a source of LPA to recruit monocytes and promote smooth-muscle cell accumulation and extracellular matrix deposition.

ADDITIONAL INTERMEDIATE SIGNALING MOLECULES

Calcium   Elevation of intracellular Ca^{2+} has a multitude of effects on platelet physiology. The concentration of Ca^{2+} in resting platelets (100 to 500 n*M*) is very low compared to the plasma concentration of Ca^{2+} (about 2 m*M*). Exposure of platelets to most agonists is accompanied by a rapid, transient rise in the intracellular free Ca^{2+} concentration to micromolar levels, followed by a quick return to normal resting levels. The cytoplasmic Ca^{2+} concentration at any given time is a result of the rates of passive Ca^{2+} influx, active Ca^{2+} extrusion across the plasma membrane, and both active release and/or uptake of Ca^{2+} by the dense tubular system (DTS), which is a Ca^{2+} storage depot in platelets analogous to the sarcoplasmic reticulum in muscle. Active Ca^{2+} extrusion and uptake of Ca^{2+} are mediated by several pumps (see Fig. 111-7). The cytosolic pool of Ca^{2+} has a rapid turnover due to a plasma membrane Na^{2+}/Ca^{2+} antiporter, whereas the dense tubular system contains a more slowly exchanging pool regulated by a Ca^{2+}/Mg^{2+} ATPase, a pump that also appears to be located in the plasma membrane.[722] During agonist stimulation, most Ca^{2+} enters the platelet cytosolic compartment through receptor-operated calcium channels (reviewed in Geiger and Walter[723]) in the plasma membrane. Release of intracellular Ca^{2+} from the DTS storage sites also occurs rapidly in response to agonist stimulation, due in large part to IP_3 that is generated as part of the phosphoinositide cycle.[724] GPIIb/IIIa may also participate in Ca^{2+} entry.[725]

Elevations of Ca^{2+} induce numerous downstream events, including activation of Ca^{2+}-sensitive forms of PLA_2[726] and PKC[727]; calmodulin-dependent enzymes such as myosin light-chain kinase, which phosphorylates myosin light chain[728] and promotes cytoskeletal rearrangements required for platelet shape change; and gelsolin, which facilitates actin severing and rearrangement, secretion, and aggregation. In addition, Ca^{2+} probably plays a direct role in the membrane fusion events that result in degranulation and the release reaction. Calcium-dependent proteases or calpains also become activated and play an important role in post aggregation events (see below).

Phosphoinositide 3-Kinases   Phosphoinositide 3 kinases (PI3 kinases) are a family of lipid kinases that phosphorylate the D-3 hydroxy group of the myo-inositol ring of phosphoinositides (reviewed in Zhang et al[729] and Rittenhouse[730]). Class I PI3 kinases are heterodimeric proteins containing both adaptor and catalytic subunits, which utilize phosphatidylinositol (PtdIns), PtdIns(4)P, and PtdIns(4,5)P_2 as substrates to form PtdIns(3)P, PtdIns(3,4)P_2, and PtdIns(3,4,5)P_3 respectively. Platelets contain two isoforms of PI3 kinase, designated *class Ia* and *class Ib*, that have distinct subunits and regulatory features. The catalytic subunit of class Ia PI3 kinases is an M_r 110,000 to 120,000 protein; the adaptor subunit, p85, has two SH2 domains, a breakpoint cluster region homology domain, a proline-rich region, and a single SH3 domain. Members of this class of PI3 kinases possess intrinsic serine-threonine protein kinase activity in addition to lipid kinase activity, and they appear to be regulated, at least in part, by binding of the p85 subunit to tyrosine-phosphorylated proteins. Following platelet activation, PI3 kinase can be coimmunoprecipitated with the tyrosine kinases Src and Syk. Class Ib PI3 kinases have been isolated from platelets and neutrophils and contain a catalytic subunit, p110γ, that is activated by the $\beta\gamma$ subunit of heterodimer G proteins. Both isoforms of PI3 kinase appear to associate with the cytoskeleton in agonist-activated platelets.

In platelets, 3-phosphorylated phosphoinositides are produced in response to a variety of agonists, including thrombin, TXA$_2$, LPA, ADP, and collagen, and may mediate early signaling events that precede GPIIb/IIIa activation as well as late events involved in stabilizing fibrinogen binding and platelet aggregation.[729-731] Thrombin stimulates rapid accumulation of PtdIns(3,4,5)P_3 and PtdIns(3,4)P_2[732] and late production of PtdIns(3,4)P_2; the latter requires fibrinogen binding to GPIIb/IIIa and calpain activity.[733] Collagen promotes the association of the p85 adaptor subunit via its SH2 domains with tyrosine-phosphorylated forms of FcRγ chain and the regulatory protein, linker-for-activator of T cells (LAT), and may thereby modulate PI 3-kinase activity.[734] FcγRIIA-induced platelet aggregation required PI3 kinase activity, which appears to be upstream of PLCγ2 in the pathway.[735]

Many of the biological actions of PI3 kinases are mediated by their phospholipid products, which bind to specific sequences in proteins. The pleckstrin homology (PH) domains (about 100 amino acids long) present in pleckstrin and other platelet proteins involved in signal transduction, recognize either PI(3,4)P_2 or PI(3,4,5)P_3 (reviewed in Leevers, Vanhaesebroeck, and Waterfield[736]). Binding of PI(3,4,5)P_3 to the amino terminal PH domain in PLCγ enhances its activity.[737] PI(3,4,5)P_3 binding to PH domains in BTK[738] targets BTK to the plasma membrane, where it is further phosphorylated and activated.[739] PI(3,4)P_2 or PI(3,4,5)P_3 binding to the PH domains in the serine/threonine kinase AKT (or protein kinase B) changes the conformation of AKT, permitting it to become activated by phosphorylation on serine and threonine by AKT-kinase (PDK1).[740,741] AKT activation is biphasic, occurring before and after platelet aggregation[733]; AKT may therefore play multiple roles in platelet activation.[733]

Small G Proteins   Some members of the Ras superfamily of small GTPases modulate integrin receptor activation.[742] Small GTPases, like their large G-protein counterparts, cycle between a resting, GDP-bound state, and an active, GTP-bound state. In their active state, small GTPases can interact with, and activate downstream signaling molecules, thus acting as molecular switches. One small GTPase, R-Ras, has been shown to activate GPIIb/IIIa when both are expressed in CHO cells—cells that are normally unable to activate this integrin by a signal transduction cascade.[743]

The small G-protein, RhoA has an established role in stress fiber formation in nucleated cells.[744] In platelets RhoA is required for vinculin-dependent focal adhesion formation in platelets adherent to fibrinogen[745], but not for GPIIb/IIIa activation.[745]

Preliminary data suggest that a third small G-protein, H-Ras, may function to suppress integrin activation.[746] H-Ras in other cells is often part of a pathway involving the serine/threonine kinases Raf, MEK and MAPK. Whether a Ras/Raf/MEK/MAPK pathway is inhibitory in platelets is not entirely clear, however, since a soluble MEK inhibitor attenuates rather than enhances platelet aggregation to low concentra-

tions of collagen and arachidonic acid.[747] Moreover, Ras is activated by platelet agonists[748], so the exact role of Ras in platelet activation remains to be determined. Based on studies in nucleated cells, PEA-15, a small protein that contains a death effector domain (DED),[749] may act in concert with an R-Ras dependent pathway, to oppose the inhibitory effects of H-Ras on integrin function. Thus it appears that the small G-proteins have the capacity to up- and down-regulate the activation state of GPIIb/IIIa.

CALCIUM-DEPENDENT PROTEASES (CALPAINS)

After ligand binding, integrin clustering, and platelet aggregation, calcium-dependent proteases or calpains become activated. Calpain activation also requires a rise in intracellular calcium. The most important and well-studied class of calpains in platelets are the μ-calpains, which are activated by micromolar concentrations of calcium, although m-calpains, which require millimolar concentrations of calcium for activation, also exist. Each form of calpain consists of an M_r 80,000 catalytic subunit paired with an M_r 30,000 subunit. Activated μ-calpains cleave numerous molecules in cells that affect platelet function, including actin binding protein (releasing GPIb, talin, and the cytoplasmic domain of GPIIIa from the membrane skeleton), and some forms of PKC (reviewed in[250]). In addition, calpain appears to be upstream of, and able to induce, the activation of the small G-proteins Rac and RhoA.[250] These small G-proteins have profound effects on cytoskeletal structure, Rac being involved in lamellipodia formation[750] and Rho being linked to stress fiber formation.[744] Thus calpains, by their effects on structural and signaling molecules, appear to affect the signaling and cytoskeletal rearrangements that occur following platelet aggregation.

MECHANISM OF ACTIVATION OF GPIIb/IIIa IN RESPONSE TO AGONIST-INDUCED SIGNAL TRANSDUCTION

The cytoplasmic domains of GPIIb and GPIIIa appear to control the activation state of the GPIIb/IIIa receptor. When recombinant GPIIb/IIIa that either lacks the GPIIb cytoplasmic domain entirely, or contains mutations in the highly conserved GFFKR sequence in the cytoplasmic domain is expressed in a cell line, the GPIIb/IIIa is in an active conformation that can bind ligand.[751,752] This activation probably occurs because of a disruption of an interaction between the two cytoplasmic domains and/or with associated proteins that maintains the integrin in a resting conformation. Evidence for an interaction between the GPIIb and GPIIIa cytoplasmic domains comes from studies suggesting that there is a salt bridge between Arg995 in GPIIb and Asp723 in GPIIIa[751] and that peptides from specific regions of the GPIIb and GPIIIa cytoplasmic domains (amino acids 999–1008 of GPIIb and 721–740 of GPIIIa) can bind to each other.[753] Interestingly, the GPIIb and GPIIIa peptide complex also binds Ca^{2+}.[753] Finally, introduction into platelets of a lipid-modified GPIIb cytoplasmic domain peptide (amino acids 989–995) activates GPIIb/IIIa and initiates platelet activation and TXA$_2$ formation.[754] Presumably this peptide displaces the normal GPIIb from its complex with GPIIIa, and thus these data support the hypothesis that disruption of the normal interaction between the cytoplasmic domains of GPIIb and GPIIIa facilitates integrin activation.

The state of GPIIb/IIIa activation may also be affected by molecules associated with the integrin. Thus, overexpression of the GPIIIa cytoplasmic domain in cells suppresses integrin activation, presumably because it competes with the normal GPIIIa for binding of molecules necessary to induce the activated state. CD98 may be one of the molecules involved in this process.[755] The interaction of GPIIb/IIIa with cytoskeletal elements has been proposed to maintain the integrin in a resting conformation; in this model, platelet activation releases these constraints and allows GPIIb/IIIa to assume its active conformation. Numerous molecules have been identified that appear to associate directly with the GPIIb or GPIIIa cytoplasmic domains or with other parts of the integrin. For example, CIB, an M_r 22,000 Ca^{2+} binding protein associates with the GPIIb cytoplasmic domain and may play a role in ligand-induced signaling through GPIIb/IIIa.[755a,755b,756] $\beta3$-endonexin[757] and the cytoskeletal proteins talin[758] and myosin[759] have been reported to bind to the GPIIIa cytoplasmic domain, and $\beta3$-endonexin[757] and talin[760] have been reported to activate GPIIb/IIIa. In addition, integrin-associated protein, a five-transmembrane-spanning molecule,[685] CD9[761,762] and CD151 (PETA-3),[763] members of the tetraspanin receptor family, likely associate with other portions of GPIIb/IIIa and coisolate with the integrin. Thrombospondin binding to IAP[683,685] and antibody-mediated cross-linking of either CD9 or CD151 to the platelet Fc receptor cause platelet activation[764] with resultant activation of GPIIb/IIIa.

SIGNALING EVENTS INDUCED BY LIGAND BINDING TO GPIIb/IIIa AND THE EARLY PHASES OF PLATELET AGGREGATION THAT LEAD TO IRREVERSIBLE AGGREGATION AND CLOT RETRACTION

Platelet aggregation is commonly described as progressing through two phases, an initial reversible aggregation phase, which is often the response observed with low concentrations of agonists, followed by a stronger, irreversible phase. The irreversible phase of aggregation correlates with TXA_2 production and platelet secretion of ADP. Fibrinogen binding to GPIIb/IIIa and the platelet-platelet contacts that occur during the initial phase of aggregation initiate specific signal transduction events, resulting in positive feedback loops that promote irreversible aggregation, maintain secretion, and initiate later events like clot retraction.[765]

Fibrinogen or vWf binding to the extracellular region of GPIIb/IIIa transmits long-range conformational changes to the integrin cytoplasmic domains that induce signaling from outside the platelet to inside the platelet (outside-in signaling).[766,767] These conformational changes, along with integrin clustering,[768] are likely to be the bases for outside-in signal transduction through GPIIb/IIIa, perhaps by altering the association of the cytoplasmic domains with one another and presumably initiating recruitment of proteins with enzymatic acitivity into cytoplasmic complexes.

When platelets are aggregated in response to one of multiple agonists, the GPIIIa cytoplasmic domain becomes phosphorylated on tyrosine.[759,769] Two sites of potential tyrosine phosphorylation exist on the GPIIIa cytoplasmic domain, and both may be utilized. Several molecules have been identified that bind specifically to the tyrosine-phosphorylated cytoplasmic domain of GPIIIa. A synthetic GPIIIa cytoplasmic domain peptide containing phosphate groups on the two candidate tyrosines binds to the contractile protein myosin,[759] and this interaction may facilitate the transmission of cytoskeletal tension from inside the platelet to outside and thus initiate clot retraction (see above). Recombinant, mutated GPIIIa that cannot be phosphorylated is unable to support extensive clot retraction when expressed in a cell line.[759] Other proteins that bind to the diphosphorylated GPIIIa cytoplasmic domain include the adapter protein SHC,[770] which also becomes tyrosine-phosphorylated during platelet aggregation.[770] Therefore, it is possible that SHC may link diphosphorylated GPIIIa to the Ras/Raf/MAPK pathway.[770,771]

Mice containing mutated GPIIIa molecules that cannot be phosphorylated exhibit a mild bleeding disorder as evidenced by occasional rebleeding of tail cuts. Moreover platelets derived from these mice form abnormally loose thrombi when activated by shear forces.[765]

Other GPIIIa cytoplasmic domain binding proteins have been described, including skelemin, a member of a family of proteins that regulate myosin,[772] and talin, which has binding sites on both GPIIb

and GPIIIa, providing another potential linkage of GPIIb/IIIa to cytoskeletal elements.[758]

Some signaling events that occur downstream of GPIIb/IIIa require only integrin clustering, whereas other events require clustering, ligand binding, and/or platelet aggregation. For example, the tyrosine kinase Syk becomes activated in response to GPIIb/IIIa clustering, independent of cytoskeletal assembly, whereas activation of the tyrosine kinase FAK requires integrin clustering, ligand binding to GPIIb/IIIa, and cytoskeletal assembly.[772a] Activation of Syk downstream of GPIIb/IIIa leads to phosphorylation of Vav1, a guanine nucleotide exchange factor for Rac, and lamellipodia formation in a cell line. Syk and Vav1 cooperate to activate Jun N-terminal kinase or JNK, extracellular-signal-regulated kinase 2 (ERK2) and AKT.[772a] These pathways are also likely to be involved in postaggregation events in the platelet.

INHIBITORY PATHWAYS IN PLATELETS

Prostaglandins   Prostaglandins that inhibit platelet activation include prostaglandin PGE_2 and PGI_2 (also called *prostacyclin*) (reviewed in Majerus[773] and Moncada and Whittle[774]). In the vasculature, the endothelium produces PGI_2 and PGE_2, which help to maintain vascular patency.[775] Inhibition is initiated by the binding of these prostaglandins to their own specific G-protein-coupled receptors. Prostaglandin receptor occupancy converts $G\alpha s$ to the GTP-bound, active form, which activates adenylyl cyclase. Adenylyl cyclase catalyzes the formation of cAMP. The exact amount of cAMP present in the cell is also determined by its rate of breakdown by phosphodiesterase (PDE). Therefore, agents that inhibit PDE such as theophilline, caffeine, and the drug cilostazol also elevate cAMP levels in platelets and other cells. Cyclic AMP then activates protein kinase A, which phosphorylates specific target proteins. The exact mechanism by which PKA inhibits platelet activation probably involves more than one pathway. One mechanism may involve phosphorylation and inhibition of the IP_3 receptor, which would repress agonist-induced intracellular Ca^{2+}-mobilization.[776] Phosphoinositide metabolism is also affected, since the activities of both PLC and PLA_2 are suppressed.[777] PGE_1 phosphorylation of $GPIb\beta$ also inhibits actin polymerization (see above). Moreover, cAMP also inhibits Raf kinase.[778] Finally, the small G-protein, Rap 1b, is phosphorylated by PKA.[779] However, the functions of Raf kinase and Rap1b in platelets are unclear.

Nitric Oxide   Nitric oxide (NO) is synthesized from L-arginine by NO synthase in endothelial cells, platelets, and other cells. The formation of NO is enhanced at sites of shear stress and by platelet agonists (e.g., thrombin or ADP),[780] and it readily diffuses into platelets.[781,782] Similar to PGI_2 or PGE_2, NO pretreatment of platelets inhibits platelet activation and can reverse platelet aggregation soon after initiation. However, NO works not by elevating cAMP but instead by increasing cGMP.[783] NO synthase activity in platelets increases during platelet activation, suggesting that NO production is a normal mechanism to limit platelet aggregation. NO and PGI_2 act together synergistically to inhibit platelet activation.[784]

CD39 (ATP Diphosphohydrolase; ADPase)   Vascular endothelium regulates platelet function by producing prostacyclin and nitric oxide, as well as by expressing CD39, a plasma-membrane-associated ATP diphosphohydrolase (ATPDase; ecto-ADPase) that converts extracellular ATP and ADP to AMP.[42,785] CD39 limits the platelet-activating effects of ADP released by damaged tissues, red blood cells, and activated platelets; furthermore, AMP generated by CD39 is degraded by ecto-5' nucleotidase to adenosine, an antagonist of ADP-induced platelet activation. CD39 is an M_r 95,000 cell-surface glycoprotein expressed on endothelial cells, activated NK cells, B cells, and T cells. It contains two putative transmembrane regions separated by an extracellular domain with six glycosylation sites and apyrase-like regions that confer the ATPDase activity. A soluble recombinant form of CD39 inhibits platelet aggregation and recruitment in vitro and may have potential as an antithrombotic agent in vivo.[608]

REFERENCES

1. White JG: Anatomy and structural organization of the platelet, in *Hemostasis and Thrombosis: Basic Principles and Clinical Practice*, edited by RW Colman, J Hirsh, VJ Marder, EW Salzman, 3rd ed, p 397. JB Lippincott, Philadelphia, 1993.

2. Coller BS: Biochemical and electrostatic considerations in primary platelet aggregation. *Ann NY Acad Sci* 416:693, 1984.

3. Schick PK: Megakaryocyte and platelet lipids, in *Hemostasis and Thrombosis: Basic Principles and Clinical Practice*, edited by RW Colman, J Hirsh, VJ Marder, EW Salzman, 3rd ed, p 574. JB Lippincott, Philadelphia, 1993.

4. Walsh PN, Schmaier AH: Platelet-coagulant protein interactions, in *Hemostasis and Thrombosis: Basic Principles and Clinical Practice*, edited by RW Colman, J Hirsh, VJ Marder, EW Salzman, 3rd ed, p 629. JB Lippincott, Philadelphia, 1993.

5. Sims PJ, Faioni EM, Wiedmer T, Shattil SJ: Complement proteins C5b-9 cause release of membrane vesicles from the platelet surface that are enriched in the membrane receptor for coagulation factor Va and express prothrombinase activity. *J Biol Chem* 263:18205, 1988.

6. Sims PJ, Wiedmer T, Esmon CT, et al: Assembly of the platelet prothrombinase complex is linked to vesiculation on the platelet plasma membrane. Studies in Scott syndrome: an isolated defect in platelet procoagulant activity. *J Biol Chem* 264:137, 1989.

7. Bevers EM, Tilly RHJ, Senden JMG, et al: Exposure of endogenous phosphatidylserine at the outer surface of stimulated platelets is reversed by restoration of aminophospholipid translocase activity. *Biochemistry* 28:2382, 1989.

8. Tuszynski GP, Mauco GP, Koshy A, et al: The platelet cytoskeleton contains elements of the prothrombinase complex. *J Biol Chem* 259:6947, 1984.

9. Comfurius P, Bevers EM, Zwaal RFA: The involvement of cytoskeleton in the regulation of transbilayer movement of phospholipids in human blood platelets. *Biochim Biophys Acta* 815:143, 1985.

10. Hartwig JH, Barkalow K, Azim A, Italiano J: The elegant platelet: signals controlling actin assembly. *Thromb Haemost* 82:392, 1999.

11. Fox JE: The platelet cytoskeleton. *Thromb Haemost* 70:884, 1993.

12. Fox JEB: Linkage of a membrane skeleton to integral membrane glycoproteins in human platelets. Identification of one of the glycoproteins as glycoprotein Ib. *J Clin Invest* 76:1673, 1985.

13. Nurden P, Heilmann E, Pannocchia A, Nurden AT: Two-way trafficking of membrane glycoproteins on thrombin-activated human platelets. *Semin Hematol* 31:240, 1994.

14. Cramer EM, Norol F, Guichard J, et al: Ultrastructure of platelet formation by human megakaryocytes cultured with the Mpl ligand. *Blood* 89:2336, 1997.

15. Castle AG, Crawford N: Platelet microtubule subunit proteins. *Thromb Haemost* 42:1630, 1979.

16. Crawford N, Scrutton MC: Biochemistry of the blood platelet, in *Haemostis and Thrombosis*, 3 ed, p 89. Churchill Livingstone, England, 1994.

17. Hartwig JH: Platelet morphology, in *Thrombosis and Hemorrhage*, 2nd ed, Loscalzo J, Schafer AI (editors). p 207. Williams & Wilkins, Baltimore, 1999.

18. Kenney DM, Linck RW: The cystoskeleton of unstimulated blood platelets: structure and composition of the isolated marginal microtubular band. *J Cell Sci* 78:1, 1985.

19. Sheetz MP: Microtubule motor complexes moving membranous organelles. *Cell Struct Funct* 21:369, 1996.

20. Daniel JL: Platelet contractile proteins, in *Hemostasis and Thrombosis: Basic Principles and Clinical Practice*, edited by RW Colman, J Hirsh, VJ Marder, EW Salzman, 3rd ed, p 557. JB Lippincott, Philadelphia, 1993.

21. Van den BH, de Vet EC, Zomer AW: The role of peroxisomes in ether lipid synthesis. Back to the roots of PAF. *Adv Exp Med Biol* 416:33, 1996.

22. Wanders RJ, van Weringh G, Schrakamp G, Tager JM, van den BH, Schutgens RB: Deficiency of acyl-CoA:dihydroxyacetone phosphate acyltransferase in thrombocytes of Zellweger patients: a simple postnatal diagnostic test. *Clin Chim Acta* 151:217, 1985.

23. Van den BH, Schrakamp G, Hardeman D, Zomer AW, Wanders RJ, Schutgens RB: Ether lipid synthesis and its deficiency in peroxisomal disorders. *Biochimie* 75:183, 1993.

24. Holmsen H: Platelet secretion and energy metabolism, in *Hemostasis and Thrombosis: Basic Principles and Clinical Practice*, edited by RW Colman, J Hirsh, VJ Marder, EW Salzman, 3rd ed, p 524. JB Lippincott, Philadelphia, 1993.

25. Schapira AH: Mitochondrial dysfunction in neurodegenerative disorders. *Biochim Biophys Acta* 1366:225, 1998.

26. Lenaz G, Bovina C, Castelluccio C, et al: Mitochondrial complex I defects in aging. *Mol Cell Biochem* 174:329, 1997.

27. Holmsen H, Kaplan KL, Dangelmaier CA: Differential energy requirements for platelet responses: a simultaneous study of aggregation three secretory processes, arachidonate liberation, phosphatidylinositol turnover and phosphatidate production. *Biochem J* 208:9, 1982.

28. Verhoeven AJM, Mommersteeg ME, Akkerman JWN: Quantification of energy consumption in platelets during thrombin-induced aggregation and secretion: tight coupling between platelet responses and the increment in energy consumption. *Biochem J* 221:777, 1984.

29. Nieuwenhuis HK, van Osterhout JJG, Rozemuller E, van Iwaarden F, Sixma JJ: Studies with a monoclonal antibody against activated platelets: evidence that a secreted 53,000 molecular weight lysosome-like granule protein is exposed on the surface of activated platelets in the circulation. *Blood* 70:838, 1987.

30. Abrams C, Shattil SJ: Immunological detection of activated platelets in clinical disorders. *Thromb Haemost* 65:467, 1991.

31. Castellot JJ, Favreau LV, Karnovsky MJ, Rosenberg RD: Inhibition of vascular smooth muscle cell growth by endothelial cell derived heparin. Possible role of a platelet endoglucosidase. *J Biol Chem* 257:11256, 1982.

32. McNicol A, Israels SJ: Platelet dense granules: structure, function and implications for Haemostis. *Thromb Res* 95:1, 1999.

33. Ugurbil K, Holmsen H, Shulman RG: Adenine nucleotide storage pools and secretion in platelets as studied by 31P nuclear magnetic resonance. *Proc Natl Acad Sci USA* 76:2227, 1979.

34. Ugurbil K, Fukami MH, Holmsen H: 31P-NMR studies of nucleotide and amine storage in the dense granules of pig platelets. *Biochemistry* 23:4097, 1984.

35. Oh J, Bailin T, Fukai K, et al: Positional cloning of a gene for Hermansky-Pudlak syndrome, a disorder of cytoplasmic organelles. *Nat Genet* 14:300, 1996.

36. Nagle DL, Karim MA, Woolf EA, et al: Identification and mutation analysis of the complete gene for Chediak-Higashi syndrome. *Nat Genet* 14:307, 1996.

37. FitzGerald GA: Dipyridamole. *N Engl J Med* 316:1247, 1987.

38. Marcus AJ, Safier LB, Hajjar KA, et al: Inhibition of platelet function by an aspirin-insensitive endothelial cell ADPase. Thromboregulation by endothelial cells. *J Clin Invest* 88:1690, 1991.

39. Naik UP, Kornecki E, Ehrlich YH: Phosphorylation and dephosphorylation of human platelet surface proteins by an ecto-protein kinase/phosphatase system. *Biochim Biophys Acta* 1092:256, 1991.

40. Kalafatis M, Rand MD, Jenny RJ, Ehrlich YH, Mann KG: Phosphorylation of factor Va and factor VIIIa by activated platelets. *Blood* 81:704, 1993.

41. Hatmi M, Gavaret JM, Elalamy I, Vargaftig BB, Jacquemin C: Evidence for cAMP-dependent platelet ectoprotein kinase activity that phosphorylates platelet glycoprotein IV (CD36). *J Biol Chem* 271:24776, 1996.

42. Marcus AJ, Broekman MJ, Drosopoulos JH, et al: The endothelial cell ecto-ADPase responsible for inhibition of platelet function is CD39. *J Clin Invest* 99:1351, 1997.

43. Harrison P, Cramer EM: Platelet α granules. *Blood Rev* 7:52, 1993.

44. Hayward CP, Furmaniak-Kazmierczak E, Cieutat AM, et al: Factor V is complexed with multimerin in resting platelet lysates and colocalizes with multimerin in platelet alpha-granules. *J Biol Chem* 270:19217, 1995.

45. George JN: Platelet immunoglobulin G: its significance for the evaluation of thrombocytopenia and for understanding the origin of alpha-granule protein. *Blood* 76:859, 1990.

46. George JN: Platelet IgG: measurement, interpretation, and clinical significance. *Prog Hemost Thromb* 10:97, 1991.

47. Niewiarowski S, Holt JC, Cook JJ: Biochemistry and physiology of secreted platelet proteins, in *Hemostasis and Thrombosis: Basic Princi-*

ples and Clinical Practice, edited by RW Colman, J Hirsh, VJ Marder, EW Salzman, 3rd ed, p 546. JB Lippincott, Philadelphia, 1993.

48. Niewiarowski S: Secreted platelet proteins, in *Haemostis and Thrombosis*, edited by AL Bloom, CD Forbes, DP Thomas, EGD Tuddenham, 3rd ed, p 167. Churchill Livingstone, Edinburgh, 1994.

49. Kawahara RS, Deuel TF: Platelet-derived growth factor-inducible gene JE is a member of a family of small inducible genes related to platelet factor 4. *J Biol Chem* 264:679, 1989.

50. Brown KD, Zurawski SM, Mosmann TR, Zurawski G: A family of small inducible proteins secreted by leukocytes are members of a new super-family that includes leukocyte and fibroblast-derived inflammatory agents, growth factors, and indicators of various activation processes. *J Immunol* 142:679, 1989.

51. Oppenheim JJ, Zachariae COC, Mukaida N, Matsushima K: Properties of the novel proinflammatory supergene "intercrine" cytokine family. *Ann Rev Immunol* 9:617, 1991.

52. Rollins BJ: Chemokines. *Blood* 90:909, 1997.

53. Handin RI, Cohen HJ: Purification and binding properties of human platelet factor 4. *J Biol Chem* 58:731, 1976.

54. Loscalzo J, Melnick B, Handin RI: The interaction of platelet factor 4 and glycosaminoglycans. *Arch Biochem Biophys* 240:446, 1985.

55. Rucinski B, Niewiarowski S, Strzyzewski M, Holt JC, Mayo KH: Human platelet factor 4 and its C-terminal peptides: heparin binding and clearance from the circulation. *Thromb Haemost* 63:493, 1990.

56. Barber AG, Kaser-Glanzmann R, Jakabova M, Luscher EF: Chromatography of chondroitin sulfate proteoglycan carrier for heparin neutralizing activity (platelet factor 4) released from human blood platelets. *Biochim Biophys Acta* 286:312, 1972.

57. Huang SS, Huang JS, Deuel TF: Proteoglycan carrier of human platelet factor 4: isolation and characterization. *J Biol Chem* 257:11546, 1982.

58. Cowan SW, Bakshi EN, Machim KJ, Isaacs NW: Binding of heparin to human platelet factor 4. *Biochem J* 234:485, 1986.

59. Busch C, Dawes J, Pepper DW, Wasteson A: Binding of platelet factor 4 to cultured human umbilical vein endothelial cells. *Thromb Res* 19:129, 1980.

60. Visentin GP, Ford SE, Scott JP, Aster RH: Antibodies from patients with heparin-induced thrombocytopenia/thrombosis are specific for platelet factor 4 complexed with heparin or bound to endothelial cells. *J Clin Invest* 93:81, 1994.

61. Rucinski B, Stewart GJ, DeFeo PA, Boden G, Niewiarowski S: Uptake and processing of human platelet factor 4 by hepatocytes. *Proc Soc Exp Biol Med* 186:361, 1987.

62. Deuel TF, Senior RM, Change D, Griffin GL, Heinrikson RL, Kaiser ET: Platelet factor 4 is chemotactic for neutrophils and monocytes. *Proc Natl Acad Sci USA* 78:4854, 1981.

63. Maione TE, Gray GS, Petro J, et al: Inhibition of angiogenesis by recombinant human platelet factor-4 and related peptides. *Science* 247:77, 1990.

64. Brindley LL, Sweet JM, Goetzl EJ: Stimulation of histamine release from human basophils by human platelet factor 4. *J Clin Invest* 72:1218, 1983.

65. Maione TE, Gray GS, Petro J, et al: Inhibition of angiogenesis by recombinant human platelet factor-4 and related peptides. *Science* 247:77, 1990.

66. Gewirtz AM, Calabretta B, Rucinski B, Niewiarowski S, Xu W-Y: Inhibition of human megakaryocytopoiesis in vitro by platelet factor 4 and a synthetic C-terminal PF4 peptide. *J Clin Invest* 83:1477, 1989.

67. Han ZC, Sensebe L, Abgrall JF, Briere J: Platelet factor 4 inhibits human megakaryocytopoiesis in vitro. *Blood* 75:1234, 1990.

68. Katz IR, Thorbecke GJ, Bell MK, Yin J-Z, Clarke D, Zucker MB: Protease-induced immunoregulatory activity of platelet factor 4. *Proc Natl Acad Sci USA* 83:3491, 1986.

69. Beyth RJ, Culp LA: Complementary adhesive responses of human skin fibroblasts to the cell-binding domain of fibronectin and the heparin sulfate-binding protein, platelet factor 4. *Exp Cell Res* 155:537, 1984.

70. Capitanio AM, Niewiarowski S, Rucinski B, et al: Interaction of platelet factor 4 with human platelets. *Biochim Biophys Acta* 839:161, 1985.

71. Dumenco LL, Everson B, Culp LA, Ratnoff OD: Inhibition of the activation of Hageman factor (Factor XII) by platelet factor 4. *J Lab Clin Med* 112:394, 1988.

72. Engstad CS, Lia K, Rekdal O, Olsen JO, Osterud B: A novel biological effect of platelet factor 4 (PF4): enhancement of LPS-induced tissue factor activity in monocytes. *J Leuk Biol* 58:575, 1995.

73. Aziz KA, Cawley JC, Zuzel M: Platelets prime PMN via released PF4: mechanism of priming and synergy with GM-CSF. *Br J Haematol* 91:846, 1995.

74. Castor CW, Miller JW, Walz D: Structural and biological characteristics of connective tissue activating peptide (CTAP III), a major human platelet-derived growth factor. *Proc Natl Acad Sci USA* 80:765, 1983.

75. Holt JC, Harrie ME, Holt AM, Lange E, Henschen A, Niewiarowski S: Characterization of human platelet basic protein, a precursor form of low-affinity platelet factor 4 and beta-thromboglobulin. *Biochemistry* 25:1988, 1986.

76. Walz A, Dewald B, von Tscharner V, Baggiolini M: Effects of the neutrophil-activating peptide NAP-2, platelet basic protein, connective tissue-activating peptide III and platelet factor 4 on human neutrophils. *J Exp Med* 170:1745, 1989.

77. Bastl CP, Musial J, Kloczewiak M, Guzzo J, Berman I, Niewiarowski S: Role of kidney in the catabolic clearance of human platelet antiheparin proteins from rat circulation. *Blood* 57:233, 1981.

78. Hayward CP: Multimerin: a bench-to-bedside chronology of a unique platelet and endothelial cell protein—from discovery to function to abnormalities in disease. *Clin Invest Med* 20:176, 1997.

79. Polgar J, Magnenat E, Wells TN, Clemetson KJ: Platelet glycoprotein Ia* is the processed form of multimerin—isolation and determination of N-terminal sequences of stored and released forms. *Thromb Haemost* 80:645, 1998.

80. Hayward CP, Cramer EM, Song Z, et al: Studies of multimerin in human endothelial cells. *Blood* 91:1304, 1998.

81. Harrison P: Platelet α-granular fibrinogen. *Platelets* 3:1, 1992.

82. Coller BS, Seligsohn U, West SM, Scudder LE, Norton KJ: Absence of the γ-Leu 427 (γ′) variant in the platelet alpha-granular fibrinogen pool supports the role of glycoprotein IIb/IIIa in mediating fibrinogen uptake in platelets/megakaryocytes. *Blood* 79:3394, 1992.

83. Coller BS, Seligsohn U, West SM, Scudder LE, Norton KJ: Platelet fibrinogen and vitronectin in Glanzmann thrombasthenia: evidence consistent with specific roles for glycoprotein IIb/IIIa and αVβ3 integrins in platelet protein trafficking. *Blood* 78:2603, 1991.

84. Fay WP, Parker AC, Ansari MN, Zheng X, Ginsburg D: Vitronectin inhibits the thrombotic response to arterial injury in mice. *Blood* 93:1825, 1999.

85. Baenziger NL, Brodie GN, Majerus PW: A thrombin-sensitive protein of human platelet membranes. *Proc Natl Acad Sci USA* 68:240, 1971.

86. Lawler J, Hynes RO: The structure of human thrombospondin, an adhesive glycoprotein with multiple calcium-binding sites and homologies with several different proteins. *J Cell Biol* 103:1635, 1986.

87. Mosher DF, Doyle MJ, Jaffe EA: Synthesis and secretion of thrombospondin by cultured human endothelial cells. *J Cell Biol* 93:343, 1982.

88. Schwartz BS: Monocyte synthesis of thrombospondin. *J Biol Chem* 264:7512, 1989.

89. Plow EF, McEver RP, Coller BS, Marguerie GA, Ginsburg MH: Related binding mechanisms for fibrinogen, fibronectin, von Willebrand factor and thrombospondin on thrombin-stimulated human platelets. *Blood* 66:724, 1985.

90. Lawler J, Hynes RO: An integrin receptor on normal and thrombasthenic platelets which binds thrombospondin. *Blood* 74:2022, 1989.

91. Asch AS, Liu I, Briccetti FM, et al: Analysis of CD36 binding domains: ligand specificity controlled by dephosphorylation of an ectodomain. *Science* 262:1436, 1993.

92. Aiken ML, Ginsberg MH, Byers-Ward V, Plow EF: Effects of OKM5, a monoclonal antibody to glycoprotein IV, on platelet aggregation and thrombospondin surface expression. *Blood* 76:2501, 1990.

93. Chung J, Wang XQ, Lindberg FP, Frazier WA: Thrombospondin-1 acts via IAP/CD47 to synergize with collagen in alpha2beta1-mediated platelet activation. *Blood* 94:642, 1999.

94. Chung J, Gao AG, Frazier WA: Thrombospondin acts via integrin-associated protein to activate the platelet integrin alphaIIbbeta3. *J Biol Chem* 272:14740, 1997.

95. Leung LLK, Nachman RL: Complex formation of platelet thrombospondin with fibrinogen. *J Clin Invest* 70:542, 1982.

96. Tuszynski GP, Srivastava S, Switalska HI, Holt JC, Cierniewski CS, Niewiarowski S: The interaction of human platelet thrombospondin with fibrinogen. *J Biol Chem* 260:12240, 1985.

97. Dardik R, Lahav J: Functional changes in the conformation of thrombo-

spondin-1 during complexation with fibronectin or heparin. *Exp Cell Res* 248:407, 1999.

98. Leung LLK: Role of thrombospondin in platelet aggregation. *J Clin Invest* 74:1764, 1984.

99. Silverstein RL, Leung LLK, Harpel PC, Nachman RL: Complex formation of platelet thrombospondin with plasminogen. *J Clin Invest* 74:1625, 1984.

100. Schultz-Cherry S, Murphy-Ullrich JE: Thrombospondin causes activation of latent transforming growth factor-beta secreted by endothelial cells by a novel mechanism. *J Cell Biol* 122:923, 1993.

101. Brown E, Hooper L, Ho T, Gresham H: Integrin-associated protein: a 50-kD plasma membrane antigen physically and functionally associated with integrins. *J Cell Biol* 111:2785, 1990.

102. Gao AG, Lindberg FP, Finn MB, Blystone SD, Brown EJ, Frazier WA: Integrin-associated protein is a receptor for the C-terminal domain of thrombospondin. *J Biol Chem* 271:21, 1996.

103. Tracy PB, Eide LC, Bowie EJW, Mann KG: Radioimmunoassay of factor V in human plasma and platelets. *Blood* 60:59, 1982.

104. Chesney CM, Pifer D, Colman RW: Subcellular localization and secretion of factor V from human platelets. *Proc Natl Acad Sci USA* 78:5180, 1981.

105. Chiu HC, Schick P, Colman RW: Biosynthesis of coagulation factor V by megakaryocytes. *J Clin Invest* 75:339, 1985.

106. Gewirtz A, Keefer M, Memoli M, et al: Biology of human megakaryocyte factor V. *Blood* 67:1639, 1986.

107. Kane WH, Mruk JS, Majerus PW: Activation of coagulation factor V by a platelet protease. *J Clin Invest* 70:1092, 1982.

108. Tracy PB, Nesheim ME, Mann KG: Proteolytic alterations of factor Va bound to platelets. *J Biol Chem* 662:669, 1983.

109. Tracy PB, Giles AR, Mann KG, et al: Factor V (Quebec): a bleeding diathesis associated with a qualitative platelet factor V deficiency. *J Clin Invest* 74:1221, 1984.

110. Nesheim ME, Nichols WL, Cole TL, et al: Isolation and study of an acquired inhibitor of human coagulation factor V. *J Clin Invest* 405:415, 1986.

111. Bode AP, Sandberg H, Dombrose FA, Lentz BR: Association of factor V activity with membranous vesicles released from human platelets: requirement for platelet stimulation. *Thromb Res* 39:49, 1985.

112. Deuel TF, Huang SS, Huang JS: Platelet derived growth factor: purification, characterization and role in normal and abnormal cell growth, in *Biochemistry of Platelets*, edited by DR Phillips, MA Shuman, p 347. Academic, London, 1986.

113. Heldin C-H, Westermark B: Platelet-derived growth factor: three isoforms and two receptor types. *Trends in Genetics* 5:108, 1989.

114. Ross R: Peptide regulatory factors. Platelet-derived growth factor. *Lancet* 1:1179, 1989.

115. Madtes DK, Raines EW, Ross R: Modulation of local concentrations of platelet-derived growth factor. *Am Rev Resp Dis* 140:1118, 1989.

116. Berk BC, Alexander RW: Vasoactive effects of growth factors. *Biochem Pharmacol* 38:219, 1989.

117. Waterfield MD, Scrace GT, Whittle N, et al: Platelet-derived growth factor is structurally related to the putative transforming protein p28-sis of simian sarcoma virus. *Nature* 304:35, 1983.

118. Doolittle RF, Hunkapiller MW, Hood LE, et al: Simian sarcoma virus onc gene, v-sis, is derived from the gene (or genes) encoding a platelet-derived growth factor. *Science* 22:275, 1983.

119. Williams LT: Signal transduction by the platelet-derived growth factor receptor. *Science* 24:1564, 1989.

120. King GL, Buchwald S: Characterization and partial purification of an endothelial cell growth factor from human platelets. *J Clin Invest* 73:392, 1984.

121. Maloney JP, Silliman CC, Ambruso DR, Wang J, Tuder RM, Voelkel NF: In vitro release of vascular endothelial growth factor during platelet aggregation. *Am J Physiol* 275:H1054, 1998.

122. Weltermann A, Wolzt M, Petersmann K, et al: Large amounts of vascular endothelial growth factor at the site of hemostatic plug formation in vivo. *Arterioscler Thromb Vasc Biol* 19:1757, 1999.

123. Webb NJ, Bottomley MJ, Watson CJ, Brenchley PE: Vascular endothelial growth factor (VEGF) is released from platelets during blood clotting: implications for measurement of circulating VEGF levels in clinical disease. *Clin Sci (Colch)* 94:395, 1998.

124. Mohle R, Green D, Moore MA, Nachman RL, Rafii S: Constitutive

production and thrombin-induced release of vascular endothelial growth factor by human megakaryocytes and platelets. *Proc Natl Acad Sci USA* 94:663, 1997.

125. Amirkhosravi A, Amaya M, Siddiqui F, Biggerstaff JP, Meyer TV, Francis JL: Blockade of GPIIb/IIIa inhibits the release of vascular endothelial growth factor (VEGF) from tumor cell-activated platelets and experimental metastasis. *Platelets* 10:285, 1999.

126. Katoh O, Tauchi H, Kawaishi K, Kimura A, Satow Y: Expression of the vascular endothelial growth factor (VEGF) receptor gene, KDR, in hematopoietic cells and inhibitory effect of VEGF on apoptotic cell death caused by ionizing radiation. *Cancer Res* 55:5687, 1995.

127. Wartiovaara U, Salven P, Mikkola H, et al: Peripheral blood platelets express VEGF-C and VEGF which are released during platelet activation. *Thromb Haemost* 80:171, 1998.

128. Salven P, Orpana A, Joensuu H: Leukocytes and platelets of patients with cancer contain high levels of vascular endothelial growth factor. *Clin Cancer Res* 5:487, 1999.

129. Verheul HM, Pinedo HM: Tumor growth: A putative role for platelets? *Oncologist* 3:II, 1998.

130. Solovey A, Gui L, Ramakrishnan S, Steinberg MH, Hebbel RP: Sickle cell anemia as a possible state of enhanced anti-apoptotic tone: survival effect of vascular endothelial growth factor on circulating and unanchored endothelial cells. *Blood* 93:3824, 1999.

131. Cao J, Mathews MK, McLeod DS, Merges C, Hjelmeland LM, Lutty GA: Angiogenic factors in human proliferative sickle cell retinopathy. *Br J Ophthalmol* 83:838, 1999.

132. Kiuru J, Viinikka L, Myllyla G, Pesonen K, Perheentupa J: Cytoskeleton-dependent release of human platelet epidermal growth factor. *Life Sci* 49:1997, 1991.

133. Busch AI, Martins RN, Rumble B, et al: The amyloid precursor protein of Alzheimer's disease is released by human platelets. *J Biol Chem* 265:15977, 1990.

134. Van Nostrand WE, Schmaier AH, Farrow JS, Cines DB, Cunningham DD: Protease nexin-2/amyloid beta-protein precursor in blood is a platelet-specific protein. *Biochem Biophys Res Commun* 175:15, 1991.

135. Rosenberg RN, Baskin F, Fosmire JA, et al: Altered amyloid protein processing in platelets of patients with Alzheimer disease. *Arch Neurol* 54:139, 1997.

136. Schmaier AH, Dahl LD, Rozemuller AJM, et al: Protease nexin-2/amyloid β protein precursor. A tight-binding inhibitor of coagulation factor IXa. *J Clin Invest* 92(5):2540, 1993.

137. Schmaier AH, Dahl LD, Hasan AA, Cines DB, Bauer KA, Van Nostrand WE: Factor IXa inhibition by protease nexin-2/amyloid beta-protein precursor on phospholipid vesicles and cell membranes. *Biochemistry* 34:1171, 1995.

138. Scandura JM, Zhang Y, Van Nostrand WE, Walsh PN: Progress curve analysis of the kinetics with which blood coagulation factor XIa is inhibited by protease nexin-2. *Biochemistry* 36:412, 1997.

139. McDonagh J, McDonagh RP Jr, Delage JM, Wagner RH: Factor XIII in human plasma and platelets. *J Clin Invest* 48:940, 1969.

140. Devine DV, Bishop PD: Platelet-associated factor XIII in platelet activation, adhesion, and clot stabilization. *Semin Thromb Hemost* 22:409, 1996.

141. Rifkin DB, Kojima S, Abe M, Harpel JG: TGF-β: structure, function, and formation. *Thromb Haemost* 70:177, 1993.

142. Wakefield LM, Smith DM, Flanders KC, Sporn MB: Latent transforming growth factor β from human platelets. A high molecular weight complex containing precursor sequences. *J Biol Chem* 263:7646, 1988.

143. Massague J: The transforming growth factor-beta family. *Annu Rev Cell Biol* 6:597–641:597, 1990.

144. Lin HY, Wang XF, Ng-Eaton E, Weinberg RA, Lodish HF: Expression cloning of the TGF-beta type II receptor, a functional transmembrane serine/threonine kinase. *Cell* 68:775, 1992.

145. Sakamaki S, Hirayama Y, Matsunaga T, et al: Transforming growth factor-beta1 (TGF-beta1) induces thrombopoietin from bone marrow stromal cells, which stimulates the expression of TGF-beta receptor on megakaryocytes and, in turn, renders them susceptible to suppression by TGF-beta itself with high specificity. *Blood* 94:1961, 1999.

146. Kronemann N, Bouloumia A, Bassus S, Kirchmaier CM, Busse R, Schini-Kerth VB: Aggregating human platelets stimulate expression of vascular endothelial growth factor in cultured vascular smooth muscle cells

through a synergistic effect of transforming growth factor-beta(1) and platelet-derived growth factor(AB). *Circulation* 100:855, 1999.

147. Fuhrman B, Brook GJ, Aviram M: Proteins derived from platelet alpha granules modulate the uptake of oxidized low density lipoprotein by macrophages. *Biochim Biophys Acta* 1127:15, 1992.

148. Ts'ao CH: Rough endoplasmic reticulum and ribosomes in blood platelets. *Scand J Haematol* 8:134, 1971.

149. Booyse FM, Hoveke TP, Rafelson ME Jr: Studies on human platelets. II. Protein synthetic activity of various platelet populations. *Biochim Biophys Acta* 157:660, 1968.

150. Newman PJ, Derbes RS, Aster RH: The human platelet alloantigens, PlA1 and PlA2, are associated with a leucine33/proline33 amino acid polymorphism in membrane glycoprotein IIIa, and are distinguishable by DNA typing. *J Clin Invest* 83:1778, 1989.

151. Ginsburg D, Konkle BA, Gill JC, et al: Molecular basis of human von Willebrand disease: analysis of platelet von Willebrand factor mRNA. *Proc Natl Acad Sci USA* 86:3723, 1989.

152. Weyrich AS, Dixon DA, Pabla R, et al: Signal-dependent translation of a regulatory protein, Bcl-3, in activated human platelets. *Proc Natl Acad Sci USA* 95:5556, 1998.

153. Pabla R, Weyrich AS, Dixon DA, et al: Integrin-dependent control of translation: engagement of integrin alphaIIbbeta3 regulates synthesis of proteins in activated human platelets. *J Cell Biol* 144:175, 1999.

154. Behnke O: The morphology of blood platelet membrane systems. *Semin Haematol* 3:3, 1970.

155. White JG: Electron microscopic studies of platelet secretion. *Prog Hem Thromb* 2:49, 1974.

156. Stenberg PE, Shuman MA, Levine SP, Bainton D: Redistribution of a granules and their contents in thrombin-stimulated platelets. *J Cell Biol* 98:748, 1984.

157. Ginsberg MH, Taylor L, Painter RG: The mechanism of thrombin-induced platelet factor 4 secretion. *Blood* 55:661, 1980.

158. George JN, Pickett EB, Saucerman S, et al: Platelet surface glycoproteins. Studies on resting and activated platelets and platelet membrane microparticles in normal subjects, and observations in patients during adult respiratory distress syndrome and cardiac surgery. *J Clin Invest* 78:340, 1986.

159. Michelson AD: Thrombin-induced down-regulation of the platelet membrane glycoprotein Ib-IX complex. *Semin Thromb Hemost* 18:18, 1992.

160. Michelson AD, Barnard MR: Plasmin-induced redistribution of platelet glycoprotein Ib. *Blood* 76:2005, 1990.

161. Suzuki H, Nakamura S, Itoh Y, Yamazaki H, Tanoue K: Immunocytochemical evidence for the translocation of α-granule membrane glycoprotein IIb/IIIa (integrin αIIbβ3) of human platelets to the surface membrane during the release reaction. *Histochemistry* 97:381, 1992.

162. Breton-Gorius J, Guichard J: Ultrastructural localization of peroxidase activity in human platelets and megakaryocytes. *Am J Pathol* 66:277, 1972.

163. White JG: Interaction of membrane systems in blood platelets. *Am J Pathol* 66:295, 1972.

164. Robblee LS, Shepro D, Belamarich FA: Calcium uptake and associated adenosine triphosphate activity of isolated platelet membranes. *J Gen Physiol* 61:462, 1973.

165. Menashi S, Davis C, Crawford N: Calcium uptake associated with an intracellular membrane fraction prepared from human blood platelets by high-voltage, free-flow electrophoresis. *FEBS Lett* 140:298, 1982.

166. Michalak M, Mariani P, Opas M: Calreticulin, a multifunctional Ca2+ binding chaperone of the endoplasmic reticulum. *Biochem Cell Biol* 76:779, 1998.

167. Kaser-Glanzmann R, Jakabova M, George JN, Luscher EF: Further characterization of calcium accumulating vesicles from human blood platelets. *Biochim Biophys Acta* 542:357, 1978.

168. Tertyshnikova S, Fein A: Inhibition of inositol 1,4,5-trisphosphate-induced Ca2+ release by cAMP-dependent protein kinase in a living cell. *Proc Natl Acad Sci USA* 95:1613, 1998.

169. Gerrard JM, White JG, Rao GHR, Townsend D: Localization of platelet prostaglandin production in the platelet dense tubular system. *Am J Pathol* 83:283, 1976.

170. Picot D, Loll PJ, Garavito RM: The X-ray crystal structure of the membrane protein prostaglandin H2 synthase-1. *Nature* 367:243, 1994.

171. Badimon L, Badimon JJ, Turitto VT, Vallabhajosula S, Fuster V: Platelet thrombus formation on collagen type I. A model of deep vessel injury.

Influence of blood rheology, von Willebrand factor, and blood coagulation. *Circulation* 78:1431, 1988.

172. Coller BS: Platelets in cardiovascular thrombosis and thrombolysis; in *The Heart and Cardiovascular System*, 2d ed, p 219. Raven, New York, 1991.

173. Weiss HJ, Turitto VT, Baumgartner HR, Nemerson Y, Hoffmann T: Evidence for the presence of tissue factor activity on subendothelium. *Blood* 73:968, 1989.

174. Wilcox JN, Smith KM, Schwartz SM, Gordon D: Localization of tissue factor in the normal vessel wall and in the atherosclerotic plaque. *Proc Natl Acad Sci USA* 86:2839, 1989.

175. Goldsmith HL, Turitto VT: Rheological aspects of thrombosis and haemostasis: basic principles and applications. *Thromb Haemost* 55:415, 1986.

176. Giesen PL, Rauch U, Bohrmann B, et al: Blood-borne tissue factor: another view of thrombosis. *Proc Natl Acad Sci USA* 96:2311, 1999.

177. Roth GJ: Developing relationships: arterial platelet adhesion, glycoprotein Ib, and leucine rich glycoproteins. *Blood* 77:5, 1991.

178. Sixma JJ: Interaction of blood platelets with the vessel wall, in *Haemostasis and Thrombosis*, edited by AL Bloom, CD Forbes, DP Thomas, EGD Tuddenham, 3rd ed, p 259. Churchill Livingstone, Edinburgh, 1994.

179. Ruggeri ZM: Structure and function of von Willebrand factor. *Thromb Haemost* 82:576, 1999.

180. Andrews RK, Shen Y, Gardiner EE, Dong J, Lopez JA, Berndt MC: The glycoprotein Ib-IX-V complex in platelet adhesion and signaling. *Thromb Haemost* 82:357, 1999.

181. Moake JL, Turner NA, Stathopoulos NA, Nolasco LH, Hellums JD: Involvement of large plasma von Willebrand factor (vWF) multimers and unusually large vWF forms derived from endothelial cells in shear stress-induced platelet aggregation. *J Clin Invest* 78:1456, 1986.

182. Ikeda Y, Handa M, Kawano K, et al: The role of von Willebrand factor and fibrinogen in platelet aggregation under varying shear stress. *J Clin Invest* 87:1234, 1991.

183. Ruggeri ZM: Mechanisms of shear-induced platelet adhesion and aggregation. *Thromb Haemost* 70:119, 1993.

184. Coller BS: Platelet von Willebrand factor interactions, in *Platelet Glycoproteins*, edited by J George, D Phillips, p 215. Plenum, New York, 1985.

185. Rand JH, Patel ND, Schwartz E, Zhou SL, Potter BJ: 150-kD von Willebrand factor binding protein extracted from human vascular subendothelium is type VI collagen. *J Clin Invest* 88:253, 1991.

186. Goto S, Ikeda Y, Saldivar E, Ruggeri ZM: Distinct mechanisms of platelet aggregation as a consequence of different shearing flow conditions. *J Clin Invest* 101:479, 1998.

187. Coller BS: Interaction of normal, thrombasthenic, and Bernard-Soulier platelets with immobilized fibrinogen: defective platelet-fibrinogen interaction in thrombasthenia. *Blood* 55:169, 1980.

188. Savage B, Ruggeri ZM: Selective recognition of adhesive sites in surface-bound fibrinogen by glycoprotein IIb-IIIa on nonactivated platelets. *J Biol Chem* 266:11227, 1991.

189. Santoro SA: Molecular basis of platelet adhesion to collagen, in *Platelet Membrane Receptors: Molecular Biology, Immunobiology, Biochemistry and Pathology*, edited by GA Jamieson, p 291. Alan R. Liss, New York, 1988.

190. Chiang TM, Rinaldy A, Kang AH: Cloning, characterization, and functional studies of a nonintegrin platelet receptor for type I collagen. *J Clin Invest* 100:514, 1997.

191. Clemetson JM, Polgar J, Magnenat E, Wells TN, Clemetson KJ: The platelet collagen receptor glycoprotein VI is a member of the immunoglobulin superfamily closely related to FcalphaR and the natural killer receptors. *J Biol Chem* 274:29019, 1999.

192. Clemetson KJ: Platelet collagen receptors: a new target for inhibition? *Haemostas* 29:16, 1999.

193. Coller BS, Beer JH, Scudder LE, Steinberg MH: Collagen-platelet interactions: evidence for a direct interaction of collagen with platelet GPIa/IIa and an indirect interaction with platelet GPIIb/IIIa mediated by adhesive proteins. *Blood* 74:182, 1989.

194. Saelman EU, Nieuwenhuis HK, Hese KM, et al: Platelet adhesion to collagen types I through VIII under conditions of stasis and flow is mediated by GPIa/IIa (α2β1-integrin). *Blood* 83:1244, 1994.

195. Watson SP: Collagen receptor signaling in platelets and megakaryocytes. *Thromb Haemost* 82:376, 1999.

196. Nakamura T, Kambayashi J, Okuma M, Tandon NN: Activation of the GP IIb-IIIa complex induced by platelet adhesion to collagen is mediated by both alpha2beta1 integrin and GP VI. *J Biol Chem* 274:11897, 1999.

197. Matsuno K, Diaz-Ricart M, Montgomery RR, Aster RH, Jamieson GA, Tandon NN: Inhibition of platelet adhesion to collagen by monoclonal anti-CD36 antibodies. *Br J Haematol* 92:960, 1996.

198. Ruggeri ZM, Dent JA, Saldivar E: Contribution of distinct adhesive interactions to platelet aggregation in flowing blood. *Blood* 94:172, 1999.

199. Savage B, Almus-Jacobs F, Ruggeri ZM: Specific synergy of multiple substrate-receptor interactions in platelet thrombus formation under flow. *Cell* 94:657, 1998.

200. Santos MT, Valles J, Marcus AJ, et al: Enhancement of platelet reactivity and modulation of eicosanoid production by intact erythrocytes. A new approach to platelet activation and recruitment. *J Clin Invest* 87:571, 1991.

201. Coller BS, Kutok JL, Scudder LE, et al: Studies of activated GPIIb/IIIa receptors on the luminal surface of adherent platelets. Paradoxical loss of luminal receptors when platelets adhere to high density fibrinogen. *J Clin Invest* 92:2796, 1993.

202. Shattil S: Regulation of platelet anchorage and signaling by integrin $\alpha IIb\beta 3$. *Thromb Haemost* 70:224, 1993.

203. Weiss HJ, Turitto VT, Baumgartner HR: Further evidence that glycoprotein IIb-IIIa mediates platelet spreading on subendothelium. *Thromb Haemost* 65:202, 1991.

204. Shattil SJ: Signaling through platelet integrin $\alpha IIb\beta 3$: inside-out, outside-in and sideways. *Thromb Haemost* 82:318, 1999.

205. Denis CC, Methia N, Frenette PS, et al: A mouse model of severe von Willebrand disease: Defects in hemostasis and thrombosis. *Proc Nat Acad Sci USA* 95:9524, 1998.

206. Loscalzo J, Inbal A, Handin RI: von Willebrand protein facilitates platelet incorporation into polymerizing fibrin. *J Clin Invest* 78:1112, 1986.

207. Michelson AD, Barnard MR: Thrombin-induced changes in platelet membrane glycoproteins Ib, IX, and IIb-IIIa complex. *Blood* 70:1673, 1987.

208. McEver RP, Beckstead JH, Moore KL, et al: GMP-140, a platelet-granule membrane protein, is also synthesized by vascular endothelial cells and is localized in Weibel-Palade bodies. *J Clin Invest* 84:92, 1989.

209. McEver RP: Properties of GMP-140, an inducible granule membrane protein of platelets and endothelium. *Blood Cells* 16:73, 1990.

210. Harwell DW, Wagner DD: New discoveries with mice mutant in endothelial and platelet selectins. *Thromb Haemost* 82:850, 1999.

211. Henn V, Slupsky JR, Grafe M, et al: CD40 ligand on activated platelets triggers an inflammatory reaction of endothelial cells. *Nature* 391:591, 1998.

212. Barry OP, FitzGerald GA: Mechanisms of cellular activation by platelet microparticles. *Thromb Haemost* 82:794, 1999.

213. Smith JA, Henderson AH, Randall MD: Endothelium-derived relaxing factor, prostanoids and endothelins, in *Haemostasis and Thrombosis*, edited by AL Bloom, CD Forbes, DP Thomas, EGD Tuddenham, 3rd ed, p 183. Churchill Livingstone, Edinburgh, 1994.

214. Valles J, Santos MT, Marcus AJE, et al: Down-regulation of human platelet reactivity by neutrophils. Participation of lipoxygenase derivatives and adhesive proteins. *J Clin Invest* 1993.

215. Selak MA: Cathepsin G and thrombin: evidence for two different platelet receptors. *Biochem J* 297:269, 1994.

216. Molino M, Di Lallo M, Martelli N, de Gaetano G, Cerletti C: Effects of leukocyte-derived cathepsin G on platelet membrane glycoprotein Ib-IX and IIb-IIIa complexes: a comparison with thrombin. *Blood* 82:2442, 1993.

217. Peerschke EI: Ca^{2+} mobilization and fibrinogen binding of platelets refractory to adenosine diphosphate stimulation. *J Lab Clin Med* 106:111, 1985.

218. Murray R, FitzGerald GA: Regulation of thromboxane receptor activation in human platelets. *Proc Natl Acad Sci USA* 86:124, 1989.

219. Coughlin SR: Protease-activated receptors and platelet function. *Thromb Haemost* 82:353, 1999.

220. Phillips DR, Charo IF, Parise LV, Fitzgerald LA: The platelet membrane glycoprotein IIb-IIIa complex. *Blood* 71:831, 1988.

221. Plow EF, Ginsberg MH: Cellular adhesion: GPIIb-IIIa as a prototypic adhesion receptor. *Prog Hemost Thromb* 9:117, 1989.

222. Peerschke EI: The platelet fibrinogen receptor. *Semin Hematol* 22:241, 1985.

223. Weiss HJ, Hawiger J, Ruggeri ZM, Turitto VT, Thiagarajan P, Hoffman T: Fibrinogen-independent platelet adhesion and thrombus formation on subendothelium mediated by glycoprotein IIb-IIIa complex at high shear rate. *J Clin Invest* 83:288, 1989.

224. Bennett JS: The platelet-fibrinogen interaction, in *Platelet Membrane Glycoproteins*, edited by JN George, AT Nurden, DR Phillips, p 193. Plenum, New York, 1985.

225. Grant JA, Scrutton MC: Positive interaction between agonists in the aggregation response of human platelets: Interaction between ADP, adrenaline and vasopressin. *Br J Haematol* 44:109, 1980.

226. Steen VM, Holmsen H: Synergism between thrombin and epinephrine in human platelets: Different dose-response relationships for aggregation and dense granule secretion. *Thromb Haemost* 54:680, 1985.

227. Folts JD, Rowe GG: Epinephrine potentiation of in vivo stimuli reverses aspirin inhibition of platelet thrombus formation in stenosed canine coronary arteries. *Thromb Res* 50:507, 1988.

228. Folts JD, Bonebrake FC: The effects of cigarette smoke and nicotine on platelet thrombus formation in stenosed dog coronary arteries: Inhibition with phentolamine. *Circulation* 65:465, 1989.

229. Hjemdahl P, Chronos NA, Wilson DJ, Bouloux P, Goodall AH: Epinephrine sensitizes human platelets in vivo and in vitro as studied by fibrinogen binding and P-selectin expression. *Arterioscler Thromb* 14:77, 1994.

230. Moake JL, Turner NA, Stathopoulos NA, Nolasco LH, Hellums JD: Shear-induced platelet aggregation can be mediated by vWF released from platelets, as well as by exogenous large or unusually large vWF multimers, requires adenosine diphosphate, and is resistant to aspirin. *Blood* 71:1366, 1988.

231. Karpatkin S, Langer RM: Biochemical energetics of simulated platelet plug formation: effect of thrombin, adenosine diphosphate, and epinephrine on intra- and extracellular adenine nucleotide kinetics. *J Clin Invest* 47:2158, 1968.

232. Akkerman JWN, Gorter G, Schrama L, Holmsen H: A novel technique for rapid determination of energy consumption in platelets: determination of different energy consumption associated with three secretory responses. *Biochem J* 210:145, 1983.

233. Akkerman JWN, Holmsen H: Interrelationships among platelet responses: studies on the burst in protein liberation, lactate production and oxygen uptake during platelet aggregation and Ca++ secretion. *Blood* 57:956, 1981.

234. Akkerman JWN, Verhoeven AJM: Energy metabolism and function, in *Platelet Responses and Metabolism*, edited by H Holmsen, 3rd ed, p 69. CRC Press, Boca Raton, 1987.

235. Holmsen H, Farstad M: Energy metabolism, in *Platelet Responses and Metabolism*, edited by H Holmsen, 2nd ed, p 245. CRC Press, Boca Raton, 1987.

236. Shimizu T, Murphy S: Roles of acetate and phosphate in the successful storage of platelet concentrates prepared with an acetate-containing additive solution. *Transfusion* 33:304, 1993.

237. Simons ER, Greenberg-Sperssky SM: Transmembrane monovalent cation gradients, in *Platelet Responses and Metabolism*, edited by H Holmsen, 3rd ed, p 31. CRC Press, Boca Raton, 1987.

238. Dean WL: Structure, function and subcellular localization of a human platelet Ca^{++}-ATPase. *Cell Calcium* 10:289, 1989.

239. Daniel JL, Molish IR, Robkin L, et al: Nucleotide exchange between cytosolic ATP and F-actin-bound ADP may be a major ATP-utilizing process in unstimulated platelets. *Eur J Biochem* 156:677, 1986.

240. Verhoeven AJM, Tysnes O-B, Aarbakke GM, et al: Turnover of the phosphomonoester groups of polyphosphoinositol lipids in unstimulated platelets. *Eur J Biochem* 166:3, 1987.

241. Frelinger AL 3d, Cohen I, Plow EF, et al: Selective inhibition of integrin function by antibodies specific for ligand-occupied receptor conformers. *J Biol Chem* 265:6346, 1990.

242. Furman MI, Gardner TM, Goldschmidt-Clermont: Mechanisms of cytoskeletal reorganization during platelet activation. *Thromb Haemost* 70:229, 1993.

243. Nachmias VT, Yoshida K: The cytoskeleton of the blood platelets: a dynamic structure. *Adv Cyclic Nucleotide Res* 2:181, 1999.

244. Fox JEB, Boyles JK, Reynolds CC, Phillips DR: Actin filament content and organization in unstimulated platelets. *J Cell Biol* 98:1985, 1984.

245. Escolar G, Krumwiede M, White JG: Organization of the actin cytoskeleton of resting and activated platelets in suspension. *Am J Pathol* 123:86, 1986.

246. Nachmias VT: Cytoskeleton of human platelets at rest and after spreading. *J Cell Biol* 86:795, 1980.

247. Gonnella PA, Nachmias VT: Platelet activation and microfilament bundling. *J Biol Chem* 89:146, 1981.

248. Phillips DR, Jennings LK, Edwards HH: Identification of membrane proteins mediating the interaction of human platelets. *J Cell Biol* 86:77, 1980.

249. Shattil SJ, Brugge JS: Protein tyrosine phosphorylation and the adhesive functions of platelets. *Curr Opin Cell Biol* 3:869, 1991.

250. Fox JEB: On the role of calpain and Rho proteins in regulating integrin-induced signaling. *Thromb Haemost* 82:391, 1999.

251. Fox JEB, Goll DE, Reynolds CC, Phillips DR: Identification of two proteins (actin-binding protein and P235) that are hydrolyzed by endogenous Ca^{++}-dependent protease during platelet aggregation. *J Biol Chem* 260:1060, 1985.

252. Fox JE, Reynolds CC, Phillips DR: Calcium-dependent proteolysis occurs during platelet aggregation. *J Biol Chem* 258:9973, 1983.

253. Fox JE, Taylor RG, Taffarel M, Boyles JK, Goll DE: Evidence that activation of platelet calpain is induced as a consequence of binding of adhesive ligand to the integrin, glycoprotein IIb-IIIa. *J Cell Biol* 120:1501, 1993.

254. Fox JEB, Austin CD, Reynolds CC, et al: Evidence that agonist-induced activation of calpain causes the shedding of procoagulant-containing microvesicles from the membrane of aggregating platelets. *J Biol Chem* 266:13289, 1991.

255. Dachary-Prigent J, Freyssinet J-M, Pasquet J-M, et al: Annexin V as a probe of aminophospholipid exposure and platelet membrane vesiculation: a flow cytometry study showing a role for free sulfhydryl groups. *Blood* 81:2554, 1993.

256. Nachmias VT: Platelet and megakaryocyte shape change: triggered alterations in the cytoskeleton. *Sem Hematol* 20:261, 1983.

257. Heemskerk JW, Vuist WM, Feijge MA, Reutelingsperger CP, Lindhout T: Collagen but not fibrinogen surfaces induce bleb formation, exposure of phosphatidylserine, and procoagulant activity of adherent platelets: evidence for regulation by protein tyrosine kinase-dependent Ca^{2+} responses. *Blood* 90:2615, 1997.

258. Ma AD, Abrams CS: Pleckstrin homology domains and phospholipid-induced cytoskeletal reorganization. *Thromb Haemost* 82:399, 1999.

259. Olorundare OE, Simmons SR, Albrecht RM: Cytochalasin D and E: effects on fibrinogen receptor movement and cytoskeletal reorganization in fully spread, surface-activated platelets: a correlative light and electron microscopic investigation. *Blood* 79:99, 1992.

260. White JG: Induction of patching and its reversal on surface-activated human platelets. *Br J Haematol* 76:108, 1990.

261. Bennett JS, Zigmond S, Vilaire G, Cunningham ME, Bednar B: The platelet cytoskeleton regulates the affinity of the integrin alpha(IIb)-beta(3) for fibrinogen. *J Biol Chem* 274:25301, 1999.

262. Lemons PP, Chen D, Bernstein AM, Bennett MK, Whiteheart SW: Regulated secretion in platelets: identification of elements of the platelet exocytosis machinery. *Blood* 90:1490, 1997.

263. Karniguian A, Zahraoui A, Tavitian A: Identification of small GTP-binding rab proteins in human platelets: thrombin-induced phosphorylation of rab3B, rab6, and rab8 proteins. *Proc Natl Acad Sci USA* 90:7647, 1993.

264. Morimoto T, Ogihara S: ATP is required in platelet serotonin exocytosis for protein phosphorylation and priming of secretory vesicles docked on the plasma membrane. *J Cell Sci* 109 (Pt 1):113, 1996.

265. Gerrard JM, Beattie LL, Park J, et al: A role for protein kinase C in the membrane fusion necessary for platelet granule secretion. *Blood* 74:2405, 1989.

266. Augustine GJ, Burns ME, DeBello WM, Pettit DL, Schweizer FE: Exocytosis: proteins and perturbations. *Annu Rev Pharmacol Toxicol* 36:659, 1996.

267. Budtz-Olsen OE: *Clot Retraction*. Charles Thomas, Springfield, 1951.

268. Kunitada S, FitzGerald GA, Fitzgerald DJ: Inhibition of clot lysis and decreased binding of tissue-type plasminogen activator as a consequence of clot retraction. *Blood* 79:1420, 1992.

269. Pollard TD, Fujiwara K, Handin R, Weiss G: Contractile proteins in platelet activation and contraction. *Ann NY Acad Sci* 283:218, 1977.

270. Cohen I, Gerrard JM, White JG: Ultrastructure of clots during isometric contraction. *J Cell Biol* 91:775, 1982.

271. Cohen I: The mechanism of clot retraction, in *Platelet Membrane Glyco-*

proteins, edited by JN George, AT Nurden, DR Phillips, p 299. Plenum, New York, 1985.

272. Carr ME Jr, Carr SL, Hantgan RR, Braaten J: Glycoprotein IIb/IIIa blockade inhibits platelet-mediated force development and reduces gel elastic modulus. *Thromb Haemost* 73:499, 1995.

273. Leistikow EA: Platelet internalization in early thrombogenesis. *Semin Thromb Hemost* 22:289, 1996.

274. Ward CM, Kestin AS, Newman PJ: A Leu262Pro mutation in the integrin beta(3) subunit results in an alpha(IIb)-beta(3) complex that binds fibrin but not fibrinogen. *Blood* 96:161, 2000.

275. Coller BS, Peerschke EI, Scudder LE, Sullivan CA: A murine monoclonal antibody that completely blocks the binding of fibrinogen to platelets produces a thrombasthenic-like state in normal platelets and binds to glycoproteins IIb and/or IIIa. *J Clin Invest* 72:325, 1983.

276. Rooney MM, Farrell DH, van Hemel BM, de Groot PG, Lord ST: The contribution of the three hypothesized integrin-binding sites in fibrinogen to platelet-mediated clot retraction. *Blood* 92:2374, 1998.

277. Rooney MM, Parise LV, Lord ST: Dissecting clot retraction and platelet aggregation. Clot retraction does not require an intact fibrinogen gamma chain C terminus. *J Biol Chem* 271:8553, 1996.

278. Solum NO: Procoagulant expresion in platelets and defects leading to clinical disorders. *Arterioscler Thromb Vasc Biol* 19:2841, 1999.

279. Bevers EM, Comfurius P, Dekkers DW, Zwaal RF: Lipid translocation across the plasma membrane of mammalian cells. *Biochim Biophys Acta* 1439:317, 1999.

280. Zhou Q, Zhao J, Stout JG, Luhm RA, Wiedmer T, Sims PJ: Molecular cloning of human plasma membrane phospholipid scramblase. A protein mediating transbilayer movement of plasma membrane phospholipids. *J Biol Chem* 272:18240, 1997.

281. Zhou Q, Sims PJ, Wiedmer T: Identity of a conserved motif in phospholipid scramblase that is required for Ca^{2+}-accelerated transbilayer movement of membrane phospholipids. *Biochemistry* 37:2356, 1998.

282. Thiagarajan P, Tait JF: Collagen-induced exposure of anionic phospholipid in platelets and platelet-derived microparticles. *J Biol Chem* 266:24302, 1991.

283. Reverter JC, Beguin S, Kessels H, Kumar R, Hemker HC, Coller BS: Inhibition of platelet-mediated, tissue factor-induced, thrombin generation by the mouse/human chimeric 7E3 antibody: potential implications for the effect of c7E3 Fab treatment on acute thrombosis and "clinical restenosis." *J Clin Invest* 98:863, 1996.

284. Miyazaki Y, Nomura S, Miyake T, et al: High shear stress can initiate both platelet aggregation and shedding of procoagulant containing microparticles. *Blood* 88:3456, 1996.

285. Lee DH, Warkentin TE, Denomme GA, Hayward CP, Kelton JG: A diagnostic test for heparin-induced thrombocytopenia: detection of platelet microparticles using flow cytometry. *Br J Haematol* 95:724, 1996.

286. Beguin S, Kumar R, Keularts I, Seligsohn U, Coller BS, Hemker HC: Fibrin-dependent platelet procoagulant activity requires GPIb receptors and von Willebrand factor. *Blood* 93:564, 1999.

287. George JN, Pickett EB, Saucerman S, et al: Platelet surface glycoproteins. Studies on resting and activated platelets and platelet membrane microparticles in normal subjects, and observations in patients during adult respiratory distress syndrome and cardiac surgery. *J Clin Invest* 78:340, 1986.

288. Siljander P, Carpen O, Lassila R: Platelet-derived microparticles associate with fibrin during thrombosis. *Blood* 87:4651, 1996.

289. Shcherbina A, Remold-O'Donnell E: Role of caspase in a subset of human platelet activation responses. *Blood* 93:4222, 1999.

290. Wolf BB, Goldstein JC, Stennicke HR, et al: Calpain functions in a caspase-independent manner to promote apoptosis-like events during platelet activation. *Blood* 94:1683, 1999.

291. Zucker MB, McPherson J: Reactions of platelets near surfaces in vitro: lessons from the platelet retention test. *Ann NY Acad Sci* 283:128, 1977.

292. Mann KG, Tracy PB, Kirshnaswamy S: Platelets and coagulation, in *Thrombosis and Haemostasis*, edited by M Verstrate, LH Vermylen, J Arnout, p 505. Leuven University Press, Leuven, Belgium, 1987.

293. Zwaal RFA, Comfurius P, Bevers EM: Platelet procoagulant activity and microvesicle formation. Its putative role of hemostasis and thrombosis. *Biochim Biophys Acta* 1180:1, 1992.

294. Weiss HJ: Scott syndrome—a disorder of platelet coagulant activity. *Semin Hematol* 31:312, 1994.

295. Swords NA, Tracy PB, Mann KG: Intact platelet membranes, not plate-

let-released microvesicles, support the procoagulant activity of adherent platelets. *Arterioscler Thromb* 13:1613, 1993.

296. Weiss HJ, Lages B: Platelet prothrombinase activity and intracellular calcium responses in patients with storage pool deficiency, glycoprotein IIb-IIIa deficiency, or impaired platelet coagulant activity—a comparison with Scott syndrome. *Blood* 89:1599, 1997.

297. Hultin MB: Modulation of thrombin-mediated activation of factor VIII:C by calcium ions, phospholipid, and platelets. *Blood* 66:53, 1985.

298. Nesheim ME, Furmaniak-Kazmierczak E, Henin C, Cote G: On the existence of platelet receptors for factors V(a) and factor VIII (a). *Thromb Haemost* 70:80, 1993.

299. Osterud B, Rapaport SI, Lavine KK: Factor V activity of platelets: evidence for an activated factor V molecule and for a platelet activator. *Blood* 49:834, 1977.

300. Toti F, Satta N, Fressinaud E, Meyer D, Freyssinet JM: Scott syndrome, characterized by impaired transmembrane migration of procoagulant phosphatidylserine and hemorrhagic complications, is an inherited disorder. *Blood* 87:1409, 1996.

301. Zhou Q, Sims PJ, Wiedmer T: Expression of proteins controlling transbilayer movement of plasma membrane phospholipids in the B lymphocytes from a patient with Scott syndrome. *Blood* 92:1707, 1998.

302. Martincic D, Kravtsov V, Gailani D: Factor XI messenger RNA in human platelets. *Blood* 94:3397, 1999.

303. Walsh PN: Platelets and factor XI bypass the contact system of blood coagulation. *Thromb Haemost* 82:234, 1999.

304. Lopez JA: The platelet glycoprotein Ib-IX complex. *Blood Coagul Fibrinolysis* 5:97, 1994.

305. Rajagopalan V, Essex DW, Shapiro SS, Konkle BA: Tumor necrosis factor-alpha modulation of glycoprotein Ib-alpha expression in human endothelial and erythroleukemia cells. *Blood* 80:153, 1992.

306. Wu G, Essex DW, Meloni FJ, et al: Human endothelial cells in culture and in vivo express on their surface all four components of the glycoprotein Ib/IX/V complex. *Blood* 90:2660, 1997.

307. Hynes RO: Integrins: a family of cell surface receptors. *Cell* 48:549, 1987.

308. Peerschke EIB: Platelet membranes and receptors, in *Thrombosis and Hemorrhage*, edited by AI Schafer, p 219. Blackwell, Boston, 1994.

309. Bennett JS: The molecular biology of platelet membrane proteins. *Semin Hematol* 27:186, 1990.

310. Wagner CL, Mascelli MA, Neblock DS, Weisman HF, Coller BS, Jordan RE: Analysis of GPIIb/IIIa receptor number by quantification of 7E3 binding to human platelets. *Blood* 88:907, 1996.

311. Woods VL, Jr, Wolff LE, Keller DM: Resting platelets contain a substantial centrally located pool of glycoprotein IIb-IIIa complexes which may be accessible to some but not other extracellular proteins. *J Biol Chem* 261:15242, 1986.

312. Cramer ER, Savidge GF, Vainchenker W, et al: α granule pool of glycoprotein IIb-IIIa in normal and pathologic platelets and megakaryocytes. *Blood* 75:1220, 1990.

313. Youssefian T, Masse JM, Rendu F, Guichard J, Cramer EM: Platelet and megakaryocyte dense granules contain glycoproteins Ib and IIb-IIIa. *Blood* 89:4047, 1997.

314. Carrell NA, Fitzgerald LA, Steiner B, Erickson HP, Phillips DR: Structure of human platelet membrane glycoproteins IIb and IIIa as determined by electron microscopy. *J Biol Chem* 260:1743, 1985.

315. Calvete JJ, Mann K, Alvarez MV, Lopez MM, Gonzalez-Rodriguez J: Proteolytic dissection of the isolated platelet fibrinogen receptor, integrin GPIIb/IIIa. Localization of GPIIb and GPIIIa sequences putatively involved in the subunit interface and in intrasubunit and intrachain contacts. *Biochem J* 282 (Pt 2):523, 1992.

316. Poncz M, Eisman R, Heidenreich R, et al: Structure of the platelet membrane glycoprotein IIb. Homology to the alpha subunits of the vitronectin and fibronectin membrane receptors. *J Biol Chem* 262:8476, 1987.

317. Fitzgerald LA, Steiner B, Rall SC Jr, Lo SS, Phillips DR: Protein sequence of endothelial glycoprotein IIIa derived from a cDNA clone. Identity with platelet glycoprotein IIIa and similarity to "integrin." *J Biol Chem* 262:3936, 1987.

318. Bray PF, Barsh G, Rosa JP, Luo XY, Magenis E, Shuman MA: Physical linkage of the genes for platelet membrane glycoproteins IIb and IIIa. *Proc Natl Acad Sci USA* 85:8683, 1988.

319. Thornton MA, Poncz M, Korostishevsky M, et al: The human platelet alphaIIb gene is not closely linked to its integrin partner beta3. *Blood* 94:2039, 1999.

320. Steiner B, Parise LV, Leung B, Phillips DR: Ca^{+2} dependent structural transitions of the platelet glycoprotein IIb-IIIa complex. Preparation of stable glycoprotein IIb and IIIa monomers. *J Biol Chem* 266:14986, 1991.

321. Duperray A, Troesch A, Berthier R, et al: Biosynthesis and assembly of platelet GPIIb-IIIa in human megakaryocytes: evidence that assembly between pro-GPIIb and GPIIIa is a prerequisite for expression of the complex on the cell surface. *Blood* 74:1603, 1989.

322. O'Toole TE, Loftus JC, Plow EF, Glass AA, Harper JR, Ginsberg MH: Efficient surface expression of platelet GPIIb-IIIa requires both subunits. *Blood* 74:14, 1989.

323. McEver RP, Baenziger JU, Majerus PW: Isolation and structural characterization of the polypeptide subunits of membrane glycoprotein IIb-IIIa from human platelets. *Blood* 59:80, 1982.

324. Wencel-Drake JD: Plasma membrane GPIIb/IIIa. Evidence for a cycling receptor pool. *Am J Clin Pathol* 136:61, 1990.

325. Coller BS: Activation-specific platelet antigens, in *Platelet Immunobiology: Molecular and Clinical Aspects*, edited by TJ Kunicki, p 166. JB Lippincott, Philadelphia, 1989.

326. Sims PJ, Ginsberg MH, Plow EF, Shattil SJ: Effect of platelet activation on the conformation of the plasma membrane glycoprotein IIb-IIIa complex. *J Biol Chem* 266:7345, 1991.

327. O'Toole TE, Mandelman D, Forsyth J, Shattil SJ, Plow EF, Ginsberg MH: Modulation of the affinity of integrin αIIbβ3 (GPIIb-IIIa) by the cytoplasmic domain of alpha IIb. *Science* 254:845, 1991.

328. O'Toole TE, Katagiri Y, Faull RJ, et al: Integrin cytoplasmic domains mediate inside-out signal transduction. *J Cell Biol* 124:1047, 1994.

329. D'Souza SE, Ginsberg MH, Burke TA, et al: Localization of an Arg-Gly-Asp recognition site within an integrin adhesion receptor. *Science* 242:91, 1988.

330. D'Souza SE, Ginsberg MH, Burke TA, Plow EF: The ligand binding site of the platelet integrin receptor GPIIb-IIIa is proximal to the second calcium binding domain of its α-subunit. *J Biol Chem* 265:3440, 1990.

331. D'Souza SE, Ginsberg MH, Matsueda G, Plow EF: A discrete sequence in a platelet integrin is involved in ligand recogntion. *Nature* 350:66, 1991.

332. Charo IF, Nannizzi L, Phillips DR, Hsu MA, Scarborough RM: Inhibition of fibrinogen binding to GPIIb-IIIa by a GPIIIa peptide. *J Biol Chem* 266:1415, 1991.

333. Tozer EC, Liddington RC, Sutcliffe MJ, Smeeton AH, Loftus JC: Ligand binding to integrin αIIbβ3 is dependent on a MIDAS-like domain in the beta3 subunit. *J Biol Chem* 271:21978, 1996.

334. Lin EK, Ratnikov BI, Tsai PM, et al: Evidence that the integrin beta3 and beta5 subunits contain a metal ion- dependent adhesion site-like motif but lack an I domain. *J Biol Chem* 272:14236, 1997.

335. Springer TA: Folding of the N-terminal, ligand-binding region of integrin α-subunits into a β-propeller domain. *Proc Natl Acad Sci USA* 94:65, 1997.

336. Coller BS, Cheresh DA, Asch E, Seligsohn U: Platelet vitronectin receptor expression differentiates Iraqi-Jewish from Arab patients with Glanzmann thrombasthenia in Israel. *Blood* 77:75, 1991.

337. Hynes RO: Integrins: a family of cell surface receptors. *Cell* 48:549, 1987.

338. Ruoslahti E: Fibronectin and its receptors. *Annu Rev Biochem* 57:375, 1988.

339. Doolittle RF, Watt KWK, Cottrell BA, Strong DD, Riley M: The amino acid sequence of the alpha-chain of human fibrinogen. *Nature* 280:464, 1979.

340. Hawiger J: Adhesive interactions of platelets and their blockade. *Ann NY Acad Sci* 614:270, 1991.

341. Cheresh DA, Berliner SA, Vicente V, Ruggeri ZM: Recognition of distinct adhesive sites on fibrinogen by related integrins on platelets and endothelial cells. *Cell* 58:945, 1989.

342. Farrell DH, Thiagarajan P, Chung DW, Davie EW: Role of fibrinogen α and γ chain sites in platelet aggregation. *Proc Natl Acad Sci USA* 89:10729, 1992.

343. Farrell DH, Thiagarajan P: Binding of recombinant fibrinogen mutants to platelets. *J Biol Chem* 269:226, 1994.

344. Topol EJ, Byzova TV, Plow EF: Platelet GPIIb-IIIa blockers. *Lancet* 353:227, 1999.

345. Wencel-Drake JD, Boudignon-Proudhon C, Dieter MG, Criss AB, Parise

LV: Internalization of bound fibrinogen modulates platelet aggregation. *Blood* 87:602, 1996.

346. Peerschke EIB: Events occurring after thrombin-induced fibrinogen binding to platelets. *Semin Thromb Hemost* 18:34, 1992.

347. Zamarron C, Ginsberg MH, Plow EF: A receptor-induced binding site in fibrinogen elicited by its interaction with platelet membrane glycoprotein IIb-IIIa. *J Biol Chem* 266:17106, 1991.

348. Ugarova TP, Budzynski AZ, Shattil SJ, Ruggeri ZM, Ginsberg MH, Plow EF: Conformational changes in fibrinogen elecited by its interaction with platelet membrane glycoprotein GPIIb-IIIa. *J Biol Chem* 268:21080, 1993.

349. Heilmann E, Hourdille P, Pruvost A, Paponneau A, Nurden AT: Thrombin-induced platelet aggregates have a dynamic structure: time-dependent redistribution of GPIIb/IIIa complexes and secreted adhesive proteins. *Arterioscler Thromb* 11:704, 1991.

350. Weisel JW, Nagaswami C, Vilaire G, Bennett JS: Examination of the platelet membrane glycoprotein IIb-IIIa complex and its interaction with fibrinogen and other ligands by electron microscopy. *J Biol Chem* 267:16637, 1992.

351. Isenberg WM, McEver RP, Phillips DR, Shuman MA, Bainton DF: The platelet fibrinogen receptor: an immunogold-surface replica study of agonist-induced ligand binding and receptor clustering. *J Cell Biol* 104:1655, 1987.

352. Asch E, Podack E: Vitronectin binds to activated human platelets and plays a role in platelet aggregation. *J Clin Invest* 85:1372, 1990.

353. Haverstick DM, Cowan JF, Yamada KM, Santoro SA: Inhibition of platelet adhesion to fibronectin, fibrinogen, and von Willebrand factor substrates by a synthetic tetrapeptide derived from the cell-binding domain of fibronectin. *Blood* 66:946, 1985.

354. Plow EF, D'Souza SE, Ginsberg MH: Ligand binding to GPIIb-IIIa: a status report. *Semin Thromb Hemost* 18:324, 1992.

355. Schullek J, Jordan J, Montgomery RR: Interaction of von Willebrand factor with human platelets in the plasma milieu. *J Clin Invest* 73:421, 1984.

356. Kieffer N, Fitzgerald LA, Wolf D, Cheresh DA, Phillips DR: Adhesive properties of the $\beta 3$ integrins. Comparison of GPIIb-IIIa and the vitronectin receptor individually expressed in human melanoma cells. *J Cell Biol* 113:451, 1991.

357. Moskowitz KA, Kudryk B, Coller BS: Fibrinogen coating density affects the conformation of immobilized fibrinogen: implications for platelet adhesion and spreading. *Thromb Haemost* 79:824, 1998.

358. Hatton MW, Moar SL, Richardson M: Deendothelialization in vivo initiates a thrombogenic reaction at the rabbit aorta surface. Correlation of uptake of fibrinogen and antithrombin III with thrombin generation by the exposed subendothelium. *Am J Pathol* 135:499, 1989.

359. Miles LA, Ginsberg MH, White JG, Plow EF: Plasminogen interacts with human platelets through two distinct mechanisms. *J Clin Invest* 77:2001, 1986.

360. Cox AD, Devine DV: Factor XIIIa binding to activated platelets is mediated through activation of glycoprotein IIb-IIIa. *Blood* 83:1006, 1994.

361. Peerschke EI, Grant RA, Zucker MB: Decreased association of 45-calcium with platelets unable to aggregate due to thrombasthenia or prolonged calcium deprivation. *Br J Haematol* 46:247, 1980.

362. Powling MJ, Hardisty RM: Glycoprotein IIb-IIIa complex and Ca^{++} influx into stimulated platelets. *Blood* 66:731, 1985.

363. Rybak MEM, Renzulli LA: Effect of calcium channel blockers on platelet GPIIb-IIIa as a calcium channel in liposomes: comparison with effects on the intact platelet. *Thromb Haemost* 67:131, 1991.

364. Ameisen JC, Joseph M, Caen JP, et al: A role for glycoprotein IIb-IIIa complexes in the binding of IgE to human platelets and platelet IgE-dependent cytolytic function. *Br J Haematol* 64:21, 1986.

365. Coburn J, Barthold SW, Leong JM: Diverse Lyme disease spirochetes bind integrin alpha IIb beta 3 on human platelets. *Infect Immun* 62:5559, 1994.

366. Pischel KD, Hemler MD, Huang C, Bluestein HG, Woods VL: Use of the monoclonal antibody 12F1 to characterize the differentiation antigen VLA-2. *J Immunol* 138:226, 1987.

367. Kunicki DJ, Nugent DJ, Staats SJ, et al: The human fibroblast II extracellular matrix receptor mediates platelet adhesion to collagen and is identical to the platelet glycoprotein Ia-IIa complex. *J Biol Chem* 263:4516, 1988.

368. Staatz WD, Rajpara SM, Wayner EA, Carter WG, Santoro SA: The membrane glycoprotein Ia-IIa (VLA-2) complex mediates the Mg^{++}-dependent adhesion of platelets to collagen. *J Cell Biol* 108:1917, 1989.

369. Barnes MJ, Knight CG, Farndale RW: The collagen-platelet interaction. *Curr Opin Hematol* 5:314, 1998.

370. Takada Y, Hemler ME: The primary structure of the VLA-2/collagen receptor $\alpha 2$ subunit (platelet GPIa): homology to other integrins and the presence of a possible collagen-binding domain. *J Cell Biol* 109:397, 1987.

371. Staatz WD, Walsh JJ, Pexton T, Santoro SA: The $\alpha 2\beta 1$ integrin cell surface collagen receptor binds to the $\alpha 1(I)$-CB3 peptide of collagen. *J Biol Chem* 265:4778, 1990.

372. Knight CG, Morton LF, Onley DJ, et al: Identification in collagen type I of an integrin alpha2 beta1-binding site containing an essential GER sequence. *J Biol Chem* 273:33287, 1998.

373. Santoro SA, Walsh JJ, Staatz WD, Baranski KJ: Distinct determinants on collagen support $\alpha 2\beta 1$ integrin-mediated platelet adhesion and platelet activation. *Cell Regul* 2:905, 1991.

374. Verkleij MW, Ijsseldijk MJ, Heijnen-Snyder GJ, et al: Adhesive domains in the collagen III fragment alpha1(III)CB4 that support alpha2beta1-von Willebrand factor-mediated platelet adhesion under flow conditions. *Thromb Haemost* 82:1137, 1999.

375. Nieuwenhuis HK, Akkerman JWN, Houdijk WPM, Sixma JJ: Human blood platelets showing no response to collagen fail to express surface glycoprotein Ia. *Nature* 318:470, 1985.

376. Kritzik M, Savage B, Nugent DJ, Santoso S, Ruggeri ZM, Kunicki TJ: Nucleotide polymorphisms in the alpha2 gene define multiple alleles that are associated with differences in platelet alpha2 beta1 density. *Blood* 92:2382, 1998.

377. Bray PF: Integrin polymorphisms as risk factors for thrombosis. *Thromb Haemost* 82:337, 1999.

378. Moshfegh K, Wuillemin WA, Redondo M, et al: Association of two silent polymorphisms of platelet glycoprotein Ia/IIa receptor with risk of myocardial infarction: a case-control study. *Lancet* 353:351, 1999.

379. Santoso S, Kunicki TJ, Kroll H, Haberbosch W, Gardemann A: Association of the platelet glycoprotein Ia C807T gene polymorphism with nonfatal myocardial infarction in younger patients. *Blood* 93:2449, 1999.

380. Carlsson LE, Santoso S, Spitzer C, Kessler C, Greinacher A: The alpha2 gene coding sequence T807/A873 of the platelet collagen receptor integrin alpha2beta1 might be a genetic risk factor for the development of stroke in younger patients. *Blood* 93:3583, 1999.

381. Elices MJ, Hemler ME: The integrin VLA-2 can be a laminin as well as a collagen receptor. *Proc Natl Acad Sci USA* 86:9906, 1989.

382. Kirchhofer D, Languinol R, Ruoslahti E, Pierschbacher MD: $\alpha 2\beta 1$ integrins from different cell types show different binding specificities. *J Biol Chem* 265:615, 1990.

383. Piotrowicz RS, Orchekowski RP, Nugent DJ, Yamada KY, Kunicki TJ: Glycoprotein Ic-IIa functions as an activation-independent fibronectin receptor on human platelets. *J Cell Biol* 106:1359, 1988.

384. Wayner EA, Carter WG, Piotrowicz RS, Kunicki TJ: The function of multiple extracellular matrix receptors in mediating cell adhesion to extracellular matrix: preparation of monoclonal antibodies to the fibronectin receptor that specifically inhibit cell adhesion of fibronectin and react with platelet glycoproteins Ic-IIa. *J Cell Biol* 107:1881, 1988.

385. Vuillet-Gaugler MH, Breton-Gorius J, Vainchenker W, et al: Loss of attachment to fibronectin with terminal human erythroid differentiation. *Blood* 75:865, 1990.

386. Sonnenberg A, Modderman PW, Hogervorst F: Laminin receptor on platelets is the integrin VLA-6. *Nature* 336:487, 1988.

387. Hindriks G, Ijsseldijk MJ, Sonnenberg A, Sixma JJ, de Groot PG: Platelet adhesion to laminin: role of Ca2+ and Mg2+ ions, shear rate, and platelet membrane glycoproteins. *Blood* 79:928, 1992.

388. Tandon NN, Holland EA, Kralisz U, Kleinman HK, Robey FA, Jamieson GA: Interaction of human platelets with laminin and identification of the 67 kDa laminin receptor on platelets. *Biochem J* 274:535, 1991.

389. Fitzgerald LA, Poncz M, Steiner B, Rall Jr SC, Bennett JS, Phillips DR: Comparison of cDNA-derived protein sequences of the human fibronectin and vitronectin receptor a subunits and platelet glycoprotein IIb. *Biochemistry* 26:8158, 1987.

390. Lam SC, Plow EF, D'Souza SE, Cheresh DA, Frelinger AL, III, Ginsberg MH: Isolation and characterization of a platelet membrane protein related to the vitronectin receptor. *J Biol Chem* 264:3742, 1989.

391. Charo IF, Bekeart LS, Phillips DR: Platelet glycoprotein IIb-IIIa-like proteins mediate endothelial cell attachment to adhesive proteins and the extracellular matrix. *J Biol Chem* 262:9935, 1987.

392. Bennett JS, Chan C, Vilaire G, Mousa SA, DeGrado WF: Agonist-activated alphavbeta3 on platelets and lymphocytes binds to the matrix protein osteopontin. *J Biol Chem* 272:8137, 1997.

393. Beckstead JH, Stenberg PE, McEver RP, Shuman MA, Bainton DF: Immunohistochemical localization of membrane and alpha-granule proteins in human megakaryocytes: application to plastic-embedded bone marrow biopsy specimens. *Blood* 67:285, 1986.

394. Davies J, Warwick J, Totty N, Philip R, Helfrich M, Horton M: The osteoclast functional antigen, implicated in the regulation of bone resorption is biochemically related to the vitronectin receptor. *J Cell Biol* 109:1817, 1989.

395. Savill J, Dransfield I, Hogg N, Haslett C: Vitronectin receptor-mediated phagocytosis of cells undergoing apoptosis. *Nature* 343:170, 1990.

396. Brooks PC, Clark RA, Cheresh DA: Requirement of vascular integrin $\alpha V\beta 3$ for angiogenesis. *Science* 264:569, 1994.

397. Varner JA, Cheresh DA: Integrins and cancer. *Curr Opin Cell Biol* 8:724, 1996.

398. Choi ET, Engel L, Callow AD, et al: Inhibition of neointimal hyperplasia by blocking $\alpha_v\beta_3$ integrin with a small peptide antagonist *Gpen*GRGDS-PCA. *J Vasc Surg* 19:125, 1994.

399. Lopez JH, Chung DW, Fujikawa K, Hagen FS, Davie EW, Roth GJ: The α and β chains of human platelet glycoprotein Ib are both transmembrane proteins containing a leucine-rich amino acid sequence. *Proc Natl Acad Sci USA* 85:2135, 1988.

400. Lopez JA, Andrews RK, Afshar-Kharghan V, Berndt MC: Bernard-Soulier syndrome. *Blood* 91:4397, 1998.

401. Lopez JA, Ludwig EW, McCarthy BJ: Polymorphism of human glycoprotein Ibα results from a variable number of repeats of a 13-amino acid sequence in the mucin-like macroglycopeptide region. Structure function implications. *J Biol Chem* 267:10055, 1992.

402. Murata M, Matsubara Y, Kawano K, et al: Coronary artery disease and polymorphisms in a receptor mediating shear stress-dependent platelet activation. *Circulation* 96:3281, 1997.

403. Gonzalez-Conejero R, Lozano ML, Rivera J, et al: Polymorphisms of platelet membrane glycoprotein Ib associated with arterial thrombotic disease. *Blood* 92:2771, 1998.

404. Carlsson LE, Greinacher A, Spitzer C, Walther R, Kessler C: Polymorphisms of the human platelet antigens HPA-1, HPA-2, HPA-3, and HPA-5 on the platelet receptors for fibrinogen (GPIIb/IIIa), von Willebrand factor (GPIb/IX), and collagen (GPIa/IIa) are not correlated with an increased risk for stroke. *Stroke* 28:1392, 1997.

405. Kaski S, Kekomaki R, Partanen J: Systematic screening for genetic polymorphism in human platelet glycoprotein Ibalpha. *Immunogenetics* 44:170, 1996.

406. Suzuki K, Hayashi T, Akiba J, et al: StyI polymorphism at nucleotide 1610 in the human platelet glycoprotein Ib alpha gene. *Jpn J Hum Genet* 41:419, 1996.

407. Afshar-Kharghan V, Li CQ, Khoshnevis-Asl M, Lopez JA: Kozak sequence polymorphism of the glycoprotein (GP) Ibalpha gene is a major determinant of the plasma membrane levels of the platelet GP Ib-IX-V complex. *Blood* 94:186, 1999.

408. Tsuj T, Tsunehisa S, Watanabe Y, Yamamoto K, Tohyama H, Osawa T: The carbohydrate moiety of human platelet glycocalicin. The structure of the major ser/thr sugar chain. *J Biol Chem* 258:6335, 1983.

409. Fox JEB, Aggerbeck LP, Berndt MC: Structure of the glycoprotein Ib-IX complex from platelet membranes. *J Biol Chem* 263:4882, 1988.

410. Solum NO, Hagen I, Filion-Myklebust C, Staback T: Platelet glycocalicin: its membrane association in solvent and aqueous media. *Biochim Biophys Acta* 597:235, 1990.

411. Coller BS, Kalomiris EL, Steinberg M, Scudder LE: Evidence that glycocalicin circulates in normal plasma. *J Clin Invest* 73:794, 1984.

412. Steinberg MH, Kelton JG, Coller BS: Plasma glycocalicin: an aid in the classification of thrombocytopenic disorders. *N Engl J Med* 317:1037, 1987.

413. Beer JH, Buchi L, Steiner B: Glycocalicin: a new assay—the normal plasma levels and its potential usefulness in selected diseases. *Blood* 83:691, 1994.

414. Kalomiris EL, Coller BS: Thiol-specific probes indicate that the alpha chain of platelet glycoprotein Ib is a transmembrane protein with a reactive endofacial sulfhydryl group. *Biochemistry* 24:5430, 1985.

415. Fox JEB, Berndt MC: Cyclic AMP-dependent phosphorylation of glycoprotein Ib inhibits collagen-induced polymerization of actin in platelets. *J Biol Chem* 264:9520, 1989.

416. Andrews RK, Fox JE: Identification of a region in the cytoplasmic domain of the platelet membrane glycoprotein Ib-IX complex that binds to purified actin-binding protein. *J Biol Chem* 267:18605, 1992.

417. Coller BS: Inhibition of von Willebrand factor-dependent platelet function by increased platelet cyclic AMP and its prevention by cytoskeleton-disrupting agents. *Blood* 57:846, 1981.

418. Coller BS: Effects of tertiary amine local anesthetics on von Willebrand factor-dependent platelet function: alteration of membrane reactivity and degradation of GPIb by a calcium-dependent protease(s). *Blood* 248:1355, 1982.

419. Dong JF, Li CQ, Sae-Tung G, Hyun W, Afshar-Kharghan V, Lopez JA: The cytoplasmic domain of glycoprotein (GP) Ibalpha constrains the lateral diffusion of the GP Ib-IX complex and modulates von Willebrand factor binding. *Biochemistry* 36:12421, 1997.

420. Muzbarek L, Laposata M: Glycoprotein Ib and glycoprotein IX in human platelets are acylated with palmitic acid through thioester linkages. *J Biol Chem* 264:9716, 1989.

421. Sullam PM, Hyun WC, Szollosi J, Dong J, Foss WM, Lopez JA: Physical proximity and functional interplay of the glycoprotein Ib-IX-V complex and the Fc receptor FcgammaRIIA on the platelet plasma membrane. *J Biol Chem* 273:5331, 1998.

422. Falati S, Edmead CE, Poole AW: Glycoprotein Ib-V-IX, a receptor for von Willebrand factor, couples physically and functionally to the Fc receptor γ-chain, Fyn, and Lyn to activate human platelets. *Blood* 94:1648, 1999.

423. Du X, Beutler L, Ruan C, Castaldi PA, Berndt MC: Glycoprotein Ib and glycoprotein IX are fully complexed in the intact platelet membrane. *Blood* 69:1524, 1987.

424. Hickey MJ, Williams SA, Roth GJ: Human platelet GPIX: An adhesive prototype of leucine-rich glycoproteins with flank-center-flank structures. *Proc Natl Acad Sci USA* 86:6773, 1989.

425. Hickey MJ, Deaven LL, Roth GJ: Human platelet glycoprotein IX. Characterization of cDNA and localization of the gene to chromosome 3. *FEBS Lett* 274:189, 1991.

426. Lopez JA, Leung B, Reynolds CC, Li CQ, Fox JEB: Efficient plasma membrane expression of a functional platelet glycoprotein Ib-IX complex requires the presence of its three subunits. *J Biol Chem* 267:12851, 1992.

427. Kobe B, Deisenhofer J: Crystal structure of porcine ribonuclease inhibitor, a protein with leucine-rich repeats. *Nature* 366:751, 1993.

428. Vincente V, Houghten RA, Ruggeri ZM: Identification of a site in the α chain of platelet glycoprotein Ib that participates in von Willebrand binding. *J Biol Chem* 265:274, 1990.

429. Katagiri Y, Hayashi Y, Yamamoto K, Tanoue K, Kosaki G, Yamazaki H: Localization of von Willebrand factor and thrombin-interactive domains in human platelet glycoprotein Ib. *Thromb Haemost* 63:122, 1990.

430. Murata M, Ware J, Ruggeri ZM: Site-directed mutagenesis of a soluble recombinant fragment of platelet glycoprotein Ib alpha demonstrating negatively charged residues involved in von Willebrand factor binding. *J Biol Chem* 266:15474, 1991.

431. Hess D, Schaller J, Rickli EE, Clemetson KJ: Identification of the disulphide bonds in human platelet glycocalicin. *Eur J Biochem* 199:389, 1991.

432. Scott JP, Montgomery RR, Retzinger GS: Dimeric ristocetin flocculates proteins, binds to platelets, and mediates von Willebrand factor-dependent agglutination of platelets. *J Biol Chem* 266:8149, 1991.

433. Andrews RK, Booth WJ, Gorman JJ, Castaldi PA, Berndt MC: Purification of botrocetin from Bothrops jararaca venom. Analysis of the botrocetin-mediated interaction between von Willebrand factor and the human platelet membrane glycoprotein Ib-IX complex. *Biochemistry* 28:8317, 1989.

434. Olson JD, Zaleski A, Herrmann D, Flood PA: Adhesion of platelets to purified solid-phase von Willebrand factor: effect of wall shear rate, ADP, thrombin, and ristocetin. *J Lab Clin Med* 114:6, 1989.

435. Parker RI, Gralnick HR: Fibrin monomer induces binding of endogenous vWF to the glycocalicin portion of platelet glycoprotein Ib. *Blood* 70:1589, 1987.

436. Sakariassen KS, Fressinaud E, Grima JP, Meyer D, Baumgartner HR: Role of platelet membrane glycoproteins and von Willebrand factor in adhesion of platelets to subendothelium and collagen. *Ann NY Acad Sci* 516:52, 1987.

437. Sakariassen KS, Nievelstein PFEM, Coller BS, Sixma JJ: The role of platelet membrane glycoproteins Ib and IIb-IIIa in platelet adherence to human artery subendothelium. *Br J Haematol* 63:681, 1986.

438. Ikeda Y, Murata M, Araki Y, et al: Importance of fibrinogen and platelet membrane glycoprotein IIb/IIIa in shear-induced platelet aggregation. *Thromb Res* 51:157, 1988.

439. Siediecki CA, Lestini BJ, Kottke-Marchant KK, Eppell SJ, Wilson DL, Marchant RE: Shear-dependent changes in the three-dimensional structure of human von Willebrand factor. *Blood* 88:2939, 1996.

440. Jamieson GA: The activation of platelets by thrombin: a model for activation by high and moderate affinity receptor pathways. *Prog Clin Biol Res* 283:137, 1988.

441. Ruggeri Z: The platelet glycoprotein Ib-IX complex. *Prog Hem Thromb* 10:35, 1991.

442. Harmon JT, Jamieson GA: The glycocalicin portion of platelet glycoprotein Ib expresses both high and moderate affinity receptor sites of thrombin. A soluble radioreceptor assay for the injection of thrombin with platelets. *J Biol Chem* 261:13224, 1986.

443. Frenette PS, Moyna C, Hartwell DW, Lowe JB, Hynes RO, Wagner DD: Platelet-endothelial interactions in inflamed mesenteric venules. *Blood* 91:1318, 1998.

444. Berndt MC, Phillips DR: Purification and preliminary physiochemical characterization of human platelet membrane glycoprotein V. *J Biol Chem* 256:59, 1981.

445. Zafar RS, Walz DA: Platelet membrane glycoprotein V: characterization of the thrombin-sensitive glycoprotein from human platelets. *Thromb Res* 53:31, 1989.

446. Shimomura T, Fujimura K, Maehama S, et al: Rapid purification and characterization of human platelet glycoprotein V: the amino acid sequence contains leucine-rich repetitive modules as in glycoprotein Ib. *Blood* 75:2349, 1990.

447. Lanza F, Morales M, De La Salle C, et al: Cloning and characterization of the gene encoding the human platelet glycoprotein V. A member of the leucine-rich glycoprotein family cleaved during thrombin-induced platelet activation. *J Biol Chem* 268:20801, 1993.

448. Modderman PW, Admiraal LG, Sonnenberg A, von dem Borne AEGKr: Glycoproteins V and Ib-IX form a noncovalent complex in the platelet membrane. *J Biol Chem* 267:364, 1992.

449. Dong JF, Gao S, Lopez JA: Synthesis, assembly, and intracellular transport of the platelet glycoprotein Ib-IX-V complex. *J Biol Chem* 273:31449, 1998.

450. McGowan EB, Ding A, Detwiler TC: Correlation of thrombin-induced glycoprotein V hydrolysis and platelet activation. *J Biol Chem* 258:11243, 1983.

451. Ramakrishnan V, Reeves PS, DeGuzman F, et al: Increased thrombin responsiveness in platelets from mice lacking glycoprotein V. *Proc Natl Acad Sci* 96:13336, 1999.

452. Newman PJ, Berndt MC, Gorski J, White GC, Paddock LS, Muller WA: PECAM-1 (CD31) cloning and relation to adhesion molecules of the immunoglobulin gene superfamily. *Science* 247:1219, 1990.

453. Metzelaar MJ, Korteweg J, Sixma JJ, Nieuwenhuis HK: Biochemical characterization of PECAM-1 (CD31 antigen) on human platelets. *Thromb Haemost* 66:700, 1991.

454. Varon D, Jackson DE, Shenkman B, et al: Platelet/endothelial cell adhesion molecule-1 serves as a costimulatory agonist receptor that modulates integrin-dependent adhesion and aggregation of human platelets. *Blood* 91:500, 1998.

455. Jackson DE, Ward CM, Wang R, Newman PJ: The protein-tyrosine phosphatase SHP-2 binds platelet/endothelial cell adhesion molecule-1 (PECAM-1) and forms a distinct signaling complex during platelet aggregation. Evidence for a mechanistic link between PECAM-1- and integrin-mediated cellular signaling. *J Biol Chem* 272:6986, 1997.

456. Albelda SM, Muller WA, Buck CA, Newman PJ: Molecular and cellular properties of PECAM-1 (endoCAM/CD31): a novel vascular cell-cell adhesion molecule. *J Cell Biol* 114:1059, 1991.

457. DeLisser HM, Yan HC, Newman PJ, Muller WA, Buck CA, Albelda SM: Platelet/endothelial cell adhesion molecule-1 (CD31)-mediated cellular aggregation involves cell surface glycosaminoglycans. *J Biol Chem* 268:16037, 1993.

458. Gumina RJ, el Schultz J, Yao Z, et al: Antibody to platelet/endothelial cell adhesion molecule-1 reduces myocardial infarct size in a rat model of ischemia-reperfusion injury. *Circulation* 94:3327, 1996.

459. Qiu WQ, de Bruin D, Brownstein BH, Pearse R, Ravetch JV: Organization of the human and mouse low-affinity Fc gamma R genes: duplication and recombination. *Science* 248:732, 1990.

460. Parren PW, Warmerdam PA, Boeije LC, et al: On the interaction of IgG subclasses with the low affinity Fc gamma RIIa (CD32) on human monocytes, neutrophils, and platelets. Analysis of a functional polymorphism to human IgG2. *J Clin Invest* 90:1537, 1992.

461. Rosenfeld SI, Looney RJ, Leddy JP, Phipps DC, Abraham GN, Anderson CL: Human platelet Fc receptor for immunoglobulin G. Identification as a 40,000-molecular-weight membrane protein shared by monocytes. *J Clin Invest* 76:2317, 1985.

462. Rosenfeld SI, Ryan DH, Looney RJ, Anderson CL, Abraham GN, Leddy JP: Human Fc receptors: stable inter-donor variation in quantitative expression on platelets correlates with functional responses. *J Immunol* 138:2869, 1987.

463. Anderson GP, van de Winkel JG, Anderson CL: Anti-GPIIb/IIIa (CD41) monoclonal antibody-induced platelet activation requires Fc receptor-dependent cell-cell interaction. *Br J Haematol* 79:75, 1991.

464. Hildreth JE, Derr D, Azorsa DO: Characterization of a novel self-associating Mr 40,000 platelet glycoprotein. *Blood* 77:121, 1991.

465. Gratacap MP, Payrastre B, Viala C, Mauco G, Plantavid M, Chap H: Phosphatidylinositol 3,4,5-trisphosphate-dependent stimulation of phospholipase C-gamma2 is an early key event in FcgammaRIIA-mediated activation of human platelets. *J Biol Chem* 273:24314, 1998.

466. Chong BH, Pilgrim RL, Cooley MA, Chesterman CN: Increased expression of platelet IgG Fc receptors in immune heparin- induced thrombocytopenia. *Blood* 81:988, 1993.

467. Denomme GA, Warkentin TE, Horsewood P, Sheppard JA, Warner MN, Kelton JG: Activation of platelets by sera containing IgG1 heparin-dependent antibodies: an explanation for the predominance of the Fc gammaRIIa ''low responder'' (his131) gene in patients with heparin-induced thrombocytopenia. *J Lab Clin Med* 130:278, 1997.

468. Carlsson LE, Santoso S, Baurichter G, et al: Heparin-induced thrombocytopenia: new insights into the impact of the FcgammaRIIa-R-H131 polymorphism. *Blood* 92:1526, 1998.

469. Williams Y, Lynch S, McCann S, Smith O, Feighery C, Whelan A: Correlation of platelet Fc gammaRIIA polymorphism in refractory idiopathic (immune) thrombocytopenic purpura. *Br J Haematol* 101:779, 1998.

470. Torti M, Bertoni A, Canobbio I, Sinigaglia F, Lapetina EG, Balduini C: Rap1B and Rap2B translocation to the cytoskeleton by von Willebrand factor involves FcgammaII receptor-mediated protein tyrosine phosphorylation. *J Biol Chem* 274:13690, 1999.

471. Peerschke EI, Ghebrehiwet B: C1q augments platelet activation in response to aggregated Ig. *J Immunol* 159:5594, 1997.

472. Gibbins J, Asselin J, Farndale R, Barnes M, Law CL, Watson SP: Tyrosine phosphorylation of the Fc receptor gamma-chain in collagen-stimulated platelets. *J Biol Chem* 271:18095, 1996.

473. Reth M: Antigen receptor tail clue. *Nature* 338:383, 1989.

474. Flaswinkel H, Barner M, Reth M: The tyrosine activation motif as a target of protein tyrosine kinases and SH2 domains. *Semin Immunol* 7:21, 1995.

475. Tsuji M, Ezumi Y, Arai M, Takayama H: A novel association of Fc receptor gamma-chain with glycoprotein VI and their co-expression as a collagen receptor in human platelets. *J Biol Chem* 272:23528, 1997.

476. Chacko GW, Duchemin AM, Coggeshall KM, Osborne JM, Brandt JT, Anderson CL: Clustering of the platelet Fc gamma receptor induces noncovalent association with the tyrosine kinase p72syk. *J Biol Chem* 269:32435, 1994.

477. Gibbins JM, Briddon S, Shutes A, et al: The p85 subunit of phosphatidylinositol 3-kinase associates with the Fc receptor gamma-chain and linker for activitor of T cells (LAT) in platelets stimulated by collagen and convulxin. *J Biol Chem* 273:34437, 1998.

478. Gross BS, Melford SK, Watson SP: Evidence that phospholipase C-gamma2 interacts with SLP-76, Syk, Lyn, LAT and the Fc receptor gamma-chain after stimulation of the collagen receptor glycoprotein VI in human platelets. *Eur J Biochem* 263:612, 1999.

479. Diacovo TG, deFougerolles AR, Bainton DF, Springer TA: A functional integrin ligand on the surface of platelets: intercellular adhesion molecule-2. *J Clin Invest* 94:1243, 1994.

480. Larsen E, Celi A, Gilbert GE, et al: PADGEM protein: a receptor that mediates the interaction of activated platelets with neutrophils and monocytes. *Cell* 59:305, 1989.

481. Haskard DO: Adhesive proteins, in *Haemostasis and Thrombosis*, edited by AL Bloom, CD Forbes, DP Thomas, EGD Tuddenham, 3rd ed, p 233. Churchill Livingstone, Edinburgh, 1994.

482. Hamburger SA, McEver RP: GMP-140 mediates adhesion of stimulated platelets to neutrophils. *Blood* 75:550, 1990.

483. Geng JG, Bevilacqua P, Moore KL, et al: Rapid neutrophil adhesion to activated endothelium mediated by GMP-140. *Nature* 343:757, 1990.

484. Handa K, Nudelman ED, Stroud MR, Shiozawa T, Hakomori S: Selectin GMP-140 (CD62;PADGEM) binds to sialosyl-Le(a) and sialosyl-Le(x), and sulfated glycans modulate this binding. *Biochem Biophys Res Commun* 181:1223, 1991.

485. Polley MJ, Phillips ML, Wayner E, et al: CD62 and endothelial cell-leukocyte adhesion molecule I (ELAM-1) recognize the same carbohydrate ligand, sialyl-Lewis^x. *Proc Natl Acad Sci USA* 88:6224, 1991.

486. Aruffo A, Kolanus W, Walz G, Fredman P, Seed B: CD62/P-selectin recognition of myeloid and tumor cell sulfatides. *Cell* 67:35, 1991.

487. Stone JP, Wagner DD: P-selectin mediates adhesion of platelets to neuroblastoma and small cell lung cancer. *J Clin Invest* 92:804, 1993.

488. Sako D, Chang XJ, Barone KM, et al: Expression cloning of a functional glycoprotein ligand for P-selectin. *Cell* 75:1179, 1993.

489. Yang J, Furie BC, Furie B: The biology of P-selectin glycoprotein ligand-1: its role as a selectin counterreceptor in leukocyte-endothelial and leukocyte-platelet interaction. *Thromb Haemost* 81:1, 1999.

490. McEver RP, Cummings RD: Perspectives series: cell adhesion in vascular biology. Role of PSGL-1 binding to selectins in leukocyte recruitment. *J Clin Invest* 100:485, 1997.

491. Celi A, Pellegrini G, Lorenzet R, et al: P-selectin induces the expression of tissue factor on monocytes. *Proc Natl Acad Sci USA* 91:8767, 1994.

492. Mayadas TN, Johnson RC, Rayburn H, Hynes RO, Wagner DD: Leukocyte rolling and extravasation are severely compromised in P selectin-deficient mice. *Cell* 74:541, 1993.

493. Palabrica T, Lobb R, Furie BC, et al: Leukocyte accumulation promoting fibrin deposition is mediated in vivo by P-selectin on adherent platelets. *Nature* 359:848, 1992.

494. Chong BH, Murray B, Berndt MC, Dunlop LC, Brighton T, Chesterman CN: Plasma P-selectin is increased in thrombotic consumptive platelet disorders. *Blood* 83:1535, 1994.

495. Boucheix C, Benoit P, Frachet P, et al: Molecular cloning of the CD9 antigen. A new family of cell surface proteins. *J Biol Chem* 266:117, 1991.

496. Lanza F, Wolf D, Fox CF, et al: cDNA cloning and expression of platelet p24/CD9. Evidence for a new family of multiple membrane-spanning proteins. *J Biol Chem* 266:10638, 1991.

497. Hato T, Ikeda K, Yasukawa M, Watanabe A, Kobayashi Y: Exposure of platelet fibrinogen receptors by a monoclonal antibody to CD9 antigen. *Blood* 72:224, 1988.

498. Brisson C, Azorsa DO, Jennings LK, Moog S, Cazenave JP, Lanza F: Co-localization of CD9 and GPIIb-IIIa (alpha IIb beta 3 integrin) on activated platelet pseudopods and alpha-granule membranes. *Histochem J* 29:153, 1997.

499. Jennings LK, Fox CF, Kouns WC, McKay CP, Ballou LR, Schultz HE: The activation of human platelets mediated by anti-human platelet p24/CD9 monoclonal antibodies. *J Biol Chem* 265:3815, 1990.

500. Hato T, Sumida M, Yasukawa M, Watanabe A, Okuda H, Kobayashi Y: Induction of platelet Ca^{2+} influx and mobilization by a monoclonal antibody to CD9 antigen. *Blood* 75:1087, 1990.

501. Worthington RE, Carroll RC, Boucheix C: Platelet activation by CD9 monoclonal antibodies is mediated by the Fc gamma II receptor. *Br J Haematol* 74:216, 1990.

502. Slupsky JR, Seehafer JG, Tang SC, Masellis-Smith A, Shaw AR: Evidence that monoclonal antibodies against CD9 antigen induce specific association between CD9 and the platelet glycoprotein IIb-IIIa complex. *J Biol Chem* 264:12289, 1989.

503. Nishibori M, Cham B, McNicol A, Shalev A, Jain N, Gerrard JM: The protein CD63 is in platelet dense granules, is deficient in a patient with Hermansky-Pudlak syndrome, and appears identical to granulophysin. *J Clin Invest* 91:1775, 1993.

504. Metzelaar MJ, Wijngaard PL, Peters PJ, Sixma JJ, Nieuwenhuis HK, Clevers HC: CD63 antigen. A novel lysosomal membrane glycoprotein, cloned by a screening procedure for intracellular antigens in eukaryotic cells. *J Biol Chem* 266:3239, 1991.

505. Roberts JJ, Rodgers SE, Drury J, Ashman LK, Lloyd JV: Platelet activation induced by a murine monoclonal antibody directed against a novel tetra-span antigen. *Br J Haematol* 89:853, 1995.

506. Fitter S, Tetaz TJ, Berndt MC, Ashman LK: Molecular cloning of cDNA encoding a novel platelet-endothelial cell tetra-span antigen, PETA-3. *Blood* 86:1348, 1995.

507. Sincock PM, Mayrhofer G, Ashman LK: Localization of the transmembrane 4 superfamily (TM4SF) member PETA-3 (CD151) in normal human tissues: comparison with CD9, CD63, and alpha5beta1 integrin. *J Histochem Cytochem* 45:515, 1997.

508. Tandon NN, Lipsky RH, Burgess WH, Jamieson GA: Isolation and characterization of platelet glycoprotein IV (CD36). *J Biol Chem* 264:7570, 1989.

509. Legrand C, Pidard D, Beiso P, et al: Interaction of a monoclonal antibody to glycoprotein IV (CD36) with human platelets and its effect on platelet function. *Platelets* 2:99, 1991.

510. Daviet L, McGregor JL: Vascular biology of CD36: roles of this new adhesion molecule family in different disease states. *Thromb Haemost* 78:65, 1997.

511. Thorne RF, Meldrum CJ, Harris SJ, et al: CD36 forms covalently associated dimers and multimers in platelets and transfected COS-7 cells. *Biochem Biophys Res Commun* 240:812, 1997.

512. Thibert V, Bellucci S, Cristofari M, Gluckman E, Legrand C: Increased platelet CD36 constitutes a common marker in myeloproliferative disorders. *Br J Haematol* 91:618, 1995.

513. Asch AS, Barnwell J, Silverstein RL, Nachman RL: Isolation of the thrombospondin membrane receptor. *J Clin Invest* 79:1054, 1987.

514. Tandon NN, Kralisz U, Jamieson GA: Identification of glycoprotein IV (CD36) as a primary receptor for platelet-collagen adhesion. *J Biol Chem* 264:7576, 1989.

515. Diaz-Ricart M, Tandon NN, Gomez-Ortiz G, et al: Antibodies to CD36 (GPIV) inhibit platelet adhesion to subendothelial surfaces under flow conditions. *Arterioscler Thromb Vasc Biol* 16:883, 1996.

516. Yamamoto N, Ikeda H, Tandon NN, et al: A platelet membrane glycoprotein (GP) deficiency in healthy blood donors: Nak^a-platelets lack detectable GPIV (CD36). *Blood* 76:1698, 1990.

517. Wun T, Paglieroni T, Field CL, et al: Platelet-erythrocyte adhesion in sickle cell disease. *J Invest Med* 47:121, 1999.

518. Oquendo P, Hundt E, Lawler J, Seed B: CD36 directly mediates cyto-adherence of Plasmodium falciparum infected erythrocytes. *Cell* 58:95, 1989.

519. Nozaki S, Tanaka T, Yamashita S, et al: CD36 mediates long-chain fatty acid transport in human myocardium: complete myocardial accumulation defect of radiolabeled long-chain fatty acid analog in subjects with CD36 deficiency. *Mol Cell Biochem* 192:129, 1999.

520. Huang MM, Bolen JB, Barnwell JW, Shattil SJ, Brugge JS: Membrane glycoprotein IV (CD36) is physically associated with the Fyn, Lyn, and Yes protein-tyrosine kinases in human platelets. *Proc Natl Acad Sci USA* 88:7844, 1991.

521. Aiken JW, Ginsberg MH, Plow EF: Mechanisms for expression of thrombospondin on the platelet surface. *Semin Thromb Hemost* 13:307, 1987.

522. Silverstein RL, Febbraio M: Identification of lysosome-associated membrane protein-2 as an activation-dependent platelet surface glycoprotein. *Blood* 80:1470, 1992.

523. Peerschke EIB, Ghebrehiwet B: Human blood platelets possess specific binding sites for C1q. *J Immunol* 138:1537, 1987.

524. Peerschke EI, Ghebrehiwet B: Platelet receptors for the complement component C1q: implications for hemostasis and thrombosis. *Immunobiology* 199:239, 1998.

525. Ghebrehiwet B, Lim BL, Peerschke EI, Willis AC, Reid KB: Isolation, cDNA cloning, and overexpression of a 33-kD cell surface glycoprotein that binds to the globular "heads" of C1q. *J Exp Med* 179:1809, 1994.

526. Herwald H, Dedio J, Kellner R, Loos M, Muller-Esterl W: Isolation and characterization of the kininogen-binding protein p33 from endothelial cells. Identity with the gC1q receptor. *J Biol Chem* 271:13040, 1996.

527. Nepomuceno RR, Tenner AJ: C1qRP, the C1q receptor that enhances phagocytosis, is detected specifically in human cells of myeloid lineage, endothelial cells, and platelets. *J Immunol* 160:1929, 1998.

528. Peerschke EI, Reid KB, Ghebrehiwet B: Platelet activation by C1q results in the induction of alpha IIb/beta 3 integrins (GPIIb-IIIa) and the expression of P-selectin and procoagulant activity. *J Exp Med* 178:579, 1993.

529. Peerschke EI, Ghebrehiwet B: Platelet membrane receptors for the complement component C1q. *Semin Hematol* 31:320, 1994.

530. Metzelaar MJ, Heijnen HF, Sixma JJ, Nieuwenhuis HK: Identification of a 33-Kd protein associated with the alpha-granule membrane (GMP-33) that is expressed on the surface of activated platelets. *Blood* 79:372, 1992.

531. Rosenstein Y, Park JK, Hahn WC, Rosen FS, Bierer BE, Burakoff SJ: CD43, a molecule defective in Wiskott-Aldrich syndrome, binds ICAM-1. *Nature* 354:233, 1991.

532. Coller BS: Platelets and thrombolytic therapy. *N Engl J Med* 322:33, 1990.

533. Coller BS: Augmentation of thrombolysis with antiplatelet drugs. Overview. *Coron Art Dis* 6:911, 1995.

534. Korbut R, Gryglewski RJ: Platelets in fibrinolytic system. *J Physiol Pharmacol* 46:409, 1995.

535. Thorsen S, Brakman P, Astrup T: Influence of platelets on fibrinolysis: a critical review, in *Hematologic Reviews*, edited by JL Ambrole, 3rd ed, p 123. Marcel Dekker, New York, 1972.

536. Carroll RC, Radcliffe RD, Taylor FB, Gerrard JM: Plasminogen, plasminogen activator and platelets in the regulation of clot lysis. *J Lab Clin Med* 100:986, 1982.

537. Miles LA, Plow EF: Binding and activation of plasminogen on the platelet surface. *J Biol Chem* 260:4303, 1985.

538. Stricker RB, Wong D, Shiu DT, Reyes PT, Shuman MA: Activation of plasminogen by tissue plasminogen activator on normal and thrombasthenic platelets: effects on surface proteins and platelet aggregation. *Blood* 68:275, 1986.

539. Jeanneau C, Sultan Y: Tissue plasminogen activator in human megakaryocytes and platelets: immunocytochemical localization, immunoblotting and zymographic analysis. *Thrombosis Haemost* 19:529, 1988.

540. Park S, Harker LA, Marzec UM, Levin EG: Demonstration of single chain urokinase-type plasminogen activator on human platelet membrane. *Blood* 73:1421, 1989.

541. Plow EF, Collen D: The presence and release of α_2-antiplasmin from human platelets. *Blood* 58:1069, 1981.

542. Smariga PE, Maynard JR: Purification of a platelet protein which stimulates fibrinolytic inhibition and tissue factor in human fibroblasts. *J Biol Chem* 257:11960, 1982.

543. Erickson LA, Ginsberg MH, Loskutoff DJ: Detection and partial characterization of an inhibitor of plasminogen activator in human platelets. *J Clin Invest* 74:1465, 1984.

544. Kruithof EKO, Tran-Thang C, Bachmann F: Studies on the release of plasminogen activator inhibitor from human platelets. *Thromb Haemost* 55:201, 1986.

545. Francis CW, Marder VJ: Rapid formation of large molecular weight alpha-polymers in cross-linked fibrin induced by high factor XIII concentrations: role of platelet factor XIII. *J Clin Invest* 80:1459, 1987.

546. Fay WP, Eitzman DT, Shapiro AD, Madison EL, Ginsburg D: Platelets inhibit fibrinolysis in vitro by both plasminogen activator inhibitor-1 dependent and independent mechanisms. *Blood* 83:351, 1994.

547. Jang I-K, Gold HK, Ziskind AA, et al: Differential sensitivity of erythrocyte-rich and platelet-rich arterial thrombi to lysis with recombinant tissue-type plasminogen activator. A possible explanation for resistance to coronary thrombolysis. *Circulation* 79:920, 1989.

548. Ohlstein EH, Storer B, Fujita T, Shebuski RJ: Tissue-type plasminogen activator and streptokinase induce platelet hyperaggregability in the rabbit. *Thromb Res* 46:575, 1987.

549. Fitzgerald DJ, Catella F, Roy L, FitzGerald GA: Marked platelet activation in vivo after intravenous streptokinase in patients with acute myocardial infarction. *Circulation* 77:142, 1988.

550. Shebuski RJ: Principles underlying the use of conjunctive agents with plasminogen activators. *Ann NY Acad Sci* 667:382, 1992.

551. Rudd MA, George D, Amarante P, Vaughan DE, Loscalzo J: Temporal effects of thrombolytic agents on platelet function in vivo and their modulation by prostaglandins. *Circ Res* 67:1175, 1990.

552. Kerins DM, Roy L, FitzGerald GA, Fitzgerald DJ: Platelet and vascular function during coronary thrombolysis with tissue-type plasminogen activator. *Circulation* 80:1718, 1990.

553. Fitzgerald DJ, Wright F, FitzGerald GA: Increased thromboxane biosynthesis during coronary thrombolysis: evidence that platelet activation and thromboxane A_2 modulate the response to tissue-type plasminogen activator in vivo. *Circ Res* 65:83, 1989.

554. Penny WF, Ware JA: Platelet activation and subsequent inhibition by plasmin and recombinant tissue-type plasminogen activator. *Blood* 79:91, 1992.

555. Niewiarowski S, Senyi AF, Gillies P: Plasmin-induced platelet aggregation and platelet release reaction. *J Clin Invest* 52:1647, 1973.

556. Schafer AI, Maas AK, Ware JA, Johnson PC, Rittenhous SE, Salzman EW: Platelet protein phosphorylation, elevation of cytostolic calcium, and inositol phospholipid breakdown in platelet activation induced by plasmin. *J Clin Invest* 78:73, 1986.

557. Eisenberg PR, Sherman LA, Jaffe AS: Paradoxic elevation of fibrinopeptide A after streptokinase: evidence for continued thrombosis despite intense fibrinolysis. *J Am Coll Cardiol* 10:527, 1987.

558. Owen J, Friedman KD, Grossman BA, Wilkins C, Berke AD, Powers ER: Thrombolytic therapy with tissue plasminogen activator or streptokinase induces transient thrombin activity. *Blood* 72:616, 1988.

559. Leopold JA, Loscalzo J: Platelet activation by fibrinolytic agents: a potential mechanism for resistance to thrombolysis and reocclusion after successful thrombolysis. *Coron Artery Dis* 6:923, 1995.

560. Szczeklik A: Thrombin generation in myocardial infarction and hypercholesterolemia: effects of aspirin. *Thromb Haemost* 74:77, 1995.

561. Weitz JI, Cruickshank MK, Though D, et al: Human tissue-type plasminogen activator releases fibrinopeptides A and B from fibrinogen. *J Clin Invest* 82:1700, 1988.

562. Coller BS: Inhibitors of the platelet glycoprotein IIb/IIIa receptor as conjunctive therapy for coronary artery thrombolysis. *Coron Artery Dis* 3:1016, 1992.

563. Antman EM, Giugliano RP, Gibson CM, et al: Abciximab facilitates the rate and extent of thrombolysis: results of the thrombolysis in myocardial infarction (TIMI) 14 trial. *Circulation* 99:2720, 1999.

564. Eccleston D, Topol EJ: Inhibitors of platelet glycoprotein IIb/IIIa as augmenters of thrombolysis. *Coron Artery Dis* 6:947, 1995.

565. O'Donnell CJ, Jonas MA, Hennekens CH: Aspirin augmentation of the efficacy of thrombolysis. *Coron Artery Dis* 6:936, 1995.

566. Kowalski E, Kopeć M, Wegrzynowicz A: Influence of fibrinogen degradation products (FDP) on platelet aggregation, adhesiveness and viscous metamorphosis. *Thromb Diath Haemorrh* 10:406, 1963.

567. Schafer AL, Adelman B: Plasmin inhibition of platelet function and of arachidonic acid metabolism. *J Clin Invest* 75:456, 1985.

568. Adelman B, Michelson AD, Loscalzo J, Greenberg J, Handin RI: Plasmin effect on platelet glycoprotein Ib-von Willebrand factor interactions. *Blood* 64:32, 1985.

569. Loscalzo J, Vaughan DE: Tissue plasminogen activator promotes platelet disaggregation in plasma. *J Clin Invest* 79:1749, 1987.

570. Schafer AL, Zavoico GB, Loscalzo J, Maas AK: Synergistic inhibition of platelet activation by plasmin and prostaglandin I_2. *Blood* 69:1504, 1987.

571. Adnot S, Ferry N, Nanoune J, Lacombe ML: Plasmin: a possible physiological modulator of human platelet adenylate cyclase system. *Clin Sci* 72:467, 1987.

572. Gimple LW, Gold HK, Leinbach RC, et al: Correlation between template bleeding times and spontaneous bleeding during treatment of acute myocardial infarction with recombinant tissue-type plasminogen activator. *Circulation* 80:581, 1989.

573. Michelson AD, Gore JM, Rybak ME, Cola CA, Barnard MR: Effect of in vivo infusion of recombinant tissue-type plasminogen activator on platelet glycoprotein Ib. *Thromb Res* 60:421, 1990.

574. Federici AB, Berkowitz SD, Mannucci PM, Lotto A, Italian P.A.I.M.S.-Group, Zimmerman TS: Proteolysis of von Willebrand factor in patients undergoing thrombolytic therapy. *Circulation* 78(suppl.II):II-120, 1988.

575. Johnstone MT, Andrews T, Ware JA, et al: Bleeding time prolongation with streptokinase and its reduction with 1-desamino-8-D-arginine vasopressin. *Circulation* 82:2142, 1990.

576. Kamat SG, Schafer AI: Antiplatelet effects of fibrinolytic agents: a potential contributor to the hemostatic defect after thrombolysis. *Coron Artery Dis* 6:930, 1995.

577. Coller BS: Binding of abciximab to $\alpha V\beta 3$ and activated $\alpha M\beta 2$ receptors:

with a review of platelet-leukocyte interactions. *Thromb Haemost* 82:326, 1999.

578. Yeo EL, Sheppard JA, Feuerstein IA: Role of P-selectin and leukocyte activation in polymorphonuclear cell adhesion to surface adherent activated platelets under physiologic shear conditions (an injury vessel wall model). *Blood* 83:2498, 1994.

579. Diacovo TG, Roth SJ, Buccola JM, Bainton DF, Springer TA: Neutrophil rolling, arrest, and transmigration across activated, surface-adherent platelets via sequential action of P-selectin and the beta 2-integrin CD11b/CD18. *Blood* 88:146, 1996.

580. Sheikh S, Nash GB: Continuous activation and deactivation of integrin CD11b/CD18 during de novo expression enables rolling neutrophils to immobilize on platelets. *Blood* 87:5040, 1996.

581. Kirchhofer D, Riederer MA, Baumgartner HR: Specific accumulation of circulating monocytes and polymorphonuclear leukocytes on platelet thrombi in a vascular injury model. *Blood* 89:1270, 1997.

582. Konstantopoulos K, Neelamegham S, Burns AR, et al: Venous levels of shear support neutrophil-platelet adhesion and neutrophil aggregation in blood via P-selectin and beta2-integrin. *Circulation* 98:873, 1998.

583. Altieri DC, Plescia J, Plow EF: The structural motif glycine 190-valine 202 of the fibrinogen gamma chain interacts with CD11b/CD18 integrin (alpha M beta 2, Mac-1) and promotes leukocyte adhesion. *J Biol Chem* 268:1847, 1993.

584. Ugarova TP, Solovjov DA, Zhang L, et al: Identification of a novel recognition sequence for integrin alphaM beta2 within the gamma-chain of fibrinogen. *J Biol Chem* 273:22519, 1998.

585. Weber C, Springer TA: Neutrophil accumulation on activated, surface-adherent platelets in flow is mediated by interaction of Mac-1 with fibrinogen bound to alphaIIbbeta3 and stimulated by platelet-activating factor. *J Clin Invest* 100:2085, 1997.

586. Silverstein RL, Asch AS, Nachman RL: Glycoprotein IV mediates thrombospondin-dependent platelet-monocyte and platelet-U937 cell adhesion. *J Clin Invest* 84:546, 1989.

587. Farb A, Sangiorgi G, Carter AJ, et al: Pathology of acute and chronic coronary stenting in humans. *Circulation* 99:44, 1999.

588. Merhi Y, Provost P, Chauvet P, Theoret JF, Phillips ML, Latour JG: Selectin blockade reduces neutrophil interaction with platelets at the site of deep arterial injury by angioplasty in pigs. *Arterioscler Thromb Vasc Biol* 19:372, 1999.

589. Ott I, Neumann FJ, Gawaz M, Schmitt M, Schomig A: Increased neutrophil-platelet adhesion in patients with unstable angina. *Circulation* 94:1239, 1996.

590. Mickelson JK, Lakkis NM, Villarreal-Levy G, Hughes BJ, Smith CW: Leukocyte activation with platelet adhesion after coronary angioplasty: a mechanism for recurrent disease? *J Am Coll Cardiol* 28:345, 1996.

591. Marcus AJ, Safier LB: Thromboregulation: multicellular modulation of platelet reactivity in hemostasis and thrombosis. *FASEB J* 7:516, 1993.

592. Alderson MR, Armitage RJ, Tough TW, Strockbine L, Fanslow WC, Spriggs MK: CD40 expression by human monocytes: regulation by cytokines and activation of monocytes by the ligand for CD40. *J Exp Med* 178:669, 1993.

593. Yellin MJ, Brett J, Baum D, et al: Functional interactions of T cells with endothelial cells: the role of CD40L-CD40-mediated signals. *J Exp Med* 182:1857, 1995.

594. Pawelczyk T: Isozymes delta of phosphoinositide-specific phospholipase C. *Acta Biochim Pol* 46:91, 1999.

595. Hers I, Donath J, van Willigen G, Akkerman JW: Differential involvement of tyrosine and serine/threonine kinases in platelet integrin alphaIIbbeta3 exposure. *Arterioscler Thromb Vasc Biol* 18:404, 1998.

596. Murphy CT, Westwick J: Selective inhibition of protein kinase C. Effect on platelet-activating-factor-induced platelet functional responses. *Biochem J* 283:159, 1992.

597. Si-Tahar M, Renesto P, Falet H, Rendu F, Chignard M: The phospholipase C/protein kinase C pathway is involved in cathepsin G-induced human platelet activation: comparison with thrombin. *Biochem J* 313:401, 1996.

598. Kunapuli SP: Functional characterization of platelet ADP receptors. *Platelets* 9:343, 1998.

599. Henderson DJ, Elliot DG, Smith GM, Webb TE, Dainty IA: Cloning and characterisation of a bovine P2Y receptor. *Biochem Biophys Res Commun* 212:648, 1995.

600. Lon C, Hechler B, Vial C, et al: Platelets from P2Y1 receptor knockout

601. Offermanns S, Toombs CF, Hu YH, Simon MI: Defective platelet activation in G alpha(q)-deficient mice. *Nature* 389:183, 1997.

602. MacFarlane DE, Srivastava PC, Mills DC: 2-Methylthioadenosine[beta-32P]diphosphate. An agonist and radioligand for the receptor that inhibits the accumulation of cyclic AMP in intact blood platelets. *J Clin Invest* 71:420, 1983.

603. Mills DC: ADP receptors on platelets. *Thromb Haemost* 76:835, 1996.

604. Jin J, Daniel JL, Kunapuli SP: Molecular basis for ADP-induced platelet activation. II. The P2Y1 receptor mediates ADP-induced intracellular calcium mobilization and shape change in platelets. *J Biol Chem* 273:2030, 1998.

605. Mills DC, Puri R, Hu CJ, et al: Clopidogrel inhibits the binding of ADP analogues to the receptor mediating inhibition of platelet adenylate cyclase. *Arterioscler Thromb* 12:430, 1992.

606. MacKenzie AB, Mahaut-Smith MP, Sage SO: Activation of receptor-operated cation channels via P2X1 not P2T purinoceptors in human platelets. *J Biol Chem* 271:2879, 1996.

607. Valera S, Hussy N, Evans RJ, et al: A new class of ligand-gated ion channel defined by P2x receptor for extracellular ATP. *Nature* 371:516, 1994.

608. Gayle RB3, Maliszewski CR, Gimpel SD, et al: Inhibition of platelet function by recombinant soluble ecto-ADPase/CD39. *J Clin Invest* 101:1851, 1998.

609. Banga HS, Simons ER, Brass LF, Rittenhouse SE: Activation of phospholipases A and C in human platelets exposed to epinephrine: role of glycoproteins IIb/IIIa and dual role of epinephrine. *Proc Natl Acad Sci USA* 83:9197, 1986.

610. Shattil SJ, Budzynski A, Scrutton MC: Epinephrine induces platelet fibrinogen receptor expression, fibrinogen binding, and aggregation in whole blood in the absence of other excitatory agonists. *Blood* 73:150, 1989.

611. Lanza F, Beretz A, Stierle A, Hanau D, Kubina M, Cazenave JP: Epinephrine potentiates human platelet activation but is not an aggregating agent. *Am J Physiol* 255:1276, 1988.

612. Ware JA, Johnson PC, Smith M, Salzman EW: Effect of common agonists on cytoplasmic ionized calcium concentration in platelets. Measurement with 2-methyl-6-methoxy 8-nitroquinoline (quin2) and aequorin. *J Clin Invest* 77:878, 1986.

613. Owen NE, Feinberg H, Le Breton GC: Epinephrine induces Ca2+ uptake in human blood platelets. *Am J Physiol* 239:H483, 1980.

614. Sweatt JD, Connolly TM, Cragoe EJ, Limbird LE: Evidence that Na+/H+ exchange regulates receptor-mediated phospholipase A2 activation in human platelets. *J Biol Chem* 261:8667, 1986.

615. Homcy CJ, Graham RM: Molecular characterization of adrenergic receptors. *Circ Res* 56:635, 1985.

616. Haslam RJ, Davidson MM, Fox JE, Lynham JA: Cyclic nucleotides in platelet function. *Thromb Haemost* 40:232, 1978.

617. Salzman EW, Ware JA: Ionized calcium as an intracellular messenger in blood platelets. *Prog Hemost Thromb* 9:177, 1989.

618. Regan JW, Nakata H, DeMarinis RM, Caron MG, Lefkowitz RJ: Purification and characterization of the human platelet alpha 2- adrenergic receptor. *J Biol Chem* 261:3894, 1986.

619. Kobilka BK, Matsui H, Kobilka TS, et al: Cloning, sequencing, and expression of the gene coding for the human platelet alpha 2-adrenergic receptor. *Science* 238:650, 1987.

620. Marcus A: Platelet eicosanoid metabolism, in *Hemostasis and Thrombosis: Basic Principles and Clinical Practice*, edited by RW Colman, J Hirsh, VJ Marder, EW Salzman, 2 ed, p 676. JB Lippincott, Philadelphia, 1987.

621. Puri RN: Phospholipase A2: its role in ADP- and thrombin-induced platelet activation mechanisms. *Int J Biochem Cell Biol* 30:1107, 1998.

622. Crofford LJ: COX-1 and COX-2 tissue expression: implications and predictions. *J Rheumatol* 24:15, 1997.

623. Svensson J, Hamberg M, Samuelsson B: On the formation and effects of thromboxane A2 in human platelets. *Acta Physiol Scand* 98:285, 1976.

624. Parise LV, Venton DL, Le Breton GC: Arachidonic acid-induced platelet aggregation is mediated by a thromboxane A2/prostaglandin H2 receptor interaction. *J Pharmacol Exp Ther* 228:240, 1984.

625. Weber AA, Zimmermann KC, Meyer-Kirchrath J, Schror K: Cyclooxy-

mice do not aggregate in response to ADP. *Thromb Haemost* 82:1331, 1999.

genase-2 in human platelets as a possible factor in aspirin resistance. *Lancet* 353:900, 1999.

626. Dubois RN, Abramson SB, Crofford L, et al: Cyclooxygenase in biology and disease. *FASEB J* 12:1063, 1998.

627. Smith JB, Willis AL: Aspirin selectively inhibits prostaglandin production in human platelets. *Nat New Biol* 231:235, 1971.

628. Takahara K, Murray R, FitzGerald GA, Fitzgerald DJ: The response to thromboxane A2 analogues in human platelets. Discrimination of two binding sites linked to distinct effector systems. *J Biol Chem* 265:6836, 1990.

628a. Hirata T, Ushikubi F, Kakizuka A, Okuma M, Narumiya S: Two thromboxane A2 receptor isoforms in human platelets. Opposite coupling to adenylyl cyclase with different sensitivity to Arg60 to Leu mutation. *J Clin Invest* 97:949, 1996.

629. Parent JL, Labrecque P, Orsini MJ, Benovic JL: Internalization of the TXA2 receptor alpha and beta isoforms. Role of the differentially spliced COOH terminus in agonist-promoted receptor internalization. *J Biol Chem* 274:8941, 1999.

630. Habib A, FitzGerald GA, Maclouf J: Phosphorylation of the thromboxane receptor alpha, the predominant isoform expressed in human platelets. *J Biol Chem* 274:2645, 1999.

631. Komiotis D, Wencel-Drake JD, Dieter JP, Lim CT, Le Breton GC: Labeling of human platelet plasma membrane thromboxane A2/prostaglandin H2 receptors using SQB, a novel biotinylated receptor probe. *Biochem Pharmacol* 52:763, 1996.

632. Kim SO, Lim CT, Lam SC, et al: Purification of the human blood platelet thromboxane A2/prostaglandin H2 receptor protein. *Biochem Pharmacol* 43:313, 1992.

633. Ushikubi F, Nakajima M, Hirata M, Okuma M, Fujiwara M, Narumiya S: Purification of the thromboxane A2/prostaglandin H2 receptor from human blood platelets. *J Biol Chem* 264:16496, 1989.

634. Djellas Y, Manganello JM, Antonakis K, Le Breton GC: Identification of Galpha13 as one of the G-proteins that couple to human platelet thromboxane A2 receptors. *J Biol Chem* 274:14325, 1999.

635. Allan CJ, Higashiura K, Martin M, et al: Characterization of the cloned HEL cell thromboxane A2 receptor: evidence that the affinity state can be altered by G alpha 13 and G alpha q. *J Pharmacol Exp Ther* 277:1132, 1996.

636. Nakahata N, Miyamoto A, Ohkubo S, et al: Gq/11 communicates with thromboxane A2 receptors in human astrocytoma cells, rabbit astrocytes and human platelets. *Res Commun Mol Pathol Pharmacol* 87:243, 1995.

636a. Offermanns S, Laugwitz KL, Spicher K, Schultz G: G proteins of the G12 family are activated via thromboxane A2 and thrombin receptors in human platelets. *Proc Natl Acad Sci USA* 91:504, 1994.

637. Ushikubi F, Nakamura K, Narumiya S: Functional reconstitution of platelet thromboxane A2 receptors with Gq and Gi2 in phospholipid vesicles. *Mol Pharmacol* 46:808, 1994.

638. Thomas DW, Mannon RB, Mannon PJ, et al: Coagulation defects and altered hemodynamic responses in mice lacking receptors for thromboxane A2. *J Clin Invest* 102:1994, 1998.

639. Knezevic I, Dieter JP, Le Breton GC: Mechanism of inositol 1,4,5-trisphosphate-induced aggregation in saponin-permeabilized platelets. *J Pharmacol Exp Ther* 260:947, 1992.

640. Pulcinelli FM, Ashby B, Gazzaniga PP, Daniel JL: Protein kinase C activation is not a key step in ADP-mediated exposure of fibrinogen receptors on human platelets. *FEBS Lett* 364:87, 1995.

641. Ofosu FA, Liu L, Freedman J: Control mechanisms in thrombin generation. *Semin Thromb Hemost* 22:303, 1996.

642. Phillips DR: Thrombin interaction with human platelets. Potentiation of thrombin-induced aggregation and release by inactivated thrombin. *Thromb Diath Haemorrh* 32:207, 1974.

643. Hung DT, Vu TK, Wheaton VI, Ishii K, Coughlin SR: Cloned platelet thrombin receptor is necessary for thrombin-induced platelet activation. *J Clin Invest* 89:1350, 1992.

644. Vu T-K, Hung DT, Wheaton VI, Coughlin SR: Molecular cloning of a functional thrombin receptor reveals a novel proteolytic mechanism of receptor activation. *Cell* 64:1057, 1991.

645. Furman MI, Liu L, Benoit SE, Becker RC, Barnard MR, Michelson AD: The cleaved peptide of the thrombin receptor is a strong platelet agonist. *Proc Natl Acad Sci USA* 95:3082, 1998.

646. Ishihara H, Connolly AJ, Zeng D, et al: Protease-activated receptor 3 is a second thrombin receptor in humans. *Nature* 386:502, 1997.

647. Kahn ML, Zheng YW, Huang W, et al: A dual thrombin receptor system for platelet activation. *Nature* 394:690, 1998.

648. Kahn ML, Nakanishi-Matsui M, Shapiro MJ, Ishihara H, Coughlin SR: Protease-activated receptors 1 and 4 mediate activation of human platelets by thrombin. *J Clin Invest* 103:879, 1999.

649. Ishihara H, Zeng D, Connolly AJ, Tam C, Coughlin SR: Antibodies to protease-activated receptor 3 inhibit activation of mouse platelets by thrombin. *Blood* 91:4152, 1998.

650. Hoxie JA, Ahuja M, Belmonte E, Pizarro S, Parton R, Brass LF: Internalization and recycling of activated thrombin receptors. *J Biol Chem* 268:13756, 1993.

651. Trejo J, Coughlin SR: The cytoplasmic tails of protease-activated receptor-1 and substance P receptor specify sorting to lysosomes versus recycling. *J Biol Chem* 274:2216, 1999.

652. McIntyre TM, Zimmerman GA, Prescott SM: Biologically active oxidized phospholipids. *J Biol Chem* 274:25189, 1999.

653. Prescott SM, Zimmerman GA, McIntyre TM: Platelet-activating factor. *J Biol Chem* 265:17381, 1990.

654. Honda Z, Nakamura M, Miki I, et al: Cloning by functional expression of platelet-activating factor receptor from guinea-pig lung. *Nature* 349:342, 1991.

655. Nakamura M, Honda Z, Izumi T, et al: Molecular cloning and expression of platelet-activating factor receptor from human leukocytes. *J Biol Chem* 266:20400, 1991.

656. Carlson SA, Chatterjee TK, Fisher RA: The third intracellular domain of the platelet-activating factor receptor is a critical determinant in receptor coupling to phosphoinositide phospholipase C-activating G proteins. Studies using intracellular domain minigenes and receptor chimeras. *J Biol Chem* 271:23146, 1996.

657. Chao W, Liu H, Hanahan DJ, Olson MS: Protein tyrosine phosphorylation and regulation of the receptor for platelet-activating factor in rat Kupffer cells. Effect of sodium vanadate. *Biochem J* 288:777, 1992.

658. De Clerck F, Xhonneux B, Leysen J, Janssen PA: Evidence for functional 5-HT2 receptor sites on human blood platelets. *Biochem Pharmacol* 33:2807, 1984.

659. Leysen JE, Eens A, Gommeren W, van Gompel P, Wynants J, Janssen PA: Identification of nonserotonergic [3H]ketanserin binding sites associated with nerve terminals in rat brain and with platelets; relation with release of biogenic amine metabolites induced by ketans. *J Pharmacol Exp Ther* 244:310, 1988.

660. Cook EH Jr, Fletcher KE, Wainwright M, Marks N, Yan SY, Leventhal BL: Primary structure of the human platelet serotonin 5-HT2A receptor: identify with frontal cortex serotonin 5-HT2A receptor. *J Neurochem* 63:465, 1994.

661. Roth BL, Willins DL, Kristiansen K, Kroeze WK: 5-Hydroxytryptamine2-family receptors (5-hydroxytryptamine2A, 5-hydroxytryptamine2B, 5-hydroxytryptamine2C): where structure meets function. *Pharmacol Ther* 79:231, 1998.

662. Ozaki N, Manji H, Lubierman V, et al: A naturally occurring amino acid substitution of the human serotonin 5-HT2A receptor influences amplitude and timing of intracellular calcium mobilization. *J Neurochem* 68:2186, 1997.

663. Arora RC, Meltzer HY: Serotonin2 receptor binding in blood platelets of schizophrenic patients. *Psychiatry Res* 47:111, 1993.

664. Coccaro EF, Kavoussi RJ, Sheline YI, Berman ME, Csernansky JG: Impulsive aggression in personality disorder correlates with platelet 5-HT2A receptor binding. *Neuropsychopharmacology* 16:211, 1997.

665. Pandey GN: Altered serotonin function in suicide. Evidence from platelet and neuroendocrine studies. *Ann NY Acad Sci* 836:182, 1997.

666. Wolfe BE, Metzger E, Jimerson DC: Research update on serotonin function in bulimia nervosa and anorexia nervosa. *Psychopharmacol Bull* 33:345, 1997.

667. Tomiyoshi R, Kamei K, Muraoka S, Muneoka K, Takigawa M: Serotonin-induced platelet intracellular Ca^{2+} responses in untreated depressed patients and imipramine responders in remission. *Biol Psychiatry* 45:1042, 1999.

668. Cho R, Kapur S, Du L, Hrdina P: Relationship between central and peripheral serotonin 5-HT2A receptors: a positron emission tomography study in healthy individuals. *Neurosci Lett* 261:139, 1999.

669. de Chaffoy de Courcelles D, Leysen JE, De Clerck F, Van Belle H, Janssen PA: Evidence that phospholipid turnover is the signal transduc-

ing system coupled to serotonin-S2 receptor sites. *J Biol Chem* 260:7603, 1985.

670. Erne P, Pletscher A: Rapid intracellular release of calcium in human platelets by stimulation of 5-HT2-receptors. *Br J Pharmacol* 84:545, 1985.

671. Li N, Wallen NH, Ladjevardi M, Hjemdahl P: Effects of serotonin on platelet activation in whole blood. *Blood Coagul Fibrinolysis* 8:517, 1997.

672. Houston DS, Shepherd JT, Vanhoutte PM: Aggregating human platelets cause direct contraction and endothelium-dependent relaxation of isolated canine coronary arteries. Role of serotonin, thromboxane A2, and adenine nucleotides. *J Clin Invest* 78:539, 1986.

673. Golino P, Ashton J, Glas-Grewaalt P, McNatt J, Buja LM, Willerson JT: Mediation or reocclusion by thromboxane A2 and serotonin after thrombolysis with tissue-type plasminogen activator in a canine preparation of coronary thrombosis. *Circulation* 77:678, 1988.

674. Haslam RJ, Rosson GM: Aggregation of human blood platelets by vasopressin. *Am J Physiol* 223:958, 1972.

675. Pollock WK, MacIntyre DE: Desensitization and antagonism of vasopressin-induced phosphoinositide metabolism and elevation of cytosolic free calcium concentration in human platelets. *Biochem J* 234:67, 1986.

676. Thomas ME, Osmani AH, Scrutton MC: Some properties of the human platelet vasopressin receptor. *Thromb Res* 32:557, 1983.

677. Thibonnier M, Roberts JM: Characterization of human platelet vasopressin receptors. *J Clin Invest* 76:1857, 1985.

678. Siess W, Stifel M, Binder H, Weber PC: Activation of V1-receptors by vasopressin stimulates inositol phospholipid hydrolysis and arachidonate metabolism in human platelets. *Biochem J* 233:83, 1986.

679. Thibonnier M, Goraya T, Berti-Mattera L: G protein coupling of human platelet V1 vascular vasopressin receptors. *Am J Physiol* 264:C1336, 1993.

680. Berrettini WH, Post RM, Worthington EK, Casper JB: Human platelet vasopressin receptors. *Life Sci* 30:425, 1982.

681. Siess W: Molecular mechanisms of platelet activation. *Physiol Rev* 69:58, 1989.

682. Wun T, Paglieroni T, Lachant NA: Physiologic concentrations of arginine vasopressin activate human platelets in vitro. *Br J Haematol* 92:968, 1996.

683. Chung J, Gao AG, Frazier WA: Thrombspondin acts via integrin-associated protein to activate the platelet integrin alphaIIbbeta3. *J Biol Chem* 272:14740, 1997.

684. Dorahy DJ, Thorne RF, Fecondo JV, Burns GF: Stimulation of platelet activation and aggregation by a carboxyl–terminal peptide from thrombospondin binding to the integrin-associated protein receptor. *J Biol Chem* 272:1323, 1997.

685. Lindberg FP, Gresham HD, Schwarz E, Brown EJ: Molecular cloning of integrin-associated protein: an immunoglobulin family member with multiple membrane-spanning domains implicated in alpha v beta 3-dependent ligand binding. *J Cell Biol* 123:485, 1993.

686. Wang XQ, Frazier WA: The thrombospondin receptor CD47 (IAP) modulates and associates with alpha2 beta1 integrin in vascular smooth muscle cells. *Mol Biol Cell* 9:865, 1998.

687. Frazier WA, Gao AG, Dimitry J, et al: The thrombospondin receptor integrin-associated protein (CD47) functionally couples to heterotrimeric Gi. *J Biol Chem* 274:8554, 1999.

688. Huang MM, Bolen JB, Barnwell JW, Shattil SJ, Brugge JS: Membrane glycoprotein IV (CD36) is physically associated with the Fyn, Lyn, and Yes protein-tyrosine kinases in human platelets. *Proc Natl Acad Sci USA* 88:7844, 1991.

689. van Zanten GH, de Graaf S, Slootweg PJ, et al: Increased platelet deposition on atherosclerotic coronary arteries. *J Clin Invest* 93:615, 1994.

690. van der Rest M, Garrone R: Collagen family of proteins. *FASEB J* 5:2814, 1991.

691. Saelman EU, Kehrel B, Hese KM, de Groot PG, Sixma JJ, Nieuwenhuis HK: Platelet adhesion to collagen and endothelial cell matrix under flow conditions is not dependent on platelet glycoprotein IV. *Blood* 83:3240, 1994.

692. Ichinohe T, Takayama H, Ezumi Y, et al: Collagen-stimulated activation of Syk but not c-Src is severely compromised in human platelets lacking membrane glycoprotein VI. *J Biol Chem* 272:63, 1997.

693. Ishibashi T, Ichinohe T, Sugiyama T, Takayama H, Titani K, Okuma M: Functional significance of platelet membrane glycoprotein p62 (GP VI), a putative collagen receptor. *Int J Hematol* 62:107, 1995.

694. Kehrel B, Wierwille S, Clemetson KJ, et al: Glycoprotein VI is a major collagen receptor for platelet activation: it recognizes the platelet-activating quaternary structure of collagen, whereas CD36, glycoprotein IIb/IIIa, and von Willebrand factor do not. *Blood* 91:491, 1998.

695. Poole A, Gibbins JM, Turner M, et al: The Fc receptor gamma-chain and the tyrosine kinase Syk are essential for activation of mouse platelets by collagen. *EMBO J* 16:2333, 1997.

696. Chiang TM: Collagen-platelet interaction: platelet non-integrin receptors. *Histol Histopathol* 14:579, 1999.

697. Keely PJ, Parise LV: The alpha2beta1 integrin is a necessary co-receptor for collagen-induced activation of Syk and the subsequent phosphorylation of phospholipase Cgamma2 in platelets. *J Biol Chem* 271:26668, 1996.

698. Sugiyama T, Okuma M, Ushikubi F, Sensaki S, Kanaji K, Uchino H: A novel platelet aggregating factor found in a patient with defective collagen-induced platelet aggregation and autoimmune thrombocytopenia. *Blood* 69:1712, 1987.

699. Briddon SJ, Watson SP: Evidence for the involvement of p59fyn and p53/56lyn in collagen receptor signalling in human platelets. *Biochem J* 338:203, 1999.

700. Fujii C, Yanagi S, Sada K, Nagai K, Taniguchi T, Yamamura H: Involvement of protein-tyrosine kinase p72syk in collagen-induced signal transduction in platelets. *Eur J Biochem* 226:243, 1994.

701. Shattil SJ, Ginsberg MH, Brugge JS: Adhesive signaling in platelets. *Curr Opin Cell Biol* 6:695, 1994.

702. Soriano P, Montgomery C, Geske R, Bradley A: Targeted disruption of the c-src proto-oncogene leads to osteopetrosis in mice. *Cell* 64:693, 1991.

703. Daniel JL, Dangelmaier C, Smith JB: Evidence for a role for tyrosine phosphorylation of phospholipase Cγ2 in collagen-induced platelet cytosolic calcium mobilization. *Biochem J* 302:617, 1994.

704. Quek LS, Bolen J, Watson SP: A role for Bruton's tyrosine kinase (Btk) in platelet activation by collagen. *Curr Biol* 8:1137, 1998.

704a. Nakamura T, Jamieson GA, Okuma M, Kambayashi J, Tandon NN: Platelet adhesion to native type I collagen fibrils. Role of GPVI in divalent cation-dependent and -independent adhesion and thromboxane A2 generation. *J Biol Chem* 273:4388, 1998.

704b. Daniel JL, Dangelmaier C, Strouse R, Smith JB: Collagen induces normal signal transduction in platelets deficient in CD36 (platelet glycoprotein IV). *Thromb Haemost* 71:353, 1994.

705. Smith JB, Selak MA, Dangelmaier C, Daniel JL: Cytosolic calcium as a second messenger for collagen-induced platelet responses. *Biochem J* 288:925, 1992.

706. Greenwalt DE, Tandon NN: Platelet shape change and Ca2+ mobilization induced by collagen, but not thrombin or ADP, are inhibited by phenylarsine oxide. *Br J Haematol* 88:830, 1994.

707. Chow TW, Hellums JD, Moake JL, Kroll MH: Shear stress-induced von Willebrand factor binding to platelet glycoprotein Ib initiates calcium influx associated with aggregation. *Blood* 80:113, 1992.

708. Kroll MH, Harris TS, Moake JL, Handin RI, Schafer AI: von Willebrand factor binding to GPIb initiates signals for platelet activation. *J Clin Invest* 88:1568, 1991.

709. Calverley DC, Kavanagh TJ, Roth GJ: Human signaling protein 14-3-3zeta interacts with platelet glycoprotein Ib subunits Ibalpha and Ibbeta. *Blood* 91:1295, 1998.

710. Du X, Harris SJ, Tetaz TJ, Ginsberg MH, Berndt MC: Association of a phospholipase A2 (14-3-3 protein) with the platelet glycoprotein Ib-IX complex. *J Biol Chem* 269:18287, 1994.

711. Du X, Fox JE, Pei S: Identification of a binding sequence for the 14-3-3 protein within the cytoplasmic domain of the adhesion receptor, platelet glycoprotein Ib alpha. *J Biol Chem* 271:7362, 1996.

712. Gu M, Du X: A novel ligand-binding site in the zeta-form 14-3-3 protein recognizing the platelet glycoprotein Ibalpha and distinct from the c-Raf-binding site. *J Biol Chem* 273:33465, 1998.

713. Wardell MR, Reynolds CC, Berndt MC, Wallace RW, Fox JE: Platelet glycoprotein Ib beta is phosphorylated on serine 166 by cyclic AMP-dependent protein kinase. *J Biol Chem* 264:15656, 1989.

714. Fox JE, Berndt MC: Cyclic AMP-dependent phosphorylation of glycoprotein Ib inhibits collagen-induced polymerization of actin in platelets. *J Biol Chem* 264:9520, 1989.

715. Moolenaar WH, Kranenburg O, Postma FR, Zondag GC: Lysophosphatidic acid: G-protein signalling and cellular responses. *Curr Opin Cell Biol* 9:168, 1997.

716. Yatomi Y, Yamamura S, Ruan F, Igarashi Y: Sphingosine 1-phosphate induces platelet activation through an extracellular action and shares a platelet surface receptor with lysophosphatidic acid. *J Biol Chem* 272:5291, 1997.

717. Goetzl EJ, An S: Diversity of cellular receptors and functions for the lysophospholipid growth factors lysophosphatidic acid and sphingosine 1-phosphate. *FASEB J* 12:1589, 1998.

718. Gaits F, Fourcade O, Le Balle F, et al: Lysophosphatidic acid as a phospholipid mediator: pathways of synthesis. *FEBS Lett* 410:54, 1997.

719. Fourcade O, Simon MF, Viode C, et al: Secretory phospholipase A2 generates the novel lipid mediator lysophosphatidic acid in membrane microvesicles shed from activated cells. *Cell* 80:919, 1995.

720. Fourcade O, Le Balle F, Fauvel J, Simon MF, Chap H: Regulation of secretory type-II phospholipase A2 and of lysophosphatidic acid synthesis. *Adv Enzyme Regul* 38:99, 1998.

721. Siess W, Zangl KJ, Essler M, et al: Lysophosphatidic acid mediates the rapid activation of platelets and endothelial cells by mildly oxidized low density lipoprotein and accumulates in human atherosclerotic lesions. *Proc Natl Acad Sci USA* 96:6931, 1999.

722. Johansson JS, Haynes DH: Deliberate quin2 overload as a method for in situ characterization of active calcium binding: application to the human platelet. *J Membr Biol* 104:147, 1988.

723. Geiger J, Walter U: Properties and regulation of human platelet cation channels. *Exs* 66:281, 1993.

724. Jones GD, Gear AR: Subsecond calcium dynamics in ADP- and thrombin-stimulated platelets: a continuous-flow approach using indo-1. *Blood* 71:1539, 1988.

725. Rybak ME, Renzulli LA: Effect of calcium channel blockers on platelet GPIIb-IIIa as a calcium channel in liposomes: comparison with effects on the intact platelet. *Thromb Haemost* 67:131, 1992.

726. Dessen A, Tang J, Schmidt H, et al: Crystal structure of human cytosolic phospholipase A2 reveals a novel topology and catalytic mechanism. *Cell* 97:349, 1999.

727. Khan WA, Blobe G, Halpern A, et al: Selective regulation of protein kinase C isoenzymes by oleic acid in human platelets. *J Biol Chem* 268:5063, 1993.

728. Scholey JM, Taylor KA, Kendrick-Jones J: Regulation of non-muscle myosin assembly by calmodulin-dependent light chain kinase. *Nature* 287:233, 1980.

729. Zhang J, Zhang J, Shattil SJ, Cunningham MC, Rittenhouse SE: Phosphoinositide 3-kinase gamma and p85/phosphoinositide 3-kinase in platelets. Relative activation by thrombin receptor or beta-phorbol myristate acetate and roles in promoting the ligand-binding function of alphaIIbbeta3 integrin. *J Biol Chem* 271:6265, 1996.

730. Rittenhouse SE: Phosphoinositide 3-kinase activation and platelet function. *Blood* 88:4401, 1996.

731. Hartwig JH, Kung S, Kovacsovics T, et al: D3 phosphoinositides and outside-in integrin signaling by glycoprotein IIb-IIIa mediate platelet actin assembly and filopodial extension induced by phorbol 12-myristate 13-acetate. *J Biol Chem* 271:32986, 1996.

732. Kucera GL, Rittenhouse SE: Human platelets form 3-phosphorylated phosphoinositides in response to alpha-thrombin, U46619, or GTP gamma S. *J Biol Chem* 265:5345, 1990.

733. Banfic H, Downes CP, Rittenhouse SE: Biphasic activation of PKBalpha/Akt in platelets. Evidence for stimulation both by phosphatidylinositol 3,4-bisphosphate, produced via a novel pathway, and by phosphatidylinositol 3,4,5-trisphosphate. *J Biol Chem* 273:11630, 1998.

734. Gibbins JM, Briddon S, Shutes A, et al: The p85 subunit of phosphatidylinositol 3-kinase associates with the Fc receptor gamma-chain and linker for activitor of T cells (LAT) in platelets stimulated by collagen and convulxin. *J Biol Chem* 273:34437, 1998.

735. Gratacap MP, Payrastre B, Viala C, Mauco G, Plantavid M, Chap H: Phosphatidylinositol 3,4,5-trisphosphate-dependent stimulation of phospholipase C-gamma2 is an early key event in FcgammaRIIA-mediated activation of human platelets. *J Biol Chem* 273:24314, 1998.

736. Leevers SJ, Vanhaesebroeck B, Waterfield MD: Signalling through phosphoinositide 3-kinases: the lipids take centre stage. *Curr Opin Cell Biol* 11:219, 1999.

737. Bae YS, Cantley LG, Chen CS, Kim SR, Kwon KS, Rhee SG: Activation

738. Salim K, Bottomley MJ, Querfurth E, et al: Distinct specificity in the recognition of phosphoinositides by the pleckstrin homology domains of dynamin and Bruton's tyrosine kinase. *EMBO J* 15:6241, 1996.

739. Li Z, Wahl MI, Eguinoa A, Stephens LR, Hawkins PT, Witte ON: Phosphatidylinositol 3-kinase-gamma activates Bruton's tyrosine kinase in concert with Src family kinases. *Proc Natl Acad Sci USA* 94:13820, 1997.

740. Alessi DR, James SR, Downes CP, et al: Characterization of a 3-phosphoinositide-dependent protein kinase which phosphorylates and activates protein kinase Balpha. *Curr Biol* 7:261, 1997.

741. Stokoe D, Stephens LR, Copeland T, et al: Dual role of phosphatidylinositol-3,4,5-trisphosphate in the activation of protein kinase B. *Science* 277:567, 1997.

742. Sethi T, Ginsberg MH, Downward J, Hughes PE: The small GTP-binding protein R-Ras can influence integrin activation by antagonizing a Ras/Raf-initiated integrin suppression pathway. *Mol Biol Cell* 10:1799, 1999.

743. Zhang Z, Vuori K, Wang H, Reed JC, Ruoslahti E: Integrin activation by R-ras. *Cell* 85:61, 1996.

744. Ridley AJ, Hall A: The small GTP-binding protein rho regulates the assembly of focal adhesions and actin stress fibers in response to growth factors. *Cell* 70:389, 1992.

745. Leng L, Kashiwagi H, Ren XD, Shattil SJ: RhoA and the function of platelet integrin alphaIIbbeta3. *Blood* 91:4206, 1998.

746. Hughes PE, Renshaw MW, Pfaff M, et al: Suppression of integrin activation: a novel function of a Ras/Raf-initiated MAP kinase pathway. *Cell* 88:521, 1997.

747. McNicol A, Philpott CL, Shibou TS, Israels SJ: Effects of the mitogen-activated protein (MAP) kinase kinase inhibitor 2-(2′-amino-3′-methoxyphenyl)-oxanaphthalen-4-one (PD98059) on human platelet activation. *Biochem Pharm* 55:1759, 1998.

748. Shock DD, He K, Wencel-Drake JD, Parise LV: Ras activation in platelets after stimulation of the thrombin receptor, thromboxane A2 receptor or protein kinase C. *Biochem J* 321:525, 1997.

749. Ramos JW, Kojima TK, Hughes PE, Fenczik CA, Ginsberg MH: The death effector domain of PEA-15 is involved in its regulation of integrin activation. *J Biol Chem* 273:33897, 1998.

750. Nobes CD, Hall A: Rho, rac, and cdc42 GTPases regulate the assembly of multimolecular focal complexes associated with actin stress fibers, lamellipodia, and filopodia. *Cell* 81:53, 1995.

751. Hughes PE, Diaz-Gonzalez F, Leong L, et al: Breaking the integrin hinge. A defined structural constraint regulates integrin signaling. *J Biol Chem* 271:6571, 1996.

752. O' Toole TE, Mandelman D, Forsyth J, Shattil SJ, Plow EF, Ginsberg MH: Modulation of the affinity of integrin alpha IIb beta 3 (GPIIb-IIIa) by the cytoplasmic domain of alpha IIb. *Science* 254:845, 1991.

753. Haas TA, Plow EF: The cytoplasmic domain of alphaIIb beta3. A ternary complex of the integrin alpha and beta subunits and a divalent cation. *J Biol Chem* 271:6017, 1996.

754. Stephens G, O'Luanaigh N, Reilly D, et al: A sequence within the cytoplasmic tail of GPIIb independently activates platelet aggregation and thromboxane synthesis. *J Biol Chem* 273:20317, 1998.

755. Fenczik CA, Sethi T, Ramos JW, Hughes PE, Ginsberg MH: Complementation of dominant suppression implicates CD98 in integrin activation. *Nature* 390:81, 1997.

755a. Shock DD, Naik UP, Brittain JE, Alahari SK, Sondek J, Parise LV: Calcium-dependent properties of CIB binding to the integrin alphaIIb cytoplasmic domain and translocation to the platelet cytoskeleton. *Biochem J* 342:729, 1999.

755b. Naik UP, Patel PM, Parise LV: Identification of a novel calcium-binding protein that interacts with the integrin alphaIIb cytoplasmic domain. *J Biol Chem* 272:4651, 1997.

756. Vallar L, Melchior C, Plancon S, et al: Divalent cations differentially regulate integrin alphaIIb cytoplasmic tail binding to beta3 and to calcium- and integrin-binding protein. *J Biol Chem* 274:17257, 1999.

757. Kashiwagi H, Schwartz MA, Eigenthaler M, Davis KA, Ginsberg MH, Shattil SJ: Affinity modulation of platelet integrin alphaIIbbeta3 by beta3- endonexin, a selective binding partner of the beta3 integrin cytoplasmic tail. *J Cell Biol* 137:1433, 1997.

758. Knezevic I, Leisner TM, Lam SCT: Direct binding of the platelet integrin

alphaIIbbeta3 (GPIIb-IIIa) to talin. Evidence that interaction is mediated through the cytoplasmic domains of both alphaIIb and beta3. *J Biol Chem* 271:16416, 1996.

759. Jenkins AL, Nannizzi-Alaimo L, Silver D, et al: Tyrosine phosphorylation of the beta3 cytoplasmic domain mediates integrin-cytoskeletal interactions. *J Biol Chem* 273:13878, 1998.

760. Calderwood DA, Zent R, Grant R, et al: The talin head domain binds to integrin {beta} subunit cytoplasmic tails and regulates integrin activation. *J Biol Chem* 274:28071, 1999.

761. Indig FE, Diaz-Gonzalez F, Ginsberg MH: Analysis of the tetraspanin CD9-integrin alphaIIbbeta3 (GPIIb-IIIa) complex in platelet membranes and transfected cells. *Biochem J* 327:291, 1997.

762. Slupsky JR, Seehafer JG, Tang SC, Masellis-Smith A, Shaw AR: Evidence that monoclonal antibodies against CD9 antigen induce specific association between CD9 and the platelet glycoprotein IIb-IIIa complex. *J Biol Chem* 264:12289, 1989.

763. Fitter S, Sincock PM, Jolliffe CN, Ashman LK: Transmembrane 4 superfamily protein CD151 (PETA-3) associates with beta 1 and alpha IIb beta 3 integrins in haemopoietic cell lines and modulates cell-cell adhesion. *Biochem J* 338:61, 1999.

764. Jennings LK, Fox CF, Kouns WC, McKay CP, Ballou LR, Schultz HE: The activation of human platelets mediated by anti-human platelet p24/CD9 monoclonal antibodies. *J Biol Chem* 265:3815, 1990.

765. Law DA, DeGuzmann FR, Heiser P, Ministri-Madrid K, Phillips DR: Integrin cytoplasmic tyrosine motif is required for outside-in alphaIIb-beta3 signalling and platelet function. *Nature* 401:808, 1999.

766. Du X, Gu M, Weisel JW, et al: Long range propagation of conformational changes in integrin alpha IIb beta 3. *J Biol Chem* 268:23087, 1993.

767. Leisner TM, Wencel-Drake JD, Wang W, Lam SC: Bidirectional transmembrane modulation of integrin alphaIIbbeta3 conformations. *J Biol Chem* 274:12945, 1999.

768. Hato T, Pampori N, Shattil SJ: Complementary roles for receptor clustering and conformational change in the adhesive and signaling functions of integrin alphaIIb beta3. *J Cell Biol* 141:1685, 1998.

769. Law DA, Nannizzi-Alaimo L, Phillips DR: Outside-in integrin signal transduction. Alpha IIb beta 3-(GP IIb IIIa) tyrosine phosphorylation induced by platelet aggregation. *J Biol Chem* 271:10811, 1996.

770. Cowan KJ, Law DA, Phillips DR: SHC identified as the primary protein associated with the beta 3 diphosphorylated cytoplasmic tail peptide of alphaIIb beta3 (GPIIbIIIa) in human platelets. *Thromb Haemost* 1999.

771. Kumar G, Wang S, Gupta S, Nel A: The membrane immunoglobulin receptor utilizes a Shc/Grb2/hSOS complex for activation of the mitogen-activated protein kinase cascade in a B-cell line. *Biochem J* 307:215, 1995.

772. Reddy KB, Gascard P, Price MG, Negrescu EV, Fox JEB: Identification of an interaction between the m-band protein skelemin and beta-integrin subunits. Colocalization of a skelemin-like protein with beta1- and beta3-integrins in non-muscle cells. *J Biol Chem* 273:35039, 1998.

772a. Miranti CK, Leng L, Maschberger P, Brugge JS, Shattil SJ: Identification of a novel integrin signaling pathway involving the kinase Syk and the guanine nucleotide exchange factor Vav1. *Curr Biol* 8:1289, 1998.

773. Majerus PW: Arachidonate metabolism in vascular disorders. *J Clin Invest* 72:1521, 1983.

774. Moncada S, Whittle BJ: Biological actions of prostacyclin and its pharmacological use in platelet studies. *Adv Exp Med Biol* 192:337, 1985.

775. Marcus AJ: The role of lipids in platelet function: with particular reference to the arachidonic acid pathway. *J Lipid Res* 19:793, 1978.

776. Cavallini L, Coassin M, Borean A, Alexandre A: Prostacyclin and sodium nitroprusside inhibit the activity of the platelet inositol 1,4,5-trisphosphate receptor and promote its phosphorylation. *J Biol Chem* 271:5545, 1996.

777. Nishimura T, Yamamoto T, Komuro Y, Hara Y: Antiplatelet functions of a stable prostacyclin analog, SM-10906 are exerted by its inhibitory effect on inositol 1,4,5-trisphosphate production and cytosolic Ca^{2+} increase in rat platelets stimulated by thrombin. *Thromb Res* 79:307, 1995.

778. Cook SJ, McCormick F: Inhibition by cAMP of Ras-dependent activation of Raf. *Science* 262:1069, 1993.

779. Fischer TH, Collins JH, Gatling MN, White GC2: The localization of the cAMP-dependent protein kinase phosphorylation site in the platelet rat protein, rap 1B. *FEBS Letters* 2832:173, 1991.

780. Luscher TF, Diederich D, Siebenmann R, et al: Difference between endothelium-dependent relaxation in arterial and in venous coronary bypass grafts. *N Engl J Med* 319:462, 1988.

781. Goretski J, Hollocher TC: Trapping of nitric oxide produced during denitrification by extracellular hemoglobin. *J Biol Chem* 263:2316, 1988.

782. Loscalzo J, Welch G: Nitric oxide and its role in the cardiovascular system. *Prog Cardiovasc Dis* 38:87, 1995.

783. Mellion BT, Ignarro LJ, Ohlstein EH, Pontecorvo EG, Hyman AL, Kadowitz PJ: Evidence for the inhibitory role of guanosine 3′, 5′-monophosphate in ADP-induced human platelet aggregation in the presence of nitric oxide and related vasodilators. *Blood* 57:946, 1981.

784. Radomski MW, Palmer RM, Moncada S: Modulation of platelet aggregation by an L-arginine-nitric oxide pathway. *Trends Pharmacol Sci* 12:87, 1991.

785. Kaczmarek E, Koziak K, Sevigny J, et al: Identification and characterization of CD39/vascular ATP diphosphohydrolase. *J Biol Chem* 271:33116, 1996.

786. White JG: Platelet ultrastructure, in *Hemostasis and Thrombosis*, edited by AL Forbes, CD PT Duncan, EGD Tuttenham, 3rd ed, p 49. Churchill Livingstone, Edinburgh, 1994.

786a. Coller BS, Anderson KM, Weisman HF: Inhibitors of platelet aggregation: GPIIb/IIIa antagonists, in *Heart Disease*, edited by E Braunwald, Update 4, p 1. W. B. Saunders, Philadelphia, 1995.

786b. Coller BS: Antiplatelet agents in the prevention and therapy of thrombosis. *Ann Rev Med* 43:171, 1992.

787. McEver RP: Selectins: novel receptors that mediate leukocyte adhesion during inflammation. *Thromb Haemost* 65:223, 1991.

787a. Vu T-K, Wheaton VI, Hung DT, Charo I, Coughlin SR: Domains specifying thrombin-receptor interaction. *Nature* 353:674, 1991.

788. Coller BS: Disorders of platelets, in Ratnoff OD, Forbes CD, *Disorders of Hemostasis*, p 73. Grune & Stratton, Orlando, FL, 1984.

789. Holmsen H, Weiss HJ: Secretable storage pools in platelets. *Annu Rev Med* 30:119, 1979.

790. Pollard TD: Actin. *Curr Opin Cell Biol* 2:33, 1990.

791. Vandekerckhove J: Actin-binding proteins. *Curr Opin Cell Biol* 2:41, 1990.

792. Weeds AG, Gooch J, Pope B, Harris HE: Preparation and characterization of pig plasma and platelet gelsolins. *Eur J Biochem* 161:69, 1986.

793. Weber A, Nachmias VT, Pennise CR, Pring M, Safer D: Interaction of thymosin-β-4 with muscle and platelet actin. Implications for actin sequestration in resting platelets. *Biochemistry* 31:6179, 1992.

794. Smillie LB: Structure and function of tropomyosins from muscle and non-muscle. *Trends Biochem Sci* 4:151, 1981.

795. Vandekerckhove J: Structural principles of actin-binding proteins. *Curr Opin Cell Biol* 1:15, 1989.

796. Lind SE, Stossel TP: The microfilament network of the platelet. *Prog Hemost Thromb* 6:63, 1982.

797. Chen M, Stracher A: In situ phosphorylation of platelet actin-binding protein by cAMP-dependent protein kinase stabilizes it against proteolysis by calpain. *J Biol Chem* 264:14282, 1989.

798. O'Halloran T, Beckerle MC, Burridge K: Identification of talin as a major cytoplasmic protein implicated in platelet activation. *Nature* 317:449, 1985.

799. Koteliansky VE, Gneushev GN, Glukhova MA, Venyaminov SY, Muszbek L: Identification and isolation of vinculin from platelets. *FEBS Lett* 165:26, 1984.

800. Langer B, Gonnella PA, Nachmias VT: α-actinin and vinculin in normal and thrombasthenic platelets. *Blood* 63:606, 1984.

801. Lucas RC, Rosenberg S, Shafiq S, Stracher A, Lawrence J: The isolation and characterization of a cytoskeleton and a contractile apparatus from platelets, in *Protides of Biological Fluids*, edited by H Peeters, p 465. Pergamon, New York, 1975.

802. Wang L-L, Bryan J: Isolation of calcium-dependent platelet proteins that interact with actin. *Cell* 25:637, 1981.

803. Hathaway DR, Adelstein RS: Human platelet myosin light chain kinase requires the calcium binding protein calmodulin for activity. *Proc Natl Acad Sci USA* 76:1653, 1979.

804. Wolff DJ, Brostrom CO: Proteties and functions of the calcium-dependent regulator protein. *Adv Cyclic Nucleotide Res* 11:27, 1979.

805. Hartwig JH: Platelet morphology, in Thrombosis and Hemorrhage, edited by J. Loscalzo and A.I. Schafer, 2nd ed, p. 207, Williams & Wilkins, Baltimore, 1999.

MOLECULAR BIOLOGY AND BIOCHEMISTRY OF THE COAGULATION FACTORS AND PATHWAYS OF HEMOSTASIS

HAROLD R. ROBERTS

DOUGALD M. MONROE III

MAUREANE HOFFMAN

Blood coagulation is a very delicately balanced system. When it functions as it should, the blood is maintained in a fluid state in the vasculature, yet rapidly clots to seal an injury. When hemostatic functions fail, hemorrhage or thromboembolic phenomena result. This chapter addresses molecular and biochemical features of the proteins of the coagulation system and how they interact with cells and with one another to provide hemostasis in the living organism. We have grouped the coagulation factors as (1) the vitamin K–dependent zymogens (prothrombin; factors VII; IX, and X; and protein C); (2) the soluble cofactors [protein S, factor V, factor VIII, and von Willebrand factor (vWf)]; (3) factor XI and the other ''contact'' factors; (4) cell-associated cofactors (tissue factor and thrombomodulin); (5) fibrinogen; (6) factor XIII; and (7) the plasma coagulation protease inhibitors. Major features of the coagulation factors addressed in this chapter are shown in Table 112-1. A model of the coagulation pathway is presented that is based on current understanding of cell–cell and cell–protein interactions that regulate hemostasis. This scheme emphasizes the importance of cellular localization and plasma protease inhibitors in confining the coagulation reactions to a specific site of injury.

MOLECULAR BIOLOGY, BIOCHEMISTRY, AND LIFE SPAN OF THE COAGULATION FACTORS

VITAMIN K–DEPENDENT ZYMOGENS (PROTHROMBIN; FACTORS VII, IX, AND X; AND PROTEIN C)

COMMON STRUCTURAL AND FUNCTIONAL FEATURES

The vitamin K–dependent coagulation zymogens are inert precursors of serine proteases that must be proteolytically activated to express their enzymatic activity. They all share a similar protein domain struc-

ture (Fig. 112-1). Each of the mature vitamin K–dependent coagulation zymogen proteins has an amino-terminal γ-carboxyglutamic acid (Gla) domain with 9 to 12 Gla residues. This is followed by a hydrophobic region. All except prothrombin have two epidermal growth factor (EGF)–like domains, and all have a serine protease domain in their carboxy-terminal regions. Prothrombin has two kringle domains instead of EGF-like domains. Specific functions are associated, at least in part, with specific domains.

In addition to the functional modules found in the mature protein, each vitamin K–dependent factor is synthesized with an amino-terminal signal sequence directing it to the endoplasmic reticulum, followed by a 19– to 25–amino acid propeptide that is recognized by the γ-glutamylcarboxylase, which catalyzes carboxylation of glutamic acid residues in the amino-terminal portion of the molecule. Following translocation into the endoplasmic reticulum, the signal sequence is removed by a microsomal signal peptidase. The propeptide is cleaved following carboxylation before the mature protein is secreted.

Not only are the proteins homologous, but their gene structures are highly similar as well. The coding regions of the vitamin K–dependent factors are quite similar in size. However, the intron lengths vary substantially and account for the differences in the overall size of the genes (20 kb for prothrombin, 13 kb for factor VII, 33 kb for factor IX, 25 kb for factor X, and 10 kb for protein C). Although the cDNA of all of the vitamin K–dependent factors has been sequenced, the noncoding regions have only been characterized to varying degrees of detail. The vitamin K–dependent coagulation zymogens are synthesized primarily by the liver, and thus they all have regulatory elements that direct liver-specific expression. The regulatory elements vary, however, among the proteins.

In factors VII, IX, and X and protein C, the introns occur in identical positions in the genes,[1,2] suggesting that these enzymes evolved by duplication of a common ancestral precursor gene. The regions of the molecules that are thought of as functional domains tend to be encoded in their entirety by a single exon; that is, the signal peptide by one exon, the propeptide and Gla region by the next exon, and so on. This ''modular'' design suggests how ''exon shuffling'' could splice together intact functional units of different proteins to give rise to new proteins with novel properties.

The Gla domain that is characteristic of these proteins mediates interaction of the protein with lipid membranes. The Gla domain is named for the modified amino acids found among the first 42 residues of the mature protein. Gla residues are produced by the posttranslational modification of glutamic acid residues carried out by a specific γ-glutamylcarboxylase in the endoplasmic reticulum (Fig. 112-2). The propeptide sequence is required for γ-carboxylation to take place and is highly conserved among the vitamin K–dependent factors. Amino acids at positions −18, −17, −16, −15, and −10 are critical for recognition by the carboxylase.[3,4] This carboxylase requires oxygen, carbon dioxide, and the reduced form of vitamin K for its action. For each glutamyl residue that is carboxylated, one molecule of reduced vitamin K is converted to the epoxide form. A separate enzyme complex, vitamin K epoxide reductase, is required to convert the epoxide form of vitamin K back to the reduced form. Warfarin inhibits the activity of vitamin K epoxide reductase and prevents recycling of vitamin K back to the reduced form. The effect of warfarin is, therefore, to inhibit γ-glutamylcarboxylation, with the result that a heterogeneous population of undercarboxylated forms of the Gla-containing factors appears in circulation. These undercarboxylated forms have reduced activity. Since warfarin blocks the epoxide reductase (rather than blocking the carboxylase) and prevents recycling of vitamin K, the effects of warfarin poisoning can be reversed by administration of vitamin K. Mutations of the carboxylase can lead to low levels of all of the Gla-containing factors.[5]

Acronyms and abbreviations that appear in this chapter include: ATIII, antithrombin III; BiP, immunoglobulin-binding protein; C/EB, CCAAT/enhancer-binding protein; EGF, epidermal growth factor; Gla, γ-carboxyglutamic acid; HK, high-molecular-weight kininogen; HNF, hepatic nuclear factor; IL, interleukin; PK, prekallikrein; PS, phosphatidylserine; SCR, short consensus repeat; TAFI, thrombin-activatable fibrinolytic inhibitor; TF, tissue factor; TFPI, tissue factor pathway inhibitor; TM, thrombomodulin; vWf, von Willebrand factor.

TABLE 112-1   CHARACTERISTICS OF COAGULATION PROTEINS

PROTEIN	CONCENTRATION, μG/ML	PLASMA HALF-LIFE, H	CHROMOSOME
Zymogens			
Gla			
Prothrombin (factor II)	100–150	60–70	11p11–q12
Factor VII	0.5	3–6	13q34
Factor IX	4–5	18–24	Xq27.1–q27.2
Factor X	8–10	30–40	13q34
Protein C	4–5	6	2q13–q14
Non-Gla			
Factor XI	5	52	4q32–q35
Factor XII	30	60	5q33
Prekallikrein	50	35	4q35
Factor XIII-A chain*	10	240	6p24–p25
Factor XIII-B chain*	22		1q31–q32.1
Cofactors			
Soluble			
Factor V†	5–10	12	1q21–q25
Factor VIII	0.1–0.2	8–12	Xq28
vWf	10	12	12p13.2
Protein S	25‡	42	3p11.1–q11.2
Protein Z	2–3	60	
High-molecular-weight Kininogen	70	150	3q26
Cellular			
Tissue factor	—	—	1p21–p22
Thrombomodulin	—	—	20p12–cen
Structural protein			
Fibrinogen	2000–4000	72–120	
Aα chain			4q23–q32
Bβ chain			4q23–q32
γ chain			4q23–q32
Inhibitors			
Antithrombin III	150–400	72	1q23–q25
Tissue factor pathway Inhibitor	0.1		2q31–q32.1
Protein Z–dependent Protease inhibitor (ZPI)	1–1.6		

*All of the factor XIII-A chain is in complex with factor XIII-B chain; only half of factor XIII-B chain is in complex with factor XIII-A chain, the rest is free in plasma.
†Platelets carry significant amounts of factor XIIIa (roughly half of the total factor XIII activity) and factor V (20% of circulating factor V).
‡About 60% of the protein S is in complex with C4b binding protein.

The calcium-bound form of the Gla domain is responsible for mediating association with phospholipid membranes. Lipids with negatively charged head groups, primarily phosphatidylserine (PS), are required for this binding. Even in the absence of the appropriate protein cofactor, binding to phospholipids increases the proteolytic activity of Gla-containing proteases. Phosphatidylserine is required for activity on synthetic phospholipid membranes. The role of PS in mediating coagulation reactions on cellular membranes is more complex. PS is not normally exposed on the outer membrane leaflet of cells in contact with flowing blood. Further, activation of cells (particularly platelets) is often accompanied by exposure of PS on the outer leaflet of cell membranes. Since this activation enhances the ability to support coagulation reactions, it has often been assumed that exposure of PS on the outer surface of cells is sufficient to account for the ability of a cell to support coagulation reactions. However, other studies have shown that the level of coagulant activity on cells does not directly correlate with the amount of PS exposure. This result is in direct contrast to studies with phospholipid membranes in which the level of coagulant

activity is directly related to the amount of PS expressed. From these studies, we conclude that PS exposure is necessary for cells to support coagulation reactions, and that other features, such as cell receptors and/or binding proteins, are also necessary.

There is very high homology in the amino acid sequence in the first 42 residues of the Gla-containing proteins. This implies that the three-dimensional structure is highly conserved and that few specific interactions are determined by this region. It was once thought that the binding of Gla-containing proteins to phospholipids was mediated by calcium ion "bridging" between the Gla residues and the negatively charged phospholipid. This mechanism provided a good explanation for why both calcium and negatively charged phospholipid were required for binding. It is currently believed, however, that binding of Gla-containing factors to lipid surfaces is mediated by membrane insertion of hydrophobic residues in the first ten amino acids of the Gla domain. Calcium is essential for this to occur because calcium binding to the Gla residues induces a dramatic conformational change that exposes the hydrophobic amino acid residues in a "patch" on the surface of the protein. This patch allows the protein to insert into the phospholipid membrane (Fig. 112-3).

The striking degree of homology among the Gla domains of the vitamin K–dependent clotting factors would suggest that the affinity of the calcium–Gla complexes for phospholipids would also be very similar. However, this turns out not to be the case. Factor IX and factor X bind much more strongly ($K_d \approx 0.25~\mu$M) to phosphatidylcholine- and PS-containing vesicles than does factor VII ($K_d = 17~\mu$M).[8] The reasons for these marked differences are not clear.

The first EGF domain of the vitamin K–dependent proteins has a calcium ion–binding site that does not involve Gla residues but does involve a β-hydroxyaspartic acid. This conserved aspartic acid residue is modified posttranslationally by a β-hydroxylase about which little is known. Binding of calcium to this EGF-1 site appears to be important in activity and probably serves to orient the Gla domain relative to the rest of the molecule. The EGF-1 and EGF-2 domains serve, at least in part, to space the serine protease domain above the lipid membrane surface. Factor VIIa interaction with its cofactor, tissue factor, is mediated to some degree by direct interaction between tissue factor and both EGF domains of factor VIIa.

All of the zymogen Gla-containing factors undergo activation by cleavage of at least one peptide bond (see Fig. 112-1). Activation is indicated by appending the letter "a" to the name of the factor, except

FIGURE 112-1   Comparison of the Gla-containing zymogens showing their basic structural elements. Each circle is an amino acid. The pre-pro leader sequence contains the signal peptide as well as elements that direct carboxylation of glutamyl residues. Cleavage of the leader sequence is indicated by a slight separation from the mature protein. All have a Gla domain, with the Gla residues indicated by filled blue circles. Prothrombin has a finger loop followed by two kringle domains. Factors VII, IX, and X and protein C have EGF-like domains. Prothrombin, factor VII, and factor IX circulate as single-chain molecules. Factor X and protein C circulate as two chains that are disulfide linked. All have a catalytic domain that is homologous among the Gla-containing zymogens. The active-site His, Asp, and Ser residues are indicated by the black circles in the catalytic domain. Cleavages that convert the zymogen to an active enzyme are indicated by the arrows. In factor IX, factor X, and protein C, the released activation peptide is indicated by the gray circles. After cleavage, all of the factors are two-chain disulfide-linked molecules. The disulfide connecting the catalytic domain with the rest of the molecule is shown by the heavy bond. All catalytic domains except that of prothrombin remain attached to the Gla domain following activation.

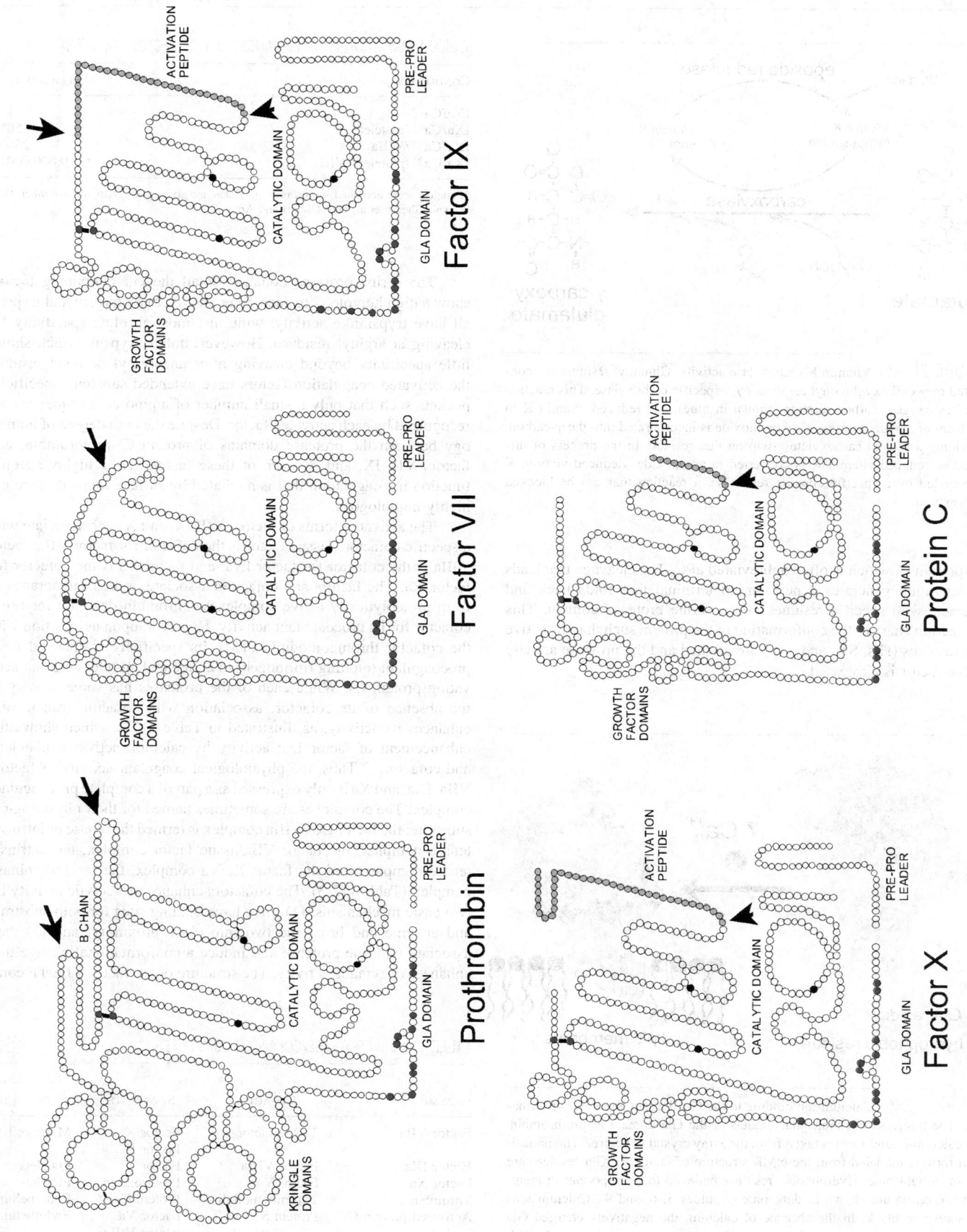

1411

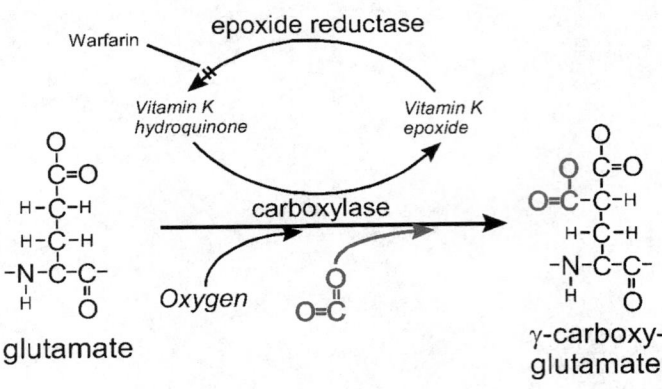

FIGURE 112-2   Vitamin K carboxylase activity. Glutamyl residues are converted to γ-carboxyglutamyl residues by a specific carboxylase. This reaction requires oxygen, carbon dioxide (shown in blue), and reduced vitamin K in the form of a hydroquinone. Carbon dioxide is incorporated into the γ-carbon, providing a second carboxylate group on that residue. In the process of this reaction, reduced vitamin K is converted to an epoxide. Reduced vitamin K is recycled by a specific epoxide reductase, a reaction that can be blocked by warfarin.

for protein C, which is often abbreviated aPC. The cleavage that leads to activation generates a new amino terminal that folds back and interacts with specific residues in the serine protease domain. This interaction changes the conformation of the protein such that the active site residues (His, Ser, and Asp) are aligned and the protease activity of the factor is expressed.

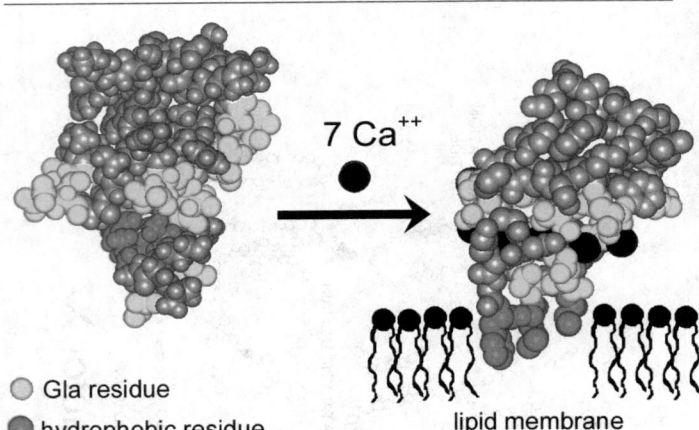

FIGURE 112-3   Calcium-ion binding to the Gla domain alters its conformation. The figure shows molecular models of the Gla domain of prothrombin. The calcium-bound form is taken from the x-ray crystal structure.[6] The noncalcium form is modeled from the NMR structure of factor X.[7] Gla residues are shown in light blue. Hydrophobic residues believed to be important in membrane insertion are shown in dark blue (residues 5, 6, and 9). Calcium ions are shown in black. In the absence of calcium, the negatively charged Gla residues are exposed to the solution, and the hydrophobic residues are buried. Calcium-ion binding to the Gla residues provides sufficient energy to alter the overall conformation of the Gla domain and expose the hydrophobic residues. In this view, only four of the seven bound calcium ions can be seen. Insertion of the hydrophobic residues into a membrane is illustrated schematically.

TABLE 112-2   COFACTOR ENHANCEMENT OF FACTOR IXa ACTIVITY

CONDITIONS	RELATIVE RATE
IXa/Ca^{++}	1
IXa/Ca^{++}/platelet*	150[†]
IXa/Ca^{++}/VIIIa	250[‡]
IXa/Ca^{++}/platelet*/VIIIa	9,000,000[†]

*Platelets were activated with thrombin. Rates are given as k_{cat}/Km and are taken from [†]Rawala-Sheikh et al[9] and [‡]Gilbert and Arena.[10]

The serine protease domains of all the Gla-containing factors show a high homology to each other and to chymotrypsin and trypsin; all have trypsinlike activity, with an almost absolute specificity for cleaving at arginyl residues. However, unlike trypsin, which shows little specificity beyond cleaving after an arginyl or lysyl residue, the activated coagulation factors have extended substrate specificity pockets such that only a small number of amino acid sequences are recognized by each activated factor. Despite the high degree of homology between the protease domains of protein C, prothrombin, and factors VII, IX, and X, each of these factors has a highly specific function in coagulation that is mediated by surface loops that are not highly homologous.

The activated forms of factors VII, IX, and X each associate with a specific cofactor. Tissue factor is the cofactor for factor VIIa; factor VIIIa is the cofactor for factor IXa; and factor Va is the cofactor for factor Xa. The factors and cofactors associate on cell membranes to form proteolytically active complexes. Thrombin does not require a cofactor for its procoagulant activity. However, upon association with the cofactor thrombomodulin (TM), its specificity is changed from procoagulant (clotting fibrinogen) to anticoagulant (cleaving and activating protein C). While each of the proteases has some activity in the absence of its cofactor, association with cofactor dramatically enhances its activity, as illustrated in Table 112-2, which shows the enhancement of factor IXa activity by calcium, activated platelets, and cofactor.[9,10] Thus, the physiological coagulant activity of factors VIIa, IXa, and Xa is only expressed as a part of a complete procoagulant complex. The complexes are sometimes named for their physiological substrate: the factor IXa/VIIIa complex is termed the tenase or intrinsic tenase complex; the factor VIIa/tissue factor complex, the extrinsic tenase complex; and the factor Xa/Va complex, the prothrombinase complex (Table 112-3). The cofactors enhance proteolytic activity by two basic mechanisms: (1) They have binding sites for both substrate and enzyme and bring the two into close proximity; and (2) they associate with the protease and induce a conformational change that enhances enzymatic activity. The structure of the factor VIIa/TF com-

TABLE 112-3   PROTEASE/COFACTOR COMPLEXES

ENZYME	COFACTOR	SUBSTRATE	CELLULAR LOCATION
Factor VIIa	Tissue factor	Factor X Factor IX	Many cells*
Factor IXa	Factor VIIIa	Factor X	Platelets
Factor Xa	Factor Va	Prothrombin	Platelets[†]
Thrombin	Thrombomodulin	Protein C	Endothelium
Activated protein C	Protein S	Factor Va Factor VIIIa	Endothelium

*TF is constitutively expressed on many extravascular cells (e.g., stromal cells, epithelial cells, astrocytes) and induced by inflammatory mediators in many other cells (e.g., monocytes, endothelial cells).
[†]Many other cells have low levels of factor Xa/factor Va activity.

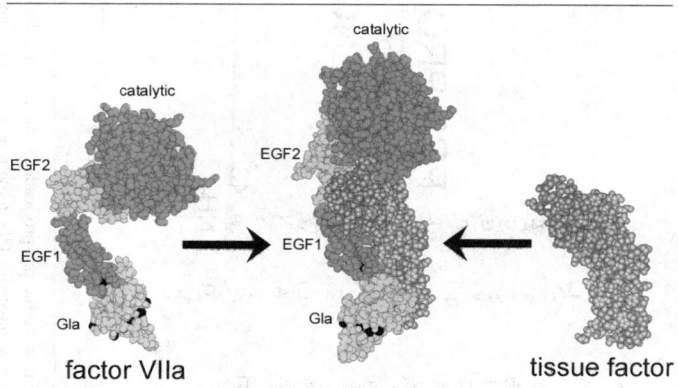

FIGURE 112-4   Complex of factors VIIa and TF. The crystal structure of TF[12] and the TF complex[13] are shown, along with a model of the free structure of factor VIIa (based on the crystal structure of factor IXa[14]). The Gla domain, EGF domains, and catalytic domain of factor VIIa are indicated. Calcium ions are shown in black. Binding to TF alters the overall structure of factor VIIa. The orientation of the EGF1 domain is identical in factor VIIa in the modeled free structure and in complex with TF. The crystal structure of the complex shows multiple close contacts between TF and multiple domains of factor VIIa.

plex has been determined by x-ray crystallography.[11] Figure 112-4 illustrates the projected change in conformation of the factor VIIa molecule when it binds to its cofactor, tissue factor. The factor IXa/VIIIa and Xa/Va complexes have not been crystallized, but it is likely that similar conformational changes occur during formation of these complexes.

PROTHROMBIN (FACTOR II)

Protein Structure   Like the other vitamin K–dependent zymogens, plasma prothrombin is primarily synthesized in the liver. It circulates as a single-chain zymogen with a M_r of approximately 72,000 and a plasma half-life of about 60 h. A schematic representation is shown in Fig. 112-5. Prothrombin has 10 Gla residues, and instead of the EGF region present in most vitamin K–dependent zymogens, it has two kringle domains. Kringle domains are structures held together by three disulfide bonds that schematically resemble a Danish pastry called a kringle. The primary function of kringle structures appears to be to bind other proteins, such as activators, substrates, cofactors, or receptors.[15]

Molecular Biology   The human prothrombin gene has been localized to chromosome 11, near the centromere.[16] It has been completely sequenced and is composed of 14 exons separated by 13 introns (Fig. 112-6). The 5′-flanking region of the prothrombin gene contains the promoter region and two or more cis-acting enhancer sequences. Cis-acting sequences are portions of the DNA that act as promoters, enhancers, or silencers. Unlike many other promoters, the promoter region of the prothrombin gene does not contain a TATA box. It has multiple potential sites of transcription initiation extending from 3 to 38 bp upstream from the initial methionine. The site at −31 is the most likely start site. The region between −887 and −875 is likely to be a binding site for hepatic nuclear factor-1 (HNF-1), a DNA-binding protein that plays a role in the liver-specific expression of a number of genes.[17] HNF-1 is an example of a trans-acting factor, a molecule that binds to a DNA sequence and affects expression of the associated gene. An additional site in the prothrombin promoter region with non-tissue-specific enhancer activity lies just upstream to the HNF-1 site.

One unusual feature of the prothrombin gene is the presence of many repetitive sequences in its 5′-flanking region.[18] About 41 percent of the gene and upstream sequence consists of Alu repeats. The function of these repetitive sequences, if any, is not known.

Several polymorphisms of the prothrombin gene have been described, and one of these is now recognized to have important functional consequences. This G-to-A transition in the 3′-untranslated region (20210 G→A) of the prothrombin gene is associated with higher than normal levels of plasma prothrombin.[19] Increased prothrombin levels have been associated with an increased risk of thromboembolic phenomena (see Chap. 127).

Activation and Activity   Prothrombin is cleaved by the factor Xa/Va complex in two places (Arg271 and Arg320), as shown in Fig. 112-7.[6,20-22] The catalytic domain (thrombin), M_r 36,600, is released from the remainder of the molecule (prothrombin fragment 1.2). Since one molecule of prothrombin fragment 1.2 is released for each molecule of thrombin, assays for fragment 1.2 reflect the level of prothrombin activation.

Thrombin cleaves a number of biologically important substrates. It removes fibrinopeptides A and B from fibrinogen to form fibrin monomers, which then spontaneously polymerize to form a fibrin clot (see Chap. 124). The anion-binding exosite spans residues 387 through 398 and is involved in binding to fibrinogen, thrombomodulin, hirudin, heparin cofactor II, and the proteolytically activated thrombin receptors. It is interesting to note that this region of thrombin is identical in human, bovine, rat, and mouse.[23] In addition to directly clotting fibrinogen, thrombin has a procoagulant effect by participating in positive feedback loops by activating platelets and coagulation factors V, VIII, XI, and XIII.

Thrombin is a potent platelet activator through at least two types of receptors. These include the G-protein-linked, proteolytically activated receptors PAR-1 and PAR-4, as well as platelet glycoprotein Ibα (see Chap. 111).

Another function of thrombin is to activate a procarboxypeptidase-B–like enzyme to its active state, a reaction enhanced by thrombomodulin. The active carboxypeptidase inhibits plasmin-mediated fibrinolysis by removing carboxyl-terminal lysine residues, which facilitate plasminogen binding, from partially degraded fibrin. Thus, the carboxypeptidase has been termed thrombin-activatable fibrinolytic inhibitor (TAFI).[24]

In addition to its procoagulant activity, thrombin also has an anticoagulant function. Thus, thrombin binds to the cofactor thrombomodulin on endothelial cells, which allows it to activate protein C.[25] Thrombin also has growth factor and cytokinelike activities that may play a role in atherosclerosis, wound healing, and inflammation.[26]

The primary plasma inhibitor of thrombin in coagulation is antithrombin III (ATIII). Heparin cofactor II also inhibits thrombin and may serve as an extravascular thrombin inhibitor that regulates the growth factor and cytokinelike activities of thrombin.[26]

FACTOR VII

Protein Structure   Factor VII circulates as a single-chain zymogen of M_r 50,000. It has the shortest half-life of the procoagulant factors, about 3.5 h (see Table 112-1) and has 10 Gla residues.

Molecular Biology   The human factor VII gene is located on chromosome 13, very close to the gene for factor X. The gene consists of eight exons and seven introns, with an overall size of about 13 kb and an organization similar to that of the other vitamin K–dependent factors (Fig. 112-8).[1,2]

The major transcription start site in the factor VII gene is at −51. Three other minor start sites have been described.[27] A hormone-responsive element and binding sites for the trans-acting factors HF-4 and Sp-1 are present between −233 and −58 in the promoter region of the factor VII gene.

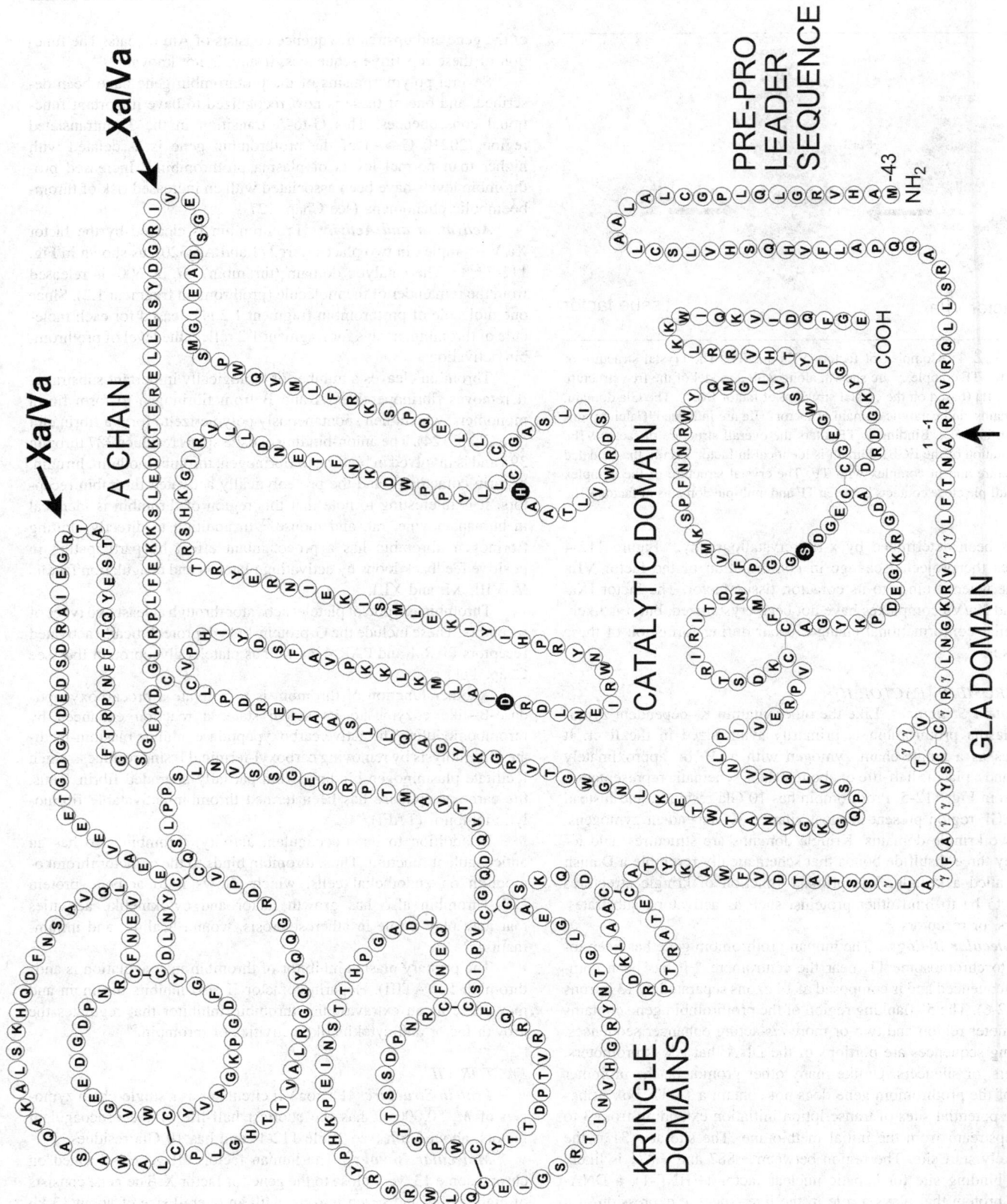

FIGURE 112-5 Domains of prothrombin. Each amino acid in prothrombin is shown. Gla residues are indicated by γ. The cleavage site to remove the pre-pro leader sequence is indicated by an arrow. The active-site His, Asp, and Ser are shown by black circles. Cleavage sites for factor Xa/factor Va are shown by arrows. Cleavage removes the Gla domain and kringles, leaving thrombin composed of a small A-chain disulfide linked to the B chain (catalytic domain).

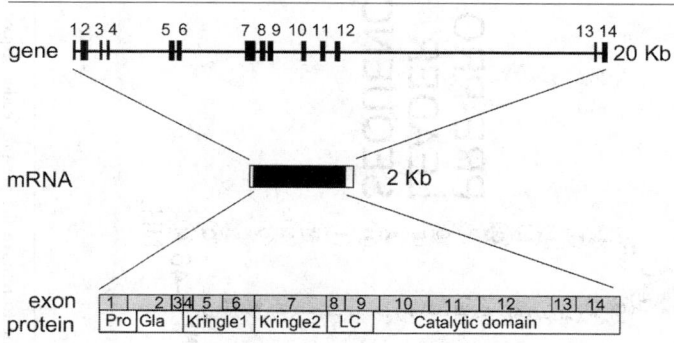

FIGURE 112-6   Relationship between gene structure and protein structure in prothrombin. The exons, introns, mRNA, and protein structure are as indicated. Promoter elements upstream from exon 1 are not shown but are discussed in the text. The mRNA is 2 kb, with small 5'- and 3'-untranslated regions. In the protein, Pro indicates the pre-pro leader sequence. Kringle 1 and 2 are shown. LC, light chain or A chain.

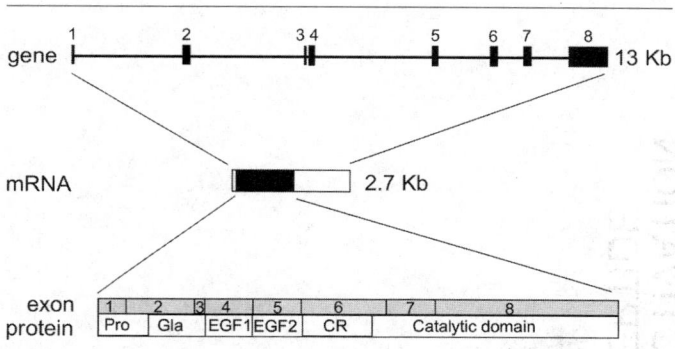

FIGURE 112-8   Relationship between gene structure and protein structure in factor VII. The exons, introns, mRNA, and protein structure are as indicated. Promoter elements upstream from exon 1 are not shown but are discussed in the text. The mRNA is 2.7 kb, with a small 5'-untranslated region and a relatively large 3'-untranslated region. In the protein, Pro indicates the pre-pro leader sequence. CR, connecting region; EGF, epidermal growth factor–like domains.

Activation and Activity   Factor VII binds to tissue factor with a K_d in the subnanomolar range. Once bound to its cofactor, factor VII can be activated by a number of different proteases that cleave between Arg152 and Ile153. The physiological activator of factor VII is thought to be factor Xa. Unlike prothrombin, the catalytic domain of factor VII is linked to the rest of the molecule by a disulfide bond, so no portion is cleaved from the protein (see Fig. 112-1). The factor VIIa/TF complex activates both factors IX and X. It is inhibited by tissue factor pathway inhibitor (TFPI) in complex with factor Xa. It is also inhibited by ATIII, but only in the presence of heparin.

FACTOR IX

Protein Structure   Factor IX, also synthesized in hepatocytes, circulates as a single-chain zymogen of M_r 57,000 and a plasma half-life of 18 to 24 h. It has 12 Gla residues. Only about 40 percent of factor IX molecules are hydroxylated at Asp64 in the EGF-1 domain. All the other Gla-containing zymogens have complete hydroxylation of the homologous residues (Fig. 112-9). Factor IX contains N- and O-linked carbohydrate moieties found mostly in the activation peptide. In the mature molecule the Tyr residue at position 155 is sulfated, while the Ser residue at position 158 is phosphorylated.

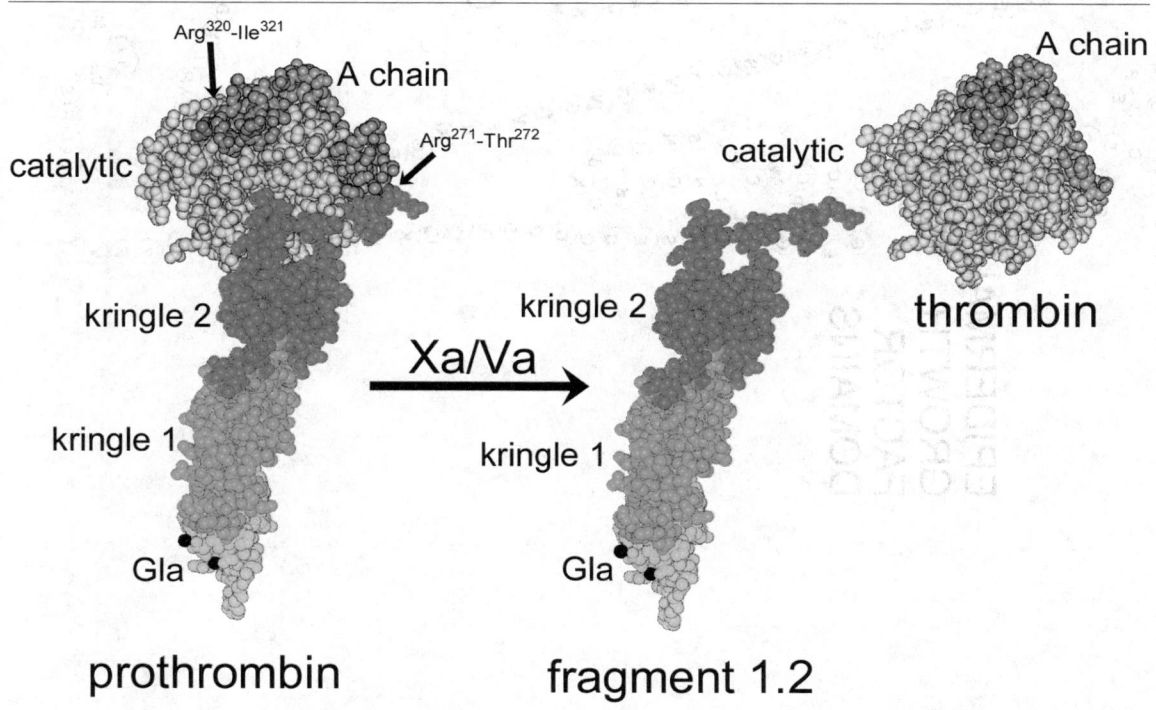

FIGURE 112-7   Activation of prothrombin. A model of prothrombin constructed from four crystal structures is shown.[6,20–22] The Gla domain, both kringle domains, and the catalytic domain are indicated. Calcium ions are shown in black. Cleavage by factor Xa/factor Va releases thrombin from the rest of the molecule, fragment 1.2.

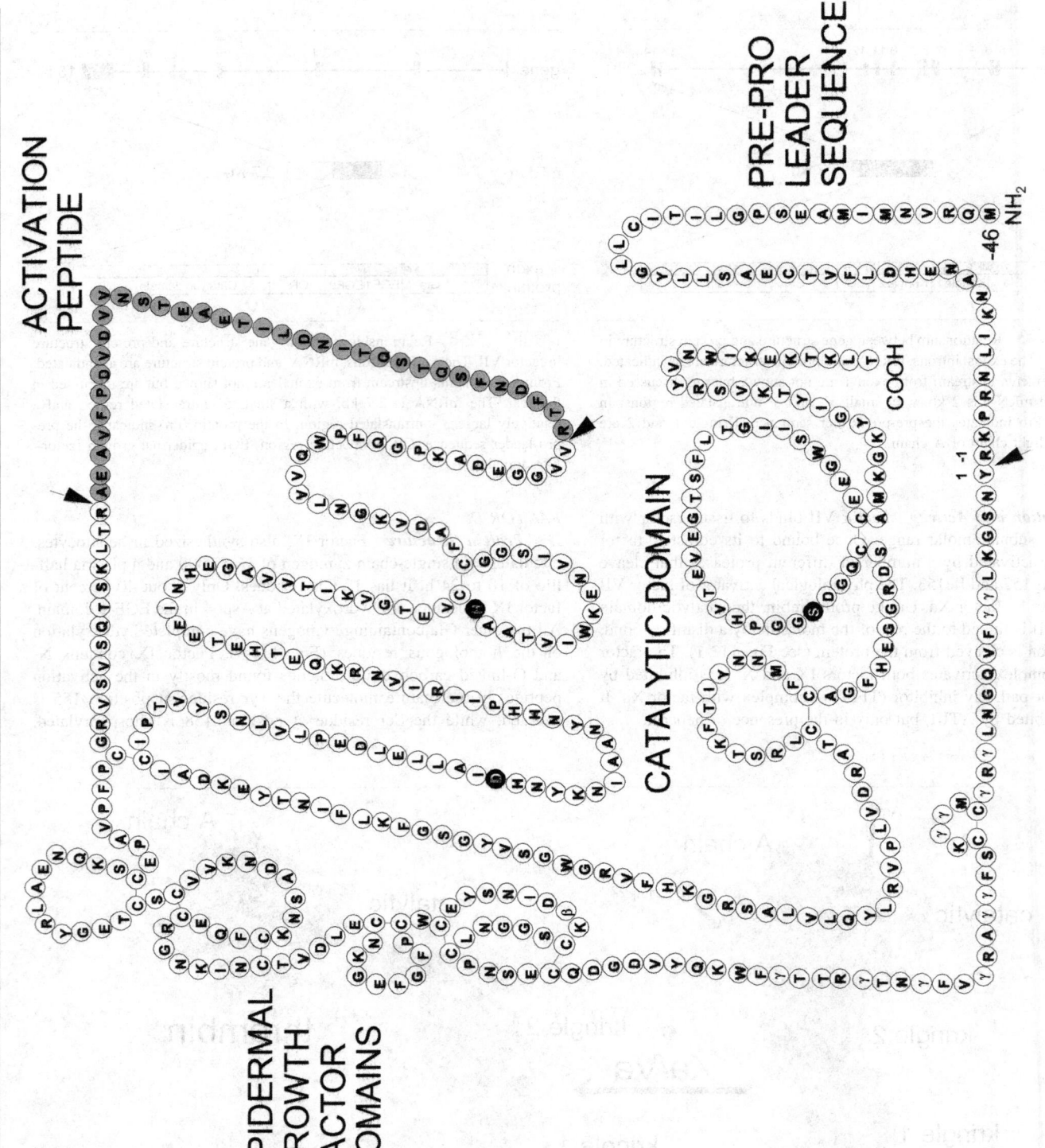

FIGURE 112-9 Domains of factor IX. Each amino acid in factor IX is shown. Gla residues are indicated by γ. The cleavage site to remove the pre-pro leader sequence is indicated by an arrow. The active-site His, Asp, and Ser are shown by black circles. Cleavage sites for factor XIa and factor VIIa/TF are indicated by arrows.

Factor IX, unlike other vitamin–K dependent factors, has been shown to bind effectively to collagen IV in vitro.[28] The molecule appears to bind to collagen IV in vivo and may account for the observation that, when factor IX is infused into hemophilia B patients, recovery is only 50 percent of that expected (see Chap. 123).[29] The physiological relevance of this observation remains to be determined.

Molecular Biology   The gene for factor IX is located on the tip of the long arm of the X chromosome at position Xq27.1–q27.2.[30] Therefore, deficiency of factor IX (hemophilia B) is sex linked. The gene contains eight exons, seven introns, and a long 1.4-kb 3'-untranslated region, with an overall size of 33 kb (Fig. 112-10).

Eight polymorphisms have been described within or flanking the factor IX gene. These polymorphisms can be useful for antenatal diagnosis and carrier detection of hemophilia B by restriction fragment length polymorphism analysis.[31]

The promoter activity of the 5'-untranslated region of the factor IX gene resides 274 bp upstream of the major transcription start site.[32] Binding sites for several *trans*-acting factors have been identified, including sites for CCAAT/enhancer-binding protein (C/EBP),[33] D-site binding protein,[34] HNF-4,[35] and HNF-1.[36]

Activation and Activity   Factor IX can be activated either by factor XIa or by the factor VIIa/TF complex. Full activation requires cleavage of two bonds (Arg145 and Arg180), releasing an activation peptide of M_r of approximately 10,000 (see Fig. 112-9).

In complex with its cofactor, factor VIIIa, on a phospholipid membrane surface, factor IXa activates factor X. Physiologically this activity is primarily expressed on the surface of activated platelets, and there is evidence suggesting that platelets express a receptor-binding protein for factor IXa that promotes assembly of the factor IXa/VIIIa complex.[37]

The primary plasma inhibitor of factor IXa appears to be ATIII. Inhibition of factor IXa by ATIII is slow compared to ATIII inhibition of thrombin. However, it is enhanced in the presence of heparin.

FACTOR X

Protein Structure   Factor X circulates as a two-chain, disulfide-linked zymogen of M_r 59,000 (see Fig. 112-1) and has a plasma half-life of about 34 to 40 h. A three amino acid sequence (Arg180-Lys181-Arg182) is cleaved from the protein during intracellular processing. The light-chain M_r is approximately 17,000, and the heavy-chain M_r

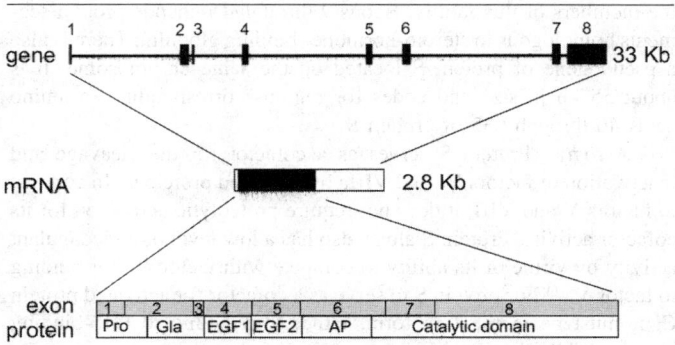

FIGURE 112-10   Relationship between gene structure and protein structure in factor IX. The exons, introns, mRNA, and protein structure are as indicated. Promoter elements upstream from exon 1 are not shown but are discussed in the text. The mRNA is 2.8 kb, with a small 5'-untranslated region and a relatively large 3'-untranslated region. In the protein, Pro indicates the pre-pro leader sequence. AP indicates the activation peptide, which is released after cleavage of two bonds.

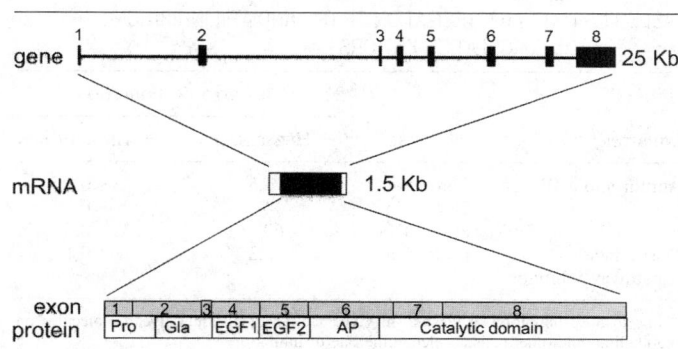

FIGURE 112-11   Relationship between gene structure and protein structure in factor X. The exons, introns, mRNA, and protein structure are as indicated. Promoter elements upstream from exon 1 are not shown but are discussed in the text. The mRNA is 1.5 kb with a relatively large 5'-untranslated region and a small 3'-untranslated region. In the protein, Pro indicates the pre-pro leader sequence. AP, activation peptide.

is approximately 40,000. The light chain contains the Gla domain with its 11 Gla residues, and the two EGF domains. The heavy chain contains the catalytic domain and the activation peptide. Like all other vitamin K–dependent factors, it is synthesized in the liver.

Molecular Biology   The gene for human factor X is on chromosome 13q34–qter[39] in close proximity to the factor VII gene. It is composed of eight exons and seven introns,[1] with a size of approximately 25 kb (Fig. 112-11). The 3'-untranslated region is unusually short, being only 10 base pairs. A number of potentially useful polymorphisms have been identified.[40]

The factor X promoter region has been sequenced and characterized. It lacks a typical TATA box but contains a CCAAT sequence at −120 to −116. Factor X appears to have multiple start sites of transcription.[41] This finding is consistent with the multiple start sites reported for other promoters lacking a TATA box. Like the factor IX gene, a binding site for HNF-4 has been identified.[42] However, unlike the factor IX gene, there does not appear to be a binding site for C/EBP.

Activation and Activity   Factor X can be activated by factor VIIa/TF or factor IXa/VIIIa by cleavage at the Arg194-Ile195 bond. It can be autocatalytically cleaved near the carboxyl terminus of the heavy chain to yield ''β-Xa,'' which is also enzymatically active.

Factor Xa in complex with factor Va on a phospholipid membrane surface activates prothrombin to thrombin by cleaving two peptide bonds. Factor Xa may also play a physiological role in activation of factors VII,[43] VIII,[44] and V.[45] While any membrane surface that expresses anionic phospholipid can support prothrombinase complex assembly, the activated platelet surface is especially well suited for this purpose. Prothrombinase assembly on platelets is not strictly a function of phospholipid composition, but is coordinated by one or more specific binding proteins.[46]

Like thrombin, factor X has biological activities not directly related to coagulation. It is reported to have mitogenic activity for smooth muscle cells.[47] Factor Xa also possesses receptor-mediated proinflammatory activities.[48] The primary plasma inhibitor of factor Xa is ATIII, and the inhibition by ATIII is accelerated by heparin. Tissue factor pathway inhibitor is also a potent inhibitor of factor Xa, as shown in Table 112-4.

PROTEIN C

Protein Structure   Protein C, unlike the other vitamin K–dependent zymogens, is not a procoagulant but controls coagulation by inactivating factors Va and VIIIa. It circulates as a two-chain

TABLE 112-4   CHARACTERIZATION OF TFPI AND ATIII INHIBITION OF
                        COAGULATION FACTORS

| INHIBITOR | PROTEASE | TIME TO 50% INHIBITION* | |
		− HEPARIN, MIN	+ HEPARIN, MIN
Antithrombin III	Thrombin	1.5	<0.1
	Factor Xa	4	<0.1
	Factor IXa	60	0.6
Tissue factor pathway inhibitor	Factor Xa	0.3	<0.1

*Time to 50% inhibition in plasma. In vivo, natural glycosaminoglycan molecules on endothelium and other cells accelerate the rate of inhibition.

disulfide-linked zymogen with 9 Gla residues (see Fig. 112-1). It has an M_r of 59,000 and a short plasma half-life of about 6 h (see Chap. 113).

Molecular Biology   The gene for human protein C is on chromosome 2q13–14.[49] It was originally described as being composed of eight exons with a size of approximately 10 kb.[50] Other workers have described it as having nine exons and eight introns,[51] with the first exon corresponding to the 5′-noncoding region (Fig. 112-12). Thus, the first exon is transcribed from the gene into mRNA but is not translated into protein. The gene structure is very similar to the other vitamin K–dependent factors, with especially close homology to factor IX.

Activation and Activity   Protein C is activated by the thrombin–thrombomodulin complex. A single cleavage at Arg169-Leu170 releases a 12 amino acid activation peptide, leading to activated protein C with a M_r of 56,000.

Activated protein C, in complex with its cofactor protein S, proteolytically inactivates factors Va and VIIIa. It has also been reported that factor V can act as a cofactor for the inactivation of factors Va and VIIIa by activated protein C.[52] The primary inhibitor of activated protein C is protein C inhibitor, also known as plasminogen activator inhibitor-3.[53]

SOLUBLE COFACTORS (PROTEIN S, FACTOR V, FACTOR VIII, AND VON WILLEBRAND FACTOR)

PROTEIN S

Protein Structure   Protein S is a single-chain plasma glycoprotein cofactor with a M_r of approximately 75,000 and a plasma half-life of about 42 h. It contains 11 Gla residues in the amino-terminal

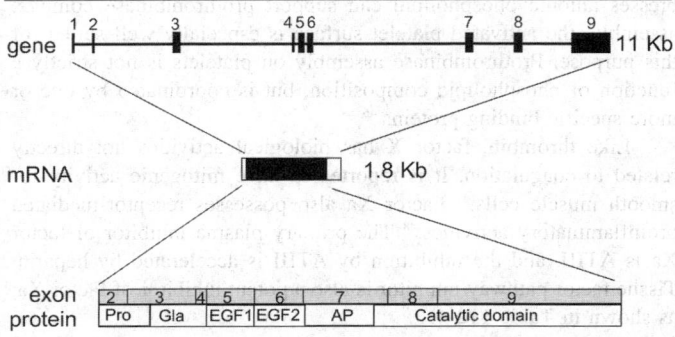

FIGURE 112-12   Relationship between gene structure and protein structure in protein C. The exons, introns, mRNA, and protein structure are as indicated. The mRNA is 1.8 kb, with a small 5′-untranslated region coded for by exon 1 and a relatively small 3′-untranslated region. In the protein, Pro indicates the pre-pro leader sequence. AP, activation peptide.

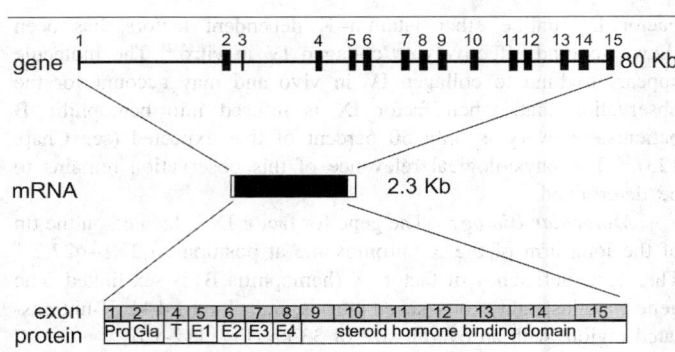

FIGURE 112-13   Relationship between gene structure and protein structure in protein S. The exons, introns, mRNA, and protein structure are as indicated. The mRNA is 2.3 kb, with a small 5′- and 3′-untranslated region. E, EGF-like domains; T, thrombin-sensitive finger region.

region. Its structure is somewhat different from that of the Gla-containing zymogens (Fig. 112-13). Protein S is organized into a Gla domain, a thrombin-sensitive finger region, four EGF domains, and a region with homology to steroid-binding proteins. Unlike the other vitamin K–dependent factors, it does not contain a serine protease domain and so does not have the potential to catalyze reactions. Each EGF domain contains a modified amino acid, either β-hydroxyaspartic acid or β-hydroxyasparagine. Protein S circulates both in the free form (≈40% of the total amount) and in a form bound to C4b-binding protein. The steroid-hormone–binding globulinlike region of protein S is involved in binding to the alpha subunit of C4b-binding protein. Protein S is inactive when bound to C4b-binding protein.[54] Like the Gla-containing zymogens, protein S is synthesized with a signal peptide that directs it to the endoplasmic reticulum and a propeptide that binds to the γ-glutamylcarboxylase. The signal sequence and propeptide are removed before the mature protein is secreted.

Protein S is synthesized primarily by hepatocytes[55] but also by endothelial cells,[56] megakaryocytes,[57] Leydig cells,[58] and osteoblasts.[59]

Molecular Biology   The human protein S gene is on chromosome 3, spanning the centromere from p11.1 to q11.2. It is over 80 kb in length and contains 15 exons and 14 introns (see Fig. 112-13).[60] Exons 1 through 8 encode protein domains that are homologous to the Gla-containing zymogens. The intron–exon structure is typical of the members of this family. Exons 9 through 15 encode protein segments homologous to steroid-hormone–binding globulin. There is also a pseudogene of protein S located on the same chromosome. It is about 55 kb in size and codes for regions corresponding to amino acids 46 through 635 of protein S.

Activity   Protein S serves as a cofactor for the cleavage and inactivation of factors Va and VIIIa by activated protein C. In contrast to factors V and VIII, it does not require proteolytic activation for its cofactor activity. Protein S alone also has a low level of anticoagulant activity by virtue of its ability to compete with factor Xa for binding to factor Va.[61] For protein S to serve as a cofactor for activated protein C, it must be in the free form, rather than bound to C4b-binding protein. While the C4b-binding protein is an acute-phase reactant, its alpha subunit, which binds protein S, is not increased in inflammatory states; thus, the free protein S concentration is not affected by the acute-phase response.

FACTOR V

Protein Structure   Factors V and VIII are homologous in their gene structures, amino acid sequences, and protein domain structures. Factor V is a large glycoprotein with a M_r of approximately 330,000

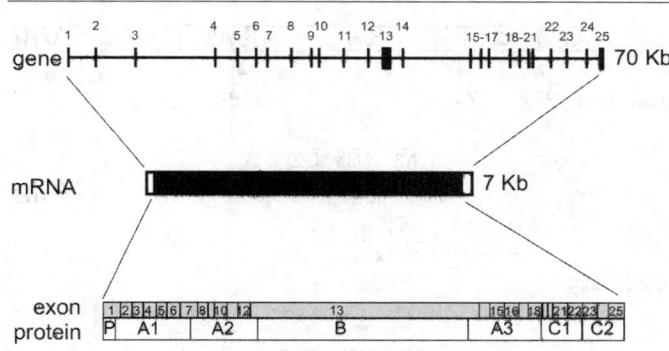

FIGURE 112-14 Relationship between gene structure and protein structure in factor V. The exons, introns, mRNA, and protein structure are as indicated. The mRNA is 7 kb, with some 5′- and 3′-untranslated sequence. In the protein, P indicates the propeptide leader sequence.

and a plasma half-life of about 12 h, with some reports of a half-life of up to 36 h.[62] It has the following domain organization: A1-A2-B-A3-C1-C2 (Fig. 112-14). The three A domains have significant homology to the copper-binding plasma protein ceruloplasmin. The C domains have some homology to fat globule proteins. The C2 domain of factor V mediates binding to lipid membranes.[63] The A and C domains of factor V are approximately 40 percent identical to the homologous regions in factor VIII. In contrast, the B domains show little homology between the two proteins and are not known to be homologous to any other proteins. In factor V, unlike factor VIII, sequences in the B domain appear to be important in promoting its activation by thrombin.

The acidic regions of factor V have a high proportion of Asp and Glu residues. These regions are thought to be important in promoting activation, possibly by providing a site of interaction with the anion-binding exosite of thrombin.

Factor V shows five potential sites for tyrosine sulfation, at residues 696, 698, 1494, 1510, and 1565. Sulfation of factor V also plays a role in the protein's activity by enhancing activation by thrombin and by promoting maximal factor Xa activation of prothrombin.[64] Factor V contains both N-linked and O-linked carbohydrate moieties, most of which are clustered in the B domain.

Molecular Biology The gene for factor V is located on chromosome 1q21–q25. It is located very close to the genes for the selectin family of leukocyte adhesion molecules. The factor V gene spans about 70 kb and consists of 25 exons (see Fig. 112-14). The gene structure is very similar to that of the factor VIII gene, with exon–intron boundaries occurring at exactly the same location in 21 of 24 cases.[65] The mechanisms governing factor V gene transcription and translation are not clear.

Activation and Activity Factor V circulates in plasma as a single-chain molecule. As much as 20 percent of the circulating factor V is found in platelet alpha granules. However, platelet factor V is heterogeneous because of proteolysis within the B domain. Platelet proteases, including calpain, are able to cleave the B domain and produce a partially activated form of factor V (see Chap. 122).

In platelets, but not in plasma, the factor V is complexed to a large multimeric protein called multimerin.[66] Multimerin has a massive repeating structure, with some of the multimers having molecular weights of several million. Multimerin has structural features that suggest it may mediate adhesive interactions. While multimerin appears functionally similar to vWf, the two proteins share no structural homology.

Full factor V cofactor activity is achieved only after cleavage at several bonds (Fig. 112-15). Factor V is believed to be primarily

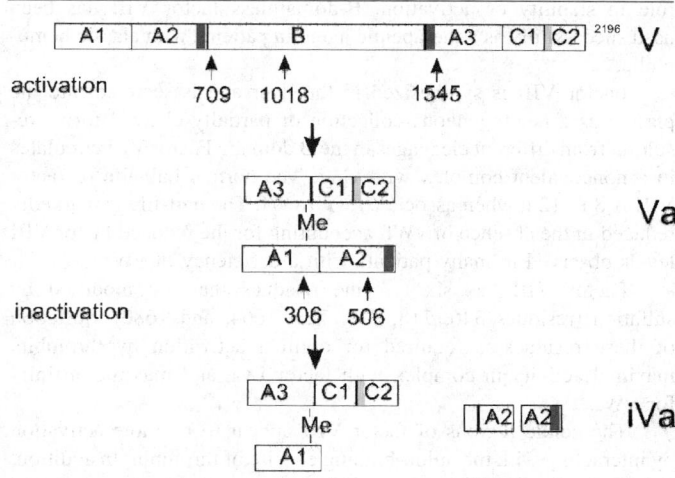

FIGURE 112-15 Activation and inactivation of factor V. For full cofactor activity, factor V requires cleavage by thrombin or factor Xa. The acidic domains, shown in dark blue, are believed to bind to the anion-binding exosite in thrombin and enhance thrombin activation of factor V. Cleavage of residue 1018 enhances cleavage at residue 1545. Heavy and light chains are held together by noncovalent interactions mediated by metal ions (Me). Membrane binding is mediated through a site in the C2 domain (shown in light blue). Cleavages at residues 306 and 506 by activated protein C inactivate factor V by releasing two A2 fragments (iVa).

activated by thrombin in vivo, although it can be activated by factor Xa as well.[45] Thrombin cleaves factor V at Arg709 and Arg1545 to produce a two-chain heterodimeric molecule consisting of an A1-A2 heavy chain (M_r 110,000) that is associated with an A3-C1-C2 light chain (M_r 73,000). The two chains are noncovalently linked through metal ions (probably calcium). Activated factor V is inactivated by activated protein C cleavage at Arg306 and Arg506, followed by dissociation of the cleaved A2 fragments.[62] A common Arg506Gln change confers activated protein C resistance that has been associated with an increased risk of venous thromboembolism.[67]

FACTOR VIII

Protein Structure The domain organization of the factor VIII protein is A1-A2-B-A3-C1-C2, like that of factor V (Fig. 112-16). In factor VIII, the B domain does not appear to play a significant

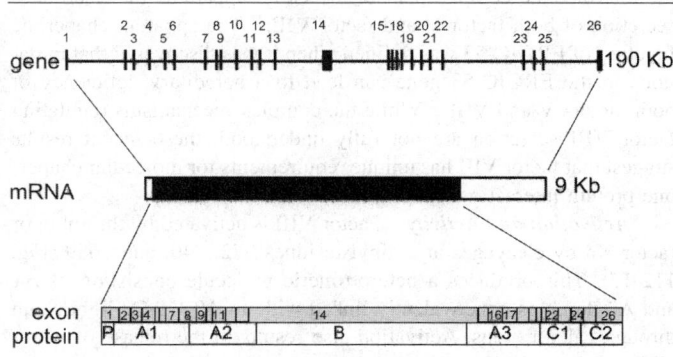

FIGURE 112-16 Relationship between gene structure and protein structure in factor VIII. The exons, introns, mRNA, and protein structure are as indicated. Promoter elements upstream from exon 1 are not shown but are discussed in the text. The mRNA is 9 kb, with some 5′-untranslated sequence and a large 3′-untranslated region. In the protein, P indicates the propeptide leader sequence.

role in stability or activation. B-domainless factor VIII has been used successfully as a therapeutic agent in patients with classic hemophilia.

Factor VIII is synthesized in the liver and is secreted into the plasma as a heterogeneous collection of partially cleaved forms resulting from different cleavages in the B domain. Factor VIII circulates in a noncovalent complex with vWf. The normal half-life of factor VIII is 8 to 12 h when associated with vWf. The half-life is markedly reduced in the absence of vWf, accounting for the reduced factor VIII levels observed in many patients with a deficiency of vWf.

Factor VIII has six tyrosine residues that are modified by sulfation (residues 346, 718, 719, 723, 1664, and 1680). Sulfation of these residues is required for optimal activation by thrombin, maximal activity in complex with factor IXa, and maximal affinity for vWf.

The acidic regions of factor VIII appear to promote activation by interacting with the anion-binding exosite of thrombin. In addition, the site for factor VIII binding to vWF is in the acidic domain in the light chain of factor VIII.[68]

Molecular Biology　The factor VIII gene is on the X chromosome at q28. Deficiency of factor VIII results in classic sex-linked hemophilia A. The factor VIII gene contains 26 exons (see Fig. 112-16), one more than factor V. Exon 5 of factor V corresponds to exons 5 and 6 of the factor VIII gene.[69] The gene for factor VIII is much larger than that for factor V, spanning about 190 kb. This is largely because six of the introns in the factor VIII gene are much larger than the corresponding introns in the factor V gene. The mRNA for factor VIII is also much larger than that for factor V because of a 1.8-kb 3′-untranslated region in the factor VIII message.

Attempts to produce factor VIII in cell culture for therapeutic use have recently led to advances in understanding its intracellular processing in the endoplasmic reticulum and Golgi apparatus. Factor VIII is not secreted very efficiently from the cell. Several molecular chaperone proteins have been identified that appear to play a role in regulating transit of the factor VIII protein through secretory and/or degradative pathways. Calnexin and calreticulin are chaperone proteins that preferentially interact with glycoproteins containing monoglycosylated N-linked oligosaccharides. These proteins bind to the heavily glycosylated B domain of factor VIII and enhance both its intracellular degradation and secretion.[70] Factor V associates with calreticulin but not calnexin. Factor VIII, but not factor V, also interacts through its A1 domain with another chaperone protein, immunoglobulin-binding protein (BiP). Association with BiP appears to enhance the stability of factor VIII, but also retards its secretion.[71]

The mannose-binding protein ERGIC-53 is a protein found in the intermediate compartment of the Golgi apparatus that facilitates secretion of both factor V and factor VIII.[72] The apparent chaperone function of ERGIC-53 was defined when it was discovered that mutations in the ERGIC-53 gene can lead to a hereditary deficiency of both factors V and VIII.[73] While the complex mechanisms regulating factor VIII secretion are not fully understood, these recent results suggest that factor VIII has unique requirements for molecular chaperone protein interactions for its intracellular processing.

Activation and Activity　Factor VIII is activated by thrombin or factor Xa by cleavages at arginyl residues 372, 740, and 1689 (Fig. 112-17). This produces a heterotrimeric molecule consisting of A1 and A2 domains noncovalently linked with an A3-C1-C2 light chain through calcium ions. Activation also results in the release of factor VIIIa from vWf. The factor VIIIa molecule is thermodynamically unstable, and dissociation of the A2 domain results in the spontaneous loss of activity. Factor VIIIa is also inactivated by thrombin or activated protein C (aPC) through additional cleavages at arginyl residues 336 and 562 (see Fig. 112-17).

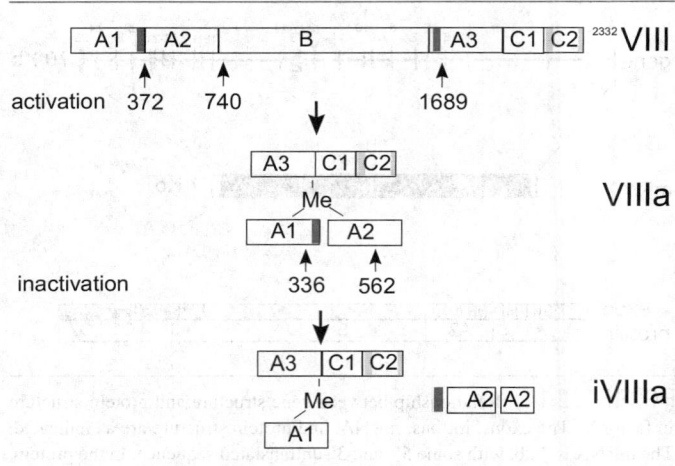

FIGURE 112-17　Activation and inactivation of factor VIII. For full cofactor activity, factor VIII requires cleavage by thrombin or factor Xa. The acidic domains, shown in dark blue, are believed to bind to the anion-binding exosite in thrombin and enhance thrombin activation of factor VIII. The acidic region in the A3 domain mediates vWf binding. The chains of factor VIIIa are held together by noncovalent interactions mediated by metal ions (Me). Factor VIIIa is thermodynamically unstable because the A2 domain can spontaneously dissociate from the complex. Membrane binding is mediated through sites in the C2 domain (shown in light blue). Cleavages at residues 336 and 562 inactivate factor VIIIa, releasing the A2 fragments (iVIIIa).

VON WILLEBRAND FACTOR

The structure, molecular biology, and activities of vWf are discussed in greater detail in Chap. 135.

Protein Structure and Activity　von Willebrand factor is a large multimeric glycoprotein that serves as a carrier for factor VIII and is required for normal platelet adhesion to components of the vessel wall. It is synthesized as a prepropolypeptide with a 22 amino acid signal sequence, a 741 amino acid precursor polypeptide called vWf antigen II, and the mature vWf polypeptide chain.[74] The mature vWf protein contains three A domains, three B domains, two C domains, and four D domains. The A domains are structurally homologous to a family of proteins involved in extracellular matrix or cell adhesive functions.[75] Factor VIII binds to the amino-terminal region of vWf, within the first 272 amino acids of the mature protein subunit.[76]

In the endoplasmic reticulum, the pro-vWf monomers form disulfide-stabilized dimers. The dimers move to the Golgi apparatus, where they assemble into high-molecular-weight multimers, which are also held together by disulfide bonds. The propeptide is essential for multimerization to occur. It is usually removed before secretion of the mature vWf multimers. The circulating vWf multimers range in size from M_r of approximately 500,000 to over 20,000,000.[77] The higher-molecular-weight multimers are most effective in promoting platelet adhesion. However, all multimers can bind factor VIII and enhance its stability. The plasma half-life of vWF is about 12 h.

Molecular Biology　The vWF gene is located on chromosome 12 and spans about 180 kb. It contains 52 exons.[78] von Willebrand factor is synthesized only in endothelial cells and megakaryocytes, but how tissue-specific expression is regulated is not known.

FACTOR XI AND THE CONTACT FACTORS

FACTOR XI

Protein Structure　Factor XI, along with factor XII, high-molecular-weight kininogen (HK), and prekallikrein (PK), are sometimes

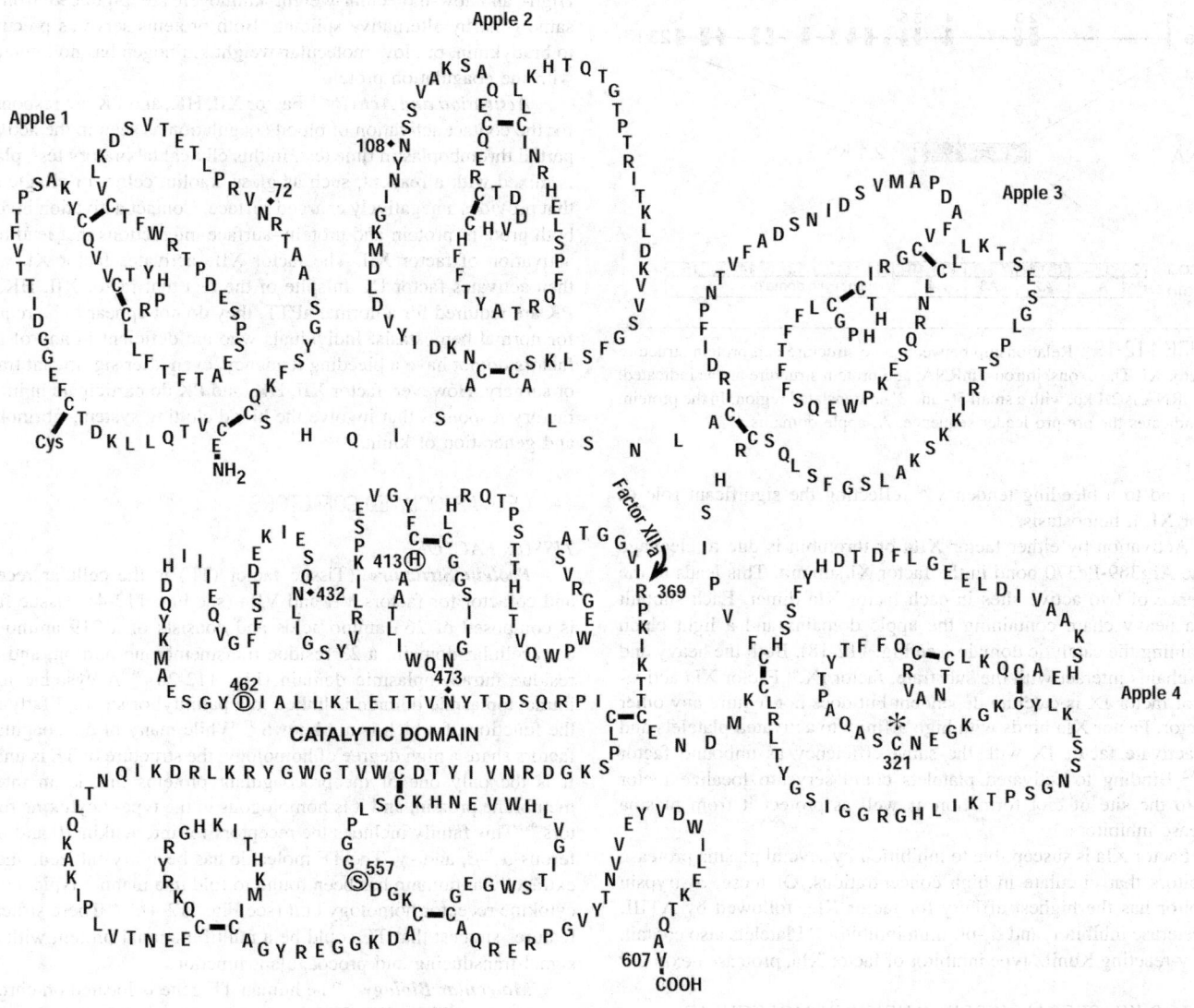

FIGURE 112-18   Domains of factor XI monomer. Each amino acid in circulating factor XI is shown. The apple 1 through 4 domains are named for their appearance in this scheme. The disulfide bond that links the factor XI homodimers is indicated by the Cys residue in the first apple domain. Cys321 in the apple 4 domain is also needed for dimerization. The active-site His, Asp, and Ser residues are circled. The cleavage site for factor XIIa is shown by the arrow.

referred to as the contact factors. Factor XI is a zymogen precursor of a serine protease. Factor XI circulates in complex with the nonenzymatic cofactor HK.

Factor XI is synthesized in the liver and has a plasma mean half-life of 52 h.[79] Although synthesized as a single chain, it circulates as a homodimer held together by a disulfide bond.[80] Each subunit has a M_r of approximately 80,000, including about 5 percent carbohydrate. Each factor XI subunit contains four repeats of a structural motif called an apple domain, as shown in Fig. 112-18. Each apple domain contains 90 or 91 amino acids held together by three disulfide bonds. Specific functions have been assigned to the different apple domains within factor XI,[81–84] including sites for binding to HK, prothrombin, platelets, factor IX, thrombin, and factor XIIa.

Molecular Biology   The human factor XI gene is 23 kb in length and is localized to chromosome 4q32–35.[85] It consists of 15 exons and 14 introns (Fig. 112-19).[86] The transcription initiation site has not

yet been determined. Exon 1 encodes a 5′-untranslated region that is transcribed into mRNA but not translated into protein. The signal peptide is encoded in exon 2. Each of the four apple domains is encoded in two exons. The light chain is encoded in five exons, with an organization similar to that of the homologous proteins PK, tissue plasminogen activator, urokinase, and factor XII.

Activation and Activity   Factor XI can be activated by more than one mechanism in vitro. There is some controversy as to the mechanism of factor XI activation in vivo. In vitro, factor XI can be activated by factor XIIa. In the fluid phase and on charged surfaces, thrombin can activate factor XI even in the absence of the other contact factors.[87,88] Factor XI can also be activated by thrombin on the surface of activated platelets, and this pathway is perhaps the most likely mechanism of activation in vivo.[89] It seems possible that more than one mechanism operates under certain circumstances, but definitive proof is lacking.

In contrast to the other contact factors, deficiencies of factor XI

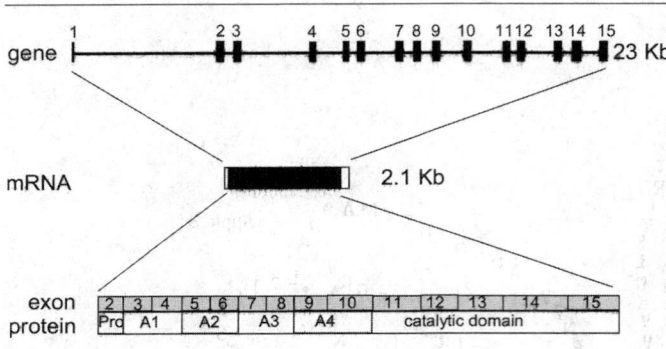

FIGURE 112-19   Relationship between gene structure and protein structure in factor XI. The exons, introns, mRNA, and protein structure are as indicated. The mRNA is 2.1 kb, with a small 5'- and 3'-untranslated region. In the protein, Pro indicates the pre-pro leader sequence. A, apple domains.

may lead to a bleeding tendency,[90] reflecting the significant role of factor XI in hemostasis.

Activation by either factor XIIa or thrombin is due to cleavage of the Arg369-Ile370 bond in the factor XI subunit. This leads to the presence of two active sites in each factor XIa dimer. Each subunit has a heavy chain containing the apple domains and a light chain containing the catalytic domain (see Fig. 112-18). Both the heavy and light chains interact with the substrate, factor IX.[91] Factor XIa activation of factor IX is calcium dependent but does not require any other cofactor. Factor XIa binds with high affinity to activated platelets and can activate factor IX with the same efficiency as unbound factor XIa.[92] Binding to activated platelets could serve to localize factor XIa to the site of clot formation as well as protect it from plasma protease inhibitors.

Factor XIa is susceptible to inhibition by several plasma protease inhibitors that circulate in high concentrations. Of these, α_1-trypsin inhibitor has the highest affinity for factor XIa, followed by ATIII, C1-esterase inhibitor, and α_2-plasmin inhibitor.[93] Platelets also contain a slow-reacting Kunitz-type inhibitor of factor XIa, protease nexin 2.[94]

FACTOR XII, PREKALLIKREIN, AND HIGH-MOLECULAR-WEIGHT KININOGEN

Protein Structure   Factor XII and PK are zymogen precursors of proteases. Prekallikrein has four apple domains and is highly homologous to factor XI. Factor XII is homologous to plasminogen activators. High-molecular-weight kininogen (HK) is a nonenzymatic cofactor that circulates in complex with factor XI and with PK. In addition to its nonenzymatic role in contact activation, HK acts as a thiol protease inhibitor and as an anti-adhesive protein. High-molecular-weight kininogen is cleaved at two sites by kallikrein to release the bioactive nonapeptide bradykinin, a potent vasodilator. The plasma levels, plasma half-lives, and chromosomal locations of factor XII, PK, and HK are shown in Table 112-1.[95] All three proteins are synthesized in the liver.

Molecular Biology   The gene for factor XII is located on chromosome 5q33–qter and spans about 12 kb. It contains 14 exons. The intron–exon structure of the gene is similar to that of the plasminogen activator family of serine proteases. Portions of the gene are homologous to domains found in fibronectin and tissue-type plasminogen activator. The gene for PK is located on chromosome 4q35, close to the factor XI gene. The precise gene structure of the human PK gene has not yet been determined. The rat PK gene spans 22 kb, has 15 exons, and is homologous to the human factor XI gene. The gene for HK is located on chromosome 3, contains 11 exons, and spans 27 kb.

High- and low-molecular-weight kininogen are produced from the same gene by alternative splicing. Both proteins serve as precursors to bradykinin, but low-molecular-weight kininogen has no interaction with the coagulation proteins.

Activation and Activity   Factor XII, HK, and PK are responsible for the contact activation of blood coagulation as seen in the activated partial thromboplastin time test. In this clinical laboratory test, plasma is mixed with a reagent, such as glass, kaolin, celite, or ellagic acid, that provides a negatively charged surface. Contact activation involves both protein–protein and protein–surface interactions that lead to the activation of factor XII. The factor XIIa activates factor XI, which then activates factor IX. In spite of the fact that factor XII, HK, and PK are required for a normal aPTT, they do not appear to be required for normal hemostasis. Individuals who are deficient in any of these factors do not have a bleeding tendency, even after significant trauma or surgery. However, factor XII, HK, and PK do participate in inflammatory responses that involve the blood clotting system, fibrinolysis, and generation of kinins.

CELL-ASSOCIATED COFACTORS

TISSUE FACTOR

Protein Structure   Tissue factor (TF) is the cellular receptor and cofactor for factors VII and VIIa (see Fig. 112-4). Tissue factor is composed of 263 amino acids and consists of a 219 amino acid extracellular domain, a 23 residue transmembrane portion, and a 21 residue intracytoplasmic domain (Fig. 112-20).[96] A cysteine in the intracytoplasmic domain is linked to a palmityl or stearoyl fatty acid, the function of which is not known.[97] While many of the coagulation factors share a high degree of homology, the structure of TF is unique. It is the only one of the procoagulant proteins that is an integral membrane protein, and it is homologous to the type-2 cytokine receptors.[98] This family includes the receptors for interleukin-10 and interferons-α, -β, and -γ. The TF molecule has been crystallized, and the extracellular domain has been found to fold in a manner typical of the cytokine receptor homology unit (see Fig. 112-4).[13,99] These structural features suggest that TF could be a multifunctional protein with both signal-transducing and procoagulant functions.

Molecular Biology   The human TF gene is located on chromosome 1p21–p22.[100] The DNA sequence of the TF gene has been determined and consists of 6 exons and 5 introns that span about 13 kb.[101] The first exon codes for the signal peptide, whereas the second through fifth encode the extracellular domain. The sixth exon codes

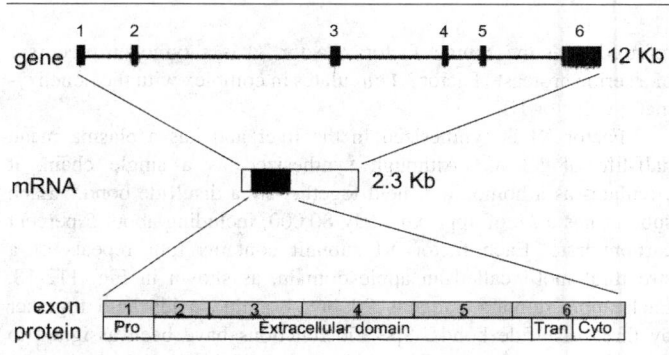

FIGURE 112-20   Relationship between gene structure and protein structure in TF. The exons, introns, mRNA, and protein structure are as indicated. The mRNA is 2.3 kb, with a 5'-untranslated region and a large 3'-untranslated region. Cyto, cytoplasmic domain; Pro, pre-pro leader sequence; Tran, transmembrane region.

for the transmembrane and cytoplasmic domains, as well as a relatively long 3'-untranslated region.

The initiation site for transcription of the TF gene has been well defined, and the region with promoter activity has been found to be from −383 to −121 bp relative to the start site.[102] The promoter contains a serum response element with a putative binding site for Sp-1, and a lipopolysaccharide-responsive element with AP-1 and NF-κB-like sites.

Tissue factor is expressed constitutively on many extravascular tissues. While TF is not normally expressed by cells in contact with flowing blood, TF expression can be induced on blood monocytes and vascular endothelial cells by bacterial products, inflammatory cytokines, and engagement of P-selectin glycoprotein ligand-1 on monocytes.[103–106] Expression of intravascular TF may contribute to the procoagulant state associated with inflammation or infection.

Activation and Activity   The factor VIIa/TF complex is thought to be the major physiologic initiator of blood coagulation. Tissue factor is normally expressed in the adventitia of blood vessels and by epidermal, stromal, and glial cells.[107,108] It has also been shown that leukocytes, which normally have no TF activity, can express TF when exposed to vessel media or collagen.[109] The process of coagulation is initiated when an injury ruptures a vessel and allows blood to come into contact with extravascular TF. When circulating factor VII binds to TF, it is rapidly converted to the active protease, factor VIIa.[43] The factor VIIa/TF complex can activate both factor IX and factor X.[110]

The binding of factor VIIa to TF enhances its proteolytic activity by almost three orders of magnitude.[111,112] However, unlike binding of factor IXa or Xa to their cofactors, binding of factor VIIa to TF does not strictly require calcium,[113] and the affinity of the interaction is only slightly enhanced by the presence of anionic phospholipid.[114,115] However, the cleavage of factor IX or X by factor VIIa/TF is enhanced by anionic phospholipid.[115] This effect is due to the enhanced binding of the substrate rather than to any effect of the phospholipid on the catalytic efficiency of the VIIa/TF complex.

Reported K_d values for factor VIIa binding to TF on cells range from approximately 20 to 80 p*M*. This broad range of values may reflect the effects of the local cellular environment on the affinity of TF for factor VIIa. Binding of factor VIIa to TF that is reconstituted into synthetic phospholipid vesicles always results in enhanced factor VIIa proteolytic activity. However, binding of factor VIIa to cellular sources of TF does not always correlate with enhanced enzymatic activity. This suggests that cells can regulate the cofactor activity of TF in a manner that is not reproduced by synthetic phospholipid vesicles.

Tissue factor does not require proteolytic activation to express its activity. However, it appears that TF can occur in a latent, or "encrypted," form[116,117]; that is, TF detected as antigen on the cell surface may not express cofactor activity. It has been hypothesized that the TF could form dimers that block access to the substrate binding site on TF. Dimerized ("encrypted") TF could still bind factor VII but would be inactive because it could not bind factor IX or X. The physiologic regulators that control TF encryption are not clear, and it remains to be determined whether this is an important regulatory mechanism in vivo.

THROMBOMODULIN

Protein Structure   Thrombomodulin is a transmembrane protein of M_r 78,000.[118] It is the cellular cofactor for thrombin.[119] Thrombomodulin has a leader sequence followed by lectinlike domains homologous to the asialoglycoprotein receptor (Fig. 112-21).[120] However, TM has no known lectinlike activity. Following the lectinlike domain are six EGF-like domains, the fourth, fifth, and sixth of which are responsible for both thrombin-binding and protein-C–activating activities (see Fig. 112-21).[121] A serine- and threonine-rich region follows the EGF

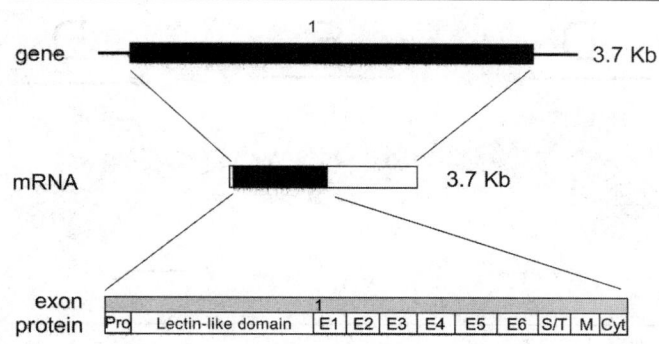

FIGURE 112-21   Relationship between gene structure and protein structure in TM. The TM gene has no introns. It covers 3.7 kb on chromosome 20 (p12–centromere). The mRNA is the same size, with a small 5'-untranslated region and a large 3'-untranslated region. In the protein, Pro indicates the pre-pro leader sequence. Cyt, cytoplasmic domain; E, EGF-like domains; M, transmembrane region; S/T, serine-, threonine-rich region.

domains and is the site of O-linked glycosylation. A chondroitin sulfate moiety, which enhances TM anticoagulant activity, is attached to Ser492 in this region.[122] The 23 amino acid transmembrane domain follows the serine- and threonine-rich region, followed by a short cytoplasmic tail.

Molecular Biology   The human TM gene is located on chromosome 20p12–cen[123] and spans about 3.5 kb. It consists of a single exon (see Fig. 112-21). Intronless genes are uncommon and include rhodopsin, angiogenin, mitochondrial genes, interferons-α and -β, and β-adrenergic receptors. The functional significance of the lack of introns is not known.

Activation and Activity   Thrombin can cleave a number of substrates without a cofactor, such as fibrinogen, factors V and VIII, and the proteolytically activated thrombin receptors. However, binding to the cofactor TM localizes thrombin to endothelial cell surfaces and induces a conformational change such that its ability to activate protein C is enhanced 1000- to 2000-fold. Thrombin bound to TM no longer activates platelets, nor does it cleave fibrinogen or activate factor V or factor VIII.[124] Thus, TM changes the activity of thrombin from procoagulant to anticoagulant. Thrombomodulin also enhances the ability of thrombin to activate the thrombin-activatable inhibitor of fibrinolysis (TAFI)[24]

Thrombomodulin is expressed on the surface of vascular endothelial cells and appears to play a major role in preventing thrombosis from occurring on intact endothelium in the microcirculation.[125] Thrombomodulin has also been detected in mesothelial cells,[126] mononuclear phagocytes,[127] squamous epithelium,[128] megakaryocytes, and malignant cells,[25,129] where its function is unknown. The level of TM expression differs among endothelial cells from different sites.[130] Endothelial TM and TF expression are regulated by inflammatory cytokines in a reciprocal fashion. Thus, thrombosis may be favored at sites of inflammation by a concurrent elevation of endothelial TF and depression of endothelial TM.

Protein C inhibitor has recently been shown to be an effective inhibitor of the thrombin–TM complex.[131]

FIBRINOGEN

PROTEIN STRUCTURE

Fibrinogen forms the structural meshwork that consolidates an initial platelet plug into a solid hemostatic clot. The physiologic importance of fibrinogen is underscored by the bleeding diathesis associated with

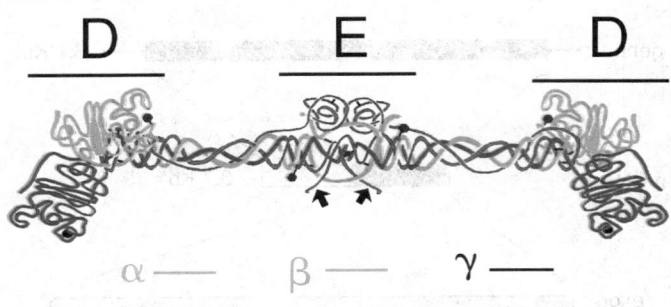

FIGURE 112-22   Structure of fibrinogen. Fibrinogen is a dimer. Each dimer consists of three chains: Aα, shown in gray; Bβ, shown in blue; and γ, shown in black. The disulfides that link the two dimers are in the central E domain. The D domains consist primarily of the carboxyl-terminal regions of the Bβ and γ chains. The helical region connecting the two domains consists of all three chains intertwined.[139]

afibrinogenemia[132,133] and some dysfibrinogenemias[134] (see Chap. 124). Other dysfibrinogenemias are associated with thromboembolic disease.[135]

Fibrinogen is a dimeric glycoprotein whose dominant form has a M_r of 340,000. It is found in plasma and in platelet α-granules. Each of the two subunits contains three disulfide-linked polypeptide chains[136] that are referred to as the Aα (M_r 66,500), Bβ (M_r 52,000), and γ (M_r 46,500) chains. Fibrinopeptides A and B are released from the amino termini of the Aα and Bβ chains by thrombin cleavage of the Arg16-Gly17 and Arg14-Gly15 bonds, respectively.[137] The central globular domain of fibrinogen is called the E domain. It includes the disulfide-linked amino termini of all six polypeptide chains, referred to as the N-terminal disulfide knot.[138] The E domain is linked by helical, coiled-coil domains to the carboxyl-terminal globular domains of the three chains, designated the D domains. A trinodular model of fibrinogen structure has been proposed based on its electron microscopic appearance (Fig. 112-22). N-linked glycosylation occurs at Asn364 of the Bβ chain and Asn52 of the γ chain.

In normal individuals the plasma half-life of fibrinogen is 3 to 5 days,[140] with only a small proportion of the catabolism due to consumption. Plasma fibrinogen is synthesized in the liver. Fibrinogen is an acute-phase reactant, and its synthesis can be increased up to 20-fold with a strong inflammatory stimulus.[141,142] Interleukin-6 (IL-6) is an important mediator of increased fibrinogen synthesis during an acute-phase response,[143] and IL-6 secretion can be upregulated by fibrin- or fibrinogen-degradation products.

MOLECULAR BIOLOGY

The genes for the three chains of fibrinogen are found within a 50-kb length of DNA on chromosome 4 at q23–q32 (Fig. 112-23);[144] have all been sequenced. The genomic sequences show a high degree of homology, suggesting they were derived through duplication of a common ancestral gene.[145,146] The homology extends to sites upstream of the gene, suggesting that common regulatory elements may reside in these areas, thus helping to coordinate synthesis of the three chains.[147]

Studies of tissue-specific expression and acute-phase regulation of the mRNA of the fibrinogen chains have revealed some surprises. The expression of the γ chain is regulated by ubiquitous factors, such as SP1, while transcription of the Aα and Bβ genes requires the liver-specific factor HNF-1.[148] The Bβ-chain promoter contains an IL-6 responsive element that appears to be present in the upstream sequences of the other chains as well.[149] Because of the differences in the promoter regions of the genes for the three chains, the tissue distribution differs. The highest levels of mRNA for all three chains are found in the liver. However, γ-chain transcripts have been found in a number of organs that lack transcripts of the other chains. Messenger RNA for Aα and Bβ has been found in the kidney, consistent with the presence of HNF-1 in kidney.[150]

Because of the presence of fibrinogen in the alpha granules of platelets, it was initially assumed that megakaryocytes synthesized fibrinogen. However, while some γ-chain transcripts are present in marrow precursors, it appears that most of the fibrinogen found within platelets is taken up from the plasma by endocytosis (see Chap. 111).[151,152]

ACTIVATION AND ACTIVITY

Thrombin binds to the central domain of fibrinogen and proteolytically releases two fibrinopeptides A (Aα 1–16) and two fibrinopeptides B (Bβ 1–14) from each fibrinogen molecule.[153] Release of the fibrinopeptides exposes binding sites in the E domain that have complementary sites in the D domains of other fibrin monomers.[154,155] These complementary binding sites lead to the initial formation of two-stranded protofibrils with a half-staggered overlap configuration (Fig. 112-24). Protofibrils then aggregate into thick fibers consisting of 14 to 22 protofibrils that branch into a meshwork of interconnected thick fibers.[156] The half-staggered overlap of the fibrin monomers gives a characteristic cross-banded pattern on electron micrographs.[157] Calcium appears to enhance lateral fiber growth by binding to sites on human fibrinogen.[158,159]

During fibrin monomer polymerization, other plasma proteins also bind to the surface of the developing meshwork. These include elements of the fibrinolytic system and a variety of adhesive proteins, including fibronectin, thrombospondin, and vWf. These surface proteins influence the generation, cross-linking, and lysis of fibrin. Fibrin or fibrinogen also has specific integrin-binding sites that are essential for platelet binding (for additional details see Chap. 111). The thrombin that initiates fibrin polymerization also activates factor XIII, which stabilizes the fibrin polymer by cross-linking. Factor XIIIa also cross-links other bound proteins, such as plasminogen activator-1, vitronectin, fibronectin, and α₂-antiplasmin, to the fibrin network.

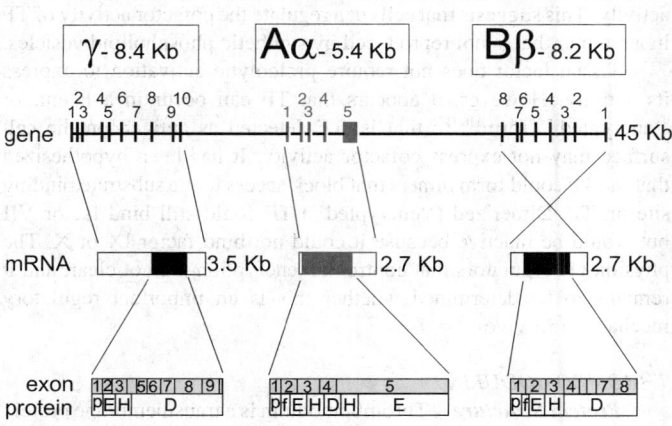

FIGURE 112-23   Relationship between gene structure and protein structure in fibrinogen. The exons, introns, mRNA, and protein structure for the three chains of fibrinogen are shown. The Bβ chain is translated in the opposite direction from the Aα and γ chains. In the proteins, P designates the pre-pro leader sequence. D, residues in the D domain; E, residues in the E domain; H, residues in the helical connecting region; f, fibrinopeptide residues.

Once formed, the fibrin mesh can be degraded by the fibrinolytic system. Plasmin cleaves fibrin and fibrinogen in an ordered sequence at arginyl and lysyl bonds, giving rise to a series of soluble degradation products.[160] The plasmin digestion of fibrinogen initially cleaves the $A\alpha$ polar appendage and the $B\beta$ 1–42 fragment, generating fragment X (M_r 250,000), which can still form a clot, albeit slowly. Further action of plasmin releases a D fragment (M_r 100,000) from fragment X to form fragment Y (M_r 150,000). Fragment Y is further cleaved to form another fragment D and a fragment E (M_r 50,000). Similar fragments are generated during plasmin digestion of cross-linked fibrin, with two exceptions: (1) the $B\beta$ 15–42 is released from the des 1–14 $B\beta$ chain of fibrin, and (2) D-dimer and other covalently cross-linked degradation products are cleaved from the cross-linked fibrin polymer. Monoclonal antibodies recognizing the fibrin D-dimer fragments can help to discriminate fibrin degradation products from fibrinogen degradation products.[161]

Although the large X fragment can still polymerize into a weak clot,[162] the smaller Y and D fragments inhibit normal fibrin monomer polymerization.[163] The inhibition of polymerization can prolong the thrombin time and lead to spuriously low values of fibrinogen when measured in clotting assays.

FACTOR XIII

PROTEIN STRUCTURE

Factor XIII is a 320,000 M_r glycoprotein composed of A and B subunits with a plasma half-life of about 10 days. It is a protransglutaminase that is activated by thrombin in the presence of calcium.[164] The A chain contains the cysteine-active site, while the B chain is not enzymatically active and functions as a carrier protein. The cDNA and protein sequences of both subunits have been determined.[165–167]

The factor XIII A chain is a unique member of the transglutaminase family, which is composed of calcium- and thiol-dependent enzymes found in all human tissues and fluids. Factor XIIIa cross-links proteins between the γ-carbon of glutamine in one protein and the ε amino group of lysine in the other. The A chain contains 731 amino acids and has a M_r of approximately 83,000 (Fig. 112-25). There is no typical signal sequence to direct secretion, and thus the mechanism of secretion of the A chain is not known.

The B chain is homologous to complement-regulatory proteins. It is synthesized as a chain of 661 amino acids starting with a signal peptide. The mature B chain is composed of 641 amino acids[167] and has a M_r of appproximately 76,500, including 8.5 percent carbohydrate. The B chain contains 10 short consensus repeat units (SCR, also called GP-1 or Sushi domains; Fig. 112-26). Each SCR contains 60 to 70 amino acids, containing four conserved cysteine residues with a characteristic pattern of disulfide bonds.[168] Short consensus repeat sequences are found in other complement-related proteins, including factor H; C4-b–binding protein; CR1; decay-accelerating factor; and the complement factors C1r, C1s, C2, factor B, C6, and C7. Short consensus repeat units are also present in the interleukin-2 receptor, endothelial leukocyte adhesion molecule 1, and β_2-glycoprotein 1.

In addition to plasma, factor XIII also is found in platelets, monocytes, and monocyte-derived macrophages. While the plasma factor is a heterotetramer consisting of paired A and B subunits (A2B2), its cellular counterpart lacks the B subunits and is a homodimer of A subunits (A2). Monocytes-macrophages can synthesize factor XIII,[169]

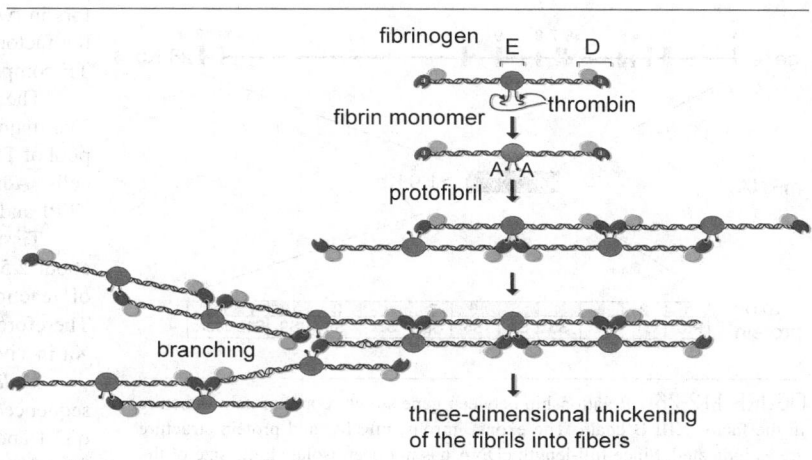

FIGURE 112-24   Cleavage of fibrinogen and polymerization of fibrin. The structure of fibrinogen is indicated schematically. Cleavage sites for fibrinopeptide A by thrombin are shown. Cleavage of the B peptide is not shown in this figure. Release of fibrinopeptide A exposes binding sites in the E domain that match complementary sites in the D domain. Fibrin monomers polymerize by half-staggered overlaps. Polymerization can also lead to branched structures.[139]

and the factor XIII found in platelets is probably synthesized by megakaryocytes.[170] Cells of marrow origin seem to be the primary site for the synthesis of subunit A in plasma factor XIII, but hepatocytes might also contribute.[164] The B subunit of plasma factor XIII is synthesized in the liver.

MOLECULAR BIOLOGY

The factor XIII A-chain gene has been localized to chromosome 6 p24–p25.[171] It contains 15 exons and 14 introns and is over 160 kb in size (see Fig. 112-25).[166] The fibrin-binding domain is encoded by exons 2 thorugh 12. The active site, with its reactive thiol at Cys314, is present in exon 7. The structure of the factor XIII A-chain gene is quite similar to that of other transglutaminases. The transcription initiation site for the A chain is unknown, but three potential sites have been described, at −170, −150, and −40 relative to the inital methionine.[166]

The factor XIII B chain has been localized to chromosome 1q31– q32.1. It has 12 exons separated by 11 introns and is about 28 kb in

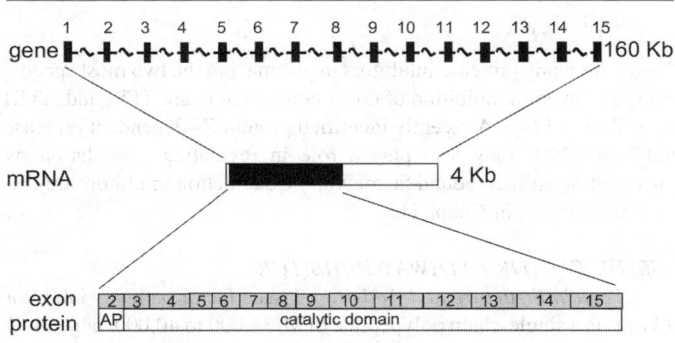

FIGURE 112-25   Relationship between gene structure and protein structure in the factor XIII A chain. The exons, mRNA, and protein structure for the factor XIII A chain are shown. The size of the introns in the factor XIII A chain has not been published. The mRNA is 4 kb, with some 5′-untranslated sequence coded in exon 1 and a large 3′-untranslated region. In the protein, AP indicates the activation peptide.

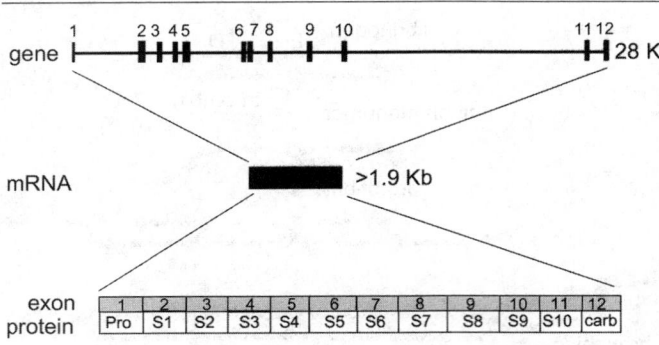

FIGURE 112-26   Relationship between gene structure and protein structure in the factor XIII B chain. The exons, introns, mRNA, and protein structure are as indicated. Since full-length cDNA has not been isolated, the size of the mRNA is not known. In the protein, Pro indicates the propeptide. Carb; carboxyl-terminal region; S, Sushi (SCR) domains.

size (see Fig. 112-26).[172] Each SCR is encoded by a single exon. The regulation of the factor XIII B-chain expression is poorly understood. A total of 30 potential start sites are located upstream of the initial methionine.

ACTIVATION AND ACTIVITY

Plasma factor XIII circulates in association with its substrate, fibrinogen. The key step in the activation of plasma factor XIII is thrombin cleavage of the Arg37-Gly38 bond in the A chain to release a M_r 4500 activation peptide. This leads to dissociation of the A and B subunits and exposure of the active site on the free A subunits. Cellular factor XIII in platelets becomes activated through a nonproteolytic process. When intracytoplasmic Ca^{2+} is elevated during platelet activation, the zymogen, in the absence of the B chain, becomes an active configuration.[164] The main physiological function of plasma factor XIIIa is to cross-link the α and γ chains of fibrin to stabilize the fibrin plug. In the absence of factor XIII, a clot forms, but it is inadequate for hemostasis. Additional protein substrates of factor XIIIa include components of the clotting and fibrinolytic system, as well as multiple adhesive and contractile proteins. Factor XIIIa also protects fibrin from fibrinolysis by cross-linking it to α_2-antiplasmin. Plasma factor XIII is also involved in wound healing and tissue repair, and is essential for maintaining pregnancy.

INHIBITORS

There are many protease inhibitors in plasma, but the two most specifically involved in inhibition of coagulation factors are TFPI and ATIII (see Table 112-4). A recently identified protein-Z–dependent protease inhibitor (PZI) may also play a role in regulating coagulation by inactivating surface-bound factor Xa.[173] Coagulation inhibitors are discussed in detail in Chap. 113.

TISSUE FACTOR PATHWAY INHIBITOR

Protein Structure and Activity   Tissue factor pathway inhibitor (TFPI) is a single-chain polypeptide of M_r 34,000 to 40,000, depending upon the degree of proteolysis of the carboxyl-terminal region. Tissue factor pathway inhibitor contains three Kunitz-type protease inhibitor domains. The second Kunitz domain binds and inhibits factor Xa, and this interaction is required for the first Kunitz domain to bind and inhibit the factor VIIa/TF complex. The function of the third Kunitz domain is not clear, but it may be involved in binding to glycosaminoglycans. Thus, TFPI is unique among the coagulation protease inhibi-

tors in two respects: (1) It has inhibitory sites for both factor Xa and the factor VIIa/TF complex, and (2) it cannot inhibit the factor VIIa/TF complex unless it has also bound factor Xa.[174,175]

The primary site of plasma TFPI synthesis is endothelial cells.[176] The majority of circulating TFPI is bound to lipoproteins. A second pool of TFPI is bound to heparian sulfates on the surface of endothelial cells. Administration of heparin releases the endothelial-cell–bound TFPI and raises the plasma level severalfold.[177]

Tissue factor pathway inhibitor is only present in the plasma at about 2.5 nM, compared to ATIII, at about 2 μM. However, its rate of reaction with factor Xa in plasma is similar to that of ATIII. Therefore, TFPI contributes significantly to the inhibition of factor Xa in vivo.

Molecular Biology   The gene for TFPI has not been completely sequenced. However, it is known to be located on chromosome 2q31–q32.1 and has nine exons that span 70 kb.[178] The first two exons code for a 5′-untranslated region. No TATA box is present in the promoter region of the TFPI gene. DNA sequences that are consistent with binding sites for the transcription factors GATA-2, AP-1, and NF-1 are present in the 5′-untranslated region of the TFPI gene. It is thought that GATA-2 binding is necessary for constitutive expression of TFPI by endothelial cells.[176]

An alternatively spliced form of TFPI has also been described. This form, TFPI-β, lacks the third Kunitz domain and instead has a unique carboxyl terminal of unknown function. It is found in plasma and has inhibitory activity similar to that of full-length TFPI.[179]

ANTITHROMBIN III

Protein Structure and Activity   Antithrombin III (ATIII) is a member of the large family of serine protease inhibitors (serpins). These inhibitors act as "suicide" substrates for their target proteases through a surface-exposed structure termed a reactive site loop. An amino acid sequence in the reactive site loop is recognized by the target protease; it forms a one-to-one complex that blocks the active site of the protease. The primary proteases targeted by ATIII are thrombin, factor Xa, and factor IXa, while factor VIIa is resistant to inhibition by ATIII[180–182] unless it is complexed to TF in the presence of heparin. All these reactions are enhanced by heparin (see Table 112-4). While the reaction between ATIII and the serine proteases is reversible, dissociation is probably insignificant under physiological conditions. The protease–serpin complex is cleared from the circulation by receptor-mediated endocytosis in the liver.[183] Antithrombin III is an important physiological inhibitor of the blood coagulation proteases, since its deficiency leads to a significantly increased risk of thrombosis.

Molecular Biology   The gene for ATIII is on the long arm of chromosome 1. The gene has seven exons and spans about 13.5 kb. Little is known about transcriptional regulation of ATIII. The region from −89 to −68 has been implicated in the binding of transcription factors from rat liver,[184] but the specific transcription factors involved are not clear.

PATHWAYS OF HEMOSTASIS

EARLY MODELS OF COAGULATION

In the 1960s two groups proposed a model of coagulation that envisioned a sequential series of steps in which activation of one clotting factor led to the activation of another, finally leading to a burst of thrombin generation.[185,186] Each clotting factor was thought to exist as a proenzyme that could be converted to an active enzyme.

The original cascade models were subsequently modified to include the observation that some procoagulants were cofactors and did

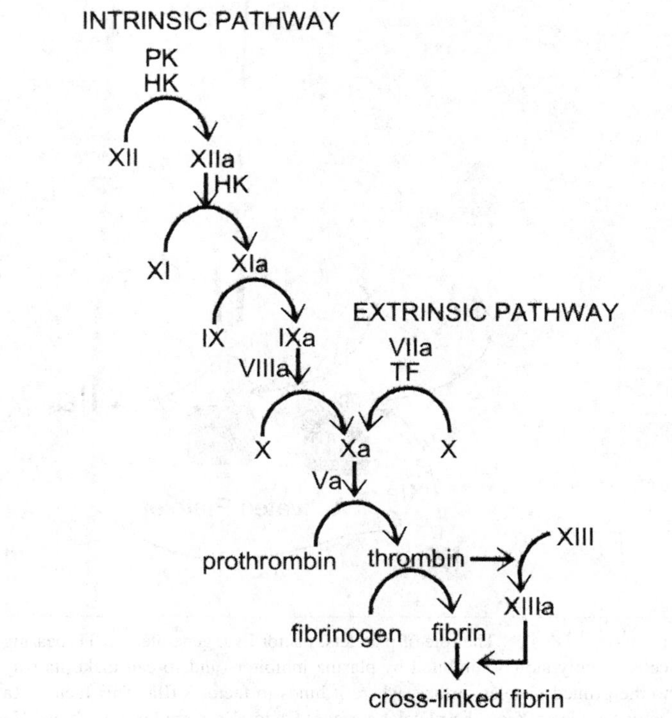

INTRINSIC PATHWAY

```
        PK
        HK
          ↓
   XII → XIIa
          ↓ HK
          ↓
    XI → XIa        EXTRINSIC PATHWAY
          ↓
   IX → IXa      VIIa
 VIIIa ↓          TF
          ↓      ↓  ↓
       X    Xa     X
          Va ↓
          ↓
prothrombin  thrombin →        XIII
          ↓              ↓
fibrinogen   fibrin     XIIIa
                  ↓
          cross-linked fibrin
```

FIGURE 112-27 Cascade model of coagulation. This model shows successive activation of coagulation factors proceeding from the top of the schematic to thrombin generation and fibrin formation at the bottom. The intrinsic and extrinsic pathways are as indicated.

not possess enzymatic activity. In addition, the clotting sequences were divided into so-called extrinsic and intrinsic systems, as shown in Fig. 112-27. The extrinsic system consisted of factor VIIa and TF, the latter being viewed as extrinsic to the circulating blood. The factors in the so-called intrinsic system were all viewed as being intravascular. Both pathways could activate factor X, which, in complex with its cofactor Va, could convert prothrombin to thrombin. While these earlier concepts of coagulation were extremely valuable, several groups recognized that the intrinsic and extrinsic systems could not operate independently of one another and that all the clotting factors were somehow interrelated. Only in this way could hemostasis in vivo be explained.

REVISION OF THE COAGULATION MODELS

Key observations made by several groups have led to a revision of earlier models of coagulation. A major observation was that a complex of factor VIIa/TF activated not only factor X but also factor IX.[110] Other important observations led to the conclusion that the major initiating event in hemostasis in vivo was the formation of a factor VIIa/TF complex at the site of injury.[187–189] This led to the belief that factor VIII and IX deficiencies, which resulted in hemophilia A and B respectively were, in fact, abnormalities of the VIIa/TF pathway, even though factors IX and VIII were considered components of the intrinsic system. It was also recognized that in vivo coagulation was regulated by control mechanisms, one of which was the localization of the coagulation reactions to cell surfaces. In addition, earlier and more recent observations emphasized the importance of plasma inhibitors of each step of the coagulation process. These include TFPI, which inhibits the factor VIIa/TF/Xa complex[175,190]; proteins C and S,

which inactivate factors Va and VIIIa[125,191,192]; and ATIII, which inhibits thrombin and other coagulation proteases.[193]

A CELL-BASED MODEL OF COAGULATION

ROLE OF THE TF-BEARING CELL

The goal of hemostasis is to produce a fibrin clot to seal a site of injury or rupture in the blood vessel wall. This process is initiated when TF-bearing cells are exposed to blood at a site of injury. TF is anchored to cells via a transmembrane domain and acts as a receptor for plasma factor VII. Once bound to TF, zymogen factor VII is rapidly converted to factor VIIa through mechanisms not yet completely understood. The resulting factor VIIa/TF complex, localized by cells to the site of injury, catalyzes two very important reactions: (1) activation of factor X to factor Xa, and (2) activation of factor IX to IXa. The factors Xa and IXa formed on the TF-bearing cells have very distinct and separate functions in the process of blood coagulation.

The factor Xa formed on the TF-bearing cell interacts with its cofactor Va to form a prothrombinase complex sufficient to generate a very small amount of thrombin in the vicinity of the TF cells (Fig. 112-28). Although this amount of thrombin may not be sufficient to clot fibrinogen, it is sufficient to initiate events that "prime" the clotting system for a subsequent burst of thrombin generation. Experiments using a cell-based model have shown that minute amounts of thrombin are formed in the milieu of TF-bearing cells exposed to plasma concentrations of procoagulants, even in the absence of platelets. The small amounts of factor Va required for prothrombinase assembly on the TF-bearing cells are activated by factor Xa[45] or by noncoagulation proteases elaborated by the cells.[194] The small amounts of thrombin generated on the TF-bearing cells are capable of accomp-

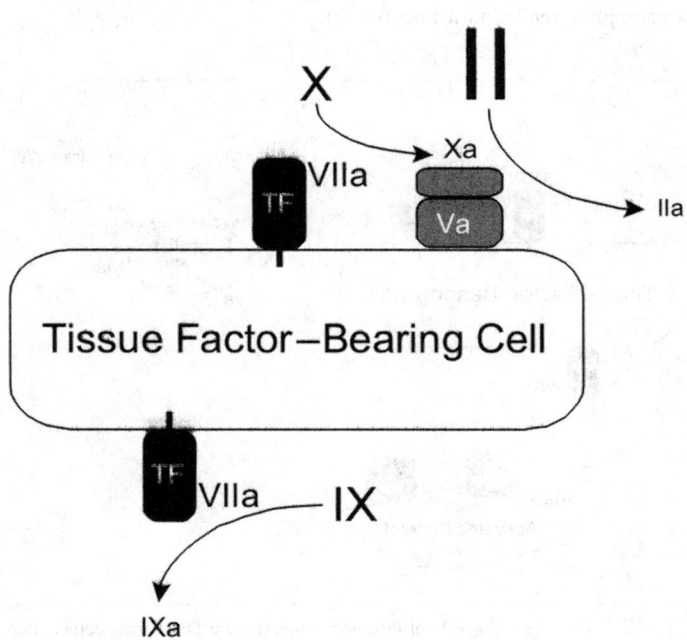

FIGURE 112-28 The role of TF-bearing cells. Factor VIIa bound to TF can activate both factor X and factor IX. Factor Xa and factor IXa activated by factor VIIa/TF play distinct roles in coagulation. Factor Xa is assembled into a prothrombinase complex on the surface of the TF-bearing cell. This generates a small amount of thrombin.

lishing the following[89,195]: (1) activating platelets, (2) activating factor V, (3) activating factor VIII and dissociating factor VIII from vWf, and (4) activating factor XI (Fig. 112-29). The activity of the factor Xa formed by the factor VIIa/TF complex is restricted to the TF-bearing cell. Factor Xa that diffuses off the cell surface is rapidly inhibited by TFPI or ATIII.

Unlike factor Xa, the primary site of activity of the factor IXa formed by factor VIIa/TF is on activated platelets in close proximity to the TF-bearing cell. Factor IXa can diffuse to adjacent cell surfaces because it is not inhibited by TFPI and is inhibited much more slowly by ATIII than is factor Xa (see Table 112-4).

ROLE OF ACTIVATED PLATELETS

Platelets also play a major role in localizing clotting reactions to the site of injury since they adhere and aggregate at the same sites where TF is exposed. Platelet localization and activation are mediated by vWf, thrombin, platelet receptors, and vessel wall components such as collagen (see Chap. 111).

Once platelets are activated, the cofactors Va and VIIIa are rapidly localized to the platelet membrane surface (see Fig. 112-29). Cofactor binding is mediated in part by the exposure of PS on the platelet membrane, a process resulting from a flip-flop mechanism whereby PS on the inner leaflet of the membrane bilayer flips to the outside.[196] In addition, it appears that the cofactors bind to the platelet surface before the binding of the respective enzymes.[197]

The factor IXa formed by the factor VIIa/TF complex binds to the surface of activated platelets (Fig. 112-30). Specific sites on the activated platelets bind factor IXa and promote formation of active factor IXa/VIIIa complexes.[198,199] Once the platelet ''tenase'' complex is assembled, factor X is recruited from the plasma and is activated to factor Xa on the platelet surface. Factor Xa then associates with factor Va on the surface to generate a burst of thrombin sufficient to clot fibrinogen and form a hemostatic plug (see Fig. 112-30). Factor XIII, activated by thrombin, cross-links fibrin and stabilizes the hemostatic plug, rendering it impermeable.

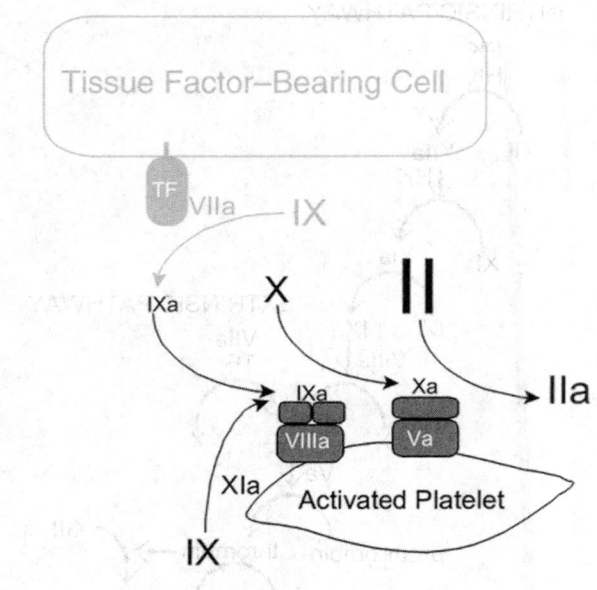

FIGURE 112-30   The role of platelets. Factor IXa, generated on TF-bearing cells, is only slowly inhibited by plasma inhibitors and so can make its way to the primed platelet surface, where it binds to factor VIIIa. This factor IXa activates factor X on the platelet surface. Factor Xa complexes to factor Va and activates prothrombin, leading to the burst of thrombin generation responsible for cleaving fibrinogen. Additional factor IXa is supplied by factor XIa on the platelet surface.

Factor XIa, formed by thrombin activation of the zymogen, also associates with the platelet surface, where it can activate more factor IX to IXa.[89,92] Thus, it appears that factor XIa activation enhances the platelet tenase activity and serves as a ''booster'' mechanism to enhance thrombin generation.

The role of factor XI in hemostasis has been a point of major interest, since even severe factor XI deficiency does not result in a hemorrhagic tendency comparable to that seen in severe factor VIII or IX deficiency. This observation can be explained if factor XI is viewed as an enhancer, or booster, of thrombin generation. In factor VIII and IX deficiency, the individual has a markedly decreased ability to generate factor Xa on the platelet surface. Thus, one would expect that patients with a severe deficiency of either factor VIII or factor IX would generate insufficient thrombin for hemostasis, since the tenase, and hence prothrombinase, activity would be markedly reduced. In contrast, patients with factor XI deficiency would always possess baseline tenase activity. Such patients only lack the ability to boost platelet surface factor X activation by producing extra factor IXa. Without the boost in thrombin generation by factor XI, there may be decreased activation of thrombin activatable fibrinolysis inhibitor (TAFI) resulting in enhanced fibrinolysis that may contribute to the bleeding tendency seen in factor-XI–deficient patients.[200] Even though each step of the model has been depicted as an isolated set of reactions, they should be viewed as an overlapping continuum of events, as illustrated in Fig. 112-31.

ROLE OF ENDOTHELIAL CELLS

Once a fibrin–platelet clot is formed over an area of injury, the clotting process must be terminated to avoid thrombotic occlusion in adjacent normal areas of the vasculature. If the coagulation mechanism were not controlled, clotting could occur throughout the entire vascular tree after even a modest procoagulant stimulus. Endothelial cells play a

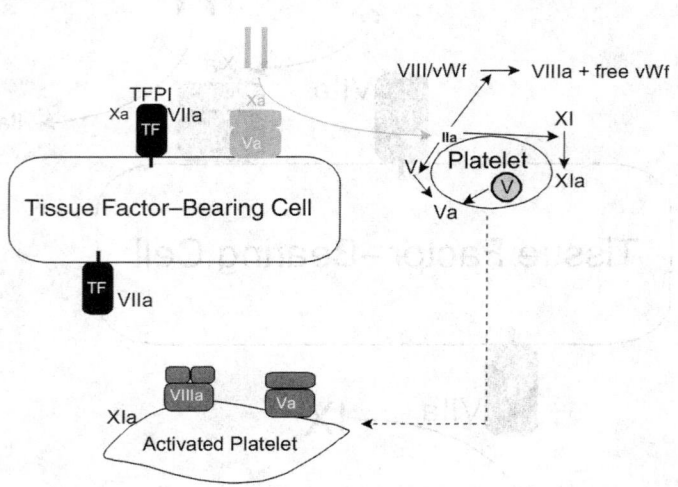

FIGURE 112-29   The role of thrombin generated by TF-bearing cells. After the initial generation of factor Xa on TF-bearing cells, subsequent factor Xa generation is shut down when TFPI reacts with factor Xa to inactivate the factor VIIa/TF complex. The small amount of thrombin generated on the TF-bearing cells plays a critical role in priming platelets for subsequent coagulation steps. This thrombin activates platelets, releases factor V from alpha granules, activates factor V, activates factor VIII and releases it from vWf, and activates factor XI.

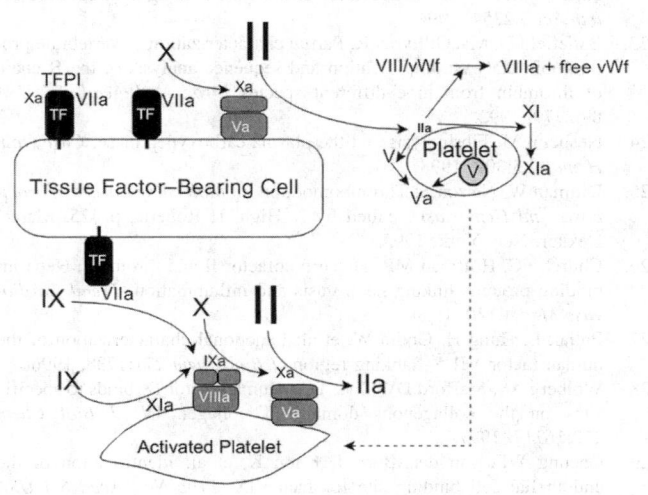

FIGURE 112-31   A cell-based model of hemostasis. The sequence of events shown in previous figures is summarized here.

major role in confining the coagulation reactions to a site of injury and preventing clot extension to areas where an intact endothelium is present (see Chap. 114). Endothelial cells have two major types of anticoagulant-antithrombotic activities as illustrated in Fig. 112-32. The protein C–protein S–TM system is activated in response to thrombin generation. Some of the thrombin formed during the coagulation process can diffuse away or be swept downstream from a site of injury. When thrombin reaches an intact endothelial cell, it binds to TM on the endothelial surface. The thrombin–TM complex then activates protein C, which binds to its cofactor protein S and inactivates any factor Va or VIIIa that finds its way to the adjacent endothelial cell membranes. This prevents the generation of additional thrombin in the vasculature. The endothelial cell also posseses other anticoagulant features. The protease inhibitors ATIII and TFPI are always present, bound to heparan sulfates expressed on the endothelial surface, where they can inactivate proteases near an intact endothelium.[201] Endothelial cells also inhibit platelet activation by releasing the inhibitors prostacyclin and nitric oxide, as well as digesting ADP by their membrane ecto-ADPase, CD39.[202]

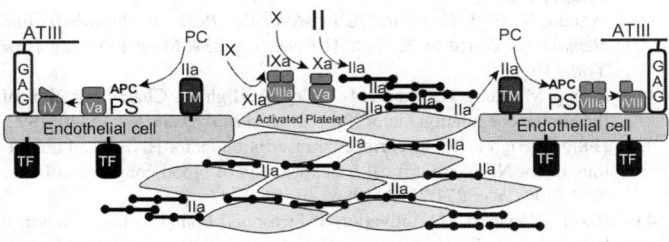

FIGURE 112-32   The role of endothelial cells. Activated coagulation proteins generated on platelets localized to a site of an injury are confined to the site. Activated coagulation factors that move to an endothelial cell surface are rapidly inhibited by ATIII associated with glycosaminoglycans (GAG) on the endothelial surface. Further, thrombin that reaches the endothelial cell surface binds to TM. Once bound, thrombin can no longer cleave fibrinogen. Instead, thrombin activates protein C, leading to the formation of activated protein C (aPC)/protein S (PS) complexes on the endothelial cell, which inactivate factors Va and VIIIa (iV, iVIII).

ROLE OF PLASMA PROTEASE INHIBITORS

Like cell-based coagulation, circulating protease inhibitors are also critical in localizing the coagulation reactions to specific cell surfaces by directly inhibiting proteases that escape into the fluid phase (see Fig. 112-32). Not only are the plasma protease inhibitors key players in confining a clot to the proper location, but they also impose a threshold effect on the coagulation process.[203] Thus, in the presence of inhibitors, coagulation does not proceed unless procoagulant factors are generated in sufficient amounts to overcome the effects of inhibitors. If the triggering event is not sufficiently strong, the system returns to baseline rather than continuing through the coagulation process. Under pathological conditions, the trigger for clotting may be so strong as to overwhelm the control of inhibitors and lead to disseminated intravascular coagulation or thrombosis (see Chap. 126).

ROLE OF FIBRINOLYSIS

Once a hemostatic clot has been formed, some provision must be made for its eventual removal as wound healing takes place. Dissolution of clots is accomplished by the fibrinolytic system, as discussed in detail in Chap. 116.

THE CONCEPT OF BASAL COAGULATION AND ANTICOAGULATION

A low level of basal coagulation factor activation probably occurs at all times.[204] It was shown over 20 years ago that fibrinopeptides are continuously cleaved from fibrinogen at low levels in normal individuals.[205] It has also been shown that there are low levels of circulating factor VIIa and of the activation peptides from factors IX and X in the blood of normal individuals.[206–208] This has been called basal coagulation and may occur as a result of the minor injuries to vessels that occur during normal daily activities or perhaps when the lower-molecular-weight coagulation factors percolate through the extravascular spaces. This process does not lead to clot formation under normal circumstances. The coagulation process only proceeds when enough thrombin is generated on or near the TF-bearing cell to trigger activation of platelets and cofactors. One wonders, however, whether minute hemostatic plugs are not constantly formed throughout the body to maintain the integrity of the vascular tree. This basal coagulation must be balanced by activity of the anticoagulation and fibrinolytic systems. This is evidenced by the presence of low levels of the protein C activation peptide and tissue plasminogen activator activity in normal individuals.[209]

BLOOD COAGULATION AS A PART OF THE HOST DEFENSE MECHANISM

The process of hemostasis is only a small part of the overall host response to injury. While different parts of the host response are presented as though they were truly separate processes, in fact coagulation, fibrinolysis, inflammation, the immune response, and wound healing are interrelated parts of the overall response to injury.

There are many ways in which coagulation factors or byproducts play important roles in the response to injury. One clear example is the multiple roles of thrombin. It acts not only as a procoagulant to clot fibrinogen, but also as a growth factor and cytokine that promotes monocyte, fibroblast, and endothelial cell influx into an area of recent injury and sets the stage for removal of damaged tissue and for wound healing.[26] Platelets also have multiple roles in the response to injury. They release several growth factors and cytokines upon activation, some of which play key roles in wound healing and atherosclerosis. Factor Xa, TF, and fibrinogen fragments, similarly, seem to have roles as inflammatory mediators and cell growth regulators. In addition, the contact factors (factor XII, PK, and HK) may play a role as a bridge between the coagulation reactions and other host defense mechanisms.

No doubt the list of multifunctional molecules will grow as understanding of the blood clotting mechanism increases.

REFERENCES

1. Leytus S, Foster D, Kurachi K, Davie E: Gene for human factor X, a blood coagulation factor whose gene organization is essentially identical with that of factor IX and protein C. *Biochemistry* 25:5098, 1986.
2. Yoshitake S, Schach BG, Foster DC, et al: Nucleotide sequence of the gene for human factor IX (antihemophilic factor B). *Biochemistry* 24:3736, 1985.
3. Jorgensen M, Cantor A, Furie B, et al: Recognition site directing vitamin K–dependent γ-carboxylation residues on the propeptide of factor IX. *Cell* 48:185, 1987.
4. Huber P, Schmitz T, Griffin J, et al: Identification of amino acids in the γ-carboxylation recognition site on the propeptide of prothrombin. *J Biol Chem* 265:12467, 1990.
5. Brenner B, Sanchez-Vega B, Wu SM, et al: A missense mutation in γ-glutamyl carboxylase gene causes combined deficiency of all vitamin K–dependent blood coagulation factors. *Blood* 92:4554, 1998.
6. Soriano-Garcia M, Padmanabhan K, de Vos AM, Tulinsky A: The Ca^{2+} ion and membrane binding structure of the Gla domain of Ca-prothrombin fragment 1. *Biochemistry* 31:2554, 1992.
7. Sunnerhagen M, Forsen S, Hoffren AM, et al: Structure of the Ca(2+)-free Gla domain sheds light on membrane binding of blood coagulation proteins. *Nature Struct Biol* 2:504, 1995.
8. Nelsestuen G, Kisiel W, Di Scipio RG: Interaction of vitamin K–dependent proteins with membranes. *Biochemistry* 17:2134, 1978.
9. Rawal-Sheikh R, Ahmad SS, Ashby B, Walsh PN: Kinetics of coagulation factor X activation by platelet-bound factor IXa. *Biochemistry* 29:2606, 1990.
10. Gilbert GE, Arena AA: Partial activation of the factor VIIIa-factor IXa enzyme complex by dihexanoic phosphatidylserine at submicellar concentrations. *Biochemistry* 36:10768, 1997.
11. Kirchhofer D, Guha A, Nemerson Y, et al: Activation of blood coagulation factor VIIa with cleaved tissue factor extracellular domain and crystallization of the active complex. *Proteins* 22:419, 1995.
12. Muller Y, Ultsch M, de Vos A: The crystal structure of the extracellular domain of human tissue factor refined to 1.7 Å resolution. *J Mol Biol* 256:144, 1996.
13. Banner DW, D'Arcy A, Chene C, et al: The crystal structure of the complex of blood coagulation factor VIIa with soluble tissue factor. *Nature* 380:41, 1996.
14. Brandstetter H, Bauer M, Huber R, et al: X-ray structure of clotting factor IXa: active site and module structure related to Xase activity and hemophilia B. *Proc Natl Acad Sci USA* 92:9796, 1995.
15. Patthy L, Trexler M, Vali Z, et al: Kringles: Modules specialized for protein binding. Homology of the gelatin-binding region of fibronectin with the kringle structure of proteases. *FEBS Lett* 171:131, 1984.
16. Royle N, Irwin D, Koschinsky ML, et al: Human genes encoding prothrombin and ceruloplasmin map to 11p11–q12 and 3q21–24, respectively. *Somat Cell Mol Genet* 13, 1987.
17. Chow BK, Ting V, Tufaro F, MacGillivray R: Characterization of a novel liver-specific enhancer in the human prothrombin gene. *J Biol Chem* 266:18927, 1991.
18. Degen S: The prothrombin gene and its liver-specific expression. *Semin Thromb Hemost* 18:230, 1992.
19. Poort S, Rosendaal F, Reitsina P, Bertina R: A common genetic variant in the 3′-untranslated region of the prothrombin gene is associated with elevated plasma prothrombin levels and an increase in venous thrombosis. *Blood* 88:3698, 1996.
20. Bode W, Mayr I, Baumann U, et al: The refined 1.9 Å crystal structure of human alpha-thrombin: interaction with D-Phe-Pro-Arg chloromethylketone and significance of the Tyr-Pro-Pro-Trp insertion segment. *EMBO J* 8:3467, 1989.
21. Martin PD, Malkowski MG, Box J, et al: New insights into the regulation of the blood clotting cascade derived from the X-ray crystal structure of bovine meizothrombin des F1 in complex with PPACK. *Structure* 5:1681, 1997.
22. Vijayalakshmi J, Padmanabhan KP, Mann KG, Tulinsky A: The isomorphous structures of prethrombin 2, hirugen-, and PPACK-thrombin:

changes accompanying activation and exosite binding to thrombin. *Protein Sci* 3:2254, 1994.
23. Banefield D, MacGillivray R: Partial characterization of vertebrate prothrombin cDNAs: amplification and sequence analysis of the B chain of thrombin from nine different species. *Proc Natl Acad Sci USA* 89:2779, 1992.
24. Nesheim M: Fibrinolysis and the plasma carboxypeptidase. *Curr Opin Hematol* 5:309, 1998.
25. Dittman W, Nelson S: Thrombomodulin, in *Molecular Basis of Thrombosis and Hemostasis,* edited by K High, H Roberts, p 425. Marcel Dekker, New York, 1995.
26. Church FC, Hoffman MR: Heparin cofactor II and thrombin: Heparin-binding proteins linking hemostasis and inflammation. *Trend Cardiovasc Med* 4:140, 1994.
27. Pollak E, Hung H, Godin W, et al: Functional characterization of the human factor VII 5′-flanking region. *J Biol Chem* 271:1738, 1996.
28. Wolberg AS, Stafford DW, Erie DA: Human factor IX binds to specific sites on the collagenous domain of collagen IV. *J Biol Chem* 272:16717, 1997.
29. Cheung WF, van den Born J, Kuhn K, et al: Identification of the endothelial cell binding site for factor IX. *Proc Natl Acad Sci USA* 93:11068, 1996.
30. Camerino G, Grzeschik K, Jaye M, et al: Regional localization on the human X chromosome and polymorphism of the coagulation factor IX gene (hemophilia B locus). *Proc Natl Acad Sci USA* 81:498, 1984.
31. Winship P, Rees D, Alkan M: Detection of polymorphisms at cytosine phosphoguanadine dinucleotides and diagnosis of haemophilia B carriers. *Lancet* 1:631, 1989.
32. High K, Roberts H: Factor IX, in *Molecular Basis of Thrombosis and Hemostasis,* edited by K High, H Roberts, p 215. Marcel Dekker, New York, 1995.
33. Graves B, Johnson P, McKnight S: Homologous recognition of a promoter domain common to the MSV LTR and the HSV tk gene. *Cell* 44:565, 1986.
34. Mueller C, Maire P, Schibler U: DBP, a liver-enriched transcriptional activator, is expressed late in ontogeny and its tissue specificity is determined posttranslationally. *Cell* 61:279, 1990.
35. Sladek F, Zhong W, Lai E, Darnell J: Liver-enriched transcription factor HNF-4 is a novel member of the steroid hormone receptor superfamily. *Gene Dev* 4:2353, 1990.
36. Paonessa G, Gounari F, Frank R, Cortese R: Purification of a NF1-like DNA-binding protein from rat liver and cloning of the corresponding cDNA. *EMBO J* 7:3115, 1988.
37. London FS, Walsh PN: Activation dependent appearance of a platelet protein that recognizes coagulation factor IXa. *Circulation* 86:I465, 1992.
38. DiScipio RG, Hermodson M, Yates S, Davie E: A comparison of human prothrombin, factor IX (Christmas factor), factor X (Stuart factor) and protein S. *Biochemistry* 16:698, 1977.
39. Scambler P, Williamson R: The structural gene for human coagulation factor X is located on chromosome 13q34. *Cytogenet Cell Genet* 39:231, 1985.
40. Watzke H, High K: Factor X, in *Molecular Basis of Thrombosis and Hemostasis,* edited by K High, H Roberts, p 239. Marcel Dekker, New York, 1995.
41. Huang M, Hung H, Stanfield-Oakley S, High K: Characterization of the human coagulation factor X promoter. *J Biol Chem* 267:15440, 1992.
42. Hung H, High K: Liver-enriched transcription factor HNF-4 and ubiquitous factor NF-Y are critical for expression of blood coagulation factor X. *J Biol Chem* 271:2323, 1996.
43. Rao L, Rapaport SI: Activation of factor VII bound to tissue factor: a key early step in the tissue factor pathway of blood coagulation. *Proc Natl Acad Sci USA* 85:6687, 1988.
44. Neuenschwander PF, Jesty J: Thrombin-activated and factor Xa-activated human factor VIII: differences in cofactor activity and decay rate. *Arch Biochem Biophys* 296:426, 1992.
45. Monkovic DD, Tracy PB: Activation of human factor V by factor Xa and thrombin. *Biochemistry* 29:1118, 1990.
46. Bouchard BA, Catcher CS, Thrash BR, et al: Effector cell protease receptor-1, a platelet activation-dependent membrane protein, regulates prothrombinase-catalyzed thrombin generation. *J Biol Chem* 272:9244, 1997.

47. Gasic GP, Arenas CP, Gasic TB, Gasic GJ: Coagulation factors X, Xa, and protein S as potent mitogens of cultured aortic smooth muscle cells. *Proc Natl Acad Sci USA* 89:2317, 1992.

48. Altieri DC, Edgington TS: Identification of effector cell protease receptor-1: a leukocyte-distributed receptor for the serine protease factor Xa. *J Immunol* 145:246, 1990.

49. Patracchini P, Aiello V, Palazzi P, et al: Sublocalization of the human protein C gene on chromosome 2q13–q14. *Hum Genet* 81:191, 1989.

50. Foster D, Yoshitake S, Davie E: The nucleotide sequence of the gene for human protein C. *Proc Natl Acad Sci USA* 82:4673, 1985.

51. Plutzky J, Hoskins J, Long G, Crabtree G: Evolution and organization of the human protein C gene. *Proc Natl Acad Sci USA* 83:546, 1986.

52. Shen L, Dahlback B: Factor V and protein S as synergistic cofactors to activated protein C in degradation of factor VIIIa. *J Biol Chem* 269:18735, 1994.

53. Cooper S, Church F: PCI: protein C inhibitor? *Adv Exp Med Biol* 425:45, 1997.

54. Dahlback B: Inhibition of protein Ca, a cofactor function of human and bovine protein S by C4b-binding protein. *J Biol Chem* 261:12022, 1986.

55. Fair D, Marlar R: Biosynthesis and secretion of factor VII, protein C, protein S and the protein C inhibitor from a human hepatoma cell line. *Blood* 67:64, 1986.

56. Fair D, Marlar R, Levin E: Human endothelial cells synthesize protein S. *Blood* 67:1168, 1986.

57. Ogura M, Tanabe N, Nishioka J, et al: Biosynthesis and secretion of functional protein S by a human megakaryoblastic cell line. *Blood* 70:301, 1987.

58. Dahlback B: Protein S and C4b-binding protein: components involved in the regulation of the protein C anticoagulant system. *Thromb Haemostas* 66:49, 1991.

59. Maillard C, Berruyer M, Serre C, et al: Protein S, a vitamin K–dependent protein, is a bone matrix component synthesized and secreted by osteoblasts. *Endocrinology* 130:1599, 1992.

60. Edenbrandt C-M, Lundvall A, Wydro R, Stenflo J: Molecular analysis of the gene for vitamin K–dependent protein S and its pseudogene. Cloning and partial characterization. *Biochemistry* 29:7861, 1990.

61. Hackeng T, van't Veer C, Meijers J, Bouma B: Human protein S inhibits prothrombinase complex activity on endothelial cells and platelets via direct interactions with factors Va and Xa. *J Biol Chem* 269:21051, 1994.

62. Ortel T, Keller F, Kane W: Factor V, in *Molecular Basis of Thrombosis and Hemostasis,* edited by K High, H Roberts, p 119. Marcel Dekker, New York, 1995.

63. Ortel TL, Quinn-Allen MA, Keller FG, et al: Localization of functionally important epitopes within the second C-type domain of coagulation factor V using recombinant chimeras. *J Biol Chem* 269:15898, 1994.

64. Pittman DD, Tomkinson KN, Michnick D, et al: Posttranslational sulfation of factor V is required for efficient thrombin cleavage and activation and for full procoagulant activity. *Biochemistry* 33:6592, 1994.

65. Cripe L, Moore K, Kane W: Structure of the gene for human coagulation factor V. *Biochemistry* 31:3777, 1992.

66. Hayward C: Multimerin: a bench-to-bedside chronology of a unique platelet and endothelial cell protein—from discovery to function to abnormalities in disease. *Clin Invest Med* 20:176, 1997.

67. Bertina RM, Koeleman BP, Koster T, et al: Mutation in blood coagulation factor V associated with resistance to activated protein C. *Nature* 369:64, 1994.

68. Lollar P, Hill-Eubanks D, Parker C: Association of the factor VIII light chain with von Willebrand factor. *J Biol Chem* 263:10451, 1988.

69. Gitschier J, Wood W, Goralka T, et al: Characterization of the human factor VIII gene. *Nature* 312:326, 1984.

70. Pipe S, Morris J, Shah J, Kaufman R: Differential interaction of coagulation factor VIII and factor V with protein chaperones calnexin and calreticulin. *J Biol Chem* 273:8537, 1998.

71. Swaroop M, Moussalli M, Pipe S, Kaufman R: Mutagenesis of a potential immunoglobulin-binding protein-binding site enhances secretion of coagulation factor VIII. *J Biol Chem* 272:24121, 1997.

72. Moussalli M, Pipe S, Nichols W, et al: Mistargeting of the lectin ERGIC-53 to the endoplasmic reticulum impairs the secretion of coagulation factors V and VIII. *Blood* 92:474a, 1998.

73. Nichols W, Seligsohn U, Zivelin A, et al: Mutations in the ER-Golgi intermediate compartment protein ERGIC-53 cause combined deficiency of coagulation factors V and VIII. *Cell* 93:61, 1998.

74. Bonthron D, Handin R, Kaufman R, et al: Structure of pre-pro-von Willebrand factor and its expression in heterologous cells. *Nature* 324:270, 1986.

75. Colombatti A, Bonaldo P: The superfamily of proteins with von Willebrand factor type A-domains: one theme common to components of extracellular matrix, hemostasis, cellular adhesion, and defense mechanisms. *Blood* 77:2305, 1991.

76. Foster P, Fulcher C, Marti T, et al: A major factor VIII binding domain resides within the amino-terminal 272 amino acid residues of von Willebrand factor. *J Biol Chem* 262:8443, 1987.

77. Zimmerman T, Roberts J, Edgington T: Factor-VIII-related antigen: multiple molecular forms in human plasma. *Proc Natl Acad Sci USA* 72:5121, 1975.

78. Mancuso D, Tuley E, Westfield L, et al: Structure of the gene for human von Willebrand factor. *J Biol Chem* 264:19514, 1989.

79. Bolton-Maggs PH, Wensley RT, Kernoff PB, et al: Production and therapeutic use of a factor XI concentrate from plasma. *Thromb Haemost* 67:314, 1992.

80. Fujikawa K, Chung DW: Factor XI, in *Molecular Basis of Thrombosis and Hemostasis,* edited by K High, H Roberts, p 257. Marcel Dekker, New York, 1995.

81. Baglia FA, Seaman FS, Walsh PN: The apple 1 and apple 4 domains of factor XI act synergistically to promote the surface-mediated activation of factor XI by factor XIIa. *Blood* 85:2078, 1995.

82. Baglia FA, Jameson BA, Walsh PN: Identification and characterization of a binding site for platelets in the apple 3 domain of coagulation factor XI. *J Biol Chem* 270:6734, 1995.

83. Baglia FA, Jameson BA, Walsh PN: Identification and characterization of a binding site for factor XIIa in the apple 4 domain of coagulation factor XI. *J Biol Chem* 268:3838, 1993.

84. Baglia FA, Walsh PN: A binding site for thrombin in the apple 1 domain of factor XI. *J Biol Chem* 271:3652, 1996.

85. Kato A, Asakai R, Davie E, Aoki N: Factor XI gene (F11) is located on the distal end of the long arm of human chromosome 4. *Cytogenet Cell Genet* 52:77, 1989.

86. Asakai R, Davie E, Chung D: Organization of the gene for human factor XI. *Biochemistry* 26:7221, 1987.

87. Gailani D, Broze GJ Jr: Factor XI activation in a revised model of blood coagulation. *Science* 253:909, 1991.

88. Naito K, Fujikawa K: Activation of human blood coagulation factor XI independent of factor XII. Factor XI is activated by thrombin and factor XIa in the presence of negatively charged surfaces. *J Biol Chem* 266:7353, 1991.

89. Oliver J, Monroe D, Roberts H, Hoffman M: Thrombin activates factor XI on activated platelets in the absence of factor XII. *Arterioscler Thromb Vasc Biol* 19:170, 1999.

90. Ragni MV, Sinha D, Seaman F, et al: Comparison of bleeding tendency, factor XI coagulant activity, and factor XI antigen in 25 factor XI-deficient kindreds. *Blood* 65:719, 1985.

91. Sinha D, Seaman FS, Walsh PN: Role of calcium ions and the heavy chain of factor XIa in the activation of human coagulation factor IX. *Biochemistry* 26:3768, 1987.

92. Sinha D, Seaman FS, Koshy A, et al: Blood coagulation factor XIa binds specifically to a site on activated human platelets distinct from that for factor XI. *J Clin Invest* 73:1550, 1984.

93. Walsh PN, Sinha D, Kueppers F, et al: Regulation of factor XIa activity by platelets and alpha 1-protease inhibitor. *J Clin Invest* 80:1578, 1987.

94. Cronlund AL, Walsh PN: A low molecular weight platelet inhibitor of factor XIa: Purification, characterization, and possible role in blood coagulation. *Biochemistry* 31:1685, 1992.

95. Saito H, Kojima T: Factor XII, prekallikrein and high-molecular-weight kininogen, in *Molecular Basis of Thrombosis and Hemostasis,* edited by K High, H Roberts, p 269. Marcel Dekker, New York, 1995.

96. Morrissey JH, Fakhrai H, Edgington TS: Molecular cloning of the cDNA for tissue factor, the cellular receptor for the initiation of the coagulation protease cascade. *Cell* 50:129, 1987.

97. Bach R, Konigsberg W, Nemerson Y: Human tissue factor contains thioester-linked palmitate and stearate on the cytoplasmic half cysteine. *Biochemistry* 27:4227, 1988.

98. Martin D, Boys C, Ruf W: Tissue factor: molecular recognition and cofactor function. *FASEB J* 9:852, 1995.

99. Mueller BM: Different roles for plasminogen activators and metalloproteinases in melanoma metastasis. *Curr Top Microbiol Immunol* 213:65, 1996.

100. Kao FT, Hartz J, Horton R, et al: Regional assignment of human tissue factor gene (F3) to chromosome 1p21–p22. *Somat Cell Mol Genet* 14:407, 1988.

101. Mackman N, Morrissey JH, Fowler B, Edgington TS: Complete sequence of the human tissue factor gene, a highly regulated cellular receptor that initiates the coagulation protease cascade. *Biochemistry* 28:1755, 1989.

102. Mackman N, Fowler B, Edgington TS, Morrissey JH: Functional analysis of the human tissue factor promoter and induction by serum. *Proc Natl Acad Sci USA* 87:2254, 1990.

103. Gregory SA, Morrissey JH, Edgington TS: Regulation of tissue factor gene expression in the monocyte procoagulant response to endotoxin. *Mol Cell Biol* 9:2752, 1989.

104. Schecter AD, Rollins BJ, Zhang YJ, et al: Tissue factor is induced by monocyte chemoattractant protein-1 in human aortic smooth muscle and THP-1 cells. *J Biol Chem* 272:28568, 1997.

105. Conway EM, Bach R, Rosenberg RD, Konigsberg WH: Tumor necrosis factor enhances expression of tissue factor mRNA in endothelial cells. *Thromb Res* 53:231, 1989.

106. Hoffman M, Cooper S: Thrombin enhances monocyte secretion of tumor necrosis factor and interleukin-1 beta by two distinct mechanisms. *Blood Cell Mol Dis* 21:156, 1995.

107. Drake TA, Morrissey JH, Edgington TS: Selective cellular expression of tissue factor in human tissues. Implications for disorders of hemostasis and thrombosis. *Am J Pathol* 134:1087, 1989.

108. Eddleston M, de la Torre J, Oldstone M, et al: Astrocytes are the primary source of tissue factor in the murine central nervous system. A role for astrocytes in cerebral hemostasis. *J Clin Invest* 92:349, 1993.

109. Giesen PLA, Rauch U, Bohrmann B, et al: Blood-borne tissue factor: Another view of thrombosis. *Proc Natl Acad Sci USA* 96:2311, 1999.

110. Østerud B, Rapaport SI: Activation of factor IX by the reaction product of tissue factor and factor VII: additional pathway for initiating blood coagulation. *Proc Natl Acad Sci USA* 74:5260, 1977.

111. Shigematsu Y, Miyata T, Higashi S, et al: Expression of human soluble tissue factor in yeast and enzymatic properties of its complex with factor VIIa. *J Biol Chem* 267:21329, 1992.

112. Lawson JH, Butenas S, Mann KG: The evaluation of complex-dependent alterations in human factor VIIa. *J Biol Chem* 267:4834, 1992.

113. Neuenschwander PF, Morrissey JH: Roles of the membrane-interactive regions of factor VIIa and tissue factor. The factor VIIa Gla domain is dispensable for binding to tissue factor but important for activation of factor X. *J Biol Chem* 269:8007, 1994.

114. Neuenschwander PF, Morrissey JH: Deletion of the membrane anchoring region of tissue factor abolishes autoactivation of factor VII but not cofactor function. Analysis of a mutant with a selective deficiency in activity. *J Biol Chem* 267:14477, 1992.

115. Krishnaswamy S, Field KA, Edgington TS, et al: Role of the membrane surface in the activation of human coagulation factor X. *J Biol Chem* 267:26110, 1992.

116. Bach R, Moldow C: Mechanism of tissue factor activation on HL-60 cells. *Blood* 89:3270, 1997.

117. Bach R, Rifkin DB: Expression of tissue factor procoagulant activity: regulation by cytosolic calcium. *Proc Natl Acad Sci USA* 87:6995, 1990.

118. Wen D, Dittman W, Ye R, et al: Human thrombomodulin: complete cDNA sequence and chromosome localization of the gene. *Biochemistry* 26:4350, 1987.

119. Esmon N, Owen W, Esmon C: Isolation of a membrane-bound cofactor for thrombin-catalyzed activation of protein C. *J Biol Chem* 257:859, 1982.

120. Patthy L: Detecting distant homologies of mosaic proteins. Analysis of sequences of thrombomodulin, thrombospondin complement components C9, C8 alpha, and C8 beta, vitronectin and plasma cell membrane glycoprotein PC-1. *J Mol Biol* 202:689, 1988.

121. Stearns D, Kurosawa S, Esmon C: Microthrombomodulin. Residues 310–486 from the epidermal growth factor precursor homology domain of thrombomodulin will accelerate protein C activation. *J Biol Chem* 264:3352, 1989.

122. Parkinson J, Vlahos C, Yan S, Bang N: Recombinant human thrombomodulin. Regulation of cofactor activity and anticoagulant function by a glycosaminoglycan side chain. *Biochem J* 283:151, 1992.

123. Espinosa R, Sadler J, LeBeau M: Regional localization of the human thrombomodulin gene to 20p12-cen. *Genomics* 5:649, 1989.

124. Esmon C, Esmon N, Harris K: Complex formation between thrombin and thrombomodulin inhibits both thrombin-catalyzed fibrin formation and factor V activation. *J Biol Chem* 257:7944, 1982.

125. Cadroy Y, Diquelou A, Dupouy D, et al: The thrombomodulin/protein C/protein S anticoagulant pathway modulates the thrombogenic properties of the normal resting and stimulated endothelium. *Arterioscler Thromb Vasc Biol* 17:520, 1997.

126. Verhagen HJ, Heijnen-Snyder GJ, Pronk A, et al: Thrombomodulin activity on mesothelial cells: perspectives for mesothelial cells as an alternative for endothelial cells: for cell seeding on vascular grafts. *Br J Haematol* 95:542, 1996.

127. McCachren SS, Diggs J, Weinberg JB, Dittman WA: Thrombomodulin expression by human blood monocytes and by human synovial tissue lining macrophages. *Blood* 78:3128, 1991.

128. Raife TJ, Demetroulis EM, Lentz SR: Regulation of thrombomodulin expression by all-*trans*-retinoic acid and tumor necrosis factor-alpha: differential responses in keratinocytes and endothelial cells. *Blood* 88:2043, 1996.

129. Ishii H, Nakana M, Tsubouchi J, et al: Distribution of thrombomodulin in human tissues and characterization of thrombomodulin in plasma. *Acta Haematol Jpn* 51:1218, 1998.

130. Dichek D, Quertermous T: Variability in messenger RNA levels in human umbilical vein endothelial cells of different lineage and time in culture. *In Vitro Cell Dev Biol* 25:289, 1989.

131. Rezaie A, Cooper S, Church F, Esmon C: Protein C inhibitor is a potent inhibitor of the thrombin-thrombomodulin complex. *J Biol Chem* 270:25336, 1995.

132. Yamagata S, Mori K, Kayaba T, et al: A case of congenital afibrinogenemia and review of reported cases in Japan. *Tohoku J Exp Med* 96:15, 1968.

133. Egbring R, Andrassy K, Egli H, Meyer-Lindenberg J: Diagnostische und therapeutische probleme bei kongenitale afibrinogenamia. *Blut* 22, 1971.

134. Carrell N, McDonagh J: Functional defects in abnormal fibrinogens, in *Fibrinogen: Structural Variants and Interaction,* edited by A Henschen, B Hesse, J McDonagh, T Saldeen, p 155. Walter DeGruyter, Berlin, 1985.

135. Egeberg O: Inherited fibrinogen abnormality causing thrombophilia. *Thromb Diath Haemorrh* 17:176, 1967.

136. Gardlund B, Hessel B, Marguerie G, et al: Primary structure of human fibrinogen: Characterization of disulfide-containing cyanogen-bromide fragments. *Eur J Biochem* 77:595, 1977.

137. Blomback B: Studies on the action of thrombotic enzymes on bovine fibrinogen as measured by N-terminal analysis. *Avkiv Kem* 12:321, 1958.

138. Blomback B, Blomback M, Henschen A, et al: N-terminal disulphide knot of human fibrinogen. *Nature* 218:130, 1968.

139. Côté HF, Lord ST, Pratt KP: γ-Chain dysfibrinogenemias: Molecular structure-function relationships of naturally occurring mutations in the γ-chain of human fibrinogen. *Blood* 92:2195, 1998.

140. Collen D, Tytgat C, Claeys H, Piessens R: Metabolism and distribution of fibrinogen: I. Fibrinogen turnover in physiological conditions in humans. *Br J Haematol* 22:681, 1972.

141. Reeve K, Franks J: Fibrinogen synthesis, distribution and degradation. *Semin Thromb Hemost* 1:129, 1974.

142. Fuller G, Otto J, Woloski B, et al: The effects of hepatocyte-stimulating factor on fibrinogen biosynthesis in hepatocyte monolayers. *J Cell Biol* 101:1481, 1985.

143. Huber P, Laurent M, Dalmon J: Human β-fibrinogen gene expression. Upstream sequences involved in its tissue specific expression and its dexamethasone and interleukin-6 stimulation. *J Biol Chem* 265:5695, 1990.

144. Chung D, Harris I, Davie E: Nucleotide sequences of the three genes coding for human fibrinogen. *Adv Exp Med Biol* 281:39, 1990.

145. Doolittle R, Cottrell B, Strong D, Watt K: The amino acid sequence of the α-chain of human fibrinogen. *Nature* 280:464, 1979.

146. Kant I, Fornace A, Saxe D, et al: Evolution and organization of the fibrinogen locus on chromosome 4: gene duplication accompanied by transposition and inversion. *Proc Natl Acad Sci USA* 82:2344, 1985.

147. Morgan J, Courtois G, Fourel G: Sp 1, a CAAT-binding factor, and the adenovirus major late promoter transcription factor interact with functional regions of the gamma-fibrinogen promoter. *Mol Cell Biol* 8:2628, 1988.

148. Courtois G, Morgan J, Campbell L, et al: Interaction of a liver-specific nuclear factor with the fibrinogen and α-1-antitrypsin promoters. *Science* 238:688, 1987.

149. Dalmon J, Laurent M, Courtois G: The human β fibrinogen promoter contains a hepatocyte nuclear factor 1-dependent interleukin-6-responsive element. *Mol Cell Biol* 13:1183, 1993.

150. Haidaris P, Courtney M: Tissue-specific and ubiquitous expression of fibrinogen γ-chain mRNA. *Blood Coag Fibrinol* 1:433, 1990.

151. Handagama PJ, Shuman MA, Bainton DF: In vivo defibrination results in markedly decreased amounts of fibrinogen in rat megakaryocytes and platelets. *Am J Pathol* 137:1393, 1990.

152. Louache F, Debili N, Cramer E, et al: Fibrinogen is not synthesized by human megakaryocytes. *Blood* 77:311, 1991.

153. Vali Z, Scheraga H: Localization of the binding site on fibrin for the secondary binding site of thrombin. *Biochemistry* 27:1956, 1988.

154. Olexa S, Budzynski A: Evidence for four different polymerization sites involved in human fibrin formation. *Proc Natl Acad Sci USA* 77:1374, 1980.

155. Kaczmarek E, McDonagh J: Thrombin binding to the Aα-, Bβ-, and gamma-chains of fibrinogen and to their remnants contained in fragment E. *J Biol Chem* 263:13896, 1988.

156. Weisel J, Phillips G, Cohen C: The structure of fibrinogen and fibrin: II. Architecture of the fibrin clot. *Ann NY Acad Sci* 408:367, 1983.

157. Hantgan R, Fowler W, Erickson H, Hermans J: Fibrin assembly: a comparison of electron microscopic and light scattering results. *Thromb Haemost* 44:119, 1980.

158. Dang C, Shin C, Bell W, Nagaswami C, Weisel J: Fibrinogen sialic acid residues are low affinity calcium-binding sites that influence fibrin assembly. *J Biol Chem* 264:15104, 1989.

159. Nieuwenhuizen W, van Ruijven-Vermneer J, Nooijen W, et al: Recalculation of calcium-binding properties of human and rat fibrin(ogen) and their degradation products. *Thromb Res* 22:653, 1981.

160. Marder V, Budzynski A: Degradation products of fibrinogen and cross linked fibrin-projected clinical applications. *Thromb Diath Haemorrh* 32:49, 1974.

161. Elms M, Bunce I, Bundesen P, et al: Measurement of cross-linked fibrin degradation products: an immunoassay using monoclonal antibodies. *Thromb Haemostas* 50:591, 1983.

162. Hermans J, McDonagh J: Fibrin: Structure and interactions. *Semin Thromb Hemost* 8:11, 1982.

163. Williams J, Hantgan R, Hermanns J, McDonagh J: Characterization of the inhibition of fibrin assembly by fibrinogen fragment D. *Biochem J* 197:661, 1981.

164. Lai T-S, Greenberg C: Factor XIII, in *Molecular Basis of Thrombosis and Hemostasis,* edited by K High, H Roberts, p 287. Marcel Dekker, New York, 1995.

165. Bottenus R, Ichinose A, Davie E: Nucleotide sequence of the gene for the b subunit of human factor XIII. *Biochemistry* 29:11195, 1990.

166. Ichinose A, Davie E: Characterization of the gene for the α subunit of human factor XIII (plasma transglutaminase), a blood coagulation factor. *Proc Natl Acad Sci USA* 85:5829, 1988.

167. Ichinose A, McMillen B, Fujikawa K, Davie E: Amino acid sequence of the B subunit of human factor XIII, a protein composed of ten repetitive segments. *Biochemistry* 25:4633, 1986.

168. Ichinose A, Bottenus R, Davie E: Structure of transglutaminases. *J Biol Chem* 265:13411, 1990.

169. Henricksson P, Becker S, Lynch G, McDonagh J: Identification of intracellular factor XIII in human monocytes and macrophages. *J Clin Invest* 76:528, 1985.

170. McDonagh J, McDonagh R, Deleage J, Wagner R: Factor XIII in human plasma and platelets. *J Clin Invest* 48:940, 1969.

171. Weisberg L, Shiu D, Greenberg C, et al: Localization of the gene for coagulation factor XIII a-chain to chromosome 6 and identification of sites of synthesis. *J Clin Invest* 79:649, 1987.

172. Bottenus R, Ichinose A, Davie E: Nucleotide sequence of the gene for the b subunit of human factor XIII. *Biochemistry* 29:11195, 1990.

173. Han X, Fiehler R, Broze GJ: Isolation of a protein Z-dependent plasma protease inhibitor. *Proc Natl Acad Sci USA* 95:9250, 1998.

174. Broze GJ Jr, Warren LA, Novotny WF, et al: The lipoprotein-associated coagulation inhibitor that inhibits the factor VII-tissue factor complex also inhibits factor Xa: insight into its possible mechanism of action. *Blood* 71:335, 1988.

175. Warn-Cramer B, Rao L, Maki S, Rapaport SI: Modifications of extrinsic pathway inhibitor (EPI) and factor Xa that affect their ability to interact and to inhibit factor VIIa/tissue factor: evidence for a two-step model of inhibition. *Thromb Haemostas* 60:453, 1988.

176. Ameri A, Kuppuswamy M, Basu S, Bajaj S: Expression of tissue factor pathway inhibitor by cultured endothelial cells in response to inflammatory mediators. *Blood* 79:3219, 1992.

177. Sandset P, Abildgaard U, Larsen M: Heparin induces release of extrinsic coagulation pathway inhibitor (EPI). *Thromb Res* 50:803, 1988.

178. Girard T, Eddy R, Wesselschmidt R, et al: Structure of the human lipoprotein-associated coagulation inhibitor gene: Intron/exon organization and localization of the gene to chromosome 2. *J Biol Chem* 266:5036, 1991.

179. Chang JY, Monroe DM, Oliver JA, Roberts HR: TFPIβ, a second product from the mouse tissue factor pathway inhibitor (TFPI) gene. *Thromb Haemost* 81:45, 1999.

180. Griffith MJ: Measurement of the heparin enhanced-antithrombin III/thrombin reaction rate in the presence of synthetic substrate. *Thromb Res* 25:245, 1982.

181. Fuchs HE, Trapp HG, Griffith MJ, et al: Regulation of factor IXa in vitro in human and mouse plasma and in vivo in the mouse. Role of the endothelium and the plasma proteinase inhibitors. *J Clin Invest* 73:1696, 1984.

182. Sheffield W, Wu Y, Blajchman M: Antithrombin: Structure and function, in *Molecular Basis of Thrombosis and Hemostasis,* edited by K High, H Roberts, p 355. Marcel Dekker, New York, 1995.

183. Pizzo S: Serpin receptor 1: a hepatic receptor that mediates the clearance of antithrombin III-protease complexes. *Am J Med* 87:10S, 1989.

184. Ochoa A, Brunel F, Mendelson D, et al: Different liver nuclear proteins bind to similar DNA sequences in the 5' flanking regions of three hepatic genes. *Nucleic Acids Res* 17:119, 1989.

185. Macfarlane RG: An enzyme cascade in the blood clotting mechanism, and its function as a biological amplifier. *Nature* 202:498, 1964.

186. Davie EW, Ratnoff OD: Waterfall sequence for intrinsic blood clotting. *Science* 145:1310, 1964.

187. Nemerson Y, Esnouf MP: Activation of a proteolytic system by a membrane lipoprotein: mechanism of action of tissue factor. *Proc Natl Acad Sci USA* 70:310, 1973.

188. Nemerson Y: The tissue factor pathway of blood coagulation. *Semin Hematol* 29:170, 1992.

189. Repke D, Gemmell CH, Guha A, et al: Hemophilia as a defect of the tissue factor pathway of blood coagulation: effect of factors VIII and IX on factor X activation in a continuous-flow reactor. *Proc Natl Acad Sci USA* 87:7623, 1990.

190. Broze GJ Jr, Girard TJ, Novotny WF: Regulation of coagulation by a multivalent Kunitz-type inhibitor. *Biochemistry* 29:7539, 1990.

191. Hockin MF, Kalafatis M, Shatos M, Mann KG: Protein C activation and factor Va inactivation on human umbilical vein endothelial cells. *Arterioscler Thromb Vasc Biol* 17:2765, 1997.

192. Fay PJ, Smudzin TM, Walker FJ: Activated protein C-catalyzed inactivation of human factor VIII and VIIIa. Identification of cleavage sites and correlation of proteolysis with cofactor activity. *J Biol Chem* 266:20139, 1991.

193. Pieters J, Willems G, Hemker HC, Lindhout T: Inhibition of factor IXa and factor Xa by antithrombin III/heparin during factor X activation. *J Biol Chem* 263:15313, 1988.

194. Allen DH, Tracy PB: Human coagulation factor V is activated to the functional cofactor by elastase and cathepsin G expressed at the monocyte surface. *J Biol Chem* 270:1408, 1995.

195. Monroe DM, Hoffman M, Roberts HR: Transmission of a procoagulant signal from tissue factor-bearing cell to platelets. *Blood Coagul Fibrinol* 7:459, 1996.

196. Williamson P, Bevers EM, Smeets EF, et al: Continuous analysis of the mechanism of activated transbilayer lipid movement in platelets. *Biochemistry* 34:10448, 1995.

197. Monroe DM, Roberts HR, Hoffman M: Platelet procoagulant complex assembly in a tissue factor-initiated system. *Br J Haematol* 88:364, 1994.

198. Ahmad SS, Rawala-Sheikh R, Walsh PN: Platelet receptor occupancy with factor IXa promotes factor X activation. *J Biol Chem* 264: 20012, 1989.

199. Ahmad SS, Rawala-Sheikh R, Ashby B, Walsh PN: Platelet receptor-mediated factor X activation by factor IXa: High-affinity factor IXa receptors induced by factor VIII are deficient on platelets in Scott syndrome. *J Clin Invest* 84:824, 1989.

200. Bouma BN, von dem Borne PAK, Meijers JCM: Factor XI and protection of the fibrin clot against lysis—a role for the intrinsic pathway of coagulation in fibrinolysis. *Thromb Haemost* 80:24, 1998.

201. de Agostini A, Watkins S, Slayter H, et al: Localization of the anticoagulantly active heparan sulfate proteoglycans in vascular endothelium: antithrombin binding on cultured endothelial cells and perfused rat aorta. *J Cell Biol* 111:1293, 1990.

202. Marcus AJ, Broekman MJ, Drosopoulos JH, et al: The endothelial cell ecto-ADPase responsible for inhibition of platelet function is CD39. *J Clin Invest* 99:1351, 1997.

203. Jesty J, Beltrami E, Willems G: Mathematical analysis of a proteolytic positive-feedback loop: dependence of lag time and enzyme yields on the initial conditions and kinetic parameters. *Biochemistry* 32:6266, 1993.

204. Brakman P, Albrechtsen OK, Astrup T: A comparative study of coagulation and fibrinolysis in blood from normal men and women. *Br J Haematol* 12:74, 1966.

205. Nossel H, Yudelman I, Canfield RE: Measurement of fibrinopeptide A in human blood. *J Clin Invest* 54:43, 1974.

206. Bauer KA, Kass BL, ten Cate H, et al: Factor IX is activated in vivo by the tissue factor mechanism. *Blood* 76:731, 1990.

207. Bauer KA, Kass BL, ten Cate H, et al: Detection of factor X activation in humans. *Blood* 74:2007, 1989.

208. Morrissey JH: Tissue factor modulation of factor VIIa activity: use in measuring trace levels of factor VIIa in plasma. *Thromb Haemostas* 74:185, 1995.

209. Conard J, Bauer KA, Gruber A, et al: Normalization of markers of coagulation activation with a purified protein C concentrate in adults with homozygous protein C deficiency. *Blood* 82:1159, 1993.

CONTROL OF COAGULATION REACTIONS

JOHN H. GRIFFIN

Normally, the blood coagulation system is active, but idling, and is poised for explosive generation of thrombin. The requirement for positive feedback activation of clotting factors (e.g., factors V, VIII, XI, and VII) imparts special threshold properties to the blood coagulation pathways, making the coagulant response nonlinearly responsive to stimuli. Analysis of blood coagulation as a threshold system suggests all-or-none responses to various levels of stimuli, depending on the ensemble of reactions that determine up-regulation and down-regulation of thrombin generation. Because of synergies between cellular and humoral anticoagulant mechanisms, the presence of multiple coagulation inhibitors with complementary modes of action prevents massive thrombin generation in the absence of a substantial procoagulant stimulus. This chapter highlights plasma mechanisms that inhibit blood coagulation, with an emphasis on mechanisms whose defects cause hereditary thrombophilias. The majority of hereditary defects involves the anticoagulant protein C pathway, which includes protein C and protein S as anticoagulant factors, thrombomodulin and endothelial protein C receptor as cofactors for activation of protein C, and factors Va and VIIIa as substrates for activated protein C. Variant factor V containing Gln506 in place of Arg506 causes activated protein C resistance by impairing the efficiency of the protein C pathway. Plasma protease inhibitors are essential to block clotting proteases. Antithrombin neutralizes all proteases of the intrinsic coagulation pathway, including thrombin and factors Xa, IXa, XIa, and XIIa, in reactions stimulated by glycosaminoglycans. Tissue factor pathway inhibitor neutralizes the extrinsic coagulation pathway factors VIIa and Xa. Other plasma protease inhibitors can also neutralize various coagulation proteases, although the clinical significance of these reactions is less apparent than the reaction of antithrombin with thrombin.

INTRODUCTION

Control of coagulation reactions is essential for normal hemostasis. As part of the tangled web of host defense systems that respond to vascular injury, the blood coagulation factors act in concert with the endothelium and platelets to generate a protective fibrin-platelet clot, forming a hemostatic plug. Pathologic thrombosis occurs when the

Acronyms and abbreviations that appear in this chapter include: APC, activated protein C; C4BP, C4b-binding protein; DIC, disseminated intravascular coagulation; EPCR, endothelial cell protein C receptor; EPI, extrinsic pathway inhibitor; Gla, γ-carboxyglutamic acid; HDL, high-density lipoprotein; LACI, lipoprotein-associated coagulation inhibitor; SHBG, sex-hormone-binding globulin–like region; TFPI, tissue factor pathway inhibitor; previously also described as, TSR, thrombin-sensitive region.

protective clot is extended beyond its beneficial size, when a clot occurs inappropriately at sites of vascular disease, or when a clot embolizes to other sites in the circulatory bed. For normal hemostasis, both procoagulant and anticoagulant factors must interact with the vascular components and cell surfaces, including the vessel wall (see Chap. 114) and platelets (see Chaps. 111 and 112). Moreover, the action of the fibrinolytic system must be integrated with coagulation reactions for timely formation and dissolution of blood clots (see Chap 116). For extensive discussion of regulation of coagulation, the reader is referred to recent books that focus only on hemostasis and thrombosis.[1,2] This chapter on control of coagulation highlights the major physiologic mechanisms for down-regulation of blood coagulation reactions and the plasma proteins that inhibit blood coagulation, with an emphasis on those mechanisms whose defects are clinically significant based on insights gleaned from consideration of the hereditary thrombophilias (see Chap 127).

BLOOD COAGULATION PATHWAYS AND PROTEIN C ANTICOAGULANT PATHWAY

Although more than 40 years have elapsed since the elaboration of the cascade model for blood coagulation pathways,[3,4] the basic outline of sequential conversions of protease zymogens to active serine proteases is still useful, albeit with important modifications, to represent blood coagulation reactions (Fig. 113-1). The major conceptual advances in the past two decades emphasize both positive and negative feedback reactions as depicted in Fig. 113-1.

In positive feedback reactions, procoagulant thrombin activates platelets and factors V, VIII, and XI[5–10] (see Chap. 112). Small amounts of thrombin can be generated by trace amounts of tissue factor via the extrinsic pathway. Subsequently, thrombin can activate factors XI, VIII, and V, thereby stimulating each of the steps in the intrinsic pathway and thus amplifying thrombin generation. In negative feedback reactions that involve the protein C pathway, binding of thrombin to thrombomodulin converts the bound thrombin to an anticoagulant enzyme that converts the protein C zymogen to the anticoagulant serine protease, activated protein C (APC) (Fig. 113-1). This surface-dependent reaction is enhanced by the endothelial cell protein C receptor (EPCR).[7,11,12] In a subsequent negative feedback loop, APC with the aid of its nonenzymatic cofactor, protein S, inactivates factors Va and VIIIa by highly selective proteolysis, yielding inactive (i) cofactors, factors V_i and VIII_i. Protein S also can directly inhibit factors VIIIa, Xa, and Va.[13–19] Thus, APC and protein S inhibit multiple steps in the intrinsic coagulation pathway. At each step in the coagulation pathways, each clotting protease can be inhibited by one or more protease inhibitors. Given the highly nonlinear nature of the coagulation pathways with both positive and negative feedback reactions, synergy between the protein C pathway and plasma protease inhibitors is important for regulating thrombin generation.

Plasma from all normal subjects contains circulating active enzymes, factor VIIa,[20,21] and APC,[22] as well as various polypeptide fragments generated by the action of clotting proteases, namely fibrinopeptides,[23,24] prothrombin fragment 1+2,[25] and activation peptides for factors IX and X.[26,27] Thus, there is continuous activation of coagulation factors at a basal physiologic low level. The presence of multiple clotting factors that require positive feedback activation (e.g., factors V, VIII, XI, and VII) imparts special threshold properties to the blood coagulation pathways, making the coagulant response nonlinearly responsive to stimuli. Theoretical analysis of blood coagulation as a threshold system suggests there can be an all-or-none response to various levels of stimulation, depending on the ensemble of activating and inhibitory reactions that defines up-regulation and down-regulation of thrombin generation.[28,29] It appears that the coagulation system is active, but idling, and is poised for extensive and explosive generation

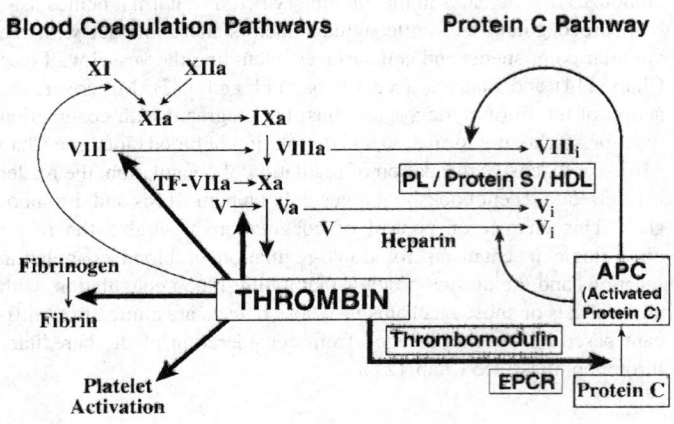

FIGURE 113-1　Blood coagulation and protein C pathways. Thrombin can be either procoagulant (*left*) or anticoagulant (*right*) depending on cofactors and surfaces. Coagulant thrombin clots fibrinogen and activates platelets, factor V, factor VIII, factor XI, and factor XIII. Conversion of zymogen protein C to anticoagulant APC by thrombomodulin-bound thrombin is enhanced by endothelial protein C receptor (EPCR). APC with its nonenzymatic cofactor, protein S, inactivates factors Va and VIIIa by highly selective proteolysis (e.g., at Arg506 and Arg306 in factor Va), yielding inactivated (i) factors V_i and VIII_i. This anticoagulant action may be enhanced by platelets, endothelial cells, or their microparticles. HDL can also provide protein S-dependent anticoagulant APC-cofactor activity. The direct actions of protein S inhibiting generation of thrombin by directly reacting with factors Va and Xa are also indicated. Adapted from Griffin with permission.[308]

of thrombin. Because of synergy among various cellular and humoral anticoagulant mechanisms that establish a threshold system, the presence of multiple coagulation inhibitors with complementary modes of action prevents massive thrombin generation in the absence of a substantial procoagulant stimulus.

HEREDITARY DEFICIENCIES ASSOCIATED WITH THROMBOTIC DISEASE

Evidence for the physiologic importance of specific factors for controlling coagulation reactions comes from clinical observations and animal model studies. Major identified genetic risk factors for venous thrombosis involve protein structural defects in factor V, protein C, protein S, and antithrombin. There are also gene regulatory defects associated with thrombotic disease such as the nt G20210A polymorphism in the prothrombin gene that causes elevated levels of prothrombin and the defects in protein C regulatory elements that decrease the expression of protein C (see Chap. 127). Deficiencies of thrombomodulin are less well established as clinically significant, but they may be associated with increased risk of arterial thrombosis (see Chap 127). Hereditary abnormalities of EPCR have not yet been definitively linked to increased risks of thrombosis.

PROTEIN C PATHWAY COMPONENTS

Schematic representations of the structures of protein C, protein S, thrombomodulin, and EPCR are shown in Fig. 113-2. These proteins contain multiple domains, each of which may mediate different molecular functions. Values for the molecular weight, normal plasma concentration, chromosomal location, and gene structures of these factors are given in Table 113-1. Factors Va and VIIIa, as substrates of APC, are also participants in the reactions of the protein C pathway. Moreover, certain forms of factor V can also act as an APC cofactor,[30,31] as detailed below.

PROTEIN C

In 1976, Stenflo designated a bovine plasma vitamin-K-dependent protein that eluted in the third peak (peak C) from an anion exchange column as bovine "protein C."[32] Protein C was found to be identical to a previously identified anticoagulant factor, autoprothrombin II-A.[33,34] Biochemical studies showed that protein C is a zymogen that can be isolated from either bovine or human plasma and that can be converted to an anticoagulantly active serine protease by the action of thrombin.[35,36]

Protein C is synthesized in the liver as a polypeptide precursor of 461 residues, with a prepropeptide of 42 amino acids that contains the signal for carboxylation of Glu residues by a carboxylase that forms 9 γ-carboxyglutamic acid (Gla) residues and secretion of the mature protein.[37–40] The mature glycoprotein of M_r 62,000 contains 419 residues (Fig. 113-2) and N-linked carbohydrate, and the majority of the secreted protein C molecules are cleaved by a furin-like endoprotease that releases Lys156-Arg157 and generates a two-chain zymogen that circulates in plasma at 70 nM (4 μg/ml).[41–43] The heavy and light chains of plasma protein C are covalently linked by a disulfide bond that keeps the serine protease globular domain (residues 170–419) covalently tethered to the N-terminal string of three domains, the Gla domain and the epidermal growth-factor-like domains EGF1 and EGF2 (Fig. 113-2).[37–40,44–46]

The Gla domain of protein C (residues 1–42) and of APC is important for a number of functions, including binding of these proteins to phospholipid-containing membranes, thrombomodulin, and EPCR; thus, incomplete carboxylation impairs the functional anticoagulant activity of APC.[47–52] The EGF1 domain undergoes an unusual posttranslational modification resulting in β-hydroxyaspartic acid at residue 71, and this modification appears essential for full anticoagulant activity.[53,54] The two EGF modules in the light chain may also contribute to interactions of APC with protein S and of protein C with thrombomodulin. The C-terminus of the light chain is implicated in binding of APC to its substrate, factor Va.[55]

The serine protease domain of protein C is homologous to other chymotrypsin-like proteases, and three-dimensional modeling[56,57] and x-ray crystallographic structures[46] reflect the structural similarity of APC to members of the serine protease family. The serine protease domain of APC exerts its trypsin-like anticoagulant activity by highly specific interactions with factors Va and VIIIa followed by cleavage at only two Arg-containing peptide bonds (see below). APC residues 390 to 404 and 311 to 325 appear to contribute to specific recognition of factor Va.[58,59]

Purified protein C concentrates have been successfully used to treat patients with thrombotic episodes.[60–63]

PROTEIN C GENE

The protein C gene, comprising nine exons and eight introns, is located on chromosome 2q14-21 and spans 11 kb (see Fig. 112-12, Table 113-1).[64–69] The protein C gene is homologous to the genes for factors VII, IX, and X (see Chap. 112).

PROTEIN C MUTATIONS

Many different mutations in the protein C gene have been identified that cause protein C deficiency associated with thrombosis, and a database of more than 100 different mutations was published.[70] Based on three-dimensional models of the protease domain of protein C, the structural basis for protein C defects has been rationalized.[57,71,72] Most mutations that cause type I protein C deficiency, characterized by parallel reductions in activity and antigen, involve amino acid residues that form the hydrophobic cores of the two folded globulin-like domains that are characteristic of serine proteases. These mutations destabilize either the process or the product of protein folding, and they result in unstable molecules that are poorly secreted and/or exhibit a very short circulatory half-life. In contrast, most mutations that cause type II defects (reduced activity but normal antigen levels), i.e., circulating dysfunctional molecules, involve polar surface residues that do not affect polypeptide folding or thermodynamic stability; these polar residues presumably are involved in protein-protein interactions important for expression of anticoagulant activity.

A murine model of severe protein C deficiency due to homozygous knockout of the mouse protein C gene showed a similar phenotype as severe human protein C deficiency (Chap. 127), with perinatal consumptive coagulopathy in the brain and liver and either death or massive thrombosis that occurred either intrauterine or shortly after birth.[73]

PROTEIN S

Protein S was first purified from plasma by DiScipio and colleagues who named it *protein S* in honor of Seattle, the city of its discovery.[74,75] It is a vitamin-K-dependent glycoprotein that is synthesized by hepatocytes, neuroblastoma cells, kidney cells, testis, megakaryocytes, and endothelial cells[76–80] and is found in platelet α-granules.[81] Protein S is inducible by IL-4 in T cells.[82]

Protein S is synthesized as a precursor protein of 676 amino acids which gives rise to a mature secreted single-chain glycoprotein of 635 residues with three *N*-linked carbohydrate side chains (Fig. 113-2, Table 113-1).[83–86] Eleven Gla residues in the N-terminal region of mature protein S contribute to Ca^{2+}-mediated binding of the protein to phospholipid membranes. The thrombin-sensitive region (TSR), residues 47 to 72, follows the Gla-domain (Fig. 113-2). Four EGF modules each contain one unusual residue of β-hydroxyaspartic acid or β-hydroxyasparagine whose function has not been established, although they likely contribute to Ca^{2+}-binding.[84,87–89]

The C-terminal region of protein S, residues 270 to 635, the sex-hormone-binding globulin (SHBG)-like region contains binding sites for C4b-binding protein (C4BP) (see below)[90,91] and for factor V as well as factor Va.[92,93] Thus, different domains of protein S exhibit a number of different binding sites for different plasma proteins.

PROTEIN S GENE

The protein S gene, comprising 15 exons and 14 introns, is located on chromosome 3p11.1-11.2 and spans 80 kb (see Fig. 112-13, Table 113-1).[68,94–101] The protein S gene has limited homology with other genes for vitamin-K-dependent factors in the Gla and EGF domains (see Chap. 112) and notable homology of the region coding for residues 240 to 635 with genes of the SHBG family. Because humans contain a protein S pseudogene that contains several stop codons and is not translated, the normal active gene is designated as the protein S 1 or protein Sα gene, and the pseudogene is protein S 2 or protein Sβ gene. The pseudogene is 97 percent homologous with the normal gene and is located very near the normal protein S gene on chromosome 3.

PROTEIN S MUTATIONS

Many different mutations in the protein S gene have been identified that cause protein S deficiency associated with thrombosis, and a

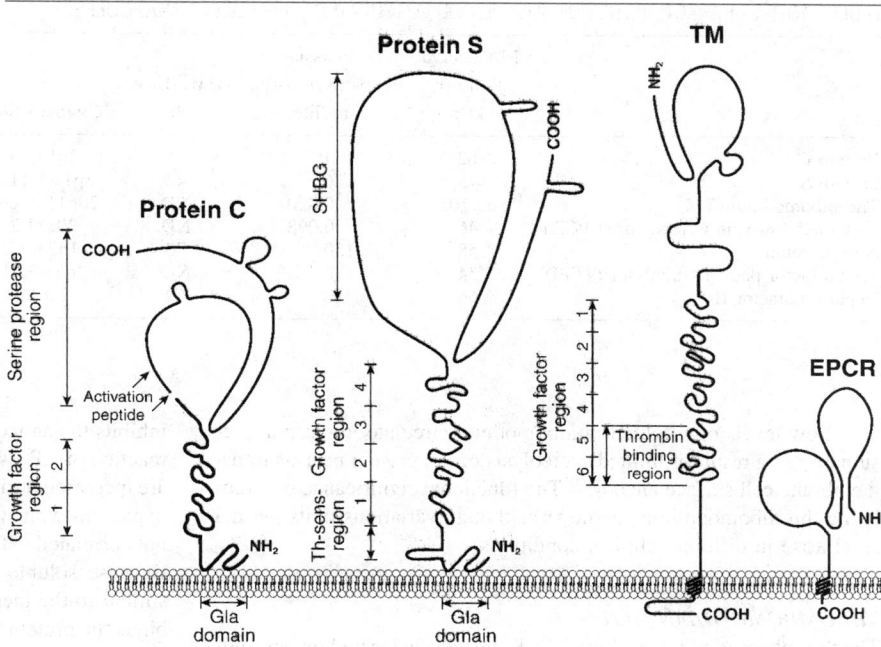

FIGURE 113-2 Membrane-bound protein C, protein S, thrombomodulin, and the endothelial cell protein C receptor (EPCR). Each protein is a multidomain protein that extends above the surface of cell membranes, and different domains mediate different functions of each protein. Protein C and protein S can bind reversibly to phospholipid membranes through their NH$_2$-terminal domains which contain 9 or 11 γ-carboxyglutamic acid (Gla) residues that bind 4 to 6 Ca^{2+} ions. Thrombomodulin and EPCR are integral membrane proteins that are embedded in cell membranes by a single hydrophobic transmembrane sequence. Adapted from Esmon with permission.[108]

database of more than 100 different mutations was published.[102] One protein S polymorphism present in less than 1 percent of Caucasians causes replacement of Ser460 by Pro and results in absence of *N*-linked carbohydrate on Asn458 in the variant, designated protein S Heerlen.[103] The functional consequences of the absence of this carbohydrate or of the presence of Pro460 for protein S functions have not been established.

THROMBOMODULIN

Thrombomodulin was discovered and named by Esmon and Owen, who demonstrated that endothelial cell surfaces possess a nonenzymatic cofactor that accelerates protein C activation by thrombin.[104,105] Moreover, binding of thrombin to thrombomodulin converts thrombin from a procoagulant enzyme to an anticoagulant enzyme because thrombomodulin-bound thrombin loses its normal ability to clot fibrinogen or activate platelets.[106,107] Thrombomodulin is a multidomain transmembrane protein comprising an N-terminal lectin-like domain, six EGF domains, a Ser/Thr-rich region, a single membrane-spanning sequence, and an intracellular C-terminal tail (Fig. 113-2).[108–113] Much is known about structure-function relationships of this protein.[108,114–119] EGF domains 4, 5, and 6 are essential for activation of protein C, with the latter two domains binding thrombin and the first domain binding protein C. The mature protein has 557 amino acid residues and variable amounts of *N*-linked and *O*-linked carbohydrates that cause variability in molecular size. Glycosaminoglycans, notably chondroitin sulfate, covalently attached to the Ser/Thr-rich region, contribute to the functional properties of thrombomodulin by enhancing either protein C activation by thrombin or by accelerating neutralization of thrombin by protease inhibitors. Modulation of the substrate specificity of thrombin by thrombomodulin involves conformational changes in thrombin caused by binding of thrombomodulin.[120,121]

TABLE 113-1   CHARACTERISTICS OF SOME BLOOD COAGULATION REGULATORY MOLECULES

	MOLECULAR WEIGHT, kDa	PLASMA CONCENTRATION, mg/liter	HALF-LIFE, h	CHROMOSOME	GENE, kb	EXONS, N	FUNCTION
Protein C	62	4	6	2q13-14	11	9	Anticoagulant protease
Protein S	75	26	42	3p11.1-11.2	80	15	APC-cofactor coagulation inhibitor
Thrombomodulin (TM)	60-105	0.020	ND	20p11.2–cen	3.7	1	Receptor for thrombin/protein C
Endothelial protein C receptor (EPCR)	46	0.098	ND	20q11.2	6	4	Receptor for protein C/APC
Antithrombin	58	150	70	1q23-25	14	7	Protease inhibitor
Tissue factor pathway inhibitor (TFPI)	34	0.1	ND	2q31-32.1	85	9	Protease inhibitor
Heparin cofactor II	66	70	60	22q11	16	5	Protease inhibitor

Low levels of soluble thrombomodulin circulate in plasma, presumably as a result of limited proteolysis of the protein near its transmembrane cell surface anchor.[122] The functional significance of circulating thrombomodulin is unknown, although variations in its plasma level arise in different clinical conditions.

THROMBOMODULIN GENE

The thrombomodulin gene, which lacks introns, is located on chromosome 20p12 and spans 3.7 kb (Fig. 112-21) (Table 113-1).[111,112,123,124] Down-regulation of the thrombomodulin gene is stimulated by a variety of inflammatory agents, including endotoxin, IL-1, and TNF-α and is up-regulated by retinoic acid (see Esmon[125]). In general, agents that down-regulate thrombomodulin expression usually up-regulate tissue factor expression in a manner consistent with the general concept that these cellular factors exert opposing activities on the hemostatic balance.

THROMBOMODULIN MUTATIONS

Inherited deficiencies of thrombomodulin are not well established as clinically significant, but they may be associated with increased risk of thrombosis.[126–128]

ENDOTHELIAL PROTEIN C RECEPTOR

An endothelial cell protein C receptor (EPCR) that binds both protein C and APC was cloned by Fukudome and Esmon in 1994.[129] Subsequent studies, especially those by Esmon's laboratory, have defined many properties of the murine, bovine, and human EPCR.[52,130–140]

The mature EPCR glycoprotein contains 221 amino acid residues and N-linked carbohydrate, giving an Mr of 46,000. EPCR is an integral membrane protein that is homologous to CD1/MHC class I molecules. The N-terminus is part of an extracellular domain which is connected to a single transmembrane sequence that is followed by a short Arg-Arg-Cys-COOH cytoplasmic tail (Fig. 113-2). The cytoplasmic tail can be palmitoylated, and this modification may localize EPCR to caveolae.[140] EPCR binds protein C and APC equally well and appears to do so through their Gla domains. EPCR is mainly located on the surface of large vessels, in contrast to the predominant localization of thrombomodulin in the microcirculation. EPCR on endothelial surfaces enhances by fivefold the rate of activation of protein C by thrombin:thrombomodulin, as depicted in Fig. 113-3. Based on the homology between EPCR and CD1/MHC class I molecules, a three-dimensional model of EPCR was constructed, allowing speculation about EPCR structure-function relationships.[141]

Soluble EPCR is found in normal human plasma at 100 ng/ml; in purified reaction mixtures, soluble EPCR at relatively high levels inhibits the anticoagulant action of APC against factor Va but not the reaction of APC with protease inhibitors.[131,142] Levels of soluble EPCR are increased during disseminated intravascular coagulation (DIC) and in patients with systemic lupus erythematosus, and EPCR increases are not correlated with alterations in circulating thrombomodulin levels.[143] Because soluble EPCR binds protein C and APC with an affinity similar to the membrane-bound molecule, it is speculated that EPCR binds the protein C and the APC Gla domains without thermodynamically significant contributions from membrane phospholipids.

APC is thought to exert anti-inflammatory activity that is independent of its anticoagulant activity[144,145] (for review, see Esmon[140]). It is possible that EPCR in APC:EPCR complexes modulates the biologic activity of APC by shifting its proteolytic specificity toward currently unknown substrates. Currently, the involvement of EPCR in physiologic hemostasis is unknown.

EPCR GENE

The EPCR gene, comprising four exons and three introns, is located on chromosome 20q11.2 and spans 6 kb.[146]

ACTIVATION OF PROTEIN C

Protein C is converted to an active serine protease due to cleavage by thrombin at the Arg169-Leu170 peptide bond in a Ca^{2+}-dependent reaction that is accelerated by orders of magnitude by thrombomodulin (see above).[35,36,105]

Proof that thrombin is a physiologic activator of protein C includes the demonstrations that thrombin infusions into baboons generate anticoagulant activity due to APC.[147,148] Interestingly, thrombin infusion

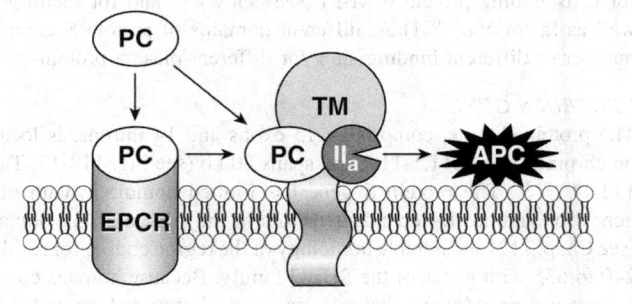

FIGURE 113-3   Thrombin-dependent activation of protein C on cell surface. On an endothelial surface, protein C (PC) is activated by limited proteolysis by the thrombin:thrombomodulin complex (IIa:TM) which liberates a dodecapeptide (residues 158–169) from protein C to generate the anticoagulant serine protease, activated protein C (APC). This proteolytic activation of protein C is accelerated fivefold by the endothelial cell protein C receptor (EPCR). Based on the scheme of van de Poel with permission.[256]

into hyperlipidemic monkeys with atherosclerosis generated less APC and caused a poorer ex vivo response to APC compared with normolipidemic control monkeys,[149] showing that hyperlipidemia and vascular disease can affect protein C activation.

Proof that thrombomodulin is a physiologic antithrombotic cofactor comes from studies of mice containing a targeted point mutation in thrombomodulin that markedly impairs its ability to activate protein C. Mice with a specific Glu to Pro mutation in the loop between EGF4 and EGF5 in thrombomodulin have a hypercoagulable state, fibrin deposition, and a severely reduced ability to activate protein C.[150,151] However, thrombomodulin has additional biologic functions, including a critical as yet undefined role in fetal development, because complete knockout of the thrombomodulin gene is associated with embryonic lethality before development of an intact cardiovascular system.[152] Factor Va also enhances the rate of activation of protein C by thrombin, although the physiologic significance of this reaction has not been assessed.[153]

Proof that ischemia causes protein C activation in vivo comes from several studies. Even a brief occlusion of the left anterior descending coronary artery in pigs results in APC generation.[154] During cerebral ischemia in humans undergoing routine endarterectomy, APC increases in the venous cerebral blood.[155] Protein C is significantly activated during cardiopulmonary bypass, mainly during the minutes immediately after aortic unclamping in the ischemic vascular beds.[156] Streptokinase therapy for acute myocardial infarction increases circulating APC.[157]

Circulating APC concentration in normal human subjects is highly correlated with circulating levels of protein C zymogen.[158] Based on protein C infusion studies in protein-C-deficient subjects, it appears that basal activation of protein C is strongly determined by the concentration of protein C.[159]

Although EPCR has not yet been shown to contribute to physiologic protein C activation, in vitro studies of thrombin-dependent protein C activation using purified EPCR and thrombomodulin in reconstituted phospholipid vesicles shows that EPCR without negatively charged phospholipids can provide the surface for protein C activation by thrombin:thrombomodulin, suggesting that EPCR concentration in different vascular beds will determine the effectiveness of the thrombin:thrombomodulin complex.[135] This concept for protein C activation is presented in Fig. 113-3, which schematically indicates phospholipid-independent activation of protein C. This model for protein C activation allows EPCR to substitute for negatively charged phospholipids, and it also implies that a cellular response to a specific stimulus might bring EPCR and thrombomodulin in close proximity such that protein C activation is enhanced by a specific agonist that itself does not generate thrombin or up-regulate thrombomodulin (see Fig. 113-3).

Thrombomodulin is abundantly present in the small blood vessels but less so in large vessels, whereas EPCR is more abundant in large vessels than in small vessels.[125] Thrombomodulin levels vary markedly in different tissues,[160] with significant consequences for a variable tendency for fibrin deposition in different organs.[108,140,150,151] In contrast to an initial report that thrombomodulin is absent in brain,[161] low levels are expressed in brain,[162–165] and brain-specific activation of protein C in humans occurs during carotid occlusion.[155]

Proteolytic cleavage and activation of protein C can also be effected by meizothrombin, plasmin, or factor Xa.[166–169] On the surface of cultured endothelial cells, negatively charged sulfated polysaccharides in the presence of phospholipid vesicles containing phosphatidyl ethanolamine can enhance the rate of protein C activation by factor Xa to approach the protein C activation rate of thrombin:thrombomodulin.[169] No data have indicated whether protein C activation by plasmin or factor Xa is physiologically relevant.

EXPRESSION OF ACTIVATED PROTEIN C ACTIVITY

The mechanism of APC anticoagulant activity involves factors V and VIII, the two homologous coagulation cofactors that circulate as inactive molecules and are converted to active cofactors by limited proteolysis (see Chap. 112 and Figs. 112-15 and 112-17). APC circulates at 40 pM in normal humans, and there is an inverse correlation between fibrinopeptide A and APC levels in healthy nonsmoking adults, suggesting APC is a significant regulator of basal thrombin activity.[22,170] In contrast to the availability of substantial information about the modes of action of APC and protein S as anticoagulant factors, no specific molecular mechanisms for the expression of anti-inflammatory activity by APC and/or protein S have been demonstrated.

Factors V and VIII are synthesized as large single-chain precursor coagulation cofactors of M_r 330,000, consisting of three homologous A domains (A1, A2, and A3) and two homologous C domains (C1 and C2) with a very large intervening, generally nonhomologous domain, designated the *B domain*, that connects the A2 and A3 domains. In factors Va and VIIIa, the A domains form heterotrimeric structures like ceruloplasmin, while the C domains form head-to-tail heterodimeric structures.[171–174] As depicted in Fig. 113-4, activation of factor V is accomplished by limited proteolysis at Arg709, Arg1018, and Arg1545 by thrombin, factor Xa, or other proteases; cleavage at Arg1545 is the key step for generating factor Va. The various forms of factor Va (Fig. 113-4) are composed of two polypeptide chains, one bearing the A1-A2 domains and the other bearing the A3-C1-C2 domains. The noncovalent interactions between the two chains are stabilized by Ca^{2+} ions because these chains dissociate in the absence of divalent metal ions. Although generally similar to factor V activation, factor VIII activation (Fig. 112-17) involves formation of a heterotrimer of polypeptide chains, one each containing the A1 domain, the A2 domain, and the A3-C1-C2 domains respectively. In contrast to heterodimeric factor Va, heterotrimeric factor VIIIa is intrinsically unstable due to spontaneous dissociation of the A2 domain.[175]

FACTORS Va AND VIIIa AS SUBSTRATES AND APC RESISTANCE

Irreversible proteolytic inactivation of factors Va and VIIIa by APC can be accomplished by proteolysis at Arg506 and Arg306 in factor Va and Arg562 and Arg362 in factor VIIIa[8,175–181] (Figs. 112-15, 112-17, 112-5). Currently, the most common identifiable venous thrombosis risk factor involves a mutation of Arg506 to Gln in factor V that results in APC resistance (see Chap. 127). The complexities of APC-dependent inactivation of factor Va and VIIIa are compounded by the number of different molecular forms of Va and VIIIa that can be generated by limited proteolysis by a variety of proteases and by their differing susceptibilities to APC and to the different APC cofactors. While some elements of these complexities are clear, most details are not presently well understood, and APC resistance can be caused by a number of molecular defects in APC cofactors or in APC's substrates.

APC RESISTANCE

APC resistance is defined as an abnormally reduced anticoagulant response of a plasma sample to APC (see Chap. 127) and can be caused by many potential abnormalities in the protein C pathway. Such abnormalities could include defective APC cofactors, defective APC substrates, or antibodies or other agents that interfere with the normal functioning of the protein C pathway.

A report of familial venous thrombosis associated with APC resistance without any identifiable defect led to an intensive search for a genetic explanation[182] that was soon found to involve replacement of G by A at nucleotide 1691 in exon 10 of the factor V gene which

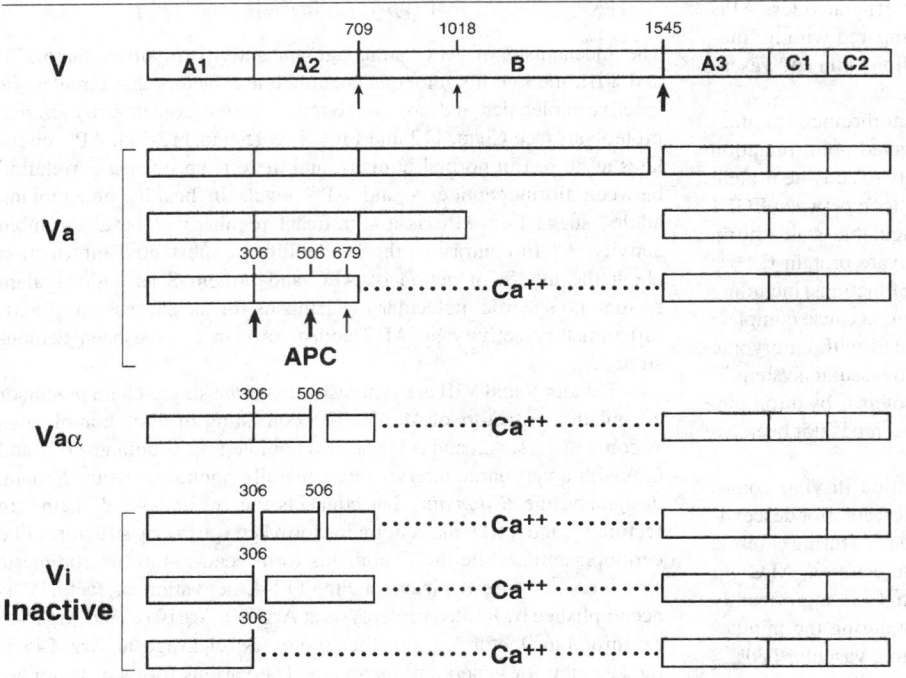

FIGURE 113-4   Proteolytic activation and inactivation of factors V and Va. Lines represent polypeptide structures of factor V, active factor Va species, and inactive factor V$_i$. Activation of factor V by thrombin, factor Xa, or Russell's viper's venom is associated with cleavages at Arg709, Arg1018, and Arg1545. Inactivation of factor Va by APC involves cleavages at Arg506, Arg306, and Arg679. If factor Va is cleaved by APC only at Arg506, designated as *factor Vaα*, it exhibits approximately 70 percent procoagulant activity. Cleavage at Arg306 is the most important cleavage for full inactivation of factor Va and is markedly phospholipid-dependent and enhanced approximately 20-fold by protein S. Protein S–dependent cleavage at Arg306 by APC is also enhanced by HDL. The bottom line indicates that dissociation of the A2 domain is associated with inactivation of factor Va. Based on an unpublished scheme of T. Hackeng with permission.

causes the amino acid replacement of Arg506 by Gln.[8,183–185] This factor V variant, which arose in a single Caucasian founder some 21,000 to 34,000 years ago,[186] is known as *Gln506-factor V* or *factor V Leiden*. This mutation is currently a common, but not the only, cause of APC resistance.

The molecular mechanism for APC resistance of Gln506-factor V is based on the fact that the variant molecule is inactivated 10 times slower than normal Arg506-factor Va.[185,187–191] The variant factor Va exhibits only a partial resistance to APC because cleavage at Arg306 in factor Va also occurs, causing complete loss of factor Va activity. This finding helps explain why APC resistance due to Gln506-factor V is a rather mild risk factor for venous thrombosis and why a combination of genetic risk factors or a combination of a genetic and acquired risk factors for venous thrombosis is found in a significant fraction of symptomatic patients (see Chap. 127). Another possibility to help explain the mild risk of venous thrombosis associated with Gln506-factor V is that factor Va may be inactivated in vivo by proteases other than APC that cleave at sites other than residue Arg506.

A factor V haplotype, designated R2, has also been associated with mild APC resistance,[192] although it appears that the R2 haplotype may only be a risk factor when present along with a Gln506-factor V allele.[193]

Plasma and recombinant factor V can exist in two biochemically distinct forms, designated *factor V1* and *factor V2*.[194–197] Factor V1 has *N*-linked carbohydrate on Asn2181, near the phospholipid binding region of the C2 domain, whereas factor V2 has none. Because the *N*-linked carbohydrate appears to decrease the apparent affinity of

factor V1 or Va1 for phospholipid, it reduces the specific clotting activity and susceptibility to APC. Normal plasma contains a mixture of factors V1 and V2. Removal of the carbohydrate attached to factor V increases the rate of inactivation of factor Va by APC, although the clinical significance of this phenomenon is unknown.[198]

APC resistance with no identifiable genetic or acquired abnormalities is well described in patients with venous and arterial thrombosis.[199–203] Further studies are needed to identify the causes of APC resistance in these patients, and further work is needed to develop and compare various APC resistance assays that have different sensitivities to different physiologic variable or plasma components. For example, APTT-based assays are not equivalently sensitive as are dilute tissue-factor-based assays to plasma HDL levels or oral contraceptive use.[204,205] Plasma variables, such as prothrombin levels, may affect the response to APC by inhibiting APC action.[206]

VARIABLE PROTEOLYZED FORMS OF FACTORS Va AND VIIIa

Proteolytic activation of factors Va and VIIIa can generate different forms of each active cofactor that differ in specific activity. For example, factor VIIIa generated by factor Xa has lower specific activity and longer half-life than that generated by thrombin,[175,207] and factor Va generated by cleavage only at Arg709 and Arg1018 (without cleavage at Arg1545) has a lower specific activity than that generated after cleavage at Arg1545.[208] Factor Va can be cleaved at Arg1765, and this could generate forms of factor Va with differing specific activities.[209] Factor VIIa:tissue factor complexes can cleave factor V at novel sites to produce a form of factor V that can be destroyed by APC without the requirement for full activation of the cofactor precursor.[210]

APC COFACTORS

APC anticoagulant activity is enhanced by a number of factors that are termed APC cofactors; these include certain Ca^{2+} ions, phospholipids, protein S, factor V, and HDL.

Phospholipids as APC Cofactors   Certain phospholipids such as phosphatidyl serine, phosphatidyl ethanolamine, and cardiolipin enhance the anticoagulant activity of APC.[211–214]

Protein S   Protein S forms a 1:1 complex with APC[215] and enhances by 10- to 20-fold the rate of APC's cleavage at Arg306 in factor Va but not the Arg506 cleavage.[190] Part of the mechanism for this activity of protein S may be related to its ability to bring the active site of APC closer to the plane of the phospholipid membrane on which the APC:protein S complex is located when the complex is formed.[216,217] Protein S also facilitates the action of APC against factor VIIIa.[218,219] Protein S enhances APC's action, in part at least, by ablating the ability of factor Xa to protect factor Va from APC.[220] The TSR and EGF domains of protein S are implicated in binding APC for expression of anticoagulant activity by the APC:protein S complex.[221–226] Cleavage of the TSR by thrombin abolishes normal binding of protein S to phospholipid and its APC-cofactor anticoagulant activity.[227–230]

Factor V Factor V apparently can have anticoagulant as well as procoagulant properties because it enhances the anticoagulant action of APC against factor VIIIa in a reaction in which protein S acts synergistically with factor V.[30,31,231–233] Cleavage at Arg1545, which optimizes factor Va procoagulant activity, ablates the molecule's anticoagulant cofactor activity. However, when factor V is cleaved at Arg506 by APC, its APC cofactor activity is increased 10-fold. This suggests that Gln506-factor V has two potential prothrombotic defects, namely, resistance of the variant factor Va to APC inactivation and resistance of the variant factor V to activation of its APC cofactor function.[232]

High-Density Lipoprotein High-density lipoprotein (HDL) enhances the anticoagulant activity of APC both in plasma and in purified reaction mixtures. This APC cofactor activity requires protein S and involves, at least in part, stimulation of APC's cleavage at Arg306 in factor Va.[204] In animal models, HDL inhibits DIC induced by endotoxin infusion in baboons and ferric chloride–induced arterial thrombosis in rats.[234,235] HDL is heterogeneous in both protein and lipid composition, and the components responsible for this activity have not been identified. The clinical significance of this anticoagulant property of HDL is unknown.

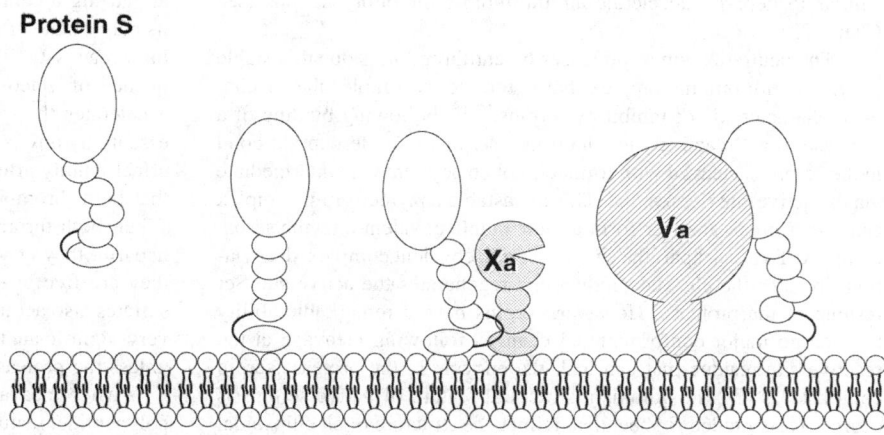

FIGURE 113-5   Protein S direct inhibition of prothrombin activation. Protein S inhibits directly the activity of the prothrombinase complex by reversibly binding to factor Va and/or factor Xa. On the left, protein S is depicted in solution and bound to a phospholipid (PL) membrane surface. On the right, inactive complexes of factors Va:PS and Xa:PS are depicted.[14–16] It is possible that ternary complexes of protein S:fVa:fXa also can exist.[248] Protein S can also bind factor VIIIa and inhibit activation of factor X by factor IXa:VIIIa complexes (not shown).[18] Based on an unpublished scheme of S. Yegneswaran with permission.

INHIBITION OF ACTIVATED PROTEIN C

APC is a normal component of circulating blood, and it likely contributes to antithrombotic surveillance mechanisms.[22] Circulating APC levels are determined by the balance of mechanisms for APC generation compared with mechanisms for APC inhibition and clearance. Determinants of APC generation include: (1) protein C zymogen levels; (2) endogenous thrombin generation; and (3) thrombomodulin and EPCR availability. Clearance of APC appears to be mainly caused by inhibition of APC by protease inhibitors.[236,237] The major plasma inhibitors of APC include α_1-antitrypsin, protein C inhibitor, and α_2-macroglobulin.[236,238–247]

PROTEIN S ANTICOAGULANT ACTIVITY

Protein S has both indirect and direct anticoagulant activity because of its ability to serve as a nonenzymatic APC cofactor (see above and Fig. 113-1) and because, independent of APC, it inhibits coagulation reactions by directly binding to procoagulant factors. APC-independent activity is based on the ability of protein S to inhibit directly the activity of the prothrombinase complex by reversibly binding to factor Va and/or factor Xa (Fig. 113-5).[14–16] As depicted in Fig. 113-5, protein S can bind factors Xa or Va to form inactive complexes. It is possible that ternary complexes of protein S:fVa:fXa might be formed.[248] The TSR and the EGF3 domains of protein S are thought to bind factor Xa, contributing to APC-independent anticoagulant activity.[222,249] Protein S can also bind factor VIIIa and inhibit activation of factor X by factor IXa:VIIIa complexes.[18,250]

C4b-binding protein is a plasma protein that enhances inactivation of the complement cascade by binding to C4b and promoting proteolytic inactivation of C4b by factor I. C4b-binding protein reversibly binds protein S with high affinity,[251–253] and formation of this complex affects some of the anticoagulant activities of protein S (see review by Dahlbäck[12]). When factor Va is the targeted substrate, the APC-cofactor activity of protein S is neutralized by its binding to C4b-binding protein.[254,255] However, the association of C4b-binding protein with protein S does not ablate its ability to serve as an APC cofactor when the substrate is factor VIIIa[256] or its ability to inhibit the prothrombinase complex. This latter observation is explained by the ability of C4b-binding protein to block binding of protein S to factor Va but not to factor Xa. C4b-binding protein in plasma is a heteropolymer containing two different kinds of disulfide-linked polypeptides, six or seven α chains and a single β chain, and the latter chain is responsible for binding protein S.[257–259] Residues 30 to 45 of the β chain bind to the SHBG domain of protein S.[90,260,261] Because the affinity of protein S for C4b-binding protein is so high, the amount of free protein S in plasma is determined by the absolute concentrations of the two proteins, such that normally there is approximately 240 nM protein S:C4b-binding protein complexes and 120 nM free protein S.[253] During an acute phase reaction, the level of the C4b-binding protein α chain but not the β chain is increased, so that the change in total C4b-binding protein does not alter the level of free and bound protein S.[262]

INHIBITION OF COAGULATION PROTEASES

Antithrombin, initially designated *antithrombin III*, is the clinically most important inhibitor of clotting factor proteases (see Chap 127). Antithrombin can neutralize all proteases of the intrinsic coagulation pathway, including thrombin and factors Xa, IXa, XIa, and XIIa, in reactions that are enhanced by heparin and related glycosaminoglycans (see Chap 112). Tissue factor pathway inhibitor (TFPI), previously also described as lipoprotein-associated coagulation inhibitor (LACI), can neutralize factors VIIa and Xa, proteases of the extrinsic coagulation pathway. In addition, other plasma protease inhibitors can neutralize various coagulation proteases, although the clinical significance of these reactions is less well defined than the reaction of antithrombin with thrombin.

ANTITHROMBIN

Antithrombin is synthesized in the liver and is present in plasma at 150 μg/ml. Antithrombin is a typical member of the serine protease inhibitor (serpin) superfamily.[263] Heparin and endogenous endothelial heparan sulfates, which are heterogeneous but structurally similar to heparin, accelerate antithrombin's inhibitory actions (see Chap 133).

The neutralization of proteases by antithrombin is due to a stable enzyme:antithrombin complex that is formed by a molecular mechanism characteristic of inhibitory serpins.[263-269] Following binding of a protease to a ''reactive site'' loop in a serpin, a single peptide bond in the serpin is cleaved with formation of an acyl-enzyme intermediate via the active site Ser residue. This metastable enzyme:serpin complex can either break apart or form a more stable covalent enzyme:serpin complex. To break apart the enzyme:serpin covalent complex, deacylation liberates the cleaved product and regenerates the active site Ser residue of the protease. However, serpins have a remarkable ability to undergo major conformational changes following cleavage at the reactive site residue that can lock the enzyme in the protease:serpin complex.[263,267-269] The dominant structural feature of native serpins is a large five-stranded β-sheet that defines the structure of an ellipsoidal protein. Following cleavage at the reactive center residue in the reactive center loop by a protease, this extended loop is able to partially or completely insert itself into the five-stranded β-sheet, forming a very stable six-stranded β-sheet. If this insertion reaction proceeds before deacylation occurs, then the protease remains covalently attached to the reactive center P1 residue through the protease's active site Ser residue, and a stable covalent protease:inhibitor complex is formed.

Heparin enhancement of the rate of reaction between antithrombin and thrombin is caused by two distinct effects of heparin, one involving conformational effects on antithrombin and the other involving ''approximation'' effects on both thrombin and antithrombin.[270-275] For the first effect, a particular pentasaccharide within heparin is most potent at causing a conformational change that converts antithrombin from its native state of moderate reactivity to a conformation with relatively high reactivity. This pentasaccharide contains a specific sulfated sequence of glucosamine and iduronic acid residues,[270,274,276,277] and it accelerates the reaction of antithrombin with not only thrombin but essentially any target protease. On the other hand, the approximation effect mainly affects its reaction with thrombin and is due to the fact that both thrombin and antithrombin have high affinity for heparin. When both thrombin and antithrombin are simultaneously bound to heparin, they encounter each other much more frequently than when they are free in solution, thus increasing the reaction rate. Heparan sulfates also act in this manner. This approximation mechanism is not very significant for proteases other than thrombin (e.g., factor Xa) unless the protease has a very high affinity for heparin.

After cleavage of a propeptide from a 464-residue precursor polypeptide, mature antithrombin contains 432 amino acid residues.[278] It has four sites for N-linked carbohydrate attachment, one of which (Asn135) is variably glycosylated, giving rise to a β-isoform that has higher affinity for heparin.[279,280] Heparin binding to antithrombin is mediated by a number of positively charged Arg and Lys residues that are located in the N-terminal sequence of the protein within residues 41 to 49 and 107 to 156, whereas the reactive center loop containing the scissile peptide bond at Arg393-Ser394 is near the C-terminus.

ANTITHROMBIN GENE

The antithrombin gene comprising seven exons and six introns spans 13.4 kb and is located on chromosome 1q23-25.[281-284]

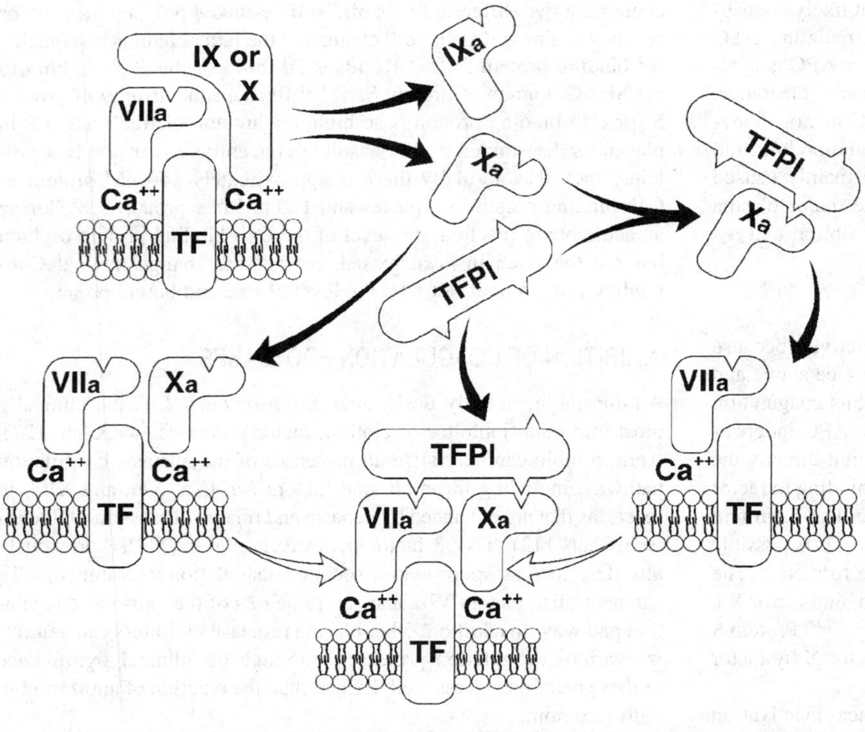

ANTITHROMBIN MUTATIONS

Hereditary deficiencies of antithrombin are well recognized as risk factors for venous thrombosis (see Chap 127). Over a hundred different mutations have been reported to be associated with thrombosis, and a complete database of mutations is published and is available on the world wide web through the courtesy of Lane and colleagues[285] at http://www.med.ic.ac.uk/dd/ddhc. Mutations that cause antithrombin deficiency are scattered throughout the molecule. Defects can be classified as type I, characterized by parallel decreases in antigen and activity, or type II, characterized by circulating dysfunctional molecules such that plasma has decreased activity but normal or near-normal antigen levels. Type II defects are further classified based on whether the dysfunction involves only reactive center defects (tested in the absence of heparin), only heparin-binding defects, or both of these properties (pleiotropic effects). Reactive center defects carry the largest risk of thrombosis, while heparin-binding defects are associated with less risk of venous thrombosis (see Chap 127).

FIGURE 113-6   Feedback inhibition of factor VIIa by TFPI in factor Xa:TFPI complexes. Surface-bound factor VIIa:tissue factor (TF) complexes generate factors IXa and Xa (*upper left*). Free TFPI is a multivalent protease inhibitor containing three Kunitz-type protease inhibitor domains. After factor Xa complexes with and is inhibited by the Kunitz-2 domain of TFPI, the Xa:TFPI complex (*right side*) can bind to and inhibit a TF:factor VIIa complex, forming a quaternary complex (*lower center*). Alternatively, TFPI might combine with a surface-bound ternary complex of TF:VIIa:Xa (*lower left*) to form a final quaternary complex (*lower center*). Adapted from Broze with permission.[9]

TISSUE FACTOR PATHWAY INHIBITOR

The mature TFPI protein, previously known as *lipoprotein-associated coagulation inhibitor* (LACI) or *extrinsic pathway inhibitor* (EPI), has an M_r of 34,000 and contains an acidic N-terminal sequence, three homologous but distinct Kunitz-type protease inhibitor domains, and a C-terminal positively charged basic amino acid sequence.[9,286]

Although present at only 100 ng/ml in normal plasma, TFPI is a significant inhibitor of the extrinsic coagulation pathway that functions synergistically with the protein C pathway and antithrombin to suppress thrombin generation. TFPI is synthesized by endothelial cells and smooth muscle cells.[9,287] Approximately half of TFPI in plasma is associated with lipoproteins, mainly LDL, and a substantial amount of TFPI is released when heparin is infused.[288,289]

Studies from the laboratories of Broze and others support the reaction scheme for neutralization of factors Xa and VIIa by TFPI depicted in Fig. 113-6.[9,99,290–293] Initially, the second Kunitz domain of TFPI reacts with and inhibits the active site of factor Xa. Subsequently, this binary complex reacts with factor VIIa in the TF:VIIa complex to form a quaternary protein complex on a membrane. TFPI can react with factor VIIa in the absence of factor Xa, but at a much slower rate. Interestingly, TFPI can neutralize factor Xa when the enzyme is bound in a prothrombinase complex, i.e., in a Xa:Va:phospholipid complex. Because TFPI requires factor Xa for kinetically favorable reactions with factor VIIa, TFPI does not shut off the initiation of the extrinsic pathway by tissue factor until some significant amount of factor Xa is generated. Then TFPI provides negative feedback inhibition of the generation of factor Xa by the VIIa:tissue factor complex. For hemostasis, amplification of an initiating signal generated by tissue factor then requires extensive thrombin generation by the intrinsic pathway that is caused by the positive feedback action of thrombin (see Fig. 113-1 and Chap. 112).

Proof that TFPI functions physiologically as an inhibitor of coagulation comes from animal model studies showing that depletion of TFPI predisposes animals to endotoxin-induced DIC and the generalized Schwarzman reaction and that treatment of animals with TFPI reduces mortality from *E. coli* septic shock.[294–296] Mice carrying complete deficiency of TFPI in gene knockout studies do not survive beyond the neonatal period and die of hemorrhage with signs of fibrin formation, suggestive of consumptive coagulopathy.[297]

TFPI GENE

The sequence of TFPI was established from cloning of its cDNA and the TFPI gene that contains 9 exons, spans 85 kb, and is located on chromosome 2q31-32.1.[286,298,299]

TFPI MUTATIONS

Hereditary abnormalities of TFPI have not yet been definitively associated with an increased risk of thrombosis, although one recent report has suggested a linkage to venous thrombosis.[300]

OTHER PROTEASE INHIBITORS

Thrombin in plasma can be inhibited not only by antithrombin but also by α_2-macroglobulin, an acute phase reactant. Heparin cofactor II, a serpin whose inhibitory activity is greatly enhanced by dermatan sulfate, also inhibits thrombin in vivo and in vitro by an approximation mechanism.[301,302] In purified reaction mixtures, protein C inhibitor also efficiently neutralizes thrombin in the presence of thrombomodulin.[303,304] Hereditary defects of protease inhibitors other than antithrombin have not yet been linked to an increased risk of thrombosis, although several reports linking heparin cofactor II deficiency to venous thrombosis have appeared.[305–307]

REFERENCES

1. Loscalzo J, Schafer AI: *Thrombosis and Hemorrhage*, edited by J Loscalzo, AI Schafer. Williams & Wilkins, Baltimore, 1998.
2. Colman RW, Hirsh J, Marder VJ, Salzman EW: *Hemostasis and Thrombosis*, edited by RW Colman, J Hirsh, VJ Marder, EW Salzman. Lippincott, Philadelphia, 1994.
3. MacFarlane RG: An enzyme cascade in the blood clotting mechanism and its function as a biological amplifier. *Nature* 202:498, 1964.
4. Davie EW, Ratnoff OD: Waterfall sequence for intrinsic blood clotting. *Science* 145:1310, 1964.
5. Davie EW, Fujikawa K, Kisiel W: The coagulation cascade: initiation, maintenance, and regulation. *Biochemistry* 30:10363, 1991.
6. Furie B, Furie BC: The molecular basis of blood coagulation. *Cell* 53:505, 1988.
7. Lammle B, Griffin JH: Formation of the fibrin clot: the balance of procoagulant and inhibitory factors. *Clin Haematol* 14:281, 1985.
8. Kane WH, Davie EW: Blood coagulation factors V and VIII: structural and functional similarities and their relationship to hemorrhagic and thrombotic disorders. *Blood* 71:539, 1988.
9. Broze GJ Jr: Tissue factor pathway inhibitor and the revised theory of coagulation. *Annu Rev Med* 46:103, 1995.
10. Bouma BN, dem Borne PA, Meijers JC: Factor XI and protection of the fibrin clot against lysis—a role for the intrinsic pathway of coagulation in fibrinolysis. *Thromb Haemost* 80:24, 1998.
11. Esmon CT: The regulation of natural anticoagulant pathways. *Science* 235:1348, 1987.
12. Dahlbäck B, Stenflo J: The protein C anticoagulant system, in *The Molecular Basis of Blood Diseases*, p 599. Saunders, Philadelphia, 1994.
13. Mitchell CA, Kelemen SM, Salem HH: The anticoagulant properties of a modified form of protein S. *Thromb Haemost* 60:298, 1988.
14. Heeb MJ, Mesters RM, Tans G, Rosing J, Griffin JH: Binding of protein S to factor Va associated with inhibition of prothrombinase that is independent of activated protein C. *J Biol Chem* 268:2872, 1993.
15. Heeb MJ, Rosing J, Bakker HM, et al: Protein S binds to and inhibits factor Xa. *Proc Natl Acad Sci USA* 91:2728, 1994.
16. Hackeng TM, van't Veer C, Meijers JCM, Bouma BN: Human protein S inhibits prothrombinase complex activity on endothelial cells and platelets via direct interactions with factors Va and Xa. *J Biol Chem* 269:21051, 1994.
17. Van't Veer C, Hackeng TM, Biesbroeck D, Sixma JJ, Bouma BN: Increased prothrombin activation in protein S-deficient plasma under flow conditions on endothelial cell matrix: an independent anticoagulant function of protein S in plasma. *Blood* 85:1815, 1995.
18. Koppelman SJ, Hackeng TM, Sixma JJ, Bouma BN: Inhibition of the intrinsic factor X activating complex by protein S: evidence for a specific binding of protein S to factor VIII. *Blood* 86:1062, 1995.
19. Van't Veer C, Butenas S, Golden NJ, Mann KG: Regulation of prothrombinase activity by protein S. *Thromb Haemost* 82:80, 1999.
20. Wildgoose P, Nemerson Y, Hansen LL, et al: Measurement of basal levels of factor VIIa in hemophilia A and B patients. *Blood* 80:25, 1992.
21. Morrissey JH, Macik BG, Neuenschwander PF, Comp PC: Quantitation of activated factor VII levels in plasma using a tissue factor mutant selectively deficient in promoting factor VII activation. *Blood* 81:734, 1993.
22. Gruber A, Griffin JH: Direct detection of activated protein C in blood from human subjects. *Blood* 79:2340, 1992.
23. Nossel HL, Yudelman I, Canfield RE, et al: Measurement of fibrinopeptide A in human blood. *J Clin Invest* 54:43, 1974.
24. Nossel HL: Radioimmunoassay of fibrinopeptides in relation to intravascular coagulation and thrombosis. *N Engl J Med* 295:428, 1976.
25. Bauer KA, Rosenberg RD: The pathophysiology of the prethrombotic state in humans: insights gained from studies using markers of hemostatic system activation. *Blood* 70:343, 1987.
26. Bauer KA, Kass BL, ten Cate H, et al: Detection of factor X activation in humans. *Blood* 74:2007, 1989.
27. Bauer KA, Kass BL, ten Cate H, Hawiger JJ, Rosenberg RD: Factor IX is activated in vivo by the tissue factor mechanism. *Blood* 76:731, 1990.
28. Jesty J, Beltrami E, Willems G: Mathematical analysis of a proteolytic positive-feedback loop: dependence of lag time and enzyme yields on the initial conditions and kinetic parameters. *Biochemistry* 32:6266, 1993.
29. Beltrami E, Jesty J: Mathematical analysis of activation thresholds in enzyme-catalyzed positive feedbacks: application to the feedbacks of blood coagulation. *Proc Natl Acad Sci USA* 92:8744, 1995.
30. Shen L, Dahlbäck B: Factor V and protein S as synergistic cofactors to activated protein C in degradation of factor VIIIa. *J Biol Chem* 269:18735, 1994.
31. Shen L, He X, Dahlbäck B: Synergistic cofactor function of factor V

and protein S to activated protein C in the inactivation of the factor VIIIa-Factor IXa complex. *Thromb Haemost* 78:1030, 1997.

32. Stenflo JA: A new vitamin K-dependent protein: purification from bovine plasma and preliminary characterization. *J Biol Chem* 251:355, 1976.

33. Seegers WH, Novoa E, Henry RL, Hassouna HI: Relationship of "new" vitamin K-dependent protein C and "old" autoprothrombin II-A. *Thromb Res* 8:543, 1976.

34. Marciniak E: Inhibitor of human blood coagulation elicited by thrombin. *J Lab Clin Med* 79:924, 1972.

35. Kisiel W, Canfield WM, Ericsson LH, Davie EW: Anticoagulant properties of bovine plasma protein C following activation by thrombin. *Biochemistry* 16:5824, 1977.

36. Kisiel W: Human plasma protein C. Isolation, characterization and mechanism of activation by α-thrombin. *J Clin Invest* 64:761, 1979.

37. Long GL, Balagje RM, MacGillivray RTA: Cloning and sequencing of liver cDNA coding for bovine protein C. *Proc Natl Acad Sci USA* 81:5653, 1984.

38. Foster D, Davie EW: Characterization of a cDNA coding for human protein C. *Proc Natl Acad Sci USA* 81:4766, 1984.

39. Beckman RJ, Schmidt RJ, Santerre RF, et al: The structure and evolution of a 461 amino acid human protein C precursor and its messenger RNA, based upon the DNA sequence of cloned human liver cDNA's. *Nucl Acids Res* 13:5233, 1985.

40. Foster DC, Rudinski MS, Schach BG, et al: Propeptide of human protein C is necessary for γ-carboxylation. *Biochemistry* 26:7003, 1987.

41. Hay CR: Factor VIII inhibitors in mild and moderate-severity haemophilia A. *Haemophilia* 4:558, 1998.

42. Heeb MJ, Schwarz HP, White T, et al: Immunoblotting studies of the molecular forms of protein C in plasma. *Thromb Res* 52:33, 1988.

43. Griffin JH, Evatt B, Zimmerman TS, Kleiss AJ, Wideman C: Deficiency of protein C in congenital thrombotic disease. *J Clin Invest* 68:1370, 1981.

44. Fernlund P, Stenflo JA: Amino acid sequence of the light chain of bovine protein C. *J Biol Chem* 257:12170, 1982.

45. Stenflo JA, Fernlund P: Amino acid sequence of the heavy chain of bovine protein C. *J Biol Chem* 257:12180, 1982.

46. Mather T, Oganessyan V, Hof P, et al: The 2.8 Å crystal structure of Gla-domainless activated protein C. *EMBO J* 15:6822, 1996.

47. Kurosawa S, Galvin JB, Esmon NL, Esmon CT: Proteolytic formation and properties of functional domains of thrombomodulin. *J Biol Chem* 262:2206, 1987.

48. Zhang L, Castellino FJ: A gamma-carboxyglutamic acid variant (gamma⁶D, gamma⁷D) of human activated protein C displays greatly reduced activity as an anticoagulant. *Biochemistry* 29:10828, 1990.

49. Zhang L, Castellino FJ: Role of the hexapeptide disulfide loop present in the gamma-carboxyglutamic acid domain of human protein C in its activation properties and in the in vitro anticoagulant activity of activated protein C. *Biochemistry* 30:6696, 1991.

50. Jhingan A, Zhang L, Christiansen WT, Castellino FJ: The activities of recombinant gamma-carboxyglutamic-acid-deficient mutants of activated human protein C toward human coagulation factor Va and factor VIII in purified systems and in plasma. *Biochemistry* 33:1869, 1994.

51. Zhang L, Castellino FJ: The binding energy of human coagulation protein C to acidic phospholipid vesicles contains a major contribution from leucine 5 in the gamma-carboxyglutamic acid domain. *J Biol Chem* 269:3590, 1994.

52. Regan LM, Mollica JS, Rezaie AR, Esmon CT: The interaction between the endothelial cell protein C receptor and protein C is dictated by the gamma-carboxyglutamic acid domain of protein C. *J Biol Chem* 272:26279, 1997.

53. Drakenberg T, Fernlund P, Roepstorff P, Stenflo J: Beta-hydroxyaspartic acid in vitamin K-dependent protein C. *Proc Natl Acad Sci USA* 80:1802, 1983.

54. Ohlin AK, Landes G, Bourdon P, et al: Beta-hydroxyaspartic acid in the first epidermal growth factor-like domain of protein C. Its role in Ca²⁺ binding and biological activity. *J Biol Chem* 263:19240, 1988.

55. Mesters RM, Heeb MJ, Griffin JH: A novel exosite in the light chain of human activated protein C essential for interaction with blood coagulation factor Va. *Biochemistry* 32:12656, 1993.

56. Fisher CL, Greengard JS, Griffin JH: Models of the serine protease domain of the human antithrombotic plasma factor activated protein C and its zymogen. *Protein Sci* 3:588, 1994.

57. Greengard JS, Fisher CL, Villoutreix B, Griffin JH: Structural basis for type I and type II deficiencies of antithrombotic plasma protein C: patterns revealed by three-dimensional molecular modeling of mutations of the protease domain. *Proteins* 18:367, 1994.

58. Mesters RM, Houghten RA, Griffin JH: Identification of a sequence of human activated protein C (residues 390-404) essential for its anticoagulant activity. *J Biol Chem* 266:24514, 1991.

59. Mesters RM, Heeb MJ, Griffin JH: Interactions and inhibition of blood coagulation factor Va involving residues 311–325 of activated protein C. *Protein Sci* 2:1482, 1993.

60. Dreyfus M, Magny JF, Bridey F, et al: Treatment of homozygous protein C deficiency and neonatal purpura fulminans with a purified protein C concentrate. *N Engl J Med* 325:1565, 1991.

61. Rivard GE, David M, Farrell C, Schwarz HP: Treatment of purpura fulminans in meningococcemia with protein C concentrate. *J Pediatr* 126:646, 1995.

62. Gerson WT, Dickerman JD, Bovill EG, Golden E: Severe acquired protein C deficiency in purpura fulminans associated with disseminated intravascular coagulation: treatment with protein C concentrate. *Pediatrics* 91:418, 1993.

63. Rintala E, Seppala OP, Kotilainen P, Pettila V, Rasi V: Protein C in the treatment of coagulopathy in meningococcal disease. *Crit Care Med* 26:965, 1998.

64. Foster DC, Yoshitake S, Davie EW: The nucleotide sequence of the gene for human protein C. *Proc Natl Acad Sci USA* 82:4673, 1985.

65. Esmon CT, Fukudome K: Cellular regulation of the protein C pathway. *Semin Cell Biol* 6:259, 1995.

66. Rocchi M, Roncuzzi L, Santamaria R, et al: Mapping through somatic cell hybrids and cDNA probes of protein C to chromosome 2, factor X to chromosome 13, and alpha 1-acid glycoprotein to chromosome 9. *Hum Genet* 74:30, 1986.

67. Kato A, Miura O, Sumi Y, Aoki N: Assignment of the human protein C gene (PROC) to chromosome region 2q14-q21 by in situ hybridization. *Cytogenet Cell Genet* 47:46, 1988.

68. Long GL, Marshall A, Gardner JC, Naylor SL: Genes for human vitamin K-dependent plasma proteins C and S are located on chromosomes 2 and 3, respectively. *Somat Cell Mol Genet* 140:93, 1988.

69. Patracchini P, Aiello V, Palazzi P, Calzolari E, Bernardi F: Sublocalization of the human protein C gene on chromosome 2q13-q14. *Hum Genet* 81:191, 1989.

70. Reitsma PH, Bernardi F, Doig RG, et al: Protein C deficiency: a database of mutations, 1995 update. On behalf of the Subcommittee on Plasma Coagulation Inhibitors of the Scientific and Standardization Committee of the ISTH. *Thromb Haemost* 73:876, 1995.

71. Greengard JS, Griffin JH, Fisher CL: Possible structural implications of 20 mutations in the protein C protease domain. *Thromb Haemost* 72:869, 1994.

72. Wacey AI, Pemberton S, Cooper DN, Kakkar VV, Tuddenham EGD: A molecular model of the serine protease domain of activated protein C: application to the study of missense mutations causing protein C deficiency. *Br J Haematol* 84:290, 1993.

73. Jalbert LR, Rosen ED, Moons L, et al: Inactivation of the gene for anticoagulant protein C causes lethal perinatal consumptive coagulopathy in mice. *J Clin Invest* 102:1481, 1998.

74. DiScipio RG, Hermodson MA, Yates SG, Davie EW: A comparison of human prothrombin, factor IX (Christmas factor), factor X (Stuart factor), and protein S. *Biochemistry* 16:698, 1977.

75. DiScipio RG, Davie EW: Characterization of protein S, a gamma-carboxyglutamic acid containing protein from bovine and human plasma. *Biochemistry* 18:899, 1979.

76. Fair DS, Marlar RA: Biosynthesis and secretion of factor VII, protein C, protein S, and the protein C inhibitor from a human hepatoma cell line. *Blood* 67:64, 1986.

77. Phillips DJ, Greengard JS, Fernández JA, et al: Protein S, an antithrombotic factor, is synthesized and released by neural tumor cells. *J Neurochem* 61:344, 1993.

78. Stern D, Brett J, Harris K, Nawroth P: Participation of endothelial cells in the protein C-protein S anticoagulant pathway: the synthesis and release of protein S. *J Cell Biol* 102:1971, 1986.

79. Malm J, He XH, Bjartell A, et al: Vitamin K-dependent protein S in Leydig cells of human testis. *Biochem J* 302:845, 1994.

80. Fair DS, Marlar RA, Levin EG: Human endothelial cells synthesize protein S. *Blood* 67:1168, 1986.

81. Schwarz HP, Heeb MJ, Wencel-Drake JD, Griffin JH: Identification and characterization of protein S in human platelets. *Blood* 66:1452, 1985.

82. Smiley ST, Boyer SN, Heeb MJ, Griffin JH, Grusby MJ: Protein S is inducible by interleukin 4 in T cells and inhibits lymphoid cell procoagulant activity. *Proc Natl Acad Sci USA* 94:11484, 1997.

83. Lundwall A, Dackowski W, Cohen E, et al: Isolation and sequence of the cDNA for human protein S, a regulator of blood coagulation. *Proc Natl Acad Sci USA* 83:6716, 1986.

84. Dahlbäck B, Lundwall A, Stenflo JA: Primary structure of bovine vitamin K-dependent protein S. *Proc Natl Acad Sci USA* 83:4199, 1986.

85. Ploos van Amstel HK, van der Zanden L, Reitsma PH, Bertina RM: Human protein S cDNA encodes Phe-16 and Tyr 222 in consensus sequences for the post-translational processing. *FEBS Lett* 222:186, 1987.

86. Hoskins J, Norman DK, Beckmann RJ, Long GL: Cloning and characterization of human liver cDNA encoding a protein S precursor. *Proc Natl Acad Sci USA* 84:349, 1987.

87. Stenflo JA, Lundwall A, Dahlbäck B: βHydroxyasparagine in domains homologous to the epidermal growth factor precursor in vitamin K-dependent protein S. *Proc Natl Acad Sci USA* 84:368, 1987.

88. Dahlbäck B, Hildebrand B, Linse S: Novel type of very high affinity calcium-binding sites in β-hydroxy-asparagine-containing epidermal growth factor-like domains in vitamin K-dependent protein S. *J Biol Chem* 265:18481, 1990.

89. Nelson RM, VanDusen WJ, Friedman PA, Long GL: α-Hydroxyaspartic acid and α-hydroxyasparagine residues in recombinant human protein S are not required for anticoagulant cofactor activity or for binding to C4b-binding protein. *J Biol Chem* 266:20586, 1991.

90. Fernández JA, Heeb MJ, Griffin JH: Identification of residues 413–433 of plasma protein S as essential for binding to C4b-binding protein. *J Biol Chem* 268:16788, 1993.

91. Chang GTG, Maas BHA, Ploos van Amstel HK, et al: The carboxy terminal loop of human protein S is involved in the interaction with C4b-binding protein. *Blood* 78 suppl: 277a, 1991.

92. Heeb MJ, Kojima Y, Tans G, Rosing J, Griffin JH: C-terminal residues 621–635 of protein S are essential for binding to factor Va. *J Biol Chem* 274:36187, 1999.

93. Nyberg P, Dahlback B, Garcia DF: The SHBG-like region of protein S is crucial for factor V-dependent APC-cofactor function. *FEBS Lett* 433:28, 1998.

94. Ploos van Amstel JK, Van der Zanden AL, Bakker E, Reitsma PH, Bertina RM: Two genes homologous with human protein S cDNA are located on chromosome 3. *Thromb Haemost* 58:982, 1987.

95. Watkins PC, Eddy R, Fukushima Y, et al: The gene for protein S maps near the contromere of human chromosome 3. *Blood* 71:238, 1988.

96. Gershagen S, Fernlund P, Lundwall A: A cDNA coding for human sex hormone binding globulin: Homology to vitamin K-dependent protein S. *FEBS Lett* 220:129, 1987.

97. Baker ME, French FS, Joseph DR: Vitamin K-dependent protein S is similar to rat androgen-binding protein. *Biochem J* 243:293, 1987.

98. Schmidel DK, Tatro AV, Phelps LG, Tomczak JA, Long GL: Organization of the human protein S gene. *Biochemistry* 29:7845, 1990.

99. Rapaport SI: Inhibition of factor VIIa/tissue factor-induced blood coagulation: with particular emphasis upon a factor Xa-dependent inhibitory mechanism. *Blood* 73:359, 1989.

100. Edenbrandt C-M, Lundwall A, Wydro R, Stenflo JA: Molecular analysis of the gene for vitamin K-dependent protein S and its pseudogene. Cloning and partial gene organization. *Biochemistry* 29:7861, 1990.

101. Gershagen S, Fernlund P, Edenbrandt C-M: The genes for SHBG/ABP and the SHBG-like region of vitamin K-dependent protein S have evolved from a common ancestral gene. *J Steroid Biochem Mol Biol* 40(4-6):763, 1991.

102. Gandrille S, Borgel D, Ireland H, et al: Protein S deficiency: a database of mutations. For the Plasma Coagulation Inhibitors Subcommittee of the Scientific and Standardization Committee of the International Society on Thrombosis and Haemostasis. *Thromb Haemost* 77:1201, 1997.

103. Bertina RM, Ploos van Amstel HK, van Wijngaarden A, et al: Heerlen polymorphism of protein S, an immunologic polymorphism due to dimorphism of residue 460. *Blood* 76:538, 1990.

104. Esmon CT, Owen WG: Identification of an endothelial cell cofactor for thrombin-catalyzed activation of protein C. *Proc Natl Acad Sci USA* 78:2249, 1981.

105. Owen WG, Esmon CT: Functional properties of an endothelial cell cofactor for thrombin-catalyzed activation of protein C. *J Biol Chem* 256:5532, 1981.

106. Esmon CT, Esmon NL, Harris KW: Complex formation between thrombin and thrombomodulin inhibits both thrombin-catalyzed fibrin formation and factor V activation. *J Biol Chem* 257:7944, 1982.

107. Esmon NL, Carroll RC, Esmon CT: Thrombomodulin blocks the ability of thrombin to activate platelets. *J Biol Chem* 258:12238, 1983.

108. Esmon CT: The roles of protein C and thrombomodulin in the regulation of blood coagulation. *J Biol Chem* 264:4743, 1989.

109. Jackman RW, Beeler DL, VanDeWater L, Rosenberg RD: Characterization of a thrombomodulin cDNA reveals structural similarity to the low density lipoprotein receptor. *Proc Natl Acad Sci USA* 83:8834, 1986.

110. Suzuki K, Kusumoto H, Deyashiki Y, et al: Structure and expression of human thrombomodulin, a thrombin receptor on endothelium acting as a cofactor for protein C activation. *EMBO J* 6:1891, 1987.

111. Jackman RW, Beeler DL, Fritze L, Soff G, Rosenberg RD: Human thrombomodulin gene is intron depleted: nucleic acid sequences of the cDNA and gene predict protein structure and suggest sites of regulatory control. *Proc Natl Acad Sci USA* 84:6425, 1987.

112. Wen D, Dittman WA, Ye RD, et al: Human thrombomodulin: complete cDNA sequence and chromosome localization of the gene. *Biochemistry* 26:4350, 1987.

113. Petersen TE: The amino-terminal domain of thrombomodulin and pancreatic stone protein are homologous with lectins. *FEBS Lett* 231:51, 1988.

114. Sadler JE, Lentz SR, Sheehan JP, Tsiang M, Wu Q: Structure-function relationships of the thrombin-thrombomodulin interaction. *Haemostasis* 23 (suppl 1):183, 1993.

115. Ye J, Esmon CT, Johnson AE: The chondroitin sulfate moiety of thrombomodulin binds a second molecule of thrombin. *J Biol Chem* 268:2373, 1993.

116. Bourin MC, Ohlin AK, Lane DA, Stenflo J, Lindahl U: Relationship between anticoagulant activities and polyanionic properties of rabbit thrombomodulin. *J Biol Chem* 263:8044, 1988.

117. Nawa K, Sakano K, Fujiwara H, et al: Presence and function of chondroitin-4-sulfate on recombinant human soluble thrombomodulin. *Biochem Biophys Res Commun* 171:729, 1990.

118. Suzuki K, Hayashi T, Nishioka J, et al: A domain composed of epidermal growth factor-like structures of human thrombomodulin is essential for thrombin binding and for protein C activation. *J Biol Chem* 264:4872, 1989.

119. Koyama T, Parkinson JF, Aoki N, et al: Relationship between post-translational glycosylation and anticoagulant function of secretable recombinant mutants of human thrombomodulin. *Br J Haematol* 78:515, 1991.

120. Musci G, Berliner LJ, Esmon CT: Evidence for multiple conformational changes in the active center of thrombin induced by complex formation with thrombomodulin: an analysis employing nitroxide spin-labels. *Biochemistry* 27:769, 1988.

121. Ye J, Esmon NL, Esmon CT, Johnson AE: The active site of thrombin is altered upon binding to thrombomodulin. *J Biol Chem* 266:23016, 1991.

122. Takano S, Kimura S, Ohdama S, Aoki N: Plasma thrombomodulin in health and diseases. *Blood* 76:2024, 1990.

123. Shirai T, Shiojiri S, Ito H, et al: Gene structure of human thrombomodulin, a cofactor for thrombin-catalyzed activation of protein C. *J Biochem* 103:281, 1988.

124. Espinosa R III, Sadler JE, Le Beau MM: Regional localization of the human thrombomodulin gene to 20p12-cen. *Genomics* 5:649, 1989.

125. Esmon CT: Cell mediated events that control blood coagulation and vascular injury. *Annu Rev Cell Biol* 9:1, 1993.

126. Ohlin AK, Marlar RA: The first mutation identified in the thrombomodulin gene in a 45-year-old man presenting with thromboembolic disease. *Blood* 85:330, 1995.

127. Norlund L, Holm J, Zoller B, Ohlin AK: A common thrombomodulin amino acid dimorphism is associated with myocardial infarction. *Thromb Haemost* 77:248, 1997.

128. Ireland H, Kunz G, Kyriakoulis K, Stubbs PJ, Lane DA: Thrombomodulin gene mutations associated with myocardial infarction. *Circulation* 96:15, 1997.

129. Fukudome K, Esmon CT: Identification, cloning, and regulation of a novel endothelial cell protein C–activated protein C receptor. *J Biol Chem* 269:26486, 1994.

130. Fukudome K, Esmon CT: Molecular cloning and expression of murine and bovine endothelial cell protein C–activated protein C receptor (EPCR). The structural and functional conservation in human, bovine, and murine EPCR. *J Biol Chem* 270:5571, 1995.

131. Regan LM, Stearns-Kurosawa DJ, Kurosawa S, et al: The endothelial cell protein C receptor. Inhibition of activated protein C anticoagulant function without modulation of reaction with proteinase inhibitors. *J Biol Chem* 271:17499, 1996.

132. Fukudome K, Kurosawa S, Stearns-Kurosawa DJ, et al: The endothelial cell protein C receptor. Cell surface expression and direct ligand binding by the soluble receptor. *J Biol Chem* 271:17491, 1996.

133. Stearns-Kurosawa DJ, Kurosawa S, Mollica JS, Ferrell GL, Esmon CT: The endothelial cell protein C receptor augments protein C activation by the thrombin-thrombomodulin complex. *Proc Natl Acad Sci USA* 93:10212, 1996.

134. Laszik Z, Mitro A, Taylor FB Jr, Ferrell G, Esmon CT: Human protein C receptor is present primarily on endothelium of large blood vessels: implications for the control of the protein C pathway. *Circulation* 96:3633, 1997.

135. Xu J, Esmon NL, Esmon CT: Reconstitution of the human endothelial cell protein C receptor with thrombomodulin in phosphatidylcholine vesicles enhances protein C activation. *J Biol Chem* 274:6704, 1999.

136. Fukudome K, Ye X, Tsuneyoshi N, et al: Activation mechanism of anticoagulant protein C in large blood vessels involving the endothelial cell protein C receptor. *J Exp Med* 187:1029, 1998.

137. Liang Z, Rosen ED, Castellino FJ: Nucleotide structure and characterization of the murine gene encoding the endothelial cell protein C receptor. *Thromb Haemost* 81:585, 1999.

138. Ye X, Fukudome K, Tsuneyoshi N, et al: The endothelial cell protein C receptor (EPCR) functions as a primary receptor for protein C activation on endothelial cells in arteries, veins, and capillaries. *Biochem Biophys Res Commun* 259:671, 1999.

139. Simmonds RE, Lane DA: Structural and functional implications of the intron/exon organization of the human endothelial cell protein C–activated protein C receptor (EPCR) gene: comparison with the structure of CD1/major histocompatibility complex alpha1 and alpha2 domains. *Blood* 94:632, 1999.

140. Esmon CT, Xu J, Gu JM, et al: Endothelial protein C receptor. *Thromb Haemost* 82:251, 1999.

141. Villoutreix BO, Blom AM, Dahlback B: Structural prediction and analysis of endothelial cell protein C–activated protein C receptor. *Protein Eng* 12:833, 1999.

142. Kurosawa S, Stearns-Kurosawa DJ, Hidari N, Esmon CT: Identification of functional endothelial protein C receptor in human plasma. *J Clin Invest* 100:411, 1997.

143. Kurosawa S, Stearns-Kurosawa DJ, Carson CW, et al: Plasma levels of endothelial cell protein C receptor are elevated in patients with sepsis and systemic lupus erythematosus: lack of correlation with thrombomodulin suggests involvement of different pathological processes [letter]. *Blood* 91:725, 1998.

144. Taylor FB, Chang A, Esmon CT, et al: Protein C prevents the coagulopathic and lethal effects of *Escherichia coli* infusion in the baboon. *J Clin Invest* 79:918, 1987.

145. Taylor F, Chang A, Ferrel G, et al: C4b-binding protein exacerbates the host response to *Escherichia coli*. *Blood* 78:357, 1991.

146. Hayashi T, Nakamura H, Okada A, et al: Organization and chromosomal localization of the human endothelial protein C receptor gene. *Gene* 238:367, 1999.

147. Comp PC, Jacocks RM, Ferrell GL, Esmon CT: Activation of protein C in vivo. *J Clin Invest* 70:127, 1982.

148. Hanson SR, Griffin JH, Harker LA, et al: Antithrombotic effects of thrombin-induced activation of endogenous protein C in primates. *J Clin Invest* 92:2003, 1993.

149. Lentz SR, Fernandez JA, Griffin JH, et al: Impaired anticoagulant response to infusion of thrombin in atherosclerotic monkeys associated

150. with acquired defects in the protein C system. *Arterioscler Thromb Vasc Biol* 19:1744, 1999.

150. Weiler-Guettler H, Christie PD, Beeler DL, et al: A targeted point mutation in thrombomodulin generates viable mice with a prethrombotic state. *J Clin Invest* 101:1983, 1998.

151. Christie PD, Edelberg JM, Picard MH, et al: A murine model of myocardial microvascular thrombosis. *J Clin Invest* 104:533, 1999.

152. Healy AM, Rayburn HB, Rosenberg RD, Weiler H: Absence of the blood-clotting regulator thrombomodulin causes embryonic lethality in mice before development of a functional cardiovascular system. *Proc Natl Acad Sci USA* 92:850, 1995.

153. Salem HH, Esmon NL, Esmon CT, Majerus PW: Effects of thrombomodulin and coagulation factor Va-light chain on protein C activation in vitro. *J Clin Invest* 73:968, 1984.

154. Snow TR, Deal MT, Dickey DT, Esmon CT: Protein C activation following coronary artery occlusion in the in situ porcine heart. *Circulation* 84:293, 1991.

155. Macko RF, Killewich LA, Fernandez JA, et al: Brain-specific protein C activation during carotid artery occlusion in humans. *Stroke* 30:542, 1999.

156. Petaja J, Pesonen E, Fernandez JA, et al: Cardiopulmonary bypass and activation of antithrombotic plasma protein C. *J Thorac Cardiovasc Surg* 118:422, 1999.

157. Gruber A, Pal A, Kiss RG, Sas G, Griffin JH: Generation of activated protein C during thrombolysis. Lancet 342:1275, 1993.

158. Macko RF, Ameriso SF, Gruber A, et al: Impairments of the protein C system and fibrinolysis in infection-associated stroke. *Stroke* 27:2005, 1996.

159. Conard J, Bauer KA, Gruber A, et al: Normalization of markers of coagulation activation with a purified protein C concentrate in adults with homozygous protein C deficiency. *Blood* 82:1159, 1993.

160. Bajaj MS, Kuppuswamy MN, Manepalli AN, Bajaj SP: Transcriptional expression of tissue factor pathway inhibitor, thrombomodulin and von Willebrand factor in normal human tissues. *Thromb Haemost* 82:1047, 1999.

161. Ishii H, Salem HH, Bell CE, Laposata EA, Majerus PW: Thrombomodulin, an endothelial anticoagulant protein, is absent from the human brain. *Blood* 67:362, 1986.

162. Wong VL, Hofman FM, Ishii H, Fisher M: Regional distribution of thrombomodulin in human brain. *Brain Res* 556:1, 1991.

163. Boffa MC, Jackman RW, Peyri N, Boffa JF, George B: Thrombomodulin in the central nervous system. *Nouv Rev Fr Hematol* 33:423, 1991.

164. Tran ND, Wong VL, Schreiber SS, Bready JV, Fisher M: Regulation of brain capillary endothelial thrombomodulin mRNA expression. *Stroke* 27:2304, 1996.

165. Wang L, Tran ND, Kittaka M, et al: Thrombomodulin expression in bovine brain capillaries. Anticoagulant function of the blood-brain barrier, regional differences, and regulatory mechanisms. *Arterioscler Thromb Vasc Biol* 17:3139, 1997.

166. Hackeng TM, Tans G, Koppelman SJ, et al: Protein C activation on endothelial cells by prothrombin activation products generated in situ: Meizothrombin is a better protein C activator than α-thrombin. *Biochem J* 319:399, 1996.

167. Varadi K, Philapitsch A, Santa T, Schwarz HP: Activation and inactivation of human protein C by plasmin. *Thromb Haemost* 71:615, 1994.

168. Haley PE, Doyle MF, Mann KG: The activation of bovine protein C by factor Xa. *J Biol Chem* 264:16303, 1989.

169. Rezaie AR: Rapid activation of protein C by factor Xa and thrombin in the presence of polyanionic compounds. *Blood* 91:4572, 1998.

170. Fernandez JA, Petaja J, Gruber A, Griffin JH: Activated protein C correlates inversely with thrombin levels in resting healthy individuals. *Am J Hematol* 56:29, 1997.

171. Pemberton S, Lindley P, Zaitsev V, et al: A molecular model for the triplicated A domains of human factor VIII based on the crystal structure of human ceruloplasmin. *Blood* 89:2413, 1997.

172. Villoutreix BO, Dahlback B: Structural investigation of the A domains of human blood coagulation factor V by molecular modeling. *Protein Sci* 7:1317, 1998.

173. Pellequer JL, Gale AJ, Griffin JH, Getzoff ED: Homology modeling of factor Va, a cofactor of the prothrombinase complex. *Protein Sci* 7:159, 1998;

174. Pellequer JL, Gale AJ, Griffin JH, Getzoff ED: Homology models of

the C domains of blood coagulation factors V and VIII: a proposed membrane binding mode for FV and FVIII C2 domains. *Blood Cell Mol Dis* 24:448, 1998.

175. Fay PJ: Regulation of factor VIIIa in the intrinsic factor Xase. *Thromb Haemost* 82:193, 1999.

176. Walker FJ, Sexton PW, Esmon CT: The inhibition of blood coagulation by activated protein C through the selective inactivation of activated factor V. *Biochim Biophys Acta* 571:333, 1979.

177. Marlar RA, Kleiss AJ, Griffin JH: Mechanism of action of human activated protein C, a thrombin-dependent anticoagulant enzyme. *Blood* 59:1067, 1982.

178. Suzuki K, Stenflo JA, Dahlbäck B, Teodorsson B: Inactivation of human coagulation factor V by activated protein C. *J Biol Chem* 258:1914, 1983.

179. Fulcher CA, Gardiner JE, Griffin JH, Zimmerman TS: Proteolytic inactivation of activated human factor VIII procoagulant protein by activated protein C and its analogy to factor V. *Blood* 63:486, 1984.

180. Guinto ER, Esmon CT: Loss of prothrombin and of factor Xa-factor Va interactions upon inactivation of factor Va by activated protein C. *J Biol Chem* 259:13986, 1984.

181. Kalafatis M, Rand MD, Mann KG: The mechanism of inactivation of human factor V and human factor Va by activated protein C. *J Biol Chem* 269:31869, 1994.

182. Dahlbäck B, Carlsson M, Svensson PJ: Familial thrombophilia due to a previously unrecognized mechanism characterized by poor anticoagulant response to activated protein C: Prediction of a cofactor to activated protein C. *Proc Natl Acad Sci USA* 90:1004, 1993.

183. Bertina RM, Koeleman BPC, Koster T, et al: Mutation in blood coagulation factor V associated with resistance to activated protein C. *Nature* 369:64, 1994.

184. Greengard JS, Sun X, Xu X, et al: Activated protein C resistance caused by Arg506Gln mutation in factor Va. *Lancet* 343:1361, 1994.

185. Sun X, Evatt B, Griffin JH: Blood coagulation factor Va abnormality associated with resistance to activated protein C in venous thrombophilia. *Blood* 83:3120, 1994.

186. Zivelin A, Griffin JH, Xi X, et al: A single genetic origin for a common Caucasian risk factor for venous thrombosis. *Blood* 89:397, 1997.

187. Heeb MJ, Kojima Y, Greengard J, Griffin JH: Activated protein C resistance: Molecular mechanisms based on studies using purified Gln^{506}-factor V. *Blood* 85:3405, 1995.

188. Kalafatis M, Bertina RM, Rand MD, Mann KG: Characterization of the molecular defect in factor V^{R506Q}. *J Biol Chem* 270:4053, 1995.

189. O'Brien LM, Medved LV, Fay PJ: Localization of factor IXa and factor VIIIa interactive sites. *J Biol Chem* 27045:27087, 1995.

190. Rosing J, Hoekema L, Nicolaes GAF, et al: Effects of protein S and factor Xa on peptide bond cleavages during inactivation of factor Va and factor Va^{R506Q} by activated protein C. *J Biol Chem* 270:27852, 1995.

191. Rosing J, Tans G: Coagulation factor V, an old star shines again. *Thromb Haemost* 78:427, 1997.

192. Bernardi F, Faioni EM, Castoldi E, et al: A factor V genetic component differing from factor V R506Q contributes to the activated protein C resistance phenotype. *Blood* 90:1552, 1997.

193. Faioni EM, Franchi F, Bucciarelli P, et al: Coinheritance of the HR2 haplotype in the factor V gene confers an increased risk of venous thromboembolism to carriers of factor V R506Q (Factor V Leiden). *Blood* 94:3062, 1999.

194. Rosing J, Bakker H, Thomassen MC, et al: Characterization of two forms of human factor Va with different cofactor activities. *J Biol Chem* 268:21130, 1993.

195. Hoekema L, Nicolaes GA, Hemker HC, Tans G, Rosing J: Human factor Va1 and factor Va2: properties in the procoagulant and anticoagulant pathways. *Biochemistry* 36:3331, 1997.

196. Kim SW, Ortel TL, Quinn-Allen MA, et al: Partial glycosylation at asparagine-2181 of the second C-type domain of human factor V modulates assembly of the prothrombinase complex. *Biochemistry* 38:11448, 1999.

197. Nicolaes GA, Villoutreix BO, Dahlback B: Partial glycosylation of Asn2181 in human factor V as a cause of molecular and functional heterogeneity. Modulation of glycosylation efficiency by mutagenesis of the consensus sequence for N-linked glycosylation. *Biochemistry* 38:13584, 1999.

198. Fernández JA, Hackeng TM, Kojima K, Griffin JH: The carbohydrate moiety of factor V modulates inactivation by activated protein C. *Blood* 8912:4348, 1997.

199. Fisher M, Fernández JA, Ameriso SF, et al: Activated protein C resistance in ischemic stroke not due to factor V arginine^{506}→glutamine mutation. *Stroke* 27:1163, 1996.

200. Van der Bom JG, Bots ML, Haverkate F, et al: Reduced response to activated protein C is associated with increased risk for cerebrovascular disease. *Ann Intern Med* 125:265, 1996.

201. De Visser MC, Rosendaal FR, Bertina RM: A reduced sensitivity for activated protein C in the absence of factor V Leiden increases the risk of venous thrombosis. *Blood* 93:1271, 1999.

202. Rodeghiero F, Tosetto A: Activated protein C resistance and factor V Leiden mutation are independent risk factors for venous thromboembolism. *Ann Intern Med* 130:643, 1999.

203. Kiechl S, Muigg A, Santer P, et al: Poor response to activated protein C as a prominent risk predictor of advanced atherosclerosis and arterial disease. *Circulation* 99:614, 1999.

204. Griffin JH, Kojima K, Banka CL, Curtiss LK, Fernandez JA: High-density lipoprotein enhancement of anticoagulant activities of plasma protein S and activated protein C. *J Clin Invest* 103:219, 1999.

205. Curvers J, Thomassen MC, Nicolaes GA, et al: Acquired APC resistance and oral contraceptives: differences between two functional tests. *Br J Haematol* 105:88, 1999.

206. Smirnov MD, Safa O, Esmon NL, Esmon CT: Inhibition of activated protein C anticoagulant activity by prothrombin. *Blood* 94:3839, 1999.

207. Neuenschwander P, Jesty J: A comparison of phospholipid and platelets in the activation of human factor VIII by thrombin and factor Xa, and in the activation of factor X. *Blood* 72:1761, 1988.

208. Keller FG, Ortel TL, Quinn-Allen MA, Kane WH: Thrombin-catalyzed activation of recombinant human factor V. *Biochemistry* 34:4118, 1995.

209. Thorelli E, Kaufman RJ, Dahlbäck B: Cleavage requirements for activation of factor V by factor Xa. *Eur J Biochem* 247:12, 1997.

210. Safa O, Morrissey JH, Esmon CT, Esmon NL: Factor VIIa/tissue factor generates a form of factor V with unchanged specific activity, resistance to activation by thrombin, and increased sensitivity to activated protein C. *Biochemistry* 38:1829, 1999.

211. Bakker HM, Tans G, Jannssen-Claessen T, et al: The effect of phospholipids, calcium ions and protein S on rate constants of human factor Va inactivation by activated human protein C. *Eur J Biochem* 208:171, 1992.

212. Smirnov M, Esmon C: Phosphatidylethanolamine incorporation into vesicles selectively enhances factor Va inactivation by activated protein C. *J Biol Chem* 269:816, 1994.

213. Smirnov MD, Triplett DT, Comp PC, Esmon NL, Esmon CT: On the role of phosphatidylethanolamine in the inhibition of activated protein C activity by antiphospholipid antibodies. *J Clin Invest* 95:309, 1995.

214. Fernández JA, Kojima K, Hackeng TM, Griffin JH: Cardiolipin, a protein C pathway cofactor: Implications for anticardiolipin antibody syndrome. *Thromb Haemost* 73(6):1392, 1995.

215. Nishioka J, Suzuki K: Inhibition of cofactor activity of protein S by a complex of protein S and C4b-binding protein: Evidence for inactive ternary complex formation between protein S, C4b-binding protein, and activated protein C. *J Biol Chem* 265:9072, 1990.

216. Yegneswaran S, Wood GM, Esmon CT, Johnson AE: Protein S alters the active site location of activated protein C above the membrane surface. A fluorescence resonance energy transfer study of topography. *J Biol Chem* 272:25013, 1997.

217. Yegneswaran S, Smirnov MD, Safa O, et al: Relocating the active site of activated protein C eliminates the need for its protein S cofactor. A fluorescence resonance energy transfer study. *J Biol Chem* 274:5462, 1999.

218. Gardiner JE, McGann MA, Berridge CW, et al: Protein S as a cofactor for activated protein C in plasma and in the inactivation of purified factor VIII:C. *Circulation* 70:205a, 1984.

219. Koedam JA, Meijers JCM, Sixma JJ, Bouma BN: Inactivation of human factor VIII by activated protein C. Cofactor activity of protein S and protective effect of von Willebrand factor. *J Clin Invest* 82:1236, 1988.

220. Solymoss S, Tucker MM, Tracy PB: Kinetics of inactivation of membrane-bound factor Va by activated protein C: protein S modulates factor Xa protection. *J Biol Chem* 263:14884, 1988.

221. Dahlback B, Hildebrand B, Malm J: Characterization of functionally important domains in human vitamin K-dependent protein S using monoclonal antibodies. *J Biol Chem* 265:8127, 1990.

222. Yegneswaran S, Hackeng T, Johnson AE, Griffin JH: Phospholipid-dependent protein S interaction with factor Xa mediated through the thrombin-sensitive region of protein S. *Thromb Haemost* 82:428, 1999.

223. Leroy-Matheron C, Gouault-Heilmann M, Aiach M, Gandrille S: A mutation of the active protein S gene leading to an EGF1-lacking protein in a family with qualitative (type II) deficiency. *Blood* 91:4608, 1998.

224. He X, Shen L, Villoutreix BO, Dahlback B: Amino acid residues in thrombin-sensitive region and first epidermal growth factor domain of vitamin K-dependent protein S determining specificity of the activated protein C cofactor function. *J Biol Chem* 273:27449, 1998.

225. Stenberg Y, Drakenberg T, Dahlback B, Stenflo J: Characterization of recombinant epidermal growth factor (EGF)-like modules from vitamin-K-dependent protein S expressed in *Spodoptera* cells-the cofactor activity depends on the N-terminal EGF module in human protein S. *Eur J Biochem* 251:558, 1998.

226. He X, Shen L, Dahlbäck B: Expression and functional characterization of chimeras between human and bovine vitamin-K-dependent protein-S-defining modules important for the species specificity of the activated protein C cofactor activity. *Eur J Biochem* 227:433, 1995.

227. Dahlbäck B, Hildebrand B: Degradation of human complement component C4b in the presence of the C4b-binding protein-protein S complex. *Biochem J* 209:857, 1983.

228. Suzuki K, Nishioka J, Hashimoto S: Regulation of activated protein C by thrombin-modified protein S. *J Biochem* 94:699, 1983.

229. Walker FJ: Regulation of vitamin K-dependent protein S: inactivation by thrombin. *J Biol Chem* 259:10335, 1984.

230. Dahlbäck B, Lundwall A, Stenflo JA: Localization of thrombin cleavage sites in the amino-terminal region of bovine protein S. *J Biol Chem* 261:5111, 1986.

231. Váradi K, Rosing J, Tans G, et al: Factor V enhances the cofactor function of protein S in the APC-mediated inactivation of factor VIII: Influence of the factor V^{R506Q} mutation. *Thromb Haemost* 76:208, 1996.

232. Thorelli E, Kaufman RJ, Dahlback B: Cleavage of factor V at Arg 506 by activated protein C and the expression of anticoagulant activity of factor V. *Blood* 93:2552, 1999.

233. Thorelli E: Mechanisms that regulate the anticoagulant function of coagulation factor V. *Scand J Clin Lab Invest Suppl* 229:19, 1999.

234. Pajkrt D, Lerch PG, van der Poll T, et al: Differential effects of reconstituted high-density lipoprotein on coagulation, fibrinolysis and platelet activation during human endotoxemia. *Thromb Haemost* 77:303, 1997.

235. Li D, Weng S, Yang B, et al: Inhibition of arterial thrombus formation by ApoA1 Milano. *Arterioscler Thromb Vasc Biol* 19:378, 1999.

236. Heeb MJ, Gruber A, Griffin JH: Identification of divalent metal ion-dependent inhibition of activated protein C by α_2-macroglobulin and α_2-antiplasmin in blood and comparisons to inhibition of factor Xa, thrombin, and plasmin. *J Biol Chem* 226:17606, 1991.

237. Okajima K, Koga S, Kaji M, et al: Effect of protein C and activated protein C on coagulation and fibrinolysis in normal human subjects. *Thromb Haemost* 63:48, 1990.

238. Heeb MJ, Griffin JH: Physiologic inhibition of human activated protein C by α_1-antitrypsin. *J Biol Chem* 263:11613, 1988.

239. Heeb MJ, España F, Geiger M, et al: Immunological identity of heparin-dependent plasma and urinary protein C inhibitor and plasminogen activator inhibitor-3. *J Biol Chem* 262:15813, 1987.

240. Heeb MJ, España F, Griffin JH: Inhibition and complexation of activated protein C by two major inhibitors in plasma. *Blood* 73:446, 1989.

241. España F, Griffin JH: Determination of functional and antigenic protein C inhibitor and its complexes with activated protein C in plasma by ELISAs. *Thromb Res* 55:671, 1989.

242. España F, Vicente V, Tabernero D, Scharrer I, Griffin JH: Determination of plasma protein C inhibitor and of two activated protein C-inhibitor complexes in normals and in patients with intravascular coagulation and thrombotic disease. *Thromb Res* 59:593, 1990.

243. España F, Gilabert J, Aznar J, et al: Complexes of activated protein C with α_1-antitrypsin in normal pregnancy and in severe preeclampsia. *Am J Obstet Gynecol* 164:1310, 1991.

244. Hoogendoorn H, Nesheim ME, Giles AR: A qualitative and quantitative analysis of the activation and inactivation of protein C in vivo in a primate model. *Blood* 75:2164, 1990.

245. España F, Gruber A, Heeb MJ, et al: In vivo and in vitro complexes of activated protein C with two inhibitors in baboons. *Blood* 77:1754, 1991.

246. Hoogendoorn H, Toh CH, Nesheim ME, Giles AR: α_2-Macroglobulin binds and inhibits activated protein C. *Blood* 78:2283, 1991.

247. Scully MF, Toh CH, Hoogendoorn H, et al: Activation of protein C and its distribution between its inhibitors, protein C inhibitor, α_1-antitrypsin and α_2-macroglobulin, in patients with disseminated intravascular coagulation. *Thromb Haemost* 69:448, 1993.

248. Hayashi T, Nishioka J, Suzuki K: Molecular mechanism of the dysfunction of protein S(Tokushima) (Lys155→Glu) for the regulation of the blood coagulation system. *Biochim Biophys Acta* 1272:159, 1995.

249. Stenberg Y, Muranyi A, Steen C, et al: EGF-like module pair 3-4 in vitamin K-dependent protein S: modulation of calcium affinity of module 4 by module 3 and interaction with factor X. *J Mol Biol* 293:653, 1999.

250. Koppelman SJ, van't Veer C, Sixma JJ, Bouma BN: Synergistic inhibition of the intrinsic factor X activation by protein S and C4b-binding protein. *Blood* 86:2653, 1995.

251. Dahlbäck B: Purification of human C4b-binding protein and formation of its complex with vitamin K-dependent protein S. *Biochem J* 209:847, 1983.

252. Nelson RM, Long GL: Solution-phase equilibrium binding interaction of human protein S with C4b-binding protein. *Biochemistry* 30:2384, 1991.

253. Griffin JH, Gruber A, Fernández JA: Reevaluation of total, free and bound protein S and C4b-binding protein levels in plasma anticoagulated with citrate or hirudin. *Blood* 79:32003, 1992.

254. Comp PC, Nixon RR, Cooper MR, Esmon CT: Familial protein S deficiency is associated with recurrent thrombosis. *J Clin Invest* 74:2082, 1984.

255. Dahlbäck B: Inhibition of the protein Ca cofactor function of human and bovine protein S by C4b-binding protein. *J Biol Chem* 261:12022, 1986.

256. Van de Poel R: Regulation of the protein C anticoagulant pathway by C4b-binding protein. Ph.D. Thesis, University of Utrecht, 1999.

257. Hillarp A, Dahlbäck B: Novel subunit in C4b-binding protein required for protein S binding. *J Biol Chem* 263:12759, 1988.

258. Hillarp A, Hessing M, Dahlbäck B: Protein S binding in relation to the subunit composition of human C4b-binding protein. *FEBS Lett* 259:53, 1989.

259. Hillarp A, Dahlbäck B: Cloning of cDNA coding for the beta chain of human complement component C4b-binding protein: Sequence homology with the alpha chain. *Proc Natl Acad Sci USA* 87:1183, 1990.

260. Fernández JA, Griffin JH: A protein S binding site on C4b-binding protein involves β chain residues 31-45. *J Biol Chem* 269:2535, 1994.

261. Fernández JA, Griffin JH, Chang GTG, et al: Involvement of amino acid residues 423-429 of human protein S in binding to C4b-binding protein. *Blood Cell Mol Dis* 24:101, 1998.

262. García de Frutos P, Alim RI, Härdig Y, Zöller B, Dahlbäck B: Differential regulation of α and β chains of C4b-binding protein during acute-phase response resulting in stable plasma levels of free anticoagulant protein S. *Blood* 84:815, 1994.

263. Huber R, Carrell RW: Implications of the three-dimensional structure of α_1-antitrypsin for structure and function of serpins. *Biochemistry* 28:8951, 1989.

264. Schreuder HA, de Boer B, Dijkema R, et al: The intact and cleaved human antithrombin III complex as a model for serpin-proteinase interactions. *Nat Struct Biol* 1:48, 1994.

265. Mourey L, Samama JP, Delarue M, et al: Crystal structure of cleaved bovine antithrombin III at 3.2 Å resolution. *J Mol Biol* 232:223, 1993.

266. Carrell RW, Stein PE, Fermi G, Wardell MR: Biological implications of a 3 Å structure of dimeric antithrombin. *Structure* 2:257, 1994.

267. Whisstock J, Skinner R, Lesk AM: An atlas of serpin conformations. *Trends Biochem Sci* 23:63, 1998.

268. Skinner R, Abrahams JP, Whisstock JC, et al: The 2.6 Å structure of antithrombin indicates a conformational change at the heparin binding site. *J Mol Biol* 266:601, 1997.

269. Whisstock J, Lesk AM, Carrell R: Modeling of serpin-protease complexes: antithrombin-thrombin, α_1-antitrypsin (358Met→Arg)-thrombin, α_1-antitrypsin (358Met→Arg)-trypsin, and antitrypsin-elastase. *Proteins* 26:288, 1996.

270. Rosenberg RD, Rosenberg JS: Natural anticoagulant mechanisms. *J Clin Invest* 74:1, 1984.

271. Carrell RW, Christey PB, Boswell DR: Serpins: antithrombin and other inhibitors of coagulation and fibrinolysis evidence from amino acid sequences, in *Thrombosis and Haemostasis*, p 1. International Society

on Thrombosis and Haemostasis and Leuvin University Press, Leuven, 1987.

272. Rosenberg RD, Damus PS: The purification and mechanism of action of human antithrombin-heparin cofactor. *J Biol Chem* 248:6490, 1973.

273. Olson ST, Bjork I, Sheffer R, et al: Role of the antithrombin-binding pentasaccharide in heparin acceleration of antithrombin-proteinase reactions. Resolution of the antithrombin conformational change contribution to heparin rate enhancement. *J Biol Chem* 267:12528, 1992.

274. Gettins P, Patston PA, Schapira M: Structure and mechanism of action of serpins. *Hematol Oncol Clin North Am* 6:1393, 1992.

275. Gettins PG, Fan B, Crews BC, et al: Transmission of conformational change from the heparin binding site to the reactive center of antithrombin. *Biochemistry* 32:8385, 1993.

276. Choay J, Petitou M, Lormeau JC, et al: Structure-activity relationship in heparin: a synthetic pentasaccharide with high affinity for antithrombin III and eliciting high anti-factor Xa activity. *Biochem Biophys Res Commun* 116:492, 1983.

277. Bourin MC, Lindahl U: Glycosaminoglycans and the regulation of blood coagulation. *Biochem J* 289:313, 1993.

278. Olds RJ, Lane DA, Chowdhury V, et al: Complete nucleotide sequence of the antithrombin gene: evidence for homologous recombination causing thrombophilia. *Biochemistry* 32:4216, 1993.

279. Picard V, Ersdal-Badju E, Bock SC: Partial glycosylation of antithrombin III asparagine-135 is caused by the serine in the third position of its N-glycosylation consensus sequence and is responsible for production of the beta-antithrombin III isoform with enhanced heparin affinity. *Biochemistry* 34:8433, 1995.

280. Turko IV, Fan B, Gettins PG: Carbohydrate isoforms of antithrombin variant N135Q with different heparin affinities. *FEBS Lett* 335:9, 1993.

281. Bock SC, Wion KL, Vehar GA, Lawn RM: Cloning and expression of the cDNA for human antithrombin III. *Nucleic Acids Res* 10:8113, 1982.

282. Bock SC, Harris JF, Balazs I, Trent JM: Assignment of the human antithrombin III structural gene to chromosome 1q23-25. *Cytogenet Cell Genet* 39:67, 1985.

283. Chandra T, Stackhouse R, Kidd VJ, Woo SL: Isolation and sequence characterization of a cDNA clone of human antithrombin III. *Proc Natl Acad Sci USA* 80:1845, 1983.

284. Prochownik EV, Markham AF, Orkin SH: Isolation of a cDNA clone for human antithrombin III. *J Biol Chem* 258:8389, 1983.

285. Lane DA, Bayston T, Olds RJ, et al: Antithrombin mutation database: 2nd (1997) update. For the Plasma Coagulation Inhibitors Subcommittee of the Scientific and Standardization Committee of the International Society on Thrombosis and Haemostasis. *Thromb Haemost* 77:197, 1997.

286. Wun TC, Kretzmer KK, Girard TJ, Miletich JP, Broze GJ Jr: Cloning and characterization of a cDNA coding for the lipoprotein-associated coagulation inhibitor shows that it consists of three tandem Kunitz-type inhibitory domains. *J Biol Chem* 263:6001, 1988.

287. Caplice NM, Mueske CS, Kleppe LS, et al: Expression of tissue factor pathway inhibitor in vascular smooth muscle cells and its regulation by growth factors. *Circ Res* 83:1264, 1998.

288. Lesnik P, Vonica A, Guerin M, Moreau M, Chapman MJ: Anticoagulant activity of tissue factor pathway inhibitor in human plasma is preferentially associated with dense subspecies of LDL and HDL and with Lp(a). *Arterioscler Thromb* 13:1066, 1993.

289. Sandset PM, Abildgaard U, Larsen ML: Heparin induces release of extrinsic coagulation pathway inhibitor (EPI). *Thromb Res* 50:803, 1988.

290. Girard TJ, Warren LA, Novotny WF, et al: Functional significance of the Kunitz-type inhibitory domains of lipoprotein-associated coagulation inhibitor. *Nature* 338:518, 1989.

291. Broze GJ Jr, Warren LA, Novotny WF, et al: The lipoprotein-associated coagulation inhibitor that inhibits the factor VII-tissue factor complex also inhibits factor Xa: insight into its possible mechanism of action. *Blood* 71:335, 1988.

292. Rao LV, Rapaport SI: Studies of a mechanism inhibiting the initiation of the extrinsic pathway of coagulation. *Blood* 69:645, 1987.

293. Baugh RJ, Broze GJ Jr, Krishnaswamy S: Regulation of extrinsic pathway factor Xa formation by tissue factor pathway inhibitor. *J Biol Chem* 273:4378, 1998.

294. Sandset PM, Warn-Cramer BJ, Rao LV, Maki SL, Rapaport SI: Depletion of extrinsic pathway inhibitor (EPI) sensitizes rabbits to disseminated intravascular coagulation induced with tissue factor: evidence supporting a physiologic role for EPI as a natural anticoagulant. *Proc Natl Acad Sci USA* 88:708, 1991.

295. Sandset PM, Warn-Cramer BJ, Maki SL, Rapaport SI: Immunodepletion of extrinsic pathway inhibitor sensitizes rabbits to endotoxin-induced intravascular coagulation and the generalized Shwartzman reaction. *Blood* 78:1496, 1991.

296. Creasey AA, Chang AC, Feigen L, et al: Tissue factor pathway inhibitor reduces mortality from *Escherichia coli* septic shock. *J Clin Invest* 91:2850, 1993.

297. Huang ZF, Broze G Jr: Consequences of tissue factor pathway inhibitor gene-disruption in mice. *Thromb Haemost* 78:699, 1997.

298. Van der Logt CP, Reitsma PH, Bertina RM: Intron-exon organization of the human gene coding for the lipoprotein-associated coagulation inhibitor: the factor Xa dependent inhibitor of the extrinsic pathway of coagulation. *Biochemistry* 30:1571, 1991.

299. Girard TJ, Eddy R, Wesselschmidt RL, et al: Structure of the human lipoprotein-associated coagulation inhibitor gene. Intron/exon gene organization and localization of the gene to chromosome 2. *J Biol Chem* 266:5036, 1991.

300. Kleesiek K, Schmidt M, Gotting C, et al: The 536C→T transition in the human tissue factor pathway inhibitor (TFPI) gene is statistically associated with a higher risk for venous thrombosis. *Thromb Haemost* 82:1, 1999.

301. Tollefsen DM, Majerus DW, Blank MK: Heparin cofactor II. Purification and properties of a heparin-dependent inhibitor of thrombin in human plasma. *J Biol Chem* 257:2162, 1982.

302. Andersson TR, Sie P, Pelzer H, et al: Elevated levels of thrombin-heparin cofactor II complex in plasma from patients with disseminated intravascular coagulation. *Thromb Res* 66:591, 1992.

303. Suzuki K, Deyashiki Y, Nishioka J, et al: Characterization of a cDNA for human protein C inhibitor: a new member of the plasma serine protease inhibitor superfamily. *J Biol Chem* 262:611, 1987.

304. Rezaie AR, Cooper ST, Church FC, Esmon CT: Protein C inhibitor is a potent inhibitor of the thrombin-thrombomodulin complex. *J Biol Chem* 270:25336, 1995.

305. Sie P, Dupouy D, Pichon J, Boneu B: Constitutional heparin cofactor II deficiency associated with recurrent thrombosis. *Lancet* 20:415, 1985.

306. Tran TH, Marbet GA, Duckert F: Association of hereditary heparin cofactor II deficiency with thrombosis. *Lancet* 20:413, 1985.

307. Bertina RM, van der Linden IK, Engesser L, Muller HP, Brommer EJP: Hereditary heparin cofactor II deficiency and the risk of development of thrombosis. *Thromb Haemost* 57:196, 1987.

308. Griffin JH: The thrombin paradox. *Nature* 378:337, 1995.

CHAPTER 114

VASCULAR FUNCTION IN HEMOSTASIS

KATHERINE A. HAJJAR

NAOMI L. ESMON

AARON J. MARCUS

WILLIAM A. MULLER

Blood vessels play a critical role in the control of hemostasis, thrombosis, and inflammation. Endothelial cells, which form the lining of all blood vessels, are particularly important in this process because of their intimate association with flowing blood. Endothelial cells have the unique capability to express and elaborate thromboregulatory molecules, which can be classified as early or late with respect to an endothelial cell stimulus. In addition, pro-inflammatory leukocyte adhesion molecules are expressed upon endothelial cell perturbation (Table 114-1).

Thromboregulators acting at the initial stages of thrombus formation interfere with platelet deposition or regulate the contractile state of the blood vessel. They include nitric oxide, eicosanoids, and the ectoADPase/CD39. Nitric oxide is a highly reactive, and therefore evanescent, gas produced by endothelium that acts as a potent vasodilator and inhibitor of platelet aggregation. The endothelial cell eicosanoids, similarly, are fatty-acid-derived hydrocarbons that block platelet aggregation and induce vascular relaxation. The endothelins are a family of endothelium-derived peptides that strongly stimulate vascular constriction over prolonged periods of time. Endothelial cell ectoADPase is a membrane-associated protein that metabolizes adenosine diphosphate (ADP) in the primary platelet releasate, thus preventing recruitment of additional platelets to the initial hemostatic plug.

The late thromboregulators act to regulate thrombin generation, neutralize thrombin, or lyse thrombi. Endothelin is a long-acting vasoconstrictor. Antithrombin III, a natural anticoagulant, is a circulating inhibitor of thrombin and factor Xa, which employs endothelial cell heparan proteoglycans as cofactors. Tissue factor pathway inhibitor is a protein that inhibits factor VIIa tissue factor activity. The

Acronyms and abbreviations that appear in this chapter include: ADP, adenosine diphosphate; APC, activated protein C; Apo(a), apolipoprotein(a); ApoE, apolipoprotein(e); ATIII, antithrombin III; cAMP, adenosine 3',5'-cyclic phosphate; CAMs, cell adhesion molecules; DDAVP, desmopressin acetate; EDRF, endothelium-derived relaxing factor; EGF, epidermal growth factor; EPCR, endothelial cell protein C receptor; ET-1, endothelin-1; ICAM-1, intercellular adhesion molecule 1; LDL, low-density lipoprotein; LFA-3, lymphocyte-function-associated antigen-3; Lp(a), lipoprotein(a); LPS, lipopolysaccharide; MAdCAM-1, mucosal addressin cell adhesion molecule 1; NK cells, natural killer cells; NO, nitric oxide; NOS, nitric-oxide synthase; PAF, platelet activating factor; PAI, plasminogen activator inhibitor; PCI, protein C inhibitor; PSGL-1, P-selectin glycoprotein ligand 1; TAFI, T thrombin activatable fibrinolysis inhibitor; TF, tissue factor; TFPI, tissue factor pathway inhibitor; TGF-β, transforming growth factor beta; TM, thrombomodulin; TNF-α, tumor necrosis factor alpha; tPA, tissue plasminogen activator; uPA, urokinase plasminogen activator; uPAR, uPA receptor; VCAM-1, vascular adhesion molecule 1; VEGF, vascular endothelial growth factor; VLDL, very low density lipoprotein; vWF, von Willebrand factor.

thrombomodulin/endothelial cell protein C receptor (EPCR)/protein C system of the vascular wall is integrally involved in the regulation of hemostasis through direct anticoagulant effects on thrombin. Cellular signals resulting from thrombin-mediated activation of protein C and interaction of activated protein C with the EPCR appear to be linked to the inflammatory system. The fibrinolytic system is inextricably intertwined with the vascular endothelium, as endothelial cells not only synthesize and secrete elements of the fibrinolytic system under specific circumstances but also regulate the formation of plasmin. Impairment of fibrinolytic synthetic and assembly systems may play a central role in the etiology of occlusive vascular disease.

In the setting of inflammation, alterations in thromboregulatory balance are evidenced by increased expression of tissue factor and modulation of the thrombomodulin/EPCR/protein C system. Under the same circumstances, endothelial cell adhesion molecules, in addition, constitute a special class of glycoproteins that mediate physical interactions between endothelial cells and leukocytes. Such glycoproteins include members of two molecular families, the cell adhesion molecules (CAMs—MadCAM-1, ICAM-1, VCAM-1, and PECAM-1) and the selectins (P- and E-selectin). In concert, these molecules create a dynamic and changeable interface that modulates a panoply of interactions between the endothelium and various classes of circulating leukocytes.

ENDOTHELIAL CELLS AND HEMOSTASIS

The endothelium acts as a dynamic interface between flowing blood and the vessel wall. It is subject to unique physical forces, circulating factors, and cell–cell interactions that create region-specific phenotypes. In addition to its role in maintaining vascular permeability, the endothelium serves to regulate the fluid state of blood by displaying thromboresistance and profibrinolytic properties.

In vivo, endothelial cells are highly heterogeneous. They undergo "transdifferentiation," a process whereby they acquire specialized characteristics in response to signals from the local microenvironment. Thus, small- and large-vessel endothelial cells in vivo, and even endothelial cells from different tissues within the same organ, may express distinct surface molecules, show different membrane specializations such as fenestrae, and exhibit varying synthetic capabilities.

Since the early 1970s, endothelial cells cultivated in vitro, mainly from large-vessel umbilical veins, have served as an important and informative model in vascular biology. However, cultured endothelial cells have significant limitations. First, they exist in an active, replicative mode compared to their in vivo counterparts. In addition, cultured endothelial cells tend to lose their specific regional characteristics and acquire dedifferentiated properties with repeated passage. With the introduction of transgenic animal models, comparisons can be made between in vivo and in vitro studies.

THROMBOREGULATION BY VASCULAR ENDOTHELIAL CELLS

Thromboregulation[1,2] refers to a group of processes by which blood cells in the circulation and cells of the vessel wall interact to facilitate or inhibit thrombus formation. It is accomplished through cell proximity or contact and can be cell-associated or involve released compounds generated during agonist exposure. Thromboregulatory systems function to prevent or reverse platelet accumulation, activation of coagulation factors, and formation of fibrin, thereby maintaining blood fluidity[1-10] (Fig. 114-1).

The physiologic defense systems that render endothelial surfaces antithrombotic can be overwhelmed by excessive shear stress, injury, increased turbulence, and inflammation.[11] The endothelial cells are thereby transformed into a prothrombotic and antifibrinolytic phenotype.[12] This transformation is accompanied by up-regulation of leuko-

TABLE 114-1   ENDOTHELIAL CELL THROMBOREGULATORS

Early thromboregulators
  Nitric oxide (NO)
  Eicosanoids (prostacyclin, PGI_2, and PGD_2)
  Endothelial cell ecto-ADPase (CD39)
  Endothelin
Late thromboregulators
  Endothelin
  Antithrombin III
  Endothelial cell/heparan proteoglycans
  Tissue factor pathway inhibitor
  Thrombomodulin-protein C-protein S pathway
  Fibrinolytic system (plasminogen activators, inhibitors, and receptors)
Inflammatory thromboregulators
  Tissue factor pathway inhibitor
  Thrombomodulin-protein C-protein S pathway
  Cellular adhesion molecules
  Selectins

cyte and endothelial cell adhesion molecules,[13] increased expression of tissue factor, and accumulation of monocytes/macrophages in the vessel wall.[11] Such events commonly occur at the site of fissured or fractured atherosclerotic plaques in the coronary and cerebrovascular circulation[9,11] and involve exposure of tissue factor to the blood.[14]

The early thromboregulatory systems are the eicosanoids (PGI_2, PGD_2), nitric oxide (NO), and the ecto-ADPase/CD39 systems. Because they operate very early in the hemostatic/thrombotic cascade, they represent attractive targets for therapeutic intervention, including up-regulation, administration, and gene therapy.

PROSTACYCLIN AS A THROMBOREGULATOR

The discovery of thromboxanes by Hamberg, Svensson, and Samuelsson in 1975 initiated a new era in platelet biochemistry and physiol-

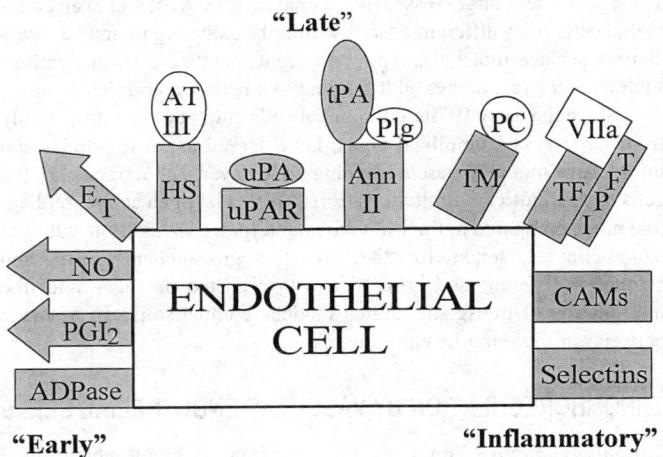

FIGURE 114-1   Schematic depiction of some endothelial cell thromboregulatory properties. Secreted products are represented as arrows. Cell-surface-associated molecules appear as boxes. Endothelial cell synthetic products are shaded. "Early" thromboregulators modulate activation of platelets and blood vessel contractility. "Late" thromboregulators modify activation of the coagulation cascade or fibrinolytic system. "Inflammatory" thromboregulators are those whose expression or activity are directed by inflammatory mediators. ADPase, endothelial cell ectoADPase; PGI_2, prostacyclin; NO, nitric oxide; ET, endothelin; HS, heparan sulfate; AT III, antithrombin III; uPA, urokinase plasminogen activator; uPAR, uPA receptor; Ann II, annexin II; tPA, tissue plasminogen activator; Plg, plasminogen; TM, thrombomodulin; PC, protein C; TF, tissue factor; VIIa, factor VIIa; TFPI, tissue factor pathway inhibitor; CAMs, cellular adhesion molecules.

ogy.[15] It meant that the activated platelet releasate contains two vasoconstrictors (thromboxane and serotonin) and an agonist for platelet aggregation (thromboxane), operative through ADP release. Subsequently, an agent derived from endothelium that caused vasodilatation and inhibited aggregation was discovered. Initially named PGX, it was later designated as PGI_2, or prostacyclin.[16–18]

BIOSYNTHESIS OF PROSTACYCLIN IN ENDOTHELIAL CELLS

There is a wide range of agonists for eicosanoid production in endothelial cells. They can be hormonal, biochemical, or physical, such as shear stress. Exposure to stimuli increases intracellular calcium levels, which in turn activates phospholipases such as A_2 and C. The phospholipases catalyze formation of free arachidonate from membrane phospholipids. In some tissues, activity of phospholipase A_2 may be rate limiting for eicosanoid production. Oxygenation and cyclization of free arachidonate are catalyzed by a microsomal enzyme known as PGH synthase-1 (also known as cyclooxygenase or COX-1). A cyclic endoperoxide, PGG_2, then forms and is reduced to PGH_2 via peroxidase activity in COX-1. Although endoperoxides are biochemically active, they are transformed to eicosanoid end products within 5 min. The major and most important COX-1 product of endothelial cells is prostacyclin (PGI_2), which is catalyzed by the isomerase PGI-synthase. Other endothelial cell isomerases catalyze formation of PGE_2, $PGF_{2\alpha}$, and PGD_2. PGD_2 acts in a manner similar to PGI_2, and on the same receptor. With a half-life of 3 min, PGI_2 undergoes chemical hydrolysis to 6-keto-$PGF_{1\alpha}$. The synthesis of PGG_2/H_2 is common to many tissues, but subsequent processing is specific for a given tissue. For example, in platelets, thromboxane-synthase catalyzes metabolism of PGH_2 to thromboxane A_2 (Fig. 114-2).[2,10,15–19] Endothelial cells do not contain cytosolic enzymes that catalyze oxygenation of arachidonate to lipid hydroperoxides, i.e., the lipoxygenases. However, via transcellular metabolism, endothelial cells take part in production of lipoxygenase products.[1,2,19]

THE TWO ISOFORMS OF PROSTACYCLIN G/H SYNTHASE

The cloning of an early response gene from 3T3 fibroblasts demonstrated that the cDNA was highly homologous to COX-1.[20] It then became apparent that there are two forms of COX, COX-1 (constitutive) and COX-2 (induced as an intermediate-early gene in monocytes, macrophages, neutrophils, and endothelial cells).[21] COX-2 is inducible in endothelial cells by prothrombotic, inflammatory, or mitogenic stimuli and in neutrophils by inflammatory stimuli.[22–28] In a given species, there is approximately 60 percent homology between deduced amino acid sequences. COX-1 contains 576 residues as compared to 587 for COX-2. There is a C-terminal sequence of 18 amino acids in COX-2 that is absent in COX-1. Antibodies directed at this C-terminal sequence can identify COX-2 by Western blot. The catalytic activities of both COX enzymes are similar, and all amino acids critical for COX-1 activity are conserved in COX-2. The active site in COX-1 is, however, slightly larger than that of COX-2, which is important for design of COX inhibitors. COX-2 contains mannose and an additional N-glycosylation site at the 18–amino acid C-terminal sequence. An N-glycosylation site at Asn410 is required for COX-1 to fold into an active conformation. The gene for COX-1 is located on chromosome 9 and is 22 kb long, and the gene for COX-2 is located on chromosome 1 and is 8 kb long. Transcription of COX-2 proceeds via several signaling mechanisms, including cAMP/protein kinase A, protein kinase C, tyrosine kinases, and pathways activated by growth factors, endotoxin, and cytokines.[21,29,30]

AUTACOID FUNCTIONS OF PROSTACYCLIN (PGI_2)

Activity of PGI_2 as a muscle relaxant can be demonstrated following infusion of the parent molecule or its analogs. The inhibitory action

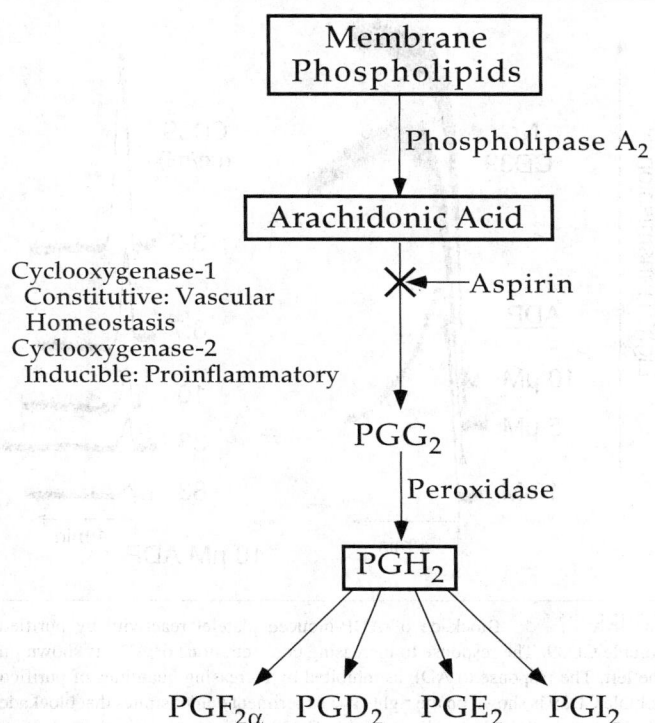

FIGURE 114-2 Transformation of released arachidonate to prostaglandins and prostacylin in endothelial cells as catalyzed by cyclooxygenase enzymes.[29,284] In response to prothrombotic or inflammatory stimuli, the essential fatty acid arachidonate is released from cell membrane phospholipids by phospholipase A_2 (PLA_2). Regulatory enzymes of this pathway are the cyclooxygenase, COX-1, which functions mainly in the endoplasmic reticulum, and COX-2 which functions principally in the nucleus. COX-1 and COX-2 catalyze insertion of two molecules of oxygen into arachidonate to form endoperoxide PGG_2, which is then peroxidized to the endoperoxide PGH_2. The latter is the precursor common to all eicosanoids. The endothelial eicosanoids are depicted herein.

of PGI_2 and analogs is due to an interaction with its receptor on vascular smooth muscle cells and platelets. The biochemical effects of PGI_2 are mediated mainly through G proteins and result in an increase in intraplatelet concentrations of cyclic AMP[9] that lead to abolition of shape change, absence of platelet secretion, and impaired binding of von Willebrand factor and fibrinogen to the platelet surface. PGI_2 also inhibits platelet adhesion to subendothelium—especially at high shear rates.[9] Decreased PGI_2 production has been described in thrombotic thrombocytopenic purpura (TTP).[31] Thus far, it has not been possible to utilize prostacyclin or its analogs as therapeutic agents because of side effects, such as diarrhea.[17]

NITRIC OXIDE, AN ENDOTHELIAL VASODILATOR AND INHIBITOR OF PLATELET FUNCTION

Nitric oxide is a colorless gas, slightly soluble in water and highly reactive with O_2 to form nitrogen dioxide, NO_2. It has a half-life of about 6 s and can also form the stable cation NO^+. NO is the first gas to be characterized as an intracellular messenger. Nitric oxide accounts for the action of what was originally termed the endothelium-derived relaxing factor (EDRF).[32,33] Upon release from endothelial cells, NO induces vasodilation, regulates normal vascular tone, and inhibits platelet aggregation. Overproduction of NO may be involved in the hypotension that accompanies endotoxic shock. In the pulmonary

bed, abnormally low levels of NO may contribute to the etiology of pulmonary hypertension.[34]

In vascular endothelial cells, NO is formed from L-arginine by nitric-oxide synthase (NOS) in the presence of NADPH and oxygen.[33] L-arginine is then converted to citrulline and nitric oxide. In endothelial cells, the isoform of NO synthase (eNOS or the NOS3 gene product) functions constitutively, but is further activated by receptor-dependent agonists that elevate intracellular calcium. Important stimuli include ADP, thrombin, bradykinin, and shear stress.[9] Shear forces induce transcriptional activation of the eNOS gene because its promoter contains a shear response consensus sequence (GAGACC).[9] The NO that forms activates guanylate cyclase, thereby generating cyclic GMP. NO is then oxidized to nitrite and then to nitrate, which can be measured in blood samples. Nitric oxide in the circulation is rapidly inactivated by erythrocytes.[34] Inhalation of nitric oxide has a vasodilatory effect on the pulmonary vasculature. In patients with congestive heart failure and pulmonary congestion, NO inhalation decreases pulmonary hypertension and increases pulmonary ventilation.[35]

Interestingly, production of NO by endothelial cells appears to be impaired in the presence of the thiol-containing amino acid, homocysteine. Cynomolgus monkeys with diet-induced hyperhomocysteinemia (11 μM) showed reduced blood flow in the lower extremity and an impaired response to endothelial-cell-dependent vasodilators.[36] Similarly, production of NO by endothelial cells in vitro is significantly inhibited in the presence of homocysteine,[37] possibly by a mechanism involving impairment of the enzyme glutathione peroxidase.[38]

STRUCTURE AND BIOCHEMICAL PROPERTIES OF NOS

There are two groups of isoforms of NOS: One is constitutively synthesized and regulated by Ca^{2+} and calmodulin. The second is cytokine-inducible and posttranscriptionally regulated.[32] Most NOSs are cytosolic, whether inducible or constitutive. A membrane-bound, constitutive NOS isoform containing a myristoylation consensus sequence has been isolated from bovine aortic endothelial cells.[32] Endothelial NOS is M_r 144,000 and shares 57 percent amino acid sequence identity with neuronal NOS. The cofactor (6R)-tetrahydro-L-biopterin (H_4B) participates in inducible and constitutive NOS isoform reactions. It is thought that H_4B stabilizes the enzyme in a manner allowing for maximum activity of the NOS subunit to which the pterin binds.[32] Biological reactions controlled by NO include vasodilation, regulation of normal vascular tone, and inhibition of platelet aggregation.[39]

BLOCKADE OF PLATELET AGGREGATION AND SECRETION BY NO

Platelet aggregation and serotonin secretion in response to thrombin can be blocked via formation of endothelial NO.[40] This action of NO as an inhibitor is unaffected by aspirin, indicating that it is not due to participation of endothelial eicosanoids.[40]

In addition to the constitutive isoform of NOS (eNOS, the NOS3 gene product), endothelial cells stimulated by agonists such as cytokines will express the inducible form of NO synthase, iNOS, which is the NOS2 gene product. In this manner, NO can further inhibit platelet reactivity and reduce basal vessel tone via relaxation of vascular smooth muscle. In biochemical terms, this is due to binding of NO to the heme prosthetic group of guanylyl cyclase. The inhibitory effect of NO on platelet secretion can be monitored by surface expression of P-selectin. The ability of NO to inhibit mobilization of intracellular platelet calcium results in reduction of the conformational changes in platelet membrane GPIIb/IIIa—a requirement for fibrinogen binding and subsequent aggregation. Other effects of NO, such as inhibition of leukocyte adhesion to the endothelial surface, inhibition of smooth muscle cell migration, and reduction of smooth muscle cell proliferation, all suggest that secretion of NO into the microenvironment is a major component of the response to vascular injury.[9,11]

ENDOTHELIN (ET)

In addition to producing two important vasodilators (PGI$_2$, NO), endothelial cells also synthesize endothelins—potent vasoconstrictors. Endothelins are a group of 21-amino acid peptides, produced in a broad spectrum of cells.[9] Endothelin-1 (ET-1) is not stored in the cell but forms from an inactive precursor, preproendothelin-1. Shear stress, hypoxia, or ischemia induce transcription of the gene encoding preproendothelin-1. Preproendothelin-1 is cleaved by an ET-1-converting enzyme, thereby forming the active peptide. ET-1 emerging from the activated endothelial cell binds to a G-protein-coupled receptor in smooth muscle. This binding increases the cytosolic calcium concentration, thus promoting smooth muscle contraction. When concentrations of other thromboregulators, such as NO, are decreased, the action of ET-1 may be amplified and produce greater vasoconstriction.

Excessive ET-1 has also been implicated in the hepatorenal syndrome—a form of renal failure observed in patients with severe liver disease. This disorder is characterized by intense and prolonged renal vasoconstriction. The hypoxia, oxidant injury, and endotoxemia that commonly characterize end-stage liver disease are probably the stimuli for endothelin production. The renal vasoconstriction has been attributed to activation of the sympathetic and renin-angiotensin systems in the kidney.[9,41,42]

INHIBITION OF PLATELET FUNCTION BY ECTO-ADPASE/CD39

In addition to the platelet inhibition by PGI$_2$ and NO, endothelial cells can inhibit platelet function by the action of endothelial cell CD39, an ectoenzyme with ADPase and ATPase activities.[7,43] The enzyme belongs to the E-type ATP diphosphohydrolase (ATPase) family, members of which degrade nucleotide tri- and/or diphosphates (apyrase, EC3.6.1.5).[1,6–8,43] A soluble CD39 molecule has been generated by removing the NH$_2$-terminal and COOH-terminal portions of CD39, including the two transmembrane regions.[8] ADP released from activated platelets is metabolized by CD39, thereby inhibiting ADP-induced platelet activation, release, and aggregation (Fig. 114-3). Recombinant soluble CD39 can also inhibit ADP-induced platelet aggregation in vitro, and intravenous injection in mice decreases platelet aggregation in response to ADP and other agonists. It thus has potential as an antithrombotic agent.

THE PROTEIN C PATHWAY

The protein C pathway plays a critical role in the prevention of thrombosis as described in detail in Chap. 113. This pathway is initiated on the endothelial cell surface when thrombin combines with the endothelial receptor protein thrombomodulin (TM). Although thrombin is capable of slowly activating protein C, this reaction is markedly inhibited in the presence of physiologic concentrations of calcium ions. Once thrombin is bound to TM, the rate of protein C activation is dramatically enhanced[44] and is dependent on the presence of calcium. The detailed biochemistry of this activation reaction has been reviewed elsewhere.[45,46] In large vessels, an additional protein, the endothelial cell protein C receptor, can bind protein C and further augment its activation by the thrombin–TM complex.[47] Presumably the activated protein C (APC) can dissociate from EPCR and interact with protein S on either the endothelial cell or platelet surface to exert its function. The function of APC per se will not be discussed here, as it can be found in detail elsewhere in this book (see Chap. 113) and in other reviews.[45,46,48]

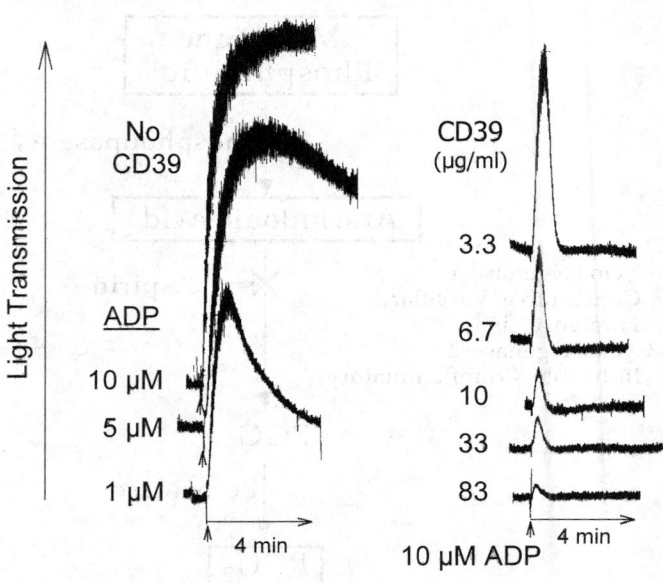

FIGURE 114-3 Blockade of ADP-induced platelet reactivity by purified soluble CD39. The response to increasing concentrations of ADP is shown on the left. The response to ADP as inhibited by increasing quantities of purified soluble CD39 is shown on the right. The experiment demonstrates that blockade of platelet reactivity by purified soluble CD39 is far greater than the reduction of platelet activation when ADP as an agonist is diluted 10-fold. Thus, in the presence of only 3.3 μg/ml soluble CD39 platelet aggregation induced by 10 μM ADP was abruptly terminated, with the curve rapidly returning to baseline.[8]

THROMBOMODULIN

FUNCTIONS OF THROMBOMODULIN

In addition to functioning as a cofactor for protein C activation, TM has many other effects on thrombin. When thrombin is bound to TM, it is no longer able to clot fibrinogen, activate platelets, activate factors V and VIII,[45] or interact with the protease-activated receptors.[49,50] Thus, TM acts as a direct anticoagulant. The rates of inactivation of thrombin by its inhibitors antithrombin III (ATIII) and protein C inhibitor (PCI) are also enhanced when thrombin is complexed with TM.[51] This leads to an estimated half-life of thrombin in the complex of 2 to 3 s.

TM also has functions that appear to oppose its many anticoagulant functions. TM promotes the activation of a procarboxypeptidase B by thrombin. This carboxypeptidase, also referred to as *thrombin activatable fibrinolysis inhibitor* or *TAFI*,[52] causes partial inhibition of fibrin degradation by plasmin, presumably by removing carboxy-terminal lysine residues from fibrin, thereby decreasing the binding of fibrin to certain forms of plasminogen and plasmin (see Chap. 116). The carboxypeptidase B may also inactivate other vasoactive substances by a similar mechanism. TM also accelerates the proteolytic inactivation of prourokinase by thrombin,[53,54] which may affect both fibrinolysis and tissue remodeling.[55] Despite these antifibrinolytic affects of TM, many in vivo experiments have demonstrated that soluble TM infusion results in a net antithrombotic and/or anti-inflammatory effect.[51] Thus, the physiological effect of thrombin–TM mediated activation of TAFI or inactivation of prourokinase remains unknown at this time.

There is intriguing evidence that, independent of its effect on hemostasis, TM plays a crucial role in development. Thus, when the TM gene is deleted by homologous recombination in mice, embryos die on day 8.5, prior to the development of a functional cardiovascular system,[56] implying that TM has functions in addition to its anticoagulant and fibrinolytic properties. In support of this proposal, animals carrying mutations of TM that greatly reduce protein C activation, but leave other regions of the molecule intact, are viable.[57] Strong expression of TM has also been observed on neural crest cells of the developing mouse embryo[58,59] and on keratinocytes,[60,61] indicating other possible roles outside of the cardiovascular system.

POTENTIAL ROLE OF THROMBOMODULIN IN ATHEROTHROMBOTIC DISEASE

Either on the cell surface or after cleavage from the surface, TM may have pro-atherogenic properties. A soluble form has been found to be mitogenic for Swiss 3T3 fibroblasts[62] and smooth muscle cells[63] in culture. Although the expression of TM is usually limited to vascular endothelial cells, TM has been observed histochemically on vascular smooth muscle cells and monocytes within the vessel wall of atherosclerotic lesions.[63] In this milieu, in which anticoagulation may not be a major function, the reported mitogenic properties of TM may dominate, leading to increased smooth muscle cell proliferation and exacerbation of the atherosclerotic lesion. Concurrently, atherogenic stimuli, such as oxidized LDL,[64] have been reported to transcriptionally downregulate TM in endothelial cells. Homocysteine, another atherogenic stimulus, has multiple effects on endothelial TM expression, both at the nucleic acid and protein level (reviewed in Lentz[65]), which overall appear to downregulate TM function. These effects may increase the thrombotic damage in the area of the atheroma, leading to extension of the lesion at the luminal surface.

TM expression on smooth muscle cells can also be protective. In cases of injury in which the endothelial layer is removed, such as in rupture of an atheroma, the underlying smooth muscle cells can act as a site for focal clot formation. However, within a relatively short period of time, the cells undergo passivation, i.e., they no longer support platelet adhesion or fibrin formation.[66] Evidence is accumulating that a contributor to this phenomenon may be the induction of TM expression on the smooth muscle cells.[66–68] In this case, in the presence of flowing blood, the anticoagulant properties dominate, limiting thrombus formation until the wound is reendothelialized. Smooth muscle cell TM may also desensitize the smooth muscle cells to the mitogenic properties of thrombin.[49]

THROMBOMODULIN STRUCTURE AND RELATION TO FUNCTION

The domain structure of TM, as shown in Fig. 114-4,[51,69,70] was deduced from the cloned cDNA for the protein. The gene for TM is intronless and is located on chromosome 20. The amino-terminal 226 residues of the mature protein show weak homology to lectinlike domains, such as the one found in the asialoglycoprotein receptor, and may be involved in the constitutive internalization of the receptor. This region is followed by six epidermal growth factor (EGF)-b type repeats. EGF domains 5 and 6, in particular EGF5, contribute most of the binding affinity for thrombin and can block fibrinogen cleavage by thrombin, although this region is not able to support protein C activation. It has been speculated that EGF5 does not exhibit the canonical disulfide bonding pattern.[71] However, this is based on protein expressed in yeast, and the bonding pattern of mammalian expressed protein has not been determined. Since all isomers are capable of binding thrombin, there is uncertainty as to the disulfide bond pattern in native TM. Although EGF45 can promote activation of protein C by thrombin, rates approaching those of the intact TM molecule require the linkage region between EGF3 and EGF4, in addition to the entire fourth, fifth, and sixth EGF modules. EGF3 is required for catalysis of TAFI activation.[72] Human TM contains a methionine in position 388 (between the fourth and fifth EGF domains) which is quite sensitive to oxidation, leading to inactivation of the molecule.[73]

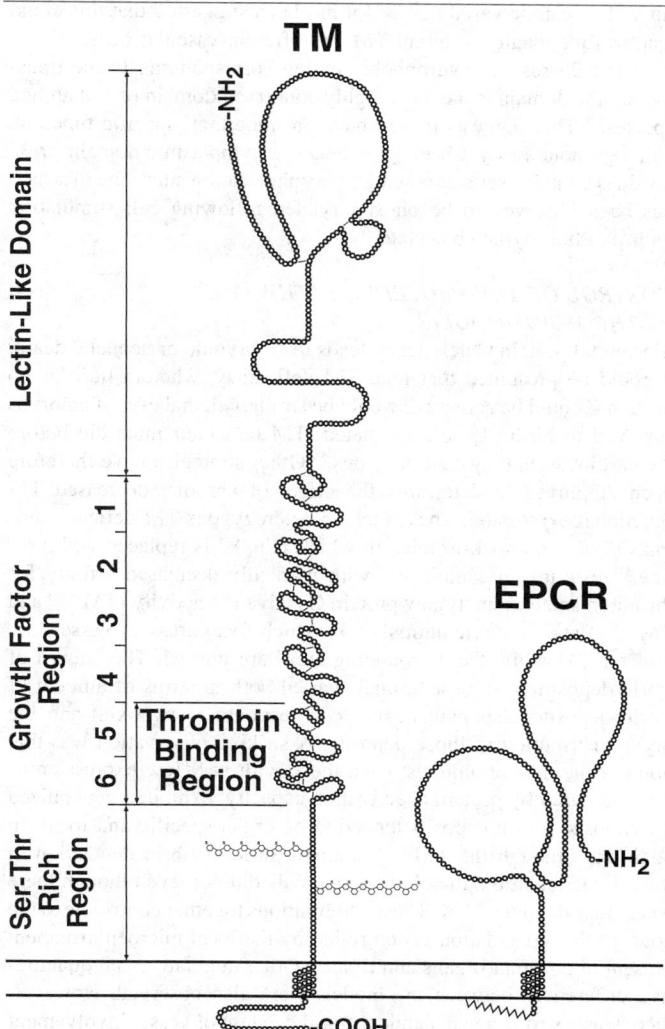

FIGURE 114-4   Structure of the endothelial cell receptors involved in the protein C pathway. The domain structure of thrombomodulin (TM) and the endothelial protein C receptor (EPCR) are illustrated. Structures shown on the Ser-Thr-rich region of TM represent chondroitin sulfate attachment. The zigzag structure at the carboxyl terminus of EPCR represents the palmitic acid modification. See text for detailed descriptions. (Modified figure reprinted with permission from *J Biol Chem* 264:4743, 1989; copyright the American Society of Biochemistry and Molecular Biology, Inc., 1989.)

Following the EGF domains is a 34-residue region rich in serine and threonine. This domain contains several *O*-linked glycosylation sites as well as two potential chondroitin sulfate attachment sites. This region is apparently elongated and serves the function of a spacer, positioning the binding sites of TM appropriately above the cell surface. The presence of chondroitin sulfate in this region has several functional consequences. It enhances the affinity of TM for thrombin, facilitates inhibition of thrombin by ATIII and PCI, modulates the calcium dependence of protein C activation, and is directly involved in platelet factor 4 modulation of protein C activation.[70] Both biochemical[74] and electron microscopic[75] experiments indicate that the glycosaminoglycan chain can bind a second molecule of thrombin. There was debate for some time as to whether naturally occurring human TM contains chondroitin sulfate.[76] However, human placental TM has now been found to contain chondroitin sulfate.[77] Addition of chondroitin sulfate can be variable,[78] and it has been suggested that this could lead to functionally different TMs in different vascular beds.[78,79]

The 23-residue hydrophobic region corresponding to the transmembrane domain is the most highly conserved domain of TM among species.[80] This suggests it may have an important, specific function, although none has yet been detected. The cytoplasmic domain of 38 residues contains several potential phosphorylation sites, one of which has been observed to be phosphorylated following cell stimulation with phorbol myristate acetate.[81]

CONTROL OF THE PROTEIN C PATHWAY BY THROMBOMODULIN

Since total protein C deficiency leads to embryonic or neonatal death, it could be presumed that total TM deficiency, wherein little or no protein C could be activated, would be similarly lethal even if embryos survived to birth. As already stated, TM knockout mice die before the cardiovascular system develops.[56] Other strategies have therefore been employed to determine the effect of chronic, decreased TM functional expression. These include heterozygous TM-deficient animals (TM$^{-/+}$), knock-in mice in which Glu387 is replaced with proline,[57] resulting in a molecule with markedly decreased affinity for thrombin and extremely low protein C activation activity (TM$^{-/Pro}$ and TM$^{Pro/Pro}$) and chimeric animals,[82] in which focal areas of vessels are null for TM while the surrounding areas are normal. The pattern of fibrin deposition in these animals varied both in terms of amount of fibrin deposited (spontaneously or in response to hypoxia) and the organ distribution of those deposits. A striking observation was that none of the mutant animals, even those with very low expression of TM measured by protein C activation capacity, exhibited generalized thrombosis. Fibrin deposits tended to be organ specific and focal. In addition, although the TM$^{Pro/Pro}$ animals showed fibrin deposition in the microcirculation, the chimeric animals did not, even though there were areas devoid of TM. These observations together contribute to the concept that coagulation is controlled by the local microenvironment present in different organs and tissues. Other qualitative and quantitative differences between the models were also observed. However, there was a strong age dependence of the extent of vessel involvement and reactivity in the chimeric animals, supporting the hypothesis that age-related alterations in the vasculature and/or coagulation system can predispose individuals to thrombosis. It is not known whether age played a significant role in the TM$^{Pro/Pro}$ or heterozygous null animals. It must be noted that both the direct antithrombin and the protein C activation functions of TM are compromised in all these animals. It is not known whether one or several TM properties are responsible for the observed phenotypes.

CONTROL OF THROMBOMODULIN EXPRESSION

The TM gene contains both a cAMP-responsive element in its 3' untranslated region[83] and a retinoic acid response element in its 5' untranslated region.[84,85] Agents that increase cAMP levels intracellularly increase TM expression,[83,86,87] as do retinoids. In addition, these same effectors, as well as IL-4[88] and vascular endothelial growth factor (VEGF),[89] will blunt, if not totally block, the effect of suppressors of TM expression.[85,90] It is unclear whether protein kinase C-controlled pathways are involved in regulation of TM.[87,91,92] The effects of active phorbol esters are biphasic.[87] Heat shock also leads to a biphasic response.[93] The TM gene contains several tandem heat shock elements in its 5' untranslated region. Although TM antigen does not change early in response to heat in human umbilical vein endothelial culture, the message decreases significantly for 6 h before it rises dramatically and then continues for at least 48 h. An increase in surface activity can be observed by 18 h of treatment. This is in marked contrast to the normal response of heat-responsive genes, in which the response

occurs within 1 h of stress. In addition, the TM response does not attenuate as classic heat shock protein expression does. This would suggest that multiple regulatory mechanisms are operative. This augmentation of TM synthesis may serve to protect the vasculature from further thrombotic damage during an inflammatory response. In line with this concept, histamine,[94] an additional inflammatory mediator, has also been reported to enhance TM synthesis.

Inflammatory mediators, in general, tend to decrease the function of TM, thereby sensitizing at least the involved areas of injury to thrombosis. These mediators include endotoxin, IL-1, tumor necrosis factor alpha (TNF-α),[87] transforming growth factor beta (TGF-β),[95] and viral infection.[96] Hypoxia also leads to a decrease in TM expression,[97] apparently through the cAMP-responsive element.[98] Since hypoxia also increases VEGF production,[99] which has been reported to induce TM expression,[90] it is difficult to predict which pathway would dominate in any specific microenvironment in vivo.

Another mechanism by which TM expression can be attenuated is through endothelial cell interaction with activated leukocytes, such as those present during inflammation. TM is sensitive to proteolytic release products,[100] and neutrophil elastase is the enzyme most commonly implicated in this process. TNF treatment increases the release of TM from endothelial cells by neutrophil elastase.[101–103] Because of the proteolysis of TM in response to inflammation or endothelial injury, measurements of TM in plasma are believed to reflect endothelial injury in various disease states.[104,105]

Leukocytes may also modulate TM activity by oxidation of the critical methionine in the molecule.[73,100] The major basic protein from the granules of eosinophils can also interact with TM to inhibit its protein C activation potential.[106] The cationic protein released from platelet granules, platelet factor 4, seems to have opposite effects on TM. At least in vitro, platelet factor 4 can both inhibit the direct anticoagulant functions of TM[107] and enhance protein C activation.[108] Whether either of these effects are of significance in vivo is unknown.

THE ENDOTHELIAL PROTEIN C RECEPTOR

The EPCR[109] is a 220–amino acid, type 1 transmembrane protein.[110,111] EPCR has two extracellular domains that show structural homology with the α and β domains of MHC class 1 molecules. Since there are 3 Cys residues in the extracellular domain, the possibility of crosslinking with another protein exists. The transmembrane domain contains two Gly-Gly sequences that are not commonly found in this region of membrane proteins. The cytoplasmic domain of human EPCR is only three amino acids long, Arg-Arg-Cys. The terminal Cys can be acylated with palmitate and this appears to have functional consequences.

The binding of protein C or APC to EPCR is mediated through the Gla domain of the ligands and requires nearly complete carboxylation of the Gla residues.[51,70,110,111] Both proteins are bound with similar affinity, about 30 nM.[109] Binding requires the presence of calcium and is tightened by the presence of magnesium ions. EPCR augments protein C activation by the thrombin–TM complex, primarily through decreasing the K_m for protein C.[112,113] Recombinant soluble EPCR binds the ligands with the same affinity as the cellular form and the soluble form can compete for binding by cellular EPCR, thereby inhibiting protein C activation on cells expressing EPCR. The enhanced activation observed on cells can be recapitulated by incorporation of both receptors (TM and EPCR) into phosphatidylcholine vesicles, indicating that additional cellular proteins or architecture are not required.[77]

When APC is bound to soluble EPCR, it is no longer capable of inactivating factor Va.[114] Due to technical difficulties, it is not known whether APC bound to cellular or membrane-bound EPCR can still bind protein S or function as an anticoagulant. The APC–EPCR complex can still be inhibited by its protein inhibitors, PCI and α_1-antitrypsin.[114] Based on analogy with the thrombin–TM complex, it is tantalizing to hypothesize that a similar switch in substrate specificity occurs in the APC–EPCR complex, changing APC from an anticoagulant into an anti-inflammatory agent.[115,116] The new substrates remain to be identified.

CONTROL OF EPCR EXPRESSION

Control of the expression of EPCR is quite complex and is only beginning to be understood. The gene structure has recently been reported,[117] and, although the entire promoter region has not yet been detailed, some of the regulatory elements in the 5'-flanking region have been described.[48,110,111] Reporter genes driven by the proximal 220 bases of the promoter region show essentially endothelial-cell–specific expression. A potential thrombin response element is present at -337 to -343. When the region from -1080 to -700 is included in the reporter construct, expression is observed only in cells derived from large-vessel endothelium, not in those derived from microvascular or capillary beds. This is consistent with the observation that EPCR is expressed primarily on the endothelium of large vessels.

Inflammatory mediators affect EPCR expression and can result in the generation of soluble forms of the receptor.[110,111] Endotoxin increases EPCR mRNA when given to rats, and the increase can be blocked by co-infusion of hirudin, indicating that the rise is most likely due to stimulation through the thrombin response element. Paradoxically, tissue culture experiments showed that although EPCR message was increased in response to thrombin, cellular EPCR protein was not. Instead, soluble EPCR produced by the action of a metalloproteinase could be recovered from the cell supernatants. When the rat system was reexamined, endotoxin was found to increase EPCR levels in the plasma, and this rise was blocked by hirudin. Soluble EPCR has also been found in significant levels in humans, and the concentration appears to be increased in certain disease states.[118] The solubilization of EPCR could potentially decrease protein C function by: (1) decreasing the rate of protein C activation in large vessels because of the loss of endothelial cell TM enhancement and (2) competing for protein C binding to the surface of all endothelium. It is still possible that protein C activation is maintained by the very high concentration of TM in the microcirculation. Ectodomain shedding of membrane proteins is being recognized as a mechanism for the regulated release of bioactive agents,[119] and it is possible that the released EPCR–APC complex may serve other functions.

TISSUE FACTOR PATHWAY INHIBITOR

Tissue factor pathway inhibitor (TFPI) is a serine protease inhibitor synthesized by microvascular endothelial cells.[120] Three pools of TFPI exist in vivo—about 3 percent is platelet associated, about 10 percent circulates in plasma in association with lipoproteins, and about 85 percent remains associated with the endothelial cell surface.[121] TFPI has a heterogeneous molecular mass (M_r of 34,000 to 42,000) owing to its susceptibility to proteolytic cleavage by neutrophil elastase. The protein consists of three tandem Kunitz-type inhibitory domains, and its major function appears to be to inhibit factor Xa as well as factor VIIa/tissue factor. Inherited deficiency states of TFPI have not been reported in humans, although low levels of heparin-releasable TFPI have been reported in young individuals with thrombosis.[122] Absence of TFPI in genetically engineered mice results in embryonic lethality between days E9.5 and E11.5 due to yolk sac hemorrhage.[123] Interestingly, this lethality is overcome in mice who simultaneously lack tissue factor.[124] Although cytokines and endotoxin upregulate tissue factor in endothelial cells, these agents have only a slight stimulatory

effect upon TFPI so that the prothrombotic effect of elevated tissue factor expression remains relatively unopposed.[121]

THE ENDOTHELIAL CELL FIBRINOLYTIC SYSTEM

Plasmin, the major clot-dissolving protease, is formed upon the cleavage of a single peptide bond within the zymogen plasminogen (see Chap. 116). This tightly regulated reaction is strongly influenced by endothelial cells that produce plasminogen activators, plasminogen activator inhibitors, and fibrinolytic receptors. In this section, we will consider the role of the blood vessel wall in the regulation of plasmin generation and examine the possible roles that the endothelial cell fibrinolytic system may play in maintaining the patency of blood vessels.

ENDOTHELIAL CELL PRODUCTION OF FIBRINOLYTIC PROTEINS

In 1958, Todd demonstrated that fibrinolytic activity in human tissues is focally distributed, relating consistently to blood vessels, especially veins and venous sinusoids and, to a lesser extent, arteries.[125] Todd later showed that this activity was localized to the wall of the blood vessel rather than its contents.[126] Pandolfi later showed that plasminogen activator activity can be associated with certain individual extravascular cells.[127]

Cultured endothelial cells derived from umbilical vein, umbilical artery, pulmonary artery, and vena cava all synthesize tissue plasminogen activator (tPA), and the endothelial cell appears to be the principal source of tPA in blood.[128] However, the pattern of tPA expression in vivo appears to be highly restricted to specific types of vessels and anatomic locations. This pattern of expression likely reflects the extreme heterogeneity of endothelial cells in vivo.[129] In the baboon, neither tPA antigen nor tPA mRNA were detected in femoral artery or vein, carotid artery, or aorta, whereas positive signals were apparent in precapillary arterioles, postcapillary venules, and the vasa vasora ranging in diameter from 7 to 30 μm.[130] In the mouse lung, similarly, all bronchial blood vessels displayed endothelial-cell–associated tPA antigen, whereas pulmonary blood vessels were uniformly negative.[131] Expression of tPA at branch points of pulmonary blood vessels may reflect stimulation by laminar shear stress.[132]

Although in vitro studies suggest that tPA expression in cultured endothelial cells is regulated by a wide array of factors, only a few of these have been evaluated in vivo. Thrombin,[133] histamine,[134,135] oxygen radicals,[136] phorbol myristate acetate,[137] DDAVP,[138] and butyric acid liberated from dibutyryl cAMP[139] all increase tPA mRNA in the cultured endothelial cell. Both thrombin and histamine appear to act via a receptor-mediated activation of the protein kinase C pathway.[128] Laminar shear stress stimulates both tPA secretion[140] and steady-state mRNA levels.[141] Hyperosmotic stress and repetitive stretch also enhance tPA expression.[142,143] In addition, differentiating agents such as retinoids[144,145] and butyrate[139] stimulate transcription of tPA in endothelial cells in vitro.

In vivo, the circulating half-life of tPA is approximately 5 min. Infusion of DDAVP, bradykinin, platelet activating factor (PAF), endothelin, or thrombin is associated with an acute release of tPA, and a burst of fibrinolytic activity can be detected within minutes.[128] In the mouse lung, exposure to hyperoxia leads to 4.5-fold up-regulation of tPA mRNA in small-vessel endothelial cells.[131] In humans, infusion of TNF into patients with malignancy is associated with an increase in tPA,[146] while treatment of cultured endothelial cells with TNF either has no effect or decreases tPA production.[147] Deficient release of tPA in response to venous occlusion in humans has been associated with deep venous thrombotic vascular disease,[148] as well as atrophie blanche and other cutaneous vasculitides.[149]

In vivo, urokinase plasminogen activator (uPA) is not a product of resting endothelium,[150] but is produced primarily by renal tubular epithelium.[151] Expression of uPA mRNA in endothelium, however, is strongly stimulated during wound repair and physiologic angiogenesis within ovarian follicles, corpus luteum, and maternal decidua.[152] Endothelial cells passaged in culture do synthesize uPA,[153] and expression of its mRNA is stimulated by TNF by 5- to 30-fold.[154] Small increases in uPA have also been observed in vitro in response to IL-1 and lipopolysaccharide (LPS).[155–157]

The association of uPA with the blood vessel wall may be at least partly reflective of uPA's association with the uPA receptor, uPAR. In the adult mouse, uPAR mRNA is not normally detected by in situ hybridization in the endothelium of either large or small blood vessels.[158] However, upon stimulation with endotoxin, expression is detected in endothelium lining aorta, arteries, veins, and capillaries of a variety of organs including heart, kidney, brain, and liver,[158] whereas the same stimulus leads to a dramatic decrease in expression in the renal tubules.[151]

Plasminogen activator inhibitor (PAI)-1 is likely to function as a major regulator of plasmin generation in the vicinity of the endothelial cell. In vitro, PAI-1 appears to be associated mainly with the substratum of cultured human umbilical vein endothelial cells, rather than the external face of the plasma membrane.[159,160] Thrombin, IL-1, TGF-β, TNF, and endotoxin all induce dramatic increases in steady-state PAI-1 message levels.[133,155,156,161] In addition, the low-density lipoprotein-like particle, lipoprotein(a) [Lp(a)], which contains an apoprotein homologous to plasminogen, also induces a two- to fourfold increase in PAI-1 mRNA without affecting mRNA for tPA.[162] Heparin-binding growth factor 1 (endothelial cell growth factor) is recognized as a down-regulator of PAI-1 mRNA production by cultured endothelial cells; this agent has no effect on tPA.[163] These studies suggest that in vitro synthesis and secretion of PAI-1 by the endothelial cell may be regulated independently of tPA.

In vivo, quiescent endothelial cells express little or no PAI-1, the liver being the major source of plasma PAI-1. During in vivo decidual neovascularization in the ovary, PAI-1 seems to be expressed near capillary sprouts that also express uPA.[152] In addition, inflammatory cytokines are powerful stimuli for induction of PAI-1 in a variety of tissues, including liver.[164] In both rats and humans with active malignancy, injection of TNF results in a striking increase in plasma concentrations of PAI-1.[128,146]

In contrast, the endothelial cell coreceptor for tPA and plasminogen, annexin II, appears to be expressed constitutively in vivo in association with blood vessels in a wide variety of tissues. In the adult chicken, endothelial cells of vessels in the dermis, lung, renal glomeruli, pancreas, liver, and meninges stain intensely positive by immunohistology.[165] Blood vessels of the developing mouse brain are also strongly cross-reactive,[166] and in both rats[167] and humans,[168] vascular endothelial cells are positive for annexin II in all tissues studied so far.

NONFIBRINOLYTIC FUNCTIONS OF PLASMIN

PLASMIN AND ANTICOAGULANT FUNCTION

Accumulating evidence suggests a potential anticoagulant role for plasmin based on its ability to specifically modify cofactors important in the thrombin-generating cascade. Plasmin has been shown to inactivate bovine factor Va in vitro by cleaving both the heavy and light chains of this M_r 168,000 protein.[169] This lipid-dependent inactivation results in a series of plasmin-specific cleavages that are distinct from those produced by activated protein C.[170] The inactivation of human factor V by plasmin may be preceded by transient generation of procoagulant fragments that are subsequently degraded to inactive form.[171] Plasmin can also inactivate factor VIIIa, another coagulant cofactor

that is structurally homologous to factor Va.[172] Factor X, finally, is subject to a well-defined pattern of cleavage events, some of the products of which may stimulate tPA-dependent plasminogen activation.[173]

PLASMIN AND PLATELET FUNCTION

The effects of plasmin on in vitro platelet function are complex. Platelet glycoproteins IIb/IIIa and Ib, the cell surface receptors for fibrinogen and von Willebrand factor respectively, are both plasmin substrates.[174,175] Thus, plasmin formation in the vicinity of a hemostatic plug could lead to impaired adhesion and poor aggregation in response to agonists. Plasmin generation has been shown to be associated with both platelet activation[176,177] and platelet inhibition[178] or disaggregation.[179] The ultimate effect of plasmin appears to depend upon the incubation conditions, particularly the dose and duration of plasmin treatment. These findings are of potential significance in view of reports that plasminogen can interact with platelets in a manner that is enhanced upon thrombin-mediated conversion of platelet fibrinogen to fibrin.[180,181] In vivo, prolonged bleeding times were found in patients 90 min after tPA infusion for thrombolysis, suggesting early impairment of platelet function upon plasmin generation.[182] However, there is also evidence that platelets may play a role in thrombotic reocclusion following successful thrombolytic therapy.[183]

FIBRINOLYTIC FUNCTION AND VASCULAR DISEASE

Several types of evidence suggest that dysfunction of the fibrinolytic system may be associated with atherosclerotic vascular disease. Elevated levels of circulating PAI-1, for example, have been epidemiologically connected to risk for myocardial infarction.[148] uPA receptor expression appears to be significantly up-regulated in the intima versus media of atherosclerotic coronary arteries, suggesting a role for plasmin in smooth muscle cell migration.[184] Circulating levels of TGF-β are reduced in individuals with atherosclerosis, possibly reflecting impaired activation by plasmin.[185] However, the exact role of plasmin and its activators in occlusive vascular disease remains to be elucidated.

PLASMINOGEN DEFICIENCY

The role of plasmin in the evolution of the atherosclerotic lesion is presently unclear. Plasminogen deficiency in mice (PLG $-/-$) is associated with impaired healing of cutaneous wounds[186] and reduced migration of monocytes to sites of inflammation.[187] Such wound healing responses appear to depend largely on the fibrinolytic action of plasmin, since loss of fibrinogen rescues this defect.[188] Upon electrical injury to the femoral artery of wild-type mice, a wound-healing response is initiated such that a neointima forms consisting mainly of smooth muscle cells that migrate to the intima from the media. In PLG $-/-$ mice, this response is significantly attenuated. These results lead to the conclusion that plasminogen plays a significant role in vascular wound healing and arterial neointima formation, possibly by mediating cellular migration.[189] On the other hand, mice doubly deficient in plasminogen and apolipoprotein(e) [ApoE] show a predisposition to atherosclerosis compared to animals deficient in either ApoE or plasminogen alone.[190] Thus, plasmin may also play an important protective role, possibly related to degradation of fibrin. Thus, the role of plasmin in either accelerating or preventing vascular disease appears to be both complex and highly context-dependent.

IMPAIRMENT OF FIBRINOLYTIC ASSEMBLY IN VASCULAR DISEASE

As discussed in Chap. 116, there is abundant in vitro evidence to support the concept that plasminogen and plasminogen activators can assemble on cell surfaces and that assembly enhances the potential

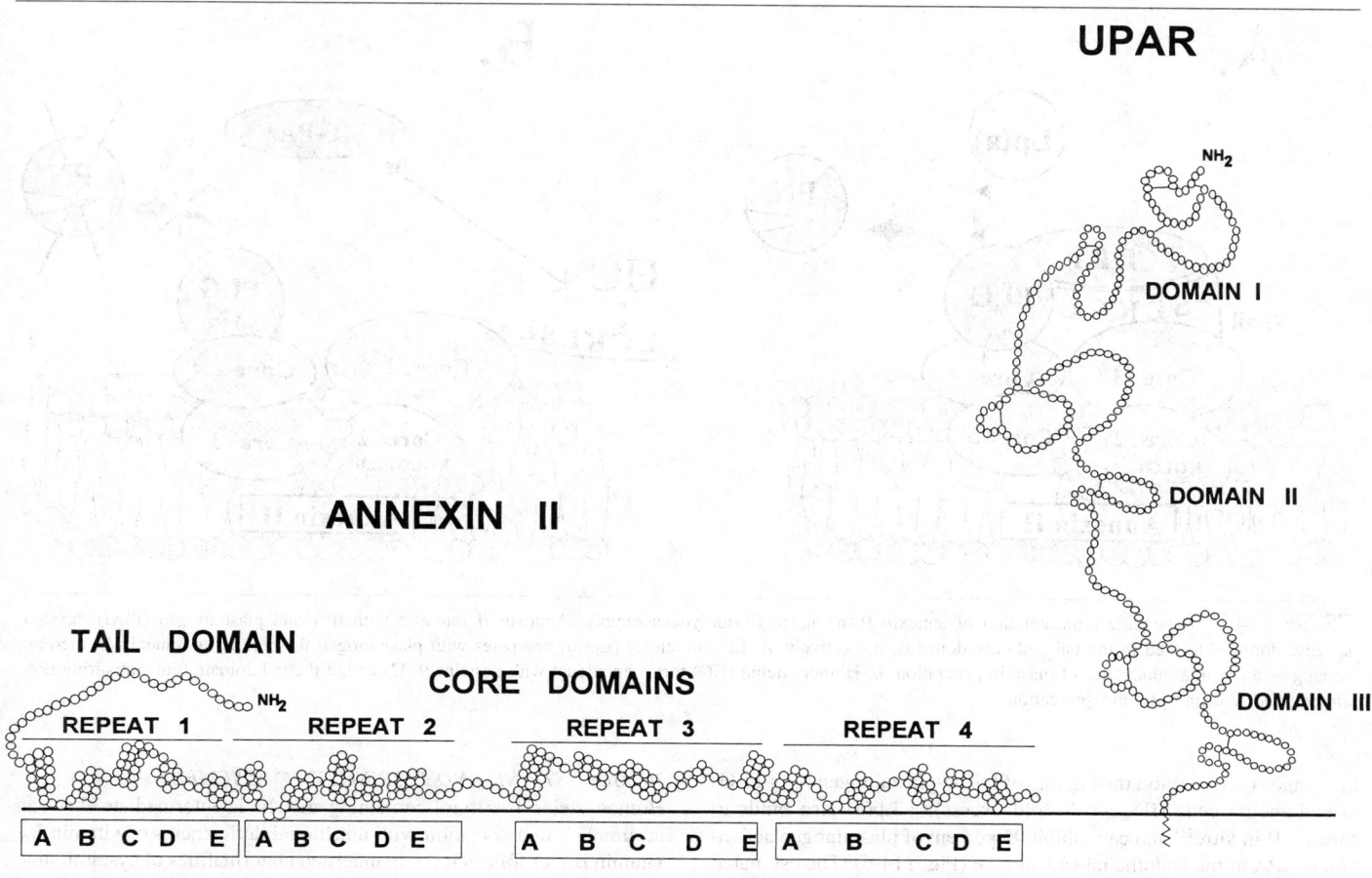

FIGURE 114-5 Two-dimensional representation of the major endothelial cell fibrinolytic receptors. Annexin II consists of an amino-terminal tail domain (~3 kDa) and a carboxyl-terminal core domain (~33 kDa).[285,286] The tail domain contains a binding site for tPA. The core domain is composed of four homologous annexin repeats, each consisting of five α-helical regions (*A* through *E*) that contribute to potential calcium-dependent phospholipid binding sites. Current evidence indicates that repeat 2 is important for the interaction of annexin II with the endothelial cell surface while plasminogen binds to lysine residue 307 within helix C of repeat 4. UPAR is a 55- to 60-kDa, glycosylphosphatidylinositol-linked protein that consists of three disulfide-linked domains.[287] Domain I contains the uPA-binding sequences, while domains II and III appear to mediate the receptor's interaction with matrix proteins such as vitronectin.

for plasmin activation. The major endothelial cell fibrinolytic receptors are uPAR and annexin II (Fig. 114-5); uPA bound to uPAR on endothelial cells is relatively protected from PAI-1 and PAI-2. However, there are as yet no known human states of deficiency or dysfunction of uPAR that relate to vascular disease. On the other hand, the profibrinolytic function of annexin II, an endothelial cell coreceptor for plasminogen and tPA, is attenuated by two atherothrombotic agents, Lp(a) and homocysteine. The assembly of tPA and plasminogen on annexin II is reviewed in detail in Chap. 116.

LIPOPROTEIN(A) AND FIBRINOLYTIC ASSEMBLY

Lp(a) is a low-density lipoprotein (LDL)-like particle that is an independent risk factor for atherosclerosis.[191–194] Lp(a) contains, in addition to apolipoprotein B-100, a disulfide-linked moiety called *apolipoprotein (a)* [Apo(a)]. Apo(a) shares a remarkable degree of homology with plasminogen, including multiple tandem repeats of domains similar to kringle IV, a single region resembling kringle V, and a pseudoprotease segment.[195] Plasminogen and Apo(a), furthermore, are genetically linked on chromosome 6 and may have arisen from a common ancestral gene.[196]

While Lp(a) levels are, at best, only transiently responsive to diet, heredity may play a more important role in regulating fibrinolytic potential at the endothelial cell surface.[197–202] In general, plasma Lp(a)

concentrations seem to correlate inversely with the ratio of kringle IV to kringle V encoding domains within the Apo(a) gene.[203] Thus, the larger the Apo(a) gene product, reflected in a greater number of kringle IV domains, the lower the concentration of Apo(a) in plasma. In addition, Lp(a) appears to represent an acute phase reactant in the postsurgical and postmyocardial infarction setting[200] and in patients with cancer,[201] suggesting a role for soluble inflammatory mediators in regulating its synthesis or assembly. The high-affinity lysine-binding site within kringle 1 of plasminogen possesses a crucial tetrad of amino acids consisting of anionic Asp55 and Asp57 plus cationic Arg34 and Arg71.[204] Kringle 4 of plasminogen, which lacks one of the four key residues (Arg34),[205] contains a lysine-binding site of intermediate affinity.[204,206–208] Kringle 37 of the originally cloned ApoA resembles plasminogen kringle 4 in that it possesses amino acids corresponding to three of the four lysine binding site residues (Asp55, Asp57, and Arg71), and many isoforms of Lp(a) have been found to have moderate lysine-binding affinity.[209] In vitro, Lp(a) binds to plasmin-treated fibrin[210] and colocalizes histologically with fibrin in atheromatous tissue.[211] Since the cell-binding activity of plasminogen is lysine-binding-site-related, kringle 37 may play a role in the interaction of Lp(a) with cell surfaces as well.

There are three potential mechanisms whereby Lp(a) may exert a prothrombotic effect by inhibiting generation of plasmin: First, both

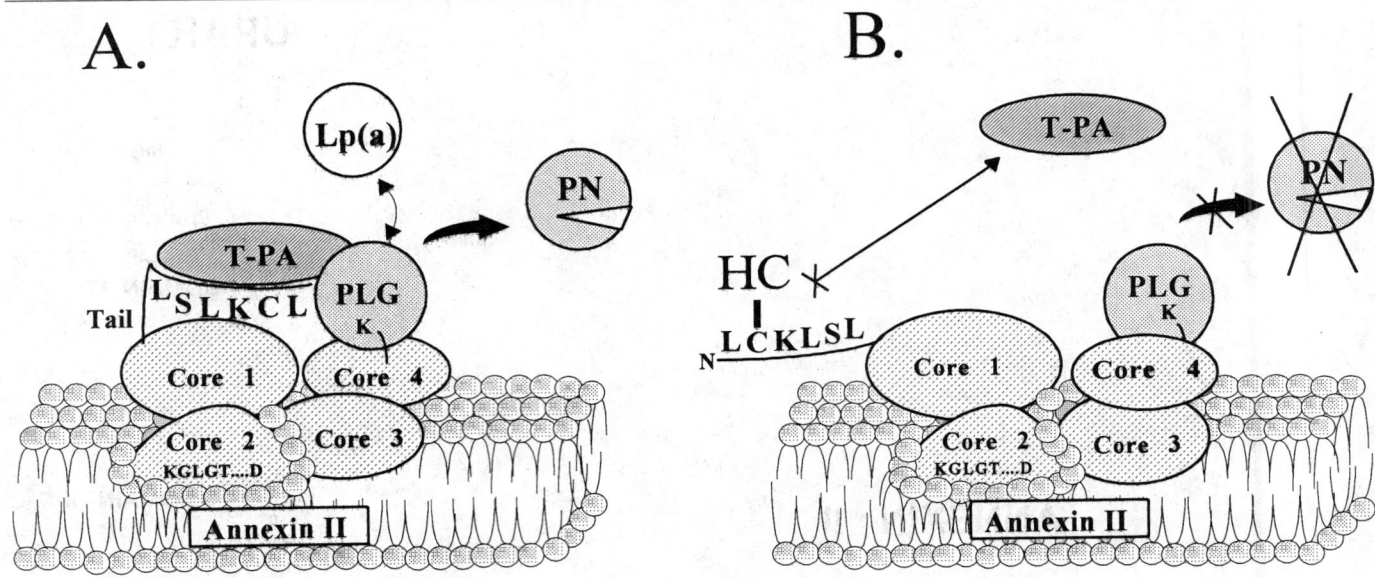

FIGURE 114-6   Schematic representation of annexin II–mediated fibrinolytic assembly. Annexin II interacts with tPA and plasminogen (PLG) through specific domains located in the tail and core domains, respectively. *A.* Lipoprotein(a) [Lp(a)] competes with plasminogen for binding to annexin II, thereby serving as a potential modulator of plasmin generation. *B.* Homocysteine (HC) forms an adduct with cysteine 9 (C) within the tail domain, thus impairing tPA binding and reducing plasmin generation.

Lp(a) and Apo(a) inhibit the binding of lysine-plasminogen (Lys-PLG) to endothelial cells (ID$_{50}$ = 36-fold excess).[212] Lp(a) also binds to annexin II in vitro[213] and can inhibit 95 percent of plasminogen activation by tPA at the endothelial cell surface (Fig. 114-6). The estimated dissociation constants for Apo(a) and plasminogen with respect to the endothelial cell surface are comparable. This finding suggests that receptor occupancy in vivo is largely determined by the ambient level of Lp(a), since plasminogen concentrations do not appear to change significantly.[212,214,215] Furthermore, anti-Lp(a) cross-reactive material can be detected within atherosclerotic lesions.[212]

Second, treatment of cultured endothelial cells with Lp(a) is associated with enhanced functional, antigenic, and transcript levels of PAI-1 without a concomitant change in plasminogen activator activity or steady-state mRNA levels for tPA. Increases in PAI-1 were not found with LDL, Lp(-), or plasminogen[162] but have been reported for very low density lipoprotein (VLDL).[216]

Third, Lp(a) may act as an inhibitor of plasminogen activators. In vitro, Lp(a) attenuates the plasmin-generating activity of streptokinase, a frequently employed thrombolytic agent, by a mechanism that involves direct competition with plasminogen for binding to streptokinase.[217,218] In addition, Lp(a) can impair plasminogen activation by tPA by acting as a competitive inhibitor of tPA in the presence of fibrinogen,[219] or as an uncompetitive inhibitor of the fibrin-dependent enhancement of tPA-induced plasmin generation.[220] Experiments in transgenic mice suggest that cell-associated plasmin activity is reduced when Apo(a) is overexpressed[221] and that these mice are resistant to lysis of an artificial thrombus by tPA.[222]

Lp(a) is not expressed in mammals other than primates and hedgehogs. However, when Lp(a) was overexpressed in mice receiving a high-fat diet, atherosclerotic lesions containing both lipid and anti-Apo(a) cross-reactive material were observed.[223] Deposition of both lipid and Apo(a) was reduced in mice expressing ApoA in which lysine binding sites had been mutated.[224] These data indicate that lysine binding sites of ApoA play a role in its atherogenicity in vivo, possibly by competing with plasminogen for cell surface binding sites.

HOMOCYSTEINE AND FIBRINOLYTIC ASSEMBLY

Homocysteine is a thiol-containing metabolic intermediate that can accumulate in association with nutritional deficiencies of vitamin B$_6$, vitamin B$_{12}$, or folic acid, or in inherited abnormalities of cystathionine β-synthase, methylene tetrahydrofolate reductase, or methionine synthase.[225] A meta-analysis of 27 studies including approximately 4000 patients showed homocysteine to be an independent risk factor for atherosclerosis of coronary, cerebral, and peripheral arteries.[226] Of 10 subsequent prospective studies, 8 demonstrated an increased risk of coronary heart disease, venous thromboembolism, cardiovascular complications, and death in individuals with elevated homocysteine levels.[227]

Several in vitro studies suggest that homocysteine induces dysfunction of the endothelial cell, which is highly susceptible to oxidative stress. Evidence that homocysteine impairs the intrinsic fibrinolytic system of the endothelial cell comes from experiments in which homocysteine-treated endothelial cells bound about 50 percent less tPA than untreated cells, and activated about 50 percent less plasminogen.[228] Electrospray ionization mass spectrometry studies indicate that homocysteine directly disables the tPA-binding domain of annexin II by forming a covalent adduction product with cysteine 9 within the tail domain of purified annexin II.[229] Direct disulfide-mediated complex formation between homocysteine and annexin II can also be demonstrated in cultured endothelial cells. Homocysteine treatment of annexin II further inhibits its ability to bind tPA with half-maximal effect observed at about 11 μM, a value close to the upper limit of normal for homocysteine in plasma (14 μM). Thus, inhibition of tPA–annexin II assembly on the endothelial cell may contribute to the prothrombotic effect of homocysteine in vivo.

ROLE OF ADHESION MOLECULES

A proinflammatory environment is also prothrombotic. Endothelial cells express molecules that regulate binding of leukocytes to their surface during inflammation. These interactions have both direct and indirect roles in hemostasis and thrombosis, as many of the cytokines and bioactive molecules that promote the inflammatory response also trigger the former. Moreover, the inflammatory response itself results in the expression of adhesion molecules and mediators that secondarily promote hemostasis.

MOLECULAR CHANGES IN AN INFLAMMATORY MILIEU

IMMEDIATE CHANGES

Histamine produced locally at the site of inflammation by degranulation of resident tissue mast cells stimulates the overlying endothelial cells to express P-selectin on their surfaces. This change occurs within minutes and is due to the rapid fusion of Weibel-Palade bodies with the plasma membrane bringing P-selectin to the surface. Along with P-selectin expression, fusion of the Weibel-Palade bodies with the membrane also results in the release of von Willebrand factor (vWF) into the local environment. In addition to its ability to induce exocytosis of platelet α granules and expression of P-selectin on the surface of platelets, thrombin can also trigger the release of P-selectin on the endothelial cell surface at sites of inflammation.

P-selectin serves as a receptor for P-selectin glycoprotein ligand 1 [PSGL-1] and probably other unidentified ligands located on leukocytes. PSGL-1 is a specific sialomucin containing sialylated, fucosylated O-linked oligosaccharides as well as an unusual sulfated tyrosine residue motif.[230] Dimerization of PSGL-1 may be required for optimal recognition of P-selectin.[231] Adhesive interactions between P-selectin and its ligands result in the tethering of passing leukocytes to, and rolling on, the surface of the endothelial cell—the first step in leukocyte emigration. L-selectin, another member of the selectin family of adhesion molecules, is constitutively expressed on the surfaces of most leukocytes. It binds to sialylated, fucosylated glycoprotein ligands expressed by endothelial cells in response to inflammation, as well as to CD34 constitutively expressed by cells of the high endothelial venules in peripheral lymph nodes.

The low-affinity reversible adhesions of leukocytes to the endothelium at the site of inflammation result in their rolling along the luminal surface. This stage serves to slow down the movement of leukocytes and bring them into contact with a variety of chemical mediators that trigger the next stage of leukocyte emigration—tight adhesion to the endothelial surface. These mediators include surface-bound chemokines,[232] new adhesion molecules expressed by the endothelium in response to inflammatory cytokines,[233] PAF,[234] soluble chemokines,[235] and ligands that cross-link leukocyte CD31.[236-238] The variety of chemical signals that can trigger tight adhesion is large[239] and may vary according to the nature of the inflammatory stimulus, the tissue involved, and the chronology of the response. However, they all seem to work by stimulating the activation of leukocyte integrin adhesion molecules by so-called inside-out signaling. This involves a conformational change and/or clustering of the two chains of these heterodimeric surface molecules such that the affinity or avidity respectively for their ligands on the surfaces of endothelial cells is increased.[240] Where these ligands have been identified, they are members of a third family of adhesion molecules, the immunoglobulin gene superfamily.[241] While immunoglobulin gene superfamily members have not been shown to undergo conformational change, there is evidence that the active form of intercellular adhesion molecule 1 (ICAM-1) is dimerized.[242,243]

Table 114-2 lists some of the more common leukocyte/endothelial cell adhesion molecule pairs participating in the inflammatory response. It is interesting to note that the mucosal addressin MAdCAM-1, a unique molecule expressed by endothelial cells of high endothelial venules of mesenteric lymph nodes and Peyer's patches, has structural features of both a mucin and an Ig superfamily molecule. It can bind both L-selectin and the leukocyte integrin $\alpha_4\beta_7$, expressed by a subset of memory T cells. It is believed to interact with L-selectin through its mucin [carbohydrate] domain and with $\alpha_4\beta_7$ through its Ig domains. However, identified protein ligands for L-selectin [MAdCAM-1 and CD34] have been demonstrated to bind to L-selectin only in the context of lymphocyte homing. Their role in leukocyte rolling and adhesion in postcapillary venules during an inflammatory response has not been demonstrated.

In addition to being made and secreted acutely by leukocytes and mast cells at the site of inflammation, PAF is rapidly made and expressed on the surfaces of stimulated endothelial cells. PAF [1-alkyl-2-acetyl-sn-glycero-3-phosphocholine] is produced enzymatically from phosphatidyl choline in the plasma membrane. While its role in this environment as an activator of neutrophils has been established,[234] it appears to be a relatively weak agonist of platelet activation in this location.

Examination of the rolling phenomenon in vivo by intravital microscopy shows that leukocytes may roll on other leukocytes that are already tightly adherent. These interactions, which are promoted through L-selectin and PSGL-1 on the leukocytes, amplify the inflammatory process.[243,244]

Adherent leukocytes migrate to nearby interendothelial junctions by repeated cycles of adhesion in the front and disadhesion in the rear.[239,245] At the junction, yet another distinct molecular interaction between leukocytes and endothelial cells regulates transendothelial migration for the vast majority of neutrophils, monocytes, and natural killer (NK) cells. Platelet/endothelial cell adhesion molecule-1 (PECAM/CD31) on the leukocyte contacts the same molecule concentrated at the endothelial junctions in a homophilic manner.[246-248] The relevant signals transduced by this interaction have not been worked out. However, a transient rise in the intracellular calcium ion content of the endothelial cell cytoplasm accompanies transmigration and is required for the process to proceed.[249] Blocking the function of either leukocyte or endothelial cell PECAM-1 arrests the leukocyte poised over the junction, tightly adherent to the apical side of the endothelial cell,[246,250,251] a phenotype very similar to that seen when the rise in endothelial cell intracellular calcium was blocked by the intracellular chelator, bis(2-amino-5-methylphenoxy)ethane-N,N,N′,N′-tetraacetic acid tetraacetoxymethyl ester (MAPTAM).[249]

Anti-PECAM reagents never block diapedesis completely, however, and PECAM-1-deficient mice do not have a significant defect in inflammation.[252] Therefore, PECAM-1 independent pathways of transendothelial migration must exist. The leukocyte integrin $\alpha_4\beta_1$ (VLA-4) and the $\alpha_L\beta_2/\alpha_M\beta_2$ (LFA1/Mac-1), and their endothelial counterreceptors, vascular adhesion molecule 1 (VCAM-1) and ICAM-1, have been implicated in transmigration.[239] In addition, under certain specialized conditions, there appear to be pathways across the endothelial cell that bypass the intercellular junction.[253]

At the onset of most acute inflammatory responses there is a transient increase in vascular permeability due to histamine release. The endothelial junctions are soon reestablished, and the leukocytes that arrive at the scene over the next hour find the junctions closed. During diapedesis, leukocytes migrate in ameboid fashion across the junction between tightly apposed endothelial cells. Studies performed both in vivo and in vitro indicate that during diapedesis leukocytes penetrate the vessel wall without breaching the vascular permeability barrier.[249,254] This prevents exposure of subendothelial collagen and vWF deposits to circulating platelets. While there is no known role for PECAM-1 in binding platelets to endothelial cells, it has been hypothesized to maintain the tight apposition of endothelial cells and leukocytes during diapedesis.[248]

TABLE 114-2　COMMON LEUKOCYTE-ENDOTHELIAL CELL ADHESION MOLECULE PAIRS IN INFLAMMATION

Leukocyte Molecule	CD and Integrin Nomenclature	Leukocytes Expressing*	Action	Endothelial Counter Ligand	CD Nomenclature
L-selectin	CD62L	PMN, Mo, T, B, NK	Tethering, rolling	MAdCAM-1† Gp105-120	Pending CD34
PSGL-1	CD162	PMN, Mo, T, B, NK	Tethering, rolling	P-selectin	CD62P
Sialyl Lewis^x ESL-1, CLA‡	CD15s	PMN, Mo, T, B, NK	Tethering, rolling	E-selectin	CD62E
LFA-1	CD11a/CD18 ($\alpha_L\beta_2$)	PMN, Mo, T, B, NK	Tight adhesion	ICAM-1 ICAM-2 ICAM-3	CD54 CD102 CD50
Mac-1	CD11b/CD18 ($\alpha_M\beta_2$)	PMN, Mo, NK	Tight adhesion	ICAM-1	CD54
VLA-4	CD49d/CD29 ($\alpha_4\beta_1$)	Mo, B, Eo> NK, T¶	Tight adhesion§ Rolling	VCAM-1	CD106
PECAM-1	CD31	PMN, Mo, NK Subsets of T	Diapedesis	PECAM-1	CD31

*PMN, neutrophils; Mo, monocytes; T, T lymphocytes; B, B lymphocytes; NK, natural killer cells; Eo, eosinophils.
†MAdCAM-1 (mucosal addressin cell adhesion molecule 1) and CD34 have been shown to be important for homing of T cells to lymph nodes via high endothelial venules. The protein structures bearing the L-selectin ligands, including CD15s, at sites of inflammation have not been identified.
‡ESL-1, E-selectin ligand, a protein with homology to fibroblast growth factor receptor has been identified in mice. CLA, cutaneous lymphocyte antigen, a molecule on the surface of skin-homing T cells related to PSGL-1, directs them to skin via E-selectin expressed on dermal venules.
¶Expression of VLA-4 on granulocytes is limited to eosinophils and basophils. Adult human neutrophils do not express it under normal circumstances.
§Although VLA-4–VCAM-1 interactions are generally thought to be important for tight adhesion of leukocytes to endothelium, there are reports[277,278] that leukocytes can use VLA-4 to roll on endothelial VCAM-1, as well.

ACUTE CHANGES

In addition to stimulating immediate responses by endothelial cells, cytokines and inflammatory mediators released at the site of inflammation activate the surrounding endothelial cells to initiate new genetic programs. De novo synthesis of mRNA and protein leads to the establishment of an inflammatory phenotype within several hours of exposure to adequate levels of the mediator. The changes result in the endothelial cell developing a procoagulant and proadhesive phenotype.

Stimulated by inflammatory cytokines like TNF-α or IL-1, vascular endothelial cells express several important cell adhesion molecules on their surface. E-selectin expression is induced within hours of cytokine stimulation. Expression peaks at 4 to 6 h in vitro, but in the presence of interferon gamma (IFNγ), and in vivo, expression is maintained over several days.[255,256] E-selectin mediates rolling of leukocytes bearing sialylated, fucosylated carbohydrate receptors similar to sialylated Lewis^x antigen. This molecule is important for the slow rolling seen in some vascular beds.[257] While P-selectin expression on the endothelial cell surface stimulated by thrombin or histamine is transient, expression of P-selectin can be prolonged by IL-3,[258] IL-4, or oncostatin M stimulation[259] of human endothelium, and by TNF-α stimulation of murine, but not human, endothelium.[260,261] Expression is often seen to last for hours to days. This prolonged expression requires de novo message and protein synthesis.

In general, expression of the immunoglobulin superfamily members ICAM-1 and VCAM-1 is induced by the same stimuli that induce E-selectin. Some specializations exist, at least in vitro. For example, IL-4 induces VCAM-1 but not E-selectin or ICAM-1 in microvascular endothelial cells.[262,263] These molecules serve as counterreceptors for the leukocyte integrins in the tight adhesion step, as discussed above.

CHRONIC CHANGES

Prolonged stimulation of endothelial cells with interferon γ leads to expression of MHC class II molecules (HLA-DR and DQ) on their surfaces. This takes several days in vitro. In human tissues such as skin and gut, class II is commonly seen even in the absence of overt inflammation and is thought to be due to chronic exposure of these sites to subclinical inflammation and antigenic stimulation. Cytokines can also induce the expression of CD40 ligand on endothelial cells.

The significance of class II expression on endothelial cells is that when costimulatory molecules such as CD40, ICAM-1, or lymphocyte-function-associated antigen-3 (LFA-3) are also induced by inflammatory stimuli, the endothelial cell becomes capable (at least in vitro) of acting as an antigen-presenting cell that can stimulate CD4+ memory T cells. While this may not be a major threat in the normal host, when the endothelium belongs to an organ graft with foreign MHC class II, this mechanism may well stimulate graft rejection by the host.[264-266]

The expression of the adhesion molecule ICAM-2 does not change in response to inflammatory mediators. PECAM-1 shows a unique expression pattern in response to IFNγ in vitro[267] (also Muller, unpublished) and in vivo.[268] The distribution, but not absolute amount, of PECAM on the surface changes as the molecule is no longer concentrated at intercellular borders but becomes expressed diffusely over the surface of the cell. In vitro chronic exposure of human umbilical vein endothelial cells to a combination of IFN-γ and TNF-α at relatively high doses leads to a decrease in total PECAM-1 expression.[269] It is possible that such a cytokine milieu could exist in vivo, but a similar phenotype has not been described to date.

ADHESION MOLECULES IN A THROMBOTIC MILIEU

In addition to the adhesive interactions germane to thrombosis and hemostasis, such an environment exposes leukocytes to ligands that promote their adhesion and recruitment to the vessel wall. For example, in vitro thrombin has been shown to induce E-selectin expression and IL-8 secretion by human umbilical vein endothelial cells.[270] These changes are classically induced by inflammatory cytokines such as IL-1 and TNF-α. Table 114-3 lists some mediators that could have dual roles in inflammation and hemostasis/thrombosis.

LEUKOCYTE–PLATELET INTERACTIONS

Activated platelets bind to circulating lymphocytes in a P-selectin-dependent manner. This interaction can facilitate rolling on the endothelium[271] and can even allow homing of lymphocytes to peripheral lymph nodes in the absence of L-selectin, since P-selectin on the adherent platelets will interact with the peripheral lymph node addressin.[272] In vitro, neutrophils have been shown to be capable of rolling

TABLE 114-3   DUAL ROLES OF INFLAMMATORY MEDIATORS IN THROMBOSIS/HEMOSTASIS

MEDIATOR	ROLE IN INFLAMMATION	ROLE IN THROMBOSIS OR HEMOSTASIS
Histamine, thrombin	P-selectin expression induced on vascular endothelium	Degranulation of Weibel-Palade bodies; extrusion of von Willebrand factor
Platelet activating factor	Activation of leukocyte integrins	Activation of platelets
Expression of P-selectin glycoprotein ligand [PSGL-1]	Adhesion of leukocytes to endothelial P-selectin	Adhesion of platelets to adherent leukocytes via P-selectin
Adherent platelets	Leukocyte rolling on platelet P-selectin; tight adhesion to platelet membrane component	Thrombosis
Fibrinogen	Adhesion of leukocytes to fibrinogen via $\alpha_M\beta_2$ (CD11b/CD18)	Bridging of platelets to vWF and matrix via GPIIb/IIIa; Adhesion of leukocytes to adherent platelets
Thrombin	Induction of E-selectin expression and IL-8 secretion by endothelial cells	Conversion of fibrinogen to fibrin
Leukocyte integrin $\alpha_M\beta_2$ (CD11b/CD18)	Adhesion of leukocytes to endothelium and activated platelets; phagocytosis	Binding and activation of factor X

on immobilized platelets that have undergone the release reaction via PSGL-1 on the leukocyte interacting with P-selectin on the platelet surface.[273] Moreover, following P-selectin-dependent rolling, $\alpha_M\beta_2$ (CD11b/CD18)-dependent arrest and tight adhesion of neutrophils to bound platelets has been described.[273,274] The platelet ligand for this is not known. ICAM-2 has been found on the surface of activated platelets,[274] but it is not a ligand for $\alpha_M\beta_2$, and in fact, antibodies against neither ICAM-2 nor its neutrophil receptor α_L (CD11) blocked this adhesion.[275] On the other hand, neutrophil $\alpha_M\beta_2$ has been reported to bind to fibrinogen, which may be present on the surfaces of activated platelets bound to $\alpha_{IIb}\beta_3$ (GPIIb/IIIa).

LEUKOCYTE–ENDOTHELIAL CELL–MATRIX INTERACTIONS THAT PROMOTE COAGULATION

The same proinflammatory stimuli that stimulate de novo expression of E-selectin and VCAM-1, and augment expression of ICAM-1 for the recruitment of leukocytes, stimulate synthesis and expression of tissue factor (TF) by the endothelial cells.[276] Furthermore, interaction of monocytes with endothelium stimulates production of TF in monocytes. Adhesion of monocytic cell lines to cytokine-activated endothelial cells in culture leads to a rapid increase in procoagulant activity due to induction of TF. This effect is partially blocked by a monoclonal antibody directed against E-selectin on endothelium and is mimicked by cross-linking Le^X on the monocyte cell lines.[277] A similar increase in TF gene expression can be induced by cross-linking α_4 or β_1 integrin chains, the components of VLA-4 on monocytic cell lines.[278]

A study of prolonged interaction of peripheral blood monocytes with human endothelial cells showed that within a few hours of transendothelial migration, monocytes in the collagen matrix expressed functional TF on their surfaces.[279] Furthermore, over the next several days, approximately half of these monocytes had differentiated into immature dendritic cells, bearing even higher levels of TF, migrated back across the intact endothelial monolayer in the abluminal-to-luminal direction. Tissue factor on the surface of monocytes was involved in this migration, since it could be blocked by soluble fragments of TF. The same TF fragments blocked adhesion of endothelial cells to TF in vitro. Therefore, it was hypothesized that TF expressed by the emigrating dendritic cells is directly involved in an adhesive step of this process in addition to any procoagulant role it may play.[279]

Leukocytes bound to P-selectin exposed on the surfaces of platelets on adherent thrombi promote the conversion of fibrinogen to fibrin.[280] The leukocyte integrin $\alpha_M\beta_2$ has been shown to bind fibrinogen.[281] The same integrin has a conformational form that binds coagulation factor X.[282] Monocytic cells are capable of activating the bound factor X to Xa when activated,[283] defining a pathway for activation of X that is independent of tissue factor.

REFERENCES

1. Marcus AJ, Safier LB: Thromboregulation: multicellular modulation of platelet reactivity in hemostasis and thrombosis. *FASEB J* 7:516, 1993.
2. Marcus AJ: Platelets: their role in hemostasis, thrombosis, and inflammation, in *Inflammation: Basic Principles and Clinical Correlates*, edited by JI Gallin, R Snyderman, p 77. Lippincott Williams & Wilkins, Philadelphia, 1999.
3. Marcus AJ, Hajjar DP: Vascular transcellular signalling. *J Lipid Res* 34:2017, 1993.
4. Marcus AJ, Broekman MJ, Safier LB, Ullman HL, Serhan CN, Rutherford LE: Formation of leukotrienes and other hydroxy acids during platelet-neutrophil interactions in vitro. *Biochem Biophys Res Commun* 109:130, 1982.
5. Weksler BB, Marcus AJ, Jaffe EA: Synthesis of prostaglandin I$_2$ (prostacyclin) by cultured human and bovine endothelial cells. *Proc Natl Acad Sci USA* 74:3922, 1977.
6. Marcus AJ, Safier LB, Hajjar KA, et al: Inhibition of platelet function by an aspirin-insensitive endothelial cell ADPase. Thromboregulation by endothelial cells. *J Clin Invest* 88:1690, 1991.
7. Marcus AJ, Broekman MJ, Drosopoulos JHF, et al: The endothelial cell ecto-ADPase responsible for inhibition of platelet function is CD39. *J Clin Invest* 99:1351, 1997.
8. Gayle RB, Maliszewski CR, Gimpel SD, et al: Inhibition of platelet function by recombinant soluble ecto-ADPase/CD39. *J Clin Invest* 101:1851, 1998.
9. Cines DB, Pollak ES, Buck CA, et al: Endothelial cells in physiology and in the pathophysiology of vascular disorders. *Blood* 91:3527, 1998.
10. Marcus AJ, Weksler BB, Jaffe EA, Broekman MJ: Synthesis of prostacyclin from platelet-derived endoperoxides by cultured human endothelial cells. *J Clin Invest* 66:979, 1980.
11. Ross R: Atherosclerosis: an inflammatory disease. *N Engl J Med* 340:115, 1999.
12. Garlanda C, Dejana E: Heterogeneity of endothelial cells: specific markers. *Arterioscler Thromb* 17:1193, 1999.
13. Taubman MB, Fallon JT, Schecter AD, et al: Tissue factor in the pathogenesis of atherosclerosis. *Thromb Haemost* 78:200, 1997.
14. Dong ZM, Wagner DD: Leukocyte-endothelium adhesion molecules in atherosclerosis. *J Lab Clin Med* 132:369, 1999.
15. Hamberg M, Svensson J, Samuelsson B: Thromboxanes: a new group of biologically active compounds derived from prostaglandin endoperoxides. *Proc Natl Acad Sci USA* 72:2994, 1975.
16. Piper PJ, Vane JR: Release of additional factors in anaphylaxis and its antagonism by anti-inflammatory drugs. *Nature* 223:29, 1969.
17. Moncada S, Gryglewski R, Bunting S, Vane JR: An enzyme isolated from arteries transforms prostaglandin endoperoxides to an unstable substance that inhibits platelet aggregation. *Nature* 263:663, 1976.
18. Whittaker N, Bunting S, Salmon J, et al: The chemical structure of prostaglandin X (prostacyclin). *Prostaglandins* 12:915, 1976.
19. Maclouf J, Folco G, Patrono C: Eicosanoids and isoeicosanoids: constitutive, inducible and transcellular biosynthesis in vascular disease. *Thromb Haemost* 79:691, 1998.
20. Herschman HR: Prostaglandin synthase 2. *Biochim Biophys Acta* 1299:125, 1996.

21. McAdam BF, Catella-Lawson F, Mardini IA, Kapoor S, Lawson JA, Fitzgerald GA: Systemic biosynthesis of prostacyclin by cyclooxygenase (COX)-2: the human pharmacology of a selective inhibitor of COX-2. *Proc Natl Acad Sci USA* 96:272, 1999.

22. Yaksh TL, Dirig DM, Malmberg AB: Mechanism of action of nosteroidal anti-inflammatory drugs. *Cancer Invest* 16:509, 1998.

23. DeWitt DL, Smith WL: Cloning of sheep and mouse prostaglandin endoperoxide synthases. *Methods Enzymol* 187:469, 1990.

24. Xie WL, Chipman JG, Robertson DL, Erikson RL, Simmons DL: Expression of a mitogen-responsive gene encoding prostaglandin synthase is regulated by mRNA splicing. *Proc Natl Acad Sci USA* 88:2692, 1991.

25. Kurumbail RG, Stevens Am, Gierse JK, et al: Structural basis for selective inhibition of cyclooxygenase-2 by anti-inflammatory agents [published erratum appears in *Nature* 1997 Feb 6; 385 (6616): 555]. *Nature* 384:644, 1996.

26. Smith WL, DeWitt DL: Prostaglandin endoperoxide H synthases1 and 2. *Adv Immunol* 62:167, 1996.

27. Loll PJ, Picot D, Garavito RM: The structural basis of aspirin activity inferred from the crystal structure of inactivated prostaglandin H2 synthase. *Nature Struct Biol* 2:1, 1995.

28. Pouliot M, Gilbert C, Borgeat P, et al: Expression and activity of prostaglandin endoperoxide synthase2 in agonist-activated human neutrophils. *FASEB J* 12:1109, 1998.

29. Dubois RN, Abramson SB, Crofford L, et al: Cyclooxygenase in biology and disease. *FASEB J* 12:1063, 1998.

30. Lipsky LPE, Abramson SB, Crofford L, Dubois RN, Simon LS, Van de Putte LB: The classification of cyclooxygenase inhibitors. *J Rheumatol* 25:2298, 1998.

31. Wu KK: Role of prostacyclin in the pathogenesis and therapy of thrombotic thrombocytopenic purpura, in *Hemolytic Uremic Syndrome and Thrombotic Thrombocytopenic Purpura*, edited by BS Kaplan, RS Trompeter, JL Moake, p 483. Marcel Dekker, New York, 1992.

32. Marletta MA: Nitric oxide synthase structure and mechanism. *J Biol Chem* 268:12231, 1993.

33. Moncada S, Higgs EA: Molecular mechanisms and therapeutic strategies related to nitric oxide. *FASEB J* 9:1319, 1995.

34. Moncada S, Palmer RMJ, Higgs EA: Nitric oxide: physiology, pathophysiology, and pharmacology. *Pharmacol Rev* 43:109, 1991.

35. Matsumoto A, Momomura S, Sugiura S, et al: Effect of inhaled nitric oxide on gas exchange in patients with congestive heart failure. *Ann Intern Med* 130:40, 1999.

36. Lentz SR, Sobey CG, Peigors DJ, et al: Vascular dysfunction in monkeys with diet-induced hyperhomocyst(e)inemia. *J Clin Invest* 98:24, 1996.

37. Stamler JS, Osborne JA, Jaraki O, et al: Adverse effects of homocysteine are modulated by endothelium-derived relaxing factor and related oxides of nitrogen. *J Clin Invest* 91:308, 1993.

38. Upchurch GR, Welch GN, Fabian AJ, et al: Homocyst(e)ine decreases bioavailable nitric oxide by a mechanism involving glutathione peroxidase. *J Biol Chem* 272:17012, 1997.

39. Loscalzo J, Welch G: Nitric oxide and its role in the cardiovascular system. *Prog Cardiovasc Dis* 38:87, 1995.

40. Broekman MJ, Eiroa AM, Marcus AJ: Inhibition of human platelet reactivity by endothelium-derived relaxing factor from human umbilical vein endothelial cells in suspension. Blockade of aggregation and secretion by an aspirin-insensitive mechanism. *Blood* 78:1033, 1991.

41. Epstein M: The hepatorenal syndrome newer perspectives. *N Engl J Med* 327:1810, 1992.

42. Moore K, Wendon J, Frazer M, Karani J, Williams R, Badr K: Plasma endothelin immunoreactivity in liver disease and the hepatorenal syndrome. *N Engl J Med* 327:1774, 1992.

43. Maliszewski CR, Delespesse GJ, Schoenborn MA, et al: The CD39 lymphoid cell activation antigen. Molecular cloning and structural characterization. *J Immunol* 153:3574, 1994.

44. Esmon CT, Owen WG: Identification of an endothelial cell cofactor for thrombin-catalyzed activation of protein C. *Proc Natl Acad Sci USA* 78:2249, 1981.

45. Esmon CT: The roles of protein C and thrombomodulin in the regulation of blood coagulation. *J Biol Chem* 264:4743, 1989.

46. Esmon CT: Anticoagulant properties of vascular cells: Thrombomodulin and protein C activation pathway, in *Vascular Control of Hemostasis*, edited by VWM Van Hinsbergh, p 9. Harwood Academic, The Netherlands, 1996.

47. Esmon CT, Ding W, Yasuhiro K, et al: The protein C pathway: new insights. *Thromb Haemost* 78:70, 1997.

48. Esmon CT: Natural anticoagulants and their pathways, in *Handbook of Experimental Pharmacology*, edited by GVR Born, P Cuatrecasas, D Ganten, H Herken, K Starke, P Taylor, p 447. Springer-Verlag, New York, 1999.

49. Grinnell BW, Berg DT: Surface thrombomodulin modulates thrombin receptor responses on vascular smooth muscle cells. *Am J Physiol* 270:H603, 1996.

50. Lafay M, Laguna R, Le Bonniec BF, Lasne D, Aiach M, Rendu F: Thrombomodulin modulates the mitogenic response to thrombin of human umbilical vein endothelial cells. *Thromb Haemost* 79:848, 1998.

51. Esmon CT: Anticoagulant protein C/thrombomodulin pathway, in *The Metabolic and Molecular Bases of Inherited Disease*, edited by CR Scriver, AL Beaudet, WS Sly, D Valle. McGraw-Hill, Montreal, 1999.

52. Bajzar L, Manuel R, Nesheim M: Purification and characterization of TAFI, a thrombin activable fibrinolysis inhibitor. *J Biol Chem* 270:14477, 1995.

53. De Munk GAW, Groeneveld E, Rijken DC: Acceleration of the thrombin inactivation of single chain urokinase-type plasminogen activator (prourokinase) by thrombomodulin. *J Clin Invest* 88:1680, 1991.

54. Molinari A, Giogetti C, Lansen J, et al: Thrombomodulin is a cofactor for thrombin degradation of recombinant single-chain urokinase plasminogen activator in vitro and in a perfused rabbit heart model. *Thromb Haemost* 67:226, 1992.

55. Preissner KT, May AE, Wohn KD, Germer M, Kanse SM: Molecular crosstalk between adhesion receptors and proteolytic cascades in vascular remodeling. *Thromb Haemost* 78:88, 1997.

56. Healy AM, Rayburn HB, Rosenberg RD, Weiler H: Absence of the blood-clotting regulator thrombomodulin causes embryonic lethality in mice before development of a functional cardiovascular system. *Proc Natl Acad Sci USA* 92:850, 1995.

57. Weiler-Guettler H, Christie PD, Beeler DL, et al: A targeted point mutation in thrombomodulin generates viable mice with a prethrombotic state. *J Clin Invest* 101:1983, 1998.

58. Imada S, Yamaguchi H, Nagumo M, Katayanagi S, Iwasaki H, Imada M: Identification of fetomodulin, a surface marker protein of fetal development, as thrombomodulin by gene cloning and functional assays. *Dev Biol* 140:113, 1990.

59. Imada M, Imada S, Iwasaki H, Kume A, Yamaguchi H, Moore EE: Fetomodulin: marker surface protein of fetal development which is modulatable by cyclic AMP. *Dev Biol* 122:483, 1987.

60. Mizutani H, Hayashi T, Nouchi N, et al: Functional and immunoreactive thrombomodulin expressed by keratinocytes. *J Invest Dermatol* 103:825, 1994.

61. Raife TJ, Lager DJ, Madison KC, et al: Thrombomodulin expression by human keratinocytes. Induction of cofactor activity during epidermal differentiation. *J Clin Invest* 93:1846, 1994.

62. Hamada H, Ishii H, Sakyo K, Horie S, Nishiki K, Kazama M: The epidermal growth factor-like domain of recombinant human thrombomodulin exhibits mitogenic activity for Swiss 3T3 cells. *Blood* 86:225, 1995.

63. Tohda G, Oida K, Okada Y, et al: Expression of thrombomodulin in atherosclerotic lesions and mitogenic activity of recombinant thrombomodulin in vascular smooth muscle cells. *Arterioscler Thromb Vasc Biol* 18:1861, 1998.

64. Ishii H, Kizaki K, Horie S, Kazama M: Oxidized low density lipoprotein reduces thrombomodulin transcription in cultured human endothelial cells through degradation of the lipoprotein in lysosomes. *J Biol Chem* 271:8458, 1996.

65. Lentz SR: Homocysteine and vascular dysfunction. *Life Sci* 61:1205, 1997.

66. Ma SF, Garcia JGN, Reuning U, Little SP, Bang NU, Dixon EP: Thrombin induces thrombomodulin mRNA expression via the proteolytically activated thrombin receptor in cultured bovine smooth muscle cells. *J Lab Clin Med* 129:611, 1997.

67. Fink LM, Eidt JF, Johnson K, et al: Thrombomodulin activity and localization. *Int J Dev Biol* 37:221, 1993.

68. Soff GA, Jackman RW, Rosenberg RD: Expression of thrombomodulin by smooth muscle cells in culture: different effects of tumor necrosis factor and cyclic adenosine monophosphate on thrombomodulin expres-

sion by endothelial cells and smooth muscle cells in culture. *Blood* 77:515, 1991.

69. Sadler JE: Thrombomodulin structure and function. *Thromb Haemost* 78:392, 1997.

70. Esmon CT: Protein C, protein S, and thrombomodulin, in *Hemostasis and Thrombosis: Basic Principles and Clinical Practice*, edited by RW Colman, J Hirsh, VJ Marder, A Clowes, JN George. Lippincott-Raven, Philadelphia, 2000.

71. White CE, Hunter MJ, Meininger DP, Garrod S, Komives EA: The fifth epidermal growth factor-like domain of thrombomodulin does not have an epidermal growth factor-like disulfide bonding pattern. *Proc Natl Acad Sci USA* 93:10177, 1996.

72. Kokami K, Zheng X, Sadler JE: Activation of thrombin-activatable fibrinolysis inhibitor requires epidermal growth factor-like domain 3 of thrombomodulin and is inhibited competitively by protein C. *J Biol Chem* 273:12135, 1998.

73. Glaser CB, Morser J, Clarke JH, et al: Oxidation of a specific methionine in thrombomodulin by activated neutrophil products blocks cofactor activity. *J Clin Invest* 90:2565, 1992.

74. Ye J, Esmon CT, Johnson AE: The chondroitin sulfate moiety of thrombomodulin binds a second molecule of thrombin. *J Biol Chem* 268:2373, 1993.

75. Weisel JW, Nagaswami C, Young TA, Light DR: The shape of thrombomodulin and interactions with thrombin as determined by electron microscopy. *J Biol Chem* 271:31485, 1996.

76. Parkinson JF, Koyama T, Bang NU, Preissner KT: Thrombomodulin: an anticoagulant cell surface proteoglycan with physiologically relevant glycosaminoglycan moiety. *Adv Exp Med Biol* 313:177, 1992.

77. Xu J, Esmon NL, Esmon CT: Reconstitution of the human endothelial cell protein C receptor with thrombomodulin in phosphatidylcholine vesicles enhances protein C activation. *J Biol Chem* 274:6704, 1999.

78. Lin JH, McLean K, Morser J, et al: Modulation of glycosaminoglycan addition in naturally expressed and recombinant human thrombomodulin. *J Biol Chem* 269:25021, 1994.

79. Parkinson JF, Garcia JGN, Bang NU: Decreased thrombin affinity of cell-surface thrombomodulin following treatment of cultured endothelial cells with β-D-xylose. *Biochem Biophys Res Commun* 169:177, 1990.

80. Dittman WA, Majerus PW: Structure and function of thrombomodulin: a natural anticoagulant. *Blood* 75:329, 1990.

81. Dittman WA, Kumada T, Sadler JE, Majerus PW: The structure and function of mouse thrombomodulin. Phorbol myristate acetate stimulates degradation and synthesis of thrombomodulin without affecting mRNA levels in hemangioma cells. *J Biol Chem* 263:15815, 1988.

82. Healy AM, Hancock WW, Christie PD, Rayburn HB, Rosenberg RD: Intravascular coagulation activation in a murine model of thrombomodulin deficiency: effects of lesion size, age, and hypoxia on fibrin deposition. *Blood* 92:4188, 1998.

83. Tazawa R, Yamamoto K, Suzuki K, Hirokawa K, Hirosawa S, Aoki N: Presence of functional cyclic AMP responsive element in the 3' untranslated region of the human thrombomodulin gene. *Biochim Biophys Res Commun* 200:1391, 1994.

84. Dittman WA, Nelson SC, Greer PK, Horton ET, Palomba ML, McCachren SS: Characterization of thrombomodulin expression in response to retinoic acid and identification of a retinoic acid response element in the human thrombomodulin gene. *J Biol Chem* 269:16925, 1994.

85. Ishii H, Horie S, Kizaki K, Kazama M: Retinoic acid counteracts both the downregulation of thrombomodulin and the induction of tissue factor in cultured human endothelial cells exposed to tumor necrosis factor. *Blood* 80:2556, 1992.

86. Ohdama S, Takano S, Ohashi K, Miyake S, Aoki N: Pentoxifylline prevents tumor necrosis factor-induced suppression of endothelial cell surface thrombomodulin. *Thromb Res* 62:745, 1991.

87. Hirokawa K, Aoki N: Regulatory mechanisms for thrombomodulin expression in human umbilical vein endothelial cells in vitro. *J Cell Physiol* 147:157, 1991.

88. Kapiotis S, Besemer J, Bevec D, et al: Interleukin 4 counteracts pyrogen-induced downregulation of thrombomodulin in cultured human vascular endothelial cells. *Blood* 78:410, 1991.

89. Calnek DS, Grinnell BW: Thrombomodulin-dependent anticoagulant activity is regulated by vascular endothelial growth factor. *Exp Cell Res* 238:294, 1998.

90. Miyake S, Ohdama S, Tazawa R, Aoki N: Retinoic acid prevents cyto-

91. kine-induced suppression of thrombomodulin expression on surface of human umbilical vascular endothelial cells in vitro. *Thromb Res* 68:483, 1992.

91. Herbert JM, Savi P, Laplace MC, Dumas A, Dol F: Chelerythrine, a selective protein kinase C inhibitor, counteracts pyrogen-induced expression of tissue factor without effect on thrombomodulin down-regulation in endothelial cells. *Thromb Res* 71:487, 1993.

92. Yang HL, Hseu YC, Lu FJ, Tsai HD: Humic acid reduces protein C-activating cofactor activity of thrombomodulin of human umbilical vein endothelial cells. *Br J Haematol* 101:16, 1998.

93. Conway EM, Liu L, Nowakowski B, Steiner-Mosonyi M, Jackman RW: Heat shock of vascular endothelial cells induces an up-regulatory transcriptional response of the thrombomodulin gene that is delayed in onset and does not attenuate. *J Biol Chem* 269:22804, 1994.

94. Hirokawa K, Aoki N: Up-regulation of thrombomodulin by activation of histamine H1 receptors in human umbilical-vein endothelial cells in vitro. *Biochem J* 276:739, 1991.

95. Ohji T, Urano H, Shirahata A, et al: Transforming growth factor beta 1 and beta 2 induce downmodulation of thrombomodulin in human umbilical vein endothelial cells. *Thromb Haemost* 73:812, 1995.

96. Key NS, Vercellotti GM, Winkelmann JC, et al: Infection of vascular endothelial cells with herpes simplex virus enhances tissue factor activity and reduces thrombomodulin expression. *Proc Natl Acad Sci USA* 87:7095, 1990.

97. Dufourcq P, Seigneur M, Pruvost A, et al: Membrane thrombomodulin levels are decreased during hypoxia and restored by cAMP and IBMX. *Thromb Res* 77:305, 1994.

98. Seigneur M, Dufourcq P, Belloc F, Lenoble M, Renard M, Boisseau MR: Influence of pentoxifylline on membrane thrombomodulin levels in endothelial cells submitted to hypoxic conditions. *J Cardiovasc Pharmacol* 25(suppl 2):S85, 1995.

99. Zachary I: Vascular endothelial growth factor. *Int J Biochem Cell Biol* 60:1169, 1998.

100. MacGregor IA, Perrie AM, Donnelly SC, Haslett C: Modulation of human endothelial thrombomodulin by neutrophils and their release products. *Am J Respir Crit Care Med* 155:47, 1997.

101. Boehme MWJ, Deng Y, Raeth U, et al: Release of thrombomodulin from endothelial cells by concerted action of TNFα and neutrophils: in vivo and in vitro studies. *Immunology* 87:134, 1996.

102. Key NS, Vercellotti GM, Esmon NL, Esmon CT, Jacob HS: Neutrophils enhance procoagulant effects of tumor necrosis factor on endothelium by accelerating thrombomodulin loss: role in endotoxin shock. *Clin Res* 37:601a (Abstr), 1989.

103. Abe H, Okajima K, Okabe H, Takatsuki K, Binder BR: Granulocyte proteases and hydrogen peroxide synergistically inactivate thrombomodulin of endothelial cells in vitro. *J Lab Clin Med* 123:874, 1994.

104. Boffa MC: Considering cellular thrombomodulin distribution and its modulating factors can facilitate the use of plasma thrombomodulin as a reliable endothelial marker? *Hemostasis* 26:233, 1996.

105. Blann A, Seigneur M: Soluble markers of endothelial cell function. *Clin Hemorheol Microcirc* 17:3, 1997.

106. Slungaard A, Vercellotti GM, Tran T, Gleich GJ, Key NS: Eosinophil cationic granule proteins impair thrombomodulin function. A potential mechanism for thromboembolism in hypereosinophilic heart disease. *J Clin Invest* 91:1721, 1993.

107. Bourin MC, Ohlin AK, Lane DA, Stenflo J, Lindahl U: Relationship between anticoagulant activities and polyanionic properties of rabbit thrombomodulin. *J Biol Chem* 263:8044, 1988.

108. Dudek AZ, Pennell CA, Decker TD, Young TA, Key NS, Slungaard A: Platelet factor 4 binds to glycanated forms of thrombomodulin and to protein C. A potential mechanism for enhancing generation of activated protein C. *J Biol Chem* 272:31785, 1997.

109. Fukudome K, Esmon CT: Identification, cloning, and regulation of a novel endothelial cell protein C/activated protein C receptor. *J Biol Chem* 269:26486, 1994.

110. Esmon CT, Gu J, Xu J, Qu D, Stearns-Kurosawa DJ, Kurosawa S: Regulation and functions of the protein C anticoagulant pathway. *Haematologica* 84:363, 1999.

111. Esmon CT, Xu J, Gu J, et al: Endothelial protein C receptor. *Thromb Haemost* 82:251, 1999.

112. Stearns-Kurosawa DJ, Kurosawa S, Mollica JS, Ferrell GL, Esmon CT: The endothelial cell protein C receptor augments protein C activation

by the thrombin-thrombomodulin complex. *Proc Natl Acad Sci USA* 93:10212, 1996.

113. Fukudome K, Ye X, Tsuneyoshi N, et al: Activation mechanism of anticoagulant protein C in large blood vessels involving the endothelial cell protein C receptor. *J Exp Med* 187:1029, 1998.

114. Regan LM, Stearns-Kurosawa DJ, Kurosawa S, Mollica J, Fukudome K, Esmon CT: The endothelial cell protein C receptor: inhibition of activated protein C anticoagulant function without modulation of reaction with proteinase inhibitors. *J Biol Chem* 271:17499, 1996.

115. Esmon CT, Taylor FB Jr, Snow TR: Inflammation and coagulation: linked processes potentially regulated through a common pathway mediated by protein C. *Thromb Haemost* 66:160, 1991.

116. Esmon CT, Schwarz HP: An update on clinical and basic aspects of the protein C anticoagulant pathway. *Trends Cardiovasc Med* 5:141, 1995.

117. Simmonds RE, Lane DA: Structural and functional implications of the intron/exon organization of the human endothelial cell protein C/activated protein C receptor (EPCR) gene: comparison with the structure of CD1/major histocompatibility complex α1 and α2 domains. *Blood* 94:632, 1999.

118. Kurosawa S, Stearns-Kurosawa DJ, Hidari N, Esmon CT: Identification of functional endothelial protein C receptor in human plasma. *J Clin Invest* 100:411, 1997.

119. Peschon JJ, Slack JL, Reddy P, et al: An essential role for ectodomain shedding in mammalian development. *Science* 282:1281, 1998.

120. Broze GJ: Tissue factor pathway inhibitor and the revised theory of coagulation. *Annu Rev Med* 46:103, 1995.

121. Bajaj MS, Bajaj SP: Tissue factor pathway inhibitor: potential therapeutic applications. *Thromb Haemost* 78:471, 1997.

122. Ariens RA, Alberio G, Moia M, Mannucci PM: Low levels of heparin-releasable tissue factor pathway inhibitor in young patients with thrombosis. *Thromb Haemost* 81:203, 1999.

123. Huang ZF, Higuchi D, Lasky N, Broze GJ: Tissue factor pathway inhibitor gene disruption produces intrauterine lethality in mice. *Blood* 90:944, 1997.

124. Chan JCY, Carmeliet P, Moons L, et al: Factor VII deficiency rescues the intrauterine lethality in mice associated with a tissue factor pathway inhibitor deficit. *J Clin Invest* 103:475, 1999.

125. Todd AS: Fibrinolysis autographs. *Nature* 181:495, 1958.

126. Todd AS: Localization of fibrinolytic activity in tissues. *Br Med Bull* 20:210, 1964.

127. Pandolfi M: Histochemistry of tissue plasminogen activator. *Thromb Diath Haemorrh* 34:661, 1975.

128. Van Hinsbergh VWM, Kooistra T, Emeis JJ, Koolwijk P: Regulation of plasminogen activator production by endothelial cells: role in fibrinolysis and local proteolysis. *Int J Radiat Biol* 60:261, 1991.

129. Augustin HG, Kozian DH, Johnson RC: Differentiation of endothelial cells: analysis of the constitutive and activated endothelial cell phenotypes. *BioEssays* 16:901, 1994.

130. Levin EG, del Zoppo GJ: Localization of tissue plasminogen activator in the endothelium of a limited number of vessels. *Am J Pathol* 144:855, 1994.

131. Levin EG, Santell L, Osborn KG: The expression of endothelial tissue plasminogen activator in vivo: a function defined by vessel size and anatomic location. *J Cell Sci* 110:139, 1997.

132. Levin EG, Osborn KG, Schleuning WD: Vessel-specific gene expression in the lung: tissue plasminogen activator is limited to bronchial arteries and pulmonary vessels of discrete size. *Chest* 114:68S, 1998.

133. Dichek D, Quertermous T: Thrombin regulation of mRNA levels of tissue plasminogen activator inhibitor 1 in cultured human umbilical vein endothelial cells. *Blood* 74:222, 1989.

134. Hanss M, Collen D: Secretion of tissue-type plasminogen activator and plasminogen activator inhibitor by cultured human endothelial cells: modulation by thrombin, endotoxin, and histamine. *J Lab Clin Med* 109:97, 1987.

135. Levin EG, Santell L: Stimulation and desensitization of tissue plasminogen activator release from human endothelial cells. *J Biol Chem* 263:9360, 1988.

136. Shatos MA, Doherty JM, Orfeo T, Hoak JC, Collen D, Stump DC: Modulation of the fibrinolytic response of cultured human vascular endothelium by extracellularly generated oxygen radicals. *J Biol Chem* 267:597, 1992.

137. Levin EG, Marotti KR, Santell L: Protein kinase C and the stimulation

138. Cugno M, Uziel L, Fabrizi I, Bottasso B, Maggiolini F, Agostoni A: Fibrinolytic response in normal subjects to venous occlusion and DDAVP infusion. *Thromb Res* 56:625, 1989.

139. Kooistra T, Van den Berg J, Tons A, Platenburg G, Rijken DC, Van den Berg E: Butyrate stimulates tissue-type plasminogen activator synthesis in cultured human endothelial cells. *Biochem J* 247:605, 1987.

140. Diamond SL, Eskin SG, McIntire LV: Fluid flow stimulates tissue plasminogen activator secretion by cultured human endothelial cells. *Science* 243:1483, 1989.

141. Diamond SL, Sharefkin JB, Dieffenbach C, Frasier-Scott K, McIntire LV, Eskin SG: Tissue plasminogen activator messenger RNA levels increase in cultured human endothelial cells exposed to laminar shear stress. *J Cell Physiol* 143:364, 1990.

142. Levin EG, Santell L, Saljooque F: Hyperosmotic stress stimulates tissue plasminogen activator expression by a PKC-dependent pathway. *Am J Physiol* 265:C387, 1993.

143. Iba T, Shin T, Sonoda T, Rosales O, Sumpio BE: Stimulation of endothelial secretion of tissue-type plasminogen activator by repetitive stretch. *J Surg Res* 50:457, 1991.

144. Thompson EA, Nelles L, Collen D: Effect of retinoic acid on the synthesis of tissue-type plasminogen activator and plasminogen activator inhibitor 1 in human endothelial cells. *Eur J Biochem* 201:627, 1991.

145. Bulens F, Ibanez-Tallon I, Van Acker P, et al: Retinoic acid induction of human tissue-type plasminogen activator gene expression via a direct repeat element (DR5) located at 7 kilobases. *J Biol Chem* 270:7167, 1995.

146. Van Hinsbergh VWM, Bauer KA, Kooistra T, et al: Progress of fibrinolysis during tumor necrosis factor infusions in humans. Concomitant increase in tissue-type plasminogen activator, plasminogen activator inhibitor type 1, and fibrin(ogen) degradation products. *Blood* 76:2284, 1990.

147. Schleef RR, Bevilaqua MP, Sawdey M, Gimbrone MA, Loskutoff DJ: Cytokine activation of vascular endothelium: effects on tissue-type plasminogen activator and type 1 plasminogen activator inhibitor. *J Biol Chem* 263:5797, 1988.

148. Hamsten A, Wiman B, De Faire U, Blomback M: Increased plasma levels of a rapid inhibitor of tissue plasminogen activator in young survivors of myocardial infarction. *N Engl J Med* 313:1557, 1985.

149. Pizzo SV, Murray JC, Gonias SL: Atrophie blanche: a disorder associated with defective release of tissue plasminogen activator. *Arch Pathol Lab Med* 110:517, 1986.

150. Kristensen P, Larson LI, Nielsen LS, Grondahl-Hansen J, Andreasen PA, Dano K: Human endothelial cells contain one type of plasminogen activator. *FEBS Lett* 168:33, 1984.

151. Yamamoto K, Loskutoff DJ: Fibrin deposition in tissues from endotoxin-treated mice correlates with decreases in the expression of urokinase-type but not tissue-type plasminogen activator. *J Clin Invest* 97:2440, 1996.

152. Bacharach E, Itin A, Keshet E: In vivo patterns of expression of urokinase and its inhibitor PAI1 suggest a concerted role in regulating physiological angiogenesis. *Proc Natl Acad Sci USA* 89:10686, 1992

153. Booyse FM, Scheinbuks J, Radek J, Osikowicz G, Feder S, Quarfoot AJ: Immunological identification and comparison of plasminogen activator forms in cultured normal human endothelial cells and smooth muscle cells. *Thromb Res* 24:495, 1981.

154. Van Hinsbergh VWM, Van den Berg EA, Fiers W, Dooijewaard G: Tumor necrosis factor induces the production of urokinase-type plasminogen activator by human endothelial cells. *Blood* 75:1991, 1990.

155. Sawdey M, Podor TJ, Loskutoff DJ: Regulation of type 1 plasminogen activator inhibitor gene expression in cultured bovine aortic endothelial cells. *J Biol Chem* 264:10396, 1989.

156. Van den Berg EA, Sprengers ED, Jaye M, Burgess W, Maciag T, Van Hinsbergh VWM: Regulation of plasminogen activator inhibitor 1 mRNA in human endothelial cells. *Thromb Haemost* 60:63, 1988.

157. Ellis V, Scully MF, Kakkar VV: Plasminogen activation by single-chain urokinase in functional isolation. *J Biol Chem.* 262:14998, 1987.

158. AlmusJacobs F, Varki N, Sawdey MS, Loskutoff DJ: Endotoxin stimulates expression of the murine urokinase receptor gene in vivo. *Am J Pathol* 147:688, 1995.

159. Schleef RR, Podor TJ, Dunne E, Mimuro J, Loskutoff DJ: The majority of type 1 plasminogen activator inhibitor associated with cultured human endothelial cells is located under the cells and is accessible to solution-phase tissue-type plasminogen activator. *J Cell Biol* 110:155, 1990.

160. Levin EG, Santell L: Association of a plasminogen activator inhibitor (PAI1) with the growth substratum and membrane of human endothelial cells. *J Cell Biol* 105:2543, 1987.

161. Medina R, Socher SH, Han JH, Friedman PA: Interleukin 1, endotoxin, or tumor necrosis factor/cachectin enhance the level of plasminogen activator inhibitor messenger RNA in bovine aortic endothelial cells. *Thromb Res* 54:41, 1989.

162. Etingin OR, Hajjar DP, Hajjar KA, Harpel PC, Nachman RL: Lipoprotein(a) regulates plasminogen activator inhibitor 1 expression in endothelial cells. *J Biol Chem* 266:2459, 1990.

163. Konkle B, Ginsburg D: The addition of endothelial cell growth factor and heparin to human endothelial cell cultures decrease plasminogen activator. *J Clin Invest* 82:579, 1988.

164. Sawdey MS, and Loskutoff DJ: Regulation of murine type 1 plasminogen activator inhibitor gene expression in vivo: Tissue specificity and induction by lipopolysaccharide, tumor necrosis factors, and interleukin 1. *J Clin Invest* 88:1346, 1999.

165. Greenberg ME, Brackenbury R, Edelman GM: Changes in the distribution of the 34-k-Dalton tyrosine kinase substrate during differentiation and maturation of chicken tissues. *J Cell Biol* 98:473, 1984.

166. Hamre KM, Chepenik KP, Goldowitz D: The annexins: specific markers of midline structures and sensory neurons in the developing murine central nervous system. *J Comp Neurol* 352:421, 1995.

167. Gould KL, Cooper JA, Hunter T: The 46,000-Dalton tyrosine kinase substrate is widespread, whereas the 36,000-Dalton substrate is only expressed at high levels in certain rodent tissues. *J Cell Biol* 98:487, 1984.

168. Dreier R, Schmid KW, Gerke V, Riehemann K: Differential expression of annexins I, II, and IV in human tissues: an immunohistochemical study. *Histochem Cell Biol* 110:137, 1998.

169. Omar MN, Mann KG: Inactivation of factor Va by plasmin. *J Biol Chem* 262:9750, 1987.

170. Esmon CT: The regulation of natural anticoagulant pathways. *Science* 235:1348, 1987.

171. Lee CD, Mann KG: Activation/inactivation of human factor V by plasmin. *Blood* 73:185, 1989.

172. McKee PA, Anderson JC, Switzer ME: Molecular structural studies of human factor VIII. *Ann NY Acad Sci* 240:8, 1975.

173. Pryzdial ELG, Lavigne N, Dupuis N, Kessler G: Plasmin converts factor X from coagulation zymogen to fibrinolysis cofactor. *J Biol Chem* 274:8500, 1999.

174. Stricker RB, Wong D, Shiu DT, Reyes PT, Shuman MA: Activation of plasminogen by tissue plasminogen activator on normal and thrombasthenic platelets: effects on surface proteins and platelet aggregation. *Blood* 68:275, 1986.

175. Adelman B, Michelson AD, Greenberg J, Handin RI: Proteolysis of platelet glycoprotein by plasmin is facilitated by plasmin lysine-binding regions. *Blood* 68:1280, 1986.

176. Schafer AI, Adelman B: Plasmin inhibition of platelet function and of arachidonate metabolism. *J Clin Invest* 75:456, 1985.

177. Puri RN, Zhou FX, Colman RF, Colman RW: Plasmin-induced platelet aggregation is accompanied by cleavage of aggregin and indirectly mediated by calpain. *Am J Physiol* 259:C862, 1990.

178. Schafer AI, Maas AK, Ware JA, Johnson PC, Rittenhouse SE, Salzman EW: Platelet protein phosphorylation, elevation of cytosolic calcium, and inositol phospholipid breakdown in platelet activation induced by plasmin. *J Clin Invest* 78:73, 1986.

179. Loscalzo J, Vaughan DE: Tissue plasminogen activator promotes platelet disaggregation. *J Clin Invest* 79:1749, 1986.

180. Miles LA, Ginsberg MA, White JG, Plow EF: Plasminogen interacts with platelets through two distinct mechanisms. *J Clin Invest* 77:2001, 1986.

181. Maciag T, Hoover GR, Stemerman MB, Weinstein R: Serial propagation of human endothelial cells in vitro. *J Cell Biol* 91:420, 1981.

182. Gimple LW, Gold HK, Leinbach RC, et al: Correlation between template bleeding times and spontaneous bleeding during treatment of acute myocardial infarction with recombinant tissue-type plasminogen activator. *Blood* 80:581, 1989.

183. Coller BS: Platelets and thrombolytic therapy. *N Engl J Med* 322:33, 1990.

184. Raghunath PN, Tomaszewski JE, Brady ST, Caron RJ, Okada SS, Barnathan ES: Plasminogen activator system in human coronary atherosclerosis. *Arterioscler Thromb Vasc Biol* 15:1432, 1995.

185. Grainger DJ, Kemp PR, Metcalfe JC, et al: The serum concentration of active transforming growth factor b is severely depressed in advanced atherosclerosis. *Nature Med* 1:74, 1995.

186. Romer J, Bugge TH, Pyke C, Lund LR, Flick MJ, Degen JL, Dano K: Impaired wound healing in mice with a disrupted plasminogen gene. *Nature Med* 2:287, 1996.

187. Ploplis VA, French EL, Carmeliet P, Collen D, Plow EF: Plasminogen deficiency differentially affects recruitment of inflammatory cell populations in mice. *Blood* 91:2005, 1998.

188. Bugge TH, Kombrinck KW, Flick MJ, Daugherty CC, Danton MJS, Degen JL: Loss of fibrinogen rescues mice from the pleiotropic effects of plasminogen deficiency. *Cell* 87:709, 1996.

189. Carmeliet P, Moons L, Ploplis VA, Plow EF, Collen D: Impaired arterial neointima formation in mice with disruption of the plasminogen gene. *J Clin Invest* 99:200, 1997.

190. Xiao Q, Danton MJS, Witte DP, et al: Plasminogen deficiency accelerates vessel wall disease in mice predisposed to atherosclerosis. *Proc Natl Acad Sci USA* 94:10335, 1997.

191. Scanu AM, Fless GM: Lipoprotein(a) heterogeneity and biologic relevance. *J Clin Invest* 85:1709, 1990.

192. Utermann G: The mysteries of lipoprotein(a). *Science* 246:904, 1989.

193. Loscalzo J: Lipoprotein(a), a unique risk factor for atherothrombotic disease. *Arteriosclerosis* 10:672, 1990.

194. Hajjar KA, Nachman RL: The role of lipoprotein(a) in atherogenesis and thrombosis. *Annu Rev Med* 47:423, 1996.

195. McLean JW, Tomlinson JE, Kuang WJ, et al: cDNA sequence of human apolipoprotein(a) is homologous to plasminogen. *Nature* 330:132, 1987.

196. Weitkamp LR, Guttormsen SA, Schultz JS: Linkage between the loci for the Lp(a) lipoprotein (Lp) and plasminogen (PLG). *Hum Genet* 79:80, 1988.

197. Neven L, Khalil A, Pfaffinger D, Fless GM, Jackson E, Scanu AM: Rhesus monkey model of familial hypercholesterolemia: relation between plasma Lp(a) levels, apo(a) isoforms and LDL-receptor function. *J Lipid Res* 31:633, 1990.

198. Pfaffinger D, Schuelke J, Kim C, Fless GM, Scanu AM: Relationship between apo(a) isoforms and Lp(a) density in subjects with different apo(a) phenotype: a study before and after a fatty meal. *J Lipid Res* 32:679, 1991.

199. Utermann G, Menzel HJ, Kraft HG, Duba HC, Kemmler HG, Seitz C: Lp(a) glycoprotein phenotypes. *J Clin Invest* 80:458, 1987.

200. Maeda S, Abe A, Seishima M, Makino K, Noma A, Kawade M: Transient changes of serum lipoprotein(a) as an acute phase protein. *Atherosclerosis* 78:145, 1989.

201. Wright LC, Sullivan DR, Muller M, et al: Elevated apolipoprotein(a) levels in cancer patients. *Int J Cancer* 43:241, 1989.

202. Gavish D, Azrolan N, Breslow JL: Fish oil reduces plasma Lp(a) levels and affects postprandial association of apo(a) with triglyceride-rich lipoproteins. *J Clin Invest* 84:2021, 1989.

203. Koschinsky ML, Beisiegel U, HenneBruns D, Eaton DL, Lawn RM: Apolipoprotein(a) size heterogeneity is related to variable number of repeat sequences in its mRNA. *Biochemistry* 29:640, 1990.

204. Lerch PG, Rickli EE, Lergier W, Gillessen D: Localization of individual lysine-binding regions in human plasminogen and investigations on their complex-forming properties. *Eur J Biochem* 107:7, 1980.

205. Plow EF, Collen D: Immunochemical characterization of a low-affinity lysine binding site within plasminogen. *J Biol Chem* 256:10864, 1982.

206. Vali Z, Patthy L: Location of the intermediate and high-affinity omega-aminocarboxylic acid binding sites in human plasminogen. *J Biol Chem* 257:2104, 1982.

207. Cole KR, Castellino FJ: The binding of antifibrinolytic amino acids to kringle-4–containing fragments of plasminogen. *Arch Biochem Biophys* 229:568, 1984.

208. Tulinksy A, Park CH, Mao B, Llinas M: Lysine/fibrin binding sites of kringles modeled after the structure of kringle 1 of prothrombin. *Proteins* 3:85, 1988.

209. Armstrong VW, Harrach B, Robenek H, Helmhold M, Walli AK, Seidel D: Heterogeneity of human lipoprotein Lp(a): Cytochemical and biochemical studies on the interaction of two Lp(a) species with the LDL receptor. *J Lipid Res* 31:429, 1990.

210. Harpel PC, Gordon BR, Parker TS: Plasmin catalyzes binding of lipoprotein(a) to immobilized fibrinogen and fibrin. *Proc Natl Acad Sci USA* 56:3847, 1989.

211. Wolf K, Rith M, Niendorf A, Biesegel U, Dietel M: Thrombosis: cellular elements of the vasculature. *Circulation* 80:522, 1989.

212. Hajjar KA, Gavish D, Breslow J, Nachman RL: Lipoprotein(a) modulation of endothelial cell surface fibrinolysis and its potential role in atherosclerosis. *Nature* 339:303, 1989.

213. Hajjar KA: The endothelial cell tissue plasminogen activator receptor: specific interaction with plasminogen. *J Biol Chem* 266:21962, 1991.

214. Gonzales-Gronow M, Edelberg JM, Pizzo SV: Further characterization of the cellular plasminogen binding site: evidence that plasminogen 2 and lipoprotein(a) compete for the same site. *Biochemistry* 28:2374, 1989.

215. Miles LA, Fless GM, Levin EG, Scanu AM, Plow EF: A potential basis for the thrombotic risks associated with lipoprotein(a). *Nature* 339:301, 1989.

216. Stiko-Rahm A, Wiman B, Hamsten A, Nilsson J: Secretion of plasminogen activator inhibitor 1 from cultured human umbilical vein endothelial cells is induced by very low density lipoprotein. *Arteriosclerosis* 10:1067, 1990.

217. Karadi I, Kostner GM, Gries A, Nimpf J, Romics L, Malle E: Lipoprotein(a) and plasminogen are immunochemically related. *Biochim Biophys Acta* 960:91, 1988.

218. Edelberg JM, Gonzalez-Gronow M, Pizzo SV: Lipoprotein(a) inhibits streptokinase-mediated activation of human plasminogen. *Biochemistry* 28:2370, 1989.

219. Edelberg JM, Gonzalez-Gronow M, Pizzo SV: Lipoprotein(a) inhibition of plasminogen activation by tissue-type plasminogen activator. *Thromb Res* 57:155, 1990.

220. Loscalzo J, Weinfeld M, Fless G, Scanu AM: Lipoprotein(a), fibrin binding, and plasminogen activation. *Arteriosclerosis* 10:240, 1990.

221. Grainger DJ, Kemp PR, Liu AC, Lawn RM, Metcalfe JC: Activation of transforming growth factor-beta is inhibited in transgenic apolipoprotein(a) mice. *Nature* 370:460, 1994.

222. Palabrica TM, Liu AC, Aronovitz MJ, Furie B, Lawn RM, Furie BC: Antifibrinolytic activity of apolipoprotein(a) *in vivo*: human apolipoprotein(a) transgenic mice are resistant to tissue plasminogen activator-mediated thrombolysis. *Nature Med* 1:256, 1995.

223. Lawn RM, Wade DP, Hammer RE, Chiesa G, Verstuyft JG, Rubin EM: Atherogenesis in transgenic mice expressing human apolipoprotein(a). *Nature* 360:670, 1992.

224. Boonmark NW, Lou XJ, Schwartz K, Zhang JL, Rubin EM, Lawn RM: Modification of apolipoprotein(a) lysine binding site reduces atherosclerosis in transgenic mice. *J Clin Invest* 100:558, 1997.

225. Kraus JP: Molecular basis of phenotype expression in homocystinuria. *J Inher Metab Dis* 17:383, 1994.

226. Boushey CJ, Beresford SAA, Omenn GS, Motulsky AG: A quantitative assessment of plasma homocysteine as a risk factor for vascular disease. *JAMA* 274:1049, 1995.

227. Refsum H, Ueland PM, Nygard O, Vollset SE: Homocysteine and cardiovascular disease. *Annu Rev Med* 49:31, 1998.

228. Hajjar KA: Homocysteine-induced modulation of tissue plasminogen activator to its endothelial cell membrane receptor. *J Clin Invest* 91:2873, 1993.

229. Hajjar KA, Mauri L, Jacovina AT, et al: Tissue plasminogen activator binding to the annexin II tail domain: direct modulation by homocysteine. *J Biol Chem* 273:9987, 1998.

230. Wilkins PP, Moore KL, McEver RP, Cummings RD: Tyrosine sulfation of P-selectin glycoprotein ligand 1 is required for high affinity binding to P-selectin. *J Biol Chem* 270:22677, 1995.

231. Snapp KR, Craig R, Herron M, Nelson RD, Stoolman LM, Kansas GS: Dimerization of P-selectin glycoprotein ligand 1 (PSGL1) required for optimal recognition of P-selectin. *J Cell Biol* 142:263, 1998.

232. Tanaka Y, Adams DH, Hubscher S, Hirano H, Siebenlist U, Shaw S: T-cell adhesion induced by proteoglycan-immobilized cytokine MIP1 beta. *Nature* 361:79, 1993.

233. Lo SK, Lee S, Ramos RA, et al: Endothelial leukocyte adhesion molecule 1 stimulates the adhesive activity of leukocyte integrin CD3 [CD11b/CD18, Mac1, alpha m beta 2] on human neutrophils. *J Exp Med* 173:1493, 1991.

234. Lorant DE, Patel KD, McIntyre TM, McEver RP, Prescott SM, Zimmerman GA: Coexpression of GMP140 and PAF by endothelium stimulated by histamine or thrombin: a juxtacrine system for adhesion and activation of neutrophils. *J Cell Biol* 115:223, 1991.

235. Huber AR, Kunkel SL, Todd RF, Weiss SL: Regulation of transendo-thelial neutrophil migration by endogenous interleukin-8. *Science* 254:99, 1991.

236. Tanaka Y, Albelda SM, Horgan KJ, et al: CD31 expressed on distinctive T cell subsets is a preferential amplifier of beta 1 integrin-mediated adhesion. *J Exp Med* 176:245, 1992.

237. Piali L, Albelda SM, Baldwin HS, Hammel P, Gisler RH, Imhof BA: Murine platelet endothelial cell adhesion molecule (PECAM1/CD31) modulates beta-2 integrins on lymphokine-activated killer cells. *Eur J Immunol* 23:2464, 1993.

238. Berman ME, Muller WA: Ligation of platelet/endothelial cell adhesion molecule 1 (PECAM1/CD31) on monocytes and neutrophils increases binding capacity of leukocyte CR3 (CD11b/CD18). *J Immunol* 154:299, 1995.

239. Carlos TM, Harlan JM: Leukocyte-endothelial cell adhesion molecules. *Blood* 84:2068, 1994.

240. Hynes RO: Integrins: versatility, modulation, and signalling in cell adhesion. *Cell* 69:11, 1992.

241. Miller J, Knorr R, Ferrone M, Houdei R, Carron CP, Dustin ML: Intercellular adhesion molecule 1 dimerization and its consequences for adhesion mediated by lymphocyte function–associated molecule-1. *J Exp Med* 182:1231, 1995.

242. Reilly PL, Woska RJR, Jeanfavre DD, McNally E, Rothlein R, Bormann BJ: The native structure of intercellular adhesion molecule 1 (ICAM1) is a dimer. Correlation with binding to LFA1. *J Immunol* 155:529, 1995.

243. Bargatze RF, Kurk S, Butcher EC, Jutila MA: Neutrophils roll on adherent neutrophils bound to cytokine-induced endothelial cells via L-selectin on the rolling cells. *J Exp Med* 180:1785, 1994.

244. Walcheck B, Moore KL, McEver RP, Kishimoto TK: Neutrophil–neutrophil interactions under hydrodynamic shear stress involve L-selectin and PSGL1. *J Clin Invest* 98:1081, 1996.

245. Muller WA: Migration of leukocytes across the vascular intima. Molecules and mechanisms. *Trends Cardiovasc Med* 5:15, 1995.

246. Muller WA, Ratti CM, McDonnell SL, Cohn ZA: A human endothelial cell-restricted, externally disposed plasma-lemmal protein enriched in intercellular junctions. *J Exp Med* 170:399, 1989.

247. Newman PJ, Berndt MC, Gorski J, et al: PECAM 1 [CD31] cloning and relation to adhesion molecules of the immunoglobulin gene superfamily. *Science* 247:1219, 1990.

248. Muller WA, Weigl SA, Deng X, Phillips DM: PECAM1 is required for transendothelial migration of leukocytes. *J Exp Med* 178:449, 1993.

249. Huang AJ, Manning JE, Bandak TM, Ratau MC, Hanser KR, Silverstein SC: Endothelial cell cytosolic free calcium regulates neutrophil migration across monolayers of endothelial cells. *J Cell Biol* 120:1371, 1993.

250. Liao F, Huynh HK, Eiroa A, Greene T, Polizzi E, Muller WA: Migration of monocytes across endothelium and passage through extracellular matrix involve separate molecular domains of PECAM1. *J Exp Med* 182:1337, 1995.

251. Liao F, Ali J, Greene T, Muller WA: Soluble domain 1 of platelet-endothelial cell adhesion molecule (PECAM) is sufficient to block transendothelial migration in vitro and in vivo. *J Exp Med* 185:1349, 1997.

252. Duncan GS, Andrew DP, Takimoto H, et al: Genetic evidence for functional redundancy of platelet/endothelial cell adhesion molecule-1 (PECAM1): CD31-deficient mice reveal PECAM1-dependent and PECAM1-independent functions. *J Immunol* 162:3022, 1999.

253. Feng D, Nagy JA, Pyne K, Dvorak HF, Dvorak AM: Neutrophils emigrate from venules by a transendothelial cell pathway in response to fMLP. *J Exp Med* 187:903, 1999.

254. Marchesi VT, Florey HW: Electron micrographic observations on the emigration of leukocytes. *J Exp Physiol* 45:343, 1960.

255. Leeuwenberg JFM, Von Asmuth EJ, Jeunhomme TM, Buurman WA: IFN-gamma regulates the expression of the adhesion molecule ELAM1 and IL6 production by human endothelial cells in vitro. *J Immunol* 145:2110, 1990.

256. Strindall J, Lundblad A, Pahlsson P: Interferon gamma enhancement of E-selectin expression on endothelial cells is inhibited by monensin. *Scand J Immunol* 46:338, 1997.

257. Ley K, Arbones ML, Bosse R, Vestweber D, Tedder TF, Beaudet AL: Sequential contribution of L- and P-selectin to leukocyte rolling in vivo. *J Exp Med* 181:669, 1995.

258. Khew-Goodall Y, Butcher E, Litwin MS, et al: Chronic expression of P-selectin on endothelial cells stimulated by the T-cell cytokine, interleukin-3. *Blood* 87:1432, 1999.

259. Yao L, Pan J, Setiadi H, Patel KD, McEver RP: Interleukin-4 or onco-statin M induces a prolonged increase in P-selectin mRNA and protein in human endothelial cells. *J Exp Med* 184:81, 1996.

260. Jung U, Ley K: Regulation of E-selectin, P-selectin, and intercellular adhesion molecule 1 expression in mouse cremaster vasculature. *Microcirculation* 4:311, 1997.

261. Pan J, Xia L, Yao L, McEver RP: Tumor necrosis factor-alpha or lipopolysaccharide induced expression of the murine P-selectin gene in endothelial cells involves novel kappa-B sites and a variant activating transcription factor/cAMP response element. *J Biol Chem* 273:10067, 1998.

262. Masinovsky B, Urdal D, Gallatin WM: IL4 acts synergistically with IL1 beta to promote lymphocyte adhesion to microvascular endothelium by induction of vascular cell adhesion molecule 1. *J Immunol* 145:2886, 1990.

263. Blease K, Seybold J, Adcock IM, Hellewell PG, Burke-Gaffney A: Interleukin-4 and lipopolysaccharide synergize to induce vascular adhesion molecule 1 expression in human lung microvascular endothelial cells. *Am J Respir Cell Mol Biol* 18:620, 1998.

264. Pober JS, Collins T, Gimbrone MA Jr, Libby P, Reiss CS: Inducible expression of class I major histocompatibility complex antigens and the immunogenicity of vascular endothelium. *Transplantation* 41:141, 1986.

265. Savage COS, Hughes CCW, McIntyre BW, Picard JK, Pober JS: Human CD4+ cells proliferate to HLADR+ allogeneic vascular endothelium. Identification of accessory interactions. *Transplantation* 56:128, 1993.

266. Pober JS, Orosz CG, Rose ML, Savage COS: Can graft endothelial cells initiate a host antigraft immune response? *Transplantation* 61:343, 1996.

267. Romer LH, McLean NV, Horng-Chin Y, Daise M, Sun J, Delisser HM: IFN gamma and TNF alpha induce redistribution of PECAM-1 [CD31] on human endothelial cells. *J Immunol* 154:6582, 1995.

268. Tang Q, Hendricks RL: Interferon gamma regulates platelet endothelial cell adhesion molecule 1 expression and neutrophil infiltration into herpes simplex virus–infected mouse corneas. *J Exp Med* 184:1435, 1996.

269. Rival Y, Del Maschio A, Rabiet MJ, Dejana E, Duperray A: Inhibition of platelet endothelial cell adhesion molecule 1 synthesis and leukocyte transmigration in endothelial cells by the combined action of TNFα and IFNγ. *J Immunol* 157:1233, 1996.

270. Kaplanski G, Fabrigoule M, Boulay V, et al: Thrombin induces endothelial type II activation in vitro: IL1 and TNF-alpha-independent IL-8 secretion and E-selectin expression. *J Immunol* 158:5435, 1997.

271. Diacovo TG, Puri KD, Warnock RA, Springer TA, Von Adrian UH: Platelet-mediated lymphocyte delivery to high endothelial venules. *Science* 273:252, 1996.

272. Diacovo TG, Catalina MD, Siegelman MH, Von Adrian UH: Circulating activated platelets reconstitute lymphocyte homing and immunity in L-selectin-deficient mice. *J Exp Med* 187:197, 1998.

273. Buttrum SM, Hatton R, Nash GB: Selectin-mediated rolling of neutrophils on immobilized platelets. *Blood* 82:1165, 1993.

274. Diacovo TG, Roth SJ, Buccola JM, Bainton DF, Springer TA: Neutrophil rolling, arrest, and transmigration across activated, surface-adherent platelets via sequential action of P-selectin and the beta 2–integrin CD11b/CD18. *Blood* 88:146, 1996.

275. Diacovo TG, de Fougerolles AR, Bainton DF, Springer TA: A functional integrin ligand on the surface of platelets: intercellular adhesion molecule 2. *J Clin Invest* 94:1243, 1994.

276. Altieri D: Coagulation assembly on leukocytes in transmembrane signaling and cell adhesion. *Blood* 81:569, 1993.

277. Lo SK, Cheung A, Zheng Q, Silverstein RL: Induction of tissue factor on monocytes by adhesion to endothelial cells. *J Immunol* 154:4768, 1995.

278. Fan ST, Mackman N, Cui MZ, Edgington TS: Integrin regulation of an inflammatory effector gene: direct induction of the tissue factor promoter by engagement of β-1 or α4 integrin chains. *J Immunol* 154:3266, 1995.

279. Randolph GJ, Luther T, Albrecht S, Magdolen V, Muller WA: Role of tissue factor adhesion of mononuclear phagocytes to and trafficking through endothelium. *Blood* 92:4167, 1998.

280. Palabrica T, Lobb R, Furie BC, et al: Leukocyte accumulation promoting fibrin deposition is mediated in vivo by P-selectin on adherent platelets. *Nature* 359:848, 1992.

281. Wright SD, Weitz JI, Huang AJ, Sevin SM, Silverstein SC, Loike JD: Complement receptor type 3 [CR3, CD11b/CD18] of human polymorphonuclear leukocytes recognizes fibrinogen. *Proc Natl Acad Sci USA* 85:7734, 1988.

282. Altieri DC, Morrisey JH, Edgington TS: Adhesive receptor Mac1 coordinates the activation of factor X on stimulated cells of monocytic and myeloid differentiation: an alternative initiation of the coagulation protease cascade. *Proc Natl Acad Sci USA* 85:7462, 1988.

283. Altieri DC, Edgington TS: The saturable high affinity association of factor X to ADP-stimulated monocytes defines a novel function of the Mac1 receptor. *J Biol Chem* 263:7007, 1988.

284. Serhan CN, Haeggstrom JZ, Leslie CC: Lipid mediator networks in cell signaling: update and impact of cytokines. *FASEB J* 10:1147, 1996.

285. Huber R, Berendes R, Burger A, Schneider M, Karshikov A, Luecke H: Crystal and molecular structure of human annexin V after refinement: implications for structure, membrane binding and ion channel formation of the annexin family of proteins. *J Mol Biol* 223:683, 1992.

286. Huang KS, Wallner BP, Mattaliano RJ, et al: Two human 35-kd inhibitors of phospholipase A2 are related to substrates of pp60 vsrc and of the epidermal growth factor receptor/kinase. *Cell* 46:191, 1986.

287. Blasi F, Conese M, Moller LB, et al: The urokinase receptor: structure, regulation and inhibitor-mediated internalization. *Fibrinolysis* 8:182, 1994.

CLASSIFICATION, CLINICAL MANIFESTATIONS AND EVALUATION OF DISORDERS OF HEMOSTASIS

URI SELIGSOHN
BARRY S. COLLER

> Evaluation of a hemostatic disorder is commonly initiated when: (1) A patient or a referring physician suspects a bleeding tendency; (2) a bleeding tendency is discovered in one or more family members; (3) an abnormal coagulation assay result is obtained in an individual as part of a routine examination; (4) an abnormal assay result is obtained in a patient during preparation for surgery; (5) a patient has unexplained diffuse bleeding during or after surgery or following trauma. The evaluation of a possible hemostatic disorder in each one of these scenarios is a stepwise process that requires knowledge of the various classes of hemostatic disorders commonly found under the particular circumstances. The history of the patient, the physical examination, and an initial set of hemostatic tests usually enable one to establish a tentative diagnosis. More specific tests, however, are commonly necessary to make a definitive diagnosis. In this chapter these steps will be reviewed.

CLASSIFICATION OF HEMOSTATIC DISORDERS

Hemostatic disorders can conveniently be classified as either hereditary or acquired (Table 115-1). Alternatively, they can be classified according to the mechanism of the defect. Of the acquired disorders, the thrombocytopenias are by far the most frequent entities encountered. Thrombocytopenias can result from reduced production of platelets, excessive destruction caused by antibodies or disseminated intravascular coagulation, or pooling of platelets in the spleen as in hypersplenism (see Chap 117).

THE BLEEDING HISTORY

The bleeding history is a crucial element in the evaluation of a patient with a hemorrhagic disorder, helping to define both the subsequent diagnostic approach as well as the likelihood of future bleeding. Eliciting and interpreting all of the relevant information requires a systematic and methodical approach. The following points are worth considering.

1. Patients vary in their responses to hemorrhagic symptoms, with some ignoring significant symptoms and others being very sensitive to even minor symptoms. Thus, when asked in standardized questionnaires, many normal, healthy people indicate that they have excessive bleeding or bruising.[1,2] Women are more likely to respond that they have excessive bleeding or bruising than men.

2. Patients with severe hemorrhagic disorders invariably have very abnormal bleeding histories.

3. The diagnostic value of any specific symptom varies in the different disorders, and so it is important to recognize typical patterns of bleeding (Table 115-2). Thus, unprovoked hemarthroses and muscle hemorrhages suggest one of the hemophilias, whereas mucocutaneous bleeding (epistaxis, gingival bleeding, and menorrhagia) are more characteristic of patients with qualitative platelet disorders, thrombocytopenia, or von Willebrand disease.

4. It is important to assess the extent of hemorrhage against the background of any trauma or provocation that may have elicited the hemorrhage. If a patient has never had a significant hemostatic challenge such as surgery, trauma, or childbirth, the lack of a significant bleeding history is much less valuable in excluding a mild hemorrhagic disorder. Thus, for example, a significant percentage of patients with mild von Willebrand disease or mild forms of hemophilia may have negative bleeding histories,[1] even though they may be at considerable risk of excessive bleeding after surgery or other interventions. Thus, one needs to consider these diagnoses even in elderly patients if their first severe hemostatic challenge occurs at that age.

5. It is valuable to try to obtain objective confirmation of the subjective information conveyed in the bleeding history. Objective data include: (a) previous hospital or physician visits for bleeding symptoms, along with the results of previous laboratory evaluations, (b) previous transfusions of blood products, and (c) a history of anemia and/or previous treatment with iron.

6. Although self-administered questionnaires may provide useful background information, they are not a substitute for a dialogue between physician and patient. Thus, history taking in general, but most especially in the often subtle histories related to hemostatic disorders, is an intellectually active process involving data collection, hypothesis development, new question formulation, additional data gathering, and new hypothesis development.

7. A medication history is a crucial component of the bleeding history, with particular attention to nonprescription drugs, such as aspirin, that may affect bleeding symptoms. A medication history is especially important in patients with thrombocytopenia, since drug-induced thrombocytopenia is common (see Chap. 117 and Table 115-1). Medication may also affect hemostasis through effects on the liver or kidney (see Chap. 125). The increased use of herbal and alternative medicines poses particular problems since patients may not readily share information about what they are taking and the dose they are taking of any particular active ingredient may be very difficult to determine. Resources for assessing the effects and side effects of such therapies are limited, but books (e.g., PDR for herbal medicines), papers,[3] and internet-based databases[4] are now available.

8. A nutrition history should be obtained to assess the likelihood of: (a) vitamin K deficiency, especially if the patient is also taking broad spectrum antibiotics; (b) vitamin C deficiency, especially if the patient has skin bleeding consistent with scurvy; and (c) general malnutrition and/or malabsorption. In patients on oral anticoagulants, it is important to counsel the patient to try to maintain a consistent level of vitamin K intake. Thus, major alterations in diet should be discouraged unless accompanied by more frequent monitoring of the prothrombin time. Similarly,

TABLE 115-1   CLASSIFICATION OF DISORDERS OF HEMOSTASIS

MAJOR TYPES	DISORDERS	EXAMPLES
Acquired	The thrombocytopenias	Auto- and alloimune, drug-induced, hypersplenism, hypoplastic (primary, suppressive, myelophthisic), DIC (see Chap. 117)
	Liver diseases	Cirrhosis, acute hepatic failure, liver transplantation (see Chap. 125)
	Renal failure	
	Vitamin K deficiency	Malabsorption syndrome, hemorrhagic disease of the newborn, prolonged antibiotic therapy, malnutrition, prolonged biliary obstruction (see Chaps. 125 and 132)
	Hematological disorders	Acute leukemias (particularly promyelocytic), myelodysplasias, monoclonal gammopathies, essential thrombocythemia (see Chaps. 92, 93, and 118)
	Acquired antibodies against coagulation factors	Neutralizing antibodies against factors V, VIII, and, XIII; accelerated clearance of antibody-factor complexes, e.g., acquired von Willebrand disease, hypoprothrombinemia associated with antiphospholipid antibodies (see Chaps. 122, 135, 128)
	Disseminated intravascular coagulation	Acute (sepsis, malignancies, trauma, obstetric complications) and chronic (malignancies, giant hemangiomas, missed abortion) (see Chap. 126)
	Drugs	Antiplatelet agents, anticoagulants, antithrombins, and thrombolytic, myelosuppressive, hepatotoxic, and nephrotoxic agents (see Chaps. 131, 132, 133, and 134)
	Vascular	Nonpalpable purpura ("senile," solar, and factitious purpura), use of corticosteroids, vitamin C deficiency, child abuse, thromboembolic, purpura fulminans; palpable-purpura (Henoch-Schönlein, vasculitis, dysproteinemias) (see Chap. 121)
Inherited	Deficiencies of coagulation factors	Hemophilia A (factor VIII deficiency), hemophilia B (factor IX deficiency), deficiencies of factors II, V, VII, X, XI, and XIII and von Willebrand disease (see Chaps. 123, 122, and 135)
	Platelet disorders	Glanzmann thrombasthenia, Bernard-Soulier syndrome, platelet granule disorders, etc. (see Chap. 119)
	Fibrinolytic disorders	α_2-antiplasmin deficiency, plasminogen activator inhibitor-1 deficiency (see Chaps. 116 and 136)
	Vascular	Hemorrhagic telangiectasias (see Chap. 121)
	Connective tissue disorders	Ehlers-Danlos syndrome (see Chap. 121)

new vitamins and food supplements should be checked for their vitamin K content.

9. Several tissues have high local levels of fibrinolytic activity, including the urinary tract, endometrium, and mucous membranes of the nose and oral cavity. These sites are particularly likely to have prolonged oozing of blood after trauma in patients with hemostatic abnormalities, and excessive bleeding following tooth extraction is one of the most common manifestations (see below).

10. Bleeding isolated to a single organ or system (e.g., hematuria, hematemesis, hemoptysis) is less likely to be due to a hemostatic abnormality than a local cause such as a neoplasm, an ulcer, or angiodysplasia, and thus one should perform a careful anatomic evaluation of the involved organ or system.

11. Bleeding or excessive hemorrhage may result from blood vessel disorders as well as disorders of platelets or coagulation proteins. Thus, it is important to consider hereditary hemorrhagic telangiectasias, Cushing's disease, scurvy, Ehlers-Danlos syndrome, and vasculitis in the differential diagnosis. Many primary dermatologic disorders may also have a purpuric or hemorrhagic component, and these need to be considered as well (see Chap. 121).

12. A family history is particularly important when hereditary disorders are considered. Patients will not usually spontaneously offer a history of consanguinity, and so specific inquiry should be made about this possibility. A diagram of the patient's genealogic tree, extending back at least one generation, should be included to document that genetic disorders were considered. A sex-linked pattern of inheritance is consistent with hemophilia A or B (see Chap. 123); an autosomal dominant pattern is characteristic of most forms of von Willebrand disease; and an autosomal recessive pattern is typical for all other coagulation factor deficiencies (see Chap. 122), inherited platelet disorders (see Chap. 119), and the rare severe, type 3 von Willebrand disease. Population genetic information may also be helpful, as for example, the higher prevalence of factor XI deficiency in Ashkenazi Jews (see Chap. 122).

13. The history should include information on diseases and organs that may also affect hemostasis, such as cirrhosis, renal insufficiency, essential thrombocythemia, acute leukemia, systemic lupus erythematosus, and Gaucher disease (Table 115-1).

Individual hemorrhagic symptoms often require detailed analysis before one can judge their significance with regard to the patient's diagnosis or proper therapy. Some of the more common symptoms are discussed below.

Epistaxis is one of the most common symptoms of platelet disorders and von Willebrand disease; it also is the most common symptom of hereditary hemorrhagic telangiectasias. In the latter condition, epistaxis almost always becomes more severe with advancing age. Epistaxis is not uncommon in normal children, but it usually resolves before puberty.

TABLE 115-2   CLINICAL MANIFESTATIONS TYPICALLY ASSOCIATED WITH SPECIFIC HEMOSTATIC DISORDERS

CLINICAL MANIFESTATIONS	HEMOSTATIC DISORDERS
Mucocutaneous bleeding	Thrombocytopenias, platelet dysfunction, von Willebrand disease
Cephalhematomas in newborns, hemarthroses, hematuria, and intramuscular, intracerebral and retroperitoneal hemorrhages	Severe hemophilias A and B, severe deficiencies of factor VII, factor X, or factor XIII, severe type 3 von Willebrand disease, and afibrinogenemia
Injury-related bleeding and mild spontaneous bleeding	Mild and moderate hemophilias A and B, severe factor XI deficiency, moderate deficiencies of fibrinogen and factors II, V, VII, or X, combined factors V and VIII deficiency, and α_2-antiplasmin deficiency
Bleeding from stump of umbilical cord and habitual abortions	Afibrinogenemia, hypofibrinogenemia, dysfibrinogenemia, or factor XIII deficiency
Impaired wound healing	Factor XIII deficiency
Facial purpura in newborns	Glanzmann thrombasthenia, severe thrombocytopenia
Recurrent severe epistaxis and chronic iron deficiency anemia	Hereditary hemorrhagic telangiectasias

Dry air heating systems can provoke epistaxis even in otherwise normal individuals. If bleeding is confined to a single nostril, it is more likely due to a local vascular problem than a systemic coagulopathy.

Gingival hemorrhage is also very common in patients with both qualitative and quantitative platelet abnormalities and von Willebrand disease. Occasional gum bleeding occurs in normal individuals, especially with tooth brushing using a hard bristle tooth brush and dental hygiene procedures, and thus it may be difficult to establish whether the bleeding is excessive. Even frequent gingival hemorrhage can occur in individuals with normal hemostasis if they have gum disease.

Oral mucous membrane bleeding in the form of blood blisters is a common manifestation of severe thrombocytopenia. It usually has a predilection for sites where teeth may traumatize the inner surface of the cheek.

Skin hemorrhage in the form of petechiae, purpura, and ecchymoses are common manifestations of hemostatic disorders, but skin hemorrhage is also common among individuals without hemostatic disorders. Excessive bruising is more common in women than men; moreover, women frequently note that the severity of their bruising varies with the phase of their menstrual cycle, although the most severe phase of the cycle may differ in different women. When such bruising is an isolated finding and no systemic bleeding diathesis is present, the condition is called *purpura simplex*. Features that help establish the severity of the skin hemorrhage include the size of the bruises; their frequency; whether they occur spontaneously or only with trauma; and their appearance on regions of the body that usually are not traumatized, such as the trunk and back. The color of the bruise may also yield information, with red bruises on the extensor surfaces of the arms and hands indicative of loss of supporting tissues, as is found in Cushing syndrome, gluococorticoid therapy, senile purpura, and damage due to chronic sun exposure. Jet black bruises may be due to warfarin-induced skin necrosis and similar disorders.

Tooth extractions are common hemostatic challenges and so may be helpful in defining the risk of bleeding. Molar extractions are greater hemostatic challenges than extractions of other teeth. Objective data regarding excessive bleeding based on the need for blood products or the need to have the extraction site packed or sutured are very valuable.

Excessive bleeding in response to razor nicks is common in patients with platelet disorders or von Willebrand disease. If patients indicate that they use an electric razor or a depilatory, it may be valuable to ask if they ever used a blade razor, and if so, why they switched.

Hemoptysis is virtually never the presenting symptom of a bleeding disorder and is rare even in patients with serious bleeding disorders. Blood-tinged sputum in association with upper respiratory tract infections may, however, be more common in patients with hemostatic disorders.

Hematemesis, like hemoptysis, is virtually never the presenting symptom of a hemostatic disorder, but a hemostatic disorder may exacerbate hematemesis due to an anatomic abnormality. Some hemostatic disorders are more likely to result in hematemesis as a result of a combination of effects, such as liver disease with esophageal varices and aspirin ingestion with gastritis.

Hematuria also is rarely the presenting symptom of a hemostatic disorder, but hemostatic disorders can exacerbate hematuria caused by other disorders, including simple urinary tract infections.

Hematochezia in individuals with normal hemostasis is most often due to hemorrhoids, but von Willebrand disease and platelet disorders may contribute to repeated episodes of hematochezia when associated with any one of a number of different underlying causes, including diverticuli, hemorrhoids, and angiodyplasia. Not infrequently, it is difficult to identify the precise site of bleeding. Melena is also only rarely the presenting symptom of a hemorrhagic disorder, but repeated episodes of melena may occur in patients with hemorrhagic disorders. Objective data about gastrointestinal bleeding include the number of previous endoscopic evaluations and any previous need for blood products.

Menstrual bleeding is typically excessive in amount and duration in women with platelet disorders and von Willebrand disease, but it may be difficult to establish this by history. In general, menstrual bleeding can be considered excessive if the patient indicates that she has heavy flow for more than three days or total flow for more than six or seven days. Objective data regarding menstrual bleeding includes whether a previous physician prescribed birth control pills to suppress menses; treated the patient with blood products; told the patient she was anemic; prescribed iron; performed a dilatation and curettage; performed an emergency hysterectomy to secure hemostasis; or performed an elective hysterectomy or other procedure to prevent excessive bleeding.

Childbirth poses a considerable hemostatic challenge, and so it is important to obtain a detailed history of each pregnancy, including data on excessive bleeding and the need for transfusion, dilatation and curettage, hysterectomy, or iron therapy. Repeated spontaneous abortions raise the possibility that the patient has a quantitative or qualitative abnormality of fibrinogen (see Chap. 124), factor XIII deficiency or the antiphospholipid syndrome (see Chap. 128).

Hemarthroses are the hallmark abnormality in the hemophilias and are otherwise rare except in severe von Willebrand disease. Since discoloration of the skin overlying the joint is unusual with hemarthroses, patients may not recognize that their symptoms are due to bleeding into their joints; it is more valuable, therefore, to inquire about recurrent pain, swelling, and limitation of motion.

Excessive hemorrhage in response to surgical procedures provides vital prognostic information. Specific inquiry about tonsillectomy, which presents a significant hemostatic challenge, is important, since often patients forget having had this procedure. If possible, the hospital records should be obtained because they commonly contain information that the patient does not have. Delays in discharge from the hospital or the need for blood products are especially important facts to inquire about.

Excessive bleeding in response to circumcision is common in males with hemophilia A or B, and this is often the patient's first symptom. Delayed bleeding after circumcision or from the umbilical stump may also be observed in patients with hemophilia A or B, but it is said to be particularly characteristic of bleeding due to factor XIII deficiency.

Patients with vascular disorders secondary to connective tissue abnormalities such as Ehlers-Danlos syndrome may give a history of easily distensible skin or extraordinary ligament laxness ("double-jointed"). Manifestations of Cushing syndrome include rounded facies, purple striae, truncal obesity, and fat deposition at the back of the neck. Old photographs may be very helpful in establishing a change in the patient's appearance.

PHYSICAL EXAMINATION

On physical examination one should look for signs of bleeding or their sequelae and for signs of a possible underlying disorder that can cause the hemostatic derangement (Table 115-1). Careful examination of the skin is essential for detection of petechiae and ecchymoses. These signs may be prominent on the legs, where the hydrostatic pressure is greatest.

Telangiectasias may range from pinpoint erythematous dots that blanch with pressure to classic cherry angiomata ranging in size up to several centimeters. Many normal individuals develop increasing numbers of telangiectasias with aging. Patients with hereditary hemorrhagic telangiectasias have more florid lesions that characteristically affect the vermilion border of the lips and the tongue (including the underside of the tongue), but not all patients have these classic features. Thus, a systematic search of the integument is necessary. Spider telangiectasias found in patients with liver disease have a more splotchy and serpigenous appearance than the telangiectasias associated with hereditary hemorrhagic telangiectasias; in addition, they tend to be concentrated on the shoulders, chest, and face.

The differential diagnosis of nonpalpable purpuras and palpable purpuras is detailed elsewhere (see Chap. 121). Hematomas, ecchymoses, and protacted oozing should be looked for at sites of venipunctures, injections, and arterial and venous catheter insertion sites. Joint deformities and limited joint mobility are suggestive of severe deficiency of factor VII, VIII, IX, or X, or severe von Willebrand disease (Chaps. 122, 123, and 135). Hyperelasticity of the skin and hyperextensibility of joints are typical of Ehlers-Danlos syndrome, and hyperextensibility only of the thumb probably represents one of its variants.[5]

EVALUATION BASED ON THE BLEEDING HISTORY AND INITIAL HEMOSTATIC TESTS

The patient's history and physical examination provide important information on the likelihood of the patient having a hemostatic defect, and the possible cause of the defect if one is present. It is, however, important to also perform an initial set of tests, including a prothrombin time (PT), an activated partial thromboplastin time (APTT), and platelet count, to broadly assess the major components of the hemostatic system, because: (1) the patient's history is sometimes unreliable, (2) the patient may have a mild hemostatic abnormality that has not previously manifested itself for lack of hemostatic challenge, (3) the patient may have developed an acquired hemostatic defect that has remained asymptomatic, and (4) the tests may reveal more than one abnormality.[6] Figure 115-1 shows a series of algorithms that integrate the patient's bleeding history and the results of the initial hemostatic tests. A prolonged APTT as a sole abnormality can be caused by a deficiency of factors VIII, IX, XI, or XII, or by an inhibitor, which can either be factor-specific (e.g., an antibody against factor VIII), or factor nonspecific (e.g., heparin or a lupus-type anticoagulant) Fig. 115-1, A. A prolonged PT as the sole finding can be indicative of a deficiency of factor VII or the presence of an inhibitor Fig. 115-1, B. When both the PT and APTT are abnormal, there may be an abnormality in fibrinogen, prothrombin, factor V, or factor X, an inhibitor to one of these components, or a combined deficiency of coagulation factors Fig. 115-1, C.

To distinguish between a deficiency state and the presence of an inhibitor it is useful to repeat the PT and APTT using a 1:1 mixture of patient's plasma and normal plasma. When such a mixture normalizes or nearly normalizes the prolonged PT or APTT, a deficiency state is likely. When, however, the mixture still yields a significantly prolonged PT or APTT, an inhibitor is probably present. Some inhibitors, such as antibodies to factor VIII, require a period of time to inhibit the assay, whereas other inhibitors, such as lupus-type anticoagulants and heparin, do not. It is desirable, therefore, to incubate the mixture for a period of time, commonly 2 h at 37°C (98.6°F), before performing the coagulation assay.

When none of the initial tests (PT, APTT, and platelet count) is abnormal and the patient exhibits bleeding manifestations, the bleeding time (BT), ristocetin cofactor (RCF) activity, and examination of the blood film can be helpful in distinguishing between various candidate hemostatic abnormalities. An algorithm that includes these secondary tests is shown in Fig. 115-2. It should be noted that not infrequently patients with type 1 and type 2 von Willebrand disease will have

normal results in the initial laboratory tests, since the factor VIII levels may be sufficiently high (>30 U/dl) to have a normal APTT (see Chap. 135). Examination of the blood film is helpful in distinguishing between Bernard-Soulier syndrome and von Willebrand disease since giant platelets are characteristic of the former (see Chap. 119). To distinguish type 2B and platelet-type von Willebrand disease from the other types of von Willebrand disease, the ristocetin-induced platelet aggregation test is useful. In type 2B and platelet-type von Willebrand disease, there is an enhanced response to low concentrations of ristocetin, whereas in the other types of von Willebrand disease, a decreased response is found. Total absence of platelet aggregates in a blood film prepared from nonanticoagulated blood, and absent clot retraction, are characteristic of Glanzmann thrombasthenia (see Chap. 119).

Another simple test that may be useful for distinguishing among hemostatic disorders is the thrombin time (i.e., the time for plasma to clot after adding thrombin). The thrombin time is prolonged in: (1) afibrinogenemia, hypofibrinogenemia, and dysfibrinogenemias (Chap. 124), (2) the presence of heparin, (3) disseminated intravascular coagulation (DIC) due to increased levels of fibrin(ogen) degradation products inhibiting fibrin monomer polymerization (Fig. 115-1, D) (Chap. 126), and (4) patients with amyloidosis and an immunoglobulin inhibitor of thrombin.[7]

PREOPERATIVE ASSESSMENT OF HEMOSTASIS

Surgical procedures constitute a great challenge to the hemostatic system, and therefore it is important to carefully assess the risk of bleeding in every patient. The assessment is based on the history of bleeding, the underlying disorder if any, the initial hemostatic tests (PT, APTT, and platelet count), and the type of surgery that is planned. Table 115-3 lists low- and high-risk conditions. For the high-risk conditions a critical analysis of each potential cause of bleeding should be undertaken.

In addition to the extent of the surgical trauma, the magnitude of the fibrinolytic activity at the site of surgery has to be considered; prostatectomy, for example, carries considerable risk of prolonged bleeding because of the presence of high fibrinolytic activity in urine. Some surgical procedures can be anticipated to cause hemostatic abnormalities, such as operations in which extracorporeal circulation is employed (since the extracorporeal circuits and/or the anticoagulation cause platelet dysfunction) and operations on patients with extensive malignancies or brain injury (which can give rise to disseminated intravascular coagulation). Finally, the ability to institute local hemostatic measures should be considered. Thus, liver and kidney biopsies, though considered minor procedures, have a significant risk of bleeding because it is not possible to use local measures, such as direct pressure, to control bleeding.

The initial hemostatic tests may also give other important information in managing patients undergoing surgery, providing: (1) baseline values for future comparison if bleeding occurs, and (2) information about deficiencies of factor XII, prekallikrein, or high-molecular-weight kininogen, for which no treatment is necessary, or the lupus anticoagulant, for which anticoagulant prophylaxis may be indicated.

SPECIFIC ASSAYS FOR ESTABLISHING THE DIAGNOSIS

By following the stepwise process of evaluation outlined in Figs. 115-1 and 115-2, a tentative diagnosis can be made. Further testing is usually required, however, to establish a definitive diagnosis.

THROMBOCYTOPENIAS

When the laboratory reports an abnormally low platelet count, it is essential to look at the blood film to exclude pseudothrombocytopenia.[8]

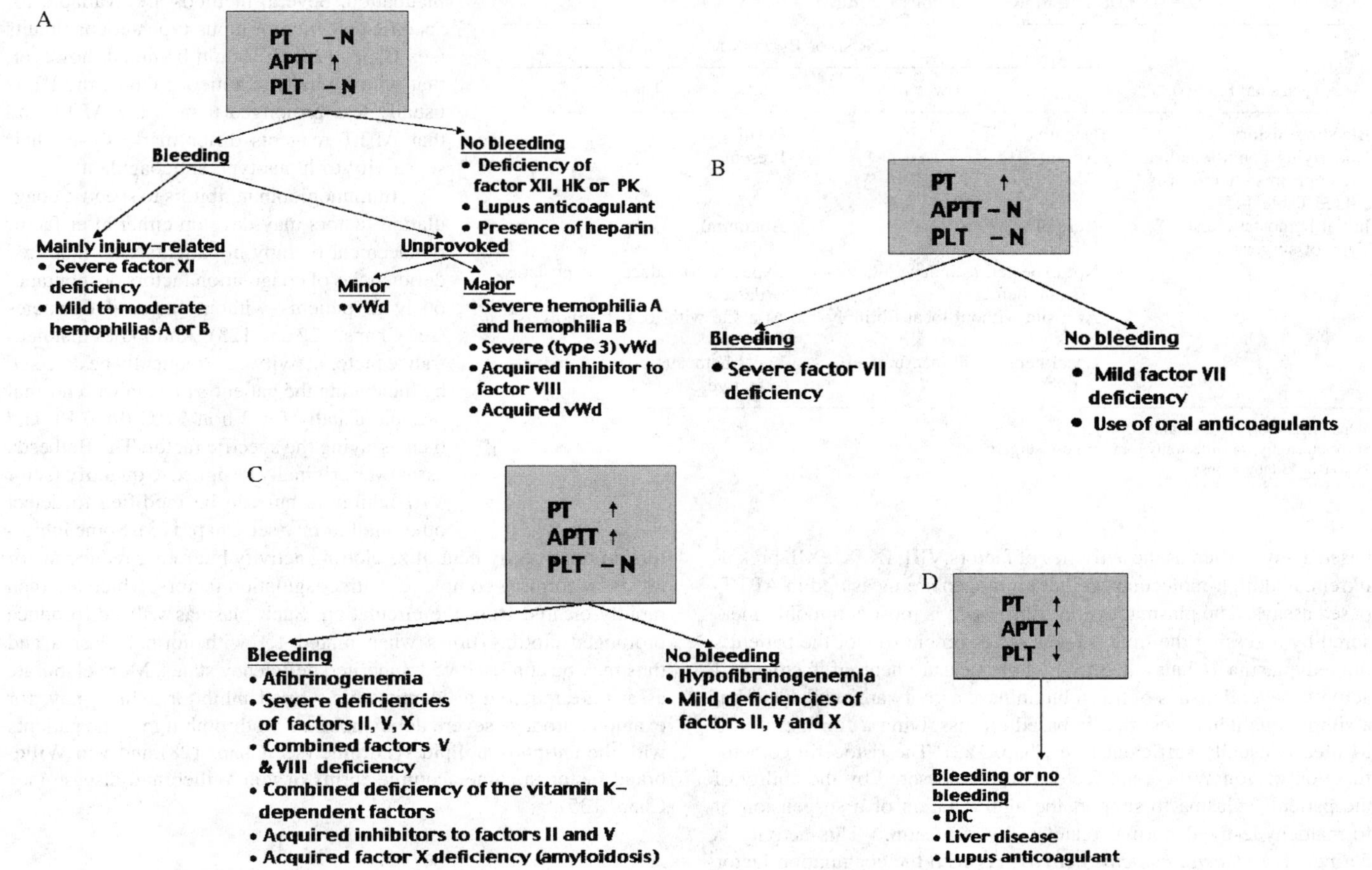

A
PT – N
APTT ↑
PLT – N
Bleeding
No bleeding
• Deficiency of factor XII, HK or PK
• Lupus anticoagulant
• Presence of heparin
Mainly injury-related
• Severe factor XI deficiency
• Mild to moderate hemophilias A or B
Unprovoked
Minor
• vWd
Major
• Severe hemophilia A and hemophilia B
• Severe (type 3) vWd
• Acquired inhibitor to factor VIII
• Acquired vWd
B
PT ↑
APTT – N
PLT – N
Bleeding
• Severe factor VII deficiency
No bleeding
• Mild factor VII deficiency
• Use of oral anticoagulants
C
PT ↑
APTT ↑
PLT – N
Bleeding
• Afibrinogenemia
• Severe deficiencies of factors II, V, X
• Combined factors V & VIII deficiency
• Combined deficiency of the vitamin K-dependent factors
• Acquired inhibitors to factors II and V
• Acquired factor X deficiency (amyloidosis)
No bleeding
• Hypofibrinogenemia
• Mild deficiencies of factors II, V and X
D
PT ↑
APTT ↑
PLT ↓
Bleeding or no bleeding
• DIC
• Liver disease
• Lupus anticoagulant

FIGURE 115-1 Measures to establish a tentative diagnosis of a hemostatic disorder by using initial tests of hemostasis and the patient's history of bleeding. APTT, activated partial thromboplastin time; BT, bleeding time; DIC, disseminated intravascular coagulation; HK, high-molecular-weight kininogen; N, normal; PK, prekallikrein; PLT-platelets; PT, prothrombin time; vWd, von Willebrand disease.

Examination of the blood film can also reveal the presence of: giant platelets, as in some inherited thrombocytopenias; giant platelets and Döhle bodies in leukocytes, as in May-Hegglin anomaly; moderately enlarged platelets, as occurs in immune thrombocytopenia or other conditions associated with shortened platelet survival; small platelets, as found in Wiskott-Aldrich syndrome; schistocytes and burr cells, as in the hemolytic-uremic syndrome and thrombotic thrombocytopenic purpura, and occasionally in disseminated intravascular coagulation; rouleaux formation, as in monoclonal gammopathies; macrocytosis and/or hypersegmentation, as in vitamin B_{12} or folic acid deficiency; and abnormal white blood cells as in leukemias and myeloproliferative disorders. Further discussion of the evaluation and differential diagnosis of the thrombocytopenias is presented in Chaps. 117 and 119.

FACTOR DEFICIENCIES

Coagulation factors are usually assayed by measuring their clotting acitvity. The most common assays analyze the ability of dilutions of the patient's plasma to correct the clotting time of a plasma known to be deficient in the factor to be measured (substrate plasma). The results are then compared to the ability of dilutions of a normal reference plasma to correct the abnormality in the substrate plasma. The activities of factors II, V, VII, and X are usually determined in PT-

Bleeding and:
PT – N
APTT – N
PLT – N
BT–N
• Factor XIII deficiency
• α_2-antiplasmin deficiency
• Dysfibrinogenemia
• Hereditary hemorrhagic telangiectasias
BT ↑
RCF ↓
• vWd
RCF–N
CR ↑
• Glanzmann thrombasthenia
CR–N
• Hereditary and acquired platelet disorders

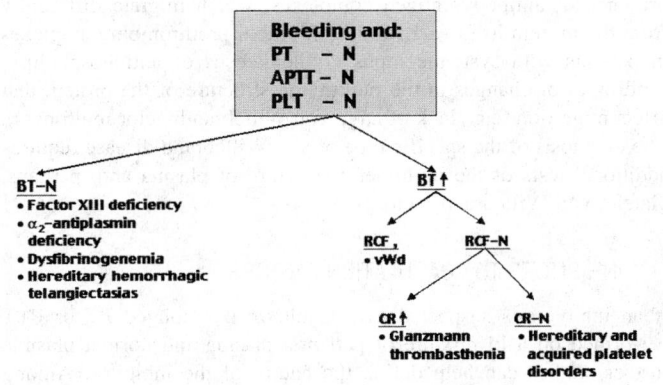

FIGURE 115-2 The tentative diagnoses in patients with bleeding manifestations and normal primary hemostatic tests, by using secondary tests: Bleeding time (BT), ristocetin cofactor activity (RCF), and clot retraction (CR). vWd, von Willebrand disease.

TABLE 115-3   EVALUATION OF THE RISK OF BLEEDING DURING SURGERY

| ASSESSED FACTOR | RISK OF BLEEDING | |
	LOW	HIGH
Bleeding history	Negative	Positive
Underlying conditions that compromise hemostasis (see Table 115-1)	Absent	Present
Initial hemostatic tests	Normal	Abnomral
Type of surgery:	Minor	Major
	Not expected to induce a hemostatic defect	Expected to induce a hemostatic defect*
	At a site without local fibrinolysis	At a site with local fibrinolysis†
	Local hemostatic measures effective	Local hemostatic measures ineffective‡

*Open heart surgery or brain surgery.
†Prostatectomy, tonsillectomy, oral or nose surgery.
‡Liver or kidney biopsy.

based assays, whereas the activities of factors VIII, IX, XI, XII, prekallikrein, and high-molecular-weight kininogen are measured in APTT-based assays. The plasma level of fibrinogen is most commonly measured by assessing the time it takes for thrombin to clot the patient's diluted plasma (Clauss method).[9] For measurement of factor XIII activity, several assays of transglutaminase activity are available,[10] but a simple qualitative test that is based on dissolving a fibrin clot in 5 M urea is usually sufficient (see Chap. 122). The ristocetin cofactor function of von Willebrand factor can be measured by the ability of the patient's plasma to support the agglutination of a suspension of formaldehyde-fixed normal platelets by ristocetin.[11] This activity is defined as *ristocetin cofactor activity*. As with the coagulation factor assays, the results using patient plasma are compared to those obtained with a normal reference plasma.

To determine whether a coagulation factor activity deficiency is due to a quantitative decrease in protein or a qualitative abnormality in the protein, immunological assays can be employed using specific polyclonal or monoclonal antibodies to assess the presence of the protein, independent of its function. Electroimmunoassays, enzyme-linked immunosorbent assays (ELISAs), and immunoradiometric assays have all been employed successfully. Crossed immunoelectrophoresis measures both the immunologic reactivity and the mobility of the protein in an electric field, and thus it can detect protein abnormalities that affect electrophoretic migration. These can include the presence of antibody-antigen complexes, which migrate differently from the protein itself (e.g., antiprothrombin-prothrombin complexes in patients with systemic lupus erythematosus or antiphospholipid syndrome) or changes in the multimeric structure of the protein that affect migration (e.g., lack of large von Willebrand factor multimers). The diagnosis of the specific type of von Willebrand disease requires additional tests of the multimeric structure of plasma and, perhaps, platelet von Willebrand factor.

INHIBITORS TO COAGULATION FACTORS

If an inhibitor is suspected as a result of a prolonged PT or PTT performed on a 1:1 mixture of patient's plasma and normal plasma, further studies can help define the nature of the inhibitor. Among inhibitors that do not require incubation (i.e., immediate-type), perhaps the most common cause is the presence of heparin in the sample. This can be verified by finding a prolonged thrombin time test on the patient's plasma that corrects with toluidine blue or other agents that neutralize heparin. The lupus-type anticoagulant also does not require

incubation. Several methods are available for specific detection of lupus-type anticoagulants (see Chap. 128). It should be noted, however, that with lupus-type anticoagulants, the PT is usually less prolonged than is the APTT and that APTT reagents differ markedly in their sensitivity to lupus-type anticoagulants.

Immunoglobin inhibitors to specific coagulation factors may develop either after factor replacement therapy in patients with inherited deficiencies of coagulation factors or spontaneously in patients without factor deficiencies (see Chaps. 122 and 123). Antibodies that neutralize factor activity can frequently be detected by incubating the patient's plasma with normal plasma, usually for 2 h at 37°C (98.6°F), and then assaying the specific factor. The Bethesda assay was originally designed to quantify factor VIII inhibitors but can be modified to detect other inhibitors[12] (see Chap. 123). Some inhibitors do not directly neutralize clotting activity but rather reduce factor levels by forming complexes with coagulation factors, which are then rapidly cleared from the circulation. Such plasmas will not produce prolonged clotting times when mixed 1:1 with normal plasma and thus may be confused with inherited deficiency states. More elaborate assays are required to identify this type of inhibitor, which may, for example, produce severe deficiencies of prothrombin in some patients with the antiphospholipid syndrome (see Chap. 128) and von Willebrand factor in some acquired forms of von Willebrand disease (see Chap. 135).[13]

PLATELET FUNCTION DISORDERS

A prolonged bleeding time is suggestive of a platelet function disorder (inherited or acquired) or von Willebrand disease; the use of the ristocetin cofactor activity assay, platelet aggregation, and/or clot retraction are useful for the initial assessment of whether the patient has von Willebrand disease or a platelet function disorder (Fig. 115-2). Chapter 119 contains a flow diagram of the steps required to diagnose the different qualitative disorders of platelet function. Additional platelet function assays and glycoprotein analysis may be required to establish the diagnosis.

REFERENCES

1. Miller CH, Graham JB, Goldin LR, Elston RC: Genetics of classic von Willebrand's disease. II. Optimal assignment of the heterozygous genotype (diagnosis) by discriminant analysis. *Blood* 54:137, 1979.
2. Wahlberg T, Blomback M, Hall P, Axelsson G: Application of indicators, predictors and diagnostic indices in coagulation disorders. I. Evaluation of a self-administered questionnaire with binary questions. *Methods Inf Med* 19:194, 1980.
3. Miller LG: Herbal medicinals: selected clinical considerations focusing on known or potential drug-herb interactions. *Arch Intern Med* 158:2200, 1998.
4. Horton RM: Alternative medicine resources on the internet. *Curr Pract Med* 1:71, 1998.
5. Kaplinsky C, Kenet G, Seligsohn U, Rechavi G: Association between hyperflexibility of the thumb and an unexplained bleeding tendency: is it a rule of thumb? *Br J Haematol* 101:260, 1998.
6. Rapaport SI: Preoperative hemostatic evaluation: which tests, if any? *Blood* 61:229, 1983.
7. Gastineau DA, Gertz MA, Daniels TM, Kyle RA, Bowie EJ: Inhibitor of the thrombin time in systemic amyloidosis: a common coagulation abnormality. *Blood* 77:2637, 1991.

8. Payne BA, Pierre RV. Pseudothrombocytopenia: A laboratory artifact with potentially serious consequences. *Mayo Clin Proc* 59:123, 1984.

9. Clauss A: Gerinnungsphysiologische schnell methodes zur des fibrinogens. *Acta Haematol* 17:327, 1957.

10. Fickenscher K, Aab A, Stuber W: A photometric assay for blood coagulation factor XIII. *Thromb Haemost* 65:535, 1991.

11. McFarlane DE, Stibbe J, Kirby EP, et al: A method for assaying von Willebrand factor (ristocetin cofactor). *Thromb Diath Haemorrh* 34:306, 1975.

12. Kasper CK, Aledort L, Aronson D, et al: Proceedings: a more uniform measurement of factor VIII inhibitors. *Thromb Diath Haemorrh* 34:612, 1975.

13. Inbal A, Bank I, Zivelin A, et al: Acquired von Willebrand disease in a patient with angiodysplasia resulting from immune-mediated clearance of von Willebrand factor. *Br J Haematol* 96:179, 1997.

MOLECULAR MECHANISMS OF FIBRINOLYSIS

KATHERINE A. HAJJAR

In recent years, several fundamental advances have enriched our understanding of the molecular mechanisms of fibrinolysis. Molecular characterization of the genes for all the major fibrinolytic proteins has led to an understanding of serine protease stucture and function, a regard for the regulatory role of cellular receptors and other cofactors, and an appreciation of mechanisms regulating transcriptional and posttranscriptional gene expression. The development of genetically engineered animals deficient in one or more fibrinolytic proteins has suggested unexpected roles for these proteins in both intravascular and extravascular settings. In addition, genetic analysis of human deficiency syndromes has revealed specific mutations that result in human disorders reflective of either fibrinolytic deficiency with thrombosis or fibrinolytic excess with hemorrhage. Finally, elucidation of acquired disorders of fibrinolysis, as seen in pregnancy, in the newborn infant, and in certain malignancies, has also served to clarify the role of the fibrinolytic system in both health and disease.

BASIC CONCEPTS OF FIBRINOLYSIS

Fibrin, the insoluble end product of the action of thrombin on fibrinogen, is found in both intravascular and extravascular settings. In response to injury, cross-linked fibrin, the final product of the coagulation cascade, is deposited in tissues and blood vessels. Once fibrin is no longer needed, the fibrinolytic system is activated, converting fibrin to its soluble degradation products through the action of the serine protease plasmin (Fig. 116-1a).

Under physiologic conditions, fibrinolysis is precisely regulated by the measured participation of activators, inhibitors, and cofactors.[1] In addition, cell surface receptors provide specialized, protected environments where plasmin can be generated without compromise by circulating inhibitors (Fig. 116-1b).[2] Endothelial cells, platelets, monocytes, macrophages, myeloid cells, and some tumor cells express protein receptor sites for plasminogen, tissue plasminogen activator (t-PA), and/or urokinase. The broad in vitro substrate specificity of plasmin suggests that it may play an important role in such extravascular events as the modification of growth and differentiation factors, matrix proteins, and procoagulant molecules. This chapter reviews the

fundamental features of plasmin generation and considers the major clinical disorders resulting from defects in this system.

COMPONENTS OF THE FIBRINOLYTIC SYSTEM

PLASMINOGEN

Synthesized primarily in the liver,[3,4] plasminogen is an approximately 92,000-M_r single-chain proenzyme that circulates in plasma at a concentration of approximately 1.5 μM (Table 116-1).[5] The plasma half-life of plasminogen in adult males is approximately 2 days.[6] Its 791 amino acids are cross-linked by 24 disulfide bridges, 16 of which give rise to 5 homologous triple-loop structures called kringles (Fig. 116-2).[7] The first (K1) and fourth (K4) of these 80–amino acid, approximately 10,000-M_r structures impart high- and low-affinity lysine binding, respectively.[8] The lysine-binding domains of plasminogen appear to mediate its specific interactions with fibrin, cell surface receptors, and other proteins including its circulating inhibitor α_2-antiplasmin.[9–13]

Posttranslational modification of plasminogen results in two glycosylation variants: forms 1 and 2 (see Table 116-1).[14,15] O-linked oligosaccharide, consisting of sialic acid, galactose, and galactosamine resident on Thr345, is common to both forms. Only form 2, however, contains N-linked oligosaccharide on Asn288, composed of sialic acid, galactose, glucosamine, and mannose. The carbohydrate portion of plasminogen appears to regulate its affinity for cellular receptors and may also specify its physiologic degradation pathway.

Activation of plasminogen results from cleavage of a single Arg-Val peptide bond at position 560-561,[16] giving rise to the active protease plasmin (see Table 116-1). Plasmin contains a typical serine protease catalytic triad (His602, Asp645, and Ser740)[5] but exhibits broad substrate specificity compared to other proteases of this class.[17] The circulating form of plasminogen, amino-terminal glutamic acid plasminogen (Glu-PLG), is readily converted by limited proteolysis to several modified forms known collectively as Lys-PLG.[18,19] Hydrolysis of the Lys77-Lys78 peptide bond gives rise to a conformationally modified form of the zymogen that more readily binds fibrin, displays two- to threefold higher avidity for cellular receptors, and is activated 10 to 20 times more rapidly than is Glu-PLG.[10,16,20] Lys-PLG does not normally circulate in plasma[16] but has been identified on cell surfaces.[21]

Spanning 52.5 kb of DNA on chromosome 6q26-27, the plasminogen gene consists of 19 exons[22,23] and directs expression of a 2.7-kb mRNA (see Fig. 116-2).[7] The 5′ upstream region of the plasminogen gene contains two regulatory elements common to genes for acute-phase reactants (CTGGGA) and six interleukin-6 (IL-6)-responsive elements.[23] Plasminogen gene activity, moreover, is stimulated by the acute-phase mediator IL-6 both in vitro and in vivo.[24] The gene is closely linked and structurally related to that of apolipoprotein(a), an apoprotein associated with the highly atherogenic low-density lipoprotein–like particle lipoprotein(a)[25] and more distantly related to other kringle-containing proteins, such as t-PA, urokinase plasminogen activator (u-PA), hepatocyte growth factor, and macrophage-stimulating protein.[26–30] The significance of the latter two proteins to the fibrinolytic system remains to be determined.

THE PHYSIOLOGIC FUNCTIONS OF PLASMINOGEN

The development of the plasminogen-deficient mouse has contributed significantly to our understanding of the physiologic function of the serine protease plasmin. Mice made completely plasminogen deficient through gene targeting undergo normal embryogenesis and development, are fertile, and survive to adulthood (Table 116-2).[31,32] In addition to runting and ligneous conjunctivitis,[33] these animals display a predisposition to thrombosis, with spontaneous thrombi appearing in liver, stomach, colon, rectum, lung, and pancreas; fibrin deposition in the

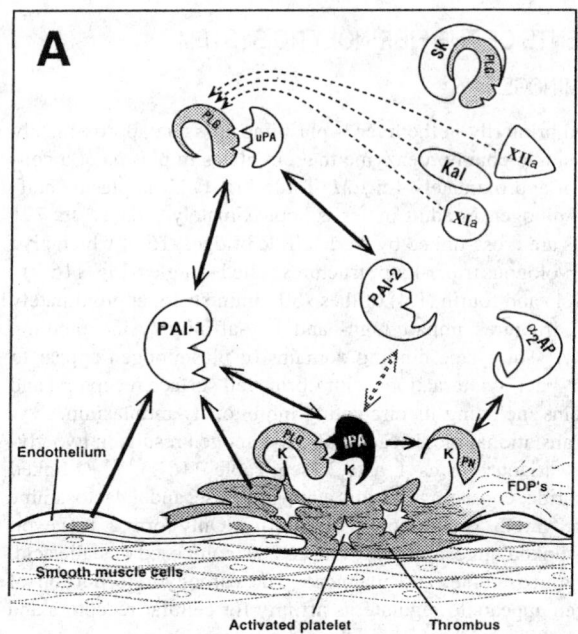

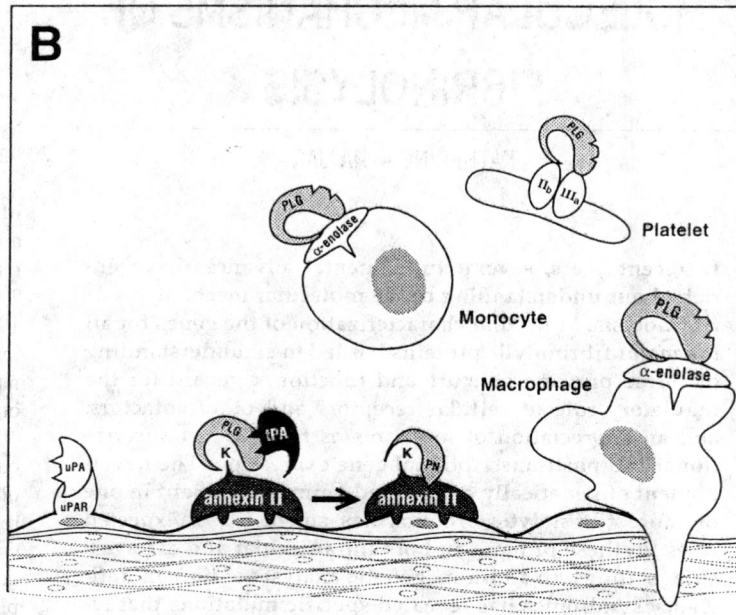

FIGURE 116-1 Overview of the fibrinolytic system. *(a)* Fibrin-based plasminogen activation. The zymogen plasminogen (PLG) is converted to the active serine protease plasmin (PN) through the action of tissue plasminogen activator (t-PA) or urokinase (u-PA). The activity of t-PA is greatly enhanced by its assembly with PLG through lysine residues (K) on a fibrin-containing thrombus. u-PA acts independently of fibrin. Both t-PA and u-PA can be inhibited by plasminogen-activator inhibitor-1 (PAI-1), which is released by endothelial cells and activated platelets. PAI-2, on the other hand, neutralizes u-PA more efficiently than t-PA. By binding to fibrin, plasmin is protected from its major inhibitor, α_2-antiplasmin (α_2-AP). Bound plasmin degrades cross-linked fibrin, giving rise to soluble fibrin degradation products (FDPs). Streptokinase (SK) is a bacterial protein that forms a complex with plasminogen, allowing it to activate other plasminogen molecules. Minor plasminogen activators include kallikrein (Kal), factor XI (XIa), and factor XII (XIIa). *(b)* Probable sites of cell surface plasminogen activation. On the blood vessel wall, endothelial cells, like monocytes and macrophages, express the u-PA receptor as well as annexin II, a coreceptor for t-PA and PLG that augments the efficiency of plasmin generation. Circulating monocytes and macrophages have cell surface α-enolase, and resting platelets express the glycoprotein IIb/IIIa complex, both of which represent potential receptors for PLG. (From KA Hajjar[1] with permission.)

liver; and ulcerative lesions in the gastrointestinal tract and rectum. These results suggest that plasminogen is not strictly required for normal development but does play a crucial role in postnatal intra- and extravascular fibrinolysis.

PLASMINOGEN ACTIVATORS

TISSUE PLASMINOGEN ACTIVATOR

One of two major endogenous plasminogen activators, t-PA consists of 527 amino acids comprising a glycoprotein of M_r approximately 72,000 (see Table 116-1).[34] t-PA contains five structural domains, including a fibronectin-like "finger," an epidermal growth factor–like domain, two kringle structures homologous to those of plasmino- gen, and a serine protease domain (see Fig. 116-2). Cleavage of the Arg275-Ile276 peptide bond by plasmin converts t-PA to a disulfide- linked, two-chain form.[34] While single-chain t-PA is less active than two-chain t-PA in the fluid phase, both forms demonstrate equivalent activity when fibrin bound.[35]

The two glycosylation forms of t-PA are distinguishable by the presence (type 1) or absence (type 2) of a complex *N*-linked oligosac- charide moiety on Asn184[36,37] (see Table 116-1). Both types, however, contain high mannose carbohydrate on Asn117, complex oligosaccha- ride on Asn448, and an *O*-linked α-fucose residue on Thr61.[38] The carbohydrate moieties of t-PA may modulate its functional activity, regulate its binding to cell surface receptors, and specify degradation pathways. Located on chromosome 8p12-q11.2, the gene for human

t-PA is encoded by 14 exons spanning a total of 36.6 kb[39–41] (see Fig. 116-2). Although exon 1 encodes a 58-nucleotide mRNA leader sequence, each of the structural domains of t-PA is encoded by 1 or 2 of the remaining 13 exons. This suggests that the t-PA gene arose by an evolutionary process called exon shuffling, whereby functionally related genes evolved through rearrangement of exons encoding auton- omous domains. Consistent with this hypothesis, deletion of exons encoding the fibronectin-like finger or kringle 2, but not kringle 1, domains of t-PA results in expression of mutants resistant to the cofactor activity of fibrin, while catalytic activity in the absence of fibrin remains intact.[42]

The proximal promoter of the human t-PA gene contains binding sequences for potentially important transcriptional factors, including AP1, NF1, SP1, and AP2[43,44] as well as a potential cyclic adenosine monophosphate (cAMP)-responsive element (CRE).[45] In vitro, many agents have been shown to exert small effects on the expression of t-PA mRNA, but relatively few enhance t-PA synthesis without augmenting plasminogen-activator inhibitor-1 (PAI-1) synthesis as well. Agents that regulate t-PA gene expression independently of PAI-1 include histamine, butyrate, retinoids, arterial levels of shear stress, and dexa- methasone.[46–49] Forskolin, which increases intracellular cAMP levels, has been reported to decrease synthesis of both t-PA and PAI-1.[44,50]

t-PA is synthesized and secreted primarily by endothelial cells, and its release is governed by a variety of stimuli, such as thrombin, histamine, bradykinin, epinephrine, acetylcholine, arginine vasopres- sin, gonadotropins, exercise, venous occlusion, and shear stress.[47,51]

TABLE 116-1   FIBRINOLYTIC PROTEINS

PROTEASES

Property	Plasminogen	t-PA	u-PA
Molecular mass	92,000	72,000	54,000
Amino acids	791	527	411
Chromosome	6	8	10
Site of synthesis	Liver	Endothelium	Endothelium, kidney
Plasma concentration			
nM	1500	0.075	0.150
μg/ml	140	0.005	0.008
Plasma half-life	48 h	5 min	8 min
N-glycosylation, %	2	13	7
Form 1	–	Asn117, Asn184, Asn448	Asn302
Form 2	Asn288	Asn117, –, Asn448	–
O-Glycosylation			
α-Fucose	–	Thr61	Thr18
Complex	Thr345	–	–
Two-chain cleavage site	Arg560-Val561	Arg275-Ile276	Lys158-Ile159
Heavy-chain domains			
Finger	No	Yes	No
Growth factor	No	Yes	Yes
Kringles (number)	5	2	1
Light-chain catalytic triad	His602, Asp645, Ser740	His322, Asp371, Ser478	His204, Asp255, Ser356

MAJOR SERPIN INHIBITORS

Property	α_2-AP	PAI-1	PAI-2
Molecular mass	70,000	52,000	60,000 (glycosylated) 47,000 (nonglycosylated)
Amino acids	452	402	393
Chromosome	18	7	18
Sites of synthesis	Kidney, liver	Endothelium Monocytes/macrophages Hepatocytes Adipocytes	Placenta Monocytes/macrophages Tumor cells
Plasma concentration			
nM	900	0.1–0.4	ND
μg/ml	50	0.02	ND
Serpin reactive site	Arg364-Met365	Arg346-Met347	Arg358-Thr359
Specificity	Plasmin	u-PA = t-PA	u-PA > t-PA

SOME PROPOSED RECEPTORS

Property	u-PAR	Annexin II	LRP	Mannose Receptor
Molecular mass	55,000–60,000	36,000	600,000	175,000
Amino acids	313	339	4544	1456
Chromosome	19	15	12	10
Source	Endothelial cells Monocytes/macrophages Fibroblasts Tumor cells	Endothelial cells Monocytes/macrophages Myeloid cells Smooth muscle cells	Hepatocytes Monocytes/macrophages Fibroblasts	Macrophages
Ligand(s)	u-PA	t-PA, plasminogen	u-PA/PAI-1; u-PA/PAI-2; t-PA/PAI-1; PN/α_2-AP	t-PA

ABBREVIATIONS: α_2-AP, α_2-antiplasmin; LRP, low-density lipoprotein receptor–like protein; ND, not determined; PAI-1, plasminogen-activator inhibitor-1; PAI-2, plasminogen activator inhibitor-2; PN, plasmin; t-PA, tissue plasminogen activator; u-PA, urokinase plasminogen activator; u-PAR, urokinase plasminogen activator receptor.

Its circulating half-life is exceedingly short (≈5 min). Functionally, t-PA is a poor activator of plasminogen. However, in the presence of fibrin, the catalytic efficiency of t-PA–dependent plasmin generation (k_{cat}/K_m) increases by at least two orders of magnitude.[20] This is due to a dramatic increase in affinity (decreased K_m) between t-PA and its substrate plasminogen in the presence of fibrin. Although it is expressed by endothelial cells, t-PA appears to represent the major circulating activator of plasminogen.[17]

UROKINASE

The second endogenous plasminogen activator, single-chain u-PA or prourokinase, is an approximately 54,000-M_r glycoprotein consisting of 411 amino acids (see Table 116-1). u-PA contains an epidermal growth factor–like domain and a single plasminogen-like kringle and possesses a classical catalytic triad (His204, Asp255, and Ser356) within its serine protease domain[52] (see Fig. 116-2). Cleavage of the Lys158-Ile159 peptide bond by plasmin or kallikrein converts single-chain u-PA to a disulfide-linked two-chain derivative.[53] Located on chromosome 10, the human u-PA gene is encoded by 11 exons spanning 6.4 kb and expressed by endothelial cells, macrophages, renal epithelial cells, and some tumor cells.[54,55] Its intron-exon structure is closely related to that of the t-PA gene.

There is circumstantial evidence that u-PA may be induced during neoplastic transformation, possibly through a mechanism involving

PLASMINOGEN

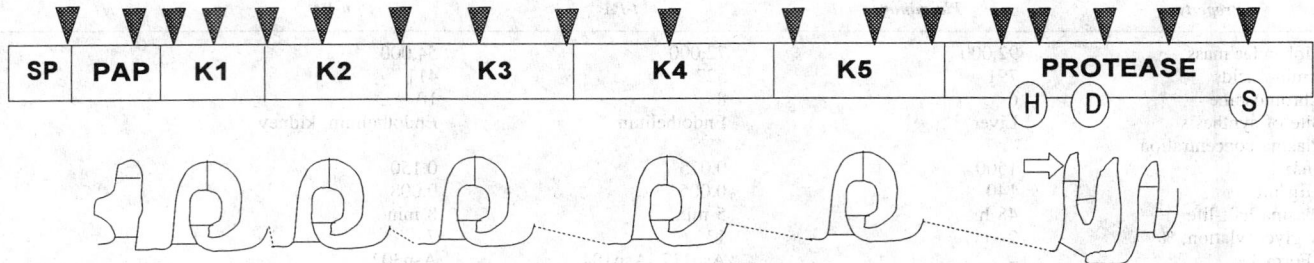

TISSUE PLASMINOGEN ACTIVATOR

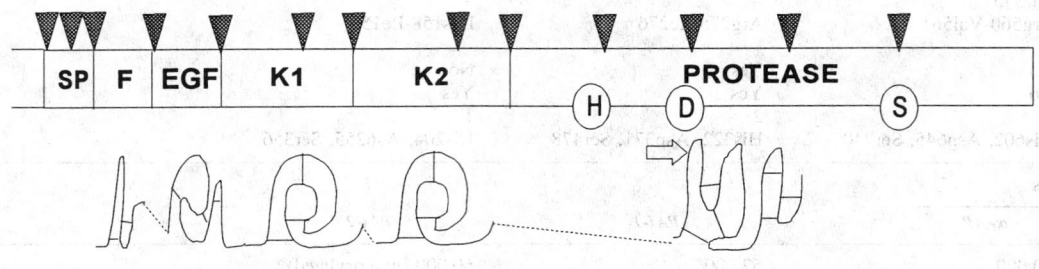

UROKINASE

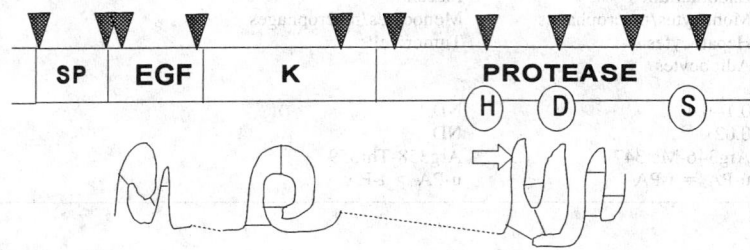

FIGURE 116-2   Structure-function relationships of plasminogen, t-PA, and u-PA. Alignment of the intron-exon structure of plasminogen, t-PA, and u-PA genes with functional protein domains. Protein domains are labeled signal peptide (SP), preactivation peptide (PAP), kringle domains (K), fibronectin-like "finger" (F), epidermal growth factor–like domain (EGF), and protease. The positions of catalytic triad amino acids histidine (H), aspartic acid (D), and serine (S) are shown within individual protease domains. The positions of individual introns relative to amino acid–encoding exons are indicated with inverted triangles (▼).

transcription factors AP1 and AP2.[56] Other agents that appear to induce expression of u-PA in vitro include hormones, growth factors, and cAMP.[49] Inflammatory cytokines such as interleukin-1 and lipopolysaccharide induce only small increments in u-PA expression, while tumor necrosis factor and transforming growth factor β (TGF-β) have a more dramatic (five- to thirtyfold) effect.[57–59]

Two-chain u-PA occurs in both high- (M_r 54,000) and low-molecular-weight (M_r 33,000) forms, which differ by the presence or absence, respectively, of a 135-residue amino-terminal fragment released by plasmin cleavage between Lys135 and Lys136.[60,61] Although both forms are capable of activating plasminogen, only the high-molecular-weight form binds to the u-PA receptor. u-PA has much lower affinity for fibrin than does t-PA and is an effective plasminogen activator both in the presence and in the absence of fibrin.[62,63] The extent to which prourokinase possesses intrinsic plasminogen-activating capacity is controversial.[64,65]

ACCESSORY PLASMINOGEN ACTIVATORS

Under certain conditions, proteases traditionally classified within the intrinsic arm of the coagulation cascade have been shown to be capable of activating plasminogen directly. These include kallikrein, factor XIa, and factor XIIa.[66,67] These proteases, however, normally account for no more than 15 percent of total plasmin-generating activity in plasma.[68]

PHYSIOLOGIC FUNCTION OF THE PLASMINOGEN ACTIVATORS

Although abnormalities of the t-PA release mechanism have been reported,[69] there are no clinical examples of complete deficiency of t-PA or u-PA in humans. Thus, the most compelling studies of the physiologic functions of these proteins come from gene-disruption analyses (see Table 116-2).[70] Both u-PA and t-PA null deletion mice exhibit normal fertility and embryonic development. However, u-PA

TABLE 116-2   GENETIC MOUSE MODELS RELEVANT TO FIBRINOLYSIS

Genotype	Phenotype
	GENE DELETION MODELS
Plasminogen	
PLG −/−	Spontaneous thrombosis, runting, premature death[31,253]
	Fibrin in liver, lungs, stomach; gastric ulcers[31,253]
	Impaired wound healing; ligneous conjunctivitis[33,200]
	Impaired monocyte recruitment[202]
	Impaired neointima formation after electrical injury[203]
	Impaired dissemination of *Borrelia burgdorferi*[204]
	Reduced excitotoxic neuronal cell death in brain[205]
Plasminogen activators	
t-PA −/−	Reduced lysis of fibrin clot[70]
	Increased endotoxin-induced thrombosis[70]
u-PA −/−	Occasional fibrin in liver/intestine[70]
	Rectal prolapse, ulcers of eyelids, face, ears[70]
	Reduced macrophage degradation of fibrin[70]
	Increased endotoxin-induced thrombosis[70]
u-PA −/−, t-PA −/−	Reduced growth, fertility, and life span; cachexia[70]
	Fibrin deposits in liver, gonads, lungs[70]
	Ulcers in intestine, skin, ears; rectal prolapse[70]
	Impaired clot lysis[70]
Inhibitors	
PAI-1 −/−	Mildly increased lysis of fibrin clot[104]
	Resistance to endotoxin-induced thrombosis[254]
LRP −/−	Embryonic lethal day 13.5 postconception[157,158]
Receptors	
u-PAR −/−	Essentially normal[255]
	Reduced macrophage PLG activation in vitro[255]
	Normal matrix degradation[255]
	OVEREXPRESSION MODELS
Apo(a) +/+	Atherosclerotic lesions with high-fat diet[256]
	Reduced cell-associated plasmin and activation of TGF-β[257]
	Resistance to t-PA−mediated clot lysis[258]
Apo(a)ΔLBS +/+	Reduced lipid deposition[259]
PAI-1 +++/+++	Venous thrombosis[103]
	Tail necrosis, hind foot edema
u-PA +++/+++	Fatal neonatal hemorrhage[260]
	Impaired learning[261]

Apo(a), Apolipoprotein(a).

−/− mice developed rectal prolapse, nonhealing ulcerations of the face and eyelids, and occasional fibrin deposition in tissues. Although they show normal rates of pulmonary clot lysis, endotoxin-induced thrombus formation is significantly enhanced. t-PA−deficient mice display a normal spontaneous phenotype. However, these animals have a decreased rate of lysis of artificially induced pulmonary thrombi as well as enhanced thrombus formation in response to injection of endotoxin. Doubly deficient (t-PA−/−, u-PA−/−) mice exhibit rectal prolapse, nonhealing ulceration, runting, and cachexia, with extensive fibrin deposition in liver, intestine, gonads, and lung. It is not surprising that clot lysis is markedly impaired. These findings demonstrate that t-PA and u-PA are not essential for normal embryologic development but do play crucial roles in lysis of artificially induced thrombi and in fibrinolytic surveillance.

INHIBITORS OF FIBRINOLYSIS

PLASMIN INHIBITORS

The action of plasmin is negatively modulated by a family of serine protease inhibitors, called serpins (see Table 116-1).[71] All serpins have a common mechanism of action by forming an irreversible complex with the active-site serine of the target protease following proteolytic cleavage of the inhibitor by the target protease. Within such a complex, both protease and inhibitor lose their activity.

A single-chain glycoprotein with a M_r of approximately 70,000, α_2-antiplasmin (α_2-AP) circulates in plasma at relatively high concentrations ($\approx 0.9 \ \mu M$) and enjoys a plasma half-life of 2.4 days[72] (see Table 116-1). This serpin contains about 1 percent carbohydrate by mass and consists of 452 amino acids with two disulfide bridges.[73] In humans, the gene is located on chromosome 18 and contains 10 exons distributed over 16 kb of DNA.[74] The promoter region of the α_2-AP gene contains a hepatitis B−like enhancer element that directs tissue-specific expression in the liver.[73] α_2-AP is also a constituent of platelet α granules.[75] Plasmin released into flowing blood or in the vicinity of a platelet-rich thrombus is immediately neutralized upon forming an irreversible 1:1 stoichiometric, lysine binding site−dependent complex with α_2-AP. Interaction with plasmin is accompanied by cleavage of the Arg364-Met365 peptide bond, and the resulting covalent complexes are cleared in the liver.

Several additional proteins can act as plasmin inhibitors (see Table 116-1). α_2-Macroglobulin is a 725,000-M_r dimeric protein synthesized by endothelial cells and macrophages and found in platelet α granules. This nonserpin inhibits plasmin with approximately 10 percent of the efficiency exhibited by α_2-AP[76] by forming noncovalent complexes with several distinct serine proteases. C_1-esterase inhibitor can also serve as an inhibitor of t-PA in plasma.[69] Protease nexin may function as a noncirculating cell surface inhibitor of trypsin,[77] thrombin, factor Xa, urokinase, or plasmin, resulting in protease-inhibitor complexes that are endocytosed via a specific nexin receptor.[78]

PLASMINOGEN-ACTIVATOR INHIBITORS

Plasminogen-Activator Inhibitor-1   Of the two major plasminogen-activator inhibitors[79] (see Table 116-1), PAI-1 is the most abundant. This approximately 52,000-M_r, single-chain, cysteine-less glycoprotein is released by endothelial cells, monocytes, macrophages, hepatocytes, adipocytes, and platelets.[80–82] Release of PAI-1 is stimulated by many cytokines, growth factors, and lipoproteins common to the global inflammatory response.[58,83,84] The PAI-1 gene consists of 9 exons, spanning 12.2 kb on chromosome 7q21.3-q22.[85] The serpin-reactive site is located at Arg346-Met347, and activity of this labile serpin is stabilized upon complex formation with vitronectin, a component of plasma and pericellular matrix.[86,87]

The upstream regulatory region of the human PAI-1 gene contains a strong endothelial cell- or fibroblast-specific element within the first 187 bp of the 5′-flanking region,[88,89] a glucocorticoid-responsive enhancer between positions −90 and +75,[89] and TGF-β−responsive elements between bases −791 and −546 and bases −328 and −186.[90] TGF-β is known to stimulate fos and jun, the two components of the AP1 complex, and an AP1 binding site (GGAGTCA) is located at −672 to −666 upstream of the PAI-1 cap site.[91] Agents that have been shown to enhance expression of PAI-1 at the message level, the protein level, or both, without affecting t-PA synthesis include the inflammatory cytokines lipopolysaccharide, interleukin-1, tumor necrosis factor-α,[57,58,83,92–94] TGF-β and basic fibroblast growth factor,[59,90,93,95] very low-density lipoprotein and lipoprotein(a),[96,97] angiotensin II,[98] thrombin,[99,100] and phorbol esters.[101] In addition, endothelial cell PAI-1 is down-regulated by forskolin[43,50] and by endothelial cell growth factor in the presence of heparin.[102]

PAI-1 is the most important and rapidly acting physiologic inhibitor of both t-PA and u-PA. Transgenic mice that overexpress PAI-1 exhibit thrombotic occlusion of tail veins and swelling of hindlimbs within 2 weeks of birth (see Table 116-2).[103] Mice deficient in PAI-1, on the other hand, exhibit normal fertility, viability, tissue histology, and development, and show no evidence of hemorrhage.[104] These observations contrast with the moderately severe bleeding disorder observed in a human patient with complete PAI-1 deficiency.[105]

Plasminogen-Activator Inhibitor-2 Originally purified from human placenta,[79,106] plasminogen activator inhibitor-2 (PAI-2) is a 393–amino acid member of the serpin family whose reactive site is the Arg358-Thr359 peptide bond[106] (see Table 116-1). The gene encoding PAI-2 is located on chromosome 18q21–23, spans 16.5 kb, and contains 8 exons.[107] PAI-2 exists as both a 47,000-M_r nonglycosylated intracellular form and a 60,000-M_r glycosylated form secreted by leukocytes and fibrosarcoma cells. Functionally, PAI-2 inhibits both two-chain t-PA and two-chain u-PA with comparable efficiency (second-order rate constant 10^5 $M^{-1}s^{-1}$). However, it is less effective toward single-chain t-PA (second-order rate constant 10^3 $M^{-1}s^{-1}$) and does not inhibit prourokinase.

Significant levels of PAI-2 are found in human plasma only during pregnancy. The 5′-untranslated region of the gene has not yet been characterized.[106] The 3′-downstream sequences include the TTATTTAT motif, which has been identified with inflammatory mediators.[108,109] In macrophages in vitro, secretion of PAI-2 is enhanced by endotoxin and phorbol esters,[109,110] and dexamethasone decreases PAI-2 expression in HT-1080 cells.[49]

CELLULAR RECEPTORS

Although structurally diverse, cell surface fibrinolytic receptors can be classified into two groups whose integrated actions are likely to be essential for homeostatic control of plasmin activity[2] (see Table 116-1). "Activation" receptors localize and potentiate plasminogen activation, while "clearance" receptors eliminate plasmin and plasminogen activators from the blood or focal microenvironments.

Activation Receptors There are three types of activation receptors: plasminogen receptors, the u-PA receptor (u-PAR), and annexin II.

Plasminogen receptors are a diverse group of proteins expressed on a wide array of cell types.[2] Reported receptors include α-enolase, glycoprotein IIb/IIIa complex, the Heymann nephritis antigen, amphoterin, and annexin II, which are expressed primarily on monocytoid cells,[111] platelets,[112] renal epithelial cells,[113] neuroblastoma cells,[114] and endothelial cells,[115,116] respectively. These binding proteins commonly interact with the kringle structures of plasminogen through carboxyl-terminal lysine residues.[111]

u-PAR is expressed on monocytes, macrophages, fibroblasts, endothelial cells, and a variety of tumor cells[2] (see Table 116-1). u-PAR cDNA was cloned and sequenced from a human fibroblast cDNA library[117] and encodes a protein of 313 amino acids with a 21-residue signal peptide. The gene consists of 7 exons distributed over 23 kb of genomic DNA and places this glycoprotein within the Ly-1/elapid venom toxin superfamily of cysteine-rich proteins.[118,119] u-PAR is anchored to the plasma membrane through glycosylphosphatidylinositol linkages.[120] u-PA bound to its receptor maintains its activity and susceptibility to the physiologic inhibitor PAI-1.[121] Formation of u-PA–PAI-1 complexes appears to hasten clearance of u-PA by hepatic or monocytoid cells.[121–123]

u-PAR appears to play a novel role in cellular signaling and adhesion events.[124] u-PAR binds the adhesive glycoprotein vitronectin at a site distinct from the u-PA binding domain,[125,126] and u-PA transfected renal epithelial cells acquire enhanced adhesion to vitronectin while they lose their adhesion to fibronectin.[127] u-PAR, furthermore, colocalizes with integrins in focal contacts and at the leading edge of migrating cells[128] and also associates with caveolin, a major component of caveolae, structures abundant in endothelial cells and thought to participate in signaling events.[129–131] Thus, integrin function may be regulated by u-PAR, signifying an integrated relationship between cellular adhesion and proteolysis.

Annexin II is a widely distributed, highly conserved, 36,000-M_r peripheral membrane protein expressed abundantly on endothelial cells,[132–135] macrophages,[136] myeloid cells,[137] and some tumor cells.[138–140] It belongs to a 20-member superfamily of calcium-dependent, phospholipid-binding proteins[141] that have in common a conserved C-terminal "core" region preceded by a more variable N-terminal "tail."[142] The human annexin II gene consists of 13 exons distributed over 40 kb of genomic DNA on chromosome 15 (15q21).[143]

Annexin II possesses the unique property of binding both plasminogen (K_d 114 nM)[115] and t-PA (K_d 30 nM),[116] but not u-PA.[116] Purified native human annexin II stimulates the catalytic efficiency of t-PA–dependent plasminogen activation by sixtyfold in the fluid phase.[144] This effect is completely inhibited in the presence of lysine analogs or upon treatment of annexin II with carboxypeptidase B, an agent that removes basic carboxyl-terminal amino acids. Although it lacks a classical signal peptide, within 16 h of its biosynthesis, annexin II is constitutively translocated to the endothelial cell surface, where it binds phospholipid via core repeat 2 containing the linear sequence KGLGT and downstream aspartate residue (Asp161).[145] Annexin II heterotetramer, composed of two annexin monomers and two p11 subunits, may have even greater stimulatory effects on t-PA–dependent plasmin generation.[134]

Lys307 appears to be crucial for the effective interaction of plasminogen with annexin II. "Activation" of the receptor with respect to plasminogen binding apparently requires cleavage at Lys307-Arg308 by a plasmin-like protease and subsequent exposure of the carboxyl-terminal Lys307 residue.[144] Lipoprotein(a), an atherogenic low-density lipoprotein (LDL)–like particle, competes with plasminogen for binding to annexin II[146] and reduces cell surface plasmin generation. This mechanism may contribute to atherogenesis by reducing fibrinolytic surveillance at the blood vessel wall.

t-PA binding to annexin II requires a separate domain consisting of residues 8 through 13 (LCKLSL) within the amino-terminal "tail" domain of the receptor.[147] This sequence is a target for homocysteine (HC), a thiol-containing amino acid that accumulates in association with nutritional deficiencies of vitamin B_6, vitamin B_{12}, or folic acid, or in inherited abnormalities of cystathionine β-synthase, methylenetetrahydrofolate reductase, or methionine synthase,[148] and is associated with atherothrombotic disease.[148–150] In vitro, HC impairs the intrinsic fibrinolytic system of the endothelial cell by approximately 50 percent[151] by forming a covalent derivative with Cys9, thus preventing its interaction with t-PA.[147] The half-maximal dose of HC for inhibition of t-PA binding to annexin II is approximately 11 μM HC, a value close to the upper limit of normal for HC in plasma (14 μM).

CLEARANCE RECEPTORS

Both u-PA and t-PA are cleared from the circulation via the liver.[152] In vitro, clearance of t-PA–PAI-1 complexes appears also to be mediated by a large two-chain receptor called the LDL-receptor–related protein (LRP).[153–155] This complex interaction requires both growth factor and finger domains of t-PA. An additional 39,000-M_r "receptor-associated protein" copurifies with LRP and may regulate the binding and uptake of LRP ligands.[156] It is interesting to note that LRP knockout embryos undergo developmental arrest by 13.5 days after conception, suggesting that regulation of serine protease activity may be crucial for early embryogenesis.[157,158]

Although several PAI-1–independent clearance pathways for t-PA have been proposed,[152] involving the large LRP subunit,[159] the mannose receptor,[160] or an α-fucose–specific receptor,[161] in vivo studies in mice suggest that LRP and the mannose receptor play a dominant role in t-PA clearance.[162]

THE FIBRINOLYTIC ACTIONS OF PLASMIN

DEGRADATION OF FIBRINOGEN AND FIBRIN

FIBRINOGEN

Fibrinogen possesses distinct proteolytic cleavage sites for plasmin and thrombin (Fig. 116-3). While plasmin cleaves carboxyl-terminal Aα and N-terminal fibrinopeptide B moieties, thrombin primarily releases fibrinopeptide A, exposing the Gly-Pro-Arg tripeptide sequence and allowing fibrinogen to polymerize and form insoluble fibrin.[163] Plasmin cleavage of fibrinogen (M_r 340,000) initially produces carboxyl-terminal fragments from the α chain within the D domain of fibrinogen (Aα fragment).[164,165] Simultaneously but more slowly, the N-terminal segments of the β chains are cleaved, releasing a peptide containing fibrinopeptide B. The resulting approximately 250,000-M_r molecule is termed fragment X and represents a clottable form of fibrinogen. Additional cleavage events may release the Bβ fragment from the α chain carboxyl terminus, and, in a series of subsequent reactions, plasmin cleaves the three polypeptide chains that connect the D and E domains, giving rise to free D domain (M_r $\approx$100,000) plus the binodular D-E fragment known as fragment Y (M_r $\approx$150,000). Finally, domains D and E are separated from each other, and some of the N-terminal fibrinopeptide A sites on domain E are also modified. Although fragment X can be converted to fibrin by thrombin, the fragments Y, D, and E are all nonclottable and in fact may inhibit the spontaneous polymerization of fibrinogen[166] (see Chap. 124).

FIBRIN

Plasmin degradation of fibrin leads to a distinct set of molecular products.[167] Species similar to fragments Y, D, and E but lacking fibrinopeptide sites are released from non–cross-linked fibrin. If fibrin has been extensively cross-linked by factor XIII, however, the resulting D fragments are cross-linked to an E domain fragment. Assay of cross-linked D-dimer fragments is employed clinically to identify disseminated intravascular coagulation states associated with excessive plasmin-mediated fibrinolysis (see Chap. 126). Several biologic activities, including inhibition of platelet function,[168] potentiation of the hypotensive effects of bradykinin,[169] chemotaxis,[170] and immune modulation have been ascribed to fibrin breakdown products.[171]

T-PA–MEDIATED PLASMINOGEN ACTIVATION

With or without fibrin, t-PA–mediated activation of plasminogen follows Michaelis-Menten kinetics.[20] In the absence of fibrin, t-PA is a weak activator of plasminogen. However, in the presence of fibrin, the catalytic efficiency (k_{cat}/K_m) of t-PA–dependent plasminogen activation is enhanced by at least two orders of magnitude. This is the basis for its specificity as a lytic agent in the treatment of thrombosis

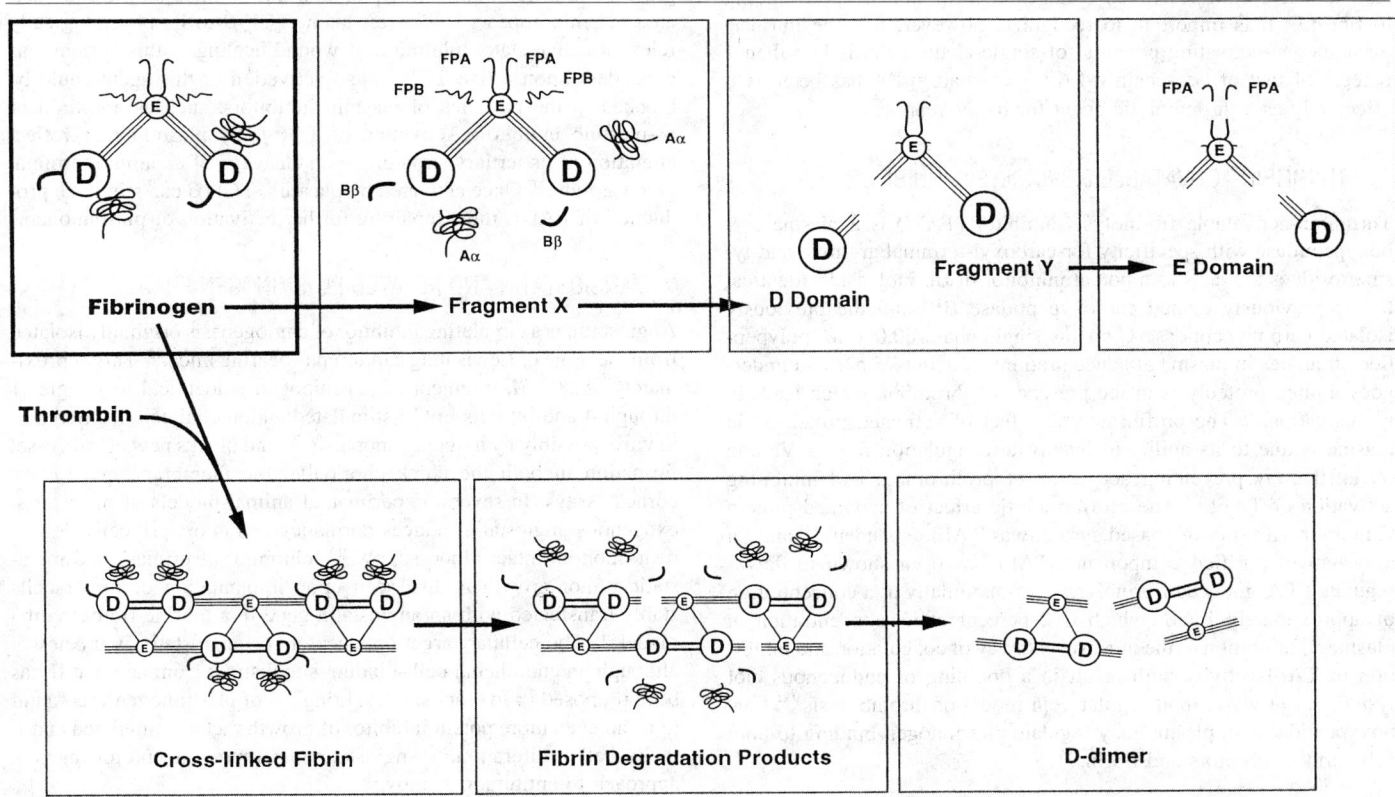

FIGURE 116-3   Degradation of fibrinogen and cross-linked fibrin by plasmin. *(Top panel)* Plasmin initially cleaves the C-terminal regions of the α and β chains within the D domain of fibrinogen, releasing the Aα and Bβ fragments. In addition, a fragment containing fibrinopeptide B (FPB) from the N-terminal region of the fibrinogen β-chain is also released, giving rise to the intermediate fragment known as fragment X. Subsequently, plasmin cleaves the three polypeptide chains connecting the D and E domains, giving rise to fragments D, E, and Y. *(Bottom panel)* Fibrinogen can also be polymerized by thrombin to form fibrin. When degrading cross-linked fibrin, plasmin initially cleaves the C-terminal region of the α and β chains within the D domain. Subsequently, some of the connecting regions between the D and E domains are severed. Fibrin is ultimately solubilized upon hydrolysis of additional peptide bonds within the central portions of the coiled-coil connectors, giving rise to fibrin degradation products such as D-dimer. (From KA Hajjar[1] with permission.)

(see Chap. 134). The affinity between t-PA and plasminogen in the absence of fibrin is low (K_m 65 μM) but increases significantly in its presence (K_m 0.16 μM), even though the catalytic rate constant remains essentially unchanged ($k_{cat} \approx 0.05$ s^{-1}). When plasmin forms on the fibrin surface, both its lysine-binding sites and its active site are occupied. Thus, it is relatively protected from its physiologic inhibitor, α_2-AP.[172] The interaction of t-PA with fibrin is probably initiated by its "finger" domain. However, once fibrin is modified by plasmin, carboxyl-terminal lysine residues are generated, and these become binding sites for kringle 2 of t-PA and kringles 1 and 4 of plasminogen.[173] Therefore, fibrin accelerates its own destruction by (1) enhancing the catalytic efficiency of plasmin formation by t-PA, (2) protecting plasmin from its physiologic inhibitor, α_2-AP, and (3) providing new binding sites for plasminogen and t-PA once its degradation has begun.

U-PA–MEDIATED PLASMIN GENERATION

For the activation of Glu-plasminogen by u-PA in a fibrin-free system, reported Michaelis constants (K_m) vary from 1.4 to 200 μM, while catalytic rate constants (k_{cat}) range from 0.26 to 1.48 s^{-1}.[1] It is interesting to note that activation of Glu-plasminogen by two-chain u-PA is increased in the presence of fibrin by about tenfold even though u-PA does not bind to fibrin.[174] In contrast, single-chain u-PA has considerable fibrin specificity. This may reflect neutralization by fibrin of components in plasma that impair plasminogen activation.[175] It may also reflect a conformational change in plasminogen upon binding to fibrin.[176] It is important to recognize, however, that the intrinsic plasminogen-activating potential of single-chain u-PA is less than 1 percent of that of two-chain u-PA.[1] Two-chain u-PA has been used effectively as a thrombolytic agent for many years.[177]

THROMBIN-ACTIVATABLE FIBRINOLYSIS INHIBITOR

Thrombin-activatable fibrinolysis inhibitor (TAFI) is a plasma carboxypeptidase with specificity for carboxyl-terminal arginine and lysine residues that acts as a potent inhibitor of fibrinolysis.[178] Identical to the previously cloned carboxypeptidase B[179] and the previously isolated carboxypeptidase U,[180] this single-chain 60,000-M_r polypeptide circulates in plasma at concentrations of about 75 nM and undergoes limited proteolysis in the presence of thrombin, which leads to its activation.[181] The profibrinolytic effect of activated protein C in plasma is due to its ability to inactivate coagulation factors Va and VIIIa, thereby preventing activation of prothrombin and inhibiting activation of TAFI.[178] The profibrinolytic effect of activated protein C in an in vitro plasma-based system was TAFI dependent,[182] and, in a system of purified components, TAFI has been shown to downregulate t-PA–induced fibrinolysis half-maximally at a concentration of approximately 1 nM, which is 2 percent of its concentration in plasma.[183] Inhibition of the intrinsic pathway of coagulation and inhibition of TAFI activity both result in a doubling of endogenous clot lysis in an in vivo rabbit jugular vein model of thrombolysis.[184] Carboxypeptidases in plasma may regulate plasminogen binding to both cell surface receptors and fibrin.[185]

THE NONFIBRINOLYTIC ACTIONS OF PLASMIN

PLASMIN AS A TISSUE REMODELER

A large number of in vitro studies suggest a role for plasmin in tissue remodeling. Basement membrane proteins, such as thrombospondin,[186] laminin,[187] fibronectin,[188] and fibrinogen,[189] are readily degraded by plasmin in vitro, suggesting possible roles in inflammation,[190] tu-

mor cell invasion,[191] embryogenesis,[192] ovulation,[193] neurodevelopment,[194,195] and prohormone activation.[196,197] Plasmin also activates matrix metalloproteinases (MMPs) types 1, 3, 7, and 10,[198] thereby facilitating the degradation of matrix proteins, such as the collagens, laminin, fibronectin, vitronectin, elastin, aggrecan, and tenascin C.[198] On the other hand, MMP activation can apparently proceed in the absence of plasminogen, possibly providing the basis for the mild phenotype observed in plasminogen null homozygote animals.[199]

A role for plasmin in tissue remodeling is further supported by in vivo observations in plasminogen-deficient mice (see Table 116-2). Impaired wound healing is observed in the plasminogen knockout[200] and is reversed upon simultaneous deletion of fibrinogen.[201] Plasminogen-deficient mice also display diminished recruitment of monocytes in response to intraperitoneal thioglycolate[202] and impaired neointima formation following electrical injury to blood vessels.[203] In studies involving *Borrelia burgdorferi*, the agent of Lyme disease, dissemination of the spirochete within its arthropod vector *Ixodes dammini* is absolutely dependent upon host plasminogen even though the deer tick contains no fibrin.[204] Further, kainate-induced excitotoxicity and attendant neuronal cell dropout in the hippocampus are not observed in plasminogen knockout mice but do occur in fibrinogen-deficient animals.[205] The latter two studies may define new roles for plasmin that appear to be unrelated to degradation of fibrin.

Plasmin may play a role in the activation of growth factors and in the proliferative response of the blood vessel to injury. TGF-β is a 25,000-M_r homodimeric polypeptide whose effects on vascular cell growth and differentiation are pleiomorphic.[206] In culture, cell-associated plasmin appears to convert latent TGF-β to its physiologically relevant active state. Inhibition of wound healing in this system was dependent upon active TGF-β, and activation of this agent could be blocked in the presence of plasmin inhibitors, such as aprotinin or α_2-plasmin inhibitor. Activation of TGF-β by plasmin may reflect alteration of its tertiary structure upon cleavage of an amino-terminal glycopeptide.[207] Once activated by plasmin, TGF-β can stimulate production of PAI-1, thus impairing further activation of plasminogen.

ANGIOSTATIN AND RELATED PLASMINOGEN FRAGMENTS

Angiostatin is a circulating inhibitor of angiogenesis originally isolated from the urine of Lewis lung carcinoma–bearing mice.[208] This approximately 38,000 M_r fragment of plasminogen is identical to kringles 1 through 4 and inhibits bFGF-stimulated endothelial cell proliferation in vitro, possibly by inducing apoptosis,[209] and blocks new blood vessel formation in both the chick chorioallantoic membrane and mouse cornea assays. In several experimental animal models of metastasis, exogenous angiostatin induces dormancy of tumors critically dependent upon an intact blood supply.[210] Inhibition of primary and metastatic tumor growth is also seen upon implantation of tumor cells stably transfected with an angiostatin gene in a murine fibrosarcoma model.[211] The cellular target or receptor for angiostatin is unknown, although an endothelial cell–binding site distinct from annexin II has been proposed.[212] In other studies, kringle 5 of plasminogen was found to be an even more potent inhibitor of growth factor–stimulated endothelial cell proliferation.[213] Angiostatin may represent a promising new approach to antitumor therapy.[214]

The mechanism of angiostatin formation is a topic of intense investigation. Lewis lung carcinoma–associated macrophages stimulated with tumor-derived GM-CSF express high levels of metalloelastase,[215] which can produce angiostatin from the parent molecule plasminogen.[215] Alternatively, angiostatin can form in vitro upon exposure of plasmin to a plasmin reductase followed by an unidentified serine protease secreted by cultured CHO or HT1080 cells.[216] Matrix metalloproteinases 7 and 9,[217] as well as urokinase in the presence of free sulfhydryl donors,[218] have also been proposed as angiostatin-generating agents. These studies suggest the possibility of multiple pathways for the generation of angiostatin.

DISORDERS OF PLASMIN GENERATION

FIBRINOLYTIC DEFICIENCY AND THROMBOSIS

Partial human plasminogen deficiency was first described in a 31-year-old male with a history of repeated episodes of thrombophlebitis, intracranial and mesenteric venous thrombosis, and pulmonary embolism.[219] Reduced plasminogen activity (50% of normal) in his plasma was traced to a Ala601Thr point mutation, and several additional patients with this defect or related substitutions have now been described.[220] Acquired plasminogen deficiency, as may occur in liver disease, sepsis, and Argentine hemorrhagic fever due to decreased synthesis and/or increased catabolism, has frequently been associated with thrombotic vascular occlusion.[221]

Congenital plasminogen deficiency has been classified into two types.[222] In type I, the concentration of immunoreactive plasminogen is reduced in parallel with functional activity. Although no examples of complete aplasminogenemia have been reported in humans, type I mutations giving rise to reduced synthesis of plasminogen are well defined (e.g., Ser572Pro).[223] In a study of consecutive patients with thrombophilia, the prevalence of plasminogen deficiency was 1.9 percent.[224] Approximately half of these individuals had other risk factors, such as deficiency of antithrombin III, protein C, or protein S, or resistance to activated protein C. Among 93 patients with type I plasminogen deficiency, the prevalence of thrombosis was 24 percent, or 9 percent when the propositi were excluded.[225] These data suggest that, compared with other thrombophilic conditions, congenital plasminogen deficiency is associated with a lower risk of thrombosis.[225]

In one well-documented case of type I plasminogen deficiency, an infant with less than 1 percent of normal plasminogen antigen and activity presented with hydrocephalus, central nervous system malformations, poor wound healing, recurrent respiratory infections, but no family history of thrombosis. His severe ligneous conjunctivitis (i.e., the development of fibrinous membrane over the eyes) resolved completely upon infusion of Lys-plasminogen.[226] This case illustrates the importance of plasminogen in extravascular fibrinolysis and underscores the role of plasminogen deficiency as a relatively weak predisposing risk factor for thrombosis.[222]

In type II plasminogen deficiency, immunoreactive protein is normal, while functional activity is reduced.[220] In a study of a Japanese cohort, 94 percent of 129 families with type II dysplasminogenemia had the Ala601Thr mutation, while 3 percent and 1 percent had the Val355Phe and Asp676Asn, respectively.[227] In this study, approximately 27 percent of individuals with dysplasminogenemia had a clinical history of thrombosis. A number of additional plasminogen polymorphisms[228,229] and clinically significant dysplasminogenemias[230] have also been reported.

Mutations in tissue plasminogen activator or urokinase have not been clinically linked to thrombophilia. However, defects in plasminogen activator release from the vessel wall as well as increased inhibition of t-PA by PAI-1 have both been associated with a thrombotic diathesis.[231,232] Increased circulating PAI-1 appears to represent an independent risk factor for vascular reocclusion in young survivors of myocardial infarction.[233] In addition, increased levels of PAI-1 have been associated with deep vein thrombosis in patients undergoing hip replacement surgery[234] and in individuals with insulin resistance.[235] With regard to the latter studies, however, one should bear in mind that PAI-1 is itself an acute-phase reactant and thus may not be directly responsible for the observed prothrombotic tendency.[236]

ENHANCED FIBRINOLYSIS AND BLEEDING

Enhanced fibrinolysis due to congenital or acquired loss of fibrinolytic inhibitor activity is associated with a bleeding diathesis.[237] Patients with congenital deficiency of α_2-AP may present with a severe hemorrhagic disorder due to impaired inactivation of plasmin and premature lysis of the hemostatic plug.[238] Acquired α_2-AP deficiency may be seen in patients with severe liver disease due to decreased synthesis, disseminated intravascular coagulation due to consumption, or nephrotic syndrome due to urinary loss, or during thrombolytic therapy, which induces excessive utilization of the inhibitor.[238]

Patients with acute promyelocytic leukemia demonstrate excessive expression of annexin II on their developmentally arrested promyelocytes. Bleeding in this disorder is accompanied by evidence of high levels of plasmin generation and depletion of α_2-antiplasmin. Bleeding resolves upon initiation of all-trans-retinoic acid therapy, which eliminates expression of promyelocyte annexin II, probably through a transcriptional mechanism.[137]

Complete loss of PAI-1 expression, resulting in hemorrhage in a 9-year-old child, was associated with severe hemorrhage in the setting of trauma or surgery.[105] This autosomal recessive trait reflected a frameshift mutation within exon 4 that induced a premature stop codon. This case demonstrates that the function of PAI-1 in humans is apparently limited to the regulation of fibrinolysis.

DEVELOPMENTAL REGULATION OF THE FIBRINOLYTIC SYSTEM

In the resting, nonstressed state, the plasmin-generating potential in the newborn is significantly less than that of the adult.[239] Although the amino acid composition and apparent molecular mass of neonatal plasminogen are indistinguishable from those of the adult protein,[240,241] plasma concentrations of plasminogen in the neonate are approximately 50 percent of those observed in adults.[240,242,243] On the other hand, levels of histidine-rich glycoprotein, a carrier protein that may limit the interaction of plasminogen with fibrin, are reduced by 50 to 80 percent in healthy, term newborns.[244] Finally, plasminogen in the neonate is heavily glycosylated, less readily activated by tissue plasminogen activator, and only weakly bound to the endothelial cell surface.[241]

Although t-PA antigen and activity levels in the healthy newborn are reduced by 63 and 75 percent, respectively, compared with adult values,[243] stressed infants, such as those with severe congenital heart disease or respiratory distress syndrome, may have t-PA antigen levels that are increased by up to eightfold.[245,246] In contrast, the principal plasmin inhibitors undergo only minimal change from birth to adulthood.[242,247,248] Thus, reduced fibrinolytic activity may contribute to the thrombogenic state commonly observed in the newborn,[249] but this predilection may be reversed under conditions of physiologic stress.

FIBRINOLYTIC ACTIVITY DURING PREGNANCY AND PUERPERIUM

Pregnancy is a hypofibrinolytic state.[250] Both plasminogen and fibrinogen levels in plasma increase by 50 to 60 percent in the third trimester. Overall fibrinolytic activity, as reflected by euglobulin lysis activity, is reduced, and increased fibrin deposition is suggested by increasing D-dimer levels throughout pregnancy.[251] Between the twentieth week of pregnancy and term, PAI-1 levels increase to three times their normal level, while PAI-2 levels rise to 25 times their level in early pregnancy.[250] Less dramatic increases in both u-PA and t-PA levels are also observed. Within 1 h of delivery, concentrations of both PAI-1 and PAI-2 begin to decrease, and they return to normal within 3 to 5 days.[250]

In preeclampsia, the hemostatic and fibrinolytic imbalances seen in pregnancy are further exaggerated.[252] Circulating PAI-1 levels exceed those in normal pregnancy, and fibrin deposition is seen in glomerular capillaries and spiral arteries of the placenta. It is interesting to note that levels of PAI-2, a marker of placental function, are reduced during preeclampsia compared with normal pregnancy, and this decrease correlates with intrauterine growth retardation of the fetus.

REFERENCES

1. Hajjar KA: The molecular basis of fibrinolysis, in *Hematology of Infancy and Childhood*, 5th ed, edited by DG Nathan, SH Orkin, p 1557. Saunders, Philadelphia, 1998.
2. Hajjar KA: Cellular receptors in the regulation of plasmin generation. *Thromb Haemost* 74:294, 1995.
3. Raum D, Marcus D, Alper CA, Levey R, Taylor PD, Starzl TE: Synthesis of human plasminogen by the liver. *Science* 208:1036, 1980.
4. Bohmfalk J, Fuller G: Plasminogen is synthesized by primary cultures of rat hepatocytes. *Science* 209:408, 1980.
5. Castellino FJ: Biochemistry of human plasminogen. *Sem Thromb Hemost* 10:18, 1984.
6. Collen D, Tytgat G, Claeys H, Verstraete M, Wallen P: Metabolism of plasminogen in healthy subjects: effect of tranexamic acid. *J Clin Invest* 51:1310, 1972.
7. Forsgren M, Raden B, Israelsson M, Larsson K, Heden LO: Molecular cloning and characterization of a full-length cDNA clone for human plasminogen. *FEBS Lett* 213:254, 1987.
8. Miles LA, Dahlberg CM, Plow EF: The cell-binding domains of plasminogen and their function in plasma. *J Biol Chem* 263:11656, 1988.
9. Markus G, De Pasquale JL, Wissler FC: Quantitative determination of the binding of epsilon-aminocaproic acid to native plasminogen. *J Biol Chem* 253:727, 1978.
10. Markus G, Priore RL, Wissler FC: The binding of tranexamic acid to native (glu) and modified (lys) human plasminogen and its effect on conformation. *J Biol Chem* 254:1211, 1979.
11. Hajjar KA, Harpel PC, Jaffe EA, Nachman RL: Binding of plasminogen to cultured human endothelial cells. *J Biol Chem* 261:11656, 1986.
12. Miles LA, Plow EF: Cellular regulation of fibrinolysis. *Thromb Haemost* 66:32, 1991.
13. Rakoczi I, Wiman B, Collen D: On the biologic significance of the specific interaction between fibrin, plasminogen, and antiplasmin. *Biochim Biophys Acta* 540:295, 1978.
14. Hayes ML, Castellino FJ: Carbohydrate of the human plasminogen variants: I. Carbohydrate composition, glycopeptide isolation, and characterization. *J Biol Chem* 254:8768, 1979.
15. Hayes ML, Castellino FJ: Carbohydrate of the human plasminogen variants: III. Structure of the O-glycosidically-linked oligosacchraide unit. *J Biol Chem* 254:8777, 1979.
16. Holvoet P, Lijnen HR, Collen D: A monoclonal antibody specific for lys-plasminogen. *J Biol Chem* 260:12106, 1985.
17. Saksela O: Plasminogen activation and regulation of proteolysis. *Biochim Biophys Acta* 823:35, 1985.
18. Wallen P, Wiman B: Characterization of human plasminogen: I. On the relationship between different molecular forms of plasminogen demonstrated in plasma and found in purified preparations. *Biochim Biophys Acta* 221:20, 1970.
19. Wallen P, Wiman B: Characterization of human plasminogen: II. Separation and partial characterization of different molecular forms of human plasminogen. *Biochim Biophys Acta* 157:122, 1972.
20. Hoylaerts M, Rijken DC, Lijnen HR, Collen D: Kinetics of the activation of plasminogen by human tissue plasminogen activator: Role of fibrin. *J Biol Chem* 257:2912, 1982.
21. Hajjar KA, Nachman RL: Endothelial cell-mediated conversion of glu-plasminogen to lys-plasminogen: further evidence for assembly of the fibrinolytic system on the endothelial cell surface. *J Clin Invest* 82:1769, 1988.
22. Murray JC, Buetow KH, Donovan M, et al: Linkage disequilibrium of plasminogen polymorphisms and assignment of the gene to human chromosome 6q26-6q27. *Am J Hum Genet* 40:338, 1987.
23. Petersen TE, Martzen MR, Ichinose A, Davie EW: Characterization of the gene for human plasminogen, a key proenzyme in the fibrinolytic system. *J Biol Chem* 265:6104, 1990.
24. Jenkins GR, Seiffert D, Parmer RJ, Miles LA: Regulation of plasminogen gene expression by interleukin-6. *Blood* 89:2394, 1997.
25. McLean JW, Tomlinson JE, Kuang WJ, et al: cDNA sequence of human apolipoprotein(a) is homologous to plasminogen. *Nature* 330:132, 1987.
26. Nakamura T, Nishizawa T, Hagiya M, et al: Molecular cloning and expression of human hepatocyte growth factor. *Nature* 342:440, 1989.
27. Weissbach L, Treadwell BV: A plasminogen-related gene is expressed in cancer cells. *Biochem Biophys Res Commun* 186:1108, 1992.
28. Yoshimura T, Yuhki N, Wang MH, Skeel A, Leonard EJ: Cloning, sequencing, and expression of human macrophage stimulating protein (MSP, MST 1) confirms MSP as a member of the family of kringle proteins and locates the MSP gene on chromosome 3. *J Biol Chem* 268:15461, 1993.
29. Byrne CD, Schwartz K, Meer K, Cheng JF, Lawn RM: The human apolipoprotein(a)/plasminogen gene cluster contains a novel homologue transcribed in liver. *Arterioscler Thromb* 14:534, 1994.
30. Ichinose A: Multiple members of the plasminogen-apolipoprotein(a) gene family associated with thrombosis. *Biochemistry* 31:3113, 1992.
31. Bugge TH, Flick MJ, Daugherty CC, Degen JL: Plasminogen deficiency causes severe thrombosis but is compatible with development and reproduction. *Genes Develop* 9:794, 1995.
32. Carmeliet P, Collen D: Gene targeting and gene transfer studies of the plasminogen/plasmin system: Implications in thrombosis, hemostasis, neointima formation, and atherosclerosis. *FASEB J* 9:934, 1995.
33. Drew AF, Kaufman AH, Kombrinck KW, Danton MJS, Degen JL, Bugge TH: Ligneous conjunctivitis in plasminogen-deficient mice. *Blood* 91:1616, 1998.
34. Pennica D, Holmes WE, Kohr WJ, et al: Cloning and expression of human tissue-type plasminogen activator cDNA in *E. coli*. *Nature* 301:214, 1983.
35. Tate KM, Higgins DL, Holmes WE, Winkler ME, Heyneker HL, Vehar GL: Functional role of proteolytic cleavage at arginine-275 of human tissue plasminogen activator as assessed by site-directed mutagenesis. *Biochemistry* 26:338, 1987.
36. Pohl G, Kenne L, Nilsson B, Einarsson M: Isolation and characterization of three different carbohydrate chains from melanoma tissue tissue plasminogen activator. *Eur J Biochem* 170:69, 1987.
37. Spellman MW, Basa LJ, Leonard CK, Chakel JA: Carbohydrate structures of tissue plasminogen activator expressed in Chinese hamster ovary cells. *J Biol Chem* 264:14100, 1989.
38. Harris RJ, Leonard CK, Guzzetta AW: Tissue plasminogen activator has an O-linked fucose attached to threonine-61 in the epidermal growth factor domain. *Biochemistry* 30:2311, 1991.
39. Ny T, Elgh F, Lund B: Structure of the human tissue-type plasminogen activator gene: Correlation of intron and exon structures to functional and structural domains. *Proc Natl Acad Sci USA* 81:5355, 1984.
40. Browne MJ, Tyrrell AWR, Chapman CG, et al: Isolation of a human tissue-type plasminogen activator genomic clone and its expression in mouse L cells. *Gene* 33:279, 1985.
41. Degen SJF, Rajput B, Reich E: The human tissue plasminogen activator gene. *J Biol Chem* 261:6872, 1986.
42. Van Zonnefeld A, Veerman H, Pannekoek H: Autonomous functions of structural domains on human tissue-type plasminogen activator. *Proc Natl Acad Sci USA* 83:4670, 1986.
43. Feng P, Ohlsson M, Ny T: The structure of the TATA-less rat tissue-type plasminogen activator gene. *J Biol Chem* 265:2022, 1990.
44. Kooistra T, Bosma PJ, Toet K, et al: Role of protein kinase C and cyclic adenosine monophosphate in the regulation of tissue-type plasminogen activator, plasminogen activator inhibitor-1, and platelet-derived growth factor mRNA levels in human endothelial cells: Possible involvement of proto-oncogenes c-jun and c-fos. *Arterioscler Thromb* 11:1042, 1991.
45. Medcalf RL, Ruegg M, Schleuning WD: A DNA motif related to the cAMP-responsive element and an exon-located activator protein-2 binding site in the human tissue-type plasminogen activator gene promoter cooperate in basal expression and convey activation by phorbol ester and cAMP. *J Biol Chem* 265:14618, 1990.
46. Kooistra T, Van den Berg J, Tons A, Platenburg G, Rijken DC, Van den Berg E: Butyrate stimulates tissue type plasminogen activator synthesis in cultured human endothelial cells. *Biochem J* 247:605, 1987.

47. Diamond SL, Eskin SG, McIntire LV: Fluid flow stimulates tissue plasminogen activator secretion by cultured human endothelial cells. *Science* 243:1483, 1989.

48. Hanss M, Collen D: Secretion of tissue-type plasminogen activator and plasminogen activator inhibitor by cultured human endothelial cells: Modulation by thrombin, endotoxin, and histamine. *J Lab Clin Med* 109:97, 1987.

49. Medcalf RL, Van den Berg E, Schleuning WD: Glucocorticoid-modulated gene expression of tissue- and urinary-type plasminogen activator and plasminogen activator inhibitor-1 and -2. *J Cell Biol* 106:971, 1988.

50. Santell L, Levin EG: Cyclic AMP potentiates phorbol ester stimulation of tissue plasminogen activator release and inhibits secretion of plasminogen activator inhibitor-1 from human endothelial cells. *J Biol Chem* 263:16802, 1988.

51. Dichek D, Quertermous T: Thrombin regulation of mRNA levels of tissue plasminogen activator inhibitor-1 in cultured human umbilical vein endothelial cells. *Blood* 74:222, 1989.

52. Kasai S, Arimura H, Nishida M, Suyama T: Primary structure of single-chain pro-urokinase. *J Biol Chem* 260:12382, 1985.

53. Gunzler WA, Steffens GJ, Otting F, Buse G, Flohe L: Structural relationship between high and low molecular mass urokinase. *Physiol Chem* 363:133, 1982.

54. Riccio A, Grimaldi G, Verde P, Sebastio G, Boast S, Blasi F: The human urokinase-plasminogen activator gene and its promoter. *Nucleic Acids Res* 13:2759, 1985.

55. Holmes WE, Pennica D, Blaber M, et al: Cloning and expression of the gene for pro-urokinase in *Escherichia coli*. *Biotechnology* 3:923, 1985.

56. Schmitt M, Wilhelm O, Janicke F, et al: Urokinase-type plasminogen activator (uPA) and its receptor (CD87): A new target in tumor invasion and metastasis. *J Obstet Gynaecol* 21:151, 1995.

57. Van Hinsbergh VWM, Van den Berg EA, Fiers W, Dooijewaard G: Tumor necrosis factor induces the production of urokinase-type plasminogen activator by human endothelial cells. *Blood* 10:1991, 1990.

58. Medina R, Socher SH, Han JH, Friedman PA: Interleukin-1, endotoxin, or tumor necrosis factor/cachectin enhance the level of plasminogen activator inhibitor messenger RNA in bovine aortic endothelial cells. *Thromb Res* 54:41, 1989.

59. Gerwin BI, Keski-Oja J, Seddon M, Lechner JF, Harris CC: TGF beta 1 modulation of urokinase and PAI-1 expression in human bronchial epithelial cells. *Am J Pathol* 259:262, 1990.

60. Stump DC, Lijnen HR, Collen D: Purification and characterization of a novel low molecular weight form of single-chain urokinase-type plasminogen activator. *J Biol Chem* 261:17120, 1986.

61. Steffens GJ, Gunzler WA, Olting F, Frankus E, Flohe L: The complete amino acid sequence of low molecular mass urokinase from human urine. *Physiol Chem* 363:1043, 1982.

62. Lijnen HR, Zamarron C, Blaber M, Winkler M, Collen D: Activation of plasminogen by pro-urokinase. *J Biol Chem* 261:1253, 1986.

63. Gurewich V, Pannell R, Louie S, Kelley P, Suddith RL, Greenlee R: Effective and fibrin-specific clot lysis by a zymogen precursor from urokinase (pro-urokinase): A study in vitro and in two animal species. *J Clin Invest* 73:1731, 1984.

64. Lijnen HR, Van Hoef B, DeCock F, Collen D: The mechanism of plasminogen activation and fibrin dissolution by single chain urokinase-type plasminogen activator in a plasma milieu in vitro. *Blood* 73:1864, 1989.

65. Petersen LC, Lund LR, Nielsen LS, Dano K, Skriver L: One-chain urokinase-type plasminogen activator from human sarcoma cells is a precursor with little or no intrinsic activity. *J Biol Chem* 263:11189, 1988.

66. Colman RW: Activation of plasminogen by human plasma kallikrein. *Biochem Biophys Res Commun* 35:273, 1968.

67. Goldsmith GH, Saito H, Ratnoff OD: The activation of plasminogen by Hageman factor (factor XII) and Hageman factor fragments. *J Clin Invest* 62:54, 1978.

68. Ouimet H, Loscalzo J: Fibrinolysis, in *Thrombosis and Hemorrhage*, edited by J Loscalzo, AI Schafer, p 127. Blackwell Scientific, Boston, 1994.

69. Huisman LG, Van Griensven JM, Kluft C: On the role of C1-inhibitor as inhibitor of tissue-type plasminogen activator in human plasma. *Thromb Haemost* 73:466, 1995.

70. Carmeliet P, Schoonjans L, Kieckens L, et al: Physiological consequences of loss of plasminogen activator gene function in mice. *Nature* 368:419, 1994.

71. Travis J, Salvesan GS: Human plasma proteinase inhibitors. *Annu Rev Biochem* 52:655, 1983.

72. Aoki N: Genetic abnormalities of the fibrinolytic system. *Sem Thromb Haemost* 10:42, 1984.

73. Holmes WE, Nelles L, Lijnen HR: Primary structure of human alpha₂-antiplasmin, a serine protease inhibitor (serpin). *J Biol Chem* 262:1659, 1987.

74. Hirosawa S, Nakamura Y, Miura O, Sumi Y, Aoki N: Organization of the human alpha₂-antiplasmin inhibitor gene. *Proc Natl Acad Sci USA* 85:6836, 1988.

75. Plow EF, Collen D: The presence and release of alpha-2-antiplasmin from human platelets. *Blood* 58:1069, 1981.

76. Aoki N, Moroi M, Tachiya K: Effects of alpha-2-plasmin inhibitor on fibrin clot lysis: Its comparison with alpha-2-macroglobulin. *Thromb Haemost* 39:22, 1978.

77. Scott RW, Bergman BL, Bajpai A, et al: Protease nexin: Properties and a modified purification procedure. *J Biol Chem* 260:7029, 1985.

78. Cunningham DD, Van Nostrand WE, Farrell DH, Campbell CH: Interactions of serine proteases with cultured fibroblasts. *J Cell Biochem* 32:281, 1986.

79. Sprengers ED, Kluft D: Plasminogen activator inhibitors. *Blood* 69:381, 1987.

80. Ny T, Sawdey M, Lawrence D, Millan JL, Loskutoff DJ: Cloning and sequence of a cDNA coding for the human beta-migrating endothelial-cell-type plasminogen activator inhibitor. *Proc Natl Acad Sci USA* 83:6776, 1986.

81. Kruithof EKO: Plasminogen activator inhibitor type 1: Biochemical, biological, and cinical aspects. *Fibrinolysis* 2:59, 1988.

82. Samad F, Yamamoto K, Loskutoff DJ: Distribution and regulation of plasminogen activator inhibitor-1 in murine adipose tissue in vivo. *J Clin Invest* 97:37, 1996.

83. Van Hinsbergh VWM, Kooistra T, Van den Berg EA, et al: Tumor necrosis factor increases the production of plasminogen activator inhibitor in human endothelial cells in vitro and in rats in vivo. *Blood* 72:1467, 1988.

84. Van den Berg EA, Sprengers ED, Jaye M, Burgess W, Maciag T, Van Hinsbergh VW: Regulation of plasminogen activator inhibitor-1 mRNA in human endothelial cells. *Thromb Haemost* 60:63, 1988.

85. Loskutoff DJ, Linders M, Keijer J, Veerman H, Van Heerikhauizen H, Pannekoek H: Structure of the human plasminogen activator inhibitor-1 gene: Non-random distribution of introns. *Biochemistry* 26:3763, 1987.

86. Mottonen J, Strand A, Symersky J, et al: Structural basis of latency in plasminogen activator inhibitor-1. *Nature* 355:270, 1992.

87. Declerck PJ, De Mol M, Alessi MC, et al: Purification and characterization of a plasminogen activator inhibitor-1 binding protein from human plasma: Identification as multimeric form of S protein (vitronectin). *J Biol Chem* 263:15454, 1988.

88. Bosma PJ, Van den Berg EA, Kooistra T, Siemieniak DR, Slightom JL: Human plasminogen activator inhibitor-1 gene: Promoter and structural nucleotide sequences. *J Biol Chem* 263:9129, 1988.

89. Van Zonnefeld AJ, Curriden SA, Loskutoff DJ: Type 1 plasminogen activator inhibitor gene: Functional analysis and glucocorticoid regulation of its promoter. *Proc Natl Acad Sci USA* 85:5525, 1988.

90. Westerhausen DR, Hopkins WE, Billadello JJ: Multiple transforming growth factor beta-inducible elements regulate expression of the plasminogen activator inhibitor type-1 gene in HepG2 cells. *J Biol Chem* 266:1092, 1991.

91. Keeton MR, Curriden SA, Van Zonneveld AJ, Loskutoff DJ: Identification of regulatory sequences in the type 1 plasminogen activator inhibitor gene responsive to transforming growth factor. *J Biol Chem* 266:23048, 1991.

92. Emeis JJ, Kooistra T: Interleukin 1 and lipopolysaccharide induce an inhibitor of tissue-type plasminogen activator in vivo and in cultured endothelial cells. *J Exp Med* 163:1260, 1986.

93. Sawdey M, Podor TJ, Loskutoff DJ: Regulation of type-1 plasminogen activator inhibitor gene expression in cultured bovine aortic endothelial cells. *J Biol Chem* 264:10396, 1989.

94. Schleef RR, Bevilaqua MP, Sawdey M, Gimbrone MA, Loskutoff DJ: Cytokine activation of vascular endothelium: Effects on tissue-type plas-

minogen activator and type 1 plasminogen activator inhibitor. *J Biol Chem* 263:5797, 1988.

95. Craik CS, Rutter WJ, Fletternick R: Splice junctions: Association with variation in protein structure. *Science* 220:1125, 1983.

96. Stiko-Rahm A, Wiman B, Hamsten A, Nilsson J: Secretion of plasminogen activator inhibitor-1 from cultured human umbilical vein endothelial cells is induced by very low density lipoprotein. *Arteriosclerosis* 10:1067, 1990.

97. Etingin OR, Hajjar DP, Hajjar KA, Harpel PC, Nachman RL: Lipoprotein(a) regulates plasminogen activator inhibitor-1 expression in endothelial cells. *J Biol Chem* 266:2459, 1990.

98. Vaughan DE, Shen C, Lazo S: Angiotensin II induces plasminogen activator inhibitor synthesis in vitro. *Circulation* 86:I-557, 1992.

99. Gelehrter TD, Scyncer-Laszuk R: Thrombin induction of plasminogen activator-inhibitor synthesis in vitro. *J Clin Invest* 77:165, 1986.

100. Van Hinsbergh VWM, Sprengers ED, Kooistra T: Effect of thrombin on the production of plasminogen activators and PA inhibitor-1 by human foreskin microvascular endothelial cells. *Thromb Haemost* 57:148, 1987.

101. Scarpati EM, Sadler JE: Regulation of endothelial cell coagulant properties: Modulation of tissue factor, plasminogen activator inhibitors, and thrombomodulin by phorbol 12-myristate 13-acetate and tumor necrosis factor. *J Biol Chem* 264:20705, 1989.

102. Konkle BA, Kollros PR, Kelly MD: Heparin-binding growth factor-1 modulation of plasminogen activator inhibitor-1 expression. *J Biol Chem* 265:21867, 1990.

103. Erickson LA, Fici GJ, Lund JE, Boyle TP, Polites HG, Marotti KR: Development of venous occlusions in transgenic mice for the plasminogen activator inhibitor-1 gene. *Nature* 346:74, 1990.

104. Carmeliet P, Kieckens L, Schoonjans L, et al: Plasminogen activator inhibitor-1 gene-deficient mice: I. Generation by homologous recombination and characterization. *J Clin Invest* 92:2746, 1993.

105. Fay WP, Shapiro AD, Shih JL, Schleef RR, Ginsburg D: Complete deficiency of plasminogen activator inhibitor type 1 due to a frameshift mutation. *N Engl J Med* 327:1729, 1992.

106. Ye RD, Wun T, Sadler JE: cDNA cloning and expression in *Escherichia coli* of a plasminogen activator inhibitor from human placenta. *J Biol Chem* 262:3718, 1987.

107. Ye RD, Aherns SM, Le Beau MM, Lebo RV, Sadler JE: Structure of the gene for human plasminogen activator inhibitor-2: The nearest mammalian homologue of chicken ovalbumin. *J Biol Chem* 264:5495, 1989.

108. Antalis TM, Clok MA, Barnes T, et al: Cloning and expression of a cDNA coding for a human monocyte-derived plasminogen activator inhibitor. *Proc Natl Acad Sci USA* 85:985, 1988.

109. Schleuning WD, Medcalf RL, Hession C, Rothenbuhler R, Shaw A: Plasminogen activator inhibitor 2: Regulation of gene transcription during phorbol ester-mediated differentiation of U-937 human histiocytic lymphoma cells. *Mol Cell Biol* 7:4564, 1987.

110. Chapman HA, Stone OL: A fibrinolytic inhibitor of human alveolar macrophages: Induction with endotoxin. *Am Rev Respir Dis* 132:569, 1985.

111. Miles LA, Dahlberg CM, Plescia J, Felez J, Kato K, Plow EF: Role of cell surface lysines in plasminogen binding to cells: Identification of alpha-enolase as a candidate plasminogen receptor. *Biochemistry* 30:1682, 1991.

112. Miles LA, Ginsberg MA, White JG, Plow EF: Plasminogen interacts with platelets through two distinct mechanisms. *J Clin Invest* 77:2001, 1986.

113. Kanalas JJ, Makker SP: Identification of the rat Heymann nephritis autoantigen (GP330) as a receptor site for plasminogen. *J Biol Chem* 266:10825, 1991.

114. Barnathan ES, Kuo A, Van der Keyl H, McCrae KR, Larsen GR, Cines DB: Tissue-type plasminogen activator binding to human endothelial cells: Evidence for two distinct binding sites. *J Biol Chem* 263:7792, 1988.

115. Hajjar KA: The endothelial cell tissue plasminogen activator receptor: Specific interaction with plasminogen. *J Biol Chem* 266:21962, 1991.

116. Hajjar KA, Hamel NM: Identification and characterization of human endothelial cell membrane binding sites for tissue plasminogen activator and urokinase. *J Biol Chem* 265:2908, 1990.

117. Roldan AL, Cubellis MV, Masucci MT, et al: Cloning and expression of the receptor for human urokinase plasminogen activator, a central

118. molecule in cell surface, plasmin-dependent proteolysis. *EMBO J* 9:467, 1990.

118. Casey JR, Petranka JG, Kottra J, Fleenor DE, Rosse WF: The structure of the urokinase-type plasminogen activator receptor gene. *Blood* 84:1151, 1994.

119. Behrendt N, Ronne E, Ploug M, et al: The human receptor for urokinase plasminogen receptor. *J Biol Chem* 265:6453, 1990.

120. Ploug M, Ronne E, Behrendt N, Jensen AL, Blasi F, Dano K: Cellular receptor for urokinase plasminogen activator: Carboxyl-terminal processing and membrane anchoring by glycosylphosphatidylinositol. *J Biol Chem* 266:1926, 1991.

121. Cubellis MV, Andreasson P, Ragno P, Mayer M, Dano K, Blasi F: Accessibility of receptor-bound urokinase to type-1 plasminogen activator inhibitor. *Proc Natl Acad Sci USA* 86:4828, 1989.

122. Cubellis MV, Wun TC, Blasi F: Receptor-mediated internalization and degradation of urokinase is caused by its specific inhibitor PAI-1. *EMBO J* 9:1079, 1990.

123. Ellis V, Behrendt N, Dano K: Plasminogen activation by receptor-bound urokinase. *J Biol Chem* 266:12752, 1991.

124. Chapman HA: Plasminogen activators, integrins, and the coordinated regulation of cell adhesion and migration. *Curr Opin Cell Biol* 9:714, 1997.

125. Waltz DA, Chapman HA: Reversible cellular adhesion to vitronectin linked to urokinase receptor occupancy. *J Biol Chem* 269:14746, 1994.

126. Wei Y, Waltz DA, Rao N, Drummond RJ, Rosenberg S, Chapman HA: Identification of the urokinase receptor as an adhesion receptor for vitronectin. *J Biol Chem* 269:32380, 1994.

127. Wei Y, Lukashev M, Simon DI, et al: Regulation of integrin function by the urokinase receptor. *Science* 273:1551, 1996.

128. Xue W, Kindzelskii AL, Todd RF, Petty HR: Physical association of complement receptor type 3 and urokinase-type plasminogen activator in neutrophil membranes. *J Immunol* 152:4630, 1994.

129. Stahl A, Mueller BM: The urokinase-type plasminogen activator receptor, a GPI-linked protein, is localized in caveolae. *J Cell Biol* 129:335, 1995.

130. Anderson RG: Caveolae: Where incoming and outgoing messengers meet. *Proc Natl Acad Sci USA* 90:10909, 1993.

131. Okamoto T, Schlegel A, Scherer PE, Lisanti MP: Caveolins, a family of scaffolding proteins for organizing "preassembled signaling complexes" at the plasma membrane. *J Biol Chem* 273:5419, 1998.

132. Chung CY, Erickson HP: Cell surface annexin II is a high affinity receptor for the alternatively spliced segment of tenascin-C. *J Cell Biol* 126:539, 1994.

133. Wright JF, Kurosky A, Wasi S: An endothelial cell-surface form of annexin II binds human cytomegalovirus. *Biochem Biophys Res Commun* 198:983, 1994.

134. Kassam G, Choi KS, Ghuman J, et al: The role of annexin II tetramer in the activation of plasminogen. *J Biol Chem* 273:4790, 1998.

135. Siever DA, Erickson HP: Extracellular annexin II. *Int J Biochem Cell Biol* 29:1219, 1997.

136. Falcone DJ, Borth W, Faisal Khan KM, Layne T, Hajjar KA: Annexin II, a constitutively expressed plasminogen receptor, mediates matrix invasion and degradation by macrophages [abstr]. *FASEB J* 1997.

137. Menell JS, Cesarman GM, Jacovina AT, McLaughlin MA, Lev EA, Hajjar KA: Annexin II and bleeding in acute promyelocytic leukemia. *N Engl J Med* 340:994, 1999.

138. Tressler RJ, Updyke TV, Yeatman TJ, Nicolson GL: Extracellular annexin is associated with divalent cation-dependent tumor cell adhesion of metastatic RAW 117 large-cell lymphoma cells. *J Cell Biochem* 53:265, 1993.

139. Yeatman TJ, Updyke TV, Kaetzel MA, Dedman JR, Nicolson GL: Expression of annexins on the surfaces of non-metastatic human and rodent tumor cells. *Clin Exp Metastasis* 11:37, 1993.

140. Tressler RJ, Nicolson GL: Butanol-extractable and detergent-solubilized cell surface components from murine large cell lymphoma cells associated with adhesion to organ microvessel endothelial cells. *J Cell Biochem* 48:162, 1992.

141. Raynal P, Pollard HB: Annexins: The problem of assessing the biologic role for a gene family of multifunctional calcium- and phospholipid-binding proeins. *Biochim Biophys Acta* 1197:63, 1994.

142. Swairjo MA, Seaton BA: Annexin structure and membrane interactions: A molecular perspective. *Ann Rev Biophys Biomol Struct* 23:193, 1994.

143. Spano F, Raugei G, Palla E, Colella C, Melli M: Characterization of the human lipocortin-2-encoding multigene family: Its structure suggests the existence of a short amino acid unit undergoing duplication. *Gene* 95:243, 1990.

144. Cesarman GM, Guevara CA, Hajjar KA: An endothelial cell receptor for plasminogen/tissue plasminogen activator: II. Annexin II-mediated enhancement of t-PA-dependent plasminogen activation. *J Biol Chem* 269:21198, 1994.

145. Hajjar KA, Guevara CA, Lev E, Dowling K, Chacko J: Interaction of the fibrinolytic receptor, annexin II, with the endothelial cell surface: Essential role of endonexin repeat 2. *J Biol Chem* 271:21652, 1996.

146. Hajjar KA, Gavish D, Breslow J, Nachman RL: Lipoprotein(a) modulation of endothelial cell surface fibrinolysis and its potential role in atherosclerosis. *Nature* 339:303, 1989.

147. Hajjar KA, Mauri L, Jacovina AT, et al: Tissue plasminogen activator binding to the annexin II tail domain: Direct modulation by homocysteine. *J Biol Chem* 273:9987, 1998.

148. Kraus JP: Molecular basis of phenotype expression in homocystinuria. *J Inher Metab Dis* 17:383, 1994.

149. Boushey CJ, Beresford SAA, Omenn GS, Motulsky AG: A quantitative assessment of plasma homocysteine as a risk factor for vascular disease. *JAMA* 274:1049, 1995.

150. Refsum H, Ueland PM, Nygard O, Vollset SE: Homocysteine and cardiovascular disease. *Ann Rev Med* 49:31, 1998.

151. Hajjar KA: Homocysteine-induced modulation of tissue plasminogen activator to its endothelial cell membrane receptor. *J Clin Invest* 91:2873, 1993.

152. Bu G, Warshawsky I, Schwartz AL: Cellular receptors for the plasminogen activators. *Blood* 83:3427, 1994.

153. Beiseigel U, Weber W, Ihrke G, Herz J, Stanley KK: The LDL-receptor-related protein, LRP, is an apolipoprotein E-binding protein. *Nature* 341:162, 1989.

154. Brown MS, Herz J, Kowal RC: The low-density lipoprotein receptor-related protein: Double agent or decoy? *Curr Opin Lipidol* 2:65, 1991.

155. Orth K, Madison EL, Gething MJ, Sambrook JF: Complexes of tissue-type plasminogen activator and its serpin inhibitor plasminogen-activator inhibitor type 1 are internalized by means of the low-density lipoprotein receptor–related protein/alpha-2-macroglobulin receptor. *Proc Natl Acad Sci USA* 89:7422, 1992.

156. Herz J, Goldstein JL, Strickland DK, Ho YK, Brown MS: 39-kDa protein modulates binding of ligands to low-density lipoprotein receptor–related protein/alpha-2-macroglobulin receptor. *J Biol Chem* 266:21232, 1991.

157. Herz J, Clouthier DE, Hammer RE: LDL receptor–related protein internalizes and degrades uPA–PAI-1 complexes and is essential for embryo implantation. *Cell* 71:411, 1992.

158. Herz J, Clouthier DE, Hammer RE: Correction: LDL receptor–related protein internalizes and degrades uPA–PAI-1 complexes and is essential for embryo implantation. *Cell* 73:428, 1993.

159. Bu G, Morton PA, Schwartz AL: Identification and partial characterization by chemical cross-linking of a binding protein for tissue-type plasminogen activator (t-PA) on rat hepatoma cells. *J Biol Chem* 267:15595, 1992.

160. Otter M, Barrett-Bergshoeff MM, Rijken DC: Binding of tissue type plasminogen activator by the mannose receptor. *J Biol Chem* 266:13931, 1991.

161. Hajjar KA, Reynolds CM: α-Fucose-mediated binding and degradation of tissue plasminogen activator by HepG2 cells. *J Clin Invest* 93:703, 1994.

162. Narita M, Bu G, Herz J, Schwartz AL: Two receptor systems are involved in the plasma clearance of tissue-type plasminogen activator (t-PA) in vivo. *J Clin Invest* 96:1164, 1995.

163. Bailey K, Bettelheim FR, Lorand L, Middlebrook WR: Action of thrombin in the clotting of fibrinogen. *Nature* 167:233, 1951.

164. Doolittle RF: The molecular biology of fibrin, in *The Molecular Basis of Blood Diseases*, edited by G Stamatoyannopoulos, AW Nienhuis, PW Majerus, H Varmus, p 701. Saunders, Philadelphia, 1994.

165. Gaffney PJ, Dobos P: A structural aspect of human fibrinogen suggested by its plasmin degradation. *FEBS Lett* 15:13, 1971.

166. Latallo ZS, Flether AP, Alkjaersig N, Sherry S: Inhibition of fibrin polymerization by fibrinogen proteolysis products. *Am J Physiol* 202:681, 1962.

167. Pizzo SV, Schwartz ML, Hill RL, McKee PA: The effect of plasmin on the subunit structure of human fibrin. *J Biol Chem* 248:4574, 1973.

168. Culasso DE, Donati MB, DeGaetano G, Vermylen J, Verstraete M: Inhibition of human platelet aggregation by plasmin digests of human and bovine preparations: Role of contaminating factor VIII–related material. *Blood* 44:169, 1974.

169. Buluk K, Malofiegen M: The pharmacologic properties of fibrinogen degradation products. *Br J Pharmacol* 35:79, 1969.

170. Richardson DL, Pepper DS, Kay AB: Chemotaxis for human monocytes by fibrinogen degradation products. *Br J Haematol* 32:507, 1976.

171. Girmann G, Pees H, Schwarze G, Scheulen PG: Immunosuppression by micromolecular fibrin-fibrinogen degradation products in cancer. *Nature* 259:399, 1976.

172. Wiman B, Collen D: On the kinetics of the reaction between human antiplasmin and plasmin. *Eur J Biochem* 84:573, 1978.

173. Van Zonnefeld AJ, Veerman H, Pannekoek H: On the interaction of the finger and the kringle-2 domain of tissue-type plasminogen activator with fibrin: Iinhibition of kringle-1 binding to fibrin by epsilon-amino-caproic acid. *J Biol Chem* 261:14214, 1986.

174. Camiolo SM, Thorsen S, Astrup T: Fibrinogenolysis and fibrinolysis with tissue plasminogen activator, urokinase, streptokinase-activated human globulin and plasmin. *Proc Soc Exp Biol Med* 138:277, 1971.

175. Lijnen HR, Zamarron C, Blaber M, Winkler ME, Collen D: Activation of plasminogen by prourokinase: I. Mechanism. *J Biol Chem* 261:1253, 1986.

176. Pannell R, Black J, Gurewich V: Complementary modes of action of tissue-type plasminogen activator and pro-urokinase by which their synergistic effect on clot lysis may be explained. *J Clin Invest* 81:853, 1988.

177. Bell W: Fibrinolytic therapy: Indications and management, in *Hematology: Basic Principles and Practice*, edited by R Hoffman, EJ Benz, SJ Shattil, B Furie, HJ Cohen, LE Silberstein, p 1814. Churchill Livingstone, New York.

178. Nesheim M, Wang W, Boffa M, Nagashima M, Morser J: Thrombin, thrombomodulin and TAFI in the molecular link between coagulation and fibrinolysis. *Thromb Haemost* 78:386, 1997.

179. Eaton DL, Malloy BE, Tsai SP, Henzel W, Drayna D: Isolation, molecular cloning, and partial characterization of a novel carboxypeptidase B from plasma. *J Biol Chem* 269:21833, 1991.

180. Wang W, Hendriks DF, Scharpe SS: Carboxypeptidase U, a plasma carboxypeptidase with high affinity for plasminogen. *J Biol Chem* 269:15937, 1994.

181. Bajzar L, Manuel R, Nesheim M: Purification and characterization of TAFI, a thrombin activatable fibrinolysis inhibitor. *J Biol Chem* 270:14477, 1995.

182. Bajzar L, Nesheim ME, Tracy PB: The profibrinolytic effect of activated protein C in clots formed from plasma is TAFI-dependent. *Blood* 88:2093, 1996.

183. Bajzar L, Morser J, Nesheim M: TAFI, or plasma procarboxypeptidase B, couples the coagulation and fibrinolytic cascades thorugh the thrombin-thrombomodulin complex. *J Biol Chem* 271:16603, 1996.

184. Minnema MC, Friederich PW, Levi M, et al: Enhancement of rabbit jugular vein thrombolysis by neutralization of factor XI: In vivo evidence for a role of factor XI as an anti-fibrinolytic factor. *J Clin Invest* 101:10, 1998.

185. Redlitz A, Tan AK, Eaton D, Plow EF: Plasma carboxypeptidases as regulators of the plasminogen system. *J Clin Invest* 96:2534, 1995.

186. Coligan JE, Slayter HS: Structure of thrombospondin. *J Biol Chem* 259:3944, 1984.

187. Ott U, Odermatt E, Engel J, Furthmayr H, Timpl R: Protease resistance and conformation of laminin. *Eur J Biochem* 123:63, 1982.

188. Aplin JD, Hughes RC: Complex carbohydrates of the extracellular matrix structures, interactions, and biologic roles. *Biochim Biophys Acta* 694:375, 1982.

189. Marder VJ, Sherry S: Thrombolytic therapy: Current status. *N Engl J Med* 318:1512, 1988.

190. Unkeless JC, Gordon S, Reich E: Secretion of plasminogen activator by stimulated macrophages. *J Exp Med* 834, 1974.

191. Ossowski L, Reich E: Antibodies to plasminogen activator inhibit human tumor metastasis. *Cell* 35:611, 1983.

192. Strickland SE, Reich E, Sherman MI: Plasminogen activator in early embryogenesis: Enzyme production by trophoblast and parietal endoderm. *Cell* 9:231, 1976.

193. Strickland SE, Beers WH: Studies on the role of plasmingen activator in ovulation. *J Biol Chem* 254:5694, 1976.

194. Moonen G, Grau-Wagemans MP, Selak I: Plasminogen activator-plasmin system and neuronal migration. *Nature* 298:753, 1982.

195. Pittman RN, Ivins JK, Buettner HM: Neuronal plasminogen activators: Cell surface binding sites and involvement in neurite outgrowth. *J Neurosci* 9:4269, 1989.

196. Virji MA, Vassalli JD, Estensen D, Reich E: Plasminogen activator of islets of Langerhans: Modulation by glucose and correlation with insulin production. *Proc Natl Acad Sci USA* 77:875, 1980.

197. Russell J, Schneider AB, Katzhendler J, Kowalski K, Sherwood LM: Modification of human placental lactogen with plasmin. *J Biol Chem* 254:2296, 1979.

198. Nagase H: Activation mechanisms of matrix metalloproteinases. *Biol Chem* 378:151, 1997.

199. Hiraoka N, Allen E, Apel IJ, Gyetko MR, Weiss SJ: Matrix metalloproteinases regulate neovascularization by acting as pericellular fibrinolysins. *Cell* 95:365, 1998.

200. Romer J, Bugge TH, Pyke C, et al: Impaired wound healing in mice with a disrupted plasminogen gene. *Nature Med* 2:287, 1996.

201. Bugge TH, Kombrinck KW, Flick MJ, Daugherty CC, Danton MJS, Degen JL: Loss of fibrinogen rescues mice from the pleiotropic effects of plasminogen deficiency. *Cell* 87:709, 1996.

202. Ploplis VA, French EL, Carmeliet P, Collen D, Plow EF: Plasminogen deficiency differentially affects recruitment of inflammatory cell populations in mice. *Blood* 91:2005, 1998.

203. Carmeliet P, Moons L, Ploplis VA, Plow EF, Collen D: Impaired arterial neointima formation in mice with disruption of the plasminogen gene. *J Clin Invest* 99:200, 1997.

204. Coleman JL, Gebbia JA, Piesman J, Degen JL, Bugge TH, Benach JL: Plasminogen is required for efficient dissemination of *B. burgdorferi* in ticks and for enhancement of spirochetemia in mice. *Cell* 89:1111, 1997.

205. Chen ZL, Strickland SE: Neuronal cell death in the hippocampus is promoted by plasmin-catalyzed degradation of laminin. *Cell* 91:917, 1997.

206. Sporn MB, Roberts AB, Wakefield LM, Assoian RK: Transforming growth factor-beta: Biological function and chemical structure. *Science* 233:532, 1986.

207. Lyons RM, Gentry LE, Purchio AF, Moses HL: Mechanism of activation of latent recombinant transforming growth factor beta1 by plasmin. *J Cell Biol* 110:1361, 1990.

208. O'Reilly MS, Holmgren L, Shing Y, et al: Angiostatin: A novel angiogenesis inhibitor that mediates the suppression of metastases by a Lewis lung carcinoma. *Cell* 79:315, 1995.

209. Lucas R, Holmgren L, Garcia I, et al: Multiple forms of angiostatin induce apoptosis in endothelial cells. *Blood* 92:4730, 1998.

210. O'Reilly MS, Holmgren L, Chen C, Folkman J: Angiostatin induces and sustains dormancy of human primary tumors in mice. *Nature Med* 2:689, 1996.

211. Cao Y, O'Reilly MS, Marshall B, Flynn E, Ji RW, Folkman J: Expression of angiostatin cDNA in a murine fibrosarcoma suppresses primary tumor growth and produces long-term dormancy of metastases. *J Clin Invest* 101:1055, 1998.

212. Moser TL, Pizzo SV, Enghild JJ, Hubchak S, Stack MS: Isolation of an angiostatin receptor from the membranes of human umbilical vein endothelial cells. *Fibrinol Proteol* 11:39, 1997.

213. Cao Y, Chen A, Seong SSA, Ji RW, Davidson D, Llinas M: Kringle 5 of plasminogen is a novel inhibitor of endothelial cell growth. *J Biol Chem* 272:22924, 1997.

214. Griscelli F, Li H, Bennaceur-Griscelli A, et al: Angiostatin gene transfer: Inhibition of tumor growth in vivo by blockage of endothelial cell proliferation associated with a mitosis arrest. *Proc Natl Acad Sci USA* 95:6367, 1998.

215. Dong Z, Kumar R, Yang X, Fidler I: Macrophage-derived metalloelastase is responsible for the generation of angiostatin in Lewis lung carcinoma. *Cell* 88:801, 1997.

216. Stathakis P, Fitzgerald M, Matthias LJ, Chesterman CN, Hogg PJ: Generation of angiostatin by reduction and proteolysis of plasmin: Catalysis by a plasmin reductase secreted by cultured cells. *J Biol Chem* 272:20641, 1997.

217. Patterson BC, Sang QXA: Angiostatin-converting enzyme activities of human matrilysin (MMP-7) and gelatinase B/type IV collagenase (MMP-9). *J Biol Chem* 272:28823, 1997.

218. Gately S, Twardowski P, Stack MS, et al: The mechanism of cancer-mediated conversion of plasminogen to the angiogenesis inhibitor angiostatin. *Proc Natl Acad Sci USA* 94:10868, 1998.

219. Aoki N, Moroi M, Sakata Y, Yoshida N, Matsuda M: Abnormal plasminogen: A hereditary molecular abnormality found in a patient with recurrent thrombosis. *J Clin Invest* 61:1186, 1978.

220. Ichinose A, Espling ES, Takamatsu J, et al: Two types of abnormal genes for plasminogen in families with a predisposition for thrombosis. *Proc Natl Acad Sci USA* 88:115, 1991.

221. Lijnen HR, Collen D: Congenital and acquired deficiencies of components of the fibrinolytic system and their relationship to bleeding or thrombosis. *Fibrinolysis* 3:67, 1989.

222. Robbins KC: Dysplasminogenemia. *Prog Cardiovasc Dis* 34:295, 1992.

223. Azuma H, Mima N, Shirakawa M, et al: Molecular pathogenesis of type I congenital plasminogen deficiency: Expression of recombinant human mutant plasminogens in mammalian cells. *Blood* 89:183, 1997.

224. Demarmels Biasiutti F, Sulzer I, Stucki B, Wuillemin WA, Furlan M, Lammle B: Is plasminogen deficiency a thrombotic risk factor? A study on 23 thrombophilic patients and their family members. *Thromb Haemost* 80:167, 1998.

225. Sartori MT, Patrassi GM, Theodoridis P, Perin A, Pietrogrande F, Girolami A: Heterozygous type I plasminogen deficiency is associated with an increased risk for thrombosis: A statistical analysis of 20 kindreds. *Blood Coagul Fibrinol* 5:889, 1994.

226. Schott D, Dempfle CE, Beck P, et al: Therapy with a purified plasminogen concentrate in an infant with ligneous conjunctivitis and homozygous plasminogen deficiency. *N Engl J Med* 339:1679, 1998.

227. Tsutsumi S, Saito T, Sakata T, Miyata T, Ichinose A: Genetic diagnosis of dysplasminogenemia: Detection of an Ala601-Thr mutation in 118 out of 125 families and identification of a new Asp676-Asn mutation. *Thromb Haemost* 76:135, 1996.

228. Summaria L, Arzadon L, Bernabe P, Robbins KC: Studies on the isolation of the multiple molecular forms of human plasminogen and plasmin by isoelectric focusing methods. *J Biochem Biophys* 247:4691, 1972.

229. Raum D, Marcus D, Alper CA: Genetic polymorphism of human plasminogen. *Am J Hum Genet* 32:681, 1980.

230. Robbins KC: Classification of abnormal plasminogens: Dysplasminogenemias. *Semin Thromb Haemost* 16:217, 1990.

231. Rakoczi I, Chamone D, Collen D, Verstraete M: Prediction of postoperative leg vein thrombosis in gynaecological patients. *Lancet* 1:509, 1978.

232. Juhan-Vague I, Valadier J, Alessi MC, et al: Deficient t-PA release and elevated PA inhibitor levels in patients with spontaneous or recurrent leg thrombosis. *Thromb Haemost* 57:67, 1987.

233. Hamsten A, Wiman B, De Faire U, Blomback M: Increased plasma levels of a rapid inhibitor of tissue plasminogen activator in young survivors of myocardial infarction. *N Engl J Med* 313:1557, 1985.

234. Paramo JA, Alfaro MJ, Rocha E: Postoperative changes in the plasmatic levels of tissue-type plasminogen activator and its fast-acting inhibitor: Relationship to deep vein thrombosis and influence of prophylaxis. *Thromb Haemost* 54:713, 1985.

235. Juhan-Vague I, Roul C, Alessi MC, Ardissone JP, Heim M, Vague P: Increased plasminogen activator inhibitor activity in non-insulin dependent diabetic patients: Relationship with plasma insulin. *Thromb Haemost* 61:370, 1989.

236. Juhan-Vague I, Alessi MC, Joly P, et al: Plasma plasminogen activator inhibitor-1 in angina pectoris: Influence of plasma insulin and acute-phase response. *Arteriosclerosis* 9:362, 1989.

237. Stump DC, Taylor FB, Nesheim ME, Giles AR, Dzik WH, Bovill EG: Pathologic fibrinolysis as a cause of clinical bleeding. *Semin Thromb Hemost* 16:260, 1990.

238. Saito H: Alpha-2-plasmin inhibitor and its deficiency states. *J Lab Clin Med* 112:671, 1988.

239. Suarez CR, Walenga J, Mangogna LC, Fareed J: Neonatal and maternal fibrinolysis: Activation at time of birth. *Am J Hematol* 19:365, 1985.

240. Summaria L: Comparison of human normal, full-term, fetal and adult plasminogen by physical and clinical analyses. *Haemostasis* 19:266, 1989.

241. Edelberg JM, Enghild JJ, Pizzo SV, Gonzales-Gronow M: Neonatal plasminogen displays altered cell surface binding and activation kinetics:

Correlation with increased glycosylation of the protein. *J Clin Invest* 86:107, 1990.

242. Andrew M, Brooker L, Leaker M, Paes B, Weitz J: Fibrin clot lysis by thrombolytic agents is impaired in newborns due to a low plasminogen concentration. *Thromb Haemost* 68:325, 1992.

243. Corrigan JJ, Sleeth JJ, Jeter MA, Lox CD: Newborn's fibrinolytic mechanism: Components and plasmin generation. *Am J Hematol* 32:273, 1989.

244. Corrigan JJ, Jeter MA: Histidine-rich glycoprotein and plasminogen plasma levels in term and preterm newborns. *Am J Dis Child* 144:825, 1990.

245. Corrigan JJ, Jeter MA: Tissue-type plasminogen activator, plasminogen activator inhibitor, and histidine-rich glycoprotein in stressed human newborns. *Pediatrics* 89:43, 1992.

246. Brus F, Van Oeveren W, Okkern A, Oetomo SB: Activation of the plasma clotting, fibrinolytic, and kinin-kallikrein system in preterm infants with severe idiopathic respiratory distress syndrome. *Pediatr Res* 36:647, 1994.

247. Cederholm-Williams SA, Spencer JAD, Wilkerson AR: Plasma levels of selected haemostatic factors in newborn babies. *Thromb Res* 23:555, 1981.

248. Andrew M, Massicotte-Nolan PM, Karpatkin M: Plasma protease inhibitors in premature infants: Influence of gestational age, postnatal age, and health status. *Proc Soc Exp Biol Med* 173:495, 1983.

249. Corrigan JJ: Thrombosis and thromboembolism, in *Hemorrhagic and Thrombotic Disease in Childhood and Adolescence*, edited by JJ Corrigan, p 147. Churchill Livingstone, New York, 1985.

250. Bonnar J, Daly L, Sheppard BL: Changes in the fibrinolytic system during pregnancy. *Semin Thromb Hemost* 16:221, 1990.

251. Hellgren M: Hemostasis during pregnancy and puerperium. *Haemostasis* 26:244, 1996.

252. Schjetlein R, Haugen G, Wisloff F: Markers of intravascular coagulation and fibrinolysis in preeclampsia: Association with intrauterine growth retardation. *Acta Obstet Gynecol Scand* 76:541, 1997.

253. Ploplis VA, Carmeliet P, Vazirzadeh S, et al: Effects of disruption of the plasminogen gene on thrombosis, growth, and health in mice. *Circulation* 92:2585, 1995.

254. Carmeliet P, Stassen JM, Schoonjans L, et al: Plasminogen activator inhibitor-1 gene-deficient mice: II. Effects on hemostasis, thrombosis, and thrombolysis. *J Clin Invest* 92:2756, 1993.

255. Dewerchin M, Van Nuffelen A, Wallays G, et al: Generation and characterization of urokinase receptor-deficient mice. *J Clin Invest* 97:870, 1996.

256. Lawn RM, Wade DP, Hammer RE, Chiesa G, Verstuyft JG, Rubin EM: Atherogenesis in transgenic mice expressing human apolipoprotein(a). *Nature* 360:670, 1992.

257. Grainger DJ, Kemp PR, Liu AC, Lawn RM, Metcalfe JC: Activation of transforming growth factor-beta is inhibited in transgenic apolipoprotein(a) mice. *Nature* 370:460, 1994.

258. Palabrica TM, Liu AC, Aronovitz MJ, Furie B, Lawn RM, Furie BC: Antifibrinolytic activity of apolipoprotein(a) in vivo: Human apolipoprotein(a) transgenic mice are resistant to tissue plasminogen activator-mediated thrombolysis. *Nature Med* 1:256, 1995.

259. Boonmark NW, Lou XJ, Schwartz K, Zhang JL, Rubin EM, Lawn RM: Modification of apolipoprotein(a) lysine binding site reduces atherosclerosis in transgenic mice. *J Clin Invest* 100:558, 1997.

260. Heckel JL, Sandgren EP, Degen JL, Palmiter RD, Brinster RL: Neonatal bleeding in transgenic mice expressing urokinase-type plasminogen activator. *Cell* 62:447, 1990.

261. Meiri N, Masos T, Rosenblum K, Miskin R, Dudai Y: Overexpression of urokinase-type plasminogen activator in transgenic mice is correlated with impaired learning. *Proc Natl Aca Sci USA* 91:3196, 1994.

THROMBOCYTOPENIA

JAMES N. GEORGE

MUJAHID A. RIZVI

This chapter describes the pathogenesis, clinical features, and management of patients with thrombocytopenia, defined as a platelet count less than 150,000/μl (150 × 10⁹/ liter). Since a number of different artifacts can produce pseudothrombocytopenia, the initial step in evaluating patients is to establish that the patient truly has thrombocytopenia. Thereafter, the thrombocytopenia can be categorized according to inheritance and whether there are defects in platelet production, platelet removal from the circulation, and/or platelet sequestration in the spleen. Platelet kinetic studies have provided useful information on determining the mechanism(s) of thrombocytopenia, but they remain research tools. It is important to construct a broad differential diagnosis for thrombocytopenia, since relatively rare, inherited disorders may be mistaken for autoimmune thrombocytopenia and result in inappropriate therapy.

Hereditary thrombocytopenias include a variety of disorders such as Fanconi anemia, thrombocytopenia with absent radii, May-Hegglin anomaly, Alport syndrome, and Wiskott-Aldrich syndrome. Thrombocytopenia can also be due to a variety of viral, bacterial, and parasitic infections; HIV infection commonly results in thrombocytopenia through multiple mechanisms. Nutritional deficiencies and alcohol ingestion can also cause thrombocytopenia.

TTP-HUS causes thrombocytopenia and ischemic vascular damage as a result of microvascular platelet-mediated thrombosis. The precise mechanism remains unknown, but abnormalities in von Willebrand factor proteolytic processing appear to contribute to some forms of the disorder. TTP-HUS has been associated with Shiga-toxin-producing *Escherichia coli* infection, especially in children, as well as other infections (including HIV), drugs, marrow transplantation, cancer, autoimmune disease, and pregnancy. Plasma exchange has dramatically improved the outcome of TTP-HUS and is the mainstay of therapy.

A number of different disorders may result in thrombocytopenia in pregnancy, including gestational thrombocytopenia, preeclampsia, and the HELLP syndrome. ITP is usually an acute, self-limited disorder in children. In adults, it is more often a chronic disorder commonly associated with other autoimmune phenomena. Glucocorticoids, IVIg, anti-Rh(D) globulin, and splenectomy are usually effective in securing hemostatically adequate platelet counts in patients with ITP.

Many different drugs can cause thrombocytopenia, and, even though the mechanisms remain obscure, most patients respond well to discontinuing the drug. Heparin-induced thrombocytopenia, which appears to be due to antibodies directed against the heparin-platelet factor 4 complex in most cases, can be associated with both venous and arterial thrombosis, as well as disseminated intravascular coagulation.

Neonatal alloimmune thrombocytopenia, caused by the transplacental passage of maternal antibodies to fetal platelet protein polymorphisms inherited from the father, can cause profound thrombocytopenia and severe hemorrhage both in utero and in the neonatal period. Posttransfusion purpura, in which the platelet count decreases dramatically 5 to 15 days after a blood transfusion, also involves an immune response to platelet protein polymorphisms, but it is complicated by a poorly understood mechanism that results in clearance of the patient's own platelets.

A systematic evaluation of patients with thrombocytopenia almost always reveals the etiology, thus laying the groundwork for instituting appropriate therapy.

Thrombocytopenia is defined as a platelet count less than 150,000/μl (150 × 10⁹/liter). Multiple mechanisms can cause, or contribute to, the development of thrombocytopenia, including decreased platelet production, increased platelet removal from the circulation, and abnormal sequestration of platelets in the spleen. In many cases of thrombocytopenia, more than one mechanism may be operative. In addition, a number of phenomena can result in a spuriously low platelet count (pseudothrombocytopenia) as measured by automated platelet counters. Disorders causing thrombocytopenia may be due to inherited and/or acquired abnormalities. This chapter first discusses platelet kinetic measurements, the major method for determining the mechanism of thrombocytopenia, and then discusses the disorders that can cause thrombocytopenia based on a combination of whether the disorder is inherited or acquired and the dominant mechanism of thrombocytopenia.

PLATELET KINETICS

There are three fundamental mechanisms of thrombocytopenia: decreased platelet production, increased platelet destruction, and pooling of a larger than normal fraction of platelets within the spleen. Platelet kinetic studies help to define the mechanism responsible for thrombocytopenia.

Studies employing an acidified citrate anticoagulant and ⁵¹Cr-chromate to label platelets yield platelet survival patterns that are nearly linear, indicating that senescence is the major mechanism of platelet removal from the circulation. However, the slight deviation from a linear equation supports the current view that while the majority of platelets survive to senescence, some are randomly removed from the circulation, presumably in the support of vascular endothelium.[1] During the 1970s, ⁵¹Cr was replaced by ¹¹¹In-oxine as the radiolabel of choice for platelet kinetic studies because of the latter's greater labeling efficiency, greater isotope energy, and shorter half-life, and it remains the current standard for measurement of platelet recovery and survival.[2,3] Current methods still require platelet isolation from whole blood, a centrifugation process that usually results in the loss of approximately one-third of the platelets,[4] and the recovered platelets

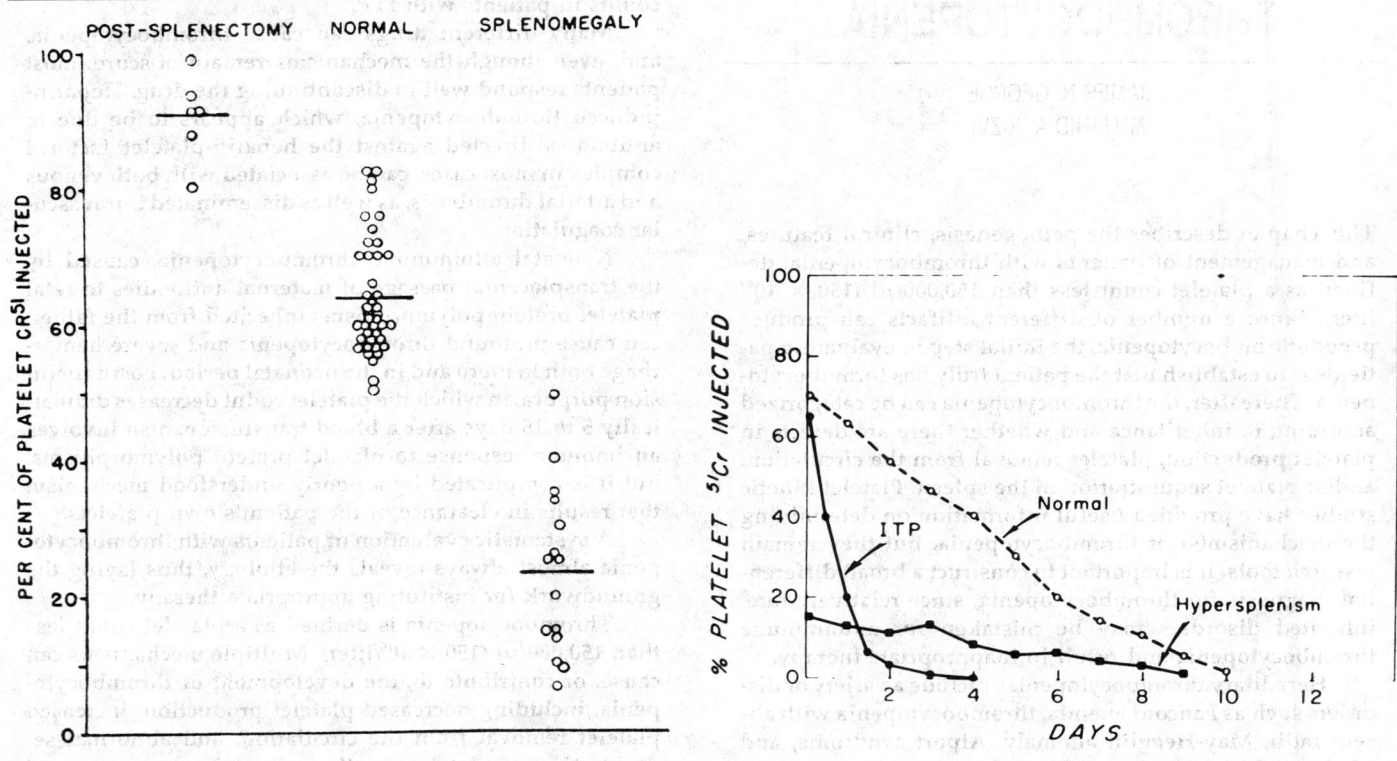

FIGURE 117-1   Platelet recovery and survival in patients with splenomegaly and hypersplenism. *Left:* recovery of ⁵¹Cr-labeled platelets in the circulation 2 h after injection of autologous radiolabeled platelets. Among the 15 patients with splenomegaly, 11 had liver cirrhosis; others had chronic lymphocytic leukemia, infectious mononucleosis, and polycythemia vera. *Right:* survival pattern of autologous ⁵¹Cr-labeled platelets in a normal subject, a patient with ITP, and a patient with hypersplenism due to congestive splenomegaly. (From Aster[5] and Ginsberg AD, Aster RH: *Disease-a-Month,* September, 1970.)

may be activated by the labeling procedure. These variables are difficult to standardize and may profoundly affect platelet recovery and survival. Therefore platelet kinetic measurements remain investigational and are not used for clinical evaluation of thrombocytopenic patients.

PLATELET DISTRIBUTION IN THE BODY

In normal subjects, about one-third of radiolabeled, reinfused platelets are sequestered in the spleen,[5] indicating that at any time about one-third of the total body platelet mass is in the spleen. In contrast, approximately 100 percent of infused platelets remain in the circulation in splenectomized subjects (Fig. 117-1).[5,6] Platelets within the spleen are in equilibrium with the peripheral circulation,[7] as demonstrated by both the transience of the sequestration of radiolabeled platelets upon reinfusion[8] and the shift of platelets from the splenic pool following removal of peripheral blood platelets by apheresis.[5,7,9,10] The normal spleen receives about 5 percent of the total blood flow; some passes directly through capillaries to splenic veins, but most is diverted into the sluggish circulation of the splenic sinusoids in the red pulp before returning to the venous system.[11] Based on the initial time required for equilibration of radiolabeled platelets, the time required for platelets to pass through the normal spleen has been estimated as 10 to 12 min.[8,12,13] This slow transport may simply be a function of the platelets' smaller size, or it may reflect a specific interaction between platelets and the splenic architecture. Epinephrine infusion can increase the platelet count by 30 to 40 percent in normal subjects by α-adrenergic stimulation that diminishes splenic blood flow.[5,11] In contrast, β-adrenergic stimulation by isoprenaline causes a slight decrease in the platelet

count.[14] After splenectomy, a transient thrombocytosis is common, but the steady-state platelet count in splenectomized subjects is not usually dramatically elevated unless anemia persists.[15]

PLATELET SURVIVAL AND SENESCENCE

The most commonly utilized method for analyzing platelet survival curves is the "multiple-hit model,"[1] implying that the platelet is subject to multiple environmental events before it is removed from the circulation. The combined effects of intrinsic senescence and random platelet removal can be appreciated from clinical observations. During the acute thrombocytopenic phase of quinidine-induced thrombocytopenia, platelet disappearance is rapid and not linear, consistent with immune injury and destruction.[16] Immediately after clearance of the quinidine, the newly produced platelets survive for about 7 days and then are cleared in a short period of time (Fig. 117-2).[16] This observation on a cohort of young platelets is consistent with aging as the major factor in platelet disappearance. Platelet survival after normalization of the platelet count demonstrated the typical, nearly linear disappearance pattern. On the other hand, the contribution of random removal of platelets in the process of hemostasis is emphasized in patients who are thrombocytopenic due to marrow failure. Figure 117-3 demonstrates that among patients with aplastic anemia, platelet survival is nearly normal when platelet counts are nearly normal, but that with increasingly severe thrombocytopenia platelet survival is progressively decreased. These data suggest a fixed requirement of approximately 7000 platelets/μl per day (7 × 10⁹/liter per day) for support of vascular integrity and provide an explanation for observations of decreased platelet survival in thrombocytopenic patients whose primary disorder is failure of platelet production.[17,18] As the total number of platelets diminishes with thrombocytopenia of any cause, the number that are removed to maintain vascular integrity represents a greater fraction of the total, resulting in a nonlinear disappearance in labeling studies. In a normal individual with a platelet count of 300,000/μl (300 × 10^9/liter), the fixed consumption of 7000/μl (7 × 10^9/liter) per day of platelets is only a small fraction of the daily turnover ascribable to senescence, approximately 40,000/μl (40 × 10^9/liter) per day. In contrast, when the platelet count drops below about 80,000/μl, the fixed consumption of 7000 platelets per μl actually exceeds the number of platelets that would be removed by a mechanism exclusively based on senescence.

PLATELET HETEROGENEITY

An indirect measure of platelet production, analogous to the reticulocyte count to assess red cell production, is the flow cytometric assay for platelet RNA content.[19,20] This assay assumes that platelets are similar to reticulocytes, in that only the youngest cells still have detectable intracellular RNA. Increased concentrations of α-granule IgG (as well as albumin and other plasma proteins) may also correlate with younger mean platelet age, and this may be an explanation for the consistent observation of high total platelet IgG concentrations in patients with thrombocytopenia due to increased platelet destruction by either immunologic or nonimmunologic mechanisms.[21]

Clinical evidence suggests that young platelets are more hemostatically effective than old platelets. For example, a patient with ITP and severe thrombocytopenia often will not have serious bleeding, suggesting that the young platelets present in these patients are more hemostatically capable than the mixed-aged population found in normal individuals. These clinical observations are supported by experi-

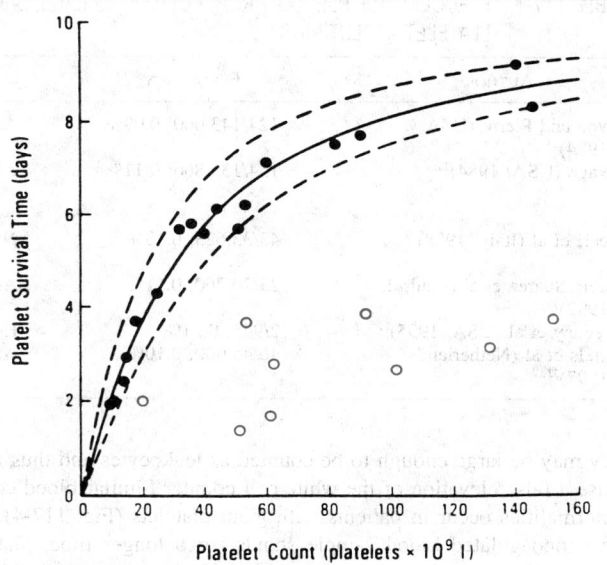

FIGURE 117-3   The relationship between the survival time of ^{111}In-oxine-labeled autologous platelets and the circulating platelet count. The closed circles are data from patients with megakaryocytic hypoplasia; the open circles are data from patients with ITP. Platelet survival strongly correlates with platelet count in patients with megakaryocytic hypoplasia but not in patients with ITP. Analysis of the data is consistent with a fixed requirement of platelets for support of vascular integrity. (Reproduced from Tomer et al.[17])

mental evidence in dogs that aged platelets are less responsive to thrombin than younger platelets.[41]

SPURIOUS THROMBOCYTOPENIA (PSEUDOTHROMBOCYTOPENIA)

The initial observation of thrombocytopenia, based on a platelet count reported by an automated particle counter, must be confirmed by microscopic examination of the blood film. False diagnoses of thrombocytopenia have led to serious problems: postponed surgery, discontinued medications, and even unnecessary glucocorticoid therapy and splenectomy.[22] Pseudothrombocytopenia occurs in both healthy subjects and patients, and it need not be associated with any particular disorder or medication.[23]

The most common artifact causing pseudothrombocytopenia is in vitro clumping of platelets in blood samples collected into EDTA anticoagulant. Alternatively, instead of clumping one to another, platelets may attach to leukocytes (platelet-leukocyte rosettes, platelet satellitism, or platelet-leukocyte adherence phenomenon). Platelet satellitism is not truly distinct from simple platelet agglutination, as some patients incorporate neutrophils within EDTA-dependent platelet clumps, and the adherence to leukocytes usually requires EDTA anticoagulant and low temperatures.[24,25] Typically platelets bind around the periphery of neutrophils (rosette), but they may also form rosettes with monocytes.[26]

Table 117-1 presents data from six surveys that reported a consistent incidence of pseudothrombocytopenia of 0.09 to 0.21 percent.[27-32] Platelet clumping is detected by examination of the blood film made from the EDTA-anticoagulated sample, demonstrating more platelets than expected from the reported count, with many in large clumps (Fig. 117-4). Cell counters merely define platelets as particles between 2 and 20 fl. Platelet clumps often appear in the leukocyte size histogram as particles less than 35 fl, the size of the smallest lymphocytes, but

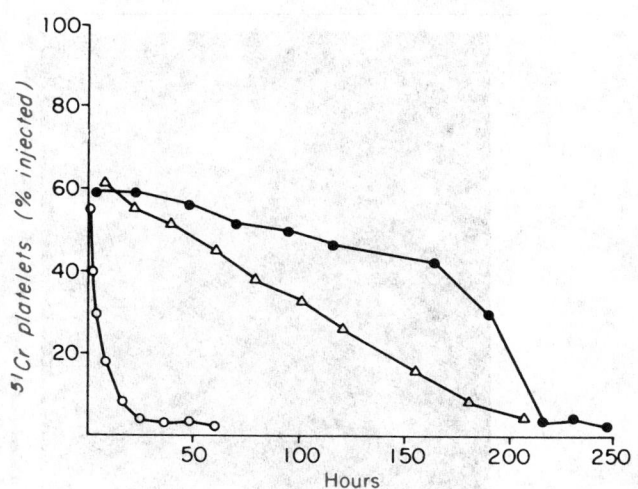

FIGURE 117-2   Platelet survival studies in patients with quinidine-induced thrombocytopenia. A patient with a quinidine-associated antibody was observed for survival of ^{51}Cr-labeled platelets on three separate occasions. The open circles demonstrate the survival of platelets immediately after quinidine administration, with dramatically shortened life span. The closed circles demonstrate the survival after recovery from drug-induced thrombocytopenia, when most of the circulating platelets will have been recently produced, and indicates the survival of a young cohort. The triangles show the platelet survival in the patient after recovery, which is a normal, linear survival curve. (Reprinted from Harker[16] with permission.)

TABLE 117-1   FREQUENCY OF PSEUDOTHROMBOCYTOPENIA CAUSED BY EDTA-DEPENDENT PLATELET AGGLUTININS

AUTHOR	FREQUENCY	COMMENT
Payne and Pierre (USA, 1984)[27]	124/143,000; 0.09%	All platelet counts for 1 year at Mayo Clinic
Savage (USA, 1984)[28]	154/135,806; 0.11%	All 154 abnormal samples were from 93,095 hospitalized patients
Vicari et al (Italy, 1988)[29]	43/33,623; 0.13%	No correlation with presence or absence of disease
Garcia Suarez et al (Madrid, 1992)[30]	23/20,760; 0.11%	Ambulatory outpatients
Sweeney et al (USA, 1995)[31]	2/945; 0.21%	Healthy apheresis donors
Bartels et al (Netherlands, 1997)[32]	46/45,000; 0.10%	Ambulatory outpatients

they may be large enough to be counted as leukocytes and thus may cause a false elevation of the white cell count.[30] Similar blood count abnormalities occur in patients with giant platelets (Fig. 117-4). As the anticoagulated blood sample stands for a longer time, platelet clumping increases; this may make the artifact more recognizable or the leukocyte histogram artifact may disappear as the clumps become too large to be recorded.[28]

Correct platelet counts may be obtained by collecting the blood sample in citrate, a weaker chelator of calcium, but some platelet agglutinins are active in any anticoagulant.[23] Therefore in some patients an accurate count can only be obtained by sampling blood directly into ammonium oxalate diluting fluid and manually counting the platelets by phase microscopy.

Typically the artifact is most prominent in the presence of EDTA, whether the abnormality is platelet clumping or platelet satellitism.[24,25] In most series, some patients also demonstrate some platelet clumping in other anticoagulants, such as citrate, acid-citrate dextrose, oxalate, and heparin.[23,28,30] In most patients, the clumping activity is greater at

temperatures less than 37°C, with maximum activity at 22°C or 4°C.[23,25] Platelet clumping occurs within a few minutes and increases over 60 to 90 min in most patients, but one report described three patients in whom no platelet clumping occurred until after 90 min.[29] Patients whose platelet-clumping activity is more pronounced at lower temperatures are often described as having "platelet cold agglutinins," although temperature dependence is also a property of many agglutinins described only as EDTA-dependent.

Platelet clumping is caused by an immunoglobulin, presumably an antibody recognizing an epitope exposed on platelets by the in vitro conditions in anticoagulated blood. The antibodies are usually IgG, though both IgA and IgM antibodies have been described.[22,23,33] The antibody titers are typically low, but in one patient[12] a monoclonal IgM protein agglutinated platelets at a titer of 1:16,384.[33] Direct interaction with platelet antigen is demonstrated by the activity of F(ab')$_2$ fragments.[22] The platelet epitope appears to be on GPIIb/IIIa in many, if not all, patients, as demonstrated by the absence of clumping with platelets from patients with Glanzmann thrombasthenia[24,34] and by immunochemical techniques.[35] These observations are consistent with the ability of EDTA to remove calcium from the GPIIb/IIIa complex[36] and expose neoepitopes on GPIIb.[37] It is unlikely that the EDTA needs to dissociate the GPIIb/IIIa complex, since the GPIIb/IIIa complex is more stable in EDTA at lower temperatures, whereas clumping is facilitated at low temperatures.[36] In one series of 88 patients with EDTA-dependent pseudothrombocytopenia, 56 also had anticardiolipin antibodies; adsorption of these sera on cardiolipin removed the EDTA-dependent platelet clumping activity, suggesting that there may be additional epitopes on platelets.[38] Antibodies mediating platelet-neutrophil satellitism appear to be able to

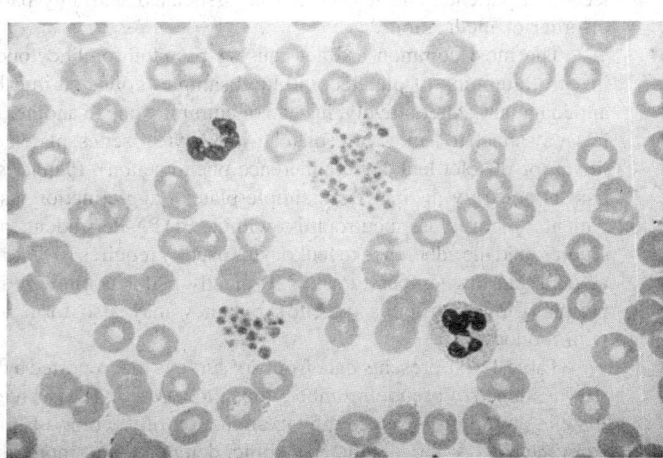
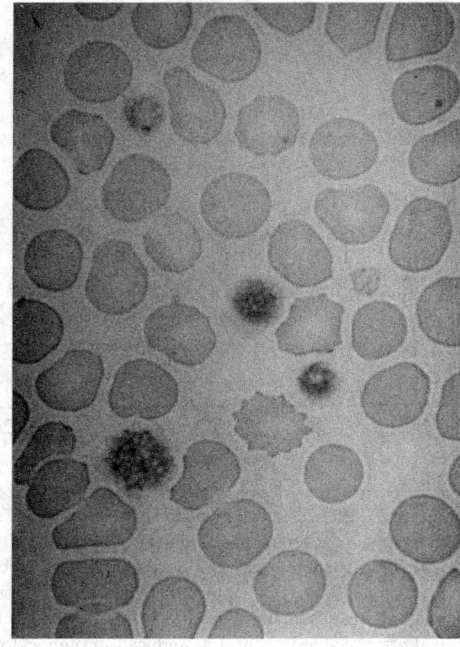

FIGURE 117-4   Blood films of platelet abnormalities associated with pseudothrombocytopenia. *Left:* clumped platelets from EDTA-anticoagulated blood with an EDTA-dependent platelet agglutinin. *Right:* giant platelets from a patient with Bernard-Soulier syndrome. (Reproduced with permission from Hoffbrand AV, Pettit JE: *Sandoz Slide Atlas of Clinical Hematology,* Sandoz Pharmaceutical Corp, 1990.)

react with both an epitope on platelet GPIIb/IIIa and the neutrophil FcγIII receptor, presumably via the Fab and Fc regions of the molecule, respectively.[24]

Platelet agglutinins appear to have no clinical importance; no abnormalities of hemostasis or thrombosis have been reported.[23] There are no complications when platelet agglutinins are discovered during pregnancy.[39] Neonatal pseudothrombocytopenia due to an EDTA-dependent agglutinin was observed in one infant born to a mother with pseudothrombocytopenia, while two other infants born to other women with pseudothrombocytopenia had normal platelet counts in EDTA.[39] Although some reports have suggested that the occurrence of these agglutinins is more frequent in ill, hospitalized patients, or in patients with autoimmune disorders,[27,28,40] others have found no correlation with any illness or even with the presence or absence of illness.[23,29,30] Sex and age incidences probably merely reflect the populations studied. Serial observations have usually demonstrated persistence of the platelet clumping.[23,28,29,40]

THROMBOCYTOPENIA DUE TO SPLENIC POOLING (SEQUESTRATION)

ETIOLOGY AND PATHOGENESIS

Platelet kinetic studies have demonstrated the reversible pooling of a large fraction, up to 90 percent, of the total body platelets within the spleen as contributory to the thrombocytopenia in patients with splenomegaly.[5,8] This process may be described as an exaggeration of the normal splenic pooling of approximately one-third of the platelet mass. Splenic pooling is demonstrated by the disappearance of radiolabeled platelets from the circulation during the first minutes after injection and their accumulation by the spleen.[5] Following equilibration within the splenic circulation, platelet survival is often normal (Fig. 117-1) or may be moderately reduced.[42] Even though the peripheral blood platelet count may be only 20 percent of normal, the total number of platelets in the circulation, counting those pooled in the spleen, is normal (Table 117-2). Platelet production, estimated by dividing the total body platelet mass by the platelet life span, is usually normal.[5] Therefore the thrombocytopenia of hypersplenism can be described as the displacement of a majority of platelets from the peripheral circulation into a slowly exchangeable splenic pool. Splenic pooling must be distinguished from increased removal of platelets in the spleen, as occurs in idiopathic thrombocytopenic purpura. Selective transient sequestration of platelets, in contrast to red cells, may result from a sieving effect that causes platelets, because of

TABLE 117-2   TOTAL BODY PLATELET MASS IN NORMAL SUBJECTS AND PATIENTS WITH THROMBOCYTOPENIA DUE TO SPLENIC POOLING*

DIAGNOSIS[†]	PLATELET MASS[‡] (PLATELETS/kg BODY WEIGHT)
Normal (30)	2.97×10^{10} (1.80–5.20)
Liver cirrhosis with congestive splenomegaly (11)	2.75×10^{10} (2.17–6.12)
Chronic lymphocytic leukemia with splenomegaly (2)	2.89×10^{10} (1.92–3.86)

*Platelet mass is estimated from the peripheral platelet count, fractional recovery of radiolabeled platelets in the circulation, and the blood volume.
[†]The number of subjects studied is given in parentheses. The mean platelet count was about 110,000/μl for the patients with liver cirrhosis and about 40,000/μl for the patients with chronic lymphocytic leukemia.
[‡]Mean values; the range of all values is given in parentheses.
SOURCE: Data are adapted from Aster.[5]

their small size, to take a more tortuous course through the splenic sinusoids, or platelets may transiently and reversibly adhere to splenic macrophages.[8,43]

Evidence supporting splenic pooling as a mechanism of thrombocytopenia is compelling. (1) The fraction of radiolabeled platelets that can be recovered from the circulation after infusion into patients with hypersplenism is very small, from 10 to 30 percent, in contrast to values of 60 to 80 percent in normal subjects and 90 to 100 percent in asplenic patients (Fig. 117-1).[5,4] (2) Intravenous epinephrine causes constriction of the splenic artery, with a fivefold decrease in splenic blood flow and passive emptying of the spleen. This results in an immediate increase in platelet count in patients with hypersplenism that is proportionately greater than the 30 to 40 percent increase seen in normal subjects.[5,11,15] Epinephrine causes a significant but minimal increase in platelet counts in asplenic subjects.[15] The epinephrine effect appears to be mediated by α-adrenergic receptors. Stimulation of β-receptors with isoprenaline infusion causes a slight decrease in the platelet count that is inhibited by β-adrenergic blockade with metoprolol or propranolol; β blockade itself causes a slight increase in the platelet count.[14] (3) Large quantities of platelets, three to seven times the number present in the peripheral circulation, can be flushed from enlarged spleens after surgical removal.[5] Removal of large numbers of platelets from the peripheral circulation by apheresis is rapidly and effectively followed by replenishment from the splenic pool, without resulting in thrombocytopenia.[8,10]

The lack of an increase in platelet production in response to the thrombocytopenia associated with increased splenic pooling indicates that the feedback mechanisms controlling platelet production do not respond to the peripheral platelet count. This is consistent with a mechanism involving clearance of the major growth factor controlling platelet production, thrombopoietin, by platelet binding and internalization, in which case the total platelet mass (which is normal in states associated with splenic pooling) is the controlling factor (see Chap. 110).

Transient thrombocytopenia occurs during hypothermia, at body temperatures below 25°C, in both animals and humans.[45] Thus, there is less severe thrombocytopenia in cardiac surgery patients supported by normothermic systemic perfusion (35° to 37°C) compared to moderately hypothermic systemic perfusion (25° to 29°C).[46] In hypothermic dogs, radiolabeled platelets are sequestered in the spleen, liver, and other organs; the platelets return to the circulation when normal body temperature is restored.[45,47] Pooling of platelets in splenic sinusoids occurs in hibernating, hypothermic ground squirrels.[48] The clinical relevance of these observations is illustrated by reports of patients, often elderly, who are hypothermic after periods of unconsciousness in inadequately heated rooms. In one report, a 69-year-old woman had 13 admissions over an 8-year period with repeated hypothermia, 31° to 34°C, and she was thrombocytopenic (platelet counts of 7000/μl to 39,000/μl) on each admission; with no therapy other than rewarming, platelet counts returned to normal in 4 to 10 days.[49] However, a review of 75 patients admitted with a diagnosis of hypothermia and temperatures of 26° to 35°C demonstrated that only three patients were thrombocytopenic.[49]

CLINICAL FEATURES

Thrombocytopenia associated with hypersplenism is often of no clinical importance; signs and symptoms are related to the primary disorder, and bleeding manifestations are usually primarily the result of coagulation abnormalities caused by the primary liver disease. This is consistent with the relatively moderate degree of thrombocytopenia, the near-normal total body content of platelets (Table 117-2),[5] and the ability to mobilize platelets from the spleen to replenish losses.[10]

The most common disorder causing thrombocytopenia due to splenic pooling is chronic liver disease with portal hypertension and congestive splenomegaly (see Chap. 125). In patients with cirrhosis and portal hypertension, moderate thrombocytopenia is the rule. Any other disease associated with an enlarged, congested spleen can similarly be associated with mild or moderate thrombocytopenia, such as in homozygous sickle cell disease in young children (before splenic atrophy occurs as a result of repeated infarctions); hemoglobin C and SC diseases; thalassemia major; chronic infections; Gaucher disease; myelofibrosis; and lymphoma. The degree of thrombocytopenia is usually correlated with the size of the spleen,[5,50,51] and the spleen is usually palpable. However, in some patients an enlarged spleen may not be palpable, and some experts believe that thrombocytopenia may be attributed to hypersplenism even in the absence of an enlarged spleen. In some of these disorders, relative failure of platelet production may contribute to the thrombocytopenia, either due to marrow involvement or due to severe liver disease with decreased thrombopoietin synthesis.[52]

LABORATORY FEATURES

The platelet count is rarely less than 40,000/μl. In patients with very large spleens and more severe thrombocytopenia, a marrow infiltrative process or severe liver disease may be present, contributing an additional component of decreased platelet production. More severe thrombocytopenia should also trigger a search for additional etiologies, such as sepsis.

TREATMENT AND PROGNOSIS

Since thrombocytopenia due to splenic pooling is rarely of clinical importance, no treatment is indicated. When splenectomy is performed for another purpose, however, the platelet count predictably returns to normal and thrombocytosis may even occur.[5] Platelet counts may also return to normal in patients following surgical correction of portal hypertension by portal-systemic shunting.[53] Platelet transfusions are usually not needed and rarely produce significant increases in the peripheral platelet count since as many as 90 percent of the transfused platelets may be sequestered in the spleen.

THROMBOCYTOPENIA ASSOCIATED WITH MASSIVE TRANSFUSION

In the era before routine platelet transfusion, thrombocytopenia often accompanied severe hemorrhage with transfusion of stored blood.[54] The severity of thrombocytopenia is related to the number of red cell transfusions but is not simply a function of the dilution factor of massive transfusion. Platelet counts may be higher than predicted, possibly by release of platelets from the splenic pool, or they may be less than predicted, because of consumption in microvascular lesions.[55] A deficiency of fibrinogen develops earlier than thrombocytopenia when major loss is replaced by red cell concentrates and plasma substitutes.[56] A study of patients requiring massive transfusion, defined as 10 or more red cell units within 24 h, demonstrated that mild thrombocytopenia (47,000/μl to 100,000/μl) occurred in all after transfusion of 15 red cell units, and more severe thrombocytopenia (25,000/μl to 61,000/μl) developed after 20 red cell units.[56,57] Disseminated intravascular coagulation, triggered by the disease responsible for the blood loss or the hypotension that commonly occurs with massive blood loss, may also contribute to the thrombocytopenia. Management of the thrombocytopenia depends on the clinical condition and the severity of the thrombocytopenia. It does not appear to be desirable to routinely transfuse platelets in a fixed ratio to packed red blood cells.

HEREDITARY AND CONGENITAL THROMBOCYTOPENIAS

Thrombocytopenia at birth or during infancy may be caused by acquired disorders (e.g., congenital syphilis); developmental abnormalities that affect platelet survival (e.g., the Kasabach-Merritt syndrome); or inherited disorders of platelet production, structure, and/or function. Table 117-3 lists the recognized disorders in the latter two categories. Thrombocytopenia may be the only abnormality or it may be associated with other abnormalities. In the Bernard-Soulier syndrome, the thrombocytopenia is associated with a well-characterized abnormality in the membrane glycoprotein Ib/IX complex, resulting in abnormal platelet functions (see Chap. 119). The descriptions of platelet function abnormalities in the other disorders are less well defined and of uncertain clinical importance. In some patients, thrombocytopenia is discovered in infancy; in others it may not be discovered until a later age, even adulthood. In these older patients a mistaken diagnosis of ITP is often made, resulting in inappropriate glucocorticoid treatment and splenectomy. Hereditary thrombocytopenia should be particularly suspected in children with moderate thrombocytopenia in whom the initial impression is chronic refractory ITP.[58] Family studies can be particularly helpful in establishing the diagnosis.

FANCONI ANEMIA

ETIOLOGY AND PATHOGENESIS

Fanconi anemia is an autosomal recessive disorder characterized by severe aplastic anemia in more than 90 percent of homozygotes, usually beginning at age 8 to 9 years.[59,60] Cells from homozygous patients demonstrate increased sensitivity to the induction of chromosomal breakage by DNA cross-linking agents such as diepoxybutane and mitomycin C. Diverse congenital abnormalities may occur, including short stature, skin hyperpigmentation, skeletal anomalies including hypoplasia of the thumb and radius (similar to the thrombocytopenia with absent radius syndrome described below), and anomalies of the genitourinary, cardiac, and central nervous systems.[59] In patients over 16 years of age, the most common anomalies are short stature and skin hyperpigmentation, but these may not be initially recognized in patients presenting with hypoplastic thrombocytopenia or pancytopenia. For example, three siblings with Fanconi anemia diagnosed at ages 22 to 36 years had no physical anomalies.[61] Patients with Fanconi anemia are at increased risk of developing leukemia and other malignancies.[62] The disorder is generally fatal unless corrected by allogeneic marrow transplantation.[63]

THROMBOCYTOPENIA WITH ABSENT RADIUS (TAR) SYNDROME

The syndrome of thrombocytopenia with absent radius (often referred to by its acronym, TAR) is usually noted at birth because of the skeletal anomalies; the thrombocytopenia may not be severe and thus may be overlooked until adulthood.[64]

ETIOLOGY AND PATHOGENESIS

Family members may be affected in a pattern suggesting an autosomal recessive trait, but the lack of consanguinity and occasional reports of affected persons in consecutive generations[65] implies a more complex pattern of inheritance, such as double heterozygosity.[66-68] The syndrome is two to three times as common as Fanconi syndrome,[67] suggesting that the gene frequency may be sufficiently high in the population as to occur often without consanguinity. Thrombopoietin production is normal, and the thrombopoietin receptor is present on platelets, but signal transduction in response to thrombopoietin is defective.[69]

CLINICAL FEATURES

The syndrome is defined by the absence of both radii, but other skeletal anomalies are common: Ulnas are absent or abnormal in most patients, and the humeri, bones of the shoulder girdle, and bones of the feet are abnormal in many patients.[68,70] One-third of patients will have congenital heart anomalies, most commonly tetralogy of Fallot and atrial septal defects.[70] Allergy to cow's milk is common, with resulting gastrointestinal symptoms.[67]

LABORATORY FEATURES

Platelet counts are variable. The most severe thrombocytopenia occurs during infancy, and most babies have purpura at birth.[70] In the initial review describing 40 patients, only 2 were older than age 4 months at diagnosis (these patients were 2 and 21 years old). During the first year of life, platelet counts are typically 15,000 to 30,000/μl, but they may decrease during periods of stress, such as surgery and infection. It is during these periods of more severe thrombocytopenia that leukemoid responses, white cell counts over 35,000/μl, with immature granulocytes, occur in more than half of infants.[67] Eosinophilia is also common, probably related to the milk allergy.[67] Marrow examination demonstrates diminished or absent megakaryocytes, and erythroid hypoplasia may also be present.[70]

TREATMENT, COURSE, AND PROGNOSIS

Treatment with glucocorticoids, splenectomy, or intravenous IgG usually has no effect.[70] Among the 15 deaths reported in the initial review of 40 patients, 10 occurred before age 4 months and 4 others occurred between ages 4 and 14 months; 13 of these deaths were due to hemorrhage, 8 from intracranial hemorrhage. One death occurred later from sepsis in a splenectomized patient.[70] If patients can be sustained during the first year or two of life, the platelet count usually recovers and survival is normal.[67] In a review of 77 patients, only one death related to thrombocytopenia occurred after the age of 14 months.[68] Platelet counts may vary during adulthood, but symptoms other than menorrhagia are unusual.[67,70] Rare patients may present as adults, with significant numbers of marrow megakaryocytes; splenectomy may be effective.[71]

MISCELLANEOUS THROMBOCYTOPENIAS INHERITED AS AUTOSOMAL RECESSIVE TRAITS

The Bernard-Soulier and gray platelet syndromes are primarily characterized by their abnormalities of platelet structure and function and are discussed in Chap. 119 (Fig. 117-4). Many isolated kindreds with hereditary or congenital thrombocytopenia have been reported. In this latter group, marrow megakaryocytes were either reduced[72] or increased,[73] and platelet survival was either decreased[73] or normal.[74] Splenectomy was effective in one family.[73]

MAY-HEGGLIN ANOMALY

ETIOLOGY AND PATHOGENESIS

The May-Hegglin anomaly is defined by autosomal dominant inheritance of giant platelets and characteristic leukocyte inclusion bodies; thrombocytopenia is common but may be absent. Thus, in an early

TABLE 117-3   HEREDITARY AND CONGENITAL THROMBOCYTOPENIAS

SYNDROME	CLINICAL FEATURES
Autosomal recessive traits	
Fanconi syndrome[59,60,62]	Typically fatal aplastic anemia presenting in childhood with other congenital anomalies. May present as isolated hypoplastic thrombocytopenia in adults with short stature and increased skin pigmentation.
Thrombocytopenia with absent radius (TAR)[64,67-70]	Severe amegakaryocytic thrombocytopenia in infancy, spontaneously recovering after age 1. May cause mild, intermittent thrombocytopenia in adults with major skeletal anomalies.
Bernard-Soulier syndrome	Giant platelets and abnormal GPIb, IX, and V complex. Heterozygotes are asymptomatic with normal platelet number and function, but large platelets.
Gray platelet syndrome	Large, pale platelets with diminished endogenous alpha granule proteins.
Isolated thrombocytopenia	May have giant platelets.
Autosomal dominant traits	
May-Hegglin anomaly[75,76]	Asymptomatic; giant platelets, occasional true thrombocytopenia, characteristic leukocyte inclusions.
Alport syndrome variants[81,82]	Giant platelets, often severe thrombocytopenia, associated with hearing loss and interstitial nephritis. Morbidity and mortality due to progressive renal failure.
Isolated thrombocytopenia[58]	Usually mild thrombocytopenia due to ineffective platelet production. May have giant platelets.
X-linked traits	
Wiskott-Aldrich syndrome[91]	Immune deficiency, eczema, and thrombocytopenia with very small platelets. Death due to infection, hemorrhage, or malignancy.
Isolated thrombocytopenia[92]	Adults with moderate thrombocytopenia, possible variants of the Wiskott-Aldrich syndrome.
Kasabach-Merritt syndrome[93,98]	Platelet consumption by localized intravascular coagulation within a congenital vascular tumor.

comprehensive review, only 10 of 25 patients were thrombocytopenic. Since the disorder is commonly asymptomatic, the diagnosis may not be made until adulthood, as in 4 of the 25 patients in the early review.[75] A later report of 15 patients found that thrombocytopenia was rarely severe, most patients had no symptoms and were discovered incidentally, and no patients died as a result of this disorder.[76] In these and other patients with giant platelets, the total platelet mass (estimated by the product of platelet number and platelet volume) is more normal than the platelet count, and total platelet mass may more accurately predict hemostatic competence. Coexpression of May-Hegglin anomaly with hereditary nephritis in one family[77] suggests an overlap with variants of Alport syndrome, described in "Alport Syndrome and Its Variants," below. With the current use of automated cell counters, it is likely that more patients will be discovered, primarily by falsely low platelet counts and abnormal platelet histograms resulting from the presence of giant platelets (Fig. 117-4).

LABORATORY FEATURES

Since automated platelet counters may not identify giant platelets as platelets, patients may have true thrombocytopenia, pseudothrombocytopenia, neither, or both. Platelet ultrastructure is normal. In one analysis of platelet volume, most were between 30 and 80 fl, with about 25 percent even larger than red cells[78]; therefore the mean platelet volume reported by routine clinical laboratory analysis will be inaccurate. Platelet membrane proteins are normal[78]; marrow megakaryocytes are normal in number and appearance[75]; and bleeding times are normal or prolonged.[76] The defining abnormality is the unique inclusion body found in most neutrophils and eosinophils, and some monocytes, which is similar in appearance on routine blood smears to toxic Döhle bodies that occur during acute infections. However, in contrast to Döhle bodies, which contain segments of rough endoplasmic reticulum arranged in parallel stacks, the May-Hegglin inclusions are composed of parallel 7- to 10-nm filaments oriented as spindle-shaped bodies.[76,79]

TREATMENT, COURSE, AND PROGNOSIS

Usually no treatment is needed, and surgery, pregnancies, and deliveries are uncomplicated, though platelet transfusions are commonly given.[75,76] Glucocorticoids, IVIg, and splenectomy have all been tried, usually because of an initial mistaken diagnosis of ITP, without effect.[76]

ALPORT SYNDROME AND ITS VARIANTS

Alport syndrome is the association of hereditary nephritis and deafness.[80] In a number of families, this syndrome has been associated with thrombocytopenia and giant platelets.[81] In one family, nephritis, deafness, and macrothrombocytopenia were accompanied by congenital cataracts (another potential feature of Alport syndrome) and leukocyte inclusions resembling Döhle bodies and the May-Hegglin inclusions.[79]

Severe thrombocytopenia is common. Platelets are large, with mean diameters of 4 to 12 μm and mean volumes of 20 to 27 fl,[79,81,82] but their ultrastructure is normal.[81,82] Marrow megakaryocytes are normal.[81,82] Bleeding times are normal or slightly prolonged; the latter may be caused by uremia rather than thrombocytopenia.[81] Platelet aggregation was abnormal in one report[81] and normal in another.[79]

Treatment with glucocorticoids and splenectomy has no effect on platelet counts. In all patients, the major cause of morbidity and mortality is progressive renal failure.[81,82]

MISCELLANEOUS THROMBOCYTOPENIAS INHERITED AS AUTOSOMAL DOMINANT TRAITS

Many families have been reported with the autosomal dominant inheritance of isolated thrombocytopenia, some with as many as 22 affected family members spanning five generations[83] and 18 family members spanning six generations.[84] The clinical data are heterogeneous, but most patients have only moderate thrombocytopenia with minimal symptoms, normal platelet morphology, and normal bone marrow megakaryocytes.[83,85,86] In some families large platelets have been observed,[86,87] and some patients have abnormal platelet function studies.[83,87] One report described a family with Wiskott-Aldrich syndrome inherited in an autosomal dominant manner.[88] In most patients platelet function is normal,[83] platelet survival is normal, and the thrombocytopenia is caused by ineffective platelet production.[83,87,89] Most patients are discovered as adults and have minimal or no bleeding symptoms, though some have severe hemorrhagic episodes.[84] A benign syndrome of uncertain inheritance with mild thrombocytopenia, large platelets, and no clinical symptoms has been described in persons of Mediterranean ethnic origin.[90]

Patients with inherited thrombocytopenia may not be rare. One report describes 83 patients who were typically referred with the diagnosis of refractory ITP, but in whom family studies demonstrated autosomal dominant thrombocytopenia.[58] All patients had large platelets, normal marrow megakaryocytes, and normal platelet survival; none had Döhle bodies. Sixty-three of the 83 patients were initially discovered to be thrombocytopenic when they were over 15 years old. Bleeding symptoms were minimal, platelet counts were greater than 50,000/μl in 59 patients, and treatment with glucocorticoids (28 patients), splenectomy (10 patients), and other modalities for the presumed diagnosis of ITP had no effect.

WISKOTT-ALDRICH SYNDROME

Wiskott-Aldrich syndrome is an X-linked immunodeficiency syndrome originally described with thrombocytopenia, eczema, and im-

munodeficiency.[91] However, only a minority of identified cases have the classic clinical triad of thrombocytopenia with small platelets, recurrent otitis media, and eczema. Since the platelets of patients with Wiskott-Aldrich syndrome have qualitative abnormalities, this entity is discussed in Chap. 119.

MISCELLANEOUS THROMBOCYTOPENIAS INHERITED AS X-LINKED TRAITS

Other families with X chromosome–linked thrombocytopenia have been reported, but all may be variants of the Wiskott-Aldrich syndrome.[92] In most patients, the thrombocytopenia is mild and has been discovered incidentally during family studies.

KASABACH-MERRITT SYNDROME

Thrombocytopenia associated with giant cavernous angiomas is most often described in infants with congenital lesions,[93,94] but thrombocytopenia may first become apparent in adults.[95–97]

ETIOLOGY AND PATHOGENESIS

The principal lesion in Kasabach-Merritt syndrome is not a true capillary hemangioma, which typically regresses during childhood, but rather a distinctive vascular tumor, described as a tufted angioma or kaposiform hemangioendothelioma with lymphaticlike vessels.[98] This distinction is important because the lesion can infiltrate aggressively and require intensive therapy.[98] Hypofibrinogenemia is common in association with thrombocytopenia, consistent with the etiology of platelet consumption within the tumor being due to intravascular coagulation.[96–98]

CLINICAL AND LABORATORY FEATURES

The hemangiomas are usually present at birth, and neonatal thrombocytopenia may be present.[98] The angiomas may be initially small and inapparent, but many grow suddenly and become painful.[98] Angiomas are usually solitary and superficial but may involve any internal organ site. Cardiac failure may occur as a result of high-volume arteriovenous shunting through the hemangioma; a bruit over the lesion may support this diagnosis.

Thrombocytopenia may be severe, red cell fragmentation may be marked,[97] and laboratory parameters typical of disseminated intravascular coagulation are usually present[93,95–97] (see Chap. 126).

TREATMENT, COURSE, AND PROGNOSIS

Treatment is often necessary because of severe bleeding or growth of the tumor.[98] Surgical resection can eliminate accessible lesions, but many angiomas are unresectable.[93,95–97] Radiation therapy may be effective.[94] Correction of the hemostatic abnormalities has been achieved by thrombosis of the lesion using aminocaproic acid and intraarterial embolization,[95–97] but these may also be ineffective.[98] Ticlopidine plus aspirin[98] and high doses of glucocorticoid[93] have been effective in correcting thrombocytopenia in isolated cases.

ACQUIRED THROMBOCYTOPENIAS DUE TO DECREASED PLATELET PRODUCTION

MEGAKARYOCYTIC APLASIA

Thrombocytopenia due to pure aplasia or hypoplasia of megakaryocytes is a rare disorder. Patients with amegakaryocytic thrombocytopenia associated with subtle abnormalities of other lineages, such as macrocytosis or dyserythropoiesis, are less rare, and these abnormalities are more likely to be a prodrome for myelodysplasia or aplastic anemia.[99–101] In patients with acquired pure megakaryocytic aplasia, the etiology appears to be autoimmune suppression of megakaryocyte development. The mechanism of thrombocytopenia is probably analogous to that in acquired pure red cell aplasia and in some patients with aplastic anemia,[102] namely, the development of autoantibodies to thrombopoietin[103] or to megakaryocytes.[104] Patients in whom an autoimmune mechanism is operative may respond to treatment with cyclosporine and antithymocyte globulin, achieving durable remissions.[105]

INFECTION

Possibly the most common cause of thrombocytopenia is infection. Thrombocytopenia occurs during the course of many diverse viral infections, such as cytomegalovirus,[106] Epstein-Barr virus,[107] and hantavirus[108]; it also occurs predictably in children receiving the measles virus vaccine (Fig. 117-5).[109] Thrombocytopenia also occurs with many other infectious diseases, such as mycoplasma,[110] mycobacteria,[111] Ehrlichiosis,[112] and malaria.[113] In most cases the etiology appears to be decreased platelet production,[109,114] although immune-mediated platelet destruction has been postulated in some patients.[115] Thrombocytopenia is common in critically ill patients with sepsis, in whom the dominant cause is platelet phagocytosis mediated by increased M-CSF.[116–118]

THROMBOCYTOPENIA ASSOCIATED WITH HIV INFECTION

Thrombocytopenia is common in patients with HIV infection. Among 738 HIV-positive patients with hemophilia, the cumulative frequency of thrombocytopenia at 6 years after seroconversion was 16 percent for children and 18 percent for adults; at 10 years the frequency increased to 27 percent in children and 43 percent in adults.[117] In another study the frequency of thrombocytopenia was 16 percent among 103 homosexual men and 37 percent among 182 intravenous drug users with a new diagnosis of HIV infection.[120] Thrombocytopenia was also common among the HIV-negative homosexual men (3%) and intravenous drug users (9%) in this last study, possibly related to the common occurrence of hepatitis.[120] HIV-infected, thrombocytopenic patients (except those with hemophilia) rarely have clinically important bleeding; platelet counts are rarely less than 50,000/μl; the mild thrombocytopenia often spontaneously resolves; and the presence of thrombocytopenia does not increase the risk of progression of AIDS.[119,121,122] Although many HIV-infected patients do not have symptoms related to their immunodeficiency when the thrombocytopenia is discovered, the occurrence of thrombocytopenia correlates with plasma viral load and CD4 cell depletion.[122,123]

ETIOLOGY AND PATHOGENESIS

The principal cause of thrombocytopenia is ineffective platelet production caused by HIV infection of the auxiliary cells of the marrow that facilitate hematopoiesis, such as macrophages and microvascular endothelial cells, resulting in diminished hematopoietic support by the marrow stroma. Direct HIV infection of hematopoietic progenitor cells is probably not responsible for the thrombocytopenia.[124–126] In addition to decreased platelet production, platelet survival is decreased, but the decease is less than in patients with chronic ITP (Table 117-4).[125,127,128] Patients with HIV-associated thrombocytopenia also have lower-than-normal initial intravascular recoveries of injected radiolabeled autologous platelets but no increased spleen or liver sequestration. This contrasts with the results in ITP patients who have normal initial platelet recoveries but subsequently demonstrate increased splenic sequestration.[125,127] The increased platelet destruction may be a result of immune platelet injury. Patients may have true autoantibodies to the specific platelet membrane glycoprotein complexes Ib/IX and IIb/

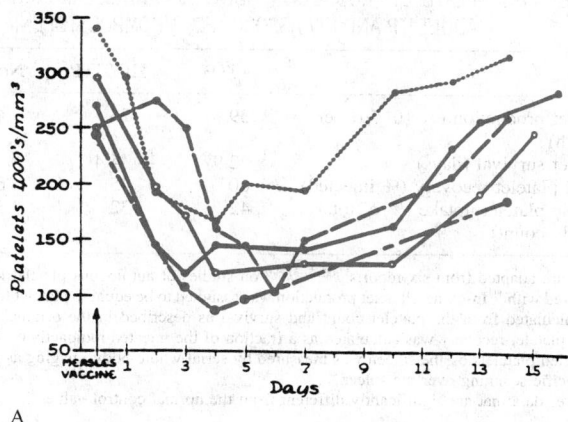

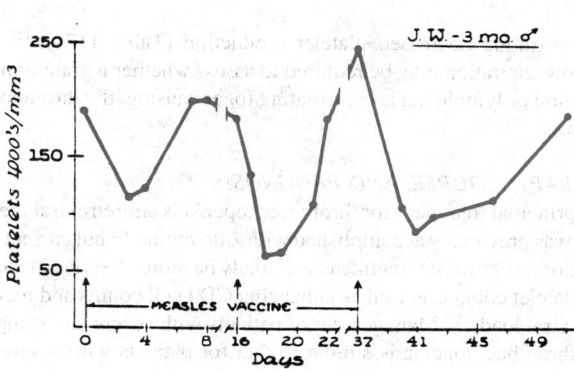

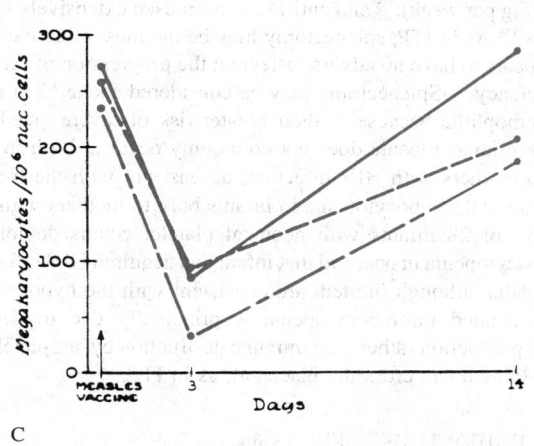

FIGURE 117-5 Thrombocytopenia caused by live measles vaccine: (*A*) Course of platelet counts in five infants after immunization. (*B*) Repeated decreases in platelet counts after three immunizations in one infant. (*C*) Changes in marrow megakaryocyte number in three infants after immunization. (Reproduced from Oski and Naiman.[109])

IIIa, but some anti-HIV antibodies appear to cross-react nonspecifically with unidentified sites on normal platelets.[125,129,130] HIV-infected patients also may have circulating immune complexes that contain antiplatelet GPIIIa antibodies.[131]

CLINICAL AND LABORATORY FEATURES

The thrombocytopenia is typically mild and is often discovered as a result of routine blood testing.[121,132] The marrow demonstrates normal or increased numbers of megakaryocytes in spite of the kinetic studies

TABLE 117-4 PLATELET PRODUCTION, SURVIVAL, AND CLEARANCE IN ADULT ITP AND HIV-ASSOCIATED THROMBOCYTOPENIA*

	ITP	HIV-ITP	NORMAL
Platelet production ($\times 10^{-3}/\mu l$ per 24 h)	39	23[†]	45
Platelet survival (days)	2.9[†]	4.4[†]	8.0
Initial platelet recovery (% injected)	60	45[†]	63
Splenic platelet uptake (% of total body count)	42[†]	32	34

*Data are adapted from six reports[17,127,357–359,407] on studies of autologous platelet kinetics measured with ^{111}In-oxine. Platelet production was assumed to be equal to platelet turnover and calculated from the platelet count and survival as described in the original report. Initial platelet recovery was calculated as a fraction of the injected radioactivity. Uptake of labeled platelets by the spleen was measured by serial whole-body imaging as well as by specific scanning over the spleen.
[†]Denotes data that are significantly different from the normal control values.

demonstrating decreased platelet production (Table 117-4).[125] Bone marrow aspiration may be required to assess whether a granulomatous infection or lymphoma is contributing to, or causing, the thrombocytopenia.

THERAPY, COURSE, AND PROGNOSIS

The principal treatment for thrombocytopenia is antiretroviral therapy. This was previously accomplished with zidovudine,[122] but current combination antiretroviral regimens will likely be more effective in increasing platelet counts, as well as enhancing CD4 cell counts and reducing HIV viral loads.[133] Management of patients with severe and symptomatic thrombocytopenia is similar to that for patients with severe ITP: Prednisone (1 mg/kg per day) is effective[122]; short courses of dexamethasone are also effective.[134] IVIg may be effective in low weekly doses (0.04 g/kg per week),[135] and anti-D has been used extensively for these patients.[136] As in ITP, splenectomy may be the most effective therapy and appears to have no adverse effect on the progression of the immunodeficiency.[137] Splenectomy may be considered sooner[119] in patients with hemophilia because of their greater risk of severe bleeding. Of note, thrombocytopenia does not commonly occur at birth in infants born to mothers with HIV infection, at least not with the frequency reported for thrombocytopenia in infants born to mothers with ITP.[138] A report of 28 infants with neonatal platelet counts demonstrated thrombocytopenia in one, and that infant had acquired HIV infection.[139] These data, although limited, are consistent with the hypothesis that HIV-associated thrombocytopenia is principally due to decreased platelet production rather than immune destruction by antiplatelet antibodies (which can cross the placenta), as in ITP.

NUTRITIONAL DEFICIENCIES AND ALCOHOL-INDUCED THROMBOCYTOPENIA

Mild thrombocytopenia occurs in about 20 percent of patients with megaloblastic anemia due to vitamin B_{12} deficiency[140]; the frequency may be higher in patients with folic acid deficiency because of the common accompanying alcoholism. Occasionally thrombocytopenia can be severe in the megaloblastic anemias, and when this coincides with fever and splenomegaly,[141] the presenting features may suggest acute leukemia. The primary mechanism for thrombocytopenia is ineffective platelet production[142]; bone marrow megakaryocytes are normal or increased in number. Abnormalities of megakaryocyte morphology are much less distinctive than the characteristic erythroid and myeloid defects, but larger size and dispersed nuclear segments, rather than polyploid single nuclei, may be seen.[143]

Thrombocytopenia in alcoholic patients is almost always due to liver cirrhosis with congestive splenomegaly or to folic acid deficiency,

but in some patients acute thrombocytopenia may occur in the absence of nutritional deficiency or splenomegaly, apparently as a result of direct marrow suppression of platelet production.[144] Ingestion of large amounts of alcohol for 5 to 10 days is required to produce sustained thrombocytopenia, which is associated with decreased numbers of marrow megakaryocytes; following withdrawal of alcohol, platelet counts return to normal in 5 to 21 days and transient thrombocytosis often occurs.[144]

Iron deficiency typically causes thrombocytosis, but it has also been reported to cause severe thrombocytopenia.[145]

ACQUIRED THROMBOCYTOPENIA DUE PRIMARILY TO SHORTENED PLATELET SURVIVAL

THROMBOTIC THROMBOCYTOPENIC PURPURA-HEMOLYTIC UREMIC SYNDROMES

IDIOPATHIC THROMBOTIC THROMBOCYTOPENIC PURPURA-HEMOLYTIC UREMIC SYNDROME

TTP[146,147] and HUS[148,149] were described initially as distinct disorders. Although some reports continue to distinguish them, they will be discussed here as a single clinical syndrome. Many diverse clinical features may be present in patients with TTP-HUS, but the minimum criteria are thrombocytopenia and microangiopathic hemolytic anemia without another clinically apparent cause.[150,151] Thrombi consisting primarily of platelets (hyaline thrombi) in terminal arterioles and capillaries[152] are consistently present, but these pathologic features are not specific for TTP-HUS, being also present in patients with malignant hypertension and nephrosclerosis, scleroderma, acute renal allograft rejection, and preeclampsia.[152] Since some clinical features of these other conditions may be similar to TTP-HUS, the distinction may be difficult.

Furthermore, the types of patients currently diagnosed as having TTP-HUS may differ from the patients who made up earlier reports, as the definition of TTP-HUS has changed since the original descriptions[146,148] and the classic review in 1966[153] which defined the pentad of clinical features: (1) microangiopathic hemolytic anemia, (2) thrombocytopenia, (3) neurologic symptoms and signs, (4) renal function abnormalities, and (5) fever. In that review,[153] the diagnosis of TTP was supported by pathologic demonstration of hyaline thrombi in 93 percent of patients and 90 percent of the patients died. In the past 20 years, the availability of curative plasma exchange treatment has created an urgency for the diagnosis, which in turn has resulted in less stringent diagnostic criteria, leading inevitably to a broader spectrum of disorders diagnosed as TTP-HUS. The availability of effective treatment has also revealed new features of the long-term clinical course.

A current classification of presenting clinical features and disease associations is presented in Table 117-5. Epidemic HUS in young children appears to be distinct from the adult syndromes, but this disorder also is different from the original description of HUS in 1955.[148] Descriptions of the childhood syndrome most commonly encountered today only began in 1982 with the appearance of Shiga-toxin-producing E. coli (typically E. coli 0157:H7).[154–157] Though children infected with this organism who have HUS all have, by definition, microangiopathic hemolytic anemia and thrombocytopenia, their predominant clinical problems are acute renal failure following hemorrhagic colitis. Most recover with only supportive care. In contrast, most adults are treated with plasma exchange upon diagnosis, regardless of presenting features or possible etiology, because of a presumption of a very high mortality based on extrapolations from the era prior to plasma exchange treatment.[153]

TABLE 117-5 THROMBOTIC THROMBOCYTOPENIC PURPURA-HEMOLYTIC UREMIC SYNDROME (TTP-HUS): A CLASSIFICATION OF CLINICAL PRESENTATIONS AND DISEASE ASSOCIATIONS

Childhood epidemic HUS
  Association with hemorrhagic colitis (typically *E. coli* 0157:H7 infection)
Adult syndromes
  Idiopathic
  Associations with other conditions:
    Hemorrhagic colitis and other infections
    Drug-induced TTP-HUS
      Quinine, ticlopidine, mitomycin C, cyclosporine
    Allogeneic bone marrow transplantation
    Metastatic carcinoma
    Pregnancy
    Autoimmune diseases (systemic lupus erythematosus,
      antiphospholipid syndrome, scleroderma)

This presentation will initially focus on the classic idiopathic adult syndrome. Specific characteristics of TTP-HUS syndromes associated with other conditions and apparent etiologies will be discussed in separate sections below.

Etiology and Pathogenesis The common pathologic features of all TTP-HUS syndromes suggest a common underlying mechanism of disease. This postulate is consistent with the hypothesis that vWf abnormalities are central to the formation of the platelet thrombi[158]; vWf is a multimeric glycoprotein synthesized in endothelial cells and megakaryocytes.[159] Endothelial vWf is secreted both into the plasma and abluminally, and the latter becomes a component of the subendothelial matrix along with other proteins such as collagen and fibronectin. Subendothelial vWf is important for platelet adhesion at sites of endothelial injury mediated by the platelet GPIb/IX receptor, and vWf secreted into the plasma is processed into smaller multimers that do not interact with unstimulated circulating platelets. The platelet cofactor activity of vWf correlates with multimer size, with larger multimers more effective in supporting platelet-platelet interactions. In 1982 Moake and colleagues observed unusually large vWf multimers in the plasma of patients with chronic relapsing TTP[160] which were comparable in size to the unprocessed vWf found in endothelial cells and platelets. These unusually large vWf multimers could directly agglutinate platelets, especially when the mixtures were subjected to high shear stress, which can unfold vWf.[161] Regions of high shear stress may well occur in the vasculature of patients with TTP-HUS due to partial arteriolar obstruction and could augment platelet reactivity with vWF.[162] Additional evidence for a role for vWf is that increased amounts of vWf are found on circulating platelets, as well as circulating aggregated platelets, in patients with TTP-HUS,[163] and immunohistochemical studies of platelet thrombi in TTP-HUS demonstrate that they are enriched in vWf and contain less fibrin, distinct from the fibrin-rich thrombi of disseminated intravascular coagulation.[158] These observations provide an explanation for the disseminated platelet agglutination, which appears to be the primary pathogenetic mechanism of TTP-HUS. Red cell fragmentation, the other cardinal clinical manifestation of TTP-HUS, is then due to passage of erythrocytes through partially obstructed blood vessels in the microcirculation under conditions of high shear stress.

Enzymatic processing of plasma vWf following endothelial synthesis and secretion may be the result of both reduction of the disulfide bonds that link the vWf monomers and specific proteolysis of vWf monomers themselves by a metalloprotease present in normal plasma.[164] Proteolysis of vWf is enhanced by shear stress; therefore the same forces that can modify plasma vWf structure and induce platelet reactivity also make the vWf molecule vulnerable to proteolysis.[164]

The importance of these observations for the etiology of TTP-HUS has been supported by the demonstration of deficient activity of the vWf-cleaving protease activity in patients with TTP-HUS. The deficiency may be inherited, as appears to be common in patients with familial or chronic, relapsing TTP-HUS,[165,166] or may be caused by autoantibody inhibition of protease activity in patients with acquired, sporadic TTP-HUS.[164,166,167] Although these reports distinguish TTP from HUS, the clinical and laboratory data presented were indistinguishable. Therefore the conclusion that the vWf-cleaving protease activity is deficient in patients diagnosed with TTP but not deficient in patients diagnosed with HUS remains unclear. Two separate reports on a total of 67 patients documented deficient vWf-cleaving protease activity.[164,166] In most patients with nonfamilial TTP, a serum inhibitor of the vWf-cleaving protease (presumably an autoantiantibody) was demonstrated[164,166]; no patients with familial TTP had a demonstrable inhibitor.[166] vWf-cleaving protease activity returned to normal in these patients when they were in clinical remission.[164,166] Plasma vWf-cleaving protease activity was normal in patients with a variety of other hematologic disorders.[164]

The deficiency of vWf-cleaving protease is assumed to result in the accumulation of the unusually large vWf multimers, which then cause platelet agglutination and microvascular thrombi.[159,161] However, in another study of 30 patients (in whom TTP and HUS were considered as a single syndrome), unusually large vWf multimers were demonstrated in 8 of 10 patients with recurrent idiopathic TTP-HUS (both during the acute episode and during remission) but in none of 15 patients with familial TTP-HUS and none of 5 patients with acute, single episodes of TTP-HUS.[168] In sharp contrast to the other studies, in this study, all patients demonstrated enhanced proteolysis of vWf, with accumulation of abnormal low-molecular-weight forms that persisted throughout remission in patients with familial TTP-HUS but corrected to normal during remission in patients with non-familial TTP-HUS.[168] These observations suggest that multiple abnormalities of vWf may occur in patients with TTP-HUS.

Other abnormal protease activities have been demonstrated in these patients. Cysteine protease activity, not normally present in plasma, has been demonstrated in sera from TTP patients and can cause platelet aggregation and secretion.[169,170] Plasma from TTP patients can also cause neutrophil-platelet aggregates,[171] and activated neutrophils may be a source of increased plasma protease activity. It has been postulated that one mechanism by which the Shiga toxin of *E. coli* 0157:H7 can cause diffuse endothelial damage and result in HUS is by mediating neutrophil adhesion to endothelial cells with resulting neutrophil activation and secretion.[172]

Endothelial cell damage appears to be a central phenomenon in the pathogenesis of TTP-HUS. Direct evidence for this is the demonstration that plasma from patients with both TTP and sporadic HUS (distinguished from childhood epidemic diarrhea-associated HUS) can cause apoptosis of microvascular endothelial cells.[173] Apoptosis occurred in endothelial cell cultures from organs typically affected by TTP-HUS (kidney, brain) but not in endothelial cells from organs not commonly affected (lung, liver).[173] Apoptosis was also demonstrated in microvascular endothelial cells from spleens removed from TTP patients but not from spleens removed from patients with ITP or trauma.[174] Complement regulation abnormalities have also been observed in patients with TTP and HUS, which may cause increased susceptibility for the development of postinfectious HUS or may enhance endothelial injury after initiation of a microangiopathic process.[175] TTP-HUS has also occurred with bee sting[176] and after cardiovascular surgery,[177,178] conditions that may also affect complement.

Thus, TTP-HUS remains a clinical syndrome that can be triggered by multiple distinct events and may be associated with multiple other disorders. The presence of the characteristic pathologic lesions of

TABLE 117-6   EVOLUTION OF DIAGNOSTIC CRITERIA FOR TTP-HUS

	PERCENT OF PATIENTS		
CLINICAL SIGN	1925–1964*	1964–1980†	1982–1989‡
Microangiopathic hemolytic anemia	96	98	100
Thrombocytopenia	96	96	100
Neurologic symptoms	92	84	63
Renal disease	88	76	59
Fever	98	59	24

*Data from Amorosi and Ultmann[153] on 271 patients. Platelet counts were often not done, and thrombocytopenia was inferred from symptoms of purpura and hemorrhage. The most common neurologic symptoms were headache (34%) and coma (31%). Renal abnormalities included proteinuria, hematuria, casts, or azotemia.
†Data from Ridolfi and Bell[184] on 258 patients. The most common neurologic symptoms were confusion (37%) and headache (31%). Renal abnormalities included principally microscopic hematuria and proteinuria.
‡Data from Rock et al[150] on 102 patients. Entry criteria for this prospective study were microangiopathic hemolytic anemia and thrombocytopenia. Neurologic symptoms were present in 63% of patients at diagnosis and another 8% of patients during the course of their disease. Renal disease was defined as an elevated BUN and/or creatinine level.

thrombotic microangiopathy in other disorders[152,180] that have distinct etiologies and outcomes, and the observation of unusually large vWf multimers in other clinically distinct disorders, such as Henoch-Schönlein purpura,[181] emphasize the inherent heterogeneity of TTP-HUS.

Clinical Features   Before the era of effective treatment, TTP was diagnosed by the defining classic pentad of symptoms and physical findings documented in the review of Amorosi and Ultmann.[153] Few patients did not have all five criteria at presentation or during the unrelenting, fatal course of the disease. However, because of the urgent need to initiate plasma exchange treatment, recent studies have required only the presence of microangiopathic hemolytic anemia and thrombocytopenia, without another clinically apparent cause, to establish the diagnosis.[150,151,182,183] The drift from the classic pentad to the current dyad is illustrated in Table 117-6 by the clinical findings at diagnosis in three consecutive large series of patients spanning 64 years.[150,153,184] The most common presenting symptoms are neurologic abnormalities, hemorrhage, fatigue (probably related to severe anemia), and abdominal pain. The duration of disease prior to initiating therapy was 1 day to 2 weeks in two series[185,186] and a median of 3 days in another study.[187]

Among neurologic abnormalities, headache and confusion are the most common findings, followed by visual symptoms, seizures, dysphasia, and paresis.[153,184] Coma was present some time during the illness in 31 percent of patients reported in 1964[153] and in 20 percent of patients reported from 1964 to 1980,[184] but it is much less common now. Brain CT and MRI scans are often normal even in the presence of severe abnormalities such as hemiparesis, seizures, and coma, consistent with global ischemia due to microvascular obstruction and the frequency of complete recovery.[188–190] New neurologic abnormalities may occur during the course of TTP-HUS.[152] Fluctuating neurologic signs may be caused by nonconvulsive status epilepticus and respond to anticonvulsant therapy.[190] Hemorrhagic symptoms are those expected from thrombocytopenia: epistaxis, hematuria, gastrointestinal bleeding, and menorrhagia.[151]

The cause of severe abdominal pain as a major presenting symptom is less obvious, but this is prominent in many series. It presumably reflects bowel ischemia due to microvascular obstruction. Amorosi and Ultmann noted nausea, vomiting, diarrhea, and abdominal pain as chief complaints in 35 percent of their patients, nearly as frequent as chief complaints of the classic presentations of neurologic abnormalities (60 percent) and purpura or hemorrhage (44 percent).[153] These

three presenting complaints were noted in an identical frequency in a subsequent review,[184] and another series noted that abdominal or flank pain was the most common presenting symptom.[185] These symptoms have not been explained by pancreatitis except in isolated cases.[191] Adults may present with severe abdominal pain and bloody diarrhea, similar to the typical presentation of epidemic childhood HUS, that may initially be mistaken for ischemic colitis.

Case series of patients with TTP-HUS consistently report a female predominance of 60 to 70 percent.[150,153,192,193] The significance of this is unknown. This female predominance may be consistent with an autoimmune etiology, but other disorders have a female predominance without immunologic involvement (e.g., cholecystitis).

Even after patients recover from the active, life-threatening phase of TTP-HUS, mild thrombocytopenia and other subtle abnormalities may persist. The risk of relapse exists for all patients, but it is uncertain whether those with chronic thrombocytopenia are at higher risk of relapse.[194]

Laboratory Features   The defining features of TTP are usually apparent from the initial blood counts and examination of the blood film; however, earlier diagnosis, especially in patients with recurrent episodes, has caused a change in the presenting laboratory features. In one series,[185] 9 of 26 patients had normal hematocrits, although anemia rapidly developed in all. Another series of 17 patients[186] included two who were not anemic at diagnosis but whose hematocrits dropped to 20 percent within several days. Similarly, red cell fragmentation may be minimal or inapparent initially.[195,196] Thrombocytopenia is an essential component of the diagnosis, and, if absent at presentation, it usually develops rapidly.[197] Consistent with the severe hemolysis, the serum indirect bilirubin and LDH levels are increased. LDH levels are often very high, with mean values of over 1000 units per liter in most series[150,151,186,192] and values up to 6000 units per liter in some cases.[197] Isoenzyme analysis has demonstrated that the increased LDH reflects not only hemolysis but also ischemic injury to multiple organs.[198] Most patients will have microscopic hematuria and proteinuria; some may have acute, oliguric renal failure.

In contrast to the era before plasma exchange treatment, tissue biopsy is not required to establish the diagnosis. Biopsies are performed only when different diagnoses are considered that require different management, such as lupus erythematosus. The characteristic lesions of TTP-HUS are arteriolar and capillary thrombi composed primarily of platelets, but also with vWf and some fibrin (Fig. 117-6).[152,158] Subendothelial hyaline deposits and periarteriolar concentric fibrosis are also common features. Renal biopsies demonstrate platelet thrombi that may occlude the lumens of glomerular capillaries and interlobular and afferent arterioles. The glomerular endothelial cells may be swollen, possibly even to the extent of occluding the capillary lumen in a pattern indistinguishable from preeclampsia. Fibrin and red cells may permeate the arterial wall and be associated with a process of mucoid intimal hyperplasia.[152] These changes are characteristic of TTP-HUS but also may be identical to the pathology of some patients with preeclampsia, malignant hypertension, acute scleroderma, and renal allograft rejection.[152] Electron microscopy of renal biopsies consistently demonstrates widening of the subendothelial space, which is pale and contains "fluffy" electron-dense material. Renal biopsies may be especially important to distinguish TTP-HUS from other forms of rapidly progressive glomerulonephritis.[152]

Differential Diagnosis   The spectrum of TTP-HUS has become wider and differential diagnosis more challenging as making the diagnosis with fewer criteria has become accepted. With plasma exchange treatment so effective, appropriate management is to err on the side of initiating plasma exchange rather than delaying treatment in an attempt to establish the diagnosis with greater certainty. Other disorders that can cause similar clinical and laboratory findings include

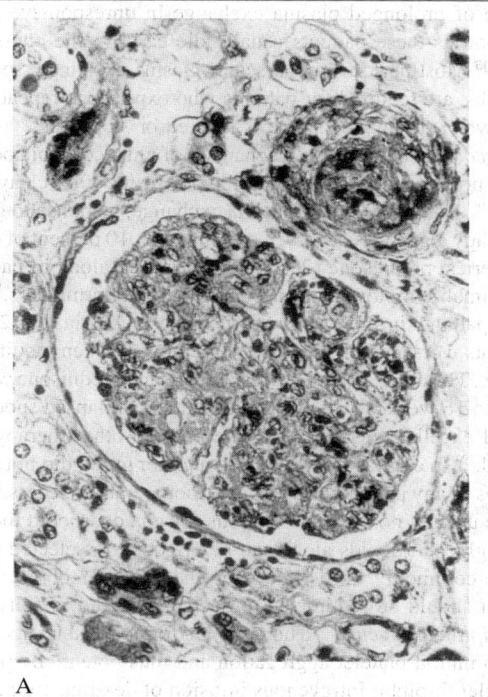

A

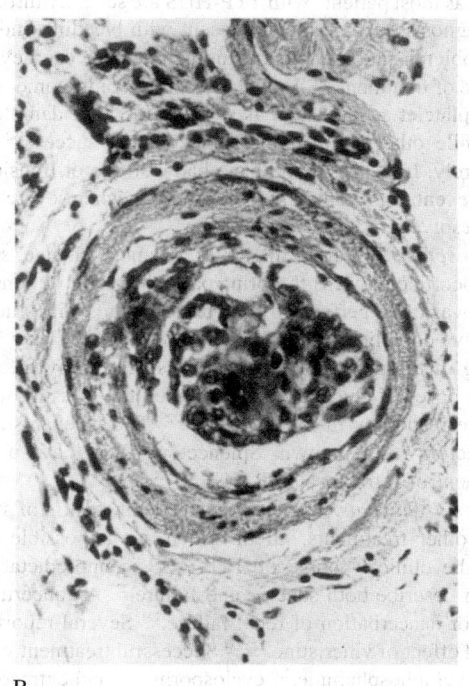

B

FIGURE 117-6   Pathology of TTP-HUS. (*A*) Renal biopsy demonstrating hyaline thrombi obstructing most capillary lumens and thrombosis occluding a preglomerular arteriole. No significant inflammatory changes are seen in the glomerulus. [Reproduced with permission from Habib R in *Hemolytic Uremic Syndrome and Thrombotic Thrombocytopenic Purpura,* Kaplan B, Trompeter R, Moake J (eds), Marcel Dekker, New York, 1992, p 324.] (*B*) Pulmonary arteriole from autopsy of a patient with gastric adenocarcinoma. The lumen is nearly obstructed by a tumor embolus. Tumor cells have also penetrated between layers of intimal proliferation. No fibrin or platelets are present. (Reproduced with permission from Antman KH et al, *Medicine* 58:377, 1979.)

sepsis, autoimmune disorders, pregnancy-related conditions (preeclampsia, HELLP syndrome), malignant hypertension, and unrecognized metastatic carcinoma. Sepsis (bacterial, fungal, viral, or rickettsial) should be considered in an acutely ill patient with chills, fever, and dysfunction of multiple organs. DIC is typically present in sepsis and should raise concern for diagnoses other than TTP-HUS. Evidence of DIC may be present in patients with TTP-HUS, resulting from tissue ischemia, but coagulation abnormalities are not usually severe[199] (see Chap. 126). An example of infection mimicking TTP-HUS is bacterial endocarditis, which can present with anemia, thrombocytopenia, fever, and neurologic and renal abnormalities. TTP-HUS can share both clinical and pathological features with systemic lupus erythematosus, catastrophic antiphospholipid syndrome, and scleroderma.[152,200–205] Moreover, TTP-HUS may occur in association with an underlying autoimmune disorder. Evan's syndrome, the concomitant presence of autoimmune hemolytic anemia and ITP, may initially be indistinguishable from TTP-HUS, but microangiopathic erythrocyte changes are uncommon in Evan's syndrome. The demonstration of a positive direct antiglobulin test is the distinguishing feature, but it may be negative in autoimmune hemolysis.[206] TTP-HUS may be initially confused with megaloblastic anemia or myelodysplasia thrombocytopenia because red cell poikilocytosis and high serum LDH may be present in all three entities.

Treatment   During the past 20 years plasma exchange has become the primary treatment for TTP-HUS. This has profoundly affected the prognosis; the mortality rate has decreased from >90% before 1964[153] to <20% in current series. Ironically, effective treatment has revealed a new spectrum of chronic relapsing disease among many of the survivors. Less intensive therapies such as prednisone alone[192] or plasma infusion alone[185] have been used for some patients with minimal disease, but the unpredictability of TTP-HUS and the continued presence of patients with unrelenting and fatal disease in every case series support the prompt initiation of plasma exchange treatment.[207] Although some reports suggest that patients defined as having HUS respond to plasma exchange treatment less well than patients with TTP, most reports describe no difference.[182]

Plasma Exchange.   With the wide availability of portable equipment, plasma exchange can be performed in almost any place at any time. Rapid initial therapy with plasma exchange is essential since anemia, thrombocytopenia, and neurologic complications may worsen in the initial days after diagnosis,[150] and about half of the deaths in patients with TTP-HUS occur in the first week of illness. Why plasma exchange is effective remains unknown. Theories of the pathogenesis of TTP-HUS could support either the removal of a harmful plasma component (such as the unusually large vWf multimers or antibodies that inhibit the vWf-cleaving metalloproteinase) or the replacement of a deficient component (such as the vWf-cleaving protease or low-molecular-weight vWf multimers). The latter idea is supported by the efficacy in some patients of merely infusing plasma.[208] A randomized, controlled trial documented that plasma infusions are less effective than plasma exchange, but this may simply have been because the patients treated with plasma exchange received threefold as much plasma.[150] The risks of plasma exchange are real and include complications associated with inserting a large central venous catheter; infectious and thrombotic complications of the indwelling catheter; allergic reactions to the plasma; infectious complications from the plasma; and alkalosis symptoms due to the infused citrate. One prospective study of 65 courses of plasma exchange in 59 patients with TTP-HUS documented that 40 percent of courses were free of complications, 30 percent had minor complications, and 30 percent had major complications, including two deaths and eight episodes of bacteremia.[209] Each procedure requires several hours and costs about $2000.

Plasma exchange is performed once daily until a response is achieved, defined by resolution of the neurologic abnormalities, a normal platelet count, and a normal or nearly normal LDH concentration.[183] Thrombocytopenia and high LDH levels usually resolve within 1 or 2 weeks; neurologic abnormalities, such as headache, confusion, and seizures, usually resolve earlier.[151] Deep coma may be completely reversible with plasma exchange.[189] One plasma volume (40 ml/kg) is the recommended volume of plasma to exchange. Larger volumes have lower efficiency as more of the infused plasma is promptly removed. An increased "dose" of plasma is one parameter to adjust if the patient does not promptly respond, and this is best achieved by increasing the frequency of plasma exchange to twice daily.

Patient plasma is routinely replaced with fresh frozen plasma, but some reports recommend "cryoprecipitate-poor" or "cryosupernatant" plasma, the fraction recovered after removal of the cryoprecipitate, which contains a significant amount of vWf, factor VIII, and fibrinogen. Theories that unusually large vWf multimers are involved in the pathogenesis of TTP-HUS suggest that infusion of vWf may retard recovery,[161] and it has been suggested that use of cryosupernatant plasma improved the response of patients who were initially refractory to plasma exchange.[209,210] However, the only data from a controlled randomized comparison of whole plasma versus cryosupernatant plasma demonstrated equivalent responses.[211] The deficiencies of factor VIII and fibrinogen in cryosupernatant plasma may necessitate the use of some whole plasma.

The optimal duration of plasma exchange treatment is unknown and the range in published series is great.[212,213] The earliest signs of recovery are improvement of neurologic abnormalities, decreased serum LDH concentration, and increased platelet count.[151] The rate of these responses may predict the clinical outcome and duration of required treatment.[212,214] An initial response may occur within minutes after beginning the first exchange or may not be observed for over 1 month.[192] Typically an initial response is seen during the first week, and recovery is nearly complete within 3 weeks.[213] Nearly all case series have some patients, however, who require more than a month of plasma exchange to achieve a successful, durable response. A prompt correction of the LDH concentration and thrombocytopenia is a good prognostic sign.[214] In one series, the serum creatinine level became normal only after a median of 90 days[197]; in another series, 26 percent of patients had creatinine clearances less than 40 ml/min 1 year after diagnosis.[215] It is unknown if continued plasma exchange after neurologic and hematologic recovery affects recovery of renal function.

Plasma exchange is continued daily until neurologic signs resolve and the platelet count is normal; then plasma exchange is often continued at increasing time intervals for another week or two.[213] The rationale for such a "tapering" regimen is that it may prevent an exacerbation of active TTP-HUS. Recurrence of the signs of TTP-HUS occurred in 58 of 70 patients in one series when plasma exchange was discontinued.[192] In other series, exacerbations occurred in 24 to 39 percent of patients[151,212,213,215,216] and required resumed daily plasma exchange before achieving a durable remission. The frequency of exacerbations supports a more prolonged initial course of plasma exchange. Substitution of plasma infusion for plasma exchange has been tried in patients who required prolonged treatment, but in one study exacerbations occurred in 22 of 36 patients treated with plasma infusion.[192]

No other treatment modality approaches the efficacy of plasma exchange, and so the role of other treatments is uncertain[217]; therefore, there is risk in discontinuing plasma exchange in favor of another treatment. Remissions may occur after as long as 8 months of plasma exchange treatment.[185] Twice-daily plasma exchange[185,192,218] and the use of cryosupernatant plasma as the replacement product[209] should be tried before plasma exchange is considered ineffective. In practice,

the issue of prolonged plasma exchange in unresponsive patients is uncommon as these patients usually die early in the course of their disease.[213] Most prolonged courses of plasma exchange, some lasting for months, are required for patients who experience repeated exacerbations when plasma exchange is tapered or stopped.

Glucocorticoids. The mechanism of glucocorticoid benefit may be immunosuppression of autoantibodies to the vWf-cleaving protease.[164,166,167] Before the era of plasma exchange, response to glucocorticoid therapy alone was observed only in about 10 percent of patients.[219] In one series, prednisone (200 mg/d) was used alone in patients who had minimal symptoms and no neurologic abnormalities.[192] Half of the 108 patients in this series fulfilled these criteria, but 24 of these 54 patients worsened on prednisone therapy and then required plasma exchange. The other 30 patients responded, and prednisone was tapered over 11 to 16 weeks. Two of these 30 patients relapsed suddenly after an initial excellent response and died before other therapy could be instituted.[192] In contrast to this report, another group did not use glucocorticoids in any patients and achieved comparable success.[150,182] Since there are usually no contraindications for glucocorticoid therapy, and because glucocorticoids alone can be effective in selected patients,[192] they are commonly used. However the duration of glucocorticoid treatment should be minimized to decrease steroid toxicity.

Antiplatelet Agents. The rationale for antiplatelet agents is their ability to inhibit platelet aggregation and thus potentially prevent microvascular thrombi. Intravenous infusion of dextran, 1 g per day, has been used as an antiplatelet agent in combination with high doses of prednisone and splenectomy.[151] A risk for these agents is increased bleeding, as most patients with TTP-HUS are severely thrombocytopenic at diagnosis, many patients present with bleeding and purpura as major problems, and life-threatening hemorrhage can develop during the course of treatment.[151] As with glucocorticoids, some case series[150] used antiplatelet agents, such as aspirin and dipyridamole, in all patients, while others with comparable clinical success[192] used these agents rarely. In patients who have had a stroke or transient cerebral ischemic event, aspirin therapy is appropriate when severe thrombocytopenia resolves.

Splenectomy. Before the era of plasma exchange, splenectomy and glucocorticoids were the principal therapeutic options, and splenectomy was often performed soon after diagnosis in spite of the risk of operative complications in critically ill patients.[220] By 1982, at the beginning of the plasma exchange era, splenectomy in combination with high doses of glucocorticoids and dextran infusion was reported to achieve responses in most patients.[220] The mechanism of benefit of splenectomy is unknown. Splenectomy may have a role in the management of refractory TTP-HUS.[151,220,221]

Other Treatments. There are anecdotal reports of success with multiple other treatments, all of which are impossible to evaluate because the clinical course of TTP-HUS is unpredictable. Reports with IVIg describe both success and failure.[222] A concern for IVIg is the risk for exacerbation of renal failure.[223] Several reports suggest a beneficial effect of vincristine.[222,224] Successful treatment with azathioprine,[225] cyclophosphamide,[226] cyclosporine,[227] and extracorporeal immunoabsorption[228] has been reported.

Platelet Transfusion. Platelet transfusions have been reported to exacerbate TTP-HUS, which is consistent with disseminated platelet aggregation as the principal pathogenesis of TTP-HUS. Cases have been reported with acute deterioration and death following platelet transfusion[192,229]; others have associated platelet transfusions with increased mortality.[230] However, most case series do not mention platelet transfusions or do not comment on adverse reactions. Thus, the risks, if any, of platelet transfusions remain unknown. The requirement for an invasive procedure in a patient with severe thrombocytopenia and risk for major bleeding is an appropriate indication for platelet transfusion, but the patient should be carefully monitored for signs and symptoms of clinical deterioration. Severe thrombocytopenia in the absence of clinically important bleeding is not an indication for platelet transfusion.

Treatment Summary. Plasma exchange is the most important treatment modality and should be continued until a durable remission is achieved. For patients who do not respond or deteriorate during the first week of daily plasma exchange, twice-daily plasma exchange may provide dramatic benefit. Both whole plasma and cryosupernatant plasma are effective. Although other treatments are commonly used, especially in patients with prolonged courses, their efficacy is uncertain.

Course and Prognosis Improved survival is the most striking feature of TTP-HUS compared to three decades ago. Of 271 patients diagnosed before 1964, only 27 (10 percent) survived.[153] Current survival is about 80 percent. Although plasma exchange has revolutionized the management and prognosis of TTP-HUS, some patients continue to have severe, refractory disease; most deaths occur early in the course of the illness or before treatment can be initiated.

With effective treatment, a new spectrum of TTP has been revealed. Acute exacerbations occur when initial daily plasma exchange is decreased in frequency in many if not most patients.[150,192,212,213,215,216] Relapses, defined as occurring after a complete hematologic remission on treatment for over 1 month, occur in approximately one-third of patients within 10 years.[230,231] Clinical features of the initial episode may predict which patients are at risk for relapse. For example, TTP-HUS occurring as an adverse reaction to quinine or ticlopidine appears to be unlikely to recur without reexposure to the drug. TTP-HUS occurring after hemorrhagic colitis does not appear to recur,[193] in accord with the lack of relapses in children following recovery from epidemic HUS caused by *E. coli* 0157:H7. No maintenance therapy appears to prevent relapses. Patients who recover from TTP-HUS and then have a late relapse predictably recover if treated,[212] though rare deaths have occurred.[230,231] Asymptomatic patients with moderate thrombocytopenia and/or poikilocytosis present difficult management dilemmas; careful observation alone, glucocorticoid treatment, or plasma exchange may each be appropriate.

The frequency of long-term sequelae after TTP-HUS is unknown but may be significant. Permanent neurologic deficits are not commonly reported. One report documented renal failure in 26 percent of patients 1 year after diagnosis,[215] comparable to the 23 to 66 percent frequency of abnormalities of renal function and blood pressure in children 10 years after an episode of epidemic HUS.[232–238]

EPIDEMIC HEMOLYTIC UREMIC SYNDROME IN CHILDREN CAUSED BY SHIGA-TOXIN-PRODUCING E. coli

Epidemic HUS of young children is a distinct disorder from the other syndromes described as TTP-HUS (Table 117-5) with regard to etiology, treatment, and prognosis. It is commonly referred to as *epidemic, enteropathic,* or simply *D⁺ HUS,* designating the prodrome of diarrhea.[154,155,239] This disorder follows acute enteric infection caused by *E. coli* or *Shigella dysenteriae* serotypes that produce Shiga toxin. Although this disorder typically occurs in young children, it can also occur in adults; in adults the course and prognosis may be more severe, similar to the other adult TTP-HUS syndromes.[239] In children, 85 to 90 percent of HUS is preceded by diarrhea; the disease in the other 10 to 15 percent of children is similar to the typical idiopathic TTP-HUS of adults, exhibiting no seasonal incidence variation, more neurologic symptoms, and a greater risk for relapse.[240] These children, in contrast to children with diarrhea-associated HUS, may require plasma exchange treatment.[241]

Epidemiology In 1982 enterohemorrhagic strains of *E. coli* (predominantly *E. coli* 0157:H7) that acquired a plasmid containing the

Shiga toxin were first recognized as human pathogens,[154,155,239] and 1 year later the association between Shiga-toxin-producing *E. coli* 0157:H7 and HUS was documented.[154] This appeared to be a new disease, since retrospective analysis of over 3000 *E. coli* cultures from 1973 to 1982 found only one isolate with serotype 0157:H7, from a woman with bloody diarrhea in 1975.[239] Serologic evidence suggests that all *E. coli* 0157 isolates from patients with colitis are derived from one particularly adaptive clone of *E. coli* that has spread throughout the world.[242] The occurrence of gastrointestinal infections caused by *E. coli* 0157:H7 is increasing dramatically,[155] but HUS can also follow diarrhea caused by Shiga-toxin-producing *E. coli* serotypes other than 0157:H7[239] and may even follow infections other than colitis.[243,244]

Epidemiologic studies have defined the features of *E. coli* 0157:H7 infections and childhood HUS.[154,156,239,245] The occurrence of colitis in persons consuming infected food is estimated to be 4 to 8 percent in community outbreaks but was 33 percent in a nursing home epidemic, which also included person-to-person transmission.[239] Progression of *E. coli* 0157:H7 infection to HUS is estimated to occur in 2 to 7 percent of sporadic cases but up to 30 percent in some epidemics.[154,239,246] *E. coli* 0157:H7 is present in the intestines of about 1 percent of healthy cattle,[155] and most outbreaks are traced to undercooked beef. However, contamination of unpasteurized milk, juices, fruits, vegetables, and water have all been implicated in outbreaks of colitis.[154,155,239,245] Person-to-person transmission is a particular problem in day-care and chronic-care facilities.[154] The peak age of infection is 6 months to 5 years, reflecting the period after weaning and maximum exposure to enteric pathogens and further suggests that older children and adults may acquire immunity to the Shiga toxin.[154,155,239] In contrast to the female predominance in adults with TTP-HUS, boys and girls are equally affected.[239] Consistent with the association with enteric pathogens, over 80 percent of cases occur between April and September.[154,155,245]

Etiology In addition to the Shiga toxin, *E. coli* 0157:H7 contains factors that promote mucosal attachment and colitis.[154] The toxic effects of the released Shiga toxin are focused on glomerular endothelial cells because of their rich display of glycosphingolipid receptors for the toxins.[157] Once bound, the toxin can initiate production of endothelin-1, which can induce vasoconstriction and provoke acute renal failure.[247]

Clinical and Laboratory Features The clinical presentation is dominated by diarrhea, which is bloody in most patients. The average duration of symptoms before diagnosis of HUS is 6 days; antimicrobial treatment of the initial diarrhea does not appear to influence the clinical course.[154,155,239] The symptoms may be severe enough to mimic ischemic colitis and require colectomy. Most patients are oliguric at the time of admission and require dialysis support.[154,237,244,247] Fever and hypertension are common. Extrarenal involvement, including pancreatitis (20 percent) and seizures (20 percent) may be prominent.[248] The most prominent laboratory features are abnormalities of acute renal failure, microangiopathic hemolytic anemia, and thrombocytopenia.

Treatment, Course, and Prognosis Plasma exchange, the cornerstone of treatment for adult TTP-HUS, appears to have minimal or no benefit.[154] Treatment is supportive; dialysis is necessary in about half of children.[154] In contrast to TTP-HUS in adults before the era of plasma exchange, epidemic childhood HUS is an acute and severe illness, but the mortality is only 3 to 10 percent.[154,239] However, HUS occurring during outbreaks of *E. coli* 0157:H7 colitis among elderly subjects may have up to 88 percent mortality.[245] Relapses are not mentioned in studies with long-term follow-up, but 23 to 66 percent of patients have abnormal renal function at evaluations many years after their acute childhood HUS.[232–238] Children who had more severe renal disease with their initial HUS[232,237] or atypical HUS had a greater risk for developing renal failure.

THROMBOTIC THROMBOCYTOPENIC PURPURA-HEMOLYTIC UREMIC SYNDROME ASSOCIATED WITH INFECTIONS OTHER THAN SHIGA-TOXIN-PRODUCING E. coli

Anecdotal reports have described TTP-HUS associated with infections caused by bacteria, rickettsiae, and viruses. Some of these infectious agents are thought to cause TTP-HUS, others may merely mimic TTP-HUS, and still others may exacerbate established TTP-HUS.[249] Distinguishing among these possibilities may be difficult. With the exception of *Shigella dysenteriae* type I, which carries the same Shiga toxin as *E. coli* 0157:H7, none of these infections is as clearly associated with the cause of TTP-HUS as the enterohemorrhagic *E. coli*. Misdiagnosis of TTP-HUS may cause a delay in the treatment of an infectious disease, and so it is important to have a high index of suspicion for infection.

Enteric Bacterial Infections   TTP-HUS following infection with *Shigella dysenteriae* type I has been described in children and in adults with TTP-HUS.[250] *Shigella dysenteriae* is uncommon among *Shigella* species causing gastroenteritis. Other reported associations with TTP-HUS include *Yersinia enterocolitica*,[251] *Campylobacter* species,[252] and *Clostridium difficile*.[253] Shiga-toxin-producing *E. coli* other than 0157:H7 strain may also be responsible for causing TTP-HUS, and these are not so easily distinguished from nonpathogenic *E. coli*.[245]

Other Bacterial Infections   TTP-HUS has been reported following *Streptococcus pneumoniae* pneumonia, bacteremia, and meningitis in children[254] and adults.[255] In one patient TTP-HUS occurred simultaneously with *Borrelia burgdorferi* infection,[256] and another had meningococcemia.[153] Five adult patients were reported with TTP-HUS and *Bartonella*-like red cell inclusions; treatment with doxycycline appeared to be effective.[257]

Rickettsial Infections   A patient with ehrlichiosis was described who was initially misdiagnosed with TTP-HUS because of acute, critical illness with coma, renal failure, and severe thrombocytopenia.[258]

Viral Infections   Over 100 patients have been reported with a TTP-HUS-like syndrome during the course of infection with HIV.[180] These patients have been identified both by the observation of unanticipated positive tests for anti-HIV antibodies in patients with a primary diagnosis of TTP-HUS[259,260] and by evaluating patients with HIV infection for signs of TTP-HUS.[261] In one series, 11 of 50 serum samples from TTP-HUS patients demonstrated anti-HIV antibodies, suggesting an epidemiologic relationship.[260] A role for HIV infection in the pathogenesis of TTP-HUS has been postulated to be related to HIV infection of endothelial cells.[262] The clinical features of patients with TTP-HUS associated with HIV infection are distinct from the features characteristic of patients with idiopathic TTP-HUS: Patients usually have a gradual onset of the disorder, survive for weeks to months without plasma exchange, have many concurrent medical problems that could account for abnormalities attributed to TTP-HUS, and have a less predictable response to plasma exchange.[180] These clinical features are similar to the reports of TTP-HUS in patients following bone marrow transplantation (described below). In these immunocompromised patients, a superimposed systemic infection, such as cytomegalovirus,[263,264] could mimic TTP-HUS.

DRUG-INDUCED THROMBOTIC THROMBOCYTOPENIC PURPURA-HEMOLYTIC UREMIC SYNDROME

TTP-HUS can be an idiosyncratic, acute adverse reaction to a drug, mediated by drug-dependent antibodies to platelets and other cells. Quinine is the best described example.[265] TTP-HUS associated with mitomycin C appears to be dose-dependent. Recognition of drug-induced TTP-HUS is critical because withdrawal of the offending drug is essential for both recovery and avoidance of recurrence.

Quinine   Acute, severe TTP-HUS has been reported following quinine ingestion,[265] and quinine ingestion was associated with 5 percent of all patients diagnosed with TTP-HUS in one recent series.[227] These patients may have quinine-dependent antiplatelet antibodies, and some may also have quinine-dependent antineutrophil antibodies, causing severe neutropenia.[265,266] Abdominal pain with nausea and vomiting are prominent presenting features, as is common in TTP-HUS.[265] Most patients require hemodialysis in addition to plasma exchange, but the prognosis is good for recovery of normal renal function. Repeated ingestion of quinine or even quinine water ("tonic")[267] can cause an immediate recurrence of TTP-HUS.

Ticlopidine   Acute, severe TTP-HUS following a short course of ticlopidine, usually less than 4 weeks, has been reported in 60 patients.[268] The frequency of TTP-HUS due to ticlopidine following coronary artery stent placement has been estimated to be approximately 1 in 1600 patients[269] in one study and somewhat lower in another.[270] Since ticlopidine is now routinely used in the estimated 400,000 patients per year in the United States who undergo coronary intervention involving a stent,[270] the above estimate corresponds to about 250 cases of TTP-HUS in the United States each year. Whether TTP-HUS is associated with clopidogrel, an analog of ticlopidine, remains to be assessed.[269]

Mitomycin C and Other Cancer Chemotherapeutic Agents   Data from a registry of cancer-associated HUS established in the 1980s identified an association between mitomycin C and TTP-HUS,[233] and a review in 1987 documented 128 cases of mitomycin-C-associated TTP-HUS.[272] Mitomycin C, an alkylating agent, is most commonly used in combination with 5-fluorouracil and doxorubicin for gastric and pancreatic carcinoma.[273,274] In this regimen, mitomycin C is administered at a dose of 10 mg/m^2 on the first day of each 8-week cycle, and the cycles are continued as long as a response occurs, which may last for more than a year.[274] Most episodes of TTP-HUS occur in patients with gastric carcinoma, but they may also occur in patients receiving adjuvant chemotherapy who have no evidence of carcinoma at autopsy.[275-278] TTP-HUS, like renal toxicity,[279] appears to be a dose-related toxicity of mitomycin C. In one review, 75 of 84 patients with TTP-HUS had received at least 60 mg[271]; in another study, all of 24 patients had received at least 1.2 mg/kg[275]; and another review reported that all patients had received at least 30 mg/m^2, equivalent to about 0.75 mg/kg.[280] Even at these total doses, however, fewer than 10 percent of patients develop the clinical features of TTP-HUS.[280,281] Renal pathology is identical to that of other TTP-HUS syndromes (Fig. 117-6).[278] Most patients who develop TTP-HUS following mitomycin C therapy die from their cancer or of renal failure.[271,272,276] The efficacy of plasma exchange treatment is uncertain.[276] The occurrence of TTP-HUS following cancer treatment with chemotherapy regimens not containing mitomycin C is uncommon; TTP-HUS associated with treatment with cisplatin, bleomycin, or pentostatin has been reported.[271,277]

Cyclosporine A   The major toxicity of cyclosporine is dose-related renal toxicity; seizures and other neurotoxic effects also occur.[282,283] A syndrome of severe renal failure, microangiopathic hemolytic anemia, and thrombocytopenia associated with cyclosporine were first reported in patients following allogeneic marrow transplantation.[284] Allogeneic marrow transplantation itself has been reported to cause a syndrome resembling TTP-HUS (see "Thrombotic Thrombocytopenic Purpura-Hemolytic Uremic Syndrome Associated with Marrow Transplants"), and thus a specific association with cyclosporine administration is difficult to establish. For example, in one report the occurrence of microangiopathy correlated with the severity of acute graft-versus-host disease, which alone can cause many clinical features similar to those of TTP-HUS.[285] Although the early reports suggested that TTP-HUS may be a common complication of cyclosporine,[285-287] the diagnosis is now much less common in spite of the wide use of cyclosporine in patients receiving marrow and solid organ allografts. This may simply be related to better regulation of cyclosporine doses and less toxicity. Tacrolimus has also been reported to cause TTP-HUS,[288] but the interpretation of these reports is difficult because the patients usually have complicated illnesses. Cyclosporine-induced TTP-HUS is almost always reversible when cyclosporine is discontinued, and in some patients cyclosporine is restarted without toxicity.[286] The efficacy of plasma exchange treatment is uncertain.

Other Drugs   Other drugs that have been associated with TTP-HUS include metronidazole,[289] cocaine,[290] simvastatin,[291] pentostatin,[292] and ecstasy (3,4-methylenedroxy methamphetamine).[293]

THROMBOTIC THROMBOCYTOPENIC PURPURA-HEMOLYTIC UREMIC SYNDROME ASSOCIATED WITH MARROW TRANSPLANTS

Although TTP-HUS has been diagnosed following autologous marrow or peripheral blood stem cell transplantation, most reported patients have undergone allogeneic marrow transplantation.[282,283,294,295] The diagnosis of TTP-HUS has been principally based on the unexpected appearance of microangiopathic hemolytic anemia, characterized by prominent red cell fragmentation and a persistent increase in serum LDH.[282,294] The diagnosis is supported when other features of TTP-HUS, thrombocytopenia, neurologic abnormalities, and renal failure seem unexplained by other complications of marrow transplantation.[283] However, since patients following bone marrow transplantation are frequently critically ill with multiorgan dysfunction, it may be difficult to establish the diagnosis of TTP-HUS. This diagnostic uncertainty has probably led to the extreme variations in the reported frequencies of TTP-HUS (2 to 76 percent among patients with allografts; 0 to 27 percent among patients with autografts) and in reported mortality (0 to 87 percent).[282] All features of TTP-HUS could be caused by more predictable complications of marrow transplantation: graft-versus-host disease, radiation toxicity, and systemic infections. Nephrotoxicity and neurotoxicity of cyclosporine may also be complicating factors.[282] Therefore it is understandable that TTP-HUS is most often diagnosed in the most complicated patients, who are at greatest risk for developing graft-versus-host disease: patients who have received transplants from matched, unrelated donors, and patients who had an HLA antigen mismatched donor.[294,296,297] Also, total body irradiation as part of the preparative regimen is correlated with the subsequent diagnosis of TTP-HUS.[294,297]

The immediate and critical decision is whether a patient may benefit from plasma exchange treatment. In contrast to patients with idiopathic TTP-HUS, delay in initiating plasma exchange treatment while alternative etiologies are assessed may be an appropriate decision. Some patients demonstrate hematologic improvement following plasma exchange,[297–299] sometimes apparently requiring the use of cryosupernatant plasma or immunoabsorption by protein A columns, but most patients do not respond.[297,299] Even in responsive patients, plasma exchange may not affect the clinical outcome.[300]

THROMBOTIC THROMBOCYTOPENIC PURPURA-HEMOLYTIC UREMIC SYNDROME ASSOCIATED WITH CANCER

Patients with extensive metastatic carcinoma who developed syndromes indistinguishable from TTP-HUS have been reported.[272,301,302] Although the full syndrome of TTP-HUS is rare, red cell poikilocytosis occurs in about 5 percent of patients with metastatic cancer,[301,303] and prospective analyses suggest that metastatic carcinoma accounts for the majority of patients (excluding patients with renal failure) who are noted to have red cell poikilocytosis.[303] The occurrence of TTP-HUS has been associated with a variety of carcinomas, but over half of the patients have had gastric carcinoma.[272,301,302] In fact, microangio-

pathic hemolytic anemia may be the sign that initiates the discovery of occult metastatic carcinoma.[301] In addition to red cell fragmentation and thrombocytopenia, a leukoerythroblastic reaction indicating marrow involvement by tumor is frequently observed.[272,301] DIC may be triggered by mucin-producing adenocarcinomas,[304] but laboratory evidence of DIC is present in only a minority of patients with metastatic carcinoma who have microangiopathic hemolysis and thrombocytopenia.[301,302] The characteristic pathological feature is widespread occurrence of microvascular tumor emboli with associated proliferation of the vascular intima, most commonly in the pulmonary circulation (Fig. 117-6).[272,301,302,305] In a retrospective search, diffuse involvement of pulmonary arterioles with tumor emboli was found in only 7 of 800 autopsies performed on patients with carcinoma.[302] Therapy, course, and prognosis are determined by the metastatic carcinoma; in patients responsive to chemotherapy, the syndrome resolves.[302] There appears to be no role for plasma exchange treatment.

THROMBOTIC THROMBOCYTOPENIC PURPURA-HEMOLYTIC UREMIC SYNDROME ASSOCIATED WITH AUTOIMMUNE DISORDERS

An association of TTP-HUS with autoimmune disorders such as SLE has been described,[153] but the diagnosis of TTP-HUS may be difficult to establish, since the signs and symptoms of SLE can mimic those of TTP-HUS.[212–214] Further complicating this association is the presence in some SLE patients of opportunistic central nervous system infections (aspergillus, candida, cytomegalovirus) and cerebral emboli from verrucous endocarditis.[212] Patients with TTP-HUS have been found to have antiphospholipid antibodies,[306] and the clinical features of catastrophic antiphospholipid syndrome may be identical to those of TTP-HUS.[215] Acute scleroderma can also be clinically[216,217] and pathologically[152,217] indistinguishable from TTP-HUS. The differential diagnosis between TTP-HUS and autoimmune disorders may be irrelevant, as all of these acute, severe autoimmune disorders have been reported to respond to plasma exchange treatment.[215,216,307] However, patients with SLE and TTP-HUS appear to have a higher mortality than patients with idiopathic TTP-HUS.[183,205]

THROMBOTIC THROMBOCYTOPENIC PURPURA-HEMOLYTIC UREMIC SYNDROME ASSOCIATED WITH PREGNANCY

In many case series of TTP-HUS, 10 to 25 percent of patients are pregnant or in the postpartum period.[153,183,308] The incidence of TTP-HUS among all pregnancies, however, is only 1 in 25,000.[309] Several case series and reviews focus on the specific issues related to the diagnosis and management of TTP-HUS during pregnancy.[309–312] The clinical and pathologic similarity to preeclampsia[309,310,312] suggests a relationship between these disorders. The recognized risk for stroke as a complication of preeclampsia further blurs its distinction from TTP-HUS.[313] Recurrent TTP-HUS has developed during successive pregnancies, and TTP-HUS that initially occurred in nonpregnant women has relapsed during a subsequent pregnancy.[308,309,311] If the disease is severe and the fetus is viable, delivery should be induced, since this will resolve preeclampsia and may[151,311,314] or may not[312] cause resolution of TTP-HUS. The possible therapeutic response to termination of the pregnancy further blurs the distinction between TTP-HUS and preeclampsia. However, termination of the pregnancy may not be necessary. In one series of 108 patients, 9 women were in their third trimester at the time of initial presentation of TTP-HUS, and all nine successfully completed their pregnancies, with delivery of 10 infants who remained healthy throughout 2 months of observation.[204] Others have reported successful completion of pregnancies with delivery of healthy infants.[153,308,310,311] There has been no report of transmission of TTP to the infant,[204,308–310] although intrauterine fetal

TABLE 117-7   INCIDENCE OF MATERNAL AND FETAL THROMBOCYTOPENIA IN 15,471 CONSECU-
TIVE WOMEN ADMITTED FOR LABOR AND DELIVERY, 1986–1992[A]

Mother's Health Status	Maternal Platelet Count <150,000/μl	Infant Platelet Count at Birth <50,000/μl
Normal (13,925)	756[b] (15%)	1[b] (0.01%)
Preeclampsia (1414) (9%)	216 (15%)	5[c] (0.35%)
ITP	31 (67%)	4[d] (8.7%)
Normal, infant at risk for neonatal alloimmune thrombocytopenia (18)[e39]	3 (17%)	9[e] (50%)
Other (68%)[f]	21 (31%)	0

[a]Data from Burrows and Kelton.[322]
[b]Two-thirds of the thrombocytopenic mothers had platelet counts of 130,000–150,000/μl. The infant had trisomy 21 and congenital marrow dysplasia.
[c]All 5 infants were premature and delivered by caesarian section; 1 had trisomy 13; 3 had birth weights <10th percentile for gestational age (2 of 3 had intracranial hemorrhage); one was normal birth weight for gestational age.
[d]Platelet counts on these 4 infants were 20,000–49,000/μl. None had clinically important bleeding.
[e]These 18 women had maternal-paternal platelet alloantigen mismatch diagnosed because of a previous thrombocytopenic fetus or were sisters of women who had infants with alloimmune thrombocytopenia; 6 of 9 infants had platelet counts <20,000/μl, and these were the only infants in this study with platelet counts <20,000/μl; 3 had intracranial hemorrhage in utero; 1 died. The thrombocytopenia in the 3 mothers was assumed to be the incidental thrombocytopenia of pregnancy.
[f]Women with other hematologic or medical disorders, not further specified.

death may occur due to placental infarction caused by thrombosis of the decidual arterioles.[315] Five of the nine women described above subsequently had a normal pregnancy and delivery,[204] and in another study most subsequent deliveries were successful.[311] Nevertheless, after recovery from TTP-HUS, subsequent pregnancies must be considered to carry a risk for recurrence.

THROMBOCYTOPENIA IN PREGNANCY

Thrombocytopenia is a common diagnostic and management issue during pregnancy. Asymptomatic thrombocytopenia occurs near term or in the peripartum period in about 5 percent of normal pregnancies, and thrombocytopenia, sometimes severe, occurs in about 15 percent of women with preeclampsia, which itself occurs in about 9 percent of all pregnancies (Table 117-7). Platelet counts during pregnancy are normal in most women,[316] but the mean may be slightly lower than in healthy nonpregnant women.[317] Serial platelet counts during pregnancy may[318] or may not[319] demonstrate a significant decrease during pregnancy, but the mean values of groups may not reflect both increases as well as decreases that occur in individual, otherwise normal patients.[320] This discussion focuses on two issues: (1) thrombocytopenia discovered incidentally during a normal pregnancy and its distinction from ITP, and (2) thrombocytopenia associated with preeclampsia and its distinction from TTP-HUS.

GESTATIONAL THROMBOCYTOPENIA
Incidental thrombocytopenia of pregnancy, also termed *gestational thrombocytopenia*, is defined by the following five criteria: (1) the presence of mild and asymptomatic thrombocytopenia, (2) lack of a past history of thrombocytopenia (except possibly during a previous pregnancy), (3) occurrence during late gestation, (4) lack of association with fetal thrombocytopenia, and (5) spontaneous resolution after delivery.[321] Platelet counts are typically greater than 70,000/μl, with about two-thirds being between 130,000 and 150,000/μl.[322,323] The frequency of gestational thrombocytopenia in the largest series of consecutive women admitted for labor and delivery is 5 percent (Table 117-7).[322] In this series neonatal thrombocytopenia did not occur in infants born to mothers with gestational thrombocytopenia (except in one infant with congenital myelodysplasia); therefore, it is considered to be benign, and any change from routine obstetrical care is discouraged.[324–326]

Etiology   The cause of gestational thrombocytopenia is unknown. Many, if not all, of its features are similar to those of mild ITP. Therefore an immunologic etiology for gestational thrombocytopenia, as part of a spectrum including ITP, has been suspected. Supporting this hypothesis was the unexpected observation that 160 women with gestational thrombocytopenia (defined by the criteria stated above) could not be distinguished from 90 women with ITP by assays for antiplatelet antibodies; both groups had higher than normal values.[327] Another study of 50 women with thrombocytopenia during pregnancy also reported that 21 had positive results for one or more antiplatelet autoantibodies,[328] although some of these women could have had a clinical diagnosis of ITP. Patients with ITP not uncommonly have more severe thrombocytopenia during pregnancy, with improvement after delivery.[329] The lack of thrombocytopenia in infants born to women with gestational thrombocytopenia, in contrast to the 5 to 10 percent occurrence of neonatal thrombocytopenia in ITP (Table 117-7),[138] may simply reflect absence of neonatal thrombocytopenia in infants born to mothers with mild ITP compared to more severe ITP.[330,331] Therefore whether gestational thrombocytopenia is truly distinct from ITP remains unknown.

Differential Diagnosis   In women with mild thrombocytopenia, the distinction from ITP is impossible, except possibly in retrospect. If the infant's platelet count is normal and the mother's platelet count returns to normal following delivery, gestational thrombocytopenia is considered the appropriate diagnosis. When thrombocytopenia is initially encountered during pregnancy, ITP is the more likely diagnosis if thrombocytopenia occurs early during pregnancy or if the platelet count is very low (<50,000/μl) during the third trimester or at term.[321]

Treatment   For both mother and infant, normal obstetric management is appropriate.[321,326,332] Epidural anesthesia is considered to be safe in women with gestational thrombocytopenia and platelet counts >50,000/μl.[333] Many women at delivery safely have epidural anesthesia with no platelet count performed, and some are likely to be mildly thrombocytopenic,[334] prompting the interesting, but controversial, suggestion that platelet counts should be avoided in asymptomatic pregnant women.[335] Delivery should be managed according to routine obstetrical practice.[332]

Course and Prognosis   The immediate concern is for fetal thrombocytopenia and the resulting risk for intracranial hemorrhage at delivery. The large case series summarized in Table 117-7 suggests that there is no risk.[322] However, other reports of selected women who had more severe thrombocytopenia than the women reported in Table 117-7 (and therefore may have had a clinical diagnosis of ITP) described severe neonatal thrombocytopenia. One report of 41 pregnancies described two infants with mild thrombocytopenia (platelet counts, 75,000 and 80,000/μl) and one with severe thrombocytopenia (12,000/μl); none had clinically important bleeding.[336] However, most of the mothers had platelet counts less than 100,000/μl, different from the women described in Table 117-7. Another study of 50 women referred for thrombocytopenia discovered during pregnancy described 63 pregnancies; 24 (38 percent) infants were thrombocytopenic either at birth or during the first two weeks of life.[328] Only one infant had clinically important bleeding, a scalp hematoma. These observations contrast not only with the data in Table 117-7 but also with the frequency of neonatal thrombocytopenia in infants born to mothers with documented ITP.[138,321,330,331] But the women in this study actually had more severe and persistent thrombocytopenia than the women described in Table 117-7, with half having platelet counts less than 70,000/μl and half having persistent thrombocytopenia after delivery.[328] Therefore, many of these women probably had ITP; these data are consistent with observations that the risk of neonatal thrombocytopenia correlates with the severity of maternal ITP.[330,331]

Although the large study of consecutive women at delivery (Table 117-7)[322] defined the frequency of thrombocytopenia, no follow-up of these women was performed, and no comparable study has defined long-term outcomes. Smaller studies of selected patients have demonstrated that thrombocytopenia in some women does not resolve for many months.[325,328,336] For those women whose platelet counts recover, and who therefore fulfill the current definition of gestational thrombocytopenia, recurrent thrombocytopenia with a subsequent pregnancy may be expected.[325]

PREECLAMPSIA

Definition   Pregnancy-induced hypertension and preeclampsia are common syndromes, especially among nulliparous women, and are a major cause of maternal and fetal morbidity and mortality.[337] Prevalence is variable in different parts of the world, but an estimate of 5 to 10 percent of all pregnancies is generally accepted (Table 117-7).[322,337] Pregnancy-induced hypertension appears after 20 weeks' gestation and disappears following delivery; *preeclampsia* is the presence of hypertension plus significant proteinuria and/or edema. *Eclampsia* is defined by the occurrence of acute neurologic abnormalities in a preeclamptic woman in the peripartum period[337-339]; its incidence is about 0.05 percent in developed countries but as high as 1 percent in underdeveloped countries.[337,339] Headache, hyperflexia, and visual disturbances can occur in patients who do not progress beyond preeclampsia, whereas seizures are the diagnostic hallmark of eclampsia; aphasia, paresis, and coma may then occur.[337,339] The additional renal pathologic features usually seen in preeclampsia are indistinguishable from TTP-HUS: thrombi and mucoid intimal hyperplasia of the afferent arterioles, glomerular capillary thrombi, and subendothelial "fluffy" deposits seen with electron microscopy.[152]

Platelet counts are lower in preeclamptic women than in women with uncomplicated pregnancies,[319] with the incidence of thrombocytopenia estimated to be approximately 15 percent (Table 117-7).[322,337] Severe thrombocytopenia, with platelet counts less than 50,000/μl, probably occurs in less than 5 percent of preeclamptic women, though the frequency and severity of thrombocytopenia increase with the severity of preeclampsia. The frequency and severity of thrombocytopenia are greater with eclampsia. If 9 percent of women have preeclampsia and 15 percent of them become thrombocytopenic (Table 117-7), thrombocytopenia due to preeclampsia will occur in about 14 of 1000 deliveries.

Etiology, Laboratory Features, and Differential Diagnosis   Preeclampsia is caused by a disorder of placental cytotrophoblast invasion of the uterine wall, resulting in shallow placental anchoring, circulatory abnormalities, and ischemia.[337] Placental ischemia triggers a systemic response causing vasoconstriction and endothelial abnormalities.[337] Vasoconstriction may also be caused by stimulatory autoantibodies to the angiotensin receptor (AT$_1$).[340] Typically, the systemic signs resolve within hours to days following delivery. In severe preeclampsia and eclampsia, thrombocytopenia and microangiopathic hemolytic anemia combined with seizures and other organ dysfunction to produce a disorder clinically indistinguishable from TTP-HUS.

The combination of thrombocytopenia and microangiopathic hemolysis, the current diagnostic dyad of TTP-HUS (Table 117-6), is characteristic of patients with severe preeclampsia, particularly patients with the HELLP syndrome, an acronym for microangiopathic hemolysis (H), elevated liver enzymes (EL), and low platelet (LP) counts.[341]

HELLP occurs in 5 to 20 percent of women with severe preeclampsia, but it may also become manifest near term without preceding hypertension.[337] Symptoms and signs of liver disease may predominate in the HELLP syndrome, representing the spectrum of acute fatty liver of pregnancy, which itself is part of the preeclampsia syndrome.[342] Thrombocytopenia and hemolysis can be severe, and serum LDH levels can be extremely high.[341] The distinction between preeclampsia/HELLP syndrome and TTP-HUS is further obscured by: (1) the oliguric acute renal failure that can occur in preeclampsia and can be exacerbated by hemorrhage and DIC resulting from placental abruption[337,341] (see Chap. 126), and (2) the occurrence of stroke during pregnancy, which is associated with pregnancy-related hypertension.[313]

Therapy, Course, and Prognosis   Delivering the fetus is the most effective method of treating preeclampsia, eclampsia, and the HELLP syndrome; advances in the care of premature neonates allow this to be performed at increasingly early time points. The platelet count nadir and the peak serum LDH may occur postpartum, during the first postpartum day in most patients, but as late as 5 to 7 days in some. For patients with severe thrombocytopenia and microangiopathic hemolytic anemia, plasma exchange is indicated if the fetus cannot be delivered or if improvement does not follow delivery. The third postpartum day is often considered the limit for only supportive therapy in anticipation of a spontaneous recovery.[341] If thrombocytopenia and hemolysis (as assessed by serum LDH levels) continue to worsen beyond this time, intervention with plasma exchange is appropriate for the presumed diagnosis of TTP-HUS. At this point TTP-HUS cannot be distinguished from atypical preeclampsia/eclampsia/HELLP syndrome, for which plasma exchange treatment may also be beneficial.[341] Earlier intervention with plasma exchange is indicated for more severe clinical problems, such as neurologic abnormalities or acute, anuric renal failure.

Infants born to mothers with preeclampsia are not at increased risk for thrombocytopenia, except for the risks related to prematurity (Table 117-7). Management of the delivery is guided by obstetrical, not hematologic, considerations.[329]

As with TTP-HUS, recurrence of HELLP syndrome in subsequent pregnancies is a concern. In the absence of persistent hypertension between pregnancies, HELLP syndrome is uncommon in subsequent pregnancies (3%), but less severe complications are more common in subsequent pregnancies: preeclampsia (19%) and preterm delivery (21%).[343]

IDIOPATHIC THROMBOCYTOPENIC PURPURA

Idiopathic thrombocytopenic purpura (ITP, also known as *primary immune thrombocytopenic purpura*) is an acquired disease of children and adults defined as isolated thrombocytopenia with no clinically apparent associated conditions or other causes of thrombocytopenia.[321] No specific criteria establish the diagnosis of ITP; the diagnosis relies on the exclusion of other causes of thrombocytopenia.[321]

The clinical syndromes of ITP are distinct between children and adults: Childhood ITP characteristically is acute in onset and resolves spontaneously in most cases within 6 months, whereas adult ITP typically has an insidious onset and rarely resolves spontaneously (Table 117-8). The incidence of ITP appears to be greater in children than in adults, and in children both sexes are equally affected[344,345] in contrast to the female predominance in adults. However, among older adults, the sex incidence may be equivalent.[346] With the expanding practice of routinely reporting platelet counts with all requests for blood counts, the apparent incidence of ITP has increased.[346] Currently 30 to 40 percent of adult patients with ITP are asymptomatic and diagnosed only incidentally.[346-348] The incidence of ITP in children is estimated to be approximately 46 new cases per million population

TABLE 117-8   CLINICAL FEATURES OF ITP IN CHILDREN AND ADULTS

	CHILDREN	ADULTS
Occurrence		
Peak age (years)	2–4	15–40
Sex (F:M)	Equal	2.6:1
Presentation		
Onset	Acute (most with symptoms <1 week)	Insidious (most with symptoms >2 months)
Symptoms	Purpura (<10% with severe bleeding)	Purpura (typically bleeding not severe)
Platelet count	Most <20,000/μl	Most <20,000/μl[a]
Course		
Spontaneous remission	83%[b]	2%[c]
Chronic disease	24%[d]	43%[d]
Response to splenectomy	71%[e]	66%[e]
Eventual complete recovery	89%[f]	64%[f]
Morbidity and mortality[g]		
Cerebral hemorrhage	<1%	3%
Hemorrhagic death	<1%	4%
Mortality of chronic, refractory disease	2%	5%

NOTE: These data are a summary of the data presented in George and colleagues.[321]
[a]Although the mean platelet counts at presentation for both children and adults were <20,000/μl in most series, some series of adults have a larger number of patients with platelet counts >30,000/μl.
[b]The frequency of spontaneous remission in children is overestimated because of the selection of patients with ITP of shorter duration and less severity for no treatment.
[c]The frequency of spontaneous remission in adults may be underestimated because in most series all patients are treated initially with steroids.
[d]Chronic disease in children is defined as thrombocytopenia persisting for longer than 6–12 months. In adults, chronic disease is defined as the lack of a permanent complete remission following steroid therapy and splenectomy. This frequency of patients with chronic, refractory disease is an overestimate, since some patients counted as not responding were lost to follow-up.
[e]Splenectomy in children was typically performed only if the symptomatic thrombocytopenia persisted for longer than 1 year. Most adults had splenectomy within 6 months of diagnosis.
[f]"Eventual" complete recovery is strongly dependent on the duration of follow-up.
[g]These data are difficult to estimate, as few series describe clinical outcomes with long-term follow-up. The increased morbidity and mortality in adults presumably reflects the longer course of ITP as well as the greater susceptibility of older adults[347,351] for serious and fatal complications.

per year,[349] and in adults it is estimated to be approximately 38 new cases per million population per year.[346]

ADULT IDIOPATHIC THROMBOCYTOPENIC PURPURA

Adult ITP may be more common in young women,[350] a group in which other autoimmune disorders are also relatively common, but recognition of ITP in older patients is increasing.[346] Because of greater risks for bleeding, the clinical manifestations and management of ITP in older adults deserve special consideration.[347,351]

Etiology and Pathogenesis   Harrington and coworkers demonstrated in 1951 that infusion of whole blood or plasma from patients with ITP into normal volunteers caused thrombocytopenia, and subsequent studies identified the active principal in ITP plasma as gamma globulin.[352,353] When ITP patients' plasmas were infused into normal subjects, the ability to induce thrombocytopenia was greatest in the plasmas of patients with severe thrombocytopenia refractory to splenectomy; it was substantially less in the plasmas of patients whose thrombocytopenia responded to therapy.[354] Increasing doses of ITP plasma infused into a normal recipient caused progressively more severe thrombocytopenia, while much higher doses were required to cause thrombocytopenia in a splenectomized recipient, suggesting that splenic removal, rather than intravascular destruction, was the major mechanism of platelet loss from the circulation[354] (Fig. 117-7). Infusion of ITP plasma into patients with hereditary spherocytosis resulted in less thrombocytopenia despite their larger spleens and accelerated red cell destruction, suggesting that platelet removal is reduced when reticuloendothelial clearance is saturated—an observation relevant to the use of intravenous gamma globulin (IVIg) and anti-Rh(D) globulin

therapy 20 years later (see "Therapy, Course and Prognosis," below). Administration of prednisone to normal subjects also diminished thrombocytopenia following infusion of ITP plasma but was less effective than splenectomy[354] (Fig. 117-7). Therefore, splenectomy not only removes a major source of antiplatelet antibody production, probably important for long-term remissions, but also removes a major site of platelet destruction, providing the commonly observed immediate response. The normal spleen contains one-third of the body's platelets, and altered microcirculation associated with lymphoid hyperplasia in ITP may allow greater platelet phagocytosis.[355] Macrophage-mediated platelet destruction may be influenced by plasma levels of M-CSF, which are significantly higher than normal in patients with ITP.[356] The positive response to splenectomy in the majority of patients with ITP further supports a central role for the spleen in the pathogenesis of ITP (Table 117-8).

Platelet Production and Destruction. Platelet kinetic studies using radiolabeled autologous platelets have demonstrated shortened intravascular survival, consistent with peripheral platelet destruction as the primary mechanism of thrombocytopenia (Table 117-4). This is consistent with the marrow finding of normal or increased megakaryocytes.[357,358] Body surface imaging with ^{111}In-oxine–labeled platelets has demonstrated splenic sequestration as the major site of platelet clearance in ITP.[357–359] These studies have also demonstrated the common occurrence of inappropriate marrow response to thrombocytopenia, with most patients having either normal or diminished platelet production[36,127,357,358] in spite of the presence of normal or increased numbers of megakaryocyte progenitors with increased cell cycle activity.[357] In several studies, the platelet production rate in patients with ITP varied from decreased to increased, with the average being approximately normal (Table 117-4). Earlier platelet survival studies found shorter platelet survival in ITP patients, suggesting greater platelet turnover and production,[357] but these studies are now considered less accurate because they employed homologous rather than autologous platelets. Ineffective thrombocytopoiesis may be due to the effect of antiplatelet antibodies on megakaryocytes or their progenitors.[360] The marrow contains normal or increased numbers of megakaryocytes.[363,364]

Antiplatelet Antibodies.   The initial tests used in studies of ITP were designed to measure the effect of patient plasma on the function of normal platelets, such as induction of platelet aggregation or secretion, similar to the tests currently used in studies of heparin-induced thrombocytopenia (see "Heparin-Induced Thrombocytopenia"). These assays were relatively insensitive to the abnormalities in ITP. When quantitative measurements of platelet IgG were developed, high values were noted in patients with ITP.[361] It was assumed that all platelet IgG was antiplatelet antibody and was located on the platelet surface. These assumptions, both of which were inaccurate, caused many difficulties in the interpretation of platelet-associated IgG measurements over the next 25 years. Normal platelets contain two distinct pools of IgG: only about 100 molecules of IgG are normally on the surface, while α granules contain about 20,000 IgG molecules.[21]

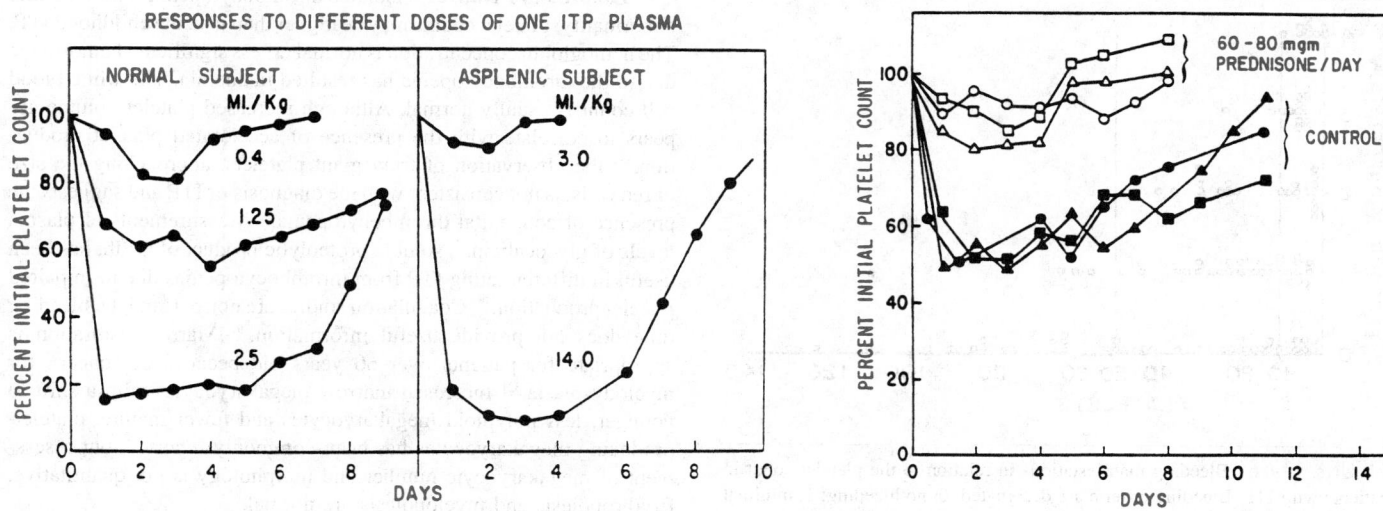

FIGURE 117-7   Response to infusions of plasma from ITP patients into normal subjects. The *left* two panels illustrate the occurrence of thrombocytopenia in a normal subject following different doses of plasma from a patient with ITP, and the results of infusion of the same ITP plasma into a splenectomized subject. Note that the ITP plasma dose that did not produce thrombocytopenia in the splenectomized subject was greater than the dose that produced marked thrombocytopenia in the normal subject. The *right* panel illustrates the effect of prednisone on the response to ITP plasma. Plasma from one ITP patient was infused into three normal subjects without and with treatment with prednisone, 60–80 mg per day. Prednisone was begun 3 h, 1 day, or 3 days before the plasma infusion and continued for a minimum of 7 days. The control infusions were given 1 and 2 months prior to, and 3 weeks after, the infusion with prednisone. (Adapted from Shulman et al,[354] with permission.)

Total platelet IgG is increased in patients with ITP, and the magnitude of increase is greater in patients with more severe thrombocytopenia.[21,362] Many patients with nonimmune thrombocytopenia, however, also have high platelet concentrations of IgG.[21,362] The concentrations of the plasma proteins, IgG, IgA, and albumin in normal platelet α granules mirror the plasma concentrations of these proteins,[363] supporting the hypothesis that these proteins are taken up by pinocytosis. In patients with ITP, platelets contain more IgG, IgA, IgM, and albumin than do normal platelets,[363] but this can be largely accounted for by increased thrombopoietic stimulation and increased platelet volume.[364,365] Thus, total platelet IgG measurements in thrombocytopenic patients may reflect only platelet size, which is known to be increased in response to thrombopoietic stress.[365] This is consistent with the observation of an increased number of younger platelets produced by thrombopoietic stress and defined by their RNA content in patients with ITP.[366] Patients with nonimmune thrombocytopenia due to increased peripheral platelet removal have increased total platelet IgG, whereas patients with thrombocytopenia due to marrow failure have normal values.[40] Exceptions to this interpretation are patients who have disorders with increased plasma IgG concentrations, such as those with IgG myeloma, liver disease, or chronic inflammatory or infectious diseases. In these patients, increased total platelet IgG content merely reflects their increased plasma IgG.[363]

Recent techniques to measure antibodies that bind to platelets or to specific platelet membrane glycoproteins detect antibodies in most patients with ITP, primarily with specificity for GPIIb/IIIa and/or GPIb/IX.[357,367,368] Titers vary inversely with the degree of thrombocytopenia during the course of the disease.[374] In one study, antibody concentrations decreased with improved platelet counts following treatment with glucocorticoid, splenectomy, cyclophosphamide, or combination chemotherapy; antibody concentrations did not change with improved platelet counts following vincristine and danazol.[369] These data suggest that the former modalities act primarily by decreasing antibody production, while the latter agents act primarily by decreasing platelet sequestration.

The clinical value of tests for antiplatelet antibodies remains uncertain. Some methods are not readily adaptable to routine clinical laboratories, and there are inconsistencies in results among reference laboratories.[370] Few studies have addressed the correlation between antiplatelet antibody tests results and clinical diagnosis. In one such study, ITP could not be distinguished from gestational thrombocytopenia[327]; in another, ITP could not be distinguished from thrombocytopenias with a demonstrable alternative etiology.[371] A third study reported that 6 of 18 patients with thrombocytopenia of apparent nonimmune etiology had serum antibodies to GPIIb/IIIa,[372] perhaps because neoepitopes can be exposed on membrane proteins during accelerated platelet destruction by any mechanism. Indeed, many plasma antibodies to GPIIb/IIIa in patients with ITP react with normally concealed cytoplasmic epitopes.[373]

In spite of problems with their measurement and interpretation, autoantibodies certainly appear to be involved in the pathogenesis of ITP. However, laboratory assays for antiplatelet antibodies in ITP remain investigational; they have not yet been demonstrated to be important for either diagnosis or management.[321]

Platelet Function.   The bleeding times of patients with ITP are usually shorter than expected for the degree of thrombocytopenia,[374] suggesting that the circulating platelets, which tend to be larger and younger than normal, have enhanced hemostatic activity. However, some patients appear to have impaired platelet function. Autoantibodies to GPIIb/IIIa and GPIb/IX can cause functional platelet disorders indistinguishable from Glanzmann thrombasthenia[375] and Bernard-Soulier syndrome,[376] but these are rare complications. Antiplatelet antibodies may also impair the aggregation of normal platelets in a manner similar to that of aspirin,[377] or inhibit platelet adhesion to subendothelial matrix.[378] Whether these observations are clinically important is unknown.

Association with Autoimmune Diseases and Other Disorders. ITP is associated with a variety of immunologic disorders. Patients in whom the thrombocytopenia is part of a clinically overt autoimmune disease are considered distinct from ITP, because the course of the

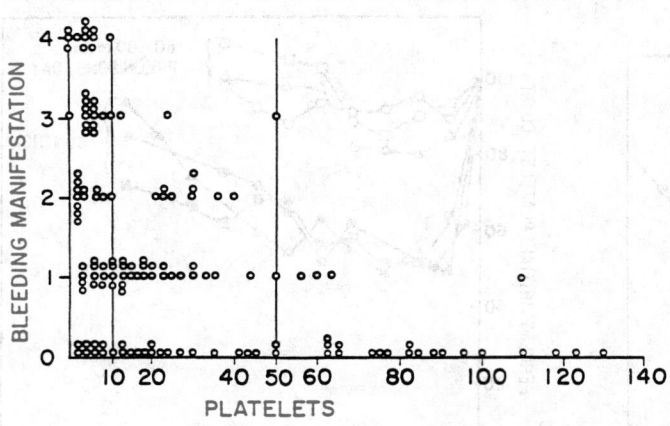

FIGURE 117-8   Bleeding manifestations in relation to the platelet count in patients with ITP. Bleeding criteria are designated: 0, no bleeding; 1, minimal bleeding after trauma; 2, spontaneous but self-limited bleeding; 3, spontaneous bleeding requiring special attention, such as nasal packs for epistaxis; and 4, severe, life-threatening bleeding. (Reproduced from Lacy and Penner[389] with permission.)

illness is primarily determined by the primary disease.[321] For example, thrombocytopenia is common in patients with SLE,[379] and management is directed principally at treating the systemic manifestations. Similarly, several case series have described the association of autoimmune thyroid disorders and thrombocytopenia[380,381]; in these patients the thrombocytopenia often resolves with effective treatment of the hyperthyroidism.[380,382] However, patients with abnormal serologic tests (e.g., antinuclear or antiphospholipid antibodies), but without a clinically evident disease such as SLE, are included within the definition of ITP because these positive serologic tests are frequently encountered in patients with typical ITP.[383–385]

Clinical Features   Most adults present with long-standing histories of purpura, which differs from the more acute presentation typical in children. An increasing number of patients are being diagnosed incidentally as a result of routine platelet counting.[346] One-third of patients in a recent case series had platelet counts greater than $30,000/\mu l$ at diagnosis; they were not treated and had no significant bleeding symptoms during 30 months of observation.[347]

The history and physical examination are normal except for the symptoms and signs of bleeding. Petechiae are not palpable and occur most commonly in dependent regions. The distribution of petechiae is also influenced by the tissue turgor, with none on the palms and soles and more in mucous membranes where hemorrhagic bullae may occur when severe thrombocytopenia is present. Symptoms and signs are predictable from the known pattern of bleeding associated with congenital platelet function disorders: purpura, menorrhagia, epistaxis, and gingival bleeding are common; gastrointestinal bleeding and hematuria are less common.[386] Intracerebral hemorrhage is uncommon, but it is the most common cause of death and may occur at any time during a prolonged course.[387,388] Older patients may be at greater risk for intracerebral hemorrhage.[347,351] Bleeding symptoms are rare unless the thrombocytopenia is severe, i.e., less than $10,000/\mu l$ $(10 \times 10^9/$ liter), and even at this level most patients do not experience major bleeding episodes (Fig. 117-8).[389]

A palpable spleen strongly suggests that ITP is not the etiology for the thrombocytopenia. One large study found that fewer than 3 percent of patients had an enlarged spleen, both by physical examination and by weight at splenectomy.[390]

Laboratory Features   Isolated thrombocytopenia is the essential abnormality. Platelet counts may be higher than in acute childhood ITP. The hemoglobin concentration is normal unless significant hemorrhage due to the thrombocytopenia has resulted in anemia. The white blood cell count is usually normal. Although increased platelet volume appears to correlate with the presence of accelerated platelet production,[364] the observation of truly giant platelets, approaching the size of red cells, is not consistent with the diagnosis of ITP and suggests the presence of congenital thrombocytopenia.[58] Measurements of plasma levels of glycocalicin, a soluble proteolytic product of GPIb, has been useful in differentiating ITP from thrombocytopenias due to impaired platelet production.[391] Coagulation studies are normal, and the bleeding time does not provide useful information.[392] Marrow aspiration is appropriate for patients over 60 years old because of concern for myelodysplasia.[321] Increased marrow megakaryocytes with a shift to younger, less polyploid megakaryocytes and fewer mature, platelet-producing megakaryocytes has been commonly reported, but assessment of megakaryocyte number and morphology is not quantitative. Erythropoiesis and myelopoiesis are normal.

Differential Diagnosis   The diagnosis of ITP is made by excluding other causes of thrombocytopenia. First, true thrombocytopenia must be distinguished from pseudothrombocytopenia caused by innocent antibodies such as EDTA-dependent agglutinins [see ''Spurious Thrombocytopenia (pseudothrombocytopenia),'' above]. Patients have been inappropriately treated with glucocorticoids and have even been subjected to splenectomy even though true thrombocytopenia never existed.[1,393] Other conditions that can mimic ITP at presentation are acute infectious illness, chronic liver disease with hypersplenism, myelodysplastic syndromes,[394,395] and chronic DIC.[396] The distinction from inherited thrombocytopenia is especially important, and recent observations suggest that inherited thrombocytopenias are not rare among patients with presumed chronic refractory ITP.[58] Drug-induced thrombocytopenia may account for some of the acute thrombocytopenias that appear to resolve spontaneously.[397,398]

Therapy, Course, and Prognosis   The clinical data on adult ITP can be estimated from 12 published series, representing 1761 patients.[321] The responses to therapy and the percentages of patients who had a complete remission at the time of the latest follow-up are remarkably consistent. Since glucocorticoids were not available until 1950, reports including patients before that time can provide information on the natural history of untreated patients. Of the ten patients with symptoms suggestive of chronic ITP, only one had a remission, and that was after 3 years; in contrast, of the 16 patients with symptoms suggestive of acute ITP, 12 had complete recovery within 3 months. Spontaneous remissions were uncommon in patients with thrombocytopenia lasting more than 100 days.[399] These observations suggest that patients at any age who have an abrupt, acute onset are more likely to have a spontaneous remission, and it may be these patients who have complete responses to glucocorticoid therapy in current practice.

More than one-third of adults with ITP fail to achieve a remission with steroids and splenectomy. Table 117-8 provides data on the frequency of spontaneous remissions and mortality in these patients, but these data are imprecise because long-term follow-up was not an objective of most reports. The mortality of patients with chronic, refractory ITP due to hemorrhage or the complications of therapy is approximately 5 percent over the lifetime of the patient. In another report of 312 patients with chronic ITP (ages 7 to 91 years), seven deaths occurred, five due to intracranial hemorrhage and two due to gastrointestinal hemorrhage.[400] Thus, the mortality in these patients is low, spontaneous remissions occur, and the reported success of many modalities does not differ greatly from the estimated frequency of spontaneous remissions.

At equivalent platelet counts, major hemorrhagic complications are more common in patients with ITP who are over 60 years of age.[347] In one study, all three hemorrhagic deaths occurred in patients 75 to 85 years old.[401] A review of 40 patients, ages 45 to 93, demonstrated more complications, greater mortality, and fewer responses to treatment in older patients.[351] Ten patients presented with life-threatening hemorrhage, and 14 others had significant gastrointestinal bleeding. Only 12 patients had a complete response to therapy, and 14 patients (35%) died of bleeding or of complications of treatment.[351]

Emergency Treatment of Acute Bleeding Due to Severe Thrombocytopenia. In patients with severe bleeding, in addition to conventional critical care measures, appropriate treatment includes platelet transfusions, high-dose parenteral glucocorticoids, and IVIg.[321] Despite presumably having short platelet survival, some patients have substantial increments in their platelet counts for many hours or even days following platelet transfusion.[402] Even if the increment is negligible, hemostasis may be achieved, at least temporarily. There are no adverse effects of platelet transfusion in patients with ITP beyond those associated with platelet transfusions in general. High doses of glucocorticoids, such as 1 g of methylprednisolone given by intravenous infusion daily for 3 days, may also cause a rapid increase of the platelet count and may ameliorate bleeding even if platelet counts remain low due to an effect on the vasculature. IVIg alone, given as 1 g/kg per day for 2 days, will increase the platelet count in most patients within 3 days.[321] A single infusion of IVIg, 0.4 to 1.0 g/kg, may increase the response to platelet transfusion and prolong the duration of response.[403] Finally, aminocaproic acid (5 g initially, then 1 g every 4 h, given orally or intravenously) has been reported to be effective in controlling acute, severe bleeding in ITP after failure of oral prednisone and platelet transfusions.[404]

Initial Management. Observation: Most patients who are incidentally discovered to have asymptomatic mild or moderate thrombocytopenia can safely be followed with no treatment. The risk that more severe thrombocytopenia will subsequently develop is estimated by one case series to be 15 percent; in this series another 15 percent of patients with asymptomatic, incidentally discovered ITP recovered spontaneously; the remaining 70 percent of patients had persistent asymptomatic thrombocytopenia.[348] Patients with platelet counts over $50,000/\mu l$ (50×10^9/liter) usually do not have spontaneous, clinically important bleeding[389] and may undergo invasive procedures.[405] Patients with platelet counts over $30,000/\mu l$ (30×10^9/liter) may also be observed without treatment and without significant risk from hemorrhage.[347]

Glucocorticoids. The proposed mechanisms of therapeutic effect of glucocorticoids in ITP are diverse. Severe thrombocytopenia may cause thinning and fenestrations of the microvascular endothelium, and glucocorticoids appear to reverse this abnormality.[406] This may explain why symptomatic purpura often improves before the platelet count increases or even without an increase in platelet count. The increased platelet count appears to reflect increased platelet production[407] as well as diminished platelet sequestration and destruction of antibody-sensitized platelets (Fig. 117-7).[354]

Prednisone, typically given in a dose of 1 mg/kg per day as a single dose, is indicated for all patients with symptomatic thrombocytopenia and probably for all patients with platelet counts below 30,000 to $50,000/\mu l$ (30 to 50×10^9/liter) who may be at increased risk for hemorrhagic complications.[321] Approximately 60 percent of patients will increase their platelet count to over $50,000/\mu l$. However, in most patients, thrombocytopenia will recur when prednisone is tapered or discontinued. The goal of prednisone therapy is to promptly lower the risk for acute hemorrhagic complications and to allow time for a spontaneous remission to occur. About one-fourth of patients will achieve a complete recovery from their ITP coincident with prednisone

therapy.[321] How long to continue prednisone therapy before considering splenectomy in refractory patients depends upon the severity of the bleeding symptoms, the dose of prednisone required to maintain an adequate response, and the risks of surgery in the individual patient. The insidious onset of osteoporosis, often within 3 months of beginning treatment, is a serious side effect of glucocorticoids.[408,409] Patients should be considered promptly for splenectomy if severe bleeding complications due to thrombocytopenia do not respond to prednisone. A common practice is to consider splenectomy in patients with persistent severe thrombocytopenia despite 4 to 6 weeks of optimal therapy.[321] Initial treatment with IVIg has no advantage over prednisone.[410]

IVIg. Following the observed disappearance of thrombocytopenia in two children with ITP who were treated with IVIg for congenital agammaglobulinemia, intravenous immunoglobulin preparations have become a standard therapy for ITP.[411] In adults, IVIg is used primarily when clinical situations require a transient increase of the platelet count or when the use of glucocorticoids is contraindicated.[412] The mechanism of action is postulated to be saturation of phagocytic Fc receptors or perhaps neutralization of antiplatelet autoantibodies by anti-idiotypic antibodies present in the IVIg.[413] The initial dose is 2 g/kg given over 2 to 5 days, and a typical response is for the platelet count to increase several days after the infusions are initiated and to return to the pretreatment level within several weeks. Comparable responses may occur with half this dose or a single dose of 0.8 g per kg.[414] In adult patients who were maintained on intermittent infusions of IVIg when platelet counts fell below $20,000/\mu l$ (20×10^9/liter), a single infusion of 60 g seemed adequate.[412] The principal side effects are fever, headache, nausea, and vomiting, which occur in 16 to 34 percent of patients,[414,415] with aseptic meningitis in 10 percent.[416] These symptoms can mimic intracerebral hemorrhage in severely thrombocytopenic patients, and often a CT scan of the head is required to determine the diagnosis. Other side effects include acute renal failure, which may be caused by the hypertonic sucrose in the IVIg preparation,[235] and hemolysis caused by alloantibodies.[417]

Anti-Rh(D) Immune Globulin. Infusion of anti-Rh(D) antiserum was tried because it was postulated that IVIg may contain red cell alloantibodies and that the mechanism of its therapeutic effect was the induction of mild hemolysis, diverting macrophages from destruction of antibody-coated platelets. Clinical trials have demonstrated that platelet counts above $50,000/\mu l$ (50×10^9/liter) could be sustained with intermittent treatment of Rh(D)$^+$ children to defer splenectomy.[418] A large experience with anti-Rh(D) has demonstrated that children with ITP respond better than adults, but that 70 percent of patients respond with an increase in platelet count of greater than $20,000/\mu l$, with half having an increase in platelet count of $>50,000/\mu l$.[136] In most patients, the response lasts more than 3 weeks.[136] These data and a retrospective study of treated children[417] suggest that the efficacy of anti-Rh(D) may be equivalent to IVIg, except that anti-Rh(D) is not effective in Rh(D)$^-$ patients (about 15 percent of the population) and is ineffective following splenectomy.[136] The only clinically important side effect of anti-Rh(D) is the predictable alloimmune hemolysis. At a dose of 50 μg/kg, few patients will have a hemoglobin decrease greater than 2 g/dl, which is not greater than the hemolysis associated with IVIg.[136,417] Other side effects, such as headache, nausea, chills, and fever, are rare (3%[136]), compared to IVIg (16 to 34 percent of patients[414,415]). Anti-Rh(D) immune globulin can be administered more rapidly than IVIg (5 to 10 min versus several hours) and is considerably less expensive.

Splenectomy. Splenectomy was a well-recognized treatment for adults with ITP for over 30 years before the introduction of glucocorticoids in 1950.[390] The success of splenectomy in achieving complete and apparently permanent responses in two-thirds of patients is reported in many case series,[321] but with longer follow-up thrombocytopenia recurs in many patients.[419] Case series that reported greater success rates may have been biased by the inclusion of children and the performance of splenectomy soon after diagnosis.[185,390] The major effects of splenectomy are twofold: (1) removal of the major site of destruction of antibody-sensitized platelets (Fig. 117-7),[354] which accounts for the frequent prompt recovery of thrombocytopenia,[390] and (2) removal of a major site of antibody synthesis.

The timing of splenectomy in adults requires judgment about the course and severity of the disease as well as the risks of glucocorticoid side effects. Surgical complications may be greater in patients who have had prolonged glucocorticoid therapy.[390] Some studies have suggested that an initial response to glucocorticoid therapy predicts a good response to splenectomy,[420] but other studies have found no relationship with the response to glucocorticoid therapy.[390,421,422] One report suggested that response to IVIg correlates with subsequent response to splenectomy,[423] but other studies have not found a correlation.[424] Attempts to predict the response to splenectomy by measuring the pattern of splenic versus hepatic sequestration with radiolabeled platelets have suggested a correlation in some studies[425] but not in others.[354,358,407,426] The overall experience with splenectomy indicates that no clinical parameters are helpful in predicting response, except that younger patients respond better.[422,426-428]

Although the immediate risks of operative and postoperative hemorrhage with splenectomy are remarkably small, even in the face of severe thrombocytopenia, it is prudent to have platelet preparations available for transfusion if bleeding is excessive during surgery. IVIg can induce a transient remission of thrombocytopenia within several days in most patients, so it can be used for preoperative preparation of patients with severe thrombocytopenia. Laparoscopic splenectomy has the disadvantage of less effective visualization to provide hemostasis in severely thrombocytopenic patients, but it offers less morbidity for patients with adequate platelet counts.[429,430]

Splenectomy is associated with a small but significantly increased risk for severe infectious complications[431]; therefore the Advisory Committee on Immunization Practices of the Centers for Disease Control and Prevention recommends that all patients should be immunized with polyvalent pneumococcal vaccine, *Haemophilus influenzae* b vaccine and quadrivalent meningococcal polysaccharide vaccine at least 2 weeks before splenectomy.[432] In addition, children are routinely placed on penicillin prophylaxis[433]; this is not routine care for adults.

Most patients who will respond to splenectomy do so within several days; responses after 10 days are unusual.[390,427] The rapidity and extent of platelet recovery appears to correlate with the durability of the response.[422,426,427] Of patients who initially respond to splenectomy and subsequently have recurrent thrombocytopenia, half will relapse within 6 months.[427] Some patients develop dramatic thrombocytosis, with platelet counts over 1,000,000/μl (1000 × 10^9/liter), but there appears to be a low risk for thrombosis.[434]

Removal of Accessory Spleens.   Accessory spleens are found and removed at the time of splenectomy in 15 to 20 percent of patients.[435-437] Additional accessory spleens may be found in as many as 10 percent of patients who are refractory to splenectomy or who relapse after splenectomy.[438] In spite of frequent reports of the efficacy of surgical removal of accessory spleens in patients with refractory or recurrent ITP, complete and durable remissions have not been documented in adults.[438] Children may have a higher frequency of partial transient responses.[438]

Splenic Irradiation and Embolization.   For patients who are poor surgical candidates, a short course (1 to 6 weeks) of radiation therapy to the spleen (total dose, 75 to 1370 cGy) may be a safe alternative treatment. In two studies, 13 of 19 patients who had platelet counts of less than 50,000/μl (<50 × 10^9/liter) responded with an increase in platelet count; in only one patient, however, was the platelet count

sustained for 6 months at a normal level.[439,440] Another alternative to splenectomy may be splenic artery embolization.[441]

Chronic Refractory ITP.   The proper management of adult patients who have not responded to glucocorticoids and splenectomy is a dilemma. Many different treatment modalities have been published, each with reports of success. However, in contrast to the results of splenectomy, results with these modalities have been inconsistent. Further, many of these additional treatments have significant risks.

Observation.   The goal of treatment is to achieve a platelet count that ensures hemostasis, not necessarily a normal platelet count. Therefore, it is appropriate to withhold treatment in patients with platelet counts greater than 30,000/μl who have no bleeding symptoms.[321] Patients who are asymptomatic with platelet counts less than 30,000/μl[389,442,443] may also be safely observed. Treatment decisions must include assessment of lifestyle and other medical conditions that may influence the relative risks of bleeding and of immunosuppressive treatment.

Glucocorticoids.   In some patients a safe platelet count can be maintained with very low doses of prednisone or intermittent doses of glucocorticoids. However, even daily prednisone doses that are equivalent to or even less than physiologic cortisol secretion (e.g., 2.5 to 5 mg per day) can cause osteoporosis by impairing normal diurnal cortisol secretion.[408,409] One report described success in 10 selected patients treated with a regimen adapted from management of multiple myeloma: dexamethasone, 40 mg per day for 4 days, repeated every 4 weeks.[444] Six of these 10 patients had failed splenectomy, and all apparently had a complete response. However, others have been unable to duplicate this success rate, and serious adverse events have been reported with this regimen.[445,446]

Azathioprine.   Azathioprine was the first agent reported to be effective in patients refractory to glucocorticoid treatment and splenectomy.[447,448] Approximately 20 percent of patients may have a complete response, defined as a normal platelet count sustained on no therapy. An additional 40 percent of patients may have a partial response, defined as an increased platelet count but only with continued treatment. The typical initial dose of azathioprine is 150 mg, or 1 to 2 mg/kg daily. Although complete responses have been seen after as many as 26 months of treatment, all responding patients increased their platelet count within 4 months.[447]

Azathioprine is relatively free of side effects, but a major concern, particularly in young patients who may require prolonged treatment, is the risk for developing a malignancy. Acute leukemia and myelodysplastic syndromes have been reported in 30 patients treated with azathioprine for nonneoplastic diseases.[449] Two patients developed leukemia and lymphoma, respectively, after prolonged treatment of ITP with azathioprine.[450,451] Risks for fetal malformations when azathioprine is taken during early pregnancy are suspected but undocumented.[452]

Cyclophosphamide.   The response to cyclophosphamide is similar to the response to azathioprine. Approximately 20 percent of patients have a complete response and 30 percent have a partial response.[448,453] A daily oral dose of 1 to 2 mg/kg per day, adjusted for leukopenia, may be given; complete responses have occurred after 1 to 6 months of treatment.[448,453] Alternatively, cyclophosphamide can be administered in larger, intermittent intravenous doses. One case series of 20 selected patients used a regimen of 1000 mg/m^2, repeated at 4-week intervals for one to five doses, and reported complete responses in 8 patients.[454] This regimen is similar to the use of cyclophosphamide in other severe autoimmune disorders.[455]

Cyclophosphamide has greater risks than azathioprine. Dose-related marrow suppression, infertility[456,457] and teratogenicity,[458] have been reported; alopecia is common; hemorrhagic cystitis occurs in about 10 percent of patients; and bladder fibrosis may occur in 25 percent.[458] The incidence of bladder cancer also appears to be increased.[449] Of greatest concern is the increased incidence of acute myelocytic leukemia and myelodysplastic syndromes. Alkylating agents are associated with a greater risk of causing malignancies than antimetabolites such as azathioprine, and daily oral doses of alkylating agents have higher risks than intermittent parenteral therapy.[449] The risk for development of acute leukemia appears to have a threshold at a total dose of 20 g.[459] Four patients have been reported who developed acute myelocytic leukemia 23 to 44 months after treatment with cyclophosphamide for chronic ITP.[451,460]

Vinca Alkaloids (Vincristine, Vinblastine). The rationale for the use of vinca alkaloids in ITP was based on their efficacy in lymphoproliferative disorders[461] and observations that vinblastine and vincristine can cause thrombocytosis in humans and experimental animals.[462,463] Vinca alkaloids have been administered either by intravenous bolus injection or intravenous infusion over several hours. Results of treatment are similar with both agents by both methods of administration. The most common regimen is vincristine, 2 mg per week by intravenous bolus, for 3 to 6 weeks. The typical platelet count response is an increase within several days and then a return to the pretreatment level within a few days to weeks. Case series vary greatly in their reports of success, with complete remissions achieved in as few as 3 percent or as many as 30 percent of patients.[464–466]

The major side effect of vincristine is dose-related peripheral neuropathy; paralytic ileus may also be a severe problem. The major side effect of vinblastine is dose-related marrow suppression. An increased frequency of second malignancies after vinca alkaloid therapy has not been reported. Vincristine causes alopecia in about 20 percent of patients; this occurs less often with vinblastine.

Danazol. In 1980, it was reported that patients treated with danazol for endometriosis had increased platelet counts.[468] Three years later, danazol was reported to increase the platelet count in patients with ITP.[467] Doses used in patients with ITP vary between 50 mg per day[469] to 800 mg per day[467]; it is unknown if there are any therapeutic differences between these regimens. When patients respond to danazol, the response is slow, occurring over a period of weeks to months. Typically, responses endure only while danazol is administered. Its major therapeutic benefit is to sustain partial remissions from symptomatic thrombocytopenia. Many patients appear to have no response.[470,471]

Side effects include headache, nausea, breast tenderness,[472] maculopapular rash,[473] and liver function abnormalities.[474] Hepatic adenomas and carcinomas have been reported in patients treated with danazol, and thus periodic ultrasound evaluations may be appropriate. Seborrhea (30 percent) and acne (20 percent) are common, and hirsutism and voice changes occur in about 7 percent of women.[471] Amenorrhea or oligomenorrhea are common and may be beneficial in symptomatic women.[471] Acute thrombocytopenia has been reported in five patients given danazol for endometriosis or to stimulate erythropoiesis; in two of these patients acute thrombocytopenia recurred with readministration of danazol.[475,476] One patient has been reported in whom thrombocytopenia worsened during treatment for ITP.[477] Acute pulmonary fibrosis has also been reported.[478]

Plasma Exchange. Plasma exchange has been used in patients who are unresponsive to other regimens with reports of limited, transient success.[479,480]

Colchicine. Colchicine treatment was tried because it has pharmacologic similarity to the vinca alkaloids, but without the latter's severe toxicities. One case series reported on 14 patients treated with colchicine,[481] 12 of whom had chronic refractory ITP. Colchicine was given in doses of 0.6 to 1.2 mg/day, adjusted from higher initial doses to avoid diarrhea. No patients had a complete response, and three had partial responses.

Vitamin C. Vitamin C was studied following a serendipitous observation of an increased platelet count in a patient who initiated taking vitamin C supplements.[482] This initial report was followed by multiple case series reporting a few patients with limited responses.[321]

Combination Chemotherapy. One report described the use of various regimens adapted from the treatment of patients with malignant lymphoma in 10 patients; 5 had a complete response.[483] Recent reports describe 4 patients treated with even more intensive chemotherapy, either with[484,485] or without[486] peripheral blood stem cell support. Of these 4 patients, 2 had complete sustained remissions,[484] 1 had no response,[485] and 1 died.[486]

Other Modalities. Seventy-two patients were treated with immunoadsorption by ex vivo perfusion of plasma through a protein A column; 16 patients (22 percent) responded with a platelet count of greater than 100,000/μl for more than 2 months.[487] However, others have reported much less favorable results and significantly greater toxicity, including severe vasculitis.[488,489] Seven patients treated with 2-chlorodeoxyadenosine had no response.[490] Reports describing patients treated with interferon-α-2b have described some success, but higher platelet counts were not sustained after interferon was discontinued.[491,492] Interferon therapy may also exacerbate thrombocytopenia.[493] Other reports have suggested benefit from treatment with cyclosporine[494] and dapsone.[495]

Treatment of ITP during Pregnancy and Delivery. The first decision is to estimate the likelihood that thrombocytopenia is due to ITP rather than gestational thrombocytopenia (Table 117-7). Tests for antiplatelet antibodies do not distinguish these presumably distinct disorders (see ''Antiplatelet Antibodies'').[327] ITP may worsen during pregnancy and improve after delivery.[329]

Early in pregnancy the management of ITP is the same as if the patient were not pregnant, using prednisone as initial therapy to treat patients whose platelet counts are less than 30,000 to 50,000/μl (30 to 50 $\times$ 10^9/liter), depending on symptoms.[321] Splenectomy should be deferred if possible, because the severity of thrombocytopenia may spontaneously improve after delivery. Splenectomy may increase the risk of fetal death and premature labor in early pregnancy, and uterine enlargement presents technical problems in performing a splenectomy later during pregnancy. IVIg is an alternative therapy that may help to delay splenectomy, although splenectomy remains the most effective treatment for severe, symptomatic, ITP.

The greatest concern for ITP during pregnancy is the risk of thrombocytopenia in the newborn infant. Although published data vary widely on the risk of thrombocytopenia in infants born to mothers with ITP,[321] a summary of published case series suggests that there is a 10 percent risk of having a platelet count of less than 50,000/μl and a 4 percent chance of having a platelet count of less than 20,000/μl.[144] The severity of ITP in the mother appears to correlate with the risk for thrombocytopenia in the infant. Neonatal thrombocytopenia is more frequent when the mother has had a splenectomy and when her platelet count has been less than 50,000/μl at some time during the pregnancy.[330,331] The occurrence of neonatal thrombocytopenia is similar among siblings.[331] Despite reports to the contrary, prednisone given for several weeks before delivery or IVIg closer to term do not seem to affect the fetal platelet count; treatment should be given only as indicated for management of the mother's thrombocytopenia.[329] Some authors recommend percutaneous umbilical blood sampling at 38 weeks' gestation to determine the fetal platelet count and recommend cesarean section delivery if the platelet count is less than 50,000/μl (50 $\times$ 10^9/liter).[324] However, this procedure has risks for fetal hemorrhage and death.[326,330,496] Direct determination of the fetal platelet count from a scalp vein when the cervix is dilated and the fetal head engaged has also been recommended, but this procedure is subject to artifacts causing either falsely low or falsely high platelet counts.[326] Current recommendations are to manage the delivery in a conventional manner, with cesarean delivery only for obstetrical indications.[321,326,332]

Neonatal intracerebral hemorrhage at birth is very rare and has not been reported among case series describing 10 or more patients with platelet counts performed at birth.[138,330,331] However, it is critical to carefully monitor the infant's platelet counts through the first several days of life, as severe thrombocytopenia and major hemorrhage can develop after delivery.[321,328,330,331,497]

CHILDHOOD ITP

Clinical Features   The peak incidence of childhood ITP occurs between ages 2 and 4 with equal incidence in boys and girls.[344,345,498] After age 10, the female predominance characteristic of adult ITP begins; therefore, ITP in adolescents, particularly adolescent girls, may be similar to the more chronic disease typically found in adults.[344]

The characteristic clinical features of childhood ITP are presented in Table 117-8 and in a summary of 12 case series reported on 1693 children.[321] Since these reports are from referral children's hospitals, they are probably biased to more severely affected patients. Children typically present with a short history of acute purpura, most often with symptoms of less than 1 or 2 weeks' duration. Bruises and petechiae are the nearly universal presenting clinical symptom. Other bleeding manifestations characteristic of thrombocytopenia, epistaxis, gingival bleeding, and gastrointestinal bleeding are uncommon.[345] A palpable spleen is present in 12 percent of patients. This difference from adults is probably related to the greater frequency of a palpable spleen in normal children, estimated to be about 10 percent.[321]

Laboratory Features   Most children present with platelet counts below 20,000/μl (20 × 10^9/liter).[321,345] Marrow aspiration has been recommended before beginning glucocorticoid treatment to exclude the possibility of acute lymphocytic leukemia, which may partially respond to glucocorticoids and thereby be masked, but this may not be necessary if the presenting clinical features are compatible with ITP and do not include atypical findings.[321] A study of 332 children with typical presentations of ITP found none to have leukemia.[499] Most U.S. pediatric hematologists perform a bone marrow aspiration before beginning glucocorticoid treatment[500]; most British pediatric hematologists do not.[345]

Course and Prognosis   Eighty-three percent of patients have a complete response within 6 months without steroid treatment or splenectomy.[321] This figure is higher than the overall response at 6 months because patients are often selected for no specific treatment based on good prognostic features: a short duration of disease with an abrupt onset and mild symptoms.[349] Most of the patients who will eventually respond develop no new purpuric symptoms after the first week. The time until the platelet count becomes normal is typically 2 to 8 weeks; approximately half of all patients who spontaneously recover do so within 4 weeks. A history of purpura longer than 2 to 4 weeks before diagnosis is the best predictor of a chronic course. Other risk factors are female sex, age over 10 years, and a higher platelet count at presentation.[498] The fate of children with chronic ITP is uncertain, but most children have a spontaneous remission when follow-up is carried on for over 15 years.[349]

Very few children with ITP have critical complications, and even fewer die or have residual disability. Among the 1693 patients in 12 case series, only 16 (1 percent) had intracerebral hemorrhage, and the risk is probably even lower with current practice.[321] Of 29 reported cases of intracerebral hemorrhage in children,[321,387] 12 occurred within the first 12 days of diagnosis, and two of these patients had a history of head trauma. The intracerebral hemorrhages in the other 17 patients occurred between 1 month and 5 years after diagnosis, typically after failure of steroids and splenectomy to induce a remission.

Most series emphasize the benign nature of childhood ITP, even for patients with chronic, symptomatic thrombocytopenia for many years.[349]

Treatment   Initial treatment is appropriate for children with platelet counts less than 10,000/μl and symptoms of minor purpura, but opinions among pediatric hematologists are sharply divided.[321] For children presenting with only bruising, without mucosal or more severe bleeding, no specific treatment is reasonable regardless of the severity of thrombocytopenia.[501] In practice, most children receive treatment, and IVIg is more widely used than glucocorticoids[500]; IVIg (0.8 g/kg as a single dose, or 2 g/kg in divided doses) can increase the platelet count slightly more rapidly than glucocorticoids, and more rapidly by several days than no treatment.[414,502] The importance of these differences is, however, uncertain, since treatment has not been shown to decrease the risk of bleeding or death.[503]

Because most children will recover completely and permanently without splenectomy and because splenectomy in children, particularly those less than 4 years of age, is associated with an increased risk of severe infection,[431,433] splenectomy is deferred for at least 6 to 12 months following the diagnosis of ITP. Even then, splenectomy is recommended only for children who have severe thrombocytopenia with significant bleeding symptoms. Splenectomy is clearly efficacious for these patients. Among the 1693 patients, only 178 underwent a splenectomy, and 126 (71 percent) had a continuous complete remission for the duration of the follow-up.[321] In a later series, only 3 of 427 children with ITP had a splenectomy.[345] In addition to all routine immunizations, polyvalent pneumococcal vaccine, *Haemophilus influenzae* b, and quadrivalent meningococcal polysaccharide vaccines should be given at least 2 weeks prior to splenectomy to achieve a maximal antibody response. The effect of these immunizations is unpredictable in children less than 2 years old. Penicillin is routinely given as prophylaxis until age 5 years.[433] Even with these precautions, splenectomized children and their parents need to be aware of the potential seriousness of febrile illnesses so that they rapidly seek medical attention.

Fewer than 10 percent of children have ITP refractory to splenectomy.[321] The efficacy of any measure beyond splenectomy is uncertain. Since the mortality for ITP in children is very low and spontaneous remissions occur even after many years,[349] potentially harmful agents must be used only in children who have symptomatic bleeding and substantial risk for death or morbidity from hemorrhage. Specific issues for the management of chronic refractory ITP are discussed above with the adult disease.

CYCLIC THROMBOCYTOPENIA

The etiology of cyclic thrombocytopenias is unknown, but many of the features suggest that these rare syndromes are unusual presentations of idiopathic (autoimmune) thrombocytopenic purpura: They occur predominantly in young women; platelet survival is shortened at the time of decreasing platelet counts; antibodies to platelet membrane glycoproteins are commonly present; cyclic thrombocytopenia can develop during the course of ITP[494,504]; and, while spontaneous remissions may occur, the cyclic occurrences of thrombocytopenia are chronic in most patients. In other patients, cyclic thrombocytopenia may be a prodrome for marrow failure.[505]

Oscillations of platelet counts within the normal range may occur in normal subjects; in some normal women oscillations appear to correlate with the menstrual cycle, with lower platelet counts preceding menstruation.[506] These observations correlate with the rare occurrence of symptomatic cyclic thrombocytopenia, which was first described in 1936 in three young women, ages 26 to 40, who had repeated episodes of severe thrombocytopenia at the onset of menses.[507] In these patients, platelet counts recovered to normal by midcycle, and the disorder spontaneously remitted after three to seven episodes. This pattern of menstrual cyclic thrombocytopenia continues to be reported,[504,508–510] though in some women the platelet cycle does not correlate with the menstrual cycle.[504,511] Less commonly, cyclic thrombocytopenia occurs in postmenopausal women and men.[505,512–514] In some patients, there are parallel cycles of neutrophils,[512] eosinophils, and lymphocytes.[507] The pathogenesis of these syndromes is varied; in some patients autoimmune platelet destruction is predominant[510,511]; in other patients, cyclic decreases in platelet production are responsible,[504,505] which may be mediated by cyclic decreases of thrombopoietin.[513,514] Another mechanism may be increased platelet phagocytosis mediated by cyclic increases of M-CSF.[513]

Management of these patients has been difficult. Prednisone often fails to correct the defect but in some patients provides a temporary remission; IVIg and splenectomy have not been effective.[505,508,511,515] Danazol induces a temporary remission in some patients with cessation of menses,[508] but oophorectomy has been ineffective.[504] Some women with menstrual cyclic thrombocytopenia have responded to birth control pills.[509]

DRUG-INDUCED THROMBOCYTOPENIA

HEPARIN-INDUCED THROMBOCYTOPENIA

Definition and History   Heparin-induced thrombocytopenia deserves particular attention because of its frequency and the variability of its clinical manifestations, which include minor and transient decreases in platelet count to severe thrombocytopenia that may be accompanied by severe thrombosis and DIC.[536–539] These complications are particularly important because of the clinical settings in which they typically occur; thus, thrombocytopenia can increase the risk of bleeding from heparin anticoagulation, and thrombosis may exacerbate the underlying thromboembolic disease for which heparin was prescribed.

Heparin was in wide clinical use for many years before thrombocytopenia was first established as an adverse reaction by the initial prospective study which documented thrombocytopenia in 16 of 52 treated patients.[540] This remarkable observation stimulated many more prospective analyses, but the 31 percent incidence of heparin-induced thrombocytopenia in the initial survey[540] has never been duplicated, and, despite multiple case reports, heparin-induced thrombosis has not been documented among more than 2000 patients in prospective studies.[541] Complicating the interpretation of the occasional occurrence of severe thrombocytopenia is the much more common occurrence of mild transient thrombocytopenia, which often resolves even with continued heparin treatment.[541] Studies of normal subjects receiving either subcutaneous[542] or intravenous[543] heparin demonstrate that platelet counts fall predictably and progressively during the first 10 days of treatment, with prompt recovery when heparin is discontinued. The heterogeneity among heparin preparations may have contributed to the inconsistency in clinical observations over the past 30 years. For example, heparin derived from beef lung probably causes more thrombocytopenia than heparin derived from porcine intestinal mucosa,[541] and differences in the occurrence of heparin-induced thrombocytopenia may even occur among different lots of heparin from the same manufacturer.[544]

Etiology and Pathogenesis   The observation that heparin predictably decreases the platelet count in normal subjects suggests a direct interaction of heparin with platelets, and this has been demonstrated in many ways. Heparin can bind to a single class of saturable sites on platelets with an apparent dissociation constant similar to the therapeutic level in plasma (0.1 to 0.4 U/ml).[545] Higher-molecular-weight fractions of heparin bind with higher affinity, probably because

of their increased total negative charge.[546] Similarly, higher-molecular-weight fractions of heparin, at therapeutic concentrations, are more active in causing platelet aggregation in plasma and enhancing aggregation and secretion induced by physiologic agonists. The platelet response varies widely, however, among normal subjects.[547–549] With higher concentrations of heparin, platelet aggregates form in blood samples in some (but not all) normal individuals. Platelet counts measured with automated counters decrease soon after heparin administration in most patients.[550,551] These observations offer a mechanism for the common observation of diminished platelet counts with heparin therapy and raise the possibility that development of antibodies to heparin may be a ubiquitous event.

Assays for heparin-dependent antiplatelet antibodies are well described but not yet immediately available in most clinical settings. In part, this is due to the complexity and unpredictability of the principal components of platelet-based assays: patient serum, normal donor platelets, and heparin. Platelets from different normal donors may or may not aggregate in the presence of patient serum and heparin[552,553]; platelets from some normal donors are aggregated by heparin without patient sera, and some patient sera can aggregate normal platelets without heparin[552]; heparin can be replaced by subaggregating concentrations of agonists such as epinephrine[552]; and the interactions are dependent on the heparin concentration, with higher concentrations inhibiting some platelet responses[554] but also causing nonspecific platelet responses in other studies.[555] In spite of these complexities, assays based on platelet secretion (^{14}C-serotonin release) have been standardized in experienced laboratories and have increased our understanding of the pathogenesis of heparin-induced thrombocytopenia.[537,539,556]

Heparin-induced thrombocytopenia appears to be due to the presence of an IgG antibody specific for complexes of heparin and the heparin-binding cationic protein, platelet factor 4 (PF4),[557,558] which is secreted from platelet α-granules and is then bound to platelet[559] and endothelial cell[560] surfaces. Antibodies may bind to heparin complexed with PF4 on platelets or endothelial cells,[561] or bind to heparin-PF4 complexes in plasma with the resulting trimolecular complex then binding to platelet surface FcγIIa receptor (FcγRIIa).[562] An attractive feature of the latter hypothesis is that these immune complexes have the ability to activate platelets and generate procoagulant membrane microparticles,[563,564] which may contribute to the thrombotic complications of heparin-induced thrombocytopenia. It is the thrombotic risk that distinguishes heparin-induced thrombocytopenia from other drug-induced thrombocytopenias.

Immune complexes activate platelets by cross-linking the FcγRIIa molecules on the platelet surface. A His/Arg polymorphism at amino acid 131 in the FcγRIIa molecule affects the binding affinity for IgG and has therefore been investigated as a possible predisposing factor for developing heparin-induced thrombocytopenia and thrombosis.[565] Thus, platelets from individuals with the His/His and His/Arg genotypes respond more to sera from patients with heparin-induced thrombocytopenia than do platelets from patients with Arg/Arg.[566,567] However, the results from five clinical studies designed to test whether this polymorphism is of clinical importance have yielded conflicting results: Three studies found that the FcγRIIa His/His genotype was overrepresented among patients with heparin-induced thrombocytopenia, consistent with the in vitro data[567–569]; one study found the opposite, an overrepresentation of the FcγRIIa Arg/Arg genotype[565]; one study found no difference.[570] The difficulty of precisely defining criteria for the diagnosis of heparin-induced thrombocytopenia and thrombosis may be responsible, at least in part, for these inconsistencies.

In addition to, or as an alternative to, the development of circulating immune complexes composed of antibody, heparin, and PF4, it has been proposed that antibodies can bind to heparin that is already bound to PF4 on the platelet surface.[561] This could enhance platelet aggregation by activating platelets and initiating the release reaction, which is consistent with data from studies demonstrating that patient sera induce release of serotonin from dense granules and initiate microparticle formation. ADP appears to be involved in this process, presumably because it is released from platelets and augments platelet aggregation.[571] The final mechanism of platelet aggregation appears to require the GPIIb/IIIa receptor, since antagonists of this receptor can inhibit platelet aggregation induced by the sera.

Clinical Features   Thrombocytopenia can occur with any heparin preparation[537]: unfractionated heparin, low-molecular-weight heparins,[572] chondroitin sulfatelike glycosaminoglycan agents,[573] and heparinlike compounds such as pentosan[574] and danaparoid.[575–577] In vitro studies of the effects of these agents on platelet activation and aggregation suggest that the higher-molecular-weight fractions of heparin interact more readily with platelets and thereby cause more thrombocytopenia,[546,547] and this has been confirmed with the demonstration of a lower incidence of thrombocytopenia in patients treated with low-molecular-weight heparin.[578] But also consistent with in vitro data, any polyanionic molecule can mimic the heparin and cause thrombocytopenia.[573] Thrombocytopenia has been reported with all routes of administration, including heparin flushes of indwelling intravenous catheters,[579] but most patients have received therapeutic doses of intravenous heparin[579] or prophylactic doses of subcutaneously administered heparin.[536]

Heparin-induced thrombocytopenia is commonly described as two syndromes, although the clinical distinction is often unclear.[537] Minimal thrombocytopenia, with platelet counts not less than 50,000/μl, may begin soon after heparin therapy is initiated; it is usually associated with large intravenous doses of heparin and may resolve even while heparin is continued. This could represent the common, possibly ubiquitous occurrence of diminished platelet counts seen in studies of normal subjects,[542,543] probably caused by the direct agglutinating effect of heparin on platelets. Tests for heparin-dependent antiplatelet antibodies are negative in these patients with mild transient thrombocytopenia.[537] Severe thrombocytopenia caused by heparin is much less common. It typically occurs after 5 to 8 days of heparin therapy, unless the patient has previously been treated with heparin, in which case it can occur immediately on administration. It may be accompanied by thrombosis or disseminated intravascular coagulation, is associated with heparin-dependent antibodies, and may recur upon readministration of heparin. Even in patients with the more severe, immunologic form of heparin-induced thrombocytopenia, platelet counts are not as low as in reports of other drug-induced thrombocytopenias; nadir platelet counts averaged 46,000 to 62,000/μl in one study.[579] Bleeding is rarely an issue; the major clinical problem is thrombosis.[536,579] The mechanism for the thrombosis is platelet activation by heparin-dependent antibodies, as described above.

Thrombosis with potentially severe and fatal complications is the most serious adverse reaction to heparin,[536,579] but the frequency of this complication is unknown. Among over 2000 patients in a group of prospective studies, only 2 had thrombotic complications, and their relation to heparin therapy was uncertain[541]; a later prospective study of 358 patients demonstrated only one patient (0.3%) with heparin-induced thrombocytopenia who also had thrombosis, and that was at the site of a femoral venous catheter used for hemodialysis.[531] A review of 23,520 consecutive patients hospitalized on an internal medicine service over 9 years, 8261 (35%) of whom were treated with heparin, demonstrated 13 (0.16%) with possible heparin-induced thrombocytopenia; the thrombocytopenia was severe in 2 patients, one of whom probably had heparin-induced arterial thrombosis (0.01%).[538] In spite of the low frequency recorded in these studies, retrospective reviews

describe many patients with heparin-induced thrombocytopenia with thrombosis: 127 patients in 14 years in a single community[536] and 32 patients in 4 years at a single hospital.[579]

Venous thrombosis is more common than arterial thrombosis in patients with heparin-induced thrombocytopenia.[536,579] In the two retrospective reviews, 29 percent and 53 percent of patients with heparin-induced thrombocytopenia developed thrombotic complications.[536,579] Deep venous thrombosis and pulmonary embolism were the most common events. Arterial thrombotic events included limb ischemia, myocardial infarction, and stroke.[536,579] Most thrombotic events occurred within the first week after diagnosis of heparin-induced thrombocytopenia.[536] Patients who developed thrombosis had a high mortality and morbidity: In a review of 32 such patients, 5 died and 3 additional patients required limb amputation.[579]

Warfarin treatment after heparin has been stopped has been reported to cause venous limb gangrene, presumably as a result of protein C depletion.[580] However, these complications may have been related to excessive warfarin doses that caused rapid declines in protein C before producing anticoagulation by reducing the plasma levels of the longer-lived procoagulants prothrombin and factor X.[581] Heparin-induced thrombocytopenia with thormbosis is probably best avoided by beginning warfarin and heparin simultaneously at the initiation of anticoagulant treatment. This allows therapeutic warfarin anticoagulation to become established in about 5 days, which is before heparin-induced thrombocytopenia is likely to occur.[581]

Rare occurrences have been reported of other allergic responses occurring simultaneously with the onset of heparin-induced thrombocytopenia, such as severe anaphylaxis with cardiopulmonary arrest.[582]

Laboratory Features   Two general types of laboratory assays have been described: (1) functional assays, based on end points of platelet aggregation or secretion, and (2) antigen assays based on ELISA using heparin-PF4 as the target antigen.[537] The principle of the functional assays is straightforward. Patient serum plus heparin are incubated with normal platelets, and an aggregation or secretion response of the platelets is measured. However, the execution of the assays may be difficult, since platelet responsiveness varies among different normal donors, with platelets from some normal donors being completely unresponsive.[537,547–549] Apparent spontaneous platelet aggregation or secretion in these assays may be caused by the presence of trace amounts of residual thrombin in the sera.

The most widely described tests are functional assays using as end points aggregation or the secretion of ^{14}C-serotonin from normal platelets preincubated with ^{14}C-serotonin.[537] Two concentrations of heparin are used in these assays: 0.1 to 0.3 U/ml, to stimulate platelet activation in the presence of platelet-dependent antibodies, and 10 to 100 U/ml, which should not cause platelet activation with sera from patients with heparin-induced thrombocytopenia, because the high heparin concentration decreases the number of heparin molecules that have more than one PF4 molecule attached and thus decreases the ability to form complexes that can cluster receptors on the platelet surface. The higher concentration is thus a control for nonspecific direct heparin activation of the normal donor platelets.[537] Although these assays can support a clinical diagnosis of heparin-induced thrombocytopenia, they may also be positive in patients with no thrombocytopenia, even patients with no history of heparin exposure.[530,532] These assays have not been adapted to routine clinical laboratories.

ELISA assays are easily adaptable to routine clinical laboratories, but their clinical value is uncertain. Direct comparison of the ELISA assay with functional assays, ^{14}C-serotonin secretion[556] or aggregation,[583,584] demonstrated general agreement, and, in each study, the ELISA identified more patients as positive, suggesting greater sensitivity. However, multiple studies have reported these antibodies in patients with no thrombocytopenia, even patients with no history of heparin exposure.[529,530,532,556,585] Thus, at present, the positive and negative predictive values of these tests remains unknown. In the few patients who had positive functional tests but negative ELISA tests, their antibodies may have been formed against heparin complexed to one or more heparin-binding chemokines (interleukin-8, neutrophil-activating peptide-2) rather than PF4 itself.[586]

Other laboratory assays are being developed to demonstrate heparin-dependent antiplatelet antibodies,[587,588] but the role of laboratory testing in clinical decision making remains unclear. When heparin-induced thrombocytopenia is suspected, heparin must be stopped. No laboratory test has been validated by demonstrating the safety of continuing heparin when a negative result is reported. Similarly, a positive ELISA assay does not necessarily confer a high risk of developing thrombocytopenia. For example, in three studies, 5 to 22 percent of patients tested before cardiac surgery were found to have positive or indeterminate results, and yet none developed the syndrome of heparin-induced thrombocytopenia.[529,532,585]

Prevention, Diagnosis, and Therapy   Awareness of the potential for thrombocytopenia with heparin use, with frequent performance of platelet counts, is the most important preventive measure. The occurrence of heparin-associated thrombocytopenia may be decreasing because of the current use of shorter courses of heparin therapy with concurrent initiation of warfarin and the increasing use of low-molecular-weight heparin.[537,581] The diagnosis of heparin-induced thrombocytopenia should be made on the basis of a platelet count less than $100,000/\mu$l, a platelet count decrease by greater than 50 percent that is not explained by other causes, or a new thromboembolic event in the absence of other etiologies.[537] If the platelet count drops below $50,000/\mu$l or there is any evidence of thrombosis, heparin should be discontinued. Since there are many reports of asymptomatic patients with platelet counts of 50,000 to $100,000/\mu$l who spontaneously recovered while continuing heparin,[541] the decision as to when to stop heparin in asymptomatic patients is complex and needs to weigh the indication for heparin and the patient's comorbidities. Evidence for disseminated intravascular coagulation should be assessed, which may itself be caused by the heparin.[540] All heparin-associated platelet and coagulation changes should reverse within several days of stopping heparin. If laboratory assays for heparin-dependent antibodies are available, they may provide supportive information, but they are unlikely to alter clinical decisions.

In most patients, the thrombocytopenia will be mild and self-limited and will be discovered at a time in the course of therapy when heparin can be safely discontinued. In the uncommon patients when alternative antithrombotic therapy is required, available options include danaparoid and recombinant hirudin[539]; investigational agents available for clinical trials or compassionate use include ancrod and argatroban.[539] Warfarin can be continued and may be sufficient. Warfarin should not be initiated with high loading doses in a patient with heparin-induced thrombocytopenia in whom heparin has been stopped, since a rapid decrease in protein C may exacerbate thrombosis.[580] Treatment for severe thrombocytopenia with thrombosis may include the use of plasma exchange.[589] There are no reports of adverse reactions to platelet transfusions, but their use in the presence of an antibody that may aggregate platelets could theoretically result in thrombosis, as has been described in thrombotic thrombocytopenic purpura.[192,229]

A difficult problem is the management of patients with a history of heparin-induced thrombocytopenia who require a procedure that routinely involves heparin anticoagulation.[590] Hemodialysis can successfully be performed without heparin.[591] Patients have undergone uncomplicated cardiac surgery with limited heparin exposure even in the presence of preoperative positive results for heparin-dependent antibodies,[529,531,585] though none of these patients had a documented clinical diagnosis of previous heparin-induced thrombocytopenia.

When heparin must be avoided during cardiac surgery, successful anticoagulation has been achieved with danaparoid,[592,593] recombinant hirudin,[594] and ancrod[590,595]; however, danaparoid dosing is difficult, and heparin-dependent antibodies may cross-react with danaparoid, resulting in thrombocytopenia and thrombosis.[575,576]

OTHER DRUG-INDUCED THROMBOCYTOPENIAS

The assessment of isolated thrombocytopenia in a patient taking several medications needs to be systematic, with drug-induced thrombocytopenia considered before establishing a diagnosis of ITP.[321] This section will discuss drugs, other than heparin and its analogs, that cause isolated thrombocytopenia by immune platelet destruction; heparin is discussed in the preceding section. Drug-induced TTP-HUS is discussed previously in this chapter; drug-induced aplastic anemia with thrombocytopenia is discussed in Chap. 31.

Etiology and Pathogenesis   Reviews of drug-induced thrombocytopenia often contain such extensive lists of implicated drugs, many of which are commonly used, that they are not helpful for decisions of which therapy to interrupt first. To address the issue of which drugs are most likely to cause thrombocytopenia, a systematic review of all published case reports defined levels of evidence to document the causal relation between the drug and the thrombocytopenia.[398] This review distinguished drugs with definite or probable causal relationships from those for which the evidence is weaker.[398] Table 117-9 presents a list of the drugs for which there is definite evidence of a causal role in producing thrombocytopenia (which includes recurrent thrombocytopenia with rechallenge in the same patient) and drugs for which the causal relation to thrombocytopenia has been validated by at least two reports with probable evidence (thus meeting all of the criteria for definite evidence except for the lack of rechallenge). Quinidine is by far the most commonly cited drug; other commonly cited drugs are similar to drugs documented in a case-control study.[397] A remarkable observation from the systematic review was how many case reports did not provide sufficient clinical information to allow a determination of even a probable causal relation.[398]

Thrombocytopenia is assumed to be the result of immune platelet destruction by drug-dependent antiplatelet antibodies. Initial experimental observations suggested that drug-antibody complexes bound to platelets via the platelet Fc-gamma receptor. This mechanism has been confirmed for heparin-induced thrombocytopenia (see below), but for other drugs, the drug-dependent antibodies appear to bind to platelets via their Fab regions.[516] The antigen on the platelet surface is formed by drug binding to a membrane glycoprotein receptor, creating a structural change that initiates antibody formation in susceptible subjects. The new antigen may be a newly revealed sequence of a surface glycoprotein or may be a complex composed of the drug and a platelet surface protein. Most experimental studies have used drug-dependent antibodies isolated from patients with quinidine or quinine-induced thrombocytopenia (Table 117-9). The antigen targets are the major platelet surface glycoproteins (GPIb/IX and GPIIb/IIIa). Different drugs may provoke drug-dependent antibodies that preferentially react with one of these glycoproteins, or drug-dependent antibodies from a single patient may react with multiple epitopes on both glycoproteins. For example, a study of sera from 15 patients with quinine-induced thrombocytopenia demonstrated that in the presence of quinine, the antibodies bound to two distinct domains on GPIb/IX, one on GPIbα and one on GPIX.[517] Some patients had only one of the antibodies; some had both. The same domains on GPIb/IX also appear to be the antigenic targets for quinidine[518,519] and ranitidine-dependent[520] antiplatelet antibodies. Definition of the specific epitope involved in patient reactions with drug-dependent antibodies may not only elucidate the mechanism of drug-induced thrombocytopenia but also identify polymorphisms in GPIb/IX that cause sensitivity for producing

DRUG	NUMBER OF PATIENT CASE REPORTS		SEVERITY OF BLEEDING	
	LEVEL I	LEVEL II	MAJOR	MINOR
Quinidine (Quiniglute, Cardioquin)	15	23	3	11
Quinine (Quinamm, Quindan)	4	3	2	4
Rifampin (Rifadin, Rimactane)	4	3	1	3
Trimethoprim/Sulfamethoxazole (Bactrim, Septra)	3	7	4	2
Methyldopa (Aldomet)	3	3	0	1
Acetaminophen (Tylenol, Panadol)	3	2	2	1
Digoxin (Lanoxin)	3	0	0	2
Danazol (Danocrine)	2	4	0	4
Diclofenac (Cataflam, Voltaren)	2	2	0	2
Aminoglutethimide (Cytadren)	2	1	1	1
Amphotericin B (Amphocin, Fungizone)	2	1	1	0
Aminosalicylic Acid (Paser)	2	1	1	1
Oxprenolol (Trasicor)	2	1	0	1
Vancomycin (Vancoled)	2	1	1	1
Levamisole (Ergamisol)	2	0	0	0
Meclofenamate (Meclodium)	2	0	0	0
Diatrizoate Meglumine/Diatrizoate Sodium (Hypaque Meglumine)	2	0	0	0
Amiodarone (Cordarone)	2	0	0	0
Naldixic Acid (Negram)	1	5	0	1
Cimetidine (Tagamet)	1	5	0	1
Chlorothiazide (Diuril)	1	2	0	1
Diatrizoate Meglumine (Urografin)	1	2	0	2
Interferon Alpha (Roferon A, Intron A)	1	2	0	1
Sulfasalazine (Azulfidine)	1	2	0	0
Ethambutol (Myambutol)	1	1	1	0
Iopanoic Acid (Telepaqye)	1	1	0	1
Sulfisoxazole (Gantrisin)	1	0	0	1
Tamoxifen (Nolvadex)	1	0	0	0
Thiothixene (Navane)	1	0	0	0
Naphazoline (Privine, Vasocon-A)	1	0	0	0
Amrinone (Inocor)	1	0	0	0
Lithium (Lithonate, Eskalith)	1	0	0	0
Diazepam (Valium)	1	0	0	0
Haloperidol (Haldol)	1	0	0	0
Alprenolol (Aptin)	1	0	0	1
Tolmetin (Tolectin)	1	0	0	0
Nitroglycerine (Nitrogard, Nitroglyn)	1	0	0	0
Minoxidil (Loniten)	1	0	0	1
Diazoxide (Proglycem, Hyperstat)	1	0	0	0
Chlorpromazine (Thorazine)	1	0	0	0
Isoniazid (Nydrazid)	1	0	0	0
Cephalothin (Keflin)	1	0	0	0
Difluormethylornithine (Eflornithine, Ornidyl)	1	0	0	0
Piperacillin (Pipracil)	1	0	0	1
Diethylstilbestrol (Stilphostrol)	1	0	0	0
Methicillin (Staphcillin)	1	0	0	1
Deferoxamine (Desferal)	1	0	0	0
Novobiocin (Albamycin)	1	0	0	0
Gold (Ridaura, Solganol)	0	11	3	3
Procainamide (Pronestyl)	0	7	0	0
Carbamazepine (Tegretol)	0	5	0	0
Hydrochlorothiazide (Aquazide-H, Esidrix)	0	4	0	2
Ranitidine (Zantac)	0	4	0	0
Chlorpropamide (Diabinese)	0	3	0	1
Oxyphenbutazone (Tandearil, Oxalid)	0	2	0	2
Sulindac (Clinoril)	0	2	0	1
Ibuprofen (Motrin)	0	2	0	2
Phenytoin (Dilantin)	0	2	0	0
Oxytetracycline (Terramycin)	0	2	0	0
Glibenclamide (Diabeta, Micronase)	0	2	0	1
Fluconazole (Diflucan)	0	2	0	0
Captopril (Capoten)	0	2	0	0
Ampicillin (Omnipen, Totacillin)	0	2	1	1

*The full list of articles reviewed and the database established by this review, as well as the methodology for establishing levels of evidence, are available at http://moon.ouhsc.edu/jgeorge, which can be accessed through the *Williams Hematology* 6th edition web page. Reprinted from George and colleagues.[398]

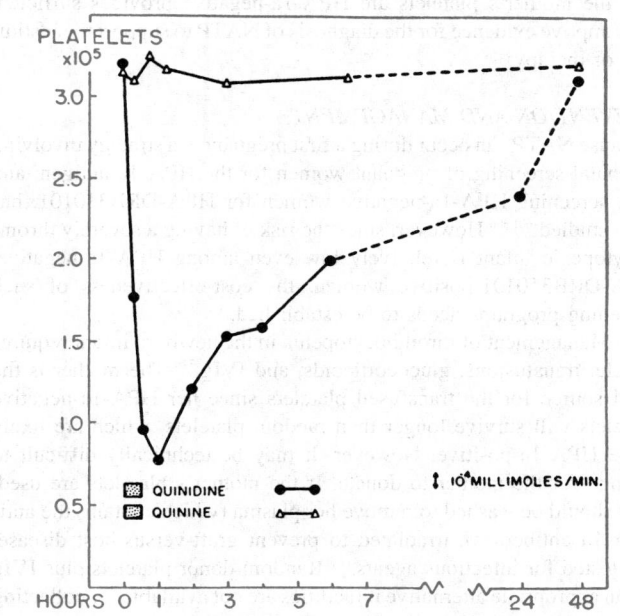

FIGURE 117-9   Induction of thrombocytopenia by infusion of a total of 1.3 mg of quinidine over a 24-min period in a patient with quinidine-dependent antibody. A lower dose of quinidine administered earlier was without effect. (From Shulman NR: *J Exp Med* 107:711, 1958.)

drug-dependent antiplatelet antibodies. Sulfonamides, along with quinidine and quinine, are frequent causes of drug-induced thrombocytopenia (Table 117-7). Studies of sera from 15 patients with thrombocytopenia caused by sulfamethoxazole or sulfisoxazole demonstrated that the antigenic epitope was not on GPIb/IX but on GPIIb/IIIa.[521] Some antibodies from patients with quinidine and quinine-dependent antiplatelet antibodies also react with GPIIb/IIIa.[522]

In addition to specificity for discrete epitopes on platelet surface glycoproteins, drug-dependent antibodies are highly specific for the structure of the drug; for example, no cross-reactivity occurs between quinidine and quinine-dependent antibodies (Fig. 117-9) or between sulfamethoxazole and sulfisoxazole-dependent antibodies, even though both pairs of drugs have similar structures.[521] Therefore the neoantigens produced by drug binding to platelets create discrete epitopes that are sensitive to minor changes in drug structure.

The implications of this mechanism for platelet destruction are apparent. A patient with prior sensitivity to the drug will have preformed antibodies that immediately react with the altered platelets upon repeat drug exposure, as demonstrated in Fig. 117-9. An exception to this is the immediate acute thrombocytopenia that may occur with the initial administration of the new class of antithrombotic agents that block the platelet fibrinogen receptor, GPIIb/IIIa.[523,524] It has been postulated that these patients have preformed antibodies to epitopes exposed on GPIIb/IIIa by drug binding; these could be the same antibodies that cause in vitro EDTA-dependent platelet agglutination and pseudothrombocytopenia.[34,35,525]

Diagnosis   The diagnosis can only be made by recovery from thrombocytopenia and can only be confirmed by recurrent thrombocytopenia with rechallenge of the drug. Prompt recovery is predictable, within 5 to 7 days.[398] Gold-induced thrombocytopenia is an exception, as gold salts are retained for a long time within the body and thrombocytopenia can persist for months, becoming indistinguishable from ITP.[526] Rechallenge with a suspected drug may be considered but can be dangerous, as severe thrombocytopenia can rapidly develop with

even very small doses (Fig. 117-9). However, when any one of multiple drugs may be involved and all are important for management, it may be appropriate to reintroduce them individually, followed by several days of close observation. For common drugs, especially those that can be purchased without a prescription, it may be safer to supervise a rechallenge and unequivocally document risk rather than risk future, unintentional use.

Laboratory assays can detect drug-dependent antibodies, and positive results can support a clinical diagnosis. However, the laboratory role remains largely investigational, since results are not promptly available when a clinical decision must be made about discontinuing a drug. Furthermore, no laboratory test has been validated by continuing a suspected drug with no adverse effects following a negative laboratory test.

Drug-dependent antibodies can be detected by flow cytometry techniques,[521] MAIPA,[527] and SPRCA.[528] Strongly positive tests are apparent, but distinction of positive from negative tests is arbitrary and not yet clinically validated. Positive tests for heparin-dependent antibodies have been reported in patients without thrombocytopenia,[529–532] and patients with clinical evidence for drug-induced thrombocytopenia may have negative tests using multiple techniques.[520,521]

Clinical and Laboratory Features   In patients with newly discovered thrombocytopenia, all medications should be identified. It is important to document not only prescription medications but also nonprescription drugs, such as products with acetaminophen (Table 117-9),[398] and drinks that may include quinine ("tonic water").[533,534]

Drug-induced thrombocytopenia typically produces profoundly low platelet counts. Among the 247 patient case reports with evidence for a definite or probable causal relation of the drug to thrombocytopenia, 23 patients (9%) had major bleeding, including two patients who died from bleeding,[398] and 68 patients (28%) had overt but minor bleeding; 96 patients (39%) had only purpura or trivial bleeding, and the remainder had no bleeding.[398] The time from beginning the drug to the initial occurrence of thrombocytopenia varies from 1 day to 3 years, but the median time is only 14 days.[398] With rechallenge, acute thrombocytopenia may occur within minutes but almost always within 3 days (Fig. 117-9).[398] Patients may also have other signs and symptoms of drug sensitivity: nausea and vomiting, rash, fever, and abnormal liver function tests.[535] Laboratory data may also demonstrate leukopenia, indicating multiple cell targets of the drug-dependent antibodies.[535] Patients who have systemic adverse reactions manifesting TTP-HUS are described in the above section on TTP-HUS.

Treatment   Withdrawal of the offending drug is the most important therapeutic measure. Prednisone is commonly given, as the distinction from ITP is never initially clear; however, it does not appear to influence recovery.[535] In patients with major bleeding, emergent treatment should be the same as for ITP: platelet transfusions, high doses of parenteral methylprednisolone, and possibly also IVIg.[321]

NEONATAL ALLOIMMUNE THROMBOCYTOPENIA

ETIOLOGY AND PATHOGENESIS

Approximately 0.14 percent of all newborns have platelet counts less than 50,000/μl (Table 117-7),[322,596,597] and alloimmunization is responsible for about one-half of these cases. These data are consistent with the risk for fetal-maternal incompatibility of platelet alloantigens, the risk for maternal antibody formation in response to incompatible fetal platelets, and the risk for neonatal thrombocytopenia when maternal alloantibodies are present. In NATP, fetal platelets are destroyed by transplacentally acquired maternal antibodies against fetal platelet alloantigens inherited from the father. NATP is comparable to neonatal alloimmune hemolytic anemia due to maternal immunization by Rh(D)$^+$ fetal red cells (see Chap. 58), except that NATP frequently occurs during the first pregnancy, indicating that maternal immunization with fetal platelets can occur during pregnancy, not only at delivery, when red cell immunization occurs.

In NATP the dominant alloantigen is HPA-1a (Pl[A1]). In an analysis of 348 infants with suspected NATP, the diagnosis was confirmed by demonstration of antibodies to platelet-specific alloantigens in 117 (34%) of the mothers; 78 percent of the alloantibodies were anti-HPA-1a, 19 percent were anti-HPA-5b (Br[a]), and 3 percent were other alloantigens, including anti-HPA-1b (Pl[A2]) and anti-HPA-3a (Bak[a]).[598] Only 2.5 percent of the Caucasian population is HPA-1a-negative, but in this study[598] 144 (41%) of the mothers of newborns with NAPT were HPA-1a-negative. Since the frequency of NATP due to HPA-1a incompatibility (about 0.05%) is much lower than the frequency of HPA-1a negativity in the Caucasian maternal population (2.5%), it is clear that not all mothers who are at risk routinely develop antibodies. An association between HLA-DRB3*0101 (DR52a) in the mother and NATP suggests that this HLA determinant is important in permitting an immune response to be mounted. The frequency of this allele in the population is 32 percent.[599] In a prospective study of 24,417 consecutive pregnant women (essentially all Caucasian, 55% multiparous, but only one with a previously thrombocytopenic child), 678 (2.8%) were HPA-1a-negative, of whom 385 were observed throughout pregnancy.[599] Antibodies to HPA-1a were detected in 46 of the 385 women (12%), all but one of whom was HLA-DRB3*0101 (DR52a)-positive, yielding an odds ratio of 140. Twenty-six of the 46 women had persistent antenatal antibodies and HPA-1a-positive infants; of these infants, 9 had severe thrombocytopenia (platelet count <50,000/μl).[599] Severe NATP was significantly associated with a third-trimester anti-HPA-1a titer of greater than 1:32; severe NATP did not occur in infants of women with either transient or postnatal-only antibodies.[599] These data are consistent with the observations of NATP in other case series (Table 117-7)[322,596,597]: HPA-1a alloimmunization complicates 1/350 unselected pregnancies, resulting in severe thrombocytopenia in 1/1200 (0.08%).[599] Since only 0.5 percent of Americans of African descent are HPA-1a-negative, their incidence of NATP is less than that of the Caucasian population.[600]

Among other platelet alloantibodies identified in NATP, most are anti-HPA-5b (Br), and these infants are less severely affected.[598,601] Other alloantibodies may cause NATP but are rarely important.[326] Since allelic gene frequencies vary among different racial and ethnic groups, the etiology of NATP will also vary. For example, among Japanese the gene frequency for HPA-1b is much lower than in Caucasian populations (0.02 vs. 0.15), and the gene frequency of HPA-4b is much higher (0.0083 vs. <0.001).[602] As expected, therefore, anti-HPA-1a has not been shown to cause NATP in the Japanese population, while antibodies to HPA-4b are the most common.[603]

CLINICAL AND LABORATORY FEATURES

In contrast to neonatal alloimmune hemolytic anemia, about half of infants with NATP are born to primiparous mothers.[326,598] The risk for NATP in a subsequent fetus of alloimmunized mothers is 85 to 90 percent,[604] and generally the second neonate's thrombocytopenia is similar to, or more severe, than that found in the first neonate.[326] In a case series of 88 infants with NATP due to anti-HPA-1a antibodies, 90 percent of infants had purpura, 66 percent had hematomas, 30 percent had gastrointestinal bleeding, and 14 percent had intracerebral hemorrhages.[598] Five of the intracerebral hemorrhages occurred in utero.[598] Bleeding may also occur following birth as the platelet count usually falls further during the first several days of life.[598] Death or neurologic impairment may occur in up to 25 percent of infants.[605] Platelet counts recover to normal in 1 to 2 weeks.[598]

In every respect, NATP is more severe than thrombocytopenia in infants born to mothers with ITP.[138] As a result, determination

that the mother's platelets are HPA-1a-negative provides sufficient presumptive evidence for the diagnosis of NATP to support the institution of therapy.

PREVENTION AND MANAGEMENT

Because NATP can occur during a first pregnancy, a strategy involving antenatal screening of pregnant women for the HPA-1a antigen, and then screening HPA-1a-negative women for HLA-DRB3*0101, has been studied.[601,606] However, since the risk of having a severely thrombocytopenic infant is relatively low even among HPA-1a-negative, HLA-DRB3*0101-positive women, the cost-effectiveness of such screening programs needs to be established.

Management of thrombocytopenia in the newborn infant requires platelet transfusions, glucocorticoids, and IVIg.[326] The mother is the ideal source for the transfused platelets since her HPA-1a-negative platelets will survive longer than random platelets, which are likely to be HPA-1a-positive. However, it may be technically difficult to arrange for the mother to donate. If the mother's platelets are used, they should be washed to remove her plasma (which contains the anti-HPA-1a antibodies), irradiated to prevent graft-versus-host disease, and tested for infectious agents.[607] Random donor platelets plus IVIg are an appropriate alternative if facilities are not available for collecting and preparing maternal platelets.

The management of subsequent pregnancies presents several interesting challenges. A prospective study of 107 fetuses whose older siblings had NATP found that at the initial in utero sampling (which took place before 24 weeks of gestation in almost 50 percent of the pregnancies), only 4 percent had normal platelet counts, 70 percent had platelet counts less than 50,000/μl, and 50 percent had platelet counts less than 20,000/μl.[604] The median initial platelet count was 18,000/μl in the 97 fetuses with HPA-1a incompatibility compared with 60,000/μl in the 10 fetuses with other antigen incompatibilities. Determination of fetal platelet counts by percutaneous blood sampling from the umbilical cord (cordocentesis) has significant risks, including hemorrhage and death of the fetus.[496] Treatment of NATP includes administration of IVIg and glucocorticoids to the mother,[608] which appears to reduce the frequency of in utero fetal intracerebral hemorrhage[604,608] but is not effective in all patients.[605] In some infants, serial in utero platelet transfusions are required.[26] Delivery by scheduled cesarean section, without labor, may reduce the risk for neonatal intracerebral hemorrhage.[609]

POSTTRANSFUSION PURPURA

Acute, severe thrombocytopenia occurring about 5 to 15 days after a blood transfusion and associated with a high titer of platelet-specific alloantibodies is a rare but well-recognized disorder defined as *posttransfusion purpura* (PTP).[600] Patients have been described who also have alloantibodies against red cells and granulocytes.[610]

Etiology and Pathogenesis   Although the sequence of events leading to PTP is clear, the etiology and pathogenesis remain obscure. Platelet destruction is caused by an alloantibody to a platelet-specific antigen; as with NATP, anti-HPA-1a (Pl[A1]) is implicated in about 80 percent of cases, but PTP due to alloimmunization to most other platelet-specific antigens has been reported.[600] Therefore, PTP occurs predominantly among HPA-1a-negative individuals who constitute 2.5 percent of Caucasians and 0.5 percent of Americans of African descent. Most patients are women, and most women are multiparous.[600]

The initial alloantibody formation to transfused HPA-1a-positive platelets is well-documented though uncommon and possibly dependent on linkage to the HLA-DRB3*0101 genotype, as in NATP.[599] What remains obscure is how the alloantibodies destroy the patient's own (HPA-1a-negative) platelets. Several hypotheses have been proposed, with varying degrees of experimental support. Soluble HPA-

1a antigen on platelet membrane microparticles is present in blood products[611] and may adsorb to the patient's platelets, providing the target antigen.[612,613] This hypothesis also provides a potential explanation for the protracted persistence of PTP for 4 to 6 weeks in some patients, since recycling of soluble antigen from platelet to platelet may occur. A second hypothesis is that immune complexes of soluble HPA-1a antigen and anti-HPA-1a alloantibodies mediate autologous platelet destruction.[600] A third hypothesis is that an autoantibody forms in parallel with the alloantibody, recognizing a conserved structural determinant adjacent to the specific antigen polymorphic site, and this antibody then destroys autologous platelets.[604]

Clinical and Laboratory Features   Case reports of PTP describe severe thrombocytopenia (platelet counts <5,000/μl) with major bleeding. Often a febrile reaction accompanies the initial presentation, inciting transfusion and subsequent transfusions.[600] Deaths from intracerebral hemorrhage have been reported.[600] Since PTP, by definition, follows transfusion of a blood product (usually packed red cells), patients are typically hospitalized and often acutely ill; therefore sepsis and drug-induced thrombocytopenia are always included in the differential diagnosis. Excluding other causes of thrombocytopenia in patients following marrow transplantation can be particularly difficult.[615]

Antibodies to a platelet-specific alloantigen, which can be distinguished from antibodies to HLA antigens, can be detected by a number of different available assays. The patient's own platelet type will only be evaluable after recovery; then documentation that the patient is HPA-1a-negative further supports the diagnosis of PTP.

Treatment, Course, and Prognosis   Because of the severity of the thrombocytopenia, treatment often needs to be initiated without having a firm diagnosis. Platelet transfusions are usually ineffective in achieving a platelet count increment and may cause severe systemic reactions[600]; nevertheless, if the patient has severe, active bleeding, platelet transfusion support is essential. Even HPA-1a-negative platelets may be rapidly destroyed, though some reports describe satisfactory responses.[615] Glucocorticoids and IVIg are usually effective. Plasma exchange is reported to be effective in 80 percent of patients.[600] Thrombocytopenia begins to resolve in several days following treatment in most patients, though it may be persistent and severe in some.[600] Anti-HPA-1a antibodies may persist in some patients following recovery,[616] but interestingly PTP may not recur with subsequent transfusion of HPA-1a-positive blood products.[617]

REFERENCES

1. Murphy EA, Francis ME: The estimation of blood platelet survival: II. The multiple hit theory. *Thromb Diath Haemorrh* 25:52, 1971.

2. International Committee for Standardization in Hematology: Panel on diagnostic application of radioisotopes in hematology. Recommended methods for radioisotope platelet survival studies. *Blood* 50:1137, 1977.

3. International Committee for Standardization in Hematology: Panel on diagnostic applications of radionuclides. Recommended method for indium-111 platelet survival studies. *J Nucl Med* 29:564, 1988.

4. Savage B, McFadden PR, Hanson SR, Harker LA: The relation of platelet density to platelet age: survival of low- and high-density [111]Indium-labeled platelets in baboons. *Blood* 68:386, 1986.

5. Aster RH: Pooling of platelets in the spleen: role in the pathogenesis of "hypersplenic" thrombocytopenia. *J Clin Invest* 45:645, 1966.

6. Heyns ADP, Lotter MG, Badenhorst PN, et al: Kinetics and fate of ^{111}In-oxime labeled platelets in asplenic subjects. *Thromb Haemost* 44:100, 1980.

7. Aster RH: Studies of the mechanism of "hypersplenic" thrombocytopenia in rats. *J Lab Clin Med* 70:736, 1967.

8. Wadenvik H, Denfors I, Kutti J: Splenic blood flow and intrasplenic platelet kinetics in relation to spleen volume. *Br J Haematol* 67:181, 1987.

9. Lee EJ, Schiffer CA: Evidence for rapid mobilization of platelets from the spleen during intensive plateletpheresis. *Am J Hematol* 19:161, 1985.

10. Heyns ADP, Badenhorst PN, Lotter MG: Kinetics and mobilization from the spleen of indium-111-labeled platelets during platelet apheresis. *Transfusion* 25:215, 1985.

11. Wadenvik H, Kutti J: The effect of an adrenaline infusion on the splenic blood flow and intrasplenic platelet kinetics. *Br J Haematol* 67:187, 1987.

12. Aster RH, Jandl JH: Platelets sequestration in man: I. Methods. *J Clin Invest* 43:843, 1964.

13. Heyns ADP, Lotter MG, Badenhorst PN, et al: Kinetics of distribution and sites of destruction of ^{111}In-labeled human platelets. *Br J Haematol* 44:269, 1980.

14. Freden K, Vilen L, Lundborg P: The peripheral platelet count and the isoprenaline-induced splenic platelet pooling in response to beta-adrenoceptor blockade. *Scand J Haematol* 23:245, 1979.

15. Vilen L, Freden K, Kutti J: Presence of a non-splenic platelet pool in man. *Scand J Haematol* 24:137, 1980.

16. Harker LA: The kinetics of platelet production and destruction in man. *Clin Haematol* 6:671, 1977.

17. Tomer A, Hanson SR, Harker LA: Autologous platelet kinetics in patients with severe thrombocytopenia: discrimination between disorders of production and destruction. *J Lab Clin Med* 118:546, 1991.

18. Hanson SR, Slichter SJ: Platelet kinetics in patients with bone marrow hypoplasia: evidence for a fixed platelet requirement. *Blood* 66:1105, 1985.

19. Rinder HM, Munz UJ, Ault KA, et al: Reticulated platelets in the evaluation of thrombopoietic disorders. *Arch Pathol Lab Med* 117:606, 1993.

20. Ault KA, Rinder HM, Mitchell J, et al: The significance of platelets with increased RNA content (reticulated platelets). *Amer J Clin Path* 98:637, 1992.

21. George JN: Platelet immunoglobulin G: its significance for the evaluation of thrombocytopenia and for understanding the origin of alpha-granule proteins. *Blood* 76(5):859, 1990.

22. Onder O, Weinstein A, Hoyer LW: Pseudothrombocytopenia caused by platelet agglutinins that are reactive in blood anticoagulated with chelating agents. *Blood* 56:177, 1980.

23. Bizzaro N: EDTA-dependent pseudothrombocytopenia: a clinical and epidemiological study of 112 cases, with 10-year follow-up. *Am J Hematol* 50:103, 1995.

24. Bizzaro N, Goldschmeding R, Von dem Borne AEGK: Platelet satellitism is Fcgamma RIII (CD16) receptor-mediated. *Am J Clin Pathol* 103:740, 1995.

25. Bizzaro N: Platelet satellitosis to polymorphonuclears: cytochemical, immunological, and ultrastructural characterization of eight cases. *Am J Hematol* 36:235, 1991.

26. Dialdetti M, Fishman P: Satellitism of platelets to monocytes in a patient with hypogammaglobulinaemia. *Scand J Haematol* 21:305, 1978.

27. Payne BA, Pierre RV: Pseudothrombocytopenia: a laboratory artifact with potentially serious consequences. *Mayo Clin Proc* 59:123, 1984.

28. Savage RA: Pseudoleukocytosis due to EDTA-induced platelet clumping. *Am J Clin Pathol* 81:317, 1984.

29. Vicari A, Banfi G, Bonini PA: EDTA-dependent pseudothrombocytopaenia: a 12-month epidemiological study. *Scand J Clin Lab Invest* 48:537, 1988.

30. Garcia Suarez J, Calero MA, Ricard MP, et al: EDTA-dependent pseudothrombocytopenia in ambulatory patients: clinical characteristics and role of new automated cell-counting in its detection. *Am J Hematol* 39:146, 1992.

31. Sweeney JD, Holme S, Heaton WAL, et al: Pseudothrombocytopenia in plateletpheresis donors. *Transfusion* 35:46, 1995.

32. Bartels PCM, Schoorl M, Lombarts AJPF: Screening for EDTA-dependent deviations in platelet counts and abnormalities in platelet distribution histograms in pseudothrombocytopenia. *Scand J Clin Lab Invest* 57:629, 1997.

33. Hoyt RH, Durie BGM: Pseudothrombocytopenia induced by a monoclonal IgM kappa platelet agglutinin. *Am J Hematol* 31:50, 1989.

34. Casonato A, Bertomoro A, Pontara E, et al: EDTA dependent pseudothrombocytopenia caused by antibodies against the cytoadhesive receptor of platelet GpIIb-IIIa. *J Clin Pathol* 47:625, 1994.

35. Fiorin F, Steffan A, Pradella P, et al: IgG platelet antibodies in EDTA-dependent pseudothrombocytopenia bind to platelet membrane glycoprotein IIb. *Amer J Clin Path* 110:178, 1998.

36. Pidard D, Didry D, Kunicki TJ, Nurden AT: Temperature-dependent effects of EDTA on the membrane glycoprotein IIb-IIIa complex and platelet aggregability. *Blood* 67:604, 1986.

37. Ginsberg MH, Lightsey A, Kunicki TJ, et al: Divalent cation regulation of the surface orientation of platelet membrane glycoprotein IIb. Correlation with fibrinogen binding function and definition of a novel variant of Glanzmann's thrombasthenia. *J Clin Invest* 78:1103, 1986.

38. Bizzaro N, Brandalise M: EDTA-dependent pseudothrombocytopenia: Association with antiplatelet and antiphospholipid antibodies. *Am J Clin Pathol* 103:103, 1995.

39. Solanki DL, Blackburn BC: Spurious thrombocytopenia during pregnancy. *Obstet Gynecol* 65:14S, 1985.

40. Berkman N, Michaeli Y, Or R, Eldor A: EDTA-dependent pseudothrombocytopenia: a clinical study of 18 patients and a review of the literature. *Am J Hematol* 36:195, 1991.

41. Peng J, Friese P, Heilmann E, et al: Aged platelets have an impaired response to thrombin as quantitated by P-selectin expression. *Blood* 83:161, 1994.

42. Hill-Zobel RL, McCandless B, Kang SA, et al: Organ distribution and fate of human platelets: Studies of asplenic and splenomegalic patients. *Am J Hematol* 23:231, 1986.

43. Weiss L: A scanning electron micrographic study of the spleen. *Blood* 43:665, 1974.

44. Toghill PJ, Green S, Ferguson R: Platelet dynamics in chronic liver disease with special reference to the role of the spleen. *J Clin Path* 30:367, 1977.

45. Villalobos TJ, Adelson E, Riley PA, Crosby WH: A cause of thrombocytopenia and leukopenia that occurs in dogs during deep hypothermia. *J Clin Invest* 37:1, 1958.

46. Yau TM, Carson S, Weisel RD, et al: The effect of warm heart surgery on postoperative bleeding. *J Thorac Cardiovasc Surg* 103:1155, 1992.

47. Pina-Cabral JM, Ribeiro da Silva A, Almeida-Dias A: Platelet sequestration during hypothermia in dogs treated with sulphinpyrazone and ticlopidine—reversibility accelerated after intra-abdominal rewarming. *Thromb Haemost* 54:838, 1985.

48. Reddick RL, Poole BL, Penick GD: Thrombocytopenia of hibernation: Mechanism of induction and recovery. *Lab Invest* 28:270, 1973.

49. Chan KM, Beard K: A patient with recurrent hypothermia associated with thrombocytopenia. *Postgrad Med J* 69:227, 1993.

50. Kutti J, Weinfeld W, Westin J: The relationship between splenic platelet pool and spleen size. *Scand J Haematol* 9:351, 1972.

51. El-Khishen MA, Henderson JM, Millikan WJ: Splenectomy is contraindicated for thrombocytopenia secondary to portal hypertension. *Surg Gynecol Obstet* 160:223, 1985.

52. Martin TG III, Somberg KA, Meng YG, et al: Thrombopoietin levels in patients with cirrhosis before and after orthotopic liver transplantation. *Ann Intern Med* 127:285, 1997.

53. Lawrence SP, Lezotte DC, Durham JD, et al: Course of thrombocytopenia of chronic liver disease after transjugular intrahepatic portosystemic shunts (TIPS): a retrospective analysis. *Dig Dis Sci* 40:1575, 1995.

54. Jackson DP, Krevans JR, Conley CL: Mechanism of the thrombocytopenia that follows multiple whole blood transfusions. *Trans Assoc Am Phys* 69:155, 1956.

55. Reed RLI, Heimbach DM, Counts RB: Prophylactic platelet administration during massive transfusion: a prospective, randomized, double-blind clinical study. *Ann Surg* 203:40, 1986.

56. Hiippala ST, Myllylä GJ, Vahtera EM: Hemostatic factors and replacement of major blood loss with plasma-poor red cell concentrates. *Anesth Analg* 81:360, 1995.

57. Leslie SD, Toy PTCY: Laboratory hemostatic abnormalities in massively transfused patients given red blood cells and crystalloid. *Am J Clin Pathol* 96:770, 1991.

58. Najean Y, Lecompte T: Hereditary thrombocytopenias in childhood. *Semin Thromb Hemost* 21:294, 1995.

59. Young NS, Alter BP: Clinical features of Fanconi's anemia, in *Aplastic Anemia: Acquired and Congenital*, p 275. Philadelphia: Saunders, 1994.

60. D'Andrea AD, Grompe M: Molecular biology of Fanconi anemia: Implications for diagnosis and therapy. *Blood* 90:1725, 1997.

61. Liu JM, Auerbach AD, Young NS: Fanconi anemia presenting unexpectedly in an adult kindred with no dysmorphic features. *Am J Med* 91:555, 1991.

62. Butturini A, Gale RP, Verlander PC, et al: Hematologic abnormalities in Fanconi anemia: an international Fanconi anemia registry study. *Blood* 84:1650, 1994.

63. Flowers MED, Zanis J, Pasquini R, et al: Marrow transplantation for Fanconi anaemia: Conditioning with reduced doses of cyclophosphamide without radiation. *Br J Haematol* 92:699, 1996.

64. Young NS, Alter BP, Blanche P: Thrombocytopenia absent radii, in *Aplastic Anemia: Acquired and Congenital*, p 395. Philadelphia: Saunders, 1994.

65. Schnur RE, Eunpu DL, Zackai EH: Thrombocytopenia with absent radius in a boy and his uncle. *Am J Med Genet* 28:117, 1987.

66. Edelberg SB, Cohn J, Brandt NJ: Congenital hypomegakaryocytic thrombocytopenia associated with bilateral absence of the radius—the TAR syndrome: intra-family variation of the clinical picture. *Hum Hered* 27:147, 1977.

67. Hall JG: Thrombocytopenia and absent radius (TAR) syndrome. *J Med Genet* 24:79, 1987.

68. Hedberg VA, Lipton JM: Thrombocytopenia with absent radii. A review of 100 cases. *Am J Pediatr Hematol Oncol* 10:51, 1988.

69. Ballmaier M, Schulze H, Strauss G, et al: Thrombopoietin in patients with congenital thrombocytopenia and absent radii: Elevated serum levels, normal receptor expression, but defective reactivity to thrombopoietin. *Blood* 90:612, 1997.

70. Hall JG, Levin J, Kuhn JP, et al: Thrombocytopenia with absent radius (TAR). *Medicine* 48:411, 1969.

71. Armitage JO, Hoak JC, Elliott TE, Fry GL: Syndrome of thrombocytopenia and absent radii: qualitatively normal platelets with remission following splenectomy. *Scand J Haematol* 20:25, 1978.

72. Myllyla G, Pelkonen R, Ikkala E, Apajalahti J: Hereditary thrombocytopenia: report of three families. *Scand J Haematol* 4:441, 1967.

73. Cullum C, Cooney DP, Schrier SL: Familial thrombocytopenic thrombocytopathy. *Br J Haematol* 13:147, 1967.

74. Murphy S, Oski FA, Naiman L: Platelet size and kinetics in hereditary and acquired thrombocytopenia. *N Engl J Med* 286:499, 1972.

75. Oski FA, Naiman JL, Allen DM, Diamond LK: Leukocyte inclusions—Dohle bodies—associated with platelet abnormality (the May-Hegglin anomaly). Report of a family and review of the literature. *Blood* 20:657, 1962.

76. Noris P, Spedini P, Belletti S, et al: Thrombocytopenia, giant platelets, and leukocyte inclusion bodies (May-Hegglin anomaly): clinical and laboratory findings. *Am J Med* 104:355, 1998.

77. Bepler G, Melhus O, Gunnells JC: Coexpression of May-Hegglin anomaly and hereditary nephritis in a family. *South Med J* 87:202, 1994.

78. Coller BS, Zarrabi MH: Platelet membrane studies in the May-Hegglin anomaly. *Blood* 58:279, 1981.

79. Peterson LC, Rao KV, Crosson JT, White JG: Fechtner syndrome—a variant of Alport's syndrome with leukocyte inclusions and macrothrombocytopenia. *Blood* 65:397, 1985.

80. Alport CA: Hereditary familial congenital haemorrhagic nephritis. *Br Med J* 1:504, 1927.

81. Epstein CJ, Sahud MA, Piel CF, et al: Hereditary macrothrombocytopathia, nephritis, and deafness. *Am J Med* 52:299, 1972.

82. Clare NM, Montiel MM, Lifschitz MD, Bannayan GA: Alport's syndrome associated with macrothrombopathic thrombocytopenia. *Am J Clin Path* 72:111, 1979.

83. Dowton SB, Beardsley D, Jamison D: Studies of a familial platelet disorder. *Blood* 65:557, 1985.

84. Quick AJ, Hussey CV: Hereditary thrombopathic thrombocytopenia. *Am J Med Sci* 245:643, 1963.

85. Bithell TC, Didisheim P, Cartwright GE, Wintrobe MM: Thrombocytopenia inherited as an autosomal dominant trait. *Blood* 25:231, 1965.

86. Fabris F, Cordiano I, Salvan F, et al: Chronic isolated macrothrombocytopenia with autosomal dominant transmission: a morphological and qualitative platelet disorder. *Eur J Haematol* 58:40, 1997.

87. Breton-Gorius J, Favier R, Guichard J, et al: A new congenital dysmegakaryopoietic thrombocytopenia (Paris-Trousseau) associated with giant platelet a-granules and chromosome 11 deletion at 11q23. *Blood* 85:1805, 1995.

88. Rocca B, Bellacosa A, De Cristofaro R, et al: Wiskott-Aldrich syndrome: report of an autosomal dominant variant. *Blood* 87:4538, 1996.

89. Erslev AJ, Palascak JE, Shaikh BS, Martinez J: Platelet kinetics in autosomal dominant macrothrombocytopenia. *J Lab Clin Med* 131:488, 1998.

90. Von Behrens WE: Splenomegaly, macrothrombocytopenia and stomatocytosis in healthy Mediterranean subjects. *Scand J Haematol* 14:258, 1975.

91. Sullivan KE, Mullen CA, Blaese RM, Winkelstein JA: A multiinstitutional survey of the Wiskott-Aldrich syndrome. *J Pediatr* 125:876, 1994.

92. Zhu QL, Zhang M, Blaese RM, et al: The Wiskott-Aldrich syndrome and X-linked congenital thrombocytopenia are caused by mutations of the same gene. *Blood* 86:3797, 1995.

93. Sadan N, Wolach B: Treatment of hemangiomas of infants with high doses of prednisone. *J Pediatr* 128:141, 1996.

94. Mitsuhashi N, Furuta M, Sakurai H, et al: Outcome of radiation therapy for patients with Kasabach-Merritt syndrome. *Int J Radiat Oncol Biol Phys* 39:467, 1997.

95. Stahl RL, Henderson JM, Hooks MA, et al: Therapy of the Kasabach-Merritt syndrome with cryoprecipitate plus intra-arterial thrombin and aminocaproic acid. *Am J Hematol* 36:272, 1991.

96. Warrell RP, Kempin SJ: Treatment of severe coagulopathy in the Kasabach-Merritt syndrome with animocaproic acid and cryoprecipitate. *N Engl J Med* 313:309, 1985.

97. Ortel TL, Onorato JJ, Bedrosian CL, Kaufman RE: Antifibrinolytic therapy in the management of the Kasabach Merritt syndrome. *Am J Hematol* 29:44, 1988.

98. Enjolras O, Wassef M, Mazoyer E, et al: Infants with Kasabach-Merritt syndrome do not have "true" hemangiomas. *J Pediatr* 130:631, 1997.

99. Manoharan A, Williams NT, Sparrow R: Acquired amegakaryocytic thrombocytopenia: report of a case and review of literature. *Q J Med* 70:243, 1989.

100. Hoffman R: Acquired pure amegakaryocytic thrombocytopenic purpura. *Semin Hematol* 28:303, 1991.

101. King JAC, Elkhalifa MY, Latour LF: Rapid progression of acquired amegakaryocytic thrombocytopenia to aplastic anemia. *South Med J* 90:91, 1997.

102. Young NS, Barrett AJ: The treatment of severe acquired aplastic anemia. *Blood* 85:3367, 1995.

103. Shiozaki H, Kuwaki T, Hagiwara T, et al: Presence of autoantibodies that can neutralize the biological activity of thrombopoietin in a patient with amegakaryocytic thrombocytopenic purpura. *Blood* 92:472a, 1998.

104. Lozano ML, Curtis BR, Hansen RM, et al: A GPIIb/IIIa-specific autoantibody from a patient with acquired amegakaryocytic thrombocytopenia appears to be the first example of a human ligand mimetic immunoglobulin. *Blood* 92:175a, 1998.

105. Leach JW, Hussein KK, George JN: Acquired pure megakaryocytic aplasia: report of two cases with long-term responses to antithymocyte globulin and cyclosporine. *Am J Hematol* 62:115, 1999.

106. Arruda VR, Rossi CL, Nogueira E, et al: Cytomegalovirus infection as cause of severe thrombocytopenia in a nonimmunosuppressed patient. *Acta Haematol* 98:228, 1997.

107. Pipp ML, Means ND, Sixbey JW, et al: Acute Epstein-Barr virus infection complicated by severe thrombocytopenia. *Clin Infect Dis* 25:1237, 1997.

108. Duchin JS, Koster FT, Peters CJ, et al: Hantavirus pulmonary syndrome: A clinical description of 17 patients with a newly recognized disease. *N Engl J Med* 330:949, 1994.

109. Oski FA, Naiman JL: Effect of live measles vaccine on the platelet count. *N Engl J Med* 275:352, 1966.

110. Isoyama K, Yamada K: Previous mycoplasma pneumoniae infection causing severe thrombocytopenic purpura. *Am J Hematol* 47:252, 1994.

111. Levin M: Acute hypersplenism and thrombocytopenia: a new presentation of disseminated mycobacterial infection in patients with acquired immunodeficiency syndrome. *Acta Haematol* 91:28, 1994.

112. Standaert SM, Dawson JE, Schaffner W, et al: Ehrlichiosis in a golf-oriented retirement community. *N Engl J Med* 333:420, 1995.

113. Yamaguchi S, Kubota T, Yamagishi T, et al: Severe thrombocytopenia suggesting immunological mechanisms in two cases of vivax malaria. *Am J Hematol* 56:183, 1997.

114. Zucker-Franklin D: The effect of viral infections on platelets and megakaryocytes. *Semin Hematol* 31:329, 1994.

115. Ronchi F, Cecchi P, Falcioni F, et al: Thrombocytopenic purpura as adverse reaction to recombinant hepatitis B vaccine. *Arch Dis Child* 78:273, 1998.

116. Francois B, Trimoreau F, Vignon P: Thrombocytopenia in the sepsis syndrome: role of hemophagocytosis and macrophage colony-stimulating factor. *Am J Med* 103:114, 1997.

117. Stephan F, Thioliere B, Verdy E, Tulliez M: Role of hemophagocytic histiocytosis in the etiology of thrombocytopenia in patients with sepsis syndrome or septic shock. *Clin Infect Dis* 25:1159, 1997.

118. Baker GR, Levin J: Transient thrombocytopenia produced by administration of macrophage colony-stimulating factor: investigations of the mechanism. *Blood* 91:89, 1998.

119. Ehmann WC, Rabkin CS, Eyster ME, Goedert JJ: Thrombocytopenia in HIV-infected and uninfected hemophiliacs. *Am J Hematol* 54:296, 1997.

120. Mientjes GHC, Van Ameijden EJC, Mulder JW, et al: Prevalence of thrombocytopenia in HIV-infected and non-HIV infected drug users and homosexual men. *Br J Haematol* 82:615, 1992.

121. Peltier JY, Lambin P, Doinel C, et al: Frequency and prognostic importance of thrombocytopenia in symptom-free HIV-infected individuals: a 5-year prospective study. *AIDS* 5:381, 1991.

122. Glatt AE, Anand A: Thrombocytopenia in patients infected with human immunodeficiency virus: treatment update. *Clin Infect Dis* 21:415, 1995.

123. Nicolle M, Levy S, Amrhein ES, et al: Normal platelet numbers correlate with plasma viral load and $CD4^+$ cell counts in HIV-1 infection. *Eur J Haematol* 61:216, 1998.

124. Bahner I, Kearns K, Coutinho S, et al: Infection of human marrow stroma by human immunodeficiency virus-1 (HIV-1) is both required and sufficient for HIV-1–induced hematopoietic suppression in vitro: demonstration by gene modification of primary human stroma. *Blood* 90:1787, 1997.

125. Cole JL, Marzec UM, Gunthel CJ, et al: Ineffective platelet production in thrombocytopenic human immunodeficiency virus-infected patients. *Blood* 91:3239, 1998.

126. Moses A, Nelson J, Bagby GC Jr: The influence of human immunodeficiency virus-1 on hematopoiesis. *Blood* 91:1479, 1998.

127. Ballem PJ, Belzberg A, Devine DV, et al: Kinetic studies of the mechanism of thrombocytopenia in patients with human immunodeficiency virus infection. *N Engl J Med* 327:1779, 1992.

128. Williams SB, Sano M, Smith N, et al: Glycocalicin levels in the plasma of HIV+ patients: an indicator of platelet turnover. *J Lab Clin Med* 132:303, 1998.

129. Gonzalez-Conejero R, Rivera J, Rosillo MC, et al: Association of autoantibodies against platelet glycoproteins Ib/IX and IIb/IIIa, and platelet-reactive anti-HIV antibodies in thrombocytopenic narcotic addicts. *Br J Haematol* 93:464, 1996.

130. Chia WK, Blanchette V, Mody M, et al: Characterization of HIV-1-specific antibodies and HIV-1-crossreactive antibodies to platelets in HIV-1-infected haemophiliac patients. *Br J Haematol* 103:1014, 1998.

131. Karpatkin S, Nardi MA, Hymes KB: Sequestration of anti-platelet GPIIIa antibody in rheumatoid factor immune complexes of human immunodeficiency virus 1 thrombocytopenic patients. *Proc Natl Acad Sci USA* 92:2263, 1995.

132. Eyster ME, Rabkin CS, Hilgartner MW, et al: Human immunodeficiency virus-related conditions in children and adults with hemophilia: rates, relationship to CD4 counts, and predictive value. *Blood* 81:828, 1993.

133. Aboulafia DM, Bundow D, Waide S, Bennett CL: Platelet enhancing effects of highly active antiretroviral therapy (HAART) among 10 patients with HIV-associated ITP. *Blood* 92:81b, 1998.

134. Ramratnam B, Parameswaran J, Newstein M, et al: Short course dexamethasone for thrombocytopenia in AIDS. *Am J Med* 100:117, 1996.

135. Majluf-Cruz A, Luna-Castaños G, Huitrón S, Nieto-Cisneros L: Usefulness of a low-dose intravenous immunoglobulin regimen for the treatment of thrombocytopenia associated with AIDS. *Am J Hematol* 59:127, 1998.

136. Scaradavou A, Woo B, Woloski BMR, et al: Intravenous Anti-D treatment of immune thrombocytopenic purpura: experience in 272 patients. *Blood* 89:2689, 1997.

137. Lord RV, Coleman MJ, Milliken ST: Splenectomy for HIV-related immune thrombocytopenia—comparison with results of splenectomy for non-HIV immune thrombocytopenic purpura. *Arch Surg* 133:205, 1998.

138. Burrows RF, Kelton JG: Pregnancy in patients with idiopathic thrombocytopenic purpura: Assessing the risks for the infant at delivery. *Obstet Gynecol Surv* 48:781, 1993.

139. Mandelbrot L, Schlienger I, Bongain A, et al: Thrombocytopenia in pregnant women infected with human immunodeficiency virus: maternal and neonatal outcome. *Am J Obstet Gynecol* 171:252, 1994.

140. Stabler SP, Allen RH, Savage DG, Lindenbaum J: Clinical spectrum and diagnosis of cobalamin deficiency. *Blood* 76:871, 1990.

141. Beck WS, Ferry JA: Megaloblastic anemia: case records of the Massachusetts General Hospital. *N Engl J Med* 325:1791, 1991.

142. Slichter SL, Harker LA: Thrombocytopenia: Mechanisms and management of defects in platelet production. *Clin Haematol* 7:523, 1978.

143. Epstein RD: Cells of the megakaryocytic series in pernicious anemia: in particular, the effect of specific therapy. *Am J Pathol* 25:239, 1949.

144. Sullivan LW: Effect of alcohol on platelet production. *Platelet Kinetics* 247, 1972.

145. Berger M, Brass LF: Severe thrombocytopenia in iron deficiency anemia. *Am J Hematol* 24:425, 1987.

146. Moschcowitz E: An acute febrile pleiochromic anemia with hyaline thrombosis of the terminal arterioles and capillaries. *Arch Intern Med* 36:89, 1925.

147. Marcus AJ: in *Hemolytic Uremic Syndrome and Thrombotic Thrombocytopenic Purpura*, edited by BS Kaplan, RS Trompeter, JL Moake, pp 19–27. New York, Marcel Dekker, 1992.

148. Gasser C, Gautier E, Steck A, et al: Hamolytisch-uramische Syndrome: Bilaterale Nierenrindennekrosen bei akuten erworbenen hamolytischen Anamien. *Schweiz Med Woch* 85:905, 1955.

149. Gautier E, Siebenmann RE: The birth of the hemolytic uremic syndrome, in *Hemolytic Uremic Syndrome and Thrombotic Thrombocytopenic Purpura*, edited by BS Kaplan, RS Trompeter, JL Moake, pp 1–17. New York, Marcel Dekker, 1992.

150. Rock GA, Shumak KH, Buskard NA, et al: Comparison of plasma exchange with plasma infusion in the treatment of thrombotic thrombocytopenic purpura. *N Engl J Med* 325:393, 1991.

151. Thompson CE, Damon LE, Ries CA, Linker CA: Thrombotic microangiopathies in the 1980s: clinical features, response to treatment, and the impact of the human immunodeficiency virus epidemic. *Blood* 80:1890, 1992.

152. Laszik Z, Silva F: Hemolytic-uremic syndrome, thrombotic thrombocytopenia purpura, and systemic sclerosis (systemic scleroderma), in *Hepinstall's Pathology of the Kidney*, 5th ed, edited by JC Jennett, JL Olson, MM Schwartz, FG Silva, pp 1003–57. Philadelphia, Lippincott-Raven, 1998.

153. Amorosi EL, Ultmann JE: Thrombotic thrombocytopenic purpura: report of 16 cases and review of the literature. *Medicine* 45:139, 1966.

154. Mead PS, Griffin PM: *Escherichia coli* 0157:H7. *Lancet* 352:1207, 1998.

155. Boyce TG, Swerdlow DL, Griffin PM: *Escherichia coli* 0157:H7 and the hemolytic-uremic syndrome. *N Engl J Med* 333:364, 1995.

156. Arbus GS: Association of verotoxin-producing *E. coli* and verotoxin with hemolytic uremic syndrome. *Kidney Int* 51:S91, 1997.

157. Keusch GT, Acheson DWK: Thrombotic thrombocytopenic purpura associated with Shiga toxins. *Semin Hematol* 34:106, 1997.

158. Asada Y, Sumiyoshi A, Hayashi T, et al: Immunohistochemistry of vascular lesions in thrombotic thrombocytopenic purpura, with special reference to factor VIII related antigen. *Thromb Res* 38:469, 1985.

159. Moake JL, Chow TW: Increased von Willebrand Factor (vWf) binding to platelets associated with impaired vWf breakdown in thrombotic thrombocytopenic purpura. *J Clin Apheresis* 13:126, 1998.

160. Moake JL, Rudy CK, Troll JH, et al: Unusually large plasma factor VII: von Willebrand factor multimers in chronic relapsing thrombotic thrombocytopenic purpura. *N Engl J Med* 307:1432, 1982.

161. Moake J: Studies on the pathophysiology of thrombotic thrombocytopenic purpura. *Semin Hematol* 34:83, 1997.

162. Kroll MH, Hellums JD, McIntire LV, et al: Platelets and shear stress. *Blood* 88:1525, 1996.

163. Chow TW, Turner NA, Chintagumpala M, et al: Increased von Willebrand factor binding to platelets in single episode and recurrent types of thrombotic thrombocytopenic purpura. *Am J Hematol* 57:293, 1998.

164. Tsai H-M, Lian ECY: Antibodies to von-Willebrand factor-cleaving protease in acute thrombotic thrombocytopenic purpura. *N Engl J Med* 339:1585, 1998.

165. Furlan M, Robles R, Solenthaler M, et al: Deficient activity of von Willebrand factor-cleaving protease in chronic relapsing thrombotic thrombocytopenic purpura. *Blood* 89:3097, 1997.

166. Furlan M, Robles R, Galbusera M, et al: Von Willebrand factor-cleaving protease in thrombotic thrombocytopenic purpura and the hemolytic-uremic syndrome. *N Engl J Med* 339:1578, 1998.

167. Furlan M, Robles R, Solenthaler M, Lämmle B: Acquired deficiency of von Willebrand factor-cleaving protease in a patient with thrombotic thrombocytopenic purpura. *Blood* 91:2839, 1998.

168. Galbusera M, Noris M, Rossi C, et al: Increased fragmentation of von Willebrand factor, due to abnormal cleavage of the subunit, parallels disease activity in recurrent hemolytic uremic syndrome and thrombotic thrombocytopenic purpura and discloses predisposition in families. *Blood* 94:610, 1999.

169. Kelton JG, Moore JC, Warkentin TE, Hayward CPM: Isolation and characterization of cysteine proteinase in thrombotic thrombocytopenic purpura. *Br J Haematol* 93:421, 1996.

170. Consonni R, Falanga A, Barbui T: Further characterization of platelet-aggregating cysteine proteinase activity in thrombotic thrombocytopenic purpura. *Br J Haematol* 87:321, 1994.

171. Valant PA, Jy W, Horstmann LL, et al: Thrombotic thrombocytopenic purpura plasma enhances platelet-leucocyte interaction *in vitro*. *Br J Haematol* 100:24, 1998.

172. Morigi M, Micheletti G, Figliuzzi M, et al: Verotoxin-1 promotes leukocyte adhesion to cultured endothelial cells under physiologic flow conditions. *Blood* 86:4553, 1995.

173. Mitra D, Jaffe EA, Weksler B: Thrombotic thrombocytopenic purpura and sporadic hemolytic- uremic syndrome plasmas induce apoptosis in restricted lineages of human microvascular endothelial cells. *Blood* 89:1224, 1997.

174. Dang CT, Magid MS, Weksler B, et al: Enhanced endothelial cell apoptosis in splenic tissues of patients with thrombotic thrombocytopenic purpura. *Blood* 93:1264, 1999.

175. Noris M, Remuzzi G: Are HUS and TTP genetically determined? *Kidney Int* 53:1085, 1998.

176. Jones MB, Armitage JO, Stone DB: Self-limited TTP-like syndrome after bee sting. *JAMA* 242:2212, 1979.

177. Chang JC, Shipstone A, Llenado-Lee MA: Postoperative thrombotic thrombocytopenic purpura following cardiovascular surgeries. *Am J Hematol* 53:1, 1996.

178. Pavlovsky M, Weinstein R: Thrombotic thrombocytopenic purpura following coronary artery bypass graft surgery: prospective observations of an emerging syndrome. *J Clin Apheresis* 12:159, 1997.

179. Moake J, Chintagumpala M, Turner N, et al: Solvent/detergent-treated plasma suppresses shear-induced platelet aggregation and prevents episodes of thrombotic thrombocytopenic purpura. *Blood* 84:490, 1994.

180. Bell WR, Chulay JD, Feinberg JE: Manifestations resembling thrombotic microangiopathy in patients with advanced human immunodeficiency virus (HIV) disease in a cytomegalovirus prophylaxis trial (ACTG 204). *Medicine* 76:369, 1997.

181. Casonato A, Pontara E, Bertomoro A, et al: Abnormally large von Willebrand Factor multimers in Henoch-Schonlein Purpura. *Am J Hematol* 51:7, 1996.

182. Rock G, Shumak K, Kelton J, et al: Thrombotic thrombocytopenic purpura: Outcome in 24 patients with renal impairment treated with plasma exchange. *Transfusion* 32:710, 1992.

183. George JN, Gilcher RO, Smith JW: Thrombotic thrombocytopenia purpura-hemolytic uremic syndrome: Diagnosis and management. *J Clin Apheresis* 13:120, 1998.

184. Ridolfi RL, Bell WR: Thrombotic thrombocytopenic purpura. Report of 25 cases and review of the literature. *Medicine* 60:413, 1981.

185. Taft EG: Advances in the treatment of TTP. *Prog Clin Biol Res* 337:151, 1990.

186. Blitzer JB, Granfortuna JM, Gottlieb AJ, et al: Thrombotic thrombocytopenic purpura: treatment with plasmapheresis. *Am J Hematol* 24:329, 1987.

187. Pisciotto P, Rosen D, Silver H, et al: Treatment of thrombotic thrombocytopenic purpura. Evaluation of plasma exchange and review of the literature. *Vox Sang* 45:185, 1983.

188. Kay AC, Solberg LA, Nichols DA, Petitt RM: Prognostic significance of computed tomography of the brain in thrombotic thrombocytopenic purpura. *Mayo Clin Proc* 66:602, 1991.

189. Vianelli N, Sermasi G, D'Alessandro R, et al: Prompt plasma exchange treatment and coma reversibility in two patients with thrombotic thrombocytopenic purpura. *Haematologia* 76:72, 1991.

190. Blum AS, Drislane FW: Nonconvulsive status epilepticus in thrombotic thrombocytopenic purpura. *Neurology* 47:1079, 1996.

191. Silva VA: Thrombotic thrombocytopenic purpura/hemolytic uremic syndrome secondary to pancreatitis. *Am J Hematol* 50:53, 1995.

192. Bell WR, Braine HG, Ness PM, Kickler TS: Improved survival in thrombotic thrombocytopenic purpura—hemolytic uremic syndrome. *N Engl J Med* 325:398, 1991.

193. Melnyk AMS, Solez K, Kjellstrand CM: Adult hemolytic-uremic syndrome—a review of 37 cases. *Arch Intern Med* 155:2077, 1995.

194. Fearing MK, Spar MD, Kahn MJ: Chronic thrombotic thrombocytopenic purpura masquerading as other disease entities. *J La State Med Soc* 150:29, 1998.

195. Fava S, Galizia AC: Thrombotic thrombocytopenic purpura-like syndrome in the absence of schistocytes. *Br J Haematol* 89:643, 1995.

196. Brilliant SE, Lester PA, Ohno AK, et al: Hemolytic-uremic syndrome without evidence of microangiopathic hemolytic anemia on peripheral blood smear. *South Med J* 89:342, 1996.

197. Roberts AW, Gillett EA, Fleming SJ: Hemolytic uremic syndrome/thrombotic thrombocytopenic purpura: Outcome with plasma exchange. *J Clin Apheresis* 6:150, 1991.

198. Cohen JD, Brecher ME, Bandarenko N: Cellular source of serum lactate dehydrogenase elevation in patients with thrombotic thrombocytopenia purpura. *J Clin Apheresis* 13:16, 1998.

199. Takahashi H, Tatewaki W, Nakamura T, et al: Coagulation studies in thrombotic thrombocytopenic purpura, with special reference to von Willebrand factor and protein S. *Am J Hematol* 30:14, 1989.

200. Devinsky O, Petito CK, Alonso DR: Clinical and neuropathological findings in systemic lupus erythematosus: the role of vasculitis, heart emboli, and thrombotic thrombocytopenic purpura. *Ann Neurol* 23:380, 1988.

201. Jorfén M, Callejas JL, Formiga F, et al: Fulminant thrombotic thrombocytopenic purpura in systemic lupus erythematosus. *Scand J Rheumatol* 27:76, 1998.

202. Jain R, Chartash E, Susin M, Furie R: Systemic lupus erythematosus complicated by thrombotic microangiopathy. *Semin Arthritis Rheum* 24:173, 1994.

203. Asherson RA, Piette JC: The catastrophic antiphospholipid syndrome 1996: acute multi-organ failure associated with antiphospholipid antibodies: a review of 31 patients. *Lupus* 5:414, 1996.

204. Miller A, Ryan PFJ, Dowling JP: Vasculitis and thrombotic thrombocytopenic purpura in a patient with limited scleroderma. *J Rheumatol* 24:598, 1997.

205. Kapur A, Ballou SP, Renston JP, et al: Recurrent acute scleroderma renal crisis complicated by thrombotic thrombocytopenic purpura. *J Rheumatol* 24:2469, 1997.

206. Gilliland BC, Baxter E, Evans RS: Red-cell antibodies in acquired hemolytic anemia with negative antiglobulin serum tests. *N Engl J Med* 285:252, 1971.

207. Colflesh CR, Agarwal R, Knochel JP: Timing of plasma exchange therapy for thrombotic thrombocytopenia purpura: A brief clinical observation. *Am J Med Sci* 311:167, 1996.

208. Byrnes JJ, Khurana M: Treatment of thrombotic thrombocytopenic purpura with plasma. *N Engl J Med* 297:1386, 1977.

209. Rizvi MA, Vesely SK, George JN: Plasma exchange complications: a review of 59 consecutive thrombotic thrombocytopenic purpura-hemolytic uremic syndrome (TTP-HUS) patients. *Thromb Haemost* 1066a, 1999.

210. Rock G, Shumak KH, Sutton DMC, et al: Cryosupernatant as replacement fluid for plasma exchange in thrombotic thrombocytopenic purpura. *Br J Haematol* 94:383, 1996.

211. North American TTP Group, Ziegler Z, Gryn JF, et al: Cryopoor plasma does not improve early response in primary adult thrombotic thrombocytopenic purpura (TTP). *Blood* 92:707a, 1998.

212. Sarode R, Gottschall JL, Aster RH, McFarland JG: Thrombotic thrombocytopenic purpura: Early and late responders. *Am J Hematol* 54:102, 1997.

213. Bandarenko N, Brecher ME, Members of the US TTP ASG: United States Thrombotic Thrombocytopenic Purpura Apheresis Study Group (US TTP ASG): Multicenter survey and retrospective analysis of current efficacy of therapeutic plasma exchange. *J Clin Apheresis* 13:133, 1998.

214. Patton JF, Manning KR, Case D, Owen J: Serum lactate dehydrogenase and platelet count predict survival in thrombotic thrombocytopenic purpura. *Am J Hematol* 47:94, 1994.

215. Vesely SK, George JN, Raskob GE: Thrombotic thrombocytopenic purpura-hemolytic uremic syndrome (TTP-HUS): A 10 year prospective cohort study. *Thromb Haemost* 2341a, 1999.

216. Onundarson PT, Rowe JM, Heal JM, Francis CW: Response to plasma exchange and splenectomy in thrombotic thrombocytopenic purpura. *Arch Intern Med* 152:791, 1992.

217. Hayward CPM, Sutton DMC, Carter WH Jr, et al: Treatment outcomes in patients with adult thrombotic thrombocytopenic purpura-hemolytic uremic syndrome. *Arch Intern Med* 154:982, 1994.

218. Taft EG: Thrombotic thrombocytopenic purpura and dose of plasma exchange. *Blood* 54:842, 1979.

219. Bukowski RM, Hewlett JS, Reimer RR, et al: Therapy of thrombotic thrombocytopenic purpura: an overview. *Semin Thromb Hemost* 7:1, 1981.

220. Cuttner J: Thrombotic thrombocytopenic purpura: a ten-year experience. *Blood* 56:302, 1980.

221. Crowther MA, Heddle N, Hayward CPM, et al: Splenectomy done during hematologic remission to prevent relapse in patients with thrombotic thrombocytopenic purpura. *Ann Intern Med* 125:294, 1996.

222. Durand JM, Lefevre P, Kaplanski G, Soubeyrand J: Ineffectiveness of high-dose intravenous gammaglobulin infusion in thrombotic thrombocytopenic purpura. *Am J Hematol* 42:234, 1993.

223. Epstein JS, Zoon KC: FDA Important Drug Warning: Acute renal failure associated with the administration of immune globulin intravenous (Human IgIV) products. FDA Warning Letter to Physicians. 1998.

224. Gutterman LA: Treatment of thrombotic thrombocytopenic purpura and hemolytic uremic syndrome: the role of vincristine, in *Hemolytic Uremic Syndrome and Thrombotic Thrombocytopenic Purpura,* edited by BS Kaplan, RS Trompeter, JL Moake, pp 513–30. New York, Marcel Dekker, 1992.

225. Moake JL, Rudy CK, Troll JH, et al: Therapy of chronic relapsing thrombotic thrombocytopenic purpura with prednisone and azathioprine. *Am J Hematol* 20:73, 1985.

226. Bird JM, Cummins D, Machin SJ: Cyclophosphamide for chronic relapsing thrombotic thrombocytopenic purpura. *Lancet* 336:565, 1990.

227. Kierdorf H, Maurin N, Heintz B: Cyclosporine for thrombotic thrombocytopenic purpura. *Ann Intern Med* 118:987, 1993.

228. Mittelman A, Puccio T, Ahmed T, et al: Response of refractory thrombotic thrombocytopenic purpura to extracorporeal immunoadsorption. *N Engl J Med* 326:711, 1992.

229. Gordon LI, Kwaan HC, Rossi EC: Deleterious effects of platelet transfusions and recovery thrombocytosis in patients with thrombotic microangiopathy. *Semin Hematol* 24:194, 1987.

230. Rose M, Eldor A: High incidence of relapses in thrombotic thrombocytopenic purpura. *Am J Med* 83:437, 1987.

231. Shumak KH, Rock GA, Nair RC: Canadian Apheresis Group: Late relapses in patients successfully treated for thrombotic thrombocytopenic purpura. *Ann Intern Med* 122:569, 1995.

232. de Jong M, Monnens L: Haemolytic-uraemic syndrome: A 10-year follow-up study of 73 patients. *Nephrol Dial Transplant* 3:379, 1988.

233. Siegler RL, Milligan MK, Burningham TH, et al: Long-term outcome and prognostic indicators in the hemolytic-uremic syndrome. *J Pediatr* 118:195, 1991.

234. Fitzpatrick MM, Shah V, Trompeter RS, et al: Long-term renal outcome of childhood haemolytic uraemic syndrome. *Brit Med J* 303:489, 1991.

235. Tönshoff B, Sammet A, Sanden I, et al: Outcome and prognostic determinants in the hemolytic uremic syndrome of children. *Nephron* 68:63, 1994.

236. Kelles A, Van Dyck M, Proesmans W: Childhood haemolytic uraemic syndrome: long-term outcome and prognostic features. *Eur J Pediatr* 153:38, 1994.

237. Gagnadoux MF, Habib R, Gubler MC, et al: Long-term (15–25 years) outcome of childhood hemolytic-uremic syndrome. *Clin Nephrol* 46:39, 1996.

238. Moghal NE, Ferreira MA, Howie AJ: The late histologic findings in diarrhea-associated hemolytic uremic syndrome. *J Pediatr* 133:220, 1998.

239. Su C, Brandt LJ: *Escherichia coli* 0157:H7 infection in humans. *Ann Intern Med* 123:698, 1995.

240. Siegler RL, Pavia AT, Hansen FL: Atypical hemolytic-uremic syndrome: A comparison with postdiarrheal disease. *J Pediatr* 128:505, 1996.

241. Lawlor ER, Webb DWM, Hill A, Wadsworth LD: Thrombotic thrombocytopenic purpura: A treatable cause of childhood encephalopathy. *J Pediatr* 130:313, 1997.

242. Goldwater PN, Bettelheim KA: New perspectives on the role of *Esche-*

richia coli O157:H7 and other enterohaemorrhagic *E. coli* serotypes in human disease. *J Med Microbiol* 47:1039, 1998.

243. Tarr PI, Fouser LS, Stapleton AE, et al: Hemolytic-uremic syndrome in a six-year-old girl after a urinary tract infection with shiga-toxin-producing *Escherichia coli* O103:H2. *N Engl J Med* 335:635, 1996.

244. Starr M, Bennett-Wood V, Bigham AK, et al: Hemolytic-uremic syndrome following urinary tract infection with enterohemorrhagic *Escherichia coli*: case report and review. *Clin Infect Dis* 27:310, 1998.

245. Slutsker L, Ries AA, Greene KD: *Escherichia coli* O157:H7 diarrhea in the United States: clinical and epidemiologic features. *Ann Intern Med* 126:505, 1997.

246. Rowe PC, Orrbine E, Lior H, et al: Risk of hemolytic uremic syndrome after sporadic *Escherichia coli* O157:H7 infection: Results of a Canadian collaborative study. *J Pediatr* 132:777, 1998.

247. Bitzan MM, Wang Y, Lin J, Marsden PA: Verotoxin and ricin have novel effects on preendothelin-1 expression but fail to modify nitric oxide synthase (ecNOS) expression and NO production in vascular endothelium. *J Clin Invest* 101:372, 1998.

248. Siegler RL: Spectrum of extrarenal involvement in postdiarrheal hemolyticuremic syndrome. *J Pediatr* 125:511, 1994.

249. Creager AJ, Brecher ME, Bandarenko N: Thrombotic thrombocytopenic purpura that is refractory to therapeutic plasma exchange in two patients with occult infection. *Transfusion*. 38:419, 1998.

250. Bloom PD, MacPhail AP, Klugman K, et al: Haemolytic-uraemic syndrome in adults with resistant *Shigella dysenteriae* type I. *Lancet* 344:206, 1994.

251. Tsukahara H, Hayashi S, Nakamura K, et al: Haemolytic uraemic syndrome associated with Yersinia enterocolitica infection. *Pediatr Nephrol* 2:309, 1988.

252. Carter JE, Cimolai N: Hemolytic-uremic syndrome associated with acute *Campylobacter upsaliensis* gastroenteritis. *Nephron* 74:489, 1996.

253. Mogyorosi A, Carley MD: Hemolytic-uremic syndrome associated with pseudomembranous colitis caused by *Clostridium difficile*. *Nephron* 76:491, 1997.

254. Cabrera GR, Fortenberry JD, Warshaw BL: Hemolytic uremic syndrome associated with invasive *Streptococcus pneumoniae* infection. *Pediatrics* 101:699, 1998.

255. Myers KA, Marrie TJ: Thrombotic microangiopathy associated with *Streptococcus pneumoniae* bacteremia: Case report and review. *Clin Infect Dis* 17:1037, 1993.

256. Schröder S, Spyridopoulos I, König J, et al: Thrombotic thrombocytopenic purpura (TTP) associated with a *Borrelia burgdorferi* infection. *Am J Hematol* 50:72, 1995.

257. Tarantolo SR, Landmark JD, Iwen PC: *Bartonella*-like erythrocyte inclusions in thrombotic thrombocytopenic purpura. *Lancet* 350:1602, 1997.

258. Marty AM, Dumler JS, Imes G, et al: Ehrlichiosis mimicking thrombotic thrombocytopenic purpura. Case report and pathological correlation. *Hum Pathol* 26:920, 1995.

259. Rarick MU, Espina B, Mocharnuk R, et al: Thrombotic thrombocytopenic purpura in patients with human immunodeficiency virus infection: A report of three cases and review of the literature. *Am J Hematol* 40:103, 1992.

260. Ucar A, Fernandez HF, Byrnes JJ, et al: Thrombotic microangiopathy and retroviral infections: a 13-year experience. *Am J Hematol* 45:304, 1994.

261. Moore RD: Schistocytosis and a thrombotic microangiopathy-like syndrome in hospitalized HIV-infected patients. *Am J Hematol* 60:116, 1999.

262. Hymes KB, Karpatkin S: Human immunodeficiency virus infection and thrombotic microangiopathy. *Semin Hematol* 34:117, 1997.

263. Neau D, Bonnet F, Viallard JF, et al: Thrombotic thrombocytopenic purpura and cytomegalovirus infection in an immunocompetent adult. *Clin Infect Dis* 25:1495, 1997.

264. Jeejeebhoy FM, Zaltzman JS: Thrombotic microangiopathy in association with cytomegalovirus infection in a renal transplant patient—a new treatment strategy. *Transplantation* 65:1645, 1998.

265. Gottschall JL, Neahring B, McFarland JG, et al: Quinine-induced immune thrombocytopenia with hemolytic uremic syndrome: Clinical and serological findings in nine patients and review of literature. *Am J Hematol* 47:283, 1994.

266. Stroncek DF, Vercellotti GM, Hammerschmidt DE, et al: Characterization of multiple quinine-dependent antibodies in a patient with episodic hemolytic uremic syndrome and immune agranulocytosis. *Blood* 80:241, 1992.

267. Gottschall JL, Elliot W, Lianos E, et al: Quinine-induced immune thrombocytopenia associated with hemolytic uremic syndrome: A new clinical entity. *Blood* 77:306, 1991.

268. Bennett CL, Weinberg PD, Rozenberg-Ben-Dror K, et al: Thrombotic thrombocytopenic purpura associated with ticlopidine—a review of 60 cases. *Ann Intern Med* 128:541, 1998.

269. Bennett CL, Kiss JE, Weinberg PD, et al: Thrombotic thrombocytopenic purpura after stenting and ticlopidine. *Lancet* 352:1036, 1998.

270. Steinhubl SR, Tan WA, Foody JM, Topol EJ: Incidence and clinical course of thrombotic thrombocytopenic purpura due to ticlopidine following coronary stenting. *JAMA* 281:806, 1999.

271. Lesesne JB, Rothschild N, Erickson B, et al: Cancer-associated hemolytic-uremic syndrome: Analysis of 85 cases from a national registry. *J Clin Oncol* 7:781, 1989.

272. Murgo AJ: Thrombotic microangiopathy in the cancer patient including those induced by chemotherapeutic agents. *Semin Hematol* 24:161, 1987.

273. Doll DC, Weiss RB, Issell BF: Mitomycin: Ten years after approval for marketing. *J Clin Oncol* 3:276, 1985.

274. MacDonald JS, Schein PS, Woolley PV, et al: 5–Fluorouracil, doxorubicin, and mitomycin (FAM) combination chemotherapy for advanced gastric cancer. *Ann Intern Med* 93:533, 1980.

275. Hanna WT, Krauss S, Regester RF, Murphy WM: Renal disease after mitomycin C therapy. *Cancer* 48:2583, 1981.

276. Cantrell JE, Phillips TM, Schein PS: Carcinoma-associated hemolytic-uremic syndrome: A complication of mitomycin C chemotherapy. *J Clin Oncol* 3:723, 1985.

277. Sheldon R, Slaughter D: A syndrome of microangiopathic hemolytic anemia, renal impairment, and pulmonary edema in chemotherapy-treated patients with adenocarcinoma. *Cancer* 58:1428, 1986.

278. Giroux L, Bettez P: Mitomycin-C nephrotoxicity: A clinico-pathologic study of 17 cases. *Am J Kidney Dis* 6:28, 1985.

279. Loprinzi CLL: Mitomycin C-induced pulmonary and renal toxicities. *Wis Med J* 83:16, 1984.

280. Verwey J, de Vries J, Pinedo HM: Mitomycin C-induced renal toxicity, a dose-dependent side effect? *Eur J Cancer* 23:195, 1987.

281. Fielding JWL, Fagg SL, Jones BG, et al: An interim report of a prospective, randomized, controlled study of adjuvant chemotherapy in operable gastric cancer: British Stomach Cancer Group. *World J Surg* 7:390, 1983.

282. Pettitt AR, Clark RE: Thrombotic microangiopathy following bone marrow transplantation. *Bone Marrow Transplant* 14:495, 1994

283. Schriber JR, Herzig GP: Transplantation-associated thrombotic thrombocytopenic purpura and hemolytic uremic syndrome. *Semin Hematol* 34:126, 1997.

284. Shulman H, Striker G, Deeg HJ: Nephrotoxicity of cyclosporin A after allogeneic marrow transplantation. *N Engl J Med* 305:1392, 1981

285. Holler E, Kolb HJ, Hiller E, et al: Microangiopathy in patients on cyclosporine prophylaxis who developed acute graft-versus-host disease after HLA-identical bone marrow transplantation. *Blood* 73:2018, 1989.

286. Hows JM, Chipping PM, Fairhead S, et al: Nephrotoxicity in bone marrow transplant recipients treated with cyclosporin A. *Br J Haematol* 54:69, 1983.

287. Atkinson K, Biggs JC, Hayes J, et al: Cyclosporin A associated nephrotoxicity in the first 100 days after allogeneic bone marrow transplantation: three distinct syndromes. *Br J Haematol* 54:59, 1983.

288. Mach-Pascual S, Samii K, Beris P: Microangiopathic hemolytic anemia complicating FK506 (tacrolimus) therapy. *Am J Hematol* 52:310, 1996.

289. Powell HR, Davidson PM, McCredie DA, et al: Haemolytic-uraemic syndrome after treatment with metronidazole. *Med J Aust* 149:222, 1988.

290. Tumlin JA, Sands JM, Someren A: Hemolytic-uremic syndrome following "crack" cocaine inhalation. *Am J Med Sci* 299:366, 1990.

291. McCarthy LJ, Porcu P, Fausel CA, et al: Thrombotic thrombocytopenic purpura and simvastatin. *Lancet* 352:1284, 1998.

292. Leach JW, Pham T, Diamandidis D, George JN: Thrombotic thrombocytopenic purpura-hemolytic uremic syndrome (TTP-HUS) following treatment with deoxycoformycin in a patient with cutaneous T cell lymphoma (Sezary Syndrome): A case report. *Am J Hematol* 61:268, 1999.

293. Schirren CA, Berghaus TM, Sackmann M: Thrombotic thrombocytopenic purpura after ecstasy-induced acute liver failure. *Ann Intern Med* 130:163, 1999.

294. Zeigler ZR, Shadduck RK, Nemunaitis J, et al: Bone marrow transplant-associated thrombotic microangiopathy: a case series. *Bone Marrow Transplant* 15:247, 1995.

295. Van Ojik H, Biesma DH, Fijnheer R, et al: Cyclosporin for thrombotic thrombocytopenic purpura after autologous bone marrow transplantation. *Br J Haematol* 96:641, 1997.

296. Paquette RL, Tran L, Landaw EM: Thrombotic microangiopathy following allogenic bone marrow transplantation is associated with intensive graft-versus-host disease prophylaxis. *Bone Marrow Transplant* 22:351, 1998.

297. Rizvi MA, Vesely SK, Roy V, George JN: Thrombotic thrombocytopenic purpura-hemolytic uremic syndrome (TTP-HUS) following bone marrow transplantation (BMT). *Thromb Haemost* 1937a, 1999.

298. Zeigler ZR, Shadduck RK, Nath R, Andrews DF III: Pilot study of combined cryosupernatant and protein A immunoadsorption exchange in the treatment of grade 3–4 bone marrow-associated thrombotic microangiopathy. *Bone Marrow Transplant* 17:81, 1996.

299. Sarode R, McFarland JG, Flomenberg N, et al: Therapeutic plasma exchange does not appear to be effective in the management of thrombotic thrombocytopenic purpura/hemolytic uremic syndrome following bone marrow transplantation. *Bone Marrow Transplant* 16:271, 1995.

300. Alam A, Ford L, Nagubandi M, et al: Treatment of thrombotic thrombocytopenic purpura-hemolytic uremic syndrome (TTP-HUS) associated with allogeneic BMT: lack of impact on final outcome. *Blood* 92:516a, 1998.

301. Lohrmann HP, Adam W, Heymer B, Kubanek B: Microangiopathic hemolytic anemia in metastatic carcinoma. *Ann Intern Med* 79:368, 1973.

302. Antman KH, Skarin AT, Mayer RJ, et al: Microangiopathic hemolytic anemia and cancer: a review. *Medicine* 58:377, 1979.

303. Forshaw J, Harwood L: Poikilocytosis associated with carcinoma. *Arch Intern Med* 117:203, 1966.

304. Pineo CF, Regoeczi E, Hatton MWC, Brain MC: Activation of coagulation by extracts of mucus: a possible pathway of intravascular coagulation accompanying adenocarcinoma. *J Lab Clin Med* 82:255, 1973.

305. Brain MC, Azzopardi JG, Baker LRI, et al: Microangiopathic hemolytic anaemia and mucin-forming adenocarcinoma. *Br J Haematol* 18:183, 1970.

306. Trent K, Neustater BR, Lottenberg R: Chronic relapsing thrombotic thrombocytopenic purpura and antiphospholipid antibodies: a report of two cases. *Am J Hematol* 54:155, 1997.

307. Nesher G, Hanna VE, Moore TL, et al: Thrombotic microangiopathic hemolytic anemia in systemic lupus erythematosus. *Semin Arthritis Rheum* 24:165, 1994.

308. Ezra Y, Rose M, Elder A: Therapy and prevention of thrombotic thrombocytopenic purpura during pregnancy: a clinical study of 16 pregnancies. *Am J Hematol* 51:1, 1996.

309. Dashe JS, Ramin SM, Cunningham FG. The long-term consequences of thrombotic microangiopathy (thrombotic thrombocytopenic purpura and hemolytic uremic syndrome) in pregnancy. *Obstet Gynecol* 91:662, 1998.

310. Egerman RS, Witlin AG, Friedman SA, Sibai BM: Thrombotic thrombocytopenic purpura and hemolytic uremic syndrome in pregnancy: Review of 11 cases. *Am J Obstet Gynecol* 175:950, 1996.

311. Mokrzycki MH, Rickles FR, Kaplan AA, Kohn OF: Thrombotic thrombocytopenic purpura in pregnancy: successful treatment with plasma exchange. *Blood Purif* 13:271, 1995.

312. McCrae KR, Cines DB: Thrombotic microangiopathy during pregnancy. *Semin Hematol* 34:148, 1997.

313. Lanska DJ, Kryscio RJ:. Stroke and intracranial venous thrombosis during pregnancy and puerperium. *Neurology* 51:1622, 1998.

314. Natelson EA, White D: Recurrent thrombotic thrombocytopenic purpura in early pregnancy: effect of uterine evacuation. *Obstet Gynecol* 66:54S, 1985.

315. Wurzel JM: TTP lesions in the placenta but not in the fetus. *N Engl J Med* 301:503, 1979.

316. Giles C, Inglis TCM: Thrombocytopenia and macrothrombocytosis in gestational hypertension. *Br J Obstet Gynaecol* 88:1115, 1981.

317. Matthews JH, Benjamin S, Gill DS, Smith NA: Pregnancy-associated thrombocytopenia: definition, incidence and natural history. *Acta Haematol* 84:24, 1990.

318. Verdy E, Bessous V, Dreyfus M, et al: Longitudinal analysis of platelet count and volume in normal pregnancy. *Thromb Haemost* 77:806, 1997.

319. Ahmed Y, Van Iddekinge B, Paul C, et al: Retrospective analysis of platelet numbers and volumes in normal pregnancy and in pre-eclampsia. *Br J Obstet Gynaecol* 100:216, 1993.

320. Minakami H, Kuwata T, Sato I: Gestational thrombocytopenia: is it new? *Am J Obstet Gynecol* 175:1676, 1996.

321. George JN, Woolf SH, Raskob GE, et al: Idiopathic thrombocytyopenic purpura: A practice guideline developed by explicit methods for the American Society of Hematology. *Blood* 88:3, 1996.

322. Burrows RF, Kelton JG: Fetal thrombocytopenia and its relation to maternal thrombocytopenia. *N Engl J Med* 329:1463, 1993.

323. Burrows RF, Kelton JG: Platelets and pregnancy. *Curr Obstet Med* 2:83, 1993.

324. Ballem PJ: Diagnosis and management of thrombocytopenia in obstetric syndromes, in *Obstetric Transfusion Practice,* edited by RA Sacher, ME Brecher, pp 49–76. Bethesda, American Association of Blood Banks, 1993.

325. Anteby E, Shalev O: Clinical relevance of gestational thrombocytopenia of <100,000/ml. *Am J Hematol* 47:118, 1994.

326. Letsky EA, Greaves M: Guidelines on the investigation and management of thrombocytopenia in pregnancy and neonatal alloimmune thrombocytopenia. *Br J Haematol* 95:21, 1996.

327. Lescale KB, Eddleman KA, Cines DB, et al: Antiplatelet antibody testing in thrombocytopenic pregnant women. *Am J Obstet Gynecol* 174:1014, 1996.

328. Ajzenberg N, Dreyfus M, Kaplan C, et al: Pregnancy-associated thrombocytopenia revisited: Assessment and follow-up of 50 cases. *Blood* 92:4573, 1998.

329. Moise KJ: Autoimmune thrombocytopenic purpura in pregnancy. *Clin Obstet Gynecol* 34:51, 1991.

330. Payne SD, Resnik R, Moore TR, et al: Maternal characteristics and risk of severe neonatal thrombocytopenia and intracranial hemorrhage in pregnancies complicated by autoimmune thrombocytopenia. *Am J Obstet Gynecol* 177:149, 1997.

331. Valat AS, Caulier MT, Devos P, et al: Relationships between severe neonatal thrombocytopenia and maternal characteristics in pregnancies associated with autoimmune thrombocytopenia. *Br J Haematol* 103:397, 1998.

332. Silver RM, Branch DW, Scott JR: Maternal thrombocytopenia in pregnancy: Time for a reassessment. *Am J Obstet Gynecol* 173:479, 1995.

333. Shalev O, Anteby E: Epidural anesthesia can be safely performed in gestational thrombocytopenia of >50,000/ul. *Blood* 88:62a, 1996.

334. Simon L, Santi TM, Sacquin P, Hamza J: Preanaesthetic assessment of coagulation abnormalities in obstetric patients: usefulness, timing and clinical implications. *Br J Anaesth* 78:678, 1997.

335. Rouse DJ, Owen J, Goldenberg RL: Routine maternal platelet count: An assessment of a technologically driven screening practice. *Am J Obstet Gynecol* 179:573, 1998.

336. Ruggeri M, Schiavotto C, Castaman G, et al: Gestational thrombocytopenia: a prospective study. *Haematologica* 82:341, 1997.

337. Mushambi MC, Halligan AW, Williamson K: Recent developments in the pathophysiology and management of pre-eclampsia. *Br J Anaesth* 76:133, 1996.

338. Leitch CR, Cameron AD, Walker JJ: The changing pattern of eclampsia over a 60-year period. *Br J Obstet Gynaecol* 104:917, 1997.

339. Thomas SV: Neurological aspects of eclampsia. *J Neurol Sci* 155:37, 1998.

340. Wallukat G, Homuth V, Fischer T, et al: Patients with preeclampsia develop agonistic autoantibodies against the angiotensin AT1 receptor. *J Clin Invest* 103:945, 1999.

341. Martin JN Jr, Files JC, Blake PG, et al: Postpartum plasma exchange for atypical preeclampsia-eclampsia as HELLP (hemolysis, elevated liver enzymes, and low platelets) syndrome. *Am J Obstet Gynecol* 172:1107, 1995.

342. Knox TA, Olans LB: Liver disease in pregnancy. *N Engl J Med* 335:569, 1996.

343. Sibai BM, Ramadan MK, Chari RS, Friedman SA: Pregnancies complicated by HELLP syndrome (hemolysis, elevated liver enzymes, and low platelets): Subsequent pregnancy outcome and long-term prognosis. *Am J Obstet Gynecol* 172:125, 1995.

344. Hedman A, Henter JI, Hedlund I, Elinder G: Prevalence and treatment of chronic idiopathic thrombocytopenic purpura of childhood in Sweden. *Acta Paediatr* 86:226, 1997.

345. Bolton-Maggs PHB, Moon I: Assessment of UK practice for management of acute childhood idiopathic thrombocytopenic purpura against published guidelines. *Lancet* 350:620, 1997.

346. Frederiksen H, Schmidt K: The incidence of ITP in adults increases with age. *Blood* 94:909, 1999.

347. Cortelazzo S, Finazzi G, Buelli M, et al: High risk of severe bleeding in aged patients with chronic idiopathic thrombocytopenic purpura. *Blood* 77:31, 1991.

348. Stasi R, Stipa E, Masi M, et al: Long-term observation of 208 adults with chronic idiopathic thrombocytopenic purpura. *Am J Med* 98:436, 1995.

349. Reid MM: Chronic idiopathic thrombocytopenic purpura: incidence, treatment, and outcome. *Arch Dis Child* 72:125, 1995.

350. George JN, El-Harake MA, Raskob GE: Chronic idiopathic thrombocytopenic purpura. *N Engl J Med* 331:1207, 1994.

351. Guthrie TH, Brannan DP, Prisant LM: Idiopathic thrombocytopenic purpura in the older adult patient. *Am J Med Sci* 296:17, 1988.

352. Harrington WJ, Minnich V, Hollingsworth JW, Moore CV: Demonstration of a thrombocytopenic factor in the blood of patients with thrombocytopenic purpura. *J Lab Clin Med* 38:1, 1951.

353. Altman LK: Black and blue at the flick of a feather, in *Anonymous, Who Goes First?* pp 273–282. New York, Random House, 1987.

354. Shulman NR, Weinrach RS, Libre EP, Andrews HL: The role of the reticuloendothelial system in the pathogenesis of idiopathic thrombocytopenic purpura. *Trans Assoc Am Phys* 78:374, 1965.

355. Schmidt EE, MacDonald IC, Groom AC: Changes in splenic microcirculatory pathways in chronic idiopathic thrombocytopenic purpura. *Blood* 78:1485, 1991.

356. Zeigler ZR, Rosenfeld CS, Numanaitis JJ, et al: Increased macrophage colony-stimulating factor levels in immune thrombocytopenic purpura. *Blood* 81:1251, 1993.

357. Ballem PJ, Segal GM, Stratton JR, et al: Mechanisms of thrombocytopenia in chronic autoimmune thrombocytopenia purpura. Evidence for both impaired platelet production and increased platelet clearance. *J Clin Invest* 80:33, 1987.

358. Siegel RS, Rae JL, Barth S, et al: Platelet survival and turnover: important factors in predicting response to splenectomy in immune thrombocytopenic purpura. *Am J Hematol* 30:206, 1989.

359. Stratton JR, Ballem PJ, Gernsheimer T, et al: Platelet destruction in autoimmune thrombocytopenic purpura: kinetics and clearance of Indium-111–labeled autologous platelets. *J Nucl Med* 30:629, 1989.

360. Takahashi R, Sekine N, Nakatake T: Influence of monoclonal antiplatelet glycoprotein antibodies on in vitro human megakaryocyte colony formation and proplatelet formation. *Blood* 93:1951, 1999.

361. Dixon R, Rosse WF, Ebbert L: Quantitative determination of antibody in idiopathic thrombocytopenic purpura. *N Engl J Med* 292:230, 1975.

362. Kelton JG, Powers P, Carter C: A prospective study of the usefulness of the measurement of platelet-associated IgG for the diagnosis of idiopathic thrombocytopenic purpura. *Blood* 60:1050, 1982.

363. George JN, Saucerman S: Platelet IgG, IgA, IgM, and albumin: correlation of platelet and plasma concentrations in normal subjects and in patients with ITP or dysproteinemia. *Blood* 72:362, 1988.

364. Levin J, Bessman JD: The inverse relation between platelet volume and platelet number. *J Lab Clin Med* 101:295, 1983.

365. Tavassoli M: Stress platelet: a platelet equivalent of stress reticulocyte. *Blood Cells* 18:295, 1992.

366. Takubo T, Yamane T, Hino M, et al: Usefulness of determining reticulated and large platelets in idiopathic thrombocytopenic purpura. *Acta Haematol* 99:109, 1998.

367. He R, Reid DM, Jones CE, Shulman NR: Spectrum of Ig classes, specificities, and titers of serum antiglycoproteins in chronic idiopathic thrombocytopenic purpura. *Blood* 83:1024, 1994.

368. Berchtold P, Wenger M: Autoantibodies against platelet glycoproteins in autoimmune thrombocytopenic purpura: their clinical significance and response to treatment. *Blood* 81:1246, 1993

369. Fujisawa K, Tani P, Piro L, McMillan R: The effect of therapy on platelet-associated autoantibody in chronic immune thrombocytopenic purpura. *Blood* 81:2872, 1993.

370. Berchtold P, Müller D, Beardsley D, et al: International study to compare antigen-specific methods used for the measurement of antiplatelet autoantibodies. *Br J Haematol* 96:477, 1997.

371. Raife TJ, Olson JD, Lentz SR: Platelet antibody testing in idiopathic thrombocytopenic purpura. *Blood* 89:1112, 1997.

372. Kekomaki R, Dawson B, McFarland J, Kunicki TJ: Localization of human platelet autoantigens to the cysteine-rich region of glycoprotein IIIa. *J Clin Invest* 88:847, 1991.

373. Fujisawa K, O'Toole TE, Tani P, et al: Autoantibodies to the presumptive cytoplasmic domain of platelet glycoprotein IIIa in patients with chronic immune thrombocytopenic purpura. *Blood* 77:2207, 1991.

374. Harker LA, Slichter SJ: The bleeding time as a screening test for evaluation of platelet function. *N Engl J Med* 287:155, 1972.

375. Balduini CL, Bertolino G, Noris P, et al: Defect of platelet aggregation and adhesion induced by autoantibodies against platelet glycoprotein IIIa. *Thromb Haemost* 68:208, 1992.

376. Varon D, Gitel SN, Varon N, et al: Immune Bernard Soulier-like syndrome associated with anti-glycoprotein-IX antibody. *Am J Hematol* 41:67, 1992.

377. Heyns AD, Fraser J, Retief FP: Platelet aggregation in chronic idiopathic thrombocytopenic purpura. *J Clin Path* 31:1239, 1978.

378. Nieuwenhuis HK, Zwaginga JJ, Sixma JJ: Analysis of patients with a prolonged bleeding time. *Thromb Haemost* 58:527, 1987.

379. Nojima J, Suehisa E, Kuratsune H, et al: High prevalence of thrombocytopenia in SLE patients with a high level of anticardiolipin antibodies combined with lupus anticoagulant. *Am J Hematol* 58:55, 1998.

380. Aggarwal A, Doolittle G: Autoimmune thrombocytopenic purpura associated with hyperthyroidism in a single individual. *South Med J* 90:933, 1997.

381. Cordiano I, Betterle C, Spadaccino CA, et al: Autoimmune thrombocytopenia (AITP) and thyroid autoimmune disease (TAD): overlapping syndromes? *Clin Exp Immunol* 113:373, 1998.

382. Hofbauer LC, Spitzweg C, Schmauss S, Heufelder AE: Graves disease associated with autoimmune thrombocytopenic purpura. *Arch Intern Med* 157:1033, 1997.

383. Kurata Y, Miyagawa S, Kosugi S, et al: High-titer antinuclear antibodies, anti-SSA/Ro antibodies and anti-nuclear RNP antibodies in patients with idiopathic thrombocytopenic purpura. *Thromb Haemost* 71:184, 1994.

384. Stasi R, Stipa E, Masi M, et al: Prevalence and clinical significance of elevated antiphospholipid antibodies in patients with idiopathic thrombocytopenic purpura. *Blood* 84:4203, 1994.

385. Lipp E, Von Felten A, Sax H, et al: Antibodies against platelet glycoproteins and antiphospholipid antibodies in autoimmune thrombocytopenia. *Eur J Haematol* 60:283, 1998.

386. George JN, Caen JP, Nurden AT: Glanzmann's thrombasthenia: the spectrum of clinical disease. *Blood* 75:1383, 1990.

387. Woerner SJ, Abildgaard CF, French BN: Intracranial hemorrhage in children with idiopathic thrombocytopenic purpura. *Pediatrics* 67:453, 1981.

388. Lee MS, Kim WC: Intracranial hemorrhage associated with idiopathic thrombocytopenic purpura: Report of seven patients and a meta-analysis. *Neurology* 50:1160, 1998.

389. Lacey JV, Penner JA: Management of idiopathic thrombocytopenic purpura in the adult. *Semin Thromb Hemost* 3:160, 1977.

390. Doan CA, Bouroncle BA, Wiseman BK: Idiopathic and secondary thrombocytopenic purpura: clinical study and evaluation of 381 cases over a period of 28 years. *Ann Intern Med* 53:861, 1960.

391. Steffan A, Pradella P, Cordiano I, et al: Glycocalicin in the diagnosis and management of immune thrombocytopenia. *Eur J Haematol* 61:77, 1998.

392. Rodgers RPC, Levin J: A critical reappraisal of the bleeding time. *Semin Thromb Hemost* 16:1, 1990.

393. Mayan H, Salomon O, Pauzner R, Farfel Z: EDTA-induced pseudo-thrombocytopenia. *South Med J* 85:213, 1992.

394. Najean Y, Lecompte T: Chronic pure thrombocytopenia in elderly patients: An aspect of the myelodysplastic syndrome. *Cancer* 64:2506, 1989.

395. Menke DM, Colon-Otero G, Cockerill KJ, et al: Refractory thrombocytopenia: A myelodysplastic syndrome that may mimic immune thrombocytopenic purpura. *Am J Clin Pathol* 98:502, 1992.

396. Mosesson MW, Colman RW, Sherry S: Chronic intravascular coagulation syndrome. Report of a case with special studies of an associated plasma cryoprecipitate ("Cryofibrinogen"). *N Engl J Med* 278:815, 1968.

397. Kaufman DW, Kelly JP, Johannes CB, et al: Acute thrombocytopenic purpura in relation to the use of drugs. *Blood* 82:2714, 1993.

398. George JN, Raskob GE, Shah SR, et al: Drug-induced thrombocytopenia:

A systematic review of published case reports. *Ann Intern Med* 129:886, 1998.

399. Watson-Williams EJ, Macpherson AIS, Davidson S: The treatment of idiopathic thrombocytopenic purpura. *Lancet* 2:221, 1958.

400. Stefanini M: Idiopathic thrombocytopenic purpura (ITP): an analysis of 1122 cases. *Nouv Rev Fr Hematol* 32:129, 1990.

401. Ikkala E, Kivilaakso E, Kotilainen M, Hastbacka J: Treatment of idiopathic thrombocytopenic purpura in adults. *Ann Clin Res* 10:83, 1978.

402. Carr JM, Kruskall MS, Kaye JA, Robinson SH: Efficacy of platelet transfusions in immune thrombocytopenia. *Am J Med* 80:1051, 1986.

403. Baumann MA, Menitove JE, Aster RH, Anderson T: Urgent treatment of idiopathic thrombocytopenic purpura with single-dose gammaglobulin infusion followed by platelet transfusion. *Ann Intern Med* 104:808, 1986.

404. Bartholomew JR, Salgia R, Bell WR: Control of bleeding in patients with immune and nonimmune thrombocytopenia with aminocaproic acid. *Arch Intern Med* 149:1959, 1989.

405. McVay PA, Toy PTCY: Lack of increased bleeding after liver biopsy in patients with mild hemostatic abnormalities. *Am J Clin Pathol* 94:747, 1990.

406. Kitchens CS, Pendergast JF: Human thrombocytopenia is associated with structural abnormalities of the endothelium that are ameliorated by glucocorticosteroid administration. *Blood* 67:203, 1986.

407. Gernsheimer T, Stratton J, Ballem PJ, Slichter SJ: Mechanisms of response to treatment in autoimmune thrombocytopenic purpura. *N Engl J Med* 320:974, 1989.

408. Lukert BP, Raisz LG: Glucocorticoid-induced osteoporosis: Pathogenesis and management. *Ann Intern Med* 112:352, 1990.

409. Reid IR: Glucocorticoid osteoporosis: mechanisms and management. *Eur J Endocrinol* 137:209, 1997.

410. Jacobs P, Wood L, Novitzky N: Intravenous gammaglobulin has no advantages over oral corticosteroids as primary therapy for adults with immune thrombocytopenia: a prospective randomized clinical trial. *Am J Med* 97:55, 1994.

411. Imbach P, d'Apuzzo V, Hirt A, et al: High-dose intravenous gammaglobulin for idiopathic thrombocytopenic purpura in childhood. *Lancet* 1:1228, 1981.

412. Bussel JB, Pham LC, Aledort L, Nachman R: Maintenance treatment of adults with chronic refractory immune thrombocytopenic purpura using repeated intravenous infusions of gammaglobulin. *Blood* 72:121, 1988.

413. Yu Z, Lennon VA: Mechanisms of intravenous immune globulin therapy in antibody-mediated autoimmune diseases. *N Engl J Med* 340:227, 1999.

414. Blanchette V, Imbach P, Andrew M, et al: Randomised trial of intravenous immunoglobulin G, intravenous anti-D, and oral prednisone in childhood acute immune thrombocytopenic purpura. *Lancet* 344:703, 1994.

415. Kattamis AC, Shankar S, Cohen AR: Neurologic complications of treatment of childhood acute immune thrombocytopenic purpura with intravenously administered immunoglobulin G. *J Pediatr* 130:281, 1997.

416. Sekul EA, Cupler EJ, Dalakas MC: Aseptic meningitis associated with high-dose intravenous immunoglobulin therapy: Frequency and risk factors. *Ann Intern Med* 121:259, 1994.

417. Tarantino MD, Madden RM, Fennewald L, et al: Treatment of childhood acute immune thrombocytopenic purpura with anti-D immune globulin or pooled immune globulin. *J Pediatr* 134:21, 1999.

418. Andrew M, Blanchette VS, Adams M, et al: A multicenter study of the treatment of childhood chronic idiopathic thrombocytopenic purpura with anti-D. *J Pediatr* 120:522, 1992.

419. Rovo A, Penchasky D, Korin J, et al: Splenectomy in idiopathic thrombocytopenic purpura (ITP). Effective, yes, but for how long. *Blood* 92:177a, 1999.

420. Rocco MV, Stein RS: Prognostic factors for splenectomy response in adult idiopathic thrombocytopenic purpura. *South Med J* 77:983, 1984.

421. Coon WW: Splenectomy for idiopathic thrombocytopenic purpura. *Surg Gynecol Obstet* 164:225, 1987.

422. Fabris F, Zanatta N, Casonato A, et al: Response to splenectomy in idiopathic thrombocytopenic purpura: prognostic value of the clinical and laboratory evaluation. *Acta Haematol* 81:28, 1989.

423. Law C, Marcaccio M, Tam P, et al: High-dose intravenous immune globulin and the response to splenectomy in patients with idiopathic thrombocytopenic purpura. *N Engl J Med* 336:1494, 1997.

424. Schneider P, Wehmeier A, Schneider W: High-dose intravenous immune globulin and the response to splenectomy in patients with idiopathic thrombocytopenic purpura. *N Engl J Med* 337:1087, 1997.

425. Najean Y, Rain JD, Billotey C: The site of destruction of autologous ^{111}In-labelled platelets and the efficiency of splenectomy in children and adults with idiopathic thrombocytopenic purpura: A study of 578 patients with 268 splenectomies. *Br J Haematol* 97:547, 1997.

426. Fenaux P, Caulier MT, Hirschauer C, et al: Reevaluation of the prognostic factors for splenectomy in chronic idiopathic thrombocytopenic purpura (ITP): A report on 181 cases. *Eur J Haematol* 42:259, 1989.

427. Julia A, Araguas C, Rossello J, et al: Lack of useful clinical predictors of response to splenectomy in patients with chronic idiopathic thrombocytopenic purpura. *Br J Haematol* 76:250, 1990.

428. Shaw JHF, Clark MA: Splenectomy for immune thrombocytopenic purpura: Auckland experience 1979–1987. *Aust NZ J Surg* 59:123, 1989.

429. Watson DI, Coventry BJ, Chin T, et al: Laparoscopic versus open splenectomy for immune thrombocytopenic purpura. *Surgery* 121:18, 1997.

430. Tsiotos G, Schlinkert RT: Laparoscopic splenectomy for immune thrombocytopenic purpura. *Arch Surg* 132:642, 1997.

431. Schilling RF: Estimating the risk for sepsis after splenectomy in hereditary spherocytosis. *Ann Intern Med* 122:187, 1995.

432. Centers for Disease Control and Prevention: Recommendations of the Advisory Committee on Immunization Practices: Use of vaccines and immune globulins in persons with altered immunocompetence. *MMWR.* 42:1, 1993.

433. Lortan JE: Clinical annotation. Management of asplenic patients. *Br J Haematol* 84:566, 1993.

434. Boxer MA, Braun J, Ellman L: Thromboembolic risk of postsplenectomy thrombocytosis. *Arch Surg* 113:808, 1978.

435. Akwari OE, Itani KMF, Coleman RE, Rosse WF: Splenectomy for primary and recurrent immune thrombocytopenic purpura. *Ann Surg* 206:529, 1987.

436. Aspnes GT, Pearson HA, Spencer RP, Pickett LK: Recurrent idiopathic thrombocytopenia purpura with "accessory" splenic tissue. *Pediatrics* 55:131, 1975.

437. Eraklis AJ, Fillwe RM: Splenectomy in childhood: a review of 1413 cases. *J Pediatr Surg* 7:382, 1972.

438. Facon T, Caulier MT, Fenaux P, et al: Accessory spleen in recurrent chronic immune thrombocytopenic purpura. *Am J Hematol* 41:184, 1992.

439. Calverley DC, Jones GW, Kelton JG: Splenic radiation for corticosteroid-resistant immune thrombocytopenia. *Ann Intern Med* 116:977, 1992.

440. Caulier MT, Darloy F, Rose C, et al: Splenic irradiation for chronic autoimmune thrombocytopenic purpura in patients with contra-indications to splenectomy. *Br J Haematol* 91:208, 1995.

441. Lagares FM, Fuertes FF, Cabrero TH, et al: Complete splenic embolization in the treatment of immune thrombocytopenic purpura. *Br J Haematol* 103:894, 1998.

442. Wandt H, Frank M, Ehninger G, et al: Safety and cost effectiveness of a 10×10^9/L trigger for prophylactic platelet transfusions compared with the traditional 20×10^9/L trigger: a prospective comparative trial in 105 patients with acute myeloid leukemia. *Blood* 91:3601, 1998.

443. Rebulla P, Finazzi G, Marangoni F, et al: The threshold for prophylactic platelet transfusions in adults with acute myeloid leukemia. *N Engl J Med* 337:1870, 1997.

444. Andersen JC: Response of resistant idiopathic thrombocytopenic purpura to pulsed high-dose dexamethasone therapy. *N Engl J Med* 330:1560, 1994.

445. Caulier MT, Rose C, Roussel MT, et al: Pulsed high-dose dexamethasone in refractory chronic idiopathic thrombocytopenic purpura: a report on 10 cases. *Br J Haematol* 91:477, 1995.

446. Demiroglu H, Dündar S: High-dose pulsed dexamethasone for immune thrombocytopenia. *N Engl J Med* 337:425, 1997.

447. Quiquandon I, Fenaux P, Caulier MT, et al: Re-evaluation of the role of azathioprine in the treatment of adult chronic idiopathic thrombocytopenic purpura: a report on 53 cases. *Br J Haematol* 74:223, 1990.

448. Pizzuto J, Ambriz R: Therapeutic experience on 934 adults with idiopathic thrombocytopenic purpura: multicentric trial of the cooperative Latin American group on hemostasis and thrombosis. *Blood* 64:1179, 1984.

449. Kyle RA, Gertz MA: Second malignancies after chemotherapy, in *The*

Chemotherapy Sourcebook, edited by MC Perry, pp 689–702. Baltimore, Williams and Wilkins, 1992.

450. Nord E, Douer D, Kessler E, et al: Sclerosing reticulum cell sarcoma following prolonged treatment with azathioprine for idiopathic thrombocytopenic purpura. *Scand J Haematol* 17:321, 1976.

451. Smith AG, Prentice AG, Lucie NP, et al: Acute myelogenous leukaemia following cytotoxic therapy: five cases and a review. *Q J Med* 51:227, 1982.

452. Doll DC, Ringenberg QS, Yarbro JW: Antineoplastic agents and pregnancy. *Semin Oncol* 16:337, 1989.

453. Verlin M, Laros RK, Penner JA: Treatment of refractory thrombocytopenic purpura with cyclophosphamide. *Am J Hematol* 1:97, 1976.

454. Reiner A, Gernsheimer T, Slichter SJ: Pulse cyclophosphamide therapy for refractory autoimmune thrombocytopenic purpura. *Blood* 85:351, 1995.

455. Dawisha SM, Yarboro CH, Vaughan EM, et al: Outpatient monthly oral bolus cyclophosphamide therapy in systemic lupus erythematosus. *J Rheumatol* 23:273, 1996.

456. Fairley KF, Barrie JU, Johnson W: Sterility and testicular atrophy related to cyclophosphamide therapy. *Lancet* 1972;568.

457. Warne GL, Fairley KF, Hobbs JB, Martin FIR: Cyclophosphamide-induced ovarian failure. *N Engl J Med* 289:1159, 1973.

458. Johnson WW, Meadows DC: Urinary-bladder fibrosis and telangiectasia associated with long-term cyclophosphamide therapy. *N Engl J Med* 284:290, 1971.

459. Curtis RE, Boice JD, Stovall M, et al: Risk of leukemia after chemotherapy and radiation treatment for breast cancer. *N Engl J Med* 326:1745, 1992.

460. Krause JR: Chronic idiopathic thrombocytopenic purpura (ITP): development of acute nonlymphocytic leukemia subsequent to treatment with cyclophosphamide. *Med Pediatric Oncol* 10:61, 1982.

461. Carbone PP, Bono V, Frei E, Brindley CO: Clinical studies with vincristine. *Blood* 21:640, 1963.

462. Hwang YF, Hamilton HE, Sheets RF: Vinblastine-induced thrombocytosis. *Lancet* 2:1075, 1969.

463. Robertson JH, Crozier EH, Woodend BE: The effect of vincristine on the platelet count in rats. *Br J Haematol* 19:331, 1970.

464. Ahn YS, Harrington WJ, Mylvaganam R, et al: Slow infusion of vinca alkaloids in the treatment of idiopathic thrombocytopenic purpura. *Ann Intern Med* 100:192, 1984.

465. Fenaux P, Quiquandon I, Caulier MT, et al: Slow infusions of vinblastine in the treatment of adult idiopathic thrombocytopenic purpura: a report on 43 cases. *Blut* 60:238, 1990.

466. Facon T, Caulier MT, Wattel E, et al: A randomized trial comparing vinblastine in slow infusion and by bolus i.v. injection in idiopathic thrombocytopenic purpura: a report on 42 patients. *Br J Haematol* 86:678, 1994.

467. Ahn YS, Harrington WJ, Simon SR, et al: Danazol for the treatment of idiopathic thrombocytopenic purpura. *N Engl J Med* 308:1396, 1983.

468. Fraser IS, Burridge J: Danazol treatment and platelet function. *Med J Aust* 1:313, 1980.

469. Ahn YS, Mylvaganam R, Garcia RO, et al: Low-dose danazol therapy in idiopathic thrombocytopenic purpura. *Ann Intern Med* 107:177, 1987.

470. McVerry BA, Auger M, Bellingham AJ: The use of danazol in the management of chronic immune thrombocytopenic purpura. *Br J Haematol* 61:145, 1985.

471. Ambriz R, Pizzuto J, Morales M, et al: Therapeutic effect of danazol on metrorrhagia in patients with idiopathic thrombocytopenic purpura (ITP). *Nouv Rev Fr Hematol* 28:275, 1986.

472. Almagro D: Danazol in idiopathic thrombocytopenic purpura. *Acta Haematol* 74:120, 1985.

473. Marino C, Cook P: Danazol for lupus thrombocytopenia. *Arch Intern Med* 145:2251, 1985.

474. Pignon J-M, Poirson E, Rochant H: Danazol in autoimmune haemolytic anaemia. *Br J Haematol* 83:343, 1993.

475. Arrowsmith JB, Dreis M: Thrombocytopenia after treatment with Danazol. *N Engl J Med* 314:585, 1986.

476. Rabinowe SN, Miller KB: Danazol-induced thrombocytopenia. *Br J Haematol* 65:383, 1987.

477. Flores A, Carles J, Junca J, Abella E: Danazol therapy in chronic immune thrombocytopenic purpura. *Eur J Haematol* 45:109, 1990.

478. Grange MJ, Dombret MC, Fantin B, Gougerot-Pocidalo MA: Fatal acute pulmonary fibrosis in a patient treated by danazol for thrombocytopenia. *Am J Hematol* 53:149, 1996.

479. Bussel JB, Saal S, Gordon B: Combined plasma exchange and intravenous gammaglobulin in the treatment of patients with refractory immune thrombocytopenic purpura. *Transfusion* 28:38, 1988.

480. Blanchette VS, Hogan VA, McCombie NE, et al: Intensive plasma exchange therapy in ten patients with idiopathic thrombocytopenic purpura. *Transfusion.* 24:388, 1984.

481. Strother SV, Zuckerman KS, LoBuglio AF: Colchicine therapy for refractory idiopathic thrombocytopenic purpura. *Arch Intern Med* 144:2198, 1984.

482. Brox AG, Howson-Jan K, Fauser AA: Treatment of idiopathic thrombocytopenic purpura with ascorbate. *Br J Haematol* 70:341, 1988.

483. Figueroa M, Gehlsen J, Hammond D, et al: Combination chemotherapy in refractory immune thrombocytopenic purpura. *N Engl J Med* 328:1226, 1993.

484. Lim SH, Kell J, Al-Sabah A, et al: Peripheral blood stem-cell transplantation for refractory autoimmune thrombocytopenic purpura. *Lancet* 349:475, 1997.

485. Skoda RC, Tichelli A, Tyndall A, et al: Autologous peripheral blood stem cell transplantation in a patient with chronic autoimmune thrombocytopenia. *Br J Haematol* 99:56, 1997.

486. Brodsky R, Petri M, Smith BD, et al: Immunoablative high-dose cyclophosphamide without stem cell rescue for refractory, severe autoimmune disease. *Ann Intern Med* 129:1031, 1998.

487. Snyder HW, Cochran SK, Balint JP, et al: Experience with protein A-immunoadsorption in treatment-resistant adult immune thrombocytopenic purpura. *Blood* 79:2237, 1992.

488. Cahill MR, Macey MG, Cavenagh JD, Newland AC: Protein A immunoadsorption in chronic refractory ITP reverses increased platelet activation but fails to achieve sustained clinical benefit. *Br J Haematol* 100:358, 1998.

489. Kabisch A, Kroll H, Wedi B, et al: Severe adverse effects of protein A immunoadsorption. *Lancet* 343:116, 1994.

490. Figueroa M, McMillan R: 2-chlorodeoxyadenosine in the treatment of chronic refractory immune thrombocytopenic purpura. *Blood* 81:3484, 1993.

491. Fujimura K, Takafuta T, Kuriya S, et al: Recombinant human interferon a-2b (rh IFNa-2b) therapy for steroid resistant idiopathic thrombocytopenic purpura (ITP). *Am J Hematol* 51:37, 1996.

492. Dubbeld P, Hillen HFP, Schouten HC: Interferon treatment of refractory idiopathic thrombocytopenic purpura (ITP). *Eur J Haematol* 52:233, 1994.

493. Cavanna L, Vallisa D, Berte R, et al: Severe immune thrombocytopenic purpura relapse after alpha-interferon in chronic myeloid leukemia, successfully treated with cyclosporine. *Am J Hematol* 47:255, 1994.

494. Shirota T, Yamamoto H, Fujimoto H, et al: Cyclic thrombocytopenia in a patient treated with cyclosporine for refractory idiopathic thrombocytopenic purpura. *Am J Hematol* 56:272, 1997.

495. Godeau B, Durand JM, Roudot-Thoraval F, et al: Dapsone for chronic autoimmune thrombocytopenic purpura: A report of 66 cases. *Br J Haematol* 97:336, 1997.

496. Paidas MJ, Berkowitz RL, Lynch L, et al: Alloimmune thrombocytopenia: Fetal and neonatal losses related to cordocentesis. *Am J Obstet.Gynecol* 172:475, 1995.

497. Burrows RF, Kelton JG: Low fetal risks in pregnancies associated with idiopathic thrombocytopenic purpura. *Am J Obstet Gynecol* 163:1147, 1990.

498. Kurtzberg J, Stockman JAI: Idiopathic autoimmune thrombocytopenia purpura. *Adv Pediatr* 41:111, 1994.

499. Calpin C, Dick P, Poon A, Feldman W: Is bone marrow aspiration needed in acute childhood idiopathic thrombocytopenic purpura to rule out leukemia? *Arch Pediatr Adolesc Med* 152:345, 1998.

500. Vesely S, Buchanan GR, George JN, et al: Self-reported diagnostic and management strategies in childhood idiopathic thrombocytopenic purpura: Results of a survey of practicing pediatric hematology/oncology specialists. *Am J Pediatr Hematol Oncol* (in press) 1999.

501. Eden OB, Lilleyman JS, British Paediatric Haematology Group: Guidelines for management of idiopathic thrombocytopenic purpura. *Arch Dis Child* 67:1056, 1997.

502. Blanchette VS, Luke B, Andrew M, et al: A prospective, randomized trial of high-dose intravenous immune globulin G therapy, oral prednisone

therapy, and no therapy in childhood acute immune thrombocytopenic purpura. *J Pediatr* 123:989, 1993.

503. Medeiros D, Buchanan GR: Major hemorrhage in children with idiopathic thrombocytopenic purpura: Immediate response to therapy and long-term outcome. *J Pediatr* 133:334, 1998.

504. Nagasawa T, Hasegawa Y, Kamoshita M, et al: Megakaryopoiesis in patients with cyclic thrombocytopenia. *Br J Haematol* 91:185, 1995.

505. Balduini CL, Stella CC, Rosti V, et al: Acquired cyclic thrombocytopenia-thrombocytosis with periodic defect of platelet function. *Br J Haematol* 85:718, 1993.

506. Cederblad G, Hahn L, Korsan-Bengtsen K: Variations in blood coagulation, fibrinolysis, platelet function and various plasma proteins during the menstrual cycle. *Thromb Haemost* 6:294, 1977.

507. Minot GR: Purpura hemorrhagica and lymphocytosis: acute type and intermittent menstrual type. *Am J Med Sci* 192:445, 1936.

508. Tomer A, Schreiber AD, McMillan R, et al: Menstrual cyclic thrombocytopenia. *Br J Haematol.* 71:519, 1989.

509. Helleberg C, Taaning E, Hansen PB: Cyclic thrombocytopenia successfully treated with low dose hormonal contraception. *Am J Hematol* 48:62, 1995.

510. Kosugi S, Tomiyama Y, Shiraga M, et al: Cyclic thrombocytopenia associated with IgM anti-GPIIb-IIIa autoantibodies. *Br J Haematol* 88:809, 1994.

511. Yanabu M, Nomura S, Fukuroi T, et al: Periodic production of antiplatelet autoantibody directed against GPIIIa in cyclic thrombocytopenia. *Acta Haematol* 89:155, 1993.

512. Tefferi A, Solberg LA, Petitt RM, Willis LG: Adult-onset cyclic bicytopenia: a case report and review of treatment of cyclic hematopoiesis. *Am J Hematol* 30:181, 1989.

513. Kimura F, Nakamura Y, Sato K, et al: Cyclic change of cytokines in a patient with cyclic thrombocytopenia. *Br J Haematol* 94:171, 1996.

514. Oh H, Nakamura H, Yokota A, et al: Serum thrombopoietin levels in cyclic thrombocytopenia. *Blood* 87:4918, 1996.

515. Williamson LM, Poole J, Redman C, et al: Transient loss of proteins carrying Kell and Lutheran red cell antigens during consecutive relapses of autoimmune thrombocytopenia. *Br J Haematol* 87:805, 1994.

516. Christie DJ, Mullen PC, Aster RH: Fab-mediated binding of drug-dependent antibodies to platelets in quinidine- and quinine-induced thrombocytopenia. *J Clin Invest* 75:310, 1985.

517. Burgess JK, Lopez JA, Berndt MC, et al: Quinine-dependent antibodies bind a restricted set of epitopes on the glycoprotein Ib-IX complex: characterization of the epitopes. *Blood* 92:2366, 1998.

518. Chong BH, Du X, Berndt MD, et al: Characterization of the binding domains on platelet glycoproteins Ib-IX and IIb/IIIa complexes for the quinine/quinidine-dependent antibodies. *Blood* 77:2190, 1991.

519. López JA, Li CQ, Weisman S, Chambers M: The glycoprotein Ib-IX complex-specific monoclonal antibody SZ1 binds to a conformation-sensitive epitope on glycoprotein IX: Implications for the target antigen of quinine/quinidine-dependent autoantibodies. *Blood* 85:1254, 1995.

520. Gentilini G, Curtis BR, Aster RH: An antibody from a patient with ranitidine-induced thrombocytopenia recognizes a site on glycoprotein IX that is a favored target for drug-induced antibodies. *Blood* 92:2359, 1998.

521. Curtis BR, McFarland JG, Wu G-G, et al: Antibodies in sulfonamide-induced immune thrombocytopenia recognize calcium-dependent epitopes on the glycoprotein IIb/IIIa Complex. *Blood* 84:176, 1994.

522. Visentin GP, Newman PJ, Aster RH: Characteristics of quinine- and quinidine-induced antibodies specific for platelet glycoproteins IIb and IIIa. *Blood* 77:2668, 1991.

523. Berkowitz SD, Harrington RA, Rund MM, Tcheng JE: Acute profound thrombocytopenia after c7E3 Fab (abciximab) therapy. *Circulation* 95:819, 1997.

524. Berkowitz SD, Sane DC, Sigmon KN, et al: Occurrence and clinical significance of thrombocytopenia in a population undergoing high-risk percutaneous coronary revascularization. *J Am Coll Cardiol* 32:311, 1998.

525. Cancio LC, Cohen DJ: Heparin-induced thrombocytopenia and thrombosis. *J Am Coll Surg* 186:76, 1998.

526. Coblyn JS, Weinblatt M, Holdsworth D, Glass D: Gold-induced thrombocytopenia. *Ann Intern Med* 95:178, 1981.

527. Nieminen U, Kekomäki R: Quinidine-induced thrombocytopenic pur-

528. Leach MF, Cooper LK, AuBuchon JP: Detection of drug-dependent, platelet-reactive antibodies by solid-phase red cell adherence assays. *Br J Haematol* 97:755, 1997.

529. Visentin GP, Malik M, Cyganiak KA, Aster RH: Patients treated with unfractionated heparin during open heart surgery are at high risk to form antibodies reactive with heparin: platelet factor 4 complexes. *J Lab Clin Med* 128:376, 1996.

530. Boon DMS, van Vliet HHDM, Zietse R, Kappers-Klunne MC: The presence of antibodies against a PF4–heparin complex in patients on haemodialysis. *Thromb Haemost* 76:480, 1996.

531. Kappers-Klunne MC, Boon DMS, Hop WCJ, et al: Heparin-induced thrombocytopenia and thrombosis: a prospective analysis of the incidence in patients with heart and cerebrovascular diseases. *Br J Haematol* 96:442, 1997.

532. Bauer TL, Arepally G, Konkle BA, et al: Prevalence of heparin-associated antibodies without thrombosis in patients undergoing cardiopulmonary bypass surgery. *Circulation* 95:1242, 1997.

533. Belkin GA: Cocktail purpura: An unusual case of quinine sensitivity. *Ann Intern Med* 66:583, 1967.

534. Siroty RR: Purpura on the rocks—with a twist. *JAMA* 235:2521, 1976.

535. Pedersen-Bjergaard U, Andersen M, Hansen PB: Drug-induced thrombocytopenia: Clinical data on 309 cases and the effect of corticosteroid therapy. *Eur J Clin Pharmacol* 52:183, 1997.

536. Warkentin TE, Kelton JG: A 14-year study of heparin-induced thrombocytopenia. *Am J Med* 101:502, 1996.

537. Warkentin TE, Chong BH, Greinacher A: Heparin-induced thrombocytopenia: toward consensus. *Thromb Haemost* 79:1, 1998.

538. Killer S, Zoppi M, Künzi UP, et al: Heparin-induced thrombocytopenia (HIT)—Results of the Comprehensive Hospital Drug Monitoring project (Berne, St Gallen). *Schweiz Med Woch* 125:2518, 1995.

539. Hirsh J, Warkentin TE, Raschke R, et al: Heparin and low-molecular-weight heparin. *Chest* 114:489s, 1998.

540. Bell WR, Tomasulo PA, Alving BA, Duffy TP: Thrombocytopenia occurring during the administration of heparin. A prospective study of 52 patients. *Ann Intern Med* 85:155, 1976.

541. George JN:. Heparin-associated thrombocytopenia, in *Disorders of Thrombosis*, edited by R Hull, GF Pineo, pp 359–73. Philadelphia, Saunders, 1996.

542. Saffle JR, Russo J, Dukes GE, Warden GD: The effect of low-dose heparin therapy on serum platelet and transaminase levels. *J Surg Res* 28:297, 1980.

543. Schwartz KA, Royer G, Kaufman DB, Penner JA: Complications of heparin administration in normal individuals. *Am J Hematol* 19:355, 1985.

544. Stead RB, Schafer AI, Rosenberg RD, et al: Heterogeneity of heparin lots associated with thrombocytopenia and thromboembolism. *Am J Med* 77:185, 1984.

545. Horne MK III, Chao ES: Heparin binding to resting and activated platelets. *Blood* 74:238, 1989.

546. Horne MKI, Chao ES: The effect of molecular weight on heparin binding to platelets. *Br J Haematol* 74:306, 1990.

547. Salzman EW, Rosenberg RD, Smith MH, et al: Effect of heparin and heparin fractions on platelet aggregation. *J Clin Invest* 65:64, 1980.

548. Saba HI, Saba SR, Morelli GA: Effect of heparin on platelet aggregation. *Am J Hematol* 17:2, 1984.

549. Westwick J, Scully MF, Poll C, Kakkar VV: Comparison of the effects of low molecular weight heparin and unfractionated heparin on activation of human platelets in vitro. *Thromb Res* 42:435, 1986.

550. Eika C: Platelet refractory state induced by heparin. *Scand J Haematol* 9:665, 1972.

551. Shojania AM, Turnbull G: Effect of heparin on platelet count and platelet aggregation. *Am J Hematol* 26:255, 1987.

552. Pfueller SL, David R: Different platelet specificities of heparin-dependent platelet aggregating factors in heparin-associated immune thrombocytopenia. *Br J Haematol* 64:149, 1986.

553. Warkentin TE, Hayward CPM, Smith CA, et al: Determinants of donor platelet variability when testing for heparin-induced thrombocytopenia. *J Lab Clin Med* 120:371, 1992.

554. Kelton JG, Sheridan D, Santos A: Heparin-induced thrombocytopenia: Laboratory studies. *Blood* 72:925, 1988.

555. Cines DB, Kaywin P, Bina M, et al: Heparin-associated thrombocytopenia. *N Engl J Med* 303:788, 1980.

556. Arepally G, Reynolds C, Tomaski A, et al: Comparison of PF4/heparin ELISA assay with the ^{14}C-serotonin release assay in the diagnosis of heparin-induced thrombocytopenia. *Am J Clin Path* 104:648, 1995.

557. Suh JS, Aster RH, Visentin GP: Antibodies from patients with heparin-induced thrombocytopenia/thrombosis recognize different epitopes on heparin:platelet factor 4. *Blood* 91:916, 1998.

558. Ziporen L, Li ZQ, Park KS, et al: Defining an antigenic epitope on platelet factor 4 associated with heparin-induced thrombocytopenia. *Blood* 92:3250, 1998.

559. George JN, Onofre AR: Human platelet surface binding of endogenous secreted factor VIII-von Willebrand factor and platelet factor 4. *Blood* 59:194, 1982.

560. Visentin GP, Ford SE, Scott JP, Aster RH: Antibodies from patients with heparin-induced thrombocytopenia/thrombosis are specific for platelet factor 4 complexed with heparin or bound to endothelial cells. *J Clin Invest* 93:81, 1994.

561. Horne MK III, Alkins BR: Platelet binding of IgG from patients with heparin-induced thrombocytopenia. *J Lab Clin Med* 127:435, 1996.

562. Newman PM, Swanson RL, Chong BH: Heparin-induced thrombocytopenia: IgG binding to PF4-heparin complexes in the fluid phase and cross-reactivity with low molecular weight heparin and heparinoid. *Thromb Haemost* 80:292, 1998.

563. Chong BH, Murray B, Berndt MC, et al: Plasma P-selectin is increased in thrombotic consumptive platelet disorders. *Blood* 79:1, 1994.

564. Warkentin TE, Hayward CPM, Boshkov LK, et al: Sera from patients with heparin-induced thrombocytopenia generate platelet-derived microparticles with procoagulant activity: An explanation for the thrombotic complications of heparin-induced thrombocytopenia. *Blood* 84:3691, 1994.

565. Carlsson LE, Santoso S, Baurichter G, et al: Heparin-induced thrombocytopenia: New insights into the impact of the FcgammaRIIa-R-H131 polymorphism. *Blood* 92:1526, 1998.

566. Bachelot-Loza C, Saffroy R, Lasne D, et al: Importance of the FcgammaRIIa-Arg/His-131 polymorphism in heparin-induced thrombocytopenia diagnosis. *Thromb Haemost* 79:523, 1998.

567. Denomme GA, Warkentin TE, Horsewood P, et al: Activation of platelets by sera containing IgG1 heparin-dependent antibodies: an explanation for the predominance of the FcgammaRIIa "low responder" (his[131]) gene in patients with heparin-induced thrombocytopenia. *J Lab Clin Med* 130:278, 1997.

568. Burgess JK, Lindeman R, Chesterman CN, Chong BH: Single amino acid mutation of Fc gamma receptor is associated with the development of heparin-induced thrombocytopenia. *Br J Haematol* 91:761, 1995.

569. Brandt JT, Isenhart CE, Osborne JM, Ahmed A: On the role of platelet FcgammaRIIa phenotype in heparin-induced thrombocytopenia. *Thromb Haemost* 74:1564, 1995.

570. Arepally G, McKenzie SE, Jiang XM, et al: FcgammaRIIA H/R[131] polymorphism, subclass-specific IgG anti-heparin/platelet factor 4 antibodies and clinical course in patients with heparin-induced thrombocytopenia and thrombosis. *Blood* 89:370, 1997.

571. Polgár J, Eichler P, Greinacher A, Clemetson KJ: Adenosine diphosphate (ADP) and ADP receptor play a major role in platelet activation/aggregation induced by sera from heparin-induced thrombocytopenia patients. *Blood* 91:549, 1998.

572. Hull RD, Raskob GE, Pineo GF, et al: Subcutaneous low-molecular-weight heparin compared with continous intravenous heparin in the treatment of proximal-vein thrombosis. *N Engl J Med* 326:975, 1992.

573. Greinacher A, Michels I, Schafer M, et al: Heparin-associated thrombocytopenia in a patient treated with polysulphated chondroitin sulphate: evidence for immunological crossreactivity between heparin and polysulphated glycosaminoglycan. *Br J Haematol* 81:252, 1992.

574. Goad KE, Horne MK, Gralnick HR: Platelet heparin binding in pentosan induced thrombocytopenia. *Blood* 80:62a, 1992.

575. Tardy-Poncet B, Mahul P, Beraud A-M, et al: Failure of Orgaran therapy in a patient with a previous heparin-induced thrombocytopenia syndrome. *Br J Haematol* 90:969, 1995.

576. Insler SR, Kraenzler EJ, Bartholomew JR, et al: Thrombosis during the use of the heparinoid Organon 10172 in a patient with heparin-induced thrombocytopenia. *Anesthesiology* 86:495, 1997.

577. Tardy B, Tardy-Poncet B, Viallon A, et al: Fatal danaparoid-sodium induced thrombocytopenia and arterial thromboses. *Thromb Haemost* 80:530, 1998.

578. Warkentin TE, Levine MN, Hirsh J, et al: Heparin-induced thrombocytopenia in patients with low-molecular-weight heparin or unfractionated heparin. *N Engl J Med* 332:1330, 1995.

579. Nand S, Wong W, Yuen B, et al: Heparin-induced thrombocytopenia with thrombosis: Incidence, analysis of risk factors, and clinical outcomes in 108 consecutive patients treated at a single institution. *Am J Hematol* 56:12, 1997.

580. Warkentin TE, Elavathil LJ, Hayward CPM, et al: The pathogenesis of venous limb gangrene associated with heparin-induced thrombocytopenia. *Ann Intern Med* 127:804, 1997.

581. Raskob GE, George JN: Thrombotic complications of antithrombotic therapy: A paradox with implications for clinical practice. *Ann Intern Med* 127:839, 1997.

582. Hewitt RL, Akers DL, Leissinger CA, et al: Concurrence of anaphylaxis and acute heparin-induced thrombocytopenia in a patient with heparin-induced antibodies. *J Vasc Surg* 28:561, 1998.

583. Look KA, Sahud M, Flaherty S, Zehnder JL: Heparin-induced platelet aggregation *vs* platelet factor 4 enzyme-linked immunosorbent assay in the diagnosis of heparin-induced thrombocytopenia-thrombosis. *Am J Clin Path* 108:78, 1997.

584. Eichler P, Budde U, Haas S, et al: First workshop for detection of heparin-induced antibodies: Validation of the heparin-induced platelet-activation test (HIPA) in comparison with a PF4/heparin ELISA. *Thromb Haemost* 81:625, 1999.

585. Jackson MR, Gillespie DL, Chang AS, et al: The incidence of heparin-induced antibodies in patients undergoing vascular surgery: a prospective study. *J Vasc Surg* 28:439, 1998.

586. Amiral J, Marfaing-Koka A, Wolf M, et al: Presence of aoutoantibodies to interleukin-8 or neutrophil-activating peptide-2 in patients with heparin-associated thrombocytopenia. *Blood* 88:410, 1996.

587. Lee DH, Warkentin TE, Denomme GA, et al: A diagnostic test for heparin-induced thrombocytopenia: Detection of platelet microparticles using flow cytometry. *Br J Haematol* 95:724, 1996.

588. Tomer A: A sensitive and specific functional flow cytometric assay for the diagnosis of heparin-induced thrombocytopenia. *Br J Haematol* 98:648, 1997.

589. Poullin P, Pietri PA, Lefevre P: Heparin-induced thrombocytopenia with thrombosis: Successful treatment with plasma exchange. *Br J Haematol* 102:630, 1998.

590. Slaughter TF, Greenberg CS: Heparin-associated thrombocytopenia and thrombosis—Implications for perioperative management. *Anesthesiology* 87:667, 1997.

591. Sepulveda S, Davis L, Schwab SJ: Blood transfusion during heparin-free hemodialysis. *Kidney Int* 51:2018, 1997.

592. Wilhelm MJ, Schmid C, Kececioglu D, et al: Cardiopulmonary bypass in patients with heparin-induced thrombocytopenia using Org 10172. *Ann Thorac Surg* 61:920, 1996.

593. Gillis S, Merin G, Zahger D, et al: Danaparoid for cardiopulmonary bypass in patients with previous heparin-induced thrombocytopenia. *Br J Haematol* 98:657, 1997.

594. Koster A, Kuppe H, Hetzer R, et al: Emergent cardiopulmonary bypass in five patients with heparin-induced thrombocytopenia type II employing recombinant hirudin. *Anesthesiology* 89:777, 1998.

595. Kanagasabay RR, Unsworth-White MJ, Robinson G, et al: Cardiopulmonary bypass with danaparoid sodium and ancrod in heparin-induced thrombocytopenia. *Ann Thorac Surg* 66:567, 1998.

596. De Moerloose P, Boehlen F, Extermann P, Hohlfeld P: Neonatal thrombocytopenia: incidence and characterization of maternal antiplatelet antibodies by MAIPA assay. *Br J Haematol* 100:735, 1998.

597. Dreyfus M, Kaplan C, Verdy E, et al: Frequency of immune thrombocytopenia in newborns: A prospective study. *Blood* 89:4402, 1997.

598. Mueller-Eckhardt C, Kiefel V, Grubert A, et al: Three hundred forty-eight cases of suspected neonatal alloimmume thrombocytopenia. *Lancet* 1:363, 1989.

599. Williamson LM, Hackett G, Rennie J, et al: The natural history of fetomaternal alloimmunization to the platelet-specific antigen HPA-1a (P1[A1], Zw[a]) as determined by antenatal screening. *Blood* 92:2280, 1998.

600. McCrae KR, Herman JH: Posttransfusion purpura: Two unusual cases and a literature review. *Am J Hematol* 52:205, 1996.

601. Panzer S, Auerbach L, Cechova E, et al: Maternal alloimmunization

against fetal platelet antigens: A prospective study. *Br J Haematol* 90:655, 1995.

602. Warkentin TE, Smith JW: The alloimmune thrombocytopenic syndromes. *Trans Med Rev* 11:296, 1997.

603. Shibata Y, Matsuda I, Miyaji T, Ichikawa Y: Yuk[a], a new platelet antigen involved in two cases of neonatal alloimmune thrombocytopenia. *Vox Sang* 50:177, 1986.

604. Bussel JB, Zabusky MR, Berkowitz RL, McFarland JG: Fetal alloimmune thrombocytopenia. *N Engl J Med* 337:22, 1997.

605. Kaplan C, Murphy MF, Kroll H, Waters AH: Feto-maternal alloimmune thrombocytopenia: antenatal therapy with IvIgG and steroids—more questions than answers. *Br J Haematol* 100:62, 1998.

606. Doughty HA, Murphy MF, Metcalfe P, Waters AH: Antenatal screening for fetal alloimmune thrombocytopenia: The results of a pilot study. *Br J Haematol* 90:321, 1995.

607. Win N, Ouwehand WH, Hurd C: Provision of platelets for severe neonatal alloimmune thrombocytopenia. *Br J Haematol* 97:930, 1997

608. Bussel JB, Berkowitz RL, Lynch L, et al: Antenatal management of alloimmune thrombocytopenia with intravenous gamma-globulin: A randomized trial of the addition of low-dose steroid to intravenous gamma-globulin. *Am J Obstet Gynecol* 174:1414, 1996.

609. Shankaran S, Bauer CR, Bain R, et al: Prenatal and perinatal risk and protective factors for neonatal intracranial hemorrhage. *Arch Pediatr Adolesc Med* 150:491, 1996.

610. Puig N, Sayas MJ, Montoro JA: Post-transfusion purpura as the main manifestation of a trilineal transfusion reaction, responsive to steroids: flow-cytometric investigation of granulocyte and platelet antibodies. *Ann Hematol* 62:232, 1991.

611. George JN, Pickett EB, Heinz R: Platelet membrane microparticles in blood bank fresh frozen plasma and cryoprecipitate. *Blood* 68:307, 1986.

612. Kickler TS, Ness PM, Herman JH, Bell WR: Studies on the pathophysiology of posttransfusion purpura. *Blood* 68:347, 1986.

613. Dieleman LA, Brand A, Claas FHJ: Acquired Zw[a] antigen on Zw[a] negative platelets demonstrated by Western blotting. *Br J Haematol* 72:539, 1989.

614. Minchinton RM, Cunningham I, Cole-Sinclair M: Autoreactive platelet antibody in post-transfusion purpura. *Aust NZ J Med* 20:111, 1990.

615. Evenson DA, Stroncek DF, Pulkrabek S, et al: Posttransfusion purpura following bone marrow transplantation. *Transfusion* 35:688, 1995.

616. Lau P, Sholtis CM, Aster RH: Post-transfusion purpura: an enigma of alloimmunization. *Am J Hematol* 9:331, 1980.

617. Budd JL, Wiegers SE, O'Hara JM: Relapsing post-transfusion purpura. A preventable disease. *Am J Med* 78:361, 1985.

THROMBOCYTOSIS AND ESSENTIAL THROMBOCYTHEMIA

ANDREW I. SCHAFER

The three major pathophysiological causes of thrombocytosis are (1) clonal, including essential (or primary) thrombocythemia and other myeloproliferative disorders; (2) familial, including rare cases of nonclonal myeloproliferation due to thrombopoietin mutations; and (3) reactive, in which thrombocytosis occurs secondary to a variety of acute and chronic clinical conditions. Essential thrombocythemia is often discovered incidentally on blood counts in asymptomatic individuals and is largely a diagnosis of exclusion. Major causes of morbidity and mortality are bleeding and thrombotic complications, the latter most commonly involving the arterial circulation. Reactive thrombocytosis usually does not cause these complications and does not require treatment. The indications for therapeutic intervention in essential thrombocythemia remain unsettled. Chemotherapy to reduce the platelet count in essential thrombocythemia is generally indicated in patients with previous bleeding or thrombotic episodes or those who are at high risk for such complications. The most commonly used drugs for cytoreduction of the platelet count are hydroxyurea, anagrelide, and recombinant interferon-α. The use of antiplatelet agents is indicated in patients with essential thrombocythemia who have had arterial thrombotic or ischemic problems.

DEFINITION AND HISTORY

The upper limit of the normal platelet count is generally considered to be between 350,000/μl (350 $\times$ 10^9/liter) and 450,000/μl (450 $\times$ 10^9/liter), varying in different laboratories. The causes of thrombocytosis, in which the platelet count exceeds this upper limit, can be broadly categorized as (1) clonal, including essential thrombocythemia and other myeloproliferative disorders; (2) familial; and (3) reactive, or secondary (Table 118-1).

Essential (primary) thrombocythemia is one of a group of related chronic myeloproliferative disorders that also includes polycythemia vera, chronic myelogenous leukemia, and myeloid metaplasia with or without myelofibrosis. The earliest descriptions of essential thrombocythemia by di Guglielmo in 1920 and by Epstein and Goedel in 1934[2] represented, in retrospect, thrombocytosis in association with other disorders. This historical misclassification underscores the diagnostic uncertainty that may occur in patients with thrombocytosis.[3] In 1960 essential thrombocythemia was established as a separate disease entity on a clinicopathologic basis.[4,5]

Acronyms and abbreviations that appear in this chapter include: CML, chronic myelogenous leukemia; IL, interleukin.

ETIOLOGY AND PATHOGENESIS

ESSENTIAL THROMBOCYTHEMIA (CLONAL THROMBOCYTOSIS)

As one of the myeloproliferative syndromes, essential thrombocythemia is a clonal disorder of the multipotential hemopoietic stem cell. The clonal nature of essential thrombocythemia was established by the finding of a single glucose-6-phosphate dehydrogenase (G-6-PD) isoenzyme expressed in all blood cell lines of women with thrombocythemia who were coincidentally heterozygous for two types of G-6-PD, enzymes "A" and "B."[6] Furthermore, the same cytogenetic abnormality was found in both the erythroid and the granulocytic precursors of a patient with thrombocythemia.[7] More recently, clonality in essential thrombocythemia and the other myeloproliferative disorders was confirmed by X-chromosome inactivation analysis of restriction fragment length polymorphisms (RFLP).[8–10]

In view of the multipotential stem cell origin of essential thrombocythemia, the reason for its predominant phenotypic expression in the megakaryocyte-platelet lineage is unclear. It may be due to the preferential responsiveness of the abnormal clone to regulatory factors that favor its differentiation into the megakaryocyte-platelet line.[11] Alternatively, the mutation(s) may occur in a single multipotent hemopoietic stem cell, the lineage potential of which has become restricted to differentiation primarily into platelets.[12]

Increased numbers of colony-forming units composed of megakaryocytes (CFU-MEG) have been cultured from the blood or marrow of patients with essential thrombocythemia, compared with control subjects or patients with secondary thrombocytosis.[13–19] Furthermore, megakaryocyte colony growth in the absence of exogenously added growth factor is usually present in patients with essential thrombocythemia, although it is unclear if this represents truly autonomous megakaryocytopoiesis or only increased sensitivity of the abnormal thrombocythemia clone to exogenous sources of megakaryocyte colony-stimulating activity.[13–20] These quantitative changes may be accompanied by abnormal CFU-MEG colony size and nuclear endoreduplication.[16]

Thrombopoietin,[21] the ligand for the megakaryocytic growth factor receptor, *c-mpl*, the human homolog of the *v-mpl* ("murine myeloproliferative leukemia virus"), is now recognized as the major humoral regulator of megakaryocytopoiesis and platelet production. While thrombopoietin supports the entire continuum of megakaryocyte development from stem cell to platelet production, other cytokines (e.g., steel factor, IL-3, IL-6, IL-11) also exert actions at different stages, probably in synergy with thrombopoietin (see Chap. 111). Plasma concentrations of thrombopoietin vary inversely with the platelet count in patients with marrow failure.[22] Mature platelets themselves appear to have an important role in regulating plasma thrombopoietin levels. Platelets have receptors for thrombopoietin *(c-mpl)* and remove it from plasma. Thus, in thrombocytopenic states, the high free plasma thrombopoietin levels that result from reduced thrombopoietin binding by the reduced circulating platelet mass should stimulate megakaryocytopoiesis; conversely, in states of thrombocytosis, depletion of free plasma thrombopoietin should decrease megakaryocytopoiesis. In both cases this modulatory mechanism is designed to restore steady-state platelet production. However, unlike the relationship between polycythemia vera and erythropoietin levels, thrombopoietin levels are normal or even elevated in essential thrombocythemia[23–26] despite the increased platelet and megakaryocyte mass. The deregulated circulating plasma levels of thrombopoietin in essential thrombocythemia may result from overproduction of endogenous thrombopoietin and/or abnormal thrombopoietin binding and consumption by the defective platelets and megakaryocytes of essential thrombocythemia.[27] In support of the latter, the expression of platelet *c-mpl* has been found to be strikingly reduced in essential thrombocythemia.[28]

TABLE 118-1   MAJOR CAUSES OF THROMBOCYTOSIS

1. Clonal thrombocytosis
   a. Essential (primary) thrombocythemia
   b. Other myeloproliferative disorders (polycythemia vera, chronic mye-
      logenous leukemia, myeloid metaplasia, myelofibrosis)
2. Familial thrombocytosis
3. Reactive (secondary) thrombocytosis
   a. Acute blood loss
   b. Iron deficiency
   c. Postsplenectomy, asplenic states
   d. Recovery from thrombocytopenia (''rebound'')
   e. Malignancies
   f. Chronic inflammatory and infectious diseases (inflammatory bowel
      disease, connective tissue disorders, temporal arteritis, tuberculosis,
      chronic pneumonitis)
   g. Acute inflammatory and infectious diseases
   h. Response to exercise
   i. Response to drugs (vincristine, epinephrine, all-*trans*-retinoic acid,
      cytokines, and growth factors)
   j. Hemolytic anemia

FAMILIAL THROMBOCYTOSIS

Rare cases of familial occurrence of thrombocytosis have been reported, generally inherited by autosomal dominant transmission. Specific mutations in the thrombopoietin gene, including exon skipping
and a single-base deletion in the 5'-untranslated region of the gene,
have been described in these families; these mutations lead to markedly
elevated plasma thrombopoietin levels.[29,30] Thus, these cases are probably *nonclonal* myeloproliferative disorders. Indeed, it is possible that
the inappropriately elevated thrombopoietin levels in some cases of
apparently essential thrombocythemia may also be due to thrombopoietin gene mutations.

REACTIVE (SECONDARY) THROMBOCYTOSIS

The mechanisms of reactive thrombocytosis are not well defined and
are likely to be as complex and diverse as the underlying disorders
that cause it. For example, increased megakaryocytopoiesis and
thrombocytosis may result from the elevated levels of IL-6 and other
cytokines that accompany many inflammatory disorders.[31] Catechol-
amine-mediated thrombocytosis may result from the release of platelets
from the spleen.[32,33] Thrombocytosis associated with the conditions
listed in Table 118-1 may persist for prolonged periods of time and
resolve only with effective treatment for the disorder or elimination of
the inciting stimulus. ''Rebound'' thrombocytosis following recovery
from bone marrow suppression generally peaks 10 to 14 days after
withdrawal of the offending drug (e.g., alcohol[34]) or replacement therapy for the cause of thrombocytopenia (e.g., for cobalamin deficiency[35]). The platelet count may also transiently rise above normal
limits with effective treatment for immune thrombocytopenic purpura.[36] Following splenectomy for any condition, the platelet count
typically rises within the first week to 1,000,000/μl or higher and
then gradually returns to normal within about 2 months. Reasons for
persistent or extreme postsplenectomy thrombocytosis include persistent anemia or unmasking of previously unrecognized essential thrombocythemia and other myeloproliferative disorders.

CLINICAL FEATURES

CLINICAL PRESENTATION

In the past, essential thrombocythemia was considered to be the least
common of the myeloproliferative disorders, typically affecting patients between the ages of 50 and 70, with an equal sex distribution.

However, with frequent inclusion of platelet counts in automated blood
analysis, more asymptomatic patients are being uncovered with the
incidental finding of thrombocytosis. Furthermore, the diagnosis of
essential thrombocythemia is being made increasingly in younger individuals. The disease is occasionally found in childhood,[37] and as noted
above, rare familial cases have been reported.[29,30,38] In contrast to some
of the other myeloproliferative disorders, constitutional or hypermetabolic symptoms such as fever, sweats, and weight loss are very uncommon in essential thrombocythemia.

Physical findings are limited usually to mild splenomegaly, which
is present in about 40 percent of the patients. Echocardiography may
reveal aortic and mitral valvular lesions, including leaflet thickening
and vegetations, similar to those described in nonbacterial thrombotic
endocarditis.[39] The relationship of cardiac valve lesions to thromboembolic complications in essential thrombocythemia is unclear.

BLEEDING AND THROMBOTIC COMPLICATIONS

Bleeding and thrombotic complications are major causes of morbidity
and mortality in essential thrombocythemia, as in the other myeloproliferative disorders.[40-44] The incidence of these hemostatic complications is unknown; it varies markedly in different series. Some symptomatic patients may exhibit an exclusive pattern of either bleeding
or thrombotic problems, whereas others appear to be paradoxically
predisposed to both types of complications during the course of their
disease. Some studies have suggested that older patients are at markedly increased risk of hemostatic complications,[45,46] while younger
patients are relatively protected from these problems.[47] However, other
reports have documented no age-related differences[48,49] and have noted
serious bleeding and thrombotic episodes in younger patients.[50,51]

Therapeutic intervention in essential thrombocythemia (see
''Therapy, Course, and Prognosis,'' below) should be guided by the
underlying risk of thrombotic or bleeding complications in any individual patient. Table 118-2 summarizes the emerging consensus of risks
of either thrombosis or bleeding, as previously reviewed.[52-55] Risks of
thrombosis in essential thrombocythemia include a previous history
of thrombosis, associated cardiovascular risk factors (e.g., smoking),
and probably advanced age. Risks of bleeding in these patients include
extreme thrombocytosis (platelet count >2,000,000/μl) and the use
of aspirin and possibly other nonsteroidal antiinflammatory drugs.
Thrombohemorrhagic complications may occur less frequently in certain populations, such as in China.[56]

BLEEDING COMPLICATIONS
Bleeding complications of essential thrombocythemia are similar in
nature to those seen in platelet or vascular disorders, occurring in

TABLE 118-2   RISKS OF THROMBOHEMORRHAGIC COMPLICATIONS IN
ESSENTIAL THROMBOCYTHEMIA

	THROMBOSIS	BLEEDING
Increased risk	Previous history of throm- bosis Associated cardiovascular risk factors (especially smoking) Advanced age (>60 years) Inadequate control of thrombocytosis (in high- risk patients)	Use of aspirin and other nonsteroidal anti- inflammatory drugs Extreme thrombocytosis (platelet count >2,000,000/μl)
No associated risk	Degree of thrombocytosis In vitro platelet function	Prolonged bleeding time In vitro platelet function

SOURCE: Modified from Schafer.[52]

superficial locations either spontaneously or after minimal trauma. The most common sites of hemorrhage are mucosal and gastrointestinal, although cutaneous, genitourinary tract, and postoperative bleeding are also seen.[43] The use of aspirin, which has been found to cause exaggerated prolongations of the bleeding time in patients with myeloproliferative disorders,[57] may lead to serious bleeding complications in occasional cases.[58]

THROMBOTIC COMPLICATIONS

Arterial thrombotic complications occur more frequently than venous thrombosis in essential thrombocythemia, although about 25 percent of all thrombotic events in these patients are deep vein thrombosis of the lower extremities.[43] The most common sites of arterial thrombosis in essential thrombocythemia involve the cerebrovascular, peripheral vascular, and coronary arterial circulations. Patients are particularly predisposed to certain specific types of thrombotic events, as described below.

Erythromelalgia and Digital Microvascular Ischemia   Erythromelalgia is characterized by intense burning or throbbing pain in a patchy distribution in the extremities, most prominently involving the feet.[59–62] The pain tends to be exacerbated by heat, exercise, and dependency and to be relieved by cold exposure and elevation of the extremity. It is often accompanied by warmth, duskiness, and mottled erythema of the involved areas, sometimes resembling livedo reticularis. Erythromelalgia may be occasionally confused with Raynaud syndrome, reflex sympathetic dystrophy, shoulder-hand syndrome, or causalgia.[62] Histopathologic examination of biopsies of the affected areas typically shows arterial endothelial swelling, fibromuscular intimal proliferation, and vascular occlusion caused predominantly by platelet thrombi.[63,64]

Signs of digital microvascular ischemia, primarily involving the toes, may develop in essential thrombocythemia independently of erythromelalgia. Painful vascular insufficiency may progress to frank gangrene and necrosis of the digits unless treatment is promptly instituted. Since thrombosis involves the small vessels, physical examination usually reveals normal peripheral pulses, and arteriography shows patent major vessels.[65] Erythromelalgia and digital ischemia in patients often respond promptly and dramatically to aspirin and reduction of the elevated platelet count.[65–67]

Cerebrovascular ischemia   A wide spectrum of neurologic manifestations in essential thrombocythemia may be caused by cerebrovascular ischemia.[43,68–73] Central nervous system involvement may take the form of nonspecific symptoms, such as headache and dizziness; a vague sense of a decrease in mental acuity; or focal neurologic signs, such as anterior or posterior cerebral artery transient ischemic attacks, seizures, or retinal artery occlusion. Ischemic stroke may be the presenting manifestation of essential thrombocythemia.[74] As in the digital ischemia syndromes, cerebrovascular ischemia may be relieved by aspirin and platelet reduction.

Recurrent Abortions and Fetal Growth Retardation   Multiple placental infarctions, presumably caused by platelet thrombi, may result in placental insufficiency in some pregnant women with essential thrombocythemia.[75,76] This may lead to recurrent spontaneous abortions, fetal growth retardation, premature deliveries, or abruptio placentae.[75–78] These serious consequences have led to the use of aspirin during pregnancy in women with essential thrombocythemia.[77] However, the successful outcome of pregnancy in the absence of any specific therapy[79,80] and the lack of clinical trials to evaluate treatment modalities make specific recommendations difficult. No correlation has been found between the outcome of the pregnancy and the degree of maternal thrombocytosis, presence of disease complications, or specific therapy for thrombocythemia. To reduce the risk of maternal or neonatal bleeding complications, aspirin should be avoided for at least one week prior to delivery. Pregnancy does not adversely affect the natural history of essential thrombocythemia.[81]

Hepatic and Portal Vein Thromboses   The myeloproliferative disorders are the most frequently identifiable underlying etiologies in patients who present with hepatic vein thrombosis (Budd-Chiari syndrome).[82,83] The incidence of myeloproliferative disorders associated with either hepatic or portal vein thrombosis may, in fact, be underestimated; such patients have been shown to have erythropoietin-independent erythroid colony growth in marrow cultures, a diagnostic marker of a stem cell abnormality, even in the absence of any overt clinical or hematologic manifestations of a myeloproliferative disorder.[83–85] Hepatic and portal vein thromboses are most commonly associated with polycythemia vera, but a number of cases associated with essential thrombocythemia have also been described.[42]

LABORATORY FEATURES

BLOOD AND MARROW FINDINGS

Untreated patients with essential thrombocythemia have platelet counts that may range from only slightly above the normal limits to several million per microliter. Some patients may have mild leukocytosis and mild anemia. Platelet morphology on blood films shows large, pale blue staining, hypogranular platelets, and occasional nucleated megakaryocyte fragments that may have a lymphoblastoid appearance. Increased platelet turnover in essential thrombocythemia is indicated by the finding of increased reticulated platelets (young platelets) in the circulation, which can be detected by flow cytometric analysis of platelet RNA. While both the percentage and the absolute number of reticulated platelets in blood are elevated in patients with essential thrombocythemia compared with healthy individuals, it is unclear whether or not this finding can distinguish essential thrombocythemia from secondary (reactive) thrombocytosis.[86,87]

As noted above, serum thrombopoietin levels are generally normal or even elevated in clonal thrombocythemia; thrombopoietin levels do not correlate with platelet count in these patients. Serum thrombopoietin levels are also usually elevated in reactive thrombocytosis, and it is not clear whether or not this test can discriminate these patients from those with essential thrombocythemia.[24,25] Plasma levels of IL-6 and C-reactive protein are low or undetectable in clonal thrombocythemia, while they may be elevated in secondary thrombocytosis, which often accompanies acute and chronic inflammatory states.[31]

Pseudohyperkalemia may be found in patients with extreme thrombocytosis or leukocytosis. It is diagnosed in thrombocytosis states when the serum potassium concentration exceeds the plasma potassium concentration and is caused by the release of intracellular potassium during the process of blood clotting in vitro.[88]

Marrow pathology in essential thrombocythemia characteristically reveals increased cellularity with megakaryocytic hyperplasia. There are frequently giant megakaryocytes with increased ploidy that occur in clusters.[89,90] Significant dysplasia of the megakaryocytes is unusual, but large masses of platelet debris (''platelet drifts'') are typically seen in marrow samples.[91] Most patients with essential thrombocythemia have no cytogenetic abnormalities using conventional techniques.[92] However, some patients who otherwise meet the diagnostic criteria of essential thrombocythemia are found to have the Philadelphia chromosome on cytogenetic analysis of the marrow.[93] Such patients generally do not have pronounced leukocytosis or other characteristic clinical features of CML. However, the natural history of their disease is more like that of CML than that of essential thrombocythemia. Some patients with essential thrombocythemia are found to have the *bcr/abl* gene rearrangement in the absence of the Philadelphia chromosome, although the clinical implications of this are not clear at present.[94]

CLINICAL TESTS OF HEMOSTASIS

The bleeding time is prolonged in fewer than 20 percent of patients with essential thrombocythemia.[40,72,78] This test generally does not correlate with the degree of thrombocytosis or specific platelet function abnormalities and it has not been found to predict reliably either a bleeding or a thrombotic tendency in patients with essential thrombocythemia.[95–97]

The platelet aggregation abnormalities in patients are variable. Reduced platelet responses to collagen, ADP, and arachidonic acid occur in less than one-third of cases.[42] A characteristic aggregation abnormality is complete loss of platelet responsiveness to epinephrine. In contrast to platelet release defects (e.g., storage pool deficiency or aspirinlike defect), in which only the second wave of platelet aggregation is absent, even the primary wave of epinephrine-stimulated aggregation is often lost in essential thrombocythemia. An abnormal epinephrine-induced platelet response is the most frequent and sometimes the only abnormality on aggregometry; this unusual abnormality is also observed in other myeloproliferative disorders.[40,42,72,78] Some patients have platelet hyperaggregability or spontaneous aggregation in vitro.[72,98–100]

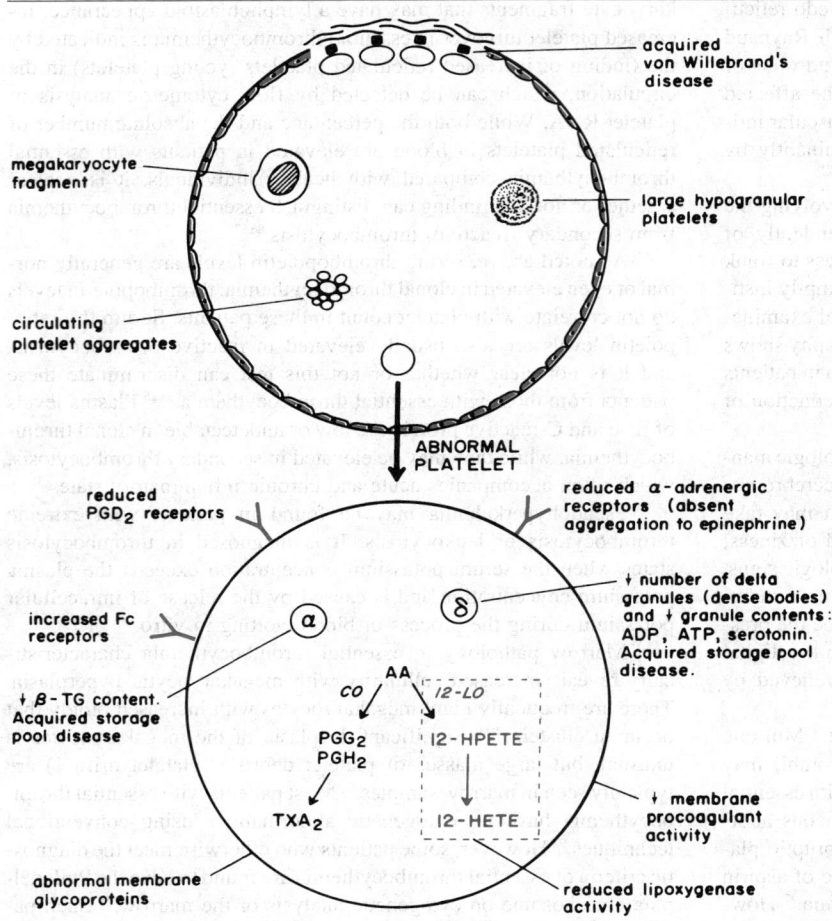

FIGURE 118-1   Structural, biochemical, and metabolic abnormalities of platelets in essential thrombocythemia. At top is a schematic of a transected vessel wall; at bottom is a schematic of a single platelet. Abbreviations: PGD$_2$, prostaglandin D$_2$; β-TG, beta-thromboglobulin; AA, arachidonic acid; CO, cyclooxygenase; 12-LO, 12-lipoxygenase; PGG$_2$ and PGH$_2$, prostaglandins G$_2$ and H$_2$; TxA$_2$, thromboxane A$_2$; 12-HETE and 12-HPETE, 12-hydroxy- and hydroperoxy-5,8,10,14-eicosatetraenoic acid. (Reprinted with permission from Schafer.[42])

SPECIFIC QUALITATIVE PLATELET ABNORMALITIES

A wide array of specific morphological, biochemical, and metabolic platelet defects has been described in patients with essential thrombocythemia.[41] These abnormalities, shown in Fig. 118-1, include acquired von Willebrand disease,[101–103] reduced α-adrenergic receptors associated with absent aggregation to epinephrine,[104] acquired storage pool disease,[97,105–108] impaired membrane procoagulant activity,[95,109] selective deficiency of 12-lipoxygenase,[110,111] abnormal membrane glycoproteins,[112,113] increased Fc receptors,[114] and reduced prostaglandin D$_2$ receptors.[115] Only some of these abnormalities are specific for the myeloproliferative disorders, and none of them have been directly demonstrated to be pathogenetically linked to clinical hemostatic complications.

DIFFERENTIAL DIAGNOSIS

DIAGNOSTIC CRITERIA FOR ESSENTIAL THROMBOCYTHEMIA

There are no tests that can be used to establish the diagnosis of essential thrombocythemia with certainty. The disease remains largely a diagnosis of exclusion. For these reasons, a set of diagnostic criteria for essential thrombocythemia (Table 118-3) has been proposed.[116] The minimum platelet count of 600,000/μl to establish the diagnosis of essential thrombocythemia has been subsequently challenged.[117] Thrombocythemia-related complications may occur in individual patients with only slight thrombocytosis or even with platelet counts in the upper normal range, and the natural history of these early stage essential thrombocythemia patients is comparable to that of patients who meet the original diagnostic criteria.[117]

Most of the diagnostic criteria listed in Table 118-3 were designed to differentiate essential thrombocythemia from other myeloproliferative disorders associated with thrombocytosis. Polycythemia vera with thrombocytosis can usually be readily distinguished from essential thrombocythemia by the finding of erythrocytosis and an elevated red cell mass. This disease may be masked by concomitant iron deficiency, which can further increase the platelet count, but a trial of iron therapy in such cases typically raises the hematocrit to polycythemic levels. As noted above, chronic myelogenous leukemia with associated thrombocytosis is sometimes misdiagnosed as essential thrombocythemia until its diagnostic cytogenetic or DNA abnormality is revealed. Myeloid metaplasia and myelofibrosis are characterized by more marked, frequently massive, splenomegaly; furthermore, in contrast to essential thrombocythemia, the blood film in myelofibrosis typically shows myelophthisic or leukoerythroblastic changes and the marrow biopsy shows fibrosis. Despite these characteristic distinctions in clinical presentation, however, some myeloproliferative disorders represent "overlap" syndromes that cannot be clearly categorized. Finally, essential thrombocythemia cannot be diagnosed without excluding possible causes of reactive (or secondary) thrombocytosis.

REACTIVE (SECONDARY) THROMBOCYTOSIS

A large number of diverse processes have been associated with reactive thrombocytosis (see Table 118-1).

TABLE 118-3   DIAGNOSTIC CRITERIA FOR ESSENTIAL THROMBOCYTHEMIA

1. Platelet count >600,000/μl.
2. Hemoglobin (13 g/dl or normal red cell mass (males <36 ml/kg, females <32 ml/kg).
3. Stainable iron in marrow or failure of iron trial (<1 g/dl rise in hemoglobin after 1 month of iron therapy).
4. No Philadelphia chromosome.
5. Collagen fibrosis of marrow
   a. Absent; or
   b. <1/3 biopsy area without both splenomegaly and leukoerythroblastic reaction.
6. No known cause for reactive thrombocytosis.

SOURCE: From Murphy et al.[116]

While many of these are active systemic diseases which dominate the clinical picture in these patients, in some individuals subclinical disorders (e.g. occult cancer) may be responsible for the secondary thrombocytosis. In the latter cases, reactive thrombocytosis is particularly difficult to distinguish from essential thrombocythemia.

Patients with reactive thrombocytosis generally do not have splenomegaly, unless enlargement of the spleen results from the underlying disease. It is now recognized that extreme thrombocytosis (platelet count >1,000,000/μl) by no means excludes a reactive or secondary process as its etiology. In fact, in a review of 280 consecutive hospitalized patients with reported platelet counts of greater than 1,000,000/μl, 82 percent were found to have reactive thrombocytosis and only 14 percent had myeloproliferative disorders.[118] Platelet morphology and platelet function are typically normal in reactive thrombocytosis, in contrast to essential thrombocythemia. In general, reactive thrombocytosis, even when extreme, does not cause thrombotic or bleeding complications and hence does not require treatment (see "Therapy, Course, and Prognosis," below).

THERAPY, COURSE, AND PROGNOSIS

The therapeutic options described below are designed specifically for patients with clonal thrombocytosis (essential thrombocythemia and thrombocytosis associated with other myeloproliferative disorders), not for those with secondary or reactive thrombocytosis. Many reports have attempted to link reactive thrombocytosis with thrombotic complications; however, the thrombotic events in these cases can be usually attributed to the underlying systemic disease (e.g., cancer, postoperative state) rather than to the secondary thrombocytosis per se. One exception might be the increased risk of thrombosis in patients who develop thrombocytosis following splenectomy for hemolytic anemias, most notably thalassemia, that are incompletely resolved by the surgical procedure.[119,120] While it is important to identify and attempt to treat the underlying systemic disease, there is no convincing evidence that either therapy to reduce the platelet count or antiplatelet therapy is beneficial in patients with reactive thrombocytosis.

CYTOREDUCTION

INDICATIONS
The pivotal therapeutic decision in essential thrombocythemia is whether or not treatment is required to reduce the elevated platelet count. This issue is controversial because of the paucity of prospective, controlled trials to determine the impact of platelet cytoreduction on morbidity and mortality in clonal thrombocytosis.

Although an association has been suggested between the platelet count in thrombocythemia and the occurrence of thrombotic complications,[73] most retrospective studies have failed to support such a correlation.[42,43,46,48,72,121] Nevertheless, one prospective study of "high-risk"

patients with essential thrombocythemia (age over 60 and/or previous episodes of thrombosis) found that control of the platelet count to levels below 600,000/μl with hydroxyurea significantly reduced the incidence of thrombotic episodes over a median follow-up period of 27 months.[54] In contrast to the unsettled indications for prophylactic platelet cytoreduction in asymptomatic patients with essential thrombocythemia, there is general consensus that lowering the platelet count in patients with active or recurrent bleeding or thrombosis may result in symptomatic improvement. The indication for prompt cytoreduction is particularly strong in patients who have microvascular digital[65,66] or cerebrovascular[71] ischemia syndromes.

THERAPEUTIC MODALITIES
When reduction of the platelet count is indicated, plateletpheresis[122–124] is generally reserved for selected cases of acute and threatening thrombotic and hemostatic problems. Reduction of the platelet count by this method is transient and may be followed by a rebound increase in the thrombocytosis. Radiophosphorus and alkylating agents (e.g., melphalan, busulfan) have been largely abandoned because of their leukemogenic potential.[125]

Hydroxyurea, a nonalkylating myelosuppressive agent, is highly effective as initial therapy for essential thrombocythemia. Doses required to control thrombocytosis are generally 10 to 30 mg/kg per day. Blood counts should be checked within 7 days of initiating therapy and monitored frequently thereafter, since hydroxyurea can cause rapid myelosuppression. Maintenance doses should be individually adjusted according to blood counts. Continuous, orally administered daily treatment with this drug reduces the platelet count to less than 500,000/μl within 8 weeks in 80 percent of patients and provides long-term control without severe marrow toxicity or serious side effects.[126] Painful but reversible leg ulceration may occur with long-term treatment with hydroxyurea.[127] Hydroxyurea was not initially considered to be leukemogenic, although a statistically insignificant trend to an increased incidence of acute leukemia with its use was noted by the Polycythemia Vera Study Group.[128] The leukemogenic potential of hydroxyurea, although not as great as with radiophosphorus or alkylating agents, has been confirmed in more recent studies[129,130]; this is an important consideration in deciding on long-term use of this drug in younger patients with essential thrombocythemia.

Anagrelide is effective in platelet cytoreduction in essential thrombocythemia, and is now an alternative first-line therapy. This quinazoline derivative can be given orally and reduces platelet counts by inhibiting marrow megakaryocyte maturation.[131,132] The recommended starting dose is 0.5 mg q.i.d. or 1 mg b.i.d., with dosage adjustments made at weekly intervals when needed. The dose required to control the platelet count in average-sized adults is approximately 2.0 to 3.0 mg/day.[133] The time to 50 percent reduction in the platelet count after the start of anagrelide therapy is approximately 11 days. Anagrelide reduces the platelet count without affecting the white blood count, although a small reduction in the hematocrit may be seen. Platelet counts are well controlled while patients are taking the drug, but its discontinuation leads to a rapid rise in the platelet count in most patients. Important adverse reactions that have been noted include neurologic and gastrointestinal symptoms, palpitations, and fluid retention.[133,134]

Recombinant interferon-α has also been demonstrated to be effective therapy for essential thrombocythemia.[135–138] This drug suppresses proliferation of the abnormal megakaryocyte clone and results in a decrease in megakaryocyte size and ploidy during therapy. Platelet counts are reduced to the normal or near-normal range in most patients within 1 month of starting interferon therapy. An effective regimen has been to initially administer interferon subcutaneously at a dose of 3,000,000 units daily, with doses subsequently adjusted according to individual tolerance and response.[139–142] Thereafter, suppression of the platelet count can be maintained for several years using lower doses of interferon administered by subcutaneous injection three times per week.[139,141] Relapse of the thrombocytosis occurs after discontinuation of interferon.[141] Severe flulike side effects are not infrequent but generally can be ameliorated by reduction of the interferon dose and by the use of acetaminophen. Interferon therapy is often accompanied by some reduction in the white blood count as well as the platelet count, but generally no effect on the hematocrit is noted. Although it is nonleukemogenic, the toxicity and cost associated with the long-term use of interferon-α make it unlikely to be used as first-line therapy in "low-risk" patients with essential thrombocythemia.[143]

ANTIPLATELET AGENTS

Aspirin may be highly effective adjunctive therapy in patients with essential thrombocythemia who have recurrent thrombotic complications, particularly digital or cerebrovascular ischemia. Aspirin (but not warfarin) improves the increased platelet turnover and the clinical symptoms of erythromelalgia.[144] However, aspirin may also cause marked prolongation of the bleeding time and the unpredictable occurrence of serious bleeding in some patients with thrombocythemia.[57,58] A short-term pilot study using low-dose (40 mg daily) aspirin in polycythemia vera patients showed no excess bleeding complications,[145] and larger trials of low-dose aspirin in myeloproliferative disorders are under way.[146] The use of aspirin in patients with essential thrombocythemia is controversial at present, with some recommending caution[40] but others recommending routine use to prevent thrombosis unless patients have a specific contraindication, such as a history of bleeding.

COURSE AND PROGNOSIS

The major causes of morbidity and mortality in essential thrombocythemia are thrombosis and hemorrhage. In rare cases, essential thrombocythemia may transform to another myeloproliferative disorder as part of the natural history of the disease.[147] Although the other myeloproliferative disorders have the potential, to a greater or lesser degree, to spontaneously convert to acute leukemia, this association is less clear in essential thrombocythemia.[135,148] The use of radiophosphorus or alkylating agents, and probably also hydroxyurea, to treat essential thrombocythemia is likely to enhance the leukemic potential of the disease. A high proportion of patients with essential thrombocythemia who develop acute myeloid leukemia and myelodysplastic syndromes with hydroxyurea treatment have chromosome 17p deletions and other characteristics of the 17p− syndrome.[130] The survival curve for patients with essential thrombocythemia has been shown to be similar to that of a normal age-matched population.[149]

REFERENCES

1. Di Guglielmo G: Erithroleucemia e piastrinemia. *Folia Med* 1:36, 1920.
2. Epstein E, Goedel A: Hämorrhagische thrombozythämie bei vaskulärer Schrumpfmilz. *Virchows Arch Pathol Anat* 292:233, 1934.
3. Fanger H, Cella LJ Jr, Lichtman H: Thrombocytemia. Report of three cases and review of literature. *N Engl J Med* 250:456, 1954.
4. Gunz FW: Hemorrhagic thrombocythemia: A critical review. *Blood* 15:706, 1960.
5. Ozer FL, Truax WE, Miesch DC, Levin WC: Primary hemorrhagic thrombocythemia. *Am J Med* 28:807, 1960.
6. Fialkow PJ, Faguet GB, Jacobsen RJ, Vaidya K, Murphy S: Evidence that essential thrombocythemia is a clonal disorder with origin in a multipotent cell. *Blood* 58:916, 1981.
7. Knuutila S, Tuutu T, Partanen S, Vuopio P: Chromosome 1q+ in ery-
throid and granulocyte-monocyte precursors in a patient with essential thrombocythemia. *Cancer Genet Cytogenet* 9:245, 1983.
8. Blanchard KL, Gilliland DG, Bunn HF: Clonality in myeloproliferative disorders. *Am J Med Sci* 304:125, 1992.
9. Tsukamoto N, Morita K, Maehara T, et al: Clonality in chronic myeloproliferative disorders defined by X-chromosome linked probes: demonstration of heterogeneity in lineage involvement. *Br J Haematol* 86:253, 1994.
10. El-Kassar N, Hetet G, Brière J, Grandchamp B: Clonality analysis of hematopoiesis in essential thrombocythemia: advantages of studying T lymphocytes and platelets. *Blood* 89:128, 1997.
11. Adamson JW, Fialkow PJ: The pathogenesis of myeloproliferative syndromes. *Br J Haematol* 38:299, 1978.
12. Ogawa M: Cellular mechanisms of myeloproliferative disorders. *Br J Haematol* 58:563, 1984.
13. Ash RC, Llindquist D, McEver RP, Zanjani ED: Differential erythroid and megakaryocytic progenitor cell growth in vitro as a diagnostic discriminant in myeloproliferative disorders. *Clin Res* 30:310A, 1982.
14. Gerwitz AM, Bruno E, Elwell J: In vitro studies of megakaryocytopoiesis in thrombocytotic disorders of man. *Blood* 61:384, 1983.
15. Komatsu N, Suda T, Eguchi M, Kaji K, Saito M, Miura Y: Megakaryocytopoiesis in vitro of patients with essential thrombocythaemia: Effect of plasma and serum of megakaryocytic colony formation. *Br J Haematol* 64:241, 1986.
16. Mazur EM, Cohen JL, Bogart L: Growth characteristics of circulating hematopoietic progenitor cells from patients with essential thrombocythemia. *Blood* 71:1544, 1988.
17. Han ZC, Abgrall JF, et al: Spontaneous formation of megakaryocyte progenitors (CFU-MK) in primary thrombocythaemia. *Acta Haematol* 78:51, 1987.
18. Juvonen E, Partanen S, Ruutu T: Colony formation by megakaryocytic progenitors in essential thrombocythaemia. *Br J Haematol* 66:161, 1987.
19. Kimura H, Ishibashi T, Sato T, Matsuda S, Uchida T, Kariyone S: Megakaryocytic colony formation (CFU-Meg) in essential thrombocythemia: Quantitative and qualitative abnormalities of bone marrow CFU-Meg. *Am J Hematol* 24:23, 1987.
20. Eridani S, Dudley JM, Sawyer BM, Pearson TC: Erythropoietic colonies in a serum-free system: Results in primary proliferative polycythaemia and thrombocythaemia. *Br J Haematol* 67:387, 1987.
21. Kaushansky K: Thrombopoietin. *N Engl J Med* 339:746, 1998.
22. Nichol JL, Hokom MM, Hornkohl A, et al: Megakaryocyte growth and development factor: analysis of in vitro effects on human megakaryopoiesis and endogenous serum levels during chemotherapy-induced thrombocytopenia. *J Clin Invest* 95:2973, 1995.
23. Pitcher L, Taylor K, Nichol J, et al: Thrombopoietin measurement in thrombocytosis: dysregulation and lack of feedback inhibition in essential thrombocythaemia. *Br J Haematol* 99:929, 1997.
24. Cerutti A, Custodi P, Duranti M, Noris P, Balduini CL: Thrombopoietin levels in patients with primary and reactive thrombocytosis. *Br J Haematol* 99:281, 1997.
25. Wang JC, Chen C, Novetsky AD, Lichter SM, Ahmed F, Friedberg NM: Blood thrombopoietin levels in clonal thrombocytosis and reactive thrombocytosis. *Am J Med* 104: 451, 1998.
26. Kiladjian JJ, Elkassar N, Hetet G, Brière J, Grandchamp B, Gardin C: Study of the thrombopoietin receptor in essential thrombocythemia. *Leukemia* 11:1821, 1997.
27. Griesshammer M, Bangerter M, Schrezenmeier H: A possible role for thrombopoietin and its receptor c-mpl in the pathobiology of essential thrombocythemia. *Semin Thromb Hemostas* 23:419, 1997.
28. Horikawa Y, Matsumura I, Hashimoto K, et al: Markedly reduced expression of platelet c-mpl receptor in essential thrombocythemia. *Blood* 90:4031, 1997.
29. Wiestner A, Schlemper RJ, van der Maas APC, Skoda RC: An activating splice donor mutation in the thrombopoietin gene causing hereditary thrombocythemia. *Nature Genetics* 18:49, 1998.
30. Kondo T, Okabe M, Sanada M, et al: Familial essential thrombocythemia associated with one-base deletion in the 5′-untranslated region of the thrombopoietin gene. *Blood* 92:1091, 1998.
31. Tefferi A, Ho TC, Ahmann GJ, Katzmann JA, Greipp PR: Plasma interleukin-6 and C-reactive protein levels in reactive versus clonal thrombocytosis. *Am J Med* 97:374, 1994.
32. McClure PD, Ingram GJC, Vaughan-Jones R: Platelet changes after

adrenaline infusions with and without adrenaline blockers. *Thromb Diath Haemorrh* 13:136, 1965.

33. Libre EP, Cowan DH, Watkins SP Jr, Shulman NR: Relationships between spleen, platelets and factor VIII levels. *Blood* 31:358, 1968.

34. Numminen H, Hillbom M, Juvela S: Platelets, alcohol consumption, and onset of brain infarction. *J Neurol Neurosurg Psychiatry* 61:376, 1996.

35. Ogston D, Dawson AA: Thrombocytosis following thrombocytopenia in man. *Postgrad Med J* 45:754, 1969.

36. Bierling P, Divine M, Farcet JP, Wallet P, Duedari N: Persistent remission of adult chronic autoimmune thrombocytopenic purpura after treatment with high-dose intravenous immunoglobulin. *Am J Haematol* 25:271, 1987.

37. Linch DC, Hutton R, Cowan D, et al: Primary thrombocythaemia in childhood. *Scand J Haematol* 28:72, 1982.

38. Eyster ME, Saletan SL, Rabellino EM, et al: Familial essential thrombocythemia. *Am J Med* 80:497, 1986.

39. Reisner SA, Rinkevich D, Markiewicz W, Tatarsky L, Brenner B: Cardiac involvement in patients with myeloproliferative disorders. *Am J Med* 93:498, 1992.

40. Schafer AI: Bleeding and thrombosis in the myeloproliferative disorders. *Blood* 64:1, 1984.

41. Schafer AI: The primary and secondary hypercoagulable states, in *Molecular Mechanisms of Hypercoagulable States*, edited by AI Schafer, p 1. Landes, Austin, TX, 1997.

42. Schafer AI: Essential thrombocythemia. *Prog Hemost Thromb* 10:69, 1991.

43. Randi ML, Stocco F, Rossi C, Tison T, Girolami A: Thrombosis and hemorrhage in thrombocytosis: Evaluation of a large cohort of patients (357 cases). *J Med* 22:213, 1991.

44. Ravandi-Kashani F, Schafer AI: Microvascular disturbances, thrombosis, and bleeding in thrombocythemia: current concepts and perspectives. *Semin Thromb Hemostas* 23:479, 1997.

45. Wasserman LR, Goldberg JD, Balcerzak SP, et al: Influence of therapy on causes of death in polycythemia vera. *Clin Res* 29:573A, 1981.

46. Kessler CM, Klein HG, Havlik RJ: Uncontrolled thrombocytosis in chronic myeloproliferative disorders. *Br J Haematol* 50:157, 1982.

47. Hoagland HC, Silverstein MN: Primary thrombocythemia in the young patient. *Mayo Clin Proc* 53:578, 1978.

48. Grossi A, Rosseti S, Vannucchi AM, Rafanelli D, Ferrini PR: Occurrence of haemorrhagic and thrombotic events in myeloproliferative disorders: A retrospective study of 108 patients. *Clin Lab Haematol* 10:167, 1988.

49. Randi ML, Casonato A, Fabris F, Vio C, Girolami A: The significance of thrombocytosis in old age. *Acta Hematol* 78:41, 1987.

50. Davis RB: Acute thrombotic complications of myeloproliferative disorders in young adults. *Am J Clin Pathol* 84:180, 1985.

51. Mitus AJ, Barbui T, Shulman LN, et al: Hemostatic complications in young patients with essential thrombocythemia. *Am J Med* 88:371, 1990.

52. Schafer AI: Management of thrombocythemia. *Curr Opin Hematol* 3:341, 1996.

53. Tefferi A, Silverstein MN, Hoagland HC: Primary thrombocythemia. *Semin Oncol* 22:334, 1995.

54. Cortelazzo S, Finazzi G, Ruggeri M, et al: Hydroxyurea for patients with essential thrombocythemia and a high risk of thrombosis. *N Engl J Med* 332:1132, 1995.

55. Barbui T, Finazzi G: Risk factors and prevention of vascular complications in polycythemia vera. *Semin Thromb Hemostas* 23: 455, 1997.

56. Kwong YL, Liang RH, Chiu EK, et al: Essential thrombocythemia: a retrospective analysis of 39 cases. *Am J Hematol* 49:39, 1995.

57. Barbui T, Buelli M, Cortelazzo S, Viero P, De Gaetano G: Aspirin and risk of bleeding in patients with thrombocythemia. *Am J Med* 83:265, 1987.

58. Tartaglia AP, Goldberg JD, Berk PD, Wasserman LR: Adverse effects of antiaggregating platelet therapy in the treatment of polycythemia vera. *Semin Hematol* 23:172, 1986.

59. Mitchell SW: On a rare vaso-motor neurosis of the extremities, and on the maladies with which it may be confounded. *Am J Med Sci* 76:2, 1878.

60. Babb RR, Alarcon-Segovia D, Fairbairn JF II: Erythermalgia: review of 51 cases. *Circulation* 29:136, 1964.

61. Kurzrock R, Cohen PR: Erythromelalgia: review of clinical characteristics and pathophysiology. *Am J Med* 91:416, 1991.

62. Michiels JJ: Erythromelalgia and vascular complications in polycythemia vera. *Semin Thromb Hemostas* 23:441, 1997.

63. Michiels JJ, ten Kate FWJ, Vuzevski VD, Abels J: Histopathology of erythromelalgia in thrombocythaemia. *Histopathology* 8:669, 1984.

64. Redding KG: Thrombocythemia as a cause of erythermalgia. *Arch Dermatol* 113:468, 1977.

65. Singh AK, Wetherley-Mein G: Microvascular occlusive lesions in primary thrombocythaemia. *Br J Haematol* 36:553, 1977.

66. Preston FE, Emmanuel IG, Winfield DA, Malia RG: Essential thrombocythaemia and peripheral gangrene. *Br Med J* 3:548, 1974.

67. Preston FE: Essential thrombocythaemia (letter). *Lancet* 1:1021, 1982.

68. Levine J, Swanson PD: Idiopathic thrombocytosis: A treatable cause of transient ischemia attacks. *Neurology* 18:711, 1968.

69. Korenman G: Neurologic syndromes associated with primary thrombocythemia. *J Mt Sinai Hosp* 36:317, 1969.

70. Singer G: Migrating emboli of retinal arteries in thrombocythaemia. *Br J Ophthalmol* 53:279, 1969.

71. Jabaily J, Iland JF, Laszlo J, et al: Neurologic manifestations of essential thrombocythemia. *Ann Intern Med* 99:513, 1983.

72. Hehlmann R, Jahn M, Baumann B, Köpcke W: Essential thrombocythemia. Clinical characteristics and course of 61 cases. *Cancer* 61:2487, 1988.

73. Lahuerta-Palacios JJ, Bornstein R, Fernandez-Debora FJ, et al: Controlled and uncontrolled thrombocytosis: Its clinical role in essential thrombocythemia. *Cancer* 61:1207, 1988.

74. Arboix A, Besses C, Acin P, et al: Ischemic stroke as first manifestation of essential thrombocythemia. Report of six cases. *Stroke* 26:1463, 1995.

75. Falconer J, Pineo G, Blahey W, Bowen T, Docksteader B, Jadusingh I: Essential thrombocythemia associated with recurrent abortions and fetal growth retardation. *Am J Hematol* 25:345, 1987.

76. Mercer B, Drouin J, Jolly E, d'Anjou G: Primary thrombocythemia in pregnancy: A report of two cases. *Am J Obstet Gynecol* 159:127, 1988.

77. Snethlage W, ten Cate JW: Thrombocythaemia and recurrent late abortions: Normal outcome of pregnancies after antiaggregating treatment. Case report. *Br J Obstet Gynaecol* 93:386, 1986.

78. Bellucci S, Janvier M, Tobelem G, et al: Essential thrombocythemias. Clinical evolutionary and biological data. *Cancer* 58:2440, 1986.

79. Jones EC, Mosesson MW, Thomason JL, Jackson TC: Essential thrombocythemia in pregnancy. *Obstet Gynecol* 71:501, 1988.

80. Sanada M: Three successful pregnancies in a woman with essential thrombocythemia. *Eur J Haematol* 42:215, 1989.

81. Beressi AH, Tefferi A, Silverstein MN, Petitt RM, Hoagland HC: Outcome analysis of 34 pregnancies in women with essential thrombocythemia. *Arch Intern Med* 155:1217, 1995.

82. Mahmoud AE, Mendoza A, Meshikhes AN, et al: Clinical spectrum, investigations and treatment of Budd-Chiari syndrome. *QJM* 89:37, 1996.

83. De Stefano V, Teofili L, Leone G, Michiels JJ: Spontaneous erythroid colony formation as the clue to an underlying myeloproliferative disorder in patients with Budd-Chiari syndrome or portal vein thrombosis. *Semin Thromb Hemostas* 23:411, 1997.

84. Valla D, Casadevall N, Lacombe C, et al: Primary myeloproliferative disorder and hepatic vein thrombosis. A prospective study of erythroid colony formation in vitro in 10 patients with Budd-Chiari syndrome. *Ann Intern Med* 103:329, 1985.

85. Valla D, Casadevall N, Huisse MG, et al: Etiology of portal vein thrombosis in adults. A prospective evaluation of primary myeloproliferative disorders. *Gastroenterology* 94:1063, 1988.

86. Rinder HM, Schuster JE, Rinder CS, Wang C, Schweidler HJ, Smith BR: Correlation of thrombosis with increased platelet turnover in thrombocytosis. *Blood* 91:1288, 1998.

87. Robinson MSC, Harrison C, Mackie IJ, Machin SJ, Harrison P: Reticulated platelets in primary and reactive thrombocytosis. *Br J Haematol* 101:338, 1998.

88. Graber M, Subramani K, Corish D, Schwab A: Thrombocytosis elevates serum potassium. *Am J Kidney Dis* 12:116, 1988.

89. Burkhardt R, Bartl R, Jager K, et al: Working classification of chronic myeloproliferative disorders based on histological, haematological and clinical findings. *J Clin Pathol* 39:237, 1986.

90. Thiele J, Schneider G, Hoeppner B, et al: Histomorphometry of bone marrow biopsies in chronic myeloproliferative disorders with associated thrombocytosis—features of significance for the diagnosis of primary (essential) thrombocythaemia. *Virchows Archiv [A]* 413:407, 1988.

91. Wolf BC, Neiman RS: The bone marrow in myeloproliferative and dysmyelopoietic syndromes. *Hematol Oncol Clin North Am* 2:669, 1988.

92. Third International Workshop on Chromosomes in Leukemia, 1980: Report of essential thrombocythemia. *Cancer Genet Cytogenet* 4:138, 1981.

93. Emilia G, Luppi M, Ferrari MG, et al: Chronic myeloid leukemia with thrombocythemic onset may be associated with different BCR/ABL variant transcripts. *Cancer Genet Cytogenet* 101:75, 1998.

94. Blickstein D, Aviram A, Luboshitz J, et al: BCR-ABL transcripts in bone marrow aspirates of Philadelphia-negative essential thrombocythemia patients: clinical presentation. *Blood* 90:2768, 1997.

95. Walsh PN, Murphy S, Barry WE: The role of platelets in the pathogenesis of thrombosis and hemorrhage in patients with thrombocytosis. *Thromb Haemost* 38:1085, 1977.

96. Murphy S, Davis J, Walsh PN, Gardner FH: Template bleeding time and clinical hemorrhage in myeloproliferative disorders. *Arch Intern Med* 138:1251, 1978.

97. Pareti FI, Gugliotta L, Mannucci L, Guarini A, Mannucci PM: Biochemical and metabolic aspects of platelet dysfunction in chronic myeloproliferative disorders. *Thromb Haemost* 47:84, 1982.

98. Wu KK: Platelet hyperaggregability and thrombosis in patients with thrombocythemia. *Ann Intern Med* 88:7, 1978.

99. Cortelazzo S, Barbui T, Bassan R, Dini E: Abnormal aggregation and increased size of platelets in myeloproliferative disorders. *Thromb Haemost* 43:127, 1980.

100. Fabris F, Randi M, Sbrojavacca R, Casonato A, Girolami A: The possible value of platelet aggregation studies in patients with increased platelet number. *Blut* 43:279, 1981.

101. Budde U, Schaefer G, Mueller N, et al: Acquired von Willebrand's disease in the myeloproliferative syndrome. *Blood* 64:981, 1984.

102. Budde U, van Genderen PJJ: Acquired von Willebrand disease in patients with high platelet counts. *Semin Thromb Hemostas* 23:425, 1997.

103. Fabris F, Casonato A, Del Ben MG, DeMarco L, Girolami A: Abnormalities of von Willebrand factor in myeloproliferative disease: A relationship with bleeding diathesis. *Br J Haematol* 63:75, 1986.

104. Kaywin P, McDonough M, Insel P, Shattil SJ: Platelet function in essential thrombocythemia: Decreased epinephrine responsiveness associated with a deficiency of platelet α-adrenergic receptors. *N Engl J Med* 299:505, 1978.

105. Maldonado JE, Pintado T, Pierre RV: Dysplastic platelets and circulating megakaryocytes in chronic myeloproliferative diseases. I. The platelets: Ultrastructure and peroxidase reaction. *Blood* 43:797, 1974.

106. Gerrard JM, Stoddard SF, Shapiro RS, et al: Platelet storage pool deficiency and prostaglandin synthesis in chronic granulocytic leukaemia. *Br J Haematol* 40:597, 1978.

107. Caranobe C, Sie P, Nouvel C, Laurent G, Pris J, Boneu B: Platelets in myeloproliferative disorders. *Scand J Haematol* 25:289, 1980.

108. Russell NH, Salmon J, Keenan JP, Bellingham AJ: Platelet adenine nucleotides and arachidonic acid metabolism in the myeloproliferative disorders. *Thromb Res* 22:389, 1981.

109. Semeraro N, Cortellazzo S, Colucci M, Barbui T: A hitherto undescribed defect of platelet coagulant activity in polycythaemia vera and essential thrombocythaemia. *Thromb Res* 16:795, 1979.

110. Okuma M, Uchino H: Altered arachidonate metabolism by platelets in patients with myeloproliferative disorders. *Blood* 54:1258, 1979.

111. Schafer AI: Deficiency of platelet lipoxygenase activity in myeloproliferative disorders. *N Engl J Med* 306:381, 1982.

112. Clezardin P, McGregor JL, Dechavanne M, Clemetson KJ: Platelet membrane glycoprotein abnormalities in patients with myeloproliferative disorders and secondary thrombocytosis. *Br J Haematol* 60:331, 1985.

113. Thibert V, Bellucci S, Cristofari M, Gluckman E, Legrand C: Increased platelet CD36 constitutes a common marker in myeloproliferative disorders. *Br J Haematol* 91:618, 1995.

114. Moore A, Nachman RL: Platelet Fc receptor: Increased expression in myeloproliferative disease. *J Clin Invest* 67:1064, 1981.

115. Cooper B, Schafer AI, Puchalsky D, Handin RI: Platelet resistance to prostaglandin D_2 in patients with myeloproliferative disorders. *Blood* 52:618, 1978.

116. Murphy S, Iland H, Rosenthal D, Laszlo J: Essential thrombocythemia: An interim report from the Polycythemia Vera Study Group. *Semin Hematol* 23:177, 1986.

117. Lengfelder E, Hochhaus A, Kronawitter U, et al: Should a platelet limit of $600 \times 10^9/l$ be used as a diagnostic criterion in essential thrombocythaemia? An analysis of the natural course including early stages. *Br J Haematol* 100:15, 1998.

118. Buss DH, Cashell AW, O'Connor ML, Richards F II, Case LD: Occurrence, etiology, and clinical significance of extreme thrombocytosis: a study case of 280 cases. *Am J Med* 96:247, 1994.

119. Hirsh J, Dacie JV: Persistent post-splenectomy thrombocytosis and thromboembolism: a consequence of continuing anaemia. *Br J Haematol* 12:44, 1966.

120. Borgna Pignatti C, Carnelli V, Caruso V, et al: Thromboembolic events in beta thalassemia major: an Italian multicenter study. *Acta Hematol* 99:76, 1998.

121. Buss DH, Stuart JJ, Lipscomb GE: The incidence of thrombotic and hemorrhagic disorders in association with extreme thrombocytosis: An analysis of 129 cases. *Am J Hematol* 20:365, 1985.

122. Taft EG, Babcock RB, Scharman WB, Tartaglia AP: Plateletpheresis in the management of thrombocytosis. *Blood* 50:927, 1977.

123. Younger J, Umlas J: Rapid reduction of platelet count in essential hemorrhagic thrombocythemia by discontinuous flow plateletpheresis. *Am J Med* 64:659, 1978.

124. Orlin JB, Berkman EM: Improvement of platelet function following plateletpheresis in patients with myeloproliferative diseases. *Transfusion* 20:540, 1980.

125. Sedlacek SM, Curtis JL, Weintraub J, Levin J: Essential thrombocythemia and leukemic transformation. *Medicine* 65:353, 1986.

126. Löfvenberg E, Wahlin A: Management of polycythaemia vera, essential thrombocythaemia and myelofibrosis with hydroxyurea. *Eur J Haematol* 41:375, 1988.

127. Best PJ, Daoud MS, Pittelkow MR, Pettit RM: Hydroxyurea-induced leg ulceration in 14 patients. *Ann Intern Med* 128:29, 1998.

128. Kaplan ME, Mack K, Goldberg JD, Donovan PB, Berk PD, Wasserman LR: Long-term management of polycythemia vera with hydroxyurea: A progress report. *Semin Hematol* 23:167, 1986.

129. Weinfeld A, Swolin B, Westin J: Acute leukemia after hydroxyurea therapy in polycythaemia vera and allied disorders: prospective study of efficacy and leukaemogenicity with therapeutic implications. *Eur J Haematol* 52:134, 1994.

130. Sterkers Y, Preudhomme C, Lai J-L, et al: Acute myeloid leukemia and myelodysplastic syndromes following essential thrombocythemia treated with hydroxyurea: high proportion of cases with 17p deletion. *Blood* 91:616, 1998.

131. Silverstein MN, Petitt RM, Solberg LA Jr, Fleming JS, Knight RC, Schacter LP: Anagrelide: a new drug for treating thrombocytosis. *N Engl J Med* 318:1292, 1988.

132. Solberg LA, Tefferi A, Oles KJ, Tarach JS, Petitt RM, Forstrom LA: The effects of anagrelide on human megakaryocytopoiesis. *Br J Haematol* 99:174, 1997.

133. Anagrelide Study Group: Anagrelide, a therapy for thrombocythemic states: experience in 577 patients. *Am J Med* 92:69, 1992.

134. Petitt RM, Silverstein MN, Petrone ME: Anagrelide for control of thrombocythemia in polycythemia and other myeloproliferative disorders. *Semin Hematol* 34:51, 1997.

135. Gugliotta L, Macchi S, Catani L, et al: Recombinant α-2a interferon (α-IFN) in the treatment of essential thrombocythaemia. Preliminary report. *Haematologica* 72:277, 1987.

136. Giles FJ, Singer CR, Gray AG, et al: Alpha-interferon therapy for essential thrombocythaemia. *Lancet* 2:70, 1988.

137. Tichelli A, Gratwohl A, Berger C, et al: Treatment of thrombocytosis in myeloproliferative disorders with interferon alpha-2a. *Blut* 58:15, 1989.

138. Ludwig H, Linkesch W, Gisslinger H, et al: Interferon alfa corrects thrombocytosis in patients with myeloproliferative disorders. *Cancer Immunol Immunother* 25:266, 1987.

139. Yataganas X, Meletis J, Plata E, et al: Alpha interferon treatment of essential thrombocythemia and other myeloproliferative disorders with excessive thrombocytosis. *Eur J Cancer* 27(suppl 4):S69, 1991.

140. Giralt M, Rubio D, Cortes MT, et al: Alpha interferon in the management of essential thrombocythaemia. *Eur J Cancer* 27(suppl 4):S72, 1991.

141. Gisslinger H, Chott A, Scheithauer W, Gilly B, Linkesch W, Ludwig H: Interferon in essential thrombocythaemia. *Br J Haematol* 79(suppl 1): 42, 1991.

142. Gilles FJ: Maintenance therapy in the myeloproliferative disorders: the current options. *Br J Haematol* 79(suppl 1):92, 1991.

143. Elliott MA, Tefferi A: Interferon-α therapy in polycythemia vera and essential thrombocythemia. *Semin Thromb Hemostas* 23:463, 1997.

144. van Genderen PJJ, Michiels JJ, van Strik R, Lindemans J, van Vilet HHDM: Platelet consumption in thrombocythemia complicated by erythromelalgia: reversal by aspirin. *Thromb Haemost* 73:210, 1995.

145. Gruppo Italiano Studio Policitemia Vera: Low-dose aspirin in polycythaemia vera. A pilot study. *Br J Haematol* 97:453, 1997.

146. Landolfi R, Marchioli R (on behalf of the ECLAP investigators): European Collaboration on Low-dose Aspirin in Polycythemia Vera (ECLAP): a randomized trial. *Semin Thromb Hemostas* 23:473, 1997.

147. Silverstein MN: Myeloproliferative disorders. *Postgrad Med* 61:206, 1977.

148. Geller SA, Shapiro E: Acute leukemia as a natural sequel to primary thrombocythemia. *Am J Clin Pathol* 77:353, 1982.

149. Rozman C, Giralt M, Feliu E, Rubio D, Cortes MT: Life expectancy of patients with chronic nonleukaemic myeloproliferative disorders. *Cancer* 67:2658, 1991.

HEREDITARY QUALITATIVE PLATELET DISORDERS

BARRY S. COLLER
DEBORAH L. FRENCH

Abnormalities of platelet function manifest themselves primarily as excessive hemorrhage at mucocutaneous sites, with ecchymoses, petechiae, epistaxis, gingival hemorrhage, and menorrhagia most common. Both quantitative and qualitative platelet abnormalities can produce these symptoms, so it is necessary to exclude thrombocytopenia by performing a platelet count (see Chap. 117). A prolonged bleeding time in a patient with a normal platelet count is indicative of a qualitative platelet abnormality, von Willebrand disease (see Chap. 135), or afibrinogenemia (see Chap. 124). Acquired qualitative platelet abnormalities are discussed in Chap. 120, and the hereditary qualitative platelet abnormalities are the subject of this chapter.

The hereditary qualitative platelet disorders can be classified according to the major locus of the defect (Table 119-1; Fig. 119-1). Thus, abnormalities of platelet glycoproteins, platelet granules, and signal transduction and secretion can all result in hemorrhagic diatheses and prolonged bleeding times. Glanzmann thrombasthenia results from abnormalities in either GPIIb or GPIIIa, resulting in loss of GPIIb/IIIa receptor function. This results in a profound defect in platelet aggregation and secondary defects in platelet adhesion and platelet coagulant activity. Loss of the platelet GPIb/IX/V complex due to abnormalities in GPIbα, GPIbβ, or GPIX results in the Bernard-Soulier syndrome, which is characterized by giant platelets and thrombocytopenia. The major defect is in platelet adhesion due to a decrease in platelet interactions with von Willebrand factor, but abnormalities in thrombin-induced aggregation are also present. Other defects in platelet GPIa/IIa (α2β1) and GPVI, as well as isolated defects in agonist receptors or proteins involved in signal transduction may also produce hemorrhagic symptoms, but these disorders are less well characterized. Abnormalities of platelet coagulant activity, that is, the ability of platelets to facilitate thrombin generation (see Chaps. 111 and 112), can also lead to a hemorrhagic diathesis, but this platelet defect is unique in not usually producing mucocutaneous hemorrhage or a prolonged bleeding time.

The following abbreviations and acronyms are used in this chapter: CMV, cytomegalovirus; ICAM-1, intercellular adhesion molecule 1; PCR, polymerase chain reaction; WASP, Wiskott-Aldrich syndrome protein.

GLYCOPROTEIN ABNORMALITIES

GLYCOPROTEIN IIB/IIIA ($\alpha IIb\beta 3$; CD41/CD61) - GLANZMANN THROMBASTHENIA

DEFINITION AND HISTORY

Glanzmann thrombasthenia is an inherited hemorrhagic disorder characterized by a severe reduction in, or absence of, platelet aggregation in response to multiple physiologic agonists due to qualitative or quantitative abnormalities of platelet glycoprotein (GP) IIb (αIIb; CD 41) and/or GPIIIa ($\beta 3$; CD61).

Glanzmann, a Swiss pediatrician, described a group of patients with hemorrhagic symptoms and "weak" platelets (i.e., thrombasthenia) in 1918.[1] Subsequent studies demonstrated that platelets from thrombasthenic patients failed to aggregate in response to physiologic agonists such as ADP, epinephrine, collagen, and thrombin[2-5]; had markedly reduced[2,4-6] levels of platelet fibrinogen; and had reduced or absent clot retraction.[7] In the mid-1970s, Nurden and Caen[8] and Phillips and colleagues[9] discovered that thrombasthenic platelets were deficient in both GPIIb and GPIIIa. Later studies demonstrated that GPIIb and GPIIIa form a calcium-dependent complex in the platelet membrane that functions as a receptor for fibrinogen and other adhesive glycoproteins.[10-13] Cloning and sequencing of the cDNAs for GPIIb[14] and GPIIIa[15] identified them as separate protein subunits that are members of the integrin receptor superfamily[16] and permitted the molecular biological characterization of the disorder in affected patients. Identification of the DNA defects in selected patients has provided information on the structure-function relationships of the GPIIb/IIIa receptor and permitted DNA-based carrier detection and prenatal diagnosis.[17-58]

ETIOLOGY AND PATHOGENESIS

Glanzmann thrombasthenia is a rare disorder characterized by autosomal recessive inheritance with a worldwide distribution. In regions where consanguineous matings are common, groups of patients with the disorder have been identified, and in several populations founder mutations have been identified by analyzing polymorphisms in the DNA surrounding the affected mutation. These include 42 patients from South India; 39 patients from the Iraqi-Jewish population in Israel; 46 Arab patients from Israel, Jordan, and Saudi Arabia; and a smaller number of patients from three Gypsy families.[6,24,41,59-63] An analysis of the gene frequency for the more common mutation causing Glanzmann thrombasthenia in the Iraqi-Jewish population revealed 6 of 700 individuals to be carriers.[41]

The platelet GPIIb/IIIa receptor is required for platelet aggregation induced by all of the agonists thought to operate in vivo (ADP, epinephrine, thrombin, collagen, thromboxane A_2) (see Chap. 111).[10-12] Consequently, abnormalities in the receptor result in a failure of platelet plug formation at sites of vascular injury, leading to excessive bleeding and bruising.

The GPIIb/IIIa receptor is also responsible for the uptake of fibrinogen from plasma into platelet α granules,[64-67] so patients with Glanzmann thrombasthenia have markedly reduced levels of platelet fibrinogen.[2,4,5,68,69] Clot retraction requires platelets with intact GPIIb/IIIa receptors,[70-72] presumably to make contact with fibrin, and so patients with Glanzmann thrombasthenia usually have abnormal clot retraction.[2,7]

Defects in either GPIIb or GPIIIa result in the same functional defect because both subunits are required for receptor function (see Chap. 111). Biosynthetic studies indicate that GPIIb and GPIIIa form a complex soon after protein synthesis in the rough endoplasmic reticulum[73-75]; subsequent posttranslational processing[76] and transport to the platelet membrane require that the complex be intact (Fig. 119-2).[77,78] Complex formation protects the glycoproteins from proteolytic digestion,[73-76] so if either GPIIb or GPIIIa is absent or unable to form a

TABLE 119-1　INHERITED DISORDERS OF PLATELET FUNCTION

I. Glycoprotein abnormalities
　Glycoprotein IIb/IIIa (αIIbβ3; CD41/CD61): Glanzmann thrombasthenia
　Glycoproteins Ib (CD42b,c), IX (CD42a), and V: Bernard-Soulier syndrome
　Glycoprotein Ib (CD42b,c): Platelet-type (pseudo–) von Willebrand disease
　Glycoprotein Ia/IIa (α2β1; VLA-2; CD49b/CD29)
　Glycoprotein IV (CD36)
　Glycoprotein VI
II. Abnormal membrane-cytoskeleton interactions
　Wiskott-Aldrich syndrome (Wiskott-Aldrich syndrome protein; WASP)
III. Abnormalities of platelet granules
　δ-Storage pool deficiency
　α, δ-Storage pool deficiency
　Gray platelet syndrome: α-storage pool deficiency
　Quebec platelet disorder
IV. Abnormalities of platelet coagulant activity
V. Abnormalities of signal transduction and secretion
　Defects in platelet agonist receptors or agonist-specific signal transduction
　Defects in arachidonic acid metabolism and thromboxane production
　Defects in phospholipase C, Gαq, calcium mobilization, and calcium responsiveness

SOURCE: Adapted from Coller[496] with permission.

normal complex, the other subunit will be rapidly degraded. Thus, a deficiency in either glycoprotein produces a deficiency in both. Since complex formation and vesicular transport are also required for proteolytic processing of pro-GPIIb into its constituent GPIIbα and GPIIbβ subunits,[76] if complex formation and/or vesicular transport does not occur normally, the very small amount of residual GPIIb will be pro-GPIIb, not mature GPIIb.[79]

GPIIIa (β3) can also combine with the αV-integrin (CD51) subunit to form the αVβ3 "vitronectin" receptor[15,80,81] (Fig. 119-3) (see Chap. 111). Despite its common name, this receptor can bind many of the same adhesive glycoproteins as GPIIb/IIIa, although there are some differences in ligand preference and binding sequences.[81–85] A small number of αVβ3 receptors are present on platelets (50 to 100 per platelet)[84,86,87]; osteoclasts, endothelial cells, and uterine cells, among others, also have αVβ3 receptors.[88–90] Glanzmann thrombasthenia patients with defects in GPIIIa also are deficient in αVβ3, whereas patients with defects in GPIIb have either normal or increased numbers of platelet αVβ3 receptors.[19,20,35,84,87,89] At present, there is no evidence that patients who lack αVβ3 receptors in addition to lacking GPIIb/IIIa receptors have a more severe hemorrhagic diathesis or suffer from any other abnormalities, perhaps because alternative receptors containing αV associated with other β-subunits can substitute for αVβ3.[87]

The molecular biological abnormalities in more than 60 patients with Glanzmann thrombasthenia have been identified, and they are listed in an internet database that is updated continuously[40] (http://med.mssm.edu/glanzmanndb) and can be reached through the Williams Hematology website (http://www.williamshematology.com). Table 119-2 and Figs. 119-4 and 119-5 contain information on mutations of particular interest. Of note, about 40% of the patients with identified mutations are compound heterozygotes rather than homozygotes, indicating that a sizable number of silent carriers are present in the population. Where consanguinity is common, the disorder is more likely to be due to a homozygous mutation arising in a founder,

FIGURE 119-1　Evaluation of patients for abnormalities in platelet number or function and related disorders.

A reduced platelet count occurs in patients with purely quantitative platelet disorders (inherited or acquired) as well as in patients who have inherited qualitative platelet disorders associated with thrombocytopenia. Platelet size (determined from the blood film and/or the mean platelet volume) helps to separate the inherited quantitative platelet syndromes from the acquired thrombocytopenias and the inherited combined quantitative and qualitative thrombocytopenias (see Chap. 117). Very small platelets are characteristic of the Wiskott-Aldrich syndrome. Large platelets that lack purple granules are observed in the gray platelet syndrome (α-storage pool deficiency), but one needs to be certain that the stain is working properly and that there is no plasma factor producing platelet degranulation such as an abnormal immunoglobulin. Confirmation of the diagnosis of gray platelet syndrome is obtained with biochemical analysis of α-granule contents. Patients with platelet-type (pseudo–) von Willebrand disease (vWd) and type 2B vWd have moderate thrombocytopenia and large platelets. Studies of GPIb function and biochemistry are required to establish the diagnosis. The platelets in Bernard-Soulier syndrome are truly giant, with many larger than erythrocytes; the diagnosis is confirmed with biochemical and functional analyses of the GPIb/IX/V complex.

The bleeding time is prolonged in virtually all patients with qualitative platelet disorders (although to various extents) except in platelet coagulant activity disorders, in which the serum prothrombin time is the preferred screening assay. Other tests of platelet coagulant activity are used to establish the diagnosis. Platelet aggregation can separate patients into those with defects in the primary wave of platelet aggregation (dependent on fibrinogen, von Willebrand factor, or their respective receptors) and those with defects in the secondary wave of aggregation. Enhanced ristocetin-induced platelet aggregation at low concentrations of ristocetin has been identified in patients with platelet-type vWd (who have a defect in the GPIb receptor that facilitates von Willebrand factor binding) and in patients with type 2B von Willebrand disease (who have an intrinsic defect in von Willebrand factor) (see Chap. 135). These two diseases can be distinguished by analyzing the binding of the patient's von Willebrand factor to normal platelets, or the ability of cryoprecipitate or asialo–von Willebrand factor to aggregate patient platelets; confirmation of the diagnosis of platelet-type von Willebrand disease requires analysis of GPIb.

Neither ristocetin nor the snake venom botrocetin induces platelet aggregation if the plasma lacks functional von Willebrand factor, as in most cases of von Willebrand disease (see Chap. 135), or if the platelets lack functional GPIb/IX complexes, as in Bernard-Soulier syndrome. The defect in von Willebrand disease, but not in Bernard-Soulier syndrome, can be corrected by adding normal plasma. Direct analysis of von Willebrand factor and the platelet GPIb/IX complex will confirm the diagnosis.

Patients whose plasma lacks fibrinogen (afibrinogenemia) (see Chap. 124) or whose platelets cannot bind fibrinogen because of abnormal GPIIb/IIIa receptors (Glanzmann thrombasthenia) will have no primary wave of platelet aggregation in response to ADP or epinephrine. Analysis of plasma fibrinogen and platelet GPIIb/IIIa receptors can differentiate between these two groups. Isolated defects in the primary response to collagen have been observed in patients with abnormalities in platelet GPIa/IIa (α2β1) or GPVI. Platelet glycoprotein analysis can separate these from each other. Other isolated defects in one or more of the ADP receptors or the thromboxane A$_2$ receptor will result in decreased ADP-induced platelet aggregation, whereas isolated defects in the receptors for epinephrine or platelet-activating factor lead to defects in primary aggregation in response to these agonists.

A heterogeneous group of platelet defects can result in an abnormal secondary wave of platelet aggregation in response to ADP and epinephrine, and diminished response to low concentrations of collagen and thrombin, but they can be broadly separated into granule defects and defects in the platelet release reaction. These two groups can be distinguished on the basis of their release of granule contents in response to high concentrations of thrombin: platelets from patients with release reaction abnormalities will release normal amounts of granule contents whereas patients with reduced granule contents will release abnormally small amounts of granule contents. α-granule contents and dense body contents can be measured immunologically and biochemically; electron microscopy can confirm the diagnosis of granule defects. Release reaction abnormalities can be subcategorized by analysis of the response to arachidonic acid or a thromboxane A$_2$ analogue, as well as by measuring release of arachidonic acid, calcium fluxes, and phosphoinositide metabolism. (Adapted from Coller,[496] reprinted with permission.)

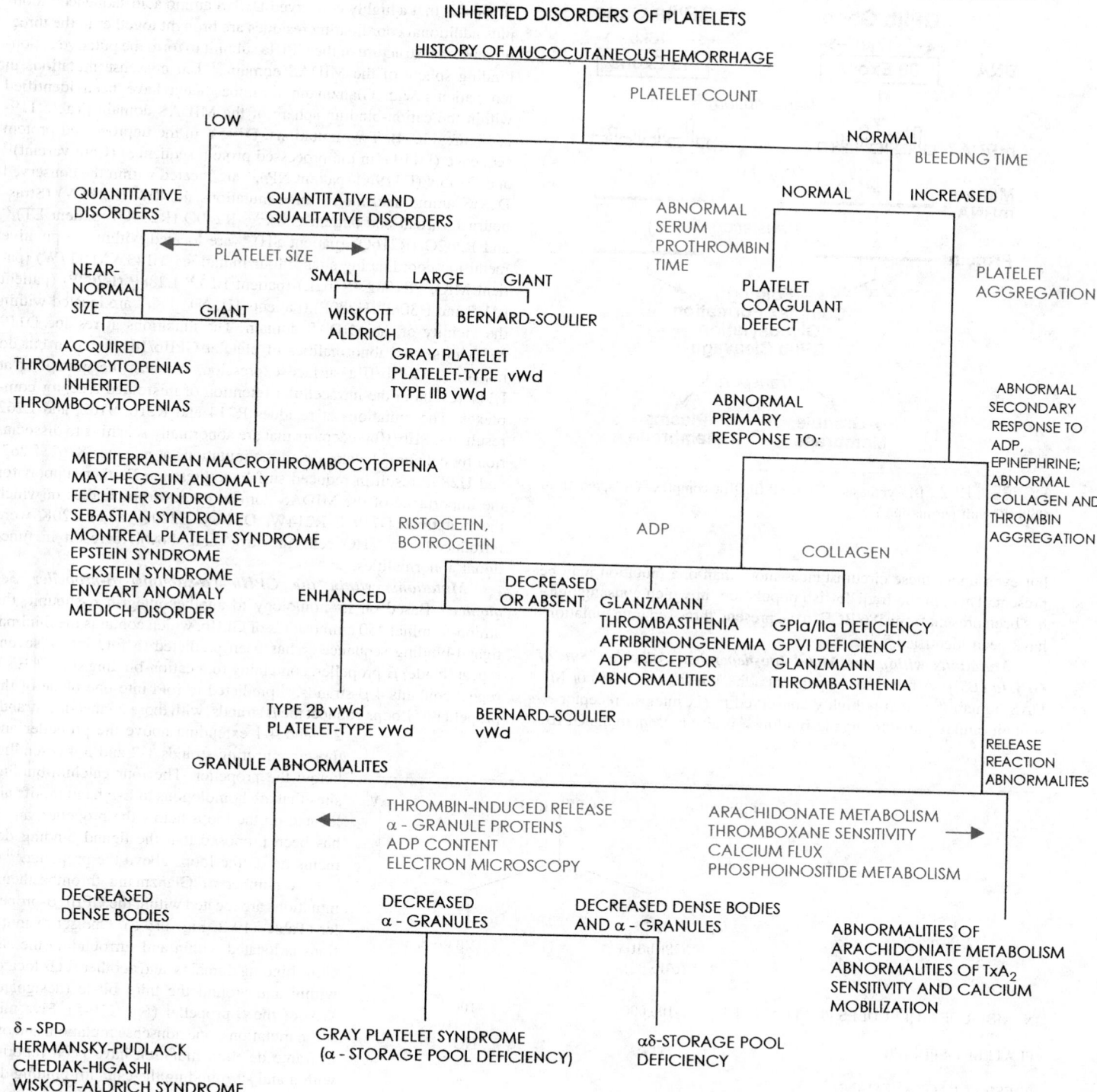

INHERITED DISORDERS OF PLATELETS

HISTORY OF MUCOCUTANEOUS HEMORRHAGE

PLATELET COUNT

LOW   NORMAL

                                              BLEEDING TIME

                                    NORMAL   INCREASED

QUANTITATIVE   QUANTITATIVE AND
DISORDERS   QUALITATIVE DISORDERS   ABNORMAL
                                          SERUM
        ← PLATELET SIZE →   PROTHROMBIN
                                          TIME   PLATELET
NEAR-   SMALL   LARGE   GIANT   PLATELET   AGGREGATION
NORMAL   COAGULANT
SIZE   GIANT   WISKOTT   DEFECT
                      ALDRICH   BERNARD-SOULIER
ACQUIRED
THROMBOCYTOPENIAS   GRAY PLATELET
INHERITED   PLATELET-TYPE vWd
THROMBOCYTOPENIAS   TYPE IIB vWd
                                              ABNORMAL   ABNORMAL
                                              PRIMARY   SECONDARY
                                              RESPONSE TO: RESPONSE TO
                                                                      ADP,
MEDITERRANEAN MACROTHROMBOCYTOPENIA   EPINEPHRINE;
MAY-HEGGLIN ANOMALY   ABNORMAL
FECHTNER SYNDROME   COLLAGEN AND
SEBASTIAN SYNDROME   THROMBIN
MONTREAL PLATELET SYNDROME   RISTOCETIN,   ADP   AGGREGATION
EPSTEIN SYNDROME   BOTROCETIN
ECKSTEIN SYNDROME   COLLAGEN
ENVEART ANOMALY   ENHANCED   DECREASED   GLANZMANN
MEDICH DISORDER   OR ABSENT   THROMBASTHENIA   GPIa/IIa DEFICIENCY
                                           AFRIBRINONGENEMIA GPVI DEFICIENCY
                                           ADP RECEPTOR   GLANZMANN
                                           ABNORMALITIES   THROMBASTHENIA

                      TYPE 2B vWd   BERNARD-SOULIER
                      PLATELET-TYPE vWd   vWd
                                                                      RELEASE
GRANULE ABNORMALITES   REACTION
                                                                      ABNORMALITES
            THROMBIN-INDUCED RELEASE   ARACHIDONATE METABOLISM
            α - GRANULE PROTEINS   THROMBOXANE SENSITIVITY
        ←   ADP CONTENT   CALCIUM FLUX   →
            ELECTRON MICROSCOPY   PHOSPHOINOSITIDE METABOLISM

DECREASED   DECREASED   DECREASED DENSE BODIES
DENSE BODIES   α - GRANULES   AND α - GRANULES   ABNORMALITIES OF
                                                          ARACHIDONATE METABOLISM
                                                          ABNORMALITIES OF TxA$_2$
                                                          SENSITIVITY AND CALCIUM
                                                          MOBILIZATION
δ - SPD
HERMANSKY-PUDLACK   GRAY PLATELET SYNDROME   αδ-STORAGE POOL
CHEDIAK-HIGASHI   (α - STORAGE POOL DEFICIENCY)   DEFICIENCY
WISKOTT-ALDRICH SYNDROME

Abbreviations: vWd = von WILLEBRAND DISEASE
                 SPD = STORAGE POOL DEFICIENCY

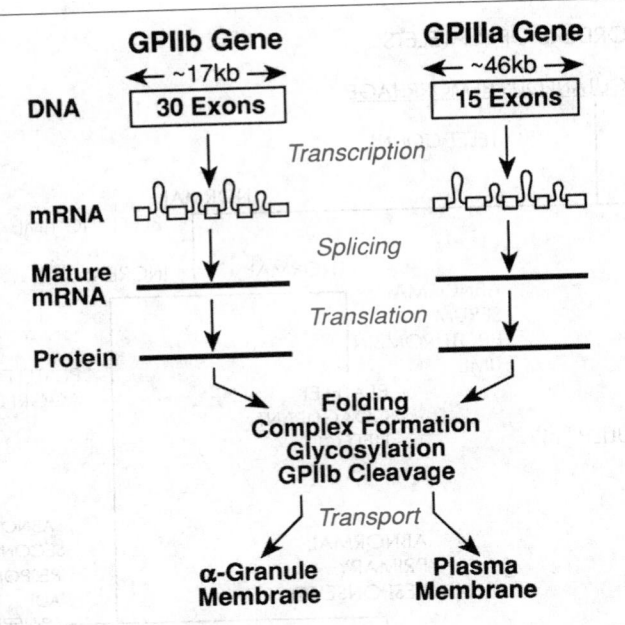

GPIIb Gene   **GPIIIa Gene**

DNA   ← ~17kb →   ← ~46kb →
             [30 Exons]   [15 Exons]

                    Transcription

mRNA

                    Splicing

Mature
mRNA

                    Translation

Protein

                    Folding
                 Complex Formation
                   Glycosylation
                  GPIIb Cleavage

                    Transport

          α-Granule   Plasma
          Membrane   Membrane

FIGURE 119-2 Biosynthesis of the GPIIb/IIIa complex. (Adapted from Coller[496] with permission.)

(β3) subunit.[94] Mutagenesis and molecular modeling experiments have suggested that a highly conserved DxSxS amino acid sequence[95] motif plus additional coordinating residues are brought together in the three-dimensional structure of the GPIIIa subunit to form the putative cation-binding sphere of the MIDAS domain.[92] Ten missense mutations in ten patients with Glanzmann thrombasthenia have been identified within the cation-binding sphere of the MIDAS domain (Table 119-2, Figure 119-4). Two mutations, D145Y in the unprocessed protein sequence (D119Y in the processed protein sequence) (Cam variant)[18] and D145N (D119N) (patient NR),[96] are located within the conserved DxSxS amino acid motif; three mutations, R240W (R214W) (Strasbourg I variant and patient CM),[25,33] R240Q (R214Q) (patient ET),[23] and R242Q (R216Q) (patient SH),[97] are located within the putative metal ion coordinating sites[23]; four mutations, L143W (L117W) (patient MK),[98] S188L (S162L) (patient BL),[55] L288P (L262P) (patient LD)[46] and H306P (H280P) (patients HJ, NT, TK)[47] are located within the vicinity of the MIDAS domain. The mutations at residue D119 result in severe abnormalities of platelet GPIIb/IIIa function but do not affect GPIIb/IIIa surface expression, whereas the mutations at L117 results in the intracellular retention of misfolded receptor complexes. The mutations at residues R214 and R216, S162, and L262 result in GPIIb/IIIa receptors that are abnormally sensitive to dissociation by calcium chelation, and the mutations at residues S162, L262, and H280P result in reduced surface expression. Further support for the importance of the MIDAS domain comes from studies in which the mutations D119N, R214W, D217N, E220Q, and E220K were introduced into CHO cells in vitro[99] and shown to result in functional abnormalities.

Mutations within the GPIIb (α-subunit) β-propeller Sequence Based on its homology to another integrin α-subunit, the amino-terminal 450 amino acids of GPIIb, which contains the minimal ligand-binding sequence,[100] has been predicted to fold into a seven-repeat (blade) β-propeller, containing four cation-binding sites.[101] Each repeat contains 4 β-strands,[102] predicted to fold into one blade of the propeller.[101] Loops connect the β strands, with those connecting strands 2-3 and 4-1 extending above the propeller and those connecting strands 1-2 and 3-4 extending below the propeller. The four calcium-binding sites that are homologous to E-F hand motifs are located on the loops below the propeller, and it has been proposed that the ligand binding domains lie on the loops above the propeller.[101]

A number of Glanzmann thrombasthenia mutations are located within the GPIIb β-propeller (Table 119-2; Fig. 119-5). One set of mutations is located within and surrounding the calcium-binding domains, and another set is located within and around the third blade (designated W3) of the β-propeller (Fig. 119-5). Five missense mutations, one nonsense mutation, and one in-frame deletion mutation have been reported within and surrounding the calcium-binding domains in a total of 10 patients. Many of these mutations affect transport of the GPIIb/IIIa complex to the cell surface. These mutations include a G273D (G242D) substitution (patient FLD)[35] which precedes the first calcium-binding domain; a F320S (F289S) (Japanese-1)[48] which precedes the second calcium-binding domain; a E355K (E324K) substitution (patients FL, Swiss, and Japanese-2)[36,48,56] located between the second and third calcium-binding domains; a R358H (R327H) substitution (patients KJ and Mila-

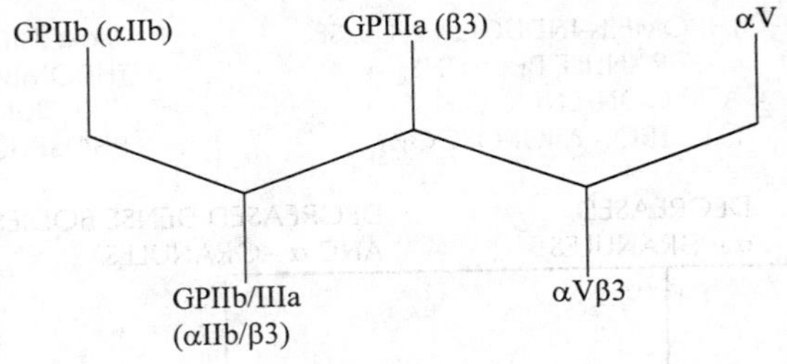

but even under these circumstances more than one mutation may be present. Thus, in the Iraqi Jewish population, in which consanguinity has been present from 586 BCE to the present, three separate mutations have been identified.[41,91]

Mutations within the Metal Ion-dependent Adhesion Site of GPIIIa (β3) A metal ion-dependent adhesion site (MIDAS) or MIDAS domain,[92] which is highly conserved in six integrin receptor α-subunits and required for ligand-binding,[93] is also present in the GPIIIa

	GPIIb/IIIa (αIIb/β3)	αVβ3
NUMBER OF MOLECULES PER PLATELET	~100,000	~100
PLATELET-SPECIFIC	YES	NO
PRESENT IN GLANZMANN THROMBASTHENIA PATIENTS WITH DEFECT IN GPIIb (αIIb)	NO	YES
PRESENT IN GLANZMANN THROMBASTHENIA PATIENTS WITH DEFECT IN GPIIIa (β3)	NO	NO

FIGURE 119-3 The relationship between the GPIIb/IIIa (αIIbβ3) and αVβ3 receptors. Both receptors share the common β-integrin subunit GPIIIa (β3). GPIIb/IIIa is present at high density on platelets, is platelet-specific, and is abnormal in all patients with Glanzmann thrombasthenia. The αVβ3 receptor is expressed at very low levels on platelets, is not platelet-specific, and is only decreased in Glanzmann thrombasthenia patients whose defects are in GPIIIa (β3).

TABLE 119-2   SELECTED MOLECULAR BIOLOGIC ABNORMALITIES IN GLANZMANN THROMBASTHENIA

MUTATIONS WITHIN THE GPIIb β-PROPELLER DOMAIN

PATIENT	GENOTYPE	EXON	MUTATION[1]	MUTATION[2] PHENOTYPE	AMINO ACID SUBSTITUTION[3]	REF
Mennonite	Homozygote	4	526C→G	Missense	P176A(P145A)	44
JF	Compound	4	526C→G	Missense	P176A(P145A)	44
	Heterozygote	28	2929C→T	Nonsense	R977X(R946X)	
Chinese-14	Compound	4	527C→T	Missense	P176L(P145L)	44
	Heterozygote	16	IVS15(-1)del	Unknown	Unknown	
KO	Homozygote	5	575-580Ins	Ins: in frame	R192T193(R161T162)	51
LW	Homozygote	6	641T→C	Missense	L214P(L183P)	54
FLD	Homozygote	8	818G→A	Missense	G273D(G242D)	35
Japanese-1	Compound	11	959T→C	Missense	F320S(F289S)	48
	Heterozygote		Unknown	Unknown	Unknown	
FL	Homozygote	12	1063G→A	Missense	E355K(E324K)	36
Swiss	Compound	12	1063C→A	Missense	E355K(E324K)	56
	Heterozygote	18	1787T→C	Missense	I596T(I565T)	
KJ	Homozygote	12	1073G→A	Missense	R358H(R327H)	37
Mila-1	Homozygote	12	1073G→A	Missense	R358H(R327H)	38
Japanese-2	Compound	12	1063G→A	Missense	E355K(E324K)	48
	Heterozygote		Unknown	Unknown	Unknown	
LM	Homozygote	13	1346G→A	Missense	G449D(G418D)	34
LeM	Compound	13	1366-1371del	Del: in frame	V(425)D(426)del	39
	Heterozygote		Unknown	Unknown	Unknown	
DV and SV	Compound	14	1413C→G	Nonsense	Y471X(Y440X)	53
	Heterozygote	29	3015insG	Ins: out of frame	Frameshift	

MUTATIONS WITHIN THE GPIIIa (β3) MIDAS DOMAIN

PATIENT	GENOTYPE	EXON[1]	MUTATION[2]	MUTATION PHENOTYPE	AMINO ACID SUBSTITUTION[3]	REF
MK	Homozygote	4	428T→G	Missense	L143W(L117W)	98
Cam	Homozygote	4	433G→T	Missense	D145Y(D119Y)	18
NR	Homozygote	4	433G→A	Missense	D145N(D119N)	96
BL	Homozygote	4	563C→T	Missense	S188L(S162L)	55
Strasbourg I	Homozygote	5	718C→T	Missense	R240W(R214W)	25
CM	Homozygote	5	718C→T	Missense	R240W(R214W)	33
ET	Homozygote	5	719G→A	Missense	R240Q(R214Q)	23
SH	Homozygote	5	725G→A	Missense	R242Q(R216Q)	97
LD	Compound	6	847delGC	Del: out of frame	Premature termination	46
	Heterozygote	6	863T→C	Missense	L288P(L262P)	
NT	Homozygote	6	917A→C	Missense	H306P(H280P)	47

MUTATIONS AFFECTING RECEPTOR ACTIVATION

PATIENT	GENOTYPE	EXON[1]	MUTATION[2]	MUTATION PHENOTYPE	AMINO ACID SUBSTITUTION[3]	Ref
RM	Compound	11	1791delT	Del: out of frame	Premature termination	45
	Heterozygote	14	2248C→T	Nonsense	R750X(R724X)	
Paris I	Compound	15	2332T→C	Missense	S778P(S752P)	22
	Heterozygote		Unknown	Unknown	No transcript	

[1]Numbering for GPIIb according to Heidenreich et al: *Biochemistry* 29:1232, 1990. Numbering for GPIIIa (β3) is modified according to Villa-Garcia et al: *Blood* 83:668, 1994.
[2]Nomenclature is based on recommendations by Beaudet et al: *Hum Mutat* 8:197, 1996; ibid, 203. The cDNA nucleotide numbering begins with the A nucleotide of the ATG start codon according to Poncz et al: *J Biol Chem* 262:8476, 1987 for GPIIb and Fitzgerald et al: *J Biol Chem* 262:3936, 1987 for GPIIIa (β3). Nucleotide substitutions: cDNA nucleotide number followed by nucleotide→nucleotide substitution. Abbreviations: del, deletion; ins, insertion; inv, inversion; IVS, intervening sequence.
[3]Amino acid numbering begins with methionine of the ATG start codon according to references listed in footnote 2. Amino acid codon numbers including and excluding (in parentheses) the leader sequence are provided. Amino acid substitution are designated by amino acid-codon number-amino acid. Single letter amino acid code: C, cysteine; D, aspartate; E, glutamate; K, lysine; L, leucine; M, methionine; N, asparagine; P, proline; Q, glutamine; R, arginine; S, serine; V, valine; W, tryptophane; Y, tyrosine; X, nonsense mutation.

1)[37,38] also located between the second and third calcium-binding domains; a G449D (G418D) substitution (patient LM)[34] which precedes the fourth calcium-binding domain; a V425D426 deletion (patient LeM)[39] at the beginning of the fourth calcium-binding domain; and a Y471X (Y440X) nonsense mutation just following the fourth calcium-binding domain.[53]

Another set of mutations are located within the vicinity of the third blade (W3) of the β-propeller, which contains a predicted β-turn structure that has been implicated in ligand binding to GPIIb/IIIa and other integrin receptors.[103,104] Three missense mutations and one insertion found in five patients result in functionally defective receptors. P176A (P145A) (Mennonite and patient JF) and P176L (P145L) (Chinese-14)[44] substitutions and an R192T193 (R161T162) (patient KO)[51] insertion are located within the 4-1 connecting hairpin

loop between the second (W2) and third (W3) blades of the propeller. A L214P (L183P) substitution (patient LW)[54] is located at the end of the second β-strand near the 2-3 connecting hairpin loop. Independent support for the functional importance of this region comes from in vitro CHO cell expression system data[99] indicating that a D255V (D224V) mutation,[105] located within the 4-1 connecting hairpin loop between the third and fourth blades of the propeller, disrupts receptor ligand binding.

Mutations That Affect Receptor Activation   The cytoplasmic domain of GPIIIa plays a functional role in integrin activation and the regulation of ligand binding.[22,106,107] Two Glanzmann thrombasthenia mutations have been identified in this region (Table 119-2). One is a R750X (R724X) nonsense mutation (patient RM)[45] that results in the deletion of the carboxy-terminal 39 residues of GPIIIa, and the other

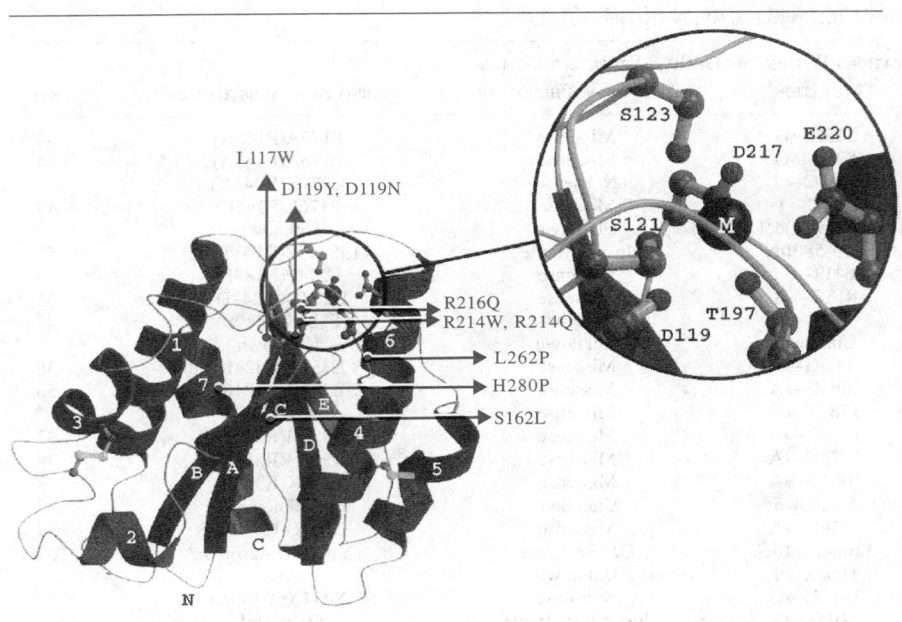

FIGURE 119-4   Glanzmann thrombasthenia mutations located within the vicinity of the metal ion–dependent adhesion site (MIDAS) of GPIIIa (β3). A ribbon diagram of the MIDAS domain located within GPIIIa (β3) is shown and represents the minimal ligand-binding region of this integrin subunit. The cation-binding $D^{119}xS^{121}xS^{123}$ motif and coordinating residues D^{217} and E^{220} are shown in the highlighted circle. The location of Glanzmann thrombasthenia mutations within and surrounding the MIDAS domain are shown. (Adapted from Tozer[94] with permission.)

is a S778P (S752P) missense mutation (patient P or Paris I).[22,107,108] This latter patient is unusual in that he had no history of excessive hemorrhage, but he did have a prolonged bleeding time and his platelets did not aggregate in response to ADP. These mutations do not severely affect surface expression of platelet GPIIb/IIIa complexes, but both mutant receptors are unresponsive to agonist stimulation. Mammalian cell expression studies show normal adhesion to immobilized fibrinogen but abnormal cell spreading. Cells expressing the S778P (S752P) mutant receptors have reduced focal adhesion plaque formation and cells expressing the R750X (R724X) mutant receptors have undetectable tyrosine phosphorylation of focal adhesion kinase, pp125^{FAK}. These mutations provide evidence for the role of the GPIIIa cytoplasmic tail in inside-out signaling (i.e., platelet signals that lead to GPIIb/IIIa adopting a high-affinity ligand binding conformation) and outside-in signaling (i.e., signaling to the interior of the platelet as a result of GPIIb/IIIa binding ligand).

CLINICAL FEATURES

The clinical manifestations of a total of 232 patients with Glanzmann thrombasthenia have been the subject of two reviews, and Table 119-3 summarizes data from 177 of these patients.[6,24] Menorrhagia occurs in nearly all patients, especially at the time of menarche. Purpura can be present immediately after birth but often is not dramatic. Petechiae of the face and subconjunctival hemorrhage associated with crying may be the first symptoms in neonates and babies. Epistaxis is a common symptom and can be life-threatening.[6,24,109] It usually abates in adulthood. Gingival bleeding can be a chronic source of blood (and iron) loss, especially if the teeth are not kept in good repair. Gastrointestinal bleeding was only present in 12 percent of patients in one review[6] but was present in 49 percent of patients in another.[24] Gastrointestinal bleeding is usually intermittent, and it is often difficult to identify the bleeding site.

Hemarthroses are very rare, and spontaneous ones even rarer, distinguishing Glanzmann thrombasthenia from the hemophilias and related illnesses. The platelet abnormality in Glanzmann thrombasthenia undoubtedly increases the risk of excessive bleeding when there is trauma to the central nervous system, but it is remarkable that spontaneous central nervous system bleeding is so rare.[6,24]

Patients with Glanzmann thrombasthenia do not appear to bleed excessively during pregnancy, but immediate postpartum hemorrhage is very common unless platelet transfusions are administered.[6] Delayed postpartum hemorrhage can also be severe; it may be less likely to occur in patients delivered by cesarean section.[6] Surgical procedures, including oral surgery, are usually complicated by excessive bleeding unless prophylactic platelet transfusions are administered.[6,24,110]

The hemorrhagic diathesis in Glanzmann thrombasthenia is notable for its variability and the lack of correlation between the biochemical platelet abnormalities and clinical severity.[6] Even within groups of patients such as the Iraqi Jews, most of whom share the same genetic abnormality and have very similar platelet function and biochemical profiles, there is a wide spectrum of clinical severity.[24,41] Moreover, the severity of bleeding symptoms can vary significantly during the lifetime of individual patients. Thus, factors other than the platelet defect itself play important roles in determining the risk of bleeding.

Carriers of Glanzmann thrombasthenia appear to be asymptomatic and generally have normal results in platelet function tests,[6,24] but a prolonged bleeding time has been reported in at least one heterozygote.[57]

LABORATORY FEATURES

Characteristic laboratory data in patients with Glanzmann thrombasthenia are given in Table 119-4. Patients have normal platelet counts and morphology, prolonged bleeding times, decreased or absent clot retraction, and abnormal platelet aggregation responses to physiologic stimuli (Fig. 119-6). Platelets of patients with Glanzmann thrombasthenia have a normal (or near-normal) initial slope of ristocetin-induced aggregation, reflecting the normal levels of plasma von Willebrand factor and the normal platelet GPIb/IX content; the reduced second wave of aggregation at low doses of ristocetin reflects the impaired GPIIb/IIIa function,[111] and the interesting cyclical aggregation at higher doses of ristocetin[112] probably reflects a complex interaction between ristocetin-induced binding of von Willebrand factor to GPIb/IX and inhibition of this interaction by released ADP.[113] In each case, the abnormalities reflect the inability of the platelets to bind fibrinogen and/or other adhesive glycoproteins. Platelets undergo normal shape change in response to ADP and thrombin, demonstrating their ability to undergo metabolic and cytoskeletal changes in response to these agents. Similarly, high doses of thrombin and collagen produce normal release of dense body and α-granule contents[2,4,114]; the release reaction abnormalities observed with lower doses of these agents reflect the lack of augmentation of the release reaction normally produced by platelet aggregation.[2,111,115–117]

Platelets in whole blood or platelet-rich plasma adhere to glass because fibrinogen first becomes deposited on the glass and the platelets then adhere to the immobilized fibrino-gen.[118,119] Platelets from patients with Glanz-mann thrombasthenia fail to adhere to glass,[2,4,118] and this forms the basis of their abnormality in the glass bead retention assay.[120] Platelet coagulant activity has been variably reported as normal or abnor-mal,[2-5,121–123] probably as a result of variations in the assays used to assess this activity or individual patient differences. A defect in platelet microparticle formation and support of thrombin generation has been identified in some patients,[122–125] but not all patients appear to share this abnormality.[126] GPIIb/IIIa and αVβ3 have been shown to bind prothrombin, probably accounting for some of the abnor-malities identified.[127,128]

In flow chamber studies, thrombasthenic platelets adhere normally to deendothelialized blood vessels at low and intermediate shear rates but do not spread normally or form plate-let thrombi.[129–131] A defect in adhesion occurs at higher shear rates. A paradoxical increase in fibrin formation on these surfaces has been observed with thrombasthenic platelets, but the explanation for this phenomenon re-mains unknown.[132]

Platelet GPIIb/IIIa and αVβ3 can be quantitated by any one of several techniques, including, monoclonal antibody binding (us-ing flow cytometry or radiolabeled binding), immunoblotting, and surface labeling fol-lowed by sodium dodecyl-sulfate polacrylam-ide gel electrophoresis (SDS-PAGE) (Fig. 119-7). Based on the results of such studies, patients with Glanzmann thrombasthenia have been subcategorized by GPIIb/IIIa content into those with less than 5 percent of normal GPIIb/IIIa (type I), 5 to 20 percent (type II), or 50 percent or more (variants).[6,133] In one review of 64 patients, 78 percent were type I, 14 percent were type II, and 8 percent were variants.[6] The subtyping of Glanzmann throm-basthenia into type I, type II, and variants predated the identification of GPIIb/IIIa ab-normalities as the cause of Glanzmann throm-basthenia and was based on functional data. With current methods of more precise labora-tory analysis and the recognition of the diverse clinical and functional abnormalities present in Glanzmann thrombas-thenia, this categorization provides only limited information.

Although there are very few αVβ3 receptors per platelet, they can be reliably measured by radiolabeled antibody binding and by flow cytometry[87]; they can also be measured on patient lymphocytes after transformation with Epstein-Barr virus.[134] The αVβ3 level is very useful in making a preliminary assessment of whether the patient has a defect in GPIIb or GPIIIa, since patients who lack GPIIIa also lack αVβ3 receptors.[135]

Fibrinogen-binding studies assess the function of the GPIIb/IIIa complex.[10,11] The most common method is to add radiolabeled fibrino-gen to platelets suspended in buffer (prepared either by washing or gel filtration) and then measure the binding of radioactivity when the platelets are stimulated with ADP[10,11] or a similar agonist. Fibrinogen

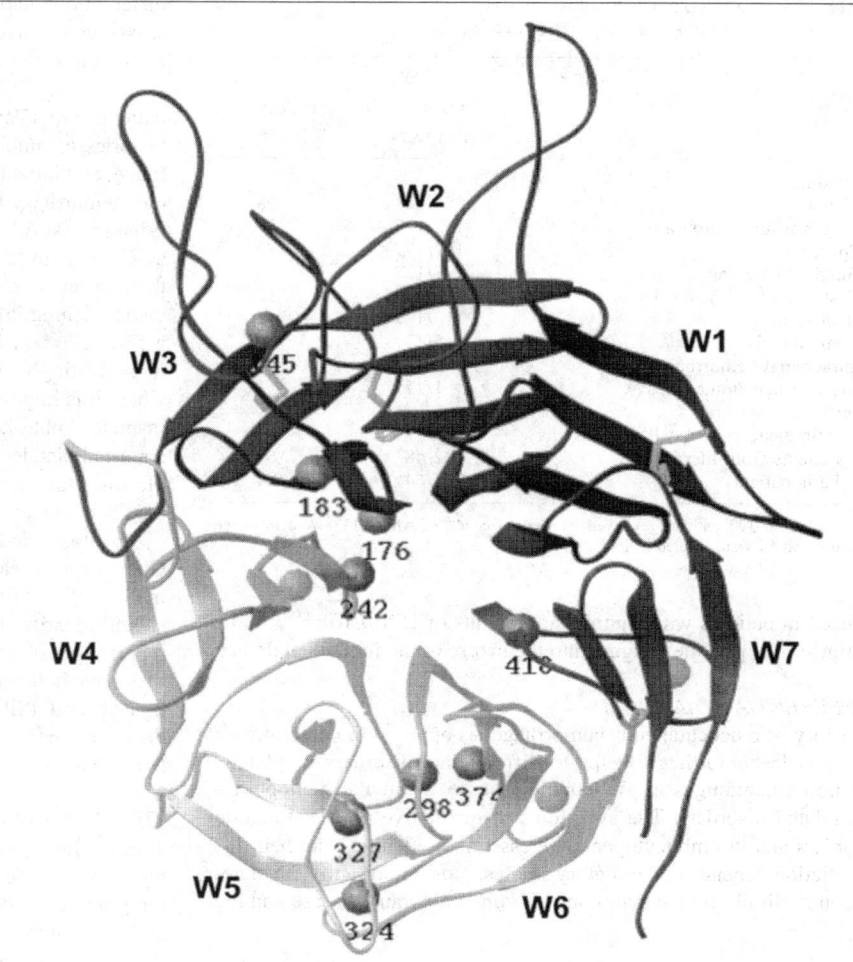

FIGURE 119-5   Glanzmann thrombasthenia mutations located within the β-propeller structure of GPIIb. A is the view from the top and B is the view from the side. This structure was deduced from the amino acid sequence of the αIIb integrin subunit. A ribbon diagram of a seven blade (W1-W7) β-propeller structure is shown. Each blade is comprised of anti-parallel β-strands (numbered 1-4 from the inside to the outside) that are connected by hairpin loops. The hairpin loops connecting β-strands 1-2 and 3-4 are located at the bottom of the structure and the loops connecting strands 3-4 and 4-1, which are hypothesized to support ligand binding, are located on the top of the structure. The calcium-binding domains are located within the 1-2 connecting loops in blades W4-7, and thus lie on the bottom of the structure; the location of three of the four calcium ions is shown as turquoise spheres. The location of selected Glanzmann thrombasthenia mutations within and surrounding the calcium-binding domains and within the third blade of the propeller are shown. (Adapted from Springer[101] with permission.) A 3-dimensional version of this figure is available from the Williams Hematology website (http://www.williamshematology.com).

can also be labeled with a fluorescent molecule, and then flow cytome-try can be used to measure fibrinogen binding. These techniques are most useful in detecting qualitative abnormalities of GPIIb/IIIa in patients with variant Glanzmann thrombasthenia. The binding of a monoclonal antibody (PAC1) to platelets gives similar information because the antibody only binds to the activated form of GPIIb/IIIa.[136]

Carriers of Glanzmann thrombasthenia have essentially normal platelet function.[59] Their platelets, however, only contain about 60 percent of the normal number of GPIIb/IIIa receptors.[137] Carrier detec-tion is most accurately performed by DNA analysis when the defect is known, and advances in PCR technology allows this to be performed even with DNA obtained from cells in random urine samples.[21]

Platelet fibrinogen is reduced to about 10 percent of normal in patients with marked reductions in GPIIb/IIIa[2,5,68,69] but is variably

TABLE 119-3   BLEEDING IN PATIENTS WITH
GLANZMANN THROMBASTHENIA

	No. of Affected Patients	Frequency, %
Symptoms		
Menorrhagia	54/55	98
Easy bruising, purpura	152/177	86
Epistaxis	129/177	73
Gingival bleeding	97/177	55
Gastrointestinal hemorrhage	22/177	12
Hematuria	10/177	6
Hemarthrosis	5/177	3
Intracranial hemorrhage	3/177	2
Visceral hematoma	1/177	1
Severity		
Requirement for red cell transfusions		
Patients from literature*	32/48	67
Paris patients	54/64	84

*Data are from 177 patients reviewed by George et al,[6] of whom 113 were from the literature and 64 were studied in Paris.

reduced in patients with significant amounts of GPIIb/IIIa.[133,138,139] Its presence may provide insights into the nature of the functional defect.

DIFFERENTIAL DIAGNOSIS

A history of mucocutaneous hemorrhage, as opposed to hemarthroses and muscle hemorrhage, helps to differentiate disorders of platelet function (including von Willebrand disease) from the hemophilias and related disorders. The symptoms of qualitative platelet function disorders and thrombocytopenia are essentially identical, so their differentiation depends on laboratory studies, most importantly the platelet count. Similarly, the symptoms of von Willebrand disease and the

TABLE 119-4   LABORATORY FEATURES OF GLANZMANN THROMBASTHENIA

I. Platelet count: normal
II. Bleeding time: markedly prolonged
III. Tests of platelet function
   A. Platelet aggregation in response to:
     1. Epinephrine—no observable response
     2. ADP and thrombin—shape change, but no aggregation
     3. Collagen—shape change followed by variable increase in light transmission due most likely to progressive adhesion to collagen fibers (pseudoaggregation).
     4. Ristocetin—normal initial slope of aggregation; at low concentrations, inhibition of second wave; at high concentrations, cyclical aggregation–disaggregation.
   B. Clot retraction: absent or reduced (rarely normal)
   C. Platelet release reaction: decreased with epinephrine and low concentrations of ADP, thrombin and collagen; normal with high concentrations of thrombin and collagen.
   D. Interaction with glass (platelet retention test): absent or reduced.
   E. Platelet coagulant activity: variably abnormal.
   F. Microparticle formation: variably abnormal.
   G. Ex vivo interaction with deendothelialized blood vessels in flow chambers: marked abnormality in platelet thrombus formation and defective platelet spreading; decreased platelet adhesion at high shear rates.
IV. Tests of GPIIb/IIIa and $\alpha V\beta 3$ receptors: number and functional integrity.
   A. GPIIb/IIIa content: reduced or absent, except in variants.
   B. $\alpha V\beta 3$ content: reduced or absent in patients with GPIIIa ($\beta 3$) defects; normal or increased in patients with GPIIb defects.
   C. Platelet binding of fibrinogen and other adhesive glycoproteins to GPIIb/IIIa: reduced or absent.
   D. Platelet fibrinogen content: markedly reduced, except in some variants.

different qualitative platelet disorders are often indistinguishable, and so assays of factor VIII, von Willebrand factor, and platelet function are required to make the definitive diagnosis. Although patients with afibrinogenemia have platelet aggregation studies similar to those of patients with Glanzmann thrombasthenia, they are more likely to have histories of umbilical stump bleeding, fetal wastage, muscle hemorrhage, and intraabdominal hemorrhage in addition to the mucocutaneous hemorrhage typical of Glanzmann thrombasthenia. A plasma fibrinogen assay establishes the diagnosis. Hereditary disorders, such as Glanzmann thrombasthenia, are usually present at birth or have their onset in early childhood. Thus, the history can be helpful in distinguishing inherited from acquired abnormalities. Figure 119-1 is a flow diagram that depicts a logical series of steps one may take in evaluating patients with mucocutaneous hemorrhage. In situations where it is important to rapidly ascertain whether a patient has Glanzmann thrombasthenia, a tentative diagnosis can be established based on a normal platelet count, reduced or absent clot retraction, a prolonged bleeding time, and the lack of platelet clumps when a specimen of unanticoagulated blood is used to make a blood smear.

Autoantibodies to GPIIb/IIIa may produce the phenotype of Glanzmann disease and many of the characteristic laboratory abnormalities.[140–144] Mixing studies using patient plasma and normal platelets should identify these acquired autoimmune disorders. A preliminary report suggested that some patients with acute promyelocytic leukemia may have deficiencies of platelet GPIIb/IIIa,[145] perhaps due to disruption of the GPIIb and GPIIIa genes, both at 17q21.32, as a result of the common translocations affecting chromosome 17 in this disorder[146] (see Chap. 93).

THERAPY, COURSE, AND PROGNOSIS

Therapy involves both preventive measures and treatment of specific bleeding episodes. Dental hygiene is especially important in minimizing gingival hemorrhage. Antiplatelet agents should be avoided. Iron and folate may be needed in patients with sufficient ongoing hemorrhage to cause anemia and iron depletion. Hepatitis B vaccine should be administered early in life, using a small-gauge needle and with prolonged direct pressure to the injection site to prevent excessive bleeding. Hormonal therapy can control menorrhagia in virtually all patients. Since menorrhagia is often most severe at the time of menarche, and can result in the need for emergency hysterectomy,[147] it may be justified to initiate hormonal therapy before menarche,[6] but the possibility of premature cessation of bone growth needs to be considered as well.

Antifibrinolytic agents may be useful in patients with gingival bleeding or who are undergoing tooth extractions. Either epsilon aminocaproic acid (40 mg/kg PO given four times daily)[6] or tranexamic acid (0.5 to 1.0 g PO given three or four times daily)[148,149] have been recommended based on studies in patients with hemophilia A or B; tranexamic acid usually produces fewer gastrointestinal side effects than epsilon aminocaproic acid. These agents are contraindicated if disseminated intravascular coagulation is present. A tranexamic acid mouthwash (10 ml of a 5 percent solution used four times daily) is effective in controlling gum bleeding in patients treated with oral anticoagulants and in patients with hemophilia,[150] and the author has found this helpful in Glanzmann thrombasthenia. Desmopressin (DDAVP) (see Chap. 135) usually does not normalize the bleeding time in patients with Glanzmann thrombasthenia,[6,151] but exceptions have been reported.[152] Anecdotal reports suggest that it may improve hemostasis, even without normalizing the bleeding time.[152,153]

Topical agents can also help arrest bleeding in Glanzmann thrombasthenia patients. Gelfoam (a form of resolvable, oxidized, regenerated cellulose) soaked in either tranexamic acid or topical thrombin, or any one of several fibrin sealants prepared from a source of fibrinogen and a source of thrombin, with or without antifibrinolytic agents or other components,[155,156] have been used in patients with coagulopathies, with the latter being particularly effective. Bovine thrombin, however, has induced antibody formation to itself and contaminating factors V and XI; at least some antibodies to factor V have cross-reacted with human factor V and caused serious hemorrhage.[157,158] IgE-mediated anaphylaxis has also been reported with bovine topical thrombin.[159] A microfibrillar collagen hemostatic agent of bovine origin has been used to secure hemostasis in bleeding normal individuals. However, antibodies to bovine (and rabbit) tissue factor have been identified in some patients treated with this hemostatic agent, but these did not cross-react with human tissue factor nor did they induce a hemorrhagic diathesis.[160] For dental procedures, custom splints of soft acrylic help prevent excessive hemorrhage.[161]

Control of epistaxis can be particularly difficult. A step-wise approach has been described that involves the following: elevation of the head and local pressure; topical vasoconstriction with cottonoid pledgets and oxymetazoline; cauterization with silver nitrate or trichloroacetic acid; anterior packing; posterior packing; and, finally, arterial ligation or embolic occlusion of the internal maxillary artery.[109] When the simple topical measures fail to control bleeding, platelet transfusions are administered.

Postpartum hemorrhage may benefit from administration of low concentrations of prostaglandin E_2 or $F_{2\alpha}$ via continuous intrauterine irrigation[162a]; this experimental technique has been effective in normal patients with severe postpartum hemorrhage, but additional data are required about its effectiveness in patients with platelet disorders.

Erythropoietin was reported to improve the bleeding time and platelet retention in one patient with Glanzmann thrombasthenia, even without producing a significant increase in hemoglobin concentration.[152] A positive effect of erythropoietin on platelet function, independent of an effect on hemoglobin, has also been reported in uremia.[163,164]

Transfusion of platelets (see Chap. 142) is the mainstay of therapy for serious bleeding in Glanzmann thrombasthenia and as prophylaxis prior to surgery or other major hemostatic stresses. Since patients are likely to need transfusions throughout their lifetimes, hepatitis B vaccine should be administered at an early age, and all transfusions of both platelets and packed red blood cells should be given with leukocyte depletion filters to decrease the risk of alloimmunization[165] and cytomegalovirus (CMV) transmission.[166] Febrile transfusion reactions can be diminished by leukodepletion at the time of blood collection.[167] Even in patients who are refractory to platelets, leukocyte depletion filters may improve the recovery of transfused platelets in the circulation.[168] Females of childbearing potential who are Rh negative should not be given Rh-positive platelets. It may also be justified to use only HLA-matched platelets, even early in the patient's course, to minimize the risk of alloimmunization.[169] The use of family members' platelets may be convenient, but if consideration is given to marrow transplantation from a family member, it may be advisable to avoid donations from family members. Similarly, if bone marrow transplantation is considered, and the patient has not already developed

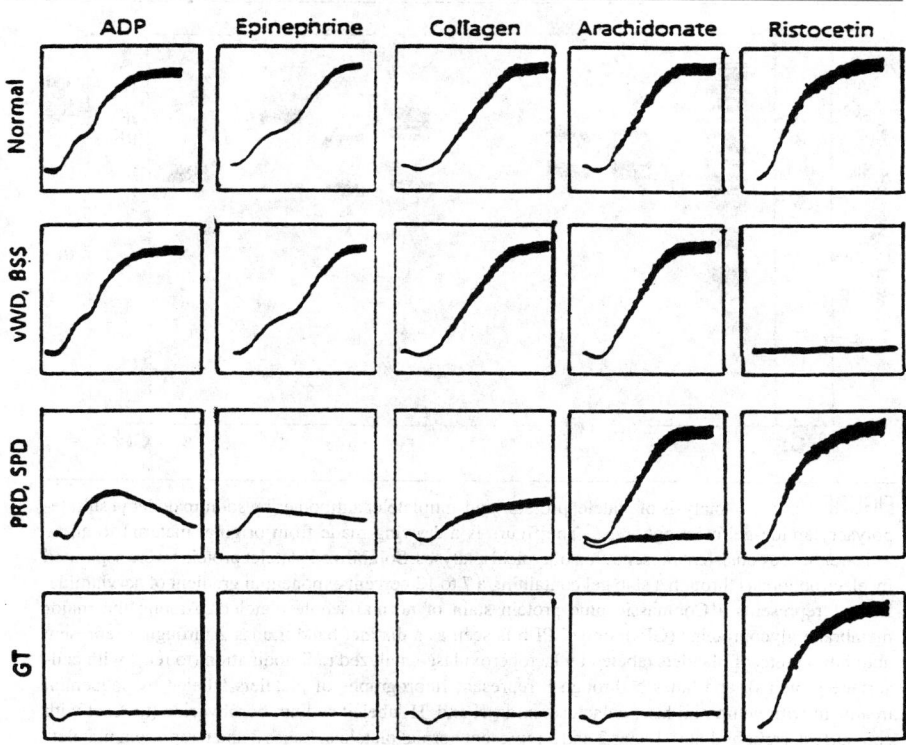

FIGURE 119-6   Patterns of platelet aggregation in response to several agonists in different disease states, including von Willebrand disease (vWD); Bernard-Soulier syndrome (BSS); platelet release defects (PRD), including aspirin ingestion; storage pool disease (SPD); and Glanzmann thrombasthenia (GT). Note that patients with platelet release defects have abnormal arachidonic acid–induced aggregation whereas those with storage pool deficiency have nearly normal responses to arachidonate. (Courtesy of Dr. Robert Handin, with permission.)

CMV infection, it may be desirable to select blood from donors who do not have evidence of CMV infection.

Platelet alloimmunization poses several different problems in patients with Glanzmann thrombasthenia, depending upon the antigen involved. In addition to antibodies directed at platelet proteins other than GPIIb/IIIa, such as HLA determinants, patients can make several different types of antibodies to GPIIb and/or GPIIIa. These include antibodies to: (1) the well-recognized polymorphic alloantigens on GPIIb and IIIa[170] (see Chap. 138); (2) other regions of GPIIb/IIIa that are not involved in ligand binding; and (3) the ligand-binding regions of GPIIb/IIIa. Since the platelets from most patients with Glanzmann thrombasthenia lack GPIIb/IIIa alloantigens, antibodies against these determinants, as well as against other nonligand-binding domains of GPIIb/IIIa, could theoretically be produced either as a result of transfusions or pregnancy. Such antibodies could result in refractoriness to platelet transfusions, a predisposition to developing posttransfusion purpura, or a predisposition to having children with neonatal isoimmune thrombocytopenia (see Chap. 117).[170] One possible case of neonatal thrombocytopenia based on such a mechanism has been reported, but an autoantibody could not be excluded.[171]

The development of antibodies that inhibit GPIIb/IIIa function has the potential to make further transfusions ineffectual, even if the platelets circulate. Several such cases have been reported.[6,171–174] The antibodies produced by the patients induce a thrombasthenic defect in normal platelets. If patients with antibodies to GPIIb/IIIa that block ligand binding have severe hemorrhage, it is reasonable to try plasmapheresis to remove the offending antibodies, but the efficacy of such treatment is not defined, and at best it provides only short-term bene-

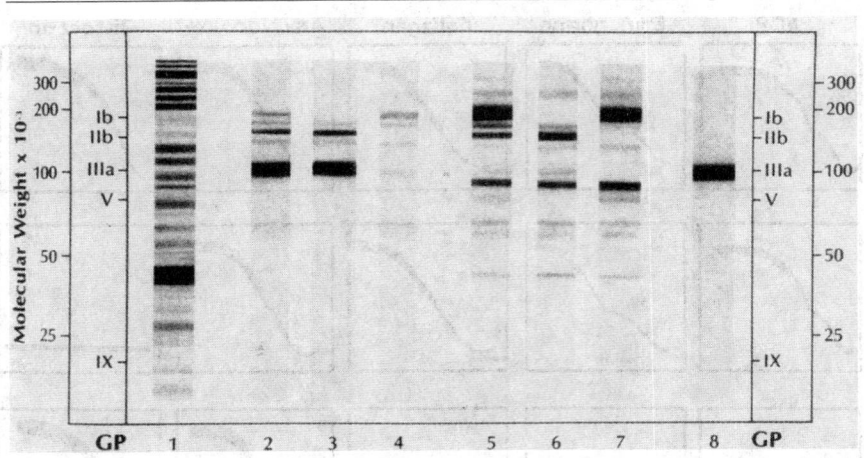

FIGURE 119-7   Analysis of platelet proteins and antiplatelet antibodies by sodium dodecyl sulfate-polyacrylamide-gel electrophoresis. The figure is a drawing made from original material to allow a clearer, more consistent presentation of typical analyses. Solubilized platelet proteins were separated by electrophoresis through a slab gel containing a 7 to 12 percent exponential gradient of acrylamide. Lane 1 represents a Coomassie blue protein stain of normal whole platelets. Among the major membrane glycoproteins (GPs), only GPIIb is seen as a distinct band. Lanes 2 through 4 represent autoradiographs of platelets labeled by lactoperoxidase-catalyzed radioiodination (to react with cell-surface proteins), and lanes 5 through 8 represent fluorographs of platelets labeled by sequential treatment with neuraminidase, galactose oxidase, and ^{3}H-labeled sodium borohydride (to react with cell-surface carbohydrate). Lanes 2 and 5 represent normal platelets. Lanes 3 and 6 represent platelets from a patient with the Bernard-Soulier syndrome. The absence of GPIb can be seen with both techniques, and the absence of GPV, GPIX, and a high-molecular-weight band that may contain complexes of GPIb can be seen in lane 6. Lanes 4 and 7 represent platelets from a patient with Glanzmann thrombasthenia, demonstrating the absence of GPIIb and IIIa. Lane 8 is an immunoblot. Normal platelet proteins were transferred from the gel section to nitrocellulose paper that was first incubated with anti-P1^{A1} (a human alloantibody that reacts with GPIIIa) and then ^{125}I-labeled staphylococcal protein A; the radiolabeled protein was finally developed by autoradiography. (From George JN, Nurden AT, Phillips DR: Molecular defects in interactions of platelets with the vessel wall. N Eng J Med 311: 1084, 1984 with permission).

fit.[175] It is notable that at least one patient has been reported to have had an inhibitory antibody for more than 15 years without significant hemorrhage.[6,176]

Allogeneic marrow transplantation has been reported in two patients with Glanzmann thrombasthenia. The first was a 5-year-old male who had several severe gastrointestinal hemorrhages.[177] His bleeding diathesis was cured, and 9 years after the transplant he was alive and well, but with mild graft-versus-host disease.[6] The second patient, who required multiple hospital admissions to control bleeding but had only received a platelet transfusion once, was transplanted at age 2.5 years from an HLA-identical sibling who was heterozygous for Glanzmann thrombasthenia.[178] She was well 19 months after the transplant.

Recombinant factor VIIa has been used to treat at least seven patients with Glanzmann thrombasthenia, two of whom had antibodies to HLA antigens or GPIIb/IIIa.[179–182] Although the preliminary reports have indicated favorable results in securing hemostasis, in one case thromboembolism occurred 6 days after the termination of a 15-day continuous infusion. Thus, at the time of writing, this treatment is experimental.

Progress has been made in gene therapy approaches to correcting the genetic defect in Glanzmann thrombasthenia,[183] and a GPIIIa-deficient mouse model of Glanzmann thrombasthenia provides a useful animal system for assessing the potential of gene therapy for human treatment.[184] Since methods of marrow transplantation and gene transfer therapy are likely to improve, it will be important to reassess the risk:benefit ratios of these therapies for individual patients with Glanzmann thrombasthenia.

Although Glanzmann thrombasthenia is a severe disease, the prognosis for survival is generally good. In one series, 2 of 64 patients died of hemorrhage and in another, 3 of 43 patients died of hemorrhage.[6,24] A nationwide survey in Japan identified 98 Glanzmann thrombasthenia patients in 1976 and 192 in 1991.[185] The mortality rate in 1976 was 6.8 percent, which was slightly higher than for hemophilia. By 1991, the mortality rate decreased to 4.9 percent. The age-adjusted standardized mortality ratio decreased from 1.76 to 0.83 over the same time, and the percentage of patients over 30 years old increased from 4.5 percent to 24.5 percent. These data indicate that the prognosis improved significantly during the study period.

GLYCOPROTEIN Ib (CD42b,c), IX (CD42a), AND V—BERNARD-SOULIER SYNDROME

DEFINITION AND HISTORY
Bernard-Soulier syndrome is an inherited disorder characterized by thrombocytopenia, giant platelets, and a failure of the platelets to undergo selective von Willebrand factor–dependent platelet interactions as a result of abnormalities in the platelet GPIb/IX complex (CD42). Defective interactions between platelets and thrombin may also be present.

In 1948 Bernard and Soulier described two children from a consanguineous family who had a severe bleeding disorder characterized by mucocutaneous hemorrhage.[186,187] Evaluation of the patients' blood revealed variable thrombocytopenia and giant platelets. Beginning in the early 1970s, Bernard-Soulier syndrome platelets were shown to have a functional defect in von Willebrand factor–dependent platelet adhesion and agglutination.[188–190] In 1975 Nurden and Caen identified an abnormality in platelet GPIb as the cause of the functional defect.[191] Later studies confirmed the defect in von Willebrand factor-GPIb interactions[192–194] and identified additional defects in platelet GPV and GPIX.[195,196] A mouse model of Bernard-Soulier syndrome has been produced by gene targeting of GPIbα.[197]

ETIOLOGY AND PATHOGENESIS
Epidemiology   This rare disease, with a prevalence estimated as less than 1 in 1 million has been reported from countries around the world.[187,195,198–248] Consanguinity is common in the families with affected children[187] because the disorder is usually inherited as an autosomal recessive trait and because spontaneous mutations appear infrequently. However, an autosomal dominant form of the disease has been reported.[221]

Causes of Hemorrhage   Four different features of Bernard-Soulier syndrome may contribute to the hemorrhagic diathesis: thrombocytopenia, abnormal platelet interactions with von Willebrand factor, abnormal platelet interactions with thrombin, and abnormal platelet coagulant activity.

The pathophysiology of the thrombocytopenia is uncertain. Early studies suggested a marked shortening of platelet survival, presumably due to the decrease in platelet surface charge resulting from the GPIb defect.[249,250] Later studies using ^{111}In-oxine to label platelets reported more modest or no shortening of platelet survival, indicating that ineffective thrombopoiesis and/or decreased thrombopoiesis may contribute to the thrombocytopenia.[251,252] Irregularities in the demarcation membrane system have been identified in Bernard-Soulier syndrome megakaryocytes and may contribute to abnormal platelet production.[253] Based on observations in other giant platelet syndromes (see Chap. 117), the large size of Bernard-Soulier platelets would tend to diminish the adverse hemostatic effects of the thrombocytopenia because the platelet mass is better preserved. However, in fact, the bleeding diathesis with Bernard-Soulier syndrome is more severe than expected from the thrombocytopenia, reinforcing the conclusion that the qualitative platelet defect is clinically significant.[176,187]

The platelet GPIb/IX complex functions as a receptor for von Willebrand factor (see Chaps. 111 and 135).[241,254,255] This interaction is crucial in the adhesion of platelets to subendothelial surfaces, especially under high shear conditions, where von Willebrand factor acts as a bridge between the subendothelial matrix and the platelet.[130,131] The relative roles of subendothelial von Willebrand factor, plasma von Willebrand factor, and platelet von Willebrand factor have not been completely defined, but they probably all contribute.[255]

GPIb/IX–von Willebrand factor interactions can also occur in platelet suspensions at high shear rates; this can lead to platelet activation, with subsequent aggregation mediated by GPIIb/IIIa.[255–258] Whether the shear rates in vivo ever reach the levels required to initiate von Willebrand factor binding, however, is not established.

The platelets of patients with Bernard-Soulier syndrome have a decreased response to platelet activation by thrombin, especially at limiting concentrations of thrombin.[259–262] Bernard-Soulier platelets are deficient in two different proteins that interact with thrombin, namely GPIbα, which binds thrombin,[254,263–265] and GPV, which is a thrombin substrate (see Chap. 111). Paradoxically, mice deficient in GPV actually have increased sensitivity to thrombin activation.[266] Thus, the GPIbα defect in thrombin binding seems to override the enhanced sensitivity to thrombin expected from the GPV defect. Since thrombin is one of the major physiologic activators of platelets, this abnormality may also contribute to the hemorrhagic diathesis.

Bernard-Soulier platelets appear defective in supporting thrombin generation as judged by the serum prothrombin time,[267] a test performed with whole blood, but in other tests of platelet coagulant activity, Bernard-Soulier platelets support coagulation as well as or better than normal platelets.[121,268] Defects in collagen-induced coagulant activity and the association of factors V, VIII, and XI with Bernard-Soulier platelets have been described,[268] but their significance is unclear. Abnormal membrane lipids have also been reported.[269] Binding of von Willebrand factor to GPIb/IX has been implicated in fibrin-dependent, but not fibrin-independent, augmentation of platelet coagulant activity, and thus fibrin-dependent coagulant activity is likely to be abnormal in Bernard-Soulier syndrome.[123] This finding might be able to partially reconcile the above observations, since the serum prothrombin time is one of the few assays used to assess platelet coagulant activity in which fibrin forms.

The mechanisms producing the giant platelets in Bernard-Soulier syndrome have not been identified, but since giant platelets are found in Bernard-Soulier syndrome variants in which GPIb/IX is present, but unable to bind ligand, it has been proposed that the abnormality is due to the inability of GPIb/IX to bind a postulated novel bone marrow ligand.[241] It cannot be due to an inability to bind von Willebrand factor, since patients lacking von Willebrand factor do not have large platelets. A defect in GPIb/IX-mediated signaling due to a deficiency of phospholipase C has been described, and it has been proposed that this abnormality may be the cause of the large platelets.[241,270] A mechanical alteration in the plasma membrane of Bernard-Soulier platelets has been identified by micropipette experiments, showing the plasma membranes to be more deformable than normal.[271] The increased deformability may reflect the loss of the normal interaction of GPIb/IX with the cytoskeleton via actin-binding protein (filamin-1) (see Chap. 111).

Bernard-Soulier platelets are deficient not only in GPIbα, GPIbβ, and GPIX, but also in GPV, and all of these proteins are thought to exist in a complex (see Chap. 111).[196,241,272] It is of considerable interest that all of these proteins share highly conserved leucine-rich regions.[241,254,255] One possible explanation for the loss of surface expression of all the proteins is that they need to form a complex during biosynthesis in order to be transported to the surface[255]; evidence supports the need for GPIbα, GPIbβ, and GPIX to all be present for optimal surface expression,[273] but data from mice deficient in GPV indicate that this glycoprotein is not required for surface expression of the GPIb/IX complex.[266]

At the molecular level, the platelets from different patients with Bernard-Soulier syndrome are heterogeneous, with many having no detectable GPIb and others having variable amounts, up to 50 percent of normal.[208,210,215,217,241,270,274,275] There also is variability in the degree of concordance in the reduction of GPIb and the other deficient proteins.[223,276]

Molecular Biological Defects   The molecular biological basis of Bernard-Soulier syndrome has been determined in a number of patients, and data on some of these patients are given in Table 119-5. Defects have been identified in GPIbα, GPIbβ, and GPIX, but not in GPV. Nearly one-half of the defects affect the leucine-rich repeats or the conserved flanking sequences, supporting the importance of these structural elements in the biogenesis and surface expression of the GPIb/IX/V complex. Three patients have been described who are homozygous for a deletion in the last 2 bases of codon 492 of GPIbα (nucleotides 1523 and 1524) resulting in a frame shift that alters the membrane-spanning region and results in premature termination, and another patient has been described who is heterozygous for this deletion and a missense mutation of GPIbα.[236,238,239,247] The defect in the transmembrane domain appears to result in a poorly anchored GPIbα, as indicated by the presence of GPIbα antigen in plasma. Haplotype analysis indicated that the mutations in these 4 apparently unrelated patients may, in fact, have derived from a common founder. Two reported defects in GPIbβ are of particular interest because in both cases one of the GPIbβ genes, and several nearby genes on chromosome 22, were deleted, resulting in the patients having the DiGeorge/Velo-cardio-facial syndrome.[231,232,245] In other studies of patients with the Velo-cardio-facial syndrome due to heterozygous deletions of 22q11, giant platelets and relative thrombocytopenia, but no bleeding disorder or abnormal platelet function were observed, consistent with the patients being heterozygous for GPIb/IX deficiency.[243]

Several variants of Bernard-Soulier syndrome have been described. An autosomal dominant form has been ascribed to a heterozygous mutation in the second leucine-rich repeat of GPIbα (Leu57-Phe).[221] Presumably, the abnormal GPIbα interferes with the function of the normal ones. The affected patients have moderate bleeding symptoms, moderate thrombocytopenia, and giant platelets. The GPIb is unusually susceptible to proteolysis and functions ineffectively with regard to its interactions with von Willebrand factor. The "Bolzano" defect, which has been described in two patients, involves the sixth leucine-rich repeat of GPIbα (Ala156Val). This mutation results in a GPIbα molecule that cannot bind von Willebrand factor but can bind thrombin. In one patient, the Bolzano defect was homozygous, and the patient had nearly normal levels of GPIb/IX/V complex.[216] In the other, it coexisted with a 12 amino acid deletion and an amino acid substitution (Glu181Lys); GPIbα platelet expression was markedly reduced in this patient.[248] A Japanese patient heterozygous for 2 mutations in GPIbβ, one of which produced an additional Cys at amino acid 88, had a mild bleeding disorder, significant amounts of functional platelet GPIb/IX/V complex, and very large platelets; of note, the

TABLE 119-5   MOLECULAR BIOLOGIC ABNORMALITIES IN BERNARD-SOULIER SYNDROME

GPIBα MUTATIONS

PATIENT DESIGNATION	GENOTYPE	MUTATION[1,2]	PHENOTYPE	AMINO ACID SUBSTITUTION[3]	AFFECTED LEUCINE REPEATS	REF
Caucasian Male	Homozygous	103Adel	Del: Out of frame	Premature termination	N-Flank	233
Caucasian Male	Heterozygous Autosomal Dominant	217C→T	Missense	L57F	II	221
Caucasian Male	Homozygous	275Tdel	Del: Out of frame	Premature termination	IV	225
African-Am Male	Homozygous	434T→C	Missense	L129P	V	228
Finnish Female	Compound	434T→C	Missense	L129P	V	247
	Heterozygous	1523ATdel	Del: Out of frame	Premature termination		
Bolzano variant Male	Homozygous	515C→T	Missense	A156V	VI	224
Female	Compound	515C→T	Missense	A156V	VI	248
	Heterozygous	554-589del	Del: In frame	N169-Q180del→E181K	VII	
Nancy I variant Male	Homozygous	583CTCdel	Del: In frame	L179del	VII	229
Spanish Male	Homozygous	673T→A	Missense	C209S	C-Flank	226
Japanese Female	Homozygous	930TGdel	Del: Out of frame	Premature termination		235
Male	Compound	1077G→A	Nonsense	W343X		218
	Heterozygous	Unknown				
Japanese Male	Compound	1376Tins	Ins: Out of frame	Premature termination		235
	Heterozygous	1396Adel	Del: Out of frame	Premature termination		
BSS Kagoshima	Homozygous	1379C→A	Nonsense	S444X		227
Japanese Female	Homozygous	1396Adel	Del: Out of frame	Premature termination		230
Finnish Female	Homozygous	1523ATdel	Del: Out of frame	Premature termination		247
Caucasian Female	Homozygous	1523ATdel	Del: Out of frame	Premature termination		236
Caucasian Female	Homozygous	1523ATdel	Del: Out of frame	Premature termination		237
Karlstad variant Swedish Male	Homozygous	1542G→A	Nonsense	W498X		238

GPIbβ MUTATIONS

PATIENT DESIGNATION	GENOTYPE	MUTATION[1,2]	PHENOTYPE	AMINO ACID SUBSTITUTION[3]	REF
Male	Compound	-133C→G	Promoter base change	GATA site	231
	Heterozygote	Deletion	Allele deleted		
Japanese Female	Compound	338A→G	Missense	Y88C	239
	Heterozygote	457G→C	Missense	A108P	
African-American Male	Compound	314Cdel	Del: Out of frame	Premature termination	245
	Heterozygote	Deletion	Allele deleted		

GPIX MUTATIONS

PATIENT DESIGNATION	GENOTYPE	MUTATION[1,2]	PHENOTYPE	AMINO ACID SUBSTITUTION[3]	AFFECTED LEUCINE REPEATS	REF
Female	Compound	110A→G	Missense	D21G	N-Flank	223
	Heterozygote	182A→G	Missense	N45S	I	
Caucasion Male	Homozygote	182A→G	Missense	N45S	I	494
Finnish 5 families 3 Female, 2 Male	Homozygote	182A→G	Missense	N45S	I	246
Male	Homozygote	167T→C	Missense	L40P	I	242
Male	Homozygote	212T→C	Missense	F55S	I	240
Japanese Female	Homozygote	266G→A	Missense	C73Y	C-Flank	495
Japanese Male	Homozygote	266G→A	Missense	C73Y	C-Flank	495
Japanese Female	Homozygote	426G→A	Nonsense	W126X		230

[1]Nucleotide numbering begins with the A of the ATG start codon as +1. The amino acid number (including the leader sequence) is multiplied by 3 and the nucleotide number within the codon is determined. Amino acid numbering for GPIbα is according to Lopez et al, *Proc Natl Acad Sci USA* 84:5615, 1987, for GPIbβ is according to Lopez et al, *Proc Natl Acad Sci USA* 85:2135, 1988, and for GPIX is according to Hickey et al, *FEBS Lett* 274:189, 1990.
[2]Abbreviations used: del and DEL, deletion; Ins, insertion; N-Flank, region containing the amino-terminal flanking sequence of the leucine-rich repeats; C-Flank, region containing the carboxy-terminal flanking sequence of the leucine-rich repeats.
[3]Amino acid numbering begins with the first amino acid of the mature protein (excluding the leader sequence) as +1 (according to the references in footnote 1 above). Amino acid numbers including the leader sequence are determined by adding 16 residues for GPIbα, 25 residues for GPIbβ, and 16 residues for GPIX.

patient did not have thrombocytopenia. A defect in GPIbβ cross-linking to GPIbα was proposed as the cause of the abnormality.[239]

CLINICAL FEATURES

Epistaxis is the most common symptom of Bernard-Soulier syndrome (70 percent), with ecchymoses (58 percent), menometrorrhagia (44 percent), gingival hemorrhage (42 percent), and gastrointestinal bleeding (22 percent) also common.[187] Hemorrhagic symptoms that occur with lower frequency include posttraumatic bleeding (13 percent), hematuria (7 percent), cerebral hemorrhage (4 percent), and retinal hemorrhage (2 percent). There is considerable variability in symptoms

among patients,[176] even among patients within a single family.[241,277] A review that includes brief descriptions of the clinical features of 55 patients, reported through 1998, has been published.[241]

LABORATORY FEATURES

Platelet Number and Morphology   Thrombocytopenia is present in nearly all patients but is variable in its severity, ranging from about 20,000 platelets/μl to near normal levels. Platelets are large on smear, with more than one-third usually having diameters greater than 3.5 μm and some being as large or larger than lymphocytes. The platelets display only minor variations in vesicular structures and the open canalicular system by electron microscopy.[187] The membrane of Bernard-Soulier platelets appears to be more deformable than normal,[271] perhaps because GPIb ordinarily interacts with the platelet cytoskeleton (see Chap. 111).[278]

Bleeding Time   The bleeding time is almost always prolonged, but the degree of prolongation is variable.

Platelet Aggregation   The hallmark findings in the Bernard-Soulier syndrome are the failure of platelets to aggregate in response to ristocetin[189] or botrocetin,[192,279] agents that require von Willebrand factor–GPIb interactions (Fig. 119-6). In von Willebrand disease, but not Bernard-Soulier syndrome, this defect can be corrected by adding normal plasma (or von Willebrand factor).

Although, the large size of the platelets in Bernard-Soulier syndrome and the thrombocytopenia make it technically difficult to perform platelet aggregation studies, in general, aggregation induced by ADP, epinephrine, or collagen is either normal or enhanced.[190,219,280] The response to thrombin is usually dose-dependent, with essentially a normal response at high doses of thrombin[260] but with a prolonged lag phase and a diminished response at low doses of thrombin.[259,281]

Platelet Coagulant Activity   The coagulant activity of Bernard-Soulier platelets has been variably reported as reduced, normal, or increased.[121,267,268] The variable presence of fibrin in the different assays used to assess platelet coagulant activity may account for these inconsistent results, since GPIb-von Willebrand factor interactions enhance platelet coagulant activity when fibrin is present but not when it is absent.[123]

Platelet GPIb/IX/V Content   Platelet surface GPIb, GPIX, and GPV are usually decreased or absent in Bernard-Soulier syndrome. This can be established by monoclonal antibody binding or by biochemical and immunologic assessment of solubilized platelet proteins (Fig. 119-7).

Platelet-Thrombin Interactions   GPIb may be responsible for the high-affinity binding of thrombin to platelets, but since there are only 50 high-affinity thrombin-binding sites per platelet and 25,000 GPIb molecules per platelet, perhaps only a subpopulation of GPIb molecules are involved.[254] The relationship, if any, between GPIb and the seven-transmembrane domain thrombin receptors (PAR-1 and PAR-4) present on platelets remains to be defined (see Chap. 111), but it appears that both GPIb and the seven-transmembrane domain receptors are required for maximal response to thrombin.[281] GPV, which is missing from the platelet surface in Bernard-Soulier syndrome, is cleaved by thrombin, but the cleavage does not appear to be necessary or sufficient for thrombin-induced platelet activation.[266,282,283] As noted above, platelets of mice lacking GPV have increased responsiveness to thrombin.[266]

Ex Vivo Interaction with Subendothelial Surfaces   Bernard-Soulier platelets demonstrate defective adhesion to subendothelial surfaces, especially at shear rates greater than 650 s^{-1}.[130,131,188,284] The results are similar to those in patients with von Willebrand disease.

Shear-Induced Platelet Aggregation   Unlike normal platelets, Bernard-Soulier platelets are not aggregated by high shear rates.[256,257] The initial interaction in this process appears to be binding of von Willebrand factor to GPIb,[255] with subsequent activation of GPIIb/IIIa, perhaps through signaling via the protein 14-3-3ζ associated with the cytoplasmic domain of GPIbα[258,285] or either Fcγ receptor IIA or the Fc receptor γ chain, both of which have been identified as linked to the GPIb/IX complex and both of which are capable of initiating signal transduction (see Chap. 111).[286,287]

DIFFERENTIAL DIAGNOSIS

This is discussed in the section on the differential diagnosis of Glanzmann thrombasthenia above. Acquired Bernard-Soulier syndrome has been reported due to autoantibodies,[288–292] as part of a juvenile myelo-

dysplastic syndrome,[293,294] and in association with acute myelogenous leukemia.[294]

THERAPY, COURSE, AND PROGNOSIS

The therapy of Bernard-Soulier syndrome is essentially identical to that for Glanzmann thrombasthenia (see above). Splenectomy has been performed when the diagnosis of immune thrombocytopenia was mistakenly made, but this usually does not normalize the platelet count or improve the bleeding diathesis.[248] Oral contraceptives can control menorrhagia.[295] Desmopressin (DDAVP) has been variably effective in decreasing the bleeding time.[153,207,209,219,234,242,296–298] Platelet transfusions are effective when needed but carry a risk of alloimmunization, including the production of antibodies to the functional region of GPIb.[299,300] A preliminary report indicates that factor VIIa infusion may be beneficial, but such therapy is experimental.[301] Patients have had successful pregnancies and deliveries, but serious delayed bleeding can occur, and emergency hysterectomy has been required to control the hemorrhage.[199,202,212,222,244,300] Neonatal thrombocytopenia presumed to be due to maternal alloimmunization has been reported.[300]

As with Glanzmann thrombasthenia, the prognosis of patients with Bernard-Soulier syndrome has improved as platelet transfusion support has become more readily available and other supportive measures have become more effective.

GPIB (CD42B,C)—PLATELET-TYPE (PSEUDO-) VON WILLEBRAND DISEASE

DEFINITION AND HISTORY

A heterogeneous group of patients has been described with mild to moderate bleeding symptoms, variably enlarged platelets, variable thrombocytopenia, and diminished plasma high-molecular-weight von Willebrand factor multimers. The fundamental defect in these patients is thought to be an enhanced interaction between an abnormal platelet GPIb/IX receptor and normal plasma von Willebrand factor.[302–307] Since these patients have some of the hallmarks of von Willebrand disease, but the defect is in platelet GPIb/IX, it has been termed both *pseudo-von Willebrand disease* and *platelet-type von Willebrand disease*.

ETIOLOGY AND PATHOGENESIS

A qualitative abnormality in GPIb is thought to be responsible for this disorder, with ongoing in vivo binding of high-molecular-weight von Willebrand multimers to platelets causing depletion of the plasma high-molecular-weight multimers. In addition, the binding of von Willebrand factor to platelets may lead to shortened platelet survival, perhaps accounting for the variable thrombocytopenia. Inheritance appears to be autosomal dominant.

Abnormalities in the M_r of GPIb were identified in two families,[307] but these may have resulted from a now-recognized polymorphism in GPIb (see Chap. 111) rather than being related to the functional disorder. Heterozygous point mutations in the GPIbα DNA (Gly233 → Val and Met239 → Val) have been found in several different families.[308–311] Both of these mutations are in the carboxy terminal flanking sequence of the leucine-rich repeats, a region implicated in ligand binding,[241,254,255] (see Fig. 111-11) and molecular modeling suggests that the M239V substitution produces a significant conformational change in the molecule.[312]

CLINICAL FEATURES

Patients have mild to moderate mucocutaneous hemorrhage.

LABORATORY FEATURES AND DIFFERENTIAL DIAGNOSIS

The bleeding time is often, but not invariably, prolonged. Mild thrombocytopenia and somewhat enlarged platelets are present in some, but not all, patients. Plasma von Willebrand factor levels are mildly reduced, with a disproportionate reduction in the high-molecular-weight multimers.

The most characteristic laboratory finding in platelet-type von Willebrand disease is enhanced platelet aggregation in response to low concentrations of ristocetin[302–306] or botrocetin.[313] This same abnormality is present in patients with type IIb von Willebrand disease, as is selective depletion of plasma high-molecular-weight von Willebrand factor multimers (see Chap. 135). In platelet-type von Willebrand disease, however, the defect is in platelet GPIbα, whereas in type IIb von Willebrand disease, the defect is in the von Willebrand factor molecule. Several assays can help differentiate between these abnormalities[304,314–316]: (1) normal von Willebrand factor (in cryoprecipitate or purified) will aggregate platelets from patients with platelet-type von Willebrand disease, but not platelets from patients with type IIb von Willebrand disease; (2) isolated platelets from patients with platelet-type von Willebrand disease will bind normal von Willebrand factor at lower concentrations of ristocetin than will normal platelets or platelets from patients with type IIb von Willebrand disease; (3) plasma von Willebrand factor from patients with type IIb von Willebrand disease will bind to normal platelets at lower-than-normal concentrations of ristocetin, whereas higher-than-normal concentrations of ristocetin are required to get the plasma von Willebrand factor from patients with platelet-type von Willebrand factor to bind to normal platelets[315]; and (4) von Willebrand factor lacking sialic acid residues (asialo–von Willebrand factor) will agglutinate platelets from patients with platelet-type von Willebrand disease in the presence of EDTA.[317]

THERAPY, COURSE, AND PROGNOSIS

Since normal von Willebrand factor (especially the high-molecular-weight forms) can bind excessively to the platelets of patients with platelet-type von Willebrand disease and potentially lead to rapid platelet clearance from the circulation, increasing the von Willebrand factor level by any means (desmopressin infusion or von Willebrand replacement with cryoprecipitate or von Willebrand factor concentrates) poses a potential risk of inducing thrombocytopenia.[314,318] It may be possible to estimate this risk by assessing whether the patient's platelets aggregate ex vivo in response to von Willebrand factor (as in cryoprecipitate).[303] Low-dose cryoprecipitate has successfully supported hemostasis, without inducing thrombocytopenia in patients at risk of having thrombocytopenia.[305,318,319] Consideration should also be given to platelet transfusion if thrombocytopenia is severe. A preliminary report indicates that factor VIIa infusion may be beneficial, but this therapy is experimental.[321]

GLYCOPROTEIN IA/IIA ($\alpha2\beta1$; VLA-2; CD49B/CD29)

GPIa/IIa ($\alpha2\beta1$) can mediate platelet adhesion to collagen and platelet activation under certain conditions (see Chap. 111). Nieuwenhuis and coworkers[321,322] reported a female patient with excessive posttraumatic bruising and menorrhagia, but no epistaxis, gum bleeding, or excessive bleeding after tonsillectomy or appendectomy, whose platelets selectively failed to aggregate or undergo shape change in response to collagen. The bleeding time was markedly prolonged, and the patient's platelets failed to adhere and spread normally on subendothelial surfaces. The patient's platelets only contained about 15 to 25 percent of the normal amount of GPIa,[321,323] and a reduction in GPIIa was also apparent.[321] It is difficult to draw conclusions about the physiologic role of GPIa/IIa in platelet function from this patient, since her GPIa/IIa deficiency was incomplete, her bleeding symptoms were mild, and some of the platelet function abnormalities (e.g., abnormal platelet-collagen interactions in the presence of the divalent chelating agent EDTA) are difficult to ascribe to the deficiency in GPIa/IIa.[321,324]

Another patient with GPIa deficiency has been described.[325] She had a history of mucocutaneous and postoperative bleeding. Her bleeding time was prolonged, and platelet aggregation in response to collagen was selectively reduced but not absent. In addition to her GPIa defect, she also had little or no intact thrombospondin, and exogenous thrombospondin corrected the defect in platelet aggregation. The patient's hemorrhagic symptoms and platelet defects disappeared when she reached menopause. Of note, the above patient reported by Nienwenhuis and coworkers also was reported to improve at the time of menopause.[326]

GPIV (CD36)

Approximately 3 percent of the Japanese population, about 2.4 percent of the African-American population, and 0.3 percent of the Caucasian population of the United States have platelets that lack GPIV.[327,328] Although GPIV has been implicated in platelet interactions with collagen and thrombospondin,[329,330] as well as in platelet-monocyte interactions,[331] individuals lacking GPIV do not have a hemorrhagic diathesis. Platelets from these patients can bind thrombospondin via alternative receptors[332] and there is controversy as to whether they have even a mild defect in adhesion to collagen.[333,334] Two forms of GPIV (CD36) deficiency have been described: type I in which both platelets and monocytes are deficient, and type II in which only platelets are deficient.[335] A C478T substitution leading to a Pro90Ser substitution and abnormal posttranslational modification is a common abnormality contributing to both type I and type II deficiencies in the Japanese population. In the type I form, patients are homozygous for the abnormality, whereas in type II deficiency, patients are doubly heterozygous for the Pro90Ser abnormality and an unidentified platelet-specific expression defect.[335,336] Other abnormalities that have been associated with type I deficiency include a dinucleotide deletion (539-540) in exon 5, a 161 bp deletion (331–491) corresponding to loss of exon 4, and a nucleotide insertion at position 1159 in codon 317, leading to a frameshift and premature stop.[337,338]

GPIV (CD36) deficiency can result in refractoriness to platelet transfusions due to isoimmunization (see Chap. 138) and has been implicated in post-tranfusion purpura (see Chap. 117).[339] GPIV (CD36) has also been implicated in monocyte binding of oxidized LDL and myocardial uptake of long-chain fatty acids.[340] Individuals with type I GPIV (CD36) deficiency have profound abnormalities in myocardial long-chain fatty acid uptake as judged by nuclear medicine studies, and there may be an association with hypertrophic cardiomyopathy.[340,341]

GPVI

GPVI can mediate platelet adhesion to collagen and is important in collagen-induced signal transduction (see Chap. 111). Two patients with mild bleeding disorders and deficiencies of platelet GPVI have been described.[342,343] Both patients had selective abnormalities in platelet-collagen interactions. An acquired defect in GPVI due to an autoantibody has also been described[344]; platelets from this patient also had abnormal collagen-induced platelet aggregation.

ABNORMAL MEMBRANE-CYTOSKELETAL INTERACTIONS

WISKOTT-ALDRICH SYNDROME

DEFINITION AND HISTORY

The Wiskott-Aldrich syndrome, which affects four of every million males worldwide, is an X-chromosome-linked inherited disorder characterized by small platelets, thrombocytopenia, recurrent infections, and eczema, although only a minority of patients have all of the classic manifestations (see Chap. 88).[345–347] In addition, a variety of immunologic abnormalities affecting T-lymphocyte function, immunoglobulin levels, cellular immunity, and responsiveness to polysaccharide antigens are commonly present.[345,347] The immune deficiency is probably responsible for an increase in lymphoreticular malignancies associated with the disorder. Death from infection, hemorrhage, or malignancy is common before adulthood.

ETIOLOGY AND PATHOGENESIS

The Wiskott-Aldrich syndrome protein (WASP) has been identified and its amino acid sequence deduced from the cDNA. The protein contains a unique Wiskott homology domain, which is also present in a number of other genes that convey signals from the surface of cells to the actin cytoskeleton. The other domains, and their interactions with other proteins, are schematically depicted in Fig. 119-8.[345] WASP is found in all hematopoietic stem-cell-derived lineages. It is likely that signals from G-protein-coupled receptors can initiate actin bundling via WASP. Not all patients with Wiskott-Aldrich syndrome have mutations in the WASP gene,[345] and so other genes may be involved. An international database of WASP mutations[348] is available and can be accessed via the *Williams Hematology* webpage.

A defect in the surface glycoprotein sialophorin (CD43, gp115, leukosialin) has also been described in Wiskott-Aldrich syndrome.[349] CD43 is a carbohydrate-rich protein found in one form on T lymphocytes, B cells, and monocytes, and in another form on neutrophils and platelets. The CD43 abnormalities are most likely a reflection of aberrant *O*-linked oligosaccharide biosynthesis,[350] but the connection between the WASP defect and aberrant *O*-linked glycosidation is unknown. CD43 can bind intercellular adhesion molecule 1 (ICAM-1), a protein implicated in immune function,[351] and so the CD43 abnormality may contribute to the immunodeficiency. Moreover, transgenic animals with overexpression of *O*-glycan Core 2 GlcNAc transferase (an enzyme that modifies CD43 and is increased in Wiskott-Aldrich platelets and resting T lymphocytes) have defects in T-cell function.[352] Deficiencies in platelet GPIb, perhaps also due to aberrant *O*-linked oligosaccharide synthesis, have been described in some patients with the Wiskott-Aldrich syndrome,[349,350] but this is not an invariant finding.[352,353] Deficiencies in GPIa have also been recorded in some, but not all, patients.[349] Similarly, decreases in platelet GPIIb/IIIa and GPIV have been reported based on flow cytometry studies, even after adjustment of the data for platelet size.[352]

The thrombocytopenia in Wiskott-Aldrich syndrome was initially ascribed to shortened platelet survival due to an intrinsic platelet defect, since autologous platelet survival was found to be short and transfused normal platelets were reported to have normal survival.[354–356] A later study, however, found normal autologous platelet recovery and only a modest decrease in platelet survival.[357] Since bone marrow megakaryocytes were not decreased, this indicated that ineffective thrombopoiesis was also contributing to the thrombocytopenia.[347] The normal level of reticulated platelets found in Wiskott-Aldrich syndrome de-

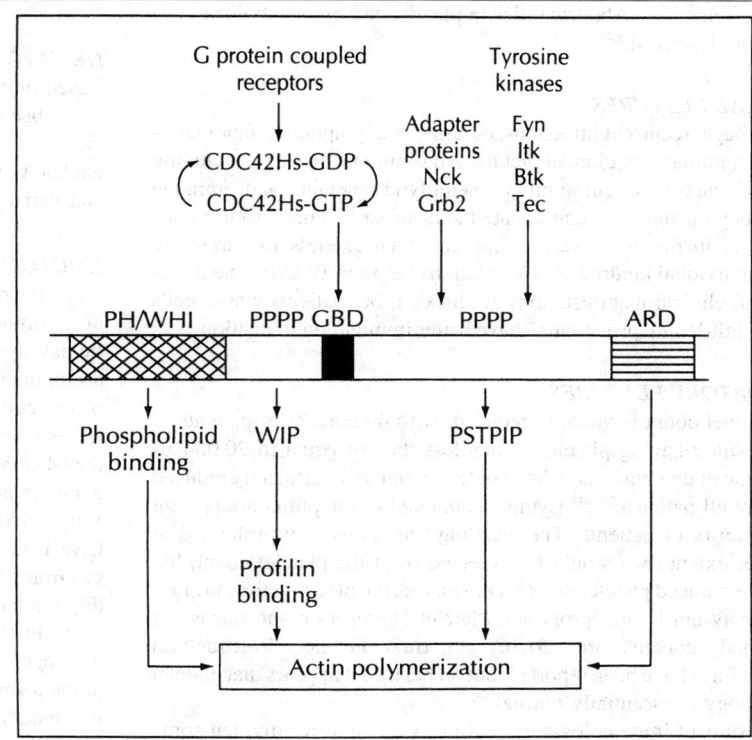

FIGURE 119-8   Domain structure of the Wiskott-Aldrich syndrome protein and identification of molecules that interact with the protein. There is a second Wiskott homology domain just before the actin regulatory domain (ARD), which is not included in the figure. PSTPIP is a cytoskeletal-associated protein.[345] PH, pleckstrin homology domain; WH1, Wiskott homology 1; PPPP, polyproline regions; GBD, GTPase binding domain; WIP, WASP-interacting protein; ARD, actin regulatory domain. Reproduced with permission from Sullivan.[345]

spite the thrombocytopenia, also indicates that ineffective thrombopoiesis may be contributing to the thrombocytopenia.[352] The alterations in platelet glycoproteins may contribute to these phenomena, but so might the elevated platelet-associated IgG levels founds on the platelets of patients with Wiskott-Aldrich syndrome.[352] Splenectomy consistently improves the platelet count,[358,359] which supports shortened survival as a major mechanism of thrombocytopenia. Postsplenectomy, immune thrombocytopenia has been reported to be a common cause of recurrent severe thrombocytopenia and hemorrhage.[345,347,360]

The cause of the small size of the platelets is unknown, but it is reasonable to presume that it is related to an abnormality in the connection between the membrane and the cytoskeleton caused by the defect in the WASP. The spleen appears to play a complex role in the platelet size defect, since platelet size increases soon after splenectomy to near normal values but then decreases to below normal again over a period of months.[355,358,361] Thrombocytopenia and small platelet size have been used to determine whether a fetus is affected with the syndrome, but a false-negative result has been reported, raising the possibility that the platelet abnormalities develop late in gestation.[362]

Variant forms of Wiskott-Aldrich syndrome characterized by thrombocytopenia and X-chromosome-linked inheritance have been reported.[363]

Platelets from most patients with Wiskott-Aldrich syndrome have qualitative as well as quantitative abnormalities. Most common is a deficiency in the storage pool of adenine nucleotides, producing a reduced positive feedback mechanism during platelet activation and aggregation.[354,356,363] Abnormalities in platelet energy metabolism have also been described.[356,364]

CLINICAL FEATURES

Hemorrhage, recurrent infections, eczema, and lymphoreticular malignancies dominate the clinical picture. Autoimmune diseases, including arthritis, vasculitis, autoimmune hemolytic anemia, and immune thrombocytopenia, may complicate the disorder.[360] There is enormous variability in disease severity, and this even extends to variability within individual kindreds.[345] Correlations between WASP gene mutations and clinical manifestations are inexact, but patients whose cells express full-length protein may have better immunologic function.[345,348]

LABORATORY FEATURES

The platelet count is variably reduced, with 44 percent of patients in a large study having platelet counts less than or equal to 20,000/μl at the time of diagnosis, and the platelet volume is significantly reduced in nearly all patients.[346,347] Lymphopenia and eosinophilia are present in a minority of patients. The bleeding time is usually prolonged to a greater extent than would be expected from the platelet count, but when the reduced platelet mass is considered, the bleeding time prolongation may not be inappropriate. Platelet aggregation and release of dense body contents are variably abnormal. Platelet ultrastructural abnormalities have been reported, but on balance it appears that platelet morphology is essentially normal.[365]

Results of immunologic evaluations vary significantly, but some patients have decreased numbers of CD8 T cells.[346] Serum levels of IgG are usually normal, whereas serum levels of IgM are usually depressed and serum levels of IgA and IgE are usually elevated.[347] Variable deficiencies in immune response to antigenic challenge, especially polysaccharide antigens, are common.[347]

THERAPY, COURSE, AND PROGNOSIS

Splenectomy usually, but not invariably, improves the thrombocytopenia and usually partially corrects the defect in platelet size, at least temporarily.[346,358,359] It may also improve platelet function. Thus, splenectomy should be considered in patients with excessive hemorrhage. Opportunistic infections present serious problems.[345,347,358] There is an increased risk of overwhelming bacterial sepsis after splenectomy, but this can be reduced by the use of pneumococcal, meningococcal, and Haemophilius influenza vaccines, as well as prophylactic antibiotics and intravenous immunoglobulin. Patients with Wiskott-Aldrich syndrome tend to have hypercatabolism of IgG and thus may require a higher dose and more frequent dosing of IgG.[347] If platelet transfusion is required to stop hemorrhage, the platelets should be irradiated to prevent transfusion-related graft-versus-host disease. It is preferable to obtain platelets from donors who are free of cytomegalovirus.[3]

Bone marrow transplantation can cure the disorder.[345,359] Since the prognosis is otherwise very poor, transplantation before the onset of significant immunodeficiency has been recommended when a histocompatible donor is available.[345,359] Transplantation from matched unrelated donors can be successful in young patients, but the success rate declines after 5 to 6 years of age.[347] Cord blood cells may be a useful alternative source of stem cells for transplantation.

GRANULE ABNORMALITIES

A heterogeneous group of disorders involving platelet granules has been described. They are broadly categorized into defects affecting dense granules (δ-storage pool deficiency), α granules (α-storage pool deficiency, or gray platelet syndrome), or both dense bodies and α-granules ($\alpha\delta$-storage pool deficiency).

δ-STORAGE POOL DEFICIENCY

DEFINITION AND HISTORY

Based on the original description of Weiss and coworkers in 1969[366] and subsequent studies by other investigators,[367,368] δ-storage pool deficiency is a heterogeneous disorder characterized by a mild bleeding tendency, abnormalities in the second wave of platelet aggregation, and variable deficiencies of the contents of platelet dense granules.

ETIOLOGY AND PATHOGENESIS

δ-storage pool deficiency can be a primary, inherited platelet disorder or a component of a multisystem disorder, such as the Hermansky-Pudlak syndrome[369,370] (variable oculocutaneous albinism, excessive accumulation of ceroid-like material in lysosomes in monocyte-macrophage cells in bone marrow and other tissues, variable pulmonary fibrosis, inflammatory bowel disease, and a hemorrhagic diathesis), the Chediak-Higashi syndrome[371-374] (partial oculocutaneous albinism, giant lysosomal granules, and frequent pyogenic infections), and the Wiskott-Aldrich syndrome (see above and Chap. 88). Other diseases have been associated with δ-storage pool deficiency (Ehlers-Danlos syndrome, osteogenesis imperfecta, thrombocytopenia with absent radii), but the relationship is less well established.[368] The mode of inheritance in the primary form is not well defined,[368] but an autosomal dominant pattern has been identified in some patients. The inheritance of the forms associated with multisystem disorders follows the autosomal recessive and X-linked patterns characteristic of those disorders.

An association between platelet granule defects and other inherited platelet abnormalities, and a predisposition to hematologic malignancies has been reported in several different families.[375] Defects in platelet function and platelet granules in leukemia and myeloproliferative disorders have been reported[376] but were originally presumed to be secondary to abnormalities of the leukemic clone or in vivo activation of platelets. However, since families have been reported whose members have a platelet abnormality prior to developing the hematologic malignancy, it is possible that the platelet abnormality and the leukemia may both be related to an underlying abnormality. Since several oncogenes appear to act via changes in signal transduction, this may be a link between the two phenomena.[377] Monosomy 7 has been reported in more than one family.[377]

The etiology of primary human δ-storage pool deficiency is unknown, but based on data from animal models it is most likely due to a defect intrinsic to hematopoietic precursors. In δ-storage pool deficiency associated with Hermansky-Pudlak syndrome, there may be a total failure of δ-granule formation as judged by electron microscopy of platelets and megakaryocytes[365] and the absence of CD63 (ME491; limp-1; lamp-3; granulophysin), a lysosomal and dense granule membrane protein of M_f 40,000 that is also found in melanosomes (see Chap. 111).[370,378] The disorder is unusually common in patients from northwest Puerto Rico, and linkage analysis of patients from this area led to the identification of the HPS gene, which is abnormal in these patients. The gene codes for a 700 amino acid protein of unknown function that is not homologous to other proteins.[370] The mutation in the Puerto Rican kindreds is a 16-bp duplication in exon 15; other mutations of the same gene have been identified in patients from other ethnic groups.[370] Mutations in the beta 3A subunit of the heterotetrameric AP3-complex, a protein involved in protein sorting to lysosomes, have also been identified in patients with Hermansky-Pudlack syndrome.[379]

In other forms of δ-storage pool disease, data obtained with uranaffin, a dye that specifically stains amine-containing granules, indicate that dense granule membranes are formed but are not properly filled.[368,380,381] The defects in the different substances contained in dense granules are also heterogeneous, with some patients able to secrete significant amounts of calcium and pyrophosphate even when adenine nucleotide secretion is nearly completely absent.[368]

The heterogeneity of human δ-storage pool deficiency is matched by a similar heterogeneity among animals with disorders associated with abnormal platelet dense granules. Thus, 14 separate inherited mouse defects have been reported to include dense granule deficiencies[382-384]; one of these (pale ear or *ep*) has been linked to the mouse equivalent of the *HPS* gene,[383] whereas another (pearl or *pe*) has been linked to the mouse equivalent of the beta 3A subunit of AP-3 complex.[385] Another mouse mutation (the pallid mutation) has been genetically linked to protein 4.2.[382] The beige mouse and rat serve as models for Chediak-Higashi syndrome, and the beige gene and a gene associated with Chediak-Higashi syndrome have been identified[386] (see Chap. 111). Thus, cytoskeletal and membranoskeletal proteins may be important in δ-granule formation and function. Several of these animal disorders are also characterized by abnormalities in lysosomes, pigment, and inner ear function.[382,383]

CLINICAL FEATURES

Patients with δ-storage pool deficiency as part of the Hermansky-Pudlak syndrome may have severe, or even lethal, hemorrhage.[370,387] For all other forms of the disorder, the bleeding tendency is only mild to moderate.[368]

Mucocutaneous hemorrhage is most common, with excessive bruising and epistaxis as well as increased bleeding after delivery, tooth extractions, and surgical procedures. The bleeding symptoms can be considerably more severe, however, if patients are taking aspirin or other antiplatelet agents.[367,368]

LABORATORY FEATURES

The results of platelet function tests are variable from patient to patient, and even in the same patient over time, making it difficult to provide precise criteria.[365,366-368,388-391] The bleeding time is usually prolonged, and there may be some correlation between the severity of dense granule deficiency and the bleeding time prolongation[392]; however, patients with δ-storage pool deficiency may have normal bleeding times.

Platelet aggregation abnormalities are characteristic (Fig. 119-6). ADP and epinephrine induce normal primary waves of aggregation, but the secondary waves are variably abnormal, with the defects ranging from minor to major. The concentration of collagen used affects the results obtained in patients with δ-storage pool deficiency; low concentrations accentuate the abnormality and high concentrations obscure it. It is important, therefore, to use the lowest concentration that gives a strong response with normal platelets.[368] If aspirin treatment of normal platelets results in a diminished aggregation response, the concentration of collagen is probably low enough to detect the abnormality in δ storage pool–deficient platelets. Thrombin at high concentrations causes maximal release of platelet dense body contents, even when platelets have been treated with aspirin or have an intrinsic release reaction abnormality. Therefore, this reagent can distinguish between δ-storage pool deficiency (diminished release) and abnormalities of the platelet release reaction (normal release). Release of ATP from platelets can be measured by luminescence simultaneously with platelet aggregation using specially designed aggregometers.[115]

More sophisticated tests can define further the extent of the platelet abnormality. The total platelet content of adenine nucleotides is reduced, and the ratio of total platelet ATP to ADP is increased because it more closely reflects the ratio in the cytoplasmic, "metabolic" pool of adenine nucleotides (about 8:1) than in the "storage" pool in dense granules (about 2:3) (see Chap. 111).[368,388,392] Platelet serotonin is variably reduced, with the lowest levels found in patients with Hermansky-Pudlak syndrome.[393] Serotonin can be taken up by platelets

of patients with δ-storage pool deficiency, but since it cannot be stored in dense granules it is rapidly catabolized.[393] Abnormalities in platelet secretion and arachidonic acid metabolism have been identified but are quite variable, and it is not clear whether they result from the aggregation abnormalities.[368,394-396] Reduced levels of plasma and platelet von Willebrand factor activity in association with a decrease in plasma high-molecular-weight multimers and an increase in low-molecular-weight multimers has been reported in Hermansky-Pudlak syndrome.[397,398] Combined δ-storage pool disease in Hermansky-Pudlak syndrome and reduced von Willebrand factor activity may result in more severe bleeding,[397] but in one study no association between bleeding and von Willebrand factor levels could be identified.[398]

The decrease or absence of platelet dense bodies can be confirmed by electron microscopy, using either whole mounts[399,400] or thin sections of platelets fixed in the presence of calcium.[365] Some patients have abnormal granules.[381,390,401] Uranaffin and osium may help to identify dense granules.[380,402] The fluorescent amine mepacrine can be used to quantify dense bodies by fluorescent microscopy.[403]

Platelet thrombus formation on subendothelial surfaces is decreased in δ-storage pool deficiency, and a hematocrit-related defect in platelet adhesion has also been noted.[131]

DIFFERENTIAL DIAGNOSIS

See "Differential Diagnosis" for Glanzmann thrombasthenia.

THERAPY, COURSE, AND PROGNOSIS

The general principles of patient management are similar to those described for Glanzmann thrombasthenia. Patients should be specifically instructed to avoid aspirin or other antiplatelet agents. Short courses of glucocorticoids before surgery may reduce the operative risk,[368,404] but the effectiveness of this therapy is not clear. Desmopressin normalizes the bleeding time in only some patients, but it is possible that it improves hemostasis without complete bleeding time normalization.[151,405-409] Cryoprecipitate can correct the bleeding time in patients with δ-storage pool deficiency[410]; although this correction may be due to an increase in plasma von Willebrand factor, it is also possible that it is due to the infusion of platelet fragments and microparticles found in cryoprecipitate.[411,412] Platelet transfusions should be effective in treating hemorrhage in patients with δ-storage pool deficiency, but the mildness of the disorder rarely makes this necessary.

GRAY PLATELET SYNDROME (α-GRANULE DEFICIENCY)

DEFINITION AND HISTORY

Raccuglia[413] reported the first patient with gray platelet syndrome, an 11-year-old female with a lifelong bleeding tendency, in 1971. Since then a number of additional patients with isolated abnormalities in platelet α-granules have been reported,[414-427] including one patient with Goldenhar syndrome,[414] and one patient with Marfan syndrome.[426] A Japanese family with 24 affected members has also been reported,[428] but these patients were atypical in having only about 50 percent reduction in platelet factor 4 and only a partial loss of platelet granularity; they also had apparently coincidental reductions in von Willebrand factor.

ETIOLOGY AND PATHOGENESIS

Studies utilizing antibodies to the α-granule membrane protein P-selectin (CD62P) and other α-granule membrane proteins indicate that gray platelets contain α-granule membranes, but the membranes form abnormal vesicular structures rather than α granules.[429,430] The P-selectin (CD62P) molecules join the plasma membrane when platelets are stimulated with thrombin, indicating that the membranes are able to fuse with the plasma membrane. Antibodies specific for proteins contained in α granules, such as fibrinogen and von Willebrand factor, identify small and misshapen α granules in gray platelets, further supporting a defect in packaging.[431] Plasma levels of the α-granule proteins β-thromboglobulin and platelet factor 4 are normal or increased, indicating that the defect is not in the synthesis of α-granule proteins.[414] Studies of the megakaryocytes in patients with the gray platelet syndrome identified von Willebrand factor, platelet-derived growth factor, and platelet factor 4 in early megakaryocytes, but a failure of the proteins to be retained in α granules as the megakaryocytes matured.[272] It has been postulated that the leakage of platelet-derived growth factor, and perhaps collagenase, from platelet α granules may be responsible for the mild reticulin fibrosis that has been observed in some patients,[417,419,427,432] leading to splenomegaly in at least one patient.[427] The fibrosis does not, however, appear to be progressive. An association with pulmonary fibrosis has also been reported,[424] raising the possibility of leakage of growth factors from megakaryocytes in the lung, but this remains speculative.

The primary defect responsible for abnormal granule formation has not been identified, but it could involve membrane production, protein targeting, granule formation, or protein retention. The evidence for a constant recycling of α granules to and from the plasma membrane adds additional loci where defects may result in abnormalities in α granules.[433]

CLINICAL FEATURES
Hemorrhagic manifestations are usually mild in the gray platelet syndrome, but severe bleeding has been noted in a patient with head trauma.[420]

LABORATORY FEATURES
Platelets appear as larger-than-normal, pale, ghostlike, oval forms on blood films. Often they can be extremely difficult to identify. Thrombocytopenia is common and can be moderately severe, with the count dropping below $50,000/\mu l$. Platelet aggregation abnormalities are present, but the reported abnormalities vary considerably. ADP and epinephrine-induced aggregation is normal or nearly normal. Collagen and thrombin-induced aggregation tends to be more abnormal, but this is not a consistent finding.[421,425,434] The abnormal thrombin-induced aggregation was studied further in one patient; abnormal platelet aggregation in response to thrombin receptor activating peptide and normal numbers of thrombin PAR-1 receptors were found.[425] Additional abnormalities in phosphoinositide metabolism, protein phosphorylation, calcium mobilization, platelet factor Va, and platelet secretion have been described.[435–437] Thus, it is unclear whether the α-granule protein deficiency, the defects in signal transduction, or both are responsible for the platelet aggregation abnormalities. The failure of α-granule proteins to fully correct the aggregation defects suggests that the signal transduction defects may be significant.[421]

Gray platelets are deficient in α-granule contents, including fibrinogen, von Willebrand factor, thrombospondin, platelet factor 4, β-thromboglobulin, and platelet derived growth factor; these can be analyzed by immunologic assays or polyacrylamide gel electrophoresis. Platelet IgG and albumin are less severely affected. Electron microscopy confirms a selective absence of α granules, with normal numbers of dense granules.[365,419,431]

DIFFERENTIAL DIAGNOSIS
See ''Differential Diagnosis'' for Glanzmann thrombasthenia. Degranulated platelets are sometimes observed in myelodysplastic and myeloproliferative disorders, but the clinical setting should provide enough information to establish the diagnosis. Some EDTA-dependent phenomena can cause platelets to degranulate in vitro and appear gray on smear.[438]

THERAPY, COURSE, AND PROGNOSIS
The general measures for treating this disorder are similar to those for Glanzmann thrombasthenia. Desmopressin produces inconsistent correction of the bleeding time,[418,439] but hemostasis after a tooth extraction was acceptable after desmopressin treatment in one patient, even without correction of the bleeding time.[418] Antifibrinolytic therapy may also be beneficial.[420] Platelet transfusions are rarely needed but should be given for serious hemorrhage.

Thrombocytopenia can contribute to the hemostatic defect. Glucocorticoid therapy may or may not increase the platelet count but usually does not result in a normal count.[413,418] The mechanism for this effect is unknown, but it raises the possibility that an immune mechanism may contribute to the thrombocytopenia in some patients. Splenectomy resulted in normalization of the platelet count in two patients soon after the surgery,[413,427] but in one of them the count slowly decreased thereafter.[414]

α,δ-STORAGE POOL DEFICIENCY

This rare disorder is characterized by moderate to severe defects in both α and δ granules, with heterogeneous expression in the few patients in whom it has been reported.[368,440] One severely affected patient also had decreased platelet P-selectin (CD62P), a point of distinction from other patients with the disorder and patients with gray platelet syndrome.[441] Clinical and laboratory features are similar to those of δ-storage pool deficiency. In general, the defect in dense granules is more severe than the defect in α granules. Decreased α 2-adrenergic receptors[442] and increased platelet GPIV (CD36)[443] have been reported in isolated cases, as has an association with hematologic malignancy.[377]

QUEBEC PLATELET DISORDER

Originally described as *factor V Quebec*, the early description of this autosomal dominant disorder included severe bleeding after trauma, mild thrombocytopenia, decreased functional platelet factor V, and normal plasma factor V (see Chap. 122).[444,445] Subsequent studies demonstrated that the platelets of these patients had markedly reduced levels of multimerin and thrombospondin (see Chap. 111), and both reduced levels and proteolysis of a number of α-granule proteins, including factor V, fibrinogen, von Willebrand factor, and osteonectin.[446] Platelet factor 4 and β-thromboglobulin, which are also α-granule proteins, did not, however, show evidence of proteolysis. Thus, these patients' platelets have a generalized defect that results in excessive proteolysis of select α-granule proteins. The mechanism of the defect in these patients, and whether the multimerin deficiency plays an etiologic role, remain unknown. Since the platelet factor V abnormality is prominent, this defect may also be classified as a defect in platelet coagulant activity (see ''Abnormalities of Platelet Coagulant Activity'' below).

ABNORMALITIES OF PLATELET COAGULANT ACTIVITY

DEFINITION AND HISTORY

Patients whose platelets fail to facilitate thrombin generation are defined as having defects in platelet coagulant activity (see Chap. 111). Only a few patients have been described with isolated defects in platelet coagulant activity,[447–451] but minor defects in coagulant activity secondary to abnormalities in platelet aggregation are more common.

The patient Scott, described by Weiss and colleagues in 1979, has been studied in detail,[447,448] and thus patients with isolated abnormalities in platelet coagulant activity are commonly referred to as having *Scott syndrome.*[449–451]

ETIOLOGY AND PATHOGENESIS

The primary abnormality in the patient Scott appears to be a failure of platelets to undergo normal microvesiculation in response to several different stimuli.[448,452] This is thought to be responsible for the decreased translocation of phosphatidylserine to the platelet's outer membrane leaflet, which in turn is presumed to be responsible for decreased binding of factors Va-Xa and VIIIa-IXa.[452–455] Without platelet binding of these intermediates in blood coagulation, the reactions do not proceed at their normal rate. This patient's defect was not confined to platelets, since her erythrocytes demonstrated a similar defect in microvesicle formation.[456]

Complementation studies using the patient's lymphocytes and a myeloma cell line suggested that the patient's cells lack a functional gene product.[457] Two other patients with sporadic defects in platelet coagulant activity have been described, and in both cases, the most significant abnormality was in collagen + thrombin-induced prothrombinase activity in the absence of added factor Va. In one of these patients, this may have been due to a defect in α granule factor V distinct from the abnormality found in the Quebec platelet syndrome (see "Quebec Platelet Syndrome" above).[450] A French family with Scott syndrome has been reported in which the propositus, who had a significant bleeding diathesis, was the product of a first-cousin mating; her two sisters had already died from hemorrhage and thus could not be studied. Her platelets and transformed lymphocytes demonstrated severe abnormalities in platelet coagulant activity, whereas platelets from her son and daughter, who were asymptomatic, had partial abnormalities in platelet coagulant activity. This suggests an autosomal recessive inheritance in this family.[449] The propositus' platelets were found to have a defect in protein tyrosine phosphorylation in response to thrombin and collagen + thrombin, especially of an M_r 40,000 protein, suggesting that a defect in signal transduction may be responsible for the abnormality in coagulant activity.[451]

CLINICAL FEATURES

Platelet coagulant defects differ from other platelet function disorders in that the hemorrhagic manifestations are not primarily mucocutaneous. For example, the patient Scott[447,448] did not have easy bruising or excessive bleeding after superficial cuts. She did, however, have variably severe bleeding after tooth extractions, menorrhagia, severe postpartum hemorrhage requiring transfusions and hysterectomy, and a spontaneous pelvic hematoma. Bleeding after surgery was present in the two sporadic cases, but epistaxis and easy bruising were only present in one of the two patients.[450] In the French family, the 71-year-old female propositus had epistaxis, trauma-related hematomas, and bleeding after tooth extractions and childbirth.[449] Her two older sisters died from hemorrhage during childbirth.

LABORATORY FEATURES

The bleeding time is usually normal, which distinguishes platelet coagulant defects from other qualitative platelet abnormalities.[448–450] The serum prothrombin time, which reflects the completeness of clotting of whole blood as reflected in consumption of prothrombin, is consistently abnormal and serves as a convenient screening assay.[447,449,450] More specific assays of "platelet factor 3," the phenomenologic designation of all of the platelet's contributions to accelerat-

ing clot formation, are also abnormal. There are a number of different techniques used to measure platelet factor 3, however, and so the results vary considerably.[458]

The patient Scott[452,454,455,459] had normal platelet aggregation, normal platelet phospholipid content, normal to enhanced platelet adhesion to subendothelium with diminished thrombus formation, severely impaired fibrin formation on subendothelium, diminished factor Va binding to platelets and platelet microparticles, diminished platelet acceleration of both factor X activation and prothrombin activation, decreased microparticle formation, and decreased activation-dependent exposure of negatively charged phospholipids. Platelet calpain and aminophospholipid translocase, enzymes that might potentially contribute to the functional abnormalities, were normal. Abnormalities in exposure of negatively charged phospholipids and shedding of microparticles, measured by any one of several techniques, including the binding of annexin V to the surface of platelets and microparticles, have been consistent findings in all of the patients described.[449–451]

DIFFERENTIAL DIAGNOSIS

The normal bleeding time, abnormal serum prothrombin time, and in several of the reported cases, the lack of the characteristic mucocutaneous pattern of bleeding, distinguish platelet coagulant defects from the other qualitative platelet disorders. See "Differential Diagnosis" for Glanzmann thrombasthenia.

THERAPY, COURSE, AND PROGNOSIS

Platelet or whole blood transfusions have been effective as prophylaxis and as therapy for bleeding episodes.[447–450] Prothrombin complex concentrates, which may contain activated coagulation species that can bypass some of the activation steps, have also been reported to be effective in the patient Scott.[368] These preparations may induce thrombosis, however, and thus should be reserved for serious hemorrhagic episodes.

ABNORMALITIES OF PLATELET AGONIST RECEPTORS, SIGNAL TRANSDUCTION, AND SECRETION

Platelet activation is a complex phenomenon involving agonist binding to receptors; signal transduction through G-protein-coupled receptors and other types of receptors; phosphoinositol metabolism resulting in calcium mobilization and phosphorylation of target proteins; arachidonic acid metabolism leading to thromboxane A_2 production; activation of the GPIIb/IIIa receptor, and release of granule contents (see Chap. 111). Defects involving any of these phenomena can result in impaired platelet function.[368,460]

Abnormalities in signal transduction usually produce only a minor hemorrhagic tendency, comparable to that caused by aspirin ingestion. Therapy is not usually necessary, but if it is, desmopressin may be helpful. It is likely, therefore, that many patients with these defects do not come to medical attention. In addition, only a small percentage of patients with defects in signal transduction have had their abnormalities defined at the molecular level.

DEFECTS IN PLATELET AGONIST RECEPTORS OR AGONIST-SPECIFIC SIGNAL TRANSDUCTION

THROMBOXANE A_2
A mutation in the thromboxane A_2 receptor (Arg60Leu) has been described as causing a dominantly inherited bleeding disorder in two unrelated families from Japan.[461] The mutation is in the first cytoplasmic loop of the receptor, and studies with recombinant mutated

receptor indicate a defect in signal initiation rather than ligand binding. The proposed dominant inheritance suggests the possibility that the abnormal receptor acts in a dominant negative fashion.

ADP

Abnormalities in one or more of the ADP receptors on platelets, or ADP-specific signal transduction, have been described in patients with bleeding disorders.[462-464]

EPINEPHRINE

Abnormalities of α-adrenergic receptors or α-adrenergic-specific signal transduction have been described in several patients.[460,465-467]

PLATELET-ACTIVATING FACTOR

A defect in the platelet activating factor receptor or platelet activating factor–specific signal transduction has been reported.[468]

DEFECTS IN SIGNAL TRANSDUCTION

DEFECTS IN ARACHIDONIC ACID METABOLISM AND THROMBOXANE PRODUCTION

Arachidonic Acid Release from Phospholipids   Several patients have been described whose platelets aggregated normally in response to arachidonic acid but not to ADP, epinephrine, and/or collagen. The patients' platelets did not release arachidonic acid normally in response to thrombin but appeared to have normal phospholipase A2 activity, suggesting a defect in moblizing sufficient calcium to activate the phopholipase.[469,470] A patient with Hermansky-Pudlak syndrome whose platelets had δ-storage pool deficiency and abnormal phospholipase A2 activity has also been reported.[471] Another patient whose platelets failed to release arachidonic acid normally has also been identified.[472]

Cyclooxygenase (Prostaglandin H_2 Synthase-1) Deficiency   Deficient platelet cyclooxygenase (prostaglandin H_2 synthase-1) activity leading to impaired platelet function has been identified in a number of patients.[473-478] Platelets from such patients cannot make thromboxane from arachidonic acid but can make it from cyclic endoperoxides. If cyclooxygenase activity is also deficient in endothelial cells, prostacyclin production will also be impaired, as was demonstrated in one patient.[475] The clinical manifestations of patients with cyclooxygenase deficiency are, therefore, of considerable interest, since they presumably reflect the competing influences of thromboxane A_2 and prostacyclin. One patient had a mild bleeding disorder,[475] whereas another[476] had evidence of a thrombotic vascular disease, including a transient ischemic attack.

Thromboxane Synthase Deficiency   Presumed platelet thromboxane synthase deficiencies have been identified in two families based on the failure of cyclic endoperoxides to be converted into thromboxane A_2.[479,480] An otherwise mild bleeding disorder associated with one life-threatening hemorrhage and a variably prolonged bleeding time was found in one patient.[480]

DEFECTS IN PHOSPHOLIPASE C, Gα Q, CALCIUM MOBILIZATION, AND CALCIUM RESPONSIVENESS

Defects in platelet secretion and the second wave of platelet aggregation with weak agonists such as epinephrine and ADP, but not strong agonists such as high-dose collagen or thrombin, are commonly encountered. When aspirin ingestion is excluded and the platelets are found to be capable of making thromboxane A_2 in response to the weak agonists, it has been inferred that the platelets' diminished response is due to one or more abnormalities of the thromboxane A_2 receptor (discussed above), the signal transduction pathway involved in calcium mobilization, or the calcium-responsive mechanisms involved in plate-

let activation.[460,465,470,481-488] Since ADP acts synergistically with thromboxane A_2, some of these abnormalities may reflect a contribution from diminished ADP secretion or responsiveness as well.[470]

A defect in phospholipase C activation[489] has been described as has a primary selective deficiency in phospholipase C-β2.[490] In addition, a selective deficiency of Gαq, a G protein implicated in signal transduction, has been described in association with a mild bleeding disorder and abnormal platelet aggregation and secretion.[491] This last defect is of particular interest, since mice lacking Gαq also have been reported to have abnormal platelet function.[492]

REFERENCES

1. Glanzmann E: Hereditäre hämmorhagische thrombasthenie. *Beitr Pathologie Bluplätchen J Kinderkt* 88:113, 1918.
2. Caen JP, Castaldi PA, Leclerc JC, et al: Congenital bleeding disorders with long bleeding time and normal platelet count. I. Glanzmann's thrombasthenia. *Am J Med* 41:4, 1966.
3. Hardisty RM, Dormandy KM, Hutton RA: Thrombasthenia: studies on three cases. *Br J Haematol* 10:371, 1964.
4. Zucker MB, Pert JH, Hilgartner MW: Platelet function in a patient with thrombasthenia. *Blood* 28:524, 1966.
5. Weiss HJ, Kochwa S: Studies of platelet function and proteins in 3 patients with Glanzmann's thrombasthenia. *J Lab Clin Med* 71:153, 1968.
6. George JN, Caen JP, Nurden AT: Glanzmann's thrombasthenia: the spectrum of clinical disease. *Blood* 75:1383, 1990.
7. Caen JP: Glanzmann's thrombasthenia. *Clin Haematol* 1:383, 1972.
8. Nurden AT, Caen JP: An abnormal platelet glycoprotein pattern in three cases of Glanzmann's thrombasthenia. *Br J Haematol* 28:253, 1974.
9. Phillips DR, Jenkins CS, Luscher EF, Larrieu M: Molecular differences of exposed surface proteins on thrombasthenic platelet plasma membranes. *Nature* 257:599, 1975.
10. Peerschke EI: The platelet fibrinogen receptor. *Sem Hematol* 22:241, 1985.
11. Bennett JS: The platelet-fibrinogen interaction, in *Platelet Membrane Glycoproteins,* edited by JN George, AT Nurden, DR Phillips. p 193. Plenum, New York, 1985.
12. Phillips DR, Charo IF, Parise LV, Fitzgerald LA: The platelet membrane glycoprotein IIb-IIIa complex. *Blood* 71:831, 1988.
13. Plow EF, Ginsberg MH: Cellular adhesion: GPIIb-IIIa as a prototypic adhesion receptor. *Prog Hem Thromb* 9:117, 1989.
14. Poncz M, Eisman R, Heidenreich R, et al: Structure of the platelet membrane glycoprotein IIb. Homology to the alpha subunits of the vitronectin and fibronectin membrane receptors. *J Biol Chem* 262:8476, 1987.
15. Fitzgerald LA, Steiner B, Rall SC, Jr., Lo SS, Phillips DR: Protein sequence of endothelial glycoprotein IIIa derived from a cDNA clone. Identity with platelet glycoprotein IIIa and similarity to "integrin." *J Biol Chem* 262:3936, 1987.
16. Hynes RO: Integrins: a family of cell surface receptors. *Cell* 48:549, 1987.
17. Bray PF, Shuman MA: Identification of an abnormal gene for the GPIIIa subunit of the platelet fibrinogen receptor resulting in Glanzmann's thrombasthenia. *Blood* 75:881, 1990.
18. Loftus JC, O'Toole TE, Plow EF, Glass A, Frelinger AL, Ginsberg MH: A β3 integrin mutation abolishes ligand binding and alters divalent cation-dependent conformation. *Science* 249:915, 1990.
19. Newman PJ, Seligsohn U, Lyman S, Coller BS: The molecular genetic basis of Glanzmann thrombasthenia in the Iraqi-Jewish and Arab populations in Israel. *Proc Natl Acad Sci USA* 88:3160, 1991.
20. Burk CD, Newman PJ, Lyman S, Gill J, Coller BS, Poncz M: A deletion in the gene for glycoprotein IIb associated with Glanzmann's thrombasthenia. *J Clin Invest* 87:270, 1991.
21. Peretz H, Seligsohn U, Zwang E, Coller BS, Newman PJ: Detection of the Glanzmann's thrombasthenia mutations in Arab and Iraqi-Jewish patients by polymerase chain reaction and restriction analysis of blood or urine samples. *Thromb Haemostas* 66:500, 1991.
22. Chen Y-P, Djaffar I, Pidard E, et al: Ser752Pro mutation in the cytoplasmic domain of integrin β3 subunit and defective activation of platelet

integrin αIIbβ3 (glycoprotein IIb-IIIa) in a variant of Glanzmann throm-basthenia. *Proc Natl Acad Sci USA* 89:10169, 1992.

23. Bajt ML, Ginsberg MH, Frelinger AL, III, Berndt MC, Loftus JC: A spontaneous mutation of integrin αIIbβ3 (platelet glycoprotein IIb-IIIa) helps define a ligand binding site. *J Biol Chem* 267:3789, 1992.

24. Seligsohn U, Peretz H, Newman PJ, Coller BS: Glanzmann thrombas-thenia in Israel: clinical, biochemical and molecular genetic characteriza-tion, in *Genetic Diversity Among Jews*, edited by B Bonné-Tamir, A Adam, p 275. Oxford University Press, New York, 1992.

25. Lanza F, Stierle A, Fournier D, et al: A new variant of Glanzmann's thrombasthenia (Strasbourg I). Platelets with functionally defective gly-coprotein IIb-IIIa complexes and a glycoprotein IIIa Arg214Trp muta-tion. *J Clin Invest* 89:1995, 1992.

26. Kato A, Yamamoto K, Miyazaki S, Jung SM, Moroi M, Aoki N: Molecu-lar basis for Glanzmann's thrombasthenia (GT) in a compound heterozy-gote with glycoprotein IIb gene: a proposal for the classification of GT based on the biosynthetic pathway of glycoprotein IIb-IIIa complex. *Blood* 79:3212, 1992.

27. Gu J-M, Xu W-F, Wang X-D, Wu Q-Y, Chi C-W, Ruan C-G: Identifica-tion of a nonsense mutation at amino acid 584-arginine of platelet glycoprotein IIb in patients with type I Glanzmann thrombasthenia. *Br J Haematol* 83:442, 1993.

28. Simsek S, Heyboer H, de Bruijne-Admiraal LG, Goldschmeding R, Cuijpers HThM, von dem Borne AEGKr: Glanzmann's thrombasthenia caused by homozygosity for a splice defect that leads to deletion of the first coding exon of the glycoprotein IIIa mRNA. *Blood* 81:2044, 1993.

29. Djaffar I, Caen JP, Rosa JP: A large alteration in the human platelet glycoprotein IIIa (integrin beta 3) gene associated with Glanzmann's thrombasthenia. *Hum Mol Genet* 2:2183, 1993.

30. Babu R, Nibu K, Jablonski L, Poncz M: Rapid diagnosis of Glanzmann thrombasthenia using a single-stranded conformational polymorphism analysis. *Thromb Haemost* 69:1018, 1993.

31. Li L, Bray PF: Homologous recombination among three intragene Alu sequences causes an inversion-deletion resulting in the hereditary bleed-ing disorder Glanzmann thrombasthenia. *Am J Hum Genet* 53:140, 1993.

32. Jin Y, Dietz HC, Nurden A, Bray PF: Single-strand conformation poly-morphism analysis is a rapid and effective method for the identification of mutations and polymorphisms in the gene for glycoprotein IIIa. *Blood* 82:2281, 1993.

33. Djaffar I, Rosa JP: A second case of variant of Glanzmann's thrombas-thenia due to substitution of platelet GPIIIa (integrin beta 3) Arg214 by Trp. *Hum Mol Genet* 2:2179, 1993.

34. Wilcox DA, Wautier JL, Pidard D, Newman PJ: A single amino acid substitution flanking the fourth calcium binding domain of alpha IIb prevents maturation of the alpha IIb beta 3 integrin complex. *J Biol Chem* 269:4450, 1994.

35. Poncz M, Rifat S, Coller BS, et al: Glanzmann thrombasthenia secondary to a Gly273Asp mutation adjacent to the first calcium-binding domain of platelet glycoprotein IIb. *J Clin Invest* 93:172, 1994.

36. Bourre R, Peyruchaud O, Bray PF, Combrie R, Nurden P, Nurden AT: A point mutation in the gene for platelet GPIIb leads to a substitution in a highly conserved amino acid located between the second and third Ca++-binding domain. *Blood* 86: 452a, 1995.

37. Wilcox DA, Paddock CM, Lyman S, Gill JC, Newman PJ: Glanzmann thrombasthenia resulting from a single amino acid substitution between the second and third calcium-binding domains of GPIIb. Role of the GPIIb amino terminus in integrin subunit association. *J Clin Invest* 95:1553, 1995.

38. Ferrer M, Fernandez-Pinel M, Gonzalez-Manchon C, Gonzalez J, Ayuso MS, Parrilla R: A mutant (Arg327 His) GPIIb associated to thrombas-thenia exerts a dominant negative effect in stably transfected CHO cells. *Thromb Haemost* 76:292, 1996.

39. Basani RB, Vilaire G, Shattil SJ, Kolodziej MA, Bennett JS, Poncz M: Glanzmann thrombasthenia due to a two amino acid deletion in the fourth calcium-binding domain of alpha IIb: demonstration of the importance of calcium-binding domains in the conformation of alpha IIb beta 3. *Blood* 88:167, 1996.

40. French DL, Coller BS: Hematologically important mutations: Glanz-mann thrombasthenia. *Blood Cells Mol Dis* 23:39, 1997.

41. Rosenberg N, Yatuv R, Orion Y, et al: Glanzmann thrombasthenia caused by an 11.2-kb deletion in the glycoprotein IIIa (beta3) is a second

mutation in Iraqi Jews that stemmed from a distinct founder. *Blood* 89:3654, 1997.

42. Milet S, Bourre F, Peyruchaud O, et al: Amino acid substitution Cys457 to Tyr in the β3 subunit of αIIbβ3 is involved in an atypical case of Glanzmann thrombasthenia. *Thromb Haemostas* 77:360, 1997.

43. French DL, Coller BS, Usher S, et al: Prenatal diagnosis of Glanzmann thrombasthenia using the polymorphic markers BRCA1 and THRA1 on chromosome 17. *Br J Haematol* 102:582, 1998.

44. Basani RB, French DL, Vilaire G, Brown DL, et al: A naturally-occurring mutation near the amino terminus of αIIb defines a new region involved in ligand binding to αIIbβ3. *Blood* 95:180, 2000.

45. Wang R, Shattil SJ, Ambruso DR, Newman PJ: Truncation of the cytoplasmic domain of β3 in a variant form of Glanzmann thrombas-thenia abrogates signaling through the integrin αIIBβ3 complex. *J Clin Invest* 100:2393, 1997.

46. Ward CM, Kestin AS, Newman PJ: A Leu262Pro mutation in the integrin β3 subunit results in an αIIbβ3 complex that binds fibrin but not fibrino-gen. *Blood* 96:161, 2000.

47. Ambo H, Kamata T, Handa M, et al: Three novel integrin beta3 subunit missense mutations (H280P, C560F, and G579S) in thrombasthenia, including one (H280P) prevalent in Japanese patients. *Biochem Biophys Res Commun* 251:763, 1998.

48. Ambo H, Kamata T, Handa M, et al: Novel point mutations in the alphaIIb subunit (Phe289 Ser, Glu324 Lys and Gln747 Pro) causing thrombasthenic phenotypes in four Japanese patients. *Br J Haematol* 102:829, 1998.

49. Peyruchaud O, Nurden AT, Milet S, et al: R to Q amino acid substitution in the GFFKR sequence of the cytoplasmic domain of the integrin IIb subunit in a patient with a Glanzmann's thrombasthenia-like syndrome. *Blood* 92:4178, 1998.

50. Tadokoro S, Tomiyama Y, Honda S, et al: A Gln747 Pro substitution in the IIb subunit is responsible for a moderate IIbbeta3 deficiency in Glanzmann thrombasthenia. *Blood* 92:2750, 1998.

51. Honda S, Tomiyama Y, Shiraga M, et al: A two-amino acid insertion in the Cys146-Cys167 loop of the αIIb subunit is associated with a variant of Glanzmann thrombasthenia. *J Clin Invest* 102:1183, 1998.

52. Ferrer M, Tao J, Sanchez-Ayuso M, et al: Truncation of glycoprotein (GP)IIa (616-762) prevents complex formation with GPIIb: Novel muta-tion in exon 11 of GPIIIa associated with thrombasthenia. *Blood* 92:4712, 1998.

53. Scott JP, III, Scott JP, Chao YL, Newman PJ, Ward CM: A frameshift mutation at Gly975 in the transmembrane domain of GPIIb prevents GPIIb-IIIa expression—analysis of two novel mutations in a kindred with type I glanzmann thrombasthenia. *Thromb Haemost* 80:546, 1998.

54. Grimaldi CM, Chen F, Wu C, Weiss HJ, Coller BS, French DL: Glyco-protein IIb Leu214Pro mutation produces Glanzmann thrombasthenia with both quantitative and qualitative abnormalities in GPIIb/IIIa. *Blood* 91:1562, 1998.

55. Jackson DE, White MM, Jennings LK, Newman PJ: A Ser162 Leu mutation within glycoprotein (GP) IIIa (integrin beta3) results in an unstable alphaIIbbeta3 complex that retains partial function in a novel form of type II Glanzmann thrombasthenia. *Thromb Haemost* 80:42, 1998.

56. Ruan J, Peyruchaud O, Alberio L, et al: Double heterozygosity of the GPIIb gene in a Swiss patient with Glanzmann's thrombasthenia. *Br J Haematol* 102:918, 1998.

57. Ruan J, Schmugge M, Clemetson KJ, et al: Homozygous Cys542 Arg substitution in GPIIIa in a Swiss patient with type I Glanzmann's throm-basthenia. *Br J Haematol* 105:523, 1999.

58. Gonzalez-Manchon C, Fernandez-Pinel M, Arias-Salgado EG, et al: Molecular genetic analysis of a compound heterozygote for the glycopro-tein (GP) IIb gene associated with Glanzmann's thrombasthenia: disrup-tion of the 674-687 disulfide bridge in GPIIb prevents surface exposure of GPIIb-IIIa complexes. *Blood* 93:866, 1999.

59. Reichert N, Seligsohn U, Ramot B: Clinical and genetic studies of Glanzmann's thrombasthenia in Israel. *Thromb Diath Haemorrh* 34: 806, 1975.

60. Awidi AS: Increased incidence of Glanzmann's thrombasthenia in Jor-dan as compared with Scandinavia. *Scand J Haematol* 30:218, 1983.

61. Khanduri U, Pulimood R, Sudarsanam A, Carman RH, Jadhav M, Pereira S: Glanzmann's thrombasthenia. A review and report of 42 cases from South India. *Thromb Haemost* 46:717, 1981.

62. Ahmed MA, Al Sohaibani MO, Al Mohaya SA, Sumer T, Al Sheikh EH, Knox-Macaulay H: Inherited bleeding disorders in the eastern province of Saudi Arabia. *Acta Haematol* 79:202, 1988.

63. Awidi AS: Rare inherited bleeding disorders secondary to coagulation factors in Jordan: a nine-year study. *Acta Haematol* 88:11, 1992.

64. Handagama PJ, Shuman MA, Bainton DF: Incorporation of intravenously injected albumin, immunoglobulin G, and fibrinogen in guinea pig megakaryocyte granules. *J Clin Invest* 84:73, 1989.

65. Harrison P, Wilbourn BR, Debili N, et al: Uptake of plasma fibrinogen into the alpha granules of human megakaryocytes and platelets. *J Clin Invest* 84:1320, 1989.

66. Handagama P, Rappolee DA, Werb Z, Levin J, Bainton DF: Platelet alpha-granule fibrinogen, albumin, and immunoglobulin G are not synthesized by rat and mouse megakaryocytes. *J Clin Invest* 86:1364, 1990.

67. Harrison P: Platelet α-granular fibrinogen. *Platelets* 3:1, 1992.

68. Coller BS, Seligsohn U, West SM, Scudder LE, Norton KJ: Platelet fibrinogen and vitronectin in Glanzmann thrombasthenia: evidence consistent with specific roles for glycoprotein IIb/IIIa and αVβ3 integrins in platelet protein trafficking. *Blood* 78:2603, 1991.

69. Disdier M, Legrand C, Bouillot C, Dubernard V, Pidard D, Nurden AT: Quantitation of platelet fibrinogen and thrombospondin in Glanzmann's thrombasthenia by electroimmunoassay. *Thromb Res* 53:521, 1989.

70. Degos L, Dautigny A, Brouet JC, et al: A molecular defect in thrombasthenic platelets. *J Clin Invest* 56:236, 1975.

71. Cohen I, Gerrard JM, White JG: Ultrastructure of clots during isometric contraction. *J Cell Biol* 91:775, 1982.

72. Gartner TK, Ogilvie ML: Peptides and monoclonal antibodies which bind to platelet glycoproteins IIb and/or IIIa inhibit clot retraction. *Thromb Res* 49:43, 1988.

73. Duperray A, Troesch A, Berthier R, et al: Biosynthesis and assembly of platelet GPIIb-IIIa in human megakaryocytes: evidence that assembly between pro-GPIIb and GPIIIa is a prerequisite for expression of the complex on the cell surface. *Blood* 74:1603, 1989.

74. Bodary SC, Napier MA, McLean JW: Expression of recombinant platelet glycoprotein IIbIIIa results in a functional fibrinogen-binding complex. *J Biol Chem* 264:18859, 1989.

75. O'Toole TE, Loftus JC, Plow EF, Glass AA, Harper JR, Ginsberg MH: Efficient surface expression of platelet GPIIb-IIIa requires both subunits. *Blood* 74:14, 1989.

76. Kolodziej MA, Vilaire G, Gonder D, Poncz M, Bennett JS: Study of the endoproteolytic cleavage of platelet glycoprotein IIb using oligonucleotide-mediated mutagenesis. *J Biol Chem* 266:23499, 1991.

77. Bennett JS: The molecular biology of platelet membrane proteins. *Sem Hematol* 27:186, 1990.

78. Kieffer N, Phillips DR: Platelet membrane glycoproteins: functions in cellular interactions. *Annu Rev Cell Biol* 6:329, 1990.

79. Seligsohn U, Coller BS, Zivelin A, Plow EF, Ginsberg MH: Immunoblot analysis of platelet GPIIb in patients with Glanzmann thrombasthenia in Israel. *Br J Haematol* 72:415, 1989.

80. Zimrin AB, Eisman R, Vilaire G, Schwartz E, Bennett JS, Poncz M: Structure of platelet glycoprotein IIIa. A common subunit for two different membrane receptors. *J Clin Invest* 81:1470, 1988.

81. Cheresh DA: Human endothelial cells synthesize and express an Arg-Gly-Asp-directed adhesion receptor involved in attachment to fibrinogen and von Willebrand factor. *Proc Natl Acad Sci USA* 84:6471, 1987.

82. Smith JW, Cheresh DA: The Arg-Gly-Asp binding domain of the vitronectin receptor. *J Biol Chem* 263:18726, 1988.

83. Cheresh DA, Berliner SA, Vicente V, Ruggeri ZM: Recognition of distinct adhesive sites on fibrinogen by related integrins on platelets and endothelial cells. *Cell* 58:945, 1989.

84. Lawler J, Hynes RO: An integrin receptor on normal and thrombasthenic platelets which binds thrombospondin. *Blood* 74:2022, 1989.

85. Yokoyama K, Zhang XP, Medved L, Takada Y: Specific binding of integrin alpha v beta 3 to the fibrinogen gamma and alpha E chain C-terminal domains. *Biochemistry* 38:5872, 1999.

86. Lam SC, Plow EF, D'Souza SE, Cheresh DA, Frelinger AL, III, Ginsberg MH: Isolation and characterization of a platelet membrane protein related to the vitronectin receptor. *J Biol Chem* 264:3742, 1989.

87. Coller BS, Cheresh DA, Asch E, Seligsohn U: Platelet vitronectin receptor expression differentiates Iraqi-Jewish from Arab patients with Glanzmann thrombasthenia in Israel. *Blood* 77:75, 1991.

88. Beckstead JH, Stenberg PE, McEver RP, Shuman MA, Bainton DF: Immunohistochemical localization of membrane and alpha-granule proteins in human megakaryocytes: application to plastic-embedded bone marrow biopsy specimens. *Blood* 67:285, 1986.

89. Krissansen GW, Elliott MJ, Lucas CM, et al: Identification of a novel integrin beta subunit expressed on cultured monocytes (macrophages). *J Biol Chem* 265:823, 1990.

90. Byzova TV, Rabbani R, D'Souza SE, Plow EF: Role of integrin alpha(v)beta3 in vascular biology. *Thromb Haemost* 80:726, 1998.

91. Yatuv R, Rosenberg N, Dardik R, Brenner B, Seligsohn U: Glanzmann thrombasthenia in two Iraqi-Jewish siblings is caused by a novel splice junction mutation in the glycoprotein IIb. *Blood Coagul Fibrinol* 9:285, 1998.

92. Lee JO, Rieu P, Arnaout MA, Liddington R: Crystal structure of the A domain from the alpha subunit of integrin CR3 (CD11b/CD18). *Cell* 80:631, 1995.

93. Michishita M, Videm V, Arnaout MA: A novel divalent cation-binding site in the A domain of the beta 2 integrin CR3 (CD11b/CD18) is essential for ligand binding. *Cell* 72:857, 1993.

94. Tozer EC, Liddington RC, Sutcliffe MJ, Smeeton AH, Loftus JC: Ligand binding to integrin αIIbβ3 is dependent on a MIDAS-like domain in the beta3 subunit. *J Biol Chem* 271:21978, 1996.

95. Bajt ML, Loftus JC: Mutation of a ligand binding domain of beta 3 integrin. Integral role of oxygenated residues in alpha IIb beta 3 (GPIIb-IIIa) receptor function. *J Biol Chem* 269:20913, 1994.

96. Ward CM, Chao YL, Kato GJ, Casella J, Bray PF, Newman PJ: Substitution of Asn, but not Tyr, for Asp119 of the β3 integrin subunit preserves fibrin binding and clot retraction. *Blood* 90:26a, 1997.

97. Newman PJ, Weyerbusch-Bottum S, Visentin GP, Gidwitz S, White GC: Type II Glanzmann thrombasthenia due to a destablizing amino acid substitution in platelet membrane glycoprotein IIIa. *Thromb Haemost* 69:1017, 1993.

98. Basani RB, Brown DL, Vilaire G, Bennett JS, Poncz M: A Leu117 Trp mutation within the RGD-peptide cross-linking region of beta3 results in Glanzmann thrombasthenia by preventing alphaIIb beta3 export to the platelet surface. *Blood* 90:3082, 1997.

99. Baker EK, Tozer EC, Pfaff M, Shattil SJ, Loftus JC, Ginsberg MH: A genetic analysis of integrin function: Glanzmann thrombasthenia in vitro. *Proc Natl Acad Sci USA* 94:1973, 1997.

100. Loftus JC, Halloran CE, Ginsberg MH, Feigen LP, Zablocki JA, Smith JW: The amino-terminal one-third of alpha IIb defines the ligand recognition specificity of integrin alpha IIb beta 3. *J Biol Chem* 271:2033, 1996.

101. Springer TA: Folding of the N-terminal, ligand-binding region of integrin α-subunits into a β propeller domain. *Proc Natl Acad Sci USA* 94:65, 1997.

102. Tuckwell DS, Humphries MJ, Brass A: A secondary structure model of the integrin alpha subunit N-terminal domain based on analysis of multiple alignments. *Cell Adhes Commun* 2:385, 1994.

103. Irie A, Kamata T, Puzon-McLaughlin W, Takada Y: Critical amino acid residues for ligand binding are clustered in a predicted β-turn of the third N-terminal repeat in the integrin α4 and α5 subunits. *EMBO J* 14:5550, 1995.

104. Kamata T, Irie A, Tokuhira M, Takada Y: Critical residues of integrin αIIb subunit for binding of αIIbβ3 (glycoprotein IIb-IIIa) to fibrinogen and ligand-mimetic antibodies (PAC-1, OP-G2, and LJ-CP3). *J Biol Chem* 271:18610, 1996.

105. Tozer EC, Baker EK, Ginsberg MH, Loftus JC: A mutation in the alpha subunit of the platelet integrin alphaIIbbeta3 identifies a novel region important for ligand binding. *Blood* 93:918, 1999.

106. Ylanne J, Chen Y, O'Toole TE, Loftus JC, Takada Y, Ginsberg MH: Distinct functions of integrin alpha and beta subunit cytoplasmic domains in cell spreading and formation of focal adhesions. *J Cell Biol* 122:223, 1993.

107. Ylanne J, Huuskonen J, O'Toole TE, Ginsberg MH, Virtanen I, Gahmberg CG: Mutation of the cytoplasmic domain of the integrin beta 3 subunit. Differential effects on cell spreading, recruitment to adhesion plaques, endocytosis, and phagocytosis. *J Biol Chem* 270:9550, 1995.

108. Chen YP, O'Toole TE, Ylanne J, Rosa JP, Ginsberg MH: A point mutation in the integrin beta 3 cytoplasmic domain (S752→P) impairs bidirectional signaling through alpha IIb beta 3 (platelet glycoprotein IIb-IIIa). *Blood* 84:1857, 1994.

109. Guarisco JL, Cheney ML, Ohene-Frempong K, LeJeune FE, Jr., Blair

PA: Limited septoplasty as treatment for recurrent epistaxis in a child with Glanzmann's thrombasthenia. *Laryngoscope* 97:336, 1987.

110. Seligsohn U, Rososhansky S: A Glanzmann's thrombasthenia cluster among Iraqi Jews in Israel. *Thromb Haemost* 52:230, 1984.

111. Coller BS, Peerschke EI, Scudder LE, Sullivan CA: A murine monoclonal antibody that completely blocks the binding of fibrinogen to platelets produces a thrombasthenic-like state in normal platelets and binds to glycoproteins IIb and/or IIIa. *J Clin Invest* 72:325, 1983.

112. Chediak J, Telfer MC, Vander LB, Maxey B, Cohen I: Cycles of agglutination-disagglutination induced by ristocetin in thrombasthenic platelets. *Br J Haematol* 43:113, 1979.

113. Grant RA, Zucker MB, McPherson J: ADP-induced inhibition of von Willebrand factor-mediated platelet agglutination. *Am J Physiol* 230: 1406, 1976.

114. Malmsten C, Kindahl H, Samuelsson B, Levy-Toledano S, Tobelem G, Caen JP: Thromboxane synthesis and the platelet release reaction in Bernard-Soulier syndrome, thrombasthenia Glanzmann and Hermansky-Pudlak syndrome. *Br J Haematol* 35:511, 1977.

115. Charo IF, Feinman RD, Detwiler TC: Interrelations of platelet aggregation and secretion. *J Clin Invest* 60:866, 1977.

116. Heptinstall S, Taylor PM: The effects of citrate and extracellular calcium ions on the platelet release reaction induced by adenosine diphosphate and collagen. *Thromb Haemost* 42:778, 1979.

117. Caen JP, Cronberg S, Levy-Toledano S, Kubisz P, Pinkhas JP: New data on Glanzmann's thrombasthenia. *Proc Soc Exp Biol Med* 136: 1082, 1971.

118. Zucker MB, Vroman L: Platelet adhesion induced by fibrinogen adsorbed onto glass. *Proc Soc Exp Biol Med* 131:318, 1969.

119. Stanford MF, Munoz PC, Vroman L: Platelets adhere where flow has left fibrinogen on glass. *Ann N Y Acad Sci* 416:504, 1983.

120. Zucker MB, McPherson J: Reactions of platelets near surfaces in vitro: lessons from the platelet retention test. *Ann N Y Acad Sci* 283:128, 1977.

121. Bevers EM, Comfurius P, Nieuwenhuis HK, et al: Platelet prothrombin converting activity in hereditary disorders of platelet function. *Br J Haematol* 63:335, 1986.

122. Reverter JC, Beguin S, Kessels H, Kumar R, Hemker HC, Coller BS: Inhibition of platelet-mediated, tissue factor-induced, thrombin generation by the mouse/human chimeric 7E3 anibody: Potential implications for the effect of c7E3 Fab treatment on acute thrombosis and "clinical restenosis." *J Clin Invest* 98:863, 1996.

123. Beguin S, Kumar R, Keularts I, Seligsohn U, Coller BS, Hemker HC: Fibrin-dependent platelet procoagulant activity requires GPIb receptors and von Willebrand factor. *Blood* 93:564, 1999.

124. Gemmell CH, Sefton MV, Yeo EL: Platelet-derived microparticle formation involves glycoprotein IIb-IIIa. Inhibition by RGDS and a Glanzmann's thrombasthenia defect. *J Biol Chem* 268:14586, 1993.

125. Nomura S, Komiyama Y, Matsuura E, et al: Participation of $\alpha_{IIb}\beta_3$ in platelet microparticle generation by collagen plus thrombin. *Thromb Haemostis* 26:31, 1996.

126. Nomura S, Komiyama Y, Murakami T, et al: Flow cytometric analysis of surface membrane proteins on activated platelets and platelet-derived microparticles from healthy and thrombasthenic individuals. *Int J Hematol* 58:203, 1993.

127. Byzova TV, Plow EF: Networking in the hemostatic system. Integrin alphaIIbbeta3 binds prothrombin and influences its activation. *J Biol Chem* 272:27183, 1997.

128. Byzova TV, Plow EF: Activation of alphaVbeta3 on vascular cells controls recognition of prothrombin. *J Cell Biol* 143:2081, 1998.

129. Tschopp TB, Weiss HJ, Baumgartner HR: Interaction of thrombasthenic platelets with subendothelium: normal adhesion, absent aggregation. *Experientia* 31:113, 1975.

130. Sakariassen KS, Nievelstein PFEM, Coller BS, Sixma JJ: The role of platelet membrane glycoproteins Ib and IIb-IIIa in platelet adherence to human artery subendothelium. *Br J Haematol* 63:681, 1986.

131. Weiss HJ, Turitto VT, Baumgartner HR: Platelet adhesion and thrombus formation on subendothelium in platelets deficient in glycoproteins IIb-IIIa, Ib, and storage granules. *Blood* 67:322, 1986.

132. Weiss HJ, Turitto VT, Baumgartner HR: The role of shear rate and platelets in promoting fibrin formation on rabbit subendothelium: studies utilizing patients with quantitative and qualitative platelet defects. *J Clin Invest* 78:1072, 1986.

133. Lee H, Nurden AT, Thomaidis A, Caen JP: Relationship between fibrino-

gen binding and platelet glycoprotein deficiencies in Glanzmann's thrombasthenia type I and type II. *Br J Haematol* 48:47, 1981.

134. Rosenberg N, Dardik R, Rosenthal E, Zivelin A, Seligsohn U: Mutations in the alphaIIb and beta3 genes that cause Glanzmann thrombasthenia can be distinguished by a simple procedure using transformed B-lymphocytes. *Thromb Haemost* 79:244, 1998.

135. Coller BS, Seligsohn U, Peretz H, Newman PJ: Glanzmann thrombasthenia: new insights from an historical perspective. *Semin Hematol* 31: 301, 1994.

136. Shattil SJ, Hoxie JA, Cunningham M, Brass LF: Changes in the platelet membrane glycoprotein IIb.IIIa complex during platelet activation. *J Biol Chem* 260:11107, 1985.

137. Coller BS, Seligsohn U, Zivelin A, Zwang E, Lusky A, Modan M: Immunologic and biochemical characterization of homozygous and heterozygous Glanzmann's thrombasthenia in Iraqi-Jewish and Arab populations of Israel: comparison of techniques for carrier detection. *Br J Haematol* 62:723, 1986.

138. Karpatkin M, Howard L, Karpatkin S: Studies of the origin of platelet-associated fibrinogen. *J Lab Clin Med* 104:223, 1984.

139. Grimaldi CM, Chen F, Scudder LE, Coller BS, French DL: A Cys374Tyr homozygous mutation of platelet glycoprotein IIIa (beta3) in a Chinese patient with Glanzmann's thrombasthenia. *Blood* 88:1666, 1996.

140. Diminno G, Coraggio F, Cerbone AM, et al: A myeloma paraprotein with specificity for platelet glycoprotein IIIa in a patient with a fatal bleeding disorder. *J Clin Invest* 77:157, 1986.

141. Niessner H, Clemetson KJ, Panzer S, Mueller-Eckhardt C, Santoso S, Bettelheim P: Acquired thrombasthenia due to GPIIb/IIIa-specific platelet autoantibodies. *Blood* 68:571, 1986.

142. Kubota T, Tanoue K, Murohashi I, et al: Autoantibody against platelet glycoprotein IIb/IIIa in a patient with non-hodgkin's lymphoma. *Thromb Res* 53:379, 1989.

143. Malik U, Dutcher JP, Oleksowicz L: Acquired Glanzmann's thrombasthenia associated with Hodgkin's lymphoma: a case report and review of the literature. *Cancer* 82:1764, 1998.

144. Macchi L, Nurden P, Marit G, et al: Autoimmune thrombocytopenic purpura (AITP) and acquired thrombasthenia due to autoantibodies to GP IIb-IIIa in a patient with an unusual platelet membrane glycoprotein composition. *Am J Hematol* 57:164, 1998.

145. Chen Y, Wu Q-Y, Wang Z: Abnormalities of platelet membrane glycoproteins in acute non-lymphomblastic leukemia. *Thromb Haemost* 62:176, 1989.

146. Bray PF, Barsh G, Rosa JP, Luo XY, Magenis E, Shuman MA: Physical linkage of the genes for platelet membrane glycoproteins IIb and IIIa. *Proc Natl Acad Sci USA* 85:8683, 1988.

147. Markovitch O, Ellis M, Holzinger M, Goldberger S, Beyth Y: Severe juvenile vaginal bleeding due to Glanzmann's thrombasthenia: case report and review of the literature. *Am J Hematol* 57:225, 1998.

148. Ratnoff OD: Some therapeutic agents influencing hemostasis, in *Hemostasis and Thrombosis: Basic Principles and Clinical Practice*, edited by RW Colman, J Hirsh, VJ Marder, EW Salzman, 2d ed, p 1026. Lippincott, Philadelphia, 1987.

149. Berliner S, Horowitz I, Martinowitz U, Brenner B, Seligsohn U: Dental surgery in patients with severe factor XI deficiency without plasma replacement. *Blood Coagul Fibrinol* 3:465, 1992.

150. Sindet-Pedersen S, Ramstrom G, Bernvil S, Blomback M: Hemostatic effect of tranexamic acid mouthwash in anticoagulant-treated patients undergoing oral surgery. *N Engl J Med* 320:840, 1989.

151. Mannucci PM: Desmopressin (DDAVP) for treatment of disorders of hemostasis. *Prog Hem Thromb* 8:19, 1986.

152. Lethagen S, Karlsson MK: Erythropoietin and desmopressin obviated transfusion in a thromboasthenic Jehovah's witness undergoing scoliosis surgery. *Thromb Haemost* 2:11, 1996.

153. DiMichele DM, Hathaway WE: Use of DDAVP in inherited and acquired platelet dysfunction. *Am J Hematol* 33:39, 1990.

154. Tengborn L, Petruson B: A patient with Glanzmann thrombasthenia and epistaxis successfully treated with recombinant factor VIIa. *Thromb Haemost* 75:981, 1996.

155. Tock B, Drohan W, Hess J, Pusateri A, Holcomb J, MacPhee M: Haemophilia and advanced fibrin sealant technologies. *Haemophilia* 4:449, 1998.

156. Martinowitz U, Varon D, Heim M: The role of fibrin tissue adhesives in surgery of haemophilia patients. *Haemophilia* 4:443, 1998.

157. Cmolik BL, Spero JA, Magovern GJ, Clark RE: Redo cardiac surgery: late bleeding complications from topical thrombin-induced factor V deficiency. *J Thorac Cardiovasc Surg* 105:222, 1993.

158. Banninger H, Hardegger T, Tobler A, et al: Fibrin glue in surgery: frequent development of inhibitors of bovine thrombin and human factor V. *Br J Haematol* 85:528, 1993.

159. Tudokoro K, Ohtoshi T, Takafuji S, et al: Topical thrombin-induced IgE-mediated anaphylaxis: RAST analysis and skin test studies. *J Allergy Clin Immunol* 88:620, 1991.

160. Tsuda H, Higashi S, Iwanaga S, Kubota T, Morita T, Yanaga K: Development of antitissue factor antibodies in patients after liver surgery. *Blood* 82:96, 1993.

161. Jasmin JR, Dupont D, Velin P: Multiple dental extractions in a child with Glanzmann's thrombasthenia: report of case. *ASDC J Dent Child* 54:208, 1987.

162. Peyser MR, Kuperminc MJ: Management of severe postpartum hemorrhage by intrauterine irrigation with prostaglandin E2. *Am J Obstet Gynecol* 162:694, 1990.

162a. Kuperminc MJ, Gall I, Bar-Am A, et al: Intrauterine irrigation with prostaglandin F2-alpha for management of severe postpartum hemorrhage. *Acta Obstet Gynecol Scand* 77:548, 1998.

163. Cases A, Escolar G, Reverter JC, et al: Recombinant human erythropoietin treatment improves platelet function in uremic patients. *Kidney Int* 42:668, 1992.

164. Tsao CJ, Kao RH, Cheng TY, Huang CC, Chang SL, Lee FN: The effect of recombinant human erythropoietin on hemostatic status in chronic uremic patients. *Int J Hematol* 55:197, 1992.

165. Sniecinski I, O'Donnell MR, Nowicki B, Hill LR: Prevention of refractoriness and HLA-alloimmunization using filtered blood products. *Blood* 71:1402, 1988.

166. Andreu G: Role of leukocyte depletion in the prevention of transfusion-induced cytomegalovirus infection. *Semin Hematol* 28:26, 1991.

167. Heddle NM, Klama L, Singer J, et al: The role of the plasma from platelet concentrates in transfusion reactions. *N Engl J Med* 331:625, 1994.

168. Saarinen UM, Kekomaki R, Siimes MA, Myllyla G: Effective prophylaxis against platelet refractoriness in multitransfused patients by use of leukocyte-free blood components. *Blood* 75:512, 1990.

169. Slichter SJ: Platelet transfusions a constantly evolving therapy. *Thromb Haemost* 66:178, 1991.

170. Newman PJ, McFarland JG, Aster RH: The alloimmune thrombocytopenias, in *Thrombosis and Hemorrhage,* edited by J Loscalzo, AI Schafer, p 531. Blackwell Scientific, Boston, 1994.

171. Jallu V, Pico M, Chevaleyre J, Vezon G, Kunicki TJ, Nurden AT: Characterization of an antibody to the integrin beta 3 subunit (GP IIIa) from a patient with neonatal thrombocytopenia and an inherited deficiency of GP IIb-IIIa complexes in platelets (Glanzmann's thrombasthenia). *Hum Antibodies Hybridomas* 3:93, 1992.

172. Levy-Toledano S, Tobelem G, Legrand C, et al: Acquired IgG antibody occurring in a thrombasthenic patient: its effect on human platelet function. *Blood* 51:1065, 1978.

173. Rosa JP, Kieffer N, Didry D, Pidard D, Kunicki TJ, Nurden AT: The human platelet membrane glycoprotein complex GP IIb-IIIa expresses antigenic sites not exposed on the dissociated glycoproteins. *Blood* 64:1246, 1984.

174. Coller BS, Peerschke EI, Seligsohn U, Scudder LE, Nurden AT, Rosa J-P: Studies on the binding of an alloimmune and two murine monoclonal antibodies to the platelet glycoprotein IIb-IIIa complex receptor. *J Lab Clin Med* 107:384, 1986.

175. Ito K, Yoshida H, Hatoyama H, et al: Antibody removal therapy used successfully at delivery of a pregnant patient with Glanzmann's thrombasthenia and multiple anti-platelet antibodies. *Vox Sang* 61:40, 1991.

176. George JN, Nurden AT: Inherited disorders of the platelet membrane: Glanzmann's thrombasthenia and Bernard-Soulier syndrome, in *Hemostasis and Thrombosis: Basic Principles and Clinical Practice,* edited by RW Colman, J Hirsh, VJ Marder, EW Salzman, p 726. Lippincott, Philadelphia, 1987.

177. Bellucci S, Devergie A, Gluckman E, et al: Complete correction of Glanzmann's thrombasthenia by allogeneic bone marrow transplantation. *Br J Haematol* 59:635, 1985.

178. Johnson A, Goodall AH, Downie CJ, Vellodi A, Michael DP: Bone marrow transplantation for Glanzmann's thrombasthenia. *Bone Marrow Transplant* 14:147, 1994.

179. Poon MC, Demers C, Jobin F, Wu JW: Recombinant factor VIIa is effective for bleeding and surgery in patients with Glanzmann thrombasthenia. *Blood* 94:3951, 1999.

180. Wielenga JJ, Siebel Y, van Buuren HR: Use of recombinant factor VIIa and HLA matched platelets to prevent bleeding during and after major surgery in a patient with Glanzmann's thrombasthenia. *Haemophilia* 4:299, 1998.

181. Schulman S, d'Oiron R, Martinowitz U, et al: Experiences with continuous infusion of recombinant activated factor VII. *Blood Coagul Fibrinol* 9(Suppl 1):S97, 1998.

182. Méanart C, Trzeciak MC, Attali O, Négrier C: Continuous infusion of NovoSeven® during colectomy in a Glanzmann thrombasthenia patient with anti-glycoprotein IIb-IIIa antibody. *Haemophilia* 4:299, 1998.

183. Wilcox DA, Olsen JC, Ishizawa L, Griffith M, White GC: Integrin alphaIIb promoter-targeted expression of gene products in megakaryocytes derived from retrovirus-transduced human hematopoietic cells. *Proc Natl Acad Sci USA* 96:9654, 1999.

184. Hodivala-Dilke KM, Tsakiris DA, Rayburn H, et al: Beta3-integrin-deficient mice are a model for Glanzmann thrombasthenia showing placental defects and reduced survival. *J Clin Invest* 103:229, 1999.

185. Yasunaga K, Nomura S: Statistical analysis of Glanzmann's thrombasthenia in Japan. *Acta Haematol* 89:165, 1993.

186. Bernard J, Soulier J-P: Sur une nouvelle variete de dystrophie thrombocytaire-hemorragipare congenitale. *Semin Hop Paris* 24:3217, 1948.

187. Bernard J: History of congenital hemorrhagic thrombocytopathic dystrophy. *Blood Cells* 9:179, 1983.

188. Weiss HJ, Tschopp TB, Baumgartner HR, Sussman II, Johnson MM, Egan JJ: Decreased adhesion of giant (Bernard-Soulier) platelets to subendothelium. Further implications on the role of the von Willebrand factor in hemostasis. *Am J Med* 57:920, 1974.

189. Howard MA, Hutton RA, Hardisty RM: Hereditary giant platelet syndrome: a disorder of a new aspect of platelet function. *Br Med J* 2:586, 1973.

190. Bithell TC, Parekh SJ, Strong RR: Platelet-function studies in the Bernard-Soulier syndrome. *Ann N Y Acad Sci* 201:145–60:145, 1972.

191. Nurden AT, Caen JP: Specific roles for platelet surface glycoproteins in platelet function. *Nature* 255:720, 1975.

192. Howard MA, Perkin J, Salem HH, Firkin BG: The agglutination of human platelets by botrocetin: evidence that botrocetin and ristocetin act at different sites on the factor VIII molecule and platelet membrane. *Br J Haematol* 57:25, 1984.

193. Moake JL, Olson JD, Troll JH, Tang SS, Funicella T, Peterson DM: Binding of radioiodinated human von Willebrand factor to Bernard–Soulier, thrombasthenic and von Willebrand's disease platelets. *Thromb Res* 19:21, 1980.

194. Zucker MB, Kim SJ, McPherson J, Grant RA: Binding of factor VIII to platelets in the presence of ristocetin. *Br J Haematol* 35:535, 1977.

195. Berndt MC, Gregory C, Chong BH, Zola H, Castaldi PA: Additional glycoprotein defects in Bernard-Soulier's syndrome: confirmation of genetic basis by parental analysis. *Blood* 62:800, 1983.

196. Clemetson KJ, McGregor JL, James E, Dechavanne M, Lusher EF: Characterization of the platelet membrane glycoprotein abnormalities in Bernard-Soulier syndrome and comparison with normal by surface-labeling techniques and high-resolution two-dimensional gel electrophoresis. *J Clin Invest* 70:304, 1982.

197. Ware J, Russell S, Ruggeri ZM: Generation and rescue of a murine model of platelet dysfunction: the Bernard-Soulier syndrome. *Proc Natl Acad Sci (USA)* 97:2803, 2000.

198. McGill M, Jamieson GA, Drouin J, Cho MS, Rock GA: Morphometric analysis of platelets in Bernard-Soulier syndrome: size and configuration in patients and carriers. *Thromb Haemost* 52:37, 1984.

199. Michalas S, Malamitsi-Puchner A, Tsevrenis H: Pregnancy and delivery in Bernard-Soulier syndrome. *Acta Obstet Gynecol Scand* 63:185, 1984.

200. Suhasini G, Nanivadekar SA, Sawant PD, Agarwal MB, Bichile LS, Bavdankar PY: Bernard-Soulier syndrome presenting as recurrent exsanguinating haematemesis. *Indian J Gastroenterol* 5:137, 1986.

201. Heslop HE, Hickton CM, Laird E, Tait JD, Doig JR, Beard EJ: Twin pregnancy and parturition in a patient with the Bernard Soulier syndrome. *Scand J Haematol* 37:71, 1986.

202. De Marco L, Fabris F, Casonato A, et al: Bernard-Soulier syndrome: diagnosis by an ELISA method using monoclonal antibodies in 2 new unrelated patients. *Acta Haematol* 75:203, 1986.

203. Sheffer R, Ilan Y, Eldor A: Bernard-Soulier syndrome. *Harefuah* 111:119, 1986.

204. Ingerslev J, Stenbjerg S, Taaning E: A case of Bernard-Soulier syndrome: study of platelet glycoprotein Ib in a kindred. *Eur J Haematol* 39:182, 1987.

205. Oki Y, Yoshioka K, Konishi M, et al: A case of Bernard-Soulier syndrome. *Nippon Naika Gakkai Zasshi* 76:1414, 1987.

206. deMoerloose P, Vogel JJ, Clemetson KJ, Petite J, Bienz D, Bouvier CA: Bernard-Soulier syndrome in a Swiss family. *Schweiz Med Wochenschr* 117:1817, 1987.

207. Cuthbert RJ, Watson HH, Handa SI, Abbott I, Ludlam CA: DDAVP shortens the bleeding time in Bernard-Soulier syndrome. *Thromb Res* 49:649, 1988.

208. Drouin J, McGregor JL, Parmentier S, Izaguirre CA, Clemetson KJ: Residual amounts of glycoprotein Ib concomitant with near-absence of glycoprotein IX in platelets of Bernard-Soulier patients. *Blood* 72:1086, 1988.

209. Mant MJ: DDAVP in Bernard-Soulier syndrome. *Thromb Res* 52:77, 1988.

210. Stevens MC, Blanchette VS, Freedman MH, Sparling C, Kunicki TJ: A variant form of Bernard-Soulier syndrome: mild haemostatic defect associated with partial platelet GPIb deficiency. *Clin Lab Haematol* 10:443, 1988.

211. Shimamoto Y, Kaneoka H, Matsuzaki M, et al: Genetic markers and thrombin reaction in a family of Bernard-Soulier syndrome. *Nippon Ketsueki Gakkai Zasshi* 52:1155, 1989.

212. Peaceman AM, Katz AR, Laville M: Bernard-Soulier syndrome complicating pregnancy: a case report. *Obstet Gynecol* 73:457, 1989.

213. Nichols WL, Kaese SE, Gastineau DA, Otteman LA, Bowie EJ: Bernard-Soulier syndrome: whole blood diagnostic assays of platelets. *Mayo Clin Proc* 64:522, 1989.

214. Ware J, Russell SR, Vicente V, et al: Nonsense mutation in the glycoprotein Ib alpha coding sequence associated with Bernard-Soulier syndrome. *Proc Natl Acad Sci USA* 87:2026, 1990.

215. Finch CN, Miller JL, Lyle VA, Handin RI: Evidence that an abnormality in the glycoprotein Ib alpha gene is not the cause of abnormal platelet function in a family with classic Bernard-Soulier disease. *Blood* 75:2357, 1990.

216. De Marco L, Mazzucato M, Fabris F, et al: Variant Bernard-Soulier syndrome type Bolzano. A congenital bleeding disorder due to a structural and functional abnormality of the platelet glycoprotein Ib-IX complex. *J Clin Invest* 86:25, 1990.

217. Poulsen LO, Taaning E: Variation in surface platelet glycoprotein Ib expression in Bernard-Soulier syndrome. *Haemostis* 20:155, 1990.

218. Ware J, Russell SR, Vicente V, et al: Nonsense mutation in the glycoprotein Ibalpha coding sequence associated with Bernard-Soulier syndrome. *Proc Natl Acad Sci USA* 87:2026, 1990.

219. Waldenstrom E, Holmberg L, Axelsson U, Winqvist I, Nilsson IM: Bernard-Soulier syndrome in two Swedish families: effect of DDAVP on bleeding time. *Eur J Haematol* 46:182, 1991.

220. Humphries JE, Yirinec BA, Hess CE: Atherosclerosis and unstable angina in Bernard-Soulier syndrome. *Am J Clin Pathol* 97:652, 1992.

221. Miller JL, Lyle VA, Cunningham D: Mutation of leucine-57 to phenylalanine in a platelet glycoprotein Ib alpha leucine tandem repeat occurring in patients with an autosomal dominant variant of Bernard-Soulier disease. *Blood* 79:439, 1992.

222. Avila MA, Jacyntho C, Santos ML, et al: Bernard-Soulier syndrome and pregnancy: a case report. *J Gynecol Obstet Biol Reprod (Paris)* 21:73, 1992.

223. Wright SD, Michaelides K, Johnson DJ, West NC, Tuddenham EG: Double heterozygosity for mutations in the platelet glycoprotein IX gene in three siblings with Bernard-Soulier syndrome. *Blood* 81:2339, 1993.

224. Ware J, Russell SR, Marchese P, et al: Point mutation in a leucine-rich repeat of platelet glycoprotein Ibalpha in the Bernard-Soulier syndrome. *J Clin Invest* 92:1213, 1993.

225. Simsek S, Admiraal LG, Modderman PW, van der Schoot CE, von dem Borne AEGK: Identification of a homozygous single base pair deletion in the gene coding for the human platelet glycoprotein Ibalpha causing Bernard-Soulier syndrome. *Thromb Haemost* 72:444, 1994.

226. Simsek S, Noris P, Lozano M, et al: Cys209Ser mutation in the platelet membrane glycoprotein Ibalpha gene is associated with Bernard Soulier syndrome. *Br J Haematol* 88:839, 1994.

227. Kunishima S, Miura G, Fukutani H, et al: Bernard-Soulier syndrome Kagoshima: Ser 444-Stop mutation of glycoprotein (GP) Ibalpha resulting in circulating truncated GPIbalpha and surface expression of GPIbbeta and GPIX. *Blood* 84:3356, 1994.

228. Li C, Martin SE, Roth GJ: The genetic defect in two well-studied cases of Bernard-Soulier syndrome: A point mutation in the fifth leucine-rich repeat of platelet glycoprotein Ibα. *Blood* 86:3805, 1995.

229. De La Salle C, Baas M-J, Lanza F, et al: A three-base deletion removing a leucine residue in a leucine-rich repeat of platelet glycoprotein Ibalpha associated with a variant of Bernard-Soulier syndrome (Nancy I). *Br J Haematol* 89:386, 1995.

230. Noda M, Fujimura K, Takafuta T, et al: Heterogenous expression of glycoprotein Ib, IX and V in platelets from two patients with Bernard-Soulier syndrome caused by different genetic abnormalities. *Thromb Haemost* 74:1411, 1995.

231. Budarf ML, Konkle BA, Ludlow LB, et al: Identification of a patient with Bernard-Soulier syndrome and a deletion in the DiGeorge/Velocardio-facial chromosomal region in 22q11.2. *Hum Mol Genet* 4:763, 1995.

232. Ludlow LB, Schick BP, Budarf ML, et al: Identification of a mutation in a GATA binding site of the platelet glycoprotein Ibbeta promoter resulting in the Bernard-Soulier syndrome. *J Biol Chem* 271:22076, 1996.

233. Li C, Pasquale DN, Roth GJ: Bernard-Soulier syndrome with severe bleeding: absent platelet glycoprotein Ib alpha due to a homozygous one-base deletion. *Thromb Haemost* 76:670, 1996.

234. Martinez-Murillo C, Quintana-Gonzalez S, Ambriz-Fernandez R, Arzate-Hernandez G, Gutierrez-Romero M, Gaminio-Gomez E: Utility of desmopression in 4 cases of thrombocytopathies associated with giant platelets. *Rev Invest Clin* 49:281, 1997.

235. Kanaji T, Okamura T, Kuroiwa M, et al: Molecular and genetic analysis of two patients with Bernard-Soulier syndrome: identification of new mutations in glycoprotein Ibalpha gene. *Thromb Haemost* 77:1055, 1997.

236. Kenny D, Newman PJ, Morateck PA, Montgomery RR: A dinucleotide deletion results in defective membrane anchoring and circulating soluble glycoprotein Ibalpha in a novel form of Bernard-Soulier syndrome. *Blood* 90:2626, 1997.

237. Afshar-Kharghan V, Lopez JA: Bernard-Soulier syndrome caused by a dinucleotide deletion and reading frameshift in the region encoding the glycoprotein Ibalpha transmembrane domain. *Blood* 90:2634, 1997.

238. Holmberg L, Karpman D, Nilsson I, Olofsson T: Bernard-Soulier syndrome Karlstad: Trp 498-Stop mutation resulting in a truncated glycoprotein Ibalpha that contains part of the transmembrane domain. *Br J Haematol* 98:57, 1997.

239. Kunishima S, Lopez JA, Kobayashi S, et al: Missense mutations of the glycoprotein (GP) Ib beta gene impairing the GPIb alpha/beta disulfide linkage in a family with giant platelet disorder. *Blood* 89:2404, 1997.

240. Noris P, Simsek S, Stibbe J, von dem Borne AEGK: A phenylalanine-55 to serine aminoacid substitution in the human glycoprotein IX leucine-rich repeat is associated with Bernard-Soulier syndrome. *Br J Haematol* 97:312, 1997.

241. Lopez JA, Andrews RK, Afshar-Kharghan V, Berndt MC: Bernard-Soulier syndrome. *Blood* 91:4397, 1998.

242. Noris P, Arbustini E, Spedini P, Belletti S, Balduini CL: A new variant of Bernard-Soulier syndrome characterized by dysfunctional glycoprotein (GP) Ib and severely reduced amounts of GPIX and GPV. *Br J Haematol* 103:1004, 1998.

243. Van Geet C, Devriendt K, Eyskens B, Vermylen J, Hoylaerts MF: Velocardiofacial syndrome patients with a heterozygous chromosome 22q11 deletion have giant platelets. *Pediatr Res* 44:607, 1998.

244. Khalil A, Seoud M, Tannous R, Usta I, Shamseddine A: Bernard-Soulier syndrome in pregnancy: case report and review of the literature. *Clin Lab Haematol* 20:125, 1998.

245. Kenny D, Morateck PA, Gill JC, Montgomery RR: The critical interaction of glycoprotein (GP) Ibβ with GPIX-a genetic cause of Bernard-Soulier syndrome. *Blood* 93:2968, 1999.

246. Koskela S, Javela K, Jouppila J, et al: Variant Bernard-Soulier syndrome due to homozygous Asn45Ser mutation in the platelet glycoprotein (GP) IX in seven patients of five unrelated Finnish families. *Eur J Haematol* 62:256, 1999.

247. Koskela S, Partanen J, Salmi TT, Kekomaki R: Molecular characteriza-

tion of two mutations in platelet glycoprotein (GP) Ibalpha in two Finnish Bernard-Soulier syndrome families. *Eur J Haematol* 62:160, 1999.

248. Margaglione M, D'Andrea G, Grandone E, Brancaccio V, Amoriello A, Di Minno G: Compound heterozygosity (554-589 del, C515-T transition) in the platelet glycoprotein Ib alpha gene in a patient with a severe bleeding tendency. *Thromb Haemost* 81:486, 1999.

249. Grottum KA, Solum NO: Congenital thrombocytopenia with giant platelets: a defect in the platelet membrane. *Br J Haematol* 16:277, 1969.

250. Greenberg JP, Packham MA, Guccione MA, Rand ML, Reimbers HJ, Mustard JF: Survival of rabbit-platelets treated in vitro with chymotrypsin, plasmin, trypsin, and neuraminidase. *Blood* 53:916, 1979.

251. Heyns Ad, Badenhorst PN, Wessels P, Pieters H, Lotter MG: Kinetics, in vivo redistribution and sites of sequestration of indium–111-labelled platelets in giant platelet syndromes. *Br J Haematol* 60:323, 1985.

252. Tomer A, Scharf RE, McMillan R, Ruggeri ZM, Harker LA: Bernard-Soulier syndrome: quantitative characterization of megakaryocytes and platelets by flow cytometric and platelet kinetic measurements. *Eur J Haematol* 52:193, 1994.

253. Nurden P, Nurden A: Giant platelets, megakaryocytes and the expression of glycoprotein Ib-IX complexes. *C R Acad Sci III* 319:717, 1996.

254. Ruggeri Z: The platelet glycoprotein Ib-IX complex. *Prog Hem Thromb* 10:35, 1991.

255. Roth GJ: Developing relationships: arterial platelet adhesion, glycoprotein Ib, and leucine-rich glycoproteins. *Blood* 77:5, 1991.

256. Ikeda Y, Handa M, Kawano K, et al: The role of von Willebrand factor and fibrinogen in platelet aggregation under varying shear stress. *J Clin Invest* 87:1234, 1991.

257. Peterson DM, Stathopoulos NA, Giorgio TD, Hellums JD, Moake JL: Shear-induced platelet aggregation requires von Willebrand factor and platelet membrane glycoproteins Ib and IIb-IIIa. *Blood* 69:625, 1987.

258. Ruggeri ZM: Mechanisms of shear-induced platelet adhesion and aggregation. *Thromb Haemost* 70:119, 1993.

259. Jamieson GA, Okumura T: Reduced thrombin binding and aggregation in Bernard-Soulier platelets. *J Clin Invest* 61:861, 1978.

260. Nurden AT, George JN, Phillips DR: Human platelet membrane glycoproteins, in *Biochemistry of the Platelet,* edited by M Shuman. DR Phillips, p 159. Academic, New York, 1986.

261. Jandrot-Perrus M, Rendu F, Caen JP, Levy-Toledano S, Guillin MC: The common pathway for alpha- and gamma-thrombin-induced platelet activation is independent of GPIb: a study of Bernard-Soulier platelets. *Br J Haematol* 75:385, 1990.

262. De Marco L, Mazzucato M, Masotti A, Fenton JW, Ruggeri ZM: Function of glycoprotein Ib alpha in platelet activation induced by alpha-thrombin. *J Biol Chem* 266:23776, 1991.

263. Larsen NE, Simons ER: Preparation and application of a photoreactive thrombin analogue: binding to human platelets. *Biochemistry* 20:4141, 1981.

264. Hagen I, Brosstad F, Solum NO, Korsmo R: Crossed immunoelectrophoresis using immobilized thrombin in intermediate gell. A method for demonstration of thrombin-binding platelet proteins. *J Lab Clin Med* 97:213, 1981.

265. Harmon JT, Jamieson GA: The glycocalicin portion of platelet glycoprotein Ib expresses both high and moderate affinity receptor sites of thrombin. A soluble radioreceptor assay for the injection of thrombin with platelets. *J Biol Chem* 261:13224, 1986.

266. Ramakrishnan V, Reeves PS, DeGuzman F, Deshpands U, Ministri-Madrid K, Phillips DR: Gene targeting of glycoprotein V indicates that this glycoprotein is a negative modulator of platelet function. *Thromb Haemost* 82:209, 1999.

267. Caen J, Bellucci S: The defective prothrombin consumption in Bernard-Soulier syndrome. Hypotheses from 1948 to 1982. *Blood Cells* 9:389, 1983.

268. Walsh PN, Mills DC, Pareti FI, et al: Hereditary giant platelet syndrome. Absence of collagen-induced coagulant activity and deficiency of factor-XI binding to platelets. *Br J Haematol* 29:639, 1975.

269. Perret B, Levy-Toledano S, Platavid M: Abnormal phospholipid organization in Bernard-Soulier platelets. *Thromb Res* 31:529, 1983.

270. McNicol A, Drouin J, Clemetson KJ, Gerrard JM: Phospholipase C activity in platelets from Bernard-Soulier syndrome patients. *Arterioscler Thromb* 13:1567, 1993.

271. White JG, Burris SM, Hasegawa D, Johnson M: Micropipette aspiration of human blood platelets: a defect in Bernard-Soulier's syndrome. *Blood* 63:1249, 1984.

272. Nurden AT: Congenital abnormalities of platelet membrane glycoproteins., in *Platelet Immunobiology, Molecular and Clinical Aspects,* p 95. Lippincott, Philadelphia, 1989.

273. Lopez JA, Leung B, Reynolds CC, Li CQ, Fox JEB: Efficient plasma membrane expression of a functional platelet glycoprotein Ib-IX complex requires the presence of its three subunits. *J Biol Chem* 267:12851, 1992.

274. Nurden AT, Didry-Dupies V, Rosa JP: Molecular defects of platelets in Bernard Soulier syndrome. *Blood Cells* 9:333, 1983.

275. Nurden AT: Inherited abnormalities of platelets. *Thromb Haemost* 82:468, 1999.

276. Nurden AT, Jallu V, Hourdille P: GP Ib and Bernard-Soulier platelets. *Blood* 73:2225, 1989.

277. George JN, Reimann TA, Moake JL, Morgan RK, Cimo PL, Sears DA: Bernard-Soulier disease: a study of four patients and their parents. *Br J Haematol* 48:459, 1981.

278. Fox JEB: Linkage of a membrane skeleton to integral membrane glycoproteins in human platelets. Identification of one of the glycoproteins as glycoprotein Ib. *J Clin Invest* 76:1673, 1985.

279. Eaton LA Jr., Read MS, Brinkhous KM: Glycoprotein Ib bioassays. Activity levels in Bernard-Soulier syndrome and in stored blood bank platelets. *Arch Pathol Lab Med* 115:488, 1991.

280. Evensen SA, Solum NO, Grottum KA, Hovig T: Familial bleeding disorder with a moderate thrombocytopenia and giant blood platelets. *Scand J Haematol* 13:203, 1974.

281. Greco NJ, Tandon NN, Jones GD, et al: Contributions of glycoprotein Ib and the seven transmembrane domain receptor to increases in platelet cytoplasmic $[Ca^{2+}]$ induced by α-thrombin. *Biochemistry* 35:906, 1996.

282. McGowan EB, Ding A, Detwiler TC: Correlation of thrombin-induced glycoprotein V hydrolysis and platelet activation. *J Biol Chem* 258:11243, 1983.

283. Bienz D, Schnippering W, Clemetson KJ: Glycoprotein V is not the thrombin activation receptor on human blood platelets. *Blood* 68:720, 1986.

284. Caen JP, Nurden AT, Jeanneau C, et al: Bernard-Soulier syndrome: a new platelet glycoprotein abnormality. Its relationship with platelet adhesion to subendothelium and with the factor VIII von Willebrand protein. *J Lab Clin Med* 87:586, 1976.

285. Andrews RK, Harris SJ, McNally T, Berndt MC: Binding of purified 14-3-3 zeta signaling protein to discrete amino acid sequences within the cytoplasmic domain of the platelet membrane glycoprotein Ib-IX-V complex. *Biochemistry* 37:638, 1998.

286. Sullam PM, Hyun WC, Szollosi J, Dong J, Foss WM, Lopez JA: Physical proximity and functional interplay of the glycoprotein Ib-IX-V complex and the Fc receptor FcgammaRIIA on the platelet plasma membrane. *J Biol Chem* 273:5331, 1998.

287. Falati S, Edmead CE, Poole AW: Glycoprotein Ib-V-IX, a receptor for von Willebrand factor, couples physically and functionally to the Fc receptor γ-chain, Fyn, and Lyn to activate human platelets. *Blood* 94:1648, 1999.

288. Stricker RB, Wong D, Saks SR, Crash L, Shuman MA: Acquired Bernard-Soulier syndrome. Evidence for the role of a 210,000- molecular weight protein in the interaction of platelets with von Willebrand factor. *J Clin Invest* 76:1274, 1985.

289. Deckmyn H, Vanhoorelbeke K, Peerlinck K: Inhibitory and activating human antiplatelet antibodies. *Baillieres Clin Haematol* 11:343, 1998.

290. Devine DV, Currie MS, Rosse WF, Greenberg CS: Pseudo-Bernard-Soulier syndrome: thrombocytopenia caused by autoantibody to platelet glycoprotein Ib. *Blood* 70:428, 1987.

291. Varon D, Gitel SN, Varon N, et al: Immune Bernard Soulier-like syndrome associated with anti-glycoprotein IX antibody. *Am J Hematol* 41:67, 1992.

292. Beales IL: An acquired-pseudo Bernard Soulier syndrome occurring with autoimmune chronic active hepatitis and anti-cardiolipin antibody. *Postgrad Med J* 70:305, 1994.

293. Berndt MC, Kabral A, Grimsley P, Watson N, Robertson TI, Bradstock KF: An acquired Bernard-Soulier-like platelet defect associated with juvenile myelodysplastic syndrome. *Br J Haematol* 68:97, 1988.

294. Hicsonmez G, Gumruk F, Cetin M, Ozbek N, Tuncer M, Gursel T: Bernard-Soulier-like functional platelet defect in myelodysplastic syn-

drome and in acute myeloblastic leukemia associated with trilineage myelodysplasia. *Turk J Pediatr* 37:425, 1995.

295. Sharma JB, Buckshee K, Sharma S: Puberty menorrhagia due to Bernard Soulier syndrome and its successful treatment by Ovral hormonal tablets. *Aust N Z J Obstet Gynaecol* 31:369, 1991.

296. Greinacher A, Potzsch B, Kiefel V, White JG, Muller-Berghaus G, Mueller-Eckhardt C: Evidence that DDAVP transiently improves hemostasis in Bernard-Soulier syndrome independent of von Willebrand-factor. *Ann Hematol* 67:149, 1993.

297. Kemahli S, Canatan D, Uysal Z, Akar N, Cin S, Arcasoy A: DDAVP shortens bleeding time in Bernard-Soulier syndrome. *Thromb Haemost* 71:675, 1994.

298. Saade G, Homsi R, Seoud M: Bernard-Soulier syndrome in pregnancy; a report of four pregnancies in one patient, and review of the literature. *Eur J Obstet Gynecol Reprod Biol* 40:149, 1991.

299. Degos L, Tobelem G, Lethielleux P, Levy-Toledano S, Caen J, Colombani J: Molecular defect in platelets from patients with bernard-soulier syndrome. *Blood* 50:899, 1977.

300. Peng TC, Kickler TS, Bell WR, Haller E: Obstetric complications in a patient with Bernard-Soulier syndrome. *Am J Obstet Gynecol* 165:425, 1991.

301. Peters M, Heijboer H: Treatment of a patient with Bernard-Soulier syndrome and recurrent nosebleeds with recombinant factor VIIa. *Thromb Haemost* 80:352, 1998.

302. Takahashi H: Studies on the pathophysiology and treatment of von Willebrand's disease. IV. Mechanism of increased ristocetin-induced platelet aggregation in von Willebrand's disease. *Thromb Res* 19:857, 1980.

303. Krizek DM, Rick ME, Williams SB, Gralnick HR: Cryoprecipitate transfusion in variant von Willebrand's disease and thrombocytopenia. *Ann Intern Med* 98:484, 1983.

304. Weiss HJ, Meyer D, Rabinowitz R, et al: Pseudo-von Willebrand's disease. An intrinsic platelet defect with aggregation by unmodified human factor VIII/von Willebrand factor and enhanced adsorption of its high-molecular-weight multimers. *N Engl J Med* 306:326, 1982.

305. Miller JL, Castella A: Platelet-type von Willebrand's disease: characterization of a new bleeding disorder. *Blood* 60:790, 1982.

306. Gralnick HR, Williams SB, Shafer BC, Corash L: Factor VIII/von Willebrand factor binding to von Willebrand's disease platelets. *Blood* 60:328, 1982.

307. Takahashi H, Handa M, Watanabe K, et al: Further characterization of platelet-type von Willebrand's disease in Japan. *Blood* 64:1254, 1984.

308. Miller JL, Cunningham D, Lyle VA, Finch CN: Mutation in the gene encoding the alpha chain of platelet glycoprotein Ib in platelet-type von Willebrand disease. *Proc Natl Acad Sci USA* 88:4761, 1991.

309. Russell SD, Roth GJ: Pseudo-von Willebrand disease: a mutation in the platelet glycoprotein Ib alpha gene associated with a hyperactive surface receptor. *Blood* 81:1787, 1993.

310. Takahashi H, Murata M, Moriki T, et al: Substitution of Val for Met at residue 239 of platelet glycoprotein Ib alpha in Japanese patients with platelet-type von Willebrand disease. *Blood* 85:727, 1995.

311. Kunishima S, Heaton DC, Naoe T, et al: De novo mutation of the platelet glycoprotein Ib alpha gene in a patient with pseudo-von Willebrand disease. *Blood Coagul Fibrinolysis* 8:311, 1997.

312. Pincus MR, Carty RP, Miller JL: Structural implications of the substitution of Val for Met at residue 239 in the alpha chain of human platelet glycoprotein Ib. *J Protein Chem* 13:629, 1994.

313. Takahashi H, Nagayama R, Hattori A, Shibata A: Botrocetin- and polybrene-induced platelet aggregation in platelet-type von Willebrand disease. *Am J Hematol* 18:179, 1985.

314. Miller JL, Kupinski JM, Castella A, Ruggeri ZM: von Willebrand factor binds to platelets and induces aggregation in platelet-type but not type IIB von Willebrand disease. *J Clin Invest* 72:1532, 1983.

315. Scott JP, Montgomery RR: The rapid differentiation of type IIb von Willebrand's disease from platelet-type (pseudo) von Willebrand's disease by the ''neutral'' monoclonal antibody binding assay. *Am J Clin Pathol* 96:723, 1991.

316. Miller JL: Sorting out heightened interactions between platelets and von Willebrand factor. ''IIB or not IIB?'' is becoming an increasingly answerable question in the molecular era. *Am J Clin Pathol* 96:681, 1991.

317. Miller JL, Ruggeri ZM, Lyle VA: Unique interactions of asialo von

318. Willebrand factor with platelets in platelet-type von Willebrand disease. *Blood* 70:1804, 1987.

319. Takahashi H: Replacement therapy in pletelet-type von Willebrand disease. *Am J Hematol* 18:351, 1985.

319. Miller JL: Platelet-type von Willebrand's disease. *Clin Lab Med* 4:319, 1984.

320. Fressinaud E, Signaud-Fiks M, Le Boterff C, Piot B: Use of recombinant factor VIIa (NovoSeven®) for dental extraction in a patient affected by platelet-type (pseudo) von Willebrand disease. *Haemophilia* 4:299, 1998.

321. Nieuwenhuis HK, Akkerman JWN, Houdijk WPM, Sixma JJ: Human blood platelets showing no response to collagen fail to express surface glycoprotein Ia. *Nature* 318:470, 1985.

322. Nieuwenhuis HK, Sakariassen KS, Houdijk WPM, Nievelstein PFEM, Sixma JJ: Deficiency of platelet membrane glycoprotein Ia associated with a decreased platelet adhesion to subendothelium: a defect in platelet spreading. *Blood* 68:692, 1986.

323. Beer JH, Nieuwenhuis HK, Sixma JJ, Coller BS: Deficiency of antibody 6F1 binding to the platelets of a patient with an isolated defect in platelet-collagen interaction. *Circulation* (Suppl.)78:II-308, 1988.

324. Coller BS, Beer JH, Scudder LE, Steinberg MH: Collagen-platelet interactions: evidence for a direct interaction of collagen with platelet GPIa/IIa and an indirect interaction with platelet GPIIb/IIa mediated by adhesive proteins. *Blood* 74:182, 1989.

325. Kehrel B, Balleisen L, Kokott R, et al: Deficiency of intact thrombospondin and membrane glycoprotein Ia in platelets with defective collagen-induced aggregation and spontaneous loss of disorder. *Blood* 71:1074, 1988.

326. Clemetson KJ: Platelet collagen receptors: a new target for inhibition? *Haemostasis* 29:16, 1999.

327. Yamamoto N, Ikeda H, Tandon NN, et al: A platelet membrane glycoprotein (GP) deficiency in healthy blood donors: Nak^a-platelets lack detectable GPIV (CD36). *Blood* 76:1698, 1990.

328. Curtis BR, Aster RH: Incidence of the Nak(a)-negative platelet phenotype in African Americans is similar to that of Asians. *Transfusion* 36:331, 1996.

329. Asch AS, Barnwell J, Silverstein RL, Nachman RL: Isolation of the thrombospondin membrane receptor. *J Clin Invest* 79:1054, 1987.

330. Tandon NN, Kralisz U, Jamieson GA: Identification of glycoprotein IV (CD36) as a primary receptor for platelet-collagen adhesion. *J Biol Chem* 264:7576, 1989.

331. Silverstein RL, Asch AS, Nachman RL: Glycoprotein IV mediates thrombospondin-dependent platelet-monocyte and platelet-U937 cell adhesion. *J Clin Invest* 84:546, 1989.

332. Kehrel B, Kronenberg A, Schwippert B, et al: Thrombospondin binds normally to glycoprotein IIIb deficient platelets. *Biochem Biophys Res Commun* 179:985, 1991.

333. Tandon NN, Ockenhouse CF, Greco NJ, Jamieson GA: Adhesive functions of platelets lacking glycoprotein IV (CD36). *Blood* 78:2809, 1991.

334. Saelman EU, Kehrel B, Hese KM, de Groot PG, Sixma JJ, Nieuwenhuis HK: Platelet adhesion to collagen and endothelial cell matrix under flow conditions is not dependent on platelet glycoprotein IV. *Blood* 83:3240, 1994.

335. Kashiwagi H, Tomiyama Y, Honda S, et al: Molecular basis of CD36 deficiency. Evidence that a 478C→T substitution (proline90→serine) in CD36 cDNA accounts for CD36 deficiency. *J Clin Invest* 95:1040, 1995.

336. Kashiwagi H, Tomiyama Y, Kosugi S, et al: Family studies of type II CD36 deficient subjects: linkage of a CD36 allele to a platelet-specific mRNA expression defect(s) causing type II CD36 deficiency. *Thromb Haemost* 74:758, 1995.

337. Kashiwagi H, Tomiyama Y, Kosugi S, et al: Identification of molecular defects in a subject with type I CD36 deficiency. *Blood* 83:3545, 1994.

338. Kashiwagi H, Tomiyama Y, Nozaki S, et al: A single nucleotide insertion in codon 317 of the CD36 gene leads to CD36 deficiency. *Arterioscler Thromb Vasc Biol* 16:1026, 1996.

339. Bierling P, Godeau B, Fromont P, et al: Posttransfusion purpura-like syndrome associated with CD36 (Naka) isoimmunization. *Transfusion* 35:777, 1995.

340. Nozaki S, Tanaka T, Yamashita S, et al: CD36 mediates long-chain fatty acid transport in human myocardium: complete myocardial accumulation defect of radiolabeled long-chain fatty acid analog in subjects with CD36 deficiency. *Mol Cell Biochem* 192:129, 1999.

341. Okamoto F, Tanaka T, Sohmiya K, Kawamura K: CD36 abnormality and impaired myocardial long-chain fatty acid uptake in patients with hypertrophic cardiomyopathy. *Jpn Circ J* 62:499, 1998.

342. Moroi M, Jung SM, Okuma M, Shinmyozu K: A patient with platelets deficient in glycoprotein VI that lack both collagen-induced aggregation and adhesion. *J Clin Invest* 84:1440, 1989.

343. Ryo R, Yoshida A, Sugano W, et al: Deficiency of P62, a putative collagen receptor, in platelets from a patient with defective collagen-induced platelet aggregation. *Am J Hematol* 39:25, 1992.

344. Sugiyama T, Okuma M, Ushikubi F, Sensaki S, Kanaji K, Uchino H: A novel platelet aggregating factor found in a patient with defective collagen-induced platelet aggregation and autoimmune thrombocytopenia. *Blood* 69:1712, 1987.

345. Sullivan KE: Recent advances in our understanding of Wiskott-Aldrich syndrome. *Curr Opin Hematol* 6:8, 1999.

346. Sullivan KE, Mullen CA, Blaese RM, Winkelstein JA: A multiinstitutional survey of the Wiskott-Aldrich syndrome. *J Pediatr* 125:876, 1994.

347. Ochs HD: The Wiskott-Aldrich syndrome. *Springer Semin Immunopathol* 19:435, 1998.

348. Zhu Q, Watanabe C, Liu T, et al: Wiskott-Aldrich syndrome/X-linked thrombocytopenia: WASP gene mutations, protein expression, and phenotype. *Blood* 90:2680, 1997.

349. Parkman R, Remold-O'Donnell E, Kenney DM, Perrine S, Rosen FS: Surface protein abnormalities in lymphocytes and platelets from patients with Wiskott-Aldrich syndrome. *Lancet* 2:1387, 1981.

350. Higgins EA, Siminovitch KA, Zhuang DL, Brockhausen I, Dennis JW: Aberrant *O*-linked oligosaccharide biosynthesis in lymphocytes and platelets from patients with the Wiskott-Aldrich syndrome. *J Biol Chem* 266:6280, 1991.

351. Rosenstein Y, Park JK, Hahn WC, Rosen FS, Bierer BE, Burakoff SJ: CD43, a molecule defective in Wiskott-Aldrich syndrome, binds ICAM-1. *Nature* 354:233, 1991.

352. Semple JW, Siminovitch KA, Mody M, et al: Flow cytometric analysis of platelets from children with the Wiskott-Aldrich syndrome reveals defects in platelet development, activation and structure. *Br J Haemotal* 97:747, 1997.

353. Pidard D, Didry D, Le Deist F, et al: Analysis of the membrane glycoproteins of platelets in the Wiskott-Aldrich syndrome. *Br J Haematol* 69:529, 1988.

354. Grottum KA, Hovig T, Holmsen H, Abrahamsen AF, Jeremic M, Seip M: Wiskott-Aldrich syndrome: qualitative platelet defects and short platelet survival. *Br J Haematol* 17:373, 1969.

355. Murphy S, Oski FA, Naiman JL, Lusch CJ, Goldberg S, Gardner FH: Platelet size and kinetics in hereditary and acquired thrombocytopenia. *N Engl J Med* 286:499, 1972.

356. Baldini MG: Nature of the platelet defect in the Wiskott-Aldrich syndrome. *Ann N Y Acad Sci* 201:437, 1972.

357. Ochs HD, Slichter SJ, Harker LA, Von Behrens WE, Clark RA, Wedgwood RJ: The Wiskott-Aldrich syndrome: studies of lymphocytes, granulocytes, and platelets. *Blood* 55:243, 1980.

358. Litzman J, Jones A, Hann I, Chapel H, Strobel S, Morgan G: Intravenous immunoglobulin, splenectomy, and antibiotic prophylaxis in Wiskott-Aldrich syndrome. *Arch Dis Child* 75:436, 1996.

359. Mullen CA, Anderson KD, Blaese RM: Splenectomy and/or bone marrow transplantation in the management of the Wiskott-Aldrich syndrome: long-term follow-up of 62 cases. *Blood* 82:2961, 1993.

360. Akman IO, Ostrov BE, Neudorf S: Autoimmune manifestations of the Wiskott-Aldrich syndrome. *Semin Arthritis Rheum* 27:218, 1998.

361. Lum LG, Tubergen DG, Corash L, Blaese RM: Splenectomy in the management of the thrombocytopenia of the Wiskott-Aldrich syndrome. *N Engl J Med* 302:892, 1980.

362. Lorenz P, Bollmann R, Hinkel GK, et al: False-negative prenatal exclusion of Wiskott-Aldrich syndrome by measurement of fetal platelet count and size. *Prenat Diagn* 11:819, 1991.

363. Stormorken H, Hellum B, Egeland T, Abrahamsen TG, Hovig T: X-linked thrombocytopenia and thrombocytopathia: attenuated Wiskott-Aldrich syndrome. Functional and morphological studies of platelets and lymphocytes. *Thromb Haemost* 65:300, 1991.

364. Verhoeven AJ, van Oostrum IE, van Haarlem H, Akkerman JW: Impaired energy metabolism in platelets from patients with Wiskott-Aldrich syndrome. *Thromb Haemost* 61:10, 1989.

365. White JG: Inherited abnormalities of the platelet membrane and secretory granules. *Hum Pathol* 18:123, 1987.

366. Weiss HJ, Chervenick PA, Zalusky R, Factor A: A familial defect in platelet function associated with impaired release of adenosine diphosphate. *N Engl J Med* 281:1264, 1969.

367. Nieuwenhuis HK, Akkerman JW, Sixma JJ: Patients with a prolonged bleeding time and normal aggregation tests may have storage pool deficiency: studies on one hundred six patients. *Blood* 70:620, 1987.

368. Weiss HJ: Inherited disorders of platelet granules and signal transduction, in *Hemostasis and Thrombosis: Basic Principles and Clinical Practice,* RW Colman, J Hirsh, VJ Marder, EW Salzman 3rd ed, p 673. Lippincott, Philadelphia, 1993.

369. Hermansky F, Pudlak P: Albinism associated with hemorrhagic diathesis and unusual pigmented reticular cells in the bone marrow: report of two cases with histochemical studies. *Blood* 14:162, 1959.

370. Gahl WA, Brantly M, Kaiser-Kupfer MI, et al: Genetic defects and clinical characteristics of patients with a form of oculocutaneous albinism (Hermansky-Pudlak syndrome). *N Engl J Med* 338:1258, 1998.

371. Buchanan GR, Handin RI: Platelet function in the Chediak-Higashi syndrome. *Blood* 47:941, 1976.

372. Costa JL, Fauci AS, Wolff SM: A platelet abnormality in the Chediak-Higashi syndrome of man. *Blood* 48:517, 1976.

373. Boxer GJ, Holmsen H, Robkin L, et al: Abnormal platelet function in Chediak-Higashi syndrome. *Br J Haematol* 35:521, 1977.

374. Apitz-Castro R, Cruz MR, Ledezma E, et al: The storage pool deficiency in platelets from humans with the Chediak-Higashi syndrome: study of six patients. *Br J Haematol* 59:471, 1985.

375. Gerrard JM, Israels ED, Biship AJ, et al: Inherited platelet-storage pool deficiency associated with a high incidence of acute myeloid leukaemia. *Br J Haematol* 79:246, 1991.

376. Cowan DH, Graham RC Jr., Baunach D: The platelet defect in leukemia. Platelet ultrastructure, adenine nucleotide metabolism, and the release reaction. *J Clin Invest* 56:188, 1975.

377. Gerrard JM, McNicol A: Platelet storage pool deficiency, leukemia, and myelodysplastic syndromes. *Leuk Lymphoma* 8:277, 1992.

378. Nishibori M, Cham B, McNicol A, Shalev A, Jain N, Gerrard JM: The protein CD63 is in platelet dense granules, is deficient in a patient with Hermansky-Pudlak syndrome, and appears identical to granulophysin. *J Clin Invest* 91:1775, 1993.

379. Dell'Angelica EC, Shotelersuk V, Aguilar RC, Gahl WA, Bonifacino JS: Altered trafficking of lysosomal proteins in Hermansky-Pudlak syndrome due to mutations in the beta 3A subunit of the AP-3 adaptor. *Mol Cell* 3:11, 1999.

380. Payne CM: A qualitative ultrastructural evaluation of the cell organelle specificity of the uranaffin reaction to normal human platelets. *Am J Clin Pathol* 31:62, 1984.

381. Weiss HJ, Lages B, Vicic W, et al: Heterogeneous abnormalities of platelet dense granule ultrastructure in 20 patients with congenital storage pool deficiency. *Br J Haematol* 83:282, 1993.

382. White RA, Peters LL, Adkison LR, Korsgren C, Cohen CM, Lux SE: The murine pallid mutation is a platelet storage pool disease associated with the protein 4.2 (pallidin) gene. *Nat Genet* 2:80, 1992.

383. Swank RT, Novak EK, McGarry MP, Rusiniak ME, Feng L: Mouse models of Hermansky Pudlak syndrome: a review. *Pigment Cell Res* 11:60, 1998.

384. Shotelersuk V, Gahl WA: Hermansky-Pudlak syndrome: models for intracellular vesicle formation. *Mol Genet Metab* 65:85, 1998.

385. Zhen L, Jiang S, Feng L, et al: Abnormal expression and subcellular distribution of subunit proteins of the AP-3 adaptor complex lead to platelet storage pool deficiency in the pearl mouse. *Blood* 94:146, 1999.

386. Spritz RA: Genetic defects in Chediak-Higashi syndrome and the beige mouse. *J Clin Immunol* 18:97, 1998.

387. Hardisty RM, Mills DC, Ketsa-Ard K: The platelet defect associated with albinism. *Br J Haematol* 23:679, 1972.

388. Pareti FI, Day HJ, Mills DC: Nucleotide and serotonin metabolism in platelets with defective secondary aggregation. *Blood* 44:789, 1974.

389. Holmsen H, Weiss HJ: Hereditary defect in the platelet release reaction caused by a deficiency in the storage pool of platelet adenine nucleotides. *Br J Haematol* 19:643, 1970.

390. White JG, Witkop CJ: Studies of platelets in a variant of the Hermansky-Pudlak syndrome. *Am J Pathol* 63:319, 1971.

391. Holmsen H, Weiss HJ: Further evidence for a deficient storage pool of

adenine nucleotides in platelets from some patients with thrombocyto-pathia—"storage pool disease." *Blood* 39:197, 1972.

392. Akkerman JW, Nieuwenhuis HK, Mommersteeg-Leautaud ME, Gorter G, Sixma JJ: ATP-ADP compartmentation in storage pool deficient platelets: correlation between granule-bound ADP and the bleeding time. *Br J Haematol* 55:135, 1983.

393. Weiss HJ, Tschopp TB, Rogers J, Brand H: Studies of platelet 5-hydroxytryptamine (serotonin) in storage pool disease and albinism. *J Clin Invest* 54:421, 1974.

394. Willis AL, Weiss HJ: A congenital defect in platelet prostaglandin production associated with impaired hemostasis in storage pool disease. *Prostaglandins* 4:783, 1973.

395. Holmsen H, Setkowsky CA, Lages B, Day HJ, Weiss HJ, Scrutton MC: Content and thrombin-induced release of acid hydrolases in gel-filtered platelets from patients with storage pool disease. *Blood* 46:131, 1975.

396. Weiss HJ, Lages B: Platelet malondialdehyde production and aggrega-tion responses induced by arachidonate, prostaglandin-G2, collagen, and epinephrine in 12 patients with storage pool deficiency. *Blood* 58:27, 1981.

397. Witkop CJ, Jr., Bowie EJ, Krumwiede MD, Swanson JL, Plumhoff EA, White JG: Synergistic effect of storage pool deficient platelets and low plasma von Willebrand factor on the severity of the hemorrhagic diathe-sis in Hermansky-Pudlak syndrome. *Am J Hematol* 44:256, 1993.

398. McKeown LP, Hansmann KE, Wilson O, et al: Platelet von Willebrand factor in Hermansky-Pudlak syndrome. *Am J Hematol* 59:115, 1998.

399. Israels SJ, McNicol A, Robertson C, Gerrard JM: Platelet storage pool deficiency: diagnosis in patients with prolonged bleeding times and normal platelet aggregation. *Br J Haematol* 75:118, 1990.

400. Witkop CJ, Krumwiede M, Sedano H, White JG: Reliability of absent platelet dense bodies as a diagnostic criterion for Hermansky-Pudlak syndrome. *Am J Hematol* 26:305, 1987.

401. Weiss HJ, Ames RP: Ultrastructural findings in storage-pool disease and aspirin-like defects in platelets. *Am J Pathol* 71:447, 1973.

402. Richards JG, DaPrada M: Uranaffin reaction: a new cytochemical tech-nique for the localization of adenine nucleotides in organelles storing biogenic amines. *J Histochem Cytochem* 25:1322, 1977.

403. Lorez HP, Richards JG, Da Prada M, et al: Storage pool disease: compar-ative fluorescence microscopical, cytochemical and biochemical studies on amine-storing organelles of human blood platelets. *Br J Haematol* 43:297, 1979.

404. Mielke CH Jr., Levine PH, Zucker S: Preoperative prednisone therapy in platelet function disorders. *Thromb Res* 21:655, 1981.

405. Kobrinsky NL, Israels ED, Gerrard JM, et al: Shortening of bleeding time by 1-deamino-8-D-arginine vasopressin in various bleeding disorders. *Lancet* 1:1145, 1984.

406. Nieuwenhuis HK, Sixma JJ: 1-Desamino-8-D-arginine vasopressin (des-mopressin) shortens the bleeding time in storage pool deficiency. *Ann Intern Med* 108:65, 1988.

407. Wijermans PW, van Dorp DB: Hermansky-Pudlak syndrome: correction of bleeding time by 1-desamino-8D-arginine vasopressin. *Am J Hematol* 30:154, 1989.

408. Van Dorp DB, Wijermans PW, Meire F, Vrensen G: The Hermansky-Pudlak syndrome. Variable reaction to 1-desamino-8D-arginine vaso-pressin for correction of the bleeding time. *Ophthal Paediatr Genet* 11:237, 1990.

409. Castaman G, Rodeghiero F: Consistency of responses to separate desmo-pressin infusion in patients with storage pool disease and isolated pro-longed bleeding time. *Thromb Res* 69:407, 1993.

410. Gerritsen SW, Akkerman JW, Sixma JJ: Correction of the bleeding time in patients with storage pool deficiency by infusion of cryoprecipitate. *Br J Haematol* 40:153, 1978.

411. Coller BS, Hirschman RJ, Gralnick HR: Studies of the factor VIII/von Willebrand factor antigen on human platelets. *Thromb Res* 6:469, 1975.

412. George JN, Pickett EB, Heinz R: Platelet membrane microparticles in blood bank fresh frozen plasma and cryoprecipitate. *Blood* 68:307, 1986.

413. Raccuglia G: Gray platelet syndrome. A variety of qualitative platelet disorder. *Am J Med* 51:818, 1971.

414. Gerrard JM, Phillips DR, Rao GH, et al: Biochemical studies of two patients with the gray platelet syndrome. Selective deficiency of platelet alpha granules. *J Clin Invest* 66:102, 1980.

415. Levy-Toledano S, Caen JP, Breton-Gorius J, et al: Gray platelet syn-

416. Nurden AT, Kunicki TJ, Dupuis D, Soria C, Caen JP: Specific protein and glycoprotein deficiencies in platelets isolated from two patients with the gray platelet syndrome. *Blood* 59:709, 1982.

417. Coller BS, Hultin MB, Nurden AT: Isolated alpha-granule deficiency (gray platelet syndrome) with slight increase in bone marrow reticulin and possible glycoprotein and/or protease defect. *Thromb Haemost* 50:211, 1983.

418. Kohler M, Hellstern P, Morgenstern E, et al: Gray platelet syndrome: selective alpha-granule deficiency and thrombocytopenia due to in-creased platelet turnover. *Blut* 50:331, 1985.

419. Berndt MC, Castaldi PA, Gordon S, Halley H, McPherson VJ: Morpho-logical and biochemical confirmation of gray platelet syndrome in two siblings. *Aust N Z J Med* 13:387, 1983.

420. Gootenberg JE, Buchanan GR, Holtkamp CA, Casey CS: Severe hemor-rhage in a patient with gray platelet syndrome. *J Pediatr* 109:1017, 1986.

421. Srivastava PC, Powling MJ, Nokes TJ, Patrick AD, Dawes J, Hardisty RM: Grey platelet syndrome: studies on platelet alpha-granules, lyso-somes and defective response to thrombin. *Br J Haematol* 65:441, 1987.

422. Berrebi A, Klepfish A, Varon D, et al: Gray platelet syndrome in the elderly. *Am J Hematol* 28:270, 1988.

423. Wills EJ: Gray platelet syndrome. *Ultrastruct Pathol* 13:451, 1989.

424. Facon T, Goudemand J, Caron C, et al: Simultaneous occurrence of grey platelet syndrome and idiopathic pulmonary fibrosis: a role for abnormal megakaryocytes in the pathogenesis of pulmonary fibrosis? *Br J Haematol* 74:542, 1990.

425. Lages B, Sussman II, Levine SP, Coletti D, Weiss HJ: Platelet alpha granule deficiency associated with decreased P-selectin and selective impairment of thrombin-induced activation in a new patient with gray platelet syndrome (alpha-storage pool deficiency). *J Lab Clin Med* 129:364, 1997.

426. Martinez-Murillo C, Payns BE, Arzate HG, et al: Gray-platelet syndrome associated with Marfan disease in a Mexican family. *Sangre (Barc)* 39:287, 1994.

427. Jantunen E, Hanninen A, Naukkarinen A, Vornanen M, Lahtinen R: Gray platelet syndrome with splenomegaly and signs of extramedullary hematopoiesis: a case report with review of the literature. *Am J Hematol* 46:218, 1994.

428. Mori K, Suzuki S, Sugai K: Electron microscopic and functional studies on platelets in gray platelet syndrome. *Tohoku J Exp Med* 143:261, 1984.

429. Berger G, Masse JM, Cramer EM: Alpha-granule membrane mirrors the platelet plasma membrane and contains the glycoproteins Ib, IX, and V. *Blood* 87:1385, 1996.

430. Rosa JP, George JN, Bainton DF, Nurden AT, Caen JP, McEver RP: Gray platelet syndrome. Demonstration of alpha granule membranes that can fuse with the cell surface. *J Clin Invest* 80:1138, 1987.

431. Cramer EM, Vainchenker W, Vinci G, Guichard J, Breton-Gorius J: Gray platelet syndrome: immunoelectron microscopic localization of fibrinogen and von Willebrand factor in platelets and megakaryocytes. *Blood* 66:1309, 1985.

432. Caen JP, Deschamps JF, Bodevin E, Bryckaert MC, Dupuy E, Wasteson A: Megakaryocytes and myelofibrosis in gray platelet syndrome. *Nouv Rev Fr Hematol* 29:109, 1987.

433. Wencel-Drake JD: Plasma membrane GPIIb/IIIa. Evidence for a cycling receptor pool. *Am J Clin Pathol* 136:61, 1990.

434. Greenberg-Sepersky SM, Simons ER, White JG: Studies of platelets from patients with the grey platelet syndrome. *Br J Haematol* 59:603, 1985.

435. Rendu F, Marche P, Hovig T, et al: Abnormal phosphoinositide metabo-lism and protein phosphorylation in platelets from a patient with the grey platelet syndrome. *Br J Haematol* 67:199, 1987.

436. Baruch D, Lindhout T, Dupuy E, Caen JP: Thrombin-induced platelet factor Va formation in patients with a gray platelet syndrome. *Thromb Haemost* 58:768, 1987.

437. Enouf J, Lebret M, Bredoux R, Levy-Toledano S, Caen JP: Abnormal calcium transport into microsomes of grey platelet syndrome. *Br J Haematol* 65:437, 1987.

438. Cockbill SR, Burmester HB, Heptinstall S: Pseudo grey platelet syn-drome—grey platelets due to degranulation in blood collected into EDTA. *Eur J Haematol* 41:326, 1988.

439. Pfueller SL, Howard MA, White JG, Menon C, Berry EW: Shortening

of bleeding time by 1-deamino-8-arginine vasopressin (DDAVP) in the absence of platelet von Willebrand factor in Gray platelet syndrome. *Thromb Haemost* 58:1060, 1987.

440. Weiss HJ, Witte LD, Kaplan KL, et al: Heterogeneity in storage pool deficiency: studies on granule-bound substances in 18 patients including variants deficient in alpha- granules, platelet factor 4, beta-thromboglobulin, and platelet-derived growth factor. *Blood* 54:1296, 1979.

441. Lages B, Shattil SJ, Bainton DF, Weiss HJ: Decreased content and surface expression of alpha-granule membrane protein GMP-140 in one of two types of platelet alpha delta storage pool deficiency. *J Clin Invest* 87:919, 1991.

442. Weiss HJ, Lages B: The response of platelets to epinephrine in storage pool deficiency-Evidence pertaining to the role of adenosine diphosphate in mediating primary and secondary aggregation. *Blood* 72:1717, 1988.

443. Jamieson GA, Okumura T, Fishback B, et al: Platelet membrane glycoproteins in thrombasthenia, Bernard-Soulier syndrome, and storage pool disease. *J Lab Clin Med* 93:652, 1979.

444. Tracy PB, Giles AR, Mann KG, Eide LL, Hoogendoorn H, Rivard GE: Factor V (Quebec): a bleeding diathesis associated with a qualitative platelet factor V deficiency. *J Clin Invest* 74:1221, 1984.

445. Janeway CM, Rivard GE, Tracy PB, Mann KG: Factor V Quebec revisited. *Blood* 87:3571, 1996.

446. Hayward CP, Rivard GE, Kane WH, et al: An autosomal dominant, qualitative platelet disorder associated with multimerin deficiency, abnormalities in platelet factor V, thrombospondin, von Willebrand factor, and fibrinogen and an epinephrine aggregation defect. *Blood* 87:4967, 1996.

447. Weiss HJ, Vicic WJ, Lages BA, Rogers J: Isolated deficiency of platelet procoagulant activity. *Am J Med* 67:206, 1979.

448. Weiss HJ: Scott syndrome—a disorder of platelet coagulant activity. *Sem Hematol* 31:312, 1994.

449. Toti F, Satta N, Fressinaud E, Meyer D, Freyssinet JM: Scott syndrome, characterized by impaired transmembrane migration of procoagulant phosphatidylserine and hemorrhagic complications, is an inherited disorder. *Blood* 87:1409, 1996.

450. Weiss HJ, Lages B: Platelet prothrombinase activity and intracellular calcium responses in patients with storage pool deficiency, glycoprotein IIb-IIIa deficiency, or impaired platelet coagulant activity—a comparison with Scott syndrome. *Blood* 89:1599, 1997.

451. Dachary-Prigent J, Pasquet JM, Fressinaud E, Toti F, Freyssinet JM, Nurden AT: Aminophospholipid exposure, microvesiculation and abnormal protein tyrosine phosphorylation in the platelets of a patient with Scott syndrome: a study using physiologic agonists and local anaesthetics. *Br J Haematol* 99:959, 1997.

452. Sims PJ, Wiedmer T, Esmon CT, et al: Assembly of the platelet prothrombinase complex is linked to vesiculation on the platelet plasma membrane. Studies in Scott syndrome: an isolated defect in platelet procoagulant activity. *J Biol Chem* 264:137, 1989.

453. Miletich JP, Kane WH, Hofmann SL, Stanford N, Majerus PW: Deficiency of factor Xa-factor Va binding sites on the platelets of a patient with a bleeding disorder. *Blood* 54:1015, 1979.

454. Rosing J, Bevers EM, Comfurius P, et al: Impaired factor X and prothrombin activation associated with decreased phospholipid exposure in platelets from a patient with a bleeding disorder. *Blood* 65:1557, 1985.

455. Ahmad SS, Rawala-Sheikh R, Ashby B, Walsh PN: Platelet receptor-mediated factor X activation by factor IXa. High-affinity factor IXa receptors induced by factor VIII are deficient on platelets in Scott syndrome. *J Clin Invest* 84:824, 1989.

456. Bevers EM, Wiedmer T, Comfurius P, et al: Defective Ca(2+)-induced microvesiculation and deficient expression of procoagulant activity in erythrocytes from a patient with a bleeding disorder: a study of the red blood cells of Scott syndrome. *Blood* 79:380, 1992.

457. Kojima H, Newton-Nash D, Weiss HJ, Zhao J, Sims PJ, Wiedmer T: Production and characterization of transformed B-lymphocytes expressing the membrane defect of Scott syndrome. *J Clin Invest* 94:2237, 1994.

458. Weiss HJ: Platelet aggregation, adhesion and adenosine diphosphate release in thrombopathia (platelet factor 3 deficiency). A comparison with Glanzmann's thrombasthenia and von Willebrand's disease. *Am J Med* 43:570, 1967.

459. Zhou Q, Sims PJ, Wiedmer T: Expression of proteins controlling transbilayer movement of plasma membrane phospholipids in the B lymphocytes from a patient with Scott syndrome. *Blood* 92:1707, 1998.

460. Rao AK: Congenital disorders of platelet function: disorders of signal transduction and secretion. *Am J Med Sci* 316:69, 1998.

461. Hirata T, Kakizuka A, Ushikubi F, Fuse I, Okuma M, Narumiya S: Arg60 to Leu mutation of the human thromboxane A2 receptor in a dominantly inherited bleeding disorder. *J Clin Invest* 94:1662, 1994.

462. Cattaneo M, Lecchi A, Randi AM, McGregor JL, Mannucci PM: Identification of a new congenital defect of platelet function characterized by severe impairment of platelet responses to adenosine diphosphate. *Blood* 80:2787, 1992.

463. Cattaneo M, Lombardi R, Zighetti ML, et al: Deficiency of (33P)2MeS-ADP binding sites on platelets with secretion defect, normal granule stores and normal thromboxane A2 production. Evidence that ADP potentiates platelet secretion independently of the formation of large platelet aggregates and thromboxane A2 production. *Thromb Haemost* 77:986, 1997.

464. Nurden P, Savi P, Heilmann E, et al: An inherited bleeding disorder linked to a defective interaction between ADP and its receptor on platelets. Its influence on glycoprotein IIb-IIIa complex function. *J Clin Invest* 95:1612, 1995.

465. Scrutton MC, Clare KA, Hutton RA, Bruckdorfer KR: Depressed responsiveness to adrenaline in platelets from apparently normal human donors: a familial trait. *Br J Haematol* 49:303, 1981.

466. Tamponi G, Pannocchia A, Arduino C, et al: Congenital deficiency of alpha-2-adrenoceptors on human platelets: description of two cases. *Thromb Haemost* 58:1012, 1987.

467. Rao AK, Willis J, Kowalska MA, Wachtfogel YT, Colman RW: Differential requirements for platelet aggregation and inhibition of adenylate cyclase by epinephrine. Studies of a familial platelet alpha 2-adrenergic receptor defect. *Blood* 71:494, 1988.

468. Pelczar-Wissner CJ, McDonald EG, Sussman II: Absence of platelet activating factor (PAF) mediated platelet aggregation: a new platelet defect. *Am J Hematol* 16:419, 1984.

469. Wu KK: Bleeding disorders due to abnormalities in platelet prostaglandins, in *Prostaglandins in Clinical Medicine,* edited by KK Wu, EC Rossi, p 81. Year Book, Chicago, 1982.

470. Rao AK: Congenital disorders of platelet function. *Hematol Oncol Clin North Am* 4:65, 1990.

471. Rendu F, Breton-Gorius J, Trugnan G, et al: Studies on a new variant of the Hermansky-Pudlak syndrome: qualitative, ultrastructural, and functional abnormalities of the platelet-dense bodies associated with a phospholipase A defect. *Am J Hematol* 4:387, 1978.

472. Holmsen H, Walsh PN, Koike K, et al: Familial bleeding disorder associated with deficiencies in platelet signal processing and glycoproteins. *Br J Haematol* 67:335, 1987.

473. Malmsten C, Hamberg M, Svensson J, Samuelsson B: Physiological role of an endoperoxide in human platelets: hemostatic defect due to platelet cyclo-oxygenase deficiency. *Proc Natl Acad Sci USA* 72:1446, 1975.

474. Lagarde M, Byron PA, Vargaftig BB, Dechavanne M: Impairment of platelet thromboxane A2 generation and of the platelet release reaction in two patients with congenital deficiency of platelet cyclo-oxygenase. *Br J Haematol* 38:251, 1978.

475. Pareti FI, Mannucci PM, D'Angelo A, Smith JB, Sautebin L, Galli G: Congenital deficiency of thromboxane and prostacyclin. *Lancet* 1:898, 1980.

476. Rak K, Boda Z: Haemostatic balance in congenital deficiency of platelet cyclo-oxygenase. *Lancet* 2:44, 1980.

477. Horellou MH, Lecompte T, Lecrubier C, et al: Familial and constitutional bleeding disorder due to platelet cyclo-oxygenase deficiency. *Am J Hematol* 14:1, 1983.

478. Rao AK, Koike K, Day HJ, Smith JB, Holmsen H: Bleeding disorder associated with albumin-dependent partial deficiency in platelet thromboxane production. Effect of albumin on arachidonate metabolism in platelets. *Am J Clin Pathol* 83:687, 1985.

479. Defreyn G, Machin SJ, Carreras LO, Dauden MV, Chamone DA, Vermylen J: Familial bleeding tendency with partial platelet thromboxane synthetase deficiency: reorientation of cyclic endoperoxide metabolism. *Br J Haematol* 49:29, 1981.

480. Mestel F, Oetliker O, Beck E, Felix R, Imbach P, Wagner HP: Severe bleeding associated with defective thromboxane synthetase. *Lancet* 1:157, 1980.

481. Wu KK, Minkoff IM, Rossi EC, Chen YC: Hereditary bleeding disorder

due to a primary defect in platelet release reaction. *Br J Haematol* 47:241, 1981.

482. Wu KK, Le Breton GC, Tai HH, Chen YC: Abnormal platelet response to thromboxane A2. *J Clin Invest* 67:1801, 1981.

483. Lages B, Malmsten C, Weiss HJ, Samuelsson B: Impaired platelet response to thromboxane-A2 and defective calcium mobilization in a patient with a bleeding disorder. *Blood* 57:545, 1981.

484. White JG: Structural defects in inherited and giant platelet disorders. *Adv Hum Genet* 19:133, 1990.

485. Samama M, Lecrubier C, Conard J, et al: Constitutional thrombocytopathy with subnormal response to thromboxane A2. *Br J Haematol* 48:293, 1981.

486. Lages B, Weiss HJ: Heterogeneous defects of platelet secretion and responses to weak agonists in patients with bleeding disorders. *Br J Haematol* 68:53, 1988.

487. Lages B, Weiss HJ: Impairment of phosphatidylinositol metabolism in a patient with a bleeding disorder associated with defects of initial platelet responses. *Thromb Haemost* 59:175, 1988.

488. Rao AK, Kowalska MA, Disa J: Impaired cytoplasmic ionized calcium mobilization in inherited platelet secretion defects. *Blood* 74:664, 1989.

489. Yang X, Sun L, Ghosh S, Rao AK: Human platelet signaling defect characterized by impaired production of inositol-1,4,5-triphosphate and phosphatidic acid and diminished Pleckstrin phosphorylation: evidence for defective phospholipase C activation. *Blood* 88:1676, 1996.

490. Lee SB, Rao AK, Lee KH, Yang X, Bae YS, Rhee SG: Decreased expression of phospholipase C-beta 2 isozyme in human platelets with impaired function. *Blood* 88:1684, 1996.

491. Gabbeta J, Yang X, Kowalska MA, Sun L, Dhanasekaran N, Rao AK: Platelet signal transduction defect with Galpha subunit dysfunction and diminished Galphaq in a patient with abnormal platelet responses. *Proc Natl Acad Sci USA* 94:8750, 1997.

492. Offermanns S, Toombs CF, Hu YH, Simon MI: Defective platelet activation in G alpha(q)-deficient mice. *Nature* 389:183, 1997.

493. Coller BS: Inherited disorders of platelet function, in *Hemostasis and Thrombosis,* edited by AL Bloom, CD Forbes, DP Thomas, EGD Tuddenham, p 721. Churchill Livingstone, Edinburgh, 1992.

494. Clemetson JM, Kyrle PA, Brenner B, Clemetson KJ: Variant Bernard-Soulier syndrome associated with a homozygous mutation in the leucine-rich domain of glycoprotein IX. *Blood* 84:1124, 1994.

495. Noda M, Fujimura K, Takafuta T, et al: A point mutation in glycoprotein IX coding sequence (Cys73(TGT) to Tyr (TAT)) causes impaired surface expression of GPIb-IX-V complex in two families with Bernard-Soulier syndrome. *Thromb Haemost* 6:874, 1996.

ACQUIRED QUALITATIVE PLATELET DISORDERS DUE TO DISEASES, DRUGS, AND FOODS

SANFORD J. SHATTIL

CHARLES S. ABRAMS

JOEL S. BENNETT

Acquired qualitative platelet disorders are frequent causes of abnormal platelet function in vitro, prolonged bleeding times, and occasionally mild bleeding diatheses. However, their clinical importance increases in the presence of thrombocytopenia or additional disorders of hemostasis. Acquired disorders of platelet function can be conveniently classified into those that result from systemic diseases, hematologic diseases, and the effect of drugs. Of the systemic diseases, renal failure is most prominently associated with abnormal platelet function due to the retention of platelet inhibitory compounds. Platelet function may also be abnormal in the presence of antiplatelet antibodies, following cardiopulmonary bypass, and in association with liver disease or disseminated intravascular coagulation. Hematologic diseases associated with abnormal platelet function include marrow processes in which platelets may be intrinsically abnormal, such as the myeloproliferative disorders, acute and chronic leukemias, and myelodysplastic syndromes; dysproteinemias in which abnormal plasma proteins can impair platelet function; and acquired forms of von Willebrand disease. Drugs are the most frequent cause of acquired qualitative platelet dysfunction. Aspirin is the most notable drug in this regard because of its frequent use, its irreversible effect on platelet prostaglandin synthesis, and its documented effect on hemostatic competency, although this effect is minimal in normal individuals. Other nonsteroidal anti-inflammatory drugs reversibly inhibit platelet prostaglandin synthesis and usually have little effect on hemostasis. The antiplatelet effect of a number of drugs has proven useful in preventing arterial thrombosis, but, as would be anticipated, excessive bleeding can be a complication of their use. In addition to aspirin, these drugs include the thienopyridines ticlopidine and clopidogrel, which primarily antagonize ADP-stimulated platelet aggregation, and drugs that specifically inhibit the platelet glycoprotein (GP) IIb/IIIa receptor. Other drugs used to treat thrombosis, such as heparin and fibrinolytic agents,

can also impair platelet function in vitro and ex vivo, but the clinical significance of these observations is uncertain. High doses of the β-lactam antibiotics can impair platelet function in vitro and prolong the bleeding time, while clinically significant bleeding is unusual in the absence of a coexisting hemostatic defect. Similarly, a number of miscellaneous drugs, including a variety of psychotropic, chemotherapeutic, and anesthetic agents, as well as a number of foods and food additives, have been reported to affect platelet function in vitro, but these effects do not appear to be of clinical significance.

Platelet function may be adversely affected by drugs and by hematologic and nonhematologic disorders. Because the use of aspirin and other nonsteroidal anti-inflammatory agents is pervasive in our society, acquired platelet dysfunction is much more frequent than inherited platelet dysfunction. Acquired disorders of platelet function can be classified according to the underlying clinical condition with which they are associated (Table 120-1).

It is important to have a balanced view of the clinical significance of these disorders. On the one hand, their severity is usually mild. On the other hand, there are important exceptions to this rule, particularly when platelet dysfunction is associated with other hemostatic defects. If the patient does not present with a history of bleeding, it may be difficult to predict the risk of future bleeding. This is not surprising, since even patients with thrombocytopenia may experience little or no spontaneous bleeding until their platelet count is less than $10,000/\mu l$. Furthermore, clinical assessment of these disorders is made problematic by difficulties in standardization and interpretation of the two most frequently used laboratory tests of platelet function: the bleeding time and platelet aggregometry. These tests appear more useful in diagnosing platelet dysfunction than in predicting the risk of bleeding.[1,2]

SYSTEMIC DISORDERS ASSOCIATED WITH ABNORMAL PLATELET FUNCTION

UREMIA

DEFINITION AND HISTORY

Bleeding may be a serious complication of acute and chronic renal failure.[3] In the predialysis era, hemorrhage was a cause of morbidity in approximately 50 percent of uremic patients and a cause of death in approximately 30 percent.[4] Spontaneous bleeding in patients with renal failure can involve the skin and the gastrointestinal and genitourinary tracts.[5] Bleeding into the central nervous system (e.g., subdural hematoma or subarachnoid hemorrhage), pericardial and pleural spaces, anterior chamber of the eye, retroperitoneum, or internal organs is less common. Gastrointestinal hemorrhage is common in patients with acute renal failure, and patients with chronic renal failure account for a significant proportion of patients requiring endoscopy for upper gastrointestinal bleeding.[6] It is noteworthy, however, that 90 percent of patients with renal failure and gastrointestinal bleeding have an anatomic diagnosis at endoscopy, most commonly angiodysplasia or peptic ulceration. Rectal ulcers in uremic individuals can cause sudden and massive lower gastrointestinal hemorrhage.

With the advent of dialysis, the frequency of severe, spontaneous hemorrhage has decreased. Experience with percutaneous renal biopsy in several thousand patients with renal disease supports the notion that the hemostatic defect in patients with renal disease is usually mild. Although the incidence of small perirenal hematomas following biopsy may be as high as 85 percent when patients are examined by computed tomography, gross hematuria is observed in only 5 to 10

TABLE 120-1   ACQUIRED QUALITATIVE PLATELET DISORDERS

Systemic Disorders Associated with Abnormal Platelet Function
  Uremia
  Antiplatelet antibodies
  Cardiopulmonary bypass
  Liver disease
  Disseminated intravascular coagulation
Hematologic Disorders Associated with Abnormal Platelet Function
  Chronic myeloproliferative disorders
  Leukemias and myelodysplastic syndromes
  Dysproteinemias
  Acquired von Willebrand disease
Drugs That Affect Platelet Function
  Nonsteroidal anti-inflammatory drugs
  Antibiotics
  Thienopyridines (ticlopidine and clopidogrel)
  GPIIb/IIIa receptor antagonists
  Drugs that increase platelet cyclic AMP
  Anticoagulants and fibrinolytic agents
  Cardiovascular drugs
  Volume expanders
  Psychotropic agents and anesthetics
  Oncologic drugs
  Foods and food additives

percent of cases and is usually transient.[7,8] Severe bleeding following biopsy requiring surgical intervention is even less common and usually can be attributed to factors other than a uremic hemostatic defect, such as needle lacerations of the kidney or spleen, anomalous vessels, heparin anticoagulation, or the presence of amyloid in the kidney.

ETIOLOGY AND PATHOGENESIS

The hemostatic defect in uremia has been attributed to abnormal platelet function.[5] Defects in every phase of platelet function—adhesion, aggregation, and procoagulant activity—have been reported in uremia. Adhesion of platelets to subendothelial tissues is defective in uremia.[9–11] In theory, an adhesion defect might be caused by factors in the circulating blood, by defects intrinsic to the platelet, or by abnormalities of the vessel wall. One major factor is anemia. In patients with renal disease, the severity of anemia correlates with the severity of renal failure.[12] In an ex vivo perfusion system, a lowered hematocrit causes a platelet adhesion defect that can be corrected by increasing the hematocrit to ≥ 30 percent.[9] Furthermore, in uremic patients, successful treatment of anemia with red blood cell transfusion or recombinant human erythropoietin results in partial or complete correction of the bleeding time.[13] This "beneficial" effect is seen when the hematocrit is corrected to the level of 27 to 32 percent.[5,14–17] The influence of red blood cells on primary hemostasis is not unique to uremia. In normal individuals, the bleeding time correlates with the hematocrit even though both sets of values are in the normal range.[18] Furthermore, bleeding times can be prolonged in patients with severe anemia of any etiology.[18,19] This effect of red cells may be explained, in part, on rheological grounds, inasmuch as they displace platelets to the periphery of a column of circulating blood.[20] In addition, red cells have been found to enhance the reactivity of platelets in vitro.[21] Thus, anemia appears to play a significant role in the platelet adhesion defect and in the prolonged bleeding times of uremic individuals.

Since correction of anemia does not return the bleeding time to normal in all uremic individuals, there are likely other factors that impair platelet adhesion.[9] Normal platelet adhesion requires initial platelet contact followed by platelet spreading upon the subendothelial matrix. At high shear rates, such as those found in the capillary circulation, contact is dependent on the binding of von Willebrand factor (vWf) to the platelet GPIb-IX complex.[22,23] This interaction is also necessary for ristocetin-induced platelet aggregation in vitro. Since

the latter may be decreased in uremia, it has been suggested that uremia is associated with a quantitative or qualitative abnormality of vWf or GPIb-IX. However, vWf levels in plasma, measured either immunologically or functionally by ristocetin cofactor activity, are normal or elevated in renal failure,[24] and qualitative abnormalities of vWf have not been uniformly observed.[10,25,26] Moreover, studies in which uremic platelets were mixed with normal plasma or normal platelets were mixed with uremic plasma have failed to demonstrate consistent quantitative or qualitative abnormalities in GPIb-IX.[10,26,27]

On the other hand, uremic plasma can inhibit platelet adhesion to everted, de-endothelialized human umbilical artery segments, while uremic platelets adhere normally in the presence of normal plasma. High levels of vWf present in uremic plasma could compensate for this relative adhesion defect.[10] The component of uremic plasma responsible for this defect remains to be identified. In another perfusion system using rabbit vessels, uremic platelets exhibited markedly reduced spreading on the subendothelium, attributed to impaired interaction of vWf with platelet GPIIb/IIIa.[28] Since vWf can bind to GPIIb/IIIa only after platelet activation, this suggests that platelet activation may be defective in uremia.

A number of observations support the existence of a "platelet activation defect" in uremia. For example, uremic platelets exhibit reduced fibrinogen binding, aggregation, and secretion in response to a variety of agonists. This abnormality may be retained by platelets after their separation from uremic plasma, and in some cases uremic plasma has been shown to impart the defect to normal platelets.[29] The ability of activated platelets to provide a procoagulant surface for the generation of activated factor X and thrombin (referred to in the past as platelet factor 3) is consistently reduced in uremia.[30] Uremic platelets may also exhibit a reduction in several of the biochemical responses necessary for aggregation, secretion, and procoagulant activity, including a rise in cytoplasmic free calcium levels,[31] release of arachidonic acid from platelet phospholipids,[4] and conversion of arachidonic acid to prostaglandin endoperoxides and thromboxane A_2.[32–34] A decrease in the dense-granule content of ADP and serotonin has been observed in uremia,[35] as has an increase in the level of cyclic AMP.[36] Since ADP and serotonin are platelet agonists and cyclic AMP is an inhibitor of platelet function, decreased platelet ADP and serotonin stores could contribute to an activation defect.

The cause of the platelet activation defects in uremia remains to be defined. Both dialyzable and nondialyzable substances in uremic plasma may be responsible. For example, platelet aggregation in vitro can be inhibited by small dialyzable substances, such as guanidinosuccinic acid and phenolic acids, and by poorly characterized "middle molecules" at concentrations found in uremic plasma.[37] Reduced ex vivo aggregation responses may improve after the patient is placed on dialysis.[38,39] However, venous and arterial segments from uremic patients produce more prostacyclin than their normal counterparts, and this is not corrected by dialysis.[40,41] Moreover, in a rat model of uremia, prolonged bleeding times were normalized by treatment with an inhibitor of nitric oxide formation,[42] suggesting that this inhibitor of platelet function, which is produced and released from endothelial cells, is responsible, at least in part, for the defect in uremic platelets.[43] Some substances found in high concentrations in uremic plasma, such as urea and parathyroid hormone, appear to play no role in the platelet dysfunction.

Two additional factors should be considered when a patient with renal failure exhibits a bleeding tendency: concurrent medications and thrombocytopenia. Aspirin can prolong the bleeding time inordinately in uremia. It is surprising to note that, unlike the effect of aspirin on cyclooxygenase, this effect is transient and correlates with blood levels of aspirin.[44,45] Bleeding in uremia may be potentiated by the administration of heparin during hemodialysis. In these cases, the use of an ethylene–vinyl alcohol copolymer hollow-fiber dialyzer or intermittent saline infusion and high blood flow rates may eliminate the need for heparin.[3] Beta-lactam antibiotics that prolong the bleeding time may have a greater effect in uremic patients and increase the occurrence of bleeding, particularly if renal clearance of the antibiotic is reduced.[46]

Mild thrombocytopenia has been reported in chronic renal failure due to both diminished marrow production and platelet survival.[47] Although a slight reduction in the number of normal platelets would not be expected to prolong the bleeding time, the mean platelet volume may also be decreased in uremia. This decreases the "circulating platelet mass" (platelet count × mean platelet volume). It is of interest, therefore, that the circulating platelet mass is inversely related to the bleeding time in uremic individuals.[48] A platelet count below $100 \times 10^5/\mu l$ should alert the physician that the renal failure may be due to a systemic disease or medication that can also cause thrombocytopenia, such as multiple myeloma, systemic vasculitis, hemolytic-uremic syndrome, eclampsia, renal allograft rejection, or heparin.

CLINICAL AND LABORATORY FEATURES

Although a lesser problem than in the past, abnormal platelet function in uremic patients remains a clinical issue for several reasons. First, it may contribute to serious bleeding in some patients with renal failure, particularly following surgical procedures or trauma or in conjunction with anatomic lesions of the gastrointestinal tract. Second, it is often associated with a prolongation of the bleeding time. This test measures the adhesion and aggregation of platelets in a skin wound, usually on the volar surface of the forearm. The bleeding time is subject to a number of technical variables that affect its sensitivity. When a sensitive version of the test is performed in uremic individuals, most patients exhibit a prolonged bleeding time.[3,40,49] Because the bleeding time is the only readily available in vivo test of platelet function, reliance has been placed on it as an indicator of hemorrhagic risk in uremia. However, recent critical reviews of the published literature indicate that insufficient data are available for the bleeding time to be used for this purpose.[1,2,50] Although a less sensitive "thigh" bleeding time has been introduced in the hopes of better correlating with clinical bleeding in uremia,[51] it has yet to be evaluated sufficiently to recommend its routine use. Finally, in specific circumstances where therapy for a uremic bleeding diathesis is necessary, the uremic platelet defect can usually be successfully treated.

THERAPY

The first principle of management is to determine, by a careful history and examination of the patient, if an increased risk for clinically significant bleeding is present. Abnormal platelet aggregation and a prolonged bleeding time are common in uremic patients, but they are not, by themselves, indications for therapeutic intervention. The frequency of excessive bleeding after biopsies or other surgical procedures in uremic patients who have not received specific treatment is not known, but it may be uncommon. If bleeding does complicate a procedure, a rapid but thorough search for causes of bleeding should be initiated without assuming that uremia is the etiology. Several therapeutic maneuvers can either partially or completely correct an abnormal bleeding time in uremic patients (see below), and anecdotal observations indicate that they may also improve hemostasis. Apart from inducing remission of the renal disease or successful renal transplantation, these maneuvers are not uniformly effective. Because prospective studies comparing various treatment regimens have not been performed, the choice of therapy should be based on considerations such as the severity of the bleeding, the anticipated severity of the hemostatic stress imposed by surgery or trauma, the predicted duration of the therapeutic effect, and the risks of therapy.

Dialysis Intensive dialysis can correct the bleeding time and

bleeding diathesis in many patients, but is only partially effective in others.[39,52] Peritoneal dialysis and hemodialysis are equally effective.[53,54] If a patient undergoing dialysis bleeds, it may be worthwhile to increase the intensity of the dialysis.

Desmopressin Desmopressin (1-desamino-8-D-arginine vasopressin, DDAVP) is a vasopressin analog whose pressor effects (on V_1 vasopressin receptors) are substantially less than its antidiuretic effects (on V_2 vasopressin receptors). DDAVP causes the release of vWf from tissue stores, predominantly endothelial cells, and it has been reported to shorten the bleeding time in 50 to 75 percent of patients with uremia. In many cases, surgery has been carried out safely after administration of this drug, although no controlled trial has been performed.[55] DDAVP is usually administered intravenously in saline solution in a dose of 0.3 μg/kg over 15 to 30 min (maximum dose 20 μg), but it is also effective at this dose when given subcutaneously.[55] The drug can also be given as an intranasal spray.[56] Improvement in the bleeding time is seen within 30 to 60 min of administration, lasts for approximately 4 h, and roughly correlates with the rise in the plasma levels of vWf and the appearance in the circulation of high-molecular-weight vWf multimers.[57] However, DDAVP is also efficacious in patients whose plasma contains normal or increased amounts of vWf, suggesting that mechanisms in addition to changes in the quantity or quality of circulating vWf may be involved in the DDAVP effect.[58] In some patients, the drug has been given repeatedly at 12- to 24-h intervals, although tachyphylaxis can occur.[59]

At the recommended dose, side effects of DDAVP have been mild and uncommon and have included a 10 to 15 percent decrease in mean arterial pressure, a 20 to 30 percent increase in pulse rate, facial flushing, water retention, and hyponatremia leading to seizures, the latter more common after repeated administration and when fluids are given freely.[55,60] Water retention and hyponatremia have not been observed in patients whose kidneys cannot respond to the hormone. Several uremic and nonuremic individuals with atherosclerosis have been reported to develop stroke or myocardial infarction after DDAVP administration, although such complications appear to be rare.[61–63] If dialysis is not effective, DDAVP is the treatment of choice for uremic bleeding, particularly if only a short-term effect is required.[57]

Transfusion of Red Blood Cells Increasing the hematocrit, either through red blood cell transfusion or treatment with recombinant human erythropoietin, is associated with correction of the bleeding time and a suggestion of diminished clinical bleeding in uremic individuals. Improvement or normalization of the bleeding time is observed at hematocrits ≥ 32 percent.[5,14–17] The beneficial effects of red cells and DDAVP may be additive.[64] Correction of the bleeding time by increasing the red cell mass would be expected to be more durable than correction with DDAVP. The widespread use of recombinant erythropoietin in patients with chronic renal failure should eliminate the contribution of anemia to the hemorrhagic diathesis in these patients.[13] Moreover, a number of reports suggest that erythropoietin has an effect on platelets that is independent of an increase in hematocrit,[13] perhaps the result of an increase in the number of young platelets in the circulation.[65] In addition, except in emergencies, any potential hemostatic advantage to be gained by transfusion of red blood cells is likely be outweighed by the inherent risks of transfusion.

Conjugated Estrogens Conjugated estrogens have been reported to shorten the bleeding time in most, but not all, uremic individuals, both in uncontrolled studies and in randomized, double-blind studies.[25,66–68] In addition, estrogen therapy appears to be useful in some patients with uremia who bleed from gastrointestinal telangiectasia.[69] The drug is usually administered in a dose of 0.6 mg/kg intravenously for 5 days. Shortening of the bleeding time may be seen within 72 h of the first dose; the maximal effect occurs within 5 to 7 days, and it can persist for up to 14 days. Lower doses have not been effective.[67] One report suggests that oral conjugated estrogens are effective at a dose of 50 mg/day, but this regimen has not been compared with the parenteral regimen in a controlled study.[70] Conjugated estrogens have been well tolerated. No changes in the plasma levels or multimer distribution of vWf have been noted with this treatment. It has been postulated that the active component in conjugated estrogens is 17β-estradiol and that it works through an estrogen receptor mechanism.[71] While endothelial cells contain such receptors, platelets do not. Thus, the mechanism by which estrogens affect hemostasis remains obscure. Since the reported response to conjugated estrogens is more durable than the response to DDAVP, this therapy may have a role in certain clinical situations.

Cryoprecipitate   In uncontrolled studies of uremic patients, the infusion of cryoprecipitate has been reported to correct the bleeding time and to ameliorate bleeding.[72,73] However, others have reported inconsistent results.[74] It is conceivable that hemostasis is promoted by either the vWf or the platelet microparticles found within cryoprecipitate preparations.[75] The uncertain efficacy of this blood product coupled with the risks inherent in its administration argue against its routine use for uremic bleeding.

ANTIPLATELET ANTIBODIES

DEFINITION AND HISTORY

The α-granules of normal platelets contain approximately 20,000 molecules of IgG, but only about 100 IgG molecules are present on the platelet surface.[76] Until recently, measurements of increased IgG on the platelet surface have included IgG that is not necessarily pathogenic or even specific for platelet antigens, making it difficult to assess from the older literature the potential adverse effect of antiplatelet antibodies on platelet function and survival. This should be kept in mind when considering studies that report that increased antibody binding to the platelet surface (with or without complement binding) has been detected in several pathologic conditions, including idiopathic thrombocytopenic purpura (ITP), systemic lupus erythematosus (SLE), and platelet alloimmunization, and can result in platelet destruction (see Chap. 117). In most instances, the surviving platelets function normally. In some cases of ITP, however, bleeding times may be shorter than expected for the degree of thrombocytopenia,[77] although some individuals with circulating antiplatelet antibodies have impaired platelet function. Accordingly, while a platelet count above $50,000/\mu l$ is generally regarded as "safe,"[78] this cannot always be assumed to be the case in patients with immune thrombocytopenia.

ETIOLOGY AND PATHOGENESIS

While the mechanism by which autoantibodies or alloantibodies impair platelet function is usually not apparent, antibody binding to specific structures on the platelet membrane has been shown to be responsible in a number of cases. Most antibodies are directed against the GPIIb/IIIa complex, but antibodies directed against GPIb/IX/V, GPIa/IIa (integrin $\alpha_2\beta_1$), and GPIV have been detected as well.[79] In most cases, the in vivo consequences of antibody-mediated platelet dysfunction are obscured by the presence of thrombocytopenia (see Chap. 117). In some cases, the antibody has actually been demonstrated to have no effect on platelet function in vitro.[80] However, in several patients with normal platelet counts and autoantibodies against GPIIb/IIIa, there was absent platelet aggregation and a bleeding diathesis reminiscent of Glanzmann thrombasthenia.[81-84] Similarly, two IgG autoantibodies against GPIb have been reported that selectively inhibited ristocetin-induced platelet aggregation. In one patient, lymphadenopathy and polyclonal hypergammaglobulinemia were associated with a prolonged bleeding time and clinical bleeding.[85] In the second case, the clinical significance of the antibody's selective effect on GPIb function

was obscured by severe thrombocytopenia.[86] In two other patients, impaired collagen-induced platelet aggregation was associated with autoantibodies directed against one of the platelet collagen receptors GPIa/IIa.[87,88] Finally, a human monoclonal antibody derived from a patient with SLE was shown to react with a 32-kDa antigen on the surface of activated platelets and inhibit the second wave of platelet aggregation induced by ADP or a thromboxane A_2 analog.[89]

Besides interfering with the function of membrane components, some antibodies can activate platelets and induce aggregation and secretion. In vitro, antibodies can activate platelets through immune complex binding to platelet Fc receptors, by depositing sublytic quantities of the membrane attack complex of complement (C5b-9) on the cell surface[90] or by binding to a specific membrane antigen.[91] If antibodies are able to activate platelets in vivo in a similar fashion, the platelets might be expected to be refractory to agonists and to exhibit storage pool deficiency. While the activation of platelets in vivo is a possible explanation for the acquired storage pool disease seen in ITP or SLE, alternative mechanisms must also be considered. For example, some antibodies might affect the uptake of substances into platelet granules during megakaryocytopoiesis.[92]

CLINICAL AND LABORATORY FEATURES

Platelet dysfunction should be suspected in any patient with ITP or SLE who has mucocutaneous bleeding with a platelet count that is not ordinarily associated with this complication (e.g., $\geq 50,000/\mu l$). In such cases, the bleeding time may be longer than expected for the platelet count.[93,94] The clinical spectrum of autoimmune platelet dysfunction may also include some individuals, usually women, with "easy bruising" and a normal platelet count. These patients may have ITP with "compensated thrombocytolysis," since a substantial proportion of them have circulating antiplatelet antibodies and megathrombocytes.[95]

Patients with antiplatelet antibodies may exhibit defective platelet function in vitro even if they do not manifest a prolonged bleeding time or excessive bleeding. In two series, 13 of 19 patients with ITP demonstrated impaired platelet aggregation to ADP, epinephrine, or collagen.[96,97] Similarly, 22 of 35 patients with SLE were found to have reduced platelet aggregation in response to these agonists.[98,99] The functional abnormalities appeared to be antibody mediated, because IgG purified from the plasma or eluted from the platelets of some of the patients inhibited the aggregation of normal platelets.

Several aspects of platelet function may be impaired by antiplatelet antibodies. Some antiplatelet antibodies may inhibit the adhesion of platelets to the subendothelial matrix.[100] However, the most frequently reported abnormality is absence of platelet aggregation in response to low concentrations of collagen and absence of the second wave of aggregation in response to ADP or epinephrine. This pattern of abnormalities is identical to that seen in individuals with congenital storage pool disease. In fact, both ITP and SLE may be associated with an acquired form of storage pool disease manifested by a reduced platelet content of dense and α-granule components.[93,101] In one report, platelets in ITP also exhibited an activation defect manifested by impaired conversion of arachidonic acid to thromboxane A_2.[94]

THERAPY

Antibody-mediated platelet dysfunction and bleeding almost always occur in the setting of immune thrombocytopenia. The treatment for ITP is discussed in Chap. 117.

CARDIOPULMONARY BYPASS

DEFINITION AND HISTORY

Circulation of blood through an extracorporeal bypass circuit during cardiac surgery elicits a variety of hemostatic defects. The most significant challenges to the hemostatic system result from thrombocytopenia, defects in platelet function, and hyperfibrinolysis.[102,103] At its extreme, this can lead to significant postoperative bleeding that can last hours to days after bypass. It is estimated that excessive postoperative bleeding occurs in 5 percent of patients after extracorporeal bypass; roughly half of this due to surgical causes, and most of the remainder is attibutable to qualitative platelet defects and hyperfibrinolysis.

ETIOLOGY AND PATHOGENESIS

Thrombocytopenia is a consistent feature of bypass surgery.[103,104] Typically, platelet counts decrease to 50 percent of presurgical levels approximately 25 min after initiation of bypass, but thrombocytopenia may occur within 5 min and can persist for as long as several days.[102,105,106] Although the thrombocytopenia is mostly attributable to hemodilution from priming the pump with colloid or crystalloid solutions, it is often more profound than can be accounted for by hemodilution alone.[105–107] Platelet adhesion to artificial surfaces in the circuit has been demonstrated by scanning electron micrographs.[108] The mechanism of this interaction is uncertain but probably involves the deposition of fibrinogen onto the bypass circuit and platelet adhesion mediated by the fibrinogen receptor GPIIb/IIIa.[109,110] Less common causes of thrombocytopenia during bypass are disseminated intravascular coagulation, sequestration of damaged platelets in the liver, and heparin-induced thrombocytopenia.[111]

Qualitative platelet defects are the primary nonstructural hemostatic defects induced by the bypass circuit[112,113] and manifest as prolonged bleeding times, abnormal ex vivo platelet aggregation in response to several agonists, decreased platelet agglutination in response to ristocetin, deficiency of both α and dense granules, and the generation of platelet microparticles.[102,105,106,110,114–116] The severity of these abnormalities correlates with the duration of extracorporeal bypass, and they generally resolve within 2 to 24 h.[112]

The bypass-induced defects in platelet function likely result from platelet activation and fragmentation[116,117] due to hypothermia, contact with fibrinogen-coated synthetic surfaces, contact with the blood-air interface, damage caused by blood suctioning, and exposure to traces of thrombin, plasmin, ADP, or complement.[110,118–120] Exposure to thrombin during bypass has been reported to reduce subsequent platelet response to the thrombin-activating peptide TRAP and to be associated with increased postoperative blood loss.[121] Drugs such as heparin, protamine, and aspirin, as well as the production of fibrin degradation products, can also impair platelet function.[103,122,123] Controversy exists about the significance of these defects in vivo. At one extreme, some investigators have suggested that the entire qualitative platelet defect is due to the use of heparin during bypass surgery and its inhibitory effect on thrombin activity[122]; however, this would not account for the bleeding diathesis that can exist hours after reversal of heparin.

Hyperfibrinolysis may also contribute to the bleeding diathesis associated with cardiopulmonary bypass.[124,125] This is likely due to thrombus formation in the pericardial cavity followed by local, and subsequently systemic, fibrinolysis.[125] The relevance of hyperfibrinolysis to postbypass bleeding is bolstered by the efficacy of antifibrinolytic therapy in minimizing cardiopulmonary bypass surgery blood loss, as discussed below.

THERAPY

A preoperative evaluation of cardiac surgical candidates should include a history of bleeding in either the patient or a family member. Some authors recommend a screening prothrombin time, partial thromboplastin time, and bleeding time, even in individuals with no history of bleeding.[126] However, the validity of this approach is controversial.[127] Regardless, prophylactic transfusion of allogeneic blood components, be they platelets, whole blood, red cells, fresh-frozen plasma, or cryo-

precipitate, is not indicated.[112,128,129] Studies of the preoperative use of recombinant human erythropoietin in anemic, or erythropoietin plus autologous blood donation in nonanemic, patients suggest that these approaches are reasonable.[130–132] Cell savers are now often used during bypass surgery, and the collected washed autologous red blood cells are reinfused after completion of the cardiopulmonary bypass. In addition, blood collected from chest tube drainage has been reinfused to minimize allogeneic transfusion.[133] The safety of transfusing large quantities of blood by this technique has not fully been established.[134]

Several pharmacologic maneuvers have been tried to assist in the management of postoperative bleeding. Postoperative patients with a prolonged bleeding time and excessive blood loss may respond to DDAVP, as evidenced by a shortening of the bleeding time. However, results of trials using this agent have been contradictory, some studies showing a reduced blood loss and others showing no benefit.[135,136] These differences may be attributable to the observation that vWf is frequently elevated in postoperative patients.[135,136] Based on the assumption that platelet activation during bypass surgery could be a major cause of postoperative platelet dysfunction, infusion of platelet activation inhibitors such as prostaglandin E_1 (PGE_1), prostacyclin, or stable prostacyclin analogs has been carried out in animal models and in humans. By increasing platelet cyclic AMP and reducing platelet responsiveness, these agents prevent bypass-induced thrombocytopenia and platelet dysfunction. However, randomized trials using prostacyclin and its analog, Iloprost, did not show a clear overall benefit, in part due to significant toxicity, including hypotension.[137,138]

Evidence suggests that the protease inhibitor aprotinin can reduce mediastinal blood loss and transfusion requirements.[139,140] Although some studies suggest that aprotinin exerts a protective effect on platelets,[139,141] others do not support this hypothesis.[142,143] Aprotinin does inhibit hyperfibrinolysis, and this may be its sole beneficial activity at low dosage.[142,144] Treatment with aprotinin is usually started preoperatively and continued for the duration of surgery, with reported reductions of blood loss of 50 percent.[141,145] There is little evidence to support the concern that aprotinin causes a postoperative hypercoagulable state leading to coronary graft occlusion.[146] Its major toxicities include allergic reactions, particularly in patients who have received the drug within the past 6 months, and pancreatitis.[147,148] Other antifibrinolytic agents that may have a role in minimizing postoperative blood loss include ε-aminocaproic acid and tranexamic acid.[149,150]

The most important determinant of blood loss following cardiopulmonary surgery is the surgical procedure itself (i.e., minimal time on the bypass apparatus and rigorous hemostatic technique). If excessive nonsurgical postoperative bleeding occurs, one should verify that the patient is no longer hypothermic and that heparin has been fully reversed. At this point, the administration of pharmacologic agents, along with judicious transfusions of platelets, cryoprecipitate, fresh-frozen plasma, and red blood cells, is appropriate.

MISCELLANEOUS DISORDERS

Chronic liver disease of various etiologies has been reported to cause a prolonged bleeding time and reduced platelet aggregation and procoagulant activity.[151,152] The prolonged bleeding time in such patients may respond to infusion of DDAVP.[153] However, the existence of a platelet function defect specific to liver disease was placed in doubt by a study of 60 patients with cirrhosis in whom aggregation studies and bleeding times were compatible with the degree of thrombocytopenia.[154] The etiology of the bleeding diathesis associated with fulminant or end-stage liver disease is multifactorial and includes decreased coagulation factor production, fibrinolysis, dysfibrinogenemia, thrombocytopenia due to hypersplenism, and occasionally disseminated intravascular coagulation (DIC; see Chaps. 125 and 126). Thus, the prolonged bleeding time reported in some patients with severe liver disease may be due to multiple factors, including thrombocytopenia, hypofibrinogenemia, and anemia, none of which imply an intrinsic defect in platelet function.[155]

Patients with DIC may exhibit reduced platelet aggregation and acquired storage pool deficiency (see Chap. 126).[156,157] These result from platelet activation in vivo by thrombin or other agonists. Alternatively, elevated levels of fibrin(ogen) degradation products and low fibrinogen levels that accompany DIC may also contribute to the platelet defect. Although purified low-molecular-weight fibrinogen degradation products can impair platelet aggregation, this effect requires concentrations of degradation products unlikely to occur in vivo.[158] Furthermore, hypofibrinogenemia would contribute to a defect in aggregation only in extreme cases because the fibrinogen concentration in normal plasma is at least 15-fold greater than that required to saturate platelet fibrinogen receptors.[159] Finally, it is difficult to assess the significance of platelet dysfunction in most patients with DIC due to the simultaneous presence of thrombocytopenia and other hemostatic defects.

A prolonged bleeding time and decreased platelet aggregation and secretion in response to epinephrine or ADP has been reported in Bartter syndrome. It has been suggested that the platelet abnormalities are due to an inhibitory plasma factor, possibly a prostaglandin.[160] The paradoxical ability of aspirin to correct the prolonged bleeding time supports this contention.

There are isolated reports of a slight prolongation of the bleeding time and/or ex vivo platelet function defects in a number of other clinical conditions. These include nonthrombocytopenic purpura with eosinophilia,[161,162] atopic asthma and hay fever,[163] acute respiratory failure,[164] and Wilms tumor elaborating hyaluronic acid.[165] The clinical significance of these associations is not clear.

HEMATOLOGIC DISORDERS ASSOCIATED WITH ABNORMAL PLATELET FUNCTION

CHRONIC MYELOPROLIFERATIVE DISORDERS

DEFINITION AND HISTORY
Bleeding and thrombosis are significant causes of morbidity and mortality in the chronic myeloproliferative disorders: essential thrombocythemia, polycythemia rubra vera, myelofibrosis with myeloid metaplasia, and chronic myelogenous leukemia.[166] Thrombocytosis is a constant finding in essential thrombocythemia (see Chap. 118) and may be seen in each of the other disorders.

ETIOLOGY AND PATHOGENESIS
Several factors contribute to the hemostatic abnormalities in the myeloproliferative disorders. These include:

1. Increased whole-blood viscosity in polycythemia vera. The engorgement of blood vessels associated with polycythemia is a risk factor for bleeding, particularly in postoperative situations.[167,168]
2. Intrinsic defects in platelet function. A number of intrinsic platelet defects have been reported in the myeloproliferative disorders. However, the bleeding time is prolonged in only a minority of patients, and bleeding can occur in individuals with normal bleeding times.[169]
3. Elevated platelet counts. The contribution of an elevated platelet count, by itself, to the risk of hemorrhage and thrombosis is controversial.[170–174] A number of retrospective studies indicate that the risk of abnormal hemostasis cannot be confidently predicted from the degree of thrombocytosis.[169]

Under the light or electron microscope, platelets in these disorders may be larger or smaller than normal, may be abnormally shaped, and may exhibit a reduction in the number of storage granules.[175] In essential thrombocythemia, platelet survival may be modestly reduced.[176] A number of functional and biochemical abnormalities have been described in platelets from patients with myeloproliferative disorders. The most frequently encountered functional abnormality is a decrease in platelet aggregation and secretion in response to epinephrine, ADP, or collagen.[169] The defect in epinephrine-induced aggregation often includes absence of the primary wave of aggregation, which is unusual in other conditions. This is not simply due to an elevated platelet count, because it is not encountered in reactive thrombocytosis.[177] Thus, loss of platelet responsiveness to epinephrine may have utility in confirming the presence of a myeloproliferative disorder. Reduced aggregation and secretion has been associated with one or more of the following: decreased agonist-induced release of arachidonic acid from membrane phospholipids[178,179]; reduced conversion of arachidonic acid to prostaglandin endoperoxides or lipoxygenase products[180]; reduced platelet responsiveness to thromboxane A_2[181,182]; deficiency of dense or α-granules[183,184]; deficiency of GPIa/IIa ($\alpha_2\beta_1$), resulting in platelet unresponsiveness to collagen[185]; and decreased numbers of α_2-adrenergic receptors, leading to reduced or absent platelet responses to epinephrine.[186,187] On the other hand, spontaneous platelet aggregation in a patient with essential thrombocythemia[188] and thrombosis has been reported, as has increased thromboxane biosynthesis by platelets from patients with essential thrombocythemia[189] and polycythemia vera.[190]

Reduction in platelet procoagulant activity has also been reported in some patients with myeloproliferative disorders and thrombocytosis,[191] as have specific platelet membrane abnormalities, including decreased amounts of the GPIb-IX complex, resulting in an acquired form of Bernard-Soulier syndrome[192]; decreased numbers of receptors for PGD_2[193]; increased numbers of receptors for the Fc portion of IgG[194]; an increase in GPIV (CD36) with[195,196] or without[197] a corresponding decrease in GPIb; and impaired expression of thrombopoietin receptors.[198] An acquired form of von Willebrand disease has been observed in several individuals with chronic myelogenous leukemia and other myeloproliferative syndromes.[199] In these cases, there was a reduction in the plasma level of the high-molecular-weight vWf multimers[200]; in some, the vWf abnormality was corrected transiently by infusion of DDAVP.[196,201] In others, the abnormalities were partially or completely corrected by cytoreductive therapy.[199,202]

CLINICAL AND LABORATORY FEATURES
Bleeding occurs in about one-third of patients with myeloproliferative disorders and contributes to mortality in 10 percent. Thrombosis also occurs in one-third of cases, contributing to mortality in 15 to 40 percent.[203] Most symptomatic patients experience either bleeding or thrombosis; however, some develop both complications during the course of their disease. Bleeding usually involves the skin or mucous membranes but may also occur after surgery or trauma. Thrombosis may involve arteries or veins and may occur in unusual locations, such as the hepatic, portal, and mesenteric circulations.[203–205] Indeed, full-blown or latent myeloproliferative disorders account for a substantial proportion of patients with the Budd-Chiari syndrome.[205,206] Individuals with essential thrombocythemia may experience ischemia and necrosis of the fingers and toes due to digital artery thrombosis, microvascular occlusion in the coronary circulation, and transient neurologic symptoms due to cerebrovascular occlusion.[207] A syndrome of redness and burning pain in the extremities, termed erythromelalgia, is strongly associated with essential thrombocythemia and polycythemia vera and is thought to be due to arteriolar platelet thrombi.[208] It has been difficult to predict the risk of bleeding or thrombosis in asymptomatic

patients,[209] but an increased number of reticulated platelets in patients with thrombocytosis, thought to reflect an increase in platelet turnover, has been associated with an increased risk for thrombosis.[210] Vascular complications are also more likely to occur in patients older than 60 and in patients with other risk factors for vascular disease.[211]

Several features of these platelet functional defects require emphasis. First, none is unique to a particular myeloproliferative disorder. Second, their relative frequency has varied widely in reported series. Third, none has been predictive of bleeding or thrombosis. Fourth, although the myeloproliferative disorders comprise several distinct clinicopathologic entities, they represent clonal abnormalities of hematopoiesis. Therefore, platelets may acquire structural and biochemical abnormalities as they develop from a clone of abnormal megakaryocytes.

THERAPY

Therapy should be considered for the symptomatic patient and for the patient about to undergo surgery. Treatment includes correction of polycythemia and maintenance of the hematocrit below 45 percent[212] as well as treatment of the underlying disorder. Platelet count reduction in patients with thrombocytosis, either by plateletpheresis or cytoreductive agents, has generally been associated with clinical improvement.[203] Effective cytoreductive agents include the ribonuclease reductase inhibitor hydroxyurea[213] and anagrelide.[214] Anagrelide, an imidazoquinazolin derivative, is thought to decrease platelet counts by specifically impairing megakaryocyte maturation.[215] Anagrelide has essentially no effect on red and white cell counts and is not known to be leukemogenic. Nevertheless, 10 to 20 percent of patients experience neurologic, gastrointestinal, and cardiac side effects, in particular, fluid retention, necessitating discontinuation of the drug. During an episode of acute bleeding, DDAVP infusion may temporarily improve hemostasis if the patient has an acquired storage pool defect or acquired von Willebrand disease.[184,201] Aspirin (300–600 mg/day) may be useful in patients with thrombosis, particularly those with erythromelalgia or with digital or cerebrovascular ischemia.[216,217] However, aspirin can exacerbate a bleeding tendency in patients with myeloproliferative disorders.[218]

LEUKEMIAS AND MYELODYSPLASTIC SYNDROMES

CLINICAL AND LABORATORY FEATURES

The most frequent cause of bleeding in these disorders is thrombocytopenia. However, abnormal platelet function in vitro has been described in acute myelogenous leukemia, and in some patients this may be clinically significant. In acute myelogenous leukemia and its variants, platelets may be larger than normal, abnormally shaped, and exhibit a marked variation in the number of granules. There may be decreased aggregation and serotonin release in response to ADP, epinephrine, or collagen, as well as decreased platelet procoagulant activity. The functional abnormalities may be due to either acquired storage pool deficiency or a defect in the process of platelet activation.[219-221] These defects are intrinsic to the platelet and are probably related to the fact that the megakaryocytes from which platelets are derived have originated from a leukemic stem cell. Bleeding in the acute leukemias usually responds to platelet transfusions and to treatment of the underlying disease. Identical platelet abnormalities may be seen in the myelodysplastic syndromes (preleukemias).[219,222] In these syndromes platelets appear to be less uniformly affected, perhaps because there is a residual population of normal platelets admixed with those from the malignant clone.

Reduced platelet aggregation has been reported in children with acute lymphocytic leukemia.[220] Unless the leukemia is biphenotypic, it is difficult to ascribe the platelet defect to the leukemic process itself. Platelets are normal in children with lymphoblastic leukemia in complete remission.[223] Hairy-cell leukemia is a lymphoproliferative disease in which platelet dysfunction may rarely complicate the clinical picture. Bleeding is responsible for death in 8 percent of patients, but it is usually due to thrombocytopenia rather than platelet dysfunction.[224] Some patients may exhibit storage pool deficiency or a defect in the process of platelet activation, and these abnormalities have been reported to disappear following splenectomy.[225-229] However, this should be interpreted with caution because splenectomy usually corrects the thrombocytopenia as well. A single case of acquired von Willebrand disease in association with hairy-cell leukemia has been reported.[230]

DYSPROTEINEMIAS

DEFINITION AND HISTORY

Platelet dysfunction is observed in approximately one-third of patients with IgA myeloma or Waldenström macroglobulinemia, 15 percent of patients with IgG multiple myeloma, and occasionally in patients with monoclonal gammopathy of undetermined significance.[231] In addition to platelet dysfunction, other causes of bleeding should be considered in these patients, including the hyperviscosity syndrome,[232] thrombocytopenia, complications of amyloidosis (e.g., amyloid angiopathy[233] or acquired factor X deficiency[234,235]), and, rarely, a circulating heparin-like anticoagulant[236,237] or systemic fibrin(ogen)olysis.[238,239] The myeloma protein may also affect in vitro coagulation tests by interfering with fibrin polymerization and with the function of other coagulation proteins.[231]

ETIOLOGY AND PATHOGENESIS

The bleeding time may be prolonged in patients with dysproteinemias, even in the absence of clinical bleeding. The platelet defect is caused by the monoclonal protein. It has been suggested that some monoclonal immunoglobulins interact with the platelet surface to interfere nonspecifically with platelet adhesion or stimulus-response coupling. This concept is supported by the observations that platelet dysfunction is more common when the concentration of the paraprotein in plasma or on the platelet membrane is very high[240]; that platelet aggregation, secretion, clot retraction, and platelet procoagulant activity may all be affected; and that normal platelets acquire these defects when incubated with the purified monoclonal immunoglobulin.[241]

In some cases, specific interactions of the monoclonal protein with platelets have been described. One IgA myeloma protein inhibited the ability of a suspension of aortic connective tissue to aggregate normal platelets.[242] The bleeding time and bleeding diathesis of the patient from whom this myeloma protein was obtained were corrected by removal of the protein by plasmapheresis. In another patient, an IgG myeloma protein bound specifically to platelet GPIIIa. Both the intact immunoglobulin and its F(ab')₂ fragment inhibited the binding of fibrinogen to activated platelets, thus inducing a thrombasthenic-like state.[243] Several patients with myeloma, benign monoclonal gammopathy, or chronic lymphocytic leukemia have been reported to have an acquired form of von Willebrand disease in which the plasma level of vWf is reduced or the high-molecular-weight multimers of vWf are lacking (see below).[244-246]

THERAPY

When clinically significant platelet dysfunction occurs in a patient with a dysproteinemia, cytoreductive therapy should be considered as a means to reduce the production and plasma level of the monoclonal immunoglobulin.[231] Plasmapheresis can also control bleeding by reducing the level of the abnormal protein, and it can be lifesaving during acute bleeds.[247,248] Cryoprecipitate, DDAVP, intravenous gamma globulin, and/or plasmapheresis may be transiently effective in patients with acquired von Willebrand disease (see below).[244,245,249,250]

ACQUIRED VON WILLEBRAND DISEASE

Although inherited von Willebrand disease is common (1–3% worldwide), acquired von Willebrand disease is a relatively rare disorder that typically occurs in the setting of an autoimmune or clonal hematologic disease. The latter include multiple myeloma,[251,252] Waldenström's macroglobulinemia,[253] low-grade non-Hodgkin's lymphoma,[254,255] chronic lymphocytic leukemia,[256] and myeloproliferative disorders.[257] In many hematologic disorders, a specific anti-vWf antibody is present,[249,251,252,258] while in autoimmune disorders, anti-vWF antibodies are part of a generalized autoimmune response.[259] When acquired von Willebrand disease occurs in other clinical situations, such as cancer or hypothyroidism, it may result from the nonspecific direct absorption of vWf onto tumor cells[230,260,261] or decreased vWf production.[262,263]

Mucocutaneous bleeding and a prolonged bleeding time should raise the suspicion of acquired von Willebrand disease in patients without a prior personal or family history of bleeding. This is especially important in patients with known autoimmune disease or lymphoproliferative or myeloproliferative disorders.[264] Diagnostic evaluation includes measurements of factor VIII coagulant activity, vWf antigen, and ristocetin cofactor activity. The presence of an in vitro inhibitor may or may not be detected, depending on whether the antibody binds to vWf and neutralizes its function or merely leads to accelerated vWf clearance by the reticuloendothelial system.[264] Patient management includes infusions of desmopressin,[252,256,259] vWf-containing factor VIII concentrates,[265] or high-dose intravenous immunoglobulin.[266,267] The latter has been efficacious in patients when acquired von Willebrand disease is associated with a lymphoproliferative disorder or monoclonal paraprotein and most likely acts by delaying vWf clearance via reticuloendothelial cell blockade, although other mechanisms have been postulated.[268–270] Treatment of the underlying associated disease is only sometimes helpful.[264]

DRUGS THAT AFFECT PLATELET FUNCTION

Drugs represent the most common cause of platelet dysfunction (Table 120-2).[271] For example, in an analysis of 72 hospitalized patients with a prolonged bleeding time, 54 percent were receiving large doses of antibiotics known to prolong the bleeding time and 10 percent were taking aspirin or other nonsteroidal anti-inflammatory drugs.[272] Some drugs can prolong the bleeding time and either cause or exacerbate a bleeding diathesis. Other drugs may prolong the bleeding time but not cause bleeding, while others may only affect platelet function ex vivo or when added to platelets in vitro. It is important for the hematologist to understand the clinical significance of these distinctions.

ASPIRIN AND OTHER NONSTEROIDAL ANTI-INFLAMMATORY DRUGS

ASPIRIN
Aspirin inhibits platelets by acetylating and irreversibly inactivating the enzyme PG endoperoxide H synthase-1 (PGHS-1, cyclooxygenase-1; see Chap. 131 for the use of aspirin as an antithrombotic agent).[273] Inactivation of PGHS-1 prevents platelet synthesis of PG endoperoxides and the subsequent synthesis of thromboxane A_2 by thromboxane synthase, thereby inhibiting platelet responses that require these substances. Thus, platelet responses to ADP, epinephrine, arachidonic acid, and low doses of collagen and thrombin are affected, while responses to higher doses of collagen or thrombin are not.[274,275] Platelet

TABLE 120-2   DRUGS THAT INHIBIT PLATELET FUNCTION

Nonsteroidal Anti-inflammatory Drugs
   Aspirin, sulfinpyrazone, indomethacin, ibuprofen, sulindac, naproxen, phenylbutazone, meclofenamic acid, mefenamic acid, diflunisal, piroxicam, tolmetin, zomepirac

Antibiotics
   Penicillins
      Penicillin G, carbenicillin, ticarcillin, methicillin, ampicillin, piperacillin, azlocillin, mezlocillin, apalcillin, sulbenicillin, temocillin
   Cephalosporins
      Cephalothin, moxalactam, cefoxitin, cefotaxime, cefazolin
   Nitrofurantoin
   Miconazole

Thienopyridines
   Ticlopidine, clopidogrel

GPIIb/IIIa Antagonists
   Abciximab, tirofiban, eptifibatide

Drugs That Affect Platelet cAMP Levels or Function
   Prostacyclin, iloprost, dipyridamole, cilostazol

Anticoagulants, Fibrinolytic Agents, and Antifibrinolytic Agents
Heparin
   Streptokinase, tissue plasminogen activator, urokinase
   ε-Aminocaproic acid

Cardiovascular Drugs
   Nitroglycerin, isosorbide dinitrate, propranolol, nitroprusside, nifedipine, verapamil, diltiazem, quinidine

Volume Expanders
   Dextran, hydroxyethyl starch

Psychotropic Drugs and Anesthetics
   Psychotropic drugs
      Imipramine, amitriptyline, nortriptyline, chlorpromazine, promethazine, flufenazine, trifluoperazine, haloperidol
   Anesthetics
      Local
         Dibucaine, tetracaine, metycaine, cyclaine, butacaine, nupercaine, procaine, cocaine, plaquenil
      General
         Halothane

Oncologic Drugs
   Mithramycin, daunorubicin, BCNU

Miscellaneous Drugs
   Ketanserin
   Antihistamines
      Diphenhydramine, chlorpheniramine, mepyramine
   Radiographic contrast agent
      Iopamidol, iothalamate, ioxalate, meglumine diatrizoate, sodium diatrizoate

Foods and Food Additives
   ω_3 Fatty acids, ethanol, Chinese black tree fungus, onion extract, ajoene, cumin, turmeric

prostaglandin synthesis in an adult is nearly completely inhibited by a single 100-mg dose of aspirin or by 30 mg taken daily for 7 to 10 days.[276] Although small doses of aspirin inhibit both platelet and endothelial cell cyclooxygenase irreversibly,[277] they have no lasting effect on prostacyclin production by endothelial cells.[278] This is likely due to the ability of endothelial cells to synthesize additional cyclooxygenase unaffected by aspirin.[279] In vitro studies also suggest that the presence of erythrocytes contributes to agonist-stimulated platelet reactivity,[21] an effect that can be inhibited by aspirin at doses greater than those required to inhibit platelet PGHS-1.[280]

Aspirin is one of the few drugs that prolong the bleeding time in humans and appear to act by blocking aggregation rather than adhesion. In normal individuals, the effect on the bleeding time is slight (generally no more than 1.2 to 2.0 times the preaspirin bleeding time),[281,282] observed in both males and females, and requires that almost all the cyclooxygenase in the circulating platelets be inhibited.[281] The sensitivity of the bleeding time to aspirin is dependent on such technical variables as the direction of the incision on the forearm and the degree of hydrostatic pressure applied to the arm.[283] The bleeding time may remain prolonged for 1 to 4 days after the aspirin has been discontinued, and platelet aggregation test results may remain abnormal for up to a week until the affected platelets are replaced by newly formed ones.[284]

The significance of aspirin ingestion for the hemostatic competency of normal individuals appears to be minimal. Nevertheless, patients chronically taking aspirin report a significant increase in bruising, epistaxis, and gastrointesinal blood loss.[285] The latter appears to be due to a direct effect of the drug on the gastric mucosa.[286,287] Moreover, there was a slight, but not statistically significant, increase in hemorrhagic strokes in a group of otherwise healthy physicians who took aspirin chronically as primary prophylaxis against myocardial infarction.[285] Aspirin may also increase bleeding in the mother and the neonate during parturition.[288] In addition, some, but not all, studies have shown that aspirin taken preoperatively increases the amount of blood loss following cardiothoracic surgery (see Chap. 131).[289,290] On the other hand, a retrospective analysis has documented the safety of performing epidural and spinal anesthesia in patients who had ingested aspirin.[291] While aspirin may increase the amount of blood loss following general surgery,[292] the significance of aspirin ingestion in this clinical setting has never been tested in a prospective, randomized, double-blind study with objective end points. Many surgeons ask their patients to avoid aspirin, particularly prior to cardiothoracic, plastic, or neurosurgical procedures, in which the limits of tolerable bleeding are narrow.[293] Aspirin causes a marked prolongation of the bleeding time and precipitates hemorrhage in individuals with preexistent hemostatic defects such as von Willebrand disease, hemophilia A, warfarin ingestion, uremia, or other disorders of platelet function.[44,45,294] While ingestion of ethanol has no direct effect on the bleeding time, it can potentiate the effect of aspirin.[295,296] Infusion of DDAVP has been effective in correcting a prolonged bleeding time due to aspirin.[297,298]

OTHER NONSTEROIDAL ANTI-INFLAMMATORY DRUGS
Nonsteroidal anti-inflammatory drugs such as indomethacin, ibuprofen, naproxen, phenylbutazone, and sulfinpyrazone also inhibit platelet cyclooxygenase.[299] In contrast to aspirin, their effect is reversible and generally short-lasting (<4 h). An exception is piroxicam, whose effect may last for days due to its prolonged half-life.[300] These drugs may cause a transient prolongation of the bleeding time when given in therapeutic doses; however, this is usually not clinically significant.[301–303] Indeed, ibuprofen has been given safely to patients with hemophilia A.[304,305] However, care must be taken when ibuprofen is given to patients with hemophilia and HIV infection receiving zidovudine, since increased bleeding has been reported in this circumstance.[306] Analgesics such as acetaminophen, sodium or choline salicylate, and narcotics neither inhibit cyclooxygenase nor prolong the bleeding time.[304,307,308] Drugs that inhibit thromboxane synthetase (e.g., OKY-1581) may impair platelet secretion and second-wave aggregation in response to ADP; however, these effects have not been observed in every subject.[309,310]

ANTIBIOTICS

Various penicillins contain a β-lactam ring and a unique side chain. Most penicillins cause a dose-dependent prolongation of the bleeding time in normal volunteers.[311] Because they reduce platelet aggregation and secretion as well as ristocetin-induced platelet agglutination, they may affect both platelet adhesion and platelet activation. Results of tests of platelet aggregation are abnormal in at least 50 to 75 percent of individuals receiving large doses (at least several grams per day) of carbenicillin, penicillin G, ticarcillin, ampicillin, nafcillin, and azlocillin and in 25 to 50 percent of patients taking piperacillin, azlocillin, apalcillin, or mezlocillin.[311–313] Differences in the antiplatelet effects

of these antibiotics probably relate to differences in blood levels and drug potency. Their effect on platelets is maximal after 1 to 3 days of administration and may remain for several days after the antibiotic has been stopped, suggesting that the effect of these antibiotics on platelets in vivo is irreversible.

Penicillins may impair the interaction of agonists and vWf with the platelet membrane.[314] Indeed, when many penicillins are incubated with washed platelets, albeit at concentrations higher than those attained in vivo, they inhibit the interaction of vWf and agonists, such as ADP and epinephrine, with their platelet receptors.[315] The relative in vitro antiplatelet potency of the penicillins correlates well with their lipid solubility and with the inhibitory potency of the isolated side chains.[316,317] Moreover, the inhibitory effect of penicillin G on platelet function in vitro is potentiated by the presence of probenecid.[318] When platelet function was tested after intravenous administration of penicillin, oxacillin, or mezlocillin for 3 to 17 days to patients or normal volunteers, irreversible inhibition of agonist-induced aggregation was noted, along with a 40 percent reduction in low-affinity thromboxane A_2 receptors.[319] Thus, penicillins probably inhibit platelet function by binding to one or more membrane components necessary for adhesive interactions with the vessel wall or for stimulus-response coupling.

Although clinically significant bleeding has been associated with the use of carbenicillin, penicillin G, ticarcillin, and nafcillin, it is far less common than prolongation of the bleeding time.[311,320] Patients with coexisting hemostatic defects (e.g., thrombocytopenia, vitamin K deficiency, or uremia) may be particularly prone to this complication. On the other hand, high doses of penicillin G did not increase gastrointestinal blood loss in a thrombocytopenic rabbit model.[321] In our experience, bleeding due to antibiotic-induced platelet dysfunction is uncommon and unpredictable. Since β-lactam–induced platelet dysfunction resolves with time following cessation of the drug, this class of drugs should be considered as a potential cause of bleeding in the appropriate clinical setting. A similar pattern of platelet dysfunction has been reported with some cephalosporins or related antibiotics but not with others.[311,322,323] Broad-spectrum antibiotics can also cause a bleeding diathesis attributable to vitamin K deficiency. Nitrofurantoin, a structurally unrelated antibiotic, may cause a mild prolongation of the bleeding time and impair platelet aggregation when blood levels of the drug are higher than 20 μM.[324] Miconazole, an antifungal agent, has been shown to inhibit human and rabbit platelet cyclooxygenase in vitro and rabbit platelet cyclooxygenase after intravenous infusion.[325]

THIENOPYRIDINES

The thienopyridines ticlopidine and clopidogrel are used as antithrombotic agents in arterial diseases (see Chap. 131). They may be more effective than aspirin in the secondary prevention of cerebrovascular and cardiovascular events.[326–330] The antithrombotic effects of thienopyridines and aspirin may be additive, especially in preventing thrombotic complications after coronary artery stent placement.[329,331]

Ticlopidine and clopidogrel differ from aspirin in the mechanism of their antiplatelet activity and in their toxicity profile. Both appear to be prodrugs that depend on metabolites for their effects.[326] Ticlopidine at 250 mg by mouth twice a day or clopidogrel at 75 mg once per day has been shown to inhibit platelet aggregation ex vivo and to prolong the bleeding time in humans. The degree of prolongation of the bleeding time is equivalent to or greater than that of aspirin, and the effect of thienopyridines and aspirin appears additive.[332] Effects of ticlopidine and clopidogrel on platelet aggregation and the bleeding time may be seen within 24 to 48 h of the first dose but are not maximal for 4 to 6 days. Moreover, the effects may last for 4 to 10 days after the drugs have been discontinued. This may be explained by their extended half-life after multiple dosing or by irreversible effects on platelets.[326]

Ex vivo studies indicate that ticlopidine and clopidogrel impair fibrinogen binding to its platelet receptor, GPIIb/IIIa, and inhibit platelet aggregation in response to many agonists, particularly ADP. The effect on ADP-induced platelet aggregation seems to account for the observed decrease in responses to low concentrations of other agonists, since ADP released from dense granules plays a role in those responses. Indeed, aggregation in response to high concentrations of thrombin or collagen are normal.[326,333,334] ADP-induced platelet shape change and calcium transients are unimpaired, implying that the drugs do not affect the binding of ADP to receptors involved in these particular responses. Thus, the major effect of ticlopidine may be impairment of stimulus-response coupling between one or more ADP receptors and the fibrinogen receptor. Platelets contain at least three different ADP receptors (P2Y1, $P2_{AC}$, and P2X),[335,336] and the thienopyridines may selectively block the $P2_{AC}$ receptor.[337,338] These drugs may work through noncompetitive inhibition of ADP binding to the receptor.[339]

Ticlopidine administration has been associated with potentially serious hematologic complications, including neutropenia ($<1200/\mu l$ in 2.4 percent of individuals)[326,340,341] and, less commonly, aplastic anemia, thrombotic thrombocytopenic purpura, and thrombocytopenia.[342,346] Results from a large clinical trial suggest that these complications may be less common with clopidogrel[327] but continued assessment is warranted.[327a]

GPIIB/IIIA RECEPTOR ANTAGONISTS

Drugs that specifically impair the function of platelet GPIIb/IIIa have been developed for use as antithrombotic agents in the setting of ischemic coronary artery disease.[347] Because inherited GPIIb/IIIa abnormalities result in the bleeding disorder Glanzmann thrombasthenia,[348] it is not surprising that these drugs can predispose to bleeding. In EPIC, a clinical trial of the efficacy of abciximab, a chimeric human-murine anti-GPIIb/IIIa monoclonal antibody Fab fragment, in patients undergoing percutaneous coronary angioplasty, 14 percent of patients given abciximab experienced major bleeding, compared with 7 percent of patients given placebo.[349] However, the patients were also given aspirin and heparin, and when the heparin dose was decreased in the subsequent EPILOG trial, the incidence of major bleeding in patients receiving abciximab decreased to 2.0 percent, compared with 3.1 percent in the control group receiving heparin and aspirin alone.[350] Nonetheless, in both EPIC and EPILOG, minor bleeding was significantly more frequent in patients given abciximab and standard-dose heparin compared with patients given standard-dose heparin alone, attesting to the ability of a GPIIb/IIIa antagonist to impair normal hemostasis. In the PRISM-PLUS and PURSUIT trials of the synthetic low-molecular-weight GPIIb/IIIa inhibitors tirofiban and eptifibatide, respectively, major and minor bleeding were slightly more frequent in patients receiving the study drug than in control subjects.[351,352] Similarly, patients receiving the oral GPIIb/IIIa inhibitors xemilofiban and sibrafiban for 30 and 28 days, respectively, frequently experienced mucocutaneous bleeding similar to that experienced by patients with thrombasthenia.[353,354]

The risk of bleeding in patients undergoing percutaneous coronary interventions given GPIIb/IIIa antagonists can be minimized by using low-dose heparin (e.g., 70 units/kg, as in EPILOG[350]), by avoiding treatment of patients who are receiving warfarin at therapeutic doses, by early vascular sheath removal, and by meticulous care of vascular puncture sites.[355] Platelet transfusions appear to rapidly reverse the defect in platelet function in patients receiving abciximab, primarily by decreasing the extent of GPIIb/IIIa blockade. The ability of platelet transfusion to reverse the effects of the other GPIIb/IIIa antagonists

is less clear, but these drugs have short half-lives if renal and hepatic function are normal.

Thrombocytopenia occurring within 24 h of initiating therapy has been observed in small numbers of patients following the administration of all types of GPIIb/IIIa antagonists.[351,352,354,356] In the EPIC trial, the incidences of platelet counts less than $100,000/\mu l$ and less than $50,000/\mu l$ in patients receiving abciximab for the first time were 3.9 percent and 0.9 percent, respectively.[356] There are also anecdotal reports of acute profound thrombocytopenia (platelet counts $<20,000$).[357,358] The mechanism responsible for the decrease in platelet count is uncertain, but it may be related to the presence of preexisting anti-GPIIb/IIIa antibodies that recognize epitopes on GPIIb/IIIa exposed by binding of the GPIIb/IIIa antagonist.[359] The thrombocytopenia usually reverses readily when the drug is stopped, but it may also be reversed by platelet transfusion if clinically indicated.[355] Thrombocytopenia in patients receiving GPIIb/IIIa antagonists must be differentiated from pseudothrombopenia due to drug-induced platelet clumping, from heparin-induced thrombocytopenia in patients receiving heparin concurrently, and from other causes of thrombocytopenia, depending on the clinical circumstances. It is particularly important to identify thrombocytopenia early, since GPIIb/IIIa antagonists are administered as long infusions, and the drug should be stopped as soon as true thrombocytopenia has been confirmed. In most cases of profound thrombocytopenia, a platelet count obtained 2 to 4 h after initiating therapy will provide evidence of a significant decrease in platelet count.

DRUGS THAT AFFECT PLATELET CYCLIC NUCLEOTIDE LEVELS OR FUNCTION

The pyrimidopyrimidine derivative dipyridamole inhibits platelet function in vitro, but the clinical utility of this drug is controversial.[360,361] Dipyridamole inhibits cyclic nucleotide phosphodiesterase, resulting in the intracellular accumulation of cAMP. Dipyridamole may also inhibit the breakdown of cGMP, resulting in the potentiation of a nitric oxide effect.[362] Although several clinical trials failed to demonstrate a benefit of dipyridamole,[361] the European Stroke Prevention Study 2 (ESPS 2) did show benefit from receiving dipyridamole in preventing stroke and transient ischemic attack, although there was no difference in mortality between patients taking dipyridamole and those taking placebo or among patients taking dipyridamole plus aspirin and those taking either agent alone.[363] The basis for the different outcomes of the various trials is unclear but could be due to higher dipyridamole dosage or the sustained-release dipyridamole preparation used in ESPS 2.

Intravenous infusions of PGE_1, prostacyclin, or stable analogs of prostacyclin stimulate platelet adenylyl cyclase, causing an increase in platelet cAMP levels and a decrease in platelet responsiveness.[137,309,364] These agents cause a transient prolongation of the bleeding time and inhibit platelet shape change, aggregation, and secretion. However, their clinical utility is limited by their short half-life and side effects, which include peripheral vasodilatation.[137,138] Cilostazol, a member of a new class of phosphodiesterase III inhibitors, has been approved in the United States for the treatment of peripheral vascular disease[365] and may have utility in the prevention of cardiac stent occlusion.[366] Nitric oxide and organic nitrates such as nitroglycerin inhibit platelet function in vitro, probably by activating guanylyl cyclase, thereby increasing cGMP.[367] Their effect on in vivo platelet function is uncertain. High concentrations of caffeine and theophylline also inhibit platelet phosphodiesterases in vitro.

ANTICOAGULANTS, FIBRINOLYTIC AGENTS, AND ANTIFIBRINOLYTIC AGENTS

Heparin predisposes to bleeding primarily through its anticoagulant effect, but it may also affect platelet function. For example, a bolus injection of heparin (100 units/kg) can cause a significant prolongation of the bleeding time in normal subjects and in patients prior to cardio-pulmonary bypass, suggesting that therapeutic doses of heparin may impair platelet function.[103] Heparin likely impairs platelet function by inhibiting the generation and action of thrombin, a potent platelet agonist. In vitro studies also suggest that heparin can enhance platelet aggregation induced by other platelet agonists.[368] Heparin binds to a single class of high-affinity binding sites on resting platelets and to an additional class of lower-affinity binding sites on fully activated platelets.[369] High heparin doses have also been found to impair vWf-dependent platelet function, possibly by binding to the heparin-binding domain of vWf.[370] The contribution of these effects on platelet function to the bleeding complications of heparin therapy are uncertain.

Bleeding during fibrinolytic therapy is due predominantly to the combined effects of structural lesions in blood vessels and the fibrin(ogen)olytic activity of the agent used. However, pharmacologic doses of streptokinase, urokinase, and tissue plasminogen activator (t-PA) can affect platelet function.[371] High concentrations of plasmin ex vivo cause platelet aggregation.[372] Moreover, marked increases in the urinary excretion of the thromboxane A_2 metabolite 2,3-dinor-TxB_2 have been detected in patients receiving streptokinase or t-PA for coronary thrombolysis, suggesting that in vivo platelet activation had occurred during infusion of the drug.[373,374] Nevertheless, several in vitro studies indicate that plasmin generation has an inhibitory effect on platelet function. First, very high levels of fibrin(ogen) degradation products coupled with very low levels of fibrinogen may impair platelet aggregation.[375] Second, plasminogen can bind to platelets[376] and, after its conversion to plasmin, enzymatically degrades platelet GPIb, impairing the interaction of platelets with vWf.[377,378] Third, plasmin can inhibit platelet arachidonic acid metabolism.[379] Fourth, t-PA promotes the disaggregation of platelet aggregates, presumably by inducing lysis of the fibrinogen that mediates aggregate formation.[380] Finally, after initial activation, platelets incubated with plasmin and recombinant t-PA in vitro become refractory to activation by other agonists.[381] Whether any of the in vitro and ex vivo observations apply to the in vivo situation and are clinically significant remains to be determined.[382] The antifibrinolytic drug ε-aminocaproic acid can increase the bleeding time when administered for several days at doses greater than 24 g/day.[383]

CARDIOVASCULAR DRUGS

Administration of nitroprusside (which increases platelet cGMP),[384,385] nitroglycerin,[386] and propranolol[387,388] can decrease platelet aggregation and secretion ex vivo; nitroprusside can increase the bleeding time twofold when administered at infusion rates of 6 to 8 μg/kg per minute, whereas trimethaphan, another effective parenteral antihypertensive agent, does not.[384,389] Inhalation of nitric oxide, advocated for the treatment of pulmonary hypertension and the adult respiratory distress syndrome, can impair agonist-induced platelet aggregation ex vivo, although effects on the bleeding time have been variable.[390-392] The clinical significance of these observations is unclear. Organic "calcium channel blockers," such as verapamil, nifedipine, and diltiazem, inhibit platelet aggregation when added at very high concentrations to washed platelets.[393] This effect is seen primarily with epinephrine-induced aggregation and does not appear to be related to calcium channel blockade. For example, verapamil can act as an β_2-adrenergic receptor antagonist at concentrations that inhibit platelet function.[394] At therapeutic doses, calcium channel blockers do not prolong the bleeding time, although one agent, nisoldipine, has been reported to inhibit agonist-induced calcium transients and platelet aggregation after 10 days of oral administration.[395] At high concentrations, the antiarrhythmic drug quinidine has been reported to cause a mild prolongation of the bleeding time and potentiate the effect of aspirin.[396]

VOLUME EXPANDERS

Dextran is a neutral polysaccharide that is heterogeneous in molecular size. Two preparations with average molecular weights of 40,000 and 70,000 are in clinical use. Although dextran infusions may prolong the bleeding time in normal subjects and in patients with von Willebrand disease, this has not been observed in most of the normal subjects.[397-399] Infused dextran adsorbs to the platelet surface and can impair platelet aggregation, secretion, and procoagulant activity. The maximal effect of dextran may require several hours, suggesting that larger molecules with a slower rate of clearance are responsible.[397] Curiously, the drug has no effect when added to platelet-rich plasma.[397] Dextran infusion produces a modest reduction in plasma vWf antigen and ristocetin cofactor activity.[398] Despite these effects on primary hemostasis and the use of dextran in the operative setting as a volume expander or for antithrombotic prophylaxis, prospective studies indicate that dextran is not associated with significant postoperative bleeding unless it is administered together with low-dose heparin.[400,401] Hydroxyethyl starch, another volume expander, while generally safe, may prolong the bleeding time and predispose to hemorrhage, particularly if it is administered in doses of a 6% solution exceeding 20 ml/kg. It may predispose to bleeding in lower doses if administered simultaneously with low-dose heparin or if given to patients with a preexistent hemostatic defect or after major cardiothoracic surgery.[402-404] Different hydroxyethyl starch preparations vary in the average number of hydroxymethyl groups per glucose unit, and this may affect both intravascular survival and effects on hemostasis.[405]

PSYCHOTROPIC DRUGS, ANESTHETICS, AND COCAINE

Platelets from patients taking antidepressants or phenothiazines may exhibit impaired aggregation responses, but this is not associated with bleeding.[406,407] The effect on aggregation has been attributed to inhibition of intracellular signaling molecules, such as PKC.[408] Fluoxetine does not appear to impair in vitro platelet aggregation and has only rarely been associated with clinical bleeding.[409,410] General anesthesia with halothane may cause a slight prolongation of the bleeding time, most likely due to an effect on calcium signaling, but this has no adverse effect on surgical hemostasis.[411] In addition to an association with thrombocytopenia, cocaine has been reported to either inhibit platelet function[412,413] or to induce platelet activation.[414] The clinical relevance of these observations is unknown.

ONCOLOGIC DRUGS

Administration of mithramycin to a total dose of 6 to 21 mg has been associated with mucocutaneous bleeding, an increase in the bleeding time, and decreased platelet aggregation.[415] An ex vivo defect in platelet secretion and secondary aggregation has been reported in patients with solid tumors within 48 h of receiving infusions of autologous marrow and high-dose chemotherapy consisting of cisplatin, cyclophosphamide, and either BCNU or melphelan.[416] Both daunorubicin and BCNU can inhibit platelet aggregation and secretion when added to platelet-rich plasma, but as single agents they have not been shown to cause clinically significant platelet dysfunction.[417-419] Administration of recombinant forms of thrombopoietin to thrombocytopenic patients with cancer results in the production of normally functioning platelets.[420,421]

MISCELLANEOUS AGENTS

The immunosuppressive drug cyclosporine A has been reported to enhance ADP-stimulated platelet aggregation in vitro.[422-424] A relationship of this effect to the thrombosis often suffered by patients receiving the drug is unclear. Antihistamines,[425] the serotonin antagonist ketanserin,[426] and some radiographic contrast agents[427,428] can impair platelet aggregation responses ex vivo by unknown mechanisms.

FOODS AND FOOD ADDITIVES

The effect of certain foods and food additives on platelet function must be considered. For example, a diet rich in fish oils containing ω_3 fatty acids (eicosapentaenoic acid and docosahexaenoic acid) causes a slight prolongation of the bleeding time.[429] These fatty acids act by reducing the platelet content of arachidonic acid and by competing with arachidonic acid for cyclooxygenase.[430,431] Easy bruising noted after eating Chinese food has been attributed to an antiplatelet effect of the black tree fungus.[432] A component of extract of onion can inhibit platelet arachidonic acid metabolism.[433] Ajoene, a component of garlic, is an inhibitor of fibrinogen binding and platelet aggregation.[434,435] Extracts of two commonly used spices, cumin and turmeric, inhibit platelet aggregation and eicosanoid biosynthesis.[436]

REFERENCES

1. Rodgers RPC, Levin J: A critical reappraisal of the bleeding time. *Semin Thromb Hemost* 16:1, 1990.
2. Lind SE: The bleeding time does not predict surgical bleeding. *Blood* 77:3547, 1991.
3. Remuzzi G: Bleeding disorders in uremia: Pathophysiology and treatment. *Adv Nephrol* 18:171, 1989.
4. Rao AK: Uraemic platelets. *Lancet* 1:913, 1986.
5. Weigert AL, Schafer AI: Uremic bleeding: Pathogenesis and therapy. *Am J Med Sci* 316:94, 1998.
6. Akmal M, Sawelson S, Karubian F, Gadallah M: The prevalence and significance of occult blood loss in patients with predialysis advanced renal failure (CRF), or receiving dialytic therapy. *Clin Nephrol* 42:198, 1994.
7. Rosenbaum R, Hoffstein PE, Stanley RJ, Klahr S: Use of computerized tomography to diagnose complications of percutaneous renal biopsy. *Kidney Int* 14:87, 1978.
8. Diaz-Buxo JA, Donadio JVJ: Complications of percutaneous renal biopsy: An analysis of 1000 consecutive biopsies. *Clin Nephrol* 4:223, 1975.
9. Castillo R, Lozano T, Escolar G, et al: Defective platelet adhesion on vessel subendothelium in uremic patients. *Blood* 68:337, 1986.
10. Zwaginga JJ, Ijsseldijk MJW, Beeser-Visser N, et al: High von Willebrand factor concentration compensates a relative adhesion defect in uremic blood. *Blood* 75:1498, 1990.
11. Zwaginga JJ, Ijsseldijk I, de Groot PG, et al: Defects in platelet adhesion and aggregate formation in uremic bleeding disorder can be attributed to factors in plasma. *Artertiosc Thromb* 11:733, 1991.
12. Gordge MP, Faint RW, Rylance PB, Neild GH: Platelet function and the bleeding time in progressive renal failure. *Thromb Haemost* 60:83, 1988.
13. Tang WW, Stead RA, Goodkin DA: Effects of epoetin alfa on hemostasis in chronic renal failure. *Am J Nephrol* 18:263, 1998.
14. Fernandez F, Goudable C, Sie P, et al: Low haematocrit and prolonged bleeding time in uraemic patients: Effect of red cell transfusions. *Br J Haematol* 59:139, 1985.
15. Livio M, Gotti E, Marchesi D, et al: Uraemic bleeding: Role of anaemia and beneficial effect of red cell transfusions. *Lancet* 2:1013, 1982.
16. Moia M, Mannucci PM, Vizzotto L, et al: Improvement in the haemostatic defect of uraemia after treatment with recombinant human erythropoietin. *Lancet* 2:1227, 1987.
17. Vigano G, Benigni A, Mendogni D, et al: Recombinant human erythropoietin to correct uremic bleeding. *Am J Kidney Dis* 18:44, 1991.
18. Small M, Lowe GDO, Cameron E, Forbes CD: Contribution of the hematocrit to the bleeding time. *Haemostasis* 13:379, 1983.
19. Anonymous: The bleeding time and the haematocrit. *Lancet* 1:997, 1984.
20. Turrito VT, Weiss HJ: Red blood cells: Their dual role in thrombus formation. *Science* 207:541, 1980.
21. Marcus AJ, Safier LB: Thromboregulation: Multicellular modulation of platelet reactivity in hemostasis and thrombosis. *FASEB J* 7:516, 1993.
22. Weiss JH, Turrito VT, Baumgartner HR: Effect of shear rate in platelet interaction with subendothelium in citrated native blood: Shear-depen-dent increase in adherence in von Willebrand's disease and the Bernard-Soulier syndrome. *J Lab Clin Med* 92:750, 1978.
23. Sakariassen KS, Bolhuis PA, Sixma JJ: Platelet adherence to subendothelium of human arteries in pulsatile and steady flow. *Thromb Res* 19:547, 1980.
24. Deykin D: Uremic bleeding. *Kidney Int* 24:698, 1983.
25. Livio M, Mannucci PM, Vigano G, et al: Conjugated estrogens for the management of bleeding associated with renal failure. *N Engl J Med* 315:731, 1986.
26. Sloand EM, Sloand JA, Prodouz K, et al: Reduction of platelet glycoprotein Ib in uremia. *Br J Haematol* 77:375, 1991.
27. Gralnick HR, McKeown LP, Williams SB, et al: Plasma and platelet von Willebrand factor defects in uremia. *Am J Med* 85:806, 1988.
28. Escolar G, Cases A, Bastida E, et al: Uremic platelets have a functional defect affecting the interaction of von Willebrand factor with glycoprotein IIb-IIIa. *Blood* 76:1336, 1990.
29. Di Minno G, Cerbone A, Usberti M, et al: Platelet dysfunction in uremia: II. Correction by arachidonic acid of the impaired exposure of fibrinogen receptors by adenosine diphosphate or collagen. *J Lab Clin Med* 108:246, 1986.
30. Rabiner SF, Hrodek O: Platelet factor 3 in normal subjects and patients with renal failure. *J Clin Invest* 47:901, 1968.
31. Ware JA, Clark BA, Smith M, Salzman EW: Abnormalities of cytoplasmic Ca^{2+} in platelets from patients with uremia. *Blood* 73:172, 1989.
32. Remuzzi G, Benigni A, Dodesini P, et al: Reduced platelet thromboxane formation in uremia: Evidence for a functional cyclooxygenase defect. *J Clin Invest* 71:762, 1983.
33. Winter M, Frampton G, Bennett A, Machin SJ, et al: Synthesis of thromboxane B₂ in uraemia and the effects of dialysis. *Thromb Res* 30:265, 1983.
34. Bloom A, Greaves M, Preston FE, Brown CB: Evidence against a platelet cyclooxygenase defect in uraemic subjects on chronic haemodialysis. *Br J Haematol* 62:143, 1986.
35. Eknoyan G, Brown CH: Biochemical abnormalities of platelets in renal failure: Evidence for decreased platelet serotonin, adenosine diphosphate and Mg-dependent adenosine triphosphatase. *Am J Nephrol* 1:17, 1981.
36. Vlachoyannis J, Schoeppe W: Adenylate cyclase activity and cAMP content of human platelets in uraemia. *Eur J Clin Invest* 12:379, 1982.
37. Bazilinski N, Shaykh M, Dunea G, et al: Inhibition of platelet function by uremic middle molecules. *Nephron* 40:423, 1985.
38. Remuzzi G, Livio M, Marchiaro G, et al: Bleeding in renal failure: Altered platelet function in chronic uraemia only partially corrected by haemodialysis. *Nephron* 22:347, 1978.
39. Castaldi PA, Sydney MB: The bleeding disorder of uraemia. *Lancet* 2:66, 1966.
40. Livio M, Benigni A, Remuzzi G: Coagulation abnormalities in uremia. *Semin Nephrol* 5:82, 1985.
41. Remuzzi G, Cavenaghi AE, Mecca G, et al: Prostacyclin-like activity and bleeding in renal failure. *Lancet* 2:1195, 1977.
42. Remuzzi G, Perico N, Zoja C, et al: Role of endothelium-derived nitric oxide in the bleeding tendency of uremia. *J Clin Invest* 86:1768, 1990.
43. Aiello S, Noris M, Todeschini M, et al: Renal and systemic nitric oxide synthesis in rats with renal mass reduction. *Kidney Int* 52:171, 1997.
44. Livio M, Benigni A, Vigano G, et al: Moderate doses of aspirin and risk of bleeding in renal failure. *Lancet* 1:414, 1986.
45. Gaspari F, Vigano G, Orisio S, et al: Aspirin prolongs bleeding time in uremia by a mechanism distinct from platelet cyclooxygenase inhibition. *J Clin Invest* 79:1788, 1987.
46. Andrassy K, Ritz E: Uremia as a cause of bleeding. *Am J Nephrol* 5:313, 1985.
47. George CRP, Slichter SJ, Quadracci LJ: A kinetic evaluation of hemostasis in renal disease. *N Engl J Med* 291:1111, 1974.
48. Michalak E, Walkowiak B, Paradowski M, Cieriewski CS: The decreased circulating platelet mass and its relation to bleeding time in chronic renal failure. *Thromb Haemost* 65:11, 1991.
49. Mannucci PM, Remuzzi G, Pusineri F, et al: Deamino-8-arginine vasopressin shortens the bleeding time in uremia. *N Engl J Med* 308:8, 1983.
50. Peterson P, Hayes TE, Arkin CF, et al: The preoperative bleeding time test lacks clinical benefit. *Arch Surg* 133:134, 1998.
51. Liu YK, Goldstein DM, Arora K, et al: Thigh bleeding time as a valid indicator of hemostatic competency during surgical treatment of patients with advanced renal disease. *Surg Gynecol Obstet* 172:269, 1991.

52. Hutton RA, O'Shea MJ: Haemostatic mechanism in uraemia. *J Clin Pathol* 21:406, 1968.

53. Stewart JH, Castaldi PA: Uraemic bleeding: A reversible platelet defect corrected by dialysis. *Q J Med* 36:409, 1967.

54. Lindsay RM, Friesen M, Koens F, et al: Platelet function in patients on long-term peritoneal dialysis. *Clin Nephrol* 6:335, 1976.

55. Mannucci PM: Desmopressin: A non-transfusional form of treatment for congenital and acquired bleeding disorders. *Blood* 72:1449, 1988.

56. Rose EH, Aledort LM: Nasal spray desmopressin (DDAVP) for mild hemophilia A and von Willebrand disease. *Ann Intern Med* 114:563, 1991.

57. Mannucci PM: Desmopressin (DDAVP) for treatment of disorders of hemostasis. *Prog Hemost Thromb* 8:19, 1986.

58. Mannucci PM: Desmopressin (DDAVP) in the treatment of bleeding disorders: The first 20 years. *Blood* 90:2515, 1997.

59. Canavese C, Salomone M, Pacitti A, et al: Reduced response of uraemic bleeding time to repeated doses of desmopressin. *Lancet* 1:867, 1985.

60. Bichet DG, Razi M, Lonegran M, Arthur M-F: 1-Desamino [8-D-arginine] vasopressin (dDAVP) decreases blood pressure and increases pulse rate in normal individuals. *Thromb Haemost* 60:348, 1988.

61. Byrnes JJ, Larcada A, Moake JL: Thrombosis following desmopressin for uremic bleeding. *Am J Hematol* 28:63, 1988.

62. Anonymous: Desmopressin and arterial thrombosis. *Lancet* 1:938, 1989.

63. Mannucci PM: Desmopressin and thrombosis. *Lancet* 2:675, 1989.

64. Gotti E, Mecca G, Valentino C, et al: Renal biopsy in patients with acute renal failure and prolonged bleeding time. *Lancet* 2:978, 1984.

65. Tassies D, Reverter JC, Cases A, et al: Effect of recombinant human erythropoietin treatment on circulating reticulated platelets in uremic patients: Association with early improvement in platelet function. *Am J Hematol* 59:105, 1998.

66. Liu YK, Kosfeld RE, Marcum SG: Treatment of uremic bleeding with conjugated estrogen. *Lancet* 2:887, 1984.

67. Vigano G, Gaspari F, Locatelli M, et al: Dose-effect and pharmacokinetics of estrogens given to correct bleeding time in uremia. *Kidney Int* 34:853, 1988.

68. Heistinger M, Stockenhuber F, Schneider B, et al: Effect of conjugated estrogens on platelet function and prostacyclin generation in CRF. *Kidney Int* 38:1181, 1990.

69. Bronner MH, Pate MD, Cunningham JT: Estrogen-progesterone therapy for bleeding of gastrointestinal telangiectasias in chronic renal failure. *Ann Intern Med* 105:371, 1986.

70. Shemin D, Elnour M, Amarantes B, Abuelo JG: Oral estrogens decrease bleeding time and improve clinical bleeding in patients with renal failure. *Am J Med* 89:436, 1990.

71. Vigano G, Zoja C, Corna D, et al: 17 β-estradiol is the most active component of the conjugated estrogen mixture active on uremic bleeding by a receptor mechanism. *Mol Pharmacol* 252:344, 1990.

72. Juhl A: DDAVP, cryoprecipitate and highly "purified" factor VIII concentrate in uremia. *Nephron* 43:305, 1986.

73. Janson PA, Jubelirer SJ, Weinstein MS, Deykin D: Treatment of bleeding tendency in uremia with cryoprecipitate. *N Engl J Med* 303:1318, 1980.

74. Triulzi DJ, Blumber N: Variability in response to cryoprecipitate treatment for hemostatic defects in uremia. *Yale J Biol Med* 63:1, 1990.

75. George JN: Platelet membrane microparticles in blood bank fresh frozen plasma and cryoprecipitate. *Blood* 68:307, 1986.

76. George JN: Platelet IgG: Measurement, interpretation, and clinical significance. *Prog Hemost Thromb* 10:97, 1991.

77. Thompson AR, Harker LA: *Approach to Bleeding Disorders: Manual of Hemostasis and Thrombosis,* 3rd ed, p 57. FA Davis, Philadelphia, 1983.

78. George JN, Woolf SH, Raskob GE, et al: Idiopathic thrombocytopenic purpura: A practice guideline developed by explicit methods for the American Society of Hematology. *Blood* 88:3, 1996.

79. George JN, El-Harake MA, Raskob GE: Chronic idiopathic thrombocytopenic purpura. *N Engl J Med* 331:1207, 1994.

80. Uesugi Y, Fuse I, Toba K, et al: Acquired immune thrombocytopenia caused by IgG antiglycoprotein Ib antibody in a patient with Hodgkin's disease. *Acta Haematol* 98:217, 1997.

81. Meyer M, Kirchmaier CM, Schirmer A, et al: Acquired disorder of platelet function associated with autoantibodies against membrane glycoprotein IIb-IIIa complex-1: Glycoprotein analysis. *Thromb Haemost* 65:491, 1991.

82. Balduini CL, Grignani G, Sinigaglia F, et al: Severe platelet dysfunc-

tion in a patient with autoantibodies against membrane glycoproteins IIb-IIIa. *Haemostasis* 7:98, 1987.

83. Balduini CL, Bertolino G, Noris P, et al: Defect of platelet aggregation and adhesion induced by autoantibodies against platelet glycoprotein IIIa. *Thromb Haemost* 68:208, 1992.

84. Fuse I, Higuchi W, Narita M, et al: Overproduction of antiplatelet antibody against glycoprotein IIb after splenectomy in a patient with Evans syndrome resulting in acquired thrombasthenia [comments]. *Acta Haematol* 99:83, 1998.

85. Stricker RB, Wong D, Saks SR, et al: Acquired Bernard-Soulier syndrome: Evidence for the role of a 210,000–molecular weight protein in the interaction of platelets with von Willebrand factor. *J Clin Invest* 76:1274, 1985.

86. Devine DV, Currie MS, Rosse WF, Greenberg CS: Pseudo-Bernard-Soulier syndrome: Thrombocytopenia caused by autoantibody to platelet glycoprotein Ib. *Blood* 70:428, 1987.

87. Deckmyn H, Zhang J, Van Houtte E, Vermylen J: Production and nucleotide sequence of an inhibitory human IgM autoantibody directed against platelet glycoprotein Ia/IIa. *Blood* 84:1968, 1994.

88. Dromigny A, Triadou P, Lesavre P, et al: Lack of platelet response to collagen associated with autoantibodies against glycoprotein (GP) Ia/IIa and Ib/IX leading to the discovery of SLE. *Hematol Cell Ther* 38:355, 1996.

89. Xu H, Frojmovic MM, Wong T, Rauch J: p32, a platelet autoantigen recognized by an SLE-derived autoantibody that inhibits platelet aggregation. *J Autoimmun* 8:97, 1995.

90. Wiedmer T, Ando B, Sims PJ: Complement C5b-9-stimulated platelet secretion is associated with a calcium-initiated activation of cellular protein kinases. *J Biol Chem* 262:13674, 1987.

91. Sugiyama T, Okuma M, Ushikubi F, et al: A novel platelet aggregating factor found in a patient with defective collagen-induced platelet aggregation and autoimmune thrombocytopenia. *Blood* 69:1712, 1987.

92. Handagama PJ, George JN, Shuman MA, et al: Incorporation of a circulating protein into megakaryocyte and platelet granules. *Proc Nat Acad Sci USA* 84:861, 1987.

93. Weiss HJ, Rosove MH, Lages BA, Kaplan KL: Acquired storage pool deficiency with increased platelet-associated IgG. *Am J Med* 69:711, 1980.

94. Stuart MJ, Kelton JG, Allen JB: Abnormal platelet function and arachidonate metabolism in chronic idiopathic thrombocytopenic purpura. *Blood* 58:326, 1981.

95. Lackner H, Karpatkin S: On the "easy bruising" syndrome with normal platelet count: A study of 75 patients. *Ann Intern Med* 83:190, 1975.

96. Clancy R, Jenkins E, Firkin B: Qualitative platelet abnormalities in idiopathic thrombocytopenic purpura. *N Engl J Med* 286:622, 1972.

97. Heyns DA, Fraser J, Retief FP: Platelet aggregation in chronic idiopathic thrombocytopenic purpura. *J Clin Pathol* 31:1239, 1978.

98. Regan MG, Lackner H, Karpatkin S: Platelet function and coagulation profile in lupus erythematosus. *Am J Med* 81:462, 1974.

99. Dorsch CA, Meyerhoff J: Mechanisms of abnormal platelet aggregation in systemic lupus erythematosus. *Arthritis Rheum* 25:966, 1982.

100. Nieuwenhuis HK, Zwaginga JJ, Sixma JJ: Analysis of patients with a prolonged bleeding time. *Thromb Haemost* 58:527, 1987.

101. Meyerhoff J, Dorsch CA: Decreased platelet serotonin levels in systemic lupus erythematosus. *Arthritis Rheum* 24:1495, 1981.

102. Harker LA, Malpass TW, Branson HE, et al: Mechanism of abnormal bleeding in patients undergoing cardiopulmonary bypass: Acquired transient platelet dysfunction associated with selective alpha-granule release. *Blood* 56:824, 1980.

103. Khuri SF, Valeri CR, Loscalzo J, et al: Heparin causes platelet dysfunction and induces fibrinolysis before cardiopulmonary bypass [comments]. *Ann Thorac Surg* 60:1008, 1995.

104. Colman RW: Platelet and neutrophil activation in cardiopulmonary bypass. *Ann Thorac Surg* 49:32, 1990.

105. Mammen EF, Koets MH, Washington BC, et al: Hemostasis changes during cardiopulmonary bypass surgery. *Semin Thromb Hemost* 11:281, 1985.

106. Khuri SF, Wolfe JA, Josa M, et al: Hematologic changes during and after cardiopulmonary bypass and their relationship to the bleeding time and nonsurgical blood loss. *J Thorac Cardiovasc Surg* 104:94, 1992.

107. Martin JF, Daniel TD, Trowbridge EA: Acute and chronic changes

in platelet volume and count after cardiopulmonary bypass induced thrombocytopenia in man. *Thromb Haemost* 57:55, 1987.

108. Chandler AB, Hutson MS: Platelet plug formation in an extracorporeal unit. *Am J Clin Pathol* 64:101, 1975.

109. Uniyal S, Brash JL: Patterns of adsorption of proteins from human plasma onto foreign surfaces. *Thromb Haemost* 47:285, 1982.

110. Lindon JN, McManama, Kushner L: Does the conformation of adsorbed fibrinogen dictate platelet interactions with artificial surfaces? *Blood* 68:355, 1986.

111. Singer RL, Mannion JD, Bauer TL, et al: Complications from heparin-induced thrombocytopenia in patients undergoing cardiopulmonary bypass. *Chest* 104:1436, 1993.

112. Woodman RC, Harker LA: Bleeding complications associated with cardiopulmonary bypass. *Blood* 76:1680, 1990.

113. Bick RL: Hemostasis defects associated with cardiac surgery, prosthetic devices, and other extracorporeal circuits. *N Engl J Med* 22:1446, 1986.

114. McKenna R, Bachmann F, Whittaker B, et al: The hemostatic mechanism after open heart surgery: II. Frequency of abnormal platelet functions during and after extracorporeal circulation. *J Thorac Cardiovasc Surg* 70:298, 1975.

115. Beurling-Harbury C, Galvan CA: Acquired decrease in platelet secretory ADP associated with increased post-operative bleeding in post-cardio-pulmonary bypass patients and in patients with severe valvular heart disease. *Blood* 52:13, 1978.

116. Abrams CS, Ellison N, Budzynski AZ, Shattil S: Direct detection of activated platelets and platelet-derived microparticles in humans. *Blood* 75:128, 1990.

117. George JN, Pickett EB, Saucerman S, et al: Platelet surface glycopro-teins: Studies on resting and activated platelets and platelet membrane microparticles in normal subjects, and observations in patients during adult respiratory distress syndrome and cardiac surgery. *J Clin Invest* 78:340, 1986.

118. Bachmann F, McKenna R, Cole ER, Najafi H: The hemostatic mecha-nism after open heart surgery: I. Studies on plasma coagulation factors and fibrinolysis in 512 patients after extracorporeal circulation. *J Thorac Cardiovasc Surg* 70:76, 1975.

119. Gluszko P, Ricinski B, Musial J, et al: Fibrinogen receptors in platelet adhesion to surfaces of extracorporeal circuit. *Am J Physiol* 252: H615, 1987.

120. van den Dungen JJ, Karliczek GF, Brenken U, et al: Clinical study of blood trauma during perfusion with membrane and bubble oxygenators. *Thorac Cardiovasc Surg* 83:108, 1982.

121. Ferraris VA, Ferraris SP, Singh A, et al: The platelet thrombin receptor and postoperative bleeding. *Ann Thorac Surg* 65:352, 1998.

122. Kestin AS, Valeri CR, Khuri SF, et al: The platelet function defect of cardiopulmonary bypass. *Blood* 82:107, 1993.

123. Weksler BB, Pett SB, Alonso D, et al: Differential inhibition of aspirin of vascular prostaglandin synthesis in atherosclerotic patients. *N Engl J Med* 308:800, 1983.

124. Hunt BJ, Parratt RN, Segal HC, et al: Activation of coagulation and fibrinolysis during cardiothoracic operations. *Ann Thorac Surg* 65:712, 1998.

125. Tabuchi N, de Haan J, Boonstra PW, van Oeveren W: Activation of fibrinolysis in the pericardial cavity during cardiopulmonary bypass. *J Thorac Cardiovasc Surg* 106:828, 1993.

126. Rapaport SI: Preoperative hemostatic evaluation: which tests, if any? *Blood* 61:229, 1983.

127. Magovern JA, Sakert T, Benckart DH, et al: A model for predicting transfusion after coronary artery bypass grafting. *Ann Thorac Surg* 61:27, 1996.

128. Simon TA, Akl BF, Murphy W: Controlled trial of routine administration of platelet concentrates in cardiopulmonary bypass surgery. *Ann Thorac Surg* 37:359, 1987.

129. Wasser MNJM, Houbiers JGA, D'Amaro J, et al: The effect of fresh versus stored blood on post-operative bleeding after coronary bypass surgery: A prospective randomized study. *Br J Haematol* 72:81, 1989.

130. Sowade O, Warnke H, Scigalla P, et al: Avoidance of allogeneic blood transfusions by treatment with epoetin beta (recombinant human erythro-poietin) in patients undergoing open-heart surgery. *Blood* 89:411, 1997.

131. Shimpo H, Mizumoto T, Onoda K, et al: Erythropoietin in pediatric cardiac surgery: Clinical efficacy and effective dose. *Chest* 111:1565, 1997.

132. Schmoeckel M, Nollert G, Mempel M, et al: Effects of recombinant human erythropoietin on autologous blood donation before open heart surgery. *Thorac Cardiovasc Surg* 41:364, 1993.

133. Axford TC, Dearani JA, Ragno G, et al: Safety and therapeutic effective-ness of reinfused shed blood after open heart surgery. *Ann Thorac Surg* 57:615, 1994.

134. Griffith LD, Billman GF, Daily PO, Lane TA: Apparent coagulopathy caused by infusion of shed mediastinal blood and its prevention by washing of the infusate. *Ann Thorac Surg* 47:400, 1989.

135. Hackmann T, Gascoyne R, Naiman SC, et al: A trial of desmopressin to reduce blood loss in uncomplicated cardiac surgery. *N Engl J Med* 321:1437, 1989.

136. Seear MD, Wadsworth LD, Rogers PC, et al: The effect of desmopressin acetate (DDAVP) on postoperative blood loss after cardiac operations in children [comments]. *J Thorac Cardiovasc Surg* 98:217, 1989.

137. Walker ID, Davidson JF, Faichney A, et al: A double-blind study of prostacyclin in cardiopulmonary bypass surgery. *Br J Haematol* 49: 415, 1981.

138. Fish KJ, Sarnquist FH, van Steennis C, et al: A prospective, randomized study of the effects of prostacyclin on platelets and blood loss during coronary bypass operations. *J Thorac Cardiovasc Surg* 91:436, 1986.

139. van Oeveren W, Harder MP, Roozendaal KJ, et al: Aprotinin protects platelets against the initial effect of cardiopulmonary bypass. *J Thorac Cardiovasc Surg* 99:788, 1990.

140. Hardy J-F, Desroches J: Natural and synthetic antifibrinolytics in cardiac surgery. *Can J Anesthesiol* 39:353, 1992.

141. Speekenbrink RG, Wildevuur CR, Sturk A, Eijsman L: Low-dose and high-dose aprotinin improve hemostasis in coronary operations. *J Thorac Cardiovasc Surg* 112:523, 1996.

142. Orchard MA, Goodchild CS, Prentice CR, et al: Aprotinin reduces cardiopulmonary bypass-induced blood loss and inhibits fibrinolysis without influencing platelets. *Br J Haematol* 85:533, 1993.

143. Wahba A, Black G, Koksch M, et al: Aprotinin has no effect on platelet activation and adhesion during cardiopulmonary bypass. *Thromb Hae-most* 75:844, 1996.

144. Mastroroberto P, Chello M, Zofrea S, Marchese AR: Suppressed fibrino-lysis after administration of low-dose aprotinin: Reduced level of plas-min-alpha$_2$-plasmin inhibitor complexes and postoperative blood loss. *Eur J Cardiothorac Surg* 9:143, 1995.

145. Rich JB: The efficacy and safety of aprotinin use in cardiac surgery. *Ann Thorac Surg* 66:S6, 1998.

146. Bidstrup BP, Underwood SR, Sapsford RN, Streets EM: Effect of aproti-nin (Trasylol) on aorta-coronary bypass graft patency. *J Thorac Cardio-vasc Surg* 105:147, 1993.

147. Dietrich W, Spath P, Ebell A, Richter JA: Prevalence of anaphylactic reactions to aprotinin: Analysis of two hundred forty-eight reexposures to aprotinin in heart operations. *J Thorac Cardiovasc Surg* 113:194, 1997.

148. Miller JM: Trasylol in primary acute pancreatitis [letter]. *Br J Surg* 65: 887, 1978.

149. Pinosky ML, Kennedy DJ, Fishman RL, et al: Tranexamic acid reduces bleeding after cardiopulmonary bypass when compared to epsilon amino-caproic acid and placebo. *J Cardiac Surg* 12:330, 1997.

150. Penta de Peppo A, Pierri MD, Scafuri A, et al: Intraoperative antifibrino-lysis and blood-saving techniques in cardiac surgery: Prospective trial of 3 antifibrinolytic drugs. *Tex Heart Inst J* 22:231, 1995.

151. Krauss JS, Jonah MH: Platelet dysfunction (thrombocytopathy) in extra-hepatic biliary obstruction. *South Med J* 75:506, 1982.

152. Hillbom M, Muuronen A, Neiman J: Liver disease and platelet function in alcoholics. *Br Med J* 295:581, 1987.

153. Mannucci PM, Vicente V, Vianello L, et al: Controlled trial of desmo-pressin in liver cirrhosis and other conditions associated with a prolonged bleeding time. *Blood* 67:1148, 1986.

154. Stein SF, Harker LA: Kinetic and functional studies of platelets, fibrino-gen, and plasminogen in patients with hepatic cirrhosis. *J Lab Clin Med* 99:217, 1982.

155. Violi F, Leo R, Vezza E, et al: Bleeding time in patients with cirrhosis: Relation with degree of liver failure and clotting abnormalities. Coagula-tion Abnormalities in Cirrhosis Study Group. *J Hepatol* 20:531, 1994.

156. Pareti FI, Capitanio A, Mannucci L: Acquired storage pool disease in platelets during disseminated intravascular coagulation. *Blood* 48:511, 1976.

157. Pareti FI, Capitanio A, Mannucci L, et al: Acquired dysfunction due to the circulation of "exhausted" platelets. *Am J Med* 69:235, 1980.

158. Solum NO, Rigollot C, Budzynski A, Marder VJ: A quantitative evaluation of the inhibition of platelet aggregation by low molecular weight degradation products of fibrinogen. *Br J Haematol* 24:619, 1973.

159. Bennett JS, Vilaire G: Exposure of platelet fibrinogen receptors by ADP and epinephrine. *J Clin Invest* 64:1393, 1979.

160. Stoff JS, Stemerman M, Steer M, et al: A defect in platelet aggregation in Bartter's syndrome. *Am J Med* 68:171, 1980.

161. Lim SH, Tan CE, Agasthian T, Chew LS: Acquired platelet dysfunction with eosinophilia: Review of seven adult cases. *J Clin Pathol* 42:950, 1989.

162. Poon MC, Ng SC, Coppes MJ: Acquired platelet dysfunction with eosinophilia in white children. *J Pediatr* 126:959, 1995.

163. Szczeklik A, Milner PC, Birch J, et al: Prolonged bleeding time, reduced platelet aggregation, altered PAF-acether sensitivity and increased platelet mass are a trait of asthma and hay fever. *Thromb Haemost* 56:283, 1986.

164. Carvalho AC, Quinn DA, DeMarinis SM, et al: Platelet function in acute respiratory failure. *Am J Hematol* 25:377, 1987.

165. Bracey AW, Wu AH, Aceves J, et al: Platelet dysfunction associated with Wilms tumor and hyaluronic acid. *Am J Hematol* 24:247, 1987.

166. Landolfi R, Rocca B, Patrono C: Bleeding and thrombosis in myeloproliferative disorders: Mechanisms and treatment. *Crit Rev Oncol Hematol* 20:203, 1995.

167. Murphy S: Polycythemia vera. *Dis Mon* 38:165, 1992.

168. Wasserman LR, Gilbert H: Complications of polycythemia vera. *Semin Hematol* 3:199, 1966.

169. Schafer AI: Essential thrombocythemia. *Prog Hemost Thromb* 10:69, 1991.

170. Mitus AJ, Barbui T, Shulman LN, et al: Hemostatic complications in young patients with essential thrombocythemia. *Am J Med* 88:371, 1990.

171. Lahuerta-Palacios JJ, Bornstein R, Fernandez-Debora FJ, et al: Controlled and uncontrolled thrombocytosis: Its clinical role in essential thrombocytosis. *Cancer* 61:1207, 1988.

172. Kessler CM, Klein HG, Havlik RJ: Uncontrolled thrombocytosis in chronic myeloproliferative disorders. *Br J Haematol* 50:157, 1982.

173. McIntyre KJ, Hoagland HC, Silverstein MN, Petitt RM: Essential thrombocythemia in young adults. *Mayo Clin Proc* 66:149, 1991.

174. Bellucci S, Janvier M, Tobelem G, et al: Essential thrombocythemias: Clinical evolutionary and biological data. *Cancer* 58:2440, 1986.

175. Maldonado JE, Pintado T, Pierre RV: Dysplastic platelets and circulating megakaryocytes in chronic myeloproliferative diseases: I. The platelets: Ultrastructure and peroxidase reaction. *Blood* 43:797, 1974.

176. Bautista AP, Buckler PW, Towler HM, et al: Measurement of platelet life-span in normal subjects and patients with myeloproliferative disease. *Br J Haematol* 58:679, 1984.

177. Ginsberg AD: Platelet function in patients with high platelet counts. *Ann Intern Med* 82:506, 1975.

178. Jubilirer SJ, Russell F, Faillacourt R, Deykin D: Platelet arachidonic acid metabolism and platelet function in ten patients with chronic myelogenous leukemia. *Blood* 56:728, 1980.

179. Pareti FI, Gugliotta L, Mannucci L, et al: Biochemical and metabolic aspects of platelet dysfunction in chronic myeloproliferative disorders. *Thromb Haemost* 47:84, 1982.

180. Schafer AI: Deficiency of platelet lipoxygenase activity in myeloproliferative disorders. *N Engl J Med* 306:381, 1982.

181. Okuma M, Takayama H, Uchino H: Subnormal platelet response to thromboxane A_2 in a patient with chronic myeloid leukaemia. *Br J Haematol* 51:469, 1982.

182. Ushikubi F, Okuma M, Kanaji K, et al: Hemorrhagic thrombocytopathy with platelet thromboxane A_2 receptor abnormality: Defective signal transduction with normal binding activity. *Thromb Haemost* 57:158, 1987.

183. Malpass TW, Savage B, Hanson SR, et al: Correlation between prolonged bleeding time and depletion of platelet dense granule ADP in patients with myelodysplastic and myeloproliferative disorders. *J Lab Clin Med* 103:894, 1984.

184. Mohri H: Acquired von Willebrand disease and storage pool disease in chronic myelocytic leukemia. *Am J Hematol* 22:391, 1986.

185. Handa M, Wantanabe K, Kawai Y, et al: Platelet unresponsiveness to collagen: Involvement of glycoprotein Ia-IIa ($\alpha_2\beta_1$ integrin) deficiency associated with a myeloproliferative disorder. *Thromb Haemost* 73: 521, 1995.

186. Kaywin P, McDonough M, Insel PA, Shattil SJ: Platelet function in essential thrombocythemia: Decreased epinephrine responsiveness associated with a deficiency of platelet alpha-adrenergic receptors. *N Engl J Med* 299:505, 1978.

187. Swart SS, Pearson D, Wood JK, Barnett DB: Functional significance of the platelet alpha$_2$-adrenoceptor: Studies in patients with myeloproliferative disorders. *Thromb Res* 33:531, 1984.

188. Nurden P, Bihour C, Smith M, et al: Platelet activation and thrombosis: Studies in a patient with essential thrombocythemia. *Am J Hematol* 51:79, 1996.

189. Rocca B, Ciabattoni G, Tartaglione R, et al: Increased thromboxane biosynthesis in essential thrombocythemia. *Thromb Haemost* 74:1225, 1995.

190. Landolfi R, Ciabattoni G, Patrignani P, et al: Increased thromboxane biosynthesis in patients with polycythemia vera: Evidence for aspirin-suppressible platelet activation in vivo. *Blood* 80:1965, 1992.

191. Walsh PN, Murphy S, Barry WE: The role of platelets in the pathogenesis of thrombosis and hemorrhage in patients with thrombocytosis. *Thromb Haemost* 38:1085, 1977.

192. Berndt MC, Kabral A, Grimsley P, et al: An acquired Bernard-Soulier-like platelet defect associated with juvenile myelodysplastic syndrome. *Br J Haematol* 68:97, 1988.

193. Cooper B, Schafer AI, Puchalsky D, Handin RI: Platelet resistance to prostaglandin D_2 in patients with myeloproliferative disorders. *Blood* 52:618, 1978.

194. Moore A, Nachman RL: Platelet Fc receptor: Increased expression in myeloproliferative disease. *J Clin Invest* 67:1064, 1981.

195. Bolin RB, Okumura T, Jamieson GA: Changes in distribution of platelet membrane glycoproteins in patients with myeloproliferative disorders. *Am J Hematol* 3:63, 1977.

196. Eche N, Sie P, Caranobe C, et al: Platelets in myeloproliferative disorders: III. Glycoprotein profile in relation to platelet function and platelet density. *Scand J Haematol* 26:123, 1981.

197. Thibert V, Bellucci S, Cristofari M, et al: Increased platelet CD36 constitutes a common marker in myeloproliferative disorders. *Br J Haemtol* 91:618, 1995.

198. Moliterno AR, Hankins D, Spivak JL: Impaired expression of the thrombopoietin receptor by platelets from patients with polycythemia vera. *N Engl J Med* 338:572, 1998.

199. Budde U, Schaefer G, Mueller N, et al: Acquired von Willebrand's disease in the myeloproliferative syndrome. *Blood* 64:981, 1984.

200. van Genderen PJJ, Budde U, Michiels JJ, et al: The reduction in large von Willebrand factor multimers in plasma in essential thrombocythemia is related to platelet count. *Br J Haematol* 93:962, 1996.

201. Mohri H, Ohkubo T: Acquired von Willebrand's syndrome due to an inhibitor of IgG specific for von Willebrand's factor in polycythemia rubra vera. *Acta Haematol* 78:258, 1987.

202. van Genderen PJJ, Prins FJ, Lucas IS, et al: Decreased half-life of plasma von Willebrand factor collagen binding activity in essential thrombocythemia: Normalization after cytoreduction of the increased platelet count. *Br J Haematol* 99:832, 1997.

203. Schafer AI: Bleeding and thrombosis in the myeloproliferative disorders. *Blood* 64:1, 1984.

204. Murphy S: Thrombocytosis and thrombocythaemia. *Clin Haematol* 12:89, 1983.

205. Mitchell MC, Boitnott JK, Kaufman S, et al: Budd-Chiari syndrome: Etiology, diagnosis and management. *Medicine* 61:199, 1982.

206. Valla D, Casadevall N, Huisse MG, et al: Etiology of portal vein thrombosis in adults: A propspective evaluation of primary myeloproliferative disorders. *Gastroenterology* 94:1063, 1988.

207. Singh AK, Wetherley-Mein G: Microvascular occlusive lesions in primary thrombocythaemia. *Br J Haematol* 36:553, 1977.

208. van Genderen PJJ, Michiels JJ, van Strik R, et al: Platelet consumption in thrombocythemia complicated by erythromelalgia: reversal by aspirin. *Thromb Haemost* 73:210, 1995.

209. Kessler CM, Klein HG, Havlik RJ: Uncontrolled thrombocytosis in chronic myeloproliferative disorders. *Br J Haematol* 50:157, 1982.

210. Rinder HM, Schuster JE, Rinder CS, et al: Correlation of thrombosis with increased platelet turnover in thrombocytosis. *Blood* 91:1288, 1998.

211. Besses C, Cervantes F, Pereira A, et al: Major vascular complications

in essential thrombocythemia: A study of the predictive factors in a series of 148 patients. *Leukemia* 13:150, 1999.

212. Kaplan ME, Mack K, Goldberg JD: Long-term management of polycythemia vera with hydroxyurea: A progress report. *Semin Hematol* 23:167, 1986.

213. Cortelazzo S, Finazzi G, Ruggeri M, et al: Hydroxyurea for patients with essential thrombocythemia and a high risk of thrombosis. *N Engl J Med* 332:1132, 1995.

214. Group AS: Anagrelide, a therapy for thrombocythemic states: Experience in 577 patients. *Am J Med* 92:69, 1992.

215. Solberg LA, Tefferi A, Oles KJ, et al: The effects of anagrelide on human megakaryocytopoiesis. *Br J Haematol* 99:174, 1997.

216. Preston FE: Aspirin, prostaglandins, and peripheral gangrene. *Am J Med* 74(suppl):55, 1983.

217. Michiels JJ, Abels J, Steketee J, et al: Erythromelalgia caused by platelet-mediated arteriolar inflammation and thrombosis in thrombocythemia. *Ann Intern Med* 102:466, 1985.

218. van Genderen PJJ, Mulder PGH, Waleboer M, et al: Prevention and treatment of thrombotic complications in essential thrombocythemia: Efficacy and safety of aspirin. *Br J Haematol* 97:179, 1997.

219. Sultan Y, Caen JP: Platelet dysfunction in preleukemic states and in various types of leukemia. *Ann NY Acad Sci* 201:300, 1972.

220. Cowan DH, Haut JJ: Platelet function in acute leukemia. *J Lab Clin Med* 79:893, 1972.

221. Cowan DH, Graham RR Jr, Baunach D: The platelet defect in leukemia, platelet ultrastructure, adenine nucleotide metabolism and the release reaction. *J Clin Invest* 56:188, 1975.

222. Meschengieser S, Blanco A, Maugeri N, et al: Platelet function and intraplatelet von Willebrand factor antigen and fibrinogen in myelodysplastic syndromes. *Thromb Res* 46:601, 1987.

223. Pui C-H, Jackson CW, Chesney C: Normal platelet function after therapy for acute lymphocytic leukemia. *Arch Intern Med* 143:73, 1983.

224. Westbrook CA, Golde DW: Clinical problems in hairy cell leukemia: Diagnosis and management. *Semin Oncol* 11:514, 1984.

225. Levine PH, Katayama I: The platelet in leukemic reticuloendotheliosis. *Cancer* 36:1353, 1975.

226. Feiner AS, Myers AM, Moore GE: Leukemic reticuloendotheliosis: Loss of platelet defect after splenectomy. *J Am Med Assoc* 241:1684, 1979.

227. Sweet DL, Golomb HM: Correction of platelet defect after splenectomy in hairy cell leukemia. *J Am Med Assoc* 241:1684, 1979.

228. Zuzel M, Cawley JC, Paton RC, et al: Platelet function in hairy-cell leukaemia. *J Clin Pathol* 32:814, 1979.

229. Rosove MH, Naeim F, Harwig S, Zighelboim J: Severe platelet dysfunction in hairy cell leukemia with improvement after splenectomy. *Blood* 55:903, 1980.

230. Roussi JH, Houbouyan LL, Alterescu R, et al: Acquired von Willebrand's syndrome associated with hairy cell leukemia. *Br J Haematol* 46:503, 1980.

231. Lackner H: Hemostatic abnormalities associated with dysproteinemias. *Semin Hematol* 10:125, 1973.

232. Perkins HA, McKenzie MR, Fudenberg HH: Hemostatic defects in dysproteinemias. *Blood* 35:695, 1970.

233. Rapoport M, Yona R, Kaufman S, et al: Unusual bleeding manifestations of amyloidosis in patients with multiple myeloma. *Clin Lab Haematol* 16:349, 1994.

234. Furie B, Greene E, Furie BC: Syndrome of acquired factor X deficiency and systemic amyloidosis. *N Engl J Med* 297:81, 1977.

235. McPherson RA, Onstad JW, Ugoretz RJ, Wolf PL: Coagulopathy in amyloidosis: Combined deficiency of factors IX and X. *Am J Hematol* 3:225, 1977.

236. Palmer RN, Rick ME, Rick PD, et al: Circulating heparan sulfate anticoagulant in a patient with a fatal bleeding disorder. *N Engl J Med* 310:1696, 1984.

237. Chapman GS, George CB, Danley DL: Heparin-like anticoagulant associated with plasma cell myeloma. *Am J Clin Pathol* 83:764, 1985.

238. Liebman H, Chinowsky M, Valdin J, et al: Increased fibrinolysis and amyloidosis. *Arch Intern Med* 143:678, 1983.

239. Meyer K, Williams EC: Fibrinolysis and acquired alpha-2 plasmin inhibitor deficiency in amyloidosis. *Am J Med* 79:394, 1985.

240. McGrath KM, Stuart JJ, Richards F II: Correlation between serum IgG, platelet membrane IgG and platelet function in hypergammaglobulinemic states. *Br J Haematol* 42:585, 1979.

241. Kasturi J, Saraya AK: Platelet functions in dysproteinemia. *Acta Haematol* 59:104, 1978.

242. Vigliano EM, Horowitz HI: Bleeding syndrome in a patient with IgA myeloma: Interaction of protein and connective tissue. *Blood* 29:823, 1967.

243. DiMinno G, Coraggio F, Cerbone AM, et al: A myeloma paraprotein with specificity for platelet glycoprotein IIIa in a patient with a fatal bleeding disorder. *J Clin Invest* 77:157, 1986.

244. Mohri H, Noguchi T, Kodama F, et al: Acquired von Willebrand disease due to inhibitor of human myeloma protein specific for von Willebrand factor. *J Clin Pathol* 87:663, 1987.

245. Takahashi H, Nagayama R, Tanabe Y, et al: DDAVP in acquired von Willebrand syndrome associated with multiple myeloma. *Am J Hematol* 22:421, 1986.

246. Mannucci PM, Lombardi R, Bader R, et al: Studies of the pathophysiology of acquired von Willebrand's disease in seven patients with lymphoproliferative disorders or benign monoclonal gammopathies. *Blood* 64:614, 1984.

247. Wallace MR, Simon SR, Ershler WB, Burns SL: Hemorrhagic diathesis in multiple myeloma. *Acta Haematol* 72:340, 1984.

248. Hyman BT, Westrick MA: Multiple myeloma with polyneuropathy and coagulopathy. *Arch Intern Med* 146:993, 1986.

249. Bovill EG, Ershler WB, Golden EA, et al: A human myeloma-produced monoclonal protein directed against the active subpopulation of von Willebrand factor. *Am J Clin Pathol* 85:115, 1986.

250. Silberstein LE, Abrahm J, Shattil SJ: The efficacy of intensive plasma exchange in acquired von Willebrand's disease. *Transfusion* 27:234, 1987.

251. Bovill EG, Ershler WB, Golden EA, et al: A human myeloma-produced monoclonal protein directed against the active subpopulation of von Willebrand factor. *Am J Clin Pathol* 85:115, 1986.

252. Mohri H, Noguchi T, Kodama F, et al: Acquired von Willebrand disease due to inhibitor of human myeloma protein specific for von Willebrand factor. *Am J Clin Pathol* 87:663, 1987.

253. Mazurier C, Parquet-Gernez A, Descamps J, et al: Acquired von Willebrand's syndrome in the course of Waldenstrom's disease. *Thromb Haemost* 44:115, 1980.

254. van Genderen PJ, Vink T, Michiels JJ, et al: Acquired von Willebrand disease caused by an autoantibody selectively inhibiting the binding of von Willebrand factor to collagen. *Blood* 84:3378, 1994.

255. Handin RI, Martin V, Moloney WC: Antibody-induced von Willebrand's disease: A newly defined inhibitor syndrome. *Blood* 48:393, 1976.

256. Goudemand J, Samor B, Caron C, et al: Acquired type II von Willebrand's disease: Demonstration of a complexed inhibitor of the von Willebrand factor-platelet interaction and response to treatment. *Br J Haematol* 68:227, 1988.

257. Budde U, Schaefer G, Mueller N, et al: Acquired von Willebrand's disease in the myeloproliferative syndrome. *Blood* 64:981, 1984.

258. Mohri H, Hisanaga S, Mishima A, et al: Autoantibody inhibits binding of von Willebrand factor to glycoprotein Ib and collagen in multiple myeloma: recognition sites present on the A1 loop and A3 domains of von Willebrand factor. *Blood Coag Fibrinol* 9:91, 1998.

259. Igarashi N, Miura M, Kato E, et al: Acquired von Willebrand's syndrome with lupus-like serology. *Am J Pediatr Hematol Oncol* 11:32, 1989.

260. Scott JP, Montgomery RR, Tubergen DG, Hays T: Acquired von Willebrand's disease in association with Wilm's tumor: Regression following treatment. *Blood* 48:665, 1981.

261. Rao KP, Kizer J, Jones TJ, et al: Acquired von Willebrand's syndrome associated with an extranodal pulmonary lymphoma. *Arch Pathol Lab Med* 112:47, 1988.

262. Levesque H, Borg JY, Cailleux N, et al: Acquired von Willebrand's syndrome associated with decrease of plasminogen activator and its inhibitor during hypothyroidism. *Eur J Med* 2:287, 1993.

263. Aylesworth CA, Smallridge RC, Rick ME, Alving BM: Acquired von Willebrand's disease: A rare manifestation of postpartum thyroiditis. *Am J Hematol* 50:217, 1995.

264. Tefferi A, Nichols WL: Acquired von Willebrand disease: Concise review of occurrence, diagnosis, pathogenesis, and treatment. *Am J Med* 103:536, 1997.

265. Joist JH, Cowan JF, Zimmerman TS: Acquired von Willebrand's disease: Evidence for a quantitative and qualitative factor VIII disorder. *N Engl J Med* 298:988, 1978.

266. Macik BG, Gabriel DA, White GC 2d, et al: The use of high-dose intravenous gamma-globulin in acquired von Willebrand syndrome. *Arch Pathol Lab Med* 112:143, 1988.

267. White LA, Chisholm M: Gastro-intestinal bleeding in acquired von Willebrand's disease: efficacy of high-dose immuno-globulin where substitution treatments failed. *Br J Haematol* 84:332, 1993.

268. Rinder MR, Richard RE, Rinder HM: Acquired von Willebrand's disease: A concise review. *Am J Hematol* 54:139, 1997.

269. van Genderen PJJ, Terpstra W, Michiels JJ, et al: High-dose intravenous immunoglobulin delays clearance of von Willebrand factor in acquired von Willebrand disease. *Thromb Haemost* 73:890, 1995.

270. van Genderen PJJ, Papatsonis DNM, Michiels JJ, et al: High-dose intravenous immunoglobulin therapy for acquired von Willebrand disease. *Postgrad Med J* 70:916, 1994.

271. George J, Shattil SJ: The clinical importance of acquired abnormalities of platelet function. *N Engl J Med* 324:27, 1991.

272. Wisloff F, Godal HC: Prolonged bleeding time with adequate platelet count in hospital patients. *Scand J Haematol* 27:45, 1981.

273. Smith WL, Garavito RM, DeWitt DL: Prostaglandin endoperoxide H synthases (cyclooxygenases)-1 and -2. *J Biol Chem* 271:33157, 1996.

274. Weiss HJ, Aledort LM: Impaired platelet/connective tissue reaction in man after aspirin ingestion. *Lancet* 2:495, 1967.

275. O'Brien JR: Effect of salicylates on human platelets. *Lancet* 1:779, 1968.

276. Patrono C: Aspirin as an antiplatelet drug. *N Engl J Med* 330:1287, 1994.

277. Kyrle PA, Eichler HG, Jager U, Lechner K: Inhibition of prostacyclin and thromboxane A_2 generation by low-dose aspirin at the site of plug formation in man in vivo. *Circulation* 75:1025, 1987.

278. Clarke RJ, Mayo G, Price P, FitzGerald GA: Suppression of thromboxane A_2 but not systemic prostacyclin by controlled-release aspirin. *N Engl J Med* 325:1137, 1991.

279. Jaffe EQ, Weksler BB: Recovery of endothelial cell prostacyclin production after inhibition by low doses of aspirin. *J Clin Invest* 63:532, 1979.

280. Santos MT, Valles J, Aznar J, et al: Prothombotic effects of erythrocytes on platelet reactivity. *Circulation* 95:63, 1997.

281. Kallmann R, Nieuwenhuis HK, de Groot PG, et al: Effects of low doses of aspirin, 10 mg and 30 mg daily, on bleeding time, thromboxane production and 6-keto-PGF1a excretion in healthy subjects. *Thromb Res* 45:355, 1987.

282. Nakajima H, Takami H, Yamagata K, et al: Aspirin effects on colonic mucosal bleeding. *Dis Colon Rectum* 40:1484, 1997.

283. Mielke CH Jr: Aspirin prolongation of the template bleeding time: Influence of venostasis and direction of incision. *Blood* 60:1139, 1982.

284. Hirsh J, Salzman EW, Harker L, et al: Aspirin and other platelet active drugs: Relationship among dose, effectiveness, and side effects. *Chest* 95:12S, 1989.

285. Steering Committee of the Physicians' Health Study Research Group: Final report on the aspirin component of the ongoing Physicians' Health Study. *N Engl J Med* 321:129, 1989.

286. Page IH: Salicylate damage to the gastric mucosal barrier. *N Engl J Med* 276:1307, 1967.

287. Leonards JR, Levy G: The role of dosage form in aspirin-induced gastrointestinal bleeding. *Clin Pharmacol Ther* 8:400, 1969.

288. Stuart MJ, Gross SJ, Elrad H, Graeber JE: Effects of acetylsalicylic acid ingestin on maternal and neonatal hemostasis. *N Engl J Med* 307:909, 1982.

289. Ferraris VA, Ferraris S, Lough FC, Berry WR: Preoperative aspirin ingestion increases operative blood loss after coronary artery bypass grafting. *Ann Thorac Surg* 45:71, 1988.

290. Sethi GK, Copeland JG, Goldman S, et al: Implications of preoperative administration of aspirin in patients undergoing coronary artery bypass grafting: Department of Veterans Affairs cooperative study of antiplatelet therapy. *J Am Coll Cardiol* 15:15, 1990.

291. Horlocker TT, Wedel DJ, Offord KP: Does preoperative antiplatelet therapy increase the risk of hemorrhagic complications associated with regional anesthesia? *Anesth Analg* 70:631, 1990.

292. Kitchen L, Erichson RB, Sideropoulos H: Effect of drug-induced platelet dysfunction on surgical bleeding. *Am J Surg* 143:215, 1982.

293. Kennedy BM: Aspirin and surgery: A review. *Ir Med J* 77:363, 1984.

294. Chesbro JH, Fuster V, Elveback LR, et al: Trial of combined warfarin plus dipyridamole or aspirin therapy in prosthetic heart valve replacement: Danger of aspirin compared to dipyridamole. *Am J Cardiol* 51:1537, 1983.

295. Deykin D, Janson P, McMahon L: Ethanol potentiation of aspirin-induced prolongation of the bleeding time. *N Engl J Med* 306:852, 1982.

296. Rosove HH, Harwig SSL: Confirmation that ethanol potentiates aspirin-induced prolongation of the bleeding time. *Thromb Res* 31:525, 1983.

297. Kobrinsky NL, Israels ED, Gerrard JM, et al: Shortening of bleeding time by 1-deamino-8-arginine vasopressin in various bleeding disorders. *Lancet* 1:1145, 1984.

298. Lethagen S, Rugarn P: The effect of DDAVP and placebo on platelet function and prolonged bleeding time induced by oral acetyl salicylic acid intake in healthy volunteers. *Thromb Haemost* 67:185, 1992.

299. Simon SL, Mills JA: Non-steroidal anti-inflammatory drugs. *N Engl J Med* 302:1119, 1980.

300. McAueen EG, Facoory B: Non-steroidal anti-inflammatory drugs and platelet function. *NZ Med J* 99:358, 1986.

301. Buchanan GR, Martin V, Levine PH, et al: The effects of "anti-platelet" drugs on bleeding time and platelet aggregation in normal human subjects. *Am J Clin Pathol* 68:355, 1977.

302. Nadell J, Bruno J, Varady J, Segre EJ: Effect of naproxen and of aspirin on bleeding time and platelet aggregation. *J Clin Pharmacol* 14:176, 1974.

303. Mielke CH Jr, Kahn SB, Muschek LL, et al: Effects of zomepirac on hemostasis in healthy adults and on platelet function in vitro. *J Clin Pharmacol* 20:409, 1980.

304. Thomas P, Hepburn B, Kim HC, Saidi P: Nonsteroidal anti-inflammatory drugs in the treatment of hemophilic arthropathy. *Am J Hematol* 12:131, 1982.

305. McIntyre BA, Philip RB, Inwood JJ: Effect of ibuprofen on platelet function in normal subjects and hemophiliac patients. *Clin Pharmacol Ther* 24:616, 1978.

306. Ragni MV, Miller BJ, Whalen R, Ptachcinski R: Bleeding tendency, platelet function, and pharmacokinetics of ibuprofen and zidovudine in HIV(+) hemophilic men. *Am J Hematol* 40:176, 1992.

307. Kasper CK, Rapaport SI: Bleeding times and platelet aggregation after analgesics in hemophilia. *Ann Intern Med* 77:189, 1972.

308. Mielke CH Jr: Comparative effects of aspirin and acetaminophen on hemostasis. *Arch Intern Med* 141:305, 1981.

309. Huddleston CB, Wareing TH, Clanton JA, Bender HW Jr: Amelioration of the deleterious effects of platelets activated during cardiopulmonary bypass: Comparison of a thromboxane synthetase inhibitor and a prostacylin analogue. *J Thorac Cardiovasc Surg* 89:190, 1985.

310. Ito T, Ogawa K, Sakai K, et al: Effects of a selective inhibitor of thromboxane synthetase (OKY-1581) in humans. *Adv Prostaglandin Thromboxane Leukotriene Res* 11:245, 1983.

311. Sattler FR, Weitekamp MR, Ballard JO: Potential for bleeding with the new beta-lactam antibiotics. *Ann Intern Med* 105:924, 1986.

312. Pillgram-Larsen J, Wisloff F, Jorgensen JJ, et al: Effect of high-dose ampicillin and cloxacillin on bleeding time and bleeding in open-heart surgery. *Scand J Thorac Cardiovasc Surg* 19:45, 1985.

313. Fass RJ, Copelan EA, Brandt JT, et al: Platelet-mediated bleeding caused by broad-spectrum penicillins. *J Infect Dis* 155:1242, 1987.

314. Cazenave JP, Packman MA, Guccione MA, Mustard JF: Effects of penicillin G on platelet aggregation, release and adherence to collagen. *Proc Soc Exp Biol Med* 142:159, 1973.

315. Shattil SJ, Bennett JS, McDonough M, Turnbull J: Carbenicillin and penicillin G inhibit platelet function in vitro by impairing the interaction of agonists with the platelet surface. *J Clin Invest* 65:329, 1980.

316. Henry D, Audet P, Shattil SJ: Relationships between the structure of penicillins and their anti-platelet activity. *Blood* 54(suppl 1):243a, 1979.

317. Fletcher C, Pearson C, Choi SC, et al: In vitro comparison of antiplatelet effects of β-lactam penicillins. *J Lab Clin Med* 108:217, 1986.

318. Packham MA, Rand ML, Perry DW, et al: Probenecid inhibits platelet responses to aggregating agents in vitro and has a synergistic inhibitory effect with penicillin G. *Thromb Haemost* 76:239, 1996.

319. Burroughs SF, Johnson GJ: β-Lactam antibiotic-induced platelet dysfunction: Evidence for irreversible platelet activation in vitro and in vivo after prolonged exposure to penicillin. *Blood* 75:1473, 1990.

320. Sattler FR, Weitekamp MR, Sayegh A, Ballard JO: Impaired hemostasis caused by beta-lactam antibiotics. *Am J Surg* 155:30, 1988.

321. Giles AR, Greenwood P, Tinlin S: A platelet release defect induced by aspirin or penicillin G does not increase gastrointestinal blood loss in thrombocytopenic rabbits. *Br J Haematol* 57:17, 1984.

322. Andrassy K, Koderisch J, Trenk D, et al: Hemostasis in patients with

normal and inpaired renal function under treatment with cefodizime. *Infection* 15:348, 1987.

323. Brown RB, Klar J, Lemeshow S, et al: Enhanced bleeding with cefoxitin or moxalactam: statistical analysis within a defined population of 1,493 pateints. *Arch Intern Med* 146:2159, 1986.

324. Rossi EC, Levin NW: Inhibition of primary ADP-induced platelet aggregation in normal subjects after the administration of nitrofurantoin (Furadantin). *J Clin Invest* 52:2457, 1973.

325. Ishikawa S, Manabe S, Wada O: Miconazole inhibition of platelet aggregation by inhibiting cyclooxygenase. *Biochem Pharmacol* 35:1787, 1986.

326. McTavish D, Faulds D, Goa KL: Ticlopidine: An updated review of its pharmacology and therapeutic use in platelet-dependent disorders. *Drugs* 40:238, 1992.

327. CAPRIE Steering Committee: A randomized, blinded, trial of clopidogrel versus aspirin in patients at risk of ischaemic events (CAPRIE). *Lancet* 48:1329, 1996.

327a. Bennett CL, Connors JM, Carwile JM, et al: Thrombotic thrombocytopenic purpura associated with clopidogrel. *N Engl J Med* 342:1773, 2000.

328. Rupprecht HJ, Darius H, Borkowski U, et al: Comparison of antiplatelet effects of aspirin, ticlopidine, or their combination after stent implantation. *Circulation* 97:1046, 1998.

329. Leon MB, Baim DS, Popma JJ, et al: A clinical trial comparing three antithrombotic-drug regimens after coronary-artery stenting: Stent Anticoagulation Restenosis Study investigators [comments]. *N Engl J Med* 339:1665, 1998.

330. Sharis PJ, Cannon CP, Loscalzo J: The antiplatelet effects of ticlopidine and clopidogrel. *Ann Intern Med* 129:394, 1998.

331. Bossavy JP, Thalamas C, Sagnard L, et al: A double-blind randomized comparison of combined aspirin and ticlopidine therapy versus aspirin or ticlopidine alone on experimental arterial thrombogenesis in humans. *Blood* 92:1518, 1998.

332. De Caterina R, Sicari R, Bernini W, et al: Benefit/risk profile of combined antiplatelet therapy with ticlopidine and aspirin. *Thromb Haemost* 65: 504, 1991.

333. Hardisty RM, Powling MJ, Nokes TJC: The action of ticlopidine on human platelets: Studies on aggregation, secretion, calcium mobilization and membrane glycoproteins. *Thromb Haemost* 64:150, 1990.

334. Humbert M, Nurden P, Bihour C, et al: Ultrastructural studies of platelet aggregates from human subjects receiving clopidogrel and from a patient with an inherited defect of an ADP-dependent pathway of platelet activation. *Arteriosc Thromb Vasc Biol* 16:1532, 1996.

335. Daniel JL, Dangelmaier C, Jin JG, et al: Molecular basis for ADP-induced platelet activation: I. Evidence for three distinct ADP receptors on human platelets. *J Biol Chem* 273:2024, 1998.

336. Jantzen HM, Gousset L, Bhaskar V, et al: Evidence for two distinct G-protein-coupled ADP receptors mediating platelet activation. *Thromb Haemost* 81:111, 1999.

337. Hechler B, Eckly A, Ohlmann P, et al: The P2Y1 receptor, necessary but not sufficient to support full ADP-induced platelet aggregation, is not the target of the drug clopidogrel. *Br J Haematol* 103:858, 1998.

338. Geiger J, Honig-Liedl P, Schanzenbacher P, Walter U: Ligand specificity and ticlopidine effects distinguish three human platelet ADP receptors. *Eur J Pharmacol* 351:235, 1998.

339. Savi P, Laplace MC, Maffrand JP, Herbert JM: Binding of [3H]-2-methylthio ADP to rat platelets: Effect of clopidogrel and ticlopidine. *J Pharmacol Exp Ther* 269:772, 1994.

340. Hass WK, Easton JD, Adams HP, et al: A randomized trial comparing ticlopidine hydrochloride with aspirin for the prevention of stroke in high-risk patients. *N Engl J Med* 321:501, 1989.

341. Gent M, Blakely JA, Easton JD, et al: The Canadian American Ticlopidine Study (CATS) in thromboembolic stroke. *Lancet* 1:1215, 1989.

342. Mataiz R, Ojeda E, Perez MDC, Jiminez S: Ticlopidine and severe aplastic anemia. *Br J Haematol* 80:125, 1992.

343. Garnier G, Taillan B, Pesce A, et al: Ticlopidine and severe aplastic anemia. *Br J Haematol* 81:459, 1992.

344. Bennett CL, Weinberg PD, Rozenberg-Ben-Dror K, et al: Thrombotic thrombocytopenic purpura associated with ticlopidine: A review of 60 cases [comments]. *Ann Intern Med* 128:541, 1998.

345. Steinhubl SR, Tan WA, Foody JM, Topol EJ: Incidence and clinical course of thrombotic thrombocytopenic purpura due to ticlopidine

following coronary stenting: EPISTENT investigators evaluation of platelet IIb/IIIa inhibitor for stenting. *J Am Med Assoc* 281:806, 1999.

346. Chen DK, Kim JS, Sutton DM: Thrombotic thrombocytopenic purpura associated with ticlopidine use: A report of 3 cases and review of the literature. *Arch Intern Med* 159:311, 1999.

347. Lefkovits J, Plow EF, Topol EJ: Platelet glycoprotein IIb/IIIa receptors in cardiovascular medicine. *N Engl J Med* 332:1553, 1995.

348. George JN, Caen JP, Nurden AT: Glanzmann's thrombasthenia: The spectrum of clinical disease. *Blood* 75:1383, 1990.

349. The EPIC Investigators: Use of a monoclonal antibody directed against the platelet glycoprotein IIb/IIIa receptor in high risk coronary angioplasty. *N Engl J Med* 330:956, 1994.

350. The EPILOG Investigators: Platelet glycoprotein IIb/IIIa receptor blockade and low-dose heparin during percutaneous coronary revascularization. *N Engl J Med* 336:1689, 1997.

351. Platelet Receptor Inhibition in Ischemic Syndrome Management in Patients Limited by Unstable Signs and Symptoms (PRISM PLUS) Study Investigators: Inhibition of the platelet glycoprotein IIb/IIIa receptor with tirofiban in unstable angina and non-Q-wave myocardial infarction. *N Engl J Med* 338:1488, 1998.

352. The PURSUIT Trial Investigators: Inhibition of platelet glycoprotein IIb/IIIa with eptifibatide in patients with acute coronary syndromes. *N Engl J Med* 339:436, 1998.

353. Simpfendorfer C, Kottke-Marchant K, Lowrie M, et al: First chronic platelet glycoprotein IIb/IIIa blockade: A randomized, placebo-controlled pilot study of xemilofiban in unstable angina with percutaneous coronary interventions. *Circulation* 96:76, 1997.

354. Cannon CP, McCabe CH, Borzak S, et al: Randomized trial of an oral platelet glycoprotein IIb/IIIa antagonist, sibrafiban, in patients after an acute coronary syndrome. *Circulation* 97:340, 1998.

355. Ferguson JJ, Kereiakes DJ, Adgey J, et al: Safe use of platelet GP IIb/IIIa inhibitors. *Am Heart J* 135:577, 1998.

356. Berkowitz SD, Sane DC, Sigmon KN, et al: Occurrence and clinical significance of thrombocytopenia in a population undergoing high-risk percutaneous coronary revascularization. *J Am Coll Cardiol* 32:311, 1998.

357. Kereiakes DJ, Essell JH, Abbottsmith CW, et al: Abciximab-associated profound thrombocytopenia: Therapy with immunoglobulin and platelet transfusion. *Am J Cardiol* 78:1161, 1996.

358. Berkowitz SD, Harrington RA, Rund MM, Tcheng JE: Acute profound thrombocytopenia after c7E3 Fab (abciximab) therapy. *Circulation* 95:809, 1997.

359. Bednar B, Cook JJ, Holahan MA, et al: Fibrinogen receptor antagonist-induced thrombocytopenia in chimpanzee and rhesus monkeys associated with preexisting drug-dependent antibodies to platelet glycoprotein IIb/IIIa. *Blood* 94:1, 1999.

360. Gresele P, Arnout J, Deckmyn H, Vermylen J: Mechanism of the antiplatelet action of dipyridamole in whole blood: Modulation of adenosine concentration and activity. *Thromb Haemost* 55:12, 1986.

361. FitzGerald GA: Dipyridamole. *N Engl J Med* 316:1247, 1987.

362. Ivy DD, Kinsella JP, Ziegler JW, Abman SH: Dipyridamole attenuates rebound pulmonary hypertension after inhaled nitric oxide withdrawal in postoperative congenital heart disease. *J Thorac Cardiovasc Surg* 115:875, 1998.

363. Diener HC, Cunha L, Forbes C, et al: European Stroke Prevention Study: II. Dipyridamole and acetylsalicylic acid in the secondary prevention of stroke. *J Neurol Sci* 143:1, 1996.

364. Fisher CA, Kappa JR, Sinha AK, et al: Comparison of equimolar concentratons of iloprost, prostacyclin, and prostaglandin E_1 on human platelet function. *J Lab Clin Med* 109:184, 1987.

365. Sorkin EM, Markham A: Cilostazol. *Drugs Aging* 14:63, 1999.

366. Yoshitomi Y, Kojima S, Sugi T, et al: Antiplatelet treatment with cilostazol after stent implantation. *Heart* 80:393, 1998.

367. Loscalzo J, Welch G: Nitric oxide and its role in the cardiovascular system. *Prog Cardiovasc Dis* 38:87, 1995.

368. Salzman EW, Rosenberg RD, Smith MH, et al: Effect of heparin and heparin fractions on platelet aggregation. *J Clin Invest* 65:64, 1980.

369. Horne MKI, Chao ES: Heparin binding to resting and activated platelets. *Blood* 74:238, 1989.

370. Sobel M, McNeill PM, Carlson PL, et al: Heparin inhibition of von Willebrand factor-dependent platelet function in vitro and in vivo. *J Clin Invest* 87:1787, 1991.

371. Coller BS: Platelets and thrombolytic therapy. *N Engl J Med* 322:33, 1990.

372. Niewiarowski S, Senyi AF, Gillies P: Plasmin-induced platelet aggregation and platelet release reaction. *J Clin Invest* 52:1647, 1973.

373. Fitzgerald DJ, Catella F, Roy L, FitzGerald GA: Marked platelet activation in vivo after intravenous streptokinase in patients with acute myocardial infarction. *Circulation* 77:142, 1988.

374. Kerins DM, Roy L, FitzGerald GA, Fitzgerald DJ: Platelet and vascular function during coronary thrombolysis with tissue-type plasminogen activator. *Circulation* 80:1718, 1989.

375. Thorsen LI, Brosstad F, Gogstad G, et al: Competitions between fibrinogen with its degradation products for interactions with the platelet-fibrinogen receptor. *Thromb Res* 44:611, 1986.

376. Miles LA, Ginsberg MH, White JG, Plow EF: Plasminogen interacts with human platelets through two distinct mechanisms. *J Clin Invest* 77:2001, 1986.

377. Adelman B, Michaelson AD, Loscalzo J, et al: Plasmin effect on platelet glycoprotein Ib-von Willebrand factor interactions. *Blood* 65:32, 1985.

378. Stricker RB, Wong D, Shiu DT, et al: Activation of plasminogen by tissue plasminogen activator on normal and thrombasthenic platelets: Effects on surface proteins and platelet aggregation. *Blood* 68:275, 1986.

379. Schafer AI, Adelman B: Plasmin inhibition of platelet function and of arachidonic acid metabolism. *J Clin Invest* 75:456, 1985.

380. Loscalzo J, Vaughn DE: Tissue plasminogen activator promotes platelet disaggregation in plasma. *J Clin Invest* 79:1749, 1987.

381. Penny WF, Ware JA: Platelet activation and subsequent inhibition by plasmin and recombinant tissue-type plasminogen activator. *Blood* 79:91, 1992.

382. Winters KJ, Eisenberg PR, Jaffe AS, Santoro SA: Dependence of plasmin-mediated degradation of platelet adhesive receptors on temperature and Ca^{2+}. *Blood* 76:1546, 1990.

383. Green D, Tsao C-H, Cerullo L, et al: Clinical and laboratory investigation of the effects of ε-aminocaproic acid on hemostasis. *J Lab Clin Med* 105:321, 1985.

384. Hines R, Barash PG: Infusion of sodium nitroprusside induces platelet dysfunction in vitro. *Anesthesia* 70:611, 1989.

385. Kroll MH, Schafer AI: Biochemical mechanisms of platelet activation. *Blood* 74:1181, 1989.

386. Schafer AI, Alexander RW, Handin RI: Inhibition of platelet function by organic nitrate vasodilators. *Blood* 55:649, 1980.

387. Weksler B, Gillick M, Pink J: Effect of propranolol on platelet function. *Blood* 49:185, 1977.

388. Leon R, Tiarks CY, Pechet L: Some observations on the in vivo effect of propranolol on platelet aggregation and release. *Am J Hematol* 5:117, 1978.

389. Hines R: Preservation of platelet function during trimethaphan infusion. *Anesthesia* 72:834, 1990.

390. Hogman M, Frostell C, Arnberg H, Hedenstierna G: Bleeding time prolongation and NO inhalation. *Lancet* 341:1664, 1993.

391. Samama CM, Diaby M, Fellahi JL, et al: Inhibition of platelet aggregation by inhaled nitric oxide in patients with acute respiratory distress syndrome. *Anesth* 83:56, 1995.

392. Gries A, Bode C, Peter K, et al: Inhaled nitric oxide inhibits human platelet aggregation, P-selectin expression, and fibrinogen binding in vitro and in vivo. *Circulation* 97:1481, 1998.

393. Ring ME, Corrigan JJ Jr, Fenster PE: Effects of oral diltiazem on platelet function: Alone and in combination with ''low dose'' aspirin. *Thromb Res* 44:391, 1986.

394. Barnathan E, Addonizio VP, Shattil SJ: Interaction of verapamil with human platelet alpha-adrenergic receptors. *Am J Physiol* 242:H19, 1982.

395. Fujinishi A, Takahara K, Ohba C, et al: Effects of nisoldipine on cytosolic calcium, platelet aggregation, and coagulation/fibrinolysis in patients with coronary artery disease. *Angiology* 48:515, 1997.

396. Lawson D, Mehta J, Mehta P, et al: Cumulative effects of quinidine and aspirin on bleeding time and platelet α_2-adrenoceptors: Potential mechanism of bleeding diathesis in patients receiving this combination. *J Lab Clin Med* 108:581, 1986.

397. Weiss HJ: The effect of clinical dextran on platelet aggregation, adhesion, and ADP release in man: In vivo and in vitro studies. *J Lab Clin Med* 69:37, 1967.

398. Aberg M, Hedner U, Bergentz S-E: Effect of dextran 70 on factor VIII and platelet function in von Willebrand's disease. *Thromb Res* 12:629, 1978.

399. Mishler JM IV: Synthetic plasma volume expanders: Their pharmacology, safety and clinical efficacy. *Clin Haematol* 13:75, 1984.

400. Kelton JG, Hirsh J: Bleeding associated with antithrombotic therapy. *Semin Hematol* 17:259, 1980.

401. Korttila K, Lauritsalo K, Särmö A: Suitability of plasma expanders in patients receiving low-dose heparin for prevention of venous thrombosis after surgery. *Acta Anaesthesiol Scand* 27:104, 1983.

402. Cope JT, Banks D, Mauney MC, et al: Intraoperative hetastarch infusion impairs hemostasis after cardiac operations. *Ann Thorac Surg* 63:78, 1997.

403. Ruttmann TG, James MF, Aronson I: In vivo investigation into the effects of haemodilution with hydroxyethyl starch (200/0.5) and normal saline on coagulation. *Br J Anaesth* 80:612, 1998.

404. Roberts JS, Bratton SL: Colloid volume expanders: Problems, pitfalls and possibilities. *Drugs* 55:621, 1998.

405. Treib J, Haass A, Pindur G: Coagulation disorders caused by hydroxyethyl starch. *Thromb Haemost* 78:974, 1997.

406. Rysanek R, Svelha S, Spankova H, Mlejnkova M: The effect of tricyclic antidepressive drugs on adrenaline and adenosine diphosphate induced platelet aggregation. *J Pharmacol* 18:616, 1966.

407. Warlow C, Ogston D, Douglas AS: Platelet function after administration of chlorpromazine to human subjects. *Haemostasis* 5:21, 1976.

408. Morishita S, Aoki S, Watanabe S: Different effect of desipramine on protein kinase C in platelets between bipolar and major depressive disorders. *Psychiatry Clin Neurosci* 53:11, 1999.

409. Alderman CP, Seshadri P, Ben-Tovim DI: Effects of serotonin reuptake inhibitors on hemostasis. *Ann Pharmacother* 30:1232, 1996.

410. Pai VB, Kelly MW: Bruising associated with the use of fluoxetine. *Ann Pharmacother* 30:786, 1996.

411. Corbin F, Blaise G, Sauve R: Differential effect of halothane and forskolin on platelet cytosolic Ca^{2+} mobilization and aggregation. *Anesthesiology* 89:401, 1998.

412. Heesch CM, Negus BH, Steiner M, et al: Effects of in vivo cocaine administration on human platelet aggregation. *Am J Cardiol* 78:237, 1996.

413. Jennings LK, White MM, Sauer CM, et al: Cocaine-induced platelet defects. *Stroke* 24:1352, 1993.

414. Togna G, Graziani M, Sorrentino C, Caprino L: Prostanoid production in the presence of platelet activation in hypoxic cocaine-treated rats. *Haemostasis* 26:311, 1996.

415. Ahr DJ, Scialla SJ, Kimball DB Jr: Acquired platelet dysfunction following mithramycin therapy. *Cancer* 41:448, 1978.

416. Panella TJ, Peters W, White JG, et al: Platelets acquire a secretion defect after high-dose chemotherapy. *Cancer* 65:1711, 1990.

417. Pogliani EM, Fantasia R, Lambertenghi-Deliliers G, Cofranesco E: Daunorubicin and platelet function. *Thromb Haemost* 45:38, 1981.

418. McKenna R, Ahmad T, Ts'ao C-H, Frischer H: Glutathione reductase deficiency and platelet dysfunction induced by 1,3-bis(2-chloroethyl)-1-nitrosourea. *J Lab Clin Med* 102:102, 1983.

419. Karolak L, Chandra A, Kahn W, et al: High-dose chemotherapy-induced platelet defect: Inhibition of platelet signal transduction pathways. *Mol Pharmacol* 43:37, 1993.

420. O'Malley CJ, Rasko JEJ, Basser RL, et al: Administration of pegylated recombinant human megakaryocyte growth and development factor in humans stimulates the production of functional platelets that show no evidence of in vivo activation. *Blood* 88:3288, 1996.

421. Vadhan-Rai S, Murray LJ, Bueso-Ramos C, et al: Stimulation of megakaryocyte and platelet production by a single dose of recombinant human thrombopoietin in patients with cancer. *Ann Intern Med* 126:673, 1997.

422. Vanrentenghem Y, Roels L, Lerut T, et al: Thromboembolic complications and hemostatic changes in cylcosporine-treated cadaveric kidney allograft recipients. *Lancet* 1:999, 1985.

423. Cohen H, Neild GH, Patel R, et al: Evidence for chronic platelet hyperaggregability and in vivo platelet activation in cyclosporine treated renal allograft recipients. *Thromb Res* 49:91, 1988.

424. Grace AA, Barradus MA, Mikhailidis DP, et al: Cyclosporine A enhances platelet aggregation. *Kidney Int* 32:889, 1987.

425. Thomson C, Forbes CD, Prentice CRM: A comparison of the effects of antihistamines on platelet function. *Thromb Diath Haemorrh* 30:547, 1973.

426. Group TPT: Platelet function during long-term treatment with ketanserin of claudicating patients with peripheral atherosclerosis: A multicenter, double-blind, placebo-controlled trial. *Thromb Res* 55:13, 1989.

427. Parvez Z, Moncada R, Fareed J, Messmore HL: Antiplatelet action of intravascular contrast media. *Invest Radiol* 19:208, 1984.

428. Rao AK, Rao VM, Willis J, et al: Inhibition of platelet function by contrast media: Iopamidol and Hexabrix are less inhibitory than Conray-60. *Radiology* 156:311, 1985.

429. Goodnight SH, Harris WS, Conner WE: The effects of ω_3 fatty acids on platelet composition and function in man: A prospective, controlled study. *Blood* 58:880, 1981.

430. Moncada S, Higgs EA: Arachidonate metabolism in blood cells and the vessel wall. *Clin Haematol* 15:273, 1986.

431. Leaf A, Weber PC: Cardiovascular effects of ω-3 fatty acids. *N Engl J Med* 318:549, 1988

432. Hammerschmidt DE: Szechwan purpura. *N Engl J Med* 302:1191, 1980.

433. Srivastava KC: Onion exerts antiaggregatory effects by altering arachidonic acid metabolism in platelets. *Prostaglandins Leukotrienes Med* 24:43, 1986.

434. Apitz-Castro R, Ledezma E, Escalante J, Jain MK: The molecular basis of the antiplatelet action of ajoene: Direct interaction with the fibrinogen receptor. *Biochem Biophys Res Commun* 141:145, 1986.

435. Apitz-Castro R, Escalante J, Vargas R, Jain MK: Ajoene, the antiplatelet principle of garlic, synergistically potentiates the antiaggregatory action of prostacylin, forskolin, indomethacin and dipyridamole on human platelets. *Thromb Res* 42:303, 1986.

436. Srivastava KC: Extracts from two frequently consumed spices—cumin (*Cuminum cyminum*) and turmeric (*Curcuma longa*)—inhibit platelet aggregation and alter eicosanoid biosynthesis in human blood platelets. *Prostaglandins Leukotrienes Essential Fatty Acids* 37:57, 1993.

THE VASCULAR PURPURAS

PAUL I. SCHNEIDERMAN

Petechiae, purpura, and ecchymoses (collectively referred to as *purpura*) are all caused by the extravasation of red blood cells from the vasculature into the skin and/or subcutaneous tissue. Hemostatic disorders can cause petechiae, purpura, and ecchymoses but so can autoimmune, drug-induced, infiltrative, inflammatory, metabolic, neoplastic, primary cutaneous, and vascular disorders. Moreover, primary cutaneous and vascular lesions can simulate petechiae, purpura, and ecchymoses. The general category of purpuras can be conveniently divided into those in which the lesions are nonpalpable and those in which the lesions are palpable. Palpable lesions are more commonly due to vasculitic and/or inflammatory damage to blood vessels, but nonpalpable lesions may be due to hemostatic disorders, bland vascular damage, or vasculitic and/or inflammatory damage. The identification and classification of purpuric lesions can provide important diagnostic information.

Purpura, or skin hemorrhage, is defined as the extravasation of red cells from the vasculature into the skin and/or subcutaneous tissue. Blood leaking in minute amounts produces pinpoint red lesions less than 2 mm in size (petechiae), and blood leaking in larger amounts produces purpuric lesions (2 mm to 1 cm) or ecchymoses (>1 cm).[1] Conventional usage often groups purpuric lesions and ecchymoses under the term *purpura,* and the general group of disorders that produces such lesions, including petechiae, is often referred to as *the purpuras.* All of these hemorrhagic lesions can be differentiated from erythema (reddened skin due to increased blood flow to superficial blood vessels) and telangiectasias (dilated superficial capillaries), in which the blood remains confined within the vasculature and which blanch on direct pressure. Blanching of lesions with pressure can be demonstrated using a glass slide or hand lens (diascopy) (see Plates XXV-1 and XXV-2). Purpura may demonstrate partial blanching, but a nonblanchable component will remain. Superficial lesions of the purpuras are bright red or deep red; deeper lesions have more of a purple appearance. With time, purpuric lesions evolve into deep purple, brown, orange, or blue-green discolorations.

Extravasation of blood from the vasculature depends upon the integrity of blood vessels, which in turn depends upon: (1) the competence of the hemostatic mechanism to combat the basal level of ongoing vascular trauma, (2) the strength of the blood vessel and its surrounding tissues, and (3) the transmural pressure gradient tending to drive blood out of the vessel. Even if these systems are functioning normally, serious trauma may be sufficient to cause hemorrhagic extravasation.

A classification of disorders producing skin hemorrhage is given in Table 121-1.[2,3] It is organized primarily according to etiology but

Acronyms and abbreviations that appear in this chapter include: CREST, calcinosis, Raynaud phenomenon, esophageal motor dysfunction, sclerodactyly, and telangiectasia; DIC, disseminated intravascular coagulation; MELAS, *mitochondrial encephalopathy, lactic acidosis, strokelike*; PAI-1, plasminogen activator inhibitor 1; TGF-β, transforming growth factor beta.

is subdivided on the basis of the physical finding of palpability because palpability can be determined at the bedside; thus this finding can aid in developing a differential diagnosis. Palpability is most likely due to extravascular fibrin deposition. Presumably, the generalized increase in vascular permeability secondary to an inflammatory process results in marked extravasation of plasma proteins including fibrinogen and other coagulation factors, and cytokine activation of inflammatory cells triggers coagulation by causing the cells to express tissue factor. This palpable induration can be experimentally diminished in delayed hypersensitivity reactions by the administration of oral anticoagulants, supporting a major role for the coagulation mechanism.[4] Palpability also may be secondary to extensive cellular infiltration as in certain inflammatory or malignant disorders.

Purpuric lesions secondary to hemostatic defects are described elsewhere (see Chap. 115).

NONPALPABLE PURPURA

INCREASED TRANSMURAL PRESSURE GRADIENT

Any activity or event that results in a dramatic increase in intrathoracic pressure can produce the clinical picture of minute petechiae of the face ("mask phenomenon"), neck, and upper chest, with a sharp demarcation at the nipple line, accompanying cervicofacial cyanosis and edema, and bilateral subconjunctival hemorrhage. Among the many causes are prolonged Valsalva maneuvers, coughing, vomiting,[5] labor and delivery, weight lifting, vigorous exercise, generalized seizures,[6] severe crush injury of the thorax or upper abdomen (thoracoabdominal compression), and child abuse.[7–10] Eyelid and conjunctival petechiae are characteristic findings of neck compression (strangling).[11] The clinical picture of acute increased transmural pressure gradient is caused by the reflux of blood from the heart retrograde through the valveless superior vena cava and great veins of the head and neck, causing the overlying capillaries to become engorged, with resultant egress of erythrocytes. These findings are similar to those observed in patients with the superior vena cava syndrome or in newborns with umbilical cord strangulation. Basilar skull fracture needs to be considered in the differential diagnosis of subconjunctival hemorrhage, but with this entity, periorbital ecchymosis and/or epistaxis are common.

Suction purpura encompasses a diverse collection of petechial and purpuric eruptions that result from the generation of negative pressure on the surface of the body. Well-demarcated, annular lesions are commonly produced by this mechanism, whether by vacuum extractors at the time of delivery, rubber suction cups on toys, cupping, ECG leads, kissing, or wearing a gas mask.[12]

Lesions on the lower extremities, especially in the elderly, may be due to acute venous stasis due to tight clothing or stockings. Occasionally such dependent purpura may be palpable, even in the absence of microscopic inflammation. Acute compression of the inferior vena cava, as, for example, by a large but unruptured aortic aneurysm, can produce edema and purpura of the lower extremities. In addition, common cutaneous disorders (drug rash, contact dermatitis,[13] and sunburn) often progress to become petechial and purpuric after the first 24 h.

CHRONIC

Chronic venous stasis of the lower extremity, due either to venous valvular incompetence or chronic use of tight-fitting stockings or garments, can convert subclinical insults of diverse etiologies into frank purpura. Thus, it is common for the first signs of petechiae due to thrombocytopenia to appear at the ankles. Chronic venous stasis accompanied by recurrent episodes of extravasation of red cells leads to the development of purpuric and yellow-brown macules ("brown

TABLE 121-1   THE PURPURAS

I   Hemostatic defects
   A   Platelet abnormalities
     1   Quantitative
     2   Qualitative
   B   Coagulation abnormalities
II   Nonhemostatic defects—the vascular purpuras
   A   Nonpalpable purpura
     1   Increased transmural pressure gradient
      a   Acute (Valsalva, coughing, vomiting, childbirth, weight lifting, suction purpura)
      b   Chronic—venous stasis
      c   High altitude
     2   Decreased mechanical integrity of microcirculation and supporting tissues
      a   Senile purpura—due to aging and chronic ultraviolet radiation
      b   Glucocorticoid excess—Cushing syndrome, topical glucocorticoids
      c   Vitamin C deficiency—scurvy
      d   Abnormal connective tissue—Ehlers-Danlos syndrome, pseudoxanthoma elasticum
      e   Amyloid infiltration of blood vessels
      f   ?Hormonal—female easy bruising syndrome (purpura simplex)
      g   MELAS syndrome
     3   Trauma to blood vessels
      a   Physical
       (1)   Injuries
       (2)   Child abuse
       (3)   Factitial purpura
       (4)   Coma bullae
      b   Ultraviolet radiation
       (1)   Purpuric sunburn
       (2)   Solar purpura
      c   Infectious
       (1)   Bacterial
       (2)   Fungal
       (3)   Viral
       (4)   Parasitic
      d   Embolic
       (1)   Infectious organisms*
       (2)   Atheroemboli (cholesterol crystal emboli)
       (3)   Fat emboli
       (4)   Tumor emboli
       (5)   Calciphylaxis (cutaneous vascular calcification)
      e   Neoplastic*
      f   Allergic and/or inflammatory
       (1)   Serum sickness
       (2)   Pigmented purpuric eruptions
       (3)   Contact dermatitis
       (4)   Dysproteinemias*
       (5)   Pyoderma gangrenosum
       (6)   Visceral inflammatory disease
      g   Toxic—chemicals, arthropod bites
      h   Thrombotic
       (1)   Disseminated intravascular coagulation
       (2)   Coumarin skin necrosis
       (3)   Heparin-associated skin necrosis
       (4)   Protein C or S deficiency
       (5)   Purpura fulminans
       (6)   Paroxysmal nocturnal hemoglobinuria*
       (7)   "Antiphospholipid" antibody syndrome
      i   Drug-related
     4   Unknown
      a   Psychogenic purpura
      b   Purpura of familial Mediterranean fever

TABLE 121-1   THE PURPURAS (CONTINUED)

   B   Palpable purpura
     1   Cutaneous vasculitis
      a   Henoch-Schönlein purpura
      b   Acute hemorrhagic edema of infancy
      c   Collagen vascular disease†
      d   Systemic vasculitis
      e   Hypersensitivity vasculitis including drug-induced vasculitis
      f   Infectious vasculitis (not embolic)
      g   Paraneoplastic vasculitis
     2   Dysproteinemias
      a   Cryoglobulinemia
      b   Hyperglobulinemic purpura of Waldenström
      c   Cryofibrinogenemia
      d λ light-chain vasculopathy
     3   Primary cutaneous diseases
     4   Unknown—papular-purpuric "gloves and socks" syndrome

DISORDERS SIMULATING PURPURA

I   Disorders with telangiectasias
   A   "Petechial" cherry angiomata
   B   Hereditary hemorrhagic telangiectasia (Osler-Weber-Rendu disease)
   C   CREST syndrome
   D   Chronic actinic telangiectasia
   E   Chronic liver disease
   F   AIDS-associated telangiectasia
   G   Pregnancy-related telangiectasia
   H   Ataxia telangiectasia
   I   Other
II   Kaposi sarcoma‡
III   Fabry disease (angiokeratoma corporis diffusum)
IV   Extramedullary hematopoiesis ("blueberry muffin" baby)
V   Angioma serpiginosum

*May also have a palpable purpuric component.
†May also have a nonpalpable purpuric component.
‡May also have a purpuric component, either nonpalpable or palpable.

for this purpura may be increased transmural pressure due to reduced extravascular pressure, rather than increased intravascular pressure.

CONDITIONS AFFECTING THE INTEGRITY OF THE BLOOD VESSEL WALL AND ITS SUPPORTING TISSUES

ACTINIC PURPURA (SENILE PURPURA)

Chronic solar damage and decreased collagen, elastin, and ground substance due to aging may result in characteristic red to purple irregular purpuric patches on the extensor surfaces of the forearms and hands (see Plates XXV-3 and XXV-4).[15] The skin in solar purpura is thin and lacks elasticity, making it particularly susceptible to tears induced by shearing forces.[16] These purpuric changes occur after minor or inapparent trauma and may take months to resolve. Syndromes of premature aging such as the Hutchinson-Gilford syndrome (progeria), Werner's syndrome (pangeria), acrogeria, and others may all give rise to acral purpuric changes identical to those of senile purpura.[17]

GLUCOCORTICOID EXCESS

The patches of purpura in Cushing syndrome may appear on both the flexor and extensor aspects of both the upper and lower extremities. As with actinic purpura, shearing stress is a common precipitating event, and the patches may last for weeks to months. The lesions have a characteristic bright red or purple appearance, and the skin is thin and fragile.[2] Glucocorticoids administered parenterally, orally, or by inhalation all may produce similar dermal thinning and purpura.[18]

The use of potent fluorinated topical glucocorticoids, especially if applied under occlusive dressings, may result in cutaneous striae, atrophy, and purpura. If the atrophy is severe enough, ulceration with extrusion of fat to the surface of the skin (fat herniation) may ensue.

patches"), with the latter due to the persistent presence of hemosiderin, the hemoglobin breakdown product.

HIGH ALTITUDE

An increase in cutaneous petechiae has been noted in mountain climbers ascending higher than 3800 m above sea level.[14] The mechanism

Microscopic evaluation of the skin in glucocorticoid atrophy usually reveals loss of dermal connective tissue with thinning of the epidermis.

VITAMIN C (ASCORBIC ACID) DEFICIENCY (SCURVY)

Vitamin C is required for the formation of collagen and ground substance in the skin. Deficiency of vitamin C can develop after 2 to 3 months of inadequate intake[19] and is characterized by the presence of horny keratinous plugs in the orifices of the hair follicles (follicular keratosis), petechiae, and perifollicular purpura with entrapped "corkscrew" hairs on the upper arms, legs, back, and buttocks (see Plate XXV-5). Initially, swelling, pain, and purpura are present. Large ecchymoses on the legs and mucous membrane purpura are seen in more severe cases, often produced by mild trauma. Hemorrhagic gingivitis, stomatitis, conjunctivitis, myalgias, arthralgias, and bone pain due to hemorrhage into muscles, joints, and bones may also occur.[20] Chronic ascorbate deficiency may present with woody edema and hyperpigmentation of the lower extremities.[21] Therefore, scurvy is characterized by the four H's—hemorrhagic signs, hyperkeratosis of hair follicles, hypochondriasis (weakness and arthralgias), and hematologic abnormalities (impaired platelet aggregation).[19] Alcoholics, the elderly, food faddists, and patients on dialysis have a higher risk for developing scurvy.

EHLERS-DANLOS SYNDROME AND PSEUDOXANTHOMA ELASTICUM

Easy bruising is one of the most prominent features of Ehlers-Danlos syndrome types IV and V (ecchymotic and X-linked), but it may also be seen in types I to III (gravis, mitis, and benign hypermobile) (see Plate XXV-6). Milder forms of Ehlers-Danlos syndrome have recently been described that also demonstrate mild to moderate bruising.[22] An association between thumb hyperextensibility and purpura has been reported, and the hyperextensibility may be an indicator of Ehlers-Danlos syndrome.[23] In evaluating patients for this heterogeneous group of connective tissue disorders, it is important to assess the elasticity of the skin, the extensibility of the joints, and the presence of other abnormalities such as high-arched palate and pectus excavatum. In pseudoxanthoma elasticum, recurrent mucous membrane hemorrhages may be a prominent physical finding. Patients with Marfan's syndrome and Noonan's syndrome may also demonstrate mild bleeding tendencies and increased capillary fragility.[24]

AMYLOID INFILTRATION OF BLOOD VESSELS

Mucocutaneous manifestations may be prominent in primary systemic amyloidosis associated with multiple myeloma or other paraproteinemias. Tissue biopsy reveals light-chain (AL) deposits of amyloid extensively infiltrating blood vessel walls and/or present diffusely throughout the dermis, resulting in increased vascular fragility. As a result, minimal trauma can produce hemorrhagic lesions ("pinch purpura"). Petechiae occur readily when there is an increase in transmural pressure (e.g., after a Valsalva maneuver or after proctoscopy), especially when the amyloidosis involves the eyelids and face (see Plates XXV-7 and XXV-8). Other cutaneous lesions are seen on the face, neck, scalp, or anogenital region in approximately one-third of patients with primary amyloidosis, and so the presence of these lesions may help to suggest the diagnosis; these include brown- to tan-colored translucent papules, plaques, nodules, bullae, xanthoma-like nodules, and sclerodermoid plaques that may become hemorrhagic either spontaneously or following trauma. Macroglossia with central irregular enlargement and peripheral indentations secondary to pressure from the adjacent teeth (scalloped tongue); diffuse eyelid and bulbar conjunctival swelling; alopecia and nail changes; smooth, waxy infiltration of the palms and volar fingertips[25]; and a rim of purpura ("purpuric halo") surrounding cherry angiomas have all been described in amyloidosis.[26]

COLLOID MILIUM

Colloid milium is characterized clinically by yellow papules and plaques, and histologically by the deposition of upper dermal amorphous material (similar to amyloid). Lesions of colloid milium may become purpuric after trauma.[27]

FEMALE EASY-BRUISING SYNDROME

The female predominance and the frequent association with phases of the menstrual cycle suggest that the female easy-bruising syndrome (purpura simplex) is due to hormonal effects on the blood vessel and/or its surrounding tissues.[2] Concomitant use of nonsteroidal anti-inflammatory medications may inhibit platelet function and contribute to the severity of the symptoms. Patients complain of frequent purpuric and ecchymotic lesions on the thighs ("devil's pinches") with minimal trauma. Patients with this entity who do not have other platelet or coagulation disorders do not appear to be at increased risk of hemorrhage from more severe hemostatic challenges such as surgery.

ADMINISTRATION OF LORENZO'S OIL

Purpura from a defect in vessel wall function has been seen in a patient receiving Lorenzo's oil (glycerol trioleate and glycerol trierucate).[28]

MELAS SYNDROME

Mitochondrial encephalomyopathy encompasses a group of disorders characterized by one or more enzymatic defects of aerobic metabolism leading to morphologic abnormalities of mitochondria in skeletal and cardiac muscle, the central nervous system, kidneys, liver, and endocrine organs. A 6-month-old boy with MELAS syndrome who demonstrated recurrent crops of purpuric macules on the palms and soles has been described.[29]

TRAUMA TO BLOOD VESSELS

PHYSICAL

Traumatic injury, if severe enough, causes skin hemorrhage even in normal individuals. It is thus important to know in detail the extent of an injury before deciding whether the skin hemorrhage is consistent with the magnitude of the trauma.[7] Traumatic lesions usually have well-defined margins. Depending on the etiology, the pattern may be annular or circumferential (e.g., hardball injury), linear or loop-shaped (e.g., child beating), periorbital (swim goggle purpura),[30] subungual (e.g., running shoe injury) (see Plate XXV-9), pinpoint (e.g., black dot heel, or talon noire), or genital (e.g., pinch marks from child abuse). The lesions associated with child abuse often include both cutaneous purpura, due to bruising from fingertip or hand pressure, and petechiae of the bulbar and palpebral conjunctivae, due to strangulation and/or smothering.[31,32]

Patients with factitial, or self-inflicted, purpura usually have medium- to large-sized ecchymotic lesions on the lower extremities, but the trunk or upper extremities may also be involved. These patients characteristically express indifference to the bruises.

Patients manifesting "coma bullae" present with irregular, clear or hemorrhagic bullae at sites of prolonged external pressure. Histologically, sweat gland necrosis is the diagnostic finding.

Purpura characteristically occurs after treatment of vascular anomalies with the 585-nm pulsed dye laser.[33]

ULTRAVIOLET RADIATION

Acute sunburn can have a petechial component if the damage is severe enough. Patients have been described who developed petechial lesions on the legs and trunk after suberythemal exposures to natural sunlight (solar purpura); these lesions were attributed to hypersensitivity to long-wave ultraviolet light [UVA (320 to 400 nm) or UVB (280 to 320 nm)]. Leukocytoclastic vasculitis was observed histologically in one patient.[34–36]

A syndrome has been reported in which transfused neonates with hyperbilirubinemia developed purpuric patches at sites of maximal exposure to blue light phototherapy.[37] The eruptions resolved in 2 to 7 days after discontinuation of the ultraviolet light therapy. The etiology of this purpuric phototherapy-induced eruption in neonates may be elevated plasma porphyrins (coproporphyrin and protoporphyrin).

INFECTIOUS

Bacterial, fungal, viral, rickettsial, protozoal, and parasitic infections may produce purpura.[38,39] The pathogenesis of infectious purpura is often complex and may include direct vascular invasion by the organism, disseminated intravascular coagulation, purpura fulminans, immune complex vasculitis, Shwartzman-like phenomena, septic emboli, direct effects of toxins released by the infecting organisms on the vasculature, and thrombocytopenia. Although characteristic patterns of purpura have been described for different infectious agents, overlap between the patterns is quite common.

Bacterial sepsis, including acute and subacute bacterial endocarditis due to gram-positive or gram-negative organisms, may cause a wide variety of dermatologic changes, including petechial or purpuric macules or papules; hemorrhagic bullae, erosions, or ulcers; or widespread ecchymoses and ischemic infarction of the skin (purpura fulminans, see below). The full syndrome of purpura fulminans can develop during bacterial infections, including streptococcal, staphylococcal, pneumococcal, and meningococcal bacteremias, and during scarlet fever, *Haemophilus* influenza, Rocky Mountain spotted fever, leptospirosis, and disease caused by *Vibrio parahaemolyticus* and dysgonic fermenter type 2. It is less common for it to follow viral (rubella, varicella, and roseola) or fungal (*Candida* spp.) infections. Asplenic patients with overwhelming pneumococcal sepsis may have facial petechiae and purpura, acral cyanosis, and/or livedo reticularis as their presenting symptoms.[40] About 20 percent of children admitted to the hospital with fever and petechiae[41] have documented invasive bacterial disease due to a variety of organisms, including *N. meningitidis, H. influenzae, Streptococcus pneumoniae, Staphylococcus aureus,* and *Escherichia coli*. Enteroviral and adenoviral pathogens can also be isolated on occasion. It has been reported that about 7 percent of children with fever and petechiae seen in emergency room departments have meningococcemia.[42] Palpable purpuric lesions associated with bacterial endocarditis may be an indication of immune complex formation. Splinter hemorrhages of the nails, historically associated with subacute bacterial endocarditis, occur in healthy individuals and in association with a variety of illnesses and thus are of little specific diagnostic value.[43]

Gram-negative sepsis with *Pseudomonas* species, *Klebsiella* species, *Aeromonas hydrophila,* or *E. coli* in the setting of severe immunocompromise may produce characteristic lesions of ecthyma gangrenosum (see Plate XXV-10). These lesions, which are seen in about 5 percent of patients with *Pseudomonas* sepsis, begin as erythematous or purpuric macules, then progress to plaquelike edema and erythema with nodule formation surmounted by irregular purpura. Within 48 h, these lesions develop into hemorrhagic or necrotic vesicles or bullae, surrounded by concentric areas of normal skin and a thin band of erythema.[44,45] Still later, the lesions evolve into edematous hemorrhagic plaques and then indurated painless ulcers. Lesions may be single or multiple and occur most often on the legs, abdomen, axillae, and anogenital areas. The palms and soles may occasionally be involved. The differential diagnosis of ecthyma gangrenosum includes fungal sepsis due to *Candida* species,[46] drug eruptions, cryoglobulinemia (see below), pyoderma gangrenosum, necrotizing vasculitis, polyarteritis nodosa, hyperviscosity syndrome, Sweet's syndrome, and leukemic infiltrates.

Meningococcemia initially produces erythematous papules, but these soon evolve into widespread petechiae with stellate purple to slate-gray purpuric lesions (see Plate XXV-11). These cutaneous lesions are the presenting sign in the vast majority of patients.[47] The purpura of meningococcemia may be due to direct vascular invasion by the organism or to an endotoxin-induced Shwartzman reaction. Acrocyanosis and symmetrical peripheral gangrene may ensue and are thought to be due to ischemic damage secondary to fibrin deposition as a result of disseminated intravascular coagulation. Purpura fulminans then rapidly follows.[47] The combination of purulent meningitis and petechiae strongly suggests that *Neisseria meningitidis* is the etiologic agent.[48] The presence of a rash in meningococcal infections indicates that there is a high likelihood of a fatal outcome.[49] Adult patients with meningococcemia and purpura fulminans have markedly depressed levels of proteins C and S and moderately decreased antithrombin III levels. Plasminogen activator inhibitor 1 (PAI-1), an acute phase protein inhibitor of tissue plasminogen activator, is increased in meningococcal purpura fulminans. Administration of antithrombin III concentrates,[50] recombinant tissue plasminogen activator,[51] or protein C[52,53] have been reported to result in rapid clinical improvement in select patients (see Chap. 126).

In chronic, intermittent meningococcemia an immune complex dermatitis may develop, manifesting itself as a poorly defined erythema with or without hemorrhagic papulovesicles over the joints.

A clinical presentation nearly identical to that of acute meningococcemia is seen in children with Brazilian purpuric fever,[54] a syndrome described in children aged 1 to 10. Purulent conjunctivitis caused by *Haemophilus aegyptius* heralds the syndrome, followed by purpura fulminans with fever, vomiting, abdominal pain, shock, and death. Bacterial endotoxin is probably the cause of this illness; treatment with antibiotics has been reported to improve the outcome.

In streptococcal pharyngitis, the erythrogenic toxin of *S. pyogenes* causes the classic rash of scarlet fever with associated linear purpuric lines in the skin folds (Pastia's lines). Streptococcal pharyngitis without scarlet fever can produce perioral, neck, and truncal petechiae in 2 percent of patients.[55]

Rickettsial infections, including Rocky Mountain spotted fever and epidemic typhus, produce cutaneous changes; urticarial macules may be seen initially and then evolve into petechiae (see Plate XXV-12), ecchymoses, focal hemorrhagic bullae, and/or more extensive areas of hemorrhagic necrosis (see Plate XXV-13).

The characteristic lesion of Lyme borreliosis is a nonpurpuric annular expanding plaque (erythema migrans). The lesion may contain a central purpuric macule or papule, or a hemorrhagic bulla (see Plate XXV-14).

Patients with either disseminated fungal infections [e.g., caused by *Cryptococcus, Candida* (see Plate XXV-15), *Zygomycetes, Aspergillus* (see Plate XXV-16), *Histoplasma, Alternaria,* or *Fusarium*][56,57] or locally invasive fungal diseases (e.g., mucormycosis, aspergillosis) may have hemorrhagic necrosis, purpura, and/or petechiae early in the course of the illness[58]; they may also demonstrate ecthyma gangrenosum-like lesions (e.g., with *Candida* or *A. niger* infections).

Viral infections occasionally have primary purpuric eruptions as their presenting manifestation. Parvovirus B19 infection may result in a petechial or confluent purpuric rash on the buttocks, axilla, and/or chest[59] (see Plate XXV-17). The papular-purpuric gloves and socks syndrome,[47,60–62] a disorder of adolescents and young adults, is characterized by well-demarcated symmetrical pruritic or painful acral edema and erythema; confluent petechial/purpuric papules and plaques of the hands and feet (including the palms and soles); oral erythema and erosions; swelling of the lips and tongue; and angular or erosive cheilitis. Palatal petechiae are common. Other areas of involvement include the inner thighs, inguinal region, buttocks, elbows, and knees. Systemic manifestations include fever, fatigue, myalgias, anorexia, lymphadenopathy, and arthralgias. This syndrome has been associated with infections caused by parvovirus B19, measles virus,[63] cytomegalovirus, Coxsackie B6 virus, and human herpes virus 6 (HHV-6).

Hemorrhagic fever with renal syndrome comprises a constellation of findings including fever, acute renal failure, headache, vomiting, and prostration associated with mucocutaneous petechiae, ecchymoses, facial flushing, periorbital edema, and both conjunctival and palatal petechiae.[64] This disorder is caused by Hantaan virus and is transmitted to humans by wild rodents; it is endemic to the former Soviet Union, Asia, Scandinavia, and Europe.

Parasitic infections, especially in the immunocompromised host, may produce purpura. Migration of filariform larvae of *Strongyloides stercoralis* typically produces rapidly progressive periumbilical and abdominal "thumb-print," linear, and reticulated purpura on a background of petechiae (see Plate XXV-18).[65–67] Disseminated cutaneous *Pneumocystis carinii* infection in patients with AIDS may demonstrate purpuric papules and nodules that closely resemble lesions of Kaposi sarcoma (see below).[68] Schistosomal cercarial dermatitis may begin as erythematous macules and urticarial lesions, which then develop central hemorrhage or vesiculation.

EMBOLIC

Atheroemboli with prominent cholesterol crystals, usually originating from atherosclerotic lesions in the aorta, can cause acral petechiae and purpura, acral livedo reticularis, nodules, unilateral peripheral ulcers, and bilateral cyanosis and gangrene[69] (see Plates XXV-19 and XXV-20). Distal pulses are present because these emboli are usually small and thus lodge in small blood vessels. Atheroemboli originating in the aortic arch or carotid arteries may affect the cerebral circulation and occasionally can be directly visualized in retinal arteries as refractile interruptions in the column of arterial blood. Transesophageal echocardiography is useful in identifying such lesions in the aorta.[70] Atheroemboli occur most frequently in older men (>50 years old) after diagnostic or vascular repair procedures. There is also an association with oral anticoagulant use, presumably as a result of increased lesion friability due to diminished fibrin support. Cholesterol embolization to the pancreas makes elevations of serum amylase levels a common accompanying laboratory finding. Livedo reticularis in an elderly patient is the most common presentation of cholesterol embolization.

Fat embolism may occur 2 to 3 days after severe trauma or following liposuction. The initial findings include petechiae of the upper extremity, thorax, and/or conjunctivae. The full syndrome includes hyperthermia, respiratory distress, retinal fat emboli, neurologic symptoms, and pulmonary infiltrates (see Chap. 126).[71,72]

Emboli from left atrial myxomas may cause acral purpura (nonblanching serpiginous and annular violaceous lesions of the fingertips), splinter hemorrhages, acral necrosis, and palpable purpura, as well as nonpurpuric manifestations including acral red papules with claudication, peripheral cyanosis, acral livedo reticularis, leg ulcers, and Raynaud's phenomenon.[73]

Calciphylaxis is defined as a syndrome of subcutaneous and vascular calcification in patients with secondary hyperparathyroidism due to end-stage renal failure. Hemorrhagic necrosis in a livedoid (vascular) pattern may be observed in these patients. The subcutaneous and vascular calcification following infusion of calcium gluconate or in chronic hypercalcemia may result in cutaneous necrosis and hemorrhage in a speckled or vascular pattern.

NEOPLASTIC

Infiltration of the skin in Langerhans cell histiocytosis (Chap. 78) can result in the development of a papular and crusted dermatitis of the scalp and intertriginous areas (see Plate XXV-21). Although these lesions usually simulate seborrheic dermatitis, they may have both petechial and purpuric features. Early cutaneous T-cell lymphoma may produce cutaneous lesions mimicking those seen in the pigmented purpuric eruptions. Similarly, skin infiltrations in patients with leukemias (see Plate XXV-27), lymphomas, and plasma cell disorders can be purpuric or can simulate purpura.[74,75]

ALLERGIC AND/OR INFLAMMATORY

In serum sickness, occurring either in association with drugs or infections, morbilliform or urticarial eruptions are the most common cutaneous manifestations. Petechiae, palpable purpura, and erythema multiforme lesions may occur. Linear or serpiginous bands of erythema may be seen at the margins of the palmar and/or plantar surfaces[76] (see Plate XXV-22). If the patients are thrombocytopenic, purpura usually appears within these linear bands. This eruption often heralds the onset of the syndrome. Direct immunofluorescence of involved skin demonstrates immunoglobulin and complement deposits.

The pigmented purpuric eruptions,[77–79] including Schamberg's disease, Majocchi's disease, and others, are a poorly understood group of disorders characterized by pinpoint petechiae and purpura on a background of red-brown or orange hyperpigmentation (see Plate XXV-23). Scaling, lichenification, and/or atrophy are occasionally seen. Itching may or may not be present. These eruptions characteristically involve the lower extremities, but they may be seen on the arms, trunk, and even the palms and soles.[80] Unilateral, linear, and zosteriform variants of pigmented purpuric eruptions have been identified.[81] The pigmented purpuric eruptions are not associated with any systemic manifestations. There is clinical overlap among these disorders, and a patient may have features of more than one pigmented purpuric eruption. Histologically, extravasation of red blood cells, hemosiderin deposits within macrophages, and a perivascular lymphohistiocytic (helper T cell)[82] infiltrate with endothelial cell swelling are seen. The pathogenesis of these disorders is not established but may include increased capillary dilatation with increased fragility and subsequent rupture of the capillaries in the papillary dermis, aneurysmal dilatation of the microvasculature, and possibly abnormal cellular immune responses to an unknown antigen.[83] Involved skin has been demonstrated to contain activated helper T cells along with keratinocytes positive for antigenic markers associated with receptors for effector immune cells.[84] Decreased aggregation of platelets in response to collagen has been reported.[85] Cutaneous T-cell lymphoma has been reported to produce lesions simulating those found in the pigmented purpuric eruptions, and so this disorder needs to be considered in the differential diagnosis.[86] Other disorders included in the differential diagnosis are drug hypersensitivity,[87] purpuric clothing dermatitis, sensitivity to food additives,[88] and hyperglobulinemic purpura of Waldenström.

Purpuric eruptions can result from allergic or irritant contact dermatitis to benzoyl peroxide,[89] clothing, cobalt, rubber, woolen garments, elastic dyes, Balsam of Peru,[90] local anesthetic (EMLA) cream,[91,92] or detergent whiteners, and these may simulate the pigmented purpuric eruptions.[93]

Pyoderma gangrenosum is a destructive, necrotizing ulceration of the skin presenting as a nodule, pustule, or hemorrhagic bulla (see Plate XXV-24). These furuncular nodules and pustules occur on the calves, thighs, buttocks, and face; they ulcerate rapidly, developing an undermined violaceous or blue border with surrounding erythema. The necrotic base is erythematous and edematous. Lesions heal with atrophic and cribriform scars. Systemic toxicity and high fever may accompany lesions of pyoderma gangrenosum. Clinical associations of these lesions include inflammatory bowel disease, rheumatoid arthritis, other polyarthritis syndromes, monoclonal gammopathies, hypogammaglobulinemia, blood dyscrasias, myeloma, lymphoma, and acute leukemia. Although any lesion of pyoderma gangrenosum may develop hemorrhagic necrosis, a specific superficial hemorrhagic bullous form with giant bullae is often associated with acute leukemia or other myeloproliferative disorder.

VISCERAL INFLAMMATORY DISEASE OR HEMORRHAGE

Intraabdominal inflammatory disease such as acute pancreatitis, ruptured ectopic pregnancy, or perforated duodenal ulcer may result in periumbilical purpura (Cullen's sign) (see Plate XXV-25). Purpura or ecchymosis on the flanks may be an indicator of retroperitoneal hemorrhage (Grey-Turner sign) (see Plate XXV-26).

THROMBOTIC

Disseminated intravascular coagulation (DIC) may result from a variety of different insults (see Chap. 126). Since there is potential for both thrombotic and hemorrhagic manifestations in DIC, it is not surprising that the skin manifestations are diverse. The most common skin findings are acral cyanosis with variably associated petechial, purpuric, and ecchymotic lesions, but in severe cases hemorrhagic gangrene of fingers and toes can occur.[49] The competence of the fibrinolytic system to digest deposited fibrin determines the extent of tissue compromise. The presence of peripheral gangrene may be an important consideration in the often difficult decision as to whether heparin is indicated in treating the syndrome[39] (see Plate XXV-28). The administration of antithrombin III[50] or protein C concentrate[52] appears to be of therapeutic benefit in some patients with disseminated intravascular coagulation due to meningococcemia, and recombinant tissue plasminogen activator has been reported to restore perfusion in this syndrome.[51]

COUMARIN SKIN NECROSIS

This thrombotic disorder affects about 1 in 500 patients receiving coumarin, with clinical lesions appearing between days 2 and 14 of coumarin administration.[94] Patients deficient in protein C are at a higher risk of developing coumarin necrosis because activated protein C functions as an anticoagulant, and it is one of the vitamin K–dependent factors that is most rapidly reduced by coumarin administration.[95] Coumarin necrosis begins suddenly as painful erythematous patches (see Plate XXV-29) that rapidly become edematous and progress to irregularly shaped hemorrhagic and necrotic plaques, nodules, and bullae; eventually large tumid indurations and infarcts occur with eschar formation and sloughing.[96] Coumarin necrosis is more common in women, with lesions occurring most often in fatty areas, such as the buttocks, thighs, and breasts. Acral areas, such as the fingers, toes, and penis, can occasionally be involved.[97] Lesions may be symmetric and widely distributed and on occasion may require surgical intervention.[98] Histologically, fibrin and platelet thrombi are observed in the dermal and subcutaneous vasculature. In one study, tumor necrosis factor was identified in the lesions, and endothelial cell adhesion molecules were upregulated.[99] The syndrome of coumarin necrosis is usually easily differentiated from hemorrhage due to excessive anticoagulation, since the latter usually occurs in association with excessive anticoagulation, has no sex predilection, is unrelated to the onset of therapy, is corrected with vitamin K, is worsened by continuation of coumarin or heparin, and is not associated with necrosis histologically. In addition, the lesions of coumarin necrosis contain the black eschar in the center of the necrotic zone.

Skin necrosis due to subcutaneous or intravenous heparin administration also has been described.[99] Necrosis of the skin may occur at the site of subcutaneous heparin injection or in a more widespread

distribution. Skin lesions represent a hypersensitivity reaction to heparin and appear 6 to 14 days following initiation of therapy. This syndrome is to be differentiated from heparin-induced thrombocytopenia, which may also be associated with purpuric skin lesions, or even skin necrosis if disseminated intravascular coagulation is part of the syndrome.

PURPURA FULMINANS

Purpura fulminans is a syndrome characterized by a triad of fever, disseminated intravascular coagulation with acral purpura and ecchymoses, and hypotension (see Chap. 126).[100] Clinical features include widespread arterial and venous thrombosis. Cutaneous discomfort develops initially, followed by erythema, edema, and petechiae. Thereafter, there is rapid development of painful purpuric papules and plaques with advancing erythematous borders. Finally, there is massive widespread ecchymoses, symmetric hemorrhagic necrosis, and bulla formation, often accentuated on the upper and lower extremities, abdomen, thighs, and buttocks.[101,102] The lesions enlarge with time and progress to gangrene, often with autoamputation of the digits. In adults and children, bacterial sepsis may trigger the syndrome or it may occur without antecedent infection.[39,103] In children, purpura fulminans most commonly follows Group A streptococcal, varicella, and/or upper respiratory infections, but a wide variety of organisms have been incriminated.[104] In sepsis-associated purpura fulminans, the purpura and necrosis begin in the distal extremities, and hemorrhagic necrosis of internal organs is common. Hypotension may not, however, be present.[105] Endotoxin is the most likely initiator of sepsis-associated purpura fulminans, leading to an increase in systemic cytokines, shock, and DIC. Prostration, fever, edema of the involved extremities, and hemorrhagic necrosis of the adrenal cortex may be seen, and death is not uncommon. The differential diagnosis includes thrombotic thrombocytopenic purpura, allergic or septic vasculitis, postinfectious thrombocytopenia, dermal hemorrhage, homozygous protein C or S deficiency, coumarin necrosis, ischemia due to lupus anticoagulant, Waldenström macroglobulinemia, and paroxysmal nocturnal hemoglobinuria. Histopathology reveals hemorrhagic necrosis of the dermis, with thromboses of the capillaries and small blood vessels. Fibrinoid necrosis of vessel walls and perivascular polymorphonuclear cell infiltrates have been described. The endothelial cell may be the target of both postinfectious and idiopathic purpura fulminans, and mechanisms similar to those described for DIC may be involved (see Chap. 126).[106] Tumor necrosis factor alpha and IL-1 are the cytokines thought to be most responsible for mediating the vascular events of purpura fulminans,[104,107] including increased leukocyte adherence and inflammation (see Chap. 67).

Homozygous protein C deficiency can produce essentially the same pattern in the neonate,[101,108–111] with onset in the first 12 h of life of diffuse, symmetric purpuric and ecchymotic skin lesions (see Chap. 127). These rapidly turn red-purple and grow peripherally, evolving into irreversible hemorrhagic and necrotic lesions. Central nervous system thrombosis and blindness are common. Both the skin lesions and venous thrombosis respond rapidly to plasma therapy, and long-term anticoagulation with warfarin has been effective in preventing recurrence.[112,113] Replacement therapy with protein C concentrate has been successful, as has liver transplantation.[47] Cutaneous necrosis similar to coumarin necrosis has been observed in patients with acquired protein C deficiency due to liver disease, malabsorption, administration of antibiotics, or autoantibodies to protein C.[114] Similarly, acquired protein C deficiency has been noted in some patients with sepsis-associated purpura fulminans. Several infants with homozygous protein S deficiency have also demonstrated neonatal recurrent purpura fulminans (see Chap. 127).[115,116] Postinfectious purpura fulminans has also been reported in association with antiprotein S IgG and IgM antibodies.[117] Resistance to activated protein C due to factor V Leiden has also been reported to cause neonatal purpura fulminans.[47,118]

In idiopathic purpura fulminans, 1 to 3 months after the initial infection, indurated and painful symmetric purple-gray lesions appear that are surrounded by a thin (10 mm) advancing erythematous border. These lesions then rapidly develop hemorrhagic necrosis and bullae,[111] enlarge, and may progress to dry gangrene. Lesions most commonly occur on the lower half of the body, especially the thighs, legs, buttocks, and lower trunk. Head and neck involvement (nose and ears) occurs but is uncommon, and mucous membranes are spared. Distal extremities are not involved in idiopathic purpura fulminans, which helps to distinguish it from sepsis-associated purpura fulminans.

PAROXYSMAL NOCTURNAL HEMOGLOBINURIA (SEE CHAP. 36)

Patients with this disorder may occasionally develop erythematous patches with dusky centers that may enlarge to form large, painful plaques of erythema with central necrosis.[119] Hemorrhagic bullae, ulceration, petechiae, ecchymoses, palpable purpura, and eschar formation also have been described. Differential diagnosis of the cutaneous findings includes thrombocytopenia, Henoch-Schönlein purpura, purpura fulminans, coumarin necrosis, vasculitis, and ecthyma gangrenosum. The lesions may be painful. Intravascular thrombi in the absence of vasculitis is the histologic appearance.

"ANTIPHOSPHOLIPID" ANTIBODY SYNDROME

The "antiphospholipid" antibody syndrome is an acquired multisystem disorder characterized by the variable presence of a lupus-type anticoagulant and/or antibodies to protein-phospholipid complexes, usually in high titer, in association with a tendency to thrombosis, fetal wastage, and/or thrombocytopenia[120–122] (see Chap. 128). Major clinical manifestations include recurrent thrombotic events (arterial or venous), recurrent fetal loss, thrombocytopenia, skin lesions, and neurologic complications. Visceral vascular occlusion may occur. Cutaneous findings may include widespread cutaneous necrosis with thrombi within the microvasculature (as seen in purpura fulminans), livedo reticularis, peripheral gangrene, painful skin nodules, leg ulcers, pyoderma gangrenosum-like lesions, thrombophlebitis, subungual splinter hemorrhages, porcelain-white scars, acral red to purple macules, and ecchymoses[123] (see Plates XXV-30 and XXV-31). The proposed mechanisms of thrombosis in antiphospholipid antibody syndrome include endothelial cell damage and activation, decreased prostacyclin release from endothelial cells, impaired fibrinolytic activity, inhibition of thrombomodulin-induced activation of protein C, inhibition of annexin V binding and platelet activation.[122]

KASABACH-MERRITT SYNDROME[124]

The Kasabach-Merritt syndrome is defined by the presence of an inflammatory bruised, reddish or purple mass in a neonate or young infant in association with profound thrombocytopenia and widespread ecchymoses. The large mass is a vascular lesion, previously believed to be a hemangioma but currently thought to be either a Kaposiform hemangioendothelioma or a tufted angioma. It is postulated that the vascular anomaly triggers platelet trapping and that platelet activation within the lesions sustains the growth of the cellular component of the vascular lesion.

DRUG-RELATED

Nonthrombocytopenic petechial and purpuric reactions can be observed after administration of a variety of drugs (see Plate XXV-32).[87,125,126] The mechanism for some of these reactions is presumed to be allergic hypersensitivity.

UNKNOWN

The Gardner-Diamond syndrome (psychogenic purpura, autoerythrocyte sensitization, or painful bruising syndrome) usually affects young women and is characterized by grouped tender bruises, appearing spontaneously or after minimal trauma, that are often preceded by pain or tingling.[127–129] The bruising may be so extensive that the patient loses the use of the limb. The onset of the disorder may coincide with surgical or accidental trauma. Many of the patients have significant psychological disturbances, and some of the patients are thought to have self-inflicted trauma. Intradermal injection of erythrocytes is said to elicit an ecchymotic response, indicating an "allergic" reaction to the patient's own erythrocytes (or DNA), perhaps as a result of an immune response to altered membrane phospholipid distribution,[130] but there is considerable controversy about the specificity and significance of this test.[131] Histologically, edema and a mononuclear cell infiltrate with extravasated red blood cells are observed. Localized neurogenic release of fibrinolytic activity in the skin has been proposed as a mechanism to link the psychological and dermal components of the syndrome.[132]

Approximately 25 percent of children with familial Mediterranean fever were described as having nonspecific 1- to 2-cm petechial or slightly raised purpuric papules on the face, trunk, and extremities.[133] These lesions resolved spontaneously in 1 to 3 weeks and were the most common cutaneous findings in these children.

PALPABLE PURPURA

CUTANEOUS VASCULITIS

HENOCH-SCHÖNLEIN PURPURA

This syndrome is manifested by leukocytoclastic vasculitis that predominantly affects children between the ages of 2 and 10, with a peak between the ages of 3 and 7.[134–137] It is the most common vasculitis of childhood. Palpable purpuric cutaneous lesions, acute gastrointestinal symptoms (abdominal cramping), as well as renal (hematuria), arthritic (ankle and knee), cardiac, pulmonary, and central nervous system lesions are observed. Renal involvement in adults is more common, but the prognosis in children and adults is the same.[138,139] In children, there is an increased incidence in boys,[140] but there is no sex predilection in adults. A decreased incidence during the summer has been reported, and community outbreaks have been described. In spite of numerous reports linking various precipitating factors (infections, environmental chemicals, toxins, insect bites, complement component C2 deficiency, familial Mediterranean fever,[141,142] and malignancies) to the development of Henoch-Schönlein purpura, there is no convincing evidence supporting such associations. Genetic factors may play a role in determining susceptibility or resistance to Henoch-Schönlein purpura. Thus, the presence of DRB*01, DRB*11, DQA*0301, as well as complement 4 locus II gene deletion makes an individual more prone to develop Henoch-Schönlein purpura,[143] while DRB*07 may make one less likely to develop the disease.[144]

The clinical presentation in more than 50 percent of patients includes fever and the explosive onset over the legs and buttocks of urticarial papules, plaques, and targetoid plaques, with or without purpura, palpable purpura (see Plate XXV-33), or hemorrhagic vesicles or bullae; progression to larger stellate, reticulate, and necrotic lesions may occur. Lesions may be seen on the arms, hands, or face, but rarely on the trunk, and may recur over weeks to months. Occasionally, ecchymotic lesions resembling child abuse may be present, but, unlike the latter, the lesions of Henoch-Schönlein purpura are usually strikingly symmetric. Scrotal edema, purpura, and testicular pain may be the initial symptoms in Henoch-Schönlein purpura and must be differentiated from testicular torsion.[145] Henoch-Schönlein vasculitis involves the precapillary, capillary, and postcapillary vessels of the skin, gastrointestinal tract, joints, and kidneys. Thus, arthralgias and abdominal pain usually accompany the rash. Occasionally, the characteristic cutaneous eruption is delayed and follows the appearance of abdominal pain.[146] Melena and signs of peritonitis are common. There may be an association between decreased factor XIII activity in children with Henoch-Schönlein purpura and abdominal symptoms. Leukocytosis, elevated C-reactive protein, and thrombocytosis are significantly associated with gastrointestinal bleeding in children with Henoch-Schönlein purpura.[147] Oligoarticular arthritis of the large joints is nearly always present, and proteinuria and hematuria occur in approximately 40 percent of patients. In older children and adults, renal disease progresses in 10 to 20 percent. In a review of 57 adults with Henoch-Schönlein purpura, the presence of a recent infection, fever, and truncal purpura correlated with renal involvement.[148] Neither the presence of bullous or necrotic lesions, nor the histologic severity of the cutaneous vasculitis, were predictive of renal involvement.

Henoch-Schönlein purpura is thought to be an immune complex disease, with IgA, IgG, and C3 being deposited in the cutaneous and renal vasculature. The C5b-9 complex (membrane attack complex) is also found in cutaneous and renal vascular lesions in Henoch-Schönlein purpura,[149] and a role for complement activation in the production of the vasculitic changes has been suggested. Approximately 50 percent of patients with Henoch-Schönlein purpura produce IgA rheumatoid factor,[137,150] and IgA-containing immune complexes have been detected in the serum, especially during the early phases of the syndrome. Familial IgA nephropathy has also been described in association with Henoch-Schönlein purpura. IgA-fibronectin complexes and IgA-anticardiolipin antibodies have also been detected in serum. A stippled pattern of IgA in the dermal blood vessels is seen on direct immunofluorescence of the skin.[151,152] The IgA-fibronectin aggregates detected in the sera of patients with Henoch-Schönlein purpura with IgA nephropathy may help to explain the binding of IgA to peripheral and glomerular vessels.[153] The presence of IgA deposits in the vasculitic lesions has been correlated with a longer clinical course, a more favorable initial response to systemic glucocorticoid therapy, and a higher incidence of systemic involvement (renal and arthritic).[154] The presence of decreased factor XIII, severe abdominal symptoms, and persistent purpura correlate with an increased risk of renal involvement,[155] and the presence of high-titer IgA anti-endothelial-cell antibodies and elevated levels of soluble thrombomodulin in serum are associated with severe proteinuria and active renal disease.[156] The IL-1 receptor antagonist allele may be a genetic marker shared by patients with Henoch-Schönlein purpura and those with IgA nephropathy with gross hematuria.[157] Decreased IgA sialic acid content is found in Henoch-Schönlein purpura, a finding similar to that of patients with IgA nephropathy.[158] Serum levels of malondialdehyde, a marker of lipid peroxidation, are significantly elevated in patients with Henoch-Schönlein purpura with renal involvement. Indicators of endothelial cell damage (von Willebrand factor, soluble thrombomodulin, and tissue plasminogen activator) as well as the cytokine tumor necrosis factor alpha are all increased in a significant number of patients with Henoch-Schönlein purpura.[159-161]

Inhibitors of prostacyclin have also been suggested as playing a role in the pathogenesis of Henoch-Schönlein purpura. Monoclonal antibodies to intercellular adhesion molecule-1 (ICAM-1) on endothelial cells and to CD18 or CD11b on leukocytes block the hemorrhagic vasculitis in experimentally induced Shwartzman reactions,[162] suggesting that intravascular leukocyte aggregation can contribute to the hemorrhagic response in this disorder and perhaps related disorders such as Henoch-Schönlein purpura.

Ten percent of adults with other forms of leukocytoclastic vasculitis demonstrate livedoid superficial plaques with multifocal areas of hemorrhage or necrosis and reticulate margins connecting adjacent lesions.[163] These lesions contain IgA and C3 within the blood vessel walls. Smooth-margined purpuric papules with uniform hemorrhage show IgA but more frequently demonstrate IgG or IgM vascular deposits.

ACUTE HEMORRHAGIC EDEMA OF INFANCY

This entity is composed of a triad of fever, irislike or medallion-like large purpuric cutaneous lesions, and edema affecting infants between the ages of 4 months and 2 years.[164-168] It is heralded by the sudden onset of peripheral edema, purpuric targetoid plaques, and painful petechiae and ecchymoses, all of which resolve spontaneously within 1 to 3 weeks. Occasionally, reticulate purpura, tender necrotic lesions of the ears, and/or urticaria are observed. The cutaneous lesions and the accompanying edema are localized to the cheeks, eyelids, ears, extremities, and genitalia. As in Henoch-Schönlein purpura, lesions begin as urticarial plaques, then progress to an irislike pattern of purpura or ecchymoses. Joint or abdominal pain is very rarely seen. Histopathologic examination demonstrates leukocytoclastic vasculitis. Immunofluorescent studies of the skin reveal vascular deposits of IgG, IgM, IgA, C3, C1q, and fibrinogen. Acute hemorrhagic edema differs from Henoch-Schönlein purpura because it is found in patients under 2 years of age, it is limited to cutaneous manifestations, and the rash is more monomorphic. Acute hemorrhagic edema should be differentiated from meningococcemia, septic emboli, drug eruption, hemorrhagic erythema multiforme, Kawasaki disease, acute febrile neutrophilic dermatosis (Sweet's syndrome), and child abuse.

COLLAGEN VASCULAR DISEASES (SEE PLATE XXV-34)

These disorders may have an array of vasculitic purpuric lesions with a mixture of palpable and nonpalpable lesions, including petechiae, papules and nodules, ecchymoses, hemorrhagic bullae, hemorrhagic necrosis, purpuric ulcers, splinter hemorrhages, and periungual hemorrhage.[169-173] Other disorders with systemic large and/or small vessel vasculitis, including hypocomplementemic vasculitis, polyarteritis nodosa (including microscopic polyarteritis nodosa)[174] (see Plate XXV-35), Wegener's granulomatosis (see Plate XXV-36), Churg-Strauss angiitis, mixed connective tissue disease,[6] rheumatoid vasculitis, relapsing polychondritis, or rheumatoid arthritis with IgA immune complex vasculitis, may have a similar array of such lesions. Nonpurpuric cutaneous lesions also may be present including ulcers, subcutaneous nodules, livedo reticularis, blanchable erythema, erythematous plaques, and telangiectasia. Patients with urticarial vasculitis frequently have lesions that resolve with purpura.[175]

BEHÇET'S DISEASE

Behçet's disease is a chronic inflammatory multisystem disorder characterized by recurrent oral and genital ulcerations, cutaneous lesions, arthralgias, and gastrointestinal, vascular, and central nervous system manifestations. A review of 42 patients from Japan reported leukocytoclastic vasculitis in 17 percent of the patients, some of whom had palpable purpura and hemorrhagic bullae.[176]

HYPERSENSITIVITY VASCULITIS

The constellation of findings characteristic of this disease includes palpable purpura, joint symptoms, and leukocytoclastic vasculitis. The prognosis is excellent.[177] It may be seen as a drug reaction, in the setting of infection (e.g., staphylococcal or streptococcal, leprosy, acute or subacute bacterial endocarditis, hepatitis B or C, pulmonary or nodal tuberculosis, or HIV disease), or as a reaction to unknown antigens.[178,179]

Chronic infectious hepatitis may be associated with necrotizing vasculitis, hypocomplementemia, and cryoglobulinemia.[180,181]

Alpha-1 antitrypsin deficiency has been described in association with systemic vasculitis, including cutaneous involvement resembling that observed in microscopic polyarteritis, Wegener's granulomatosis, and Henoch-Schönlein purpura.[182]

DRUG-INDUCED LEUKOCYTOCLASTIC VASCULITIS

This entity has been reported with acebutolol, amiodarone, amphetamine, anistreplase, aspirin, captopril, cefoxitin, chlorthalidone, cimetidine, ciprofloxacin, coumadin, didanosine, diltiazem, ethacrynic acid, furosemide (see Plate XXV-37), granulocyte colony-stimulating factor, hydantoin, hydralazine, hydrochlorthiazide, insulin, interferon, iodides, nifedipine, ofloxacin, penicillin, phenacetin, phenothiazines, procainamide, propranolol, propylthiouracil, quinidine, rifampin, streptokinase, sulfonamides, tamoxifen, tartrazine, zidovudine, and others.[126,183–185]

PARANEOPLASTIC VASCULITIS

This is a syndrome of petechiae, palpable purpura, urticaria, maculopapular lesions, leg ulcers, and/or erythema multiforme seen in association with hairy-cell leukemia and other lympho- and myeloproliferative disorders.[186–188] Intense pruritus or dysesthesias accompany the dermatologic findings. The cutaneous lesions often precede or signal the recurrence of the malignancy. Carcinomas of the breast, lung, colon, cervix, prostate, nasopharynx, and kidney have all been reported in association with cutaneous vasculitis.[188,189]

LONG-DISTANCE WALKERS

Long-distance walkers may develop purpuric lesions of leukocytoclastic vasculitis on the lower legs.[190]

DYSPROTEINEMIAS

CRYOGLOBULINEMIA

Cryoglobulins are cold-precipitable proteins found in plasma or serum. Single-component cryoglobulins may be IgG, IgM, or IgA.[191] These cryoproteins may be idiopathic in origin or occur in association with Waldenström macroglobulinemia, myeloma, or lymphoma. Mixed cryoglobulins have rheumatoid-factor-like activity and are usually composed of IgG molecules complexed with IgM molecules having anti-IgG reactivity (or less frequently IgG or IgA molecules with anti-IgG reactivity). Mixed cryoglobulins may be seen as an idiopathic phenomenon or in association with a wide variety of subacute and chronic disorders, most particularly hepatitis C. The immune complex may be composed of hepatitis C virus (HCV), anti-HCV, and IgA-type rheumatoid factor[192] or HCV, IgM-like rheumatoid factor, and IgG.[193] These high-molecular-weight complexes may initiate alterations in endothelial cells resulting in increased vascular permeability, neutrophil infiltration, and vessel wall damage. Mixed cryoglobulinemia is characterized by the classical clinical triad of purpura, weakness, and arthralgias. Cutaneous findings of cryoglobulinemia are common and include the intermittent appearance of acral hemorrhagic necrosis, macular and palpable purpura (see Plate XXV-38), livedo reticularis, subungual hemorrhage (see Plate XXV-39), hemorrhagic bullae, urticaria, leg ulcerations, Raynaud's phenomenon, follicular pustular purpura, and erythema multiforme-like lesions.[194–196] Cutaneous lesions often resemble those seen in the pigmented purpuric eruptions. Mucous membrane oral and nasal lesions are occasionally observed. Arthritis, nephropathies, neuropathies, and chronic hepatitis and/or cirrhosis are prominent associated findings.[197] Treatment of hepatitis C–associated mixed cryoglobulinemia with interferon alpha may eradicate the cryoglobulins and their associated cutaneous and systemic manifestations.[198] Monoclonal cryoglobulins may crystallize and result in livedo reticularis with purpuric necrosis, destructive arthropathy, and malignant hypertension (cryocrystalglobulinemia).[199]

HYPERGLOBULINEMIC PURPURA OF WALDENSTRÖM

The characteristic cutaneous findings of benign hyperglobulinemic purpura are crops of petechiae in the same stage of development on the lower legs and ankles of young women (age 18 to 40 years).[200] These lesions can be macular and papular, discrete or confluent, with hemosiderin staining (see Plate XXV-40).[201–203] Palpable purpura is rare, and ecchymoses do not occur. Lesions may be present on the thighs, abdomen, and arms. Lymphadenopathy is common. Lesions recur at intervals of days, weeks, or months, and precipitating factors may include increased hydrostatic pressure, hyperviscosity, and low temperatures.[204] The polyclonal increase of globulins (mostly IgG) can be associated with Sjögren's syndrome, systemic lupus erythematosus, polymyositis, rheumatoid arthritis, myeloma, thymoma, sarcoid, cystic fibrosis, or multiple sclerosis. The eruption closely resembles those seen in the pigmented purpuric eruptions and cryoglobulinemia. Histologically, leukocytoclastic vasculitis or perivascular lymphocytic infiltrates, red blood cells, and variable arteriolar necrosis are found. The hypergammaglobulinemia consists of elevated levels of IgG, as well as IgA and IgM. There is a decrease in IgG_2.[205] The sedimentation rate is usually elevated. Circulating IgG-anti-IgG (only IgG_1 subclass) and/or IgA and IgM-anti-IgG immune complexes have been detected. Many patients have antibodies to Ro/SSA.[206] Lymphocytotoxic antibodies against suppressor lymphocytes with resultant lymphopenia and antimyelin antibodies have also been noted. This disorder is not to be confused with Waldenström macroglobulinemia; the latter has multiple cutaneous findings including the IgM storage papule, infiltrative plaques and/or nodules, purpuric lesions secondary to cryoglobulins, and mucocutaneous oozing and bleeding as a result of the concomitant hyperviscosity syndrome. These patients have a monoclonal IgM paraprotein spike rather than the polyclonal broad-based gammopathy seen in hyperglobulinemic purpura of Waldenström.

CRYOFIBRINOGENEMIA

Cryofibrinogenemia indicates the presence in the blood of an abnormal cold-precipitable protein derived from fibrinogen or fibrin. The most common cutaneous manifestations are sensitivity to cold, purpura, livedo reticularis, cyanosis, ulcerations, erythema, hematoma, urticaria, gangrene, and Raynaud's phenomenon. Lesions appear on the distal extremities, buttocks, nose, and ears.[207] Acral blisters have also been described. Cryofibrinogenemia may occur as a primary (essential) or secondary form, usually in association with laboratory evidence of chronic disseminated intravascular coagulation. Secondary cryofibrinogenemia may occur in association with neoplastic, thromboembolic, and infectious disorders.

LIGHT-CHAIN VASCULOPATHY

A vasculopathy with deposition in the skin of λ light-chain crystals has been described in two patients who demonstrated nonpalpable purpura, hemorrhagic vesicles, ischemic necrosis of the extremities, and rapidly progressive renal failure.[208] Intravascular λ light chains were observed on direct immunofluorescence of skin. Monoclonal λ light chains were observed in serum, and extensive crystalline deposits were present in tissues. One case of IgG κ intact paraprotein crystallization with cutaneous involvement has also been described.[209] The clinical picture closely resembles severe necrotizing vasculitis, but no histologic evidence of vasculitis was present in these cases.

PRIMARY CUTANEOUS DISEASES

Allergic contact dermatitis (purple poison ivy), drug eruptions on the lower extremities, acne vulgaris, insect bites (especially black fly bites), dermatitis herpetiformis, pityriasis rosea, and other primary cutaneous disorders may present with purpuric papules and vesicles mimicking septic and vasculitic lesions.

NONPURPURIC DISORDERS SIMULATING PURPURA

DISORDERS WITH TELANGIECTASIAS

HEREDITARY HEMORRHAGIC TELANGIECTASIA (OSLER-WEBER-RENDU DISEASE)

This is an autosomal dominant inherited disorder with an estimated frequency of 1 in 50,000 characterized by widespread dermal, mucosal, and visceral telangiectasias.[210] One form of the disorder, characterized by a high frequency of pulmonary arteriovenous malformations, has been identified as being due to abnormalities in the endothelial protein endoglin on chromosome 9, which appears to mediate the response of endothelial cells to members of the transforming growth factor beta (TGF-β) family.[210] A number of the mutations involve the production of truncated forms of the receptor, opening up the possibility of a dominant negative mechanism to explain the autosomal dominant inheritance pattern.[211] Another form of the disease has been linked to a region of chromosome 3 containing the TGF-β II receptor, and a third form has been linked to the activin-receptor-like kinase 1 gene on chromosome 12, which is a cell surface receptor for the TGF-β superfamily of ligands.[212,213] Clinically, venous lakes and papular, punctate, matlike, and linear telangiectasias appear on all areas of the skin and mucous membranes, with a predominance of lesions on the dorsum and ventral aspects of the tongue, and on the face, lips, perioral region, nasal mucosa, fingertips, toes, and trunk.[214] Recurrent epistaxis is a nearly universal finding in this disorder, with symptoms almost always becoming worse with age. It is estimated, however, that 10 percent of patients manifest no bleeding. The severity of the disorder relates to the age of onset of epistaxis, with the most severely affected patients developing recurrent nosebleeds during childhood. The cutaneous changes usually begin at puberty and progress through the third to fourth decades. Bleeding can occur in virtually every organ, with gastrointestinal, oral, and urogenital sites most common. In the gastrointestinal tract, the stomach and duodenum are more common sites of bleeding than the colon. Pulmonary arteriovenous fistulae may be seen in 20 percent of patients and may be associated with oxygen desaturation, hemoptysis, hemothorax, brain abscess, or cerebral ischemia due to paradoxical emboli. Hepatic and splenic arteriovenous fistulae, as well as intracranial, aortic, and splenic aneurysms have all been reported. Histologically, the vessels of hereditary hemorrhagic telangiectasia show a discontinuous endothelium and incomplete smooth muscle. The surrounding stroma lacks elastin. Thus, the bleeding tendencies are thought to be due to mechanical fragility of the abnormal vessels.

Therapy for hereditary hemorrhagic telangiectasias remains problematic, with laser treatment for cutaneous lesions; split-thickness skin grafting, embolization, or hormonal therapy (estrogen or estrogens plus progesterone) for epistaxis; pulmonary resection or embolization for pulmonary arteriovenous malformations; and hormonal therapy and laser coagulation for gastrointestinal lesions.[210] The antifibrinolytic agent epsilon aminocaproic acid has been reported to be beneficial in controlling hemorrhage,[215] but negative results have also been reported.[216]

OTHER TELANGIECTATIC SYNDROMES

Spiderlike telangiectatic mats seen in the CREST syndrome (calcinosis, Raynaud phenomenon, esophageal motor dysfunction, sclerodactyly, and telangiectasia) may be easily confused with the lesions of chronic actinic damage and those of hereditary hemorrhagic telangiec-

tasia. Vascular nevi, angiokeratoma corporis diffusum, ataxia telangiectasia, and spider telangiectasias from chronic liver disease also must be differentiated. Spider telangiectasias have a central, prominent, easily blanchable feeding vessel with several smaller telangiectasias emanating from this central vessel. Spider telangiectasias seen in patients with chronic liver disease are distributed from the head to the nipple line and correlate with the risk of bleeding from esophageal varices.[217] Spider and papular telangiectasias on the upper trunk and arms have been reported to be a cutaneous manifestation of AIDS.[218]

"PETECHIAL" CHERRY ANGIOMATA

Cherry angiomas are the common papular, brightly erythematous lesions seen on the trunk and extremities of middle-aged and older men and women. The lesions increase in size and number with age and may produce easy bruising, since they tend to bleed excessively with trauma. Pinpoint angiomas may be present in large numbers and may mimic a petechial eruption.

KAPOSI SARCOMA

AIDS-related Kaposi sarcoma is easily confused with purpuric and ecchymotic lesions, lichen aureus, as well as some of the other pigmented purpuric eruptions. Oral lesions of epidemic Kaposi sarcoma may mimic petechiae and purpura. Similarly, angiosarcoma may present as a purple-to-brown plaque resembling purpura.

INTRAVASCULAR LARGE-CELL LYMPHOMA

Intravascular large-cell lymphoma, previously referred to as *malignant angioendotheliomatosis,* may present with asymptomatic "purpuric" patches, ecchymotic-like plaques, or palpable purpura-like lesions.[219] Associated neurologic signs and symptoms are common.

FABRY'S DISEASE (ANGIOKERATOMA CORPORIS DIFFUSUM)

This X-linked inherited disorder of glycolipid metabolism is due to a deficiency of the enzyme alpha-galactosidase A (ceramide trihexosidase).[220] Accumulation of glycolipid throughout the body leads to cutaneous, renal, ophthalmologic, cardiac, and central nervous system manifestations. Angiokeratoma corporis diffusum lesions are pinpoint to 4-mm nonblanchable deep red, blue, or black macules or papules. The nonblanchable lesions are distributed over the trunk, extremities, and genitalia. In mild cases, lesions are localized to the thighs, scrotum, or periumbilical region. Grouping of lesions may occur. Superficial corneal dystrophy and varicosities of the bulbar conjunctivum are commonly seen. Glycolipid deposits are histochemically detected in the media and intima of small dermal blood vessels.

EXTRAMEDULLARY HEMATOPOIESIS ("BLUEBERRY MUFFIN" BABY)

These dark red, blue, or blue-gray 1- to 7-mm macules and/or papules are present at birth or within the first 48 h of life in infants with congenital rubella, cytomegalovirus, Coxsackie virus B2, parvovirus B19 infections,[221] Rh incompatibility, hereditary spherocytosis, or twin transfusion syndrome.[47] Rarely, healthy newborns may demonstrate extramedullary hematopoiesis. The lesions are most commonly found on the scalp, neck, and trunk but may be widely distributed. These lesions fade into tan- or copper-colored macules by 8 weeks of age. Adults with marrow infiltration (e.g., myelofibrosis) also may develop lesions of extramedullary hematopoiesis. Occasionally newborn infants with neoplastic or infiltrative diseases, such as neuroblastoma, rhabdomyosarcoma, leukemia, and Langerhans cell histiocytosis, can present with a blueberry-muffin-like appearance.

ANGIOMA SERPIGINOSUM

Angioma serpiginosum is a vascular nevoid lesion with pinpoint vascular ectasias on a background of erythema.[2] The lesion is partially blanchable and is not petechial. Capillary microscopy demonstrates punctate dilated capillaries. This lesion is usually seen on the legs and buttocks of women but may occur anywhere and expand in childhood and regress with age. Differential diagnosis includes the pigmented purpuric eruptions (e.g., purpura annularis telangiectoides).

GRANULOMA ANNULARE

Granuloma annulare is a cutaneous disorder characterized by annular grouping of skin-colored to erythematous papules over the extensor surfaces (elbows, knuckles, ankles, and feet). The violaceous purpuric papules may be mistaken for septic emboli. Although usually idiopathic, it has been reported in association with a childhood myelodysplastic syndrome.[222]

REFERENCES

1. Rohrer MJ, Michelotti MC, Nahrwold DL: A prospective evaluation of the efficacy of preoperative coagulation testing. *Ann Surg* 208:554, 1988.
2. Champion RH: Purpura, in *Textbook of Dermatology,* 5 ed, edited by RH Champion, JL Burton, pp 1881–1892. Blackwell Scientific, Oxford, 1992.
3. Crosby WH: Purpura, in *Clinical Dermatology,* 15th ed, edited by DJ Demis, pp 7–22. Lippincott, Philadelphia, 1988.
4. Edwards RL, Rickles FR: Delayed hypersensitivity in man: effects of systemic anticoagulation. *Science* 200:541, 1978.
5. Alcalay J, Ingber A, Sandbank M: Mask phenomenon: postemesis facial purpura. *Cutis* 38:28, 1986.
6. Magro CM, Crowson AN, Regauer S: Mixed connective tissue disease. A clinical, histologic, and immunofluorescence study of eight cases. *Am J Dermatopathol* 19:206, 1997.
7. Rasmussen JE: Puzzling purpuras in children and young adults. *J Am Acad Dermatol* 6:67, 1982.
8. Schachner LA, Hansen RC: *Neonatal Skin and Skin Disorders,* p 263. New York, Churchill Livingston, 1988.
9. Lowe L, Rapini RP, Johnson TM: Traumatic asphyxia. *J Am Acad Dermatol* 23:972, 1990.
10. Perrot LJ: Masque ecchymotique. Specific or nonspecific indicator for abuse. *Am J Forensic Med Pathol* 10:95, 1989.
11. Kondo T, Betz P, Eisenmenger W: Retrospective study on skin reddenings and petechiae in the eyelids and the conjunctivae in forensic physical examinations. *Int J Legal Med* 110:204, 1997.
12. Metzker A, Merlob P: Suction purpura. *Arch Dermatol* 128:822, 1992.
13. Fisher AA: Purpuric contact dermatitis. *Cutis* 33:346, 1984.
14. Mitchell RE: Chronic solar dermatosis: a light and electron microscopic study of the dermis. *J Invest Dermatol* 48:203, 1967.
15. Feinstein RJ, Halprin KM, Penneys NS, et al: Senile purpura. *Arch Dermatol* 108:229, 1973.
16. Beauregard S, Gilchrest BA: Syndromes of premature aging. *Dermatol Clin* 5:109, 1987.
17. Forster PJ: Microvascular fragility at high altitude. *Br Med J* 296:1004, 1988.
18. Capewell S, Reynolds S, Shuttleworth D, Edwards C, Finlay AY: Purpura and dermal thinning associated with high dose inhaled corticosteroids. *BMJ* 300:1548, 1990.
19. Wirth PB, Kalb RE: Follicular purpuric macules of the extremities. Scurvy. *Arch Dermatol* 126:385, 1990.
20. Leone J, Delhinger V, Maes D, et al: Rheumatic manifestations of scurvy. A report of two cases. *Rev Rhum Engl Ed* 64:428, 1997.
21. Walker A: Chronic scurvy. *Br J Dermatol* 80:625, 1968.
22. Holzberg M, Hewan-Lowe KO, Olansky AJ: The Ehlers-Danlos syndrome: Recognition, characterization, and importance of a milder variant

of the classic form. A preliminary study. *J Am Acad Dermatol* 19:656, 1988.
23. Kaplinsky C, Kenet G, Seligsohn U, Rechavi G: Association between hyperflexibility of the thumb and an unexplained bleeding tendency: is it a rule of thumb? *Br J Haematol* 101:260, 1998.
24. Sidhu-Malik NK, Wenstrup RJ: The Ehlers-Danlos syndromes and Marfan syndrome: inherited diseases of connective tissue with overlapping clinical features. *Semin Dermatol* 14:40, 1995.
25. Kwong C-K: Mucocutaneous manifestations in systemic amyloidosis, in *Clinics in Dermatology,* edited by C-K Kwong, SM Breathnach, pp 7–12. Elsevier, New York, 1990.
26. Schmidt CP: Purpuric halos around hemangiomas in systemic amyloidosis. *Cutis* 48:141, 1991.
27. Sevigny GM, Ford MJ: Stroke-induced purpura in lesions of colloid milium. *Cutis* 56:109, 1995.
28. Chai BC, Etches WS, Stewart MW, Siminoski K: Bleeding in a patient taking Lorenzo's oil: evidence for a vascular defect. *Postgrad Med J* 72:113, 1996.
29. Horiguchi Y, Fujii T, Imamura S: Purpuric cutaneous manifestations in mitochondrial encephalomyopathy. *J Dermatol* 18:295, 1991.
30. Jowett NI, Jowett SG: Ocular purpura in a swimmer. *Postgrad Med J* 73:819, 1997.
31. Ellerse NS: The cutaneous manifestations of child abuse and neglect. *Am J Dis Child* 133:906, 1979.
32. AMA diagnostic and treatment guidelines concerning child abuse and neglect. Council on Scientific Affairs. *JAMA* 254:796, 1985.
33. Unger WP: How ''safe'' is safe enough? *Dermatol Surg* 22:191, 1996.
34. Leung AK: Purpura associated with exposure to sunlight. *J R Soc Med* 79:423, 1986.
35. Kalivas L, Kalivas J: Solar purpura. *Arch Dermatol* 124:24, 1988.
36. Guarrera M, Parodi A, Rebora A: Solar purpura is not related to polymorphous light eruption. *Photodermatol* 6:293, 1989.
37. Paller AS, Eramo LR, Farrell EE, et al: Purpuric phototherapy-induced eruption in transfused neonates: Relation to transient porphyrinemia. *Pediatrics* 100:360, 1997.
38. Kingston ME, Mackey D: Skin clues in the diagnosis of life-threatening infections. *Rev Infect Dis* 8:1, 1986.
39. Musher DM: Cutaneous manifestations of bacterial sepsis. *Hosp Pract (Off Ed)* 24:71, 1989.
40. Rusonis PA, Robinson HN, Lamberg SI: Livedo reticularis and purpura: presenting features in fulminant pneumococcal septicemia in an asplenic patient. *J Am Acad Dermatol* 15:1120, 1986.
41. Van Nguyen Q, Nguyen EA, Weiner LB: Incidence of invasive bacterial disease in children with fever and petechiae. *Pediatrics* 74:77, 1984.
42. Baker RC, Seguin JH, Leslie N, et al: Fever and petechiae in children. *Pediatrics* 84:1051, 1989.
43. Fanning WL, Aronson M: Osler's node, Janeway lesions, and splinter hemorrhages. *Arch Dermatol* 113:648, 1977.
44. Dorff GJ, Geimer NF, Rosenthal DR, Rytel MW: Pseudomonas septicemia. Illustrated evolution of its skin lesion. *Arch Intern Med* 128:591, 1971.
45. El Baze P, Thyss A, Caldani C, et al: *Pseudomonas aeruginosa* O-11 folliculitis. Development into ecthyma gangrenosum in immunosuppressed patients. *Arch Dermatol* 121:873, 1985.
46. Fine JD, Miller JA, Harrist TJ, Haynes HA: Cutaneous lesions in disseminated candidiasis mimicking ecthyma gangrenosum. *Am J Med* 70:1133, 1981.
47. Baselga E, Drolet BA, Esterly NB: Purpura in infants and children. *J Am Acad Dermatol* 37:673, 1997.
48. Mancebo J, Domingo P, Blanch L, et al: The predictive value of petechiae in adults with bacterial meningitis. *JAMA* 256:2820, 1986.
49. Tesoro LJ, Selbst SM: Factors affecting outcome in meningococcal infections. *Am J Dis Child* 145:218, 1991.
50. Fourrier F, Lestavel P, Chopin C, et al: Meningococcemia and purpura fulminans in adults: acute deficiencies of proteins C and S and early treatment with antithrombin III concentrates. *Intensive Care Med* 16:121, 1990.
51. Aiuto LT, Barone SR, Cohen PS, Boxer RA: Recombinant tissue plasminogen activator restores perfusion in meningococcal purpura fulminans. *Crit Care Med* 25:1079, 1997.
52. Rintala E, Seppala OP, Kotilainen P, et al: Protein C in the treatment of coagulopathy in meningococcal disease. *Crit Care Med* 26:965, 1998.

53. Smith OP, White B, Vaughan D, et al: Use of protein-C concentrate, heparin, and haemodiafiltration in meningococcus-induced purpura fulminans. *Lancet* 350:1590, 1997.

54. Harrison LH, Broome CV: Brazilian purpuric fever—progress but unanswered questions. *Pediatr Infect Dis J* 8:248, 1989.

55. Braverman IM: Infections, in *Skin Signs of Systemic Disease,* 3rd ed, p 602. Saunders, Philadelphia, 1998.

56. Grossman ME, Silvers DN, Walther RR: Cutaneous manifestations of disseminated candidiasis. *J Am Acad Dermatol* 2:111, 1980.

57. Helm TN, Longworth DL, Hall GS, et al: Case report and review of resolved fusariosis. *J Am Acad Dermatol* 23:393, 1990.

58. Radentz WH: Opportunistic fungal infections in immunocompromised hosts. *J Am Acad Dermatol* 20:989, 1989.

59. Shiraishi H, Umetsu K, Yamamoto H, et al: Human parvovirus (HPV/B19) infection with purpura. *Microbiol Immunol* 33:369, 1989.

60. Harms M, Feldmann R, Saurat JH: Papular-purpuric "gloves and socks" syndrome. *J Am Acad Dermatol* 23:850, 1990.

61. Smith PT, Landry ML, Carey H, et al: Papular-purpuric gloves and socks syndrome associated with acute parvovirus B19 infection: case report and review. *Clin Infect Dis* 27:164, 1998.

62. Saulsbury FT: Petechial gloves and socks syndrome caused by parvovirus B19. *Pediatr Dermatol* 15:35, 1998.

63. Perez-Ferriols A, Martinez-Aparicio A, Aliaga-Boniche A: Papular-purpuric "gloves and socks" syndrome caused by measles virus. *J Am Acad Dermatol* 30:291, 1994.

64. Bruno P, Hassell LH, Brown J, et al: The protean manifestations of hemorrhagic fever with renal syndrome. A retrospective review of 26 cases from Korea. *Ann Intern Med* 113:385, 1990.

65. Von Kuster LC, Genta RM: Cutaneous manifestations of strongyloidiasis. *Arch Dermatol* 124:1826, 1988.

66. Kalb RE, Grossman ME: Periumbilical purpura in disseminated strongyloidiasis. *JAMA* 256:1170, 1986.

67. Ronan SG, Reddy RL, Manaligod JR, et al: Disseminated strongyloidiasis presenting as purpura. *J Am Acad Dermatol* 21:1123, 1989.

68. Litwin MA, Williams CM: Cutaneous *Pneumocystis carinii* infection mimicking Kaposi sarcoma. *Ann Intern Med* 117:48, 1992.

69. Falanga V, Fine MJ, Kapoor WN: The cutaneous manifestations of cholesterol crystal embolization. *Arch Dermatol* 122:1194, 1986.

70. Tunick PA, Lackner H, Katz ES, et al: Multiple emboli from a large aortic arch thrombus in a patient with thrombotic diathesis. *Am Heart J* 124:239, 1992.

71. Miller JD: Fat embolism: a clinical diagnosis. *Am Fam Physician* 35:129, 1987.

72. Oh WH, Mital MA: Fat embolism: current concepts of pathogenesis, diagnosis, and treatment. *Orthop Clin North Am* 9:769, 1978.

73. McAllister SM, Bornstein AM, Callen JP: Painful acral purpura. *Arch Dermatol* 134:789, 1998.

74. Francis JS, Sybert VP, Benjamin DR: Congenital monocytic leukemia: report of a case with cutaneous involvement, and review of the literature. *Pediatr Dermatol* 6:306, 1989.

75. Dreizen S, McCredie KB, Keating MJ, et al: Leukemia-associated skin infiltrates. *Postgrad Med* 85:45, 1989.

76. Bielory L, Yancey KB, Young NS, et al: Cutaneous manifestations of serum sickness in patients receiving antithymocyte globulin. *J Am Acad Dermatol* 13:411, 1985.

77. Sherertz EF: Pigmented purpuric eruptions. *Semin Thromb Hemost* 10:190, 1984.

78. Randall SJ, Kierland RR, Montgomery H: Pigmented purpuric eruptions. *Arch Dermatol* 64:177, 1951.

79. Newton RC, Raimer SS: Pigmented purpuric eruptions. *Dermatol Clin* 3:165, 1985.

80. Geary RC Jr, Marks VJ: Idiopathic pigmented purpuric eruption with palmar-plantar involvement. *Cutis* 40:109, 1987.

81. Hersh CS, Shwayder TA: Unilateral progressive pigmentary purpura (Schamberg's disease) in a 15-year-old boy. *J Am Acad Dermatol* 24:651, 1991.

82. Smoller BR, Kamel OW: Pigmented purpuric eruptions: immunopathologic studies supportive of a common immunophenotype. *J Cutan Pathol* 18:423, 1991.

83. Aiba S, Tagami H: Immunohistologic studies in Schamberg's disease. Evidence for cellular immune reaction in lesional skin. *Arch Dermatol* 124:1058, 1988.

84. Simon M Jr, Heese A, Gotz A: Immunopathological investigations in purpura pigmentosa chronica. *Acta Derm Venereol* 69:101, 1989.

85. Brozena SJ, Cohen LE, Saba HI, Fenske NA: A pigmentary purpuric eruption associated with an unusual platelet dysfunction. *Int J Dermatol* 28:537, 1989.

86. Barnhill RL, Braverman IM: Progression of pigmented purpura-like eruptions to mycosis fungoides: Report of three cases. *J Am Acad Dermatol* 19:25, 1988.

87. Horiuchi Y, Maruoka H: Petechial eruptions due to simvastatin in a patient with diabetes mellitus and liver cirrhosis. *J Dermatol* 24:549, 1997.

88. Michaelsson G, Pettersson L, Juhlin L: Purpura caused by food and drug additives. *Arch Dermatol* 109:49, 1974.

89. Van Joost T, van Ulsen J, Vuzevski VD, et al: Purpuric contact dermatitis to benzoyl peroxide. *J Am Acad Dermatol* 22:359, 1990.

90. Koch P, Baum HP, John S: Purpuric patch test reaction and venulitis due to methyl methacrylate in a dental prosthesis. *Contact Dermatitis* 34:213, 1996.

91. Calobrisi SD, Drolet BA, Esterly NB: Petechial eruption after the application of EMLA cream. *Pediatrics* 101:471, 1998.

92. De Waard-van der Spek FB, Oranje AP: Purpura caused by EMLA is of toxic origin. *Contact Dermatitis* 36:11, 1997.

93. Calnan CD, Peachey RDG: Allergic contact purpura. *Clinical Allergy* 1:287, 1971.

94. Renicu AM: Anticoagulant-induced necrosis of skin and subcutaneous tissues: report of two cases and review of the English literature. *South Med J* 69:775, 1976.

95. McGehee WG, Klotz TA, Epstein DJ, Rapaport SI: Coumarin necrosis associated with hereditary protein C deficiency. *Ann Intern Med* 101:59, 1984.

96. Horn JR, Danziger LH, Davis RJ: Warfarin-induced skin necrosis: report of four cases. *Am J Hosp Pharm* 38:1763, 1981.

97. Stone MS, Rosen T: Acral purpura: an unusual sign of coumarin necrosis. *J Am Acad Dermatol* 14:797, 1986.

98. Cole MS, Minifee PK, Wolma FJ: Coumarin necrosis—a review of the literature. *Surgery* 103:271, 1988.

99. Hermes B, Haas N, Henz BM: Immunopathological events of adverse cutaneous reactions to coumarin and heparin. *Acta Derm Venereol* 77:35, 1997.

100. Adcock DM, Hicks MJ: Dermatopathology of skin necrosis associated with purpura fulminans. *Semin Thromb Hemost* 16:283, 1990.

101. Auletta MJ, Headington JT: Purpura fulminans. A cutaneous manifestation of severe protein C deficiency. *Arch Dermatol* 124:1387, 1988.

102. Spicer TE, Rau JM: Purpura fulminans. *Am J Med* 61:566, 1976.

103. Hautekeete ML, Berneman ZN, Bieger R, et al: Purpura fulminans in pneumococcal sepsis. *Arch Intern Med* 146:497, 1986.

104. Darmstadt GL: Acute infectious purpura fulminans: pathogenesis and medical management. *Pediatr Dermatol* 15:169, 1998.

105. Carpenter CT, Kaiser AB: Purpura fulminans in pneumococcal sepsis: case report and review. *Scand J Infect Dis* 29:479, 1997.

106. Adcock DM, Brozna J, Marlar RA: Proposed classification and pathologic mechanisms of purpura fulminans and skin necrosis. *Semin Thromb Hemost* 16:333, 1990.

107. Waage A, Halstensen A, Espevik T: Association between tumour necrosis factor in serum and fatal outcome in patients with meningococcal disease. *Lancet* 1:355, 1987.

108. Gladson CL, Groncy P, Griffin JH: Coumarin necrosis, neonatal purpura fulminans, and protein C deficiency. *Arch Dermatol* 123:1701a, 1987.

109. Marlar RA, Neumann A: Neonatal purpura fulminans due to homozygous protein C or protein S deficiencies. *Semin Thromb Hemost* 16:299, 1990.

110. Kemahli S, Alhenc-Gelas M, Gandrille S, et al: Homozygous protein C deficiency with a double variant His 202 to Tyr and Ala 346 to Thr. *Blood Coagul Fibrinolysis* 9:351, 1998.

111. Griffin JH, Evatt B, Zimmerman TS, et al: Deficiency of protein C in congenital thrombotic disease. *J Clin Invest* 68:1370, 1981.

112. Branson HE, Katz J, Marble R, Griffin JH: Inherited protein C deficiency and coumarin-responsive chronic relapsing purpura fulminans in a newborn infant. *Lancet* 2:1165, 1983.

113. Sills RH, Marlar RA, Montgomery RR, et al: Severe homozygous protein C deficiency. *J Pediatr* 105:409, 1984.

114. Gruber A, Blasko G, Sas G: Functional deficiency of protein C and skin necrosis in multiple myeloma. *Thromb Res* 42:579, 1986.

115. Pegelow CH, Ledford M, Young JN, Zilleruelo G: Severe protein S deficiency in a newborn. *Pediatrics* 89:674, 1992.

116. Mahasandana C, Suvatte V, Chuansumrit A, et al: Homozygous protein S deficiency in an infant with purpura fulminans. *J Pediatr* 117:750, 1990.

117. Levin M, Eley BS, Louis J, et al: Postinfectious purpura fulminans caused by an autoantibody directed against protein S. *J Pediatr* 127:355, 1995.

118. Pipe SW, Schmaier AH, Nichols WC, et al: Neonatal purpura fulminans in association with factor V R506Q mutation. *J Pediatr* 128:706, 1996.

119. Rietschel RL, Lewis CW, Simmons RA, Phyliky RL: Skin lesions in paroxysmal nocturnal hemoglobinuria. *Arch Dermatol* 114:560, 1978.

120. Lockshin MD: Antiphospholipid antibody syndrome [clinical conference]. *JAMA* 268:1451, 1992.

121. Asherson RA, Khamashta MA, Ordi-Ros J, et al: The ''primary'' antiphospholipid syndrome: major clinical and serological features. *Medicine (Baltimore)* 68:366, 1989.

122. Viard JP, Amoura Z, Bach JF: Association of anti-beta 2 glycoprotein I antibodies with lupus-type circulating anticoagulant and thrombosis in systemic lupus erythematosus. *Am J Med* 93:181, 1992.

123. Grob JJ, Bonerandi JJ: Thrombotic skin disease as a marker of the anticardiolipin syndrome. Livedo vasculitis and distal gangrene associated with abnormal serum antiphospholipid activity. *J Am Acad Dermatol* 20:1063, 1989.

124. Sarkar M, Mulliken JB, Kozakewich HP, et al: Thrombocytopenic coagulopathy (Kasabach-Merritt phenomenon) is associated with Kaposiform hemangioendothelioma and not with common infantile hemangioma. *Plast Reconstr Surg* 100:1377, 1997.

125. Rinker MH, Sangueza OP, Davis LS: Reticulated purpura occurring with contrast medium after hysterosalpingography. *Br J Dermatol* 138:919, 1998.

126. Bruinsma W: *A Guide To Drug Eruptions,* p 40. Brussels, The Free University, 1990.

127. Gardner FH, Diamond LK: Autoerythrocyte sensitization: a form of purpura producing painful bruising following autosensitization to red blood cells in certain women. *Blood* 10:675, 1955.

128. Ratnoff OD, Agle DP: Psychogenic purpura: a re-evaluation of the syndrome of autoerythrocyte sensitization. *Medicine Baltimore* 47:475, 1968.

129. Gottlieb AJ: Autoerythrocyte and DNA sensitivity, in *Hematology,* edited by JW Williams, E Beutler, AJ Erslev, et al, pp 1441. McGraw-Hill, New York, 1990.

130. Strunecka A, Krpejsova L, Palecek J, et al: Transbilayer redistribution of phosphatidylserine in erythrocytes of a patient with autoerythrocyte sensitization syndrome (psychogenic purpura). *Folia Haematol Int Mag Klin Morphol Blutforsch* 117:829, 1990.

131. McDuffe FC, McGuire FL: Clinical and psychological patterns in autoerythrocyte sensitivity. *Ann Intern Med* 63:255, 1965.

132. Lotti T, Benci M, Sarti MG, et al: Psychogenic purpura with abnormally increased tPA dependent cutaneous fibrinolytic activity. *Int J Dermatol* 32:521, 1993.

133. Majeed HA, Quabazard Z, Hijazi Z, et al: The cutaneous manifestations in children with familial Mediterranean fever (recurrent hereditary polyserositis). A six-year study. *Q J Med* 75:607, 1990.

134. Meadow R: Schönlein-Henoch syndrome. *Arch Dis Child* 54:822, 1979.

135. Allen DM, Diamond LK, Howell DA: Anaphylactoid purpura in children (Schönlein-Henoch syndrome). *Am J Dis Child* 99:833, 1960.

136. Macke SE, Jordon RE: Leukocytoclastic vasculitis. A cutaneous expression of immune complex disease. *Arch Dermatol* 118:296, 1982.

137. Saulsbury FT: IgA rheumatoid factor in Henoch-Schönlein purpura. *J Pediatr* 108:71, 1986.

138. Blanco R, Martinez-Taboada VM, Rodriguez-Valverde V, et al: Henoch-Schönlein purpura in adulthood and childhood: two different expressions of the same syndrome. *Arthritis Rheum* 40:859, 1997.

139. Coppo R, Mazzucco G, Cagnoli L, et al: Long-term prognosis of Henoch-Schönlein nephritis in adults and children. Italian Group of Renal Immunopathology Collaborative Study on Henoch-Schönlein purpura. *Nephrol Dial Transplant* 12:2277, 1997.

140. Piette WW: What is Schönlein-Henoch purpura, and why should we care? *Arch Dermatol* 133:515, 1997.

141. Ozdogan H, Arisoy N, Kasapcapur O, et al: Vasculitis in familial Mediterranean fever. *J Rheumatol* 24:323, 1997.

142. Saatci U, Ozen S, Ozdemir S, et al: Familial Mediterranean fever in children: report of a large series and discussion of the risk and prognostic factors of amyloidosis. *Eur J Pediatr* 156:619, 1997.

143. Jin DK, Kohsaka T, Koo JW, et al: Complement 4 locus II gene deletion and DQA1*0301 gene: genetic risk factors for IgA nephropathy and Henoch-Schönlein nephritis. *Nephron* 73:390, 1996.

144. Amoroso A, Berrino M, Canale L, et al: Immunogenetics of Henoch-Schoenlein disease. *Eur J Immunogenet* 24:323, 1997.

145. Mintzer CO, Nussinovitch M, Danziger Y, et al: Scrotal involvement in Henoch-Schönlein purpura in children. *Scand J Urol Nephrol* 32:138, 1998.

146. Sharieff GQ, Francis K, Kuppermann N: Atypical presentation of Henoch-Schöenlein purpura in two children. *Am J Emerg Med* 15:375, 1997.

147. Lin SJ, Huang JL, Hsieh KH: Clinical and laboratory correlation of acute Henoch-Schönlein purpura in children. *Chung Hua Min Kuo Hsiao Erh Ko I Hsueh Hui Tsa Chih* 39:94, 1998.

148. Tancrede-Bohin E, Ochonisky S, Vignon-Pennamen MD, et al: Schönlein-Henoch purpura in adult patients. Predictive factors for IgA glomerulonephritis in a retrospective study of 57 cases. *Arch Dermatol* 133:438, 1997.

149. Kawana S, Shen GH, Kobayashi Y, Nishiyama S: Membrane attack complex of complement in Henoch-Schönlein purpura skin and nephritis. *Arch Dermatol Res* 282:183, 1990.

150. Miyagawa S, Shiiki H, Nakatani C, et al: Association of IgA immune complex vasculitis and rheumatoid arthritis. *J Am Acad Dermatol* 24:295, 1991.

151. Levinsky RJ, Barrett TM: IgA immune complexes in Henoch-Schönlein purpura. *Lancet* 11:1100, 1997.

152. Kawana S, Ohta M, Nishiyama S: Value of the assay for IgA-containing circulating immune complexes in Henoch-Schönlein purpura. *Dermatologica* 172:245, 1986.

153. Cederholm B, Linne T, Wieslander J, et al: Fibronectin-immunoglobulin complexes in the early course of IgA and Henoch-Schönlein nephritis. *Pediatr Nephrol* 5:200, 1991.

154. Mills JA, Michel BA, Bloch DA, et al: The American College of Rheumatology 1990. Criteria for the classification of Henoch-Schönlein purpura. *Arthritis Rheum* 33:1114, 1990.

155. Kaku Y, Nohara K, Honda S: Renal involvement in Henoch-Schönlein purpura: a multivariate analysis of prognostic factors. *Kidney Int* 53:1755, 1998.

156. Fujieda M, Oishi N, Naruse K, et al: Soluble thrombomodulin and antibodies to bovine glomerular endothelial cells in patients with Henoch-Schönlein purpura. *Arch Dis Child* 78:240, 1998.

157. Liu ZH, Cheng ZH, Yu YS, et al: Interleukin-1 receptor antagonist allele: is it a genetic link between Henoch-Schönlein nephritis and IgA nephropathy? *Kidney Int* 51:1938, 1997.

158. Saulsbury FT: Alterations in the O-linked glycosylation of IgA1 in children with Henoch-Schönlein purpura. *J Rheumatol* 24:2246, 1997.

159. Besbas N, Erbay A, Saatci U, et al: Thrombomodulin, tissue plasminogen activator and plasminogen activator inhibitor-1 in Henoch-Schönlein purpura. *Clin Exp Rheumatol* 16:95, 1998.

160. Wu TH, Wu SC, Huang TP, et al: Increased excretion of tumor necrosis factor alpha and interleukin 1 beta in urine from patients with IgA nephropathy and Schönlein-Henoch purpura. *Nephron* 74:79, 1996.

161. Besbas N, Saatci U, Ruacan S, et al: The role of cytokines in Henoch-Schönlein purpura. *Scand J Rheumatol* 26:456, 1997.

162. Argenbright LW, Barton RW: Interactions of leukocyte integrins with intercellular adhesion molecule 1 in the production of inflammatory vascular injury in vivo. The Shwartzman reaction revisited. *J Clin Invest* 89:259, 1992.

163. Piette WW, Stone MS: A cutaneous sign of IgA-associated small dermal vessel leukocytoclastic vasculitis in adults (Henoch-Schönlein purpura). *Arch Dermatol* 125:53, 1989.

164. Saraclar Y, Tinaztepe K, Adalioglu G, Tuncer A: Acute hemorrhagic edema of infancy (AHEI)—a variant of Henoch-Schönlein purpura or a distinct clinical entity? *J Allergy Clin Immunol* 86:473, 1990.

165. Dubin BA, Bronson DM, Eng AM: Acute hemorrhagic edema of childhood: an unusual variant of leukocytoclastic vasculitis. *J Am Acad Dermatol* 23:347, 1990.

166. Legrain V, Lejean S, Taieb A, et al: Infantile acute hemorrhagic edema of the skin: study of ten cases. *J Am Acad Dermatol* 24:17, 1991.

167. Gonggryp LA, Todd G: Acute hemorrhagic edema of childhood (AHE). *Pediatr Dermatol* 15:91, 1998.

168. Long D, Helm KF: Acute hemorrhagic edema of infancy: Finkelstein's disease. *Cutis* 61:283, 1998.

169. Fauci AS, Haynes B, Katz P: The spectrum of vasculitis: clinical, pathologic, immunologic and therapeutic considerations. *Ann Intern Med* 89:660, 1978.

170. Sams WM Jr, Thorne EG, Small P, et al: Leukocytoclastic vasculitis. *Arch Dermatol* 112:219, 1976.

171. Sams WM Jr: Necrotizing vasculitis. *J Am Acad Dermatol* 3:1, 1980.

172. Fauci AS: Vasculitis. *J Allergy Clin Immunol* 72:211, 1983.

173. McAllister SM, Bornstein AM, Callen JP: Painful acral purpura. *Arch Dermatol* 134:789, 1998.

174. Akimoto S, Ishikawa O, Tsukada Y, et al: Microscopic polyangiitis mimicking Henoch-Schönlein purpura followed by severe renal involvement: a diagnostic role for antineutrophil cytoplasmic autoantibody. *Br J Dermatol* 136:298, 1997.

175. Mehregan DR, Hall MJ, Gibson LE: Urticarial vasculitis: a histopathologic and clinical review of 72 cases. *J Am Acad Dermatol* 26:441, 1992.

176. Chen KR, Kawahara Y, Miyakawa S, Nishikawa T: Cutaneous vasculitis in Behcet's disease: a clinical and histopathologic study of 20 patients. *J Am Acad Dermatol* 36:689, 1997.

177. Martinez-Taboada VM, Blanco R, Garcia-Fuentes M, Rodriguez-Valverde V: Clinical features and outcome of 95 patients with hypersensitivity vasculitis. *Am J Med* 102:186, 1997.

178. Calabrese LH, Michel BA, Bloch DA, et al: The American College of Rheumatology 1990 criteria for the classification of hypersensitivity vasculitis. *Arthritis Rheum* 33:1108, 1990.

179. Sams WM Jr: Hypersensitivity angiitis. *J Invest Dermatol* 93:78S, 1989.

180. Daoud MS, el Azhary RA, Gibson LE, et al: Chronic hepatitis C, cryoglobulinemia, and cutaneous necrotizing vasculitis. Clinical, pathologic, and immunopathologic study of twelve patients. *J Am Acad Dermatol* 34:219, 1996.

181. Abe Y, Tanaka Y, Takenaka M, et al: Leucocytoclastic vasculitis associated with mixed cryoglobulinaemia and hepatitis C virus infection. *Br J Dermatol* 136:272, 1997.

182. Wooten MD, Jasin HE: Vasculitis and lymphoproliferative diseases. *Semin Arthritis Rheum* 26:564, 1996.

183. Reiner DM, Frishman WH, Luftschein S, Grossman M: Adverse cutaneous reactions from cardiovascular drug therapy. *NY State J Med* 92:137, 1992.

184. Pace JL, Gatt P: Fatal vasculitis associated with ofloxacin. *BMJ* 299:658, 1989.

185. Reis JJ, Kaplan PW: Postictal hemifacial purpura. *Seizure* 7:337, 1998.

186. Cupps TR, Fauci AS: Vasculitis and neoplasm. *Major Probl Intern Med* 21:116, 1981.

187. Longley S, Caldwell JR, Panush RS: Paraneoplastic vasculitis. Unique syndrome of cutaneous angiitis and arthritis associated with myeloproliferative disorders. *Am J Med* 80:1027, 1986.

188. Greer JM, Longley S, Edwards NL, et al: Vasculitis associated with malignancy. Experience with 13 patients and literature review. *Medicine (Baltimore)* 67:220, 1988.

189. Callen JP: Cutaneous leukocytoclastic vasculitis in a patient with an adenocarcinoma of the colon. *J Rheumatol* 14:386, 1987.

190. Prins M, Veraart JC, Vermeulen AH, et al: Leucocytoclastic vasculitis induced by prolonged exercise. *Br J Dermatol* 134:915, 1996.

191. Winfield JB: Cryoglobulinemia. *Hum Pathol* 14:350, 1983.

192. Agnello V, Romain PL: Mixed cryoglobulinemia secondary to hepatitis C virus infection. *Rheum Dis Clin North Am* 22:1, 1996.

193. Agnello V, Abel G: Localization of hepatitis C virus in cutaneous vasculitic lesions in patients with type II cryoglobulinemia. *Arthritis Rheum* 40:2007, 1997.

194. Brouet JC, Clauvel JP, Danon F, et al: Biologic and clinical significance of cryoglobulins. A report of 86 cases. *Am J Med* 57:775, 1974.

195. Gorevic PD, Kassab HJ, Levo Y, et al: Mixed cryoglobulinemia: clinical aspects and long-term follow-up of 40 patients. *Am J Med* 69:287, 1980.

196. Cohen SJ, Pittelkow MR, Su WP: Cutaneous manifestations of cryoglobulinemia: clinical and histopathologic study of seventy-two patients. *J Am Acad Dermatol* 25:21, 1991.

197. Ferri C, La Civita L, Longombardo G, et al: Mixed cryoglobulinaemia: a cross-road between autoimmune and lymphoproliferative disorders. *Lupus* 7:275, 1998.

198. Akriviadis EA, Xanthakis I, Navrozidou C, Papadopoulos A: Prevalence of cryoglobulinemia in chronic hepatitis C virus infection and response to treatment with interferon-alpha. *J Clin Gastroenterol* 25:612, 1997.

199. Papo T, Musset L, Bardin T, et al: Cryocrystalglobulinemia as a cause of systemic vasculopathy and widespread erosive arthropathy. *Arthritis Rheum* 39:335, 1996.

200. Finder KA, McCollough ML, Dixon SL, et al: Hypergammaglobulinemic purpura of Waldenstrom. *J Am Acad Dermatol* 23:669, 1990.

201. Ferreiro JE, Pasarin G, Quesada R, Gould E: Benign hypergammaglobulinemic purpura of Waldenstrom associated with Sjogren's syndrome. Case report and review of immunologic aspects. *Am J Med* 81:734, 1986.

202. Waldenström J: Clinical methods for determination of hyperproteinemia and their practical value for diagnosis. *Nord Med* 20:2288, 1943.

203. Strauss WG: Purpura hyperglobulinemia of Waldenström. Report of a case and review of the literature. *N Engl J Med* 260:857, 1959.

204. Kyle RA, Gleich GJ, Bayrid ED, Vaughan JH: Benign hypergammaglobulinemic purpura of Waldenström. *Medicine (Baltimore)* 50:113, 1971.

205. Oosterkamp HM, van der Pijl H, Derksen J, et al: Arthritis and hypergammaglobulinemic purpura in hypersensitivity pneumonitis. *Am J Med* 100:478, 1996.

206. Miyagawa S, Fukumoto T, Kanauchi M, et al: Hypergammaglobulinaemic purpura of Waldenstrom and Ro/SSA autoantibodies. *Br J Dermatol* 134:919, 1996.

207. Bair JS, Wu YC, Lu YC: Cryofibrinogenemia: report of a case. *J Formos Med Assoc* 90:99, 1991.

208. Stone GC, Wall BA, Oppliger IR, et al: A vasculopathy with deposition of lambda light chain crystals. *Ann Intern Med* 110:275, 1989.

209. Mullen B, Chalvardjian A: Crystalline tissue deposits on a case of multiple myeloma. *Arch Pathol Lab Med* 105:94, 1981.

210. Haitjema T, Westermann CJ, Overtoom TT, et al: Hereditary hemorrhagic telangiectasia (Osler-Weber-Rendu disease): new insights in pathogenesis, complications, and treatment. *Arch Intern Med* 156:714, 1996.

211. McAllister KA, Baldwin MA, Thukkani AK, et al: Six novel mutations in the endoglin gene in hereditary hemorrhagic telangiectasia type 1 suggest a dominant-negative effect of receptor function. *Hum Mol Genet* 4:1983, 1995.

212. Vincent P, Plauchu H, Hazan J, et al: A third locus for hereditary haemorrhagic telangiectasia maps to chromosome 12q. *Hum Mol Genet* 4:945, 1995.

213. Johnson DW, Berg JN, Baldwin MA, et al: Mutations in the activin receptor-like kinase 1 gene in hereditary haemorrhagic telangiectasia type 2. *Nat Genet* 13:189, 1996.

214. Peery WH: Clinical spectrum of hereditary hemorrhagic telangiectasia (Osler-Weber-Rendu disease). *Am J Med* 82:989, 1987.

215. Saba HI, Morelli GA, Logrono LA: Brief report: treatment of bleeding in hereditary hemorrhagic telangiectasia with aminocaproic acid. *N Engl J Med* 330:1789, 1994.

216. Phillips MD: Stopping bleeding in hereditary telangiectasia. *N Engl J Med* 330:1822, 1994.

217. Foutch PG, Sullivan JA, Gaines JA, Sanowski RA: Cutaneous vascular spiders in cirrhotic patients: correlation with hemorrhage from esophageal varices. *Am J Gastroenterol* 83:723, 1988.

218. Fauci AS, Macher AM, Longo DL, et al: NIH conference. Acquired immunodeficiency syndrome: epidemiologic, clinical, immunologic, and therapeutic considerations. *Ann Intern Med* 100:92, 1984.

219. Chang A, Zic JA, Boyd AS: Intravascular large cell lymphoma: a patient with asymptomatic purpuric patches and a chronic clinical course. *J Am Acad Dermatol* 39:318, 1998.

220. Desnick RJ, Bishop DF: Fabry disease: α-galactosidase deficiency and Schindler disease: α-N-acetylgalactosaminidase deficiency, in *The Metabolic Basis of Inherited Disease*, 6th ed, edited by CR Scriver, AL Beaudet, WS Sly, et al, pp 1751–1796. McGraw-Hill, New York, 1989.

221. Fine JD, Arndt KA: Torch syndrome, in *Clinical Dermatology*, 15th ed, edited by DJ Demis, p 1. Lippincott, Philadelphia, 1988.

222. Jones MA, Laing VB, Files B, Park HK: Granuloma annulare mimicking septic emboli in a child with myelodysplastic syndrome. *J Am Acad Dermatol* 38:106, 1998.

INHERITED DEFICIENCIES OF COAGULATION FACTORS II, V, VII, XI, AND XIII AND THE COMBINED DEFICIENCIES OF FACTORS V AND VIII AND OF THE VITAMIN K-DEPENDENT FACTORS

URI SELIGSOHN
GILBERT C. WHITE, II

Bleeding tendencies caused by inherited deficiencies of one or more coagulation factors are rare disorders distributed worldwide. Homozygotes or compound heterozygotes for the mutant genes responsible for these defects exhibit bleeding manifestations that are of variable severity and usually related to the extent of the decreased activity of the particular coagulation factor. Heterozygotes for the various deficiencies very rarely display a bleeding tendency. Numerous mutations have been identified in genes encoding coagulation factors II, V, VII, X, XI, and XIII. For some factors, such as factors II, VII, and X, mutations giving rise to dysfunctional proteins are common, while for other factors, such as factors V, XI, and XIII, true deficiencies are more common. Combined factor V and factor VIII deficiency, inherited as an autosomal recessive trait, can result from mutations in the gene encoding a transport protein of the endoplasmic reticulum–Golgi intermediate compartment. The very rare combined deficiency of the vitamin K–dependent coagulation factors can be caused by mutations in the gene that encodes for a carboxylase that γ-carboxylates glutamic acid residues in these proteins. Treatment of patients with the various coagulation factor deficiencies may be necessary during spontaneous bleeding episodes, during and after surgical procedures, and to prevent intracranial hemorrhage. In most deficiency states, plasma replacement has been used, but specific concentrates of all the vitamin K–dependent factors and of factors VII, XI, and XIII are also available.

Acronyms and abbreviations that appear in this chapter include: aPTT, activated partial thromboplastin time; BHK, baby hamster kidney; CRM−, cross-reacting material negative; CRM+, cross-reacting material positive; CRM^{red}, cross-reacting material reduced; DIC, disseminated intravascular coagulation; EGF, epidermal growth factor; ERGIC-53, endoplasmic reticulum–Golgi intermediate compartment 53; Gla, γ-carboxyglutamic acid; HK, high-molecular-weight kininogen; PK, prekallikrein; PT, prothrombin time; TAFI, thrombin-activatable fibrinolysis inhibitor; TAFIa, activated TAFI.

INTRODUCTION

Inherited deficiencies of coagulation factors other than factor VIII (hemophilia A) and factor IX (hemophilia B) are rare bleeding disorders that have been described in most populations. The severity of the bleeding manifestations in affected patients, who are usually homozygotes or compound heterozygotes for a mutant gene, is variable and usually relates to the extent of the deficiency. While some patients may only have mild bruising or display excessive bleeding only following trauma, others, such as patients with less than 1 percent of normal factor VII, XIII, or X activities, may exhibit intracranial hemorrhages and hemarthroses similar to those of patients with severe hemophilia A and B.

The study of these disorders has significantly advanced the understanding of the pathophysiology of blood coagulation mechanisms (see Chap. 112). Following the characterization of the genes encoding for the coagulation factors, a host of mutations causing the various deficiencies have been identified. The use of molecular genetic techniques has established the molecular basis for two disorders that have constituted enigmas for several decades. Thus, the inherited combined deficiency of factors V and VIII was shown in most instances to be caused by mutations in a gene encoding for a transport protein carrying factors V and VIII from the endoplasmic reticulum to the Golgi apparatus, and the combined deficiency of all vitamin K–dependent factors was shown to result from a mutated gene encoding for the carboxylase that introduces γ-carboxyl groups into these coagulation factors.

This chapter reviews the clinical, biochemical, and genetic aspects of the inherited deficiencies of coagulation factors that cause bleeding tendencies other than the hemophilias (see Chap. 123) and von Willebrand disease (see Chap. 135).

FACTOR II (PROTHROMBIN) DEFICIENCY

DEFINITION

Inherited hypoprothrombinemia and dysprothrombinemia are rare, genetically heterogeneous, autosomal recessive disorders characterized by mild to moderate bleeding. Both abnormalities of prothrombin impair the generation of thrombin, the central enzyme of the blood coagulation system.

MOLECULAR FEATURES AND BIOCHEMISTRY

Prothrombin is a protein of approximately 72,000 M_r that is structurally homologous with other members of the vitamin K–dependent proteins; factors VII, IX, and X; protein C; protein S; and bone γ-carboxyglutamic acid (Gla) protein. Prothrombin is synthesized in the liver as a pre-propeptide of 622 amino acids and is composed of the following domains: propeptide (residues −43 to −1), Gla (residues 1–40), kringle (residues 41–271), and catalytic (residues 272–579).[1–3] The propeptide domain is responsible for protein processing, targeting, and carboxylation, and is removed prior to secretion from the cell. The Gla domain constitutes the amino terminus of the mature prothrombin molecule and contains the 10 glutamic acid residues that are posttranslationally modified through the action of vitamin K–dependent carboxylase to Gla. As a result of this modification, prothrombin acquires the capacity to bind calcium and to bind to membranes containing acidic phospholipids. The kringle domain contains two extensively folded, disulfide-bonded kringle motifs, each consisting of approximately 79 amino acids,[4] that are present in diverse proteins and are thought to mediate protein-protein interactions. The second kringle mediates the interaction of prothrombin with activated factor V.[5] The catalytic domain contains the enzyme's active site, which is responsible for cleavage of fibrinogen. The residues characteristic for the serine protease family, His363, Asp419, and Ser525, constitute a charge relay system responsible for bond cleavage.

The prothrombin gene is located on chromosome 11 near the centromere.[6] The organization of the 26,930-bp gene consists of a 6544-bp upstream 5′ flanking sequence, a 20,241-bp coding region composed of 14 exons separated by 13 intervening sequences, and a 145-bp 3′ flanking sequence.[7] A comparison of the organization of the prothrombin gene shows homology with the organization of other vitamin K–dependent serine protease genes, with the highest degree of homology in the part encoding the Gla domain. An unusual feature of the prothrombin gene is the presence of 41 copies of Alu-repetitive sequences in the upstream and intervening sequences.[7,8] The function, if any, of these sequences is unknown.

Prothrombin plays a central role in coagulation, functioning in both tissue factor- and surface-activated pathways. Prothrombin is converted to its proteolytically active form, thrombin, by activated factor X in the presence of activated factor V and phospholipid surfaces provided by platelets and other cells (see Chap. 112). In addition to conversion of fibrinogen to fibrin (see Chap. 124) thrombin also (1) induces aggregation of platelets; (2) activates coagulation factor XIII, resulting in cross-linking of fibrin; (3) converts plasminogen to plasmin, thereby activating the fibrinolytic system; (4) activates thrombin-activatable fibrinolysis inhibitor; (5) activates coagulation factors V, VIII, and XI, promoting generation of additional thrombin; and (6) activates protein C in the presence of thrombomodulin (see Chap. 113). Thrombin also stimulates wound healing through its action as a growth factor and regulates vascular tone.

GENETICS

Abnormalities of prothrombin are inherited in an autosomal recessive manner. Among individuals with true prothrombin deficiency, heterozygotes exhibit prothrombin levels that are approximately 50 percent of normal, while homozygotes display levels that are typically less than 10 percent of normal. Prothrombin activity and antigen levels are reduced concordantly in these patients, and they are therefore designated as cross-reacting material negative (CRM−). Heterozygotes for dysprothrombinemias exhibit prothrombin activity levels that are around 50 percent of normal, with antigen levels that are normal or nearly normal. Prothrombin activity in homozygotes for dysprothrombinemia varies between 1 and 20 percent of normal, while antigen levels are either normal (CRM+) or partially reduced (CRM^red). Compound heterozygotes bearing one prothrombin deficiency allele and one dysprothrombin allele have been reported and typically have prothrombin activity levels between 1 and 20 perecnt, with antigen levels between 13 and 50 percent of normal.

The molecular defects responsible for inherited prothrombin deficiency have not been extensively studied. In contrast, dysprothrombinemias have been shown to result almost exclusively from missense mutations. These mutations can be further divided into (1) mutations in which the defect results in abnormally slow activation of prothrombin and (2) mutations in which prothrombin activation is normal but the thrombin formed is abnormal and has an altered ability to clot fibrinogen. Table 122-1 lists examples of each type of inherited dysprothrombinemia.[9–31] Mutations in which prothrombin activation is abnormal include prothrombin San Juan, where there is an inability to bind calcium; prothrombins Madrid and Barcelona, where cleavage by activated factor X is abnormal; and prothrombin Segovia, where there is a possible defect in prothrombin fragment 2.[11] Missense mutations that affect the function of thrombin encode for defects that interfere with the catalytic activity of thrombin or its interaction with fibrinogen. In prothrombins Molise, Tokushima, and Metz, point mutations are present in the catalytic domain, resulting in production of defective thrombin molecules. The activation of prothrombin by factor Xa is normal, but the thrombin that is generated is unable to cleave fibrinogen and exhibits abnormal catalytic activity toward small peptide substrates. In prothrombin Molise and Tokushima, Arg418 is replaced by tryptophan.[22,23] This amino acid is located next to the aspartic acid of the catalytic site, and the substitution appears to interfere with the catalytic activity of thrombin. In prothrombin Quick I, where Arg382 is replaced by cysteine,[27] and in prothrombin Quick II, where Gly558 is replaced by valine,[30] the catalytic activity of thrombin toward small peptide substrates is intact, yet there is defective interaction with fibrinogen.

A number of polymorphisms have been identified in the prothrombin gene. One of these, a G-to-A change at nucleotide 20210 in the 3′-untranslated region of the prothrombin gene, is associated with increased plasma levels of prothrombin and an increased tendency to venous thrombosis.[32–36] Its effect on the risk of arterial thrombosis is controversial.[37–39] The prothrombin 20210 G→A polymorphism appears to be common in Caucasian populations,[40,41] and evidence was provided for a founder effect.[42] The polymorphism is very rare in individuals of African and Asian descent.[40,41]

CLINICAL MANIFESTATIONS

Inherited hypoprothrombinemia and dysprothrombinemia are characterized by mild to moderate mucocutaneous and soft-tissue bleeding that usually correlates with the degree of

TABLE 122-1   INHERITED DYSPROTHROMBINEMIAS

Name of Mutation and Reference	Mutation	Activity/Antigen, U/dl	Defect
Dysprothrombinemias Characterized by Abnormal Activation			
Canberra[9]	E157K		Pro-region
Cardeza[10]	ND	50/100	Prothrombin 2 region
Segovia[11]	ND	10/100	Fragment 2 defect?
Madrid, Obihiro[12,13]	R271C	12/100	Factor Xa cleavage
Barcelona[14]	R273C		Factor Xa cleavage
Padua[15,16] (Dhahran)	R271H	50/100	Factor Xa cleavage
Clamart[17]	R321I	50/100	Factor Xa cleavage
Houston[18]	ND	5/51	Factor Xa cleavage
Gainesville[19]	ND	23/70	Factor Xa cleavage
Perija[20]	ND	2/70	Factor Xa cleavage
San Juan[21]	ND	20/93	Calcium-binding site
Dysprothrombinemias Characterized by Abnormal Thrombin			
Molise[22,23] (Tokushima)	R418W	11/45	Defective catalytic region
Metz[24]	ND	10/50	Defective catalytic region
Greenville[25]	R517Q	51/102	Defective catalytic region
Quick I*,[16,27] (Corpus Christi)	R382C	<2/34	Defective fibrinogen binding
Himi I*,[26]	M337T	10/88	Defective fibrinogen binding
Himi II*,[26]	R388H		Defective fibrinogen binding
Salakta[28,29] (Frankfurt)	E466A	16/100	Defective fibrinogen binding
Quick II*,[30]	G558V		Defective fibrinogen binding

*Prothrombins Quick I and II and prothrombins Himi I and II were identified in two compound heterozygotes, respectively.
ABBREVIATION: ND, not determined.
SOURCE: Modified Girolami et al.[31] Updated information can be found on the internet.[83]

functional prothrombin deficiency. With prothrombin levels of less than 1 percent of normal, bleeding may occur spontaneously or following trauma. Surgical bleeding may be significant. Menstrual bleeding in females, epistaxis, gingival bleeding, easy bruising, and subcutaneous hematomas may occur. Hemarthroses can occur but are less frequent than in the hemophilias. In patients with prothrombin activities of 2 to 5 percent of normal, bleeding may be quite variable. Some individuals may bleed following minimal trauma, while others may be asymptomatic. Patients with prothrombin activity of 5 to 50 percent usually bleed only following major trauma and surgery, or do not bleed at all.

DIFFERENTIAL DIAGNOSIS

The activated partial thromboplastin time (aPTT) and prothrombin time (PT) are variably prolonged in inherited hypoprothrombinemia and dysprothrombinemia, but thrombin time is normal. The diagnosis of a prothrombin abnormality is established by the demonstration of decreased functional levels of prothrombin. Both functional and antigenic levels of prothrombin should be determined in cases of possible prothrombin deficiency in order to establish the presence of a dysprothrombinemia. Although acquired prothrombin deficiency is infrequent (e.g., in patients with antiphospholipid antibodies who have a bleeding tendency), family studies are helpful in establishing the diagnosis of an inherited deficiency.

Prothrombin can be activated by several snake venoms, and the pattern of activation by these enzymes may provide clues to the nature of the prothrombin abnormality. Activation of prothrombin by Taipan viper venom and by *Pseudonaja textilis* venom is independent of factor V. Thus, a normal Taipan viper venom or *Pseudonaja textilis* venom time with an abnormal classical one-stage assay for prothrombin implies a defect in the region of prothrombin that binds factor V. *Echis carinatus* venom activates prothrombin in the absence of factor V, phospholipid, and calcium and can therefore be used together with other prothrombin activators to test the requirement for each of these components. Plasma prothrombin immunoelectrophoresis is also useful in the diagnosis of dysprothrombinemias. Prothrombins Canberra, Segovia, and Denver show reduced anodic migration, while prothrombins Barcelona, San Juan, and Habana show enhanced anodic migration.

Prolonged aPTT and PT with a normal thrombin time are also seen in inherited factor V and factor X deficiency, in acquired conditions such as vitamin K deficiency, with therapeutic or surreptitious use of warfarin, in liver disease, and with lupus anticoagulants. These various disorders are readily distinguished by taking the patient's history and by performing additional factor assays (see Chap. 115).

THERAPY

Replacement therapy in patients with inherited prothrombin deficiency and dysprothrombinemia is with prothrombin complex concentrates containing coagulation factors II, VII, IX, and X. These concentrates are heated or treated with solvent-detergent, processes that remove HIV, hepatitis B, hepatitis C, and other viruses but do not remove parvovirus, hepatitis A virus,[43–46] and other possible bloodborne agents, such as Creutzfeldt-Jakob disease and its new variant. Thus, these concentrates are not without risk. In addition to the zymogen forms of factors II, VII, IX, and X, prothrombin complex concentrates also contain small amounts of activated forms of some of these factors. As a result, their administration may cause venous thromboembolism, myocardial infarction, or stroke.[47] The risk of thrombosis appears to increase with the dose, and, thus, repeated administration of small doses is probably safer.

Fresh-frozen plasma is also effective but confers a very low, but measurable, risk of HIV and hepatitis B and C virus transmission. Solvent-detergent-treated fresh-frozen plasma has been developed and can provide increased safety from these infections. However, since it is prepared from large pools of plasma, it may increase the risk of transmitting agents that are not destroyed by solvent-detergent treatment.

In many cases, the decision is not what to use for treatment but whether treatment is needed. Bruises and mild superficial bleeding do not generally require replacement therapy. Since the biologic half-life of prothrombin is approximately 3 days, in many cases a single treatment is all that is needed.

FACTOR VII DEFICIENCY

DEFINITION AND HISTORY

Hereditary deficiency of factor VII, first described by Alexander et al in 1951,[48] is a rare autosomal recessive disorder that occurs throughout the world. Its prevalence is not precisely known, except for that of one mutation responsible for the disease that is frequently observed among Iranian and Moroccan Jews (see below). The disorder is symptomatic only in homozygotes or compound hererozygotes, and the symptoms vary greatly from mild to severe. A presumptive diagnosis can be easily established, since factor VII deficiency is the only coagulation disorder that produces a prolonged PT and a normal aPTT.

BIOCHEMISTRY AND MOLECULAR FEATURES

Human factor VII is a single-chain glycoprotein ($M_r \approx 50,000$) that is secreted from the liver parenchymal cells as a zymogen. The mature protein consists of 406 amino acids and is organized in three main domains: a Gla domain at the N terminus, a growth factor domain in the center, and a serine protease domain at the C terminus.[49] Vitamin K is required for the formation of the Gla residues that bind calcium ions and permit interactions with phospholipid membranes. The factor VII gene spans about 12.8 kb[50] and is located on chromosome 13q34,[51,52] 2.8 kb upstream from the factor X gene.[53] The gene contains one exon that encodes for a preprotein leader sequence and eight exons that encode for the mature protein. Promoter and silencer elements of the 5' flanking region have been characterized.[54,55] Factor VII zymogen circulates in blood at an extremely low concentration (≈ 500 ng/ml)[56] and has the shortest half-life of all coagulation factors (5 h).[57]

Factor VII is converted to activated factor VII (factor VIIa) by cleavage of an Arg152-Ile153 bond, resulting in a two-chain molecule held together by a disulfide bond. This cleavage can be caused by factor Xa,[58] factor IXa,[59] factor XIIa,[59,60] thrombin,[58] and factor VIIa in an autoactivation process.[61] Binding of factor VII to tissue factor strikingly enhances these reactions.[62–66]

Factor VIIa can be detected in plasma by a sensitive assay employing a recombinant soluble form of tissue factor.[67] The mean concentration of plasma factor VIIa is 3.6 ng/ml in normal individuals, which represents 0.76 percent of the total factor VII mass in plasma. The half-life of factor VIIa is relatively long (≈ 2.5 h)[68] compared to other activated coagulation factors. Factor IXa is probably responsible for the basal levels of plasma factor VIIa in normal individuals, since patients with severe hemophilia B, unlike patients with severe hemophilia A, have a very low concentration of circulating factor VIIa.[69,70] Moreover, hemophilia B patients acquire normal levels of factor VIIa within a few hours of infusion of purified factor IX.[71]

Current theories are that blood coagulation is initiated when blood is exposed to tissue factor present in the subendothelium, in the tissues, or on the surface of stimulated monocytes (see Chap. 112). The exposed tissue factor forms a complex with circulating factor VIIa, which can activate factors X and factor IX.[72] The rate of factor X activation by this pathway is, however, 50 times lower than the rate achieved by the combined effects of factor IXa, factor VIIIa, phospholipid, and calcium ions.[73] It thus seems that factor VIIa plays a role in maintaining a low-key coagulant activity in the normal state and in the initial generation of thrombin once tissue factor becomes exposed. The sources of factor Va, which is essential for thrombin formation, and factor IXa, which is essential for maintaining the basal levels of factor VIIa, are unclear.[74]

When factor VII is completely lacking, as in knock-out mice, fatal hemorrhage occurs perinatally.[75] It is interesting to note that mice lacking tissue factor die during the embryonal phase due to abnormalities in the vascular wall,[76] while transgenic mice, rescued by incorporation of about 1 percent human tissue factor activity, develop normally and exhibit normal hemostasis.[77]

GENETICS

Factor VII deficiency is inherited as an autosomal recessive trait. The disorder manifests only in homozygotes or compound heterozygotes, of whom some are also homozygotes for polymorphisms associated with reduced factor VII levels.[78,79]

The heterogeneity of factor VII deficiency was already apparent in 1971, when two of four patients studied were found to have dysfunctional factor VII demonstrable by the presence of antibody-neutralizing material.[80] Later studies confirmed these observations and classified subjects with factor VII deficiency into CRM−, CRM+ (having normal levels of factor VII antigen), and CRM^{red}.[81,82] The latter two categories predominated.[82] Further complexity emanated from observations of variable reactivities of plasma from individuals with factor VII deficiency to bovine, rabbit, and human tissue factor.[82] Following the characterization of the factor VII gene, the heterogeneity of factor VII deficiency was confirmed. Thirty-five mutations were reviewed in 1997,[64] and many additional mutations have been published via the internet.[83] Most of the mutations are single-base substitutions that are distributed throughout the gene. The majority of them are missense mutations, with a few splice-site and nonsense mutations. Short deletions have also been described.[64] Two interesting single-base substitutions were recently described in the promoter region of the gene that disrupt the hepatocyte nuclear factor 4 and SP1 binding sites, respectively.[84,85] Both probands bearing the respective mutations are homozygotes and exhibit a very severe bleeding tendency.

Most mutations causing factor VII deficiency have been observed in individual patients. However, one missense mutation Ala244Val, was detected in 23 unrelated subjects with factor VII deficiency studied in Israel.[79] Most subjects were of Iranian and Moroccan Jewish origin and were found to share an identical haplotype, consistent with a founder effect. In the general Iranian Jewish and Moroccan Jewish populations, the prevalences of the Ala244Val allele are 0.023 and 0.025, respectively.[79]

Although the Dubin-Johnson syndrome was found to be associated with factor VII deficiency in Iranian and Moroccan Jews,[86] this is probably simply a reflection of high consanguinity rates in these populations, since the gene of the canalicular multispecific organic anion transporter, which is impaired in Dubin-Johnson syndrome,[87] is on chromosome 10q24,[88] while the gene for factor VII is on chromosome 13q34.[51,52]

Three polymorphisms in the factor VII gene have been found to be associated with reduced plasma levels of factor VII. Since an increased level of factor VII was established as a risk factor for coronary heart disease in middle-aged men[89] and was particularly

found to be associated with fatal coronary events,[90] the three polymorphisms have become the subject of intensive research. The first polymorphism, an Arg353Gln substitution, results in impaired secretion of factor VII from cells[91] and gives rise to a 20 to 25 percent decrease in plasma factor VII level in heterozygotes and a 40 to 50 percent decrease in homozygotes.[92,93] The allele frequency of the Arg353Gln polymorphism varies significantly in different populations. For example, in Japanese subjects the observed frequency is only 3.5 percent,[94] while in Afro-Caribbeans it is 8 percent,[95] in northern Europeans it is 9 percent,[95] and in Italians it is 21 percent.[96] The highest allele frequencies are in Gujaratis (25 percent) and Dravidian Indians (29 percent).[97] While in all these studies an association between the 353Gln allele and reduced levels of factor VII and factor VIIa was evident,[98] conflicting data exist regarding the relationship between the finding of the Arg353Gln polymorphism and the risk of coronary heart disease.[96,99,100] Conceivably, the significant effects on factor VII level exerted by dietary intake of fats,[101] serum cholesterol and triglyceride levels,[102] body mass,[103] age,[103,104] and gender[104] confound the effect conferred by the polymorphism. The second polymorphism associated with a diminished factor VII level is a decanucleotide insertion upstream from the 5′ end of the gene at −323. The insertion was shown to confer a 33 percent decrease in the promoter activity.[55] The relative effects of this polymorphism and the Arg353Gln polymorphism on factor VII level are difficult to assess, since linkage disequilibrium exists between these markers.[93] A third polymorphism associated with factor VII level is a hypervariable region 4 polymorphism in intron 7.[105] The variable number of tandem repeats (five to eight copies of 37 bp) apparently influences the splicing efficiency. Although the effect of the variable repeats on factor VII level is less conspicuous than the decanucleotide insertion at the promoter region and the Arg353Gln polymorphism, a recent study showed that subjects bearing alleles with seven repeats, who had reduced factor VII levels, manifested a lower risk of myocardial infarction.[96]

CLINICAL FEATURES

Bleeding manifestations only occur in homozygotes and in compound heterozygotes for factor VII deficiency. Heterozygotes who have partial factor VII deficiency do not exhibit hemorrhagic manifestations, even following trauma.[57,106] Patients who have factor VII levels of less than 1 percent frequently present with a disease that is indistinguishable from severe hemophilia A or hemophilia B. Such patients are afflicted by hemarthrosis, leading to severe arthropathy,[57,107] and can present with life-threatening intracerebral hemorrhage.[57,108] Patients with slightly higher levels of factor VII have also been reported to manifest such severe bleeding episodes, but this seems to be exceptional, since most patients with factor VII levels of 5 percent or more have a much milder disease, characterized by epistaxis, gingival bleeding, menorrhagia, and easy bruising. Dental extractions, tonsillectomy, and surgical procedures involving the urogenital tracts are frequently accompanied by bleeding when no prior therapy is instituted.[57] In contrast, surgical procedures such as laparotomy, herniorrhaphy, appendectomy, and hysterectomy have been uneventful.[57] This apparent discrepancy can be explained by different extents of local fibrinolysis exhibited by the respective traumatized tissues. Factor VII levels rise during pregnancy in healthy females[109] but do not change in homozygous patients with the deficiency.[110] Nevertheless, postpartum hemorrhage has not been observed in patients with factor VII deficiency, except for a few instances.[57,111]

Inhibitors to factor VII have not been described in patients with inherited factor VII deficiency. A spontaneous, acquired inhibitor to factor VII causing cerebral hemorrhage was, however, reported in one patient; this patient responded to immunosuppression.[112]

Venous thromboembolism has been described in several patients.[113] This indicates that the deficiency of factor VII, like deficiencies of other coagulation factors, is not protective against venous thromboembolism.

LABORATORY FEATURES

A normal aPTT and a prolonged PT in a patient with a lifelong history of a mild or severe bleeding tendency is consistent with the diagnosis of factor VII deficiency (see Chap. 115). The prolonged PT is correctable by normal serum (containing factor VII) but not by absorbed plasma (devoid of factor VII). Making the diagnosis depends on a specific assay of factor VII activity using known factor VII–deficient plasma. Factor VII antigen can be measured by a radioimmunoassay.[56,82] Factor VIIa is measurable by a clotting assay using soluble tissue factor, which is insensitive to native factor VII,[67] or by an enzyme-linked immunoabsorbent assay using an antibody that exhibits 3000-fold greater reactivity with factor VIIa than with factor VII.[114] Heterozygous carriers have reduced mean levels of factor VII activity, but the range of activity overlaps with normal values. Factor VII activity can also be decreased when the subject under investigation has vitamin K deficiency, which occurs quite frequently. Detection of heterozygotes can be facilitated by concomitant measurements of factor VII activity and antigen levels following administration of vitamin K. Since most factor VII deficiency states have been shown to be CRM+ or CRM[red],[81,82] a finding of reduced factor VII activity and significantly higher factor VII antigen level is consistent with heterozygosity.[115] A more definitive approach is identification of the mutant gene in the involved family and tracking it among family members.

DIFFERENTIAL DIAGNOSIS

Before the diagnosis of inherited factor VII deficiency is made, the common causes for acquired factor VII deficiency must be excluded. These include liver disease, vitamin K deficiency, and use of warfarin and related anticoagulants. Very rare hereditary defects that need to be distinguished from factor VII deficiency are the combined deficiency of all vitamin K–dependent factors (see below), combined deficiency of factors VII and X,[116] and combined deficiency of factors VII and IX.[117]

THERAPY

For minor bleeding episodes, replacement therapy is unnecessary. Local hemostasis for skin lacerations and administration of an antifibrinolytic agent for menorrhagia, epistaxis, and gingival hemorrhage are usually sufficient to arrest bleeding. Replacement therapy is essential in patients who present with severe hemorrhage, such as hemarthrosis or intracerebral bleeding. When surgery is required, the following should be considered:

1. The tissue involved during surgery. Dental extractions, tonsillectomy, nose surgery, and urological interventions are likely to be associated with bleeding because of local fibrinolysis.
2. The history of bleeding. Patients who have experienced hemarthroses, intracerebral hemorrhage, or other severe bleeding episodes have a much higher risk of bleeding than do those who have not had such symptoms.
3. The basic level of factor VII. Patients with very low activities (<3 percent of normal) are more likely to bleed.
4. A trough factor VII level of 20 to 25 percent of normal is probably sufficient, even when extensive trauma is inflicted.[57,106,118]

5. Volume overload is to be expected if plasma is used as the replacement material.
6. The half-life of factor VII is short ($\approx$5 h).[57]
7. The safety of the blood component to be used.

When plasma is used for major surgery, a loading dose of 15 ml/kg should be administered, followed by 4 ml/kg every 6 h for 7 to 10 days. Diuretics or even plasmapheresis might be necessary because of volume overload.[118] Prothrombin complex concentrates containing activated clotting factors[68] can be used, but they confer a risk of thrombosis.[119] Specific factor VII concentrates have been successfully used in series of patients.[120–122] Another option is the use of recombinant factor VIIa, which was successfully used during seven surgical procedures in two patients with severe factor VII deficiency.[123]

FACTOR X DEFICIENCY

DEFINITION

Factor X deficiency, which is usually characterized by moderate to severe bleeding, is an autosomal recessive disorder first reported by Telfer and colleagues and by Hougie and coworkers.[124,125]

BIOCHEMISTRY AND MOLECULAR FEATURES

The gene encoding factor X is located on chromosome 13q34-qter, adjacent to the gene encoding for factor VII.[126,127] The gene spans approximately 25 kb and is composed of eight exons.[128] The factor X gene shows significant homology with the genes of other vitamin K–dependent serine proteases, suggesting that all of these multidomain genes have evolved from a common ancestral gene.[129]

The protein encoded by the factor X gene is 488 amino acids in length. At the N terminus is a 23–amino acid signal peptide, which targets factor X as a secretory protein and is removed by a signal peptidase. The Gla domain forms the N terminus of the mature protein and contains 11 Gla residues,[130] which are responsible for calcium and phospholipid binding. Adjacent to the Gla domain is a short stack of predominantly hydrophobic amino acids, followed by the epidermal growth factor (EGF) domain, which contains two EGF motifs that are believed to mediate protein-protein interactions. The heavily glycosylated 52–amino acid activation peptide of factor X separates the EGF domain and the C-terminus catalytic domain.

Factor X undergoes proteolytic processing in the endoplasmic reticulum so that circulating factor X is a two-chain, disulfide-linked protein consisting of a 17-kDa light chain composed of the Gla and EGF domains, and a 40-kDa heavy chain composed of the activation and the catalytic domains.[131] Factor X can be activated by a complex of phospholipid, factor IXa, and factor VIIIa through the intrinsic pathway of coagulation or by membrane-bound factor VIIa–tissue factor through the extrinsic pathway of coagulation.[132] Factor X can also be activated by a component of Russell's viper venom,[133] by trypsin, and, in an autocatalytic reaction, by factor Xa. In each case, the activation of factor X is accomplished by proteolytic cleavage and subsequent removal of the activation peptide. Activated factor X, in turn, activates prothrombin to thrombin in a reaction that requires a phospholipid surface, divalent cations, and thrombin-activated factor V.

GENETICS

Factor X deficiency is inherited in an autosomal recessive manner, with males and females equally affected. Heterozygotes have factor X levels that are approximately 50 percent of normal and are generally asymptomatic. The genetic defects that cause a deficiency of factor

TABLE 122-2   INHERITED FACTOR X DEFICIENCY*

NAME OF MUTATION AND REFERENCE	MUTATION	ACTIVITY/ANTIGEN, U/dl	DEFECT
Deletion Mutations			
134	Del exon VII/VIII	<1/<1	Deletion of catalytic domain
135	Del exon VII/VIII	<1/<1	Deletion of catalytic domain
San Antonio[136]	DelC814		Termination frameshift
Missense Mutations			
Santo Domingo[137,138]	G-20R	<1/<5	Abnormal signal peptide removal
St. Louis II[139]	E7G	1/100	Reduced phospholipid binding
Vorarlberg[140]	E14K	5/20	Reduced phospholipid binding
Ketchikan[141,142]	E14G	5/20	Reduced phospholipid binding
	E102K		
Frankfurt I[143]	E25K	56/66	Reduced conversion to Xa
Malmö[144]	E26D	35/100	Reduced phospholipid binding
Wenatchee II[145]	N57T	10/30	
Öckerö[146]	G114R	25/?	
Wenatchee I[145]	R139C	10/30	Abnormal cleavage of factor X by IXa
Stockton[147]	D282N	43/101	Reduced catalytic activity of factor X
Prower pedigree[148]	R287W	6/?	
Stuart pedigree	V298M	<1/<1	Defective secretion
Roma[149]	T318M	3/80	Abnormal intrinsic activation of factor X
San Antonio[136]	R326C	14/36	Defect in anion-binding exosite
Marseille[142]	S334P	21/100	Reduced activation of factor X
Friuli[150]	P343S	9/100	Abnormal substrate binding
Vienna[151,152]	E201G	<1/<5	
	H383Q	6/?	
	W421R	6/?	

*Updated information can be found on the internet.[83]

X may be quantitative or qualitative and are classified as CRM+, CRM^red, and CRM− according to the functional and immunological analysis of the abnormal factor X molecule.

As shown in Table 122-2, the molecular defects associated with factor X deficiency consist of large deletions, small frameshift deletions, nonsense mutations, and missense mutations.[134–152] The deletion mutations result in the absence of protein synthesis or in the synthesis of unstable or dysfunctional proteins. CRM+ variants may affect factor X function in several ways. Activation through the intrinsic pathway may be preferentially affected, as with factor X Roma[149] and factor X San Antonio,[136] and activation by both pathways may be affected, as with factor X Friuli[150] and some of the mutations in the Gla residues, such as factor X St. Louis II.[139] Activation by Russell's viper venom may be relatively preserved. For example, with factor X Friuli, there is 25 percent activation with Russell's viper venom but only 3 percent activation through the intrinsic and extrinsic pathways. Similarly, with factor X Roma, there is full activation with Russell's viper venom but impaired activation through the intrinsic and, to a lesser extent, extrinsic pathways. Missense mutations may also affect synthesis or secretion, thus producing CRM− phenotypes, as with factor X Santo Domingo[138] and the Stuart mutation.

CLINICAL MANIFESTATIONS

The clinical manifestations of factor X deficiency are related to the functional levels of factor X. Individuals with severe factor X deficiency having functional factor X levels less than 1 percent of normal bleed spontaneously and following trauma. Bleeding is primarily into joints and soft tissues and from mucous membranes.[153] More unusual bleeding may also occur, including central nervous system hemorrhage; intramural intestinal bleeding, which can produce symptoms like those of an acute abdomen; urinary tract bleeding; and soft-tissue bleeding with the development of hemorrhagic pseudocysts or

pseudotumors. Menorrhagia may be especially problematic in women with factor X deficiency. Umbilical cord bleeding after delivery is also common. In individuals with moderate or mild deficiencies of factor X and in heterozygotes, bleeding is less common, usually occurring only after trauma or during or after surgery. Such patients may experience easy bruising as the only clinical manifestation.

DIFFERENTIAL DIAGNOSIS

The diagnosis of factor X deficiency is suggested by the demonstration of prolonged PT and aPTT assays. The Russell's viper venom time, which is based on the activation of factor X by the venom, is also prolonged. The thrombin time is normal. The diagnosis of factor X deficiency depends on the demonstration of an isolated deficiency of factor X by a specific factor X assay.

Prolonged PT and aPTT assays in conjunction with a normal thrombin time can also be observed in patients with prothrombin deficiency, factor V deficiency, multiple factor deficiencies, vitamin K deficiency, liver disease, and lupus anticoagulants. Factor X deficiency is distinguished from these disorders by measurements of the levels of factor X and other specific factors, including factors II, V, VII, and IX (see Chap. 115).

Inherited factor X deficiency must also be differentiated from various acquired causes of isolated factor X deficiency, such as systemic amyloidosis.[154–157] Factor X deficiency that sometimes occurs in this disorder can be due to (1) selective binding of factor X to the amyloid fibrils that can be erroneously attributed to the presence of an inhibitor when exogenously infused factor X is rapidly removed from the circulation,[155,156] or (2) presence of abnormal factor X molecules with reduced activity versus antigen level.[157] Amyloidosis associated with factor X deficiency due to both causes is generally of the primary type. Acquired isolated factor X deficiency has also been reported in association with respiratory infections, spindle cell thymoma, fungicide exposure, renal and adrenal adenocarcinoma, acute myelogenous leukemia, and use of methylbromide. Acquired inhibitors of factor X have also been reported.[158]

THERAPY

The treatment of inherited factor X deficiency is usually with heated and solvent-detergent-treated prothrombin complex concentrates that contain factor X in addition to factors II, VII, and IX. The use of these concentrates carries a low risk of transmission of bloodborne viruses. There is, however, a risk of thrombosis, including venous thromboembolism, disseminated intravascular coagulation, and myocardial infarction,[47,159] which is thought to be dose dependent. As a result, administration of doses over 2000 units is not recommended. If a larger dose is needed, it is recommended that divided doses be used.

For soft-tissue, mucous membrane, and joint hemorrhages, the aim of treatment should be to maintain a factor X level of at least 30 percent of normal. For more serious hemorrhages, a factor X level of 50 to 100 percent should be the goal. The biologic half-life of factor X is 24 to 40 h.[160,161] Based on this, if continued treatment is needed, prothrombin complex concentrates should be administrated every 24 h until hemostasis is achieved. Fresh-frozen plasma that contains factor X at a concentration of 1 unit/ml can also be used to treat patients with factor X deficiency. The issue of volume overload with plasma and the relative merits of using solvent-detergent-treated plasma are discussed above (see "Therapy" under "Factor II and Factor VII Deficiency").

COMBINED DEFICIENCY OF THE VITAMIN K-DEPENDENT FACTORS

In 1966 McMillan and Roberts reported the first case of severe hereditary deficiency of coagulation factors II, VII, IX, and X.[162] The combined deficiency of these vitamin K–dependent factors is a very rare autosomal recessive disorder that can be manifested by a mild or severe bleeding tendency. Protein C and protein S levels have also been reduced in cases where these proteins were assayed.[163,164] Evidence for impaired γ-carboxylation of the affected factors was described in 1979,[165] and a missense mutation in the γ-glutamylcarboxylase gene was identified in one case as the cause of the combined deficiency in 1998.[166]

Administration of large doses of vitamin K has resulted in improved hemostasis and partial correction of the factors' levels in several cases.[162,164] In patients who do not respond to vitamin K administration, fresh-frozen plasma should be used for replacement therapy.[167]

FACTOR V DEFICIENCY

DEFINITION

Hereditary factor V deficiency, initially described as parahemophilia,[168] is a rare autosomal recessive disorder that is manifested in homozygotes as a moderate bleeding tendency. The prevalence of the disorder is unknown, and no specific ethnic or population clusters have been reported.

BIOCHEMISTRY AND MOLECULAR FEATURES

Human plasma factor V is a high-molecular-weight ($M_r \approx 330,000$) single-chain glycoprotein that consists of 2196 amino acids.[169,170] Analysis of the approximately 7-kb factor V cDNA showed that the protein is organized according to the following domain structure: A_1-A_2-B-A_3-C_1-C_2.[171] The A and C domains have approximately 40 percent

homology with analogous domains in factor VIII. The large B domain shows no homology with the corresponding B domain of factor VIII. The gene contains 25 exons[171] and was mapped to chromosome 1q21-25.[172] Factor V is converted to its activated form following several proteolytic cleavages by thrombin[173] or factor Xa.[174] These cleavages remove the B domain and yield factor Va, consisting of a heavy chain (A_1-A_2 domains) associated by Ca^{2+} with a light chain (A_3-C_1-C_2 domains).[169,170] The light chain contains the binding sites for membrane phospholipids, prothrombin, and activated protein C; both light and heavy chains are probably necessary for binding factor Xa.[170]

The assembly of factor Va and factor Xa on the phospholipid membrane of platelets in the presence of Ca^{2+} forms the prothrombinase complex, which catalyzes the conversion of prothrombin to thrombin.[169] The exclusion of factor Va from the prothrombinase complex reduces the rate of thrombin generation by four orders of magnitude.[169] Factor V is synthesized by the liver[175] and by megakaryocytes.[176] Its plasma concentration is appproximately 7 μg/ml,[177] and its half-life is 12 to 15 h.[178] About 20 percent of factor V in whole blood is localized in the α granules of platelets,[179] where it is complexed with an extremely large protein multimerin.[180] Platelet factor V is partially fragmented,[179] but full activity is preserved. Its release from platelets upon their activation exerts an important hemostatic effect, since patients with an inherited defect of α-granule proteins, including platelet factor V, have a severe bleeding tendency.[181,182]

Factor Va is inactivated by activated protein C through limited proteolysis in the presence of protein S, Ca^{2+}, and either platelet or endothelial cell membrane phospholipids.[183] Partial protection from this cleavage is provided by factor Xa when factor Xa is bound to factor Va.[184] Partial resistance to inactivation by activated protein C occurs when the cleavage sites of factor Va (Arg306 and Arg506) are mutated (see Chap. 127).

GENETICS

Factor V deficiency is inherited as an autosomal recessive trait. Heterozygotes whose plasma factor V activity ranges between 26 and 60 percent of normal are usually asymptomatic.[185]

Assays of factor V antigen have shown that most homozygotes have a true deficiency. Only 2 of 21 patients examined in one study[169] and 4 of 14 patients examined in another study[186] were shown to possess dysfunctional factor V.

Candidate mutations responsible for factor V deficiency were reported only in a few unrelated subjects. In one report, two siblings were found to bear an Ala221Val missense mutation that seemed to code for a factor V molecule with reduced functional activity.[187] In another study, a patient with partial factor V deficiency was found to bear a nt 5509 G→A change in exon 16 that predicted an Ala1779Thr substitution and perhaps a splicing abnormality.[188] The third mutation identified was a 4-bp deletion in exon 13 that introduced a frameshift and a stop codon, which should lead to synthesis of a truncated form of factor V that lacks part of the B domain and domains A_3, C_1, and C_2.[189] It is remarkable that the homozygous proband, whose factor V antigen and activity were approximately 1 percent of normal, had only a mild bleeding tendency.

Subjects who are compound heterozygotes for factor V Arg506Gln (factor V Leiden) and for a factor V null allele have normal hemostasis (despite reduced factor V clotting activity), but since they are phenotypically homozygous for activated protein C resistance, they may present with thrombosis.[188,190–193]

Among several polymorphisms detected in the factor V gene, the His1299Arg in exon 13 is of particular interest, since it is associated with a reduced plasma factor V level.[194] Moreover, in two heterozygotes for factor V R506Q (factor V Leiden) who presented with thrombosis, reduced factor V activity due to the His1299Arg polymorphism conferred a pseudohomozygous phenotype for activated protein C resistance.[194]

Factor V Quebec was initially described as an autosomal dominant disorder with severe bleeding manifestations.[195] Affected patients had platelet factor V activity of 2 to 4 percent of normal, slightly reduced platelet factor V antigen, moderately decreased plasma factor V activity, and mild thrombocytopenia. The inactive platelet factor V in these patients is caused by abnormal proteolysis of several platelet α-granule proteins,[181,182,196] including fibrinogen, von Willebrand factor, thrombospondin, and factor V complexed with multimerin.[180] Thus, factor V Quebec, described in two unrelated families,[195,196] is a deficiency of platelet factor V activity secondary to a generalized platelet defect.

CLINICAL MANIFESTATIONS

Gene-targeting experiments in mice have shown that total deficiency of factor V is incompatible with life.[197] Mice die either during embryogenesis from vascular abnormalities or reach term but die within hours from massive hemorrhage. Homozygous patients whose factor V level ranges from less than 1 to 10 percent of normal exhibit a lifelong bleeding tendency. Manifestations include, in decreasing order of frequency, ecchymoses, epistaxis, gingival bleeding, hemorrhage following minor lacerations, and menorrhagia.[178] Bleeding from other sites is less common, but instances of hemarthroses unrelated to trauma, and intracerebral hemorrhage have been reported.[178,198] Trauma, dental extractions, and surgery confer a high risk of excessive bleeding.

Venous and arterial thromboses have been described in patients with factor V levels ranging between 2 and 14 percent of normal.[199–201] These observations indicate that factor V deficiency, like deficiencies of other coagulation factors, does not provide protection against thrombosis.[202] Factor V deficiency deprives activated protein C of one of its essential substrates, thereby down-regulating the inhibitory function of the protein C system. As already discussed, this is highlighted in patients with thrombosis who are compound heterozygotes for a factor V deficiency allele and an allele bearing the factor V Leiden mutation.[188,190–193]

DIFFERENTIAL DIAGNOSIS

Hereditary factor V deficiency must be distinguished from hereditary combined factor V and factor VIII deficiency, from acquired factor V deficiency associated with severe liver dysfunction or disseminated intravascular coagulation (DIC), and from a deficiency related to an acquired inhibitor to factor V. In both factor V and combined factor V and VIII deficiencies, the PT and aPTT assays are prolonged, inheritance is autosomal recessive, and bleeding manifestations are similar. An assay of factor VIII is therefore essential for distinction between these entities (see Chap. 115). The clinical manifestations of severe liver disease or DIC are sufficient for easy distinction between acquired and inherited factor V deficiency.

Acquired inhibitors to factor V are of three major classes: spontaneous, after transfusion in factor V–deficient patients, and after exposure to preparations of bovine thrombin. Belonging to the first class are spontaneously occurring inhibitors of unknown etiology that have been rarely reported in patients following surgery or in patients treated by aminoglycoside antibiotics or other drugs.[203,204] Inhibitors in this class that were characterized were either IgGs or IgMs.[204] Patients who develop such inhibitors are either asymptomatic or present with a severe bleeding tendency that, in at least two instances, was fatal.[205,206] In most cases these inhibitors disappear spontaneously.[203] Inhibitors in the second class have been reported in two patients with hereditary factor V deficiency, who developed the inhibitors following transfusions of plasma.[207,208] In one of the patients, the inhibitor disappeared, while in the other patient a low titer of the inhibitor persisted.[208] The third class of inhibitors consists of antibodies that develop in patients exposed to topical bovine thrombin.[209] The afflicted patients may react not only to the bovine thrombin but also to bovine factor V that is present in the commercial preparations of bovine thrombin.[210] The anti–bovine factor V antibodies cross-react with endogenous factor V and can cause an extremely low level of factor V.[210,211] Bleeding manifestations are variable in such patients. In a review of 17 patients, 5 were asymptomatic, and 12 had bleeding manifestations ranging from minimal to life-threatening.[212] A prolonged thrombin time with bovine thrombin that shortens when using human thrombin is consistent with the diagnosis of anti–bovine thrombin antibodies, and prolonged PT and aPPT suggest the presence of factor V inhibitors.

A recent study of 12 patients who developed autoantibodies of the first class or bovine thrombin–induced antibodies of the third class demonstrated that, in those patients who had significant bleeding manifestations, the antibodies reacted with a common epitope at the N-terminal region of the C_2 domain of factor V.[213] This domain was previously shown to be required for binding factor Va to phosphatidylserine, which is essential for the generation of prothombinase activity.[214]

THERAPY

Patients with epistaxis and gingival bleeding may respond to tranexamic acid (1g q.i.d), and local hemostatic measures may suffice for minor lacerations. If these measures fail, if severe spontaneous bleeding occurs, or if surgery is performed, fresh-frozen plasma replacement should be given. The following should be considered when planning plasma replacement therapy: (1) the half-life of factor V is approximately 12 to 14 h; (2) a factor V level of 25 percent is usually adequate even for major surgery[215,216]; and (3) surgical procedures at sites such as the urogenital tract, oral cavity, and nose, with high local fibrinolytic activity, are likely to result in excessive bleeding, and late bleeding may occur. Infusion of a loading dose of 20 ml/kg of fresh-frozen plasma followed by 5 to 10 ml/kg every 12 h for 7 to 10 days is usually adequate to ensure hemostasis during and after surgery.

Patients with inhibitors to factor V from any class may present a serious therapeutic challenge. Successful management of bleeding has been achieved in this situation in one patient by platelet transfusions, apparently due to greater hemostatic effects of platelet factor V,[217] perhaps as a result of decreased access of the inhibitor to the factor V. Immunosuppressive therapy with or without plasma exchange was successful in elimination of the inhibitor in two patients,[218,219] but it failed in another patient, who died of hemorrhage.[206]

COMBINED DEFICIENCY OF FACTORS V AND VIII

DEFINITION

Combined deficiency of factors V and VIII, first described in 1954,[220] is a rare, moderate bleeding disorder that is transmitted as an autosomal recessive trait.[221] Affected homozygotes have plasma levels of factors V and VIII in the range of 5 to 30 percent of normal.[222] The disorder results in most cases from a deficiency of an intracellular protein found in the endoplasmic reticulum–Golgi intermediate compartment (ERGIC-53) that is required for the transport of factors V and VIII through the cellular secretory pathway.[223] The disorder has been detected in many populations, but a relatively high frequency was observed among Tunisian and Middle Eastern Jews residing in Israel[221] and among Iranians.[224]

BIOCHEMISTRY AND MOLECULAR FEATURES

Factor V and factor VIII are essential coagulation factors that circulate in plasma as precursors. Upon limited proteolysis by thrombin or by factor Xa, and in concert with negatively charged phospholipid surfaces, factor V and factor VIII exhibit profound cofactor activities for the activation of factor X by factor IXa and for the activation of prothrombin by factor Xa, respectively. Inactivation of factors Va and VIIIa is accomplished by activated protein C in the presence of protein S and phospholipids through several proteolytic cleavages at distinct sites. Factors V and VIII have similar domain organizations with partial homology (see ''Factor V Deficiency'' and Chap. 112), and both are synthesized by liver parenchymal cells.[225,226] Distinct genes that encode for factor V and factor VIII are located on chromosomes 1 and X, respectively.[227,228] Mutations in the factor VIII gene result in hemophilia A, afflicting about 1 : 5000 males, and mutations in the factor V gene cause hereditary factor V deficiency, which is a rare autosomal recessive disorder.

The pathogenesis of combined deficiency of factors V and VIII has puzzled investigators for more than 40 years. The original hypothesis was that the disorder represents impaired synthesis of a precursor protein for both factors V and VIII.[220] However, transfusion studies excluded this possibility.[229,230] Accelerated degradation of factors V and VIII by activated protein C due to a deficiency of protein C inhibitor was proposed as an alternative mechanism for the disease[231] but was incompatible with observations of a normal rate of factor VIII disappearance in patients with the combined deficiency following transfusion of cryoprecipitate and desmopressin infusion.[222] Moreover, measurements of protein C inhibitor levels in plasma of affected patients disclosed normal values, thereby excluding a deficiency state.[232,233] Functional impairments of factors V and VIII, presumably due to posttranslational processing, was also entertained. However, plasma factor V and factor VIII clotting activities in affected patients corresponded very well with antigen levels,[234,235] and both factors were activated by thrombin as anticipated.[236] Homozygosity mapping in nine unrelated Jewish families demonstrated that the gene for the deficiency of factors V and VIII was localized on the long arm of chromosome 18.[237,238] Genetic linkage studies and recombination analysis localized the gene to an approximately 2.5 cm region,[237] and ultimately the involved protein was identified as ERGIC-53,[223] a 53-kDa transmembrane protein located in the intermediate compartment between the endoplasmic reticulum and Golgi.[239,240] Analysis of ERGIC-53 mRNA in three affected patients disclosed two mutations predicting truncation of the protein, and indeed the protein was totally absent from EBV-transformed lymphocytes from the patients.[223] ERGIC-53 may be involved in transport of glycoproteins from the endoplasmic reticulum to Golgi.[241] Since no other protein abnormalities (including ceruloplasmin, which is partially homologous to factors V and VIII) have been identified in patients with combined factor V and factor VIII deficiency,[222] it appears that the function of ERGIC-53 is confined to the transport of factors V and VIII. It seems likely that ERGIC-53, previously shown to exhibit affinity to mannose residues,[242] interacts with the extensively glycosylated B domains of factors V and VIII by a lectin-like function.[243]

Since all patients with the combined deficiency have residual plasma levels of factors V and VIII ranging between 5 and 30 percent of normal, alternative mechanisms of intracellular transport of factors V and VIII probably exist. Moreover, other genetic defects are also likely to cause the combined deficiency, since no genetic linkage to the ERGIC-53 locus could be found in at least two of the afflicted families.[244]

GENETICS

The defect is inherited as an autosomal recessive trait, and thus, as expected, consanguinity in affected families is common.[221,222,244] Coincidental association between hemophilia A and factor V deficiency is estimated to be extremely rare[245] and has indeed been reported in only five families.[246–250]

In five unrelated families of Tunisian Jewish origin, a GT→GC change was detected at a donor splice site of the ERGIC-53 gene leading to loss of splicing and predicting a truncated protein.[223] In five additional families of Middle Eastern Jewish origin (Iraq, Iran, and Egypt), a G insertion was identified in a stretch of four guanines from bases 86 to 89, predicting a frameshift and also leading to a truncated ERGIC-53. Allele-specific oligonucleotide hybridization analyses clearly distinguished between homozygotes and heterozygotes for each mutation.[223] Distinct founder haplotypes were found for patients of Tunisian Jewish and Middle Eastern Jewish origin.[237] Recently, 16 additional mutations were detected in 54 families studied.[244,251]

CLINICAL MANIFESTATIONS

Homozygous patients exhibit spontaneous as well as posttraumatic bleeding manifestations. Commonly observed are menorrhagia, epistaxis, easy bruising, and gingival hemorrhage.[222,224] Hemarthrosis unrelated to trauma was described in about 20 percent of the cases.[222,224] Less common are hematuria and gastrointestinal hemorrhage. Spontaneous intracranial hemorrhage was reported only in 1 patient.[224] Dental extractions and surgical procedures are almost always accompanied by excessive bleeding when no replacement of the missing factors is provided. It is interesting that bleeding was noted only in 1 of 6 Jewish patients who underwent circumcision on the eighth day of life.[221] In contrast, Muslim patients bled excessively following circumcision performed at age 5 to 7 years.[224] Postpartum hemorrhage was noted in 13 of 17 women.[222,224]

Heterozygotes exhibit slight but significantly reduced mean levels of factor V and factor VIII.[221] In a literature survey of 161 heterozygotes, 22 were reported to have significant bleeding manifestations.[252] There was no correlation between factor V or VIII level and the bleeding tendency.[222,252]

DIFFERENTIAL DIAGNOSIS

Hemophilia A can be easily distinguished from combined deficiency of factors V and VIII by the X-linked mode of inheritance and by the normal PT observed in patients affected by hemophilia A. Hereditary factor V deficiency can be confused with combined deficiency of factors V and VIII, since both entities are inherited as autosomal recessive traits, have similar manifestations, and are characterized by prolonged PT and aPTT assays. Assays of factors V and VIII are therefore essential for making the distinction (see also Chap. 115). A coincidental association between mild or moderate hemophilia A and hereditary factor V deficiency should be borne in mind. Other features that are helpful in distinguishing between the two entities are (1) consanguinity, which is frequently present in parents of patients with the combined deficiency; (2) independent segregation of factor V and factor VIII deficiency among immediate relatives of patients with the coincidental association; and (3) concordant reductions in levels of factors V and VIII, which are more likely in patients afflicted by the combined deficiency.

THERAPY

An antifibrinolytic agent such as tranexamic acid or ε-aminocaproic acid can be helpful in patients who exhibit menorrhagia, epistaxis, or gingival bleeding. Patients with severe bleeding episodes or patients undergoing surgical procedures, including dental extractions, should receive fresh-frozen plasma for replacement of factor V, and cryoprecipitate or factor VIII concentrate as a source of factor VIII. Desmopressin can also be used for achieving an increase of endogenous plasma factor VIII level,[222] but this treatment sometimes fails.[253] As with other clotting factor deficiencies, replacement therapy in patients undergoing major surgery should last for 7 to 10 days after the operation. Hemostatically safe levels of factor V and VIII have not been established, but given the significant bleeding experienced by patients with factor V and VIII levels of up to 30 percent of normal, it is reasonable to aim for trough factor levels of greater than 50 percent of normal during and after surgery. Volume overload can be a serious problem but can be circumvented by plasma exchange and concomitant use of a factor VIII concentrate.[253]

FACTOR XI DEFICIENCY

DEFINITION AND HISTORY

Factor XI deficiency was initially described as a "new hemophilia" in 1953 by Rosenthal et al[254] in two sisters and their maternal uncle, and was erroneously thought to be transmitted as an autosomal dominant disorder with variable expressivity. Later studies, however, clearly established that the mode of transmission of factor XI deficiency is autosomal recessive.[255,256] The disorder is exhibited in homozygotes or compound heterozygotes as a mild to moderate bleeding tendency that is mainly injury related. Affected subjects are rarely encountered in most populations, except for Jews, particularly of Ashkenazi origin, among whom the deficiency is common.[256]

Until recently, factor XI was regarded as one of the "contact" coagulation factors, functioning in the initiation of the intrinsic coagulation system. Numerous studies showed that, when blood or plasma is exposed to negatively charged surfaces in vitro, a series of reactions involving factor XII, high-molecular-weight kininogen (HK), and prekallikrein (PK) take place that yield α factor XIIa. Alpha factor XIIa then activates factor XI, and factor XIa, in turn, propagates the intrinsic coagulation system by activating factor IX in the presence of calcium ions. All attempts to ascribe to the contact activation pathway an essential function in vivo have been futile, since, unlike factor XI deficiency, severe deficiencies of factor XII, HK, and PK have not been shown to cause any hemostatic derangement. Recent studies demonstrated that factor XI can be activated by thrombin,[257,258] thereby bypassing the contact reactions. This finding and new observations on the involvement of factor XI in the intrinsic coagulation system (see Chap. 112) and in the fibrinolytic system (see below) explain why factor XI is important for hemostasis, whereas factor XII, HK, and PK are probably not.

BIOCHEMISTRY AND MOLECULAR FEATURES

Factor XI is a glycoprotein that consists of two identical polypeptide chains of 80 kDa linked together by a disulfide bond.[259] Each subunit contains 607 amino acids with a serine protease domain at the C terminus and 4 tandem repeats of 90 or 91 amino acids, designated apple domains, at the N terminus. A disulfide bond is formed between Cys321 residues, which are contained in the fourth apple domain of each monomer.[260] In blood, factor XI is complexed noncovalently with HK through a binding region in the first apple domain.[261] The normal plasma concentration of factor XI is about 4 μg/ml. The 23-kb gene

encoding for factor XI consists of 15 exons and 14 introns[262] and is on chromosome 4q34-35.[263]

Activation of factor XI involves cleavage of the Arg369-Ile370 bond, yielding a heavy chain containing the four apple domains linked by a disulfide bond to a light chain containing the catalytic domain.[259] Each activated molecule thus contains two catalytic sites. Factor XI adhered to negatively charged surfaces by HK can be activated by α factor XIIa or through autoactivation by factor XIa.[264] However, it is doubtful whether these reactions occur in vivo. The major activator of factor XI in vivo is probably thrombin,[257,258] and the reaction can take place in the fluid phase,[265] on the surface of platelets (see Chap. 112), or on the fibrin surface after a clot is formed.[266] Once factor XIa is generated, it activates factor IX by limited proteolysis of two peptide bonds in the presence of calcium ions.[267] Factor IXa then activates factor X in the presence of factor VIIIa, negatively charged phospholipids, and calcium ions. Thus, through thrombin-mediated activation of factor XI, additional thrombin is generated.

The presence of factor XI is also essential for activation of procarboxypeptidase B by thrombin. This protein, also named thrombin-activatable fibrinolysis inhibitor (TAFI), was first described in 1990[268] and later fully characterized.[269,270] Activated TAFI (TAFIa) removes terminal lysine residues from fibrin, leading to impaired binding of certain forms of plasminogen to fibrin, thereby disrupting the process of tissue plasminogen activator–induced plasmin generation in the blood clot.[271] TAFIa is thus a strong inhibitor of fibrinolysis. Large amounts of thrombin are necessary for TAFI activation, but the reaction is substantially augmented when thrombin is bound to thrombomodulin.[272] It follows that impaired generation of thrombin, for example, in inherited deficiencies of factors VIII, IX, or XI, not only delays clot formation but enhances premature lysis of clots.[273] Activation of factor XI by thrombin, particularly within the blood clot, is essential for adequate TAFI activation and protection of the clot from lysis in vitro[274,275] and in vivo.[276] These data fit well with the clinical observations of bleeding in factor XI–deficient patients occurring commonly at sites rich in local fibrinolytic activity[277] and with the effective prevention of such episodes by antifibrinolytic agents (see below).[278]

Factor XI is synthesized in the liver, and a case has been described of acquired factor XI deficiency due to liver transplantation from a donor who, in retrospect, was found to have the deficiency.[279] A small amount of a 230-kDa protein with factor XI activity was found in platelets and was suggested to be derived from an alternatively spliced transcript found in megakaryocytes.[280] However, another study showed a normally spliced transcript in platelets.[281]

GENETICS

INHERITANCE

Factor XI deficiency is inherited as an autosomal recessive trait that is characterized by plasma factor XI levels of less than 15 percent of normal in homozygotes and compound heterozygotes.[255,277] In heterozygotes, factor XI levels frequently range between 25 and 70 percent of normal but can even be higher.[256,282] Factor XI deficiency due to a dysfunctional molecule is exceedingly rare. In a study of 125 patients from various ethnic origins, none was found to have discordant levels of factor XI activity and antigen.[283] Only two cases with severe deficiency of factor XI activity and seemingly normal antigen levels have been described.[284,285]

MUTATIONS

Three mutations, designated types I, II, and III, were first described in 1989 in six Ashkenazi Jewish patients who had severe factor XI deficiency.[286] The type I mutation is a G-to-A change at the splice site of the last intron of the gene; type II is a G-to-T change in exon

5 at Glu117 leading to a stop codon TAA; and type III is a T-to-C change in exon 9 that results in a substitution of Phe283 by Leu in the fourth apple domain of the protein. A fourth mutation, designated type IV, was later identified in another Ashkenazi Jewish patient and was found to consist of a 14-bp deletion at the intron N–exon 14 junction.[287] Of the four mutations among Jews, the predominant mutations are the type II and type III mutations (see below). Additional mutations have been reported in non-Jewish patients.[83,260,288–294]

The majority of mutations so far described are point mutations at the coding region or at intron-exon boundaries. Of six missense mutations that were expressed in BHK cells[260,295] or COS-7 cells,[288] five mutations involving the fourth apple domain of the protein exhibited impaired secretion of factor XI from the cells. Pulse chase experiments used in two of these studies identified impaired intracellular dimerization of factor XI as the probable cause for retarded secretion and intracellular degradation of the oligomers.[260,295]

ETHNIC DISTRIBUTION AND PREVALENCE

Most patients with factor XI deficiency are Jewish.[255,256,277,282] Sporadically, patients have been described who are of English, German, Italian, French, Basque, Chinese, Japanese, Indian, Arab, and African American origin.[282,283,296–298] Several instances of vertical transmission of severe factor XI deficiency in Ashkenazi Jewish families (consistent with pseudodominance) suggested that the gene frequency in this segment of Jews is very high. This indeed was found in two surveys of this population performed in Israel.[256]

Type II and type III are the predominant mutations causing factor XI deficiency in Ashkenazi Jews.[277,296] Of 250 mutant alleles analyzed in 125 unrelated subjects with severe deficiency, 246 were either of the type II (123 alleles) or the type III (123 alleles).[299] Screening the general Ashkenazi Jewish population for these mutations disclosed allele frequencies of 0.0217 for type II mutation and 0.0254 for type III mutation. Hence, the estimated frequency of subjects with severe factor XI deficiency in Ashkenazi Jews is 1:450 and of heterozygotes for both types of mutation, 1:11. These data indicate that factor XI deficiency is the most frequent hereditary disorder in this population. It is interesting to note that the type II mutation has also been observed in Iraqi Jews with a similar allele frequency, 0.0167,[299] in Palestinian Arabs with a frequency of 0.0065, and in Sephardic and other Middle Eastern Jews with a frequency of 0.0027.[300] In sharp contrast, the type III mutation was not detected in 1343 Jews of non-Ashkenazi origin or in 313 Palestinian Arabs.[300]

FOUNDER EFFECTS FOR THE TYPE II AND TYPE III MUTATIONS

Haplotype analysis based on examination of factor XI gene polymorphisms disclosed distinct founder effects for type II and type III mutations.[300] In view of the similar prevalences of the type II mutation in Iraqi and Ashkenazi Jews, its presence in Palestinian Arabs and Sephardic Jews, and the historical information about the divergence of these populations 2000 to 2500 years ago, the type II mutation seems to have occurred in ancient times. Type III mutation, which is confined to Ashkenazi Jews, probably stemmed from a founder who lived in more recent times. Evidence supporting these hypotheses has been presented.[301]

CLINICAL FEATURES

BLEEDING MANIFESTATIONS IN HOMOZYGOTES AND COMPOUND HETEROZYGOTES

Most bleeding manifestations in homozygotes and compound heterozygotes are related to injuries. Excessive bleeding can occur at the time of injury or begin several hours or days following trauma. Some patients with severe factor XI deficiency may not bleed at all following trauma,[255] and in others the bleeding tendency may vary from one hemostatic challenge to another.[277,282] These apparent inconsistencies can now be partially explained by the genotype of the patient, which affects the extent of the deficiency, as well as by the variable sites of injury.[282,302,303] Homozygotes for the type III missense mutation, whose mean factor XI level was 9.7 percent of normal, had significantly fewer injury-related bleeding events than did homozygotes for the type II mutation, with a mean factor XI level of 1.2 percent of normal. Surgical procedures that involve tissues with high fibrinolytic activity (the urinary tract, tonsils, nose, and tooth sockets) are frequently associated with excessive bleeding in patients with severe factor XI deficiency irrespective of the genotype.[277] A significantly lower frequency of bleeding complications follows surgical interventions at sites without excessive local fibrinolysis, such as appendectomy, cholecystectomy, circumcision, and orthopedic surgery.[277,303] This site-related bleeding tendency can now be understood in light of the demonstrated function of factor XI in preventing clot lysis (see above).

Spontaneous bleeding manifestations such as menorrhagia, gingival bleeding, ecchymoses, and epistaxis do occur in patients with severe factor XI deficiency but are uncommon.[302,303] Postpartum hemorrhage can occur but is infrequent; only three episodes were observed following delivery of 28 children in 14 women.[282]

BLEEDING MANIFESTATIONS IN HETEROZYGOTES

Whether or not heterozygotes exhibit a bleeding tendency has been a matter of debate. In one extensive study, heterozygotes had almost no bleeding complications following a variety of surgical procedures, including operations at sites with enhanced local fibrinolysis.[255] In another study, all heterozygotes who underwent urologic surgery did well, except for one patient, whose factor XI level was 25 percent of normal.[304] Contrasting with these observations are studies that identified a bleeding tendency, particularly following injury in 33 percent,[282] 48 percent,[302] and 20 percent[303] of heterozygotes. Variable definitions of what constitutes a bleeding tendency[305] can only partially explain this discrepancy. A more likely explanation for the variable manifestations in heterozygotes is the coexistence of additional hemostatic abnormalities in those patients who do bleed. Thus, heterozygotes who were defined as bleeders tended to have lower levels of factor VIII and von Willebrand factor, and possess blood group O, known to be associated with reduced von Willebrand factor levels. Moreover, in another study, most heterozygotes who presented with a bleeding tendency also had a platelet function abnormality.[306] It can be concluded that heterozygotes for factor XI deficiency may display a risk of bleeding that is significantly lower than the risk of bleeding exhibited by homozygotes and compound heterozygotes. This statement is supported by a recent study that assessed the risk of bleeding in patients from 45 families.[303] The odds ratio for bleeding was 13.0 in homozygotes and compound heterozygotes and only 2.6 in heterozygotes.

THROMBOSIS

Although factor XI plays an essential role in blood coagulation and fibrinolysis, a severe deficiency state does not protect patients from venous or arterial thrombosis. Patients with severe factor XI deficiency have been reported to have acute myocardial infarction[307] and pulmonary embolism.[308] Thrombotic events have also been described in patients following infusion of factor XI concentrates (see "Therapy," below).

ASSOCIATION OF FACTOR XI DEFICIENCY WITH OTHER DISORDERS

Factor XI deficiency was described in patients with Gaucher disease.[309–311] In view of the independent segregation of the two disorders,[309] it seems that the coincidental occurrence of Gaucher disease and hereditary factor XI deficiency stems from the high frequency of the respective mutant genes in the Ashkenazi Jewish population. Patients with Noonan syndrome were reported to exhibit factor XI deficiency and a bleeding tendency.[312] Recent studies, however, showed that, in addition to factor XI deficiency, patients with Noonan syndrome display several other abnormalities in coagulation factors and platelet function for which no explanation has been provided.[313,314] A variety of other inherited disorders of hemostasis have been described in association with factor XI deficiency, including von Willebrand disease,[315,316] factor VIII deficiency,[282,317,318] and factor VII deficiency.[319] Due to the high prevalence of factor XI deficiency in Jews, these associations are expected to be quite frequent.

ACQUIRED INHIBITORS

Inhibitors that neutralize factor XI activity have been described in patients with hereditary factor XI deficiency.[320–328] Most patients had severe factor XI deficiency and received transfusions of plasma prior to the development of the inhibitor. The inhibitory activity was associated with polyclonal IgG antibodies in eight patients studied.[321,323,325,326] The antibodies bound to various parts of factor XI, interfering with its activation, complex formation with HK, and catalytic activity. It is interesting to note that spontaneous bleeding manifestations did not seem to be aggravated by the development of the inhibitors, except for one patient, in whom the titer of the antibody was extremely high.[321] Securing hemostasis during and after surgery in such cases is a serious problem (see "Therapy," below).

LABORATORY FEATURES

Patients with factor XI deficiency have prolonged aPTT and normal PT (see Chap. 115). All homozygotes and compound heterozygotes have aPTTs that are longer than two standard deviations above the normal mean.[329] However, aPTT values in heterozygotes substantially overlap the normal range.[277,329] Consequently, screening of patients for a hemostatic abnormality prior to surgery (which is recommended for Jewish patients because of the high prevalence of factor XI deficiency) will identify all patients with a severe factor XI deficiency. The diagnosis is established by a clotting assay using a modified aPTT system and factor XI–deficient plasma.[255] Factor XI antigen can be measured by radioimmunoassay.[283] Analysis of DNA polymerase chain reaction and restriction enzyme digestion can identify the patients' genotype.[277,286,291,296] Mean factor XI levels and aPTT values in type II homozygotes are 1.2 percent of normal and 108 s, respectively; in compound heterozygotes for the type II and type III mutations the values are 3.3 percent of normal and 85 s, respectively; and in type III homozygotes the values are 9.7 percent of normal and 67 s, respectively.[277,296] Although it has been reported that heterozygotes for the type II mutation have a significantly lower mean factor XI level than do heterozygotes for the type III mutation,[277] in another study similar values were found in patients bearing these two genotypes.[296]

THERAPY

PATIENTS WITH A SEVERE DEFICIENCY

Patients with severe factor XI deficiency who have to undergo a surgical procedure should be carefully evaluated and meticulously prepared for the operation. A negative history of bleeding complications following previous procedures does not exclude the possibility of an increased bleeding tendency. Other hemostatic abnormalities and the presence of an inhibitor to factor XI should be excluded.

Aspirin and other antiplatelet agents should be avoided for 1 week prior to surgery.

In choosing the treatment modality and the intensity of treatment, the following considerations should be taken into account:

1. The age of the patient and history of cardiovascular disease. Use of plasma may create volume overload, and use of a factor XI concentrate can induce thrombosis (see below).
2. The baseline plasma level of factor XI. Homozygotes with levels of approximately 10 percent of normal have a low risk of bleeding (except for procedures at sites high in local fibrinolytic activity) compared to homozygotes or compound heterozygotes, who have lower levels.[277]
3. Presence of an inhibitor to factor XI. In such patients, plasma or factor XI concentrate cannot be used.
4. The site of surgery. In patients operated on at a site with high local fibrinolytic activity, as in dental surgery and urologic surgery, the risk of bleeding is high, and the use of an antifibrinolytic agent should be considered.
5. Safety. Transmission of infectious agents and allergic reactions are more common following plasma transfusion than after infusion of factor XI concentrate; concentrates, however, can induce thrombosis.
6. The half-life of factor XI. A mean half-life of 52 h was recorded following infusion of a factor XI concentrate[330] and 45 h following plasma transfusion.[331]

Patients undergoing dental extractions do not need replacement therapy. Tranexamic acid (1 g q.i.d) from 12 h before surgery until 7 days after surgery is effective in preventing bleeding.[278] Epsilon-aminocaproic acid (5–6 g q.i.d.) given similarly is expected to achieve the same results. For major surgery or surgery at sites with high levels of local fibrinolysis, transfusion of fresh-frozen plasma should be given for 10 to 14 days, aiming at trough factor XI levels of 45 percent of normal.[332] For surgery at tissues not displaying high levels of local fibrinolysis, fresh-frozen plasma can be transfused for 5 to 7 days, targeting at trough factor XI levels of 30 percent of normal. Following prostatectomy and bladder operations, continuous flushing of the bladder with saline solution containing tranexamic acid 0.5 to 1 g/liter can be helpful for hemostasis. For nose surgery and tonsillectomy, apart from replacement therapy, tranexamic acid or ε-aminocaproic acid, given as for dental extraction, should be considered.

Two viral-inactivated factor XI concentrates have been used for treatment of patients with factor XI deficiency.[330,333,334] However, infusions of both concentrates give rise to laboratory signs of DIC.[335,336] Pulmonary embolism and arterial thrombosis, including fatal cases, have also been reported in patients receiving the concentrates,[337,338] albeit mostly in elderly patients who had preexisting cardiovascular disease and who were given a dose exceeding 30 units/kg. Consequently, at the present time these concentrates must be used with great caution.

PATIENTS WITH PARTIAL FACTOR XI DEFICIENCY

Heterozygotes who have a negative history of a bleeding tendency, who do not exhibit any additional hemostatic abnormality, and whose plasma factor XI level is more than 40 percent of normal probably do not need any treatment while undergoing surgery.[304] If, however, a positive bleeding history is elicited in such patients, a detailed investigation of the hemostatic system should be performed. If an additional abnormality is found, adequate measures should be taken to correct it, in addition to the use of replacement therapy for 5 days, aiming at trough factor XI levels of 45 percent of normal. Desmopressin may be useful in the prevention of bleeding, but only a limited number of patients receiving this therapy have been reported.[339,340] The beneficial effect of desmopressin may be related to the increase in the plasma levels of von Willebrand factor and factor VIII.

PATIENTS WITH AN INHIBITOR TO FACTOR XI

Most reported patients have not exhibited an aggravation of their bleeding tendency following the development of an inhibitor. Consequently, when such patients undergo dental extraction, use of tranexamic acid and fibrin glue may be sufficient,[341] but limited evidence to support this contention is available. Uneventful surgery was described in a patient who underwent plasmapheresis and was given an antifibrinolytic agent.[324] Another patient underwent uneventful tonsillectomy after receiving only an antifibrinolytic drug.[342] Activated prothrombin complex[321,328] and recombinant factor VIIa[343] have also been successfully used for major surgical procedures.

FACTOR XIII DEFICIENCY

DEFINITION

Factor XIII (fibrin-stabilizing factor) is a transglutaminase that crosslinks and thereby stabilizes fibrin monomers. Deficiency of factor XIII, first described by Duckert et al in 1960, results in a moderate to severe hemorrhagic disorder and sometimes in abnormal wound healing.[344]

BIOCHEMISTRY AND MOLECULAR FEATURES

Plasma factor XIII is a heterotetramer with a M_r of aproximately 340,000 composed of two a chains and two b chains linked together through noncovalent bonds. The a chain ($M_r \approx 82,000$) contains the catalytic site of factor XIII, an activation peptide, and a calcium-binding site.[345] The factor XIII a chain is structurally homologous with the a chain of tissue transglutaminase,[346] the a chain of keratinocyte transglutaminase,[347] and band 4.2 of erythrocytes,[348] although the latter lacks tansglutaminase activity. At the N terminus of the factor XIII a chain is an activation peptide that is removed by thrombin cleavage during thrombin-catalyzed activation.[349,350] An active-site sulfhydryl residue, which is characteristic for this class of enzymes, is located at Cys298. Two calcium-binding domains flank the active-site cysteine.

The two b chains of factor XIII function as carrier proteins for the a chains,[351,352] stabilizing the a chains in the circulation and regulating the calcium-dependent activation of factor XIII. The b chain, M_r approximately 76,500, is composed of ten homologous consensus, or ''sushi,'' repeats.[353] Each repeat is approximately 60 amino acids in length and contains four disulfide bonds, with Cys1 linked to Cys3 and Cys2 linked to Cys4. The function of these repeats is unknown.

The gene for the factor XIII a chain is located on chromosome 6p24-p25.[354,355] The gene spans 142 kb and is composed of 15 exons ranging in size from 63 to 1688 bp. In general, there is conservation among genes of the transglutaminase family. For example, the sequences encompassing the active site thiol is encoded by exon VII; the calcium-binding sequences are encoded by exons VI and XI; and the fibrin-binding sequences are encoded by exons III and V. Where the transglutaminases diverge is at the N terminus in the sequences encoded by exon II; in factor XIII a chain, exon II encodes the activation domain, and, in keratinocyte transglutaminase, exon II encodes sequences that localize the protein intracellularly.

The b chain has been localized to chromosome 1q31-q32.1.[356] It is interesting to note that a number of other genes encoding for proteins with sushi repeats are also located on chromosome 1. The gene for

the b chain spans 28 kb and is composed of 12 exons.[353] The first exon encodes the leader sequence, while exons II through XI each encode a single sushi repeat. Exon XII encodes the C terminus of the b chain.

The site of synthesis of the a chain is uncertain. The protein has been identified in monocytes and platelets[357–359] and, variably, in the liver.[358,360,361] The b chain is synthesized in the liver.[357,361] The assembly of the factor XIII tetramer probably occurs in the circulation.

Factor XIII circulates in plasma as an inactive precursor that is activated by thrombin. Thrombin cleaves an Arg37-Gly38 bond at the N terminus of the a chain, releasing a 4500-kDa activation peptide.[349] Following thrombin-mediated removal of the activation peptide and binding of calcium, the active-site sulfhydryl residue becomes exposed and factor XIII becomes proteolytically active.[350] The b-chain dimer subsequently dissociates from the complex to produce the fully active a-chain dimer.

Factor XIIIa catalyzes the formation of peptide bonds between adjacent molecules of fibrin monomer and thus imparts chemical and mechanical stability to a clot. The peptide bond that is formed consists of an amide bond between the γ-carbonyl group of glutamine and the ε-amino group of lysine. In fibrin, this amide bond is between a-chain sequences and between γ-chain sequences. The γ-chain links occur between Glu398 on the γ chain of one fibrin molecule and Lys406 on the γ chain of another fibrin molecule.[362] Cross-linking sites in the a chain have been identified as Glu328, Glu366, Lys508, Lys556, and Lys562, but the linking residues are not certain.[363] Factor XIIIa also cross-links a2-antiplasmin to the a chain of fibrin,[364] thereby increasing the resistance of fibrin to plasmin degradation, and cross-links fibronectin to the a chain of fibrin,[365] thereby affecting the mechanical properties of the clot and increasing cell adhesion. A number of other proteins are also substrates for factor XIIIa, including collagen, thrombospondin, von Willebrand factor, vinculin, vitronectin, actin, myosin, and lipoprotein(a),[365–374] but the physiologic significance of these reactions is less clear.

Tissue transglutaminase consisting only of two a chains is present in the soluble fraction of a variety of cells, particularly platelets and monocytes.[375–378] Upon activation by thrombin, tissue transglutaminase cross-links fibrin in a manner that is similar to the effect of activated factor XIII.

GENETICS

Inherited factor XIII deficiency is transmitted in an autosomal recessive manner. Parents of affected individuals are typically asymptomatic, and consanguinity is common. Deficiency of the factor XIII a chain is the predominant abnormality and occurs at a frequency of approximately 1 in 2 million. Approximately 200 unrelated cases have been described. The molecular defects responsible for the a chain deficiency are presented in Table 122-3,[379–394] and an updated listing is available on the internet.[83] Missense mutations are the most common mutations of the a chain gene. Deficiency of the b chain as a cause of factor XIII deficiency has been reported in only three cases.[395–398]

CLINICAL MANIFESTATIONS

Factor XIII deficiency causes formation of blood clots that are less stable and more susceptible to fibrinolytic degradation by plasmin. As a result, affected individuals have an increased tendency to bleed. Bleeding from the umbilical cord in the first few days of life is common. Patients with factor XIII deficiency have a higher incidence of intracranial hemorrhage than do patients with other inherited bleed-

TABLE 122-3   INHERITED FACTOR XIII DEFICIENCIES*

REFERENCE	MUTATION	DEFECT
Subunit a Mutations		
Nonsense mutations		
380	Del exons 3–11	
381	Del 13 bp exon III	Frameshift mutation
382	Del AG E43	Frameshift mutation
379	Del T F8	Frameshift mutation
383	Ins C exon 9	Frameshift mutation
Nagoya I 384	Del 20 bp exon I	Splice defect
379	G→A exon XIV	Splice defect
378	Ins T intron D	Splice defect
380	G→A intron E	Splice defect
387	R171Stop	Termination mutation
388	Y441Stop	Termination mutation
389	R661Stop	Termination mutation
Missense mutations		
388	N60K	Decreased dansylcadaverine incorporation
389	M242T	Decreased [¹⁴C] putrescine incorporation
379	R252I	Decreased [¹⁴C] putrescine incorporation
384	R260C	Decreased coagulant activity
379	R326Q	Decreased [¹⁴C] putrescine incorporation
391	N344 del	Decreased catalytic activity
	A394V	Decreased coagulant activity
380	R408Q	Decreased coagulant activity
392	V414F	Decreased coagulant activity
379	L498P	Decreased [¹⁴C] putrescine incorporation
388	G501R	Decreased dansylcadaverine incorporation
393	L660P	Decreased coagulant activity
Calgary³⁹⁴	L667P	Decreased coagulant activity
Subunit b Mutations		
398	Ins AAC	Insertion of stop mutation
396	Del A	Splice defect
397	C430F	

*Updated information can be found in the internet.[83]

ing disorders. This is the basis for recommending prophylaxis against intracranial hemorrhage by regular replacement therapy. Ecchymoses, hematomas, and prolonged bleeding following trauma are also characteristic. Hemarthroses and bleeding into the muscles are less common, however, than in the hemophilias. In some patients, bleeding following trauma may be delayed for 12 to 36 h, while in other patients immediate bleeding occurs. Habitual abortions and poor wound healing have also been described.

DIFFERENTIAL DIAGNOSIS

The PT, aPTT, and thrombin time are normal in factor XIII deficiency (see Chap. 115). Because of increased fibrin breakdown, levels of fibrin degradation products may be increased and result in a minimally prolonged thrombin time. This may be the only clue to the diagnosis based on simple coagulation screening tests. The diagnosis of factor XIII deficiency is established by the demonstration of increased clot solubility in 5 M urea, dilute monochloroacetic acid, or acetic acid. Factor XIIIa may also be determined quantitatively by measuring its ability to catalyze the incorporation of fluorescent or radioactive amines into proteins such as casein.

The disorder is easily differentiated from other deficiencies of plasma coagulation factors by the demonstration of normal screening coagulation test results and the demonstration of increased fibrin solubility. Deficiency of α₂-antiplasmin may also cause an increased tendency to bleed, normal screening test results, and increased clot solubility. A specific assay for α₂-antiplasmin is required to distinguish between the two disorders. Patients with α₂-antiplasmin deficiency,

however, appear to have a milder bleeding disorder and do not manifest umbilical cord and intracranial hemorrhages. Acquired factor XIII deficiency may occur during DIC, during primary fibrinolysis, or in the presence of an inhibitor against factor XIII. Disseminated intravascular coagulation and fibrinolysis are usually easy to distinguish from inherited factor XIII deficiency because of the reduced fibrinogen levels and other abnormalities (see Chap. 126). A family history and a lifelong history of bleeding help to distinguish inherited factor XIII deficiency from an acquired inhibitor or other causes for the deficiency.

THERAPY

Replacement therapy for factor XIII deficiency is highly satisfactory because of the small quantities of factor XIII needed for effective hemostasis and the long half-life of factor XIII, which is approximately 19 days. Plasma-derived, virus-inactivated concentrates of factor XIII are available[399] and are the treatment of choice. Fresh-frozen plasma can also be used where the concentrates are unavailable. Transfusion of only 2 to 3 ml of plasma per kilogram of body weight will produce hemostasis for periods of up to 4 weeks. Prophylactic therapy using infusions of plasma every 3 to 4 weeks has been successful in achieving normal hemostasis and preventing habitual abortions.

REFERENCES

1. Walz DA, Hewett-Emmett D, Seegers WH: Amino acid sequence of human prothrombin fragments 1 and 2. *Proc Natl Acad Sci USA* 74:1969, 1977.
2. Butkowski J, Elion J, Downing MR, Mann KG: Primary structure of human prothrombin 2 and alpha-thrombin. *J Biol Chem* 252:4942, 1977.
3. Degen SJ, McGillivray RT, Davie EW: Characterization of the complementary deoxyribonucleic acid and gene coding for human prothrombin. *Biochemistry* 22:2087, 1983.
4. Magnusson S, Stotrup-Jensen L, Petersen TE, et al: Homologous "kringle" structures common to plasminogen and prothrombin: Substrate specificity of enzymes activating prothrombin and plasminogen, in *Proteolysis and Physiological Regulation*, edited by DW Ribbons, K Brew, p 203. Academic Press, New York, 1976.
5. Bajaj SP, Butkowski RJ, Mann KG: Prothrombin fragments: Ca²⁺ binding and activation kinetics. *J Biol Chem* 250:2150, 1975.
6. Royle NJ, Irwin DM, Koschinsky ML, et al: Human genes encoding prothrombin and ceruloplasmin map to 11p11-q12 and 3q21-24, respectively. *Somat Cell Mol Genet* 13:285, 1987.
7. Degen SJ, Davie EW: Nucleotide sequence of the gene for human prothrombin. *Biochemistry* 26:6165, 1987.
8. Bancroft JD, Schaefer LA, Degen SJ: Characterization of the Alu-rich 5'-flanking region of the human prothrombin-encoding gene: Identification of a positive *cis* -acting element that regulates liver-specific expression. *Gene* 95:253, 1990.
9. Board PG, Shaw DC: Determination of the amino acid substitution in human prothrombin type 3 (157 Glu leads to Lys) and the localization of a third thrombin cleavage site. *Br J Haematol* 54:245, 1983.
10. Shapiro SS, Martinez J, Holburn RR: Congenital dysprothrombinemia: An inherited structural disorder of human prothrombin. *J Clin Invest* 48:2251, 1969.
11. Rocha E, Paramo JA, Bascones C, et al: Prothrombin Segovia: A new congenital abnormality of prothrombin. *Scand J Haematol* 36:444, 1986.

12. Diuguid DL, Rabiet MJ, Furie BC, Furie B: Molecular defects of factor IX Chicago-2 (Arg145His) and prothrombin Madrid (Arg271Cys): Arginine mutations that preclude zymogen activation. *Blood* 74:193, 1989.

13. Miyata T, Zheng YZ, Kato A, Kato H: A point mutation (Arg271→Cys) of a homozygote for dysfunctional prothrombin, prohrombin Obihiro, which has a region of high sequence variability. *Br J Haematol* 90:688, 1995.

14. Rabiet MJ, Furie BC, Furie B: Molecular defect of prothrombin Barcelona: Substitution of cysteine for arginine at residue 273. *J Biol Chem* 261:15045, 1986.

15. James HL, Kim DJ, Zheng DQ, Girolami A: Prothrombin Padua I: Incomplete activation due to an amino acid substitution at a factor Xa cleavage site. *Blood Coag Fibrinol* 5:841, 1994.

16. O'Marcaigh AS, Nichols WL, Hassinger NL, et al: Genetic analysis and functional characterization of prothrombins Corpus Christi (Arg382-Cys), Dhahran (Arg271-His), and hypoprothrombinemia. *Blood* 88:2611, 1996.

17. Huisse MG, Dreyfus M, Guillin MC: Prothrombin Clamart: Prothrombin variant with defective Arg320-Ile cleavage by factor Xa. *Thromb Res* 44:11, 1986.

18. Weinger RS, Rudy C, Moake JL, et al: Prothrombin Houston: A dysprothrombin identifiable by crossed immunoelectrofocusing and abnormal *Echis carinatus* venom activation. *Blood* 55:811, 1980.

19. Smith LG, Coone LA, Kitchens CS: Prothrombin Gainesville: A dysprothrombinemia in a pair of identical twins. *Am J Hematol* 11:223, 1981.

20. Ruiz-Saez A, Luengo J, Rodriguez A, et al: Prothrombin Perija: A new congenital dysprothrombinemia in an Indian family. *Thromb Res* 44:587, 1986.

21. Shapiro SS, McCord S: Prothrombin. *Prog Hemost Thromb* 4:177, 1978.

22. Girolami A, Coccheri S, Palareti G, et al: Prothrombin Molise: A "new" congenital dysprothrombinemia, double heterozygosis with an abnormal prothrombin and "true" prothrombin deficiency. *Blood* 52:115, 1978.

23. Miyata T, Moita T, Inomoto T, et al: Prothrombin Tokushima, a replacement of arginine-418 by tryptophan that impairs the fibrinogen clotting activity of derived thrombin Tokushima. *Biochemistry* 26:1117, 1987.

24. Josso F, Rio Y, Beguin S: A new variant of human prothrombin: Prothrombin Metz, demonstration in a family showing double heterozygosity for congenital hypoprothrombinemia and dysprothrombinemia. *Haemostasis* 12:309, 1982.

25. Henriksen RA, Dunham CK, Miller LD, et al: Prothrombin Greenville, Arg517→Gln, identified in an individual heterozygous for dysprothrombinemia. *Blood* 91:2026, 1998.

26. Morishita E, Saito M, Kumabashiri I, et al: Prothrombin Himi: A compound heterozygote for two dysfunctional prothrombin molecules (Met-337→Thr and Arg-388→His). *Blood* 80:2275, 1992.

27. Henriksen RA, Mann KG: Identification of the primary structural defect in the dysthrombin thrombin Quick I: Substitution of cysteine for arginine-382. *Biochemistry* 27:9160, 1988.

28. Miyata T, Aruga R, Umeyama H, et al: Prothrombin Salakta: Substitution of glutamic acid-466 by alanine reduces the fibrinogen clotting activity and the esterase activity. *Biochemistry* 31:7457, 1992.

29. Degen SJ, McDowell SA, Sparks LM, Scharrer I: Prothrombin Frankfurt: A dysfunctional prothrombin characterized by substitution of Glu-466 by Ala. *Thromb Haemost* 73:203, 1995.

30. Henriksen RA, Mann KG: Substitution of valine for glycine-558 in the congenital dysthrombin thrombin Quick II alters primary substrate specificity. *Biochemistry* 28:2078, 1989.

31. Girolami A, Scarano L, Saggiorato G, et al: Congenital deficiencies and abnormalities of prothrombin. *Blood Coag Fibrinol* 9:557, 1998.

32. Poort SR, Rosendaal FR, Reitsma PH, Bertina RM: A common genetic variation in the 3′-untranslated region of the prothrombin gene is associated with elevated plasma prothrombin levels and an increase in venous thrombosis. *Blood* 88:3698, 1996.

33. Cumming AM, Keeney S, Salden A, et al: The prothrombin gene G20210A variant: Prevalence in a U.K. anticoagulant clinical population. *Br J Haemtol* 98:353, 1997.

34. Hillarp A, Zoller B, Svensson PJ, Dahlback B: The 20210A allele of the prothrombin gene is a common risk factor among Swedish outpatients with verified deep venous thrombosis. *Thromb Haemost* 78:990, 1997.

35. Brown K, Luddington R, Williamson D, et al: Risk of venous thromboembolism associated with a G to A transition at position 20210 in the 3′-untranslated region of the prothrombin gene. *Br J Haematol* 98:907, 1997.

36. Howard TE, Marusa M, Channell C, Duncan A: A patient homozygous for a mutation in the prothrombin gene 3′-untranslated region associated with massive thrombosis. *Blood Coagul Fibrinol* 8:316, 1997.

37. Corral J, Gonzalez-Conejero R, Lozano ML, et al: The venous thormbosis risk factor 20210A allele of the prothrombin gene is not a major risk factor for arterial thrombotic disease. *Br J Haematol* 99:304, 1997.

38. Ferraresi P, Marchetti G, Legnani C, et al: The heterozygous 20210 G/A prothrombin genotype is associated with early venous thrombosis in inherited thrombophilias and is not increased in frequency in artery disease. *Arterioscler Thromb Vasc Biol* 17:2418, 1997.

39. Watzle HH, Schuttrumpf J, Graf S, et al: Increased prevalence of a polymorphism in the gene coding for human prothrombin in patients with coronary heart disease. *Thromb Res* 87:521, 1997.

40. Franco RF, Santos SE, Elion J, et al: Prevalence of the G20210A polymorphism in the 3′-untranslated region of the prothrombin gene in different human populations. *Acta Haematol* 100:9, 1998.

41. Rosendaal FR, Doggen CJ, Zivelin A, et al: Geographic distribution of the 20210 G to A prothrombin variant. *Thromb Haemost* 79:706, 1998.

42. Zivelin A, Rosenberg N, Faier S, et al: A single genetic origin for the common prothrombotic G20210A polymorphism in the prothrombin gene. *Blood* 92:1119, 1998.

43. Mannucci PM: Outbreak of hepatitis A among Italian patients with haemophilia. *Lancet* 339:819, 1992.

44. Gerritzen A, Schneweis KE, Brackmann HH, et al: Acute hepatitis A in haemophilias. *Lancet* 340:1231, 1992.

45. Ragni MV, Koch WC, Jorda JA: Parvovirus B19 infection in patients with hemophilia. *Transfusion* 36:238, 1996.

46. Yee TT, Cohen BJ, Pasi KJ, Lee CA: Transmission of symptomatic parvovirus B19 infection by clotting factor concentrate. *Br J Haematol* 93:457, 1996.

47. Lusher JM: Thrombogenicity associated with factor IX complex concentrates. *Semin Hematol* 28:3, 1991.

48. Alexander B, Goldstein R, Landwehr G, Cook CD: Congenital SPCA deficiency: A hitherto unrecognized coagulation defect with hemorrhage rectified by serum and serum fractions. *J Clin Invest* 30:596, 1951.

49. Hagen FS, Gray CL, O'Hara P, et al: Characterization of a cDNA coding for human factor VII. *Proc Natl Acad Sci USA* 83:2412, 1986.

50. O'Hara PJ, Grant FJ, Haldeman BA, et al: Nucleotide sequence of the gene coding for human factor VII, a vitamin K-dependent protein participating in blood coagulation. *Proc Natl Acad Sci USA* 84:5158, 1987.

51. Ott R, Pfeiffer RA: Evidence that activities of coagulation factors VII and X are linked to chromosome 13 (q34). *Hum Hered* 34:123, 1984.

52. Gilgenkrantz S, Briquel ME, Andre E, et al: Structural genes of coagulaton factors VII and X located on 13q34. *Ann Genet* 29:32, 1986.

53. Miao CH, Leytus SP, Chung DW, Davie EW: Liver-specific expression of the gene coding for human factor X, a blood coagulation factor. *J Biol Chem* 267:7395, 1992.

54. Greenberg D, Miao CH, Ho WT, et al: Liver-specific expression of the human factor VII gene. *Proc Natl Acad Sci USA* 92:12347, 1995.

55. Pollak ES, Hung HL, Godin W, et al: Functional characterization of the human factor VII 5′-flanking region. *J Biol Chem* 271:1738, 1996.

56. Fair DS: Quantitation of factor VII in the plasma of normal and warfarin-treated individuals by radioimmunoassay. *Blood* 62:784, 1983.

57. Marder VJ, Shulman NR: Clinical aspects of congenital factor VII deficiency. *Am J Med* 37:182, 1964.

58. Radcliffe R, Nemerson Y: Activation and control of factor VII by activated factor X and thrombin: Isolation and characterization of a single chain form of factor VII. *J Biol Chem* 250:388, 1975.

59. Seligsohn U, Osterud B, Brown SF, et al: Activation of human factor VII in plasma and in purified systems: Roles of activated factor IX, kallikrein, and activated factor XII. *J Clin Invest* 64:1056, 1979.

60. Radcliffe R, Bagdasarian A, Colman R, Nemerson Y: Activation of bovine factor VII by Hageman factor fragments. *Blood* 50:611, 1977.

61. Nakagaki T, Foster DC, Berkner KL, Kisiel W: Initiation of the extrinsic pathway of blood coagulation: Evidence for the tissue factor dependent autoactivation of human coagulation factor VII. *Biochemistry* 30:10819, 1991.

62. Rapaport SI, Rao LV: The tissue factor pathway: How it has become a "prima ballerina." *Thromb Haemost* 74:7, 1995.

63. Banner DW, D'Arcy A, Chene C, et al: The crystal structure of the complex of blood coagulation factor VIIa with soluble tissue factor. *Nature* 380:41, 1996.

64. Cooper DN, Millar DS, Wacey A, et al: Inherited factor VII deficiency: Molecular genetics and pathophysiology. *Thromb Haemost* 78:151, 1997.

65. Edgington TS, Dickinson CD, Ruf W: The structural basis of function of the TF-VIIa complex in the cellular initiation of coagulation. *Thromb Haemost* 78:401, 1997.

66. Morrissey JH, Neuenschwander PF, Huang Q, et al: Factor VIIa–tissue factor: Functional importance of protein-membrane interactions. *Thromb Haemost* 78:112, 1997.

67. Morrissey JH, Macik BG, Neuenschwander PF, Comp PC: Quantitation of activated factor VII levels in plasma using a tissue factor mutant selectively deficient in promoting factor VII activation. *Blood* 81:734, 1993.

68. Seligsohn U, Kasper CK, Osterud B, Rapaport SI: Activated factor VII: Presence in factor IX concentrates and persistence in the circulation after infusion. *Blood* 53:828, 1979.

69. Miller BC, Hultin MB, Jesty J: Altered factor VII activity in hemophilia. *Blood* 65:845, 1985.

70. Wildgoose P, Nemerson Y, Hansen LL, et al: Measurement of basal levels of factor VIIa in hemophilia A and B patients. *Blood* 80:25, 1992.

71. Eichinger S, Mannucci PM, Tradati F, et al: Determinants of plasma factor VIIa levels in humans. *Blood* 86:3021, 1995.

72. Osterud B, Rapaport SI: Activation of factor IX by the reaction product of tissue factor and factor VII: Additional pathway for initiating blood coagulation. *Proc Natl Acad Sci USA* 74:5260, 1977.

73. Butenas S, Van't Veer C, Mann KG: Evaluation of the initiation phase of blood coagulation using ultrasensitive assays for serine proteases. *J Biol Chem* 272:21527, 1997.

74. Bauer KA: Activation of the factor VII-tissue factor pathway. *Thromb Haemost* 78:108, 1997.

75. Rosen ED, Chan JC, Idusogie E, et al: Mice lacking factor VII develop normally but suffer fatal perinatal bleeding. *Nature* 390:290, 1997.

76. Carmeliet P, Mackman N, Moons L, et al: Role of tissue factor in embryonic blood vessel development. *Nature* 383:73, 1996.

77. Parry GC, Erlich JH, Carmeliet P, et al: Low levels of tissue factor are compatible with development and hemostasis in mice. *J Clin Invest* 101:560, 1998.

78. Arbini AA, Bodkin D, Lopaciuk S, Bauer KA: Molecular analysis of Polish patients with factor VII deficiency. *Blood* 84:2214, 1994.

79. Tamary H, Fromovich Y, Shalmon L, et al: Ala244Val is a common, probably ancient mutation causing factor VII deficiency in Moroccan and Iranian Jews. *Thromb Haemost* 76:283, 1996.

80. Goodnight SH Jr, Feinstein DI, Osterud B, Rapaport SI: Factor VII antibody-neutralizing material in hereditary and acquired factor VII deficiency. *Blood* 38:1, 1971.

81. Mariani G, Mazzucconi MG, Hermans J, et al: Factor VII deficiency: Immunological characterization of genetic variants and detection of carriers. *Br J Haematol* 48:7, 1981.

82. Triplett DA, Brandt JT, Batard MA, et al: Hereditary factor VII deficiency: Heterogeneity defined by combined functional and immunochemical analysis. *Blood* 66:1284, 1985.

83. http://www.uwcm.ac.uk//uwcm/mg/hgmd0.html

84. Arbini AA, Pollak ES, Bayleran JK, et al: Severe factor VII deficiency due to a mutation disrupting a hepatocyte nuclear factor 4 binding site in the factor VII promoter. *Blood* 89:176, 1997.

85. Carew JA, Pollak ES, High KA, Bauer KA: Severe factor VII deficiency due to a mutation disrupting an Ap1 binding site in the factor VII promoter. *Blood* 92:1639, 1998.

86. Seligsohn U, Shani M, Ramot B, et al: Dubin-Johnson syndrome in Israel: II. Association with factor VII deficiency. *Q J Med* 39:569, 1970.

87. Paulusma CC, Kool M, Bosma PJ, et al: A mutation in the human canalicular multispecific organic anion transporter gene causes the Dubin-Johnson syndrome. *Hepatolology* 25:1539, 1997.

88. Van Kuijck MA, Kool M, Merkx GF, et al: Assignment of the canalicular multispecific organic anion transporter gene (CMOAT) to human chromosome 10q24 and mouse chromosome 19D2 by fluorescent in situ hybridization. *Cytogenet Cell Genet* 77:285, 1997.

89. Meade TW, Mellows S, Brozovic M, et al: Haemostatic function and ischaemic heart disease: Principal results of the Northwick Park Heart Study. *Lancet* 2:533, 1986.

90. Ruddock V, Meade TW: Factor-VII activity and ischaemic heart disease: Fatal and non-fatal events. *Q J Med* 87:403, 1994.

91. Hunault M, Arbini AA, Lopaciuk S, et al: The Arg[353] Gln polymorphism reduces the level of coagulation factor VII: In vivo and in vitro studies. *Arterioscler Thromb Vasc Biol* 17:2825, 1997.

92. Green F, Kelleher C, Wilkes H, et al: A common genetic polymorphism associated with lower coagulation factor VII levels in healthy individuals. *Arterioscler Thromb* 11:540, 1991.

93. Bernardi F, Marchetti G, Pinotti M, et al: Factor VII gene polymorphisms contribute about one-third of the factor VII level variation in plasma. *Arterioscler Thromb Vasc Biol* 16:72, 1996.

94. Kario K, Narita N, Matsuo T, et al: Genetic determinants of plasma factor VII activity in the Japanese. *Thromb Haemost* 73:617, 1995.

95. Lane A, Cruickshank JK, Mitchell J, et al: Genetic and environmental determinants of factor VII coagulant activity in ethnic groups at differing risk of coronary heart disease. *Atherosclerosis* 94:43, 1992.

96. Ia coviello L, Di Castelnuovo A, DeKnijff P, et al: Polymorphisms in the coagulation factor VII gene and the risk of myocardial infarction. *N Engl J Med* 338:79, 1998.

97. Saha N, Liu Y, Hong CK, et al: Association of factor VII genotype with plasma factor VII activity and antigen levels in healthy Indian adults and interaction with triglycerides. *Arterioscler Thromb* 14:1923, 1994.

98. Bernardi F, Arcieri P, Bertina RM, et al: Contribution of factor VII genotype to activated FVII levels: Differences in genotype frequencies between northern and southern European populations. *Arterioscler Thromb Vasc Biol* 17:2548, 1997.

99. Lane A, Green F, Scarabin PY, et al: Factor VII Arg/Gln353 polymorphism determines factor VII coagulant activity in patients with myocardial infarction (MI) and control subjects in Belfast and in France but is not a strong indicator of MI risk in the ECTIM study. *Atherosclerosis* 119:119, 1996.

100. Doggen CJ, Manger C, Bertina RM, et al: A genetic propensity to high factor VII is not associated with the risk of myocardial infarction in men. *Thromb Haemost* 80:281, 1998.

101. Miller GJ: Effects of diet composition on coagulation pathways. *Am J Clin Nutr* 67(suppl 3):542S, 1998.

102. Hoffman CJ, Miller RH, Hultin MB: Correlation of factor VII activity and antigen with cholesterol and triglycerides in healthy young adults. *Arterioscler Thromb* 12:267, 1992.

103. Balleisen L, Assmann G, Bailey J, et al: Epidemiological study on factor VII, factor VIII and fibrinogen in an industrial population: II. Baseline data on the relation to blood pressure, blood glucose, uric acid, and lipid fractions. *Thromb Haemost* 54:721, 1985.

104. Folsom AR, Wu KK, Davis CE, et al: Population correlates of plasma fibrinogen and factor VII, putative cardiovascular risk factors. *Atherosclerosis* 91:191, 1991.

105. Marchetti G, Gemmati D, Patracchini P, et al: PCR detection of a repeat polymorphism within the F7 gene. *Nucleic Acids Res* 19:4570, 1991.

106. Hall CA, Rapaport SI, Ames SB, et al: A clinical and family study of hereditary proconvertin (factor VII) deficiency. *Am J Med* 37:172, 1964.

107. Mariani G, Mazzucconi MG: Factor VII congenital deficiency: Clinical picture and classification of the variants. *Haemostasis* 13:169, 1983.

108. Ragni MV, Lewis JH, Spero JA, Hasiba U: Factor VII deficiency. *Am J Hematol* 10:79, 1981.

109. de Moerloose P, Amiral J, Vissac AM, Reber G: Longitudinal study on activated factors XII and VII levels during normal pregnancy. *Br J Haematol* 100:40, 1998.

110. Seligsohn U, Peyser MR, Toaff R, et al: Severe hereditary deficiency of factor VII during pregnancy: Evidence for the absence of transplacental diffusion of factor VII. *Thromb Diath Haemorrh* 24:146, 1970.

111. Robertson LE, Wasserstrum N, Banez E, et al: Hereditary factor VII deficiency in pregnancy: Peripartum treatment with factor VII concentrate. *Am J Hematol* 40:38, 1992.

112. Delmer A, Horellou MH, Andreu G, et al: Life-threatening intracranial bleeding associated with the presence of an antifactor VII autoantibody. *Blood* 74:229, 1989.

113. Solanki DL, Corn M: Thromboembolism in patients with hereditary deficiency of coagulation factors. *South Med J* 73:944, 1980.

114. Philippou H, Adami A, Amersey RA, et al: A novel specific immunoas-

say for plasma two-chain factor VIIa: Investigation of FVIIa levels in normal individuals and in patients with acute coronary syndromes. *Blood* 89:767, 1997.

115. Mariani G, Hermans J, Orlando M, et al: Carrier detection in factor VII congenital deficiency. *Br J Haematol* 60:687, 1985.

116. Boxus G, Slacmeulder M, Ninane J: Combined hereditary deficiency in factors VII and X revealed by a prolonged partial thromboplastin time. *Arch Pediatr* 4:44, 1997.

117. Hall C, London AR, Moynihan AC, Dodds WJ: Hereditary factor VII and IX deficiencies in a large kindred. *Br J Haematol* 29:319, 1975.

118. Briet E, Onvlee G: Hip surgery in a patient with severe factor VII deficiency. *Haemostasis* 17:273, 1987.

119. Cederbaum AI, Blatt PM, Roberts HR: Intravascular coagulation with use of human prothrombin complex concentrates. *Ann Intern Med* 84:683, 1976.

120. Rivard GE, Kovac I, Kunschak M, Thone P: Clinical study of recovery and half-life of vapor-heated factor VII concentrate. *Transfusion* 34:975, 1994.

121. Eikenboom JC, Bos CF, Briet E: Peri-operative replacement therapy with factor VII concentrate in a patient with severe factor VII deficiency. *Thromb Haemost* 67:285, 1992.

122. Cohen LJ, McWilliams NB, Neuberg R, et al: Prophylaxis and therapy with factor VII concentrate (human) immuno, vapor heated in patients with congenital factor VII deficiency: A summary of case reports. *Am J Hematol* 50:269, 1995.

123. Ingerslev J, Knudsen L, Hvid I, et al: Use of recombinant factor VIIa in surgery in factor-VII-deficient patients. *Haemophilia* 3:215, 1997.

124. Telfer TP, Denson KW, Wright DW: A "new" coagulation defect. *Br J Haematol* 2:308, 1956.

125. Hougie C, Barrow EM, Graham JB: Stuart clotting defect: I. Segregation of an hereditary hemorrhagic state from the heterogenous group heretofore called "stable factor" (SPCA, proconvertin, factor VII) deficiency. *J Clin Invest* 36:485, 1957.

126. Scambler PJ, Williamson R: The structural gene for human coagulation factor X is located on chromosome 13q34. *Cytogenet Cell Genet* 39:231, 1985.

127. Royle NJ, Fung MR, McGillivray RT, Hamerton JL: The gene for clotting factor 10 is mapped to 13q32-qter. *Cytogenet Cell Genet* 41:185, 1986.

128. Leytus SP, Foster DC, Kurachi K, Davie EW: Gene for human factor X: A blood coagulation factor whose gene organization is essentially identical with that of factor IX and protein C. *Biochemistry* 25:5098, 1986.

129. Neurath H: Evolution of proteolytic enzymes. *Science* 224:350, 1984.

130. McMullen BA, Fujikawa K, Kisiel W, et al: Complete amino acid sequence of the light chain of human blood coagulation factor X: Evidence for identification of residue 63 as beta-hydroxyaspartic acid. *Biochemistry* 22:2875, 1983.

131. Jackson CM: Characterization of two glycoprotein variants of bovine factor X and demonstration that the factor X zymogen contains two polypeptide chains. *Biochemistry* 11:4873, 1972.

132. Fujikawa K, Coan MH, Legaz ME, Davie EW: The mechanism of activation of bovine factor X (Stuart factor) by intrinsic and extrinsic pathways. *Biochemistry* 13:5290, 1974.

133. Fujikawa K, Legaz ME, Davie EW: Bovine factor X (Stuart factor): Mechanism of activation by protein from Russell's viper venom. *Biochemistry* 11:4892, 1972.

134. Bernardi F, Marchetti G, Patracchini P, et al: Partial gene deletion in a family with factor X deficiency. *Blood* 73:2123, 1989.

135. Wieland K, Millar DS, Grundy CB, et al: Molecular genetic analysis of factor X deficiency: Gene deletion and germline mosaicism. *Hum Genet* 86:273, 1991.

136. Reddy SV, Zhou ZQ, Rao KJ, et al: Molecular chatacterization of human factor X San Antonio. *Blood* 74:1486, 1989.

137. Racchi M, Watzke HH, High KA, Lively MO: Human coagulation factor X deficiency caused by a mutant signal peptide that blocks cleavage by signal peptidase but not targeting and translocation to the endoplasmic reticulum. *J Biol Chem* 268:5735, 1993.

138. Watzke HH, Wallmark A, Hamaguchi N, et al: Factor X Santo Domingo: Evidence that the severe clinical phenotype arises from a mutation blocking secretion. *J Clin Invest* 88:1685, 1991.

139. Rudolph AE, Mullane MP, Porche-Sorbet R, et al: Factor X St. Louis II. Identification of a glycine substitution at residue 7 and characterization of the recombinant protein. *J Biol Chem* 271:28601, 1996.

140. Watzke HH, Lechner K, Roberts HR, et al: Molecular defect (Gla+14-Lys) and its functional consequences in a hereditary factor X deficiency (factor X "Vorarlberg"). *J Biol Chem* 265:11982, 1990.

141. Kim DJ, Thompson AR, James HL: Factor X Ketchikan: A variant molecule in which Gly replaces a Gla residue at position 14 in the light chain. *Hum Genet* 95:212, 1995.

142. Marchetti G, Castaman G, Pinotti M, et al: Molecular bases of CRM+ factor X deficiency: A frequent mutation (Ser334Pro) in the catalytic domain and a substitution (Glu102Lys) in the second EGF-like domain. *Br J Haematol* 90:910, 1995.

143. Nobauer-Huhmann IM, Holler W, Krinninger B, et al: Molecular and functional characterization of a hereditary factor X deficiency (Gla+25 to Lys). *Blood Coag Fibrinol* 9:143, 1998.

144. Wallmark A, Larson P, Ljung R: Molecular defect (Gla26-Asp) and its functional consequences in a hereditary factor X deficiency (factor X "Malmö 4"). *Blood* 78:60a, 1991.

145. Kim DJ, Thompson AR, Nash DR, James HL: Factors X Wenatchee I and II: Compound heterozygosity involving two variant proteins. *Biochim Biophys Acta* 1271:327, 1995.

146. Wallmark A, Ho C, Monroe DM, et al: Molecular defect in F. X. "Öckerö," a mild congenital F. X. deficiency. *Thromb Haemost* 65:1263, 1991.

147. Messier TL, Wong CY, Bovill EG, et al: Factor X Stockton: A mild bleeding diathesis associated with an active site mutation in factor X. *Blood Coag Fibrinol* 7:5, 1996.

148. Cooper DN, Millar DS, Wacey A, et al: Inherited factor X deficiency: Molecular genetics and pathophysiology. *Thromb Haemost* 78:161, 1997.

149. De Stefano V, Leone G, Ferrelli R, et al: Factor X Roma: A congenital factor X variant defective at different degrees in the intrinsic and the extrinsic activation. *Br J Haematol* 69:387, 1988.

150. Girolami A, Molaro G, Lazzarin M, et al: A "new" congenital haemorrhagic condition due to the presence of an abnormal factor X (factor X Friuli): Study of a large kindred. *Br J Haematol* 19:179, 1970.

151. Watzke HH, Krinninger G, Lechner K, High KA: Molecular analysis and in vitro expression of a hereditary CRM-negative factor X variant: FX Vienna. *Blood* 80(suppl 1):365a, 1992.

152. Odom MW, Leone G, De Stefano V, et al: Five novel point mutations: two causing haemophilia B and three causing factor X deficiency. *Mol Cell Probes* 8:63, 1994.

153. Peyvandi F, Mannucci PM, Lak M, et al: Congenital factor X deficiency: Spectrum of bleeding symptoms in 32 Iranian patients. *Br J Haematol* 102:626, 1998.

154. Howell M: Acquired factor X deficiency associated with systemic amyloidosis: A report of a case. *Blood* 21:739, 1963.

155. Furie B, Greene E, Furie BC: Syndrome of acquired factor X deficiency and systemic amyloidosis: In vivo studies of the metabolic fate of factor X. *N Engl J Med* 297:81, 1977.

156. Furie B, Voo L, McAdam KP, Furie BC: Mechanism of factor X deficiency in systemic amyloidosis. *N Engl J Med* 304:827, 1981.

157. Fair DS, Edgington TS: Heterogeneity of hereditary and acquired factor X deficiencies by combined immunochemical and functional analyses. *Br J Haematol* 59:235, 1985.

158. Rao LV, Zivelin A, Iturbe I, Rapaport SI: Antibody-induced acute factor X deficiency: Clinical manifestations and properties of the antibody. *Thromb Haemost* 72:363, 1994.

159. Blatt PM, Lundblad RL, Kingdon HS, et al: Thrombogenic materials in prothrombin complex concentrates. *Ann Intern Med* 81:766, 1974.

160. Biggs R, Denson KWE: The fate of prothrombin and factors VII, IX, and X tansfused to patients deficient in these factors. *Br J Haematol* 9:532, 1963.

161. Roberts HR, Lechler E, Webster WP, Penick GD: Survival of transfused factor X in patients with Stuart disease. *Thromb Diath Haemorrh* 18:305, 1965.

162. McMillan CW, Roberts HR: Congenital combined deficiency of coagulation factors II, VII, IX and X: Report of a case. *N Engl J Med* 274:1313, 1966.

163. Samama M, Bertina RM, Conard J, Horellou MH: Combined congenital deficiency in protein C and in factors II, VII, IX, and X. *Thromb Haemost* 50:359, 1983.

164. Brenner B, Tavori S, Zivelin A, et al: Hereditary deficiency of all vitamin K–dependent procoagulants and anticoagulants. *Br J Haematol* 75:537, 1990.

165. Chung KS, Bezeaud A, Goldsmith JC, et al: Congenital deficiency of blood clotting factors II, VII, IX, and X. *Blood* 53:776, 1979.

166. Brenner B, Sanchez-Vega B, Wu SM, et al: A missense mutation in gamma-glutamyl carboxylase gene causes combined deficiency of all vitamin K–dependent blood coagulation factors. *Blood* 92:4554, 1998.

167. Goldsmith GH, Pence RE, Ratnoff OD, et al: Studies on a family with combined deficiencies of vitamin K–dependent coagulation factors. *J Clin Invest* 69:1253, 1982.

168. Owren PA: Parahemophilia: Hemorrhagic diathesis due to absence of a previously unknown factor. *Lancet* 1:446, 1947.

169. Tracy PB, Mann KG: Abnormal formation of the prothrombinase complex: Factor V deficiency and related disorders. *Hum Pathol* 18:162, 1987.

170. Kane WH, Davie EW: Blood coagulation factors V and VIII: Structural and functional similarities and their relationship to hemorrhagic and thrombotic disorders. *Blood* 71:539, 1988.

171. Cripe LD, Moore KD, Kane WH: Structure of the gene for human coagulation factor V. *Biochemistry* 31:3777, 1992.

172. Wang H, Riddell DC, Guinto ER, et al: Localization of the gene encoding human factor V to chromosome 1q21-25. *Genomics* 2:324, 1988.

173. Suzuki K, Dahlback B, Stenflo J: Thrombin-catalyzed activation of human coagulation factor V. *J Biol Chem* 257:6556, 1982.

174. Foster WB, Nesheim ME, Mann KG: The factor Xa-catalyzed activation of factor V. *J Biol Chem* 258:13970, 1983.

175. Wilson DB, Salem HH, Mruk JS, et al: Biosynthesis of coagulation factor V by human hepatocellular carcinoma cell line. *J Clin Invest* 73:654, 1983.

176. Gewirtz AM, Keefer M, Doshi K, et al: Biology of human megakaryocyte factor V. *Blood* 67:1639, 1986.

177. Tracy PB, Eide LL, Bowie EJ, Mann KG: Radioimmunoassay of factor V in human plasma and platelets. *Blood* 60:59, 1982.

178. Seeler RA: Parahemophilia: Factor V deficiency. *Med Clin North Am* 56:119, 1972.

179. Viskup RW, Tracy PB, Mann KG: The isolation of human platelet factor V. *Blood* 69:1188, 1987.

180. Hayward CP, Furmaniak-Kazmierczak E, Cieutat AM, et al: Factor V is complexed with multimerin in resting platelet lysates and colocalizes with multimerin in platelet alpha-granules. *J Biol Chem* 270:19217, 1995.

181. Hayward CP, Rivard GE, Kane WH, et al: An autosomal dominant, qualitative platelet disorder associated with multimerin deficiency, abnormalities in platelet factor V, thrombospondin, von Willebrand factor, and fibrinogen and an epinephrine aggregation defect. *Blood* 87:4967, 1996.

182. Janeway CM, Rivard GE, Tracy PB, Mann KG: Factor V Quebec revisited. *Blood* 87:3571, 1996.

183. Suzuki K, Stenflo J, Dahlback B, Teodorsson B: Inactivation of human coagulation factor V by activated protein C. *J Biol Chem* 258:1914, 1983.

184. Nesheim ME, Canfield WM, Kisiel W, Mann KG: Studies of the capacity of factor Xa to protect factor Va from inactivation by activated protein C. *J Biol Chem* 257:1443, 1982.

185. Mitterstieler G, Muller W, Geir W: Congenital factor V deficiency: A family study. *Scand J Haematol* 21:9, 1978.

186. Chiu HC, Whitaker E, Colman RW: Heterogeneity of human factor V deficiency: Evidence for the existence of antigen-positive variants. *J Clin Invest* 72:493, 1983.

187. Murray JM, Rand MD, Egan JO, et al: Factor V New Brunswick: Ala221-to-Val substitution results in reduced cofactor activity. *Blood* 86:1820, 1995.

188. Guasch JF, Lensen RP, Bertina RM: Molecular characterization of a type I quantitative factor V deficiency in a thrombosis patient that is "pseudohomozygous" for activated protein C resistance. *Thromb Haemost* 77:252, 1997.

189. Guasch JF, Cannegieter S, Reitsma PH, et al: Severe coagulation factor V deficiency caused by a 4 bp deletion in the factor V gene. *Br J Haematol* 101:32, 1998.

190. Simioni P, Scudeller A, Radossi P, et al: "Pseudohomozygous" activated protein C resistance due to double heterozygous factor V defects (factor V Leiden mutation and type I quantitative factor V defect)

191. associated with thrombosis: Report of two cases belonging to two unrelated kindreds. *Thromb Haemost* 75:422, 1996.

191. Zehnder JL, Jain M: Recurrent thrombosis due to compound heterozygosity for factor V Leiden and factor V deficiency. *Blood Coag Fibrinol* 7:361, 1996.

192. Girolami A, Simioni P, Venturelli U, et al: Factor V antigen levels in APC resistance, in factor V deficiency and in combined APC resistance and factor V deficiency (pseudohomozygosis for APC resistance). *Blood Coag Fibrinol* 8:245, 1997.

193. Delahousse B, Iochmann S, Pouplard C, et al: Pseudo-homozygous activated protein C resistance due to coinheritance of heterozygous factor V Leiden mutation and type I factor V deficiency: Variable expression when analyzed by different activated protein C resistance functional assays. *Blood Coag Fibrinol* 8:503, 1997.

194. Lunghi B, Iacoviello L, Gemmati D, et al: Detection of new polymorphic markers in the factor V gene: Association with factor V levels in plasma. *Thromb Haemost* 75:45, 1996.

195. Tracy PB, Giles AR, Mann KG, et al: Factor V (Quebec): A bleeding diathesis associated with a qualitative platelet factor V deficiency. *J Clin Invest* 74:1221, 1984.

196. Hayward CP, Cramer EM, Kane WH, et al: Studies of a second family with the Quebec platelet disorder: Evidence that the degradation of the alpha-granule membrane and its soluble contents are not secondary to a defect in targeting proteins to alpha-granules. *Blood* 89:1243, 1997.

197. Cui J, O'Shea KS, Purkayastha A, et al: Fatal haemorrhage and incomplete block to embryogenesis in mice lacking coagulation factor V. *Nature* 384:66, 1996.

198. Yoon SG, Cho ST, Park SK, et al: A case of coagulation factor V deficiency complicated with intracranial hemorrhage. *Korean J Intern Med* 12:80:1997.

199. Miller SP: Coagulation dynamic in factor V deficiency: A family study with a note on the occurrence of thrombophlebitis. *Thromb Diath Haemorrh* 13:500, 1965.

200. Reich NE, Hoffman GC, de Wolfe VG, Van Ordstrand HS: Recurrent thrombophlebitis and pulmonary emboli in congenital factor 5 deficiency. *Chest* 69:113, 1976.

201. Manotti C, Quintavalla R, Pini M, et al: Thromboembolic manifestations and congenital factor V deficiency: A family study. *Haemostasis* 19:331, 1989.

202. Goodnough LT, Saito H, Ratnoff OD: Thrombosis or myocardial infarction in congenital clotting factor abnormalities and chronic thormbocytopenias: A report of 21 patients and a review of 50 previously reported cases. *Medicine (Baltimore)* 62:248, 1983.

203. Feinstein DI: Acquired inhibitors of factor V. *Thromb Haemost* 39:663, 1978.

204. Nesheim ME, Nichols WL, Cole TL, et al: Isolation and study of an acquired inhibitor of human coagulation factor V. *J Clin Invest* 77:405, 1986.

205. Bryning K, Leslie J: Factor V inhibitor and bullous pemphigoid. *Br Med J* 2:677, 1977.

206. Coots MC, Muhleman AF, Glueck HI: Hemorrhagic death associated with a high titer factor V inhibitor. *Am J Hematol* 4:193, 1978.

207. Fratantoni JC, Hilgartner M, Nachman RL: Nature of the defect in congenital factor V deficiency: Study in a patient with an acquired circulating anticoagulant. *Blood* 39:751, 1972.

208. Mazzucconi MG, Solinas S, Chistolini A, et al: Inhibitor to factor V in severe factor V congenital deficiency: A case report. *Nouv Rev Fr Hematol* 27:303, 1985.

209. Stricker RB, Lane PK, Leffert JD, et al: Development of antithrombin antibodies following surgery in patients with prosthetic cardiac valves. *Blood* 72:1375, 1988.

210. Zehnder JL, Leung LL: Development of antibodies to thrombin and factor V with recurrent bleeding in a patient exposed to topical bovine thrombin. *Blood* 76:2011, 1990.

211. Rapaport SI, Zivelin A, Minow RA, et al: Clinical significance of antibodies to bovine and human thrombin and factor V after surgical use of bovine thrombin. *Am J Clin Pathol* 97:84, 1992.

212. Ortel TL, Charles LA, Keller FG, et al: Topical thrombin and acquired coagulation factor inhibitors: Clinical spectrum and laboratory diagnosis. *Am J Hematol* 45:128, 1994.

213. Ortel TL, Moore KD, Quinn-Allen MA, et al: Inhibitory anti-factor V

antibodies bind to the factor V C2 domain and are associated with hemorrhagic manifestations. *Blood* 91:4188, 1998.

214. Ortel TL, Devore-Carter D, Quinn-Allen MA, Kane WH: Deletion analysis of recombinant human factor V: Evidence for a phosphatidylserine binding site in the second C-type domain. *J Biol Chem* 267:4189, 1992.

215. Webster WP, Roberts HR, Penick GD: Hemostasis in factor V deficiency. *Am J Med* Sci248:194, 1964.

216. Tanis BC, van der Meer FJ, Bloem RM, Vlasveld LT: Successful excision of a pseudotumour in a congenitally factor V deficient patient. *Br J Haematol* 100:380, 1998.

217. Chediak J, Ashenhurst JB, Garlick I, Desser RK: Successful management of bleeding in a patient with factor V inhibitor by platelet transfusion. *Blood* 56:835, 1980.

218. Smid WM, de Wolf JT, Nijland JH, et al: Severe bleeding caused by an inhibitor to coagulation factor V: A case report. *Blood Coag Fibrinol* 5:133, 1994.

219. Fu YX, Kaufman R, Rudolph AE, et al: Multimodality therapy of an acquired factor V inhibitor. *Am J Hematol* 51:315, 1996.

220. Oeri J, Matter M, Isenschmid H, et al: Angeborener Mangel an Faktor V (Parahaemophilie) verbunden mit echter Haemophilie A bein zwei Brudern. *Med Probl Paediatr* 1:575, 1954.

221. Seligsohn U, Zivelin A, Zwang E: Combined factor V and factor VIII deficiency among non-Ashkenazi Jews. *N Engl J Med* 307:1191, 1982.

222. Seligsohn U: Combined factor V and factor VIII deficiency, in *Factor VIII: Von Willebrand Factor*, vol 2, edited by J Seghatchian, GT Savidge, p 89. CRC Press, Boca Raton, FL, 1989.

223. Nichols WC, Seligsohn U, Zivelin A, et al: Mutations in the ER-Golgi intermediate compartment protein ERGIC-53 cause combined deficiency of coagulation factors V and VIII. *Cell* 93:61, 1998.

224. Peyvandi F, Tuddenham EG, Akhtari AM, et al: Bleeding symptoms in 27 Iranian patients with the combined deficiency of factor V and factor VIII. *Br J Haematol* 100:773, 1998.

225. Wilson DB, Salem HH, Mruk JS, et al: Biosynthesis of coagulation factor V by a human hepatocellular carcinoma cell line. *J Clin Invest* 73:654, 1984.

226. Wion Kl, Kelly D, Summerfield JA: Distribution of factor VIII mRNA and antigen in human liver and other tissues. *Nature* 317:726, 1985.

227. Wang H, Riddell DC, Guinto ER, et al: Localization of the gene encoding human factor V to chromosome 1q21-25. *Genomics* 2:324, 1988.

228. Gitschier J, Wood WI, Goralka TM, et al: Characterization of the human factor VIII gene. *Nature* 312:326, 1984.

229. Seligsohn U, Ramot B: Combined factor-V and factor-VIII deficiency: Report of four cases. *Br J Haematol* 16:475, 1969.

230. Saito H, Katsumi O: Congenital combined deficiency of factor V and factor VIII: A case report and the effect of transfusion of normal plasma and hemophilic blood. *Thromb Diath Haemorrh* 22:316, 1969.

231. Marlar RA, Griffin JH: Deficiency of protein C inhibitor in combined factor V/VIII deficiency disease. *J Clin Invest* 66:1186, 1980.

232. Canfield MW, Kisiel W: Evidence of normal functional levels of activated protein C inhibitor in combined factor V/VIII deficiency disease. *J Clin Invest* 70:1260, 1982.

233. Susuki K, Nishioka J, Hashimoto S, et al: Normal titer of functional and immunoreactive protein-C inhibitor in plasma of patients with congenital combined deficiency of factor V and factor VIII. *Blood* 62:1266, 1983.

234. Seligsohn U, Zivelin A, Zwang E: Decreased factor VIII clotting antigen levels in the combined factor V and VIII deficiency. *Thromb Res* 33:95, 1984.

235. Tracy PB, Mann KG: Abnormal formation of the prothrombinase complex: Factor V deficiency and related disorders. *Hum Pathol* 18:162, 1987.

236. Hultin MB, Eyster ME: Combined factor V-VIII deficiency: A case report with studies of factor V and VIII activation by thrombin. *Blood* 58:1103, 1981.

237. Nichols WC, Seligsohn U, Zivelin A, et al: Linkage of combined factors V and VIII deficiency to chromosome 18q by homozygosity mapping. *J Clin Invest* 99:596, 1997.

238. Neerman-Arbez M, Antonarakis SE, Blouin JL, et al: The locus for combined factor V-factor VIII deficiency (F5F8D) maps to 18q21, between D18S849 and D18S1103. *Am J Hum Genet* 61:143, 1997.

239. Schindler R, Itin C, Zerial M, et al: ERGIC-53, a membrane protein of the ER-Golgi intermediate compartment, carries an ER retention motif. *Eur J Cell Biol* 61:1, 1993.

240. Schweizer A, Fransen JA, Bachi T, et al: Identification, by a monoclonal antibody, of a 53-kD protein associated with a tubulo-vesicular compartment at the *cis*-side of the Golgi apparatus. *J Cell Biol* 107:1643, 1988.

241. Kappeler F, Klopfenstein DR, Foguet M, et al: The recycling of ERGIC-53 in the early secretory pathway: ERGIC-53 carries a cytosolic endoplasmic reticulum-exit determinant interacting with COPII. *J Biol Chem* 272:31801, 1997.

242. Itin C, Roche AC, Monsigny M, Hauri HP: ERGIC-53 is a functional mannose-selective and calcium-dependent human homologue of leguminous lectins. *Mol Biol* Cell 7:483, 1996.

243. Moussalli M, Pile SW, Nichols WC, et al: Mistargeting of the lectin ERGIC-53 to the endoplasmic reticulum impairs the secretion of coagulation factors V and VIII. *Blood* 92:474a, 1998.

244. Nichols WC, Terry VH, Matthew MA, et al: ERGIC-53 gene structure and mutation analysis in 19 combined factors V and VIII deficiency families. *Blood* 93:2261, 1999.

245. Soff GA, Levin J, Bell WR: Familial multiple coagulation factor deficiencies: I. Review of the literature: Differentiation of single hereditary disorders associated with multiple factor deficiencies from coincidental concurrence of single factor deficiency state. *Semin Thromb Hemost* 7:112, 1981.

246. Gobbi F: Heredity of combined deficiency of AHG and proaccelerin. *Scand J Haematol* 3:222, 1966.

247. Girolami A, Gastaldi G, Patrassi G, Galletti A: Combined congenital deficiency of factor V and factor VIII: Report of a further case with some considerations on the hereditary transmission of this disorder. *Acta Haematol* 55:234, 1976.

248. Mazzone D, Fichera A, Pratico G, Sciacca F: Combined congenital deficiency of factor V and factor VIII. *Acta Haematol* 68:337, 1982.

249. Bartlett JA, Sweeney JD, Sadowsky D: Exodontia in combined factor V and factor VIII deficiency. *J Oral Maxillofac Surg* 43:537, 1985.

250. Tsurumi H, Takahashi T, Moriwaki H, Muto Y: Congenital combined deficiency of factor V and factor VIII with acquired ichthyosis, epidermodysplasia verruciformis, and immunological abnormalities. *Am J Hematol* 40:320, 1992.

251. Neerman-Arbez M, Johnson KM, Morris MA, et al: Molecular analysis of the ERGIC-53 gene in 35 families with combined factor V-factor VIII deficiency (F5F8D). *Blood* 93:2253, 1999.

252. Fischer RR, Giddings JC, Roisenberg I: Hereditary combined deficiency of clotting factors V and VIII with involvement of von Willebrand factor. *Clin Lab Haematol* 10:53, 1988.

253. Sallah AS, Angchaisuksiri P, Roberts HR: Use of plasma exchange in hereditary deficiency of factor V and factor VIII. *Am J Hematol* 52:229, 1996.

254. Rosenthal RL, Dreskin OH, Rosenthal N: A new hemophilia like disease caused by deficiency of a third plasma thromboplastin factor. *Proc Soc Exp Biol Med* 82:171, 1953.

255. Rapaport SI, Proctor RR, Patch NJ, Yettra M: The mode of inheritance of PTA deficiency: Evidence for the existence of major PTA deficiency and minor PTA deficiency. *Blood* 18:149, 1961.

256. Seligsohn U: High gene frequency of factor XI (PTA) deficiency in Ashkenazi-Jews. *Blood* 51:1223, 1978.

257. Gailani D, Broze GJ Jr: Factor XI activation in a revised model of blood coagulation. *Science* 253:909, 1991.

258. Naito K, Fujikawa K: Activation of human blood coagulation factor XI independent of factor XII: Factor XI is activated by thrombin and factor XIa in the presence of negatively charged surfaces. *J Biol Chem* 266:7353, 1991.

259. McMullen BA, Fujikawa K, Davie EW: Location of the disulfide bonds in human coagulation factor XI: The presence of tandem apple domains. *Biochemistry* 30:2056, 1991.

260. Meijers JCM, Mulvihill ER, Davie EW, Chung DW: Apple four in human blood coagulation factor XI mediates dimer formation. *Biochemistry* 31: 4680, 1992.

261. Seaman FS, Baglia FA, Gurr JA, et al: Binding of high-molecular-mass kininogen to the apple 1 domain of factor XI is mediated in part by Val64 and Ile77. *Biochem J* 304:715, 1994.

262. Asakai R, Davie EW, Chung DW: Organization of the gene for human factor XI. *Biochemistry* 26:7221, 1987.

263. Kato A, Asakai R, Davie EW, Aoki N: Factor XI gene (F11) is located on the distal end of the long arm of human chromosome 4. *Cytogenet Cell Genet* 52:77, 1989.

264. Bouma BN, Griffin JH: Human blood coagulation factor XI: Purification, properties, and mechanism of activation by activated factor XII. *J Biol Chem* 252:6432, 1977.

265. Von dem Borne PA, Koppelman SJ, Bouma BN, Meijers JC: Surface independent factor XI activation by thrombin in the presence of high molecular weight kininogen. *Thromb Haemost* 72:397, 1994.

266. Von dem Borne PA, Meijers JC, Bouma BN: Effect of heparin on the activation of factor XI by fibrin-bound thrombin. *Thromb Haemost* 76:347, 1996.

267. Osterud B, Bouma BN, Griffin JH: Human blood coagulation factor IX: Purification, properties, and mechanism of activation by activated factor XI. *J Biol Chem* 253:5946, 1978.

268. Hendriks D, Wang W, Scharpe S, et al: Purification and characterization of a new arginine carboxypeptidase in human serum. *Biochem Biophys Acta* 1034:86, 1990.

269. Eaton DL, Malloy BE, Tsai SP, et al: Isolation, molecular cloning, and partial characterization of a novel carboxypeptidase B from human plasma. *J Biol Chem* 266:21833, 1991.

270. Bajzar L, Manuel R, Nesheim ME: Purification and characterization of TAFI, a thrombin-activatable fibrinolysis inhibitor. *J Biol Chem* 270:14477, 1995.

271. Nesheim M, Wang W, Boffa M, et al: Thrombin, thrombomodulin and TAFI in the molecular link between coagulation and fibrinolysis. *Thromb Haemost* 78:386, 1997.

272. Bajzar L, Morser J, Nesheim M: TAFI, or plasma procarboxypeptidase B, couples the coagulation and fibrinolytic cascades through the thrombin-thrombomodulin complex. *J Biol Chem* 271:16603, 1996.

273. Broze GJ Jr, Higuchi DA: Coagulation-dependent inhibition of fibrinolysis: Role of carboxypeptidase-U and the premature lysis of clots from hemophilic plasma. *Blood* 88:3815, 1996.

274. Von dem Borne PA, Meijers JC, Bouma BN: Feedback activation of factor XI by thrombin in plasma results in additional formation of thrombin that protects fibrin clots from fibrinolysis. *Blood* 86:3035, 1995.

275. Von dem Borne PA, Bajzar L, Meijers JC, et al: Thrombin-mediated activation of factor XI results in a thormbin-activatable fibrinolysis inhibitor-dependent inhibition of fibrinolysis. *J Clin Invest* 99:2323, 1997.

276. Minnema MC, Friederich PW, Levi M, et al: Enhancement of rabbit jugular vein thombolysis by neutralization of factor XI: In vivo evidence for a role of factor XI as an anti-fibrinolytic factor. *J Clin Invest* 101:10, 1998.

277. Asakai R, Chung DW, Davie EW, Seligsohn U: Factor XI deficiency in Ashkenazi Jews in Israel. *N Engl J Med* 325:153, 1991.

278. Berliner S, Horowitz I, Martinowitz U, et al: Dental surgery in patients with severe factor XI deficiency without plasma replacement. *Blood Coag Fibrinol* 3:465, 1992.

279. Clarkson K, Rosenfeld B, Fair J, et al: Factor XI deficiency acquired by liver transplantation. *Ann Intern Med* 115:877, 1991.

280. Hu CJ, Baglia FA, Mills DC, et al: Tissue-specific expression of functional platelet factor XI is independent of plasma factor XI expression. *Blood* 91:3800, 1998.

281. Martincic D, Kravtsov V, Gailani D: Factor XI messenger RNA in human platelets. *Blood* 94:3397, 1999.

282. Bolton-Maggs PH, Young Wan-Yin B, McCraw AH, et al: Inheritance and bleeding in factor XI deficiency. *Br J Haematol* 69:521, 1988.

283. Saito H, Ratnoff OD, Bouma BN, Seligsohn U: Failure to detect variant (CRM+) plasma thromboplastin antecedent (factor XI) molecules in hereditary plasma thromboplastin antecedent deficiency: A study of 125 patients of several ethnic backgrounds. *J Lab Clin Med* 106:718, 1985.

284. Mannhalter C, Hellstern P, Deutsch E: Identification of a defective factor XI cross-reacting material in a factor XI-deficient patient. *Blood* 70:31, 1987.

285. Hayashi T, Satoh S, Suzuki K, et al: Cross-reacting material positive (CRM+) factor XI deficiency, XI Yamagata, with a GT→AT transition at donor splicing site of an intron J of the factor XI gene. *Thromb Haemost* suppl 77:1883a, 1997.

286. Asakai R, Chung DW, Ratnoff OD, Davie EW: Factor XI (plasma thromboplastin antecedent) deficiency in Ashkenazi Jews is a bleeding disorder that can result from three types of point mutations. *Proc Natl Acad Sci USA* 86:7667, 1989.

287. Peretz H, Zivelin A, Usher S, Seligsohn U: A 14-bp deletion (codon

288. Pugh RE, McVey JH, Tuddenham EGD, Hancock JF: Six point mutations that cause factor XI deficiency. *Blood* 85:1509, 1995.

289. Ventura C, Santos AIM, Tavares A, et al: Molecular pathology of factor XI deficiency in the Portuguese population. *Thromb Haemost* suppl:859a, 1997.

290. Imanaka Y, Lal K, Nishimura T, et al: Identification of two novel mutations in non-Jewish factor XI deficiency. *Br J Haematol* 90:916, 1995.

291. Alhaq A, Mitchell MJ, Sethi M, et al: Identification of a novel mutation in a non-Jewish factor XI-deficient kindred. *Blood* 90:2075a, 1997.

292. Martincic D, Zimmerman SA, Ware RE, Gailani D: Identification of a mutation and polymorphisms in the factor XI gene of an African-American family by dideoxy fingerprinting. *Blood* 90:2076a, 1997.

293. Wistinghausen B, Reischer A, Oddoux C, et al: Severe factor XI deficiency in an Arab family associated with a novel mutation in exon 11. *Br J Haematol* 99:575, 1997.

294. McVey JH, Imanaka Y, Nishimura T, et al: Identification of a novel mechanism of human genetic disease: A missense mutation causing FXI deficiency through a change in mRNA stability. *Thromb Haemost* 73:2071a, 1995.

295. Meijers JC, Davie EW, Chung DW: Expression of human blood coagulation factor XI: Characterization of the defect in factor XI type III deficiency. *Blood* 79:1435, 1992.

296. Hancock JF, Wieland K, Pugh RE, et al: A molecular genetic study of factor XI deficiency. *Blood* 77:1942, 1991.

297. Bauduer F, Dupreuilh F, Ducout L, Marti B: Factor XI deficiency in the French Basque country. *Br J Haematol* 102:137a, 1998.

298. Awidi AS: Rare inherited bleeding disorders secondary to coagulation factors in Jordan: A nine-year study. *Acta Haematol* 88:11, 1992.

299. Shpilberg O, Peretz H, Zivelin A, et al: One of the two common mutations causing factor XI deficiency in Ashkenazi Jews (type II) is also prevalent in Iraqi Jews, who represent the ancient gene pool of Jews. *Blood* 85:429, 1995.

300. Peretz H, Mulai A, Usher S, et al: The two common mutations causing factor XI deficiency in Jews stem from distinct founders: One of ancient Middle Eastern origin and another of more recent European origin. *Blood* 90:2654, 1997.

301. Goldstein DB, Reich DE, Bradman N, et al: Age estimates of two common mutations causing factor XI deficiency: Recent genetic drift is not necessary for elevated disease incidence among Ashkenazi Jews. *Am J Hum Genet* 64:1071, 1999.

302. Bolton-Maggs PH, Patterson DA, Wensley RT, Tuddenham EG: Definition of the bleeding tendency in factor XI-deficient kindreds: A clinical and laboratory study. *Thromb Haemost* 73:194, 1995.

303. Brenner B, Laor A, Lupo H, et al: Bleeding predictors in factor-XI-deficient patients. *Blood Coag Fibrinol* 8:511, 1997.

304. Sidi A, Seligsohn U, Jonas P, Many M: Factor XI deficiency: Detection and management during urological surgery. *J Urol* 119:528, 1978.

305. Eikenboon JC, Rosendaal FR, Briet E: Value of the patient interview: All but consensus among haemostasis experts. *Haemostasis* 22:221, 1992.

306. Peter MK, Meili EO, von Felten A: Factor XI deficiency: Do patients with hemorrhagic diathesis also have hemostasis defects? *Shweiz Med Wochenschr* 126:999, 1996.

307. Goodnough LT, Saito H, Ratnoff OD: Thrombosis or myocardial infarction in congenital clotting factor abnormalities and chronic thrombocytopenias: A report of 21 patients and a review of 50 previously reported cases. *Medicine (Baltimore)* 62:248, 1983.

308. Brodsky JB, Burgess GE: Pulmonary embolism with factor XI deficiency. *JAMA* 534:1156, 1975.

309. Seligsohn U, Zitman D, Many A, Klibansky C: Coexistence of factor XI (plasma thromboplastin antecedent) deficiency and Gaucher's disease. *Isr J Med Sci* 12:1448, 1976.

310. Berrebi A, Malnick SD, Vorst EJ, Stein D: High incidence of factor XI deficiency in Gaucher's disease. *Am J Hematol* 40:153, 1992.

311. Billett HH, Rizvi S, Sawitsky A: Coagulation abnormalities in patients with Gaucher's disease: Effect of therapy. *Am J Hematol* 51:234, 1996.

312. Kitchens CS, Alexander JA: Partial deficiency of coagulation factor XI as a newly recognized feature of Noonan syndrome. *J Pediatr* 102:224, 1983.

554 del AAGgtaacagagtg) at exon 14/intron N junction of the coagulation factor XI gene disrupts splicing and causes severe factor XI deficiency. *Hum Mutat* 8:77, 1996.

313. Sharland M, Patton MA, Talbot S, et al: Coagulation-factor deficiencies and abnormal bleeding in Noonan's syndrome. *Lancet* 339:19, 1992.

314. Singer ST, Hurst D, Addiego JE Jr: Bleeding disorders in Noonan syndrome: Three case reports and review of the literature. *J Pediatr Hematol Oncol* 19:130, 1997.

315. Chediak J, Lambert E, Johnson EI, Telfer MC: Combined severe factor XI deficiency and von Willebrand's disease. *Am J Clin Pathol* 74:108, 1980.

316. Tavori S, Brenner B, Tatarsky I: The effect of combined factor XI deficiency with von Willebrand factor abnormalities on haemorrhagic diathesis. *Thromb Haemost* 63:36, 1990.

317. Lian EC, Deykin D, Harkness DR: Combined deficiencies of factor VIII (AHF) and factor XI (PTA). *Am J Hematol* 1:319, 1976.

318. Berg LP, Varon D, Martinowitz U, et al: Combined factor VII/factor VIII/factor XI deficiency may cause intra-familial clinical variability in haemophilia A among Ashkenazi Jews. *Blood Coag Fibrinol* 5:59, 1994.

319. Berube C, Ofosu FA, Kelton JG, Blajchman MA: A novel congenital haemostatic defect: Combined factor VII and factor XI deficiency. *Blood Coag Fibrinol* 3:357, 1992.

320. Josephson AM, Lisker R: Demonstration of a circulating anticoagulant in plasma thromboplastin antecedent deficiency. *J Clin Invest* 37:148, 1958.

321. Stern DM, Nossel HL, Owen J: Acquired antibody to factor XI in a patient with congenital factor XI deficiency. *J Clin Invest* 69:1270, 1982.

322. Morgan K, Schiffman S, Feinstein D: Acquired factor XI inhibitors in two patients with hereditary factor XI deficiency. *Thromb Haemost* 51:371, 1984.

323. Goldsmith GH Jr, Sliverman P: Inhibitors of plasma thormboplastin antecedent (factor XI): Studies on mechanism of inhibition. *J Lab Clin Med* 106:279, 1985.

324. Schnall SF, Duffy TP, Clyne LP: Acquired factor XI inhibitors in congenitally deficient patients. *Am J Hematol* 26:323, 1987.

325. De La Cadena RA, Baglia FA, Johnson CA, et al: Naturally occurring human antibodies against two distinct functional domains in the heavy chain of FXI/FXIa. *Blood* 2:1748, 1988.

326. Musclow CE, Amato D, Ofosu F, et al: Transfusion-induced specific anti-factor XI inhibitor in a patient with previously unrecognized factor XI deficiency. *Am J Pathol* 89:418, 1988.

327. Ginsberg SS, Clyne LP, McPhedran P, et al: Successful childbirth by a patient with congenital factor XI deficiency and an acquired inhibitor. *Br J Haematol* 84:172, 1993.

328. Connelly NR, Brull SJ: Anesthetic management of a patient with factor XI deficiency and factor XI inhibitor undergoing a cesarean section. *Anesth Analg* 76:1365, 1993.

329. Seligsohn U, Modan M: Definition of the population at risk of bleeding due to factor XI deficiency in Ashkenazic Jews and the value of activated partial thromboplastin time in its detection. *Isr J Med Sci* 17:413, 1981.

330. Bolton-Maggs PHB, Wensley RT, Kernoff PBA, et al: Production and therapeutic use of a factor XI concentrate from human plasma. *Thromb Haemost* 67:314, 1992.

331. Inbal A, Epstein O, Blickstein D, et al: Evaluation of solvent/detergent treated plasma in the management of patients with hereditary and acquired coagulation disorders. *Blood Coag Fibrinol* 4:599, 1993.

332. Seligsohn U: Factor XI deficiency. *Thromb Haemost* 70:68, 1993.

333. De Raucourt MH, Aurousseau MH, Denninger MH, et al: Use of a factor XI concentrate in three severe factor XI-deficient patients. *Blood Coag Fibrinol* 6:486, 1995.

334. Aledort LM, Forster A, Maksoud J, Isola L: BPL factor XI concentrate: Clinical experience in the USA. *Haemophilia* 3:59, 1997.

335. Mannucci PM, Bauer KA, Santagostino E, et al: Activation of the coagulation cascade after infusion of a factor XI concentrate in congenitally deficient patients. *Blood* 84:1314, 1994.

336. Richards EM, Makris MM, Cooper P, Preston FE: In vivo coagulation activation following infusion of highly purified factor XI concentrate. *Br J Haematol* 96:293, 1997.

337. Bolton-Maggs PHB, Colvin BT, Satchi G, et al: Thrombogenic potential of factor XI concentrate. *Lancet* 344:748, 1994.

338. Briggs N, Harman C, Dash CH: A decade of experience with factor XI concentrate. *Haemophilia* 2:14, 1996.

339. Castaman G, Ruggeri M, Rodeghiero F: Clinical usefulness of desmopressin for prevention of surgical bleeding in patients with symptomatic heterozygous factor XI deficiency. *Br J Haematol* 94:168, 1996.

340. Bauduer F, Bendriss P, Freyburger G, et al: Use of desmopressin for prophylaxis of surgical bleeding in factor XI-deficient patients. *Acta Haematol* 99:52, 1998.

341. Rakocz M, Mazar A, Varon D, et al: Dental extractions in patients with bleeding disorders. *Oral Surg Oral Med Oral Pathol* 75:280, 1993.

342. McKenna R, Cole ER, Jones P: Lack of bleeding after tonsillectomy in a patient with a specific factor XI inhibitor [abstract]. *Thromb Haemost* 65:1167, 1991.

343. Hedner U: Factor VIIa in the treatment of haemophilia. *Blood Coag Fibrinol* 1:307, 1990.

344. Duckert F, Jung E, Sherling DH: An undescribed congenital haemorrhagic diathesis probably due to fibrin stabilizing factor deficiency. *Thromb Diath Haemorrh* 5:179, 1960.

345. Chung SI, Lewis MS, Folk JE: Relationships of the catalytic properties of human plasma and platelet transglutaminases (activated blood coagulation factor XIII) to their subunit structures. *J Biol Chem* 249:940, 1974.

346. Gentile V, Saydak M, Chiocca EA, et al: Isolation and characterization of cDNA clones to mouse macrophage and human endothelial cell tissue transglutaminases. *J Biol Chem* 266:478, 1991.

347. Phillips MA, Stewart BE, Qin Q, et al: Primary structure of keratinocyte transglutaminase. *Proc Natl Acad Sci USA* 87:9333, 1990.

348. Sung LA, Chien S, Chang LS, et al: Molecular cloning of human protein 4.2: A major component of the erythrocyte membrane. *Proc Natl Acad Sci USA* 87:955, 1990.

349. Takagi T, Doolittle RF: Amino acid sequence studies on factor XIII and the peptide released during its activation by thrombin. *Biochemistry* 13:750, 1974.

350. Curtis CG, Brown KL, Credo RB, et al: Calcium-dependent unmasking of active center cysteine during activation of fibrin stabilizing factor. *Biochemistry* 13:3774, 1974.

351. Lorand L, Gray AJ, Brown K, Credo RB, et al: Dissociation of the subunit structure of fibrin stabilizing factor during activation of the zymogen. *Biochem Biophys Commun* 56:914, 1974.

352. Mary A, Achyuthan KE, Greenberg CS: b-Chains prevent the proteolytic inactivation of the a-chains of plasma factor XIII. *Biochem Biophys Acta* 966:328, 1988.

353. Bottenus RE, Ichinose A, Davie EW: Nucleotide sequence of the gene for the b subunit of human factor XIII. *Biochemistry* 29:11195, 1990.

354. Board PG, Webb GC, McKee J, Ichinose A: Localization of the coagulation factor XIII A subunit gene (F13A) to chromosome bands 6p24-p25. *Cytogenet Cell Genet* 48:25, 1988.

355. Weisberg LJ, Shiu DT, Greenberg CS, et al: Localization of the gene for coagulation factor XIII a-chain to chromosome 6 and identification of sites of synthesis. *J Clin Invest* 79:649, 1987.

356. Webb GC, Coggan M, Ichinose A, Board PG: Localization of the coagulation factor XIII B subunit gene (F13B) to chromosome bands 1q31-32.1 and restriction fragment length polymorphism at the locus. *Hum Genet* 81:157, 1989.

357. Wolpl A, Lattke H, Board PG, et al: Coagulation factor XIII A and B subunits in bone marrow and liver transplantation. *Transplantation* 43:151, 1987.

358. Weisberg LJ, Shiu DT, Conkling PR, Shuman MA: Identification of normal human peripheral blood monocytes and liver as sites of synthesis of coagulation factor XIII a-chain. *Blood* 70:579, 1987.

359. Poon MC, Russell JA, Lowe S, et al: Hemopoietic origin of factor XIII A subunits in platelets, monocytes, and plasma: Evidence from bone marrow transplantation studies. *J Clin Invest* 84:787, 1989.

360. Grundmann U, Amann E, Zettlmeissl G, Kupper HA: Characterization of cDNA coding for human factor XIIIa. *Proc Natl Acad Sci USA* 83:8024, 1986.

361. Nagy JA, Kradin RL, McDonagh J: Biosynthesis of factor XIII A and B subunits. *Adv Exp Med Biol* 231:29, 1988.

362. Varadi A, Scheraga HA: Localization of segments essential for polymerization and for calcium binding in the gamma-chain of human fibrinogen. *Biochemistry* 25:519, 1986.

363. McKee PA, Mattock P, Hill RL: Subunit structure of human fibrinogen, soluble fibrin, and cross-linked insoluble fibrin. *Proc Natl Acad Sci USA* 66:738, 1970.

364. Sakata Y, Aoki N: Cross-linking of alpha 2-plasmin inhibitor to fibrin by fibrin-stabilizing factor. *J Clin Invest* 65:290, 1980.

365. Mosher DF, Schad PE, Vann JM: Cross-linking of collagen and fibronec-

tin by factor XIIIa: Localization of participating glutaminyl residues to a tryptic fragment of fibronectin. *J Biol Chem* 255:1181, 1980.

366. Bale MD, Westrick LG, Mosher DF: Incorporation of thrombospondin into fibrin clots. *J Biol Chem* 260:7502, 1985.

367. Lynch GW, Slayter HS, Miller BE, McDonagh J: Characterization of thrombospondin as a substrate for factor XIII transglutaminase. *J Biol Chem* 262:1772, 1987.

368. Bockenstedt P, McDonagh J, Handin RI: Binding and covalent cross-linking of purified von Willebrand factor to native monomeric collagen. *J Clin Invest* 78:551, 1986.

369. Hada M, Kaminski M, Bockenstedt P, McDonagh J: Covalent crosslinking of von Willebrand factor to fibrin. *Blood* 68:95, 1986.

370. Asijee GM, Muszbek L, Kappelmayer J, et al: Platelet vinculin: A substrate of activated factor XIII. *Biochem Biophys Acta* 954:303, 1988.

371. Sane DC, Moser TL, Pippen AM, et al: Vitronectin is a substrate for transglutaminases. *Biochem Biophys Res Commun* 157:115, 1988.

372. Mui PT, Ganguly P: Cross-linking of actin and fibrin by fibrin-stabilizing factor. *Am J Physiol* 233:H346, 1977.

373. Cohen I, Young-Bandala L, Blankenberg TA, et al: Fibrinoligase-catalyzed cross-linking of myosin from platelet and skeletal muscle. *Arch Biochem Biophys* 192:100, 1979.

374. Borth W, Chang V, Bishop P, Harpel PC: Lipoprotein(a) is a substrate for factor XIIIa and tissue transglutaminase. *J Biol Chem* 266:18149, 1991.

375. Schwartz ML, Pizzo SV, Hill RL, McKee PA: Human factor XIII from plasma and platelets: Molecular weights, subunit structures, proteolytic activation, and cross-linking of fibrinogen and fibrin. *J Biol Chem* 248:1395, 1973.

376. Lopaciuk S, Lovette KM, McDonagh J, et al: Subcellular distribution of fibrinogen and factor XIII in human blood platelets. *Thromb Res* 8:453, 1976.

377. Henriksson P, Becker S, Lynch G, McDonagh J: Identification of intracellular factor XIII in human monocytes and macrophages. *J Clin Invest* 76:528, 1985.

378. Adany R, Belkin A, Vasilevskaya T, Muszbek L: Identification of blood coagulation factor XIII in human peritoneal macrophages. *Eur J Cell Biol* 38:171, 1985.

379. Mikkola H, Yee VC, Syrjälä M, et al: Four novel mutations in deficiency of coagulation factor XIII: Consequences to expression and structure of the A-subunit. *Blood* 87:141, 1996.

380. Anwar R, Miloszewski KJ, Markham AF: Identification of a large deletion, spanning exons 4 to 11 of the human factor XIIIa gene, in a factor XIII-deficient family. *Blood* 91:149, 1998.

381. Aslam S, Bowen DJ, Mandalaki T, et al: Factor XIII(A) subunit deficiency due to a homozygous 13-base pair deletion in exon 3 of the A subunit gene. *Am J Hematol* 53:77, 1996.

382. Kamura T, Okamura T, Murakawa M, et al: Deficiency of coagulation factor XIII A subunit caused by the dinucleotide deletion at the 5' end of exon III. *J Clin Invest* 90:315, 1992.

383. Aslam S, Standen GR, Bruce LJ, et al: A novel insertion mutation (1286insC) in exon 9 of the factor XIII-A subunit gene. *Blood Coag Fibrinol* 9:441, 1998.

384. Izumi T, Nagaoka U, Saito T, et al: Novel deletion and insertion mutations cause splicing defects, leading to severe reduction in mRNA levels of the A subunit in severe factor XIII deficiency. *Thromb Haemost* 79:479, 1998.

385. Board P, Coggan M, Miloszewski K: Identification of a point mutation in factor XIII A subunit deficiency. *Blood* 80:937, 1992.

386. Vreken P, Niessen RW, Peters M, et al: A point mutation in an invariant splice acceptor site results in a decreased mRNA level in a patient with severe coagulation factor XIII subunit A deficiency. *Thromb Haemost* 74:584, 1995.

387. Standen GR, Bowen DJ: Factor XIII A Bristol 1: Detection of a nonsense mutation (Arg171→stop codon) in factor XIII A subunit deficiency. *Br J Haematol* 85:769, 1993.

388. Coggan M, Baker R, Miloszewski K, et al: Mutations causing coagulation factor XIII subunit A deficiency: Characterization of the mutant proteins after expression in yeast. *Blood* 85:2455, 1995.

389. Mikkola H, Syrjala M, Rasi V, et al: Deficiency in the A-subunit of coagulation factor XIII: Two novel point mutations demonstrate different effects on transcript levels. *Blood* 84:517, 1994.

390. Ichinose A, Tsukamoto H, Izumi T, et al: Arg260-Cys mutation in severe factor XIII deficiency: Conformational change of the a subunit is predicted by molecular modeling and mechanics. *Br J Haematol* 101:264, 1998.

391. Kangsadalampai S, Chelvanayagam G, Baker RT, et al: A novel Asn344 deletion in the core domain of coagulation factor XIII A subunit: Its effects on protein structure and function. *Blood* 92:481, 1998.

392. Aslam S, Yee VC, Narayanan S, et al: Structural analysis of a missense mutation (Val141Phe) in the catalytic core domain of the factor XIII(A) subunit. *Br J Haematol* 98:346, 1997.

393. Inbal A, Yee VC, Kornbrot N, et al: Factor XIII deficiency due to a Leu660Pro mutation in the factor XIII subunit-a gene in three unrelated Palestinian Arab families. *Thromb Haemost* 77:1062, 1997.

394. Aslam S, Poon MC, Yee VC, et al: Factor XIIIA Calgary: A candidate missense mutation (Leu667Pro) in the beta barrel 2 domain of the factor XIIIA subunit. *Br J Haematol* 91:452, 1995.

395. Saito M, Asakura H, Yoshida T, et al: A familial factor XIII subunit B deficiency. *Br J Haematol* 74:290, 1990.

396. Hashiguchi T, Saito M, Morishita E, et al: Two genetic defects in a patient with complete deficiency of the b-subunit for coagulation factor XIII. *Blood* 82:145, 1993.

397. Hashiguchi R, Ichinose A: Molecular and cellular basis of deficiency of the b subunit for factor XIII secondary to a Cys430-Phe mutation in the seventh sushi domain. *J Clin Invest* 95:1002, 1995.

398. Izumi T, Hashiguchi T, Castaman G, et al: Type I factor XIII deficiency is caused by a genetic defect of its b subunit: Insertion of triplet AAC in exon III leads to premature termination in the second sushi domain. *Blood* 87:2769, 1996.

399. Gootenberg JE: Factor concentrates for the treatment of factor XIII deficiency. *Curr Opin Hematol* 5:372, 1998.

HEMOPHILIA A AND HEMOPHILIA B

HAROLD R. ROBERTS

MAUREANE HOFFMAN

The clinical manifestations of hemophilia A and B due to deficiency of factors VIII and IX, respectively, are clinically indistinguishable and occur in mild, moderate, and severe forms. They are the only blood clotting disorders inherited in a sex-linked recessive pattern. The severe forms of both hemophilia A and B are characterized by frequent hemarthroses, leading to chronic crippling hemarthropathy when not treated very early or prophylactically. Highly purified concentrates, prepared from human plasma or manufactured by recombinant technology, are available for treatment and are considered to be both safe and effective. In addition, prophylactic treatment is recommended, when feasible, for all severely affected patients. The main complication of treatment is the development of antibody inhibitors against either factor VIII or factor IX, which are more common in patients with hemophilia A than in patients with hemophilia B.

HEMOPHILIA A (CLASSIC HEMOPHILIA, FACTOR VIII DEFICIENCY)

DEFINITION AND HISTORY

Hemophilia A is an X-linked hereditary disorder that is due to defective and/or deficient factor VIII molecules. It is less common than von Willebrand disease (vWD), but it is more common than other inherited clotting factor abnormalities. However, hemophilia A is still rare, with an estimated incidence of only 1 in every 10,000 live male births. It is found in all ethnic groups in all parts of the world.[1]

Sex-linked hemophilia was recognized in the second century, when a rabbi correctly deduced that sons of hemophilic carriers were at risk for bleeding following circumcision.[2] In the nineteenth century, several authors noted the sex-linked inheritance pattern of the disease and ascribed the hemorrhagic episodes to delayed blood coagulation. Morawitz developed the classical theory of blood coagulation, which recognized two major reactions: conversion of prothrombin to thrombin by a tissue substance that Morawitz termed *thrombokinase* and conversion of fibrinogen to fibrin by thrombin.[3] In 1911, Addis demonstrated that thrombin formed more slowly in hemophilic blood than normal blood and that the defect could be corrected by small amounts of normal plasma.[4] However, he incorrectly theorized that hemophilia was due to prothrombin deficiency. As protein purification techniques

Acronyms and abbreviations that appear in this chapter include: AAV, adeno-associated vector; aPTT, activated partial thromboplastin time; CJD, Creutzfeldt-Jakob disease; DDAVP, 1,8-desamino-D-arginine vasopressin, desmopressin; PTC, plasma thromboplastin component; PT, prothrombin time; PTT, partial thromboplastin time; RFLP, restriction fragment length polymorphism; vWD, von Willebrand disease; vWF, von Willebrand factor.

improved throughout the 1930s and 1940s, thrombokinase was resolved into several distinct components. Brinkhous demonstrated that the prothrombin content of hemophilic plasma was normal and that the basic defect in hemophilia was the delayed conversion of prothrombin to thrombin.[5] The defect could be corrected by a fraction of normal plasma that contained the antihemophilic factor, later named *factor VIII*. In 1947 Pavlovsky observed that when blood from one patient with hemophilia he was studying was transfused into another, the prolonged clotting time in the recipient was corrected.[6] At the time, Pavlovsky did not recognize that he was dealing with two different types of hemophilia. This was recognized by Aggeler and coworkers in 1952, when they described a patient deficient in "plasma thromboplastin component," a blood-clotting factor different from factor VIII.[7] A deficiency of "plasma thromboplastin component," later termed factor IX, is expressed clinically as hemophilia B.[8]

In 1964 a proposal was put forth to organize the growing number of coagulation factors into a cascade, or waterfall, mechanism.[9,10] In this scheme each zymogen clotting factor was activated to a protease that subsequently acted on the next zymogen until thrombin was ultimately produced. In this scheme both factor VIII and factor IX were considered to be proenzymes. Later, however, it was shown that factor VIII was not a proenzyme but rather a cofactor, which, when activated by thrombin, acted as an essential cofactor for factor IXa. Recently, the cascade hypothesis has been modified so that the primary role of the tissue factor/factor VII complex in the initiation of coagulation is emphasized (see Chap. 112).[11]

ETIOLOGY AND PATHOGENESIS

Hemophilia A is a heterogeneous disorder resulting from defects in the factor VIII gene that leads to a reduction in the circulating levels of functional factor VIII. The reduction in activity can be due to a decreased amount of factor VIII protein, the presence of a functionally abnormal protein, or a combination of both. For factor VIII to be an effective cofactor for factor IXa, it must first be activated by thrombin, a reaction that results in the formation of a heterotrimer composed of the A_1, A_2, and A_3, $-C_1$, $-C_2$ domains of factor VIII in a complex with calcium (see Chap. 112).[12] Activated factor VIII (VIIIa) and activated factor IX (IXa) associate on the surface of activated platelets to form a functional factor X-activating complex ("tenase" or "Xase").[13] In the presence of factor VIIIa, the rate of factor X activation by factor IXa is dramatically enhanced. It is not surprising that hemophilia A and B have similar clinical manifestations, since both factor VIIIa and factor IXa are required to form the Xase complex. The lack of either leads to a similar lack of platelet Xase activity. In patients with hemophilia, clot formation is delayed because thrombin generation is markedly decreased. The clot that is formed is friable and easily dislodged, leading to excessive bleeding.

GENETICS

Hemophilia A is an X-linked recessive disorder that occurs almost exclusively in males. About 30 percent of the mutations arise de novo. The inheritance pattern of both hemophilia A and B is shown in Fig. 123-1. Note that all the sons of affected hemophilic males are normal, while all the daughters are obligatory carriers of the factor VIII defect. Sons of carriers have a 50 percent chance of being affected, while daughters of carriers have a 50 percent chance of being carriers themselves.

The factor VIII gene is very large, about 186 kb, with about 9 kb of exons. It contains 26 exons and 25 intervening sequences or introns. The size and complexity of the gene have made it difficult to pinpoint, on a routine basis, specific mutations that result in hemo-

Inheritance Patterns for Hemophilia A and B

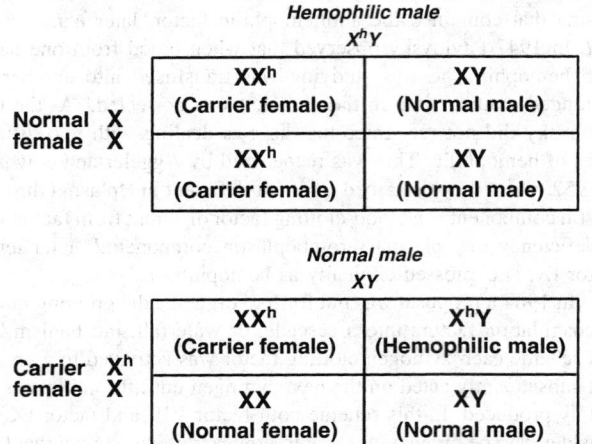

FIGURE 123-1   Inheritance pattern of hemophilia A. X is normal; X^h is an abnormal X chromosome with the hemophilic gene; Y is normal; XX is a normal female; XY is a normal male; XX^h is a carrier female; X^hY is a hemophilic male.

philia. Nevertheless, the factor VIII gene has now been cloned and sequenced, and numerous specific mutations have been described.[14]

Hemophilia A can be due to multiple alterations in the factor VIII gene, including gene rearrangements; missense mutations, in which there is a single base substitution leading to an amino acid change in the molecule; nonsense mutations, which result in a stop codon; abnormal splicing of the gene; deletions of all or portions of the gene; or insertions of genetic elements.[14] A review of the genetic defects leading to hemophilia A can be found on the Internet.[15] A summary of the different mutations as of 1996 are shown in Table 123-1.[16]

One of the most common mutations, accounting for 40 to 50 percent of patients, is a unique combined gene inversion and crossing-over that disrupts the factor VIII gene.[17,18] The factor VIII gene is schematically represented in Figs. 123-2 and 123-3. Within intron 22 are two other genes, one called *F8A*, which is transcribed in the 5' direction, and *F8B*, which is transcribed in the 3' direction of the factor VIII gene. In addition, the hatched boxes in Fig. 123-3 show two other homologous sequences (a_2,a_3) 5' to the *F8A* gene that lies within intron 22 (a_1). The presence of an extragenic *F8A* sequence 5' to the *F8A* gene within intron 22 is central to the inversion and translocation of the factor VIII gene from exon 1 to exon 22. The mechanism is homologous recombination between the *F8A* gene sequence that lies within intron 22 and one of the homologous sequences of the *F8A* gene 5' to the factor VIII gene. During meiosis, there is crossing-over of homologous sequences between the *F8A* gene nested in intron 22 and the extragenic *F8A* sequence 5' to intron 22 so that transcription of the complete factor VIII sequence is interrupted as shown in Fig. 123-3. Many of the patients with an inversion are susceptible to development of antifactor VIII inhibitor antibodies.

Of the different insertions in the factor VIII gene that have been reported, a few are LINE (L_1) elements which are transposon sequences, i.e., sequences that have been inserted frequently throughout the genome.[19] Most insertions result in severe hemophilia.

Mutations in hemophilia A occur frequently at CpG dinucleotides (see Chap. 9).[19] Since TaqI recognizes the sequence TCGA, CpG mutations at this site can be directly detected by the loss of a TaqI cleavage site. Codons for the amino acid arginine (CGA) are frequently affected by mutations at CG doublets. A C→T transition often results in a stop codon as shown in Fig. 123-4. A stop codon results in synthesis of a truncated factor VIII molecule and is usually associated with severe hemophilia.

A G→A transition results in a missense mutation, which often leads to a dysfunctional factor VIII molecule and may be associated with mild, moderate, or severe hemophilia. Some missense mutations result in the production of normal or near-normal amounts of factor VIII antigen, while the coagulant activity may be dramatically or only slightly reduced. Many other single base substitutions have been described, resulting in hemophilia of varying degrees of severity.

Large deletions in the factor VIII gene are almost always associated with severe hemophilia. However, cases have been described in which a small deletion that does not change the reading frame of the gene results in milder disease. Patients with large deletions who have no detectable factor VIII antigen are also thought to be more susceptible to the development of anti-factor VIII antibodies, although it is clear that antibodies also occur in patients without deletions.[14,19]

TABLE 123-1   SUMMARY OF DIFFERENT MUTATIONS REPORTED FOR HEMOPHILIA A

	Point Mutations			Deletions		
EXON	MISSENSE*	NONSENSE (STOP)	SPLICING ≅	SMALL	LARGE	INSERTIONS
1	9	1	1	1	—	—
2	2	—	—	2	—	1
3	13	—	1	2	—	—
4	10	2	2	1	—	—
5	6	—	3	—	—	—
6	1	—	2	1	—	—
7	19	1	—	4	—	—
8	12	3	—	7	—	—
9	3	1	1	2	—	—
10	5	—	—	1	—	—
11	10	1	3	—	—	1
12	8	3	1	—	—	1
13	12	2	—	3	—	1
14	22	9	1	24	—	13
15	5	1	1	—	—	—
16	11	3	1	3	—	—
17	10	1	—	2	—	2
18	11	3	—	2	—	3
19	4	1	—	1	—	—
20	2	1	—	—	—	—
21	2	1	—	—	—	—
22	8	1	—	—	—	—
23	11	1	—	2	—	—
24	6	1	—	4	—	1
25	8	1	1	1	—	—
26	8	2	—	1	—	—
Total	218	40	18	64	92	23

*Including 5 missense mutations which are predicted to affect splice junctions.
≅In the case of intronic substitutions, splice mutations are referred to the preceding exon.
Reprinted by permission of the publisher from Review of haemophilia A molecular biology, *HAMPSTeRS* Website, MRC Clinical Sciences Center, Imperial College Medical School, Hammersmith Hospital, London.

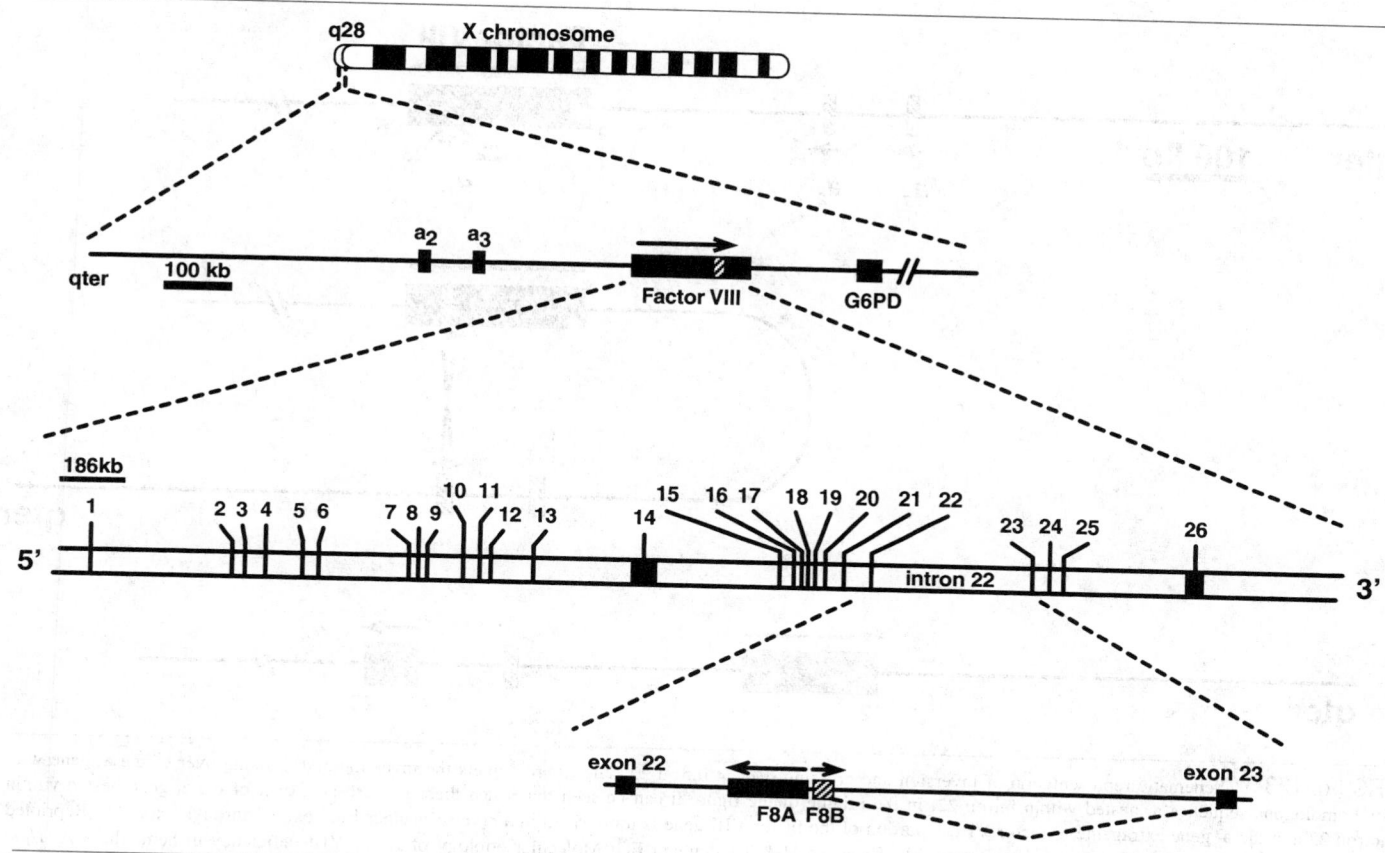

FIGURE 123-2   A schematic representation of the factor VIII gene. The factor VIII gene is located at q28 on the X chromosome. The figure shows the region of factor VIII gene to be enlarged on the second line. Notice that there are two genes designated a_2 and a_3 5' to the factor VIII gene. The hatched area in factor VIII gene corresponds to intron 22 shown in the third line. Notice within intron 22 (fourth line) two nested genes, one of which is designated *F8A*, which is transcribed in a direction opposite that of the whole factor VIII gene and is homologous to the a_2 a_3 genes shown in line 2. (Reprinted with permission of the publisher from "Hemophilia A and Parahemophilia," in the *Metabolic and Molecular Basis of Inherited Diseases*, 7th ed, vol 3, edited by CR Scriver, AL Beaudet, WS Sly, D Valle, p 3247. McGraw-Hill, New York, 1995.)

Hemophilia A in females is extremely rare, although affected female offspring from an affected father and carrier mother have been reported. Hemophilia A may also occur in females with X-chromosomal abnormalities such as Turner syndrome, X mosaicism, and other X-chromosomal defects.[20,21] If a carrier female has the normal X chromosome inactivated disproportionately ("imbalanced X-inactivation"), she may have factor VIII levels sufficiently low to cause bleeding manifestations. Usually, these are mild but may be serious during surgical procedures or in instances of significant trauma.

PRENATAL DIAGNOSIS AND CARRIER DETECTION

A careful and complete family history is important for carrier detection.[22] All the daughters of a hemophilic father will be obligatory carriers of the hemophilic defect. If a known carrier has a daughter, there is a 50 percent chance that the daughter will be a carrier.

Carrier detection becomes important when a daughter of a known carrier or a female offspring of a patient with hemophilia wishes to become pregnant. If resources for advanced carrier detection are not available, one can take a careful family history and measure both factor VIII coagulant activity and the vWF antigen. The ratio of vWF to factor VIII is higher in carrier females than noncarriers, and, thus, determining the ratio adds to the sensitivity of the test. Carriers generally have 50 percent or less of the normal factor VIII level. When these data are added to the family history, one can calculate the probability of whether a woman is a carrier.[23,24]

Carriers who carry the intron 22 inversion can be identified using the Southern blot technique. Where the capability exists, analysis of the complete coding region can be performed using gradient gel electrophoresis and single strand conformation polymorphism (SSCP) technology.[22]

The use of markers for restriction fragment length polymorphism (RFLP) is simpler than direct sequencing of the coding region of the factor VIII gene, but the use of this technique requires that the pedigree analysis include at least one hemophilic male whose mother is heterozygous for one or more RFLP markers. An example of RFLP analysis is shown in Fig. 123-5.[25,26] The polymorphic markers include the variable number of tandem repeats (VNTR) in introns 13 and 22, as well as Bcl I and Xba I restriction sites. One can readily see that the female III-2 has the same polymorphic marker in intron 13 and the same Xba I restriction site as her hemophilic brother, carrier mother, and hemophilic grandfather. In contrast, the female III-1 inherits markers that are not linked with hemophilia.

Prenatal diagnosis of hemophilia can now be carried out almost routinely. If a carrier female has a fetus that can be identified as a female by chromosomal analysis of cells obtained by amniocentesis (about the sixteenth week), or by chorionic villus sampling at the tenth week of gestation, it is usually of little worry whether the female fetus

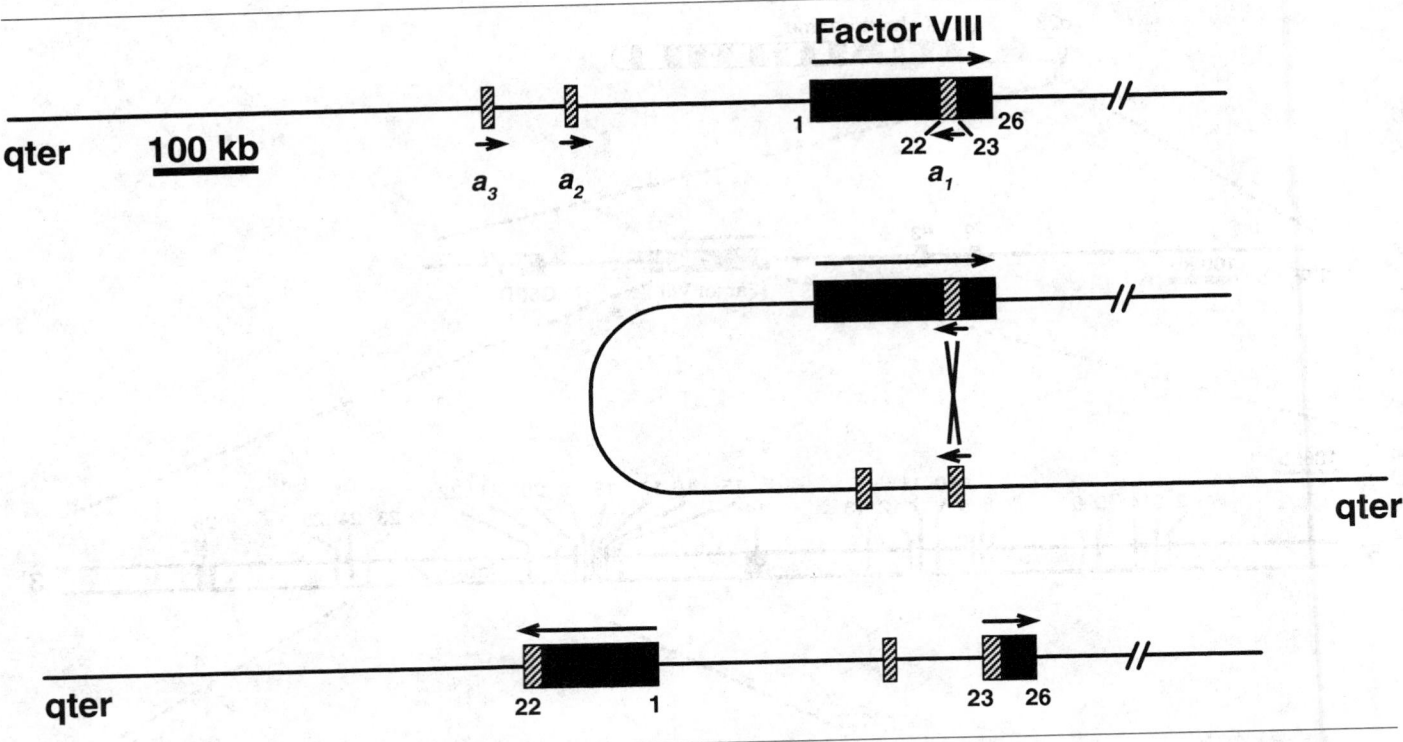

FIGURE 123-3 Schematic representation of inversion and crossing-over at intron 22. The figure depicts the inversion and crossing-over of the a₃ gene with its homologous sequence a₁ nested within intron 22. In the middle of the figure it can be seen that when there is a crossing-over of the a₁ gene nested within intron 22 and the a₃ gene extragenic to factor VIII, a portion of the factor VIII gene is transcribed in a reverse manner from exon 1 through exon 22. (Reprinted with permission of the publisher from: Antonarakis SE, Kazazian HH, Tuddenham EG: Molecular etiology of factor VIII deficiency in hemophilia A. *Hum Mutat* 5:1, 1995.)

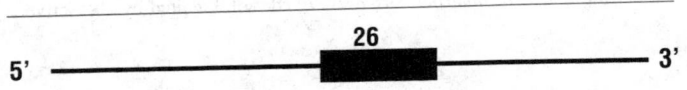

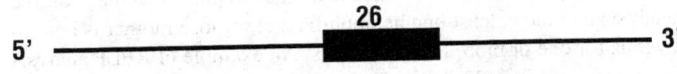

FIGURE 123-4 Examples of mutations and CG doublets. In this figure the black box denotes exon 26. Note that a C to T transition results in a stop codon (TGA) while a G to A transition results in a substitution of a glutamine for an arginine residue.

is a carrier, since carriers usually have no bleeding tendency. If the fetus is male, sufficient cells can be obtained to carry out DNA analysis using the methods described above. A decision as to whether an affected fetus is carried to term is one that should be decided by the parents after they are provided with all the necessary information.

CLINICAL FEATURES

Hemophilia A is characterized by excessive bleeding into various parts of the body. Soft-tissue hematomas and hemarthroses leading to severe, crippling hemarthropathy are highly characteristic of the disease. The disease has been broadly classified as *mild, moderate,* and *severe,* although there is overlap between categories. Table 123-2 shows a classification based on the severity of clinical manifestations. A range of plasma factor VIII concentrations in percentages of normal and in units per milliliter is given for each category of severity. Occasionally, some patients with very low factor VIII clotting activity will be mildly affected clinically. It has been suggested that some patients with factor VIII levels compatible with severe hemophilia may exhibit mild symptoms because of the coinheritance of the factor V Leiden mutation (R506Q) with the hemophilic gene.[27] However, in some patients with "severe" hemophilia with a "milder" bleeding diathesis, neither the factor V Leiden mutation nor other known "prothombotic" markers have been found.[28] Severely affected patients (less than 1 percent factor VIII) frequently experience bleeding without known trauma other than that associated with the usual day-to-day activities. Without effective treatment, recurrent hemarthroses, resulting in chronic hemophilic arthropathy, occur by young adulthood and are highly characteristic of the severe form of the disorder. Severely affected patients are also subject to serious hemorrhages that may dissect through tissue planes, ultimately leading to compromise of vital organs. However, bleeding episodes are intermittent, and some patients go for weeks or months without hemorrhage. Except for intracranial bleeding, sudden death due to hemorrhage is rare.

Moderately affected patients with hemophilia have occasional hematomas and hemarthroses usually, but not always, associated with known trauma. These patients have greater than 1 to 5 percent factor VIII activity. Although hemarthroses occur in moderately affected patients, hemarthropathy is less disabling than that occurring in severely affected patients.

Mildly affected patients with hemophilia (6 to 30 percent factor VIII) have infrequent bleeding episodes, and the disease may go undiagnosed, only to be discovered because of excessive hemorrhage postoperatively, following trauma, or after the toss and tumble of contact sports.

Most carriers have roughly 50 percent factor VIII activity and experience no bleeding difficulty, even with surgical procedures. Carriers with factor VIII levels below 50 percent, usually due to extremely imbalanced X-inactivation, may experience excessive bleeding after trauma (e.g., childbirth or surgery), and therefore a factor VIII level should be obtained in all carriers.

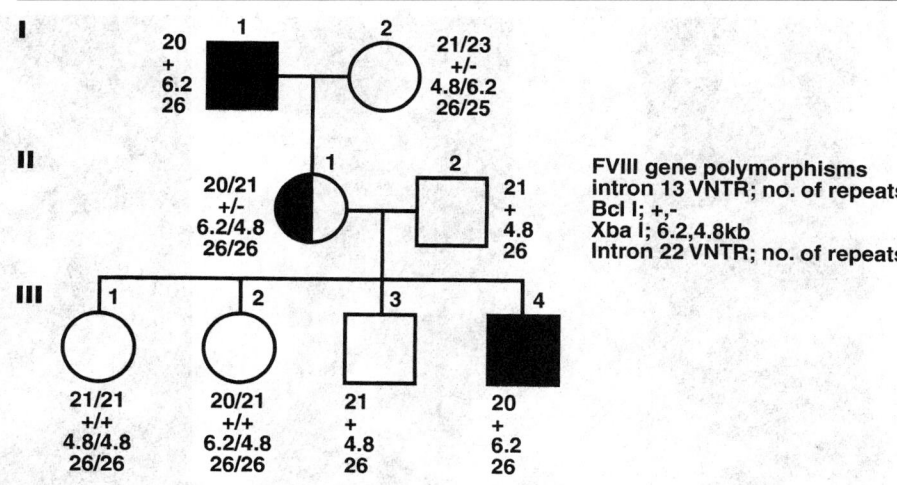

FIGURE 123-5 Use of RFLP and VNTR for carrier diagnosis of hemophilia. The carrier female (II-1) is informative for polymorphisms at intron 13 and the Xba I site but not informative for markers on Bcl I or on intron 22. As can be seen III-2 is a carrier of the hemophilic trait with markers similar to the hemophilic grandfather (I-1) and hemophilic brother (III-4). *VNTR* stands for variable number of tandem repeats, while the Bcl I and Xba I are sites cleaved by these restriction endonucleons. (Reprinted with permission of the publisher from Diagnosis of hemophilia A and B carriers, in *Hemophilia*, edited by CD Forbes, LM Aledort, R Madhok, p. 68. 1997.)

HEMARTHROSES

Bleeding into joints accounts for about 75 percent of bleeding episodes in severely affected patients with hemophilia A.[29] The normal synovium has few cells, but below the synovial layer are numerous capillaries that can be damaged by the mechanical trauma associated with day-to-day use of joints. The joints most frequently involved, in decreasing order of frequency, are knees, elbows, ankles, shoulders, wrists, and hips. Hinge joints are much more likely to be involved than ball and socket joints. Hemarthroses usually occur when an affected child begins to walk.

Hemarthroses are sometimes heralded by an aura of mild discomfort, which, over a period of minutes to hours, becomes progressively painful. The joint usually swells, becomes warm, and exhibits limited motion. Occasionally the patient experiences a mild fever. Significant and sustained fever, however, suggests an infected joint. Bleeding in the knee joint is more easily detected by physical findings than bleeding into either the elbow or shoulder. When bleeding stops, the blood resorbs, and the symptoms subside over a period of several days. If hemarthroses are treated early and the joint is not chronically involved, pain usually subsides in 6 to 8 h and disappears in 12 to 24 h. However, repeated hemorrhage into the joints eventually results in extensive destruction of articular cartilage, synovial hyperplasia, and other reactive changes in the adjacent bone and tissues. Acute bleeding into a chronically affected joint may be difficult to distinguish from the pain of degenerative arthritis.

One of the major complications of repeated hemarthroses is joint deformity complicated by muscle atrophy and soft tissue contractures (Fig. 123-6). The various radiologic stages of progressive destruction of joint cartilage and adjacent bone are shown in Figure 123-7. Osteoporosis and cystic areas in the subchondral bone may develop, and there is progressive loss of joint space.

Repeated bleeding into a joint results in synovial hypertrophy and inflammation. The synovium is thickened and folded, leading to limitation of joint motion. This results in a tendency for repeated hemorrhages leading to a so-called target joint. The joints most often involved are the knees, ankles, and elbows, which become chronically swollen. Bleeding into such a joint with significant synovial hypertrophy is usually less painful than bleeding into a normal joint, but pain, nevertheless, may occur. Chronic synovitis may persist for months or years unless adequately treated.

Infection of hemophilic joints is not common but must be suspected in all patients with fever, leukocytosis, or other systemic manifestations. Rapid diagnosis is mandatory, since infection of such joints leads to rapid loss of joint architecture and function. A painful swollen joint may require aspiration, which should be performed by experienced personnel using meticulous aseptic techniques and appropriate factor replacement therapy.

HEMATOMAS

Hematomas are characteristic of blood clotting factor deficiencies. They are usually not seen, for example, in uncomplicated thrombocytopenia. Hemorrhage into subcutaneous connective tissues or into muscles may occur with or without known trauma. Once formed, hematomas may stabilize and slowly resorb without treatment. However, in

TABLE 123-2   CLINICAL CLASSIFICATION OF HEMOPHILIA

CLASSIFICATION	FACTOR VIII LEVEL	CLINICAL FEATURES
Severe	≤ 1% of normal (≤ 0.01 U/ml)	1. Spontaneous hemorrhage from early infancy 2. Frequent spontaneous hemarthroses and other hemorrhages, requiring clotting factor replacement
Moderate	1–5% of normal (0.01–0.05 U/ml)	1. Hemorrhage secondary to trauma or surgery 2. Occasional spontaneous hemarthroses
Mild	6–30% of normal (0.06–0.30 U/ml)	1. Hemorrhage secondary to trauma or surgery 2. Rare spontaneous hemorrhage

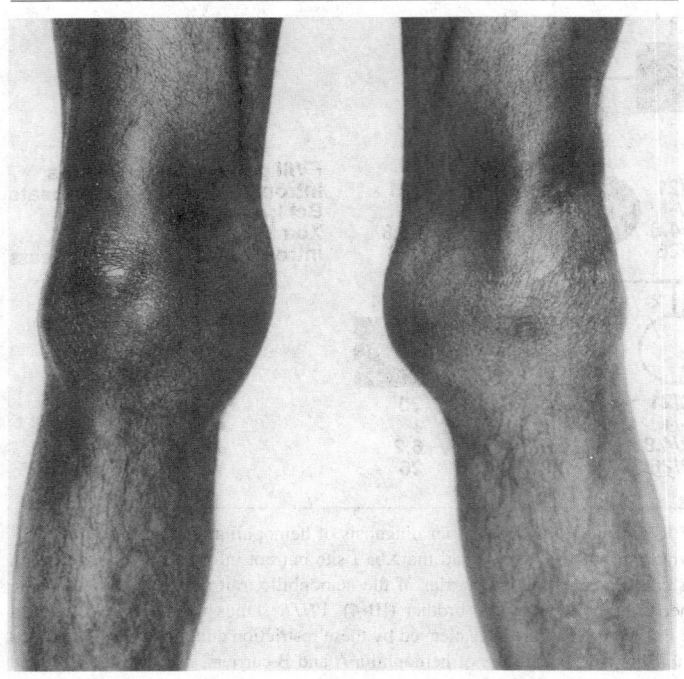

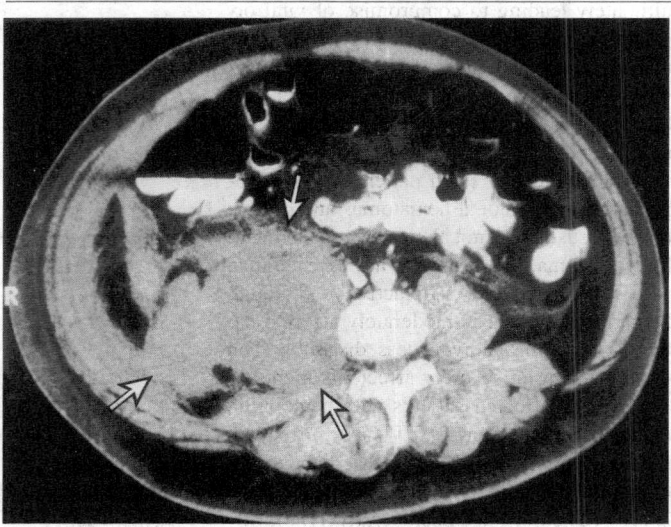

FIGURE 123-8 CT scan of a retroperitoneal hematoma in a patient with severe hemophilia A. The arrows depict the extent of the hematoma.

FIGURE 123-6 Hemophilic arthropathy. The chronic effects of a repeated hemorrhage into the knee of a severely affected hemophilic.

moderately and severely affected patients, hematomas have a tendency to enlarge progressively and to dissect in all directions. Retroperitoneal hematomas have been known to dissect through the diaphragm, into the chest, and into the soft tissues of the neck, resulting in compromise of the airway. They may also compromise renal function by causing ureteral obstruction. The computed tomographic (CT) scan of a retroperitoneal hemorrhage is shown in Fig. 123-8. Other hematomas may expand locally and cause compression of adjacent organs, blood vessels, and nerves. A rare, and often fatal, complication of an abdominal hematoma is perforation and drainage into the colon. Subcutaneous hematomas have also been known to dissect into muscle. Pharyngeal and retropharyngeal hematomas, sometimes complicating simple colds, may enlarge and obstruct the airway. Hemorrhage in or around

the airway is a potentially life-threatening situation that requires prompt administration of factor VIII. Hemorrhages occur into muscle in the following order of frequency: calf, thigh, buttocks, and forearm. Bleeding into the iliopsoas muscle is also frequent. Hematomas in these areas may lead to muscle contractures, nerve palsies, and muscle atrophy. Bleeding into the tongue or frenulum is particularly frequent in young children and is usually due to trauma. Bleeding into the myocardium is extremely unusual.

PSEUDOTUMORS (BLOOD CYSTS)

Pseudotumors are blood cysts that occur in soft tissues or bone. They are rare but dangerous complications of hemophilia.[30] They are classified into three types. One is a simple cyst that is confined by tendinous attachments within the fascial envelope of a muscle. The second type initially develops as a simple cyst in soft tissues such as a tendon, but it interferes with the vascular supply to the adjacent bone and periosteum, resulting in cyst formation and resorption of bone. The third type is thought to result from subperiosteal bleeding that separates

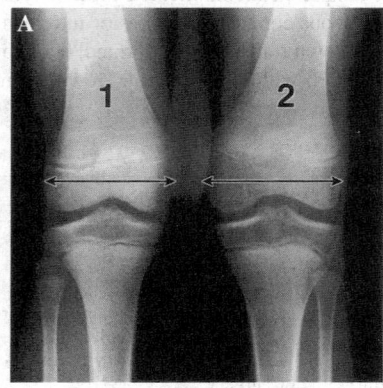
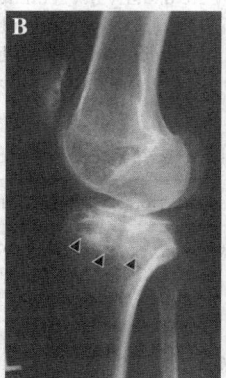
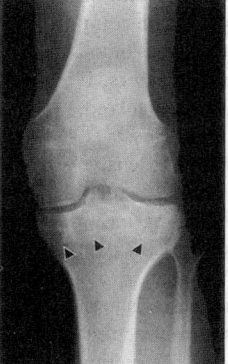
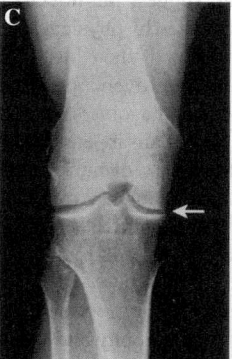
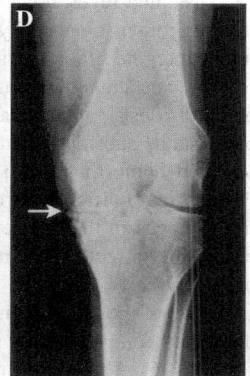

FIGURE 123-7 Various radiologic stages of hemophilic arthropathy. The stages 0 (normal joint) and 1 (fluid in the joint) are not shown. *A*: Stage 2 shows some osteoporosis and epiphyseal overgrowth in knee 2. The arrows show that the epiphysis is wider in knee 2 then in knee 1. *B*: In Stage 3 subchondral bone cysts are identified by arrows, and joint spaces exhibit irregularities. *C*: Stage 4. Prominent bone cysts with marked narrowing of joint space is denoted by the arrow. *D*: Stage 5. Obliteration of joint space with epiphyseal overgrowth is shown denoted by the arrow.

the periosteum from the bony cortex (Fig. 123-9). The extent of periosteal stripping is limited by the aponeurotic or tendinous attachments. Most pseudotumors are not associated with pain unless there is rapid growth or nerve compression. As the volume of the cyst increases, it compresses and destroys the adjacent muscle, nerve, and/ or bone. Pseudotumors usually contain either serosanguinous fluid or a viscous brownish material surrounded by a fibrous membrane. They have a tendency to expand over a period of several years and eventually become multiloculated. Some reach enormous size and involve so many structures as to be inoperable. Erosion through surrounding tissues and penetration into viscera or through the skin can occur, usually as a late event. Sinus tracts from the pseudotumor predispose to infection and septicemia. Pseudotumors develop primarily in the lower half of the body, usually in the thigh, buttock, or pelvis, but may occur anywhere, including the temporal bone. The small bones of the hands or feet are most frequently affected in younger patients. Computerized tomography or magnetic resonance imaging (MRI) are useful in diagnosis. Needle biopsies of pseudotumors should be avoided because of the risk of infection and hemorrhage. The only reliable treatment is operative removal of the entire mass. Unless the pseudotumor is completely removed, it is likely to reform.

HEMATURIA

Virtually all severely affected patients with hemophilia experience episodes of hematuria. The urine may be brown or red, depending

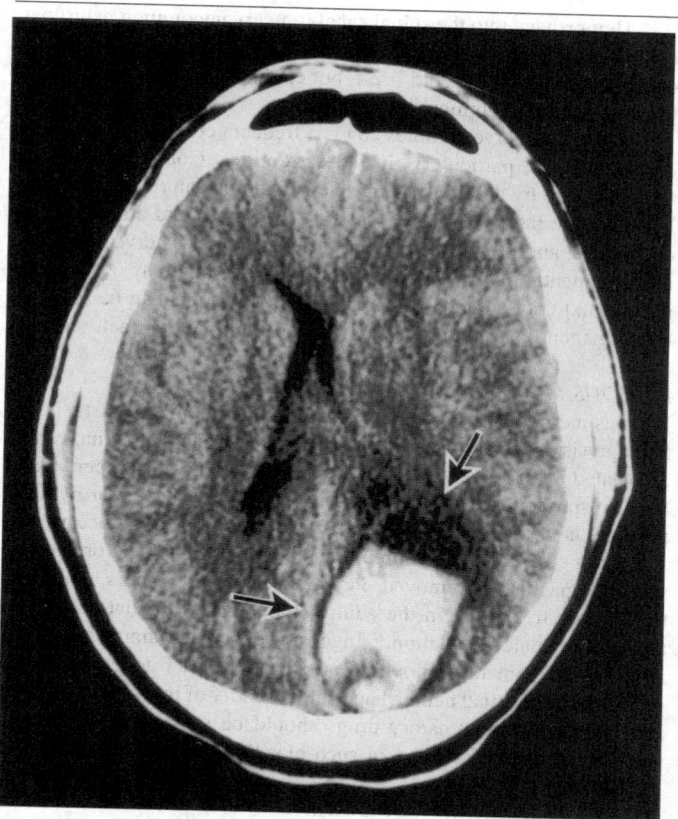

FIGURE 123-10 CT scan of a intracerebral hematoma in a severely affected hemophilic. The arrows point to the lesion. Notice compression of the ventricles.

upon the rate of bleeding. Most bleeding arises from the renal pelvis, usually from one kidney, but occasionally from both. One should consider a structural lesion as a cause of hematuria. Initially, when necessary, intravenous pyelography, ultrasound, or other appropriate studies of the genitourinary tract should be used for diagnosis, although frequently no lesions are detected except for filling defects caused by clots. If the hematuria clears upon urination, bleeding from the lower genitourinary tract should be suspected. Severe renal colic may occur when clots obstruct the ureters. If the hematuria is minimal and painless, and the patient's past history suggests no genitourinary pathology, the physician is justified in waiting a few days for bleeding to cease. If bleeding continues, treatment with factor VIII may be necessary.

NEUROLOGIC COMPLICATIONS

Intracranial bleeding is the most dangerous hemorrhagic event in hemophilic patients.[31] Hemorrhage into the central nervous system may be "spontaneous" but usually follows trauma, which may be trivial. Symptoms often occur soon after trauma, but sometimes bleeding is delayed. Symptoms of a subdural hematoma, for example, may be delayed for several weeks. Hemophilic patients with unusual headaches should always be suspected of having hemorrhage into the brain parenchyma, a subdural or an epidural hematoma (Fig. 123-10). When intracranial bleeding is suspected, the patient should be treated immediately with factor VIII. Diagnostic procedures, such as CT scans or MRI studies, should be delayed until after initiation of treatment. Although lumbar puncture has been performed safely in severe hemophilic patients without replacement therapy, it is safer to replace factor VIII to a level of about 50 percent of normal prior to the procedure.

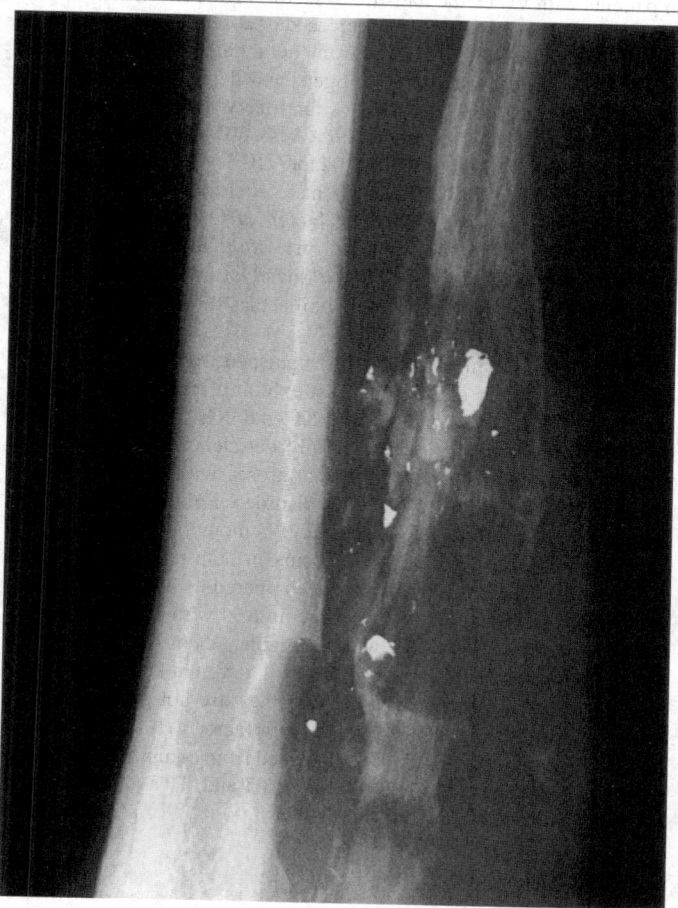

FIGURE 123-9 Pseudotumor of the fibula in a severely affected hemophilic. Notice the virtual destruction with cysts and calcifications. There is also involvement of the tibia.

Hemorrhage into the spinal canal is a very uncommon neurologic complication in hemophilia but can result in paraplegia. Bleeding may occur within the spinal cord itself, but epidural bleeding compressing the cord is more common.[31]

Peripheral nerve compression is a frequent complication of muscle hematomas, particularly in the extremities. Compression of the femoral nerve by an iliopsoas muscle hematoma can result in sensory loss over the lateral and anterior thigh, weakness and atrophy of the quadriceps, and loss of the patellar reflex. The ulnar nerve is the next most frequently involved peripheral nerve. Bleeding may occur in any muscle and may compress local neural supply. This can be followed by permanent neuromuscular defects and multiple contractures.

MUCOUS MEMBRANE HEMORRHAGE

Mucous membrane bleeding is common in hemophilia. Epistaxis and hemoptysis, often resulting from allergic reactions or trauma, can be associated with local structural lesions involving the upper and/or lower respiratory tract. Treatment of epistaxis by cautery or by nasal packing is sometimes followed by recurrent bleeding because of sloughing of the cauterized area or dislodging of a poorly formed clot when the packing is removed. Peptic ulcer disease occurs about five times more frequently in the adult hemophilia A population than in the general male population.[32] Ingestion of anti-inflammatory drugs for relief of pain of hemophilic arthropathy is a frequent cause of upper gastrointestinal hemorrhage, and a history of ingestion of aspirin and other anti-inflammatory drugs should be specifically addressed when assessing the etiology of such bleeding.[33]

DENTAL AND SURGICAL BLEEDING

Severe hemophilia is usually diagnosed in childhood, and so patients are treated pre- and postoperatively to prevent bleeding. Mildly, or sometimes moderately, affected patients, however, may go unrecognized until surgery results in excessive bleeding at the surgical site. Bleeding may be delayed for several hours or, occasionally, for several days. Surgery in such patients is characterized by poor wound healing due to poor clot formation. Prolonged bleeding and subsequent infection of the wound hematoma may further complicate healing. With appropriate factor VIII replacement therapy, intra- and postoperative hemorrhages can be prevented.

Dental extraction is the most frequent surgical procedure performed on hemophilic patients. Loss of deciduous teeth is seldom the cause of excessive bleeding, but extraction of permanent teeth may result in excessive hemorrhage that can persist intermittently for several days to weeks unless appropriate treatment is administered. In the untreated patient with severe hemophilia, life-threatening, dissecting pharyngeal and/or sublingual hematomas may result from dental procedures or even from administration of regional block anesthesia.

LABORATORY FEATURES

Patients with severe hemophilia A characteristically have a prolonged activated partial thromboplastin time (aPTT). The prothrombin time (PT), thrombin-clotting time (TCT), and bleeding time (BT) are normal, although minor increases in BT have been reported by some investigators. Different combinations of aPTT reagents and instrumentation exhibit varying sensitivities to factor VIII levels. In mild hemophilia, the aPTT may be only slightly prolonged or at the upper limit of normal, especially if the factor VIII activity is at or above 20 percent of normal. The aPTT is corrected when hemophilic plasma is mixed with an equal volume of normal plasma and not corrected when mixed with plasma of a known patient with hemophilia A. If the hemophilic plasma contains an inhibitor antibody against factor VIII, the aPTT on a similar mixture will be prolonged, although incubation of the

mixture for 1 or 2 h at 37°C may be required to detect a prolongation. A definitive diagnosis of hemophilia A should be based on a specific assay for factor VIII activity.

Functional factor VIII coagulant activity is measured by one-stage clotting assays based on aPTT.[34] Chromogenic assays for factor VIII activity are also used widely but do not always agree with one-stage assays.[34] Factor VIII antigen is measured by immunologic assays, which will detect normal and most abnormal factor VIII molecules. If the factor VIII antigen level is normal but the clotting activity is reduced, the patient has a dysfunctional factor VIII molecule. Such patients have antigen-positive hemophilia, also referred to as cross-reacting material–positive (CRM+).[35] In other patients, both the factor VIII antigen and activity are nearly undetectable. These patients are CRM-negative.

Factor VIII activity is expressed as percent of normal or as units per milliliter of plasma. By definition, 1 unit of factor VIII is equal to the amount in 1 ml of pooled fresh normal human plasma. Also by definition, 1 unit of factor VIII/ml is 100 percent of normal.

DIFFERENTIAL DIAGNOSIS

von Willebrand disease can sometimes be confused with hemophilia A. The basic defect in vWD is reduced activity of von Willebrand factor (vWF), which acts as a carrier of factor VIII in vivo (see Chap. 135). Thus, in vWD, factor VIII levels are reduced, although there is considerable variability. Although factor VIII is synthesized normally in patients with vWD, the half-life of factor VIII is shortened because the vWF "carrier" molecule is decreased or absent. Other abnormalities in vWD that distinguish it from hemophilia A are prolonged bleeding time, decreased vWF antigen, and decreased ristocetin-induced platelet agglutination. One variant of vWD that is particularly difficult to distinguish from hemophilia A is vWD-Normandy, in which the vWF activities are normal but factor VIII levels are low. Several mutations causing vWD-Normandy have been described, but all of them result in decreased binding of factor VIII to vWF. This results in a shortening of the intravascular survival of factor VIII and thus reduced factor VIII activity. The Normandy variant should be suspected in patients with mild hemophilia that do not exhibit a sex-linked recessive inheritance pattern.[36]

Hemophilia A must also be distinguished from other hereditary blood-clotting factor deficiencies that exhibit a prolonged aPTT, including deficiencies of factors IX, XI, and XII; prekallikrein; and high-molecular-weight kininogen. Only deficiencies of factors VIII and IX cause chronic crippling hemarthroses with a family history suggestive of an X-linked bleeding disorder. Hemophilia A can be distinguished from factor IX deficiency (hemophilia B) only by specific assays. Factor XI deficiency occurs in both males and females and is a milder hemorrhagic disorder compared to severe hemophilia A or B. Factor XI deficiency can be confused with mild hemophilia A or B, but specific assays will distinguish them. Deficiencies of factor XII, prekallikrein, and high-molecular-weight kininogen can be distinguished from hemophilia because they are not associated with clinical bleeding. Mild hemophilia A, with factor VIII levels of about 15 percent of normal, must be distinguished from combined deficiency of both factor V and factor VIII.[37] Both the PT and aPTT are moderately prolonged in the combined disorder.

THERAPY

GENERAL

General principles applicable to the therapy of hemophilia A patients include the avoidance of aspirin, nonsteroidal anti-inflammatory drugs, and other agents that interfere with platelet aggregation. There are, however, exceptions to this rule. In view of the pain of hemophilic arthropathy, nonsteroidal anti-inflammatory agents are required. In these instances the physician should choose the agent that causes the least amount of increased bleeding. Usually this requires trying agents by trial and error to find the one most suitable for the patient. Patients should be advised of the numerous over-the-counter analgesics that contain aspirin or other antiplatelet agents. Addictive narcotic agents should be used with great caution and only when clearly indicated, since drug dependency can be a major problem in this disease. In general, intramuscular injections should be avoided. In the absence of prophylactic therapy, it is important to treat patients with hemophilia A as early as possible to avoid complications of bleeding. Surgical procedures on hemophilic patients should be scheduled early in the week to avoid "weekend crises." Ample supplies of factor VIII should be available in the blood bank or pharmacy to ensure rapid access to treatment when needed. All hemophilic patients should have access to home treatment and periodic examinations at a comprehensive hemophilia diagnostic and treatment center. Prophylactic therapy should be considered in all severely affected patients.

FACTOR VIII REPLACEMENT THERAPY

Hemorrhagic episodes in patients with hemophilia A can be managed by replacing factor VIII. Several plasma products are available for use in raising factor VIII to hemostatic levels. Fresh-frozen plasma and cryoprecipitate both contain factor VIII and were once the only products available for treatment. A disadvantage of plasma is that large volumes must be infused to achieve and maintain even minimal levels of factor VIII. The highest factor VIII level that can be achieved with plasma is about 20 percent of normal, and this is not always attainable nor sufficient for hemostasis. Cryoprecipitate can be used to attain normal levels of factor VIII, but individual bags of cryoprecipitate must be pooled, the factor VIII dose can only be estimated, and the product must be stored frozen. Several commercial lyophilized factor VIII concentrates, using cryoprecipitate of pooled normal human plasmas as starting material (2000 to 20,000 donors), are now available and do not have the disadvantages of plasma and cryoprecipitate (Table 123-3). Factor VIII concentrates have been sterilized, either by heating in solution, superheating to 80°C after lyophilization, or by exposure to organic solvent-detergents that inactivate enveloped viruses including HIV and hepatitis B and C viruses but do not inactivate parvovirus nor hepatitis A.[38,39] Parvovirus infection is not frequent in hemophilia A patients, since it is transmitted by cellular elements of the blood. Nevertheless, seroconversion to B19 parvovirus has been observed in patients receiving plasma-derived concentrates undergoing solvent-detergent extraction or pasteurization. Hepatitis A has also occurred in patients receiving plasma-derived concentrates inactivated by solvent-detergent techniques.[40]

Some of these products contain significant amounts of vWF (Table 123-3). Plasma-derived factor VIII concentrates prepared by monoclonal antibody techniques, and subjected to one of the procedures mentioned above, are highly purified and, barring breakdown in manufacturing techniques, are generally safe in terms of transmission of viral diseases.

Factor VIII produced by recombinant DNA techniques is now available and is both safe and effective (Table 123-3).[41] In addition to human factor VIII, porcine factor VIII is also commercially available for human use. Porcine factor VIII may be of great benefit in hemophilic patients with factor VIII antibodies, since the human anti-factor VIII antibody may not cross-react with porcine factor VIII. A comprehensive list of factor VIII concentrates can be found on the Internet.[42,43]

The dose of factor VIII can be ascertained as follows: If one unit of factor VIII per milliliter of plasma is considered to be 100 percent of normal, the dose required to raise the level to a given value is

TABLE 123-3   CURRENTLY AVAILABLE FACTOR VIII PRODUCTS[a]

	ORIGIN	VIRAL INACTIVATION
Intermediate purity		
Humate P[b]	Plasma	Pasteurization[c]
Profilate SD[b]	Plasma	Solvent detergent[d]
High purity		
Koate HP[b]	Plasma	Solvent detergent[d]
Beriate	Plasma	Pasteurization[c]
Immunate	Plasma	Vapor heating[e]
Hyate C	Porcine plasma	
Ultrapure[f]		
Hemofil M	Plasma	Solvent detergent[d]
Monoclate P	Plasma	Pasteurization[c]
Recombinant		
Recombinate[f]	CHO cells[g]	
Kogenate[f]	BHK cells[h]	
Refacto[i]	CHO cells[g]	
(B-domain deleted)		

[a]Additional concentrates are available in Europe.
[b]Contains vWF.
[c]Pasteurization at 60°C for 10 h.
[d]Solvent-detergent: TNBP + polysorbate 88.
[e]Vapor heating at 60°C for 10 h and 80°C for 1 h.
[f]Human albumin added; insignificant vWF.
[g]Chinese hamster ovarian cells.
[h]Baby hamster kidney cells.
[i]Not yet available.
NOTE: Helixate and Bioclate marketed by Centeon are the same as Kogenate and Recombinate, respectively.
SOURCE: Reprinted from *Hematology 1997*, p 36, American Society of Hematology, Washington, DC, 1997.

dependent upon the patient's plasma volume (roughly 5 percent of body weight in kilograms) and the level to which factor VIII is to be raised. Thus, the plasma volume of a 70-kg adult is roughly equivalent to 3500 ml (5% × 70 kg = 3.5 kg = 3500g, roughly equivalent to 3500 ml). To achieve normal factor VIII levels of 1 U/ml (100 percent), 3500 U of factor VIII should be given. This assumes a 100 percent recovery of the administered dose. In recent studies recovery approaches 100 percent, but this depends upon the method of assay and the factor VIII standard used for comparison.[44] After the initial dose of factor VIII, further doses of factor VIII are based on a half-life of 8 to 12 h. Thus, after a loading dose of 3500 U of factor VIII, a dose of 1750 U could be given in 12 h. However, for practical purposes, the dose of factor VIII is based on the knowledge that 1 unit of factor VIII per kilogram of body weight will raise the circulating factor VIII level about 0.02 U/ml. Thus, to raise the factor VIII level to 100 percent, that is, 1 U/ml, the dose of factor VIII required would be about 50 U per kilogram body weight, assuming that the patient's baseline factor VIII level is less than 1 percent of normal. The site and severity of hemorrhage determine the frequency and dose of factor VIII to be infused. Table 123-4 summarizes the recommended doses of factor VIII for various types of hemorrhage. These doses are not based on rigorous randomized studies, and recommendations vary from one hemophilia center to another. Given the high cost of factor VIII, some physicians prefer the lower doses.

Factor VIII can also be given as a constant infusion. Following a loading dose to raise factor VIII to the desired level, 150 to 200 U of factor VIII per hour can be infused. Factor VIII levels can be conveniently monitored from blood obtained from veins other than the one in which factor VIII is infused. In selected patients, factor VIII can be given outside the hospital in a continuous infusion using pump devices.[45]

DDAVP (1,8-DESAMINO-D-ARGININE VASOPRESSIN, DESMOPRESSIN)

During the 1970s, it was found that DDAVP caused a transient rise in factor VIII in normal subjects as well as in those with mild to

TABLE 123-4   DOSES OF FACTOR VIII FOR TREATMENT OF HEMORRHAGE*

Site of Hemorrhage	Desired Factor VIII Level, % of Normal	Factor VIII Dose, Units/kg Body Weight†	Frequency of Dose,‡ q Hours	Duration, Days
Hemarthroses	30–50	~25	12–24	1–2
Superficial intramuscular hematoma	30–50	~25	12–24	1–2
Gastrointestinal tract	~50	~25	12	7–10
Epistaxis	30–50	~25	12	Until resolved
Oral mucosa	30–50	~25	12	Until resolved
Hematuria	30–100	~25–50	12	Until resolved
Central nervous system	50–100	50	12	At least 7–10 days
Retropharyngeal	50–100	50	12	At least 7–10 days
Retroperitoneal	50–100	50	12	At least 7–10 days

*Mild or moderately affected patients may respond to DDAVP, which should be used in lieu of blood or blood products whenever possible.
†The factor VIII may be administered in a continuous infusion if the patient is hospitalized. After initial bolus, about 150 units factor VIII per hour is usually sufficient in an average-sized adult. Doses are given every 12 to 24 h.
‡Both the frequency of dosing and duration of therapy may be adjusted in keeping with the severity and duration of each patient's bleeding episode.

moderate hemophilia. Patients with severe hemophilia A do not respond.[46] After a dose of DDAVP, 0.3 μg per kilogram body weight, factor VIII levels increase two- to threefold above baseline in most, but not all, mildly or moderately affected hemophilia A patients. A concentrated intranasal spray of DDAVP can also be used (150 mg in each nostril).[47] The degree of response to the drug should always be determined in patients before a bleeding episode, since occasionally mildly or moderately affected patients will not respond. The peak response to DDAVP usually occurs 30 to 60 min postinfusion. In patients with mild or moderate hemophilia A, and in carriers whose baseline factor VIII levels are lower than 0.5 U/ml, DDAVP should be used in lieu of blood products. The mechanism by which DDAVP causes an increase in factor VIII is unknown.

Repeated administration of DDAVP results in a diminished response to the agent (tachyphylaxis). In many patients the response to the second dose of DDAVP is, on the average, 30 percent less than the response to the first dose, and after further doses the response rate may be even less.[48] DDAVP is a potent antidiuretic, and as a result, hyponatremia has been reported in some patients whose water intake exceeds about 1 liter per 24 h. There has been no convincing evidence that administration of DDAVP is associated with thrombosis in hemophilic patients.

ANTIFIBRINOLYTIC AGENTS

Antifibrinolytic agents, e.g., epsilon-aminocaproic acid (EACA) and tranexamic acid, have been used to enhance hemostasis in patients with hemophilia A.[49,50] Fibrinolytic inhibitors may be given as adjunctive therapy for bleeding from mucous membranes and are particularly valuable as adjunctive therapy for dental procedures. The usual dose of tranexamic acid for adults is 1 g four times daily. Unfortunately, tranexamic acid is not available in the United States for oral therapy. EACA can be given as a loading dose of 4 to 5 g followed by 1 g/h in adults. Another regimen is 4 g every 4 to 6 h orally for 2 to 8 days depending upon the severity of the bleeding episode. Antifibrinolytic agents are particularly useful as adjunctive therapy. However, it should be emphasized that antifibrinolytic therapy is contraindicated in the presence of hematuria.

FIBRIN GLUE

Fibrin glue, otherwise known as *fibrin tissue adhesives*, has been used as adjunctive therapy to factor VIII in hemophilic patients.[51] Briefly, fibrin glue contains fibrinogen, thrombin, and factor XIII. In some commercial products fibrinolytic inhibitors are added. The fibrinogen-factor XIII mixture is placed on the site of injury and clotted with a thrombin solution containing calcium. As a result, the fibrin clot is cross-linked and anchored to tissue. It is especially useful for hemosta-sis in patients undergoing dental surgery, who receive a preextraction bolus of factor VIII followed by application of fibrin glue to the tooth socket. Fibrin glue has also been used as adjunctive therapy to factor VIII following orthopedic procedures and circumcision. It has been of particular value for controlling bleeding when applied to the bed of a surgical wound following removal of large pseudotumors. Some hemophilia centers prepare their own "homemade" fibrin glue using cryoprecipitate as a source of fibrinogen and factor XIII. In some cases bovine thrombin preparations are used for clotting the fibrinogen solution. Bovine thrombin can result in complications, since it is contaminated with small amounts of bovine factor V. As a result, human antibodies to bovine factor V and thrombin may develop in patients receiving such products. These antibodies may cross-react with human factor V and/or human thrombin, resulting in a transient hemorrhagic disorder.[52]

TREATMENT OF MINOR OR MODERATE HEMORRHAGE

On occasion, superficial cuts and abrasions are managed with local measures, i.e., application of pressure sometimes suffices to control bleeding, even though oozing may continue off and on for several hours. Topical thrombin is of no value in this type of bleeding. In general, cautery should be avoided, since bleeding may restart when the cauterized area sloughs.

When replacement therapy for epistaxis is needed, the factor VIII level should be raised to about 0.5 U/ml (50 percent of normal). For treatment of hematuria, patients should be instructed to drink large quantities of fluids. If hematuria is mild, uncomplicated, and painless, factor VIII replacement is not necessary unless it persists. Gross or protracted hematuria may require replacement therapy, and, in these patients, factor VIII levels of at least 50 percent of normal are needed and should be continued until bleeding stops.

Hemophilic patients needing endoscopic procedures should first be treated with factor VIII to raise levels to at least 0.5 U/ml. Only one dose may be necessary if endoscopy is uncomplicated. In cases of severe abrasions or perforations following endoscopy, factor VIII replacement should be continued until healing of the lesion is complete. In the case of expanding soft-tissue hematomas, factor VIII therapy should be started immediately and maintained until the hematoma begins to resolve. With effective therapy the patient usually experiences rapid relief from pain. For treatment of acute hemarthroses, prompt administration of factor VIII decreases the occurrence of extensive degenerative joint changes, as well as deformity and muscle wasting. For chronic synovitis and for bleeding into "target" joints, daily administration of factor VIII to raise levels to 100 percent of normal for 6 to 8 weeks may be indicated.

TREATMENT OF MAJOR NONSURGICAL HEMORRHAGES

Any hemorrhage in a patient with hemophilia A may become major, but the following are common and frequently life-threatening: retropharyngeal; retroperitoneal; and central nervous system bleeding, whether subdural, subarachnoid, or into the brain parenchyma.[53]

For treatment of retropharyngeal bleeding, in particular that associated with a sensation of tightness in the throat, pain in the neck, dysphagia, or difficulty breathing, patients should receive factor VIII immediately in doses sufficient to raise factor VIII levels to normal (1.0 U/ml). Near-normal levels should be maintained until bleeding has ceased and the hematoma begins to resolve. For retroperitoneal hemorrhage, early treatment is required, and therapy should be continued for 7 to 10 days; otherwise bleeding may recur upon resumption of activity. Immediate administration of factor VIII, sufficient to raise the level to normal, should be started with the first sign of an intracranial hemorrhage or following a history of head trauma. Even asymptomatic patients with a history of head trauma should receive at least one dose of factor VIII as a prophylactic measure, and this should be given before diagnostic procedures such as a CT scan. Treatment of a known intracranial hemorrhage should be maintained for a minimum of 7 to 10 days, and the circulating factor VIII level should be kept normal throughout this period. Evacuation of subdural hematomas and surgical removal of hematomas involving the brain parenchyma can be carried out depending upon location. Despite aggressive replacement therapy, however, mortality from central nervous system bleeding is high.

REPLACEMENT OF FACTOR VIII
FOR SURGICAL PROCEDURES

For major surgical procedures, factor VIII should be raised to normal levels before operation and maintained for 7 to 10 days, or until healing is well underway. Treatment can be begun a few hours prior to surgery and continued intraoperatively. Postoperatively, factor VIII levels should be monitored at least once or twice daily to ensure that adequate levels are maintained. Since factor VIII may be "consumed" during surgery, doses of factor VIII higher than normal are sometimes required. Thus, factor VIII levels should be measured during surgery as well as in the postoperative period. Bone and joint surgery may require longer periods of factor VIII coverage. Replacement of knee, hip, and elbow joints is now possible, and several weeks of replacement therapy may be needed.[54]

HOME THERAPY

Home therapy using available factor VIII concentrates was introduced in the United States in 1977 and represented a major advance in the treatment of all forms of hemophilia.[55] Children as young as 3 years of age can be treated at home by parents or other reliable adults. Patients 6 years and older can be taught to treat themselves with factor VIII in the correct dose for an appropriate length of time. The training of patients and their families for home therapy is best accomplished in a regional comprehensive hemophilia diagnostic and treatment center or an affiliate of one of these centers. Patients are given an adequate supply of factor concentrates along with the paraphernalia required for intravenous administration. The prompt treatment of hemarthroses and hematomas made possible by home therapy resulted in a marked improvement in morbidity and mortality associated with hemophilia. In addition, the quality of life of hemophilia A patients was dramatically improved.[56,57]

PROPHYLACTIC THERAPY

The advent of stable and safe factor VIII concentrates has made prophylactic therapy for severely affected hemophilia A patients feasible. The administration of 50 U factor VIII/kg body weight three times weekly markedly decreases the frequency of hemophilic arthropathy and other long-term effects of hemorrhagic episodes.[58,59] In 1997, the Medical and Scientific Advisory Council of the National Hemophilia Foundation recommended prophylactic therapy for severely affected patients. For prophylactic therapy to be successful, patients should be selected for reliability in managing central venous catheter devices.[60,61] An analysis of the economic impact of prophylactic therapy, weighing the benefits against the high costs of factor VIII concentrates, suggests that the clinical benefit of prophylaxis is warranted as evidenced by significant improvement in the clinical condition of patients and improvement in the quality of life.[62]

LIVER TRANSPLANTATION AND GENE THERAPY

Normal livers have been transplanted successfully into patients with hemophilia, with resulting cure of the hemophilic condition.[63,64] However, donor livers are not widely available, so this procedure is rarely performed. As advances in modulation of graft-versus-host disease continue, the use of liver transplantation for the cure of hemophilia may increase.

Gene replacement therapy may offer ideal prophylactic treatment for hemophilia A. (See also Chap 19.) Recent advances in molecular biology have made gene insertion therapy a real possibility. Gene replacement therapy for factor VIII and factor IX has been shown to be possible in animal models using retroviral, adeno-associated, and adenoviral vectors. The early problems included low levels of expression and short duration of expression. Immune-mediated inhibition of retroviral and adenoviral vectors has also been a problem.[65] Improvements in vectors promise advances in gene therapy for hemophilia A. In addition, factors that have retarded efficient expression of factor VIII in transduced cells have been elucidated.[66] In addition, it has been possible to improve the passage of factor VIII through the endoplasmic reticulum by mutation of factor VIII residues involved in interaction with BiP, a protein chaperone within the endoplasmic reticulum.[67] Nonviral vectors are also being developed for gene therapy of factor VIII.[68] Mouse and dog models of hemophilia A exist, thus as improvements in vectorology continue, small and large animal models are available for testing as a prelude to clinical trials in humans. Human trials using gene transfer therapy (with B-domainless factor VIII in a retroviral vector) for hemophilia A have begun, but definitive results from these studies are not yet available.

COURSE AND PROGNOSIS

After the advent of factor VIII concentrates in the 1960s, there was a significant reduction in the morbidity and mortality from bleeding in hemophilia, at least until the AIDS crisis that began in the late 1970s until 1985.[69] The lifespan of hemophilia A patients began to approach that of normal individuals by the late 1970s. However, the use of replacement therapy has not been without significant complications. Common and serious adverse side effects of treatment include the following: the development of antibodies (inhibitors, circulating anticoagulants) against factor VIII; liver disease resulting from hepatitis B and C; and from about 1978, infection with HIV.[70] Factor VIII concentrates, prepared from many thousands of donors, were contaminated with HIV from about 1978 until about 1985. The vast majority of severely affected patients became infected with HIV during this period. With the introduction of heat-treated concentrates in 1985, contamination of these products with HIV has been eliminated for all practical purposes. However, AIDS is now a leading cause of death in older patients with hemophilia.[71] Chronic liver disease in hemophilia A patients resulting from transfusion-related hepatitis B and C may be accelerated by HIV infection and by the associated hepatotoxicity of antiviral drug therapy.[72] Fortunately, patients treated after 1985 can

TABLE 123-5   RISK FACTORS FOR THE DEVELOPMENT OF ANTI-FACTOR-VIII ANTIBODIES IN HEMOPHILIA A PATIENTS

- Disease severity: 80% of hemophilia A patients with inhibitors have <1% factor VIII activity.
- Exposure to factor VIII concentrates: the majority of high-titer inhibitors develop after <90 days of exposure to factor VIII.
- Genetic factors
  1. Family history of inhibitor development
  2. Negative correlation with HLA Cw5 antigen
  3. Molecular defects: the inversion and crossing-over defect in intron 22, gene deletions and nonsense point mutations resulting in patients without factor VIII antigen
- Method of purification of factor VIII concentrate

Reprinted by permission of the publisher from Inhibitors and their management, in *Haemophilia & Other Bleeding Disorders*, edited by C Rizza, G Lowe, p. 371, W. B. Saunders, New York, 1997.

expect to have virtually normal life spans free of the complications of hepatitis, AIDS, and other currently recognized blood-borne viral diseases.

FACTOR VIII INHIBITORS

Other than the transmission of viral diseases by factor VIII infusions, the main complication of hemophilia A is the development of specific inhibitor antibodies that neutralize factor VIII.[73] There is current debate about the true frequency of antifactor VIII inhibitors in severe hemophilia A patients, but in one study the frequency of inhibitors in a large group of patients after 18 years of follow-up was 20 percent.[74] This analysis included only patients treated with low- or intermediate-purity factor VIII concentrates. Frequent testing for inhibitors in previously untreated patients receiving newer highly purified factor VIII products from plasma or by recombinant technology revealed the frequent occurrence of transient inhibitors to factor VIII, many of which were of low titer and did not necessitate cessation of treatment with the same product. Although still a matter of uncertainty, it does not appear that the risk of inhibitors is higher when using highly purified plasma or recombinant products than that reported in earlier studies using products of lower purity.[75] This is not to say that development of factor VIII inhibitors may not be related to the nature of factor VIII product.[76] At least one outbreak of inhibitors appeared to be related to treatment with a specific plasma-derived factor VIII product of intermediate purity; fortunately inhibitors disappeared from the affected patients when use of the product was stopped.[77]

Factors related to the development of inhibitors are depicted in Table 123-5. As can be seen, they arise most frequently in severely affected patients, many of whom have gross gene rearrangements or inversion of the factor VIII gene. Inhibitors usually appear early in life, after about 100 exposure days to factor VIII replacement.

Factor VIII inhibitors are antibodies, most often of the IgG class and frequently restricted to the IgG$_4$ subclass.[76] Antibodies against the A$_2$ and C domains of factor VIII are most common. These antibodies interfere with the interaction of factor VIII with its cofactors and activators.[78]

The early diagnosis of factor VIII inhibitors is essential. While the presence of an inhibitor can be suspected on clinical grounds, as, for example, when a patient does not respond to conventional doses of factor VIII, laboratory diagnosis is required for confirmation. Factor VIII inhibitors are time- and temperature-dependent. The prolonged aPTT of the plasma of a patient without an inhibitor is corrected when mixed 1:1 with normal plasma even after incubation at 37°C for 1 to 2 h. In contrast, the partial thromboplastin time (PTT) on a 1:1 mixture of a patient with an inhibitor and normal plasma is prolonged after incubation at 37°C for 1 to 2 h. Specific diagnosis

rests upon the demonstration that an appropriate dilution of the patient's plasma, when added to normal plasma, neutralizes specifically factor VIII and not other blood-clotting factors that influence the PTT (i.e., factors IX, XI, XII, PK, HK). The demonstration that the inhibitor is specific for factor VIII will distinguish it from inhibitors of other clotting factors, the lupus anticoagulant, and nonspecific inhibitors. A common assay for an inhibitor is the Bethesda assay, in which the patient's plasma is diluted to a point that, when mixed with an equal volume of normal pooled human plasma and incubated for 2 h, will decrease the factor VIII activity in the mixture by 50 percent.[79] A modification of the Bethesda assay is the Nijmegen assay in which the pH of the sample over the 2-h period of incubation is controlled.[80]

There are several approaches to the treatment of factor VIII inhibitors[81] (Table 123-6). These require knowledge of whether the patient with an inhibitor is a "high" or "low" responder and whether the bleeding episode requiring treatment is considered minor or major.

High-Responder Patients   About 60 percent of patients who have inhibitors are high responders. *High responders* are defined as those patients whose inhibitor titer is higher than 10 Bethesda units (BU) at baseline, or whose inhibitor titers rise to greater than 10 BU after administration of factor VIII. Thus, high responders who are not treated with factor VIII for long periods of time may have a sustained high level of inhibitor or may have a very low to undetectable level of inhibitor before they are challenged with factor VIII.

As depicted in Table 123-6, major bleeding episodes in a high-responder patient whose initial inhibitor titer is below 10 BU should be treated with either human or porcine factor VIII. The rationale is that when the initial titer is low, sufficient factor VIII can be administered to neutralize the inhibitor and to attain adequate factor VIII levels for hemostasis. Although factor VIII inhibitor bypassing agents can be used (see below), they are not as reliable in achieving hemostasis as factor VIII, and their effect cannot be adequately monitored with specific laboratory tests. If human factor VIII is used, a loading dose of 10,000 to 15,000 U may be required and followed by up to 1000 U factor VIII per hour depending upon the factor VIII level. All patients with inhibitors should be tested to determine whether their inhibitor cross-reacts with porcine factor VIII, as measured in a Bethesda assay, in which porcine factor VIII replaces human factor VIII. If the inhibitor does not cross-react with porcine factor VIII, it can be administered in doses of 50 to 100 U/kg per body weight every 8 to 12 h.

In high-responder patients whose initial inhibitor is less than 10 BU and who experience a minor bleeding episode, the agent of choice would be a factor VIII inhibitor bypassing agent. Recombinant factor VIIa in doses of 90 to 120 μg/kg per body weight every 2 to 3 h has been recently introduced and is safe and effective in most hemorrhagic episodes. If this agent is not available, activated or unactivated prothrombin complex concentrates may be used. Factor VIII can also be used but should be avoided in most instances in view of an anamnestic response of the inhibitor to factor VIII.

High-responder patients whose initial inhibitor titer is greater than 10 BU usually do not respond to even high doses of human factor VIII. If the inhibitor cross-reacts with porcine factor, this product too may be ineffective. Thus, in high-responder patients whose initial inhibitor titer is greater than 10 BU, and who experience a major or minor bleeding episode, recombinant factor VIIa is considered by many to be the treatment of choice. If this agent is not available, activated or unactivated prothrombin complex concentrates should be used as noted in Table 123-6.

Low-Responder Patients   *Low-responder patients* are arbitrarily defined as those whose inhibitor titer is less than 10 BU even after challenge with factor VIII. For major bleeding episodes, high doses of human factor VIII or porcine factor VIII may be used as recommended above. For minor bleeds, recombinant factor VIIa, prothrombin complex concentrates (activated or unactivated), are recommended, since some ''low'' responders will convert to high responders when challenged repeatedly with factor VIII.

Nonactivated or activated prothrombin complex concentrates contain variable amounts of activated factors, including factors VIIa, IXa, and Xa. The activated products have higher concentrations of activated factors than unactivated products. It is not known how these agents ''bypass'' the inhibitors, but it is postulated that they enhance the tissue factor-factor VIIa pathway of coagulation. Both products have been used successfully for the therapy of hemophilic patients with inhibitors to factor VIII or factor IX.

One of the newer agents for treating patients with inhibitors is recombinant factor VIIa.[82] This product has been reported to be more effective than other bypassing agents. Factor VIIa is recommended in doses of approximately 90 to 120 μg/kg per body weight every 2 to 3 h. The dosing frequency is based on a plasma half-life of factor VIIa that is about 2 to 3 h. The mechanisms of action of factor VIIa have been investigated using in vitro techniques. In the recommended doses it is hypothesized that factor VIIa can activate factor X on the surface of activated platelets in the absence of tissue factor.[83] Factor Xa can then associate with factor Va and convert prothrombin to thrombin. Since activated platelets are localized to the site of vessel injury, thrombin generation by factor VIIa is localized to the site of bleeding. This may account for the reported safety of factor VIIa.[82]

Other approaches to the treatment of inhibitors include: immunosuppression; removal of the antibody by plasmapheresis; adsorption of the antibody on an affinity column during plasma exchange; and administration of intravenous gamma globulin. The Malmo protocol uses nearly all of these approaches in combination, including extracorporeal adsorption of antibody to a sepharose A column; the administration of cyclophosphamide; daily administration of factor VIII; and intravenous gamma globulin.[84]

The most promising approach to eradication of an inhibitor is the use of immune tolerance regimens. The basis of this approach is to administer daily doses of factor VIII until the inhibitor titer is undetectable.[85] Low-dose and high-dose regimens have been described as shown in Table 123-7. Factor VIII inhibitor bypassing agents are used for acute bleeds that occur during immune tolerance induction. Various approaches to the treatment of factor VIII inhibitors can be found on the Internet.[86]

INFECTIOUS COMPLICATIONS (SEE ALSO CHAP. 139)

Hepatitis Almost all multitransfused patients with hemophilia treated before 1985 were infected with one or more agents of viral hepatitis. While many infected patients did not suffer acute symptoms, at least 50 percent can be expected to develop chronic persistent or chronic active hepatitis that may lead to frank cirrhosis.[87] Hepatitis C and B viruses are commonly associated with chronic liver disease.

About 90 percent of adult hemophilic patients have antibodies to hepatitis B surface antigen (HBsAg), and at least 10 percent of severely affected adult patients have circulating HBsAg. The antigen-positive adult patients frequently have a superimposed infection with the delta agent, leading to severe active hepatitis and cirrhosis and an increased risk of hepatocellular carcinoma.[88–90] Therapy with recombinant interferon α can improve biochemical markers of hepatocellular damage and liver histology in some patients with chronic hepatitis C,[91] but the long-term benefits of α-interferon therapy are not established.

HIV Currently, about 80 percent of older, severely affected hemophilia A patients have antibodies to HIV, indicating infection with the virus. The incidence of HIV antibodies in mildly affected patients is much lower and correlates with treatment with factor VIII concentrates before viral inactivation procedures were used. In one study, 14 percent of patients treated only with cryoprecipitate during the period from 1979 to 1985 were infected with HIV, while 88 percent of patients treated with factor VIII concentrates became infected.[92] Screening of donor populations and new techniques for preparing factor VIII concentrates since 1985 have nearly eliminated the risk of HIV transmission. Many HIV-infected patients with hemophilia developed AIDS, and treatment of AIDS has become an integral part of the management of severe hemophilia. In one report, AIDS was the primary cause of deaths in hemophilia A patients between the years 1976 and 1991.[71] Bleeding was responsible for only 5 percent of deaths.

TABLE 123-6   TREATMENT OF INHIBITORS IN HEMOPHILIA A PATIENTS

TYPE OF PATIENT	INITIAL TITER	MINOR HEMORRHAGE*	MAJOR HEMORRHAGE*
High responder	<10 BU	Recombinant factor VIIa; prothrombin complex concentrates; activated prothrombin complex concentrates	Human factor VIII; recombinant factor VIIa; porcine factor VIII, prothrombin complex concentrates; activated prothrombin complex concentrates
High responder	>10 BU	Recombinant factor VIIa; prothrombin complex concentrates; activated prothrombin complex concentrates	Porcine factor VIII, recombinant factor VIIa; prothrombin complex concentrates; plasma exchange + high-dose factor VIII
Low responder	<10 BU	Recombinant factor VIIa; prothrombin complex concentrates; activated prothrombin complex concentrates	High-dose human factor VIII; recombinant factor VIIa; porcine factor VIII, activated prothrombin complex concentrates

*A choice of agents for the treatment of major and minor hemorrhage is listed below. Some physicians will choose the first product listed as the agent of choice, but the choice varies from physician to physician.

SOURCE: Reprinted by permission of the publisher from Inhibitors and their management, in *Haemophilia & Other Bleeding Disorders*, edited by C Rizza, G Lowe, p 376, W. B. Saunders, New York, 1997.

TABLE 123-7   EXAMPLES OF TOLERANCE PROTOCOLS FOR HEMOPHILIA A INHIBITOR PATIENTS

IMMUNE TOLERANCE PROTOCOLS	DOSE	INITIAL RESPONSE
High-dose regimen	100 U/kg factor VIII twice a day until antibody reaches 1 BU/ml. Then 150 U/kg Factor VIII per day until Factor VIII half-life is normal	In 16 of 21 patients, titer fell to <1 BU/ml
Low-dose regimen	50 U/kg factor VIII per day	9 of 12 patients responded
Netherlands protocol	25 U/kg factor VIII per day	11 of 18 patients responded

SOURCE: Reprinted by permission of the publisher from Inhibitors and their management, in *Haemophilia & Other Bleeding Disorders*, edited by C Rizza, G Lowe, p 379, W. B. Saunders, New York, 1997.

Perhaps related to HIV infection, immune suppression has been observed in many recipients of blood products, including factor VIII concentrates.[93] Evidence of a depressed cellular immune system can be found in most patients with hemophilia A who have been treated with factor concentrates.[94] There is often a reduced ratio of T-helper lymphocytes to T-suppressor lymphocytes, in addition to a decrease in natural killer cells. Anergy to cutaneously applied antigens is also a common finding in patients who have been multiply transfused. The degree of immune suppression may be related in part to the purity of the transfused product.[95,96] Improved methods of purification have led to the development of products that appear to be less immunosuppressive.

Risk of Transmission of Viral Diseases by New Factor VIII Products   Available factor VIII concentrates are considered to be safe and effective, and there is virtually no risk of transmitting currently known viral diseases with these products. There have, however, been occasional exceptions. For example, solvent-detergent extraction does not inactivate viruses without lipid envelopes, including hepatitis A virus and parvovirus. As a result, outbreaks of hepatitis A have been reported in patients receiving some solvent-detergent-treated products. These outbreaks of viral diseases are usually related to breakdowns during the manufacturing process.

Prions   Prions are infectious particles that consist of proteinaceous material that is devoid of a nucleic acid genome.[97] They are thought to be variant forms of a normal protein with an altered conformation. The ''infectious'' nature of prions may be due to their ability to bind to other proteins and induce similar conformational changes in them such that new ''infectious'' particles can be generated. Prions are responsible for several neurodegenerative disorders including Creutzfeldt-Jakob disease (CJD) in humans, scrapie in sheep, and spongiform encephalopathy in cows. Prions are resistant to all currently available viral inactivation techniques. Although prion diseases are generally transmitted by ingestion of infected neural tissues, there is a new variant of CJD which appears to occur in people who have eaten beef from cows infected with a form of prion causing bovine spongiform encephalopathy.[98] This form of CJD has been reported mainly in the United Kingdom and has been related to the bovine disease. For example, prions have been found in tonsillar tissue of patients with new-variant CJD, heightening the concern about whether prions of this type might be transmitted by blood products. To date there is no evidence that new variant CJD or, for that matter, the usual form of CJD is transmitted in this way. However, conclusive data are lacking, since the incubation period for the disease may be many years. For this reason certain plasma products prepared from blood of donors in the United Kingdom have been withdrawn until more data are available. There is, however, encouraging preliminary data in that autopsies of 33 hemophilics in the United Kingdom showed no evidence of prion disease.[98]

HEMOPHILIA B (FACTOR IX DEFICIENCY, CHRISTMAS FACTOR DEFICIENCY)

DEFINITION AND HISTORY

Hemophilia B is clinically indistinguishable from hemophilia A. It is a sex-linked, recessive hemorrhagic disease characterized by a decrease in factor IX clotting activity. In 1952 Aggeler and colleagues and Biggs and colleagues observed the existence of another X-linked bleeding disorder that was clinically similar to classic hemophilia.[7,99] The deficient factor has been designated as *factor IX*, and the disease is called *hemophilia B*. Other synonyms for factor IX include *plasma thromboplastin component* (PTC) and *Christmas factor*, named after the family in which it was described.

ETIOLOGY AND PATHOGENESIS

Hemophilia B occurs in 1 out of every 25,000 to 30,000 male births. Just as with hemophilia A, hemophilia B is found in all ethnic groups and has no geographic predilection.

Factor IX is a vitamin-K-dependent, single-chain glycoprotein consisting of 415 amino acids. It is activated by the factor VIIa/tissue factor complex, or factor XIa, to form the active enzyme, factor IXa. Once activated, factor IXa activates factor X in the presence of activated factor VIII, phospholipid (activated platelets), and calcium. Factor VIIIa is a necessary cofactor for the activity of factor IXa. Therefore, deficiency of either factor IX or VIII leads to a similar lack of factor X-activating activity. Factor Xa converts prothrombin to thrombin in the presence of activated factor V phospholipid and calcium. Thus, deficiency of factor IX results in delayed conversion of prothrombin to thrombin, which is the cause of the bleeding tendency. Hemophilia B can result from either the absence or dysfunction of factor IX molecules. Clinical severity of hemophilia B is roughly correlated with factor IX functional activity.

GENETICS AND MOLECULAR BIOLOGY

The factor IX gene is on the long arm of the X chromosome and is approximately 33 kb in length, much smaller than the gene for factor VIII.[100] Because it is less complex, the factor IX gene has been studied in greater detail than the factor VIII gene. A schematic diagram of the gene and the protein product is depicted in Fig. 123-11. The protein consists of a signal peptide that targets the protein for secretion from the hepatocyte to the circulation. The propeptide is necessary for posttranslational modification of 12 amino-terminal glutamic acid residues by an intracellular vitamin-K-dependent carboxylase. The propeptide is cleaved from the mature protein before it enters the circulation. The next domain contains the 12 γ-carboxyglutamic acid (Gla) residues that are necessary for calcium-dependent lipid binding. The activation peptide is cleaved from the zymogen form of factor IX either by factor VIIa/TF or by factor XIa, resulting in a two-chain active enzyme, factor IXaβ. The catalytic triad (histidine 221, aspartic acid 229, and serine 365) resides on the heavy chain.

Many genetic variants of hemophilia B have been described. They include point mutations, frameshifts, deletions, and other abnormalities that cause structural and/or functional changes in the factor IX protein.[101–103] Several hundred unique mutations have been reported, and a database of mutations has been developed and is updated yearly.[104] It can also be found on the Internet.[105]

Over 30 percent of factor IX mutations occur at CG dinucleotides. These mutations often involve critical arginine residues that result in a dysfunctional molecule.[106–109] Many mutations have been reported in more than one kindred, and some of these derive from the same ''founder.''[109,110] As predicted by genetic theory of X-linked recessive disorders, approximately one-third of mutations resulting in hemophilia B arise de novo.

Mutations in regulatory regions of the factor IX gene have also been identified. Particularly interesting examples are mutations in the 5′ promoter region that lead to the hemophilia B Leiden phenotype (Table 123-8). This disorder is characterized by very low levels of factor IX antigen and activity at birth and during early childhood. The levels gradually rise to 60 percent of normal or greater following puberty, apparently in response to endogenous androgen synthesis. Several different mutations in the promoter region of the factor IX gene disrupt binding of transcription factors, resulting in reduced transcription of the factor IX gene.[111–113] The hormonal changes occurring at puberty are apparently able to overcome the transcription defect and maintain hemostatically adequate levels of factor IX.

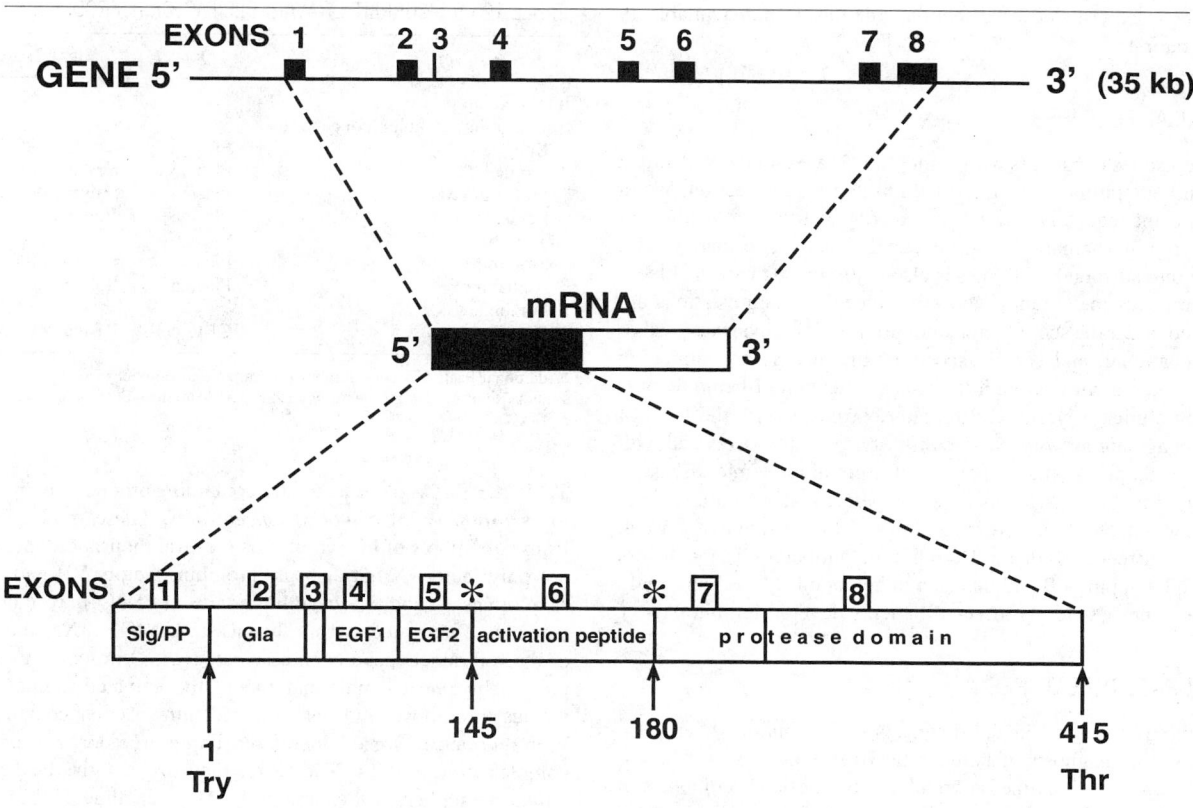

FIGURE 123-11   Schematic diagram of the factor IX gene, the messenger RNA, and the protein. The exons are depicted by the black boxes. The white 3' portion of the RNA is untranslated. The diagram of the protein shows the domains and the exons that encode each portion of the protein. The cleavage sites by factor XIa or factor VIIa/tissue factor are depicted by asterisks.

Hemophilia Bm is characterized by a deficiency of factor IX clotting activity and a prolonged ox-brain prothrombin time. The original hemophilia B patient with a prolonged ox-brain prothrombin time had the surname Martin and this led to the term *hemophilia Bm.*[102,114] A number of missense mutations affecting amino acid residues at positions 180, 181, and 182 of the protein as well as several residues close to the active site region have been identified in the patients having the characteristic findings of hemophilia Bm. These mutations result in a factor IX molecule that exhibits abnormal interaction with ox-brain tissue factor.[114]

Hemophilia B inheritance is similar to that of hemophilia A. All daughters of affected males are obligatory carriers, while all sons are normal. Female carriers may have factor IX levels ranging from less than 10 to 100 percent of normal, but the mean level is about 50 percent of normal. Carriers of hemophilia B are usually asymptomatic, except in the cases of extreme X-chromosome inactivation, X-mosaicism, Turner syndrome, or testicular feminization.[115] When the level of factor IX activity is less than 25 percent of normal, abnormal bleeding may occur, especially after trauma.

CARRIER DETECTION AND PRENATAL DIAGNOSIS

Carrier detection and genetic screening are sometimes possible through the use of DNA probes to directly identify mutations. As with factor VIII, mutations at CpG nucleotide pairs disrupt TaqI cleavage sites and can therefore be directly detected by restriction endonuclease mapping. More commonly, RFLP analysis is used. Prenatal diagnosis has been reliably accomplished by RFLP analysis of DNA obtained by chorionic villus sampling as early as 8 to 10 weeks after conception.[116] This procedure can also be performed on fetal cells obtained by amniocentesis and is more accurate than fetal blood sampling for factor IX activity and factor IX antigenic material. Direct sequencing of the factor IX gene

TABLE 123-8   MUTATIONS IN THE PUTATIVE PROMOTER REGION OF THE FACTOR IX GENE

Nucleotide Substitution	Nucleotide Change	F IX % Activity	F IX % Antigen	Comments
−21	T→G	<1–70	—	Disruption of HNF-4 binding site; F IX activity increases after puberty
−20	T→A	<1–60	<1–60	*
−20	T→C	9	—	*
−6	G→A	13–70	—	*
−5	A→T	3	—	*
6	T→A	<2–20	—	*
8	T→C	1–32	—	C/EBP binding site: F IX clotting activity increases after puberty
13	A→G	<1–60	<1–60	†
13	delete 1	<1–60	<1–60	†

*F IX activity increases after puberty.
†C/EBP binding site: F IX clotting activity increases after puberty.
SOURCE: Reprinted with permission of the publisher from HR Roberts: Molecular biology of hemophilia B. *Thromb Haemos* 70(1):3, 1993.

can also be used for carrier detection, but this is not available in most laboratories.

CLINICAL FEATURES

Bleeding episodes in patients with hemophilia B are clinically identical to those in hemophilia A, as described in the previous section. When patients are inadequately treated, repeated hemarthroses leading to chronic, crippling hemarthropathy occur. Hematoma formation with dissection into surrounding tissues is also common. Hematuria, bleeding from mucous membranes, and other bleeding manifestations are as described under the section on hemophilia A. The physical, psychological, vocational, and social aspects of the disease are similar to those encountered with hemophilia A. Classification of hemophilia B is based on clinical severity and roughly correlates with the level of factor IX coagulant activity. Severe disease is usually associated with factor IX levels of less than 1 percent of normal; moderate disease is associated with factor IX levels of 1 to 5 percent; and mild disease is associated with factor IX levels ranging from 5 to 40 percent of normal.

The occurrence of factor IX inhibitor antibodies is much less common in hemophilia B patients than in hemophilia A patients. Only about 3 percent of severely affected patients develop inhibitors.

LABORATORY FEATURES

The screening tests used in the diagnosis of hemophilia A are also employed in the diagnosis of hemophilia B. In most cases of hemophilia B, the prothrombin time is normal, and the partial thromboplastin time is prolonged. However, specific assay of factor IX coagulant activity is required for the definitive diagnosis. The most commonly used test is a one-stage clotting assay based on the PTT. Determination of factor IX antigen levels is of value in further classification of the disorder. Even though prothrombin times are usually normal in hemophilia B, they are occasionally prolonged, especially when ox-brain thromboplastin is the source of tissue factor. The factor IX in patients with hemophilia Bm competes with factor X for activation by the factor VIIa/tissue factor complex, thus resulting in a long PT.[117] Since most American prothrombin time reagents contain rabbit brain tissue factor, the prothrombin times recorded for American patients with hemophilia Bm are usually normal, and the hemophilia Bm subtype will not be identified. In all forms of hemophilia B, the bleeding time is normal.

DIFFERENTIAL DIAGNOSIS

Hemophilia B must be distinguished from hemophilia A. Both are inherited as X-linked recessive disorders, and both have virtually identical hemorrhagic manifestations. The only way to differentiate hemophilia B from hemophilia A is to perform specific assays for factors VIII and IX on the patient's plasma.

Inherited and acquired deficiencies of other vitamin-K-dependent factors, liver disease, and warfarin overdose must also be distinguished from hemophilia B. In these cases, not only factor IX but all other vitamin-K-dependent clotting factors will be decreased including prothrombin, factor VII, and factor X. Acquired antibodies specific for factor IX occur in nonhemophilic patients, but these are very rare.

THERAPY

FACTOR IX REPLACEMENT

The basic treatment of hemophilia B is replacement of factor IX. There are several products available for use, and they are listed in

TABLE 123-9　CURRENTLY AVAILABLE FACTOR IX PRODUCTS*

	ORIGIN	VIRAL INACTIVATION
Intermediate purity (prothrombin complex concentrates)		
Konyne 80	Plasma	Dry heat 80°C
Proplex T	Plasma	Dry heat 60°C
Profilnine SD	Plasma	Solvent detergent
Bebulin VH	Plasma	Vapor heating
High purity		
Mononine	Plasma	Ultra filtration; chemical
Alphanine	Plasma	Solvent detergent
Recombinant		
BeneFix	CHO cells	Pasteurization

*Additional Factor IX concentrates are available in Europe.
SOURCE: Reprinted from *Hematology 1997*, p 36, American Society of Hematology, Washington, DC, 1997.

Table 123-9. The older factor-IX-containing products are often referred to as *prothrombin complex concentrates*. These products, prepared from large pools of human plasma (several thousand donors), contain not only factor IX but also prothrombin, factors VII and X, as well as proteins C and S. In addition, the products may contain small amounts of activated factors such as factors VIIa, IXa, and Xa. Some of these products have been associated with thromboembolic events, presumably due to contamination with the activated components. Deep venous thrombosis and disseminated intravascular coagulation have been reported in some patients receiving large doses of prothrombin complex concentrates. Therefore, they are not the best choice for replacement therapy in hemophilia B, even though they are much cheaper than the highly purified factor IX concentrates. When prothrombin complex concentrates are used for replacement therapy, factor IX levels of greater than 50 percent of normal should not be exceeded in order to minimize the risk of thrombosis. The use of these products in factor-IX-deficient patients with liver dysfunction is especially hazardous, since it has been shown that activated factors contaminating these preparations are not cleared efficiently by a diseased liver and as a result thrombosis can be induced.

The highly purified factor IX products are also listed in Table 123-9. Some are prepared from human plasma while one product (BeneFix) is produced by recombinant DNA technology. Although all available factor IX concentrates are now considered to be safe and effective, the recombinant product undergoes a final viral inactivation step. In addition, it is not exposed to human albumin or bovine serum during preparation. Thus, even the theoretical risk of transmission of prion diseases is averted with this preparation. Some clinicians consider the recombinant product to be the agent of choice, although it has a major drawback in that the intravascular recovery of factor IX is generally lower than the recovery of highly purified factor IX product prepared from plasma.[118]

DOSING OF FACTOR IX

The dose calculations for all factor IX products are different from those used in hemophilia A. The reason is that intravascular recovery of factor IX is usually only about 50 percent, and, in the case of the recombinant product, the recovery is even lower. The reason for this is unclear, but it has been proposed that factor IX binds to elements on the vessel wall. In fact, factor IX binds specifically to collagen type IV, a component of the vessel wall.[119] The dose of factor IX can be estimated by assuming that one unit of factor IX per kilogram body weight will increase circulating factor IX by 1 percent of normal or 0.01 U/ml. Thus, in a severely affected patient, to achieve a level of 100 percent of normal (using only highly purified factor IX products), 100 U of factor IX per kilogram body weight should be given as a bolus, followed by one-half this amount every 12 to 18 h. Dosing should be monitored by assays of factor IX before and after bolus administration. Factor IX can also be administered as a constant infusion after the bolus administration. The dose of factor IX to be infused per hour can be estimated on the basis of a factor IX half-life of 12 to 18 h. Thus, in a 60-kg adult, who receives highly purified factor IX, 6000 U of the factor should raise the factor IX level to about 100 percent of normal. Over the next 12 to 18 h, the level will decrease by about 50 percent, and thus the patient will need about 3000 U of factor IX during that period or 250 U of factor IX per hour as an infusion. These calculations are only estimates of average responses, and so factor IX dosing should be monitored by factor IX assays and the dose adjusted appropriately. Prophylactic therapy for hemophilia B can also be attempted in individuals selected in the same manner as that described for hemophilia A patients. The dose of factor IX is 25 to 40 U/kg of body weight twice weekly.

Although currently available factor IX concentrates are safe in terms of transmission of HIV and hepatitis B and C viruses, patients treated prior to 1985 may have been infected with these agents.

COURSE AND PROGNOSIS

Unless treated properly, hemophilia B is fraught with the same complications of recurrent hemorrhages as hemophilia A. Thus, in inadequately treated patients, hemarthroses and chronic hemophilic arthropathy are common. In addition to joint deformities, chronic active hepatitis and chronic persistent hepatitis are common in patients treated before 1985. About 50 percent of older and severely affected patients are now HIV-positive. Patients treated after 1985 are unlikely to have contracted HIV and can expect to have a relatively normal life span.

Patients with severe hemophilia B may develop inhibitory antibodies against factor IX, making treatment very difficult.[120,121] About 3 percent of patients with severe hemophilia B develop specific inhibitor antibodies, frequently restricted in immunoglobulin composition to the IgG$_4$ subclass and kappa light chains.[122] Most inhibitors can be detected when the aPTT on a mixture of normal and patient's plasma is prolonged. In contrast to the inhibitors in hemophilia A patients, inhibitor antibodies against factor IX are not time- and temperature-dependent, and, thus, it is usually not necessary to incubate the mixtures for 2 h at 37°C. Inhibitors to factor IX can be quantitated by modifying the Bethesda method for detecting factor VIII inhibitors. Many patients with inhibitors have mutations that result in the absence of circulating factor IX antigen, most commonly deletions and nonsense mutations.

TREATMENT OF FACTOR IX INHIBITORS

When the inhibitor titer is below 10 BU/ml, it is sometimes possible to neutralize the factor IX inhibitor using large doses of highly purified factor IX concentrates. However, when the inhibitor titer is greater than 10 BU/ml, acute bleeding in patients should be treated with the same agents used to bypass factor VIII inhibitors as shown in Table 123-6. Recombinant factor VIIa in doses of 90 to 120 μg/kg body weight intravenously every 2 to 3 h may be used. Alternatively, activated or nonactivated prothrombin complex concentrates can be used as noted in Table 123-6.

Induction of immune tolerance can also be tried in hemophilia B patients using daily infusions of highly purified factor IX preparations. However, significant adverse reactions have been reported in severely affected patients, including anaphylaxis and the nephrotic syndrome.[123] Of the reported cases, many patients were less than 12 years of age and suffered from severe hemophilia B due to large deletions of the factor IX gene. The nephrotic syndrome may be transient and remit upon cessation of factor IX replacement. The etiology of the nephrotic

syndrome is not known. Patients with hemophilia B and factor IX antibodies who experience anaphylaxis with factor IX infusions should be treated with factor VIIa concentrates.

GENE THERAPY FOR HEMOPHILIA B

Long-term correction of hemophilia B has been achieved in animal models.[124–126] Transduction of muscle cells by an adeno-associated viral (AAV) vector containing a factor IX construct resulted in phenotypic correction of the clotting defect in hemophilia B dogs for greater than 17 months.[124] Likewise, transduction of hepatocytes with an AAV vector containing factor IX DNA has also been reported to correct the hemophilia defect in hemophilia B mice and dogs for about 7 and 8 months, respectively. Sustained factor IX levels of up to 25 percent of normal were obtained in one study in mice,[125] while levels exceeding 100 percent were achieved in another study.[126] The results in animals are encouraging and suggest that permanent corrections of the hemophilic defect using gene transfer technology in humans may be possible (see also Chap. 19). Clinical trials of gene transfer therapy for hemophilia B using adeno-associated viral vectors containing factor IX cDNA have been started, but the studies are preliminary.[127]

REFERENCES

1. Brinkhous KM: A short history of hemophilia, with some comments on the word "hemophilia," in *Handbook of Hemophilia*, edited by KM Brinkhous, HC Hemker, p 3. Elsevier, New York, 1975.
2. Katznelson JL: Hemophilia, with special reference to the Talmud. *Heb Med J* 1:165, 1956.
3. Morawitz P: Die Chemie der Blutgerinnung. *Ergebnisse Physiol* 4:307, 1905.
4. Addis T: The pathogenesis of hereditary haemophilia. *J Pathol Bacteriol* 15:427, 1911.
5. Brinkhous KM: A study of the clotting defect in hemophilia. The delayed formation of thrombin. *Am J Med Sci* 198:509, 1939.
6. Pavlovsky A: Contribution to the pathogenesis of hemophilia. *Blood* 2:185, 1947.
7. Aggeler PM, White SG, Glendenning MB: Plasma thromboplastin component (PTC) deficiency: A new disease resembling hemophilia. *Proc Soc Exp Biol Med* 79:692, 1952.
8. Wright IS: The nomenclature of blood clotting factors. *Thromb Diath Haemorr* 7:381, 1962.
9. Macfarlane RG: An enzyme cascade in the blood clotting mechanism, and its function as a biological amplifier. *Nature* 202:498, 1964.
10. Davie EW, Ratnoff OD: Waterfall sequence for intrinsic blood clotting. *Science* 145:1310, 1964.
11. Broze GR Jr: Tissue factor pathway inhibitor and the revised theory of coagulation. *Annu Rev Med* 46:103, 1995.
12. Fay PJ: Reconstitution of human factor VIII from isolated subunits. *Arch Biochem Biophys* 262:525, 1988.
13. Roberts HR, Monroe DM, Oliver JA, et al: Newer concepts of blood coagulation. *Haemophilia* 4:331, 1998.
14. Tuddenham EGD: Factor VIII, in *Molecular Basis of Thrombosis and Hemostasis*, edited by High KA and Roberts HR, p 167. Marcel Dekker, New York, 1995.
15. http://europium.csc.mrc.ac.uk: Hemophilia A mutation, structure, test and resource site (HAMSTeRS).
16. Tuddenham EGD, Cooper DN, Gitschier J, et al: Haemophilia A: database of nucleotide substitutions, deletions, insertions and rearrangements of the factor VIII gene. *Nucleic Acids Res* 22:4851, 1996.
17. Lakich D, Kazazian HH, Antonarakis SE, Gitschier J: Inversions disrupting the factor VIII gene are a common cause of severe hemophilia A. *Nat Genet* 5:236, 1993.
18. Higuchi M, Kazazian HH Jr, Kasch L, et al: Molecular characterization of severe hemophilia A suggests that about half the mutations are not within the coding regions and splice junctions of the factor VIII gene. *Proc Natl Acad Sci USA* 88(16):7405, 1991.
19. Antonarakis SE, Youssoufian H, Kazazian H: Molecular genetics of hemophilia in man (factor VIII deficiency). *Mol Biol Med* 4:81, 1987.

20. Mori PG, Pasino M, Vadala CR, et al: Haemophilia 'A' in a 46Xi(Xq) female. *Br J Haematol* 43:143, 1979.

21. Gitschier J, Kogan S, Diamond C, Levinson B: Genetic basis of hemophilia A. *Thromb Haemost* 66:37, 1991.

22. Peake IR Molecular genetics and counseling in haemophilia. *Thromb Haemost* 74:40, 1995.

23. Peake IR, Lillicrap DP, Boulyjenkov V, et al: Report of a joint WHO/WFH meeting on control of haemophilia: carrier detection and prenatal diagnosis. *Blood Coagul Fibrinolysis* 4:313, 1993.

24. Graham JB: Evolution of methods for carrier detection in hemophilia. *Prog Clin Biol Res* 324:29, 1990.

25. Goodeve AC, Peake IR: Diagnosis of hemophilia A and B carriers and prenatal diagnosis, in *Haemophilia*, edited by CD Forbes, L Aledort, R Madhok, p 63. Chapman & Hall, London, 1997.

26. Poon MC, Hoar DI, Low S, et al: Hemophilia A carrier detection by restriction fragment length polymorphism analysis and discriminant analysis based on ELISA of factor VIII and vWf. *J Lab Clin Med* 119:751, 1992.

27. Nichols WC, Amano K, Cacheris PM, et al: Moderation of hemophilia A phenotype by the factor V R506Q mutation. *Blood* 88:1183, 1996.

28. Arbini AA, Mannucci PM, Bauer K: Low prevalence of the factor V Leiden mutation among "severe" hemophiliacs with a "milder" bleeding diathesis. *Thromb Haemost* 74:1255, 1995.

29. R Madhok: Musculoskeletal bleeding in hemophilia, in *Hemophilia*, edited by CD Forbes, L Aledort, R Madhok, p 115. Chapman & Hall, London, 1997.

30. Gilbert MS: The hemophilic pseudotumor. *Prog Clin Biol Res* 324:257, 1990.

31. Hanley JP, Ludlam CA: Central and peripheral nervous system bleeding, in *Hemophilia*, edited by CD Forbes, L Aledort, R Madhok, p 87. Chapman & Hall, London, 1997.

32. Carron DB, Boon TH, Walker FC: Peptic ulcer in the haemophiliac and its relation to gastrointestinal bleeding. *Lancet* 2:1036, 1965.

33. Griffin PH, Chopra S: Spontaneous intramural gastric hematoma: a unique presentation for hemophilia. *Am J Gastroenterol* 80:430, 1985.

34. Cinotti S, Longo G, Messori A, et al: Reproducibility of one-stage, two-stage and chromogenic assays of factor VIII activity: a multi-center study. *Thromb Res* 61(4):385, 1991.

35. Hoyer LW, Breckenridge RT: Immunologic studies of antihemophilic factor (AHF, factor VIII): cross-reacting material in a genetic variant of hemophilia A. *Blood* 32:962, 1968.

36. Tully EA, Gaucher C, Jorieux S, et al: Expression of von Willebrand factor "Normandy." An autosomal mutation that mimics hemophilia A. *Proc Natl Acad Sci USA* 88:6377, 1991.

37. Ginsburg D, Nichols WC, Zivelin A, et al: Combined factors V and VIII deficiency—the solution. *Haemophilia* 4:677, 1998.

38. Santagostino E, Mannucci PM, Gringeri A, et al: Transmission of parvovirus B19 by coagulation factor concentrates exposed to 100 degrees C of heat after lyophilization. *Transfusion* 37:517, 1997.

39. Robertson BH, Alter MJ, Bell BP, et al: Hepatitis A virus sequence detected in clotting factor concentrates associated with disease transmission. *Biologicals* 26:95, 1998.

40. Souci JM, Robertson BH, Bell BP, et al: Hepatitis A virus infections associated with clotting factor concentrate in the United States. *Transfusion* 38:573, 1998.

41. White GC, Pickens EM, Liles DK, Roberts HR: Mammalian recombinant coagulation proteins: structure and function. *Trans Sci* 19:177, 1998.

42. http://www.wfh.org.

43. http://www.med.unc.edu/isth/welcome.

44. Prowse CV: In vivo recovery of factor VIII following transfusion: a survey of recent data and publications to assess the influence of standards used for potency assignment. On behalf of the Subcommittee on Factor VIII and IX of the Scientific and Standardization Committee of the ISTH. *Thromb Haemost* 74:1191, 1995.

45. Martinowitz U, Shulman S: Review of pumps for continuous infusion of coagulation factor concentrates: what are the options? *Blood Coagul Fibrinolysis* suppl 1:S27, 1996.

46. Rodeghiero F, Castaman G, Di Bona E, Ruggeri M: Consistency of responses to repeated DDAVP infusions in patients with von Willebrand's disease and hemophilia A. *Blood* 74:1997, 1989.

47. Lusher JM: Response to 1-deamino-8-D-arginine vasopressin in von Willebrand disease. *Haemostasis* 24:276, 1994.

48. Mannucci PM, Bettega D, Cattaneo M: Patterns of development of tachyphylaxis in patients with haemophilia and von Willebrand disease after repeated doses of desmopressin (DDAVP). *Br J Haematol* 82:87, 1992.

49. Forbes CD, Barr RD, Reid G, et al: Tranexamic acid in control of haemorrhage after dental extraction in haemophilia and Christmas disease. *Br Med J* 2:311, 1972.

50. Walsh PN, Rizza CR, Matthews JM, et al: Epsilon-aminocaproic acid therapy for dental extractions in haemophilia and Christmas disease: a double blind controlled trial. *Br J Haematol* 20:463, 1971.

51. Martinowitz U, Saltz R: Fibrin sealant. *Curr Opin Haematol* 3:395, 1996.

52. Ortel TL, Charles LA, Keller FG, et al: Topical thrombin and acquired coagulation factor inhibitors: clinical spectrum and laboratory diagnosis. *Am J Hematol* 45:128, 1994.

53. Eyster ME, Gill FM, Blatt PM, et al: Central nervous system bleeding in hemophiliacs. *Blood* 51:1179, 1978.

54. DeGnore LT, Wilson FC: Surgical management of hemophilic arthropathy. *Instr Course Lec* 38:383, 1989.

55. Rabiner SF, Telfer MC: Home transfusion for patients with hemophilia A. *New Engl J Med* 283:1011, 1977.

56. Aledort LM: Lessons from hemophilia. *New Engl J Med* 306:607, 1982.

57. Hilgartner MW, Cardi D, Goldberg J: Home therapy, in *Hemophilia*, edited by CD Forbes, LM Aledort, R Madhok, p 171. Chapman & Hall, London, 1997.

58. Nilsson IM, Berntorp E, Lofqvist T, Pettersson H: Twenty-five years' experience of prophylactic treatment in severe haemophilia A and B. *J Intern Med* 232:25, 1992.

59. Aledort LM: Prophylaxis: the next haemophilia treatment (editorial comment). *J Intern Med* 232:1, 1992.

60. Collins PW, Khair KS, Leisner R, Hann IM: Complications experienced with central venous catheters in children with congenital bleeding disorders. *Br J Haematol* 99:206, 1997.

61. Lofqvist T, Nilsson IM, Berntorp E, Pettersson H: Haemophilia prophylaxis in young patients—a long-term follow-up. *J Intern Med* 241:395, 1997.

62. Bohn RL, Avorn T, Glynn RT, et al: Prophylactic use of factor VIII: an economic evaluation. *Thromb Haemost* 79:932, 1998.

63. Bontempo FA, Lewis JH, Gorenc TJ, et al: Liver transplantation in hemophilia A. *Blood* 69:1721, 1987.

64. Delorme MA, Adams PC, Grant D, et al: Orthotopic liver transplantation in a patient with combined hemophilia A and B. *Am J Hematol* 33:136, 1990.

65. Thompson AR: Progress towards gene therapy for the hemophilias. *Thromb Haemost* 74:45, 1995.

66. Hoeben RC, Fallaux FJ, Schagen FHE, et al: Factors impeding efficient expression of factor VIII complementary DNA minigenes. *Blood Coagul Fibrinolysis* 8:S15, 1997.

67. Kaufman RJ, Pipe SW, Tagliavacca L, et al: Biosynthesis, assembly, and secretion of coagulation factor VIII. *Blood Coagul Fibrinolysis* 8:S3, 1997.

68. Lollo CP, Kwoh DY, Mockler TC, et al: Non-viral gene delivery: vehicle and delivery characterization. *Blood Coagul Fibrinolysis* 8:S31, 1997.

69. Jones P: HIV infection and haemophilia. *Arch Dis Child* 66:364, 1991.

70. Levetow LB, Sox HCJ, Stoto MA: *HIV and the Blood Supply: An Analysis of Crisis Decision Making, Institute of Medicine*, pp 1–235. National Academy Press, Washington, DC, 1994.

71. Eyster ME, Schaefer JH, Ragni MV, et al: Changing causes of death in Pennsylvania's hemophiliacs 1976 to 1991: impact of liver disease and acquired immunodeficiency syndrome (letter). *Blood* 79:2494, 1992.

72. Ragni MV: Progression of HIV in haemophilia. *Haemophilia* 4:601, 1998.

73. Hoyer LW: Factor VIII inhibitors. *Curr Opin Haematol* 2:365, 1995.

74. Briet E, Rosendaal FR, Kreuz W, et al: High titer inhibitors in severe hemophilia A. A meta-analysis based on eight long-term follow-up studies concerning inhibitors associated with crude or intermediate purity factor VIII products. *Thromb Haemost* 72:162, 1994.

75. Hoyer LW: Inhibitors in hemophilia, in *Hemophilia*, edited by CD Forbes, LM Aledort, R Madkoh, p 213. Chapman & Hall, London, 1997.

76. Roberts HR: Immunology of inhibitors to clotting factors, in *Autoimmune Disorders of Blood*, edited by LE Silberstein, p 151. American Association of Blood Banks, 1996.

77. Peerlinck K, Arnout J, Gilles JH, et al: A higher than expected incidence of factor VIII inhibitors in multitransfused haemophilia A patients treated with an intermittent purity pasteurized factor VIII concentrate. *Thromb Haemost* 69:115, 1993.

78. Scandella D, Mattingly M, de Graafe S, Fulcher CA: Localization of epitopes for human factor VIII inhibitor antibodies by immunoblotting and antibody neutralization. *Blood* 74:1618, 1989.

79. Kasper CK: Laboratory tests for factor VIII inhibitors, their variation, significance and interpretation. *Blood Coagul Fibrinolysis* 2:S7, 1991.

80. Verbruggen B, Novakova I, Wessels H, et al: The Nijmegen modification of the Bethesda assay for factor VIII:C inhibitors: improved specificity and reliability and specificity. *Thromb Haemost* 73:247, 1995.

81. White GC II, Roberts HR: The treatment of factor VIII inhibitors—a general overview. *Vox Sanguinis* 70:19, 1996.

82. Lusher J, Ingerslev J, Roberts HR, Hedner U: Clinical experience with recombinant factor VIIa. *Blood Coagul Fibrinolysis* 9:119, 1998.

83. Monroe DM, Hoffman M, Oliver JA, Roberts HR: A possible mechanism of action of activated factor VII independent of tissue factor. *Blood Coagul Fibrinolysis* 9:S21, 1998.

84. Nilsson IM, Berntorp E, Freiberghaus C: Treatment of patients with factor VIII and IX inhibitors. *Thromb Haemost* 70:56, 1993.

85. Brackmann HH, Effenberger W, Heiss L, et al: Immune tolerance induction: a role for recombinant activated factor VII (rVIIa)? *Eur J Haematol* 63:18, 1998.

86. http://www.haemophilia-forum.org.

87. Triger DR, Preston FE: Chronic liver disease in haemophiliacs. *Br J Haematol* 74:241, 1990.

88. Lemon SM, Becherer PR, Wang JG, et al: Hepatitis delta infection among multiply-transfused hemophiliacs. *Prog Clin Biol Res* 364:351, 1991.

89. Rosina F, Saracco G, Rizzetto M: Risk of post-transfusion infection with the hepatitis delta virus. A multicenter study. *N Engl J Med* 312:1488, 1985.

90. Gerritzen A, Brackmann H, van Loo B, et al: Chronic delta hepatitis in haemophiliacs. *J Med Virol* 34:188, 1991.

91. Makris M, Preston FE, Triger DR, et al: A randomized controlled trial of recombinant interferon-alpha in chronic hepatitis C in hemophiliacs. *Blood* 78:1672, 1991.

92. Gjerset GF, Clements MJ, Counts RB, et al: Treatment type and amount influenced human immunodeficiency virus seroprevalence of patients with congenital bleeding disorders. *Blood* 78:1623, 1991.

93. Schulman S: Effects of factor VIII concentrates on the immune system in hemophilic patients. *Ann Hematol* 63:145, 1991.

94. Gomperts ED, de Biasi R, De Vreker R: The impact of clotting factor concentrates on the immune system in individuals with hemophilia. *Transfus Med Rev* 6:44, 1992.

95. Pasi KJ, Hill FG: In vitro and in vivo inhibition of monocyte phagocytic function by factor VIII concentrates: correlation with concentrate purity [published erratum appears in *Br J Haematol* 77:570, 1991].

96. Farrugia A: Purity of factor VIII concentrates and immune function in hemophiliacs (letter; comment). *Blood* 79:2800, 1992.

97. Prusiner SB: Molecular biology of prion diseases. *Science* 252:1515, 1991.

98. Lee CA, Ironside JW, Bell JE, et al: Retrospective neuropathological review of prion disease in UK haemophilic patients. *Thromb Haemost* 80:909, 1998.

99. Biggs R, Douglas AS, Macfarlane RG: Christmas disease: a condition previously mistaken for hemophilia. *Br Med J* 12:1373, 1952.

100. Kurachi K, Davie EW: Isolation and characterization of a cDNA coding for factor IX. *Proc Natl Acad Sci USA* 79:6461, 1982.

101. Noyes CM, Griffith MJ, Roberts HR, Lundblad RL: Identification of the molecular defect in factor IX Chapel Hill: substitution of a histidine for an arginine at position 145. *Proc Natl Acad Sci USA* 80:4200, 1983.

102. Brown PE, Hougie C, Roberts HR: The genetic heterogeneity of hemophilia B. *N Engl J Med* 283:61, 1970.

103. Roberts HR: Molecular biology of hemophilia B. *Thromb Haemost* 70:1, 1993.

104. Giannelli F, Green PM, Sommer SS, et al: Haemophilia B: database of point mutations and short additions and deletions—eighth edition. *Nucleic Acids Res* 26:265, 1998.

105. http://www.umds.ac.uk/molgen/haemBdatabase.html.

106. Monroe DM, McCord DM, Huang MN, et al: Functional consequences of an arginine 180 to glutamine mutation in factor IX Hilo. *Blood* 73:1540, 1989.

107. Bertina RM, van der Linden IK, Mannucci PM, et al: Mutations in hemophilia Bm occur at the Arg 180-Val activation site or in the catalytic domain of factor IX. *J Biol Chem* 265:10876, 1990.

108. Bottema CD, Ketterling RP, Ii S, et al: Missense mutations and evolutionary conservation of amino acids: evidence that many of the amino acids in factor IX function as ''spacer'' elements. *Am J Hum Genet* 49:820, 1991.

109. Ludwig M, Sabharwal AK, Brackmann HH, et al: Hemophilia B caused by five different nondeletion mutations in the protease domain of factor IX. *Blood* 79:1225, 1992.

110. Ketterling RP, Bottema CD, Phillips JA III, Sommer SS: Evidence that descendants of three founders constitute about 25% of hemophilia B in the United States. *Genomics* 10:1093, 1991.

111. Briet E, Bertina RM, van Tilburg NH, Veltkamp JJ: Hemophilia B Leyden: a sex-linked hereditary disorder that improves after puberty. *N Engl J Med* 306:788, 1982.

112. Crossley M, Ludwig M, Stowell KM, et al: Recovery from hemophilia B Leyden: an androgen-responsive element in the factor IX promoter. *Science* 257:377, 1992.

113. Reijnen MJ, Sladek FM, Bertina RM, Reitsma PH: Disruption of a binding site for hepatocyte nuclear factor 4 results in hemophilia B Leyden. *Proc Natl Acad Sci USA* 89:6300, 1992.

114. Hamaguchi N, Roberts HR, Stafford DW: Mutations in the catalytic region of factor IX that are related to the subclass hemophilia Bm. *Biochem* 32:6324, 1993.

115. Lusher JM, McMillan CW: Severe factor VIII and factor IX deficiency in females. *Am J Med* 65:637, 1978.

116. McGraw RA, Davis LM, Lundblad RL, et al: Structure and function of factor IX: defects in haemophilia B. *Clin Haematol* 14:359, 1985.

117. Bertina RM: Factor IX variants, in *Haemostasis and Thrombosis*, edited by AL Bloom, D Thomas, p 437. Churchill Livingstone, London, 1987.

118. White GC, Bebe A, Nielsen B: Recombinant factor IX. *Thromb Haemost* 78:261, 1997.

119. Wolberg AS, Stafford DW, Erie DA: Human factor IX binds to specific sites on the collagenous domain of collagen IV. *J Biol Chem* 272:16717, 1997.

120. Kim HC, McMillan CW, White GC, et al: Purified factor IX using monoclonal immunoaffinity technique: clinical trials in hemophilia B and comparison to prothrombin complex concentrates. *Blood* 79:568, 1992.

121. Briet E, Reisner HM, Roberts HR: Inhibitors in Christmas disease, in *Factor VIII Inhibitors*, edited by LW Hoyer, p 408. Alan R. Liss, New York, 1984.

122. High KA: Factor IX, in *Inhibitors to Coagulation Factors*, edited by LM Aledort, LW Hoyer, JM Lusher, et al, p 79. Plenum, New York, 1995.

123. Warrier I, Ewenstein BM, Koerper MA, et al: Factor IX inhibitors and anaphylaxis in hemophilia B. *J Ped Hematol Oncol* 19:23, 1997.

124. Herzog RW, Yang EY, Couto LB, et al: Long term correction of hemophilia B by gene transfer of blood coagulation factor IX mediated by adeno-associated viral vector. *Nature Med* 5:56, 1999.

125. Synder RO, Miao C, Meuse L, et al: Correction of hemophilia B in canine and murine models using recombinant adeno-associated viral vectors. *Nature Med* 5:64, 1999.

126. Wang L, Takabe K, Bidlingmaier SM, et al: Sustained correction of bleeding disorder in hemophilia B mice by gene therapy. *Proc Natl Acad Sci USA* 96:3906, 1999.

127. Kay MA, Manno CS, Ragni PJ, et al: Evidence for gene transfer and expression of factor IX in haemophilia B patients treated with AAV vector. *Nat Genet* 24:257, 2000.

HEREDITARY ABNORMALITIES
OF FIBRINOGEN

MICHAEL W. MOSESSON

There are two general overlapping classes of hereditary fibrinogen disorders, *afibrinogenemia* and *dysfibrinogenemia*. Afibrinogenemia is inherited as an autosomal recessive trait and is associated with a variable degree of bleeding ranging from minimal to catastrophic. The underlying mechanism for this condition is not well established but is probably due to failure of hepatic fibrinogen synthesis and/or secretion. A related form of this disorder is manifested as *hypofibrinogenemia* associated with hepatic storage disease, in which liver secretion of a mutant fibrinogen is impaired. *Hereditary dysfibrinogenemia* is characterized by the biosynthesis of a structurally abnormal fibrinogen molecule that exhibits altered functional properties. Although most dysfibrinogenemics are asymptomatic, the disorder is commonly associated with bleeding, thrombophilia, or with fibrinogen-related organ pathology such as amyloidosis. Dysfibrinogenemic disorders can be grouped into functionally distinguishable subcategories that are exemplified in each of the phases of the fibrinogen-fibrin conversion: (1) Abnormal fibrinopeptide release, or a defective E_A or E_B site; (2) defects in D domains involving the Da site, Db site, D:D site, γ_{XL} site, or the αC domain. Defects in these regions are usually associated with distinctive functional abnormalities, and bleeding or thrombophilia are found in almost all categories. Some αC domain defects are associated with hereditary renal amyloidosis, in which an abnormal fragment of the Aα chain is deposited in the kidneys. *Hypodysfibrinogenemia* is a subcategory characterized by low circulating levels of abnormal fibrinogen levels, a category that overlaps with hypofibrinogenemia manifested as hepatic storage disease. The pathophysiological basis for hypodysfibrinogenemia includes hypercatabolism, reduced synthesis, or impaired secretion, but in most cases neither the genetic basis nor the structural abnormality is known.

INTRODUCTION

Fibrinogen is a 340-kD plasma protein that circulates at a concentration of 1.5 to 3.5 mg/ml. Each fibrinogen molecule is about 45 nm in length and comprises a symmetrical disulfide-bridged dimer consisting of two outer D domains and a central E domain that are joined through coiled-coil regions[1,2] (Fig. 124-1). Electron microscopy has confirmed its tridomainal structure and additionally shows a twofold axis of symmetry perpendicular to the long axis.[3–5] Each half-molecule consists of two sets of three different polypeptide chains, Aα, Bβ, and

γ, that are joined in their amino terminal regions by disulfide bridges to form the E domain.[1,6–8] The Aα chain consists of 610, the Bβ chain of 461, and the major form of the γ chain, γA, 411 residues[1]. A minor γ chain variant termed γ', amounting to about 8 percent of the total,[9] is comprised of 427 residues and has a unique acidic amino acid sequence[10] after position 407. Carbohydrate side chain groups are attached to the Bβ and γ chains and are linked through N-acetylglucosamine to Asp52 of each γ chain, and Asp364 of each Bβ chain.[11]

Fibrinogen is synthesized by hepatocytes[12,13] and chain synthesis is under the coordinated control of three separate genes located on chromosome 4.[14–17] Subsequent to hepatic assembly of the constituent polypeptide chains and the addition of carbohydrate side chains, the mature molecule is secreted into the circulation, where it manifests a half-life of 4 days and a fractional catabolic rate of 25 percent per day.[18,19] In addition to the fibrinogen in plasma, blood contains an intracellular fibrinogen pool that is stored within platelet α-granules. Both megakaryocytes and platelets are capable of internalizing plasma fibrinogen via the fibrinogen glycoprotein(GP)IIb/IIIa ($\alpha_{IIb}\beta_3$) receptor[20–22] (see Chap. 111). This absorptive process is specifically dependent upon GPIIb/IIIa binding to the C-terminal platelet recognition sequence that is present on γA chains, but absent from γchains. Thus, internalized platelet fibrinogen molecules contain only γA chains.[22–25] This phenomenon is especially interesting in relation to the abnormal γ chains in fibrinogen Paris I ($\gamma_{Paris I}$), which are not found in platelets,[26] a subject that is discussed more fully in a later section.

Fibrin(ogen) participates in numerous physiological processes, most of which are listed below. *Fibrinogen when converted by thrombin into fibrin, forms an insoluble fibrin clot; it supports platelet aggregation, and it binds to vascular endothelial and other cells. Fibrinogen also binds to plasma or tissue matrix proteins such as fibronectin, to peptide growth factors, and it serves as a carrier protein for factor XIII. Fibrin provides a template for the assembly and activation of the fibrinolytic system, has binding sites for tissue matrix components such as glycosaminoglycans, and possesses non-substrate thrombin binding sites. Both fibrinogen and fibrin serve as substrates for factor XIIIa and other transglutaminases, which catalyze covalent cross-linking.*

CONVERSION AND ASSEMBLY

Conversion of fibrinogen into fibrin has three distinct phases: (1) enzymatic cleavage by thrombin to produce fibrin; (2) fibrin self-assembly to an organized polymeric structure; (3) covalent cross-linking of fibrin by factor XIIIa. In the first phase of conversion to fibrin, cleavage of fibrinogen at Aα16R-17G* and later Bβ14R-15G results in release of two fibrinopeptides A (FPA) and two fibrinopeptides B (FPB),[27–29] and exposure of E_A and E_B polymerization sites, respectively. One portion of the E_A site is located at the amino terminal end of the fibrin α chain comprising the amino terminal Aα17-20 GPRV sequence.[30,31] Another portion of this site is in the amino terminal region of the fibrinogen Bβ chain, specifically in the β15-42 sequence.[32–36] The E_A site in fibrin interacts with a constitutive complementary association site, Da, in the D domain of another molecule (the so-called D:E interaction) to initiate and accelerate the fibrin assembly process.[29,37–39] This site is situated in a segment of the D domain encompassed by γ337-379.[40–42]

The initial assembly of a fibrin clot involves Da:E_A associations that result in formation of double-stranded fibrils in which fibrin

---

*A one letter abbreviation for amino acids is used in this chapter. A, alanine; C, cysteine; D, aspartic acid; E, glutamic acid; F, phenylalanine; G, glycine; H, histidine; I, isoleucine; K, lysine; L, leucine; M, methionine; N, asparagine; P, proline; Q, glutamine; R, arginine; S, serine; T, threonine; V, valine; W, tryptophan; Y, tyrosine.

Acronyms and abbreviations that appear in this chapter include: ADP, adenosine 5' diphosphate; HRA, hereditary renal amyloidosis.

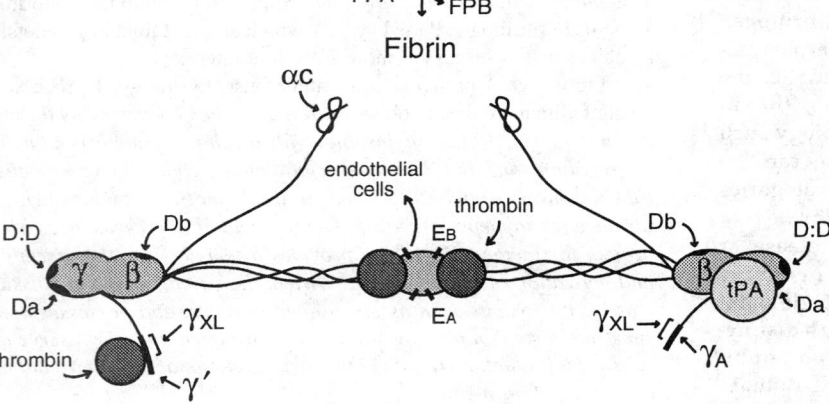

Fibrinogen

D Domain

αC   FPB   I-9

E Domain

$$SO_3 \quad SO_3$$
398 QQHHLGGAKQ**VRPEHPAETEYDSLYPEDDL**427   398 QQHHLGGAKQ**AGDV**411

platelets

thrombin

FPA → FPB

Fibrin

αC

endothelial
cells

thrombin

FIGURE 124-1   Diagram of fibrinogen and fibrin showing the major domains and the intermolecular association sites that participate in fibrin polymerization and cross-linking.

Enzymatic conversion of fibrinogen to fibrin by thrombin results in release of fibrinopeptides A (FPA) and B (FPB) and exposure of E_A and E_B polymerization sites, respectively. Structural features within the D domains of this model include two separate self-association sites, γ_{XL} and D:D. Other constitutive association sites are Da, which interacts with an available E_A site in fibrin (i.e., the fibrin D:E interaction), and Db, which interacts with an E_B site in fibrin. γ_{XL} overlaps the factor XIIIa cross-linking site in the C-terminal region of γ_A or γ' chains, which are known γ chain variants. Their C-terminal sequences (nonidentical residues in bold) and the residues used by XIIIa for cross-linking are shown. Only γ_A chains contain the platelet fibrinogen receptor $\alpha_{IIb}\beta_3$ binding sequence. D:D site interaction promotes end-to-end alignment of fibrin or fibrinogen molecules in assembling fibrils. The Aα chain cleavage site that produces plasma fraction I-9 fibrinogen is indicated. The αC domain in the C-terminal region of the Aα chain emerges from the D domain and is shown dissociating from its noncovalent association with the fibrin E domain as a result of thrombin cleavage of FPB. The two locations of thrombin binding in fibrin and tPA binding at fibrin-specific epitopes in fibrin are also shown, as is the endothelial cell binding site (β15-42) that becomes exposed by cleavage of FPB. (Reproduced with permission from ref. 2.)

molecules become aligned in an end-to-middle domain staggered overlapping arrangement[43–46] (Fig. 124-2). Subsequently fibrils undergo branching and lateral fibril associations that result in fiber networks.[47,48] Two types of fibril branching occur, the first of which, called a *tetramolecular junction*, consists of two fibrils that converge to form a four-stranded fibril.[47,49] The second, termed a trimolecular junction, consists of three fibrils which converge at a junction comprised of three D:E interacting molecules to form a symmetrical three-armed structure. Progressive lateral fibril associations result in formation of thick fiber bundles and large fiber branches.

FPB (Bβ1-14) release occurs more slowly than release of FPA[27–29] and exposes an independent polymerization site, E_B,[50,51] beginning with the β15-18 sequence, GHRP.[30,31] FPB cleavage is accelerated by fibrin polymerization whereas fibrinopeptide cleavage at the Aα site is independent of fibrin polymerization, per se.[52–54] E_B is utilized through interactions with a complementary binding pocket, Db, located in the β chain segment of the D domain encompassed by β397-432.[55,56] The interaction is evidently not required for lateral fibril and fiber association but contributes to this process through cooperative interactions resulting from alignment of D domains in the fibrin polymer.[50,51]

In addition to the Da:E_A site interactions that guide fibrin assembly, there are other distinct D domain self-association sites termed 'γ_{XL}' and 'D:D', respectively,[57–59] that contribute to this process. Interactions between D:D sites, which are situated at the distal ends of D domains, promote end-to-end alignment of fibrin molecules in assembling polymers.[57,58] The interface for this site lies between γ275R and γ300S,[42] but other nearby γ chain residues contribute to the site, as evidenced by impaired D:D interactions in dysfibrinogenemic molecules such as fibrinogen Kurashiki I (γG268E).[60]

The so-called γ_{XL} assembly site is situated in the C-terminal region of each γ chain. It contains the factor XIIIa crosslinking sequence between γ398/399 Gln and γ406 Lys and overlaps the platelet fibrinogen receptor $\alpha_{IIb}\beta_3$ binding site at γ400-411 of γ_A chains.[61,62] The γ' variant chain also contains this cross-linking peptide sequence and therefore undergoes factor-XIIIa-mediated cross-linking normally.[63] γ' chains, however, lack a functional $\alpha_{IIb}\beta_3$ platelet binding site and instead they contain an acidic C-terminal sequence beginning at γ'408 and ending at γ'427.[10] By binding to factor XIII B subunits via its unique γ' sequence, fibrinogen serves as a carrier protein for factor XIII in plasma.[64] Fibrin γ' chains also bind to thrombin with high affinity.[65]

Still another association site that plays a role in fibrin assembly and other functions is located in the C-terminal region of the Aα chain and is commonly referred to as the 'αC' domain. This segment of the molecule originates in the D domain at residue 111 and ends at residue 610.[1] Fibrin formed from circulating fibrinogen "catabolite" molecules (e.g., fraction I-9) lacking a C-terminal portion of the αC domain manifests a prolonged thrombin time and reduced turbidity development and produces thinner fibrin fibers.[66,67] In fibrinogen molecules, the αC domains tend to be noncovalently tethered at the E domain[4,68,69] but become dissociated from it as a result of FPB cleavage.[68,69] This event evidently makes the αC domain available for noncovalent interaction with other αC domains, a process that promotes lateral fibril associations and fibrin network assembly. A considerable number of symptomatic dysfibrinogenemias are associated with irregularities in this region of the molecule.

Besides its role in mediating fibrin polymerization, the β chain of fibrin participates in cell-matrix interactions. Exposure of the β15-42 sequence by release of FPB promotes platelet spreading,[70] fibroblast proliferation,[71] endothelial cell spreading, proliferation and capillary

tube formation,[71–73] and release of von Willebrand factor.[74,75] Endothelial cell binding is a
heparin- or proteolglycan-dependent process,[76,77] that correlates with exposure of a heparin-binding domain in β15-42.[78]

CROSS-LINKING

In the presence of factor XIIIa, fibrin undergoes
intermolecular covalent cross-linking by virtue
of forming ε-(γ-glutamyl)lysine isopeptide
bonds.[79,80] The resulting cross-linked clot exhibits almost perfect elastic behavior and becomes more rigid and resistant to deforma-
tion.[81] Cross-linking of γ chains first involves
formation of γ dimers,[82] which occur as reciprocal bridges between lysine at position 406 of
one γ chain and glutamine at position 398 or
399 of another.[83–85] Slower cross-linking among
α chains creates α chain oligomers and polymers.[86] Cross-linking also occurs between α
chains and γ chains,[47,87] and other plasma proteins, notably α_2-plasmin inhibitor and fibronectin, become cross-linked to α chains.[88–91]
Oligomeric forms of crosslinked γ chains also
occur, namely γ trimers and γ tetramers.[47,87]
They form more slowly than γ dimers or even
α polymers,[47,92] and contribute to development
of resistance to fibrinolysis.[92] Because there is a
single donor lysine residue at γ406,[83,85] trimeric
and tetrameric cross-linked structures form by
utilization or reutilization of that same lysine
406 residue. Whereas γ dimers usually lie in
a transverse position between the strands of
each fibril,[57,59,93–95] trimeric and tetrameric structures form through *interfibrillar* interactions
subsequent to intrafibrillar γ chain dimerization (see Fig. 124-2).

THROMBIN BINDING TO FIBRIN(OGEN)

Thrombin binds to its substrate, fibrinogen, at
N-terminal sites on Aα and Bβ chains through
an anion-binding fibrinogen recognition site in
thrombin termed *exosite I*.[96,97] Substrate binding
leads to proteolytic cleavage and release of FPA and FPB, respectively.
The binding site for FPA cleavage is contained within residues 1 to
51 of the N-terminal Aα chain, whereas the binding site for FPB
cleavage is at least in part in the N-terminal Bβ chain.[52,65,98] Other
evidence for a thrombin binding sequence in the Bβ chain comes from
studies of two dysfibrinogenemic Bβ chain mutant molecules, New
York I (des Bβ9-72)[32,99] and Naples (BβA68T),[100,101] both of which
showed impaired thrombin binding. These dysfibrinogenemias are
discussed in subsequent sections.

There are two classes of nonsubstrate thrombin binding sites in
fibrin, one of high affinity and the other of low affinity,[65,102] and each
class has a distinct location.[65] The low-affinity binding sites are in the
fibrin E domain and represent, at least in part, a residual aspect of
fibrinogen substrate recognition. The α27-50 sequence in fibrin contributes to the low-affinity site.[103,104] The high-affinity site is located
exclusively on γ' chains of fibrin(ogen)[65] and probably competes for
thrombin binding at thrombin exosite-dependent sites in other proteins

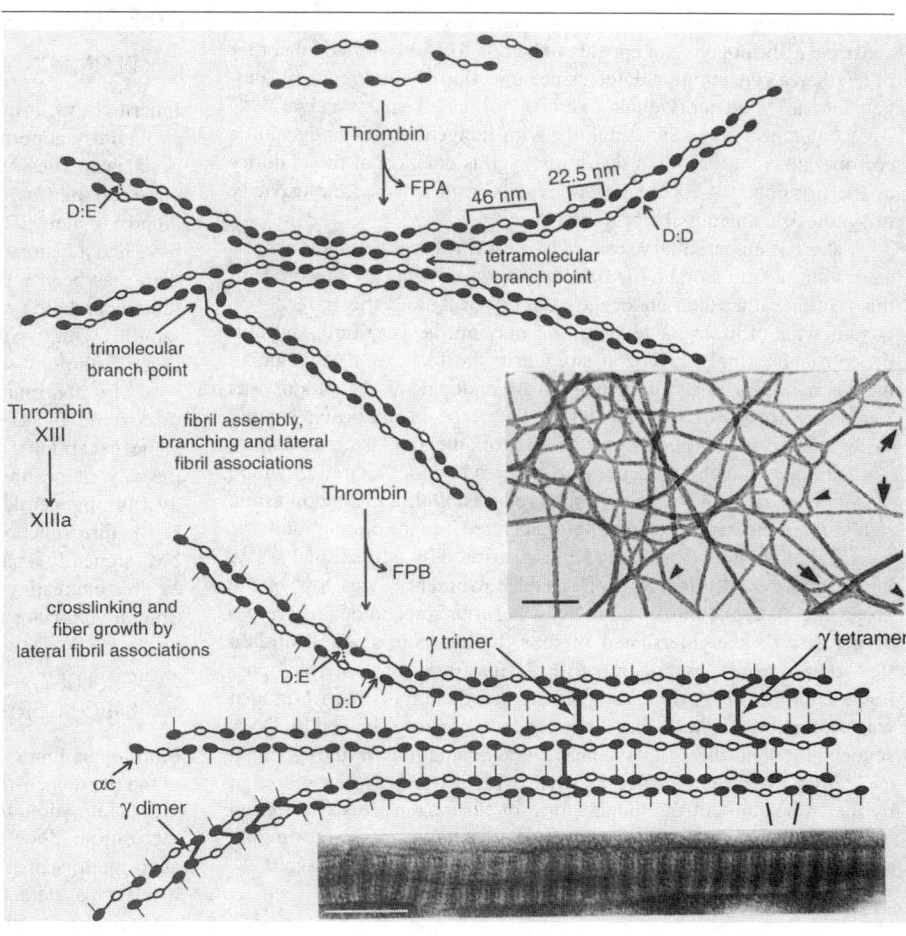

FIGURE 124-2   Schematic diagram of fibrin assembly and cross-linking.
Fibrin assembly begins after FPA release with noncovalent D:E interactions between the E$_A$ and
D$_A$ sites (dotted lines) to form end-to-middle staggered overlapping double-stranded fibrils (upper). Fibrils
also branch and undergo lateral associations to form wider fibrils and fibers [Inset, Critical point dried
fibril matrix containing trimolecular (arrows) and tetramolecular (arrowheads) junctions; bar, 100 nm].
After cleavage of FPB (lower), αC domains become available for self-association with other αC domains,
thereby promoting lateral fibril association and fiber assembly [Inset, negatively contrasted fibrin fiber
showing 22.5 nm periodicity; bar, 100 nm]. Activation of factor XIII to XIIIa by thrombin results in
introduction of ε-(γ-glutamyl) lysine cross-links among C-terminal γ_{XL} sites (thick lines between D
domains) mainly between the strands of each fibril to form γ dimers. γ trimers and γ tetramers form by
interfibril γ chain cross-linking. (Reproduced with permission from ref. 2.)

or cells (e.g., the platelet/endothelial cell thrombin receptor) or even
at fibrinogen substrate sites.

AFIBRINOGENEMIA AND HYPOFIBRINOGENEMIA

DEFINITION, HISTORY, AND CLINICAL FEATURES

Congenital afibrinogenemia is a rare disorder that has been described
in more than 150 families.[105,106] In the classical disorder the disease is
inherited as an autosomal recessive trait. Consanguinity is common.
Typically, low levels of plasma fibrinogen in both parents supports a
recessive inheritance pattern. Clinical expression in terms of hemmor-
hagic manifestations ranges widely from minimal to catastrophic.[105,106]
Umbilical cord bleeding may be the first manifestation, and it can be
the cause of death in newborns. Later in life, such problems as gum
bleeding, epistaxis, menorrhagia, gastrointestinal hemorrhage, muscle
hemorrhage, spontaneous abortions, and hemarthrosis can present,

but the leading cause of hemorrhagic death is intracranial bleeding. Classical afibrinogenemia appears to be due to a biosynthetic disorder rather than a consumptive defect, since injection of autologous fibrinogen into affected individuals exhibits normal plasma survival.[107–109] A recent report on a Swiss family with congenital afibrinogenemia corroborates that idea[109a] in that homozygous deletion of the majority of the fibrinogen A$\alpha\alpha$ chain gene results in absence of the capacity to synthesize functional fibrinogen.

There is an hereditary form of hypofibrinogenemia that is associated with hepatic storage disease,[110–113] and including that disorder in this section rather than under the category of hypodysfibrinogenemia is somewhat arbitrary. The condition may not be very rare, and evidence of abnormal fibrinogen storage in the form of PAS-negative inclusion bodies in the cisternae of the endoplasmic reticulum was found in 9 of 700 liver biopsies.[113] This type of abnormal hepatic storage of fibrinogen fulfills the criteria for an endoplasmic reticulum storage disease such as occurs in α1-antitrypsin deficiency in which an abnormal α1-antitrypsin variant is retained within the endoplasmic reticulum of the liver instead of being secreted into the circulation.[114–116]

The circulating fibrinogen level, measured by a functional assay, in the kindred reported by Callea and coworkers[112] was low in the propositus (0.2–0.4 mg/ml), in two of her four sons, in her sister, two of her sister's daughters, and in four of her sister's grandchildren (0.4–0.85 mg/ml). Immunoreactive plasma fibrinogen in the propositus was higher (1.0 mg/ml) suggesting that the circulating fibrinogen was dysfunctional. George and coworkers[117] recently showed by DNA sequencing that there is a heterozygous mutation in the γ chain (γG284R) of fibrinogen Brescia that evidently impairs its secretion by the liver. None of the mutant form of fibrinogen Brescia is found in plasma, but the secreted fibrinogen is hypersialated, suggesting an explanation for the presence of dysfunctional plasma fibrinogen.

LABORATORY FEATURES

All tests based upon the appearance of a fibrin clot are abnormal in afibrinogenemic and hypofibrinogenemic subjects. These include the whole blood clotting time, partial thromboplastin time, prothrombin time, and thrombin and reptilase times. These abnormalities are correctable by the addition of normal plasma or purified fibrinogen. The diagnosis is established by immunological measurements of fibrinogen concentration.[118,119] The platelet fibrinogen content in most cases is negligible.[118] Related coagulation abnormalities include a prolonged bleeding time and abnormal platelet aggregation, especially with ADP. These abnormalities can be corrected by infusion of plasma or fibrinogen concentrates.[119–121]

THERAPY, COURSE, AND PROGNOSIS

Patients with afibrinogenemia or hypofibrinogenemia may require replacement therapy to control bleeding episodes or in preparation for surgery. Many patients receive fibrinogen replacement in the form of cryoprecipitate, a plasma-derived fibrinogen concentrate that contains approximately 300 mg fibrinogen per unit. An afibrinogenemic adult with a plasma volume of 3 liters will require 12 units of cryoprecipitate to increase the fibrinogen level to an adequate hemostatic level of 1 mg/ml.[122] Since the fractional catabolic rate of fibrinogen is 25 percent per day, patients should receive one-third of the initial loading dose daily for as long as fibrinogen level elevation is desired. Cryoprecipitate is also used during pregnancy to prevent spontaneous abortion and to assist in carrying pregnancies to term.[123] Development of antifibrinogen antibodies has been reported,[124] and some patients undergoing replacement therapy have experienced thrombosis.[125–127]

DYSFIBRINOGENEMIA

DEFINITION AND HISTORY

Inherited dysfibrinogenemia is characterized by the biosynthesis of a structurally abnormal fibrinogen molecule that exhibits altered functional properties. More than 260 cases of congenital dysfibrinogenemia were reported by 1994,[128] and now that number is in excess of 300. Approximately 25 percent of the reported cases of dysfibrinogenemia have had a history of bleeding, and in about 20 percent of the families there has been a tendency toward thrombosis (thrombophilia),[128] the remainder being clinically asymptomatic in these regards. In some families with dysfibrinogenemia there is associated fibrinogen-related organ pathology such as amyloidosis or hepatic storage disease.

The abnormality in blood is most commonly but not always discovered by a prolonged thrombin-mediated clotting time. With some exceptions, the various mutants described carry the name of the city of origin of the patient. The main focus for discussion of dysfibrinogenemia in this chapter is placed on abnormalities for which a structure/function correlation can be made, whose dysfunction can be assigned to a particular domain or region in the molecule, or which exhibit interesting or unique clinical or pathophysiological features. Some dysfibrinogens are discussed under more than one subtopic.

ETIOLOGY, PATHOGENESIS, CLINICAL AND LABORATORY FEATURES

Fibrinogen abnormalities are usually reflected in one or more phases of the fibrinogen-fibrin conversion and fibrin assembly process including: (1) impaired release of fibrinopeptides, (2) defects in fibrin polymerization, (3) defective cross-linking by factor XIIIa. Other important abnormalities involve other aspects of fibrin(ogen) function or metabolism such as defective intrahepatic assembly, storage and/or secretion, catabolism, abnormal deposition in tissues, defective assembly of the fibrinolytic system, abnormal interactions with platelets, endothelial cells, or calcium binding.

ABNORMAL FIBRINOPEPTIDE RELEASE, OR A DEFECTIVE E$_A$ OR E$_B$ SITE

Fibrinogen Detroit was the first abnormal fibrinogen in which a specific amino acid substitution was identified (AαR19S)[129]; this mutation is at the fibrin E$_A$ polymerization site (i.e., GPRV) and results in impaired fibrin polymerization and a bleeding tendency. Amino acid substitutions at this site in other kindreds are associated with bleeding in some (Munich I, AαR19N[128]; Mannheim I, AαR19G[128]) and with thrombosis in others (Aarhus, AαR19G[128]; Kumamoto, AαR19G[130]). As pointed out in the section on thrombophilia, there may be coexisiting as yet undetermined genetic or environmental risk factors in some patients that account for such seemingly paradoxical clinical manifestations. Substitution of Aα18 Pro with Leu (Kyoto II)[131] is also associated with a bleeding tendency due to a defective E$_A$ site. In fibrinogen Canterbury (AαV20D),[132] the E$_A$ polymerization site is missing as well as the entire FPA sequence (i.e., Aα1 to 19). This arises because the AαV20D mutation creates a cleavage site at R19 (RGPRD) for the intracellular enzyme furin, and the mutant Aα chain is cleaved at that site prior to secretion to create a sequence beginning with Aα20D. A mild bleeding tendency exists with this situation. Fibrinogen Nijmegen (BβR44C)[133] exhibits abnormal polymerization (consistent with an abnormal E$_A$ polymerization site) plus abnormal tPA-induced plasminogen activation and binding[134] but does not exhibit impaired fibrinopeptide release like fibrinogen Naples (BβA68T).[100,101,135]

Thrombin binds to fibrinogen and cleaves each Aα chain at 16R/17G to release FPA. The most common mutation is at Aα16, with Arg replacement leading to delayed (R→H) or absent (R→C) FPA release. Most of these subjects, especially those who are heterozygous, have no bleeding tendencies. Some patients with a bleeding tendency are homozygous for the defect (Metz[136]; Giessen I[137]; Bicêtre I[128]) or have other demonstrable abnormalities, such as an abnormal von Willebrand factor[138] or impaired cross-linking.[139] Substitution of V for G at Aα17 (Bremen I[140]) results in delayed FPA release as well as a modest impairment of fibrin monomer polymerization, indicating that there is also a defect at the E_A polymerization site resulting from the change of GPRV to VPRV. This defect is associated with a bleeding tendency and delayed wound healing.

Dysfibrinogenemias with a structural alteration in Aα 7-12 segment of the FPA sequence (Lille, Mitaka II, Rouen I[128]) exhibit defective substrate binding with thrombin and impaired FPA release. There is a bleeding tendency only with Mitaka II. Delayed FPA release is also associated with dysfibrinogens manifesting a structural defect in the N-terminal region of the Bβ chain, including fibrinogen New York I (Bβ9-72 deletion[32]), fibrinogen Naples (BβA68T[100,101,135]), and dysfibrinogenemias involving substitutions at the FPB cleavage site, BβR14C (Table 124-1) or BβG15C (Ise[128]; Fukuoka II[141]).

FPB release results in exposure of the E_B polymerization site,[50,51] but does not occur in mutant Bβ chains with Cys substitutions at the FPB cleavage site, BβR14C (Table 124-1) and in fibrinogen New York I, which exhibits deletion of Bβ9-72, corresponding to exon 2 of the Bβ chain gene.[32] Impaired FPB release also occurs in dysfibrinogenemias having a mutation at the FPB cleavage site BβG15C (Ise[128]; Fukuoka II[141]) and in fibrinogen Naples I (BβA68T[100,101,135]). Fibrinogen Nijmegen (BβR44C[133]) does not exhibit impaired fibrinopeptide release but rather abnormal polymerization (consistent with an abnormal E_A polymerization site). Further details on Bβ chain defective dysfibrinogenemic families exhibiting thromboembolic disorders, such as fibrinogens New York I, Naples I, and Nijmegen, are contained in the section on thrombophilia.

POLYMERIZATION DEFECTS IN THE D DOMAINS

Fibrin assembly initially involves Da:E_A site interactions that drive the formation of staggered overlapping end-to-middle molecular associations resulting in double-stranded fibrils. In addition, there are two other distinct association sites in each D domain, termed 'γ_{XL}' and 'D:D', respectively. In the following sections we consider each of these sites in terms of known congenital abnormalities of fibrinogen. These structural changes have been reviewed.[142,143]

Da Site   D domain mutations are associated with defective fibrin polymerization, and many are located in a region of the Da site, covering a rather large stretch of the γ chain. These include fibrinogen Matsumoto I (γD364H[144]) and fibrinogen Melun I (γD364V[145]); the latter is associated with thrombophilia. Other dysfibrinogenemias that induce functional changes at the Da site include: Kyoto III (γD330Y[146]), Milano I (γD330V[147]), Nagoya I (γQ329R[148]), Osaka V (γR375G[149]), and Bern I (γN337K[150]). Fibrinogen Milano VII (γS358C-albumin) molecules, which are disulfide-linked to albumin[151] displayed a marked polymerization defect. It is not clear how this abnormality relates to abnormal polymerization, since the location itself does not appear to contribute to Da site function, and removal of albumin did not normalize the defect. None of these last-mentioned dysfibrinogens have thrombotic or bleeding manifestations.

Db Site   To date, no dysfibrinogenemias have been described involving this region of the D domain. The substitution in fibrinogen Pontoise (BβA335T[152]) results in a new glycosylation site in the β chain portion of its D domain, and the molecule exhibits defective polymerization. The defect may be related to a steric or a charge effect on the polymerization process, but it is not likely to be directly related to an abnormality in the GHRP binding pocket, per se.

D:D Site   The interface for the D:D site lies between γ275R and γ300S, with γ280T contacting γ275R at the D:D interface.[42] The nearby γ chain residues also contribute to the site, as evidenced by functional impairment of D:D interactions in molecules such as fibrinogen Kurashiki I (γG268E[60,153]).

Fibrinogen Tokyo II[58,154] is one of many reported clinically asymptomatic γR275C-substituted dysfibrinogens and was the first to be characterized in terms of its D:D site defect. Several others have Arg substituted by His and one by Ser (Table 124-1). Tokyo II fibrin displayed normal D:E associations and normal γ chain cross-linking. Factor XIIIa-cross-linked fibrinogen polymers were defective in that otherwise linear double-stranded fibrils were disorganized due to failure of normal end-to-end molecular associations. For the same reason, Tokyo II fibrin showed increased fiber branching.[58] The same type of abnormal fibrin branching has been shown for fibrinogen Haifa I (γR275H[155]), a case in which thrombophilia was prominent. Fibrinogen Banks Penninsula (γY280C[156]) which is associated with mild bleeding, shows the same polymerization defect as described above for Tokyo II fibrinogen, because the Cys substitution at γ280 disrupts the normal D:D contact with γ275R.

Fibrinogen Baltimore I (γG292V[128]) may represent another example of defective D:D site function, although its characteristics are not identical to those of fibrinogen Tokyo II. The Baltimore I patient had a history of recurrent thrombosis, pulmonary embolism, and mild bleeding.[157] Electron microscopy of fibrin networks showed thinner, relatively more branched fibers. Cross-linking of γ chains was evidently normal, as seems to be characteristic of purely D:D defective molecules, but α-polymer formation was also delayed, though correctable. There are other γ chain mutations that may also cause abnormal D:D site function. These include mutations at γ308 N to I (Baltimore III[158]) or N to K (Kyoto I[159]; Bicêtre II[160]; Matsumoto II[161]), and glycosylation at γ308N due to a γM310T mutation (Asahi I[162]).

γ_{XL} Site   The γ_{XL} association site contains the factor XIIIa cross-linking sequence and overlaps the platelet fibrinogen receptor $\alpha_{IIb}\beta_3$ binding site. There are no reported changes specifically involving this region of the molecule, although markedly impaired to absent γ chain cross-linking at this site has been documented in fibrinogen Asahi I[162] and in fibrinogen Paris I (see below).[163] Fibrinogen Asahi I has a carbohydrate group incorporated at γ308N that may sterically interfere with cross-linking at the γ_{XL} site, although it does not interfere with factor-XIIIa-mediated incorporation of amine donors at γ398Q. A dysfibrinogen with the same γ310 Met to Thr substitution as Asahi I (Frankfurt VII[164]) has been reported to display abnormal ADP-induced platelet aggregation, probably by sterically hindering the C-terminal platelet-binding sequence at the γ_{XL} site. Fibrinogen Vlissingen (γdel 319N,320D[165]) also displayed abnormal platelet aggregation,[164] evidently resulting from disruption of its calcium binding site. These molecules are also discussed in the section on thrombophilia.

The fibrinogen Paris I abnormality is characterized by markedly impaired fibrin polymerization and clot retraction[166] but is not associated with either clinical bleeding or thrombophilia. The propositus, however, displayed surgical wound dehiscence. The defect (γ350/insert/γG351S) involves a point mutation in intron 8 that results in insertion of a 15 amino acid sequence after γ350 and substitution of S for G at γ351.[167] The $\gamma_{Paris I}$ chains have a normal C-terminal sequence beyond γ351,[167,168] yet despite this, the γ_{XL} site does not participate in factor-XIIIa-mediated γ chain cross-linking nor can amine donors be incorporated into $\gamma_{Paris I}$ chains.[163] Furthermore, $\gamma_{Paris I}$ chains manifest defective ADP-induced platelet aggregation,[168] and $\gamma_{Paris I}$-containing molecules are not incorporated into platelets.[26] This suggests that marked conformational changes have occurred in the Paris I D domain that make the C-terminal γ_A chain sequence unavailable for any function attributable to the γ_{XL} site.

TABLE 124-1 DYSFIBRINOGENS WITH KNOWN STRUCTURAL DEFECTS OR WITH DEFEND FUNCTIONAL CHARACTERISTICS

Molecular Defect	Name	Organ Pathology	Hypofibrinogenemia	Bleeding	Thrombophilia	Literature Refs
Aα chain:						
D7N	Lille	0	0	0	0	128
E11G	Mitaka II	0	0	yes	0	128
G12V	Rouen	0	0	0	0	128
R16H	Bicêtre I, Giessen I, etc. (>30)	0	0	yes/variable	0	128, 137–139
R16C	Metz I, Zurich I, etc. (>15)	0	0	yes/variable	0	128, 136
G17V	Bremen I	0	0	yes	0	140
P18L	Kyoto II	0	0	yes	0	131
R19S	Detroit	0	0	yes	0	128, 129
R19N	Munich I	0	0	yes	0	128
R19G	Mannheim I	0	0	yes	0	128
R19G	Aarhus I, Kumamoto	0	0	0	yes	128, 130
V20D/Aα 1-19del	Canterbury	0	0	yes	0	132
R141S-139N-glycosylation	Lima I	0	0	0	0	180
R268Q/frameshift/271P stop	Otago	0	0	yes	0	218
S434N-glycosylation	Caracas II	0	yes	yes	0	178, 179
451 insert/453 stop-albumin	Milano III	0	0	0	yes	170, 171
461 stop-albumin	Marburg I	0	0	yes	yes	169, 192
522 del/frame shift/547 stop	none	Amyloidosis-renal	yes	yes	yes	186
524del/frame shift/547 stop	none	Amyloidosis-renal	0	0	0	185
E526V	none	Amyloidosis-renal	0	0	0	183, 184
S532C	Caracas V	0	0	0	yes	194, 210, 211
R554C-albumin	Dusart, Chapel Hill III	0	0	0	yes	128, 172–177, 209
R554L	none	Amyloidosis-renal	0	0	0	182
abnormal FPA release	Giessen II	0	yes	yes	0	128
Bβ chain:						
R14C	Ijmuiden	0	0	0	yes	133
R14C	Christchurch II	0	0	yes	0	128
R14C	Seattle I	0	0	0	0	128
G15C	Ise, Fukuoka II	0	0	0	yes	128, 141
9-72del	New York I	0	0	0	yes	32, 99, 128
R44C	Nijmegen	0	0	0	yes	133, 134
A68T	Naples I	0	0	0	yes	100, 101, 135
A335T	Pontoise	0	0	0	0	152
abnormal FPB release	Baltimore II	0	0	yes	0	191
Bβ chain	Oslo I	0	0	0	yes	128
γ chain:						
G268E	Kurashiki I	0	0	0	0	60, 153
R275C	Baltimore IV, Milano V, Morioka I, Osaka II, Tochigi I, Tokyo II, Villajoyosa I	0	0	0	0	58, 128, 154, 196, 214
R275C	Bologna I, Cedar Rapids	0	0	0	yes	194, 195
R275H	Barcelona IV, Claro I, Essen I, Osaka III, Perugia I, Saga I	0	0	0	0	128, 197, 198, 216
R275H	Haifa I, Barcelona III, Bergamo II	—	—	0	yes	128, 155, 196, 197, 198
R275S	Kamogawa	0	0	0	0	215
Y280C	Banks Penninsula	0	0	yes	0	156
G284R	Brescia	hepatic storage	yes	0	0	112, 117
G292V	Baltimore I	0	0	yes	yes	128, 157
N308I	Baltimore III	0	0	0	0	128, 158
N308K	Kyoto I	0	0	0	0	128, 159
N308K	Bicêtre II	0	0	0	yes	128, 160
N308K	Matsumoto II	0	0	yes	0	161
M310T-N308 glycosylation	Asahi I, Frankfurt VII	0	0	yes	0	128, 162, 164
D318G	Giessen IV	0	0	yes	yes	128, 194
del319N,320D	Vlissingen I	0	0	0	yes	164, 165
Q329R	Nagoya I	0	0	0	0	148
D330V	Milano I	0	0	0	0	147
D330Y	Kyoto III	0	0	0	0	146
N337K	Bern I	0	0	0	0	26, 163, 166–168
350/insert/G351S	Paris I	0	0	0	0	217
A357T	Frankfurt I	0	yes	yes	0	151
S358C	Milano VII-albumin	0	0	0	0	144
D364H	Matsumoto I	0	0	0	0	145
D364V	Melun I	0	0	0	yes	149
R375G	Osaka V	0	0	0	0	212, 213
K380N	Kaiserslautern	0	0	0	yes	189
Unknown site:						
—	Bethesda III	0	yes	yes	0	190
—	Chapel Hill I	0	yes	0	0	193
—	Malmöe I	0	yes	0	yes	187
—	Parma	0	yes	yes	0	188
—	Philadelphia I	0	yes	yes	0	

THE D DOMAIN SEGMENT OF THE Aα CHAIN AND THE αC DOMAIN

Fibrinogen Marburg[169] is a homozygous hypodysfibrinogenemia lacking amino acid residues Aα461-610. This abnormality is covered in the section on thrombophilia, as is another Aα chain truncation mutant, fibrinogen Milano III.[170,171] Fibrinogen Dusart (AαR554C-albumin[172-177]) is also covered in that section. Fibrinogen Otago[217] a hypodysfibrinogenemic Aα chain truncation mutant, is discusssed in the section on hypodysfibrinogenemia.

Fibrinogen Caracas II (AαS434N-glycosylated[178]) is characterized by impaired fibrin gelation that is related to N-glycosolation. The fibrin ultrastructure shows thinner, less well-ordered fibers.[179] The carbohydrate group may interfere with fibrin polymerization in the same way as the bulky albumin group does in the case of fibrinogen Dusart, or possibly the problem may be related to repulsive forces generated by its negative charge. In contrast to several other thrombophilic dysfibrinogenemias that are located in this region of the molecule, this dysfibrinogenemia is asymptomatic.

Fibrinogen Lima (AαR141S,Aα139N-glycosylation[180]) is a homozygous dysfibrinogenemia discovered in a family without a history of bleeding or thrombosis. The glycosolation site is located in the proximal portion of the D domain and evidently does not interefere with D:E or D:D interactions, nor with fibrin-dependent plasminogen activation by tPA. It most likely interferes with lateral fibril associations due to the bulky carbohydrate group or to the repulsive negative charge on the carbohydrate group.

Amyloidosis Hereditary amyloidosis is an autosomal dominant trait characterized by progressive extracellular deposition of an amyloid protein in various organs. Hereditary forms of amyloidosis are associated with mutants of several plasma proteins: transerythretin, gelsolin, apolipoprotein A1, lysozyme, and, most recently, fibrinogen.[181] Transerythretin-associated amyloidoses, the most common form, have peripheral neuropathy and cardiomyopathy as major clinical manifestations, but patients have also developed gastrointestinal dysfunction, nephropathy, sexual impotence, vitreous opacification, and cerebral hemorrhage. In amyloidosis related to apolipoprotein A1, lysozyme, and fibrinogen, renal amyloid deposition has been the major finding. In 1993, amyloid fibrils obtained from the kidney of a patient with hereditary renal amyloidosis (HRA) were found to contain an extractable fragment of the fibrinogen Aα chain covering residues 499 through 580 and containing an Aα R554L mutation.[182] The propositus in this family developed nephrotic syndrome and azotemia at the age of 36, requiring cadaveric renal transplantation at the age of 40. A second renal transplantation for the same condition was done at the age of 50. After death from septicemia, an autopsy revealed the same amyloid deposition in the transplanted kidney as had been found in the original and first transplanted kidneys. A sibling had died at the age of 28 with nephrotic syndrome, and the propositus' son died at the age of 24 with azotemia and renal amyloidosis. It is important to note that substitution of Cys for Arg at position 554 in the Aα chain, namely fibrinogens Dusart and Chapel Hill III (AαR554C), does not result in amyloidosis such as occurs in the R554L mutation but instead causes a different functional impairment and clinical picture (see "Thrombophilia").

Other mutations in the Aα chain gene in families with HRA have been reported. Four kindreds were described with an AαE526V mutation with HRA manifested clinically in the fifth to seventh decades of life.[183,184] In one study[184] plasma fibrinogen levels were found to be within the normal range as were the thrombin times, and the distribution of normal and mutant Aα chains was equal, indicating a heterozygous defect.

Another kindred with clinical recognition of HRA in the fourth to fifth decade of life and low plasma fibrinogen levels has been described.[185] DNA sequence analysis showed a nucleotide deletion causing a frame shift after position Aα524 that produced an abnormal sequence and Aα chain termination after position 547. The abnormal peptide sequence was found in amyloid deposits in the kidneys but was not present in plasma fibrinogen. A similar frame shift mutation in the Aα chain gene in another kindred with the onset of kidney disease as early as the second decade resulted in renal deposition of a 49-residue hybrid peptide whose N-terminal 23 amino acids were identical to Aα499 to 521.[186] The remaining 26 C-terminal amino acids in the peptide resulting from a frame shift at codon 522 had a unique sequence that terminated at position 547.

Therapy and Course Renal transplantation is at best a temporizing solution to the problem of renal failure in fibrinogen-related HRA, since amyloid deposits accumulate in transplanted kidneys, just as in the original kidneys, causing eventual destruction of the allograft.[182,186] Liver transplantation would seem to be preferable to renal transplantation, but has not yet been attempted to our knowledge.

HYPODYSFIBRINOGENEMIA

Inherited hypodysfibrinogenemia includes cases of dysfibrinogenemia in which plasma fibrinogen levels are less than 1.5 mg/ml, as measured immunochemically or by other physical methods. Clottable protein measurements are not a reliable indicator of fibrinogen concentration, since functionally abnormal molecules are not always incorporated into a clot. Eighteen cases of hypodysfibrinogenemia have been described.[128,217,218] In the first described case, fibrinogen Parma,[187] the patient had a severe bleeding disorder that was corrected by infusing normal fibrinogen, which itself seemed to exhibit normal plasma survival. Fibrinogens Philadelphia I[188] and Bethesda III[189] possess the same properties, including normal fibrinopeptide release, defective fibrin polymerization, increased catabolic rate of the autologous protein, but normal survival of infused fibrinogen. These findings suggest that hypercatabolism is caused by an intrinsic molecular defect of the mutant fibrinogen that accounts for the hypofibrinogenemia. In the case of fibrinogen Chapel Hill I,[190] homologous and autologous fibrinogen turnover were normal or nearly normal, suggesting a different mechanism for the hypofibrinogenemia than in Philadelphia I or Bethesda III. In fibrinogen Baltimore II,[191] FPB release was delayed, and autologous fibrinogen synthesis was reduced, but homologous and autologous catabolism were normal. A better understanding of the cause for this abnormality awaits details on the exact structural anomaly.

Fibrinogen Frankfurt I (γA357T) is a heterozygously transmitted dysfibrinogen associated with hypofibrinogenemia, bleeding, impaired fibrin polymerization, and decreased support of platelet aggregation.[217] Fibrinogen Otago, a homozygous hypodysfibrinogenemia (AαR268Q/frameshift/271Pstop), is associated with mild bleeding, multiple spontaneous first trimester abortions, and abnormal scar formation,[218] a behavior consistent with that of patients with afibrinogenemia. Cryoprecipitate infusion during one pregnancy in the propositus resulted in a normal birth. The data suggest that there is decreased hepatic assembly and/or secretion of molecules with truncated Aα chains. Fibrinogens Marburg I[169] and Malmöe I[193] are discussed in the section on thrombophilia.

Management of these conditions with plasma or fibrinogen concentrates is generally the same as that described for afibrinogenemia.

DYSFIBRINOGENEMIA AND THROMBOPHILIA

Dysfibrinogenemia associated with thrombosis occurs in about 20 percent of dysfibrinogenemic families.[128,194] Among such families, there has been a high incidence of thrombotic problems related to pregnancy, in particular spontaneous abortion and post partum thromboembolism. Most of the thrombophilic familes that have been identified to date are listed in Table 124-1, and those with defined or potential mechanisms for the thrombophilic condition are discussed below.

Fibrinogens Nijmegen and Ijmuiden   Fibrinogen Nijmegen is associated with abnormal tPA-induced plasminogen activation but normal fibrinopeptide release.[133,134] Abnormal high-molecular-weight fibrinogen complexes and albumin-linked fibrinogen molecules were also found. Fibrinogen Ijmuiden was similar to Nijmegen in these respects, and in addition showed abnormal FPB release.[133] The polymerization abnormality that both fibrinogens show may cause abnormal tPA-mediated plasminogen activation, which in turn may contribute to the thrombophilia.

Fibrinogen Cedar Rapids   Of the numerous dysfibrinogenemic families which are characterized by an amino acid substitution at position 275R of the normal γ chain, either R to C, R to H, or R to S (Table 124-1), all but five are asymptomatic. Of the families reporting thrombophilia, there are two with γR275C, Bologna I[194] and Cedar Rapids[195] and three with γR275H substitutions. The γR275H Haifa I patient[196] presented at the age of 30 with arterial occlusions, Barcelona III with venous thrombosis,[197] and Bergamo II with pulmonary embolism associated with pregnancy.[198] Clearly there is no simple direct linkage between this type of structural abnormality and thromboembolism, and other contributory conditions must be sought.

Several genetic risk factors are important in the pathogenesis of venous thromboembolism, and these include abnormalities of protein C, protein S, antithrombin III, plasminogen, prothrombin, fibrinogen, plasma homocysteine levels, and most recently, factor V.[199,200] The aforementioned defect was manifested as resistance to activated protein C due to a mutation in the factor V gene resulting in substitution of Gln for Arg at position 506, commonly referred to as factor V Leiden.[201-204]

Fibrinogen Cedar Rapids is a heterozygous dysfibrinogenemia in which thromboembolic disease was associated with pregnancy in three second-generation family members.[195] Each affected member of the family was heterozygous for the factor V Leiden defect, whereas the parents and their siblings manifested either the factor V Leiden defect (paternal) or fibrinogen Cedar Rapids (maternal) and were asymptomatic. These observations suggest that coexpression of factor V Leiden and fibrinogen Cedar Rapids is associated with thrombophilia. Another possible example of such concurrent conditions is to be found in fibrinogen Giessen IV (γD318G[194]). The exact mechanism by which two coexisting conditions contribute to the thrombophilic state is not clear, but such conditions may ultimately be found in certain families with thrombophilia, especially those with variable clinical expression of thromboembolic disease among families or individuals (e.g., fibrinogens Kumamoto, Melun I, Kaiserslautern). This subject is covered in detail in Chap. 127.

Defects in the Calcium Binding Site of the γ Chain   A high-affinity calcium binding site in the γ chain is located between residues 311 and 336, and involves residues at γ318D, γ320D, γ322F, γ324G, and γ328E.[165,205] The calcium site is important for the structural integrity of the D domain and provides a protective effect against plasmin cleavage of the γ chain.[206] Fibrinogen Vlissingen (γdel319N,320D[165]) was identified in a woman who had been hospitalized because of pulmonary embolism. Fibrin polymerization was delayed both in the presence or absence of calcium. The deletion of γ chain residues 319 and 320 resulted in defective calcium binding and probable allosterically mediated dysfunction of the Da polymerization site and possibly the D:D site as well. Abnormal ADP-induced platelet aggregation has also been reported for this abnormal fibrinogen,[164] implying impaired function at the γ$_{XL}$ site. The functional relationship between the calcium-binding defect and thrombophilia, as in many situations, is not clear. Similarly, the fibrinogen Giessen IV (γD318G)[194] defect results in defective calcium binding and polymerization and was reported in an 18-year-old woman with recurrent venous thrombosis as well as mild bleeding, who also was heterozygous for the factor V Leiden defect.

Truncation Mutations Involving the Aα Chain   Fibrinogen Marburg[169] is a homozygous hypodysfibrinogenemia lacking amino acid residues Aα461-610 due to a stop codon at position 461 of the Aα chain. Its unpaired cysteine residue at position 442 forms a disulfide bridge with albumin and other substances.[192] The Marburg patient suffered from severe uterine bleeding after caesarian section, pelvic vein thrombosis, and recurrent thromboembolic disease. Another homozygous truncation mutant, fibrinogen Milano III,[170,171] is also associated with recurrent venous thrombosis. Unlike fibrinogen Marburg, this mutant fibrinogen circulates at normal levels. The abnormality is associated with defective lateral fibril association and comes about by a single base insertion after Aα451, resulting in a premature stop at 453S. Because of premature Aα chain termination, there is an unpaired Cys residue at position 442, and like Marburg, this is associated with covalent linkage of albumin to the Aα chain. The thrombophilia may be causally related to formation of fine fibrin clots, which reportedly are resistant to fibrinolysis.[177,207,208]

The Dusart Syndrome   Fibrinogen Dusart (AαR554C-albumin[172-177]) manifests marked thrombophilia and has been studied extensively. The defect is the same as that in fibrinogen Chapel Hill III,[128,209] which also presented with thrombophilia. Dusart fibrinogen displays reduced plasminogen binding,[173,176] impaired fibrin-dependent tPA activation,[173] and abnormal fibrin polymerization and clot structure[172,174,175,177] that is normalized by removing the affected region of the molecule.[175] In addition to these abnormalities, fibrinogen Dusart molecules show an enhanced self-association tendency that is directly related to the Aα chain defect, and the fibrinogen cross-linking rate is accelerated.[176] It has been suggested that the thrombophilia is attributable to hypofibrinolysis caused by the abnormal clot structure itself,[177] but the other factors mentioned above may be just as important in causing the syndrome.

The fibrinogen Caracas V abnormality (AαS532C[194]) is located in about the same region of the Aα chain as the Dusart and Chapel Hill III anomalies. This dysfibrinogenemia has been associated with both venous and arterial thrombotic diseases in several members of the kindred.[210] Electron microscopy of Caracas V fibrin revealed no differences from normal,[211] suggesting that expression of the defect is different from that of Dusart.

Thrombin Binding Defects   Low-affinity nonsubstrate thrombin-binding sites are in the fibrin E domain and represent, at least in part, a residual aspect of fibrinogen substrate recognition.[65] Both fibrinogen New York I (desBβ9-72)[99] and fibrinogen Naples I (BβA68T),[100,101] presented with striking thromboembolic disease, and both fibrins showed impaired thrombin binding, seemingly at the low-affinity thrombin binding site. Fibrinogen New York I exhibited recurrent venous thrombosis and fatal pulmonary embolism. Homozygous members of the fibrinogen Naples I kindred suffered juvenile arterial stroke, thrombotic abdominal aortic occlusions, and postoperative deep venous thrombosis. Fibrinogens Kumamoto and Aarhus I (both AαR19G) are each associated with thrombosis, and reduced thrombin binding to fibrin has been reported for Kumamoto.[130] However, fibrinogen Mannheim I, with the same Aα chain defect, has a bleeding tendency and no thrombosis.[128]

Melun I   The defect in fibrinogen Melun I (D364V[145]) is situated in a position that interferes with Da site function. This family has a pervasive history of venous thromboembolic disease in the heterozygous state. One may presume that defective Da:Ea site interactions contribute to the thrombophilia that has been observed. However, an anomaly (D364H) at the same site (fibrinogen Matsumoto I)[144] is not associated with thrombophilia. As in other situations of this kind, more information will be needed to solve this paradoxical situation.

Oslo I The Oslo I dysfibrinogenemia involves a Bβ chain defect and is associated with a shortened thrombin time and increased fibrinogen activity as a cofactor for platelet aggregation.[128] This augmented behavior of fibrinogen may be presumed to be causally related to the thrombophilic state, but until the structural defect is known, it will not be clear how the anomaly brings about these effects.

Kaiserslautern Fibrinogen Kaiserslautern (γK380N-glycosylated[212,213]) was described in a 34-year-old woman who developed a cerebral sinus thrombosis after caesarean section and is included in the thrombophilia section for that reason, even though other members of her family with the functional defect were asymptomatic. The site of the abnormality is quite removed from either the Da polymerization pocket or the D:D association site. The polymerization defect is normalized with calcium or by removing sialic acid residues, and thus appears to be due to electrostatic repulsion between condensing fibrils. The mechanism for the thrombophilia is unclear.

Therapy Patients with thrombophilic dysfibrinogenemias are heterogeneous both with respect to their molecular abnormalities as well as their thromboembolic problems. Bleeding, especially when associated with hypofibrinogenemia (e.g., fibrinogen Marburg), may be managed by infusing fibrinogen concentrates as well as by blood replacement. Patients with potentially life-threatening thrombophilic manifestations, such as occurs with fibrinogen Cedar Rapids,[195] have been successfully managed with plasma exchange prior to major surgery. However, there is insufficient evidence to suggest that this type of treatment is more effective than more general measures for managing potential thromboembolism, such as treatment with anticoagulants. Long-term management strategies for thrombophilic dysfibrinogenemia are the same as those in patients with recurrent thromboembolism and include life-long anticoagulation with vitamin K antagonists.

REFERENCES

1. Henschen A, Lottspeich F, Kehl M, Southan C: Covalent structure of fibrinogen. *Ann NY Acad Sci* 408:28, 1983.

2. Mosesson MW: Fibrinogen and fibrin polymerization: Appraisal of the binding events that accompany fibrin generation and fibrin clot assembly. *Blood Coag Fibrinol* 8:257, 1997.

3. Slayter HS: Electron microscopic studies of fibrinogen structure: historical perspectives and recent experiments. *Ann NY Acad Sci* 408:131, 1983.

4. Mosesson MW, Hainfeld JF, Haschemeyer RH, Wall JS: Identification and mass analysis of human fibrinogen molecules and their domains by scanning transmission electron microscopy. *J Mol Biol* 153:695, 1981.

5. Williams RC: Morphology of fibrinogen monomers and of fibrin polymers. *Ann NY Acad Sci* 408:180, 1983.

6. Blombäck B, Hessel B, Hogg D: Disulfide bridges in NH$_2$-terminal part of human fibrinogen. *Thromb Res* 8:639, 1976.

7. Huang S, Cao Z, Davie EW: The role of amino-terminal disulfide bonds in the structure and assembly of human fibrinogen. *Biochem Biophys Res Comm* 190:488, 1993.

8. Zhang J-Z, Redman CM: Role of interchain disulfide bonds on the assembly and secretion of human fibrinogen. *J Biol Chem* 269: 652, 1994.

9. Finlayson JS, Mosesson MW: Heterogeneity of human fibrinogen. *Biochemistry* 2:42, 1963

10. Wolfenstein-Todel C, Mosesson MW: Carboxy-terminal amino acid sequence of a human fibrinogen γ chain variant (γ'). *Biochemistry* 20: 6146, 1981.

11. Townsend RR, Hilliker E, Li YT, Laine RA, Bell WR, Lee YC: Carbohydrate structure of human fibrinogen. *J Biol Chem* 257:9704, 1982.

12. Barnhart MI, Cress DC, Noonan SM, Walsh RT: Influence of fibrinolytic products on hepatic release and synthesis of fibrinogen. *Thromb Haemostas* (suppl 39): 143, 1970

13. Fuller GM, Nickerson JM, Adams MA: Translation and cotranslational events in fibrinogen synthesis. *Ann NY Acad Sci* 408:440, 1983.

14. Olaisen B, Teissberg P, Gedde-Dahl T Jr: Fibrinogen γ chain locus is on chromosome 4 in man. *Hum Genet* 61:24, 1982.

15. Chung DW, Rixon MW, Que BG, Davie EW: Cloning of fibrinogen genes and their cDNA. *Ann NY Acad Sci* 408:449, 1983.

16. Crabtree GR, Kant JA, Fornace AJ Jr, Rauch CA, Fowlkes DM: Regulation and characterization of the mRNAs for the Aα, Bβ, and γ chains of fibrinogen. *Ann NY Acad Sci* 408:457, 1983.

17. Kant J, Fornace AJ Jr, Saxe D, Simon MI, McBride OW, Crabtree GR: Organization and evolution of the human fibrinogen locus on chromosome four. *Proc Natl Acad Sci (USA)* 82:2344, 1985.

18. Collen D, Tytgat GN, Claeys H, Piessens R: Metabolism and distribution of fibrinogen. I. Fibrinogen turnover in physiological conditions in humans. *Br J Haematol* 22:681, 1972.

19. Martinez J, Holburn RR, Shapiro SS, Erslev AJ: Fibrinogen Philadelphia. A hereditary hypodysfibrinogenemia characterized by fibrinogen hypercatabolism. *J Clin Invest* 53:600, 1974.

20. Harrison P, Wilbourn B, Debili N, et al: Uptake of plasma fibrinogen into the alpha granules of human megakaryocytes and platelets. *J Clin Invest* 84:1320, 1989.

21. Handagama P, Scarborough RM, Shuman MA, Bainton DF: Endocytosis of fibrinogen into megakaryocyte and platelet α-granules is mediated by α$_{IIb}$β$_3$ (glycoprotein IIb-IIIa). *Blood* 82:135, 1993.

22. Handagama P, Amrani DL, Shuman MA: Endocytosis of fibrinogen into hamster megakaryocyte α granules is dependent on a dimeric γA configuration. *Blood* 85:1790, 1995.

23. Mosesson MW, Homandberg GA, Amrani DL: Human platelet fibrinogen gamma chain structure. *Blood* 63:990, 1984.

24. Francis CW, Nachman RL, Marder VJ: Plasma and platelet fibrinogen differ in gamma chain content. *Thromb Haemost* 51:84, 1984.

25. Kunicki TJ, Newman PJ, Amrani DL, Mosesson MW: Human platelet fibrinogen: Purification and hemostatic properties. *Blood* 66:808, 1985.

26. Jandrot-Perrus M, Mosesson MW, Denninger MH, Ménaché D: Studies of platelet fibrinogen from a subject with a congenital plasma fibrinogen abnormality (fibrinogen Paris I). *Blood* 54:1109, 1979.

27. Scheraga HA, Laskowski M, Jr : The fibrinogen-fibrin conversion. *Adv Prot Chem* 12: 1, 1957.

28. Blombäck B: Studies on the action of thrombic enzymes on bovine fibrinogen as measured by N-terminal analysis. *Arkiv Kemi* 12: 321, 1958.

29. Blombäck B, Hessel B, Hogg D, Therkildsen L: A two-step fibrinogen-fibrin transition in blood coagulation. *Nature (London)* 275:501, 1978.

30. Laudano AP, Doolittle RF: Studies on synthetic peptides that bind to fibrinogen and prevent fibrin polymerization. *Proc Natl Acad Sci (USA)* 75:3085, 1978.

31. Laudano AP, Doolittle RF: Studies on synthetic peptides that bind to fibrinogen and prevent fibrin polymerization: structural requirements and species differences. *Biochemistry* 19:1013, 1980.

32. Liu CY, Koehn JA, Morgan FJ: Characterization of fibrinogen New York I. A dysfunctional fibrinogen with a deletion of Bβ 9-72 corresponding exactly to exon 2 of the gene. *J Biol Chem* 260:4390, 1985.

33. Pandya BV, Cierniewski CS, Budzynski AZ: Conservation of human fibrinogen conformation after cleavage of the Bβ chain NH$_2$-terminus. *J Biol Chem* 260:2994, 1985.

34. Shimizu A, Saito Y, Inada Y: Distinctive role of histidine-16 of the Bβ chain of fibrinogen in the end-to-end association of fibrin. *Proc Natl Acad Sci (USA)* 83:591, 1986.

35. Siebenlist KR, DiOrio JP, Budzynski AZ, Mosesson MW: The polymerization and thrombin-binding properties of des-(Bβ1-42)-fibrin. *J Biol Chem* 265:18650, 1990.

36. Pandya BV, Gabriel JL, O'Brien JO, Budzynski AZ: Polymerization site in the β chain of fibrin: mapping of the Bβ1-55 sequence. *Biochemistry* 30:162, 1991.

37. Kudryk B, Reuterby J, Blombäck B: Adsorption of plasmic fragment D to thrombin modified fibrinogen-sepharose. *Thromb Res* 2:297, 1973.

38. Kudryk B, Collen D, Woods KR, Blombäck B: Evidence for localization of polymerization sites in fibrinogen. *J Biol Chem* 1974; 249:3322, 1974.

39. Olexa SA, Budzynski AZ: Evidence for four different polymerization sites involved in human fibrin formation. *Proc Natl Acad Sci (USA)* 1980; 77:1374, 1980.

40. Shimizu A, Nagel GM, Doolittle RF: Photoaffinity labeling of the primary fibrin polymerization site: Isolation of a CNBr fragment corresponding to γ 337-379. *Proc Natl Acad Sci (USA)* 89:2888, 1992.

41. Yamazumi K, Doolittle RF: Photoaffinity labeling of the primary fibrin

polymerization site: localization of the label to γ-chain tyr-363. *Proc Natl Acad Sci (USA)* 89:2893, 1992.

42. Spraggon G, Everse SJ, Doolittle RF: Crystal structures of fragment D from human fibrinogen and its crosslinked counterpart from fibrin. *Nature* 389:455, 1997.

43. Ferry JD: The mechanism of polymerization of fibrinogen. *Proc Natl Acad Sci (USA)* 38: 566, 1952.

44. Krakow W, Endres GF, Siegel BM, Scheraga HA: An electron microscopic investigation of the polymerization of bovine fibrin monomer. *J Mol Biol* 71:95, 1972.

45. Fowler WE, Hantgan RR, Hermans J, Erickson HP: Structure of the fibrin protofibril. *Proc Natl Acad Sci (USA)* 78:4872, 1981.

46. Hantgan R, McDonagh J, Hermans J: Fibrin assembly. *Ann NY Acad Sci* 408:344, 1983.

47. Mosesson MW, Siebenlist KR, Amrani DL, DiOrio JP: Identification of covalently linked trimeric and tetrameric D domains in crosslinked fibrin. *Proc Natl Acad Sci (USA)* 86:1113, 1989.

48. Hewat EA, Tranqui L, Wade RH: Electron microscope structural study of modified fibrin and a related modified fibrinogen aggregate. *J Mol Biol* 170:203, 1983.

49. Mosesson DiOrio JP, Siebenlist KR, Wall JS, Hainfeld JF: Evidence for a second type of branch point in fibrin polymer networks, the trimolecular junction. *Blood* 82:1517, 1993.

50. Shainoff JR, Dardik BN: Fibrinopeptide B in fibrin assembly and metabolism: physiologic significance in delayed release of the peptide. *Ann NY Acad Sci* 408:254, 1983.

51. Shainoff JR, Dardik BN: Fibrinopeptide B and aggregation of fibrinogen. *Science* 1979; 204:200, 1979.

52. Martinelli RA, Scheraga HA: Steady-state kinetic study of the bovine thrombin-fibrinogen interaction. *Biochemistry* 19:2343, 1980.

53. Hurlet-Jensen A, Cummins HZ, Nossel HL, Liu CY: Fibrin polymerization and release of fibrinopeptide B by thrombin. *Thromb Res* 27: 419, 1982.

54. Ruf W, Bender A, Lane DA, Preissner KT, Selmayr E, Müller-Berhaus G: Thrombin-induced fibrinopeptide B release from normal and variant fibrinogens: influence of inhibitors of fibrin polymerization. *Biochim Biophys Acta* 965:169, 1988.

55. Medved LV, Litvinovich SV, Ugarova TP, Lukinova NI, Kilikhevich VN, Ardemasova ZA: Localization of a fibrin polymerization site complementary to Gly-His-Arg sequence. *FEBS Lett* 320:239, 1993.

56. Everse SJ, Spraggon G, Veerapandian L, Riley M, Doolittle RF: Crystal structure of fragment double-D from human fibrin with two different bound ligands. *Biochemistry* 37:8637, 1998.

57. Mosesson MW, Siebenlist KR, Hainfeld JF, Wall JS: The covalent structure of factor XIIIa-crosslinked fibrinogen fibrils. *J Struct Biol* 115:88, 1995.

58. Mosesson MW, Siebenlist KR, DiOrio JP, Matsuda M, Hainfeld JF, Wall JS: The role of fibrinogen D domain intermolecular association sites in the polymerization of fibrin and fibrinogen Tokyo II (γ275 arg→cys). *J Clin Invest* 96:1053, 1995.

59. Siebenlist KR, Meh DA, Wall JS, Hainfeld JF, Mosesson MW: Orientation of the C-terminal regions of fibrin γ chain dimers determined from the crosslinked products formed in mixtures of fibrin, fragment D, and factor XIIIa. *Thromb Haemostas* 74:1113, 1995.

60. Niwa K, Takebe M, Sugo T, et al: A γ Gly-268 to Glu substitution is responsible for impaired fibrin assembly in a homozygous dysfibrinogen Kurashiki I. *Blood* 87:4686, 1996.

61. Kloczewiak M, Timmons S, Hawiger J: Recognition site for the platelet receptor is present on the 15-residue carboxy-terminal fragment of the γ chain of human fibrinogen and is not involved in the fibrin polymerization reaction. *Thromb Res* 29:249, 1983.

62. Kloczewiak M, Timmons S, Lucas TJ, Hawiger J: Platelet receptor recognition site on human fibrinogen. Synthesis and structure-function relationship of peptides corresponding to the carboxy-terminal segment of the γ chain. *Biochemistry* 23:1767, 1984.

63. Wolfenstein-Todel C, Mosesson MW: Human plasma fibrinogen heterogeneity: Evidence for an extended carboxyl-terminal sequence in a normal fibrinogen variant (γ). *Proc Natl Acad Sci (USA)* 77:5069, 1980.

64. Siebenlist KR, DA Meh, Mosesson MW: Plasma factor XIII binds specifically to fibrinogen molecules containing γ′ chains. *Biochemistry* 35:10448, 1996.

65. Meh DA, Siebenlist KR, Mosesson MW: Identification and characterization of the thrombin binding sites on fibrin. *J Biol Chem* 271:23121, 1996.

66. Mosesson MW, Sherry S: Preparation and properties of human fibrinogen of relatively high solubility. *Biochemistry* 5:2829, 1966.

67. Hasegawa N, Sasaki S: Location of the binding site "b" for lateral polymerization of fibrin. *Thromb Res* 57:183, 1990.

68. Veklich YI, Gorkun OV, Medved LV, Nieuwenhuizen W, Weisel JW: Carboxyl-terminal portions of the α chains of fibrinogen and fibrin. *J Biol Chem* 268:13577, 1993.

69. Gorkun OV, Veklich YI, Medved LV, Henschen A, Weisel JW: Role of the αC domains of fibrin in clot formation. *Biochemistry* 33:6986, 1994.

70. Hamaguchi M, Bunce LA, Sporn LA, Francis CW: Spreading of platelets on fibrin is mediated by the amino terminus of the β chain including peptide β15-42. *Blood* 81:2348, 1993.

71. Sporn LA, Bunce LA, Francis CW: Cell proliferation on fibrin: Modulation by fibrinopeptide cleavage. *Blood* 86:1801, 1995.

72. Chalupowicz DG, Chowdhury ZA, Bach TL, Barsigian C, Martinez J: Fibrin II induces endothelial cell capillary tube formation. *J Cell Biol* 130:207, 1995.

73. Bach TL, Barsigian C, Yaen CH, Martinez J: Endothelial cell VE-cadherin functions as a receptor for the β15-42 sequence of fibrin. *J Biol Chem* 273:30719, 1998

74. Ribes JA, Bunce LA, Francis CW: Mediation of fibrin-induced release of von Willebrand factor from cultured endothelial cells by the fibrin β chain. *J Clin Invest* 84:435, 1989.

75. Francis CW, Bunce LA, Sporn LA: Endothelial cell responses to fibrin mediated by FPB cleavage and the amino terminus of the β chain. *Blood Cells* 19:291, 1993.

76. Odrljin TM, Frances CW, Sporn LA, Bunce LA, Marder VJ, Simpson-Haidaris PJ: Heparin binding domain of fibrin mediates its binding to endothelial cells. *Arterioscler Thromb Vasc Biol* 16:1544, 1996.

77. Erban JK, Wagner DD: A 130-kDa protein in endothelial cells binds to amino acids 15-42 of the Bβ chain of fibrinogen. *J Biol Chem* 267:2451, 1992.

78. Odrljin TM, Shainoff JR, Lawrence SO, Simpson-Haidaris PJ: Thrombin cleavage enhances exposure of a heparin binding domain in the N-terminus of the fibrin β chain. *Blood* 88:2050, 1996.

79. Matačić S, Loewy AG: The identification of isopeptide crosslinks in insoluble fibrin. *Biochem Biophys Res Commun* 30:356, 1968.

80. Pisano JJ, Finlayson JS, Peyton MP: Crosslink in fibrin polymerized by factor XIII: ε-(γ-glutamyl)lysine. *Science* 160:892, 1968.

81. Shimizu A, Ferry JD: Ligation of fibrinogen by factor XIIIa with dithiothreitol: mechanical properties of ligated fibrinogen gels. *Biopolymers* 27:703, 1988.

82. Chen R, Doolittle RF: Identification of the polypeptide chains involved in the cross-linking of fibrin. *Proc Natl Acad Sci USA* 63:420, 1969.

83. Chen R, Doolittle RF: γ-γ cross-linking sites in human and bovine fibrin. *Biochemistry* 10:4486, 1971.

84. Doolittle RF, Chen R, Lau F: Hybrid fibrin: proof of the intermolecular nature of γ-γ crosslinking units. *Biochem Biophys Res Comm* 44:94, 1971.

85. Purves LR, Purves M, Brandt W: Cleavage of fibrin-derived D-dimer into monomers by endopeptidase from puff adder venom (bitis arietans) acting at cross-linked sites of the γ-chain. Sequence of carboxy-terminal cyanogen bromide γ-chain fragments. *Biochemistry* 26:4640, 1987.

86. McKee PA, Mattock P, Hill RL: Subunit structure of human fibrinogen, soluble fibrin, and cross-linked insoluble fibrin. *Proc Natl Acad Sci USA* 66:738, 1970.

87. Shainoff JR, Urbanic DA, DiBello PM: Immunoelectrophoretic characterization of the cross-linking of fibrinogen and fibrin by factor XIIIa and tissue transglutaminase. *J Biol Chem* 166:6429, 1991.

88. Stathakis NE, Mosesson MW, Chen AB, Galanakis DK: Cryoprecipitation of fibrin-fibrinogen complexes induced by the cold-insoluble globulin of plasma. *Blood* 51:1211, 1978.

89. Tamaki T, Aoki N: Cross-linking of α₂-plasmin inhibitor and fibronectin to fibrin by fibrin-stabilizing factor. *Biochim Biophys Acta* 661:280, 1981.

90. Sobel JH, Ehrlich PH, Birken S, Saffron AJ, Canfield RE: Monoclonal antibody to the region of fibronectin involved in cross-linking to human fibrin. *Biochemistry* 22:4175, 1983.

91. Kimura S, Aoki N: Cross-linking site in fibrinogen for α₂-plasmin inhibitor. *J Biol Chem* 261:15591, 1986.

92. Siebenlist KR, Mosesson MW: Factors affecting γ-chain multimer formation in cross-linked fibrin. *Biochemistry* 31:936, 1992.

93. Selmayr E, Thiel W, Müller-Berghaus G: Crosslinking of fibrinogen to immobilized des AA-fibrin. *Thromb Res* 39:459, 1985.

94. Selmayr E, Deffner M, Bachmann L, Müller-Berghaus G: Chromatography and electron microscopy of cross-linked fibrin polymers—A new model describing the cross-linking at the DD-trans contact of the fibrin molecules. *Biopolymers* 27:1733. 1988.

95. Mosesson MW, Siebenlist KR, Meh DA, Wall JS, Hainfeld JF: The location of the carboxy-terminal region of γ chains in fibrinogen and fibrin D domains. *Proc Natl Acad Sci (USA)* 95:10511, 1998.

96. Fenton JW, II, Olson TA, Zabinski MP, Wilner GD: Anion-binding exosite of human α-thrombin and fibrin(ogen) recognition. *Biochemistry* 27:7106, 1988.

97. Stubbs MT, Bode W: A player of many parts: the spotlight falls on thrombin's structure. *Thromb Res* 69:1, 1993.

98. Scheraga HA: Interaction of thrombin and fibrinogen and the polymerization of fibrin monomer. *Ann NY Acad Sci* 408:330, 1983.

99. Liu CY, Wallen P, Handley DA: Fibrinogen New York I: the structural, functional, and genetic defects and an hypothesis of the role of fibrin in the regulation of coagulation and fibrinolysis, in *Fibrinogen, Fibrin Formation, and Fibrinolysis*, vol 4, edited by D Lane, A Henschen, M Jasani, p 79. Walter de Gruyter, Berlin, 1986.

100. Di Minno G, Martinez J, Cirillo F, et al: A role for platelets and thrombin in the juvenile stroke of two siblings with defective thrombin-adsorbing capacity of fibrin(ogen). *Arterioscl Thromb* 11:785, 1991.

101. Koopman J, Haverkate F, Lord ST, Grimbergen J, Mannucci PM: Molecular basis of fibrinogen Naples associated with defective thrombin binding and thrombophilia. Homozygous substitution of Bβ 68 Ala→Thr. *J Clin Invest* 90:238, 1992.

102. Liu CY, Nossel HL, Kaplan KL: The binding of thrombin by fibrin. *J Biol Chem* 254:10421, 1979.

103. Vali Z, Scheraga HA: Localization of the binding site on fibrin for the secondary binding site of thrombin. *Biochemistry* 27:1956, 1988.

104. Binnie CG, Lord ST: A synthetic analog of fibrinogen α27-50 is an inhibitor of thrombin. *Thromb Haemost* 65:165, 1994.

105. Mammen EF: Fibrinogen abnormalities. *Semin Thromb Hemost* 9:1, 1983.

106. Almondhiry H, Ehmann WC: Congenital afibrinogenemia. *Am J Hematol* 46:343, 1994.

107. Gitlin D, Borges WH: Studies on the metabolism of fibrinogen in two patients with congenital afibrinogenemia. *Blood* 8:679, 1953.

108. Hardisty RM, Pinniger JL: Congenital afibrinogenemia: further observations on the blood coagulation mechanism. *Br J Haematol* 2:139, 1956.

109. Tytgat GN, Collen D, Vermylen J: Metabolism and distribution of fibrinogen. II. Fibrinogen turnover in polycythemia, thrombocytosis, haemophilia A, congenital afibrinogenemia and during streptokinase therapy. *Br J Haematol* 22:701, 1972.

109a. Neerman-Arbez M, Honsberger A, Antonarakis SE, Morris MA: Deletion of the fibrogen alpha-chain gene (FGA) causes congenital afibrogenemia. *J Clin Invest* 103:215, 1999.

110. Pfeifer U, Ormanns W, Klinge O: Hepatocellular fibrinogen storage in familial hypofibrinogenemia. *Virchows Arch B Cell Pathol* 36:247, 1981.

111. Wehinger H, Klinge O, Alexandrakis F, Schurmann J, Witt J, Seydowitz HH: Hereditary hypofibrinogenemia with fibrinogen storage in the liver. *Eur J Pediatr* 141:109, 1983.

112. Callea F, De Vos R, Pinackat J: Hereditary hypofibrinogenemia with hepatic storage of fibrinogen: a new endoplasmic reticulum storage disease, in *Fibrinogen 2. Biochemistry, Physiology, and Clinical Relevance*, edited by GDO Lowe, JT Douglas, CD Forbes, A Henschen, p 75. Elsevier, Amsterdam, 1987.

113. Callea F, Tortora O, Kojima T, et al: Hypofibrinogenemia and fibrinogen storage disease, in *Fibrinogen 3. Biochemistry, Biological Functions, Gene Regulation and Expression*, edited by MW Mosesson, DL Amrani, KR Siebenlist, JP DiOrio, p 247. Elsevier, Amsterdam, 1988.

114. Sharp HL, Bridges RA, Krivit W, Freier EF: Cirrhosis associated with alpha1-antitrypsin deficiency: a previously unrecognized inherited disorder. *J Lab Clin Med* 73:934, 1969.

115. Eriksson S: Liver disease in alpha₁-antitrypsin deficiency. *Scand J Gastroenterol* 20:907, 1985.

116. Nukiwa T, Satoh K, Brantly ML, et al: Identification of a second mutation in the protein-coding sequence of the Z type Alpha 1-antitrypsin gene. *J Biol Chem* 261:15989, 1986.

117. George P, Wyatt J, Callea F, Brennan S: Fibrinogen Brescia: Hypofibrinogenemia and hepatic fibrinogen storage are associated with a gamma chain substitution (284 Gly→Arg) and hypersialylation of the circulating fibrinogen. *Blood Coag Fibrinol* 9:698, 1998.

118. Base W, Barsigian C, Schaeffer A, et al: Influence of branched-chain amino acids and branched-chain keto acids on protein synthesis in isolated hepatocytes. *Hepatology* 7:234, 1987.

119. Weiss HJ, Rogers J: Fibrinogen and platelets in the primary arrest of bleeding: studies in two patients with congenital afibrinogenemia. *N Engl J Med* 285:369, 1971.

120. Girolami A, De Marco L, Virgolini L, et al: Platelet adhesiveness and aggregation in congenital afibrinogenemia. An investigation of three patients with post-transfusion cross-correction studies between them. *Blut* 30:87, 1975.

121. Cattaneo M, Bettega D, Lombardi R, et al: Sustained correction of the bleeding time in an afibrinogenemic patient after infusion of fresh frozen plasma. *Br J Haematol* 82:388, 1992.

122. Salzman EW: Hemostatic problems in surgical patients, in *Hemostasis and Thrombosis: Basic Principles and Clinical Practice*, 2nd ed, edited by RW Colman, J Hirsch, VJ Marder, ED Salzman, p 920. Lippincott, Philadelphia, 1987.

123. Inamoto Y, Terao T: First report of a case of congenital afibrinogenemia with successful delivery. *Am J Obstet Gynecol* 153:803, 1985.

124. De Vries A, Rosenberg T, Kochwa S, Boss JH: Precipitating antifibrinogen antibodies appearing after fibrinogen infusions in a patient with congenital afibrinogenemia. *Am J Med* 30:486, 1961.

125. Caen J, Faur J, Ineeman S, et al: Nécrose ischémique bilatérale dans un cas de grande hypofibrinogénémie congénitale. *Nouv Rev Fr Hematol* 4:321, 1964.

126. Ingram GIC, McBrien DJ, Spencer H: Fatal pulmonary embolus in congenital fibrinopenia. Report of two cases. *Acta Hematol* 35:56, 1966.

127. MacKinnon HH, Fekete JF: Congenital afibrinogenemia: vascular changes and multiple thromboses induced by fibrinogen infusions and contraceptive medication. *Can Med Assoc J* 140:597, 1971.

128. Ebert R: *Index of Variant Human Fibrinogens*, pp 1–423. CRC Press, Boca Raton, FL, 1994.

129. Blombäck M, Blombäck B, Mammen EF, Prasad AS: Fibrinogen Detroit—A molecular defect in the N-terminal disulphide knot of human fibrinogen. *Nature* 218:134, 1968.

130. Yamaguchi FI, Sugo T, Hashimoto Y, Kimura K, Okajima K, Matsuda M: Fibrinogen Kumamoto with an Aα Arg19→Gly substitution associated clinically with thrombosis. *Fibrinolysis* 10(suppl 4):23, 1996.

131. Yoshida N, Okuma M, Hirata H, Matsuda M, Yamazumi K, Asakura S: Fibrinogen Kyoto II, a new congenitally abnormal molecule, characterized by replacement of Aα proline-18 by leucine. *Blood* 78:149, 1991.

132. Brennan SO, Hammonds B, George PM: Aberrant hepatic processing causes removal of activation peptide and primary polymerization site from fibrinogen Canterbury (Aα20 Val→Asp). *J Clin Invest* 96:2854, 1995.

133. Koopman J, Haverkate F, Grimbergen J: Abnormal fibrinogens Ijmuiden (BβArg14→Cys) and Nijmegen (BβArg44→Cys) form disulfide-linked fibrinogen-albumin complexes. *Proc Natl Acad Sci (USA)* 89:3478, 1992.

134. Engesser L, Koopman J, de Munk G: Fibrinogen Nijmegen: Congenital dysfibrinogenemia associated with impaired t-PA-mediated plasminogen activation and decreased binding of t-PA. *Thromb Haemostas* 60:113, 1988.

135. Lord ST, Strickland E, Jayjock E: Strategy for recombinant multichain protein synthesis: fibrinogen Bβ-chain variants as thrombin substrates. *Biochemistry* 35:2342, 1996.

136. Soria J, Soria C, Samama M, Henschen A, Southan C: Detection of fibrinogen abnormality in dysfibrinogenemia: Special report on fibrinogen Metz characterized by an amino acid substitution located at the peptide bond cleaved by thrombin, in *Fibrinogen-Recent Biochemical and Medical Aspects*, edited by A Henschen, H Graeff, F Lottspeich, p 129. W de Gruyter, Berlin, 1982.

137. Alving BM, Henschen AH. Fibrinogen Giessen I: A congenital homozygously expressed dysfibrinogenemia with Aα-16 Arg-His substitution. *Am J Hematol* 25:479, 1987.

138. Siebenlist KR, Prchal JT, Mosesson MW: Fibrinogen Birmingham: a

heterozygous dysfibrinogenemia (Aα16 Arg→His) containing heterodimeric molecules. *Blood* 71:613, 1988.

139. Carrell N, McDonagh J: Fibrinogen Chapel Hill II: defective in reactions with thrombin, factor XIIIa, and plasmin. *Br J Haematol* 52:35, 1982.

140. Wada Y, Niwa K, Maekawa H, et al: A new type of congenital dysfibrinogen, fibrinogen Bremen, with an Aα Gly-17 to Val substitution associated with hemorrhagic diathesis and delayed wound healing. *Thromb Haemost* 70:397, 1993.

141. Kamura T, Tsuda H, Yae Y, et al: An abnormal fibrinogen Fukuoka II (Gly B beta 15→Cys) characterized by defective fibrin lateral association and mixed disulfide formation. *J Biol Chem* 270:29392, 1995.

142. Côté HCF, Lord ST, Pratt KP: γ-chain dysfibrinogenemias: Molecular structure-function relationships of naturally occurring mutations in the γ chain of human fibrinogen. *Blood* 92:2195, 1998.

143. Everse SJ, Spraggaon G, Doolittle RF: A three-dimensional consideration of variant human fibrinogens. *Thromb Haemostas* 80:1, 1998.

144. Okumura N, Furihata K, Terasawa F, Nakogoshi R, Ueno I, Katsuyama T: Fibrinogen Matsumoto I: A γ364 Asp→His (GAT→CAT) substitution associated with defective fibrin polymerization. *Thromb Haemost* 75:887, 1996.

145. Bentolila S, Samama MM, Conard J, Horellou MH, French P: Association of dysfibrinogenemia and thrombosis. Apropos of a family (fibrinogen Melun) and review of the literature. *Ann Med Interne* 146:575, 1995.

146. Terukina S, Yamazumi K, Okamoto K, Yamashita H, Ito Y, Matsuda M: Fibrinogen Kyoto III: a congenital dysfibrinogenemia with a γaspartic acid-330 to tyrosine substitution. *Blood* 74:2681, 1989.

147. Reber P, Furlan M, Rupp C, et al: Characterization of fibrinogen Milano I: amino acid exchange γ330 Asp→Val impairs fibrin polymerization. *Blood* 67:1751, 1986.

148. Miyata T, Furukawa K, Iwanaga S, Takamatsu J, Saito H: Fibrinogen Nagoya, a replacement of glutamine-329 by arginine in the γ-chain that impairs polymerization of fibrin monomer. *J Biochem (Tokyo)* 105:10, 1989.

149. Yoshida N, Hirata H, Morigami Y, et al: Characterization of an abnormal fibrinogen Osaka V with the replacement of γ-arginine 375 by glycine. The lack of high-affinity calcium binding to D-domains and the lack of protective effect of calcium on fibrinolysis. *J Biol Chem* 267:2753, 1992.

150. Steinmann C, Reber P, Jungo M, et al: Fibrinogen Bern I: substitution γ337 Asn→Lys is responsible for defective fibrin monomer polymerization. *Blood* 82:2104, 1993.

151. Steinmann C, Bögli C, Jungo M et al: A new substitution, γ358 Ser→Cys, in fibrinogen Milano VIII causes defective fibrin polymerization. *Blood* 84:1874, 1994.

152. Kaudewitz H, Henschen A, Soria J, Soria C: Fibrinogen Pontoise—A genetically abnormal fibrinogen with defective fibrin polymerization but normal fibrinopeptide release, in *Fibrinogen, Fibrin Formation and Fibrinolysis*, edited by DA Lane, A Henschen, MK Jasani, p 91. W de Gruyter, Berlin, 1986.

153. DiOrio JP, Mosesson MW, M Matsuda: Fibrinogen Kurashiki (γG268E) fibrin network structure. *Microscopy Microanal* 4(suppl 2):1160,1998.

154. Matsuda M, Baba M, Morimoto K, Nakamikawa C: "Fibrinogen Tokyo II." An abnormal fibrinogen with an impaired polymerization site on the aligned DD domain of fibrin molecules. *J Clin Invest* 72:1034, 1983.

155. Siebenlist KR, Mosesson MW, DiOrio JP, Tavori S, Tatarsky I, Rimon A: The polymerization of fibrin prepared from fibrinogen Haifa (γ275 arg→his). *Thromb Haemost* 62:875, 1989.

156. Fellowes AP, Brennan SO, Ridgway HJ, Heaton DC, George PM: Electrospray ionization mass spectrometry identification of fibrinogen Banks Penninsula (γ280Tyr→Cys): A new variant with defective polymerization. *Br J Haematol* 101:24, 1998.

157. Beck EA, Charache P, Jackson DP: A new inherited coagulation disorder caused by an abnormal fibrinogen ('Fibrinogen Baltimore'). *Nature (London)* 208:143, 1965.

158. Bantia S, Bell WR, Dang CV: Polymerization defect of fibrinogen Baltimore III due to a γAsn[308]→Ile mutation. *Blood* 75:1659, 1990.

159. Yoshida N, Terukina S, Okuma M, Moroi M, Aoki N, Matsuda M: Characterization of an apparently lower molecular weight γ-chain variant in fibrinogen Kyoto I. *J Biol Chem* 263:13848, 1988.

160. Grailhe P, Boyer-Neumann C, Haverkate F, Grimbergen J, Larrieu MJ, Anglés-Cano E: The mutation in fibrinogen Bicêtre II (γAsn[308]→Lys) does not affect the binding of t-PA and plasminogen to fibrin. *Blood Coag Fibrinol* 4:679, 1993.

161. Okumura N, Furihata K, Terasawa F, Ishikawa S, Ueno I, Katsuyama T: Fibrinogen Matsumoto II: γ[308]Asn→Lys (AAT→AAG) mutation associated with bleeding tendency. *Br J Haemat* 94:526, 1996.

162. Yamazumi K, Shimura K, Terukina S, Takahashi N, Matsuda M: A γ methionine-310 to threonine substitution and consequent N-glycosolation at asparagine-308 identified in a congenital dysfibrinogenemia associated with posttraumatic bleeding, fibrinogen Asahi. *J Clin Invest* 83:1590, 1989.

163. Mosesson MW. Amrani DL, Ménaché D. Studies on the structural abnormality of fibrinogen Paris I. *J Clin Invest* 57:782, 1976.

164. Galanakis DK, Spitzer SG, Scharrer I, Peerschke EI: Impaired platelet aggregation support by two dysfibrinogens: A γ319-320 deletion and a γ310Met→Thr substitution. *Thromb Haemost* 69:2564(abs), 1993.

165. Koopman J, Haverkate F, Briët E, Lord ST: A congenitally abnormal fibrinogen (Vlissingen) with a 6-base deletion in the γ-chain gene, causing defective calcium binding and impaired fibrin polymerization. *J Biol Chem* 266:13456, 1991.

166. Ménaché D. Constitutional and familial abnormal fibrinogen. *Thromb Diath Haemorrh* (suppl 13):173, 1964.

167. Rosenberg JB, Newman PJ, Mosesson MW, Guillin M-C, Amrani DL: Paris I dysfibrinogenemia: a point mutation in intron 8 results insertion of a 15 amino acid sequence in the fibrinogen γ-chain. *Thromb Haemostas* 69:217, 1993.

168. Denninger M-H, Jandrot-Perrus M, Elion J, et al: ADP-induced platelet aggregation depends on the conformation or availability of the terminal gamma chain sequence of fibrinogen. Study of the reactivity of fibrinogen Paris I. *Blood* 70:558, 1987.

169. Koopman J, Haverkate F, Grimbergen J, Egbring R, Lord ST: Fibrinogen Marburg: a homozygous case of dysfibrinogenemia, lacking amino acid Aα 461-610 (Lys 461→AAA Stop TAA). *Blood* 80:1972, 1992.

170. Furlan M, Steinmann C, Jungo M, et al: A frameshift mutation in exon V of the Aα-chain gene leading to truncated Aα-chains in the homozygous dysfibrinogen Milano III. *J Biol Chem* 269:33129, 1994.

171. Furlan M, Steinmann C, Lämmle B: Binding of calcium ions and their effect on clotting of fibrinogen Milano III, a variant with truncated Aα-chains. *Blood Coag Fibrinol* 7:331, 1996.

172. Soria J, Soria C, Caen JP: A new type of congenital dysfibrinogenemia with defective fibrin lysis-Dusard syndrome: possible relationship to thrombosis. *Br J Haematol* 53:575, 1983.

173. Lijnen HR, Soria J, Soria C, Collen D, Caen JP: Dysfibrinogenemia (fibrinogen Dusard) associated with impaired fibrin-enhanced plasminogen activation. *Thromb Haemost* 51:108, 1984.

174. Koopman J, Haverkate F, Grimbergen J, et al: Molecular basis for fibrinogen Dusart (Aα 544 Arg→Cys) and its association with abnormal fibrin polymerization and thrombophilia. *J Clin Invest* 91:1637, 1993.

175. Siebenlist KR, Mosesson MW, DiOrio JP, Soria J, Soria C, Caen JP: The polymerization of fibrinogen Dusart (Aα 554 Arg→Cys) after removal of carboxy-terminal regions of Aα chains. *Blood Coag Fibrinol* 4:61, 1993.

176. Mosesson MW, Siebenlist KR, Hainfeld JF, et al: The relationship between the fibrinogen D domain self-association/cross-linking site (γXL) and the fibrinogen Dusart abnormality (Aα R544C-albumin). Clues to thrombophilia in the "Dusart Syndrome." *J Clin Invest* 97:2342, 1996.

177. Collet J-P, Soria J, Mirshahi M, et al: Dusart Syndrome: A new concept of the relationship between fibrin clot architecture and fibrin clot degradability: Hypofibrinolysis related to an abnormal clot structure. *Blood* 82:2462, 1993.

178. Maekawa H, Yamazumi K, Maramatsu S, et al: An Aα Ser-434 to N-glycosylated Asn substitution in a dysfibrinogen, fibrinogen Caracas II, characterized by impaired fibrin gel formation. *J Biol Chem* 266:11575, 1991.

179. Woodhead JL, Nagaswami C, Matsuda M, Arocha-Piñango CL, Weisel JW: The ultrastructure of fibrinogen Caracas II molecules, fibers, and clots. *J Biol Chem* 271:4946, 1996.

180. Maekawa H, Yamazumi K, Muramatsu S, et al: Fibrinogen Lima: A homozygous dysfibrinogen with an Aα-arginine-141 to serine substitution associated with extra, N-glycolsolation at Aα-asparagine-139. *J Clin Invest* 90:67, 1992.

181. Benson MD: Amyloidosis, in *The Metabolic Basis of Inherited Disease*, 7th ed, edited by CR Scriver, AL Beaudet, WS Sly, DV Valle, p 4159. McGraw-Hill, New York, 1995.

182. Benson MD, Liepnieks J, Uemichi T, Wheeler G, Correa R: Hereditary

renal amyloidosis associated with a mutant fibrinogen α-chain. *Nature (Genetics)* 3:252, 1993.

183. Uemichi T, Liepnieks JJ, Alexander F, Benson MD: The molecular basis of renal amyloidosis in Irish-American and Polish-Canadian kindreds.*Q J Med* 89:745, 1996.

184. Uemichi T, Liepnieks JJ, Benson M: Hereditary renal amyloidosis with a novel variant fibrinogen. *J Clin Invest* 93:731, 1994.

185. Uemichi T, Liepnieks JJ, Yamada T, Gertz MA, Bang N, Benson MD: A frame shift mutation in the fibrinogen Aα chain gene in a kindred with renal amyloidosis. *Blood* 87:4197, 1996.

186. Asi HL, Liepnieks JJ, Uemichi T, et al: Renal amyloidosis with a frame shift mutation in fibrinogen Aα-chain gene producing a novel amyloid protein. *Blood* 90:4799, 1997.

187. Imperato C, Dettori AG: Ipofibrinogenemia congenita con fibrinoastenia. *Helv Pediatr Acta* 4:380, 1958.

188. Martinez J, Holburn RR, Shapiro SS, Erslev AJ: Fibrinogen Philadelphia. A hereditary hypodysfibrinogenemia characterized by fibrinogen hypercatabolism. *J Clin Invest* 53:600, 1974.

189. Gralnick HR, Coller BS, Fratantoni JC, Martinez J: Fibrinogen Bethesda III: A hypodysfibrinogenemia. *Blood* 53:28, 1979.

190. McDonagh RP, Carrell NA, Roberts HR, Blatt PM, McDonagh J: Fibrinogen Chapel Hill: hypodysfibrinogenemia with a tertiary polymerization defect. *Am J Hematol* 9:23, 1980.

191. Ebert RF, Bell WR: Fibrinogen Baltimore II: Congenital hypo-dysfibrinogenemia with delayed release of fibrinopeptide B and decreased rate of fibrinogen synthesis. *Proc Natl Acad Sci (USA)* 80:7318, 1983.

192. Sugo T, Nakamikawa C, Takebe M, Kohno I, Egbring R, Matsuda M: Factor XIIIa cross-linking of the Marburg fibrin: Formation of αmχγn-heteromultimers and the α-chain-linked albuminχγ complex, and disturbed protofibril assembly resulting in acquisition of plasmin resistance relevant to thrombophilia. *Blood* 91:3282, 1998.

193. Soria J, Soria C, Hedner U, Nilsson IM, Bergqvist D, Samama M: Episodes of increased fibronectin level observed in a patient suffering from recurrent thrombosis related to congenital hypodysfibrinogenemia (fibrinogen Malmöe). *Br J Haematol* 61:727, 1985.

194. Haverkate F, Samama M: Familial Dysfibrinogenemia and Thrombophilia. Report on a study of the SSC subcommittee on fibrinogen. *Thromb Haemostas* 73:151, 1995.

195. Mosesson MW, KR Siebenlist, JD Olson: Thrombophilia associated with dysfibrinogenemia [fibrinogen Cedar Rapids (γR275C)] and a heterozygous factor V Leiden defect. *Thromb Haemostas (suppl)* 382 abs, 1997.

196. Brook JG, Tabori S, Tatarsky I, Hashmonai M, Schramek A: Fibrinogen 'Haifa—a new fibrinogen variant. *Haemostas* 13:277, 1983.

197. Borrell M, Garí M, Coll C, et al: Abnormal polymerization and normal binding of plasminogen and t-PA in three new dysfibrinogenemias: Barcelona III and IV (γ275Arg→His) and Villajoyosa (γ275Arg→Cys): *Blood Coag Fibrinol* 6:198, 1995.

198. Reber P, Furlan M, Henschen A, et al: Three abnormal fibrinogen variants with the same amino acid substitution (γ275Arg→His): Fibrinogens Bergamo II, Essen and Perugia. *Thromb Haemostas* 56:401, 1986.

199. Bick RL, Kaplan H. Syndromes of thrombosis and hypercoagulability: congenital and acquired thrombophilias. *Clin Appl Thromb/Hemostas* 4:25, 1998.

200. Dahlbäck B: Inherited thrombophilia: Resistance to activated protein C as a pathogenic factor of venous thromboembolism. *Blood* 85:607, 1995.

201. Bertina RM, Koeleman BPC, Koster T, et al: Mutation in blood coagulation V associated with resistance to activated protein C. *Nature* 369:64, 1994.

202. Zöller B, Dahlbäck B: Linkage between inherited resistance to activated protein C and factor V gene mutation in venous thrombosis. *Lancet* 343:1536, 1994.

203. Greengard JS, Sun X, Xu X, Fernandez JA, Griffin JH, Evatt B: Activated protein C resistance caused by Arg506Gln mutation in factor Va. *Lancet* 343:1362, 1994.

204. Voorberg J, Roelse J, Koopman R, et al: Association of idiopathic thromboembolism with single point mutation at Arg506 of factor V. *Lancet* 343:1535, 1994.

205. Dang CV, Ebert RF, Bell WR: Localization of a fibrinogen calcium binding site between γ-subunit positions 311 and 336 by terbium fluorescence. *J Biol Chem* 260:9713, 1985.

206. Haverkate F, Timan G: Protective effect of calcium in the plasmin degradation of fibrinogen and fibrin fragments. *Thromb Res* 10:803, 1977.

207. Gabriel DA, Muga K, Boothroyd EM: The effect of fibrin structure in fibrinolysis. *J Biol Chem* 267:24259, 1992.

208. Carr ME Jr, Alving BM: Effect of fibrin structure on plasmin-mediated dissolution of plasma clots. *Blood Coag Fibrinol* 6:567, 1995.

209. Wada Y, Lord ST: A correlation between thrombotic disease and a specific fibrinogen abnormality (Aα 554 Arg→Cys) in two unrelated kindred, Dusart and Chapel Hill III. *Blood* 84:3709, 1994.

210. Arocha-Piñango CL, Torres A, Marchi R, et al: A new thrombotic dysfibrinogenemia present in several members of a Venezuelan family. *Thromb Haemstas* 58:149(abs), 1987.

211. Marchi R, Arocha-Piñango CL, Gil F: Electron microscopy studies of 7 patients with dysfibrinogenemia and some of their relatives. *Rev Iberoamer Thromb Hemostasia* 3:185, 1990.

212. Brennan SO, Loreth RM, George PM: Oligosaccharide configuration of fibrinogen Kaiserslautern: electrospray ionization analysis of intact γ chains. *Thromb Haemost* 80:263, 1998.

213. Ridgway HJ, Brennan SO, Loreth RM, George PM: Fibrinogen Kaiserslautern (γ380 Lys to Asn): a new glycosolated variant with delayed polymerization. *Br J Haematol* 99:562, 1997.

214. Steinmann C, Bögli C, Jungo M, et al: Fibrinogen Milano V: a congenital dysfibrinogenemia with a γ275 Arg→Cys substitution. *Blood Coag Fibrinol* 5:463, 1994.

215. Niwa K, Kawata Y, Madoiwa S, et al: Fibrinogen Kamogawa: a new type of γArg-275 to ser substitution characterized by delayed fibrin gel formation. *Thromb Haemostas* 73:1229 (abs), 1995.

216. Steinmann C, Jungo M, Beck EA, Lämmle B, Furlan M: Fibrinogen Claro—another dysfunctional fibrinogen variant with γ 275 arginine→histidine substitution. *Thromb Res* 81:145, 1996.

217. Galanakis DK, Peerschke EI, Spitzer S, Scharrer I. Fibrinogen Frankfurt I, a γ357 Ala→Thr substitution associated with impaired fibrin polymerization and decreased platelet aggregation support. *Blood* 86 (suppl 1):76a, 1995.

218. Fibrinogen Otago: A major α chain truncation associated with severe hypofibrinogenaemia and recurrent miscarriage. *Br J Haematol* 98:632, 1997

HEMOSTATIC DYSFUNCTION RELATED TO LIVER DISEASES AND LIVER TRANSPLANTATION

EBERHARD F. MAMMEN

Liver diseases are frequently associated with hemostatic derangements that can lead to spontaneous and injury-related bleeding manifestations. The hemostatic abnormalities are complex and can include thrombocytopenia, platelet dysfunction, diminished plasma levels of coagulation factors, enhanced fibrinolysis, dysfibrinogenemia, and/or sometimes disseminated intravascular coagulation. The extent of the hemostatic abnormalities usually correlates with the magnitude of liver dysfunction. Careful laboratory evaluation of the hemostatic systems is essential in patients with liver disease who bleed or in whom surgical procedures are planned. Treatment consists mainly of plasma, cryoprecipitate, and platelet transfusions. Other treatment modalities include infusion of coagulation factor concentrates and administration of antifibrinolytic drugs, but both confer a risk of thrombosis.

Profound hemostatic failure accompanies the different stages of orthotopic liver transplantation and invariably leads to excessive bleeding. The main cause for the hemostatic defect in such patients is accelerated fibrinolysis, and several studies have shown that the use of antifibrinolytic agents, together with replacement therapy by blood components, can ameliorate bleeding.

INTRODUCTION

The liver plays a central role in hemostasis. Liver parenchymal cells are the site of synthesis of many coagulation factors as well as many of the physiological inhibitors of coagulation (e.g., protein C, protein S, and antithrombin III) and essential components of the fibrinolytic system (e.g., plasminogen and α_2-antiplasmin). The liver also regulates hemostasis and fibrinolysis by clearing activated coagulation factors from the circulation and plasminogen activators. When significant liver dysfunction occurs, the supervening outcome is usually a bleeding tendency that is related to the decreased levels of procoagulants and enhanced fibrinolysis. Thrombosis due to decreased synthesis of inhibitors of coagulation, although a theoretical possibility, is in fact uncommon. The bleeding tendency can also stem from thrombocytopenia, platelet dysfunction, decreased vitamin K availability, dysfibrinogenemia, and disseminated intravascular coagulation (DIC) associated with secondary fibrinolysis.

Acronyms and abbreviations that appear in this chapter include: aPTT, activated partial thromboplastin time; DIC, disseminated intravascular coagulation; FDP, fibrin degradation products; PAI-1, plasminogen activator inhibitor 1; PT, prothrombin time; t-PA, tissue plasminogen activator; TT, thrombin time; vWF, von Willebrand factor.

Patients with acute viral or toxic hepatitis usually do not present with a bleeding tendency unless the disorder is fulminant. In contrast, patients with chronic liver disease frequently present with spontaneous bleeding or with injury-related hemorrhage. This chapter reviews the hemostatic abnormalities that occur in patients with chronic liver disease and in patients undergoing orthotopic liver transplantation.

HEMOSTATIC DEFECTS IN CHRONIC LIVER DISEASE

BLEEDING MANIFESTATIONS

Patients with chronic liver disease may present with purpura, epistaxis, gingival bleeding, and/or menorrhagia. Minor or major surgical procedures at sites where there is a high level of local fibrinolysis (e.g., oral mucosa, urogenital tract) are particularly prone to excessive bleeding. Bleeding can also follow head trauma and soft-tissue trauma.

PATHOGENESIS

DECREASED SYNTHESIS OF COAGULATION FACTORS

The progressive loss of liver parenchymal cells is associated with diminished synthesis of all coagulation factors except for von Willebrand factor (vWF), which is produced by endothelial cells and megakaryocytes (see Chap. 135), and factor VIII, whose levels in plasma are increased for an unknown reason.[1] The vitamin K–dependent factors, particularly factor VII, are sensitive to liver dysfunction. Thus, decreased plasma activity of factors II, VII, X, and, to lesser extent, factor IX[2] can result not only from the decreased synthetic capacity of the liver cells but also from diminished γ-carboxylation due to reduced vitamin K availability. Common causes for a limited supply of vitamin K in patients with liver disease include diminished intestinal absorption due to cholestasis, malnutrition, prolonged gut sterilization by antibiotics, and intestinal malabsorption. Plasma factor V is frequently decreased, and the extent of the deficiency correlates well with the magnitude of liver dysfunction.[3] Plasma fibrinogen concentrations are usually in the normal range unless liver dysfunction is advanced[4] or the patient has DIC.

THROMBOCYTOPENIA

The leading cause of thrombocytopenia in patients with chronic liver disease is congestive splenomegaly or ''hypersplenism.'' Up to 90 percent of the total platelet mass may be in the massively enlarged spleen, compared with about 33 percent in a normal spleen.[5,6] Patients with cirrhosis have shortened platelet survival, which may contribute to the thrombocytopenia.[5,7] Thrombocytopenia can also be related to an autoimmune mechanism. Thus, patients with primary biliary cirrhosis, but not patients with alcoholic cirrhosis, were shown to have antibodies against the glycoprotein (GP)Ib/IX complex and against GPIIb/IIIa.[8] Additional potential causes for thrombocytopenia are DIC, folic acid deficiency, and decreased megakaryopoiesis.[9]

PLATELET DYSFUNCTION

In a study of 60 patients with severe, but stable, cirrhosis, mean values of bleeding time, platelet adhesion, and platelet aggregation induced by collagen, epinephrine, or ADP were in the normal range.[5] In contrast, other studies have demonstrated a platelet storage pool defect,[10] reduced thromboxane A_2 synthesis,[11] impaired signal transduction,[12] and diminished adhesion under flow conditions.[13] Studies of the interaction of platelet GPIb/IX complex vWF in patients with cirrhosis have yielded different results. Thus, one group of investigators observed a diminished number of GPIb/IX complexes on platelets, decreased platelet binding of vWF, and reduced ristocetin–induced platelet agglutination.[14] In sharp contrast, another group showed an increased number of GPIb molecules and enhanced botrocetin-induced platelet agglutination.[15] Increased plasma levels of vWF antigen and activity have been described,[15,16] albeit with a reduction of the high-molecular-weight vWF multimers which are hemostatically most active.[15,17] The decrease in the large vWF multimers, which has been attributed to enhanced proteolysis, has been proposed to give rise to excessive bleeding during orthotopic liver transplantation[17] (see Liver Transplantation, below). Thus, when judged in its entirety, it is unclear whether platelet dysfunction contributes significantly to the hemostatic diathesis in chronic liver disease.

ENHANCED FIBRINOLYSIS

The enhanced fibrinolysis observed in patients with chronic liver disease is thought to be caused by impaired control of the fibrinolytic system. Thus, the synthesis of α_2-antiplasmin is decreased,[18] there is diminished clearance of tissue plasminogen activator (t-PA),[19] and for unknown reasons there are reduced plasma levels of plasminogen activator inhibitor 1 (PAI-1), which is synthesized by endothelial cells.[20] These defects lead to increased plasma levels of t-PA and urokinase[21] and to a decreased half-life of plasminogen.[5,22] Enhanced fibrinolysis was also shown to be secondary to low-grade DIC in patients with cirrhosis due to endotoxemia[23] and was implicated in another group of patients in whom a shortened half-life of plasminogen was corrected by administration of heparin.[22]

DYSFIBRINOGENEMIA

Dysfibrinogenemia characterized by impaired fibrin polymerization and a prolonged thrombin time is commonly observed in patients with chronic liver disease.[24,25] The dysfibrinogenemia is due to an increased content of sialic acid in fibrinogen synthesized by the affected liver.[26] Removal of the excess sialic acid from the aberrant fibrinogen by neuraminidase results in correction of the thrombin time and normalization of fibrin monomer aggregation.[27] It is unknown, however, whether the dysfibrinogenemia contributes to the bleeding tendency exhibited by patients with chronic liver disease.

DIC

Patients with chronic liver disease are prone to develop DIC, and when it occurs they have a diminished capacity to contain the process. These defects stem from: (1) reduced plasma levels of the physiological inhibitors of coagulation, protein C, protein S, and antithrombin III; (2) diminished capacity of the liver to clear activated coagulation factors; and (3) impaired capacity to replenish coagulation factors that have been consumed by DIC. In addition, the secondary fibrinolysis that is associated with DIC may be particularly excessive due to the defective control mechanisms of fibrinolysis displayed by patients with chronic liver disease (see Chap. 126).

LABORATORY FEATURES

Patients with chronic liver disease who present with bleeding or are candidates for surgical intervention need to undergo laboratory evaluation for hemostatic abnormalities. The changes in hemostatic parameters that can be observed are summarized in Table 125-1. Frequently, the degree of the changes is related to the extent of liver dysfunction.[1]

The essential tests that need to be performed are: prothrombin time (PT), activated partial thromboplastin time (aPTT), thrombin time (TT), platelet count, fibrinogen, whole blood or euglobulin clot lysis time, D-dimer and fibrin degradation products (FDP). Results of these tests should allow one to establish whether thrombocytopenia, fibrinolysis, DIC, or deficiency of coagulation factors is present. More subtle interpretation may also be possible. For example, a prolonged TT in

TABLE 125-1   POSSIBLE HEMOSTATIC CHANGES IN CHRONIC LIVER DISEASE

Coagulation System		Fibrinolytic System	
Prothrombin time	↑	Whole blood clot lysis time	↓
aPTT	↑	Euglobulin clot lysis time	↓
Thrombin time	↑	Fibrin(ogen) degradation products	↑
Factors II, VII, IX, X	↓	D-dimer	↑
Factor V	↓	α_2-antiplasmin	↓
Factor VIII	↑	Plasminogen activator inhibitor 1	↓
vWF	↑		
Fibrinogen	↑		

Inhibitory Factors		Platelets	
Protein C	↓	Number	↓
Protein S	↓	Aggregation	↓ or N
Antithrombin III	↓	Adhesion	↓ or N
TFPI	N	Bleeding time	↑ or N

ABBREVIATIONS: aPTT, activated partial thromboplastin time; vWF, von Willebrand factor; N, normal; TFPI, tissue factor pathway inhibitor.

the presence of normal plasma fibrinogen and normal FDP suggests the presence of a dysfibrinogenemia.

Assays of factors V, VII, and VIII can be helpful in further evaluation of the hemostatic abnormalities. Thus, decreased levels of factors V and VII with a normal or increased level of factor VIII is consistent with liver dysfunction; decreased levels of factor VII with normal levels of factors V and VIII is consistent with vitamin K deficiency, and decreased levels of factors V, VII, VIII, and fibrinogen suggest the presence of DIC.

THERAPY

The various hemostatic defects associated with chronic liver disease may constitute the main cause of spontaneous and injury-related bleeding. Alternatively, they can enhance bleeding from esophageal varices, erosive gastritis, or hemorrhoids. The treatment strategy should be based on careful clinical evaluation of the causes of bleeding and assessment of the major hemostatic abnormalities involved. Thus, in patients with esophageal varices, sclerotherapy or therapy to decrease the pressure in the portal system are the primary targets, whereas attempts to correct the hemostatic defects are secondary. In patients who bleed spontaneously, in patients who bleed following trauma, or in patients predicted to bleed following surgery, the primary goal of treatment would be correction of the hemostatic defects.

FRESH-FROZEN PLASMA

Transfusion of fresh-frozen plasma replenishes all the deficient coagulation factors and physiological inhibitors of the coagulation and fibrinolytic systems. The correction of the levels of these components, however, is brief for factors like factor VII that have a short half-life so that repeated transfusion of relatively large volumes of fresh-frozen plasma is necessary for maintenance of adequate levels of these coagulation factors. As a consequence, volume overload can become a serious limiting factor. In extreme circumstances, plasma exchange can be employed. Another drawback of plasma replacement therapy is the risk of transmission of viral diseases, although the risk of transmitting HIV and hepatitis B and C can be diminished by using solvent-detergent-treated plasma.

PROTHROMBIN COMPLEX CONCENTRATES

Prothrombin complex concentrates provide all the vitamin K–dependent factors, which are frequently diminished in the plasma of patients with chronic liver disease. The use of these concentrates, however, does not correct the level of factor V, and since the deficiency of this factor may significantly enhance bleeding, concomitant transfusion of fresh-frozen plasma may be necessary. Administration of prothrombin complex concentrates can result in thrombosis, since activated coagulation factors present in the concentrates are not adequately cleared by the affected liver (see Chaps. 122, 123, 126). In addition, the use of prothrombin complex concentrates may be associated with a risk of transmitting viruses like hepatitis A virus or parvovirus (see Chaps. 122 and 123).

VITAMIN K ADMINISTRATION

When decreased vitamin K availability is suggested, as in patients with intra- or extrahepatic cholestasis, patients who have received antibiotics for a long time, or patients whose factor VII level is markedly decreased but factor V level is normal, administration of vitamin K_1 (10 mg) is warranted. Vitamin K_1 given intravenously can correct or improve the PT and aPTT within 8 to 24 h. The dose can be repeated daily until correction is complete and then as maintenance doses if the cause of the deficiency is ongoing.

PLATELET TRANSFUSION

When serious or life-threatening bleeding occurs in patients with chronic liver disease or when it is anticipated during surgical procedures, platelet transfusion should be used with the aim of increasing their number to $75,000/\mu L$ or more. In patients with severe splenomegaly this may not be possible to attain. The number of platelet units to be used depends on the platelet count prior to transfusion but is difficult to assess accurately, since the extent of sequestration of platelets by the spleen is unpredictable. Performing a platelet count 1 h after transfusion provides valuable information on the degree of sequestration.

CRYOPRECIPITATE

Since fibrinogen levels are usually not decreased to levels likely to cause bleeding, it is usually unnecessary to use cryoprecipitate in patients with chronic liver disease who bleed. The plasma level of fibrinogen may be decreased when DIC occurs, and in such conditions administration of cryoprecipitate may be warranted (see Chap. 126).

ANTIFIBRINOLYTIC AGENTS

Tranexamic acid or ε-aminocaproic acid have been successfully used in patients with chronic liver disease who underwent dental extractions.[28] Since hyperfibrinolysis is one of the significant causes for the hemostatic abnormalities in liver disease, the use of these agents can be beneficial for achieving hemostasis in other circumstances as well. However, if DIC is associated with liver disease, the use of antifibrinolytic agents can induce thromboembolism. Consequently, before using an antifibrinolytic agent, DIC has to be excluded.

LIVER TRANSPLANTATION

Orthotopic liver transplantation is associated with profound disturbances in hemostasis that lead to excessive bleeding during the procedure.[29,30] The patient is initially always hemostatically compromised, surgical trauma is extensive, there is an obligatory anhepatic phase during which coagulation factors are not produced, and there is excessive fibrinolysis during both the anhepatic phase and early reperfusion phase.

During the anhepatic phase, t-PA released from the endothelial cells of the recipient is not cleared from the circulation, resulting in a profound increase in plasma t-PA level. Since PAI-1 levels are low, the t-PA produces marked conversion of plasminogen to plasmin[31];

moreover, since α_2-antiplasmin levels are low, the plasmin can act relatively unopposed.[18,20]

During the reperfusion phase there is a second fibrinolytic "burst" due to massive t-PA release from the stored organ.[32,33] This is accompanied by generation of other proteolytic enzymes, such as elastases, trypsin, and cathepsin B,[34] that may also contribute to the overall proteolytic state and the associated bleeding.[35] Proteolytic breakdown of vWF also appears to contribute to the severe bleeding during this phase of transplantation.[17]

Thromboelastography has been used during transplantation to monitor the hemostatic status of the patient during the various phases of surgery, including ex vivo clot formation, clot strength, and fibrinolysis.[36] The availability of these data in the operating room allows the anaesthesiologists and surgeons to evaluate and follow the effects of replacement therapy and antifibrinolytic treatment.[33] The excessive bleeding during liver transplantation has been ameliorated by the use of aprotinin, a broad-spectrum serine protease inhibitor, in several[37,38] but not all studies.[39] Thus, in some studies, administration of aprotinin reduced the need for transfusion of blood components[37,38] and was associated with decreased plasma levels of t-PA and D-dimer and increased levels of α_2-antiplasmin.[38] In another study, however, the use of aprotinin failed to reduce the requirement for blood component replacement.[39] Large doses of tranexamic acid have also been reported to reduce blood loss and transfusion requirement.[40]

REFERENCES

1. Lechner K, Niessner H, Thaler E: Coagulation abnormalities in liver disease. *Semin Thromb Hemost* 4:40, 1977.
2. Rapaport SI, Ames SB, Mikkelsen S, Goodman JR: Plasma clotting factors in chronic hepatocellular disease. *N Engl J Med* 263:278, 1960.
3. Deutsch E: Blood coagulation changes in liver diseases. *Prog Liver Dis* 2:69, 1965.
4. Dymock IW, Tucher JS, Woolf IL, et al: Coagulation studies as a prognostic index in acute liver failure. *Br J Haematol* 29:385, 1975.
5. Stein SF, Harker LA: Kinetic and functional studies of platelets, fibrinogen, and plasminogen in patients with hepatic cirrhosis. *J Lab Clin Med* 99:217, 1986.
6. Schmidt KG, Rasmussen J, Bekker C, Madsen PE: Kinetics and in vivo distribution of indium-111 labeled autologous platelets in chronic hepatic disease: Mechanisms of thrombocytopenia. *Scand J Haematol* 34:39, 1985.
7. Aoki Y, Hirai K, Tanikawa K: Mechanisms of thrombocytopenia in liver cirrhosis: Kinetics of indium-111 tropolone labelled platelets. *Eur J Nucl Med* 20:123, 1993
8. Feistauer SM, Penner E, Mayr WR, Panzer S: Target platelet antigens of autoantibodies in patients with primary biliary cirrhosis. *Hepatology* 25:1343, 1997.
9. Cowan DH: Effect of alcoholism on hemostasis. *Semin Hematol* 17:137, 1980.
10. Laffi G, Marra F, Gresele P, et al: Evidence for a storage pool defect in platelets from cirrhotic patients with defective aggregation. *Gastroenterology* 103:641, 1992.
11. Laffi G, Cominelli F, Ruggiero M, et al: Altered platelet function in cirrhosis of the liver. Impairment of inositol lipid and arachidonic acid metabolism in response to agonists. *Hepatology* 8:1620, 1988.
12. Laffi G, Marra F, Ruggiero M, et al: Defective signal transduction in platelets from cirrhotics is associated with increased cyclic nucleotides. *Gastroenterology* 105:148, 1993.
13. Ordinas A, Escolar G, Cirera I, et al: Existence of a platelet-adhesion defect in patients with cirrhosis independent of hematocrit: studies under flow conditions. *Hepatology* 24:1137, 1996.
14. Sanchez-Roig MJ, Rivera J, Moraleda JM, Garcia UV: Quantitative defects of glycoprotein Ib in severe cirrhotic patients. *Am J Hematol* 45:10, 1994.
15. Beer JH, Clerici N, Baillod P, von Felten A, Schlappritzi E, Büchi L: Quantitative and qualitative analysis of platelet GPIb and von Willebrand factor in liver cirrhosis. *Thromb Haemost* 73:601, 1995.

16. Green AJ, Ratnoff OD: Elevated antihemophilic factor (AHF, factor VIII) procoagulant activity and AHF-like antigen in alcoholic cirrhosis of the liver. *J Lab Clin Med* 83:189, 1974.

17. Lattuade A, Mannucci PM, Chen C, Legnani C, Palaretti G: Transfusion requirements are correlated with the degree of proteolysis of von Willebrand factor during orthotopic liver transplantation. *Thromb Haemost* 78:813, 1997.

18. Aoki NM, Yamanaka T: The α_2-plasmin inhibitor levels in liver disease. *Clin Chim Acta* 84:99, 1978.

19. Tytgat G, Collen D, De Vreker RR, Verstraete M: Investigations on the fibrinolytic system in liver cirrhosis. *Acta Haematol* (Basel) 40:265, 1968.

20. Hersch SL, Kunelis T, Francis RB: The pathogenesis of accelerated fibrinolysis in liver cirrhosis: a critical role for tissue plasminogen activator inhibitor. *Blood* 69:1315, 1987.

21. Booth NA, Anderson JA, Bennett B: Plasminogen activators in alcoholic cirrhosis: demonstration of increased tissue type and urokinase type activator. *J Clin Pathol* 37:777, 1984.

22. Collen D, Bouvier J, Chamone DAF, Verstraete M: Turnover of radiolabelled plasminogen and prothrombin in cirrhosis of the liver. *Eur J Clin Invest* 8:185, 1978.

23. Violi F, Ferro D, Basili S, et al: Association between low-grade disseminated intravascular coagulation and endotoxemia in patients with liver cirrhosis. *Gastroenterology* 109:531, 1995.

24. Green G, Thomson JM, Dymock IW, Poller L: Abnormal fibrin polymerization in liver disease. *Br J Haematol* 34:427, 1976.

25. Palascak JE, Martinez J: Dysfibrinogenemia associated with liver disease. *J Clin Invest* 60:89, 1977.

26. Martinez J, Palascak JE, Kwasniak D: Abnormal sialic acid content of the dysfibrinogenemia associated with liver disease. *J Clin Invest* 61:535, 1978.

27. Martinez J, MacDonald KA, Palascak JE: The role of sialic acid in the dysfibrinogenemia associated with liver disease: distribution of sialic acid on the constituent chains. *Blood* 61:1196, 1983.

28. Francis RB, Feinstein DI: Clinical significance of accelerated fibrinolysis in liver disease. *Haemostasis* 14:460, 1984.

29. Neuhaus P: Hemostasis in liver transplantation. The surgeon's view. *Semin Thromb Hemost* 19:183, 1993.

30. Porte RJ: Coagulation and fibrinolysis in orthotopic liver transplantation. Current views and insights. *Semin Thromb Hemost* 19:191, 1993.

31. Lewis JH, Bontempo FA, Awad SA, et al: Liver transplantation: intraoperative changes in coagulation factors in 100 first transplants. *Hepatology* 9:710, 1989.

32. Porte RJ, Bontempo FA, Knot EA, et al: Systemic effects of tissue plasminogen activator-associated fibrinolysis and its relation to thrombin generation in orthotopic liver transplantation. *Transplantation* 47:478, 1989.

33. McNicol PL, Liu G, Harely ID, et al: Patterns of coagulopathy during liver transplantation: experience with the first 75 cases using thromboelastography. *Anaesth Intensive Care* 22:659, 1994.

34. Legnani C, Palareti G, Rodorigo G, et al: Protease activities, as well as plasminogen activators, contribute to the "lytic" state during orthotopic liver transplantation. *Transplantation* 56:568, 1993.

35. Ries H, Jochum M, Machleidt W, et al: Possible role of the phagocytic proteinases, cathepsin B and elastase in orthotopic liver transplantation. *Transplant Proc* 23:1947, 1991.

36. Kang YG, Martin DJ, Marquez J, et al: Intraoperative changes in blood coagulation and thromboelastographic monitoring in liver transplantation. *Anesth Analg* 64:888, 1985.

37. Scudamore CH, Randall TE, Jewesson PJ, et al: Aprotinin reduces the need for blood products during liver transplantation. *Am J Surg* 169:546, 1995.

38. Llamas P, Cabrera R, Gomez-Arnau J, Fernandez MN: Hemostasis and blood requirements in orthotopic liver transplantation with and without high-dose aprotinin. *Haematologica* 83:338, 1998.

39. Garcia-Huete L, Domenech P, Sabate A, Martinez-Brotons F, Jaurrieta E, Figueras J: The prophylactic effect of aprotinin on intraoperative bleeding in liver transplantation: a randomized clinical study. *Hepatology* 26:1143, 1997.

40. Boylan JF, Klinck JR, Sandler AN, et al: Tranexamic acid reduces blood loss, transfusion requirements, and coagulation factor use in primary orthotopic liver transplantation. *Anesthesiology* 85:1043, 1996.

COLOR PLATES

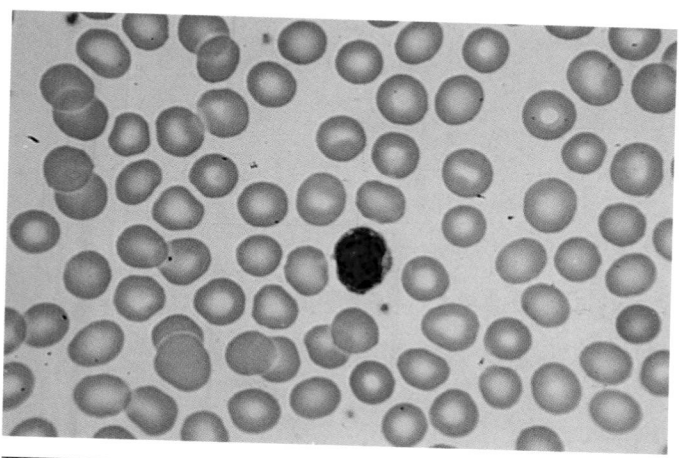

PLATE I-1   Normal erythrocytes

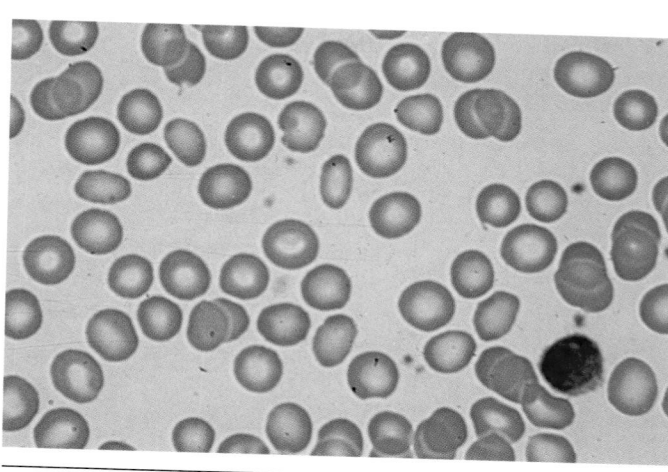

PLATE I-2   Slight hypochromia and microcytosis in early iron deficiency anemia

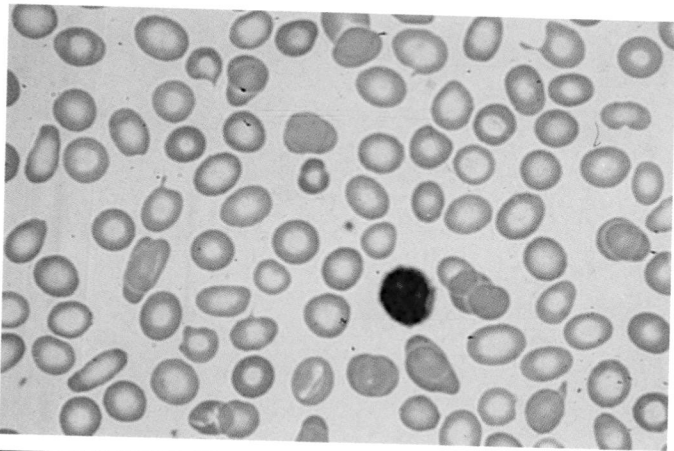

PLATE I-3   Severe hypochromia and microcytosis in iron deficiency anemia

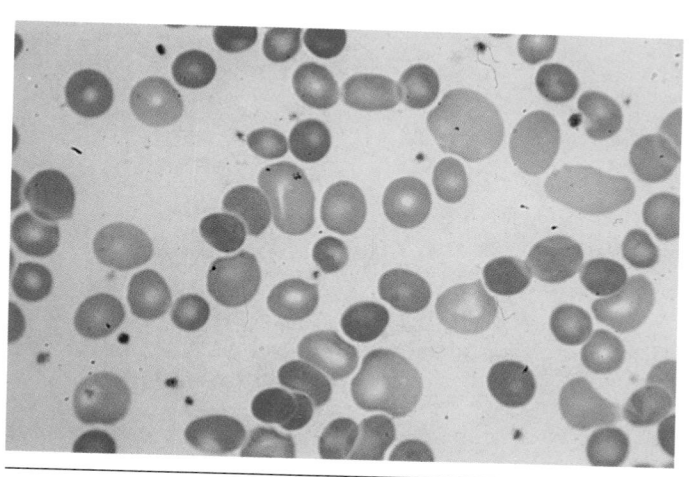

PLATE I-4   Polychromatophilia

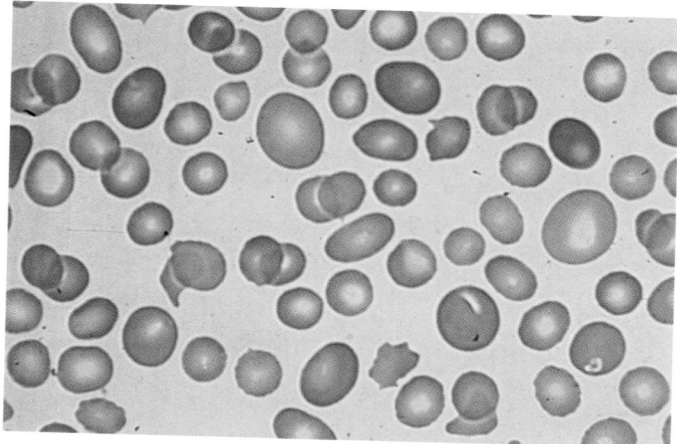

PLATE I-5   Macrocytosis

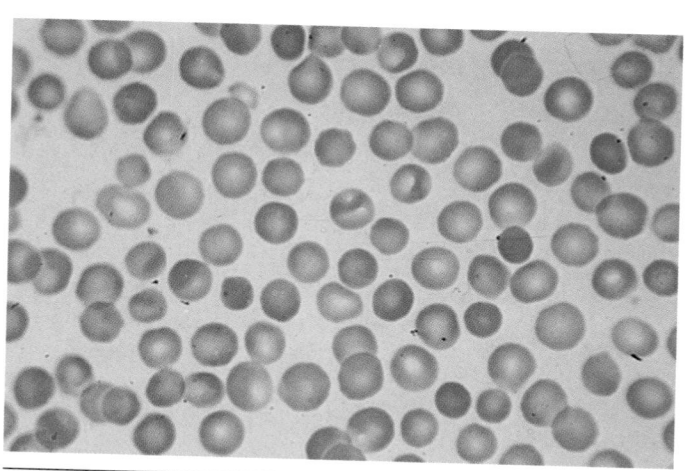

PLATE I-6   Spherocytosis

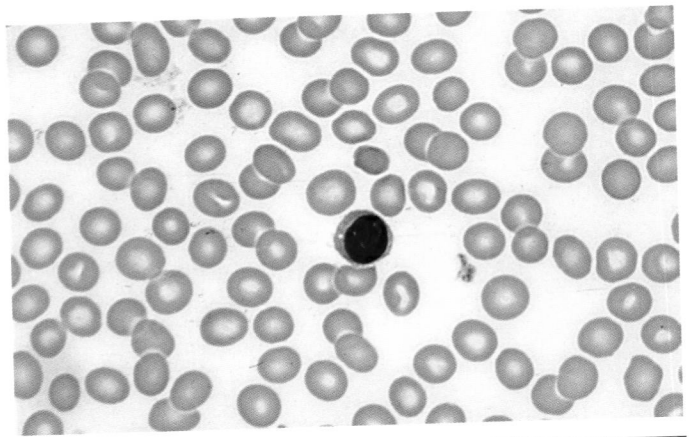

PLATE I-7 Normal red cell distribution

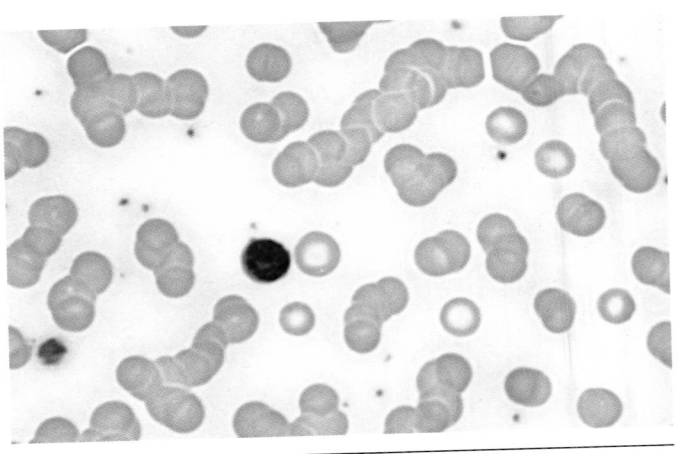

PLATE I-8 Rouleaux formation

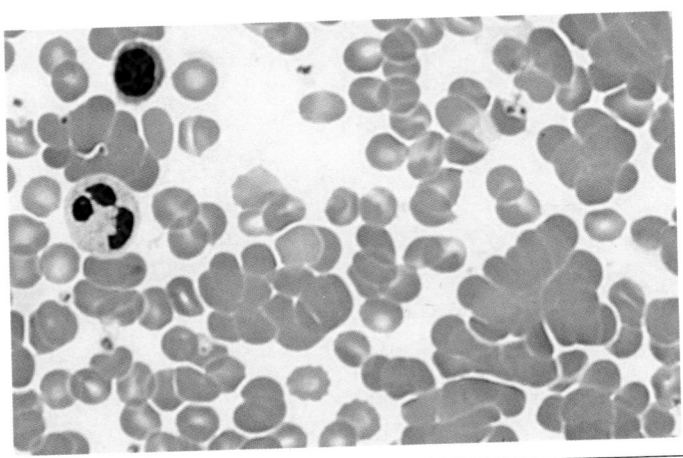

PLATE I-9 Erythrocyte agglutination

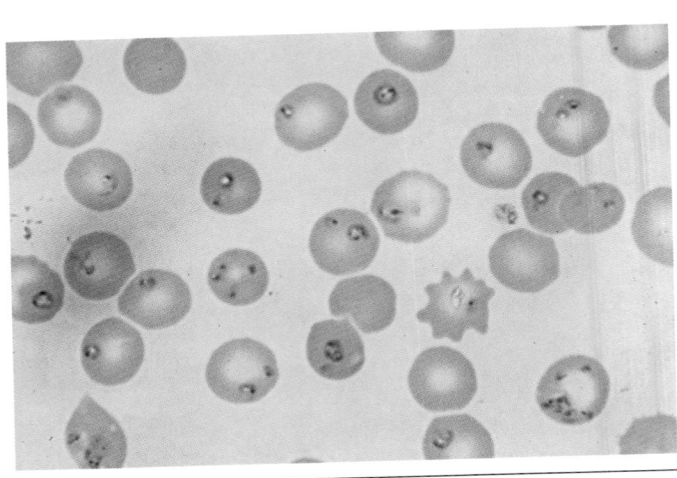

PLATE I-10 Red cell containing *Babesia microti*

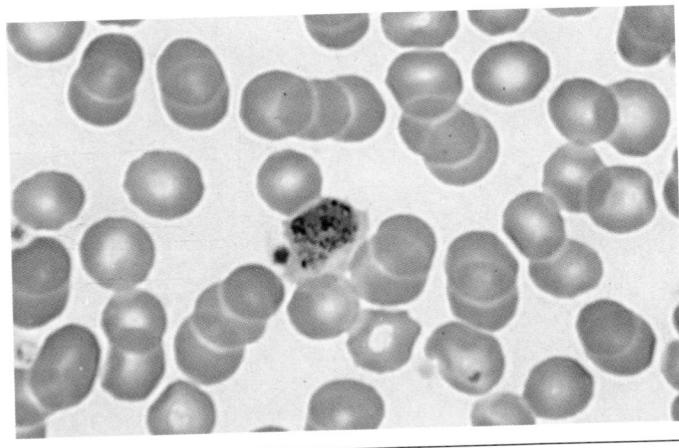

PLATE I-11 A red cell containing a trophozoite of *Plasmodium vivax*

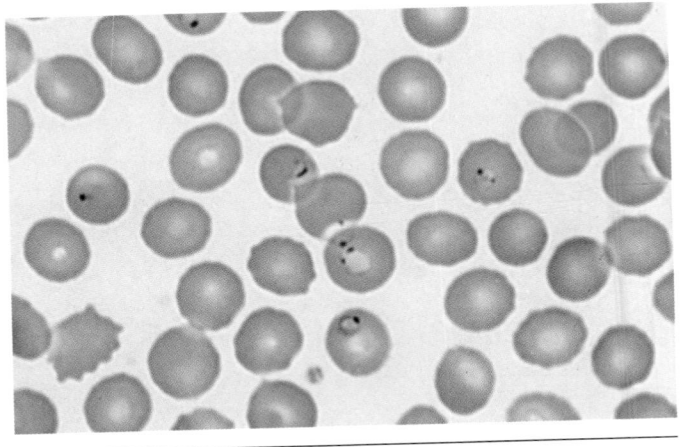

PLATE I-12 Red cells containing *Plasmodium falciparum* ring forms

(I-1 through I-12 are blood films)

PLATE II
RED CELL MORPHOLOGY

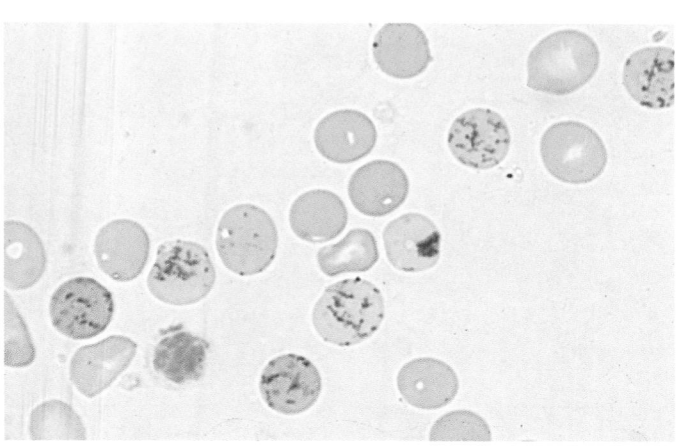

PLATE II-1   Red cells stained supravitally with new methylene blue. Reticulocytes retain intracellular stained precipitates of ribosomal RNA

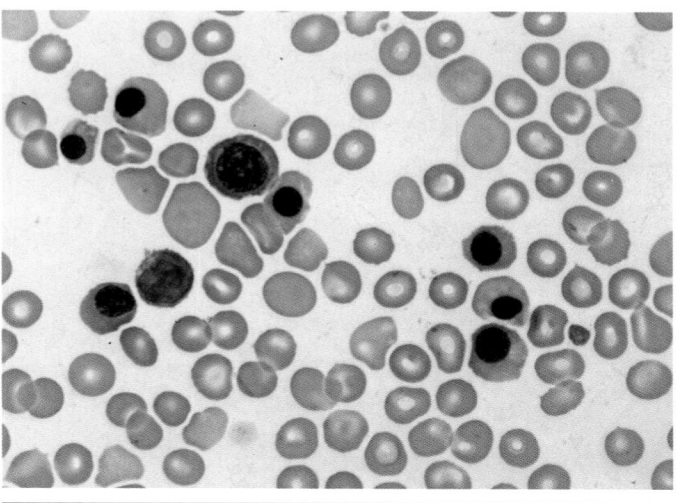

PLATE II-2   Hemolytic disease of the newborn (erythroblastosis fetalis). Polychromatophilic cells, spherocytes, and circulating erythroblasts

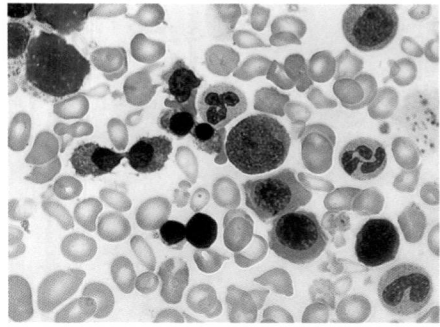

PLATE II-3   Marrow film. Congenital dyserythropoietic anemia. Red cell shape abnormalities and nuclear anomalies of the erythroblasts (bridging)

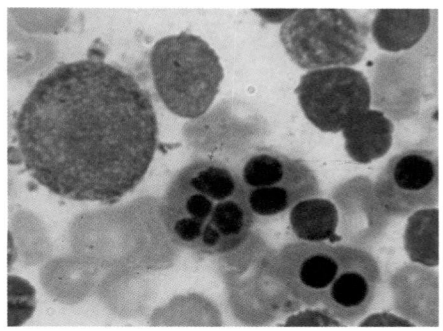

PLATE II-4   Marrow film. Erythroblastic multinuclearity

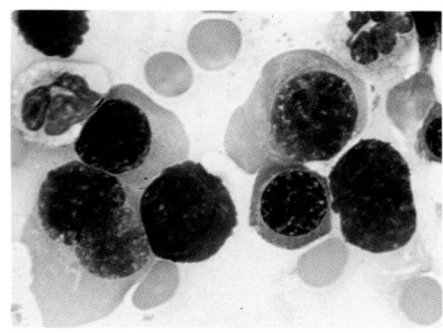

PLATE II-5   Marrow film. Congenital dyserythropoietic anemia. Note giant erythroblasts and binucleated erythroblast

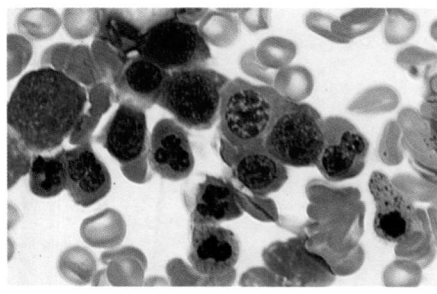

PLATE II-6   Chronic arsenic poisoning. Marrow film. Marked dyserythropoiesis

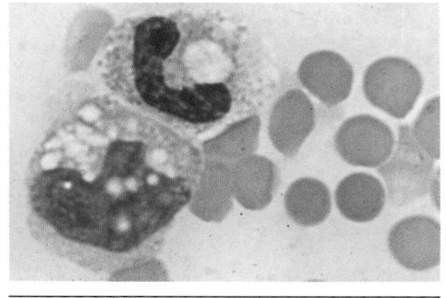

PLATE II-7   Clostridium septicemia. Erythrophagocytosis by a macrophage and neutrophil. Microspherocytes and profound decrease in red cells

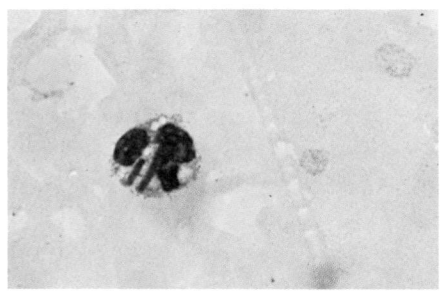

PLATE II-8   Clostridial septicemia. *Clostridium* bacilli in a neutrophil

PLATE III
RED CELL MORPHOLOGY

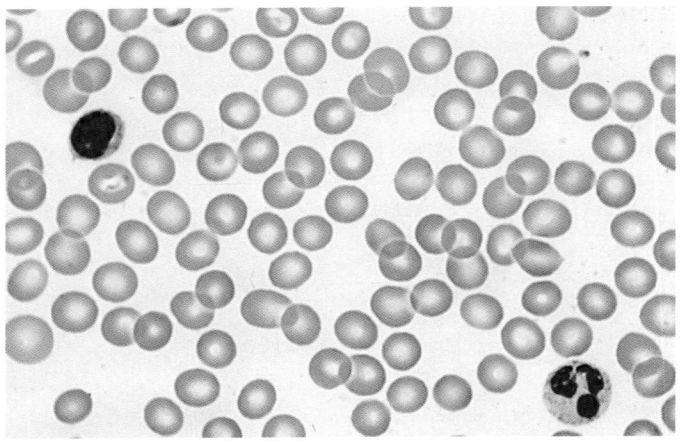

PLATE III-1 Normal blood film

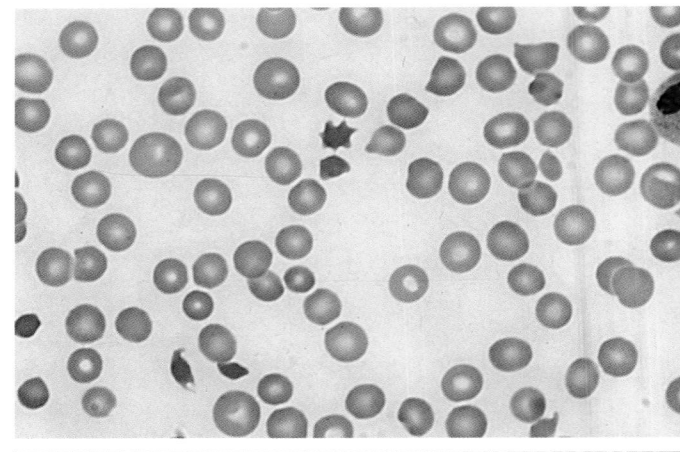

PLATE III-2 Fragmented red cells: Disseminated intravascular coagulation

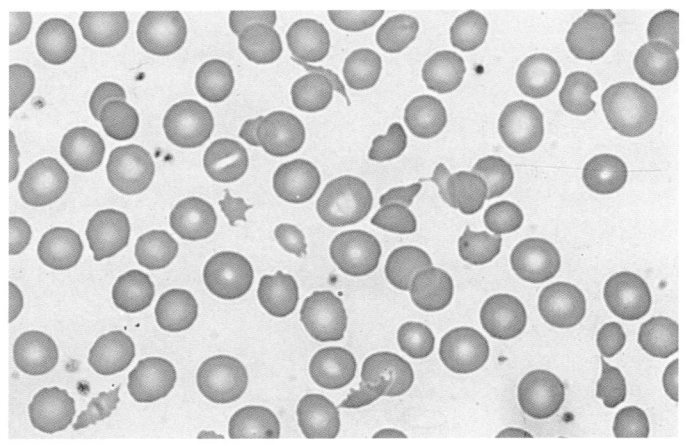

PLATE III-3 Fragmented red cells: Heart valve hemolysis

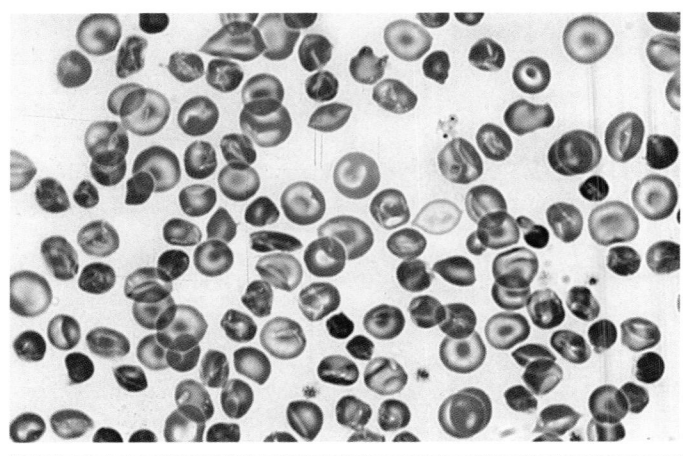

PLATE III-4 Target cells: Hemoglobin C disease

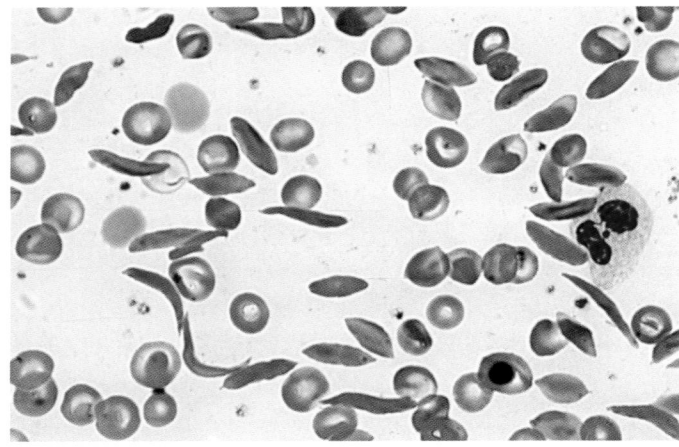

PLATE III-5 Sickle cells: Homozygous sickle cell disease

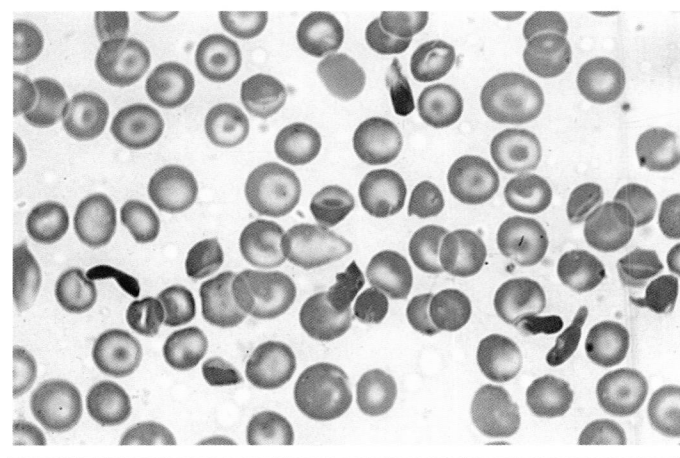

PLATE III-6 Target cells and sickle cells: Hemoglobin SC disease

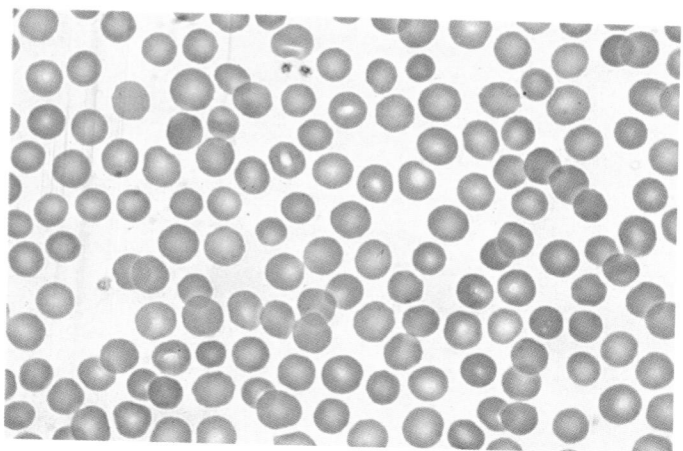

PLATE III-7 Spherocytes: Hereditary spherocytosis

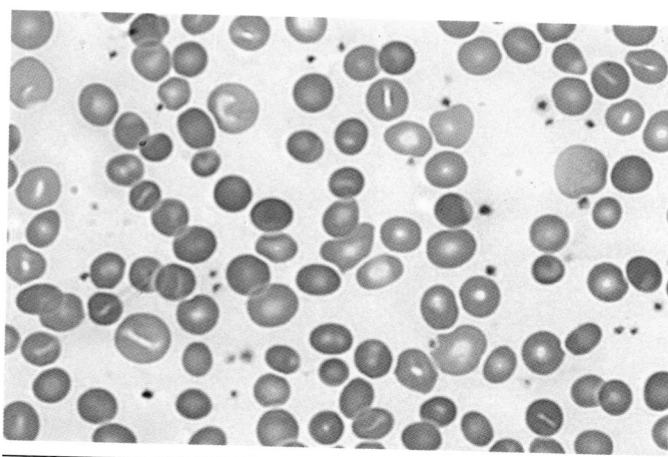

PLATE III-8 Spherocytes: Autoimmune hemolytic anemia

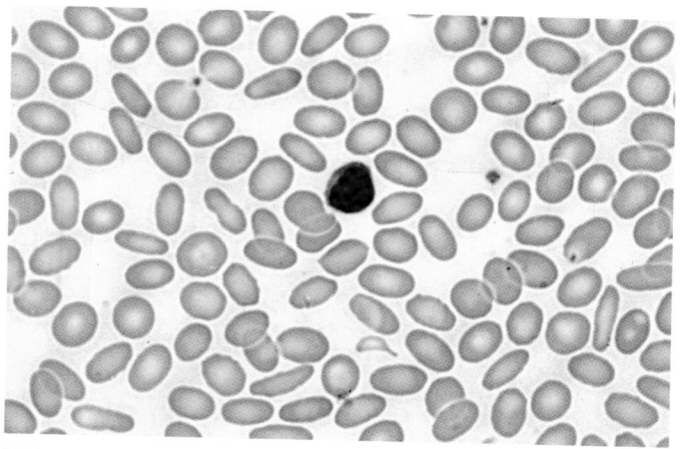

PLATE III-9 Elliptocytosis

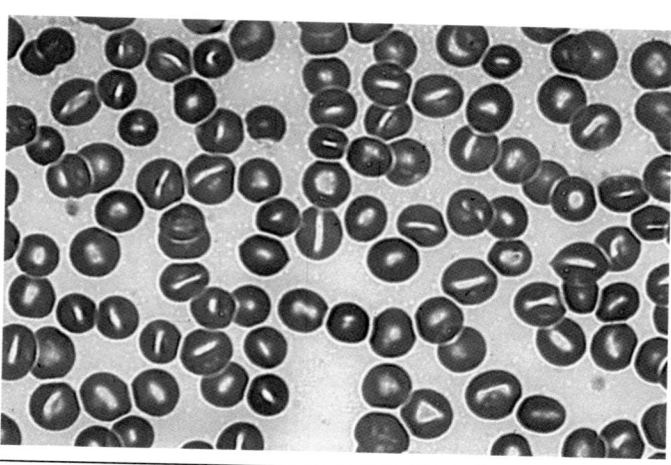

PLATE III-10 Stomatocytosis

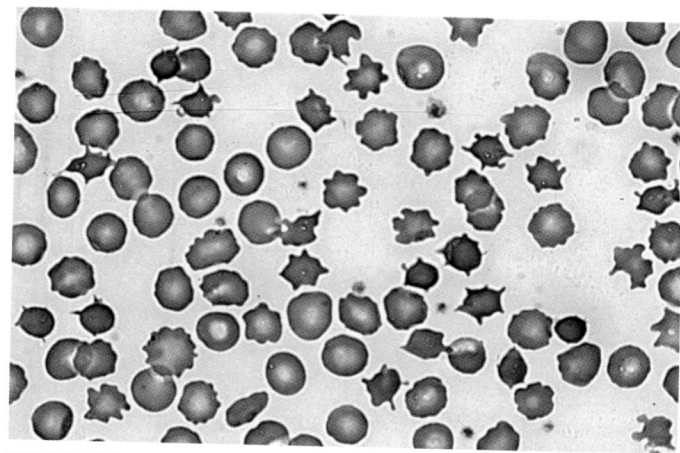

PLATE III-11 Acanthocytosis

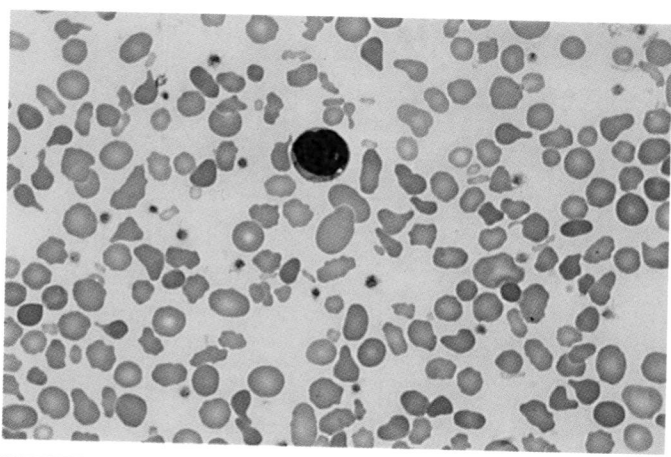

PLATE III-12 Poikilocytes: Hereditary Pyropoikilocytosis

(III-1 through III-12 are blood films)

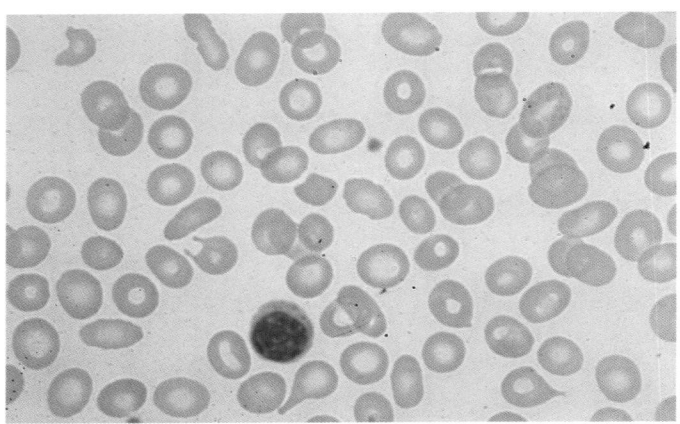

PLATE IV-1   Thalassemia minor. Mild hypochromia, poikilocytosis, and stippled red cell

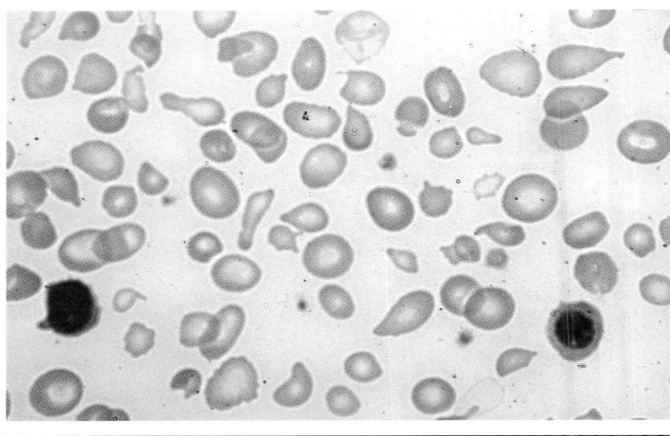

PLATE IV-2   Thalassemia major. Severe poikilocytosis, mild hypochromia, nucleated red cell

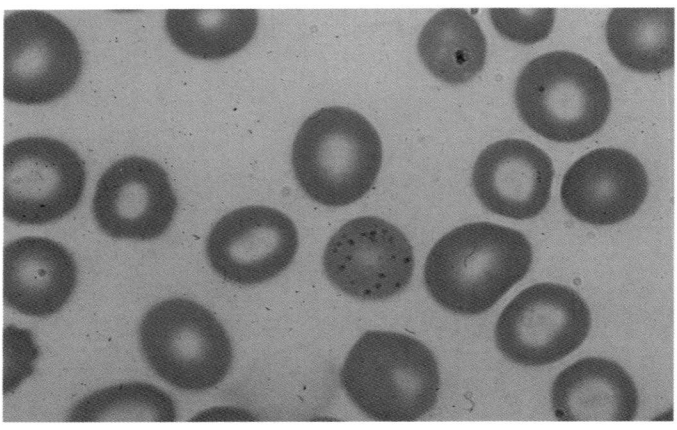

PLATE IV-3   Lead poisoning. Mild hypochromia. Coarsely stippled red cell

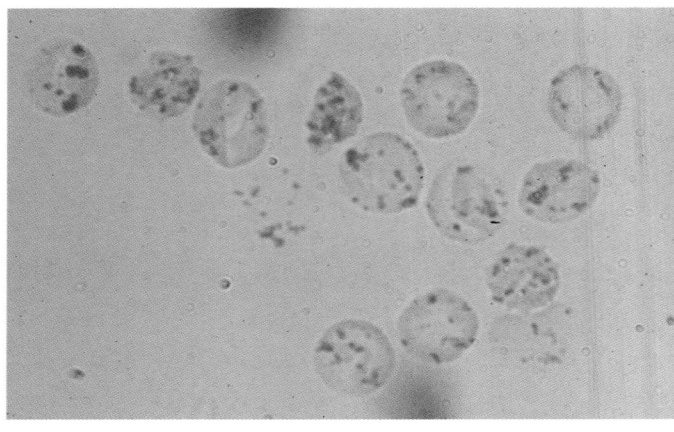

PLATE IV-4   Heinz bodies. Blood mixed with hypotonic solution of crystal violet. Precipitates of denatured hemoglobin within the cells

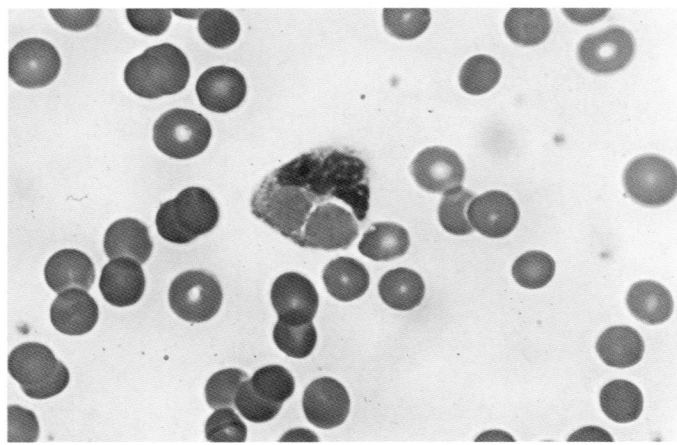

PLATE IV-5   Severe autoimmune hemolytic anemia. Scant red cells on film, frequent microspherocytes, erythrophagocytosis by blood monocyte

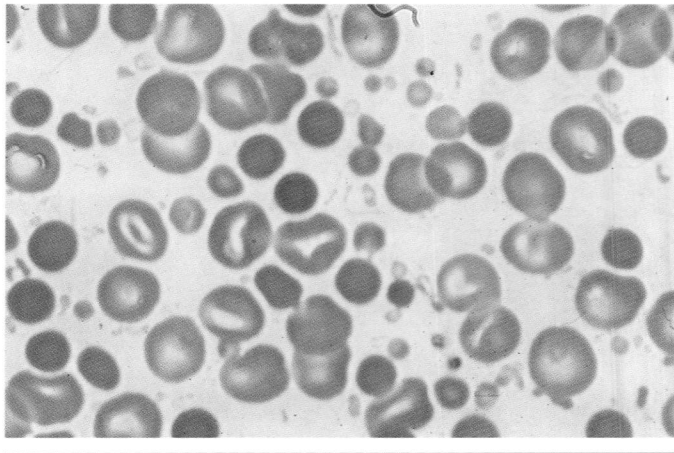

PLATE IV-6   Extensive third degree burns. Spherocytosis, including extremely small spherical "cells"

P L A T E   V
NORMAL ERYTHROPOIESIS

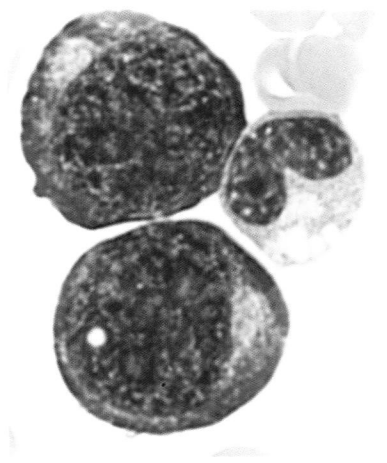

PLATE V-1 Proerythroblasts

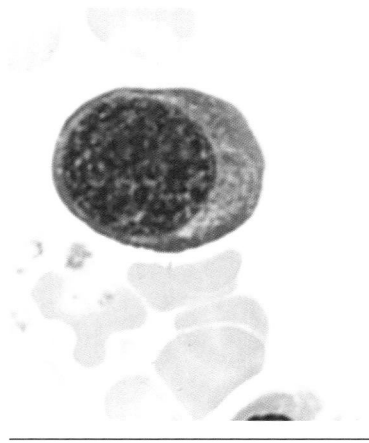

PLATE V-2 Basophilic erythroblasts

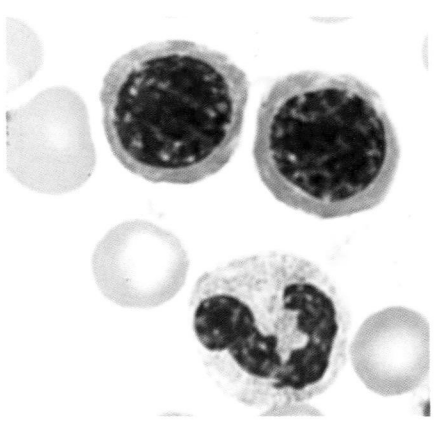

PLATE V-3 Polychromatophilic erythroblasts

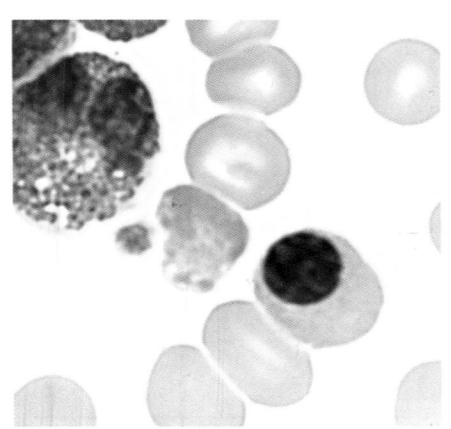

PLATE V-4 Orthochromatic erythroblast

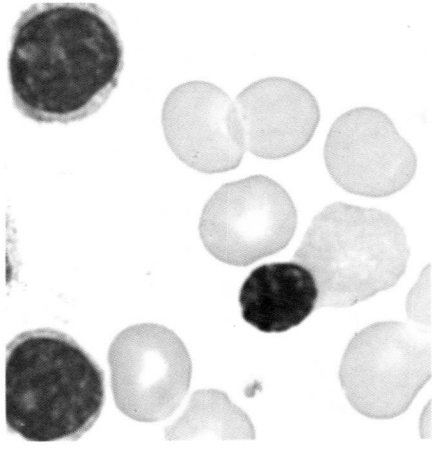

PLATE V-5 Enucleation of orthochromatic erythroblast

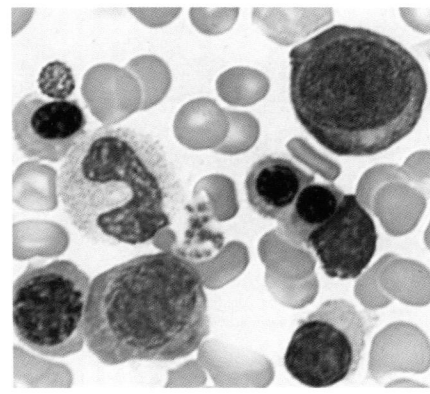

PLATE V-7 Proerythroblast, basophilic erythroblast, polychromatophilic erythroblast, orthochromatic erythroblasts (also, note small plasma cell)

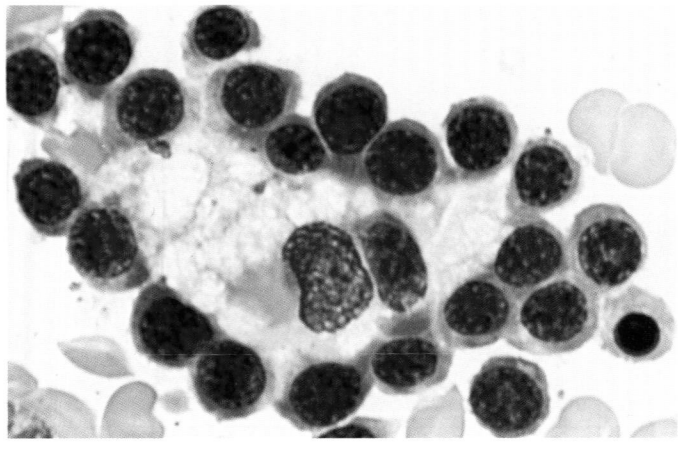

PLATE V-6 Erythroid islet: Central macrophage with surrounding erythroblasts

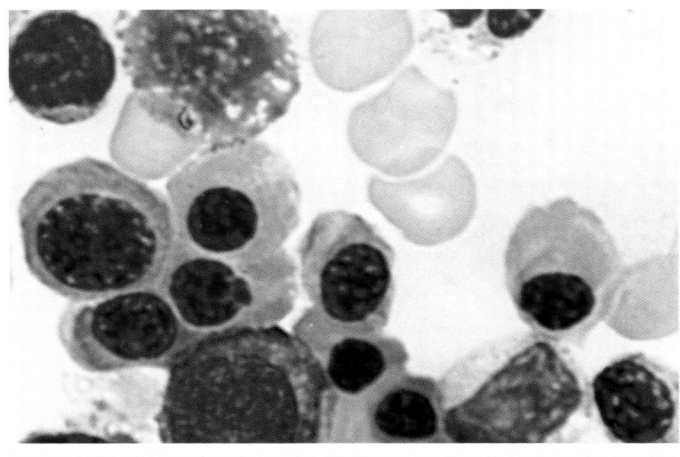

PLATE V-8 Basophilic, polychromatophilic, and orthochromatic erythroblasts

(V-1 through V-8 are marrow cells)

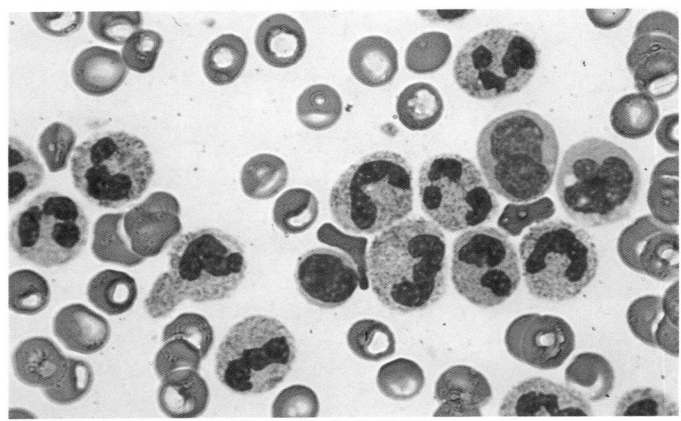

PLATE VIII-1   Extreme neutrophilia (leukemoid reaction)

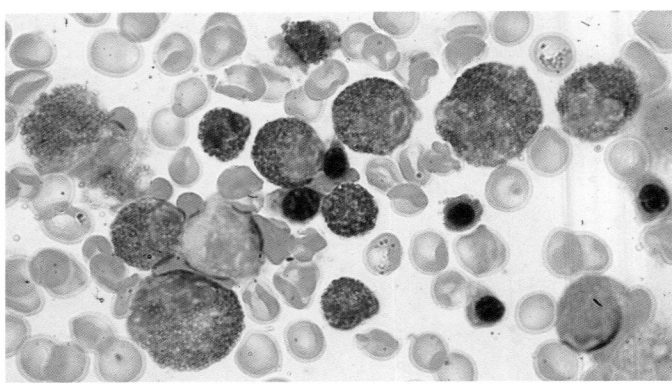

PLATE VIII-2   Hypereosinophilic syndrome. Intense marrow eosinophilia. Eosinophilic myelocytes and segmented forms

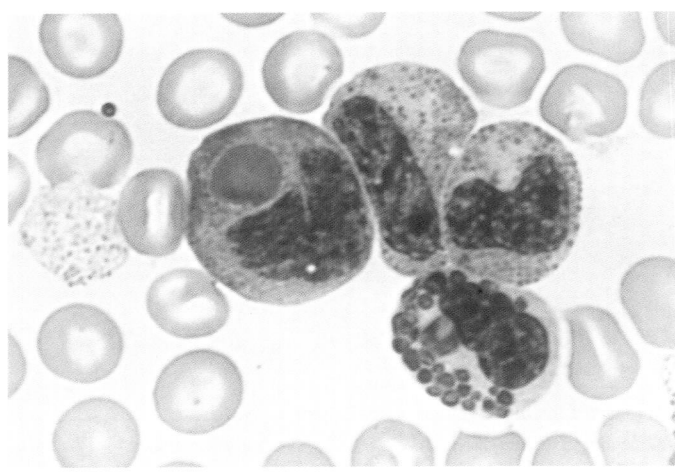

PLATE VIII-3   Chédiak-Higashi disease. Note monstrous granule in monocyte and giant granules in band neutrophil

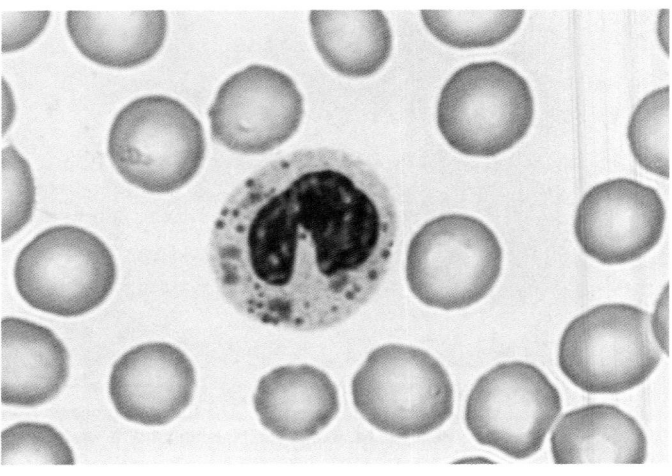

PLATE VIII-4   Chédiak-Higashi disease. Note giant granules in neutrophil

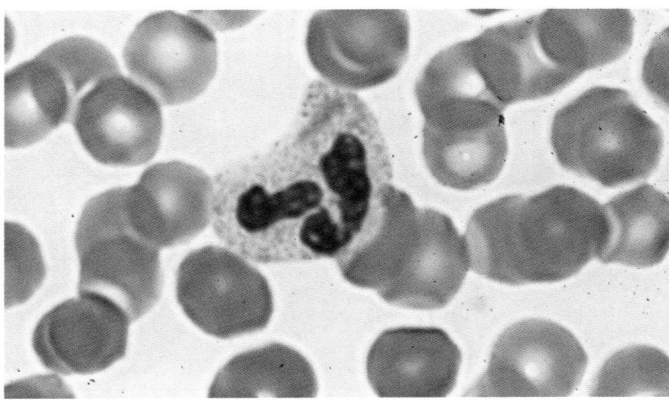

PLATE VIII-5   May-Hegglin anomaly. Note violaceous inclusion Döhle body-like in neutrophil

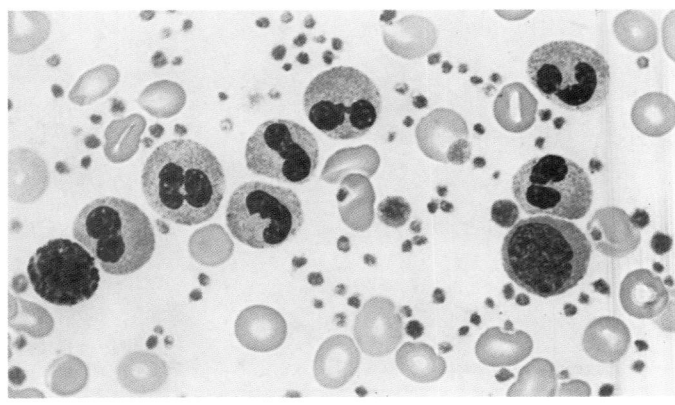

PLATE VIII-6   Heterozygote for the Pelger-Huët anomaly of leukocyte nuclei. Bilobed (pince-nez shape) nuclei (buffy coat)

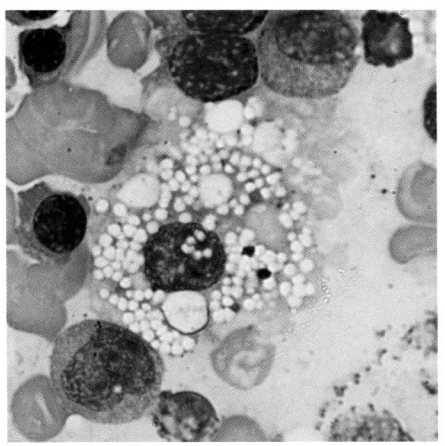

PLATE IX-1   Active macrophage

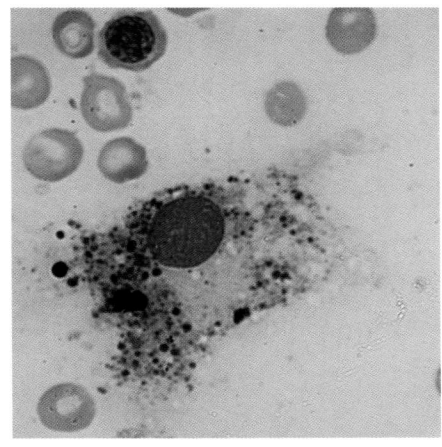

PLATE IX-2   Macrophage with iron particles, Wright stain

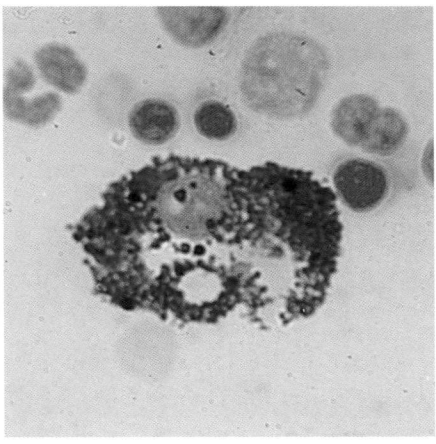

PLATE IX-3   Macrophage with iron particles, Prussian blue stain

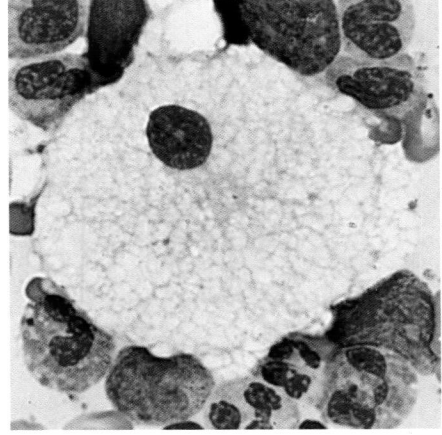

PLATE IX-4   Niemann-Pick cell

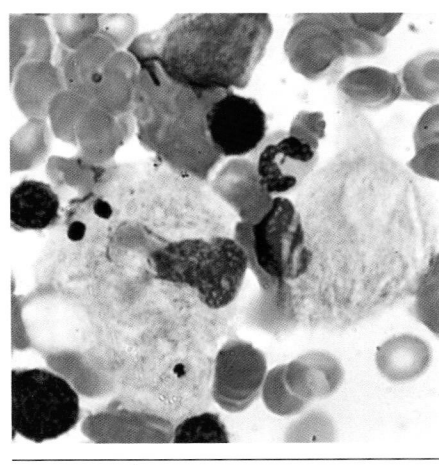

PLATE IX-5   Gaucher cells in the adult form of the disease

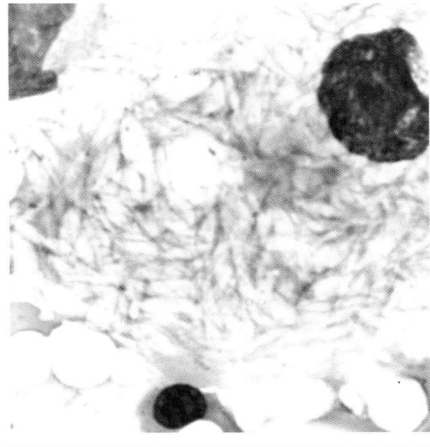

PLATE IX-6   Pseudo-Gaucher cell in a patient with chronic myelogenous leukemia

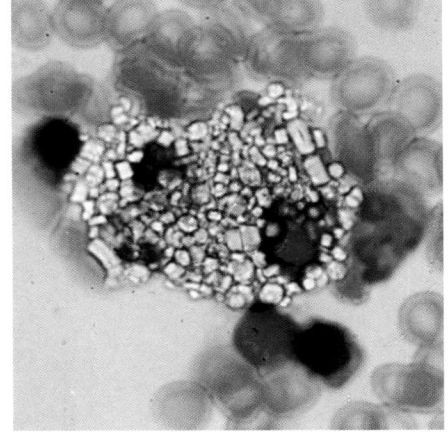

PLATE IX-7   Macrophage engorged with cystine crystals

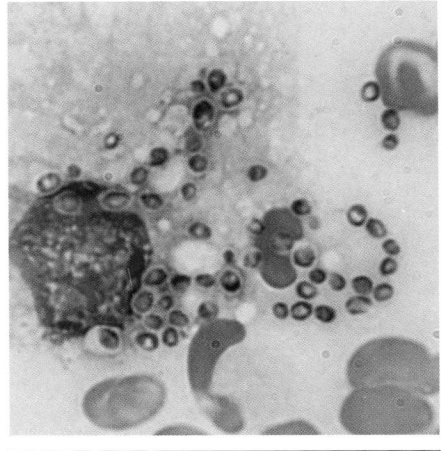

PLATE IX-8   Macrophage containing *Histoplasma capsulatum*

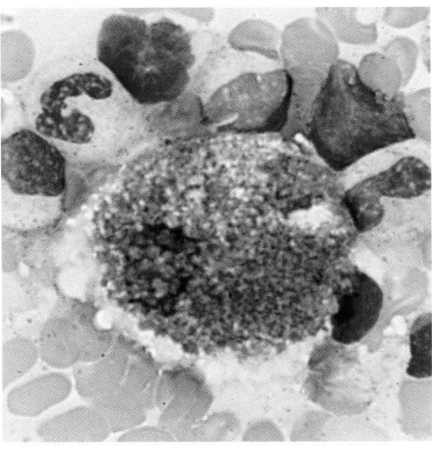

PLATE IX-9   Macrophage in sea blue histiocytosis

(IX-1 through IX-9 are marrow macrophages)

NORMAL NEUTROPHILOPOIESIS

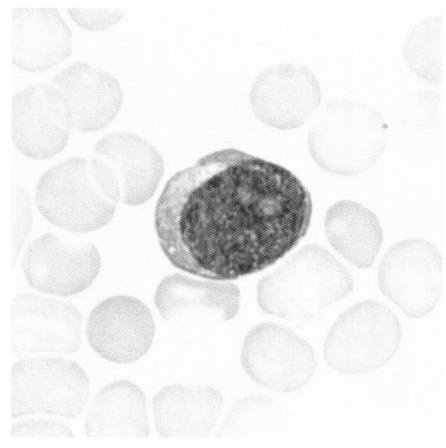

PLATE X-1 Myeloblast

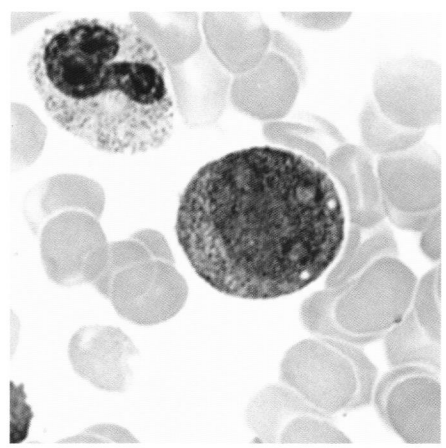

PLATE X-2 Promyelocyte

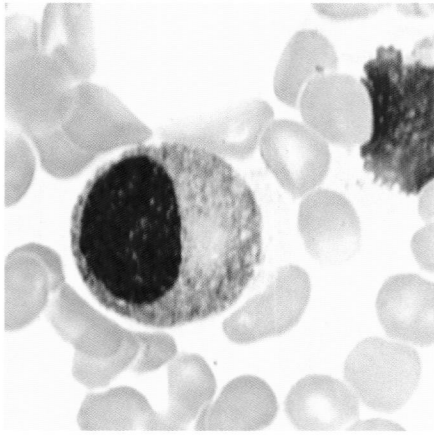

PLATE X-3 Early neutrophilic myelocyte

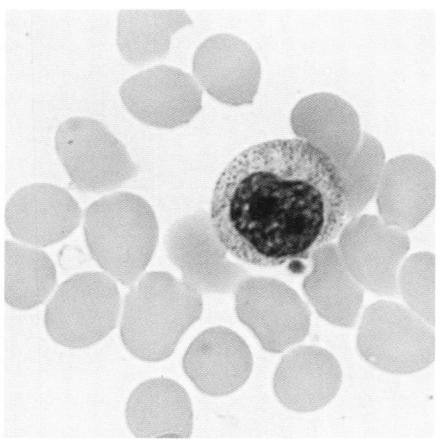

PLATE X-4 Late neutrophilic myelocyte

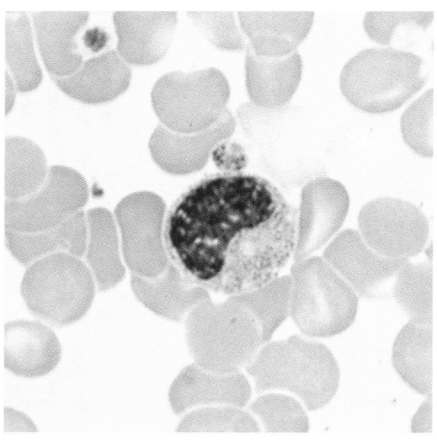

PLATE X-5 Neutrophilic metamyelocyte

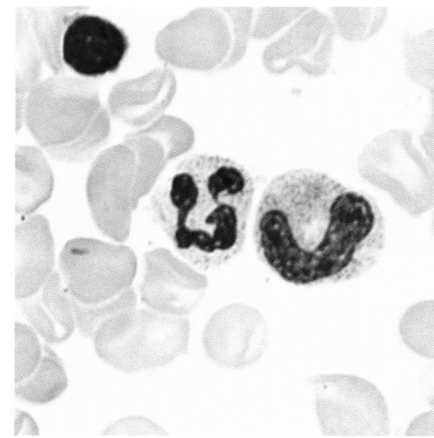

PLATE X-6 Band and segmented neutrophils

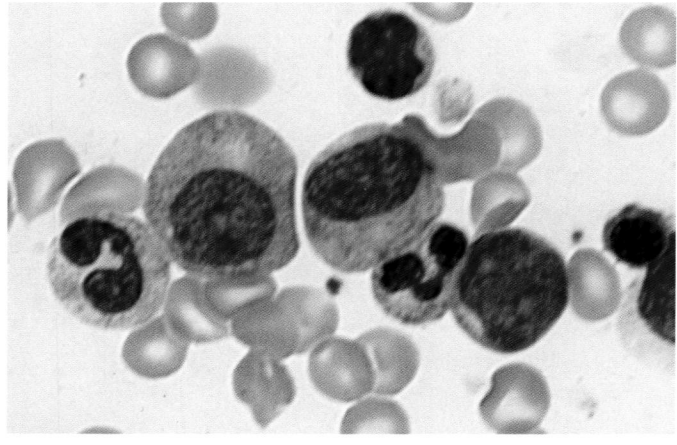

PLATE X-7 Myeloblast, early myelocytes, band and segmented neutrophils

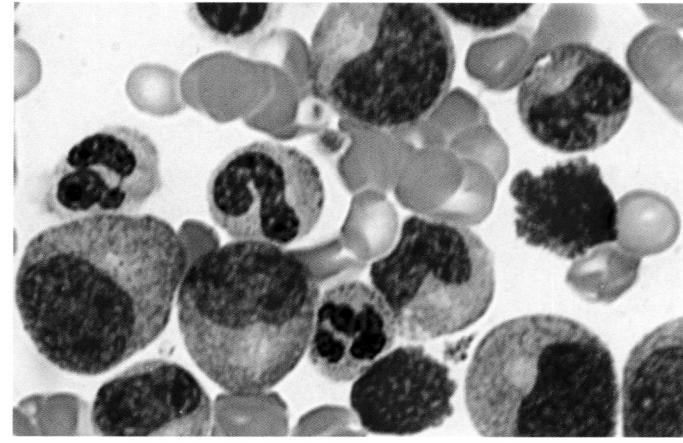

PLATE X-8 Promyelocyte, early myelocytes, metamyelocytes, band and segmented neutrophils

(X-1 through X-8 are marrow films)

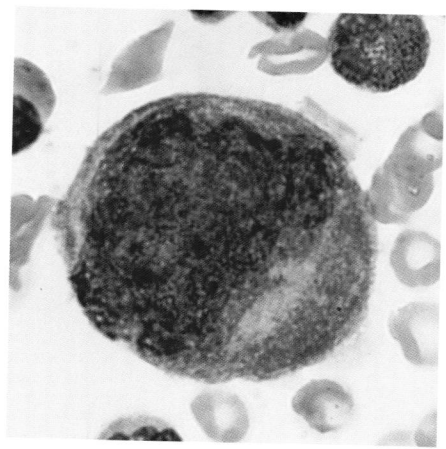

PLATE XI-1 Immature megakaryocyte

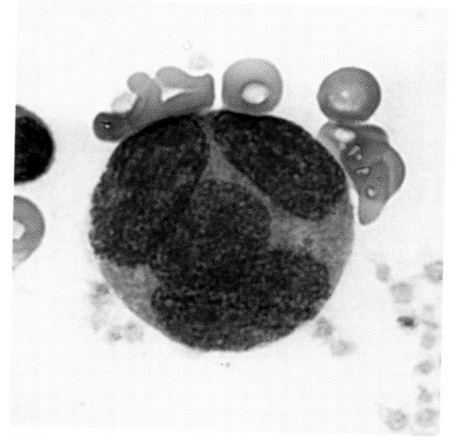

PLATE XI-2 Immature megakaryocyte

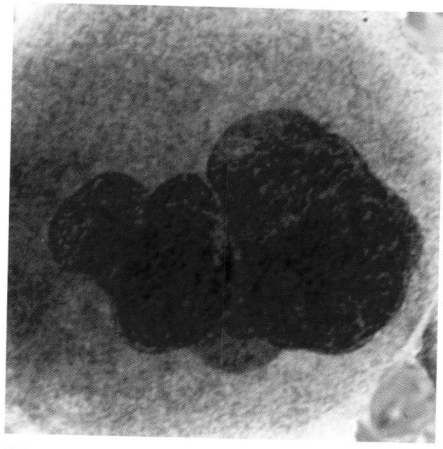

PLATE XI-3 Mature megakaryocyte

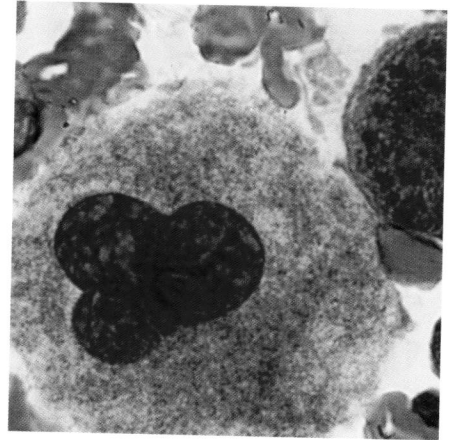

PLATE XI-4 Mature megakaryocyte

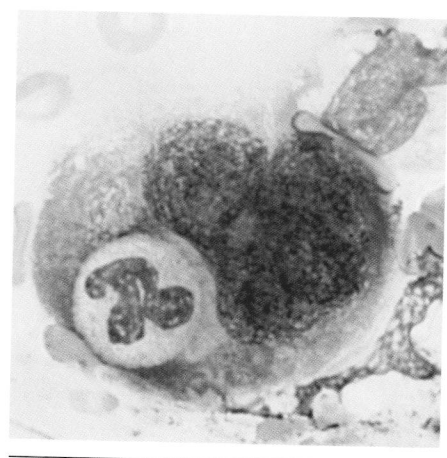

PLATE XI-5 Emperipolesis, the migration of a neutrophil into the canalicular system of megakaryocyte cytoplasm

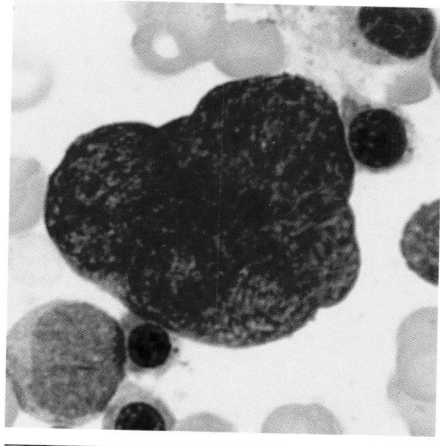

PLATE XI-6 The residue of a megakaryocyte nucleus

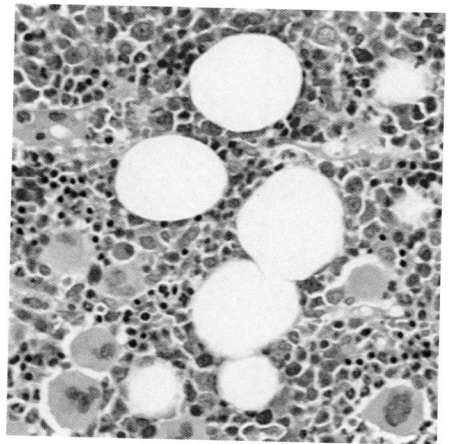

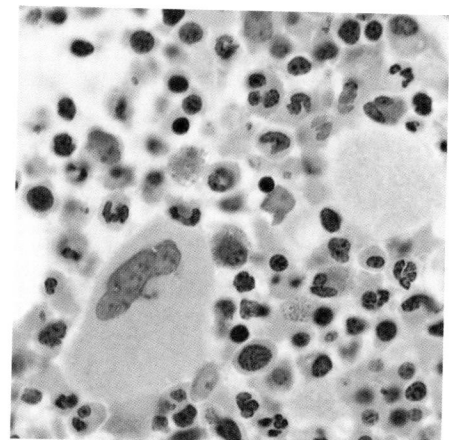

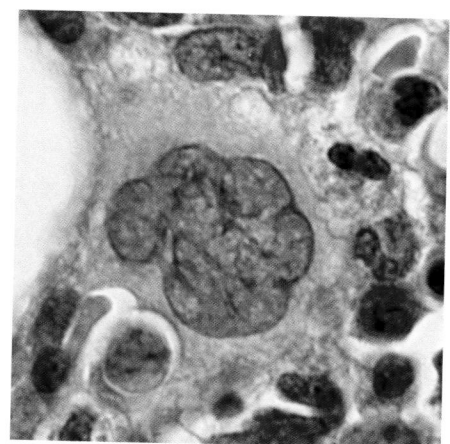

PLATE XI-7, 8, 9 Marrow biopsies demonstrating megakaryocytes

(XI-1 through XI-6 are marrow films)

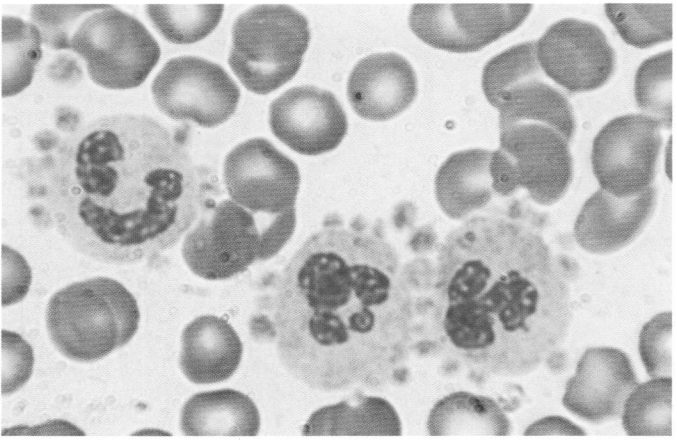

PLATE XII-1 Platelet satellitism

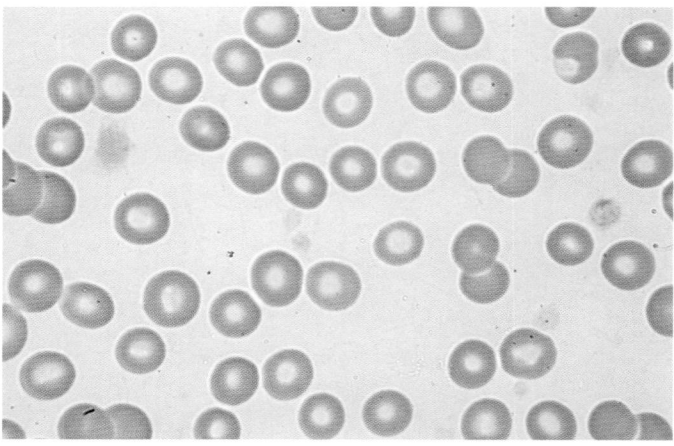

PLATE XII-2 Gray platelet syndrome

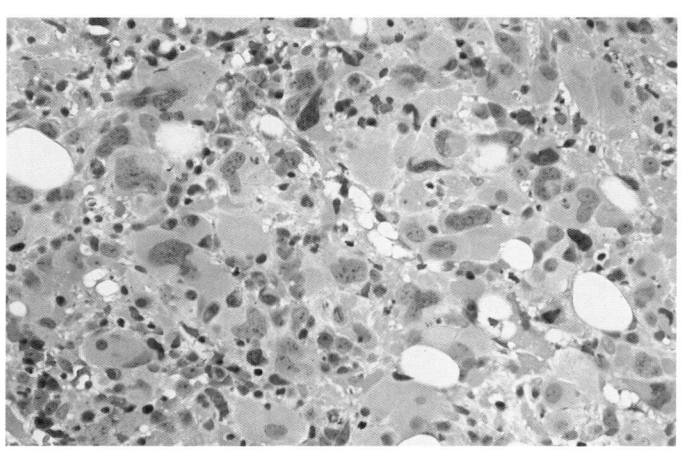

PLATE XII-3 Acute megakaryocytic leukemia. Marrow section

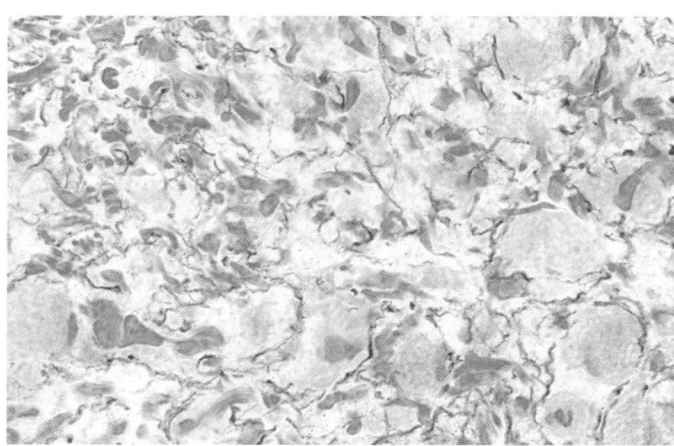

PLATE XII-4 Acute megakaryocytic leukemia. Marrow section. Silver stain demonstrating increased reticulin fibers.

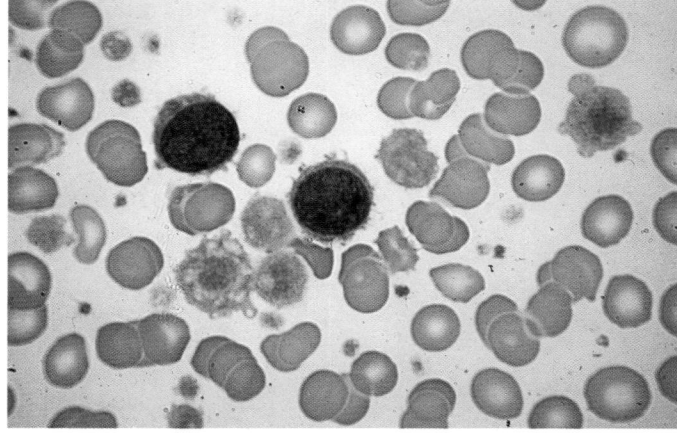

PLATE XII-5 Idiopathic myelofibrosis (agnogenic myeloid metaplasia) and probable megakaryocytic leukemic conversion. Dwarfed megakaryocyte and enormous platelets (megakaryocytic cytoplasmic fragments)

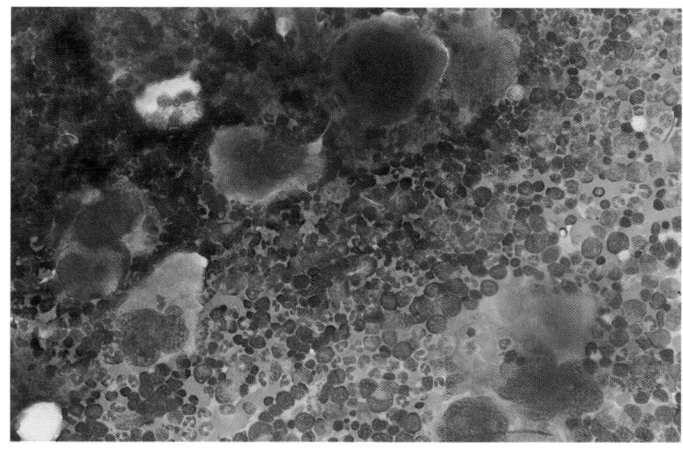

PLATE XII-6 Essential thrombocythemia. Marrow film. Marked increase in megakaryocytes

P L A T E   X I I I
NORMAL AND ABNORMAL PLATELETS

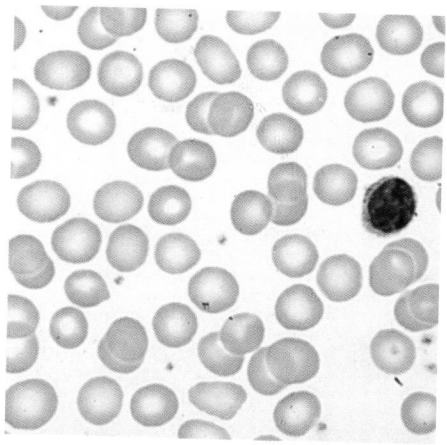

PLATE XIII-1   Normal platelets

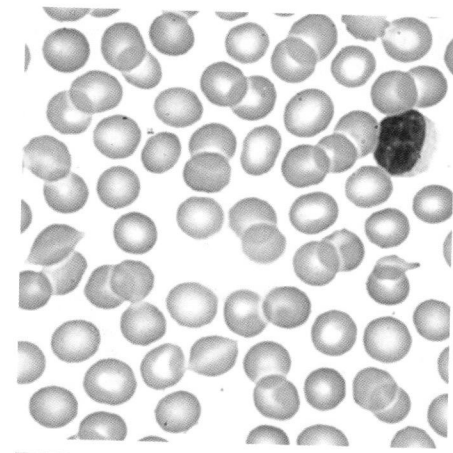

PLATE XIII-2   Thrombocytopenia

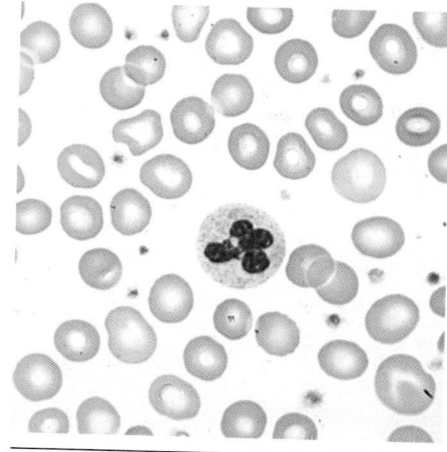

PLATE XIII-3   Reactive thrombocytosis

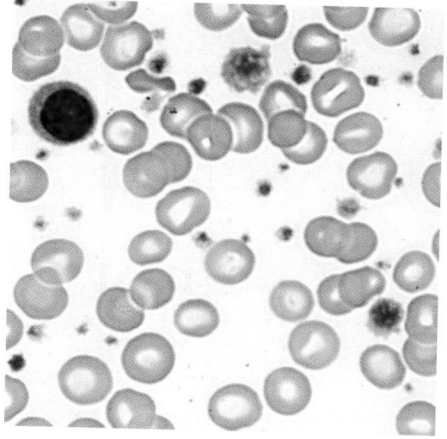

PLATE XIII-4   Thrombocythemia: Increased number of platelets and large abnormal platelets

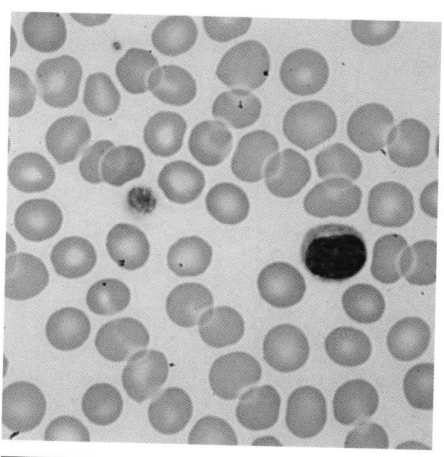

PLATE XIII-5   Giant platelets (megathrombocyte)

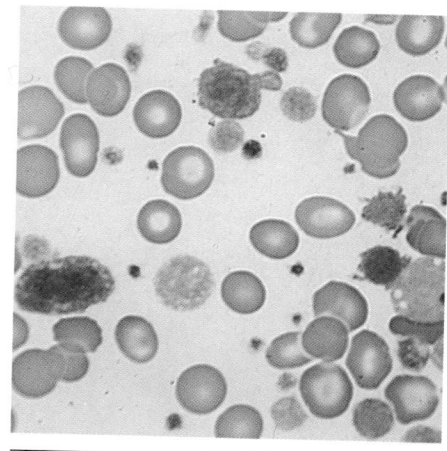

PLATE XIII-6   Giant platelets characteristic of myeloproliferative diseases: All of the blue-staining elements in the film are platelets

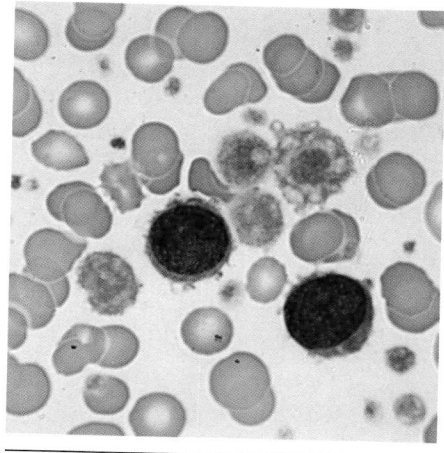

PLATE XIII-7   Dwarf megakaryocytes and giant platelets

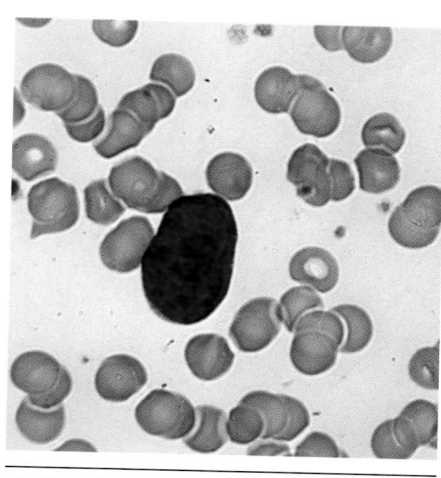

PLATE XIII-8   Megakaryocyte nucleus

(XIII-1 through XIII-8 are blood films)

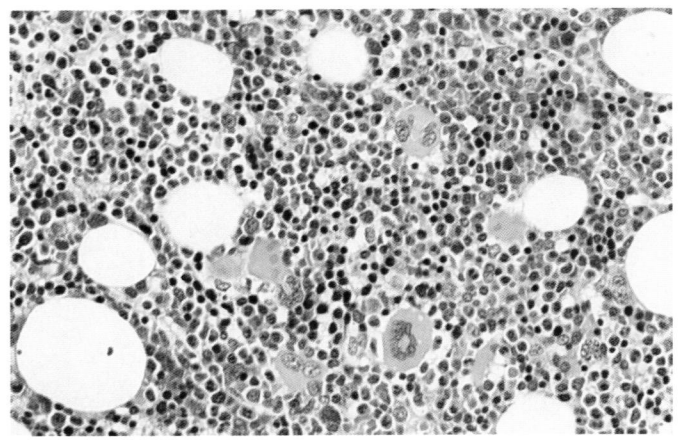

PLATE XIV-1 Normal

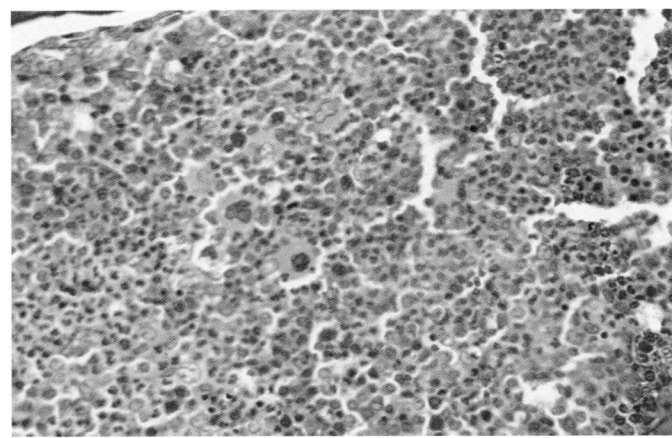

PLATE XIV-2 Hypercellular

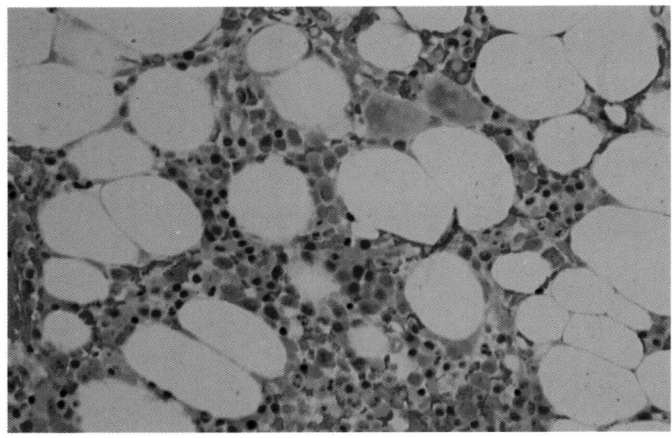

PLATE XIV-3 Hypocellular

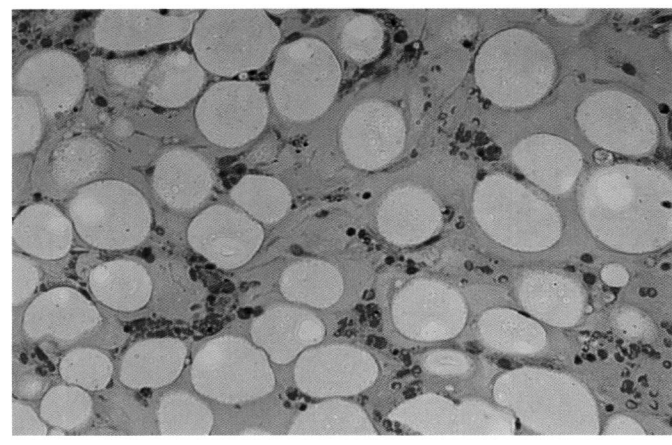

PLATE XIV-4 Aplasia

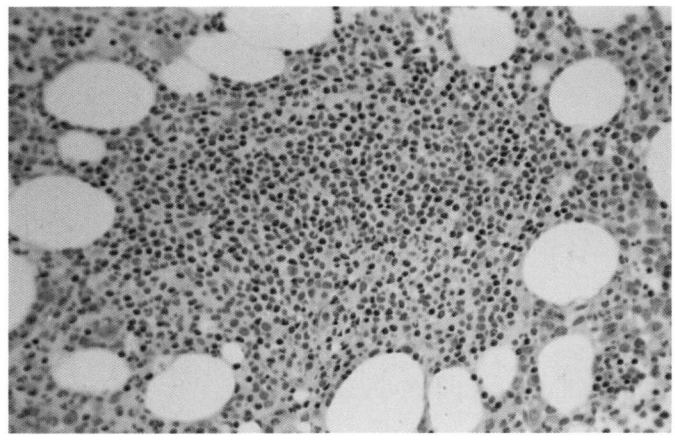

PLATE XIV-5 Lymphoid aggregate: Uncertain significance

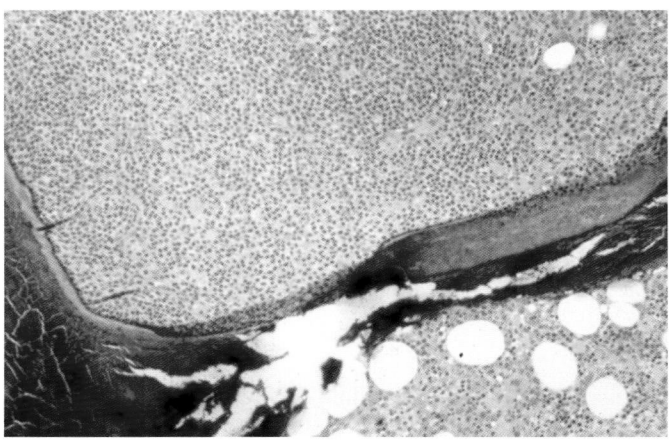

PLATE XIV-6 Lymphoma in marrow: Note paratrabecular location

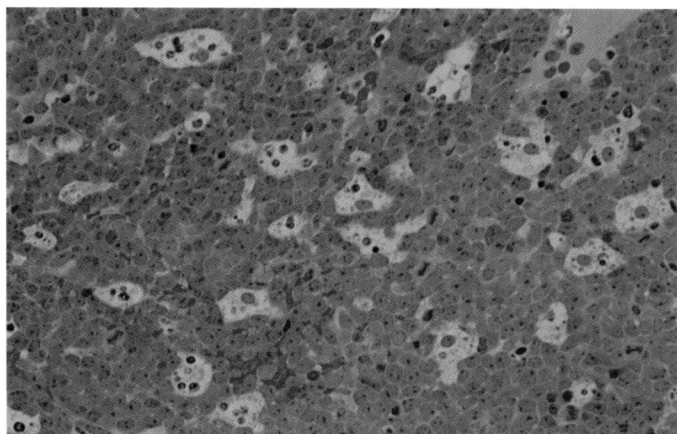

PLATE XIV-7 Burkitt lymphoma: Note the starry sky appearance as a result of the interspersed macrophages

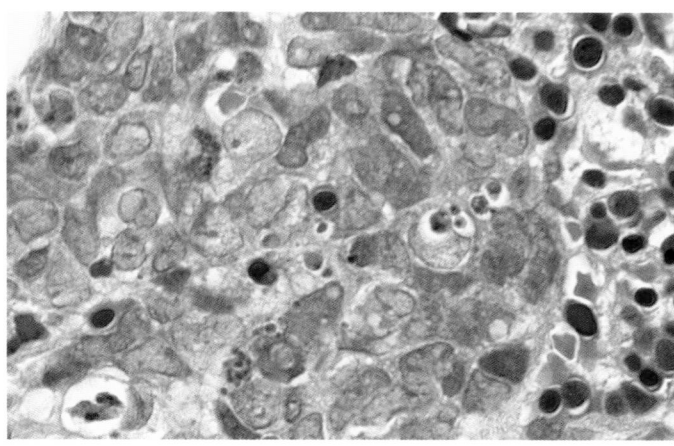

PLATE XIV-8 Metastatic carcinoma

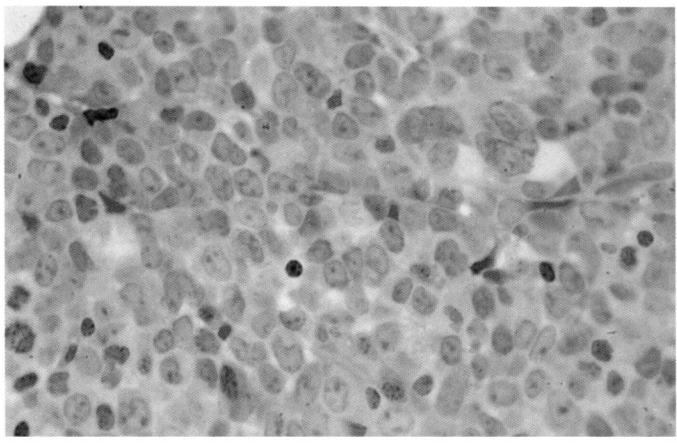

PLATE XIV-9 Acute myelogenous leukemia

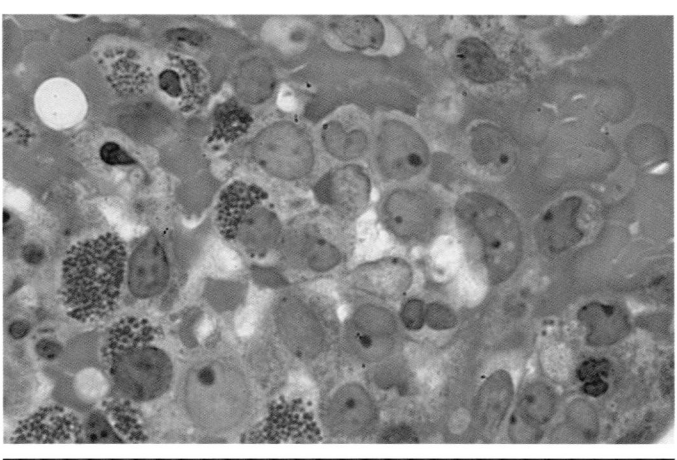

PLATE XIV-10 Acute myelogenous leukemia with marked increase in eosinophils

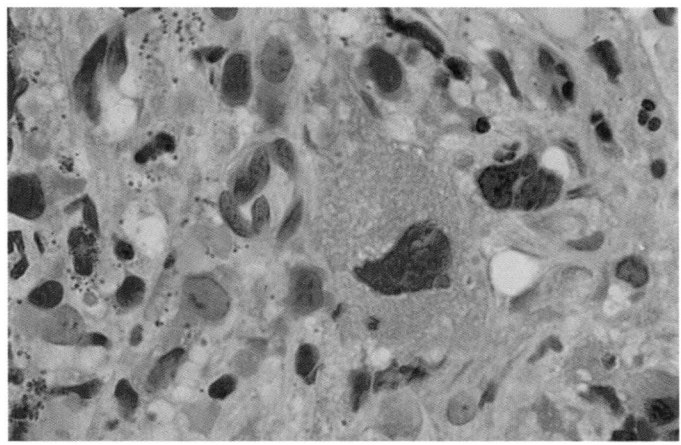

PLATE XIV-11 Myelofibrosis: Increased numbers of megakaryocytes and decreased marrow cellularity

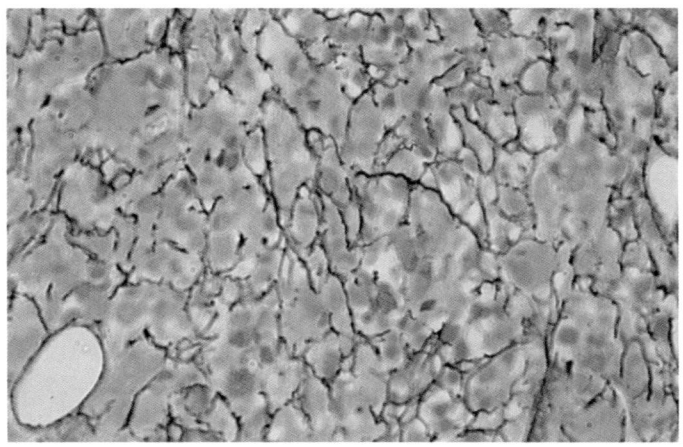

PLATE XIV-12 Myelofibrosis: Silver stain showing increased reticulin

(XIV-1 through XIV-12 are marrow biopsies)

PLATE XV
NON-HEMATOPOIETIC CELLS IN MARROW

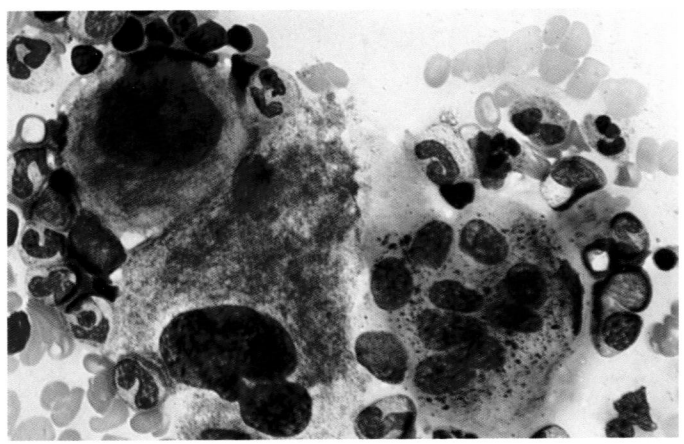

PLATE XV-1 Osteoclast

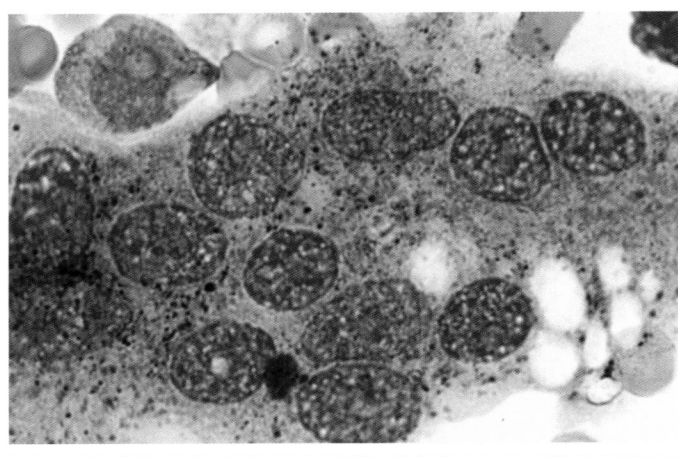

PLATE XV-2 Osteoclast

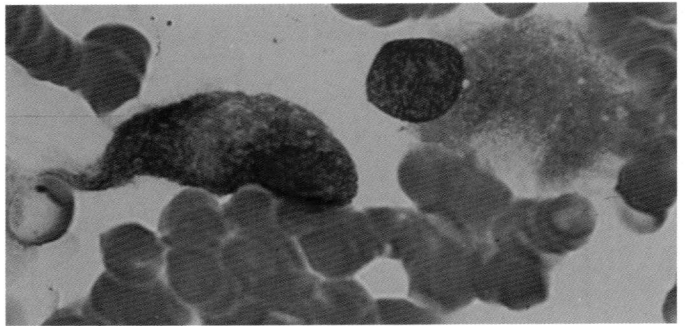

PLATE XV-3 Osteoblasts

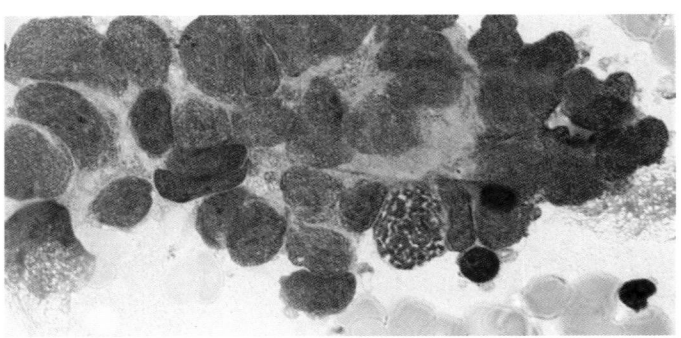

PLATE XV-4 Aggregate of metastatic lung carcinoma cells

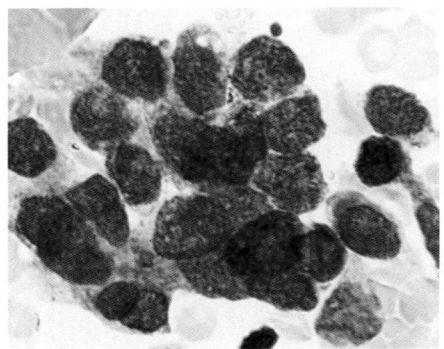

PLATE XV-5 Aggregate of metastatic prostate carcinoma cells

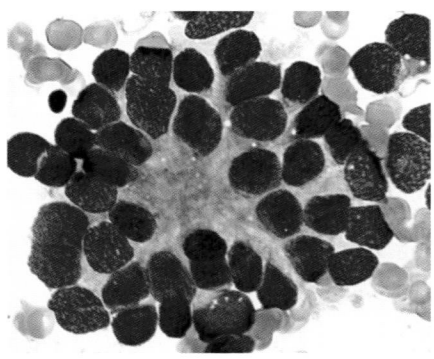

PLATE XV-6 Metastatic neuroblastoma cells: Note the characteristic rosette appearance

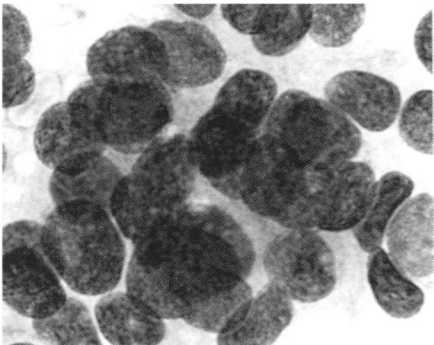

PLATE XV-7 Metastatic breast carcinoma cells

(XV-1 through XV-7 are marrow films)

PLATE XVI
ACUTE MYELOGENOUS LEUKEMIA

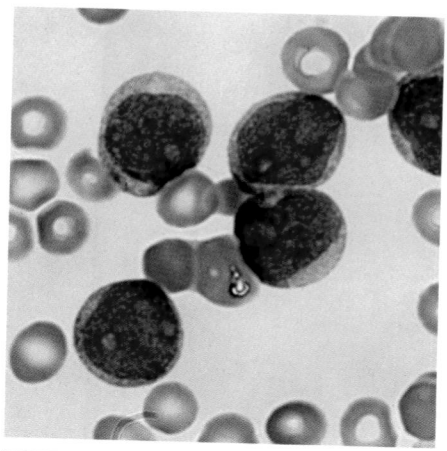

PLATE XVI-1   Leukemic myeloblasts

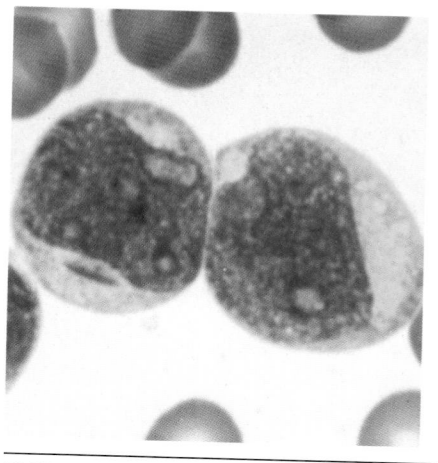

PLATE XVI-2   Leukemic myeloblasts with an Auer rod

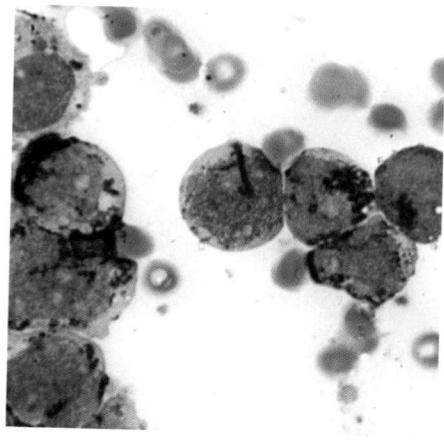

PLATE XVI-3   Leukemic myeloblasts stained with peroxidase: Note the staining of an Auer rod

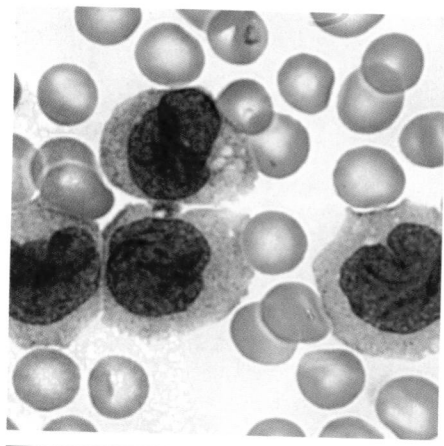

PLATE XVI-4   Leukemic monocytes

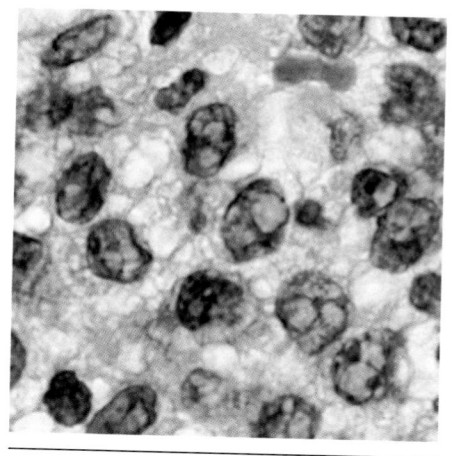

PLATE XVI-5   A skin biopsy showing infiltration of leukemic monocytes

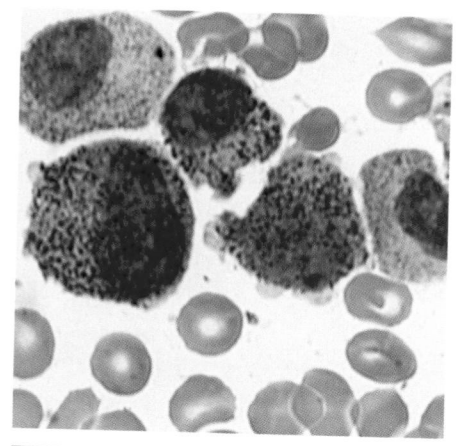

PLATE XVI-6   Leukemic promyelocytes

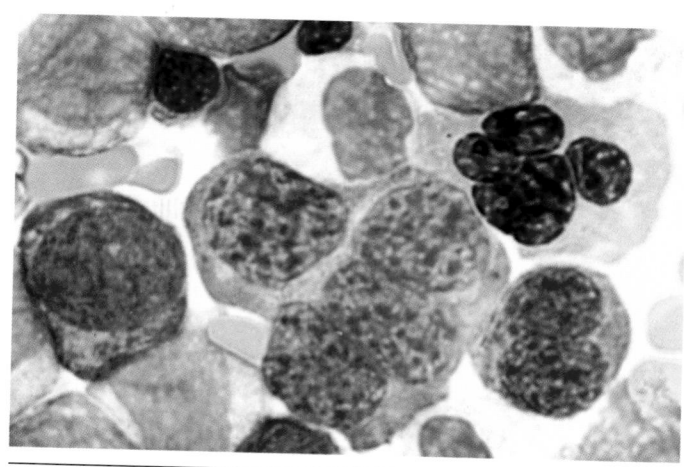

PLATE XVI-7   Erythroleukemia cells

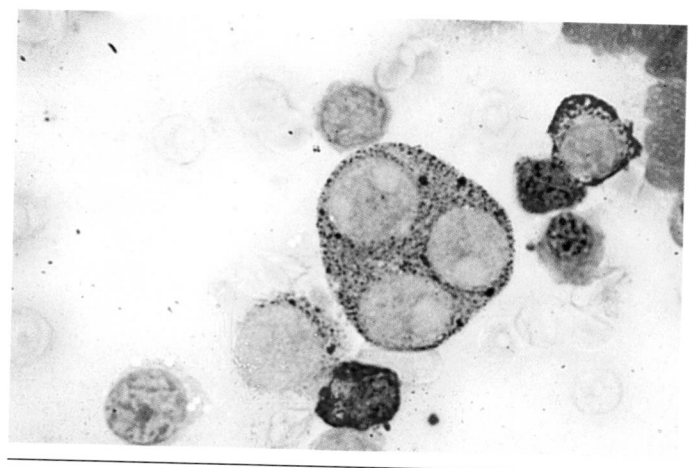

PLATE XVI-8   Erythroleukemia cells stained with periodic acid-Schiff

(XVI-1 through XVI-8 are marrow films)

ACUTE MYELOGENOUS LEUKEMIA

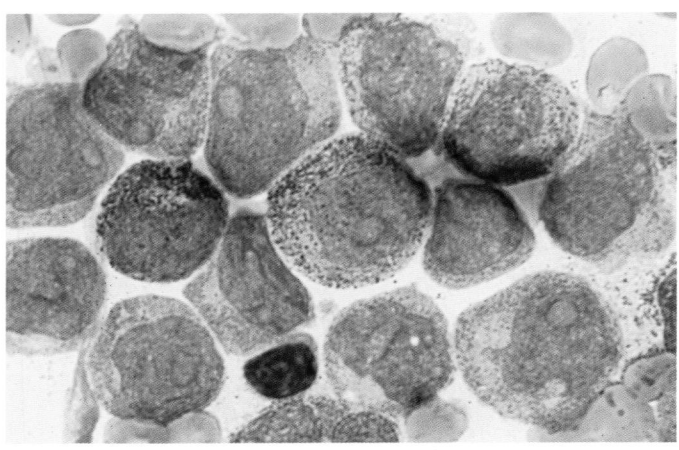

PLATE XVII-1 Acute promyelocytic leukemia. Marrow film. Predominance of promyelocytes, many with large nucleoli

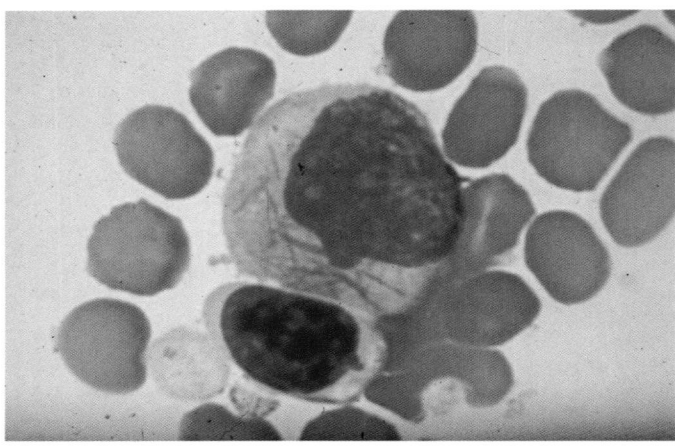

PLATE XVII-2 Acute promyelocytic leukemia. Marrow film. Multiple Auer rods in leukemic cell

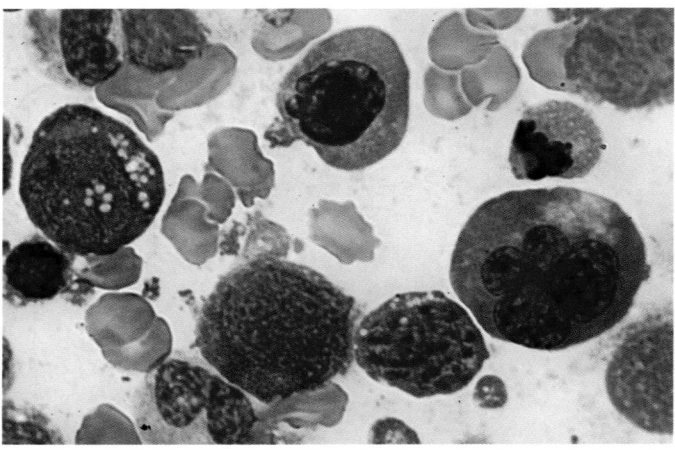

PLATE XVII-3 Acute erythroid leukemia. Marrow film. Large erythroblasts with bizarre nuclear morphology

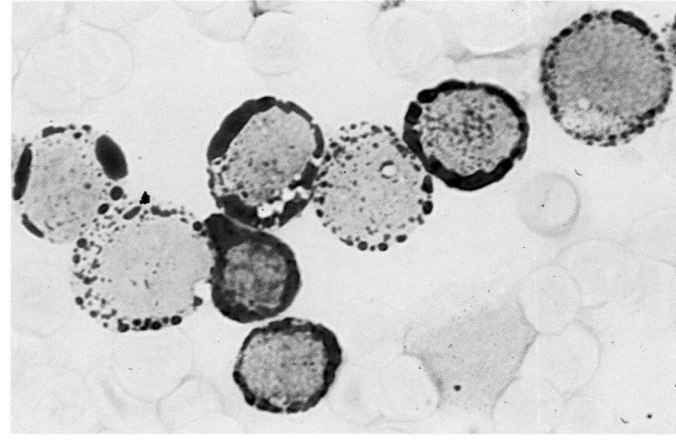

PLATE XVII-4 Acute erythroid leukemia. Marrow film stained with periodic acid Schiff reagent. Intense PAS-positive staining of leukemic erythroblasts

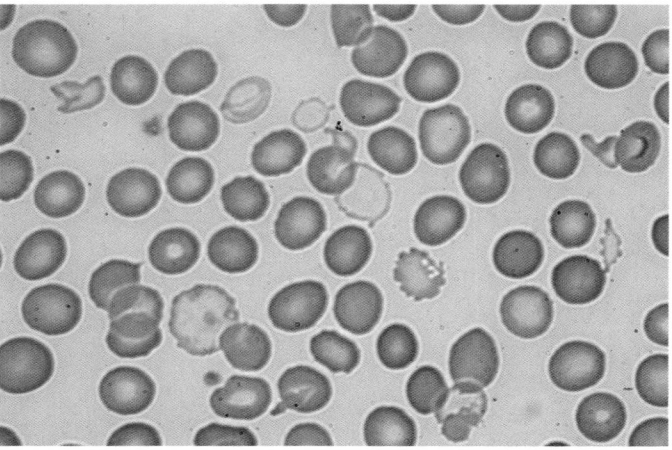

PLATE XVII-5 Acute erythroid leukemia. Blood film. Striking anisochromia and poikilocytosis. Some red cells are so poorly hemoglobinized that they mimic red cell ghosts

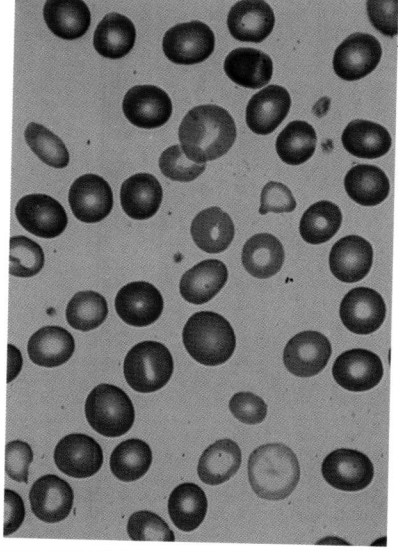

PLATE XVIII-1 Erythrocyte abnormalities: Anisocytosis, poikilocytosis, anisochromia

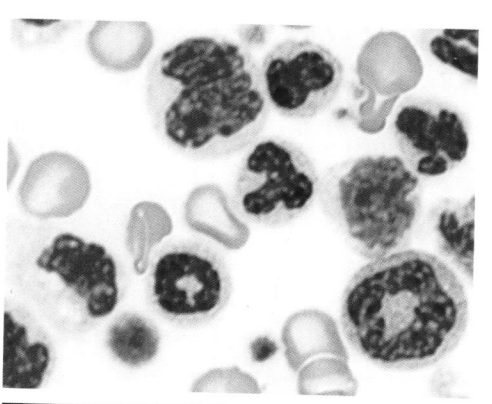

PLATE XVIII-2 Buffy coat showing neutrophil abnormalities including ringed nuclei, hyperdense nuclear pattern, and decreased nuclear segmentation

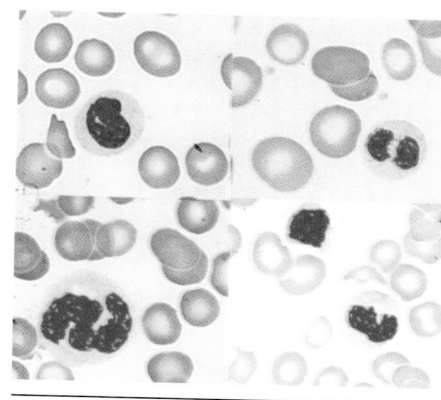

PLATE XVIII-3 Hyposegmented neutrophils, acquired Pelger-Huët abnormality

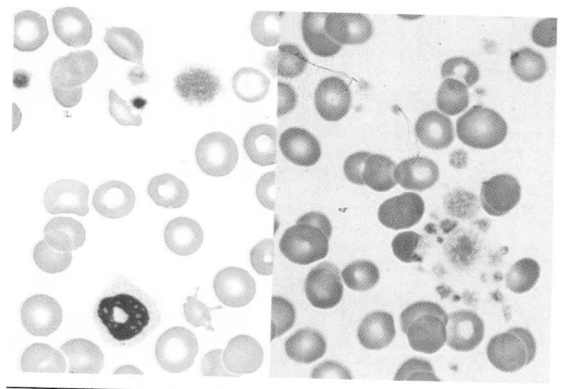

PLATE XVIII-4 Giant platelets, red cell abnormalities, and neutrophil with ringed nucleus

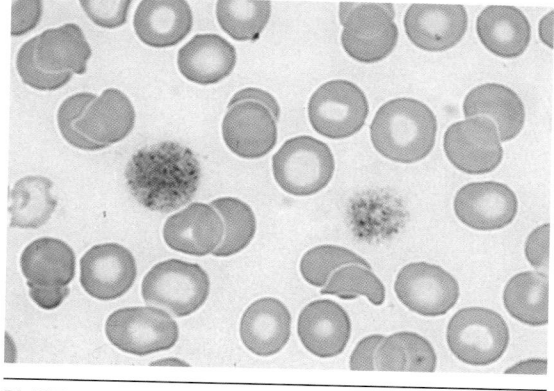

PLATE XVIII-5 Giant platelets

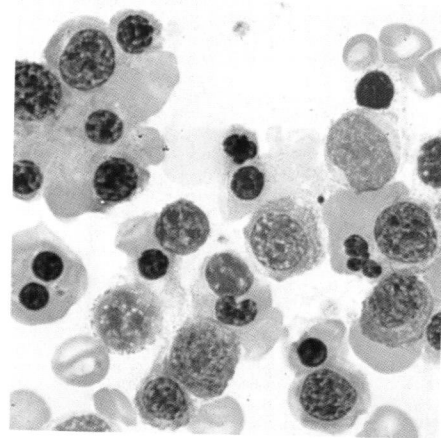

PLATE XVIII-6 Dyserythropoiesis with binucleate and fragmented erythroblastic nuclei, and ineffective erythropoiesis

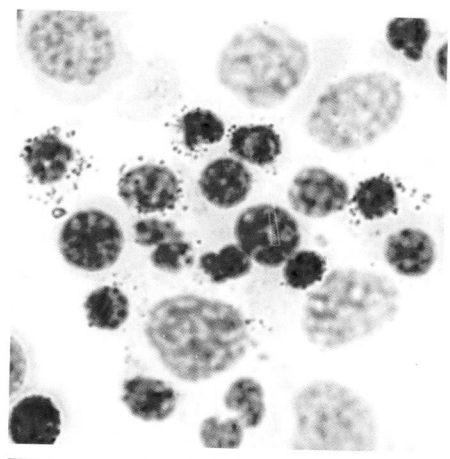

PLATE XVIII-7 Sideroblasts stained with Prussian blue: Increased siderotic granules and circumnuclear rings (ringed sideroblasts)

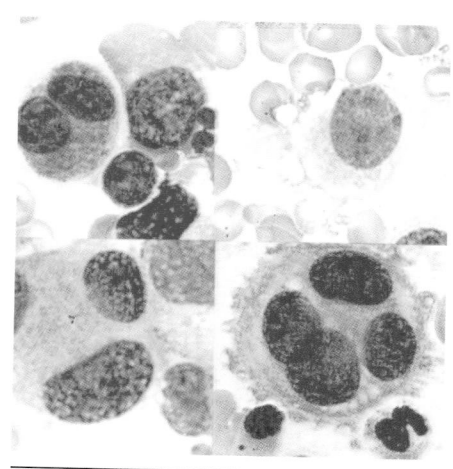

PLATE XVIII-8 Abnormal megakaryocytes

(XVIII-1, XVIII-3 through XVIII-5 are blood films; XVIII-6 through XVIII-8 are marrow films)

CHRONIC MYELOGENOUS LEUKEMIA

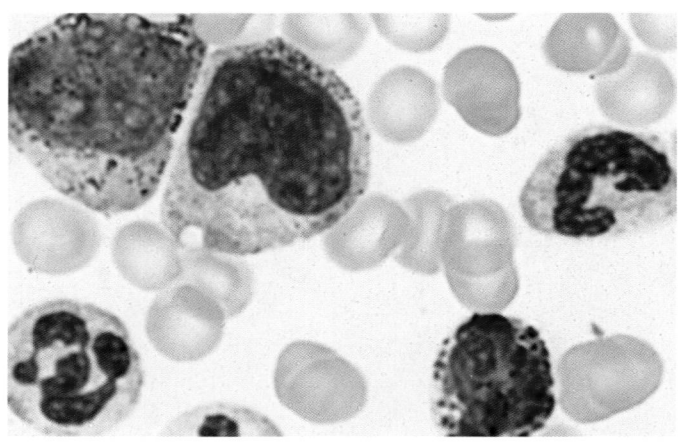

PLATE XIX-1 Myelocytes, neutrophils, and a basophil

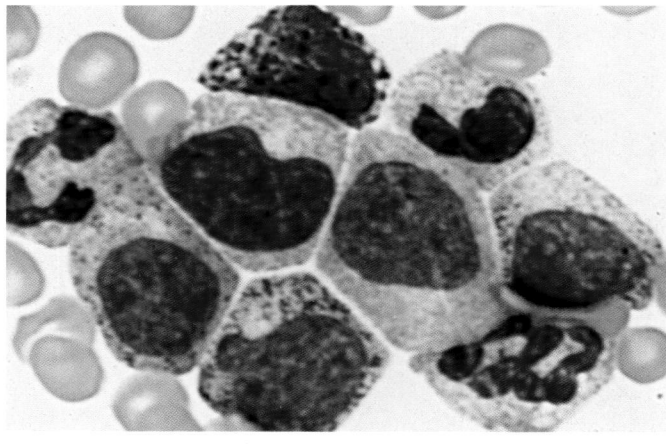

PLATE XIX-2 Myelocytes, neutrophils, and a basophil

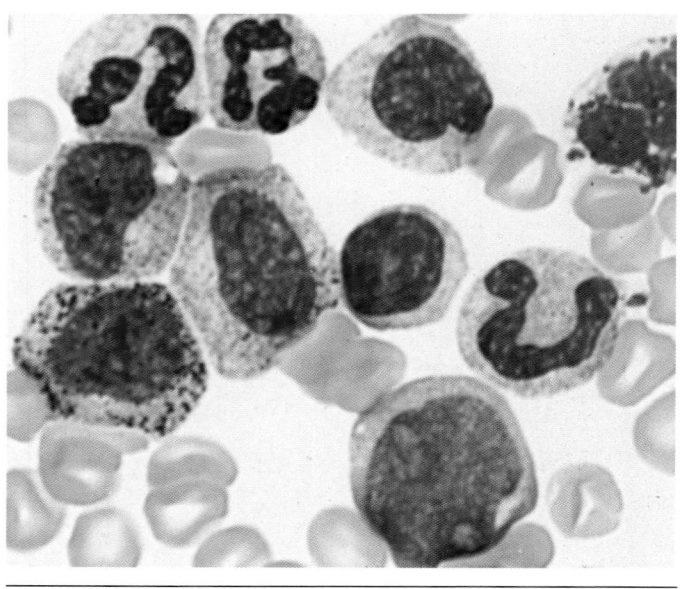

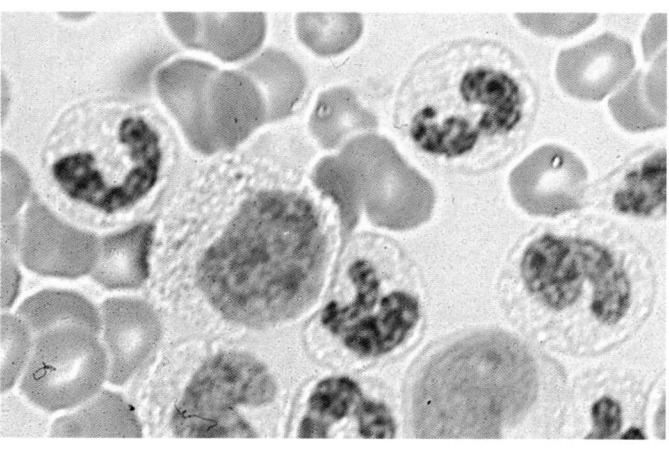

PLATE XIX-4 Absence of leukocyte alkaline phosphatase staining of the neutrophils from a patient with chronic myelogenous leukemia

PLATE XIX-3 Myeloblast, myelocytes, and neutrophils

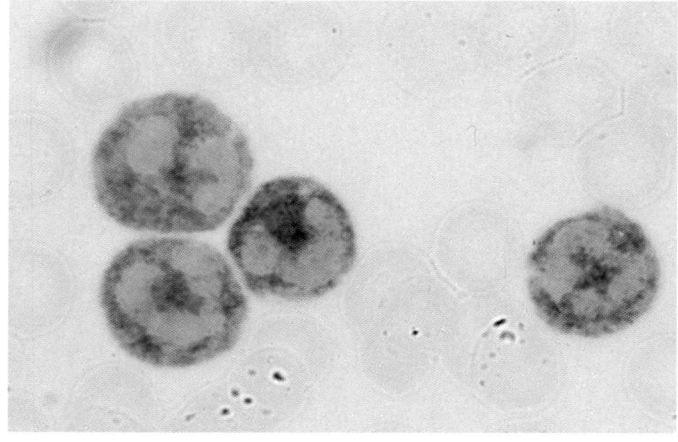

PLATE XIX-5 Leukocyte alkaline phosphatase staining of inflammatory neutrophils

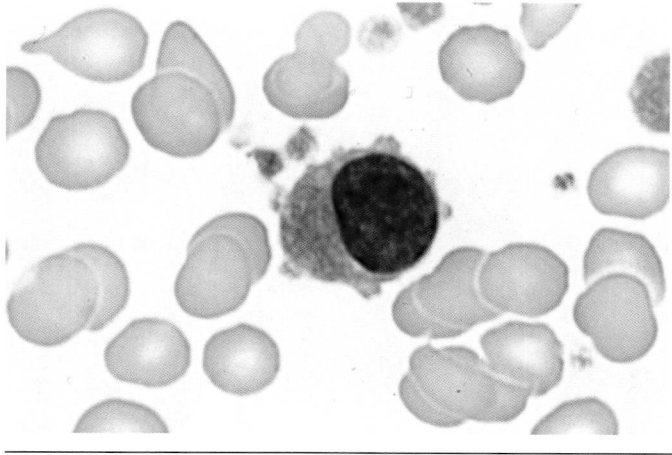

PLATE XIX-6 Micromegakaryocyte in a patient with chronic myelogenous leukemia undergoing acute transformation

(XIX-1 through XVI-6 are blood films)

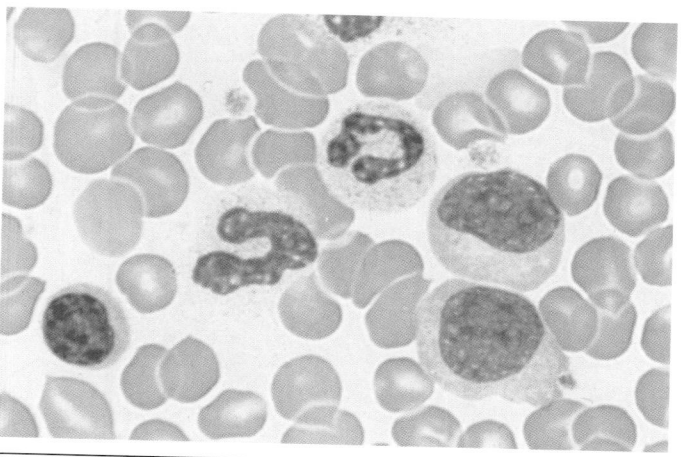

PLATE XX-1 Buffy coat from patient with infectious mononucleosis: Two large reactive lymphocytes

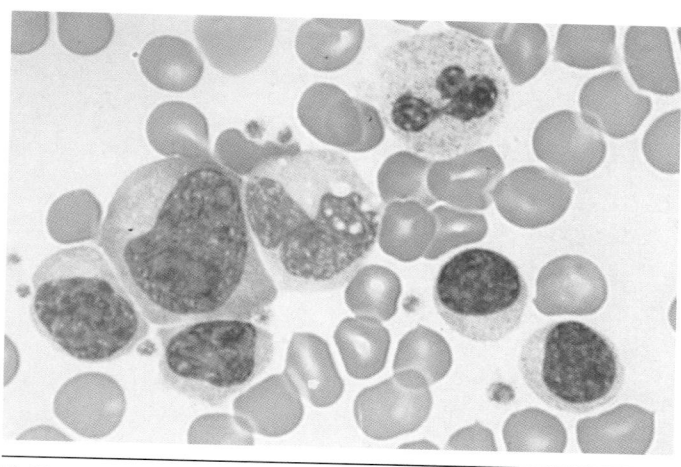

PLATE XX-2 Buffy coat from patient with infectious mononucleosis: Reactive lymphocytes, plasmacytoid lymphocytes, and monocyte

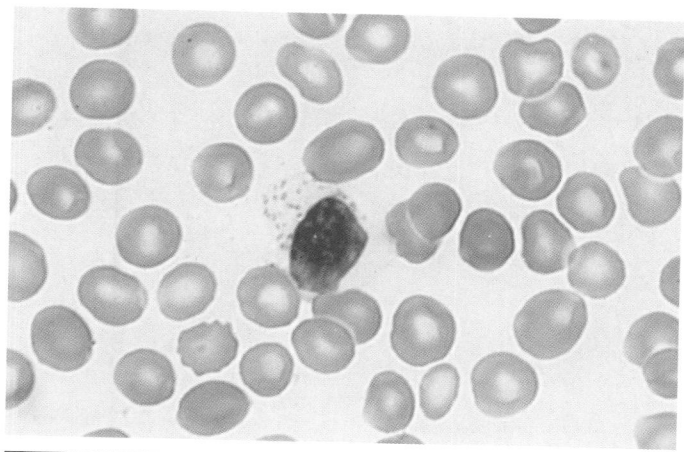

PLATE XX-3 Large granular lymphocyte

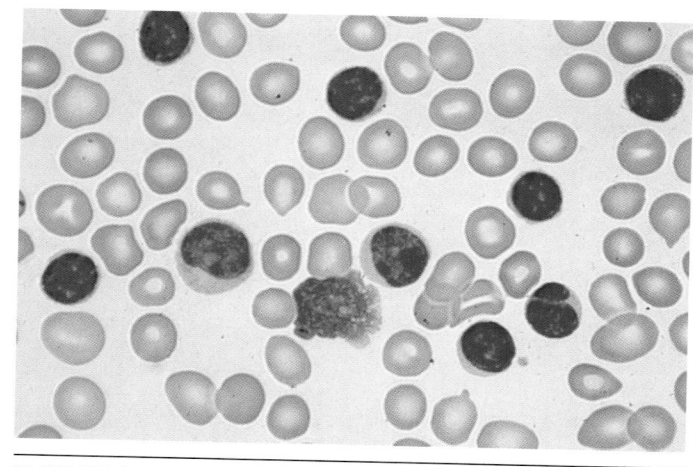

PLATE XX-4 Chronic lymphocytic leukemia

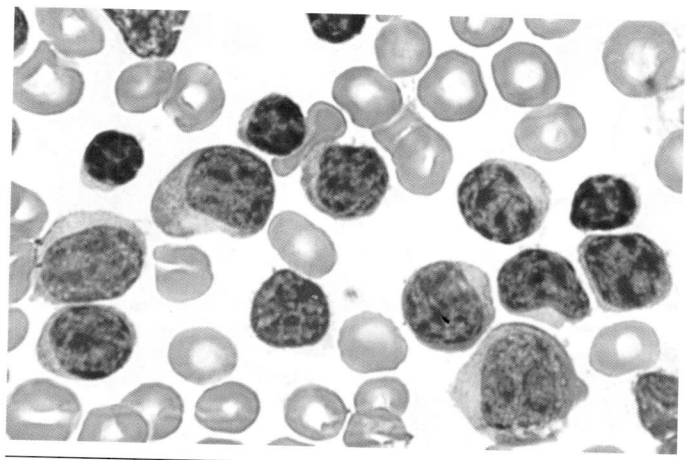

PLATE XX-5 Chronic lymphocytic leukemia

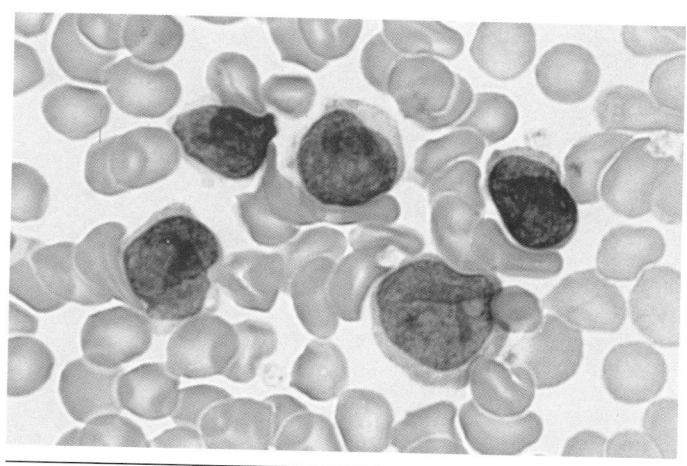

PLATE XX-6 Sézary cell leukemia

(XX-1 through XX-6 are blood films)

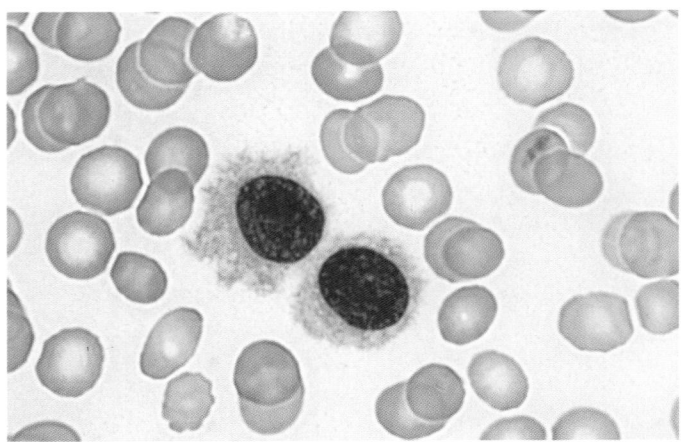

PLATE XX-7 Hairy cell leukemia

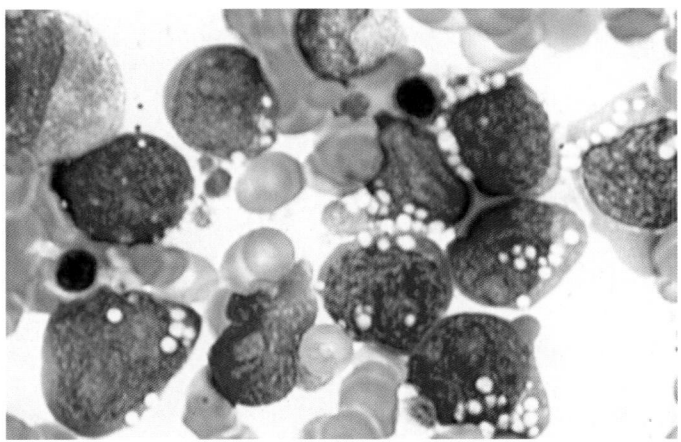

PLATE XX-8 Burkitt cell leukemia

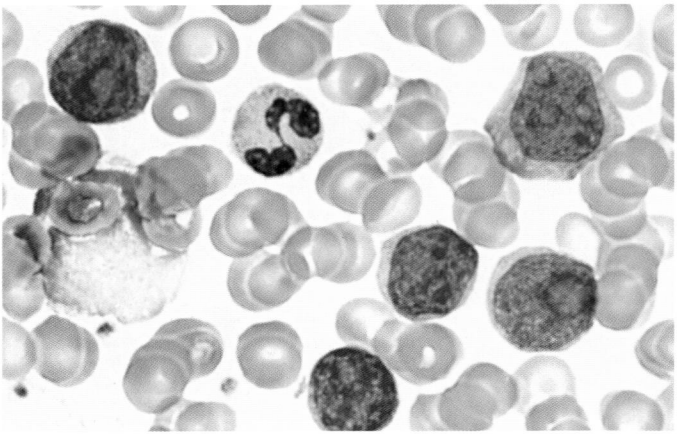

PLATE XX-9 Acute prolymphocytic leukemia

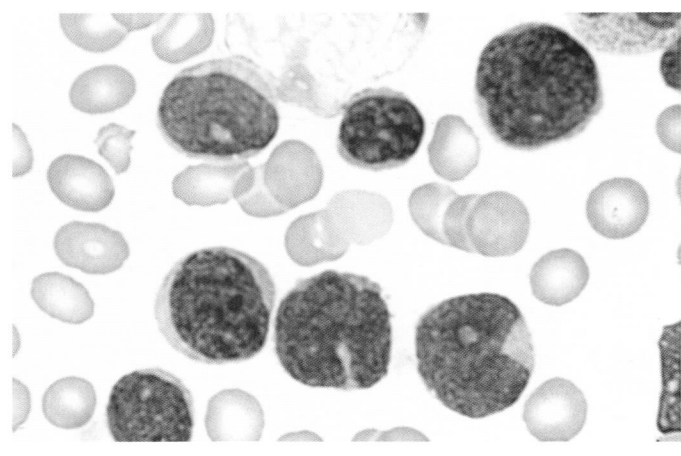

PLATE XX-10 Leukemic phase of small cell, cleaved follicular lymphoma

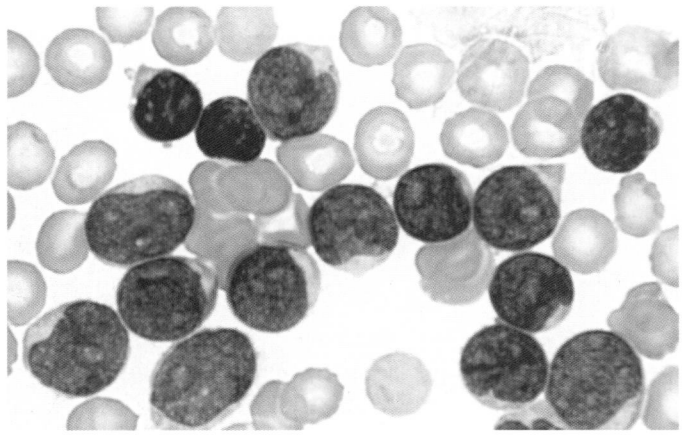

PLATE XX-11 Acute lymphocytic leukemia

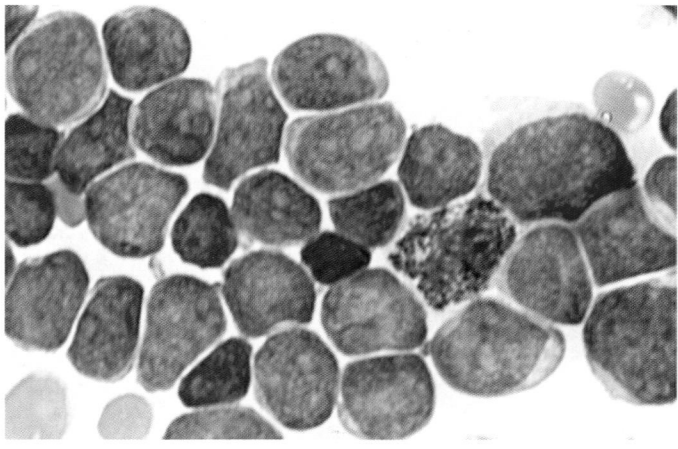

PLATE XX-12 Acute lymphocytic leukemia stained with peroxidase: Note that the blast cells are unreactive and the neutrophil is stained

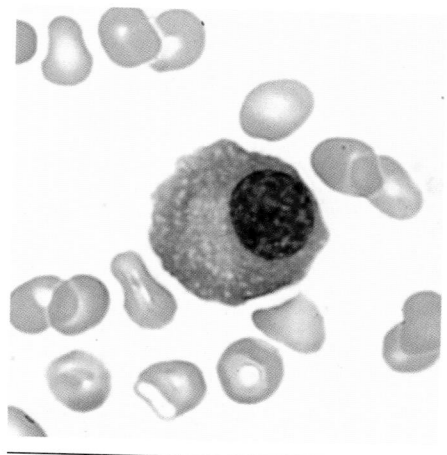

PLATE XXI-1 Plasma cell

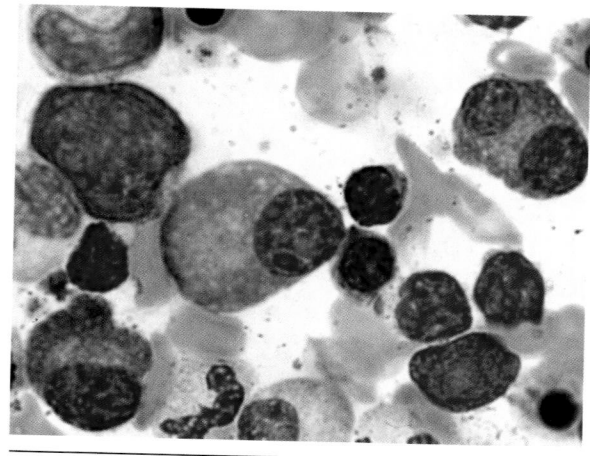

PLATE XXI-2 Plasma cells

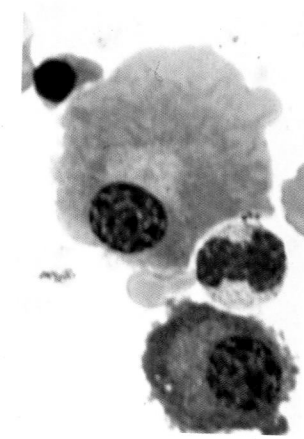

PLATE XXI-3 Plasma cells

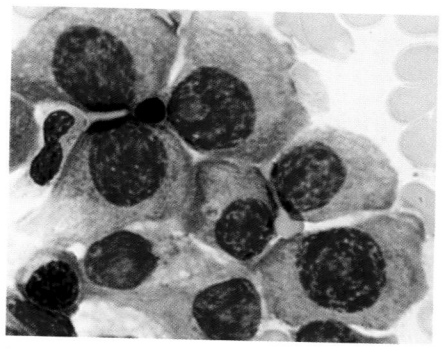

PLATE XXI-4 Myeloma cells

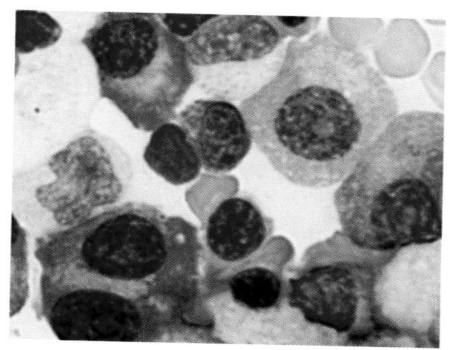

PLATE XXI-5 Myeloma cells

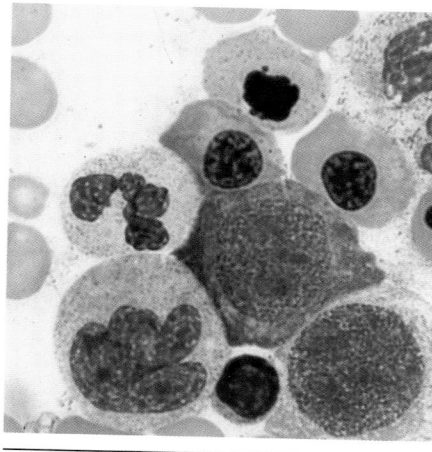

PLATE XXI-6 Blood film of patient with plasma cell leukemia

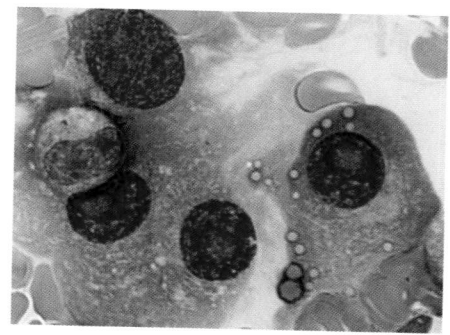

PLATE XXI-7 Myeloma cells

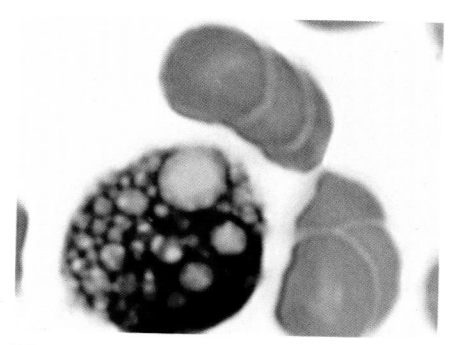

PLATE XXI-8 Mott cells

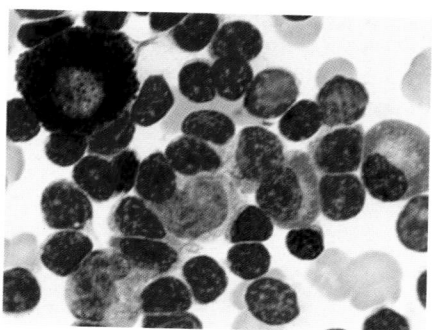

PLATE XXI-9 Waldenström macroglobulinemia: Increased lymphocytes, occasional plasma cells, and a mast cell

(XXI-1 through XXI-9 are marrow films)

LYMPH NODE BIOPSIES

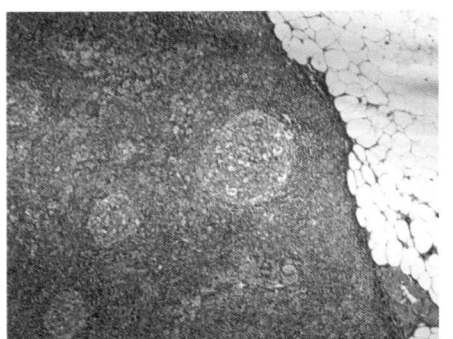

PLATE XXII-1   Normal lymph node

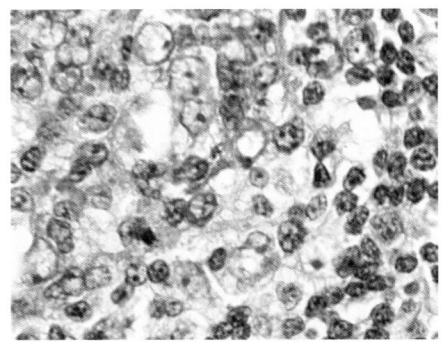

PLATE XXII-2   Normal lymph node

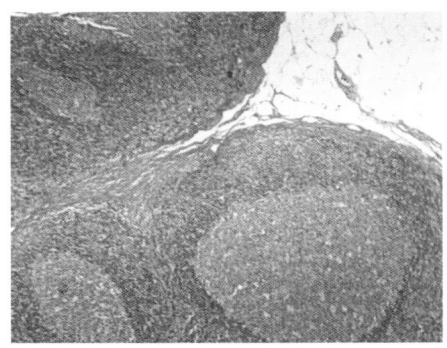

PLATE XXII-3   Benign follicular hyperplasia

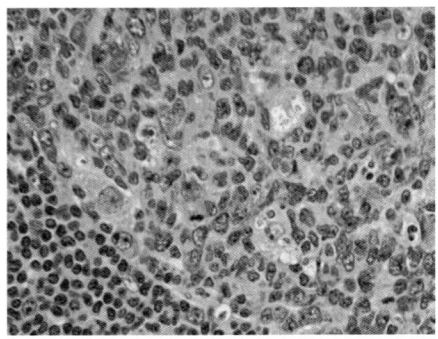

PLATE XXII-4   Follicular hyperplasia: Reactive germinal center

PLATE XXII-5   Malignant lymphoma, small lymphocytic type

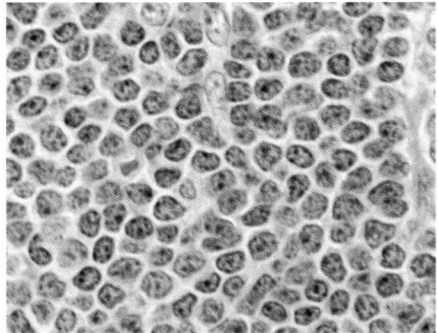

PLATE XXII-6   Malignant lymphoma, small lymphocytic type

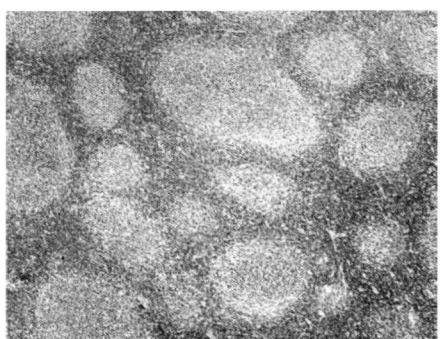

PLATE XXII-7   Malignant lymphoma, follicular, small cleaved cell type

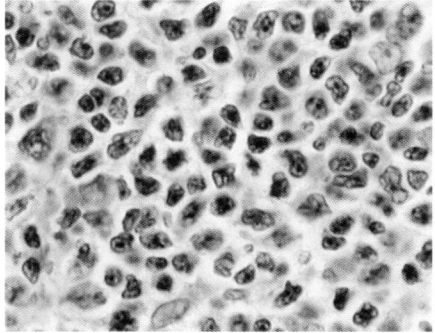

PLATE XXII-8   Malignant lymphoma, follicular, small cleaved cell type

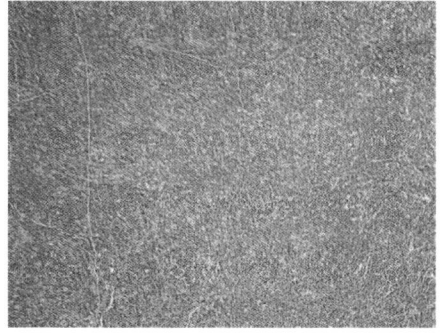

PLATE XXII-9   Malignant lymphoma, diffuse, large cell type

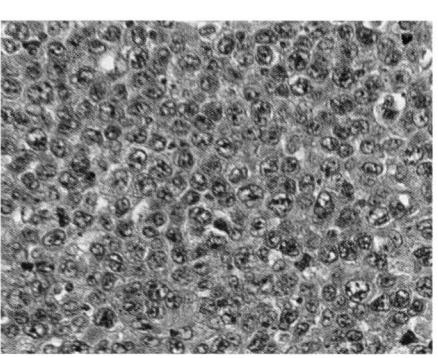

PLATE XXII-10   Malignant lymphoma, diffuse, large cell type

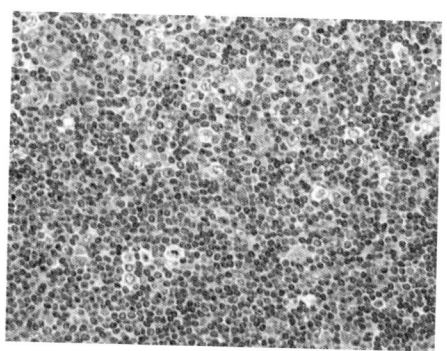

PLATE XXII-11   Hodgkin disease: Lymphocyte predominance

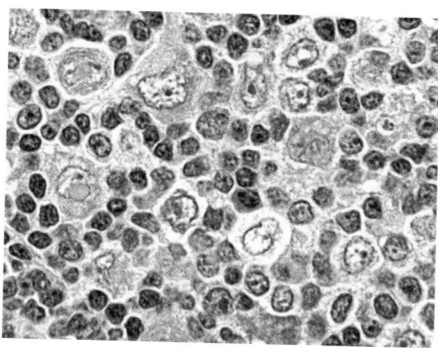

PLATE XXII-12   Hodgkin disease: Lymphocyte predominance

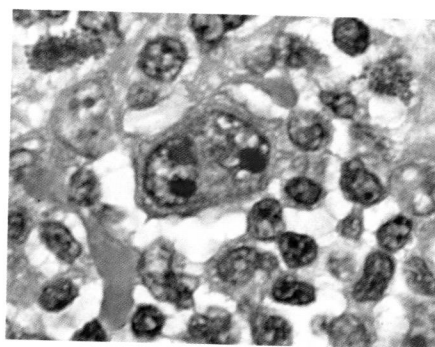

PLATE XXII-13   Hodgkin disease: Reed-Sternberg cell

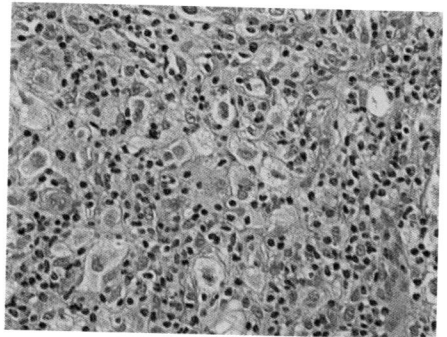

PLATE XXII-14   Hodgkin disease: Nodular sclerosing type

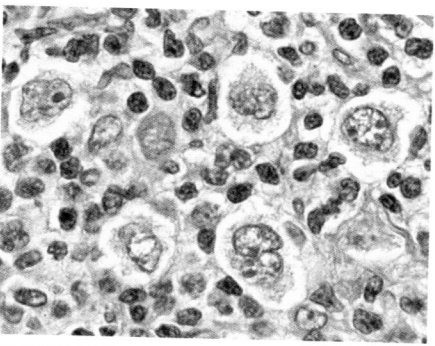

PLATE XXII-15   Hodgkin disease: Nodular sclerosing type

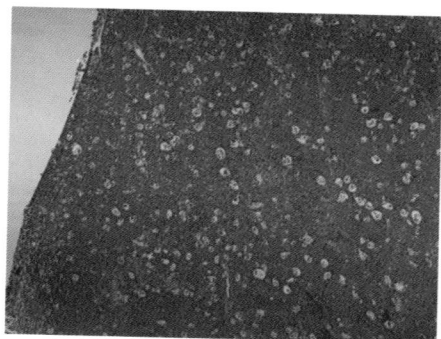

PLATE XXII-16   Burkitt lymphoma: Note starry sky appearance from the interspersed macrophages

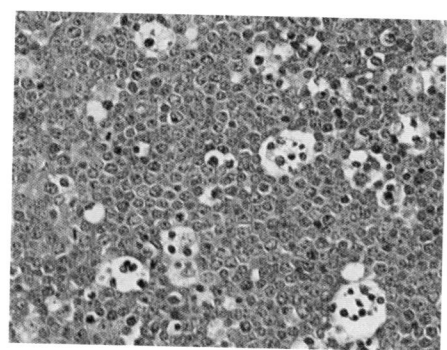

PLATE XXII-17   Burkitt lymphoma

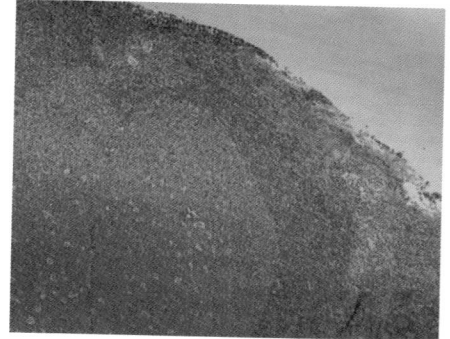

PLATE XXII-18   Lymphoid hyperplasia in acquired immunodeficiency syndrome

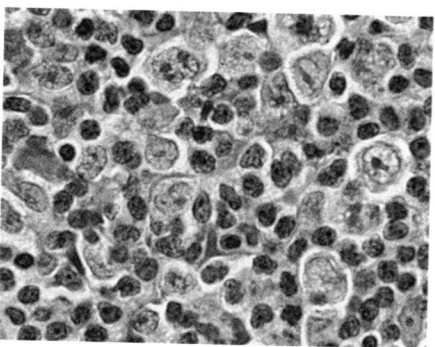

PLATE XXII-19   Lymphoid hyperplasia in acquired immunodeficiency syndrome

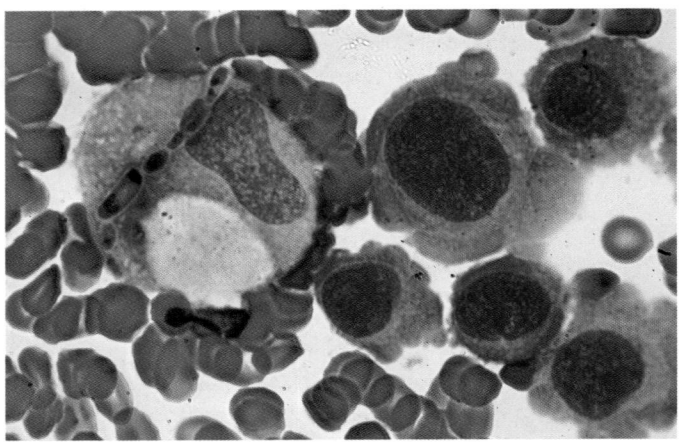

PLATE XXIII-1 Candidiasis. Pleural fluid film. Macrophage with ingested Candida. Adjacent mesothelial cells

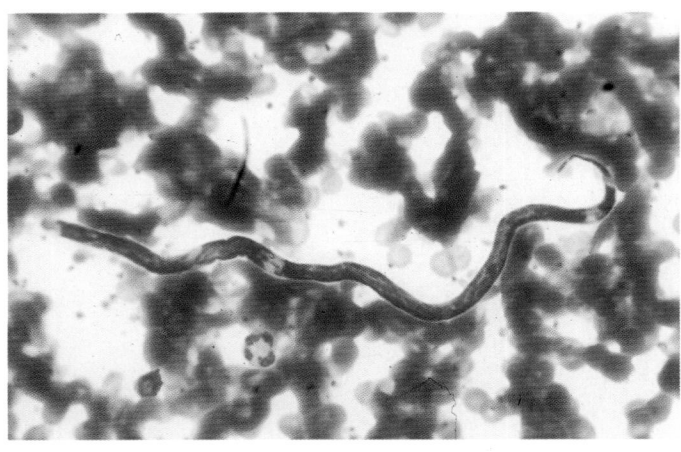

PLATE XXIII-2 Microfilaria of *Loa loa*. Blood film

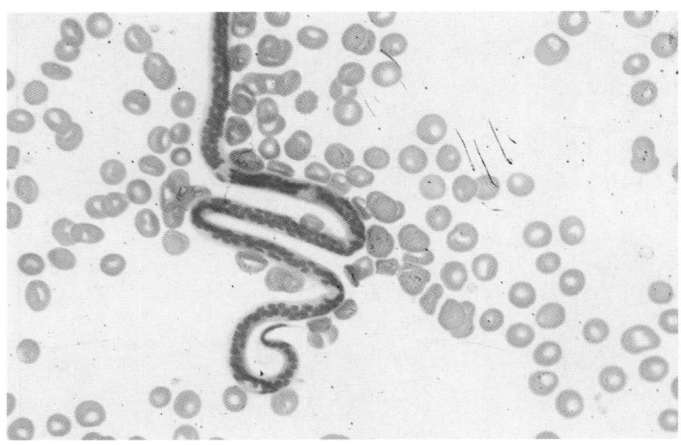

PLATE XXIII-3 Microfilaria of *Wuchereria bancrofti*. Blood film

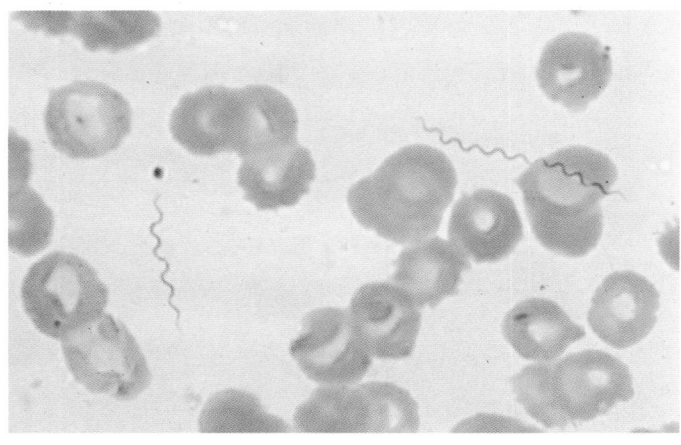

PLATE XXIII-4 Spirochetes of *Borrelia* species. Blood film

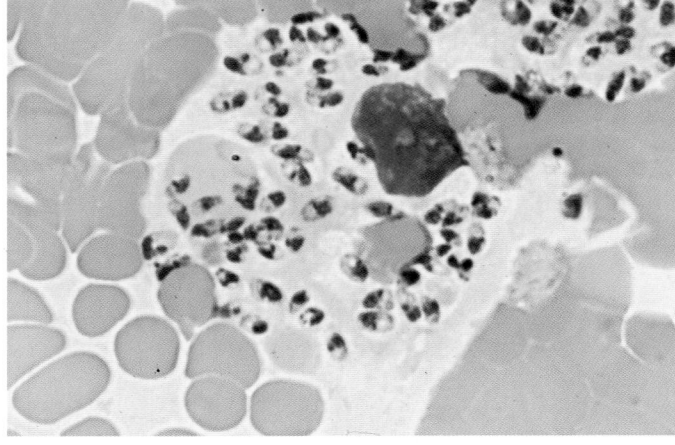

PLATE XXIII-5 Macrophage loaded with the amastiogotes of *Leishmania* species. Pleural fluid film. The "T" shapes are in contrast to those of Histoplasma capsulatum (see Plate VI-8)

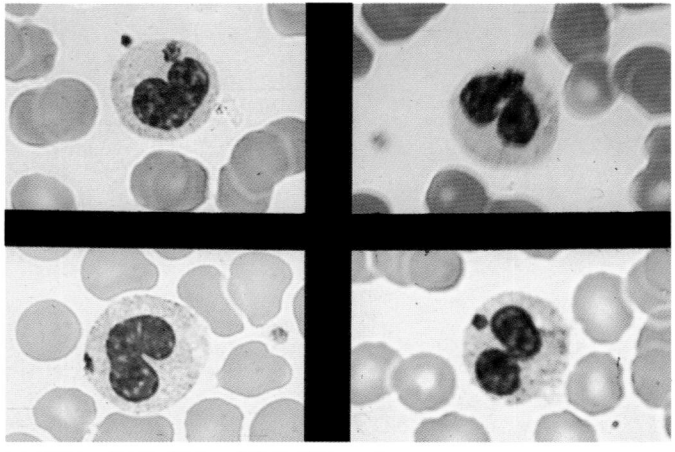

PLATE XXIII-6 Ehrlichiosis. Blood film. The intracellular *Ehrlichia* are evident

FLOURESCENCE IN SITU HYBRIDIZATION (FISH) FOR CYTOGENETIC ANALYSIS

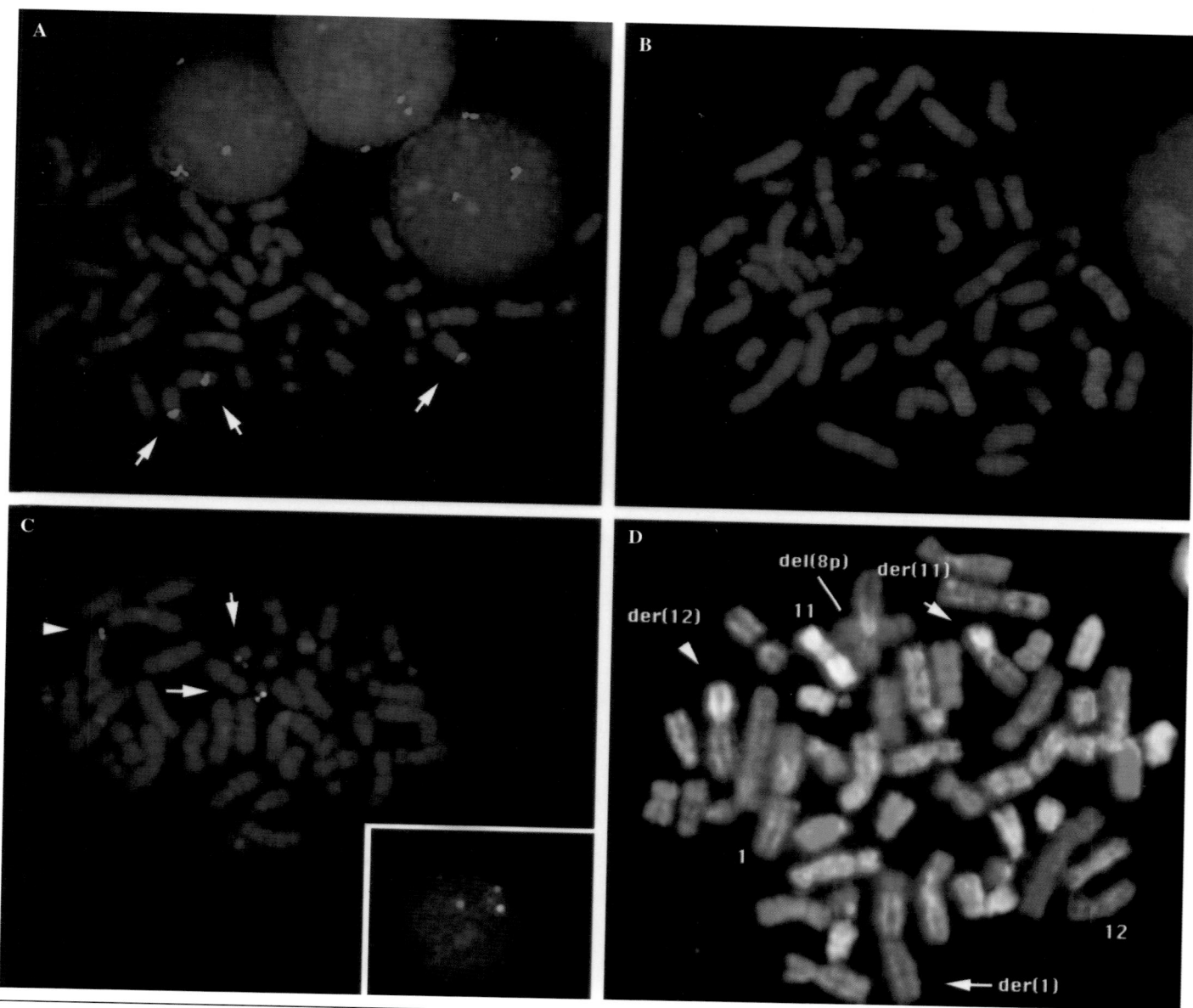

PLATE XXIV Fluorescence in situ Hybridization (FISH) for Cytogenetic Analysis (A–D) Photomicrographs of metaphase and interphase cells following FISH. In panels A–C, the cells are counterstained with 4,6-diamidino-2-phenylindole-dihydrochloride (DAPI). (A) Hybridization of a directly labeled centromere-specific probe for chromosome 8 (CEP8 Spectrum Green, Vysis Inc.) to metaphase and interphase cells from an AML with trisomy 8. Centromere-specific probes hybridize to the repetitive DNA sequences that are present at the centromeres of human chromosomes. The chromosome 8 homologs are identified with arrows. (B) Hybridization of a directly labeled chromosome 8-specific painting probe (WCP8 Spectrum Green, Vysis Inc.) to a metaphase cell with trisomy 8 from an AML. (C) Hybridization of a locus-specific probe for the detection of a recurring translocation, the t(9;22)(q34;q11.2) in CML. The probe is a mixture of digoxigenin-labeled DNA probes (detected with rhodamine-labeled antibodies) for the major break-point cluster region of the BCR gene at 22q11.2, and biotin-labeled probes (detected with FITC-avidin) for the ABL gene at 9q34 (M-bcr/abl probe, Oncor). In cells with the t(9;22), only one green signal (arrowhead) and one red signal (short arrow) is observed on the normal 9 and 22 homologs, and a yellow fusion signal (long arrow) is observed on the Ph chromosome as a result of the juxtaposition of the ABL and BCR sequences. (D) Spectral karyotyping analysis of a metaphase cell from an AML-M7. Twenty-four differentially labeled probes, each representing one human chromosome, are cohybridized, and imaging analysis software assigns a unique color to each. A complex karyotype was identified by conventional cytogenetic analysis, including a derivative chromosome 1 with additional material of unknown origin on 1p, a deletion of 8p, a derivative chromosome 11 resulting from an unbalanced translocation involving 1 and 11, and a derivative chromosome 12, consisting of 11q and 12q. The results of spectral karyotyping confirmed the identity of the rearranged chromosome 12 (arrowhead) and clarified the other abnormalities. The additional material on 1p was derived from chromosome 8 (long arrow, blue signal), and the der(11) actually consisted of material from chromosomes 1, 11, and 12 (short arrow, 11p white signal; chromosome 12 brown signal; 1p blue-pink signal).

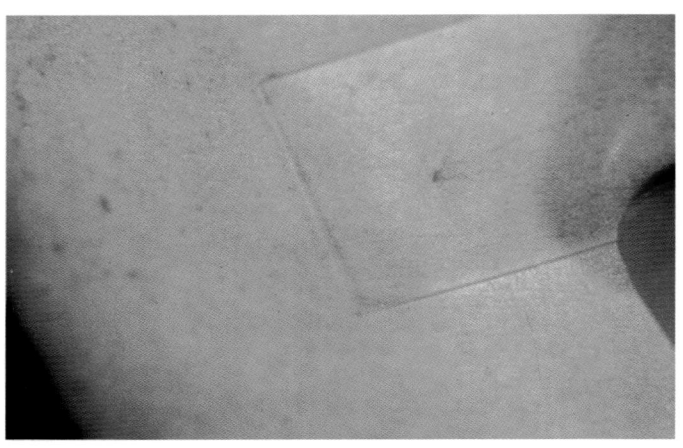

PLATE XXV-1   Spider telangiectasia

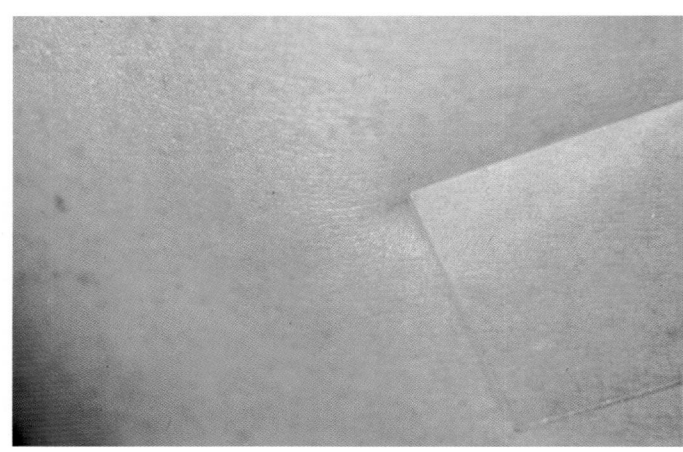

PLATE XXV-2   Blanching of spider telangiectasia

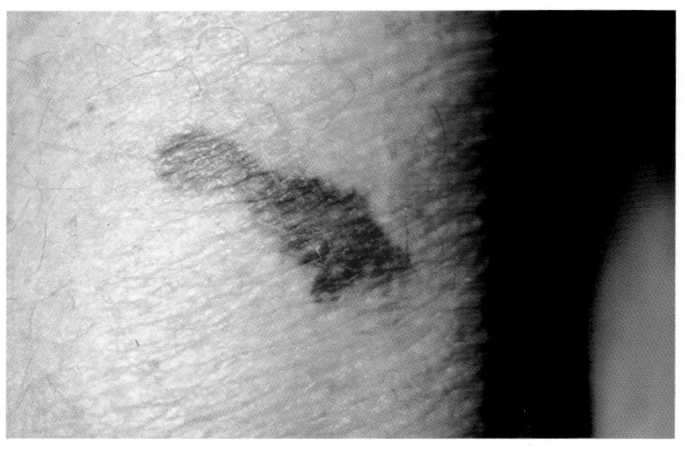

PLATE XXV-3   Senile purpura

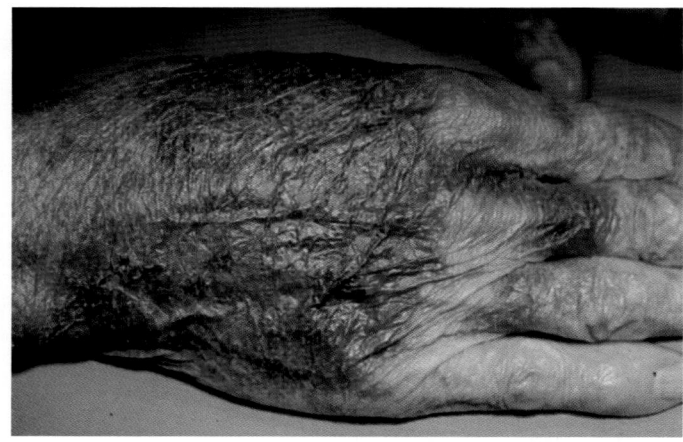

PLATE XXV-4   Senile purpura

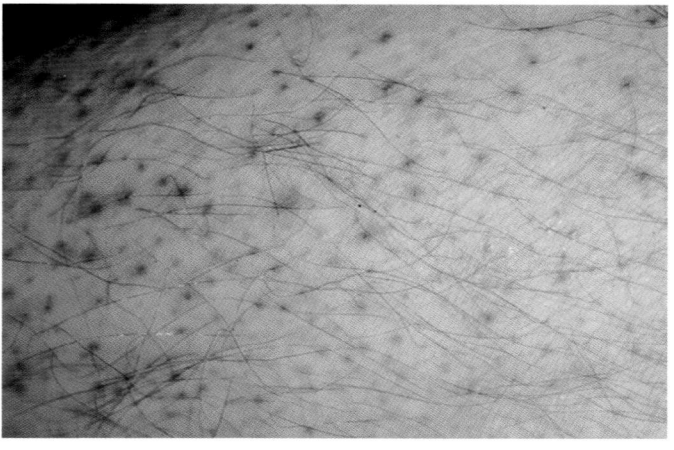

PLATE XXV-5   Parafollicular hemorrhages of scurvy

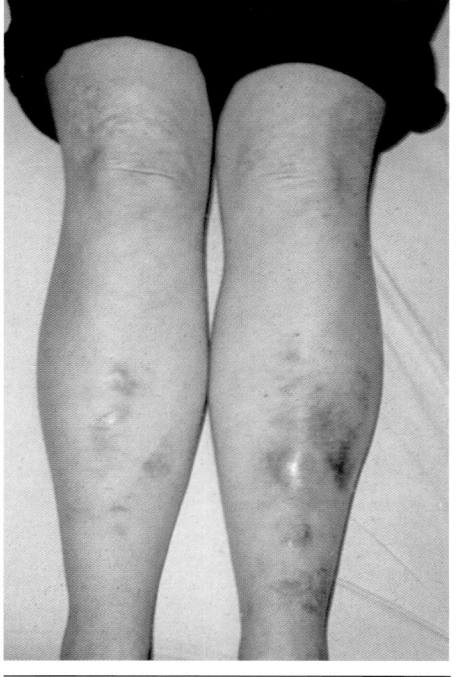

PLATE XXV-6 Purpura associated with Ehlers-Danlos Syndrome

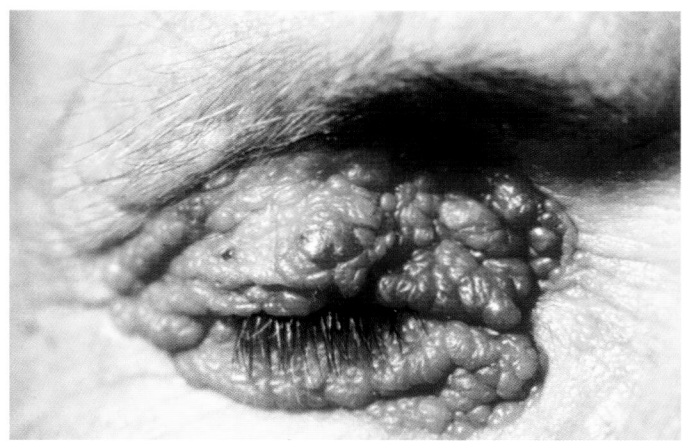

PLATE XXV-7 Amyloidoses

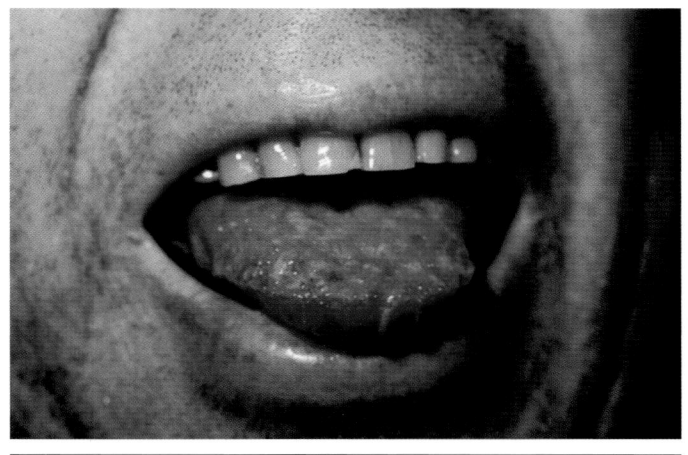

PLATE XXV-8 Amyloidoses

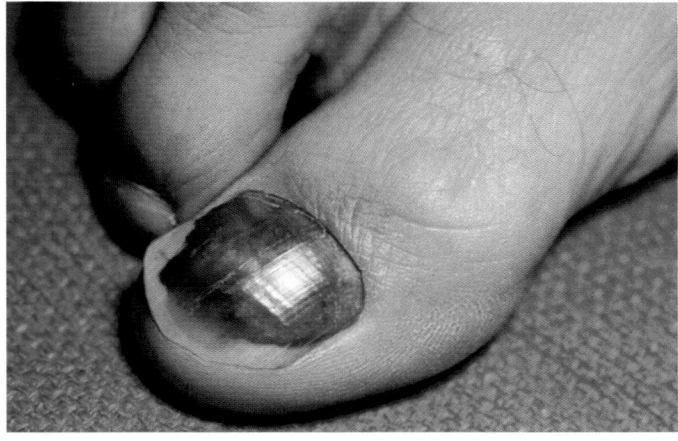

PLATE XXV-9 Tennis toe: Subungual hemorrhage

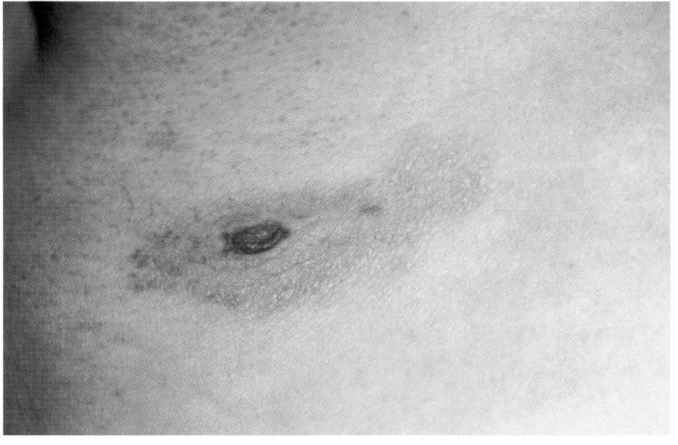

PLATE XXV-10 Ecthyma gangrenosum

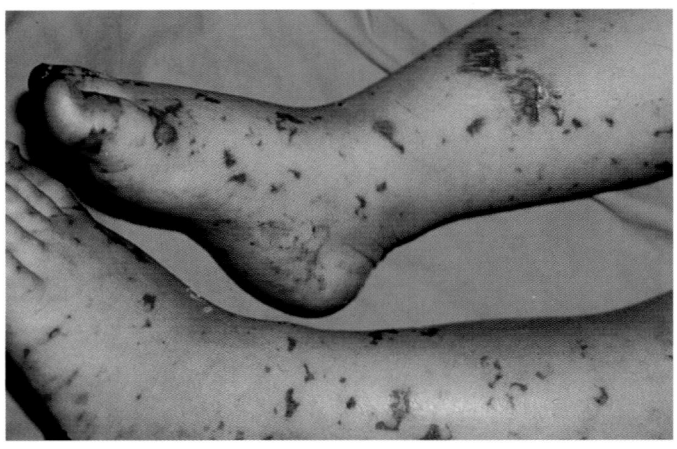

PLATE XXV-11   Meningococcemia: Stellate purpura

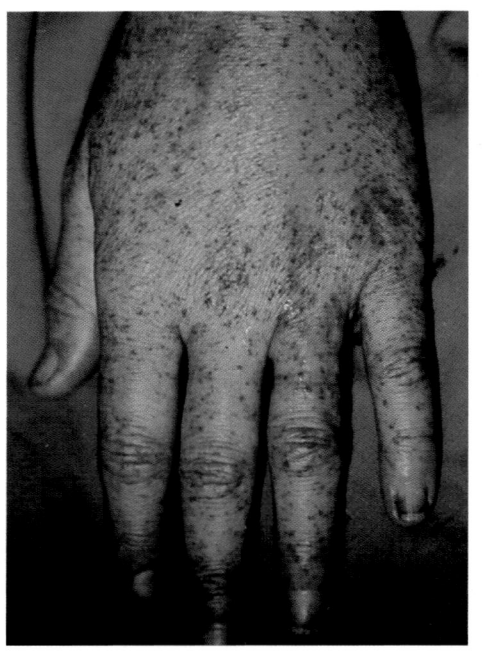

PLATE XXV-12   Rocky Mountain spotted fever:
Petechiae

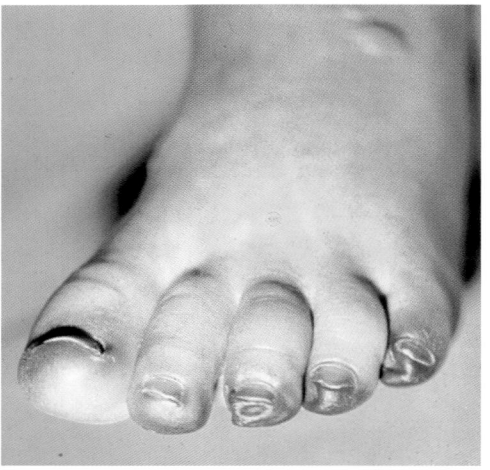

PLATE XXV-13   Rocky Mountain spotted fever:
Peripheral purpuric gangrene

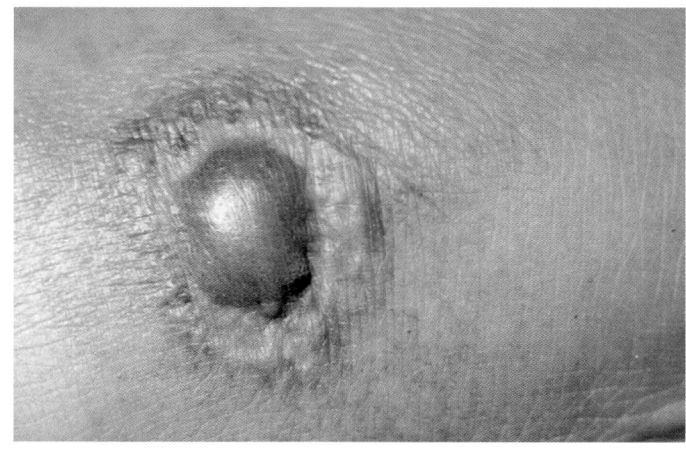

PLATE XXV-14   Lyme disease: Hemorrhagic central bulla

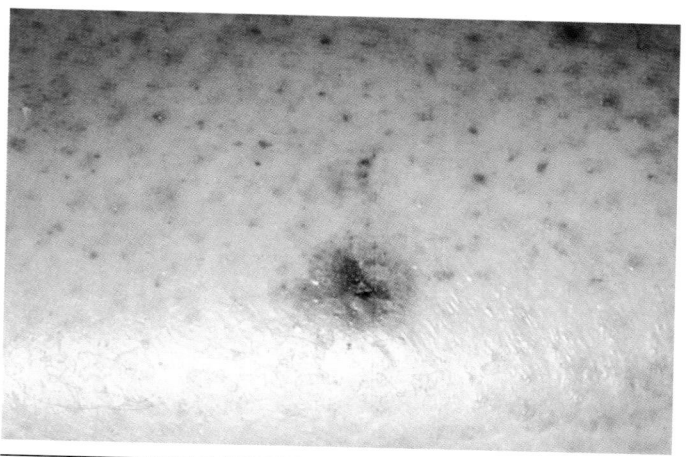

PLATE XXV-15 Candidemia: Purpuric nodule in a patient with acute myelogenous leukemia

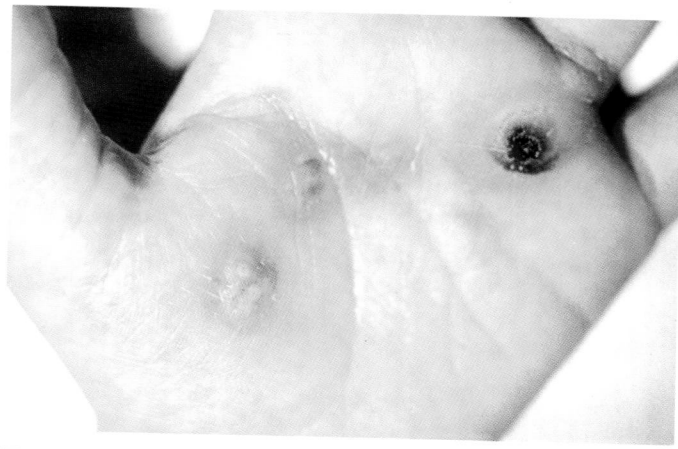

PLATE XXV-16 Aspergillosis: Primary cutaneous inoculation from contaminated armboard

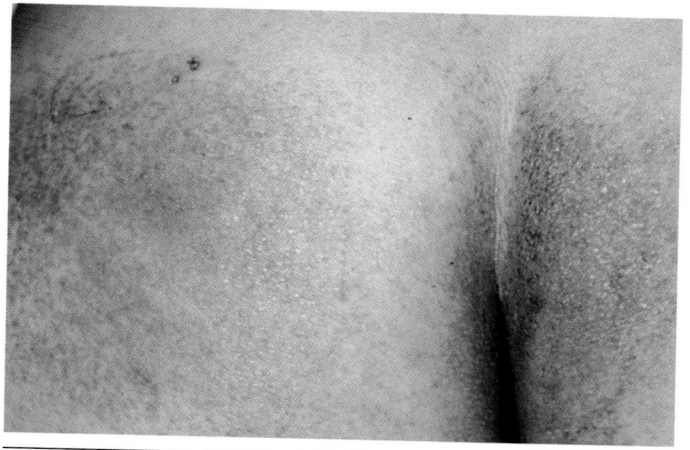

PLATE XXV-17 Parvovirus B-19

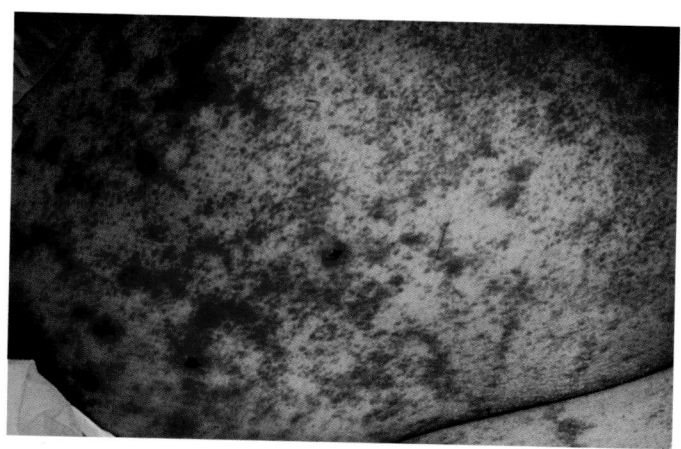

PLATE XXV-18 Disseminated strongyloidiasis

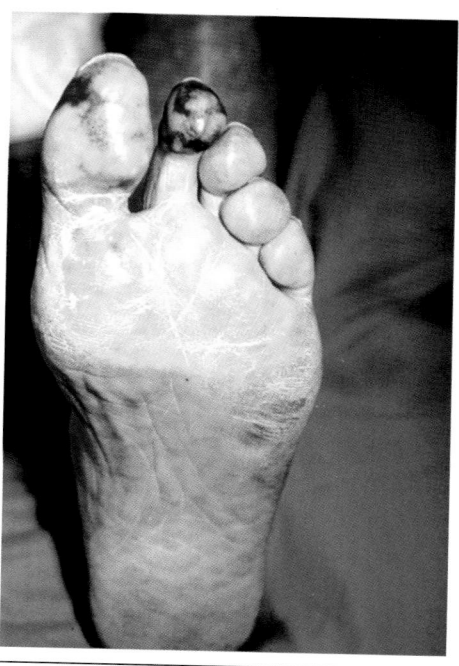

PLATE XXV-19 Cholesterol emboli

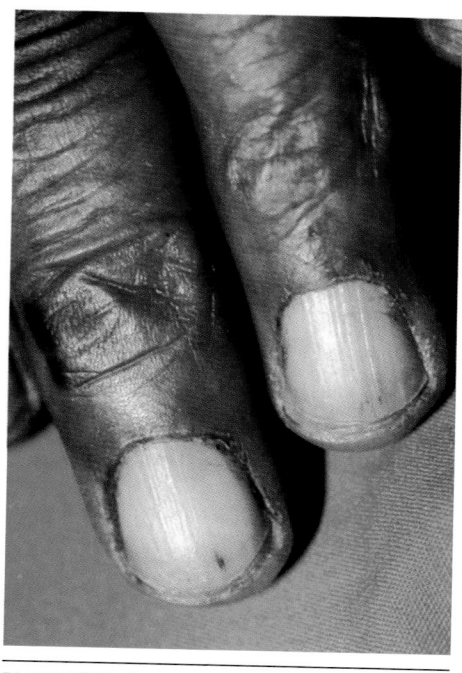

PLATE XXV-20 Cholesterol emboli: Splinter hemorrhages

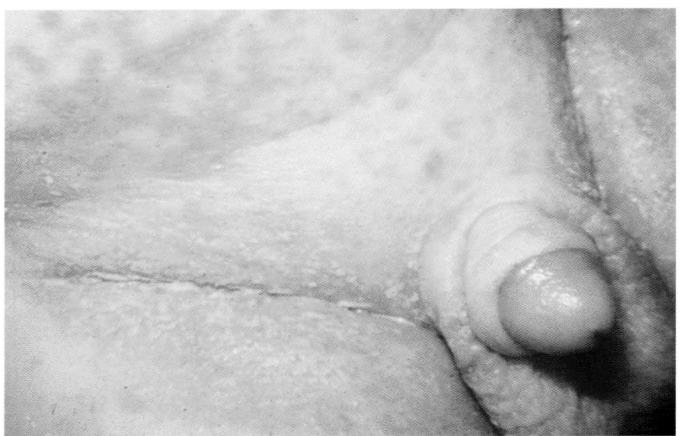

PLATE XXV-21   Langerhans cell histiocytosis

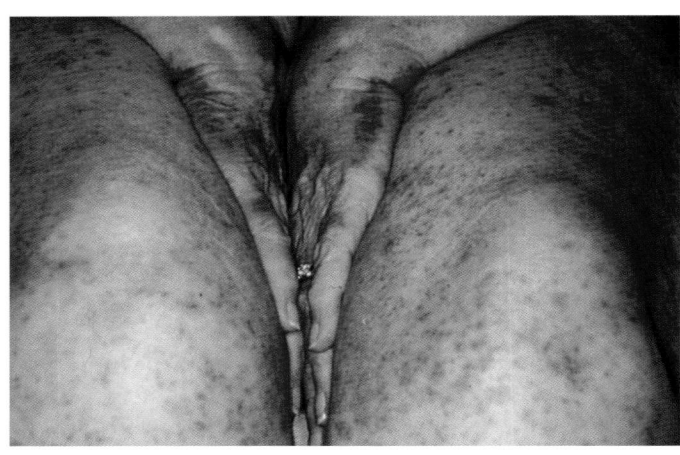

PLATE XXV-22   Serum sickness due to antithymocyte globulin

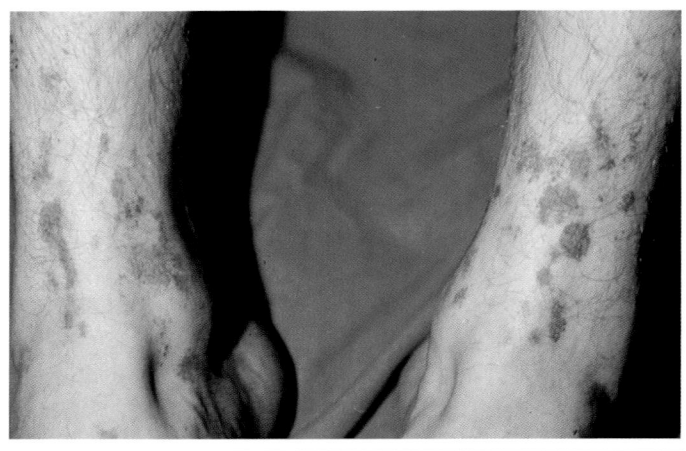

PLATE XXV-23   Schamberg disease: Pigmented purpuric eruption

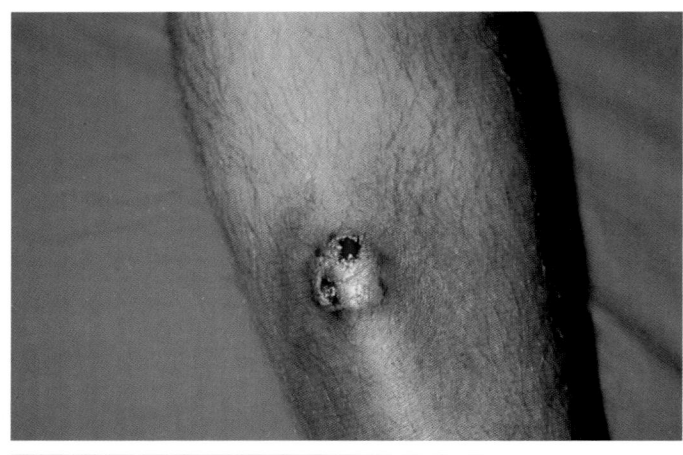

PLATE XXV-24   Pyoderma gangrenosum: Central purpuraa

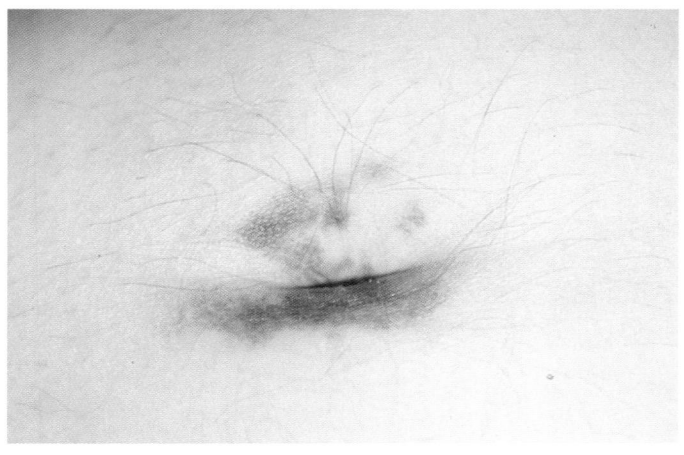

PLATE XXV-25   Cullen sign

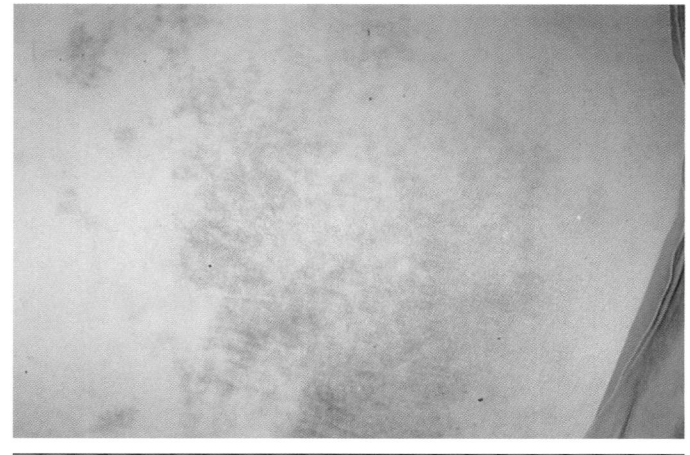

PLATE XXV-26   Grey-Turner sign

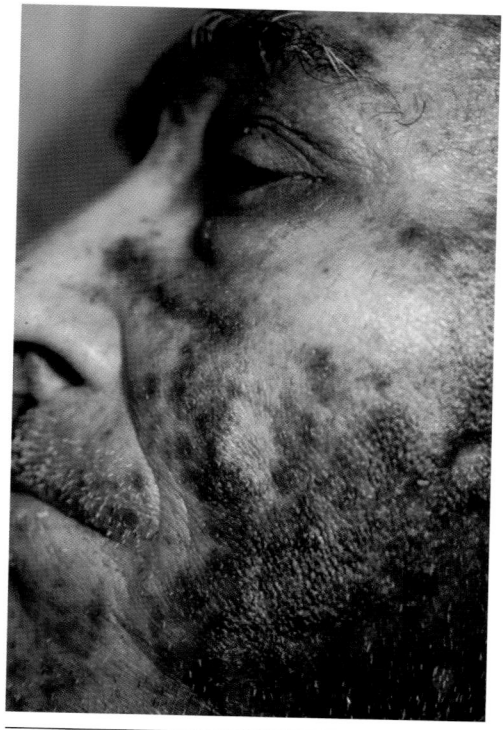

PLATE XXV-27 Cutaneous infiltration with acute myelogenous leukemia blast cells

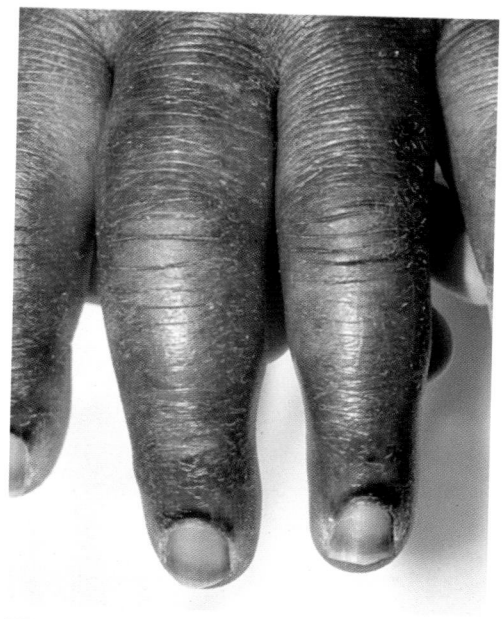

PLATE XXV-28 Disseminated intravascular coagulation

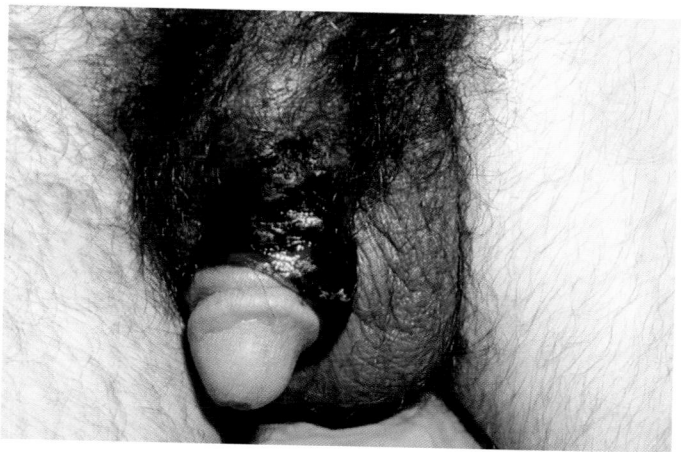

PLATE XXV-29 Coumadin necrosis

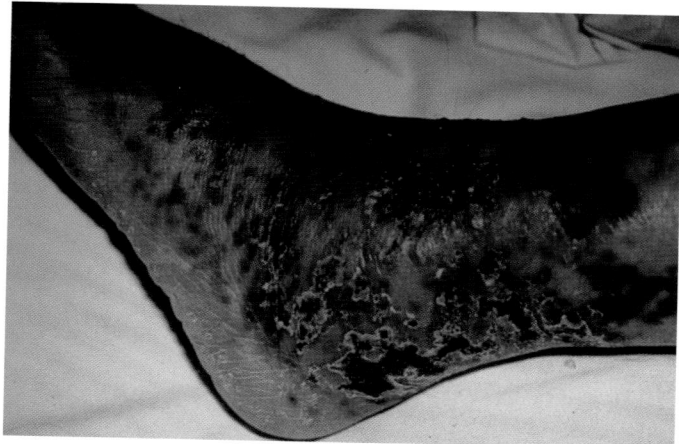

PLATE XXV-30 Antiphospholipid antibody syndrome: Anticardiolipin antibody

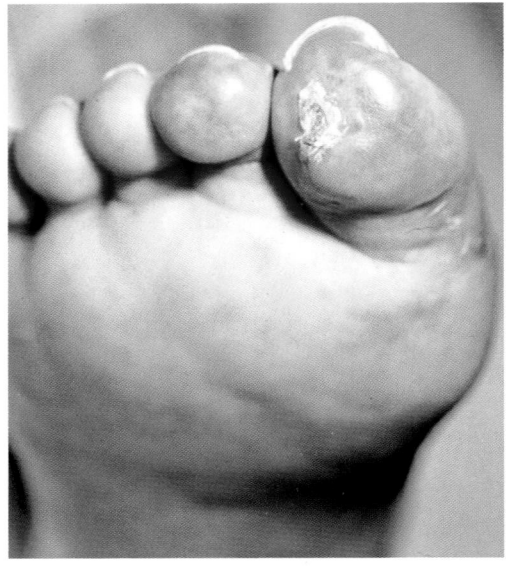

PLATE XXV-31 Antiphospholipid antibody syndrome: Lupus anticoagulant

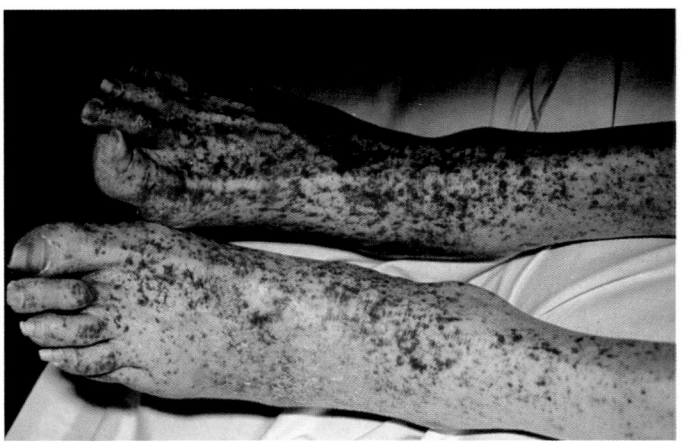

PLATE XXV-32 Quinidine purpura

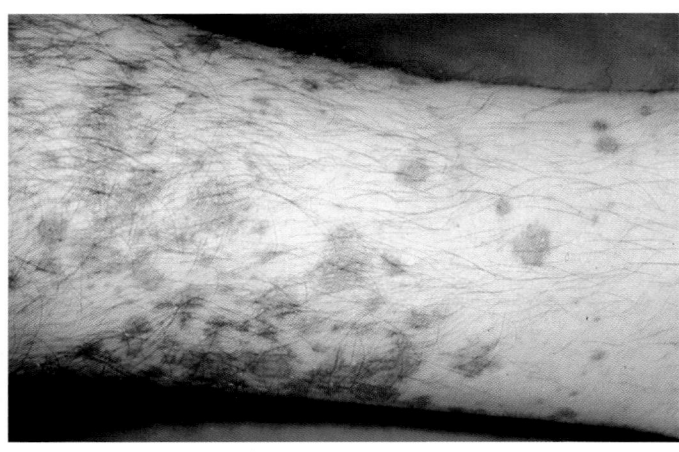

PLATE XXV-33 Schönlein-Henoch purpura

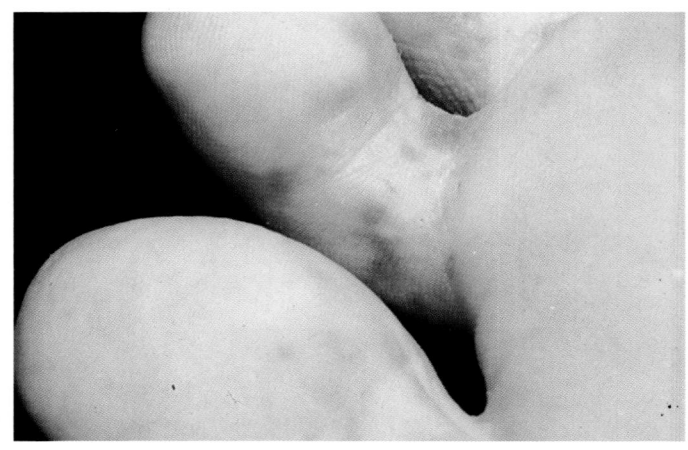

PLATE XXV-34 Systemic lupus erythematosus vasculitis

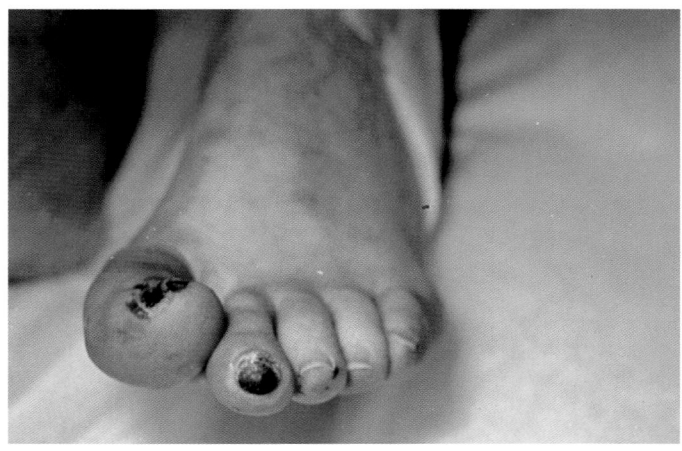

PLATE XXV-35 Polyarteritis nodosa: Acral purpura

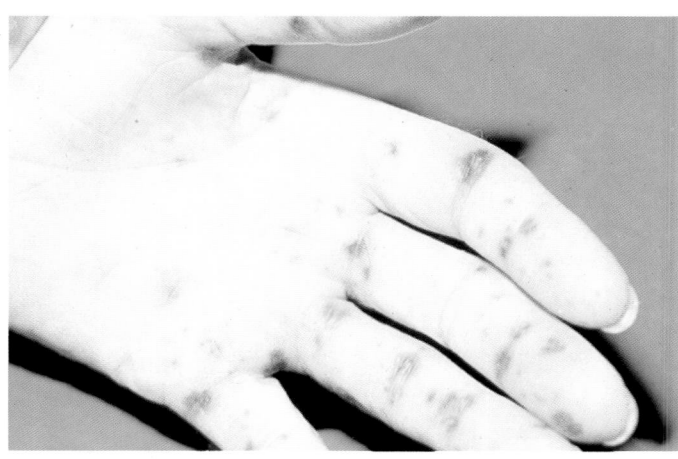

PLATE XXV-36 Wegener granulomatosis

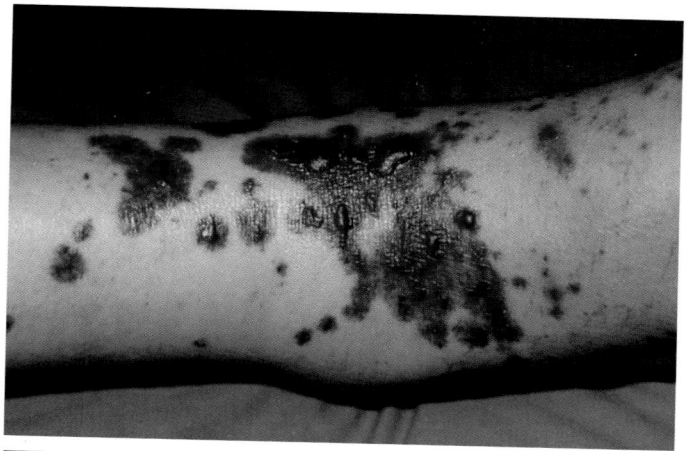

PLATE XXV-37 Leukocytoclastic vasculitis secondary to furosemide

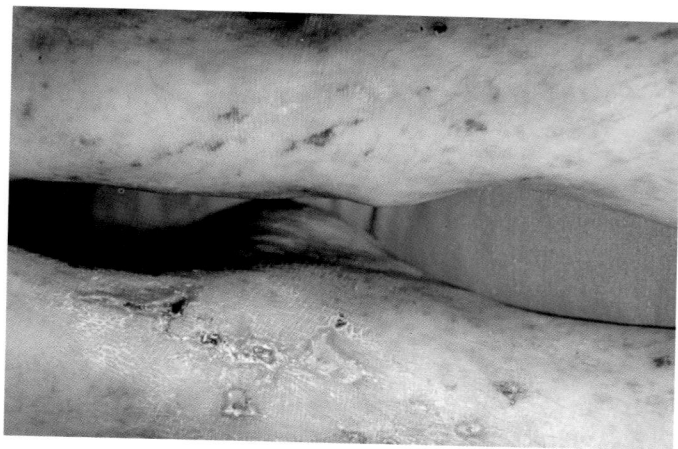

PLATE XXV-38 Cryoglobulinemia: Peripheral purpura

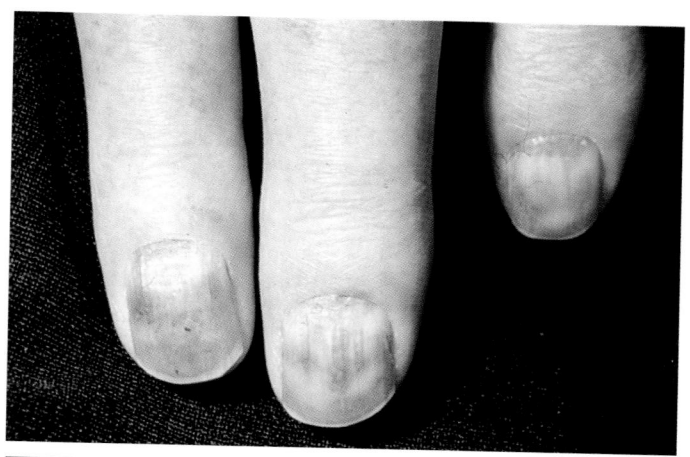

PLATE XXV-39 Cryoglobulinemia: Subungual purpura

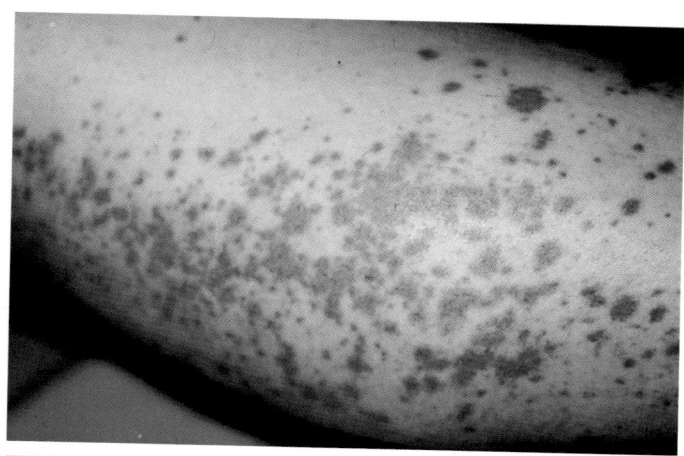

PLATE XXV-40 Waldenström hyperglobulinemic purpura

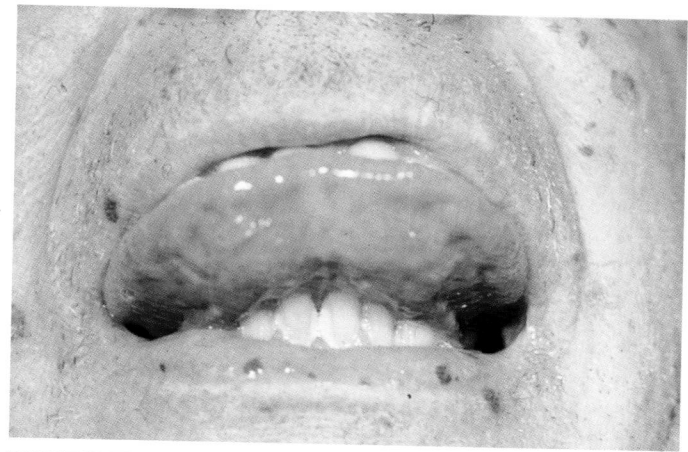

PLATE XXV-41 Hereditary hemorrhagic telangiectasia: Sublingual telangiectasia

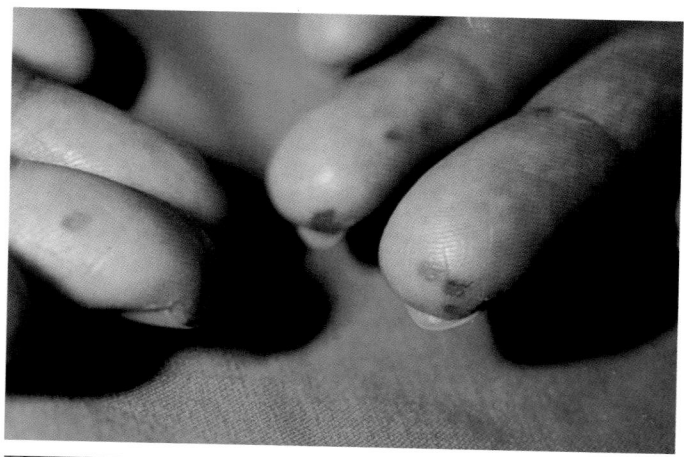

PLATE XXV-42 Hereditary hemorrhageic telangiectasia: Acral telangiectasias

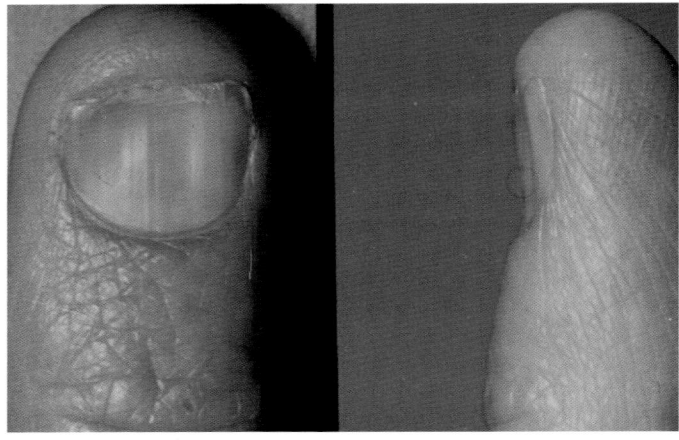

PLATE XXV-43 Koilonychia in severe iron deficiency

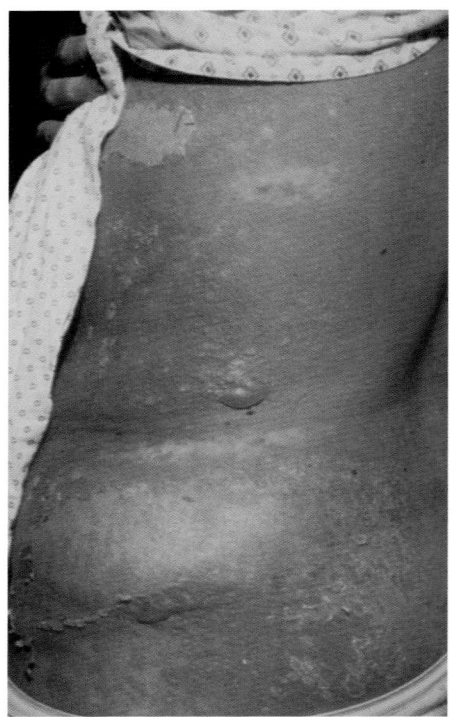

PLATE XXV-44 Grade IV graft-versus-host disease of the skin with diffuse erythroderma and bullous formation

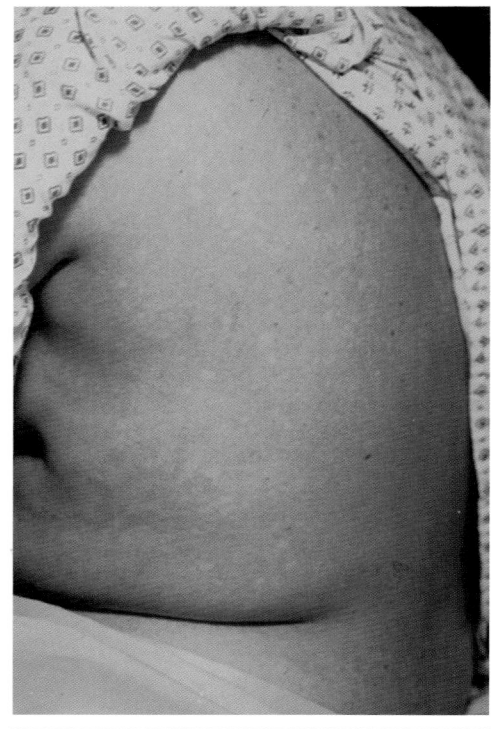

PLATE XXV-45 Complete resolution of grade IV graft-versus-host disease after therapy with high-dose glucocorticoids and antithymocyte globulin

DISSEMINATED INTRAVASCULAR COAGULATION

URI SELIGSOHN

When procoagulants are introduced or produced in the blood circulation and manage to overcome the control mechanisms of blood coagulation, widespread thrombin is generated which can lead to disseminated intravascular coagulation (DIC). The clinical manifestations of DIC include multiorgan dysfunction caused by microthrombi and bleeding caused by consumption of platelets, fibrinogen, factor V, and factor VIII, as well as secondary fibrinolysis. Tissue factor exposure to blood is the most common trigger of DIC. This can occur when monocytes and endothelial cells are induced to generate and express tissue factor during the systemic inflammatory response syndrome (e.g., gram-negative and gram-positive infections, fungemia, burns, severe trauma) or when contact is established between blood and tissue factor constitutively present on membranes of cells foreign to blood (e.g., malignant cells, placenta, brain cells, adventitia, traumatized tissues). Both DIC and the underlying disorders causing DIC contribute to a high rate of mortality. The severity of the organ dysfunction and extent of hemostatic failure, as well as increasing age, have been associated with a grave prognosis. Laboratory features include thrombocytopenia, reduced fibrinogen level, elevated levels of D-dimer and fibrin(o)gen) degradation products, and prolonged partial thromboplastin, prothrombin, and thrombin times. Several underlying disorders affect these hemostatic parameters and can lead to a false positive diagnosis of DIC (e.g., liver-disease–related coagulation abnormalities and thrombocytopenia) or to a false negative diagnosis (e.g., pregnancy-related high fibrinogen levels). Repeating the tests every 6 to 8 h can overcome these limitations. Early detection of DIC, vigorous treatment of the underlying disorder, and support of vital functions are essential for survival of affected patients. Blood component therapy is pertinent in patients who bleed excessively, whereas heparin administration is indicated in a limited number of circumstances.

DEFINITION AND HISTORY

Disseminated intravascular coagulation (DIC) is a clinicopathologic syndrome in which widespread intravascular coagulation is induced

Acronyms and abbreviations that appear in this chapter include: APL, acute promyelocytic leukemia; aPTT, activated partial thromboplastin time; ARDS, adult respiratory distress syndrome; AT, antithrombin; ATRA, all-*trans*-retinoic acid; DIC, disseminated intravascular coagulation; FDP, fibrinogen degradation products; HELLP, hemolysis, elevated liver enzymes, low platelet count; IL, interleukin; PAI, plasminogen activator inhibitor; PAP, plasmin-antiplasmin; PS, protein S; SIRS, systemic inflammatory response syndrome; TAFI, thrombin activatable fibrinolysis inhibitor; TAT, thrombin-AT; TF, tissue factor; TFPI, tissue factor pathway inhibitor; TNF, tissue necrosis factor; t-PA, tissue plasminogen activator; TT, thrombin time.

by procoagulants that are introduced or produced in the blood circulation and overcome the natural anticoagulant mechanisms. DIC may cause tissue ischemia from occlusive microthrombi as well as bleeding from both the consumption of platelets and coagulation factors and the anticoagulant effect of products of secondary fibrinolysis. DIC complicates a variety of disorders, and the complexity of its pathophysiology has made it the subject of a voluminous literature, including books,[1-7] book chapters, review articles, and case studies.[4,7-18]

In 1834, Dupuy reported that injection of brain material into animals caused widespread clots in blood vessels, thus providing the first description of DIC.[19] Trousseau, in 1865,[20] described the tendency to thrombosis, sometimes disseminated, in cachectic patients with malignancies. Naunyn, in 1873,[21] showed that disseminated thrombosis could be evoked by intravenous injection of dissolved red cells, and Wooldridge[22,23] then demonstrated that the procoagulant involved was a substance contained in the stroma of the red cells.

The mechanism by which DIC can lead to bleeding was clarified only in 1961, when Lasch and coworkers introduced the concept of consumption coagulopathy,[24] and McKay established that DIC is a pathogenetic feature of a variety of diseases.[1] Sizable series of cases were first described in 1967, following the introduction of defined laboratory criteria for DIC.[8] Yet in spite of the vast experience that has been accumulated, DIC still constitutes a major clinicopathologic and therapeutic challenge.

ETIOLOGY AND PATHOGENESIS

PATHOLOGY

Extensive data on autopsy findings in cases with DIC are available.[1,7,9,15,25-35] Common findings include diffuse multiorgan bleeding, hemorrhagic necrosis, microthrombi in small blood vessels, and thrombi in medium and large blood vessels. Not all patients who had unequivocal clinical and laboratory signs of DIC had all these postmortem findings,[15,25,27,30] and conversely, some patients in whom clinical and laboratory signs were not consistent with DIC did have the typical autopsy findings.[15,26-28] This occasional lack of correlation between the clinical, laboratory, and pathologic findings still remains unexplained.

Organs most frequently involved by diffuse microthrombi are the lungs and kidneys, followed by the brain, heart, liver, spleen, adrenals, pancreas, and gut. Acute tubular necrosis is more frequent than renal cortical necrosis in patients with DIC.[25,27,31] A significant proportion of cases with chronic DIC have nonbacterial thrombotic endocarditis involving mainly the mitral and aortic valves.[15,27,28,33,34] Moreover, in a retrospective pathologic study, about 50 percent of patients with nonbacterial thrombotic endocarditis had DIC.[32] These heart lesions can be a source of arterial embolization, leading to infarction of the brain, kidneys, and myocardium.[32,34]

PATHOGENESIS

INITIATING FACTORS

The intravascular generation of substantial amounts of thrombin via the tissue factor pathway, combined with the failure of the natural blood coagulation inhibitory mechanisms, initiates DIC in most instances. The major clinical conditions causing DIC and the presumptive initiating pathways are shown in Fig. 126-1. Tissue factor is constitutively present in cell membranes of most tissues, including the media and adventitia of blood vessels. Under normal circumstances blood is not exposed to tissue factor. When, however, blood becomes exposed to tissues (e.g., with trauma, burns, or abruptio placentae) or cells foreign to blood enter the circulation (e.g., metastasis, leukemic cells, amniotic fluid embolism), the coagulation system is ignited.

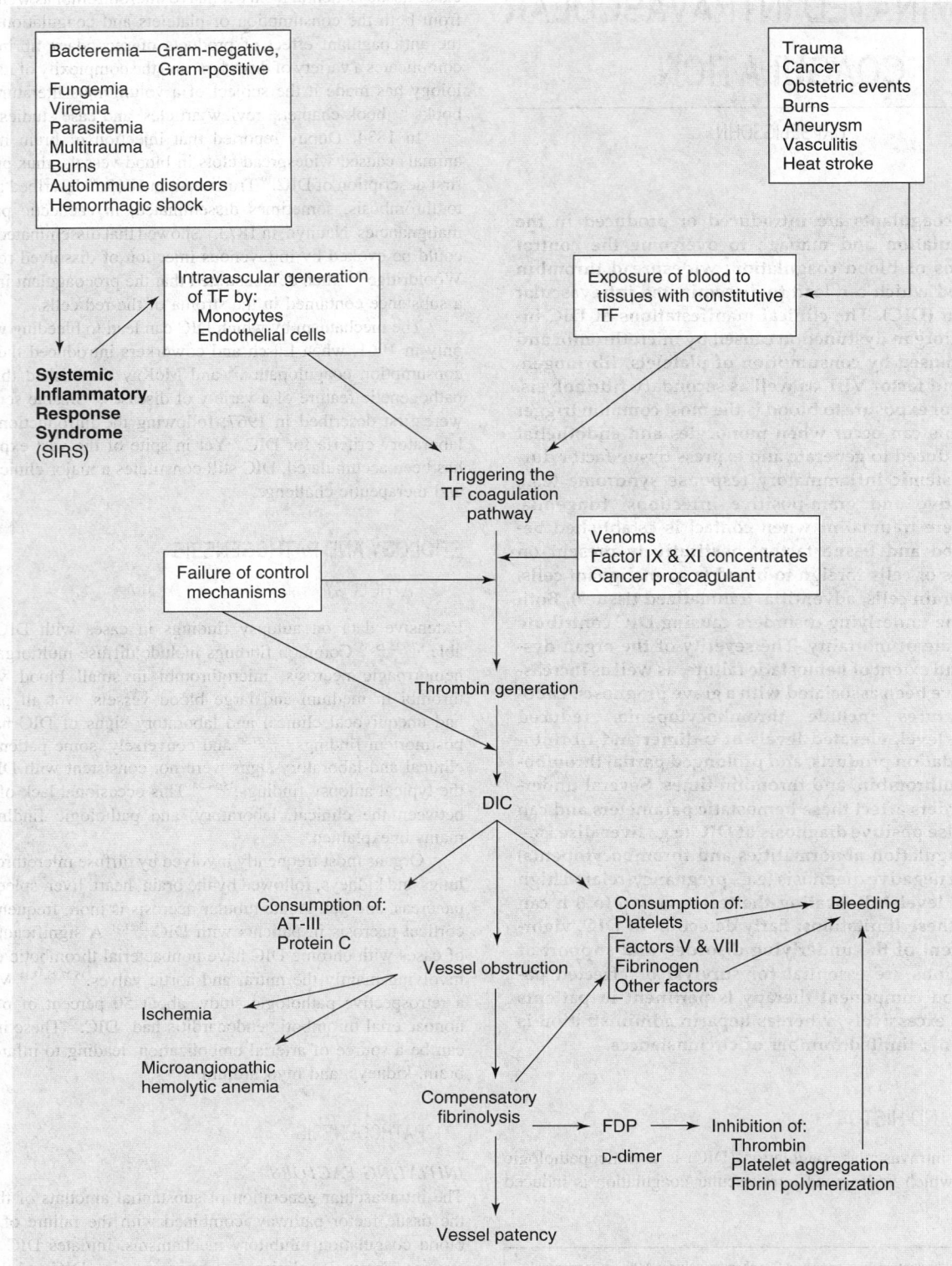

FIGURE 126-1   Initiation and consequences of DIC. TF, tissue factor; FDP, fibrinogen and fibrin degradation products.

Tissue factor can also be generated and expressed on membranes of monocytes and endothelial cells during the systemic inflammatory response syndrome (SIRS). SIRS designates a series of inflammatory events arising from a variety of infections or other insults like burns, trauma, or autoimmune disorders.[36,37] When bacteria are the cause of SIRS the severity of the syndrome can be graded as sepsis, severe sepsis, and septic shock,[36] with stepwise increases in the rates of DIC, multiorgan dysfunction, and mortality.[38–40]

The complex events that occur during SIRS involve monocytes, endothelial cells, neutrophils, and platelets; interactions among these cells; cytokines and other mediators; and activation of the complement system.[37] During these events, tissue factor can be generated and expressed by monocytes and by endothelial cells throughout the vasculature. In vitro studies and investigations of primates injected with live *Escherichia coli* and of humans injected with low doses of endotoxin have provided evidence that endotoxin can cause tissue factor exposure to blood by acting directly on monocytes and endothelial cells or by acting indirectly through monocyte secretion of tissue necrosis factor (TNF)-α, interleukin (IL)-1β, and IL-6.[41,42] Platelets can also be activated by endotoxin,[43] and activated platelets exhibiting P-selectin enhance tissue factor generation by monocytes.[44] Additional effects of endotoxin and the cytokines released in response to endotoxin include (1) down-regulation of the two major physiological inhibitory mechanisms of coagulation, endothelial cell thrombomodulin,[45] and glycosaminoglycans[46]; (2) brief enhancement of fibrinolysis by tissue plasminogen activator (t-PA) secretion from endothelial cells; and (3) longer-term profound inhibition of fibrinolysis caused by increased plasma concentrations of plasminogen activator inhibitor (PAI)-1.[42]

Initiation of DIC by activation of the contact system of coagulation during SIRS is probably unimportant. Thus, blockade of the contact system by a monoclonal antibody against factor XII does not prevent endotoxin-induced DIC,[47] and only a modest increase in factor XIIa$_\alpha$ is observed in patients with septic shock.[48] In contrast, neutrophils become activated during SIRS and release elastase, which both injures the vessel wall[49] and inactivates antithrombin.[50]

Less common initiators of DIC are: a cancer procoagulant that activates factor X, snake venoms that activate factor X or factor II, and activated coagulation factors that are variably contained in concentrates of coagulation factor IX and factor XI (see Infusion of Factor IX and Factor XI Concentrates, below).

The widespread generation of thrombin induces deposition of fibrin, which leads to vessel obstruction and consumption of substantial amounts of hemostatic factors, i.e., platelets; fibrinogen; factors V, VIII, and others; protein C (PC); and antithrombin-III (AT-III). These events result in tissue ischemia, mild microangiopathic hemolytic anemia, bleeding, and further impairment of the control mechanism of coagulation.

The intravascular thrombi and thrombin itself[51] trigger secretion of t-PA from endothelial cells, which sets off compensatory thrombolysis; this, if successful, leads to reopening of the occluded blood vessels. The by-products of thrombolysis, fibrin/fibrinogen degradation products, may, however, further enhance bleeding by interfering with platelet aggregation, fibrin polymerization, and thrombin activity (see Fig. 126-1).

CONTROL MECHANISMS

Several protective mechanisms either neutralize components that initiate DIC or correct its deleterious consequences. Thrombin generated in DIC can be effectively removed by the enormous endothelial cell surface area of the microcirculation by means of forming a complex with AT-III, which is bound to endothelial heparan sulfate,[52] and by binding to thrombomodulin on the endothelial surface. The latter interaction abolishes thrombin's procoagulant effects on fibrinogen,

factor XIII, and platelets, while enhancing activation of the anticoagulant protein PC. Activated PC, in turn, inactivates factors Va and VIIIa in the presence of protein S (PS) and exerts a profibrinolytic effect by inhibiting activation of thrombin activatable fibrinolysis inhibitor (TAFI).[53] Tissue factor pathway inhibitor (TFPI) is another line of defense at the vessel wall, although its effect is only exerted when relatively small amounts of tissue factor gain access to the circulation.[54] Thrombin binding to endothelial cells also stimulates the release of t-PA, thereby enhancing fibrinolysis.[51] Thus, as long as blood flow through the microcirculation is maintained, there is effective neutralization of procoagulant material, unless overwhelming amounts have entered the circulation.

The mononuclear phagocyte system also plays a role in protection from DIC. It can remove soluble tissue factor[55] and the soluble complexes of fibrin monomers.[56] Liver parenchymal cells also take part in the control of DIC by clearing activated factors IX, X, and XI from the circulation[57,58] and by replenishing depleted coagulation factors, plasminogen, α$_2$-antiplasmin, AT-III, and PC. The bone marrow is another tissue that plays an important role in the control of DIC by increasing the production of platelets by megakaryocytes.

The control mechanisms may be seriously compromised by the underlying disease that initiated the DIC. For example, leukemias may deplete or suppress the megakaryocyte pool, hepatic disease may impair both the synthetic and clearance functions of the liver, or shock may decrease neutralization of thrombin by decreasing blood flow through the microcirculation.

The manifestations of DIC depend on the magnitude and rate of exposure of blood to the DIC trigger. For example, the dramatic cases of "acute" DIC, characterized by severe bleeding due to excessive consumption of hemostatic components, may develop when blood is exposed to large amounts of tissue factor over a brief period of time. Such a trigger overwhelms the control mechanisms before any compensatory mechanisms have had enough time to respond. Alternatively, "chronic" DIC develops when blood is continuously or intermittently exposed to small amounts of tissue factor. In such instances, the control mechanisms have time to partially contain the DIC trigger and replenish the depleted coagulation, fibrinolytic, and inhibitory proteins by augmented production. Under these circumstances, clinical signs may be minimal or altogether absent, and most coagulation tests will be only slightly impaired. More sensitive assays such as increased turnover of platelets and fibrinogen, increased levels of D-dimer (see Laboratory Features, below), and increased levels of fibrin/fibrinogen degradation products will, however, indicate that compensated chronic DIC is occurring.

FREQUENCY OF UNDERLYING DISORDERS

Numerous disorders can provoke DIC (see Fig. 126-1), but only a few constitute major causes, as can be inferred from retrospective clinical studies.[4,7,10,12,14–16] Infectious diseases and malignant disorders together account for about two-thirds of the DIC cases in the major series, except for one study[7] that included a disproportionately large number of obstetric cases (Table 126-1). Trauma was a major cause of DIC in two series,[10,12] probably reflecting the specialized nature of the clinical material in the two centers. Two Japanese series[14,15] had a relatively high proportion of cases with malignant diseases and a relatively low number of obstetric cases.

CLINICAL FEATURES

Clinical manifestations are attributable to the disseminated intravascular coagulation, to the underlying disease, or to both. Bleeding manifestations were common in all series of DIC cases, but considerable variation existed in the relative frequency of shock and of dysfunction

TABLE 126-1   THE RELATIVE FREQUENCY (%) OF MAJOR UNDERLYING DISEASES IN SERIES OF CASES WITH DIC

REFERENCE NUMBER	N	INFECTIOUS DISEASES	MALIGNANT DISEASES	SURGERY AND TRAUMA	LIVER DISEASES	OBSTETRIC DISORDERS	MISCELLANEOUS DISEASES
4	60	41	30	2	5	2	20
10	118	40	7	24	4	4	21
12	346	26	24	19	8	—	23
14	503	15	61	2	6	4	12
15	88	7	67	—	—	—	26
16	345	16	55	—	4	5	20
7	361	15	6	14	3	38	24

of the liver, kidney, lungs, and central nervous system (Table 126-2). These variations probably reflect the different nature of the underlying disorders in the respective series.

BLEEDING

Acute DIC is frequently heralded by hemorrhage into the skin at multiple sites.[4,10] Petechiae, ecchymoses, and oozing from venipunctures, arterial lines, catheters, and injured tissues are common. Bleeding may also occur on mucosal surfaces. Hemorrhage may be life threatening, with massive bleeding into the gastrointestinal tract,[10] lungs,[4] central nervous system, or orbit.[7] Patients with chronic DIC usually exhibit only minor skin and mucosal bleeding.

THROMBOSIS AND THROMBOEMBOLISM

Extensive organ dysfunction can result from microvascular thrombi or from venous and/or arterial thromboembolism. For example, involvement of the skin can cause hemorrhagic bullae, acral necrosis, and gangrene.[4,7] Thrombosis of major veins and arteries and pulmonary embolism occur but are rare[4,10]; cerebral embolism can complicate nonbacterial thrombotic endocarditis in patients with chronic DIC.[32]

SHOCK

Both the diseases underlying DIC and DIC itself can cause shock. For example, septicemia or excessive blood loss due to trauma or to obstetric complications can by themselves cause shock. Whatever may be the cause of shock, its advent in cases with DIC is of great concern.

RENAL DYSFUNCTION

Renal cortical ischemia induced by microthrombosis of afferent glomerular arterioles and acute tubular necrosis related to hypotension are the major causes of renal dysfunction in DIC. Oliguria, anuria,

azotemia, and hematuria were observed in 25 to 67 percent of the cases in all series (see Table 126-2).

LIVER DYSFUNCTION

Hepatocellular dysfunction sufficient to cause jaundice has been reported in 22 percent[10] and 57 percent[7] of patients with DIC. Infectious diseases and prolonged hypotension contribute to hepatic dysfunction.

CENTRAL NERVOUS SYSTEM DYSFUNCTION

Microthrombi, macrothrombi, emboli, and hemorrhage in the cerebral vasculature have all been held responsible for the nonspecific neurologic symptoms and signs displayed by patients with DIC.[4,9] These include coma, delirium, transient focal neurologic symptoms, and signs of meningeal irritation. Careful exclusion of causes other than DIC is essential.

PULMONARY DYSFUNCTION

Symptoms and signs of respiratory dysfunction in DIC range from transient hypoxemia in mild cases to pulmonary hemorrhage and adult respiratory distress syndrome (ARDS) in severe cases. While pulmonary hemorrhage is specific for DIC,[4,35] ARDS is not.[59–61] Pulmonary hemorrhage is heralded by hemoptysis, dyspnea, and chest pain, and physical examination reveals rales, wheezing, and occasionally a pleural friction rub. Chest X-rays show diffuse infiltration due to excessive intra-alveolar hemorrhage. ARDS is characterized by tachypnea, auscultatory silence, hypoxemia, low lung compliance, normal wedge pressure, and "white lungs" on chest X-rays.[60] It stems from severe damage to the pulmonary vascular endothelium, which permits egress of blood components into the pulmonary interstitium and alveoli. This leads to intra-alveolar hyaline membrane formation and severe respiratory insufficiency. ARDS can be caused by septic shock, severe trauma, fat embolism, amniotic fluid embolism, and heat stroke—all

TABLE 126-2   FREQUENCY (%) OF CLINICAL MANIFESTATIONS IN SERIES OF CASES WITH DIC

REFERENCE NUMBER	N	BLEEDING	THROMBO-EMBOLISM	RENAL DYSFUNCTION	LIVER DYSFUNCTION	RESPIRATORY DYSFUNCTION	CNS MANIFES-TATIONS	SHOCK	ACRAL CYANOSIS	MISCELLANEOUS MANIFESTATIONS
4	60	87	22	67	*	78	65	*	14	8
9	89	76	23	39	*	*	11	*	0	14
10	118	64	8	25	22	16	2	14	0	22
11	47	87	47	40	†	38	†	†	†	—
12	346	77	†	†	†	†	†	†	†	—
7	361	73	11	61	57	37	13	55	13‡	—

*Difficulties in defining relationship to DIC.
†Not mentioned.
‡Including necrotizing purpura and acral gangrene.

of which can also incite DIC. Yet, only a fraction of patients with ARDS exhibit signs of DIC.[59] When DIC and ARDS are simultaneously triggered, each will aggravate the other. Regardless of the mechanism, ARDS is a serious complication in patients with DIC.

MORTALITY

Both DIC and its underlying disorders contribute to the high rate of mortality. Mortality is correlated independently with the extent of organ dysfunction,[10] the degree of hemostatic failure,[10,17] and increasing age.[10] Mortality rates in major series of patients with DIC ranged from 31 to 86 percent,[10–12,18,39,62] whether or not heparin was administered.

LABORATORY FEATURES

Knowledge of the potential underlying disorders can lead to early detection of acute and chronic DIC. Laboratory tests confirm or exclude a presumptive diagnosis of DIC, discriminate acute from chronic DIC, and distinguish between DIC associated with secondary fibrinolysis and primary fibrinogenolysis. They may also provide guidelines for treatment, help monitor therapy, and provide predictive information with regard to mortality.[10,18] The underlying diseases themselves, however, may affect the laboratory findings. For example, impairment of hemostasis, and/or thrombocytopenia unrelated to DIC, can arise from hepatic disease and from marrow involvement by leukemia; impaired hemostasis may also occur normally in the neonatal period. Conversely, the elevated levels of some hemostatic components that are normally observed during pregnancy may obscure the presence of DIC. These limitations in laboratory diagnosis of DIC can be overcome by repeating the tests every 6 to 8 h and observing the dynamics of the process.

ACUTE DIC

Patients with acute DIC are critically ill, and therefore rapid diagnosis is essential. The following tests are adequate: platelet count, prothrombin time (PT), activated partial thromboplastin time (aPTT), D-dimer, thrombin time (TT), fibrinogen level, fibrinogen degradation products (FDP), and a blood film to check for fragmented red cells. These parameters will reflect the extent of consumption of hemostatic components, the presence of by-products of in vivo thrombin generation, and the extent of secondary fibrinolysis. In most instances, changes in three or more parameters in addition to a decreased platelet count are consistent with DIC, and no further tests are necessary. A normal fibrinogen level may, however, be present relatively early in DIC since many of the underlying disorders are associated with increased fibrinogen levels, and thus the increased fibrinogen consumption may not have had sufficient time to decrease the fibrinogen below normal levels. Since the normal fibrinogen half-life time is approximately 4 days, a 50 percent or greater decrease in fibrinogen level over a 1-day period is compelling evidence supporting DIC or fibrinolysis, regardless of whether the final value is within the normal range.

Several DIC scoring systems based on laboratory data[10] or a combination of laboratory data and clinical manifestations[16] have been proposed to assess the severity of DIC. These scores have prognostic value, since good correlations have been found between the degree of abnormality of the laboratory results and the extent of organ involvement, as well as between the severity of hemostatic impairment and subsequent mortality.[10,18]

Assay of plasma D-dimer is very useful for evaluation of patients with acute DIC.[63,64] Increased levels indicate that cross-linked fibrin generated by thrombin has been digested by plasmin.

The presence of thrombin-AT-III (TAT) complexes[65] and of plasmin-antiplasmin (PAP) complexes[66] reflect the extent of activation of the coagulation and fibrinolytic systems, respectively.[67] Patients with sepsis-induced DIC usually have high levels of TAT and low levels of PAP, indicating that the balance is tipped to thrombosis rather than fibrinolysis, resulting in multiorgan dysfunction, whereas patients with acute promyelocytic leukemia may have high PAP levels associated with bleeding due to excessive fibrino(geno)lysis[67] (see Leukemia, below).

CHRONIC DIC

A continuous or intermittent slow rate of initiation of intravascular coagulation occurs in distinct clinical entities including metastatic carcinoma, giant hemangioma, or the dead fetus syndrome. In these conditions the control mechanisms may effectively prevent severe clinical manifestations by neutralizing active enzymes and by augmenting the synthesis of the consumed hemostatic components. Consequently, laboratory tests reveal variable values. For example, the platelet count may be only mildly reduced, fibrinogen levels can be normal or high, and the PT and aPTT may be within normal limits. However, there usually are increases in fibrin(ogen) degradation products and D-dimer levels. Fragmented red cells are commonly, but not universally, found in DIC, but the degree of fragmentation is almost always less than that usually observed in thrombotic thrombocytopenic purpura.

DIC ACCOMPANIED BY PRIMARY FIBRINO(GENO)LYSIS

When DIC is accompanied by primary fibrino(geno)lysis, both the coagulation and the fibrinolytic systems are triggered concomitantly, that is, thrombin and plasmin are generated independently. The typical laboratory findings are a decreased platelet count, increased levels of D-dimer, shortened whole blood clot lysis, shortened euglobulin lysis time, and very high levels of fibrin(ogen) degradation products. However, these crude parameters can also be abnormal when there is DIC and secondary fibrinolysis, and therefore the distinction between DIC with secondary fibrinolysis from DIC accompanied by primary fibrino(geno)lysis is not clear. Notwithstanding these difficult ambiguities in pathophysiology, a pattern of DIC associated with primary fibrino(geno)lysis occurs in acute promyelocytic leukemia, heat stroke, metastatic prostatic carcinoma, and amniotic fluid embolism (see the discussions of these conditions under Specific Underlying Disorders, below).

PRIMARY FIBRINOGENOLYSIS

Primary fibrinogenolysis occurs when plasmin is generated in the absence of DIC. This has been described in hepatic disorders, prostatic carcinoma, and cases without an apparent cause. At present, most cases of primary fibrinogenolysis are iatrogenically induced during thrombolytic therapy (see Chap. 134). Primary fibrinogenolysis can be distinguished from DIC by finding a normal platelet count, rapid whole blood clot lysis, shortened euglobulin lysis time, and greatly elevated fibrinogen degradation products. Theoretically, D-dimer levels should be normal, but elevated levels are often found in states of primary fibrino(geno)lysis such as t-PA therapy.

THERAPY

No controlled studies of patients with DIC have been performed. Such studies are difficult to carry out in view of the variabilities in DIC triggers, clinical presentations, and grades of severity. Fig. 126-2 shows

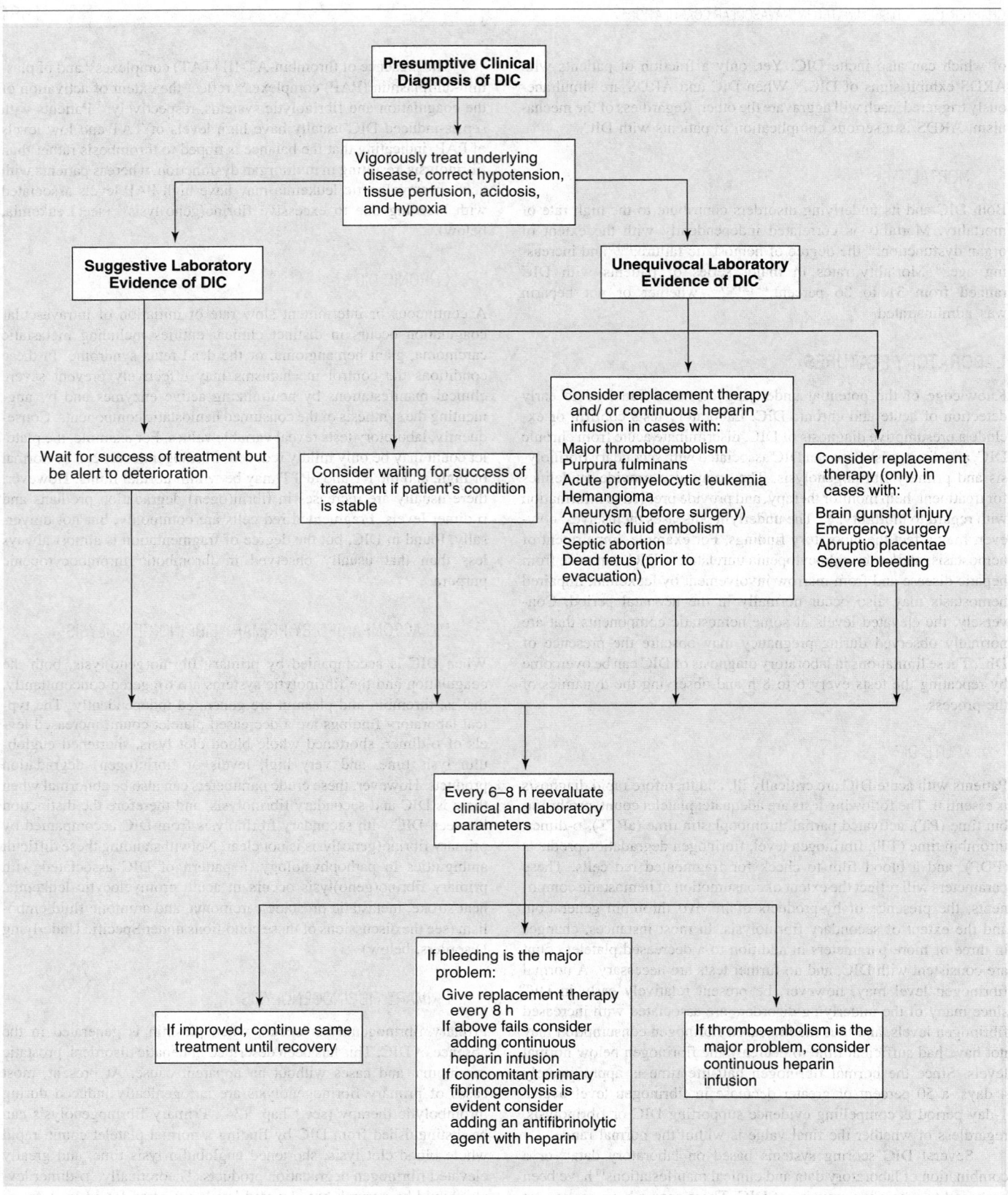

FIGURE 126-2 General guidelines for initial treatment and follow-up of patients with DIC. The success of management is related to taking rapid, vigorous measures against the underlying disease; close clinical observation; thoughtful consideration in each individual patient; availability of 24-h coagulation laboratory services; and an adequate supply of platelet concentrates, cryoprecipitate, fresh-frozen plasma, and packed red cells for replacement therapy. Heparin, when indicated, should be administered by continuous infusion. The basis and limitations of each of the outlined recommendations are detailed throughout the text.

general guidelines for management of patients with DIC, but decisions regarding treatment must be individualized after all clinically important aspects have been carefully considered.

MANAGEMENT OF UNDERLYING DISORDERS

The survival of patients with DIC depends on vigorous treatment of the underlying disorders so as to curtail the triggers of blood coagulation. Examples of such treatment are intensive antibiotic treatment in patients with gram-negative bacteremia, hysterectomy in patients with abruptio placentae, resection of an aortic aneurysm, and debridement of crushed tissues.

The underlying disease and DIC itself frequently compromise the patient's vital functions. This results in further aggravation of DIC, and therefore intensive support of vital functions is required. Volume replacement and correction of hypotension and oxygenation will improve blood flow through the microcirculation, thus restoring the functions of blood coagulation inhibitory systems. Careful monitoring of pulmonary, cardiac, and renal function enables prompt institution of supportive measures, such as use of a respirator for better oxygenation, inotropic drugs for improvement of cardiac output, and maintenance of electrolyte balance.

BLOOD COMPONENT THERAPY

Although commonly quoted as fact, the hypothesis that hemostatic replacement therapy in DIC "fuels the fire" has never been proved. Platelet concentrates, cryoprecipitate, and fresh-frozen plasma contain the hemostatic factors and inhibitors of blood coagulation commonly depleted in patients with DIC. In general, patients should be transfused with blood components only when they have bleeding and depleted hemostatic factors. Also eligible are patients being prepared for emergency surgery and patients with gunshot-induced brain injury. Replacement therapy for thrombocytopenia should consist of 6 to 10 units of platelet concentrate, ideally attempting to raise the platelet count to more than 50,000 to 100,000/μl; for hypofibrinogenemia (<100 mg/dl), 8 to 10 units of cryoprecipitate; and for depletion of other coagulation factors, 1 to 2 units of fresh-frozen plasma depending on the severity of the depletion and the patient's body weight. Replacement therapy may need to be repeated every 8 h, with adjustment of doses according to the platelet count, PT, aPTT, fibrinogen level, and volume status. Fibrin(ogen) degradation products and D-dimer are not very useful for monitoring therapy because their clearance can be delayed, especially in cases of renal dysfunction, and because fibrinogen degradation products can be elevated due to earlier transfusion of stored plasma products. Infusions should be stopped as soon as normal or near-normal values of hemostatic factors are attained. Prothrombin complex concentrates are contraindicated in view of their potential prothrombotic effect.

HEPARIN ADMINISTRATION

In most clinical circumstances, patients with DIC are seen when the process is already well established. None of the clinical reports has shown a reduction in mortality in patients with DIC treated with heparin; heparin has, at best, improved the levels of hemostatic factors in the treated patients.[68] In contrast, heparin administration can seriously aggravate bleeding in such patients,[9,11] especially when the patients have severe hemostatic failure due to consumption and when there is hepatic or renal dysfunction. Moreover, heparin can exacerbate bleeding from sites of traumatic injury. Heparin may, in fact, have reduced anticoagulant effect in DIC, since AT-III is commonly de-

pleted and fibrin monomers, which are produced during DIC, protect thrombin from inactivation by heparin-AT-III complex.[69]

Notwithstanding these considerations, administration of heparin is beneficial in some categories of chronic DIC, e.g., metastatic carcinomas, purpura fulminans, dead fetus syndrome (at time of removal), and aortic aneurysm (prior to resection). Heparin is also indicated for treating thromboembolic complications in large vessels and before surgery in patients with chronic DIC (see Fig. 126-2). Heparin administration may also be helpful in patients with acute DIC when intensive blood component replacement fails to improve excessive bleeding, or when thrombosis threatens to cause irreversible tissue injury (e.g., acute cortical necrosis of the kidney or digital gangrene).

Heparin should be used cautiously in all the above conditions. In chronic DIC a continuous infusion of heparin, 500 to 750 U/h without a bolus injection, may be sufficient. If no response is obtained within 24 h, escalating dosages can be used. In hyperacute DIC cases, such as mismatched transfusion, amniotic fluid embolism, septic abortion, and purpura fulminans, an intravenous bolus injection of 5000 to 10,000 units of heparin may be given simultaneously with replacement therapy with blood products; some experts would not give a bolus dose of heparin even under these circumstances. A continuous infusion of 500 to 1000 U/h of heparin may be necessary to maintain the benefit until the underlying disease responds to treatment.

ANTITHROMBIN-III CONCENTRATE

AT-III concentrate infusion has been used in the treatment of patients with DIC, either alone or in combination with heparin,[70,71] but only small numbers of patients have been studied. In one double-blind controlled study of patients with DIC and septic shock, large doses of AT-III concentrate caused a shortening of the duration of DIC and lowered the mortality by 44 percent, but this decline did not reach statistical significance.[72] Two additional trials that await completion show similar trends.[73] Thus, no definitive recommendations regarding the clinical use of AT-III concentrate can be made at present.

INHIBITORS OF FIBRINOLYSIS

Patients with DIC should not be treated with antifibrinolytic agents like ϵ-aminocaproic acid or tranexamic acid since these drugs block the secondary fibrinolysis that accompanies DIC and presumably helps to preserve tissue perfusion. Indeed, the use of these agents in patients with DIC has been complicated by severe thrombosis.[74,75]

A different situation prevails in patients with DIC accompanied by primary fibrino(geno)lysis, as in some cases of acute promyelocytic leukemia, giant hemangioma, heat stroke, amniotic fluid embolism, some forms of liver disease, and metastatic carcinoma of the prostate. In these conditions the use of fibrinolytic inhibitors can be considered, provided that (1) the patient is bleeding profusely and has not responded to replacement therapy; and (2) excessive fibrino(geno)lysis is observed, i.e., rapid whole blood clot lysis or a very short euglobulin lysis time. In such circumstances the use of antifibrinolytic agents should be preceded by replacement of depleted blood components and continuous heparin infusion.

OTHER TREATMENT MODALITIES

Gabexate mesilate and nafamostat mesilate[76,77] are synthetic serine protease inhibitors that have been used in Japan for the treatment of patients with DIC. A study of 395 DIC patients given gabexate mesilate for 1 week demonstrated improvement in 58 percent of the cases, mainly in their hemostatic factors.[18] Other preparations have been successfully tested in animals and in a few patients. For example, a protein C concentrate appeared to be helpful in four children with DIC induced by meningococcemia.[78] Other agents, such as anti-tissue-factor antibodies[79,80] or active-site-inhibited factor VIIa,[81] have been shown in experimental animals not only to prevent endotoxin-induced DIC but also to attenuate the lethal inflammatory effects of *E. coli*. Similarly, recombinant tissue factor pathway inhibitor (TFPI) produced good results in animals, and clinical trials are in progress.[82] Clinical trials employing antiendotoxin monoclonal antibodies in patients with gram-negative septicemia have been described, but the efficacy of this treatment modality is inconclusive.[83–85] More promising results have been obtained with recombinant IL-10 in human subjects injected with small doses of endotoxin.[86] IL-10 not only inhibited the release of TNF-α and IL-1β, but was found to inhibit the coagulant and fibrinolytic responses.[86]

SPECIFIC UNDERLYING DISORDERS

INFECTIOUS DISEASES

Bacterial infections are among the most common causes of DIC. Certain clinical conditions make patients particularly vulnerable to infection-induced DIC. For instance, pregnant women, who have reduced plasma PS levels and diminished fibrinolytic activity, are predisposed to severe infection-induced DIC; asplenic patients have a tendency to develop fulminant DIC, which is related to their inability to clear bacteria, particularly pneumococci[87]; and newborns have a similar vulnerability, which is probably related to immaturity of their coagulation inhibitory systems. Infections are also frequently superimposed on trauma and malignancies, which are themselves potential triggers of DIC. In addition, infections can aggravate bleeding and thrombosis by directly inducing thrombocytopenia, hepatic dysfunction, and shock, with diminished blood flow in the microcirculation.

GRAM-NEGATIVE INFECTIONS

Meningococcemia is a fulminant gram-negative infection characterized by extensive hemorrhagic necrosis, DIC, and shock. The extent of the hemostatic derangement in patients with meningococcemia correlates with prognosis.[88,89] Heparin treatment is of questionable benefit in meningococcemia.

More frequent gram-negative infections associated with DIC are caused by *Pseudomonas aeruginosa, E. coli,* and *Proteus vulgaris.* Patients affected by such bacteremias may have only laboratory signs of DIC[10] or may have severe DIC, especially when shock develops.[90] Under the latter conditions, persistently low levels of AT-III and PC predict a fatal outcome.[72] The presentation in extreme cases may be reminiscent of the generalized Shwartzman reaction.[91] Mortality is very high, even if vigorous antibiotic therapy and supportive measures are promptly instituted. Heparin administration has, so far, not been shown to have a clear benefit. Some investigators failed to demonstrate any effect of heparin on mortality, though they did show a slight improvement in laboratory findings,[18,68] while others[62] found an increased rate of survival in patients who had received heparin. In view of these conflicting reports, heparin therapy should only be considered in special cases such as pregnant women with gram-negative septicemia[92] and patients who present with skin necrosis.

GRAM-POSITIVE INFECTIONS

Staphylococcus aureus bacteremia can cause DIC[48] accompanied by renal cortical and dermal necrosis.[93] The mechanism by which DIC is produced may be related to an α toxin that activates platelets and induces IL-1 secretion by macrophages.[94] *Streptococcus pneumoniae* infection has been associated with the Waterhouse-Friderichsen syn-

drome[95] and with acral gangrene,[96] particularly in asplenic patients.[87] Initiation of DIC in these conditions is ascribed to the capsular antigen of the bacterium and to antigen-antibody complex formation.[97]

Other gram-positive bacteria that can cause DIC are the anaerobic clostridia. Clostridial bacteremia is a highly lethal disease characterized by septic shock, DIC, renal failure, and hemolytic anemia.[98,99]

OTHER INFECTIONS

Common viral infections such as influenza, varicella, rubella, and rubeola have rarely been associated with DIC.[100] However, purpura fulminans associated with DIC has been reported in patients with infections and either hereditary thrombophilias[101] or acquired antibodies to PS.[102] Other viral infections can cause ''hemorrhagic fevers'' characterized by fever, hypotension, bleeding, and renal failure. Laboratory evidence of DIC can accompany Korean and dengue-related hemorrhagic fevers[103,104] but apparently not the Argentine hemorrhagic fever.[105] Release of tissue factor from cells in which viruses replicate[106] and increased levels of TNF-α have been suggested as mechanisms for initiation of the tissue factor pathway in these conditions.[107]

Fungal infections[108,109] and miliary tuberculosis[110] have also at times been associated with DIC. In falciparum malaria, thrombocytopenia is common but overt DIC is very rare.[111] However, activation of the coagulation system with elevated levels of TAT complexes has been reported.[112]

PURPURA FULMINANS

Purpura fulminans is a severe, often lethal form of DIC in which extensive areas of the skin over the extremities and buttocks undergo hemorrhagic necrosis. The disease affects infants and children predominantly[113,114] but occasionally also adults.[115] Biopsy of the skin lesions reveals diffuse microthrombi in small blood vessels and vasculitis. Its onset can be within 2 to 4 weeks of a mild infection such as scarlet fever, varicella, or rubella or can occur during an acute viral or bacterial infection in patients with acquired[114] or hereditary thrombophilias[101] affecting the PC inhibitory pathway. Homozygous PC deficiency presents in neonates soon after birth as purpura fulminans,[116] with or without thrombosis.[117]

Patients affected by purpura fulminans are acutely ill with fever, hypotension, and hemorrhage from multiple sites; they frequently have typical laboratory signs of DIC.[113,114] Full heparinization can be beneficial in these patients[113,114] and should be supplemented by transfusion of the depleted hemostatic components. PC concentrate has been reported to be beneficial both in cases due to inherited deficiency of PC and in cases in which acquired PC deficiency accompanies purpura fulminans.[78,114] Excision of necrotic skin areas and grafting are indispensable at a later stage.

SOLID TUMORS

Trousseau was the first to describe the propensity to thrombosis of patients with cancerous cachexia,[20] and evidence for malignancy-related primary fibrino(geno)lysis and/or DIC was provided 70 years ago.[118] A recent review of the subject is available.[119]

In 182 patients with malignant disorders, excessive bleeding was recorded in 75 cases, venous thrombosis in 123, migratory thrombophlebitis in 96, arterial thrombosis in 45, and arterial embolism due to nonbacterial thrombotic endocarditis in 31.[120] Multifocal hemorrhagic infarctions of the brain, caused by fibrin microemboli and manifested as disorders of consciousness, have also been described.[121] Patients with solid tumors and DIC are more prone to thrombosis than to bleeding, while patients with leukemia and DIC are more prone to hemorrhage.

Both bleeding and thromboembolism stem from the DIC that is initiated by exposure of the blood to tissue factor present in carcinomas.[122-125] A factor X–activating procoagulant present in the mucin secreted by adenocarcinomas was postulated as a cause of DIC in some patients,[126] but this observation could not be confirmed.[125] A third postulated mechanism for triggering the coagulation system is via activation of factor X by a cysteine proteinase or "cancer procoagulant."[127] However, this material was found to contain tissue factor and to exert only a weak effect on activation of factor X.[125]

Depending on the rate and quantity of exposure or influx of shed vesicles from tumors containing tissue factor,[128] a decompensated, compensated, or overcompensated hemostatic state develops.[126] For instance, a patient may be asymptomatic or present with venous thromboembolism (Trousseau syndrome) if the tumor cells expose or release tissue factor slowly or intermittently and the ensuing utilization of fibrinogen and platelets is compensated by increased production of these components. Conversely, massive thrombosis[130] or severe bleeding[9,11] may supervene in a patient whose circulation is deluged by tissue factor.

Patients with solid tumors are vulnerable to additional triggers of DIC that can aggravate thromboembolism and bleeding. These triggers include septicemia, immobilization, suppression of platelet production by chemotherapy, and involvement by metastases of the liver, which impede the role of the liver in the control of DIC.

Microangiopathic hemolytic anemia is frequently induced by DIC in patients with malignancies and is particularly severe in patients with widespread intravascular metastases of mucin-secreting adenocarcinomas.[131]

Chronic DIC associated with malignancy can be treated successfully by heparinization.[120,125] The indications include arterial or venous thrombosis, significant bleeding, preparation for surgery, and prophylaxis before institution of intensive chemotherapy. Replacement of depleted blood components may be required during initial heparinization, but once appropriate anticoagulation has been achieved DIC usually abates. Treatment can then be followed by subcutaneous unfractionated heparin[125] or low molecular weight heparin,[132] but not warfarin.[125] Patients with neoplastic disorders who develop acute severe DIC can also be treated by heparinization, but the results are only partially successful.[9] Patients with prostatic carcinoma exhibiting primary fibrinogenolysis or DIC with extensive secondary fibrinolysis can be treated successfully by ε-aminocaproic acid[133] or by tranexamic acid, but only after heparin has begun to mitigate the DIC. However, the diagnosis should be unequivocal in view of the hazards involved when antifibrinolytic agents are used in patients with DIC and secondary fibrinolysis,[74,75] and other precautions should be taken as well (see "Therapy").

LEUKEMIAS

In 1935, bleeding together with a low fibrinogen level was noted in a patient with acute myelocytic leukemia.[134] Since then, numerous reports have been published on DIC and fibrinolysis complicating the course of acute leukemias. Although relatively uncommon among the acute leukemias, acute promyelocytic leukemia (APL) is the entity most frequently associated with life-threatening hemorrhage. The pathogenesis of the hemostatic disturbance in APL and the implied therapeutic approach are complex.[135,136] One school of thought maintains that severe DIC accompanied by profound secondary fibrinolysis is responsible for the abnormalities, and therefore heparin should be administered during induction therapy. This hypothesis is based upon (1) postmortem examinations that showed widespread thrombosis in such patients[137-139]; (2) finding tissue factor in cells of patients with

APL,[140,141] a factor X–activating proteinase,[142] and excessive IL-1 production that induces tissue factor synthesis in monocytes and endothelial cells[143]; and (3) demonstration of increased levels of prothrombin fragment 1.2 and TAT complexes.[144] However, clinical experience in patients with APL failed to show an unequivocal advantage for heparin therapy over support by blood products[145,146] or use of antifibrinolytic agents.[146]

Other authorities regard primary fibrinogenolysis as the predominant cause of the serious bleeding in patients with APL.[147] This hypothesis is based on finding (1) urokinase-type plasminogen activator[148] and t-PA[149] in leukemic cells from patients with APL; (2) low plasma levels of α₂-antiplasmin[150]; and (3) decreased activity of plasminogen activator inhibitor.[151] Consequently, treatment with antifibrinolytic agents has been recommended.[146,147,150]

It is not unlikely that patients with APL may have concomitant DIC and primary fibrino(geno)lysis and that both processes are triggered by the leukemic cells to variable extents. Introduction of sensitive tests recording the relative magnitude of thrombin and of plasmin generation (TAT and PAP assays)[67] may provide information as to when, in a given patient, one should administer heparin, when to use an antifibrinolytic agent, or perhaps both. In any case, treatment should always include blood component replacement until balanced hemostasis is achieved.

The introduction of all-*trans*-retinoic acid (ATRA) in the treatment of patients with APL raised hopes that the APL coagulopathy might be ameliorated, since it was shown in vitro that ATRA therapy decreased the production of tissue factor by leukemic cells and increased thrombomodulin expression.[152] Indeed, in several uncontrolled studies the hemostatic abnormalities have improved when ATRA was used.[135,136] However, in a controlled study of 346 patients with APL, early mortality from hemorrhage was similar in patients whose induction therapy consisted of ATRA (6%) or chemotherapy (7%).[153] Moreover, thrombotic events were also observed by several authors in patients who received ATRA, and these events were either related or unrelated to the "ATRA syndrome."[154-157]

A high incidence of DIC, particularly during induction therapy without L-asparaginase, has also been described in adult patients with acute lymphoblastic leukemia.[158] The pathogenesis of DIC in these patients is not clear at present. Platelet transfusions and cryoprecipitate and plasma replacement seem effective in such patients.[158]

TRAUMA

When DIC complicates trauma it usually occurs in severely injured patients. Extensive exposure of tissue factor to the blood circulation and hemorrhagic shock are probably the most immediate triggers of DIC in such instances. Later, however, DIC can be induced within the framework of the systemic inflammatory response syndrome (SIRS) that not infrequently accompanies multiorgan trauma. A series of elegant studies has demonstrated that the levels of TNF-α, IL-1β, PAI-1, circulating tissue factor, plasma elastase derived from neutrophils, and soluble thrombomodulin are all elevated in patients who have signs of DIC.[159-161] Moreover, DIC is a predictor of the multiple organ dysfunction syndrome (ARDS included) and death. Careful monitoring of laboratory signs of DIC, of reduced fibrinolytic activity, and perhaps of AT-III level[162] are useful for predicting the outcome of such patients.

DIC can be aggravated in patients with severe trauma who require massive blood replacement since stored blood does not contain platelets or sufficient amounts of factors V or VIII. Moreover, infection is common in such patients and may contribute to the DIC.

The time interval between trauma and medical intervention correlates with the development and magnitude of DIC. Experience during the Vietnam war proved that fast evacuation and prompt medical care reduces the risk of DIC.[163] Debridement of damaged tissues to arrest the influx of tissue factor into the circulation is of paramount importance. Vital functions such as blood flow through the microcirculation and respiratory, cardiac, and renal performance must be monitored and supported; measures also need to be taken against potential infections. Transfusion of appropriate blood components should be given to replenish the consumed or lost clotting factors and platelets. Use of an AT-III concentrate has been tried,[70,71,164] but the limited data currently available do not provide unequivocal evidence for its efficacy.

BRAIN INJURY

Brain injury can be associated with DIC, most likely because the injury exposes the abundant tissue factor of brain tissue to blood. The DIC can cause serious bleeding,[165] but transfusion of platelets and plasma components can effectively arrest bleeding.[166] In fatal cases DIC was confirmed by the presence of microthrombi in the brain, liver, lungs, kidneys, and pancreas.[167] Studies of adults and children with head injuries have shown a high rate of mortality when DIC is present.[168] In fact, a laboratory DIC score has predictive value for prognosis of patients with head injuries, thereby supplementing the Glasgow coma score.[168,169] Hence, though bleeding in patients with DIC related to brain injury can be managed by replacement therapy, it carries a grave prognosis.

BURNS

Tissue factor exposed to blood at sites of burned tissue, the systemic inflammatory response syndrome induced by the burn, and the commonly present superimposed infections can all trigger DIC in patients with burns. Bleeding, laboratory tests indicative of DIC, and vascular microthrombi in biopsies of undamaged skin have all been described in patients with extensive burns.[170] Kinetic studies with labeled fibrinogen and labeled platelets disclosed that in addition to systemic consumption of hemostatic factors, significant local consumption also takes place in burned areas.[171] A clinicopathologic study of 139 patients who died during treatment for a severe burn disclosed that 18 percent had cerebral infarctions caused by septic arterial occlusions or DIC and about 4 percent had intracranial hemorrhage.[172]

Replacement therapy with blood components is the treatment of choice in patients with burns and bleeding, due to low levels of hemostatic components. Heparin should be avoided if possible.

LIVER DISEASES

Very complicated derangements of hemostasis occur in patients with severe liver disease and during liver transplantation (see also Chap. 125). There is reduced synthesis of most coagulation factors and natural anticoagulants (PC, PS, and AT-III) and of the main components of the fibrinolytic system (plasminogen and α_2-antiplasmin). In addition, there is decreased capacity of the liver to clear the circulation of activated factors IX, X, and XI as well as t-PA.[57,58,173] Moreover, thrombocytopenia is common as a result of hypersplenism. The similarities between the hemostatic defects observed in patients with liver disease and in patients with DIC are therefore striking and have evoked an ongoing controversy as to whether DIC contributes to hemostatic derangements associated with liver disease.[174,175]

Several laboratory and clinical observations support the hypothesis that DIC accompanies hepatic disorders. They include a shortened half-life of radiolabeled fibrinogen and prolongation of fibrinogen half-life by administration of heparin[176,177]; failure of replacement therapy to significantly increase the levels of hemostatic factors (suggesting

continuous consumption)[178]; and increased blood levels of D-dimer,[179] TAT complexes,[180,181] and fibrinopeptide A[182]—all indicative of ongoing thrombin generation.

Other observations and considerations argue against the hypothesis that DIC accompanies liver diseases. They include: (1) There is an extremely low incidence (2.2%) of microthrombosis in the tissues of patients who die of liver disease[183]; and (2) Many of the hemostatic abnormalities of patients with hepatic disorders can stem from causes other than DIC or are not consistent with DIC. Examples of alternative explanations include: (a) A prolonged thrombin time may be due to acquired dysfibrinogenemia.[184] (b) Low levels of coagulation factors and inhibitors may be due to reduced synthesis. (c) Increased FDP levels may be a consequence of primary fibrinogenolysis induced by reduced synthesis of α_2-antiplasmin and of plasminogen activator inhibitor-1 along with decreased clearance of t-PA. (d) Factor VIII levels are commonly increased rather than decreased.[185] (e) The kinetic data show that the apparently excessive consumption of fibrinogen can be explained by loss of fibrinogen into extravascular spaces.[186] (f) Fibrinogen and plasminogen do not appear to be removed rapidly when labeled endogenously by ^{75}Se-selenomethionine.[187]

A third hypothesis maintains that patients with liver disease usually do not present with DIC but are extremely sensitive to the various triggers of DIC in view of their impeded capacity to clear procoagulants and to synthesize essential components of the coagulation, inhibitory, and fibrinolytic systems. Indeed, patients with primary or metastatic liver disease who undergo a peritoneovenous shunt operation for severe ascites are more likely to develop DIC than are patients with ascites who undergo the same procedure because of other causes.[188]

What, then, should be the approach to patients with liver disease and bleeding without an apparent local cause? First, possible underlying causes of DIC should be carefully considered and identified, and then a hemostatic profile should be examined at frequent intervals in order to detect any dynamic changes that may be helpful for recognizing DIC. The sensitive assays that reflect thrombin generation (TAT complex) or concomitant thrombin and plasmin generation (D-dimer) may help to establish the diagnosis of DIC in a patient with liver disease.[189]

Given the present diagnostic limitations and therefore the uncertainty as to whether a patient is bleeding because of liver disease per se or because of superimposed DIC, the treatment should consist of replacement of hemostatic factors, and if a DIC trigger is identified specific vigorous treatment should be instituted. Prothrombin complex concentrates containing activated clotting factors should be avoided in view of their potential thrombogenic effects. Antifibrinolytic agents can be considered in patients with severe bleeding who do not respond to replacement therapy, but evidence of fibrinolysis should be obtained and treatment preceded by continuous heparin infusion.

Clinical and laboratory signs of DIC have been observed in some patients after a peritoneovenous shunt procedure (the LeVeen shunt) for ascites associated with liver disease. In an early review of 278 patients with the LeVeen shunt, DIC was observed postoperatively in only 10 cases,[190] but other investigators have reported higher frequencies, with the shunt apparently contributing to death in some cases.[191] A review reported the elimination of the postshunt DIC by careful removal of the ascites fluid at the time of surgery.[192]

HEAT STROKE

Heat stroke is a syndrome characterized by a rise in body temperature to over 42°C that follows collapse of the thermoregulatory mechanism. The following predisposing factors have been identified: a high environmental temperature, strenuous physical activity, infection, dehydration, and lack of acclimatization.[193,194] Extensive hemorrhage, unclottable blood, and venous engorgement were found as early as 1838 in postmortem examination of patients who had died of heat stroke.[195] Investigations have confirmed that a severe hemorrhagic diathesis and multiple organ failure often accompany heat stroke.[193,196–199] Diffuse fibrin deposition and hemorrhagic infarctions are found in fatal human cases[197,200] and in dogs with experimental heat stroke.[201] DIC associated with profound fibrino(geno)lysis is evident in patients with heat stroke.[199,202–204] The possible triggers of DIC in patients with heat stroke include endothelial cell damage[205] and tissue factor released from heat-damaged tissues.

Both the severity of the syndrome and the stage of its development affect the type and magnitude of hemostatic alterations.[199,203,204] Thus, in a study of 56 patients, three groups were discernible: nonbleeders, bleeders without DIC but with slight consumption of hemostatic factors, and bleeders with typical signs of DIC.[199] Prompt cooling and support of vital functions have substantially reduced the high mortality that was commonly observed in early studies.[193] Replacement of hemostatic components is the treatment of choice when bleeding occurs.[194] Heparin administration may be beneficial[206–209] but carries a high risk,[210] as does treatment with antifibrinolytic agents.

SNAKE BITES

Several species of snakes belonging to the Viperidae family produce venoms that have a wide range of activities affecting hemostasis. Prominent among these species are the *Vipera, Echis* (*E. carinatus* or *E. coloratus*), *Aspis, Crotalus, Bothrops,* and *Agkistrodon.* Several reviews are available on the biochemistry, pathophysiology, and clinical aspects of snake bites.[211–217]

Venoms of the above-mentioned snakes contain enzymes or peptides that exert the following activities: (1) thrombin-like activity, cleaving fibrinopeptide A from the Aα chain of fibrinogen (*Agkistrodon rhodostoma*); (2) activation of prothrombin even in the absence of calcium ions (*Echis carinatus*); (3) activation of factors X and V (Russell viper venom); (4) fibrinogenolytic activity (*Agkistrodon acutus*)[214]; (5) induction of thrombocytopenia by platelet aggregation[214]; (6) inhibition of platelet aggregation by the low molecular weight arginine-glycine-aspartic acid-containing peptides from a variety of snake species[218]; (7) activation of protein C[219]; and (8) activities causing damage to endothelial cells, leading to bleeding, tissue ischemia, and edema. Interestingly, victims of snake bites rarely experience excessive bleeding or thromboembolism,[211,212,215,216,220] in spite of the serious derangements in hemostatic tests and findings that are sometimes consistent with DIC.[220–222]

The major symptoms and signs, which are related to other effects of envenomation, are vomiting, diarrhea, apprehension, hypotension, local swelling, ischemia, and necrosis. Consequently, treatment for victims of snake bites should consist of immediate immobilization, administration of antivenom and fluids, and other general measures to preserve vital functions. Local incisions, cooling, and application of tourniquet should be avoided.[212,214] Two controlled trials showed no advantage of administering heparin and antivenom compared to antivenom alone.[223,224] In the event of bleeding, replacement with platelet concentrates and plasma components is advisable.

INFUSION OF FACTOR IX AND FACTOR XI CONCENTRATES

Concentrates of the vitamin K-dependent clotting factors are used to treat patients with hemophilia B and patients with other hereditary or acquired coagulation factor deficiencies. Instances of severe DIC[225,226]

have been reported in patients after the administration of these concentrates, and these reactions may be related to the presence of factors IXa, VIIa, and Xa in the concentrates.[227] Factor VIIa has a relatively long $T_{1/2}$ (2.5 h) in vivo.[228] A contributing factor in these patients is hepatic dysfunction,[225,226] which impedes the capacity of the liver to neutralize and remove factors IXa and Xa.[57,58] Newly prepared factor IX concentrates appear to be less thrombogenic[229] because they are almost completely free of activated clotting factors. Nevertheless, prothrombin complex concentrates should not be given as replacement therapy to patients with DIC, and patients with hepatic dysfunction should receive prothrombin complex concentrates only as a last resort, preferably only after their nonthrombogenicity has been established.

Two factor XI concentrates produced in England and France, respectively, have been shown to induce activation of the coagulation and fibrinolytic systems.[230,231] Infusions of these concentrates have been associated with severe thrombotic events in several patients,[232] but no instances of severe DIC have been observed. Contributing factors in the development of DIC are cardiovascular diseases, cancer, and surgery.

HEMANGIOMAS

In 1940 Kasabach and Merritt described the association between giant hemangioma and a bleeding tendency.[233] Studies employing radiolabeled fibrinogen[234,235] and platelets[236] provided evidence that within the hemangioma there is consumption of platelets and fibrinogen due to localized intravascular clotting and excessive fibrinogenolysis. Conceivably, there is concomitant local activation of the coagulation pathway, as well as release of large amounts of t-PA by the abnormal endothelium lining the tumor vessels. Microangiopathic hemolytic anemia and laboratory signs of DIC and fibrinolysis have been demonstrated in patients with giant hemangiomas.[237–239]

Accelerated growth of hemangiomas in infants is associated with augmented consumption of hemostatic factors, which can be effectively treated with irradiation, glucocorticoids, and interferon. Spontaneous mild to moderate bleeding manifestations have been observed, but severe bleeding generally occurs only after surgery.[240] Therefore, extreme caution should be exercised with invasive procedures.

Signs of DIC have also been associated with other vascular lesions, such as the Klippel-Trenaunay syndrome,[241,242] hemangioendothelioma of the liver[243] and spleen,[244] hemangioendotheliosarcoma,[245] and even hereditary hemorrhagic telangiectasis.[246]

In patients with the Kasabach-Merritt syndrome, tumor regression and improvement of hemostatic parameters have been attained by means of inducing thrombosis in the hemangioma with antifibrinolytic agents alone[247] or in combination with cryoprecipitate.[248] When successful, this results in correction of the coagulation abnormalities.

AORTIC ANEURYSM

An association between aortic aneurysm and DIC has been well documented.[249] In a series of patients with aortic aneurysm, 40 percent had elevated levels of fibrin(ogen) split products, but only 4 percent had significant bleeding and laboratory evidence of DIC.[250] Several factors predispose patients with aortic aneurysms to the development of DIC: a large surface area,[250] dissection,[249] and expansion of the aneurysm.[251] Clinical and laboratory signs of DIC should be carefully sought in patients with an aortic aneurysm since bleeding may seriously complicate surgical repair of the aneurysm.[250,252,253] The initiation of localized and generalized intravascular coagulation can be ascribed to activation of the tissue factor pathway by the abundant amounts of tissue factor present in atherosclerotic plaques.[254] Spontaneous correction of the abnormal coagulation tests can take place and is attributed to packing of the aneurysm with blood clots.[255] When patients present with significant bleeding or when surgery is planned, the hemostatic defects should be corrected by replacement therapy and continuous infusion of heparin.[256] Surgical resection produces a permanent solution.

HEMOLYTIC ANEMIAS

Early studies[22,23,257,258] described the strong in vitro and in vivo procoagulant effect of the stroma of red cells, and conversely, fibrin deposition in the vasculature induced by injections of thrombin or thromboplastin was shown to induce intravascular hemolysis.[259,260] Hence, it was suggested that a vicious cycle of DIC causing hemolysis and hemolysis aggravating DIC could develop in certain circumstances.[261] Whether this actually occurs in cases of DIC causing hemolysis has not been rigorously proved. A possible example of a relationship between DIC and hemolysis is incompatible blood transfusion, in which massive hemolysis is commonly associated with excessive bleeding and DIC, with widespread thrombosis in fatal cases.[262-264] However, the trigger of DIC in these cases could not simply be ascribed to the release of red cell stroma, since patients with massive hemolysis due to favism do not develop DIC.[265] It rather appears that the antigen-antibody reaction results in activation of monocytes (which release cytokines and express tissue factor) and complement (with the assembly of the membrane attack complex inflicting damage to endothelial cells[266]), all leading to DIC.

Microangiopathic hemolytic anemias and disseminated or localized intravascular coagulation may be initiated by disseminated cancer[131] and giant hemangioma.[238] In these circumstances hemolytic anemia may be aggravated by intravascular coagulation, but there is little to suggest that the hemolysis aggravates or initiates DIC.

DIC DURING PREGNANCY

Pregnancy predisposes patients to DIC for at least three reasons: (1) Pregnancy itself produces a hypercoagulable state, manifested by evidence of low-grade thrombin generation, with elevated levels of fibrin monomer complexes and fibrinopeptide A; (2) Pregnancy is associated with reduced fibrinolytic activity due to increased plasma levels of PAI-1; and (3) Pregnancy is associated with a decline in the plasma level of PS. DIC may be difficult to diagnose during pregnancy due to the high initial levels of coagulation factors like fibrinogen, factor VIII, and factor VII. Progressive reductions in these factors, however, can confirm or exclude the diagnosis of DIC in suspected cases.[267] Thrombocytopenia may be particularly helpful in determining whether DIC is present, provided other causes of thrombocytopenia are excluded.

ABRUPTIO PLACENTAE

The dramatic clinical presentation of abruptio placentae was first reported by DeLee in 1901,[268] but the immediate cause for sudden detachment of the placenta is still unknown. Older multiparous women or patients with one of the hypertensive disorders of pregnancy are thought to be at highest risk.[269,270] The severe hemostatic failure accompanying abruptio placentae is the result of acute DIC emanating from the introduction of large amounts of placental tissue factor into the blood circulation.[270,271]

In two large series of deliveries, abruptio placentae occurred in 0.2 to 0.4 percent of pregnancies,[269,272] and of these only 38 percent were associated with hypofibrinogenemia.[269] Thus, not all patients with abruptio placentae develop DIC, and among those who do, different grades of severity are found, with only the more severe forms resulting in shock and fetal death.

Rapid volume replenishment and evacuation of the uterus is the treatment of choice.[270] Transfusion of cryoprecipitate, fresh-frozen plasma, and platelets should be given when profuse bleeding occurs.[273,274] However, in the absence of severe bleeding, administration of blood components may not be necessary since depleted coagulation factors increase rapidly following delivery.[275] Heparin or antifibrinolytic agents are not indicated. Following a cesarean section it is advisable to give either low-dose heparin 5000 U twice a day subcutaneously or low molecular weight heparin, continuing treatment until the patient is completely mobile to prevent venous thrombosis.

AMNIOTIC FLUID EMBOLISM

This rare catastrophic disorder described by Steiner and Lushbaugh in 1941[276] occurs only in 1 in 8000 to 1 in 80,000 deliveries. A mortality rate of 86 percent was reported in a 1979 review of 272 cases.[277] A 1995 review of 46 cases found a mortality rate of 61 percent,[278] demonstrating that the mortality remains extraordinarily high. Patients predisposed to amniotic fluid embolism are multiparous women whose pregnancies are postmature with large fetuses and woman undergoing a tumultuous labor after pharmacologic or surgical induction.[276,277,279] A recent registry, however, failed to show a correlation between prolonged labor or oxytocin use and the occurrence of the syndrome.[278] Apparently, amniotic fluid is introduced into the maternal circulation through tears in the chorioamniotic membranes, rupture of the uterus, and injury of uterine veins.[277] Possible triggers of DIC are tissue factor[280] and an activator of factor X[281] present in amniotic fluid. The mechanical obstruction of pulmonary blood vessels by fetal debris, meconium, and other particulate matter in the amniotic fluid also enhances local fibrin-platelet thrombus formation and fibrinolysis. The extensive occlusion of the pulmonary arteries and an acute anaphylactoid response reminiscent of severe systemic inflammatory response syndrome[278] provoke sudden dyspnea, cyanosis, acute cor pulmonale, left ventricular dysfunction, shock, and convulsions. These symptoms are followed within minutes to several hours by severe bleeding in 37 percent of the cases.[277] Hemorrhage is particularly severe from the atonic uterus, from puncture sites, and from the gastrointestinal tract and other organs.

The best prospect for decreasing mortality lies in early elective termination of parturition in patients at high risk and prevention of hypertonic and tetanic uterine contractions during labor. When the syndrome is recognized, immediate pulmonary and cardiovascular support is essential. At present, insufficient data are available on the use of heparin or antifibrinolytic agents. Platelet concentrates, fresh-frozen plasma, and cryoprecipitate are given when bleeding and profound hemostatic impairment supervene.

PREECLAMPSIA AND ECLAMPSIA

Thrombocytopenia described in early reports of eclampsia[282] and widespread deposition of fibrin in blood vessels observed in fatal cases[283] were interpreted as evidence of DIC triggered by placental tissue factor becoming exposed to the circulation.[284] A critical analysis of the literature concluded that the thrombocytopenia in these patients stems from endothelial injury rather than DIC.[285] However, other investigators have provided evidence for significant DIC in preeclampsia and eclampsia.[286-291] Moreover, in a large series of patients there was a good correlation between the clinical severity and abnormalities in platelet counts and fibrin(ogen) degradation products.[288] Also consistent with DIC were results of assays of sensitive parameters of thrombin generation and activation of fibrinolysis, such as TAT, D-dimer, and fibrinopeptide Bβ1–42.[289-292] Despite these observations, administration of heparin to patients with preeclampsia and eclampsia has not resulted in convincing benefits.[293]

"HELLP" SYNDROME

The syndrome of hemolysis (H), elevated liver enzymes (EL), low platelet count (LP), and severe epigastric pain is a complication of pregnancy-induced hypertension[294]; 70 percent of the cases occur during the third trimester of pregnancy and 30 percent occur during the postpartum period.[295] Liver biopsy findings of fibrin deposition in hepatic blood vessels[296] and laboratory tests consistent with DIC in a significant proportion of patients[295,297,298] imply that DIC may play a role in the pathogenesis of this syndrome. Hepatic imaging in 33 patients revealed subcapsular hematomas in 13 and intraparenchymal hemorrhage in 6.[299] What actually triggers DIC in these cases is not known. Multiple organ dysfunctions manifested by acute renal failure, ascites, pulmonary edema, and severe hemorrhage due to DIC may develop, leading to a maternal mortality rate of 1.1 percent.[295] Management of patients with HELLP syndrome consists of supportive care, careful monitoring, and blood component replacement therapy. Some authors advocate immediate induction of labor, while others prefer to wait until signs of DIC develop in order to achieve greater fetal maturity.[300] In patients with postpartum HELLP syndrome persisting for more than 72 h, plasma exchange seems to be beneficial.[301] HELLP syndrome tends to recur in subsequent gestations.[302]

SEPSIS DURING PREGNANCY

Gram-negative bacteria, group A streptococci, and *Clostridium perfringens* are among the more common causes of sepsis during pregnancy. These infections are frequently associated with fulminant DIC. The pathogens gain entry into the circulation during abortion, via amnionitis that may follow invasive procedures or prolonged rupture of membranes, by endometritis developing during labor, and by way of the urinary tract. About 40 percent of bacteremic patients experience shock, which is associated with significant mortality.[303] In addition, there is a high rate of bleeding and organ dysfunction affecting the kidneys, lungs, and central nervous system. The human equivalent of the generalized Shwartzman reaction was described in such circumstances.[304,305]

Treatment of all cases of sepsis-related DIC should include antibiotics, support of vital functions, and surgical intervention to remove any local nidus of infection. Abortion or even hysterectomy may need to be considered. If bleeding is brisk or surgery is contemplated, cryoprecipitate, platelet concentrates, and fresh-frozen plasma should be given. Administration of heparin reportedly decreases the rate of DIC after septic abortion,[306,307] but controlled trials have not been conducted.

THE DEAD FETUS SYNDROME

Several weeks after intrauterine fetal death, patients may exhibit laboratory signs of DIC, occasionally accompanied by bleeding.[308] Apparently, tissue factor from the retained dead fetus or placenta slowly enters the maternal circulation and initiates DIC, which is sometimes accompanied by significant fibrinolysis.[309] Once the diagnosis of intrauterine fetal death is established, serial blood coagulation tests should be performed. A progressive deterioration in these tests calls for immediate evacuation of the uterus. Induction of labor should be preceded by continuous infusion of heparin at a rate of 1000 U/h until normal fibrinogen levels and a normal platelet count are obtained.[310,311] At this point, administration of heparin is discontinued, and 8 to 12 h later the uterus evacuated. When patients present with bleeding or induction of labor becomes urgent, replacement therapy with cryoprecipitate is useful. Platelet transfusion is rarely needed.

The entity of fetal death and DIC can occur following the demise of one of multiple gestations. If it occurs at term, therapy is begun as discussed. If it occurs prior to fetal maturity, prolonged administration of heparin can be useful.[309] Interestingly, when selective termination of the life of an anomalous fetus is performed in women with multiple pregnancies, hemostatic abnormalities develop in only approximately 3 percent of cases.[312]

ACUTE FATTY LIVER

Acute fatty liver of pregnancy is a rare disorder of unknown etiology that occurs during the third trimester of pregnancy and can lead to hepatic failure, encephalopathy, and death of the mother and fetus.[313–315] The disease is characterized by severe liver dysfunction,[314] renal failure, hypertension, and signs of DIC.[314,316] The typical histological feature is microvesicular fatty infiltration of the liver. Exceedingly low levels of AT-III and other laboratory signs of DIC were observed in a series of 28 patients, but no definite clinical benefit from AT-III concentrate infusion was achieved.[316] The primary therapy for these patients is early delivery and supportive care.

NEWBORNS

Newborns have a limited capacity to cope with triggers of DIC for several reasons: (1) Their ability to clear soluble fibrin and activated factors is reduced; (2) Their fibrinolytic potential is decreased due to low plasminogen level; and (3) Their capacity to synthesize coagulation factors and inhibitors is limited.[317,318] Criteria for the diagnosis of DIC in newborns are different from those of adults. One must take into account the physiologic hemostatic findings common at this age, which include low levels of the vitamin K–dependent factors, reduced AT-III and PC levels, and a prolonged thrombin time. The laboratory evidence of DIC in the newborn is based on the progressive decline of hemostatic parameters, thrombocytopenia, and reduced levels of fibrinogen, factor V, and factor VIII.[317,319]

DIC occurs in sick neonates and particularly in those who are premature. More than one underlying cause can usually be identified in newborns with DIC. The most frequent underlying conditions are: sepsis, hyaline membrane disease (respiratory distress syndrome), asphyxia, necrotizing enterocolitis, intravascular hemolysis, abruptio placentae, and eclampsia.[317–320]

Bleeding from multiple sites is the most common manifestation of DIC in newborns, with intracranial hemorrhage being the most life-threatening condition. In about 20 percent of neonates no clinical manifestations of DIC are apparent,[320] and thus a high index of suspicion in patients at risk is essential.

Vigorous therapeutic measures directed toward the underlying disorder, general support of vital functions, and blood component therapy are the best means to treat neonates with DIC. If bleeding persists, a two-volume exchange transfusion with fresh, heparinized whole blood is recommended by some authorities.[322] Most studies could not demonstrate any survival benefit from administration of heparin,[317,319,320,323,324] although slight improvements in bleeding[323] and in coagulation defects[324] have been reported.

REFERENCES

1. McKay DG: *Disseminated Intravascular Coagulation: An Intermediary Mechanism of Disease.* Hoeber Medical Division. Harper and Row. New York, 1965.

2. Hardaway RM: *Syndromes of Disseminated Intravascular Coagulation with Special Reference to Shock and Hemorrhage.* Charles C. Thomas, Springfield, IL, 1966.

3. Mammen EF, Anderson GF, Barnhard MI (eds): Disseminated intravascular coagulation. *Thromb Diathes Haemorrh* (suppl) 36, 1969.

4. Minna JD, Robboy SJ, Colman RW: *Disseminated Intravascular Coagulation in Man.* Charles C. Thomas, Springfield, IL, 1974.

5. Bick RL: *Disseminated Intravascular Coagulation and Related Syndromes.* CRC Press, Boca Raton, FL, 1983.

6. Abe T, Yamanaka M (eds): *Disseminated Intravascular Coagulation. Bibliotheca Haematologica,* No. 49. Karger, Basel, 1983.

7. Larcan A, Lambert H, Gerard A: *Consumption Coagulopathies.* Masson, New York, 1987.

8. Merskey C, Johnson AJ, Kleiner GJ, et al: The defibrination syndrome: clinical features and laboratory diagnosis. *Br J Haematol* 13:528, 1967.

9. Al-Mondhiry H: Disseminated intravascular coagulation. Experience in a major cancer center. *Thromb Diathes Haemorrh* 34:181, 1975.

10. Siegal T, Seligsohn U, Aghai E, Modan M: Clinical and laboratory aspects of disseminated intravascular coagulation (DIC): a study of 118 cases. *Thromb Haemost* 39:122, 1978.

11. Mant MJ, King EG: Severe, acute disseminated intravascular coagulation. A reappraisal of its pathophysiology, clinical significance and therapy based on 47 patients. *Am J Med* 67:557, 1979.

12. Spero JA, Lewis JH, Hasiba U: Disseminated intravascular coagulation. Findings in 346 patients. *Thromb Haemost* 43:28, 1980.

13. Bick RL: Disseminated intravascular coagulation: a clinical/laboratory study of 48 patients. *Ann NY Acad Sci* 370:843, 1981.

14. Matsuda M, Aoki N: Statistics on underlying and causative diseases of DIC in Japan. A cooperative study, in *Disseminated Intravascular Coagulation,* edited by T Abe, M Yamanaka, pp 15–22, Karger, Basel, 1983.

15. Tanaka K, Imamura T: Incidence and clinicopathological significance of DIC in autopsy cases, in *Disseminated Intravascular Coagulation,* edited by T Abe, M Yamakaka, pp 79–93. Karger, Basel, 1983.

16. Kobayashi N, Maekawa T, Takada M, Tanaka H: Criteria for diagnosis of DIC on the analysis of clinical and laboratory findings in 345 patients collected by the research committee on DIC in Japan, in *Disseminated Intravascular Coagulation,* edited by T Abe, M Yamanaka, pp 265–275. Karger, Basel, 1983.

17. Sharp AA: Diagnosis of disseminated intravascular coagulation, in *Disseminated Intravascular Coagulation,* edited by T Abe, M Yamanaka, pp 251–263, Karger, Basel, 1983.

18. Wada H, Wakita Y, Nakase T, et al: Outcome of disseminated intravascular coagulation in relation to the score when treatment was begun. *Thromb Haemost* 74:848, 1995.

19. Dupuy M: Injections de matière cerebral dans les veines. *Gas Med Paris* 2:524, 1834.

20. Trousseau A: Phlegmasia alba dolens. *Clin Med Hotel Dieu Paris,* p 695, 1965.

21. Naunyn C: Untersuchungen über Blutgerinnung im lebeden tiere und ihre Folgen. *Arch Exp Pathol Pharmacol,* Bd 1, 1873.

22. Wooldridge LC: Note on the relation of the red blood corpuscles to coagulation. *Practitioner* 38:187, 1886.

23. Wooldridge LC: Ueber intravasculare gerinnungen. *Arch Ant Physiol Abt (Leipzig)* p 397, 1886.

24. Lasch HG, Krecke HJ, Rodriguez-Erdman F, et al: Verbrauchskoagulopathien (Patogenese und Therapie). *Folia Haematol* 6:325, 1961.

25. Robboy SJ, Major MC, Colman RW, Minna JD: Pathology of disseminated intravascular coagulation (DIC). Analysis of 26 cases. *Hum Pathol* 3:327, 1972.

26. Kim HS, Suzuki M, Lie JT, Titus JL: Clinically unsuspected disseminated intravascular coagulation (DIC). An autopsy survey. *Am J Clin Pathol* 66:31, 1976.

27. Mori K, Hizawa K: Histopathological study of disseminated intravascular coagulation. An analysis of 114 autopsy cases. *Tokushima J Exp Med* 29:47, 1982.

28. Watanabe T, Imamura T, Nakagaki K, Tanaka K: Disseminated intravascular coagulation in autopsy cases. Its incidence and clinicopathologic significance. *Pathol Res Pract* 165:311, 1979.

29. Shimamura K, Oka K, Nakazawa M, Kojima M: Distribution patterns of microthrombi in disseminated intravascular coagulation. *Pathol Lab Med* 107:543, 1983.

30. Wilde JT, Roberts KM, Greaves M, Preston FE: Association between necropsy evidence of disseminated intravascular coagulation and coagulation variables before death in patients in intensive care units. *J Clin Pathol* 41:138, 1988.

31. Kojima M, Shimamura K, Mori N, et al: A histological study on microthrombi in autopsy cases of DIC. *Bibl Haematol* 49:95, 1983.

32. Kim HS, Suzuki M, Lie JT, Titus JL: Nonbacterial thrombotic endocarditis (NBTE) and disseminated intravascular coagulation (DIC). *Arch Pathol Lab Med* 101:65, 1977.

33. Sugiura M, Hiraoka K, Ohkawa S, et al: A clinico-pathological study on cardiac lesions in 64 cases of disseminated intravascular coagulation. *Jpn Heart J* 18:57, 1977.

34. Kuramoto K, Matsushita S, Yamanouchi H: Nonbacterial thrombotic endocarditis as a cause of cerebral and myocardial infarction. *Jpn Circ J* 48:1000, 1984.

35. Katsumura Y, Ohtsubo K: Incidence of pulmonary thromboembolism, infarction and hemorrhage in disseminated intravascular coagulation: a necroscopic analysis. *Thorax* 50:160, 1995.

36. American College of Chest Physicians/Society of Critical Care Medicine Consensus Conference: Definitions for sepsis and organ failure and guidelines for the use of innovative therapies in sepsis. *Crit Care Med* 20:864, 1992.

37. Davies MG, Hagen PO: Systemic inflammatory response syndrome. *Brit J Surg* 84:920, 1997.

38. Fourrier F, Chopin C, Goudemand J, et al: Septic shock, multiple organ failure, and disseminated intravascular coagulation. Compared patterns of antithrombin III, protein C, and protein S deficiencies. *Chest* 101:816, 1992.

39. Rangel-Frausto MS, Pittet D, Costigan M, et al: The natural history of the systemic inflammatory response syndrome (SIRS). A prospective study. *JAMA* 273:117, 1995.

40. Gando S, Kameue T, Nanzaki S, Nakanishi Y: Disseminated intravascular coagulation is a frequent complication of systemic inflammatory response syndrome. *Thromb Haemost* 75:224, 1996.

41. ten Cate JW, van der Poll T, Levi M, et al: Cytokines: triggers of clinical thrombotic disease. *Thromb Haemost* 78:415, 1997.

42. Vervloet MG, Thijs LG, Hack CE: Derangements of coagulation and fibrinolysis in critically ill patients with sepsis and septic shock. *Semin Thromb Hemost* 24:33, 1998.

43. Muller-Berghaus G: Pathophysiologic and biochemical events in disseminated intravascular coagulation: dysregulation of procoagulant and anticoagulant pathways. *Semin Thromb Hemost* 15:58, 1989.

44. Celi A, Pellegrini G, Lorenzet R, et al: P-selectin induces the expression of tissue factor on monocytes. *Proc Natl Acad Sci USA* 91:8767, 1994.

45. Moore KL, Andreoli SP, Esmon NL, et al: Endotoxin enhances tissue factor and suppresses thrombomodulin expression of human vascular endothelium in vitro. *J Clin Invest* 79:124, 1987.

46. Kobayashhi M, Shimada K, Ozawa T: Human recombinant interleukin 1-beta and tumor necrosis factor alfa-mediated suppression of heparin-like compounds on cultured porcine aortic endothelial cells. *J Cell Physiol* 144:383, 1990.

47. Pixley RA, De La Cadena R, Page JD, et al: The contact system contributes to hypotension but not disseminated intravascular coagulation in lethal bacteremia. *J Clin Invest* 91:61, 1993.

48. Mesters RM, Mannucci PM, Coppola R, et al: Factor VIIa and antithrombin III activity during severe sepsis and septic shock in neutropenic patients. *Blood* 88:881, 1996.

49. Weiss SJ: Tissue destruction by neutrophils. *N Engl J Med* 320:365, 1989.

50. Jordan RE, Nelson RM, Kilpatrick J, et al: Inactivation of human antithrombin by neutrophil elastase. Kinetics of the heparin-dependent reaction. *J Biol Chem* 264:10493, 1989.

51. Levin EG, Marzec U, Anderson J, Harker LA: Thrombin stimulates tissue plasminogen activator release from cultured endothelial cells. *J Clin Invest* 74:1988, 1984.

52. Rosenberg RD: Biochemistry of heparin antithrombin interactions and the physiologic role of this natural anticoagulant mechanism. *Am J Med* 87 (suppl 3B):2S, 1989.

53. Bajzar L, Nesheim ME, Tracy PB: The profibrinolytic effect of activated protein C in clots formed from plasma is TAFI-dependent. *Blood* 88:2093, 1996.

54. Sandset PM, Warn-Cramer BJ, Rao LVM, et al: Depletion of extrinsic pathway inhibitor (EPI) sensitizes rabbits to disseminated intravascular coagulation induced with tissue factor: evidence supporting a physiologic role for EPI as a natural anticoagulant. *Proc Natl Acad Sci USA* 88:708, 1991.

55. Spaet TH, Horowitz HHI, Zucker-Franklin D, et al: Reticuloendothelial clearance of blood thromboplastin by rats. *Blood* 19:196, 1961.

56. Sherman LA, Lee J, Jacobson A: Quantitation of the reticuloendothelial system clearance of soluble fibrin. *Br J Haematol* 37:231, 1977.

57. Deykin D: The role of the liver in serum-induced hypercoagulability. *J Clin Invest* 45:256, 1966.

58. Deykin D, Cochios F, DeCamp G, Lopez A: Hepatic removal of activated factor X by the perfused rabbit liver. *Am J Physiol* 214:414, 1968.

59. Bone RC, Francis PB, Pierce AK: Disseminated intravascular coagulation with the adult respiratory distress syndrome. *Am J Med* 61:585, 1976.

60. Rinaldo JE, Christman JW: Mechanisms and mediators of the adult respiratory distress syndrome. *Clin Chest Med* 11:621, 1990.

61. Kollef MH, Schuster DP: The acute respiratory distress syndrome. *N Engl J Med* 332:27, 1995.

62. Colman RW, Robboy SJ, Minna JD: Disseminated intravascular coagulation. A reappraisal. *Annu Rev Med* 30:359, 1979.

63. Carr JM, McKinney M, McDonagh J: Diagnosis of disseminated intravascular coagulation. Role of D-dimer. *Am J Clin Pathol* 91:280, 1989.

64. Bovill EG: Disseminated intravascular coagulation: pathophysiology and laboratory diagnosis. *Fibrinol* 7 (suppl 2):17, 1993.

65. Hoek JA, Sturk A, ten Cate JW, et al: Laboratory and clinical evaluation of an assay of thrombin-antithrombin III complexes in plasma. *Clin Chem* 34:2058, 1988.

66. Takahashi H, Hanano M, Takizawa S, et al: Plasmin-alpha 2-plasmin inhibitor complex in plasma of patients with disseminated intravascular coagulation. *Am J Hematol* 28:162, 1988.

67. Asakura H, Jokaji H, Saito M, et al: Study of the balance between coagulation and fibrinolysis in disseminated intravascular coagulation using molecular markers. *Blood Coag Fibrinol* 5:829, 1994.

68. Corrigan JJ, Jordan CM: Heparin therapy in septicemia with disseminated intravascular coagulation. *N Engl J Med* 283:778, 1970.

69. Hogg PJ, Jackson CM: Fibrin monomer protects thrombin from inactivation by heparin-antithrombin III: Implications for heparin efficacy. *Proc Natl Acad Sci USA* 86:3619, 1989.

70. Blauhut B, Kramar H, Vinazzer H, Bergmann H: Substitution of antithrombin III in shock and DIC: A randomized study. *Thromb Res* 39:81, 1985.

71. Vinazzer HA: Antithrombin III in shock and disseminated intravascular coagulation. *Clin Appl Thrombosis/Hemostasis* 1:62, 1995.

72. Fourrier F, Chopin C, Huart JJ, et al: Double-blind, placebo-controlled trial of antithrombin III concentrates in septic shock with disseminated intravascular coagulation. *Chest* 104:882, 1993.

73. Eisele B, Lamy M: Clinical experience with antithrombin III concentrates in critically ill patients with sepsis and multiple organ failure. *Semin Thromb Hemost* 24:71, 1998.

74. Naeye RL: Thrombotic state after a hemorrhagic diathesis, a possible complication of therapy with epsilon-aminocaproic acid. *Blood* 19:694, 1962.

75. Gralnick HR, Greipp P: Thrombosis with epsilon aminocaproic acid therapy. *Am J Clin Pathol* 56:151, 1971.

76. Taenaka N, Shimada Y, Hirata T, et al: Gabexate mesilate (FOY) therapy of disseminated intravascular coagulation due to sepsis. *Crit Care Med* 11:735, 1983.

77. Shibata A, Takahashi H, Aoki N, et al: Nafamostat mesilate as a therapy for disseminated intravascular coagulation (DIC): A well-controlled multicenter comparative study. *Thromb Haemost* 62:371, 1989.

78. Rivard GE, David M, Farrell C, Schwartz HP: Treatment of purpura fulminans in meningococcemia with protein C concentrate. *J Pediatr* 126:646, 1995.

79. Warr TA, Rao LVM, Rapaport SI: DIC in rabbits induced by administration of endotoxin or tissue factor: effect of antitissue factor antibodies and measurement of plasma extrinsic pathway inhibitor activity. *Blood* 75:1481, 1990.

80. Taylor FB Jr, Chang AC, Ruf W, et al: Lethal septic shock is prevented by blocking tissue factor. *Circ Shock* 33:127, 1991.

81. Taylor FB, Chang ACK, Peer G, et al: Active site inhibited factor VIIa (DEGR VIIa) attenuates the coagulant and interleukin-6 and -8, but not tumor necrosis factor responses of the baboon to LD100 *Escherichia coli*. *Blood* 91:1609, 1998.

82. Bajaj MS, Bajaj SP: Tissue factor pathway inhibitor: potential therapeutic applications. *Thromb Haemost* 78:471, 1997.

83. Warren HS, Danner RL, Munford RS: Anti-endotoxin monoclonal antibodies. *N Engl J Med* 326:1153, 1992.

84. Cross AS: Antiendotoxin antibodies: a dead end? *Ann Intern Med* 121:58, 1994.

85. Anderson MR, Blumer JL: Advances in the therapy for sepsis in children. *Pediat Clin North Am* 44:179, 1997.

86. Pajkrt D, van der Poll T, Levi M, et al: Interleukin-10 inhibits activation of coagulation and fibrinolysis during human endotoxemia. *Blood* 89:2701, 1997.

87. Bisno AL, Freeman JC: The syndrome of asplenia, pneumococcal sepsis, and disseminated intravascular coagulation. *Ann Intern Med* 72:389, 1970.

88. Vik-Mo H, Lote K, Nordoy A: Disseminated intravascular coagulation in patients with meningococcal infection: laboratory diagnosis and prognostic factors. *Scand J Infect Dis* 10:187, 1978.

89. Kornelisse RF, Hazelzet JA, Hop WC, et al: Meningococcal septic shock in children: clinical and laboratory features, outcome, and development of a prognostic score. *Clin Infect Dis* 25:640, 1997.

90. Corrigan JJ, Ray WL, May N: Changes in the blood coagulation system associated with septicemia. *N Engl J Med* 279:851, 1968.

91. Rapaport SI, Tatter D, Caeur-Barron N, Hjort PF: *Pseudomonas* septicemia with intravascular clotting leading to the generalized Shwartzman reaction. *N Engl J Med* 271:80, 1964.

92. Clarkson AR, Sage RE, Lawrence JR: Consumption coagulopathy and acute renal failure due to gram-negative septicemia after abortion. Complete recovery with heparin therapy. *Ann Intern Med* 70:1191, 1969.

93. Murray HW, Tuazon CU, Sheagren JN: Staphylococcal septicemia and disseminated intravascular coagulation. *Arch Intern Med* 137:844, 1977.

94. Bhakdi S, Muhly M, Mannhardt U, et al: Staphylococcal alpha toxin promotes blood coagulation via attack on human platelets. *J Exp Med* 168:527, 1988.

95. Ratnoff OD, Nebehay WG: Multiple coagulative defects in a patient with Waterhouse-Friderichsen syndrome. *Ann Intern Med* 56:627, 1962.

96. Stossel TP, Levy R: Intravascular coagulation associated with pneumococcal bacteremia and symmetrical peripheral gangrene. *Arch Intern Med* 125:876, 1970.

97. Rytel MW, Dee TH, Ferstenfeld JE, Hensley GT: Possible pathogenetic role of capsular antigens in fulminant pneumococcal disease with disseminated intravascular coagulation (DIC). *Am J Med* 57:889, 1974.

98. De Virgilio C, Klein S, Chang L, et al: Clostridial bacteremia: implications for the surgeon. *Am Surg* 57:388, 1991.

99. Yoshikawa T, Tanaka KR, Guze LB: Infection and disseminated intravascular coagulation. *Medicine (Baltimore)* 50:237, 1971.

100. Cosgriff TM: Viruses and hemostasis. *Rev Infect Dis* 11 (suppl 4):S672, 1989.

101. Inbal A, Kenet G, Zivelin A, et al: Purpura fulminans induced by disseminated intravascular coagulation following infection in two unrelated children with double heterozygosity for factor V Leiden and protein S deficiency. *Thromb Haemost* 77:1086, 1997.

102. Levin M, Eley BS, Louis J, et al: Postinfectious purpura fulminans caused by an autoantibody directed against protein S. *J Pediatr* 127:355, 1995.

103. Lee M, Lee JS, Kim BK: Disseminated intravascular coagulation in Korean hemorrhagic fever. *Bibl Haematol* 49:181, 1983.

104. Isarangkura PB, Pongpanich B, Pintadit P, et al: Hemostatic derangement in dengue haemorrhagic fever. *Southeast Asian J Trop Med Public Health* 18:331, 1987.

105. Molinas FC, de Bracco MM, Maiztegui JI: Hemostasis and the complement system in Argentine hemorrhagic fever. *Rev Infect Dis* 11 (suppl 4):S762, 1989.

106. Grob C: Tissue factor initiation of disseminated intravascular coagulation in filovirus infection. *Med Hypotheses* 45:380, 1995.

107. Vitarana T, de Silva H, Withana N, Gunasekera C: Elevated tumour necrosis factor in dengue fever and dengue haemorrhagic fever. *Ceylon Med J* 36:63, 1991.

108. Philippidis P, Naiman JL, Sibinga MS, Valdes-Dapnea MA: Disseminated intravascular coagulation in *Candida albicans* septicemia. *J Pediatr* 78:683, 1971.

109. Fera G, Semeraro N, De Mitrio V, Schiraldi O: Disseminated intravascular coagulation associated with disseminated cryptococcosis in a patient with acquired immunodeficiency syndrome. *Infection* 21:171, 1993.

110. Mavligit GM, Binder RA, Crosby WH: Disseminated intravascular coagulation in miliary tuberculosis. *Arch Intern Med* 130:388, 1972.

111. Rojanasthien S, Surakamolleart V, Boonpucknavig S, Isarangkura P: Hematological and coagulation studies in malaria. *J Med Assoc Thai* 75 (suppl 1):190, 1992.

112. Pukrittayakamee S, White NJ, Clemens R, et al: Activation of the

coagulation cascade in falciparum malaria. *Tans R Soc Trop Med Hyg* 83:762, 1989.

113. Hjort PF, Rapaport SI, Jorgensen L: Purpura fulminans. Report of a case successfully treated with heparin and hydrocortisone. Review of 50 cases from the literature. *Scand J Haematol* 1:69, 1964.

114. Gerson WT, Dickerman JD, Bovill EG, Golden E: Severe acquired protein C deficiency in purpura fulminans associated with disseminated intravascular coagulation: treatment with protein C concentrate. *Pediatrics* 91:418, 1993.

115. Tishler M, Abramov AL, Seligsohn U, Kahn Y: Purpura fulminans in an adult. *Isr J Med Sci* 22:820, 1986.

116. Branson HE, Katz J, Marble R, Griffin JH: Inherited protein C deficiency and a coumarin-responsive chronic relapsing purpura fulminans syndrome in a newborn infant. *Lancet* 2:1156, 1983.

117. Seligsohn U, Berger A, Abend M, et al: Homozygous protein C deficiency manifested by massive venous thrombosis in the newborn. *N Engl J Med* 310, 1984.

118. Jurgens R, Trautwein H: über Fibrinopenie (Fibrinogenopenie) beim Erwaschsenen, nebst Bemerkungen über die herkunft des Fibrinogens. *Dtsch Arch Klin Med* 169:28, 1930.

119. Goad KE, Gralnick HR: Coagulation disorders in cancer. *Hematol Oncol Clin North Am* 10:457, 1996.

120. Sack GH Jr, Levin J, Bell WR: Trousseau's syndrome and other manifestations of chronic disseminated coagulopathy in patients with neoplasms: clinical, pathophysiologic, and therapeutic features. *Medicine (Baltimore)* 56:1, 1977.

121. Collins RC, Al-Mondhiry H, Chernik NL, et al: Neurologic manifestations of intravascular coagulation in cancer: a clinicopathologic analysis of 12 cases. *Neurology* 25:795, 1975.

122. Szczepanski M, Bardadin K, Zawadzki J, Pypno W: Procoagulant activity of gastric, colorectal and renal cancer is factor VII-dependent. *J Cancer Res Clin Oncol* 114:519, 1988.

123. Gonmori H, Maekawa T, Kobayashi N, et al: The role of tissue thromboplastin in the development of DIC accompanying neoplastic diseases. *Bibl Haematol* 49:23, 1983

124. Zacharski LR, Schned AR, Sorenson GD: Occurrence of fibrin and tissue factor antigen in human small cell carcinoma of the lung. *Cancer Res* 43:3963, 1983.

125. Callander N, Rapaport SI: Trousseau's syndrome. *West J Med* 158:364, 1993.

126. Pineo GF, Regoeczi E, Hatton MWC, Brain MC: The activation of coagulation by extracts of mucus: a possible pathway of intravascular coagulation accompanying adenocarcinomas. *J Lab Clin Med* 82:255, 1973.

127. Falanga A, Gordon SG: Isolation and characterization of cancer procoagulant: a cysteine proteinase from malignant tissue. *Biochemistry* 24:5558, 985.

128. Dvorak HF, Quay SC, Orenstein NS, et al: Tumor shedding and coagulation. *Science* 212:923, 1981.

129. Owen CA Jr, Bowie EJW: Chronic intravascular coagulation syndromes, a summary. *Mayo Clin Proc* 49:673, 1974.

130. Bell WR, Starksen NF, Tong S, Proterfield JK: Trousseau's syndrome. Devastating coagulopathy in the absence of heparin. *Am J Med* 79:423, 1985.

131. Seligsohn U, Weber H, Yoran C, et al: Microangiopathic hemolytic anemia and defibrination syndrome in metastatic carcinoma of the stomach. *Isr J Med Sci* 4:69, 1968.

132. Zuger M, Demarmels Biasiutti F, et al: Subcutaneous low-molecular-weight heparin for treatment of Trousseau's syndrome. *Ann Hematol* 75:165, 1997.

133. Cooper DL, Sandler AB, Wilson LD, Duffy TP: Disseminated intravascular coagulation and excessive fibrinolysis in a patient with metastatic prostate cancer. Response to epsilon-aminocaproic acid. *Cancer* 70:656, 1992.

134. Risak E: Die Fibrinopenie. *Z Klin Med* 128:606, 1935.

135. De Loughery TG, Goodnight SH: Acute promyelocytic leukaemia in the all-*trans*-retinoic acid era. *Med Oncol* 13:233, 1996.

136. Barbui T, Finazzi G, Falanga A: The impact of all-*trans*-retinoic acid on the coagulopathy of acute promyelocytic leukaemia. *Blood* 91:3093, 1998.

137. Pittman GR, Senhauser DA, Lowney JF: Acute promyelocytic leukemia. A report of 3 autopsied cases. *Am J Clin Pathol* 46:214, 1966.

138. Polliak A: Acute promyelocytic leukemia with disseminated intravascular coagulation. *Am J Clin Pathol* 56:155, 1971.

139. Gralnick HR, Tan HK: Acute promyelocytic leukemia. A model for understanding the role of the malignant cell in hemostasis. *Hum Pathol* 5:661, 1974.

140. Gralnick HR, Abrell E: Studies of the procoagulant and fibrinolytic activity of promyelocytes in acute promyelocytic leukaemia. *Br J Haematol* 24:89, 1973.

141. Andoh K, Kubota T, Takada M, et al: Tissue factor activity in leukemia cells. Special reference to disseminated intravascular coagulation. *Cancer* 59:748, 1987.

142. Falanga A, Alessio MG, Donati MB, et al: A new procoagulant in acute leukemia. *Blood* 71:870, 1988.

143. Cozzolino F, Torcia M, Miliani A, et al: Potential role of interleukin-1 as the trigger for diffuse intravascular coagulation in acute non-lymphoblastic leukemia. *Am J Med* 84:240, 1988.

144. Bauer KA, Rosenberg RD: Thrombin generation in acute promyelocytic leukemia. *Blood* 64:791, 1984.

145. Tallman MS, Kwaan HC: Reassessing the hemostatic disorder associated with acute promyelocytic leukemia. *Blood* 79:543, 1992.

146. Rodeghiero F, Avvisati G, Castaman G, et al: Early deaths and anti-hemorrhagic treatments in acute promyelocytic leukemia. A GIMENA retrospective study in 268 consecutive patients. *Blood* 75:2112, 1990.

147. Avvisati G, ten Cate JW, Mandelli F: Acute promyelocytic leukaemia. *Br J Haematol* 81:315, 1992.

148. Bennett B, Booth NA, Croll A, et al: The bleeding disorder in acute promyelocytic leukaemia: fibrinolysis due to u-PA rather than defibrination. *Br J Haematol* 71:511, 1989.

149. Francis RB, Seyfert U: Tissue plasminogen activator antigen and activity in disseminated intravascular coagulation. Clinicopathologic correlations. *J Lab Clin Med* 110:541, 1987.

150. Schwartz BS, Williams EC, Conlan MG, Mosher DF: Epsilon-aminocaproic acid in the treatment of patients with acute promyelocytic leukemia and acquired alpha-2-plasmin inhibitor deficiency. *Ann Intern Med* 105:873, 1986.

151. Sakata Y, Murakami T, Noro A, et al: The specific activity of plasminogen activator inhibitor-1 in disseminated intravascular coagulation with acute promyelocytic leukemia. *Blood* 77:1949, 1991.

152. Koyama T, Hirosawa S, Kawamata N, et al: All-*trans*-retinoic acid upregulates thrombomodulin and downregulates tissue-factor expression in acute promyelocytic leukemia cells: distinct expression of thrombomodulin and tissue factor in human leukemic cells. *Blood* 84:3001, 1994.

153. Tallman MS, Andersen JW, Schiffer CA, et al: All-*trans*-retinoic acid in acute promyelocytic leukemia. *N Engl J Med* 337:1021, 1997.

154. Runde V, Aul C, Heyll A, Schneider W: All-*trans*-retinoic acid: not only a differentiating agent, but also an inducer of thromboembolic events in patients with M3 leukemia. *Blood* 79:534, 1992.

155. Hashimoto S, Koike T, Tatewaki W, et al: Fatal thromboembolism in acute promyelocytic leukemia during all-*trans*-retinoic acid therapy combined with antifibrinolytic therapy for prophylaxis of hemorrhage. *Leukemia* 8:1113, 1994.

156. Escudier SM, Kantarjian HM, Estey EH: Thrombosis in patients with acute promyelocytic leukemia treated with and without all-*trans*-retinoic acid. *Leuk Lymphoma* 20:435, 1996.

157. Pogliani EM, Rossini F, Casaroli I, et al: Thrombotic complications in acute promyelocytic leukemia during all-*trans*-retinoic acid therapy. *Acta Haematol* 97:228, 1997.

158. Sarris A, Cortes J, Kantarjian H, et al: Disseminated intravascular coagulation in adult acute lymphoblastic leukemia: frequent complications with fibrinogen levels less than 100 mg/dl. *Leuk Lymphoma* 21:85, 1996.

159. Gando S, Nakanishi Y, Tedo I: Cytokines and plasminogen activator inhibitor-1 in posttrauma disseminated intravascular coagulation: relationship to multiple organ dysfunction syndrome. *Crit Care Med* 23:1835, 1995.

160. Gando S, Kameue T, Nanzaki S, et al: Increased neutrophil elastase, persistent intravascular coagulation, and decreased fibrinolytic activity in patients with posttraumatic acute respiratory distress syndrome. *J Trauma* 42:1068, 1997.

161. Gando S, Kameue T, Nanzaki S, et al: Participation of tissue factor and thrombin in posttraumatic systemic inflammatory syndrome. *Crit Care Med* 25:1820, 1997.

162. Owings JT, Bagley M, Gosselin R, et al: Effect of critical injury on

plasma antithrombin activity: low antithrombin levels are associated with thromboembolic complications. *J Trauma* 41:396, 1996.

163. Simmons RL, Collins JA, Heisterkamp CA, et al: Coagulation disorders in combat casualties: I. Acute changes after wounding. II. Effect of massive transfusion. III. Post-resuscitative changes. *Ann Surg* 169:455, 1969.

164. Jochum M: Influence of high-dose antithrombin concentrate therapy on the release of cellular proteinases, cytokines, and soluble adhesion molecules in acute inflammation. *Semin Hematol* 32 (4 suppl 2):19, 1995.

165. Goodnight SH, Kenover G, Rapaport SI, et al: Defibrination after brain-tissue destruction. A serious complication of head injury. *N Engl J Med* 290:1043, 1974.

166. Scherer RU, Spangenberg P: Procoagulant activity in patients with isolated severe head trauma. *Crit Care Med* 26:149, 1998.

167. Kaufman HH, Hui KS, Mattson JC, et al: Clinicopathological correlations of disseminated intravascular coagulation in patients with head injury. *Neurosurgery* 15:34, 1984.

168. Olson JD, Kaufman HH, Moake J, et al: The incidence and significance of hemostatic abnormalities in patients with head injuries. *Neurosurgery* 24:825, 1989.

169. Selladurai BM, Vickneswaran M, Duraisamy S, Atan M: Coagulopathy in acute head injury—a study of its role as a prognostic indicator. *Br J Neurosurg* 11:398, 1997.

170. McManus WF, Eurenius K, Pruitt BA: Disseminated intravascular coagulation in burned patients. *J Trauma* 13:416, 1973.

171. Simon TL, Current PW, Harker LA: Kinetic characterization of hemostasis in thermal injury. *J Lab Clin Med* 82:702, 1977.

172. Winkelman MD, Galloway PG: Central nervous system complications of thermal burns. A postmortem study of 139 patients. *Medicine (Baltimore)* 71:271, 1992.

173. Fletcher AP, Biederman O, Moore D, et al: Abnormal plasminogen-plasmin system activity (fibrinolysis) in patients with hepatic cirrhosis: its cause and consequences. *J Clin Invest* 43:681, 1964.

174. Bloom AL: Intravascular coagulation and the liver. *Br J Haematol* 30:1, 1975.

175. Carr JM: Disseminated intravascular coagulation in cirrhosis. *Hepatology* 10:103, 1989.

176. Tytgat GN, Collen D, Verstraete M: Metabolism of fibrinogen in cirrhosis of the liver. *J Clin Invest* 50:1960, 1971.

177. Coleman M, Finlayson N, Bettigole RE, et al: Fibrinogen survival in cirrhosis: improvement by "low dose" heparin. *Ann Intern Med* 83:79, 1975.

178. Tytgat GN, Piesens J, Collen D, De Groote J: Experience with exchange transfusion in the treatment of hepatic coma. *Digestion* 1:257, 1968.

179. Carr JM, McKinney M, McDonagh J: Diagnosis of DIC: role of D-dimer. *Am J Clin Pathol* 91;280, 1989.

180. Paramo JA, Rifon J, Fernandez J, et al: Thrombin activation and increased fibrinolysis in patients with chronic liver disease. *Blood Coag Fibrinol* 2:227, 1991.

181. Van Wersch JWJ, Russel MG, Lustermans FA: The extent of diffuse intravascular coagulation and fibrinolysis in patients with liver cirrhosis. *Eur J Clin Chem Clin Biochem* 30:275, 1992.

182. Coccheri S, Mannucci PM, Palaret G, et al: Significance of plasma fibrinopeptide A and high molecular weight fibrinogen in patients with liver cirrhosis. *Br J Haematol* 52:503, 1982.

183. Oka K, Tanaka K: Intravascular coagulation in autopsy cases with liver diseases. *Thromb Haemost* 42:564, 1979.

184. Palascak JE, Martinez J: Dysfibrinogenemia associated with liver disease. *J Clin Invest* 60:89, 1977.

185. Corrigan JJ, Bennett BB, Bueffel B: The value of factor VIII levels in acquired hypofibrinogenemia. *Am J Clin Pathol* 60:897, 1973.

186. Straub PW: Diffuse intravascular coagulation in liver disease? *Semin Thromb Haemost* 4:29, 1977.

187. Canoso RT, Hutton RA, Deykin D: The hemostatic defect of chronic liver disease. Kinetic studies using ⁷⁵Se-Selenomethionine. *Gastroenterology* 76:540, 1979.

188. Tempero MA, Davis RB, Reed E, Edney J: Thrombocytopenia and laboratory evidence of disseminated intravascular coagulation after shunts for ascites in malignant disease. *Cancer* 55:2718, 1985.

189. Bakker CM, Knot EA, Stibbe J, Wilson JH: Disseminated intravascular coagulation in liver cirrhosis. *J Hepatol* 15:330, 1992.

190. LeVeen HH, Wapnick S, Grosberg S, Kinney MU: Further experience with peritoneovenous shunt for ascites. *Ann Surg* 184:574, 1976.

191. Rubinstein D, McInness I, Dudley F: Morbidity and mortality after peritoneovenous shunt surgery for refractory ascites. *Gut* 26:1070, 1985.

192. LeVeen EG, LeVeen HH: The place of the peritoneovenous shunt in the treatment of ascites. *ASAIO Trans* 35:165, 1989.

193. Shibolet S, Coll R, Gilat T, et al: Heatstroke: its clinical picture and mechanism in 36 cases. *Q J Med* 36:525, 1967.

194. Shibolet S, Lancaster MC, Danon Y: Heat stroke: a review. *Aviat Space Environ Med* 47:280, 1976.

195. Wakefield EG, Hall WW: Heat injuries: a preparatory study for experimental heat stroke. *JAMA* 89:92, 1927.

196. Gauss H, Meyer KA: Heat stroke: report of one hundred and fifty-eight cases from Cook County Hospital, Chicago. *Am J Med Sci* 154:554, 1917.

197. Malamud N, Naymaker W, Custer RP: Heat stroke. A clinicopathology study of 125 fatal cases. *Milit Surg* 99:397, 1946.

198. Hart GR, Anderson RJ, Crumpler CP, et al: Epidemic classical heat stroke: clinical characteristics and course of 28 patients. *Medicine (Baltimore)* 61:189, 1982.

199. Mustafa KY, Omer O, Khogali M, et al: Blood coagulation and fibrinolysis in heat stroke. *Br J Haematol* 61:517, 1985.

200. Chao TC, Sinniah R, Pakiam JE: Acute heat stroke deaths. *Pathology* 13:145, 1981.

201. Rosenthal T, Shapiro Y, Seligsohn U, Ramot B: Disseminated intravascular coagulation in experimental heatstroke. *Thromb Diath Haemorrh* 26:417, 1971.

202. Shibolet S, Fisher S, Gilat T, et al: Fibrinolysis and hemorrhages in fatal heatstroke. *N Engl J Med* 266:169, 1962.

203. Al-Mashhadani SA, Gader AG, al-Harthi SS, et al: The coagulopathy of heat stroke: alterations in coagulation and fibrinolysis in heat stroke patients during the pilgrimage (Haj) to Makkah. *Blood Coagul Fibrinol* 5:731, 1994.

204. Bouchama A, Bridey F, Hammami MM, et al: Activation of coagulation and fibrinolysis in heatstroke. *Thromb Haemost* 76:909, 1996.

205. Sohal RS, Sun SC, Colcolough HL, et al: Heat stroke. An electron microscopy study of endothelial cell damage and disseminated intravascular coagulation. *Arch Intern Med* 122:43, 1968.

206. Weber MB, Blakely JA: The haemorrhagic diathesis of heatstroke. A consumption coagulopathy successfully treated with heparin. *Lancet* 1:1190, 1969.

207. Cornell CJ, Fein SH, Reilly B, Cornwell GG: Heparin therapy for heat stroke. *Ann Intern Med* 81:702, 1974.

208. Perschick JS, Winkelstein A, Shadduck RK: Disseminated intravascular coagulation in heat stroke. *JAMA* 231:480, 1975.

209. Knochel JP: Disseminated intravascular coagulation in heat stroke. Response to heparin therapy. *JAMA* 231:496, 1975.

210. Shibolet S, Farfel Z: Heparin therapy for heatstroke. *Ann Intern Med* 82:857, 1975.

211. De Vries A, Cohen I: Hemorrhagic and blood coagulation disturbing action of snake venoms, in *Recent Advances in Blood Coagulation,* edited by L Poller, p 277. Churchill, London, 1969.

212. Efrati P: Snake venoms and blood coagulation, in *Snake Venoms,* edited by Chen-Yuan Lee, p 956. Springer-Verlag, Berlin, 1979.

213. Russell EF: Snake venoms and blood coagulation, in *Snake Venoms,* edited by Chen-Yuan Lee, p 978. Springer-Verlag, Berlin, 1979.

214. Seegers WH, Ouyang C: Snake venoms and blood coagulation, in *Snake Venoms,* edited by Chen-Yuan Lee, p 684. Springer-Verlag, Berlin, 1979.

215. Reid HA: Clinical hemostatic disorders caused by venoms, in *Disorders of Hemostasis,* edited by OD Ratnoff, CD Forbes, p 511. Grune and Stratton, Orlando, FL, 1984.

216. Kitchens CS: Hemostatic aspects of envenomation by North American snakes. *Hematol Oncol Clin North Am* 6:1189, 1992.

217. Hutton RA, Warrell DA: Action of snake venom components on the haemostatic system. *Blood Rev* 7:176, 1993.

218. Huang TF, Holt JC, Lukasiwic H, Niewiarowski S: Trigamin: A low molecular weight peptide inhibiting fibrinogen interaction with platelet receptors expressed on glycoprotein IIb-IIIa complex. *J Biol Chem* 262:16157, 1987.

219. Klein JD, Walker FJ: Purification of a protein C activator from the venom of the southern copperhead snake (*Agkistrodon contortrix*). *Biochemistry* 25:4175, 1986.

220. Schulchynska-Castel H, Dvilansky A, Keynan A: *Echis colorata* bites:

clinical evaluation of 42 patients. A retrospective study. *Isr J Med Sci* 22:880, 1986.

221. Weiss HJ, Phillips LL, Hopewell WS, et al: Heparin therapy in a patient bitten by a saw-scaled viper (*Echis carinatus*), a snake whose venom activated prothrombin. *Am J Med* 54:653, 1973.

222. Fainaru M, Eisenberg S, Manny N, Hershko C: The natural course of defibrination syndrome caused by *Echis colorata* venom in man. *Thromb Diath Haemorrh* 31:420, 1974.

223. Warrell DA, Pope HM, Prentice CRM: Disseminated intravascular coagulation caused by the carpet viper (*Echis carinatus*): trial of heparin. *Br Haematol* 33:335, 1976.

224. Swe TN, Lwin M, Han KE, et al: Heparin therapy in Russell's viper bite victims with disseminated intravascular coagulation: a controlled trial. *Southeast Asian J Trop Med Public Health* 23:282, 1992.

225. Blatt PM, Lundblad RL, Kingdon HS, et al: Thrombogenic materials in prothrombin complex concentrates. *Ann Intern Med* 81:766, 1974.

226. Cederbaum AI, Blatt PM, Roberts HR: Intravascular coagulation with use of human prothrombin complex concentrates. *Ann Intern Med* 84:683, 1976.

227. Hultin MB: Activated clotting factors in factor IX concentrates. *Blood* 54:1028, 1979.

228. Seligsohn U, Kasper CK, Osterud B, Rapaport SI: Activated factor VII: presence in factor IX concentrate and persistence in the circulation after infusion. *Blood* 53:828, 1979.

229. Menache D, Behre HE, Orthner Cl, et al: Coagulation factor IX concentrate: method of preparation and assessment of potential in vivo thrombogenicity in animal models. *Blood* 64:1220, 1984.

230. Mannucci PM, Bauer KA, Santagostino E, et al: Activation of the coagulation cascade after infusion of a factor XI concentrate in congenitally deficient patients. *Blood* 84:1314, 1994.

231. Richards EM, Makris MM, Cooper P, Preston FE: In vivo coagulation activation following infusion of highly purified factor XI concentrate. *Br J Haematol* 96:293, 1997.

232. Bolton-Maggs Ph, Colvin BT, Satchi BT, et al: Thrombogenic potential of factor XI concentrate. *Lancet* 344:748, 1994.

233. Kasabach HH, Merritt KK: Capillary hemangioma with extensive purpura. *Am J Dis Child* 59:1063, 1940.

234. Blix S, Aas K: Giant hemangioma, thrombocytopenia, fibrinogenopenia, and fibrinolytic activity. *Acta Med Scand* 169:63, 1961.

235. Straub PW, Kessler S, Schreiber A, Frick PG: Chronic intravascular coagulation in Kasabach-Merritt syndrome. Preferential accumulation of fibrinogen 131I in a giant hemangioma. *Arch Intern Med* 129:475, 1972.

236. Warrell RP, Kempin SJ, Benua RS, et al: Intra-tumoral consumption of indium-111 labeled platelets in a patient with hemangiomatosis and intravascular coagulation (Kasabach-Merritt syndrome). *Cancer* 52:2256, 1983.

237. Propp RP, Scharfman WB: Hemangioma-thrombocytopenia syndrome associated with microangiopathic hemolytic anemia. *Blood* 28:623, 1966.

238. Inceman S, Tangun Y: Chronic defibrination syndrome due to a giant hemangioma associated with microangiopathic hemolytic anemia. *Am J Med* 46:997, 1969.

239. Seligsohn U, Ramot B: Angiopathic hemolytic anemias: report of 5 cases and review of the literature. *J Isr Med Assoc* 74:39, 1968.

240. Gilon E, Ramot B, Sheba C: Multiple hemangiomata associated with thrombocytopenia: remarks on the pathogenesis of the thrombocytopenia in this syndrome. *Blood* 14:74, 1958.

241. D'Amico JA, Hoffman GC, Dyment PG: Klippel-Trenaunay syndrome associated with chronic disseminated intravascular coagulation and massive osteolysis. *Cleve Clin Q* 44:181, 1977.

242. Poon MC, Kloiber R, Birdsell DC: Epsilon-aminocaproic acid in the reversal of consumptive coagulopathy with platelet sequestration in a vascular malformation of Klippel-Trenaunay syndrome. *Am J Med* 87:211, 1989.

243. Alpert LI, Benesh B: Hemangioendothelioma of the liver associated with microangiopathic hemolytic anemia. *Am J Med* 48:624, 1970.

244. Shanberge JH, Tanaka K, Gruhl MC: Chronic consumption coagulopathy due to hemangiomatous transformation of the spleen. *Am J Clin Pathol* 56:723, 1971.

245. Blix S, Jacobsen CD: The defibrination syndrome in a patient with hemangio-endothelio-sarcoma. *Acta Med Scand* 173:377, 1963.

246. Bick RL: Hereditary hemorrhagic telangiectasia and disseminated intra-

vascular coagulation: a new clinical syndrome. *Ann NY Acad Sci* 370:851, 1981.

247. Bell AJ, Chisholm M, Hickton M: Reversal of coagulopathy in Kasabach-Merritt syndrome with tranexamic acid. *Scand J Haematol* 37:249, 1986.

248. Warrell RP, Kempin SJ: Treatment of severe coagulopathy in the Kasabach-Merritt syndrome with aminocaproic acid and cryoprecipitate. *N Eng J Med* 313:309, 1985.

249. Fine NL, Applebaum J, Elguezabal A, Castleman L: Multiple coagulation defects in association with dissecting aneurysm. *Arch Intern Med* 119:522, 1967.

250. Fisher DI, Yawn DH, Crawford S: Preoperative disseminated intravascular coagulation associated with aortic aneurysm. *Arch Surg* 118:1252, 1983.

251. Bieger R, Vreeken J, Stibbe J, Loeliger EA: Arterial aneurysm as a cause of consumption coagulopathy. *N Engl J Med* 285:152, 1971.

252. ten Cate JW, Timmers H, Becker AE: Coagulopathy in ruptured or dissecting aortic aneurysm. *Am J Med* 59:171, 1975.

253. Mulcare RJ, Royster TS, Phillips LL: Intravascular coagulation in surgical procedures on the abdominal aorta. *Surg Gynecol Obstet* 143:730, 1976.

254. Wilcox JN, Smith KM, Schwartz SM, Gordon D: Localization of tissue factor in the normal vessel wall and in the atherosclerotic plaque. *Proc Natl Acad Sci USA* 86:2839, 1989.

255. Straub PW, Kessler S: Umzatz und lokalisation von 1131-Fibrinogen bei chronischer intravasaler Gerinnung. *Schweiz med Wochenschr* 100:2001, 1970.

256. Goto H, Kimoto A, Kawaguchi H, et al: Surgical treatment of abdominal aortic aneurysm complicated with chronic disseminated intravascular coagulopathy. *J Cardiovasc Surg* 26:280, 1985.

257. Quick AJ, Georgatsos JG, Hussey CV: The clotting activity of human erythrocytes: theoretical and clinical implications. *Am J Med* 228:207, 1954.

258. Surgenor DM: Erythrocytes and blood coagulation. *Thromb Diathes Hemorrh* 32:247, 1974.

259. Brain MC, Esterly JR, Beck EA: Intravascular haemolysis with experimentally produced vascular thrombi. *Br J Haematol* 13:868, 1967.

260. Rubenberg ML, Regoeczi E, Bull BS, et al: Microangiopathic haemolytic anaemia: the experimental production of haemolysis and red-cell fragmentation by defibrination in vivo. *Br J Haematol* 14:627, 1968.

261. Baker LRI, Rubenberg ML, Dacie JV, Brain MC: Fibrinogen catabolism in microangiopathic haemolytic anaemia. *Br J Haematol* 14:617, 1968.

262. Drinker CK, Brittingham HH: The cause of the reactions following transfusion of citrated blood. *Arch Intern Med* 23:133, 1919.

263. Astrowe PS: Hemolysis following transfusion. *JAMA* 79:1511, 1923.

264. Krevans JR, Jackson DP, Conley Cl, Hartman RC: The nature of the hemorrhagic disorder accompanying hemolytic transfusion reactions in man. *Blood* 12:834, 1957.

265. Mannucci PM, Lobina GF, Caocci L, Dioguardi N: Effect on blood coagulation of massive intravascular haemolysis. *Blood* 33:207, 1969.

266. Hamilton K, Hattori R, Esmon C, Sims P: Complement proteins C5b-9 induce vesiculation of the endothelial plasma membrane and expose catalytic surface for assembly of the prothrombinase enzyme complex. *J Biol Chem* 265:3809, 1990.

267. Weiner CP: The obstetric patient and disseminated intravascular coagulation. *Clin Perinatol* 13:705, 1986.

268. DeLee JB: A case of fatal hemorrhagic diathesis with premature detachment of the placenta. *Am J Obstet Gynecol* 44:785, 1901.

269. Pritchard JA, Brekken AL: Clinical and laboratory studies on severe abruptio placentae. *Am J Obstet Gynecol* 97:681, 1967.

270. Eskes TK: Abruptio placentae. A "classic" dedicated to Elizabeth Ramsey. *Eur J Obstet Gynecol Reprod Biol* 75:63, 1997.

271. Schneider Cl: Fibrin embolism (disseminated intravascular coagulation) with defibrination as one of the end results during abruptio placentae. *Surg Gynecol Obstet* 92:27, 1951.

272. Diekmann WJ: Blood chemistry and renal function in abruptio placentae. *Am J Obstet Gynecol* 31:734, 1936.

273. Weiner CP: The obstetric patient and disseminated intravascular coagulation. *Clin Perinatol* 13:705, 1986.

274. Crane S, Chun B, Acker D: Treatment of obstetrical hemorrhagic emergencies. *Curr Opin Obstet Gynecol* 5:675, 1993.

275. Kleiner GJ, Merskey C, Johnson AJ, Markus WD: Defibrination in normal and abnormal parturition. *Br J Haematol* 19:159, 1970.

276. Steiner PE, Lushbaugh CC: Maternal pulmonary embolism by amniotic fluid as a cause of obstetric shock and unexpected deaths in obstetrics. *JAMA* 117:1245, 1340, 1941.

277. Morgan M: Amniotic fluid embolism. *Anaesthesia* 34:20, 1979.

278. Clark SL, Hankins GD, Dudley DA, et al: Amniotic fluid embolism: analysis of the national registry. *Am J Obstet Gynecol* 172:1158, 1995.

279. Peterson EP, Taylor HB: Amniotic fluid embolism. An analysis of 40 cases. *Obstet Gynecol* 35:787, 1970.

280. Yaffe H, Eldor A, Hornshtein E, Sadovsky E: Thromboplastic activity in amniotic fluid during pregnancy. *Obstet Gynecol* 50:454, 1977.

281. Phillips LL, Davidson EC: Procoagulant properties of amniotic fluid. *Am J Obstet Gynecol* 113:911, 1972.

282. Stahnke E: Über das Verhalten der blutplattchen bei Eklampsie. *Zentralbl Gynak* 46:391, 1922.

283. McKay DG, Marrill SJ, Weiner AE, et al: The pathologic anatomy of eclampsia, bilateral renal cortical necrosis, pituitary necrosis, and other acute fatal complications of pregnancy, and its possible relationship to the generalized Shwartzman phenomenon. *Am J Obstet Gynecol* 55:507, 1953.

284. Page EW: On the pathogenesis of pre-eclampsia and eclampsia. *J Obstet Gynecol Br Commonwealth* 79:883, 1972.

285. Gibson B, Hunter D, Neame PB, Kelton JG: Thrombocytopenia in preeclampsia and eclampsia. *Semin Thromb Haemost* 8:234, 1982.

286. McKay DG: Chronic intravascular coagulation in normal pregnancy and pre-eclampsia. *Contr Nephrol* 25:108, 1981.

287. Bonnar J, McNichol GP, Douglas AS: Coagulation and fibrinolytic systems in pre-eclampsia and eclampsia. *Br Med J* 2:12, 1971.

288. Giles C: Intravascular coagulation in gestational hypertension and pre-eclampsia: The value of haematological screening tests. *Clin Lab Haematol* 4:351, 1982.

289. Kobayashi T, Terao T: Preeclampsia as chronic disseminated intravascular coagulation. Study of two parameters–thrombin-antithrombin III complex and D-dimers. *Gynecol Obstet Invest* 24:170, 1987.

290. Metz J, Cincotta R, Francis M, et al: Screening for consumptive coagulopathy in preeclampsia. *Int J Gynaecol Obstet* 46:3, 1994.

291. Schjetlein R, Haugen G, Wisloff F: Markers of intravascular coagulation and fibrinolysis in preeclampsia: association with intrauterine growth retardation. *Acta Obstet Gynecol Scand* 76:541, 1997.

292. Borok Z, Weitz J, Owen J, et al: Fibrinogen proteolysis and platelet alpha granule release in pre-eclampsia/eclampsia. *Blood* 63:525, 1984.

293. Broughton Pipkin F, Rubin PC: Pre-eclampsia—the ''disease of theories.'' *Br Med Bull* 50:381, 1994.

294. Weinstein L: Syndrome of hemolysis, elevated liver enzymes, and low platelet count; a severe consequence of hypertension in pregnancy. *Am J Obstet Gynecol* 142:159, 1982.

295. Sibai BM, Ramadan MK, Usta I, et al: Maternal morbidity and mortality in 442 pregnancies with hemolysis, elevated liver enzymes, and low platelets. *Am J Obstet Gynecol* 169:1000, 1993.

296. Aarnoudse JG, Houthoff JH, Weits K, et al: A syndrome of liver damage and intravascular coagulation in the last trimester of normotensive pregnancy. A clinical and histopathological study. *Br J Obstet Gynaecol* 93:145, 1986.

297. De Boer K, Buller HR, ten Cate JW, et al: Coagulation studies in the syndrome of haemolysis, elevated liver enzymes and low platelets. *Br J Obstet Gynecol* 98:42, 1991.

298. Audibert F, Friedman SA, Frangieh AY, Sibai BM: Clinical utility of strict diagnostic criteria for the HELLP (hemolysis, elevated liver enzymes, and low platelets) syndrome. *Am J Obstet Gynecol* 175:460, 1996.

299. Barton JR, Sibai BM: Hepatic imaging in HELLP syndrome (hemolysis, elevated liver enzymes, and low platelet count). *Am J Obstet Gynecol* 174:1820, 1996.

300. Van Dam PA, Renier M, Backelandt M, et al: Disseminated intravascular coagulation and the syndrome of hemolysis, elevated liver enzymes, and low platelets in severe pre-eclampsia. *Obstet Gynecol* 73:97, 1989.

301. Martin JN Jr, Files JC, Blake PG, et al: Postpartum plasma exchange for atypical preeclampsia-eclampsia as HELLP (hemolysis, elevated liver enzymes, and low platelets) syndrome. *Am J Obstet Gynecol* 172:1107, 1995.

302. Sullivan CA, Magann EF, Perry KG Jr, et al: The recurrence risk of the syndrome of hemolysis, elevated liver enzymes, and low platelets (HELLP) in subsequent gestations. *Am J Obstet Gynecol* 171:940, 1994.

303. Lee W, Clark SL, Cotton DB, et al: Septic shock during pregnancy. *Am J Obstet Gynecol* 159:410, 1988.

304. McKay DC, Jewett JF, Reid DE: Endotoxin shock and the generalized Shwartzman reaction in pregnancy. *Am J Obstet Gynecol* 78:546, 1959.

305. Pfau von P, Lasch HG, Gunther O: Sanarelli-Shwartzmann-Phaenomen bei febrilen Fehlgeburten und Schweren Schock und Blutungs-zustanden in der Geburtshilfe. *Gynaecologia* 150:17, 1960.

306. Kuhn W, Graeff H: Infizierter Abort und disseminierte intravaskulare Gerinnung (DIG). *Med Welt* 22:1199, 1971.

307. Koch HH, Keller O: Unsere Erfahrungen mit den prophylaktischen massnahmen zur Verhinderung des Sanarelli-Shwartzman Phaenomen (SSP) beim infizierten Abort. *Geburtshilfe Frauenheilkd* 33:460, 1973.

308. Pritchard JA, Ratnoff OD: Studies of fibrinogen and other hemostatic factors in women with intrauterine death and delayed delivery. *Surg Gynecol Obstet* 101:467, 1955.

309. Romero R, Copel JA, Hobbins JC: Intrauterine fetal demise and hemostatic failure: the fetal death syndrome. *Clin Obstet Gynecol* 28:24, 1985.

310. Lerner R, Margolin M, Slate WG, et al: Heparin in the treatment of hypofibrinogenemia complicating fetal death in utero. *Am J Obstet Gynecol* 97:373, 1967.

311. Gallup DG, Lucas WE: Heparin treatment of consumption coagulopathy associated with intrauterine fetal death. *Obstet Gynecol* 35:690, 1970.

312. Berkowitz RL, Stone JL, Eddleman KA: One hundred consecutive cases of selective termination of an abnormal fetus in a multifetal gestation. *Obstet Gynecol* 90:606, 1997.

313. Bacq Y, Riely CA: Acute fatty liver of pregnancy: the hepatologist's view. *Gastroenterologist* 1:257, 1993.

314. Usta IM, Barton JR, Amon EA, et al: Acute fatty liver of pregnancy: an experience in the diagnosis and management of fourteen cases. *Am J Obstet Gynecol* 171:1342, 1994.

315. Pereira SP, O'Donohue J, Wendon J, Williams R: Maternal and perinatal outcome in severe pregnancy-related liver disease. *Hepatology* 26:1258, 1997.

316. Castro MA, Goodwin TM, Shaw KJ, et al: Disseminated intravascular coagulation and antithrombin III depression in acute fatty liver of pregnancy. *Am J Obstet Gynecol* 174:211, 1996.

317. Hathaway WE, Mull MM, Peschet GS: Disseminated intravascular coagulation in the newborn. *Pediatrics* 43:233, 1969.

318. Corrigan JJ: Activation of coagulation and disseminated intravascular coagulation in the newborn. *Am J Pediat Hematol Oncol* 1:245, 1979.

319. Woods WG, Luban NL, Hilgartner MW, Miller DR: Disseminated intravascular coagulation in the newborn. *Am J Dis Child* 133:44, 1979.

320. Corrigan JJ: Disseminated intravascular coagulopathy. *Pediatr Rev* 1:37, 1979.

321. Gross SJ, Filston HC, Anderson JC: Controlled study of treatment for disseminated intravascular coagulation in the neonate. *J Pediatr* 100:445, 1982.

322. Emery ML: Disseminated intravascular coagulation in the neonate. *Neonatal Netw* 11:5, 1992.

323. Markarian M, Lubchenko LO, Rosenblut E, et al: Hypercoagulability in premature infants with special reference to the respiratory distress syndrome and hemorrhage: II. The effect of heparin. *Biol Neonate* 17:98, 1971.

324. Gobel U, von Voss H, Jurgens H, et al: Efficiency of heparin in the treatment of newborn infants with respiratory distress syndrome and disseminated intravascular coagulation. *Eur J Pediatr* 133:47, 1980.

HEREDITARY THROMBOPHILIA

SCOTT H. GOODNIGHT

JOHN H. GRIFFIN

Hereditary thrombophilia is defined as a genetically determined increased likelihood of thrombosis. An emerging paradigm suggests that thromboembolism is a multicausal disease involving one or more genetic defects in conjunction with acquired risk factors such as inactivity, trauma, malignancy, inflammation, pregnancy, oral contraceptive use, or autoimmune disease. The three most common hereditary defects (found in a substantial proportion of patients presenting with venous thrombosis) include activated protein C resistance caused by replacement of Arg506 by Gln in the factor V gene (factor V Leiden), a prothrombin polymorphism (G20210A) that causes elevated plasma prothrombin levels, and hyperhomocysteinemia. Additional genetic abnormalities include deficiencies of the anticoagulant factors protein C, protein S, or antithrombin. The majority of these thrombophilic defects either enhance procoagulant reactions or hamper anticoagulant mechanisms and thus cause a prothrombotic state due to hypercoagulability of the blood. Venous thrombosis is the most common manifestation of hereditary thrombophilia, although a minority of patients, particularly those with other vascular risk factors, may develop arterial thrombi as well. Less usual presentations of venous thromboembolic disease include abdominal and cerebral vein thrombosis, along with pregnancy loss or other complications due to placental vascular insufficiency and thrombosis. Laboratory assays are now widely available to identify the great majority of patients with thrombophilia. Knowledge of these disorders affects patient management, including the duration of anticoagulant treatment, the use of clotting factor replacement therapy, the need for prophylactic antithrombotic agents, and counseling involving the relative risks of pregnancy and use of oral contraceptives or hormone replacement.

INTRODUCTION

Hereditary thrombophilia is defined as a genetically determined increased risk of thrombosis. According to Virchow's classic (and still useful) triad, risk factors for thrombosis may involve abnormalities in the vessel wall (see Chap. 114), rheology, and/or blood components. Identification of defects in specific blood components, especially plasma factors, has provided molecular insights into the pathogenesis of thrombophilia. The major defects associated with familial thrombophilia are listed in Table 127-1. The first description of hereditary thrombophilia caused by a deficiency of an anticoagulant protein was by Egeberg in 1965.[1] Members of the family described in the report

suffered from recurrent venous thrombosis, and the disorder was inherited in an autosomal dominant pattern. The plasma of affected family members had reduced amounts of an inhibitor to thrombin, antithrombin III. In 1976, Stenflo and coworkers[2] purified and characterized an anticoagulant factor, protein C, from bovine plasma, and subsequently the first patients with hereditary protein C deficiency and thrombosis were described by Griffin and colleagues.[3] Three years later protein S deficiency was reported in several families with thrombosis by Schwarz and coworkers[4] and Comp and coworkers.[5,6] In 1993 Dahlback and coworkers reported three families with venous thrombosis associated with hereditary resistance to activated protein C (APC),[7,8] and in 1994 the underlying genetic defect was simultaneously reported by three laboratories to involve the factor V mutation of Arg506 to Gln, a defect now often referred to as *factor V Leiden*.[9–11] At about the same time, mild to moderate hyperhomocysteinemia was also recognized as a risk factor for venous thrombosis,[12] although a predisposition to arterial vascular disease due to elevated levels of homocysteine had been known for some time.[13] In 1996, a mutation in the 3'-untranslated region of prothrombin was identified and linked to familial venous thromboembolism by Poort and colleagues.[14] Many important observations have come from the Leiden Thrombophilia Study of 300 to 500 Dutch consecutive patients presenting with a first episode of venous thrombosis.[15,16] With the imminent characterization of about 100,000 human genes, one can anticipate a steady stream of advances in the identification of more genetic defects responsible for hereditary thrombophilia.

Specific hereditary thrombophilias can now be identified in 30 to 50 percent of patients presenting with a first episode of venous thromboembolism, with even higher percentages found in subjects with recurrent thrombosis. Patients with hereditary thrombophilia may have more than one hereditary thrombophilia and associated acquired abnormalities such as antiphospholipid antibodies, malignancy, myeloproliferative diseases, or inflammatory disorders (Fig. 127-1). Hereditary prothrombotic states are usually associated with venous rather than arterial thrombosis; however, in association with other risk factors such as smoking or diabetes, recent data suggest that up to 10 percent of arterial thromboses are associated with hereditary thrombophilia.[17,18]

Venous thrombosis and its complications are important and common medical problems, estimated to occur at a rate of 1.2 events/ 1000 population per year.[19] Thus, for the population of the United States, there will be approximately 201,000 new cases of venous thromboembolism per year, of which 107,000 will be deep venous thrombosis and 94,000 will be pulmonary embolism.

In this chapter, we will discuss the pathogenesis and unique clinical features of each of the more common hereditary thrombophilias (see Table 127-1). Thereafter an approach to the diagnosis and subsequent treatment of these thrombophilic patients will be presented.

MAJOR HEREDITARY DEFECTS

HEREDITARY RESISTANCE TO ACTIVATED PROTEIN C

DEFINITION AND HISTORY
The term *activated protein C (APC) resistance* is defined as an abnormally reduced anticoagulant response of a subject's plasma to APC on the basis of in vitro testing. A "normal" range for response to APC is established for the various coagulation or other related assay conditions used to assess response to APC.[7,20,21] In 1989, an abnormally poor response to APC was described for several individual patients with venous thrombosis when it was shown that partially purified antibody fractions interfered with expression of APC activity.[22–24] In 1991, familial APC resistance was first reported in one kindred and was ascribed to an APC-resistant factor VIII defect.[25] Apparently this mechanism could not be confirmed, and in 1993, the description of

TABLE 127-1   MAJOR HEREDITARY DEFECTS ASSOCIATED WITH INCREASED RISK OF VENOUS THROMBOSIS

ABNORMALITY	PREVALENCE,* %	
	UNSELECTED	SELECTED
Activated protein C (APC) resistance caused by Arg506 to Gln mutation (factor V Leiden)	14–20	20–50
Prothrombin polymorphism (G20210A) causing elevated prothrombin level	4–8	10–20
Hyperhomocysteinemia*	5–10	NA
Protein C deficiency	1–4	3–12
Protein S deficiency	1–4	3–12
Antithrombin deficiency	1–3	1–6
Elevated factor VIII*	25	NA

*Unselected patients are defined as consecutive patients presenting with a first episode of venous thrombosis (under 70 years old in the Leiden Thrombosis Study), and selected patients are those under 50 years old with a personal or familial history of venous thrombosis.
†Elevated homocysteine or factor VIII is usually defined as greater than 95th percentile or greater than 150 percent of asymptomatic normal controls respectively. NA indicates data not available.

three unrelated families presenting with venous thrombosis associated with APC resistance without any identifiable defect stimulated an intensive search for genetic and molecular mechanistic explanations.[7] Three laboratories independently reported in May of 1994 that a single genetic defect was associated with APC resistance, involving replacement of G by A at nucleotide 1691 in exon 10 of the factor V gene which causes the amino acid replacement of Arg506 by Gln.[9–11] Further analysis indicated genetic linkage between APC resistance and the factor V gene.[26,27] In the published literature and in this chapter, this defect is variously termed Gln506-factor V, Q^{506}-factor V, or factor V Leiden.

ETIOLOGY AND PATHOGENESIS

APC resistance can be caused by heterogeneous molecular defects, although replacement of Arg506 by Gln in factor V is responsible for

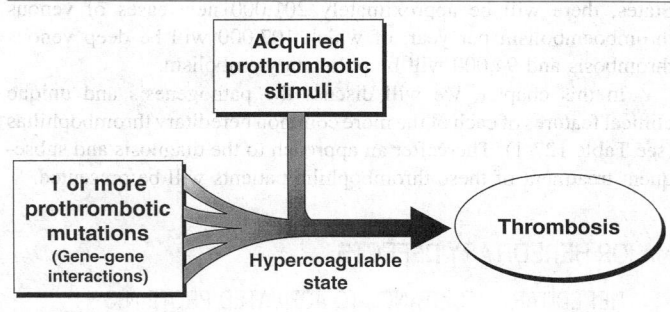

FIGURE 127-1   Paradigm for genetic contribution to venous thrombosis. Clinically significant venous thrombosis most often follows from the simultaneous presence of an acquired risk factor for thrombosis and one or more genetic factors that convey thrombotic risk. The presence of two genetic factors (i.e., gene-gene interaction) greatly increases the likelihood of thrombosis. Mild genetic risk factors include APC resistance with or without factor V Leiden; the prothrombin G20210A polymorphism causing elevated plasma prothrombin levels; and heterozygous deficiency of protein C, protein S, or antithrombin. Hyperhomocysteinemia is a mild risk factor. Elevated levels (more than 150 percent of normal) of various coagulation factors, including factors VIII, XI, and IX and fibrinogen also appear to be mild risk factors for venous thrombosis. Venous thrombosis patients frequently have two or more genetic risk factors. See Schafer,[351] Bertina,[15] Rosendaal,[16,78] and van Boven.[279] Taken from Schafer with permission.[351]

APC resistance in the great majority of patients. APC resistance is a laboratory phenotype, whereas Gln506-factor V is a genotype, and the term *APC resistance* should not be used as a synonym for *factor V Leiden*. APC resistance caused by defects other than factor V Leiden is associated with increased risk of venous thrombosis[28,29] or ischemic stroke.[30,31]

Theoretically, any genetic abnormality of a protein C pathway component that interferes with the expression of APC activity can cause APC resistance as could acquired abnormalities such as antibodies against protein C pathway components.[32,33] Although the causes of many cases of acquired APC resistance are unknown, the majority (more than 90 percent) of hereditary APC resistant subjects have the same genetic abnormality, factor V at G1691A (Arg506Gln), which arose in a single Caucasian founder some 21,000 to 34,000 years ago.[34] The molecular mechanism for APC resistance in such probands involves resistance of Gln506-factor Va to proteolytic inactivation by APC,[9,35,36] with kinetic studies showing that the Gln506-variant is inactivated 10 times slower than normal Arg506-factor Va.[36–39] Gln506-factor Va, whether activated by thrombin or factor Xa, is partially but not entirely resistant to APC, implying that inactivation of Gln506-factor Va by APC can occur in vivo, albeit at a reduced rate. Explanation for only a *partial* resistance to APC derives from the fact that cleavage of factor Va by APC at Arg306 also occurs, causing complete loss of factor Va activity, although this cleavage is slower than that at the Arg506 site.[36–40] This finding helps explain why APC resistance due to Gln506-factor V is a rather mild risk factor for venous thrombosis and why a combination of genetic risk factors or a combination of a genetic risk factor plus acquired risk factors for venous thrombosis is found in a significant fraction of symptomatic patients (see below). Another possibility to help explain the mild risk of venous thrombosis associated with Gln506-factor V is that factor Va may be inactivated in vivo by proteases other than APC that cleave at sites other than residue 506.

There are additional potential molecular defects that might contribute to thrombosis in hereditary APC resistance. In purified clotting factor reaction mixtures, factor V enhances inactivation of factor VIIIa by APC in the presence of protein S,[41] and APC resistant subjects carrying Gln506-Factor V are reportedly defective in this APC cofactor activity.[42–45] APC resistance caused by rare factor V mutations that replace Arg306 by Thr[46] or Gly[47] have been reported, although the relationship to relative risks of thrombosis have not been established.[48] A factor V haplotype, designated R2, has also been associated with mild APC resistance.[49] The molecular mechanisms and thrombotic risks associated with the R2 factor V haplotype which contains normal Arg506 remain to be defined, although it appears that the R2 haplotype is only a risk factor when present along with the Gln506-factor V allele.[50]

APC is a normal component of circulating blood that contributes to antithrombotic surveillance mechanisms and prevents thrombosis (see Chap 113).[51] Normal subjects have a mean APC concentration of 2.3 ng/ml (38 pM) in the circulation,[52] and the in vivo half-life of APC in normal adult human subjects as well as in freshly drawn whole blood is approximately 22 min.[53,54] Thus, there is continuous activation of the protein C pathway in vivo. In normal subjects, there is an inverse relationship between levels of circulating APC and of thrombin.[55] APC levels are increased when thrombin is acutely generated such as during DIC, ischemia, or surgical procedures.

Because circulating APC has such a long half-life, it provides systemic anticoagulation to down-regulate thrombin generation and to limit extension of hemostatic plugs. Hence, genetic or acquired defects that impair the response to APC are understandably prothrombotic. Elevated plasma levels of prothrombin fragment F1+2 and thrombin-antithrombin complexes are found in many subjects heterozygous or homozygous for Gln506-factor V,[56-59] presumably reflecting the impairment of the expression of APC's anticoagulant activity.

APC resistance has been associated with less intrapartum blood loss, suggesting an evolutionary advantage.[60] However, pregnancy loss is increased in some women due to thrombosis in the placental vasculature (see below). Hemophilia A patients who also inherit Gln506-factor V have been reported to have less severe hemorrhagic symptoms.[61]

CLINICAL FEATURES

The factor V Leiden mutation is present in 3 to 12 percent of Caucasians and is rare in other ethnic groups.[62-64] Deep and superficial venous thromboses are the most common manifestations of this disorder, whereas pulmonary embolism and thromboses in unusual locations appear to be relatively less frequent than in subjects with deficiencies in antithrombin, protein C, or protein S.[65-69] In patients with venous insufficiency leading to leg ulcers, approximately 25 percent were found to have APC resistance[70] or factor V Leiden.[71] Cerebral, hepatic, and other thromboses have been reported in patients with factor V Leiden.[72-74] About half the patients will have idiopathic (unprovoked) venous thromboembolism, with 20 percent occurring after surgery, and 30 percent in women who are pregnant or taking birth control pills.[75] Pregnancy loss and other obstetric complications occur at an increased rate in women with factor V Leiden (see below).

The risk of thrombosis in subjects with factor V Leiden appears to be somewhat lower than in patients from families with deficiencies of antithrombin or protein C[76,77]; nonetheless, since factor V Leiden is so common, it accounts for the largest proportion of patients presenting with a first thromboembolic event (20 to 25 percent).[78] The relative risk of venous thrombosis in patients heterozygous for factor V Leiden is increased by four to eightfold in studies from Europe and North America.[20,67,79-81] The risk of idiopathic venous thromboembolism for men increases with age, from a relative risk of 1.23 at age 40 to 50 years to 5.97 for those aged 70 years and older.[79] First-degree relatives of symptomatic carriers of the factor V mutation develop thromboses at a rate of 0.45 percent per year (0.25 percent per year in the 15- to 30-year age group, and 1.1 percent per year in those over 60).[75,77] In several studies, recurrent thrombotic events are rather frequent, occurring at a rate of 5 to 10 percent per year following a first thrombosis.[82-84] However, other investigators found no increased rates of recurrence when compared to thrombosis patients without factor V Leiden.[85-87] Homozygous carriers of factor V Leiden have an odds ratio for venous thrombosis of 50 to 100, and it is estimated that approximately half of such individuals will experience a clinically significant episode during their lives.[88] Although thromboses in homozygotes are substantially more common than in heterozygotes, the disorder is far less severe than in subjects with homozygous deficiency of protein C, or protein S.[56,88,89] Despite the increased thrombotic risk, the presence of factor V Leiden does not increase overall mortality.[90-93]

Coronary artery thrombosis has been notably associated with the factor V Leiden mutation in young women[17] and men[94] also displaying other vascular risk factors. The relative risk of myocardial infarction in carriers of V Leiden from the Netherlands is 1.4, which increased to three- to sixfold if other risk factors such as obesity, smoking, hypertension, or diabetes were present.[95] Similar findings have been reported for young women from Washington State, with odds ratios of up to 32 for myocardial infarction in V Leiden carriers who were also smokers.[17] However, other studies have failed to find a relationship between APC resistance and myocardial infarction or stroke in older individuals.[80,96-98] Factor V Leiden seems to be relatively common in children who develop cerebral infarction or venous thrombosis.[99-101]

PREDISPOSING FACTORS FOR THROMBOSIS IN SUBJECTS WITH FACTOR V LEIDEN

Although isolated factor V Leiden is associated with a relatively mild hypercoagulable state, the risk of thrombosis is greatly magnified when other prothrombotic disorders are also present (Fig. 127-1). These additional risk factors may be hereditary (e.g., protein C deficiency or the prothrombin gene mutation), acquired (antiphospholipid antibodies, hyperhomocysteinemia), physical (inactivity or surgery), due to other diseases (malignancy or inflammation), or hormonal (oral contraceptives or pregnancy).[78]

Multiple hereditary thrombophilic defects (i.e., gene-gene interaction) are quite common, and are found in up to 15 percent of patients presenting with venous thromboembolism.[102] Factor V Leiden has been reported in combination with protein C deficiency,[9,103-105] protein S deficiency,[106-108] antithrombin deficiency,[109] the prothrombin gene mutation,[110,111] and hyperhomocysteinemia.[112-114] In families with combined defects, thromboses occurred more frequently and at an earlier age in the subjects with two separate defects.

Pregnancy and estrogen-containing oral contraceptives substantially enhance the risk of thrombosis in women with factor V Leiden. Of women who develop venous thromboembolism during pregnancy, 28 to 46 percent will carry the factor V mutation.[115-117] The relative risk of developing thrombosis for heterozygotes during or after pregnancy is increased over threefold, with a higher probability of recurrence (relative risk of 3.86).[117] Several studies have examined the risks of thromboembolism in women with factor V Leiden using third-generation oral contraceptives. There is a highly significant increase of 30- to 80-fold in the odds ratio for thrombosis, with an absolute increase in risk from 0.8 to 28.5 per10,000 women per year.[118,119] Even higher risks are seen in women who are homozygous for the mutation.[120] Data are not yet available on the risk of thrombosis in women with factor V Leiden (with or without a history of thrombosis) who receive hormone replacement therapy. A major side effect of selective estrogen receptor modulators such as tamoxifen or raloxifene may also exert an increased risk of venous thrombosis. Three cases of tamoxifen-associated venous thrombosis were associated with factor V Leiden.[121]

LABORATORY ASSAYS

Coagulation assays and DNA-based assays are available for the identification of patients with APC resistance. Plasma-based coagulation tests depend on the relative prolongation of the activated partial thromboplastin time (aPTT) or other coagulation screening tests caused by the addition of purified APC. Individuals with resistance to APC have less prolongation of the aPTT than normal. Although an aPTT assay was originally used, current assays employ factor V deficient plasma,[35] which makes the test informative in most patients with lupus inhibitors, in pregnant patients, in patients with inflammatory states, and in patients on anticoagulants. The test is sensitive and specific when compared with the genetic test for factor V Leiden.[122-126] Studies using the first-generation assay (see above) have suggested that an abnormally low APC ratio is associated with venous thrombosis, in both the presence and absence of the factor V Leiden mutation[28,29] and with ischemic stroke.[30,31] Thus, there is clinically relevant information in the classic aPTT-based APC resistance test that is not obtained using factor V deficient substrate plasma. Tissue-factor-based APC resistance assays can provide additional information about plasma components that differentially modulate the protein C pathway,[127-129] such as "anticoagulant" high-density lipoprotein or as yet unidentified factors that are altered by oral contraceptive usage. The presence of platelets or platelet microparticles in plasma tested for APC resistance using aPTT assays,[130-132] as well as autoantibodies against APC,[33] can reduce the anticoagulant response to APC, indicating the need to carefully prepare plasma prior to testing.

Many DNA-based assays for the factor V Leiden polymorphism are available. Genomic DNA is isolated, amplified by polymerase chain reaction (PCR), subjected to restriction fragment length polymorphism analysis, and analyzed for G or A at nucleotide 1691.[9] Plasma coagulation tests are often used for screening patients, followed by confirmation of positive results with the DNA assay. Only DNA tests clearly distinguish factor V Leiden heterozygosity from homozygosity. ''Pseudo-homozygotes'' heterozygous for factor V Ledien and for a dysfunctional factor V allele will have very low APC-resistance ratios in the plasma test but will be heterozygous by the DNA assay for factor V Leiden.[133–135]

PROTHROMBIN G20210A GENE POLYMORPHISM

DEFINITION AND HISTORY

In 1996, Poort and colleagues reported that a polymorphism in the 3′-untranslated region of the prothrombin gene, namely nt G20210A, was associated with increased risk of venous thrombosis and with elevated levels of plasma prothrombin.[14] This polymorphism likely arose as a single mutation in a Caucasian founder,[136] and the polymorphism is currently found in 1 to 5 percent of Caucasians.[137]

ETIOLOGY AND PATHOGENESIS

Replacement of G by A at nt 20210 in the 3′-untranslated region of the prothrombin gene does not alter transcription of the gene but may increase translation, thus resulting in elevated synthesis and secretion of prothrombin by the liver. The elevated level of plasma prothrombin likely contributes directly to increased thrombotic risk by causing increased thrombin generation.

CLINICAL FEATURES

The prothrombin gene mutation is found largely in Caucasian populations.[136] In contrast to factor V Leiden, the frequency of the mutation seems to increase from northern Europe to southern Europe, i.e., only 1.7 percent of the population in northern Europe had the abnormality compared with 3 to 5 percent in the south of Europe and the Middle East.[137,138] The prothrombin gene mutation is associated with venous thrombosis in all age groups.[139] When sequential patients presenting with a first venous thromboembolism are analyzed, 4 to 8 percent of them will have the mutation, and the odds ratio for thrombosis in subjects with prothrombin 20210A is increased approximately 2- to 5.5-fold.[14,102,140–145] In patients with recurrent thromboembolism or a family history of thrombosis, as many as 15 to 18 percent will have the defect compared with 1 to 3 percent of controls in various populations.[14,146] As mentioned earlier, the prothrombin variant is associated with elevated plasma levels of prothrombin (e.g., a mean of 132 percent).[14] Increased prothrombin activity or antigen is also associated with an increased risk of thrombosis even in the absence of the mutation.[147]

As in other forms of hereditary thrombophilia, the prothrombin gene mutation has been found in patients with thrombosis in unusual sites, particularly cerebral sinus vein thrombosis.[148–153] For example, in a study of 40 patients with cerebral vein thrombosis, 20 percent had the gene defect (OR 10.2). Many of these thromboses were in young women taking oral contraceptives, which raises the likelihood of thrombosis even higher (i.e., an OR of 150).[150]

Individuals who are homozygous for the prothrombin gene mutation appear more likely than heterozygotes to develop thrombosis.[154–156] The mutation also occurs in concert with other hereditary thrombophilic states (8 percent in one study).[111,140,142,146,157] When the prothrombin variant was associated with factor V Leiden in young symptomatic

patients, overall thrombosis rates were increased as well as spontaneous events and thromboses in unusual locations.[111]

The prothrombin gene mutation appears generally not to be over-represented in unselected patients with cerebral vascular or coronary artery disease.[146,158–161] However, certain selected groups of patients with arterial thrombosis have an increased likelihood of carrying the mutation.[95,141,155,162–164] In young (younger than 50 years) patients with documented ischemic stroke but without other risk factors such as diabetes, hypertension, or hyperlipidemia, 15 percent had the prothrombin gene mutation (giving an odds ratio for ischemic stroke of 5.1).[155] The mutation also appears to be associated with an increased risk of myocardial infarction, especially in those with other major risk factors for coronary heart disease such as smoking.[95,162] Finally, a large proportion of a group of young women with acute unexplained spinal cord infarction were found to have the mutation.[165] All were taking oral contraceptives and most were smokers.

LABORATORY DIAGNOSIS

Identification of the mutation in the 3′-untranslated region of the prothrombin gene requires DNA analysis following PCR amplification of the pertinent region.[14] Although prothrombin levels are elevated, assay of prothrombin activity or prothrombin antigen is usually not sufficiently sensitive or specific to screen for the presence of the mutation or as a more effective predictor of thrombosis.[146,147,157]

HYPERHOMOCYSTEINEMIA

DEFINITION AND HISTORY

A plasma homocysteine level above the normal range defines hyperhomocysteinemia. Severe hyperhomocysteinemia, also identifiable as homocystinuria, is rare and is an autosomal recessive trait associated with severe defects in cystathionine β-synthase, 5,10-methylenetetrahydrofolate reductase (MTHFR), or possibly other enzymes that affect homocysteine metabolism.[166–168] Such severe abnormalities are associated with neurologic abnormalities, premature cardiovascular disease, stroke, and vascular thrombosis. Mild to moderate hyperhomocysteinemia is an independent risk factor for arteriosclerosis and arterial thrombosis.[13,167,169] A meta-analysis of 10 case-control studies concluded that mild hyperhomocysteinemia conveys a significant, though mild, increased risk of venous thrombosis.[170]

ETIOLOGY AND PATHOGENESIS

Homocysteine is an intermediate in the metabolism of the sulfur-containing amino acids, methionine and cysteine, and homocysteine participates in several metabolic pathways. Remethylation of homocysteine to generate methionine requires the vitamin B_{12}-dependent enzyme, methionine synthase, and 5-methyltetrahydrofolate, which are part of a metabolic pathway that recycles tetrahydrofolate, and 5-methyltetrahydrofolate and involves the enzyme methylenetetrahydrofolate reductase. For the synthesis of cysteine from homocysteine, a transulfuration pathway first involves condensation of homocysteine with serine to generate cystathionine by the vitamin B_6-dependent enzyme, cystathionine β-synthase; then deamination and cleavage of cystathionine to yield cysteine and α-ketobutyrate is accomplished by the vitamin B_6-dependent enzyme, cystathioninase. The most common known genetic cause of mild hyperhomocysteinemia involves an MTHFR gene polymorphism, nt C677T, that causes a conservative replacement of Ala222 by Val which results in a variant enzyme with reduced specific activity and increased thermolability.[113] Homozygosity for this so-called thermolabile form of MTHFR, i.e., homozygosity for TT at nt677, is associated with mild hyperhomocysteinemia.

The most common cause of rare, severe hyperhomocysteinemia is defective cystathionine β-synthase. Suboptimal levels of folate or vitamins B_6 or B_{12} can also contribute to acquired mild to moderate hyperhomocysteinemia by providing inadequate cofactor levels to support the enzymes that regulate homocysteine metabolism. Conversely, administration of folate with vitamins B_6 and B_{12} can reduce homocysteine levels.[171,172] To date, no controlled studies of vitamin therapy to reduce homocysteine levels in venous thrombosis patients have been reported nor has it been proved that this vitamin strategy reduces arterial or venous thrombotic risk.

The exact mechanisms by which hyperhomocysteinemia causes increased risk of thrombosis have not been defined, although there is strong evidence that elevated homocysteine levels cause deleterious prothrombotic alterations in a number of normal vascular functions based on animal model studies, tissue culture experiments, and clinical research (see Chap. 114).[173-175]

CLINICAL FEATURES

Hyperhomocysteinemia is commonly associated with venous thromboembolism as well as arterial disease. From 10 to 25 percent of patients with primary or recurrent venous thrombosis have plasma homocysteine concentrations that are greater than the 95th percentile of the distribution in normal individuals (i.e., greater than 17 to 22 μmol/liter).[167,169,176-180] Meta-analysis of multiple studies suggest that the odds ratio for venous thrombosis is 2.5 to 3.0 if homocysteine concentrations are elevated.[170] Coagulation activation markers such as F1.2 or plasma levels of activated protein C are increased in patients with hyperhomocysteinemia and thrombosis, suggesting the presence of hypercoagulability.[181,182]

The association of hyperhomocysteinema and venous thrombosis is stronger among women (e.g., OR 7), and it also increases with age, rising to an odds ratio of 5.5 for individuals who are older than 50 years.[176] In most but not all studies,[183] the combination of hyperhomocysteinemia in concert with other hypercoagulable states substantially increases the risk of thromboembolism.[112,114,169] For example, in the Physicians Health Study, the odds ratio for idiopathic venous thromboembolism in subjects with hyperhomocysteinemia was 3.4, for those with factor V Leiden it was 3.6, but for subjects with both disorders, the odds ratio was greatly increased to over 20.[114] Hyperhomocysteinemia is also a strong predictor of recurrent thrombosis (OR 2–3), with reported recurrence rates of up to 10 percentper year for the first 2 years after cessation of oral anticoagulants.[177,180]

The thermolabile form of MTHFR has been associated with hyperhomocysteinemia, particularly during periods of folate deficiency.[184,185] Although controversial, it appears that homozygosity alone for this enzyme defect (which occurs in 10 to 20 percent of normal individuals) is associated with either an absent or a mild increased risk of venous thromboembolism in the absence of associated thrombotic risk factors.[102,113,186-189] However, subjects who are homozygous for the MTHFR variant who also have factor V Leiden or the prothrombin gene mutation may be at a mildly to moderately increased risk of thrombosis.[102,113,186,188]

LABORATORY DIAGNOSIS

Plasma homocysteine concentrations can be measured by HPLC or an immunoassay or by performing a methionine loading test. Both fasting levels and levels after methionine loading have been used to assess hyperhomocysteinemia.[190-193] Although the methionine loading test may detect additional subjects with hyperhomocysteinemia, it is not clear that the predictive value for thrombosis is sufficiently increased to warrant the additional effort and cost of this procedure.[169,177,193,194] Blood samples for homocysteine levels should be obtained in the fasting state, kept cold, and centrifuged immediately.[190,192] Individual measurements reflect average homocysteine concentrations over time (e.g., 4 weeks) reasonably well.[190] Serum homocysteine levels are higher than plasma levels, and male values are higher than female values.[195] The thermolabile nt 677T variant of MTHFR and mutations in the cystathionine beta-synthase gene can be assessed using DNA-based molecular techniques.[196]

PROTEIN C DEFICIENCY

DEFINITION AND HISTORY

The first cases of familial heterozygous protein C deficiency (about 50 percent of normal plasma level) associated with venous thrombosis in young adulthood[3] and of severe protein C deficiency (less than 1 percent protein C activity) associated with neonatal purpura fulminans[197] were reported in 1981. Most typically, hereditary deficiency of protein C results from an autosomal trait in which affected individuals have approximately 50 percent of the normal level of functional plasma protein C. Over 150 different mutations in the protein C gene which are associated with thrombosis have now been reported.[198] Heterozygous protein C deficiency conveys a mildly increased risk of venous thrombosis. Fewer than two dozen cases of severe protein C deficiency due to homozygosity or compound heterozygosity have been reported in neonates with purpura fulminans or massive thrombosis. Type I protein C deficiency is defined as a disorder with parallel reductions in both plasma antigen and anticoagulant activity levels, whereas type II deficiency, associated with circulating dysfunctional molecules, involves normal plasma levels of antigen but low levels of anticoagulant activity.

ETIOLOGY AND PATHOGENESIS

Protein C is synthesized in the liver and circulates in plasma as a serine protease zymogen; it is activated by limited proteolysis by thrombin bound to thrombomodulin, possibly with additional acceleration by an endothelial protein C receptor (see Chap. 113). APC is a potent anticoagulant enzyme that down-regulates the blood coagulation pathways by proteolytic and irreversible inactivation of factors Va and VIIIa. Thus, decreased levels of protein C zymogen may impair the inhibition of thrombin generation and contribute to hypercoagulability.

CLINICAL FEATURES

Protein C deficiency occurs in 0.2 to 0.4 percent of normal individuals[199,200] and is found in approximately 4 to 5 percent of consecutive outpatients with objectively confirmed deep venous thrombosis.[201] Deficiency of protein C is linked to thrombosis (OR 6.5–8),[76,201] and many families with hereditary protein C deficiency and thromboembolism have been reported.[3,202-204] The mean age of first thrombosis has been reported to be similar (approximately 45 years) in patients with factor V Leiden and protein C deficiency suggesting similar thrombotic tendencies in the two types of thrombophilia.[205] When mortality rates are compared, individuals with protein C deficiency have a normal life-span.[206]

Variability in clinical expression is a hallmark of the disorder. Subjects identified by screening large numbers of normal individuals (e.g., blood donors) in most instances have neither a personal nor a family history of thromboembolism.[199,200] The discrepancy in thrombosis rates between these surveys and studies of families who have striking thrombotic symptoms can be explained in part by the coinheritance of factor V Leiden or another thrombophilic state (Fig. 127-1).[9,103-105,207,208] Polymorphisms in the promotor region of the protein C gene resulting in lower levels of protein C in some of the families could also be involved.[209] Recurrent thrombosis in affected families with protein C deficiency is quite common and is unprovoked in about 60 percent of instances.[210,211]

Deep and superficial venous thrombosis is the most common clinical presentation of protein C deficiency.[210-213] By the age of 45, up to 50 percent of heterozygous subjects in clinically affected families will have venous thromboembolism, and half of the episodes will be spontaneous.[203] Protein C deficiency has been linked to unusual sites of venous thrombosis including the cerebral and mesenteric veins.[210,214] Arterial thrombosis seems to be uncommon, although ischemic stroke and other arterial occlusive events have been reported.[76,215]

Homozygous protein C deficiency with protein C levels of less than 1 percent produces a fulminating thrombotic diathesis including the dramatic syndrome of neonatal purpura fulminans in affected infants.[197,216–219] In a similar scenario, "warfarin skin necrosis," large areas of thrombotic skin necrosis, appear over central areas of the body (breast, abdomen, genitalia) in subjects with heterozygous protein C deficiency given warfarin.[220] In this syndrome in protein C deficient patients, the vitamin K antagonist induces a fall in protein C activity from approximately 50 percent to very low levels because of the short half-life of protein C in vivo (4 to 8 h).[221] Because the half-lives of prothrombin, factor IX, and factor X are much longer, a transient hypercoagulable state may arise at the outset of vitamin K-antagonist therapy. Heparin or low-molecular-weight heparin should be used when initiating warfarin treatment in subjects known to be protein C deficient.[202]

LABORATORY DIAGNOSIS

Most laboratories screen for protein C deficiency with a protein C activity assay that employs a highly specific snake venom protease to activate protein C.[222,223] Protein C activity is best assessed with an assay that employs a coagulation rather than a chromogenic end point to identify the greatest number of patients with protein C deficiency.[224] Immunoassays are used to distinguish type I defects (reduced antigen and activity) from type II disorders (normal antigen, reduced activity).[225] Normal ranges for protein C increase with age (4 percent per decade) so that results need to be interpreted against these age-specific norms.[222] Protein C gene promotor polymorphisms also influence plasma concentrations of the protein which can vary from 94 to 106 percent,[209,226] and liver disease or oral contraceptives can lower or raise protein C levels respectively.[227] Consequently, protein C levels of less than 55 percent (in the absence of oral anticoagulants or overt liver disease) suggest protein C deficiency, but levels from 55 to 70 percent must be considered borderline, and repeated testing or family studies should be undertaken.[224] The use of DNA-based assays to identify patients with hereditary protein C deficiency is not practical because more than 150 different mutations have been described.[198]

The diagnosis of hereditary protein C deficiency in patients who are receiving warfarin is particularly difficult. Protein C antigen levels can be compared with antigen levels for other vitamin K-dependent clotting factors such as factor VII or X, but only if careful control ranges are established for the ratios of protein C to two other vitamin K-dependent factors are established.[3,202] In most situations, it is necessary to wait until at least 2 weeks after the end of anticoagulant therapy for a reliable diagnosis. Warfarin should not be restarted before laboratory results have been returned to reduce the possibility of warfarin-induced skin necrosis in patients who are later found to have protein C deficiency.

PROTEIN S DEFICIENCY

DEFINITION AND HISTORY

Familial heterozygous protein S deficiency associated with venous thrombosis was first reported in 1984.[4–6] Since then, many other families with the disorder have been identified.[76,228–232] Many different mutations in the protein S gene (over 100) associated with thrombosis have been identified.[233] Severe deficiency (less than 1 percent of normal protein S levels) due to homozygous or compound heterozygous de-

fects has been reported in only a few infants who presented with neonatal purpura fulminans.[234–236] Protein S enhances the anticoagulant activity of APC, and hence currently available functional assays of protein S measure APC-cofactor activity using protein S–depleted plasma as substrate. Type I protein S deficiency is defined as parallel reductions in both antigen and anticoagulant activity levels in plasma whereas type II deficiency, associated with circulating dysfunctional molecules, involves normal plasma levels of antigen but low levels of anticoagulant activity. Protein S reversibly associates with the plasma complement factor, C4b-binding protein (C4BP), previously known as *proline-rich lipoprotein*. In normal plasma, approximately 60 percent of protein S is bound to C4BP, and 40 percent is free; importantly, only the free form of protein S functions as a cofactor for APC. This gives rise to another type of protein S deficiency, designated *type III deficiency*, in which free protein S is low while total protein S antigen is usually in the low normal range.

ETIOLOGY AND PATHOGENESIS

Protein S is principally synthesized in the liver, but other organs may be important sites for its synthesis, including the endothelium, kidney, testes, and brain (see Chap. 113). Because protein S is a cofactor for APC (see Chap. 113), decreased levels of free protein S may impair the down-regulation of thrombin generation and contribute to hypercoagulability. Protein S also exhibits anticoagulant activity that is independent of APC by directly binding to and inhibiting factors Va, VIIIa, and Xa,[237–242] suggesting that deficiency of protein S could also contribute to hypercoagulability by failing to impair factors Va or Xa in the absence of APC. At present, only the APC-cofactor activity of protein S is routinely assayed because there is no generally available standardized assay for the anticoagulant activity of protein S that is independent of APC.

CLINICAL FEATURES

In several studies, approximately 3 percent of unselected outpatients presenting with venous thromboembolism have low levels of protein S[201,243,244]; higher prevalences are reported for patients under 50 years of age and for patients with a personal or family history of venous thrombosis. The odds ratio for thrombosis in patients with free protein S deficiency has been variably reported to be 1.6,[201] 2.4,[243] 8.5,[76] and 11.5[230] (see below). After an initial venous thrombosis, recurrence rates in protein S–deficient patients average 3.5 percent per year.[212,213,245]

Deep venous thrombosis and pulmonary embolism are the most common forms of thrombosis associated with protein S deficiency, although superficial vein thrombophlebitis and thrombosis in unusual sites also occur.[210–212] As in other forms of thrombophilia, about 50 percent of thromboses are unprovoked.[211] Arterial thrombosis has been reported in a significant number of protein S–deficient patients, particularly in those who smoke or have other thrombotic risk factors.[18,106,246,247] Neonatal purpura fulminans has been reported in rare infants with homozygous or compound heterozygous protein S deficiency and very low levels of protein S.[234–236] Warfarin-induced skin necrosis has also been reported in association with protein S deficiency.[248]

Acquired forms of protein S deficiency are rather common. Oral contraceptive usage decreases plasma protein S levels. Reduced levels of free protein S are regularly found in pregnancy (e.g., as low as 20 to 30 percent of normal),[249,250] in patients who are taking oral anticoagulants, and in disseminated intravascular coagulation, liver disease, nephrotic syndrome, inflammatory conditions, and acute thromboembolism.[251–254] Protein S deficiency can also occur in concert with the lupus anticoagulant[255,256] and as a result of autoantibodies to protein S following varicella or other infections in children.[257–261]

The likelihood of thrombosis varies widely in patients with protein S deficiency. In general, population-based case control studies yield low odds ratios for thrombosis,[201] whereas family studies show a high rate of venous thromboembolism in protein S–deficient relatives compared with nonaffected family members.[230] Some of the patients identified in the case control studies may have had an acquired deficiency of protein S which was temporary.[224] Even more important, several of the families with protein S deficiency have been found to have a second thrombophilic defect, most commonly either factor V Leiden,[106,108] or the prothrombin nt 20210A gene mutation.[157] Other risk factors, particularly smoking and obesity, also increase the risk of thrombosis in protein S–deficient family members.[18,230,231]

LABORATORY EVALUATION

Laboratory assays of plasma protein S must be chosen and interpreted with care because the protein circulates both free and bound to C4BP. Moreover, normal ranges differ for males compared with females and depend on age. Free protein S antigen or APC-cofactor anticoagulant activity are better than total protein S antigen in screening for hereditary protein S deficiency.[201,262] Free protein S antigen can be assayed using monoclonal antibodies specific for free protein S.[263,264] Protein S activity assays may be affected by coexisting APC resistance, although the second-generation assays in which factor V–deficient plasma is used as substrate have improved specificity.[265–267] Assessment of total and free protein S plus protein S activity should allow the classification of patients with protein S defects into types I, II, or III. Type I and type III deficiencies may actually be phenotypic variants of the same disease, because within families, different individuals carrying the same DNA mutation in the protein S gene can present with laboratory findings indicating either type I or type III deficiency.[262] Type II deficiency, i.e., normal free protein S antigen with reduced protein S activity, is quite uncommon[224] so that screening patients with free protein S antigen levels is clinically reasonable. In normal patients, there is an excellent correlation between free protein S antigen and anticoagulant activity. The lower limit of the normal range for free protein S is lower in females than in males (55 percent versus 65 percent)[268]; protein S is remarkably sensitive to hormonal status in females.

A coagulation assay for protein S anticoagulant activity independent of APC has been described in which the APTT is determined in the absence and presence of anti–protein S neutralizing polyclonal antibodies added to the test plasma. The APTT is shorter in the presence of antibodies, and the ratio of clotting times is indicative of protein S anticoagulant activity.[269] At present, the clinical utility of this interesting assay has not been demonstrated, and the assay is not accessible for routine laboratories.

The high frequency of acquired protein S deficiency makes identification of hereditary defects more difficult. Common acquired conditions leading to low protein S levels should be excluded and tests repeated before making a diagnosis of hereditary thrombophilia. Family studies may also be useful. Oral anticoagulant therapy markedly reduces protein S antigen and activity levels. Assays are not often useful during pregnancy, because the low concentrations of protein S normally seen at that time cause diagnostic confusion.[249] Diagnosis of hereditary protein S deficiency using DNA techniques is not favored unless the defect has previously been established in the family because there are numerous different mutations in the protein S gene causing protein S deficiency.

ANTITHROMBIN DEFICIENCY

DEFINITION AND HISTORY

Antithrombin, also known as *antithrombin III*, is a plasma protease inhibitor that neutralizes thrombin by irreversibly forming a 1:1 com-plex. The rate of inhibition of thrombin or other serine trypsinlike proteases by antithrombin is catalyzed by heparin. The first family with hereditary antithrombin deficiency and thrombosis was reported by Egeberg in 1965.[1] Since then, many more families have been described.[270–272] A database of over 250 mutations in the antithrombin gene is available[273] and can be accessed via the internet (http://www.med.ic.ac.uk/dd/ddhc). Type I antithrombin deficiency is defined by low levels of antigen and activity in the absence or presence of heparin. Type II deficiency involves the presence of dysfunctional molecules in the plasma and is defined by normal levels of antigen with defects that affect either the inhibitor's active center, which complexes with the target enzyme's active site, or the inhibitor's heparin binding site which mediates heparin-dependent acceleration of antithrombin's action. Severe deficiency of antithrombin (less than 5 percent) is very rare, involves defects in heparin-dependent enhancement of antithrombin, and is associated with severe venous and arterial thrombosis.[274–277] Type I antithrombin deficiency is found in 0.023 percent of normal individuals in Scotland, whereas type II defects, mostly in asymptomatic individuals and families, is much more common and found in 0.16 percent of people screened.[278]

ETIOLOGY AND PATHOGENESIS

Antithrombin is a major protease inhibitor that neutralizes factors Xa, IXa, XIa, and thrombin in reactions accelerated in the presence of heparin or by heparan sulfate on endothelial surfaces (see Chap. 113). Therefore, defects in antithrombin compromise the normal inhibition of the coagulation pathways and cause a hypercoagulable state. Molecular antithrombin defects can involve either the reactive center that combines with the active site of the coagulation proteases or the heparin binding region that mediates heparin-dependent acceleration of antithrombin-protease reactions (see Chap. 113).

CLINICAL FEATURES

Antithrombin deficiency is found in approximately 1 percent of consecutive outpatients under 70 years old with a first objectively documented venous thrombosis (see references[76–78]), and the odds ratio for thrombosis in patients with antithrombin deficiency is approximately 10 to 20 and is notably greater than in subjects with factor V Leiden.[76,78,201,279] Recurrence rates have been reported to be quite high in the first year after a thrombosis (12 to 17 percent) in selected patients with type I antithrombin deficiency,[213,245] but lower rates have been reported in other studies (about 4 percent per year).[211,280] There is no evidence that there are differences in clinical severity between patients with heterozygous type I defects and those with type II mutations involving the thrombin binding site. Mortality rates are not increased in these patients.[281,282] Patients with type II mutations of the heparin-binding site have few if any thrombotic episodes, although homozygous mutations affecting heparin binding are associated with thromboembolism.[280]

Venous thrombosis of the lower extremities, which occurs at an early age and peaks in the second decade of life, is the most common symptom in antithrombin deficiency.[280] Superficial venous thrombosis appears to be somewhat less common than in protein C or protein S deficiency, or in APC resistance.[76,210,211] Thrombosis in unusual sites such as the mesenteric or cerebral veins has been reported.[210,211] Arterial thrombosis occurs infrequently (about 1 percent of affected patients).[283] As previously indicated for patients with other forms of hereditary thrombophilia, gene-gene and gene-environment interactions markedly increase the risk of thrombosis in subjects with antithrombin deficiency by 5-fold and 20-fold respectively.[279] Patients with severe antithrombin deficiency, i.e., activity levels less than 5 percent, are exceedingly rare, most likely because the profound deficiency state causes fetal loss in utero. A few infants with homozygous defects involving the heparin-binding region of the molecule have survived, but most have suffered severe venous and arterial thrombosis.[274–277] No patients homozygous for reactive center defects have been identified, leading to the speculation that complete deficiency of antithrombin is incompatible with life.

Resistance to the anticoagulant effects of heparin has been observed in some patients with antithrombin deficiency. However, heparin resistance is quite common in general patients with thrombosis. Up to 40 percent of patients without antithrombin deficiency will require more than 40,000 units of heparin daily to prolong the APTT into the therapeutic range.[284] Both acute thrombosis and several days of heparin therapy can decrease antithrombin levels, occasionally to as low as 50 percent of normal, which may lead to an erroneous diagnosis of hereditary antithrombin deficiency.[285,286] Acquired conditions leading to lowered levels of antithrombin are common and include liver disease, DIC, nephrotic syndrome, chemotherapy with asparaginase, and preeclampsia.[287–291]

LABORATORY DIAGNOSIS

Antithrombin deficiency screening assays should first be performed in the presence of heparin because defects may involve either the reactive center of the inhibitor or the heparin-binding site. If initial results are abnormal, then assays that measure the ability of the inhibitor to neutralize thrombin in the absence of heparin (progressive antithrombin activity) should be done to characterize the abnormality. Antithrombin activity assays that utilize a chromogenic substrate are widely available.[292] Most laboratories now use factor Xa or bovine thrombin in their antithrombin assays to avoid the inhibitory effects of heparin cofactor II on human thrombin.[293,294] The normal range for antithrombin levels in normal plasma is quite narrow (i.e., 84 to 116 percent).[293] Antithrombin antigen measurements are used to help distinguish type I from type II defects. Crossed immunoelectrophoresis using an antithrombin antibody in the presence and absence of heparin can help identify defects in the heparin-binding portion of the molecule.[295]

In general, patients with type I deficiency and many of those with type II disorders involving the thrombin binding site will have antithrombin activity levels of 40 to 60 percent. Levels of 60 to 84 percent can be due to other type II defects but frequently are a result of acquired antithrombin deficiency such as occurs with mild liver disease, acute thrombosis, or heparin therapy. If these confounding conditions are present, measurement of levels should be repeated and family studies performed if possible.

HIGH LEVELS OF FACTOR VIII AND OTHER COAGULATION FACTORS

DEFINITION AND HISTORY

Based on analysis of the frequency of factor VIII levels that exceed 150 percent of normal values, an elevated factor VIII level has been defined as a significant independent risk factor for venous thrombosis.[296,297] Both factor VIII activity and antigen levels are increased.[297] The increased risk was similar to that of heterozygosities for factor V Leiden or prothrombin G20210A. Preliminary reports of other epidemiologic studies indicate that elevated levels (higher than 150 percent of normal) of factors XI, IX, X, and V are also risk factors for venous thrombosis.

ETIOLOGY AND PATHOGENESIS

Although factor VIII is an acute phase reactant and elevations can be caused by inflammation, it appears that factor VIII elevations in venous thrombosis patients are not commonly caused by systemic inflammation.[297,298] Therefore, elevated factor VIII levels are likely to be directly pathogenic by increasing coagulability of blood via the blood coagula-

tion pathways. Studies of factor VIII levels in different families indicate a significant genetic influence in addition to the known influences from levels of von Willebrand factor, blood group antigens, and the presence of inflammation. Elevations of factor VIII and other coagulation factors of the intrinsic coagulation pathway, e.g., factors XI, IX, X, or V, may contribute to hypercoagulability by increasing thrombin generation.

CLINICAL FEATURES

The clinical presentation of patients with elevated factor VIII levels is not known to differ from that of patients with the other genetic risk factors described in this chapter.

LABORATORY DIAGNOSIS

Factor VIII procoagulant activity is measured with routine coagulation assays commonly used to screen for hemophilia (see Chaps. 112 and 123). In venous thrombosis patients, factor VIII antigen levels correlate with activity measurements.[297]

HEREDITARY THROMBOTIC DYSFIBRINOGENEMIA

DEFINITION AND HISTORY

Dysfibrinogenemia is defined as a qualitative defect in the molecule due to a mutation in the gene for one of fibrinogen's polypeptide chains. The hereditary dysfibrinogenemias represent a heterogeneous group of abnormalities that can be asymptomatic or cause either thrombosis or bleeding. Initial reports of dysfibrinogenemias associated with thrombophilia appeared in the 1960s from several laboratories. For a detailed treatment of dysfibrinogenemia, see Chap 124.

ETIOLOGY AND PATHOGENESIS

For normal hemostasis, fibrin is formed after release of fibrinopeptides from fibrinogen due to proteolysis by thrombin and subsequent polymerization of fibrin monomers. Fibrin is then stabilized by covalent cross-links introduced by factor XIIIa. Plasmin-dependent proteolysis of fibrin either to limit formation or growth of a thrombus or to clear fibrin in a timely and normal fashion during healing is essential. Defects in fibrinogen that cause abnormal fibrinolysis cause thrombosis, either because fibrin is not cleared in a normal fashion or because the growth of a normal hemostatic plug is not limited. Specific defects causing hypofibrinolysis can involve alterations of plasmin cleavage sites in fibrin or of sites that promote assembly of components of the fibrinolytic system, e.g., binding sites for plasminogen or plasminogen activators (see Chap. 124).

CLINICAL FEATURES

Patients with hereditary thrombotic dysfibrinogenemias usually present with venous thrombosis at a young age (e.g., 27 to 32 years old).[299] An occasional patient will have both thrombosis and bleeding (usually postpartum hemorrhage).[299] An increased rate of spontaneous abortion and stillbirth is also observed.[299] Approximately 20 percent of reported cases of hereditary dysfibrinogenemia have been associated with thrombosis, whereas about 30 percent manifested bleeding, and the remainder were clinically silent.[299] As summarized in detail in Chap. 124, several dozens of reports of abnormal fibrinogens associated with thrombosis have appeared.[300] When a large number of patients presenting with thromboembolism were screened, the prevalence rate of dysfibrinogenemia was found to be 0.8 percent.[299]

LABORATORY DIAGNOSIS

Prolongation of a dilute thrombin time and/or reptilase time due to delayed fibrin polymerization is common with dysfibrinogenemia, as is a disparity between measurement of immunoreactive and clottable fibrinogen. More sophisticated testing often demonstrates abnormal fibrinogen structure or resistance of the fibrin to fibrinolysis. Unfortunately there are no assays readily available that measure the key properties of fibrinogen that are likely to cause thrombosis in patients with dysfibrinogenemia, and therefore this defect may be underdiagnosed.

Therapy relies on anticoagulants. In some instances, the administration of cryoprecipitate as a source of normal fibrinogen should be considered for surgical procedures, both to raise low concentrations of fibrinogen into a hemostatic range and possibly to reduce the risk of thrombosis by dilution of the abnormal prothrombotic fibrinogen.

OTHER POTENTIAL THROMBOPHILIC DISORDERS

Hereditary defects in the fibrinolytic system (see Chap. 116) and in thrombomodulin are potential thrombophilic risk factors. Japanese families with several hereditary dysplasminogenemias[301–303] and hypo-plasminogenemias[304] have been identified, but these abnormalities were not associated with thrombosis in subjects other than the propositus. Heterozygous plasminogen deficiency is found more often in Asian than in Caucasian populations. One kindred with elevated levels of plasminogen activator inhibitor 1 (PAI-1)and thrombosis was subsequently shown to have protein S deficiency.[231] As yet, an association between defects in the fibrinolytic system and thrombosis has not been firmly established.[305] Several mutations in the thrombomodulin gene have been discovered in families with thrombosis.[306–308] The genetic defects are scattered throughout the thrombomodulin gene and are associated with variable levels of soluble thrombomodulin in the plasma.[307] In aggregate, thrombomodulin defects appear to be relatively common, being found in approximately 5 percent of a group of 200 patients with thromboembolic disease.[307] It is not yet clear whether one or more of these mutations constitute a major risk factor, whether they may contribute to the risk of thrombosis in patients with other forms of thrombophilia such as protein S deficiency, or whether they are neutral polymorphisms. At this juncture, routine screening of thrombosis patients for fibrinolytic or thrombomodulin defects is probably not indicated.

DIAGNOSIS OF THROMBOPHILIA

Plasma or molecular assays are now widely available for each of the common hereditary hypercoagulable states (Table 127-2). Up to 50 percent of patients presenting with a first deep vein thrombosis (DVT) will be found to have an abnormal laboratory test suggesting a thrombophilic defect. Those with recurrent venous thromboembolism or a strong family history of thrombosis are even more likely to have evidence of thrombophilia. Multiple disorders in the same patient are common; e.g., in one series of patients, 16 percent had more than one type of thrombophilia.[102]

Comprehensive testing for patients with venous thromboembolism should include: an APC resistance test (followed by a factor V Leiden mutation if needed), prothrombin gene mutation analysis,

TABLE 127-2   LABORATORY EVALUATION FOR HEREDITARY THROMBOPHILIA

APC resistance ratio	Antithrombin activity
Factor V Leiden	
Prothrombin gene G20210A mutation	Protein C activity
Plasma homocysteine	Protein S activity (or free protein S antigen)
Factor VIII assay	Fibrinogen (clottable)
	Dilute thrombin time

plasma homocysteine concentration, protein C activity (by a clotting assay), protein S activity assay (or free protein S antigen), antithrombin activity, factor VIII activity assay, and fibrinogen concentration (clottable) with a dilute thrombin time ($+/-$ reptilase time) (see Table 127-2). Additional tests for antiphospholipid antibodies should also be considered in patients suspected of having acquired thrombophilia (see Chap. 128). The most appropriate tests for patients with arterial thrombosis are less clear. However, plasma homocysteine, antiphospholipid antibody studies, lipoprotein(a) concentration, and colony assays to search for covert myeloproliferative disorders should be considered. Factor V Leiden, the prothrombin gene mutation, protein S, and other tests for "venous" thrombophilia may prove useful in some patients with premature coronary heart disease or stroke, particularly if other risk factors are present such as smoking, hypertension, diabetes, or obesity. If test results for the more common disorders are normal but the likelihood of a familial hypercoagulable state is high, tests for other causes of thrombosis might be helpful. Experimental tests to consider are assays for elevated levels of factors XI, V, and IX, the 4G4G promoter polymorphism in the PAI-1 gene, a plasminogen activity assay, or perhaps molecular assays for defects in thrombomodulin.

A laboratory evaluation for thrombophilia should be considered if the results of testing could make a difference in the clinical care of the patient or family members. Examples of a potential clinical impact include:

- Changes in the duration or intensity of oral anticoagulant therapy
- Administration of specific therapy (e.g., antithrombin concentrates, vitamins for homocysteinemia)
- More intense prophylaxis for high-risk situations (e.g., surgery, acute illness, immobility)
- Better accuracy in estimates of the future risk of thrombosis in clinical settings (e.g., surgery or pregnancy)
- Counseling of women as to the risks of oral contraceptives, pregnancy, or hormone replacement therapy
- Study of family members at risk of thrombosis

Routine testing of all female family members of a patient found to have factor V Leiden prior to starting oral contraceptives is probably not indicated.[75,309] However, if the family has a strong family history of venous thromboembolism in women who were pregnant or taking birth control pills or if the patient has had an episode of venous thrombosis, then test results could help in deciding whether to recommend oral contraceptives or alternative methods of birth control.[309]

Children with venous or arterial thrombosis (particularly stroke) are also likely to have an underlying thrombophilic disorder. Of these defects, factor V Leiden is the most common, but other disorders including the prothrombin 20210A gene mutation, protein C deficiency, elevations in lipoprotein(a), and antiphospholipid antibodies have been reported.[99,100,310–313]

Laboratory testing is best performed several weeks after completion of a course of oral anticoagulants in patients with thrombosis, to avoid confounding effects of acute thrombosis or heparin or warfarin therapy on the assay results. However, stopping anticoagulants in some patients with a high risk of recurrent thromboembolism may not be advisable. With the exception of assays for protein C and protein S, all other thrombophilic factors can be assayed in patients taking oral anticoagulants. Options for assessment of protein C or protein S levels in patients requiring warfarin include comparing their relative antigen levels with other "benchmark" vitamin K-dependent clotting factors[3,202] or obtaining assays on family members. Alternatively, heparin or low-molecular-weight (LMW) heparin can be substituted for warfarin for a period of time (approximately 2 weeks) prior to drawing blood for analysis.

THERAPY OF THROMBOPHILIA

Thrombophilia patients who develop a DVT or PE are initially given standard venous thromboembolism treatment with heparin or LMW heparin for acute therapy and warfarin for longer-term protection. Warfarin has been shown to effectively prevent recurrent thromboembolism at an INR range of 2 to 3.[314,315] Higher intensities of warfarin are unnecessary and will increase the risk of bleeding. The absolute risk of major hemorrhage with oral anticoagulants in patients with venous thromboembolism averages 1 to 3 percent per year, with a fatality rate of 0.2 to 0.4 percent per year.[314,316]

The optimal duration of anticoagulant treatment in patients with thrombosis and a history of thombophilia is an important clinical question.[314,317] Warfarin therapy is usually given for 6 months[315] following a thrombotic event (see Chap. 132). However, longer treatment may be indicated in patients with hereditary thrombophilia if the risk of additional thromboemboli substantially outweighs the risk of bleeding due to oral anticoagulants. The lack of reliable data on the absolute risks of recurrent thrombosis in patients with one or more thrombophilic states makes clinical decision making more difficult.[314,317] However, several factors make recurrent thrombosis more likely, and, if present, longer-term treatment is more appropriate:

- A spontaneous rather than a provoked thrombosis or pulmonary embolism[316]
- A high odds ratio for thrombosis; e.g., antithrombin deficiency (OR = 8) versus factor V Leiden (OR = 2.5)
- A strong family history of thrombosis (suggesting the presence of multiple hereditary defects)
- A history of recurrent thromboses
- Multiple inherited or acquired risk factors (e.g., factor V Leiden + prothrombin G20210A gene mutation; or factor V Leiden + antiphospholipid antibodies)
- Permanent rather than temporary major risk factors
- Unusual or life-threatening thromboses (e.g., cerebral vein or mesenteric thrombosis; ileofemoral deep venous thrombosis with multiple pulmonary emboli).

Decisions as to long-term anticoagulant therapy are best tailored to individual patients. A thorough assessment should include: (1) an estimate of the future risk of thrombosis; (2) an estimate of the future risk of major or fatal hemorrhage; and (3) patient preferences (e.g., impact of the decision on occupational or social situations).

Prophylactic oral anticoagulation therapy is usually not warranted in subjects who have not yet suffered a thrombotic event but who are discovered to have hereditary thrombophilia because of family testing or some other reason. In this instance, the risks of hemorrhage due to warfarin (about 1 to 3 percent per year) clearly outweigh the risk of thrombosis (e.g., 0.4 percent per year in asymptomatic individuals with APC resistance). In contrast, most authorities would recommend long-term antithrombotic treatment for patients who have suffered recurrent thromboses and who have more than one hereditary or acquired hypercoagulable state. More clinical trial data are needed before persuasive clinical guidelines can be recommended for patients with narrower risk/benefit ratios; e.g., a young patient with a first spontaneous but extensive DVT and a single prothrombotic disorder such as the factor V Leiden mutation.

If oral anticoagulant therapy is not used, an alternative approach includes intensive antithrombotic prophylaxis (e.g., LMW heparin) for events with a high risk of thrombosis such as surgery, infectious (e.g., pneumonia) or inflammatory diseases (e.g., inflammatory bowel disease), or prolonged periods of inactivity. Effective prophylaxis should reduce the risk of thromboembolism by about half, since approximately 50 percent of thromboses in patients with hereditary hy-

percoagulable states can be attributed to a known provoking factor. Other recommendations include patient education as to the signs and symptoms of acute DVT or PE, facilitation of diagnostic testing should symptoms occur, and continued follow-up in case new laboratory tests or clinical recommendations appear in the future.

Specific therapies are available for some thrombophilic disorders. Antithrombin concentrates are now widely available and can be administered for surgery, major trauma, and at the time of delivery in patients with antithrombin deficiency.[318–320] Protein C and activated protein C concentrates are under development and, when available, may be useful in infants or children with homozygous protein C deficiency, or in heterozygous subjects during surgery or other major stresses.[321–323] Cryoprecipitate is a source of normal fibrinogen, which can be useful for replacement of normal fibrinogen in patients with hereditary dysfibrinogenemia. Finally, although not yet proved to prevent thrombosis in patients with hyperhomocysteinemia, B vitamins (folic acid, pyridoxine, B12) effectively lower homocysteine concentrations into the normal range.[171,172]

THROMBOPHILIA AND PREGNANCY, ORAL CONTRACEPTIVES, AND HORMONE REPLACEMENT THERAPY

MANAGEMENT OF PREGNANCY IN THROMBOPHILIC WOMEN

Pregnancy substantially increases the risk of thrombosis in women with thrombophilia.[324] To date, treatment guidelines supported by clinical trial data for the treatment of these women are not available. Screening all women for a thrombophilic state prior to pregnancy does not seem warranted based on an extremely high cost:benefit ratio.[325,326] Similarly, routine heparin prophylaxis for previously asymptomatic individuals known to carry the V Leiden gene mutation or other mild thrombophilic defects is not indicated. Prophylactic heparin (or LMW heparin if proved safe and effective in pregnancy) should be considered for women with a history of venous thromboembolism, particularly if the prior thrombosis was related to pregnancy or oral contraceptives.[324,327,328] The potential antithrombotic benefit should offset the risks of heparin-induced osteopenia, bleeding, or heparin-induced thrombocytopenia. Venous thromboembolism that occurs during pregnancy requires therapeutic doses of heparin for the remainder of the pregnancy, followed by postpartum anticoagulants for at least 4 to 6 weeks.[324] Antithrombin concentrates (along with low-dose heparin) should be considered for women with hereditary antithrombin deficiency during the peripartum period or during complications of pregnancy.

PREGNANCY LOSS DUE TO THROMBOPHILIA

Thrombophilia is a cause of fetal loss and other complications of pregnancy, most likely due to thrombosis of the placental vasculature.[326,329] Fetal loss is often manifested by stillbirth (second or third trimester) rather than first trimester miscarriage.[329] In addition, severe preeclampsia, fetal growth retardation, and placental infarction have all been linked to maternal or fetal hypercoagulable states.[330–334] Most of the hereditary thrombophilic states have been implicated. Factor V Leiden has been linked to fetal loss (OR 2–3),[329,335–338] as have protein C deficiency (OR 2.3), protein S deficiency (OR 3.3), and antithrombin deficiency (OR 5.2).[329] If combined defects are present, the odds ratio for fetal loss increases to 14.3.[329] Hyperhomocysteinemia has been associated with placental abruption, placental infarction, and stillbirth; moreover, homozygosity for the thermolabile MTHFR defect has also been linked to pregnancy complications.[330,331,334,339] Although quantitative data are not available, pregnancy loss appears to be increased in women with hereditary thrombotic dysfibrinogenemia.[299]

When adverse outcomes of pregnancy were combined, including stillbirth, preeclampsia, abruptio placentae, and fetal growth retardation, 52 percent of affected women were found to have thrombophilia compared to a rate of 17 percent in women with normal pregnancies.[330] Diagnostic studies for thrombophilia should be considered for women with recurrent midtrimester pregnancy loss or other adverse pregnancy outcomes, particularly if future studies suggest that antithrombotic treatment (e.g., low-dose heparin, LMW heparin, or aspirin) is effective.[340]

ESTROGENS: ORAL CONTRACEPTIVES AND HORMONE REPLACEMENT THERAPY

Oral contraceptives increase the risk of thrombosis in women with hereditary thrombophilia.[118,119,341–343] For example, the odds ratio for thrombosis in women with factor V Leiden who use third-generation oral contraceptives is increased 30- to 50-fold.[118,119] In absolute numbers this represents an increase in risk from 1/12,500 women per year without V Leiden to 1/400 women per year in women with factor V Leiden.[119] The thrombotic risk associated with birth control pills is greater in women who are homozygous for factor V Leiden.[120] Screening for the factor V mutation prior to the administration of oral contraceptives is probably not cost-effective. By one estimate, it would be necessary to screen 2.25 million women to detect 90,000 women with V Leiden, in order to prevent one death from venous thromboembolism by withholding the oral contraceptives.[344] However, if a woman with factor V Leiden has a history of thrombosis or is homozygous for the mutation, then avoidance of oral contraceptives would certainly be prudent.[119,120,345] Oral contraceptives probably should not be recommended for women known to be deficient in antithrombin, protein C, and possibly protein S.[341]

Whether to recommend hormone replacement therapy in women with hereditary thrombophilia is a particularly difficult question. The relative risk of venous thrombosis with replacement estrogens is significantly increased by a factor of 2 to 4 when large groups of women are studied, but the absolute risk of thrombosis is quite low; i.e., 1 excess thrombosis per 5000 women per year.[346–350] However, studies are not yet available to estimate any potential increase in the relative or absolute risk of thrombosis in women who use hormone replacement therapy and carry the factor V Leiden mutation or other genetic thrombophilic risk factors.

Use of selective estrogen receptor modulators such as tamoxifen or raloxifene increases the risk of venous thrombosis. Three cases of tamoxifen-associated venous thrombosis associated with factor V Leiden have been reported.[121] Given the increasing use of selective estrogen receptor modulators for treating or preventing breast cancer and osteoporosis, it will be important to determine whether thrombophilic genetic risk factors (e.g., those listed in Table 127-1) will increase the liklihood of selective estrogen receptor modulator–associated venous thrombosis.

REFERENCES

1. Egeberg O: Inherited antithrombin deficiency causing thrombophilia. *Thromb Diath Haemorrh* 13:516, 1963.
2. Stenflo J, Fernlund P, Egan W, Roepstorff P: Vitamin K-dependent modifications of glutamic acid residues in prothrombin. *Proc Natl Acad Sci* 71:2730, 1974.
3. Griffin JH, Evatt B, Zimmerman TS, Kleiss AJ: Deficiency of protein C in congenital thrombotic disease. *J Clin Invest* 68:1370, 1981.
4. Schwarz HP, Fischer M, Hopmeier P, Batard MA, Griffin JH: Plasma protein S deficiency in familial thrombotic disease. *Blood* 64:1297, 1984.

5. Comp PC, Nixon RR, Cooper MR, Esmon CT: Familial protein S deficiency is associated with recurrent thrombosis. *J Clin Invest* 74:2082, 1984.
6. Comp PC, Esmon CT: Recurrent venous thromboembolism in patients with a partial deficiency of protein S. *N Engl J Med* 311:1525, 1984.
7. Dahlback B, Carlsson M, Svensson PJ: Familial thrombophilia due to a previously unrecognized mechanism characterized by poor anticoagulant response to activated protein C: prediction of a cofactor to activated protein C. *Proc Natl Acad Sci* 90:1004, 1993.
8. Svensson PJ, Dahlbäck B: Resistance to activated protein C as a basis for venous thrombosis. *N Engl J Med* 330:517, 1994.
9. Bertina RM, Koeleman BPC, Koster T, et al: Mutation in blood coagulation factor V associated with resistance to activated protein C. *Nature* 369:64, 1994.
10. Greengard JS, Sun X, Xu X, et al: Activated protein C resistance caused by Arg506Gln mutation in factor Va. *Lancet* 343:1361, 1994.
11. Voorberg J, Roelse J, Koopman R, et al: Association of idiopathic venous thromboembolism with single point-mutation at Arg506 of factor V. *Lancet* 343:1535, 1994.
12. Bienvenu T, Ankri A, Chadefaux B, Montalescot G, Kamoun P: Elevated total plasma homocysteine, a risk factor for thrombosis. Relation to coagulation and fibrinolytic parameters. *Thromb Res* 70:123, 1993.
13. McCully KS: Vascular pathology of homocysteinemia: implications for the pathogenesis of arteriosclerosis. *Am J Pathol* 56:111, 1969.
14. Poort SR, Rosendaal FR, Reitsma PH, Bertina RM: A common genetic variation in the 3′-untranslated region of the prothrombin gene is associated with elevated plasma prothrombin levels and an increase in venous thrombosis. *Blood* 88:3698, 1996.
15. Bertina RM: Molecular risk factors for thrombosis. *Thromb Haemost* 82:601, 1999.
16. Rosendaal FR: Risk factors for venous thrombotic disease. *Thromb Haemost* 82:610, 1999.
17. Rosendaal FR, Siscovick DS, Schwartz SM, et al: Factor V Leiden (resistance to activated protein C) increases the risk of myocardial infarction in young women. *Blood* 89:2817, 1997.
18. Zoller B, Garcia dF, Dahlback B: A common 4G allele in the promoter of the plasminogen activator inhibitor-1 (PAI-1) gene as a risk factor for pulmonary embolism and arterial thrombosis in hereditary protein S deficiency. *Thromb Haemost* 79:802, 1998.
19. Silverstein MD, Heit JA, Mohr DN, et al: Trends in the incidence of deep vein thrombosis and pulmonary embolism: a 25-year population-based study. *Arch Intern Med* 158:585, 1998.
20. Koster T, Rosendaal FR, Deronde H, et al: Venous thrombosis due to poor anticogaulant response to activated protein-C-Leiden Thrombophilia Study. *Lancet* 342:1503, 1993.
21. Griffin JH, Evatt B, Wideman C, Fernandez JA: Anticoagulant protein C pathway defective in majority of thrombophilic patients. *Blood* 82:1989, 1993.
22. Marciniak E, Romond EH: Impaired catalytic function of activated protein C: a new in vitro manifestation of lupus anticoagulant. *Blood* 74:2426, 1989.
23. Malia RG, Kitchen S, Greaves M, Preston FE: Inhibition of activated protein C and its cofactor protein S by antiphospholipid antibodies. *Br J Haematol* 76:101, 1990.
24. Amer L, Kisiel W, Searles RP, Williams RC Jr: Impairment of the protein C anticoagulant pathway in a patient with systemic lupus erythematosus, anticardiolipin antibodies and thrombosis. *Thromb Res* 57:247, 1990.
25. Dahlback B, Carlsson M: Factor VIII defect associated with familial thrombophilia. *Thromb Haemost* 65:658, 1991.
26. Zoller B, Dahlbäck B: Linkage between inherited resistance to activated protein C and factor V gene mutation in venous thrombosis. *Lancet* 343:1536, 1994.
27. Zoller B, Svensson PJ, He X, Dahlback B: Identification of the same factor V gene mutation in 47 out of 50 thrombosis-prone families with inherited resistance to activated protein C. *J Clin Invest* 94:2521, 1994.
28. De Visser MCH, Rosendaal FR, Bertina RM: A reduced sensitivity for activated protein C in the absence of factor V Leiden increases the risk of venous thrombosis. *Blood* 93:1271, 1999.
29. Rodeghiero F, Tosetto A: Activated protein C resistance and factor V Leiden mutation are independent risk factors for venous thromboembolism. *Ann Intern Med* 130:643, 1999.
30. Fisher M, Fernandez JA, Ameriso SF, et al: Activated protein C resis-

tance in ischemic stroke not due to factor V arginine506→glutamine mutation. *Stroke* 27:1163, 1996.

31. Van der Bom JG, Bots ML, Haverkate F, et al: Reduced response to activated protein C is associated with increased risk for cerebrovascular disease. *Ann Intern Med* 125:265, 1996.

32. Oosting JD, Derksen RHWM, Bobbink IWG, et al: Antiphospholipid antibodies directed against a combination of phospholipids with prothrombin, protein C, or protein S: an explanation for their pathogenic mechanism? *Blood* 81:2618, 1993.

33. Zivelin A, Gitel S, Griffin JH, et al: Extensive venous and arterial thrombosis associated with an inhibitor to activated protein C. *Blood* 94:895, 1999.

34. Zivelin A, Griffin JH, Xu X, et al: A single genetic origin for a common caucasian risk factor for venous thrombosis. *Blood* 89:397, 1997.

35. Sun X, Evatt B, Griffin JH: Blood coagulation factor Va abnormality associated with resistance to activated protein C in venous thrombophilia. *Blood* 83:3120, 1994.

36. Heeb MJ, Kojima Y, Greengard JS, Griffin JH: Activated protein C resistance: molecular mechanisms based on studies using purified Gln506-factor V. *Blood* 85:3405, 1995.

37. Kalafatis M, Bertina RM, Rand MD, Mann KG: Characterization of the molecular defect in factor VR506Q. *J Biol Chem* 270:4053, 1995.

38. Nicolaes GAF, Tans G, Thomassen MCLGD, et al: Peptide bond cleavages and loss of functional activity during inactivation of factor Va and factor Va^{R506Q} by activated protein C. *J Biol Chem* 270:21158, 1995.

39. Rosing J, Hoekema L, Nicolaes GA, et al: Effects of protein S and factor Xa on peptide bond cleavages during inactivation of factor Va and factor VaR506Q by activated protein C. *J Biol Chem* 270:27852, 1995.

40. Kalafatis M, Rand MD, Mann KG: The mechanism of inactivation of human factor V and human factor Va by activated protein C. *J Biol Chem* 269:31869, 1994.

41. Shen L, Dahlback B: Factor V and protein S as synergistic cofactors to activated protein C in degradation of factor VIIIa. *J Biol Chem* 269:18735, 1994.

42. Dahlback B, Hildebrand B: Inherited resistance to activated protein C is corrected by anticoagulant cofactor activity found to be a property of factor V. *Proc Natl Acad Sci* 91:1396, 1994.

43. Thorelli E, Kaufman RJ, Dahlback B: Cleavage of factor V at Arg 506 by activated protein C and the expression of anticoagulant activity of factor V. *Blood* 93:2552, 1999.

44. Dahlback B: Procoagulant and anticoagulant properties of coagulation factor V: factor V Leiden (APC resistance) causes hypercoagulability by dual mechanisms. *J Lab Clin Med* 133:415, 1999.

45. Varadi K, Rosing J, Tans G, et al: Factor V enhances the cofactor function of protein S in the APC-mediated inactivation of factor VIII: influence of the factor VR506Q mutation. *Thromb Haemost* 76:208, 1996.

46. Williamson D, Brown K, Luddington R, Baglin C, Baglin T: Factor V Cambridge: a new mutation (Arg^{306}→Thr) associated with resistance to activated protein C. *Blood* 91:1140, 1998.

47. Chan WP, Lee CK, Kwong YL, Lam CK, Liang R: A novel mutation of Arg^{306} of factor V gene in Hong Kong Chinese. *Blood* 91:1135, 1998.

48. Franco RF, Maffei FH, Lourenco D, et al: Factor VArg^{306}→Thr (factor V Cambridge) and factor V Arg^{306}→Gly mutations in venous thrombotic disease. *Br J Haematol* 103:888, 1998.

49. Bernardi F, Faioni EM, Castoldi E, et al: A factor V genetic component differing from factor V R506Q contributes to the activated protein C resistance phenotype. *Blood* 90:1552, 1997.

50. Alhenc-Gelas M, Nicaud V, Gandrille S, et al: The factor V gene A4070G mutation and the risk of venous thrombosis. *Thromb Haemost* 81:193, 1999.

51. Griffin JH: Blood coagulation. The thrombin paradox [news; comment]. *Nature* 378:337, 1995.

52. Gruber A, Griffin JH. Direct detection of activated protein C in blood from human subjects. *Blood* 79:2340, 1992.

53. Okajima K, Koga S, Kaji M, et al: Effect of protein C and activated protein C on coagulation and fibrinolysis in normal human subjects. *Thromb Haemost* 63:48, 1990.

54. Heeb MJ, Gruber A, Griffin JH: Identification of divalent metal ion-dependent inhibition of activated protein C by alpha 2-macroglobulin and alpha 2-antiplasmin in blood and comparisons to inhibition of factor Xa, thrombin, and plasmin. *J Biol Chem* 266:17606, 1991.

55. Fernandez JA, Petaja J, Gruber A, Griffin JH: Activated protein C correlates inversely with thrombin levels in resting healthy individuals. *Am J Hematol* 56:29, 1997.

56. Greengard JS, Eichinger S, Griffin JH, Bauer KA: Variability of thrombosis among homozygous siblings with resistance to activated protein C due to an Arg→Gln mutation in the gene for factor V. *N Engl J Med* 331:1559, 1994.

57. Martinelli I, Bottasso B, Duca F, Faioni E, Mannucci PM: Heightened thrombin generation in individuals with resistance to activated protein C. *Thromb Haemost* 75:703, 1996.

58. Simioni P, Scarano L, Gavasso S, et al: Prothrombin fragment 1+2 and thrombin-antithrombin complex levels in patients with inherited APC resistance due to factor V Leiden mutation. *Br J Haematol* 92:435, 1996.

59. Zoller B, Holm J, Svensson P, Dahlback B: Elevated levels of prothrombin activation fragment 1+2 in plasma from patients with heterozygous Arg^{506} to Gln mutation in the factor V gene (APC-resistance) and/or inherited protein S deficiency. *Thromb Haemost* 75:270, 1996.

60. Lindqvist PG, Svensson PJ, Dahlback B, Marsal K: Factor V Q^{506} mutation (activated protein C resistance) associated with reduced intrapartum blood loss—a possible evolutionary selection mechanism. *Thromb Haemost* 79:69, 1998.

61. Nichols WC, Amano K, Cacheris PM, et al: Moderation of hemophilia A phenotype by the factor V R506Q mutation. *Blood* 88:1183, 1996.

62. Rees DC, Cox M, Clegg JB: World distribution of factor V Leiden. *Lancet* 346:1133, 1995.

63. Ridker PM, Miletich JP, Hennekens CH, Buring JE: Ethnic distribution of factor V Leiden in 4047 men and women—implications for venous thromboembolism screening. *JAMA* 277:1305, 1997.

64. Gregg JP, Yamane AJ, Grody WW. Prevalence of the factor V-Leiden mutation in four distinct American ethnic populations. *Am J Med Genet* 73:334, 1997;

65. Dahlback B: Resistance to activated protein C as risk factor for thrombosis: molecular mechanisms, laboratory investigation, and clinical management. *Sem Hematol* 34:217, 1997.

66. Turkstra F, Karemaker R, Kuijer PMM, Prins MH, Büller HR: Is the prevalence of the factor V Leiden mutation in patients with pulmonary embolism and deep vein thrombosis really different? *Thromb Haemost* 81:345, 1999.

67. Manten B, Westendorp RGJ, Koster T, Reitsma PH, Rosendaal FR: Risk factor profiles in patients with different clinical manifestations of venous thromboembolism: a focus on the factor V Leiden mutation. *Thromb Haemost* 76:510, 1996.

68. Desmarais S, De Moerloose P, Reber G, et al: Resistance to activated protein C in an unselected population of patients with pulmonary embolism. *Lancet* 347:1374, 1996.

69. Vandenbroucke JP, Bertina RM, Holmes ZR, et al: Factor V Leiden and fatal pulmonary embolism. *Thromb Haemost* 79:511, 1998.

70. Munkvad S, Jorgensen M: Resistance to activated protein C: a common anticoagulant deficiency in patients with venous leg ulceration. *Br J Dermatol* 134:296, 1996.

71. Maessen-Visch MB, Hamulyak K, Tazelaar DJ, Crombag NHCM, Neumann HAM: The prevalence of factor V Leiden mutation in patients with leg ulcers and venous insufficiency. *Arch Dermatol* 135:41, 1999.

72. Zuber M, Toulon P, Marnet L, Mas JL: Factor V Leiden mutation in cerebral venous thrombosis. *Stroke* 27:1721, 1996.

73. Lüdemann P, Nabavi DG, Junker R, et al: Factor V Leiden mutation is a risk factor for cerebral venous thrombosis—a case-control study of 55 patients. *Stroke* 29:2507, 1998.

74. Leebeek FWG, Lameris JS, Van Buuren HR, et al: Budd-Chiari syndrome, portal vein and mesenteric vein thrombosis in a patient homozygous for factor V Leiden mutation treated by TIPS and thrombolysis. *Br J Haematol* 102:929, 1998.

75. Middeldorp S, Henkens CMA, Koopman MMW, et al: The incidence of venous thromboembolism in family members of patients with factor V Leiden mutation and venous thrombosis. *Ann Intern Med* 128:15, 1998.

76. Martinelli I, Mannucci PM, De Stefano V, et al: Different risks of thrombosis in four coagulation defects associated with inherited thrombophilia: a study of 150 families. *Blood* 92:2353, 1998.

77. Bucciarelli P, Rosendaal FR, Tripodi A, et al: Risk of venous thromboembolism and clinical manifestations in carriers of antithrombin, protein C, protein S deficiency, or activated protein C resistance—a multicenter

collaborative family study. *Arterioscler Thromb Vasc Biol* 19:1026, 1999.

78. Rosendaal FR: Venous thrombosis: a multicausal disease. *Lancet* 353: 1167, 1999.

79. Ridker PM, Glynn RJ, Miletich JP, et al: Age-specific incidence rates of venous thromboembolism among heterozygous carriers of factor V Leiden mutation. *Ann Intern Med* 126:528, 1997.

80. Ridker PM, Hennekens CH, Lindpaintner K, et al: Mutation in the gene coding for coagulation facator V and the risk of myocardial infarction, stroke, and venous thrombosis in apparently healthy men. *N Engl J Med* 332:912, 1995.

81. Price DT, Ridker PM: Factor V Leiden mutation and the risks for thromboembolic disease: a clinical perspective. *Ann Intern Med* 127: 895, 1997.

82. Ridker PM, Miletich JP, Stampfer MJ, et al: Factor V Leiden and risks of recurrent idiopathic venous thromboembolism. *Circulation* 92: 2800, 1995.

83. Simioni P, Prandoni P, Lensing AWA, et al: The risk of recurrent venous thromboembolism in patients with an Arg[506]→Gln mutation in the gene for factor V (factor Leiden). *N Engl J Med* 336:399, 1997.

84. Baglin C, Brown K, Luddington R, Baglin T: Rick of recurrent venous thromboembolism in patients with the factor V Leiden (FVR 506Q) mutation: effect of warfarin and prediction by precipitating factors. *Br J Haematol* 100:764, 1998.

85. Eichinger S, Minar E, Hirschl M, et al: The risk of early recurrent venous thromboembolism after oral anticoagulant therapy in patients with the G20210A transition in the prothrombin gene. *Thromb Haemost* 81:14, 1999.

86. Rintelen C, Pabinger I, Knöbl P, Lechner K, Mannhalter C: Probability of recurrence of thrombosis in patients with and without factor V Leiden. *Thromb Haemost* 75:229, 1996.

87. Lindmarker P, Schulman S, Sten-Linder M, et al: The risk of recurrent venous thromboembolism in carriers and non-carriers of the G1691A allele in the coagulation factor V gene and the G20210A allele in the prothrombin gene. *Thromb Haemost* 81:684, 1999.

88. Rosendaal FR, Koster T, Vandenbroucke JP, Reitsma PH: High risk of thrombosis in patients homozygous for factor V Leiden (activated protein C resistance). *Blood* 85:1504, 1995.

89. Emmerich J, Alhenc-Gelas M, Aillaud MF, et al: Clinical features in 36 patients homozygous for the ARG 506→GLN factor V mutation. *Thromb Haemost* 77:620, 1997.

90. Mari D, Mannucci PM, Duca F, Bertolini S, Franceschi C: Mutant factor V (Arg506Gln) in health centenarians. *Lancet* 347:1044, 1996.

91. Heijmans BT, Westendorp RGJ, Knook DL, Kluft C, Slagboom PE: The risk of mortality and the factor V Leiden mutation in a population-based cohort. *Thromb Haemost* 80:607, 1998.

92. Hille ETM, Westendorp RGJ, Vandenbroucke JP, Rosendaal FR: Mortality and causes of death in families with the factor V Leiden mutation (resistance to activated protein C). *Blood* 89:1963, 1997.

93. Rees DC, Liu YT, Cox MJ, Elliott P, Wainscoat JS: Factor V Leiden and thermolabile methylenetetrahydrofolate reductase in extreme old age. *Thromb Haemost* 78:1357, 1997.

94. Inbal A, Freimark D, Modan B, et al: Synergistic effects of prothrombotic polymorphisms and atherogenic factors on the risk of myocardial infarction in young males. *Blood* 93:2186, 1999.

95. Doggen CJM, Cats VM, Bertina RM, Rosendaal FR: Interaction of coagulation defects and cardiovascular risk factors—increased risk of myocardial infarction associated with factor V Leiden or prothrombin 20210A. *Circulation* 97:1037, 1998.

96. Press RD, Liu XY, Beamer N, Coull BM: Ischemic stroke in the elderly—role of the common factor V mutation causing resistance to activated protein C. *Stroke* 27:44, 1996.

97. Van Bockxmeer FM, Baker RI, Taylor RR: Premature ischaemic heart disease and the gene for coagulation factor V. *Nature Med* 1:185, 1995.

98. Cushman M, Rosendaal FR, Psaty BM, et al: Factor V Leiden is not a risk factor for arterial vascular disease in the elderly: results from the Cardiovascular Health Study. *Thromb Haemost* 79:912, 1998.

99. Becker S, Heller CH, Gropp F, Scharrer I, Kreuz W: Thrombophilic disorders in children with cerebral infarction. *Lancet* 352:1756, 1998.

100. Nowak-Gottl U, Koch HG, Aschka I, et al: Resistance to activated protein C (APCR) in children with venous or arterial thromboembolism. *Br J Haematol* 92:992, 1996.

101. Sifontes MT, Nuss R, Hunger SP, et al: Activated protein C resistance and the factor V Leiden mutation in children with thrombosis. *Am J Hematol* 57:29, 1998.

102. Salomon O, Steinberg DM, Zivelin A, et al: Single and combined prothrombotic factors in patients with idiopathic venous thromboembolism—prevalence and risk assessment. *Arterioscler Thromb Vasc Biol* 19:511, 1999.

103. Gandrille S, Greengard JS, Alhenc-Gelas M, et al: Incidence of activated protein C resistance caused by the ARG 506 GLN mutation in factor V in 113 unrelated symptomatic protein C-deficient patients. The French Network on the behalf of INSERM. *Blood* 86:219, 1995.

104. Brenner B, Zivelin A, Lanir N, et al: Venous thromboembolism associated with double heterozygosity for R506Q mutation of factor V and for T298M mutation of protein C in a large family of a previously described homozygous protein C deficient newborn with massive thrombosis. *Blood* 88:877, 1996.

105. Koeleman BPC, Reitsma PH, Allaart CF, Bertina RM: Activated protein C resistance as an additional risk factor for thrombosis in protein C-deficient families. *Blood* 84:1031, 1994.

106. Zoller B, Berntsdotter A, Garcia de Frutos P, Dahlback B: Resistance to activated protein C as an additional genetic risk factor in hereditary deficiency of protein S. *Blood* 85:3518, 1995.

107. Zoller B, He X, Dahlback B: Homozygous APC-resistance combined with inherited type I protein S deficiency in a young boy with severe thrombotic disease. *Thromb Haemost* 73:743, 1995.

108. Koeleman BP, van Rumpt D, Hamulyak K, Reitsma PH, Bertina RM: Factor V Leiden: an additional risk factor for thrombosis in protein S deficient families? *Thromb Haemost* 74:580, 1995.

109. Van Boven HH, Reitsma PH, Rosendaal FR, et al: Factor V Leiden (FV R506Q) in families with inherited antithrombin deficiency. *Thromb Haemost* 75:417, 1996.

110. Tosetto A, Rodeghiero F, Martinelli I, et al: Additional genetic risk factors for venous thromboembolism in carriers of the factor V Leiden mutation. *Br J Haematol* 103:871, 1998.

111. Ehrenforth S, Prondsinski MV, Aygören-Pürsün E, Scharrer I, Ganser A: Study of the prothrombin gene 20210 GA variant in FV:Q[506] carriers in relationship to the presence or absence of juvenile venous thromboembolism. *Arterioscler Thromb Vasc Biol* 19:276, 1999.

112. Mandel H, Brenner B, Berant M, et al: Coexistence of hereditary homocystinuria and Factor V Leiden—effect on thrombosis. *N Engl J Med* 334:763, 1996.

113. Cattaneo M, Tsai MY, Bucciarelli P, et al: A common mutation in the methylenetetrahydrofolate reductase gene (C677T) increases the risk for deep-vein thrombosis in patients with mutant factor V (factor V:Q506). *Arterioscler Thromb Vasc Biol* 17:1662, 1997.

114. Ridker PM, Hennekens CH, Selhub J, et al: Interrelation of hyperhomocysteinemia, factor V Leiden, and risk of future venous thromboembolism. *Circulation* 95:1777, 1997.

115. Dizon-Townson DS, Nelson LM, Jang H, Varner MW, Ward K: The incidence of the factor V Leiden mutation in an obstetric population and its relationship to deep vein thrombosis. *Am J Obstet Gynecol* 176:883, 1997.

116. Hallak M, Senderowicz J, Cassel A, et al: Activated protein C resistance (factor V Leiden) associated with thrombosis in pregnancy. *Am J Obstet Gynecol* 176:889, 1997.

117. Bokarewa MI, Bremme K, Blomback M: Arg[506]-Gln mutation in factor V and risk of thrombosis during pregnancy. *Br J Haematol* 92:473, 1996.

118. Bloemenkamp KWM, Rosendaal FR, Helmerhorst FM, Büller HR, Vandenbroucke JP: Enhancement by factor V Leiden mutation of risk of deep-vein thrombosis associated with oral contraceptives containing third- generation progestagen. *Lancet* 346:1593, 1995.

119. Vandenbroucke JP, Koster T, Brit E, et al: Increased risk of venous thrombosis in oral-contraceptive users who are carriers of factor V Leiden mutation. *Lancet* 344:1453, 1994.

120. Rintelen C, Mannhalter C, Ireland H, et al: Oral contraceptives enhance the risk of clinical manifestation of venous thrombosis at a young age in females homozygous for factor V Leiden. *Br J Haematol* 93:487, 1996.

121. Weitz IC, Israel VK, Liebman HA: Tamoxifen-associated venous thrombosis and activated protein C resistance due to factor V Leiden. *Cancer* 79:2024, 1997.

122. Trossart M, Conard J, Horellou MH, et al: Modified APC resistance assay for patients on oral anticoagulants. *Lancet* 344:1709, 1994.

123. Svensson PJ, Zoller B, Dahlback B: Evaluation of original and modified APC-resistance tests in unselected outpatients with clinically suspected thrombosis and in healthy controls. *Thromb Haemost* 77:332, 1997.

124. Kapiotis S, Quehenberger P, Jilma B, et al: Improved characteristics of aPC-resistance assay. Coatest aPC resistance by predilution of samples with factor V deficiency plasma. *Am J Clin Pathol* 106:588, 1996.

125. Dahlback B: Resistance to activated protein C, the Arg^{506} to Gln mutation in the factor V gene, and venous thrombosis. *Thromb Haemost* 73:739, 1995.

126. Jorquera JI, Montoro JM, Fernandez MA, Aznar JA, Aznar J: Modified test for activated protein C resistance. *Lancet* 344:1162, 1994.

127. Le DT, Griffin JH, Greengard JS, Mujumdar V, Rapaport SI: Use of a generally applicable tissue factor-dependent factor V assay to detect activated protein C-resistant factor Va in patients receiving warfarin and in patients with a lupus anticoagulant. *Blood* 85:1704, 1995.

128. Griffin JH, Kojima K, Banka CL, Curtiss LK, Fernández JA: High-density lipoprotein enhancement of anticoagulant activities of plasma protein S and activated protein C. *J Clin Invest* 103:219, 1999.

129. Curvers J, Thomassen MCLG, Nicolaes GAF, et al: Acquired APC resistance and oral contraceptives: differences between two functional tests. *Br J Haematol* 105:88, 1999.

130. Stearns-Kurosawa DJ, Kurosawa S, Mollica JS, Ferrell GL, Esmon CT: The endothelial cell protein C receptor augments protein C activation by the thrombin-thrombomodulin complex. *Proc Natl Acad Sci* 93:10212, 1996.

131. Cooper PC, Abuzenadah A, Preston FE: APC resistance test, a new phenomenon—the role of platelets. *Br J Haematol* 86(suppl):33, 1999.

132. Shizuka R, Kanda T, Amagai H, Kobayashi I: False-positive activated protein C (APC) sensitivity ratio caused by freezing and by contamination of plasma with platelets. *Thromb Res* 78:189, 1995.

133. Simioni P, Scudeller A, Radossi P, et al: "Pseudo homozygous" activated protein C resistance due to double heterozygous factor V defects (factor V Leiden mutation and type I quantitative factor V defect) associated with thrombosis: report of two cases belonging to two unrelated kindreds. *Thromb Haemost* 75:422, 1996.

134. Castoldi E, Kalafatis M, Lunghi B, et al: Molecular bases of pseudo-homozygous APC resistance: the compound heterozygosity for FV R506Q and a FV Null mutation results in the exclusive presence of FV Leiden molecules in plasma. *Thromb Haemost* 80:403, 1998.

135. Kalafatis M, Bernardi F, Simioni P, et al: Phenotype and genotype expression in pseudohomozygous factor V^{LEIDEN}—the need for phenotype analysis. *Arterioscler Thromb Vasc Biol* 19:336, 1999.

136. Zivelin A, Rosenberg N, Faier S, et al: A single genetic origin for the common prothrombotic G20210A polymorphism in the prothrombin gene. *Blood* 92:1119, 1998.

137. Rosendaal FR, Doggen CJM, Zivelin A, et al: Geographic distribution of the 20210 G to A prothrombin variant. *Thromb Haemost* 79:706, 1998.

138. Souto JC, Coll I, Llobet D, et al: The prothrombin 20210A allele is the most prevalent genetic risk factor for venous thromboembolism in the Spanish population. *Thromb Haemost* 80:366, 1998.

139. Rosendaal FR, Vos HL, Poort SL, Bertina RM: Prothrombin 20210A variant and age at thrombosis. *Thromb Haemost* 79:444, 1998.

140. Leroyer C, Mercier B, Oger E, et al: Prevalence of 20210 A allele of the prothrombin gene in venous thromboembolism patients. *Thromb Haemost* 80:49, 1998.

141. Arruda VR, Annichino-Bizzacchi JM, Gonçalves MS, Costa FF: Prevalence of the prothrombin gene variant (nt20210A) in venous thrombosis and arterial disease. *Thromb Haemost* 78:1430, 1997.

142. Margaglione M, Brancaccio V, Giuliani N, et al: Increased risk for venous thrombosis in carriers of the prothrombin $G{\rightarrow}A^{20210}$ gene variant. *Ann Intern Med* 129:89, 1998.

143. Hillarp A, Zoller B, Svensson PJ, Dahlback B: The 20210 A allele of the prothrombin gene is a common risk factor among Swedish outpatients with verified deep venous thrombosis. *Thromb Haemost* 78:990, 1997.

144. Cumming AM, Keeney S, Salden A, et al: The prothrombin gene G 20210A variant: Prevalence in a U.K. anticoagulant clinic population. *Br J Haematol* 98:353, 1997.

145. Brown K, Luddington R, Williamson D, Baker P, Baglin T: The risk of venous thromboembolism associated with a G to A transition at position 20210 in the 3'-untranslated region of the prothrombin gene. *Br J Haematol* 98:907, 1997.

146. Ferraresi P, Marchetti G, Legnani C, et al: The heterozygous 20210

147. G/A prothrombin genotype is associated with early venous thrombosis in inherited thrombophilias and is not increased in frequency in artery disease. *Arterioscler Thromb Vasc Biol* 17:2418, 1997.

147. Simioni P, Tormene D, Manfrin D, et al: Prothrombin antigen levels in symptomatic and asymptomatic carriers of the 20210A prothrombin variant. *Br J Haematol* 103:1045, 1998.

148. De Stefano V, Chiusolo P, Paciaroni K, et al: Hepatic vein thrombosis in a patient with mutant prothrombin 20210A allele. *Thromb Haemost* 80:519, 1998.

149. Darnige L, Jezequel P, Amoura Z, et al: Mesenteric venous thrombosis in two patients heterozygous for the 20210 A allele of the prothrombin gene. *Thromb Haemost* 80:703, 1998.

150. Martinelli I, Sacchi E, Landi G, et al: High risk of cerebral-vein thrombosis in carriers of a prothrombin-gene mutation and in users of oral contraceptives. *N Engl J Med* 338:1793, 1998.

151. Biousse V, Conard J, Brouzes C, et al: Frequency of the 20210 G→A mutation in the 3'-untranslated region of the prothrombin gene in 35 cases of cerebral venous thrombosis. *Stroke* 29:1398, 1998.

152. Chamouard P, Pencreach E, Maloisel F, et al: Frequent factor II G20210A mutation in idiopathic portal vein thrombosis. *Gastroenterology* 116:144, 1999.

153. Reuner KH, Ruf A, Grau A, et al: Prothrombin gene G20210→A transition is a risk factor for cerebral venous thrombosis. *Stroke* 29:1765, 1998.

154. Zawadzki C, Gaveriaux V, Trillot N, et al: Homozygous G20210A transition in the prothrombin gene associated with severe venous thrombotic disease: two cases in a French family. *Thromb Haemost* 80:1027, 1998.

155. De Stefano V, Chiusolo P, Paciaroni K, et al: Prothrombin G20210A mutant genotype is a risk factor for cerebrovascular ischemic disease in young patients. *Blood* 91:3562, 1998.

156. Howard TE, Marusa M, Channell C, Duncan A: A patient homozygous for a mutation in the prothrombin gene 3″-untranslated region associated with massive thrombosis. *Blood Coagul Fibrinolysis* 8:316, 1997.

157. Makris M, Preston FE, Beauchamp NJ, et al: Co-inheritance of the 20210A allele of the prothrombin gene increases the risk of thrombosis in subjects with familial thrombophilia. *Thromb Haemost* 78:1426, 1997.

158. Corral J, Gonzalez-Conejero R, Lozano ML, et al: The venous thrombosis risk factor 20210 A allele of the prothrombin gene is not a major risk factor for arterial thrombotic disease. *Br J Haematol* 99:304, 1997.

159. Eikelboom JW, Baker RI, Parsons R, Taylor RR, Van Bockxmeer FM: No association between the 20210 G/A prothrombin gene mutation and premature coronary artery disease. *Thromb Haemost* 80:878, 1998.

160. Redondo M, Watzke HH, Stucki B, et al: Coagulation factors II, V, VII, and X, prothrombin gene 20210G→A transition, and factor V Leiden in coronary artery disease—high factor V clotting activity is an independent risk factor for myocardial infarction. *Arterioscler Thromb Vasc Biol* 19:1020, 1999.

161. Ridker PM, Hennekens CH, Miletich JP: G20210A mutation in prothrombin gene and risk of myocardial infarction, stroke, and venous thrombosis in a large cohort of US men. *Circulation* 99:999, 1999.

162. Rosendaal FR, Siscovick DS, Schwartz SM, et al: A common prothrombin variant (20210 G to A) increases the risk of myocardial infarction in young women. *Blood* 90:1747, 1997.

163. Franco RF, Trip MD, Ten Cate H, et al: The 20210 G→A mutation in the 3'-untranslated region of the prothrombin gene and the risk for arterial thrombotic disease. *Br J Haematol* 104:50, 1999.

164. Gardemann A, Arsic T, Katz N, et al: The factor II G20210A and factor V G1691A gene transitions and coronary heart disease. *Thromb Haemost* 81:208, 1999.

165. Mercier E, Quere I, Campello C, Mares P, Gris JC: The 20210A allele of the prothrombin gene is frequent in young women with unexplained spinal cord infarction. *Blood* 92:1840, 1998.

166. Mudd SH, Levy Hl, Skovby F: Disorders of transsulfuration, in Scriver CR, Beaudet AL, Sly WS, Valle D, *The metabolic and molecular bases of inherited disease*, p 1279. McGraw-Hill, New York, 1995.

167. Cattaneo M: Hyperhomocysteinemia, atherosclerosis and thrombosis. *Thromb Haemost* 81:165, 1999.

168. D'Angelo A, Selhub J: Homocysteine and thrombotic disease. *Blood* 90:1, 1997.

169. Fermo I, D'Angelo SV, Paroni R, et al: Prevaleance of moderate hyperhomocysteinemia in patients with early-onset venous and arterial occlusive disease. *Ann Intern Med* 123:747, 1995.

170. Den Heijer M, Rosendaal FR, Blom HJ, Gerrits WBJ, Bos GMJ: Hyperhomocysteinemia and venous thrombosis: a meta-analysis. *Thromb Haemost* 80:874, 1998.

171. den Heijer M, Brouwer IA, Bos GMJ, et al: Vitamin supplementation reduces blood homocysteine levels—a controlled trial in patients with venous thrombosis and healthy volunteers. *Arterioscler Thromb Vasc Biol* 18:356, 1998.

172. Woodside JV, Yarnell JWG, McMaster D, et al: Effect of B-group vitamins and antioxidant vitamins on hyperhomocysteinemia: a double-blind, randomized, factorial-design, controlled trial. *Am J Clin Nutr* 67:858, 1998.

173. Harker LA, Ross R, Slichter SJ, Scott CR: Homocystine-induced arteriosclerosis: the role of endothelial cell injury and platelet response in its genesis. *J Clin Invest* 58:731, 1976.

174. Lentz SR, Sobey CG, Piegors DJ, et al: Vascular dysfunction in monkeys with diet-induced hyperhomocyst(e)inemia. *J Clin Invest* 98:24, 1996.

175. Lentz SR: Mechanisms of thrombosis in hyperhomocysteinemia. *Curr Opin Hematol* 5:343, 1998.

176. Den Heijer M, Koster T, Blom HJ, et al: Hyperhomocysteinemia as a risk factor for deep-vein thrombosis. *N Engl J Med* 334:759, 1996.

177. Den Heijer M, Blom HJ, Gerrits WBJ, et al: Is hyperhomocysteinaemia a risk factor for recurrent venous thrombosis? *Lancet* 345:882, 1995.

178. Simioni P, Prandoni P, Burlina A, et al: Hyperhomocysteinemia and deep-vein thrombosis—a case-control study. *Thromb Haemost* 76:883, 1996.

179. Falcon CR, Cattaneo M, Panzeri D, Martinelli I, Mannucci PM: High prevalence of hyperhomocyst(e)inemia in patients with juvenile venous thrombosis. *Arterioscler Thromb* 14:1080, 1994.

180. Eichinger S, Stümpflen A, Hirschl M, et al: Hyperhomocysteinemia is a risk factor of recurrent venous thromboembolism. *Thromb Haemost* 80:566, 1998.

181. Kyrle PA, Stümpflen A, Hirschl M, et al: Levels of prothrombin fragment F1+2 in patients with hyperhomocysteinemia and a history of venous thromboembolism. *Thromb Haemost* 78:1327, 1997.

182. Cattaneo M, Franchi F, Zighetti ML, et al: Plasma levels of activated protein C in healthy subjects and patients with previous venous thromboembolism—relationships with plasma homocysteine levels. *Arterioscler Thromb Vasc Biol* 18:1371, 1998.

183. Kluijtmans LAJ, Boers GHJ, Verbruggen B, et al: Homozygous cystathionine β-synthase deficiency, combined with factor V Leiden or thermolabile methylenetetrahydrofolate reductase in the risk of venous thrombosis. *Blood* 91:2015, 1998.

184. Kang SS, Zhou J, Wong PW, Kowalisyn J, Strokosch G: Intermediate homocysteinemia: a thermolabile variant of methylenetetrahydrofolate reductase. *Am J Hum Genet* 43:414, 1988.

185. De Franchis R, Mancini FP, D'Angelo A, et al: Elevated total plasma homocysteine and 677C→T mutation of the 5,10-methylenetetrahydrofolate reductase gene in thrombotic vascular disease [letter]. *Am J Hum Genet* 59:262, 1996.

186. Margaglione M, D'Andrea G, D'Addedda M, et al: The methylenetetrahydrofolate reductase TT677 genotype is associated with venous thrombosis independently of the coexistence of the FV leiden and the prothrombin A^{20210} mutation. *Thromb Haemost* 79:907, 1998.

187. Kluijtmans LAJ, den Heijer M, Reitsma PH, et al: Thermolabile methylenetetrahydrofolate reductase and factor V Leiden in the risk of deep-vein thrombosis. *Thromb Haemost* 79:254, 1998.

188. Legnani C, Palareti G, Grauso F, et al: Hyperhomocyst(e)inemia and a common methylenetetrahydrofolate reductase mutation (Ala^{223}Val MTHFR) in patients with inherited thrombophilic coagulation defects. *Arterioscler Thromb Vasc Biol* 17:2924, 1997.

189. Tosetto A, Missiaglia E, Frezzato M, Rodeghiero F: The VITA Project: C677T mutation in the methylene-tetrahydrofolate reductase gene and risk of venous thromboembolism. *Br J Haematol* 97:804, 1997.

190. Garg UC, Zheng ZJ, Folsom AR, et al: Short-term and long-term variability of plasma homocysteine measurement. *Clin Chem* 43:141, 1997.

191. Refsum H, Fiskerstrand T, Guttormsen AB, Ueland PM: Assessment of homocysteine status. *J Inherit Metab Dis* 20:286, 1997.

192. Miner SES, Evrovski J, Cole DEC: Clinical chemistry and molecular biology of homocysteine metabolism: an update. *Clin Biochem* 30:189, 1997.

193. Van Der Griend R, Haas FJLM, Duran M, et al: Methionine loading test is necessary for detection of hyperhomocysteinemia. *J Lab Clin Med* 132:67, 1998.

194. Welch GN, Loscalzo J: Homocysteine and atherothrombosis. *N Engl J Med* 338:1042, 1998.

195. Jacobsen DW, Gatautis VJ, Green R, et al: Rapid HPLC determination of total homocysteine and other thiols in serum and plasma: sex differences and correlation with cobalamin and folate concentrations in healthy subjects [see comments]. *Clin Chem* 40:873, 1994.

196. Frosst P, Blom HJ, Milos R, et al: A candidate genetic risk factor for vascular disease: a common mutation in methylenetetrahydrofolate reductase [letter]. *Nat Genet* 10:111, 1995.

197. Branson HE, Katz J, Marble R, Griffin JH: Inherited protein C deficiency and coumarin-responsive chronic relapsing purpura fulminans in a newborn infant. *Lancet* 2:1165, 1983.

198. Reitsma PH, Bernardi F, Doig RG, et al: Protein C deficiency: a database of mutations, 1995 update. On behalf of the Subcommittee on Plasma Coagulation Inhibitors of the Scientific and Standardization Committee of the ISTH. [Review] [112 refs]. *Thromb Haemost* 73:876, 1995.

199. Miletich J, Sherman L, Broze G: Absence of thrombosis in subjects with heterozygous protein C deficiency. *N Engl J Med* 317:991, 1987.

200. Tait RC, Walker ID, Reitsma PH, et al: Prevalence of protein C deficiency in the healthy population. *Thromb Haemost* 73:87, 1995.

201. Koster T, Rosendaal FR, Briët E, et al: Protein C deficiency in a controlled series of unselected outpatients: an infrequent but clear risk factor for venous thrombosis (Leiden thrombophilia study). *Blood* 85:2756, 1995.

202. Bertina RM, Broekmans AW, van dL I, Mertens K: Protein C deficiency in a Dutch family with thrombotic disease. *Thromb Haemost* 48:1, 1982.

203. Allaart CF, Poort SR, Rosendaal FR, et al: Increased risk of venous thrombosis in carriers of hereditary protein C deficiency defect. *Lancet* 341:134, 1993.

204. Bovill EG, Bauer KA, Dickerman JD, Callas P, West B: The clinical spectrum of heterozygous protein C deficiency in a large New England kindred. *Blood* 73:712, 1989.

205. Lensen RPM, Rosendaal FR, Koster T, et al: Apparent different thrombotic tendency in patients with factor V Leiden and protein C deficiency due to selection of patients. *Blood* 88:4205, 1996.

206. Allaart CF, Rosendaal FR, Noteboom WMP, Vandenbroucke JP, Briet E: Survival in families with hereditary protein C deficiency, 1820 to 1993. *Br Med J* 311:910, 1995.

207. Hasstedt SJ, Bovill EG, Callas PW, Long GL: An unknown genetic defect increases venous thrombosis risk, through interaction with protein C deficiency. *Am J Hum Genet* 63:569, 1998.

208. Gandrille S, Priollet P, Capron L, et al: Association of inherited dysfibrinogenaemia and protein C deficiency in two unrelated families. *Br J Haematol* 68:329, 1988.

209. Spek CA, Koster T, Rosendaal FR, Bertina RM, Reitsma PH: Genotypic variation in the promoter region of the protein C gene is associated with plasma protein C levels and thrombotic risk. *Arterioscler Thromb Vasc Biol* 15:214, 1995.

210. Pabinger I, Schneider B: Thrombotic risk in hereditary antithrombin III, protein C, or protein S deficiency—a cooperative, retrospective study. *Arterioscler Thromb Vasc Biol* 16:742, 1996.

211. De Stefano V, Leone G, Mastrangelo S, et al: Clinical manifestations and management of inherited thrombophilia: retrospective analysis and follow-up after diagnosis of 238 patients with congenital deficiency of antithrombin III, protein C, protein S. *Thromb Haemost* 72:352, 1994.

212. Pabinger I, Kyrle PA, Heistinger M, et al: The risk of thromboembolism in asymptomatic patients with protein C and protein S deficiency: a prospective cohort study. *Thromb Haemost* 71:441, 1994.

213. Van den Belt AGM, Sanson BJ, Simioni P, et al: Recurrence of venous thromboembolism in patients with familial thrombophilia. *Arch Intern Med* 157:2227, 1997.

214. De Bruijn SFTM, Stam J, Koopman MMW, Vandenbroucke JP: Cerebral venous sinus thrombosis study: case-control study of risk of cerebral sinus thrombosis in oral contraceptive users who are carriers of hereditary prothrombotic conditions. *Br Med J* 316:589, 1998.

215. Camerlingo M, Finazzi G, Casto L, et al: Inherited protein C deficiency and nonhemorrhagic arterial stroke in young adults. *Neurology* 41:1371, 1991.

216. Seligsohn U, Berger A, Abend M, et al: Homozygous protein C defi-

ciency manifested by massive venous thrombosis in the newborn. *N Engl J Med* 310:559, 1984.

217. Sills RH, Marlar RA, Montgomery RR, Deshpande GN, Humbert JR: Severe homozygous protein C deficiency. *J Pediatr* 105:409, 1984.

218. Marciniak E, Wilson HD, Marlar RA: Neonatal purpura fulminans: a genetic disorder related to the absence of protein C in blood. *Blood* 65:15, 1985.

219. Monagle P, Andrew M, Halton J, et al: Homozygous protein C deficiency: Description of a new mutation and successful treatment with low molecular weight heparin. *Thromb Haemost* 79:756, 1998.

220. McGehee WG, Klotz TA, Epstein DJ, Rapaport SI: Coumarin necrosis associated with hereditary protein C deficiency. *Ann Int Med* 101:59, 1984.

221. Vigano D'A, Comp PC, Esmon CT, D'Angelo A: Relationship between protein C antigen and anticoagulant activity during oral anticoagulation and in selected disease states. *J Clin Invest* 77:416, 1986.

222. Miletich JP: Laboratory diagnosis of protein C deficiency. [Review] [31 refs]. *Semin Thromb Hemost* 16:169, 1990.

223. Francis RBJ, Seyfert U: Rapid amidolytic assay of protein C in whole plasma using an activator from the venom of Agkistrodon contortrix. *Am J Clin Pathol* 87:619, 1987.

224. Aiach M, Borgel D, Gaussem P, et al: Protein C and protein S deficiencies. *Semin Hematol* 34:205, 1997.

225. Berdeaux DH, Abshire TC, Marlar RA: Dysfunctional protein C deficiency (Type II). A report of 11 cases in 3 American families and review of the literature. *Am J Clin Pathol* 99:677, 1993.

226. Aiach M, Nicaud V, Alhenc-Gelas M, et al: Complex association of protein C gene promoter polymorphism with circulating protein C levels and thrombotic risk. *Arterioscler Thromb Vasc Biol* 19:1573, 1999.

227. Tait RC, Walker ID, Islam SI, et al: Protein C activity in healthy volunteers—influence of age, sex, smoking and oral contraceptives. *Thromb Haemost* 70:281, 1993.

228. Engesser L, Broekmans AW, Briet E, Brommer EJP, Bertina RM: Hereditary protein S deficiency: clinical manifestations. *Ann Intern Med* 106:677, 1987.

229. Reitsma PH, Ploos van Amstel HK, Bertina RM: Three novel mutations in five unrelated subjects with hereditary protein S deficiency type I. *J Clin Invest* 93:486, 1994.

230. Simmonds RE, Ireland H, Lane DA, et al: Clarification of the risk for venous thrombosis associated with hereditary protein S deficiency by investigation of a large kindred with a characterized gene defect. *Ann Intern Med* 128:8, 1998.

231. Bolan CD, Krishnamurti C, Tang DB, Carrington LR, Alving BM: Association of protein S deficiency with thrombosis in a kindred with increased levels of plasminogen activator inhibitor-1. *Ann Intern Med* 119:779, 1993.

232. Broekmans AW, Bertina RM, Reinalda-Poot J, et al: Hereditary protein S deficiency and venous thrombo-embolism. A study in three Dutch families. *Thromb Haemost* 53:273, 1985.

233. Gandrille S, Borgel D, Ireland H, et al: Protein S deficiency: a database of mutations. For the Plasma Coagulation Inhibitors Subcommittee of the Scientific and Standardization Committee of the International Society on Thrombosis and Haemostasis. *Thromb Haemost* 77:1201, 1997.

234. Mahasandana C, Suvatte V, Chuansumrit A, et al: Homozygous protein S deficiency in an infant with purpura fulminans. *J Pediatr* 117:750, 1990.

235. Pegelow CH, Ledford M, Young JN, Zilleruelo G: Severe protein S deficiency in a newborn. [Review] [26 refs]. *Pediatrics* 89:674, 1992.

236. Pung-amritt P, Poor SR, Vos HL, et al: Compound heterozygosity for one novel and one recurrent mutation in a Thai patient with severe protein S deficiency. *Thromb Haemost* 81:189, 1999.

237. Heeb MJ, Mesters RM, Tans G, Rosing J, Griffin JH: Binding of protein S to factor Va associated with inhibition of prothrombinase that is independent of activated protein C. *J Biol Chem* 268:2872, 1993.

238. Heeb MJ, Rosing J, Bakker HM, et al: Protein S binds to and inhibits factor Xa. *Proc Natl Acad Sci USA* 91:2728, 1994.

239. Hackeng TM, Van't Veer C, Meijers JCM, Bouma BN: Human protein S inhibits prothrombinase complex activity on endothelial cells and platelets via direct interactions with factors Va and Xa. *J Biol Chem* 269:21051, 1994.

240. Koppelman SJ, Hackeng TM, Sixma JJ, Bouma BN: Inhibition of the intrinsic factor X activating complex by protein S: evidence for a specific binding of protein S to factor VIII. *Blood* 86:1062, 1995.

241. Koppelman SJ, Van't Veer C, Sixma JJ, Bouma BN: Synergistic inhibition of the intrinsic factor X activation by protein S and C4b-binding protein. *Blood* 86:2653, 1995.

242. Van't Veer C, Hackeng TM, Biesbroeck D, Sixma JJ, Bouma BN: Increased prothrombin activation in protein S-deficient plasma under flow conditions on endothelial cell matrix: an independent anticoagulant function of protein S in plasma. *Blood* 85:1815, 1995.

243. Faioni EM, Valsecchi C, Palla A, et al: Free protein S deficiency is a risk factor for venous thrombosis. *Thromb Haemost* 78:1343, 1997.

244. Heijboer H, Brandjes DPM, Büller HR, Sturk A, Ten Cate JW: Deficiencies of coagulation-inhibiting and fibrinolytic proteins in outpatients with deep-vein thrombosis. *N Engl J Med* 323:1512, 1990.

245. Finazzi G, Barbui T: Different incidence of venous thrombosis in patients with inherited deficiencies of antithrombin III, protein C and protein S. *Thromb Haemost* 71:15, 1994.

246. Coller BS, Owen J, Jesty J, et al: Deficiency of plasma protein S, protein C, or antithrombin III and arterial thrombosis. *Arteriosclerosis* 7:456, 1987.

247. Allaart CF, Aronson DC, Ruys T, et al: Hereditary protein S deficiency in young adults with arterial occlusive disease. *Thromb Haemost* 64:206, 1990.

248. Grimaudo V, Gueissaz F, Hauert J, et al: Necrosis of skin induced by coumarin in a patient deficient in protein S. *Br Med J* 298:233, 1989.

249. Comp PC, Thurnau GR, Welsh J, Esmon CT: Functional and immunologic protein S levels are decreased during pregnancy. *Blood* 68:881, 1986.

250. Malm J, Laurell M, Dahlback B: Changes in the plasma levels of vitamin K-dependent proteins C and S and of C4b-binding protein during pregnancy and oral contraception. *Br J Haematol* 68:437, 1988.

251. Comp PC, Doray D, Patton D, Esmon CT: An abnormal plasma distribution of protein S occurs in functional protein S deficiency. *Blood* 67:504, 1986.

252. D'Angelo A, Vigano-D'Angelo S, Esmon CT, Comp PC: Acquired deficiences of protein S. Protein S activity during oral anticoagulation, in liver disease, and in disseminated intravascular coagulation. *J Clin Invest* 81:1445, 1988.

253. Vigano-D'Angelo S, D'Angelo A, Kaufman CE, et al: Protein S deficiency occurs in the nephrotic syndrome. *Ann Intern Med* 107:42, 1987.

254. Aadland E, Odegaard OR, Roseth A, Try K: Free protein S deficiency in patients with chronic inflammatory bowel disease. *Scand J Gastroenterol* 27:957, 1992.

255. Parke AL, Weinstein RE, Bona RD, Maier DB, Walker FJ: The thrombotic diathesis associated with the presence of phospholipid antibodies may be due to low levels of free protein S. *Am J Med* 93:49, 1992.

256. Ginsberg JS, Demers C, Brill-Edwards P, et al: Acquired free protein S deficiency is associated with antiphospholipid antibodies and increased thrombin generation in patients with systemic lupus erythematosus. *Am J Med* 98:379, 1995.

257. Levin M, Eley BS, Louis J, et al: Postinfectious purpura fulminans caused by an autoantibody directed against protein S. *J Pediatr* 127:355, 1995.

258. Blanco A, Bonduel M, Peñalva L, Hepner M, Lazzari M: Deep vein thrombosis in a 13-year-old boy with hereditary protein S deficiency and a review of the pediatric literature. *Am J Hematol* 45:330, 1994.

259. D'Angelo A, Della Valle P, Crippa L, et al: Brief report: Autoimmune protein S deficiency in a boy with severe thromboembolic disease. *N Engl J Med* 328:1753, 1993.

260. Bergmann F, Hoyer PF, Vigano D'Angelo S, et al: Severe autoimmune protein S deficiency in a boy with idiopathic purpura fulminans. *Br J Haematol* 89:610, 1995.

261. Woods CR, Johnson CA: Varicella purpura fulminans associated with heterozygosity for factor V Leiden and transient protein S deficiency. *Pediatrics* 102:1208, 1998.

262. Zoller B, Garcia de Frutos P, Dahlback B: Evaluation of the relationship between protein S and C4b-binding protein isoforms in hereditary protein S deficiency demonstrating type I and type III deficiencies to be phenotypic variants of the same genetic disease. *Blood* 85:3524, 1995.

263. Wolf M, Boyer-Neumann C, Peynaud-Debayle E, et al: Clinical applications of a direct assay of free protein S antigen using monoclonal antibodies. A study of 59 cases. *Blood Coagul Fibrinolysis* 5:187, 1994.

264. Amiral J, Grosley B, Boyer-Neumann C, et al: New direct assay of free protein S antigen using two distinct monoclonal antibodies specific for the free form. *Blood Coagul Fibrinolysis* 5:179, 1994.

265. Faioni EM, Boyer-Neumann C, Franchi F, et al: Another protein S functional assay is sensitive to resistance to activated protein C. *Thromb Haemost* 72:648, 1994.

266. Brunet D, Barthet MC, Morange PE, et al: Protein S deficiency: different biological phenotypes according to the assays used. *Thromb Haemost* 79:446, 1998.

267. Wolf M, Boyer-Neumann C, Leroy-Matheron C, et al: Functional assay of protein S in 70 patients with congenital and acquired disorders. *Blood Coagul Fibrinolysis* 2:705, 1991.

268. Gari M, Falkon L, Urrutia T, et al: The influence of low protein S plasma levels in young women, on the definition of normal range. *Thromb Res* 73:149, 1994.

269. Van Wijnen M, Van't Veer C, Meijers JCM, Bertina RM, Bouma BN: A plasma coagulation assay for an activated protein C-independent anticoagulant activity of protein S. *Thromb Haemost* 80:930, 1998.

270. Demers C, Ginsberg JS, Hirsh J, Henderson P, Blajchman MA: Thrombosis in antithrombin-III-deficient persons. Report of a large kindred and literature review. *Ann Intern Med* 116:754, 1992.

271. Van Boven HH, Lane DA: Antithrombin and its inherited deficiency states. *Semin Hematol* 34:188, 1997.

272. Blajchman MA, Austin RC, Fernandez-Rachubinski F, Sheffield WP: Molecular basis of inherited human antithrombin deficiency. *Blood* 80:2159, 1992.

273. Lane DA, Bayston T, Olds RJ, et al: Antithrombin mutation database: 2nd (1997) update. For the Plasma Coagulation Inhibitors Subcommittee of the Scientific and Standardization Committee of the International Society on Thrombosis and Haemostasis. *Thromb Haemost* 77:197, 1997.

274. Sakuragawa N, Takahashi K, Kondo S, Koide T: Antithrombin III Toyama: a hereditary abnormal antithrombin III of a patient with recurrent thrombophlebitis. *Thromb Res* 31:305, 1983.

275. Fischer AM, Cornu P, Sternberg C, et al: Antithrombin III Alger: a new homozygous AT III variant. *Thromb Haemost* 55:218, 1986.

276. Okajima K, Ueyama H, Hashimoto Y, et al: Homozygous variant of antithrombin III that lacks affinity for heparin, AT III Kumamoto. *Thromb Haemost* 61:20, 1989.

277. Boyer C, Wolf M, Vedrenne J, Meyer D, Larrieu MJ: Homozygous variant of antithrombin III: AT III Fontainebleau. *Thromb Haemost* 56:18, 1986.

278. Tait RC, Walker ID, Perry DJ, et al: Prevalence of antithrombin deficiency in the healthy population. *Br J Haematol* 87:106, 1994.

279. Van Boven HH, Vandenbroucke JP, Briët E, Rosendaal FR: Gene-gene and gene-environment interactions determine risk of thrombosis in families with inherited antithrombin deficiency. *Blood* 94:2590, 1999.

280. Hirsh J, Piovella F, Pini M: Congenital antithrombin III deficiency. Incidence and clinical features. *Am J Med* 87 [suppl 3B]:34S, 1989.

281. Rosendaal FR, Heijboer H, Briet E, et al: Mortality in hereditary antithrombin III deficiency—1830 to 1989. *Lancet* 337:260, 1991.

282. Van Boven HH, Olds RJ, Thein S-L, et al: Hereditary antithrombin deficiency: heterogeneity of the molecular basis and mortality in Dutch families. *Blood* 84:4209, 1994.

283. Coller BS, Owen J, Jesty J, et al: Deficiency of plasma protein S, protein C, or antithrombin III and arterial thrombosis. *Arteriosclerosis* 7:456, 1987.

284. Levine MN, Hirsh J, Gent M, et al: A randomized trial comparing activated thromboplastin time with heparin assay in patients with acute venous thromboembolism requiring large daily doses of heparin. *Arch Intern Med* 154:49, 1994.

285. De Boer AC, van Riel LA, den Ottolander GJ: Measurement of antithrombin III, alpha 2-macroglobulin and alpha 1-antitrypsin in patients with deep venous thrombosis and pulmonary embolism. *Thromb Res* 15:17, 1979.

286. Marciniak E, Gockerman JP: Heparin-induced decrease in circulating antithrombin-III. *Lancet* 2:581, 1977.

287. Von Kaulla E, Von Kaulla KN: Antithrombin 3 and diseases. *Am J Clin Pathol* 48:69, 1967.

288. Damus PS, Wallace GA: Immunologic measurement of antithrombin III-heparin cofactor and alpha2 macroglobulin in disseminated intravascular coagulation and hepatic failure coagulopathy. *Thromb Res* 6:27, 1975.

289. Kauffmann RH, Veltkamp JJ, van Tilburg NH, Van Es LA: Acquired antithrombin III deficiency and thrombosis in the nephrotic syndrome. *Am J Med* 65:607, 1978.

290. Buchanan GR, Holtkamp CA: Reduced antithrombin III levels during L-asparaginase therapy. *Med Pediatr Oncol* 8:7, 1980.

291. Weenink GH, Treffers PE, Vijn P, Smorenberg-Schoorl ME, Ten Cate JW: Antithrombin III levels in preeclampsia correlate with maternal and fetal morbidity. *Am J Obstet Gynecol* 148:1092, 1984.

292. Abildgaard U, Lie M, Odegard OR: Antithrombin (heparin cofactor) assay with "new" chromogenic substrates (S-2238 and Chromozym TH). *Thromb Res* 11:549, 1977.

293. Demers C, Henderson P, Blajchman MA, et al: An antithrombin III assay based on factor Xa inhibition provides a more reliable test to identify congenital antithrombin III deficiency than an assay based on thrombin inhibition. *Thromb Haemost* 69:231, 1993.

294. Bohner J, Von Pape K-W, Blaurock M: Thrombin-based antithrombin assays show over-estimation of antithrombin III activity in patients on heparin therapy due to heparin cofactor II influence. *Thromb Haemost* 71:280, 1994.

295. Sas G, Pepper DS, Cash JD: Plasma and serum antithrombin III: differentiation by crossed immunoelectrophoresis. *Thromb Res* 6:87, 1975.

296. Koster T, Blann AD, Briët E, Vandenbroucke JP, Rosendaal FR: Role of clotting factor VIII in effect of von Willebrand factor on occurrence of deep-vein thrombosis. *Lancet* 345:152, 1995.

297. O'Donnell J, Tuddenham EG, Manning R, et al: High prevalence of elevated factor VIII levels in patients referred for thrombophilia screening: role of increased synthesis and relationship to the acute phase reaction. *Thromb Haemost* 77:825, 1997.

298. Kamphuisen PW, Eikenboom JC, Vos HL, et al: Increased levels of factor VIII and fibrinogen in patients with venous thrombosis are not caused by acute phase reactions. *Thromb Haemost* 81:680, 1999.

299. Haverkate F, Samama M: Familial dysfibrinogenemia and thrombophilia. Report on a study of the SSC Subcommittee on Fibrinogen. *Thromb Haemost* 73:151, 1995.

300. Martinez J: Congenital dysfibrinogenemia. *Curr Opin Hematol* 4:357, 1997.

301. Aoki N, Moroi M, Sakata Y, Yoshida N, Matsuda M: Abnormal plasminogen. A hereditary molecular abnormality found in a patient with recurrent thrombosis. *J Clin Invest* 61:1186, 1978.

302. Miyata T, Iwanaga S, Sakata Y, Aoki N: Plasminogen Tochigi: Inactive plasmin resulting from replacement of alanine-600 by threonine in the active site. *Proc Natl Acad Sci USA* 79:6132, 1982.

303. Miyata T, Iwanaga S, Sakata Y, et al: Plasminogens Tochigi II and Nagoya: two additional molecular defects with Ala600Val replacement found in plasmin light chain variants. *J Biochem (Tokyo)* 96:277, 1984.

304. Shigekiyo T, Uno Y, Tomonari A, et al: Type I congenital plasminogen deficiency is not a risk factor for thrombosis. *Thromb Haemost* 67:189, 1992.

305. Prins MH, Hirsh J: A critical review of the evidence supporting a relationship between impaired fibrinolytic activity and venous thromboembolism. *Arch Intern Med* 151:1721, 1991.

306. Ohlin AK, Marlar RA: The first mutation identified in the thrombomodulin gene in a 45-year-old man presenting with thromboembolic disease. *Blood* 85:330, 1995.

307. Ohlin AK, Marlar RA: Thrombomodulin gene defects in families with thromboembolic disease—a report on four families. *Thromb Haemost* 81:338, 1999.

308. Ohlin AK, Norlund L, Marlar RA: Thrombomodulin gene variations and thromboembolic disease. [Review] [26 refs]. *Thromb Haemost* 78:396, 1997.

309. Walker ID: Factor V Leiden: should all women be screened prior to commencing the contraceptive pill? [Review] [22 refs]. *Blood Rev* 13:8, 1999.

310. Hagstrom JN, Walter J, Bluebond-Langner R, et al: Prevalence of the factor V leiden mutation in children and neonates with thromboembolic disease. *J Pediatr* 133:777, 1998.

311. Zenz W, Bodo Z, Plotho J, et al: Factor V Leiden and prothrombin gene G 20210 A variant in children with ischemic stroke. *Thromb Haemost* 80:763, 1998.

312. DeVeber G, Monagle P, Chan A, et al: Prothrombotic disorders in infants and children with cerebral thromboembolism. *Arch Neurol* 55:1539, 1998.

313. Nowak-Göttl U, Junker R, Hartmeier M, et al: Increased lipoprotein(a)

is an important risk factor for venous thromboembolism in childhood. *Circulation* 100:743, 1999.

314. Hirsh J, Kearon C, Ginsberg J: Duration of anticoagulant therapy after first episode of venous thrombosis in patients with inherited thrombophilia. *Arch Intern Med* 157:2174, 1997.

315. Schulman S, Rhedin AS, Lindmarker P, et al: A comparison of six weeks with six months of oral anticoagulant therapy after a first episode of venous thromboembolism. *N Engl J Med* 332:1661, 1995.

316. Kearon C, Gent M, Hirsh J, et al: A comparison of three months of anticoagulation with extended anticoagulation for a first episode of idiopathic venous thromboembolism. *N Engl J Med* 340:901, 1999.

317. Lensing AWA, Prandoni P, Prins MH, Büller HR: Deep-vein thrombosis. *Lancet* 353:479, 1999.

318. Lechner K, Kyrle PA: Antithrombin III concentrates—are they clinically useful? *Thromb Haemost* 73:340, 1995.

319. Bucur SZ, Levy JH, Despotis GJ, Spiess BD, Hillyer CD: Uses of antithrombin III concentrate in congenital and acquired deficiency states. *Transfusion* 38:481, 1998.

320. Menache D, O'Malley JP, Schorr JB, et al: Evaluation of the safety, recovery, half-life, and clinical efficacy of antithrombin III (human) in patients with hereditary antithrombin III deficiency. *Blood* 75:33, 1990.

321. Vukovich T, Auberger K, Weil J, et al: Replacement therapy for a homozygous protein C deficiency-state using a concentrate of human protein C and S. *Br J Haematol* 70:435, 1988.

322. Manco-Johnson M, Nuss R: Protein C concentrate prevents peripartum thrombosis. *Am J Hematol* 40:69, 1992.

323. Gerson WT, Dickerman JD, Bovill EG, Golden E: Severe acquired protein C deficiency in purpura fulminans associated with disseminated intravascular coagulation: treatment with protein C concentrate. *Pediatrics* 91:418, 1993.

324. Toglia MR, Weg JG: Venous thromboembolism during pregnancy. *N Engl J Med* 335:108, 1996.

325. McColl MD, Ramsay JE, Tait RC, et al: Risk factors for pregnancy associated venous thromboembolism. *Thromb Haemost* 78:1183, 1997.

326. Greer IA: Thrombosis in pregnancy: maternal and fetal issues. *Lancet* 353:1258, 1999.

327. Bauer KA: Management of patients with hereditary defects predisposing to thrombosis including pregnant women. *Thromb Haemost* 74:94, 1995.

328. Friederich PW, Sanson BJ, Simioni P, et al: Frequency of pregnancy-related venous thromboembolism in anticoagulant factor-deficient women: implications for prophylaxis. *Ann Intern Med* 125:955, 1996.

329. Preston FE, Rosendaal FR, Walker ID, et al: Increased fetal loss in women with heritable thrombophilia. *Lancet* 348:913, 1996.

330. Kupferminc MJ, Eldor A, Steinman N, et al: Increased frequency of genetic thrombophilia in women with complications of pregnancy. *N Engl J Med* 340:9, 1999.

331. Goddijn-Wessel TAW, Wouters MGAJ, Molen EFvd, et al: Hyperhomocysteinemia: a risk factor for placental abruption or infarction. *Eur J Obstet Gynecol Reprod Biol* 66:23, 1996.

332. Powers RW, Evens RW, Majors AK, et al: Plasma homocysteine concentration is increased in preeclampsia and is associated with evidence of endothelial activation. *Am J Obstet Gynecol* 179:1605, 1998.

333. Grandone E, Margaglione M, Colaizzo D, et al: Prothrombotic genetic risk factors and the occurrence of gestational hypertension with or without proteinuria. *Thromb Haemost* 81:349, 1999.

334. De Vries JIP, Dekker GA, Huijgens PC, et al: Hyperhomocysteinaemia and protein S deficiency in complicated pregnancies. *Br J Obstet Gynaecol* 104:1248, 1997.

335. Ridker PM, Miletich JP, Buring JE, et al: Factor V Leiden mutation as a risk factor for recurrent pregnancy loss. *Ann Intern Med* 128:1000, 1998.

336. Gardone E, Margaglione M, Colaizzo D, et al: Factor V Leiden is associated with repeated and recurrent unexplained fetal losses. *Thromb Haemost* 77:822, 1997.

337. Dizon-Townson D, Meline L, Nelson LM, Varner M, Ward K: Fetal carriers of the factor V Leiden mutation are prone to miscarriage and placental infarction. *Am J Obstet Gynecol* 177:402, 1997.

338. Brenner B, Mandel H, Lanir N, Younis J, Rothbart H: Activated protein C resistance can be associated with recurrent fetal loss. *Br J Haematol* 97:551, 1997.

339. Quere I, Bellet H, Hoffet M, et al: A woman with five consecutive fetal deaths: case report and retrospective analysis of hyperhomocysteinemia prevalence in 100 consecutive women with recurrent miscarriages. *Fertil Steril* 69:152, 1998.

340. Sibai BM: Thrombophilias and adverse outcomes of pregnancy—what should a clinician do? *N Engl J Med* 340:50, 1999.

341. Pabinger I, Schneider B, GTH Study Group Natural Inhibitors: Thrombotic risk of women with hereditary antithrombin III-, protein C- and protein S-deficiency taking oral contraceptive medication. *Thromb Haemost* 71:548, 1994.

342. Martinelli I, Taioli E, Bucciarelli P, Akhavan S, Mannucci PM: Interaction between the G20210A mutation of the prothrombin gene and oral contraceptive use in deep vein thrombosis. *Arterioscler Thromb Vasc Biol* 19:700, 1999.

343. Trauscht-Van Horn JJ, Capeless EL, Easterling TR, Bovill EG: Pregnancy loss and thrombosis with protein C deficiency. *Am J Obstet Gynecol* 167:968, 1992.

344. Rosendaal FR: Oral contraceptives and screening for factor V Leiden. *Thromb Haemost* 75:524, 1996.

345. Vandenbroucke JP, Van der Meer FJM, Helmerhorst FM, Rosendaal FR: Factor V Leiden: should we screen oral contraceptive users and pregnant women? *Br Med J* 313:1127, 1996.

346. Jick H, Jick SS, Gurewich V, Myers MW, Vasilakis C: Risk of idiopathic cardiovascular death and nonfatal venous thromboembolism in women using oral contraceptives with differing progestagen components. *Lancet* 346:1589, 1995.

347. Vandenbroucke JP, Helmerhorst FM: Risk of venous thrombosis with hormone-replacement therapy. *Lancet* 348:972, 1996.

348. Jick H, Derby LE, Myers MW, Vasilakis C, Newton KM: Risk of hospital admission for idiopathic venous thromboembolism among users of postmenopausal oestrogens. *Lancet* 348:981, 1996.

349. Daly E, Vessey MP, Hawkins MN, et al: Risk of venous thromboembolism in users of hormone replacement therapy. *Lancet* 348:977, 1996.

350. Douketis J, Ginsberg JS, Holbrook A, et al: A reevaluation of the risk for venous thromboembolism with the use of oral contraceptives and hormone replacement therapy. *Arch Intern Med* 157:1522, 1997.

351. Schafer AI: Hypercoagulable states: molecular genetics to clinical practice. *Lancet* 344:1739, 1994.

LUPUS ANTICOAGULANTS AND RELATED DISORDERS

JACOB H. RAND

The antiphospholipid (aPL) syndrome is an acquired disorder in which patients have thrombotic manifestations together with laboratory evidence for autoantibodies which recognize anionic phospholipid-protein complexes. The disorder is considered to be secondary when it occurs in the presence of systemic lupus erythematosus (SLE) or other major autoimmune conditions and primary in their absence. The aPL syndrome usually manifests clinically as vascular thrombosis or embolism or as recurrent spontaneous pregnancy losses. While the deep veins of the lower extremities are the most frequent sites of thrombosis, thromboembolism can involve virtually any portion of the arterial or venous circulations. Additional reported manifestations of the aPL syndrome include immune thrombocytopenia, livedo reticularis, stroke, atherosclerosis, pulmonary hypertension, and sensorineural hearing loss. Rare patients will present with a catastrophic form of the aPL syndrome caused by disseminated large- and small-vessel thrombi with accompanying multiorgan ischemia and infarction. This form of the disorder may also mimic the presentation of thrombotic thrombocytopenic purpura or disseminated intravascular coagulation.

The antigenic targets for the antibodies generated in this condition appear to be epitopes on phospholipid-binding proteins such as β_2 glycoprotein I (β_2GPI) rather than the phospholipid itself. The syndrome is recognized by laboratory evidence for the presence of antibodies against these phospholipid-protein cofactor complexes by ELISA assays (anticardiolopin, antiphosphatidyl serine, or anti-β_2GPI assays) or by coagulation assays ("lupus anticoagulants") which paradoxically report the inhibition of phospholipid-dependent coagulation reactions. Several conditions are associated with increased levels of antibodies directed against anionic phospholipids themselves but not against protein cofactors. These are not associated with an increased risk of thrombosis and include infections such as syphilis and Lyme disease, hepatitis C and alcoholic liver injury, HIV infection, and multiple sclerosis.

Patients with spontaneous vascular thrombosis and the aPL syndrome should be treated with oral anticoagulant therapy. Hydroxychloroquine may be a useful adjunct for prevention of thrombosis. The catastrophic aPL syndrome may require additional therapy with high-dose anticoagulants, plasmapheresis, and immunosuppressive agents. Patients with recurrent spontaneous pregnancy losses and the aPL syndrome require treatment with aspirin and heparin for the major portion of their pregnancies and may need additional prophylaxis against deep vein thrombosis during the postpartum period. Since aPL tests may be abnormal in conditions other than the aPL syndrome, patients should not be committed to antithrombotic therapy on the basis of laboratory tests alone. The clinician should have documented evidence-or at least a very high suspicion—for thromboembolism or pregnancy losses before treating. In patients who are treated with warfarin, care should be taken to confirm that coagulation tests for monitoring oral anticoagulant therapy reflect true reductions in the levels of coagulation proteins and that these are not artifactually affected by lupus anticoagulants.

DEFINITION AND HISTORY

DEFINITION

The aPL antibody syndrome is a disorder in which vascular thrombosis or recurrent pregnancy losses occur in patients who have laboratory evidence for antibodies against phospholipids or phospholipid-binding protein cofactors. The presence of these antibodies is detectable with immunoassays using solid phase phospholipids (the structures of several relevant phospholipids are shown in Fig. 128-1) and protein cofactors as antigenic targets, or with coagulation assays that demonstrate the inhibition of phospholipid-dependent coagulation reactions known as the lupus anticoagulant (LA) phenomenon. The syndrome was first proposed to be a distinct entity, the *anticardiolipin (aCL) syndrome*, in 1985[1] and was soon renamed the *aPL syndrome*.[2] The disorder is classified as primary if no other autoimmune condition such as systemic lupus erythematosus is concurrent, and secondary in the presence of such disorders (Fig. 128-2). There appears to be no difference in the clinical presentations or in the courses of thrombosis of patients with the primary and secondary disorders.[3,4] In view of the apparent multiplicity of antigens recognized by the antibodies (see "Antigenic Specificities" below) and the ambiguous pathophysiology, other names for the condition, such as the *aPL/cofactor syndrome*,[5] the *antibody-mediated thrombosis syndrome*,[6,7] or the eponym *Hughes syndrome*[8] have been proposed.

HISTORY

In retrospect, the first serologic evidence for the disorder was the observation of the biological false-positive serological test for syphilis (BFP syphilis test), described by Moore and Mohr in 1952.[9] This laboratory anomaly was found to often be associated with SLE[10] and with an anticoagulant phenomenon,[11] but its clinical significance was not known. In the early 1950s, the development of coagulation tests which used a phospholipid extract of animal brain (cephalin) to accelerate coagulation reactions[12] led to the recognition of abnormalities that were attributed to the presence of an anticoagulant in patients with systemic lupus eythematosus—frequently together with BFP syphilis tests. This phenomenon was named the "*lupus anticoagulant*".[13] Although the first report of patients with these anticoagulants described bleeding manifestations,[14] it became evident that these in vitro anticoagulants were associated with bleeding problems in vivo only if there were other hemostatic defects present, such as hypoprothrombinemia, thrombocytopenia, platelet function abnormalities, or specific inhibitors of blood coagulation factors.[11] It was surprising when these anticoagulants were found to be associated with thrombotic and

---

Acronyms and abbreviations that appear in this chapter include: aCL, anticardiolipin; APC, activated protein C; aPS, antibodies to phosphatidyl serine; aPL, antiphospholipid; BFP syphilis test, biological false-positive serological test for syphilis; dRVVT, dilute Russell viper venom time; GP, glycoprotein; IVF, in vitro fertilization; LA, lupus anticoagulant; LMWH, low-molecular-weight heparins; PAI-1, plasminogen activator inhibitor 1; RVV, Russell viper venom; SLE, systemic lupus erythematosus; SNAP, seronegative aPL syndrome.

Glycerol Backbone	Nomenclature	R group	Charge
	Cardiolipin (CL)	$-CH_2-CH-CH_2-P=O$	(–)
	Phosphatidylethanolamine (PE)	$-CH_2-CH_2-NH_3^+$	neutral
	Phosphatidylcholine (PC)	$-CH_2-CH_2-N^+(CH_3)_3$	neutral
	Phosphatidylserine (PS)	$-CH_2-CH-N^+H_3$	(–)
	Phosphatidylinositol (PI)		(–)
	Phosphatidic acid (PA)	– No R group	(–)

FIGURE 128-1   Phospholipid structures. (Reprinted with permission from *Obstet Gynecol Surv.*[154])

embolic manifestations[15] and with recurrent pregnancy loss.[16] A major step leading to the identification of the aPL syndrome occurred in 1983 when a quantitative test was developed to assay antibodies against the anionic phospholipid known as *cardiolipin* (diphosphatidyl glycerol), which is the primary antigen in the syphilis test reagent.[17]

As shown in Fig. 128-2, individuals having aPL antibodies include those with aPL syndrome (whether primary or secondary) and those without the clinical syndrome. The latter include completely asymptomatic normal healthy people, patients with infections that induce antibodies recognizing anionic phospholipids directly, and patients on medications such as chlorpromazine or procainamide. In the asymptomatic normal healthy population there are some individuals who are at high risk but have not yet developed the disorder (pre-aPL syndrome). There are also patients who are suspected to have a seronegative form of the disorder (SNAP—seronegative aPL syndrome).

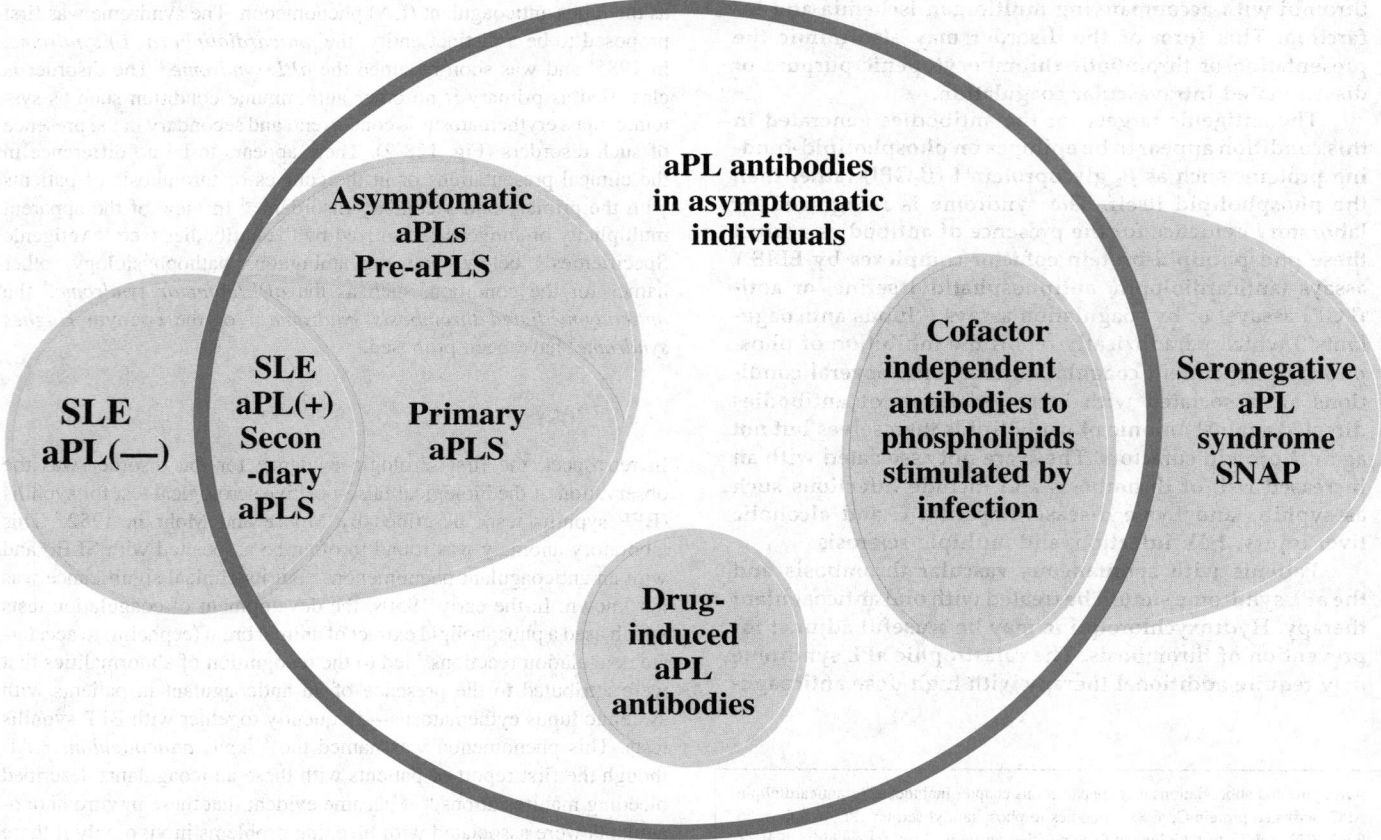

FIGURE 128-2   The conceptual distribution of patients having antibodies against phospholipid and of patients with the aPL syndrome. The large thick-walled circle includes all patients having antibodies against phospholipid. Within this group are patients with the aPL syndrome (primary, secondary, and asymptomatic) and patients having antibodies but lacking the syndrome. Outside the circle are patients with seronegative aPL syndrome ("SNAP") and patients with SLE lacking aPL antibodies.

ETIOLOGY AND PATHOGENESIS

ETIOLOGY

The genesis of the antibodies in this disorder and even their antigenic specificities are not yet understood. The disorder is generally considered to fall into the category of autoimmune conditions. While antibodies against anionic phospholipid moieties arise during the course of infections such as syphilis and Lyme disease, those antibodies are distinct from antibodies generated by patients with the syndrome, because they recognize phospholipid epitopes directly (i.e., they are not cofactor dependent) and are not associated with the clinical manifestations of the syndrome. In contrast (as described below in "Antigenic Specificities"), the antibodies generated in patients with the syndrome recognize epitopes which include protein cofactors, primarily β_2GPI, and thus are often referred to as being cofactor-dependent.

GENETIC PREDISPOSITION HLA Linkages

Familial clustering of raised aPL antibody levels[18] along with HLA-linkages[19-22] indicate that the antibodies probably occur in response to some antigenic challenge in a genetically susceptible host. One study suggested that the aPL responses in SLE and in primary aPL syndrome are immunogenetically distinct from SLE itself. The strongest association with aPL was the HLA-DR53 haplotypes, some of which include DQ7, whereas the HLA-B8, DR17, DQ2 haplotypes closely associated with SLE were significantly decreased in patients with primary and secondary aPL syndrome.[20]

POSSIBLE ETIOLOGIC AGENTS

There have been intriguing reports of the aPL syndrome arising in patients with infections (in contrast to patients having antibodies against phospholipid alone without the syndrome, whose relationship to infection has been well established). aPL antibodies have been reported in patients with postvaricella purpura fulminans[23] or venous thrombosis[24], in patients with varicella pneumonia and spontaneous tibial artery thrombosis[25] and in patients with hepatitis C.[26] An association of aPL and mesenteric and femoropopliteal thrombosis in a patient with cytomegalovirus infection has also been reported.[27] Also, β_2GPI cofactor dependent antibodies against cardiolipin, phosphatidyl serine and phosphatidyl ethanolamine have been identified in sera from patients with parvovirus B19.[28] Anticardiolipin antibodies having β_2GPI-dependence and lupus anticoagulant activity have been generated in rabbits immunized with lipid A and lipoteichoic acid, suggesting that some bacteria might contribute to the production of pathogenic aPL antibodies.[29] It has been proposed that cellular apoptosis, with the resulting exposure of anionic phospholipids on the cell surface, triggers the generation of aPL antibodies.[30-32]

PATHOGENESIS

The pathophysiologic mechanisms of this syndrome have remained obscure. In part, this is because of the apparent multiplicity of antigenic determinants recognized by the antibodies. Also, a large number of effects have been described for the antibodies in vitro and in cell culture systems, and it is difficult to determine which of these are clinically relevant. Many of these effects, including the paradoxical lupus anticoagulant (LA) phenomenon, are a consequence of the multiple roles involving phospholipids in the hemostatic system and in biologic processes in general.

RELATIONSHIP OF ANTIBODIES TO CLINICAL MANIFESTATIONS-EVIDENCE FROM ANIMAL STUDIES

Although there had been much debate about the relationship of the aPL antibodies to the disease process—i.e., whether cause, effect, or epiphenomenon—convincing evidence has accumulated from experimental animal models of the aPL syndrome to indicate that aPL antibodies can play a causal role in the development of thrombosis and pregnancy loss. Mice immunized against β_2GPI develop aPL antibodies and pregnancy wastage.[33] Mice that have been passively or actively immunized with aPL antibodies develop fetal wastage.[34,35-36] Also, mice infused with the aPL antibodies developed significantly larger thrombi in femoral veins after experimental vascular injury than mice infused with control antibodies.[37,38] Importantly, a monoclonal human anticardiolipin antibody derived from a patient with the aPL syndrome promoted thrombosis in mice.[39] Also, atherosclerosis in a susceptible mouse model (the LDL-receptor knockout mouse) was accelerated by immunization with human anticardiolipin antibodies from an aPL syndrome patient, suggesting that these antibodies may play a role in the development of atherosclerosis in patients with the aPL syndrome.[40]

A direct causal relationship between aPL antibodies and thrombotic manifestations or pregnancy losses in humans has not yet been proved. While it is clear that there are patients with aPL antibodies who manifest thrombosis and pregnancy loss, the fact that elevated levels of antibodies are detectable in a significant proportion of asymptomatic individuals[41-44] has raised questions about their predictive value.

ANTIGENIC SPECIFICITIES

While there is evidence that some aPL antibodies may recognize phospholipids directly without protein cofactors,[45] purified aPL antibodies generally do not bind directly to purified cardiolipin in the absence of a source of serum proteins.[46,47] aPL antibodies from patients with the syndrome are usually "dependent" upon a serum phospholipid-binding protein, that is known as β_2GPI or apolipoprotein H, for recognition of the phospholipid in ELISAs. In contrast, antibodies against phospholipid that arise in the course of the immunologic response to syphilis infection are not cofactor-dependent and recognize the anionic phospholipid epitopes directly.[48]

β_2GPI is a highly glycosylated single-chain plasma protein composed of 326 amino acids with a molecular weight of 50 kDa (Fig. 128-3) that appears to be the major, but not the only, cofactor for the recognition of anionic phospholipid by aPL antibodies.[49] The protein is a member of the complement control protein or short consensus repeat superfamily.[50] There is evidence that β_2GPI itself may be one of the major epitopes for aPL antibodies or may, in complex with phospholipids, form an antigenic site. aPL antibodies can recognize β_2GPI directly (i.e., in the absence of phospholipid) if the protein antigen is present on microtiter plates at a sufficient density.[51,52] The protein has repeating motifs or domains that structurally resemble multiple loops ("sushi domains"). The physiologic function of β_2GPI has not yet been established, but it has been proposed that the protein may play a scavenging role for exposed anionic phospholipid following apoptosis.[53] Work with deletional mutants demonstrated that the phospholipid recognition and an antibody recognition site are present at the protein's highly cationic fifth sushi domain.[54-56] The relationship between antibody recognition of β_2GPI and thrombosis is not yet clear; however, there is also evidence that aPL antibody recognition of the fourth sushi domain plays a role.[57]

Following the discovery of the cofactor role for β_2GPI, additional candidate cofactors and antigenic targets were identified.[58] These include prothrombin (coagulation factor II), coagulation factor V, protein C, protein S, annexin-V, high-molecular-weight kininogen, and low-molecular-weight kininogen. Interestingly, protein C can be a target of aCL in the presence of cardiolipin and β_2GPI, leading to protein C dysfunction.[59] Also, antibodies of some aPL patients have been found to cross-react with heparin and inhibit the formation of antithrombin III-thrombin complexes.[60]

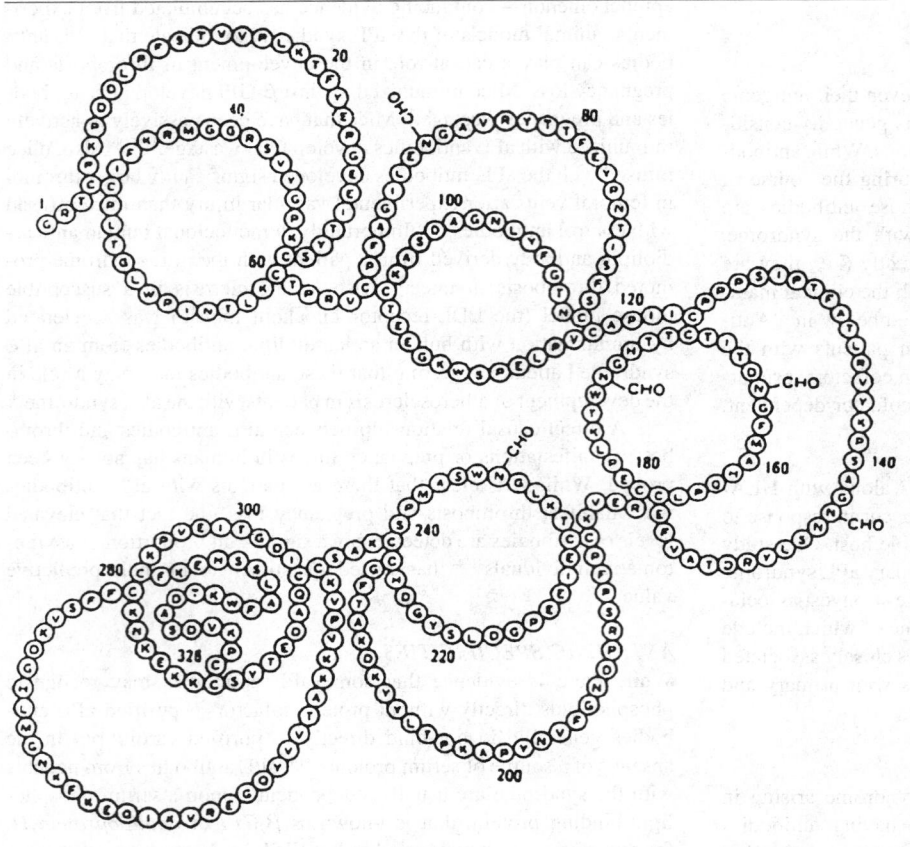

FIGURE 128-3   Amino acid sequence and location of disulfide bonds in human β_2GPI. (Reprinted with permission from Hughes et al.[8])

It has been proposed that phosphatidyl-ethanolamine reactivity is associated with thrombosis in autoimmune diseases, since a high proportion of patients with aPL syndrome also have antibodies reactive with this zwitterionic phospholipid.[61] Antibody recognition of phosphatidyl-ethanolamine appears to require kininogen or kininogen-associated proteins as cofactor.[62]

The oxidation of phosphospholipids may be necessary for aPL antibody recognition.[63,64] The epitopes for some aPL antibodies appear to be adducts of oxidized phospholipid and protein such as β_2GPI.[65] Thus, some affinity-purified cardiolipin-binding antibodies in sera from patients with systemic lupus erythematosus appear to cross-react with oxidized LDL.[66] Elevated levels of the latter antibodies have been proposed to be markers for arterial thrombosis,[67] but there is controversy on this point.[68]

Antimitochondrial M5 type antibodies have been reported to be a serological marker for the aPL syndrome distinct from anticardiolipin and anti-β_2GPI antibodies. These antibodies, unlike aCL and anti-β_2GPI IgG antibodies, are not significantly associated with thrombosis, but they are associated with thrombocytopenia and recurrent fetal loss.[69]

PROPOSED PATHOGENIC MECHANISMS

Since virtually any of the many biologic processes that involve or require phospholipids may be affected by the presence of antibodies which bind to the phospholipids (either directly or via cofactors), any proposed aPL-mediated effects that are based on in vitro studies must be evaluated for in vivo relevance. Also, any plausible explanation for the aPL syndrome needs to account for the paradox of the LA

phenomenon. The current hypotheses for pathogenic mechanisms in the aPL syndrome are summarized in Table 128-1. It is possible that several of these effects could act in concert to cause the clinical manifestations.

aPL Antibody-mediated Disruption of the Annexin-V Anticoagulant Shield
Annexin-V (placental anticoagulant protein-I, vascular anticoagulant α) has potent anticoagulant properties in vitro that are based on its high affinity for anionic phospholipids and its capacity to displace coagulation factors from phospholipid surfaces.[70] Thus far, more than 20 annexin proteins have been identified in both animal and plant cells.[71,72] These are very similar in structure, with most of the members consisting of 4 highly homologous cassette domains of about 70 amino acids each. The uniqueness of each of the proteins is believed to reside in the structure of its amino-terminal sequences.

Annexin-V significantly prolongs phospholipid-dependent coagulation reactions by forming two-dimensional clusters that displace coagulation proteins from phospholipid surfaces.[70] This clustering property is likely to be of functional importance, since it permits the formation of a protective shield of annexin-V over the phospholipid surface, blocking the phospholipids from availability for coagulation reactions.

There is evidence to suggest that annexin-V plays an antithrombotic role in physiologic conditions. Phosphatidyl serine is present on the apical membranes of syncytialized trophoblasts, where it is covered by a binding layer of annexin-V.[73–75] Treatment of a pregnant animal model with anti–annexin-V antibodies results in placental necrosis, fibrosis, and pregnancy loss.[76] Dissociation of annexin-V from the surface of human placental trophoblasts and human umbilical vein endothelial cells accelerates the coagulation of plasma exposed to those cells.[77] Thus, annexin-V may play a thrombomodulatory role on the surfaces of cells lining the placental and systemic vasculatures.

aPL antibodies may promote thrombosis by displacing annexin-V from phospholipid membrane surfaces.[78] There is a marked reduction of annexin-V on the apical membranes of human placentas of women

TABLE 128-1   MECHANISMS PROPOSED FOR THE APL SYNDROME

Disruption of annexin-V shield
Altered eicosanoid synthesis
Injury to endothelium
Induction of receptors for cell adhesion molecules on endothelium
Increase of endothelin-1
Induction of tissue factor expression on monocytes and on endothelial cells
Induction of apoptosis
Interference with protein C pathway
 aPL binding to proteins C and S
 Inhibition of activation of protein C
 Acquired activated protein C resistance
Inhibition of heparin—antithrombin III complexes
Crossreactivity to oxidized low-density lipoprotein
Increase of plasminogen activator inhibitor 1
Impairment of autoactivation of factor XII and reduced fibrinolysis
Platelet activation

with aPL antibodies as compared to placentas of women with uncomplicated term deliveries, non-aPL-related pregnancy losses and elective pregnancy-terminations.[79,80] Moreover, IgG fractions from aPL syndrome patients reduce the quantity of annexin-V on cultured trophoblasts and endothelial cells and also accelerate the coagulation of plasma exposed to these cells.[77] Similarly, a monoclonal antiphosphatidyl serine antibody reduces the level of annexin-V on a syncytialized trophoblast cell line and increases the binding of prothrombin to these cells.[75]

While the displacement of annexin-V occurs via aPL antibodies, some investigators have identified patients with antibodies that recognize annexin-V directly.[81,82] Anti–annexin-V antibodies from patients with the aPL syndrome can induce apoptosis in cultured human umbilical vein endothelial cells.[83]

Effects of aPL Antibodies on Platelets and on Eicosanoid Metabolism Some investigators have demonstrated that aPL antibodies stimulate platelet aggregation.[84,85] Also, circulating activated (CD62-positive) platelets were detected by flow cytometry in the majority of primary aPL syndrome patients with neurological disease, suggesting the existence of a relationship among activated platelet, aCL, and the neurological disorders.[86]

aPL antibodies may alter the balance of eicosanoid synthesis toward prothrombotic moieties as indicated by the presence of an increased quantity of thromboxane metabolites in the urine of aPL patients compared to controls.[87,88] However, other studies have not found aPL antibodies to affect eicosanoid metabolism.[89,90]

Effects of aPL Antibodies on Vascular Endothelial Cells aPL antibodies have been found to recognize, injure, and/or activate cultured vascular endothelial cells.[91–94] Cultured endothelial cells incubated with aPL express increased levels of cell adhesion molecules,[95] an effect that may be mediated by β_2GPI[96] and may increase the adhesion of leukocytes to the vascular wall and promote inflammation and thrombosis. Not all studies have been able, however, to demonstrate such an effect.[97] It has also been demonstrated that incubation of cultured endothelial cells with aPL results in the increased expression of tissue factor.[98,99] Significantly increased plasma levels of endothelin-1, which is thought to play a role in arterial tone, vasospasm, and thrombotic arterial occlusion, were found in aPL syndrome patients with arterial thrombosis.[100] Human monoclonal aCL-induced preproendothelin-1 mRNA levels significantly more than control monoclonal antibody.

Immune Complexes The IgG$_2$ subtype of aPL is most closely associated with thrombosis[95]; it has therefore been postulated that complement-fixation plays an important role in aPL-mediated thrombosis. High-titer anticardiolipin IgG antibodies have been shown to bind complement C5b-9, as demonstrated by a monoclonal antibody.[101] Also, it has been found that the concentration and avidity of aPL antibodies were higher in fractions which were enriched for circulating immune complexes.[102]

Induction of Tissue Factor Activity by Leukocytes In addition to the expression of tissue factor by cultured endothelial cells mentioned above,[98] aPL antibodies have also been reported to promote tissue factor synthesis by leukocytes.[103] In one study, the ability of IgG to stimulate monocyte tissue factor expression was associated with the presence of decreased free protein S and increased prothrombotic markers.[104]

Interference with the Components of the Protein C Pathway The protein C pathway, one of the important endogenous antithrombotic mechanisms (see Chap. 113), is initiated when thrombin binds to thrombomodulin on endothelial cells. This binding modifies the substrate specificity of thrombin; the enzyme loses its procoagulant specificities and cleaves protein C to activated protein C (APC). In the presence of the free form of protein S, APC proteolyzes coagulation factors Va and VIIIa. aPL antibodies can interfere with the protein C system by: (1) inhibiting the formation of thrombin; (2) decreasing the activation of protein C by the thrombomodulin-thrombin complex; (3) inhibiting the assembly of the protein C complex; (4) inhibiting the activity of protein C, directly or via its cofactor protein S, and (5) binding to factors Va and VIIIa in a manner that protects them from proteolysis by APC.[105] In addition, patients with aPL syndrome have been found to have protein S deficiency.[106,107]

Inhibition of the Antithrombin-III Pathway Antithrombin-III is a member of the serine protease inhibitors family. Individuals with inherited deficiencies of antithrombin III are at increased risk for deep vein thrombosis (see Chap. 127). The antithrombotic activity of this protein is markedly accelerated by the presence of heparin. In vivo, heparan sulfate proteoglycans may exert a thrombomodulatory effect. It has been demonstrated that at least some aPL antibodies cross-react with heparin and heparinoid molecules (which are highly polyanionic) and inhibit the acceleration of antithrombin-III activity.[60]

Additional Effects aPL antibodies may show cross-reactivity against oxidized-LDL[63,64,66] and may thereby be associated with an increased risk of atherosclerosis.[108] Also, it has been suggested that fibrinolysis may be impaired in the aPL syndrome, since females with the disorder have been described to have elevated plasminogen activator inhibitor 1 (PAI-1) levels.[106] Fibrinolysis may also be impaired via anti-β_2GPI-mediated inhibition of the autoactivation of factor XII[109] and the ensuing reductions of kallikrein and urokinase.

Although aPL antibodies are unquestionably associated with thrombosis, it is also clear that there are a significant number of individuals with positive aPL screening tests who are asymptomatic. At present, it is not possible to distinguish those asymptomatic individuals who are at increased risk for future thromboembolic events and pregnancy losses (pre-aPL syndrome) from false positives (Fig. 128-2). The current available data from animal models support a causal role for the antibodies in the development of thrombosis. However, it remains possible that the primary pathogenic process might be the exposure of thrombogenic anionic phospholipids through some other process and that the development of aPL could be the effect of autoimmune reactivity to anionic phospholipids in susceptible individuals. For example, the surfaces of apoptotic cells promote procoagulant activity,[110] and aPL antibodies have been shown to bind to phospholipid exposed by apoptotic thymocytes.[31] Thus, it is possible that aPL antibodies may be both an effect and a cause of thrombosis. Anionic phospholipids, exposed during blood clotting, could trigger immunological recognition and formation of aPL antibodies which could then promote a vicious cycle through their thrombogenic properties. Finally, it is still possible that the aPL could be an epiphenomenon or a surrogate marker and not directly involved in the cause-effect relationships of this disease process.

CLINICAL FEATURES

Patients generally present with thrombotic manifestations-i.e., evidence for vaso-occlusion or end-organ ischemia or infarction—and/or pregnancy losses and complications. The usual age of patients at the time of presentation with thrombosis is about 35 to 45,[111] with the disease rarely presenting past the age of 60.[112] Men and women are equally susceptible.[111] The thrombotic manifestations may occur in the setting of a concurrent autoimmune condition such as SLE (secondary aPL syndrome) or as an independent autoimmune disorder (primary aPL syndrome). No differences have been observed between the arterial and venous distributions of thromboses of primary and secondary aPL patients.[113]

TABLE 128-2　CLINICAL MANIFESTATIONS OF THE APL SYNDROME

Venous and arterial thromboembolism
Pregnancy losses and complications
Thrombocytopenia
Stroke
Livedo reticularis, necrotizing skin vasculitis
Coronary artery disease
Valvular heart disease
Pulmonary hypertention, acute respiratory distress syndrome
Atherosclerosis and peripheral artery disease
Retinal disease
Adrenal failure, hemorrhagic adrenal infarction
Gastrointestinal manifestations: Budd-Chiari syndrome, mesenteric and portal vein obstructions, hepatic infarction, esophageal necrosis, gastric and colonic ulceration, gall bladder necrosis.
Catastrophic aPL syndrome with microangiopathy

SYSTEMIC VASCULAR THROMBOSIS

Patients may present with spontaneous venous and/or arterial thrombosis or embolism which may involve any site in the vasculature. The syndrome should be especially suspected when unusual sites are involved or when a patient experiences recurrent thromboses with no other cause.[114] Nevertheless, most patients will present with deep vein thrombosis of the lower extremities, similar to most patients with venous thromboembolism and to patients with other thrombophilias.[115] In one study of patients with radiologic evidence of thrombosis, 59 percent had thrombi limited to the venous circulation, 28 percent had solely arterial thromboses, and 13 percent had both types of events.[114] Deep vein thrombosis of the legs was the most common finding, occurring in about half of the patients; other sites of venous thrombotic events included pulmonary embolism, thoracic veins (superior vena cava, subclavian vein, or jugular vein), and abdominal or pelvic veins.[114] Patients may also present with stroke, cerebral venous infarction, upper extremity venous thrombosis,[115] myocardial infarction, adrenal infarction, acalculous gall bladder infarction, aortic thrombosis with renal infarction,[116] and mesenteric artery thrombosis.[117]

Thrombosis may occur spontaneously or in the presence of a predisposing factor such as estrogen hormone replacement therapy, oral contraceptives,[113,118] vascular stasis, surgery, or trauma. Women are at particularly high risk for venous thrombosis during pregnancy and in the postpartum period.[113] Some patients with venous thrombosis—but generally not with arterial thrombosis[119]—will also have concurrent genetic thrombophilic conditions such as heterozygosity for the factor V Leiden polymorphism.[119–122] Having a history for a previous thromboembolic event is a major risk factor for future thromboembolism. The risk of recurrence doubles to about 30 percent in patients with a first episode of venous thromboembolism who also have aCL antibodies.[123] The risk of recurrence correlates with the titer of antibodies.[123]

A 4-year prospective study of 360 patients with aPL antibodies reported that previous thrombosis and aCL titer higher than 40 U are independent predictors of thrombosis.[124] Remarkably, other than thrombosis, hematological malignancies including non-Hodgkin lymphoma were the major causes of death in this group of patients.

LUPUS AND OTHER AUTOIMMUNE CONDITIONS

The aPL syndrome is classified within the category of autoimmune disorders. Patients may have concurrent features of other autoimmune conditions such as SLE. About 30 to 40 percent of SLE patients have elevated aPL antibodies. In one study of 47 patients with SLE and aPL antibodies who were diagnosed for the aPL syndrome, about half had thrombosis, about half had thrombocytopenia, and about 40 percent

had neuropsychiatric manifestations, consisting mainly of cerebrovascular ischemic disease.[125] Immune thrombocytopenia is probably the most common concurrent condition in patients with the aPL syndrome. aPL syndrome has also been associated with myasthenia gravis,[126] Budd-Chiari syndrome in the setting of SLE,[127] Graves' disease,[128] autoimmune hemolytic anemia, progressive systemic sclerosis,[129] Evan's syndrome,[130] and secondary Sjogren's syndrome in the presence of SLE.[131] There does not appear to be a direct association between relapsing polychondritis and the aPL syndrome.[132] Rather, the elevated aPL antibodies in patients with this disorder appear to occur in patients who also have SLE. Although patients with vaso-occlusive disease and aPL antibodies generally have thrombosis,[133] elevated aPL antibodies have also been observed in vasculitis. aCL antibodies are present early in the course of giant cell arteritis and disappear within a few weeks of initiation of corticosteroid therapy.[134] Takayasu arteritis[135] and polyarteritis nodosa[136] have also been associated with the aPL syndrome.

STROKE AND OTHER NEUROLOGIC CONDITIONS

Prospective analysis for the presence of aPL antibodies in stroke patients in the AntiPhospholipid Antibody Stroke Study (APASS) demonstrated that elevated levels of anticardiolipin antibodies are associated with increased risk for developing stroke but not with subsequent thromboembolic events.[137] The aPL syndrome should be suspected in young patients with transient ischemic attacks or stroke, particularly when the usual risk factors for cerebrovascular disease are absent.[138] aPL-associated stroke has also been reported with other medical conditions such as Crohn's disease[139] and liver transplantation.[140] Most aPL patients presenting with stroke appear to have arterial thromboembolic strokes that are clinically indistinguishable from general patients with arteriosclerotic strokes; however, a significant proportion of patients have cerebral venous infarction.[141] aPL antibodies may be an important factor contributing to development of cerebral venous thrombosis even in the presence of other potential etiologies or risk factors. The onset of cerebral venous thrombosis in the presence of aPL antibodies occurs at a relatively young age and with relatively more extensive involvement of the superficial and deep cerebral venous system.[141] In one series of 40 cases of cerebral venous thrombosis, three patients (8 percent) had elevated aPL antibodies, and two of these three also had factor V Leiden mutation.[142] Superior sagittal sinus thrombosis has been associated with the primary aPL syndrome.[143]

Additional neurologic abnormalities which have been associated with aPL antibodies include seizures, chorea, migraines, Guillain-Burrè syndrome, transient global amnesia, dementia, diabetic peripheral neuropathy, and orthostatic hypotention.[144] Recurrent acute transverse myelopathy has been described with aPL syndrome[145–149]; however, in one study of 315 SLE patients, including 10 with a history of transverse myelopathy, the disorder was not associated with aPL antibodies.[150] There is a high incidence of elevated aCL antibodies in patients with multiple sclerosis (in one series 9 percent had IgG antibodies and 44 percent had IgM antibodies).[151] However, no clinical distinction has been observed betwen aPL-positive and aPL-negative multiple sclerosis patients. An increased prevalence of LA and aCL antibodies in psychotic patients, even in the absence of taking chlorpromazine or other antipsychotic drugs, has been reported.[152] In this study, 32 percent (11/34) of the unmedicated psychotic patients had laboratory evidence for aPL antibodies.[152]

CATASTROPHIC APL SYNDROME

Rarely, patients present with a *catastrophic* form of the aPL syndrome, which is characterized by severe widespread vascular occlusions, sometimes leading to death. These patients present with evidence for severe multiorgan ischemia/infarction, usually with concurrent microvascular thrombosis. Patients with catastrophic aPL syndrome can present with massive venous thromboembolism, along with respiratory failure, stroke, abnormal liver enzymes, renal impairment, adrenal insufficiency and areas of cutaneous infarction. The respiratory failure is usually due to acute respiratory distress syndrome and diffuse alveolar hemorrhage. Laboratory evidence for disseminated intravascular coagulation is frequently present. A review of 50 patients with catastrophic aPL syndrome[153] showed that two-thirds were females, with a mean age in the late thirties, but ranging from childhood to old age. Most had primary aPL syndrome, while the minority had SLE and other autoimmune conditions including Sjogren syndrome, scleroderma and rheumatoid arthritis. Precipitating factors were thought to contribute to the development of catastrophic aPL syndrome in some of the patients. These included infections, drugs (sulfur-containing diuretics, captopril, and oral contraceptives), surgical procedures, and cessation of prior anticoagulant therapy. The patients usually presented with multiple organ failure developing over a very short period of time. Most patients manifested evidence of microangiopathy affecting predominantly small vessels of the kidney, lungs, brain, heart, and liver. Only a minority of patients experienced large-vessel occlusions. Death occurred in about half of the patients.

PREGNANCY LOSSES, OBSTETRICAL COMPLICATIONS, AND INFERTILITY

For a comprehensive review, the reader is referred to Lockwood and Rand.[154] Most studies have estimated the prevalence of aPL antibodies among general obstetric populations at about 5 percent or less; most of these patients are not clinically affected.[155] Among obstetrical patients with recurrent fetal losses, about 16 to 38 percent of patients are found to have aPL antibodies.

Female patients with the aPL syndrome often present with a history of recurrent (usually defined as three or more) pregnancy losses. Pregnancies occurring in women with aPL antibodies are at significantly increased risk of miscarriage, prematurity, intrauterine growth retardation, and preeclampsia.[156] Although pregnancy losses occurring in the middle trimester or later in pregnancy—even stillbirth—are most striking, it has been estimated that approximately half of the patients with this condition experience first-trimester losses. Pregnant patients with the aPL syndrome are also more prone to develop deep vein thrombosis during pregnancy or the puerperium. Rarely, pregnant patients develop the catastrophic form of the aPL syndrome, described above.[157,158] The best predictor for pregnancy loss in a patient testing positive for aPL antibodies is not the degree of laboratory abnormality but whether the patient has a history of previous pregnancy loss or thrombosis.[124,159]

There is evidence for increased activation of coagulation mechanisms in pregnant women with the aPL syndrome. Prothrombin activation fragment F1.2, a marker for thrombin generation, is increased in pregnant patients with aPL antibodies and a previous history of pregnancy losses, compared to control healthy non-aPL pregnant women.[160] Histologic abnormalities were found in many, but not all, placentas of aPL patients. One study did not define a morphologic lesion specific for the aPL syndrome but did describe a higher frequency of decreased vasculo-syncytial membranes, the presence of villous fibrosis, hypovascular villi, increased syncytial knots, and evidence of thrombosis or infarction.[161] Studies of placental pathology in patients with aPL antibodies but without a prior history of fetal loss showed that about half had uteroplacental vascular pathology, about half had evidence of thrombotic occlusion, and about one-third had chronic villitis and/or decidual plasma cell infiltrates.[162,163]

The thrombotic occlusions and vascular pathology may be due to the marked decrease of the placental anticoagulant protein annexin-V which has been described on the apical membranes of aPL placental syncytiotrophoblasts.[79] It has been proposed that the reduction of this protein, which normally lines the interface between the maternal and fetal circulations, may disrupt a constitutive antithrombotic mechanism within the intervillous blood circulation.[74,76] This would accelerate coagulation within the maternal side of the maternal-fetal interface.

There is controversy about whether aPL syndrome is a cause of reproductive failure (i.e., infertility) in patients undergoing in vitro fertilization (IVF). In one study of women undergoing this procedure, aPL antibodies were detected in 22 percent of women with implantation failure compared with 5 percent of controls.[164] It was noted that most of these antibodies reacted with phospholipids other than cardiolipin. Nevertheless, other investigators are not convinced that aPL antibodies play a role in infertility and IVF-failure.[165,166]

BLEEDING

A minority of patients with the aPL syndrome exhibit a bleeding tendency. In these patients, the presence of a concurrent coagulopathy needs to be excluded. Severe bleeding due to acquired hypoprothrombinemia has been reported.[167,168] This diagnosis may be missed when coagulation abnormalities are attributed only to the LA effect, and thus a specific assay for prothrombin should be performed when the prothrombin time is prolonged. Other associated bleeding causes in the aPL syndrome include acquired thrombocytopathies, thrombocytopenia (usually immune-mediated), and acquired inhibitors against specific coagulation factors, e.g., factor VIII.

CUTANEOUS MANIFESTATIONS

Cutaneous manifestations may occur as the first sign of aPL syndrome.[169] Noninflammatory vascular thrombosis is the most frequent histopathologic feature observed. These include livedo reticularis (occasionally, a necrosing form[170]), necrotizing vasculitis, livedoid vasculitis, thrombophlebitis, cutaneous ulceration and necrosis, erythematous macules, purpura, ecchymoses, painful skin nodules, and subungual splinter hemorrhages. Rarely, the aPL syndrome may also be associated with anetoderma (macular atrophy), discoid lupus erythematosus, cutaneous T-cell lymphoma, or disorders that closely resemble Sneddon or Degos syndromes. Patients with systemic sclerosis who are aCL-positive have more widespread skin and visceral involvement than those who are aCL-negative with this disorder.[171]

CORONARY ARTERY DISEASE

aPL antibodies have been associated with increased susceptibility to coronary artery disease—particularly premature atherosclerosis.[172] Antiprothrombin antibodies were reported to be a predictor of myocardial infarction in middle-aged men, and one study found that the joint effect of antiprothrombin antibodies with other known risk factors were multiplicative.[173] Coronary artery disease also appears to be associated with antibodies against oxidized LDL. The aPL sydrome should be considered in patients who lack the usual risk factors for coronary artery disease or who have evidence for thrombotic or embolic coronary occlusion without angiographic evidence of atherosclerotic disease. aPL antibodies also appear to be a risk factor for restenosis after percutaneous transluminal coronary angioplasty, where restenosis with recurrent ischaemia appears to occur earlier and more frequently.[174,175]

VALVULAR HEART DISEASE

Approximately 35 percent of patients with primary aPL syndrome have valvular abnormalities detected by echocardiography.[176] Also, about 20 percent of cardiac patients with valvular heart disease have evidence for aPL antibodies compared with about 10 percent of matched control subjects.[177] Valvular abnormalities occur in about half of patients with SLE and aPL antibodies. Valvulopathy includes leaflet thickening, vegetations, regurgitation, and stenosis.[178] The aPL syndrome valvular lesion consists mainly of superficial or intravalvular fibrin deposits in association with variable degrees of vascular proliferation, fibroblast influx, fibrosis, and calcification. This results in valve thickening, fusion, and rigidity, sometimes leading to functional abnormalities. Inflammation is not a prominent feature of this lesion.[179] Deposits of immunoglobulins including aCL antibodies, and of complement components, are common in the affected valves of patients with primary and secondary aPL syndrome.[180] One study of patients with SLE, progressive systemic sclerosis, rheumatoid arthritis, and primary aPL syndrome, however, did not find a relationship between increased aCL antibodies and valvular abnormalities.[181]

PERIPHERAL VASCULAR DISEASE

One prospective study found that about one-third of patients with peripheral arterial disease undergoing bypass grafting procedures had elevated aPL antibody levels (mostly aCL antibodies). Although these patients did not appear to be at increased risk for reocclusion, this may have been due to the higher frequency of anticoagulant therapy given in these patients.[182] An unusual pattern of premature aortoiliac atherosclerosis has been reported in women under the age of 50, which appears to be associated with the presence of aPL antibodies in about 40 percent of the patients. Intraarterial thromboembolic events are common at presentation and complicate surgical management.[183]

PULMONARY MANIFESTATIONS

In addition to pulmonary thromboembolism, patients with the aPL syndrome may present with in situ thrombosis in pulmonary vessels. aPL antibodies have been described in pulmonary hypertension.[184–186] In one prospective trial of 38 consecutive patients with precapillary pulmonary hypertension, about 30 percent had aPL antibodies with various phospholipid specificities.[185] aPL antibody syndrome has been diagnosed in patients presenting with refractory noninflammatory pulmonary vasculopathy.[187,188] The majority of patients with catastrophic aPL syndrome have dyspnea, and most of these individuals have acute respiratory distress syndrome.[153]

GASTROINTESTINAL MANIFESTATIONS

Gastrointestinal manifestations of aPL syndrome include Budd-Chiari syndrome, hepatic infarction, esophageal necrosis with perforation, intestinal ischemia and infarction, pancreatitis, and colonic ulceration. Also, primary biliary cirrhosis,[189] acute acalculous cholecystitis with gall bladder necrosis,[190,191] and giant gastric ulceration have been associated with aPL antibody syndrome.[192] There have been case reports of the primary aPL syndrome associated with mesenteric inflammatory venoocclusive disease,[193] and with mesenteric and portal venous obstruction.[194]

THROMBOCYTOPENIA

About 20 to 40 percent of patients with the aPL syndrome have varying degrees of thrombocytopenia. This is usually mild or moderate and is rarely significant enough to cause bleeding complications or to affect anticoagulant therapy.[195,196] Most cases appear to be immune-mediated. It is not yet clear whether aPL antibodies themselves can directly reduce platelet counts or whether these reflect a common autoimmune background but are mediated by different antibody populations. Antibodies directed against major platelet membrane glycoproteins may play a role in the thrombocytopenia. The majority of patients with the aPL syndrome and thrombocytopenia have antibodies against glycoprotein (GP) IIb/IIIa complex and/or GP Ib/IX complex according to one study.[197] However, in another study no correlation was found between the presence of antibodies against platelet GPIIb/IIIa, GPIb/IX, and thrombocytopenia, and the eluted platelet antibodies did not have any LA activity.[198] It thus appears that platelet antibodies may represent an independent marker for autoimmunity in these patients. Conversely, aPL antibodies and antibodies against platelet membrane glycoprotein were present simultaneously in about 70 percent of patients with immune-mediated thrombocytopenia.[199]

RETINAL ABNORMALITIES

The diagnosis of aPL antibody retinopathy should be suspected in patients with diffuse retinal vasoocclusion, particularly when characterized by involvement of both arteries and veins, neovascularization at presentation, and symptoms of systemic rheumatologic disease.[200] aPL antibodies were present in 5 to 33 percent of patients with retinal vein occlusion.[201,202] Cilioretinal artery occlusion[203] and optic neuropathy[204] have also been described with the aPL syndrome.

LIVER DISEASES

aPL antibodies are frequently elevated in patients with chronic liver disease of various causes. In one prospective study of patients with liver disease, about half of patients with alcoholic liver disease and one-third of patients with chronic hepatitis C virus hepatitis had elevated aPL antibodies; the frequency was even higher in patients with more severe cirrhosis.[205] In another study, aCL antibodies were found in 22 percent of patients with chronic hepatitis C.[26] Since hepatitis C infection has been associated with other autoimmune disorders such as rheumatoid arthritis, SLE, polymyositis, and thyroid disease,[206] it is possible that the the aPL antibodies in this condition may also be autoimmune in origin.

"SERONEGATIVE" APL SYNDROME

Some patients present with the clinical picture of this syndrome but without laboratory evidence of aPL in their serum at the time of initial presentation and are found to develop laboratory evidence for the antibodies several months later.[207]

APL AND AIDS

While patients with HIV-1 infection frequently have elevated aPL antibodies, they rarely have thrombotic manifestations. In one series, 64 percent of HIV-1 patients had elevated aCL antibodies.[208] However, most of these positive patients also had antibodies against phosphatidyl choline, and very few had antibodies to β_2GPI, antiprothrombin antibodies, LA, biological false positive test for syphilis, or thrombosis.[208]

APL SYNDROME IN CHILDREN

aPL syndrome has been reported among pediatric patients in whom diverse clinical features are common as in adults.[184] aPL-related thrombosis seems to constitute a significant proportion of childhood thromboses. About one-third of children suffering a thrombotic event have circulating aPL antibodies, and more than two-thirds of children with idiopathic cerebral ischemia have evidence for elevated aPL antibodies.[209] One study reported a high prevalence of aCL antibodies in children (7/10) who suffered acute cerebral infarction.[210] Also, a variety of neurological disorders, including migraine, benign intracranial hypertension, or unilateral movement disorders such as hemichorea and hemidystonia other than stroke have been associated with aPL antibodies in childhood.[211] The catastrophic form of the syndrome is rare in children.[212]

OTHER MANIFESTATIONS

Acute adrenal failure secondary to bilateral infarction of the adrenal glands has been reported as the first manifestation of primary aPL syndrome.[213] Adrenal hemorrhage has also been reported.[214–216] aPL antibodies has also been associated with bone marrow necrosis.[217] Sudden acute sensorineural hearing loss in patients with systemic lupus erythematosus or lupus-like syndromes may be a manifestation of the aPL syndrome.[218]

LABORATORY FEATURES

INTRODUCTION

The diagnosis of the aPL syndrome requires the presence of antibodies against phospholipids and/or relevant protein cofactors. This is most commonly obtained through immunoassays that detect aCL, antiphosphatidyl serine, anti-β_2GPI, or antiprothrombin antibodies or through evidence for interference with phospholipid-dependent coagulation assays (lupus anticoagulant phenomenon) (Table 128-3). Definitive guidelines and criteria for laboratory testing are not yet available, and thus the laboratory diagnosis of the aPL syndrome is frequently problematic. At present, no single test is sufficient for diagnosing this disorder. It is therefore recommended that when the disorder is suspected, a panel of tests, including syphilis testing, antibodies against cardiolipin, phosphatidyl serine, and β_2GPI and coagulation tests for lupus anticoagulant, should be performed.

IMMUNOASSAYS

ANTIPHOSPHOLIPID ANTIBODY AND COFACTOR ASSAYS
Most patients with the condition are identified by elevated levels of aCL antibodies. The precursor of this assay, the biologic false-positive VDRL test for syphilis, in which cardiolipin is the primary antigen, is itself a crude aPL test. High levels of aCL antibodies are predictive

TABLE 128-3   DIAGNOSTIC TESTS FOR THE APL SYNDROME

Immunoassays
Serologic test for syphilis ("biologic false positive")
Anticardiolipin antibodies
Antiphosphatidyl serine antibodies
Anti-β_2GPI antibodies
Antiprothrombin antibodies
Coagulation tests
aPTT with mixing incubation studies, aPL-sensitive and insensitive reagents
    and platelet neutralization procedure
Dilute Russell viper venom time
Kaolin clotting time
Tissue thromboplastin inhibition test
Hexagonal phase array test
Textarin/ecarin test

for an increased risk of thrombosis. During a 10-year follow-up on patients who presented with raised levels of aCL antibodies, about 50 percent of patients who presented with elevated antibodies but without clinical manifestations of the syndrome, went on to develop the syndrome.[219] Also, the presence of elevated titers of anticardiolipin antibodies 6 months after an episode of venous thromboembolism is a predictor for an increased risk of recurrence and of death.[123] Women with IgM antibodies, IgG aCL antibodies lower than 20 IgG binding units, and without a LA do not appear to be at risk for aPL-syndrome.[220] In contrast, women with an IgG aCL titer greater than 20 binding units or a positive LA were found to be more likely to develop complications.[220]

As mentioned previously, most patients with elevated aCL antibodies do not have the aPL syndrome. The prevalence of positive tests in the asymptomatic "normal" population has generally ranged from about 3 to 10 percent. In a prospective study of 2132 consecutive Spanish patients with venous thromboembolism, 4.1 percent were found to have elevated aCL antibodies (i.e., about the same prevalence as in the asymptomatic healthy population).[221] It should be borne in mind, however, that many individuals have antibodies which are elevated in response to microbial infections and are not associated with thrombotic complications. Patients with syphilis, Lyme disease, and other infections may be misdiagnosed for the aPL syndrome on the basis of elevated aCL antibodies when concurrent stroke or arterial thrombosis are present, and these must always be ruled out in susceptible patients. Also, the aCL ELISA test will be artifactually abnormal in patients with hypergammaglobulinemias unless the results of parallel assays, done on microtiterplates that are not coated with cardiolipin, are subtracted.[222]

aPL syndrome has been described primarily with elevated aCL IgG antibodies but also occurs with elevated IgM antibodies. aCL antibody isotype distributions may vary in different ethnic groups.[223] While all four IgG subclasses are found in autoimmune aCL, the presence of IgG$_2$ is significantly associated with thrombotic complications.[224] There is controversy about whether a polymorphism in the Fc gamma receptor IIA expressed on platelets, monocytes, and endothelial cells efficiently recognizing IgG$_2$ may be a genetic marker for the aPL syndrome.[225,226]

There have been some reports of patients with elevated IgA aCL antibodies with aPL syndrome. However, the determination of IgA aCL antibodies does not appear to be helpful in diagnosing the aPL syndrome or in explaining thrombotic events or fetal loss since the prevalence of true positivity to IgA anticardiolipin antibodies is extremely low; for example in one study of 795 patients, IgA aPL were found in only two patients, both of whom were also positive to IgG aPL.[227]

About 20 percent of patients taking procainamide have moderate to high levels of aCL antibodies.[228] In these patients, the antibodies are associated with anti-β_2GPI specificity. However, the predictive significance of procainamide-induced aPL is not known. Treatment with chlorpromazine is frequently associated with the development of aCL antibodies; these are rarely associated with thrombosis,[229] and it is not clear whether these are cofactor dependent.

ANTIPHOSPHATIDYL SERINE ANTIBODY ASSAY
Since cardiolipin is present in intracellular membranes and does not become exposed to coagulation proteins in vivo, it was hypothesized that tests for antibodies against phosphatidyl serine, which is normally present in the inner leaflet of the plasma membrane, may be more relevant pathophysiologically. Phosphatidyl serine is also exposed on syncytialized cells, on apoptotic cells and on activated platelets. Antibodies to phosphatidyl serine (aPS) appear to correlate more specifically with aPL syndrome than aCL antibodies.[230–233]

ASSAYS FOR ANTIBODIES AGAINST OTHER PHOSPHOLIPIDS

Antibodies against the zwitterionic phospholipid, phosphatidyl ethanolamine, have been associated with thrombosis and with activated protein C resistance.[234] Some studies have suggested that antiphosphatidyl ethanolamine antibodies can occur in the aPL syndrome in the absence of antibodies against cardiolipin or other anionic phospholipids.[235] Some investigators have advocated testing for antibodies against a panel of phospholipids other than cardiolipin,[235-238] while others have disagreed,[239] and one group recommends that a mixture of anionic and zwitterionic phospholipids be used for testing for antibodies.[240]

ANTI-β_2GPI ANTIBODY ASSAY

β_2GPI is believed to be the major protein cofactor for the aPL antibodies. ELISAs for anti-β_2GPI antibodies are considered to be more specific but less sensitive for the aPL syndrome than aCL assays.[241] While these antibodies are usually seen in patients with abnormal aCL and aPS antibodies, some patients with the aPL syndrome, whether primary or secondary, may present with antibodies to β_2GPI but without antibodies detectable in standard aPL assays.[242,243] Despite their higher specificity for the aPL syndrome (98 percent) and high positive predictive value (about 90 percent), β_2GPI antibodies cannot be relied upon alone for the diagnosis because of their low sensitivity (40 to 50 percent).[244,245] Concurrent testing for aCL and aPS antibodies and LA is therefore advised. The presence of elevated levels of anti-β_2GPI antibodies correlates well with thrombosis. In one study, elevated levels of antibodies against β_2GPI were found in 49 percent of a group of SLE patients and were significantly associated with deep venous thrombosis. Testing of antibodies against β_2GPI and prothrombin seem to be clinically useful for evaluating the risk of thrombosis.[246]

ANTIPROTHROMBIN ANTIBODY ASSAY

Prothrombin is the second major cofactor for aPL antibodies. Antiprothrombin antibodies occur in 30 percent of patients with SLE and have been significantly associated with thrombosis.[246-248] The presence of these antibodies also correlates with hypoprothrombinemia and with thrombocytopenia.[249]

COAGULATION TESTS

LUPUS ANTICOAGULANTS

One of the most perplexing features of the aPL syndrome is the frequent presence of the LA phenomenon in vitro.[250,251] Although commonly used, the term *LA* is a misnomer, since it is not restricted to patients with systemic lupus erythematosus. LAs appear to act by limiting the quantity of phospholipid available to support coagulation reactions (listed in Table 128-4), thus prolonging the coagulation times. A number of different methods have been devised to detect the LA phenomenon including modifications of the aPTT test with LA-sensitive and -insensitive reagents, the kaolin clotting time, the dilute Russell viper venom time (*dRVVT*), the tissue thromboplastin inhibition time, the hexagonal phase array test, and the platelet neutralization procedure. The common denominator for the various LA tests is that they detect the inhibition of the phospholipid-dependent blood coagulation reactions.[11]

The results of LA tests can be so variable that even specialized laboratories may frequently disagree. For example, three surveys in the United Kingdom have shown that while most laboratories can agree in their identification of plasmas containing strong positive LA activity, there is frequent disagreement about plasmas that are known to have weak LA activity (these are missed in about half the cases) and frequent misdiagnosis of factor-IX-deficient LA-negative plasmas as being LA-positive.[252]

Paradoxically, the presence of the LA activity is more predictive and more specific for the occurrence of thrombosis or pregnancy loss than the aCL ELISA assays,[44,253-256] the anti-β_2GPI assay, or the antiprothrombin assay.[254] The LA appears to be more predictive for venous thromboembolism than aCL antibodies even when only high titers of aCL are considered.[257] Thus, in a meta-analysis of the risk for aPL-associated venous thromboembolism in individuals with aPL antibodies without underlying autoimmune disease or previous thrombosis for a 15-year period, the mean odds ratios were: for aCL antibodies-1.6; for high titres of aCL -3.2, and for LA -11.0.[257] The presence of LA also appears to be a significant risk factor for arterial thrombosis.[256,258]

In addition to their role in immunoassays for aPL antibodies, protein cofactors also play a role in the LA activity.[8,259] In the case of β_2GPI, the LA activity of anti-β_2GPI antibodies appears to depend on their epitope specificity. Anti-β_2GPI mAbs directed against the third and fourth domains of β_2GPI have a LA effect, whereas anti-β_2GPI mAbs directed against the fifth domain and the carboxy-terminal region of the fourth sushi domain show no LA-like activity.[260] While LA can be due to antiprothrombin antibodies, removal of antiprothrombin antibodies does not eliminate LA activity in the majority of plasmas.[8]

It is not clear why the LA, a test for in vitro anticoagulant activity, is the marker which correlates best with in vivo thrombosis in the aPL syndrome. Conceivably, the LA effect "reports" aPL antibody-phospholipid/cofactor complexes having the highest affinities and avidities for the antigens and the most potent ability to displace endogenous phospholipid-binding anticoagulant proteins which shield anionic phospholipids from participating in coagulation reactions.[78] This explanation for the LA phenomenon and a "lupus procoagulant" mechanism has been described in detail by the author.[78] A model is presented in Fig. 128-4.

DILUTE RUSSELL VIPER VENOM TIME

DRVVT is considered to be one of the most sensitive of the LA tests. The test is performed by using Russell viper venom (RVV) in a system containing limiting quantities of diluted rabbit brain phospholipid. The RVV directly activates coagulation factor X, leading to the formation of fibrin clot. LA will prolong the dRVVT by interfering with the assembly of the prothrombinase complex. To ensure that prolongation of the clotting time is not due to a factor deficiency, the method uses mixtures of patient and control plasmas. The presence of the LA may be confirmed by addition of an excess of phospholipid which will correct the prolongation.

APTT TESTS

Prolongation of the aPTT will detect some LAs, and, in the general population, LAs are the most frequent cause of prolonged aPTT tests.[261] The various reagents available for performing aPTTs vary widely in their sensitivity to LAs, and thus it is important to know which reagents are used. The aPTT reflects the contact activation coagulation pathway. When the aPTT of a particular plasma sample is prolonged, and not "correctable" by mixture with normal plasma, the presence of an "anticoagulant" or "inhibitor" should be suspected. The LA needs to be differentiated from inhibitors of specific coagulation factors and from anticoagulants such as heparin. Besides specific assays to exclude the latter two possibilities, the clinician should check whether the aPTT is normalized when an LA-insensitive aPTT reagent is used or

---

TABLE 128-4   PHOSPHOLIPID-DEPENDENT COAGULATION REACTIONS

1. Tissue factor-factor VII (VIIa) mediated activation of factors X and IX
2. Factor IXa and factor VIIIa activation of factor X to factor IXa
3. Factor Xa and factor Va activation of prothrombin to thrombin

when the assay is done using frozen washed platelets as the source of phospholipid—also referred to as the *platelet neutralization procedure*. Also, the effects of incubation with normal plasma may be helpful in differentiating LAs from coagulation factor inhibitors. aPTTs done on mixtures of normal plasma and plasma containing a factor VIII inhibitor may show no prolongation immediately after mixing but marked prolongation with incubation at 37°C, whereas LA-containing plasmas will usually markedly prolong the aPTT immediately after mixing with normal plasmas and show no further prolongation with incubation. However, both types of anticoagulants—LA and specific coagulation factor inhibitors—may coexist in rare patients. Specific coagulation factor inhibitor assays should clarify this issue. It should also be recognized that LAs may result in artifactual decreases in coagulation factor levels using the standard assays, since they are based on aPTT. These patients can be misdiagnosed as having multiple coagulation factor deficiencies. This problem can usually be avoided by using an aPTT reagent which is insensitive to LA for the specific factor assays or by repeating the coagulation factor assays following dilution of the plasma samples. The latter will result in improved coagulation factor levels with progressive dilution.

KAOLIN CLOTTING TIME

This assay depends upon the ability of aPL antibodies to block the availability of trace quantities of phospholipid present in centrifuged plasma from participation in coagulation reactions. Some authors maintain that the kaolin clotting time–LA test reflects dependence on prothrombin as a cofactor and is less likely to be associated with thrombosis than the dRVV test, which appears to be more dependent on β_2GPI.[249,262]

TISSUE THROMBOPLASTIN INHIBITION TEST

This test is a prothrombin time assay done with diluted tissue factor-phospholipid complex. It can be performed with standard and recombinant tissue factor.[263,264] The results are expressed as a ratio of the patient:control clotting times.

HEXAGONAL PHASE ARRAY TEST

aPL antibodies can recognize phosphatidyl ethanolamine in the hexagonal phase array configuration but not in the lamellar phase. The principle of this test is that incubation of plasma with the hexagonal phase phosphatidyl ethanolamine should absorb the LA antibodies, if these are present, and therefore normalize a prolonged aPTT due to LA.

TEXTARIN/ECARIN TEST

This test depends on the different coagulation mechanisms initiated by two snake venoms—Textarin activates prothrombin via a phospholipid

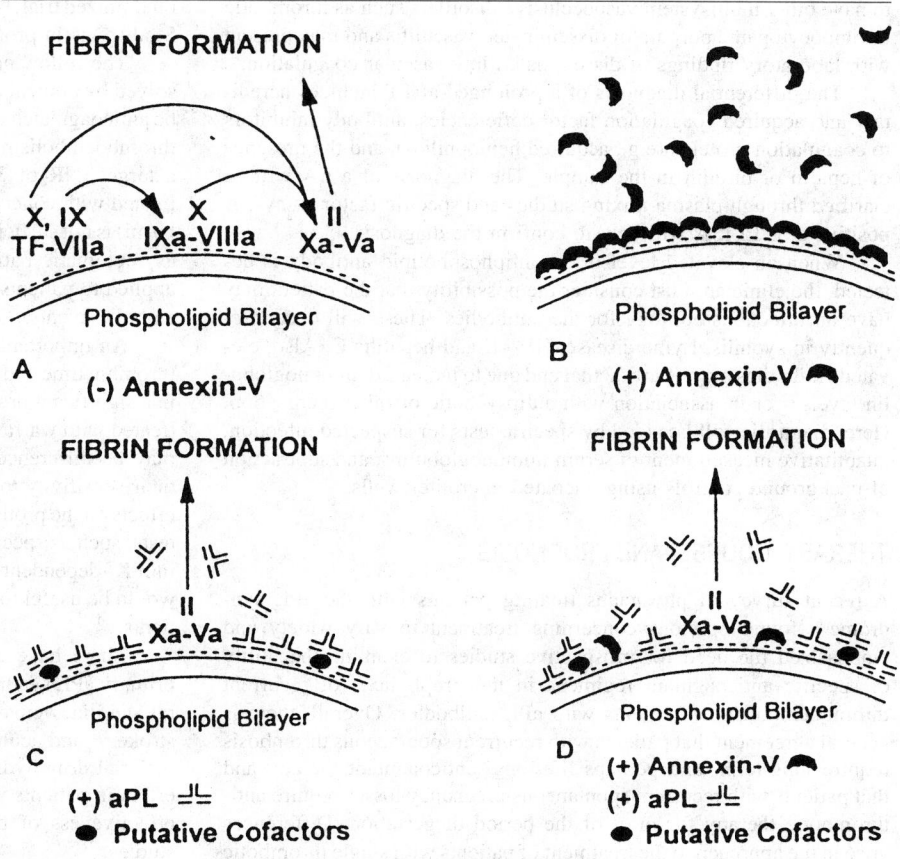

FIGURE 128-4   A model for the mechanisms of the "lupus anticoagulant effect" and for a "lupus procoagulant effect":

(A) Anionic phospholipids (negative charges), when exposed on the apical surface of the cell membrane bilayer, serve as potent cofactors for the assembly of three different coagulation complexes: the tissue factor (TF)-VIIa complex, the IXa-VIIIa complex, and the Xa-Va complex, and thereby accelerate blood coagulation. The TF complexes yield either factor IXa or factor Xa, the IXa complex yields factor Xa, and the Xa formed from both of these reactions is the active enzyme in the prothrombinase complex which yields factor IIa (thrombin), which in turn cleaves fibrinogen to form fibrin.

(B) Annexin-V, in the absence of aPL antibodies, serves as a potent anticoagulant by forming clusters which bind that high affinity to the anionic phospholipid surface and shield the surface from the assembly of the phospholipid-dependent coagulation complexes.

(C) In the absence of annexin-V, aPL antibodies can prolong the coagulation times, compared to control antibodies, by reducing the access of coagulation factors to anionic phospholipids. This may result in a "lupus anticoagulant" effect. Lupus anticoagulant tests can be designed to be sensitive by limiting the quantities of phospholipids.

(D) In the presence of annexin-V, antiphospholipid antibodies, either directly or via interaction with protein-phospholipid cofactors, disrupt the the ability of annexin-V to cluster on the phospholipid surface. This results in a net increase of the amount of anionic phospholipid available for promoting coagulation reactions. The aPL-cofactor complexes expose significantly more phospholipids by disrupting the annexin-V shield than they block by direct binding. This manifests in the net acceleration of coagulation in vitro and in thrombophilia in vivo. (Reprinted with permission from Rand and coworkers.[78])

dependent pathway, and Ecarin activates prothrombin even in the absence of phospholipid.[264]

DIFFERENTIAL DIAGNOSIS

Patients with the aPL syndrome usually present with vascular occlusion, recurrent pregnancy losses, or abnormal coagulation screening tests. When vascular occlusion occurs in the setting of a known autoimmune disorder such as SLE, then the possibility of vasculitis must be considered. Patients with the catastrophic aPL syndrome may appear to have other multisystem vasoocclusive disorders such as thrombotic thrombocytopenic purpura or disseminated vasculitis and may present with laboratory findings of disseminated intravascular coagulation.

The differential diagnosis of a prolonged aPTT includes hereditary and acquired coagulation factor deficiencies, antibody inhibitors to coagulation proteins (e.g., acquired hemophilias), and the presence of heparin or hirudin in the sample. The diagnosis of a LA will be clarified through plasma mixing studies and specific factor assays. A positive aPL ELISA will help to confirm the diagnosis.

When an elevated level of an antiphospholipid antibody is detected, the clinician must consider the possibility that the patient may have an infectious etiology for the antibodies. These will occur frequently in syphilis, Lyme disease, HIV-1, and hepatitis C. Also, elevated antibodies may be artifactual and due to increased immunoglobulin levels[222] or in association with antipsychotic or other medication. Here, diagnosis will be aided by specific tests for suspected infection, quantitative measurement of serum immunoglobulins, and subtraction of background controls using uncoated microtiter wells.

THERAPY, COURSE, AND PROGNOSIS

A recent survey of physicians treating patients with the aPL syndrome[265] found opinions concerning treatment to vary widely and emphasized the need for prospective studies to examine the utility of specific anticoagulant regimens in the prophylaxis of recurrent thromboembolism in patients with aPL antibodies. Overall, there is general agreement that patients with recurrent spontaneous thrombosis require long-term, and perhaps life-long, anticoagulant therapy and that patients with recurrent spontaneous pregnancy losses require antithrombotic therapy for most of the period of gestation. Differences arise in the approach to the treatment of patients with single thrombotic events, with significant thrombotic events in the distant past, and with thrombotic events that were not spontaneous. Opinions also vary widely on the treatment of asymptomatic pregnant women with aPL antibodies, especially if they are in an older age category or have difficulties with fertility.

THROMBOSIS

There is no evidence that the acute treatment for patients presenting with thrombosis in the aPL syndrome should be any different from that of patients with other thrombotic etiologies. For patients treated with intravenous unfractionated heparin, care must be taken to determine whether the patient might have a preexisting LA that can interfere with the aPTT monitoring of heparin levels by aPTT. If so, then the heparin concentration can be estimated with one of the LA-insensitive aPTT reagents, with a specific heparin assay, or with the activated coagulation time test, which is usually insensitive to LAs.

Patients who have experienced spontaneous thromboembolism and have evidence for the aPL syndrome should be treated with long-term oral anticoagulant therapy. Studies have yielded varying results as to the recommended intensity of anticoagulant therapy. For example, a prospective study on the treatment of venous thromboembolism concluded that an INR in the range of 2.0 to 3.0 will prevent recurrences.[44,123] A retrospective study of a variety of patients with the aPL syndrome showed that a higher intensity (INR greater than 3.0) was necessary for preventing recurrences.[266] In one retrospective study, 6 out of 16 patients (37 percent) followed over 6 to 42 months developed deep venous thrombosis in spite of oral anticoagulation (INR 1.5 to 3.0).[267] Another study of secondary aPL syndrome concluded that conventional management of thromboembolic manifestations with heparin and/or oral anticoagulants prevented neither recurrent thromboses nor fatal outcomes.[125] At the time of writing a large prospective

randomized trial, the Warfarin in Antiphospholipid Syndrome (WAPS) Study,[268] is in progress to study optimal treatment.

The following is recommended until the treatment is further resolved by clinical trial. Patients with venous thromboembolism should be anticoagulated to an INR of approximately 3.0. Patients with arterial thromboembolism should have their warfarin doses adjusted to achieve a target INR of 3.0 to 3.5 where possible. Patients should not be treated with concurrent aspirin.[269] A high titer of aCL (greater than 30 U/ml) is not sufficient to justify prophylactic anticoagulation therapy in asymptomatic patients,[267] and the same conclusion can probably be applied to patients with LAs who have not experienced thrombotic or embolic events.

An important practical consequence of the LA effect is that prothrombin time and INR results have been reported to be falsely elevated in a significant proportion of patients with the aPL syndrome and LAs treated with warfarin anticoagulant therapy.[270] As with the aPTT, there may be differences in the prothrombin time reagent with regard to their sensitivity to LAs, and different LAs vary significantly in their effects on the prothrombin time.[271] It has been suggested that alternative tests, such as specific chromogenic coagulation factor assays for vitamin K–dependent proteins or the *prothrombin and proconvertin time*, would be useful to confirm the appropriate warfarin effect in these patients.[270]

There have also been case reports of fibrinolytic treatment in primary aPL syndrome for extensive thrombosis of the common femoral and iliac veins extending to the lower vena cava,[272] acute ischemic stroke,[273] and acute myocardial infarction.[274] Treatment with the antimalarial drug hydroxychloroquine appears to have an antithrombotic effect in patients with the aPL syndrome and SLE.[275,276] The potential effectiveness of this treatment has also been supported by animal studies.[277]

Patients with the catastrophic aPL syndrome may be refractory to therapy with anticoagulation alone. A review of 50 cases showed that 70 percent of the patients recovered following management with the combination of anticoagulation, steroids, and plasmapheresis or intravenous gammaglobulins.[278]

Experimental therapies of the aPL syndrome include specific antiidiotypic or anti-CD4 antibodies, IL-3, ciprofloxacin or bromocriptine, and bone-marrow transplantation.[279]

PREGNANCY LOSS

Women with a history of three or more spontaneous pregnancy losses and evidence of aPL antibodies should be treated with a combination of low dose aspirin (75 to 81 mg daily) and unfractionated heparin (5000 units subcutaneously every 12 h).[280–282] Treatment should be started as soon as pregnancy is documented, and both medications can be stopped 1 month prior to term if there are no complications (e.g., thromboembolism, intrauterine growth retardation, oligoamnion, or fetal distress). Some practitioners extend treatment with aspirin until about 1 week before term, and some extend it until labor. For complicated pregnancies, anticoagulant therapy may be warranted until just before delivery, and in especially high risk situations, induction of early delivery may be necessary. Prophylactic doses of heparin (i.e., 5000 units every 12 h subcutaneous) should be started about 4 to 6 h after delivery, if significant bleeding has ceased, and continued until the patient is fully ambulatory. For patients who have experienced systemic thromboembolism, oral anticoagulant therapy is warranted for at least 6 weeks after delivery. Treatment with low-molecular-weight heparins (LMWH) has been described,[283–286] but at the time of writing these drugs have not been approved in the United States for use during pregnancy. The potential benefits of LMWH include once-daily injections, a decreased rate of allergic reactions, and the possibility of decreased bone loss compared to unfractionated heparins.

The presence of aPL antibodies during pregnancy, without any history of clinical problems, does not require treatment. A prospective study of an untreated general obstetric population found that 2 to 3 percent of nonpregnant patients had low-titer aCL antibodies and that there was a live birth rate of about 60 percent among these patients. The organizing group of the aPL Antibody Treatment Trial[287] randomly assigned 19 women with one or no prior spontaneous abortion and without a history of thrombosis or thrombocytopenia to low-dose aspirin or no treatment and found that both groups were at such a low risk for pregnancy losses that prophylactic therapy seemed unwarranted.

While prednisone also improves the outcomes of pregnant patients with the aPL syndrome,[34,287,288] this benefit comes along with significant toxicity.[287] Thus, both corticosteroids and intravenous IgG (see below) should probably be considered only for patients who are refractory to anticoagulant therapy or who have a severe immune thrombocytopenia or a contraindication to heparin therapy. The results of one study cast doubt on the benefit of prednisone in autoimmune-associated pregnancy losses.[289] Treatment with the combination of prednisone and heparin should be avoided, when possible, since this combination will markedly increase the risk of osteopenia and of vertebral fractures.[290] There have been preliminary reports of treatment of aPL-associated recurrent first-trimester pregnancy losses with intravenous immunoglobulin,[291] but randomized placebo-controlled trials are necessary to confirm the efficacy of this treatment.

REFERENCES

1. Hughes GR: The anticardiolipin syndrome. *Clin Exp Rheumatol* 3:285, 1985.
2. Harris EN, Hughes GRV, Gharavi AE: The antiphospholipid antibody syndrome. *J Rheumatol* 13(suppl):210, 1987.
3. Vianna JL, Khamashta MA, Ordi Ros J, et al: Comparison of the primary and secondary antiphospholipid syndrome: a European Multicenter Study of 114 patients. *Am J Med* 96:3, 1994.
4. Krnic Barrie S, O'Connor CR, Looney SW, Pierangeli SS, Harris EN: A retrospective review of 61 patients with antiphospholipid syndrome. Analysis of factors influencing recurrent thrombosis. *Arch Intern Med* 157:2101, 1997.
5. Alarcon Segovia D, Cabral AR: The concept and classification of antiphospholipid/cofactor syndromes. *Lupus* 5:364, 1996.
6. Roubey RA, Hoffman M: From antiphospholipid syndrome to antibody-mediated thrombosis. *Lancet* 350:1491, 1997.
7. Vermylen J, Hoylaerts MF, Arnout J: Antibody-mediated thrombosis. *Thromb Haemost* 78:420, 1997.
8. Hughes GR, Khamashta MA, Gharavi AE, Wilson WA, eds: *Lupus (Special Issue, 8th International Symposium on Antiphospholipid Antibodies, vol 7 Suppl 2)*. Stockton Press, Hampshire, 1998.
9. Moore JE, Mohr CF: Biologically false positive serological tests for syphilis: type, incidence, and cause. *JAMA* 150:467, 1952.
10. Moore JE, Lutz WB: Natural history of systemic lupus erythematosus: approach to its study through chronic biologic false positive reactors. *J Chronic Dis* 1:297, 1955.
11. Shapiro SS, Thiagarajan P: Lupus anticoagulants. *Prog Hemost Thromb* 6:263, 1982.
12. Bell WN, Alton HG: A brain extract as a substitute for platelet suspensions in the thromboplastin generation test. *Nature* 174:880, 1954.
13. Feinstein DI, Rapaport SI: Acquired inhibitors of blood coagulation, in *Progress in Hemostasis and Thrombosis*, p 75. Grune & Stratton, New York, 1972.
14. Conley CL, Hartmann RC: A hemorrhagic disorder caused by circulating anticoagulant in patients with disseminated lupus erythematosus. *J Clin Invest* 31:621, 1952.
15. Bowie WEJ, Thompson JH, Pascuzzi CA, Owen GA: Thrombosis in systemic erythematosus despite circulating anticoagulants. *J Clin Invest* 62:416, 1963.

16. Laurell A, Nilsson I: Hypergammaglobulinemia, circulating anticoagulant and biologic false-positive Wassermann reaction. *J Lab Clin Med* 49:694, 1957.
17. Harris EN, Gharavi AE, Boey ML, et al: Anticardiolipin antibodies: detection by radioimmunoassay and association with thrombosis in systemic lupus erythematosus. *Lancet* 2:1211, 1983.
18. Hellan M, Kuhnel E, Speiser W, Lechner K, Eichinger S: Familial lupus anticoagulant: a case report and review of the literature. *Blood Coagul Fibrinolysis* 9:195, 1998.
19. Sebastiani GD, Galeazzi M, Morozzi G, Marcolongo R: The immunogenetics of the antiphospholipid syndrome, anticardiolipin antibodies, and lupus anticoagulant. *Semin Arthritis Rheum* 25:414, 1996.
20. Goldstein R, Moulds JM, Smith CD, Sengar DP: MHC studies of the primary antiphospholipid antibody syndrome and of antiphospholipid antibodies in systemic lupus erythematosus. *J Rheumatol* 23:1173, 1996.
21. Granados J, Vargas AG, Drenkard C, et al: Relationship of anticardiolipin antibodies and antiphospholipid syndrome to HLA-DR7 in Mexican patients with systemic lupus erythematosus (SLE). *Lupus* 6:57, 1997.
22. Wilson WA, Gharavi AE: Genetic risk factors for aPL syndrome. *Lupus* 5:398, 1996.
23. Manco Johnson MJ, Nuss R, Key N, et al: Lupus anticoagulant and protein S deficiency in children with postvaricella purpura fulminans or thrombosis. *J Pediatr* 128:319, 1996.
24. Barcat D, Constans J, Seigneur M, et al: Deep venous thrombosis in an adult with varicella. *Rev Med Interne* 19:509, 1998.
25. Peyton BD, Cutler BS, Stewart FM: Spontaneous tibial artery thrombosis associated with varicella pneumonia and free protein S deficiency. *J Vasc Surg* 27:563, 1998.
26. Prieto J, Yuste JR, Beloqui O, et al: Anticardiolipin antibodies in chronic hepatitis C: implication of hepatitis C virus as the cause of the antiphospholipid syndrome. *Hepatology* 23:199, 1996.
27. Labarca JA, Rabaggliati RM, Radrigan FJ, et al: Antiphospholipid syndrome associated with cytomegalovirus infection: case report and review. *Clin Infect Dis* 24:197, 1997.
28. Loizou S, Cazabon JK, Walport MJ, Tait D, So AK: Similarities of specificity and cofactor dependence in serum antiphospholipid antibodies from patients with human parvovirus B19 infection and from those with systemic lupus erythematosus. *Arthritis Rheum* 40:103, 1997.
29. Gotoh M, Matsuda J: Induction of anticardiolipin antibody and/or lupus anticoagulant in rabbits by immunization with lipoteichoic, lipopolysaccharide and lipid A. *Lupus* 5:593, 1996.
30. Eschwege V, Freyssinet JM: The possible contribution of cell apoptosis and necrosis to the generation of phospholipid-binding antibodies. *Ann Med Interne Paris* 147 Suppl 1:33, 1996.
31. Price BE, Rauch J, Shia MA, et al: Anti-phospholipid autoantibodies bind to apoptotic, but not viable, thymocytes in a beta 2-glycoprotein I-dependent manner. *J Immunol* 157:2201, 1996.
32. Pittoni V, Isenberg D: Apoptosis and antiphospholipid antibodies. *Semin Arthritis Rheum* 28:163, 1998.
33. Garcia CO, Kanbour SA, Tang H, et al: Induction of experimental antiphospholipid antibody syndrome in PL/J mice following immunization with beta 2 GPI. *Am J Reprod Immunol* 37:118, 1997.
34. Branch DW, Dudly DJ, Mitchell MD, et al: Immunoglobulin fractions from patients with antiphospholipids antibodies cause fetal death in BALB/c mice: a model for autoimmune fetal loss. *Am J Obstet Gynecol* 163:210, 1990.
35. Blank M, Faden D, Tincani A, et al: Immunization with anticardiolipin cofactor (beta-2-glycoprotein I) induces experimental antiphospholipid syndrome in naive mice. *J Autoimmun* 7:441, 1994.
36. Krause I, Blank M, Gilbrut B, Shoenfeld Y: The effect of aspirin on recurrent fetal loss in experimental antiphospholipid syndrome. *Am J Reprod Immunol* 29:155, 1993.
37. Pierangeli SS, Harris EN: In vivo models of thrombosis for the antiphospholipid syndrome. *Lupus* 5:451, 1996.
38. Pierangeli SS, Barker JH, Stikovac D, et al: Effect of human IgG antiphospholipid antibodies on an in vivo thrombosis model in mice. *Thromb Haemost* 71:670, 1994.
39. Olee T, Pierangeli SS, Handley HH, et al: A monoclonal IgG anticardiolipin antibody from a patient with the antiphospholipid syndrome is thrombogenic in mice. *Proc Natl Acad Sci USA* 93:8606, 1996.
40. George J, Afek A, Gilburd B, et al: Atherosclerosis in LDL-receptor

knockout mice is accelerated by immunization with anticardiolipin anti-bodies. *Lupus* 6:723, 1997.

41. Shi W, Krilis SA, Chong BH, Gordon S, Chesterman CN: Prevalence of lupus anticoagulant and anticardiolipin antibodies in a healthy population. *Aust N Z J Med* 20:231, 1990.

42. Vila P, Hernandez MC, Lopez Fernandez MF, Batlle J: Prevalence, follow-up and clinical significance of the anticardiolipin antibodies in normal subjects. *Thromb Haemost* 72:209, 1994.

43. Jones JV, Eastwood BJ, Jones E, James H, Mansour M: Antiphospholipid antibodies in a healthy population: methods for estimating the distribution. *J Rheumatol* 22:55, 1995.

44. Ginsberg JS, Wells PS, Brill Edwards P, et al: Antiphospholipid antibodies and venous thromboembolism. *Blood* 86:3685, 1995.

45. Sorice M, Circella A, Griggi T, et al: Anticardiolipin and anti-beta 2-GPI are two distinct populations of autoantibodies. *Thromb Haemost* 75:303, 1996.

46. Galli M, Comfurius P, Maassen C, et al: Anticardiolipin antibodies (ACA) directed not to cardiolipin but to a plasma protein cofactor. *Lancet* 335:1544, 1990.

47. McNeil HP, Simpson RJ, Chesterman CN, Krilis SA: Anti-phospholipid antibodies are directed against a complex antigen that includes a lipid-binding inhibitor of coagulation: beta 2-glycoprotein I (apolipoprotein H). *Proc Natl Acad Sci USA* 87:4120, 1990.

48. Roubey RA, Pratt CW, Buyon JP, Winfield JB: Lupus anticoagulant activity of autoimmune antiphospholipid antibodies is dependent upon beta 2-glycoprotein I. *J Clin Invest* 90:1100, 1992.

49. Schultz DR: Antiphospholipid antibodies: basic immunology and assays. *Semin Arthritis Rheum* 26:724, 1997.

50. Goldsmith GH, Pierangeli SS, Branch DW, Gharavi AE, Harris EN: Inhibition of prothrombin activation by antiphospholipid antibodies and beta 2-glycoprotein 1. *Br J Haematol* 87:548, 1994.

51. Pengo V, Biasiolo A, Brocco T, Tonetto S, Ruffatti A: Autoantibodies to phospholipid-binding plasma proteins in patients with thrombosis and phospholipid-reactive antibodies. *Thromb Haemost* 75:721, 1996.

52. Roubey RA, Eisenberg RA, Harper MF, Winfield JB: ''Anticardiolipin'' autoantibodies recognize beta 2-glycoprotein I in the absence of phospholipid. Importance of Ag density and bivalent binding. *J Immunol* 154:954, 1995.

53. Chonn A, Semple SC, Cullis PR: Beta 2 glycoprotein I is a major protein associated with very rapidly cleared liposomes in vivo, suggesting a significant role in the immune clearance of ''non-self'' particles. *J Biol Chem* 270:25845, 1995.

54. Hunt J, Krilis S: The fifth domain of beta 2-glycoprotein I contains a phospholipid binding site (Cys281-Cys288) and a region recognized by anticardiolipin antibodies. *J Immunol* 152:653, 1994.

55. Matsuura E, Igarashi M, Igarashi Y, et al: Molecular studies on phospholipid-binding sites and cryptic epitopes appearing on beta 2-glycoprotein I structure recognized by anticardiolipin antibodies. *Lupus* 4 (suppl 1):S13, 1995.

56. Kamboh MI, Mehdi H: Genetics of apolipoprotein H (beta 2-glycoprotein I) and anionic phospholipid binding. *Lupus* 7 (suppl 2):S10, 1998.

57. Koike T, Ichikawa K, Kasahara H, et al: Epitopes on beta2-GPI recognized by anticardiolipin antibodies. *Lupus* 7 (suppl 2):S14, 1998.

58. de Groot PG, Horbach DA, Derksen RH: Protein C and other cofactors involved in the binding of antiphospholipid antibodies: relation to the pathogenesis of thrombosis. *Lupus* 5:488, 1996.

59. Atsumi T, Khamashta MA, Amengual O, et al: Binding of anticardiolipin antibodies to protein C via beta 2-glycoprotein I (beta 2-GPI): a possible mechanism in the inhibitory effect of antiphospholipid antibodies on the protein C system. *Clin Exp Immunol* 112:325, 1998.

60. Shibata S, Harpel PC, Gharavi A, Rand J, Fillit H: Autoantibodies to heparin from patients with antiphospholipid antibody syndrome inhibit formation of antithrombin III-thrombin complexes. *Blood* 83:2532, 1994.

61. Drouvalakis KA, Buchanan RR: Phospholipid specificity of autoimmune and drug induced lupus anticoagulants; association of phosphatidyletha-nolamine reactivity with thrombosis in autoimmune disease. *J Rheumatol* 25:290, 1998.

62. Sugi T, McIntyre JA: Autoantibodies to phosphatidylethanolamine (PE) recognize a kininogen- PE complex. *Blood* 86:3083, 1995.

63. Witztum JL, Horkko S: The role of oxidized LDL in atherogenesis:

immunological response and anti-phospholipid antibodies. *Ann N Y Acad Sci* 811:88, 1997.

64. Horkko S, Miller E, Dudl E, et al: Antiphospholipid antibodies are directed against epitopes of oxidized phospholipids. Recognition of cardiolipin by monoclonal antibodies to epitopes of oxidized low density lipoprotein. *J Clin Invest* 98:815, 1996.

65. Horkko S, Miller E, Branch DW, Palinski W, Witztum JL: The epitopes for some antiphospholipid antibodies are adducts of oxidized phospholipid and beta 2 glycoprotein 1 (and other proteins). *Proc Natl Acad Sci USA* 94:10356, 1997.

66. Vaarala O, Puurunen M, Lukka M, et al: Affinity-purified cardiolipin-binding antibodies show heterogeneity in their binding to oxidized low-density lipoprotein. *Clin Exp Immunol* 104:269, 1996.

67. Amengual O, Atsumi T, Khamashta MA, Tinahones F, Hughes GR: Autoantibodies against oxidized low-density lipoprotein in antiphospholipid syndrome. *Br J Rheumatol* 36:964, 1997.

68. Romero FI, Amengual O, Atsumi T, et al: Arterial disease in lupus and secondary antiphospholipid syndrome: association with anti-beta2-glycoprotein I antibodies but not with antibodies against oxidized low-density lipoprotein. *Br J Rheumatol* 37:883, 1998.

69. La-Rosa L, Covini G, Galperin C, et al: Anti-mitochondrial M5 type antibody represents one of the serological markers for anti-phospholipid syndrome distinct from anti-cardiolipin and anti-beta 2-glycoprotein I antibodies. *Clin Exp Immunol* 112:144, 1998.

70. Andree HAM, Hermens WT, Hemker HC, Willems GM: Displacement of factor Va by annexin V, in *Phospholipid Binding and Anticoagulant Action of Annexin V*, p 73. Universitaire Pers Maastricht, Maastricht, The Netherlands, 1992.

71. Morgan RO, Pilar Fernandez M: Distinct annexin subfamilies in plants and protists diverged prior to animal annexins and from a common ancestor. *J Mol Evol* 44:178, 1997.

72. Rand JH: ''Annexinopathies''—a new class of diseases. *N Engl J Med* 340:1035, 1999.

73. Lyden TW, Vogt E, Ng AK, Johnson PM, Rote NS: Monoclonal anti-phospholipid antibody reactivity against human placental trophoblast. *J Reprod Immunol* 22:1, 1992.

74. Krikun G, Lockwood CJ, Wu XX, et al: The expression of the placental anticoagulant protein, annexin V, by villous trophoblasts: immunolocalization and in vitro regulation. *Placenta* 15:601, 1994.

75. Vogt E, Ng AK, Rote NS: Antiphosphatidylserine antibody removes annexin-V and facilitates the binding of prothrombin at the surface of a choriocarcinoma model of trophoblast differentiation. *Am J Obstet Gynecol* 177:964, 1997.

76. Wang X, Campos B, Kaetzel MA, Dedman JR: Annexin V is critical in the maintenance of murine placental integrity. *Am J Obstet Gynecol* 180:1008, 1999.

77. Rand JH, Wu XX, Andree HA, et al: Pregnancy loss in the antiphospholipid-antibody syndrome—a possible thrombogenic mechanism. *N Engl J Med* 337:154, 1997.

78. Rand JH, Wu XX, Andree HAM, et al: Antiphospholipid antibodies accelerate plasma coagulation by inhibiting annexin-V binding to phospholipids: a ''lupus procoagulant'' phenomenon. *Blood* 92:1652, 1998.

79. Rand JH, Wu XX, Guller S, et al: Reduction of annexin-V (placental anticoagulant protein-I) on placental villi of women with antiphospholipid antibodies and recurrent spontaneous abortion. *Am J Obstet Gynecol* 171:1566, 1994.

80. Rand JH, Wu XX, Guller S, et al: Antiphospholipid immunoglobulin G antibodies reduce annexin-V levels on syncytiotrophoblast apical membranes and in culture media of placental villi. *Am J Obstet Gynecol* 177:918, 1997.

81. Matsuda J, Saitoh N, Gohchi K, Gotoh M, Tsukamoto M: Anti-annexin V antibody in systemic lupus erythematosus patients with lupus anticoagulant and/or anticardiolipin antibody. *Am J Hematol* 47:56, 1994.

82. Matsuda J, Gotoh M, Saitoh N, et al: Anti-annexin antibody in the sera of patients with habitual fetal loss or preeclampsia [letter]. *Thromb Res* 75:105, 1994.

83. Nakamura N, Ban T, Yamaji K, Yoneda Y, Wada Y: Localization of the apoptosis-inducing activity of lupus anticoagulant in an annexin V-binding antibody subset. *J Clin Invest* 101:1951, 1998.

84. Hughes GR, Harris NN, Gharavi AE: The anticardiolipin syndrome. *J Rheumatol* 13:486, 1986.

85. Lin YL, Wang CT: Activation of human platelets by the rabbit anticardiolipin antibodies. *Blood* 80:3135, 1992.

86. Emmi L, Bergamini C, Spinelli A, et al: Possible pathogenetic role of activated platelets in the primary antiphospholipid syndrome involving the central nervous system. *Ann N Y Acad Sci* 823:188, 1997.

87. Lellouche F, Martinuzzo M, Said P, Maclouf J, Carreras LO: Imbalance of thromboxane/prostacyclin biosynthesis in patients with lupus anticoagulant. *Blood* 78:2894, 1991.

88. Kaaja R, Julkunen H, Viinikka L, Ylikorkala O: Production of prostacyclin and thromboxane in lupus pregnancies: effect of small dose of aspirin. *Obstet Gynecol* 81:327, 1993.

89. Hasselaar P, Derksen RH, Blokzijl L, de Groot PG: Thrombosis associated with antiphospholipid antibodies cannot be explained by effects on endothelial and platelet prostanoid synthesis. *Thromb Haemost* 59:80, 1988.

90. Schinco PC, Marranca D, Bazzan M, et al: Lupus anticoagulant: interference with in vivo prostaglandin production and with platelet sensitivity to prostacyclin. *Scand J Rheumatol* 21:124, 1992.

91. Dueymes M, Levy Y, Ziporen L, et al: Do some antiphospholipid antibodies target endothelial cells? *Ann Med Interne Paris* 147 Suppl 1:22, 1996.

92. Del Papa N, Guidali L, Sala A, et al: Endothelial cells as target for antiphospholipid antibodies. Human polyclonal and monoclonal anti-beta 2-glycoprotein I antibodies react in vitro with endothelial cells through adherent beta 2-glycoprotein I and induce endothelial activation. *Arthritis Rheum* 40:551, 1997.

93. Matsuda J, Gotoh M, Gohchi K, et al: Anti-endothelial cell antibodies to the endothelial hybridoma cell line (EAhy926) in systemic lupus erythematosus patients with antiphospholipid antibodies. *Br J Haematol* 97:227, 1997.

94. Navarro M, Cervera R, Teixido M, Reverter JC, Font J, Lopez SA, Monteagudo J, Escolar G, Ingelmo M: Antibodies to endothelial cells and to beta 2-glycoprotein I in the antiphospholipid syndrome: prevalence and isotype distribution. *Br J Rheumatol* 35:523, 1996.

95. Simantov R, Lo SK, Gharavi A, Sammaritano LR, Salmon JE, Silverstein RL: Antiphospholipid antibodies activate vascular endothelial cells. *Lupus* 1996; 5:440, 1996.

96. Meroni PL, Papa ND, Beltrami B, et al: Modulation of endothelial cell function by antiphospholipid antibodies. *Lupus* 5:448, 1996.

97. Hanly JG, Hong C, Issekutz A: Beta 2-glycoprotein I and anticardiolipin antibody binding to resting and activated cultured human endothelial cells. *J Rheumatol* 23:1543, 1996.

98. Branch DW, Rodgers GM: Induction of endothelial cell tissue factor activity by sera from patients with antiphospholipid syndrome: a possible mechanism of thrombosis. *Am J Obstet Gynecol* 168:206, 1993.

99. Oosting JD, Derksen RH, Blokzijl L, Sixma JJ, de Groot PG: Antiphospholipid antibody positive sera enhance endothelial cell procoagulant activity—studies in a thrombosis model. *Thromb Haemost* 68:278, 1992.

100. Atsumi T, Khamashta MA, Haworth RS, et al: Arterial disease and thrombosis in the antiphospholipid syndrome: a pathogenic role for endothelin 1. *Arthritis Rheum* 41:800, 1998.

101. Stewart MW, Etches WS, Gordon PA: Antiphospholipid antibody-dependent C5b-9 formation. *Br J Haematol* 96:451, 1997.

102. Arfors L, Lefvert AK: Enrichment of antibodies against phospholipids in circulating immune complexes (CIC) in the anti-phospholipid syndrome (APLS). *Clin Exp Immunol* 108:47, 1997.

103. Martini F, Farsi A, Gori AM, et al: Antiphospholipid antibodies (aPL) increase the potential monocyte procoagulant activity in patients with systemic lupus erythematosus. *Lupus* 5:206, 1996.

104. Reverter JC, Tassies D, Font J, et al: Hypercoagulable state in patients with antiphospholipid syndrome is related to high induced tissue factor expression on monocytes and to low free protein s. *Arterioscler Thromb Vasc Biol* 16:1319, 1996.

105. de Groot PG, Horbach DA, Derksen RH: Protein C and other cofactors involved in the binding of antiphospholipid antibodies: relation to the pathogenesis of thrombosis. *Lupus* 5:488, 1996.

106. Ames PR, Tommasino C, Iannaccone L, et al: Coagulation activation and fibrinolytic imbalance in subjects with idiopathic antiphospholipid antibodies–a crucial role for acquired free protein S deficiency. *Thromb Haemost* 76:190, 1996.

107. Crowther MA, Johnston M, Weitz J, Ginsberg JS: Free protein S deficiency may be found in patients with antiphospholipid antibodies who do not have systemic lupus erythematosus. *Thromb Haemost* 76:689, 1996.

108. Vaarala O: Antiphospholipid antibodies and atherosclerosis. *Lupus* 5:442, 1996.

109. Schousboe I, Rasmussen MS: Synchronized inhibition of the phospholipid mediated autoactivation of factor XII in plasma by beta 2-glycoprotein I and anti-beta 2-glycoprotein I. *Thromb Haemost* 73:798, 1995.

110. Casciola Rosen L, Rosen A, Petri M, Schlissel M: Surface blebs on apoptotic cells are sites of enhanced procoagulant activity: implications for coagulation events and antigenic spread in systemic lupus erythematosus. *Proc Natl Acad Sci USA* 93:1624, 1996.

111. Stone JH, Amend WJ, Criswell LA: Outcome of renal transplantation in systemic lupus erythematosus. *Semin Arthritis Rheum* 27:17, 1997.

112. Piette JC, Cacoub P: Antiphospholipid syndrome in the elderly: caution [editorial]. *Circulation* 97:2195, 1998.

113. Krnic BS, O'Connor CR, Looney SW, Pierangeli SS, Harris EN: A retrospective review of 61 patients with antiphospholipid syndrome. Analysis of factors influencing recurrent thrombosis. *Arch Intern Med* 157:2101, 1997.

114. Provenzale JM, Ortel TL, Allen NB: Systemic thrombosis in patients with antiphospholipid antibodies: lesion distribution and imaging findings. *Am J Roentgenol* 170:285, 1998.

115. Martinelli I, Cattaneo M, Panzeri D, Taioli E, Mannucci PM: Risk factors for deep venous thrombosis of the upper extremities. *Ann Intern Med* 1997; 126:707, 1997.

116. Poux JM, Boudet R, Lacroix P, et al: Renal infarction and thrombosis of the infrarenal aorta in a 35-year-old man with primary antiphospholipid syndrome. *Am J Kidney Dis* 27:721, 1996.

117. Kojima E, Naito K, Iwai M, et al: Antiphospholipid syndrome complicated by thrombosis of the superior mesenteric artery, co-existence of smooth muscle hyperplasia. *Intern Med* 36:528, 1997.

118. Girolami A, Zanon E, Zanardi S, Saracino MA, Simioni P: Thromboembolic disease developing during oral contraceptive therapy in young females with antiphospholipid antibodies. *Blood Coagul Fibrinolysis* 7:497, 1996.

119. Montaruli B, Borchiellini A, Tamponi G, et al: Factor V Arg←Gln mutation in patients with antiphospholipid antibodies. *Lupus* 5:303, 1996.

120. Simantov R, Lo SK, Salmon JE, Sammaritano LR, Silverstein RL: Factor V Leiden increases the risk of thrombosis in patients with antiphospholipid antibodies. *Thromb Res* 84:361, 1996.

121. Schutt M, Kluter H, Hagedorn GM, Fehm HL, Wiedemann GJ: Familial coexistence of primary antiphospholipid syndrome and factor V Leiden. *Lupus* 7:176, 1998.

122. Brenner B, Vulfsons SL, Lanir N, Nahir M: Coexistence of familial antiphospholipid syndrome and factor V Leiden: impact on thrombotic diathesis. *Br J Haematol* 94:166, 1996.

123. Schulman S, Svenungsson E, Granqvist S: Anticardiolipin antibodies predict early recurrence of thromboembolism and death among patients with venous thromboembolism following anticoagulant therapy. Duration of Anticoagulation Study Group. *Am J Med* 104:332, 1998.

124. Finazzi G, Brancaccio V, Moia M, et al: Natural history and risk factors for thrombosis in 360 patients with antiphospholipid antibodies: a four-year prospective study from the Italian Registry. *Am J Med* 100:530, 1996.

125. Petrovic R, Petrovic M, Novicic SD, et al: Anticardiolipin antibodies and clinical spectrum of antiphospholipid syndrome in patients with systemic lupus erythematosus. *Vojnosanit Pregl* 55:23, 1998.

126. Shoenfeld Y, Lorber M, Yucel T, Yazici H: Primary antiphospholipid syndrome emerging following thymectomy for myasthenia gravis: additional evidence for the kaleidoscope of autoimmunity. *Lupus* 6:474, 1997.

127. Yun YY, Yoh KA, Yang HI, et al: A case of Budd-Chiari syndrome with high antiphospholipid antibody in a patient with systemic lupus erythematosus. *Korean J Intern Med* 11:82, 1996.

128. Hofbauer LC, Spitzweg C, Heufelder AE: Graves' disease associated with the primary antiphospholipid syndrome. *J Rheumatol* 23:1435, 1996.

129. Chun WH, Bang D, Lee SK: Antiphospholipid syndrome associated with progressive systemic sclerosis. *J Dermatol* 23:347, 1996.

130. Frolow M, Jankowski M, Swadzba J, Musial J: [Evan's syndrome with antiphospholipid-protein antibodies]. *Pol Merkuriusz Lek* 1:344, 1996.

131. Cervera R, Garcia CM, Font J, et al: Antiphospholipid antibodies in primary Sjogren's syndrome: prevalence and clinical significance in a series of 80 patients. *Clin Exp Rheumatol* 15:361, 1997.

132. Zeuner M, Straub RH, Schlosser U, et al: Anti-phospholipid-antibodies in patients with relapsing polychondritis. *Lupus* 7:12, 1998.

133. Lie TJ: Pathology of the antiphospholipid syndrome, in *The Antiphospholipid Syndrome*, p 89. CRC Press, Boca Raton, 1996.

134. Meyer O, Nicaise P, Moreau S, et al: Antibodies to cardiolipin and beta 2 glycoprotein I in patients with polymyalgia rheumatica and giant cell arteritis. *Rev Rhum Engl Ed* 63:241, 1996.

135. Yokoi K, Hosoi E, Akaike M, Shigekiyo T, Saito S: Takayasu's arteritis associated with antiphospholipid antibodies. Report of two cases. *Angiology* 47:315, 1996.

136. Dasgupta B, Almond MK, Tanqueray A: Polyarteritis nodosa and the antiphospholipid syndrome. *Br J Rheumatol* 36:1210, 1997.

137. The antiphospholipid antibodies and stroke study group (APASS): Anticardiolipin antibodies and the risk of recurrent thrombo-occlusive events and death. *Neurology* 48:91, 1997.

138. Weingarten K, Filippi C, Barbut D, Zimmerman RD: The neuroimaging features of the cardiolipin antibody syndrome. *Clin Imaging* 21:6, 1997.

139. Mevorach D, Goldberg Y, Gomori JM, Rachmilewitz D: Antiphospholipid syndrome manifested by ischemic stroke in a patient with Crohn's disease. *J Clin Gastroenterol* 22:141, 1996.

140. Bronster DJ, Gousse R, Fassas A, Rand JH: Anticardiolipin antibody-associated stroke after liver transplantation. *Transplantation* 63:908, 1997.

141. Carhuapoma JR, Mitsias P, Levine SR: Cerebral venous thrombosis and anticardiolipin antibodies. *Stroke* 28:2363, 1997.

142. Deschiens MA, Conard J, Horellou MH, et al: Coagulation studies, factor V Leiden, and anticardiolipin antibodies in 40 cases of cerebral venous thrombosis. *Stroke* 27:1724, 1996.

143. Nagai S, Horie Y, Akai T, Takeda S, Takaku A: Superior sagittal sinus thrombosis associated with primary antiphospholipid syndrome—case report. *Neurol Med Chir Tokyo* 38:34, 1998.

144. Brey RL, Escalante A: Neurological manifestations of antiphospholipid antibody syndrome. *Lupus* 7 (suppl 2):S67, 1998.

145. Matsushita T, Kanda F, Yamada H, Chihara K: Recurrent acute transverse myelopathy: an 83-year-old man with antiphospholipid syndrome. *Rinsho Shinkeigaku* 37:987, 1997.

146. Ruiz AG, Guzman RJ, Flores FJ, Garay MJ: Refractory hiccough heralding transverse myelitis in the primary antiphospholipid syndrome. *Lupus* 7:49, 1998.

147. Takamura Y, Morimoto S, Tanooka A, Yoshikawa J: Transverse myelitis in a patient with primary antiphospholipid syndrome—a case report. *No To Shinkei* 48:851, 1996.

148. Campi A, Filippi M, Comi G, Scotti G: Recurrent acute transverse myelopathy associated with anticardiolipin antibodies. *Am J Neuroradiol* 19:781, 1998.

149. Smyth AE, Bruce IN, McMillan SA, Bell AL: Transverse myelitis: a complication of systemic lupus erythematosus that is associated with the antiphospholipid syndrome. *Ulster Med J* 65:91, 1996.

150. Mok CC, Lau CS, Chan EY, Wong RW: Acute transverse myelopathy in systemic lupus erythematosus: clinical presentation, treatment, and outcome. *J Rheumatol* 25:467, 1998.

151. Sugiyama Y, Yamamoto T: Characterization of serum anti-phospholipid antibodies in patients with multiple sclerosis. *Tohoku J Exp Med* 178:203, 1996.

152. Schwartz M, Rochas M, Weller B, et al: High association of anticardiolipin antibodies with psychosis. *J Clin Psychiatry* 59:20, 1998.

153. Asherson RA: The catastrophic antiphospholipid syndrome, 1998. A review of the clinical features, possible pathogenesis and treatment. *Lupus* 7 (suppl 2):S55, 1998.

154. Lockwood CJ, Rand JH: The immunobiology and obstetrical consequences of antiphospholipid antibodies. *Obstet Gynecol Surv* 49:432, 1994.

155. Lockshin MD: Pregnancy loss and antiphospholipid antibodies. *Lupus* 7 (suppl 2):S86, 1998.

156. Rai R, Regan L: Obstetric complications of antiphospholipid antibodies. *Curr Opin Obstet Gynecol* 9:387, 1997.

157. Ornstein MH, Rand JH: An association between refractory HELLP syndrome and antiphospholipid antibodies during pregnancy; a report of 2 cases. *J Rheumatol* 21:1360, 1994.

158. Neuwelt CM, Daikh DI, Linfoot JA, et al: Catastrophic antiphospholipid syndrome: response to repeated plasmapheresis over three years. *Arthritis Rheum* 40:1534, 1997.

159. Ramsey-Goldman R, Kutzer JE, Kuller LH, et al: Pregnancy outcome and anti-cardiolipin antibody in women with systemic lupus erythematosus. *Am J Epidemiol* 138:1057, 1993.

160. Zangari M, Lockwood CJ, Scher J, Rand JH: Prothrombin activation fragment (F1.2) is increased in pregnant patients with antiphospholipid antibodies. *Thromb Res* 85:177, 1997.

161. Out HJ, Bruinse HW, Christiaens GC, et al: Prevalence of antiphospholipid antibodies in patients with fetal loss. *Ann Rheum Dis* 50:553, 1991.

162. Salafia CM, Cowchock FS: Placental pathology and antiphospholipid antibodies: a descriptive study. *Am J Perinatol* 14:435, 1997.

163. Salafia CM, Parke AL: Placental pathology in systemic lupus erythematosus and phospholipid antibody syndrome. *Rheum Dis Clin North Am* 23:85, 1997.

164. Coulam CB, Kaider BD, Kaider AS, Janowicz P, Roussev RG: Antiphospholipid antibodies associated with implantation failure after IVF/ET. *J Assist Reprod Genet* 14:603, 1997.

165. Kutteh WH, Yetman DL, Chantilis SJ, Crain J: Effect of antiphospholipid antibodies in women undergoing in-vitro fertilization: role of heparin and aspirin. *Hum Reprod* 12:1171, 1997.

166. Balasch J, Creus M, Fabregues F, et al: Antiphospholipid antibodies and the outcome of pregnancy after the first in-vitro fertilization and embryo transfer cycle. *Hum Reprod* 13:1180, 1998.

167. Vivaldi P, Rossetti G, Galli M, Finazzi G: Severe bleeding due to acquired hypoprothrombinemia-lupus anticoagulant syndrome. Case report and review of literature. *Haematologica* 82:345, 1997.

168. Hudson N, Duffy CM, Rauch J, Paquin JD, Esdaile JM: Catastrophic haemorrhage in a case of paediatric primary antiphospholipid syndrome and factor II deficiency. *Lupus* 6:68, 1997.

169. Gibson GE, Su WP, Pittelkow MR: Antiphospholipid syndrome and the skin. *J Am Acad Dermatol* 36:970, 1997.

170. Aronoff DM, Callen JP: Necrosing livedo reticularis in a patient with recurrent pulmonary hemorrhage. *J Am Acad Dermatol* 37:300, 1997.

171. Picillo U, Migliaresi S, Marcialis MR, Ferruzzi AM, Tirri G: Clinical setting of patients with systemic sclerosis by serum autoantibodies. *Clin Rheumatol* 16:378, 1997.

172. Vaarala O: Antiphospholipid antibodies and myocardial infarction. *Lupus* 7 (suppl 2):S132, 1998.

173. Vaarala O, Puurunen M, Manttari M, et al: Antibodies to prothrombin imply a risk of myocardial infarction in middle-aged men. *Thromb Haemost* 75:456, 1996.

174. Ludia C, Domenico P, Monia C, et al: Antiphospholipid antibodies: a new risk factor for restenosis after percutaneous transluminal coronary angioplasty? *Autoimmunity* 27:141, 1998.

175. Chambers-JD J, Haire HD, Deligonul U: Multiple early percutaneous transluminal coronary angioplasty failures related to lupus anticoagulant. *Am Heart J* 132:189, 1996.

176. Niaz A, Butany J: Antiphospholipid antibody syndrome with involvement of a bioprosthetic heart valve. *Can J Cardiol* 14:951, 1998.

177. Bouillanne O, Millaire A, De-Groote P, et al: Prevalence and clinical significance of antiphospholipid antibodies in heart valve disease: a case-control study. *Am Heart J* 132:790, 1996.

178. Nesher G, Ilany J, Rosenmann D, Abraham AS: Valvular dysfunction in antiphospholipid syndrome: prevalence, clinical features, and treatment. *Semin Arthritis Rheum* 27:27, 1997.

179. Garcia TR, Amigo MC, de-la-Rosa A, Moron A, Reyes PA: Valvular heart disease in primary antiphospholipid syndrome (PAPS): clinical and morphological findings. *Lupus* 5:56, 1996.

180. Ziporen L, Goldberg I, Arad M, et al: Libman-Sacks endocarditis in the antiphospholipid syndrome: immunopathologic findings in deformed heart valves. *Lupus* 5:196, 1996.

181. Gabrielli F, Alcini E, Prima MA, Lucifero A, Masala C: Cardiac involvement in connective tissue diseases and primary antiphospholipid syndrome: echocardiographic assessment and correlation with antiphospholipid antibodies. *Acta Cardiol* 51:425, 1996.

182. Lee RW, Taylor-LM J, Landry GJ, et al: Prospective comparison of infrainguinal bypass grafting in patients with and without antiphospholipid antibodies. *J Vasc Surg* 24:524, 1996.

183. Gagne PJ, Vitti MJ, Fink LM, et al: Young women with advanced aortoiliac occlusive disease: new insights. *Ann Vasc Surg* 10:546, 1996.

184. von-Scheven E, Athreya BH, Rose CD, Goldsmith DP, Morton L: Clinical characteristics of antiphospholipid antibody syndrome in children. *J Pediatr* 129:339, 1996.

185. Karmochkine M, Cacoub P, Dorent R, et al: High prevalence of antiphospholipid antibodies in precapillary pulmonary hypertension. *J Rheumatol* 23:286, 1996.

186. Miyashita Y, Koike H, Misawa A, et al: Asymptomatic pulmonary hypertension complicated with antiphospholipid syndrome case. *Intern Med* 35:912, 1996.

187. Kerr JE, Poe R, Kramer Z: Antiphospholipid antibody syndrome presenting as a refractory noninflammatory pulmonary vasculopathy. *Chest* 112:1707, 1997.

188. Maggiorini M, Knoblauch A, Schneider J, Russi EW: Diffuse microvascular pulmonary thrombosis associated with primary antiphospholipid antibody syndrome. *Eur Respir J* 10:727, 1997.

189. Hoffman M, Burke M, Fried M, et al: Primary biliary cirrhosis associated with antiphospholipid syndrome. *Isr J Med Sci* 33:681, 1997.

190. Date K, Shirai Y, Hatakeyama K: Antiphospholipid antibody syndrome presenting as acute acalculous cholecystitis. *Am J Gastroenterol* 92:2127, 1997.

191. Dessailloud R, Papo T, Vaneecloo S, et al: Acalculous ischemic gallbladder necrosis in the catastrophic antiphospholipid syndrome. *Arthritis Rheum* 41:1318, 1998.

192. Kalman DR, Khan A, Romain PL, Nompleggi DJ: Giant gastric ulceration associated with antiphospholipid antibody syndrome. *Am J Gastroenterol* 91:1244, 1996.

193. Gul A, Inanc M, Ocal L, et al: Primary antiphospholipid syndrome associated with mesenteric inflammatory veno-occlusive disease. *Clin Rheumatol* 15:207, 1996.

194. Lee HJ, Park JW, Chang JC: Mesenteric and portal venous obstruction associated with primary antiphospholipid antibody syndrome. *J Gastroenterol Hepatol* 12:822, 1997.

195. Galli M, Finazzi G, Barbui T: Thrombocytopenia in the antiphospholipid syndrome: pathophysiology, clinical relevance and treatment. *Ann Med Interne Paris* 147 (suppl 1):24, 1996.

196. Cuadrado MJ, Mujic F, Munoz E, Khamashta MA, Hughes GR: Thrombocytopenia in the antiphospholipid syndrome. *Ann Rheum Dis* 56:194, 1997.

197. Macchi L, Rispal P, Clofent SG, et al: Anti-platelet antibodies in patients with systemic lupus erythematosus and the primary antiphospholipid antibody syndrome: their relationship with the observed thrombocytopenia. *Br J Haematol* 98:336, 1997.

198. Panzer S, Gschwandtner ME, Hutter D, Spitzauer S, Pabinger I: Specificities of platelet autoantibodies in patients with lupus anticoagulants in primary antiphospholipid syndrome. *Ann Hematol* 74:239, 1997.

199. Lipp E, von-Felten A, Sax H, Muller D, Berchtold P: Antibodies against platelet glycoproteins and antiphospholipid antibodies in autoimmune thrombocytopenia. *Eur J Haematol* 60:283, 1998.

200. Dunn JP, Noorily SW, Petri M, et al: Antiphospholipid antibodies and retinal vascular disease. *Lupus* 5:313, 1996.

201. Coniglio M, Platania A, Di-Nucci GD, et al: Antiphospholipid-protein antibodies are not an uncommon feature in retinal venous occlusions. *Thromb Res* 83:183, 1996.

202. Glacet-Bernard A, Bayani N, Chretien P, Cochard C, Lelong F, Coscas G: Antiphospholipid antibodies in retinal vascular occlusions. A prospective study of 75 patients. *Arch Ophthal* 112:790, 1994.

203. Dori D, Gelfand YA, Brenner B, Miller B: Cilioretinal artery occlusion: an ocular complication of primary antiphospholipid syndrome. *Retina* 17:555, 1997.

204. Reino S, Munoz RF, Cervera R, et al: Optic neuropathy in the "primary" antiphospholipid syndrome: report of a case and review of the literature. *Clin Rheumatol* 16:629, 1997.

205. Biron C, Andreani H, Blanc P, et al: Prevalence of antiphospholipid antibodies in patients with chronic liver disease related to alcohol or hepatitis C virus: correlation with liver injury. *J Lab Clin Med* 131:243, 1998.

206. McMurray RW: Hepatitis C-associated autoimmune disorders. *Rheum Dis Clin North Am* 24:353, 1998.

207. Miret C, Cervera R, Reverter JC, et al: Antiphospholipid syndrome without antiphospholipid antibodies at the time of the thrombotic event: transient "seronegative" antiphospholipid syndrome? *Clin Exp Rheumatol* 15:541, 1997.

208. Abuaf N, Laperche S, Rajoely B, et al: Autoantibodies to phospholipids and to the coagulation proteins in AIDS. *Thromb Haemost* 77:856, 1997.

209. Ravelli A, Martini A: Antiphospholipid antibody syndrome in pediatric patients. *Rheum Dis Clin North Am* 23:657, 1997.

210. Baca V, Garcia RR, Ramirez LM, et al: Cerebral infarction and antiphospholipid syndrome in children. *J Rheumatol* 23:1428, 1996.

211. Angelini L, Zibordi F, Zorzi G, et al: Neurological disorders, other than stroke, associated with antiphospholipid antibodies in childhood. *Neuropediatrics* 27:149, 1996.

212. Falcini F, Taccetti G, Ermini M, Trapani S, Matucci CM: Catastrophic antiphospholipid antibody syndrome in pediatric systemic lupus erythematosus. *J Rheumatol* 24:389, 1997.

213. Marie I, Levesque H, Heron F, et al: Acute adrenal failure secondary to bilateral infarction of the adrenal glands as the first manifestation of primary antiphospholipid antibody syndrome [letter]. *Ann Rheum Dis* 56:567, 1997.

214. Caron P, Chabannier MH, Cambus JP, et al: Definitive adrenal insufficiency due to bilateral adrenal hemorrhage and primary antiphospholipid syndrome. *J Clin Endocrinol Metab* 83:1437, 1998.

215. Garris GW, Smith BD: Bilateral adrenal hemorrhage and acute addisonian crisis—a complication of antiphospholipid syndrome. *J Tenn Med Assoc* 89:120, 1996.

216. Hsu B, Udden MM, Lynch EC: Autoimmune hemolytic anemia, primary adrenal insufficiency, and the antiphospholipid syndrome. *Am J Med Sci* 314:41, 1997.

217. Paydas S, Kocak R, Zorludemir S, Baslamisli F: Bone marrow necrosis in antiphospholipid syndrome. *J Clin Pathol* 50:261, 1997.

218. Naarendorp M, Spiera H: Sudden sensorineural hearing loss in patients with systemic lupus erythematosus or lupus-like syndromes and antiphospholipid antibodies. *J Rheumatol* 25:589, 1998.

219. Shah NM, Khamashta MA, Atsumi T, Hughes GR: Outcome of patients with anticardiolipin antibodies: a 10 year follow-up of 52 patients. *Lupus* 7:3, 1998.

220. Silver RM, Porter TF, van LI, et al: Anticardiolipin antibodies: clinical consequences of "low titers." *Obstet Gynecol* 87:494, 1996.

221. Mateo J, Oliver A, Borrell M, Sala N, Fontcuberta J: Laboratory evaluation and clinical characteristics of 2,132 consecutive unselected patients with venous thromboembolism—results of the Spanish Multicentric Study on Thrombophilia (EMET-Study). *Thromb Haemost* 77:444, 1997.

222. Lenzi R, Rand JH, Spiera H: Anticardiolipin antibodies in pregnant patients with systemic lupus erythematosus [letter]. *N Engl J Med* 314:1392, 1986.

223. Molina JF, Gutierrez US, Molina J, et al: Variability of anticardiolipin antibody isotype distribution in 3 geographic populations of patients with systemic lupus erythematosus. *J Rheumatol* 24:291, 1997.

224. Sammaritano LR: Significance of aPL IgG subclasses. *Lupus* 5:436, 1996.

225. Sammaritano LR, Ng S, Sobel R, et al: Anticardiolipin IgG subclasses: association of IgG2 with arterial and/or venous thrombosis. *Arthritis Rheum* 40:1998, 1997.

226. Atsumi T, Caliz R, Amengual O, Khamashta MA, Hughes GR: Fcgamma receptor IIA H/R131 polymorphism in patients with antiphospholipid antibodies. *Thromb Haemost* 79:924, 1998.

227. Selva OA, Ordi RJ, Monegal FF, et al: IgA anticardiolipin antibodies—relation with other antiphospholipid antibodies and clinical significance. *Thromb Haemost* 79:282, 1998.

228. Merrill JT, Shen C, Gugnani M, Lahita RG, Mongey AB: High prevalence of antiphospholipid antibodies in patients taking procainamide. *J Rheumatol* 24:1083, 1997.

229. Karmochkine M, Piette JC, Mazoyer E, et al: Antiphospholipid antibodies: cause of thrombosis or an epiphenomenon? *Presse Med* 24:267, 1995.

230. Colaco CB, Male DK: Anti-phospholipid antibodies in syphilis and a thrombotic subset of SLE: distinct profiles of epitope specificity. *Clin Exp Immunol* 59:449, 1985.

231. Triplett DA: Assays for detection of antiphospholipid antibodies. *Lupus* 3:281, 1994.

232. Branch DW, Rote NS, Dostal DA, Scott JR: Association of lupus anticoagulant with antibody against phosphatidylserine. *Clin Immunol Immunopathol* 42:63, 1987.

233. Harris EN: Antiphospholipid antibodies. *Br J Haematol* 74:1, 1990.

234. Esmon NL, Smirnov MD, Esmon CT: Lupus anticoagulants and throm-
      bosis: the role of phospholipids. *Haematologica* 82:474, 1997.
235. Berard M, Chantome R, Marcelli A, Boffa MC: Antiphosphatidylethano-
      lamine antibodies as the only antiphospholipid antibodies. I. Association
      with thrombosis and vascular cutaneous diseases [see comments]. *J
      Rheumatol* 23:1369, 1996.
236. Rauch J, Janoff AS: Antibodies against phospholipids other than cardio-
      lipin: potential roles for both phospholipid and protein. *Lupus* 5:498,
      1996.
237. Yetman DL, Kutteh WH: Antiphospholipid antibody panels and recur-
      rent pregnancy loss: prevalence of anticardiolipin antibodies compared
      with other antiphospholipid antibodies. *Fertil Steril* 66:540, 1996.
238. de Maistre E, Gobert B, Bene MC, et al: Comparative assessment of
      phospholipid-binding antibodies indicates limited overlapping. *J Clin
      Lab Anal* 10:6, 1996.
239. Branch DW, Silver R, Pierangeli S, van Leeuwen I, Harris EN: Antiphos-
      pholipid antibodies other than lupus anticoagulant and anticardiolipin
      antibodies in women with recurrent pregnancy loss, fertile controls, and
      antiphospholipid syndrome. *Obstet Gynecol* 89:549, 1997.
240. Laroche P, Berard M, Rouquette AM, Desgruelle C, Boffa MC: Advan-
      tage of using both anionic and zwitterionic phospholipid antigens for
      the detection of antiphospholipid antibodies. *Am J Clin Pathol*
      106:549, 1996.
241. Amengual O, Atsumi T, Khamashta MA, Koike T, Hughes GR: Specific-
      ity of ELISA for antibody to beta 2-glycoprotein I in patients with
      antiphospholipid syndrome. *Br J Rheumatol* 35:1239, 1996.
242. Alarcon SD, Mestanza M, Cabiedes J, Cabral AR: The antiphospholipid/
      cofactor syndromes. II. A variant in patients with systemic lupus erythe-
      matosus with antibodies to beta 2-glycoprotein I but no antibodies detect-
      able in standard antiphospholipid assays. *J Rheumatol* 24:1545, 1997.
243. Cabral AR, Amigo MC, Cabiedes J, Alarcon SD: The antiphospholipid/
      cofactor syndromes: a primary variant with antibodies to beta 2-glyco-
      protein-I but no antibodies detectable in standard antiphospholipid
      assays. *Am J Med* 101:472, 1996.
244. Sanmarco M, Soler C, Christides C, et al: Prevalence and clinical signifi-
      cance of IgG isotype anti-beta 2-glycoprotein I antibodies in antiphos-
      pholipid syndrome: a comparative study with anticardiolipin antibodies.
      J Lab Clin Med 129:499, 1997.
245. Day HM, Thiagarajan P, Ahn C, et al: Autoantibodies to beta 2-glycopro-
      tein I in systemic lupus erythematosus and primary antiphospholipid
      antibody syndrome: clinical correlations in comparison with other anti-
      phospholipid antibody tests. *J Rheumatol* 25:667, 1998.
246. Puurunen M, Vaarala O, Julkunen H, Aho K, Palosuo T: Antibodies to
      phospholipid-binding plasma proteins and occurrence of thrombosis in
      patients with systemic lupus erythematosus. *Clin Immunol Immunopa-
      thol* 80:16, 1996.
247. Bertolaccini ML, Atsumi T, Khamashta MA, Amengual O, Hughes GR:
      Autoantibodies to human prothrombin and clinical manifestations in 207
      patients with systemic lupus erythematosus. *J Rheumatol* 25:1104, 1998.
248. Palosuo T, Virtamo J, Haukka J, et al: High antibody levels to prothrom-
      bin imply a risk of deep venous thrombosis and pulmonary embolism
      in middle-aged men—a nested case-control study. *Thromb Haemost*
      78:1178, 1997.
249. Galli M, Barbui T: Prothrombin as cofactor for antiphospholipids. *Lupus*
      7 (suppl 2):S37, 1998.
250. Shapiro SS: The lupus anticoagulant/antiphospholipid syndrome. *Annu
      Rev Med* 47:533, 1996.
251. Triplett DA: Lupus anticoagulants/antiphospholipid-protein antibodies:
      the great imposters. *Lupus* 5:431, 1996.
252. Jennings I, Kitchen S, Woods TA, Preston FE, Greaves M: Potentially
      clinically important inaccuracies in testing for the lupus anticoagulant:
      an analysis of results from three surveys of the UK National External
      Quality Assessment Scheme (NEQAS) for Blood Coagulation. *Thromb
      Haemost* 77:934, 1997.
253. Lockwood CJ, Romero R, Feinberg RF, et al: The prevalence and
      biologic significance of lupus anticoagulant and anticardiolipin antibod-
      ies in a general obstetric population. *Am J Obstet Gynecol* 161:369, 1989.
254. Horbach DA, van-Oort E, Donders RC, Derksen RH, de-Groot PG:
      Lupus anticoagulant is the strongest risk factor for both venous and
      arterial thrombosis in patients with systemic lupus erythematosus. Com-
      parison between different assays for the detection of antiphospholipid
      antibodies. *Thromb Haemost* 76:916, 1996.
255. Cabral AR, Cabiedes J, Alarcon Segovia D: Antibodies to phospholipid-
      free beta 2-glycoprotein-I in patients with primary antiphospholipid
      syndrome. *J Rheumatol* 22:1894, 1995.
256. Fijnheer R, Horbach DA, Donders RC, et al: Factor V Leiden, antiphos-
      pholipid antibodies and thrombosis in systemic lupus erythematosus.
      Thromb Haemost 76:514, 1996.
257. Wahl DG, Guillemin F, De-Maistre E, et al: Meta-analysis of the risk
      of venous thrombosis in individuals with antiphospholipid antibodies
      without underlying autoimmune disease or previous thrombosis. *Lupus*
      7:15, 1998.
258. Nojima J, Suehisa E, Akita N, et al: Risk of arterial thrombosis in
      patients with anticardiolipin antibodies and lupus anticoagulant. *Br J
      Haematol* 96:447, 1997.
259. Galli M, Bevers EM, Comfurius P, Barbui T, Zwaal RF: Effect of
      antiphospholipid antibodies on procoagulant activity of activated plate-
      lets and platelet-derived microvesicles. *Br J Haematol* 83:466, 1993.
260. Takeya H, Mori T, Gabazza EC, et al: Anti-beta 2-glycoprotein I (be-
      ta2GPI) monoclonal antibodies with lupus anticoagulant-like activity
      enhance the beta2GPI binding to phospholipids. *J Clin Invest*
      99:2260, 1997.
261. Kitchens CS: Prolonged activated partial thromboplastin time of un-
      known etiology: a prospective study of 100 consecutive cases referred
      for consultation. *Am J Hematol* 27:38, 1988.
262. Galli M, Finazzi G, Bevers EM, Barbui T: Kaolin clotting time and
      dilute Russell's viper venom time distinguish between prothrombin-
      dependent and beta 2-glycoprotein I-dependent antiphospholipid anti-
      bodies. *Blood* 86:617, 1995.
263. Liu HW, Wong KL, Lin CK, et al: The reappraisal of dilute tissue
      thromboplastin inhibition test in the diagnosis of lupus anticoagulant.
      Br J Haematol 72:229, 1989.
264. Forastiero RR, Cerrato GS, Carreras LO: Evaluation of recently de-
      scribed tests for detection of the lupus anticoagulant. *Thromb Haemost*
      72:728, 1994.
265. McCrae KR: Antiphospholipid antibody associated thrombosis: a con-
      sensus for treatment? *Lupus* 5:560, 1996.
266. Khamashta MA, Cuadrado MJ, Mujic F, et al: The management of
      thrombosis in the antiphospholipid-antibody syndrome. *N Engl J Med*
      332:993, 1995.
267. Urfer C, Pichler WJ, Helbling A: Antiphospholipid antibodies syndrome:
      follow-up of patients with a high antiphospholipid antibodies titer.
      Schweiz Med Wochenschr 126:2136, 1996.
268. Finazzi G, Barbui T: Feasibility of a randomized clinical trial for the
      prevention of recurrent thrombosis in the antiphospholipid syndrome:
      the WAPS project. Provisional Steering Committee of the Warfarin in
      Antiphospholipid Syndrome (WAPS) Study. *Ann Med Interne Paris*
      147 Suppl 1:38, 1996.
269. Khamashta MA, Cuadrado MJ, Mujic F, et al: The management of
      thrombosis in the antiphospholipid-antibody syndrome. *N Engl J Med*
      332:993, 1995.
270. Moll S, Ortel TL: Monitoring warfarin therapy in patients with lupus
      anticoagulants. *Ann Intern Med* 127:177, 1997.
271. Della VP, Crippa L, Safa O, et al: Potential failure of the International
      Normalized Ratio (INR) System in the monitoring of oral anticoagulation
      in patients with lupus anticoagulants. *Ann Med Interne Paris* 147 Suppl
      1:10, 1996.
272. Camps GM, Guil M, Sanchez LJ, et al: Fibrinolytic treatment in primary
      antiphospholipid syndrome. *Lupus* 5:627, 1996.
273. Julkunen H, Hedman C, Kauppi M: Thrombolysis for acute ischemic
      stroke in the primary antiphospholipid syndrome. *J Rheumatol*
      24:181, 1997.
274. Ho YL, Chen MF, Wu CC, Chen WJ, Lee YT: Successful treatment of
      acute myocardial infarction by thrombolytic therapy in a patient with
      primary antiphospholipid antibody syndrome. *Cardiology* 87:354, 1996.
275. Petri M: Thrombosis and systemic lupus erythematosus: the Hopkins
      Lupus Cohort perspective [editorial]. *Scand J Rheumatol* 25:191, 1996.
276. Wallace DJ: The use of chloroquine and hydroxychloroquine for non-
      infectious conditions other than rheumatoid arthritis or lupus: a critical
      review. *Lupus* 5 (suppl 1):S59, 1996.
277. Edwards MH, Pierangeli S, Liu X, et al: Hydroxychloroquine reverses
      thrombogenic properties of antiphospholipid antibodies in mice. *Circula-
      tion* 96:4380, 1997.
278. Asherson RA, Cervera R, Piette JC, et al: Catastrophic antiphospholipid

syndrome. Clinical and laboratory features of 50 patients. *Medicine* 77:195, 1998.

279. Krause I, Blank M, Shoenfeld Y: Immunomodulation of experimental APS: lessons from murine models. *Lupus* 5:458, 1996.

280. Rai R, Cohen H, Dave M, Regan L: Randomised controlled trial of aspirin and aspirin plus heparin in pregnant women with recurrent miscarriage associated with phospholipid antibodies (or antiphospholipid antibodies). *Br Med J* 314:253, 1997.

281. Kutteh WH: Antiphospholipid antibody-associated recurrent pregnancy loss: treatment with heparin and low-dose aspirin is superior to low-dose aspirin alone. *Am J Obstet Gynecol* 174:1584, 1996.

282. Kutteh WH, Ermel LD: A clinical trial for the treatment of antiphospholipid antibody-associated recurrent pregnancy loss with lower dose heparin and aspirin. *Am J Reprod Immunol* 35:402, 1996.

283. Hunt BJ, Doughty HA, Majumdar G, et al: Thromboprophylaxis with low molecular weight heparin (Fragmin) in high risk pregnancies. *Thromb Haemost* 77:39, 1997.

284. Granger KA, Farquharson RG: Obstetric outcome in antiphospholipid syndrome. *Lupus* 6:509, 1997.

285. Lima F, Khamashta MA, Buchanan NM, et al: A study of sixty pregnancies in patients with the antiphospholipid syndrome. *Clin Exp Rheumatol* 14:131, 1996.

286. Dulitzki M, Pauzner R, Langevitz P, et al: Low-molecular-weight heparin during pregnancy and delivery: preliminary experience with 41 pregnancies. *Obstet Gynecol* 87:380, 1996.

287. Cowchock S, Reece EA: Do low-risk pregnant women with antiphospholipid antibodies need to be treated? Organizing Group of the Antiphospholipid Antibody Treatment Trial. *Am J Obstet Gynecol* 176:1099, 1997.

288. Reece EA, Garofalo J, Zheng XZ, Assimakopoulos E: Pregnancy outcome. Influence of antiphospholipid antibody titer, prior pregnancy losses and treatment. *J Reprod Med* 42:49, 1997.

289. Laskin CA, Bombardier C, Hannah ME, et al: Prednisone and aspirin in women with autoantibodies and unexplained recurrent fetal loss. *N Engl J Med* 337:148, 1997.

290. Cowchock S: Treatment of antiphospholipid syndrome in pregnancy. *Lupus* 7 (suppl 2):S95, 1998.

291. Marzusch K, Dietl J, Klein R, et al: Recurrent first trimester spontaneous abortion associated with antiphospholipid antibodies: a pilot study of treatment with intravenous immunoglobulin. *Acta Obstet Gynecol Scand* 75:922, 1996.

VENOUS THROMBOSIS

GARY E. RASKOB
RUSSELL D. HULL
GRAHAM F. PINEO

This chapter provides an overview of the diagnosis and treatment of venous thrombosis, and its major complication, pulmonary embolism. Clinical recommendations are linked to the strength of the evidence from clinical trials. Most clinically important pulmonary emboli arise from proximal deep-vein thrombosis (thrombosis involving the popliteal, femoral, or iliac veins). Upper-extremity deep-vein thrombosis may also lead to clinically important pulmonary embolism. The clinical features of both deep-vein thrombosis and pulmonary embolism are nonspecific, and objective testing is required to confirm or exclude the presence of venous thromboembolism. Strategies for the diagnosis of venous thromboembolism include tests for the detection of pulmonary embolism (lung scanning or pulmonary angiography) and tests for deep-vein thrombosis of the legs (ultrasound, impedance plethysmography, or venography). The measurement of plasma D-dimer by a rapid ELISA technique is useful as an exclusion test in patients with clinically suspected venous thromboembolism. Spiral CT or magnetic resonance imaging (MRI) are useful tests for ruling in the diagnosis of pulmonary embolism if positive results are obtained, but the safety of withholding treatment in patients with negative results remains uncertain. Anticoagulant treatment with continuous intravenous heparin or subcutaneous low-molecular-weight heparin, followed by long-term treatment with oral warfarin sodium, is the treatment of choice for most patients with proximal deep-vein thrombosis and/or submassive pulmonary embolism. Low-molecular-weight heparin enables outpatient therapy for many patients with uncomplicated venous thromboembolism. Thrombolytic therapy is indicated for patients with pulmonary embolism who present with cardiovascular collapse or who have clinical or echocardiographic findings of right ventricular impairment. The role of thrombolytic therapy for patients with deep-vein thrombosis is limited because it remains uncertain whether systemic or catheter-directed thrombolysis will reduce the incidence of the postphlebitic syndrome. The insertion of a vena cava filter is effective for preventing major pulmonary embolism and is indicated for patients with acute venous thromboembolism who have an absolute contraindication to anticoagulant therapy or who have recurrent venous thromboembolism despite adequate anticoagulant treatment.

Acronyms and abbreviations that appear in this chapter include: APTT, activated partial thromboplastin time; DVT, deep-vein thrombosis; ELISA, enzyme-linked immunosorbent assay; HIT, heparin-induced thrombocytopenia; IPG, impedance plethysmography; LMW, low-molecular-weight; MRI, magnetic resonance imaging; PE, pulmonary embolism.

DEFINITION AND HISTORY

Venous thrombosis commonly develops in the deep veins of the leg or the arm, or in the superficial veins of these extremities. Superficial venous thrombosis is a relatively benign disorder unless extension into the deep venous system develops. Thrombosis involving the deep veins of the leg is divided into two prognostic categories: (1) calf-vein thrombosis in which thrombi remain confined to the deep calf veins, and (2) proximal-vein thrombosis in which thrombosis involves the popliteal, femoral, or iliac veins (see "Therapy, Course, and Prognosis," below).[1]

Pulmonary emboli originate from thrombi in the deep veins of the leg in 90 percent or more of patients. Other less common sources of pulmonary embolism include the deep pelvic veins, renal veins, inferior vena cava, right side of the heart, or the axillary veins. Most clinically important pulmonary emboli arise from proximal deep-vein thrombosis of the leg. Upper-extremity deep-vein thrombosis may also lead to clinically important pulmonary embolism.[2] Deep-vein thrombosis and/or pulmonary embolism are referred to collectively as *venous thromboembolism*.

Venous thromboembolism is a common disorder. The estimated annual incidence of symptomatic venous thromboembolism is 117 cases per 100,000 population.[3] This translates to more than 250,000 patients each year in the United States. The incidence of venous thromboembolism increases with each decade over the age of 60. The large proportion of the United States' population that will soon enter into the older age group will make venous thromboembolism an increasingly important national health problem.[3]

Effective prophylaxis against venous thromboembolism is now available for most high-risk patients. The use of prophylaxis is more effective for preventing death and morbidity from venous thromboembolism than is treatment of the established disease. Evidence-based recommendations for the prevention of venous thromboembolism have been published recently.[4]

Historically, venous thromboembolism usually occurred in sick hospitalized patients. More recently, the burden of illness from venous thromboembolism has shifted to the community setting such that most patients now present as outpatients to their primary care physician or the emergency room. The reason for this shift has been the greatly reduced lengths of hospital stay for most surgical procedures or medical conditions in recent years. Consequently, patients who are placed at risk for venous thromboembolism because of surgery or medical illness are discharged from the hospital either before the period of risk has ended or with subclinical venous thrombi present that subsequently evolve and lead to symptomatic deep-vein thrombosis or pulmonary embolism. The shift in burden of illness from the hospital to community setting has stimulated the development of effective, safe, and cost-effective methods for outpatient diagnosis and management.

ETIOLOGY AND PATHOGENESIS

Venous thrombi are composed mainly of fibrin and red blood cells, with variable platelet and leukocyte components. The formation, growth, and breakdown of venous thromboemboli reflect a balance between thrombogenic stimuli and protective mechanisms. The thrombogenic stimuli are (1) venous stasis, (2) activation of blood coagulation, and (3) vein damage. The protective mechanisms are (1) the inactivation of activated coagulation factors by circulating inhibitors (e.g., antithrombin III, activated protein C), (2) clearance of activated coagulation factors and soluble fibrin polymer complexes by the reticuloendothelial system and by the liver, and (3) lysis of fibrin by fibrinolytic enzymes derived from plasma, endothelial cells, and leukocytes.

Risk factors for venous thromboembolism include advancing age (greater than 40 years), a past history of venous thromboembolism, surgery or trauma, immobilization, cancer, congestive heart failure, myocardial infarction, leg paralysis, estrogens, pregnancy or postpartum state, varicose veins, obesity, antiphospholipid antibody syndrome, hyperhomocysteinemia, and several inherited prothrombotic conditions. These inherited conditions include activated protein C resistance, prothrombin 20210 A, deficiencies of antithrombin III, protein C or protein S, and several types of dysfibrinogenemia (see Chaps. 124 and 127). The risk of thromboembolism is increased when more than one predisposing factor is present.

Activated protein C resistance is the most common hereditary abnormality predisposing to venous thrombosis. The defect is due to substitution of glutamine for arginine at residue 506 in the *factor V molecule*, making factor V resistant to proteolysis by activated protein C. The gene mutation is commonly designated as *factor V Leiden* and follows autosomal dominant inheritance. Patients who are homozygous for the factor V Leiden mutation have a markedly increased risk of thromboembolism and present with clinical thromboembolism at a younger age (median 31 years) than those who are heterozygous (median age 46 years).[5] Factor V Leiden is present in approximately 5 percent of the normal Caucasian population, in 16 percent of patients with a first-episode of deep-vein thrombosis, and in up to 35 percent of patients with idiopathic deep-vein thrombosis.[6] Prothrombin 20210 A is a recently identified gene mutation predisposing to venous thromboembolism. It is present in approximately 2 to 3 percent of apparently healthy individuals and in 7 percent of those with deep-vein thrombosis.[7] In 40 percent to up to 60 percent of patients with idiopathic deep-vein thrombosis, an inherited abnormality cannot be detected, suggesting that other gene mutations are present and may have an etiologic role.

Pulmonary embolism occurs in 50 percent of patients with objectively documented proximal-vein thrombosis.[1] Many of these emboli are asymptomatic. The clinical importance of pulmonary embolism depends on the size of the embolus and the patient's cardiorespiratory reserve. Usually only part of the thrombus embolizes, and thus 30 percent to 70 percent of patients with pulmonary embolism by angiography also have detectable deep-vein thrombosis of the legs.[8] Deep-vein thrombosis and pulmonary embolism are not separate disorders but a continuous syndrome of venous thromboembolism, in which the initial clinical presentation may be symptoms of either deep-vein thrombosis or pulmonary embolism. Strategies for the detection of venous thromboembolism include tests for the detection of pulmonary embolism (lung scanning or pulmonary angiography)[8,9] and tests for deep-vein thrombosis of the legs (ultrasound, impedance plethysmography, or venography)[10–12] (see sections on "Objective Testing").

CLINICAL FEATURES

The clinical features of venous thrombosis include leg pain, tenderness, and swelling, a palpable cord (i.e., a thrombosed vessel that is palpable as a cord), discoloration, venous distention, and prominence of the superficial veins, and cyanosis. The clinical diagnosis of deep-vein thrombosis is highly nonspecific because each of the symptoms or signs may be caused by nonthrombotic disorders. The rare exception is the patient with phlegmasia cerulea dolens, in whom the diagnosis of massive ilieofemoral thrombosis is obvious. This syndrome occurs in less than 1 percent of patients with symptomatic venous thrombosis. In most patients, the symptoms and signs are nonspecific, and in 50 percent to 85 percent of patients the clinical suspicion of deep-vein thrombosis is not confirmed by objective testing.[10–12] Patients with minor symptoms and signs may have extensive deep-venous thrombi. Conversely, patients with florid leg pain and swelling, suggesting extensive deep-vein thrombosis, may have negative results by objective testing. Patients can be assigned pretest probabilities of deep-

vein thrombosis based on the patient's clinical features and history. However, these pretest probabilities are neither sufficiently high to give anticoagulant treatment or sufficiently low to withhold treatment without performing objective testing.

The clinical features of acute pulmonary embolism include the following syndromes which may overlap: (1) transient dyspnea and tachypnea in the absence of other clinical features, (2) the syndrome of pulmonary infarction or congestive atelectasis (also known as *ischemic pneumonitis* or *incomplete infarction*), including pleuritic chest pain, cough, hemoptysis, pleural effusion, and pulmonary infiltrates on chest radiograph, (3) right-sided heart failure associated with severe dyspnea and tachypnea, (4) cardiovascular collapse with hypotension, syncope, and coma (usually associated with massive pulmonary embolism), and (5) several less common and nonspecific clinical presentations including unexplained tachycardia or arrhythmia, resistant cardiac failure, wheezing, cough, fever, anxiety/apprehension, or confusion. All the above clinical features are nonspecific and may be caused by a variety of cardiorespiratory disorders. Objective testing is mandatory to confirm or exclude the presence of pulmonary embolism. Classifying patients into categories of pretest probability (low, intermediate, or high) is useful in only a minority of patients when combined with lung scan findings.

LABORATORY FEATURES

Venous thromboembolism is associated with nonspecific laboratory changes that make up the acute-phase response to tissue injury. This response includes elevated levels of fibrinogen and factor VIII, increases in the leukocyte and platelet counts, and systemic activation of blood coagulation, fibrin formation, and fibrin breakdown, with increases in the plasma concentrations of prothrombin fragment 1.2, fibrinopeptide A, complexes of thrombin-antithrombin III, and fibrin degradation products. All these changes are nonspecific and may occur as the result of surgery, trauma, infection, inflammation, or infarction. None of the reported laboratory changes can be used to predict the development of venous thromboembolism.

The fibrin breakdown fragment D-dimer can be measured by an enzyme-linked immunosorbant assay or by a latex agglutination assay. Some of these assays have a rapid turnaround time and some are quantitative. The D-dimer may be useful as an exclusionary test for patients with suspected venous thromboembolism (see sections on "Objective Testing").[13–16] A positive result is highly nonspecific.[13,14]

DIFFERENTIAL DIAGNOSIS

DIFFERENTIAL DIAGNOSIS OF DEEP-VEIN THROMBOSIS

The differential diagnosis in patients with clinically suspected deep-vein thrombosis includes muscle strain or tear, direct twisting injury to the leg, lymphangitis or lymphatic obstruction, venous reflux, popliteal cyst, cellulitis, leg swelling in a paralyzed limb, and abnormality of the knee joint. An alternate diagnosis is frequently not evident at presentation, and so, without objective testing, it is impossible to exclude deep-vein thrombosis. The cause of symptoms can often be determined by careful follow-up once deep-vein thrombosis has been excluded by objective testing. In approximately 25 percent of patients, however, the cause of pain, tenderness, and swelling remains uncertain even after careful follow-up.

OBJECTIVE TESTING FOR DEEP-VEIN THROMBOSIS

The objective tests that have a role in diagnosing patients with clinically suspected deep-vein thrombosis are ultrasound imaging, impedance plethysmography, and venography. Each of these tests has been validated by properly designed clinical trials, including prospective studies with long-term follow-up that have established the safety of withholding anticoagulant treatment in patients with negative test results.[10,11,17]

Noninvasive testing with either ultrasound imaging or impedance plethysmography is effective for identifying patients with proximal-vein thrombosis. Both tests have limited sensitivity for calf-vein thrombosis and require serial testing to detect extension of calf-vein thrombosis into the popliteal vein or more proximally. When performed serially, these tests can safely replace venography in symptomatic patients. Venography continues to have an important role in selected patients, such as those for whom serial testing is impractical, and those with abnormal noninvasive test results who have conditions known to produce false positive results.

The wide availability of ultrasound imaging has supplanted impedance plethysmography as the principal noninvasive test for deep-vein thrombosis in most centers. However, the value of impedance plethysmography for patients with suspected acute recurrent deep-vein thrombosis is underappreciated. One logical approach is to use ultrasound imaging with vein compression as the initial test for patients with suspected *first-episode* deep-vein thrombosis (Fig. 129-1) and impedance plethysmography as the preferred initial test for patients with suspected *recurrent* deep-vein thrombosis (Fig. 129-2).

Ultrasound imaging using vein compression has two practical advantages: (1) It is more sensitive than impedance plethysmography for small nonocclusive thrombi that barely extend into the popliteal vein, and this enables serial testing to be limited to a single repeat test done 5 to 7 days after presentation, and (2) it is not influenced by congestive cardiac failure or by disorders which impair deep-venous filling (e.g., peripheral arterial disease), which may produce false positive impedance plethysmography results.

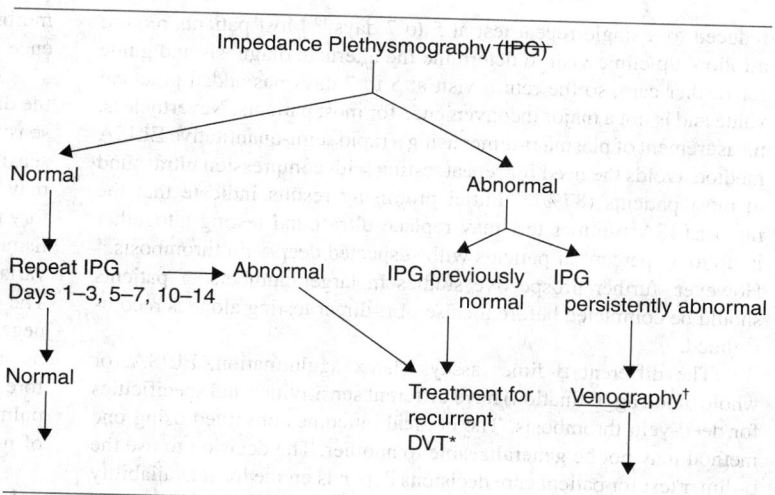

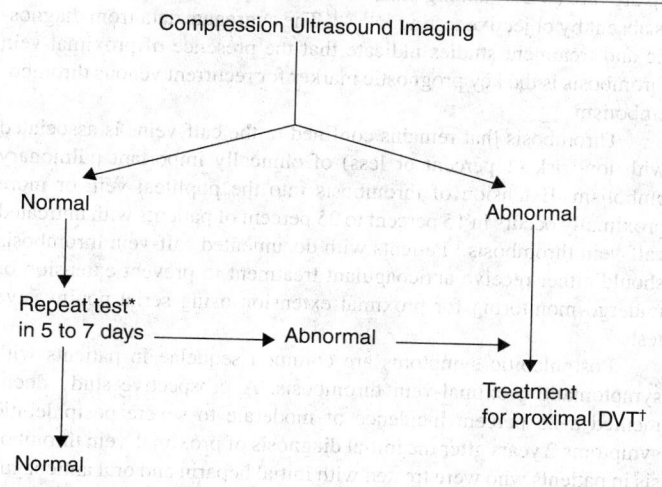

FIGURE 129-1   Diagnosis and therapy of patients with suspected first-episode deep-vein thrombosis (DVT). Imaging of the common femoral vein in the groin and of the popliteal vein in the popliteal fossa extending distally 10 cm from mid-patella.

*Repeat test can be avoided if a measurement of plasma D-dimer is negative using a rapid ELISA technique.[15]

†Perform additional testing, including venography and/or CT or MR imaging, if ultrasound is abnormal only at the common femoral vein site.

FIGURE 129-2   Diagnosis and therapy of patients with suspected recurrent deep-vein thrombosis.

*Venography should also be performed in patients with new abnormal IPG results if a concurrent condition is present that can produce falsely abnormal test results.

†The criterion for diagnosing an acute recurrent deep-vein thrombosis by venography is the finding of a new intraluminal filling defect that is constant on all films. In some patients, venography cannot establish or exclude the presence of acute recurrent deep-vein thrombosis (i.e. an indeterminate venogram), due to the presence of persistent intraluminal filling defects, non-visualized venous segments, and/or extensive collateral veins. In such patients, anticoagulant treatment should probably be given rather than risk death from massive pulmonary embolism.

In the absence of these conditions, impedance plethysmography has a similarly high positive predictive value (>90%) to compression ultrasound,[10,11] but clinical examination of the patient is required to exclude potential causes of false positive results.

Impedance plethysmography is a valuable test for patients with suspected recurrent deep-vein thrombosis because the test returns to normal earlier in patients with proximal-vein thrombosis than does compression ultrasound. Impedance plethysmography returns to normal in 65 percent of patients by 3 months, 85 percent by 6 months, and 95 percent by 1 year, compared to 30 percent, 45 percent, and 60 percent respectively for compression ultrasound. Compression ultrasound may remain abnormal for 2 years or more due to persistent noncompressibility of the vein caused by fibrous organization of the original thrombus. A normal impedance plethysmography result obtained at the time of completing anticoagulant treatment at 3 to 6 months provides a useful baseline for future comparison. An impedance plethysmography result which has changed from normal to abnormal is highly predictive of acute recurrent proximal-vein thrombosis.[12] The finding of a new noncompressible venous segment by ultrasound is probably highly predictive of acute recurrent thrombosis, but this criterion is of limited value, since many patients have persistently noncompressible venous segments due to the initial episode. To date, no criteria by ultrasound imaging for the presence or absence of acute recurrent deep-vein thrombosis have been validated by prospective follow-up studies to establish the safety of withholding anticoagulant treatment.

Studies have suggested a high negative predictive value of D-dimer for acute deep-vein thrombosis.[13–16] The measurement of plasma D-dimer is useful in patients with initially negative noninvasive test results to exclude the presence of deep-vein thrombosis and avoid the need for repeated testing.[15] However, this is less important now in patients with suspected first-episode deep-vein thrombosis because the need for repeated testing with compression ultrasound has been reduced to a single repeat test at 5 to 7 days.[10] Most patients require a follow-up clinic visit to determine the alternate diagnosis and guide for further care, so the return visit at 5 to 7 days has added practical value and is not a major inconvenience for most patients. Nevertheless, measurement of plasma D-dimer using a rapid semi-quantitative ELISA method avoids the need for repeat testing with compression ultrasound in most patients (87%).[15] Initial promising results indicate that the rapid ELISA D-dimer test may replace ultrasound testing altogether in up to 30 percent of patients with suspected deep-vein thrombosis.[16] However, further prospective studies in larger numbers of patients should be completed before the use of D-dimer testing alone is recommended.

The different D-dimer assays (latex agglutination, ELISA, or whole blood agglutination) have different sensitivities and specificities for deep-vein thrombosis. The clinical outcomes observed using one method may not be generalizeable to another. The decision to use the D-dimer test for patient care decisions depends on the local availability of an appropriate assay that has been validated by clinical outcome studies.

The value of D-dimer is potentially greater in patients with suspected acute recurrent deep-vein thrombosis. However, the safety of withholding anticoagulant treatment in such patients with negative D-dimer results has not been established by adequately designed clinical trials.

DIFFERENTIAL DIAGNOSIS OF PULMONARY EMBOLISM

The differential diagnosis in patients with suspected pulmonary embolism includes multiple cardiopulmonary disorders for each of the clinical syndromes. For the presentation of dyspnea and tachypnea these include atelectasis, pneumonia, pneumothorax, acute pulmonary edema, bronchitis, bronchiolitis, and acute bronchial obstruction. For the syndrome of pulmonary infarction (e.g., pleuritic chest pain, hemoptysis) these include pneumonia, pneumothorax, pericarditis, pulmonary or bronchial neoplasm, bronchiectasis, acute bronchitis, tuberculosis, diaphragmatic inflammation, myositis, muscle strain, and rib fracture. For the clinical presentation of right-sided heart failure, these include myocardial infarction, myocarditis, and cardiac tamponade. For cardiovascular collapse this includes myocardial infarction, acute massive hemorrhage, gram-negative septicemia, cardiac tamponade, and spontaneous pneumothorax.

OBJECTIVE TESTING FOR PULMONARY EMBOLISM

The key tests include lung scanning, pulmonary angiography, and objective testing for proximal deep-vein thrombosis. The diagnostic approach is summarized in Fig. 129-3.

Objective testing for deep-vein thrombosis is useful in patients with suspected pulmonary embolism, particularly those with nondiagnostic lung scan results (indeterminate, intermediate, or low-probability categories). The detection of proximal-vein thrombosis by objective testing provides an indication for anticoagulant treatment, regardless of the presence or absence of pulmonary embolism, and avoids the need for further testing. A negative result by objective testing for deep-vein thrombosis does not exclude the presence of pulmonary embolism.[8] If the patient has adequate cardiorespiratory reserve, then serial noninvasive testing for proximal-vein thrombosis may be used as an alternative to pulmonary angiography[18] (see Fig. 129-3). The rationale is that the clinical objective in such patients is to prevent recurrent pulmonary embolism, which is unlikely in the absence of proximal-vein thrombosis. For patients with inadequate cardiorespiratory reserve (Fig. 129-3), the clinical objective is to prevent death and

morbidity from an existing embolus, and further testing for the presence or absence of pulmonary embolism is needed.

Both spiral CT imaging and MRI are promising approaches for the diagnosis of pulmonary embolism.[19,20] Spiral CT imaging is highly sensitive for large emboli (segmental or greater arteries) but is less sensitive for emboli in subsegmental pulmonary arteries. Such emboli may be clinically important in patients with inadequate cardiorespiratory reserve. MRI appears to be highly sensitive for pulmonary embolism. However, a recent study documented significant interobserver variation in the sensitivity, ranging from 70 percent to 100 percent.[20] The safety of withholding anticoagulant treatment in patients with negative results by spiral CT imaging or MRI has not been established by prospective clinical trials incorporating long-term follow-up. Therefore, spiral CT or MRI are useful tests for ruling in the diagnosis of pulmonary embolism if positive results are obtained, but the validity of negative results remains uncertain.

The assay for plasma D-dimer is potentially useful to exclude pulmonary embolism based on a high negative predictive value reported in initial studies from centers with research expertise in measuring D-dimer.[13,14] Promising outcome results have been obtained using a rapid ELISA technique.[16] However, further studies in larger numbers of patients are required to establish the safety of withholding anticoagulant treatment in patients with suspected pulmonary embolism who have a negative D-dimer result.

THERAPY, COURSE, AND PROGNOSIS

CLINICAL COURSE OF VENOUS THROMBOEMBOLISM

Proximal deep-vein thrombosis is a serious and potentially lethal condition. Untreated proximal-vein thrombosis is associated with a 10 percent rate of fatal pulmonary embolism. Inadequately treated proximal-vein thrombosis results in a 20 percent to 50 percent risk of important recurrent venous thromboembolic events.[21-23] Prospective studies of patients with clinically suspected deep-vein thrombosis or pulmonary embolism indicate that new venous thromboembolic events on follow-up are rare (≤2%) among patients in whom proximal-vein thrombosis is absent by objective testing.[10,11,15-18] The aggregate data from diagnostic and treatment studies indicate that the presence of proximal-vein thrombosis is the key prognostic marker for recurrent venous thromboembolism.

Thrombosis that remains confined to the calf-veins is associated with low risk (1 percent or less) of clinically important pulmonary embolism. Extension of thrombosis into the popliteal vein or more proximally occurs in 15 percent to 25 percent of patients with untreated calf-vein thrombosis.[1] Patients with documented calf-vein thrombosis should either receive anticoagulant treatment to prevent extension or undergo monitoring for proximal extension using serial noninvasive tests.

Postphlebitic symptoms are common sequelae in patients with symptomatic proximal-vein thrombosis. A prospective study documented a 25 percent incidence of moderate to severe postphlebitic symptoms 2 years after the initial diagnosis of proximal-vein thrombosis in patients who were treated with initial heparin and oral anticoagulants for 3 months.[24] This study also demonstrated that ipsilateral recurrent venous thrombosis is strongly associated with the subsequent development of moderate or severe postphlebitic symptoms.

OBJECTIVES OF ANTITHROMBOTIC TREATMENT

The objectives of treatment in patients with established venous thromboembolism are (1) to prevent death from pulmonary embolism, (2)

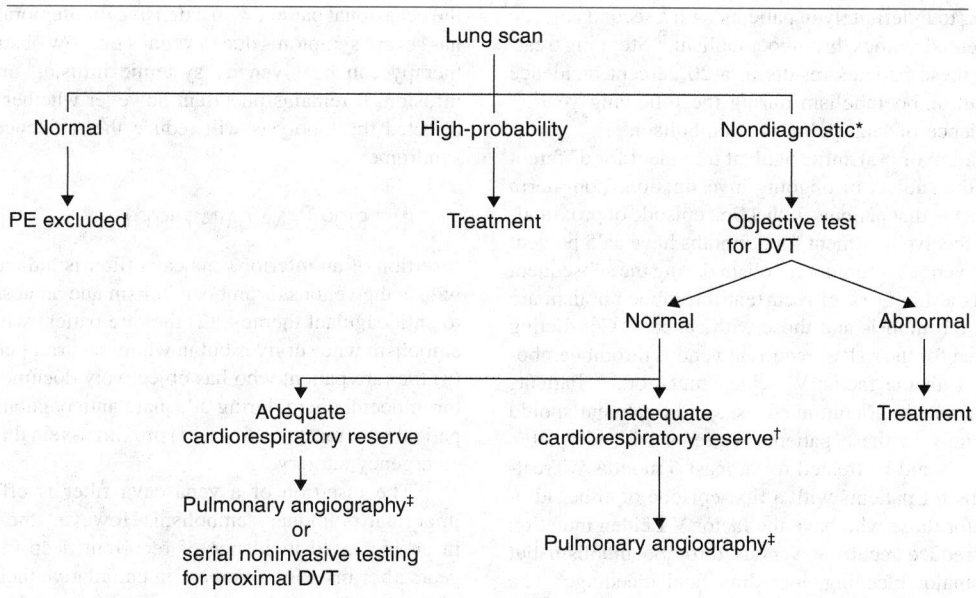

FIGURE 129-3   Diagnosis and therapy of patients with suspected pulmonary embolism (PE).

*Nondiagnostic includes the intermediate, indeterminate, and low-probability lung scan patterns.

†Cardiorespiratory reserve is "inadequate" if one or more of the following are present: syncope, hypotension (systolic blood pressure less than 90 mm Hg), pulmonary edema, clinical findings of right heart failure or echocardiographic evidence of right ventricular hypokinesis, acute tachyarrhythmia, severe hypoxemia ($PO_2 <$ 50 mm Hg), or severe respiratory insufficiency ($PCO_2 <$ 45 mm Hg, $FEV_1 <$ 1.0, vital capacity $<$ 1.5 liter).

‡CT or MR imaging may be performed before pulmonary angiography—a positive result by these imaging techniques is useful for establishing the presence of pulmonary embolism, but the safety of withholding treatment in patients with negative results by CT or MR imaging is uncertain (particularly in patients with inadequate cardiorespiratory reserve).

to prevent morbidity from recurrent venous thrombosis or pulmonary embolism, and (3) to prevent or minimize the postphlebitic syndrome.

For most patients, the first two objectives are achieved by providing adequate anticoagulant treatment. Thrombolytic therapy is indicated in selected patients with pulmonary embolism (see "Thrombolytic Therapy"). The use of an inferior vena cava filter is indicated to prevent death from pulmonary embolism in patients in whom anticoagulant treatment is absolutely contraindicated and in other selected patients (see Inferior "Vena Cava Filter").

ANTICOAGULANT THERAPY

Anticoagulant therapy is the treatment of choice for most patients with proximal-vein thrombosis or pulmonary embolism. The absolute contraindications to anticoagulant treatment include intracranial bleeding, serious active bleeding, recent brain, eye, or spinal cord surgery, and malignant hypertension. Relative contraindications include recent major surgery, recent cerebrovascular accident, active gastrointestinal tract bleeding, severe hypertension, severe renal or hepatic failure, and severe thrombocytopenia (platelets $<$ 50,000/μl).

Patients with proximal-vein thrombosis require both adequate initial anticoagulant treatment with heparin or low-molecular-weight (LMW) heparin, and adequate long-term anticoagulant therapy to prevent recurrent venous thromboembolism.[21-23] Adequate anticoagulant treatment reduces the incidence of recurrent venous thromboembolism during the first three months after diagnosis from 25 percent to 5 percent or less.[21-23]

Initial therapy with continuous intravenous heparin has been the standard approach for treatment of deep-vein thrombosis or pulmonary embolism for more than 20 years. More recently, LMW heparin given by subcutaneous injection once or twice daily has been shown to be as effective and safe as continuous intravenous heparin for the initial treatment of patients with proximal-vein thrombosis and submassive pulmonary embolism.[21] If unfractionated heparin is given for initial therapy, it is important to achieve an adequate anticoagulant effect, defined as an activated partial thromboplastin time (APTT) above the lower limit of therapeutic range within the first 24 hours.[22] Failure to achieve an adequate APTT effect early during therapy is associated with a high incidence (25%) of recurrent venous thromboembolism[22]; two-thirds of these recurrent events occur between 2 and 12 weeks after the initial diagnosis, despite treatment with oral anticoagulants.[23] The clinical trial data indicate that the initial management with either unfractionated heparin or LMW heparin is critical to the patient's long-term outcome.[23]

LMW heparin has the advantage that it does not require anticoagulant monitoring and dose finding. LMW heparin enables outpatient therapy for many patients with uncomplicated proximal-vein thrombosis. Outpatient LMW heparin therapy provides the potential for major cost savings to the health care system compared to therapy with unfractionated heparin in-hospital, without detracting from the effectiveness or safety of treatment. Further details of therapy with unfractionated heparin and LMW heparin are given in Chap. 133, including treatment regimens, monitoring, and adverse effects.

Oral anticoagulant therapy is begun together with initial heparin or LMW heparin therapy and overlapped for 4 to 5 days. Oral anticoagulant treatment is continued for 3 to 6 months in patients with a first-episode of proximal-vein thrombosis or pulmonary embolism. Stopping oral anticoagulant treatment at 4 to 6 weeks results in a high incidence (12% to 20%) of recurrent venous thromboembolism during the following 12 to 24 months.[25] Oral anticoagulant treatment should be continued for 1 year to indefinitely in patients with a second episode of objectively documented venous thromboembolism.[26] Stopping treatment at 3 months in these patients results in a 20 percent incidence of recurrent venous thromboembolism during the following year[12,26] and a 5 percent incidence of fatal pulmonary embolism.[12]

The optimal duration of oral anticoagulant treatment for different patient subgroups is the subject of ongoing investigation. Long-term follow-up studies indicate that patients with a first episode of proximal-vein thrombosis who receive treatment for 3 months have a 25 percent incidence of recurrent venous thromboembolism during the subsequent 5 years.[24] The patients at high risk of recurrent thromboembolism are those with idiopathic thrombosis and those with cancer.[24] Conflicting data have been reported for the risk of recurrent venous thromboembolism among patients with the factor V Leiden mutation.[6,27] Patients with advanced cancer remain at continued risk, and treatment should be continued indefinitely in these patients. Patients with idiopathic deep-vein thrombosis should be treated for at least 6 months.[21] Treatment beyond 6 months for patients with a first-episode of either idiopathic thrombosis or for those who have the factor V Leiden mutation has the potential to reduce recurrent venous thromboembolism but also has the risk of major bleeding, including fatal bleeding.[26] The relative risk-benefit of extending treatment beyond 6 months for selected patients with a first-episode of venous thromboembolism awaits the results of ongoing clinical trials. Further details of oral anticoagulant treatment are provided in Chap. 132.

Adjusted dose subcutaneous heparin is the long-term anticoagulant regimen of choice in pregnant patients (see Chap. 133 for further details). LMW heparin and heparinoids do not cross the placenta, and initial experience suggests these agents are safe for use in pregnant patients.[28] However, controlled clinical trials comparing the efficacy and safety of LMW heparin with unfractionated heparin in pregnant patients have not been completed. It is also uncertain if the dosing regimens for LMW heparin evaluated by clinical trials in nonpregnant patients are generalizeable to the pregnant patient. LMW heparin has the advantages of causing less thrombocytopenia and potentially less osteoporosis than unfractionated heparin. However, routine use of LMW heparin for the pregnant patient is currently not recommended because of a lack of clinical trial data documenting efficacy and safety.[28] Danaparoid is the preferred drug for pregnant patients with acute heparin-induced thrombocytopenia (HIT) or with a history of HIT who require anticoagulant treatment.[28]

LMW heparin given once daily by subcutaneous injection without monitoring is currently undergoing evaluation by clinical trials for the long-term treatment of deep-vein thrombosis.

THROMBOLYTIC THERAPY

Thrombolytic therapy is indicated for patients with pulmonary embolism who present with evidence of vascular collapse (hypotension and/or syncope) and for patients with pulmonary embolism who have clinical findings of right ventricular failure or echocardiographic evidence of right ventricular hypokinesis. Thrombolytic therapy provides more rapid lysis of pulmonary emboli and more rapid restoration of right ventricular function and pulmonary perfusion than anticoagulant treatment.[29] An effective regimen is 100 mg of rtPA by intravenous infusion over 2 h (50 mg per h). Heparin is then given by continuous infusion once the thrombin time or activated partial thromboplastin time is less than twice control.[29] The starting infusion dose is 1000 units/h. Further details of thrombolytic therapy are given in Chap. 134.

The role of thrombolytic therapy for patients with deep-vein thrombosis is currently very limited. Thrombolytic therapy may be indicated in patients with acute massive proximal-vein thrombosis (phlegmasia cerulea dolens with impending venous gangrene) or in

the occasional patient with extensive ilieofemoral vein thrombosis who has severe symptoms due to venous outflow obstruction. Thrombolytic therapy can be given by systemic infusion or by catheter-directed infusion. It remains uncertain however whether systemic or catheter-directed thrombolysis will reduce the incidence of the postphlebitic syndrome.

INFERIOR VENA CAVA FILTER

Insertion of an inferior vena cava filter is indicated for (1) the patient with acute venous thromboembolism and an absolute contraindication to anticoagulant therapy, (2) the rare patient with massive pulmonary embolism who survives but in whom recurrent embolism may be fatal, (3) the rare patient who has objectively documented recurrent venous thromboembolism during adequate anticoagulant therapy, and (4) the patient with recent (<6 weeks) proximal-vein thrombosis who requires emergency surgery.

The insertion of a vena cava filter is effective for preventing important pulmonary embolism. However, the use of a filter results in an increased incidence of recurrent deep-vein thrombosis 1 to 2 years after insertion (increase in cumulative incidence at 2 years from 12% to 21%).[30] If it is not contraindicated, long-term anticoagulant treatment should be administered after placement of a vena cava filter to prevent morbidity from recurrent deep-vein thrombosis.

REFERENCES

1. Moser KM, Lemoine JR: Is embolic risk conditioned by localization of deep venous thrombosis? *Ann Intern Med* 94:439, 1981.
2. Prandoni P, Polistena P, Bernardi E, et al: Upper-extremity deep vein thrombosis. Risk factors, diagnosis and complications. *Arch Intern Med* 157:57, 1997.
3. Silverstein MD, Heit JA, Mohr DN, Petterson TM, O'Fallon WM, Melton LJ: Trends in the incidence of deep vein thrombosis and pulmonary embolism. A 25-year population-based study. *Arch Intern Med* 158:585, 1998.
4. Clagett GP, Anderson FA, Geerts W, et al: Prevention of venous thromboembolism. *Chest* 114::531s, 1998.
5. Rosendaal FR, Koster T, Vandebroucke JP, Reitsma PH. High risk of thrombosis in patients homozygous for Factor V Leiden (activated Protein C resistance). *Blood* 85:1504, 1995
6. Simioni P, Prandoni P, Lensing AWA, et al: The risk of recurrent venous thromboembolism in patients with an Arg[506]→Gln mutation in the gene for factor V (factor V Leiden). *N Engl J Med* 336:399, 1997.
7. Rosendaal FR, Doggen CJM, Zivelin A, et al. Geographic distribution of the 20210 G to A prothrombin variant. *Thromb Haemost* 79:706, 1998.
8. Hull R, Hirsh J, Carter C, et al: Diagnostic value of ventilation-perfusion lung scanning in patients with suspected pulmonary embolism. *Chest* 88:819, 1985.
9. The PIOPED Investigators: Value of the ventilation/perfusion scan in acute pulmonary embolism: results of the Prospective Investigation of Pulmonary Embolism Diagnosis (PIOPED). *JAMA* 263:2753, 1990.
10. Birdwell BG, Raskob GE, Whitsett TL, et al: The clinical validity of normal compression ultrasonography in outpatients suspected of having deep venous thrombosis. *Ann Intern Med* 128:1, 1998.
11. Hull RD, Hirsh J, Carter CJ, et al: Diagnostic efficacy of impedance plethysmography for clinically suspected deep-vein thrombosis. *Ann Intern Med* 102:21, 1985.
12. Hull RD, Carter CJ, Jay RM, et al: The diagnosis of acute, recurrent deep-vein thrombosis: a diagnostic challenge. *Circulation* 67:901, 1983.
13. Becker DM, Philbrick JT, Bachhuber TL, Humpries JE: D-dimer testing and acute venous thromboembolism: a shortcut to accurate diagnosis? *Arch Intern Med* 156:939, 1996.
14. Turkstra F, van Beek EJR, ten Cate JW, Buller HR: Reliable rapid blood test for the exclusion of venous thromboembolism in symptomatic outpatients. *Thromb Haemost* 76:9, 1996.
15. Bernardi E, Prandoni P, Lensing AW, et al: D-dimer testing as an adjunct to ultrasonography in patients with clinically suspected deep-vein thrombosis: prospective cohort study. *BMJ* 317:1037, 1998.

16. Perrier A, Desmarais S, Miron MJ, et al: Non-invasive diagnosis of venous thromboembolism in outpatients. *Lancet* 353:190, 1999.

17. Hull R, Hirsh J, Sackett DL, et al: Clinical validity of a negative venogram in patients with clinically suspected venous thrombosis. *Circulation* 64:622, 1981.

18. Hull RD, Raskob GE, Ginsberg JS, et al: A noninvasive strategy for the treatment of patients with suspected pulmonary embolism. *Arch Intern Med* 154:289, 1994.

19. Mayo JR, Remy-Jardin M, Muller NL, et al: Pulmonary embolism: prospective comparison of spiral CT with ventilation-perfusion scintigraphy. *Radiology* 205:447, 1997.

20. Meaney JFM, Weg JG, Chenevert TL, et al: Diagnosis of pulmonary embolism with magnetic resonance angiography. *N Engl J Med* 336:1422, 1997.

21. Hyers TM, Agnelli G, Hull RD, et al: Antithrombotic therapy for venous thromboembolic disease. *Chest* 114:561s, 1998.

22. Hull RD, Raskob GE, Brant RF, Pineo GF, Valentine KA: Relation between the time to achieve the lower limit of the APTT therapeutic range and recurrent venous thromboembolism during heparin treatment for deep vein thrombosis. *Arch Intern Med* 157:2562, 1997.

23. Hull RD, Raskob GE, Brant RF, Pineo GF, Valentin KA: The importance of initial heparin treatment on long-term clinical outcomes of antithrombotic therapy: the emerging theme of delayed recurrence. *Arch Intern Med* 157:2317, 1997.

24. Prandoni P, Lensing AWA, Cogo A, et al: The long-term clinical course of acute deep venous thrombosis. *Ann Intern Med* 125:1, 1996.

25. Schulman S, Rhedin A-S, Lindmarker P, et al: A comparison of six weeks with six months of oral anticoagulant therapy after a first episode of venous thromboembolism. *N Engl J Med* 332:1661, 1995.

26. Schulman S, Granqvist S, Holmström M, et al: The duration of oral anticoagulant therapy after a second episode of venous thromboembolism. *N Engl J Med* 336:393, 1997.

27. Eichinger S, Pabinger I, Stumpflen A, et al: The risk of recurrent venous thromboembolism in patients with and without Factor V Leiden. *Thromb Haemost* 77:624, 1997.

28. Ginsberg JS, Hirsh J: Use of antithrombotic agents during pregnancy. *Chest* 114:524s, 1998.

29. Goldhaber SZ, Haire WD, Feldstein ML, et al: Alteplase versus heparin in acute pulmonary embolism: randomised trial assessing right-ventricular function and pulmonary perfusion. *Lancet* 341:507, 1993.

30. Decousus H, Leizorovicz A, Parent F, et al: A clinical trial of vena caval filters in the prevention of pulmonary embolism in patients with proximal deep-vein thrombosis. *N Engl J Med* 338:409, 1998.

CHAPTER 130

ATHEROSCLEROSIS, THROMBOSIS, AND CORONARY ARTERY DISEASE

MARK B. TAUBMAN

Atherosclerosis manifested by cardiovascular, cerebrovascular, and peripheral vascular disease is the leading underlying cause of mortality in the United States and other industrialized countries. This disease is characterized by an inflammatory and proliferative response of the arterial wall and the subsequent development of thrombosis, often in association with plaque rupture. Many of the important developments in the treatment of acute coronary syndromes, such as the use of aspirin, thrombolytic drugs, and antiplatelet agents, have targeted the thrombotic component of atherosclerosis.

Tissue factor (TF) is thought to be a key determinant of plaque thrombogenicity and of the hypercoagulable state associated with acute arterial injury. The cellular source of plaque TF is likely to be macrophages and smooth-muscle cells (SMC). However, the location of the TF most important for initiating or propagating arterial thrombosis may be extracellular, arising from cell necrosis, apoptosis, and vesiculation from the cell surface. Circulating TF may also play an important role in determining the extent of arterial thrombosis. The fibrinolytic system is thought to provide the normal arterial wall with an antithrombotic surface. However, the role of plasminogen activators in protecting injured or atherosclerotic vessels against thrombosis remains controversial. Plasmin may also be important in mediating vascular remodeling by its effects on metalloproteinase activation and SMC proliferation and migration.

INTRODUCTION: CORONARY ARTERY DISEASE AND THROMBOSIS

Atherosclerosis is the leading underlying cause of mortality in the United States and other industrialized countries.[1,2] The major manifestations of atherosclerosis are coronary artery disease (CAD) (myocardial infarction (MI), angina, sudden death), cerebrovascular disease (ischemic stroke), and peripheral vascular disease (intermittent claudication, ischemic limbs). It is estimated that more than 1.5 million MIs occur annually in the United States, with approximately 500,000 resulting in death[2]. A substantial portion of these deaths (200–300,000) occur before patients reach the hospital, largely due to arrhythmias.[2]

An additional 200,000 deaths are attributable to stroke and peripheral vascular disease. Among survivors of MI, approximately 200,000 die annually from complications of heart failure; this number is rising as the incidence of death from acute MI falls.

The association of coronary atherosclerosis with thrombosis was first made in 1912 by Herrick,[3] who noted thrombotic coronary occlusions in patients presenting with acute MI. Subsequently, the term *coronary thrombosis* entered the vernacular to describe MI. In an autopsy study of patients dying of MI in 1966, Constantinides[4] demonstrated that thrombotic occlusion was associated with fractures of the fibrous lining of atherosclerotic plaques. A series of studies by Davies and colleagues[5-7] further established the importance of plaque rupture as the cause of acute ischemic syndromes—MI, unstable angina (UA), and sudden death.

Studies demonstrating that coronary artery spasm might be an important cause of MI in patients with coronary atherosclerosis[8,9] led to a reevaluation in the 1970s of the role of thrombosis as the precipitating event in acute coronary syndromes and raised a question as to whether the thrombus seen at autopsy was deposited subsequent to a vasospastic occlusive event.

In the 1980s, the identification of thrombosis on coronary angiography,[10] and studies demonstrating the efficacy of intracoronary[11] and intravenous[12,13] thrombolysis in opening occluded coronary arteries refocused attention on thrombosis as the main cause of acute MI. The success of aspirin in the treatment of UA and in secondary prevention of MI[13,14] further helped to establish thrombosis as a major cause of acute coronary events and also suggested that platelet aggregation played a critical role. The importance of platelet aggregation has been buttressed by the success of new antiplatelet agents in the treatment of acute coronary syndromes.[15,16] Although the mechanism of coronary thrombosis remains to be fully elucidated, the inciting event in the majority of patients appears to be rupture of the atherosclerotic plaque.

The Framingham Heart Study was established in 1948 to examine factors associated with risk for CAD.[17] To date, approximately 75 percent of the original Framingham Heart Study participants have died, the leading cause of death being CAD. The Framingham Heart Study was instrumental in defining the risk factors for CAD.[18] Many other programs have subsequently provided important data to corroborate the Framingham findings and to establish additional risk factors (see Pasternak and colleagues[19] and Table 130-1).

CLINICAL PRESENTATIONS OF CORONARY ARTERY DISEASE

Angina pectoris results from reversible myocardial ischemia and is characterized by episodic chest discomfort lasting for up to 20 min. Angina is the most common presentation of CAD, with a prevalence of greater than 20 percent in men ages 65 to 69 years and greater than 13 percent in women of similar age.[2] The principal pathologic finding underlying typical angina is stenosis (>70%) of one or more coronary arteries.

UA is an acute coronary syndrome characterized by chest pain of new onset or an abrupt worsening of previously stable angina. Like stable angina, episodes are reversible and not associated with evidence of cardiac muscle damage. The risk of MI and death within a year of an episode of UA is as high as 15 percent.[20-23]

MI, death of cardiac muscle, is due to irreversible ischemia resulting from prolonged coronary artery occlusion. Sudden death is a frequent concomitant of MI and is due to the development of arrhythmias, usually ventricular fibrillation.

TABLE 130-1   RISK FACTORS FOR CORONARY ARTERY DISEASE

Increasing age
Elevated LDL cholesterol
  Decreased HDL cholesterol
  Elevated lipoprotein(a), in some populations
  Elevated triglycerides
Cigarette smoking
Diabetes mellitus
  Glucose intolerance
  Elevated serum insulin
Family history of coronary artery disease
    Hypertension (systolic pressure >140 mmHg, diastolic pressure >90 mmHg)
      Left ventricular hypertrophy
Menopause
Obesity
Physical inactivity
Male sex
Short stature
Thrombogenic risk factors
  Elevated fibrinogen
  Increased platelet aggregability (data suggestive, but not established)

PATHOPHYSIOLOGY OF ATHEROSCLEROTIC DISEASE

CLASSIFICATION OF ATHEROSCLEROTIC PLAQUES

Studies in humans have been largely confined to pathologic examination at a single point in time of vessels taken at autopsy, plaques removed during surgical or percutaneous endarterectomies, and fragments removed during coronary atherectomies. These studies have been instrumental in establishing the progression of coronary atherosclerosis over decades.

The American Heart Association has classified atherosclerotic plaques into five phases (Fig. 130-1), based upon the work of Stary

and colleagues.[24] Phase 1 (types I–III) is characterized by a small plaque, often present during the first decade of life. Type I lesions are not apparent by gross examination and are characterized by isolated foam cells in the arterial wall. Type II lesions have a more abundant accumulation of foam cells organized to form a fatty streak, the first lesion that is apparent on gross examination. Type III lesions are characterized by a raised fatty streak, comprised of foam cells, increased number of SMC, and small extracellular accumulations of lipid. Phase 2 (types IV and Va) is characterized by nonobstructive "soft" lesions. Type IV lesions are characterized by diffuse extracellular lipid. Type Va lesions also have a high extracellular lipid content; however, the lipid is more localized and surrounded by a thin cap. The type Va lesion is thought to have the highest propensity to rupture.

Phase 3 and 4 are characterized by plaque rupture (Fig. 130-1) and thrombosis (phase 3 if mural, phase 4 if occlusive) and the development of a type VI complex lesion. Organization of the thrombus by connective tissue ultimately results in severely stenotic (type Vb) or occlusive (type Vc) fibrotic lesions. In some cases, type Va lesions do not rupture and progress to type Vb and Vc lesions, characterized by thick fibrous caps comprised of SMC and collagen. These lesions become increasingly stenotic over time.

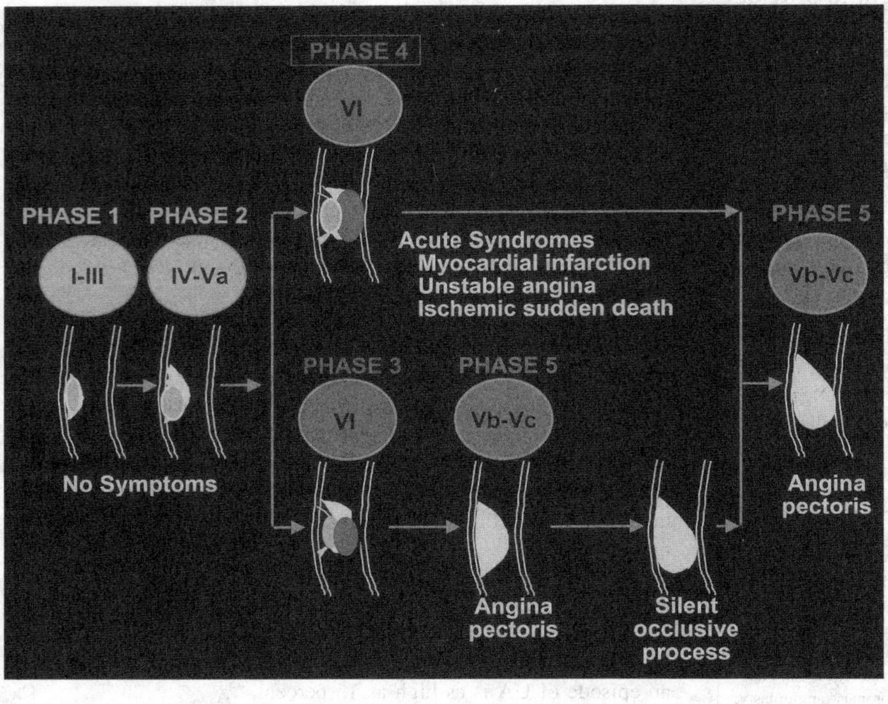

ANIMAL MODELS OF ATHEROSCLEROSIS

Most animals are resistant to atherosclerosis and do not develop plaques when raised on normal laboratory chow. Virtually all models of atherosclerosis have therefore relied on the use of high-fat, high-cholesterol diets, many of which more closely simulate the diet of individuals in industrialized countries. Normal and Watanabe heritable hyperlipidemic rabbits[25,26] primarily develop fatty streaks when kept on atherogenic diets, although prolonged feeding can result in more advanced lesions. Similarly, dietary-induced atherosclerosis in pigs[27] leads to early lesions. Hypercholesterolemic diets in nonhuman primates[28–31] generate lesions ranging from fatty streaks to more advanced fibrous plaques.

Perhaps the most important advance in the study of atherosclerosis has been the development of transgenic and knockout mouse models (reviewed in Breslow[32]). Normal mice and rats fail to develop atherosclerotic lesions, even when fed diets rich in cholesterol and fat. Mice deficient in apolipoprotein E (ApoE$^{-/-}$), the major protein constituent of HDL, have severe hypercholesterolemia and develop all lesion types, including advanced lesions with necrotic cores and fibrous caps.[33] Similarly, mice lacking the LDL receptor (LDLR$^{-/-}$) have extremely high cholesterol levels and develop severe lesions.[34] Mice overexpressing apolipoprotein B, the major protein constituent of LDL, have cholesterol levels and profiles similar to those seen in hypercholesterolemic humans but develop less severe lesions.[35] The use of these transgenic animal models has allowed investigators to study the molecular events associated with the development of atherosclerosis under conditions in which lesion progression is greatly accelerated. Furthermore, by mating these mice with those deficient in a specific gene hypothesized to be important in atherosclerosis, one can establish the role of that gene in plaque development or progression. For example, an important role for

FIGURE 130-1   Classification of atherosclerotic plaques based upon gross pathologic and clinical findings. Roman numerals and phases indicate histologic types, as classified by the Committee on Vascular Lesions of the Council on Arteriosclerosis, American Heart Association. (Reproduced with permission from Fuster V: Mechanisms leading to myocardial infarction: insights from studies of vascular biology. *Circulation* 94:2013, 1994.)

monocyte chemoattractant protein-1 (MCP-1) in plaque development has been established by generating LDLR$^{-/-}$ mice that are also lacking MCP-1,[36] or ApoE$^{-/-}$ mice lacking the MCP-1 receptor, CCR2.[37] Both mice have a 50 percent reduction in plaque size and macrophage-derived foam cell accumulation within the lesions. An even greater reduction in plaque size and foam cell accumulation has been found when the mice overexpressing apolipoprotein B are mated to the MCP-1$^{-/-}$ mice.[38] Despite the power of atherosclerotic mouse models, their lesions remain distinct from those of humans in two critical aspects: They do not rupture spontaneously, and they do not display intramural thrombosis.

RESPONSE-TO-INJURY MODEL OF ATHEROSCLEROSIS

Data derived from studies on animal models of atherosclerosis and the examination of pathologic specimens from human disease have led to a widely accepted hypothesis, first advanced by Ross and colleagues, that atherosclerosis develops as a response to injury.[39,40] This hypothesis views atherosclerosis as a normal wound-healing process designed to repair an insult to the arterial wall. The first line of defense against atherosclerosis is a normal endothelial layer. The endothelium provides a nonadherent, nonthrombogenic surface, helps in the formation of the basement membrane, and acts as a semipermeable barrier to and from the underlying media. Normal endothelium also promotes vasodilatation by the secretion of nitric oxide (NO) and prostacyclin (see Chap. 114). The atherosclerotic process is thought to begin with damage to this layer, resulting in endothelial dysfunction. Endothelial dysfunction does not require denudation or severe damage. It may occur in response to circulating factors, such as tumor necrosis factor α (TNF-α) and interleukin-1 (reviewed in Pober and Cotran[41] and Libby and coworkers[42]) or mechanical forces, such as shear stress and cyclic stretch.[43,44] Many of the established risk factors for CAD (Table 130-1) are thought to act by causing injury to the normal endothelial surface.

Table 130-2 lists some of the properties of dysfunctional endothelium.[45,46] Endothelial dysfunction is associated with a decrease in the production of vasorelaxants, such as NO, and an increase in the secretion of vasoconstrictors, such as endothelin-1. Dysfunctional endothelium also provides a more thrombogenic surface, as a result of an increase in platelet adherence, activation of the coagulation cascade, and perhaps down-regulation of fibrinolysis. "Activated" endothelial cells may also up-regulate the synthesis of SMC growth factors and may down-regulate the synthesis of factors that normally inhibit SMC growth and migration.

One of the most important properties of dysfunctional endothelium is enhanced permeability, manifested in part by transport of LDL into the vessel wall.[47] These lipids may be modified by the endothelium. The most important modification appears to be oxidation.[48] Oxidized LDL is toxic to endothelial cells (EC) and also acts as an activator of SMC and macrophages.[49–51] Oxidized LDL may also stimulate tissue factor synthesis in SMC, EC, and macrophages, thereby promoting a procoagulant state.

Another feature of dysfunctional endothelium is the up-regulation of proinflammatory molecules, including endothelial-leukocyte adhesion molecules and leukocyte chemoattractants.[45,52] One of the earliest morphologic events in the development of a plaque is the adherence of circulating leukocytes, particularly monocytes, to the endothelium.[27–29] Adherent monocytes subsequently migrate into the arterial wall, and along with some activated SMC, ingest modified lipids and lipoproteins and become lipid-filled foam cells, ultimately generating a visible type II fatty streak. Monocytes also differentiate into activated macrophages that secrete cytokines, growth factors, metalloproteinases, and procoagulant molecules. Among the cytokines are a variety of chemoattractants, such as MCP-1, that stimulate further leukocyte migration. Among the growth factors are platelet-derived growth factor (PDGF) and fibroblast growth factors (FGFs), which stimulate SMC to proliferate, migrate, and synthesize extracellular matrix, thereby enlarging the fatty streaks and ultimately generating large plaques (type III). More advanced lesions (type IV and Va) are characterized by necrosis of foam cells, leading to the development of a lipid-rich core surrounded by a thin cap comprised of SMC, macrophages, and matrix. The lipid-rich core also contains high levels of tissue factor,[53] presumably derived from activated macrophages and SMC.

THROMBOSIS AND PLAQUE RUPTURE

Thrombosis is often the final event leading to catastrophic arterial occlusion. The steps leading to acute thrombosis are not fully understood. Plaque rupture is thought to play a major role in the majority of cases (Fig. 130-2).[54–56] Plaque rupture often involves "vulnerable" plaques with large lipid cores and thin fibrous caps.[57,58] Features of plaque vulnerability include the presence of an inflammatory cell infiltrate, made up of macrophages and T lymphocytes.[59,60] These inflammatory cells, along with activated SMC, elaborate cytokines[42] and metalloproteinases.[61] The metalloproteinases are a family of enzymes (see Libby[60] for review) that degrade extracellular matrix and may thus help disrupt the fibrous cap. Mechanical stress may also play an important role in plaque rupture.[62,63] In about 25 percent of cases, thrombosis is associated with superficial erosion of the plaque surface rather than rupture.[59,64] Erosion-related thrombosis often occurs in the setting of a severely stenotic vessel dominated by a heavily

TABLE 130-2   PROPERTIES OF NORMAL AND DYSFUNCTIONAL ATHEROSCLEROTIC ENDOTHELIUM

	NORMAL ENDOTHELIUM	DYSFUNCTIONAL ENDOTHELIUM
Inflammatory properties	Absent or low levels of leukocyte adhesion molecules	Expression of leukocyte adhesion molecules (e.g., VCAM-1, ICAM-1)
	Absent or low levels of inflammatory cytokines	Expression of inflammatory cytokines (e.g., MCP-1)
Anticoagulant properties	Minimal platelet adhesion	Increased platelet adhesion
	Absent expression of procoagulant molecules (e.g., tissue factor and PAI-1)	Increased expression of procoagulant molecules*
	Active fibrinolysis (constitutive expression of plasminogen activators)	Decreased fibrinolysis*
Vasoregulatory properties	Secretion of vasodilators (e.g., NO, prostaglandin I$_2$)	Secretion of vasoconstrictors (e.g., endothelin)
		Decreased secretion of NO
Smooth muscle cell regulatory properties	Inhibitors of smooth muscle cell proliferation and migration, e.g., TGF-β	Activators of smooth muscle cell proliferation and migration (e.g., PDGF)
Regulation of vascular permeability	Minimal cholesterol transport	Increased cholesterol transport

*Denotes proposed properties, but not well established

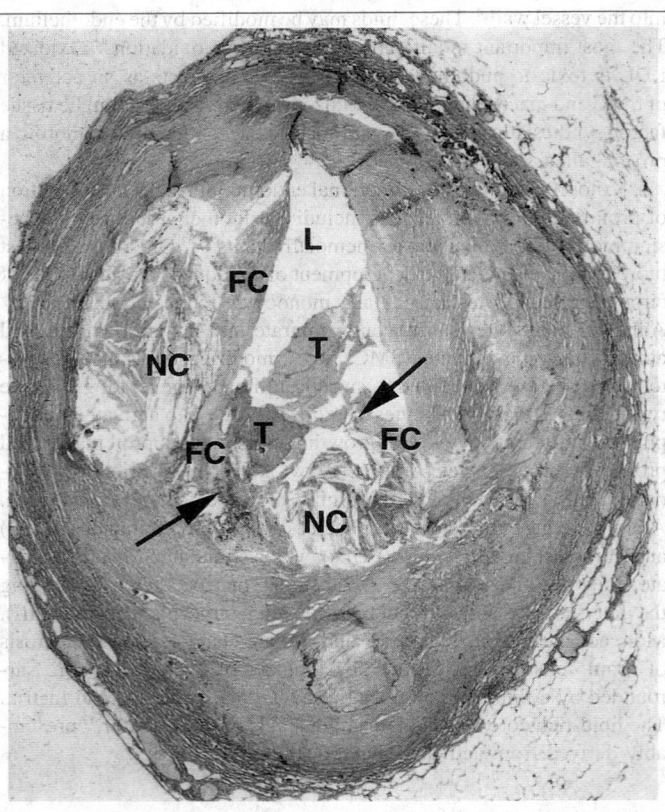

FIGURE 130-2   Morphologic characteristics of an advanced atherosclerotic plaque. Hematoxylin and eosin stain (original magnification ×25) of a human left main coronary artery, showing a necrotic core (NC) and fibrous cap (FC). Arrows depict site of plaque rupture. A thrombus (T) can be seen in the lumen (L). (Courtesy Dr. John T. Fallon, Mount Sinai School of Medicine, NY.)

calcified "stable" plaque that is rich in proteoglycan matrix and SMC and lacks a superficial lipid core.[59]

MODELS OF ACUTE ARTERIAL INJURY AND THROMBUS FORMATION

Models of acute arterial injury have been used for several decades to examine changes in the vessel wall associated with the development of atherosclerosis, but it is not clear to what extent the molecular events associated with acute injury reflect those occurring during chronic atherosclerosis. The development of percutaneous transluminal coronary angioplasty (PTCA), and more recently coronary artery stenting, to treat CAD has stimulated interest in arterial injury models, because they may reflect events associated with these procedures. In particular, the development of intimal hyperplasia in response to injury is thought to be an important contributor to restenosis after angioplasty and stenting.

Thrombus formation is commonly associated with acute arterial injury induced by PTCA[65] and stenting.[66] Although acute thrombosis can result in rapid and total occlusion of the vessel lumen, it can largely be prevented by the use of platelet inhibitors and anticoagulants. Thrombosis is also a common feature of many animal models of arterial injury. When the arterial endothelium is denuded, circulating platelets rapidly adhere to the surface, in part through the interaction between von Willebrand factor and glycoprotein (Gp)Ib (reviewed in Shafer[67]). Collagen and thrombin stimulate platelet activation, causing the release of arachidonic acid and the subsequent formation of throm-

boxane A_2. Adenosine diphosphate (ADP) is secreted by activated platelets and induces further platelet activation. This results in conformational changes in glycoprotein IIb/IIIa and platelet aggregation. Additional thrombin is generated on the platelet surface, leading to fibrin deposition.

The presence and extent of fibrin deposition varies with the degree of injury (superficial or deep), the type of vessel (carotid, femoral, aorta, or coronary), the state of the vessel prior to injury (normal, cholesterol fed, previously injured), and the species. In the pig carotid balloon injury model,[68,69] superficial injury, defined as endothelial denudation and no medial injury, is associated with platelet deposition but no fibrin generation. Deeper injury, defined by the presence of a medial tear, results in marked platelet accumulation and fibrin generation.

Balloon injury to normal rodent arteries is associated with platelet deposition without fibrin, even when medial smooth muscle injury is present.[70–74] Platelet-fibrin microthrombi are found when previously injured arteries are subjected to a second injury.[70,71,73,75,76] Treatment of these doubly injured rabbits with intravenous heparin reduces platelet accumulation by approximately 50 percent,[71] suggesting that activation of the coagulation cascade may be involved.

MOLECULAR BASIS OF THE ATHEROTHROMBOTIC STATE

A number of molecules have been implicated in the development of the athero-thrombotic state. Some of these will be discussed in detail in the following sections.

TISSUE FACTOR

TF is a low-molecular-weight transmembrane protein that initiates the extrinsic clotting cascade and is considered the major initiator of coagulation and hemostasis[77–79] (see Chap. 112). TF was first identified as a component of human atherosclerotic plaques in 1972[80] and currently is considered the major initiator of thrombosis associated with acute coronary syndromes.

TF IN THE NORMAL ARTERIAL WALL
Although EC, SMC, macrophages, and fibroblasts synthesize TF, its distribution in the normal arterial wall is not uniform. TF mRNA and antigen are abundant in the adventitia of normal arteries,[81,82] but they are minimal in normal intima and media. The constitutive expression of TF in the adventitia allows for rapid hemostasis in the event of external injury to the blood vessel and presumably evolved to prevent hemorrhage. In contrast, the expression of active TF on the luminal surface could be potentially catastrophic by initiating intraarterial thrombosis.

TF IN ATHEROSCLEROTIC PLAQUES
TF antigen has been detected in all cellular elements comprising the atherosclerotic plaque (see Fig. 130-3).[53,82–86] TF is most abundant in the foam cells, macrophages, and intimal SMC located in the fibrous cap and tissues surrounding the lipid-rich necrotic core. TF antigen is also present in the medial SMC and EC overlying the plaque. TF antigen is also abundant in the extracellular matrix of the intima and within the necrotic core.[53,86]

TF activity has been detected in 90 percent of specimens from directional coronary atherectomies[84] and may be attenuated by the presence of tissue factor pathway inhibitor (TFPI).[87] In studies employing an *ex vivo* perfusion system, the lipid rich necrotic core, an abundant source of TF, was found to be the most thrombogenic component of the plaque.[88,89] Macrophages and intimal SMC are the most likely source of the TF found in the core. This TF may derive

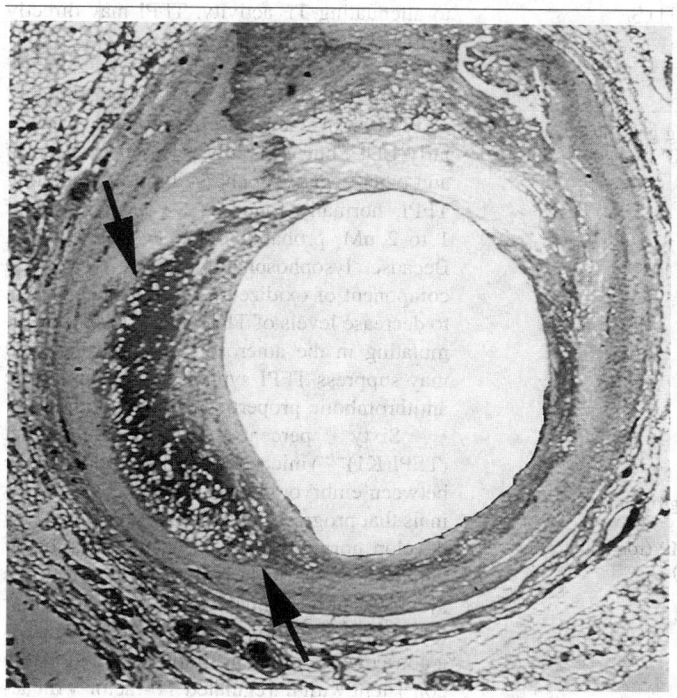

FIGURE 130-3   Expression of tissue factor in a human atherosclerotic plaque. Human coronary artery stained with an antibody to tissue factor. Staining is most prominent in the necrotic core (between arrows). Original magnification ×25. (Courtesy Dr. John T. Fallon, Mount Sinai School of Medicine, NY.)

from cell debris, may be released during apoptosis,[90] or may be shed from the plasma membrane of activated healthy cells.[91] Plaque rupture may thus expose active TF to circulating blood, leading to acute thrombosis.

TF IN ANIMAL MODELS OF ARTERIAL INJURY

TF mRNA and activity are induced in the media as an early event (1 to 2 h) after arterial balloon injury in animals,[92–95] returning to baseline levels after several days. However, TF antigen subsequently accumulates throughout the developing neointima in these animal models.[53]

Animal models of injury to normal arteries are not often associated with the deposition of fibrin or the generation of thrombi. This suggests that the induction of TF mRNA and protein in the arterial wall is not sufficient to establish arterial thrombosis. The presence of an intact internal elastic lamina separating the media from the lumen, the rapid accumulation of platelets on the luminal surface, and the rapid secretion of matrix by injured SMC may effectively prevent newly synthesized medial TF from coming into contact with circulating blood and initiating coagulation. In addition, the TF antigen and activity identified in the media may be intracellular or encrypted on the cell surface (discussed in detail below) and therefore ineffective in initiating thrombosis. TF exposed on the cell surface may also rapidly associate with TFPI or other inhibitors. Sequential arterial injury is more frequently associated with fibrin deposition and mural thrombosis.[70,71,73,75] This may be due in part to the immediate exposure of intimal TF.

A number of animal studies[93,96–100] have provided evidence that TF also plays a role in intimal hyperplasia. Studies using inhibitors of TF activity have also provided evidence that TF expression is critical to the development of platelet-fibrin thrombi after sequential arterial injury.[75,76]

CIRCULATING TF AND THROMBOSIS

TF is present in whole blood and plasma.[101–104] Plasma TF levels are elevated in patients with sickle cell disease,[103] disseminated intravascular coagulation,[101] and acute MI.[102] Circulating TF may play a primary role in the initiation or propagation of arterial thrombosis.[104] Thrombi that form on normal porcine arterial media and on collagen-coated glass slides perfused for 5 min with native human blood contain TF antigen, and antibodies against TF markedly reduce thrombus formation on both surfaces. TF antigen is most abundant in membrane vesicles that cluster near the surface of platelets. Thus circulating TF may adhere to exposed surfaces and may act alone or in concert with TF located in the injured vessel wall to propagate arterial thrombosis. The source of this circulating TF is unknown, but it is likely that it derives from blood leukocytes or endothelial cells.

REGULATION OF TF BY CELLS OF THE ARTERIAL WALL

In most models of acute arterial injury, the endothelial is denuded, and SMC are the most likely source of TF activity. In models in which injury is produced on a substrate of atherosclerosis, macrophages rapidly accumulate in the intima and media and thus provide a second source of TF. In established atherosclerotic plaques, macrophages appear to be the most abundant source of TF, followed by intimal SMC, and to a much lesser degree medial SMC and regenerating endothelium.

TF is a member of the class of "immediate early" genes, which are expressed at low levels in quiescent cells and rapidly induced by serum and growth factors.[105] Under most circumstances, the induction of TF occurs principally at the level of transcription, although increases in TF mRNA stability are also partly responsible (reviewed in Edgington and coworkers[77]). In addition to its regulation by serum and growth factors, TF is also induced by a variety of cytokines, endotoxin lipopolysaccharide (LPS), antigen-antibody complexes, lymphocyte products, and lipoproteins (see Table 130-3). Many of these agents are found in abundance in atherosclerotic plaques and in the injured arterial wall.

TF is induced in EC and monocytes by modified and oxidized forms of LDL.[106,107] This raises the possibility that hypercholesterolemia may directly promote thrombosis, even at an early stage in plaque development. TF is also induced during monocyte-macrophage differentiation in cell culture.[108] The differentiation of monocytes to macrophages is an early event in the development of atherosclerotic lesions and occurs concomitantly with migration of monocytes into the arterial wall. The induction of TF by thrombin in SMC and EC[109–111] is also intriguing, because thrombin is an end-product of TF activation. Thus, thrombin may be part of a positive feedback loop, helping to perpetuate a procoagulant state. TF is also induced by laminar shear stress in cultured EC and fibroblasts.[112,113]

Mammalian TF promoter regions share striking sequence similarities, suggesting that the mechanism of TF gene regulation is highly conserved.[114–117] Human TF gene regulation involves several elements, working either cooperatively or singly (reviewed in Mackman[118]). Basal TF gene expression is regulated by a series of Sp1 sites. Induction of TF by growth factors and cytokines in EC and monocytes is dependent upon two AP-1 sites and an NFκB-site. These sites have been implicated in the regulation of many genes by growth factors, cytokines, and mediators of inflammation. TF transcription thus appears to be part of an extensive genetic program induced by processes such as growth, inflammation, and wound healing.

TF EXPRESSION ON CELL SURFACES

Under virtually all culture conditions, the induction of TF mRNA is accompanied by the accumulation of TF protein and an increase in procoagulant activity. A critical determinant of whether TF expression

TABLE 130-3   ACTIVATORS AND INHIBITORS OF TISSUE FACTOR SYNTHESIS IN CELLS
OF THE ARTERIAL WALL

CELL TYPE	ACTIVATORS	INHIBITORS
Endothelial cells	Tumor necrosis factor α	Heparin binding growth factor
	Endotoxin lipopolysasccharide	Increased cAMP (forskolin, dibu-
		tyryl cAMP)
	Interleukin-1	
	Vascular endothelial growth factor	
	Transforming growth factor β	
	Thrombin	
	Modified/oxidized LDL	
	Phorbol esters	
Smooth muscle cells	Platelet-derived growth factor	
	Thrombin	
	Angiotensin II	
	Monocyte chemoattractant	
	protein-1	
	Serum	
	Phorbol esters	
Monocyte/macrophages	Endotoxin lipopolysaccharide	Transforming growth factor β
	Vascular endothelial growth factor	
	Immune complexes	Increased cAMP (forskolin, dibu-
		tyryl cAMP)
	Modified/oxidized LDL	
	T lymphocytes and products (e.g.,	Salicylates
	CD40)	
	Phorbol esters	Interleukin-4
		Interleukin-10
		Interleukin-13
Fibroblasts	Serum	
	Platelet-derived growth factor	
	Transforming growth factor β	

in atherosclerotic or injured vessels leads to a procoagulant state is whether the protein is present in an active state and is accessible to the circulation. Studies employing monolayers of SMC, EC, fibroblasts, and macrophages have found that, although TF protein is present on the cell surface, the majority of surface TF is not active.[91,111,119–125] This "encrypted" or "latent" TF can be activated by processes that alter the structure or phospholipid composition of the cell membrane or cause cell lysis. It is likely that much of the TF present in cells of the arterial wall or atherosclerotic plaque is similarly encrypted or intracellular. Thus, in addition to inducing *de novo* TF synthesis, arterial injury and plaque rupture may convert encrypted TF already present in the arterial wall into active TF. Release of intracellular TF as a consequence of cell necrosis or apoptosis may also be important in generating a procoagulant state within the arterial wall.

TF IN CELL-DERIVED MICROPARTICLES

A substantial amount of TF antigen in the atherosclerotic plaque appears to be located in the extracellular matrix or in the lipid-rich necrotic core. Cultured cells can release TF into the culture medium in microparticles or small vesicles.[90,91,126,127] These particles presumably bud from the cell surface as a normal consequence of cellular metabolism, rather than as a consequence of necrosis or apoptosis. TF-containing microparticles may be an important source of procoagulant activity in the arterial wall.

TISSUE FACTOR PATHWAY INHIBITOR

TFPI is an endogenous Kunitz-type proteinase inhibitor that directly inhibits activated factor X and, in a factor Xa-dependent fashion, produces feedback inhibition of the factor VIIa/TF catalytic complex (reviewed in Broze[128] and Mann and colleagues[129] and Chap. 113). The second Kunitz domain inhibits factor Xa, whereas the first Kunitz domain inhibits factor VIIa in the TF-factor VIIa complex. In addition

to attenuating TF activity, TFPI may directly inhibit SMC proliferation.[130]

TFPI is made predominantly by EC,[131,132] although SMC may provide a second source.[133] TFPI is highly bound to lipoproteins, particularly LDL, but is rapidly released by heparin and other negatively charged ions. Circulating TFPI, normally found at a concentration of 1 to 2 nM, probably modulates TF activity. Because lysophosphatidylcholine (LPC), a component of oxidized LDL, has been shown to decrease levels of TFPI in EC,[134] LPC accumulating in the atherosclerotic vascular wall may suppress TFPI synthesis, attenuating the antithrombotic properties of the endothelium.

Sixty percent of TFPI-deficient (TFPI(K1)$^{-/-}$) mice die of yolk sac hemorrhage between embryonic days 9.5 and 11.5.[135] Animals that progress beyond embryonic day 11.5 develop normally but die in late gestation of hemorrhage, particularly in the central nervous system. These animals exhibit intravascular thrombosis, suggesting that the hemorrhage is a consequence of a consumptive coagulopathy consistent with unregulated TF-factor VIIa activity.

TFPI antigen and mRNA have been detected in the adventitia of normal arteries.[136] Low levels of TFPI mRNA have also been detected in medial SMC,[136] whereas TFPI antigen has been found in medial SMC and intimal endothelium of normal human coronary arteries.[133] In contrast, high levels of TFPI antigen and mRNA have been found in EC, SMC within the fibrous cap, and macrophages within the shoulder region of human carotid endarterectomy specimens and in early fatty streaks of hypercholesterolemic rabbits.[87] Areas rich in TFPI also stain prominently for TF antigen.

In animal models, TFPI treatment has been shown to attenuate intimal hyperplasia and stenosis after balloon injury[98,100] and to prevent thrombotic arterial reocclusion after tPA-mediated thrombolysis.[137] The role of exogenous TFPI in treating human disease remains to be determined.

THE FIBRINOLYTIC SYSTEM: PLASMINOGEN ACTIVATORS

The fibrinolytic system is thought to play an important role in offsetting the effects of increased TF expression in the arterial wall. This is underscored by the success of activators of fibrinolysis in revascularization in the setting of acute MI (see below). A general scheme of the fibrinolytic system is shown in Chap. 116. Fibrinolysis requires the generation of plasmin from plasminogen, an inactive proenzyme. The active plasmin degrades fibrin, as well as other extracellular matrix proteins.

Plasminogen activators (PAs) convert plasminogen to plasmin. Plasmin cleaves fibrin, thus acting as an endogenous thrombolytic agent. Two types of plasminogen activator have been identified, tissue-type plasminogen activator (tPA) and urokinase-type plasminogen activator (uPA). EC of the normal arterial wall secrete tPA, but little or no uPA.[138–142] Low levels of tPA mRNA and antigen have also been detected in SMC of normal arteries.[142]

PLASMINOGEN ACTIVATORS IN ATHEROSCLEROTIC PLAQUES

The secretion of tPA by normal EC is thought to be important in maintaining an antithrombotic surface, but experimental data are conflicting regarding PAs in atherosclerotic lesions.[142-147] PA activity may be modulated by the presence of plasminogen activator inhibitor-1 (PAI-1).

PLASMINOGEN ACTIVATORS IN ARTERIAL INJURY

In animal models, after balloon arterial injury, uPA activity in carotid arteries rapidly increases, reaching a maximum between 16 and 24 h, whereas tPA activity appears at 3 days[148]; uPA and tPA mRNA increase steadily, reaching a maximum at 7 days. The induction of PAs, particularly uPA, may prevent fibrin accumulation. It remains to be determined whether a similar induction of PAs occurs after human coronary angioplasty.

OTHER ROLES FOR PAs IN ATHEROSCLEROSIS

The expression of PAs in atherosclerotic and injured vessels may serve functions other than fibrinolysis. Plasmin has been shown to activate latent cytokines, such as transforming growth factor beta (TGF-β) and basic FGF.[149,150] The activation of TGF-β by plasmin has been implicated in the suppression of SMC proliferation[151] and migration[152] in cell culture. Apo(a) overexpressing mice display decreased plasminogen activation and increased atherosclerosis.[153] It is thought that this is in part due to the ability of lipoprotein(a) to inhibit plasmin generation and therefore to inhibit TGF-β.

Plasmin also activates metalloproteinases, such as collagenase and stromelysin,[154] which may serve to promote SMC migration and proliferation. In the rat carotid artery injury model, most of the induced tPA is present in the media before the SMC migrated into the intima.[148] Tranexamic acid, a synthetic inhibitor of plasmin activity, reduces SMC migration by 73 percent after arterial balloon injury,[155] suggesting that in this model the effect of plasmin in promoting migration may be more important than its effect on TGF-β–mediated growth suppression. In contrast, continuous infusion of tPA for 7 days causes an 80 percent decrease in intimal hyperplasia in hypercholesterolemic animals subjected to balloon injury of the common iliac artery.[156] The administration of exogenous tPA may therefore have a significantly different effect on the arterial wall than that of endogenously regulated PAs.

PLASMINOGEN ACTIVATOR INHIBITOR 1

Plasminogen activator inhibitor 1 is the major physiologic inhibitor of tPA and uPA.[157] PAI-1 is found in the circulation largely in association with platelets and to a lesser extent in plasma.[158] Plasma PAI-1 is bound to vitronectin,[159] and its level displays a circadian rhythm, with a peak in the morning and a trough in the evening, inverse to that of tPA.[160] Higher PAI-1 levels are seen with increases in age,[161] blood pressure, triglyceride levels, and body mass[162]; the levels correlate with insulin resistance.[163] PAI-1 binds to fibrin and forms a stable complex with tPA or uPA.[164] This inhibits plasmin activation and protects the thrombus from lysis. PAI-1 may also limit the efficacy of exogenous thrombolytic agents.[165,166]

PLASMA PAI-1

Increased PAI-1 levels and/or reduced fibrinolysis have been found in patients with coronary artery disease (reviewed in Prisco and colleagues[167]), angina,[168-170] and MI.[171-173] Increased plasma PAI-1 activity has also been found in patients with stroke[174] and carotid atherosclerosis.[175] Increased circulating PAI-1 has also been shown to correlate with decreased patency of coronary arteries after thrombolytic therapy for acute MI.[173] In contrast, decreased levels of PAI-1 activity after PTCA have been associated with reduced risk of restenosis.[176]

EXPRESSION OF PAI-1 IN ATHEROSCLEROTIC PLAQUES

There is little PAI-1 in normal vessels,[157] but significant amounts are present in all three cellular components of atherosclerotic plaques: SMC, EC, and macrophages.[157,177] Highest levels are detected in SMC and macrophages around the necrotic core.[147,178,179] PAI-1 colocalizes in human atherosclerotic coronary arteries with other components of the plasminogen activator system, including tPA, uPA, and uPA receptor (uPAR). However, levels of PAI-1 appear to be substantially higher.[147,180-182]

In addition to its presence in atherosclerotic plaques, PAI-1 has also been identified in extracts of thrombi. Levels of PAI-1 antigen in these thrombi are substantially higher (as much as 2000-fold) than that found in circulating blood and also much higher than that of tPA or the tPA-PAI-1 complex.[180,181,183] This is likely due to the accumulation of platelets within the thrombus.

PAI-1 IN ARTERIAL INJURY

In animal models, PAI-1 mRNA is not detectable in uninjured carotid arteries but is rapidly induced (within 3 h) by balloon arterial injury.[184,185] PAI-1 induction is first detected in the adventitia, and within 24 h in the media. PAI-1 antigen and mRNA subsequently accumulate over time in neointimal SMC and EC. The induction of PAI-1 activity follows the same time course. PAI-1 is also increased in animal models of arterial thrombosis.[186] PAI-1 mRNA increases in EC and macrophages juxtaposed to the thrombus and in SMC adjacent to the neointima.

CELLULAR REGULATION OF PAI-1

PAI-1 is secreted by EC, SMC, fibroblasts, macrophages, and hepatocytes.[187-189] Its synthesis is upregulated in SMC and EC by cytokines (interleukin 1, TNF-α), TGF-β, basic FGF, PDGF, angiotensin II, plasminogen, and α thrombin[190-195] α-thrombin, a potent stimulator of TF, also stimulates synthesis of PAI-1 in cultured SMC.[196,197] Therefore, thrombin is part of two positive procoagulant feedback loops, potentiating the synthesis of TF and PAI-1. SMC from atherosclerotic arteries also express higher levels of PAI-1, in association with decreased levels of tPA.[198]

Lipoprotein(a), a risk factor for coronary artery disease, induces PAI-1 antigen, activity, and steady-state mRNA levels in EC.[199] SMC and macrophages may play an important role in regulating the synthesis of PAI-1 by cultured EC.[189,200] Quiescent SMC appear to inhibit PAI-1 production by EC, whereas proliferating and atherosclerotic SMC may secrete a soluble factor that stimulates PAI-1 production by EC. Differentiated macrophages also secrete a soluble factor that regulates endothelial cell PAI-1 production.

PLASMINOGEN ACTIVATOR INHIBITOR 2 (PAI-2)

A second inhibitor of PAs, PAI-2, also has been identified.[201] PAI-2 is found largely as an intracellular protein. Therefore, its role in regulating thrombosis is unclear. It is possible that under conditions of cell injury, PAI-2 is released into the extracellular matrix and can contribute to inhibiting fibrinolysis (for review see Bachmann[202]).

RECEPTOR FOR uPA

In addition to generating plasmin, PAs may also have direct effects on the arterial wall through interactions with cell surface receptors. The uPAR is a transmembrane glycoprotein, which is thought to be critical for localizing the activity of uPA to the cell surface, accelerating plasminogen activation, delaying PAI-1 inhibition of plasminogen activation,[203] and regulating the clearance of uPA.[204] uPAR is expressed by cultured EC, macrophages, and SMC.[205,206] The induction of uPAR in SMC is common to a number of growth agonists, including epidermal growth factor (EGF), TGFβ, basic FGF, PDGF, phorbol esters, and α thrombin.[206,207]

uPAR expression is also upregulated at the leading edge of migrating SMC,[208] EC,[209] and monocytes.[210] Studies suggest that uPAR may be involved in integrin-mediated cell adhesion and migration through interactions with vitronectin (reviewed in Wei and colleagues[211]) and the Mac-1 receptor (CD11b/CD18).[212,213] Binding of uPA to uPAR has also been implicated in intracellular signaling via tyrosine phosphorylation,[214,215] macrophage protease expression,[216] growth,[217,218] and chemotaxis.[214,215] These effects do not require uPA enzymatic activity and can be initiated by enzymatically inactive fragments of uPA.[219]

uPAR expression is up-regulated in SMC and macrophages of early lesions of cholesterol-fed animals.[220] The expression of uPAR is also markedly increased in the intima of human coronary atherosclerotic lesions[147,207] and in SMC and macrophages of thickened saphenous vein grafts.[207] The significance of increased uPAR in atherosclerosis is unknown.

TRANSGENIC MOUSE MODELS AND THE FIBRINOLYTIC SYSTEM

Studies of transgenic mice lacking one or more of the components of the fibrinolytic system have provided considerable insights into the role of plasminogen activation in mediating arterial thrombosis and intimal hyperplasia (reviewed in Carmeliet and Collen[221]).

PLASMINOGEN DEFICIENCY

In plasminogen-deficient (Plg$^{-/-}$) mice, wound healing (i.e., neointima formation and reendothelialization) after vascular injury is significantly impaired.[222] In Plg$^{-/-}$ mice, SMC accumulate at the uninjured borders but fail to migrate into the necrotic center. Proliferation of SMC is not affected. Analogous abnormalities in the healing of skin wounds were also noted.[223]

tPA AND uPA DEFICIENCY

uPA$^{-/-}$ mice, either alone or in combination with tPA$^{-/-}$, have less intimal hyperplasia in response to arterial injury.[224] SMC accumulate at the uninjured borders but fail to migrate into the necrotic center. Cultured uPA$^{-/-}$ SMC also demonstrated decreased migratory capacity. In contrast, tPA$^{-/-}$ mice do not exhibit altered intimal hyperplasia or SMC migration.

PAI-1 DEFICIENCY

In PAI-1$^{-/-}$ mice subjected to arterial injury, wound healing is significantly enhanced, and there is increased neointima formation.[225] Proliferation of SMC is not affected by PAI-1 deficiency. However, SMC originating from the uninjured borders migrate into the necrotic center of the arterial wound more rapidly than wild-type SMC. There are no differences in reendothelialization of the injured arteries. PAI-1 deficiency in mice is associated with increased thrombolysis.[226]

uPAR DEFICIENCY

uPAR-deficient (uPAR$^{-/-}$) mice have no abnormalities of fertility, development, or hemostasis,[227] and skin wounds heal normally.[228] They also have no abnormalities in intimal hyperplasia or SMC migration after vascular injury.[229] uPA becomes bound to the cell surface of uPAR$^{+/+}$ cells, whereas it binds to the pericellular space around uPAR$^{-/-}$cells. This suggests that binding of uPA to uPAR is not required to provide sufficient uPA-mediated plasmin proteolysis to allow SMC migration into the vascular lesion.

α2-ANTIPLASMIN

α2-antiplasmin (α$_2$-AP) is the principal inhibitor of plasmin and plays an important role in determining clot lysis.[230] α$_2$-AP circulates in the blood at a concentration of approximately 1 μM, over 1000-fold higher than PAI-1. Small amounts have been detected in human platelets.[231] α$_2$-AP can be cross-linked to fibrin via factor XIII.[232] High concentrations of PAI-1 and α$_2$-AP have been found in extracts prepared from human thrombi.[180]

FIBRINOGEN

Evidence links elevated levels of fibrinogen with coronary atherosclerosis and ischemic vascular events. Fibrinogen is synthesized in the liver and circulates at a concentration of 200 to 400 mg/dl. Increased levels of fibrinogen correlate positively with most risk factors for coronary artery disease, including menopause,[233] obesity,[233,234] elevated levels of LDL cholesterol and lipoprotein(a),[233] hypertension,[235] and diabetes mellitus.[236] Levels increase in patients who smoke[237] and may decrease with smoking cessation.[233,238] Levels also decrease with increasing levels of HDL cholesterol.[233] Levels of fibrinogen have been shown to be increased in patients with stroke and MI (reviewed in Wilhelmsen[239] and Kannel and colleagues[240]). In the Framingham Study,[240] Northwick Park Heart Study,[241] and Bezafibrate Infarction Prevention (BIP) Study,[242] an elevated fibrinogen level was found to be an independent risk factor for MI. A meta-analysis of six prospective studies found an odds ratios for cardiovascular events for the upper versus the lowest tercile of 2.3 and strengthened the concept that fibrinogen levels are an independent variable for cardiovascular disease.[243]

PROTHROMBIN FRAGMENTS 1 AND 2 AND FIBRINOPEPTIDE A

Patients with UA and MI appear to have a hypercoagulable state and display increased levels of prothrombin fragments 1 and 2 and fibrinopeptide A.[244-247] Fibrinopeptide A levels return quickly to normal, suggesting that activation may occur only during the acute thrombotic event. Levels of prothrombin fragments 1 and 2 may remain elevated for as long as 6 months,[247] suggesting that some abnormality may persist after the acute event. This appears to be independent of the extent of coronary artery disease.

HOMOCYSTEINE

Homocysteine is a sulfhydryl-containing amino acid produced by demethylation of methionine. Folate and vitamin B$_{12}$ are required for remethylation of homocysteine to methionine, and therefore levels of homocysteine are related inversely to levels of folate and B$_{12}$. Very high levels of homocysteine were initially found in the blood of patients with homocystinuria, an autosomal recessive disease characterized by skeletal abnormalities, ocular lens dislocation, mental retardation, premature atherosclerosis, and a predisposition toward thromboembolic events.[248] Most cases of homocystinuria are due to a deficiency in the enzyme, cystathionine β-synthase, which is involved in the catabolic transsulfuration of homocysteine.[249,250] More moderate elevations of homocysteine appear to be an independent risk factor for coronary artery disease, peripheral vascular disease, and stroke (reviewed in Welch and Loscalzo[251]). In some studies, the correlation extends into the "normal" range (5–15 mmol/liter) and does not appear to have a threshold. Homocysteine levels are reduced by treatment with folic acid, alone or in combination with vitamins B$_6$ or B$_{12}$.[252]

Homocysteine is toxic to cultured EC and causes endothelial damage and desquamation in animal models.[253-255] The effects of homocysteine may in part be due to its oxidation and the formation of superoxide and hydrogen peroxide.[256] Homocysteine has numerous effects on endothelial and platelet function that may promote a pro-thrombotic state. These include an increase in platelet consumption,[257] inactivation of protein C,[258] a decrease in prostacyclin synthesis and an increase in the synthesis of thromboxane A2.[259,260] Homocysteine also causes alterations in von Willebrand factor secretion,[261] increased factor V[262] and TF expression,[263] inhibition of thrombomodulin[264] and heparan sulfate expression,[265] and modulation of binding of tPA to EC.[266] Homocysteine enhances the binding of lipoprotein(a) to fibrin[267] and thus may potentiate the thrombotic properties of lipopro-tein(a).[268–270]

LIPOPROTEIN(A)

Lipoprotein(a) consists of an LDL particle complexed with apolipopro-tein(a).[271] Lipoprotein(a) is synthesized in the liver and circulates in the blood at concentrations ranging from 1 mg/dl to 100 mg/dl, but usually is less than 20 mg/dl. Levels correlate with those of LDL cholesterol.[272] Higher levels are present at menopause and in patients with diabetes mellitus and acute MI.[272,273] High levels of lipoprotein(a) have been found in patients with familial hypercholesterolemia[274] and in siblings and offspring of patients with early coronary artery dis-ease.[275] Several large studies have found that lipoprotein(a) is an inde-pendent risk factor for serious cardiovascular events, including MI and death.[276–279] Other studies, however, have failed to confirm this.[280,281] Lipoprotein(a) has also been associated with an increased incidence of coronary artery disease in Asian populations[282] but not in Ameri-can blacks.[283]

Several mechanisms have been proposed to explain the relation-ship between lipoprotein(a), atherosclerosis and thrombosis (reviewed in Harpel[284] and Hajjar and Nachman[285]). Lipoprotein(a) has been found in atherosclerotic plaques.[286,287] Lipoprotein(a) displaces plasminogen from sites on fibrin and fibrinogen and inhibits plasminogen activation by streptokinase (SK) and tPA.[288] Lipoprotein(a) may similarly inhibit endogenous fibrinolytic activity.[289] Lipoprotein(a) also increases the release of PAI-1 and down-regulates plasmin generation in EC.[199] Lipoprotein(a) may enhance the delivery of LDL cholesterol to the vessel wall[290] and thus promotes foam cell development. High levels of lipoprotein(a) may also interfere with activation of latent growth factors, such as TGFβ, which may be important in regulating SMC pro-liferation.

TREATMENT OF ACUTE CORONARY SYNDROMES

UNSTABLE ANGINA

ANTIANGINAL MEDICATION

Guidelines for the treatment of stable angina can be found in a docu-ment prepared by the task force of the European society of cardiol-ogy.[291] Treatment of unstable angina includes bed rest, supplemental O2, and pain management. Nitrates remain the choice for the immediate relief of angina.[20,292,293] However, tolerance can develop within 24 h.[294] It is important to note that "rebound" angina and even MI can occur after abrupt cessation of nitrates.[293] Although nitrates are highly effec-tive for pain management, they have not been shown to reduce the incidence of MI or death in UA. β-blockers have also been shown to be effective in relieving symptoms and in reducing the incidence of MI in patients with UA (reviewed in Yusuf and coworkers[295]). In view of their beneficial effect on secondary prevention of MI and sudden death, β-blockers are usually continued indefinitely.

ASPIRIN

Although aspirin may have limited effects on anginal pain, several large trials have demonstrated that aspirin prevents MI and death in patients with UA by as much as 50 percent.[14,296–299] Aspirin, 325 mg, is thus given immediately to most patients with UA or suspected MI and continued indefinitely at 81 mg/day or more.

ANTICOAGULATION

Intravenous heparin, most often given as a 5000-unit bolus every 6 h or as a bolus followed by a continuous infusion, is one of the preferred treatment modalities for UA.[297,298,300–302] In some studies, heparin has been shown to be effective in relieving angina.[297,302] Heparin has also been shown to reduce death and MI as compared to placebo,[300] but it is not clear whether heparin alone is more or less effective than aspirin. Several studies have suggested that the combination of heparin and aspirin is most beneficial.[298,303,304] Subcutaneous heparin has also been shown to be effective in reducing angina and ischemia.[297]

Low-molecular-weight heparins have been proposed as an alter-native to standard heparin because they are easier to administer, and there is no need to monitor therapy. Comparisons with standard heparin are conflicting, with some studies demonstrating improved efficacy for low-molecular-weight heparin,[304,305] whereas others suggest no dif-ference.[306] In these studies, most patients have also been treated with aspirin.

Although oral anticoagulation has little place in the acute treat-ment of UA, it may reduce the incidence of significant cardiac events in the longer term.[299,307] Although the ATACS study suggested a possible benefit of the combination of low-dose warfarin and aspirin at 12 weeks in patients with UA, the much larger Coumadin Aspirin Rein-farction Study (CARS) study, which examined patients after MI, failed to show such benefit.[308]

THROMBOLYSIS

Despite its role in the treatment of patients with acute MI, thrombolytic therapy does not appear to benefit patients with UA and may in fact paradoxically increase the incidence of MI.[309–314]

ANTIPLATELET THERAPY

Abciximab, a monoclonal antibody fragment to the platelet glycopro-tein IIb/IIIa receptor has been evaluated in high-risk patients (e.g., those with UA, recent MI, or high-risk angiographic lesions) undergo-ing angioplasty with or without stent placement[315–318] and was found to produce significant decreases in short- and long-term clinical events. The CAPTURE trial, which focused on patients with UA, also showed a significant benefit in clinical outcomes with abciximab treatment, even before percutaneous coronary intervention.[319]

Small molecule antagonists of glycoprotein IIb/IIIa (tirofiban, integrilin, lamifiban) have also been studied and been found safe and efficacious in the treatment of UA when combined with heparin.[320–325]

ANTITHROMBINS

Treatment of UA patients with hirudin, an antithrombin isolated from the leech, results in lower rates of death, nonfatal MI, or refractory angina as compared to heparin.[326–328] Hirulog, a synthetic antithrombin peptide has also been shown to control anginal symptoms[329] and to reduce the incidence of death and MI[330] in patients with UA. Whereas hirudin has been found to be more effective than heparin in reducing serious events after angioplasty in patients with UA,[331] hirulog has failed to show a similar benefit.[332]

REVASCULARIZATION

In many centers, intervention with PTCA and, when appropriate, stent placement, is the treatment of choice for UA, with an initial success rate of greater than 90 percent. Complication rates of interventions are high, however, and include a greater than 5 percent incidence of MI, a greater than 5 percent incidence of emergency bypass surgery, and a higher restenosis rate.[333–336] Also of note is a higher rate of acute closure, often successfully treated with thrombolytic agents.[337,338] The timing of angioplasty remains controversial, with some studies supporting the use of heparin or aspirin for 24 to 48 h prior to PTCA,[339] and others showing no benefit by waiting.[340] Prior to the advent of PTCA, bypass surgery was frequently employed for the treatment of patients with UA refractory to medical treatment.[341] Because of the relatively high 1-year mortality in patients with UA (often approaching 20 percent),[342,343] bypass surgery was also widely employed after initial medical stabilization. Because of the predilection of many centers for early angiography and PTCA in patients with UA, bypass surgery in the acute setting has been largely relegated to failed PTCA or for patients with left main or triple vessel disease. Bypass surgery after medical stabilization continues to be the procedure of choice in patients with severe disease.

ACUTE MI

Initial treatment of acute MI includes careful monitoring, supplemental O_2, and management of pain with morphine sulfate. Based upon its beneficial effects on mortality in several large trials,[13,14,296,297] aspirin, 325 mg per day, is given immediately upon diagnosis and is continued indefinitely at a dose of at least 81 mg/day. Nitrates are effective for the treatment of peri- and post-MI angina. Although early studies of nitrates in acute MI suggested a significant reduction in mortality,[344] recent large-scale trials have failed to confirm these benefits.[345,346]

THROMBOLYTIC THERAPY

Thrombolysis is the cornerstone of reperfusion therapy for acute MI and is considered in all patients with ST segment elevation who present within 12 h from the onset of symptoms. Virtually all studies have shown a significant reduction in mortality with pooled data from over 60,000 patients demonstrating an overall reduction of 18 percent.[12,13,347,348] There is an inverse relationship between the time to onset of treatment and the survival benefit, with patients treated in the first hour having the highest benefit[349] and those treated after 12 h having none.[350,351] Absolute contraindications for thrombolytic therapy are active bleeding and recent stroke, trauma, or major surgery. Relative contraindications are severe hypertension (>180/110 mm Hg), previous cerebrovascular history, prior gastrointestinal hemorrhage, active menstruation, pregnancy, prolonged cardiopulmonary resuscitation, recent surgery and recent noncompressible vascular puncture, or ongoing warfarin therapy.

Several large trials have examined the effects of different thrombolytic regimens on mortality. The GISSI-2 trial[352] found no significant difference in the 30-day mortality of 20,749 patients randomized to t-PA or SK. The ISIS-3 trial found no difference in mortality among 41,299 patients randomized to t-PA, streptokinase, or anistreplase.[353] In contrast, GUSTO-I, which evaluated 41,021 patients,[354] found that accelerated alteplase t-PA, administered over 90 min with intravenous heparin, reduced 30-day mortality by 15 percent (1 percent absolute mortality benefit) as compared to streptokinase with intravenous or subcutaneous heparin, or the combination of t-PA and streptokinase with intravenous heparin. The differences correlated with earlier complete infarct vessel patency and were maintained at 1 year of follow-up.[354,355] Based upon this study, t-PA is used in more than 75 percent of patients treated in the United States.

EMERGENT INTERVENTION

In centers that can provide short transit times to the cardiac catheterization laboratory, PTCA has been used as an alternative to thrombolysis.

PTCA is also used as a "rescue" for unsuccessful thrombolysis, particularly in patients with large MIs. Rescue PTCA has been associated with a decrease in mortality and improvement in left ventricular function, particularly in patients treated within 2 h of unsuccessful thrombolysis.[356–359] In contrast, PTCA performed immediately after successful thrombolysis is associated with a higher mortality, a more frequent need for emergency bypass surgery, and no improvement in left ventricular function.[360–362] The experience with stenting for acute MI has shown a significant reduction in death, reinfarction, or reintervention as compared with balloon dilatation alone.[363–365] Because of the success of thrombolysis, the use of bypass surgery in acute MI is limited.

TREATMENT OF THE POST-MI PATIENT

After the initial treatment of acute MI, attention focuses on "secondary" prevention. This includes aggressive risk factor modification, such as cessation of smoking, decreasing LDL cholesterol (with diet or lipid-lowering agents), weight reduction, and regular physical activity. Several pharmacologic interventions are also routinely employed.

β-blockers remain a cornerstone of post-MI treatment.[344,366–368] Angiotensin converting enzyme inhibitors have been shown to increase survival, reduce the incidence of heart failure, reduce the incidence of reinfarction, and decrease the need for revascularization in patients with acute MI and left ventricular dysfunction.[345,346,369–371]

A large number of clinical studies have supported the use of aspirin for secondary prevention after MI.[13,372–374] Although there remains some question as to the dosage necessary to provide a maximal effect on secondary prevention, regimens of 81 to 325 mg/day of aspirin is in widespread use in post-MI patients. A meta-analysis of six randomized trials calculated a 13 percent reduction in cardiovascular mortality, a 31 percent reduction in the rate of nonfatal MI, and a 42 percent reduction in nonfatal strokes with long-term aspirin treatment.[375] The CAPRIE study found a similar event rate in patients treated with clopidogrel (75 mg/day) as compared to aspirin (325 mg/day).[376]

Several studies of warfarin in post-MI patients showed a reduction in risk for death and reinfarction but an increase in serious bleeding episodes.[299,307,377] The recent CARS study found no improvement with the combination of full-dose aspirin and low-dose warfarin when compared with aspirin alone and also suggested an increase in bleeding.[308] Warfarin has been associated with decreased risk for embolic events in patients with echocardiographic evidence of left ventricular thrombus.[378,379] The use of warfarin after MI is limited largely to patients with this complication.

REFERENCES

1. Tunstall-Pedoe H, Kuulasmaa K, Amouyel P, Arveiler D, Rajakangas AM, Pajak A: Myocardial infarction and coronary deaths in the World Health Organization MONICA Project. Registration procedures, event rates, and case-fatality rates in 38 populations from 21 countries in four continents. *Circulation* 90:583, 1994.
2. *Heart and Stroke Facts:* 1997 *Statistical Supplement.* Dallas, TX: American Heart Association, 1997.
3. Herrick JB: Clinical features of sudden obstruction of the coronary arteries. *JAMA* 59:2015, 1912.
4. Constantinides P: Plaque fissures in human coronary thrombosis. *J Atheroscler Res*:1, 1966.
5. Davies MJ, Fulton WF, Robertson WB: The relation of coronary thrombosis to ischaemic myocardial necrosis. *J Pathol* 127:99, 1979.
6. Davies MJ, Thomas A: Thrombosis and acute coronary-artery lesions in sudden cardiac ischemic death. *N Engl J Med* 310:1137, 1984.
7. Davies MJ, Thomas AC: Plaque fissuring—the cause of acute myocar-

dial infarction, sudden ischaemic death, and crescendo angina. *Br Heart J* 53:363, 1985.

8. Maseri A, L'Abbate A, Baroldi G, et al: Coronary vasospasm as a possible cause of myocardial infarction. A conclusion derived from the study of ''preinfarction'' angina. *N Engl J Med* 299:1271, 1978.

9. Bertrand ME, LaBlanche JM, Tilmant PY, et al: Frequency of provoked coronary arterial spasm in 1089 consecutive patients undergoing coronary arteriography. *Circulation* 65:1299, 1982.

10. DeWood MA, Spores J, Notske R, et al: Prevalence of total coronary occlusion during the early hours of transmural myocardial infarction. *N Engl J Med* 303:897, 1980.

11. Rentrop P, Blanke H, Karsch KR, Kaiser H, Kostering H, Leitz K: Selective intracoronary thrombolysis in acute myocardial infarction and unstable angina pectoris. *Circulation* 63:307, 1981.

12. Effectiveness of intravenous thrombolytic treatment in acute myocardial infarction. Gruppo Italiano per lo Studio della Streptochinasi nell'Infarto Miocardico (GISSI). *Lancet* 1:397, 1986.

13. Randomised trial of intravenous streptokinase, oral aspirin, both, or neither among 17,187 cases of suspected acute myocardial infarction: ISIS-2. ISIS-2 (Second International Study of Infarct Survival) Collaborative Group. *Lancet* 2:349, 1988.

14. Lewis HD Jr, Davis JW, Archibald DG, et al: Protective effects of aspirin against acute myocardial infarction and death in men with unstable angina. Results of a Veterans Administration Cooperative Study. *N Engl J Med* 309:396, 1983.

15. Theroux P: Glycoprotein IIb/IIIa inhibitors in unstable angina. *Curr Opin Cardiol* 12:447, 1997.

16. Gonzalez ER: Antiplatelet therapy in atherosclerotic cardiovascular disease. *Clin Therapeut* 20:B18, 1998.

17. Dawber TR, Meadors GF, Moore FEJ: Epidemiological approaches to heart disease: the Framingham Study. *Am J Public Health* 41:279, 1951.

18. Kannel WB, Wilson PW: An update on coronary risk factors. *Med Clin North Am* 79:951, 1995.

19. Pasternak RC, Grundy SM, Levy D, Thompson PD: 27th Bethesda Conference: matching the intensity of risk factor management with the hazard for coronary disease events. Task Force 3. Spectrum of risk factors for coronary heart disease. *J Am Coll Cardiol* 27:978, 1996.

20. Krauss KR, Hutter AM Jr, DeSanctis RW: Acute coronary insufficiency. Course and follow-up. *Circulation* 45:I66, 1972.

21. Heng MK, Norris RM, Singh BM, Partridge JB: Prognosis in unstable angina. *Br Heart J* 38:921, 1976.

22. Cairns JA, Singer J, Gent M, et al: One year mortality outcomes of all coronary and intensive care unit patients with acute myocardial infarction, unstable angina or other chest pain in Hamilton, Ontario, a city of 375,000 people. *Can J Cardiol* 5:239, 1989.

23. Anderson HV, Cannon CP, Stone PH, et al: One-year results of the Thrombolysis in Myocardial Infarction (TIMI) IIIB clinical trial. A randomized comparison of tissue-type plasminogen activator versus placebo and early invasive versus early conservative strategies in unstable angina and non-Q wave myocardial infarction. *J Am Coll Cardiol* 26:1643, 1995.

24. Stary HC, Chandler AB, Dinsmore RE, et al: A definition of advanced types of atherosclerotic lesions and a histological classification of atherosclerosis. A report from the Committee on Vascular Lesions of the Council on Arteriosclerosis, American Heart Association. *Circulation* 92:1355, 1995.

25. Rosenfeld ME, Tsukada T, Chait A, Bierman EL, Gown AM, Ross R: Fatty streak expansion and maturation in Watanabe Heritable Hyperlipemic and comparably hypercholesterolemic fat-fed rabbits. *Arteriosclerosis* 7:24, 1987.

26. Rosenfeld ME, Tsukada T, Gown AM, Ross R: Fatty streak initiation in Watanabe Heritable Hyperlipemic and comparably hypercholesterolemic fat-fed rabbits. *Arteriosclerosis* 7:9, 1987.

27. Gerrity RG, Naito HK, Richardson M, Schwartz CJ: Dietary induced atherogenesis in swine. Morphology of the intima in prelesion stages. *Am J Pathol* 95:775, 1979.

28. Faggiotto A, Ross R: Studies of hypercholesterolemia in the nonhuman primate. II. Fatty streak conversion to fibrous plaque. *Arteriosclerosis* 4:341, 1984.

29. Faggiotto A, Ross R, Harker L: Studies of hypercholesterolemia in the nonhuman primate. I. Changes that lead to fatty streak formation. *Arteriosclerosis* 4:323, 1984.

30. Masuda J, Ross R: Atherogenesis during low level hypercholesterolemia in the nonhuman primate. II. Fatty streak conversion to fibrous plaque. *Arteriosclerosis* 10:178, 1990.

31. Masuda J, Ross R: Atherogenesis during low level hypercholesterolemia in the nonhuman primate. I. Fatty streak formation. *Arteriosclerosis* 10:164, 1990.

32. Breslow JL: Mouse models of atherosclerosis. *Science* 272:685, 1996.

33. Nakashima Y, Plump AS, Raines EW, Breslow JL, Ross R: ApoE-deficient mice develop lesions of all phases of atherosclerosis throughout the arterial tree. *Arterioscler Thromb* 14:133, 1994.

34. Ishibashi S, Goldstein JL, Brown MS, Herz J, Burns DK: Massive xanthomatosis and atherosclerosis in cholesterol-fed low density lipoprotein receptor-negative mice. *J Clin Invest* 93:1885, 1994.

35. Young SG: Using genetically modified mice to study apolipoprotein B. *J Atheroscler Thromb* 3:62, 1996.

36. Gu L, Okada Y, Clinton SK, et al: Absence of monocyte chemoattractant protein-1 reduces atherosclerosis in low density lipoprotein receptor-deficient mice. *Mol Cell* 2:275, 1998.

37. Boring L, Gosling J, Cleary M, Charo IF: Decreased lesion formation in CCR2$^{-/-}$ mice reveals a role for chemokines in the initiation of atherosclerosis. *Nature* 394:894, 1998.

38. Gosling J, Slaymaker S, Gu L, et al: MCP-1 deficiency reduces susceptibility to atherosclerosis in mice that overexpress human apolipoprotein B. *J Clin Invest* 103:773, 1999.

39. Ross R, Glomset JA: Atherosclerosis and the arterial smooth muscle cell: proliferation of smooth muscle is a key event in the genesis of the lesions of atherosclerosis. *Science* 180:1332, 1973.

40. Ross R: Cell biology of atherosclerosis. *Annu Rev Physiol* 57:791, 1995.

41. Pober JS, Cotran RS: Cytokines and endothelial cell biology. *Physiol Rev* 70:427, 1990.

42. Libby P, Sukhova G, Lee RT, Galis ZS: Cytokines regulate vascular functions related to stability of the atherosclerotic plaque. *J Cardiovasc Pharmacol* 25 suppl 2:S9, 1995.

43. Davies PF, Tripathi SC: Mechanical stress mechanisms and the cell. An endothelial paradigm. *Circ Res* 72:239, 1993.

44. Gimbrone MA Jr, Resnick N, Nagel T, Khachigian LM, Collins T, Topper JN: Hemodynamics, endothelial gene expression, and atherogenesis. *Ann N Y Acad Sci* 811:1, 1997.

45. Gimbrone MA Jr: Vascular endothelium: an integrator of pathophysiologic stimuli in atherosclerosis. *Am J Cardiol* 75:67B, 1995.

46. Cines DB, Pollak ES, Buck CA, et al: Endothelial cells in physiology and in the pathophysiology of vascular disorders. *Blood* 91:3527, 1998.

47. Simionescu N, Vasile E, Lupu F, Popescu G, Simionescu M: Prelesional events in atherogenesis. Accumulation of extracellular cholesterol-rich liposomes in the arterial intima and cardiac valves of the hyperlipidemic rabbit. *Am J Pathol* 123:109, 1986.

48. Henriksen T, Mahoney EM, Steinberg D: Enhanced macrophage degradation of low density lipoprotein previously incubated with cultured endothelial cells: recognition by receptors for acetylated low density lipoproteins. *Proc Natl Acad Sci USA* 78:6499, 1981.

49. Cathcart MK, Morel DW, Chisolm GM: Monocytes and neutrophils oxidize low density lipoprotein making it cytotoxic. *J Leukoc Biol* 38:341, 1985.

50. Rosenfeld ME, Palinski W, Yla-Herttuala S, Carew TE: Macrophages, endothelial cells, and lipoprotein oxidation in the pathogenesis of atherosclerosis. *Toxicol Pathol* 18:560, 1990.

51. Steinberg D: Antioxidants and atherosclerosis. A current assessment. *Circulation* 84:1420, 1991.

52. Luscinskas FW, Gimbrone MA Jr: Endothelial-dependent mechanisms in chronic inflammatory leukocyte recruitment. *Annu Rev Med* 47:413, 1996.

53. Thiruvikraman SV, Guha A, Roboz J, Taubman MB, Nemerson Y, Fallon JT: In situ localization of tissue factor in human atherosclerotic plaques by binding of digoxigenin-labeled factors VIIa and X. *Lab Invest* 75:451, 1996.

54. Fuster V, Badimon L, Badimon JJ, Chesebro JH: The pathogenesis of coronary artery disease and the acute coronary syndromes (1). *N Engl J Med* 326:242, 1992.

55. Fuster V, Badimon L, Badimon JJ, Chesebro JH: The pathogenesis of coronary artery disease and the acute coronary syndromes (2). *N Engl J Med* 326:310, 1992.

56. Kullo IJ, Edwards WD, Schwartz RS: Vulnerable plaque: pathobiology and clinical implications. *Ann Intern Med* 129:1050, 1998.

57. Davies MJ, Richardson PD, Woolf N, Katz DR, Mann J: Risk of thrombosis in human atherosclerotic plaques: role of extracellular lipid, macrophage, and smooth muscle cell content. LA - Eng. *Br Heart J* 69:377, 1993.

58. Davies MJ: Stability and instability: two faces of coronary. Paul Dudley White Lecture 1995. *Circulation* 94:2013, 1996.

59. Van der Wal AC, Becker AE, van der Loos CM, Das PK: Site of intimal rupture or erosion of thrombosed coronary atherosclerotic plaques is characterized by an inflammatory process irrespective of the dominant plaque morphology. *Circulation* 89:36, 1994.

60. Libby P: Molecular bases of the acute coronary syndromes. *Circulation* 91:2844, 1995.

61. Galis ZS, Sukhova GK, Lark MW, Libby P: Increased expression of matrix metalloproteinases and matrix degrading activity in vulnerable regions of human atherosclerotic plaques. *J Clin Invest* 94:2493, 1994.

62. Richardson PD, Davies MJ, Born GV: Influence of plaque configuration and stress distribution on fissuring of coronary atherosclerotic plaques. *Lancet* 2:941, 1989.

63. Cheng GC, Loree HM, Kamm RD, Fishbein MC, Lee RT: Distribution of circumferential stress in ruptured and stable atherosclerotic lesions. A structural analysis with histopathological correlation. *Circulation* 87:1179, 1993.

64. Davies MJ: A macro and micro view of coronary vascular insult in ischemic heart disease. *Circulation* 82: (3 Suppl):1138, 1990.

65. Losordo DW, Rosenfield K, Pieczek A, Baker K, Harding M, Isner JM: How does angioplasty work? Serial analysis of human iliac arteries using intravascular ultrasound. *Circulation* 86:1845, 1992.

66. Nath FC, Muller DW, Ellis SG, et al: Thrombosis of a flexible coil coronary stent: frequency, predictors and clinical outcome. *J Am Coll Cardiol* 21:622, 1993.

67. Schafer AI: Antiplatelet therapy. *Am J Med* 101:199, 1996.

68. Steele PM, Chesebro JH, Stanson AW, et al: Balloon angioplasty. Natural history of the pathophysiological response to injury in a pig model. *Circ Res* 57:105, 1985.

69. Heras M, Chesebro JH, Penny WJ, Bailey KR, Badimon L, Fuster V: Effects of thrombin inhibition on the development of acute platelet-thrombus deposition during angioplasty in pigs. Heparin versus recombinant hirudin, a specific thrombin inhibitor. *Circulation* 79:657, 1989.

70. Stemerman BM: Thrombogenesis of the rabbit arterial plaque. *Am J Pathol* 73:7, 1973.

71. Groves MH, Rathbone-Kinlough LR, Richardson M, Jorgensen L, Moore S, Mustard FJ: Thrombin generation and fibrin formation following injury to rabbit neointima. *Lab Invest* 46:605, 1982.

72. Clowes AW, Reidy MA, Clowes MM: Kinetics of cellular proliferation after arterial injury. I. Smooth muscle growth in the absence of endothelium. *Lab Invest* 49:327, 1983.

73. Richardson M, Kinlough-Rathbone LR, Groves HM, Jorgensen L, Mustard JF, Moore S: Ultrastructural changes in re-endothelialized and non-endothelialized rabbit aortic neointima following re-injury with a ballon catheter. *Br J Exp Path* 65:597, 1984.

74. Consigny MP, Tulenko NT, Nicosia FR: Immediate and long-term effects of angioplasty-balloon dilation on normal rabbit iliac artery. *Arteriosclerosis* 6:265, 1986.

75. Asada Y, Hara S, Tsuneyoshi A, et al: Fibrin-rich and platelet-rich thrombus formation on neointima: recombinant tissue factor pathway inhibitor prevents fibrin formation and neointimal development following repeated balloon injury of rabbit aorta. *Thromb Haemost* 80:506, 1998.

76. Courtman DW, Schwartz SM, Hart CE: Sequential injury of the rabbit abdominal aorta induces intramural coagulation and luminal narrowing independent of intimal mass: extrinsic pathway inhibition eliminates luminal narrowing. *Circ Res* 82:996, 1998.

77. Edgington TS, Mackman N, Brand K, Ruf W: The structural biology of expression and function of tissue factor. *Thromb Haemost* 66:67, 1991.

78. Nemerson Y: Tissue factor: then and now. *Thromb Haemost* 74:180, 1995.

79. Rapaport SI, Rao LV: The tissue factor pathway: how it has become a "prima ballerina." *Thromb Haemost* 74:7, 1995.

80. Zeldis SM, Nemerson Y, Pitlick FA, Lentz TL: Tissue factor (thrombo-

81. Drake TA, Morrissey JH, Edgington TS: Selective cellular expression of tissue factor in human tissues. *Am J Pathol* 134:1087, 1989.

82. Wilcox JN, Smith KM, Schwartz SM, Gordon D: Localization of tissue factor in the normal vessel wall and in the atherosclerotic plaque. *Proc Natl Acad Sci USA* 86:2839, 1989.

83. Annex BH, Denning SM, Channon KM, et al: Differential expression of tissue factor protein in directional atherectomy specimens from patients with stable and unstable coronary syndromes. *Circulation* 91:619, 1995.

84. Marmur JD, Thiruvikraman SV, Fyfe BS, et al: Identification of active tissue factor in human coronary atheroma. *Circulation* 94:1226, 1996.

85. Moreno PR, Bernardi VH, Lopez-Cuellar J, et al: Macrophages, smooth muscle cells, and tissue factor in unstable angina. Implications for cell-mediated thrombogenicity in acute coronary syndromes. *Circulation* 94:3090, 1996.

86. Hatakeyama K, Asada Y, Marutsuka K, Sato Y, Kamikubo Y, Sumiyoshi A: Localization and activity of tissue factor in human aortic atherosclerotic lesions. *Atherosclerosis* 133:213, 1997.

87. Caplice NM, Mueske CS, Kleppe LS, Simari RD: Presence of tissue factor pathway inhibitor in human atherosclerotic plaques is associated with reduced tissue factor activity. *Circulation* 98:1051, 1998.

88. Fernandez-Ortiz A, Badimon JJ, Falk E, et al: Characterization of the relative thrombogenicity of atherosclerotic plaque components: implications for consequences of plaque rupture. *J Am Coll Cardiol* 23:1562, 1994.

89. Toschi V, Gallo R, Lettino M, et al: Tissue factor modulates the thrombogenicity of human atherosclerotic plaques. *Circulation* 95:594, 1997.

90. Mallat Z, Hugel B, Ohan J, Leseche G, Freyssinet JM, Tedgui A: Shed membrane microparticles with procoagulant potential in human atherosclerotic plaques : A role for apoptosis in plaque thrombogenicity. *Circulation* 99:348, 1999.

91. Maynard JR, Heckman CA, Pitlick FA, Nemerson Y: Association of tissue factor activity with the surface of cultured cells. *J Clin Invest* 55:814, 1975.

92. Marmur JD, Rossikhina M, Guha A, et al: Tissue factor is rapidly induced in arterial smooth muscle after balloon injury. *J Clin Invest* 91:2253, 1993.

93. Pawashe AB, Golino P, Ambrosio G, et al: A monoclonal antibody against rabbit tissue factor inhibits thrombus formation in stenotic injured rabbit carotid arteries. *Circ Res* 74:56, 1994.

94. Speidel CM, Eisenberg PR, Ruf W, Edgington TS, Abendschein DR: Tissue factor mediates prolonged procoagulant activity on the luminal surface of balloon-injured aortas in rabbits. *Circulation* 92:3323, 1995.

95. Gertz SD, Fallon JT, Gallo R, et al: Hirudin reduces tissue factor expression in neointima after balloon injury in rabbit femoral and porcine coronary arteries. *Circulation* 98:580, 1998.

96. Jang IK, Gold HK, Leinbach RC, Fallon JT, Collen D, Wilcox JN: Antithrombotic effect of a monoclonal antibody against tissue factor in a rabbit model of platelet-mediated arterial thrombosis. *Arterioscler Thromb* 12:948, 1992.

97. Golino P, Ragni M, Cirillo P, et al: Antithrombotic effects of recombinant human, active site-blocked factor VIIa in a rabbit model of recurrent arterial thrombosis. *Circ Res* 82:39, 1998.

98. Jang Y, Guzman LA, Lincoff AM, et al: Influence of blockade at specific levels of the coagulation cascade on restenosis in a rabbit atherosclerotic femoral artery injury model. *Circulation* 92:3041, 1995.

99. Harker LA, Hanson SR, Wilcox JN, Kelly AB: Antithrombotic and antilesion benefits without hemorrhagic risks by inhibiting tissue factor pathway. *Haemostasis* 26 (suppl 1):76, 1996.

100. Oltrona L, Speidel CM, Recchia D, Wickline SA, Eisenberg PR, Abendschein DR: Inhibition of tissue factor-mediated coagulation markedly attenuates stenosis after balloon-induced arterial injury inminipigs. *Circulation* 96:646, 1997.

101. Fukuda C, Iijima K, Nakamura K: Measuring tissue factor (factor III) activity in plasma. *Clin Chem* 35:1897, 1989.

102. Suefuji H, Ogawa H, Yasue H, et al: Increased plasma tissue factor levels in acute myocardial infarction. *Am Heart J* 134:253, 1997.

103. Key NS, Slungaard A, Dandelet L, et al: Whole blood tissue factor procoagulant activity is elevated in patients with sickle cell disease. *Blood* 91:4216, 1998.

plastin): localization to plasma membranes by peroxidase-conjugated antibodies. *Science* 175:766, 1972.

104. Giesen PLA, Rauch U, Bohrmann B, et al: Blood-borne tissue factor: a new view of thrombosis. *Proc Natl Acad Sci USA* 99:2311, 1999.

105. Hartzell S, Ryder K, Lanahan A, Lau LF, Nathan D: A growth factor-responsive gene of murine BALB/c 3T3 cells encodes a protein homologous to human tissue factor. *Mol Cell Biol* 9:2567, 1989.

106. Drake TA, Hannani K, Fei HH, Lavi S, Berliner JA: Minimally oxidized low-density lipoprotein induces tissue factor expression in cultured human endothelial cells. *Am J Pathol* 138:601, 1991.

107. Brand K, Banka CL, Mackman N, Terkeltaub RA, Fan ST, Curtiss LK: Oxidized LDL enhances lipopolysaccharide-induced tissue factor expression in human adherent monocytes. *Arterioscler Thromb* 14:790, 1994.

108. van den Eijnden MM, Steenhauer SI, Reitsma PH, Bertina RM: Tissue factor expression during monocyte-macrophage differentiation. *Thromb Haemost* 77:1129, 1997.

109. Brox JH, Osterud B, Bjorklid E, Fenton JW: Production and availability of thromboplastin in endothelial cells: the effects of thrombin, endotoxin and platelets. *Br J Haematol* 57:239, 1984.

110. Taubman MB, Marmur JD, Rosenfield CL, Guha A, Nichtberger S, Nemerson Y: Agonist-mediated tissue factor expression in cultured vascular smooth muscle cells. Role of Ca2+ mobilization and protein kinase C activation. *J Clin Invest* 91:547, 1993.

111. Schecter AD, Giesen PL, Taby O, et al: Tissue factor expression in human arterial smooth muscle cells. TF is present in three cellular pools after growth factor stimulation. *J Clin Invest* 100:2276, 1997.

112. Grabowski EF, Zuckerman DB, Nemerson Y: The functional expression of tissue factor by fibroblasts and endothelial cells under flow conditions. *Blood* 81:3265, 1993.

113. Lin MC, Almus-Jacobs F, Chen HH, et al: Shear stress induction of the tissue factor gene. *J Clin Invest* 99:737, 1997.

114. Mackman N, Morrissey JH, Fowler B, Edgington TS: Complete sequence of the human tissue factor gene, a highly regulated cellular receptor that initiates the coagulation protease cascade. *Biochemistry* 28:1755, 1989.

115. Mackman N, Imes S, Maske WH, Taylor B, Lusis AJ, Drake TA: Structure of the murine tissue factor gene. Chromosome location and conservation of regulatory elements in the promoter. *Arterioscler Thromb* 12:474, 1992.

116. Moll T, Czyz M, Holzmuller H, et al: Regulation of the tissue factor promoter in endothelial cells. Binding of NF kappa B-, AP-1-, and Sp1-like transcription factors. *J Biol Chem* 270:3849, 1995.

117. Taby O, Rosenfield CL, Bogdanov V, Nemerson Y, Taubman MB: Cloning of the rat tissue factor cDNA and promoter: identification of a serum-response region. *Thromb Haemost* 76:697, 1996.

118. Mackman N: Regulation of the tissue factor gene. *Thromb Haemost* 78:747, 1997.

119. Drake TA, Ruf W, Morrissey JH, Edgington TS: Functional tissue factor is entirely cell surface expressed on lipopolysaccharide-stimulated human blood monocytes and a constitutively tissue factor-producing neoplastic cell line. *J Cell Biol* 109:389, 1989.

120. Le DT, Rapaport SI, Rao LV: Relations between factor VIIa binding and expression of factor VIIa/tissue factor catalytic activity on cell surfaces. *J Biol Chem* 267:15447, 1992.

121. Carson SD: Manifestation of cryptic fibroblast tissue factor occurs at detergent concentrations which dissolve the plasma membrane. *Blood Coagul Fibrinolysis* 7:303, 1996.

122. Greeno EW, Bach RR, Moldow CF: Apoptosis is associated with increased cell surface tissue factor procoagulant activity. *Lab Invest* 75:281, 1996.

123. Mulder AB, Smit JW, Bom VJ, et al: Association of smooth muscle cell tissue factor with caveolae. *Blood* 88:1306, 1996.

124. Sevinsky RJ, Rao MVL, Ruf W: Ligand-induced protease receptor translocation into caveolae: a mechanism for regulating cell surface proteolsis of the tissue factor-dependent coagulation pathway. *J Cell Biol* 133:293, 1996.

125. Bach RR, Moldow CF: Mechanism of tissue factor activation on HL-60 cells. *Blood* 89:3270, 1997.

126. Carson SD, Perry GA, Pirruccello SJ: Fibroblast tissue factor: calcium and ionophore induce shape changes, release of membrane vesicles, and redistribution of tissue factor antigen in addition to increased procoagulant activity. *Blood* 84:526, 1994.

127. Satta N, Toti F, Feugeas O, et al: Monocyte vesiculation is a possible mechanism for dissemination of membrane-associated procoagulant activities and adhesion molecules after stimulation by lipopolysaccharide. *J Immunol* 153:3245, 1994.

128. Broze GJ Jr: Tissue factor pathway inhibitor and the revised theory of coagulation. *Annu Rev Med* 46:103, 1995.

129. Mann KG, van't Veer C, Cawthern K, Butenas S: The role of the tissue factor pathway in initiation of coagulation. *Blood Coagul Fibrinolysis* 9 (suppl 1):S3, 1998.

130. Kamikubo Y, Nakahara Y, Takemoto S, Hamuro T, Miyamoto S, Funatsu A: Human recombinant tissue-factor pathway inhibitor prevents the proliferation of cultured human neonatal aortic smooth muscle cells. *FEBS Lett* 407:116, 1997.

131. Bajaj MS, Kuppuswamy MN, Saito H, Spitzer SG, Bajaj SP: Cultured normal human hepatocytes do not synthesize lipoprotein-associated coagulation inhibitor: evidence that endothelium is the principal site of its synthesis. *Proc Natl Acad Sci USA.* 87:8869, 1990.

132. Werling RW, Zacharski LR, Kisiel W, Bajaj SP, Memoli VA, Rousseau SM: Distribution of tissue factor pathway inhibitor in normal and malignant human tissues. *Thromb Haemost* 69:366, 1993.

133. Caplice NM, Mueske CS, Kleppe LS, Peterson TE, Broze GJ, Jr, Simari RD: Expression of tissue factor pathway inhibitor in vascular smooth muscle cells and its regulation by growth factors. *Circ Res* 83:1264, 1998.

134. Sato N, Kokame K, Miyata T, Kato H: Lysophosphatidylcholine decreases the synthesis of tissue factor pathway inhibitor in human umbilical vein endothelial cells. *Thromb Haemost* 79:217, 1998.

135. Broze GJ Jr: Tissue factor pathway inhibitor gene disruption. *Blood Coagul Fibrinolysis* 9(suppl 1):S89, 1998.

136. Drew AF, Davenport P, Apostolopoulos J, Tipping PG: Tissue factor pathway inhibitor expression in atherosclerosis. *Lab Invest* 77:291, 1997.

137. Haskel EJ, Torr SR, Day KC, et al: Prevention of arterial reocclusion after thrombolysis with recombinant lipoprotein-associated coagulation inhibitor . *Circulation* 84:821, 1991.

138. Gross JL, Moscatelli D, Jaffe EA, Rifkin DB: Plasminogen activator and collagenase production by cultured capillary endothelial cells. *J Cell Biol* 95:974, 1982.

139. Levin EG, Loskutoff DJ: Cultured bovine endothelial cells produce both urokinase and tissue-type plasminogen activators. *J Cell Biol* 94:631, 1982.

140. Nachman RL, Hajjar KA: Endothelial cell fibrinolytic assembly. *Ann N Y Acad Sci* 614:240, 1991.

141. Levin EG, del Zoppo GJ: Localization of tissue plasminogen activator in the endothelium of a limited number of vessels. *Am J Pathol* 144:855, 1994.

142. Lupu F, Heim DA, Bachmann F, Hurni M, Kakkar VV, Kruithof EK: Plasminogen activator expression in human atherosclerotic lesions. *Arterioscler Thromb Vasc Biol* 15:1444, 1995.

143. Ljungner H, Bergqvist D: Decreased fibrinolytic activity in human atherosclerotic vessels. *Atherosclerosis* 50:113, 1984.

144. Bjorkerud S: Impaired fibrinolysis-inducing capacity for postinjury phenotype of cultivated human arterial and human atherosclerotic intimal smooth muscle cells. *Circ Res* 62:1011, 1988.

145. Underwood MJ, De Bono DP: Increased fibrinolytic activity in the intima of atheromatous coronary arteries: protection at a price. *Cardiovasc Res* 27:882, 1993.

146. Reilly JM, Sicard GA, Lucore CL: Abnormal expression of plasminogen activators in aortic aneurysmal and occlusive disease. *J Vasc Surg* 19:865, 1994.

147. Raghunath PN, Tomaszewski JE, Brady ST, Caron RJ, Okada SS, Barnathan ES: Plasminogen activator system in human coronary atherosclerosis. *Arterioscler Thromb Vasc Biol* 15:1432, 1995.

148. Clowes AW, Clowes MM, Au YP, Reidy MA, Belin D: Smooth muscle cells express urokinase during mitogenesis and tissue-type plasminogen activator during migration in injured rat carotid artery. *Circ Res* 67:61, 1990.

149. Lyons RM, Gentry LE, Purchio AF, Moses HL: Mechanism of activation of latent recombinant transforming growth factor beta 1 by plasmin. *J Cell Biol* 110:1361, 1990.

150. Saksela O, Rifkin DB: Release of basic fibroblast growth factor-heparan sulfate complexes from endothelial cells by plasminogen activator-mediated proteolytic activity. *J Cell Biol* 110:767, 1990.

151. Grainger DJ, Kirschenlohr HL, Metcalfe JC, Weissberg PL, Wade DP,

Lawn RM: Proliferation of human smooth muscle cells promoted by lipoprotein(a). *Science* 260:1655, 1993.

152. Kojima S, Harpel PC, Rifkin DB: Lipoprotein(a) inhibits the generation of transforming growth factor beta: an endogenous inhibitor of smooth muscle cell migration. *J Cell Biol* 113:1439, 1991.

153. Grainger DJ, Kemp PR, Liu AC, Lawn RM, Metcalfe JC: Activation of transforming growth factor-beta is inhibited in transgenic apolipoprotein(a) mice. *Nature* 370:460, 1994.

154. He CS, Wilhelm SM, Pentland AP, et al: Tissue cooperation in a proteolytic cascade activating human interstitial collagenase. *Proc Natl Acad Sci USA* 86:2632, 1989.

155. Jackson CL, Reidy MA: The role of plasminogen activation in smooth muscle cell migration after arterial injury. *Ann NY Acad Sci* 667:141, 1992.

156. Kanamasa K, Ishida N, Kato H, et al: Recombinant tissue plasminogen activator prevents intimal hyperplasia after balloon angioplasty in hypercholesterolemic rabbits. *Jpn Circ J* 60:889, 1996.

157. Loskutoff DJ, Sawdey M, Keeton M, Schneiderman J: Regulation of PAI-1 gene expression in vivo. *Thromb Haemost* 70:135, 1993.

158. Booth NA, Simpson AJ, Croll A, Bennett B, MacGregor IR: Plasminogen activator inhibitor (PAI-1) in plasma and platelets. *Br J Haematol* 70:327, 1988.

159. Green F, Humphries S: Genetic determinants of arterial thrombosis. *Baillieres Clin Haematol* 7:675, 1994.

160. Lijnen HR, Bachmann F, Collen D, et al: Mechanisms of plasminogen activation. *J Intern Med* 236:415, 1994.

161. Aillaud MF, Pignol F, Alessi MC, et al: Increase in plasma concentration of plasminogen activator inhibitor, fibrinogen, von Willebrand factor, factor VIII:C and in erythrocyte sedimentation rate with age. *Thromb Haemost* 55:330, 1986.

162. Juhan-Vague I, Vague P, Alessi MC, et al: Relationships between plasma insulin triglyceride, body mass index, and plasminogen activator inhibitor 1. *Diabete Metab* 13:331, 1987.

163. Juhan-Vague I, Alessi MC, Vague P: Increased plasma plasminogen activator inhibitor 1 levels. A possible link between insulin resistance and atherothrombosis. *Diabetologia* 34:457, 1991.

164. Wagner OF, de Vries C, Hohmann C, Veerman H, Pannekoek H: Interaction between plasminogen activator inhibitor type 1 (PAI-1) bound to fibrin and either tissue-type plasminogen activator (t-PA) or urokinase-type plasminogen activator (u-PA). Binding of t-PA/PAI-1 complexes to fibrin mediated by both the finger and the kringle-2 domain of t-PA. *J Clin Invest* 84:647, 1989.

165. Vaughan DE, Declerck PJ, Van Houtte E, De Mol M, Collen D: Reactivated recombinant plasminogen activator inhibitor-1 (rPAI-1) effectively prevents thrombolysis in vivo. *Thromb Haemost* 68:60, 1992.

166. Fay WP, Eitzman DT, Shapiro AD, Madison EL, Ginsburg D: Platelets inhibit fibrinolysis in vitro by both plasminogen activator inhibitor-1-dependent and -independent mechanisms. *Blood* 83:351, 1994.

167. Prisco D, Chiarantini E, Boddi M, Rostagno C, Colella A, Gensini GF: Predictive value for thrombotic disease of plasminogen activator inhibitor-1 plasma levels. *Int J Clin Lab Res* 23:78, 1993.

168. Aznar J, Estelles A, Tormo G, et al: Plasminogen activator inhibitor activity and other fibrinolytic variables in patients with coronary artery disease. *Br Heart J* 59:535, 1988.

169. Huber K, Resch I, Stefenelli T, et al: Plasminogen activator inhibitor-1 levels in patients with chronic angina pectoris with or without angiographic evidence of coronary sclerosis. *Thromb Haemost* 63:336, 1990.

170. Zalewski A, Shi Y, Nardone D, et al: Evidence for reduced fibrinolytic activity in unstable angina at rest. Clinical, biochemical, and angiographic correlates. *Circulation* 83:1685, 1991.

171. Gram J, Kluft C, Jespersen J: Depression of tissue plasminogen activator (t-PA) activity and rise of t-PA inhibition and acute phase reactants in blood of patients with acute myocardial infarction (AMI). *Thromb Haemost* 58:817, 1987.

172. Hamsten A, de Faire U, Walldius G, et al: Plasminogen activator inhibitor in plasma: risk factor for recurrent myocardial infarction. *Lancet* 2:3, 1987.

173. Barbash GI, Hod H, Roth A, et al: Correlation of baseline plasminogen activator inhibitor activity with patency of the infarct artery after thrombolytic therapy in acute myocardial infarction. *Am J Cardiol* 64:1231, 1989.

174. Ridker PM, Hennekens CH, Stampfer MJ, Manson JE, Vaughan DE: Prospective study of endogenous tissue plasminogen activator and risk of stroke. *Lancet* 343:940, 1994.

175. Salomaa V, Stinson V, Kark JD, Folsom AR, Davis CE, Wu KK: Association of fibrinolytic parameters with early atherosclerosis. The ARIC Study. Atherosclerosis Risk in Communities Study. *Circulation* 91:284, 1995.

176. Huber K, Jorg M, Probst P, et al: A decrease in plasminogen activator inhibitor-1 activity after successful percutaneous transluminal coronary angioplasty is associated with a significantly reduced risk for coronary restenosis. *Thromb Haemost* 67:209, 1992.

177. Schneiderman J, Sawdey MS, Keeton MR, et al: Increased type 1 plasminogen activator inhibitor gene expression in atherosclerotic human arteries. *Proc Natl Acad Sci USA* 89:6998, 1992.

178. Lupu F, Bergonzelli GE, Heim DA, et al: Localization and production of plasminogen activator inhibitor-1 in human healthy and atherosclerotic arteries. *Arterioscler Thromb* 13:1090, 1993.

179. Chomiki N, Henry M, Alessi MC, Anfosso F, Juhan-Vague I: Plasminogen activator inhibitor-1 expression in human liver and healthy or atherosclerotic vessel walls. *Thromb Haemost* 72:44, 1994.

180. Robbie LA, Bennett B, Croll AM, Brown PA, Booth NA: Proteins of the fibrinolytic system in human thrombi. *Thromb Haemost* 75:127, 1996.

181. Robbie LA, Booth NA, Brown AJ, Bennett B: Inhibitors of fibrinolysis are elevated in atherosclerotic plaque. *Arterioscler Thromb Vasc Biol* 16:539, 1996.

182. Loskutoff DJ: PAI-1 inhibits neointimal formation after arterial injury in mice: a new target for controlling restenosis? *Circulation* 96:2772, 1997.

183. Fay WP, Parker AC, Condrey LR, Shapiro AD: Human plasminogen activator inhibitor-1 (PAI-1) deficiency: characterization of a large kindred with a null mutation in the PAI-1 gene. *Blood* 90:204, 1997.

184. Sawa H, Lundgren C, Sobel BE, Fujii S: Increased intramural expression of plasminogen activator inhibitor type 1 after balloon injury: a potential progenitor of restenosis. *J Am Coll Cardiol* 24:1742, 1994.

185. Hasenstab D, Forough R, Clowes AW: Plasminogen activator inhibitor type 1 and tissue inhibitor of metalloproteinases-2 increase after arterial injury in rats. *Circ Res* 80:490, 1997.

186. Sawa H, Fujii S, Sobel BE: Augmented arterial wall expression of type-1 plasminogen activator inhibitor induced by thrombosis. *Arterioscler Thromb* 12:1507, 1992.

187. Loskutoff DJ, van Mourik JA, Erickson LA, Lawrence D: Detection of an unusually stable fibrinolytic inhibitor produced by bovine endothelial cells. *Proc Natl Acad Sci USA* 80:2956, 1983.

188. Laug WE: Vascular smooth muscle cells inhibit the plasminogen activators secreted by endothelial cells. *Thromb Haemost* 53:165, 1985.

189. Tipping PG, Davenport P, Gallicchio M, Filonzi EL, Apostolopoulos J, Wojta J: Atheromatous plaque macrophages produce plasminogen activator inhibitor type-1 and stimulate its production by endothelial cells and vascular smooth muscle cells. *Am J Pathol* 143:875, 1993.

190. Gelehrter TD, Sznycer-Laszuk R: Thrombin induction of plasminogen activator-inhibitor in cultured human endothelial cells. *J Clin Invest* 77:165, 1986.

191. Saksela O, Moscatelli D, Rifkin DB: The opposing effects of basic fibroblast growth factor and transforming growth factor beta on the regulation of plasminogen activator activity in capillary endothelial cells. *J Cell Biol* 105:957, 1987.

192. Hasselaar P, Loskutoff DJ, Sawdey M, Sage EH: SPARC induces the expression of type 1 plasminogen activator inhibitor in cultured bovine aortic endothelial cells. *J Biol Chem* 266:13178, 1991.

193. Reilly CF, McFall RC: Platelet-derived growth factor and transforming growth factor-beta regulate plasminogen activator inhibitor-1 synthesis in vascular smooth muscle cells. *J Biol Chem* 266:9419, 1991.

194. Sawdey MS, Loskutoff DJ: Regulation of murine type 1 plasminogen activator inhibitor gene expression in vivo. Tissue specificity and induction by lipopolysaccharide, tumor necrosis factor-alpha, and transforming growth factor-beta. *J Clin Invest* 88:1346, 1991.

195. van Leeuwen RT, Kol A, Andreotti F, Kluft C, Maseri A, Sperti G: Angiotensin II increases plasminogen activator inhibitor type 1 and tissue-type plasminogen activator messenger RNA in cultured rat aortic smooth muscle cells. *Circulation* 90:362, 1994.

196. Noda-Heiny H, Fujii S, Sobel BE: Induction of vascular smooth muscle cell expression of plasminogen activator inhibitor-1 by thrombin. *Circ Res* 72:36, 1993.

197. Wojta J, Gallicchio M, Zoellner H, et al: Thrombin stimulates expression

of tissue-type plasminogen activator and plasminogen activator inhibitor type 1 in cultured human vascular smooth muscle cells. *Thromb Haemost* 70:469, 1993.

198. Christ G, Hufnagl P, Kaun C, et al: Antifibrinolytic properties of the vascular wall. Dependence on the history of smooth muscle cell doublings in vitro and in vivo. *Arterioscler Thromb Vasc Biol* 17:723, 1997.

199. Etingin OR, Hajjar DP, Hajjar KA, Harpel PC, Nachman RL: Lipoprotein (a) regulates plasminogen activator inhibitor-1 expression in endothelial cells. A potential mechanism in thrombogenesis. *J Biol Chem* 266:2459, 1991.

200. Christ G, Seiffert D, Hufnagl P, Gessl A, Wojta J, Binder BR: Type 1 plasminogen activator inhibitor synthesis of endothelial cells is downregulated by smooth muscle cells. *Blood* 81:1277, 1993.

201. Kruithof EK, Gudinchet A, Bachmann F: Plasminogen activator inhibitor 1 and plasminogen activator inhibitor 2 in various disease states. *Thromb Haemost* 59:7, 1988.

202. Bachmann F: The enigma PAI-2. Gene expression, evolutionary and functional aspects. *Thromb Haemost* 74:172, 1995.

203. Higazi AA, Mazar A, Wang J, et al: Single-chain urokinase-type plasminogen activator bound to its receptor is relatively resistant to plasminogen activator inhibitor type 1. *Blood* 87:3545, 1996.

204. Blasi F: The urokinase receptor and cell migration. *Semin Thromb Hemost* 22:513, 1996.

205. Barnathan ES, Kuo A, Kariko K, et al: Characterization of human endothelial cell urokinase-type plasminogen activator receptor protein and messenger RNA. *Blood* 76:1795, 1990.

206. Reuning U, Bang NU: Regulation of the urokinase-type plasminogen activator receptor on vascular smooth muscle cells is under the control of thrombin and other mitogens. *Arterioscler Thromb* 12:1161, 1992.

207. Okada SS, Golden MA, Raghunath PN, et al: Native atherosclerosis and vein graft arterialization: association with increased urokinase receptor expression in vitro and in vivo. *Thromb Haemost* 80:140, 1998.

208. Okada SS, Tomaszewski JE, Barnathan ES: Migrating vascular smooth muscle cells polarize cell surface urokinase receptors after injury in vitro. *Exp Cell Res* 217:180, 1995.

209. Pepper MS, Sappino AP, Stocklin R, Montesano R, Orci L, Vassalli JD: Upregulation of urokinase receptor expression on migrating endothelial cells. *J Cell Biol* 122:673, 1993.

210. Estreicher A, Muhlhauser J, Carpentier JL, Orci L, Vassalli JD: The receptor for urokinase type plasminogen activator polarizes expression of the protease to the leading edge of migrating monocytes and promotes degradation of enzyme inhibitor complexes. *J Cell Biol* 111:783, 1990.

211. Wei Y, Lukashev M, Simon DI, et al: Regulation of integrin function by the urokinase receptor. *Science* 273:1551, 1996.

212. Sitrin RG, Todd RF, 3rd, Albrecht E, Gyetko MR: The urokinase receptor (CD87) facilitates CD11b/CD18-mediated adhesion of human monocytes. *J Clin Invest* 97:1942, 1996.

213. Wong WS, Simon DI, Rosoff PM, Rao NK, Chapman HA: Mechanisms of pertussis toxin-induced myelomonocytic cell adhesion: role of Mac-1(CD11b/CD18) and urokinase receptor (CD87). *Immunology* 88:90, 1996.

214. Anichini E, Fibbi G, Pucci M, Caldini R, Chevanne M, Del Rosso M: Production of second messengers following chemotactic and mitogenic urokinase-receptor interaction in human fibroblasts and mouse fibroblasts transfected with human urokinase receptor. *Exp Cell Res* 213:438, 1994.

215. Resnati M, Guttinger M, Valcamonica S, Sidenius N, Blasi F, Fazioli F: Proteolytic cleavage of the urokinase receptor substitutes for the agonist-induced chemotactic effect. *Embo J* 15:1572, 1996.

216. Rao NK, Shi GP, Chapman HA: Urokinase receptor is a multifunctional protein: influence of receptor occupancy on macrophage gene expression. *J Clin Invest* 96:465, 1995.

217. Rabbani SA, Mazar AP, Bernier SM, et al: Structural requirements for the growth factor activity of the amino- terminal domain of urokinase. *J Biol Chem* 267:14151, 1992.

218. De Petro G, Copeta A, Barlati S: Urokinase-type and tissue-type plasminogen activators as growth factors of human fibroblasts. *Exp Cell Res* 213:286, 1994.

219. Higazi AA, Upson RH, Cohen RL, et al: Interaction of single-chain urokinase with its receptor induces the appearance and disappearance of binding epitopes within the resultant complex for other cell surface proteins. *Blood* 88:542, 1996.

220. Noda-Heiny H, Daugherty A, Sobel BE: Augmented urokinase receptor expression in atheroma. *Arterioscler Thromb Vasc Biol* 15:37, 1995.

221. Carmeliet P, Collen D: Molecular genetics of the fibrinolytic and coagulation systems in haemostasis, thrombogenesis, restenosis and atherosclerosis. *Curr Opin Lipidol* 8:118, 1997.

222. Carmeliet P, Moons L, Ploplis V, Plow E, Collen D: Impaired arterial neointima formation in mice with disruption of the plasminogen gene. *J Clin Invest* 99:200, 1997.

223. Romer J, Bugge TH, Pyke C, et al: Impaired wound healing in mice with a disrupted plasminogen gene. *Nat Med* 2:287, 1996.

224. Carmeliet P, Moons L, Herbert JM, et al: Urokinase but not tissue plasminogen activator mediates arterial neointima formation in mice. *Circ Res* 81:829, 1997.

225. Carmeliet P, Moons L, Lijnen R, et al: Inhibitory role of plasminogen activator inhibitor-1 in arterial wound healing and neointima formation: a gene targeting and gene transfer study in mice. *Circulation* 96:3180, 1997.

226. Farrehi PM, Ozaki CK, Carmeliet P, Fay WP: Regulation of arterial thrombolysis by plasminogen activator inhibitor-1 in mice. *Circulation* 97:1002, 1998.

227. Bugge TH, Suh TT, Flick MJ, et al: The receptor for urokinase-type plasminogen activator is not essential for mouse development or fertility. *J Biol Chem* 270:16886, 1995.

228. Bugge TH, Flick MJ, Danton MJ, et al: Urokinase-type plasminogen activator is effective in fibrin clearance in the absence of its receptor or tissue-type plasminogen activator. *Proc Natl Acad Sci USA* 93:5899, 1996.

229. Carmeliet P, Moons L, Dewerchin M, et al: Receptor-independent role of urokinase-type plasminogen activator in pericellular plasmin and matrix metalloproteinase proteolysis during vascular wound healing in mice. *J Cell Biol* 140:233, 1998.

230. Robbie LA, Booth NA, Croll AM, Bennett B: The roles of alpha 2-antiplasmin and plasminogen activator inhibitor 1 (PAI-1) in the inhibition of clot lysis. *Thromb Haemost* 70:301, 1993.

231. Plow EF, Collen D: The presence and release of alpha 2-antiplasmin from human platelets. *Blood* 58:1069, 1981.

232. Sakata Y, Aoki N: Significance of cross-linking of alpha 2-plasmin inhibitor to fibrin in inhibition of fibrinolysis and in hemostasis. *J Clin Invest* 69:536, 1982.

233. Folsom AR: Epidemiology of fibrinogen. *Eur Heart J* 16 (suppl A):21, 1995.

234. Thompson WD, Smith EB: Atherosclerosis and the coagulation system. *J Pathol* 159:97, 1989.

235. Letcher RL, Chien S, Pickering TG, Sealey JE, Laragh JH: Direct relationship between blood pressure and blood viscosity in normal and hypertensive subjects. Role of fibrinogen and concentration. *Am J Med* 70:1195, 1981.

236. Kannel WB, D'Agostino RB, Wilson PW, Belanger AJ, Gagnon DR: Diabetes, fibrinogen, and risk of cardiovascular disease: the Framingham experience. *Am Heart J* 120:672, 1990.

237. Ernst E, Matrai A, Schmolzl C, Magyarosy I: Dose-effect relationship between smoking and blood rheology. *Br J Haematol* 65:485, 1987.

238. Yarnell JW, Sweetnam PM, Rogers S, et al: Some long term effects of smoking on the haemostatic system: a report from the Caerphilly and Speedwell Collaborative Surveys. *J Clin Pathol* 40:909, 1987.

239. Wilhelmsen L, Svardsudd K, Korsan-Bengtsen K, Larsson B, Welin L, Tibblin G: Fibrinogen as a risk factor for stroke and myocardial infarction. *N Engl J Med* 311:501, 1984.

240. Kannel WB, Wolf PA, Castelli WP, D'Agostino RB: Fibrinogen and risk of cardiovascular disease. The Framingham Study. *JAMA* 258:1183, 1987.

241. Meade TW, Mellows S, Brozovic M, et al: Haemostatic function and ischaemic heart disease: principal results of the Northwick Park Heart Study. *Lancet* 2:533, 1986.

242. Barasch E, Benderly M, Graff E, et al: Plasma fibrinogen levels and their correlates in 6457 coronary heart disease patients. The Bezafibrate Infarction Prevention (BIP) Study. *J Clin Epidemiol* 48:757, 1995.

243. Ernst E: Fibrinogen as a cardiovascular risk factor—interrelationship with infections and inflammation. *Eur Heart J* 14 (suppl K):82, 1993.

244. Eisenberg PR, Sherman LA, Schectman K, Perez J, Sobel BE, Jaffe AS: Fibrinopeptide A: a marker of acute coronary thrombosis. *Circulation* 71:912, 1985.

245. Kruskal JB, Commerford PJ, Franks JJ, Kirsch RE: Fibrin and fibrino-gen-related antigens in patients with stable and unstable coronary artery disease. *N Engl J Med* 317:1361, 1987.

246. Neri Serneri GG, Gensini GF, Carnovali M, et al: Association between time of increased fibrinopeptide A levels in plasma and episodes of spontaneous angina: a controlled prospective study. *Am Heart J* 113:672, 1987.

247. Merlini PA, Bauer KA, Oltrona L, et al: Persistent activation of coagula-tion mechanism in unstable angina and myocardial infarction. *Circula-tion* 90:61, 1994.

248. McCully KS: Vascular pathology of homocysteinemia: implications for the pathogenesis of arteriosclerosis. *Am J Pathol* 56:111, 1969.

249. Finkelstein JD: The metabolism of homocysteine: pathways and regula-tion. *Eur J Pediatr* 157 (suppl 2):S40, 1998.

250. Kraus JP: Biochemistry and molecular genetics of cystathionine beta-synthase deficiency. *Eur J Pediatr* 157 (suppl 2):S50, 1998.

251. Welch GN, Loscalzo J: Homocysteine and atherothrombosis. *N Engl J Med* 338:1042, 1998.

252. Brattstrom L: Vitamins as homocysteine-lowering agents. *J Nutr* 126:1276S, 1996.

253. Harker LA, Ross R, Slichter SJ, Scott CR: Homocystine-induced arterio-sclerosis. The role of endothelial cell injury and platelet response in its genesis. *J Clin Invest* 58:731, 1976.

254. Dudman NP, Hicks C, Lynch JF, Wilcken DE, Wang J: Homocysteine thiolactone disposal by human arterial endothelial cells and serum in vitro. *Arterioscler Thromb* 11:663, 1991.

255. Ueland PM, Refsum H, Brattström L: Plasma homocysteine and cardio-vascular disease, in RBJ Francis, editor, *Atherosclerotic Cardiovascular Disease, Hemostasis, and Endothelial Function*, p 183. Marcel Dekker, New York, 1992.

256. Loscalzo J: The oxidant stress of hyperhomocyst(e)inemia. *J Clin Invest* 98:5, 1996.

257. Harker LA, Slichter SJ, Scott CR, Ross R: Homocystinemia. Vascular injury and arterial thrombosis. *N Engl J Med* 291:537, 1974.

258. Rodgers GM, Conn MT: Homocysteine, an atherogenic stimulus, re-duces protein C activation by arterial and venous endothelial cells. *Blood* 75:895, 1990.

259. Panganamala RV, Karpen CW, Merola AJ: Peroxide mediated effects of homocysteine on arterial prostacyclin synthesis. *Prostaglandins Leukot Med* 22:349, 1986.

260. Wang J, Dudman NP, Wilcken DE: Effects of homocysteine and related compounds on prostacyclin production by cultured human vascular endo-thelial cells. *Thromb Haemost* 70:1047, 1993.

261. Lentz SR, Sadler JE: Inhibition of thrombomodulin surface expression and protein C activation by the thrombogenic agent homocysteine. *J Clin Invest* 88:1906, 1991.

262. Rodgers GM, Kane WH: Activation of endogenous factor V by a homo-cysteine-induced vascular endothelial cell activator. *J Clin Invest* 77:1909, 1986.

263. Fryer RH, Wilson BD, Gubler DB, Fitzgerald LA, Rodgers GM: Homo-cysteine, a risk factor for premature vascular disease and thrombosis, induces tissue factor activity in endothelial cells. *Arterioscler Thromb* 13:1327, 1993.

264. Hayashi T, Honda G, Suzuki K: An atherogenic stimulus homocysteine inhibits cofactor activity of thrombomodulin and enhances thrombomo-dulin expression in human umbilical vein endothelial cells. *Blood* 79:2930, 1992.

265. Nishinaga M, Ozawa T, Shimada K: Homocysteine, a thrombogenic agent, suppresses anticoagulant heparan sulfate expression in cultured porcine aortic endothelial cells. *J Clin Invest* 92:1381, 1993.

266. Hajjar KA: Homocysteine-induced modulation of tissue plasminogen activator binding to its endothelial cell membrane receptor. *J Clin Invest* 91:2873, 1993.

267. Harpel PC, Chang VT, Borth W: Homocysteine and other sulfhydryl compounds enhance the binding of lipoprotein(a) to fibrin: a potential biochemical link between thrombosis, atherogenesis, and sulfhydryl compound metabolism. *Proc Natl Acad Sci USA* 89:10193, 1992.

268. Alfthan G, Pekkanen J, Jauhiainen M, et al: Relation of serum homocys-teine and lipoprotein(a) concentrations to atherosclerotic disease in a prospective Finnish population based study. *Atherosclerosis* 106:9, 1994.

269. von Eckardstein A, Malinow MR, Upson B, et al: Effects of age, lipopro-teins, and hemostatic parameters on the role of homocyst(e)inemia as a cardiovascular risk factor in men. *Arterioscler Thromb* 14:460, 1994.

270. Glueck CJ, Shaw P, Lang JE, Tracy T, Sieve-Smith L, Wang Y: Evidence that homocysteine is an independent risk factor for atherosclerosis in hyperlipidemic patients. *Am J Cardiol* 75:132, 1995.

271. Utermann G: The mysteries of lipoprotein(a). *Science* 246:904, 1989.

272. Heinrich J, Sandkamp M, Kokott R, Schulte H, Assmann G: Relationship of lipoprotein(a) to variables of coagulation and fibrinolysis in a healthy population. *Clin Chem* 37:1950, 1991.

273. Maeda S, Abe A, Seishima M, Makino K, Noma A, Kawade M: Transient changes of serum lipoprotein(a) as an acute phase protein. *Atherosclero-sis* 78:145, 1989.

274. Seed M, Hoppichler F, Reaveley D, et al: Relation of serum lipoprotein(a) concentration and apolipoprotein(a) phenotype to coronary heart disease in patients with familial hypercholesterolemia. *N Engl J Med* 322:1494, 1990.

275. Berg K, Dahlen G, Borresen AL: Lp(a) phenotypes, other lipoprotein parameters, and a family history of coronary heart disease in middle-aged males. *Clin Genet* 16:347, 1979.

276. Rosengren A, Wilhelmsen L, Eriksson E, Risberg B, Wedel H: Lipopro-tein(a) and coronary heart disease: a prospective case-control study in a general population sample of middle aged men. *Br Med J* 301:1248, 1990.

277. Sigurdsson G, Baldursdottir A, Sigvaldason H, Agnarsson U, Thorgeirs-son G, Sigfusson N: Predictive value of apolipoproteins in a prospective survey of coronary artery disease in men. *Am J Cardiol* 69:1251, 1992.

278. Schaefer EJ, Lamon-Fava S, Jenner JL, et al: Lipoprotein(a) levels and risk of coronary heart disease in men. The Lipid Research Clinics Coronary Primary Prevention Trial. *JAMA* 271:999, 1994.

279. Bostom AG, Cupples LA, Jenner JL, et al: Elevated plasma lipoprotein(a) and coronary heart disease in men aged 55 years and younger. A prospec-tive study. *JAMA* 276:544, 1996.

280. Jauhiainen M, Koskinen P, Ehnholm C, et al: Lipoprotein (a) and coro-nary heart disease risk: a nested case-control study of the Helsinki Heart Study participants. *Atherosclerosis* 89:59, 1991.

281. Ridker PM, Hennekens CH, Stampfer MJ: A prospective study of lipo-protein(a) and the risk of myocardial infarction. *JAMA* 270:2195, 1993.

282. Sandholzer C, Boerwinkle E, Saha N, Tong MC, Utermann G: Apolipo-protein(a) phenotypes, Lp(a) concentration and plasma lipid levels in relation to coronary heart disease in a Chinese population: evidence for the role of the apo(a) gene in coronary heart disease. *J Clin Invest* 89:1040, 1992.

283. Moliterno DJ, Jokinen EV, Miserez AR, et al: No association between plasma lipoprotein(a) concentrations and the presence or absence of coronary atherosclerosis in African-Americans. *Arterioscler Thromb Vasc Biol* 15:850, 1995.

284. Harpel PC, Hermann A, Zhang X, Ostfeld I, Borth W: Lipoprotein(a), plasmin modulation, and atherogenesis. *Thromb Haemost* 74:382, 1995.

285. Hajjar KA, Nachman RL: The role of lipoprotein(a) in atherogenesis and thrombosis. *Annu Rev Med* 47:423, 1996.

286. Rath M, Niendorf A, Reblin T, Dietel M, Krebber HJ, Beisiegel U: Detection and quantification of lipoprotein(a) in the arterial wall of 107 coronary bypass patients. *Arteriosclerosis* 9:579, 1989. Published erratum appears in *Arteriosclerosis* 10:1147, 1990.

287. Dangas G, Mehran R, Harpel PC, et al: Lipoprotein(a) and inflammation in human coronary atheroma: association with the severity of clinical presentation. *J Am Coll Cardiol* 32:2035, 1998.

288. Loscalzo J, Weinfeld M, Fless GM, Scanu AM: Lipoprotein(a), fibrin binding, and plasminogen activation. *Arteriosclerosis* 10:240, 1990.

289. Hervio L, Chapman MJ, Thillet J, Loyau S, Angles-Cano E: Does apolipoprotein(a) heterogeneity influence lipoprotein(a) effects on fibri-nolysis? *Blood* 82:392, 1993.

290. Bihari-Varga M, Gruber E, Rotheneder M, Zechner R, Kostner GM: Interaction of lipoprotein Lp(a) and low density lipoprotein with glyco-saminoglycans from human aorta. *Arteriosclerosis* 8:851, 1988.

291. Management of stable angina pectoris. Recommendations of the Task Force of the European Society of Cardiology. *Eur Heart J* 18:394, 1997.

292. Mulcahy R, Al Awadhi AH, de Buitleor M, Tobin G, Johnson H, Contoy R: Natural history and prognosis of unstable angina. *Am Heart J* 109:753, 1985.

293. Figueras J, Lidon R, Cortadellas J: Rebound myocardial ischaemia fol-

lowing abrupt interruption of intravenous nitroglycerin infusion in patients with unstable angina at rest. *Eur Heart J* 12:405, 1991.

294. Jugdutt BI, Warnica JW: Tolerance with low dose intravenous nitroglycerin therapy in acute myocardial infarction. *Am J Cardiol* 64:581, 1989.

295. Yusuf S, Wittes J, Friedman L: Overview of results of randomized clinical trials in heart disease. II. Unstable angina, heart failure, primary prevention with aspirin, and risk factor modification. *JAMA* 260:2259, 1988.

296. Cairns JA, Gent M, Singer J, et al: Aspirin, sulfinpyrazone, or both in unstable angina. Results of a Canadian multicenter trial. *N Engl J Med* 313:1369, 1985.

297. Theroux P, Ouimet H, McCans J, et al: Aspirin, heparin, or both to treat acute unstable angina. *N Engl J Med* 319:1105, 1988.

298. Risk of myocardial infarction and death during treatment with low dose aspirin and intravenous heparin in men with unstable coronary artery disease. The RISC Group. *Lancet* 336:827, 1990.

299. Anticoagulants in the Secondary Prevention of Events in Coronary Thrombosis (ASPECT) Research Group. Effect of long-term oral anticoagulant treatment on mortality and cardiovascular morbidity after myocardial infarction. *Lancet* 343:499, 1994.

300. Telford AM, Wilson C: Trial of heparin versus atenolol in prevention of myocardial infarction in intermediate coronary syndrome. *Lancet* 1:1225, 1981.

301. Holdright D, Patel D, Cunningham D, et al: Comparison of the effect of heparin and aspirin versus aspirin alone on transient myocardial ischemia and in-hospital prognosis in patients with unstable angina. *J Am Coll Cardiol* 24:39, 1994.

302. Neri Serneri GG, Modesti PA, Gensini GF, et al: Randomised comparison of subcutaneous heparin, intravenous heparin, and aspirin in unstable angina. Studio Epoorine Sottocutanea nell'Angina Instobile (SESAIR) Refrattorie Group. *Lancet* 345:1201, 1995.

303. Cohen M, Adams PC, Parry G, et al: Combination antithrombotic therapy in unstable rest angina and non-Q-wave infarction in nonprior aspirin users. Primary end points analysis from the ATACS trial. Antithrombotic Therapy in Acute Coronary Syndromes Research Group. *Circulation* 89:81, 1994.

304. Gurfinkel EP, Manos EJ, Mejail RI, et al: Low molecular weight heparin versus regular heparin or aspirin in the treatment of unstable angina and silent ischemia. *J Am Coll Cardiol* 26:313, 1995.

305. Theroux P, Waters D, Qiu S, McCans J, de Guise P, Juneau M: Aspirin versus heparin to prevent myocardial infarction during the acute phase of unstable angina. *Circulation* 88:2045, 1993.

306. Low-molecular-weight heparin during instability in coronary artery disease, Fragmin during Instability in Coronary Artery Disease (FRISC) study group. *Lancet* 347:561, 1996.

307. Smith P, Arnesen H, Holme I: The effect of warfarin on mortality and reinfarction after myocardial infarction. *N Engl J Med* 323:147, 1990.

308. Randomised double-blind trial of fixed low-dose warfarin with aspirin after myocardial infarction. Coumadin Aspirin Reinfarction Study (CARS) Investigators. *Lancet* 350:389, 1997.

309. Bar FW, Verheugt FW, Col J, et al: Thrombolysis in patients with unstable angina improves the angiographic but not the clinical outcome. Results of UNASEM, a multicenter, randomized, placebo-controlled, clinical trial with anistreplase. *Circulation* 86:131, 1992.

310. Karlsson JE, Berglund U, Bjorkholm A, Ohlsson J, Swahn E, Wallentin L: Thrombolysis with recombinant human tissue-type plasminogen activator during instability in coronary artery disease: effect on myocardial ischemia and need for coronary revascularization. TRIC Study Group. *Am Heart J* 124:1419, 1992.

311. Schreiber TL, Rizik D, White C, et al: Randomized trial of thrombolysis versus heparin in unstable angina. *Circulation* 86:1407, 1992.

312. Effects of tissue plasminogen activator and a comparison of early invasive and conservative strategies in unstable angina and non-Q-wave myocardial infarction. Results of the TIMI IIIB Trial. Thrombolysis in Myocardial Ischemia. *Circulation* 89:1545, 1994.

313. Ambrose JA, Almeida OD, Sharma SK, et al: Adjunctive thrombolytic therapy during angioplasty for ischemic rest angina. Results of the TAUSA Trial. TAUSA Investigators. Thrombolysis and Angioplasty in Unstable Angina trial. *Circulation* 90:69, 1994.

314. White HD, French JK, Norris RM, Williams BF, Hart HH, Cross DB: Effects of streptokinase in patients presenting within 6 hours of prolonged chest pain with ST segment depression. *Br Heart J* 73:500, 1995.

315. Abbott RD, Wilson PW, Kannel WB, Castelli WP: High density lipoprotein cholesterol, total cholesterol screening, and myocardial infarction. The Framingham Study. *Arteriosclerosis* 8:207, 1988.

316. Use of a monoclonal antibody directed against the platelet glycoprotein IIb/IIIa receptor in high-risk coronary angioplasty. The EPIC Investigation. *N Engl J Med* 330:956, 1994.

317. Topol EJ, Califf RM, Weisman HF, et al: Randomised trial of coronary intervention with antibody against platelet IIb/IIIa integrin for reduction of clinical restenosis: results at six months. The EPIC Investigators. *Lancet* 343:881, 1994.

318. Platelet glycoprotein IIb/IIIa receptor blockade and low-dose heparin during percutaneous coronary revascularization. The EPILOG Investigators. *N Engl J Med* 336:1689, 1997.

319. Randomised placebo-controlled trial of abciximab before and during coronary intervention in refractory unstable angina: the CAPTURE Study. *Lancet* 349:1429, 1997.

320. Theroux P, Kouz S, Roy L, et al: Platelet membrane receptor glycoprotein IIb/IIIa antagonism in unstable angina. The Canadian Lamifiban Study. *Circulation* 94:899, 1996.

321. Effects of platelet glycoprotein IIb/IIIa blockade with tirofiban on adverse cardiac events in patients with unstable angina or acute myocardial infarction undergoing coronary angioplasty. The RESTORE Investigators. Randomized Efficacy Study of Tirofiban for Outcomes and REstenosis. *Circulation* 96:1445, 1997.

322. Randomised placebo-controlled trial of effect of eptifibatide on complications of percutaneous coronary intervention: IMPACT-II. Integrilin to Minimise Platelet Aggregation and Coronary Thrombosis-II. *Lancet* 349:1422, 1997.

323. Inhibition of the platelet glycoprotein IIb/IIIa receptor with tirofiban in unstable angina and non-Q-wave myocardial infarction. Platelet Receptor Inhibition in Ischemic Syndrome Management in Patients Limited by Unstable Signs and Symptoms (PRISM-PLUS) Study Investigators. *N Engl J Med* 338:1488, 1998.

324. A comparison of aspirin plus tirofiban with aspirin plus heparin for unstable angina. Platelet Receptor Inhibition in Ischemic Syndrome Management (PRISM) Study Investigators. *N Engl J Med* 338:1498, 1998.

325. Alexander JH, Harrington RA: Recent antiplatelet drug trials in the acute coronary syndromes. Clinical interpretation of PRISM, PRISM-PLUS, PARAGON A and PURSUIT. *Drugs* 56:965, 1998.

326. A comparison of recombinant hirudin with heparin for the treatment of acute coronary syndromes. The Global Use of Strategies to Open Occluded Coronary Arteries (GUSTO) IIb investigators. *N Engl J Med* 335:775, 1996.

327. Comparison of the effects of two doses of recombinant hirudin compared with heparin in patients with acute myocardial ischemia without ST elevation: a pilot study. Organization to Assess Strategies for Ischemic Syndromes (OASIS) Investigators. *Circulation* 96:769, 1997.

328. Effects of recombinant hirudin (lepirudin) compared with heparin on death, myocardial infarction, refractory angina, and revascularisation procedures in patients with acute myocardial ischaemia without ST elevation: a randomised trial. Organisation to Assess Strategies for Ischemic Syndromes (OASIS-2) Investigators. *Lancet* 353:429, 1999.

329. Lidon RM, Theroux P, Juneau M, Adelman B, Maraganore J: Initial experience with a direct antithrombin, Hirulog, in unstable angina. Anticoagulant, antithrombotic, and clinical effects. *Circulation* 88:1495, 1993.

330. Fuchs J, Cannon CP: Hirulog in the treatment of unstable angina. Results of the Thrombin Inhibition in Myocardial Ischemia (TIMI) 7 trial. *Circulation* 92:727, 1995.

331. Serruys PW, Herrman JP, Simon R, et al: A comparison of hirudin with heparin in the prevention of restenosis after coronary angioplasty. Helvetica Investigators. *N Engl J Med* 333:757, 1995.

332. Bittl JA, Strony J, Brinker JA, et al: Treatment with bivalirudin (Hirulog) as compared with heparin during coronary angioplasty for unstable or postinfarction angina. Hirulog Angioplasty Study Investigators. *N Engl J Med* 333:764, 1995.

333. De Feyter PJ, Suryapranata H, Serruys PW, et al: Coronary angioplasty for unstable angina: immediate and late results in 200 consecutive patients with identification of risk factors for unfavorable early and late outcome. *J Am Coll Cardiol* 12:324, 1988.

334. Myler RK, Shaw RE, Stertzer SH, et al: Unstable angina and coronary angioplasty. *Circulation* 82 (3 Suppl):1188, 1990.

335. Bentivoglio LG, Detre K, Yeh W, Williams DO, Kelsey SF, Faxon DP: Outcome of percutaneous transluminal coronary angioplasty in subsets of unstable angina pectoris. A report of the 1985-1986 National Heart, Lung, and Blood Institute Percutaneous Transluminal Coronary Angioplasty Registry. *J Am Coll Cardiol* 24:1195, 1994.

336. Mehran R, Ambrose JA, Bongu RM, et al: Angioplasty of complex lesions in ischemic rest angina: results of the Thrombolysis and Angioplasty in Unstable Angina (TAUSA) trial. *J Am Coll Cardiol* 26:961, 1995.

337. Gulba DC, Daniel WG, Simon R, et al: Role of thrombolysis and thrombin in patients with acute coronary occlusion during percutaneous transluminal coronary angioplasty. *J Am Coll Cardiol* 16:563, 1990.

338. Schieman G, Cohen BM, Kozina J, et al: Intracoronary urokinase for intracoronary thrombus accumulation complicating percutaneous transluminal coronary angioplasty in acute ischemic syndromes. *Circulation* 82:2052, 1990.

339. Laskey MA, Deutsch E, Barnathan E, Laskey WK: Influence of heparin therapy on percutaneous transluminal coronary angioplasty outcome in unstable angina pectoris. *Am J Cardiol* 65:1425, 1990.

340. Antoniucci D, Santoro GM, Bolognese L, et al: Early coronary angioplasty as compared with delayed coronary angioplasty in patients with high-risk unstable angina pectoris. *Coron Artery Dis* 7:75, 1996.

341. Kaiser GC, Schaff HV, Killip T: Myocardial revascularization for unstable angina pectoris. *Circulation* 79:160, 1989.

342. Bertolasi CA, Tronge JE, Riccitelli MA, Villamayor RM, Zuffardi E: Natural history of unstable angina with medical or surgical therapy. *Chest* 70:596, 1976.

343. Scott SM, Deupree RH, Sharma GV, Luchi RJ: VA Study of Unstable Angina. 10-year results show duration of surgical advantage for patients with impaired ejection fraction. *Circulation* 90:(II):120, 1994.

344. Yusuf S, Peto R, Lewis J, Collins R, Sleight P: Beta blockade during and after myocardial infarction: an overview of the randomized trials. *Prog Cardiovasc Dis* 27:335, 1985.

345. GISSI-3: effects of lisinopril and transdermal glyceryl trinitrate singly and together on 6-week mortality and ventricular function after acute myocardial infarction. Gruppo Italiano per lo Studio della Sopravvivenza nell'infarto Miocardico. *Lancet* 343:1115, 1994.

346. ISIS-4: a randomised factorial trial assessing early oral captopril, oral mononitrate, and intravenous magnesium sulphate in 58,050 patients with suspected acute myocardial infarction. ISIS-4 (Fourth International Study of Infarct Survival) Collaborative Group. *Lancet* 345: 669, 1995.

347. Effect of intravenous APSAC on mortality after acute myocardial infarction: preliminary report of a placebo-controlled clinical trial. AIMS Trial Study Group. *Lancet* 1:545, 1988.

348. Wilcox RG, von der Lippe G, Olsson CG, Jensen G, Skene AM, Hampton JR: Trial of tissue plasminogen activator for mortality reduction in acute myocardial infarction. Anglo-Scandinavian Study of Early Thrombolysis (ASSET). *Lancet* 2:525, 1988.

349. Boersma E, Maas AC, Deckers JW, Simoons ML: Early thrombolytic treatment in acute myocardial infarction: reappraisal of the golden hour. *Lancet* 348:771, 1996.

350. Late Assessment of Thrombolytic Efficacy (LATE) study with alteplase 6–24 hours after onset of acute myocardial infarction. *Lancet* 342:759, 1993.

351. Randomised trial of late thrombolysis in patients with suspected acute myocardial infarction. EMERAS (Estudio Multicentrico Estreptoquinasa Republicas de America del Sur) Collaborative Group. *Lancet* 342:767, 1993.

352. GISSI-2: a factorial randomised trial of alteplase versus streptokinase and heparin versus no heparin among 12,490 patients with acute myocardial infarction. Gruppo Italiano per lo Studio della Sopravvivenza nell'Infarto Miocardico. *Lancet* 336:65, 1990.

353. ISIS-3: a randomised comparison of streptokinase vs tissue plasminogen activator vs anistreplase and of aspirin plus heparin vs aspirin alone among 41,299 cases of suspected acute myocardial infarction. ISIS-3 (Third International Study of Infarct Survival) Collaborative Group. *Lancet* 339:753, 1992.

354. The effects of tissue plasminogen activator, streptokinase, or both on coronary-artery patency, ventricular function, and survival after acute myocardial infarction. The GUSTO Angiographic Investigators. *N Engl J Med* 329:1615, 1993.

355. Califf RM, White HD, Van de Werf F, et al: One-year results from the Global Utilization of Streptokinase and TPA for Occluded Coronary Arteries (GUSTO-I) trial. GUSTO-I Investigators. *Circulation* 94:1233, 1996.

356. Topol EJ: Coronary angioplasty for acute myocardial infarction. *Ann Intern Med* 109:970, 1988.

357. Abbottsmith CW, Topol EJ, George BS, et al: Fate of patients with acute myocardial infarction with patency of the infarct-related vessel achieved with successful thrombolysis versus rescue angioplasty. *J Am Coll Cardiol* 16:770, 1990.

358. Ellis SG, da Silva ER, Heyndrickx G, et al: Randomized comparison of rescue angioplasty with conservative management of patients with early failure of thrombolysis for acute anterior myocardial infarction. *Circulation* 90:2280, 1994.

359. McKendall GR, Forman S, Sopko G, Braunwald E, Williams DO: Value of rescue percutaneous transluminal coronary angioplasty following unsuccessful thrombolytic therapy in patients with acute myocardial infarction. Thrombolysis in Myocardial Infarction Investigators. *Am J Cardiol* 76:1108, 1995.

360. Topol EJ, Califf RM, George BS, et al: A randomized trial of immediate versus delayed elective angioplasty after intravenous tissue plasminogen activator in acute myocardial infarction. *N Engl J Med* 317:581, 1987.

361. Immediate vs delayed catheterization and angioplasty following thrombolytic therapy for acute myocardial infarction. TIMI II A results. The TIMI Research Group. *JAMA* 260:2849, 1988.

362. Simoons ML, Arnold AE, Betriu A, et al: Thrombolysis with tissue plasminogen activator in acute myocardial infarction: no additional benefit from immediate percutaneous coronary angioplasty. *Lancet* 1:197, 1988.

363. Schomig A, Neumann FJ, Walter H, et al: Coronary stent placement in patients with acute myocardial infarction: comparison of clinical and angiographic outcome after randomization to antiplatelet or anticoagulant therapy. *J Am Coll Cardiol* 29:28, 1997.

364. Antoniucci D, Santoro GM, Bolognese L, Valenti R, Trapani M, Fazzini PF: A clinical trial comparing primary stenting of the infarct-related artery with optimal primary angioplasty for acute myocardial infarction: results from the Florence Randomized Elective Stenting in Acute Coronary Occlusions (FRESCO) trial. *J Am Coll Cardiol* 31:1234, 1998.

365. Rodriguez A, Bernardi V, Fernandez M, et al: In-hospital and late results of coronary stents versus conventional balloon angioplasty in acute myocardial infarction (GRAMI trial). Gianturco-Roubin in Acute Myocardial Infarction. *Am J Cardiol* 81:1286, 1998.

366. Randomised trial of intravenous atenolol among 16 027 cases of suspected acute myocardial infarction: ISIS-1. First International Study of Infarct Survival Collaborative Group. *Lancet* 2:57, 1986.

367. Mechanisms for the early mortality reduction produced by beta-blockade started early in acute myocardial infarction: ISIS-1. ISIS-1 (First International Study of Infarct Survival) Collaborative Group. *Lancet* 1:921, 1988.

368. Soumerai SB, McLaughlin TJ, Spiegelman D, Hertzmark E, Thibault G, Goldman L: Adverse outcomes of underuse of beta-blockers in elderly survivors of acute myocardial infarction . *JAMA* 277:115, 1997.

369. Ambrosioni E, Borghi C, Magnani B: The effect of the angiotensin-converting-enzyme inhibitor zofenopril on mortality and morbidity after anterior myocardial infarction. The Survival of Myocardial Infarction Long-Term Evaluation (SMILE) Study Investigators. *N Engl J Med* 332:80, 1995.

370. Kober L, Torp-Pedersen C, Carlsen JE, et al: A clinical trial of the angiotensin-converting-enzyme inhibitor trandolapril in patients with left ventricular dysfunction after myocardial infarction. Trandolapril Cardiac Evaluation (TRACE) Study Group. *N Engl J Med* 333:1670, 1995.

371. Vantrimpont P, Rouleau JL, Wun CC, et al: Additive beneficial effects of beta-blockers to angiotensin-converting enzyme inhibitors in the Survival and Ventricular Enlargement (SAVE) Study. SAVE Investigators. *J Am Coll Cardiol* 29:229, 1997.

372. Elwood PC, Sweetnam PM: Aspirin and secondary mortality after myocardial infarction. *Lancet* 2:1313, 1979.

373. The aspirin myocardial infarction study: final results. The Aspirin Myocardial Infarction Study research group. *Circulation* 62:(V):79, 1980.

374. Klimt CR, Knatterud GL, Stamler J, Meier P: Persantine-Aspirin Rein-
     farction Study. Part II. Secondary coronary prevention with persantine
     and aspirin. *J Am Coll Cardiol* 7:251, 1986.
375. Collaborative overview of randomised trials of antiplatelet therapy—I:
     Prevention of death, myocardial infarction, and stroke by prolonged
     antiplatelet therapy in various categories of patients. Antiplatelet Tri-
     alists' Collaboration. *Br Med J* 308:81, 1994.
376. A randomised, blinded, trial of clopidogrel versus aspirin in patients at
     risk of ischaemic events (CAPRIE). CAPRIE Steering Committee. *Lan-
     cet* 348:1329, 1996.
377. Goldstein RE, Andrews M, Hall WJ, Moss AJ: Marked reduction in
     long-term cardiac deaths with aspirin after a coronary event. Multicenter
     Myocardial Ischemia Research Group. *J Am Coll Cardiol* 28:326, 1996.
378. Weintraub WS, Ba'albaki HA: Decision analysis concerning the applica-
     tion of echocardiography to the diagnosis and treatment of mural thrombi
     after anterior wall acute myocardial infarction. *Am J Cardiol* 64:708,
     1989.
379. Kouvaras G, Chronopoulos G, Soufras G, et al: The effects of long-
     term antithrombotic treatment on left ventricular thrombi in patients
     after an acute myocardial infarction. *Am Heart J* 119:73, 1990.

ANTIPLATELET THERAPY

HARVEY J. WEISS

> The properties that make platelets useful in promoting the arrest of bleeding also lead them to be deposited as thrombi in blood vessels and on the surfaces of heart valves, artificial membranes, and prosthetic devices. In addition, substances produced or stored in platelets, when secreted, may be involved in vasospasm and proliferative responses, atherogenesis, and inflammation. Aspirin, the thienopyridine derivatives ticlopidine and clopidogrel, and a number of platelet glycoprotein (GP) IIb/IIIa receptor antagonists have been demonstrated to be efficacious in preventing and/or treating thrombotic vascular disease.

The term "antiplatelet" has no precise meaning at present. It has been used to describe drugs that inhibit platelet activation in vitro, modify experimentally induced thrombosis, prolong the survival of radioactively labeled platelets, or interfere with some presumed platelet-mediated pathologic processes. Drugs possessing these properties are shown in Table 131-1. The first part of this chapter will describe these agents, their mechanisms of action, and their pharmacology. The second part will describe the clinical application of these agents.

ANTIPLATELET DRUGS

ASPIRIN

Following early observations that aspirin (acetylsalicylic acid) ingestion can result in a mild hemostatic defect and prolong the bleeding time,[1,2] studies in the late 1960s demonstrated that a single, oral dose of

Acronyms and abbreviations that appear in this chapter include: ADP, adenosine diphosphate; AMIS, Aspirin in Myocardial Infarction Study; CABS, coronary artery bypass surgery; CAPRIE, Clopidogrel versus Aspirin in Patients at Risk of Ischaemic Events; CAPTURE, Chimeric 7E3 Antiplatelet in Unstable angina Refractory to standard treatment; CAST, Chinese Acute Stroke Trial; CATS, Canadian-American Ticlopidine Study; COX, cyclooxygenase; cyclic AMP (cAMP), cyclic adenosine monophosphate; cGMP, cyclic guanosine monophosphate; EPA, eicosapentaenoic acid; EPIC, Evaluation of 7E3 for the Prevention of Ischemic Complications; EPILOG, Evaluation of PTCA to Improve Long-term Outcome by c7E3 GPIIb/IIIa receptor blockade; EPISTENT, Evaluation of IIb/IIIa Platelet Inhibitor for Stenting; GP, glycoprotein; IMPACT II, Integrilin to Minimize Platelet Aggregation and Coronary Thrombosis; ISIS-2, Second International Study of Infarct Survival; ISIS-3, Third International Study of Infarct Survival; IST, International Stroke Trial; KGD sequence, lysine-glycine-aspartic acid sequence; NO, nitric oxide; NSAIDs, non-steroidal anti-inflammatory drugs; PARAGON, Platelet IIb/IIIa Antagonist for the Reduction of Acute coronary syndrome events in a Global Organization Network; Paris II, Second Persantine Aspirin Reinfarction Study; PCI, percutaneous coronary interventions; PDGF, platelet-derived growth factor; PG, prostaglandin; PGE$_1$, prostaglandin E$_1$; PGHS-1, PGH-synthase; PGI$_2$, prostacyclin; PRISM, Platelet Receptor Inhibition in Ischemic Syndrome Management; PRISM-PLUS, Platelet Receptor Inhibition in Ischemic Syndrome Management in Patients Limited by Unstable Signs and Symptoms; PTCA, percutaneous transluminal coronary angioplasty; PURSUIT, Platelet IIb/IIIa Underpinning the Receptor for Suppression of Unstable Ischemia Trial; RAPPORT, ReoPro and Primary PTCA Organization and Randomized Trial; RESTORE, Randomized Efficacy Study of Tirofiban for Outcomes and Restenosis; RGD sequence, arginine-glycine-aspartic acid sequence; RINDs, reversible ischemic neurologic deficits; TASS, Ticlopidine Aspirin Stroke Study; TIAs, transient ischemic attacks; TxA$_2$, thromboxane A$_2$.

the drug inhibited collagen-induced platelet aggregation and secondary aggregation responses to weak agonists such as ADP and epinephrine for about 7 days, whereas sodium salicylate was without effect.[3] The aspirin effect corresponded roughly to the platelet life span and suggested that aspirin induced an irreversible inhibitory effect on platelet function through some mechanism involving the acetyl group.[3] Subsequent studies demonstrated that, in platelets, aspirin inhibits the conversion of arachidonic acid to prostaglandins[1,2,4] and thromboxane A$_2$ (TxA$_2$),[5] one of the most potent platelet aggregating agents that has been described.[6] In platelets, arachidonate is released from phospholipids in the platelet membrane, principally through the action of phospholipase A$_2$, in response to a variety of agonists[7-9] (see Chap. 111). Arachidonic acid is then converted to prostaglandin (PG) H$_2$ by the enzyme PGH-synthase, PGHS-1, also referred to as cyclooxygenase (COX-1).[9,10] The latter is a homodimeric, heme-containing protein with two catalytic activities, one of which (COX) cyclizes arachidonate to PGG$_2$, while the other (peroxidase) catalyzes a two-electron reduction of PGG$_2$ to PGH$_2$.[10-12] The latter endoperoxide is then converted to TxA$_2$ by a specific isomerase called thromboxane synthase.[9,10] Aspirin selectively blocks the cyclooxygenase (but not the peroxidase) activity of COX-1 by irreversibly acetylating the hydroxyl group[12,13] of a crucial serine at position 530 (Ser530) or 529 (Ser529) in sheep[14] or human[15] platelets, respectively. Since the platelet is an anucleate cell, containing only a small amount of mRNA derived from megakaryocytes, it is unable to replace the irreversibly inactivated COX-1 through new protein synthesis, thereby accounting for the permanence of the "aspirin effect" on prostaglandin synthesis[12] and platelet function.[3] Although it was initially believed that serine 529/530 could be the active site within COX-1, later studies identified this site as tyrosine 385[16,17] and showed that the covalent binding of aspirin to Ser529/530 has the effect of sterically hindering the access of arachidonate to the tyrosine residue responsible for initiating catalysis.[16,18] Aspirin, as well as other salicylates, can also inhibit a second PGH-synthase isoenzyme, COX-2,[16] that is undetectable in most mammalian tissues (including platelets), but whose expression can be induced in monocytes and other cells in response to inflammatory and mitogenic mediators.[10] The concentration of aspirin required for inhibiting COX-2 is considerably higher than that required for inhibiting COX-1, which explains why the antiplatelet/antithrombotic dose of aspirin is so much lower than the anti-inflammatory dose.[10,16]

The antiplatelet effects of aspirin are complicated by its capacity for blocking the cyclooxygenase activity in endothelial cells, thereby inhibiting the conversion of endoperoxides to PGI$_2$ (prostacyclin).[19] The latter eicosanoid can interact with a receptor on the surface of platelets and initiate a series of changes that increase the intracellular concentration of cyclic-AMP, thereby inhibiting platelet aggregation[7,19] (see Chap. 111). In contrast to platelets, inhibition of endothelial cell cyclooxygenase is not permanent, because these cells can synthesize new enzymes, and recovery of PGI$_2$ production by cultured umbilical vein endothelial cells has been observed 2 h after aspirin treatment.[20]

The ability of aspirin to inhibit (irreversibly) the formation of both platelet TxA$_2$ (a potential prothrombotic agent) and endothelial cell PGI$_2$ (a potential antithrombotic agent) has raised the question of whether there is a dose of aspirin that will suppress TxA$_2$ synthesis without inhibiting the production of PGI$_2$. It is assumed that, if such a dose exists, it will be the optimum "antithrombotic" dose. However, several aspects of this question are unresolved. First, there is no convincing evidence that blocking the production of PGI$_2$ is prothrombotic. In addition, even if the preservation of PGI$_2$ production were desirable, a dose of aspirin that optimally inhibits the production of TxA$_2$ without affecting PGI$_2$ has not been found.[21] In addition, when PGI$_2$ production was assessed by measuring the amount of a stable metabolite, 6-keto-PGF$_{1\alpha}$, that is produced locally at the site of acute injury, as in a bleeding time wound, PGI$_2$ production was markedly

TABLE 131-1   ANTIPLATELET DRUGS USED IN CLINICAL MEDICINE

Drugs that have been used as antithrombotic agents
Aspirin
Inhibitors of thromboxane A$_2$ synthesis or binding
Prostaglandin I$_2$ (prostacyclin) and analogues
Dipyridamole
Thienopyridine derivatives (ticlopidine, clopidogrel)
GPIIb/IIIa antagonists
Dextran
Sulfinpyrazone
Heparin
Fish oils and n-3 fatty acids

Other drugs with antiplatelet effects
Nitrates
Calcium channel blockers
β-adrenergic blocking agents
Serotonin antagonists
β-lactam antibiotics
Vitamin E

inhibited by daily aspirin doses as low as 30 mg per day.[22] A controlled-release formulation of aspirin has been reported that inhibited thromboxane synthesis with only minimal inhibition of basal or bradykinin-induced PGI$_2$ production.[23] This effect is based on the observation that aspirin is rapidly deacetylated in the liver; therefore, aspirin absorbed in the stomach and intestine can acetylate platelets in the portal circulation before it is metabolized in the liver. The endothelial cells in the systemic circulation are not exposed to aspirin, but rather salicylate, which cannot acetylate cyclooxygenase. Whether this approach will also preserve local PGI$_2$ production at sites of injury remains to be determined.

Many studies have addressed the question of whether there is a dose of aspirin that will result in the optimal inhibition of TxA$_2$ production and platelet aggregation. When the TxA$_2$ production has been assessed by measuring the concentration of a stable metabolite, TxB$_2$, in clotted blood, daily aspirin doses (mg) were reported to inhibit serum TxB$_2$ production as follows: 20 mg, 95 percent[21]; 30 mg, 94 percent[24]; 100 mg, 98 percent[25]; 100 mg, 95 percent[26]; and 325 mg, 91 percent.[27] Thus, somewhere between 2 and 9 percent of serum TxB$_2$ production was preserved with those dosage schedules, and therefore, it is theoretically possible that some TxA$_2$ formation at sites of vascular injury, such as a ruptured atherosclerotic plaque, might still occur in patients receiving doses of aspirin sufficient to cause substantial, but incomplete, inhibition of its production.[28] Although relatively low daily doses of aspirin will eliminate secondary platelet aggregation in response to epinephrine, the dose-response inhibitory effects of aspirin on platelets by other agonists may be significantly different in patients with vascular disease than in normal subjects.[29] The current consensus is that clinically effective inhibition of platelet aggregation and thromboxane formation can be achieved as follows (loading dose, mg/daily maintenance dose, mg): 320/80–160,[12] 120/30–50,[10] 200–300/75–100.[30] Whether these relatively low-dose schedules are universally applicable or might have to be modified in subgroups of patients with vascular disease, such as those with atherothrombosis in the cerebral circulation, is still the subject of some dispute (see later). Finally, the recent finding that a single 500-mg dose of aspirin may be required to block a newly described red cell–mediated, thromboxane A$_2$–independent platelet reactivity could have implications for aspirin therapy in patients with vascular disorders.[31]

The possibility that aspirin, because of its platelet-inhibitory properties, might be useful as an antithrombotic agent has been studied in a variety of injury-induced thrombosis models in animals and found, in most cases, to confer some protection against thrombosis.[1,2]

In general, other nonsteroidal anti-inflammatory drugs (NSAIDs) inhibit platelet aggregation and secretion[32] through a mechanism similar to that of aspirin, i.e., through inhibition of platelet cyclooxygenase.[1,2,33] Among NSAIDs, the prolonged inhibition of platelet function may be unique to aspirin. The effect of indomethacin, for example, is short-lived, and regardless of the size of the dose, inhibition is no longer detectable after 6 h.[1,34]

INHIBITORS OF THROMBOXANE A$_2$ SYNTHESIS OR BINDING

Thromboxane synthase, the enzyme that catalyzes the synthesis of TxA$_2$ from PGH$_2$, is inhibited by a variety of pharmacologic agents, including prostaglandin endoperoxide analogues, imidazole and its derivatives, and pyridine and its derivatives[1,6,7,34,35]; administration of these compounds in human subjects can markedly reduce serum TxB$_2$ levels.[36] In theory, administration of these agents should block TxA$_2$ synthesis and also promote the transfer of platelet-derived PGH$_2$ to endothelial cells, where it could be utilized for production of PGI$_2$.[34,37] However, the value of the thromboxane synthase inhibitors that have been developed have been limited by their incomplete inhibition of TxA$_2$ synthesis, as well as the proaggregatory effects of the prostaglandin endoperoxides that accumulate after their administration.[34]

Drugs have also been described that can block the receptor for TxA$_2$, a cloned receptor that, on ligand stimulation, results in activation of phospholipase C.[10] Although some of these TxA$_2$ receptor antagonists, such as sulotroban and ifetroban, have shown antithrombotic activity in animal models of thrombosis,[10,38] they have yielded disappointing results in phase II/III clinical trials.[10,35] Drugs such as picotamide and ridogrel, which have the dual properties of blocking both thromboxane synthase and the TxA$_2$ receptor have also been developed,[10,35] based on experimental evidence suggesting a synergistic interaction between the two approaches.[10] Their role(s) as clinical antithrombotic agents is unclear.

PROSTAGLANDIN I$_2$ AND ANALOGUES

PGI$_2$ (prostacyclin) is a potent inhibitor of platelet aggregation and platelet thrombus formation ex vivo, as well as a strong vasodilator (see above and Chap. 111). The inhibitory effects of PGI$_2$, or its analogues, are due principally to their interaction with a receptor on the platelet surface that initiates a series of biochemical changes, mediated at least in part through G proteins, that increase the intra-platelet concentration of cyclic AMP, a potent inhibitor of several biochemical processes that are crucial for platelet activation (see Chap. 111). PGI$_2$ may result in hypotension and gastrointestinal symptoms at doses that inhibit platelet function. More stable analogues of PGI$_2$ (iloprost, cicaprost, beraprost) have been produced and shown to be potent inhibitors of platelet aggregation.[11,34,35,39] The current status of prostacyclin analogues as antithrombotic agents has been recently reviewed.[11,35] In general, their side effects have limited their effectiveness in preventing thrombosis.

DIPYRIDAMOLE

Dipyridamole, a pyrimidopyrimidine compound with vasodilator properties, was introduced for the treatment of angina pectoris in 1961. Its antithrombotic properties were reported in 1968 when it was shown that the drug inhibited platelet-induced thromboembolism in the cerebrocortical blood vessels of rabbits.[40] Similar results have been obtained in other experimental models, but negative results have also been reported.[1,2,41] As discussed later, dipyridamole reduces the frequency of thromboembolism when administered with warfarin in patients with prosthetic heart valves.[42] It has been administered in divided daily doses ranging from 75 to 400 mg. In general, platelet aggregation in platelet-rich plasma is not inhibited by dipyridamole, either when administered orally or when added in vitro in pharmacologic concentrations, although exceptions have been reported.[1,2,41] However, the drug has been reported to inhibit platelet aggregation when studies are performed in the presence of erythrocytes by the technique of whole blood aggregometry.[43]

The basis for the antiplatelet and antithrombotic properties of dipyridamole is not clear.[1,10,41,43] It inhibits phosphodiesterase and, in theory, could increase platelet cyclic AMP to levels at which it is inhibitory to platelet aggregation (see Chap. 111). Dipyridamole may also indirectly increase the plasma concentration of adenosine that is produced from damaged cells, such as erythrocytes, by inhibiting its subsequent uptake into cells, particularly erythrocytes and endothelial cells.[1,43] This could explain why the drug inhibits platelet aggregation and thromboembolism under circumstances where erythrocytes may be damaged, as might occur in whole blood aggregometry tests and in patients with prosthetic heart valves.[7]

TICLOPIDINE AND CLOPIDOGREL

Ticlopidine and clopidogrel are structurally related thienopyridine derivatives that, after oral administration, specifically inhibit ADP-induced platelet aggregation.[1,11,44–49] Neither drug is active in vitro, requiring metabolic activation by a liver cytochrome P 450 mechanism.[44,50] The molecular characteristics of the active metabolites have not been clearly defined.[10] After oral administration in humans, both drugs prolong the bleeding time (to a greater extent than aspirin)[10,44,51] and inhibit platelet aggregation by ADP even at high agonist concentrations.[1,44,47] Platelet aggregation by low, but not high, concentrations of collagen and thrombin are also inhibited by the drugs,[11,44,47] suggesting that these inhibitory effects are probably due to a blockade of ADP-mediated amplification of the response to these agonists. Both ticlopidine[52] and clopidogrel[53] appear to exert their antiplatelet effects by inhibiting the binding of ADP to platelets. Recent studies using radiolabeled analogues of ADP (e.g., ^{3}H-2-MeS-ADP) have shown that both ticlopidine and clopidogrel dramatically reduce the binding of ADP to a P2 purinergic receptor on platelets.[53–55] The thienopyridine drugs do not inhibit platelet shape change or calcium influx.[53] Therefore, the inhibited ADP receptor does not appear to belong to the ligand-gated ion channel or inotropic receptor designated as the P2X superfamily of purinergic receptors.[56,57] Rather, both ticlopidine and clopidogrel selectively neutralize the ability of ADP to inhibit the increase in adenyl cyclase (and hence cyclic AMP) that occurs when platelets are exposed to agents such as PGE$_1$.[56,58] Thus, the thienopyridine drugs may bind to one of the subclasses of G-protein-coupled P2 receptors, or "metabotropic" superfamily, responsible for inhibition of stimulated adenyl cyclase activity in platelets.[59] However, the exact relationship between inhibition of PGE$_1$-stimulated adenyl cyclase and platelet aggregation by ADP remains to be clarified[48] (see Chap. 111).

Both ticlopidine and clopidogrel have been found to inhibit experimentally induced thrombosis,[11] and synergism with aspirin has been described in some studies.[10] Because their effects on platelets are affected through active metabolites, there is a delay in the onset of effective treatment. Ticlopidine is usually administered orally in doses of 250 mg twice daily, and its full antiplatelet activity is only obtained after 5 to 7 days. When clopidogrel is administered to healthy volunteers in a dose of 50 to 100 mg daily, maximal steady-state inhibition of ADP-induced aggregation ($\approx$50–60 percent) is reached in 4 to 7 days.[10,46,60] Besides diarrhea and rashes, more serious side effects of ticlopidine administration include neutropenia (1 percent of patients), which is usually reversible but occasionally accompanied by serious infection[7]; thrombocytopenia aplastic anemia[61]; and thrombotic throm-

bocytopenic purpura.[62] A major advantage of clopidogrel is the relatively infrequent occurrence of serious side effects.[60]

INHIBITORS OF THE PLATELET GPIIb/IIIa RECEPTOR

Transformation of the platelet GPIIb/IIIa receptor to its high-affinity ligand binding state in activated platelets is the final common pathway by which all agonists act to initiate platelet aggregation (see Chap. 111). Platelets in which the receptor is either blocked or congenitally deficient on an inherited basis will not aggregate with any physiologic agonist, in contrast to the more limited inhibition obtained with aspirin or ticlopidine. Therefore, agents that can block the receptor function of GPIIb/IIIa may be useful in preventing platelet-induced thrombosis. This type of blockade has been achieved both with monoclonal antibodies directed against the GPIIb/IIIa complex and with a variety of peptide and nonpeptide antagonists of GPIIb/IIIa.

MONOCLONAL ANTIBODIES

Monoclonal antibodies to GPIIb/IIIa markedly inhibit thrombus formation in a variety of animal models.[7] In addition, these antibodies speed reperfusion of thrombosed coronary arteries and prevent reocclusion of the involved blood vessel in animal models of thrombolysis.[7] The first antibody to be tested in human studies was a murine monoclonal antibody 7E3[63] in which the Fc region had been removed in order to prevent the removal of antibody-coated platelets by Fc receptors on macrophages. Because initial values in humans showed that this antibody was potentially immunogenic, a human-mouse chimeric antibody fragment (c7E3 Fab) was developed which consists of the variable regions of the mouse antibody joined to the constant regions of the human antibody.[64] This antibody, now referred to as abciximab, inhibits platelet aggregation almost completely when 80 percent of the GPIIb/IIIa receptors are blocked and is a more potent inhibitor of platelet thrombus formation than aspirin.[65] Abciximab, in addition to blocking the binding of adhesive proteins to GPIIb/IIIa, also binds to the $\alpha_v\beta_3$ vitronectin receptor that is present on endothelial and smooth muscle cells and has been implicated in the processes of cell adhesion, proliferation, and migration.[66] Finally, abciximab also inhibits the prothrombinase activity of platelets,[67,68] and this property could contribute further to its antithrombotic potential beyond its capacity for inhibiting platelet aggregation. The currently recommended dosing protocol is to administer an intravenous bolus of abciximab (0.25 mg/kg) followed by an infusion of 0.125 μg/kg/min (10 μg/min maximum) for 12 h.[69] No allergic or anaphylactic reactions have been reported, but mild (<100,000 cells/μl) or severe (<50,000 cells/μl) thrombocytopenia has been reported in 2.5 to 5.6 percent and 0.9 to 1.6 percent, respectively, of patients in three clinical trials that have utilized abciximab.[70]

PEPTIDE INHIBITORS

The GPIIb/IIIa receptor recognizes the arginine-glycine-aspartic acid (RGD) sequence contained in a number of adhesive molecules such as von Willebrand factor (see Chap. 111). RGD-containing low molecular weight peptides that compete with adhesive proteins for binding to GPIIb/IIIa have been isolated from the venom of several species of the viper family.[10] These peptides, known as disintegrins, are likely to be immunogenic and have been used primarily to provide insight into the structural requirements for GPIIb/IIIa antagonism and to provide the basis for the design of synthetic low molecular weight antagonists. Although linear peptides based on the RGD sequence possess some inhibitory activity, cyclic RGD peptides are more resistant to enzymatic breakdown, have a higher affinity for GPIIb/IIIa, and are about 10 times more potent than linear analogues.[11] One cyclic peptide inhibitor (eptifibatide) that has undergone clinical trials is based on a lysine-glycine-aspartic acid (KGD) rather than an RGD sequence[71]; it is a more specific inhibitor of the GPIIb/IIIa receptor than RGD-containing peptides.[72]

NONPEPTIDE INHIBITORS

A variety of nonpeptide agents have been developed that mimic the structure and charge characteristics of the RGD sequence and thereby inhibit the binding of adhesive proteins to GPIIb/IIIa. These peptidomimetic agents may have a longer survival time than peptide inhibitors[72] and are potentially orally effective.[9] Tirofiban, a tyrosine derivative,[73] and lamifiban[74] are two such small molecule peptidomimetic agents that have recently undergone clinical evaluation. Among agents that have been shown to be orally active, xemlofibin[75] and sibrafiban[76] have recently undergone clinical trials and others are currently under investigation.[72,77,78] Thrombocytopenia has also been reported in a very small percentage of patients receiving these agents.

OTHER ANTIPLATELET AGENTS

DEXTRAN

Infusion of 60 to 100 g of dextran of M_r 66 to 72 kDa can increase the bleeding time and inhibit platelet reactivity in a variety of tests.[1,2,41] The mechanism by which dextran inhibits platelet function is not clear, but could be related to alterations in the platelet membrane, to its interaction with plasma proteins that are necessary for platelet aggregation, or by transiently decreasing the plasma levels of von Willebrand factor.[1,41] Antithrombotic properties have been described in numerous experimental and clinical studies.[1,2,41]

SULFINPYRAZONE

This uricosuric pyrazole compound related to phenylbutazone, when administered in divided oral doses of 800 mg per day or higher, is a competitive inhibitor of platelet cyclooxygenase.[1,41,79] In addition to inhibiting experimentally induced platelet thrombi[34] and normalizing platelet survival in patients with artificial heart valves,[34] the drug has been reported to limit the extent of endothelial cell injury in several experimental models.[1,41]

FISH OILS AND n-3 FATTY ACIDS

The n-3 fatty acids (also referred to as omega-3 fatty acids), such as eicosapentaenoic acid (EPA) (C20:5 n-3) and docosahexaenoic acid (C22:6 n-3), are highly unsaturated fatty acids that, in platelets, compete with arachidonic acid for cyclooxygenase and result in the formation of thromboxane A_3, a weak platelet agonist, rather than the strong agonist thromboxane A_2.[7,34,80] In addition, EPA results in the production in endothelial cells of PGI_3, a potent platelet inhibitor.[34] Supplementing an individual's diet with n-3 fatty acids results in a prolongation of the bleeding time and decreased platelet aggregation, associated with decreased production of TxA_2.[7,34,80] Administration of diets rich in n-3 fatty acids produces antithrombotic effects in animal models of thrombosis,[7] but the antithrombotic effects of such diets in humans have been questioned.[10]

NITRATES

Nitroglycerin, as well as other organic nitrate derivatives, inhibits platelet aggregation by ADP and other platelet agonists and reduces the extent of platelet-induced thrombus formation in experimental models.[81] In humans, intravenously administered nitroglycerin and nitroprusside prolong the bleeding time and inhibit platelet aggregation ex vivo.[7,81] Organic nitrates, such as the nitrovasodilators that have been used to lower blood pressure and relieve anginal attacks, are converted ultimately to nitric oxide (NO) (or an S-nitrosothiol congener thereof), thereby activating guanylate cyclase and resulting in an increase in intracellular cGMP, which is both a vasodilator and platelet inhibitor[7,81] (see Chap. 111). NO may also exert a platelet inhibitory effect by activating endothelial cell cyclooxygenase, thereby promoting the release of the potent antiplatelet antagonist PGI_2 (prostacyclin, see above).[82]

CALCIUM CHANNEL BLOCKERS

A rise in intracellular calcium concentration is required for platelet aggregation, secretion, and thromboxane A_2 production (see Chap. 111). Current evidence suggests that, in platelets, calcium channels that are involved in calcium influx are not of the voltage-regulated type,[83] but the matter is controversial.[84] In general, calcium channel blocking agents have been more effective in inhibiting platelet activation in vitro than in vivo,[85] and drug concentrations in plasma may be too low to be effective. The potential use of these agents as antithrombotic agents is unclear. In one study, oral verapamil, in a dose of 340 mg/d for 7 days, was reported to inhibit platelet thrombus formation ex vivo in patients with stable coronary disease.[86]

β-ADRENERGIC BLOCKING AGENTS

β-adrenergic blocking agents such as propranolol have been reported to reverse the enhanced ADP-induced aggregation observed in patients with angina pectoris,[41,87] but whether this effect is related to nonspecific membrane effects of the drug rather than to β-adrenergic blockade is not clear.[1,2,88] In some studies, administration of propranolol to healthy subjects had no significant effect on platelet aggregation,[89] and in one study timolol (a nonselective beta-blocker) induced a significant increase in platelet aggregation and reduction in platelet cyclic AMP,[90] whereas metoprolol had none of these effects.

OTHER DRUGS

Other drugs with antiplatelet properties that are used in clinical medicine include heparin and other antithrombins (see Chaps. 132, 133), vitamin E, serotonin antagonists, penicillin, other β-lactam antibiotics, and others.[1,2,10]

ANTIPLATELET DRUGS IN CLINICAL MEDICINE

The antiplatelet properties of drugs are frequently inferred from in vitro tests and experimental models that may not reflect accurately some, or even any, of the clinical events for which the drugs are used. A more rational basis for the clinical pharmacology of antiplatelet therapy will require further advances in understanding platelet activation mechanisms and the role of platelets in the various clinical conditions for which antiplatelet therapy may be useful. At present, a drug is usually chosen because it has been shown to have some antiplatelet property (as discussed above) in the hope that it will also prevent the (presumably) platelet-mediated clinical event or process. The topic has been the subject of many general reviews.[1,2,7,9–11,34,35,91–93]

ISCHEMIC HEART DISEASE

The clinical symptoms that are associated with a reduction of the blood supply to the heart are, in most cases, due either to the gradual narrowing of the atherosclerotic coronary arteries, or the abrupt reduction in flow due to a sudden further narrowing of a major coronary vessel by vasospasm or the deposition of an intraluminal platelet-fibrin thrombus.[1,2,94] Thus, the efficacy of an antiplatelet agent in the syndromes associated with ischemic heart disease will depend on whether, and how, platelets contribute to the process, and the extent to which the drug modifies favorably the platelet activation mechanisms involved.

ATHEROSCLEROSIS

Platelets could play a role in the development of atherosclerosis by releasing mitogens, such as platelet-derived growth factor (PDGF), or vascular permeability factors, but their importance has not been established.[7,94] Should platelets prove to be important, a useful antiplatelet drug would probably have to inhibit either platelet adhesion or the secretion of biologically active substances from adherent platelets. At present, there is no evidence that the progress of atherosclerosis can be favorably modified by any antiplatelet drug currently used in clinical medicine.

STABLE ANGINA PECTORIS

Stable angina is due primarily to increases in the myocardial oxygen demand beyond the capacity of the stenosed, atherosclerotic vessels to increase their delivery of oxygenated blood.[94] Although some studies have suggested that platelet aggregation or release of vasospastic substances such as thromboxane A_2 could play a role in precipitating anginal attacks,[1,95,96] negative findings reported in other studies[1,97,98] leave this question unresolved. In the U.S. Physicians' Trial,[99] aspirin did not affect favorably the anginal symptoms in a subset of men with this condition.[100] However, in this trial,[100] as well as in a study on 2035 patients who received a class III antiarrhythmic drug (sotalol) and either 75 mg of aspirin daily or a placebo, aspirin reduced the incidence of subsequent myocardial infarctions.[101] Aspirin will reduce the frequency of acute thrombotic events in patients with ischemic heart disease (see below), but left unresolved is whether a more potent antiplatelet agent might affect favorably the symptoms of angina pectoris or the underlying atherosclerotic process.

ACUTE CORONARY SYNDROMES AND PERCUTANEOUS CORONARY INTERVENTIONS

Angiographic, angioscopic, and pathologic studies indicate that platelets play a role in acute or subacute syndromes associated with coronary atherosclerosis.[102,103] In most cases, the thrombi formed in acute coronary syndromes are caused by the rupture of an atherosclerotic plaque,[94] exposing tissue factor and platelet-reactive materials, such as collagen. The resultant platelet-fibrin thrombus accounts for the abrupt reduction in coronary blood flow, and the nature of the clinical event (unstable angina, non-Q-wave infarction, or Q-wave infarction) is probably determined by the degree of the occlusion, the distribution of the involved vessel, the presence of collateral blood vessels, and the reversibility of the obstruction. It is generally agreed that rupture of the plaque can promote the deposition of normal platelets, but it is uncertain whether hyperresponsive platelets constitute another risk factor in patients who are predisposed to acute coronary syndromes.[1,2,7]

Platelets also play a role in precipitating acute and subacute events associated with percutaneous coronary interventions (PCI) designed to improve blood flow in coronary arteries, such as balloon angioplasty (PTCA), atherectomy, and stenting. Thus, disruption of the atherosclerotic plaque during PTCA exposes prothrombotic material that probably accounts for a significant percentage of the abrupt closure that can occur shortly after the procedure[34]; the remainder is probably due to coronary mechanical occlusion secondary to dissection and flap formation. The mechanism promoting acute occlusion after percutaneous coronary revascularization is probably different from that involved in the late restenosis which may occur after these procedures.[104] Although the mechanism responsible for late stenosis remains to be clarified, the liberation from platelets of growth factors (such as PDGF), GPIIb/IIIa-mediated platelet events involved in thrombin generation, and increased surface expression of the integrin $\alpha_v\beta_3$ on smooth muscle cells could all contribute to this process.[104]

An appreciation of the important role of platelets in the pathogenesis of acute coronary syndromes has led to the increasing use of antiplatelet agents in clinical cardiology.

UNSTABLE ANGINA, NON-Q-WAVE MYOCARDIAL INFARCTION, AND PERCUTANEOUS CORONARY INTERVENTIONS

Aspirin   Episodic increases in thromboxane A_2 biosynthesis, as reflected by plasma measurements of thromboxane B_2 in the coronary sinus or urinary 11-dehydro-thromboxane B_2 and 2,3-dinor-thromboxane B_2 excretion, have been reported in patients with unstable angina.[105,106] The results of four randomized, placebo-controlled, double-blind trials demonstrated the beneficial effects of aspirin on patients with unstable angina. Treatment with aspirin in daily doses of 75 mg[107] or 325 mg[108] for 3 months; 650 mg for 3 to 9 days[109]; and 1300 mg for 24 months[110] significantly reduced the incidence of both myocardial infarction and cardiac death by 50 to 70 percent and also reduced the symptoms of severe angina and the subsequent need for coronary revascularization.[111] Meta-analysis of six unstable angina studies suggested an additional benefit from addition of heparin.[112] Of interest, one study found that aspirin therapy in patients with unstable angina did not completely suppress the synthesis of TxA_2, possibly reflecting extraplatelet sources.[113]

The incidence of acute thrombotic occlusions and Q-wave infarction after PCI can be reduced by aspirin, alone[34,114] or in combination with dipyridamole.[114] Aspirin alone appears to be as effective as a combination of aspirin and dipyridamole.[115] Currently, the major use of aspirin in PCI is its administration, as adjunctive therapy, with heparin and more potent antiplatelet drugs (see below).

Ticlopidine   When used to treat unstable angina, ticlopidine added to "conventional" therapy with drugs (β-blockers, calcium channel antagonists, and nitrates) that alone, or in combination, could have antiplatelet properties (see above) reduced the risk for nonfatal myocardial infarction (46 percent), nonfatal plus fatal myocardial infarction (53 percent), fatal myocardial infarction and vascular death (47 percent), and total vascular events (46 percent).[116] However, its delayed onset of action (as long as 20–30 days[116]) is a very serious limitation in using ticlopidine as the sole drug to treat unstable angina. Ticlopidine, in combination with aspirin, has also been found to be superior to aspirin alone or conventional anticoagulation in preventing vascular complications after coronary stenting.[49,117]

GPIIb/IIIa Antagonists   An increasing number of studies have reported on the efficacy of GPIIb/IIIa antagonists in favorably modifying the clinical course of patients with acute coronary syndromes, such as unstable angina and evolving myocardial infarction, or in preventing ischemic vascular complications after PCI (for reviews specific to these agents, see Refs. 9, 65, 77, 78, 118–120). All patients in these studies received aspirin, and most received heparin. In the first major study [Evaluation of 7E3 for the Prevention of Ischemic Complications (EPIC)], abciximab, administered as a single bolus dose followed by a 12-h infusion, was found to reduce by 35 percent ($P = 0.008$) the primary end point of death, acute myocardial infarction, or urgent revascularization at 30 days in 2099 high-risk patients undergoing coronary angioplasty.[119,121] The incidence of major bleeding events (14 percent) in the treated group was twice that in the controls. The benefits of abciximab treatment were maintained for 6 months, due principally to a decreased need for either repeat percutaneous intervention or coronary artery bypass surgery (CABS).[122] The beneficial effect of therapy was still observable after 3 years.[123] In a subsequent study (EPILOG) on 2792 lower-risk patients undergoing coronary intervention, abciximab reduced the incidence of primary end points by 55 percent ($P < 0.001$).[124] The increase in major bleeding events associated with abciximab therapy in the EPIC study, which

TABLE 131-2　GLYCOPROTEIN IIB/IIIA ANTAGONISTS IN ACUTE CORONARY SYNDROMES (ACS)*

Antagonist	Type	Study	Reference	No. of Patients	Entry	Intervention†	Duration of Therapy (h)	End Points 30d, % Change‡
Abciximab	Chimeric	EPIC (1994)	121–123	2099	High-risk ACS	Yes	12	−35, P = 0.008
(c7E3 Fab,	Monoclonal	EPILOG (1997)	124	2792	All-risk ACS	Yes	12	−55, P < 0.001
ReoPro)	Fab fragment	CAPTURE (1997)	125	1265	Refractory UA	Yes	18–24 + 1	−29, P = 0.012
		RAPPORT (1998)	126	483	Acute MI + angio	Yes	12	−48, P = 0.030
		EPISTENT (1998)	127	2399	Elective stenting	Yes	12	−51, P = 0.001
Eptifibatide	Cyclic KGD	IMPACT II (1997)	128	4010	All-risk	Yes	20–24	−15, P = 0.06
(Integrilin)	Heptapeptide	PURSUIT (1998)	129,136	10,948	UA, non-Q MI	variable	72	−10, P = 0.04
Tirofiban	Nonpeptide	RESTORE (1997)	130	2139	UA, acute MI	Yes	36	−16, P = 0.16
(Aggrestat)		PRISM (1998)	131	3232	UA	variable	48	−17, P = 0.34
		PRISM PLUS (1998)	132	1915	UA, non-Q MI	variable	48	−17, P = 0.03
Lamifiban	Nonpeptide	CANADIAN (1996)	134	365	UA, non-Q MI	variable	72–120	−69, P = 0.003
(RO-44-9883)		PARAGON A (1998)	133	2282	UA	variable	72–120	−11, P = 0.48

*Unstable angina (UA) or evolving acute myocardial infarction (acute MI).
†Angioplasty (angio), atherectomy, or stenting.
‡For multiple dosage regimens, best results are shown.

were principally at vascular access sites, was largely eliminated in EPILOG by reducing and weight-adjusting the dose of heparin and by removing the vascular sheath shortly after the procedure. The major studies through 1998 in which patients with acute coronary syndromes were given GPIIb/IIIa antagonists, with aspirin and heparin, are outlined in Table 131-2. The best results for reducing 30-day end points have been obtained with abciximab, which reduced the primary end points at 30 days by 35 percent in EPIC (P = 0.008),[121] by 55 percent in EPILOG (P < 0.001),[124] by 29 percent in the CAPTURE study of refractory unstable angina (P = 0.012),[125] by 48 percent in the RAPPORT acute myocardial infarction/angioplasty study (P = 0.03),[126] and by 51 percent in the EPISTENT elective stenting study (P = 0.001).[127] A significant reduction, or trend in that direction, was also observed using eptifibatide in the IMPACT II all-risk coronary syndrome study (15 percent, P = 0.06)[128] and the PURSUIT study on patients with unstable angina or non-Q-wave myocardial infarction (10 percent, P = 0.04).[129] Similar trends were observed in patients receiving tirofiban in studies designated as RESTORE (16 percent, P = 0.16)[130] and PRISM (7 percent, P = 0.34),[131] and in patients entered into the PRISM-PLUS study[132] who received heparin (17 percent, P = 0.03). In one study (PARAGON A), low-dose lamifiban (with or without heparin) reduced nonsignificantly (11 percent, P = 0.48) the 30-day end points, but significantly (23 percent, P = 0.027) the 6-month end points,[133] and in one small Canadian study, lamifiban was strikingly effective in reducing end points (69 percent, P = 0.003).[134]

A recent meta-analysis of 16 clinical studies that utilized GPIIb/IIIa antagonists in ischemic heart disease evaluated the odds ratios and benefits per 1000 patients in reducing significant end points at 48 to 96 hours, 30 days, and 6 months after beginning therapy.[135] The results of this meta-analysis, summarized in Table 131-3, establish the important role of GPIIb/IIIa antagonists in managing patients with acute coronary syndromes. Whether the superior results obtained with abciximab to date are due to underdosing with the other inhibitors or to unique properties of abciximab, such as its ability to inhibit the $\alpha_v\beta_3$ vitronectin receptor (see above), remains to be determined. Further studies are also needed to determine the optimum duration of therapy with GPIIb/IIIa antagonists.

The need and dosage requirement for heparin in association with GPIIb/IIIa antagonists requires further study. In two of the studies that used either tirofiban (PRISM PLUS)[132] or eptifibatide (PURSUIT),[136] failure to administer heparin concurrently with the GPIIb/IIIa antagonist may have been detrimental. The lower than "standard" dose of heparin in the EPILOG versus EPIC studies appears to have reduced

bleeding without compromising the antithrombotic efficacy,[124] but no studies using abciximab alone in acute coronary syndromes have been reported to date. Finally, the development of oral GPIIb/IIIa antagonists opens the possibility of achieving long-term platelet inhibition in patients with clinical syndromes associated with ischemic heart disease, and several early-phase trials with these agents (sibrafiban and xemilofiban) have been reported.[137,138]

ACUTE MYOCARDIAL INFARCTION

Antiplatelet Agents Alone　In the ISIS-2 trial, which evaluated 17,187 patients, aspirin therapy (160 mg immediately and then daily for 1 month) for acute myocardial infarction decreased mortality and reinfarction when given alone, had an additive benefit when administered with streptokinase, and reduced the incidence of reinfarction that occurs after thrombolytic therapy.[139] In fact, aspirin alone decreased 35-day mortality almost as much as streptokinase alone (23 percent vs 25 percent), and aspirin + streptokinase decreased mortality by 12 percent, suggesting an additive effect of using both drugs.[139] The benefits were observed in both men and women.[139] In the subsequent ISIS-3 trial, involving over 40,000 patients, no significant advantage of adding heparin to aspirin was observed.[140] A summary of a meta-analysis[141] of the effects of antiplatelet therapy in reducing the risks of a subsequent vascular event in patients with acute myocardial infarction is shown in Table 131-4. The major uses of antiplatelet agents in acute myocardial infarction have been their administration

TABLE 131-3　CLINICAL BENEFITS FROM UTILIZING GPIIB/IIIA ANTAGONISTS IN ISCHEMIC HEART DISEASE*

End Point	Odds Ratio (benefit per 1000 patients)		
	48–96 hours	30 days	6 months
Death	0.70† (1)	0.87[NS] (3)	0.97[NS] (2)
Death or myocardial infarction (MI)	0.66† (17)	0.76‡ (20)	0.82† (20)
Death, MI, or revascularization	0.66† (27)	0.77† (30)	0.89† (23)

*Meta-analysis of 16 randomized trials (n = 32,135 patients) in which the entry criteria were either an intent to perform a percutaneous coronary procedure or symptoms of acute coronary ischemia without ST-segment elevation on the ECG.
‡P < 0.05; †P < 0.001; NS, not significant.
SOURCE: Ref. 135, with permission.

TABLE 131-4 ANTIPLATELET TRIALS IN CEREBROVASCULAR AND CARDIAC DISEASE

				% Reduction in Odds of Outcome (benefit per 1000 patients) (±SD)*				
Trial Entry Criterion	No. Trials	Rx mos	No. Patients (all trials)	Nonfatal Myocardial Infarction	Nonfatal Stroke	Vascular Death	Any Vascular Event[†]	Death from Any Cause
Cerebrovascular‡	18	33	11,707	36±11 (9±3)	23±6 (20±6)	14±7 (11±6)	22±4 (37±8)	16±6 (17±7)
Prior myocardial infarction§	11	27	19,791	31± 6 (18±4)	39±11 (6±2)	15±5 (13±5)	25± 4 (36±6)	12±5 (12±5)
Acute myocardial infarction¶	9	1	18,773	54± 8 (12±2)	40±17 (2±1)	22±4 (24±4)	29±4 (38±5)	23±4 (24±4)
Primary prevention	3	42	1360	29± 8 (5± 2)	−21±13 (−2±1)	2±10 (1±2)	10± 6 (4±3)	5± 7 (3±2)

*Data for some outcomes unavailable in some trials.
[†]Myocardial infarction, stroke, or vascular death.
‡Transient ischemic attacks/strokes; 10 trials used aspirin, alone or in combination with other drugs.
§Eight trials used aspirin, alone or with dipyridamole.
¶Most patients ($n = 17,187$) were from a single study.
Source: Ref. 141.

to patients undergoing percutaneous coronary revascularization, as reviewed above, and in conjunction with thrombolytic therapy, reviewed below.

Antiplatelet Agents in Combination with Thrombolytic Therapy Successful reperfusion of acutely occluded coronary arteries with fibrinolytic agents has been estimated to occur in 75 to 90 percent of treated patients.[7] Experimental evidence indicates that thrombi that are particularly rich in platelets, as may occur in some patients with myocardial infarction, are more resistant to lysis by thrombolytic agents[7,142] and that enhanced lysis and perfusion may be achieved when a monoclonal antibody to GPIIb/IIIa is used in conjunction with fibrinolytic therapy.[7,142] Platelets may also play a role in the reocclusion of a coronary artery that occurs after successful thrombolysis. Thrombolytic agents may paradoxically activate platelets by a variety of mechanisms, and the thrombi in reoccluded vessels may be particularly rich in platelets.[7,142] In experimental models, reocclusion has been abolished by antiplatelet agents such as aspirin, PGI_2, regimens that combine TxA_2 receptor blockade and inhibition of thromboxane synthase, and glycoprotein GPIIb/IIIa antagonists.[7,142] A meta-analysis of 32 studies of patients receiving thrombolytic therapy for acute myocardial infarction showed that the reocclusion rate assessed by angiography in 419 patients treated with aspirin was 11 percent compared with 25 percent in 513 patients without aspirin therapy ($P < 0.001$).[143] Because of the positive results obtained in experimental models and the beneficial effects of aspirin, several clinical studies have addressed the question of whether more potent antiplatelet agents, notably GPIIb/IIIa antagonists, would help to speed reperfusion and favorably affect clinical end points in patients with acute myocardial infarction undergoing thrombolytic therapy. In several relatively small studies, both abciximab[144] and eptifibatide[145] have been reported to improve reperfusion at 90 min after instituting thrombolytic therapy. Whether this type of therapy will improve clinical end points remains to be determined.

SECONDARY PREVENTION STUDIES

These studies address the question of whether antiplatelet therapy will modify the clinical course, principally by reducing mortality and myocardial infarction, of patients who have already suffered one infarction. Conceptually, the question is similar to that raised in studying patients with unstable angina, since the mechanisms that are responsible for producing the acute events (myocardial infarction and sudden death) are probably similar in both syndromes. Table 131-5 outlines seven major randomized long-term studies[146–152] with aspirin, or aspirin and dipyridamole, that have been carried out on a total of about 15,000

patients, in the majority men, who suffered one or more myocardial infarctions. These studies have differed from one another in some aspects of design that could affect the outcome, such as drug dosage, time of entry after myocardial infarction, and the decision as to whether to exclude from final analysis patients who withdrew from treatment or were otherwise deemed ineligible.[1,153] The general design and overall results of these trials are summarized in Table 131-5 and have been reviewed in detail.[1,154] Six of the trials tested aspirin alone, in a dose ranging from 300 to 1500 mg per day. In five of the studies, a trend favoring aspirin in reducing overall mortality by 17 to 30 percent was reported, but in no individual study was the reduction considered significant. In the largest study (AMIS), the mortality rate was greater (but not significantly) in the aspirin-treated group.[149] In all six studies, as well as in the study utilizing aspirin plus dipyridamole only (Paris II), there was a trend toward a reduction in the incidence of nonfatal myocardial infarction. Analysis of the pooled data on the studies in which aspirin alone was tested showed a significant risk reduction with aspirin for total mortality ($P < 0.03$), all cardiovascular deaths (16 percent; $P < 0.01$), and fatal or nonfatal myocardial infarction (21 percent; $P < 0.001$).[155]

In 1988, the Antiplatelet Trialists' Collaboration published a meta-analysis of randomized trials on patients who received antiplatelet therapy for various conditions, including secondary prevention after myocardial infarction.[156] A summary of their subsequent meta-analysis[141] of secondary prevention trials with all antiplatelet drugs, published in 1994, is shown in Table 131-4. For the 11 trials, involving almost 20,000 patients, allocation to antiplatelet treatment had no significant effect on nonvascular mortality, but reduced nonfatal myocardial infarction by 31 ± 6 percent, nonfatal stroke by 39 ± 11 percent, vascular death by 15 ± 5 percent, and death from any cause by 12 ± 5 percent, with corresponding benefits per 1000 patients treated of 18 ± 4, 6 ± 2, 13 ± 5, and 12 ± 5 respectively (Table 131-4). The weighted mean duration of antiplatelet therapy in these studies was 27 months, and allocation to antiplatelet therapy produced a highly significant reduction ($2P < 0.00001$) of about 36 per 1000 patients in the risk of suffering another vascular event, defined as myocardial infarction, stroke, or vascular death[141] (Table 131-4). In separate analyses of the secondary prevention myocardial infarction trials, sulfinpyrazone may have been better than nontreatment, but a direct comparison with aspirin showed a trend favoring aspirin.[156] There was no significant advantage to adding dipyridamole to aspirin, and no data for dipyridamole alone.[156] Finally, no particular dose of aspirin between 300 and 1500 mg per day in the secondary prevention studies seemed to be more beneficial than any other dose.[156]

TABLE 131-5   SECONDARY PREVENTION TRIALS WITH ANTIPLATELET DRUGS

								% REDUCTION OF EVENT[†]		
TRIAL	REFERENCE	DRUG	TOTAL DAILY DOSE (MG)	SEX	NUMBER RANDOMIZED	AVERAGE TIME FROM MI (MO)	AVERAGE FOLLOW-UP (MO)	OVERALL MORTALITY	SUDDEN DEATH	NONFATAL MI
Elwood I	146	ASA	300	M	1239	2.5	12	25	—	—
CDPA	147	ASA	972	M	1529	85	22	30	19	5
Breddin	148	ASA	1500	M, F	946*	1.3	24	18	33	27
AMIS	149	ASA	1000	M, F	4524	25	39	+11	+35	22
Elwood II	150	ASA	900	M, F	1682	0.3	12	18	—	35
Paris I	151	ASA	972	M, F	2026	20.2	41	18	+27	29
		ASA + DPM	972 + 225					16	16	19
Paris II	152	ASA + DPM	972 + 225	M, F	3128	2.8	23	3	+20	37

ASA, acetylsalicylic acid; DPM, dipyridamole.
*Including 320 receiving phenprocoumon.
[†] + signifies increased incidence.

The secondary prevention Clopidogrel versus Aspirin in Patients at Risk of Ischaemic Events (CAPRIE) trial[60] enrolled 19,185 patients and included, in approximately equal numbers, patients with a recent history of acute myocardial infarction or ischemic stroke, or symptomatic atherosclerotic peripheral vascular disease. After a mean follow-up of 1.9 years, the actuarial annual rate of the primary outcome events (ischemic stroke, myocardial infarction, or vascular death) was 5.83 percent in the aspirin-treated group and 5.32 percent in the clopidogrel-treated group. This was a relative risk reduction of 8.7 percent (95 percent confidence interval, 0.3–16.8, $P = 0.043$).[157]

PRIMARY PREVENTION STUDIES
The potential use of aspirin in the prophylaxis of myocardial infarction was suggested by early clinical observations[158] and case-control studies.[159] There have been two large trials employing aspirin in a population without a prior history of major vascular events, such as myocardial infarction or stroke. In one study, 22,071 male U.S. physicians received either a placebo or 325 mg of aspirin every other day.[99] During 5 years of follow-up, aspirin reduced the incidence of myocardial infarction by 44 percent ($P < 0.00001$), but there was no reduction in overall mortality. In a smaller study employing 5139 male British physicians, 500 mg of aspirin daily did not reduce either total mortality or myocardial infarction.[160] These studies have been reviewed in detail elsewhere,[160] and a summary of a meta-analysis of the trials (which also included one much smaller study) is shown in Table 131-4. In one nonrandomized study of more than 87,000 American female nurses, aspirin dosage was noted, but not controlled. Aspirin consumption was associated with a 32 percent reduction in the incidence of first myocardial infarction, as compared with those who did not take aspirin ($P = 0.0005$).[161] From all the above studies, a tentative conclusion is that aspirin may reduce the incidence of myocardial infarction in asymptomatic men and women, particularly in those over the age of 50 and with cardiovascular risk factors.[93,162] A trend toward increased risk for hemorrhagic stroke in aspirin-treated patients was also suggested by these studies.[93]

CORONARY ARTERY BYPASS SURGERY (CABS)
The different mechanisms involved in early thrombotic occlusion (less than 1 month), occlusion during the first postoperative year, and closure during the 10 subsequent years after saphenous vein grafting or internal mammary artery bypass surgery for coronary artery disease have been reviewed.[34,163] The incidence of early thrombosis after CABS can be significantly reduced with the use of antiplatelet agents (principally varying combinations of aspirin and dipyridamole) administered perioperatively, preferably before, but no later than 48 h after surgery.[34,164,165] The improvement in graft patency with aspirin alone per-

sists after 1 year.[164] Ticlopidine has also been reported to improve graft patency in several studies.[165] A meta-analysis of 20 studies utilizing various combinations of aspirin, dipyridamole, and ticlopidine has been published.[166] Among patients who had CABS, allocation to a mean scheduled duration of 7 months of antiplatelet therapy was associated with prevention of occlusion in 92 (SD ± 15) patients per 1000 (21.1 percent of antiplatelet allocated patients versus 30.3 percent of corresponding controls).

The use of antiplatelet agents may increase perioperative bleeding in patients undergoing CABS. When administered preoperatively, aspirin produced a small but significant increase in drainage from the chest tube, in perioperative transfusion requirements, and in the reoperation rate, but there was no excess mortality due to bleeding complications.[167] It has been suggested that starting antiplatelet therapy after invasive vascular procedures, including CABS, reduces the risk of bleeding while still preventing occlusion.[166,168] In support of this concept, less bleeding (transfusion requirement, reoperation), but equivalent graft occlusion rates 8 days after surgery, was observed in patients who received aspirin (325 mg daily) 6 h after CABS compared with those whose therapy was started preoperatively.[169]

Extensive data on the use of antiplatelet drugs in patients receiving internal mammary artery grafts are not available. However, limited data suggests that the patency rates after 1 year are 92 to 100 percent, whether or not antiplatelet agents are used.[165]

VALVULAR HEART DISEASE

Because of the high risk of thromboembolism in patients receiving prosthetic heart valves, antithrombotic therapy is generally recommended for these patients. Anticoagulant therapy has been effective in reducing the incidence of thromboembolism, whereas antiplatelet therapy alone has not been effective.[1,2,34,170] However, several studies have demonstrated that the addition of either aspirin (160 mg/d) or dipyridamole (400 mg/d) will confer additional protection in patients who suffer systemic thromboembolism despite adequate anticoagulation.[1,2,34,170] For patients with prosthetic heart valves at high risk of thromboembolism, combined warfarin and aspirin therapy may be beneficial compared with warfarin alone.[171] The possible use of antiplatelet agents in patients with rheumatic valvular disease (without prosthetic replacement), mitral valve prolapse, and other valvular disorders has been reviewed.[172]

There is some evidence that aspirin alone may be useful in reducing the incidence of thromboembolism in patients with atrial fibrillation (associated with both valvular and nonvalvular disorders),[173] but this therapy should probably be reserved for patients who are unable to take adjusted-dose warfarin or for those in subgroups at a relatively low risk for stroke.[174,175] In addition, the use of a regimen consisting of low-intensity, fixed-dose warfarin plus aspirin (325 mg per day) was found to be insufficient for stroke prevention in patients with atrial fibrillation at high risk for thromboembolism.[176]

CEREBROVASCULAR DISEASE

PATHOPHYSIOLOGY

Platelets are involved in the pathogenesis of ischemic syndromes involving the cerebral circulation.[1,2,41] For example, patients with transient ischemic attacks (TIAs) frequently have ulcerated atherosclerotic lesions in the extracranial portion of the basilar or internal carotid arteries, and as early as the mid-1950s it was initially suggested that these attacks might be the result of microembolization from thrombi deposited on the lesions.[177] More direct evidence came from observations of the passage of microemboli through the retinal arterioles during attacks of amaurosis fugax[178] and the histological demonstration[179] that some of these microemboli were composed of platelet aggregates. In addition, enhanced platelet activation occurs in some patients with transient ischemic attacks or after recovery from completed strokes.[1,2] Since any large clinical study of cerebrovascular disease may contain patients with cerebral ischemia of varying etiologies, a method for identifying those whose symptoms are due to platelet emboli would be of great value.

CLINICAL TRIALS

The question of whether antiplatelet drugs can reduce the incidence of TIAs, strokes, and vascular deaths has been addressed in trials that studied patients with a previous history of TIAs and/or reversible ischemic neurologic deficits (RINDs) and/or strokes. These studies have varied in their size, inclusion criteria, drug dosage, and end points, as discussed in various reviews.[1,34,91-93,180-183] The second meta-analysis of the Antiplatelet Trialists' Collaboration (see above) is shown in Table 131-4.[141] Patients with cerebrovascular symptoms were entered into 18 trials, 10 of which tested the efficacy of aspirin in daily doses ranging from 300 to 1500 mg per day. In some studies, dipyridamole or sulfinpyrazone, alone or in combination with aspirin, were also evaluated. Eleven studies entered patients with a prior myocardial infarction and nine entered patients with an acute infarction. The overall results of this analysis (summarized in Table 131-4) demonstrated the efficacy of antiplatelet therapy in preventing cerebrovascular events in patients with either prior cerebrovascular or cardiac events. For patients with prior cerebrovascular disease, the use of antiplatelet therapy resulted in a reduction in the odds ratio for nonfatal stroke by 23 ± 6 percent, for nonfatal myocardial infarction by 36 ± 11 percent, and for vascular death by 14 ± 7 percent, with corresponding benefits per 1000 patients treated of 20 ± 6, 9 ± 3, and 11 ± 6, respectively. All these reductions were highly significant. In early studies that utilized both aspirin and a combination of aspirin and dipyridamole, the addition of dipyridamole did not appear to confer any additional advantage in the cerebrovascular studies.[156] However, the combination therapy was found to be more effective in a recent study that used low-dose aspirin (50 mg daily) and a high dose (400 mg daily) of a modified-release formulation of dipyridamole with improved bioavailability.[184] Two studies have reported the beneficial effects of ticlopidine in stroke prevention.[185,186] In one study (TASS), 3069 patients with TIAs or minor stroke received ticlopidine (500 mg) or aspirin (1300 mg) daily.[185] Compared with aspirin, ticlopidine produced a significant relative risk reduction (12 percent) in the event rate for stroke or death and a 21 percent reduction for fatal or nonfatal stroke at 3 years. Subgroup analysis also showed a trend favoring ticlopidine in preventing transient ischemic attacks.[186] In another study (CATS), treatment of patients with a recent ischemic stroke with

ticlopidine (500 mg or placebo) resulted in a 30 percent reduction in stroke, myocardial infarction, or vascular death, with comparable results in males and females.[187] A subgroup analysis of the CAPRIE study[60] (see above) found that in patients with recent ischemic stroke, clopidogrel treatment was associated with a nonsignificant trend toward a lower annual rate of subsequent stroke, myocardial infarction, or vascular death compared with aspirin (7.15 percent vs 7.71 percent, $P = 0.26$).

In several studies the benefits from aspirin were confined to men, whereas this was not the case in other trials.[188] Although the issue is not completely resolved, overall analysis of the various trials suggests that the benefits of aspirin are comparable in men and women.[180,189] A second question pertains to the optimum dose of aspirin. The Antiplatelet Trialists' meta-analysis of studies utilizing aspirin in daily doses ranging from 300 to 1300 mg,[156] and two subsequently published trials of low-dose aspirin,[190,191] suggested that daily aspirin doses of 75 to 300 mg are effective, and no differences in efficacy were found in one study that compared 300 mg with 1200 mg daily.[192] However, the conclusion that dosage regimens of aspirin of 300 mg or less are as effective as those utilizing much higher doses (975 to 1300 mg) has been challenged,[193] and several studies suggested that daily doses of aspirin in excess of 300 mg may be necessary to obtain maximum antiplatelet and antithrombotic effects in a, perhaps small, subgroup of patients.[29,194,195] This conclusion has also been challenged.[196]

There have been two studies of the use of aspirin administered within 48 h of suspected acute ischemic stroke. The Chinese Acute Stroke Trial (CAST) enrolled 21,106 patients, half of whom received 160 mg of aspirin daily and the other half a placebo for up to 4 weeks,[197] and the International Stroke Trial (IST) administered 300 mg of aspirin daily to a subgroup ($n = 4858$) of patients among a large study group ($n = 19,438$) in which the efficacy of heparin was also evaluated.[198] The pooled results of the two studies indicated that aspirin produced a small, but significant, reduction of about 10 deaths or recurrent strokes per 1000 during the first few weeks.[198]

PERIPHERAL VASCULAR DISEASE

Ischemic symptoms in most patients with peripheral vascular disease are generally held to be the result of decreased blood flow consequent to occlusive atherosclerotic disease of large vessels. However, involvement of small vessels, through occlusions by platelet microaggregates, or through spasm produced by platelet-derived products, could also contribute to these symptoms. In addition, platelet-induced thrombosis probably plays a role in the acute, thromboembolic events that are frequent complications of peripheral vascular disease. The question of whether treatment with antiplatelet drugs, such as aspirin or ticlopidine, favorably affects the course of either peripheral atherosclerosis or its occlusive complications is unsettled.[1,34,91,92,199] In the U.S. Physicians' Trial, aspirin significantly reduced the need for peripheral arterial surgery, but did not affect the incidence of intermittent claudication,[200] confirming the general impression[199] that currently employed antiplatelet therapy may reduce the incidence of thrombotic complications in patients with peripheral vascular disease without affecting the basic disease process. Relief of clinical symptoms through the use of PGE_1 or PGI_2,[1,91,201] or a PGI_2 analogue (iloprost),[39] has been reported, but further studies are needed. In addition, it is not clear whether beneficial effects are related to the platelet inhibitory, vasodilatory, or other properties of these drugs. In the CAPRIE study (see above), the subgroup of patients who appeared to derive the most benefit from clopidogrel (compared with aspirin) were those with symptomatic peripheral vascular disease.[60]

Although the role of antiplatelet therapy in preventing graft occlusion after peripheral artery reconstructive surgery is controversial,[199] meta-analysis[165] suggests that vascular graft occlusions may be reduced by approximately one-third in aspirin-treated patients.[202] One study reported improved patency of infrainguinal vein bypass grafts in patients treated with ticlopidine as compared with placebo.[203]

SMALL VESSEL THROMBOTIC DISEASES (MICROANGIOPATHIES)

Platelet-fibrin thrombi in the microcirculation are involved in the pathogenesis of some glomerular disorders, transplant rejection, and a variety of other conditions broadly classified as microangiopathies.[1,2] In some experimental and clinical studies, the course of these disorders has been favorably influenced by antiplatelet drugs.

RENAL DISEASE
Platelet-fibrin thrombi play a role in the pathogenesis of membranoproliferative glomerulonephritis,[1,2,91] and favorable results have been observed using combinations of dipyridamole, aspirin, and anticoagulants.[1,2,91,92] Negative results with aspirin alone have also been reported.[1,91] Antiplatelet agents may also modify or delay the rejection of renal allografts,[1,2,91] but more data are necessary to support this conclusion. At present no definitive conclusions can be drawn about the efficacy of antiplatelet drugs in progressive renal disease.[204]

THROMBOTIC THROMBOCYTOPENIC PURPURA
Platelet microthrombi in this disorder are thought to form as a result of the presence of unusually large von Willebrand factor multimers that are released from injured endothelial cells, and not processed to smaller forms due to immune-mediated deficiency of a specific plasma protease activity (see Chap. 117). Although the efficacy of varying combinations of aspirin, dipyridamole, dextran, sulfinpyrazone, and PGI2 in modifying the course of this disorder has been suggested,[1,205] the beneficial effect of antiplatelet agents (aspirin plus dipyridamole, in particular) has been challenged[206]; in some situations, such agents may significantly increase the risk of bleeding. Present evidence favors plasma exchange as the initial therapy of choice in this disorder (see Chap. 117).

PREGNANCY-INDUCED HYPERTENSION
Enhanced platelet activation is a contributing factor in the pathogenesis of pregnancy-induced hypertension, an entity that encompasses a group of disorders previously designated as toxemia of pregnancy, preeclampsia, and eclampsia.[207] Meta-analysis of early, relatively small clinical trials suggested that administration of low-dose aspirin (60–150 mg per day) during the second and third trimesters prevented preeclampsia in high-risk patients with no associated risk to the mother or fetus,[207] but subsequent larger trials failed to confirm these findings.[208] The question of whether properly selected subgroups of patients might benefit from aspirin therapy remains a subject of debate.[209]

OTHER ARTERIAL THROMBOTIC DISORDERS

In myeloproliferative disorders, particularly essential thrombocythemia, aspirin is effective in alleviating symptoms in the subgroup of patients with the syndrome of digital ischemia and spontaneous platelet aggregation (erythromelalgia).[210] Whether antiplatelet agents (aspirin, in particular) are useful in preventing the more widespread thrombotic complications in these disorders is controversial,[210,211] and reservations have been expressed concerning their use, particularly with regard to the increased predilection to hemorrhage[210,212] (see Chap. 118). Antiplatelet therapy has also been used, with varying success, in managing patients with the lupus anticoagulant/"antiphospholid" syndrome, including those complications that occur during pregnancy[213] (see Chap. 128). At present, aspirin is used primarily in combination with heparin during pregnancy, with warfarin used for most other thrombotic indications. Antiplatelet therapy has also been used in a variety of other disorders or clinical situations where platelet-induced thrombi may play a role, such as arteriovenous shunts and fistulas used in renal hemodialysis, vascular catheters, and extracorporeal devices used for cardiopulmonary bypass.[1,2,91,165]

VENOUS THROMBOSIS

Although platelets are more important in initiating arterial than venous thrombi[1,2] (see Chap. 130), the differences in the pathophysiology of these two types of thrombi are not absolute. Early experimental and clinical evidence suggested that antiplatelet drugs (dextran, aspirin, aspirin plus dipyridamole, or sulfinpyrazone) might be useful in the prophylaxis of venous thrombosis,[1,2,41] although the results were not conclusive. The most persuasive evidence for the efficacy of aspirin, administered in doses of 900 to 1300 mg per day, in preventing venographically documented venous thrombosis, has been obtained in patients undergoing hip surgery,[1,93,214] particularly in reducing the risk of proximal vein thrombosis.[93,215] A meta-analysis of 53 trials involving a total of 8400 patients who received an average of 2 weeks of antiplatelet therapy versus control in general orthopedic surgery, and 9 trials involving 600 patients with other conditions that predisposed them to venous thrombosis, was published in 1994.[216] Overall, therapy produced a highly significant ($2P < 0.0001$) reduction in venous thrombosis (25 percent incidence in treatment vs 34 percent in the control group) and an even greater proportional reduction in pulmonary emboli (1.0 percent incidence in treatment vs 2.7 percent in the control group). The validity of recommending antiplatelet therapy as prophylaxis against venous thromboembolism based on this type of analysis has been challenged[217] and defended.[218]

REFERENCES

1. Weiss HJ: *Platelets: Pathophysiology and Antiplatelet Drug Therapy.* Alan R. Liss, New York, 1982.
2. Weiss HJ: Anti-platelet drugs: a new pharmacologic approach to the prevention of thrombosis. *Am Heart J* 92:86, 1976.
3. Weiss HJ, Aledort LM, Kochwa S: The effect of salicylates on the hemostatic properties of platelets in man. *J Clin Invest* 47:2169, 1968.
4. Smith JG, Willis AL: Aspirin selectively inhibits prostaglandin production in human platelets. *Nature* 2341:235, 1971.
5. Hamberg M, Svensson J, Samuelsson B: Thromboxanes: a new group of biologically active compounds derived from prostaglandin endoperoxides. *Proc Natl Acad Sci USA* 72:2994, 1975.
6. FitzGerald GA: Mechanisms of platelet activation: thromboxane A2 as an amplifying signal for other agonists. *Am J Cardiol* 68:11B, 1991.
7. Coller BS: Platelets in cardiovascular thrombosis and thrombolysis, in *The Heart and Cardiovascular System,* 2d ed, edited by Fozzard HA, et al, p 219. Raven Press, Ltd., New York, 1992.
8. Bills TK, Smith JB, Silver MJ: Selective release of arachidonic acid from the phospholipids of human platelets in response to thrombin. *J Clin Invest* 60:1, 1977.
9. Schafer AI: Antiplatelet therapy with glycoprotein IIb/IIIa receptor inhibitors and other novel agents. *Texas Heart Inst J* 24:90, 1997.
10. FitzGerald GA, Patrono C: Antiplatelet drugs, in *Cardiovascular Thrombosis: Thrombocardiology and Thromboneurology* 2nd ed, Edited by Verzzacia M, Fuster V, Topol EJ, p 121, Lippincott-Raven, Philadelphia, 1998.
11. Schrör K: Antiplatelet drugs. A comparative review. *Drugs* 50:7, 1995.
12. Roth GJ, Calverley DC: Aspirin, platelets, and thrombosis: Theory and practice. *Blood* 83:885, 1994.
13. Roth GJ, Siok CJ: Acetylation of the NH2-terminal serine of prostaglandin synthetase by aspirin. *J Biol Chem* 253:3782, 1978.
14. DeWitt DL, Smith WL: Primary structure of prostaglandin G/H synthase

from sheep vesicular gland determined from the complementary DNA sequence. *Proc Natl Acad Sci USA* 85:1412, 1988.

15. Funk C, Funk LB, Kennedy M, et al: Human platelet/erythroleukemia cell PGG/H synthase: cDNA cloning, expression, mutagenesis and gene chromosomal assignment. *FASEB J* 5:2304, 1991.

16. Schrör K: Aspirin and platelets: The antiplatelet action of aspirin and its role in thrombosis treatment and prophylaxis. *Semin Thromb Hemost* 23:349, 1997.

17. Shimokawa T, Kulmacz RJ, DeWitt DL, Smith WL: Tyrosine 385 of prostaglandin endoperoxide synthase is required for cyclooxygenase catalysis. *J Biol Chem* 265:20073, 1990.

18. Shimokawa T, Smith WL: Prostaglandin endoperoxide synthase: The aspirin acetylation region. *J Biol Chem* 267:12387, 1992.

19. Vane JR, Anggard EE, Botting RM: Regulatory functions of the vascular endothelium. *N Eng J Med* 323:27, 1990.

20. Jaffe EA, Weksler BB: Recovery of endothelial cell prostacyclin production after inhibition by low doses of aspirin. *J Clin Invest* 63:543, 1979.

21. FitzGerald GA, Oates JA, Hawiger J, et al: Endogenous biosynthesis of prostacyclin and thromboxane and platelet function during chronic administration of aspirin in man. *J Clin Invest* 71:676, 1983.

22. Kyrle PA, Eichler HG, Jager U, Lechner K: Inhibition of prostaglandin and thromboxane A_2 generation by low-dose aspirin at the site of plug formation in man *in vivo*. *Circulation* 75:1025, 1987.

23. Clarke RJ, Mayo G, Price P, FitzGerald GA: Suppression of thromboxane A_2 but not of systemic prostacyclin by controlled-release aspirin. *N Engl J Med* 325:1137, 1991.

24. Kallman R, Nieuwenhuis HK, de Groot PG, et al: Effects of low doses of aspirin, 10 mg and 30 mg daily, on bleeding time, thromboxane production and 6-keto-PGF1a excretion in healthy subjects. *Thromb Res* 45:355, 1987.

25. Patrono C, Ciabattoni G, Pinca E, et al: Low dose aspirin and inhibition of thromboxane B_2 production in healthy subjects. *Thromb Res* 17:317, 1980.

26. Patrignani P, Filabozzi P, Patrono C: Selective cumulative inhibition of platelet thromboxane production by low-dose aspirin in healthy subjects. *J Clin Invest* 69:1366, 1982.

27. De Caterina R, Boem A, Gazzetti P, et al: Long-term maintenance of thromboxane inhibition by two different aspirin regimens in patients with unstable angina. *Thromb Res* 60:169, 1990.

28. Reilly IAG, FitzGerald GA: Inhibition of thromboxane formation in vivo and ex vivo: implications for therapy with platelet inhibitory drugs. *Blood* 69:180, 1987.

29. Tohgi H, Konno S, Tamura K, et al: The effects of low-to-high doses of aspirin on platelet aggregability and metabolites of thromboxane A_2 and prostacyclin. *Stroke* 23:1400, 1992.

30. Patrono C: Aspirin as an antiplatelet drug. *N Engl J Med* 330:1287, 1994.

31. Valles J, Santos MT, Aznar J, et al: Erythrocyte promotion of platelet reactivity decreases the effectiveness of aspirin as an antithrombotic therapeutic modality. *Circulation* 97:350, 1998.

32. O'Brien JR, Finch W, Clark E: A comparison of an effect of different anti-inflammatory drugs on human platelets. *J Clin Pathol* 23:522, 1970.

33. Patrono C, Ciabattoni G, Patrignani P, et al: Clinical pharmacology of platelet cyclooxygenase inhibition. *Circulation* 72:1177, 1985.

34. Stein B, Fuster V, Israel D, et al: Platelet inhibitor agents in cardiovascular disease: an update. *J Am Coll Cardiol* 14:813, 1989.

35. Joseph JE, Machin SJ: New antiplatelet drugs. *Blood Reviews* 11:178, 1997.

36. Tyler HM, Saxton CAPD, Parry MJ: Administration to man of UK-37,248-01, a selective inhibitor of thromboxane synthetase. *Lancet* 1:629, 1981.

37. FitzGerald GA, Reilly IAG, Pedersen AK: The biochemical pharmacology of thromboxane synthase inhibition in man. *Circulation* 72:1194, 1985.

38. Jang I-K, Fuster V, Gold HK: Antiplatelets. *Coronary Artery Disease* 3:1030, 1992.

39. Grant SM, Goa KL: Iloprost. A review of its pharmacodynamic and pharmacokinetic properties, and therapeutic potential in peripheral vascular disease, myocardial ischaemia and extracorporeal circulation procedures. *Drugs* 43:889, 1992.

40. Emmons PR, Harrison MJG, Jonour AJ, Mitchell JRA: Effect of pyrimidopyrimidine derivative on thrombus formation, platelet adhesiveness and blood pressure in rabbits and rats. *Nature* 218:1972, 1968.

41. Weiss HJ: Antiplatelet therapy. *N Eng J Med* 298:1344 and 1403, 1978.

42. Sullivan JM, Harken DE, Gorlin R: Pharmacologic control of thromboembolic complications of cardiac-valve replacement. *N Engl J Med* 284:1391, 1971.

43. FitzGerald GA: Dipyridamole. *N Engl J Med* 316:1247, 1987.

44. Defreyn G, Bernat A, Delebasse D, Maffrand J-P: Pharmacology of ticlopidine: A review. *Semin Thromb Hemost* 15:159, 1989.

45. DiMinno G, Cerbone AM, Mattioli PL, et al: Functionally thrombasthenic state in normal platelets following administration of ticlopidine. *J Clin Invest* 75:328, 1985.

46. Herbert JM, Frehel D, Valle E, et al: Clopidogrel, a novel antiplatelet and antithrombotic agent. *Cardiovasc Drug Rev* 11:180, 1993.

47. Schrör K: The basic pharmacology of ticlopidine and clopidogrel. *Platelets* 4:252, 1993.

48. Mills DCB: ADP receptors on platelets. *Thromb Haemost* 76:835, 1996.

49. Sharis PJ, Cannon CP, Loscalzo J: The antiplatelet effects of ticlopidine and clopidogrel. *Ann Intern Med* 129:394, 1998.

50. Savi P, Combalbert J, Graich C, et al: The antiaggregating activity of clopidogrel is due to a metabolic activation by the hepatic cytochrome P450-1A. *Thromb Haemost* 72:313, 1994.

51. Mills DCB, Puri RN, Hu CJ, et al: Clopidogrel inhibits the binding of ADP analogues to the receptor mediating inhibition of platelet adenylate cyclase. *Atheroscler Thromb* 12:430, 1992.

52. Lips JPM, Sixma JJ, Schiphorst ME: The effect of ticlopidine administration to humans on the binding of adenosine diphosphate to blood platelets. *Thromb Res* 17:19, 1980.

53. Savi P, Heilmann E, Nurden P, et al: Clopidogrel: an antithrombotic drug acting on the ADP-dependent activation pathway of human platelets. *Clin Appl Thrombos/Hemost* 2:35, 1996.

54. Savi P, Laplace MC, Herbert JM: Evidence for the existence of two different ADP-binding sites on rat platelets. *Thromb Res* 76:157, 1994.

55. Savi P, Laplace MC, Maffrand JP, Herbert JM: Binding of (^{3}H)-2-methyl-thioADP to rat platelets—effect of clopidogrel and ticlopidine. *J Pharm Exp Therap* 269:772, 1994.

56. Gachet C, Hechler B, Léon C, et al: Purinergic receptors on blood platelets. *Platelets* 7:261, 1996.

57. Savi P, Bornia J, Salel V, et al: Characterization of P2x1 purinoreceptors on rat platelets: effect of clopidogrel. *Brit J Haemat* 98:880, 1997.

58. Defreyn G, Gachet C, Savi P, et al: Ticlopidine and clopidogrel (SR 25990C) selectively neutralize ADP inhibition of PGE$_1$-activated platelet adenylate cyclase in rats and rabbits. *Thromb Haemost* 65:186, 1991.

59. Gachet C, Hechler B, Léon C, et al: Activation of ADP receptors and platelet function. *Thromb Haemost* 78:271, 1997.

60. CAPRIE Steering Committee: A randomised, blinded trial of clopidogrel versus aspirin in patients at risk of ischaemic events (CAPRIE). *Lancet* 348:1329, 1996.

61. Yeh S-P, Hsueh E-J, Wu H, Wang Y-C: Ticlopidine-associated aplastic anemia. *Ann Hematol* 76:87, 1998.

62. Bennett CL, Weinberg PD, Rozenberg-Ben-Dror K, et al: Thrombotic thrombocytopenic purpura associated with ticlopidine. A review of 60 cases. *Ann Intern Med* 128:541, 1998.

63. Coller BS, Peerschke EI, Sacudder LE, Sullivan CA: A murine monoclonal antibody that completely blocks the binding of fibrinogen to platelets produces a thrombasthenic-like state in normal platelets and binds to glycoproteins IIb and/or IIIA. *J Clin Invest* 72:325, 1983.

64. Knight DM, Wagner C, Jordan R, et al: The immunogenicity of the 7E3 murine monoclonal Fab antibody fragment variable region is dramatically reduced in humans by substitution of human for murine constant regions. *Mol Immunol* 32:1271, 1995.

65. Coller BS: Platelet GPIIb/IIIa antagonists: the first anti-integrin receptor therapeutics. *J Clin Invest* 99:1467, 1997.

66. Felding-Habermann B, Cheresh DA: Vitronectin and its receptors. *Curr Opin Cell Biol* 5:864, 1993.

67. Reverter JC, Bguin S, Kessels H, et al: Inhibition of platelet-mediated, tissue factor-induced thrombin generation by the mouse/human chimeric 7E3 antibody. Potential implications for the effect of c7E3 Fab treatment on acute thrombosis and ''clinical restenosis.'' *J Clin Invest* 98:863, 1996.

68. Weiss HJ, Lages B: Platelet prothrombinase activity and intracellular calcium responses in patients with glycoprotein IIb-IIIa deficiency, granule defects, or impaired platelet coagulant activity—a comparison with Scott Syndrome. *Blood* 89:1599, 1997.

69. Chronos N, Vahanian A, Betriu A, et al: Use of abciximab in interventional cardiology. *Am Heart J* 135:S67, 1998.

70. Ferguson JJ, Kereiakes DJ, Adgey AAJ, et al: Safe use of platelet GPIIb/IIIa inhibitors. *Am Heart J* 135:S77, 1998.

71. Phillips DR, Scarborough RM: Clinical pharmacology of eptifibatide. *Am J Cardiol* 80:11B, 1997.

72. Lefkovits J, Plow EF, Topol EJ: Platelet glycoprotein IIb/IIIa receptors as an antithrombotic strategy. *N Engl J Med* 332:1553, 1995.

73. Perlinck K, DeLuperleire I, Goldberg M, et al: MK-383 (L-700,462), a selective non-peptide platelet glycoprotein IIb/IIIa antagonist, is active in man. *Circulation* 88:1512, 1993.

74. Kouns WC, Kirchhofer D, Hadvary P, et al: Reversible conformational changes induced in glycoprotein IIb/IIIa by a potent and selective peptidomimetic inhibitor. *Blood* 80:2539, 1992.

75. Szalony JA, Haas NF, Salyers AK, et al: Extended inhibition of platelet aggregation with the orally active platelet inhibitor SC-54684A. *Circulation* 91:411, 1995.

76. Weller T, Alig L, Beresini M, et al: Orally active fibrinogen receptor antagonists: 2. Amidoximes as prodrugs of amidines. *J Med Chem* 39:3139, 1996.

77. Braunwald E, Maseri A, Armstrong PW, et al: Rationale and clinical evidence for the use of GP IIb/IIIa inhibitors in acute coronary syndromes. *Am Heart J* 135:S56, 1998.

78. Van de Werf F: Clinical trials with glycoprotein IIb/IIIa receptor antagonists in acute coronary syndromes. *Thromb Haemost* 78:210, 1997.

79. Ali M, McDonald JWD: Effects of sulfinpyrazone on platelet prostaglandin synthesis and platelet release of serotonin. *J Lab Clin Med* 89:868, 1977.

80. Von Schacky C, Weber PC: Metabolism and effects on platelet function of the purified eicosapentaenoic and docosahexaenoic acids in humans. *J Clin Invest* 76:2446, 1989.

81. Loscalzo J: Antiplatelet and antithrombotic effects of organic nitrates. *Am J Card* 70:18B, 1992.

82. Salvemini D, Currie MG, Mollace V: Nitric oxide–mediated cyclooxygenase activation—a key event in the antiplatelet effects of nitrovasodilators. *J Clin Invest* 97:2562, 1996.

83. Pannocchia A, Praloran N, Arduino C, et al: Absence of (-) [3H]desmethoxyverapamil binding sites on human platelets and lack of evidence for voltage-dependent calcium channels. *Eur J Pharmacol* 142:83, 1987.

84. Pales J, Palacios-Araus L, Lopez A, Gual A: Effects of dihydropyridines and inorganic calcium blockers on aggregation and on intracellular free calcium in platelets. *Biochim Biophys Acta* 1064:169, 1991.

85. Schachter M: Do calcium antagonists affect platelets? *Eur Heart J* (Suppl K):75, 1987.

86. Lacoste LL, Lam JYT, Hung J, Waters D: Oral verapamil inhibits platelet thrombus formation in humans. *Circulation* 89:630, 1994.

87. Frishman WH, Weksler B, Christodoulo JB, et al: Reversal of abnormal platelet aggregability and change in exercise tolerance in patients with angina pectoris. *Circulation* 50:887, 1974.

88. Kutti J, Vilén L: Beta-blockers as anti-platelet drugs. *Acta Med Scand* 213:1, 1985.

89. Pamphilon DH, Boon RJ, Prentice AG, Rozkovec A: Lack of significant effect of therapeutic propranolol on measurable platelet function in healthy subjects. *J Clin Pathol* 42:793, 1989.

90. Winther K, Knudsen JB, Jorgensen EO, Eldrup E: Differential effects of timolol and metoprolol on platelet function at rest and during exercise. *Eur J Clin Pharmacol* 33:587, 1988.

91. Harker LA: Antiplatelet drugs in the management of patients with thrombotic disorders. *Sem Thromb Hemost* 12:134, 1986.

92. Webster MWI, Chesebro JH, Fuster V: Platelet inhibitor therapy. Agents and clinical implications. *Hematol/Oncol Clin North Am* 4:265, 1990.

93. Hirsh J, Dalen JE, Fuster V, et al: Aspirin and other platelet active drugs: the relationship between dose, effectiveness, and side effects. *Chest* 102:327S, 1992.

94. Fuster V, Badimon L, Badimon JJ, Chesebro JH: The pathogenesis of coronary artery disease and the acute coronary syndromes. *N Engl J Med* 326:242, 1992.

95. Hirsh PD, Hillis LD, Campbell WB, et al: Release of prostaglandins and thromboxane into the coronary circulation in patients with ischemic heart disease. *N Engl J Med* 304:685, 1981.

96. Lewy RI, Wiener L, Walinsky P, et al: Thromboxane release during

97. Verheugt FWA, Serruys PW, Van Vliet H, et al: Intracoronary platelet release in patients with and without coronary artery disease. *Thromb Haemost* 49:28, 1983.

98. Nicols AB, Gold KD, Marcella JJ, et al: Effect of pacing-induced myocardial ischemia on platelet activation and fibrin formation in the coronary circulation. *J Am Coll Cardiol* 10:40, 1987.

99. The Steering Committee of the Physicians' Health Study Research Group: Final report on the aspirin component of the ongoing Physicians' Health Study. *N Engl J Med* 321:129, 1989.

100. Ridker PM, Manson JE, Buring JE, et al: The effect of chronic platelet inhibition with low-dose aspirin on atherosclerotic progression and acute thrombosis: clinical evidence from the Physicians' Health Study. *Am Heart J* 122:1288, 1991.

101. Juul-Moller S, Edvardsson N, Jahnmatz B, et al: Double-blind trial of aspirin in primary prevention of myocardial infarction in patients with stable chronic angina pectoris. The Swedish Angina Pectoris Aspirin Trial (SAPAT) group. *Lancet* 340:1421, 1992.

102. Ambrose JA, Winters SL, Stern A, et al: Angiographic morphology and the pathogenesis of unstable angina pectoris. *J Am Coll Cardiol* 5:609, 1985.

103. Mizuno K, Satomura K, Miyamoto A, et al: Angioscopic evaluation of coronary-artery thrombi in acute coronary syndromes. *N Engl J Med* 326:287, 1992.

104. Le Breton H, Plow EF, Topol EJ: Role of platelets in restenosis after percutaneous coronary revascularization. *J Am Coll Cardiol* 28:1643, 1996.

105. Hamm CW, Lorenz RL, Bleifeld W, et al: Biochemical evidence of platelet activation in patients with unstable angina. *J Am Coll Cardiol* 10:988, 1987.

106. Vejar M, Fragasso G, Hackett D, et al: Dissociation of platelet activation and spontaneous myocardial ischemia in unstable angina. *Thromb Haemost* 63:163, 1990.

107. The RISC Group: Risk of myocardial infarction and death during treatment with low dose aspirin and intravenous heparin in men with unstable coronary artery disease. *Lancet* 336:827, 1990.

108. Lewis HD Jr, Davis JW, Archibald DG, et al: Protective effects of aspirin against acute myocardial infarction and death in men with unstable angina: results of a Veterans Administration cooperative study. *N Engl J Med* 309:396, 1983.

109. Théroux P, Ouimet H, McCans J, et al: Aspirin, heparin, or both to treat acute unstable angina. *N Engl J Med* 319:1105, 1988.

110. Cairns JA, Gent M, Singer J, et al: Aspirin, sulfinpyrazone, or both in unstable angina: results of a Canadian multicenter trial. *N Engl J Med* 313:1369, 1985.

111. Wallentin LC and the Research Group on Instability in Coronary Artery Disease in Southeast Sweden: Aspirin (75 mg/day) after an episode of unstable coronary artery disease: Long-term effects on the risk for myocardial infarction, occurrence of severe angina and the need for revascularization. *J Am Coll Cardiol* 18:1587, 1993.

112. Oler A, Whooley MA, Oler J, Grady D: Adding heparin to aspirin reduces the incidence of myocardial infarction and death in patients with unstable angina: a meta-analysis. *JAMA* 276:811, 1996.

113. Cipollone F, Patrignani P, Greco A, et al: Differential suppression of thromboxane biosynthesis by indobufen and aspirin in patients with unstable angina. *Circulation* 96:1109, 1997.

114. Barnathan ES, Schwartz JS, Taylor L, et al: Aspirin and dipyridamole in the prevention of acute coronary thrombosis complicating coronary angioplasty. *Circulation* 76:125, 1987.

115. Lembo NJ, Black AJ, Roubin GS, et al: Does the addition of dipyridamole to aspirin decrease acute coronary angioplasty complications? The results of a prosepctive randomized clinical trial (abstr). *J Am Coll Cardiol* 13(Suppl A):237A, 1988.

116. Balsano F, Rizzon P, Violi F, et al: Antiplatelet treatment with ticlopidine in unstable angina: a controlled multicenter clinical trial. *Circulation* 82:17, 1990.

117. Leon MB, Baim DS, Popma JJ, et al for the Stent Anticoagulation Restenosis Study Investigators: A clinical trial comparing three antithrombotic-drug regimens after coronary-artery stenting. *N Engl J Med* 339:1665, 1998.

118. Frishman WH, Burns B, Atac B, et al: Novel antiplatelet therapies for

pacing-induced angina: possible vaso-constrictor influence on the coronary vasculature. *Circulation* 61:1165, 1980.

treatment of patients with ischemic heart disease: Inhibitors of the platelet glycoprotein IIb/IIIa integrin receptor. *Am Heart J* 130:877, 1995.

119. Adgey AAJ: An overview of the results of clinical trials with glycoprotein IIb/IIIa inhibitors. *Am Heart J* 135:S43, 1998.

120. Tcheng JE: Platelet glycoprotein IIb/IIIa integrin blockade: recent clinical trials in interventional cardiology. *Thromb Haemost* 78:205, 1997.

121. The EPIC Investigators: Use of a monoclonal antibody directed against the platelet glycoprotein IIb/IIIa receptor in high-risk coronary angioplasty. *N Engl J Med* 330:956, 1994.

122. Topol EJ, Califf RM, Weisman HF, et al on behalf of the EPIC Investigators: Randomized trial of coronary intervention with antibody against IIb/IIIa integrin for reduction of clinical restenosis: results at six months. *Lancet* 343:881, 1994.

123. Topol EJ, Ferguson JJ, Weisman HF, et al: Long-term protection from myocardial ischemic events in a randomized trial of brief integrin β_3 blockade with percutaneous coronary intervention. *JAMA* 278:479, 1997.

124. The EPILOG Investigators: Platelet glycoprotein IIb/IIIa receptor blockade and low-dose heparin during percutaneous coronary revascularization. *N Engl J Med* 336:1689, 1997.

125. The CAPTURE Investigators: Randomized placebo-controlled trial of abciximab before and during coronary intervention in refractory unstable angina: the CAPTURE study. *Lancet* 349:1429, 1997.

126. Brener SJ, Barr LA, Burchenal JE, et al: Randomized, placebo-controlled trial of platelet glycoprotein IIb/IIIa blockade with primary angioplasty for acute myocardial infarction. ReoPro and Primary PTCA Organization and Randomized Trial (RAPPORT) Investigators. *Circulation* 98:734, 1998.

127. The EPISTENT Investigators: Randomised placebo-controlled and balloon-angioplasty-controlled trial to assess safety of coronary stenting with use of platelet glycoprotein-IIb/IIIa blockade. *Lancet* 352:87, 1998.

128. The IMPACT II Investigators: Randomized placebo-controlled trial of effect of eptifibatide on complications of percutaneous coronary intervention. *Lancet* 349:1422, 1997.

129. The PURSUIT Trial Investigators: Inhibition of platelet glycoprotein IIb/IIIa with eptifibatide in patients with acute coronary syndromes. *N Engl J Med* 339:436, 1998.

130. The RESTORE Study Group: Effects of platelet glycoprotein IIb/IIIa blockade with tirofiban on adverse cardiac events in patients with unstable angina or acute myocardial infarction undergoing coronary angioplasty. *Circulation* 96:1445, 1997.

131. The Platelet Receptor Inhibition in Ischemic Syndrome Management (PRISM) Study Investigators: A comparison of aspirin plus tirofiban with aspirin plus heparin for unstable angina. *N Engl J Med* 338:1498, 1998.

132. The Platelet Receptor Inhibition in Ischemic Syndrome Management in Patients Limited by Unstable Signs and Symptoms (PRISM-PLUS) Study Investigators: Inhibition of the platelet glycoprotein IIb/IIIa receptor with tirofiban in unstable angina and non-Q wave myocardial infarction. *N Engl J Med* 338:1488, 1998.

133. The PARAGON Investigators: An international, randomized, controlled trial of lamifiban, a platelet glycoprotein IIb/IIIa inhibitor, heparin or both in unstable angina. *Circulation* 97:2386, 1998.

134. Théroux P, Kouz S, Roy L on behalf of the Canadian Lamifiban Study Investigators: Platelet membrane receptor glycoprotein IIb/IIIa antagonism in unstable angina: The Canadian Lamifiban Study. *Circulation* 94:899, 1996.

135. Kong DF, Califf RB, Miller DP, et al: Clinical outcomes of therapeutic agents that block the platelet glycoprotein IIb/IIIa integrin in ischemic heart disease. *Circulation* 98:2829, 1998.

136. Peterson JG, Lauer MA, Sapp SK, Topol EJ: Heparin use is required for clinical benefit of GIIb/IIIa inhibitor eptifibatide in acute coronary syndromes: Insights from the PURSUIT Trial. Abstracts of the 71st Scientific Session of the American Heart Association. *Circulation* (suppl) 98:I-360, 1998.

137. Cannon CP, McCabe CH, Borzak S, et al for the TIMI 12 Investigators: Randomized trial of an oral platelet glycoprotein IIb/IIIa antagonist, sibrafiban, in patients after an acute coronary syndrome—results of the TIMI 12 trial. *Circulation* 97:340, 1998.

138. Simpfendorfer C, Kottke-Marchant K, Lowrie M, et al: First chronic platelet glycoprotein IIb/IIIa integrin blockade. A randomized, placebo-controlled pilot study of xemilofiban in unstable angina with percutaneous coronary interventions. *Circulation* 96:76, 1997.

139. ISIS-2 (Second International Study of Infarct Survival) Collaborative Group: Randomized trial of intravenous streptokinase, oral aspirin, both, or neither among 17,187 cases of suspected acute myocardial infarction: ISIS-2. *Lancet* 2:349, 1988.

140. ISIS-3 Collaborative Group: ISIS-3: a randomized comparison of streptokinase vs tissue plasminogen activator vs anistreplase and of aspirin plus heparin vs aspirin alone among 41,299 cases of suspected acute myocardial infarction. *Lancet* 339:753, 1992.

141. Antiplatelet Trialists' Collaboration: Collaborative overview of randomised trials of antiplatelet therapy: I. Prevention of death, myocardial infarction, and stroke by prolonged antiplatelet therapy in various categories of patients. *BMJ* 308:81, 1994.

142. Coller BS: Platelets and thrombolytic therapy. *N Engl J Med* 322:33, 1990.

143. Roux S, Christeller S, Lüdin E: Effects of aspirin on coronary reocclusion and recurrent ischemia after thrombolysis: a meta-analysis. *J Am Coll Cardiol* 19:671, 1992.

144. Giugliano RP, Antman EM, McCabe CH, et al: Abciximab + tPA improves coronary flow in a wide range of subgroups: results from TIMI 14. Abstracts of the 71st Scientific Session of the American Heart Association. *Circulation* 98(suppl):I560, 1998.

145. Ohman EM, Kleiman NS, Gacioch O, et al for the IMPACT-AMI Investigators: Combined accelerated tissue-plasminogen activator and platelet glycoprotein IIb/IIIa integrin receptor blockade with integrilin in acute myocardial infarction: results of a randomized placebo-controlled, dose-ranging trial. *Circulation* 95:846, 1997.

146. Elwood PC, Cochrane AL, Burr ML, et al: A randomized controlled trial of acetylsalicylic acid and the secondary prevention of mortality from myocardial infarction. *Br Med J* 1:436, 1974.

147. The Coronary Drug Project Research Group: Aspirin in coronary heart disease. *J Chronic Dis* 29:625, 1976.

148. Breddin K, Loew D, Lechner K, et al: The German-Austrian aspirin trial: a comparison of acetylsalicylic acid, placebo and phenprocoumon in secondary prevention of myocardial infarction. *Circulation* 62(Suppl V):63, 1980.

149. Aspirin Myocardial Infarction Study Research Group: A randomized controlled trial of aspirin in persons recovered from myocardial infarction. *JAMA* 243:661, 1980.

150. Elwood PC, Sweetman PM: Aspirin and secondary mortality after myocardial infarction. *Lancet* 12:1313, 1979.

151. The Persantine-Aspirin Reinfarction Study Research Group: Persantine and aspirin in coronary heart disease. *Circulation* 62:449, 1980.

152. Klimt CR, Knatterud GL, Stamler J, Meier P: Persantine-aspirin reinfarction study: II. Secondary coronary prevention with persantine and aspirin. *J Am Coll Cardiol* 7:251, 1986.

153. Canner PL: Aspirin in coronary heart disease. Comparison of six clinical trials. *Isr J Med Sci* 19:413, 1983.

154. Cairns JA, Hirsh J, Lewis HD Jr, et al: Antithrombotic agents in coronary artery disease. *Chest* 102:456S, 1992.

155. Peto R: Aspirin after myocardial infarction [editorial]. *Lancet* 1:1172, 1980.

156. Antiplatelet Trialists' Collaboration: Secondary prevention of vascular disease by prolonged antiplatelet treatment. *BMJ* 296:320, 1988.

157. Hankey GJ: Clopidogrel: a new safe and effective antiplatelet agent. But unanswered questions remain. *Med J Aust* 167:120, 1997.

158. Craven LL: Experiences with aspirin (acetylsalicylic acid) in the nonspecific prophylaxis of coronary thrombosis. *Miss Valley Med J* 75:38, 1953.

159. Boston Collaborative Drug Surveillance Group: Regular aspirin intake and acute myocardial infarction. *Br Med J* 5:269, 1975.

160. Peto R, Gray R, Collins R, et al: Randomized trial of prophylactic daily aspirin in British male doctors. *BMJ* 296:313, 1988.

161. Manson JE, Stampfer MJ, Colditz GA, et al: A prospective study of aspirin use and primary prevention of cardiovascular disease in women. *JAMA* 266:521, 1991.

162. Fuster V, Cohen M, Halperin J: Aspirin in the prevention of coronary disease. *N Engl J Med* 321:129, 1989.

163. Stein PD, Dalen JE, Goldman S, et al: Antithrombotic therapy in patients with saphenous vein and internal mammary artery bypass grafts following percutaneous transluminal coronary angioplasty. *Chest* 102:508S, 1992.

164. Goldman S, Copeland J, Moritz T, et al: Saphenous vein graft patency 1 year after coronary artery bypass surgery and effects of antiplatelet

therapy: results of a Veterans Administration cooperative study. *Circulation* 80:1190, 1989.

165. Limet R, David JL, Magotteaux P, et al: Prevention of aorta-coronary bypass graft occlusion. *J Thorac Cardiovasc Surg* 94:773, 1987.

166. Antiplatelet Trialists' Collaboration: Collaborative overview of randomised trials of antiplatelet therapy: I. Maintenance of vascular graft or arterial patency by antiplatelet therapy. *BMJ* 308:159, 1994.

167. Goldman S, Copeland JG, Moritz T, et al: Saphenous vein graft patency 1 year after coronary artery bypass surgery and effects of antiplatelet therapy: results of a Veterans Administration cooperative study. *Circulation* 80:1190, 1989.

168. Israel DH, Adams PC, Stein B, et al: Antithrombotic therapy in the coronary vein graft patient. *Clin Cardiol* 14:283, 1991.

169. Goldman S, Copeland J, Moritz T, et al: Starting aspirin therapy after operation: effects on early graft patency. *Circulation* 84:520, 1991.

170. Stein PD, Alpert JS, Copeland J, et al: Antithrombotic therapy in patients with mechanical and biological prosthetic heart valves. *Chest* 102:445S, 1992.

171. Loewen P, Sunderii R, Gin K: The efficacy and safety of combination warfarin and ASA therapy: a systemic review of the literature and update of guidelines. *Canad J Cardiol* 14:717, 1998.

172. Levine HJ, Pauker SG, Salzman EW, Eckman MH: Antithrombotic therapy in valvular heart disease. *Chest* 102:434S, 1992.

173. The Atrial Fibrillation Investigators: The efficacy of aspirin in patients with atrial fibrillation. Analysis of pooled data from 3 randomized trials. *Arch Int Med* 157:1237, 1997.

174. Alberg GW, Atwood JE, Hirsh J, et al: Stroke prevention in nonvalvular atrial fibrillation. *Ann Int Med* 115:727, 1991.

175. Lip GY, Lowe GD: Warfarin and aspirin as thromboprophylaxis in atrial fibrillation. *Brit J Clin Pharm* 41:369, 1996.

176. Anonymous: Adjusted-dose warfarin versus low-intensity, fixed-dose aspirin for high-risk patients with atrial fibrillation: Stroke prevention in atrial fibrillation III randomised clinical trial. *Lancet* 348:633, 1996.

177. Millikan CH, Siekert RG, Schick RM: Studies in cerebrovascular disease: the use of anticoagulant drugs in the treatment of intermittent insufficiency of the internal carotid arterial system. *Proc Staff Meet Mayo Clin* 30:578, 1955.

178. Fisher CM: Observations on the fundus oculi in transient monocular blindness. *Neurology* 9:33, 1959.

179. McBrien DJ, Bradley RD, Ashton N: The nature of retinal emboli in stenosis of the internal carotid artery. *Lancet* 1:697, 1963.

180. Sherman DG, Dyken ML, Fisher M, et al: Antithrombotic therapy for cerebrovascular disorders. *Chest* 102: 529S, 1992.

181. Rothrock JF, Hart RG: Antithrombotic therapy in cerebrovascular disease. *Ann Int Med* 115:885, 1991.

182. Diener HC: Antiplatelet drugs in secondary prevention of stroke. *Int J Clin Pract* 52:91, 1998.

183. Barnett HJM, Eliasziw M, Meldrum HE: Drugs and surgery in the prevention of ischemic stroke. *N Engl J Med* 332:238, 1995.

184. Diener HC, Cunha L, Forbes C, et al: European Stroke Prevention Study 2: dipyridamole and acetylsalicylic acid in the secondary prevention of stroke. *J Neurol Sci* 143:1, 1996.

185. Hass WK, Easton JD, Adams HP, et al for the Ticlopidine Aspirin Study Group: A randomised trial comparing ticlopidine hydrochloride with aspirin for the prevention of stroke in high risk patients. *N Engl J Med* 321:501, 1989.

186. Harbison JW: Ticlopidine versus aspirin for the prevention of recurrent stroke. Analysis of patients with minor stroke from the Ticlopidine Aspirin Stroke Study. *Stroke* 23:1723, 1992.

187. Gent M, Blakeley JA, Easton JD, and the CATS Group: The Canadian-American ticlopidine study (CATS) in thromboembolic stroke. *Lancet* 1:1215, 1989.

188. Hershey LA: Stroke prevention in women: role of aspirin versus ticlopidine. *Am J Med* 91:288, 1991.

189. Sivenius J, Laakso M, Penttilä IM, et al: The Europoean stroke prevention study: results according to sex. *Neurology* 41:1189, 1991.

190. The SALT Collaborative Group: Swedish aspirin low-dose trial (SALT) of 75 mg aspirin as secondary prophylaxis after cerebrovascular ischaemic events. *Lancet* 338:1345, 1991.

191. The Dutch TIA Trial Study Group: A comparison of two doses of aspirin (30 mg vs 283 mg a day) in patients after a transient ischemic attack or minor ischemic stroke. *N Engl J Med* 325:1261, 1991.

192. UK-TIA Study Group: The United Kingdom transient ischaemic attack (UK-TIA) aspirin trial: Final results. *J Neurol Neurosurg Psych* 54:1044, 1991.

193. Barnett HJM, Kaste M, Meldrum H, Eliasziw M: Aspirin dose in stroke prevention. Beautiful hypotheses slain by ugly facts. *Stroke* 27:588, 1996.

194. Bornstein NM, Karepov VG, Aronovich BD, et al: Failure of aspirin treatment after stroke. *Stroke* 24:1452, 1993.

195. Helgason CM, Bolin KM, Hoff JA, et al: Development of aspirin resistance in persons with previous ischemic stroke. *Stroke* 25:2331, 1994.

196. Patrono C, Roth GJ: Aspirin in ischemic cerebrovascular disease. How strong is the case for a different dosing regimen? *Stroke* 27:756, 1996.

197. CAST: randomized placebo-controlled trial of early aspirin use in 20,000 patients with acute ischaemic stroke. CAST (Chinese Acute Stroke Trial) Collaborative Group. *Lancet* 349:1641, 1997.

198. The International Stroke Trial (IST): A randomised trial of aspirin, subcutaneous heparin, both or neither among 19,436 patients with acute presumed ischaemic stroke. International Stroke Trial Collaborative Group. *Lancet* 349:1569, 1997.

199. Clagett GP, Graor RA, Salzman EW: Antithrombotic therapy in peripheral arterial occlusive disease. *Chest* 102:516S, 1992.

200. Goldhaber SZ, Manson JE, Stampfer MJ, et al: Low-dose aspirin and subsequent peripheral arterial surgery in the Physicians' Health Study. *Lancet* 340:143, 1992.

201. Virgoline I, Fitscha P, Weiss K, et al: Intravenous prostacyclin (PGI$_2$) infusion to 108 patients with ischaemic peripheral vascular disease: phase II-open study. *Prostaglandins* 42:9, 1991.

202. Antiplatelet Trialists Collaboration: Collaborative overview of randomised trials of antiplatelet therapy: II. Maintenance of vascular graft on arterial patency by antiplatelet therapy. *BMJ* 308:159, 1994.

203. Becquemin J-P: Effect of ticlopidine on the long-term patency of saphenous-venous bypass grafts in the legs. *N Engl J Med* 337:1726, 1997.

204. Zoja C, Remuzzi G: Role of platelets in progressive glomerular diseases. *Pediatric Nephrology* 9:495, 1995.

205. Ruggenenti P, Remuzzi G: Thrombotic thrombocytopenic purpura and related disorders. *Hemat/Onc Clinics N Amer* 4:219, 1990.

206. Rosove MH, Ho WG, Goldfinger D: Ineffectiveness of aspirin and dipyridamole in the treatment of thrombotic thrombocytopenic purpura. *Ann Intern Med* 96:27, 1982.

207. Imperiale TF, Petrulis AS: A meta-analysis of low-dose aspirin for the prevention of pregnancy-induced hypertensive disease. *JAMA* 266:260, 1991.

208. Cartis S, Sibai B, Hauth J, et al: Low-dose aspirin to prevent preeclampsia in women at high risk. *N Engl J Med* 338:701, 1998.

209. Barth W: Low-dose aspirin for preeclampsia—the unresolved question. *N Engl J Med* 338:756, 1998.

210. Metus AJ, Schafer AI: Thrombocytosis and thrombocythemia. *Hemat/Onc Clinics N Amer* 4:157, 1990.

211. Ravandi-Kashani F, Schafer AI: Microvascular disturbances, thrombosis, and bleeding in thrombocytopenia: current concepts and perspectives. *Sem Thromb Hemost* 23:479, 1997.

212. Tartaglia AP, Goldberg JD, Berk PD, Wasserman LR: Adverse effects of antiaggregating platelet therapy in the treatment of polycythemia vera. *Sem Hematol* 23:172, 1986.

213. Ginsberg JS, Hirsh J: Use of antithrombotic agents during pregnancy. *Chest* 102:385S, 1992

214. Clagett GP, Anderson FA, Levine MN, et al: Prevention of venous thromboembolism. *Chest* 102:391S, 1992.

215. Powers PJ, Gent M, Jay R, et al: A randomized trial of less intense postoperative warfarin or aspirin therapy in the prevention of venous thromboembolism after surgery for fractured hip. *Arch Int Med* 149:771, 1989.

216. Antiplatelet Trialists' Collaboration: Collaborative overview of randomised trials of antiplate therapy: III. Reduction in venous thrombosis and pulmonary embolism by antiplatelet prophylaxis among surgical and medical patients. *BMJ* 308:235, 1994.

217. Cohen AT, Skinner JA, Kakkar VV: Antiplatelet treatment for thromboprophylaxis: a step forward or backwards? *BMJ* 309:1213, 1994.

218. Collins R, Baigent C, Sandercock P, Peco R for the Antiplatelet Trialists' Collaboration: Antiplatelet therapy for thromboprophylaxis: the need for careful consideration of the evidence from randomised trials. *BMJ* 309:1215, 1994.

ORAL ANTICOAGULATION

SAM SCHULMAN

The original and principal oral anticoagulants—the vitamin K antagonists—have well-known chemistry and pharmacokinetics. The standardized calibration system for monitoring treatment with vitamin K antagonists, the international normalized ratio (INR), is widely accepted. Its use increases the reliability of comparisons of treatment intensity between laboratories and improves interpretation of results obtained in clinical trials. Portable instruments for measurement of the prothrombin time permit self-management in selected cases. Computerized decision support of drug dosing contributes to improved efficacy and safety. The large number of interactions of vitamin K antagonists with other drugs is a major problem during treatment and is often the cause of bleeding complications. Predictors for hemorrhage have been related to characteristics of the patient and underlying disease as well as treatment and hemostatic variables. The detection of mutations and polymorphisms has provided some explanations for resistance or hypersensitivity to vitamin K antagonists. Among the nonhemorrhagic complications are skin necrosis, purple toe syndrome, allergic dermatologic manifestations, hepatic dysfunction, possibly reduced bone mineral density, and teratogenicity. During the perioperative state, treatment with vitamin K antagonists is managed in various ways, depending on the nature of the surgical procedure and the condition that necessitates anticoagulation. For the main indications of treatment—artificial heart valves, nonvalvular atrial fibrillation, myocardial infarction, and venous thromboembolism—large clinical trials have documented the optimum intensity of treatment. For venous thromboembolism, the duration of treatment should be tailored individually according to characteristics of the thrombotic event and presence of prothrombotic risk factors. Minidose warfarin (1 mg/day) is effective in the prophylaxis against thrombosis in central venous catheters, major gynecologic surgery, and metastatic breast cancer. A number of new oral anticoagulants, such as glycosaminoglycans or direct and selective inhibitors of factor Xa or thrombin, are under development and may prove to be safer than vitamin K antagonists due to fewer interactions with other drugs.

HISTORY

A hemorrhagic disease in cattle caused by moldy sweet clover hay was described in 1922.[1] The absence or delay of blood clotting was correlated to a greatly diminished quantity of prothrombin. Isolation

Acronyms and abbreviations that appear in this chapter include: INR, international normalized ratio; ISI, international sensitivity index; LMWH, low-molecular-weight heparin; P&P, prothrombin and proconvertin; PT, prothrombin time; rTF, recombinant tissue factor; TURP, transurethral resection of the prostate.

and purification of the "hemorrhagic agent" confirmed that the substance was dicumarol, 3,3-methylene-bis-[4-hydroxycoumarin],[2] which was promptly made available for clinical studies. The first experiences of the prophylactic and therapeutic effects of the drug in deep vein thrombosis, as well as its hemorrhagic complications, were published in 1942.[3-5] Warfarin, an acronym for the Wisconsin Alumni Research Foundation, in recognition of its synthesis at the University of Wisconsin in 1948, or 3-(1-phenyl-3-oxobutyl)4-hydroxycoumarin, is now the most commonly used coumarin derivative worldwide. The available compounds in different countries are either coumarin derivatives or indanedione derivatives. Some of the substances are also used as rodenticides.

These drugs have traditionally been termed oral anticoagulants, but are referred to as vitamin K antagonists in this chapter to highlight their specific effect and to distinguish them from new oral anticoagulants that have other mechanisms of action.

VITAMIN K ANTAGONISTS

CHEMISTRY AND MODE OF ACTION

The coumarin derivatives have in common a 4-hydroxy–coumarin nucleus with a substituent in the 3 position (Fig. 132-1). All the 4-hydroxy–coumarin compounds have an asymmetric carbon atom, and the clinically available warfarin preparations consist of a racemic mixture of the S and R enantiomers. (S)-warfarin is four to five times more potent than (R)-warfarin as an anticoagulant and is more susceptible to interactions with other drugs.[6] The formulation of warfarin for oral administration is in a crystalline form. However, amorphous warfarin sodium, which was temporarily produced, did not turn out to be bioequivalent,[7] and this may also be the case for some of the generic warfarin formulations.[8]

The vitamin K–dependent coagulation factors II, VII, IX, and X undergo posttranslational γ-carboxylation of approximately 10 glutamic acid residues in the N-terminal Gla domain[9-11] (see Chap. 112). This modification is required for the ability of the coagulation factors to bind calcium and to localize the enzymatic processes in which they participate to a phospholipid surface, such as activated platelet membranes. A reduction of the γ-carboxylated sites by 1 to 6 residues will progressively impair the coagulation activity from 70 percent of normal to no activity at all. With therapeutic doses of warfarin, approximately 3 of 10 glutamic acid residues in prothrombin are not carboxylated.[12-14]

Simultaneously with γ-carboxylation, vitamin KH_2 is converted to vitamin K epoxide, which is converted back to KH_2 by the sequential actions of vitamin K epoxide reductase and vitamin K reductase. These two enzymes are inhibited by the coumarin derivatives, thereby precluding further γ-carboxylation.[15,16] The coagulation inhibitors protein C and protein S, as well as osteocalcin, also undergo posttranslational γ-carboxylation, and vitamin K antagonists cause the synthesis of their hypo- and acarboxylated forms. Some of the drug-related adverse effects can be explained by the reduced activity of these proteins (see "Skin Necrosis" and "Teratogenicity" under "Complications of Therapy").

PHARMACOKINETICS

Warfarin is highly water soluble and is absorbed rapidly and completely from the stomach and upper gastrointestinal tract, reaching peak concentrations in plasma 60 to 90 min after oral ingestion. Impaired absorption has been described in a case with resistance to warfarin and dicumarol but not to an indanedione derivative.[17] In the circulation, 98 to 99 percent of warfarin is bound to proteins, primarily to albumin, and therefore only a small fraction of the drug is biologically active.

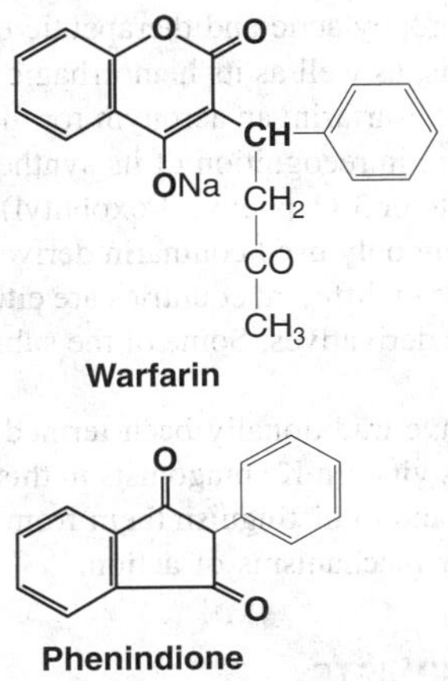

Warfarin

Phenindione

FIGURE 132-1 Structure of warfarin sodium and phenindione. Common structures for coumarin and indanedione derivatives appear in boldface.

The binding to albumin occurs at site I, which is shared with phenylbutazone and azapropazone.[18] Displacement of warfarin from albumin increases its anticoagulant activity, but at the same time the rate of elimination of the drug increases. Warfarin accumulates rapidly in the liver, mainly in the microsomes.[19]

Metabolism of warfarin is different for the two enantiomers. The biologically more potent (S)-warfarin is hydroxylated by cytochrome P_{450} 2C9 (CYP2C9) to 7-hydroxywarfarin. Mutations in the CYP2C9 gene result in three allelic variants, and a patient with very high sensitivity to warfarin was demonstrated to be homozygous for CYP2C9*3.[20] (R)-warfarin is metabolized by CYP1A2 to 6- and 8-hydroxywarfarin. The hydroxycoumarins are excreted by the kidneys. The elimination half-life of warfarin is 35 to 45 h, and the pharmacokinetics appear to be dose dependent.[21] Warfarin may also be administered intravenously, and inadvertent percutaneous absorption of a warfarin-type rat poison has been reported to cause bleeding complications.[22]

The other vitamin K antagonists have similar pharmacokinetic characteristics, except for differences in elimination.[23] Dicumarol has a lower degree of absorption from the gastrointestinal tract, and up to 36 percent of the drug can be retrieved inert in the stool.[24]

DOSING

The variability in warfarin dose requirements to achieve a given extent of anticoagulation is wide, ranging from about 1 to 20 mg/day. This may be due to differences in clearance of the drug by the liver and in target-organ sensitivity. There is a significant negative correlation between age at start of therapy and dosage, with a reduction of requirements of approximately 20 percent over a 15-year period.[25] The explanation for this finding is at least partly the decline in hepatic mass with age.[26] In children, there is an even more pronounced reduction of warfarin requirements with age, with mean doses of 0.32 and 0.09 mg/kg/day in those under 1 year of age and 11 to 18 years of age, respectively.[27] A number of algorithms and nomograms have been constructed to aid the physician in predicting the maintenance dose. They are usually based on the level of anticoagulation achieved after 2 to 4 days on a repeated loading dose.[28,29]

RESISTANCE

In rare cases, exceptionally high doses are required to achieve anticoagulation. The first hereditary form of resistance to coumarin, as well as to phenindione, with an autosomal dominant pattern was described

in 1964.[30] Mechanisms of warfarin resistance include impaired absorption,[17] high clearance of (S)-warfarin,[31] or decreased affinity of warfarin for the receptor,[32] presumably associated with a decreased sensitivity of epoxide reductase.[33] However, poor compliance, interactions with food or drugs, laboratory errors, or pharmacokinetic changes always have to be excluded.

INITIATION OF THERAPY

Vitamin K antagonists should be started concomitantly with heparin treatment[34] since it takes several days for the vitamin K antagonists to achieve an antithrombotic effect.[35] Factor VII concentration drops rapidly, reaching levels that produce a prolonged prothrombin time within 24 h, but the other vitamin K–dependent coagulation factors have longer half-lives, and an antithrombotic effect is not achieved until after 72 to 96 h.[36] Initiation of warfarin therapy within 3 days compared to after 7 days,[37] or on day 1 compared to day 5,[38] provides the same benefit with equal safety, and thus the current recommendation is to start warfarin on day 1.

The ''loading'' doses of warfarin that were used in the past frequently caused hemorrhage and have been abandoned.[39] The plasma levels of inhibitor protein C decrease much faster than the levels of factor X when warfarin is initiated at a dose of 8 mg twice a day for 2 to 3 days instead of 6 mg daily for 3 days, and it has been speculated that the higher dose produces a transient hypercoagulable state.[40] However, in a study comparing initiation of 15 mg warfarin on day 1 and 7.5 mg on days 2 and 3 with a regimen of 15 mg/day until the INR reached 1.87, both regimens were found to be safe and effective, and heparin treatment could be discontinued after 6 and 5 days, respectively.[41]

In patients with inherited deficiency of protein C or protein S, the initiation of treatment with vitamin K antagonists should be done with small doses and prolonged overlap with heparin to avoid skin necrosis (see ''Skin Necrosis,'' ''Complications of Therapy''). For patients with protein C deficiency, treatment with warfarin and protein C concentrate[42] or fresh-frozen plasma might be considered.

DISCONTINUATION OF WARFARIN

The optimal mode of cessation has likewise been a subject of debate. Indeed, there is a transient elevation of thrombin-antithrombin complexes and prothrombin fragment F1+2 after discontinuation of warfarin treatment for venous thromboembolism, with more pronounced changes after abrupt than after gradual discontinuation.[43] It has, however, been difficult to prove the clinical disadvantage of abrupt cessation in patients with venous thromboembolism. In patients treated with warfarin after thrombolysis for myocardial infarction, abrupt cessation of warfarin created a gap between the rapidly rising levels of factors VII and IX and a slow normalization of protein C and S levels, mirrored by a hypercoagulable state associated with some thromboembolic events and increased levels of fibrinopeptide A.[44]

MONITORING

LABORATORY ASSAY

Anticoagulant treatment is monitored by a one-stage prothrombin time (PT) test, the Quick thromboplastin time,[45] or a modification thereof, the prothrombin and proconvertin (P&P) method.[46] A thromboplastin extract of a tissue, providing both tissue factor and phospholipids, is added to citrated plasma, and then the plasma is recalcified to initiate the reaction. The coagulation time reflects the activity of the extrinsic and common pathway of the coagulation cascade. In the P&P method, adsorbed ox plasma as a source of factor V and fibrinogen is also added, and thus the plasma level of these factors will not have any influence on the result.

STANDARDIZED REPORTING

Due to wide variations in the sensitivities of the thromboplastins used and in the recommendations for therapeutic ranges, patients in different countries or even at different centers within a single country received substantially different intensities of anticoagulation.[47] As a result, multicenter trials and comparisons of treatment effects were impossible to perform or to interpret. For these reasons, recommendations were issued in 1985 to standardize the reporting of the PT by using the INR.[48] This is a calibration system based on a linear relationship between the logarithm of PT ratios obtained with the reference and test thromboplastins. For an individual test, the INR is calculated according to the formula $INR = (PT_{Patient} / PT_{Control})^{ISI}$, where the international sensitivity index (ISI) is a correction factor for the responsiveness of the thromboplastin to the reductions in the vitamin K–dependent coagulation factors. The precision of the INR increases with lower ISI values,[49] and hence it is important that the latter are as low as possible or, more specifically, close to 1.0, which is the ISI value of the World Health Organization international reference preparation. However, the type of instrument used will also affect the ISI value,[50] and indeed, each local reagent-instrument combination needs calibration for the achievement of reliable INR values.[51] The citrate concentration in the test tubes also affects the INR, and a single concentration should therefore be used.[52] Since pooled plasma from patients stabilized on warfarin is used for the INR model, it could be presumed that INR values obtained during the induction phase are unreliable, but in a series of 43 patients tested during the initial 5 days with five different thromboplastins, the INR system showed less variance than did the PT ratios.[53] The system is widely accepted in Europe and the United States.

REAGENTS

Due to the risk of viral contamination with tissue factor extracted from animal tissues, recombinant human tissue factor (rTF)[54,55] is the preferred reagent for monitoring treatment with vitamin K antagonists.[56,57] The presence of heparin in the patient's sample may influence the INR values, but some reagents, including the one based on rTF, are unaffected by heparin concentrations up to 1 IU/ml.[58] Similarly, the presence of a lupus anticoagulant may have a pronounced effect on the test result, leading to falsely high INR values, but this is also to some extent dependent on the sensitivity of the thromboplastin.[59,60]

Although other assays to monitor treatment have shown promising results,[61–63] none has replaced thromboplastin reagents. Assays of prothrombin fragment 1+2 and thrombin-antithrombin complexes have also been proposed for monitoring, but have not demonstrated improved ability to predict treatment failure or hemorrhagic risk.[64,65]

INSTRUMENTS

Portable instruments suitable for home use produce assay values that correlate well with results produced by laboratory instruments.[66] Training patients in capillary blood sampling and warfarin dose adjustments can permit self-management with vitamin K antagonists.[67,68] This method may also be advantageous for families with children requiring anticoagulant treatment.[69]

COMPUTERIZED DECISION SUPPORT

Anticoagulant therapy is often suboptimal in routine practice, with a high percentage of test results outside the targeted range.[70] A computerized decision support system used by physicians and nurses can improve the quality of treatment.[71,72] By collection of data via the computer system, quality control of the safety and efficacy of the anticoagulation is also facilitated. In a randomized study, computer-based control resulted in a significantly lower number of altered doses.[73]

ORGANIZATION OF ANTICOAGULANT MONITORING

The Netherlands has a nationwide organization for control of treatment with vitamin K antagonists and has documented that 80 percent of the PT of patients on long-term treatment were within the target range.[74] Centralization of patients to specialized anticoagulation clinics is likely to offer an improvement of the anticoagulant management, with a reduction of thromboembolic events, major hemorrhages, and costs of hospitalizations, as demonstrated by an overview,[75] a study of two consecutive cohorts,[76] and a small randomized trial.[77]

PROBLEMS DURING MONITORING

Unstable INRs may be due to problems with reagents, instruments, or staff. Inexperienced monitors may not wait long enough for the development of a new steady state after dose adjustments and then overshoot the desired INR. Even minor matters may affect the results. Thus, the hour of the day when the blood sample is obtained may be important, since there is a diurnal variation of the INR in patients treated with vitamin K antagonists, with the peak between 4:00 A.M. and 8:00 A.M. and the nadir between 6:00 P.M. and midnight.[78] The main uncertainty is, however, caused by the numerous interactions with vitamin K antagonists, described in the following section. It is therefore not surprising that the instability of anticoagulation increases with the number of concomitant drugs taken, irrespective of known specific interactions.[79]

INTERACTIONS

DIET

Vitamin K$_1$ (phylloquinone) is the predominant form of vitamin K present in the diet. Intake of vitamin K may cause a competition with the effect of the 4-hydroxycoumarins. Lists of foods and their vitamin K content are available from some of the manufacturers of vitamin K antagonists, but there is probably little benefit in supplying them to patients without a detailed explanation, especially since some patients may respond by omitting all vegetables from their diet. In fact, relatively few interactions between vitamin K antagonists and foods are clinically relevant, although the warfarin antagonism produced by large amounts of avocado[80] or broccoli[81] is highly probable. In the case of avocado, the vitamin K content is not high, but avocado oils seem to interfere with warfarin in some other way. Balanced advice to patients is the following[82,83]:

1. Avoid major changes in the diet. If a change is indispensable, consult the physician and increase the frequency of monitoring temporarily.
2. Avoid avocado, kale, and parsley, except as a garnish or minor ingredient, as well as the Japanese dish natto.
3. Choose up to one serving (100 g) per day from the following: broccoli, brussels sprouts, spinach, turnip greens, or other greens.
4. Discuss with the physician any substantial increase or decrease in the intake of lentils, garbanzo beans, soybeans, soybean oil, liver, or other sources rich in vitamin K.
5. Alcohol intake, other than the occasional drink, should be discouraged.
6. Supplements of vitamin E seem to cause interference with vitamin K and should be avoided. Supplements with vitamin A and C have occasionally caused an increase or decrease, respectively, of the PT, and doses higher than the recommended daily allowances should be avoided.[82]

For poorly controlled anticoagulated patients, where no drug interaction or other obvious reason can be identified, a diet with a constant vitamin K$_1$ content may be beneficial.[84,85]

TABLE 132-1   REPORTED DRUG INTERACTIONS WITH WARFARIN AND OTHER VITAMIN K ANTAGONISTS CAUSING *INCREASED* ANTICOAGULANT RESPONSE

Acarbose	Etoposide	**Oxyphenbutazone**
Acetaminophen	Felbamate	Paroxetin
Allopurinol	Feprazone	**Phenylbutazone**
Aminoglycosides	Flubiprophen	Phenyramidol
Aminosalicylic acid	**Fluconazole**	Phenytoin
Amiodarone	5-Fluorouracil	Piroxicam
Amoxicillin	**Fluoxetine**	Pravastatin
Androgens (17-alkyl)	Flutamide	Propafenone
Androgens (non-17-alkyl)	Fluvastatin	Propoxyphene
Azapropazone	Fluvoxamine	Propranolol
Azathioprine	Gemfibrozil	Quinidine
Azithromycin	**Glucagon**	Rantidine
Benzbromarone	Halofenate	**Salicylates**
Benziodarone	Hydrocodone	**(high dose)**
β-adrenergic blockers	Indomethacin	Saquinavir
Bezafibrate	Influenza vaccine	Sertralin
Bromodeoxyuridine	Interferon	Simvastatin
Carboplatin	Isoniazid	**Sulfamethoxazole-**
Cefamandole	Isoxicam	**trimethoprim**
Chloral hydrate	Itraconazole	**Sulfinpyrazone**
Chloramphenicol	Ketoconazole	Sulfonamides
Cimetidine	Ketoprophen	Sulindac
Ciprofloxacin	Levamisole	**Tamoxifen**
Citalopram	Lovastatin	Tenidap
Clarithromycin	Meclofenamate	Terbinafine
Clofibrate	Mefenamic acid	Tetracyclines
Corticosteroids	Mesna	**Thyroid hormone**
(high dose)	Methylsalicylate	Tiaprofenoic acid
Danazol	(topical)	Tolmentin
Defoperazone	**Metronidazole**	Toremiphen
Dextropropoxyphene	Miconazole	Tramadol
Diazoxide	Moricizine	Tricyclic
Diflunisal	Moxolactam	antidepressants
Disopyramide	Nalidixic acid	Vitamin E
Disulfiram	Norfloxacin	Zileuton
Erythromycin	Ofloxacin	Zolpidem
Ethacrinic acid	Omeprazole	

NOTE: Drugs with profound or frequent interactions appear in boldface.

DIARRHEA

Poor absorption of the vitamin K antagonists may occur in patients during periods with diarrhea, with use of liquid paraffin laxatives,[86] and in patients with malabsorption syndrome.

DRUGS

There is an ever-growing list of drug interactions with vitamin K antagonists (Tables 132-1 and 132-2). The vast majority of those have been reported in patients treated with warfarin, but in many cases they have been described also with at least one of the other vitamin K antagonists. At high doses, the nonsteroidal anti-inflammatory agents, as well as acetylsalicylic acid, may cause hypoprothrombinemia through inhibition of hepatic metabolism via CYP_{450} 2C9 (phenylbutazone and analogs) or protein-binding displacement.[87] Furthermore, these drugs increase the risk of bleeding by inhibiting platelet function. Finally, the risk of upper gastrointestinal hemorrhage is increased by the ulcerogenic effect of these agents.[88]

A number of different mechanisms of drug interactions with vitamin K antagonists have been described (Table 132-3). In most cases, metabolism of warfarin is inhibited, which in turn can be stereoselective for either the *R*- or *S*-enantiomer.[83]

Amitriptyline causes an unusual type of interaction with phenprocoumon during which great fluctuations of the PT have been observed.[89] Chinese herbs and traditional medicines have been reported to exert an inhibiting effect on the metabolism of warfarin, sometimes resulting in pronounced hyperanticoagulation.[90–92]

TABLE 132-2   REPORTED DRUG INTERACTIONS WITH WARFARIN AND OTHER VITAMIN K ANTAGONISTS CAUSING *DECREASED* ANTICOAGULANT RESPONSE

Aminoglutethimide	Mercaptopurine
Antipyrine	Methaqualone
Antithyroid drugs	Mianserine
Ascorbic acid	Mitotane
Azathioprine	Nafcillin
Barbiturates	Propofol
Carbamazepine	Rifampin
Cholestyramine	Simethicone
Contraceptives, oral	Spironolactone
Cyclophosphamide	Sucralfate
Dichloralphenazone	Teicoplanin
Dicloxacillin	Thiazide diuretics
Ethchlorvynol	Trazodone
Etretinate	Ubidecarone
Flucloxacillin	
Furosemide	
Glucocorticoids	
Glutethimide	
Griseofulvin	

NOTE: Drugs with profound or frequent interactions appear in boldface.

CHEMICALS

An accentuated effect of vitamin K antagonists during the summer has been reported as a result of exposure to insecticides, such as ivermectin or metidation.[93,94]

COMPLICATIONS OF THERAPY

BLEEDING

Incidence   Vitamin K antagonists cause more fatal side effects than any other drug in absolute numbers.[95] Virtually all fatalities are related to bleeding complications. The incidence of this complication varies from one study to another due to differences in intensity of anticoagulation and patient populations. In a survey of seven trials in venous thromboembolism, only one fatal hemorrhage among 1283

TABLE 132-3   MECHANISMS FOR DRUG INTERACTIONS WITH VITAMIN K ANTAGONISTS

MECHANISM	DRUG
Enhancement of vitamin K pathway	Vitamin K, lipid emulsions
Vitamin K deficiency	Antibiotics
Accelerated catabolism of coagulation factors	Thyroid hormone, androgens
Decreased synthesis of coagulation factors	Clofibrate
Decreased warfarin absorption due to binding	Cholestyramine
Increased warfarin absorption	Acarbose
Inhibition of cyclic interconversion of vitamin K generation	Second- and third-generation cephalosporins
Inhibition of cytochrome P_{450}(CYP3A4)	Clarithromycin
Inhibition of cytochrome P_{450}2C9: (*S*)-enantiomer	Sulfinpyrazone
Stereoselective inhibition of hydroxylation: (*R*)-enantiomer	Cimetidine
Nonstereoselective clearance	Amiodarone
Induction of hepatic enzymes	Barbiturates, rifampin
Displacement of protein binding	Etoposide
Potentiation of the warfarin receptor effect	Clofibrate
Antiplatelet effect	Acetylsalicylic acid

TABLE 132-4   INCIDENCE OF FATAL HEMORRHAGE IN VARIOUS PATIENT POPULATIONS

Design	Indication	Target INR	Follow-up, p-y	Fatal Bleeds per 100 p-y
Retrospective, all outpatients[276]	Atrial fibrillation	2.0–4.9	818	0.49
Randomized trial[99]	Venous thromboembolism	2.0–2.85	463	0.43
Retrospective, all outpatients, warfarin ± acetylsalicylic acid[277]	Various	2.5–4.2	4420	0.89
Inception cohort, prospective[278]	Various	Various	2008	0.25
Retrospective[279]	Various	Various	1199	0.17
Retro- and prospective cohorts[97]	Various	Various	3702	0.11

ABBREVIATION: p-y, patient years.

patients anticoagulated for 3 months was identified,[96] which illustrates the low risk observed in studies with a selected patient population. Table 132-4 compares the incidence of fatal hemorrhage in other large studies.

The definitions of major hemorrhages vary among studies. Some have specifically defined ''life-threatening'' hemorrhages, which had an incidence of 0.89 per 100 patient-years in a cohort study[97] and 0.83 in a combined cross-sectional and prospective cohort study,[98] with 7500 combined patient-years of observation. Major hemorrhages may include those with a certain drop in hemoglobin but without hospitalization, and the incidence per 100 patient-years ranged between 1.7 and 2.1 in four studies of patients with atrial fibrillation, between 0.8 and 4.1 in four trials on patients with prosthetic heart valves,[96] and between 2.2 and 7.8 in three trials on patients with venous thromboembolism, with at least 100 patient-years of follow-up.[99–101] In cohort studies, the incidence of major hemorrhages ranges from 1.2[102] to 7.0[97] per 100 patient-years.

Locations   The gastrointestinal tract is the most common site for major hemorrhages (66%),[98] and the site of bleeding, usually a peptic ulcer, can be precisely identified in 83 percent of cases.[103] However, large-bowel malignancy is another common organic lesion found in these cases, which emphasizes the importance of performing a thorough investigation to locate the source of bleeding.[104] Acute abdomen requiring laparotomy in anticoagulated patients is typically caused by intramural intestinal hematoma.[105]

Intracranial bleeding was the most common cause of fatal hemorrhage,[106] with a mortality rate of 77 percent in a prospective study of patients admitted to a department of neurosurgery.[107] A majority of these patients had intracerebral hemorrhage, whereas a minority had subdural hematoma; the latter was associated with a better prognosis.[107,108] Predictors for a poor prognosis of intracranial hemorrhage are age over 60 years, hematoma in the midline or ventricles, coma, arterial hypertension, and hyperanticoagulation at the time of bleeding.[109] The risk of developing an intracranial hematoma after an apparently minor head injury has been estimated to be 10 times higher in patients treated with warfarin.[110]

Femoral neuropathy after retroperitoneal hemorrhage,[111] radial nerve compression neuropathy after routine venipuncture,[112] and acute carpal tunnel syndrome due to intraneural hemorrhage in the median nerve[113] are rare but serious complications. Unusual sites of hemorrhage include spermatic cord hematoma,[114] spontaneous spinal epidural hematoma after a coughing spell,[115] and choroidal hemorrhage in age-related macular degeneration.[116]

Predictors   Several predictors for major hemorrhage during treatment with vitamin K antagonists have been identified (Table 132-5). Among these predictors, the influence of age has been controversial. For intracranial hemorrhage, previous ischemic cerebral events, old age, hypertension, and high intensity of anticoagulation were identified as predictors.[107,117]

Increased plasma levels of tissue plasminogen activator, its inhibitor, von Willebrand factor, and soluble thrombomodulin, all measured by immunochemical methods, have been found to correlate with the risk of hemorrhage.[118,119] These could all be markers of endothelial dysfunction and vascular disease.

Two groups have reported the interesting finding of increased bleeding in patients with missense mutations in Ala10 in the propeptide of factor IX.[120,121] The mutated protein (Ala10Val in two patients and Ala10Thr in another two) exerted a reduced affinity of the γ-glutamyl-carboxylase enzyme for the propeptide. This had no effect on plasma factor IX levels in the absence of vitamin K antagonists, but it significantly increased the patients' sensitivity to warfarin treatment, with factor IX levels dropping to less than 1 to 3 percent of normal, compared to 30 to 40 percent in patients with the wild-type factor IX. Furthermore, polymorphisms in the gene coding for cytochrome P_{450} CYP2C9, the principal catalytic enzyme for (S)-warfarin, give rise to decreased warfarin requirement and confer an increased risk of major bleeding.[122]

Treatment   In patients with a major hemorrhage, rapid reversal of the anticoagulant effect is essential. It is frequently difficult to give sufficient amounts of fresh-frozen plasma, due to volume restrictions, and some experts recommend infusion of prothrombin-complex concentrates.[123] However, these concentrates may increase the risk of thrombosis since they contain activated coagulation factors.

Minor bleeding complications have not received much attention in the literature, but a study on epistaxis during warfarin treatment showed that the medication could be continued safely, provided that the INR was within the therapeutic range and that local hemostatic measures were taken.[124]

Reversal of Overdose without Hemorrhage   In the absence of hemorrhage, hyperanticoagulation is preferably reversed by either discontinuation and careful observation or by vitamin K_1 (phytonadione) administration. An intravenous dose of 0.5 mg vitamin K_1 seems sufficient to achieve an INR in the therapeutic range in most patients within 24 h.[125] However, this route of administration should be avoided if possible, since anaphylactic reactions have been described.[126] For subcutaneous administration, an average dose of 4.9 mg vitamin K_1

TABLE 132-5   PREDICTORS FOR HEMORRHAGIC COMPLICATIONS

Risk Factor Demonstrated	Refuted by
Hyperanticoagulation[98,280,281]	
Poor anticoagulant control[279,282]	
Old age[106,278,280,281]	97,282–285
Initial phase of anticoagulation[278]	
Increasing duration of treatment[276,279]	106
Men with aortic valve prosthesis[279]	
Peripheral vascular disease[278]	
Cerebrovascular disease[278,286]	
History of alcohol abuse[282]	
Elevated thrombomodulin in plasma[119]	
Factor IX propeptide mutation[120,121]	
Polymorphisms in cytochrome 450 CYP2C9 gene[122]	

was reported as necessary,[127] whereas by the oral route, between 1 and 2.5 mg were found effective and safe, reaching a therapeutic level after 16 h.[128–130] Doses of vitamin K_1 of 10 mg or more should be avoided, since they lead to warfarin resistance for up to a week.

NONHEMORRHAGIC COMPLICATIONS

Skin Necrosis   Initially described in 1943,[131] skin necrosis occurs with a frequency of about 1 in 5000 patients treated with vitamin K antagonists,[132] although there have been occasional reports of a much higher frequency[133] (see Chap. 121). It affects predominantly women (85%) and may be related to the distribution of subcutaneous fat. Areas typically involved are breasts, thighs, and buttocks. The onset is usually within 3 to 10 days from initiation of anticoagulation, but a delay of up to 15 years has been reported.[133] Skin necrosis does not necessarily reappear with reinstitution of vitamin K antagonists.

Initial symptoms and signs are localized pain with a maculopapular rash, which within 24 to 48 h progresses to hemorrhagic lesions, hemorrhagic bullae, and necrosis, leaving an eschar that heals slowly. Plastic surgery is frequently required,[134] and when the breast is affected, mastectomy may be necessary.

It is generally believed that the pathogenic mechanism is a hypercoagulable state caused by an imbalance between severely depressed levels of protein C and protein S and only a mild reduction of coagulation factors II, IX, and X.[132,133] Preexisting deficiency of protein C or protein S, or use of large loading doses of warfarin may accentuate this imbalance. A deficiency of antithrombin may also contribute to the pathogenesis.[135] Histologically, fibrin deposits are seen in small veins and venules in the dermis and subcutaneous fat, surrounded by hemorrhage and diffuse necrosis.

Prompt administration of vitamin K has been reported to halt the progression to skin necrosis.[136] Treatment with vitamin K antagonists should be discontinued immediately in any event and reversed with plasma or, in the case of protein C deficiency, with a concentrate of protein C if available. Anticoagulation is continued with heparin until the lesions have healed, whereafter warfarin may be resumed, starting a low dose of 1 to 2 mg/day and gradually increasing it over 10 to 12 days.[133,137]

Purple Toe Syndrome   Since the first report of six patients with this complication,[138] only a few additional cases have been described (see Chap. 121). The syndrome develops 3 to 8 weeks after initiation of anticoagulation,[138] usually with bilateral burning pain and dark blue discoloration of the toes and sides of the feet, with blanching of the skin on pressure.[133] Occasionally, the hands are involved. Most of the patients have underlying cardiac disorders, diabetes mellitus, or peripheral vascular disease. It is presumed that the mechanism is cholesterol embolization from atherosclerotic plaques. Warfarin may make the plaque more friable by decreasing fibrin deposition or by hemorrhage into the plaque.[133] The burning pain, but not the discoloration, disappears on discontinuation of warfarin.[133] The safety of restoring warfarin in patients who have developed this complication is unclear.

Other Nonhemorrhagic Side Effects   Other dermatologic side effects of warfarin are maculopapular,[139] vesicular, or urticarial rashes,[140] often very itchy, occurring weeks to months after beginning anticoagulation[132] but occasionally after the first dose.[140] Eosinophilic pleurisy[141] and vasculitis[142] have been described in connection with warfarin therapy. Phenindione has also been reported to cause severe hypersensitivity.[23]

There are a few reports of toxic hepatitis induced by different vitamin K antagonists[143,144] and descriptions of intrahepatic jaundice.[145,146]

Finally, there are contradictory reports regarding the effect of warfarin on bone mineral density. Although osteocalcin is reproducibly reduced during warfarin treatment,[147–149] in combination with increased loss of calcium in urine,[147] the literature is inconsistent with regard to the effect of warfarin on reduced bone mineral density[148–152] and the incidence of fractures.[151]

TERATOGENICITY

The teratogenic effects of vitamin K antagonists consist of midface and nasal hypoplasia, stippled epiphyses, hypoplasia of the digits, optic atrophy, and mental impairment.[153] This is summarized as the warfarin embryopathy syndrome, but it can also be induced by other vitamin K antagonists given between weeks 6 and 12 of gestation. Previous estimates of the frequency of the syndrome after exposure to warfarin during weeks 6 to 12 range from 5.4 to 28.6 percent.[154,155] In more recent retrospective and prospective studies, 0 of 46[156] and 1 of 11[157] first-trimester exposures respectively resulted in embryopathy, whereas in a retrospective study of Chinese patients, 16 of 29 children had features of embryopathy, which in almost all of them was restricted to nasal hypoplasia.[158]

A similar syndrome, with nasal hypoplasia, punctate calcifications, and abnormalities of the spine, has been described in children of mothers with vitamin K deficiency due to malabsorption, in patients with epoxide reductase deficiency,[159] and in homozygotes for a point mutation in the γ-glutamylcarboxylase gene associated with a deficiency of all vitamin K–dependent coagulation factors and inhibitors.[160] With the addition of distal phalangeal hypoplasia, a similar constellation is found in X-linked, recessive chondrodysplasia punctata, where the mutations result in a deficiency of a heat-labile arylsulphatase.[161]

Vitamin K antagonist therapy during any trimester can cause central nervous system hemorrhage in approximately 1 percent of fetuses or central nervous system malformation without apparent hemorrhage in about 4 to 5 percent.[154]

Artificial Heart Valves and Pregnancy   There are numerous reports of artificial heart valve thrombosis during pregnancy, the majority of which occurred during anticoagulation with heparin, and some with fatal outcome.[156,157,162] It has therefore been considered advisable to use a vitamin K antagonist for these patients during the second and early phase of the third trimester after providing mothers with information about the risks and benefits in comparison with heparin.[154]

LACTATION

Warfarin is not contraindicated during breastfeeding, since the concentration in breast milk is less than 25 ng/ml and warfarin is not detectable in the plasma of the breastfed infants.[163]

SURGICAL MANAGEMENT

One of the frequent questions regarding treatment with vitamin K antagonists concerns the management during surgery or other invasive procedures. The possibilities range from uninterrupted anticoagulation to reversal of the vitamin K antagonism.

MINOR SURGERY

There is no need to reduce or discontinue anticoagulant treatment for cutaneous surgery[164,165] or for soft-tissue aspirations or injections.[166,167] Pacemaker surgery is also safe, provided that proper surgical technique is used.[168] For oral surgery, randomized, placebo-controlled studies have shown that unchanged anticoagulation is safe, provided that it is combined with local irrigation or a mouth rinse with a 5% solution of tranexamic acid in connection with surgery and then repeated four times daily for a week.[169–171] However, it has also been demonstrated

TABLE 132-6   DECREASE IN THE MEAN INR (±SD) AFTER DISCONTINUATION OF WARFARIN

	INR After Last Dose of Warfarin	
Steady-State INR	66 h	115 h
2.6	1.6 (1.1–2.16)	1.1 (0.8–1.4)

source: Adapted from data in RH White et al.[176]

that discontinuation of treatment with vitamin K antagonists for 2 days prior to the tooth extraction to achieve an INR of 1.5 or less may be as safe, even in patients with artificial heart valves.[172] Local anesthesia of the lower jaw with a posterior nerve block should probably be avoided.

Treatment of benign prostate hyperplasia with neodymium:YAG laser ablation has been performed without interruption of the anticoagulation, but there is a risk of major hemorrhage of approximately 15 percent.[173,174]

MAJOR SURGERY

For cardiac surgery, treatment with vitamin K antagonists can be continued, maintaining an INR of about 2.4.[175] In comparison with a reduced dose of warfarin, this regimen led to a lower heparin requirement to prolong the activated coagulation time and diminished blood loss.[175] For vascular surgery, surgeons must use meticulous hemostatic technique to allow uninterrrupted anticoagulation for prevention of occlusion of graft or operated blood vessel.

For other types of surgery, a modification of the treatment is necessary. Thus, it is useful to know the rate by which the INR decreases after discontinuation of warfarin. The results of a kinetic study in 22 patients are presented in Table 132-6. The exponential decay of INR does not start until 29 h after the last dose.[176] In case of anticoagulation after venous thromboembolism, the likelihood of a perioperative thromboembolic event during a few days is smaller than the risk of postoperative hemorrhage, and thus, brief discontinuation of warfarin is safe close to the time of planned surgery.[177] However, if thrombosis occurred close to the time of planned surgery, it is preferable to postpone surgery or to follow one of the regimens suggested for patients with artificial heart valves. In the latter patients, the risk of thrombus formation on the valve may be perceived as low during a few days of interrupted anticoagulation, since the annual risk without any antithrombotic treatment averages about 10 percent.[178] This does not take into account the increased perioperative risk due to activation of coagulation and of the fibrinolytic activity. Thus, in one study, 2 of 10 patients with mitral or combined mechanical valves had fatal strokes when anticoagulation was interrupted 3 to 5 days before surgery.[179]

A regimen that has been used for elective surgery in 197 anticoagulated patients[180] is shown in Fig. 132-2. Of 84 patients with artificial heart valves, major hemorrhage occurred in 3 who had transurethral resection of the prostate (TURP) and in 8 of 99 with major surgery, whereas 2 of the 197 patients developed ischemic stroke.[180] TURP is a procedure with a high hemorrhagic risk, and in another study, a similar regimen, but with complete interruption of heparin 4 h before and throughout surgery, was attempted.[181] Still, 1 of 12 patients had hemorrhage requiring transfusion, and 3 were readmitted for late bleeding. In general, the hemorrhagic complications have required transfusion or reoperation, whereas the ischemic strokes have resulted in chronic sequelae.

INDICATIONS

MECHANICAL HEART VALVES

The risk of thromboembolism depends on the type and position of the prosthesis and, to some extent, on patient-related factors. In a randomized study, the risk was lower with Björk-Shiley valves than with Edwards-Duro-Medics or Medtronic-Hall valves.[182] In a meta-analysis, the risk of thromboembolism was highest with a caged-ball valve (Starr-Edwards), 30 percent lower with a tilting disk valve (Björk-Shiley, Sorin, Medtronic-Hall, and Omnicarbon), and 50 percent lower with a bileaflet valve (St. Jude, DuroMedics, and CarboMedics).[178] In a cohort study, the risks with these different valves per 100 patient-years were 2.5, 0.7, and 0.5, respectively.[183] The risk is twice as high with a mitral prosthesis as with an aortic prosthesis.[178] Other factors that may increase the risk of thromboembolism are age,[183] hypertension, and smoking,[184] whereas the effects of left atrial enlargement and atrial fibrillation have been controversial.[184,185]

A retrospective cohort study of 1608 unselected patients with mechanical heart valves showed that the optimal antithrombotic effect was achieved at an INR of 2.5 to 4.9, and thus a target of 3.0 to 4.0 was recommended.[183] In one study, a target INR of 2.0 to 3.0 was as effective as an INR of 3.0 to 4.5, but there were significantly fewer minor hemorrhages in the former group.[186] The risks of thromboembolism were, however, 2.4 and 2.1 per 100 patient-years, respectively, compared to 0.71 in the cohort study; thus, whether the intensity can be lowered is controversial.

Several studies have been performed with the St. Jude Medical prosthesis with low-intensity warfarin prophylaxis (INR ≤ 2.5) in combination with dipyridamole and sometimes also acetylsalicylic acid. The incidence of thromboembolism ranged from 0.5 to 1.3 per 100 patient-years.[187–190] In a meta-analysis of five randomized trials where antiplatelet therapy or placebo was added to the prophylaxis with vitamin K antagonists, the combined regimen reduced thromboembolism by 67 percent, but at a cost of a 65 percent increase in hemorrhage and 250 percent increase in major gastrointestinal hemorrhage.[191] In a review of 16 studies with warfarin and acetylsalicylic acid compared with monotherapy with either agent, it was concluded that the combination should be reserved for patients with a high risk of thromboembolism and possibly also for those with ischemic heart disease, and that the daily dose of acetylsalicylic acid should not exceed 100 mg.[192]

Bioprosthetic heart valves also confer a risk of thromboembolism, accentuated during the first 3 months after surgery. During this period,

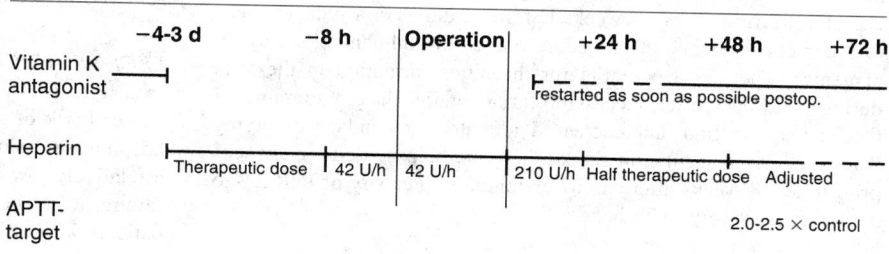

FIGURE 132-2   Example of a perioperative regimen for patients on anticoagulant therapy with a high risk of thromboembolism. The infusion rate of heparin is increased to 210 U/h when the patient returns to the ward. Heparin is discontinued when the INR is in the therapeutic range for 2 consecutive days. (Adapted from S Vigano'D'Angelo et al.[180]).

TABLE 132-7 EFFECT OF WARFARIN COMPARED TO PLACEBO IN THE PRIMARY PREVENTION OF ISCHEMIC STROKE DUE TO NONVALVULAR ATRIAL FIBRILLATION

ACRONYM	TREATMENTS	PATIENTS, N	ISCHEMIC STROKE, % PER YEAR	RRR %	MAJOR HEMORRHAGE, % PER YEAR
AFASAK[287]	Warfarin INR 2.8–4.2	335	1.94	59	3.7
	Placebo	336	4.77		0.0
BAATAF[288]	Warfarin INR 1.5–2.7	212	0.40	86	0.2
	Controls	208	2.98		0.2
SPAF[289]	Warfarin INR 2.0–3.5	210	2.3	67	1.5
	Placebo	568	6.3		1.6
CAFA[290]	Warfarin INR 2.0–3.0	187	2.11	44	2.5
	Placebo	191	3.75		0.5
SPINAF[291]	Warfarin INR 1.4–2.8	260	0.9	79	1.6
	Placebo	265	4.3		0.9

ABBREVIATION: RRR, reduction of relative risk.

it is recommended to use vitamin K antagonists, aiming at an INR 2.0 to 3.0, and to continue warfarin indefinitely in cases with atrial fibrillation, atrial thrombosis detected at echocardiography, or after a systemic embolic episode.[193]

NONVALVULAR ATRIAL FIBRILLATION

To reduce the incidence of ischemic stroke of 4.5 percent per year in chronic nonvalvular (nonrheumatic) atrial fibrillation,[194] prophylaxis is considered increasingly important. Five major placebo-controlled trials have been performed to evaluate warfarin in the primary prevention of thromboembolism (Table 132-7). A meta-analysis of these trials, including 3706 patients, showed a reduction of relative risk of ischemic stroke of 68 percent with warfarin, valid for all age groups except in those younger than 65 years of age.[195] The annual incidence of fatal bleeding ranged from 0.0 to 0.8 percent, while the annual incidence of major hemorrhages ranged from 0.2 to 2.0 percent. The recommended target INR is 2.0 to 3.0.[194] At this level, warfarin reduces the levels of prothrombin fragment 1+2, β-thromboglobulin, and fibrin D-dimer, which are elevated before treatment. Minidose warfarin does not affect these parameters[196,197] and was not shown to be clinically effective.[198]

CARDIOVERSION

Serial transesophageal echocardiography in 14 patients with atrial fibrillation demonstrated that during 4 weeks of anticoagulation with warfarin 16 of 18 atrial thrombi resolved completely and no new thrombi were formed.[199] This is in line with the experience that the use of warfarin for 3 to 4 weeks before cardioversion reduces the 1 to 3 percent incidence of procedure-related thromboembolism by 90 percent.[200] There is a potential for thrombus formation in the atria during the weeks after successful cardioversion due to stunning of mechanical function and decreased left atrial appendage emptying velocity.[201] Anticoagulation should therefore be provided for 3 weeks prior to and 4 weeks after cardioversion at an intensity of INR 2.0 to 3.0 or, alternatively, with heparin.[202,203]

SECONDARY PROPHYLAXIS AFTER CEREBRAL ISCHEMIA

In a randomized trial in patients with cerebral ischemia of presumed arterial, noncardiac origin, secondary prophylaxis with warfarin targeted at an INR of 3.0 to 4.5 was not safe and resulted in 3.0 fatal and 4.8 intracranial hemorrhages per 100 patient-years. Moreover, this

regimen was not more effective than acetylsalicylic acid, 30 mg/day.[204] In a small, nonrandomized study, patients with systemic embolization and mobile aortic atheroma had a reduced risk of stroke if they received warfarin.[205] In patients with nonvalvular atrial fibrillation, secondary stroke prevention with warfarin (target INR 2.5 to 4.0) reduced the risk of stroke from 12 to 4 percent per year without causing any intracranial bleeding event, whereas acetylsalicylic acid, 300 mg/day, was not more effective than placebo.[206] In comparison with indobufen 100 or 200 mg b.i.d., warfarin targeted at an INR of 2.0 to 3.5 was equally effective in preventing vascular complications.[207]

ISCHEMIC HEART DISEASE

Primary prevention of thrombosis in patients at high risk of ischemic heart disease is effective using the combination of a low dose of warfarin and acetylsalicylic acid.[208] Thus, warfarin targeted at an INR of 1.3 to 1.8 reduced the risk of myocardial ischemic events, and addition of low-dose acetylsalicylic acid conferred an additional benefit, although the risk of bleeding increased.[208]

In patients with unstable angina, the addition of warfarin, targeted at an INR of 2.0 to 2.5, to acetylsalicylic acid 150 mg/day reduces the risk of progression of the culprit lesion.[209] However, after aortocoronary bypass surgery, warfarin, targeted at an INR of 2.8 to 4.8, did not reduce the risk of vein graft occlusion in comparison with acetylsalicylic acid 50 mg/day.[210] Angiographic follow-up of the patency of vein grafts did not reveal any positive effect of warfarin on the progression of atherosclerosis.[211]

Patients with myocardial infarction have a 10 percent risk of suffering a reinfarction during the first year, followed by an annual risk of 5 percent.[212] Secondary prophylaxis is therefore essential; however, of the many randomized studies performed, only a few were sufficiently large to allow for firm conclusions (Table 132-8). These studies, as well as a meta-analysis,[213] demonstrated a reduction of mortality and major cardiovascular events by administration of warfarin. Although there was a significant increase in the risk of major hemorrhage, there was an overall benefit from anticoagulation.[213] Data from the largest of these trials (ASPECT) was used to estimate the optimum intensity of anticoagulation, which was between INR 2.0 and 4.0.[214] Warfarin targeted at INR 2.0 to 2.5 was not superior to acetylsalicylic acid 150 mg in the AFTER study,[215] conceivably since this intensity was insufficient. With even lower intensity of anticoagulation, using 1 or 3 mg/day of warfarin, no benefit over acetylsalicylic acid 160 mg could be detected in the CARS trial.[216]

LEFT VENTRICULAR DYSFUNCTION

In a retrospective cohort analysis the use of warfarin resulted in a reduced risk of death, primarily those due to cardiac events, and of hospital admission for heart failure.[217] Since other studies have shown a relatively low incidence of systemic embolization in chronic heart failure, it has been suggested that the use of warfarin be limited to patients with atrial fibrillation or previous embolic events.[218]

PERIPHERAL VASCULAR DISEASE

Several studies have demonstrated a benefit of long-term therapy with vitamin K antagonists after bypass surgery in the lower limb with regard to graft function, limb salvage, and patient survival.[219–221] Antiplatelet agents may, however, be at least as effective with less severe side effects for this indication.[222,223]

SURGERY

Orthopedic surgery confers a particularly high risk of venous thromboembolism, with a frequency of deep vein thrombosis as high as 70 percent. Minidose warfarin (1 mg daily), which has a negligible effect on the INR, does not provide effective prophylaxis in this situation.[224] Low-dose warfarin, which prolongs the PT about 1.2 to 1.5 times the control value, is associated with a low rate of symptomatic pulmonary embolism (0.3–0.7%) after total joint arthroplasty,[225–227] but in a randomized trial it was not more effective than acetylsalicylic acid.[225] Full-dose warfarin targeted at an INR of 2.0 to 3.0 has been compared with low-molecular-weight heparin (LMWH) in several randomized trials and the efficacy, measured as thrombosis on screening after about 7 to 9 days, was usually superior with LMWH.[228–232] In some of the studies, warfarin caused less hemorrhage than LMWH,[228,231,232] and a meta-analysis of 22 trials with combinations of warfarin, LMWH, or unfractionated heparin reiterated the relative safety of warfarin.[233] Several analyses of cost-effectiveness have, however, yielded results in favor of LMWH for arthroplasty of the hip as well as of the knee.[234–237]

A "two-step" warfarin regimen, beginning with a lower dose 10 to 14 days before arthroplasty and postoperative adjustment to reach an INR of 2.2, did not provide any advantage compared with initiation of therapy the night before surgery.[238]

Prophylaxis with warfarin after surgery for acetabular or pelvic fractures resulted in an incidence of symptomatic deep vein thrombosis and pulmonary embolism of 3 and 1 percent respectively, with minimal bleeding complications.[239]

The risk of venous thromboembolism after orthopedic surgery is not eliminated by 7 to 10 days of postoperative prophylaxis, and several studies have investigated the benefit of prolonged prophylaxis at home. In a study of 96 patients after orthopedic surgery, a fixed low dose of warfarin (2 mg/day) was compared with an adjusted higher dose given for 1 month. The regimens appeared equally effective and safe, and the fixed low dose virtually eliminated the need for monitoring.[240]

For major gynecological surgery, fixed minidose warfarin (1 mg/day) started an average of 20 days before surgery was as effective as, but safer than, warfarin targeted at an INR of 1.5 to 2.5.[241]

CENTRAL VENOUS CATHETERS

A randomized trial demonstrated that minidose warfarin reduced the risk of venous thrombosis associated with chronic central venous catheters from 38 to 10 percent during 90 days.[242] In a retrospective study of patients with central venous catheters for long-term total parenteral nutrition, minidose warfarin was not less effective than a low-dose regimen with PT prolonged to 1.2 to 1.5 times that of control subjects.[243] However, for those patients with thrombosis on minidose warfarin, a switch to the higher dose significantly reduced the risk of recurrent thrombosis.[243]

CANCER

Although it is more difficult to maintain a stable therapeutic INR (2.0–3.0) in patients with cancer than in patients without cancer,[244] the risk of warfarin-induced hemorrhage is similar.[245] For patients with metastatic breast cancer receiving chemotherapy, minidose warfarin

TABLE 132-8   EFFECT OF WARFARIN COMPARED TO PLACEBO IN THE PREVENTION OF DEATH AND NONFATAL MYOCARDIAL INFARCTION OR STROKE (=PRIMARY EVENTS) AFTER MYOCARDIAL INFARCTION

ACRONYM	TREATMENTS	PATIENTS N	PRIMARY EVENTS %	RRR %	MAJOR HEMORRHAGE %
BMRC[292]	Warfarin	195	20.9	56	8.7
	Placebo	188	47.8		0.0
VAT[293]	Warfarin	385	46.7	13	16.0
	Placebo	350	53.4		2.8
Sixty Plus[294]	Warfarin	439	17.0	38	6.1
	Placebo	439	27.5		1.1
WARIS[295]	Warfarin	607	24.8	38	1.7
	Placebo	607	39.7		0.0
ASPECT[296]	Warfarin	1700	16.9	35	4.4
	Placebo	1704	26.1		1.1

NOTE: Primary events are defined as death and nonfatal myocardial infarction and stroke.
ABBREVIATION: RRR, reduction of relative risk.

for 6 weeks, followed by adjusted low-dose warfarin targeted at an INR of 1.3 to 1.9 (mean dose 2.6 mg/day), was effective in reducing the risk of venous thromboembolism (0.7 versus 4.4% with placebo) without increasing the risk of hemorrhage.[246]

OTHER INDICATIONS FOR PRIMARY PROPHYLAXIS

In patients with membranous nephropathy, prophylaxis against thromboembolism with vitamin K antagonists appears to provide benefits that outweigh the risks.[247]

Established Venous Thromboembolism Treatment with vitamin K antagonists is started concomitantly with heparin in acute venous thromboembolism (see "Initiation of Therapy," under "Dosing"). In a randomized trial, a target INR of 2.0 to 2.5 was associated with a significant reduction of hemorrhage without any increase of thromboembolic endpoints when compared to an INR of 3.0 to 4.5.[248] A slightly wider range, of INR 2.0 to 3.0, is more convenient and often used,[101,249,250] and the incidence of major hemorrhage is 4.7 to 8.8 per 100 patient-years. With a slightly modified range of INR 2.0 to 2.85, this incidence drops to 2.4 per 100 patient-years.[99,251] This intensity is also sufficient for patients with inherited thrombophilia or venous thromboembolism in combination with antiphospholipid antibodies.[252] In patients with systemic lupus erythematosus, antiphospholipid antibodies, and venous thromboembolism, a higher intensity is, however, required[253,254] (see Chap. 128).

Multicenter trials with sufficiently large numbers of patients have shown that, if the duration of secondary prophylaxis is prolonged from 4 weeks to 3 months, the risk of recurrence during 1 year is reduced from 7.8 to 4 percent[101]; and when it is prolonged from 6 weeks to 6 months, the risk during 2 years is reduced from 18.1 to 9.5 percent.[251] These patients were included after the first event of venous thromboembolism, and the prolonged treatment did not cause any increase of major hemorrhages.[101,251] In another trial, patients with a second episode of venous thromboembolism were randomized between 6 months and indefinite duration of anticoagulation.[99] The risk of recurrence over 4 years was reduced from 20.7 to 2.6 percent, but at the cost of a trend toward more major hemorrhages: 2.7 versus 8.6 percent. After discontinuation of the secondary prophylaxis, there was a recurrence rate of 4 to 5 percent per year for several years.[99,251]

Risk factors for an increased risk of recurrence include proximal deep vein thrombosis[255]; pulmonary embolism[255]; idiopathic thromboembolism or a permanent triggering factor[255]; hereditary deficiency of antithrombin, protein C, or protein S[256]; hyperhomocysteinemia[257]; and antiphospholipid antibodies.[252] The latter are also a predictor of an increased risk of cardiovascular death, which justifies long-term secondary prophylaxis.

In pulmonary hypertension, either primary or induced by the anorectic drug aminorex, warfarin has a positive effect on survival.[258]

MISCELLANEOUS INDICATIONS

A few case reports have described a dramatic positive effect of warfarin on migraine[259] and improvement by low doses of warfarin on calcinosis in systemic sclerosis.[260] Vitamin K antagonists have been reported to improve survival in small-cell carcinoma of the lung[261,262] and to reduce the cancer incidence and mortality in patients with heart disease.[263]

NOVEL VITAMIN K ANTAGONISTS

Alcohol and ester analogs of (R)-$(+)(S)$-warfarin have reduced protein binding, which can be utilized for the development of alternative agents with a lower risk of interactions with other drugs.[264]

OTHER ORAL ANTICOAGULANTS

GLYCOSAMINOGLYCANS

The oral bioavailability of unfractionated heparin can be increased to 8 percent by addition of delivery agents that improve the gastrointestinal absorption.[265] LMWH are of a size that should make oral administration feasible. Sulodexide is composed of 80 percent iduronylglycosaminoglycan sulfate and 20 percent dermatan sulfate, and has almost complete bioavailability after oral administration and an equivalent antithrombotic effect compared with heparin.[266,267] Heparan sulfate has been given orally in a study of patients after myocardial infarction.[268]

INHIBITORS OF COAGULATION FACTOR Xa

Direct and selective factor Xa inhibitors for oral use in humans are currently under development and have shown a potent antithrombotic effect with minimal or no influence on the bleeding time in animal models.[269,270]

INHIBITORS OF THROMBIN

Several low-molecular-weight active-site inhibitors of thrombin are selective and have a high degree of bioavailablity.[271–274] A small active-site–directed thrombin inhibitor is not only a potent antithrombotic agent,[275] but by being easily incorporated into newly formed thrombi, it enhances the susceptibility of the clot to spontaneous lysis.[272] Some of these agents are currently in early-phase clinical trials. A rapid onset of activity, favorable dose-response relationships, renal excretion rather than metabolism by hepatic enzymes, and decreased potential for drug interactions via enzyme competition or protein binding could make these oral agents good candidates for replacement of both heparin and vitamin K antagonists in the prophylaxis and treatment of thrombotic disorders.

REFERENCES

1. Schofield FW: A brief account of a disease in cattle simulating hemorrhagic septicaemia due to feeding sweet clover. *Can Vet Rec* 3:74, 1922.
2. Overman RS, Stahmann MA, Sullivan WR, et al: Studies on the haemorrhagic sweet clover disease: IV. The isolation and crystallization of the haemorrhagic agent. *J Biol Chem* 141:941, 1941.
3. Allen EV, Barker NW, Waugh JM: A preparation from spoiled sweet clover (3,3'-methylene-bis-(4-hydroxycoumarin)) which prolongs coagulation and prothrombin time of the blood: A clinical study. *JAMA* 120:1009, 1942.
4. Butsch WC, Stewart JD: Clinical experience with dicoumarin, 3,3'-methylene-bis-(4-hydroxycoumarin). *JAMA* 120:10256, 1942.
5. Lehmann J: Hypoprothrombinaemia produced by methylene-bis-(hydroxycoumarin): Its use in thrombosis. *Lancet* 1:318, 1942.
6. O'Reilly RA, Aggeler PM: Determinants of the response to oral anticoagulant drugs in man. *Pharmacol Rev* 22:35, 1970.
7. Richton-Hewett S, Foster E, Apstein CS: Medical and economic consequences of a blinded oral anticoagulant brand change at a municipal hospital. *Arch Intern Med* 148:806, 1988.
8. DeCara JM, Croze S, Falk RH: Generic warfarin: A cost-effective alternative to brand-name drug or a clinical wild card? *Chest* 113:261, 1998.
9. Willingham AK, Matschiner JT: Changes in phylloquinone epoxidase activity related to prothrombin synthesis and microsomal clotting activity in the rat. *Biochem J* 140:435, 1974.
10. Stenflo J, Fernlund P, Egan W, Roepstorff P: Vitamin K dependent modifications of glutamic acid residues in prothrombin. *Proc Natl Acad Sci USA* 71:2730, 1974.
11. Magnusson S, Sottrup-Jensen L, Petersen TE, Morris HR, Dell A: Primary structure of the vitamin K–dependent part of prothrombin. *FEBS Lett* 44:189, 1974.
12. Paul B, Oxley A, Brigham K, et al: Factor II, VII, IX, and X concentrations in patients receiving long term warfarin. *J Clin Pathol* 40:94, 1987.
13. Malhotra OP: Dicumarol-induced prothrombins containing 6,7 and 8 γ-carboxyglutamic acid residues: Isolation and characterization. *Biochem Cell Biol* 67:411, 1989.
14. Esnouf MP, Prowse CV: The gamma-carboxy glutamic content of human and bovine prothrombin following warfarin treatment. *Biochim Biophys Acta* 490:471, 1977.
15. Whitlon DS, Sadowski JA, Suttie JW: Mechanisms of coumarin action: Significance of vitamin K epoxide reductase inhibition. *Biochemistry* 17:1371, 1978.
16. Fasco MJ, Hildebrandt EF, Suttie JW: Evidence that warfarin anticoagulant action involves two distinct reductase activities. *J Biol Chem* 257:11210, 1982.
17. Talstad I, Gamst ON: Warfarin resistance due to malabsorption. *J Intern Med* 236:465, 1994.
18. Rajaian H, Symonds HW, Bowmer CJ: Drug binding sites on chicken albumin: A comparison to human albumin. *J Vet Pharmacol Ther* 20:421, 1997.
19. Sutcliffe FA, MacNicoll AD, Gibson GG: Aspects of anticoaglant action: A review of the pharmacology, metabolism and toxicology of warfarin and congeners. *Rev Drug Metabol Interact* 5:225, 1987.
20. Steward DJ, Haining RL, Henne KR, et al: Genetic association between sensitivity to warfarin and expression of CYP2C9*3. *Pharmacogenetics* 7:361, 1997.
21. King SY, Joslin MA, Raudibaugh K, Pieniaszek HJ Jr, Benedek IH: Dose-dependent pharmacokinetics of warfarin in healthy volunteers. *Pharm Res* 12:1874, 1995.
22. Abell TL, Merigian KS, Lee JM, Holbert JM, McCall JW: Cutaneous exposure to warfarin-like anticoagulant causing an intracerebral hemorrhage: A case report. *J Toxicol Clin Toxicol* 32:69, 1994.
23. Shetty HG, Woods F, Routledge PA: The pharmacology of oral anticoagulants: Implications for therapy. *J Heart Valve Dis* 2:53, 1993.
24. Weiner M, Shapiro S, Axelrod J, et al: The physical disposition of dicumarol in man. *J Pharmacol Exp Ther* 99:409, 1950.
25. Wynne HA, Kamali F, Edwards C, Long A, Kelly P: Effect of ageing upon warfarin dose requirements: A longitudinal study. *Age Ageing* 25:429, 1996.
26. Wynne H, Cope L, Kelly P, Whittingham T, Edwards C, Kamali F: The influence of age, liver size and enantiomer concentrations on warfarin requirements. *Br J Clin Pharmacol* 40:203, 1995.
27. Andrew M, Marzinotto V, Brooker LA, et al: Oral anticoagulation therapy in pediatric patients: A prospective study. *Thromb Haemost* 71:265, 1994.
28. Routledge PA, Davies DM, Bell SM, Cavanagh JS, Rawlins MD: Predicting patients' warfarin requirements. *Lancet* 2:854, 1977.
29. Cazaux V, Gauthier B, Elias A, et al: Predicting daily maintenance dose of fluindione, an oral anticoagulant drug. *Thromb Haemost* 75:731, 1996.
30. O'Reilly RA, Aggeler PM, Hoag MS, et al: Hereditary transmission of exceptional resistance to coumarin anticoagulant drugs. *N Engl J Med* 271:809, 1964.
31. Hallak HO, Wedlund PJ, Modi MW, et al: High clearance of (S)-warfarin in a warfarin-resistant subject. *Br J Clin Pharmacol* 35:327, 1993.
32. Alving BM, Strickler MP, Knight RD, Barr CF, Berenberg JL, Peck

CC: Hereditary warfarin resistance: Investigation of a rare phenomenon. *Arch Intern Med* 145:499, 1985.

33. Cain D, Hutson SM, Wallin R: Warfarin resistance is associated with a protein component of the vitamin K 2,3-epoxide reductase enzyme complex in the rat liver. *Thromb Haemost* 80:128, 1998.

34. Richards RL: Venous thrombosis. *Br Med J* 2:217, 1966.

35. Deykin D, Wessler S, Reimer SM: Evidence for an antithrombotic effect of dicumarol. *Am J Physiol* 199:1161, 1960.

36. Hellemans J, Vorlat M, Verstraete M: Survival time of prothrombin and factors VII, IX and X after complete synthesis blocking doses of coumarin derivatives. *Br J Haematol* 9:506, 1963.

37. Gallus A, Jackaman J, Tillettt J: Safety and efficacy of warfarin started early after submassive venous thrombosis or pulmonary embolism. *Lancet* 2:1293, 1986.

38. Hull RD, Raskob GE, Rosenbloom D, et al: Heparin for 5 days as compared with 10 days in the initial treatment of proximal venous thrombosis. *N Engl J Med* 322:1260, 1990.

39. O'Reilly R, Aggeler PM: Studies on coumarin anticoagulant drugs: Initiation of warfarin therapy without a loading dose. *Circulation* 38:169, 1968.

40. Iguchi A, Sato K: Protein C response to induction of warfarin treatment after coronary bypass operation. *Thorac Cardiovasc Surg* 42:222, 1994.

41. Schulman S, Lockner D, Bergström K, Blombäck M: Intensive initial oral anticoagulation and shorter heparin treatment in deep vein thrombosis. *Thromb Haemost* 52:276, 1984.

42. De Stefano V, Mastrangelo S, Schwarz HP, et al: Replacement therapy with a purified protein C concentrate during initiation of oral anticoagulation in severe protein C congenital deficiency. *Thromb Haemost* 70:247, 1993.

43. Palareti G, Legnani C, Guazzaloca G, et al: Activation of blood coagulation after abrupt or stepwise withdrawal of oral anticoagulants: A prospective study. *Thromb Haemost* 72:222, 1994.

44. Grip L, Blombäck M, Schulman S: Hypercoagulable state and thromboembolism following warfarin withdrawal in post–myocardial-infarction patients. *Eur Heart J* 12:1225, 1991.

45. Quick AJ: On constitution of prothrombin. *Am J Physiol* 140:212, 1943.

46. Owren PA, Aas K: The control of dicumarol therapy and the quantitative determination of prothrombin and proconvertin. *Scand J Clin Lab Invest* 3:201, 1951.

47. Lam-Po-Tang PR, Poller L: Oral anticoagulant therapy and its control: An international survey. *Thromb Diath Haemorrh* 34:419, 1975.

48. Loeliger EA, van den Besselaar AM, Lewis SM: Reliability and clinical impact of the normalization of the prothrombin times in oral anticoagulant control. *Thromb Haemost* 53:148, 1985.

49. Taberner DA, Poller L, Thomson JM, Darby KV: Effect of international sensitivity index (ISI) of thromboplastins on precision of international normalised ratios (INR). *J Clin Pathol* 42:92, 1989.

50. Poggio M, van den Besselaar AMHP, van der Velde EA, Bertina RM: The effect of some instruments for prothrombin time testing on the international sensitivity index (ISI) of two rabbit tissue thromboplastin reagents. *Thromb Haemost* 62:868, 1989.

51. Poller L, Thomson JM, Taberner DA: Effect of automation on prothrombin time test in NEQUAS surveys. *J Clin Pathol* 42:97, 1989.

52. Danielson CF, Davis K, Jones G, Benson J, Arney K, Martin J: Effect of citrate concentration in specimen collection tubes on the international normalized ratio. *Arch Pathol Lab Med* 121:956, 1997.

53. Johnston M, Harrison L, Moffat K, Willan A, Hirsh J: Reliability of the international normalized ratio for monitoring the induction phase of warfarin: Comparison with the prothrombin time ratio. *J Lab Clin Med* 128:214, 1996.

54. Paborski LR, Tate KM, Harris RJ, et al: Purification of recombinant human tissue factor. *Biochemistry* 28:8072, 1989.

55. Rehemtulla A, Pepe M, Edgington TS: High level expression of recombinant human tissue factor in Chinese hamster ovary cells as a human thromboplastin. *Thromb Haemost* 65:521, 1991.

56. Finazzi G, Falanga A, Galli M, Cortelazzo S, Remuzzi A, Barbui T: Recombinant versus high-sensitivity conventional thromboplastin: A randomized clinical study in patients on oral anticoagulation. *Thromb Haemost* 72:804, 1994.

57. Barcellona D, Biondi G, Vannini ML, Marongiu VF: Comparison between recombinant and rabbit thromboplastin in the management of patients on oral anticoagulant therapy. *Thromb Haemost* 75:488, 1996.

58. Solomon HM, Randall JR, Simmons VL: Heparin-induced increase in the international normalized ratio: Responses of 10 commercial thromboplastin reagents. *Am J Clin Pathol* 103:735, 1995.

59. Della Valle P, Crippa L, Safa O, et al: Potential failure of the international normalized ratio (INR) system in the monitoring of oral anticoagulation in patients with lupus anticoagulants. *Ann Med Interne* 147:10, 1996.

60. Moll S, Ortel TL: Monitoring warfarin therapy in patients with lupus anticoagulants. *Ann Intern Med* 127:177, 1997.

61. Dati F, Barthels M, Conard J, et al: Multicenter evaluation of a chromogenic substrate method for photometric detection of prothrombin time. *Thromb Haemost* 58:856, 1987.

62. Kornberg A, Francis CW, Pellegrini VD Jr, Gabriel KR, Marder VJ: Comparison of native prothrombin antigen with the prothrombin time for monitoring oral anticoagulant prophylaxis. *Circulation* 88:454, 1993.

63. Smith KJ, Singaraju C, Smith LF: Factor IX metal ion-dependent antigen assays for measurement of warfarin effect. *Am J Clin Pathol* 87:370, 1987.

64. Haushofer A, Halbmayer WM, Dittel M, Prachar H, Mlczoch J, Fischer M: Course of thrombin activation markers in patients implanted with Palmaz-Schatz stents: First experiences with a post-interventional anticoagulation regimen. *Blood Coagul Fibrinol* 5:697, 1994.

65. Tripodi A, Cattaneo M, Molteni A, Cesana BM, Mannucci PM: Changes of prothrombin fragment 1+2 (F 1+2) as a function of increasing intensity of oral anticoagulation: Considerations on the suitability of F 1+2 to monitor oral anticoagulant treatment. *Thromb Haemost* 79:571, 1998.

66. Anderson DR, Harrison L, Hirsh J: Evaluation of a portable prothrombin time monitor for home use by patients who require long-term oral anticoagulant therapy. *Arch Intern Med* 153:1441, 1993.

67. Ansell JE, Patel N, Ostrovsky D, Nozzolillo E, Peterson AM, Fish L: Long-term patient self-management of oral anticoagulation. *Arch Intern Med* 155:2185, 1995.

68. Hasenkam JM, Kimose HH, Knudsen L, et al: Self management of oral anticoagulant therapy after heart valve replacement. *Eur J Cardiothorac Surg* 11:935, 1997.

69. Massicotte P, Marzinotto V, Vegh P, Adams M, Andrew M: Home monitoring of warfarin therapy in children with a whole blood prothrombin time monitor. *J Pediatr* 127:389, 1995.

70. Pell JP, McIver B, Stuart P, Malone DN, Alcock J: Comparison of anticoagulant control among patients attending general practice and a hospital anticoagulant clinic. *Br J Gen Pract* 43:152, 1993.

71. Vadher BD, Patterson DL, Leaning M: Comparison of oral anticoagulant control by a nurse-practitioner using a computer decision-support system with that by clinicians. *Clin Lab Haematol* 19:203, 1997.

72. Vadher B, Patterson DL, Leaning M: Evaluation of a decision support system for initiation and control of oral anticoagulation in a randomised trial. *Br Med J* 314:1252, 1997.

73. Ageno W, Turpie AGG: A randomized comparison of a computer-based dosing program with a manual system to monitor oral anticoagulant therapy. *Thromb Res* 91:237, 1998.

74. van den Besselaar AM, van der Meer FJ, Gerrits-Drabbe CW: Therapeutic control of oral anticoagulant treatment in The Netherlands. *Am J Clin Pathol* 90:685, 1988.

75. Ansell JE, Hughes R: Evolving models of warfarin management: Anticoagulation clinics, patient self-monitoring, and patient self-management. *Am Heart J* 132:1095, 1996.

76. Chiquette E, Amato MG, Bussey HI: Comparison of an anticoagulation clinic with usual medical care. *Arch Intern Med* 158:1641, 1998.

77. Lee YP, Schommer JC: Effect of a pharmacist-managed anticoagulation clinic on warfarin-related hospital readmissions. *Am J Health Syst Pharm* 53:1580, 1996.

78. Bleske BE, Welage LS, Warren EW, Brown MB, Shea MJ: Variations in prothrombin time and international normalized ratio over 24 hours in warfarin-treated patients. *Pharmacotherapy* 15:709, 1995.

79. Williams JRB, Griffin JP, Parkins A: Effect of concomitantly administered drugs on the control of long-term anticoagulant therapy. *Q J Med* 45:63, 1976.

80. Blickstein D, Shaklai M, Inbal A: Warfarin antagonism by avocado. *Lancet* 337:914, 1991.

81. Kempin SJ: Warfarin resistance caused by broccoli. *N Engl J Med* 308:1229, 1983.

82. Harris JE: Interaction of dietary factors with oral anticoagulants: Review and applications. *J Am Diet Assoc* 95:580, 1995.

83. Wells PS, Holbrook AM, Crowther NR, Hirsh J: Interactions of warfarin with drugs and food. *Ann Intern Med* 121:676, 1994.

84. Sorano GG, Biondi G, Conti M, Mameli G, Licheri D, Marongiu F: Controlled vitamin K content diet for improving the management of poorly controlled anticoagulated patients: A clinical practice proposal. *Haemostasis* 23:77, 1993.

85. Booth SL, Charnley JM, Sadowski JA, Saltzman E, Bovill EG, Cushman M: Dietary vitamin K₁ and stability of oral anticoagulation: Proposal of a diet with constant vitamin K₁ content. *Thromb Haemost* 77:504, 1997.

86. Reynolds JEF: Cardiovascular agents, in Martindale: *The Extra Pharmacopoeia*, 31st ed, p 965. London, Royal Pharmaceutical Society, 1996.

87. Chan TY: Adverse interactions between warfarin and nonsteroidal anti-inflammatory drugs: Mechanisms, clinical significance, and avoidance. *Ann Pharmacother* 29:1274, 1995.

88. Gabb GM: Fatal outcome of interaction between warfarin and a non-steroidal anti-inflammatory drug. *Med J Aust* 164:700, 1996.

89. Hampel H, Berger C, Muller-Spahn F: Modified oral anticoagulant potency in an amitriptyline-treated patient. *Acta Haematol* 96:178, 1996.

90. Tam LS, Chan TY, Leung WK, Critchley JA: Warfarin interactions with Chinese traditional medicines: Danshen and methyl salicylate medicated oil. *Aust NZ J Med* 25:258, 1995.

91. Yu CM, Chan JC, Sanderson JE: Chinese herbs and warfarin potentiation by "danshen." *J Intern Med* 241:337, 1997.

92. Janetzky K, Morreale AP: Probable interaction between warfarin and ginseng. *Am J Health Syst Pharm* 54:692, 1997.

93. Homeida HMA, Bagi IA, McNicholas AM, et al: Coagulation abnormalities and ivermectin. *Lancet* 1:1346, 1988.

94. Fernández MA, Ballesteros S, Aznar J: Oral anticoagulants and insecticides. *Thromb Haemost* 80:724, 1998.

95. Anonymous: ADR reporting in Sweden in 1991. *Bulletin from Swedish Adverse Drug Reaction Advisory Committee* 62:1, 1993.

96. Levine MN, Raskob G, Landefeld S, Hirsh J: Hemorrhagic complications of anticoagulant treatment. *Chest* 108:276S, 1995.

97. Fihn SD, Callahan CM, Martin DC, McDonell MB, Henikoff JG, White RH: The risk for and severity of bleeding complications in elderly patients treated with warfarin: The National Consortium of Anticoagulation Clinics. *Ann Intern Med* 124:970, 1996.

98. White RH, McKittrick T, Takakuwa J, Callahan C, McDonell M, Fihn S: Management and prognosis of life-threatening bleeding during warfarin therapy: National Consortium of Anticoagulation Clinics. *Arch Intern Med* 156:1197, 1996.

99. Schulman S, Granqvist S, Holmström M, et al: The duration of oral anticoagulant therapy after a second episode of venous thromboembolism. *N Engl J Med* 336:393, 1997.

100. Schulman S, Lockner D, Juhlin-Dannfelt A: The duration of oral anticoagulation after deep vein thrombosis: A randomized study. *Acta Med Scand* 217:547, 1985.

101. Anonymous: Optimum duration of anticoagulation for deep-vein thrombosis and pulmonary embolism: Research Committee of the British Thoracic Society. *Lancet* 340:873, 1992.

102. McKenna CJ, Galvin J, McCann HA, Sugrue DD: Risks of long-term oral anticoagulation in a non-trial medical environment. *Ir Med J* 89:144, 1996.

103. Choudari CP, Rajgopal C, Palmer KR: Acute gastrointestinal haemorrhage in anticoagulated patients: Diagnoses and response to endoscopic treatment. *Gut* 35:464, 1994.

104. Norton SA, Armstrong CP: Lower gastrointestinal bleeding during anticoagulant therapy: A life-saving complication? *Ann R Coll Surg Engl* 79:38, 1997.

105. Euhus DM, Hiatt JR: Management of the acute abdomen complicating oral anticoagulation therapy. *Am Surg* 56:581, 1990.

106. Landefeld CS, Goldman L: Major bleeding in outpatients treated with warfarin: Incidence and prediction by factors known at the start of outpatient therapy. *Am J Med* 87:144, 1989.

107. Mathiesen T, Benediktsdottir K, Johnsson H, Lindqvist M, von Holst H: Intracranial traumatic and non-traumatic haemorrhagic complications of warfarin treatment. *Acta Neurol Scand* 91:208, 1995.

108. Hylek EM, Singer DE: Risk factors for intracranial hemorrhage in outpatients taking warfarin. *Ann Intern Med* 120:897, 1994.

109. Ernestus RI, Speder B, Pakos P, Hildebrandt G, Klug N: Intracerebral hemorrhage during treatment with oral anticoagulants: Risk factors, therapy and prognosis. *Zentralbl Neurochir* 55:24, 1994.

110. Saab M, Gray A, Hodgkinson D, Irfan M: Warfarin and the apparent minor head injury. *J Accid Emerg Med* 13:208, 1996.

111. Alberty-Ryöppy A, Juntunen J, Salmi T: Femoral neuropathy following anticoagulant therapy for "economy class syndrome" in a young woman. *Acta Chir Scand* 151:643, 1985.

112. Davison BL, Kosmatka PK, Ferlic RJ: Acute radial nerve compression following routine venipuncture in an anticoagulated patient. *Am J Orthop* 25:712, 1996.

113. Bindiger A, Zelnik J, Kuschner S, Gellman H: Spontaneous acute carpal tunnel syndrome in an anticoagulated patient. *Bull Hosp Jt Dis* 54:52, 1995.

114. McKenney MG, Fietsam R Jr, Glover JL, Villalba M: Spermatic cord hematoma: Case report and literature review. *Am Surg* 62:768, 1996.

115. Maingi M, Glynn MF, Scully HE, Graham AF, Floras JS: Spontaneous spinal epidural hematoma in a patient with a mechanical aortic valve taking warfarin. *Can J Cardiol* 11:429, 1995.

116. Edwards P: Massive choroidal hemorrhage in age-related macular degeneration: a complication of anticoagulant therapy. *J Am Optom Assoc* 67:223, 1996.

117. Hart RG, Boop BS, Anderson DC: Oral anticoagulants and intracranial hemorrhage: Facts and hypotheses. *Stroke* 26:1471, 1995.

118. Brännström M, Jansson JH, Boman K, Nilsson TK: Endothelial haemostatic factors may be associated with mortality in patients on long-term anticoagulant treatment. *Thromb Haemost* 74:612, 1995.

119. Jansson JH, Boman K, Brännström M, Nilsson TK: High concentration of thrombomodulin in plasma is associated with hemorrhage. *Circulation* 96:2938, 1997.

120. Chu K, Wu SM, Stanley T, Stafford DW, High KA: A mutation in the propeptide of factor IX leads to warfarin sensitivity by a novel mechanism. *J Clin Invest* 98:1619, 1996.

121. Oldenburg J, Quenzel EM, Harbrecht U, et al: Missense mutations at ALA-10 in the factor IX propeptide: An insignificant variant in normal life but a decisive cause of bleeding during oral anticoagulant therapy. *Br J Haematol* 98:240, 1997.

122. Aithal GP, Day CP, Kesteven PJL, Daly AK: Association of polymorphisms in the cytochrome P₄₅₀ CYP2C9 with warfarin dose requirement and risk of bleeding complications. *Lancet* 353:717, 1999.

123. Makris M, Greaves M, Phillips WS, Kitchen S, Rosendaal FR, Preston EF: Emergency oral anticoagulant reversal: The relative efficacy of infusions of fresh frozen plasma and clotting factor concentrate on correction of the coagulopathy. *Thromb Haemost* 77:477, 1997.

124. Srinivasan V, Patel H, John DG, Worsley A: Warfarin and epistaxis: Should warfarin always be discontinued? *Clin Otolaryngol* 22:542, 1997.

125. Shetty HG, Backhouse G, Bentley DP, Routledge PA: Effective reversal of warfarin-induced excessive anticoagulation with low dose vitamin K₁. *Thromb Haemost* 67:13, 1992.

126. O'Reilly RA, Kearns P: Intravenous vitamin K₁ injections: Dangerous prophylaxis. *Arch Intern Med* 155:2127, 1995.

127. Fetrow CW, Overlock T, Leff L: Antagonism of warfarin-induced hypoprothrombinemia with use of low-dose subcutaneous vitamin K₁. *J Clin Pharmacol* 37:751, 1997.

128. Crowther MA, Donovan D, Harrison L, McGinnis J, Ginsberg J: Low-dose oral vitamin K reliably reverses over-anticoagulation due to warfarin. *Thromb Haemost* 79:1116, 1998.

129. Pengo V, Banzato A, Garelli E, Zasso A, Biasiolo A: Reversal of excessive effect of regular anticoagulation: Low oral dose of phytonadione (vitamin K₁) compared with warfarin discontinuation. *Blood Coagul Fibrinol* 4:739, 1993.

130. Weibert RT, Le DT, Kayser SR, Rapaport SI: Correction of excessive anticoagulation with low-dose oral vitamin K₁. *Ann Intern Med* 126:959, 1997.

131. Flood EP, Redish MH, Bociek SJ: Case report: Thrombophlebitis migrans disseminata: Report of a case in which gangrene of a breast occurred. *NY State J Med* 43:1121, 1943.

132. Gallerani M, Manfredini R, Moratelli S: Non-haemorrhagic adverse reactions of oral anticoagulant therapy. *Int J Cardiol* 49:1, 1995.

133. Sallah S, Thomas DP, Roberts HR: Warfarin and heparin-induced skin necrosis and the purple toe syndrome: Infrequent complications of anticoagulant treatment. *Thromb Haemost* 78:785, 1997.

134. Miura Y, Ardenghy M, Ramasastry S, Kovach R, Hochberg J: Coumadin necrosis of the skin: Report of four patients. *Ann Plast Surg* 37:332, 1996.

135. Colman RW, Rao AK, Rubin RN: Warfarin skin necrosis in a 33-year-old woman. *Am J Hematol* 43:300, 1993.

136. van Amstel WJ, Boekhout-Mussert MJ, Loeliger EA: Successful prevention of skin necrosis by timely administration of vitamin K. *Blut* 36:89, 1978.

137. Jillella AP, Lutcher CL: Reinstituting warfarin in patients who develop warfarin skin necrosis. *Am J Hematol* 52:117, 1996.

138. Feder W, Auerbach R: ''Purple toes'': An uncommon sequela of oral coumarin drug therapy. *Ann Intern Med* 55:911, 1961.

139. Antony SJ, Krick SK, Mehta PM: Unusual cutaneous adverse reaction to warfarin therapy. *South Med J* 86:1413, 1993.

140. Grosset AB, Allen JE, Rodgers GM: Anticoagulation with anisindione in patients who are intolerant of warfarin. *Am J Hematol* 46:138, 1994.

141. Kuwahara T, Hamada M, Inoue Y, Aono S, Hiwada K: Warfarin-induced eosinophilic pleurisy. *Intern Med* 34:794, 1995.

142. Krahn MJ, Pettigrew NM, Cuddy TE: Unusual side effects due to warfarin. *Can J Cardiol* 14:90, 1998.

143. Hautekeete M, Holvoet J, Hubens H: Cytolytic hepatitis related to the oral anticoagulant phenprocoumon. *Gastroenterol Clin Biol* 19:223, 1995.

144. Hohler T, Schnutgen M, Helmreich-Becker I, Mayet WJ, Mayer zum Buschenfelde KH: Drug-induced hepatitis: A rare complication of oral anticoagulants. *J Hepatol* 21:447, 1994.

145. Jones DB, Makepeace MC, Smith PM: Jaundice following warfarin therapy. *Postgrad Med J* 56:671, 1980.

146. Rehnqvist N: Intrahepatic jaundice due to warfarin therapy. *Acta Med Scand* 204:335, 1978.

147. Jie K-SG, Gijsbers BLMG, Knapen MHJ, Hamulák K, Frank HL, Vermeer C: Effects of vitamin K and oral anticoagulants on urinary calcium excretion. *Br J Haematol* 83:100, 1993.

148. Sato Y, Honda Y, Kunoh H, Oizumi K: Long-term oral anticoagulation reduces bone mass in patients with previous hemispheric infarction and nonrheumatic atrial fibrillation. *Stroke* 28:2390, 1997.

149. Lafforgue P, Daver L, Monties JR, Chagnaud C, de Boissezon MC, Acquaviva PC: Bone mineral density in patients given oral vitamin K antagonists. *Rev Rhum Engl Ed* 64:249, 1997.

150. Philip WJ, Martin JC, Richardson JM, Reid DM, Webster J, Douglas AS: Decreased axial and peripheral bone density in patients taking long-term warfarin. *Q J Med* 88:635, 1995.

151. Jamal SA, Browner WS, Bauer DC, Cummings SR: Warfarin use and risk for osteoporosis in elderly women: Study of Osteoporotic Fractures Research Group. *Ann Intern Med* 128:829, 1998.

152. Worcester EM, Sebastian JL, Hiatt JG, Beshensky AM, Sadowski JA: The effect of warfarin on urine calcium oxalate crystal growth inhibition and urinary excretion of calcium and nephrocalcin. *Calcif Tissue Int* 53:242, 1993.

153. Stevenson RE, Burton OM, Ferlauto GJ, Taylor HA: Hazards of oral anticoagulants during pregnancy. *JAMA* 243:1549, 1980.

154. Ginsberg JS, Hirsh J, Turner DC, Levine MN, Burrows R: Risk to the fetus of anticoagulant therapy during pregnancy. *Thromb Haemost* 61:197, 1989.

155. Iturbe-Alessio I, Del Carmen Fonseca M, Mutchinik O, Santos MA, Zajarias A, Salazar E: Risks of anticoagulant therapy in pregnant women with artificial heart valves. *N Engl J Med* 315:1390, 1986.

156. Sbarouni E, Oakley CM: Outcome of pregnancy in women with valve prostheses. *Br Heart J* 71:196, 1994.

157. Lécuru F, Desnos M, Taurelle R: Anticoagulant therapy in pregnancy: Report of 54 cases. *Acta Obstet Gynecol Scand* 75:217, 1996.

158. Wong V, Cheng CH, Chan KC: Fetal and neonatal outcome of exposure to anticoagulants during pregnancy. *Am J Med Genet* 45:17, 1993.

159. Menger H, Lin AE, Toriello HV, Bernert G, Spranger JW: Vitamin K deficiency embryopathy: A phenocopy of the warfarin embryopathy due to a disorder of embryonic vitamin K metabolism. *Am J Med Genet* 72:129, 1997.

160. Brenner B, Sanchez-Vega B, Wu SM, Lanir N, Stafford DW, Solera J: A missense mutation in gamma-glutamyl carboxylase gene causes combined deficiency of all vitamin K–dependent blood coagulation factors. *Blood* 92:4554, 1998.

161. Franco B, Meroni G, Parenti G, et al: A cluster of sulfatase genes on Xp22.3: Mutations in chondrodysplasia punctata (CDPX) and implications for warfarin embryopathy. *Cell* 81:15, 1995.

162. Salazar E, Izaguirre R, Verdejo J, Mutchinick O: Failure of adjusted doses of subcutaneous heparin to prevent thromboembolic phenomena in pregnant patients with mechanical cardiac valve prostheses. *J Am Coll Cardiol* 27:1698, 1996.

163. Orme MLE, Lewis PJ, de Swiet M, et al: May mothers given warfarin breast-feed their children? *Br Med J* 1:1564, 1977.

164. Otley CC, Fewkes JL, Frank W, Olbricht SM: Complications of cutaneous surgery in patients who are taking warfarin, aspirin, or nonsteroidal anti-inflammatory drugs. *Arch Dermatol* 132:161, 1996.

165. Billingsley EM, Maloney ME: Intraoperative and postoperative bleeding problems in patients taking warfarin, aspirin, and nonsteroidal anti-inflammatory agents: A prospective study. *Dermatol Surg* 23:381, 1997.

166. Raj G, Kumar R, McKinney WP: Safety of intramuscular influenza immunization among patients receiving long-term warfarin anticoagulation therapy. *Arch Intern Med* 155:1529, 1995.

167. Thumboo J, O'Duffy JD: A prospective study of the safety of joint and soft tissue aspirations and injections in patients taking warfarin sodium. *Arthritis Rheum* 41:736, 1998.

168. Goldstein DJ, Losquadro W, Spotnitz HM: Outpatient pacemaker procedures in orally anticoagulated patients. *Pacing Clin Electrophysiol* 21:1730, 1998.

169. Borea G, Montebugnoli L, Capuzzi P, Magelli C: Tranexamic-acid as a mouthwash in anticoagulant-treated patients undergoing oral surgery: An alternative method to discontinuing anticoagulant therapy. *Oral Surg Oral Med Oral Pathol* 75:29, 1993.

170. Ramström G, Sindet-Pedersen S, Hall G, Blombäck M, Älander U: Prevention of postsurgical bleeding in oral surgery using tranexamic acid without dose modification of oral anticoagulants. *J Oral Maxillofac Surg* 51:1211, 1993.

171. Souto JC, Oliver A, Zuazu-Jausoro I, Vives A, Fontcuberta J: Oral surgery in anticoagulated patients without reducing the dose of oral anticoagulant: A prospective randomized study. *J Oral Maxillofac Surg* 54:27, 1996.

172. Saour JN, Ali HA, Mammo LA, Sieck JO: Dental procedures in patients receiving oral anticoagulation therapy. *J Heart Valve Dis* 3:315, 1994.

173. Kingston TE, Nonnenmacher AK, Crowe H, Costello AJ, Street A: Further evaluation of transurethral laser ablation of the prostate in patients treated with anticoagulant therapy. *Aust NZ J Surg* 65:40, 1995.

174. Bolton DM, Costello AJ: Management of benign prostatic hyperplasia by transurethral laser ablation in patients treated with warfarin anticoagulation. *J Urol* 151:79, 1994.

175. Dietrich W, Dilthey G, Spannagl M, Richter JA: Warfarin pretreatment does not lead to increased bleeding tendency during cardiac surgery. *J Cardiothorac Vasc Anesth* 9:250, 1995.

176. White RH, McKittrick T, Hutchinson R, Twitchell J: Temporary discontinuation of warfarin therapy: changes in the International Normalized Ratio. *Ann Intern Med* 122:40, 1995.

177. Kearon C, Hirsh J: Management of anticoagulation before and after elective surgery. *N Engl J Med* 336:1506, 1997.

178. Cannegieter SC, Rosendaal FR, Briët E: Thromboembolic and bleeding complications in patients with mechanical heart valve prostheses. *Circulation* 89:635, 1994.

179. Katholi RE, Nolan SP, McGuire LB: Living with prosthetic heart valves: Subsequent noncardiac operations and the risk of thromboembolism or hemorrhage. *Am Heart J* 92:162, 1976.

180. Vigano D'Angelo S, Tsoureli E, Crippa L, Tomassini L, D'Angelo A: Prevalence of hemorrhagic and thrombotic complications in patients requiring oral anticoagulation and submitted to elective surgery: A study of 197 consecutive patients. *Thromb Res* 91(suppl 1):S100, 1998.

181. Chakravarti A, MacDermott S: Transurethral resection of the prostate in the anticoagulated patient. *Br J Urol* 81:520, 1998.

182. Kuntze CE, Ebels T, Eijgelaar A, Homan van der Heide JN: Rates of thromboembolism with three different mechanical heart valve prostheses: A randomised study. *Lancet* 8637:514, 1989.

183. Cannegieter SC, Rosendaal FR, Wintzen AR, van der Meer FJM, Vandenbroucke JP, Briët E: Optimal oral anticoagulant therapy in patients with mechanical heart valves. *N Engl J Med* 333:11, 1995.

184. Butchart EG, Moreno de la Santa P, Rooney SJ, Lewis PA: Arterial risk factors and ischemic cerebrovascular events after aortic valve replacement. *J Heart Valve Dis* 4:1, 1995.

185. Burchfiel CM, Hammermeister KE, Krause-Steinrauf H, et al: Left atrial

dimension and risk of systemic embolism in patients with a prosthetic heart valve. *J Am Coll Cardiol* 15:32, 1990.

186. Acar J, Iung B, Boissel JP, et al: AREVA: Multicenter randomized comparison of low-dose versus standard-dose anticoagulation in patients with mechanical prosthetic heart valves. *Circulation* 94:2107, 1996.

187. Scudicky D, Essop MR, Wisenbaugh T, et al: Frequency of prosthetic valve-related complications with very low level warfarin anticoagulation combined with dipyridamole after valve replacement using St. Jude Medical prosthesis. *Am J Cardiol* 74:1137, 1994.

188. Hayashi J, Nakazawa S, Oguma F, Miyamura H, Eguchi S: Combined warfarin and antiplatelet therapy after St. Jude Medical valve replacement for mitral valve disease. *J Am Coll Cardiol* 23:672, 1994.

189. Yamak B, Sener E, Kiziltepes U, et al: Low dose anticoagulation after St. Jude Medical prosthesis implantation in patients under 18 years of age. *J Heart Valve Dis* 4:274, 1995.

190. Kontozis L, Skudicky D, Hopley MJ, Sareli P: Long-term follow-up of St. Jude Medical prosthesis in a young rheumatic population using low-level warfarin anticoagulation: An analysis of the temporal distribution of causes of death. *Am J Cardiol* 81:736, 1998.

191. Cappelleri JC, Fiore LD, Brophy MT, Deykin D, Lau J: Efficacy and safety of combined anticoagulant and antiplatelet therapy versus anticoagulant monotherapy after mechanical heart-valve replacement: A meta-analysis. *Am Heart J* 130:547, 1995.

192. Loewen P, Sunderji R, Gin K: The efficacy and safety of combination warfarin and ASA therapy: A systematic review of the literature and update of guidelines. *Can J Cardiol* 14:717, 1998.

193. Turpie AGG: Antithrombotic therapy following heart valve replacement. *Thromb Haemost* 77:382, 1997.

194. Koefoed BG, Gulløv AL, Petersen P: Prevention of thromboembolic events in atrial fibrillation. *Thromb Haemost* 78:377, 1997.

195. Risk factors for stroke and efficacy of antithrombotic therapy in atrial fibrillation: Analysis of pooled data from five randomized controlled trials. *Arch Intern Med* 154:1449, 1994.

196. Koefoed BG, Feddersen C, Gulløv AL, Petersen P: Effect of fixed minidose warfarin, conventional dose warfarin and aspirin on INR and prothrombin fragment 1+2 in patients with atrial fibrillation. *Thromb Haemost* 77:845, 1997.

197. Lip GY, Lip PL, Zarifis J, et al: Fibrin D-dimer and beta-thromboglobulin as markers of thrombogenesis and platelet activation in atrial fibrillation: Effects of introducing ultra-low-dose warfarin and aspirin. *Circulation* 94:425, 1996.

198. Gulløv AL, Koefoed BG, Petersen P, et al: Fixed minidose warfarin and aspirin alone and in combination vs adjusted-dose warfarin for stroke prevention in atrial fibrillation: Second Copenhagen Atrial Fibrillation, Aspirin, and Anticoagulation Study. *Arch Intern Med* 158:1513, 1998.

199. Collins LJ, Silverman DI, Douglas PS, Manning WJ: Cardioversion of nonrheumatic atrial fibrillation: Reduced thromboembolic complications with 4 weeks of precardioversion anticoagulation are related to atrial thrombus resolution. *Circulation* 92:160, 1995.

200. Petersen P: Thromboembolic complications in atrial fibrillation. *Stroke* 21:4, 1990.

201. Grimm RA, Stewart WJ, Maloney JD: Impact of electrical cardioversion for atrial fibrillation on left atrial appendage function and spontaneous echo contrast: Characterisation by simultaneous transoesophageal echocardiography. *J Am Coll Cardiol* 22:1359, 1993.

202. Laupacis A, Albers G, Dalen J, Dunn M, Feinberg W, Jacobsen A: Antithrombotic therapy in atrial fibrillation: 4th ACCP Consensus Conference on Antithrombotic Therapy. *Chest* 108:352S, 1995.

203. Mayet J, Wasan B, Sutton GC: Cardioversion of atrial arrhythmias: Audit of anticoagulation management. *J R Coll Physicians Lond* 31:313, 1997.

204. Stroke Prevention in Reversible Ischemia Trial (SPIRIT) Study Group: A randomized trial of anticoagulants versus aspirin after cerebral ischemia of presumed arterial origin. *Ann Neurol* 42:857, 1997.

205. Dressler FA, Craig WR, Castello R, Labovitz AJ: Mobile aortic atheroma and systemic emboli: Efficacy of anticoagulation and influence of plaque morphology on recurrent stroke. *J Am Coll Cardiol* 31:134, 1998.

206. EAFT (European Atrial Fibrillation Trial) Study Group: Secondary prevention in non-rheumatic atrial fibrillation after transient ischaemic attack or minor stroke. *Lancet* 342:1255, 1993.

207. Morocutti C, Amabile G, Fattapposta F, et al: Indobufen versus warfarin in the secondary prevention of major vascular events in nonrheumatic

atrial fibrillation: SIFA (Studio Italiano Fibrillazione Atriale) Investigators. *Stroke* 28:1015, 1997.

208. Medical Research Council's General Practice Research Framework: Thrombosis prevention trial: Randomised trial of low-intensity oral anticoagulation with warfarin and low-dose aspirin in the primary prevention of ischaemic heart disease in men at increased risk. *Lancet* 351:233, 1998.

209. Williams MJ, Morison IM, Parker JH, Stewart RA: Progression of the culprit lesion in unstable coronary artery disease with warfarin and aspirin versus aspirin alone: Preliminary study. *J Am Coll Cardiol* 30:364, 1997.

210. van der Meer J, Hillege HL, Kootstra GJ, et al: Prevention of one-year vein-graft occlusion after aortocoronary-bypass surgery: A comparison of low-dose aspirin, low-dose aspirin plus dipyridamole, and oral anticoagulants, the CABADAS Research Group of the Interuniversity Cardiology Institute of The Netherlands. *Lancet* 342:257, 1993.

211. Post Coronary Artery Bypass Graft Trial Investigators: The effect of aggressive lowering of low-density lipoprotein cholesterol levels and low-dose anticoagulation on obstructive changes in saphenous-vein coronary-artery bypass grafts. *N Engl J Med* 336:153, 1997.

212. Mehta RH, Eagle KA: Secondary prevention in acute myocardial infarction. *Br Med J* 316:838, 1998.

213. Yusuf S, Michaelis W, Hua A, et al: Effects of oral anticoagulants on mortality, reinfarction and stroke after myocardial infarction [abstr]. *Circulation* (suppl):343, 1995.

214. Azar AJ, Cannegieter SC, Deckers JW, et al: Optimal intensity of oral anticoagulant therapy after myocardial infarction. *J Am Coll Cardiol* 27:1349, 1996.

215. Julian DG, Chamberlain DA, Pocock SJ: A comparison of aspirin and anticoagulation following thrombolysis for myocardial infarction (the AFTER study): A multicentre unblinded randomised clinical trial. *Br Med J* 313:1429, 1996.

216. Coumadin Aspirin Reinfarction Study (CARS): Randomised double-blind trial of fixed low-dose warfarin with aspirin after myocardial infarction. *Lancet* 350:389, 1997.

217. Al-Khadra AS, Salem DN, Rand WM, Udelson JE, Smith JJ, Konstam MA: Warfarin anticoagulation and survival: A cohort analysis from the Studies of Left Ventricular Dysfunction. *J Am Coll Cardiol* 31:749, 1998.

218. Cheng JW, Spinler SA: Should all patients with dilated cardiomyopathy receive chronic anticoagulation? *Ann Pharmacother* 28:604, 1994.

219. Schneider E, Brunner U, Bollinger A: Medikamentose rezidivprophylaxe nach femoropopliitealer arterienrekonstruktion. *Angio* 2:73, 1979.

220. De Smit P, van Urk H: Dutch oral anticoagulation trial. *Acta Chir Austr* 24:5, 1992.

221. Kretschmer G, Herbst F, Prager M, et al: A decade of oral anticoagulant treatment to maintain autologous vein grafts for femoropopliteal atherosclerosis. *Arch Surg* 127:1112, 1992.

222. Antiplatelet Trialist's Collaboration: Collaborative overview of randomised trials of antiplatelet therapy: II. Maintenance of vascular graft or arterial patency by antiplatelet therapy. *Br Med J* 308:159, 1994.

223. Do DD, Mahler F: Low-dose aspirin combined with dipyridamole versus anticoagulants after femoropopliteal percutaneous transluminal angioplasty. *Radiology* 193:567, 1994.

224. Fordyce MJ, Baker AS, Staddon GE: Efficacy of fixed minidose warfarin prophylaxis in total hip replacement. *Br Med J* 303:219, 1991.

225. Lotke PA, Palevsky H, Keenan AM, et al: Aspirin and warfarin for thromboembolic disease after total joint arthroplasty. *Clin Orthop* (324):251, 1996.

226. Lieberman JR, Sung R, Dorey F, Thomas BJ, Kilgus DJ, Finerman GA: Low-dose warfarin prophylaxis to prevent symptomatic pulmonary embolism after total knee arthroplasty. *J Arthroplasty* 12:180, 1997.

227. Vresilovic EJ Jr, Hozack WJ, Booth RE, Rothman RH: Incidence of pulmonary embolism after total knee arthroplasty with low-dose coumadin prophylaxis. *Clin Orthop* (286):27, 1993.

228. Hull R, Raskob G, Pineo G, et al: A comparison of subcutaneous low-molecular-weight heparin with warfarin sodium for prophylaxis against deep-vein thrombosis after hip or knee implantation. *N Engl J Med* 329:1370, 1993.

229. RD Heparin Arthroplasty Group: RD heparin compared with warfarin for prevention of venous thromboembolic disease following total hip or knee arthroplasty. *J Bone Joint Surg Am* 76:1174, 1994.

230. Leclerc JR, Geerts WH, Desjardins L, et al: Prevention of venous throm-

boembolism after knee arthroplasty: A randomized, double-blind trial comparing enoxaparin with warfarin. *Ann Intern Med* 124:619, 1996.

231. Heit JA, Berkowitz SD, Bona R, et al: Efficacy and safety of low molecular weight heparin (ardeparin sodium) compared to warfarin for the prevention of venous thromboembolism after total knee replacement surgery: A double-blind, dose-ranging study, Ardeparin Arthroplasty Study Group. *Thromb Haemost* 77:32, 1997.

232. Francis CW, Pellegrini VD Jr, Totterman S, et al: Prevention of deep-vein thrombosis after total hip arthroplasty: Comparison of warfarin and dalteparin. *J Bone Joint Surg Am* 79:1365, 1997.

233. Palmer AJ, Koppenhagen K, Kirchhof B, Weber U, Bergemann R: Efficacy and safety of low molecular weight heparin, unfractionated heparin and warfarin for thrombo-embolism prophylaxis in orthopaedic surgery: A meta-analysis of randomised clinical trials. *Haemostasis* 27:75, 1997.

234. Menzin J, Colditz GA, Regan MM, Richner RE, Oster G: Cost-effectiveness of enoxaparin vs low-dose warfarin in the prevention of deep-vein thrombosis after total hip replacement surgery. *Arch Intern Med* 155:757, 1995.

235. O'Brien BJ, Anderson DR, Goeree R: Cost-effectiveness of enoxaparin versus warfarin prophylaxis against deep-vein thrombosis after total hip replacement. *Can Med Ass J* 150:1083, 1994.

236. Garcia-Zozaya I: Warfarin vs enoxaparin for deep venous thrombosis prophylaxis after total hip and total knee arthroplasty: A cost comparison. *J Ky Med Assoc* 96:143, 1998.

237. Hawkins DW, Langley PC, Krueger KP: A pharmacoeconomic assessment of enoxaparin and warfarin as prophylaxis for deep vein thrombosis in patients undergoing knee replacement surgery. *Clin Ther* 20:182, 1998.

238. Francis CW, Pellegrini VD Jr, Leibert KM, et al: Comparison of two warfarin regimens in the prevention of venous thrombosis following total knee replacement. *Thromb Haemost* 75:706, 1996.

239. Fishmann AJ, Greeno RA, Brooks LR, Matta JM: Prevention of deep vein thrombosis and pulmonary embolism in acetabular and pelvic fracture surgery. *Clin Orthop* 305:133, 1994.

240. Wilson MG, Pei LF, Malone KM, Polak JF, Creager MA, Goldhaber SZ: Fixed low-dose versus adjusted higher-dose warfarin following orthopedic surgery: A randomized prospective trial. *J Arthroplasty* 9:127, 1994.

241. Poller L, McKernan A, Thomson JM, Elstein M, Hirsch PJ, Jones JB: Fixed minidose warfarin: A new approach to prophylaxis against venous thrombosis after major surgery. *Br Med J* 295:1309, 1987.

242. Bern MM, Lokich JJ, Wallach SR, et al: Very low doses of warfarin can prevent thrombosis in central venous catheters: A randomized prospective trial. *Ann Intern Med* 112:423, 1990.

243. Veerabagu MP, Tuttle-Newhall J, Maliakkal R, Champagne C, Mascioli EA: Warfarin and reduced central venous thrombosis in home total parenteral nutrition patients. *Nutrition* 11:142, 1995.

244. Bona RD, Sivjee KY, Hickey AD, Wallace DM, Wajcs SB: The efficacy and safety of oral anticoagulation in patients with cancer. *Thromb Haemost* 74:1055, 1995.

245. Bona RD, Hickey AD, Wallace DM: Efficacy and safety of oral anticoagulation in patients with cancer. *Thromb Haemost* 78:137, 1997.

246. Levine M, Hirsh J, Gent M, et al: Double-blind randomised trial of a very-low-dose warfarin for prevention of thromboembolism in stage IV breast cancer. *Lancet* 343:886, 1994.

247. Sarasin FP, Schifferli JA: Prophylactic oral anticoagulation in nephrotic patients with idiopathic membranous nephropathy. *Kidney Int* 45:578, 1994.

248. Hull R, Hirsh J, Jay R, et al: Different intensities of oral anticoagulant therapy in the treatment of proximal-vein thrombosis. *N Engl J Med* 307:1676, 1982.

249. Hull RD, Raskob GE, Rosenbloom D, et al: Optimal therapeutic level of heparin therapy in patients with venous thrombosis. *Arch Intern Med* 152:1589, 1992.

250. Kearon C, Gent M, Hirsh J, et al: A comparison of three months of anticoagulation with extended anticoagulation for a first episode of idiopathic venous thromboembolism. *N Engl J Med* 340:901, 1999.

251. Schulman S, Rhedin AS, Lindmarker P, et al: A comparison of six weeks with six months of oral anticoagulant therapy after a first episode of venous thromboembolism: Duration of Anticoagulation Trial Study Group. *N Engl J Med* 332:1661, 1995.

252. Schulman S, Svenungsson E, Granqvist S, Duration of Anticoagulation Trial Study Group: The predictive value of anticardiolipin antibodies in patients with venous thromboembolism. *Am J Med* 104: 332, 1998.

253. Rosove MH, Brewer PM: Antiphospholipid thrombosis: Clinical course after the first thrombotic event in 70 patients. *Ann Intern Med* 117:303, 1992.

254. Khamashta MA, Cuadrado MJ, Mujic F, Taub NA, Hunt BJ, Hughes GR: The management of thrombosis in the antiphospholipid-antibody syndrome. *N Engl J Med* 332:993, 1995.

255. Schulman S: Optimal duration of oral anticoagulant therapy in venous thromboembolism. *Thromb Haemost* 78:693, 1997.

256. Pabinger I, Schneider B: Thrombotic risk in hereditary antithrombin III, protein C, or protein S deficiency: A cooperative, retrospective study. *Arterioscler Thromb Vasc Biol* 16:742, 1996.

257. Eichinger S, Stümpflen A, Hirschl M, et al: Hyperhomocysteinemia is a risk factor of recurrent venous thromboembolism. *Thromb Haemost* 80:566, 1998.

258. Frank H, Mlczoch J, Huber K, Schuster E, Gurtner HP, Kneussl M: The effect of anticoagulant therapy in primary and anorectic drug-induced pulmonary hypertension. *Chest* 112:714, 1997.

259. Suresh CG, Neal D, Coupe MO: Warfarin treatment and migraine. *Postgrad Med J* 70:37, 1994.

260. Yoshida S, Torikai K: The effects of warfarin on calcinosis in a patient with systemic sclerosis. *J Rheumatol* 20:1233, 1993.

261. Zacharski LR, Henderson WG, Rickles FR, et al: Effect of warfarin on survival in small cell carcinoma of the lung. *JAMA* 245:831, 1980.

262. Maurer LH, Herndon JE, Hollis DR, et al: Randomized trial of chemotherapy and radiation therapy with or without warfarin for limited-stage small-cell lung cancer: A Cancer and Leukemia Group B study. *J Clin Oncol* 15:3378, 1997.

263. Carpi A, Sagripanti A, Poddighe R, Gherarducci G, Nicolini A: Cancer incidence and mortality in patients with heart disease: Effect of oral anticoagulant therapy. *Am J Clin Oncol* 18:15, 1995.

264. Kerr JS, Li HY, Wexler RS, et al: The characterization of potent novel warfarin analogs. *Thromb Res* 88:127, 1997.

265. Leone-Bay A, Paton DR, Freeman J, et al: Synthesis and evaluation of compound that facilitate the gastrointestinal absorption of heparin. *J Medic Chem* 41:1163, 1998.

266. Pinto A, Corrao S, Galati D, et al: Sulodexide versus calcium heparin in the medium-term treatment of deep vein thrombosis of the lower limbs. *Angiology* 48:805, 1997.

267. Harenberg J: Review of pharmacodynamics, pharmacokinetics, and therapeutic properties of sulodexide. *Med Res Rev* 18:1, 1998.

268. Zawilska K, Elikowski W, Turowiecka Z, et al: On the action of a heparan-like glycosaminoglycan (Hemovasal) on the mechanism of haemostasis and fibrinolysis. *Thromb Res* 78:211, 1995.

269. Sato K, Kawasaki T, Hisamichi N, et al: Antithrombotic effects of YM-60828 in three thrombosis models in guinea pigs. *Eur J Pharmacol* 350:87, 1998.

270. Morishima Y, Tanabe K, Terada Y, Hara T, Kunitada S: Antithrombotic and hemorrhagic effects of DX-9065a, a direct and selective factor Xa inhibitor: Comparison with a direct thrombin inhibitor and antithrombin III-dependent anticoagulants. *Thromb Haemost* 78:1366, 1997.

271. Lee K, Hwang SY, Hong S, et al: Structural modification of an orally active thrombin inhibitor, LB30057: Replacement of the D-pocket-binding naphthyl moiety. *Bioorg Med Chem* 6:869, 1998.

272. Mehta JL, Chen L, Nichols WW, Mattsson C, Gustafsson D, Saldeen TG: Melagatran, an oral active-site inhibitor of thrombin, prevents or delays formation of electrically induced occlusive thrombus in the canine coronary artery. *J Cardiovasc Pharmacol* 31:345, 1998.

273. Rebello SS, Miller BV, Basler GC, Lucchesi BR: CVS-1123, a direct thrombin inhibitor, prevents occlusive arterial and venous thrombosis in a canine model of vascular injury. *J Cardiovasc Pharmacol* 29:240, 1997.

274. Bajusz S, Barabas E, Fauszt I, et al: Active site-directed thrombin inhibitors: Alpha-hydroxyacyl-prolyl-arginals, new orally active stable analogues of D-Phe-Pro-Arg-H. *Semin Thromb Hemost* 22:243, 1996.

275. Eriksson BI, Carlsson S, Halvarsson M, Risberg B, Mattsson C: Antithrombotic effect of two low molecular weight thrombin inhibitors and a low-molecular weight heparin in a caval vein thrombosis model in the rat. *Thromb Haemost* 78:1404, 1997.

276. Lundström T, Rydén L: Haemorrhagic and thromboembolic complica-

tions in patients with atrial fibrillation on anticoagulant prophylaxis. *J Intern Med* 225:137, 1989.

277. Hurlen M, Erikssen J, Smith P, Arnesen H, Rollag A: Comparison of bleeding complications of warfarin and warfarin plus acetylsalicylic acid: A study in 3166 outpatients. *J Intern Med* 236:299, 1994.

278. Palareti G, Leali N, Coccheri S, et al: Bleeding complications of oral anticoagulant treatment: An inception-cohort, prospective collaborative study (ISCOAT), Italian Study on Complications of Oral Anticoagulant Therapy. *Lancet* 348:423, 1996.

279. Forfar JC: A 7-year analysis of haemorrhage in patients on long-term anticoagulant treatment. *Br Heart J* 42:128, 1979.

280. Stroke Prevention in Atrial Fibrillation Investigators: Bleeding during antithrombotic therapy in patients with atrial fibrillation. *Arch Intern Med* 156:409, 1996.

281. van der Meer FJ, Rosendaal FR, Vandenbroucke JP, Briet E: Assessment of a bleeding risk index in two cohorts of patients treated with oral anticoagulants. *Thromb Haemost* 76:12, 1996.

282. Isaacs C, Paltiel O, Blake G, Beaudet M, Conochie L, Leclerc J: Age-associated risks of prophylactic anticoagulation in the setting of hip fracture. *Am J Med* 96:487, 1994.

283. Fihn SD, McDonell M, Martin D, et al: Risk factors for complications of chronic anticoagulation: A multicenter study, Warfarin Optimized Outpatient Follow-up Study Group. *Ann Intern Med* 118:511, 1993.

284. O'Neill PA, Crossley D, Taberner DA, Fairweather DS: Safety of anticoagulation in the elderly: Reasons for discontinuing therapy. *Postgrad Med J* 68:824, 1992.

285. Schulman S: Quality of oral anticoagulant control and treatment in Sweden. Duration of Anticoagulation (DURAC) Trial Study Group. *J Intern Med* 236:143, 1994.

286. Levine MN, Raskob G, Hirsh J: Risk of haemorrhage associated with long-term anticoagulant therapy. *Drugs* 30:444, 1985.

287. Petersen P, Boysen G, Godtfredsen J, Andersen ED, Andersen B: Placebo-controlled, randomised trial of warfarin and aspirin for prevention of thromboembolic complications in chronic atrial fibrillation: The Copenhagen AFASAK study. *Lancet* 1:175, 1989.

288. Boston Area Anticoagulation Trial for Atrial Fibrillation Investigators: The effect of low-dose warfarin on the risk of stroke in patients with nonrheumatic atrial fibrillation. *N Engl J Med* 323:1505, 1990.

289. Stroke Prevention in Atrial Fibrillation Study: Final results. *Circulation* 84:527, 1991.

290. Connolly SJ, Laupacis A, Gent M, Roberts RS, Cairns JA, Joyner C: Canadian Atrial Fibrillation Anticoagulation (CAFA) Study. *J Am Coll Cardiol* 18:349, 1991.

291. Ezekowitz MD, Bridgers SL, James KE, et al: Warfarin in the prevention of stroke associated with nonrheumatic atrial fibrillation: Veterans Affairs Stroke Prevention in Nonrheumatic Atrial Fibrillation Investigators. *N Engl J Med* 327:1406, 1992.

292. British Medical Research Council: An assessment of long-term anticoagulant administration after cardiac infarction. *Br Med J* 2:837, 1964.

293. Ebert RV, Borden CW, Hipp HR, Holzman D, Lyon AF, Schnaper H: Long-term anticoagulant therapy after myocardial infarction. *JAMA* 207:2263, 1969.

294. A double-blind trial to assess long-term oral anticoagulant therapy in elderly patients after myocardial infarction: Report of the Sixty Plus Reinfarction Study Research Group. *Lancet* 2:989, 1980.

295. Smith P, Arnesen H, Holme I: The effect of warfarin on mortality and reinfarction after myocardial infarction. *N Engl J Med* 323:147, 1990.

296. Anticoagulants in the Secondary Prevention of Events in Coronary Thrombosis (ASPECT) Research Group: Effect of long-term oral anticoagulant treatment on mortality and cardiovascular morbidity after myocardial infarction: *Lancet* 343:499, 1994.

HEPARIN, HIRUDIN, AND RELATED AGENTS

GARY E. RASKOB

RUSSELL D. HULL

GRAHAM F. PINEO

This chapter provides an overview of the pharmacology and clinical use of heparin and hirudin and related antico-agulant agents including low-molecular-weight (LMW) heparin, the glycosaminoglycan mixture danaparoid, the semisynthetic hirudin fragment bivalirudin (Hirulog), and the small-molecule direct inhibitors of thrombin such as argatroban. The sections on clinical use emphasize the major indications including the treatment of venous thrombo-embolism, the treatment of acute coronary syndromes, and the treatment of patients with heparin-induced thrombocy-topenia. The recommendations for clinical use are linked to the strength of the evidence from clinical trials. Heparin has been the standard initial treatment for acute deep-vein thrombosis or pulmonary embolism for many years and has an important role in the treatment of patients with acute coronary syndromes. Heparin treatment for these indications requires laboratory monitoring of the anticoagu-lant effect and dose adjustment in the individual patient. The activated partial thromboplastin time (aPTT) is the test most commonly used to monitor heparin treatment for venous thromboembolism or acute coronary syndromes. The effectiveness of intravenous heparin for preventing recurrent venous thromboembolism depends on achieving an aPTT response above the lower limit of the therapeutic range during the first 24 h of therapy. Validated heparin protocols are more successful for establishing adequate heparinization than intuitive ordering by the clinician. LMW heparin is at least as effective and possibly more effective than unfractionated heparin for the treatment of venous thromboembolism or acute coronary syndromes. LMW heparin is given by subcutaneous injection once or twice daily and does not require laboratory monitoring of the anticoagulant effect. LMW heparin treatment enables many patients with uncomplicated venous thromboembo-lism to be treated in an outpatient setting and is more cost-effective than intravenous unfractionated heparin in such patients. LMW heparin is also cost-effective com-pared to intravenous heparin treatment of patients with acute coronary syndromes. Clinical trials of hirudin and bivalirudin in patients with acute coronary syndromes have yielded disappointing results. Hirudin has a rela-tively narrow therapeutic range. The major indication for hirudin therapy is likely to be for patients with heparin-induced thrombocytopenia who require anticoagulant treatment. Danaparoid is the drug of choice for the treatment of pregnant patients with heparin-induced thrombocytopenia who require ongoing anticoagulant therapy. The role of the small-molecule direct thrombin inhibitors remains to be determined by randomized clini-cal trials.

HEPARIN

PHARMACOLOGY

Heparin is a glycosaminoglycan composed of chains of alternating residues of D-glucosamine and iduronic acid. Heparin molecules vary in chain length and therefore in molecular mass. Heparin that is avail-able for clinical use is a mixture of molecules which vary in mass from 5000 to 30,000 daltons, with an average of 15,000 daltons. This average molecular mass corresponds to a chain length of approximately 50 monosaccharide units. The mass (chain length) of a heparin mole-cule is an important determinant of both anticoagulant activity and pharmacokinetic properties.[1]

Heparin exerts an anticoagulant effect by enhancing the inactiva-tion by antithrombin III of thrombin, factor Xa, and factor IXa. The major anticoagulant effect is due to a unique pentasaccharide which has a high affinity for binding to antithrombin III.[1] This pentasaccharide is present in only about one-third of the molecules of the heparin mixtures used in clinical practice. The pentasaccharide has been synthesized and is currently undergoing evaluation as an antithrombotic agent in clinical trials.

The inhibition of thrombin by heparin is different from the inhibi-tion of factor Xa.[1] Heparin enhances the inhibition of thrombin by forming a ternary complex in which heparin binds directly to both antithrombin III and thrombin. The inhibition of factor Xa by the heparin/antithrombin III complex does not require heparin to bind directly to factor Xa in a ternary complex. Heparin molecules that contain less than 18 saccharide units are unable to bind thrombin and antithrombin III simultaneously. These LMW heparin molecules are unable to augment the inhibition of thrombin by antithrombin III but retain the ability to augment the inhibition of factor Xa (see "LMW Heparin").

The heparin/antithrombin III complex is a weak inhibitor of thrombin bound to fibrin and of factor Xa when incorporated within the prothrombinase complex.[2] These in vitro biochemical properties have been suggested as an explanation for the limited antithrombotic efficacy of heparin in the clinical settings of high-risk coronary angi-oplasty[2,3] but remain unproved.

The pharmacokinetics of heparin after intravenous injection of a bolus dose can be described by a two-compartment model consisting of a rapid, zero-order phase, followed by a slower, first-order elimination phase.[4] The initial zero-order phase is thought to be due to rapid binding and uptake of heparin by endothelial cells and macrophages. These cells internalize the heparin and depolymerize it into LMW heparin fractions. This process is saturable within the range of heparin doses used in clinical practice, and, therefore, the half-life of heparin in plasma is dose-dependent.[4,5] The plasma half-life of heparin increases from approximately 30 min after an intravenous dose of 25 units/kg to 150 min following a dose of 400 units/kg. The second phase of heparin removal from plasma reflects the renal clearance of the LMW molecules. Heparin binds to several plasma proteins including histidine-rich glycoprotein, vitronectin, fibronectin, fibrinogen, and lipoproteins.[1] Heparin also binds to platelet factor 4 and to high-molecular-weight von Willebrand factor.

Acronyms and abbreviations that appear in this chapter include: ACT, activated clotting time; aPTT, activated partial thromboplastin time; LMW, low-molecular-weight.

LABORATORY MONITORING OF THERAPY

The aPTT is the test most commonly used in clinical practice to monitor the anticoagulant effect of heparin in patients with established venous thromboembolism or acute coronary syndromes. The aPTT is sensitive to plasma heparin concentrations of 0.1 units/ml or more. However, the different reagents used to measure aPTT and the equipment used affect the sensitivity of the assay to heparin. For this reason, it is recommended that the therapeutic range be established by each laboratory by calibrating the aPTT to a plasma heparin concentration of 0.2 to 0.4 units/ml by protamine sulfate titration or 0.3 to 0.7 units/ml by the factor Xa assay.[1] The aPTT is usually prolonged above the upper measurable limit (approximately 150 s) at plasma heparin concentrations of 1.0 units/ml or more. The activated clotting time (ACT) has a graded response to heparin concentrations of 1.0 to 5.0 units/ml. The ACT is used to monitor the effect of heparin in patients who receive high heparin doses such as those undergoing coronary angioplasty or cardiac bypass surgery.

There is considerable variation in the aPTT response to a given plasma heparin concentration among patients with venous thromboembolism or acute coronary syndromes.[1] The patient variables which influence the aPTT response include age, sex, the extent of heparin uptake by endothelial cells and macrophages, and the levels of acute-phase reactant proteins, particularly factor VIII.[1,5] For example, the aPTT response to a given heparin concentration may be diminished by elevated levels of factor VIII which can occur postoperatively or in association with acute illness, malignancy, or pregnancy.

Therefore, in patients with venous thromboembolism and acute coronary syndromes, heparin therapy must be individualized by monitoring the anticoagulant effect and adjusting the heparin dose to achieve the target aPTT therapeutic range.

CLINICAL USE

Heparin has been the standard initial therapy for acute deep-vein thrombosis or pulmonary embolism and is widely used to treat patients with acute coronary syndromes. Heparin is also used to prevent thrombosis during vascular surgery or angioplasty and to prevent ex vivo thrombi during cardiopulmonary bypass surgery. Heparin is also indicated for preventing venous thromboembolism following surgery and in medical patients.

The doses of heparin that are required to treat patients with established venous or arterial thromboembolism are greater than the doses required to prevent the development of venous thromboembolism in high-risk patients. A low dose of heparin given subcutaneously, such as 5000 units every 8 or 12 h, continues to be one of the preferred approaches for preventing venous thromboembolism in moderate- to high-risk patients undergoing general abdominal or thoracic surgery, in patients with acute ischemic stroke with leg paralysis, and in general medical patients.[6] Evidence-based reviews of the use of heparin in cardiovascular surgery[7] and coronary angioplasty[8] have been published.

VENOUS THROMBOEMBOLISM

Heparin therapy for established venous thromboembolism can be given intravenously or subcutaneously. Continuous infusion is the preferred approach for initial treatment because of the need to achieve a rapid therapeutic anticoagulant effect.[9] The appropriate regimen of subcutaneous heparin needed to ensure an adequate and rapid effect remains unknown. Two protocols for initial intravenous heparin treatment of venous thromboembolism have been validated in randomized clinical trials measuring the outcomes of recurrent thromboembolism and major bleeding.[10,11] These protocols utilize an initial intravenous bolus of 5000 units or 75 units/kg, followed by a maintenance infusion of 1250 to 1660 units/h[10] or 18 units/kg per hour.[11] The subcutaneous route of administration is used when heparin is given for the long-term treatment of venous thromboembolism or when intravenous access cannot be obtained.

An analysis of patients entered into a series of three consecutive double-blind randomized trials evaluating initial heparin therapy showed that patients who failed to achieve the lower limit of the therapeutic range for the aPTT were at increased risk of recurrent venous thromboembolism during the subsequent 3 months.[9,12] Among patients treated with an initial intravenous heparin infusion of 30,000 units per 24 h (after a bolus of 5000 units), 4 of 19 patients (21%) whose aPTTs were subtherapeutic during the initial 24 h had recurrent venous thromboembolism, compared with 24 of 392 patients (6%) who achieved an aPTT result above the lower limit of the therapeutic range within 24 h ($P = 0.03$). Of the recurrent events, 75 percent occurred between 2 and 12 weeks after the initial diagnosis, despite treatment with oral anticoagulants. These data indicate that the initial heparin treatment impacts the patient's long-term outcome for at least 3 months in the presence of adequate long-term anticoagulant therapy.[12] A previous literature review[13] was unable to document the relationship between adequate initial therapy and antithrombotic effectiveness because of missing data on the anticoagulant response or clinical outcome in many of the published reports. This literature review also reported a wide 95 percent confidence interval for the odds ratio for recurrent thromboembolism among patients who were or were not subtherapeutic during the initial 24 h of heparin treatment.[13]

The above findings are independently supported by the results of a randomized trial comparing different intensities of initial heparin treatment by continuous infusion.[11] In the patient group randomized to receive an initial heparin infusion of 1000 units/h, the aPTT results were subtherapeutic in 23 percent at 24 to 48 h, and this treatment group had a 25 percent frequency of recurrent venous thromboembolism, compared with a 5 percent recurrence rate ($P = 0.002$) in the more intense heparin infusion group who received weight-adjusted dosing, and in whom only 3 percent of patients were subtherapeutic at 24 h ($P = 0.002$). The importance of adequate initial heparin administration in patients with venous thromboembolism is summarized in Table 133-1. The results are consistent across independent studies.[11,14,15] There are similar high rates of recurrent venous thromboembolism (19% to 25%) among patients in whom the anticoagulant regimen fails to achieve an aPTT above the lower limit of the therapeutic range within 24 h, and there are consistent reductions in the rates of recurrent thromboembolism achieved by adequate heparin therapy (Table 133-1).

The use of a validated heparin protocol will lessen the likelihood of delayed adequate heparinization.[10,11] The key steps used by such protocols are adequate initial heparin infusion doses (1250 to 1600 units/h or 18 units/kg per hour) and frequent aPTT measurements in the first 24 h to identify rapidly the individual patient's heparin requirements. Although such heparin protocols are more successful in establishing adequate heparinization than intuitive ordering by the clinician,[10,11,16] some patients may still receive suboptimal therapy. This reflects a practical limitation of unfractionated heparin. The difficulties of heparin administration are compounded by the practical difficulties of standardizing aPTT testing and the therapeutic range. Therapy with LMW heparin, which does not require monitoring and dose adjustment, is the practical solution to these difficulties (see "LMW Heparin").

Adjusted-dose subcutaneous heparin is the regimen of choice for the long-term treatment of established venous thromboembolism in pregnant patients and in patients in whom warfarin cannot be used or has failed. The heparin dose is adjusted during the first few days of subcutaneous therapy to achieve an aPTT above the lower limit of the therapeutic range.[17] The subcutaneous heparin dose can be estimated from the patient's intravenous heparin requirements. A general guide is to administer two-thirds of the patient's total daily intravenous heparin dose in divided subcutaneous doses. For example, if the patient required 30,000 units per 24 h to achieve a therapeutic aPTT response, then the estimated subcutaneous regimen for long-term treatment would be 10,000 units given every 12 h. The aPTT is measured 6 h after the morning subcutaneous injection. The heparin dose is adjusted to maintain this aPTT above the lower limit of the therapeutic range.[17] Once a stable dose has been identified, the dose can be fixed for the duration of therapy, except in pregnant patients, due to changing heparin requirements throughout the course of pregnancy. The aPTT should be measured at regular intervals in pregnant patients to ensure that adequate heparin treatment is maintained. It is not uncommon for pregnant patients to develop relatively large daily heparin requirements as pregnancy progresses (e.g., 40,000 to 50,000 units daily).

ACUTE CORONARY SYNDROMES

The objectives of heparin treatment in patients with acute coronary syndromes are to reduce the risk of death, myocardial infarction, mural thrombosis, systemic embolism, and recurrent ischemia.[18]

In patients with unstable angina, intravenous heparin by continuous infusion is effective for preventing myocardial infarction and death and is more effective than aspirin alone for preventing recurrent ischemic symptoms. There is a high rate of reactivation of ischemia early after stopping intravenous heparin if aspirin is not given.[19] The reactivation of ischemia is less frequent if aspirin is given before heparin is discontinued. The combined use of heparin and aspirin is preferred in patients with unstable angina.[18] Sufficient heparin should be given to prolong the aPTT to 1.5 to 2 times control. A practical regimen is an intravenous bolus of 5000 units or 75 units/kg, followed by a continuous intravenous infusion of 1250 units/h.[18] Heparin therapy should be continued for at least 48 h or until the unstable pain pattern resolves.

Heparin is also indicated for patients with acute myocardial infarction. Every patient with acute myocardial infarction should receive at least low-dose heparin therapy to prevent venous thromboembolism.[18] However, in current practice, most patients will receive more intensive heparin therapy, either as adjunctive treatment to thrombolysis or because they are at high risk for development of mural thrombosis and systemic embolism due to large anterior Q-wave infarction, left ventricular dysfunction, echocardiographic evidence of mural thrombosis, atrial fibrillation, or a history of systemic or pulmonary embolism. The recommended regimen is intravenous heparin given as an initial bolus of 5000 units or 75 units/kg, followed by a maintenance infusion of 1250 units/h, adjusted to maintain the aPTT between 1.5 and 2 times control.[18] Heparin is continued for 48 h in patients who have received thrombolytic therapy with recombinant tissue plasminogen activator or reteplase. In patients who receive thrombolysis with streptokinase or APSAC, heparin should only be given to those patients who have risk factors for systemic embolism. Patients at high risk for developing mural thrombosis and systemic embolism because of the risk factors listed above should continue anticoagulant treatment for up to 3 months.[18] Oral anticoagulant therapy with warfarin, overlapped with heparin and adjusted to maintain the INR between 2.0 and 3.0, is the preferred approach for most patients.

TABLE 133-1   IMPORTANCE OF ADEQUATE INITIAL HEPARIN ADMINISTRATION FOR VENOUS THROMBOEMBOLISM

| | RECURRENT DVT OR PE | | |
STUDY AND YEAR	PATIENTS GIVEN ADEQUATE INTRAVENOUS HEPARIN,* n/n (%)	PATIENTS GIVEN ALTERNATIVE REGIMEN,* n/n (%)	P VALUE
Hull et al, 1986[14]	3/58 (5)	11/57 (19)	0.024
Brandjes et al, 1992[15]	4/60 (7)	12/60 (20)	0.058
Raschke et al, 1993[11]	2/41 (5)	8/32 (25)	0.02
	Patients therapeutic within 24 h, n/n (%)	Patients subtherapeutic within 24 h, n/n (%)	
Hull et al, 1997[9]	24/392 (6)	4/19 (21)	0.03

*In these trials, a regimen of intravenous heparin that achieved an adequate anticoagulant effect (aPTT ratio > 1.5) within 24 h in most patients was compared with a control group who received an alternate regimen of initial therapy that resulted in a high rate of inadequate therapy (aPTT ratio < 1.5) during the initial 24 h. These inadequate regimens were with subcutaneous heparin 15,000 units per 12 h,[14] oral anticoagulants alone,[15] and an intravenous heparin infusion of 1000 U/h.[11]

ABBREVIATIONS: aPTT, activated partial thromboplastin time; DVT, deep-vein thrombosis; PE, pulmonary embolism.

The optimal use of intravenous heparin or LMW heparin (see below) together with intravenous platelet glycoprotein (GP) IIb/IIIa receptor inhibitors is currently unknown (see Chap. 131). This issue will be increasingly important with the more widespread use of the platelet GPIIb/IIIa receptor inhibitors as initial therapy for patients with acute coronary syndromes. If abciximab is used during coronary angioplasty, less intensive intravenous heparin (bolus of 70 units/kg repeated to maintain the ACT above 200 s) reduces the risk of major bleeding without loss of antithrombotic effectiveness compared to the more intense heparin regimens traditionally used for angioplasty (bolus 10,000 to 20,000 units and maintaining ACT of 300 to 350 s).[20]

SIDE EFFECTS

The key side effects of short-term heparin therapy are bleeding and thrombocytopenia. Osteoporosis is a potential complication of long-term heparin treatment. Heparin may cause elevation of transaminase levels, but these elevations are of unknown clinical significance and usually return to normal after heparin is discontinued. Awareness of this biochemical effect is important so as to avoid unnecessary interruption of heparin therapy and unnecessary liver biopsies in patients who may develop elevated transaminases during heparin treatment. Additional rare side effects include hypersensitivity, skin reactions including necrosis, alopecia, and hyperkalemia due to hypoaldosteronism.

Bleeding complications may be categorized as major or minor according to standard international criteria.[21] Major bleeding is defined as clinically overt bleeding resulting in a decline of hemoglobin of 2 g/dl or more (or transfusion of 2 or more units of packed red cells), or bleeding which is intracranial or retroperitoneal. The rates of major bleeding reported from contemporary clinical trials of intravenous heparin treatment for venous thromboembolism range from 0 to 7 percent, and the rates of fatal bleeding range from 0 to 2 percent.[22] The presence or absence of underlying risk factors for bleeding have a marked impact on the incidence of major bleeding. Patients at high risk for major bleeding are those who have had recent surgery or trauma within the previous 14 days; those with a history of gastrointestinal bleeding, peptic ulcer disease, or genitourinary bleeding; and those with conditions predisposing to bleeding such as thrombocytopenia, liver disease, multiple invasive lines, etc. The risk of major bleeding is also increased in patients over 70 years of age. The available data indicate that the patient-related factors described above are stronger determinants of the risk of major bleeding than the heparin dose or aPTT response. Thus, the incidence of major bleeding is 10 percent among patients with one or more of these risk factors in whom the intravenous heparin infusion is begun at a dose of 1250 units/h, compared with only 1 percent among patients in whom all of the risk factors are absent, and who receive a larger initial infusion dose (1660 units/h).[23] To date, no study has definitively established a relationship between an excessively prolonged aPTT and increased risk of major bleeding for patients with venous thromboembolism or acute coronary syndromes who do not receive thrombolysis or abciximab.[1]

Heparin may cause thrombocytopenia (see Chap. 117). Two types of heparin-induced thrombocytopenia have been described: (1) early, nonimmune thrombocytopenia that often resolves while heparin is continued and does not result in clinically important consequences,[1] and (2) immune-mediated thrombocytopenia which usually occurs after 5 days of heparin treatment but may occur earlier in patients who have been previously exposed to heparin.[24] The immune form of heparin-induced thrombocytopenia may develop with prophylactic or therapeutic doses given by any route of administration. Heparin-induced immune thrombocytopenia is mediated by an immunoglobulin G (IgG) antibody directed against a complex of platelet factor 4 and heparin,[25,26] although other target antigens may also be important.[27]

The immune type of heparin-induced thrombocytopenia may be accompanied by extension of preexisting venous thromboembolism or development of new arterial thrombosis that may precede or coincide with the fall in the platelet count.[28,29] These complications have been associated with a high incidence of limb amputation and a high mortality rate.[29] Heparin in all forms should be discontinued when the diagnosis of heparin-induced thrombocytopenia is made on clinical grounds. The laboratory diagnosis of heparin-induced thrombocytopenia is often not achievable because the definitive platelet activation assays may not be available and are limited by a slow turnaround time. Most importantly, the safety of continuing heparin treatment in patients with negative results by any of the currently available assays has not been established by properly designed prospective studies. The identification of additional target antigens for heparin-induced thrombocytopenia suggests that it may not be safe to continue heparin because an ELISA assay for antibodies to the heparin/PF4 complex is negative. For patients with acute heparin-induced thrombocytopenia who require continued anticoagulant treatment, the recommended options include danaparoid sodium or recombinant hirudin (both discussed later in this chapter). LMW heparin is not recommended for anticoagulant treatment in patients with acute heparin-induced thrombocytopenia.

Osteoporosis may occur as a side effect of long-term heparin therapy (usually more than 3 months). The earliest clinical manifestation of heparin-associated osteoporosis is usually nonspecific low-back pain primarily involving the vertebrae or ribs; patients may also have spontaneous fractures in these areas. The incidence of symptomatic fractures is estimated to be about 2 percent. Up to one-third of patients treated with long-term heparin may have subclinical reductions in bone density. It is unknown if these patients are predisposed to an increased risk of future fractures.

ANTIDOTE TO HEPARIN

The anticoagulant effect of heparin can be rapidly neutralized by the intravenous injection of protamine sulfate. Protamine sulfate is indicated for selected patients with major bleeding. The appropriate neutralizing dose of protamine sulfate depends on the dose of heparin, the route of administration, and the time since the last dose was given. If protamine sulfate is used within minutes of an intravenous heparin injection, a full neutralizing dose should be given (1 mg protamine sulfate per 100 units heparin). For example, an intravenous bolus of 5000 units of heparin would require a protamine sulfate dose of 50

mg. Doses of protamine sulfate larger than 50 mg are rarely needed because heparin is cleared quickly from plasma with a half-life of approximately 60 min. After a subcutaneous injection of heparin, repeated small doses of protamine may be required because of prolonged heparin absorption from the subcutaneous depot.

LMW HEPARIN

PHARMACOLOGY

LMW heparin is prepared by depolymerization of unfractionated heparin using chemical or enzymatic methods. Several LMW heparins have been prepared for clinical use (Table 133-2). These preparations have an average molecular mass of 4000 to 6000 daltons, with a range of 1000 to 10,000 daltons.[1]

There are important pharmacologic differences between LMW heparins and unfractionated heparin. These include a reduced ability to catalyze the inhibition of thrombin in vitro while retaining the ability to inhibit the activity of factor Xa (a so-called higher anti-Xa to anti-IIa ratio).[1] The clinical relevance of this pharmacologic property is uncertain. LMW heparins exhibit less binding than unfractionated heparin to a variety of plasma proteins and to cells including platelets, endothelial cells, macrophages, and possibly osteoblasts.[1] Most plasma proteins that bind unfractionated heparin do not bind or neutralize LMW heparin. The reduced binding of LMW heparin to plasma proteins contributes to its more predictable anticoagulant dose response. The reduced binding of LMW heparin to endothelial cells and macrophages contributes to its longer plasma half-life (see below). LMW heparin causes less thrombocytopenia than unfractionated heparin[28] when given to patients who have not previously received heparin, although thrombocytopenia may still occur with LMW heparin. LMW heparin may also be less likely to cause clinically important osteoporosis than unfractionated heparin.[30]

The pharmacokinetic properties of LMW heparin make it possible to give this agent subcutaneously once or twice daily without the need for laboratory monitoring of the anticoagulant response or dose adjustment. These pharmacokinetic properties include a very high bioavailability (greater than 90%) after subcutaneous injection, a longer half-life than unfractionated heparin, and much less interindividual variation in the anticoagulant response to a given dose.[1] The anticoagulant response (anti-Xa activity) to a fixed dose of LMW heparin is highly correlated with the patient's body weight. The regimens of LMW heparin used for the treatment of patients with established venous thromboembolism or patients with acute coronary syndromes are based on units/kg body weight or on body weight range category. LMW heparin is cleared mainly by the kidneys, and therefore clearance of LMW heparin is reduced in patients with renal failure.[1] The anticoagulant (anti-Xa) effect of LMW

TABLE 133-2   LOW-MOLECULAR-WEIGHT HEPARINS

GENERIC NAME	TRADE NAME	MANUFACTURER
Enoxaparin	Lovenox	Rhone-Poulenc Rorer, Collegeville, PA
Dalteparin	Fragmin	Pharmacia-Upjohn, Kalamazoo, MI
Tinzaparin*	Innohep	Leo Pharmaceutical Products, Ballerup, Denmark and DuPont Pharmaceuticals, Wilmington, DE
Nadroparin†	Fraxiparine	Sanofi-Winthrop, New York, NY
Reviparin	Clivarin	Knoll Pharmaceutical Co, Parsippany, NJ
Certoparin	Sandoparin	Sandoz Pharmeceuticals, East Hanover, NJ

*Prepared by heparinase digestion. All others prepared by organic chemical methods.
†Ca^{2+} salt. All others are sodium salt.

TABLE 133-3   MAJOR CLINICAL OUTCOME TRIALS OF LMW HEPARIN FOR THE TREATMENT OF DEEP-VEIN THROMBOSIS AND PULMONARY EMBOLISM

STUDY	DESIGN	REGIMENS	RECURRENCE OF VTE, n/n (%)	OCCURRENCE OF MAJOR BLEEDING, n/n (%)	DEATH, n/n (%)
Prandoni et al[32]	Randomized, open	Nadroparin sc bid vs IV heparin aPTT 1.5–2.0	6/85 (7) 12/85 (14)	1/85 (1) 3/85 (4)	5/85 (6) 9/85 (11)
Hull et al[33]	Randomized, double-blind	Tinzaparin 175 Xa U/kg sc once daily vs IV heparin aPTT 1.5–2.5	6/213 (3) 15/219 (7)	1/213 (0.5)* 11/219 (5.0)	10/213 (5)* 21/219 (10)
Simmoneau et al[34]	Randomized, open	Enoxaparin 1 mg/kg sc bid vs IV heparin	0/67 2/67 (3)	0 0	3/67 (4) 2/67 (3)
Lindmarker et al[35]	Randomized, open	Dalteparin 200 Xa U/kg sc once daily vs IV heparin aPTT 1.5–3.0	5/101 (5) 3/103 (3)	0 0	2 (2) 2 (2)
Levine et al[36]	Randomized, open, home treatment†	Enoxaparin 1 mg/kg sc bid vs IV heparin aPTT 60–85 s	13/247 (5) 17/253 (7)	5/247 (2) 3/253 (1)	11/247 (4) 17/253 (7)
Koopman et al[37]	Randomized, open, home treatment†	Nadroparin‡ sc bid vs IV heparin aPTT 1.5–2.0	14/202 (7) 17/198 (9)	1/202 (0.5) 4/198 (2)	14/202 (7) 16/198 (8)
Büller et al[38]	Randomized, open	Reviparin sc bid vs IV heparin aPTT 1.5–2.5	25/510 (5) 25/511 (5)	10/510 (2) 5/511 (2)	35/510 (7) 39/511 (7)
Simmoneau et al[39]	Randomized, open	Tinzaparin 175 Xa U/kg sc once daily vs IV heparin aPTT 2.0–3.0	5/304 (2) 6/308 (2)	3/304 (1) 5/308 (2)	12/304 (4) 14/308 (5)
Charbonnier et al[40]	Randomized, double-blind	Nadroparin sc bid vs Nadroparin sc once daily	24/335 (7) 13/316 (4)	4/335 (1) 4/316 (1)	13/335 (4) 9/316 (3)

*$P < 0.05$ by comparison to intravenous (IV) heparin group.
†Patients were treated at home if they did not require hospital for management of other conditions.
‡Total daily doses were: 8200 I Xa U for patients weighing less than 50 kg, 12,300 I Xa U for patients between 50 and 70 kg, and 18,400 I Xa U for patients weighing more than 70 kg.
ABBREVIATIONS: aPTT, activated partial thromboplastin time; bid, twice daily; sc, subcutaneously; VTE, venous thromboembolism.

heparin is not completely neutralized by protamine sulfate, but treatment with protamine sulfate may still decrease the hemorrhagic effect of LMW heparin.

There are biochemical and pharmacologic differences between the LMW heparin preparations. However, the clinical relevance of these differences in terms of effectiveness or safety of treatment remains unknown. The different LMW heparin preparations are not interchangeable.[31] Each LMW heparin preparation must be evaluated by clinical trials measuring the outcomes of thromboembolism, bleeding, and mortality. The decision to use a specific LMW heparin should be based on the available clinical trial data for that preparation.

CLINICAL USE

LMW heparin has been extensively evaluated for the prevention of venous thromboembolism in high-risk patients, for the treatment of established deep-vein thrombosis and pulmonary embolism, and for the treatment of patients with acute coronary syndromes.

VENOUS THROMBOEMBOLISM

The results of the major clinical outcome studies[32–40] evaluating LMW heparin for the initial treatment of venous thromboembolism are summarized in Table 133-3. The findings indicate that LMW heparin is at least as effective and safe as intravenous unfractionated heparin. LMW heparin enables outpatient therapy for many patients with uncomplicated deep-vein thrombosis. In the two randomized trials evaluating home treatment,[36,37] 36 to 48 percent of patients receiving LMW heparin were never admitted to the hospital, and 40 percent were discharged from the hospital after a shorter hospital stay (2 to 3 days versus 5 days for intravenous unfractionated heparin). Outpatient LMW heparin provides a potential for major cost savings to the health-care system compared to therapy with intravenous heparin in the hospital.[41]

LMW heparin treatment of deep-vein thrombosis is effective when given either twice daily or once daily.[32–40,42] Treatment with once-daily subcutaneous regimens are more convenient for the patient and

the care providers. Emerging data indicate that when an equivalent total daily dose is given once daily, rather than in a divided dose twice daily, antithrombotic effectiveness may be improved.[40] Further, the only clinical trial to date suggesting superior efficacy of LMW heparin treatment to intravenous heparin utilized a once-daily regimen.[33] Treatment with LMW heparin as a single daily dose rather than divided doses maximizes the intensity of an early antithrombotic effect which was shown to be important for clinical effectiveness of unfractionated heparin.[9,12] Finally, there is no evidence from clinical trials of patients with venous thromboembolism that giving an equivalent total daily dose in divided doses rather than a single dose enhances safety in terms of bleeding complications. The regimens of LMW heparin for the treatment of established venous thromboembolism evaluated by clinical outcome studies are listed in Table 133-4.

LMW heparin has been less extensively evaluated for the initial treatment of patients with symptomatic pulmonary embolism. Two randomized trials indicate that two different LMW heparin regimens are as effective and safe as continuous intravenous unfractionated heparin in patients with submassive symptomatic pulmonary embo-

TABLE 133-4   REGIMENS OF LMW HEPARIN FOR THE TREATMENT OF VENOUS THROMBOEMBOLISM

LMW HEPARIN	REGIMEN
Enoxaparin	1.0 mg/kg bid or 1.5 mg/kg once daily
Dalteparin	200 I F Xa U/kg once daily
Tinzaparin	175 I F Xa U/kg once daily
Nadroparin	4100 I Xa U bid if < 50 kg* 6150 I Xa U bid if 50–70 kg 9200 I Xa U bid if > 70 kg
Reviparin	6300 I Xa U bid if > 60 kg 4200 I Xa U bid if 46 to 60 kg 3500 I Xa U bid if 35 to 45 kg

*Alternately, once-daily regimens of 8200 Xa U if < 50 kg, 10,250 Xa U if 50–59 kg, 12,300 if 60–69 kg, 14,350 U if 70–79 kg, 16,400 if 80–89 kg, and 18,450 if 90 kg.

lism.[38,39] The two LMW heparin regimens evaluated were reviparin twice daily in doses given according to weight category (Table 133-4) and tinzaparin 175 units/kg once daily. This regimen of tinzaparin has also been shown to be more effective than intravenous unfractionated heparin for treatment of patients with pulmonary embolism who have underlying proximal deep-vein thrombosis.[43]

ACUTE CORONARY SYNDROMES

LMW heparin is effective for treatment of patients with acute coronary syndromes.[18] The two LMW heparin regimens evaluated were enoxaparin 1 mg/kg twice daily or dalteparin 120 units/kg twice daily. The clinical trials indicate that LMW heparin is at least as effective as intravenous unfractionated heparin. Two large randomized trials indicate that the enoxaparin regimen is more effective for reducing the incidence of the composite outcome of death, myocardial infarction, or recurrent ischemia.[44,45] The enoxaparin regimen reduced the incidence of recurrent ischemic events requiring reintervention with an absolute risk reduction of 4 percent compared to intravenous unfractionated heparin. This benefit was sustained for up to 1 year. The use of enoxaparin is cost-effective by comparison to intravenous unfractionated heparin.[46]

DANAPAROID

PHARMACOLOGY

Danaparoid sodium is a mixture of glycosaminoglycans including heparan sulfate, dermatan sulfate, and chondroitin sulfate. Danaparoid was previously known as *Org 10172* and *lomoparan*. The predominant anticoagulant effect of danaparoid is due to its anti-factor-Xa activity.

Danaparoid can be given either by intravenous infusion or subcutaneous injection. The plasma half-life of the anti-factor-Xa activity of danaparoid is approximately 24 h. Danaparoid is eliminated mainly by the kidneys. There is no known antidote for danaparoid.

There may be in vitro cross-reactivity to heparin-induced thrombocytopenia antibodies with some of the glycosaminoglycans contained in danaparoid. However, this in vitro cross-reactivity is of uncertain clinical relevance because a randomized clinical trial indicates danaparoid is effective for treatment of patients with acute heparin-induced thrombocytopenia,[47] and the rate of recovery of platelet counts in patients with heparin-induced thrombocytopenia during danaparoid treatment is unrelated to the presence of in vitro cross-reactivity.[48]

CLINICAL USE

Danaparoid has been evaluated by randomized clinical trials for the prevention of deep-vein thrombosis,[6,49] for the treatment of established deep-vein thrombosis,[50] and for the treatment of patients with acute heparin-induced thrombocytopenia.[47] In this latter study, danaparoid was more effective than dextran.[47] The experience with danaparoid in a compassionate-use treatment program for heparin-induced thrombocytopenia has also been published.[51]

The major indications for danaparoid are treatment of patients with acute heparin-induced thrombocytopenia who require ongoing anticoagulation and for the prevention of thromboembolism in patients with a past history of heparin-induced thrombocytopenia. Danaparoid is the drug of choice for the prevention or treatment of thromboembolism in pregnant patients with a history of heparin-induced thrombocytopenia.

Danaparoid is given by intravenous infusion when rapid therapeutic anticoagulation is required. An intravenous bolus is given followed by a maintenance infusion. The bolus dose differs by patients' body weight category: 1500 units if less than 60 kg, 3000 units for patients 75 to 90 kg, and 3750 units for patients weighing more than 90 kg.[1] Following injection of the bolus, continuous infusion is commenced at a rate of 400 units/h for the first 4 h, then 300 units/h for the next 4 h.[1] Thereafter, a maintenance infusion of 150 to 200 units/h is given. This maintenance infusion is adjusted to maintain the plasma anti-factor Xa level between 0.5 and 0.8 units/ml. An alternative approach for maintenance treatment is to administer a subcutaneous injection of 1500 units every 8 to 12 h.

The recommended regimen when danaparoid is used for preventing the development of thromboembolism is 750 to 1500 units every 8 to 12 h depending on the patient's weight. The recommended regimens are 750 units every 12 h for patients less than 75 kg, 750 units every 8 h for patients between 75 and 90 kg, and 1500 units every 12 h for patients more than 90 kg.[1]

HIRUDIN AND DERIVATIVES

PHARMACOLOGY

Hirudin is a 65–amino acid polypeptide produced by the salivary gland of the medicinal leech *Hirudo medicinalis*. Hirudin is the most potent naturally occurring specific inhibitor of thrombin.[52] Hirudin directly inactivates thrombin by forming a 1:1 stoichiometric complex with thrombin at two specific sites: an N-terminal domain that binds to the active site of thrombin and a C-terminal domain, which binds to the main fibrinopeptide-binding region on thrombin.[52,53] Natural hirudin, recombinant hirudin, and the synthetic analogue Hirulog (bivalirudin) all contain these two binding sites.

Hirudin has been produced by recombinant DNA technology. Recombinant hirudin is not sulfated at tyrosine residue 63 and, as a result, has a tenfold reduced affinity for thrombin.[54] Bivalirudin (Hirulog) is a 20–amino acid semisynthetic peptide analogue of hirudin.[55] Bivalirudin is a potent thrombin inhibitor that differs from hirudin because it produces only transient inhibition of the active site of thrombin.

Theoretical advantages of hirudin over heparin have been proposed. Although both hirudin and heparin-antithrombin III complex inhibit thrombin enzymatic activity, hirudin is more effective in inhibiting the positive feedback mechanisms of thrombin that promote further thrombin generation, e.g., factor V activation and factor VIII activation.[52,53] Hirudin and the analogues effectively inhibit clot-bound thrombin as well as fluid-phase thrombin, whereas the heparin-antithrombin III complex is a weak inhibitor of clot-bound thrombin.[2] This may provide an advantage in suppressing the activity of thrombin after vessel injury, such as occurs in angioplasty, and inhibiting clot-bound thrombin after thrombolysis or in venous thromboemboli. Experimental studies indicate that hirudin is capable of suppressing platelet-rich arterial thrombus formation, although at much higher concentrations than are required to suppress venous thrombosis.[3] However, experimental animal studies indicate that hirudin produces more bleeding than heparin when these drugs are used in doses that achieve an equivalent aPTT ratio.[56] Moreover, since there is a very flat relationship between the hirudin concentration in plasma and the aPTT response, even a small increase in the aPTT ratio within the therapeutic range of 1.5 to 2.5 results in a marked increase in experimental bleeding with hirudin, but not with heparin.[56] These observations help to explain the results from early clinical trials with hirudin which documented very high rates of intracranial and major bleeding when hirudin was given in doses adjusted to achieve an aPTT response equivalent to the traditional therapeutic range for heparin (aPTT ratio 1.5 to 2.5).[57–59] A recombinant hirudin known as lepirudin has recently been approved for the treatment of heparin-induced thrombocytopenia. Lepirudin is given intravenously, is cleared by the kidneys, and has a plasma half-life of 1.3 h. There is no known antidote. Up to 50 percent of patients develop IgG antihirudin antibodies.[60]

The anticoagulant effect of lepirudin is monitored using the aPTT. The antihirudin antibodies may alter the anticoagulant effect, and ongoing monitoring is required in patients receiving lepirudin.

CLINICAL USE

Hirudin has been extensively evaluated by randomized clinical trials in patients with acute coronary syndromes.[57–59,61–63] It has been evaluated in patients undergoing coronary angioplasty[64] and for the prevention of deep-vein thrombosis after total hip replacement.[65] Lepirudin has been evaluated in an historical-control study for the treatment of patients with heparin-induced thrombocytopenia.[66] Bivalirudin has been evaluated by a randomized clinical trial in patients undergoing coronary angioplasty for unstable or postinfarction angina.[67]

The initial clinical trials of hirudin in patients with acute coronary syndromes documented high rates of intracranial bleeding in patients who also received thrombolytic therapy.[57–59] In these studies, hirudin was given in doses that produced an aPTT similar to that achieved with therapeutic doses of intravenous heparin. Subsequent clinical trials using lower doses of hirudin failed to demonstrate that hirudin was superior to heparin in patients with acute myocardial infarction who also received thrombolysis.[61,62] The recently completed large Oasis II trial suggests that lepirudin may be marginally more effective than heparin for preventing cardiovascular death or new myocardial infarction in patients with acute myocardial ischemia without ST-segment elevation.[63] At 7 days, the primary outcome of cardiovascular death or new myocardial infarction occurred in 4.2 percent of 5058 patients given intravenous heparin, compared with 3.6 percent of 5083 patients given lepirudin ($P = 0.077$). Long-term follow-up will be required to determine if this potential marginal benefit persists. The potential benefit was offset by an increase in major bleeding from 0.7 percent with intravenous heparin to 1.2 percent with lepirudin. The clinical trials to date indicate that hirudin is not a major advance in antithrombotic treatment of acute coronary syndromes. LMW heparin treatment has achieved larger absolute risk reductions in outcomes, and these improved outcomes persist for up to 1 year.[68] LMW heparin is easier to use, does not require anticoagulant monitoring, and is much less expensive.

The major indication for lepirudin therapy is for the treatment of patients with acute heparin-induced thrombocytopenia. An intravenous bolus of 0.4 mg/kg is given with a maintenance infusion of 0.15 mg/kg per hour. The infusion dose is adjusted to maintain an aPTT ratio of 1.5 to 2.5. The first aPTT is measured 4 h after starting the infusion, and subsequent aPTTs should be measured at least once daily. The dose should be reduced in patients with renal impairment (creatinine clearance below 60 ml/min or serum creatinine above 1.5 mg/dl). The recommended initial infusion doses for patients with renal impairment are 0.075 mg/kg per hour for a creatinine clearance of 45 to 60 ml/min, 0.045 mg/kg per hour for a creatinine clearance of 30 to 44 ml/min, and 0.0225 mg/kg per hour for creatinine clearance of 15 to 29 ml/min.

Bivalirudin has been evaluated in a randomized trial of 4098 patients undergoing angioplasty for unstable or postinfarction angina.[67] Bivalirudin was not more effective than heparin for reducing the incidence of the primary outcome, which was the cluster outcome of death in the hospital, myocardial infarction, or abrupt vessel closure. Among the prospectively stratified subgroup of patients with postinfarction angina, bivalirudin was more effective for reducing the risk of immediate ischemic complications, with a lower risk of major bleeding. However, the benefit was no longer present at 6 months.

SMALL-MOLECULE DIRECT THROMBIN INHIBITORS

Several LMW direct inhibitors of the active site of thrombin have been developed.[69] These include argatroban, napsagatran, inogatran, melagatran, and L372,460. All are potent noncovalent inhibitors of thrombin.[69] The agent L372,460 can be given orally and has a relatively long half-life.

Argatroban has been evaluated by an historical-controlled study in patients with heparin-induced thrombocytopenia.[1] This study showed a higher mortality among the patients treated with argatroban. Although this may be due to differences in the patients between the treatment groups, a possible drug effect as the cause of this excess mortality cannot be excluded. For this reason, and because alternatives are available (danaparoid sodium and lepirudin), argatroban should not be used. Further clinical trials are required to determine the therapeutic role of the small-molecule direct-acting thrombin inhibitors.

REFERENCES

1. Hirsh J, Warkentin TE, Raschke R, et al: Heparin and low-molecular-weight heparin: mechanisms of action, pharmacokinetics, dosing considerations, monitoring, efficacy, and safety. *Chest* 114:489S, 1998.
2. Weitz JL, Hudoba M, Massell D, et al: Clot-bound thrombin is protected from inhibition by heparin-antithrombin III but is susceptible to inactivation by antithrombin III-independent inhibitors. *J Clin Invest* 86:385, 1990.
3. Heras M, Chesebro JH, Webster MWI, et al: Hirudin, heparin and placebo during deep arterial injury in the pig: the in vivo role of thrombin in platelet-mediated thrombosis. *Circulation* 23:249, 1990.
4. Bjornsson TO, Wolfram BS, Kitchell BB: Heparin kinetics determined by three assay methods. *Clin Pharmacol Ther* 31:104, 1982.
5. Mungall D, Raskob G, Coleman R, et al: Pharmacokinetics and dynamics of heparin in patients with proximal-vein thrombosis. *J Clin Pharmacol* 29:896, 1989.
6. Clagett GP, Anderson FA Jr, Geerts W, et al: Prevention of venous thromboembolism. *Chest* 114:531S, 1998.
7. Jackson MR, Clagett GP: Antithrombotic therapy in peripheral arterial occlusive disease. *Chest* 114:666S, 1998.
8. Popma JJ, Weitz J, Bittl JA, et al: Antithrombotic therapy in patients undergoing coronary angioplasty. *Chest* 114:728S, 1998.
9. Hull RD, Raskob GE, Brant RF, et al: Relation between the time to achieve the lower limit of the APTT therapeutic range and recurrent venous thromboembolism during heparin treatment for deep vein thrombosis. *Arch Intern Med* 157:2562, 1997.
10. Hull RD, Raskob GE, Rosenbloom D, et al: Optimal therapeutic level of heparin therapy in patients with venous thrombosis. *Arch Intern Med* 152:1589, 1992.
11. Raschke RA, Reilly BM, Guidry JR, et al: The weight-based heparin dosing nomogram compared with a "standard care" nomogram: a randomized controlled trial. *Ann Intern Med* 119:874, 1993.
12. Hull RD, Raskob GE, Brant RF, et al: The importance of initial heparin treatment on long-term clinical outcomes of antithrombotic therapy: the emerging theme of delayed recurrence. *Arch Intern Med* 157:2317, 1997.
13. Anand S, Ginsberg JS, Kearon C, et al: The relation between the activated partial thromboplastin time response and recurrence in patients with venous thrombosis treated with continuous intravenous heparin. *Arch Intern Med* 156:1677, 1996.
14. Hull RD, Raskob GE, Hirsh J, et al: Continuous intravenous heparin compared with intermittent subcutaneous heparin in the initial treatment of proximal-vein thrombosis. *N Engl J Med* 315:1109, 1986.
15. Brandjes DPM, Heijboer H, Buller HR, et al: Acenocoumarol and heparin compared with acenocoumarol alone in the initial treatment of proximal-vein thrombosis. *N Engl J Med* 327:1485, 1992.
16. Elliot GC, Hiltunen SJ, Suchyta M, et al: Physician-guided treatment compared with a heparin protocol for deep vein thrombosis. *Arch Intern Med* 154:999, 1994.
17. Hull R, Delmore T, Carter C, et al: Adjusted subcutaneous heparin versus warfarin sodium in the long-term treatment of venous thrombosis. *N Engl J Med* 306:189, 1982.

18. Cairns JA, Théroux P, Lewis HD, et al: Antithrombotic agents in coronary artery disease. *Chest* 114:611S, 1998.

19. Theroux P, Waters D, Lam J, et al: Reactivation of unstable angina after the discontinuation of heparin. *N Engl J Med* 327:141, 1992.

20. EPILOG Investigators: Platelet glycoprotein IIb/IIIa receptor blockade and low-dose heparin during percutaneous coronary revascularization. *N Engl J Med* 336:1689, 1997.

21. Graafsma YP, Prins MH, Lensing AWA, et al: Bleeding classification in clinical trials: observer variability and clinical relevance. *Thromb Haemost* 78:1189, 1997.

22. Levine MN, Raskob G, Landefeld S, Kearon C: Hemorrhagic complications of anticoagulant treatment. *Chest* 114:511S, 1998.

23. Hull RD, Raskob GE, Rosenbloom D, et al: Heparin for 5 days as compared with 10 days in the initial treatment of proximal venous thrombosis. *N Engl J Med* 322:1260, 1990.

24. Warkentin TE, Chong BH, Greinacher A: Heparin-induced thrombocytopenia: towards consensus. *Thromb Haemost* 79:1, 1998.

25. Visentin GP, Ford SE, Scott JP, et al: Antibodies from patients with heparin-induced thrombocytopenia/thrombosis are specific for platelet factor 4 complexed with heparin or bound to endothelial cells. *J Clin Invest* 93:81, 1994.

26. Greinacher A, Pötzsch B, Amiral J, et al: Heparin-associated thrombocytopenia: isolation of the antibody and characterization of a multimolecular PF4-heparin complex as the major antigen. *Thromb Haemost* 71:247, 1994.

27. Amiral J, Marfaing-Koka A, Wolf M, et al: Presence of autoantibodies to interleukin-8 or neutrophil-activating peptide-2 in patients with heparin-associated thrombocytopenia. *Blood* 88:410, 1996.

28. Warkentin TE, Levine MN, Hirsh J, et al: Heparin-induced thrombocytopenia in patients treated with low-molecular-weight heparin or unfractionated heparin. *N Engl J Med* 332:1330, 1995.

29. Warkentin TE, Kelton JG: A 14-year study of heparin-induced thrombocytopenia. *Am J Med* 101:505, 1996.

30. Monreal M, Lafoz E, Olive A, et al: Comparison of subcutaneous unfractionated heparin with a low molecular weight heparin (Fragmin) in patients with venous thromboembolism and contraindications to coumarin. *Thromb Haemost* 71:7, 1994.

31. Nightingale SL: Appropriate use of low-molecular-weight heparin (LMWHs). *JAMA* 270:1672, 1993.

32. Prandoni P, Lensing AWA, Buller HR, et al: Comparison of subcutaneous low molecular weight heparin with intravenous standard heparin in proximal deep-vein thrombosis. *Lancet* 339:441, 1992.

33. Hull RD, Raskob GE, Pineo GF, et al: Subcutaneous low molecular weight heparin compared with continuous intravenous heparin in the treatment of proximal-vein thrombosis. *N Engl J Med* 326:975, 1992.

34. Simmoneau G, Charbonnier B, Decousus H, et al: Subcutaneous low-molecular-weight heparin compared with continuous intravenous unfractionated heparin in the treatment of proximal deep vein thrombosis. *Arch Intern Med* 153:1541, 1993.

35. Lindmarker P, Holmstron M, Granqvist S, et al: Comparison of once-daily subcutaneous Fragmin with continuous intravenous unfractionated heparin in the treatment of deep-vein thrombosis. *Thromb Haemost* 72:186, 1994.

36. Levine M, Gent M, Hirst J, et al: A comparison of low-molecular-weight heparin administered primarily at home with unfractionated heparin administered in the hospital for proximal deep-vein thrombosis. *N Engl J Med* 334:677, 1996.

37. Koopman MMW, Prandoni P, Piovell F, et al for the Tasman Study Group: Treatment of venous thrombosis with intravenous unfractionated heparin administered in the hospital as compared with subcutaneous low-molecular-weight heparin administered at home. *N Engl J Med* 334:682, 1996.

38. Büller HR, Gent M, Gallus AS, et al for the Columbus Investigators: Low-molecular-weight heparin in the treatment of patients with venous thromboembolism. *N Engl J Med* 337:657, 1997.

39. Simmoneau G, Sors H, Charbonnier B, et al for the Thèsèe Study Group: A comparison of low-molecular-weight heparin with unfractionated heparin for acute pulmonary embolism. *N Engl J Med* 337:663, 1997.

40. Charbonnier BA, Fiessinger JN, Banga JD, et al on behalf of the Fraxodi group: Comparison of a once daily with a twice daily subcutaneous low molecular weight heparin regimen in the treatment of deep vein thrombosis. *Thromb Haemost* 79:897, 1998.

41. Hull R, Raskob G, Rosenbloom D, et al: Treatment of proximal vein thrombosis with subcutaneous low-molecular-weight heparin vs. intravenous heparin: an economic perspective. *Arch Intern Med* 157:289, 1997.

42. Spiro T and the Enoxaparin Clinical Trial Group: A multicenter clinical trial comparing once- and twice-daily subcutaneous enoxaparin and intravenous heparin in the treatment of acute deep-vein thrombosis. *Thromb Haemost* 77(suppl):373, 1997.

43. Hull R, Raskob G, Brant R, et al: Subcutaneous low-molecular-weight heparin compared with continuous intravenous heparin in the treatment of patients with pulmonary embolism and underlying proximal deep-vein thrombosis. *Arch Intern Med* (in press).

44. Cohen M, Demers C, Gurfinkel EP, et al: A comparison of low-molecular-weight heparin with unfractionated heparin for unstable coronary artery disease. Efficacy and safety of Subcutaneous Enoxaparin in Non-Q-Wave Coronary Events Study Group. *N Engl J Med* 337:447, 1997.

45. Antman EM for the Thrombolysis in Myocardial Infarction (TIMI) 11B Investigators: TIMI 11B. Enoxaparin versus unfractionated heparin for unstable angina or non-Q-wave myocardial infarction: a double-blind, placebo-controlled, parallel group multicenter trial. Rationale, study design and methods. *Am Heart J* 135:S353, 1998.

46. Mark DB, Cowper PA, Berkowitz SD, et al: Economic assessment of low-molecular-weight heparin (Enoxaparin) versus unfractionated heparin in acute coronary syndrome patients: results from the ESSENCE randomized trial. *Circulation* 97:1702, 1998.

47. Chong BH: Low-molecular-weight heparinoid and heparin-induced thrombocytopenia [abstract]. *Aust NZ J Med* 26:331, 1996.

48. Warkentin TE: Danaparoid (Orgaran) for the treatment of heparin-induced thrombocytopenia (HIT) and thrombosis: effects on *in vivo* thrombin and cross-linked fibrin generation, and evaluation of the clinical significance of *in vitro* cross-reactivity (XR) of danaparoid for HIT-IgG. *Blood* 88(suppl 1):626a, 1996.

49. Gent M, Hirsh J, Ginsberg JS, et al: Low-molecular-weight heparinoid Orgaran is more effective than aspirin in the prevention of venous thromboembolism after surgery for hip fracture. *Circulation* 93:80, 1996.

50. De Valk HW, Banga JD, Wester JW, et al: Comparing subcutaneous danaparoid with intravenous unfractionated heparin for the treatment of venous thromboembolism. A randomized controlled trial. *Ann Intern Med.* 123:1, 1996.

51. Magnani HN: Heparin-induced thrombocytopenia (HIT): an overview of 230 patients treated with Orgaran (Org 10172). *Thromb Haemost* 70:554, 1993.

52. Markwardt F: The development of hirudin as an antithrombotic drug. *Thromb Res* 74:1, 1994.

53. Chari S, Chauhan VS: Hirudin-based synthetic peptides as inhibitors of thrombin. *Semin Thromb Hemost* 20:315, 1994.

54. Hofsteenga J, Stone SR, Donella-Deane A, et al: The effect of substituting phosphotyrosine for sulphotyrosine on the activity of hirudin. *Eur J Biochem* 188:55, 1990.

55. Maraganore JM, Bourdon P, Jablonski J, et al: Design and characterization of hirulogs: a novel class of bivalent peptide inhibitors or thrombin. *Biochemistry* 29:7095, 1990.

56. Klement P, Liao P, Hirsh J, et al: Hirudin causes more bleeding than heparin in a rabbit ear bleeding model. *J Lab Clin Med* 132:190, 1998.

57. The Global Use of Strategies to Open Occluded Coronary Arteries (GUSTO) IIa Investigators: Randomized trial of intravenous heparin versus recombinant hirudin for acute coronary syndromes. *Circulation* 90:1624, 1994.

58. Antman EM and TIMI 9A Investigators: Hirudin in acute myocardial infarction: safety report from the thrombolysis and thrombin inhibition in myocardial infarction (TIMI) 9A trial. *Circulation* 90:1624, 1994.

59. Neuhaus K-L, von Essen R, Tebbe U, et al: Safety observations from the pilot phase of the randomized r-hirudin for improvement of thrombolysis (HIT-III) study: a study of the Arbeitsgemeinshaft Leitender Kardiologischer Krandenausarzte (ALKK). *Circulation* 90:1638, 1994.

60. Eichler P, Greinacher A: Anti-hirudin antibodies induced by recombinant hirudin in the treatment of patients with heparin-induced thrombocytopenia (HIT). *Ann Hematol* 72(suppl):A4 (abstract), 1996.

61. GUSTO IIb Investigators: A comparison of recombinant hirudin with

heparin for the treatment of acute coronary syndromes. *N Engl J Med* 335:775, 1996.

62. Antman EM, and TIMI 9B Investigators: Hirudin in acute myocardial infarction. Thrombolysis and thrombin inhibition in myocardial infarction (TIMI) 9B trial. *Circulation* 94:911, 1996.

63. Organisation to Assess Strategies for Ischemic Syndromes (OASIS-2) Investigators: Effects of recombinant hirudin (lepirudin) compared with heparin on death, myocardial infarction, refractory angina, and revascularisation procedures in patients with acute myocardial ischaemia without ST elevation: a randomised trial. *Lancet* 353:429, 1999.

64. Serruys PW, Herrman J-PR, Simon R, et al for the Helvetica Investigators. A comparison of hirudin with heparin in the prevention of restenosis after coronary angioplasty. *N Engl J Med* 333:757, 1995.

65. Eriksson BI, Wille-Jorgenson P, Kalebo P, et al: A comparison of recombinant hirudin with a low-molecular-weight heparin to prevent thromboembolic complications after total hip replacement. *N Engl J Med* 337:1329, 1997.

66. Greinacher A, Völpel H, Janssens U, et al: Recombinant hirudin (lepirudin) provides safe and effective anticoagulation in patients with heparin-induced thrombocytopenia: a prospective study. *Circulation* 1998 (in press).

67. Bittl JA, Strony J, Brinker JA, et al for the Hirulog Angioplasty Study Investigators: Treatment with bivalirudin (Hirulog) as compared with heparin during coronary angioplasty for unstable or postinfarction angina. *N Engl J Med* 333:764, 1995.

68. Cohen M, Bigonzi F, Lotour V et al for the ESSENCE Group: One year follow-up of the ESSENCE trial (enoxaparin vs. heparin in unstable angina and non-Q-wave myocardial infarction). *J Am Coll Cardiol* 31(suppl A):79A, 1998.

69. Weitz JI, Hirsh J: New antithrombotic agents. *Chest* 114:715S, 1998.

C H A P T E R 1 3 4

FIBRINOLYTIC THERAPY

JOSEPH LOSCALZO

Fibrinolytic therapy is designed to facilitate thrombolysis and thus decrease the ischemic damage produced by thrombotic events. Currently available therapeutic agents all essentially impart proteolytic activity to the inactive plasma zymogen plasminogen. These agents either bind to and induce a conformational change in plasminogen, imparting plasmin-like protease activity to the molecule, or proteolytically cleave plasminogen into plasmin directly. Streptokinase and staphylokinase are bacterial products that can now be synthesized by recombinant DNA technology and impart proteolytic activity to plasminogen. Tissue-type plasminogen activator and urokinase-type plasminogen activators are endogenous plasminogen activators that directly activate plasminogen by converting it into plasmin. Newer agents, including reteplase, TNK-t-PA, and bat-PA, have been developed to enhance fibrinolytic specificity and the rate of lysis. This chapter will focus on the pharmacology of currently available fibrinolytic agents, provide an overview of their clinical applications in specific thrombotic disorders, and review the use of adjunctive antithrombotic therapies with thrombolytic agents in these disorders.

PLASMINOGEN ACTIVATORS

CURRENTLY AVAILABLE AGENTS

STREPTOKINASE

Biochemistry Streptokinase was first isolated in 1933[1] and subsequently demonstrated to possess fibrinolytic activity in vivo in animals and humans in the 1940s and 1950s.[2,3] A product of Lancefield group C β-hemolytic streptococci, streptokinase is a single-chain polypeptide with a molecular mass of 47 kDa. Despite its amino-terminal sequence homology to trypsinlike serine proteases, streptokinase is devoid of an active site serine residue and is thus incapable of proteolytic or amidolytic activity.[4]

Streptokinase itself has no enzymatic activity; instead plasmin-like activity is conferred upon the streptokinase-plasminogen complex without plasminogen proteolysis (see Chap. 116). Figure 134-1 illustrates the sequence of reactions that accounts for the activity and metabolism of streptokinase and the streptokinase-plasminogen complex. Stoichiometric amounts of streptokinase combine with plasminogen to form a streptokinase-plasminogen complex that possesses plasmin-like activity. This complex then reacts with uncomplexed plasminogen to convert it to plasmin directly. In addition, the streptokinase-plasminogen complex undergoes proteolytic cleavage in solution

Acronyms and abbreviations that appear in this chapter include: APSAC, anisoylated plasminogen-streptokinase activator complex; CRE, cyclic AMP-responsive element; HMW-tcu-PA, high molecular weight two-chain u-PA; LMW-tcu-PA, low molecular weight two-chain u-PA; PAI, plasmin activator inhibitor; PPACK, d-Phe-Pro-Arg-chloromethylketone; scu-PA, single-chain u-PA; TNK-t-PA, T103N,N117Q, KHRR(296–299)AAAA; t-PA, tissue-type plasminogen activator; t-PA-ΔFEK1, reteplase; u-PA, urokinase-type plasminogen activator; u-PAR, u-PA receptor.

at the Arg560-Val561 and the Lys77-Lys78 bonds of plasminogen. The complex is then itself subjected to progressive degradation into smaller fragments, resulting in the loss of plasminogen activator activity.[5–7] The activation of plasminogen by streptokinase-plasminogen obeys Michaelis-Menten kinetics[8] with a K_m of 1.4 μM and a k_{cat} of 21.8 s^{-1}. The streptokinase-plasminogen complex activates partially cleaved plasminogen (Lys-plasminogen) approximately fivefold more effectively on a molar basis than intact plasminogen (Glu-plasminogen). The relative catalytic efficiency of the streptokinase-plasminogen complex depends upon whether Glu-plasminogen or Lys-plasminogen is in the complex.

Proteolytic cleavage of both streptokinase and plasminogen in the streptokinase-plasminogen complex leads to the formation of the streptokinase-plasmin complex. The streptokinase-plasmin complex also forms when streptokinase is exposed to plasmin, and it also obeys Michaelis-Menten kinetics[8] with a K_m of 1.1 μM and a k_{cat} of 16.6 s^{-1}. As with streptokinase-plasminogen, the streptokinase-plasmin complex is approximately fivefold more efficient with Lys-plasminogen as a substrate than with Glu-plasminogen.

There are three important comparative differences between streptokinase-plasmin and free plasmin.[9–11] First, the streptokinase-plasmin complex has twice the catalytic efficiency of plasmin. Second, streptokinase-plasmin can directly convert plasminogen to plasmin, while free plasmin is only efficient at converting Glu-plasminogen to Lys-plasminogen. Third, the important plasmin inhibitors, α_2-antiplasmin and α_2-macroglobulin, are comparatively poor inhibitors of the complex.

Fibrinogen, fibrin, and the fibrin(ogen) degradation products, fragments D and E, enhance the activity of streptokinase significantly, with an overall order of efficacy of fibrin>fibrinogen>fragment D>fragment E.[9,10] Fibrin increases the catalytic efficiency of streptokinase-plasminogen-mediated activation of plasminogen 6.5-fold, while fibrinogen only induces a twofold increase in catalytic efficiency.

Pharmacology When administered in vivo to an individual bearing a thrombus, streptokinase binds to circulating plasminogen to form the streptokinase-plasminogen complex. Conversion of streptokinase-plasminogen to streptokinase-plasmin then ensues by one complex cleaving plasminogen in a second complex or by plasmin, produced by the complex acting on plasminogen, complexing with streptokinase. Fibrin binding of the streptokinase-plasmin(ogen) complex is mediated by the ''kringle'' domains of plasmin,[5] in particular kringles 1 and 4. Owing to the lack of inhibition of streptokinase-plasmin by α_2-antiplasmin,[11] this complex can activate clot-bound plasminogen directly. The subsequent generation of plasmin achieves two opposing ends. First, local degradation of fibrin leads to the elaboration of soluble fibrin(ogen) degradation products in the vicinity of the thrombus, which act to augment thrombolysis by enhancing streptokinase-plasmin activity. Second, the degradation of the streptokinase-plasmin(ogen) complex by plasmin leads to progressive attenuation of plasmin activity. In addition, circulating streptokinase-plasmin(ogen) acts upon circulating plasminogen, leading to systemic plasminemia, the proteolytic cleavage of fibrinogen into its degradation products, and the genesis of a systemic lytic state. Profound plasminemia may also lead to reduced concentrations of plasminogen within the thrombus by reequilibration, and this redistribution to plasma may attenuate rates of lysis within the thrombus (''plasminogen steal'').

Pharmacokinetic analysis shows that streptokinase is eliminated from plasma with a monophasic half-life of 18 to 30 min.[12] The biologic half-life (i.e., the half-life of the lytic effects of the plasminogen activator), by contrast, is more prolonged, ranging from 82 to 184 min.[13,14]

Clinical Application Since it was first used over 40 years ago, streptokinase has been widely employed in the treatment of a variety of

i)   Streptokinase + Plasminogen $\longrightarrow$ Streptokinase-Plasminogen

ii) Streptokinase-Plasminogen + Plasminogen $\longrightarrow$ Streptokinase-Plasminogen + Plasmin

iii) Streptokinase-Plasminogen $\longrightarrow$ Streptokinase-Plasmin

iv) Streptokinase-Plasmin $\longrightarrow$ Streptokinase-Plasmin Degradation Products

FIGURE 134-1   Sequential reactions of streptokinase and plasminogen.

thrombotic disorders (Table 134-1),[15-21] including venous thrombosis, pulmonary embolism, peripheral arterial thrombosis, cerebral embolism, thrombotic ureteral obstruction, and acute myocardial infarction. The agent has proved to be effective for lysing culprit thrombi in the majority of these disorders and to improve clinical outcomes in many. Its overall safety is somewhat limited by bleeding complications and, owing to its bacterial origin, allergic reactions including fever, hypotension, urticarial eruption, and bronchospasm. The incidence of these side effects is relatively low, with hemorrhagic complications occurring in approximately 5 percent of patients, 20 percent of which are major bleeding events; allergic reactions occurring in <1 percent of patients; and hypotensive responses requiring drug therapy occurring in 6 to 8 percent of patients. Owing to its bacterial nature, streptokinase induces antibody production in most individuals, and this may be important in patients with recent streptococcal infection. Within 3 or 4 days of administration, the level of neutralizing antibodies becomes sufficiently great to inactivate standard therapeutic doses of streptokinase. These neutralizing antibody titers persist in up to 80 percent of individuals up to 1 year following therapy and in approximately 50 percent of individuals at 2 to 4 years. For this reason, reuse of streptokinase has limited application. If reuse is contemplated, neutralizing antibody titers should first be quantified in order to ascertain the appropriate dosing strategy.

ANISOYLATED PLASMINOGEN-STREPTOKINASE ACTIVATOR COMPLEX

Biochemistry   The pronounced catalytic efficiency of the streptokinase-plasmin(ogen) complex is somewhat limited by its rapid inactivation and clearance from the blood circulation. In an effort to overcome these shortcomings, a chemically modified derivative of streptokinase was developed in which the activator is noncovalently associated with plasminogen and the active site of plasminogen is,

in turn, protected by covalent modification with a *p*-anisoyl group[22] (Fig. 134-2). This compound, termed APSAC (anisoylated plasminogen-streptokinase activator complex), binds fibrin through the plasminogen kringle domains and has a significantly prolonged half-life (94 min).

The combined molecular mass of plasminogen and streptokinase in APSAC is 131 kDa. Specific acylation of the active site Ser740 in plasminogen is achieved by the use of *p*-amidinophenyl-*p′*-anisate hydrochloride, a so-called inverse acylating agent. In the process of acylation the cationic amidino group forms an ionic bond with Asp734 at the catalytic center of plasminogen, positioning the *p*-anisoyl group near the active site serine, Ser740. An acyl transfer reaction then leads to the *p*-anisoylation of the catalytic center of the enzyme.

Pharmacology   Several important pharmacological properties are conferred on streptokinase-plasminogen as a result of *p*-anisoylation. APSAC can be administered rapidly as a single bolus without producing significant hypotension[23]; by contrast, bolus administration of streptokinase frequently leads to hypotension.[24] In addition, compared with streptokinase, APSAC has greater plasma stability, possesses a longer circulating half-life, and has greater lytic potency.

After bolus administration, deacylation of APSAC commences immediately, leading to the generation of the active streptokinase-plasminogen complex. The rate of deacylation follows first-order kinetics; in whole blood, the half-life for the process is 104 min.[25] The plasma half-life of APSAC is approximately 90 min, significantly longer than that of streptokinase.[26] The precise mechanism by which the half-life is prolonged is unclear but may be a consequence of

TABLE 134-1   DISORDERS TREATED WITH FIBRINOLYTIC THERAPY[15]

Venous thrombosis[16]
Pulmonary embolism[17]
Acute myocardial infarction[18]
Unstable angina[19]
Acute reocclusion following angioplasty
Peripheral arterial thrombosis/embolism[20]
Cerebrovascular thromboembolism[21]
Thrombosed artificial cardiac valve
Superior vena cava syndrome
Thrombosed central venous catheter
Thrombosed hemodialysis shunt or catheter
Thrombotic ureteral obstruction
Facilitation of empyema drainage

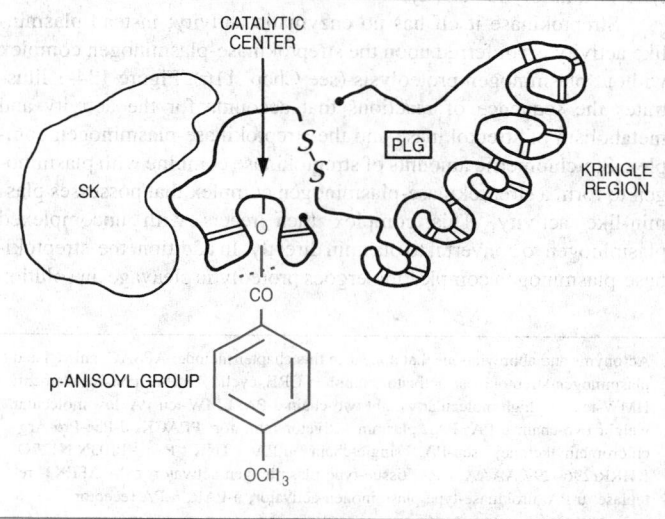

FIGURE 134-2   Structure of APSAC (SK, streptokinase; PLG, plasminogen).

slower hepatic clearance, less neutralization by plasma inhibitors, or relative resistance to proteolytic degradation in plasma.

Clinical Applications APSAC has been shown to be efficacious in acute myocardial infarction and is probably equivalent to streptokinase (see Table 134-1). Its specific benefit is ease of administration; however, hemorrhagic complications appear to be greater than with streptokinase or tissue-type plasminogen activator[27] (discussed under "Endogenous Agents" below). Bolus administration of this compound has not proven to be a critical element in the choice of agent at the current time.

Side effects of APSAC are similar to those for streptokinase, with hemorrhagic complications being of greatest concern. Again, the potential for allergic reactions remains an issue, with urticarial eruption, bronchospasm, erythema, anaphylaxis, and angioedema reported. In addition, neutralizing antibodies have been detected in patients treated with this agent.

ENDOGENOUS AGENTS

UROKINASE-TYPE PLASMINOGEN ACTIVATORS

Molecular Biology and Biochemistry The human urokinase-type plasminogen activator (u-PA) gene is located on chromosome 10, spans 6.4 kb, and contains 11 exons.[28–30] Transcription factors AP1 and AP2 may be involved in promoter modulation of u-PA expression.[30] Functional analysis of the promoter region of the human u-PA gene indicates the presence of a potential enhancer element approximately 2 kb upstream of the transcription start site as well as potential negative regulatory elements approximately 1.5 kb upstream.[31,32]

The mature gene product, single-chain u-PA (scu-PA), is a 54-kDa glycoprotein[28] isolated from urine, plasma, and conditioned cell culture media[33,34] and is synthesized in endothelial cells. scu-PA is converted to the high molecular weight two-chain derivative (HMW-tcu-PA) by limited hydrolysis of the Lys158-Ile159 bond by plasmin and kallikrein.[35] The resulting amino-terminal light chain contains 158 amino acid residues, and the carboxy-terminal heavy chain 254 amino acid residues; light and heavy chains are linked by a single disulfide bond (Cys148-Cys279).[36,37] The serine protease active site is located in the heavy chain.[29] The molecule also contains an epidermal growth factor–like domain and a kringle-type domain, both encoded by exons III to VI.[28]

HMW-tcu-PA can be converted to a low molecular weight form (LMW-tcu-PA) in which the kringle domain is removed by cleavage at Lys135-Lys136. Both the HMW-tcu-PA and this smaller 33-kDa cleavage product are used clinically.

The enzymology of u-PA is complex. scu-PA has little intrinsic plasminogen activator activity[38,39]; according to the best estimates using plasmin-resistant scu-PA mutants, the catalytic efficiency is approximately $0.00015\ \mu M^{-1}s^{-1}$, representing approximately 0.1 to 0.5 percent that of HMW-tcu-PA.[40] scu-PA is also resistant to active site inhibitors of HMW-tcu-PA. Thus, scu-PA meets the criteria for defining it as a true zymogen.

Plasminogen activation by HMW-tcu-PA follows classical Michaelis-Menten kinetics. With Glu-plasminogen as a substrate, the K_m is 50 μM and the k_{cat} is 1.0 s^{-1}.[41] With Lys-plasminogen, the catalytic efficiency has been variably reported to be increased three- to tenfold over that for Glu-plasminogen.[42] Fibrin, fibrinogen, and fibrinogen degradation fragments D and E, as well as ϵ-aminocarboxylic acids such as ϵ-aminocaproic acid or tranexamic acid, enhance the catalytic efficiency of activation of Glu-plasminogen by approximately fivefold.[39,43–45] This improved catalytic efficiency is a consequence of a conformational change in Glu-plasminogen induced by the binding of these agents to lysine-binding sites in the zymogen, which leads

to Glu-plasminogen adopting a structure similar to that of the Lys-plasminogen. As expected from this mechanism, the rate of activation of Lys-plasminogen is not affected by fibrin(ogen) or its degradation products. Importantly, scu-PA and HMW-tcu-PA do not bind to fibrin; hence, the fibrin-specificity of HMW-tcu-PA is likely to be a consequence of the enhanced catalytic efficiency of activation of fibrin-bound Glu-plasminogen that results from this fibrin-induced conformational change in the zymogen.[45–47] The cell-surface receptor for u-PA, u-PAR, serves to enhance the catalytic efficiency of u-PA up to twentyfold.[48]

Pharmacology The pharmacokinetics of u-PA is best characterized by a two-compartment model involving intravascular and interstitial compartments. In humans, scu-PA and HMW-tcu-PA are cleared differently, with initial and terminal half-lives of 69 and 27 min, respectively, for scu-PA and of 12 and 61 min for HMW-tcu-PA.[49] Studies with active-site-blocked enzymes suggest that the plasma half-life is a property of the protein itself and not a consequence of inactivation by plasma inhibitors[50]; clearance is also not dependent on glycosylation.

Clinical Applications The u-PAs have been used successfully to treat a myriad of thrombotic disorders (see Table 134-1). These include venous thrombosis, pulmonary embolism, peripheral arterial thrombosis, cerebrovascular thrombosis, unstable angina, acute myocardial infarction, and acute reocclusion following percutaneous transluminal angioplasty.

TISSUE-TYPE PLASMINOGEN ACTIVATOR

Molecular Biology and Biochemistry Tissue-type plasminogen activator (t-PA) is a 68-kDa serine protease, the cDNA for which was cloned and sequenced in 1983.[51,52] The human t-PA gene is on chromosome 8,[53,54] and approximately 36 kb of the genomic sequence have been determined.[55] The t-PA gene is complex and consists of 14 exons, with the intron-exon organization suggestive of the principle of exon shuffling in the evolution and assembly of the complete molecule. The proximal promoter sequences contain the typical TATA and CAAT sequences, and potential recognition sites for transcription factors have been identified [e.g., cyclic AMP-responsive element (CRE), AP1, NF1, SP1, and AP2], which may function in the regulation of gene expression.[56,57]

t-PA is synthesized by endothelial cells as a single-chain polypeptide.[58–60] The mature protein contains a single free cysteine, Cys83, and 17 disulfide bonds. Plasmin, kallikrein, and factor Xa are all able to cleave Arg275-Ile276 to produce the two-chain form of t-PA[61]; when compared with its single-chain precursor, the two-chain form has a lower catalytic efficiency in the absence of fibrin but an equivalent catalytic efficiency in the presence of fibrin.[62]

There are five distinct domains in the t-PA molecule (Fig. 134-3); from amino to carboxy terminus they include a fibronectin finger-like domain, an epidermal growth factor–like domain, two kringle-type domains, and a serine protease domain. Specific domains account for distinctive properties of the parent molecule, including fibrin binding, plasma clearance, cell surface binding, and fibrin stimulation of plasminogen activation; knowledge of the structure-function relationships among these domains has been provided by analyses of deletion and inclusion mutants, as well as chimeric molecules.

Plasminogen activation by the single-chain form of t-PA follows Michaelis-Menten kinetics, with a K_m of approximately 65 μM and a k_{cat} of 0.05 s^{-1}.[63] Fibrin increases the catalytic efficiency of the molecule several hundredfold and appears to be a consequence of direct binding by t-PA (K_m, 0.1 μM) to the E domain of fibrinogen through its fibronectin finger-like domain and the second kringle-type domain,[64,65] as well as to higher-ordered polymeric structures in the mature fibrin clot.[66] Fibrin-induced enhancement of t-PA activity appears to be a

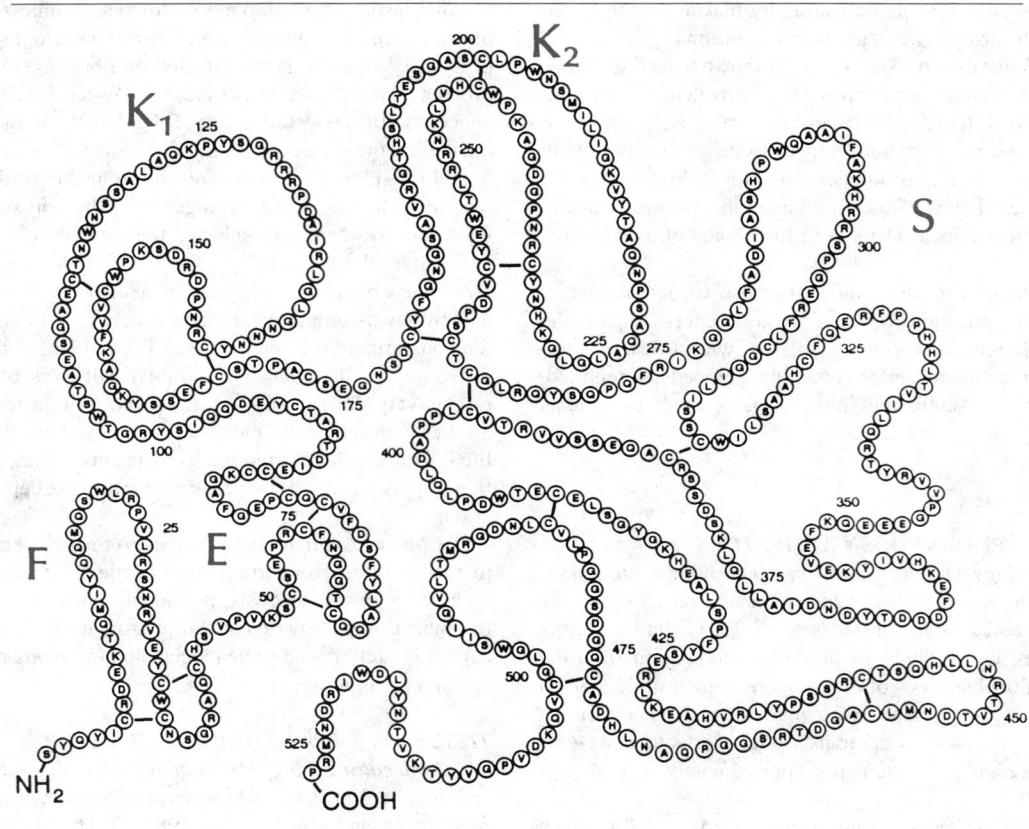

FIGURE 134-3   Structure of t-PA (F, fibronectin finger-like domain; E, epidermal growth factor–like domain; K_1, kringle 1 domain; K_2, kringle 2 domain; S, serine protease domain).

consequence of the induction of a conformational change in t-PA, in plasminogen, or both that promotes the interaction of t-PA with plasminogen on the fibrin surface.[67] Surface receptors on endothelial cells,[68] monocytes,[69] and platelets[70] also serve to enhance the catalytic efficiency of t-PA (see Chap. 116).

Pharmacology   Single- and two-chain t-PAs are cleared from plasma in a manner that is best approximated by a two-compartment model.[71] Single-chain t-PA has an initial half-life of 4.1 min and a terminal half-life of 46 min, while the two-chain form has an initial half-life of 5.2 min and a terminal half-life of 46 min. Clearance of single- and two-chain t-PA occurs in the liver, where specific hepatic receptors mediate the uptake of the molecule from plasma. The dependence of t-PA clearance on hepatic blood flow and function emphasizes the need for cautious use of this plasminogen activator in patients with intrinsic liver disease or reduced hepatic blood flow, such as in patients with significant congestive heart failure.

Clinical Applications   t-PA has been used successfully in a variety of thrombotic disorders (see Table 134-1), including venous thrombosis, pulmonary embolism, unstable angina, acute myocardial infarction, cerebrovascular thrombosis, and thrombosed artificial cardiac valves. The relative fibrin specificity of t-PA compared with other currently available plasminogen activators may not be as important as once believed. This point is particularly relevant in the treatment of thrombotic arterial occlusive disorders requiring rapid lysis to minimize tissue injury; typically, the dose of t-PA required for adequate rapidity of lysis is sufficiently high that systemic plasminemia and a lytic state are achieved. The lytic state produced by t-PA is, however, rarely as pronounced as it is with streptokinase or two-chain urokinase.

NEWER PLASMINOGEN ACTIVATORS

Staphylokinase   Staphylokinase, a 15.5-kDa protein produced by *Staphylococcus aureus,* was shown to have profibrinolytic properties more than 40 years ago.[72] Its mechanism of action is similar to that of streptokinase[73] in that staphylokinase also forms a 1:1 stoichiometric complex with plasminogen which, after conversion, forms plasmin.[74] In contrast with streptokinase, however, it can be inhibited by α_2-antiplasmin, and fibrin binding prevents inactivation by this protease inhibitor.[74] In addition, staphylokinase is much more effective at lysing platelet-rich or retracted thrombi than is streptokinase.[75]

Plasminogen activation by staphylokinase follows Michaelis-Menten kinetics. With Glu-plasminogen as the substrate, the K_m is 7 μM and the k_{cat} is 1.5 s^{-1}. Fibrin binding enhances the activity of this bacterial product approximately fourfold, primarily as a consequence of binding to plasminogen's kringle domains.

Staphylokinase is a highly efficient fibrinolytic agent, producing high rates of clot lysis without significantly influencing plasma fibrinogen, plasminogen, or α_2-antiplasmin levels. Owing to its bacterial origin, however, staphylokinase is antigenic when used in humans with neutralizing antibodies detectable 2 weeks following therapy.[76] Recent data suggest that modification of two of its three immunodominant epitopes can attenuate antigenicity without altering its potency.[77] In a preliminary clinical trial of patients with acute myocardial infarction,[76] 10 or 20 mg of staphylokinase administered over 30 min was shown to be equally efficacious and safe as weight-adjusted t-PA at restoring coronary vascular patency without depleting fibrinogen.

Mutant Tissue-Type Plasminogen Activators   Numerous attempts have been made to improve the efficacy and safety of plasminogen activators by altering the structure of the enzyme using recombinant DNA techniques. One deletion mutant, t-PAΔFEK1, or reteplase, contains only the kringle 2 and serine protease domains and demonstrates fibrin binding and plasminogen activation,[78] with a prolonged serum half-life of 58 min.[79] The efficacy and safety of this recently approved agent was best demonstrated in a recent large trial in which it was found to restore vessel patency more effectively than t-PA in patients with acute myocardial infarction; however, this benefit did not translate into a mortality benefit at 30 days, with both agents producing equivalent outcomes for this endpoint.[80]

Another t-PA mutant, TNK-t-PA, was designed to improve half-life, fibrin specificity, and resistance to inhibition by plasminogen activator inhibitor type I. Its name is derived from threonine and asparagine substitutions at positions 103 and 117, respectively, and four alanine substitutions at positions 296–299. Results of an early clinical trial confirm that the half-life of TNK-t-PA is prolonged (17 min), with equivalent efficacy as t-PA at restoring vascular patency without fibrinogenolysis.[81]

Bat-PA The vampire bat *Desmodus rotundus* secretes plasminogen activators in its saliva; the cDNAs of four of these have been cloned and sequenced, and recombinant forms have been expressed.[82] One isoform of this group of enzymes has been tested in animal models and found to be somewhat more potent than t-PA and also more fibrin-selective.[83]

Other Chemical Conjugates, Mutants, and Chimeras Given the shortcomings of currently available thrombolytic agents,[84,85] many attempts have been made to engineer an optimal agent using recombinant DNA technologies. Owing to an inability to define the "ideal" plasminogen activator (e.g., short versus long half-life, fibrin-selective versus relatively nonselective), none of the molecules designed thus far has shown significant improvement in hard clinical endpoints over "wild type" molecules.[86,87]

THROMBOLYTIC THERAPY

MONITORING THROMBOLYTIC THERAPY

In the early trials of thrombolytic therapy, investigators were careful to monitor a variety of coagulation tests as markers of thrombolytic efficacy and as possible predictors of clinical efficacy.[88] Analysis of these data, provided by many trials over the past 10 years, fails to show any distinct utility of these measurements. Prothrombin time, activated partial thromboplastin time, and thrombin time all increase with fibrinolytic therapy; fibrinogen, plasminogen, and α_2-antiplasmin are all consumed; and fibrin(ogen) degradation products are produced. None of these parameters has been shown to correlate with clinical efficacy, and only reductions in fibrinogen below 100 mg/dl (SI units) appear to be associated with an increased hemorrhagic risk. Thus, routine, repeated monitoring of these parameters is not indicated in the typical patient receiving thrombolytic therapy. One may, however, consider selected measurements to identify patients with undiagnosed hemorrhagic diatheses prior to administration of the fibrinolytic agent; to identify patients who fail to lyse as a consequence of (antibody-mediated) neutralization of the agent (seen infrequently with streptokinase use); or to monitor the adequacy of heparin therapy used adjunctively following the administration of the plasminogen activator (see "Clinical Thrombolytic Regimens"). To assess the adequacy of therapy, evidence for the elaboration of a systemic lytic state should be obtained, such as a reduction in fibrinogen, production of fibrin(ogen) degradation products, or depletion of plasminogen or α_2-antiplasmin.

TABLE 134-2 THERAPEUTIC THROMBOLYTIC REGIMENS

INDICATION	AGENT	REGIMEN
Acute MI[84,85]*	Streptokinase	1,500,000 IU over 1 h
	t-PA*	100 mg over 3 h
		(60 mg+20 mg+20 mg)
	APSAC*	30 U over 5 min
Venous thromboembolism[16]†	Streptokinase	250,000 IU loading dose,
		100,000 IU/h for 24 h
	Urokinase	2000 IU/kg (4400 IU/lb) loading dose,
		2000 IU/kg/h (4400 IU/lb/h) for 24–48 h
	t-PA	100 mg over 2 h

*MI, Myocardial infarction; t-PA, tissue-type plasminogen activator; APSAC, anisoylated plasminogen-streptokinase activator complex. †The use of thrombolytic therapy in the treatment of venous thromboembolism continues to be individualized.

CLINICAL THROMBOLYTIC REGIMENS

Although a variety of regimens have been used to administer thrombolytic therapy over the past 30 years, abundant data acquired through large clinical trials clearly show the efficacy and relative safety of specific dosing schedules in patients with acute myocardial infarction, deep venous thrombosis, and pulmonary embolism. These commonly accepted regimens are listed in Table 134-2. Fibrinolytic therapy has proven to be quite efficacious in a variety of arterial and venous thrombotic disorders as indicated in Table 134-1, and therapy has been shown to be particularly beneficial in patients with acute myocardial infarction,[18] peripheral arterial occlusion,[20] acute cerebrovascular thrombosis,[21] deep venous thrombosis,[16] and pulmonary embolism.[17]

Evidence from numerous trials over the past 15 years clearly indicates that fibrinolytic therapy with t-PA or streptokinase improves mortality and residual left ventricular function; this benefit is time-limited, and the earlier one achieves recanalization of the occluded infarct-related artery the greater the benefit.[18] An analysis of the largest trials of thrombolytic therapy indicate that approximately 12 lives are saved for every 1000 patients treated for acute myocardial infarction. Current practice involves the timely administration of t-PA or streptokinase to patients with acute myocardial infarction who present within 6 h of the onset of chest pain; those presenting within 6 to 12 h of the onset of the infarction may also receive some benefit from fibrinolytic therapy, but the advantages are somewhat outweighed by the disadvantages that are a consequence of the increased hemorrhagic risk of therapy in these patients. Absolute contraindications to fibrinolytic therapy include active internal bleeding, hemorrhagic stroke, nonhemorrhagic stroke within the past year, intracranial neoplasm, and suspected aortic dissection; relative contraindications to therapy include prolonged cardiopulmonary resuscitation, severe hypertension, trauma within the past 4 weeks, surgery within the past 3 weeks, a history of bleeding diathesis, pregnancy, and active peptic ulcer disease. As will be discussed in more detail in "Adjunctive Therapy for Fibrinolysis," it is important to recognize that when treating patients with acute myocardial infarction the adjunctive use of aspirin (325 mg chewed immediately, then daily thereafter) and of full-dose intravenous heparin (administered immediately with the infusion of t-PA or begun 2 to 4 h following infusion of streptokinase) are strongly advised. While it is clearly the case that intravenous heparin increases the rate of bleeding complications approximately twofold, the efficacy of this agent in maintaining patency of an occluded vessel is believed to outweigh the hemorrhagic risk.

u-PA has been shown to be effective in restoring patency in thrombosed peripheral arteries and does so in almost three-quarters of patients.[20] This restoration of blood flow is accompanied by a reduction in rates of both amputation and surgical revascularization.

Most recently, the benefits of fibrinolytic therapy with t-PA for patients with cerebrovascular thrombosis or embolism have been demonstrated.[21] Patients treated within 3 h of the onset of stroke with t-PA were shown to have a clear improvement in 3-month neurological status and disability compared to those treated with placebo. This benefit is tempered somewhat by the risk of intracerebral hemorrhage, although in the final analysis the benefits outweighed the risks in this population. In addition, the benefits persisted up to 24 months following therapy. Of course, patients with a hemorrhagic stroke must be excluded at the time of presentation, mandating rapid assessment by computed tomography or magnetic resonance imaging in all patients considered for therapy.

The benefits of fibrinolytic therapy in patients with venous thromboembolic disease is less dramatic than for arterial disorders. While treatment with streptokinase, u-PA, or t-PA can lyse deep venous thrombi or pulmonary emboli quite effectively, the clinical benefits over conventional therapy with heparin and warfarin have been marginal.[16,17] Only in patients with pulmonary emboli sufficiently massive to evoke right ventricular dysfunction should fibrinolytic therapy be routinely administered; however, even among this group of patients no convincing data are yet available to support an overall benefit in mortality or residual cardiopulmonary morbidity.

SHORTCOMINGS OF THROMBOLYTIC THERAPY

There are three principal shortcomings of thrombolytic therapy as it is currently used: hemorrhage, delays in times to lysis, and reocclusion. The mechanism(s) underlying these adverse outcomes of therapy are complex and require an understanding of the diverse biochemical consequences of pharmacological plasminogen activation.[89–91] Plasmin has the well-known antithrombotic effects of (1) direct fibrinolysis, (2) fibrinogenolysis leading to a reduction in blood viscosity and improvement in blood flow, (3) production of fibrin(ogen) degradation products which themselves are antithrombotic by virtue of their ability to inhibit fibrin polymerization and platelet aggregation, and (4) direct inhibition of platelet aggregation. These effects not only promote thrombolysis and vascular patency but also are at least in part responsible for the hemorrhagic complications of thrombolytic therapy. However, the actual risk of serious hemorrhage, even with the concurrent use of the antithrombotic agents described below, is in the range of 1 percent,[92,93] an incidence that must be critically compared with the serious outcomes that may result from withholding such therapy in selected patients.

Paradoxical prothrombotic effects of plasmin have also been appreciated, and these may account at least in part for the failure of thrombolytic therapy to achieve rapid lysis and prevent reocclusion.[90,91] Plasmin at relatively high concentrations (achievable during thrombolytic therapy) can activate platelets directly.[94] In addition, plasmin can lead to factor X activation and prothrombinase activity.[95,96] These two important effects of therapeutic thrombolysis, coupled with the continued exposure of the prothrombotic components of the fissured atheroma to flowing blood once thrombus is lysed, probably account for the adverse thrombotic events accompanying thrombolysis. In the current thrombolytic era these complications exceed hemorrhagic complications; for example, up to 25 percent reocclusion rates are noted for arterial thrombotic disorders following initially successful thrombolysis with t-PA.[97]

ADJUNCTIVE THERAPY FOR FIBRINOLYSIS

The complications of hemorrhage, failure to lyse, and acute reocclusion following successful lysis exemplify the complexity of mechanisms active during pharmacological fibrinolysis and provide a basis for the

TABLE 134-3   ADJUNCTIVE ANTITHROMBOTIC AGENTS USED WITH FIBRINOLYTICS

Conventional agents
Antiplatelet agent[98]
Aspirin
Antithrombin agent[99]
Heparin
Experimental agents
Antiplatelet agents[100,101]
Iloprost
Prostaglandin E$_1$
Thromboxane receptor antagonists
Thromboxane synthase inhibitors
Serotonin receptor antagonists
Platelet glycoprotein IIb/IIIa antagonists[102]
Antithrombin agents[103]
Hirudin
Bivalirudin
Argatroban
Low molecular weight heparins
D-Phe-Pro-Arg-chloromethylketone (PPACK)
Activated protein C

current approaches to combined, adjunctive therapy. Hemorrhage is prevented by limiting infusions of plasminogen activators to relatively brief periods (minutes for APSAC and up to 3 h for t-PA). By comparison with older lengthy infusions of streptokinase or urokinase for deep venous thrombosis or pulmonary embolism (24- to 72-h infusions), brief infusions are equally efficacious and associated with far less bleeding. Minimizing invasive procedures also greatly reduces hemorrhagic complications. When bleeding does occur, cessation of infusion of the plasminogen activator and mechanical compression (when possible) are the primary treatment options. In extreme cases the use of fresh-frozen plasma, platelet transfusions, or ε-aminocaproic acid should be considered. Recombinant plasminogen activator inhibitor (PAI)-1 and desmopressin may, in the future, also have a role in the treatment of hemorrhage in selected patients.

The use of antiplatelet agents such as aspirin, antiplatelet prostaglandins, or glycoprotein IIb/IIIa antagonists and of thrombin inhibitors such as heparin or hirudin greatly attenuates the thrombotic complications of thrombolytic therapy. Their combined use has been associated with increases in the vascular patency rates of thrombolytic regimens for arterial disorders in conjunction with a reduction in markers of thrombin activity (such as fibrinopeptide A) and of platelet activation. Conventional agents include aspirin and heparin. More recently, platelet glycoprotein IIb/IIIa antagonists, chief among which is the monoclonal antibody abciximab, have been shown to be superb adjunctive antiplatelet agents for patients with acute myocardial infarction treated with fibrinolytic therapy[101] or for patients with acute coronary syndromes undergoing percutaneous transluminal coronary angioplasty.[102] A host of other nonantibody glycoprotein IIb/IIIa antagonists (e.g., tirofiban, lamifiban, xemilofiban) are currently undergoing clinical evaluation and have proven to be useful adjunctive therapies in preliminary trials. However, owing to their short half-lives compared with abciximab, rebound platelet activation may occur at trough concentrations of these agents, potentially leading to recurrent thrombosis. Other experimental agents that have yet to be approved as adjunctive therapies but do provide synergism with plasminogen activators in the restoration and maintenance of vascular patency in animal models and early human trials include iloprost, prostaglandin E$_1$, thromboxane receptor antagonist and thromboxane synthase inhibitors, serotonin receptor antagonists, argatroban, activated recombinant protein C, low molecular weight heparins (e.g., enoxaparin, fraxiparin, dalteparin), D-Phe-Pro-Arg-chloromethylketone (PPACK), and the direct thrombin inhibitors hirudin and bivalirudin (Hirulog). Inasmuch as these agents can provide synergistic antithrombotic effects, they can, as well, evoke synergistic hemorrhagic complications. Clearly, in each case the antithrombotic benefit of these adjunctive agents must be weighed carefully against the hemorrhagic risk. Table 134-3[98–103] contains a listing of the currently used adjunctive therapies and newer, experimental therapies currently undergoing clinical evaluation.

REFERENCES

1. Tillett WS, Garner RL: The fibrinolytic activity of hemolytic streptococci. *J Exp Med* 58:483, 1933.
2. Tillett WS, Sherry S: The effect in patients of streptococcal fibrinolysis (streptokinase) and streptococcal deoxyribonuclease on fibrinous, purulent and sanguinous pleural exudations. *J Clin Invest* 38:1627, 1949.
3. Fletcher AP, Sherry S, Alkjaersig N, et al: The maintenance of a sustained thrombolytic state in man: II. Clinical observations on patients with myocardial infarction and other thromboembolic disorders. *J Clin Invest* 38:1111, 1959.
4. Jackson KW, Tang J: Complete amino acid sequence of streptokinase and its homology with serine proteases. *Biochemistry* 21:6620, 1982.
5. Reddy KN, Markus G: Mechanism of activation of human plasminogen by streptokinase. Presence of an active center in streptokinase-plasminogen complex. *J Biol Chem* 247:1683, 1972.
6. Summaria L, Wohl RC, Boreisha IG, Robbins KC: A virgin enzyme derived from human plasminogen. Specific cleavage of the arginyl-560 valyl peptide bond in the diisopropoxyphosphinyl virgin enzyme by plasminogen activators. *Biochemistry* 21:2056, 1982.
7. Siefring GE Jr, Castellino FJ: Interaction of streptokinase with plasminogen. Isolation and characterization of a streptokinase degradation product. *J Biol Chem* 251:3913, 1976.
8. Wohl RC, Summaria L, Arzadon L, Robbins KC: Steady state kinetics of activation of human and bovine plasminogens by streptokinase and its equimolar complexes with various activated forms of human plasminogen. *J Biol Chem* 253:1402, 1978.
9. Chibber BA, Morris JP, Castellino FJ: Effects of human fibrinogen and its cleavage products on activation of human plasminogen by streptokinase. *Biochemistry* 24:3429, 1985.
10. Takada A, Takada Y: Kinetic analyses of potentiation of plasminogen activation by streptokinase in the presence of fibrin or its degradation products. *Haemostasis* 17:1, 1987.
11. Wiman B: On the reaction of plasmin or the plasmin-streptokinase complex with aprotinin or α-antiplasmin. *Thromb Res* 17:143, 1980.
12. Mentzer RL, Budzynski AZ, Sherry S: High-dose brief-duration intravenous infusion of streptokinase in acute myocardial infarction: description of effects in circulation. *Am J Cardiol* 57:1220, 1986.
13. Grierson DS, Bjornsson TD: Pharmacokinetics of streptokinase in patients based on amidolytic activator complex activity. *Clin Pharmacol Ther* 41:304, 1987.
14. Col JJ, Col-De Beys CM, Renkin JP, Lavenne-Pardonge EM, Bachy JL, Moriau MH: Pharmacokinetics, thrombolytic efficacy and hemorrhagic risk of different streptokinase regimens in heparin-treated acute myocardial infarction. *Am J Cardiol* 63:1185, 1989.
15. Benedict CR, Mueller S, Anderson HV, Willerson JT: Thrombolytic therapy: a state of the art review. *Hosp Pract* 27:61, 1992.
16. Hyers TM, Hull RD, Weg JG: Antithrombotic therapy for venous thromboembolic disease. *Chest* 102:408S, 1992.
17. Goldhaber SZ: Evolving concepts in thrombolytic therapy for pulmonary embolism. *Chest* 101(suppl 4):183S, 1992.
18. Collins R, Peto B, Baigent C, Sleight P: Drug therapy: aspirin, heparin, and fibrinolytic therapy in suspected acute myocardial infarction. *N Engl J Med* 336:846, 1997.
19. Waters D, Lam J, Theroux P: Newer concepts in the treatment of unstable angina. *Am J Cardiol* 68:34C, 1991.
20. Clagett GP, Graor RA, Salzman EW: Antithrombotic therapy for peripheral arterial occlusive disease. *Chest* 102(suppl 4):516S, 1992.
21. Anonymous: Tissue plasminogen activator for acute ischemic stroke. The National Institute of Neurological Disorders and Stroke rt-PA Study Group. *N Engl J Med* 333:1581, 1995.
22. Smith RA, Dupe RJ, English PD, Green J: Fibrinolysis with acyl-enzymes: a new approach to thrombolytic therapy. *Nature* 290:505, 1981.
23. Green J, Dupe RJ, Smith RAG, Harris GS, English PD: Comparison of the hypotensive effects of streptokinase (human)-plasmin activator complex and BRL 26921 (*p*-anisoylated streptokinase-plasminogen activator complex) in the dog after high-dose bolus administration. *Thromb Res* 36:29, 1984.
24. Ferres H: Preclinical pharmacological evaluation of anisoylated plasminogen streptokinase activator complex. *Drugs* 33(suppl 3):33, 1987.
25. Ferres H, Hibbs M, Smith RA: Deacylation studies in vitro on anisoylated plasminogen streptokinase activator complex. *Drugs* 33(suppl 3):80, 1987.
26. Gemmill JD, Hogg KJ, Rae AP, et al: A comparison of the pharmacokinetic properties of streptokinase and anistreplase in acute myocardial infarction. *Br J Clin Pharmacol* 31:143, 1988.
27. O'Connor CM, Meese R, Carney R, et al: A randomized trial of intravenous heparin in conjunction with antistreplase (anisoylated plasminogen streptokinase activator complex) in acute myocardial infarction: the Duke University Clinical Cardiology Study (DUCCS) 1. *J Am Coll Cardiol* 23:11, 1994.
28. Holmes WE, Pernica D, Blaber M, et al: Cloning and expression of the gene for prourokinase in *E. coli*. *Biotechnology* 3:923, 1985.
29. Riccio A, Grimaldi G, Verde P, Sebastio G, Boast S, Blasi F: The human urokinase-plasminogen activator gene and its promoter. *Nucleic Acids Res* 13:2759, 1985.
30. Verde P, Stoppelli MP, Galeffi P, Di Norcera P, Blasi P: Identification and primary sequence of an unspliced human urokinase poly(A)exp(+) RNA. *Proc Natl Acad Sci USA* 81:4727, 1984.
31. Verde P, Boast S, Franze A, Robbiati F, Blasi F: An upstream enhancer and a negative element in the 5′-flanking region of the human urokinase plasminogen activator gene. *Nucleic Acid Res* 16:10699, 1988.
32. Van Hinsbergh VW, van den Berg EA, Fiers W, Dooijewaard G: Tumor necrosis factor induces the production of urokinase-type plasminogen activator by human endothelial cells. *Blood* 75:1991, 1990.
33. Hussain S, Gurewich V, Lipinski B: Purification and characterization of a single-chain high-molecular-weight form of urokinase from human urine. *Arch Biochem Biophys* 220:31, 1983.
34. Wun TC, Schleuning WD, Reich E: Isolation and characterization of urokinase from human plasma. *J Biol Chem* 257:3276, 1982.
35. Wun TC, Ossowski L, Reich E: A proenzyme form of human urokinase. *J Biol Chem* 257:7262, 1982.
36. Gunzler W, Steffens G, Otting F, et al: The primary structure of high molecular mass urokinase from human urine. The complete amino acid sequence of the A chain. *Hoppe Seyler's Z Physiol Chem* 363:1155, 1982.
37. Gunzler WA, Steffens GJ, Otting F, Buse G, Flohe L: Structural relationship between high and low molecular mass urokinase. *Hoppe Seyler's Z Physiol Chem* 363:133, 1982.
38. Ellis V, Scully MF, Kakkar VV: Plasminogen activation by single-chain urokinase in functional isolation. A kinetic study. *J Biol Chem* 262:14998, 1987.
39. Pannell R, Gurewich V: Activation of plasminogen by single-chain urokinase or by two-chain urokinase—a demonstration that single-chain urokinase has a low catalytic activity (pro-urokinase). *Blood* 69:22, 1987.
40. Nelles L, Lijnen HR, Collen D, Holmes WE: Characterization of recombinant human single chain urokinase-type plasminogen activator mutants produced by site-specific mutagenesis of lys-158. *J Biol Chem* 262:5682, 1987.
41. Collen D, Zamarron C, Lijnen HR, Hoylaerts M: Activation of plasminogen by pro-urokinase: II. Kinetics. *J Biol Chem* 261:1259, 1986.
42. Christensen U, Mullertz S: Kinetic studies on the urokinase catalyzed conversion of NH2-terminal lysine plasminogen to plasmin. *Biochem Biophys Acta* 480:275, 1977.
43. Takada A, Watahiki Y, Takada Y: Release of the N-terminal peptides from Glu-plasminogen by plasmin in the presence of fibrin. *Thromb Res* 41:819, 1986.
44. Lucas MA, Straight DL, Fretto LJ, McKee PA: The effects of fibrinogen and its cleavage products on the kinetics of plasminogen activation by urokinase and subsequent plasmin activity. *J Biol Chem* 258:12171, 1983.
45. Markus G, Priore RL, Wissler FC: The binding of tranexamic acid to native (glu) and modified (lys) plasminogen and its effect on conformation. *J Biol Chem* 254:1121, 1979.
46. Vali Z, Patthy L: The fibrin binding site of human plasminogen: arginines

32 and 34 are essential for fibrin affinity of the kringle 1 domain. *J Biol Chem* 259:13690, 1984.

47. Violand BN, Sodetz JM, Castellino FJ: The effect of epsilon-amino caproic acid on the gross conformation of plasminogen and plasmin. *Arch Biochem Biophys* 170:300, 1975.

48. Ellis V, Behrendt N, Dano N: Plasminogen activation by receptor-bound urokinase. A kinetic study with both cell-associated and isolated receptor. *J Biol Chem* 266:12752, 1991.

49. Kohler M, Sen S, Miyashita C, et al: Half-life of single-chain urokinase-type plasminogen activator (scu-PA) and two-chain urokinase-type plasminogen activator (tcu-PA) in patients with acute myocardial infarction. *Thromb Res* 62:75, 1991.

50. Collen D, De Cock F, Lijnen HR: Biological and thrombolytic properties of proenzyme and active forms of human urokinase-II. Turnover of natural and recombinant urokinase in rabbits and squirrel monkeys. *Thromb Haemost* 52:24, 1984.

51. Pennica D, Holmes WE, Kohr WJ, et al: Cloning and expression of human tissue-type plasminogen activator cDNA in *E. coli. Nature* 301:214, 1983.

52. Edlund T, Ny T, Ranby M, et al: Isolation of cDNA sequences coding for a part of human tissue plasminogen activator. *Proc Natl Acad Sci USA* 80:349, 1983.

53. Verheijen JH, Visse R, Wijnen J TH, Chang GT, Kluft C, Meerg Khan P: Assignment of the human tissue-type plasminogen activator gene (PLAT) to chromosome 8. *Hum Genet* 72:153, 1986.

54. Rajput B, Degen SF, Reich E, et al: Chromosomal locations of human tissue plasminogen activator and urokinase genes. *Science* 230:672, 1985.

55. Degen SF, Rajput B, Reich E: The human tissue plasminogen activator gene. *J Biol Chem* 261:6972, 1986.

56. Kooistra T, Bosma PJ, Toet K, et al: Role of protein kinase C and cyclic adenosine monophosphate in the regulation of tissue-type plasminogen activator, plasminogen activator inhibitor-1, and platelet-derived growth factor mRNA levels in human endothelial cells. Possible involvement in proto-oncogenes c-jun and c-fos. *Arterioscler Thromb* 11:1042, 1991.

57. Medcalf RL, Ruegg M, Schleuning WD: A DNA motif related to the cAMP-responsive element and an exon-located activator protein-2 binding site in the human tissue-type plasminogen activator gene promoter cooperate in basal expression and convey activation by phorbol ester and cAMP. *J Biol Chem* 265:14618, 1990.

58. Rijken DC, Wijngaards G, Zaal-de Jong M, Welbergen J: Purification and partial characterization of plasminogen activator from human uterine tissue. *Biochem Biophys Acta* 580:140, 1979.

59. Levine EG, Loskutoff DJ: Cultured bovine endothelial cells produce both urokinase and tissue-type plasminogen activators. *J Cell Biol* 94:631, 1982.

60. Pohl G, Einarsson M, Nilsson B, Svensson S: The size heterogeneity in melanoma tissue plasminogen activator is caused by carbohydrate differences. *Thromb Res* 50:163, 1988.

61. Ichinose A, Kisiel W, Fukikawa K: Proteolytic activation of tissue plasminogen activator by plasmin and tissue enzymes. *FEBS Lett* 175:412, 1984.

62. Loscalzo J: Structural and kinetic comparison of recombinant human single- and two-chain tissue plasminogen activator. *J Clin Invest* 82:1391, 1988.

63. Hoylaerts M, Rijken DL, Lijnen HR, Collen D: Kinetics of the activation of plasminogen by human tissue plasminogen activator. Role of fibrin. *J Biol Chem* 257:2912, 1982.

64. Nieuwenhuizen W, Voskuilen M, Vermond A, Hoegee-de Nobel B, Traas DW: The influence of fibrin(ogen) fragments on the kinetic parameters of the tissue-type plasminogen-activator-mediated activation of different forms of plasminogen. *Eur J Biochem* 174:163, 1988.

65. Suenson E, Bjerrum P, Holm A, et al: The role of fragment X polymers in the fibrin enhancement of tissue plasminogen activator-catalyzed plasmin formation. *J Biol Chem* 265:22228, 1990.

66. Rijken DL, Groeneveld E: Isolation and functional characterization of the heavy and light chains of human tissue-type plasminogen activator. *J Biol Chem* 261:3098, 1986.

67. Suensen E, Petersen LC: Fibrin and plasminogen structures essential to stimulation of plasmin formation by tissue-type plasminogen activator. *Biochem Biophys Acta* 870:510, 1986.

68. Hajjar KA, Hamel NM, Harpel PC, Nachman RL: Binding of tissue plasminogen activator to cultured human endothelial cells. *J Clin Invest* 80:1712, 1987.

69. Felez J, Chanquia CJ, Leven EG, Miles LA, Plow EF. Binding of tissue plasminogen activator to human monocytes and monocytoid cells. *Blood* 78:2318, 1991.

70. Stricker RB, Wang D, Shiu DT, Reyes PT, Shuman MA: Activation of plasminogen by tissue plasminogen activator on normal and thrombasthenic platelets: effects on surface proteins and aggregation. *Blood* 68:275, 1986.

71. Verstraete M, Su CA, Tanswell P, Feuerer W, Collen D: Pharmacokinetics and effects on fibrinolytic and coagulation parameters of two doses of recombinant tissue-type plasminogen activator in healthy volunteers. *Thromb Haemost* 56:1, 1986.

72. Lack CH: A product from *S. aureus* that is fibrinolytic. *Nature* 161:559, 1948.

73. Collen D: Staphylokinase: a potent, uniquely fibrin-selective thrombolytic agent. *Nat Med* 4:279, 1998.

74. Lijnen HR, Van Hoef B, De Cock F, et al: On the mechanism of fibrin-specific plasminogen activation by staphylokinase. *J Biol Chem* 266:11826, 1991.

75. Suehiro A, Tsujioka H, Yoshimoto H, Ueda M, Higasa S, Kakishita E: Enhancing effect of platelets on staphylokinase-mediated clot lysis and plasminogen activation. *Thromb Res* 80:135, 1995.

76. Vanderschueren S, Dens J, Kerbinchai P, et al: Randomized coronary patency trial of double-bolus recombinant staphylokinase versus front-loaded alteplase in acute myocardial infarction. *Am Heart J* 134:213, 1997.

77. Collen D, Bernaerts R, Declerck P, et al: Recombinant staphylokinase variants with altered immunoreactivity: I. Construction and characterization. *Circulation* 94:197, 1996.

78. Burck PJ, Berg DH, Warrick MW, et al: Characterization of a modified human tissue plasminogen activator comprising a kringle-2 and a protease domain. *J Biol Chem* 265:5170, 1990.

79. Jackson CV, Crowe VG, Craft TJ, et al: Thrombolytic activity of a novel plasminogen activator, LY210825, compared with recombinant tissue-type plasminogen activator in a canine model of coronary artery thrombosis. *Circulation* 82:930, 1990.

80. Anonymous. A comparison of reteplase with alteplase for acute myocardial infarction. The Global Use of Strategies to Open Occluded Arteries (GUSTO III) Investigators. *N Engl J Med* 337:1118, 1998.

81. Cannon CP, McCabe CH, Gibson CM, et al: TNK-tissue plasminogen activator in acute myocardial infarction. Results of the Thrombolysis in Myocardial Infarction (TIMI) 10A dose-ranging trial. *Circulation* 95:351, 1997.

82. Kratzschmar J, Haendler B, Langer G, et al: The plasminogen activator family from the salivary gland of the vampire bat *Desmodus rotundus*: cloning and expression. *Gene* 105:229, 1991.

83. Witt W, Baldus B, Bringmann P, Cashion L, Donner P, Schleuning WD: Thrombolytic properties of *Desmodus rotundus* (vampire bat) salivary plasminogen activator in experimental pulmonary embolism in rats. *Blood* 79:1213, 1992.

84. Granger CB, Califf RM, Topol EJ: Thrombolytic therapy for acute myocardial infarction. *Drugs* 44:293, 1992.

85. Cairns JA, Fuster V, Kennedy JW: Coronary thrombolysis. *Chest* 102:482S, 1992.

86. Haber E, Quertermous T, Matsueda GR, Runge MS: Innovative approaches to plasminogen activator therapy. *Science* 243:51, 1989.

87. Vaughan DE, Loscalzo J: New directions in thrombolytic therapy: Molecular mutants and biochemical conjugates. *Trans Cardiovasc Med* 1:36, 1991.

88. Bovill EG, Becker R, Tracy RP: Monitoring thrombolytic therapy. *Prog Cardiovasc Dis* 34:279, 1992.

89. Loscalzo J: Thrombolysis in the management of acute myocardial infarction and unstable angina. *Drugs* 37:191, 1989.

90. Coller BS: Platelets and thrombolytic therapy. *N Engl J Med* 322:33, 1990.

91. Shebuski RJ: Principles underlying the use of conjunctive agents with plasminogen activators. *Ann NY Acad Sci* 667:382, 1992.

92. Sherry S, Marder VJ: Thrombosis, fibrinolysis, and thrombolytic therapy: a perspective. *Prog Cardiovasc Dis* 34:89, 1991.

93. Califf RM, Topol EJ, George BS, Boswick JM, Abbottsmith C, Sigmon KN, et al: Hemorrhagic complications associated with the use of intrave-

nous tissue plasminogen activator in treatment of acute myocardial infarction. *Am J Med* 85:353, 1988.

94. Pasche B, Loscalzo J: Platelets and fibrinolysis. *Platelets* 2:125, 1991.

95. Eisenberg PR, Sherman LA, Jaffe AS: Paradoxic elevation of fibrinopeptide A after streptokinase: evidence for continued thrombosis despite intense fibrinolysis. *J Am Coll Cardiol* 10:527, 1987.

96. Owen J, Friedman KD, Grossman BA, Wilkins C, Berke AD, Powers ER: Thrombolytic therapy with tissue plasminogen activator or streptokinase induces transient thrombin activity. *Blood* 72:616, 1988.

97. Anonymous: Comparison of invasive and conservative strategies after treatment with intravenous tissue-type plasminogen activator in acute myocardial infarction (TIMI) phase II. *N Engl J Med* 320:618, 1989.

98. Roux S, Christeller S, Luediu E: Effects of aspirin on coronary reocclusion and recurrent ischemia after thrombolysis: A meta-analysis. *J Am Coll Cardiol* 19:671, 1992.

99. Hirsh J: Heparin and low-molecular-weight heparins. *Cor Art Dis* 3:990, 1992.

100. Ezratty A, Loscalzo J: New approaches to antiplatelet therapy. *Blood Coag Fibrinol* 2:317, 1991.

101. Coller BS: Inhibitors of platelet glycoprotein IIb/IIIa receptor as conjunctive therapy for coronary artery thrombolysis. *Cor Art Dis* 3:1016, 1992.

102. Anonymous: Platelet glycoprotein IIb/IIIa receptor blockade and low-dose heparin during percutaneous coronary revascularization. The EPILOG Investigators. *N Engl J Med* 336:1989, 1997.

103. Scharfstein J, Loscalzo J: The molecular biology of antithrombotic therapy. *Hosp Pract* 27:41, 1992.

VON WILLEBRAND DISEASE

DAVID GINSBURG

von Willebrand factor (vWF) is a central component of hemostasis, serving both as a carrier for factor VIII and as an adhesive link between platelets and the injured blood vessel wall. Abnormalities in vWF function result in von Willebrand disease (vWD), the most common inherited bleeding disorder in humans. The overall prevalence of vWD has been estimated to be as high as 1 percent of the general population, although the prevalence of clinically significant disease is probably closer to 1:1000. vWD is associated with either quantitative deficiency (type 1 and type 3) or qualitative abnormalities of vWF (type 2). The uncommon type 3 variant is the most severe form of vWD and is characterized by very low or undetectable levels of vWF, a severe bleeding diathesis, and a generally autosomal recessive pattern of inheritance. Type 1 vWD, the most common variant, is characterized by vWF that is normal in structure and function but decreased in quantity (in the range of 20 to 50 percent of normal). In type 2 vWD, the vWF is abnormal in structure and/or function. Type 2A vWD is associated with selective loss of the largest and most functionally active vWF multimers. Type 2A is further subdivided into group 1, due to mutations that interfere with biosynthesis and secretion, and group 2, in which the mutant vWF exhibits an increased sensitivity to proteolysis in plasma. Type 2N vWD is characterized by mutations within the factor VIII binding domain of vWF, leading to disproportionately decreased factor VIII and a disorder resembling mild hemophilia A, but with autosomal recessive inheritance. Type 2B vWD is due to mutations clustered within the vWF A1 domain, in a segment critical for binding to the platelet glycoprotein Ib (GPIb) receptor. These mutations produce a "gain of function" resulting in spontaneous vWF binding to platelets and clearance of the resulting platelet complexes, leading to thrombocytopenia and loss of the most active (large) vWF multimers. Type 1 vWD can often be effectively managed by treatment with DDAVP, which produces a two- to threefold increase in plasma vWF level. Response to DDAVP is generally poor in type 3 and most of the type 2 vWD variants. These disorders often require treatment with factor replacement in the form of plasma or selected factor VIII concentrates containing large quantities of intact vWF multimers.

DEFINITION AND HISTORY

In 1926, Eric von Willebrand described a bleeding disorder in 24 of 66 members of a family from the Åland Islands.[1] Both sexes were

afflicted, and the bleeding time was prolonged despite normal platelet counts and normal clot retraction. von Willebrand distinguished this condition from the other hemostatic diseases known at the time and recognized its genetic basis, calling the disorder "hereditary pseudohemophilia," but incorrectly characterizing the inheritance as X-linked dominant. von Willebrand's confusion about the inheritance pattern was probably due, at least in part, to the greater recognition of bleeding symptoms in women because of the hemostatic stresses of menstruation and parturition. The proband in the original family, Hjördis, was 5 years old at the time of von Willebrand's initial evaluation and ultimately died at age 13 during her fourth menstrual cycle. Four of Hjördis' sisters died between the ages of 2 and 4, and deaths in the family were also noted during childbirth.

An apparently similar disorder was independently reported in the United States by Minot and others in 1928. The original family in the Åland Islands was reexamined by von Willebrand and Jürgens in 1933, leading to the conclusion that the defect in this disorder was due to an impairment of platelet function. It was not until 1953 that Alexander and Goldstein demonstrated reduced levels of coagulation factor VIII in vWD patients, along with prolonged bleeding time. This observation was confirmed by others, including studies of the original von Willebrand pedigree by Nilsson and coworkers. In the late 1950s, the latter group demonstrated that a fraction of plasma referred to as "I-O" could correct the factor VIII deficiency and normalize the bleeding time, indicating that the defect in vWD was due to the deficiency of a plasma factor rather than an intrinsic platelet abnormality. Infusion of fraction I-O promptly increased the factor VIII level in a hemophilic patient, while in vWD the factor VIII level rose gradually, peaking at 5 to 8 h. Fraction I-O prepared from a hemophilia A patient was also shown to correct the defect in vWD, demonstrating that these disorders were due to deficiencies of distinct plasma factors (reviewed in refs. 2 and 3).

It was not until 1971 that Zimmerman, Ratnoff, and Powell prepared the first antibodies against what was thought to be a highly purified form of factor VIII.[4] This factor VIII–related antigen was found to be normal in hemophilia A patients but decreased in vWD. This puzzle was finally resolved with the demonstration that vWF and factor VIII are closely associated, with over 98 percent of the mass of the complex composed of vWF (see below). Thus, antibodies raised against this complex predominantly recognize vWF. The first direct assay of vWF function was based on the observation that the antibiotic ristocetin induced thrombocytopenia and the demonstration by Howard and Firkin[5] that ristocetin-induced platelet aggregation was absent in some vWD patients. Weiss and coworkers[6] used this observation to develop a quantitative assay for vWF function that remains a mainstay of laboratory evaluation for vWD to this day. In 1973, several groups succeeded in dissociating vWF from factor VIII procoagulant activity.[7,8]

Final proof that vWF and factor VIII are independent proteins encoded by distinct genes came with the cDNA cloning of the two molecules in 1984 and 1985.[9-14] These discoveries also marked the beginning of the molecular genetic era for the study of vWF and factor VIII, leading to the identification of gene mutations in many patients with hemophilia and vWD as well as considerable insight into the structure and function of these related proteins.

Table 135-1 summarizes the current nomenclature and terminology for factor VIII and vWF. vWD is a heterogenous disorder with over 20 distinct variants described. The previous complex and confusing classification has recently been consolidated and simplified,[15,16] as summarized in Table 135-2. Type 3 vWD is associated with very low or undetectable levels of vWF and severe bleeding. Type 1 vWD is characterized by concordant reductions in factor VIII activity, vWF antigen, and ristocetin cofactor activity, generally to the range of 20 to 50 percent of normal, in association with normal vWF multimer

TABLE 135-1   VON WILLEBRAND FACTOR AND FACTOR VIII TERMINOLOGY

Factor VIII
Antihemophilic factor, the protein that is reduced in plasma of patients with
    classic hemophilia A and vWD and is measured in standard coagulation
    assays
Factor VIII activity (factor VIII:C)
The coagulant property of the factor VIII protein (this term is sometimes
    used interchangeably with factor VIII)
Factor VIII antigen (VIII:Ag)
The antigenic determinant(s) on factor VIII measured by immunoassays,
    which may employ polyclonal or monoclonal antibodies
von Willebrand factor (vWF)
The large multimeric glycoprotein that is necessary for normal platelet adhe-
    sion, a normal bleeding time, and stabilizing factor VIII
von Willebrand factor antigen (vWF:Ag)
The antigenic determinant(s) on vWF measured by immunoassays, which
    may employ polyclonal or monoclonal antibodies; *inaccurate designa-
    tions of historical interest only* include factor VIII-related antigen
    (VIIIR:Ag), factor VIII antigen, AHF antigen, and AHF-like antigen
Ristocetin cofactor activity
The property of vWF that supports ristocetin-induced agglutination of
    washed or fixed normal platelets

structure. Type 2 vWD is heterogeneous and further divided into four
subtypes (2A, 2B, 2N, and 2M). Type 2A vWD is characterized by
a disproportionately low level of ristocetin cofactor activity relative
to vWF antigen and absence of large and intermediate-sized multimers.
Type 2B vWD is also associated with reduced high-molecular-weight
vWF multimers, but as the result of an abnormal vWF molecule with
increased affinity for platelet GPIb. Abnormalities in vWF that result
in decreased factor VIII binding to vWF have also been described
(type 2N) and present as mild to moderate factor VIII deficiency. Many
other subtypes have been reported, including platelet-type (pseudo-)
vWD, which is actually an intrinsic platelet disorder due to mutations
in GPIb (see Chap. 119). Finally, acquired forms of vWD also occur,
generally due to autoantibody formation.

ETIOLOGY AND PATHOGENESIS

vWF is synthesized exclusively in endothelial cells and megakaryocytes and performs two major functions in hemostasis. First, vWF
serves as the initial critical bridge between circulating platelets and
the injured blood vessel wall, accounting for the apparent defect in
platelet function and prolonged bleeding time observed in vWD pa-

tients. The vWF monomer is assembled into higher-order multimers,
a structure required for optimal adhesive function. Second, vWF serves
as the carrier in plasma for factor VIII, ensuring its stability and
localizing it to the initial platelet plug for participation in thrombin
generation and fibrin clot formation (see Chap. 112). This tight, noncovalent interaction between vWF and factor VIII accounts for the copuri-
fication of these two molecules and the resulting initial confusion as
to the origin of hemophilia and vWD. Factor VIII is encoded by the
factor VIII gene on the X chromosome (see Chaps. 112 and 123),
while vWF is encoded by a distinct gene on human chromosome 12.

THE VON WILLEBRAND FACTOR GENE AND CDNA

The vWF cDNA was initially cloned from endothelial cells[11–14] and
the corresponding gene mapped to the short arm of chromosome
12 (12p13.3).[11] The vWF mRNA is approximately 9.0 kb in length,
encoding a primary translation product of 2813 amino acid residues
with an estimated M_r of 310,000. Comparison of the primary peptide
sequence obtained from plasma vWF[17] with the vWF cDNA sequence
established the pre-propolypeptide nature of vWF.[18] Pre-propolypeptide vWF is composed of a 22–amino acid signal peptide, a 741–amino
acid precursor polypeptide (propeptide) termed *vWF antigen II*, and
the mature subunit.[11,18–21] Cleavage of the 741–amino acid propeptide
from the amino terminus produces the mature vWF subunit of 2050
amino acids (Fig. 135-1).

Analysis of the vWF sequence identifies four distinct types of
repeated domains: three A domains, three B domains, two C domains,
and four D domains.[19,22] The first pair of D domains is tandemly
arranged in the vWF propeptide, followed by a partial and full D
domain at the N terminus of the mature subunit. The final complete
D domain is separated by a segment of more than 600 amino acids
containing the triplicated A domains. The repeated domain structure
of vWF suggests that the gene may have evolved via a complex series
of partial duplications, although exon structure is not highly conserved
between homologous domains.

Comparison of the vWF amino acid sequence to other proteins
identifies a superfamily of related proteins that all share sequence
similarity with the vWF A domains.[23] The common theme among
these potentially evolutionarily related genes is a role in extracellular
matrix or adhesive function. Consistent with this notion, vWF functional domains for binding to the platelet receptor GPIb and specific
ligands within the extracellular matrix have been localized to the vWF

TABLE 135-2   CLASSIFICATION OF VON WILLEBRAND DISEASE

Type	Inheritance	Frequency	Factor VIII Activity	vWF Antigen	Ristocetin Cofactor Activity	RIPA	Plasma vWF Multimer Structure	Previous Nomenclature
Type 1	Autosomal dominant	1–30:1000; most common vWD variant (>70% of vWD)	Decreased	Decreased	Decreased	Decreased or normal	Normal	Type I
Type 3	Autosomal recessive (or codominant)	1–5:10⁶	Markedly decreased	Very low or absent	Very low or absent	Absent	Usually absent	Type III
Type 2A	Usually autosomal dominant	≈10–15% of clinically significant vWD	Decreased to normal	Usually low	Markedly decreased	Decreased	Largest and intermediate multimers absent	Type IIA, IB, I "platelet discordant," IIC–H
Type 2B	Autosomal dominant	Uncommon variant (<5% of clinical vWD)	Decreased to normal	Usually low	Decreased to normal	Increased to low concentrations of ristocetin	Largest multimers absent	Type IIB
Type 2M	Usually autosomal dominant	Rare (case reports)	Variably decreased	Variably decreased	Decreased	Variably decreased	Normal	Type B, IC, ID, Vicenza
Type 2N	Autosomal recessive	Uncommon; heterozygotes may be prevalent in some populations	Decreased	Normal	Normal	Normal	Normal	vWD Normandy
Platelet-type (pseudo-)	Autosomal dominant	Rare	Decreased to normal	Decreased to normal	Decreased	Increased to low concentrations of ristocetin	Largest multimers absent	

A repeats. A potential relationship between the vWF C domains and portions of thrombospondin and procollagen has also been proposed.[24]

The vWF gene spans approximately 180 kb and is divided into 52 exons.[25] Exons range in size from 40 bases to 1.5 kb (exon 28). The latter exon is unusually large, encoding the entire Al and A2 domains and containing nearly all of the known type 2A and type 2B vWD mutations. The concentration of these defects within one exon has facilitated the identification of human mutations responsible for these vWD variants (see Molecular Genetics of von Willebrand Disease, below). A partial, nonfunctional duplication of the vWF gene, termed a pseudogene, has been localized to human chromosome 22.[26] The pseudogene duplicates the middle portion of the vWF gene, from exons 23 to 34, and includes the intervening sequences. The pseudogene is approximately 97 percent identical in sequence to the authentic vWF gene, indicating that it is of fairly recent evolutionary origin.[27]

vWF is synthesized exclusively in megakaryocytes and endothelial cells and, as a result, has frequently been used as a specific histochemical marker to identify cells of endothelial cell origin. Although generally assumed to mark all endothelial cells, vWF is expressed at widely varying levels among endothelial cells, depending on the size and location of the associated blood vessel.[28,29] A recent careful survey in the mouse identified wide differences in the level of vWF mRNA, with 5 to 50 times higher concentrations in the lung and brain, particularly in small vessels, than in comparable vessels in the liver and kidney. In general, the higher levels of vWF mRNA and antigen were found in the endothelial cells of large vessels rather than in microvessels and in venous rather than arterial endothelial cells.[29]

Specific DNA sequences within or near the proximal promoter of the vWF gene appear to be required for endothelium-specific gene expression,[30] although it is likely that additional important regulatory elements exist outside of this region, perhaps at a great distance. A portion of the human vWF promoter from −487 to +246 has been shown to target vWF expression to blood vessels of the yolk sac and a subset of endothelial cells in the adult brain of the mouse.[31] This heterogeneity in expression level among different endothelial cell subsets has only recently been appreciated.[32]

VON WILLEBRAND FACTOR BIOSYNTHESIS

The processing steps involved in the biosynthesis of vWF are similar in megakaryocytes[33] and endothelial cells[34-36] (reviewed in ref. 37). vWF is first synthesized as a large, precursor monomer polypeptide, depicted schematically in Fig. 135-1. vWF is unusually rich in cysteine, which accounts for 8.3 percent of its amino acid content. All cysteines in the mature vWF molecule are involved in disulfide bonds.[38] Pro-vWF monomers are assembled into dimers through disulfide bonds at both C termini, and only dimers are exported from the endoplasmic reticulum (ER).[38-40]

Glycosylation begins in the ER, with 12 potential N-linked glycosylation sites present on the mature subunit and 3 on the propeptide. Extensive additional posttranslational modification of vWF occurs in the Golgi apparatus, including the addition of multiple O-linked carbohydrate structures, sulfation, and multimerization through the formation of disulfide bonds at the N termini of adjacent dimers. vWF is the only protein known to undergo extensive disulfide bond formation at this late stage, and this unique process appears to be catalyzed by a novel disulfide isomerase activity present within the vWF propeptide.[41] Mutations at either of two specific cysteines within

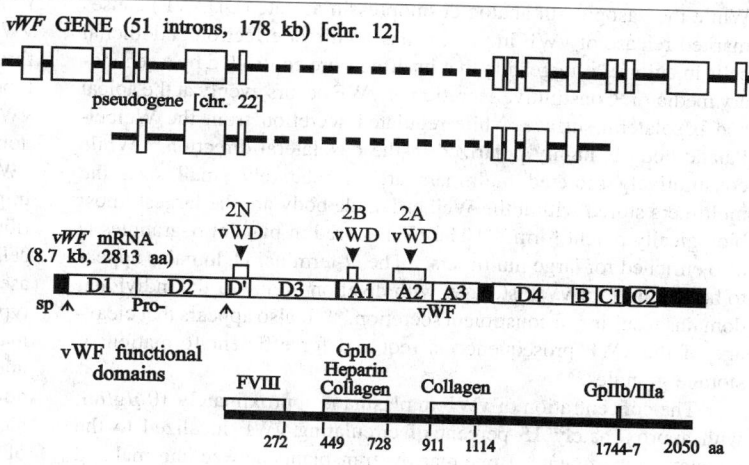

FIGURE 135-1   Schematic diagram of the human vWF gene, mRNA, and protein. The vWF gene and pseudogene are depicted at the top, with boxes representing exons and the solid black line introns. The vWF mRNA encoding the full prepro-vWF subunit is depicted in the middle as the bar and lettered boxes. The locations of signal peptide (sp) and propeptide (Pro) cleavage sites are indicated by arrowheads, and the lettered boxes denote regions of internally repeated sequence. The approximate localizations for known vWF functional domains within the mature vWF subunit are indicated at the bottom. Numbers underneath the domains refer to amino acid residues within the mature vWF subunit. The clusters of mutations responsible for type 2A, type 2B, and type 2N vWD are indicated. (aa, amino acids; chr, chromosome.) (Adapted from D Ginsburg and EJW Bowie[222] with permission.)

the propeptide that are thought to be critical for disulfide isomerase activity, or a shift in the spacing between them, results in loss of multimer formation.[41] The multimerization process appears to require the slightly acidic environment of the distal Golgi.[42] The vWF propeptide self-associates and may also serve to align vWF subunits for multimer assembly.[43] However, the propeptide facilitates multimer assembly even when coexpressed as a separate molecule from the mature vWF monomer.[44,45]

Propeptide cleavage occurs late in vWF synthesis or just prior to secretion. Cleavage occurs adjacent to two basic amino acids, Lys-Arg at positions −2 and −1. An Arg at position −4 is also required for recognition by the intracellular protease responsible for propeptide cleavage.[46] Multimerization and propeptide cleavage are not linked to each other. The multimers secreted by cultured endothelial cells contain both pro-vWF and mature subunits,[36,47] and recombinant vWF with a point mutation inhibiting propeptide cleavage is still assembled into normal multimer structures.[48] Although propeptide cleavage appears to occur primarily intracellularly, cleavage may also occur after secretion.

vWF is secreted from endothelial cells via both constitutive and regulated pathways.[37] vWF is stored in tubular structures within the α granule of platelets and within the Weibel-Palade body in endothelial cells.[49-52] Weibel-Palade bodies are derived from the Golgi apparatus and are found in most endothelial cells, though the number varies considerably. Although a number of other hemostatic proteins are also stored in the platelet α granule, the Weibel-Palade body appears to be relatively specific for vWF and its propeptide.[53,54] The transmembrane glycoprotein P-selectin is also found in the membranes of both the α granule and the Weibel-Palade body.[55] The only other known component of the Weibel-Palade body is CD63, a lysosomal protein also found on activated platelets.[56,57]

Regulated secretion of vWF from its storage site in the Weibel-Palade body is triggered by a number of secretagogues, including thrombin,[58] fibrin,[59] histamine,[60] and the C5b-9 complement complex.[61]

While the vasopressin analog desmopressin acetate (DDAVP) causes marked release of vWF in vivo, it has no direct effect on endothelial cells in culture,[62] suggesting that its effects are controlled by a secondary mediator. Constitutive secretion of vWF occurs evenly at the apical and basolateral surface, while regulated secretion from the Weibel-Palade body is highly polarized in the basolateral direction.[63] While constitutively secreted multimers are of relatively small size, the multimers stored within the Weibel-Palade body are the largest, most biologically potent form.[54,64] The vWF stored in platelet α-granules is also enriched for large multimers.[65] The N-terminal D domains appear to be required for vWF storage, with deletion of any of the individual domains resulting in constituent secretion.[66,67] It also appears that cleavage of the vWF prosequence is required for efficient formation of storage granules.[68]

The concentration of vWF in plasma is approximately 10 μg/ml, with approximately 15 percent of circulating vWF localized to the platelet compartment.[69] Bone marrow transplants between normal and vWD pigs demonstrate that platelet vWF is derived entirely from synthesis within the marrow and does not contribute to the normal plasma vWF pool.[70–72] These studies also demonstrate that both the plasma and the platelet vWF pools are required for full hemostasis, although the plasma pool appears to be more critical.

Plasma vWF appears to be further processed through cleavage by a specific protease in the circulation, resulting in reduction in the size of the largest multimers.[73,74] The major proteolytic cleavage site has been mapped to the peptide bond between Tyr842 and Met843 in the vWF A2 domain,[75] and recombinant vWF missing the A2 domain is resistant to proteolysis.[76] vWF carrying a subgroup of type 2A vWD mutations exhibits increased susceptibility to cleavage by this protease,[77] and this is the proposed mechanism for the selective loss of large vWF multimers in this group of patients (see Molecular Genetics of von Willebrand Disease, below). Recently, this specific vWF processing protease activity has been proposed to play a central role in the pathophysiology of chronic relapsing thrombotic thrombocytopenic purpura (see Chap. 117).[78–80]

THE FUNCTION OF VON WILLEBRAND FACTOR

vWF is a large multivalent adhesive protein that plays an important role in platelet attachment to subendothelial surfaces, platelet spreading, and platelet-platelet interactions, that is, aggregation at sites of vessel injury. vWF also stabilizes factor VIII. The interaction of vWF and factor VIII is important for the protection of factor VIII from inactivation or degradation. Factor VIII bound to vWF may localize to cells and/or sites where it can more readily participate in the promotion of blood coagulation and/or thrombus formation.

vWF is required for the adhesion of platelets to the subendothelium, particularly at moderate to high shear force. vWF performs this bridging function by binding to two platelet receptors, GPIb and GPIIb/IIIa, as well as to specific ligands within the exposed subendothelium at sites of vascular injury (reviewed in refs. 81–83). Binding of vWF to its platelet receptors generally does not occur in the circulation under normal conditions. However, the interaction of vWF with its ligands in the vessel wall, combined with high shear stress conditions, facilitates vWF binding to platelet GPIb and subsequent platelet adhesion and activation. Activation of platelets leads to the exposure of the GPIIb/IIIa complex, an integrin receptor that can bind to fibrinogen and other ligands, including vWF, to form the platelet-platelet bridges required for thrombus growth. Platelet adhesion to vWF immobilized at a site of injury appears to be a two-step process, with the initial tethering of the rapidly moving platelet dependent on the vWF/GPIb interaction and subsequent firm adhesion occurring through GPIIb/IIIa after platelet activation.[84,85]

von WILLEBRAND FACTOR BINDING TO THE VESSEL WALL

vWF binds to several different types of collagens, including types I through VI. Two distinct binding domains for the fibrillar collagens, types I and III, have been localized to specific segments within the vWF A1 and A3 repeats (see Fig. 135-1),[86,87] and a potential third domain has been identified in the propeptide.[88] Studies of recombinant vWF suggest that the A3 collagen-binding domain may be the most important.[89,90] The physiologic relevance of vWF interactions with fibrillar collagens has been questioned, since vWF still binds to extracellular matrix depleted of these molecules by treatment with collagenase.[91] vWF has also been shown to bind to the nonfibrillar collagen type VI, which is resistant to collagenase[92] and colocalizes with vWF in the subendothelium.[93] Type VI collagen supports the binding of vWF under high shear through cooperative interactions between binding domains within the vWF A1 and A3 repeat.[94] Although vWF binding has also been demonstrated in a number of other potential components of the subendothelium, including glycosaminoglycans[95,96] and sulfatides,[97] the biologic significance of these interactions remains to be demonstrated.

von WILLEBRAND FACTOR BINDING TO PLATELETS

vWF interacts with a receptor complex on the surface of platelets composed of the disulfide-linked GPIbα and GPIbβ chains noncovalently associated with GPIX and GPV. The binding site for vWF is within a 293–amino acid segment at the N terminus of GPIb and requires sulfation of several key tyrosine residues for optimal binding.[98] The GPIb binding domain within vWF has been mapped to the A1 segment, within the disulfide loop formed between the cysteine residues at 509 and 695 (see Fig. 135-1).[99,100] Ristocetin binds to both vWF and platelets, but the mechanism by which it enhances the vWF/GPIb interaction is still poorly understood.[101,102] The snake venom botrocetin appears to induce GPIb binding through a different alteration in the vWF A1 domain and is also used to study this interaction.[103] Scanning mutagenesis studies of recombinant vWF have characterized a number of amino acid residues within the vWF A1 domain that are critical for binding to GPIb and for interaction with botrocetin.[104] Several mutations were also identified that increase platelet binding, an effect similar to that of mutations associated with type 2B vWD (see Molecular Genetics of von Willebrand Disease, below). These natural and synthetic mutations cluster in a small area on the surface of the vWF A1 domain structure, as revealed by x-ray crystallographic studies.[105] The structure of the A1 domain closely resembles that of other previously studied A domains, including the vWF A3 domain.[106,107]

The structure of the vWF A1 domain and the mutations that cause enhanced GPIb binding, together with the observations that these mutations enhance binding to similar extents and are not additive when inserted into the same molecule, suggest an allosteric "on-off" model for vWF function.[83,108] In this model, the vWF GPIb binding domain is in an "off" configuration when at rest in the circulation. Binding to collagen (or another ligand in the vessel wall) or interaction with soluble modulators such as ristocetin or botrocetin induces a switch to the "on" conformation, resulting in platelet binding. In an alternative model, it is the immobilization of vWF on a surface, together with high shear force, that facilitates the multivalent interaction of vWF with the platelet surface, rather than a specific conformational switch within the vWF A1 domain.[82,109]

The Arg-Gly-Asp-Ser (RGDS) sequence at amino acids 1744–1747 of the mature vWF subunit serves as the binding site within vWF for GPIIb/IIIa. The latter complex, also known as α_{IIb}/β_3, is a member of the integrin family of cell surface receptors. GPIIb/IIIa undergoes a conformational change to a high-affinity ligand-binding state following platelet activation and, in addition to vWF, can bind a number of other adhesive proteins, including fibrinogen. Although vWF is present in blood at much lower concentrations than is fibrinogen, evidence suggests that vWF may be a critical ligand under flow conditions.[84,85] An RGD sequence is also present in the vWF propeptide (vWF antigen II), although its functional significance is unknown.

THE INTERACTION OF von WILLEBRAND FACTOR WITH FACTOR VIII

The noncovalent interaction between factor VIII and vWF is required for the stability of factor VIII in the circulation, as is evident from the factor VIII levels of less than 10 percent that are observed in most severe vWD patients. Although each vWF subunit appears to carry a binding site for factor VIII, the stoichiometry for the vWF/FVIII complex found in normal plasma is approximately 1 to 2 factor VIII molecules per 100 vWF monomers.[110] Factor VIII bound to vWF is also protected from proteolytic degradation by activated protein C (reviewed in refs. 83 and 111).

The factor VIII binding domain within vWF has been localized to the first 272 N-terminal amino acids of the mature subunit,[112] with antibody studies suggesting a particularly critical role for amino acids 78–96.[113,114] The mutations identified in patients with type 2N vWD, in which vWF binding to factor VIII is specifically affected (see Molecular Genetics of von Willebrand Disease, below), are all clustered in this region, including the most common type 2N mutation, at Arg91.[115] It is noteworthy that the same amino acid substitution at Arg89 is a common polymorphism that does not affect factor VIII binding.[116] The corresponding binding site for vWF on factor VIII includes an acidic region at the N terminus of the light chain (residues 1669–1689)[117] and requires sulfation of Tyr1680 for optimal binding.[118] Thrombin cleavage after Arg1689 activates and releases factor VIII from vWF. Thus, vWF may serve to efficiently deliver factor VIII to the sites of clot formation, where it can complex with factor IXa on the platelet surface.

MOLECULAR GENETICS OF VON WILLEBRAND DISEASE

vWD is an extremely heterogenous and complex disorder, with over 20 distinct subtypes reported (reviewed in refs. 83, 119, and 120). A large number of mutations within the vWF gene have now been identified (Fig. 135-2). A partial list is maintained by a consortium of vWD investigators and can be accessed through the internet at http://mmg2.im.med.umich.edu/vWF.[121,122] These findings form the basis for the simplified classification of vWD outlined in Table 135-2[15,16] and used throughout this chapter. Types 1 and 3 vWD are defined as pure quantitative deficiencies of vWF that are either partial (type 1) or complete (type 3). Type 2 vWD is characterized by qualitative abnormalities of vWF structure and/or function. The quantity of vWF found in type 2 vWD may be normal, but it is usually mildly to moderately decreased (see Table 135-2).

TYPE 3 von WILLEBRAND DISEASE

Patients with type 3 vWD have very low or undetectable levels of plasma and platelet vWF antigen and ristocetin cofactor activity and generally present early in life with severe bleeding.[123] Factor VIII coagulant activity is markedly reduced but usually detectable at levels of 3 to 10 percent of normal. Type 3 vWD appears to be inherited as an autosomal recessive trait in most families, but parents of affected individuals may have mildly reduced vWF levels and are occasionally given the diagnosis of mild type 1 vWD.

Southern blot analysis has identified gross gene deletion as the molecular mechanism for type 3 vWD in only a small subset of families[26,124–126]; however, large deletions may confer an increased risk for the development of alloantibodies against vWF.[26,126] A similar

correlation has been reported for hemophilia B (see Chap. 123). Comparative analysis of vWF genomic DNA and platelet vWF mRNA has identified nondeletion defects resulting in complete loss of vWF mRNA expression as a molecular mechanism in some patients with type 3 vWD.[127,128] A number of nonsense and frameshift mutations that would be predicted to result in loss of vWF protein expression or in expression of a markedly truncated or disrupted protein have been identified in some type 3 vWD families (see Fig. 135-2).[119,121,129,130] A frameshift mutation in exon 18 appears to be a particularly common cause of type 3 vWD in the Swedish population and has been shown to be the defect responsible for vWD in the original Åland Island pedigree.[131,132] This mutation results in a stable mRNA encoding a truncated protein that is rapidly degraded in the cell.[133] This mutation also appears to be common among type 3 vWD patients in Germany[134] but not in the United States.[133]

TYPE 1 von WILLEBRAND DISEASE

Type 1 is the most common form, accounting for approximately 70 percent of vWD patients. Type 1 vWD is generally autosomal dominant in inheritance and is associated with coordinate reductions in factor VIII, ristocetin cofactor activity, and vWF antigen with maintenance of the full complement of multimers (Fig. 135-3). Subgroups within type 1 vWD have been proposed based on the relative levels of vWF present in the plasma and platelet pools.[135–138]

Type 1 vWD is generally assumed to simply represent the heterozygous form of type 3 vWD. However, the majority of heterozygous carriers of vWF gene deletions, as well as carriers of vWF mRNA expression defects,[26,124,125,127,128] are asymptomatic and have normal vWF laboratory values, consistent with an autosomal recessive pattern of inheritance for type 3 vWD. Nonetheless, in some families with nonsense or frameshift mutations, heterozygotes with apparent type 1 vWD have been identified, indicating that some or all type 1 vWD may be due to such defects within the vWF gene (see Fig. 135-2). Mutations that give rise to defective vWF subunits that interfere in a dominant negative way with the normal allele may be particularly likely to cause symptomatic vWD in the heterozygote.[130] Mutations have been identified at several cysteine residues in the vWF D3 domain of patients with moderately severe type 1 vWD. vWF carrying one of these mutations was shown to be retained in the ER and appeared to exert a dominant negative effect on the normal vWF allele.[139]

To date, all mutation studies and genetic linkage analysis of type 1 vWD have been consistent with defects within the vWF gene (reviewed in ref. 130). However, the possibility that a subset of type 1 vWD is due to defects in genes outside of vWF (locus heterogeneity) must still be considered. Given the complex biosynthesis and processing of vWF, defects at a number of other loci could be expected to result in quantitative vWF abnormalities. However, no such example has yet been reported. It is interesting to note that a mouse model for type 1 vWD associated with an up to twentyfold reduction in plasma vWF is due to an unusual mutation in a glycosyltransferase gene, leading to aberrant posttranslation processing of vWF and accelerated clearance from plasma.[140] A similar mechanism may explain the modifying effect of the ABO blood group glycosyltransferases on plasma vWF level.[141]

TYPE 2A von WILLEBRAND DISEASE

Type 2A is the most common qualitative variant of vWD and is generally associated with autosomal dominant inheritance and selective loss of the large and intermediate vWF multimers from plasma (see Fig. 135-3). A 176-kDa proteolytic fragment present in normal individuals is markedly increased in quantity in many type 2A vWD patients. This fragment is due to proteolytic cleavage of the peptide bond between Tyr842 and Met843.[75,142] Based on this observation,

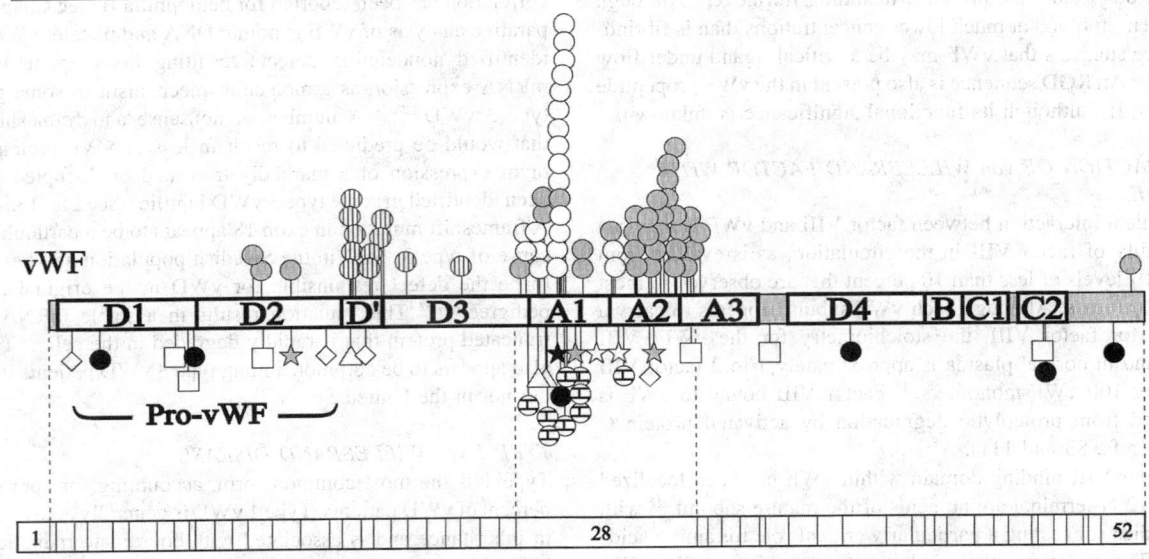

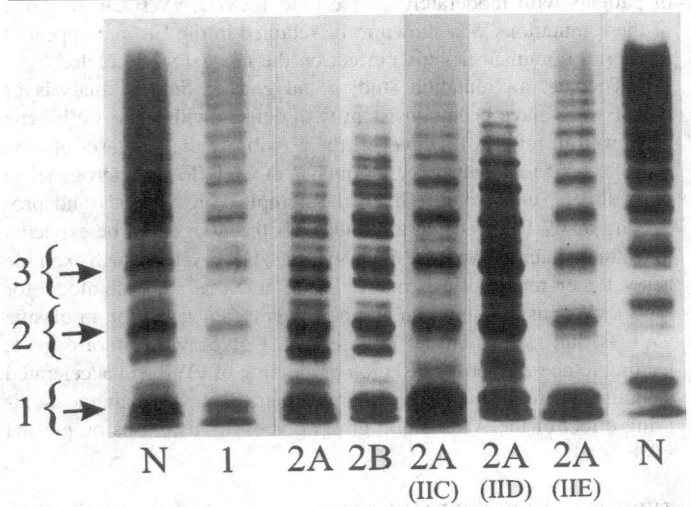

FIGURE 135-3   Agarose gel electrophoresis of plasma vWF. vWF multimers
from plasma of patients with various subtypes of vWD are shown. The brackets
to the left encompass three individual multimer subunits, including the main
band and its associate satellite bands. N indicates normal control lanes. Lanes
5 through 7 are rare variants of type 2A vWD. The former designations for
these variants are indicated in parentheses below the lanes (IIC through E).
(Adapted from SD Berkowitz et al[223] with permission.)

initial DNA sequence analysis in patients centered on vWF exon 28,
in the region encoding this segment of the vWF protein, leading to
the identification of the first point mutations responsible for vWD.[143]
Since that time, a large number of mutations have been identified,
accounting for the majority of type 2A vWD patients.[119] Most of these
mutations are clustered within a 134–amino acid segment of the vWF
A2 domain (between Gly742 and Glu875; see Fig. 135-3), and the
most common, Arg834Trp, appears to account for about one-third of
type 2A vWD patients.[119,121]

Expression of recombinant vWF containing type 2A vWD mutations has identified two distinct molecular mechanisms for the loss of
large vWF multimers characteristic of this disorder.[144] In the first
subset, classified as group 1, the type 2A vWD mutation results in a
defect in intracellular transport, with retention of mutant vWF in the
ER. In the second subset, or group 2, mutant vWF is normally processed and secreted in vitro, and thus loss of multimers in vivo presumably occurs due to increased susceptibility to proteolysis in
plasma.[75,144–147] As noted above, the protease that appears to be responsible for this cleavage has been identified.[73,74,77]

The multimer structure of platelet vWF correlates well with this
subclassification. Group 1 patients show loss of large vWF multimers
within platelets due to defective synthesis, while group 2 patients have
normal vWF multimers within the protected environment of the α
granule.[144] These observations confirm the earlier subclassification of
type 2A vWD based on platelet multimers.[135] Subclassification into
group 1 or 2 might be expected to predict response to desmopressin
therapy, although this remains to be demonstrated.

In addition to the major class of type 2A vWD described above, a number of rare variants previously classified as types IIC–H, type IB, and "platelet discordant" are now included in the new, more general type 2A category. Most of these rare variants were distinguished on the basis of subtle differences in the multimer pattern (see Fig. 135-3; reviewed in ref. 120). The IIC variant is usually inherited as an autosomal recessive trait and is associated with loss of large multimers and a prominent dimer band. Several mutations have been identified in the vWF propeptide of these patients,[148,149] presumably interfering with multimer assembly. A mutation at the C terminus of vWF, interfering with dimer formation, was recently described in a patient with the IID variant.[150] Most of the other reported variants of type 2A vWD are quite rare, often limited to single case reports.

TYPE 2B von WILLEBRAND DISEASE

Type 2B vWD is usually inherited as an autosomal dominant disorder and is characterized by thrombocytopenia and loss of large vWF multimers. The plasma vWF in type 2B vWD binds to normal platelets in the presence of lower concentrations of ristocetin than does normal vWF and often binds spontaneously. Accelerated clearance of the resulting complexes between platelets and the large, most adhesive forms of vWF accounts for the thrombocytopenia and the characteristic multimer pattern (see Fig. 135-3).

The peculiar functional abnormality characteristic of type 2B vWD suggested a molecular defect within the GPIb binding domain of vWF. For this reason, initial DNA sequence analysis focused on the corresponding portion of vWF exon 28.[151,152] Nearly all of these mutations are located within the vWF A1 domain, at one surface of the recently described crystallographic structure.[105] The four most common mutations are clustered within a 35–amino acid stretch between Arg543 and Arg578 (see Fig. 135-2); together, these account for more than 80 percent of type 2B vWD patients.[121] Functional analysis of mutant recombinant vWF[108,153–156] confirms that these single–amino acid substitutions are sufficient to account for increased GPIb binding and the resulting characteristic type 2B vWD phenotype.

Three families have been described that exhibit enhanced vWF binding to GPIb but a normal distribution of vWF multimers. These variants, previously referred to as type I New York, type I Malmö, and type I Sydney, are now all designated as type 2B vWD. Type I New York and type I Malmö have now been shown to be due to the same mutation, Pro503Leu. This mutation is located within the cluster of type 2B mutations in the vWF A1 domain and results in a similar increase in platelet GPIb binding.[157]

TYPE 2N von WILLEBRAND DISEASE

As described in Chap. 123, hemophilia A results from defects in the factor VIII gene and is inherited in an X-linked recessive manner. Rare families have been reported in which the inheritance of hemophilia appears to be autosomal, based on the occurrence of affected females or direct transmission from an affected father.[158,159] Several cases of an apparent autosomal recessive decrease in factor VIII have been shown to be due to decreased binding of factor VIII by vWF.[160–162] This disorder has also been referred to as vWD Normandy, after the province of origin of the first patient. DNA sequence analysis has identified a total of 11 mutations associated with this disorder, all located at the vWF N terminus (see Fig. 135-2).[115,120] One of these mutations, Arg91Gln, appears to be particularly common and may contribute to variability in the severity of type 1 vWD in some cases.[163]

TYPE 2M von WILLEBRAND DISEASE

This category is reserved for rare vWD variants in which a defect in vWF platelet-dependent function leads to significant bleeding but vWF multimer structure is not affected (although some have subtle multimer abnormalities). Most of these variants were previously classified as type I. The variant previously referred to as type B is associated with absent ristocetin cofactor activity but normal platelet binding with other agonists. This variant has been shown to be due to a mutation in the A1 domain (Gly561Ser).[164] Mutations have also been identified in a number of other families with normal vWF multimers and disproportionately decreased ristocetin cofactor activity.[120,165] Several families have been described with a vWD variant (vWD Vicenza) characterized by larger than normal vWF multimers.[166] Although the mutation responsible for this disorder has not been identified, genetic linkage analysis indicates that the defect lies within the vWF gene.[167]

CLINICAL FEATURES

INHERITANCE

Type 1, the most common form of vWD, is generally transmitted as an autosomal dominant disorder and accounts for approximately 70 percent of clinically significant vWD. However, disease expressivity is variable, and penetrance is incomplete.[130] Laboratory values and clinical symptoms can vary considerably, even within the same individual, and establishing a definite diagnosis of vWD is often difficult. In two large families with type 1 vWD, only 65 percent of individuals with both an affected parent and an affected descendent had significant clinical symptoms.[168] For comparison, 23 percent of the unrelated spouses of the patients, who presumably did not have a bleeding disorder, were judged to have a positive bleeding history.

A number of factors are known to modify vWF levels, including ABO blood group, Lewis antigen, estrogens, thyroid hormone, age, and stress.[169,170] ABO blood group is the best characterized of these factors. Mean vWF antigen levels for type O individuals are approximately 75 percent and for type AB individuals 123 percent when compared to a pool of normal donor plasmas. Thus, it may be difficult to differentiate between a low-normal value and mild type 1 vWD in blood group O individuals.[169] The variable expressivity and incomplete penetrance of type 1 vWD has complicated the determination of accurate incidence figures for vWD. The prevalence of type 1 vWD has been estimated to be as high as 1 percent and as low as 3 to 4 per 100,000.[171,172]

In general, the type 2 variants are more uniformly penetrant. Type 2A and type 2B vWD account for the vast majority of patients with qualitative vWF abnormalities. No accurate incidence figures are available for these subtypes, but the type 2 variants are generally felt to comprise 20 to 30 percent of all vWD diagnoses. The type 2 variants are generally autosomal dominant in inheritance, although rare cases of apparent recessive inheritance have been reported.

Estimates of prevalence for severe (type 3) vWD range from 0.5 to 5.3 per 1,000,000.[173–175] Although this variant is frequently defined as autosomal recessive in inheritance, this is not a consistent finding. As described above, one or both parents of a severe vWD patient are frequently clinically asymptomatic and often have entirely normal laboratory test results, but many families have also been reported in which one or both parents appear to be affected with classic type 1 vWD. Thus, in some families, severe vWD may represent the homozygous form of type 1 vWD. In this model, the apparent recessive inheritance in a subset of families could simply be the result of the incomplete penetrance of type 1 vWD. Alternatively, there may be a fundamental difference in the molecular mechanisms responsible for type 1 and type 3 vWD.[130]

CLINICAL SYMPTOMS

Mucocutaneous bleeding is the most common symptom in patients with type 1 vWD.[168] It is important to note that over 20 percent of normal individuals may give a positive bleeding history.[176] This observation, together with the limited sensitivity and specificity of the currently available laboratory tests (see below), makes the diagnosis of mild vWD quite difficult and probably contributes to the wide range of prevalence figures for type 1 vWD currently in the literature.

Epistaxis occurs in approximately 60 percent of type 1 vWD patients, 40 percent have easy bruising and hematomas, 35 percent have menorrhagia, and 35 percent have gingival bleeding. Gastrointestinal bleeding occurs in approximately 10 percent of patients.[177] An apparent association between hereditary hemorrhagic telangiectasia (HHT) and vWD had been reported in several families. Genetic defects causing HHT have been localized to chromosomes 3, 9, and 12 (see Chap. 123), and thus most cases are unlikely to be linked to the vWF gene on chromosome 12. However, since inheriting vWD is likely to increase the severity of bleeding from HHT, the diagnosis is more likely to be made in patients inheriting both defects.[178] Mucocutaneous bleeding is common after trauma, with about 50 percent of patients reporting bleeding after dental extraction, about 35 percent after trauma or wounds, 25 percent postpartum, and 20 percent postoperatively. Spontaneous atraumatic hemarthroses occur almost exclusively in patients with type 3 vWD. Hemarthroses in patients with moderate disease are extremely rare and are generally only encountered after major trauma.

Patients with type 3 vWD can suffer from severe clinical bleeding and experience hemarthroses and muscle hematomas, as in severe hemophilia A (see Chap. 123). The bleeding time is very prolonged. After infusion of vWF-containing plasma fractions, some of these patients develop anti-vWF antibodies that neutralize vWF. Development of antibodies has been correlated with the presence of gene deletions.[26,126]

The bleeding symptoms can be quite variable among patients within the same family and even in the same patient over time. An individual may experience postpartum bleeding with one pregnancy but not with others, and clinical symptoms in mildly to moderately affected type 1 individuals often ameliorate by the second or third decade of life. Aside from an infrequent type 3 patient, death from bleeding rarely occurs in vWD.

Thrombocytopenia is a common feature of type 2B vWD and is not seen in any other form of vWD. Most patients only experience thrombocytopenia at times of increased vWF production or secretion, such as during physical effort, in pregnancy, in newborn infants, postoperatively, or if an infection develops. The platelet count rarely drops sufficiently to contribute to clinical bleeding.[179,180] Infants with type 2B vWD may present with neonatal thrombocytopenia, which could be confused with neonatal sepsis or congenital thrombocytopenia.

Patients who are homozygous or compound heterozygous for type 2N vWD generally have normal levels of vWF antigen and ristocetin cofactor activity and normal vWF platelet adhesive function. However, factor VIII levels are moderately decreased, resulting in a mild to moderate hemophilia-like phenotype.[115] However, in contrast to patients with classic hemophilia A (factor VIII deficiency), these patients do not respond to infusion of purified factor VIII and should be treated with vWF-containing concentrates. Heterozygotes for this disorder may have mildly decreased factor VIII levels but are generally asymptomatic. Although type 2N vWD appears to be considerably less common than classic hemophilia A, it should be considered in the differential diagnosis of factor VIII deficiency, particularly if any features suggest an autosomal pattern of inheritance. Although the factor VIII level rarely drops below 5 percent, at least one type 2N vWD mutation has been associated with factor VIII levels as low as 1 percent, when coinherited with a type 3 vWD allele.[181] The latter observation suggests that a diagnosis of type 2N vWD

should also be considered in patients with marked reductions of factor VIII.

LABORATORY FEATURES

In the initial laboratory evaluation of patients suspected by history of having vWD, the following tests are routinely performed: assay of factor VIII activity, vWF antigen (vWF:Ag), and ristocetin cofactor activity. In a large epidemiologic study, the ristocetin cofactor assay was found to be more sensitive than the vWF:Ag for the diagnosis of type 1 vWD.[182] Other tests that are commonly used include the bleeding time, ristocetin-induced platelet aggregation (RIPA), and vWF multimer analysis. As noted above, results of these tests can all be normal in some patients with type 1 vWD. In addition, the wide range of normal and the considerable overlap with the levels observed in type 1 vWD make borderline levels difficult to interpret. A variety of concurrent diseases and drugs may modify the results of individual tests, including aspirin or other nonsteroidal anti-inflammatory drugs, which often prolong the bleeding time. Many conditions, such as pregnancy, time of the menstrual cycle, hypo- or hyperthyroidism, uremia, recent exercise, liver disease, infection, diabetes, estrogen therapy, or myeloproliferative syndromes, affect the factor VIII activity, vWF:Ag, and ristocetin cofactor activity levels. These values can be regarded as acute-phase reactants, and many minor illnesses can increase their levels to normal. Even controlling for many of these factors, the coefficients of variation of repeated vWF:Ag and ristocetin cofactor assays in a single person are quite large.[183] For this reason, repeated measurements are usually necessary, and the diagnosis of vWD or its exclusion should not be based on a single set of laboratory values unless they are well below or well above the limits of normal.

BLEEDING TIME

The bleeding time has long been used as a standard screening test for vWD and other abnormalities of platelet function.[184] However, results can vary considerably with the experience of the operator and a variety of other factors, and its value as a screening test has been questioned. There is now a general consensus that the bleeding time should not be used for routine patient screening in the preoperative setting.[185–187] While the bleeding time should also probably not be used as a routine screening test for vWD, it may still be of value in selected patients when taken together with the clinical history and the results of other laboratory tests. It may also be useful as a means of monitoring therapy in some settings.

FACTOR VIII

Factor VIII levels in vWD patients are generally coordinately decreased along with plasma vWF. Levels in type 3 vWD generally range from 3 to 10 percent. In contrast, the levels in type 1 and the type 2 vWD variants (other than 2N) are variable and usually only mildly or moderately decreased. The factor VIII level in type 2N vWD is more severely decreased, but rarely to less than 5 percent. The activated partial thromboplastin time (aPTT) can be prolonged in vWD, although only as a reflection of the reduced factor VIII level.

VON WILLEBRAND FACTOR ANTIGEN

Plasma vWF:Ag is usually quantitated by electroimmunoassay, radioimmunoassay, or an ELISA technique. In type 1 vWD, the vWF:Ag assay usually parallels the ristocetin cofactor activity, but it has lower specificity and sensitivity than the ristocetin cofactor assay.

In patients with type 2A vWD, the vWF:Ag is usually low but can be normal.[183]

RISTOCETIN COFACTOR ACTIVITY

The standard measure of vWF activity quantitates the ability of plasma vWF to agglutinate platelets in the presence of ristocetin,[188] also referred to as the ristocetin cofactor assay. Normal platelets washed free of plasma vWF are used either as fresh platelets or after formaldehyde fixation. This assay appears to be the most sensitive and specific single test for the detection of vWD.[182] While it is generally decreased coordinately with vWF:Ag and factor VIII in type 1 vWD patients, ristocetin cofactor activity is usually disproportionately decreased in the type 2A variants, due to the greater dependence of the latter assay on the larger vWF multimers.

A specific assay of FVIII binding to vWF has been developed and is used to confirm the diagnosis of type 2N vWD.[189] Although this assay is widely used in European hemostasis laboratories, its availability in the United States is currently limited to a few specialized reference laboratories.

A number of other assays for vWF activity have been proposed, including measurement of platelet agglutination induced by botrocetin and other snake venom proteins,[190] assays based on collagen binding,[191] and a new functional assay that measures platelet binding under high shear.[192] While the latter device shows some promise, none of these assays is currently available in the routine clinical laboratory.

RISTOCETIN-INDUCED PLATELET AGGLUTINATION (RIPA)

The addition of ristocetin to normal platelet-rich plasma causes platelet clumping. This activity is generally reduced in most vWD patients. Hyperresponsiveness to ristocetin-induced platelet agglutination results either from a type 2B vWD mutation or an intrinsic defect in the platelet (platelet-type or pseudo-vWD). In these disorders, patient platelet-rich plasma agglutinates spontaneously or at ristocetin concentrations of only 0.2 to 0.7 mg/ml. At these concentrations, normal platelet-rich plasma does not agglutinate. Type 2B and platelet-type vWD can be distinguished by RIPA experiments performed with separated patient platelets or plasma mixed with the corresponding component from a normal individual.

MULTIMER ANALYSIS

Analysis of plasma vWF multimers is critical for the proper diagnosis and subclassification of vWD (see Fig. 135-3). This is generally accomplished by agarose gel electrophoresis of plasma vWF to separate vWF multimers on the basis of molecular size, with the largest multimers migrating more slowly than the intermediate or smaller multimers. The multimers may be visualized by autoradiography after incubation with ^{125}I-monospecific anti-human vWF antibody or by nonradioactive immunologic techniques. The normal multimeric distribution is an orderly ladder of major protein bands of increasing molecular weight, going from the smallest to the largest vWF multimers (see Fig. 135-3). Each normal multimer has a fine structure consisting of one major component and two to four satellite bands.[193] Type 2B and most of the type 2A variants were initially distinguished from each other on the basis of subtle variations in the satellite band pattern.

DIFFERENTIAL DIAGNOSIS

PRENATAL DIAGNOSIS

Given the mild clinical phenotype of most patients with the common variants of vWD, prenatal diagnosis for the purpose of deciding on terminating the pregnancy is rarely performed. However, type 3 vWD patients often have a profound bleeding disorder, similar to or more severe than classic hemophilia, and so some families may request prenatal diagnosis. In those cases of vWD in which the precise mutation is known, DNA diagnosis can be performed rapidly and accurately by PCR from amniotic fluid or chorionic villus biopsies.[194] In those cases where the mutation is unknown, diagnosis can still be attempted by genetic linkage analysis using the large panel of known polymorphisms within the vWF gene.[122] One of these polymorphisms, a TCTA tetranucleotide repeat of variable length in intron 40, is particularly useful, with over 100 known polymorphic alleles. Several cases of successful prenatal diagnosis have been reported.[194–196] Although all cases of vWD analyzed to date appear to be linked to the vWF gene, the possibility of locus heterogeneity (i.e., a similar phenotype due to a mutation in a gene other than vWF) should be considered.[130]

DNA DIAGNOSIS OF VON WILLEBRAND DISEASE

With advances in understanding the molecular genetics of vWD, it is now possible to precisely diagnose and subclassify many variants of vWD on the basis of specific DNA mutations identified in the research laboratory. Unfortunately, DNA testing for vWD is not currently available in the clinical setting. As molecular testing is gradually introduced into the clinical laboratory, DNA diagnosis should be particularly straightforward for type 2B vWD, where a panel of four mutations detects over 80 percent of patients. Similar panels of mutations should be able to correctly identify the defect in the majority of type 2A and type 2N vWD. The analysis of type 3 and type 1 vWD will be more complex, since the currently known mutations account only for a small subset of these patients, except in selected populations.[131]

PLATELET-TYPE (PSEUDO-) VON WILLEBRAND DISEASE

Platelet-type (pseudo-) vWD is a platelet defect that phenotypically mimics vWD (see Chap. 119).[197] The plasma vWD lacks the largest multimers, RIPA is enhanced at low concentrations of ristocetin, and thrombocytopenia of variable degree is often present. Clinically, these patients have primarily mucocutaneous bleeding. Molecular analysis has identified mutations within the GPIbα chain as the molecular basis for pseudo-vWD. These mutations are located within the segment of GPIb thought to encode the vWF binding domain and appear to induce the conformational change complementary to that produced in the corresponding fragment of vWF by type 2B vWD mutations.[197]

The specialized RIPA test should be performed at low ristocetin concentrations to distinguish type 2B and platelet type vWD from type 2A vWD. Purified plasma vWF or cryoprecipitate causes platelet aggregation when added to platelet-rich plasma from patients with platelet-type vWD, distinguishing this disorder from type 2B vWD. In addition, type 2B vWD plasma transfers the enhanced RIPA to normal platelets, whereas plasma from patients with platelet-type vWD interacts normally with control platelets.

ACQUIRED VON WILLEBRAND DISEASE

Acquired vWD usually presents as a late-onset bleeding diathesis in a patient with no prior bleeding history and a negative family history of bleeding. Decreased levels of factor VIII, vWF:Ag, and ristocetin cofactor activity are common, and the bleeding time is usually prolonged. Acquired vWD is usually associated with another underlying disorder and has been reported to occur in patients with myeloproliferative disorders,[198] hypothyroidism,[199] benign or malignant B-cell disorders,[200] several solid tumors (particularly Wilm's tumor),[201] or certain cardiac or vascular defects,[202] or in association with several drugs, including ciprofloxacin and valproic acid.[203,204]

A variety of B-cell disorders have been associated with the development of anti-vWF autoantibodies. In most cases the acquired vWD appears to be due to rapid clearance of vWF induced by the circulating inhibitor, although these antibodies may also interfere with vWF function. Hypothyroidism results in decreased vWF synthesis,[199] and, in some cases of malignancy, the acquired vWD is thought to be due to selective adsorption of vWF to the tumor cells. In acquired vWD associated with valvular heart disease or certain drugs, vWF may be lost by accelerated destruction or proteolysis.[203,204]

The vWF multimers in acquired vWD usually exhibit a type 2A pattern, with relative depletion of the large multimer forms. Distinguishing acquired vWD from genetic vWD can be difficult, since testing for the associated autoantibodies is generally not available in the clinical setting. The diagnosis often rests on the late onset of the disease, the absence of a family history, and the identification of an associated underlying disorder.

Management of acquired vWD is generally aimed at treating the underlying disorder. vWF levels and bleeding symptoms often improve with successful treatment of hypothyroidism or an associated malignancy. Refractory patients have been treated with corticosteroids, plasma exchange, intravenous gamma globulin, DDAVP, and vWF-containing factor VIII concentrates.[204]

THERAPY, COURSE, AND PROGNOSIS

The choice of treatment in any given patient depends upon the type and severity of vWD, the clinical setting, and the type of hemostatic challenge that must be met. A previous history of trauma or surgery and the success of previous treatment are important parameters to include in assessing the risk of bleeding. In general, the goals of therapy are to normalize the factor VIII activity and the bleeding time.

DESMOPRESSIN

Epinephrine, insulin, and vasopressin given to normal volunteers induce short-lived increases in factor VIII coagulant activity and vWF levels. Desmopressin (1-desamino-8-D-arginine vasopressin, DDAVP) is an analog of antidiuretic hormone and was originally produced for the treatment of diabetes insipidus. When DDAVP is administered to healthy subjects, it causes sustained increases of factor VIII and ristocetin cofactor activity for approximately 4 h.[205] DDAVP also releases tissue plasminogen activator and plasminogen activator inhibitor, presumably from endothelial cells. Patients with type 1 vWD treated with DDAVP release unusually high-molecular-weight vWF multimers into the circulation for 1 to 3 h after the infusion.[205,206] Therapy with DDAVP increases the factor VIII activity, vWF:Ag, and ristocetin cofactor activity to two to five times the basal level and, in many instances, corrects the bleeding time of type 1 vWD patients.

DDAVP has become a mainstay for the treatment of mild hemophilia and vWD.[207] It is regularly used in the setting of mild to moderate bleeding and for prophylaxis of patients undergoing surgical procedures. DDAVP is most commonly administered at a dose of 0.3 μg/kg, with an upper limit of 20 μg. Common side effects are mild cutaneous vasodilatation resulting in a feeling of heat, facial flushing, tingling, and headaches. The potential for dilutional hyponatremia, especially in elderly and very young patients, requires appropriate attention to fluid restriction, since it may result in seizures. There have been isolated reports of acute arterial thrombosis associated with administration of DDAVP, but the risk appears to be very low when judged against the total number of patients treated.

An intranasal form of DDAVP is also available and appears to be similar in efficacy to intravenous administration,[208,209] although the response may be more variable. Patients receiving DDAVP at closely spaced intervals of less than 24 to 48 h can develop tachyphylaxis. However, in one study, 22 type 1 vWD patients showed a departure of less than 20 percent from the mean factor VIII peak level calculated from two separate infusions. In addition, the consistency of response in one patient reliably predicted the future response of that patient and other affected family members.[210] For patients requiring repeated infusions of DDAVP, the factor VIII activity and vWF responses may not be of the same magnitude as after the first infusion. Although this decay in response has considerable individual variability, after one infusion of DDAVP per day for 4 days it was found that the responses on days 2 to 4 were reduced approximately 30 percent compared to day 1.[208–211]

Approximately 80 percent of type 1 vWD patients have excellent responses to DDAVP. In patients for whom DDAVP is potentially the treatment of choice, a test dose should be given (with measurements of before and after vWF and factor VIII levels) in advance of the first required course of treatment to ensure an adequate therapeutic response. For patients with type 1 vWD who are undergoing surgical procedures, DDAVP can be administered 1 h before surgery and approximately every 12 h thereafter. The response of factor VIII and ristocetin cofactor activity should be monitored when DDAVP is administered at frequent intervals. vWF-containing factor VIII concentrates and/or cryoprecipitate should be available for transfusion as backup.

Approximately 20 to 25 percent of patients with vWD do not respond adequately to DDAVP. This includes many type 2 vWD patients and nearly all patients with type 3 vWD. The response to DDAVP of patients with type 2A vWD is variable. Although most patients respond only transiently, some patients exhibit complete hemostatic correction after DDAVP infusion.[212,213] The differences in DDAVP efficacy among type 2A patients may correspond to the type of mutation, with better responses predicted in patients with group 2 mutations, although this hypothesis remains to be tested.

Many experts consider DDAVP to be contraindicated in the treatment of type 2B vWD, as the high-molecular-weight vWF released from storage sites has an increased affinity for binding to GPIb and might be expected to induce spontaneous platelet aggregation and worsening thrombocytopenia.[214] However, there are two reports of DDAVP used successfully in type 2B vWD patients, with an associated shortening or correction of the bleeding time and variable thrombocytopenia.[215,216]

VON WILLEBRAND FACTOR REPLACEMENT THERAPY

It is important to determine the response to DDAVP for each individual in order to avoid the unnecessary use of plasma products. For type 3 vWD patients and other patients unresponsive to DDAVP, the use of selected virus-inactivated, vWF-containing factor VIII concentrates is generally safe and effective.[217] Cryoprecipitate has been successfully used in the past, but since it is not currently treated to inactivate viruses, it is less desirable. Solvent-detergent-treated plasma is available, and cryoprecipitate prepared from such plasma may be an appropriate choice. It is important to note that most standard factor VIII concentrates are not effective for vWD, presumably because the vWF is either removed or undergoes degradation during processing. Only preparations that contain large quantities of vWF with well-preserved multimer structure are suitable for use in vWD patients. A recent study reported the analysis of 11 different factor VIII concentrates.[217] Humate P and VHP are currently the two most frequently used concentrates, but only the former is available in the United States. Both of these concentrates have been shown to contain large vWF multimers resembling those found in normal plasma.[218,219]

Replacement therapy is largely empiric. In instances of serious bleeding or major surgical interventions, treatment may have to be repeated at least once a day. Although in general there is a correlation between normal hemostasis and correction of the bleeding time and factor VIII activity, this does not occur in all cases. In patients who have concomitant thrombocytopenia associated with or in addition to vWD, it may be necessary to transfuse platelets in addition to factor VIII concentrates. It is recommended that patients be treated for 7 to 10 days after major surgical procedures and for approximately 3 to 5 days after minor surgical procedures. Since postpartum hemorrhage can occur for up to a month or more after delivery, therapy may need to be prolonged in certain patients with severe disease. Sufficient therapy should be given to ensure normalization of factor VIII activity and shortening or correction of the bleeding time. If clinical bleeding continues, additional replacement therapy must be given and searches undertaken for other hemostatic defects. An occasional type 3 vWD patient will develop an alloantibody against the infused vWF, severely complicating replacement therapy.[220] The development of such a vWF inhibitor appears to be more common among type 3 vWD patients with large gene deletions.[26,126] A variety of approaches to the management of vWD inhibitors have been tried, including immunosuppression, similar to the treatment of factor VIII inhibitors in hemophilia A (see Chap. 123).

OTHER NONREPLACEMENT THERAPIES

Estrogens or oral contraceptives have been used empirically in treating menorrhagia. In addition to their effects on the ovaries and uterus, estrogens also tend to increase plasma vWF levels. Patients with vWD frequently normalize their levels of factor VIII, vWF:Ag, and ristocetin cofactor activity during pregnancy. The mechanism of action of estrogens may be related in part to the increased production of vWF through a direct effect on endothelial cells.[221] In pregnant patients with type 1 vWD, the factor VIII and ristocetin cofactor activities usually rise above 50 percent. These patients usually do not require any specific therapy at the time of parturition. In contrast, individuals who have 30 percent or less factor VIII or variant forms of vWD are more likely to require prophylactic therapy before delivery. Postpartum hemorrhage in all forms of vWD may occur as long as 1 month postpartum. Some patients are treated with plasma products prophylactically. Postpartum hemorrhage within the first few days after parturition may be related to the relatively rapid return to prepregnancy levels of factor VIII and vWF activities.

Fibrinolytic inhibitors such as ε-aminocaproic acid have been used effectively in some vWD patients. Fibrinolytic inhibitors have been suggested as an adjunct to DDAVP infusion, given the potential for enhanced fibrinolysis as a result of the release of tissue plasminogen activator along with vWF. However, fibrinolytic inhibitors are not generally used in this setting and are generally restricted to prophylactic treatment for dental procedures or empiric treatment of chronic menorrhagia or recurrent epistaxis.

REFERENCES

1. von Willebrand EA: Hereditär Pseudohemofili. *Fin Lakaresallsk Handl* 67:7, 1926.
2. Hoyer LW: von Willebrand's disease. *Prog Hemost Thromb* 3:231, 1976.
3. Nilsson IM: von Willebrand's disease: Fifty years old. *Acta Med Scand* 201:497, 1977.
4. Zimmerman TS, Ratnoff OD, Powell AE: Immunologic differentiation of classic hemophilia (factor VIII deficiency) and von Willebrand disease. *J Clin Invest* 50:244, 1971.
5. Howard MA, Firkin BG: Ristocetin: A new tool in the investigation of platelet aggregation. *Thromb Diath Haemorrh* 76:362, 1971.
6. Weiss HJ, Rogers J, Brand H: Defective ristocetin-induced platelet aggregation in von Willebrand's disease and its correction by factor VIII. *J Clin Invest* 52:2697, 1973.
7. Weiss HJ, Hoyer LW: von Willebrand factor: Dissociation from antihemophilic factor procoagulant activity. *Science* 182:1149, 1973.
8. Zimmerman TS, Edgington TS: Factor VIII coagulant activity and factor VIII–like antigen: Independent molecular entities. *J Exp Med* 138:1015, 1973.
9. Gitschier J, Wood WI, Goralka TM, et al: Characterization of the human factor VIII gene. *Nature* 312:326, 1984.
10. Toole JJ, Knopf JL, Wozney JM, et al: Molecular cloning of a cDNA encoding human antihaemophilic factor. *Nature* 312:342, 1984.
11. Ginsburg D, Handin RI, Bonthron DT, et al: Human von Willebrand factor (vWF): Isolation of complementary DNA (cDNA) clones and chromosomal localization. *Science* 228:1401, 1985.
12. Lynch DC, Zimmerman TS, Collins CJ, et al: Molecular cloning of cDNA for human von Willebrand factor: Authentication by a new method. *Cell* 41:49, 1985.
13. Sadler JE, Shelton-Inloes BB, Sorace JM, et al: Cloning and characterization of two cDNAs coding for human von Willebrand factor. *Proc Natl Acad Sci USA* 82:6394, 1985.
14. Verweij CL, de Vries CJM, Distel B, et al: Construction of cDNA coding for human von Willebrand factor using antibody probes for colony-screening and mapping of the chromosomal gene. *Nucleic Acids Res* 13:4699, 1985.
15. Sadler JE: A revised classification of von Willebrand disease. *Thromb Haemost* 71:520, 1994.
16. Sadler JE, Gralnick HR: Commentary: A new classification for von Willebrand disease. *Blood* 84:676, 1994.
17. Titani K, Kumar S, Takio K, et al: Amino acid sequence of human von Willebrand factor. *Biochemistry* 25:3171, 1986.
18. Fay PJ, Kawai Y, Wagner DD, et al: Propolypeptide of von Willebrand factor circulates in blood and is identical to von Willebrand antigen II. *Science* 232:995, 1986.
19. Bonthron DT, Handin RI, Kaufman RJ, et al: Structure of pre-pro-von Willebrand factor and its expression in heterologous cells. *Nature* 324:270, 1986.
20. Bonthron DT, Orr EC, Mitsock LM, et al: Nucleotide sequence of pre-pro-von Willebrand factor cDNA. *Nucleic Acids Res* 14:7125, 1986.
21. Shelton-Inloes BB, Broze GJ Jr, Miletich JP, Sadler JE: Evolution of human von Willebrand Factor: cDNA sequence polymorphisms, repeated domains, and relationship to von Willebrand antigen II. *Biochem Biophys Res Commun* 144:657, 1987.
22. Shelton-Inloes BB, Titani K, Sadler JE: cDNA sequences for human von Willebrand factor reveal five types of repeated domains and five possible protein sequence polymorphisms. *Biochemistry* 25:3164, 1986.
23. Colombatti A, Bonaldo P: The superfamily of proteins with von Willebrand factor type A–like domains: One theme common to components of extracellular matrix, hemostasis, cellular adhesion, and defense mechanisms. *Blood* 77:2305, 1991.
24. Hunt LT, Barker WC: von Willebrand factor shares a distinctive cysteine-rich domain with thrombospondin and procollagen. *Biochem Biophys Res Commun* 144:876, 1987.
25. Mancuso DJ, Tuley EA, Westfield LA, et al: Structure of the gene for human von Willebrand factor. *J Biol Chem* 264:19514, 1989.
26. Shelton-Inloes BB, Chehab FF, Mannucci PM, et al: Gene deletions correlate with the development of alloantibodies in von Willebrand disease. *J Clin Invest* 79:1459, 1987.
27. Mancuso DJ, Tuley EA, Westfield LA, et al: Human von Willebrand factor gene and pseudogene: Structural analysis and differentiation by polymerase chain reaction. *Biochemistry* 30:253, 1991.
28. Rand JH, Badimon L, Gordon RE, et al: Distribution of von Willebrand factor in porcine intima varies with blood vessel type and location. *Arteriosclerosis* 7:287, 1987.
29. Yamamoto K, de Waard V, Fearns C, Loskutoff DJ: Tissue distribution and regulation of murine von Willebrand factor gene expression in vivo. *Blood* 92:2791, 1998.

30. Jahroudi N, Lynch DC: Endothelial-cell-specific regulation of von Willebrand factor gene expression. *Mol Cell Biol* 14:999, 1994.

31. Aird WC, Jahroudi N, Weiler-Guettler H, et al: Human von Willebrand factor gene sequences target expression to a subpopulation of endothelial cells in transgenic mice. *Proc Natl Acad Sci USA* 92:4567, 1995.

32. Rosenberg RD, Aird WC: Vascular-bed–specific hemostasis and hypercoagulable states. *N Engl J Med* 340:1555, 1999.

33. Sporn LA, Chavin SI, Marder VJ, Wagner DD: Biosynthesis of von Willebrand protein by human megakaryocytes. *J Clin Invest* 76:1102, 1985.

34. Lynch DC, Williams R, Zimmerman TS, et al: Biosynthesis of the subunits of factor VIIIR by bovine aortic endothelial cells. *Proc Natl Acad Sci USA* 80:2738, 1983.

35. Wagner DD, Marder VJ: Biosynthesis of von Willebrand protein by human endothelial cells. *J Biol Chem* 258:2065, 1983.

36. Wagner DD, Marder VJ: Biosynthesis of von Willebrand protein by human endothelial cells: Processing steps and their intracellular localization. *J Cell Biol* 99:2123, 1984.

37. Wagner DD: Cell biology of von Willebrand factor. *Annu Rev Cell Biol* 6:217, 1990.

38. Marti T, Rosselet SJ, Titani K, Walsh KA: Identification of disulfide-bridged substructures within human von Willebrand factor. *Biochemistry* 26:8099, 1987.

39. Wagner DD, Lawrence SO, Ohlsson-Wilhelm BM, et al: Topology and order of formation of interchain disulfide bonds in von Willebrand factor. *Blood* 69:27, 1987.

40. Voorberg J, Fontijn R, Calafat J, et al: Assembly and routing of von Willebrand factor variants: The requirements for disulfide-linked dimerization reside within the carboxy-terminal 151 amino acids. *J Cell Biol* 113:195, 1991.

41. Mayadas TN, Wagner DD: Vicinal cysteines in the prosequence play a role in von Willebrand factor multimer assembly. *Proc Natl Acad Sci USA* 89:3531, 1992.

42. Mayadas TN, Wagner DD: In vitro multimerization of von Willebrand factor is triggered by low pH: Importance of the propolypeptide and free sulfhydryls. *J Biol Chem* 264:13497, 1989.

43. Wagner DD, Fay PJ, Sporn LA, et al: Divergent fates of von Willebrand factor and its propolypeptide (von Willebrand antigen II) after secretion from endothelial cells. *Proc Natl Acad Sci USA* 84:1955, 1987.

44. Verweij CL, Hart M, Pannekoek H: Expression of variant von Willebrand factor (vWF) cDNA in heterologous cells: Requirement of the propolypeptide in vWF multimer formation. *EMBO J* 6:2885, 1987.

45. Wise RJ, Pittman DD, Handin RI, et al: The propeptide of von Willebrand factor independently mediates the assembly of von Willebrand multimers. *Cell* 52:229, 1988.

46. Rehemtulla A, Kaufman RJ: Preferred sequence requirements for cleavage of pro-von Willebrand propeptide-processing enzymes. *Blood* 79:2349, 1992.

47. Lynch DC, Zimmerman TS, Ling EH, Browning PJ: An explanation for minor multimer species in endothelial cell-synthesized von Willebrand factor. *J Clin Invest* 77:2048, 1986.

48. Verweij CL, Hart M, Pannekoek H: Proteolytic cleavage of the precursor of von Willebrand factor is not essential for multimer formation. *J Biol Chem* 263:7921, 1988.

49. Weibel ER, Palade GE: New cytoplasmic components in arterial endothelia. *J Biol Chem* 23:101, 1964.

50. Wagner DD, Olmsted JB, Marder VJ: Immunolocalization of von Willebrand protein in Weibel-Palade bodies of human endothelial cells. *J Cell Biol* 95:355, 1982.

51. Cramer EM, Meyer D, le Menn R, Breton-Gorius J: Eccentric localization of von Willebrand factor in an internal structure of platelet alpha-granule resembling that of Weibel-Palade bodies. *Blood* 66:710, 1985.

52. Wagner DD: Storage and secretion of von Willebrand factor, in *Coagulation and Bleeding Disorders: The Role of Factor VIII and von Willebrand Factor,* edited by ZM Ruggeri, TS Zimmerman, p 161. Marcel Dekker, New York, 1989.

53. McCarroll DR, Levin EG, Montgomery RR: Endothelial cell synthesis of von Willebrand antigen II, von Willebrand factor, and von Willebrand factor/von Willebrand antigen II complex. *J Clin Invest* 75:1089, 1985.

54. Ewenstein BM, Warhol MJ, Handin RI, Pober JS: Composition of the von Willebrand factor storage organelle (Weibel-Palade body) isolated from cultured human umbilical vein endothelial cells. *J Cell Biol* 104:1423, 1987.

55. Bonfanti R, Furie BC, Furie B, Wagner DD: PADGEM (GMP140) is a component of Weibel-Palade bodies of human endothelial cells. *Blood* 73:1109, 1989.

56. Metzelaar MJ, Wijngaard PLJ, Peters PJ, et al: CD63 antigen: A novel lysosomal membrane glycoprotein, cloned by a screening procedure for intracellular antigens in eukaryotic cells. *J Biol Chem* 266:3239, 1991.

57. Vischer UM, Wagner DD: CD63 is a component of Weibel-Palade bodies of human endothelial cells. *Blood* 82:1184, 1993.

58. Levine JD, Harlan JM, Harker LA, et al: Thrombin-mediated release of factor VIII antigen from human umbilical vein endothelial cells in culture. *Blood* 60:531, 1982.

59. Ribes JA, Francis CW, Wagner DD: Fibrin induces release of von Willebrand factor from endothelial cells. *J Clin Invest* 79:117, 1987.

60. Hamilton KK, Sims PJ: Changes in cytosolic Ca^{2+} associated with von Willebrand factor release in human endothelial cells exposed to histamine: Study of microcarrier cell monolayers using the fluorescent probe indo-1. *J Clin Invest* 79:600, 1987.

61. Hattori R, Hamilton KK, McEver RP, Sims PJ: Complement proteins C5b-9 induce secretion of high molecular weight multimers of endothelial von Willebrand factor and translocation of granule membrane protein GMP-140 to the cell surface. *J Biol Chem* 264:9053, 1989.

62. Mannucci PM, Aberg M, Nilsson IM, Robertson B: Mechanism of plasminogen activator and factor VIII increase after vasoactive drugs. *Br J Haematol* 30:81, 1975.

63. Sporn LA, Marder VJ, Wagner DD: Differing polarity of the constitutive and regulated secretory pathways for von Willebrand factor in endothelial cells. *J Cell Biol* 108:1283, 1989.

64. Sporn LA, Marder VJ, Wagner DD: Inducible secretion of large, biologically potent von Willebrand factor multimers. *Cell* 46:185, 1986.

65. Fernandez MF, Ginsberg MH, Ruggeri ZM, et al: Multimeric structure of platelet factor VIII/von Willebrand factor: The presence of larger multimers and their reassociation with thrombin-stimulated platelets. *Blood* 60:1132, 1982.

66. Wagner DD, Saffaripour S, Bonfanti R, et al: Induction of specific storage organelles by von Willebrand factor propolypeptide. *Cell* 64:403, 1991.

67. Voorberg J, Fontijn R, Calafat J, et al: Biogenesis of von Willebrand factor-containing organelles in heterologous transfected CV-1 cells. *EMBO J* 12:749, 1993.

68. Journet AM, Saffaripour S, Cramer EM, et al: von Willebrand factor storage requires intact prosequence cleavage site. *Eur J Cell Biol* 60:31, 1993.

69. Nachman RL, Jaffe EA: Subcellular platelet factor VIII antigen and von Willebrand factor. *J Exp Med* 141:1101, 1975.

70. Bowie EJW, Solberg LA Jr, Fass DN, et al: Transplantation of normal bone marrow into a pig with severe von Willebrand's disease. *J Clin Invest* 78:26, 1986.

71. Nichols TC, Samama CM, Bellinger DA, et al: Function of von Willebrand factor after crossed bone marrow transplantation between normal and von Willebrand disease pigs: Effect on arterial thrombosis in chimeras. *Proc Natl Acad Sci USA* 92:2455, 1995.

72. André P, Brouland JP, Roussi J, et al: Role of plasma and platelet von Willebrand factor for arterial thrombogenesis and hemostasis in the pig. *Exp Hematol* 26:620, 1998.

73. Furlan M, Robles R, Lämmle B: Partial purification and characterization of a protease from human plasma cleaving von Willebrand factor to fragments produced by in vivo proteolysis. *Blood* 87:4223, 1996.

74. Tsai HM: Physiologic cleavage of von Willebrand factor by a plasma protease is dependent on its conformation and requires calcium ion. *Blood* 87:4235, 1996.

75. Dent JA, Berkowitz SD, Ware J, et al: Identification of a cleavage site directing the immunochemical detection of molecular abnormalities in type IIA von Willebrand factor. *Proc Natl Acad Sci USA* 87:6306, 1990.

76. Lankhof H, Damas C, Schiphorst ME, et al: von Willebrand factor without the A2 domain is resistant to proteolysis. *Thromb Haemost* 77:1008, 1997.

77. Tsai H-M, Sussman II, Ginsburg D, et al: Proteolytic cleavage of recombinant type 2A von Willebrand factor mutants R834W and R834Q: Inhibition by doxycycline and by monoclonal antibody VP-1. *Blood* 89:1954, 1997.

78. Furlan M, Robles R, Solenthaler M, et al: Deficient activity of von Willebrand factor–cleaving protease in chronic relapsing thrombotic thrombocytopenic purpura. *Blood* 89:3097, 1997.

79. Furlan M, Robles R, Galbusera M, et al: von Willebrand factor-cleaving protease in thrombotic thrombocytopenic purpura and the hemolytic-uremic syndrome. *N Engl J Med* 339:1578, 1998.

80. Tsai H-M, Lian ECY: Antibodies to von Willebrand factor-cleaving protease in acute thrombotic thrombocytopenic purpura. *N Engl J Med* 339:1585, 1998.

81. Ruggeri ZM: Mechanisms initiating platelet thrombus formation. *Thromb Haemost* 78:611, 1997.

82. Ruggeri ZM, Ware J, Ginsburg D: von Willebrand factor, in *Thrombosis and Hemorrhage*, 2d ed, edited by J Loscalzo, AI Schafer, p 337, Williams & Wilkins, Baltimore 1998.

83. Sadler JE: Biochemistry and genetics of von Willebrand factor. *Annu Rev Biochem* 67:395, 1998.

84. Savage B, Saldívar E, Ruggeri ZM: Initiation of platelet adhesion by arrest onto fibrinogen or translocation on von Willebrand factor. *Cell* 84:289, 1996.

85. Savage B, Almus-Jacobs F, Ruggeri ZM: Specific synergy of multiple substrate-receptor interactions in platelet thrombus formation under flow. *Cell* 94:657, 1998.

86. Kalafatis M, Takahashi Y, Girma J-P, Meyer D: Localization of a collagen-interactive domain of human von Willebrand factor between amino acid residues Gly 911 and Glu 1365. *Blood* 70:1577, 1987.

87. Pareti FI, Niiya K, McPherson JM, Ruggeri ZM: Isolation and characterization of two domains of human von Willebrand factor that interact with fibrillar collagen types I and III. *J Biol Chem* 262:13835, 1987.

88. Takagi J, Sekiya F, Kasahara K, et al: Inhibition of platelet-collagen interaction by propolypeptide of von Willebrand factor. *J Biol Chem* 264:6017, 1989.

89. Cruz MA, Yuan H, Lee JR, et al: Interaction of the von Willebrand factor (vWF) with collagen: Localization of the primary collagen-binding site by analysis of recombinant vWF A domain polypeptides. *J Biol Chem* 270:10822, 1995.

90. Lankhof H, Van Hoeij M, Schiphorst ME, et al: A3 domain is essential for interaction of von Willebrand factor with collagen type III. *Thromb Haemost* 75:950, 1996.

91. Wagner DD, Urban-Pickering M, Marder VJ: von Willebrand protein binds to extracellular matrices independently of collagen. *Proc Natl Acad Sci USA* 81:471, 1984.

92. Rand JH, Patel ND, Schwartz E, et al: 150-kD von Willebrand factor binding protein extracted from human vascular subendothelium is type VI collagen. *J Clin Invest* 88:253, 1991.

93. Rand JH, Wu X-X, Potter BJ, et al: Co-localization of von Willebrand factor and type VI collagen in human vascular subendothelium. *Am J Pathol* 142:843, 1993.

94. Mazzucato M, Spessotto P, Masotti A, et al: Identification of domains responsible for von Willebrand factor type VI collagen interaction mediating platelet adhesion under high flow. *J Biol Chem* 274:3033, 1999.

95. Fretto LJ, Fowler WE, McCaslin DR, et al: Substructure of human von Willebrand factor: Proteolysis by V8 and characterization of two functional domains. *J Biol Chem* 261:15679, 1986.

96. Fujimura Y, Titani K, Holland LZ, et al: A heparin-binding domain of human von Willebrand factor: Characterization and localization to a tryptic fragment extending from amino acid residue Val[449] to Lys[728]. *J Biol Chem* 262:1734, 1987.

97. Christophe O, Obert B, Meyer D, Girma J-P: The binding domain of von Willebrand factor to sulfatides is distinct from those interacting with glycoprotein Ib, heparin, collagen and residues between amino acid residues Leu 512 and Lys 673. *Blood* 78:2310, 1991.

98. Marchese P, Murata M, Mazzucato M, et al: Identification of three tyrosine residues of glycoprotein IB alpha with distinct roles in von Willebrand factor and alpha-thrombin binding. *J Biol Chem* 270:9571, 1995.

99. Fujimura Y, Titani K, Holland LZ, et al: von Willebrand factor: A reduced and alkylated 52/48-kDa fragment beginning at amino acid residue 449 contains the domain interacting with platelet glycoprotein Ib. *J Biol Chem* 261:381, 1986.

100. Mohri H, Fujimura Y, Shima M, et al: Structure of the von Willebrand factor domain interacting with glycoprotein Ib. *J Biol Chem* 263:17901, 1988.

101. Scott JP, Montgomery RR, Retzinger GS: Dimeric ristocetin flocculates proteins, binds to platelets, and mediates von Willebrand factor-dependent agglutination of platelets. *J Biol Chem* 266:8149, 1991.

102. Berndt MC, Du XP, Booth WJ: Ristocetin-dependent reconstitution of binding of von Willebrand factor to purified human platelet membrane glycoprotein Ib-IX complex. *Biochemistry* 27:633, 1988.

103. Andrews RK, Booth WJ, Gorman JJ, et al: Purification of botrocetin from *Bothrops jararaca* venom: Analysis of the botrocetin-mediated interaction between von Willebrand factor and the human platelet membrane glycoprotein Ib–IX complex. *Biochemistry* 28:8317, 1989.

104. Matsushita T, Sadler JE: Identification of amino acid residues essential for von Willebrand factor binding to platelet glycoprotein Ib: Charged-to-alanine scanning mutagenesis of the A1 domain of human von Willebrand factor. *J Biol Chem* 270:13406, 1995.

105. Emsley J, Cruz M, Handin RI, Liddington R: Crystal structure of the von Willebrand factor A1 domain and implications for the binding of platelet glycoprotein Ib. *J Biol Chem* 273:10396, 1998.

106. Bienkowska J, Cruz M, Atiemo A, et al: The von Willebrand factor A3 domain does not contain a metal ion-dependent adhesion site motif. *J Biol Chem* 272:25162, 1997.

107. Huizinga EG, Van der Plas RM, Kroon J, et al: Crystal structure of the A3 domain of human von Willebrand factor: Implications for collagen binding. *Structure* 5:1147, 1997.

108. Cooney KA, Ginsburg D: Comparative analysis of type 2b von Willebrand disease mutations: Implications for the mechanism of von Willebrand factor to binding platelets. *Blood* 87:2322, 1996.

109. Ruggeri ZM: von Willebrand factor. *J Clin Invest* 99:559, 1997.

110. Vlot AJ, Koppelman SJ, Van den Berg MH, et al: The affinity and stoichiometry of binding of human factor VIII to von Willebrand factor. *Blood* 85:3150, 1995.

111. Vlot AJ, Koppelman SJ, Bouma BN, Sixma JJ: Factor VIII and von Willebrand factor. *Thromb Haemost* 79:456, 1998.

112. Foster PA, Fulcher CA, Marti T, et al: A major factor VIII binding domain resides within the amino-terminal 272–amino acid residues of von Willebrand factor. *J Biol Chem* 262:8443, 1987.

113. Bahou WF, Ginsburg D, Sikkink R, et al: A monoclonal antibody to von Willebrand factor (vWF) inhibits factor VIII binding: Localization of its antigenic determinant to a nonadecapeptide at the amino terminus of the mature vWF polypeptide. *J Clin Invest* 84:56, 1989.

114. Ginsburg D, Bockenstedt PL, Allen EA, et al: Fine mapping of monoclonal antibody epitopes on human von Willebrand factor using a recombinant peptide library. *Thromb Haemost* 67:166, 1992.

115. Mazurier C: von Willebrand disease masquerading as haemophilia A. *Thromb Haemost* 67:391, 1992.

116. Cacheris PM, Nichols WC, Ginsburg D: Molecular characterization of a unique von Willebrand disease variant: A novel mutation affecting von Willebrand factor/factor VIII interaction. *J Biol Chem* 266:13499, 1991.

117. Lollar P, Hill-Eubanks DC, Parker CG: Association of the factor VIII light chain with von Willebrand factor. *J Biol Chem* 263:10451, 1988.

118. Leyte A, van Schijndel HB, Niehrs C, et al: Sulfation of Tyr1680 of human blood coagulation factor VIII is essential for the interaction of factor VIII with von Willebrand factor. *J Biol Chem* 266:740, 1991.

119. Nichols WC, Ginsburg D: von Willebrand disease. *Medicine* 76:1, 1997.

120. Nichols WC, Cooney KA, Ginsburg D, Ruggeri ZM: von Willebrand disease, in *Thrombosis and Hemorrhage,* 2d ed, edited by J Loscalzo, AI Schafer, p 729. Williams & Wilkins, Baltimore, 1998.

121. Ginsburg D, Sadler JE: von Willebrand disease: A database of point mutations, insertions, and deletions. *Thromb Haemost* 69:177, 1993.

122. Sadler JE, Ginsburg D: A database of polymorphisms in the von Willebrand factor gene and pseudogene. *Thromb Haemost* 69:185, 1993.

123. Zimmerman TS, Abildgaard CF, Meyer D: The factor VIII abnormality in severe von Willebrand's disease. *N Engl J Med* 301:1307, 1979.

124. Ngo KY, Glotz VT, Koziol JA, et al: Homozygous and heterozygous deletions of the von Willebrand factor gene in patients and carriers of severe von Willebrand disease. *Proc Natl Acad Sci USA* 85:2753, 1988.

125. Peake IR, Liddell MB, Moodie P, et al: Severe type III von Willebrand's disease caused by deletion of exon 42 of the von Willebrand factor gene: Family studies that identify carriers of the condition and a compound heterozygous individual. *Blood* 75:654, 1990.

126. Mancuso DJ, Tuley EA, Castillo R, et al: Characterization of partial gene deletions in type III von Willebrand disease with alloantibody inhibitors. *Thromb Haemost* 72:180, 1994.

127. Nichols WC, Lyons SE, Harrison JS, et al: Severe von Willebrand disease due to a defect at the level of von Willebrand factor mRNA expression: Detection by exonic PCR-restriction fragment length polymorphism analysis. *Proc Natl Acad Sci USA* 88:3857, 1991.

128. Eikenboom JCJ, Ploos van Amstel HK, Reitsma PH, Briët E: Mutations in severe, type III von Willebrand's disease in the Dutch population: Candidate missense and nonsense mutations associated with reduced levels of von Willebrand factor messenger RNA. *Thromb Haemost* 68:448, 1992.

129. Eikenboom JCJ, Castaman G, Vos HL, et al: Characterization of the genetic defects in recessive type 1 and type 3 von Willebrand disease patients of Italian origin. *Thromb Haemost* 79:709, 1998.

130. Mohlke KL, Ginsburg D: von Willebrand disease and quantitative deficiency of von Willebrand factor. *J Lab Clin Med* 130:252, 1997.

131. Zhang ZP, Falk G, Blombäck M, et al: A single cytosine deletion in exon 18 of the von Willebrand factor gene is the most common mutation in Swedish vWD type III patients. *Hum Mol Genet* 1:767, 1992.

132. Zhang ZP, Blombäck M, Nyman D, Anvret M: Mutations of von Willebrand factor gene in families with von Willebrand disease in the Åland Islands. *Proc Natl Acad Sci USA* 90:7937, 1993.

133. Mohlke KL, Nichols WC, Rehemtulla A, et al: A common frameshift mutation in von Willebrand factor does not alter mRNA stability but interferes with normal propeptide processing. *Br J Haematol* 95:184, 1996.

134. Schneppenheim R, Krey S, Bergmann F, et al: Genetic heterogeneity of severe von Willebrand disease type III in the German population. *Hum Genet* 94:640, 1994.

135. Weiss HJ, Piétu G, Rabinowitz R, et al: Heterogeneous abnormalities in the multimeric structure, antigenic properties, and plasma-platelet content of factor VIII/von Willebrand factor in subtypes of classic (type I) and variant (type IIA) von Willebrand's disease. *J Lab Clin Med* 101:411, 1983.

136. Hoyer LW, Rizza CR, Tuddenham EGD, et al: Von Willebrand factor multimer patterns in von Willebrand's disease. *Br J Haematol* 55:493, 1983.

137. Mannucci PM, Lombardi R, Bader R, et al: Heterogeneity of type I von Willebrand disease: Evidence for a subgroup with an abnormal von Willebrand factor. *Blood* 66:796, 1985.

138. Mannucci PM: Platelet von Willebrand factor in inherited and acquired bleeding disorders. *Proc Natl Acad Sci USA* 92:2428, 1995.

139. Eikenboom JCJ, Matsushita T, Reitsma PH, et al: Dominant type 1 von Willebrand disease caused by mutated cysteine residues in the D3 domain of von Willebrand factor. *Blood* 88:2433, 1996.

140. Mohlke KL, Purkayastha AA, Westrick RJ, et al: *Mvwf,* a dominant modifier of murine von Willebrand factor, results from altered lineage-specific expression of a glycosyltransferase. *Cell* 96:111, 1999.

141. Ginsburg D: Molecular genetics of von Willebrand disease. *Thromb Haemost* 82:585, 1999.

142. Berkowitz SD, Dent JA, Roberts J, et al: Epitope mapping of the von Willebrand factor subunit distinguishes fragments present in normal and type IIA von Willebrand disease from those generated by plasmin. *J Clin Invest* 79:524, 1987.

143. Ginsburg D, Konkle BA, Gill JC, et al: Molecular basis of human von Willebrand disease: Analysis of platelet von Willebrand factor mRNA. *Proc Natl Acad Sci USA* 86:3723, 1989.

144. Lyons SE, Bruck ME, Bowie EJW, Ginsburg D: Impaired intracellular transport produced by a subset of type IIA von Willebrand disease mutations. *J Biol Chem* 267:4424, 1992.

145. Dent JA, Galbusera M, Ruggeri ZM: Heterogeneity of plasma von Willebrand factor multimers resulting from proteolysis of the constituent subunit. *J Clin Invest* 88:774, 1991.

146. Gralnick HR, Williams SB, McKeown LP, et al: In vitro correction of the abnormal multimeric structure of von Willebrand factor in type IIA von Willebrand's disease. *Proc Natl Acad Sci USA.* 82:5968, 1985.

147. Kunicki TJ, Montgomery RR, Schullek J: Cleavage of human von Willebrand factor by platelet calcium-activated protease. *Blood* 65:352, 1985.

148. Schneppenheim R, Thomas KB, Krey S, et al: Identification of a candidate missense mutation in a family with von Willebrand disease type IIC. *Hum Genet* 95:681, 1995.

149. Gaucher C, Diéval J, Mazurier C: Characterization of von Willebrand factor gene defects in two unrelated patients with type IIC von Willebrand disease. *Blood* 84:1024, 1994.

150. Schneppenheim R, Brassard J, Krey S, et al: Defective dimerization of von Willebrand factor subunits due to a Cys→Arg mutation in type IID von Willebrand disease. *Proc Natl Acad Sci USA* 93:3581, 1996.

151. Cooney KA, Nichols WC, Bruck ME, et al: The molecular defect in type IIB von Willebrand disease: Identification of four potential missense mutations within the putative GpIb binding domain. *J Clin Invest* 87:1227, 1991.

152. Ribba AS, Lavergne JM, Bahnak BR, et al: Duplication of a methionine within the glycoprotein Ib binding domain of von Willebrand factor detected by denaturing gradient gel electrophoresis in a patient with type IIB von Willebrand disease. *Blood* 78:1738, 1991.

153. Cooney KA, Lyons SE, Ginsburg D: Functional analysis of a type IIB von Willebrand disease missense mutation: Increased binding of large von Willebrand factor multimers to platelets. *Proc Natl Acad Sci USA* 89:2869, 1992.

154. Ware J, Dent JA, Azuma H, et al: Identification of a point mutation in type IIB von Willebrand disease illustrating the regulation of von Willebrand factor affinity for the platelet membrane glycoprotein Ib-IX receptor. *Proc Natl Acad Sci USA* 88:2946, 1991.

155. Kroner PA, Kluessendorf ML, Scott JP, Montgomery RR: Expressed full-length von Willebrand factor containing missense mutations linked to type IIB von Willebrand disease shows enhanced binding to platelets. *Blood* 79:2048, 1992.

156. Randi AM, Jorieux S, Tuley EA, et al: Recombinant von Willebrand factor Arg[578]→Gln: A type IIB von Willebrand disease mutation affects binding to glycoprotein Ib but not to collagen or heparin. *J Biol Chem* 267:21187, 1992.

157. Holmberg L, Dent JA, Schneppenheim R, et al: von Willebrand factor mutation enhancing interaction with platelets in patients with normal multimeric structure. *J Clin Invest* 91:2169, 1993.

158. Veltkamp JJ, van Tilburg NH: Autosomal haemophilia: A variant of von Willebrand's disease. *Br J Haematol* 26:141, 1974.

159. Graham JB, Barrow ES, Roberts HR, et al: Dominant inheritance of hemophilia A in three generations of women. *Blood* 46:175, 1975.

160. Mazurier C, Gaucher C, Jorieux S, et al: Evidence for a von Willebrand factor defect in factor VIII binding in three members of a family previously misdiagnosed mild haemophilia A and haemophilia A carriers: Consequences for therapy and genetic counselling. *Br J Haematol* 76:372, 1990.

161. Mazurier C, Diéval J, Jorieux S, Delobel J, Goudemand M: A new von Willebrand factor (vWF) defect in a patient with factor VIII (FVIII) deficiency but with normal levels and multimeric patterns of both plasma and platelet vWF: Characterization of abnormal vWF/FVIII interaction. *Blood* 75:20, 1990.

162. Nishino M, Girma J-P, Rothschild C, et al: New variant of von Willebrand disease with defective binding to factor VIII. *Blood* 74:1591, 1989.

163. Eikenboom JCJ, Reitsma PH, Peerlinck KMJ, Briët E: Recessive inheritance of von Willebrand's disease type I. *Lancet* 341:982, 1993.

164. Rabinowitz I, Tuley EA, Mancuso DJ, et al: von Willebrand disease type B: A missense mutation selectively abolishes ristocetin-induced von Willebrand factor binding to platelet glycoprotein Ib. *Proc Natl Acad Sci USA* 89:9846, 1992.

165. Meyer D, Fressinaud E, Gaucher C, et al: Gene defects in 150 unrelated French cases with type 2 von Willebrand disease: From the patient to the gene. *Thromb Haemost* 78:451; 1997.

166. Mannucci PM, Lombardi R, Castaman G, et al: von Willebrand disease ''Vicenza'' with larger-than-normal (supranormal) von Willebrand factor multimers. *Blood* 71:65, 1988.

167. Randi AM, Sacchi E, Castaman GC, et al: The genetic defect of type I von Willebrand disease ''Vicenza'' is linked to the von Willebrand factor gene. *Thromb Haemost* 69:173, 1993.

168. Miller CH, Graham JB, Goldin LR, Elston RC: Genetics of classic von Willebrand's disease: I. Phenotypic variation within families. *Blood* 54:117, 1979.

169. Gill JC, Endres-Brooks J, Bauer PJ, et al: The effect of ABO blood group on the diagnosis of von Willebrand disease. *Blood* 69:1691, 1987.

170. Orstavik KH, Kornstad L, Reisner H, Berg K: Possible effect of secretor locus on plasma concentration of factor VIII and von Willebrand factor. *Blood* 73:990, 1989.

171. Rodeghiero F, Castaman G, Dini E: Epidemiological investigation of the prevalence of von Willebrand's disease. *Blood* 69:454, 1987.

172. Werner EJ, Broxson EH, Tucker EL, et al: Prevalence of von Willebrand disease in children: A multiethnic study. *J Pediatr* 123:893, 1993.

173. Weiss HJ, Ball AP, Mannucci PM: Incidence of severe von Willebrand's disease. *N Engl J Med* 307:127, 1982.

174. Berliner SA, Seligsohn U, Zivelin A, et al: A relatively high frequency of severe (type III) von Willebrand's disease in Israel. *Br J Haematol* 62:535, 1986.

175. Mannucci PM, Bloom AL, Larrieu MJ, et al: Atherosclerosis and von Willebrand factor: I. Prevalence of severe von Willebrand's disease in western Europe and Israel. *Br J Haematol* 57:163, 1984.

176. Nosek-Cenkowska B, Cheang MS, Pizzi NJ, et al: Bleeding/bruising symptomatology in children with and without bleeding disorders. *Thromb Haemost* 65:237, 1991.

177. Silwer J: von Willebrand's disease in Sweden. *Acta Paediatr Scand Suppl* 238:1, 1973.

178. Iannuzzi MC, Hidaka N, Boehnke ML, et al: Analysis of the relationship of von Willebrand disease (vWD) and hereditary hemorrhagic telangiectasia and identification of a potential type IIA vWD mutation (IIe865 to Thr). *Am J Hum Genet* 48:757, 1991.

179. Rick ME, Williams SB, Sacher RA, McKeown LP: Thrombocytopenia associated wtih pregnancy in a patient with type IIB von Willebrand's disease. *Blood* 69:786, 1987.

180. Mazurier C, Parquet-Gernez A, Goudemand J, et al: Investigation of a large kindred with type IIB von Willebrand's disease, dominant inheritance and age-dependent thrombocytopenia. *Br J Haematol* 69:499, 1988.

181. Schneppenheim R, Budde U, Krey S, et al: Results of a screening for von Willebrand disease type 2N in patients with suspected haemophilia A or von Willebrand disease type 1. *Thromb Haemost* 76:598, 1996.

182. Rodeghiero F, Castaman G, Tosetto A: von Willebrand factor antigen is less sensitive than ristocetin cofactor for the diagnosis of type I von Willebrand disease: Results based on an epidemiological investigation. *Thromb Haemost* 64:349, 1990.

183. Abildgaard CF, Suzuki Z, Harrison J, et al: Serial studies in von Willebrand's disease: Variability versus "variants." *Blood* 56:712, 1980.

184. Harker LA, Slichter SJ: The bleeding time as a screening test for evaluation of platelet function. *N Engl J Med* 287:155, 1972.

185. Lind SE: The bleeding time does not predict surgical bleeding. *Blood* 77:2547, 1991.

186. De Caterina R, Lanza M, Manca G, et al: Bleeding time and bleeding: An analysis of the relationship of the bleeding time test with parameters of surgical bleeding. *Blood* 84:3363, 1994.

187. Peterson P, Hayes TE, Arkin CF, et al: The preoperative bleeding time test lacks clinical benefit: College of American Pathologists' and American Society of Clinical Pathologists' position article. *Arch Surg* 133:134, 1998.

188. Weiss HJ, Hoyer LW, Rickles FR, et al: Quantitative assay of a plasma factor deficient in von Willebrand's disease that is necessary for platelet aggregation. *J Clin Invest* 52:2708, 1973.

189. Mazurier C, Meyer D: Factor VIII binding assay of von Willebrand factor and the diagnosis of type 2N von Willebrand disease: Results of an international survey. On behalf of the Subcommittee on von Willebrand Factor of the Scientific and Standardization Committee of the ISTH. *Thromb Haemost* 76:270, 1996.

190. Fujimura Y, Kawasaki T, Titani K: Snake venom proteins modulating the interaction between von Willebrand factor and platelet glycoprotein Ib. *Thromb Haemost* 76:633, 1996.

191. Favaloro EJ, Dean M, Grispo L, et al: von Willebrand's disease: Use of collagen binding assay provides potential improvement to laboratory monitoring of desmopressin (DDAVP) therapy. *Am J Hematol* 45:205, 1994.

192. Fressinaud E, Veyradier A, Truchaud F, et al: Screening for von Willebrand disease with a new analyzer using high shear stress: A study of 60 cases. *Blood* 91:1325, 1998.

193. Ruggeri ZM, Zimmerman TS: The complex multimeric composition of factor VIII/von Willebrand factor. *Blood* 57:1140, 1981.

194. Bignell P, Standen GR, Bowen DJ, et al: Rapid neonatal diagnosis of von Willebrand's disease by use of the polymerase chain reaction. *Lancet* 336:638, 1990.

195. Peake IR, Bowen D, Bignell P, et al: Family studies and prenatal diagnosis in severe von Willebrand disease by polymerase chain reaction amplification of a variable number tandem repeat region of the von Willebrand factor gene. *Blood* 76:555, 1990.

196. Mannhalter C, Kyrle PA, Brenner B, Lechner K: Rapid neonatal diagnosis of type IIB von Willebrand disease using the polymerase chain reaction. *Blood* 77:2538, 1991.

197. Miller JL: Platelet-type von Willebrand disease. *Thromb Haemost* 75:865, 1996.

198. Budde U, Schaefer G, Mueller N, et al: Acquired von Willebrand's disease in the myeloproliferative syndrome. *Blood* 64:981, 1984.

199. Rogers JS, Shane SR, Jencks FS: Factor VIII activity and thyroid function. *Ann Intern Med* 97:713, 1982.

200. Mannucci PM, Lombardi R, Bader R, et al: Studies of the pathophysiology of acquired von Willebrand's disease in seven patients with lymphoproliferative disorders or benign monoclonal gammopathies. *Blood* 64:614, 1984.

201. Scott JP, Montgomery RR, Tubergen DG, Hays T: Acquired von Willebrand's disease in association with Wilm's tumor: Regression following treatment. *Blood* 58:665, 1981.

202. Warkentin TE, Moore JC, Morgan DG: Aortic stenosis and bleeding gastrointestinal angiodysplasia: Is acquired von Willebrand's disease the link? *Lancet* 340:35, 1992.

203. Castaman G, Lattuada A, Mannucci PM, Rodeghiero F: Characterization of two cases of acquired transitory von Willebrand syndrome with ciprofloxacin: Evidence for heightened proteolysis of von Willebrand factor. *Am J Hematol* 49:83, 1995.

204. Tefferi A, Nichols WL: Acquired von Willebrand disease: Concise review of occurrence, diagnosis, pathogenesis, and treatment. *Am J Med* 103:536, 1997.

205. Mannucci PM, Ruggeri ZM, Pareti FI, Capitanio A: 1-Deamino-8-D-arginine vasopressin: A new pharmacological approach to the management of haemophilia and von Willebrand's diseases. *Lancet* 1:869, 1977.

206. Ruggeri ZM, Mannucci PM, Lombardi R, et al: Multimeric composition of factor VIII/von Willebrand factor following administration of DDAVP: Implications for pathophysiology and therapy of von Willebrand's disease subtypes. *Blood* 59:1272, 1982.

207. Mannucci PM: Desmopressin (DDAVP) in the treatment of bleeding disorders: The first 20 years. *Blood* 90:2515, 1997.

208. Lethagen S, Harris AS, Nilsson IM: Intranasal desmopressin (DDAVP) by spray in mild hemophilia A and von Willebrand's disease type I. *Blut* 60:187, 1990.

209. Rose EH, Aledort LM: Nasal spray desmopressin (DDAVP) for mild hemophilia A and von Willebrand disease. *Ann Intern Med* 114:563, 1991.

210. Rodeghiero F, Castaman G, Di Bona E, Ruggeri M: Consistency of responses to repeated DDAVP infusions in patients with von Willebrand's disease and hemophilia A. *Blood* 74:1997, 1989.

211. Mannucci PM, Bettega D, Cattaneo M: Patterns of development of tachyphylaxis in patients with haemophilia and von Willebrand disease after repeated doses of desmopressin (DDAVP). *Br J Haematol* 82:87, 1992.

212. de la Fuente B, Kasper CK, Rickles FR, Hoyer LW: Response of patients with mild and moderate hemophilia A and von Willebrand's disease to treatment with desmopressin. *Ann Intern Med* 103:6, 1985.

213. Gralnick HR, Williams SB, McKeown LP, et al: DDAVP in type IIa von Willebrand's disease. *Blood* 67:465, 1986.

214. Holmberg L, Nilsson IM, Borge L, et al: Platelet aggregation induced by 1-desamino-8-D-arginine vasopressin (DDAVP) in type IIB von Willebrand's disease. *N Engl J Med* 309:816, 1983.

215. Casonato A, Sartori MT, De Marco L, Girolami A: 1-Desamino-8-D-arginine vasopressin (DDAVP) infusion in type IIB von Willebrand's disease: Shortening of bleeding time and induction of a variable pseudothrombocytopenia. *Thromb Haemost* 64:117, 1990.

216. McKeown LP, Connaghan G, Wilson O, et al: 1-desamino-8-arginine-vasopressin corrects the hemostatic defects in type 2B von Willebrand's disease. *Am J Hematol* 51:158, 1996.

217. Foster PA: A perspective on the use of FVIII concentrates and cryoprecipitate prophylactically in surgery or therapeutically in severe bleeds in patients with von Willebrand disease unresponsive to DDAVP: Results of an international survey. *Thromb Haemost* 74:1370, 1995.

218. Rodeghiero F, Castaman G, Meyer D, Mannucci PM: Replacement

therapy with virus-inactivated plasma concentrates in von Willebrand disease. *Vox Sang* 62:193, 1992.

219. Mannucci PM, Tenconi PM, Castaman G, Rodeghiero F: Comparison of four virus-inactivated plasma concentrates for treatment of severe von Willebrand disease: A cross-over randomized trial. *Blood* 79:3130, 1992.

220. Mannucci PM, Ruggeri ZM, Ciavarella N, et al: Precipitating antibodies to factor VIII/von Willebrand factor in von Willebrand's disease: Effects on replacement therapy. *Blood* 57:25, 1981.

221. Harrison RL, McKee PA: Estrogen stimulates von Willebrand factor production by cultured endothelial cells. *Blood* 63:657, 1984.

222. Ginsburg D, Bowie EJW: Molecular genetics of von Willebrand disease. *Blood* 79:2507, 1992.

223. Berkowitz SD, Ruggeri ZM, Zimmerman TS: von Willebrand disease, in *Coagulation and Bleeding Disorders: The Role of Factor VIII and von Willebrand Factor,* edited by TS Zimmerman, ZM Ruggeri, p 215. Marcel Dekker, New York, 1989.

DISORDERS OF FIBRINOLYSIS AND USE OF ANTIFIBRINOLYTIC AGENTS

FEDOR BACHMANN

Under physiologic conditions the finely tuned mechanism of hemostasis, consisting of pro- and anticoagulant and pro- and antifibrinolytic components assures healing of a vascular lesion and subsequent reestablishment of normal blood flow. Excessive local or systemic fibrinolysis shifts this delicate equilibrium toward premature lysis of hemostatic plugs and bleeding.

Cases of primary, systemic hyperfibrinolysis without activation of the coagulation system are rare. They comprise the hereditary deficiencies of α_2-plasmin inhibitor and of the plasminogen activator inhibitor-1, advanced liver disease, and some cases of snake bite. Much more common is systemic hyperfibrinolysis that is secondary to the activation of the coagulation system by procoagulant factors, mainly tissue factor (as in metastatic cancer), or by artificial surfaces (as during cardiopulmonary bypass) or heart assist devices. Localized excessive fibrinolysis occurs frequently; typical examples are menorrhagia and prostatectomy. Three antifibrinolytic agents are commonly used. Aprotinin, a serine protease inhibitor, forms 1:1 stoichiometric complexes with kallikrein and plasmin and has successfully been used to reduce bleeding in cardiac surgery and liver transplantation. Epsilon-aminocaproic acid and tranexamic acid exert their antifibrinolytic effect by interfering competitively with the binding of plasmin to C-terminal lysine residues of fibrin. Both drugs have been successfully used in a wide range of conditions, including acute promyelocytic leukemia, liver transplantation, cardiac surgery, the hemophilias, factor XI deficiency, von Willebrand disease, amyloidosis, prostatectomy, and menorrhagia.

INTRODUCTION

Already during the formation of a hemostatic plug biochemical mechanisms are initiated to limit the extent of the hemostatic process and to reestablish normal blood flow. To a large extent this is accomplished by localized activation of the plasminogen-plasmin enzyme system, also called *fibrinolytic system.* To accomplish healing of a vascular lesion without compromising the stability of the hemostatic plug too

early, and to limit the activation of the fibrinolytic system to the injured area, a finely tuned mechanism is necessary, consisting of the tissue-type and of the urinary-type plasminogen activators (t-PA and u-PA, respectively), prekallikrein-kallikrein, and the fibrinolytic inhibitors α_2-antiplasmin and PAI-1 (see Chap. 116). The regulation of hemostatic and fibrinolytic processes is dynamic, representing the balance achieved between pro- and antihemostatic and pro- and antifibrinolytic mediators (Fig. 136-1). This dynamic balance can be upset if any of the components are inadequate or excessive. Excessive local or systemic activation of coagulation may result in the development of macrovascular thrombi or consumption coagulopathy. Similarly, excessive local or systemic fibrinolytic activity can result in renewed or sustained bleeding. When hemostasis is delayed as a result of either a platelet disorder or a coagulation defect, a bleeding episode may be prolonged or renewed because of the imbalance created between an abnormally slow hemostatic rate and a normal rate of fibrinolysis. For example, bleeding in a hemophilic patient following an injury may cease spontaneously but recur 24 to 48 h later, presumably as the weakened plug is dissolved by a normal fibrinolytic response. In other circumstances hemostasis is normal, but excessive local fibrinolysis may give rise to excessive bleeding, as in primary menorrhagia.[1]

Antifibrinolytic agents are useful for improving hemostasis in a wide variety of bleeding states.[2,3] There are three types of clinical conditions in which antifibrinolytic therapy has been used[4]: (1) systemic hyperfibrinolysis that follows administration of a therapeutic plasminogen activator or that stems from conditions associated with spontaneous, sustained increases in circulating plasminogen activator or lack of fibrinolytic inhibitors; (2) conditions with impaired hemostasis, e.g., hemophilia A and B; (3) excessive local fibrinolysis, as after prostatectomy where u-PA leads to premature dissolution of the hemostatic plug,[5] or as in menorrhagia where high concentrations of t-PA maintain menstrual blood in a fluid phase.[1]

PHARMACOLOGY OF ANTIFIBRINOLYTIC AGENTS

MODE OF ACTION

The stability of fibrin in the hemostatic plug depends on the availability and proper concentration of platelets, thrombin, plasminogen, thrombin-activatable fibrinolytic inhibitor, α_2-antiplasmin, and PAI-1.[6–10] Antifibrinolytic agents shift the balance toward a more stabilized hemostatic plug. The therapeutic antifibrinolytic agents fall into two categories:

1. Aprotinin, a 58-residue polypeptide (M_r 6500 Da) isolated from bovine lung parotid gland or pancreas[11]; it is a powerful inhibitor of trypsin, kallikrein, plasmin, and other serine proteases.[12,13] The three-dimensional structure of aprotinin reveals it to be a very compact molecule, probably explaining its resistance to heat, extreme pH, and proteolysis.[14] Aprotinin forms a 1:1 stoichiometric complex with several serine proteases. Lys[15] of aprotinin forms a covalent bond with the serine residue of the catalytic site of serine proteases.[15] The potency of aprotinin is expressed in kallikrein inhibitor units (KIU), where 10^6 KIU corresponds to 140 mg of the pure inhibitor.[16]

2. The synthetic lysine analogs such as 6-amino-hexanoic acid, also known as *ε-aminocaproic acid (EACA),* and tranexamic acid, also known as *trans-p-aminomethyl-cyclohexanecarboxylic acid (AMCA),* possess the ability to bind to the lysine-binding sites of plasminogen and thus inhibit competitively the binding of plasmin(ogen) to lysine residues on fibrin(ogen).[17,18] Subtle differences in the synthetic analogs can markedly affect their inhibitory potential; AMCA has a six- to tenfold higher molar potency than EACA.[19] Paradoxically, EACA and AMCA accelerate plasminogen activation in vitro by making plasminogen more susceptible

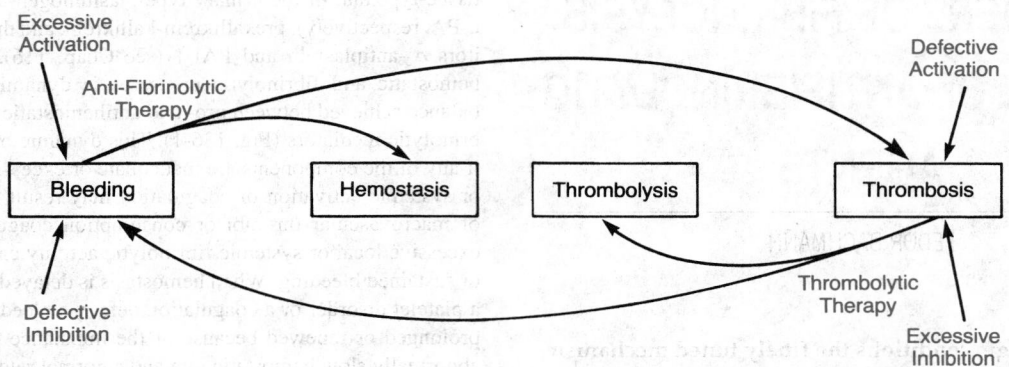

FIGURE 136-1   Disruption of the balance between the opposing forces of fibrinolysis and antifibrinolysis, leading to bleeding or thrombotic manifestations. Bleeding may result from defective inhibition or excessive activation of fibrinolysis. Conversely, defective activation or excess inhibition of fibrinolysis may result in thrombosis. Therapy with fibrinolytic agents may dissolve a thrombus, but bleeding may complicate the clinical management. Bleeding due to excess fibrinolysis may be improved by antifibrinolytic therapy but may also unmask a thrombotic predisposition. Successful therapy, that is, restoration of effective hemostasis or achievement of thrombolysis without complication, depends critically on selection of the patient to be treated. (Reproduced with permission from Francis and Marder.[209])

to proteolytic action by its activators.[20,21] However, any plasmin molecule that forms cannot bind effectively to fibrin, thereby precluding fibrinolysis.

PHARMACOKINETICS

APROTININ

Aprotinin has to be given intravenously because of gastric inactivation.[22] The drug distributes rapidly in the extracellular space, with an apparent distribution volume of 26 liters.[23] The kidney appears to be the principal organ of metabolism of aprotinin. Approximately 90 percent of the dose appears in the kidney within the first hours after infusion and remains there for 12 to 14 h. Aprotinin is filtered by the glomeruli and reabsorbed by the proximal tubules, where it is metabolized by renal lysosomes into small peptides or amino acids; from 25 to 40 percent of a single dose is excreted in the urine over 48 h, predominantly as metabolites.[23,24] The distribution $t_{1/2}\alpha$ is between 45 min to 2.5 h and the $t_{1/2}\beta$ in the range of 7 to 10 h.[4,23]

ε-AMINOCAPROIC ACID (EACA) AND TRANEXAMIC ACID (AMCA)

EACA is rapidly absorbed from the gastrointestinal tract, with peak plasma levels achieved by 2 h, after which the drug is rapidly excreted by the kidneys. Approximately 80 percent of an intravenous dose is cleared within 3 h,[25] but because EACA penetrates virtually the entire extravascular space, urinary excretion can be detected for as long as 12 to 36 h after intravenous administration. EACA is usually given as an intravenous priming dose of approximately 0.1 g per kilogram body weight over 20 to 30 min, followed by either a continuous intravenous infusion at 0.5 to 1 g/h or an equivalent intermittent dose, either orally or intravenously, every 1, 2, or 4 h. The serum half-life of AMCA is similar to that of EACA, approximately 1 to 2 h, and it is also rapidly excreted unchanged in the urine (>90 percent within 24 h).[19] When AMCA is used orally, the recommended dose is 25 mg/kg given t.i.d. or q.i.d.; when it is infused intravenously, 10 mg/kg is administered at a rate of 1 ml/min three to four times daily (commercially available ampules contain usually 500 mg/5 ml). AMCA should not be administered simultaneously with penicillin.

ADVERSE EFFECTS

APROTININ

The most common adverse effects of aprotinin are nausea, vomiting, diarrhea, muscle pain, and hypotension.[26,27] Allergic adverse effects comprise itching, rash, urticaria, and dyspnea; these are probably due to aprotinin-specific IgG and IgE antibodies.[28] Serious side effects such as cardiovascular collapse, bronchospasm, and anaphylactic shock are rare.[4,22,24] Nevertheless, the manufacturer recommends an intravenous test dose of 1 ml 10 min prior to the infusion of higher doses of aprotinin (available as infusion bottles of 500,000 KIU/50 ml and of 2,000,000 KIU/200 ml) and administration of an H_1 antagonist and an anti-H_2 drug such as cimetidine. Other, rare, adverse effects include impaired renal function,[29] perioperative myocardial infarction, and occlusion of grafts (reviewed by Robert et al[16]).

EACA AND AMCA

Both AMCA and EACA are associated with infrequent serious side effects (thrombosis, myonecrosis, hypersensitivity reactions), even with long-term administration. Minor complaints such as nasal stuffiness, abdominal discomfort, nausea, vomiting, diarrhea, conjunctival suffusion, and skin rash have been noted,[19] but their significance is questionable because they also occur in control patients in studies evaluating these agents. Myoglobinuria and muscle weakness as reflections of rhabdomyolysis require termination of therapy.[30]

Serious systemic thrombotic complications, e.g., disseminated intravascular coagulation (DIC), have occurred during antifibrinolytic therapy, but their importance has been exaggerated.[31] Antifibrinolytic therapy is most unlikely to produce thrombotic complications unless there is an ongoing or transient thrombogenic stimulus such as in DIC (see Chap. 126). The antifibrinolytic agents do not incite de novo venous thrombus formation. Thus, the incidence of clinical venous thromboembolic disease in a randomized, double-blind study after prostatic surgery was the same in control patients (17 of 256) as in patients treated with EACA (16 of 259),[32] and the incidence of a positive radioiodinated fibrinogen uptake test after retropubic prostatectomy was likewise unaffected (28 percent of 32 control patients and 30 percent of 30 patients treated with EACA).[33]

A small number of cases have been reported in which thrombotic events occurred in association with antifibrinolytic therapy, for example, in patients with metastatic prostatic carcinoma, in septic abortion, or after prolonged cardiopulmonary bypass.[2] Presumably the thrombotic process was induced by the underlying lesion or postsurgical condition, and antifibrinolytic therapy prevented the physiologic fibrinolytic response. These devastating clinical events are rarely encountered today, because antifibrinolytic therapy is administered to patients with DIC only when hemorrhage fails to respond to replacement therapy and anticoagulation (see Chap. 126).

Upper urinary tract bleeding, which can complicate hemophilia and hemoglobinopathies,[34] can lead to clots in the renal pelvis if the clot-dissolving action of urokinase is neutralized by an antifibrinolytic agent that is excreted in the urine. EACA or AMCA should therefore be avoided in such conditions. It should be noted, however, that induction of thrombosis by EACA or EACA and cryoprecipitate has been used for shrinking hemangiomas in patients with the Kasabach-Merritt syndrome.[35]

CLINICAL USE OF ANTIFIBRINOLYTIC AGENTS

Table 136-1 lists some common indications for the clinical use of antifibrinolytic agents.

SYSTEMIC HYPERFIBRIN(OGEN)OLYSIS

INHERITED DISORDERS

Hereditary deficiency of either the α_2-plasmin inhibitor[36,37] or PAI-1[38-41] may result in a lifelong bleeding disorder, presumably caused by premature lysis of hemostatic plugs at sites of vascular trauma. Inheritance is autosomal, with phenotypic manifestations of bleeding noted in homozygotes. In heterozygotes for α_2-plasmin inhibitor deficiency, bleeding has been observed to develop only at an advanced age, when vascular fragility is increased.[42] Bleeding may occur after initial hemostasis following surgery but may also be manifested spontaneously, for example, by epistaxis or ecchymoses. Given the permanent nature of the underlying defect (barring correction by gene therapy), treatment should be daily and lifelong in patients with frequent episodes of spontaneous bleeding. The oral administration of fibrinolytic inhibitors such as AMCA has been effective in normalizing hemostatic function.[37,40]

Isolated cases, and a family exhibiting increased levels of circulating active t-PA without PAI-1 deficiency, have also been described.[43,44] In one case increased t-PA levels were associated with what appeared to be an inherited deficiency of α_2-plasmin inhibitor; they returned to normal after orthotopic liver transplantation.[45]

Hereditary angioneurotic edema, due to a deficiency of the C1-inhibitor, leads to the activation of plasminogen and of the complement and the kallikrein-kinin systems during attacks.[46-48] Prophylactic treatment with EACA or AMCA reduces the incidence and severity of attacks.[49]

FIBRINOLYTIC THERAPY

Infusion of plasminogen activators such as recombinant t-PA, streptokinase, urokinase (u-PA), or anistreplase induces a plasma proteolytic state in which plasminogen is converted to plasmin, α_2-plasmin inhibitor is consumed, and the excess free plasmin variably degrades plasma fibrinogen (see Chap. 134). In addition to the desired therapeutic result of thrombolysis and vascular reperfusion, bleeding may result if hemostatic plugs at sites of vascular injury are dissolved. Following cessation of fibrinolytic treatment, the therapeutic plasminogen activators are cleared from the circulation at half-lives of 5 to 40 min,[50] after which plasma fibrinogen is regenerated by hepatic synthesis,

TABLE 136-1   ANTIFIBRINOLYTIC THERAPY WITH EACA OR AMCA IN BLEEDING STATES*

PATHOLOGIC PROCESS AND CLINICAL BLEEDING STATE	EXPERIENCE USING ANTIFIBRINOLYTIC AGENTS	COMMENT
Systemic hyperfibrinolysis		
Inherited α_2-antiplasmin or PAI-1 deficiency	Controlled with inhibitors	Rare autosomal recessive trait; prophylactic treatment indicated only in severe cases
DIC	May aggravate DIC	Treatment indicated only in rare cases with excessive activation of fibrinolysis
Fibrinolytic therapy	Usually not necessary	If bleeding is excessive antifibrinolytic agents are helpful
Malignancy (solid tumor)	Useful if bleeding is due to hyperfibrinolysis alone (rare)	Hypercoagulable state may be unmasked by antifibrinolytic treatment
Acute promyelocytic leukemia	May reduce bleeding manifestations	Coexistent thrombotic state may preclude use of antifibrinolytic agents
Liver disease and transplantation	Protracted oozing can be better controlled	An excessive hyperfibrinolytic state is present during the anhepatic and immediate postperfusion stages (Chap. 125).
Extracorporeal bypass surgery	Bleeding reduced	Intrapleural or intrapericardial clots resistant to lysis may occur with treatment
Snake venoms	Probably not useful	Most snake venoms are metalloproteinases
Localized fibrinolysis with defective hemostasis		
Hemophilia A and B, von Willebrand disease, and factor XI deficiency	Proven use for dental extractions, probable usefulness after other surgical procedures	Antifibrinolytic agents not effective as prophylaxis for hemarthrosis
Anticoagulated patients	Dental surgery blood loss decreased with administration as mouthwash	
Thrombocytopenia	Controlled trials fail to show benefit	Antifibrinolytic agents may be useful in selected patients
Amyloidosis	Proven useful	
Kasabach-Merritt syndrome	Useful for shrinking hemangioma masses if properly used	Antifibrinolytic agents may trigger systemic DIC
Localized fibrinolysis with normal hemostasis		
Prostatectomy	Reduces postoperative bleeding	Treatment indicated only for cases with severe and prolonged bleeding

(cont.)

TABLE 136-1   ANTIFIBRINOLYTIC THERAPY WITH EACA OR AMCA IN BLEEDING STATES* *(CONTINUED)*

PATHOLOGIC PROCESS AND CLINICAL BLEEDING STATE	EXPERIENCE USING ANTIFIBRINOLYTIC AGENTS	COMMENT
Renal bleeding	Effective	High risk of clots in the renal collecting system with treatment
Menorrhagia	Effectively reduces blood loss	Evaluate for underlying pathology
Upper gastrointestinal	Useful adjunctive measure to reduce bleeding	Carefully evaluate underlying lesion
Ulcerative colitis	May reduce blood loss but no effect on underlying disease	Treatment indicated for unresponsive cases only
Subarachnoid hemorrhage	Incidence of rebleeding reduced, but vasospasm is accentuated	No reduction in mortality with treatment
Orthopedic surgery	Reduces bleeding during hip and knee arthroplasty	Prophylactic treatment probably not indicated
Traumatic hyphema	Reduces the incidence of early rebleeding	No long-term benefit from treatment
Post-tonsillectomy	Incidence of rebleeding can be reduced	Prophylactic treatment may be useful in selected cases
Hereditary hemorrhagic telangiectasia	May reduce severity and frequency of epistaxis and gastrointestinal bleeding	

*DIC, disseminated intravascular coagulation; PAI-1, plasminogen activator inhibitor-1

reaching pretreatment levels at 24 to 36 h. If bleeding occurs during or immediately after treatment, therapeutic efforts at normalizing hemostasis should include correction of plasma fibrinogen with cryoprecipitate and correction of possible platelet dysfunction by platelet transfusion.[51] Although the clinical efficacy of fibrinolytic inhibitors has not been proven, these agents should be administered to inhibit residual fibrinolytic activity. Since hypofibrinogenemia persists after thrombolytic therapy for at least 12 h,[52] there is a risk of excessive bleeding during surgical trauma such as coronary artery bypass grafting.[53,54] Thus, in the TIMI II A study, percutaneous transluminal coronary angioplasty (PTCA) performed immediately after thrombolytic therapy was accompanied by increased bleeding; 20 percent of patients who underwent immediate PTCA required blood transfusions, compared to only 7 percent of patients in whom PTCA was performed 18 to 48 h after thrombolytic therapy for acute myocardial infarction.[54]

ACQUIRED PATHOLOGICAL CONDITIONS

Disseminated Intravascular Coagulation   A number of pathologic states can result in hyperplasminemia, presumably through the release of endothelial cell plasminogen activator in sufficient quantities to overcome natural inhibitors. Such states include heatstroke, hypoxia, brain injury, hypotension, thoracic surgery, and certain neoplasms and may all be associated with hemorrhage. Laboratory examinations reveal shortened euglobulin lysis time; decreased plasminogen, fibrinogen, and α_2-plasmin inhibitor levels; and elevated levels of fibrin(ogen) degradation products.[55-62] Such patients frequently have DIC as well, which can be identified if thrombocytopenia is present.

Great caution should therefore be exercised before one uses antifibrinolytic agents in these conditions (see Chap. 126).

Malignancy   Many malignant cells synthesize procoagulant components that contribute locally to tumor invasion or metastatic spread and may be associated with systemic hypercoagulable states and thrombotic manifestations.[63] The secretion of u-PA or t-PA by ovarian, breast, and prostate adenocarcinoma cells,[57,59,64-73] with or without concomitant activation of the clotting cascade, may induce a bleeding state via activation of the fibrinolytic system. The possibility that a procoagulant/thrombotic tendency may coexist with a fibrinolytic/bleeding state in patients with malignancy makes the use of fibrinolytic inhibitors especially difficult, since inhibition of fibrinolysis might unmask a prothrombic state and induce thrombosis and/or DIC. The decision to use fibrinolytic inhibitors should be based on: (1) exclusion of DIC by finding a normal and stable platelet count; (2) failure to arrest bleeding by replacement therapy or local hemostatic measures; and (3) demonstration of enhanced whole blood or euglobulin lysis times.

Acute Promyelocytic Leukemia   Promyelocytic leukemia cells produce both tissue factor and urokinase[74] and express annexin II that enhances fibrinolysis (see Chaps. 114 and 116). Thus, patients with acute promyelocytic leukemia (APL) have the potential for both thrombotic and hemorrhagic complications, which may be manifested at presentation or after induction of chemotherapy (see Chap. 126). The detection of elevated levels of thrombin-antithrombin (TAT) complexes or prothrombin fragment F_{1+2} or evidence of plasminogen activation, antiplasmin consumption, and hypofibrinogenemia provide evidence for systemic activation of coagulation and/or fibrinolysis, respectively.[75-81] Promyelocytic leukemic cells with the t(15;17) translocation express abnormally high levels of cell-surface annexin II. Annexin II is a calcium-regulated, phospholipid-binding protein on endothelial cells, macrophages, and some tumor cells. It acts as a cell surface receptor for both plasminogen and t-PA. In acute promyelocytic leukemia patients, plasmin is generated at an abnormally high rate because of the overexpression of annexin II, leading to consumption of α_2-antiplasmin and excess circulating plasmin.[82] This group of patients constitutes a therapeutic dilemma, since either bleeding or thrombotic complications or both may be apparent[82,83] and treatment of one manifestation could exacerbate or allow the development of the other. While heparin is clearly indicated for a frank thrombotic occlusion, the evidence for efficacy of heparin as prophylaxis against DIC is equivocal.[84] Similarly, there is a difference of opinion as to whether antifibrinolytic therapy is of benefit in preventing bleeding complications, which appear to be more prevalent after initiation of chemotherapy. Whereas a retrospective comparison of 268 patients managed with heparin, fibrinolytic inhibitor, or supportive treatment alone showed no difference in early hemorrhagic death with any management policy,[83] a prospective, randomized trial in 12 patients showed a significant reduction in hemorrhage and transfusion requirements with AMCA administration.[85] All-*trans*-retinoic acid, which has been successfully used for the treatment of APL, increased the expression of the urokinase receptor on the surface of APL cells and led to increased plasmin generation, whereas dexamethasone totally suppressed this effect of retinoic acid.[74] Thus, there appears to be some logic to adding dexamethasone to the chemotherapeutic regimens used for the treatment of APL.

Liver Disease and Transplantation   Increased fibrinolytic activity due to the presence of abnormal quantities of t-PA[86] and of u-PA[87] is often present in advanced liver disease, presumably due to the failure of hepatic clearance mechanisms,[88] but there may also be a component in the blood of cirrhotic patients that stimulates t-PA release from endothelial cells.[89] A cohort of 112 cirrhotic patients with esophageal varices who had not exhibited upper gastrointestinal bleeding was followed for a period of 3 years. Among the many clinical and laboratory abnormalities found in these patients, multivariate analysis revealed that hyperfibrinolysis (defined as t-PA activity and D-dimer levels above the mean ± 2 SD of 112 controls) was the only marker predictive of subsequent upper gastrointestinal bleeding.[90]

During orthotopic liver transplantation (OLT) the euglobulin lysis time greatly shortens and the levels of D-dimer, t-PA antigen and activity, and plasmin/α-plasmin inhibitor complexes increase. These changes are usually most pronounced during reperfusion of the grafted liver.[91] Several randomized studies have examined whether the administration of antifibrinolytic agents reduces blood loss and transfusion requirements during OLT. While over 10 nonrandomized studies[92] concluded that aprotinin greatly diminishes bleeding and the need for red blood cell, fresh-frozen plasma, and platelet transfusions, one randomized trial comprising 80 patients found that the administration of high-dose aprotinin (2,000,000 KIU initial dose, followed by 500,000 KIU/h) was not useful in reducing bleeding and blood product requirement. The results of this study, however, were unexpected insofar as no attenuation of the D-dimer increase during the surgical procedure was observed.[92] Also, the mean number of blood products administered during surgery exceeded 40 units, which probably led to a marked wash-out of aprotinin. Another study randomized 199 patients undergoing OLT to high-dose or low-dose aprotinin prophylaxis. No difference in blood product requirements was found.[93] Two double-blind randomized studies evaluated the effect of AMCA in OLT. High doses of 40 mg/kg/h up to a maximum of 20 g reduced the requirement of blood products from 43.5 units in control patients to 20.5 units in the AMCA-treated group ($P=0.003$),[94] whereas twentyfold smaller doses of 2 mg/kg/h had no beneficial effect[95] (see Chap. 125).

Cardiopulmonary Bypass   Extracorporeal circulation results in activation of the contact phase of the coagulation, fibrinolysis, and complement systems. Neutrophils and platelets become activated as well, and platelets are dysfunctional.[96-101] Correlations of shortened euglobulin clot lysis times with sternotomy, and with serious bleeding after open-heart surgery requiring cardiopulmonary bypass,[102] suggest that neutralization of the systemic, hyperfibrin(ogen)olytic state could be beneficial in reducing blood loss. Antifibrinolytic agents attenuate platelet activation, suggesting a potential role for plasmin-mediated platelet activation.[103,104]

Over 100 studies have been published on the blood-sparing effect of aprotinin, EACA, and AMCA in cardiac surgery, thoracoabdominal aneurysm repair, and lung transplantation, and with use of heart-assist devices. A recent meta-analysis[105] reviewed 52 randomized clinical trials of cardiac surgery published between 1985 and 1998 involving the use of aprotinin (n=46) and EACA (n=9). Compared to placebo, the mean reduction of blood losses with high-dose aprotinin (priming dose of 2,000,000 KIU, followed by 500,000 KIU/h) was 53 percent, whereas with low-dose aprotinin (usually about one-third to one-half of the high dose) and with EACA, the mean reduction was 35 percent ($P<0.001$ throughout). Less bleeding resulted in fewer re-explorations; the reduction with high-dose aprotinin was 75 percent ($P<0.001$), whereas the reduction with low-dose aprotinin was 54 percent ($P=0.048$) and the reduction with EACA 58 percent ($P=0.13$; smaller number of patients). Interestingly, there were fewer strokes occurring with all three treatment schedules ($P=$n.s.). The incidence of postoperative myocardial infarction and overall mortality was similar in the three treatment and the placebo groups.

Five randomized, double-blind studies were reported comparing AMCA to controls, with reduction in blood losses from 31 to 36 percent.[103,106-109] In a more recent trial, three different doses of AMCA (50, 100, or 150 mg/kg) were compared.[110] The most cost-effective dose was 100 mg/kg.

In general, comparative trials did not show significant differences in blood loss between low-dose aprotinin and EACA and/or AMCA, but blood loss was lower with high-dose aprotinin.[111-116] The incidence of graft occlusion after coronary artery bypass grafting was slightly but insignificantly increased[117,118] or not increased.[119]

Aspirin exposure within 7 days prior to coronary bypass surgery is associated with an increased rate of reoperation, with large increases in transfusion requirements.[120] Aprotinin counterbalances the increased risk of perioperative hemorrhage in such patients.[121,122]

Of practical importance is the fact that aprotinin, but not EACA, or AMCA prolongs the partial thromboplastin time and the activated clotting time independent of heparin, presumably by an inhibitory effect on kallikrein.[123] Thus, patients on cardiopulmonary bypass may appear to acquire a greater anticoagulant effect from heparin than actually exists.

Snake Venoms   Patients bitten by some snake or caterpillar species may develop localized or systemic bleeding. Some of these venoms are primarily procoagulants and produce DIC (see Chap. 126), whereas others activate inactive single-chain pro-UK to active two-chain UK[124] or directly degrade fibrinogen,[125-128] often without influencing the platelet count and the prothrombin time.[129] A register of snake venoms lists 67 purified fibrino(geno)lytic venom enzymes and 1 plasminogen activator enzyme.[130] Many of these enzymes are zinc-metalloproteinases. Antifibrinolytic agents probably are not useful in controlling bleeding due to these venoms.

LOCALIZED FIBRINOLYSIS WITH ABNORMAL HEMOSTASIS

HEMOPHILIA AND OTHER INHERITED BLEEDING DISORDERS

Replacement therapy is effective in providing normal hemostasis following all types of major surgical procedures in patients with hemophilia. The addition of intravenous antifibrinolytic agents to the regimen reduces bleeding and the requirement for factor VIII or factor IX concentrates, as demonstrated by studies of dental extractions.[131,132] Patients with hemophilia undergoing other surgical procedures could be similarly supported by conjoint antifibrinolytic and factor-replacement therapy. Because a hypercoagulable state may occur secondary to administration of some factor IX–rich concentrates,[133] their use along with antifibrinolytic agents in factor IX–deficient patients may present a greater risk of thrombotic complication.

Therapy of hemarthroses with small doses of factor VIII administered either early after bleeding or prophylactically to patients with hemophilia is extremely effective. EACA and AMCA do not favorably alter the long-term incidence or severity of hemarthroses in these patients.[2,134,135]

Hemophiliacs have an increased risk of developing frank renal obstruction secondary to large clots in the renal collecting system when treated with EACA.[136,137] Therefore, upper urinary tract bleeding should be managed conservatively for as long as possible, using factor replacement and high fluid intake to maintain a low urinary hematocrit and fibrinogen concentration. If bleeding lasts for weeks and requires blood transfusions, or if surgical intervention is considered, then the benefit relative to risk justifies therapy with antifibrinolytic agents.

Antifibrinolytic therapy has also been found useful following minor oral surgery[138] or major surgery[139] and in patients with menorrhagia due to von Willebrand disease.[139] Use of AMCA efficiently prevents bleeding during or after dental extractions in patients with severe factor XI deficiency (see Chap. 122).

ORAL ANTICOAGULATION THERAPY

A recent review analyzed 26 reports on dental surgical procedures and tooth extractions in patients receiving continuous anticoagulation for a prosthetic cardiac valve or vascular prosthesis.[140] The author concluded that oral anticoagulation can be safely continued in such patients with a minimal risk of bleeding. The use of an AMCA mouthwash following oral surgery was effective in reducing the incidence of bleeding episodes (without altering the dosage of anticoagulants), as compared to the bleeding in a randomized control group (1/19 versus 8/20 bleeding episodes, $P=0.01$).[141] The mouth has a high level of fibrinolytic activity due to the presence of t-PA,[142] so local inhibition of the activity may explain the efficacy of therapy for controlling bleeding.

THROMBOCYTOPENIA AND THROMBOCYTOPATHIES

Treatment with fibrinolytic inhibitors may ameliorate bleeding in patients with immune thrombocytopenic purpura who have elevated concentrations of tissue plasminogen activator.[143] Also, patients with amegakaryocytic, immune-mediated, or dyspoietic thrombocytopenia were reported to benefit from the use of fibrinolytic inhibitors.[144–146] However, in a controlled, double-blinded study of patients with amegakaryocytic thrombocytopenia (platelet count $<20\times10^9$/liter), the use of AMCA failed to decrease dependence on platelet transfusions or to reduce the incidence of cutaneous bleeding, epistaxis, or gingival hemorrhage.[147]

AMYLOIDOSIS

Several case reports describe increased levels of t-PA and/or u-PA, accompanied by decreased concentrations of plasminogen and of α_2-plasmin inhibitor in patients with amyloidosis and bleeding manifestations.[148–152] Treatment with EACA or AMCA usually was successful in controlling the bleeding. In a special variety of amyloidosis, the Dutch type of hereditary cerebral hemorrhage, the fibrinolytic activity is not increased, although high t-PA antigen levels and a low fibrinogen concentration are demonstrable.[153]

KASABACH-MERRITT SYNDROME

Patients with multiple giant hemangiomata (Kasabach-Merritt syndrome) present a particularly difficult problem, with progressive tumor enlargement that often requires extensive, dangerous, and sometimes disfiguring surgery. The variable consumption of platelets and fibrinogen suggests that thrombi are continually formed and dissolved within the hemangioma. Tumor shrinkage, improvement of laboratory evidence of intravascular coagulation, and symptomatic patient improvement have been reported when in situ thrombosis was induced by the administration of EACA, either alone or with concomitant cryoprecipitate infusion.[35,154] Local (intra-arterial) administration of EACA plus thrombin has also been successfully utilized as adjunct treatment with systemic cryoprecipitate.[155]

LOCALIZED FIBRINOLYSIS WITH NORMAL HEMOSTASIS

PROSTATECTOMY

Bleeding after prostatectomy is probably enhanced by the presence in the urine of u-PA, which diffuses into the operative site and dissolves newly formed hemostatic plugs.[156] The postoperative blood loss correlated best with the measured u-PA activity in one study.[157] Trials of systemic EACA or AMCA therapy after prostatectomy have demonstrated a significant decrease in postoperative blood loss when compared to placebo.[158,159] However, the bleeding in control patients usually is more bothersome than dangerous, and antifibrinolytic treatment probably is best applied to patients with excessive bleeding at surgery or immediately afterward. Intravesicular irrigation with EACA has not proved superior to saline irrigation for surgical bleeding, but this approach may be useful for late fibrinolytic hemorrhage, especially in patients with possible DIC.[160] Vascular thrombotic side effects in

patients treated with antifibrinolytic agents were no greater than those in control groups,[32,161] but intravesical clots that require surgical evacuation may complicate the postoperative course.[162]

RENAL BLEEDING

Antifibrinolytic therapy for prolonged spontaneous bleeding in patients with sickle cell disease and sickle cell trait can be dramatically successful.[34] Patients with renal disease who exhibit severe and protracted hematuria after renal biopsy may benefit from treatment with EACA.[163] However, there is an increased risk of significant clot formation in the renal collecting system,[164,165] which in a small number of patients is large enough to seriously impair renal function.[156] In some of these patients a trial with an intraureterally administered thrombolytic agent may be considered.[165] The abrupt appearance of extrarenal clot formation is recognized by a combination of clearing of blood from the urine, flank pain, and a nephrogram image on intravenous pyelography without dye excretion into the ureters and bladder.

UTERUS

Excessive uterine bleeding due to a variety of pathologic causes has been associated with increased local fibrinolytic activity.[166] Higher uterine t-PA activities were found in endometrial curettage samples obtained during the menstrual phase of the cycle from patients with menorrhagia compared to uterine curettings from women with normal menses.[1] Fibrinolytic activity is also increased in most patients after placement of intrauterine devices.[167] Double-blind trials of antifibrinolytic therapy show decreased bleeding in patients with menorrhagia[3,168,169] or after intrauterine device placement.[170,171] Moreover, local release of EACA from fitted silicone rubber sleeves has likewise prevented excessive bleeding associated with such devices.[172] Before instituting antifibrinolytic therapy, patients should undergo a complete gynecological, hormonal, and hemostasis evaluation. Menorrhagia is a common presenting symptom in women with von Willebrand disease.[173,174] There is no consensus on the best antifibrinolytic dosing regimen. Good results have been obtained with oral AMCA, 15 mg/kg t.i.d or q.i.d during the first 3 to 5 days of the monthly menses, but single doses of 3 to 4 g taken once daily also have been effective.[174]

The cervix contains a high concentration of t-PA, which contributes to excessive bleeding in some patients after cervical conization. The administration of AMCA was effective in reducing blood loss after such surgery and eliminating delayed bleeding during the first 5 postoperative days.[175]

GASTROINTESTINAL TRACT

Certain pathologic lesions that cause upper and lower gastrointestinal bleeding have been associated with increased fibrinolytic activity, either within the tissues themselves or in veins draining the affected organ.[176] *Helicobacter pylori* infection is associated with chronic gastritis and gastric and duodenal ulcers. Endoscopic biopsy specimens of patients with *H. pylori* infection and/or gastric and duodenal ulcers exhibited increased u-PA levels, which were highest in patients with active bleeding. In most studies, however, t-PA concentrations in these biopsies were lower than in normal mucosa. Treatment of *H. pylori* infection with omeprazole or ranitidine, and clarithromycin and metronidazole resulted in normalization of u-PA and t-PA levels.[177–179]

Prospective, controlled clinical trials[180–184] used AMCA in large groups of patients with upper gastrointestinal bleeding, with clear-cut benefit. In one trial 200 patients with acute upper gastrointestinal hemorrhage were randomized, and there was a significant difference in the requirement for surgical intervention to control bleeding (23 of 97 control patients versus only 7 of 103 AMCA-treated patients) and fewer deaths (two of the AMCA-treated patients, four of the placebo-treated patients all secondary to massive blood loss).[180] Benefit was noted in patients with esophageal varices as well as in those with gastric ulcers, gastric erosions, or miscellaneous other bleeding lesions. The favorable clinical results most likely are due to inhibition of local fibrinolysis in the mucosa of the upper gastrointestinal tract.[176,182,185]

Increased amounts of plasminogen activator are present in the rectal mucosa, and fibrin degradation products are increased in plasma of patients with active ulcerative colitis or Crohn's disease.[186–188] Clinical trials of systemic antifibrinolytic therapy in these conditions have not shown a clear benefit.[2] New approaches, such as the direct administration of an antifibrinolytic agent by enema, may ultimately prove more useful[186] without causing systemic inhibition of fibrinolysis.[189]

A marked increase of fibrinolytic activity, probably due to activation of coagulation, is also observed in hepatosplenic schistosomiasis and may contribute to bleeding from esophageal varices in these patients.[190]

SUBARACHNOID HEMORRHAGE

The cerebrospinal fluid (CSF) is usually devoid of plasminogen activator activity. After subarachnoid hemorrhage (SAH), increased fibrinolytic activity and elevated concentrations of D-dimers are found in the CSF.[191,192] However, levels of active PAI-1, of t-PA/PAI-1 complexes, and of thrombin-antithrombin complexes (a marker of thrombin generation) are also increased in the CSF, particularly in patients with severe forms of SAH and in those with subsequent cerebral infarction and/or poor outcome.[193] Elevated fibrinogen, t-PA, PAI-1, and D-dimer levels in the plasma of patients with SAH were significantly correlated with cerebral infarction and poor outcome as evaluated by the Glasgow Outcome Scale.[194]

Rebleeding occurs in 6 to 20 percent of the at-risk population, usually in the first several weeks after the initial episode and most often on the same day as the initial hemorrhage.[195] Over 30 studies have evaluated the effect of EACA or AMCA on rebleeding and outcome. Eight truly randomized controlled trials, comprising a total of 937 patients of whom 476 received antifibrinolytic drugs, 364 placebo, and 97 open control treatment, were recently reviewed by Roos et al.[196] Although antifibrinolytic therapy significantly decreased the rebleeding rate, it also clearly induced cerebral ischemia (Table 136-2). Death from all causes, and the incidences of hydrocephalus and dependency, were identical in controls and in patients treated with antifibrinolytic therapy. However, these trials were all conducted at least 10 years ago, when treatment of cerebral ischemia was not common. Modern treatment of cerebral ischemia, comprising an increase in daily fluid intake, hypervolemic hemodilution with albumin (aiming for a hematocrit of about 0.3), and the administration of nimodipine, leads to a marked decrease of cerebral ischemia, even in patients treated with AMCA.[197]

TABLE 136-2   ANTIFIBRINOLYTIC TREATMENT OF SUBARACHNOID HEMORRHAGE: META-ANALYSIS OF 8 RANDOMIZED TRIALS[196]

Event	Relative Risk	95% Confidence Interval
Death from all causes	1.03	0.86–1.22
Rebleeding rate		
All studies	0.64	0.49–0.85
Double-blind studies only	0.55	0.40–0.77
Cerebral ischemia	1.77	1.30–2.40
Hydrocephalus	1.04	0.77–1.42
Dependence, poor outcome	1.03	0.86–1.22

ORTHOPEDIC SURGERY

A few randomized studies have examined whether antifibrinolytic agents reduce blood transfusion requirements in orthopedic surgery without increasing the incidence of postoperative deep venous thrombosis. In two small total hip replacement studies, high-dose intravenous infusion of aprotinin was compared in a double-blind fashion to a placebo infusion. Total blood loss was about 30 percent lower in the aprotinin group, and the occurrence of postoperative DVT was comparable in the two groups.[198,199] AMCA reduced total blood losses by about 40 percent in a randomized, double-blind study of total knee arthroplasty.[200]

TRAUMATIC HYPHEMA

Therapy with antifibrinolytic agents is not unreasonable as a prophylactic measure against the rebleeding from traumatic hyphema, which occurs about 2 to 6 days after the initial injury in as many as 30 percent of patients. Increased local fibrinolytic activity present in circumscribed areas of the eye, specifically in the endothelium of the canal of Schlemm, is likely to contribute to the rebleeding. A favorable effect of antifibrinolytic therapy in preventing secondary bleeding following traumatic hyphema has been reported,[201–204] but on followup examination at 2 to 6 weeks there was no difference in the final visual acuity compared with that in the control group.[205]

MUCOUS MEMBRANES

Antifibrinolytic therapy in patients undergoing tonsillectomy and adenoidectomy[206] resulted in a significant decrease in blood loss, but this treatment modality is not routinely used. Treatment might reasonably be attempted in patients with unexplained serious postoperative bleeding that requires resuturing or packing, perhaps using packs impregnated with an antifibrinolytic agent.

Oral AMCA has not proved useful for adjunctive therapy of epistaxis in patients requiring hospital admission.[207]

HEREDITARY HEMORRHAGIC TELANGIECTASIA

In two patients with hereditary hemorrhagic telangiectasia experiencing recurrent epistaxis and gastrointestinal bleeding, treatment with EACA greatly reduced the frequency of bleeding episodes and improved hemoglobin levels from 70 g/liter to around 130 g/liter.[208] In other patients EACA has not proved helpful.

REFERENCES

1. Gleeson NC: Cyclic changes in endometrial tissue plasminogen activator and plasminogen activator inhibitor type 1 in women with normal menstruation and essential menorrhagia. Am J Obstet Gynecol 171:178, 1994.
2. Sherry S, Marder VJ: Therapy with antifibrinolytic agents, in Hemostasis and Thrombosis: Basic Principles and Clinical Practice, 3rd ed, edited by RW Colman, J Hirsh, VJ Marder, EW Salzman, p 335. Lippincott, Philadelphia, 1994.
3. Ogston D: Antifibrinolytic Drugs. Chemistry, Pharmacology and Clinical Usage. Wiley, New York, 1984.
4. Verstraete M: Clinical application of inhibitors of fibrinolysis. Drugs 29:236, 1985.
5. McNicol GP, Fletcher AP, Alkjaersig N, Sherry S: Impairment of hemostasis in the urinary tract: the role of urokinase. J Lab Clin Med 58:34, 1961.
6. Collen D: On the regulation and control of fibrinolysis. Thromb Haemost 43:77, 1980.
7. Bachmann F: Fibrinolysis, in Thrombosis and Haemostasis, edited by M Verstraete, J Vermylen, R Lijnen, J Arnout, p 227. Leuven University Press, Leuven, Belgium, 1987.
8. Aoki N, Harpel PC: Inhibitors of the fibrinolytic enzyme system. Semin Thromb Hemost 10:24, 1984.
9. Sprengers ED, Kluft C: Plasminogen activator inhibitors. Blood 69:381, 1987.

10. Kruithof EKO: Plasminogen activator inhibitors—a review. *Enzyme* 40:113, 1988.

11. Kunitz M, Northrop JH: Isolation from beef pancreas of crystalline trypsinogen, trypsin, a trypsin inhibitor and an inhibitor trypsin compound. *J Gen Physiol* 19:991, 1936.

12. Rühlmann A, Schramm HJ, Kukla D, Huber R: Pancreatic trypsin inhibitor (Kunitz): II. Complexes with proteinases. *Cold Spring Harb Symp Quant Biol* 36:148, 1972.

13. Wiman B: On the reaction of plasmin or plasmin streptokinase complex with aprotinin or α-antiplasmin. *Thromb Res* 17:143, 1980.

14. Huber R, Kukla D, Rühlmann A, Steigemann W: Pancreatic trypsin inhibitor (Kunitz): I. Structure and function. *Cold Spring Harb Symp Quant Biol* 36:141, 1972.

15. Rühlmann A, Kukla D, Schwager P, Bartels K, Huber R: Structure of the complex formed by bovine trypsin and bovine pancreatic trypsin inhibitor. Crystal structure determination and stereochemistry of the contact region. *J Mol Biol* 77:417, 1973.

16. Robert S, Wagner BKJ, Boulanger M, Richer M: Aprotinin. *Ann Pharmacother* 30:372, 1996.

17. Anonick PK, Vasudevan J, Gonias SL: Antifibrinolytic activities of α-N-acetyl-L-lysine methyl ester, epsilon-aminocaproic acid, and tranexamic acid. Importance of kringle interactions and active site inhibition. *Arterioscler Thromb* 12:708, 1992.

18. Fears R, Greenwood H, Hearn J, et al: Inhibition of the fibrinolytic and fibrinogenolytic activity of plasminogen activators in vitro by the antidotes ε-aminocaproic acid, tranexamic acid and aprotinin. *Fibrinolysis* 6:79, 1992.

19. Andersson L, Nilsson IM, Nilehn J-E, et al: Experimental and clinical studies on AMCA, the anti-fibrinolytic active isomer of p-aminomethylcyclohexane carboxylic acid. *Scand J Clin Lab Invest* 2:230, 1965.

20. Thorsen S, Müllertz S: Rate of activation and electrophoretic mobility of unmodified and partially degraded plasminogen. Effects of 6-aminohexanoic acid and related compounds. *Scand J Clin Lab Invest* 34:167, 1974.

21. Takada A, Sugawara Y, Takada Y: Enhancement of the activation of Glu-plasminogen by urokinase in the simultaneous presence of tranexamic acid or fibrin. *Haemostasis* 1:26, 1989.

22. Royston D: High-dose aprotinin therapy: a review of the first five years' experience. *J Cardiothorac Anesth* 6:76, 1992.

23. Levy JH, Bailey JM, Salmenperä M: Pharmacokinetics of aprotinin in preoperative cardiac surgical patients. *Anesthesiology* 80:1013, 1994.

24. Westaby S: Aprotinin in perspective. *Ann Thorac Surg* 55:1033, 1993.

25. McNicol GP, Fletcher AP, Alkjaersig N, Sherry S: The absorption, distribution and excretion of ε-aminocaproic acid following oral or intravenous administration to man. *J Lab Clin Med* 59:15, 1962.

26. Dietrich W, Barankay A, Hahnel C, Richter JA: High-dose aprotinin in cardiac surgery: three years' experience in 1,784 patients. *J Cardiothorac Vasc Anesth* 6:324, 1992.

27. Bidstrup BP, Harrison J, Royston D, Taylor KM, Treasure T: Aprotinin therapy in cardiac operations: a report on use in 41 cardiac centers in the United Kingdom. *Ann Thorac Surg* 55:971, 1993.

28. Dewachter P, Mouton C, Masson C, Gueant JL, Haberer JP: Anaphylactic reaction to aprotinin during cardiac surgery [letter]. *Anaesthesia* 48:1110, 1993.

29. Feindt PR, Walcher S, Volkmer I, et al: Effects of high-dose aprotinin on renal function in aortocoronary bypass grafting. *Ann Thorac Surg* 60:1076, 1995.

30. Kane MJ, Silverman LR, Rand JH, Paciucci PA, Holland JF: Myonecrosis as a complication of the use of epsilon amino-caproic acid: a case report and review of the literature. *Am J Med* 85:861, 1988.

31. Ratnoff OD: Epsilon aminocaproic acid—a dangerous weapon. *N Engl J Med* 280:1124, 1969.

32. Vinnicombe J, Shuttleworth KED: Aminocaproic acid in the control of haemorrhage after prostatectomy. Safety of aminocaproic acid—a controlled trial. *Lancet* 1:232, 1966.

33. Gordon-Smith IC, Hickman JA, el-Masri SH: The effect of the fibrinolytic inhibitor epsilon-aminocaproic acid on the incidence of deep-vein thrombosis after prostatectomy. *Br J Surg* 59:522, 1972.

34. Immergut MA, Stevenson T: The use of epsilon-aminocaproic acid in the control of hematuria associated with hemoglobinopathies. *Br J Urol* 93:110, 1965.

35. Warrell RP Jr, Kempin SJ: Treatment of severe coagulopathy in the Kasabach-Merritt syndrome with aminocaproic acid and cryoprecipitate. *N Engl J Med* 313:309, 1985.

36. Aoki N, Saito H, Kamiya T, Koie K, Sakata Y, Kobakura M: Congenital deficiency of α₂-plasmin inhibitor associated with severe hemorrhagic tendency. *J Clin Invest* 63:877, 1979.

37. Aoki N, Sakata Y, Matsuda M, Tateno K: Fibrinolytic states in a patient with congenital deficiency of α₂-plasmin inhibitor. *Blood* 55:483, 1980.

38. Diéval J, Nguyen G, Gross S, Delobel J, Kruithof EKO: A lifelong bleeding disorder associated with a deficiency of plasminogen activator inhibitor type 1. *Blood* 77:528, 1991.

39. Fay WP, Shapiro AD, Shih JL, Schleef RR, Ginsburg D: Complete deficiency of plasminogen-activator inhibitor type 1 due to a frameshift mutation. *N Engl J Med* 327:1729, 1992.

40. Lee MH, Vosburgh E, Anderson K, McDonagh J: Deficiency of plasma plasminogen activator inhibitor 1 results in hyperfibrinolytic breeding. *Blood* 81:2357, 1993.

41. Fay WP, Parker AC, Condrey LR, Shapiro AD: Human plasminogen activator inhibitor-1 (PAI-1) deficiency: characterization of a large kindred with a null mutation in the PAI-1 gene. *Blood* 90:204, 1997.

42. Ikematsu S, Fukutake K, Aoki N: Heterozygote for plasmin inhibitor deficiency developing hemorrhagic tendency with advancing age. *Thromb Res* 82:129, 1996.

43. Aznar J, Estellés A, Vila V, Regañón E, España F, Villa P: Inherited fibrinolytic disorder due to an enhanced plasminogen activator level. *Thromb Haemost* 52:196, 1984.

44. Booth NA, Bennett B, Wijngaards G, Grieve JHK: A new life-long hemorrhagic disorder due to excess plasminogen activator. *Blood* 61:267, 1983.

45. Humphries JE, Gonias SL, Pizzo SV, Williams ME: Life-long bleeding diathesis: effect of orthotopic liver transplantation. *Am J Clin Pathol* 102:816, 1994.

46. Cugno M, Hack CE, de Boer JP, Eerenberg AJM, Agostini A, Cicardi M: Generation of plasmin during acute attacks of hereditary angioedema. *J Lab Clin Med* 121:38, 1993.

47. Donaldson VH: Plasminogen activation in hereditary angioneurotic edema. *J Lab Clin Med* 121:13, 1993.

48. Nielsen EW, Johansen HT, Høgåsen K, Wuillemin W, Hack CE, Mollnes TE: Activation of the complement, coagulation, fibrinolytic and kallikrein-kinin systems during attacks of hereditary angioedema. *Scand J Immunol* 44:185, 1996.

49. Agostoni A, Marasini B, Cicardi M, Martignoni G, Uziel L, Pietrogrande M: Hepatic function and fibrinolysis in patients with hereditary angioedema undergoing long-term treatment with tranexamic acid. *Allergy* 33:216, 1978.

50. Marder VJ, Sherry S: Thrombolytic therapy: current status. *N Engl J Med* 318:1512,1585, 1988.

51. Coller BS: Platelets and thrombolytic therapy. *N Engl J Med* 322:33, 1990.

52. Owen J, Friedman KD, Grossman BA, Wilkins C, Berke AD, Powers ER: Quantitation of fragment X formation during thrombolytic therapy with streptokinase and tissue plasminogen activator. *J Clin Invest* 79:1642, 1987.

53. Lee KF, Mandell J, Rankin JS, Muhlbaier LH, Wechsler AS: Immediate versus delayed coronary grafting after streptokinase treatment. Postoperative blood loss and clinical results. *J Thorac Cardiovasc Surg* 95:216, 1988.

54. The TIMI Research Group: Immediate vs delayed catheterization and angioplasty following thrombolytic therapy for acute myocardial infarction. TIMI II A results. *JAMA* 260:2849, 1988.

55. Takahashi H, Urano T, Takada Y, Nagai N, Takada A: Fibrinolytic parameters as an admission prognostic marker of head injury in patients who talk and deteriorate. *J Neurosurg* 86:768, 1997.

56. Westaby S: Coagulation disturbance in profound hypothermia: the influence of anti-fibrinolytic therapy. *Semin Thorac Cardiovasc Surg* 9:246, 1997.

57. Okajima K, Kohno I, Soe G, Okabe H, Takatsuki K, Binder BR: Direct evidence for systemic fibrinogenolysis in patients with acquired α₂-plasmin inhibitor deficiency. *Am J Hematol* 45:16, 1994.

58. Bonnemaison J, Thicoïpe M, Dixmérias F, Guérin V: Coagulopathie évocatrice d'une fibrinolyse primaire après traumatisme crânien avec mort cérébrale. *Ann Fr Anesth Reanim* 17:275, 1998.

59. Walther PJ, Gore M, Pizzo SV: Increased releasable vascular plasminogen activator and a bleeding diathesis. *Am J Med* 77:566, 1984.

60. Stankiewicz AJ, Crowley JP, Steiner M: Increased levels of tissue plasminogen activator with a low plasminogen activator inhibitor-1 in a patient with postoperative bleeding. *Am J Hematol* 38:226, 1991.

61. Hunt BJ, Segal H: Hyperfibrinolysis. *J Clin Pathol* 49:958, 1996.

62. Palmer JD, Francis DA, Roath OS, Francis JL, Iannotti F: Hyperfibrinolysis during intracranial surgery: effect of high dose aprotinin. *J Neurol Neurosurg Psychiatry* 58:104, 1995.

63. Danø K, Andreasen PA, Grøndahl-Hansen J, Kristensen P, Nielsen LS, Skriver L: Plasminogen activators, tissue degradation, and cancer. *Adv Cancer Res* 44:139, 1985.

64. Davidson JF, McNicol GP, Frank GL, Anderson TJ, Douglas AS: Plasminogen-activator-producing tumour. *Br Med J* 1:88, 1969.

65. al-Mondhiry H, Manni A, Owen J, Gordon R: Hemostatic effects of hormonal stimulation in patients with metastatic prostate cancer. *Am J Hematol* 28:141, 1988.

66. Mannucci PM, Cugno M, Bottasso B, et al: Changes in fibrinolysis in patients with localized tumors. *Eur J Cancer* 26:83, 1990.

67. Zacharski LR, Memoli VA, Ornstein DL, Rousseau SM, Kisiel W, Kudryk BJ: Tumor cell procoagulant and urokinase expression in carcinoma of the ovary. *JNCI* 85:1225, 1993.

68. De Boer WA, Koolen MGJ, Roos CM, ten Cate JW: Tranexamic acid treatment of hemothorax in two patients with malignant mesothelioma. *Chest* 100:847, 1991.

69. Weltermann A, Mitterbauer GJ, Mitterbauer M, et al: Disseminierte intravasale Gerinnung (DIG) und massive Hyperfibrinolyse bei metastasierendem Uteruskarzinom. Beobachtungen über die Beeinflussusng der Gerinnunsstörung durch verschiedene Therapien (ein Fallbericht). *Wien Med Wochenschr* 110:53, 1998.

70. Webber MM, Waghray A: Urokinase-mediated extracellular matrix degradation by human prostatic carcinoma cells and its inhibition by retinoic acid. *Clin Cancer Res* 1:755, 1995.

71. López-Pedrera C, Jardí M, del Mar Malagón MD, et al: Tissue factor (TF) and urokinase plasminogen activator receptor (uPAR) and bleeding complications in leukemic patients. *Thromb Haemost* 77:62, 1997.

72. Bennett B, Croll AM, Robbie LA, Herriot R: Tumour cell u-PA as a cause of fibrinolytic bleeding in metastatic disease. *Br J Haematol* 99:570, 1997.

73. Meijer K, Smid WM, Geerards S, van der Meer J: Hyperfibrinogenolysis in disseminated adenocarcinoma. *Blood Coagul Fibrinolysis* 9:279, 1998.

74. Mustjoki S, Tapiovaara H, Sirén V, Vaheri A: Interferons and retinoids enhance and dexamethasone suppresses urokinase-mediated plasminogen activation in promyelocytic leukemia cells. *Leukemia* 12:164, 1998.

75. Bauer KA, Rosenberg RD: Thrombin generation in acute promyelocytic leukemia. *Blood* 64:791, 1984.

76. Bennett B, Booth NA, Croll A, Dawson AA: The bleeding disorder in acute promyelocytic leukaemia: fibrinolysis due to u-PA rather than defibrination. *Br J Haematol* 71:511, 1989.

77. Avvisati G, ten Cate JW, Sturk A, Lamping R, Petti MG, Mandelli F: Acquired alpha-2-antiplasmin deficiency in acute promyelocytic leukaemia. *Br J Haematol* 70:43, 1988.

78. Schwartz BS, Williams EC, Conlan MG, Mosher DF: Epsilon-aminocaproic acid in the treatment of patients with acute promyelocytic leukemia and acquired alpha-2-plasmin inhibitor deficiency. *Ann Intern Med* 105:873, 1986.

79. Falanga A, Iacoviello L, Evangelista V, et al: Loss of blast cell procoagulant activity and improvement of hemostatic variables in patients with acute promyelocytic leukemia administered all-*trans*-retinoic acid. *Blood* 86:1072, 1995.

80. Watanabe R, Murata M, Takayama N, et al: Long-term follow-up of hemostatic molecular markers during remission induction therapy with all-*trans*-retinoic acid for acute promyelocytic leukemia. Keio Hematology-Oncology Cooperative Study Group (KHOCS). *Thromb Haemost* 77:641, 1997.

81. Pogliani EM, Rossini F, Casaroli I, Maffe P, Corneo G: Thrombotic complications in acute promyelocytic leukemia during all-*trans*-retinoic acid therapy. *Acta Haematol* 97:228, 1997.

82. Menell JS, Cesarman GM, Jacovina AT, McLaughlin MA, Lev EA, Hajjar KA: Annexin II and bleeding in acute promyelocytic leukemia. *N Engl J Med* 340:994, 1999.

83. Rodeghiero F, Avvisati G, Castaman G, Barbui T, Mandelli F: Early deaths and anti-hemorrhagic treatments in acute promyelocytic leukemia. A GIMEMA retrospective study in 268 consecutive patients. *Blood* 75:2112, 1990.

84. Goldberg MA, Ginsburg D, Mayer RJ, et al: Is heparin administration necessary during induction chemotherapy for patients with acute promyelocytic leukemia? *Blood* 69:187, 1987.

85. Avvisati G, Wouter ten Cate J, Büller HR, Mandelli F: Tranexamic acid for control of haemorrhage in acute promyelocytic leukaemia. *Lancet* 2:122, 1989.

86. Booth NA, Anderson JA, Bennett B: Plasminogen activators in alcoholic cirrhosis: demonstration of increased tissue type and urokinase type activator. *J Clin Pathol* 37:772, 1984.

87. Himmelreich G, Dooijewaard G, Breinl P, et al: Evolution of urokinase-type plasminogen activator (u-PA) and tissue-type plasminogen activator (t-PA) in orthotopic liver transplantation (OLT). *Thromb Haemost* 69:56, 1993.

88. Fletcher AP, Biederman O, Moore D, Alkjaersig N, Sherry S: Abnormal plasminogen-plasmin system activity (fibrinolysis) in patients with hepatic cirrhosis: its cause and consequences. *J Clin Invest* 43:681, 1964.

89. Hayashi T, Kamogawa A, Ro S, et al: Plasma from patients with cirrhosis increases tissue plasminogen activator release from vascular endothelial cells in vitro. *Liver* 18:186, 1998.

90. Violi F, Basili V, Ferro D, et al: Association between high values of D-dimer and tissue-plasminogen activator activity and first gastrointestinal bleeding in cirrhotic patients. *Thromb Haemost* 76:177, 1996.

91. Segal HC, Hunt BJ, Cottam S, et al: Fibrinolytic activity during orthotopic liver transplantation with and without aprotinin. *Transplantation* 58:1356, 1994.

92. Garcia-Huete L, Domenech P, Sabaté A, Martinez-Brotons F, Jaurrieta E, Figueras J: The prophylactic effect of aprotinin on intraoperative bleeding in liver transplantation: a randomized clinical study. *Hepatology* 26:1143, 1997.

93. Soilleux H, Gillon M-C, Mirand A, Daibes M, Leballe F, Ecoffey C: Comparative effects of small and large aprotinin doses on bleeding during orthotopic liver transplantation. *Anesth Analg* 80:349, 1995.

94. Boylan JF, Klinck JR, Sandler AN, et al: Tranexamic acid reduces blood loss, transfusion requirements, and coagulation factor use in primary orthotopic liver transplantation. *Anesthesiology* 85:1043, 1996.

95. Kaspar M, Ramsay MA, Nguyen AT, Cogswell M, Hurst G, Ramsay KJ: Continuous small-dose tranexamic acid reduces fibrinolysis but not transfusion requirements during orthotopic liver transplantation. *Anesth Analg* 85:281, 1997.

96. McKenna R, Bachmann F, Whittaker B, Gilson JR, Weinberg M Jr: The hemostatic mechanism after open-heart surgery: II. Frequency of abnormal platelet functions during and after extracorporeal circulation. *J Thorac Cardiovasc Surg* 70:298, 1975.

97. Harker LA, Malpass TW, Branson HE, Hessel EA II, Slichter SJ: Mechanism of abnormal bleeding in patients undergoing cardiopulmonary bypass: acquired transient platelet dysfunction associated with selective alpha-granule release. *Blood* 56:824, 1980.

98. Harker LA: Bleeding after cardiopulmonary bypass. *N Engl J Med* 314:1446, 1986.

99. Wachtfogel YT, Kucich U, Hack CE, et al: Aprotinin inhibits the contact, neutrophil, and platelet activation systems during simulated extracorporeal perfusion. *J Thorac Cardiovasc Surg* 106:1, 1993.

100. Khuri SF, Valeri CR, Loscalzo J, et al: Heparin causes platelet dysfunction and induces fibrinolysis before cardiopulmonary bypass. *Ann Thorac Surg* 60:1008, 1995.

101. Williams GD, Bratton SL, Nielsen NJ, Ramamoorthy C: Fibrinolysis in pediatric patients undergoing cardiopulmonary bypass. *J Cardiothorac Vasc Anesth* 12:633, 1998.

102. Kevy SV, Glickman RM, Bernhard WF, Diamond LK, Gross RE: The pathogenesis and control of the hemorrhagic defect in open heart surgery. *Surg Gynecol Obstet* 123:313, 1966.

103. Soslau G, Horrow J, Brodsky I: Effect of tranexamic acid on platelet ADP during extracorporeal circulation. *Am J Hematol* 38:113, 1991.

104. De Haan J, Van Oeveren W: Platelets and soluble fibrin promote plasminogen activation causing downregulation of platelet glycoprotein Ib/IX complexes: protection by aprotinin. *Thromb Res* 92:171, 1998.

105. Munoz JJ, Birkmeyer NJO, Birkmeyer JD, O'Connor GT, Dacey LJ:

Is ε-aminocaproic acid as effective as aprotinin in reducing bleeding with cardiac surgery? A meta-analysis. *Circulation* 99:81, 1999.

106. Horrow JC, Hlavacek J, Strong MD, et al: Prophylactic tranexamic acid decreases bleeding after cardiac operations. *J Thorac Cardiovasc Surg* 99:70, 1990.

107. Horrow JC, Van Riper DF, Strong MD, Brodsky I, Parmet JL: Hemostatic effects of tranexamic acid and desmopressin during cardiac surgery. *Circulation* 84:2063, 1991.

108. Karski JM, Teasdale SJ, Norman P, et al: Prevention of bleeding after cardiopulmonary bypass with high-dose tranexamic acid. Double-blind, randomized clinical trial. *J Thorac Cardiovasc Surg* 110:835, 1995.

109. Horrow JC, Van Riper DF, Strong MD, Grunewald KE, Parmet JL: The dose-response relationship of tranexamic acid. *Anesthesiology* 82:383, 1995.

110. Karski JM, Dowd NP, Joiner R, et al: The effect of three different doses of tranexamic acid on blood loss after cardiac surgery with mild systemic hypothermia (32°C). *J Cardiothorac Vasc Anesth* 12:642, 1998.

111. Pugh SC, Wielogorski AK: A comparison of the effects of tranexamic acid and low-dose aprotinin on blood loss and homologous blood usage in patients undergoing cardiac surgery. *J Cardiothorac Vasc Anesth* 9:240, 1995.

112. Boughenou F, Madi-Jebara S, Massonnet-Castel S, Benmosbah L, Carpentier A, Cousin MT: Antifibrinolytiques et prévention du saignement en chirurgie cardiaque valvulaire. Comparaison de l'acide tranexamique à l'aprotinine à haute dose. *Arch Mal Coeur Vaiss* 88:363, 1995.

113. Penta de Peppo A, Pierri MD, Scafuri A, et al: Intraoperative antifibrinolysis and blood-saving techniques in cardiac surgery. Prospective trial of 3 antifibrinolytic drugs. *Tex Heart Inst J* 22:231, 1995.

114. Menichetti A, Tritapepe L, Ruvolo G, et al: Changes in coagulation patterns, blood loss and blood use after cardiopulmonary bypass: aprotinin vs tranexamic acid vs epsilon aminocaproic acid. *J Cardiovasc Surg* 37:401, 1996.

115. Landymore RW, Murphy JT, Lummis H, Carter C: The use of low-dose aprotinin, epsilon-aminocaproic acid or tranexamic acid for prevention of mediastinal bleeding in patients receiving aspirin before coronary artery bypass operations [letter]. *Eur J Cardiothorac Surg* 11:798, 1997.

116. Misfeld M, Dubbert S, Eleftheriadis S, Siemens H-J, Wagner T, Sievers HH: Fibrinolysis-adjusted perioperative low-dose aprotinin reduces blood loss in bypass operations. *Ann Thorac Surg* 66:792, 1998.

117. Lemmer JH Jr, Stanford W, Bonney SL, et al: Aprotinin for coronary bypass operations: efficacy, safety, and influence on early saphenous vein graft patency. A multicenter, randomized, double-blind, placebo-controlled study. *J Thorac Cardiovasc Surg* 107:543, 1994.

118. Laub GW, Riebman JB, Chen C, et al: The impact of aprotinin on coronary artery bypass graft patency. *Chest* 106:1370, 1994.

119. Havel M, Grabenwöger F, Schneider J, et al: Aprotinin does not decrease early graft patency after coronary artery bypass grafting despite reducing postoperative bleeding and use of donated blood. *J Thorac Cardiovasc Surg* 107:807, 1994.

120. Bashein G, Nessly ML, Rice AL, Counts RB, Misbach GA: Preoperative aspirin therapy and reoperation for bleeding after coronary artery bypass surgery. *Arch Intern Med* 151:89, 1991.

121. Klein M, Keith PR, Dauben H-P, et al: Aprotinin counterbalances an increased risk of peri-operative hemorrhage in CABG patients pretreated with aspirin. *Eur J Cardiothorac Surg* 14:360, 1998.

122. Ivert T, Intonti M, Stain-Malmgren R, Dumitrescu A, Blombäck M: Effects of aprotinin during cardiopulmonary bypass in patients treated with acetylsalicylic acid. *Scand Cardiovasc J* 32:289, 1998.

123. Dietrich W, Dilthey G, Spannagl M, Jochum M, Braun SL, Richter JA: Influence of high-dose aprotinin on anticoagulation, heparin requirement, and celite- and kaolin-activated clotting time in heparin-pretreated patients undergoing open-heart surgery. A double-blind, placebo-controlled study. *Anesthesiology* 83:679, 1995.

124. Sugiki M, Yoshida E, Anai K, Maruyama M: Activation of single-chain urokinase-type plasminogen activator by a hemorrhagic metalloproteinase, jararafibrase I, in *Bothrops jararaca* venom. *Toxicon* 36:993, 1998.

125. Coll-Sangrona E, Arocha-Piñango CL: Fibrinolytic action on fresh human clots of whole body extracts and two semipurified fractions from *Lonomia achelous* caterpillar. *Braz J Med Biol Res* 31:779, 1998.

126. Lobo de Araujo A, Donato JL, Bon C: Purification from *Bothrops*

127. Du XY, Pan H, Jin Y, Zhu H, Wu XF, Zhou YC: Purification, cDNA cloning and molecular characteristic of a fibrinolytic enzyme from the venom of *Agkistrodon acutus*. *J Nat Toxins* 7:159, 1998.

128. Siigur J, Samel M, Tonismägi K, Subbi J, Siigur E, Tu AT: Biochemical characterization of lebetase, a direct-acting fibrinolytic enzyme from *Vipera lebetina* snake venom. *Thromb Res* 90:39, 1998.

129. Premawardena AP, Seneviratne SL, Gunatilake SB, de Silva HJ: Excessive fibrinolysis: the coagulopathy following Merrem's hump-nosed viper *(Hypnale hypnale)* bites. *Am J Trop Med Hyg* 58:821, 1998.

130. Markland FS Jr: Snake venom fibrinogenolytic and fibrinolytic enzymes: an updated inventory. Registry of Exogenous Hemostatic Factors of the Scientific and Standardization Committee of the International Society on Thrombosis and Haemostasis. *Thromb Haemost* 79:668, 1998.

131. Walsh PN, Rizza CR, Matthews JM, et al: Epsilon-aminocaproic acid therapy for dental extractions in haemophilia and Christmas disease: a double blind controlled trial. *Br J Haematol* 20:463, 1971.

132. Sindet-Pedersen S, Stenbjerg S: Effect of local antifibrinolytic treatment with tranexamic acid in hemophiliacs undergoing oral surgery. *J Oral Maxillofac Surg* 44:703, 1986.

133. Lusher JM: Thrombogenicity associated with factor IX complex concentrates. *Semin Hematol* 28:3, 1991.

134. Rainsford SG, Jouhar AJ, Hall A: Tranexamic acid in the control of spontaneous bleeding in severe haemophilia. *Thromb Diath Haemorrh* 30:272, 1973.

135. Bennett AE, Ingram GIC, Inglish PJ: Antifibrinolytic treatment in haemophilia: a controlled trial of prophylaxis with tranexamic acid. *Br J Haematol* 24:83, 1973.

136. Prentice CRM, Lindsay RM, Barr RD, et al: Renal complications in haemophilia and Christmas disease. *Q J Med* 40:47, 1971.

137. van Itterbeek H, Vermylen J, Verstraete M: High obstruction of urine flow as a complication of the treatment with fibrinolysis inhibitors of haematuria in haemophiliacs. *Acta Haematol* 39:237, 1968.

138. Williamson R, Eggleston DJ: DDAVP and EACA used for minor oral surgery in von Willebrand disease. *Aust Dent J* 33:32, 1988.

139. Blombäck M, Johansson G, Johnsson H, Swedenborg J, Wabo E: Surgery in patients with von Willebrand's disease. *Br J Surg* 76:398, 1989.

140. Wahl MJ: Dental surgery in anticoagulated patients. *Arch Intern Med* 158:1610, 1998.

141. Sindet-Pedersen S, Ramström G, Bernvil S, Blombäck M: Hemostatic effect of tranexamic acid mouthwash in anticoagulant-treated patients undergoing oral surgery. *N Engl J Med* 320:840, 1989.

142. Sindet-Pedersen S, Gram J, Jespersen J: Characterization of plasminogen activators in unstimulated and stimulated human whole saliva. *J Dent Res* 66:1199, 1987.

143. Hanss M, Ville D, Dechavanne M: Increased plasma tissue-type plasminogen activator levels in patients with chronic thrombocytopenia. *Haemostasis* 20:341, 1990.

144. Gardner FH, Helmer RE: Aminocaproic acid. Use in control of hemorrhage in patients with amegakaryocytic thrombocytopenia. *JAMA* 243:35, 1980.

145. Bartholomew JR, Salgia R, Bell WR: Control of bleeding in patients with immune and nonimmune thrombocytopenia with aminocaproic acid. *Arch Intern Med* 149:1959, 1989.

146. Garewal HS, Durie BG: Anti-fibrinolytic therapy with aminocaproic acid for the control of bleeding in thrombocytopenic patients. *Scand J Haematol* 35:497, 1985.

147. Fricke W, Alling D, Kimball J, Griffith P, Klein H: Lack of efficacy of tranexamic acid in thrombocytopenic bleeding. *Transfusion* 31:345, 1991.

148. Liebman H, Chinowsky M, Valdin J, Kenoyer G, Feinstein D: Increased fibrinolysis and amyloidosis. *Arch Intern Med* 143:678, 1983.

149. Meyer K, Williams EC: Fibrinolysis and acquired alpha-2 plasmin inhibitor deficiency in amyloidosis. *Am J Med* 79:394, 1985.

150. Takahashi H, Koike T, Yoshida N, et al: Excessive fibrinolysis in suspected amyloidosis: demonstration of plasmin- α2-plasmin inhibitor complex and von Willebrand factor fragment in plasma. *Am J Hematol* 23:153, 1986.

151. Sane DC, Pizzo SV, Greenberg CS: Elevated urokinase-type plasminogen activator level and bleeding in amyloidosis: case report and literature review. *Am J Hematol* 31:53, 1989.

lanceolatus (fer de lance) venom of a fibrino(geno)lytic enzyme with esterolytic activity. *Toxicon* 36:745, 1998.

152. Liebman HA, Carfagno MK, Weitz IC, et al: Excessive fibrinolysis in amyloidosis associated with elevated plasma single-chain urokinase. *Am J Clin Pathol* 98:534, 1992.

153. Haan J, Kluft C, Leebeek FWG, de Bart ACW, Buruma OJS, Roos RAC: Hereditary cerebral hemorrhage with amyloidosis–Dutch type: a study of fibrinolysis. *Thromb Haemost* 67:16, 1992.

154. Ortel TL, Onorato JJ, Bedrosian CL, Kaufman RE: Antifibrinolytic therapy in the management of the Kasabach Merritt syndrome. *Am J Hematol* 29:44, 1988.

155. Stahl RL, Henderson JM, Hooks MA, Martin LG, Duncan A: Therapy of the Kasabach-Merritt syndrome with cryoprecipitate plus intra-arterial thrombin and aminocaproic acid. *Am J Hematol* 36:272, 1991.

156. McNicol GP, Fletcher AP, Alkjaersig N, Sherry S: The use of epsilon-aminocaproic acid, a potent inhibitor of fibrinolytic activity in the management of postoperative hematuria. *J Urol* 86:829, 1961.

157. Nielsen JD, Gram J, Holm-Nielsen A, Fabrin K, Jespersen J: Postoperative blood loss after transurethral prostatectomy is dependent on in situ fibrinolysis. *Br J Urol* 80:889, 1997.

158. Hedlund PO: Antifibrinolytic therapy with Cyklokapron in connection with prostatectomy. A double blind study. *Scand J Urol Nephrol* 3:177, 1969.

159. Vinnicombe J, Shuttleworth KED: Aminocaproic acid in the control of haemorrhage after prostatectomy. A controlled trial. *Lancet* 1:230, 1966.

160. Sharifi R, Lee M, Ray P, Millner SN, Dupont PF: Safety and efficacy of intravesical aminocaproic acid for bleeding after transurethral resection of prostate. *Urology* 27:214, 1986.

161. Smith RB, Riach P, Kaufman JJ: Epsilon aminocaproic acid and the control of post-prostatectomy bleeding: a prospective double-blind study. *J Urol* 131:1093, 1984.

162. Ward MG, Richards B: Complications of antifibrinolysis therapy after prostatectomy. *Br J Urol* 51:211, 1979.

163. Haygood TA, Atkins R, Kennedy JA, Cutler RE: Aminocaproic acid treatment of prolonged hematuria following renal biopsy. *Arch Intern Med* 127:478, 1971.

164. Pitts TO, Spero JA, Bontempo FA, Greenberg A: Acute renal failure due to high-grade obstruction following therapy with epsilon-aminocaproic acid. *Am J Kidney Dis* 8:441, 1986.

165. Wymenga LF, van der Boon WJ: Obstruction of the renal pelvis due to an insoluble blood clot after epsilon-aminocaproic acid therapy: resolution with intraureteral streptokinase instillations. *J Urol* 159:490, 1998.

166. Nilsson IM: Local fibrinolysis as a mechanism for haemorrhage. *Thromb Diath Haemorrh* 34:623, 1975.

167. Larsson B, Liedholm P, Sjöberg N-O, Åstedt B: Increased fibrinolytic activity in the endometrium of patients using copper-IUD. *Contraception* 9:531, 1974.

168. Nilsson L, Rybo G: Treatment of menorrhagia with epsilon aminocaproic acid. A double blind investigation. *Acta Obstet Gynecol Scand* 44:467, 1965.

169. Callender ST, Warner GT, Cope E: Treatment of menorrhagia with tranexamic acid. A double-blind trial. *Br Med J* 4:214, 1970.

170. Westrom L, Bengtsson LP: Effect of tranexamic acid (AMCA) in menorrhagia with intrauterine contraceptive devices. *J Reprod Med* 5:154, 1970.

171. Kasonde JM, Bonnar J: Aminocaproic acid and menstrual loss in women using intrauterine devices. *Br Med J* 4:17, 1975.

172. Tauber PF, Kloppel A, Goodpasture JC, Burns J, Ludwig H, Zaneveld LJ: Reduced menstrual blood loss by release of an antifibrinolytic agent from intrauterine contraceptive devices. *Am J Obstet Gynecol* 140:322, 1981.

173. Ewenstein BM: The pathophysiology of bleeding disorders presenting as abnormal uterine bleeding. *Am J Obstet Gynecol* 175:770, 1996.

174. Ong YL, Hull DR, Mayne EE: Menorrhagia in von Willebrand disease successfully treated with single daily dose tranexamic acid. *Haemophilia* 4:63, 1998.

175. Rybo G, Westerberg H: The effect of tranexamic acid (AMCA) on postoperative bleeding after conization. *Acta Obstet Gynecol Scand* 51:347, 1972.

176. Cox HT, Poller L, Thomson JM: Gastric fibrinolysis. A possible aetiological link with peptic ulcer. *Lancet* 1:1300, 1967.

177. Wodzinski MA, Bardhan KD, Reilly JT, Cooper P, Preston FE: Reduced tissue type plasminogen activator activity of the gastroduodenal mucosa in peptic ulcer disease. *Gut* 34:1310, 1993.

178. Götz JM, Ravensbergen JW, Verspaget HW, et al: The effect of treatment of *Helicobacter pylori* infection gastric mucosal plasminogen activators. *Fibrinolysis* 10 (suppl. 2):85, 1996.

179. Herszenyi L, Plebani M, Carraro P, et al: Impaired fibrinolysis and increased protease levels in gastric and duodenal mucosa of patients with active duodenal ulcer. *Am J Gastroenterol* 92:843, 1997.

180. Biggs JC, Hugh TB, Dodds AJ: Tranexamic acid and upper gastrointestinal haemorrhage—a double-blind trial. *Gut* 17:729, 1976.

181. Barer D, Ogilvie A, Henry D, et al: Cimetidine and tranexamic acid in the treatment of acute upper-gastrointestinal-tract bleeding. *N Engl J Med* 308:1571, 1983.

182. Bergqvist D, Dahlgren S, Hessman Y: Local inhibition of the fibrinolytic system in patients with massive upper gastrointestinal hemorrhage. *Ups J Med Sci* 85:173, 1980.

183. von Holstein CCSS, Eriksson SBS, Kallén R: Tranexamic acid as an aid to reducing blood transfusion requirements in gastric and duodenal bleeding. *Br Med J (Clin Res Ed)* 294:7, 1987.

184. Engqvist A, Broström O, von Feilitzen F, et al: Tranexamic acid in massive haemorrhage from the upper gastrointestinal tract: a double-blind study. *Scand J Gastroenterol* 14:839, 1979.

185. Oka K, Tanaka K: Local fibrinolysis of esophagus and stomach as a cause of hemorrhage in liver cirrhosis. *Thromb Res* 14:837, 1979.

186. Kondo M, Hotta T, Takemura S, Yoshikawa T, Fukumoto K: Treatment of ulcerative colitis by the direct administration of an antifibrinolytic agent as an enema. *Hepatogastroenterology* 28:270, 1981.

187. Van Bodegraven AA, Tuynman HARE, Schoorl M, Kruishoop AM, Bartels PCM: Fibrinolytic split products, fibrinolysis, and factor XIII activity in inflammatory bowel disease. *Scand J Gastroenterol* 30:580, 1995.

188. Kjeldsen J, Lassen JF, Brandslund I, Schaffalitzky de Muckadell OB: Markers of coagulation and fibrinolysis as measures of disease activity in inflammatory bowel disease. *Scand J Gastroenterol* 33:637, 1998.

189. Almer S, Andersson T, Strom M: Pharmacokinetics of tranexamic acid in patients with ulcerative colitis and in healthy volunteers after the single instillation of 2 g rectally. *J Clin Pharmacol* 32:49, 1992.

190. el-Bassiouni NE, el Bassiouny AE, el-Khayat HR, Akl MM, Omran SA: Hyperfibrinolysis in hepatosplenic schistosomiasis. *J Clin Pathol* 49:990, 1996.

191. Tsementzis SA, Honan WP, Nightingale S, Hitchcock ER, Meyer CH: Fibrinolytic activity after subarachnoid haemorrhage and the effect of tranexamic acid. *Acta Neurochir* 103:116, 1990.

192. Suzuki M, Kudo A, Otawara Y, Doi M, Kuroda K, Ogawa A: Fibrinolytic activity in the CSF and blood following subarachnoid haemorrhage. *Acta Neurochir* 139:1152, 1997.

193. Ikeda K, Asakura H, Futami K, Yamashita J: Coagulative and fibrinolytic activation in cerebrospinal fluid and plasma after subarachnoid hemorrhage. *Neurosurgery* 41:344, 1997.

194. Peltonen S, Juvela S, Kaste M, Lassila R: Hemostasis and fibrinolysis activation after subarachnoid hemorrhage. *J Neurosurg* 87:207, 1997.

195. Kassell NF, Haley EC, Torner JC: Antifibrinolytic therapy in the treatment of aneurysmal subarachnoid hemorrhage. *Clin Neurosurg* 33:137, 1986.

196. Roos YBWEM, Vermeulen M, Rinkel GJE, Algra A, van Gijn J: Systematic review of antifibrinolytic treatment in aneurysmal subarachnoid haemorrhage. *J Neurol Neurosurg Psychiatry* 65:942, 1998.

197. Vermeij FH, Hasan D, Bijvoet HWC, Avezaat CJJ: Impact of medical treatment on the outcome of patients after aneurysmal subarachnoid hemorrhage. *Stroke* 29:924, 1998.

198. Janssens M, Joris J, David JL, Lemaire R, Lamy M: High-dose aprotinin reduces blood loss in patients undergoing total hip replacement surgery. *Anesthesiology* 80:23, 1994.

199. Murkin JM, Shannon NA, Bourne RB, Rorabeck CH, Cruickshank M, Wyile G: Aprotinin decreases blood loss in patients undergoing revision or bilateral total hip arthroplasty. *Anesth Analg* 80:343, 1995.

200. Hiippala S, Strid L, Wennerstrand M, et al: Tranexamic acid (Cyklokapron) reduces perioperative blood loss associated with total knee arthroplasty. *Br J Anaesth* 74:534, 1995.

201. Jerndal T, Frisen M: Tranexamic acid (AMCA) and late hyphaema. A double blind study in cataract surgery. *Acta Ophthalmol* 54:417, 1976.

202. McGetrick JJ, Jampol LM, Goldberg MF, Frenkel M, Fiscella RG:

Aminocaproic acid decreases secondary hemorrhage after traumatic hyphema. *Arch Ophthalmol* 101:1031, 1983.

203. Deans R, Noel LP, Clarke WN: Oral administration of tranexamic acid in the management of traumatic hyphema in children. *Can J Ophthalmol* 27:181, 1992.

204. Rahmani B, Jahadi HR: Comparison of tranexamic acid and prednisolone in the treatment of traumatic hyphema. A randomized clinical trial. *Ophthalmology* 106:375, 1999.

205. Rahmani B, Jahadi HR, Rajaeefard A: An analysis of risk for secondary hemorrhage in traumatic hyphema. *Ophthalmology* 106:380, 1999.

206. Falbe-Hansen J Jr, Jacobsen B, Lorenzen E: Local application of an antifibrinolytic in tonsillectomy. A double-blind study. *J Laryngol Otol* 88:565, 1974.

207. White A, O'Reilly BF: Oral tranexamic acid in the management of epistaxis. *Clin Otolaryngol* 13:11, 1988.

208. Saba HI, Morelli GA, Logrono LA: Brief report: treatment of bleeding in hereditary hemorrhagic telangiectasia with aminocaproic acid. *N Engl J Med* 330:1789, 1994.

209. Francis CW, Marder VJ: Physiologic regulation and pathologic disorders of fibrinolysis, in *Hemostasis and Thrombosis. Basic Principles and Clinical Practice*, 3rd ed, edited by RW Colman, J Hirsh, VJ Marder, EW Salzman, p 1076. Lippincott, Philadelphia, 1994.

TRANSFUSION MEDICINE

ERYTHROCYTE ANTIGENS AND ANTIBODIES

LONI CALHOUN
LAWRENCE D. PETZ

Human red blood cells (RBC) bear numerous cell surface structures that can be recognized as antigens by the immune system of individuals who lack that particular structure. The characterization of RBC antigens and antibodies has been the basis of compatibility testing in the blood transfusion laboratory, thereby minimizing the risk of hemolytic transfusion reactions. Such knowledge has also provided the scientific basis for understanding hemolytic disease of the newborn and autoimmune hemolytic anemias. In recent years, the biochemical and molecular bases for many erythrocyte antigens have been elucidated, and this has led to further definition of their biologic functions. Blood group antigens play a critical role in susceptibility to infection by malarial parasites and also in some viral and bacterial infections. The absence of certain RBC antigens is associated with specific clinical disorders, and the recognition of these associations has led to an improved understanding of the function of antigens in the RBC membrane. Diverse inherited and acquired disorders are associated with alteration of RBC antigen expression, and these alterations often play a critical role in the clinical manifestations of these disorders. Thus, although erythrocytes have traditionally been considered relatively inert cellular containers of hemoglobin, they are in fact active in a variety of physiologic processes.

DEFINITIONS AND HISTORY

A blood group system is a group of antigens encoded by alleles at a single gene locus or at gene loci so closely linked that crossing over does not occur or is very rare. An antigen collection is a group of antigens that are phenotypically, biochemically, or genetically related, but their genes are not known to be allelic.[1]

The placement of a blood group antigen into a system or collection follows a natural progression.[2] First, its antibody is discovered, usually in the serum of a multiparous woman or a multiply transfused recipient, and found to have unique specificity. Using traditional serologic methods, the antibody can be used to study basic biochemical properties of the corresponding antigen, its pattern of inheritance, and its gene frequency, and to search for an antithetical antigen. The biochemistry and structure of the newly recognized antigen can also be evaluated using modern biochemical and molecular genetic methods. Identified characteristics are then compared to known systems and collections, and an appropriate assignment is made.

Acronyms and abbreviations that appear in this chapter include: AET, 2-aminoethyl-isothiouronium bromide; DTT, dithiothreitol; GP, glycoprotein; GPC, glycophorin C; GPD, glycophorin D; HLA, human leukocyte antigens; HEMPAS, hereditary erythroblastic multinuclearity with a positive acidified serum test; 2-ME, 2-mercapto-ethanol; RBC, red blood cell; Rh, Rhesus.

The initial naming of blood group antigens does not always follow the classical convention wherein dominant traits are given capital letters and recessive traits are designated with lower case letters. The gene in the ABO blood group system, for example, that determines the recessive O phenotype is designated *O*, while the genes *S* and *s* in the MNS system are codominant. Typically, red cell antigens are given alphabetical designations (e.g., CDE of the Rh system) and/or are named after the family of the antibody producer (e.g., Kell for Mrs. Kellacher and Fy for Mr. Duffy).

To help standardize red cell blood group terminology, the International Society of Blood Transfusion (ISBT) now uses a numerical system based on nomenclature first proposed by Rosenfield et al. Each system and collection has been given a number and letter designation, and each antigen within the system is numbered sequentially in order of discovery. To date, 23 blood group systems and 5 antigen collections are defined (Table 137-1).[1,3-5] High-incidence (or public) antigens and low-incidence (or private) antigens that are not associated with known systems or collections also are grouped into numbered series.

BLOOD GROUP SYSTEMS

See Table 137-2 for a summary of the characteristics of common erythrocyte antigens and Refs. 4 through 9 for comprehensive details.

ABO BLOOD GROUP SYSTEM

The ABO blood group system was the first system to be described and remains the most significant one in transfusion medicine. Erythrocytes from most normal individuals phenotype as A, B, AB, or O, the latter indicating a lack of A and B antigen. The sugars defining A and B antigen are found on precursor carbohydrate chains carrying the H antigen, which is produced by a gene product from another chromosome. Because H is a required precursor that becomes "hidden" when A or B sugar is added, group A or B erythrocytes appear to have less H than group O cells. Nonetheless, H is found on all human erythrocytes except in rare individuals of the O$_h$ (Bombay) phenotype, who lack the *H* (or *FUT1*) gene. This system is therefore commonly referred to as ABH.

Normal individuals who lack either A or B antigen consistently make anti-B or anti-A, respectively, within several months after birth. These antibodies can cause intravascular hemolysis of ABO incompatible erythrocytes and are associated with severe acute hemolytic transfusion reactions and death. Because these antigens also are expressed on most tissue cells, ABO compatibility is a significant consideration in solid organ transplantation. However, ABO incompatibility only rarely causes clinical hemolytic disease of the newborn, presumably because antibodies directed against the A and B antigen are predominantly IgM, which do not cross the placenta, and because A and B antigens are not well developed at birth.

RH BLOOD GROUP SYSTEM

The Rh (Rhesus) system is the second most important blood group system in transfusion medicine because antigen-positive erythrocytes so frequently immunize antigen-negative individuals through transfusion and pregnancy.

The inheritance of Rh antigens is determined by a complex of two closely linked genes: one encodes the protein carrying D antigen (RHD), the other encodes the protein carrying C or c and E or e specificity (RHCE). People who are Rh-positive have both *RHD* and *RHCE* genes, whereas Rh-negative individuals have only the *RHCE* gene. Depending on the Rh genes present on a chromosome, eight common antigen combinations or haplotypes are possible: Dce (Rh$_0$), DCe (Rh$_1$), DcE (Rh$_2$), DCE (Rh$_z$), ce (rh), Ce (rh'), cE (rh"), and CE

TABLE 137-1   INTERNATIONAL SOCIETY OF BLOOD TRANSFUSION (ISBT)–DEFINED BLOOD GROUP SYSTEMS AND ANTIGEN COLLECTIONS WITH CHROMOSOME AND GENE

CONVENTIONAL NAME	ISBT SYMBOL	ISBT NUMBER	CHROMOSOME LOCATION	GENE	TOTAL ANTIGENS
Blood group systems					
ABO	ABO	001	9q34.1-q34.2	ABO	4
MNSs	MNS	002	4q28-q31	GYPA, GYPB	40
P	P1	003	22q11.2-qter	P1	1
Rh	RH	004	1p36.13-p34.3	RHD, RHCE	45
Lutheran	LU	005	19q13.2	LU	18
Kell	KEL	006	7q33	KEL	22
Lewis	LE	007	19p13.3	FUT3	3
Duffy	FY	008	1q22-q23	FY	6
Kidd	JK	009	18q11-q12	HUT11	3
Diego	DI	010	17q12-q21	SLC4A1 (AE1)	7
Cartwright	YT	011	7q22	ACHE	2
Xg	XG	012	Xp22.32	XG	1
Scianna	SC	013	1p36.2-p22.1	SC	3
Dombrock	DO	014	Not known	DO	5
Colton	CO	015	7p14	AQP1	3
Landsteiner-Wiener	LW	016	19p13.3	LW	3
Chido/Rogers	CH/RG	017	6p21.3	C4A,C4B	9
H	H	018	19q13	FUT1	1
Kx	XK	019	Xp21.1	XK	1
Gerbich	GE	020	2q14-q21	GYPC	7
Cromer	CROMER	021	1q32	DAF	10
Knops	KN	022	1q32	CR1 (CD35)	5
Indian	IN	023	11p13	CD44	2
Antigen collections					
Cost	COST	205	—		2
Ii	I	207	—		2
Er	ER	208	—		2
(P, P$_k$, LKE)	GLOB	209	—		3
(Lewis-like: Le^c, Le^d)	—	210	—		2
Low incidence, private	—	700	—		34
High incidence, public	—	901	—		15

SOURCE: GL Daniels et al,[3] and PD Issitt and DJ Anstee.[4]

(rh^y). The letter "d" is commonly used to designate the lack of D, but there is no d antigen and anti-d has never been found.

Several nomenclatures can be used to describe Rh genes and antigens. Fisher-Race nomenclature, which uses CDE terminology, more commonly is used for antigens; Wiener nomenclature, which uses Rh designations, is favored for haplotypes and gene complexes. A person who inherits r (ce gene) from one parent and R_1 (D and Ce genes) from the other parent expresses D, C, c, and e antigens on his or her erythrocytes.

Rh is the largest blood group system, but its most important and immunogenic antigen is D (Rh$_0$ in Weiner terminology, referring to its discovery using a Rhesus monkey antibody to human erythrocytes). For most clinical purposes, it is sufficient to test individuals for the D antigen and classify them as D+ or Rh-positive, or D− or Rh-negative. Approximately 85 percent of the Caucasian population is Rh positive, and 15 percent is Rh- negative. Because most Rh-negative recipients will produce anti-D if they receive a unit of Rh-positive blood and because anti-D can cause acute hemolytic transfusion reactions and severe hemolytic disease of the newborn, all donors and recipients are routinely typed and matched for D to avoid sensitization from transfusion. Also, Rh immunoglobulin specific for D is given routinely to Rh-negative mothers bearing Rh-positive infants to prevent immunization to the D antigen.

The antigens C, c, E, and e are less immunogenic and become important in patient care only after the corresponding antibody develops or when basic Rh haplotypes must be determined. The remaining 40 antigens represent other Rh protein epitopes whose corresponding antibodies are seldom encountered. Some are encoded by variant Rh alleles and appear as antithetical antigens to C, c, E, or e or as related

"extra" antigens; others are referred to as "compound" antigens or cis gene products. For example, the protein produced by the gene ce encodes c, e, and f (or ce) antigen; other compound specificities include Ce (rh^i), cE, CE, V (ce^s), and Ce^s. Still other Rh antigens are related to the complex "mosaic" nature of D and e antigen. If immunized, individuals who lack a subpart of D or e and make antibody to the portion they lack can present with a challenging serologic picture. For example, the D+ person who lacks part of the D epitope and makes an antibody to the missing portion appears to make alloanti-D because normal D+ erythrocytes carry all D epitopes.

Some, but not all, individuals who lack part of the D antigen (partial D) have a weak expression of D on their red cells that is only detected with more sensitive antiglobulin testing. Having a C gene in transposition to a D gene (e.g., Dce/Ce or DCe/Ce genotypes) also can weaken the expression of D in some individuals. A third type of weak D expression results from inheriting a D gene that encodes all epitopes of D but in less than normal quantity.

OTHER BLOOD GROUP SYSTEMS

The other blood group systems and their antigens become important when antibody develops and transfusion is needed or when hemolytic disease of the newborn is a concern. Blood bank laboratories identify the specificity or characterize the reactivity of all antibodies detected in routine testing. Once this basic information is known, the blood bank assesses the clinical significance of the antibody and selects the most appropriate blood for transfusion. Occasionally, disease or observed red cell anomalies warrant studying red cell antigen expres-

TABLE 137-2   SUMMARY OF COMMON BLOOD GROUP SYSTEMS OR COLLECTIONS AND THEIR ANTIGENS

Blood Group (Year Recognized)	Common Antigens	Common Phenotypes	% Frequency White/Black	No. Antigen Copies on Adult RBC × 10³	Dosage (See Text)	Cord Cell Expression	Biochemistry (See Also Table 137-1 and Fig. 137-1)	Chromosome: Genes	Antigen Distribution in Blood, Fluids, and Tissues	Antigen Function	Comments
ABO (1901)	A,B	A / B / AB / O	40/27 / 11/20 / 4/4 / 45/29	AB: ~800–1000	A/B: not evident.	Weak; ~1/3 adult expression	Carbohydrate on type 1, 2, 3 and 4 precursor chains	9: ABO	RBC, lymphs, plts	Not known	Most significant antigens in transfusion and transplantation; Weak subgroups result from variant transferases; Nulls: group O (H) and O_h (Bombay) (hh)
H (1948)	H			H: ~1700	H expression depends on ABO: O>A_2> B>A_2B>A_1>A_1B			19: FUT1 (H)	Plasma, secretions; broad tissue distribution; most epi-/endothelial cells	Primary recognition antigen?	
Rh (1940)	D; C, c, C^w; E, e; f(ce); V(ce^s)	Haplotype: R_1 DCe; r ce; R_2 DcE; R_0 Dce; r' Ce; r'' cE; R_z DCE; r^y CE	42/17; 37/26; 14/11; 4/44; 2/2; 1/0; <1; <1	D on R_2R_2: 15–33; R_1R_1: 14–19; R_0r: 12–20; R_1r: 9–14; c on cc: 70–85; Cc: 37–53; e on ee: 18–24; Ee: 13–14	D: not evident; C and c: yes; E and e: yes	Normal adult	Multipass, nonglycosylated protein: 30–32 kD; 417 aa; C: serine 103/c: proline 103; E: proline 226/e: alanine 226; Forms "Rh complex" with LW, GPB, and Rh-related glycoprotein (chromosome 6)	1: RHD, RHCE	RBC specific	Possible cation transport; Possible role in RBC membrane integrity	D most significant antigen after A and B; Three causes for weak D expression (see text); Large system with many antigens; Nulls: amorphic type (r̄r̄) and regulator type (X^0r)
Lewis (1946)	Le^a, Le^b	Le(a+b−); Le(a−b+); Le(a−b−)	22/23; 72/55; 6/22; Rare	Le^b: ~3	Not evident	Weak; adult expression at age 2 years	Carbohydrate on type 1 precursor chains only; Attached to lipids in plasma and protein in secretions	19: FUT3 (Le); 19: FUT2 (Se)	Plasma and secretion antigen; on RBC, lymphs, plts only by adsorption of plasma antigen	Not known; Receptor for Helicobacter pylori	Le antigens depend on Le/Se interaction; Le/Se = Le(a−b+), ABH secretor; Le/sese = Le(a+b−), ABH nonsecretor; lele = Le(a−b−), Sese status not apparent Le(a−b+), Sese make some Le^a, do not make anti-Le^a
Ii (1956)	I, i	I adult (↑↑I↓i); I_int (↑I↓i); i cord (↓I↑i); i adult (↓↓I↑i)	Common; Rare; Common; <1:10,000	I: ~500	Not evident	Strong i; weak I. Adult expression at age 2 years	Carbohydrate on ABH active chains; lipid on RBC; protein in plasma	?	Broad tissue distribution: RBCs, plts, lymphs, granulos, monos; also in plasma, secretions (e.g., milk, saliva, urine, etc.)	Not known	Women test Le(a−b−) during pregnancy; I and i expression is inversely proportional but not products of alleles; Null: i adult
P1 / GLOB (1951)	P_1, P, P^k	P_1: P+P+P_1+; P_2: P+P+P_1−; p: P−P−P_1−; P_1^k: P^k+P−P_1+; P_2^k: P^k+P−P_1−	79/94; 21/6; Rare; Rare; Rarest	P_1: ~500; Globoside: ~15,000	Not evident, but inherited variations exist; for example, P_1 may be normal, strong, or weak.	Weak; adult expression by 7 years	Carbohydrate on RBC and plasma glycolipids; not in secretions	22: P1; ?: GLOBO	RBC, lymphs, plts, monos, fibroblasts, uroepithelial cells	Not known	P-like antigen is associated with pigeon and earthworm protein and parasitic infections; Null: p phenotype
MNS (M: 1927) (S: 1947)	M, N, S, s, U	M+N−; M+N+; M−N+; S+s−; S+s+; S−s+; S−s−U−	28/26; 50/44; 22/30; 11/3; 44/28; 45/69; 0/<1	GPA: ~800; GPB: ~200	Yes	Normal adult	Single-pass sialoglycoprotein type I; GPA: 43kD, 131 aa, carries MN; GPB: 25Kd, 72 aa, carries SsU; part of Rh complex	4: MNS 2 linked loci: GPA (MN) and GPB (Ss)	RBCs plus renal capillary epi-/endothelium	Major contributor to RBC negative charge; associated with band 3; Receptor for complement, bacteria, viruses	GPA and GPB carry multiple antigens and many genetic variants exist: variant forms of MNSs, hybrids of GPA-GPB from crossover; Nulls: see Table 137-4; can have absence of GPA, GPB, or both
Kell (1946) (Kp^a/Js^a: 1957)	K, k, Kp^a, Kp^b, Js^a, Js^b	K−k+; K+k+; K+k−; Kp(a+b−); Kp(a+b+); Kp(a−b+); Js(a+b−); Js(a+b+); Js(a−b+)	91/98; 8.8/2; 0.2/rare; 97.7/100; 2.3/rare; Rare/O; 100/80; Rare/19; 0/1	Kell: 2–6	Yes	Normal adult	Single-pass glycoprotein type II highly folded with S=S bonds: 93kD, 732 aa; K: Met 193/k: Thr 193; Kp^a: Trp 281/Kp^b: Arg 281; Js^a: Pro 597/Js^b: Leu 597	7: KEL; X: XK	Kell: RBC plus bone marrow and fetal liver tissue; not on brain, kidney, adult liver; Kx: RBC plus skeletal/heart muscle, neurologic tissue	Possible enzyme function; Structure similar to zinc neutral endopeptidases that activate/inactivate bioactive peptides	System of high- and low-frequency antigens; Common phenotype: k: Kp^b, Js^b; Kell antigen expression depends on both Kell and Xk genes; K null (K^0) lacks Kell antigens, has Kx; Kx null (XK^0) lacks Kx, has poor Kell antigen expression (McLeod phenotype); Other causes of poor Kell expression: cis Kp^a; K:-13, Ge-, K_mod autoantibody
Duffy (1950)	Fy^a, Fy^b, Fy3	Fy(a+b−)Fy3+; Fy(a+b+)Fy3+; Fy(a−b+)Fy3+; Fy(a−b−)Fy3−	17/9; 49/1; 34/22; Rare/68	Fy^a: 6–13	Yes, but not always evident due to Fy gene (see text)	Normal; adult levels at 12 weeks	Multipass glycoprotein: 35–45kD, 338 aa; Fy^a: Glycine 44; Fy^b: Asparagine 44	1: FY	RBC plus brain, colon, lung, spleen, thyroid, thymus, kidney, endothelium; not in liver or placenta tissue.	Receptor for proinflammatory chemokines (e.g., IL-8); clears proinflammatory peptides; receptor for P. vivax and P. knowlesi	Fy(a−b−) blacks do not express Fy^a on their RBC, but routinely express it on other tissues and seldom make Fy^b aby
Kidd (1951)	Jk^a, Jk^b, Jk3	Jk(a+b−)Jk3+; Jk(a+b+)Jk3+; Jk(a−b+)Jk3+; Jk(a−b−)Jk3−	28/57; 49/34; 23/9; <1% Polynesians	Jk^a: ~14	Yes	Normal adult	Multipass protein: ~43kD, 391 aa 1 potential n-glycan	18: JK (HUT11)	RBC specific	Urea transport	Important cause of DHTR; Nulls: unable to fully concentrate urine; recessive JkJk truly null; dominant inhibitor In(Jk) has weak Jk antigen
Lutheran (1951)	Lu^a, Lu^b, Lu3	Lu(a+b−)Lu3+; Lu(a+b+)Lu3+; Lu(a−b+)Lu3+; Lu(a−b−)Lu3−	0.15/−; 7.5/0; 92.3/−; Very rare	Lu^b: 1.5–4	Yes, but family variations exist	Weak; adult levels at 15 years	Single-pass glycoprotein type I: 78–85KD, 597aa 5 Ig superfamily domains: two variable, three constant	19: LU	RBC plus brain, heart, kidney, lung, pancreas, placenta, skeletal muscle	Possible role in adhesion; Possible receptor function; May mediate intracellular signaling	System of high-frequency antigens; Null: recessive type (LuLu)/true null; dominant inhibitor In(Lu)/weak antigens; X-linked inhibitor (XS2)/weak antigens; First known autosomal linkage to Se

ABBREVIATIONS: aa, amino acids; DHTR, delayed hemolytic transfusion reactions; GPA, glycophorin A; GPB, glycophorin B; granulos, granulocytes; lymphs, lymphocytes; monos, monocytes; plts, platelets; RBC, red blood cell;

sion in more detail. More extensive antigen typing sometimes offers clues to broader diagnoses.

GENERAL IMMUNOLOGY OF BLOOD GROUP ANTIGENS

An antigen is a substance that can evoke an immune response when introduced into an immunocompetent host and that can react with the antibody produced from that immune response. Its structure and stereochemical fit with its antibody are key to its specificity. An antigen can have several epitopes, or antigenic determinants, each of which is capable of eliciting an antibody response.

The ability of an antigen to stimulate an immune response is called immunogenicity, and its ability to react with an antibody is called antigenicity. These primary characteristics are affected by antigen size, shape, rigidity, and the number and location of the determinants on the red cell membrane. The ability of a host to recognize and respond to foreign antigens is influenced also by its HLA-DR alleles, as well as by genes outside the HLA system.[6]

ANTIGEN EXPRESSION

NUMBER OF ANTIGEN SITES

The number of antigen sites per erythrocyte has been estimated by measuring the uptake of[125] I-labeled antibody or of ferritin-conjugated anti-IgG.[7] Numbers vary widely among blood group systems: from 1 to 2×10^6 sites for ABH to 2 to 6×10^3 for Le^a, K, and Lu^b.

ANTIGEN DEVELOPMENT ON FETAL ERYTHROCYTES

Most erythrocyte antigens can be detected early in fetal development (ABH at 5–6 weeks' gestation and other specificities by 12 weeks), but not all are fully developed at birth. ABH, I, P$_1$, Lu^a, Lu^b, Yt^a, Xg^a, Vel, Bg, Knops, and Dombrock antigen expression is considerably weaker on cord erythrocytes than in adults, and Le^a, sometimes Le^b, Ch/Rg, AnWj, and Sd^a are not routinely detected, although 50 percent of cord samples type Le(a+) with more sensitive test methods.[6] About 2 years may pass before adult expression of ABH, I, and Lewis antigens is detected, and 7 years or more for P$_1$ and Lutheran antigens.

GENETIC VARIATION

Individuals who are homozygous for an allele typically have a greater number of antigen sites than do individuals who are heterozygous. Consequently, their erythrocytes can react more strongly with antibody. This difference in expression and antigen-antibody reactivity because of zygosity is known as dosage. For example, red cells from a homozygous *MM* individual carry a double dose of M antigen and react more strongly with anti-M than do red cells from a *MN* heterozygous individual carrying only a single dose of M. Antithetical antigens Cc, Ee, Kk, MN, Ss, and Jk^{a}Jk^b commonly show dosage.

Dosage is less obvious with D and Lu^{a}Lu^b antigens. It may be very apparent within a family but not between families because D and Lu expression and reactivity can be unique family traits. Dosage within the Duffy system also may not be serologically obvious because Fy(a+b−) or Fy(a−b+) phenotypes are seen in either homozygous (*Fy^{a}Fy^a* or *Fy^{b}Fy^b*) or heterozygous (*Fy^{a}Fy* or *Fy^{b}Fy*) individuals.

Some blood group antigens are inherited as very closely linked genes or haplotypes. Haplotype pairings and gene interaction (either *cis* or *trans*) also can effect phenotypic expression. For example, the pairing of *C* in *trans* position to *D* can result in weak expression of D (see discussion of Rh Blood Group System above), but having *E* in cis position with *D* is associated with strong D expression. Indeed, R$_2$R$_2$ red cells carry the strongest expression of D. In the Kell system, *Kp^a* is associated with weakened expression of *cis k* and Js^b.

Still other antigens are affected by regulator genes.[10] *In(Lu)*, also

called *SYN-1B*, is a dominant inhibitor gene that suppresses the expression of Lutheran antigens, P$_1$, i, and many other antigens;[11] the dominant inhibitor *In(Jk)* suppresses the expression of Jk^a and Jk^b.[12] Rare variants of the Rh regulator gene X^1 can depress or shut off the expression of the Rh antigens (see "Rh$_{null}$ Syndrome").

IMMUNOGENICITY

Immunogenicity depends on many antigen characteristics, not just the number of antigen sites. For example, a K+Fy(a+) erythrocyte carries 7 to 17×10^3 Fy^a antigen sites on its membrane, but only 3 to 6×10^3 K sites. Yet such cells are nine times more likely to stimulate the formation of anti-K than of anti-Fy^a.[6,13]

Relative immunogenicity is estimated by comparing the actual frequency with which an antibody is found to the calculated frequency of a possible immunizing event. Although numbers vary, researchers agree that after A and B, the D antigen is most immunogenic (>80 percent of Rh-negative individuals produce anti-D after receiving a single Rh-positive unit[9]), followed by K, which stimulates anti-K in 10 percent of cases.[6] The antigens c and E are three times less immunogenic than K, Fy^a is 25 times less potent, and Jk^a is 50 to 100 times less potent.[13]

BIOCHEMISTRY OF ERYTHROCYTE ANTIGENS

An antibody typically recognizes an epitope consisting of four to five amino acids or one to seven sugar residues on linear polypeptides or polysaccharides, respectively. Alternatively, the antibody-binding site may encompass a more complex three-dimensional structure with branches or folds, and recognition may depend on both amino acid and sugar moieties. Tables 137-2 and 137-3 and Fig. 137-1 provide a summary of blood group biochemistry and antigen structure.[5–8,14]

CARBOHYDRATE ANTIGENS

Polysaccharides with blood group activity are made by the sequential addition of specific sugars to specific precursors by specific transferase enzymes encoded by genes. Sugars commonly involved are D-galactose (Gal), *N*-acetyl-D-galactosamine (GalNAc), *N*-acetyl-D-glucosamine (GlcNAc), L-fucose (Fuc), and *N*-acetyl-neuraminic acid (NeuNAc, or sialic acid).

ABO, Lewis, and P blood group specificity depends on a terminal or immunodominant sugar, the polysaccharide to which the sugar is attached, and the type of linkage involved. I/i specificity is defined by a series of sugars on the inner portion of ABH oligosaccharide chains. The presence of at least two repeating Gal($\beta1 \rightarrow 4$)Glc-NAc($\beta1 \rightarrow 3$)Gal units in a linear structure defines i activity. I activity involves these same sugars in branched form. The *I* gene may actually encode the transferase responsible for branching [$\beta(1-6)$glucosaminyltransferase].

Oligosaccharide chains are attached to glycoproteins in secretion, to glycolipids in plasma, and to both on the erythrocyte membrane. About 70 percent of ABH-I antigens on the membrane are carried on glycoproteins, primarily the anion transporter band 3, but also on the glucose transporter band 4.5, the Rh glycoprotein, and others. About 10 percent are on NeuNAc-rich glycoproteins; 5 percent on simple glycolipids, and the remainder on polyglycosyl ceramide.[6] P, P^k, and P$_1$ antigens is found on glycolipids both on the membrane and in plasma; whether they are carried on membrane glycoproteins is disputed.[4]

Lewis antigens are unique in that they occur only on type 1 polysaccharide chains, precursors found in plasma and secretions but not made by erythrocytes. Hence, they are plasma and secretion antigens and only exist on red cells by adsorption of Lewis substance from plasma. The *Le* (or *FUT3*) gene encodes an α(1–4)fucosyltransferase. Whether the resulting antigen is Le^a or Le^b depends on the secretor gene, *Se* (or *FUT2*), that encodes an α(1–2)fucosyltransferase.

PROTEIN ANTIGENS

Protein structures that carry blood group antigens can be grouped into three categories: (1) those that make a single pass through the erythrocyte membrane, (2) those that make multiple passes through the membrane, and (3) those inserted into the membrane through a covalently linked lipid.

Single-pass proteins include glycophorin A with its MN antigens, glycophorin B with SsU antigens, glycophorin C and D with Gerbich antigens, and the proteins encoded by Kell, Lutheran, LW, Indian, Knops, and Xg genes. Most of these proteins have an extracellular amino terminus and an intracellular carboxyl terminus (referred to as type I). An exception to this is Kell glycoprotein, where the terminal positions are reversed: the carboxyl terminus is extracellular, and the amino terminus is intracellular (type II).

Most proteins that make multiple passes through the erythrocyte membrane have both carboxyl- and amino-terminal ends that are intracellular, are very hydrophobic, and have a transport function. Rh, Diego, Colton, Kidd, and Kx proteins are included in this category. The gene product of the Duffy gene is also a multipass protein, but it has an extracellular amino terminus and has homology with a family of cytokine receptors.

Lipid-linked proteins have their carboxyl terminus replaced with the lipid glycosylphosphoinositol and are said to be GPI-linked or anchored. Cromer, Cartwright, Dombrock, and JMH proteins belong to this category. GPI-linked proteins are of special interest to hematologists because defective synthesis of the GPI anchor is responsible for paroxysmal nocturnal hemoglobinuria.[15]

EFFECT OF ENZYMES AND OTHER CHEMICALS ON ERYTHROCYTE ANTIGENS

The biochemical structure of an antigen and its location on the RBC membrane affect its expression on erythrocytes treated with enzymes and other chemicals. These reagents are used in serologic testing to help identify complex mixtures of antibodies and to help characterize antibody specificity when identity is not apparent.

Common proteolytic enzymes, such as ficin, papain, and bromelin, cleave protein from the erythrocyte membrane. This action consequently destroys accessible protein antigens and allows carbohydrate and more protected protein antigens to react more strongly with their antibody. The reactivity of ABH, I, P, Lewis, Rh, and Kidd antigens is strongly enhanced with enzyme treatment, while MN, Fy^a, Fy^b, and many minor antigens (Xg^a, Ch, Rg, JMH, Indian, Pr, Tn, Ge2, Ge4,

TABLE 137-3 BLOOD GROUP ANTIGENS AND ANTIBODIES ASSOCIATED WITH DISEASE

SPECIFICITY	STRUCTURE	GENE
i	—Gal(β1→4)GlcNAc(β1→3)Gal(β1→4)GlcNAc(β1→3)Gal—R—	
I	—Gal(β1→4)GlcNAc(β1→6)⟍ ⟩Gal(β1→4)GlcNAc(β1→3)Gal—R —Gal(β1→4)GlcNAc(β1→3)⟋	Z*
H	Gal(β1→4 or β1→3)GlcNAc(β1→3)Gal—R | **Fuc(α1→2)**	*H(FUT1)*
A	**GalNAc(α1→3)**Gal(β1→4 or β1→3)GlcNAc(β1→3)Gal—R | Fuc(α1→2)	*A*
B	**Gal(α1→3)**Gal(β1→4 or β1→3)GlcNAc(β1→3)Gal—R | Fuc(α1→2)	*B*
Le^a	Gal(β1→3)GlcNAc(β1→3)Gal—R | **Fuc(α1→4)**	*LE (FUT3)*
Le^b	Gal(β1→3)GlcNAc(β1→3)Gal—R | | **Fuc(α1→2) Fuc(α1→4)**	*SE (FUT2)* *LE (FUT3)*
P^k	**Gal(α1→4)**Gal(β1→4)Glc-Cer	*Pk**
P	**GalNAc(β1→3)**Gal(α1→4)Gal(β1→4)Glc-Cer	*P**
P$_1$	**Gal(α1→4)**Gal(β1→4)GlcNAc(β1→3)Gal(α1→4)Gal(β1→4)Glc-Cer	*P1*
M	▽ ▽ ▽ **Ser**—Ser—Thr—Thr—**Gly**—(GPA chain: 131 amino acids)	*GPYA(M)*
N	▽ ▽ ▽ **Leu**—Ser—Thr—Thr—**GluA**—(GPA chain: 131 amino acids)	*GPYA(N)*
S	▽ ▽ ▽ Leu—Ser—Thr—Thr—GluA—**Met29**—(GPB chain: 72 amino acids)	*GPYB(S)*
s	▽ ▽ ▽ Leu—Ser—Thr—Thr—GluA—**Thr29**—(GPB chain: 72 amino acids)	*GPYB(s)*

*Proposed genes.

NOTE: Immunodominant sugars and amino acids are in bold.

ABBREVIATIONS: GPA, glycophorin A; GPB, glycophorin B; R, primary glycolipid attachment Glc-Ger; primary glycoprotein attachment GlcNAc-Asp; ▽, —Gal—GalNAc—NeuNAc

Gal—GalNAc—NeuNAc
\|
NeuNAc

and some examples of Yt^a) are destroyed. Ss can be destroyed with very strong enzyme treatment; Kell and Lutheran antigens are relatively unaffected.[4,5]

Reagents that reduce disulfide bonds, such as 2-mercaptoethanol (2-ME), dithiothreitol (DTT), and 2-aminoethylisothiouronium bromide (AET), destroy Kell blood group antigens but enhance Kx. Some researchers report that reducing reagents also denature the minor antigens LW, Scianna, Indian, JMH, and Yt^a, and weaken Lutheran, Dombrock, Cromer, Knops, AnWj, and MER2 antigens.[4,5]

Chloroquine treatment of erythrocytes at room temperature has little effect on most antigens. However, treatment for 30 min at 37°C (98.6°F) can weaken the expression of many antigens, including Fy^b, Lu^b, Yt^a, JMH, and those in the Rh, Dombrock, and Knops systems.[5]

GENETICS OF ERYTHROCYTE ANTIGENS

Protein antigens are considered direct gene products: the gene encodes a specific protein that expresses one or more antigenic epitopes. Carbo-

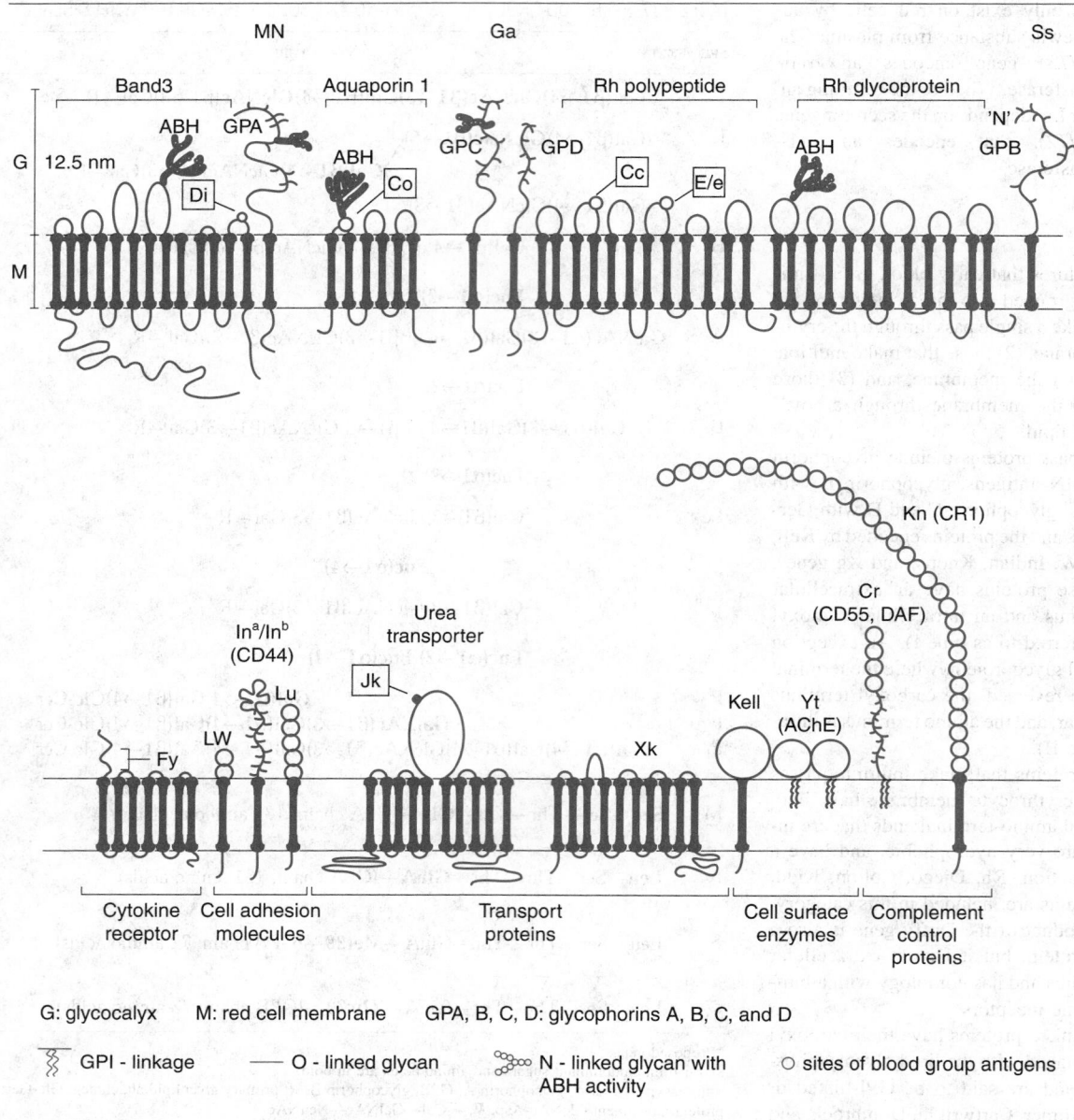

FIGURE 137-1 Erythrocyte membrane structures carrying blood group activity. (Modified from PD Issitt and DJ Anstee,[4] and PL Mollison.[6])

hydrate antigens, made by transferase action, are considered indirect gene products. Most blood group genes are located on autosomes; only two, *Xg* and *Xk*, are located on the X chromosome (see Table 137-1 for gene and chromosome location).

Most genes that encode blood group antigens have two or more alleles. Individuals who inherit two identical alleles are homozygous and make a double dose of a single gene product, while those who inherit two different alleles are heterozygous and make two gene products. Males are hemizygous for the genes located on their single X chromosome.

ALLELES

Alleles commonly arise from DNA base-pair mutations or deletions. For example, *A* and *B* alleles differ from one another by seven DNA base substitutions, which result in four amino acid substitutions in

their respective transferases.[4,5] The common *O* allele is similar to *A* except for a single base deletion at nucleotide 261 that shifts the reading frame during RNA translation. The resulting protein is truncated and has no transferase activity. Another variant *O* allele encodes a transferase identical to that of B except it has arginine instead of alanine at amino acid position 268, which also may block enzyme activity. Alleles in other blood group systems arise in similar fashion.

GENE COMPLEXES

Some blood group genes are complexes of several closely linked genes or loci that evolved through duplication of an ancestral gene. The antigens they encode are inherited within families as a packet or haplotype with few or no cross-overs. Blood group examples include the Rh system, with its genes *RHD* and *RHCE*, which encode D and CE proteins, respectively, and the MNS system, with its genes *GYPA* and *GYPB*, which encode the proteins glycophorin A and glycophorin B.

The ancestral gene for Rh is not known, but duplication appears to have taken place in early evolution in a common man-ape lineage; *RHD* and *RHCE* show remarkable homology. *GPYA* and *GPYB* probably arose by duplication of an ancestral *GPYA* gene encoding the N antigen,[16] but there is less homology between the two linked genes. The most common MNSs complex is Ns, followed by Ms, MS, and NS.

In both Rh and MNS systems, other antigens arose by further mutations, deletions, and rare cross-over within the gene complex. Unequal pairing of *GYPA* and *GYPB* during meiosis, with subsequent recombination, has resulted in hybrids such as *GYP(A-B)* (called Lepore type, in analogy with a similar hemoglobin hybrid), which encodes a protein with the amino-terminal end of glycophorin A but the carboxyl-terminal end of glycophorin B. Anti-Lepore–type hybrids *GYP(B-A-B)* and *GYP(A-B-A)* are also known. Within the Rh complex, hybrids of *RH(D-CE-D)* and *RH(CE-D-CE)* have been identified.[4,5] Such hybrids can result in altered antigen expression and new antigen epitopes.

Kell and Lutheran antigens also were thought to arise from large gene complexes of four or more loci, each having two or more alleles: K/k, $Kp^a/Kp^b/Kp^c$, Js^a/Js^b, and K^{11}/K^{17} for Kell and Lu^a/Lu^b, Lu^6/Lu^9, Lu^8/Lu^{14}, and Au^a/Au^b for Lutheran. It is more appropriate to now regard Kell and Lutheran proteins as single gene products that carry multiple antigenic epitopes. The early and still most common alleles in humans ($kKp^bJs^bK^{11}$ and $Lu^bLu^6Lu^8Au^a$) encode antigens having very high frequencies in the population. Antigens of lower frequency (K, Kp^a/Kp^c, Js^a, Lu^a, Lu9, Lu14, and Au^b) most likely arose from point mutations in different populations.

SILENT ALLELES

Some blood group alleles are said to be amorphic, or silent; that is, they do not produce a recognizable erythrocyte antigen, although they may indeed encode a product that is simply not detected with standard red cell test methods. As already discussed with regard to the ABO system, *A* and *B* genes produce transferases that add GalNAc or Gal, respectively, to the same precursors, but *O* produces no active enzyme. *AB* individuals express both A and B antigen, but *AA* and *AO* individuals express only A, and *BB* and *BO* individuals express only B. Amorphic alleles are only recognized in a homozygous state (i.e., group O individuals are *OO*), and the result is a "null" phenotype. Null phenotypes exist in all blood group systems; group O is the most common, followed by Fy(a−b−) and Le(a−b−) in Africans. All other nulls are quite rare.

The Fy(a−b−) phenotype is especially interesting. Although it was once thought that this phenotype represented the inheritance of two silent alleles, *FyFy*, it has since been shown that Fy(a−b−) Africans commonly have *Fy^b* genes that express normal Fy^b glycoprotein on tissue cells but not on erythrocytes. A mutation that disrupts the GATA-1 binding site for red cell transcription has been identified in these individuals, which helps explain why many Fy(a−b−) Africans do not make Duffy antibodies despite exposure to antigen-positive erythrocytes from transfusion.

GENE FREQUENCIES

Gene and phenotype frequencies vary widely with race and geographical boundaries.[5,9,17] This information is needed when estimating the availability of compatible blood and the probability of hemolytic disease of the newborn, and in paternity and forensic investigations.

DISTRIBUTION OF RED CELL ANTIGENS IN HEALTH AND DISEASE

EXPRESSION OF RED CELL ANTIGENS IN OTHER BODY TISSUES AND FLUIDS

Antigens in the Rh and Kidd blood group systems are present only on erythrocytes and have not been detected on platelets, lymphocytes, or granulocytes or in plasma, other body tissues, or secretions (saliva, milk, amniotic fluid, etc.).[4–6] MNSs, Lutheran, Kell, and Duffy antigens also are erythrocyte specific but have been found in other body tissues (see Table 137-2).

In contrast, ABH antigens have broad tissue distribution. In young embryos, they can be detected on all endothelial cells and all epithelial cells except those of the central nervous system. ABH, Lewis, I, and P blood group antigens are in plasma and on platelets and lymphocytes; granulocytes carry I antigen but no ABH.[6] ABH on platelets and lymphocytes may be acquired at least in part by adsorption of plasma antigen; Lewis antigen is acquired only by adsorption. Body secretions (saliva, milk, etc.) contain ABH, I, and Lewis antigen but no P system antigens. Sd^a antigen is found in most body secretions, with the greatest concentrations seen in urine.[4,6]

ASSOCIATIONS OF RED CELL ANTIGENS WITH DISEASE

ANTIGENS ASSOCIATED WITH POSSIBLE SUSCEPTIBILITY TO DISEASE

Some blood groups are statistically associated with medical conditions or disease (Table 137-4).[4–6,10,18–22] For example, blood group A is more common in persons with cancer of the salivary glands, stomach, colon, or ovary and with thrombosis (due to higher levels of factors VIII, V, and IX). Blood group O is more common in patients with duodenal and gastric ulcers, rheumatoid arthritis, and von Willebrand disease. The adult i phenotype, especially in Asians, appears genetically linked to congenital cataracts.[4,18,20] These statistical observations may not be of clinical significance.

Associations with infection arise when microorganisms carry structures with blood group activity. *Yersinia pestis* carries H-like antigen, and the smallpox virus is associated with A-like antigen, making group O and A individuals, respectively, more susceptible. The presence of blood group antibody and/or soluble blood group antigen in secretions may help confer protection. Having anti-B may offer protection against *Salmonella*, *Shigella*, *Neisseria gonorrhoeae*, and some *Escherichia coli* O_{86} infections. There is an association between nonsecretion of ABH antigen and susceptibility to *Candida albicans*, *Neisseria meningitidis*, *Streptococcus pneumoniae*, and *Haemophilus influenzae*.[20]

A number of disease associations with globoside structures have been identified. *Streptococcus suis*, which can cause meningitis and septicemia in humans, binds exclusively to P^k antigen. A class of toxins secreted by *Shigella dysenteriae*, *Vibrio cholerae*, and *Vibrio parahaemolyticus* also have binding specificity for Gal(α1→4)-Galβ(1→4). In addition, globoside is the receptor of human parvovirus B19.[8] Some strains of *E. coli* use a disaccharide receptor, Gal(α1→4)-Galβ, on uroepithelial cells to gain entry to the urinary tract receptors associated with P_1, P, and P^k antigens.[4,20,24,25] People with the rare p phenotype (P null) lack this disaccharide and are not susceptible to acute pyelonephritis from such *E. coli* strains.

PHENOTYPES ASSOCIATED WITH DISEASE RESISTANCE

Erythrocytes lacking Fy^a and Fy^b antigen are not infected by the malarial parasite *Plasmodium vivax* and the simian parasite *Plasmodium knowlesi*. The parasites attach to the red cell membrane, but junction (the joining of merizoite and erythrocyte membrane) and

TABLE 137-4   BLOOD GROUP ANTIGENS AND ANTIBODIES ASSOCIATED WITH DISEASE

	PHENOTYPES ASSOCIATED WITH DISEASE SUSCEPTIBILITY
Group A	Carcinoma of the salivary glands, stomach, colon, rectum, ovary, uterus, cervix, and bladder (T1 and T2 tumors); idiopathic thrombocytopenic purpura, coronary thrombosis, thrombosis (oral contraceptives), pernicious anemia, giardiasis, and meningococcal meningitis infections
Group B	*Escherichia coli* urinary tract infection and gonorrhea
Group O	Duodenal and gastric ulcers, rheumatoid arthritis, von Willebrand disease, typhoid, paratyphoid, and cholera
ABH nonsecretors	Duodenal ulcers, spondylarthropathies; increased susceptibility to *Candida albicans, Neisseria meningitidis, Streptococcus pneumoniae*, and *Haemophilus influenzae*
Le(a−b−)	Sjögren syndrome
Group O, Le(a−b+)	*Heliobacter pylori*
i	Congenital cataracts
Globoside	Parvovirus B19

	PHENOTYPES ASSOCIATED WITH DISEASE RESISTANCE
p (PP₁Pᵏ−)	Pyelonephritogenic infections of *E. coli*
Fy(a−b−)	*Plasmodium vivax, Plasmodium knowlesi*
Tn−, Cad−, En(a−), U−, Ge−	*Plasmodium falciparum*

	DISEASES ASSOCIATED WITH ALTERED ANTIGEN EXPRESSION
Weakened AB	Leukemia, preleukemia, Hodgkin disease, aplastic anemia, bacterial infections
Weakened MN	Bacterial infections, preleukemia, leukemia (Tn, T, Tk activation)
Enhanced i	Thalassemia, sickle cell disease, HEMPAS, Diamond-Blackfan anemia, myeloblastic or sideroblastic erythropoiesis, refractory anemia
Acquired A (Tn)	Preleukemia, acute myelogenous leukemia
Acquired B	Bacterial infections, gastrointestinal lesions or malignancies
Acquired T, Tk	Bacterial infections
Acquired K antigens	*Enterococcus faecium*
Acquired Jkᵇ antigen	*E. faecium or Micrococcus* infection
Absent Cromer-related antigens	Paroxysmal nocturnal hemoglobinuria
Weakened target antigens (Rh, Kell, Kidd, LW)	Autoimmune hemolytic anemia
Weakened I, Rh, SsU, Kpᵇ, Jkᵃ, Xgᵃ, or Enᵃ	Stomatocytic hereditary elliptocytosis

	DISEASES ASSOCIATED WITH ABSENT ANTIGENS AND NULL PHENOTYPES
Rh_null (DCEce−)	Hereditary stomatocytosis, hemolytic anemia
McLeod phenotype (Kx−)	Hereditary acanthocytosis, hemolytic anemia
Ge− (Leach type)	Hereditary elliptocytosis, hemolytic anemia

	DISEASES ASSOCIATED WITH ANTIBODY PRODUCTION
Anti-I, -IH, -i, -H, -Pr	Cold agglutinin disease
Anti-"Rh", -"Kell", -U, -Wrᵇ	Warm autoimmune hemolytic anemia
Anti-I	*Mycoplasma pneumoniae*, chronic lymphocytic leukemia, Hodgkin disease
Anti-i	Infectious mononucleosis, reticuloendothelial diseases
Anti-Iᵀ	Hodgkin disease
Anti-K	Enterocolitis, bacterial infections (*E. coli* 0125:B15, *Campylobacter jejuni* and *C. coli*)
Anti-P₁	Parasitic infections; hydatid cyst disease, liver flukes
Anti-PP₁Pᵏ	Early spontaneous abortions
Anti-P	Paroxysmal cold hemoglobinuria, early spontaneous abortions, lymphoma
Anti-NF	Renal dialysis (formaldehyde exposure)
Anti-Forssman	Neoplastic disorders
Anti-Rx	Virally-induced hemolysis
Decreased anti-A or -B	Agamma- or hypogammaglobulinemia

	"NULL" PHENOTYPES ASSOCIATED WITH BIOLOGICAL DIFFERENCES BUT NO DISEASE
Group O	Lack GalNAc or Gal on terminal Gal
Bombay	Lack Fuc on terminal Gal
Le(a−b−)	Lack Fuc on terminal GlcNAc
M−N− or En(a−)	Lack or have altered GPA
S−s−U−	Lack or have altered GPB
Wr(a−b−)	Lack GPA
Mᵏ phenotype	Lack GPA and GPB
K₀	Lack Kell glycoprotein
Jk(a−b−)	Lack or have altered Jk protein, reduced ability to concentrate urine
Lu(a−b−)	Lack or have reduced or altered Lu glycoprotein; RBC may show poikilocytosis, potassium loss, and hemolysis during storage
LW(a−b−)	Lack or have altered 40- to 47-kD KW glycoproteins
Do(a−b−), Ge(a−)	Lack a P1-linked protein
Sc: −1, −2, −3	Lack or have altered 60-kD Sc glycoprotein
Co(a−b−), Co3−	Unknown

SOURCE: Modified from ME Reid and GWG Bird,[20] and PD Issitt.[20]

penetration cannot take place. The Fy6 antigen, which Fy(a−b−) red cells lack, appears to be the critical receptor for *P. vivax* penetration.[4,21,23]

Plasmodium falciparum invasion is not dependent on Duffy antigen; instead, it is associated with red cell glycophorins and their O-linked oligosaccharides (carrying NeuNAc). Red cells with the following phenotypes have shown a decreased rate of infection: M-N- (GPA deficient), S-s-U- (GPB deficient), Ge- (Leach type or GPC deficient), and Cad- and Tn-positive red cells (with abnormal O-linked sugars).[21]

DISEASES ASSOCIATED WITH ALTERED ANTIGEN EXPRESSION

Altered antigen expression can occur with inherited and acquired disease. Inherited changes are fixed and consistent; acquired changes can disappear with remission or recovery. In some diseases, antigen expression weakens; in others, it increases or new antigens appear.

Weakened ABH expression on red cells has been noted in acute myeloid leukemias and may be due to reduced transferase activity.[4,6] Normal antigen expression returns with disease remission. Transient weakened expression of target antigen also has been reported in some cases of autoimmune hemolytic anemia. Weak Rh, Kell, and Kidd blood group activity has been reported with concurrent autoantibody.[4,6]

Increased expression of i on red cells is associated with inherited disorders, such as thalassemia, sickle cell disease, Diamond-Blackfan syndrome, or hereditary erythroblastic multinuclearity with a positive acidified serum test (HEMPAS). Increased i expression also is noted with acquired conditions that decrease the red cell maturation time in the marrow, such as myeloblastic or sideroblastic erythropoiesis, refractory anemia, or excessive phlebotomy.[6,19,20]

Expression of the crypt-antigen Tn is caused by a galactosyltransferase deficiency acquired by somatic mutation in a population of stem cells. The antigen is present on all red cells, platelets, and granulocytes arising from these stem cells. This condition (seen as persistent mixed-field agglutination because of the presence of both normal and abnormal cell clones) causes other red cell abnormalities, such as depressed MN expression, enhanced H, and reduced NeuNAc content. It is associated with preleukemia and acute myelomonocytic leukemia.[6,20] Other crypt-antigens (T, Tk) are seen as a result of infection when microbes produce enzymes that remove some sugars and expose new ones. Group A individuals can appear to acquire a B antigen when bacterial deacetylase removes the acetyl group on GalNAc.[26,27] This phenomenon is associated with severe infection, gastrointestinal lesions, or malignancies.

Red cells also may acquire new blood group activity when they adsorb membrane material from certain microorganisms.[19,20] Group B activity has been associated with *E. coli*$_{86}$ and *Proteus vulgaris* infection and K activity with *Enterococcus faecium*. Acquired Jk^b-like activity has been associated with *E. faecium* and *Micrococcus* infections, although the mechanism is not clear.

DISEASES ASSOCIATED WITH ABSENT ANTIGENS OR NULL PHENOTYPES

Rh$_{null}$ Syndrome   The Rh$_{null}$ phenotype is associated with hereditary stomatocytosis, hemolytic anemia (usually mild), and a lack of proteins carrying Rh antigen. Rh protein resides in the red cell membrane, interacts with other membrane glycoproteins and possibly the cytoskeleton, and may help regulate or organize the lipids within the red cell membrane bilayer.[22] Hence, it is important to membrane shape as well as the expression of other antigens. Rh$_{null}$ cells have depressed expression of SsU, LW, and Fy5 antigens.

Most Rh$_{null}$ red cells are stomatocytes or occasionally spherocytes and demonstrate an increased osmotic fragility, increased potassium permeability, and higher potassium pump activity. They have reduced

cation and water content and a relative deficiency of membrane cholesterol.[22] While it is assumed that these abnormalities contribute to shortened in vivo survival, Rh$_{null}$ red cells survive normally in splenectomized patients, suggesting their removal is related more to splenic clearance because of shape rather than some other intrinsic factor.[22]

Two genetic mechanisms account for the Rh$_{null}$ phenotype. Persons with the amorphic type are homozygous for the silent Rh gene $\bar{r}$ that encodes no Rh protein. Individuals with the more common regulator type of Rh$_{null}$ have normal Rh genes but are thought to be homozygous for X^0r, a rare allele of the normal Rh regulator gene X^1r that switches off Rh gene expression.[10,22]

Individuals with the Rh$_{mod}$ phenotype have similar membrane and clinical anomalies associated with Rh$_{null}$ syndrome but demonstrate some Rh antigen expression. Their hypothesized regulator gene X^Qr may represent the same recessive regulator gene of Rh$_{null}$ individuals but with less penetrance.[22]

McLeod Phenotype   More than 60 males and no females with the McLeod phenotype have been identified. Each of these individuals had acanthocytosis, decreased red cell survival, very weak expression of Kell blood group antigens, and a lack of Kx antigen on their erythrocytes. Their hemolytic anemia may be well compensated.[20,22]

Kx, a 37-kD protein encoded by the *Xk* gene on the X chromosome, interacts with the cytoskeleton and helps stabilize the membrane, much as does Rh protein. The absence of Kx is associated with a lipid deficiency in the membrane bilayer that may be critical to the Kell antigen protein and general membrane shape. Red cells with the McLeod phenotype also show a defect in water transport, increased mobility of phosphatidylcholine across the membrane, and increased phosphorylation of protein band 3 and the B band of spectrin.[28]

After age 40, patients with the McLeod phenotype develop a slowly progressive form of muscular dystrophy that is associated with areflexia, choreiform movements, and cardiomegaly, leading to cardiomyopathy. They have elevated levels of serum creatine kinase and carbonic anhydrase III. Some patients with the McLeod phenotype and X-linked granulomatous disease apparently have sustained a deletion of both the *Xk* and the *Phox-91* X-linked genes (see Chap. 72). All these anomalies may be related to a spectrum of deletions on the X chromosome near the *Xk* gene at position Xp21.

Gerbich Negative Phenotype   The *GPC* gene on chromosome 2 encodes two proteins: glycophorin C (GPC), with antigens Ge3 and Ge4 (the Ge2 portion is "hidden" by the Ge4-bearing terminal end), and its shorter partner, glycophorin D (GPD), with antigens Ge2 (now exposed) and Ge3. GPC and GPD interact with membrane skeleton proteins 4.1 and p55, which are involved in cell deformability and membrane stability.

Gerbich-negative erythrocytes of the Leach type (Ge−2, −3, and −4) lack both GPC and GPD, have reduced protein 4.1 and elliptocytosis, but exhibit normal survival in vivo.[20,22] Leach-type null red cells also have weakened expression of Kell blood group antigens.

Other Null Phenotypes   The other rare null phenotypes are not associated with red cell shape changes or hemolytic anemia.[20] However, patients with null phenotypes can develop erythrocyte antibodies that make it difficult to find compatible blood and that cause serious hemolytic transfusion reactions. For example, people with the Bombay phenotype (O$_h$ or H null) demonstrate no red cell abnormality but make potent hemolytic anti-H as well as anti-A and -B. These antibodies are incompatible with all red cells except those from other persons with the Bombay phenotype. Likewise, p individuals (PP$_1$P^k-negative) or P^k individuals (P-negative) can make hemolytic antibodies to the antigens they lack. Anti-PP$_1$P^k and anti-P also are associated with spontaneous abortions in the first trimester.[6] Women with such antibodies (notably IgG anti-P), even with a history of spontaneous abortions, have delivered viable infants after plasmapheresis.[29]

Null phenotypes in the MNSs and Lutheran systems are interesting because several types of null phenotypes are known. Within the MNSs blood group system, people may lack normal GPA [En(a−) or MN-negative], normal GPB (SsU-negative), or both (M^{k}M^k phenotype).[12,18] The rare Lu(a−b−) phenotype is caused by a dominant inhibitor called *In(Lu)* (or *SYN1−B*), the homozygous pairing of the silent allele *Lu*, or a recessive sex-linked inhibitor *XS2*.[4,6] Only the *LuLu*-type null is associated with high-prevalence antibody because the inhibitor type nulls produce very small amounts of Lutheran antigen. *In(Lu)* type Lu(a−b−) red cells have been associated with varying degrees of poikilocytosis and acanthocytosis and may hemolyze more quickly during storage, even though they demonstrate normal osmotic fragility.[30]

The Jk(a−b−) phenotype is caused by the silent alleles *JkJk* or the dominant inhibitor *In(Jk)*. Erythrocytes having the Jk(a−b−) phenotype resist lysis in 2*M* urea, a solution commonly used in automated platelet counting systems. No significant clinical abnormalities have been identified to date, although Jk(a−b−) individuals have reduced ability to concentrate urine.

ANTIERYTHROCYTE ANTIBODIES

IMMUNOLOGY OF RED CELL ANTIBODIES

Blood group antibodies are classified as autoantibodies if they are specific for self-antigens that are present on the patient's own RBC. Blood group antibodies are called alloantibodies if they react with alloantigens present on the RBC of other individuals. These antibodies also may be classified according to their mode of sensitization: naturally occurring or immune (following sensitization). A summary of common antierythrocyte antibodies is provided in Table 137-5.[4-7,31]

IMMUNOGLOBULIN CLASSES ASSOCIATED WITH BLOOD GROUP ACTIVITY

IgG IgG is the predominant antibody made in an immune response and constitutes about 80 percent of total serum immunoglobulin (see Chap. 83). When specific for erythrocyte antigens, these molecules can direct red cell destruction. Receptors on macrophages in the liver and spleen allow these cells to remove IgG-coated erythrocytes from circulation. IgG blood group antibodies also are capable of fixing complement, although some subclasses do so less efficiently than others: IgG3 > IgG1 > IgG2 > IgG4. How well an IgG antierythrocyte antibody binds complement depends also on the surface density and location of the recognized antigen. This is because the initiator of the classic complement cascade, C1q, requires that at least two IgG molecules bind the red cell within a span of 20 to 30 nm to initiate the complement cascade.[6] For example, IgG anti-D rarely binds complement, presumably because most D sites are spaced too far apart and the epitope is so small that only one anti-D molecule per epitope can bind.[6,32] Most IgG blood group antibodies do not agglutinate saline-suspended red cells, presumably because the IgG molecule is too small to span the distance between erythrocytes, although some exceptions are known (potent IgG examples of anti-A, -B, -M, and -K). Instead, most IgG antibodies sensitize red cells at 37°C (98.6°F) and are detected with the help of an antiglobulin reagent.

IgM IgM is a pentamer of five basic units (having μ: heavy chains plus a short J, or joining, chain) and makes up only about 4 percent of total serum immunoglobulin (see Chap. 83). IgM is the first class of immunoglobulin produced by a fetus and is the predominant antibody seen in an early primary immune response, but it does not cross the placenta. Because of their pentameric structure, even low-affinity IgM blood group antibodies can agglutinate red cells and activate complement very effectively. Both hemolyzing and agglutinat-

ing abilities are destroyed by the reducing reagent 2-ME or DTT. IgM blood group antibodies of very low affinity may agglutinate red cells only at temperatures below 37°C (98.6°F). Such antibodies still may fix complement onto the red cell membrane in vivo, presumably by binding to red cells at the lower temperatures of the extremities and activating the complement cascade. Because such IgM antibodies dissociate from erythrocytes at higher temperature, their reactivity may be detected in routine antiglobulin tests by virtue of the complement components that remain bound to the red cell membrane.

IgA IgA is the primary immunoglobulin in body secretions, where it exists predominantly as a dimer with a secretory component (see Chap. 83). IgA does not cross the placenta or fix complement, but aggregated IgA can activate the alternative pathway of complement, and IgA can trigger cell-mediated events. Multimeric IgA antibodies in serum are seen as hemagglutinins in blood bank tests and most often are associated with those having A, B, or Lutheran activity.

IMMUNOGLOBULIN IN THE FETUS AND NEWBORN

Young fetuses acquire low levels of maternal IgG, probably by diffusion across the placenta. These levels rise significantly between 20 and 33 weeks' gestation as a selective transport system matures and maternal IgG is actively transported across the placenta. Thus, almost all blood group antibodies detected in the fetus and newborn are from the mother and disappear within the first few months of life.

Actual fetal antibody production begins shortly before birth with low levels of IgM, followed by IgG and IgA several weeks after birth. Antibody production continues to increase with age until adult levels are reached. Anti-A and anti-B are usually detected after 2 to 6 months.

Because of this late immune response in the newborn and because maternal antibody is so predominant at birth, blood bank standards permit abbreviated testing on neonates less than 4 months old.[33] If available, the mother's serum is used (and preferred) for identifying antibodies in a newborn and for cross-matching units of blood.

NATURALLY OCCURRING ANTIBODIES

Naturally Occurring Antibodies in Development An antibody is naturally occurring when it is found in the serum of an individual who has never been exposed to the antigen through transfusion or pregnancy. These antibodies are most likely heteroagglutinins, produced in response to substances in the environment that are similar to erythrocyte antigens.

Evidence supporting this concept has come from studies on the formation of anti-B in chickens.[34] Chicks raised in a normal environment made anti-B within the first 30 days of life, while chicks raised in a germ-free environment did not make anti-B by day 60. Naturally occurring alloanti-A and -B in humans, also called isoagglutinins, can be shown to increase in titer following ingestion or inhalation of suitable bacteria.[35]

However, since many antigens that are unlikely to be present in the environment also have been associated with naturally occurring antibodies, the stimulus for naturally occurring antibodies is not clearly known and may well be spontaneous, with no stimulation.[6]

Blood Group Associations and Frequency of Naturally Occurring Antibodies Naturally occurring alloantibodies are commonly associated with the carbohydrate antigens of the ABO, Lewis, and P blood group systems. Anti-A and -B are expected in people who lack the corresponding antigens, as are antibodies specific for H, PP$_1$P^k, or P specificities. Naturally occurring antibodies reactive with A$_1$, Le^a, Le^b, or P$_1$ determinants also are seen frequently. Carbohydrate antigens, especially those with repetitive epitopes, can stimulate B cells to make specific antibody without the aid of helper T cells. Such thymus-independent immune responses typically result in antigen-specific antibodies of the IgM class.[36]

TABLE 137-5   SUMMARY OF ANTIERYTHROCYTE ANTIBODIES

Blood Group	Antibody	Ig Class		Serologic Activity			Activates Complement	Implicated In		Antigen Frequency %		Comments
		IgM	IgG	RT	37-AHG	ENZ/AET/Chlor		HTR	HDN	Whites	Blacks	
				ANTIBODIES MORE COMMONLY ENCOUNTERED								
ABO	A	M	S	M	M	I/nc/nc	Y	Y	Mild	40	27	A/B: very clinically significant, sometimes IgA
	B	M	S	M	M	I/nc/nc	Y	Y	Mild	11	20	
	A₁	M	R	M	R	I/nc/nc	R	R	N	30	—	A₁: usually not clinically significant
	H	M	R	M	R	I/nc/nc	R	R	—	>99.9	—	H: usually weak autoantibody, but strong alloantibody in O_h
Rh	D	S	M	S	M	I/nc/nc	N	Y	Sev	85	92	D: most common immune antibody
	C	F	M	—	M	I/nc/nc	N	Y	Sev	70	33	C: often found with D
	E	S	M	S	M	I/nc/nc	N	Y	Sev	30	21	Ec: often found together
	c	—	M	—	M	I/nc/nc	N	Y	Sev	80	97	Autoantibodies commonly directed against Rh protein
	e	—	M	—	M	I/nc/nc	N	Y	Mild–sev	98	99	All: clinically significant
	f(ce)	—	M	—	M	I/nc/nc	N	Y	Sev	64		
	Cʷ	S	M	—	M	I/nc/nc	N	Y	Sev	1	—	
	V	—	M	—	M	I/nc/nc	N	Y	Sev	<1	30	
Lewis	Leᵃ	M	R	M	S	I/nc/nc	Y	R	N	22	23	Common in pregnancy
	Leᵇ	M	R	M	S	I/nc/nc	Y	N	N	72	55	Not clinically significant Le(a–b–) individuals commonly make anti-Leᵃ
Ii	I	M	—	M	S	I/nc/nc	Y	R	N	>99.9	>99.9	I: common autoantibody, rare significant alloantibody
	i	M	—	M	S	I/nc/nc	Y	N	Mild	100	100	i: rare autoantibody
P	P₁	M	R	M	S	I/nc/nc	F	R	N	79	94	P₁: usually not clinically significant
(GLOB)	P	M	F	M	S	I/nc/nc	Y	Y	N–Mild	>99.9	>99.9	P: Donath-Landsteiner antibody in PNH
	PP₁Pᵏ	M	F	M	S	I/nc/nc	Y	Y	Mild–sev	>99.9	>99.9	
MNSs	M	S	S	M	F	D/nc/(nc)	N	(R)	(R)	78	70	M: common, usually not clinically significant
	N	S	S	M	R	D/nc/(nc)	N	(R)	(R)	72	74	N: rare, usually not clinically significant
	S	S	S	S	M	V/nc/(nc)	S	Y	Mild	55	31	
	s	F	M	F	M	V/nc/(nc)	N	Y	Mild–sev	89	97	SsU: clinically significant
	U	—	M	—	M	nc/nc/(nc)	R	Y	Mild–mod	100	99.7	Autoantibody specificities reported
Kell	K	S	M	F	M	nc/D/nc	R	Y	Mild–sev	9	2	K: very common immune antibody
	k	—	M	R	M	nc/D/nc	N	Y	Mild–sev	99.9	—	
	Kpᵃ	—	M	R	M	nc/D/nc	N	Y	Mild–mod	2.3	—	Autoantibodies reported
	Kpᵇ	—	M	R	M	nc/D/nc	N	Y	Mild–mod	>99.9	100	
	Jsᵃ	—	M	R	R	nc/D/nc	N	Y	Mild–sev	—	20	
	Jsᵇ	—	M	—	M	nc/D/nc	N	Y	Mild–sev	>99.9	99	
Duffy	Fyᵃ	—	M	R	M	D/nc/nc	R	Y	Mild–sev	66	10	Fyᵃ: common immune antibody
	Fyᵇ	—	M	R	M	D/nc/nc	R	Y	Mild	83	23	
Kidd	Jkᵃ	F	M	R	M	I/nc/nc	Y	Y	Mild–mod	77	92	Jkᵃ: associated with delayed HTR; hemolytic; disappears quickly from serum
	Jkᵇ	F	M	R	M	I/nc/nc	Y	Y	N–Mild	72	41	
Lutheran	Luᵃ	S	F	M	F	nc(V)/D/(nc)	N	N	N–Mild	7.7	—	Mild RBC destruction, sometimes IgA
	Luᵇ	S	S	F	M	nc(V)/D/(nc)	N	Y	Mild	99.9	—	
				ANTIBODIES LESS COMMONLY ENCOUNTERED								
Xg	Xgᵃ	S	M	R	M	D/nc/?	S	N	N	64(m) 89(f)	—	Xg: poor immunogen
Cartwright	Ytᵃ	—	M	N	M	D(V)/D(V)/nc	N	N–mod	N	99.7	—	Yt: some antibody examples clinically significant, others not
	Ytᵇ	—	M	N	M	D(V)/D/nc	N	?	N	8	—	
Ch/Rg	Ch	R	M	—	M	D/nc/nc	N	N	N	96	—	Ch/Rg: associated with C4 complement, clinically insignificant antibodies
	Rg	—	M	—	M	D/nc/nc	N	N	N	98	—	
Colton	Coᵃ	—	M	S	M	nc/nc/nc	N	N	Mild–sev	99.9	—	Co antigens found on water transport proteins
	Coᵇ	—	M	—	M	nc/nc/nc	R	N–mod	Mild	10	—	
Cost	Csᵃ	—	M	—	M	nc/nc/nc	N	N	N	96	98	
Cromer	General group	M	—	—	M	nc/D/nc	N	N–mild	N	>99.9	>99.9	CR: located on DAF molecules; associated with complement regulation
Diego	Diᵃ	—	M	S	M	nc/nc/nc	R	Y	Mild–sev	R	—	Diᵃ: antigen found in south American Indians and Asians
	Diᵇ	—	M	N	M	nc/nc/nc	N	Y	Mild	100	—	
Dombrock	Doᵃ	—	M	N	M	nc/D(V)/nc	N	Y	Mild	67	—	Doᵃ Doᵇ: poor immunogens
	Doᵇ	—	M	N	M	nc/D(V)/nc	N	Y	Mild	83	—	Hy– and Jo(a–): found only in blacks
	Hy	—	M	—	M	nc(I)/D(V)/nc	N	Y	Mild	>99	—	Gy(a–): Do nulls, found in eastern Europeans and Japanese
	Gyᵃ	—	M	—	M	nc(I)/D(V)/nc	N	Y	Mild	>99	—	
	Joᵃ	—	M	—	M	nc(I)/D(V)/nc	N	N	N	>99	—	
Gerbich	General group	—	M	—	M	D/nc/nc	Y	N–mod	(+DAT)	>99.9	>99.9	Ge: located on glycophorin C and D
Indian	Ina	—	M	—	M	D/D/nc	N	Y	(+DAT)	<0.1	<0.1	In: located on CD44 adhesion protein
	Inb	—	M	—	M	D/D/nc	N	Y	(+DAT)	99	96	
Knops	Knᵃ	—	M	—	M	D/D/nc	N	N	N	98	99	Knops antigens associated with CR1 (complement) receptor, clinically insignificant antibodies
	McCᵃ	—	M	—	M	D/D/nc	N	N	N	98	94	
	Ykᵃ	—	M	—	M	D/D/nc	N	N	N	92	98	
Scianna	Sc1	—	M	—	M	nc/D/(nc)	Y	N	Mild	>99.9	—	Sc1: some antibodies react in serum but not plasma
	Sc2	—	M	—	M	nc/D/nc	N	N	Mild	1	—	
	Sc3	—	M	—	M	nc(I)/?/nc	N	N–mild	N	>99.9	—	
High	JMH	—	M	—	M	D/D/nc	N	N	N	>99.9	>99.9	JMH: carrier protein CDw108

ABBREVIATIONS: AET, AET-treated RBC; AHG, antiglobulin phase; chlor, chloroquine-treated RBC at room temperature; D, decreased; +DAT, positive direct antiglobulin test result; ENZ, enzyme-treated RBCs; F, few; f, female; GPI, glycosylphosphatidylinositol; HDN, hemolytic disease of the newborn; HTR, hemolytic transfusion reactions; I, increased; M, most; m, male, mod, moderate; N, no; nc, no significant change using pretreated cells; R, rare; RT, room temperature; S, some; sev, severe; V, variable; Y, yes.

Within other systems,[6] anti-Sdᵃ is found in 1 to 2 percent of normal people, and anti-Vʷ and anti-Wrᵃ in about 1 percent. Other less common antibody specificities are listed in approximate order of descending frequency: M, S, N, Ge, K, Luᵃ, Diᵃ, and Xgᵃ. Rh antigens are thought to reside only on red blood cells, but naturally occurring anti-D has been reported in 0.15 percent of Rh-negative donors and anti-E in over 0.1 percent of Rh-positive donors when more sensitive enzyme detection methods are used. Examples of naturally occurring anti-C, -Cʷ, and -Cˣ also have been described.

Some naturally occurring antibodies exist as autoagglutinins (anti-

H and anti-I). Patients with autoimmune hemolytic anemia have been reported to produce many antibodies to low-frequency antigens with no specific stimulus, in addition to autoantibody.[4,6]

Characteristics of Naturally Occurring Antibodies Most naturally occurring antibodies are IgM, but some have an IgG component, and a few are predominantly IgG. Some anti-A or anti-B antibodies may even be of the IgA class. Antibodies that cause direct agglutination of saline-suspended red cells most commonly are of the IgM class. However, even IgG antibodies may cause agglutination of red cells when they bind erythrocyte antigens that are present at high density and number on the erythrocyte membrane, such as the ABO or MN antigens. With the exception of anti-A and anti-B, most common naturally occurring antibodies do not react at body temperature and are considered clinically insignificant. However, if they are found to react at 37°C (98.6°F), it is prudent to provide cross-match compatible blood for transfusion.

ANTIBODIES GENERATED IN RESPONSE TO IMMUNIZATION: IMMUNE ANTIBODIES

Immune Antibodies in Development Immune antibodies are produced following an exposure to foreign erythrocyte antigens through pregnancy or transfusion. The primary immune response is seen several weeks to several months after the first exposure to antigen. IgM usually is associated with early primary responses, but whether it is always the first antibody class made is unclear. In most individuals, IgG soon predominates. This is characteristic of a thymus-dependent immune response, where T cells help induce B cells to undergo isotype switching from IgM to IgG.[36]

In a secondary or anamnestic response, antibody concentration starts to increase several days to several weeks following exposure and may rise to very high IgG levels. Some IgG antibodies remain detectable up to 30 years after a stimulus. Others, especially Kidd antibodies, disappear after several months and are more commonly associated with delayed hemolytic transfusion reactions.[4,6]

Blood Group Associations and Frequency of Immune Antibodies Immune antibodies are found more commonly in individuals who have been multiply transfused than in multiparous women. This is because in pregnancy the immunizing dose of red cells is often too small to elicit a primary response, and the foreign antigens are limited to those of the father.[6]

Anti-D used to be the most common immune antibody found, but with the advent of Rh-matching of donors and recipients in the 1940s and the use of Rh immunoglobulin prophylaxis in the 1970s, its frequency has sharply decreased. Recent figures show anti-D to be in 0.27 to 0.56 percent of transfusion recipients, 0.10 to 0.20 percent of pregnant women, and 0.16 to 0.25 percent of healthy blood donors.[6]

In contrast, the frequency of immune antibodies other than anti-D has increased. Specificities other than D have been reported in about 0.6 percent of transfusion recipients, 0.14 percent of pregnant women, and 0.19 percent of healthy blood donors. Pooled data from three 5-year periods and approximately 300,000 patients suggest the absolute frequency of Rh antibodies other than anti-D is 0.22 percent; anti-K, 0.19 percent; anti-Fy^a, 0.05 percent; and anti-Jk^a, 0.035 percent.[6]

The rate of alloimmunization in sickle cell anemia was 18.6 percent in one survey, and 55 percent of these immunized patients made more than one antibody. The most common specificities were anti-C, -E, and -K.[6]

Characteristics of Immune Antibodies Immune antibodies are most often IgG but may be IgM and are sometimes IgA (notably Lu^a). Most immune antibodies react at body temperature and are considered clinically significant, except for those directed against Bg, Yk^a, Cs^a, McC^a, Kn^a, JMH, and sometimes Lutheran antigens.

CLINICAL SIGNIFICANCE OF ERYTHROCYTE ANTIBODIES

HEMOLYTIC TRANSFUSION REACTIONS

Clinically significant antibodies are those that are capable of destroying transfused red cells in vivo. The severity of the reaction will vary with antigen density and antibody characteristics.

Antibodies commonly associated with intravascular hemolysis include anti-A, -B, -Jk^a, and -Jk^b. ABO incompatibility is the most potent cause of immediate hemolytic reactions because A and B antigen is so strongly expressed on erythrocytes and the antibodies so efficiently bind complement. Kidd antibodies are associated more often with delayed hemolytic reactions because they typically are difficult to detect and disappear quickly from circulation. IgG anti-Jk^a appears to bind complement only when traces of IgM anti-Jk^a are also present.[6] Anti-PP$_1$P^k, -Vel, and -Le^a also have been associated with hemolysis, but such examples are rare.

Extravascular hemolysis occurs with IgG1 and IgG3 antibodies that react at body temperature, that is, immune antibodies reactive with Rh, Kidd, Kell, Duffy, or Ss antigens. Indeed, these make up the bulk of clinically significant antibodies. Antibodies not expected to cause red cell destruction are those that react only at temperatures below 37°C (98.6°F) and IgG antibodies of the IgG2 or IgG4 subclass.

HEMOLYTIC DISEASE OF THE NEWBORN

Hemolytic disease of the newborn is caused by blood group incompatibility between a sensitized mother and her fetus (see Chap. 58). Antibodies most significant in hemolytic disease of the newborn are those that cross the placenta (IgG1 and IgG3), react at body temperature to cause red cell destruction, and are directed against well-developed red cell antigens. ABO incompatibility most commonly is seen, but ABO hemolytic disease of the newborn is clinically mild, presumably because the antigens are not fully expressed at birth. Antibodies directed against the D antigen can cause severe hemolytic disease of the newborn, and fetal health should be carefully followed when anti-D titers are greater than 1:16. Hemolytic disease of the newborn severity is less predictable with other blood group antibodies and can vary from mild to severe. For example, anti-K not only causes red cell hemolysis, but it may also suppress eyrthropoiesis.

AUTOIMMUNE HEMOLYTIC ANEMIA

Autoimmune hemolytic anemia is caused by the production of "warm-" or "cold-"reactive autoantibodies directed against red cell antigens (see Chaps. 55 and 56). Production can be triggered by disease, viral infection, or drugs; from a breakdown in immune system tolerance to self antigens; or from exposure to foreign antigens that induce antibodies that cross-react with self red cell antigens.[20] Autologous specificity is not always obvious, since antigen expression can be depressed when autoantibody is present.

Warm autoantibodies react best at 37°C (98.6°F) and are primarily IgG (rarely IgM or IgA). Most are directed against the Rh protein, but Wr^b, Kell, Kidd, or MNSU blood group specificity also has been reported.

Cold-reactive autoantibodies are primarily IgM. They react best at temperatures below 25°C (77°F) but can agglutinate cells or activate complement at or near 37°C (98.6°F), causing hemolysis or vascular occlusion upon exposure to cold.[6] Most cold-reactive autoantibodies have anti-I activity. Reactivity with i, H, Pr, P, or other antigenic specificities is much less common.

The biphasic cold-reactive IgG antibody associated with paroxysmal cold hemoglobinuria (the "Donath-Landsteiner" antibody) typically reacts with the high-frequency antigen P. It attaches to cells in the cold and very efficiently activates complement before it dissociates at warmer temperatures.

DISEASES ASSOCIATED WITH ANTIBODY PRODUCTION
Table 137-4 lists diseases associated with specific antibody production. These antibodies only cause autoimmune hemolytic anemia if the patient carries the corresponding antigen.

SEROLOGIC DETECTION OF ERYTHROCYTE ANTIGENS AND ANTIBODIES

ABO

ABO grouping is the single most important test performed in the blood bank because it is the fundamental basis for determining blood compatibility. ABO grouping is determined by reacting erythrocytes with licensed antisera to identify the A or B antigens they carry (the forward, or cell, grouping) and by reacting the corresponding serum or plasma with known A and B cells to identify the antibodies present (the reverse, or serum, grouping). Positive reactions are seen as hemagglutination or hemolysis using common test methods, and the results of one test should confirm those of the other.

If results are discrepant or reactions are weaker than expected, the cause must be investigated before the ABO group can be interpreted with confidence. Discrepancies can be related to red cell anomalies, serum anomalies, or both and may be associated with disease.[4,6,9,20,31] Common causes, excluding clerical and technical error, are listed in Table 137-6.

RH

The Rh or D type is the next most important test performed for blood compatibility. Individuals who type D+ are called Rh positive, and those who type D− are called Rh negative, provided reagent and cell controls are acceptable. Blood donors and pregnant women who type D− using standard typing sera are tested further for weak D expression using more sensitive methods, such as an antiglobulin test. Those with weak D antigen are considered Rh positive. Testing for weak D is optional for transfusion recipients.[33]

EXTENDED ANTIGEN PHENOTYPING

Reagent antisera to detect other common antigens (CcEe, MNSs, Kell, Duffy, Kidd, etc.) are available but used only when identifying the

TABLE 137-6   COMMON CAUSES OF ABO DISCREPANCIES

Red cells may appear to have	
Weak or missing antigens	Weak subgroup of A or B antigen
	Excess soluble A or B antigen in plasma
	Disease-associated loss (leukemia)
	ABO nonidentical marrow transplantation
	ABO nonidentical RBC transfusions
Extra antigens	Positive direct antiglobulin test
	Antibody to reagent additive or dye
	Rouleaux or cold agglutinin on cells
	Disease-associated acquisition (polyagglutination)
Serum may appear to have	
Weak or missing antibody	Age-related (newborns or the very elderly)
	Disease-associated immunosuppression
	Congenital hypogammaglobulinemia
	ABO nonidentical marrow transplantation
Extra antibody	Alloantibodies (A_1, Le^a, Le^b, P_1, M, N)
	Autoantibodies (I, i, H, Pr, P)
	Rouleaux
	Antibodies to additives in reagents' red cells
	Passive antibody acquisition from transfusion or from passenger lymphocytes in organ transplantation

red cell phenotype is essential to antibody identification, blood compatibility, or paternity or forensic issues. Extended phenotyping is especially important to patients who are at high risk of alloimmunization from chronic blood transfusion, for example, those with sickle cell anemia or thalassemia. Ideally, the red cell phenotype of these patients should be determined prior to the initiation of transfusion therapy.

ANTIBODY SCREEN

The antibody screen, or indirect antiglobulin test, detects "atypical" or "unexpected" antibodies in the serum (i.e., other than anti-A and anti-B) using group O reagent red cells that are known to carry most common antigens. The methods used must be able to detect clinically significant antibodies. Typically, serum or plasma and screening cells are incubated at 37°C (98.6°F) with an additive to potentiate antibody-antigen reactions; then an indirect antiglobulin test is performed. Hemagglutination or hemolysis at any point is a positive reaction, indicating the presence of naturally occurring or immune alloantibody or autoantibody. The antibody screen will not detect all atypical antibodies in serum, such as antibodies to low-incidence antigens not present on screening cells and antibodies that are not apparent at 37°C (98.6°F) and in the antiglobulin phase.

DIRECT ANTIGLOBULIN TEST

The direct antiglobulin test (direct Coombs' test) detects antibody or complement bound to erythrocytes in vivo. Red cells are washed free of serum and then mixed with antiglobulin reagents that agglutinate cells coated with IgG or the C3 component of complement.

Positive direct antiglobulin test results are associated with the following: (1) transfusion reactions, where recipient alloantibody coats transfused donor red cells or transfused donor antibody coats recipient cells; (2) hemolytic disease of the newborn, where maternal antibody crosses the placenta and coats fetal red cells; (3) autoimmune hemolytic anemias, where autoantibody coats the patient's own erythrocytes; (4) drug or drug-antibody complex interactions with red cells that can sometimes lead to hemolysis; (5) passenger lymphocyte syndrome, where transient antibody produced by passenger lymphocytes from a transplanted organ coats recipient red cells; and (6) hypergammaglobulinemia, where immunoglobulins nonspecifically adsorb onto circulating red cells.

A positive direct antiglobulin test results does not always indicate decreased red cell survival. As many as 10 percent of hospital patients and between 1 in 1000 to 1 in 9000 blood donors have a positive direct antiglobulin test result with no clinical indication of hemolysis.[9]

COMPATIBILITY TESTING

Compatibility testing refers to a collection of donor and recipient tests that are performed prior to red cell transfusion. Donors are tested for ABO, Rh, and unexpected antibody by the collecting facility. However, transfusing hospitals retest the ABO (and Rh on Rh-negative units) to verify the accuracy of the blood label.[33] Routine recipient testing includes an ABO, Rh, and antibody screening on a blood sample collected within 3 days of the intended transfusion. Results are checked against historical records to verify ABO, Rh, and antibody status.

If the recipient has a negative antibody screening test result and no history of clinically significant antibodies, a serologic immediate spin cross-match between recipient serum and donor red cells or a "computer cross-match" (wherein computer software compares the ABO test results of both donor and recipient) is required to confirm ABO compatibility.[9,33]

TABLE 137-7 ABO-RH COMPATIBILITY GUIDELINES

	ANTIGEN ON RED CELLS	ANTIBODY IN SERUM	COMPATIBLE BLOOD GROUPS	
			RECIPIENT SERUM	RECIPIENT CELLS
If recipient blood group is				
A	A	Anti-B	A, O	A, AB
B	B	Anti-A	B, O	B, AB
O	O	Anti-A, Anti-B	O	O, A, B, AB
AB	A, B	None	AB, A, B, O	AB
Rh positive	D	None	Rh positive, Rh negative	Rh not considered
Rh negative	—	Anti-D only if immunized	Rh-negative	Rh not considered

NOTE: Whole blood must be identical to recipient blood group. Red blood cells must be compatible with recipient serum. Plasma should be compatible with recipient cells. Platelets/cryo should be compatible with recipient cells, but any ABO group can be given if compatible units are not available.

If clinically significant antibodies are detected in recipient serum or they have been previously identified, red cell units should test negative for the offending antigens and should be cross-match compatible at 37°C (98.6°F) and the antiglobulin phase. The frequency of finding compatible units usually reflects the antigen frequency in the general population, that is, 91 percent of units should be compatible with a patient making anti-K because 9 percent of the population is K+. This reasoning will not be valid if the local donor population varies significantly from that of the general population. To calculate the frequency of compatible units when more than one antibody is present, one must multiply the frequencies of antigen-negative units for each specificity. For example, only 21 percent of units will be compatible for the recipient having both anti-K and anti-Jka: [0.91 for K−] × [0.23 for Jk(a−)] = 0.21.

When multiple clinically significant antibodies or antibodies directed against high-frequency antigens are present, finding compatible units may be extremely difficult. Antibody producers should be encouraged to give autologous units prior to their elective blood needs. If they are not candidates for autologous donation, compatible units may be found by testing the patient's siblings or by asking regional blood suppliers to check their rare donor inventories and files. Such procurement takes additional time.

Repeat donor testing and cross-matching are not performed for plasma and platelet components, but the recipient's ABO and Rh phenotypes must be known for appropriate selection of components. General ABO-Rh compatibility guidelines are given in Table 137-7.

ANTIBODY IDENTIFICATION

All unexpected antibodies are investigated. Those detected in serum or plasma as an ABO discrepancy, a positive antibody screening result, or an incompatible cross-match are identified using a panel of 8 to 16 different group O cells that have been typed for common clinically significant antigens. Serum reactions with these cells are compared to their antigen typing to determine specificity.[9] For example, an antibody that reacts with all K+ cells but not with K− cells is most likely anti-K.

A control of autologous cells and serum is tested concurrently with panel cells. Absence of reactivity with autologous cells implies that the antibody is an alloantibody, while a positive result suggests autoantibody or a positive direct antiglobulin test result. Once the antibody specificity is identified, the subject's erythrocytes are tested for the corresponding antigen. If the alloantibody is anti-K, the cells should type K−. Such antigen typing helps to confirm serum findings.

When antibody is detected on both red cells (a positive direct antiglobulin test result) and in serum, only the antibody in serum is identified unless a review of the medical or transfusion history offers evidence that they might be different. When antibody is detected only

on red cells and hemolysis is suspected, the antibody can be eluted and tested against panel cells to identify the specificity.

REFERENCES

1. Lewis M, Anstee DJ, Bird GWG, et al: Blood group terminology 1990, from the ISBT Working Party on Terminology for Red Cell Surface Antigens. Vox Sang 58:152, 1990.
2. Rippee C, Myers J, Gindy L: Blood groups, in Clinical Practice of Transfusion Medicine, 3rd ed, edited by LD Petz, SN Swisher, S Kleinman, et al. Churchill Livingstone, New York, 1996.
3. Daniels GL, Anstee DJ, Cartron JP, et al: Blood group terminology, ISBT Working Party on Terminology for Red Cell Surface Antigens. Vox Sang 69:265, 1995.
4. Issitt PD, Anstee DJ: Applied Blood Group Serology, 4th ed. Montgomery Scientific, Miami, 1998.
5. Reid ME, Lomas-Francis C: The Blood Group Antigen Facts Book. Academic Press, San Diego, 1997.
6. Mollison PL, Engelfriet CP, Contreras M: Blood Transfusion in Clinical Medicine, 10th ed. Blackwell Scientific, Oxford, 1997.
7. Daniels GL: Human Blood Groups. Blackwell Scientific, Oxford, 1995.
8. Cartron JP, Rouger P (eds): Blood Cell Biochemistry, vol 6, Molecular Basis of Human Blood Group Antigens. Plenum Press, New York, 1995.
9. Vengelen-Tyler V (ed): Technical Manual, 12th ed. American Association of Blood Banks, Bethesda, MD, 1996.
10. Tippett P: Regulator genes affecting red cell antigens. Transfus Med Rev 4:56, 1990.
11. Marsh WL, Johnson DL, Mueller KA: Proposed new notation for the In(Lu) modifying gene. Transfusion 24:371, 1984.
12. Okubo Y, Yamaguchi H, Nagao N, et al: Heterogeneity of the phenotype Jk(a−b−) found in Japanese. Transfusion 26:237, 1986.
13. Giblett ER: A critique of the theoretical hazard of inter vs. intra-racial transfusion. Transfusion 1:23, 1961.
14. Clausen H, Hakomori S: ABH and related histo-blood group antigens: Immunochemical differences in carrier isotypes and their distribution. Vox Sang 56:1, 1989.
15. Yomtovian R, Prince GM, Medof ME: The molecular basis for paroxysmal nocturnal hemoglobinuria. Transfusion 33:852, 1993.
16. Cartron JP, Rahuel C: Human erythrocyte glycophorins: Protein and gene structure analyses. Transfus Med Rev 6:63, 1992.
17. Mourant AE, Kopec AC, Domaniewska-Sobczak K: The Distribution of Human Blood Groups and Other Polymorphisms, 2d ed. Oxford University Press, London, 1976.
18. Mourant AE, Kopec AC, Domaniewska-Sobczak K: Blood Groups and Diseases. Oxford University Press, London, 1977.
19. Garratty G (ed): Blood Group Antigens and Disease. American Association of Blood Banks, Arlington, VA, 1983.
20. Reid ME, Bird GWG: Associations between human red cell blood group antigens and disease. Transfus Med Rev 4:47, 1990.
21. Hadley TJ, Miller LH, Haynes JD: Recognition of red cells by malaria parasites: The role of erythrocyte-binding proteins. Transfus Med Rev 5:108, 1991.
22. Issitt PD: Null red cell phenotypes: Associated biological changes. Transfus Med Rev 7:139, 1993.
23. Nichols ME, Rubinstein P, Barnwell J, et al: Identification of an erythro-

cyte membrane protein complex carrying Duffy blood group antigenicity: Immunogenetics and association with susceptibility to *Plasmodium vivax. J Exp Med* 166:776, 1987.

24. Kallenius G, Mollby R, Svenson SB, et al: Occurrence of P-fimbriated *Escherichia coli* in urinary tract infection. *Lancet* 2:1369, 1981.

25. Kallenius G, Svenson S, Mollby R, Cedergren B, Hultberg H, Winberg J: Structure of carbohydrate part of receptor on human uroepithelial cells for pyelonephritogenic *Escherichia coli. Lancet* 2:604, 1981.

26. Gerbal A, Maslet C, Salmon C: Immunological aspects of the acquired B antigen. *Vox Sang* 28:398, 1975.

27. Gerbal A, Ropars C, Gerbal R, et al: Acquired B antigen disappearance by in vitro acetylation associated with A_1 activity restoration. *Vox Sang* 31:64, 1976.

28. Marsh WL, Redman CM: The Kell blood group system: A review. *Transfusion* 30:158, 1990.

29. Shirey RS et al: Plasmapheresis and successful pregnancy after fourteen miscarriages in a P_1^k with anti-P [abstr]. *Transfusion* 24:427, 1984.

30. Udden MM, Umeda M, Hirano U, et al: New abnormalities in the morphology, cell surface receptors, and electrolyte metabolism in In(Lu) erythrocytes. *Blood* 69:52, 1987.

31. Quinley ED (ed): *Immunohematology: Principles and Practice,* 2d ed. Lippincott, Philadelphia, 1998.

32. Lomas C, Tippett P, Thompson KM, et al: Demonstration of seven epitopes on the Rh antigen D using human monoclonal anti-D antibodies and red cells from D categories. *Vox Sang* 57:261, 1989.

33. Menitove JE (ed): *Standards for Blood Banks and Transfusion Services,* 18th ed. American Association of Blood Banks, Bethesda, MD, 1997.

34. Springer GF, Horton RE, Rorbes M: Origin of anti-human blood group B agglutinins in white leghorn chicks. *J Exp Med* 110:221, 1959.

35. Springer GF, Horton RE: Blood group isoantibody stimulation in man by feeding blood group-active bacteria. *J Clin Invest* 48:1280, 1969.

36. Silberstein L, Spitalnik SL: Blood group antigens and antibodies, in *Principles of Transfusion Medicine,* edited by W Rossi, TL Simon, GS Moss. Williams & Wilkins, Baltimore, 1991.

HUMAN LEUKOCYTE AND PLATELET ANTIGENS

KAREN A. SULLIVAN

THOMAS J. KIPPS

The human leukocyte histocompatibility antigens, HLA, are polymorphic cell surface glycoproteins that present antigen peptide fragments to T-cell receptors. HLA antigens are encoded by multiple, closely linked genes, located in a 4-Mb region of DNA on chromosome 6, that comprise the major histocompatibility complex (MHC) and play a central role in the regulation of immune responses. In general, the MHC genes are inherited as a single unit in simple Mendelian fashion. The products of the MHC HLA-A, HLA-B, and HLA-C genes are called *class I antigens*. Class I antigens are expressed on essentially all tissues in the body and present small peptide fragments to CD8[+] T cells. The HLA-DR, HLA-DQ, and HLA-DP genes of the MHC encode class II antigens. Class II antigens present antigen peptide fragments to CD4[+] T cells and are limited in expression primarily to B cells, monocytes, and macrophages. The HLA antigens are the principal barriers to transplantation. The degree of similarity between donor and recipient HLA antigens determines the risk of allograft rejection and, in the case of stem-cell transplantation, the risk of graft-versus-host disease (GVHD). In addition to the HLA antigens, platelets also express glycoproteins that can be recognized by autoantibodies or by antibodies made by recipients of platelet transfusions. The latter are due to platelet alloantigens that reflect polymorphism in the genes encoding major platelet glycoproteins. Immune responses to platelet alloantigens are involved in the pathogenesis of several clinical syndromes, including neonatal alloimmune thrombocytopenia, posttransfusion purpura, and refractory responses to platelet transfusion. The treatment of immune thrombocytopenia is discussed in Chap. 121. This chapter instead describes the major platelet autoantigens and outlines typing strategies used when necessary for effective platelet transfusion therapy or treatment of neonatal alloimmune thrombocytopenia.

HUMAN LEUKOCYTE ANTIGENS

DEFINITION

The human leukocyte antigens, HLA, are highly polymorphic glycoproteins encoded by a cluster of genes on the short arm of chromosome 6.[1] The genes encoding HLA antigens comprise the major histocompatibility complex. This is because, next to the ABO system, the MHC is the principal barrier to transplantation. As products of the genes influencing the outcome of transplanted tissue or organs, the HLA molecules are called *histocompatibility antigens*. The biological function of HLA molecules, however, is the presentation of antigenic peptides to T cells (see Chap. 86).

There are six major groups of HLA antigens: HLA-A, HLA-B, HLA-C, HLA-DR, HLA-DQ, and HLA-DP. These groups are divided into classes of antigens designated as *class I* and *class II*, representing the two types of HLA molecules. The HLA-A, HLA-B, and HLA-C antigens are the class I antigens. The HLA-DR, HLA-DQ, and HLA-DP antigens are the class II antigens. The class I antigens were the first and most easily identified on leukocytes by antigen and antibody reactions, i.e., serological techniques. The class II antigens were originally defined by lymphocyte proliferation assays such as the mixed lymphocyte reaction (MLR) or primed lymphocyte test (PLT) and only later were identified by serologic techniques. The antigens identified by such cellular assays were designated *HLA-Dw*. The HLA-Dw antigens (or specificities) are now known to be an in vitro measure of T-cell responses to the cumulative effects of the allotypic HLA-DR, HLA-DQ, and HLA-DP antigens. The class I antigens are ubiquitous in tissue distribution, being found on most nucleated cells of the body. HLA class II antigens have a more restricted distribution than class I. These antigens primarily are found on B lymphocytes, monocytes, macrophages, dendritic cells, and endothelial cells. However, class II antigens can be induced on other cell types through activation.[2]

Class I antigens are encoded by genes at the HLA-A, HLA-B, and HLA-C loci on chromosome 6. Class II antigens are encoded by genes at the HLA-DR, HLA-DQ, and HLA-DP loci on the chromosome. Class I and class II protein molecules are highly homologous to each other, i.e., share most of their amino acid sequences. However, the amino acid residues at small segments of the molecules vary from each other. It is these areas of variability (polymorphism) in amino acid sequences that distinguish individual HLA molecules and confer antigen specificity. Each HLA locus can code for one of many HLA antigens. Thus, each HLA locus has multiple alleles (alternative or variant forms of genes). Although there are multiple possible alleles encoding different antigens, each individual carries only one of the possible alleles at each HLA locus on each chromosome. Therefore, each person expresses only two of the many HLA-A antigens, two HLA-B antigens, and so on. A complete list of recognized antigens is provided in Table 138-1.[3]

BIOCHEMISTRY

CLASS I ANTIGENS

The HLA-A, HLA-B, and HLA-C molecules are transmembrane glycoproteins with a M_r of 56,000.[4] They are heterodimers consisting of noncovalently bound protein chains; an α heavy chain ($M_r = 45,000$) and a β light chain ($M_r = 11,000$). The α heavy chain is the polymorphic glycoprotein encoded by the HLA genes. It consists of an NH$_2$-terminal extracellular hydrophilic region, a transmembrane hydrophobic region, and an intracellular hydrophilic region, the COOH-terminus. The extracellular region of the α heavy chain consists of three domains (α_1, α_2, and α_3) based upon its folding and disulfide bonding. Each of these domains contains approximately 90 amino acids. Antigenic specificity resides in the α_1 and α_2 extracellular do-

TABLE 138-1   COMPLETE LISTING OF RECOGNIZED HLA SPECIFICITIES

A	B		C	D	DR			DQ	DP
A1	B5	B47	B77(15)	Cw1	Dw1	DR1	DR13(6)	DR51	DQ1	DPw1
A2	B7	B48	B78	Cw2	Dw2	DR103	DR14(6)	DR52	DQ2	DPw2
A203	B703	B49(21)	B81	Cw3	Dw3	DR2	DR1403	DR53	DQ3	DPw3
A210	B8	B50(21)		Cw4	Dw4	DR3	DR1404		DQ4	DPw4
A3	B12	B51(5)		Cw5	Dw5	DR4	DR15(2)		DQ5(1)	DPw5
A9	B13	B5102		Cw6	Dw6	DR5	DR16(2)		DQ6(1)	DPw6
A10	B14	B5103	Bw4	Cw7	Dw7	DR6	DR17(3)		DQ7(3)	
A11	B15	B52(5)	Bw6	Cw8	Dw8	DR7	DR18(3)		DQ8(3)	
A19	B16	B53		Cw9(w3)	Dw9	DR8			DQ9(3)	
A23(9)	B17	B54(22)		Cw10(w3)	Dw10	DR9				
A24(9)	B18	B55(22)			Dw11(w7)	DR10				
A2403	B21	B56(22)			Dw12	DR11(5)				
A25(10)	B22	B57(17)			Dw13	DR12(5)				
A26(10)	B27	B58(17)			Dw14					
A28	B2708	B59			Dw15					
A29(19)	B35	B60(40)			Dw16					
A30(19)	B37	B61(40)			Dw17(w7)					
A31(19)	B38(16)	B62(15)			Dw18(w6)					
A32(19)	B39(16)	B63(15)			Dw19(w6)					
A33(19)	B3901	B64(14)			Dw20					
A34(10)	B3902	B65(14)			Dw21					
A36	B40	B67			Dw22					
A43	B4005	B70			Dw23					
A66(10)	B41	B71(70)			Dw24v					
A68(28)	B42	B72(70)			Dw25					
A69(28)	B44(12)	B73			Dw26					
A74(19)	B45(12)	B75(15)								
A80	B46	B76(15)								

Numbers in parentheses ( ) indicate the broad antigens for which the adjacent antigen is a split (variant).

mains (see Fig. 138-1b). The β light chain is β_2-microglobulin (β_2M), a nonpolymorphic globular protein encoded by a gene on chromosome 15, which stabilizes the class I molecule on the cell surface.

CLASS II ANTIGENS

The class II antigens also are transmembrane glycoproteins formed by two noncovalently bound protein chains[5]: an α heavy chain ($M_r = 34,000$) and a β light chain ($M_r = 29,000$). Both chains are encoded by genes in the HLA region. Class II HLA molecules, like class I, also consist of an extracellular hydrophilic NH$_2$-terminal region, a hydrophobic transmembrane region, and an intracellular COOH-terminus region. Unlike class I molecules, however, the extracellular region of each chain contains only two domains. The two domains of the α chain are designated α_1 and α_2, and the two domains of the β chain are designated β_1 and β_2. The α chain of HLA-DR is constant for all HLA-DR molecules, while the β chain is polymorphic and determines the specificity of the molecule. Both the α and β chains of HLA-DQ and HLA-DP molecules are polymorphic, although the α chain is less so than the β chain. Polymorphism of class II molecules resides predominantly in the β_1 domain of the β chain. The α_2 and β_2 domains show significant amino acid homology with β_2-microglobulin, α_3 domains of HLA class I molecules, and immunoglobulin constant region domains (see Chap. 85).

STRUCTURE

The crystallization of the HLA-A2 class I antigen and, subsequently, the HLA-DR1 class II antigen, has greatly increased our knowledge of the structure and function of the HLA molecules.[6,7] The first and second α-chain domains of HLA-A2 form an interactive platform composed of a single β-pleated sheet "floor" topped by two α-helical structures with a cleft or groove between the α helices. This interactive

structure is distal to the cell surface and is supported by the α_3 domain of the HLA α heavy chain and the β_2M molecule (Fig. 138-1). The structure of HLA-DR1 is essentially similar to class I HLA molecules. In the case of class II, however, the α_1 domain of the α chain and the β_1 domain of the β chain form the interactive structure of two α helices and β-pleated sheet floor. The tertiary structure of the α_2 and β_2 domains correspond to β_2M and the class I α_3 domain respectively. Polymorphic residues of the HLA class I and class II molecules are predominantly at positions within the α helices and the floor formed by the β-pleated sheet. Antigenic peptide fragments are bound within the groove of the interactive structure for presentation to the T cell receptor[8,9] (see Chap. 86).

TISSUE DISTRIBUTION

HLA antigen expression is especially high on leukocytes. Because of their easy availability, lymphocytes are used to identify HLA types. However, class I, HLA-A, -B, and -C antigens are found on most normal tissues including platelets.[10] Although platelets express class I antigens, they often lack expression of some HLA-B antigens and most HLA-C antigens.[11] There is evidence also that some of the HLA antigens on platelets are absorbed from the plasma.[12] The class II antigens, HLA-DR, -DP, and -DQ, are more restricted in their distribution, being found primarily on B lymphocytes. Class II antigens may be found to a lesser degree on dendritic cells, endothelial cells, monocytes, and macrophages, as well as activated, but not resting, T cells.[5] Expression or increased expression of class II antigens can be induced by treatment with interferon gamma.

FUNCTION OF THE HUMAN LEUKOCYTE ANTIGENS

The function of the class I and class II molecules is to bind peptide fragments that have been derived by the intracellular degradation of

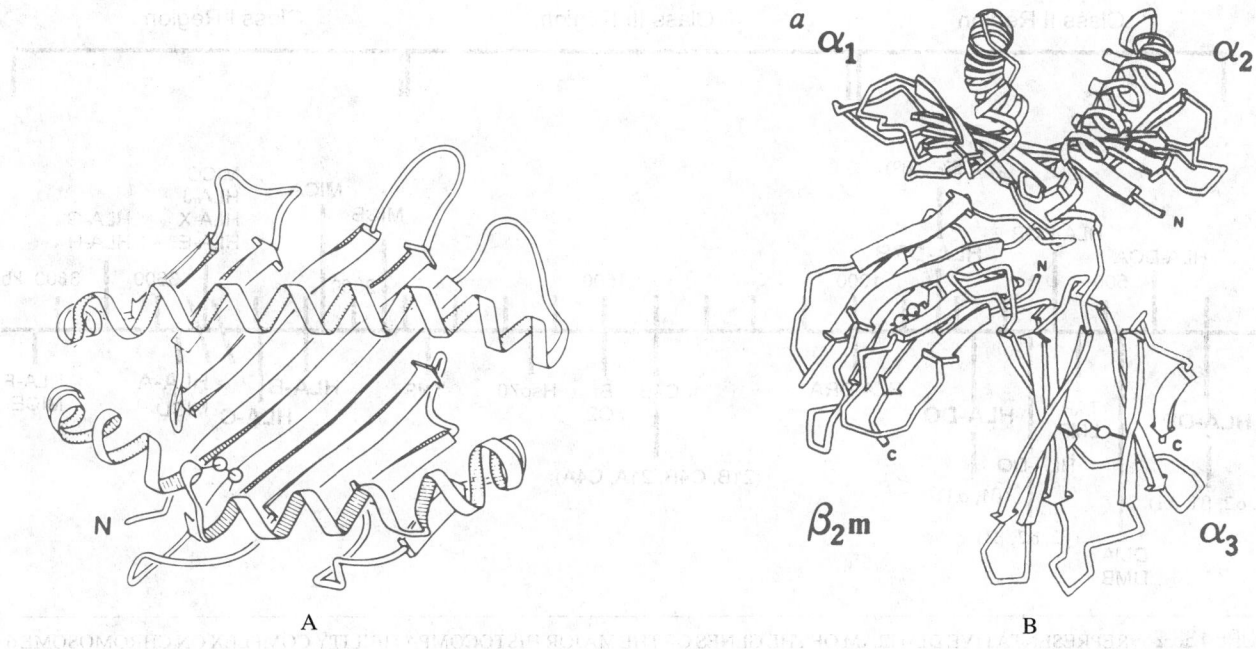

FIGURE 138-1   SCHEMATIC REPRESENTATION OF THE HLA-A2 MOLECULE

(a) The β strands are shown as broad arrows and the α helices as helical ribbons. A "pocket" or "groove" is formed by the α helices and a β-pleated sheet. The former form the rim of the pocket and the latter forms the floor. The groove holds the processed piece of antigen for presentation to the T-cell receptor in the orientation shown. N is the amino-terminus of the chain. (b) Schematic representation of the entire molecule showing the four domains of the molecule, 1 and 3. The α helices are present in the α_1 and α_2 domains. C and N represent the carboxy- and amino-termini of the two chains forming the molecule. (Both diagrams from Bjorkman and colleagues.[6] Reprinted with permission from *Nature* 329:506. Copyright 1987 Macmillan Journals Limited.)

protein antigens and present them to T cells (see Chap. 86). T-cell receptor (TCR) recognition of MHC peptide complexes is restricted by the class of HLA molecule.[13] $CD4^+$ T cells recognize antigen peptides bound by class II molecules, and $CD8^+$ T cells recognize antigen peptides bound by class I molecules (see Chap. 86). Both classes of HLA molecules bind peptide fragments in the groove or cleft formed by the β-pleated sheet floor and the two α helices of the molecule, i.e., the interactive platform[8,9] (Fig. 138-1). The class I binding groove is closed at each end with conserved amino acid residues that bind amino and carbonyl terminal peptide residues. Because the groove is closed-ended, binding peptides are restricted in length to 8 to 11 amino acid residues. The middle portions of binding peptides can bulge out toward the T-cell receptor. The class II binding groove, on the other hand, is open at each end and binds peptides of between 15 to 24 residues in an extended conformation.

Besides presenting antigen to different T-cell subsets and binding peptides of different lengths, class I and class II molecules differ in the source or type of peptide antigen that they present.[14] Class I molecules present peptides derived from endogenous proteins synthesized within the cell (cytosol), e.g., virus-encoded proteins. Class II molecules present peptides derived from exogenous antigens that are ingested by the cell, e.g., bacterial pathogens. Class I molecules are assembled in the endoplasmic reticulum (ER), and peptides must be transported into the ER to bind empty class I molecules. The genes encoding the low-molecular-weight protein (LMP) and transporter-associated-with-antigen processing (TAP) complex map within the MHC complex. The products of these genes function in antigen-peptide production (LMP) and in the transport of peptides into the ER and in the assembly of peptide-class I complexes (TAP). Class I molecules are unstable without bound peptide and can be rapidly degraded. Class

II molecules are also assembled in the ER as multimers of three class II molecules with invariant chain (Ii or CD74) proteins inserted in their grooves. The invariant chain is required in folding, transport, and peptide loading of class II molecules. The invariant protein is cleaved in the endosomes of the endocytic pathway leaving a portion of Ii in the groove (CLIP) that then is exchanged for peptides of digested exogenous antigens. The nonclassical HLA class II molecules encoded by HLA-DM genes facilitate dissociation of the invariant chain peptide, CLIP, and the loading of antigenic peptides in the groove of class II molecules. Class I and class II molecules, with their bound peptides, are subsequently transported to the cell surface.

The polymorphic nature of HLA antigens appears to be related to the need to present a huge array of different antigenic peptides. For both class I and class II molecules, the polymorphic residues clustered in their binding groove determine which antigen peptide fragments can bind. These polymorphic residues are positioned outward toward the TCR or along the α helices and form pockets along the groove that have preferences for certain amino acid side chains of peptides. Such binding pockets create unique environments characteristic of the different class I and class II alleles. As such, the pocket environment determines HLA allele-specific binding motifs and dictates which antigen peptide fragments can be bound.

GENETICS OF THE MAJOR HISTOCOMPATIBILITY COMPLEX

The genes of the major histocompatibility complex encompass a DNA segment of about 4000 kb on the short arm of chromosome 6. Along with genes encoding the HLA antigens are other genes, the protein products of which also play a role in immune responses. The α and β terminology used to describe HLA genes is the same as, but should

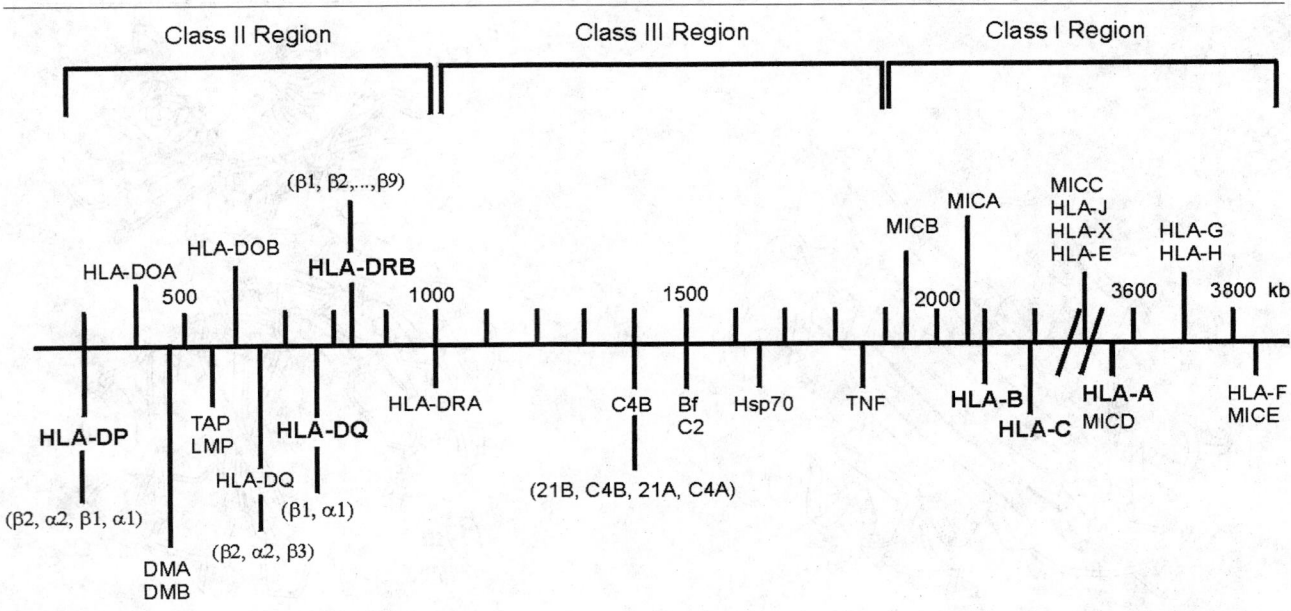

FIGURE 138-2   REPRESENTATIVE DIAGRAM OF THE GENES OF THE MAJOR HISTOCOMPATIBILITY COMPLEX ON CHROMOSOME 6
The centromere is on the left side. See text section entitled "Genetics of the Major Histocompatibility Complex." (Adapted and simplified from Campbell and Trowsdale.[15])

not be confused with, that used to designate the α heavy-chain and β light-chain structural domains of the HLA molecules. The arrangement of genes in the human MHC is depicted in Fig. 138-2.[15]

The MHC is divided into several regions of genes: the class I genes, class II genes, and a set of intervening genes called *class III genes*. The HLA class II loci are the most centromeric and encompass about 1000 kb of DNA. They are ordered sequentially, beginning with the HLA-DP genes (DPβ2, DPα2, DPβ1, and DPα1), followed by the HLA-DQ genes (DQβ2, DQα2, DQβ3, DQβ1, and DQα1), and the HLA-DR genes (DRβ1, DRβ2, DRβ3, DRβ4, DRβ5, DRβ6, DRβ7, DRβ8, DRβ9, and DRα). Genes for complement proteins (C4A, C4B, Bf, C2), 21-hydroxylase deficiency (called *21A* and *21B*), heat shock protein (HsP70), and tumor necrosis factor (TNF) separate the class II region from the class I region.[15] These genes are collectively termed *class III* and encompass about 1000 kb of DNA. The class I genes are the most telomeric covering about 2000 kb of DNA and include, in order from class III, HLA-B, HLA-C, and HLA-A genes. Interspersed within the class I and class II regions are other genes, some involved in antigen processing (LMP), some involved in peptide transport (TAP) and loading (HLA-DMA, HLA-DMB), some that are nonfunctional (i.e., pseudogenes), and some whose functions await elucidation. The currently recognized HLA genes are presented in Table 138-2.

Class I antigens are encoded by a single α chain gene at each locus, i.e., HLA-A, HLA-B, and HLA-C. Class II antigens are encoded by one α chain gene and one β chain gene. Genetic polymorphism is found in both the α and β chains of HLA-DP and HLA-DQ, although to a lesser degree in the α chain. All detected serologic specificities, however, appear to reside on the β chain. The HLA-DR molecules are unique in that the product of one α chain gene, which is not polymorphic, combines with any one of the products of the four functional β chain genes, i.e., DRB1, DRB3, DRB4, DRB5, to generate class II molecules that have different serological specificities. All HLA-DR antigens except DR51, DR52, and DR53 arise from polymorphism in the DRB1 gene. Most individuals express two β-chain gene products per chromosome or haplotype, one from DRB1 and another

from DRB3, DRB4, or DRB5. Exceptions are individuals with the DR1, DR103, DR10, and DR8 antigens in whom only the DRB1 gene is expressed. The DR51, DR52, and DR53 serological specificities are encoded by the DRB5, DRB3, and DRB4 genes respectively. Different combinations of DRB1 alleles and DRB3, DRB4, or DRB5 are expressed depending on the haplotype. DRB3 (DR52) is found on haplotypes with the DRB1 alleles encoding DR3, DR5, DR6, DR11, DR12, DR13, DR14, DR1403, DR1404, DR17, and DR18. DRB4 (DR53) is found with the DRB1 alleles encoding DR4, DR7, and DR9. DRB5 is found with DRB1 alleles encoding DR2, DR15, and DR16.

With the presence of genes that encode complement components or molecules involved in antigen processing (LMP1 and LMP7) or peptide transport into the endoplasmic reticulum (TAP1, TAP2), the MHC is a complex of genes that encode molecules that are immunologically relevant.

NOMENCLATURE

It is important to distinguish polymorphic variations that are defined serologically or by cellular assay from those that are defined by molecular techniques. Serologically and cellularly defined entities are designated as specificities or antigens, while the terms *gene* and *allele* are reserved for loci defined by nucleic acid analyses.[16] As new loci, genes, alleles, and antigens within the MHC are recognized, the terminology used is standardized by the World Health Organization through an HLA Nomenclature Committee. The reports of this committee describe the naming of new HLA genes, alleles, and serological specificities.[3,16] The most recent report also contains complete lists of all the accepted genes and alleles, as well as the serologically and cellularly defined specificities.[3] The number of MHC class I and class II gene alleles are too numerous to include here as they currently number over 900 (Table 138-3). The DNA-based, serologic-based, or cellular-based terminology is acceptable for use. Cellular terminology is used infrequently. Table 138-4 provides a comparison of serologic and DNA-based terminology.

TABLE 138-2   NAMES FOR GENES IN THE HLA REGION

NAME	PRODUCT
Class I genes:	
HLA-A	Class I α chain
HLA-B	Class I α chain
HLA-C	Class I α chain
HLA-E	Associated with class I fragment
HLA-F	Associated with class I fragment
HLA-G	Associated with class I fragment
HLA-H	Class I pseudogene
HLA-J	Class I pseudogene
HLA-K	Class I pseudogene
HLA-L	Class I pseudogene
Class II genes:	
HLA-DRA	DR α chain
HLA-DRB1	DR β1 chain determining specificities DR1, DR2, DR3, etc.
HLA-DRB2	Pseudogene with DR β-like sequences
HLA-DRB3	DR β3 chain determining DR52 and Dw24, Dw25, Dw26 specificities
HLA-DRB4	DR β4 chain determining DR53
HLA-DRB5	DR β5 chain determining DR51
HLA-DRB6	DRB pseudogene found with DR1, DR2, DR10
HLA-DRB7	DRB pseudogene found with DR4, DR7, DR9
HLA-DRB8	DRB pseudogene found with DR4, DR7, DR9
HLA-DRB9	DRB pseudogene, isolated fragment
HLA-DQA1	DQ α chain as expressed
HLA-DQB1	DQ β chain as expressed
HLA-DQA2	DQ α-chain-related sequence, not expressed
HLA-DQB2	DQ β-chain-related sequence, not expressed
HLA-DQB3	DQ β-chain-related sequence, not expressed
HLA-DOA	DO α chain
HLA-DOB	DO β chain
HLA-DMA	DM α chain
HLA-DMB	DM β chain
HLA-DPA1	DP α chain as expressed
HLA-DPB1	DP β chain as expressed
HLA-DPA2	DP α-chain-related pseudogene
HLA-DPB2	DP β-chain-related pseudogene
Other:	
TAP1	ABC (ATP binding cassette) transporter
TAP2	ABC (ATP binding cassette) transporter
LMP2	Protease-related sequence
LMP7	Protease-related sequence
MICA	Class I chain-related gene
MICB	Class I chain-related gene
MICC	Class I chain-related pseudogene
MICD	Class I chain-related pseudogene
MICE	Class I chain-related pseudogene

Adapted from Bodmer and coworkers.[3]

The HLA-A and HLA-B antigens were defined, and many antigens were named before it was recognized that the MHC is a multilocus system. Instead of changing the numbers already assigned to accepted antigens, subsequent HLA-A and HLA-B specificities and alleles continue to be numbered jointly as if they were products of a single locus, e.g., A34, B35, A36, B37. For all other HLA loci, alleles and specificities are numbered consecutively within that locus, e.g., Cw1, Cw2, etc., DR1, DR2, etc., DQ1, DQ2, etc.

GENES ENCODING HUMAN LEUKOCYTE ANTIGENS

New class I region genes are designated HLA followed by a letter in alphabetical order omitting *D*; e.g., HLA-E, HLA-F, etc. All class II genes are designated *D* followed by a letter that identifies a locus that is defined by location within the class II region of the chromosome and by the similarity of its genes, e.g., HLA-DQ, HLA-DP, etc. The locus letter is followed by the letters A or B for alpha (α) or beta (β) chain genes, and the A and B are followed by a number where there

TABLE 138-3   NUMBER OF ACCEPTED HLA ALLELES

REGION	LOCUS	NUMBER OF ALLELES
Class I		
HLA-A	A	133
HLA-B	B	275
HLA-C	Cw	77
Class II		
HLA-DR	DRB1	222
	DRB3	19
	DRB4	9
	DRB5	14
HLA-DQ	DQA1	20
	DQB1	41
HLA-DP	DPA1	17
	DPB1	85

SOURCE: references.[3,16–19]

are more than one α or β chain gene to a locus, e.g., DQA1, DQB1, DQA2, DQB2, etc. (see Table 138-2 and Fig. 138-2).

HLA ALLELES

New alleles of HLA genes are recognized through DNA sequencing of at least several clones. Alleles are designated using the gene name, e.g. DRB1, followed by an asterik (*), followed by a four-digit number. The first two digits of the number identify any previously characterized antigen, and the latter two digits identify the allele/variant. This method was chosen to maintain as much as possible the relationship between alleles and serologic specificities. As an example, *DRB1*1201* designates an allele of the protein formerly defined serologically as DR12, which itself was a serologically defined variant (split) of DR5. There are currently seven alleles that have been identified as associated with DR12. As new alleles of a gene are sequenced and accepted, they are numbered consecutively. In some cases a five-digit number is assigned to an allele. The fifth digit indicates that alleles have different DNA nucleotide sequences, but their amino acid sequences, and thus the proteins, expressed are the same. Examples of this are the DRB1*12021 and DRB1*12022 alleles.

FREQUENCIES AND RACIAL DISTRIBUTION OF HUMAN LEUKOCYTE ANTIGENS

Different races and ethnic groups can vary greatly in the frequency with which HLA antigens are found.[20,21] For example, HLA-A36 and -B42 are infrequent in Caucasians as compared to other ethnic groups. Similarly, HLA-B46, although found in other populations, has a high frequency among Asians. Similar racial or ethnic differences continue to be noted using molecular techniques.[21]

TABLE 138-4   COMPARISON OF HLA TERMINOLOGY FOR TYPING RESOLUTION

Serologic typing/antigen level
  HLA-A1, B8, Cw1, DR17, DR52, DQ2
Molecular typing
  Low resolution: gene group
    HLA-A*01, B*08, Cw*01, DRB1*03, DRB3*02, DQB1*02
  High Resolution: allele level
    HLA-A*0101, B*0801, Cw*0102, DRB1*0301, DRB3*0201, DQB1*0201
  Intermediate resolution: multiple but limited alleles*
    Class I   HLA-A*0101/0102, B*0801/0802/0803, Cw*0101/0102
    Class II HLA-DRB1*0301/0304,DRB3*0201/0202, DQB1*0201/0203

*The National Marrow Donor Program (NMDP) has established codes to identify multiple allelic possibilities in an effort to facilitate selection of possible marrow donors. For example, HLA-A*0101/0102 = HLA-A*01AB and DRB1*0301/0304 = DRB1*03AD. (www.marrow-donor.org).

HLA TYPING

Tissue typing for HLA antigens can be performed using a number of methods of varying degrees of sophistication and complexity, e.g., mixed lymphocyte culture (MLC), primed lymphocyte test, cytotoxic T lymphocyte (CTL) clones, 2-dimensional electrophoresis, isoelectric focusing, protein sequencing, and molecular assays. The most frequent procedures used in the clinical laboratory have been serological and cellular assays. However, with the advent of the polymerase chain reaction (PCR) (see Chap. 11), DNA-based typing is becoming common for class I and class II. It has essentially replaced cellular assays for the definition of HLA-DR, -DQ, and -DP (i.e., HLA-D) and, in some laboratories, has replaced serological testing completely.

SEROLOGY

Serological specificities (antigens) are recognized only if the serological reagents identify products encoded by accepted allelic DNA sequences. For example, the newer serological specificities of HLA-A2, corresponding to the allele sequences HLA-A*0203 and HLA-A*0210, are designated as HLA-A203 and HLA-A210. Similarly, the class II serologic specificity that is the product of the DRB1*0103 allele is designated DR103. Since new serological specificities are based on a correlation with an identified DNA sequence, the designation w for workshop or provisional characterization has been dropped. Exceptions to this rule are: HLA-C locus specificities, to avoid confusion with complement components, the Dw and DP specificities, defined by mixed lymphocyte reaction or the primed lymphocyte test, and Bw4 and Bw6, to distinguish them from other B locus specificities. Bw4 and Bw6 are public antigens (i.e., epitopes or serological specificities) defined by amino acid residues at positions 79, 80, and 83 on the class I α chain.[22] Public antigens are epitopes shared by multiple HLA antigens. All HLA-B α chains carry either Bw4 or Bw6, and a few HLA-A α chains carry Bw4.

The microcytotoxicity test has been the fundamental tissue typing procedure used for defining HLA antigens for over 30 years.[23] In this assay a suspension of lymphocytes is incubated with human alloantisera in a microtiter tray.[24] Rabbit serum is added as a source of complement. Cell death is measured microscopically and determined by the uptake of a vital dye or by immunofluorescence. Antibody panels generally consist of two to four sera that recognize the same specificity. This requires that patients be tested with about 150 different reagents for class I and another 80 to 150 reagents for class II. Antisera are usually obtained from multiparous women and multiply transfused individuals or can be obtained from patients who have rejected allografts. Monoclonal HLA antibodies are used occasionally along with human alloantisera. Serology for HLA-DR and -DQ requires enrichment for B lymphocytes. In addition, many antisera contain reactivity to class I antigens as well as to HLA-DR and -DQ. Before being used as anti–class II reagents, such sera must be absorbed with cells that express only class I antigens (e.g., platelets). HLA-DP antigens also may be characterized by monoclonal antibodies, although these antigens are generally not included in clinical serological typing. Serologic definition of HLA antigens is important for patients destined to receive repeated platelet transfusions. It also is important in typing patients and donors for solid organ transplantation and in the initial investigation of families of patients desiring marrow or stem cell transplantation.

CELLULAR ASSAYS

The HLA-D region of the MHC, i.e., HLA-DR, -DQ, and -DP, was initially identified by the capacity to stimulate allogeneic T cells in a mixed lymphocyte reaction.[25] Initially HLA-D was thought to be a separate locus. Although no molecule could be associated with HLA-D, a large number of HLA-D specificities have been recognized (Table 138-1). It is now clear that HLA-Dw specificity is the cumulative effect of allogeneic differences of multiple class II molecules.

Mixed Lymphocyte Reaction A mixed lymphocyte reaction involves coculturing for several days the stimulator cells from one individual with the responder lymphocytes from another. Stimulator cells are prevented from proliferating by irradiation or exposure to mitomycin C. The responder cells that recognize alloantigens expressed by stimulator cells are induced to proliferate. Stimulator cells are B cells and monocytes, i.e., antigen presenting cells. T lymphocytes are responding cells. A radioactive nucleotide, usually ³H-thymidine, is added during the last 6 to 18 h of culture to measure newly synthesized DNA. The amount of radioactive thymidine incorporated into the DNA of responder cells is generally proportional to the degree of HLA-D disparity between responder and stimulator cells. The average degree of stimulation between cells from family members that share one HLA-D haplotype is roughly half that found between cells from family members that differ for both HLA-D haplotypes. Cells from family members that share both HLA-D haplotypes, e.g., HLA identical siblings, ordinarily do not stimulate each other. Similarly, the cells from nonrelated individuals who share both HLA-D haplotypes generally stimulate each other minimally if at all.

HLA-Dw specificities are identified with the use of homozygous typing cells.[26] Homozygous typing cells (HTC) are obtained from progeny of consanguineous marriages who have inherited identical chromosomal HLA-D regions from each parent and are homozygous for all HLA-D region loci (DR, DQ, and DP). HTC do not stimulate cells from individuals who have the same HLA-D haplotype. However, they stimulate and respond to cells from individuals who are HLA-D heterozygous or fully disparate from them (see Table 138-5). Unfortunately, MLR testing for patients with hematological malignancies are often not successful, as leukemic cells generally are poor stimulators in the MLR with responder cells from almost any donor.

The results of an MLR are shown in Table 138-5. Data can be expressed as (1) gross counts per minute; (2) a stimulation index, i.e., the ratio of $A + B_x$, to $A + A_x$, where A is the responding cell and A_x and B_x are irradiated stimulating cells; or (3) a relative response, or the percentage of the maximum stimulation observed when a cell is tested against cells from an unrelated panel. Controls include cultures of cell A, A_x, B, B_x, each responder cell population alone, and cells from two unrelated individuals to gauge the ability of cells A and B to respond to and stimulate allogeneic cells.

MLR response does not require prior sensitization of the responding individual and is an in vitro measure of an in vivo allograft response. Thus, MLR measures the biological effect of multiple proteins that are intimately involved in immune response. Other biological in vitro correlates of an allograft response include the PLT and CTL assays. CTL are generated in an MLR and are the effectors of a cellular allograft response.

Primed Lymphocyte Test HLA-DP antigens were classified originally using the PLT.[27] PLT is a secondary MLR. Lymphocytes primed to antigen during an initial MLR will respond only to the priming antigen in a secondary MLR.

Although the CTL assay can be used to identify specificities and help to assess the degree of risk of allograft rejection or, graft-versus-host disease in stem-cell transplantation, it is a time-consuming and complex assay that normally is used in research laboratories.

MOLECULAR TYPING

The development of the polymerase chain reaction has radically changed the approach to HLA typing[28,29] (see Chap. 11). A number of DNA-based methods can be used in HLA typing, e.g., sequence-specific primer amplification (SSP), sequence-specific oligonucleotide

TABLE 138-5   IDENTIFICATION OF HLA-D ANTIGENS BY USE OF HOMOZYGOUS TYPING CELLS

| | | | | Stimulating Cells | | | | | |
RESPONDING CELL	FATHER$_M$*	MOTHER$_M$	CHILD1$_M$	CHILD2$_M$	CHILD5$_M$	Dw3 HTC$_M$	Dw5 HTC$_M$	Dw2 HTC$_M$	Dw6 HTC$_M$
Father(ab)†	810‡	18,450	5,140	5,400	6,800	930	750	16,700	17,750
Mother(cd)	9,250	520	3,210	2,900	3,500	8,600	9,740	640	550
Child 1(ac)	3,400	4,600	440	640	9,980	650	9,345	375	10,650
Child 2(ac)	4,100	4,800	550	550	8,760	675	8,600	460	11,120
Child 5(bd)	2,350	2,300	8,260	7,550	345	8,840	320	11,550	575

*The subscript M indicates mitomycin-treated stimulating cell.
†Genotype code.
‡Counts per minute.

probe hybridization (SSOP), restriction fragment length polymorphism (RFLP), single stranded conformational polymorphism (SSCP), heteroduplex formation, and nucleotide sequencing. All involve the amplification from genomic DNA of selected portions of HLA genes with appropriate oligonucleotide primer pairs. Generally, exons 3 and 4 of class I genes and exon 2 of class II genes are amplified. These exons are the gene fragments encoding most of the polymorphisms of the class I and class II molecules. The most common methods currently in use for HLA typing are SSP and SSOP. In typing by SSOP, genomic DNA is isolated and amplified with oligonucleotide primer pairs specific for HLA gene fragments. The amplified DNA is then analyzed using a panel of oligonucleotide probes that hybridize with specific nucleotide sequences present in the amplified gene fragment. Oligonucleotide probes are labeled either with a radioactive isotope (usually ^{32}P) or with a nonradioactive label such as biotin-avidin. Either amplified DNA is immobilized on a solid support, i.e., nylon membrane or plastic disk, and labeled probes are added (hybridization), or unlabeled probes are linked to the solid support, and amplified DNA, which is labeled during PCR, is added (reverse hybridization). Successful hybridization results in a detectable ''dot'' or band (see Figure 138-3a). Typing by SSP requires multiple independent PCR reactions. Genomic DNA is isolated and added to a panel of oligonucleotide primer pairs. Each primer pair has specificity for certain nucleotide sequences within the selected exon(s) of the HLA genes. A PCR is performed, and the resulting amplified products are analyzed by gel electrophoresis. Assignment of HLA type (i.e., genes and alleles) is based on the presence or absence of amplified product (as a band) from each reaction (see Fig. 138-3b). As with serological typing, the HLA type of the test sample is determined by the pattern with which the amplified gene fragments hybridize with the panel of different probes (SSOP) or by the pattern of products amplified in SSP.

DNA-based typing of HLA is generally performed at two levels, the first using reagents (probes or primer pairs) that detect all alleles of an HLA gene (low resolution), the second using reagents with specificity for selected alleles (high resolution). Low-resolution typing identifies the HLA gene at the serological or antigen level, e.g., HLA-A*02, HLA-DRB1*01, etc. High-resolution typing identifies specific alleles, e.g., HLA-A*0201, DRB1*0103, etc. A third level is called intermediate resolution. In intermediate resolution, more than one allele of an HLA gene could be the correct one, e.g., DRB1*0302/0303/0304/0309 (see Table 138-4). If primers or probes are unavailable, and if it is necessary to clarify the specific allele, then nucleotide sequencing of amplified product can be done. Although nucleotide sequencing is thought by many to be the definitive method, it is costly, time consuming and, as yet, a more common method in research laboratories.

Molecular typing has revealed greater polymorphism in the genes encoding HLA antigens than was previously detected.[3] For example, there are multiple alleles at HLA loci each encoding a molecule with the same serologic specificity, e.g., the HLA-A2 serologic specificity is associated with more than 20 HLA-A2 alleles. Molecular typing has also elucidated the origin of the class II public antigens, HLA-DR51, -DR52, and -DR53. Unlike the Bw4 and Bw6 class I public antigens that are due to amino acid substitutions on the class I α chain, separate DRB genes encode the HLA-DR51, -DR52, and -DR53 antigens. Furthermore, DNA-based typing has helped to reveal the relationship of HLA-DR, -DQ, and -DP to HLA-Dw specificities. For example, HLA-DR4 appeared to be one antigen, even though it was associated with several different HLA-Dw specificities. To date, 32 alleles of DR4 have been identified by molecular analysis, and each of the Dw specificities identified for DR4 is associated with a specific DR4 allele.

The use of molecular testing has a number of advantages over serologic typing. First, DNA-based typing does not require the isolation of viable lymphocyte populations but can be done using any nucleated cell source. Second, DNA-based assays have increased accuracy and specificity. HLA antigens have a high degree of homogeneity, and alloantisera produced against them can be cross-reactive. This cross-reactivity can lead to inconsistent assignment of individual specificities.

INHERITANCE OF HLA ANTIGENS

The genes of the MHC demonstrate more polymorphism than any other genetic system, i.e., multiple alleles exist for each locus. Each individual, however, has one allele for each locus per chromosome and, therefore, encodes two HLA antigens per locus. Additionally, the antigens at each HLA locus are codominant, i.e., each is expressed independently of the other. The identification of each HLA antigen of an individual is called a phenotype. Two unrelated individuals who express the same HLA antigens are HLA-phenotype identical.

Since HLA genes are closely linked on chromosome 6, recombination within the MHC is rare (less than or equal to 1 percent), and a complete set of HLA genes is usually inherited from each parent as a unit. The genes inherited from one parent are referred to as a haplotype. Maternal and paternal haplotypes can be identified through family studies. Identification of both the paternal and the maternal haplotypes in an individual provides a genotype. Siblings who inherit the same haplotypes are termed HLA-identical. Those who inherit the same haplotype from one parent but a different haplotype from the other parent are called haplo-identical. Lastly, siblings who inherit different haplotypes from each parent are HLA nonidentical. In general, family studies consist of testing for the HLA-A, -B, -C, -DR, and -DQ antigens to identify haplotypes and to rule out genetic recombination within the MHC complex. Since HLA genes are inherited together on a single chromosome, there are four possible combinations of maternal and paternal haplotypes, provided that there is no meiotic recombination between HLA genes (see Fig. 138-4). Thus, there is a

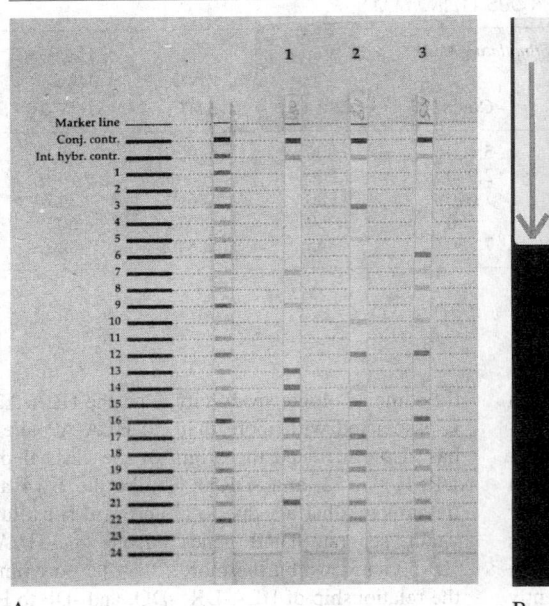
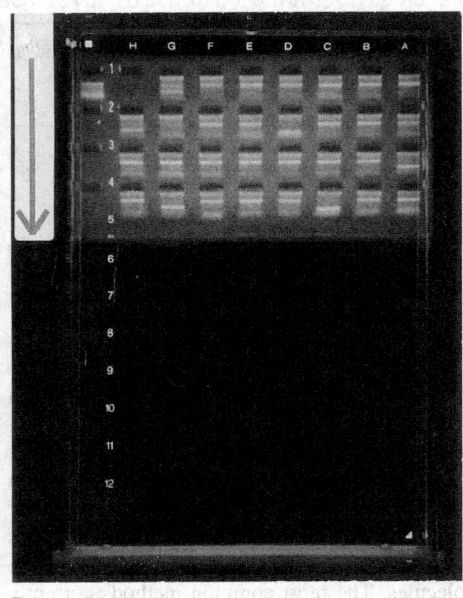

A   B

FIGURE 138-3   EXAMPLES OF SSOP AND SSP DNA-BASED TYPING

(a) SSOP: In this example, probes specific for HLA-DPB1 alleles are immobilized on nylon strips. Genomic DNA isolated from three individuals was added to oligonucleotide primer pairs that amplify all DPB1 alleles and incorporate a label into the DNA during PCR. Visible bands indicate specific hybridization of amplified DNA fragments with selected probes. The left most column identifies controls and individual probe locations on the strip. The next column is a graphical representation of the expected (typical) intensity of hybridization with each probe. Each numbered strip represents the hybridization of amplified DNA fragments from each individual with specific probes. The pattern of hybridization for the individual tested on strip 1 indicates the presence of the DPB1*0201 and DPB1*1001 alleles. The patterns of hybridization on strips 2 and 3 indicate the presence of the DPB1*2201 and DPB1*3101 alleles and the DPB1*0301 and DPB1*0401 alleles respectively. (b) SSP: This is an example of low-resolution SSP typing on one individual for class II. Isolated genomic DNA was added to a panel of oligonucleotide primer pairs specific for DRB1, DRB3, DRB4, DRB5, or DQB1 alleles. Each mixture also contains a primer pair that amplifies a non-HLA DNA nucelotide sequence that is common to all individuals as a positive control for amplification. Following PCR, each reaction mixture was analyzed by gel electrophoresis. The various bands seen at each position and moving in the direction of electrophoresis are:

- Unamplified genomic DNA (>1000 bp)
- Positive amplification control (~700 bp)—not always seen when there is a specific product
- Specific product (~75–350 bp)—Seen only in those wells that amplify the sample's alleles, i.e., 1G, 2H, 2D, 3A, 4G, 4C
- Primer dimers (usually <75 bp)—result from primer excess, and the primers form a dimer with each other. Not always seen, but some may be very bright.

Position 1H contains a negative control consisting of appropriate primer pairs but no added genomic DNA. The bands to the left of position 1H is a marker consisting of different size DNA fragments to help determine base pair product size. Analysis of the pattern of amplified specific products identify the class II type of this individual as HLA-DRB1*01, DRB1*04; DRB4*01; DQB1*03, DQB1*05, or, in serological terms, HLA-DR1, DR4; DR53; DQ3, DQ5.

1 in 4 (or 25 percent) chance that two siblings will be HLA-identical, a 2 in 4 (or 50 percent) chance that two siblings will be HLA haplo-identical and, a 1 in 4 (or 25 percent) chance that two siblings will be HLA nonidentical. All progeny are haplo-identical with their parents unless recombination has occurred.

LINKAGE DISEQUILIBRIUM

Because HLA is so highly polymorphic, the chance that two unrelated individuals would be HLA identical could be astronomical. However, the situation is somewhat alleviated because the HLA system displays a phenomenon known as *linkage disequilibrium*. That is, certain HLA alleles are inherited together on the same chromosome more often than would be predicted if HLA loci were at equilibrium. At equilibrium the

frequency of an allele at one locus is independent of the frequencies of alleles at linked loci. For example, the gene frequency of HLA-A1 in North American Caucasians is 0.138 and that of HLA-B8 is 0.09. If there were no preferential association between HLA-A1 and HLA-B8, then the frequency of the HLA-A1, B8 haplotype, predicted by equilibrium, should be 0.0124 (0.138 × 0.09 = 0.0124). However, population studies show that the actual frequency of the HLA-A1, B8 haplotype in this particular population is greater than that predicted by equilibrium, i.e., 0.0609. The degree of linkage disequilibrium is defined as the observed frequency minus its expected frequency, 0.0485 in this example. Although the particular alleles that are found in linkage disequilibria differ for various racial groups, all racial groups display significant disequilibria.

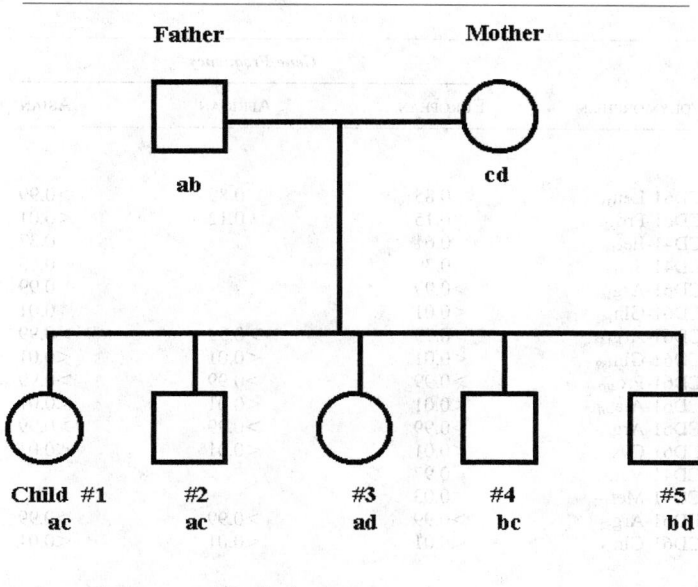

FIGURE 138-4 Representation of the inheritance of HLA. Each of the four parental chromosomes (haplotypes) is coded by a letter: *a* and *b* represent the paternal haplotypes; *c* and *d* represent the maternal haplotypes. Each child inherits one paternal haplotype (*a* or *b*) and one maternal haplotype (*c* or *d*).

CLINICAL APPLICATIONS

The HLA genes and antigens of the major histocompatibility complex play a central role in transplantation, in the regulation of immune responses, and in susceptibility to a variety of diseases. The most common application of HLA, however, is in the field of transplantation. In both solid organ and stem-cell transplantation, allografts from HLA-identical sibling donors have a significantly greater chance for survival than grafts from nonmatched family, or unrelated, donors. For solid organ transplantation, a living donor is not always available or even feasible, e.g., for heart transplantation. HLA matching is restricted to the HLA-A, -B, and -DR loci, and the level of typing is at the serologic (antigen) level or low resolution for DNA-based methods. Initially, a high degree of HLA match between potential recipients and unrelated donors was sought. However, with the increasing need for more organs and the advent of newer immunosuppressive therapies, such as cyclosporine, the level of HLA matching has declined, and some question whether HLA matching is necessary. Nonetheless, even with the newer immunosuppressive drugs, the long-term survival of allografts from HLA-matched donors exceeds that of HLA-mismatched donors.[30] Additionally, recipients of HLA-matched organs have fewer rejection episodes and fewer complications and may require less immunosuppression.

Blood or marrow stem-cell transplantation engenders problems other than allograft survival. Lymphocytes within the graft may recognize host cells as foreign. Without the ability to mount a response to such host reactive cells, patients receiving stem-cell allografts are prone to graft-versus-host disease[31,32]; see Chap. 19. With HLA-identical sibling donors, disease-free survival of 80 to 90 percent can be achieved for some malignant and nonmalignant hematological disorders.[32] However, less than 30 percent of individuals have an HLA-

identical sibling. Thus, alternative donors, such as phenotypically matched unrelated volunteers and partially matched family members, must be considered. However, the risks and incidence of graft failure and GVHD are higher than seen with HLA-identical siblings and increase with increased HLA disparity. Fortunately, molecular typing has improved the accuracy of matching unrelated donors, allowing for improved outcomes.

The HLA criteria for the selection of an appropriate stem-cell donor varies from transplant center to transplant center and, within a center, also will depend on the transplant protocol. Within families, typing for HLA-A, -B, -DR, and -DQ at the serologic or DNA-based low-resolution level is generally sufficient to identify all haplotypes, potential recombinants, and HLA-identical pairs. In those circumstances where the haplotypes are unclear, DNA-based, allele-level typing is recommended. For unrelated volunteer donors, allele-level molecular typing of HLA-A, -B, -C, -DR, and -DQ provides the best opportunity for a successful outcome and reduced GVHD. The World Marrow Donor Association (WMDA) published guidelines for the extent of HLA typing recommended for transplant centers and donor registries that participate in the exchange of stem cells for allogeneic transplantation.[33] Briefly, the WMDA recommends typing the HLA-A, -B, and -DR loci using DNA-based testing at the low-resolution level at a minimum.

PLATELET ANTIGENS

Platelets express antigens that can be recognized by autoantibodies or by antibodies made by recipients of platelet transfusions. HLA antigens are present on platelets, as judged by absorption, fluorescence, and complement fixation. In addition, platelets also possess platelet-specific antigens that are unrelated to erythrocyte or leukocyte isoantigens (see Chap. 14).

Platelet antigens can be targeted by autoantibodies, resulting in immune thrombocytopenia. A dominant platelet antigen recognized by the autoantibodies by many patients with autoimmune thrombocytopenia is the platelet glycoprotein GIIb/IIIa (otherwise called $\alpha_{IIb}\beta_3$ or CD41/CD61), although other platelet glycoproteins also may be targeted by autoantibodies.[34,35] This condition is discussed in Chap. 119.

PLATELET ALLOANTIGENS

Platelet alloantigens, also referred to as *platelet isoantigens*, are substances that induce the production of alloantibodies when platelets bearing such antigens are infused into patients who lack the specific alloantigen.[36] Immune responses to platelet alloantigens are involved in the pathogenesis of several clinical syndromes including neonatal alloimmune thrombocytopenia, posttransfusion purpura, and refractory responses to platelet transfusion.[37] In addition, immune thrombocytopenia can be an unusual complication of a type of graft-versus-host disease in which donor lymphocytes make alloantibodies specific for the platelets produced by the recipient of an organ allograft.[38]

Patients can lack a particular platelet-associated antigen altogether because they have defective alleles of the gene encoding the antigen (see Chap. 121). Such patients can make antibodies against platelets of virtually all donors that bear the platelet-associated antigen. For example, patients with Bernard-Soulier syndrome, who lack platelet GPIb-V-IX, or patients with Glanzmann thrombasthenia, who lack expression of GPIIb (CD41) and GPIIIa (CD61), can be induced to make broadly reactive antiplatelet antibodies[39,40] (see Chap. 121). Also, several percent of Japanese and approximately 0.3 percent of Caucasians are deficient in CD36, one of the major platelet glycoproteins of platelets that also is known as *GPIV*.[41] Because these patients lack a platelet antigen, they can develop antiplatelet antibodies specific for

TABLE 138-6   HUMAN PLATELET ANTIGENS

ALLOANTIGEN	CLASSIC NAME	PLATELET GLYCOPROTEIN	POLYMORPHISM	Gene Frequency		
				EUROPEAN	AFRICAN	ASIAN
GPIIb/GPIIIa ($\alpha_{IIb}\beta_3$) (CD41/CD61)						
HPA-1a	PI^{A1}, Zw^a	GPIIIa (β_3)	CD61-Leu$_{33}$	0.85	0.89	>0.99
HPA-1b	PI^{A2}, Zw^b	GPIIIa (β_3)	CD61-Pro$_{33}$	0.15	0.12	<0.01
HPA-3a	Bak^a, Lek^a	GPIIb (α_{IIb})	CD41-Ile$_{843}$	0.61		0.37
HPA-3b	Bak^b	GPIIb (α_{IIb})	CD41-Ser$_{843}$	0.39		0.63
HPA-4a	Pen^a, Yuk^b	GPIIIa (β_3)	CD61-Arg$_{185}$	>0.99		0.99
HPA-4b	Pen^b, Yuk^a	GPIIIa (β_3)	CD61-Gln$_{143}$	<0.01		0.01
HPA-6a		GPIIIa (β_3)	CD61-Arg$_{143}$	>0.99	>0.99	>0.99
HPA-6b	Ca, Tu	GPIIIa (β_3)	CD61-Gln$_{489}$	<0.01	<0.01	<0.01
HPA-7a		GPIIIa (β_3)	CD61-Pro$_{407}$	>0.99	>0.99	>0.99
HPA-7b	Mo	GPIIIa (β_3)	CD61-Ala$_{407}$	<0.01	<0.01	<0.01
HPA-8a		GPIIIa (β^3)	CD61-Arg$_{636}$	>0.99	>0.99	>0.99
HPA-8b	Sr^a	GPIIIa (β_3)	CD61-Cys$_{636}$	<0.01	<0.01	<0.01
HPA-9a	Max^a	GPIIb (α_{IIb})	CD41-Val$_{837}$	0.97		
HPA-9b	Max^b	GPIIb (α_{IIb})	CD41-Met$_{837}$	0.03		
HPA-10a	La^b	GPIIIa (β_3)	CD61-Arg$_{62}$	>0.99	>0.99	>0.99
HPA-10b	La^a	GPIIIa (β_3)	CD61-Gln$_{62}$	<0.01	<0.01	<0.01
GPIa/IIa ($\alpha_2\beta_1$) (CD49b/CD29)						
HPA-5a	Br^b Zav^b Hc^a	GPIa (α_2)	CD49b-Glu$_{505}$	0.89	0.79	0.97
HPA-5b	Br^a Zav^a Hc^b	GPIa (α_2)	CD49b-Lys$_{505}$	0.11	0.21	0.03
GPIb-IX-V (CD42/CD42d)						
HPA-2a	Ko^b Sib^b	GPIbα	CD42b-Thr$_{145}$	0.93	0.82	0.92
HPA-2b	Ko^a Sib^a	GPIbα	CD42b-Met$_{145}$	0.07	0.18	0.08

The glycoprotein associated with the alloantigen and the HPA alloantigens are listed in the far-left column. In the column marked *classic name* are the terms used prior to the HPA system for designating the alloantigen. The platelet glycoproteins on which maps the alloantigen are listed in the column labeled *platelet glycoprotein*. The column marked *polymorphism* lists the protein via the CD designation (see Chap. 14) followed by the three-letter code for the amino acid residue found at the polymorphic position (indicated in subscript). The gene frequencies for the major ethnic groups in the United States are listed in the columns marked *European, African,* or *Asian*. Listed are the approximate gene frequencies calculated from several different surveys (see text).

the deficient platelet protein after receiving transfusions of platelets from normal donors or after pregnancy.

More commonly, platelet-specific alloantigens result from genetic polymorphism in genes encoding functional platelet proteins.[36,42] These alloantigens first were defined by antiplatelet antibodies discovered in the sera of multiparous females who gave birth to infants with neonatal thrombocytopenia. Many of these subsequently were found to recognize allotypic determinants of platelet-associated membrane glycoproteins, such as GPIIb/IIIa (CD41/CD61). Each of these allotypic determinants may be generated by only a single amino acid substitution in a major platelet-associated glycoprotein (Table 138-6).[43] However, it is possible that glycosylation may contribute to or influence the expression of certain HPA epitopes, such as those associated with human platelet antigen 3 (HPA-3).[44] In any case, these amino acid substitutions generally do not appear to affect the function of platelets in vitro. However, it is conceivable that the genetic polymorphism in platelet glycoproteins may be associated with more subtle differences in platelet physiology that can contribute to the relative risk for thrombosis and/or atherosclerosis.[45–47]

A nomenclature for the human platelet alloantigens was adopted to replace the old complex "classical" nomenclatures that previously were developed independently in laboratories throughout the world (see Table 138-6). There are at least 10 HPA that have been defined at the molecular level. Each has two alleles, designated by the suffix *a* or *b*. These alleles are expressed by platelets codominantly (see Table 138-6). The *a* allele generally is the more prevalent allele. Allelic frequencies, however, vary between different racial groups[48–52] (Table 138-6). HPA-lb, for example, is expressed on platelets of approximately 15 percent of persons of European ancestry but of less than 1 percent of those of Asian ancestry.

In addition to the recognized HPA, there are several other platelet alloantigens that can be recognized by antiplatelet alloantibodies and account for neonatal alloimmune thrombocytopenia. Two, designated *Gro^a* and *Oe^a*, are associated with GPIIIa (CD61).[53,54] Another potential alloantigen, designated *Va^a*, is associated with the GPIIb/IIIa complex (CD41/CD61).[55] Two others, designated *La^a* and *Ly^a*, are localized to the GPIb-IX-V complex.[56,57] Another alloantigen results from genetic polymorphism in the gene encoding CD109 (see Chap. 14), accounting for the Gov allantigen system.[58,59] The less common allele encoding any one of these alloantigens may present at very low gene frequencies.

HPA alleles HPA-4b, -6b, -7b, -8b, -9b, and -10b also are present at gene frequencies of less than 0.1 percent, and thus are designated *private* alleles (Table 138-6). Some of these alleles, such as HPA-7b or HPA-8b,[53] are extremely rare. For this reason, the alloantigens encoded by such alleles are not likely to account for most cases of post-transfusion purpura but can be found on isolated cases of neonatal alloimmune thrombocytopenia in selected families. Alleles present at gene frequencies of greater than 2 percent within the population, on the other hand, are designated as *public* alleles. These alleles are more likely to encode the alloantigens that are targeted by antiplatelet alloantibodies.

The frequency of patients that express the more common HPA allele is greater than the gene frequency for that allele in the population. Using the classical Hardy-Weinberg equation ($a^2 + 2(ab) + b^2 = 1$), the proportion of individuals that are homozygous for the *a* allele (*a/a*) is the squared product of the gene frequency for *a* in the population (or a^2). Similarly, the proportion of cases that are homozygous for *b* is the squared product of the gene frequency for *b* (or b^2). The proportion of cases that are heterozygous (either *a/b* or *b/a*) is two times the product of the gene frequency for *a* times that for *b*. Because there are two alleles, the sum of all these products should equal 100 percent (or 1). Using such considerations for example, it is evident that persons of European ancestry will have a $(0.85)^2$, or 72 percent, chance of being homozygous for HPA-1a, a 26 percent chance of being heterozygous for HPA-1a/HPA-1b, but only a $(0.15)^2$, or 2 percent, chance of being homozygous for HPA-1b (see Table 138-6). As such, even though the gene frequency of HPA-1a is 85 percent, 98 percent of the population have at least one HPA-1a allele and will not make alloantibodies against the HPA-1a epitope. Similarly, it should be evident that it is highly unusual for anyone to be homozygous for HPA private antigens. As such, it is highly improbable that alloantibodies against HPA-4a, -6a, -7a, -8a, -9a, and -10a will account for immune thrombocytopenia. Conversely, most persons will lack the b allele of HPA private antigens and thus can potentially develop alloantibodies to HPA-4b, -6b, -7b, -8b, -9b, and -10b alloantigens.

ANTIPLATELET ANTIBODIES AFTER TRANSFUSION

Patients who are homozygous for a given allele can develop antiplatelet alloantibodies after receiving transfusions of platelets or cells that express the other allele.[60] Generally, a few transfusions of unmatched platelets can be given to patients without adverse effects. However, the risk for developing antiplatelet antibodies increases with each successive platelet transfusion. Patients receiving multiple transfusions of red blood cells also may develop antiplatelet or anti-HLA antibodies against leukocytes contaminating the red blood cell preparation.

After repeated platelet transfusions, the patient may become sensitized, possibly developing antibodies that shorten the lifespan of the transfused cells. The number of unmatched transfusions required to elicit such antibodies is variable. Some patients never make antibodies, while others become refractory after receiving only a few platelet transfusions. Others, often multiparous women, may have clinically significant antiplatelet antibodies prior to receiving any platelet transfusions. About half of all patients receiving repetitive platelet transfusions eventually produce antibodies against antigens on the transfused platelets. These antibodies may be directed against platelet-specific alloantigens, HLA antigens, or both.

Antibodies against some HPA-allelic determinants can inhibit platelet function. Anti-HPA-1 alloantibodies, for example, can inhibit clot retraction and platelet aggregation, presumably because they block the binding of GIIb/IIIa ($\alpha_{IIb}\beta_3$) to fibrinogen. Moreover, anti-HPA-4 alloantibodies can completely inhibit aggregation of HPA-4 platelets that are homozygous for allele recognized by the alloantibodies. This is because the epitope recognized by anti-HPA-4 alloantibodies is found on $_3$ at amino acid position 143 that is in close proximity to the RGD-binding domain of the $\alpha_{IIb}\beta_3$ integrin. Other anti-HPA-alloantibodies, such as alloantibodies specific for HPA-3 on the other hand, may not significantly interfere with platelet function but nonetheless can cause Fc-mediated platelet destruction and immune thrombocytopenia.

If the patient does develop anti-HLA antibodies that shorten the survival of unmatched transfused platelets, HLA-matched platelets may be more effective for subsequent transfusions. The patient and prospective platelet donors generally are matched for serological identity at the HLA-A and -B loci. Platelets derived from such HLA-matched donors generally survive longer in highly immunized patients than those received from random donors.

In some cases, it is necessary to type the platelet alloantigens of donors to provide effective platelet-transfusion therapy.[61] Different techniques for phenotyping are well established and easy to perform, but they rely on the availability of antisera.[62] The molecular genetic basis for the clinically most relevant alloantigens has been elucidated, thus facilitating widespread platelet alloantigen typing.[54]

Typing for HPA status can be achieved using the polymerase chain reaction (see Chap. 11), with subsequent analysis of the amplified gene-fragment using restriction enzymes, sequence-specific primers, dot-blot hybridization, or a fluorescent-based single-strand conformation polymorphism (F-SSCP) technique.[63-67] These techniques have proved to be highly useful in identifying the platelet genotype of fetuses at risk for neonatal alloimmune thrombocytopenia,[68] establishing the diagnosis of posttransfusion purpura, or in identifying causes of refractory responses to platelet transfusions. Molecular methods for detecting HPA status also should facilitate clinical studies on the association of certain HPA alleles with relative risk for thrombosis[46] or response to therapy for immune thrombocytopenia.[69]

REFERENCES

1. Breuning MH, Vanden Berg-Loonen EM, Bernini LF: Localization of HLA on the short arm of chromosome 6. *Hum Genet* 37:131, 1977.
2. Berrih S, ArenzanaSeidedos F, Cohen S, et al: Interferon-gamma modulates HLA class II antigen expression on cultured human thymic epithelial cells. *J Immunol* 135:1165, 1985.
3. Bodmer JB, Marsh SGE, Albert ED, et al: Nomenclature for factors of the HLA system, 1998. *Tissue Antigens* 53:407, 1999.
4. Thorsby E: Structure and function of HLA molecules. *Transplant Proc* 19:29, 1987.
5. Trowsdale J: Genetics and polymorphism: class II antigens. *Br Med Bull* 43:15, 1987.
6. Bjorkman PJ, Saper MA, Samraoui B, et al: Structure of the human class I histocompatibility antigen, HLA-A2. *Nature* 329:506, 1987.
7. Brown JH, Jardetzky TS, Gorga JC, et al: Three-dimensional structure of the human class II histocompatibility antigen HLA-DR1. *Nature* 364:33, 1993.
8. Borkman PJ, Saper MA, Samraoui B, Bennet WS, Strominger JL, Wiley DC: The foreign antigen binding site and T cell recognition regions of class I histocompatibility antigens. *Nature* 329: 512, 1987.
9. Stern LJ, Brown JH, Jardetzky TS, et al: Crystal structure of the human class II MHC protein HLA-DR-1 complexed with an influenza virus peptide. *Nature* 368:215, 1994.
10. Kostyu DD, Amos DB: The HLA complex; Genetic polymorphism and disease susceptibility, in *The Metabolic Basis of Inherited Disease*, 6ᵗʰ ed, edited by CR Scriver, AL Beaudet, WS Sly, D Valle, chap 4, p 225. McGraw-Hill, New York, 1989.
11. Mueller-Eckhardt B, Hauck M, Kayser W: HLA-C antigens on platelets. *Tissue Antigens* 16:91, 1980.
12. Lalezari P, Driscoll AM: Ability of thrombocytes to acquire HLA specificity from plasma. *Blood* 59:167, 1982.
13. Zinkernagel, RM, Doherty, PC: Restriction of in vitro T cell-mediated cytotoxicity in lymphocytic choriomeningitis within a syngeneic or semiallogeneic system. *Nature*, 248:701, 1974.
14. Mak, TW, Simard JJL: *Handbook of Immune Response Genes*. Plenum, New York, 1998.
15. Campbell RD, Trowsdale J: A map of the human major histocompatibility complex. *Immunol Today* 18:43, 1997.
16. Bodmer JB, Marsh SGE, Albert ED, et al: Nomenclature for factors of the HLA system. *Tissue Antigens* 39:161, 1992.
17. Marsh SGE: Nomenclature for factors of the HLA system, update January, 1999. *Tissue Antigens* 54:106, 1999.
18. Marsh SGE: Nomenclature for factors of the HLA system, update February, 1999. *Tissue Antigens* 54:108, 1999.
19. Marsh SGE: Nomenclature for factors of the HLA system, update March, 1999. *Tissue Antigens* 54:110, 1999.
20. Baur MP, Danilors JA: Population analysis of HLA-A, B, C, DR and other genetic markers, in *Histocompatibility Testing* 1980, edited by PA Terasaki, p 955. UCLA Tissue Typing Laboratory, Los Angeles, 1981.
21. Gjertson DW, Su-Hui, L: HLA-A/B and -DRB1/DQB1 allele level haplotype frequencies, in *HLA 1998*, edited by DW Gjertson, PI Teresaki, chap 8, p 365. American Society for Histocompatibility and Immunogenetics, Lenexa, 1998.
22. Parham P: Histocompatibility typing-Mac is back in town. *Immunol Today* 9:127, 1988.
23. Sullivan K and Amos DB: The HLA system and its detection, in *Manual*

of Clinical Laboratory Immunology, 3rd ed, edited by NR Rose, H Friedman, JL Fahey, chap 130, p 835. American Society for Microbiology, Washington, DC, 1986.

24. Terasaki P, McClelland JD: Microdroplet assay of human serum cytokines. *Nature* (London) 204:998, 1964.

25. Dupont B, Hansen JA, Yunis EJ: Human mixed lymphocyte culture reaction: genetics, specificity and biological implications. *Adv Immunol* 23:108, 1976.

26. Jorgensen F, Lamm LU, Kismeyer-Nielsen F: Mixed lymphocyte cultures with inbred individuals: an approach to MLR typing. *Tissue Antigens* 3:323, 1973.

27. Shaw SA, Johnson AH, Shearer GM: Evidence for a new segregant series of B cell antigens that are encoded in the HLA-D region and that stimulate secondary allogeneic proliferative and cytotoxic responses. *J Exper Med* 152:565, 1980.

28. Saiki RK, Gelfand DH, Stoffel S: Primer-directed enzymatic amplification of DNA with a thermostable DNA polymerase. *Science* 239:487, 1988.

29. Erlich HA, Bugawan TL: HLA class II gene polymorphism: DNA typing, evolution and relationship to disease susceptibility, in *PCR Technology: Principles and Applications* for DNA Amplification, edited by HA Erlich, p 193. Stockton, New York, 1989.

30. Dyer, PA, Taylor C, Martin S: HLA and clinical solid organ transplantation: recent publications and novel approaches, in *HLA 1998*, edited by DW Gjertson, PI Terasaki, chap 2, p 13. American Society for Histocompatibility and Immunogenetics, Lenexa, 1998.

31. Martin PJ, Gooley T, Anasetti C, Petersdorf EW, Hanson J: HLAs and risk of acute graft-vs-host disease after marrow transplantation from an HLA-identical sibling. *Biol Blood Marrow Transplant* 4:128, 1998.

32. Petersdorf EW, Gooley TA, Anasetti C, et al: Optimizing outcome after unrelated marrow transplantation by comprehensive matching of HLA class I and class II alleles in the donor and recipient. *Blood* 92:3515, 1998.

33. Hurley CK, Wade JA, Oudshoorn M, et al: A special report: histocompatibility testing guidelines for hematopoietic stem cell transplantation using volunteer donors. *Tissue Antigens* 53:394, 1999.

34. Wadenvik H, Stockelberg D, Hou M: Platelet proteins as autoantibody targets in idiopathic thrombocytopenic purpura. *Acta Paediatr Suppl* 424:26, 1998.

35. Beardsley DS, Ertem M: Platelet autoantibodies in immune thrombocytopenic purpura. *Transfus Sci* 19:237, 1998.

36. Davis GL: Platelet specific alloantigens. *Clin Lab Sci* 11:356, 1998.

37. Warkentin TE, Smith JW: The alloimmune thrombocytopenic syndromes. *Transfus Med Rev* 11:296, 1997.

38. West KA, Anderson DR, McAlister VC, et al: Alloimmune thrombocytopenia after organ transplantation. *N Engl J Med* 341:1504, 1999.

39. Bierling P, Fromont P, Elbez A, Duedari N, Kieffer N: Early immunization against platelet glycoprotein IIIa in a newborn Glanzmann type I patient. *Vox Sang* 55:109, 1988.

40. Li C, Pasquale DN, Roth GJ: Bernard-Soulier syndrome with severe bleeding: absent platelet glycoprotein Ib alpha due to a homozygous one-base deletion. *Thromb Haemost* 76:670, 1996.

41. Ikeda H: Platelet membrane protein CD36. *Hokkaido Igaku Zasshi* 74:99, 1999.

42. Newman PJ, Valentin N: Human platelet alloantigens: recent findings, new perspectives. *Thromb Haemost* 74:234, 1995.

43. Santoso S, Kiefel V: Human platelet-specific alloantigens: update. *Vox Sang* 74(suppl 2): 249, 1998.

44. Lyman S, Aster RH, Visentin GP, Newman PJ: Polymorphism of human platelet membrane glycoprotein IIb associated with the Baka/Bakb alloantigen system. *Blood* 75:2343, 1990.

45. Nurden AT: Polymorphisms of human platelet membrane glycoproteins: structure and clinical significance. *Thromb Haemost* 74:345, 1995.

46. Bray PF: Integrin polymorphisms as risk factors for thrombosis. *Thromb Haemost* 82:337, 1999.

47. Goldschmidt-Clermont PJ, Roos CM, Cooke GE: Platelet PlA2 polymorphism and thromboembolic events: from inherited risk to pharmacogenetics. *J Thromb Thrombolysis* 8:89, 1999.

48. Holensteiner A, Walchshofer S, Adler A, Kittl EM, Mayr WR, Panzer S: Human platelet antigen gene frequencies in the Austrian population. *Haemostasis* 25:133, 1995.

49. Tanaka S, Ohnoki S, Shibata H, Okubo Y, Yamaguchi H, Shibata Y: Gene frequencies of human platelet antigens on glycoprotein IIIa in Japanese. *Transfusion* 36:813, 1996.

50. Tanaka S, Taniue A, Nagao N, et al: Genotype frequencies of the human platelet antigen, Ca/Tu, in Japanese, determined by a PCR-RFLP method. *Vox Sang* 70:40, 1996.

51. Kim HO, Jin Y, Kickler TS, Blakemore K, Kwon OH, Bray PF: Gene frequencies of the five major human platelet antigens in African American, white, and Korean populations. *Transfusion* 35:863, 1995.

52. Kekomäki S, Partanen J, Kekomäki R, Platelet alloantigens HPA-1, -2, -3, -5 and -6b in Finns. *Transfus Med* 5:193, 1995.

53. Simsek S, Vlekke AB, Kuijpers RW, Goldschmeding R, von dem Borne AE: A new private platelet antigen, Groa, localized on glycoprotein IIIa, involved in neonatal alloimmune thrombocytopenia. *Vox Sang* 67:302, 1994.

54. Kroll H, Kiefel V, Santoso S: Clinical aspects and typing of platelet alloantigens. *Vox Sang* 74(suppl 2): 345, 1998.

55. Kekomäki R, Raivio P, Kero P: A new low-frequency platelet alloantigen, Vaa, on glycoprotein IIbIIIa associated with neonatal alloimmune thrombocytopenia. *Transfus Med* 2:27, 1992.

56. Peyruchaud O, Bourre F, Morel-Kopp MC, et al: HPA-10w(b) (La(a)): genetic determination of a new platelet-specific alloantigen on glycoprotein IIIa and its expression in COS-7 cells. *Blood* 89:2422, 1997.

57. Kiefel V, Vicariot M, Giovangrandi Y, et al: Alloimmunization against Iy, a low-frequency antigen on platelet glycoprotein Ib/IX as a cause of severe neonatal alloimmune thrombocytopenic purpura. *Vox Sang* 69:250, 1995.

58. Kelton JG, Smith JW, Horsewood P, Humbert JR, Hayward CP, Warkentin TE: Gova/b alloantigen system on human platelets. *Blood* 75:2172, 1990.

59. Bordin JO, Kelton JG, Warner MN, et al: Maternal immunization to Gov system alloantigens on human platelets. *Transfusion* 37:823, 1997.

60. McFarland JG: Alloimmunization and platelet transfusion. *Semin Hematol* 33:315, 1996.

61. Kekomäki R: Use of HLA- and HPA-matched platelets in alloimmunized patients. *Vox Sang* 74(suppl 2): 359, 1998.

62. Kaplan C: Evaluation of serological platelet antibody assays. *Vox Sang* 74(suppl 2): 355, 1998.

63. Unkelbach K, Kalb R, Santoso S, Kroll H, Mueller-Eckhardt C, Kiefel V: Genomic RFLP typing of human platelet alloantigens Zw(PlA), Ko, Bak and Br (HPA-1, 2, 3, 5). *Br J Haematol* 89:169, 1995.

64. Panzer S, Kaplan C: Report on the 1997 International Society of Blood Transfusion Workshop for Genotyping of Platelet Alloantigens. Platelet and granulocyte workshop ISBT. *Transfus Med* 8:125, 1998.

65. McFarland JG: Platelet and neutrophil alloantigen genotyping in clinical practice. *Transfus Clin* Biol 5:13, 1998.

66. Quintanar A, Jallu V, Legros Y, Kaplan C: Human platelet antigen genotyping using a fluorescent SSCP technique with an automatic sequencer. *Br J Haematol* 103:437, 1998.

67. Metcalfe P, Cavanagh G, Hurd C, Ouwehand WH: HPA genotyping by PCR-SSP: report of 4 exercises. *Vox Sang* 77:40, 1999.

68. Skupski DW, Bussel JB: Alloimmune thrombocytopenia. *Clin Obstet Gynecol* 42:335, 1999.

69. Nomura S, Matsuzaki T, Yamaoka M, et al: Genetic analysis of HLA- and HPA-typing in idiopathic (autoimmune) thrombocytopenic purpura patients treated with cepharanthin. *Autoimmunity* 30:99, 1999.

BLOOD PROCUREMENT AND SCREENING

JEFFREY McCULLOUGH

Blood procurement is a vital national priority that is met in the United States by volunteer donors and a pluralistic blood collection program that includes the American Red Cross, independent community blood centers, and hospitals. Over 13 million units of whole blood are collected from about 10 million donors annually. Recruitment of donors is preceded by a medical history and limited physical examination. The donated blood is subjected to as many as 15 tests that include determination of blood type, examination for red cell antibodies, and a series of studies for infectious agents that may be transmitted by blood exchange. The process usually starts with donations from random, unrelated donors but may include autologous, patient-specific, or patient-directed donors in special circumstances. In some cases, collection of platelets, leukocytes, or plasma is achieved by hemapheresis. Plasma for the subsequent manufacture of derivatives such as albumin and intravenous immunoglobulin is obtained from paid donors by for profit organizations different from those that collect whole blood and prepare blood components.

The meticulous attention to donor risk characteristics and the use of sensitive assays to detect infectious agents that may be transmitted by blood has greatly improved the safety of blood as a therapeutic product in countries that apply these practices. Nevertheless, a risk of viral infection, albeit small, remains as new improved methods are developed to move that risk from about one in thirty four thousand to a more remote possibility. The introduction of nucleic acid amplification techniques to detect microbial contaminants should further decrease the risk of acquiring an infection through transfusion.

AN OVERVIEW OF THE BLOOD BANKING SYSTEM

THE SYSTEM IN THE UNITED STATES

The United States has a pluralistic rather than a single national system of blood collection.[1,2] In the United States during 1994, approximately 13,340,000 units of blood donated by about 10,000,000 people were available for use (Table 139-1). About 92 percent of the blood was collected in 147 regional blood centers, hospitals collected 8 percent, and less than 1 percent was imported from Western Europe.[3] Approximately 7.6 percent of the units donated in the United States were autologous donations, and another 2.5 percent were directed donations—that is, blood given by family or friends for a specific patient. A single organization, the American Red Cross, collected about 45

percent of the blood through its network of about 40 regional blood centers. Community blood centers and hospitals collect the remainder. Community blood centers are individual, locally operated, nonprofit organizations, whereas the American Red Cross is a national corporation with a single FDA license and set of operating procedures for all its regional centers.

All whole blood for transfusion in the United States is donated by volunteers; however, costs are incurred in the collection, testing, production, and distribution of blood components. Blood banks are nonprofit organizations that pass on these costs to hospitals. In the past, it was sometimes possible for patients to partially reduce the cost of blood by arranging for replacement of the blood they used. This practice has generally been discontinued because of the demand it places on the patient or family during the difficult time of the illness. Instead, blood banks assume the responsibility of ensuring that the community's blood needs are met by developing public education and donor recruitment programs.

Some areas of the United States are able to provide more blood than is needed locally, and other areas are unable to collect enough blood to meet their local needs. The misalignment of blood use and blood availability is a long-standing phenomenon. Several inventory-sharing systems are used to move blood around the United States in order to alleviate the shortages, but these are complex and fragile arrangements that are not always effective. As a result, blood shortages occasionally occur in some areas of the United States.

Blood is considered a drug, and all aspects of the selection of donors, collection, processing, testing, preservation, and dispensing are regulated by the FDA as specified in the Code of Federal Regulations. The requirements in the code define the procedures, records, staff proficiency, specific testing, and donor medical requirements that blood banks must follow. Additional standard requirements are formulated by the American Association of Blood Banks, a voluntary organization that accredits blood banks. During the past decade the FDA has required that blood banks implement good manufacturing practices similar to those used by pharmaceutical manufacturers. This has had a major impact on the manner in which blood banks function.[1,2,4]

INTERNATIONAL PRACTICES

There is a considerable difference in the availability of blood and blood components throughout the world.[5-7] In general, this is related to the extent of development in the country and its health care system. For instance, in Third World countries "transfusion practice is fragmented and disorganized and it is difficult, if not impossible, to provide the five basic blood components . . . in an adequate supply."[8] These countries usually do not have an organized blood supply system, and there may be no system of obtaining a blood supply for the general community. Patients may be required to arrange for the blood they need, and thus, donors may be friends or family members of patients or even individuals who have been paid by the patient's family to donate the blood needed. There is considerable evidence that blood from paid donors is more likely to transmit disease.[9] Donor screening may not be as extensive, transmissible disease testing may be lacking, equipment may be reused, and the blood collected into containers may be unsuitable for the preparation of components. These difficulties may be compounded by the presence of endemic transfusion-transmissible diseases for which screening is difficult or expensive and thus not carried out as extensively as in more developed countries.

It was estimated that in the early 1980s about 75 million units of blood were collected worldwide, about one-third by Red Cross/Red Crescent blood programs.[10] In developed countries, especially western Europe and parts of Asia, there is usually a government agency that oversees the blood collection activities, although the extent to

TABLE 139-1   THE U.S. BLOOD SUPPLY SYSTEM IN 1994*

	NUMBER	PERCENT
Total Units Whole Blood	13,340,000	100
Blood centers (190)	12,211,000	92
Hospitals (621)	1,129,000	8
Imports	220,000	<1
RBC Transfusions	11,107,000	100
Allogeneic	10,202,000	91.8
Autologous	482,000	4.4†
Directed	105,000	0.9‡
Other		2.9
Discarded	754,000	
Platelets		
SDP collected	820,000	100
SDP transfused	714,000	87
SDP discarded	106,000	13
Platelet concentrates	3,582,000	—
Total platelets transfused*	7,866,000	—
Fresh Frozen Plasma	2,621,000	—
Cryoprecipitate	713,000	—

*Data are taken from Wallace et al.[3]
†Outdate rate 44%.
‡Outdate rate 55%.
SDP, single-donor platelet concentrate prepared by plateletpheresis. One SDP equivalent to six platelet concentrates.

which the government sets requirements and monitors or inspects the blood collection system varies.[11] Where national blood programs have been developed, usually a national blood policy is established that includes definition of the organization(s) responsible for the program, the source of funding, the type of blood donation, and regulations ensuring blood safety.[5,6] In these countries the basic processes of donor medical screening, blood collection, laboratory testing, and preparation of blood components are similar to the U.S. system. In virtually all developed countries blood is donated by volunteers and not paid donors.[12] The blood may be collected by hospitals or community-based regional blood centers or some combination of these. The supply systems and sharing among hospitals and blood centers vary with the extent of development of the country's blood supply system. The basic blood components—red cells, platelets, plasma, and cryoprecipitate—are usually available, and apheresis instruments are used to collect some platelets. Plasma derivatives such as albumin, coagulation factor VIII, and immune globulins are available. In many countries these plasma derivatives are prepared from plasma collected from volunteer donors instead of the paid-donor plasma used to prepare these derivatives in the United States. Thus, the availability of blood and its components around the world varies widely, from inadequate supplies and uncertain safety to sophisticated supply systems and component availability equal to or surpassing those of the United States.

PLASMA DERIVATIVES

The plasma industry is separate from the blood banking system described above. Plasma can be subjected to a fractionation process to produce several medically valuable products referred to as plasma "derivatives", such as albumin, fibrinogen, anti-hemophilic factor, and 19 others (see Chap. 143). Plasma fractionation is done in a manufacturing plant setting, in batches of up to 10,000 liters involving the pooling of plasma from as many as 50,000 donors. Plasma for manufacture or fractionation into derivatives can be obtained from units of whole blood, but this amount of plasma is not adequate to meet the needs for plasma derivatives. Therefore, large amounts of plasma are obtained by plasmapheresis. Because only the plasma and not red cells or platelets are removed during the plasmapheresis, individuals can donate plasma up to twice a week. Because of this

more extensive commitment to donation, plasma donors are paid and this plasma collection system is usually operated by for-profit organizations and functions separately from the system described above for whole blood donation.

Approximately 11.5 million liters of plasma is collected annually in the United States,[13] although exact figures are not known because most plasma is collected by for-profit organizations. There are 22 plasma derivatives approved for licensure by the FDA (see Chap. 143). Some derivatives are produced by only one manufacturer and others by up to six different manufacturers. Thus, disruption in the sources of plasma or in one manufacturer's plant can have serious consequences and create shortages of certain derivatives.

The remainder of this chapter will describe the blood collection system operated by voluntary community organizations to provide cellular and whole blood–derived components.

RECRUITMENT OF BLOOD DONORS

Although most Americans will require a blood transfusion at some time in their lives, less than 5 percent of the total population, or less than 10 percent of those eligible to donate, have ever done so.[13] Most donors give once or infrequently, and thus, much of the nation's blood supply comes from a small number of dedicated frequent donors.[13] Blood donors are more likely than the general population to be male, age 30 to 50, Caucasian, employed, and have more education and higher income.[13] There have been some studies of the social psychology and motivation of blood donors,[14] but the process is not well understood. It is generally believed that the most effective way to get someone to donate blood is to ask them personally. Factors such as the convenience of donation, peer pressure, receipt of blood by a family member, and perceived community needs are important factors that are superimposed onto the individual's basic social commitments. Usually blood donors are asked to give to the general community supply. Some donors are asked to give for a specific patient, and this is referred to as directed donation. Such donations may be easier to obtain and leave the donor with a stronger sense of satisfaction because of the personal nature of the donation.[13]

The heightened concerns about blood safety during the past decade have resulted in expanded requirements for the suitability for blood donation. Thus, a larger proportion of the population of potential donors is being excluded. This, along with the aging population, geographic and ethnic shifts in the population, and people's changing priorities, are causing a shrinking donor pool. Thus, it will be increasingly important to understand the motivation of blood donors and psychosocial factors that lead to blood donation.

WHOLE-BLOOD DONOR SCREENING

The approach to the selection of blood donors is designed around two themes: to insure the safety of the donor and to obtain a high-quality blood component that is as safe as possible for the recipient. Some specific steps that are taken to insure that blood is as safe as possible are the use of only volunteer blood donors, questioning of donors about their general health before their donation is scheduled, obtaining a medical history before donation, conducting a physical examination before donation, laboratory testing of donated blood, checking the donor's identity against a donor deferral registry, and providing a method by which the donor can confidentially designate the unit as unsuitable for transfusion after the donation is completed.[13]

MEDICAL HISTORY

The questions designed to protect the safety of the donor include whether the donor is under the care of a physician and has a history of cardiovascular or lung disease, seizures, present or recent pregnancy, recent donation of blood or plasma, recent major illness or surgery, unexplained weight loss, or unusual bleeding. Medications and age are also documented. Questions designed to protect the safety of the recipient include those related to the donor's general health, the presence of a bleeding disorder, a history of receipt of growth hormone, and the occurrence of or exposure to patients with hepatitis or other liver disease, AIDS (or symptoms of AIDS), Chagas disease, or babesiosis. A history is also obtained regarding the injection of drugs, receipt of coagulation factor concentrates, blood transfusion, a tattoo, acupuncture, ear piercing, an organ or tissue transplant, travel to areas endemic for malaria, recent immunizations, contact with persons with hepatitis or other transmissible diseases, ingestion of medications (especially aspirin), presence of a major illness or surgery, or previous notice of a positive test for a transmissible disease. In addition, there are several questions related to AIDS risk behavior. These include whether the potential donor has had sex with anyone with AIDS, given or received money or drugs for sex, (for males) had sex with another male, or (for females) had sex with a male who has had sex with another male. This series of sex-related questions is very specific and has changed the interaction and relationship between the donor and the blood bank.

Commonly, situations arise in which the donor's physician believes that donation would be safe but the blood bank does not accept the donor. For instance, donors with a history of cancer, other than minor skin cancer or carcinoma in situ of the cervix, are usually rejected because the genesis of malignant disease is not known. The donor is questioned about medications. Some medications may make the donor unsuitable because of the condition requiring the medication, while others may be potentially harmful to the recipient. Many other conditions must be evaluated individually by the blood bank physician, and that physician's assessment of conformance with FDA regulations, which view blood as a pharmaceutical, may not always coincide with the personal physician's view of the health of the patient who is the potential blood donor.

PHYSICAL AND LABORATORY EXAMINATION OF THE BLOOD DONOR

The examination includes determination of the temperature, pulse, blood pressure, weight, and blood hemoglobin concentration. The FDA has mandated limits for each of these. In addition, the donor's general appearance is assessed for any signs of illness or the influence of drugs or alcohol. The skin at the venipuncture site is examined for signs of intravenous drug abuse, lesions suggestive of Kaposi sarcoma, and local lesions that might make it difficult to sterilize the skin and thus lead to contamination of the blood unit during venipuncture.

COLLECTION OF WHOLE BLOOD

BLOOD CONTAINERS

Blood must be collected into single-use, sterile, FDA-licensed containers. The containers are made of plasticized material that is biocompatible with blood cells and allows diffusion of gases in order to provide optimal cell preservation (see Chap. 140 and Chap. 142). These blood containers are combinations of bags that allow separation of the whole blood into its components in a closed system, thus minimizing the chance of bacterial contamination while making storage of the components for days or weeks possible.

PREPARATION OF THE VENIPUNCTURE SITE

The blood should be drawn from an area free of skin lesions, and the phlebotomy site should be properly sterilized. The site is scrubbed with a soap solution, followed by the application of tincture of iodine or iodophor complex solution. The selection of the venipuncture site and its sterilization are very important steps, since bacterial contamination of blood can be a serious or even fatal complication of transfusion.[15,16]

VENIPUNCTURE AND BLOOD COLLECTION

The venipuncture is done with a needle that should be used only once in order to avoid contamination. The blood must flow freely and be mixed with anticoagulant frequently as it fills the container, in order to avoid the development of small clots. The actual time for collection of 450 ml is usually about 7 min and almost always less than 10 min. During blood donation there is a slight fall in cardiac output but little change in heart rate. A slight decrease in systolic pressure results, with a rise in peripheral resistance and diastolic blood pressure.[17]

Usually 450 ml ($\pm$10%) is collected, although some blood banks now collect 500 ml from larger donors. This is mixed with 63 to 70 ml of anticoagulant composed of citrate, phosphate, and dextrose (CPD). The amount of blood withdrawn must be within prescribed limits in order to maintain the proper ratio with the anticoagulant; otherwise the blood cells may be damaged and/or anticoagulation may not be satisfactory (see Chap. 140). Although the red cells could be stored in the CPD-anticoagulant solution, it is customary to remove almost all the anticoagulated plasma and resuspend the red cells in a solution that provides optimum red cell preservation (see Chap. 140).

POSTDONATION OBSERVATION AND ADVERSE REACTIONS TO BLOOD DONATION

A reaction occurs following approximately 4 percent of blood donations, but fortunately most reactions are not serious.[18,19] Donors who have reactions are more likely to be younger, unmarried, have a higher predonation heart rate and lower diastolic blood pressure, and to be first time or infrequent donors.[20] The most common reaction to blood donation involves weakness, cool skin, and diaphoresis. A more extensive but still moderate reaction involves dizziness, pallor, hypertension, and bradycardia. Bradycardia is usually taken as a sign of a vasovagal reaction rather than hypotensive or cardiovascular shock, where tachycardia would be expected. In a more severe form, this kind of reaction may progress to loss of consciousness, convulsions, and involuntary passage of urine or stool. These symptoms also are thought to be due to vasovagal reactions rather than hypovolemia.[18] Other reactions include nausea and vomiting; hyperventilation, sometimes leading to twitching or muscle spasms; hematoma at the venipuncture site; convulsions; or serious cardiac difficulties. Such serious reactions are very rare.[18,19,21] Injury of the brachial nerve and resulting pain and/or paresthesia may occur due to needle puncture of the nerve or compression from a hematoma.[22,23]

Donors are advised to drink extra fluids to replace lost blood volume and to avoid strenuous exercise for the remainder of the day of donation. This latter advice is given to avoid fainting and also to minimize the possibility that a hematoma will develop at the venipuncture site. Some donors are subject to lightheadedness or even fainting if they change position quickly. Therefore, donors are also advised not to return to work for the remainder of the day in an occupation where fainting would be hazardous to themselves or others.

SPECIAL BLOOD DONATIONS

There are several situations involving blood donation in which the blood is not being obtained for the community's general blood supply. Examples of these include autologous donation, directed donation, patient-specific donation, and therapeutic bleeding. In some of these situations the FDA requirements for blood donation may not apply.

AUTOLOGOUS DONOR BLOOD

Autologous blood donation is an old concept but was little used until the AIDS epidemic raised fears of blood transfusion both among patients and physicians. Individuals may donate blood for their own use if the need for blood can be anticipated and a donation plan developed. Most commonly this occurs with elective surgery.

Autologous blood for transfusion can be obtained by preoperative donation, acute normovolemic hemodilution, intraoperative salvage, and postoperative salvage (see also Chap. 140), but only preoperative donation will be discussed here. If patient candidates for autologous blood donation meet the usual FDA criteria for blood donation, their blood may be "crossed over," that is, used for other patients if the original autologous donor has no need for the blood. This practice is no longer allowed by AABB standards. If the autologous donor does not meet the FDA criteria for blood donation, the blood must be specially labeled, segregated during storage, and discarded if not used by that specific patient. Thus, it is important that the autologous blood donation be collected only for procedures in which there is substantial likelihood that it will be used.[24] Without this type of planning, there is a very high rate of wastage of autologous blood, estimated at 52.4 percent in 1994.[3] Thus, the cost of autologous blood is quite high.[25]

There are no age or weight restrictions for autologous donation.[13] Pregnant women may donate, but this is not recommended routinely since these patients rarely require transfusion. The autologous donor's hemoglobin may be lower (11 g/dl) than that required for routine donors (12.5 g/dl), and autologous donors may donate as often as every 72 h up to 72 h prior to the planned surgery, although usually it is only possible to obtain two to four units of blood before the hemoglobin falls below 11 g/dl. Autologous blood donors can be given erythropoietin and iron in order to increase the number of units of blood they can donate,[26] although the value of erythropoietin remains a bit unclear since this strategy has not been shown to reduce the need for allogeneic donor blood.[27] Some contraindications for autologous blood donation are bacteremia, symptomatic angina, recent seizures, and symptomatic valvular heart lesions. However, the final decision whether to withdraw blood from an autologous donor rests with the medical director of the blood bank. Often consultation between the donor's (patient's) physician and the blood bank physician is necessary in order to decide on a wise course of action.

Autologous blood must be typed for ABO and Rh antigens, and at least the first unit must be tested for transmissible diseases.[13] If any of the transmissible disease tests are positive, the unit must be labeled with a biohazard label. This is sometimes confusing or disconcerting to physicians, but it is an FDA requirement, intended to alert health care personnel to the potential hazard presented by the potentially infectious blood.

DIRECTED DONOR BLOOD

Directed donors are friends or relatives who wish to give blood for a specific patient because the patient hopes those donors will be safer than the regular blood supply. In general, the data do not indicate that directed donors have a lower incidence of transmissible disease markers,[28,29] and thus there may not be a realistic rationale for these donations. When friends or relatives are asked to donate blood, they may be reluctant to disclose risk factors that would preclude them from voluntary donation. Some blood banks refuse such donations, but most accept them as a service to the patients. However, because their blood becomes part of the community's general blood supply if

it is not used for the originally intended patient, directed donors must meet all the usual FDA requirements for routine blood donation.

PATIENT-SPECIFIC DONATION

There are a few situations in which appropriate transfusion therapy involves collecting blood from a particular donor for a particular patient. Examples are donor-specific transfusions prior to kidney transplantation, maternal platelets for a fetus projected to have alloimmune neonatal thrombocytopenia, or family members of a patient with a rare blood type. In these situations donors must meet all the usual FDA requirements, except that they may donate as often as every 3 days so long as the hemoglobin remains above the normal donor minimum of 12.5 g/dl.[13] These units must undergo all routine laboratory testing.[13]

THERAPEUTIC BLEEDING

Blood may be collected as part of the therapy of diseases such as polycythemia vera or hemochromatosis. Often the patient or the physician asks that the blood be used for transfusion as a way of comforting the patient. However, usually such blood is not used for transfusion since such donors do not meet the FDA standards for donor health.

COLLECTION AND PRODUCTION OF BLOOD COMPONENTS BY APHERESIS

Blood components can be obtained by apheresis rather than being prepared from a standard unit of whole blood. In apheresis the donor's anticoagulated whole blood is passed through an instrument in which the blood is separated into red cells, plasma, and a leukocyte/platelet fraction (see Chap. 144). Several semiautomated blood cell separator instruments are available for the collection of platelets, granulocytes, peripheral blood stem cells, mononuclear cells, or plasma.[13] All of these instruments use centrifugation to separate the blood components.[30] Some apheresis procedures involve two venipunctures with continuous flow of blood from the donor through the blood cell separator and others can be accomplished with a single venipuncture and intermittent blood withdrawal and return.

PLATELETPHERESIS

In the past most platelet concentrates have been produced from whole blood, but plateletpheresis has been used increasingly, so that by 1992, 46 percent of platelets produced in the United States were produced by plateletpheresis.[3] Plateletpheresis requires about 90 min, during which about 4000 to 5000 liters of the donor's blood is processed through the blood cell separator. This results in a platelet concentrate with a volume of about 200 ml and containing about 3.5×10^{11} platelets and less than 0.5 ml red cells. Recently manufactured blood cell separators produce a platelet concentrate that contains less than 5×10^6 leukocytes and thus can be considered leukocyte depleted. Following plateletpheresis the donor's platelet count declines by about 30 percent and does not return to pre-plateletpheresis levels for about 4 days[31] (see Chap. 142).

LEUKAPHERESIS

Leukapheresis has been used to produce a granulocyte concentrate for transfusion therapy of infections unresponsive to antibiotics.[13] In the past, leukapheresis provided only a marginally adequate dose of granulocytes for therapeutic benefit,[31] and its use had declined to very low levels (see Chap. 141). Leukapheresis is usually a more lengthy and complex procedure than plateletpheresis. Because the efficiency of granulocyte extraction from whole blood is less than for platelets, the leukapheresis procedure involves processing 6500 to 8000 ml of donor blood during about 3 h.[30] To increase the separation of granulocytes from other blood components, hydroxyethyl starch is added to the blood cell separator flow system.[30] In addition, glucocorticoids have been administered to the donor to increase the peripheral blood granulocyte count and thus increase the yield.[29] Recently, G-CSF has been administered to granulocyte donors to achieve much larger increases in granulocyte count and a much greater granulocyte yield.[32-35] Transfusion of these high-yield granulocyte concentrates results in substantial increases in the granulocyte count and has led to a renewed interest in granulocyte transfusions[36] (see Chap. 141).

PLASMAPHERESIS

Plasmapheresis can be done using sets of multiple attached bags, but this is time consuming and cumbersome and involves disconnecting the blood bags from the donor, resulting in the chance of returning the blood to the wrong donor. During the past few years semiautomated instruments have become available that require less operator involvement than the bag systems, while producing larger volumes of plasma more rapidly. The volume of plasma that can be collected depends on the size of the donor. Plasmapheresis can usually be done in about 30 min to produce up to 750 ml of plasma, depending upon the size of the donor. Very few red cells are removed. The procedure can be repeated up to twice weekly, so that theoretically a donor could provide up to about 50 liters of plasma in 1 year (see Chap. 144).

SELECTION OF APHERESIS DONORS

The selection of donors for plateletpheresis, leukapheresis, and plasmapheresis uses the same criteria as whole-blood donation.[13] Because of the unique nature of apheresis there are some additional donor requirements. Because many apheresis procedures involve two venipunctures and continuous blood flow, good venous access is important. No more than 15 percent of the donor's blood should be extracorporeal during apheresis, and thus, the donor's size is considered when making decisions about specific apheresis procedures or instruments to be used. Following plateletpheresis, the donor's platelet count declines by about 30 percent and does not return to pre-plateletpheresis levels for about 4 days.[30] Donors may undergo plateletpheresis every 48 h, although if they are donating more often than every 8 weeks a platelet count must be done to ensure that it is at least 150,000/μl (1.5 × 10^{11}/liter).[31] Following leukapheresis of G-CSF-stimulated donors the granulocyte count decreases slightly, the platelet count by 20 to 25 percent, and the hematocrit by about 1 percent.[34,35] Thus, the platelet count must be monitored in donors undergoing frequent leukaphereses. Because a plateletpheresis concentrate would be the sole source of platelets for the transfusion, the donor must not have taken aspirin for at least 3 days. For donors undergoing plasmapheresis more often than once every 8 weeks, the serum protein must be at least 6 g/dl, and every 4 months a protein electrophoresis or a quantitative immunoglobulins assay should be obtained and the results must be normal to allow further donation.[13] The amount of blood components removed from apheresis donors must be monitored. Not more than 200 ml of red cells per 2 months or approximately 1500 ml of plasma per week may be removed.[13] The laboratory testing of donors and apheresis components for transmissible diseases is the screening

TABLE 139-2   LABORATORY TESTS OF DONATED BLOOD

- ABO antigens
- Rh(D) antigen
- RBC antibody detection
- Serologic test for syphilis
- Hepatitis Bs antigen
- Hepatitis Bc antibody
- Hepatitis C antibody
- HTLV-I/II antibody
- HIV-1,2 antibody
- HIV (p24) antigen
- Alanine leucyl transferase*

Optional:
- CMV antibody
- HLA antibody
- Other RBC antigens

*No longer required for whole blood or hemapheresis donation, but still required in Europe for plasma to be manufactured into derivatives.

same as for whole-blood donation. Thus, the likelihood of disease transmission from apheresis components is the same as from whole blood.

REACTIONS IN APHERESIS DONORS

Apheresis donors can experience the same kind of reactions as whole-blood donors. In addition, apheresis donors experience a higher incidence of paresthesias, probably due to the infusion of the citrate used to anticoagulate the donor's blood while it is in the cell separator. This type of reaction is managed by slowing the flow rate of the instrument and thus slowing the rate of citrate infusion. The additional donor selection and monitoring requirements for apheresis prevent the development of reactions or complications due to excess removal of blood cells or plasma. In leukapheresis, donors may be given glucocorticoid and/or G-CSF to elevate the granulocyte count, and the sedimenting agent hydroxyethyl starch is used in the cell separator to improve the granulocyte yield. When G-CSF is used about 60 percent of donors experience side effects, usually myalgia, arthralgia, headache, or flulike symptoms.[32-35] This rate of side effects may be higher if the donors also receive glucocorticoids.[35] The major side effect of hydroxyethyl starch is blood volume expansion manifested by headache and/or hypertension.[13] Donor selection techniques are intended to minimize the likelihood of hypertension due to hydroxyethyl starch.

LABORATORY TESTING OF DONATED BLOOD

Each unit of whole blood or each apheresis component undergoes a standard battery of tests (Table 139-2), including those for the blood type, red cell antibodies, and transmissible diseases. Additional tests,

TABLE 139-3   TRANSFUSION-TRANSMITTED DISEASES*

	LACKRITZ	SLOAND	WILLIAMS	TOTAL U.S. CASES[†]
Hepatitis C		3300	103,000	117
Hepatitis B		50,000	63,000	190
HTLV-I/II		69,272	641,000	19
HIV	450,000–660,000	40,000–400,000	493,000	27
HBV and HCV			34,000	353

*Estimates of transfusion-transmitted diseases in the United States, based on data from references 38–47. One case of each disease would be expected following transfusion of the number of units of blood shown.
[†]Calculated from Schreiber GV, Busch MP, Kleinman SH: The risk of transfusion-transmitted viral infections. *N Engl J Med* 334:1685, 1996.

such as those for cytomegalovirus or HLA antibodies, may be done optionally. Eight tests, six of which have been introduced since 1985, are performed for transmissible diseases.[1] The total number of test results for each unit of donated blood is about 15, depending on the specific methodology used. In addition, since each unit of whole blood is separated into several components and there is a donor history record and two or three tubes of blood for tests, each donation generates up to 30 different data elements. All data are amalgamated in order to ensure that they are satisfactory for release of the blood into the transfusion inventory. Since busy blood collection centers deal with hundreds of donors each day, this virtual explosion of data has made it essential that blood banks operate sophisticated computer systems and, where possible, automated laboratory testing equipment. Thus, the modern blood center uses pharmaceutical-type manufacturing processes in order to ensure accuracy and cost-effectiveness.[2,4,13]

SAFETY OF THE BLOOD SUPPLY

Ironically, the improvements in blood safety have occurred at a time of increased fear of transfusion in the public and more caution in the use of blood components by physicians. The steps in donor selection and laboratory testing described above have resulted in the nation's blood supply being safer than it has ever been.[1] Each step in the overall process of donor evaluation and testing adds to blood safety in important ways. For instance, in San Francisco, changes in the medical history and donor selection criteria caused a 90 percent decrease in the HIV infectivity of the blood supply even before the introduction of a test for HIV.[37] The introduction of new tests for transmissible diseases has further reduced the proportion of infectious donors. Screening of the donor's identity against donor deferral registries detects individuals who have been previously deferred as blood donors but who for various reasons attempt to donate again. These and many other changes have resulted in the improvement in blood safety. The risk of acquiring a transfusion-transmitted disease ranges from 1 per 103,300 units for hepatitis C to 1 per 493,000 for HIV (Table 139-3). Thus, although the blood supply is safer than ever, transfusion is not risk-free and should be undertaken only after careful consideration of the patient's clinical situation and specific blood component needs (see Chap. 140).

REFERENCES

1. McCullough J: The nation's changing blood supply system. *JAMA* 269:2239, 1993.
2. McCullough J: The continuing evolution of the nation's blood supply system. *Am J Clin Pathol* 105:689, 1996.
3. Wallace EL, Churchill WH, Surgenor DM, et al: Collection and transfusion of blood and blood components in the United States, 1994. *Transfusion* 38:265, 1998.
4. Zuck TF: Current good manufacturing practices. *Transfusion* 35:95, 1995.
5. Koistinen J: Organization of blood transfusion services in developing countries. *Vox Sang* 64:247, 1994.
6. Koistinen J, Westphal R: Blood transfusion worldwide, in *Transfusion Medicine, a European Course on Blood Transfusion*, coordinated by W van Aken, B Genetet. Centre Nationale d'Enseignement à Distance, Paris, 1994.
7. Emanuel JC: Blood transfusion systems in economically restricted countries. *Vox Sang* 64:267, 1994.
8. Beal R: Transfusion science and practice in developing countries: "A high frequency of empty shelves." *Transfusion* 33:276, 1993.
9. Eastlund T: Monetary blood donation incentives and the risk of transfusion-transmitted infection. *Transfusion* 38:874, 1998.
10. Leikola J: How much blood for the world? *Vox Sang* 54:1, 1988.
11. McCullough J: National blood programs in developed countries. *Transfusion* 36:1019, 1996.
12. Barker LF, Westphal RG: Voluntary, nonremunerated blood donation: still a world health goal? *Transfusion* 38:803, 1998.
13. McCullough J: *Transfusion Medicine*. McGraw Hill, New York, 1998.
14. Piliavin JA and Callero PL (eds): *Giving Blood. The Development of an Altruistic Identity*. Johns Hopkins University Press, Baltimore, 1991.
15. Morduchowicz G, Pitlik SD, Huminer D, et al: Transfusion reactions due to bacterial contamination of blood and blood products. *Rev Infect Dis* 13:307, 1991.
16. Sazama K: Reports of 355 transfusion-associated deaths: 1976 through 1985. *Transfusion* 30:583, 1990.
17. Logic JR, Johnson SA, Smith JJ: Cardiovascular and hematologic responses to phlebotomy in blood donors. *Transfusion* 3:83, 1963.
18. Ogata H, Iinuma N, Nagashima K, Akabane T: Vasovagal reactions in blood donors. *Transfusion* 20:679, 1980.
19. Kasprisin DO, Glynn SH, Taylor F, Miller KA: Moderate and severe reactions in blood donors. *Transfusion* 32:23, 1992.
20. Callahan R, Edelman EB, Smith MS, Smith JJ: Study of the incidence and characteristics of blood donor "reactors." *Transfusion* 3:76, 1963.
21. Popovsky MA, Whitaker B, Arnold NL: Severe outcomes of allogeneic and autologous blood donation: frequency and characterization. *Transfusion* 35:734, 1995.
22. Newman BH, Waxman DA: Blood donation-related neurologic needle injury: evaluation of 2 years' worth of data from a large blood center. *Transfusion* 36:213, 1996.
23. Berry PR, Wallis WE: Venipuncture nerve injuries. *Lancet* 1:1236, 1997.
24. Axelrod FB, Pepkowitz SH, Goldfinger D: Establishment of a schedule of optimal preoperative collection of autologous blood. *Transfusion* 29:677, 1989.
25. Birkmeyer JD, Goodnough LT, AuBuchon JP, et al: The cost-effectiveness of preoperative autologous blood donation for total hip and knee replacement. *Transfusion* 33:544, 1993.
26. Goodnough LT, Rednick S, Price TH, et al: Increased preoperative collection of autologous blood with recombinant human erythropoietin therapy. *N Engl J Med* 321:1163, 1989.
27. Spivak JL: Recombinant human erythropoietin and its role in transfusion medicine. *Transfusion* 34:1, 1994.
28. Starkey NM, MacPherson JL, Bolgiano DC, et al: Markers for transfusion-transmitted disease in different groups of blood donors. *JAMA* 262:3452, 1989.
29. Williams AE, Kleinman S, Gilcher RO, et al: The prevalence of infectious disease markers in directed versus homologous blood donations (abstract). *Transfusion* 32:45S, 1992.
30. McLeod BC, Price TH, Drew MI (eds): *Apheresis: Principles and Practice*. AABB Press, Bethesda, MD, pp 27–65, 1997.
31. Lasky L, Lin A, Kahn R, McCullough J: Donor platelet response and product quality assurance in plateletpheresis. *Transfusion* 21:247, 1981.
32. Bensinger WI, Price TH, Dale DC, et al: The effects of daily recombinant human granulocyte-colony-stimulating factor administration on normal granulocyte donors undergoing leukapheresis. *Blood* 81:1883, 1993.
33. Dale DC, Liles WC, Llewellyn C, et al: Neutrophil transfusions: kinetics and functions of neutrophils mobilized with granulocyte colony-stimulating factor (G-CSF) and dexamethasone. *Transfusion* 38:713, 1998.
34. McCullough J, Clay M, Herr G, et al: Effects of granulocyte colony stimulating factor (G-CSF) on potential normal granulocyte donors. *Transfusion* 39:1136, 1999.
35. Hester J, Dignani MC, Anaissie EJ, et al: Collection and transfusion of granulocyte concentrates from donors primed with granulocyte stimulating factor and response of myelosuppressed patients with established infection. *J Clin Apheresis* 10:188, 1995.
36. Strauss RG: Neutrophil (granulocyte) transfusions in the new millennium. *Transfusion* 38:710, 1998.
37. Busch MP, Young MJ, Samson SJ, et al and the Transfusion Safety Study Group: Risk of human immunodeficiency virus (HIV) transmission by blood transfusions before the implementation of HIV-1 antibody screening. *Transfusion* 31:4, 1991.
38. Cumming PD, Wallace EL, Schorr JB, Dodd RY: Exposure of patients to human immunodeficiency virus through the transfusion of blood components that test antibody-negative. *N Engl J Med* 321:941, 1989.
39. Busch MP, Bernard EE, Khayam-Bashi H, et al: Evaluation of screened blood donations from human immunodeficiency virus type 1 infection by culture and DNA amplification of pooled cells. *N Engl J Med* 325:1, 1991.

40. Donahue JG, Munoz A, Ness PM, et al: The declining risk of post-transfusion hepatitis C virus infection. *N Engl J Med* 327:369, 1992.

41. Dodd RY: The risk of transfusion-transmitted infection. *N Engl J Med* 327:419, 1992.

42. Nelson KE, Donahue JG, Munoz A, et al: Transmission of retroviruses from seronegative donors by transfusion during cardiac surgery. *Ann Intern Med* 117:554, 1992.

43. Kleinman S, Alter H, Busch M, et al: Increased detection of hepatitis C virus (HCV)-infected blood donors by a multiple-antigen HCV enzyme immunoassay. *Transfusion* 32:805, 1992.

44. Williams AE, Thomson RA, Schreiber GB, et al: Estimates of infectious disease risk factors in US blood donors. *JAMA* 277:967, 1997.

45. Sloand EM, Pitt E, Klein HG: Safety of the blood supply. *JAMA* 274:1368, 1995.

46. Lackritz EM, Satten GA, Aberle-Grasse J, et al: Estimated risk of transmission of the human immunodeficiency virus by screened blood in the United States. *N Engl J Med* 333:1721, 1995.

47. Schreiber GB, Busch MP, Kleinman SH: The risk of transfusion-transmitted viral infections. *N Engl J Med* 334:1685, 1996.

PRESERVATION AND CLINICAL USE OF ERYTHROCYTES AND WHOLE BLOOD

ERNEST BEUTLER

Transfusion of whole blood or of red cell concentrates is important in the treatment of acute blood loss and of anemia. Red cells can be stored at 4°C for 5 weeks in media that are specially designed to maintain the physical and biochemical integrity of the erythrocytes and that maintain their viability after reinfusion. Citrate-phosphate dextrose with adenine (CPDA) is commonly used for the collection of blood. The use of whole blood as a therapeutic agent has been almost entirely replaced by the use of blood fractions. Red cells can be stored in residual plasma or in additive solutions such as AS-1, a solution containing glucose, adenine, and mannitol. Erythrocytes can also be frozen after addition of a cryoprotective agent such as glycerol, and such cells can be stored for years. A variety of "blood substitutes" based either on hemoglobin or perfluorocarbons have been designed, but all have a short intravascular half-life and have not yet been found to be clinically useful.

Transfusion of red cells can cause febrile reactions, usually due to residual leukocytes, and the transmission of infectious diseases such as HIV and hepatitis. Other adverse effects include pulmonary hypersensitivity reactions, incompatible transfusions either because of unsuspected antigens or human error, and, in immuncompromised recipients, graft-versus-host disease.

Although the association of blood with life and vitality was recognized by primitive man, the transfusion of blood was not undertaken until after Harvey had described the circulation of the blood in 1628. During the following 40 years, animal blood was transfused directly into animals and humans, sometimes with unfortunate results.[1] Interest in blood transfusion waned, and it was not until 1828 that Blundell[2] successfully treated postpartum hemorrhage by direct transfusion of human blood. However, the mortality associated with transfusion was approximately 33 percent,[3] a figure surprisingly lower than the calculated frequency of ABO incompatibility.

Safe and effective transfusion therapy had to await the discovery of red cell blood group antigens by Landsteiner[4] and the development of nontoxic anticoagulants so that blood could be stored and used for indirect transfusions.[5-7] In 1937 Fantus[8] described the establishment at Cook County Hospital in Chicago of a blood bank for the collection, storage, and compatibility testing of blood for transfusion therapy.

Acronyms and abbreviations that appear in this chapter include: ACD, acid-citrate-dextrose; AIHA, autoimmune hemolytic anemia; ATP, adenosine 5'-triphosphate; 2,3-BPG, 2,3-bisphosphoglycerate; CPD, citrate-phosphate-dextrose; CPDA-1, CPD with adenine; DIC, disseminated intravascular coagulation; IgA, immunoglobulin A; IMP, inosine monophosphate; PIP, phosphate, inosine, and pyruvate.

Extensive experience with transfusion therapy accumulated during World War II (see, for example, reference 9). Subsequently, major technical developments included the introduction of closed plastic equipment consisting of tubing and bags that minimize the risk of bacterial contamination, the availability of a practical refrigerated centrifuge that facilitates separation of components, and the introduction of automated equipment for continuous-flow cell separations.[10,11]

PRINCIPLES OF STORAGE AND PRESERVATION OF BLOOD

Erythrocytes are preserved either by liquid storage at 4°C or frozen storage with various cryoprotective agents, at either −80 or −150°C. During liquid storage, red blood cells undergo changes that lead to a loss in viability and a diminished capacity to off-load oxygen. When stored red blood cells are reinfused into the circulation, some perish within a few hours, but the remainder appear to return to an entirely normal state. The survival of those cells not removed within the first 24 h is normal.[12]

Many attempts have been made to devise a means of predicting the proportion of transfused erythrocytes that remain viable. The ATP level of the erythrocytes enjoys a reputation as a predictor of viability of red blood cells after reinfusion that is poorly deserved.[13,14] The osmotic fragility and plasma hemoglobin levels are also of little value in predicting the viability of stored red blood cells. Indeed, the increase in osmotic fragility of stored erythrocytes is almost entirely due to their becoming loaded with lactate. Not freely diffusable, this exerts an unbalanced osmotic effect when osmotic fragility is tested in saline solutions.[15]

Stored red blood cells develop multiple and complex changes in membrane structure.[16] Although it has been suggested that the exposure of phosphatidyl serine on the outer membrane, which has increasingly been implicated as a signal of red cell aging (see Chap. 29), may play a role in the loss of viability of stored erythrocytes,[17] this does not seem to be the case.[18-20] The critical changes associated with loss of viability have not been identified, so that of necessity preservative solutions are evaluated by red cell survival studies in volunteers. Licensure of preservative solutions in the United States requires that more than 70 percent of the transfused red blood cells remain in the circulation 24 h after administration.

After reinfusion, stored red blood cells need to function properly in delivering oxygen to the tissues. The loss of 2,3-bisphosphoglycerate (2,3-BPG, 2,3-DPG) (see Chap. 26) during storage results in an increase in oxygen affinity that may compromise the ability of the stored erythrocytes to deliver oxygen to the tissues.[21,22] After reinfusion the red cell 2,3-BPG level returns to half-normal in 4 h and to normal in 24 h.[23,24] Although the clinical significance of 2,3-DPG loss in stored blood is difficult to assess,[25] there is general agreement that blood with nearly normal oxygen affinity should be used for massive transfusions, particularly in infants, older patients, and patients with cardiovascular and pulmonary disease.

Ideally, preservative solutions for erythrocytes should ensure maximum viability for the longest possible storage time and should allow optimal oxygen delivery. Unfortunately, with commonly used preservative solutions optimal storage conditions for either of the two critical components, ATP and 2,3-BPG, usually produce adverse effects on the other. The effect of various preservative solutions on maintenance of ATP and 2,3-BPG levels during liquid storage is summarized in Table 140-1.

LIQUID PRESERVATION OF ERYTHROCYTES

The preservative solutions used in the past for the storage of whole blood or red blood cells contain glucose and a citrate buffer at an acid pH. The citrate ion chelates calcium and thus prevents coagulation of

TABLE 140-1   PRESERVATION OF ATP AND 2,3-BPG RED CELL CONCENTRATIONS DURING STORAGE IN DIFFERENT PRESERVATIVE SOLUTIONS

| | Storage Period, Weeks | | | | | | | |
| | 1 | | 2 | | 3 | | 4 | |
	ATP	2,3-BPG	ATP	2,3-BPG	ATP	2,3-BPG	ATP	2,3-BPG
ACD	90	60	80	10	60	5	40	5
CPD	75	120	70	85	65	40	40	10
ACD-0.5 mM adenine	85	110	85	70	80	30	65	10
CPD-0.5 mM adenine	95	100	90	40	85	10	70	5
CPD+PIP (10 mM phosphate, 5 mM inosine, 5 mM pyruvate)	70	150	60	150	55	105	45	35
Addition of PIP at 14 days					80	120	70	100

NOTE: Whole blood stored at 4°C. Values are in percent of initial values and are approximate, since there is considerable variation from donor to donor.
SOURCE: Modified from de Verdier, Åkerblom, Arturson, et al.[71,219]

the blood, glucose sustains the metabolism of red blood cells during storage, and the acid pH counteracts the marked rise of pH that occurs when blood is cooled to 4°C.[26] The two preservative solutions of this type in use until CPD-adenine was introduced in 1978 were acid-citrate-dextrose (ACD) and citrate-phosphate-dextrose (CPD) (see "ACD and CPD Whole Blood").

When whole blood or packed red blood cells are stored in either ACD or CPD, a series of well-defined biochemical changes, designated collectively as the *storage lesion,* takes place in the erythrocytes (Table 140-2). The concentration of red cell ATP falls gradually during storage.[24,26] As ATP is dephosphorylated, the levels of ADP and AMP rise at first but diminish with time as AMP is irreversibly deaminated to IMP, which is ultimately broken down to hypoxanthine.[27] When the ATP level declines to 0.4 mM or less, the capacity of red blood cells to phosphorylate glucose is impaired, and their viability is lost. The level of 2,3-BPG and consequently the hemoglobin oxygen affinity changes rapidly in ACD blood. Some 40 percent of the 2,3-BPG is lost in the first week of storage, resulting in a significant increase in oxygen affinity. After 2 weeks' storage, nearly all the 2,3-BPG has disappeared from blood stored in ACD solution. The loss of 2,3-BPG occurs more slowly in blood stored in CPD solution, because of its higher pH.[28] The oxygen affinity and 2,3-BPG levels remain nearly normal during the first week of storage, and then fall rapidly. Potassium rapidly leaks from the stored blood cells, and sodium seeps in[29] because the sodium-potassium ATPase is exquisitely sensitive to changes in temperature. The osmotic fragility of the red blood cells gradually increases, but this change is largely an artifact produced by the intracellular accumulation of lactate.[15] Some erythrocytes undergo spontaneous lysis, causing a rise of plasma hemoglobin levels. Di-(2-ethylhexyl) phthalate plasticizer leached from the polyvinyl chloride plastic in which whole blood and red cell preparations are stored retards hemolysis and improves the viability of the cells when they are reinfused.[30] Microvesicles filled with hemoglobin begin to form.[31] Erythrocytes stored at 4°C also show a progressive increase in rigidity as measured by their rate of flow through filters. Their loss of deformability correlates to some extent with the loss of ATP.[32] Because some residual leukocytes are invariably present, various cytokines are also found in

stored blood,[33] and these may play a role in some transfusion reactions. This seems particularly to be the case when certain types of apparatus are used for intraoperative salvage of erythrocytes.[34] Blood stored in ACD or CPD will yield a 70 percent 24-h survival of transfused red blood cells for up to 21 days of storage.

Major efforts have been directed toward development of preservative solutions that will maintain adequate erythrocyte levels of ATP and 2,3-BPG. Adenine and inosine are two additives that have been extensively studied. Addition of adenine to give a final concentration of 0.25 to 0.75 mM at the beginning of storage helps to prevent the loss of ATP,[35] since it can serve as a substrate for synthesis of adenine nucleotides (see Chap. 26). The addition of adenine does not prevent the loss of 2,3-BPG and may slightly hasten its depletion.

The addition of adenine alone at the end of storage is not helpful if red blood cells have lost a substantial portion of their ATP. Under these circumstances, they are unable to phosphorylate glucose and thus are unable to synthesize adenine nucleotides, or to phosphorylate ADP and AMP to ATP. If inosine is supplied, ATP formation can occur even when red cell ATP levels are very low. The phosphorolysis of inosine yields ribose-1-phosphate, which can be metabolized to yield high-energy phosphates and maintain 2,3-BPG levels (see Chap. 26). The addition of inosine either at the beginning of storage or before infusion of ATP-depleted blood markedly improves the storage viability of red blood cells,[35] but a concentration of inosine of about 10 mM is required. Infusion of inosine or of the hypoxanthine formed by its catabolism may result in dangerous hyperuricemia.

The reported capacity of ascorbic acid to maintain 2,3-BPG levels[36] is due to contaminating oxalate,[37,38] which seems to exert its function largely by inhibiting pyruvate kinase.[38] Certain xanthone derivatives exert a direct effect on the oxygen dissociation curve of hemoglobin and, in addition, elevate red cell 2,3-BPG levels[39] because of their inhibitory effect on 2,3-BPG phosphatase.[40] Dihydroxyacetone is metabolized by erythrocytes and helps to maintain 2,3-BPG levels during storage.[41–43] Periodic agitation of blood during storage improves the maintenance of 2,3-BPG levels in some preservatives, probably by preventing a localized decrease in pH in the gravity-sedimented red blood cells[44] but has little effect on red blood cells in blood collected in CPD solution.[45] Several other additives have been used experimentally to maintain or restore 2,3-BPG levels of stored red cells. The 2,3-BPG content of stored blood can be restored to normal or supranormal levels[46] by incubating the erythrocytes with phosphate, inosine, and pyruvate (PIP). Both 2,3-BPG and ATP levels in outdated blood can be restored by incubation with PIP and adenine. Phospho(enol)pyruvate can enter red blood cells when they are suspended in a slightly acidic solution, and it has also been proposed that this source of metabolic energy may be useful in red cell preservation.[47] The rejuvenated erythrocytes can be recovered by centrifugation and washing and either used for transfusion or frozen for future use.[48]

TABLE 140-2   EFFECT OF STORAGE IN ACD ON ERYTHROCYTE PROPERTIES

Alteration	ATP	2,3-BPG	Viability
↑ pH	↓	↑	↓
↓ pH	↑	↓	↑
↑ P_i[a]	↑	↑	←→
+Adenine	↑	↓	↑
+Inosine	↑	↑	↑

[a] Inorganic phosphate.

Preservative solutions that contain high concentrations of inorganic phosphate, are hypotonic, and contain ammonium have been found to maintain 2,3 BPG and ATP levels for a prolonged time.[49,50] The effects of such solutions are primarily a function of the ammonium, which relieves phosphofructokinase inhibition by ATP, and of phosphate.[51,52]

ADDITIVE SOLUTIONS

The conversion of whole blood into components requires the removal of a significant fraction of both plasma and red cell preservative solution from the red blood cells. Red cell preservation, however, can be optimized if a nutrient solution is added to the isolated red blood cells.[53] The initial blood collection can be into CPD solution or half-strength CPD (0.5 CPD).[54] The nutrient solutions that have been developed generally contain glucose as a source of energy, adenine to help support ATP levels, and mannitol to prevent hemolysis. The mechanism by which mannitol exerts this effect is unknown. Originally added to such solutions for osmotic support,[55] it has been shown that its osmotic effect is not the mechanism of action.[56] Several different additive solutions are now available in the United States (AS-3, Nutricell, Cutter Labs, Berkeley, CA; and AS-1, Adsol, Fenwall Labs, Morton Grove, IL) and in Sweden.[57] ATP levels are well maintained, and good survival is obtained after 42 days' storage with the use of additive solutions, but the 2,3-BPG level is reduced by 90 percent at 42 days.[58,59] The loss of 2,3-BPG can be prevented by incorporating bicarbonate and a CO_2 trap into the system.[60]

FROZEN STORAGE OF ERYTHROCYTES

Uncontrolled freezing and thawing of erythrocytes results in hemolysis. Freeze-thaw injury is dependent on the rate of freezing, the physical structure of ice, and the properties of water, cell membranes, and solutions at various temperatures. A current theory of freeze-thaw hemolysis suggests that slowly cooled red blood cells are damaged by osmotic dehydration as they are exposed to increasing extracellular electrolyte concentration and osmolality as water is removed by freezing.[61] Irreversible biochemical changes in the membrane may result from the prolonged exposure of the dehydrated, hypertonic red cell to temperatures insufficiently low to prevent biochemical alterations.[62] If such changes are prevented, then lysis of the red blood cells may occur on return to isotonicity, because of the excess solute content acquired during the hypertonic phase of freezing.[63] Although the precise biochemical and biophysical changes leading to hemolysis are not fully understood, empirical methods have been developed for the practical freeze-preservation of red blood cells. Preservation of erythrocytes by freezing retards or arrests the deleterious biochemical changes that occur during liquid storage.[64] Frozen cells have maintained satisfactory viability for as long as 21 years.[65] Under some conditions it is possible to preserve the metabolic activity and physical integrity of erythrocytes after lyophilization,[66,67] but the usefulness of such cells for transfusion purposes has not been documented.

Glycerol is the most commonly used cryoprotective agent for freeze-preservation of erythrocytes. Hydroxyethyl starch[68] and dextran[69] also appear to have desirable cryoprotective properties. The most commonly utilized technique currently is a slow freezing method in which the red blood cells are equilibrated with 40 to 50% glycerol and cooled to −80 to −120°C using mechanical refrigeration.[70] All methods of freeze-preservation of erythrocytes involving the use of cryoprotective agents require the technical capability for introducing and removing high concentrations of the cyoprotective agent (glycerol) under sterile conditions. Frozen red blood cells must be thawed and the glycerol removed gradually by washing in glycerol solutions of

decreasing concentration to prevent osmotic hemolysis. Under optimum conditions of processing, storage, and cell washing, over 80 percent of the freeze-preserved red blood cells from a unit of blood will survive and function normally after transfusion. Such thawed and washed red blood cells must be used within 24 h because processing breaks the closed system and introduces the possibility of bacterial contamination.

WHOLE BLOOD PREPARATIONS

Most clinical situations require the use of specific blood components, and the use of whole blood is limited to correction or prevention of hypovolemia in patients with severe acute blood loss.

ACD (ACID-CITRATE-DEXTROSE), CPD (CITRATE-PHOSPHATE-DEXTROSE), AND CPDA-1 (CPD WITH ADENINE) WHOLE BLOOD

ACD and CPD are the two preservative-anticoagulant solutions used exclusively in the past in the United States. They have been largely superseded by adenine-containing solutions. Blood is currently collected and stored in bags manufactured from plastic films.

For each 100 ml of whole blood there should be 15 ml of ACD solution or 14 ml of CPD or CPDA-1. The ACD solution (formula A) contains 8.0 g of citric acid ($C_6H_8O_7 \cdot H_2O$), 22 g of sodium citrate ($Na_3C_6H_5O_7 \cdot 2H_2O$), and 24.5 g of glucose ($C_6H_{12}O_6 \cdot H_2O$) per liter. CPD is a modified ACD solution which is slightly less acid and therefore improves the preservation of 2,3-BPG (Table 140-1). It contains 3.27 g of citric acid, 23.6 g of sodium citrate, 25.5 g of glucose, and 2.22 g of $NaH_2PO_4 \cdot H_2O$ per liter.

Adenine is incorporated into CPD or ACD preservatives in amounts sufficient to provide a concentration of 0.25 mM to 0.75 mM to increase the shelf life of the stored red blood cells.[71] CPD with adenine (CPDA-1) contains CPD, modified to contain 125 percent of the usual concentration of glucose, and adenine to provide a final concentration of 0.25 mM. Although still suboptimal, the higher glucose concentration provides an additional supply for cells packed immediately after collection so that the blood may be fractionated into components.[72,73]

A unit of whole blood may contain from 405 to 495 ml of blood.[70] The volume of each anticoagulant solution used for 450 ml of whole blood is 67.5 ml of ACD or 63 ml of CPD or CPDA-1 solution. The total fluid volume actually administered in transfusing 450 ml of whole blood is 517.5 ml of ACD and 513 ml for CPD collected blood. If the volume collected is between 300 and 405 ml, the red blood cells can be used for transfusion if they are labeled "Low Volume Unit ___ ml. Red Blood Cells."[70]

With proper collection and storage at 2 to 6°C, ACD whole blood and CPD whole blood can be used within 21 days after collection. The 21-day storage limit has been established based on survival of 70 percent of the transfused erythrocytes at 24 h after transfusion (see "Transfusion Therapy"). Blood collected in CPDA-1 is licensed for 35 days' storage.

FRESH BLOOD

Requests for "fresh" blood are usually justified by the recognition that there is a relatively rapid loss of platelets, leukocytes, and some coagulation factors with liquid storage as well as a progressive increase in the levels of undesirable products such as potassium, ammonium, and hydrogen ions.[74,75] Blood stored at 4°C over 48 h using ACD, CPD, or their adenine-containing derivatives is depleted of viable platelets.[76] Factor V remains at adequate levels (greater than 80 percent) for at least 5 days,[77] factor VIII remains above 80 percent of its original level for 1 to 2 days,[77] and factor XI activity rapidly falls to about 20 percent of its original level within the first week of storage.[78] All other clotting factors appear to be stable during liquid storage.[79–81]

Blood "freshness" cannot be precisely defined, since it depends upon the storage stability of the particular component in blood that is needed. The loss of platelets and coagulation factors in stored whole blood may be a consideration in massive transfusions following trauma or surgery. Thrombocytopenia and decreased levels of labile coagulation factors with oozing of blood may occur when more than the patient's blood volume[11] (12 to 14 units) is replaced by banked blood within a 24-h period.[82] In such cases, packed red blood cells, fresh-frozen plasma, and platelet concentrates are superior to "fresh" whole blood.

Whole blood less than 5 to 7 days old may be indicated when changes in stored blood such as increased plasma potassium and ammonium and a decreased pH must be avoided, as in patients with advanced renal or liver disease or newborn infants who are given exchange transfusions.

In a seriously ill patient massively transfused with 2- or 3-week-old banked blood, the low levels of 2,3-BPG may compromise tissue oxygenation. Although the 2,3-BPG levels are regenerated within a day or so,[23,24] it is probably prudent to administer a significant proportion of CPD blood less than 5 days old or ACD blood less than 2 days old.[21] It is also appropriate to provide patients with refractory anemias red blood cells that are less than 10 days old to avoid the infusion of nonviable cells that add unnecessarily to the patient's iron burden.

ERYTHROCYTE PREPARATIONS

Four types of erythrocyte preparations are in common use: packed red blood cells, washed red blood cells, leukocyte-reduced red blood cells, and frozen red blood cells. Washed red blood cells can be obtained from liquid-stored blood by saline washing using a continuous-flow cell separator or from frozen erythrocytes that have been extensively washed to remove the cryoprotective agent.

PACKED RED BLOOD CELLS

At any time before the expiration date of the blood, erythrocytes can be separated and recovered from ACD, CPD, or CPDA-1 whole blood by centrifugation and removal of plasma to give a hematocrit of 60 to 90 percent. Red blood cells packed to a hematocrit of less than 80 percent, or sedimented red blood cells stored at 1 to 6°C are suitable for transfusion for the full shelf life of the preservative-anticoagulant solution (21 or 35 days). Red blood cells packed to a higher hematocrit do not survive as well, chiefly because they exhaust available glucose.[72,73,83] If the blood is exposed to the external environment during preparation, the packed or sedimented red blood cells must be transfused within 24 h.[84]

Red blood cells rather than whole blood should be used for the treatment of all patients who require transfusion because of a red cell mass deficit. Packed red blood cells and balanced salt solutions appear to be as effective as whole blood in correcting the blood loss that occurs at surgery.[85]

Red blood cells are administered in the same fashion as is whole blood. The rate of administration may be slower with packed red blood cells but approaches that of whole blood if a 17-gauge or larger needle is used or if a diluting solution such as saline is used[86] or if the red blood cells have been stored in an additive solution.[87]

LEUKOCYTE-REDUCED RED BLOOD CELLS

There are three major reasons for the use of leukocyte-reduced red blood cells: (1) to prevent or avoid nonhemolytic febrile reactions due

to antibodies to white cells and platelets in the recipient exposed to previous transfusions or pregnancies (see below); (2) To prevent sensitization of patients with aplastic anemia who may be candidates for marrow transplantation; and (3) to minimize transmission of viral disease such as HIV or cytomegalovirus. To prevent febrile reactions, a unit of red blood cells should contain no more than 5×10^8 leukocytes; for the prevention of alloimmunization and to minimize transmission of viral diseases it has been recommended that no more than 5×10^6 leukocytes remain.[70]

Leukocyte-reduced blood is best prepared by passing the whole blood or packed cells through specially designed filters.[88–91] Such filters can be used either in the blood bank or at the bedside as the red blood cells are being transfused. Other methods that have been used include sedimentation, inverted centrifugation, filtration through nylon or cotton, and saline batch washing using a cell processor, frozen-thawed red blood cells, or blood filtration through a microaggregate filter.[92]

WASHED RED BLOOD CELLS

Washed red blood cells are usually obtained from whole blood. Packed red blood cells collected by centrifugation can be washed with saline using either manual batch centrifugation or continuous-flow cell separators.[93] Washed red blood cells must be used within 24 h after processing because of the risk of bacterial contamination during preparation. Frozen red blood cells are an excellent albeit expensive source of washed red blood cells.

Washed red blood cells are indicated in the rare patient who is hypersensitive to plasma. Such patients develop an allergic or febrile reaction following whole blood transfusion that can be reproduced with the injection of even a small quantity of plasma.[4] Some of these patients have a deficiency of IgA and have formed antibodies to IgA from a previous transfusion or pregnancy.[95] Saline washed red blood cells may be indicated in neonatal transfusions[96] to reduce the quantity of anticoagulant, metabolic breakdown products, extracellular potassium, and risk of cytomegalovirus infection (see "Hazards of Transfusion Therapy").

FROZEN RED BLOOD CELLS

Frozen red blood cells have a shelf life measured in years[65] rather than weeks, which simplifies the efficient management of blood inventories. These cells are somewhat leukocyte-poor and relatively free of plasma. The potential advantages of frozen red blood cells have stimulated intensive efforts to develop more practical and less costly procedures for preserving erythrocytes and other cellular blood components by freezing.

Frozen red blood cells are admirably suited for autotransfusion (see "Autologous Transfusions"). Other advantages include availability of an inventory of rare blood[97,98]; reduction in sensitization to histocompatibility antigens for potential transplant recipients as compared to unfiltered red blood cells; and more efficient inventory control. However, a unit of frozen blood costs two to three times as much as a unit stored in the liquid state.

ARTIFICIAL BLOOD SUBSTITUTES

Some functions of blood such as maintaining circulating volume and osmotic pressure can be replaced with various crystalloid and colloid macromolecules such as dextran and hydroxyethyl starch (Chap. 59). These blood substitutes, however, do not provide for oxygen transport.

Materials with the potential of supporting oxygen transport such as stroma-free hemoglobin solutions, liposome-encapsulated hemoglobin, and perfluorocarbons have been under active investigation.[99] Interest in such preparations has largely been driven by fear of transmitting microbial diseases through blood transfusion.

Perfluorochemicals are organic compounds in which all the hydrogen atoms are replaced by fluorine. Per-unit volume solutions bind almost three times the oxygen carried by blood. They are chemically inert and are not metabolized but require emulsification with surfactants to be miscible with blood. Rats survived up to 8 h following complete replacement of their blood with liquid fluorocarbon. A perfluorocarbon-hydroxyethyl starch preparation developed in Japan and marketed as Fluosol-DA (Green Corp., Osaka, Japan) that requires concurrent administration of 60 to 100 percent oxygen has been used experimentally in human volunteers and in a few patients, but no evidence of therapeutic value has been found.[100] Moreover, its use has been associated with pulmonary reactions, cytotoxicity, complement activation, retention of the fluorocarbon in the liver and spleen, and vulnerability to oxygen toxicity.

Stroma-free hemoglobin solutions have been investigated as oxygen-carrying blood substitutes.[101] Their usefulness is limited because of toxicity,[102,103] high affinity for oxygen, and a very short intravascular half-life (2 to 4 h). Hemoglobin complexes and recombinant mutant hemoglobin molecules have been prepared that will increase the intravascular life span to 10 to 12 h, and some of these have a more favorable oxygen affinity.[99] Numerous clinical studies of hemoglobin solutions have been conducted.[104] With some preparations significant hypertension occurs after infusion, and although this has been thought to be due to the binding and depletion of NO giving rise to vasospasm, the actual mechanism is not entirely clear.[105]

Hemoglobin has also been encapsulated in artificially prepared liposomes enabling the addition of 2,3 BPG to achieve near-normal oxygen-hemoglobin dissociation properties.[106,107] The relatively short life span of liposomes, problems in scaling-up the process, nonuniformity of liposome size, complement activation,[108] and difficulties in ensuring sterility make it unlikely that such encapsulated hemoglobin preparations will ever have any clinical utility.

TRANSFUSION THERAPY

A patient should be transfused only when specific, well-established indications are present and in practically all cases with blood components rather than whole blood. Informed consent should be obtained from patients except in life-threatening emergencies. Patients who are candidates for transfusion should be provided with specific information regarding the risks and benefits of the proposed transfusion therapy, and the discussion should be documented by an entry in the patient's medical record.[109]

INDICATIONS FOR TRANSFUSION THERAPY

A major clinical indication for transfusion therapy is the need to restore and maintain the volume of circulating blood to prevent or treat shock, as in hemorrhage or trauma. Probably more than 50 percent of the blood transfused is in the support of surgery.[110] Another indication is the need for specific cellular or protein components such as erythrocytes, specific coagulation factors, or platelets. Exchange transfusions may be required to remove deleterious materials from the blood, in the past primarily in infants for hemolytic disease of the newborn. Blood is also used to maintain the circulation as in extracorporeal or cardiac bypass shunts.[111,112]

HEMORRHAGE AND SHOCK

A major indication for transfusion of blood or components is existing or anticipated hemorrhage (Chap. 59). Treatment of acute blood loss should be devoted to volume support and only secondarily be con-

cerned with loss of red cell mass. A loss of approximately 1 liter of blood in a patient without cardiovascular disease can be treated with electrolyte solutions. Colloids for volume support and possibly red blood cells may be needed with losses of 1 to 2 liters. Acute blood losses in excess of 2 to 3 liters require correction of both volume deficiency and red cell mass loss.[113]

If the history and the clinical picture suggest that the patient has sustained a significant loss of blood, replacement therapy with whole blood or red blood cells is indicated. Clinical[114] and experimental[85] observations in hypovolemic (hemorrhagic) shock suggest that the combination of packed red blood cells with crystalloids or albumin is as effective as whole blood in correcting a volume deficit. Blood of any age within the usual storage limits is suitable. Many patients who have sustained blood loss do not need a whole blood transfusion and should not be exposed to the associated risks (see "Hazards of Transfusion Therapy").

SURGERY

The loss of 500 ml of blood during a surgical procedure is well tolerated by the average patient. Maintaining normovolemia with crystalloid solutions appeared to be a significant factor in preventing morbidity and mortality. One hundred patients undergoing major surgery with blood losses greater than 1000 ml were treated with Hartmann's solution (lactated Ringer's solution: NaCl, 102 meq per liter; KCl, 4 meq per liter; CaCl$_2$, 3.5 meq per liter; and sodium lactate, 27 meq per liter), using two to three times the estimated volume of blood lost. Postoperative mortality and morbidity were not affected by the use of crystalloid rather than blood, and there were no unexpected complications.[115] Even patients undergoing open heart surgery have been managed successfully without transfusions[116] despite a severe, acute decrease in red blood cell mass.

BURNS

Initially volume resuscitation is required in patients with severe burns because of the marked increase in permeability of the microcirculation in burned tissue.[117] Patients with a burn injury of more than 25 percent surface area require large volumes of balanced salt solutions during the initial 24 h.[118,119] Plasma loss, which ensues during the next 5 days, can be corrected with plasma and colloids. The progressive development of anemia during the early postburn period is best treated with packed red blood cells.

ANEMIA

Blood transfusion of patients with chronic stable anemia is probably unjustifiable if the hemoglobin level is above 7 g per 100 ml unless the patient is elderly or severe cardiac or pulmonary disease is present. There is probably significant misuse of blood transfusions in patients with chronic anemia. Data from 300 hospitals over a 1-year period (1974) revealed that 401 nonoperated patients with anemia were transfused, even though they had a hemoglobin concentration greater than 10 g per 100 ml.[120] Audit criteria for the evaluation of transfusion practice have been established.[121]

Multiple, repeated transfusions of whole blood or packed red blood cells have been used to suppress erythropoiesis in patients with thalassemia and sickle cell diseases (Chaps. 46 and 47). However, transfusional hemochromatosis (see Chap. 42) may limit the usefulness of this therapy of managing the hemoglobinopathies. One approach to the control of iron accumulation in transfusion-dependent patients with thalassemia is the use of red blood cells enriched in their content of young red blood cells, "neocytes." Young red blood cells are obtained based on size and density using a continuous-flow cell separator.[122–124] The administration of neocytes has been associated with a decreased transfusion requirement.[122,125] However, despite the fact that with modern equipment neocyte preparations can be prepared without too much difficulty,[125] they are costly and their routine use has been limited. Furthermore, the effectiveness of transfused neocytes may be less than predicted by in vitro and in vivo studies.[126]

OTHER INDICATIONS

The clinical uses of other types of blood components are presented in Chaps. 141 (leukocytes, dendritic cells, and stem cells), 142 (platelets), and 143 (plasma and plasma fractions).

MODE OF ADMINISTRATION

The most important action the physician or nurse can take before administering blood or a blood product is to read the label to verify that the unit to be used is the one selected by the laboratory for that particular patient (see ''Hazards of Transfusion Therapy'').

Blood need not be warmed before its use unless unusually large amounts must be given (more than 3 liters) at a rapid rate (greater than 100 ml per min).[127] At the usual rate of administration (500 ml in 1 to 2 h), the agglutinates that may occur in patients with high-titer cold agglutinins are usually dispersed as the transfused blood reaches body temperature.

Blood should be administered slowly during the first 30 min to minimize the amount given if an untoward reaction occurs. It is safe to transfuse 1000 ml of citrated blood within a period of 2 to 3 h to the average patient without cardiovascular disease.[127]

Drugs or medications should not be added to blood or components. Several intravenous solutions are incompatible with banked blood and should not be administered through the blood lines. Aqueous dextrose solutions cause agglomeration (clumping) and hemolysis of red blood cells, and calcium-containing solutions such as Ringer's lactate may exceed the calcium-binding capacity of the citrate in the anticoagulated blood with formation of clots.[128,129] Physiological saline is compatible with all blood components.

Most transfusion therapy is administered intravenously. A vein in the forearm or antecubital fossa is ordinarily used, although any accessible vein or a central line may be employed. Infrequently used routes for the administration of blood and components are intraarterial and intraperitoneal. Because of the hazards, transfusion into an artery should be reserved for patients who have failed to respond to rapid, large-volume intravenous transfusion. Intraperitoneal transfusions may be indicated for children in whom suitable veins are difficult to find and occasionally for the fetus in utero.[130,131]

SPECIAL SITUATIONS

SINGLE-UNIT TRANSFUSION

Single-unit transfusions have sometimes been condemned as an unwarranted use of blood.[132] However, single-unit transfusions are often justifiable. Examples include elderly surgical patients with coronary disease, patients who have sustained an acute loss of two or three units who achieve circulatory stability with one unit, and patients whose bleeding during surgery or from the gastrointestinal tract is controlled after transfusion of the first unit. Single-unit transfusion in such cases represents good judgment and therapeutic skill.[133,134]

AUTOLOGOUS TRANSFUSIONS

In autologous transfusions (autotransfusion) blood removed from a patient is returned to the patient's circulation after storage, or blood lost at or immediately after surgery is reinfused. Transfusion of autologous blood averts some problems associated with the use of homologous donor blood, such as febrile and allergic reactions, immunologic incompatibilities that may lead to hemolysis, alloimmunization, and the transmission of disease.

Three variations of autotransfusion have been used: preoperative blood collection, with storage for a variable time and retransfusion during surgery; immediate preoperative phlebotomy and hemodilution with postoperative return of the phlebotomized blood[135]; and intraoperative collection of shed blood with reinfusion during surgery.[136] Equipment designed for intraoperative autotransfusion is commercially available.[137–139]

In many elective surgical procedures the recipient can predeposit autologous blood.[140] In some patients the amount of predeposited autologous blood may be increased through the use of recombinant human erythropoietin therapy.[141] Predeposited autologous blood also may be frozen and represents the ideal product for patients with rare blood types (e.g., Rh-null) or for patients with antibodies in numbers and combinations that make it nearly impossible to find compatible units of blood.

DIRECTED OR DESIGNATED DONATIONS

Donors recruited from among family members or friends (donor-specific) contrary to expectation are no safer than volunteer blood donors. Fatal graft-versus-host reactions have been reported involving unusual HLA similarities between close relatives (see ''Graft-Versus-Host Disease'').

BLOOD FOR EXCHANGE TRANSFUSIONS

Exchange transfusions are used to treat the newborn who has severe hemolytic disease due to a feto-maternal blood group incompatibility, G6PD deficiency, or an unknown cause (Chaps. 7, 45, and 58).

Exchange transfusions have been simplified by the introduction of equipment that automatically harvests blood components from an individual (Chap. 144).

BLOOD FOR PATIENTS WITH AUTOIMMUNE HEMOLYTIC DISEASE

The provision of compatible red blood cells for patients with AIHA is one of the most difficult and challenging problems in transfusion medicine.[142] Compatibility usually cannot be assured because of the effect of autoantibodies on routine serological tests. Transfusion management of the patient with AIHA involves a risk-benefit judgment; namely: Does the need for increased oxygen-carrying capacity justify the risks of a possible hemolytic reaction? Transfusion should be avoided in these patients whenever possible.[143,144]

Ideally donor blood should be selected so that it lacks those antigens corresponding to the antibodies in the recipient, whether autoimmune or alloimmune. Patients with red cell autoantibodies are serologically incompatible with their own red blood cells and with those of most if not all donors. Such patients if previously transfused or pregnant may also have clinically significant alloantibodies difficult to detect in the presence of the autoantibody.

Usually no autoantibody specificity can be established, and it may be impossible to find serologically compatible blood. However, it may be possible to find units that react more weakly than others. A variety of time-consuming serological procedures are available to detect alloantibodies in the presence of autoantibodies, but it may require ^{51}Cr survival studies to establish compatibility. Many of these patients will tolerate hemoglobin levels of 5 to 7 g per 100 ml and should not be transfused. If life-threatening anemia is present, a transfusion may be required even in the face of serological incompatibility. In such cases blood should be selected that is at least as compatible as the patient's cells in their own serum. Packed red blood cells rather than whole blood should be used, and sometimes packed red blood cells less than 10 days old may be indicated to minimize the number and frequency of transfusions required.

BLOOD FOR EMERGENCIES

Emergencies in which no time is available to type, select, and cross-match compatible blood should be a rare occurrence, except for trauma, unexpected intraoperative hemorrhage, massive gastrointestinal bleeding, or ruptured aneurysm.[145]

If the urgency of the patient's need justifies the administration of uncross-matched blood, type O, Rh-negative blood with low plasma anti-A and anti-B titers can be used. Unfortunately, tests for donor anti-A and anti-B levels are not done routinely. The use of packed red blood cells will reduce the quantity of anti-A or -B administered. It is preferable, however, to use ABO group and Rh-type-specific blood, which is usually available within 15 min if the patient's blood is available for testing. Administration of uncross-matched group-specific blood will prevent hemolysis that may occur if a high-titered anti-A or anti-B group O blood is given to a non-O recipient. If 15 to 30 min are available, an abbreviated antibody screen can be carried out using low ionic strength conditions.[146] Group- and type-specific uncross-matched blood with a negative antibody screen provides compatibility for the recipient equivalent to that of cross-matched blood in essentially all cases.[147] The routine cross-match should be carried out retrospectively to identify any incompatibility when uncross-matched or partially cross-matched blood is administered.

BLOOD FOR TRANSPLANT RECIPIENTS

Kidney Grafts   Random donor blood transfusions can result in allogeneic immunization,[148,149] and in the early days of transplantation they were avoided in order to prevent the possibility of inducing anti-HLA antibodies in potential transplant recipients. However, a series of reports from 1973 to 1978[150-152] surprisingly demonstrated that kidney transplant patients who had received multiple blood transfusions before transplantation actually had better graft survival. This was particularly true for black and hispanic patients,[153] two groups that often demonstrate lower kidney graft survival rates than age- and gender-matched caucasian patients. While the mechanism of this apparent paradox is still not clear, the purposeful administration of random donor blood transfusions became common practice. In kidney transplant patients with living related donors, the blood transfusions were given from the related donor, a practice called "donor-specific transfusion."[154] The beneficial effect appears mediated by the HLA antigens expressed on donor leukocytes, probably monocytes but possibly also B cells.[155,156] In patients receiving donor-specific transfusions, the coadministration of low-dose azathioprine (Imuran) reduced the risk of sensitization to the donor HLA antigens from 30 percent to less than 10 percent.[157] That an immunosuppressive drug with antiproliferative effects on B cells could reduce the risk of antibody-mediated sensitization without altering the beneficial effect on graft survival supported the hypothesis that blood transfusions could generate some form of suppressor cell phenomenon presumably mediated by memory T cells. An alternative theory is that blood transfusions represent a selection process for patients prone to be "responders" to certain donor HLA antigens. In other words, if a patient is sensitized by a specific HLA antigen after a transfusion, then that antigen is avoided when matching that patient for the kidney transplant, and better graft survival results.

The current practice of blood transfusion in kidney transplantation has been changed dramatically by three developments: the introduction of cyclosporine and erythropoietin and the increasing concern over the danger of exposure to random donor transfusions. Cyclosporine is so potent an immunosuppressive drug that its use has challenged any additional beneficial effect of blood transfusions,[158,159] and the

blood transfusion effect is no longer demonstrable in kidney transplantation,[153] even in black and hispanic patients. The only possible exception is that patients transplanted under the age of 15 years still demonstrate a small transfusion effect. The widespread use of erythropoietin has ended the routine practice of blood transfusions to treat the anemia of end-stage renal disease.

Marrow Grafts   Previous blood transfusions, especially from the intended donor, are associated with a high rate of marrow graft rejection in patients with aplastic anemia but are not a serious problem in marrow transplantation of leukemic patients.[160] ABO incompatibility in otherwise histocompatible donors does not appear to affect the marrow transplant outcome.[161] There is a need to avoid an immediate transfusion reaction caused by the red blood cells in the marrow inoculum when an ABO-incompatible engraftment is carried out. Such a complication may be averted by removing anti-A or -B from the recipient by plasma exchange, by neutralization in vivo, or by removing mature red blood cells from the inoculum.[161] Indications for blood component therapy in marrow transplantation have been reviewed.[162]

Liver Grafts   Unusually large volumes of blood and the ability to recognize and correct complex hemostatic deficiencies are required for liver transplantation.[163] The demand for blood is influenced by the underlying liver disease, the nature of the preoperative coagulation defect,[164] and the intraoperative blood loss associated with handling a large vascular organ. An additional problem is that the large number of donors increases the risk of disease transmission (see "Hazards of Transfusion Therapy"). In a 1987 study the mean number of donor exposures per patient receiving a liver transplant ranged from 170 to 200 units.[163]

Blood requirements for liver transplants can be significantly reduced with intraoperative cell salvage and expansion of the blood bank erythrocyte inventory using AS-1 preservative. In 100 transplants the median intraoperative erythrocyte use was 12.6 units per transplant recipient.[165]

HAZARDS OF TRANSFUSION THERAPY

Transfusion therapy, even under ideal conditions, carries a significant risk of an adverse reaction. Such reactions are associated with significant morbidity and in some cases with a fatal outcome. Most of the reported fatalities involve human error. In one study of 70 fatalities, 56 percent were due to acute hemolytic reactions. Half of these were preventable, since they involved an ABO mismatch due to human error. Seventy-five percent of the fatalities were due to administration of correctly cross-matched blood to the wrong patient.[166] Two subsequent reviews of FDA fatality reports from 1976 to 1978[167] and from 1976 through 1985[168] continue to confirm these findings, i.e., a majority of transfusion fatalities are managerial-clerical and not technical failures.

Up to 20 percent of all transfusions may lead to some type of adverse reaction.[169] The precise risk is difficult to estimate, since many reactions may be clinically occult, accuracy of reporting is poor, the risk is influenced by the nature of the recipient population and the source of donor blood and by the diligence and expertise of the blood bank laboratory staff.

An additional problem is that about one-half of transfusions are given to anesthetized patients.[110,170] If a reaction is suspected, the transfusion should be immediately discontinued and appropriate laboratory tests and clinical studies undertaken to establish the diagnosis and institute appropriate therapy (see "Immediate Transfusion Reactions").

Transfusion reactions may be categorized as either immediate or delayed.

IMMEDIATE TRANSFUSION REACTIONS

Symptoms of an immediate reaction begin within minutes to hours and are nonspecific with respect to etiology. They may include chills, fever, urticaria, tachycardia, dyspnea, nausea and vomiting, tightness in the chest, chest and back pain, hypotension, bronchospasm, angioneurotic edema, anaphylaxis, shock, pulmonary edema, and congestive failure. In the anesthetized patient undergoing surgery, an immediate transfusion reaction may manifest itself as generalized oozing of blood from the operative site and by shock that is not corrected by the administration of blood.

Immediate transfusion reactions may be hemolytic, febrile, or may be due to contaminated blood. The symptoms may not reflect the severity of the reaction. An etiologic diagnosis usually requires additional laboratory studies.

ACUTE HEMOLYTIC TRANSFUSION REACTIONS

Hemolytic transfusion reactions may be associated with a variety of signs and symptoms such as fever, low-back pain, sensations of chest compression, hypotension, nausea, and vomiting. Two mechanisms may account for hemolysis of transfused red blood cells: (1) intravascular breakdown, most commonly due to an incompatibility in the ABO system, or (2) destruction occurring in the extravascular space, i.e., the macrophage system of the spleen, liver, and bone marrow.

Important pathogenetic mechanisms in intravascular hemolysis are DIC and a series of hemodynamic alterations leading to ischemic necrosis of tissues, notably the kidneys.[171,172] Abnormal bleeding due to a consumptive coagulopathy may develop in one-half to one-third of patients who develop major intravascular hemolysis following an incompatible transfusion.[173,174]

Infrequently an asymptomatic hemolytic transfusion reaction occurs without demonstrable antibody.[175] Such patients do not show the expected hemoglobin increment following transfusion and have hemoglobinuria and hemoglobinemia. Such reactions are rare, and the absence of demonstrable antibody requires postulating a direct cell-mediated destruction of the incompatible red blood cells.

The clinical management of a hemolytic transfusion reaction should include immediate termination of the transfusion and institution of measures to correct shock, maintain renal circulation, and correct the bleeding diathesis. The risk of serious sequelae is proportional to the volume of incompatible blood transfused. Severe complications rarely follow the transfusion of under 200 ml of red blood cells.[171] If a hemolytic reaction is suspected, therapy designed to correct bleeding and to protect the kidneys (see below) should be begun promptly without waiting for the laboratory studies to confirm its presence.

The laboratory diagnosis of an acute hemolytic reaction is based on evidence of hemolysis (hemoglobinemia and/or hemoglobinuria) and of a blood group incompatibility (antibodies in the recipient reacting with blood group antigens on transfused red blood cells). A sample of blood carefully drawn to avoid artifactual hemolysis is centrifuged for cell separation. The plasma is examined for hemoglobin (pink) or methemalbumin (brown) and is compared with the pretransfusion specimen. The urine should be examined for hemoglobin and urinary output monitored. The entire typing and cross-match procedure should be repeated to identify the blood group incompatibility. The patient and the blood transfused should be retyped, the cross-match reconfirmed, the patient's red blood cells examined for the presence of bound immunoglobulins and/or complement (antiglobulin or Coombs' test), and the patient's serum tested for the presence of blood group alloantibodies. The donor's plasma should be examined for the presence of antibodies that may react with the patient's red blood cells.

The major effort in a hemolytic reaction should be directed toward control of bleeding, if it is present, and prevention of acute tubular

necrosis. If bleeding is due to DIC (Chap. 126), heparin may be helpful, particularly in pregnant women.[174,176] Heparin therapy is not without potential risk, and its use should be restricted to cases in which a severe reaction has been confirmed. To be effective, heparin should be used early in the course of DIC.[174] When intravascular coagulation is controlled, the depleted coagulation factors can be restored by transfusing fibrinogen-rich cryoprecipitate, platelet concentrates, and fresh-frozen plasma.[177]

The prevention of renal complications relies on maintaining renal blood flow. Systolic blood pressure should be maintained above 100 torr, if necessary by administration of intravenous fluids and transfusion. Mannitol has been used by some to protect against renal failure,[178,179] but others rely solely on diuretics.[127,180] If mannitol is used, it should be given in quantities sufficient to maintain a urine flow of 100 ml per hour. Initially, 100 ml of a 20% solution are infused intravenously in 5 min. This dose can be repeated if diuresis does not occur, but not more than 100 g of mannitol should be given in a 24-h period. Diuretics such as furosemide (40–80 mg IV) or ethacrynic (50–100 mg IV) acid may be more effective in maintaining renal blood flow.

If anuria ensues, standard measures for management of the anuric patient should be instituted.

FEBRILE REACTIONS

A febrile response associated with the administration of blood may be due to a hemolytic reaction, sensitivity to leukocytes or platelets, bacterial pyrogens, or to unidentifiable causes. Febrile reactions due to bacterial pyrogens have become uncommon with the introduction of commercially manufactured disposable transfusion equipment.

The decision to stop the administration of blood in a febrile reaction is a difficult one. Many but not all febrile reactions can be tolerated by the patient with supportive care, e.g., antipyretics, antihistamines. A chill, however, may herald a more serious reaction such as a hemolytic reaction or may be due to grossly contaminated blood. Unfortunately, reliable guidelines are not available to help with this decision. The clinician should exercise his or her best judgement but should not hesitate to stop the transfusion if there is any doubt about the underlying cause of the reaction.

SENSITIVITY TO LEUKOCYTES AND PLATELETS

A frequent cause of a nonhemolytic febrile reaction is sensitization to white cell or platelet antigens.[148,181–184] Febrile reactions to buffy coat are predominantly due to leukocyte antigens.[184] Clinically there is a temperature rise during the administration of blood or shortly thereafter. The temperature continues to rise for 2 to 6 h after cessation of transfusion, and the fever may persist for 12 h. Occasionally there may be more severe manifestations and, rarely, a drop in blood pressure with nausea, vomiting, accompanied by chest and back pains. Reactions due to leukocyte antigens have a good prognosis but may be confused with a hemolytic transfusion reaction. Nonhemolytic febrile reactions account for up to 30 percent of all recognized reactions. Usually at least seven transfusions are required to induce sensitization to leukocyte antigens in men, nonparous women, or children. In gravid or parous women, reactions may occur with the first or second transfusion. Diagnosis depends on laboratory demonstration of HLA or non-HLA antibodies to white cell antigens, usually leukoagglutinins or lymphocytotoxins. Most reactions of this type are associated with sensitivity to granulocytes, but sensitivity to lymphocytes or to platelets can also cause the reaction. Treatment is supportive. Most of these reactions can be prevented if the blood or red blood cells are passed through a leukocyte filter.

PULMONARY HYPERSENSITIVITY REACTION (NONCARDIOGENIC PULMONARY EDEMA)

Occasionally, incompatibility to leukocyte antigens may also produce pulmonary edema of noncardiac origin with acute respiratory distress, chills, fever, and tachycardia usually occurring within 4 h of transfusion. Chest x-rays show bilateral diffuse, patchy pulmonary densities without cardiac enlargement.[185] Leukocyte incompatibility can be demonstrated in most cases. Sometimes recipient antibodies react with donor leukocytes,[186,187] and in other cases[188] passively transferred donor antibodies react with the recipient leukocytes or with recently transfused (interdonor) leukocytes. It is unclear why only a relatively few individuals respond to leukocyte incompatibility by the pulmonary hypersensitivity reaction instead of the usual febrile response. The reaction can also occur with platelet concentrates, fresh-frozen plasma, whole blood, and packed red blood cells. Almost 25 percent of multiparous women donors have leukoagglutinins and lymphocytotoxins that can cause these reactions. Therapy is supportive. In a healthy recipient the symptoms subside in less than 24 h, with pulmonary infiltrates clearing within 4 days. The reaction in a compromised recipient, however, can be fatal.[186] The frequency of this reaction has been estimated as 1 in 5000 transfusions.[189]

Severe pulmonary toxicity characterized by respiratory deterioration and alveolar hemorrhage has been reported in neutropenic patients receiving granulocyte transfusions and amphotericin B simultaneously. A retrospective study, however, shows that usually causes other than the concomitant administration of granulocytes and amphotericin B could account for the fatal pulmonary toxicity.[190] Moreover, it may be prudent to separate infusions of granulocytes and of amphotericin by as many hours as is practical.

A catastrophic reaction to reinfusion of blood collected with the Cell-Saver apparatus has been documented.[34] Termed "disseminated intravascular inflammation," this disorder is characterized by massive fluid accumulation, rapidly developing anemia, thrombocytopenia, and bleeding. The outcome is frequently fatal. This syndrome is believed to be due to the release of cytokines by leukocytes directly contacting the polycarbonate surface of the separating bowl used in the apparatus, and it has been suggested that it can be avoided by exercising care in the aspiration of material from the operative field, avoiding aspiration of cellular debris, irrigating fluid, and blood that has been greatly diluted into the salvage apparatus.

ALLERGIC REACTIONS

Transfusions of blood or blood products in some patients may result in generalized pruritus and urticaria. Occasionally there may be bronchospasm, angioneurotic edema, or anaphylaxis. The cause of allergic reactions is poorly understood. It has been suggested that they are due to sensitivity to plasma proteins or other agents passively transferred from the donor to the recipient. Subsequent exposure of the recipient to the antigen through medication or possibly allergens in food precipitates the reaction. Antibodies to leukocyte or platelets do not seem causally related to urticarial reactions.[191] These reactions are usually mild and respond readily to parenteral antihistamines. Serious reactions require the prompt parenteral administration of epinephrine.

ANTI-IgA IN IgA-DEFICIENT RECIPIENT

Severe anaphylactoid transfusion reactions can occur in IgA-deficient patients who have formed anti-IgA.[95] Such patients either lack or have a marked deficiency of IgA and have developed an IgG or occasionally IgM anti-IgA that may be either class-specific (IgA) or allotype-specific (Am).[192] Deficiency or absence of IgA occurs infrequently; about 1 in 650 persons lack IgA by immunodiffusion and about 1 in 886 have no demonstrable IgA.[193] The IgA present in the plasma of the transfused blood probably reacts with the anti-IgA to produce the anaphylactoid reaction. Small amounts of plasma (less than 10 ml) can produce the reaction. The reaction usually is not associated with fever but may produce dyspnea, nausea, chills, abdominal cramps, emesis, diarrhea, and profound hypotension. A fatal reaction due to anti-IgA occurring 45 min after administration of about 50 ml of blood has been reported.[194] Diagnosis requires laboratory demonstration of the absence of IgA and the presence of anti-IgA in the recipient's circulation. Reactions can usually be prevented by using washed or frozen red blood cells, since these components are prepared by procedures effective in removing donor plasma. Plasma protein components, such as albumin or plasma protein fraction, may contain sufficient IgA to produce a reaction. If platelet or granulocyte transfusions are required for IgA-deficient patients, they should be obtained from donors who lack IgA (Rare Donor File, American Association of Blood Banks).

BACTERIAL CONTAMINATION

Blood may be contaminated by cold-growing organisms (*Pseudomonas* or colon-aerogenes group). These microorganisms can utilize citrate as the primary source of carbon, and growth of blood by these microorganisms may deplete its citrate concentration sufficiently to result in clotting. Visual inspection of the blood unit may reveal clots and suggest the presence of contamination. The infusion of large numbers of gram-negative microorganisms results in a serious reaction, endotoxin shock, characterized by fever, marked hypotension, abdominal pain, vomiting, diarrhea, and the development of profound shock.[195] The reaction may start with shaking chills following a latent period of 30 min or more. As little as 10 ml of blood may contain sufficient microorganisms to produce the reaction. Rapid diagnosis is essential and can be made by drawing a small sample of residual donor blood from the container or administration tubing. The plasma obtained by slow centrifugation is smeared on a slide, fixed by heating, and Gram-stained. If the blood is heavily contaminated, several organisms can be clearly identified in most oil-immersion fields.

Septic shock is a complex disorder, and comprehensive supportive therapy is essential once the diagnosis is made. Treatment is often ineffective. The fatality rate with this type of overwhelming shock is estimated to be from 50 to 80 percent.

Bacterial contamination of blood is an uncommon complication since the introduction of disposable plastic blood bags. This transfusion hazard, however, is significant with platelet concentrates stored at room temperature (see Chap. 142).

CIRCULATORY OVERLOAD

Hypervolemia produced by administration of excess blood in patients with a compromised cardiovascular system may provoke the development of congestive heart failure and pulmonary edema. Treatment of this reaction includes administration of diuretics and in some cases rapid digitalization. Repeated phlebotomies with reinfusion of the erythrocytes as packed red blood cells may sometimes be helpful.

Patients with severe chronic anemia (hemoglobin less than 4 gm per 100 ml), such as those with pernicious anemia, who are rapidly transfused with whole blood or packed red blood cells may develop congestive failure and pulmonary edema. The slow administration of packed red blood cells appears to be well tolerated by the patient in a semiupright position. Venous pressure should be monitored in such patients, diuretics administered, and the transfusion given at a rate of 2 ml per kg of body weight per hour. It is unlikely that a transfusion will precipitate congestive heart failure if the venous pressure is normal before transfusion.[196]

AIR EMBOLISM

Air embolism is now a rare complication of transfusion therapy following the introduction of plastic equipment that provides a closed system.

Only large volumes of air and not the entry of a few bubbles results in clinically significant air embolism. Symptoms associated with air embolism include pain, cough, and sudden onset of dyspnea. Treatment consists of clamping off administration tubing; placing the patient on the left side in the head-down position with closed chest compression, so that air in the right ventricle flows away from the pulmonary outflow tract; and if possible air aspiration through a right atrial or Swan-Ganz catheter.[197]

MICROAGGREGATES IN BLOOD

Particles consisting largely of platelets and fibrin[198] form in blood stored in ACD, CPD, or CPDA-1 solutions. Such debris, consisting of particles 13 to 100 μm in size and collectively designated *microaggregates,* is not removed by the ordinary blood filter that has a pore size of about 170 μm. Microaggregates have been shown to produce pulmonary insufficiency in clinical situations involving massive transfusions of banked blood. Pulmonary complications and histologic changes in the lungs have been observed in patients receiving massive transfusions.[199,200] Infusion of nonfiltered blood resulted in a consistent increase in the pulmonary vascular resistance in experimental animals.[201] Patients transfused over 20 percent of their blood volume have increased pulmonary arteriovenous shunting when the blood is filtered with standard blood filters, but this can be prevented if microaggregate filters are used.[202]

The clinical importance of microaggregates in routine transfusions is questionable.[203] Several investigators, however, believe that microaggregate filters should be used in cardiac surgery and in critically ill patients with pulmonary insufficiency who will receive more than 3 to 5 units of banked blood in less than 12 h.[204]

REACTIONS ASSOCIATED WITH MASSIVE TRANSFUSIONS

The use of large quantities of banked blood for massive transfusions may lead to a number of complications. Among these are circulatory overload (see above), air embolism (see above), citrate intoxication, and a bleeding syndrome. Blood transfused into adults at a rate greater than a liter in 10 min will produce significant reduction in ionized calcium with myocardial depression and ECG changes. Citrate intoxication can be prevented by giving 10 ml of 10% calcium gluconate for every liter of citrated blood.

BLEEDING SYNDROMES

Bleeding may be a complication of transfusion either because an antigen-antibody reaction involving a red cell antigen initiates DIC or because coagulation factors and platelets are diluted following large-volume compatible transfusions of banked blood.[173] It should always be kept in mind that the most common cause of bleeding in surgical patients is a severed vessel.

Unexplained bleeding may be the first sign of incompatibility in the anesthetized patient and may follow the administration of 200 to 500 ml of incompatible blood. Local bleeding at the surgical site or epistaxis, bruising, or purpura due to DIC may occur following an acute hemolytic transfusion reaction. The diagnosis and management of this complication are outlined above under "Acute Hemolytic Transfusion Reactions."

Bleeding associated with transfusion of large amounts of compatible stored blood is largely due to the dilution of the intravascular volume with blood lacking in both cellular and plasma coagulation components. Since platelets do not survive in stored blood, transfusion of a volume of blood equal to that to the recipient will produce thrombocytopenia through a dilutional effect. Stored blood is deficient in platelets and in factors V, VIII, and XI. These clotting components may be depleted when a large volume transfusion is given.

DELAYED ADVERSE EFFECTS OF BLOOD TRANSFUSION

DELAYED HEMOLYTIC REACTION

In the delayed hemolytic reaction, development of previously undetected alloantibodies occurs some 4 to 14 days after transfusion of apparently compatible blood. In such cases the patient usually has been alloimmunized by a previous pregnancy or transfusion, and the concentration of antibody was below the level of serologic detection at the time of transfusion. If the transfused blood contains the corresponding antigen, an anamnestic response ensues with formation of detectable antibody that coats the transfused red blood cells and leads to their hemolysis. The principal clinical signs are onset of jaundice and absence of the expected increment in red cell mass. These reactions are associated with the development of a positive direct antiglobulin reaction (Coombs' test),[205,206] which in such patients may be confused with autoimmune hemolytic anemia,[207] or in one report with sickle-cell crisis.[208] Generally, these reactions are clinically less severe than the acute hemolytic reaction and frequently are not detected until more blood is ordered for a transfusion-unresponsive anemia. The frequency of delayed hemolytic anemia was 1 in 4000 in one report,[205] with no deaths in the 37 cases studied. Delayed hemolytic reactions, as a result, are frequently undetected.[206]

POSTTRANSFUSION PURPURA

A rare complication of transfusion therapy is posttransfusion purpura, which occurs approximately 1 week after transfusion and is associated with the development of an antibody to the platelet-specific antigen in a Pl[a1]-negative recipient (see Chap. 117).

TRANSMISSION OF DISEASE

The greatest risk to which the transfused patient is exposed is that of infection with viral agents, such as those that cause acquired immunodeficiency syndrome, lymphomas, or hepatitis, or protozoal organisms, particularly malaria. The prevention of disease transmission is discussed in Chap. 139.

GRAFT-VERSUS-HOST DISEASE

Graft-versus-host disease is an uncommon complication of transfusion therapy,[209] preventable by blood irradiation.

OTHER TYPES OF DELAYED REACTIONS

Other complications of transfusion therapy are iron overload with hemochromatosis (see Chap. 42), which occurs in patients who receive many transfusions, and alloimmunizations to red cell and histocompatibility antigens.

Alloimmunization as a transfusion complication may occur in immunocompetent transfusion-dependent recipients. Blood is matched routinely only with respect to ABO antigens and the major Rh antigen, $Rh_o(D)$. There is a high probability that the donor will have red cell antigens not present in the recipient which will result in alloimmunization. The incidence of alloimmunization is influenced by the number of units transfused, the immune status of the recipient, and probably other undefined factors. The prevalence of alloantibodies in multiply transfused patients with various hematological disorders was 11.8 percent[210]; in multiply transfused sickle cell anemia patients the prevalence has been variously reported as 36 percent,[211] 23 percent,[212] and in one series only 7.75 percent.[213] The incidence of alloimmunization in thalassemia major patients[214] is lower (5.2 percent).

More extensive pretransfusion typing including the matching for additional antigens of recipients who will require frequent transfusions appears to reduce the risk of alloimmunization. Pretransfusion matching for the major antigens (Rh, Kell, Kidd and Duffy) in patients with sickle cell anemia reduced the incidence of alloimmunization tenfold.[215] This measure alone may not be cost-effective, since not all individuals are capable of mounting an immune response to blood group antigens. A few $Rh_o(D)$-negative individuals fail to produce anti-$Rh_o(D)$ in spite of intentional immunization with the antigen.[216,217] However, 95 percent of Rh-negative individuals receiving large quantities (average 19.4 units) of Rh-positive blood during open heart surgery formed anti-D.[218] More extensive pretransfusion matching would be justifiable if a marker could be found that unequivocally identifies the responder population of recipients.

REFERENCES

1. Oberman HA: The history of transfusion medicine, in *Clinical Practice of Transfusion Medicine*, 2d ed, edited by Petz LD, Swisher SN, p 9. Churchill Livingstone, New York, 1989.
2. Blundell J: The after-management of floodings, and on transfusion. *Lancet* 13:673, 1828.
3. Routh CHF: Remarks, statistical and general, on transfusion of blood. *The Medical Times* 114, 1849.
4. Landsteiner K: Über Agglutinationserscheinungen normalen menschlichen Blutes. *Wien Klin Wochenschr* 14:1132, 1901.
5. Rous J, Turner JR: The preservation of living red blood cells in vitro: I. Methods of preservation. *J Exp Med* 23:219, 1916.
6. Rous P, Turner JR: The preservation of living red blood cells in vitro: II. The transfusion of kept cells. *J Exp Med* 23:239, 1916.
7. Robertson OH: Transfusion with preserved red blood cells. *BMJ* 1:691, 1918.
8. Fantus B: Therapy of Cook County Hospital: blood preservation. *JAMA* 109:128, 1937.
9. Churchill ED: *Surgeon to Soldiers*. Lippincott, Philadelphia, 1972.
10. Jones AL: Continuous-flow blood cell separation. *Transfusion* 8:94, 1968.
11. Hester JP, Kellogg RM, Mulzet AP, et al: Principles of blood separation and component extraction in a disposable continuous-flow single-stage channel. *Blood* 45:254, 1979.
12. Gabrio BW, Stevens AR, Finch CA: Erythrocyte preservation: III. The reversibility of the storage lesion. *J Clin Invest* 33:252, 1954.
13. Dern RJ, Brewer GJ, Wiorkowski JJ: Studies on the preservation of human blood: II. The relationship of erythrocyte adenosine triphosphate levels and other in vitro measures to red cell storageability. *J Lab Clin Med* 69:968, 1967.
14. Wood L, Beutler E: The viability of human blood stored in phosphate adenine media. *Transfusion* 7:401, 1967.
15. Beutler E, Kuhl W, West C: The osmotic fragility of erythrocytes after prolonged liquid storage and after reinfusion. *Blood* 59:1141, 1982.
16. Wolfe LC: The membrane and the lesions of storage in preserved red cells. *Transfusion* 25:185, 1985.
17. Sestier C, Sabolovic D, Geldwerth D, et al: Use of annexin V-ferrofluid to enumerate erythrocytes damaged in various pathologies or during storage in vitro. *C R Acad Sci (Paris)* 318:1141, 1995.
18. Boas FE, Forman L, Beutler E: Phosphatidylserine exposure and red cell viability in red cell ageing, storage, and in hemolytic anemia. *Blood* 90(suppl 1):272a, 1997.
19. Boas E, Forman L, Beutler E: Phosphatidyl serine exposure and red cell viability in red cell ageing and in hemolytic anemia. *Proc Natl Acad Sci USA* 85:3077, 1998.
20. Geldwerth D, Kuypers FA, Butikofer P, et al: Transbilayer mobility and distribution of red cell phospholipids during storage. *J Clin Invest* 92:308, 1993.
21. Chaplin H Jr, Beutler E, Collins JA, Giblett ER, Polesky HF: Current status of red-cell preservation and availability in relation to the developing national blood policy. *N Engl J Med* 291:68, 1974.
22. DeVerdier CH, Akerblom O, Arturson G, et al: Maintenance of oxygen transport function of stored blood, in *Transfusion and Transplantation, Proc. AABB-ISBT Transfusion Congress*, Washington, DC, 1972.
23. Beutler E, Wood L: The in vivo regeneration of red cell 2,3-diphosphoglyceric acid (DPG) after transfusion of stored blood. *J Lab Clin Med* 74:300, 1969.
24. Valeri CR, Hirsch NM: Restoration in vivo of erythrocyte adenosine triphosphate, 2,3-diphosphoglycerate, potassium ion, and sodium ion

concentrations following the transfusion of acid-citrate-dextrose-stored human red blood cells. *J Lab Clin Med* 73:722, 1969.
25. Beutler E: What is the clinical importance of alterations of the hemoglobin oxygen affinity in preserved blood—especially as produced by variations of red cell 2,3 DPG content? *Vox Sang* 34:113, 1978.
26. Beutler E, Duron O: Effect of pH on preservation of red cell ATP. *Transfusion* 5:17, 1965.
27. Bishop C: Changes in the nucleotides of stored or incubated human blood. *Transfusion* 1:349, 1961.
28. Beutler E, Meul A, Wood LA: Depletion and regeneration of 2,3-diphosphoglyceric acid in stored red blood cells. *Transfusion* 9:109, 1969.
29. Wood L, Beutler E: Temperature dependence of sodium-potassium activated erythrocyte adenosine triphosphatase. *J Lab Clin Med* 70:287, 1967.
30. AuBuchon JP, Estep TN, Davey RJ: The effect of the plasticizer Di-2-Ethylhexyl phthalate on the survival of stored RBCs. *Blood* 71:448, 1988.
31. Greenwalt TJ, McGuinness CG, Dumaswala UJ: Studies in red blood cell preservation: 4. Plasma vesicle hemoglobin exceeds free hemoglobin. *Vox Sang* 61:14, 1991.
32. Card RT, Mohandas N, Mollison PL: Relationship of post-transfusion viability to deformability of stored red cells. *Br J Haematol* 53:237, 1983.
33. Kristiansson M, Soop M, Saraste L, Sundqvist KG: Cytokines in stored red blood cell concentrates: promoters of systemic inflammation and simulators of acute transfusion reactions? *Acta Anaesthesiol Scand* 40:496, 1996.
34. Bull BS, Bull MH: Hypothesis: disseminated intravascular inflammation as the inflammatory counterpart to disseminated intravascular coagulation. *Proc Natl Acad Sci USA* 91:8190, 1994.
35. Simon ER: Adenine and purine nucleosides in human red cell preservation: a review. *Transfusion* 7:395, 1967.
36. Wood L, Beutler E: The effect of ascorbate and dihydroxyacetone on the 2,3-diphosphoglycerate and ATP levels of stored human red cells. *Transfusion* 14:272, 1974.
37. Kandler R, Grode G, Symbol R, Hickey G: Oxalate is the active component that produces increased 2,3-DPG in ascorbate stored red cells. *Transfusion* 26:563, 1986.
38. Beutler E, Forman L, West C: Effect of oxalate and malonate on red cell metabolism. *Blood* 70:1389, 1987.
39. Paterson RA, Dawson J, Hyde RM, et al: Xanthone additives for blood storage which maintains its potential for oxygen delivery: I. 2-hydroxy-ethoxy- and 2-ethoxy-6-(5-tetrazoyl) xanthones in citrate-phosphate-dextrose-adenine (CPDA-1) blood. *Transfusion* 28:34, 1988.
40. Beutler E, Forman L, West C, Gelbart T: The mechanism of improved maintenance of 2,3-diphosphoglycerate in stored blood by the xanthone compound BW A440C. *Biochem Pharmacol* 37:1057, 1988.
41. Brake JM, Deindoerfer FH: Preservation of red blood cell 2,3-diphosphoglycerate in stored blood containing dihydroxyacetone. *Transfusion* 13:84, 1973.
42. Beutler E, Guinto E: The metabolism of dihydroxyacetone by intact erythrocytes. *J Lab Clin Med* 82:534, 1973.
43. Beutler E, Guinto E: Dihydroxyacetone metabolism by human erythrocytes: demonstration of triokinase activity and its characterization. *Blood* 41:559, 1973.
44. Dern RJ, Wiorkowski JJ, Matsuda T: Studies on the preservation of human blood: V. The effect of mixing anticoagulated blood during storage on the poststorage erythrocyte survival. *J Lab Clin Med* 75:37, 1970.
45. Bensinger TA, Metro J, Beutler E: The effect of agitation on in vitro metabolism of erythrocytes stored in CPD-adenine. *Transfusion* 15:140, 1975.
46. Duhm J, Deuticke B, Gerlach E: Complete restoration of oxygen transport function and 2,3-diphosphoglycerate concentration in stored blood. *Transfusion* 11:147, 1971.
47. Matsuyama H, Niklasson F, de Verdier CH, Högman CF: Phosphoenolpyruvate in the rejuvenation of stored red cells in SAGM medium: optimal conditions and the indirect effect of methemoglobin formation. *Transfusion* 29:614, 1989.
48. Valeri CR, Zaroulis CG, Vecchione JJ, et al: Therapeutic effectiveness and safety of outdated human red blood cells rejuvenated to restore oxygen transport function to normal, frozen for 3 to 4 years at −80 C,

washed, and stored at 4 C for 24 hours prior to rapid infusion. *Transfusion* 20:159, 1980.

49. Meryman HT, Hornblower ML-S, Syring RL: Prolonged storage of red cells at 4 degrees C. *Transfusion* 26:500, 1986.

50. Greenwalt TJ, Dumaswala UJ, Dhingra N, Allen CM, Silberstein EB: Studies in red blood cell preservation: 7. In vivo and in vitro studies with a modified phosphate-ammonium additive solution. *Vox Sang* 65:87, 1993.

51. Kay A, Beutler E: The effect of ammonium, phosphate, potassium, and hypotonicity on stored red blood cells. *Transfusion* 32:37, 1992.

52. Dumaswala UJ, Oreskovic RT, Petrosky TL, Greenwalt TJ: Studies in red blood cell preservation: 5. Determining the limiting concentrations of NH_4Cl and Na_2HPO_4 needed to maintain red blood cell ATP during storage. *Vox Sang* 62:136, 1992.

53. Beutler E, Wood LA: Preservation of red cell 2,3-DPG and viability in bicarbonate-containing medium: The effect of blood-bag permeability. *J Lab Clin Med* 80:723, 1972.

54. Högman CF, Eriksson L, Gong J, et al: Half-strength citrate CPD combined with a new additive solution for improved storage of red blood cells suitable for clinical use. *Vox Sang* 65:271, 1993.

55. Beutler E: Red cell suspensions. *N Engl J Med* 300:984, 1979.

56. Beutler E, Kuhl W: Volume control of erythrocytes during storage: The role of mannitol. *Transfusion* 28:353, 1988.

57. Högman CF: Additive system approach in blood transfusion: birth of the SAG and Sagman systems. *Vox Sang* 51:339, 1986.

58. Simon TL, Marcus CS, Myhre BA, Nelson EJ: Effects of AS-3 nutrient-additive solution on 42 and 49 days of storage of red cells. *Transfusion* 27:178, 1987.

59. Beutler E, West C: Letter to the editor re: Adsol. *N Engl J Med* 312:1393, 1985.

60. Bensinger TA, Chillar R, Beutler E: Prolonged maintenance of 2,3-DPG in liquid storage: use of an internal CO_2 trap to stabilize pH. *J Lab Clin Med* 89:498, 1977.

61. Meryman HT: Freezing injury and its prevention in living cells. *Annu Rev Biophys Bioeng* 3:341, 1974.

62. Lovelock JE: Denaturation of lipid protein complexes as a cause of damage by freezing. *Proc R Soc Lond (Biol)* 147:427, 1957.

63. Lovelock JE: The haemolysis of human red blood cells by freezing and thawing. *Biochim Biophys Acta* 10:414, 1953.

64. Huggins C: Preparation and usefulness of frozen blood. *Annu Rev Med* 36:499, 1985.

65. Valeri CR, Pivacek LE, Gray AD, et al: The safety and therapeutic effectiveness of human red cells stored at $-80°C$ for as long as 21 years. *Transfusion* 29:429, 1989.

66. Goodrich RP, Sowemimo-Coker SO, Zerez CR, Tanaka KR: Preservation of metabolic activity in lyophilized human erythrocytes. *Proc Natl Acad Sci USA* 89:967, 1992.

67. Sowemimo-Coker SO, Goodrich RP, Zerez CR, Tanaka KR: Refrigerated storage of lyophilized and rehydrated, lyophilized human red cells. *Transfusion* 33:322, 1993.

68. Spieles G, Kresin M, Loges K, et al: The effect of storage temperature on the stability of frozen erythrocytes. *Cryobiology* 32:366, 1995.

69. Pellerin-Mendes C, Million L, Marchand-Arvier M, Labrude P, Vigneron C: In vitro study of the protective effect of trehalose and dextran during freezing of human red blood cells in liquid nitrogen. *Cryobiology* 35:173, 1997.

70. *Technical Manual of the American Association of Blood Banks,* Arlington, VA, 1996.

71. Åkerblom O, de Verdier CH, Finnson M, et al: Further studies on the effect of adenine in blood preservation. *Transfusion* 7:1, 1967.

72. Bensinger TA, Metro J, Beutler E: In vitro metabolism of packed erythrocytes stored in CPD-adenine. *Transfusion* 15:135, 1975.

73. Dawson RB, Hershey RT, Myers C, Holmes S: Blood preservation: XXVI. CPD-adenine packed cells: benefits of increasing the glucose. *Transfusion* 18:339, 1978.

74. Oberman HA: The indications for transfusion of freshly drawn blood. *JAMA* 199:96, 1967.

75. Heustis DW: Fresh blood: fact and fancy, in *Seminar on Current Technical Topics,* p 117. American Association of Blood Banks, Washington, DC, 1974.

76. Bolin RB, Cheney BA, Smith DJ, et al: An in vivo comparison of CPD and CPDA-2 preserved platelet concentrates after an 8-hour preprocess hold of whole blood. *Transfusion* 22:491, 1982.

77. Bowie EJW, Thompson JH, Owen CA Jr: The stability of antihemophilic globulin and labile factor in human blood. *Mayo Clin Proc* 39:144, 1964.

78. Horowitz HI, Fujimoto MM: Survival of factor XI in vitro and vivo. *Transfusion* 6:539, 1965.

79. Aggeler PM: Physiological basis for transfusion therapy in hemorrhagic disorders. *Transfusion* 1:71, 1961.

80. Mooreside DE, Graybeal FQ Jr, Langdell RD: Effects of adenine on clotting factors in fresh blood, stored blood and stored fresh frozen plasma. *Transfusion* 9:191, 1969.

81. Nilsson L, Hedner U, Nilsson IM, et al: Shelf-life of bank blood and stored plasma with special reference to coagulation factors. *Transfusion* 23:377, 1983.

82. Krevans JR, Jackson DP: Hemorrhagic disorder following massive whole blood transfusions. *JAMA* 159:171, 1955.

83. Beutler E, West C: The storage of "hard-packed" red blood cells in citrate-phosphate-dextrose (CPD) and CPD-adenine (CPDA-1). *Blood* 54:280, 1979.

84. *Standards for a Blood Transfusion Service,* American Association of Blood Banks, Washington, DC, 1987.

85. Moss GS, Proctor HJ, Homer LD, et al: Comparison of asanguineous fluids and whole blood in treatment of hemorrhagic shock. *Surg Gynecol Obstet* 129:1247, 1969.

86. Kahn RA, Staggs SD, Miller WV, Ellis FR: Use of plasma products with whole blood and packed RBCs. *JAMA* 242:2087, 1979.

87. Pineda AA, Rippetean ND, Clare DE, Bunkowske BM: Infusion flow rates of whole blood and ASH preserved erythrocytes: a comparison. *Mayo Clin Proc* 62:199, 1987.

88. Pietersz RN, Steneker I, Reesink HW, et al: Comparison of five different filters for the removal of leukocytes from red cell concentrates. *Vox Sang* 62:76, 1992.

89. Bodensteiner DC: Leukocyte depletion filters: a comparison of efficiency. *Am J Hematol* 35:184, 1990.

90. Zimmermann B, Hillringhaus I, Diekamp U: Exceptional production of leukocyte-free erythrocyte concentrates using filtration with the BPF 4 BBS leukocyte filter. *Beitr Infusionther Transfusionsmed* 32:32, 1994.

91. Krandick E, Vornwald A, Gossrau E: Leukocyte depletion by in-line-filtration. *Beitr Infusionther Transfusionsmed* 32:6, 1994.

92. Meryman HT, Hornblower M: The preparation of red cells depleted of leukocytes: review and evaluation. *Transfusion* 26:101, 1986.

93. Contreras TJ, Valleri CR: A comparison of methods to wash liquid-stored red blood cells and red blood cells frozen with high or low concentrations of glycerol. *Transfusion* 16:539, 1976.

94. Dameshek W, Neber J: Transfusion reactions to a plasma constituent of whole blood. *Blood* 5:129, 1950.

95. Leikola J, Koistinen M, Lehtinen M, Virolainen M: IgA-induced anaphylactic transfusion reaction: a report of four cases. *Blood* 42:111, 1973.

96. Sanner HE, Wooten MJ: Analysis of saline-washed red cells for transfusion to neonatal patients. *Transfusion* 25:437, 1985.

97. Grove-Rasmussen M: Selection of donors for frozen blood based on specific blood group combinations. *JAMA* 193:48, 1965.

98. Grove-Rasmussen M, Huggins CE: Selected types of frozen blood for patients with multiple blood group antibodies. *Transfusion* 13:124, 1973.

99. *Red Blood Cell Substitutes: Basic Principles and Clinical Applications,* edited by AS Rudolph, R Rabinivici, GZ Feuerstein. Marcel Dekker, New York, 1998.

100. Gould SA, Rosen AL, Sehgal LR, et al: Fluosol-DA as a red-cell substitute in acute anemia. *N Engl J Med* 314:1653, 1986.

101. De Venuto F: Modified hemoglobin solution as a resuscitation fluid. *Vox Sang* 44:129, 1983.

102. Winslow RM: *Hemoglobin-based Red Cell Substitutes,* Johns Hopkins University, Baltimore and London, 1993.

103. Winslow RM: The toxicity of hemoglobin, in *Hemoglobin-based Red Cell Substitutes,* p 136. Johns Hopkins University, Baltimore, 1992.

104. Gould SA, Moore EE, Moore FA, et al: Clinical utility of human polymerized hemoglobin as a blood substitute after acute trauma and urgent surgery. *J Trauma* 43:325, 1997.

105. Rohlfs RJ, Bruner E, Chiu A, et al: Arterial blood pressure responses to cell-free hemoglobin solutions and the reaction with nitric oxide. *J Biol Chem* 273:12128, 1998.

106. Djordjevich L, Miller IF: Synthetic erythrocytes from lipid encapsulated hemoglobin. *Exp Hematol* 8:584, 1980.

107. Hunt CA, Burnette RR, MacGregor RD, et al: Synthesis and evaluation of a prototypal artificial red cell. *Science* 230:1165, 1985.

108. Szebeni J, Wassef NM, Hartman KR, Rudolph AS, Alving CR: Complement activation in vitro by the red cell substitute, liposome-encapsulated hemoglobin: mechanism of activation and inhibition by soluble complement receptor type 1. *Transfusion* 37:150, 1997.

109. Widmann FK: Informed consent for blood transfusion: brief historical survey and summary of a conference. *Transfusion* 30:460, 1990.

110. Stehling LC, Ellison N, Faust RJ, et al: A survey of transfusion practices among anesthesiologists. *Vox Sang* 52:60, 1987.

111. Roche JK, Stengle JM: Open-heart surgery and the demand for blood. *JAMA* 225:1516, 1973.

112. Umlas J: Transfusion of patients undergoing cardiopulmonary bypass. *Hum Pathol* 14:271, 1983.

113. Hillman RS: Blood-loss anemia. *Postgrad Med* 64:88, 1978.

114. Greenwalt TJ, Perry S: Preservation and utilization of the components of human blood, in *Progress in Hematology,* edited by Brown EB and Moore CV, p 157. Grune & Stratton, New York, 1969.

115. Rigor B, Bosomworth P, Rush BJ Jr: Replacement of operative blood loss of more than 1 liter with Hartmann's solution. *JAMA* 203:229, 1968.

116. Golub S, Baily CP: Management of major surgical blood loss without transfusion. *JAMA* 198:1171, 1966.

117. Demling RH: Burns. Medical progress. *N Engl J Med* 313:1389, 1985.

118. Baxter CR: Problems and complications of burn shock resuscitation. *Surg Clin North Am* 58:1313, 1978.

119. Pruitt BA Jr: Fluid and electrolyte replacement in the burned patient. *Surg Clin North Am* 58:1291, 1978.

120. Friedman BA: Patterns of blood utilization by physicians: transfusion of nonoperated anemic patients. *Transfusion* 18:193, 1978.

121. Silberstein LE, Kruskall MS, Stehling LC, et al: Strategies for the review of transfusion practices. *JAMA* 262:1993, 1989.

122. Propper RD, Button LN, Nathan DG: New approaches to the transfusion management of thalassemia. *Blood* 55:55, 1980.

123. Keegan TE, Heaton A, Holme S, Owens M, Nelson EJ: Improved post-transfusion quality of density separated AS-3 red cells after extended storage. *Br J Haematol* 82:114, 1992.

124. Simon TL, Sohmer P, Nelson EJ: Extended survival of neocytes produced by a new system. *Transfusion* 29:221, 1989.

125. Spanos T, Ladis V, Palamidou F, et al: The impact of neocyte transfusion in the management of thalassaemia. *Vox Sang* 70:217, 1996.

126. Pisciotto P, Kiraly T, Paradis L, et al: Clinical trial of young red blood cells prepared by apheresis. *Ann Clin Lab Sci* 16:473, 1986.

127. Mollison PL, Engelfriet CP, Contreras M: *Blood Transfusion in Clinical Medicine.* Blackwell, Oxford, 1987.

128. Ryden SE, Oberman HA: Compatibility of common intravenous solutions with CPD blood. *Transfusion* 15:250, 1975.

129. Dickson DN, Gregory MA: Compatibility of blood with solutions containing calcium. *S Afr Med J* 57:785, 1980.

130. De la Luna O, Amezcua Llauger LE, Leis Marquez MT, Sanchez Solis V: Usefulness of intraperitoneal transfusion under direct ultrasound guidance. *Ginecol Obstet Mex* 59:128, 1991.

131. Harman CR, Bowman JM, Manning FA, Menticoglou SM: Intrauterine transfusion-intraperitoneal versus intravascular approach: a case-control comparison. *Am J Obstet Gynecol* 162:1053, 1990.

132. Cass RM, Blumberg N: Single-unit blood transfusion: doubtful dogma defeated. *JAMA* 257:628, 1987.

133. Reece RL, Beckett RS: Epidemiology of single-unit transfusion: a one-year experience in a community hospital. *JAMA* 195:801, 1966.

134. Allen JG: The case for the single transfusion. *N Engl J Med* 287:984, 1972.

135. Stehling L, Zander HL: Acute normovolemic hemodilution. *Transfusion* 31:857, 1991.

136. Schaff HV, Hauer JM, Brawley RK: Autotransfusion in cardiac surgical patients after operation. *Surgery* 84:713, 1978.

137. Faris PM, Ritter MA, Keating EM, Valeri CR: Unwashed filtered shed blood collected after knee and hip arthroplasties. A source of autologous red blood cells. *J Bone Joint Surg [Am]* 73A:1169, 1991.

138. Kent P, Ashley S, Thorley PJ, et al: 24-Hour survival of autotransfused red cells in elective aortic surgery: a comparison of two intraoperative autotransfusion systems. *Br J Surg* 78:1473, 1991.

139. Hall RI, Schweiger IM, Finlayson DC: Transfusion using a cell saver apparatus during surgery for coronary artery disease: is it beneficial? *Can J Anaesth* 37:S155, 1990.

140. Kruskall MS, Glazier EE, Leonard SS, et al: Utilization and efffectiveness of a hospital autologous preoperative blood donor program. *Transfusion* 26:335, 1986.

141. Goodnough LT, Rudnick S, Price TH, et al: Increased preoperative collection of autologous blood with recombinant human erythropoietin therapy. *N Engl J Med* 321:1163, 1989.

142. Masouredis SP, Chaplin H Jr: Transfusion management of autoimmune hemolytic anemia, in *Acquired Immune Hemolytic Anemias,* edited by Masouredis SP and Chaplin H Jr, p 177. Churchill Livingston, New York, 1985.

143. Rosenfield RE, Jagathambal: Transfusion therapy for autoimmune hemolytic anemia. *Semin Hematol* 13:311, 1976.

144. Petz LD: Transfusing the patient with autoimmune hemolytic anemia. *Clin Lab Med* 2:193, 1982.

145. Blumberg N, Bove JR: Uncrossmatched blood for emergency transfusion. One year's experience in a civilian setting. *JAMA* 240:2057, 1978.

146. Moore HC, Mollison PL: Use of low-ionic strength medium in manual tests for antibody detection. *Transfusion* 16:291, 1976.

147. Oberman HA, Barnes BA, Steiner EA: Role of the crossmatch in testing for serologic incompatibility. *Transfusion* 22:12, 1982.

148. Brittingham TE, Chaplin H Jr: Febrile transfusion reactions caused by sensitivity to donor leukocytes and platelets. *JAMA* 165:819, 1957.

149. Scornik JC, Ireland JE, Howard RJ, et al: Assessment of the risk for broad sensitization by blood transfusions. *Transplantation* 37:249, 1984.

150. Opelz G, Sengan DP, Mickey MR, Terasaki PI: Effect of blood transfusions on subsequent kidney transplants. *Transplant Proc* 5:253, 1973.

151. Opelz G, Terasaki PI: Improvement of kidney graft survival with increased number of transfusions. *N Engl J Med* 299:799, 1978.

152. Hourmant M, Soulillou JP, Bui-quang D: Beneficial effect of blood transfusion: role of the time interval between the last transfusion and transplantation. *Transplantation* 28:40, 1979.

153. Ahmed Z, Terasaki PI: Effect of transfusions, in *Clinical Transplant 1991,* p 305. UCLA Tissue Typing Laboratory, Los Angeles, 1992.

154. Salvatierra O Jr, Vincenti F, Amend W, et al: Deliberate donor specific blood transfusions prior to living related renal transplantation. *Ann Surg* 192:543, 1980.

155. Light JA, Metz S, Oddenino K, et al: Fresh vs. stored blood in donor specific transfusions. *Transplant Proc* 14:296, 1982.

156. Sniecinski I, O'Donnel MR, Nowicki B: Prevention of refractoriness and HLA-alloimmunization using filtered blood products. *Blood* 71:1402, 1988.

157. Salvatierra O Jr, Melzer J, Vincenti F, et al: Donor-specific blood transfusions versus cyclosporine—the DST story. *Transplant Proc* 19:160, 1987.

158. Opelz G: Improved kidney graft survival in non-transfused recipients. *Transplant Proc* 19:149, 1987.

159. Cicciarelli J: UNOS registry data: effect of transfusions, in *Clinical Transplants 1980,* p 289. UCLA Tissue Typing Laboratory, Los Angeles, 1991.

160. Thomas ED: Current status of marrow transplantation for aplastic anemia and acute leukemia. *Am J Clin Pathol* 72:887, 1979.

161. Gale RP, Feig S, Ho W, et al: ABO blood group system and bone marrow transplantation. *Blood* 50:185, 1977.

162. Brand A, Claas FHJ, Falkenburg JHF, et al: Blood component therapy in bone marrow transplantation. *Semin Hematol* 21:141, 1984.

163. Lewis JH, Bontempo FA, Cornell F, et al: Blood use in liver transplantation. *Transfusion* 27:222, 1987.

164. Owen CA, Rettke SR, Bowie EJW, et al: Hemostatic evaluation of patients undergoing liver transplantation. *Mayo Clin Proc* 62:761, 1987.

165. Motschman TL, Taswell HF, Brecher ME, et al: Blood bank support of a liver transplantation program. *Mayo Clin Proc* 64:103, 1989.

166. Schmidt PJ: Transfusion mortality: with special reference to surgical and intensive care facilities. *J Fla Med Assoc* 67:151, 1980.

167. Honig CL, Bove JR: Transfusion-associated fatalities: review of bureau of biologics reports 1976–1978. *Transfusion* 20:653, 1980.

168. Sazama K: Reports of 355 transfusion-associated deaths. 1976 through 1985. *Transfusion* 30:583, 1990.

169. Walker RH: Special report: transfusion risks. *Am J Clin Pathol* 88:374, 1987.

170. Van Dijk PM, Kleine JW: The transfusion reaction in anaesthesiological practice. *Acta Anaesthesiol Belg* 4:274, 1976.

171. Goldfinger D: Acute hemolytic transfusion reactions: a fresh look at pathogenesis and considerations regarding therapy. *Transfusion* 17:85, 1977.

172. Pineda AA, Brzica SM, Taswell HF: Hemolytic transfusion reaction: recent experience in a large blood bank. *Mayo Clin Proc* 53:378, 1978.

173. Ingram GIC: The bleeding complications of blood transfusion. *Transfusion* 5:1, 1965.

174. Rock RC, Bove JR, Nemerson Y: Heparin treatment of intravascular coagulation accompanying hemolytic transfusion reactions. *Transfusion* 9:57, 1969.

175. Harrison CR, Hayes TC, Trow LL, et al: Intravascular hemolytic transfusion reaction without detectable antibodies: a case report and review of the literature. *Vox Sang* 51:96, 1986.

176. Sack ES, Nefa OM: Fibrinogen and fibrin degradation products in hemolytic transfusion reactions. *Transfusion* 10:317, 1970.

177. Bick RL, Schmalhorst WR, Fekete L: Disseminated intravascular coagulation and blood component therapy. *Transfusion* 16:361, 1976.

178. Greenwalt TJ: Pathologenesis and management of hemolytic transfusion reactions. *Semin Hematol* 18:84, 1981.

179. Luke RG, Briggs JD, Allison MEM, et al: Factors determining response to mannitol in acute renal failure. *Am J Med Sci* 259:168, 1970.

180. Holland PV: Other adverse effects of transfusion, in *Clinical Practice of Blood Transfusion,* edited by Petz LD and Swisher SN, p 783. Churchill Livingston, New York, 1981.

181. Payne R: The association of febrile transfusion reactions with leukoagglutinins. *Vox Sang* 2:233, 1957.

182. Jensen KG: The significance of leuco-agglutinins for development of transfusion reactions. *Dan Med Bull* 9:198, 1962.

183. Perkins HA, Payne R, Ferguson J, Wood M: Nonhemolytic febrile transfusion reactions: quantitative effects of blood components with emphasis on isoantigenic incompatibility of leucocytes. *Vox Sang* 11:578, 1966.

184. Thulstrup H: The influence of leukocyte and thrombocyte incompatibility on non-haemolytic transfusion reactions: II. A prospective study. *Vox Sang* 21:434, 1971.

185. Thompson JS, Severson CD, Parmely MJ, et al: Pulmonary "hypersensitivity" reactions induced by transfusion on non-HL-A leukoagglutinins. *N Engl J Med* 284:1120, 1971.

186. Wolfe CFW, Conale VC: Fatal pulmonary hypersensitivity reaction to HL-A incompatible blood transfusion: report of a case and review of the literature. *Transfusion* 16:135, 1976.

187. Popovsky MA, Chaplin HC Jr, Moore SB: Transfusion-related acute lung injury: a neglected serious complication of hemotherapy. *Transfusion* 32:589, 1992.

188. Andrews AT, Zmijewski CM, Bowman HS, Reihart JK: Transfusion reaction with pulmonary infiltration associated with HL-A specific leukocyte antibodies. *Am J Clin Pathol* 66:483, 1976.

189. Popovsky MA, Moore SB: Diagnostic and pathogenetic considerations in transfusion-related acute lung injury. *Transfusion* 25:573, 1985.

190. Dana BW, Durie BGM, White RF, Huestis DW: Concomitant administration of granulocyte transfusions and amphotericin B in neutropenic patients: Absence of significant pulmonary toxicity. *Blood* 57:90, 1981.

191. Thulstrup H: The influence of leukocyte and thrombocyte incompatibility on non-haemolytic transfusion reactions: I. A retrospective study. *Vox Sang* 21:233, 1971.

192. Nadorp JHS, Voss M, Buys WS, et al: The significance of the presence of anti-IgA antibodies in individuals with an IgA deficiency. *Eur J Clin Invest* 3:317, 1973.

193. Vyas GN, Perkins HA, Yang Y-M, Basantani GK: Healthy blood donors with selective absence of immunoglobulin A: prevention of anaphylactic transfusion reactions caused by antibodies to IgA. *J Lab Clin Med* 85:838, 1975.

194. Pineda AA, Taswell HF: Transfusion reactions associated with anti-IgA

195. Braude AI: Transfusion reactions from contaminated blood: their recognition and treatment. *N Engl J Med* 258:1289, 1958.

196. Duke M, Herbert VD, Abelmann WH: Hemodynamic effects of blood transfusion in chronic anemia. *N Engl J Med* 271:975, 1964.

197. O'Quin RJ, Lakshminarayan S: Venous air embolism. *Arch Intern Med* 142:2173, 1982.

198. Arrington P, McNamara JJ: Mechanism of microaggregate formation in stored blood. *Ann Surg* 179:146, 1974.

199. Martin AM, Simmons RL, Heisterkamp CA: Respiratory insufficiency in combat casualties: pathological changes in the lungs of patients dying of wounds. *Ann Surg* 170:30, 1969.

200. Moseley RV, Doty DB: Death associated with multiple pulmonary emboli soon after battle injury. *Ann Surg* 171:336, 1970.

201. McNamara JJ, Buran ES, Larson E, et al: Effect of debris in stored blood on pulmonary microvasculature. *Ann Thorac Surg* 14:113, 1972.

202. Barrett J, Tahir AH, Litwin MS: Increased pulmonary arteriovenous shunting in humans following blood transfusion. *Arch Surg* 113:947, 1978.

203. Snyder EL, Bookbinder M: Role of microaggregate blood filtration in clinical medicine. *Transfusion* 23:460, 1983.

204. Hill JD, Osborn JJ, Swank RL, et al: Experience using a new Dacron wool filter during extracorporeal circulation. *Arch Surg* 101:649, 1970.

205. Pineda AA, Paswell HF, Brzica SM Jr: Delayed hemolytic transfusion reaction: an immunologic hazard of blood transfusion. *Transfusion* 18:1, 1978.

206. Moore SB, Taswell HF, Pineda AA, Sonnenberg CL: Delayed hemolytic transfusion reactions: evidence of the need for an improved pretransfusion compatibility test. *Am J Clin Pathol* 74:94, 1980.

207. Croucher BEE, Crookston MC, Crookston JH: Delayed haemolytic transfusion reaction simulating autoimmune haemolytic anemia. *Vox Sang* 12:32, 1967.

208. Diamond WJ, Brown FL, Bitterman P, et al: Delayed hemolytic transfusion reaction presenting as sickle-cell crises. *Ann Intern Med* 93:231, 1980.

209. Orlin JB, Ellis MH: Transfusion-associated graft-versus-host disease. *Curr Opin Hematol* 4:442, 1997.

210. Fluit CRMG, Kunst VAJM, Drenthe-Schonk AH: Incidence of red cell antibodies after multiple blood transfusion. *Transfusion* 30:532, 1990.

211. Orlina AR, Unger PJ, Koshy M: Post-transfusion alloimmunization in patients with sickle cell disease. *Am J Hematol* 5:101, 1978.

212. Coles SM, Klein HG, Holland PV: Alloimmunization in two multitransfused patient populations. *Transfusion* 21:462, 1981.

213. Sarnaik S, Schornack J, Lusher JM: The incidence of development of irregular red cell antibodies in patients with sickle cell anemia. *Transfusion* 26:249, 1986.

214. Sirchia G, Zanella A, Parravicini A, et al: Red cell alloantibodies in thalassemia major. Results of an Italian cooperative study. *Transfusion* 25:110, 1985.

215. Ambruso DR, Githens JH, Alcorn R, et al: Experience with donors matched for minor blood group antigens in patients with sickle cell anemia who are receiving chronic transfusion therapy. *Transfusion* 27:94, 1987.

216. Mollison PL, Frame M, Ross ME: Differences between Rh(D) negative subjects in response to Rh(D) antigen. *Br J Haematol* 19:257, 1970.

217. Barclay GR, Greiss MAM, McCann MC, et al: Rhesus immunization in male volunteers: changes in lymphocyte functions following secondary immunizations in anti-D responders and non-responders. *Br J Haematol* 53:629, 1983.

218. Cook K, Rush B: Rh(D) immunization after massive transfusion of Rh(D)-positive blood. *Med J Aust* 1:166, 1974.

219. de Verdier CH, Garby L, Hjelm M, Högman C: Adenine in blood preservation: Posttransfusion viability and biochemical changes. *Transfusion* 4:331, 1964.

COLLECTION AND TRANSFUSION OF LEUKOCYTES, DENDRITIC CELLS, AND STEM CELLS

NICHOLAS BANDARENKO

MARK E. BRECHER

The availability of blood cell components including red cells, platelets, plasma, and plasma proteins has facilitated the treatment of hematologic diseases. Preparation of an effective granulocyte product has been elusive. The advent of recombinant granulocyte-mobilizing cytokines, which recruit large numbers of granulocytes into the blood, the use of hemapheresis instruments to cull the granulocytes from up to 15 liters of blood, and the use of starches to increase the efficiency of the separation of red cells from granulocytes have combined to make granulocyte transfusion of patients with severe reversible neutropenia and serious infections possible.

Stem cell transplantation from blood products has been made possible by using chemotherapeutic agents, cytokines, or combinations of the two to mobilize stem cells from marrow into blood, allowing recovery of sufficient numbers of stem cells by hemapheresis of several blood volumes. In so doing, sufficient CD34 antigen-positive cells can be recovered to engraft an allogeneic or autogeneic recipient.

Blood mononuclear cells of several types can be harvested by hemapheresis and used for immunotherapy. T lymphocytes can be used in their native state or after lymphokine activation. CD34 antigen-positive cells can be harvested and induced to transform into antigen-presenting (dendritic) cells by in vitro treatment with several cytokines. The use of mononuclear cells for immunotherapy of lymphoma, leukemia, or myeloma is becoming more frequent, and these approaches are dependent on hemapheresis to obtain sufficient quantities of cells to have therapeutic effects.

HISTORY OF GRANULOCYTE TRANSFUSION

Granulocyte transfusion for the treatment of neutropenia was first explored in 1934 but met with little success.[1] It was not until 1953 that the first promising experiments with leukocytes were reported.[2] In these experiments, leukocytes transfused into irradiated dogs migrated to sites of infection and were capable of normal phagocytic activity.[2]

Subsequently, interest in granulocyte transfusions has been cyclical. In the 1960s there was a strong sentiment for the use of granulocyte transfusions. This enthusiasm was fueled by the ability to collect large quantities of granulocytes from patients with CML and the early success with the infusion of these cells to patients with severe granulocytopenia and life-threatening infection.[4] However, due to the unavailability of donors and concerns with transfusing malignant cells this practice was abandoned. In the 1970s, following the introduction of blood cell separators capable of harvesting large quantities of granulocytes from healthy donors, there was an overly optimistic view that granulocytes would have substantial clinical impact. However, in the 1980s disillusionment had set in following limited success with healthy-donor granulocyte therapy, and use of this therapy decreased. In the mid-1990s the introduction of recombinant cytokines capable of mobilizing large numbers of healthy-donor granulocytes led to renewed interest in granulocyte therapy.

PRECLINICAL STUDIES OF DOGS WITH GRANULOCYTE TRANSFUSION

Studies in neutropenic dogs with gram-negative sepsis,[3–7] pneumonia,[8,9] or candidemia[10–12] found increased survival with or without antibiotic therapy. A threshold dose of 2×10^8 granulocytes/kg was protective against a lethal infection with *Pseudomonas*, while there was uniform mortality when doses less than 1.5×10^8 granulocytes/kg were administered. Mean 1 h posttransfusion increments of greater than $200/\mu l$ or greater than $500/\mu l$ were seen with infusions of at least 2×10^8 and 3×10^8 granulocytes/kg, respectively. Such studies suggested that a clinical benefit from granulocyte transfusions in neutropenic septic patients would be strongly dose-dependent.

CLINICAL EXPERIENCE WITH GRANULOCYTE TRANSFUSION

GRANULOCYTE CONCENTRATES FROM CML DONORS

Cell collections from donors with CML yielded as many as 1×10^{11} phagocytic cells,[17,18] and transfusion of these concentrates increased white cell counts and led to improvement in septic neutropenic recipients.[19–21] Leukocyte transfusions from CML donors also caused a more sustained elevation of the white cell count, perhaps because of their content of granulocytic progenitors capable of cell division.[17] Patients with CML are rarely available and are not considered to be acceptable blood donors.

CONTROLLED TRIALS OF GRANULOCYTE CONCENTRATES FROM HEALTHY DONORS

There have been seven controlled clinical trials of granulocyte transfusion therapy for the treatment of bacterial sepsis in adults.[22–28] These trials were considered successful,[23,25,26] partially successful,[22,27] or unsuccessful.[24,28] A meta-analysis of these studies concluded that the dose of granulocytes transfused (greater than 1×10^{10} granulocytes transfused per day on at least four successive days) and the survival rate of controls (efficacious when the survival of the controls was under 40 percent) were primarily responsible for the disagreements across the reports.[29] When the analysis was limited to the five randomized controlled studies,[23,24–28] granulocyte therapy conferred a significant survival benefit in the following settings: (1) low survival rate of controls (RR = 8.0, 95% CI, 1.5–42), (2) adequate dose of granulocytes (RR = 4.0, 95% CI, 1.2–12), (3) timely marrow recovery; and (4) pretransfusion assessment of compatibility of granulocytes (RR = 8.0, 95% CI, 1.5–42).

Bacterial infection in the neonatal period may be life-threatening because of inadequate granulocyte function or the infant's inability to mount or sustain neutrophilia because of inadequate reserves of neutrophilic precursors. In septic neonates there have been five studies of the effects of granulocyte therapy,[30-34] four of which were randomized.[31-34] A meta-analysis of these studies found that the only significant predictor of success was a dose of cells greater than 0.5×10^9/kg (RR 18, 95% CI, 1.3–252).[29] Granulocyte therapy was not efficacious when buffy coats (as contrasted with granulocyte concentrates) which contained less than 0.5×10^9/kg granulocytes were transfused (RR = 0.74, 95% CI, 0.20–2.7). The effect of a low survival rate of controls did not reach statistical significance; however, the relative risk was large (RR = 13, 95% CI, 0.39–462). The effect of leukocyte compatibility was not assessed in the studies of neonates.

MOBILIZATION OF DONOR GRANULOCYTES AND COLLECTION

Less than five percent of the total body neutrophil pool is in the intravascular space.[36,37] These cells have a half-life of only 4 to 10 h in the intravascular compartment.[38,39] The collection of large numbers of granulocytes requires the processing of 5 to 14 liters of blood per donation, which can be accomplished within 2 to 3 h. Apheresis procedures are performed with a special centrifuge.[39-41] Donor blood is pumped through the centrifuge and separated, based on density, into three layers. The leukocyte-containing layer is harvested to form the granulocyte concentrate, and the red cells and plasma are returned to the donor. Of historical note is that an alternative, noncentrifugal method of granulocyte collection that exploited the ability of granulocytes to adhere to nylon in the presence of divalent cations was once employed.[42] Although filtration leukapheresis was simple and yielded large quantities of granulocytes,[27,39,40,42-51] the technique has been abandoned because of the need to heparinize the donor and because of reactions such as severe abdominal pain,[52] priapism,[53] complement activation in the donor,[54-58] frequent shaking chills in the recipient,[59] and poor survival, in vivo recovery, and chemotactic capability of the collected neutrophils.[18,28,60-64]

Granulocyte collections taken from healthy donors by centrifugal leukapheresis do not routinely yield adequate quantities of phagocytic cells ($0.1-0.5 \times 10^{10}$ granulocytes per liter of donor blood).[29,40] This is due to two factors: (1) the difficulty of separating granulocytes from lighter red cells and lymphocytes because of the similarity in their density, and (2) the low number of granulocytes in the circulation. The addition of a rouleaux-inducing sedimenting agent to the blood before it enters the centrifuge enhances the separation of red cells from white cells and increases yields as much as twofold. The most common rouleaux-inducing agents employed are hydroxyethyl starches.[17,19-21] Hydroxyethyl starches are branched-chain polyglucose molecules, or glucans, similar in structure to glycogen but having variable degrees of hydroxyl substitutions on the glucose residues (carbons 2, 3, and 6). Such substances are also used as a synthetic colloid volume expander. Virtually all centrifugal cell separators require the use of cell-sedimenting agents to achieve an adequate granulocyte yield. In the United States two hydroxyethyl starches, hetastarch (Hespan), sometimes referred to as high molecular weight hydroxyethyl starch or HMW-HES, and pentastarch (Pentaspan), sometimes referred to as low molecular weight hydroxyethyl starch, or LMW-HES, are approved and commercially available for human use. Pentastarch was thought to be a superior starch erythrocyte-sedimenting agent due to its lower molecular weight (average pentastarch 260 kDa, versus hetastarch 450 kDa) and consequently more rapid and complete clearance.[65] A paired controlled prospective study involving 36 donors from whom collections were alternately made with both starch sedi-

menting agents found that in 33 of 36 (92%, $P < .001$) pairs of donors, hetastarch was significantly more efficient in granulocyte collection. Overall, hetastarch provided 1.6-fold greater collections than did pentastarch.[66] Donor reactions are not common but can range from mild rashes, rhinorrhea, or paresthesias to anaphylaxis, circulatory failure, pulmonary edema, and others.

Donor granulocyte counts also can be increased prior to donation by the administration of drugs that either mobilize granulocytes from the marrow or cause a shift of granulocytes from the marginal pool to the circulating blood pool.[67,68] At present, dexamethasone or another glucocorticoid is administered either orally or by intravenous infusion to raise the donor granulocyte count prior to leukapheresis.[20,39,40,68-70] Various dose schedules have been used, but a typical regimen is 8 mg dexamethasone (or 20–30 mg prednisone) given orally 12 h prior to collection. Leukapheresis yields have increased by 50 to 100 percent after glucocorticoid administration, and their use is routine in most leukapheresis facilities. The effects of hydroxyethyl starch and glucocorticoid administration are additive, and neither has significant adverse effects on the function of the granulocytes.[60,68,71,72]

Despite the availability of glucocorticoids and erythrocyte sedimenting agents, a dose of greater than 1×10^{10} granulocytes frequently is not achieved with one apheresis collection. This level may be particularly difficult to achieve for the first collection when there has not been time to medicate the donor with glucocorticoids prior to the apheresis collection.

The introduction of cytokines such as G-CSF (Neupogen) for the mobilization of hematopoietic cells has allowed the collection of much larger numbers of granulocytes. Multiple studies employing G-CSF at a dose of 5 to 10 μg/kg per day (300–600 μg given subcutaneously) administered 12 h prior to collection will result in a blood white count in the range of $20-50 \times 10^9$/liter range with a three- to sixfold increase in the number of granulocytes collected ($4-8 \times 10^{10}$ granulocytes).[73-76] Combining glucocorticoids and cytokines results in even greater efficacy, with mean collections of $0.8-1.1 \times 10^{11}$ granulocytes.[76-78] Such doses approach the amount of granulocytes that a normal marrow produces in a day (1.5×10^9/kg).[79,80]

Use of G-CSF is not without problems. Donors complain of bone pain, headaches, fatigue, night sweats, nausea and vomiting, sleep disturbances, and redness or swelling at the injection site.[77] Comparison of multiple mobilization schemes suggests that a dose of both G-CSF and glucocorticoids given once on the day prior to collection minimizes side effects and results in a fourfold increase in granulocytes collected over the use of glucocorticoids alone.[76-78] A single dose of 300 μg of G-CSF results in nearly the same elevation in neutrophil count as a 600-μg dose 78. For repeated donations, administration of G-CSF on alternate days maintains the neutrophil count, with decreased side effects and lower cost than a daily regimen.[75] In a paired three-arm study, the use of dexamethasone alone resulted in 25 percent of donors reporting insomnia or flushing. With G-CSF, 65 percent had bone pain, headache, insomnia, fatigue, nocturia, or diaphoresis; this increased to 85 percent with combination of dexamethasone and G-CSF.[78] There are no known long-term sequelae after the transient administration of G-CSF to healthy donors.

The granulocytes collected following cytokine mobilization are not fully mature, but studies have not identified any significant dysfunction granulocyte dysfunction. Granulocytes appear activated (primed for a respiratory burst), have normal phagocytosis and staphylococcal killing capability in vitro, and have a prolonged half-life in the circulation.[73,78-81] There is evidence of degranulation and decreased postinfusion recovery (31% versus 65%), but G-CSF-stimulated granulocytes migrate into skin-window chambers and into sites of inflammation and infection.[78] After G-CSF priming of the donor, there are alterations of surface antigen expression with increased expression of adhesion molecules (CD11b, CD14, CD18) and Fc receptors (CD32, CD64).[78] The clinical significance of these changes, if any, is not known.

INDICATIONS FOR GRANULOCYTE TRANSFUSIONS

The indications for granulocyte transfusion are not well defined. In general, the patient should have (1) an absolute granulocyte count less than 500/μl (0.5 × 10^9/liter), (2) fever, (3) an identified responsible microorganism, and (4) no decrease in fever after 48 h of antibiotic treatment. Also, the prognosis without granulocyte therapy in the specific setting should be poor and the prognosis of the underlying disorder should be favorable. When possible, attempts should be made to match for leukocyte antigens and transfuse cytomegalovirus-negative, irradiated cells.

The risk of infection in granulocytopenic patients is related to the severity and duration of the cytopenia.[82] The risk of infection increases dramatically when the granulocyte count is below 500/μl (0.5 × 10^9/liter). An equally important consideration in determining the need for granulocyte transfusion is the status of the patient's marrow. If early marrow recovery is expected, granulocyte concentrates are probably superfluous. Conversely, if the neutropenia is expected to last for more than several days the patient may benefit from granulocyte transfusions when serious infection is present.

Granulocyte transfusions also have been used successfully in the treatment of infected patients with chronic granulomatous disease. In these patients granulocyte transfusion is indicated if appropriate antibiotic therapy used alone is unsuccessful.[83–86]

PROPHYLACTIC TRANSFUSION

The usefulness of giving prophylactic granulocyte transfusions to neutropenic patients without evidence of infection has been evaluated in several studies.[86–92] In a large randomized study, neutropenic patients with leukemia who received prophylactic granulocyte transfusions did not have an overall reduced incidence of infections compared with controls, although the proportion of transfused patients with bacterial septicemia was reduced. Also, prophylactic granulocyte transfusions did not improve the rates of remission, survival, or time to marrow recovery.[90] Most other studies agree with these findings. No randomized studies have been done with the G-CSF plus glucocorticoid stimulated granulocyte collections.

Two randomized studies have evaluated the use of prophylactic granulocyte transfusions in patients receiving marrow transplants. One study found fewer infections in transfused patients than in controls.[88] In contrast, the other study[89] found a decrease in bacterial septicemia in transfused patients but did not observe a reduction in overall infection; survival was not improved. Furthermore, 13 of the 18 patients receiving transfusions developed cytomegalovirus infections, compared with only 6 of 17 controls. Thus, viral infection is a significant additional hazard in severely immunosuppressed patients.

One major drawback to prophylactic granulocyte transfusion is the increased likelihood of transfusion reactions, alloimmunization, lymphocytotoxic antibodies, and refractoriness to future transfusions. Refractoriness to platelet transfusion occurs frequently in patients who are given granulocyte transfusions.[87] Although there is some reduction in the incidence of infection, the occurrence of alloimmunization and the absence of clear benefit are major deterrents to the use of prophylactic granulocyte transfusions.

G-CSF mobilized, HLA-matched, ABO compatible granulocytes provided to allogeneic bone marrow transplant recipients resulted in significant and sustained increments in the neutrophil and the platelet count.[75] The peak of the neutrophil increment was observed 4 to 12 h following infusion and the rise in the neutrophil count persisted for 25 to 37 h. Nevertheless, three of the ten recipients developed culture-proven bacterial infections during the period of granulocyte infusions.

HAZARDS

The general hazards of blood transfusion also apply to granulocyte transfusions. Hemolytic reactions may occur because there are red cells in granulocyte concentrates. ABO-compatible concentrates should be given. Recovery of granulocytes in the recipient 1 h after transfusion is adversely affected by ABO incompatibility.[22] The presence of erythrocyte antibodies in the recipient other than AB blood groups should also be ascertained prior to transfusion, but such erythrocyte incompatibilities are not an absolute contraindication to transfusion if the patient's infection is severe. If necessary, most of the erythrocytes in the concentrate can be removed by differential centrifugation prior to transfusion.

Febrile transfusion reactions occur frequently with granulocyte transfusions.[48,59] About 10 percent of recipients have chills and fever after transfusion of cells collected by a centrifugation method, as a result of antileukocytic antibodies in the recipient or pyrogen released from damaged white cells. Glucocorticoids, antihistamines, and meperidine can be given either prophylactically or therapeutically to reduce the frequency or severity of these reactions.

Acute pulmonary insufficiency has been reported with granulocyte transfusion.[93] A number of different mechanisms have been proposed. In neutropenic patients with pneumonia it has been postulated that the rapid migration of transfused granulocytes into the infected lung may induce such a reaction.[93] Leukoagglutinins in the recipient may result in leukocyte aggregates which embolize to the lung.[94] Complement activation and the generation of C5a, which results in granulocyte aggregation or adhesion to endothelial cells, also have been postulated.[95] Severe pulmonary reactions with the concomitant use of granulocyte transfusion and amphotericin B have been reported by some observers[96] but not by others.[97,98] As a precaution, however, amphotericin B and leukocyte transfusion should be administered at different times.

Severely immunosuppressed patients are at risk for other serious complications of granulocyte transfusion. Graft-versus-host disease, sometimes fatal, has occurred in patients receiving intensive chemotherapy and perhaps in neonates.[99–104] In such cases, the concentrate should be irradiated with 2500 rad prior to administration to prevent this occurrence. Severely immunosuppressed patients, especially those undergoing marrow transplantation, also may develop a cytomegalovirus infection, particularly pneumonia, that may be fatal.[89] Individuals who do not have serologic evidence of prior cytomegalovirus infection should be selected as donors for immunosuppressed patients.

STORAGE OF GRANULOCYTE CONCENTRATES

It is best to transfuse granulocytes as soon as possible after collection.[48,105] Granulocyte concentrates system should not be stored for more than 24 h.

Granulocyte chemotaxis is the first function altered during storage.[72,106–109] Changes in phagocytic function, bactericidal capacity, and biochemical functions such as fructose-6-phosphate (hexose monophosphate) shunt activity and oxygen consumption are generally less sensitive indicators of cell damage during storage.

Cell viability and bactericidal capacity seem to be well maintained at either room temperature (22°C) or during refrigerator storage (5°C) for at least 24 h,[106–111] but chemotaxis, chemotaxis-related functions, adherence to endothelial cells, and cell ATP levels are better preserved at 20–24°C.[107,108,111–117] Storage of granulocytes is associated with a tendency for hyperadherence and spontaneous aggregation that is more pronounced at 5°C.[116] Because of better preservation of function, current practice is to store granulocytes at room temperature when storage is required.

In general, granulocyte concentrates are better preserved in plasma than in other suspension fluids,[111] but it is possible that improved storage can be achieved in other optimized solutions.[118] Additional glucose may be required when the cell leukocyte count is high[119] or when there are significant numbers of contaminating platelets and red cells that compete with the granulocytes for glucose.[120] The type of plastic used in the storage bag is another important storage variable.[121] Gentle agitation was found to be beneficial in one study[122] but not in another.[111] It is unclear whether irradiation of granulocyte concentrates prior to transfusion to prevent graft-versus-host disease is associated with alteration in cell function.[123,124] The subject of granulocyte preservation has been reviewed.[125]

Cryopreservation of granulocytes would be an ideal method of storage because it would permit the "banking" of large quantities of cells that would be available when needed. Dimethyl sulfoxide is used as a cryoprotective agent, but there are no satisfactory methods for freezing granulocytes. Post-thaw recovery of viable cells, as measured by phagocytosis, rarely exceeds 25 percent.[126–128]

Granulocyte transfusion therapy has been full of promise for several decades. Now, with the ability to reliably collect G-CSF plus steroid-mobilized granulocytes from healthy donors with total doses exceeding 1×10^{11} granulocytes, large randomized trials are needed to define the efficacy, toxicity, and cost-effectiveness of granulocyte transfusions both for prophylaxis in transiently neutropenic patients and for neutropenic patients with progressive bacterial or fungal infections.[129]

APHERESIS-DERIVED PERIPHERAL BLOOD STEM CELLS

HISTORY OF PERIPHERAL BLOOD STEM CELL TRANSPLANTATION

Within the past 10 years the role of blood stem cells has evolved from research conducted in a few centers to a widely utilized therapeutic modality. Since the initial hypothesis in 1909 that hematopoietic stem cells circulate[130] and subsequently, the demonstration of hematopoietic reconstitution following myeloablative irradiation and parabiosis in rodents by Brecher and Cronkite in 1951,[131] the potential applications of blood stem cells in humans have emerged. Documentation of cell engraftment in a patient receiving granulocytes derived from a donor with chronic myelogenous leukemia in 1963[132] paved the way for the first successfully performed autologous blood stem cell transplant in a patient with chronic myelogenous leukemia in 1979.[133] In 1986, successful hematopoietic reconstitution by autologous blood stem cell transplantation was described in a patient with Burkitt lymphoma following marrow-ablative chemotherapy.[134] Initially, autologous stem cells collected by leukapheresis were used to shorten the period of pancytopenia following myeloablative chemotherapy in patients undergoing bone marrow transplantation.[135,136] Early successes with blood stem cell transplantation involved steady-state harvesting of the circulating hematopoietic stem cells by apheresis without specific mobilization strategies. Engraftment times were comparable to bone marrow transplantation.[134,137,138] Unfortunately the number of collections, time, and cost of collection and transplantation of blood stem cells were not yet optimal for the evolving technology to emerge as an alternative to marrow transplantation.[139] The development of mobilization techniques to enhance the circulating number of stem cells, optimizing of the timing of apheresis harvests, and progress on characterizing stem cells by immunophenotyping have enabled this transition to occur. Currently, autologous transplantation using blood stem cells is performed more frequently than autologous bone marrow transplants.[139–141]

Apheresis-derived blood stem cells offer several benefits over marrow transplants.[142] Apheresis collection is feasible on an outpatient basis, avoids general anesthesia, and enables the processing of multiple blood volumes per collection. Blood stem cell collection is suitable for patients whose marrow is infiltrated by disease or fibrosis or who have a history of prior pelvic radiation. Blood stem cells result in a shortened cytopenic period following myeloablative treatment, fewer infectious complications, a lower incidence of tumor cell contamination, decreased transfusion requirements, and a shortened period of hospitalization.[135,143,144] Disadvantages include a potentially longer period to obtain an adequate harvest; a greater volume to infuse; maintenance of central venous access, which predisposes to risks for infection and thrombosis[145,146]; and, in the allogeneic setting, the possibly greater risk of graft-versus-host disease due to the presence of mature lymphocytes in the stem cell suspension.

Technical advances have facilitated the application of peripheral blood stem cell transplantation. These include improved automated blood separators capable of efficient collection of mononuclear cells and the use of cryopreservation and sterile bag systems to pool components from multiple collections.[147] Innovations in mobilization techniques, quantification of appropriate stem cell doses to ensure timely engraftment, and optimization of the timing and efficiency of apheresis collections have contributed to the growing use of this stem cell collection strategy.

STEM CELL MOBILIZATION STRATEGIES

Collection of adequate numbers of stem cells from blood requires large volumes to be processed (2–4 blood volumes). Retrieval of this small population of cells is challenging, since very primitive hematopoietic cells comprise only 0.01 to 0.1 percent of circulating leukocytes and 1 to 10 percent of cells obtained from bone marrow.[148] Mobilization refers to those techniques which increase the proportion of circulating primitive cells, especially stem cells. Although the exact mechanism(s) by which mobilization occurs is unclear, glucocorticoids, endotoxin, stress, exercise, and dextran have been shown to cause alterations in the concentration of peripheral progenitor cells.[149] Mobilization strategies have significantly improved the efficiency of peripheral blood stem cell collection by apheresis and have decreased the number of procedures necessary to achieve target stem cell collection amounts. As a consequence, transplantation using blood stem cells has become an attractive alternative to marrow transplantation.

CHEMOTHERAPY

Myelosuppressive (as opposed to myeloablative) chemotherapy is associated with a recovery phase with increased concentrations in circulating hematopoietic progenitor cells.[150,151] A variety of chemotherapeutic agents/regimens can elicit mobilization, which is enhanced depending on the dose and timing of the preceding chemotherapy.[152] The effectiveness of mobilization can be assessed by in vitro clonogenic progenitor cell assays of blood. These assays have also been instrumental for quantifying the harvested stem cells after apheresis. Morphologically distinct CFU-GM, BFU-E, and CFU-GEMM colony-forming units can be quantified by colonial growth on cytokine-supplemented semisolid media after incubating 7 to 20 days. However, due to the time required for these assays they primarily provide retrospective information. Flow cytometric "real time" assessment of stem cell content using CD34 antigen has greatly enhanced the clinical utility of stem cell enumeration (see "Dose and Enumeration of Stem Cells").

Use of high-dose cyclophosphamide to mobilize progenitor cells has been effective in patients with lymphoma, myeloma, and solid tumors.[134,153,154] A 14-fold increase in the mean CFU-GM in blood of patients with lymphoma, myeloma, and solid tumors occurred two days after recovering leukocyte counts exceeded 1×10^9/liter.[154] Comparison of hematologic recovery times between autologous chemotherapy mobilized stem cell transplants and marrow autotransplants revealed significantly shorter time to attain a neutrophil count of 0.5×10^9/liter (mean of 11 days versus 22 days) and a platelet count of 50×10^9/liter (mean of 14 days versus 32 days).[144] In addition, the number of hospital days and blood component transfusions were reduced in the group that received blood stem cells.

CYTOKINES AND CHEMOTHERAPY

When mobilization regimens incorporate cytokines such as G-CSF or GM-CSF in addition to chemotherapy, progenitor cell concentrations increase dramatically over steady-state blood levels.[155] A strategy combining chemotherapy and hematopoietic growth factors offers the most effective means for mobilization of progenitor cells. This strategy was first described in the treatment of patients with sarcoma.[156] GM-CSF when combined with myelosuppressive chemotherapy produced a 63-fold elevation in circulating progenitors measured as CFU-GM by in vitro culture. GM-CSF priming alone produced a 13-fold increase in CFU-GM, and chemotherapy alone produced only a twofold rise in CFU-GM. The synergistic effect of chemotherapy plus cytokine administration becomes readily apparent when reviewing published experience. In general mobilization with chemotherapy alone affords a 20- to 50-fold increase in circulating CFU-GM. Cytokines or hematopoietic growth factors alone afford a comparable mobilization: G-CSF typically results in a 20- to 50-fold increase in CFU-GM, while GM-CSF results in a modest 10-fold increase in CFU-GM. When cytokines are combined with chemotherapy, mobilization of CFU-GM increases by approximately 70-fold (range 25 to 250 fold).[153,157-164] A median time to a platelet count of greater than 20×10^9/liter occurred in 10 days in a chemotherapy plus G-CSF mobilized stem cell transplant group, as compared to 17 days in an autologous marrow transplant group.[165] The preferred approach is to use harvested blood stem cells as the source of hematopoietic reconstitution.[140,162] However, effective mobilization of autologous stem cells in patients may be unsuccessful, depending on the extent of previous chemotherapy/radiation or involvement of the marrow in disease.[166]

STEM CELL COLLECTION FOR ALLOGENEIC TRANSPLANTATION

Blood stem cell transplantation in the allogeneic setting has evolved at a slower pace due to concerns of graft-versus-host disease that might arise from donor lymphocytes. Fortunately, experience with sibling HLA-matched donors, syngeneic donors, and a second autologous marrow transplantation revealed minimal graft-versus-host disease and few adverse effects on the donor.[167-169] Allogeneic blood stem cell transplantation results in rapid, multi-lineage engraftment following successful mobilization of donor stem cells with G-CSF. Higher doses of G-CSF enhance the progenitor cell harvest beyond that obtained by marrow harvest and have been associated with more rapid engraftment of platelets.[170] Initial enthusiasm was offset by reports of chronic graft-versus-host disease, which occurred despite the low numbers of CD3+ cells present in the blood stem-cell suspension following CD34+ cell selection.[171,172] Diminishing the graft-versus-host effect while retaining the graft-versus-leukemia effect remains a challenge.[173]

Reports of significant donor reactions have been infrequent, although cytokine mobilization has been associated with mild bone pain, headache, body aches, fatigue, nausea and vomiting, local reactions at the injection site, insomnia, night sweats, dyspnea, transient changes in serum chemistries, and thrombocytopenia.[73,74,143,174-179] Risks associated with apheresis include citrate toxicity, hypotension, fatigue, and if antecubital access is insufficient, the risks of central venous access. Large-volume leukapheresis collections are typically successful in harvesting sufficient progenitor cells in one or two collections. While clinically significant thrombocytopenia has not been described following administration of G-CSF, stem cell suspension products contain a substantial number of platelets. A drop from preapheresis platelet counts of approximately 28 percent per daily collection has been described, with recovery after about 10 days.[179] A predictable 2–4% decrease of the platelet count per liter of whole blood processed occurs in donors.[180] Close monitoring of pre-, post- and intraprocedure donor platelet counts is advisable. Strategies to minimize this problem may include shorter collections, longer recovery periods between collections, or the use of thrombopoietin. Salvaging of platelets may provide the most immediate practical solution.[181]

The long-term effects, and specifically the risk of subsequent hematologic consequences, remain a theoretical concern when exposing healthy donors to hematopoietic growth factors. Several hundred allogeneic blood stem cell donors followed for 2 to 5 years postdonation have not shown an increased risk of hematologic malignancy.[139] A prospective study of 19 donors demonstrated that one year after the administration of G-CSF their blood counts were normal and unchanged from predonation counts. Furthermore, following a second course of G-CSF the progenitor content of the peripheral blood stem-cell product was comparable to the first.[182]

DOSE AND ENUMERATION OF STEM CELLS

The CFU-GM count correlates inversely with the time to detectable engraftment, the length of hospitalization, and the amount of supportive care needed.[136,144,183] The correlation between the CFU-GM and CD34 counts reported by several independent investigators,[184-187] along with the advent of flow-cytometric quantitation of CD34 cells, has facilitated more rapid and reproducible measurement of putative stem cells in "real time."

The CD34 antigen is a glycoprotein expressed on the surface of lymphohematopoietic self-renewing stem cells, lineage-committed progenitors, some endothelial cells, embryonic fibroblasts, and marrow stromal cells. Although its functional role has yet to be definitively established, it has been suggested that the CD34 antigen assists in the adhesion and routing of primitive hematopoietic cells during hematopoiesis and differentiation.[139] Approximately 1.5 percent of the bone marrow mononuclear cells express CD34. Within this population reside the CFU-GM, BFU-E, and CFU-GEMM capable of short-term hematopoietic reconstitution,[176,188,189] as well as the pluripotential self-renewing stem cell, the exact phenotype of which remains controversial. The pluripotential stem cell presumably resides within the CD34+, thy-1^{dim}, CD38−, HLA-DR−, and lineage-specific negative subpopulation (see Chapter 14).[162]

The blood contains approximately 1 to 10 percent of the CD34+ population in the marrow in the steady state. Mobilization techniques, as discussed above, expand this circulating compartment and enable efficient collection by leukapheresis. The adequacy of a blood stem-cell collection is gauged by the number of CD34+ cells per kilogram of recipient body weight. The minimal threshold of CD34+ cells necessary for neutrophil and platelet recovery after autologous transplantation has ranged from 2 to 5×10^6 per kilogram.[166,190,191,195] Higher stem-cell doses have been associated with accelerated platelet engraftment.[170] In one study of breast cancer patients, 14 days after transplant, the probability of the platelet count being greater than 20×10^9/liter was 95, 85, 65, or 50 percent with a total infused doses of 10×10^6, 5×10^6, 2×10^6, or 1×10^6 CD34+ cells/kg, respectively. Some transplant physicians have made a distinction between an optimal cell dose for autologous versus allogeneic stem-cell grafts and recommend that the latter contain at least threefold more progenitor cells, although the necessity for this has not been proved.[139]

Increasing the total dose of CD34+ cells from apheresis-derived collections theoretically should result in a greater likelihood of enduring hematopoietic engraftment. The higher incidence of tumor cell contamination with increased numbers of apheresis collections for autologous stem-cell harvests of breast cancer patients gives pause to the notion that more is better.[193] A shortened disease-free survival was observed among breast cancer patients undergoing autologous marrow transplantation who had evidence of micrometastatic disease in the marrow harvested, as measured by immunocytochemical methods.[194]

A variety of methods for enumeration of CD34+ cells by flow cytometry have been published.[148,194–202] However, comparison of CD34 measurements from different centers is difficult due to differences in methods among laboratories. A multi-institutional study of 21 marrow and blood samples showed a twenty-fold range in results.[203] These discrepant observations confirmed results from several smaller studies[196,198,204] and emphasize the need for standardization. One approach has been suggested by the International Society for Hematotherapy and Graft Engineering (ISHAGE).[205] Counting techniques that incorporate a standard bead into the analysis or volumetric capillary cytometry hold promise for increasing accuracy and reproducibility.[206–208]

TIMING OF STEM CELL COLLECTIONS

At present, stem cell collections using continuous flow apheresis equipment depends on processing 1.5 to 4 blood volumes over several hours. Repeated daily collections over 2 to 5 days are used to reach an adequate threshold of stem cells. The adequacy of the collection is dependent on the mode of mobilization, the timing of the collection with respect to the recovering leukocytes, the volume of whole blood processed, and the amount of patient pretreatment.[162]

Recruitment of noncirculating hematopoietic progenitors during a single large-volume leukapheresis collection (2 to 3 times the donor blood volume) can occur, including a 2.5-fold increase in the CFU-GM when more than 15 liters of whole blood was processed.[186,209–211] However, such results are dependent on the patient's ability to tolerate prolonged leukapheresis, adequate mobilization, and timing.[212]

Healthy allogeneic donors treated with G-CSF have a predictable peak in circulating stem cells occurring 5 to 6 days after initiating daily subcutaneous doses of G-CSF of 5 to 10 μg/kg per day.[134,143,176,214,216]

Timing collections in the autologous setting has been more challenging. Early studies suggested that collections begin when the leukocyte count exceeded 1.0×10^9/L.[139,214] While circulating progenitor cells and the total mononuclear count begin to rise concurrently, premature cessation of cytokine administration in these studies likely led to a decrease in circulating progenitors.[139] Subsequently, cytokine administration has been continued longer throughout serial collection procedures. Peak levels of circulating progenitors have been reported 2 days after the WBC count exceeds 2×10^9/L,[213] 12 days after the WBC exceeds 10×10^9/L,[167] or when the rebounding WBC reaches 5×10^9/L.[157]

Unfortunately, the blood white cell and mononuclear cell counts do not correlate with the number of hematopoietic progenitor cells in the blood.[217,218] Quantitation of circulating CD34+ cells the day of leukapheresis is a more accurate predictor of the optimal time of stem cell harvest.[217–223] A minimum threshold greater than 10 to 30 circulating CD34+ cells per microliter will afford a satisfactory stem cell harvest, although serial collections may still be necessary to attain the appropriate CD34+ dose for transplantation.[219–221] When the circu-

lating progenitors approach or exceed 100 CD34+ cells per microliter, a single leukapheresis may provide all of the CD34+ cells necessary.

The relationship of circulating CD34+ cells with the CD34+ cell yield allows for the optimal timing of stem cell harvests. Thus, fewer collections and a lower volume of pooled product to infuse following myeloablation can be achieved. By combining microvolume fluorometry and an automated analysis, accurate CD34+ cell counts can be made in 30 min. This assay has the potential to expedite optimal timing of stem cell harvests.[207,208]

Finally, awareness of the phenotype of the patient's malignant cells is important, since lymphoblastic lymphomas and other hematologic malignancies can occasionally express the CD34 antigen and yield an erroneously high stem cell dose.

MONONUCLEAR CELLS FOR ADOPTIVE IMMUNOTHERAPY

ALLOGENEIC ADOPTIVE IMMUNOTHERAPY

Allogeneic blood cell collection and reinfusion may benefit marrow transplant patients with recurrent leukemia. This form of adoptive immunotherapy utilizes the inherent immune reactivity of apheresis-derived allogeneic leukocytes from the original marrow donor to either prevent recurrence or induce remission. With strategies that manipulate the timing and the dose of donor T lymphocytes infused following transplantation, this therapy attempts to exploit the beneficial graft-versus-leukemia effect while minimizing the risks of graft-versus-host disease. Donor lymphocytes have been used to induce cytogenetic remission in patients with CML who relapsed after transplantation.[173,224] Although the role of interferon-α in such therapy has been questioned, the antileukemia effect of reinfused donor lymphocytes in CML patients has been confirmed, yielding a composite clinical response rate of 77 percent.[225] Unfortunately, transfusion of allogeneic mononuclear cells from the original donor has not been capable of inducing a durable remission with other hematologic malignancies.[224,226] Graft-versus-host disease remains a major complication frequently accompanying this therapy. Of the CML patients who achieved remission, graft-versus-host disease developed in 73 percent (8/11) of patients receiving a total T-cell dose greater than 5×10^7/kg but only in 12.5 percent (1/8) of patients who received a total T-cell dose of 1×10^7/kg.[173] Remission in CML can result from donor leukocytes containing as few as 1×10^7 T cells/kg.

AUTOLOGOUS ADOPTIVE IMMUNOTHERAPY

Another application of mononuclear cell collection using apheresis cell separators has been in the preparation of autologous mononuclear cells with antitumor activity. Examples include the production of LAK cells,[227,228] TIL,[229] and activated dendritic cells (antigen-presenting cells). Each of these applications must be considered experimental at present.

The production of LAK cells may require pretreatment of the patient with IL-2, leukapheresis for the collection of mononuclear cells, ex vivo manipulation of the collected cells to activate and/or purify them, and reinfusion into the patient. In a study of 539 leukapheresis collections, a mean of 3.03×10^{10} lymphocytes were collected in a four-hour procedure.[230] High yields of lymphocytes in these procedures result in part from recruitment of these cells into the circulation by prior IL-2 treatment. The culturing, harvesting, and washing of these lymphocyte preparations prior to infusion, rather elaborate processes, have been described.[231–233]

Due to the limited success observed with both LAK and TIL cell therapy for metastatic cancer, attention has turned to the collection, purification, activation, and reinfusion of dendritic cells as a means for the production of tumor-specific cytotoxic T cells. Experimental evidence suggests that the presence of tumor inhibits dendritic cell maturation and activation both locally and systemically.[234] However, isolated dendritic cells (from marrow or blood) can be concentrated or cultured from CD34+ progenitor cells. These fully functional isolated dendritic cells are subjected to cytokines (such as GM-CSF, IL-4, and TNF-α) and tumor-associated antigen stimulation and have been used as a pulse therapy.[233–241] The identification of antigens such as CD83 and CMRF-44 on dendritic cells may allow the optimization of cytokine mobilization and of the timing of collection of blood dendritic cells, and possibly lead to positive selection techniques similar to those currently used for CD34+ cells.[242,243] Preliminary clinical trials with dendritic cells in low-grade B cell lymphoma, prostate cancer, and melanoma have been associated with apparent clinical responses in some patients.[239–241] These early reports, while promising, require further clinical investigation to assess the clinical efficacy.

REFERENCES

1. Strumia MM: Effect of leukocyte cream injection in treatment of neutropenias. *Am J Med Sci* 187:527, 1934.
2. Brecher G, Wilbur KM, Cronkite EP: Transfusion of separated leukocytes into irradiated dogs with aplastic marrows. *Proc Soc Exp Biol Med* 84:54, 1953.
3. Applebaum FR, Bolwes CA, Makuch RW, Deisseroth AB: Granulocyte transfusion therapy of experimental *Pseudomonas* septicemia: study of cell dose and collection technique. *Blood* 52:323, 1978.
4. Debelak KM, Epstein RB, Andersen RB: Granulocyte transfusion in leukopenic dogs: in vivo and in vitro function of granulocytes obtained by continuous-flow filtration leukopheresis. *Blood* 43:757, 1974.
5. Epstein RB, Waxman FJ, Bennett BT, Andersen BR: *Pseudomonas* septicemia in neutropenic dogs. I. Treatment with granulocyte transfusions. *Transfusion* 14:51, 1974.
6. Epstein RB, Clift RA, Thomas ED: The effect of leukocyte transfusions on experimental bacteremia in the dog. *Blood* 34:782, 1969.
7. Westrick MAMA, Debelak-Fehir KM, Epstein RB: The effect of prior whole blood transfusion on subsequent granulocyte support in leukopenic dogs. *Transfusion* 17:611, 1977.
8. Dale DC, Reynolds HY, Pennington JE, et al: Granulocyte transfusion therapy of experimental *Pseudomonas* pneumonia. *J Clin Invest* 54:664, 1974.
9. Dale DC, Reynolds HY, Pennington JE, et al: Experimental *Pseudomonas* pneumonia in leukopenic dogs: comparison of therapy with antibiotics and granulocyte transfusions. *Blood* 47:869, 1976.
10. Chow HS, Sarpel SC, Epstein RB: Pathophysiology of *Candida albicans* meningitis in normal, neutropenic, and granulocyte transfused dogs. *Blood* 55:546, 1980.
11. Chow HS, Sarpel SC, Epstein RB: Experimental candidiasis in neutropenic dogs: Tissue burden of infection and granulocyte transfusion effects. *Blood* 59:328, 1982.
12. Epstein RB, Chow HS: An analysis of quantitative relationships of granulocyte transfusion therapy in canines. *Transfusion* 21:360, 1981.
13. Buckner D, Graw RG, Eisel RJ, et al: Leukapheresis by continuous flow centrifugation (CFC) in patients with chronic myelocytic leukemia (CML). *Blood* 33:353, 1969.
14. Freireich EJ, Levin RH, Whang J, et al: The functions and fate of transfused leukocytes from donors with chronic myelocytic leukemia in leukopenic recipients. *Ann N Y Acad Sci* 113:1081, 1964.
15. Eyre HJ, Goldstein IM, Perry S, et al: Leukocyte transfusions: Function of transfused granulocytes from donors with chronic myelocytic leukemia. *Blood* 36:432, 1970.
16. Schiffer CA, Aisner J, Dutcher JP, et al: Sustained posttransfusion granulocyte count increments following transfusion of leukocytes obtained from donors with chronic myelogenous leukemia. *Am J Hematol* 15:65, 1983.
17. McCredie KB, Freireich EJ, Hester JP, et al: Increased granulocyte collection with the blood cell separator and the addition of etiocholanolone and hydroxyethyl starch. *Transfusion* 14:357, 1974.
18. Schiffer CA, Aisner J, Dutcher JP, Wiernik PH: Sustained post-transfusion granulocyte count increments following transfusion of leukocytes obtained from donors with chronic myelogenous leukemia. *Am J Hematol* 15:65, 1983.
19. Mishler JM, Hadlock DE, Fortuny IE, et al: Increased efficiency of leukocyte separation by the addition of hydroxyethyl starch to the continuous flow centrifuge. *Blood* 44:571, 1974.
20. Mishler JM, Higby DJ, Rhomberg W: Hydroxyethyl starch and dexamethasone as an adjunct to leukocyte separation with the IBM blood cell separator. *Transfusion* 14:352, 1974.
21. Mishler JM: Hydroxyethyl starch as an experimental adjunct to leukocyte separation by centrifugal means: Review of safety and efficacy. *Transfusion* 15:449, 1975.
22. Graw RG, Herzig G, Perry S, et al: Normal granulocyte transfusion therapy: Treatment of septicemia due to gram-negative bacteria. *N Engl J Med* 287:367, 1972.
23. Higby FJ, Yates JW, Henderson ES, et al: Filtration leukapheresis for granulocytic transfusion therapy. *N Engl J Med* 292:761, 1975.
24. Fortuny IE, Bloomfield CD, Hadlock DC, et al: Granulocyte transfusion. A controlled study in patients with acute non-lymphocytic leukemia. *Transfusion* 15:548, 1975.
25. Vogler WR, Wintron EF: A controlled study of the efficacy of granulocyte transfusions in patients with neutropenia. *Am J Med* 63:548, 1997.
26. Herzig RH, Herzig GP, Graw RG, et al: Successful granulocyte transfusion therapy for gram-negative septicemia: A prospectively randomized controlled study. *N Engl J Med* 296:701, 1977.
27. Alavi JB, Root RK, Djerassi I, et al: A randomized clinical trial of granulocyte transfusions for infection in acute leukemia. *N Engl J Med* 296:706, 1977.
28. Winston DJ, Ho WG, Gale RP: Therapeutic granulocyte transfusions for documented infections: A controlled trial in ninety-five infectious granulocytopenic patients with gram-negative bacteremia. *Am J Med* 68:643, 1980.
29. Vamvakas EC, Pineda A: Meta-analysis of clinical studies of the efficacy of granulocyte transfusions in the treatment of bacterial sepsis. *J Clin Apheresis* 11:1, 1996.
30. Laurenti F, Ferro R, Isacchi G, et al: Polymorphonuclear leukocyte transfusion for the treatment of sepsis in the newborn infant. *J Pediatr* 98:118, 1981.
31. Christensen RD, Rothstein G, Anstall HB, Bybee B. Granulocyte transfusions in neonates with bacterial infection, neutropenia, and depletion of mature marrow neutrophils. *Pediatrics* 70:1 1982.
32. Cairo MS, Worcester C, Rucker R, et al: Role of circulating complement and polymorphonuclear leukocyte transfusion in treatment and outcome in critically ill neonates with sepsis. *J Pediatr* 110:935, 1989.
33. Wheeler JG, Chauvenet AR, Johnson CA, Block SM, Dillard R, Abramson JS: Buffy coat transfusions in neonates with sepsis and neutrophil storage pool depletion. *Pediatrics* 79:422, 1987.
34. Baley JE, Stork EK, Warkentin PI, et al: Buffy coat transfusions in neutropenic neonates with presumed sepsis: A prospective, randomized trial. *Pediatrics* 80:712, 1987.
35. Donahue DM, Grabrio BW, Finch CA: Quantitative measurements of hematopoietic cells of the marrow. *J Clin Invest* 37:1564, 1958.
36. Donahue DM, Reiff RH, Henson ML, et al: Quantitative measurements of the erythrocytic and granulocytic cells of the marrow and blood. *J Clin Invest* 37:1571, 1958.
37. Athens JW, Haab OP, Mauer AM, et al: Leukokinetic studies. IV. The total blood circulating and marginal granulocyte pools and the granulocyte turnover rate in normal subjects. *J Clin Invest* 40:989, 1961.
38. Cartwright GE, Athens JW, Wintrobe MM: The kinetics of granulopoiesis in normal men. *Blood* 24:780, 1969.
39. MacPherson JL, Nusbacher J, Bennett JM: The acquisition of granulocytes by leukapheresis: A comparison of continuous flow centrifugation and filtration leukapheresis in normal and corticosteroid-stimulated donors. *Transfusion* 16:221, 1976.
40. Nusbacher J, McCullough J, Huestis DW: Granulocyte collection and processing, in The Granulocyte: Function and Clinical Utilization, edited by TJ Greenwalt, GA Jamieson, p 175. Liss, New York, 1977.
41. Kalmin ND, Grindon AJ: Pheresis with the IBM 2997. *Transfusion* 21:325, 1981.
42. Djerassi I, Kim JS, Suvansri U, et al: Continuous-flow filtration leukapheresis. *Transfusion* 12:75, 1972.
43. Herzig GP, Root RK, Graw RG: Granulocyte collection by continuous-flow filtration leukapheresis. *Blood* 39:554, 1972.

44. Higby DJ, Henderson ES, Burnett D, et al: Filtration leukapheresis: Effects of donor stimulation with dexamethasone. *Blood* 50:953, 1977.

45. Rubins JM, MacPherson JL, Nusbacher J, et al: Granulocyte kinetics in donors undergoing filtration leukapheresis. *Transfusion* 16:56, 1976.

46. Debalak KM, Epstein RB, Anderson BR: Granulocyte transfusions in leukopenic dogs: In vivo and in vitro function of granulocytes obtained by continuous-flow filtration leukapheresis. *Blood* 43:757, 1974.

47. Harris M, Djerassi I, Schwartz E: Polymorphonuclear leukocytes prepared by continuous flow filtration leukapheresis: Viability and function. *Blood* 44:707, 1974.

48. Higby DH, Burnette D: Granulocyte transfusions: Current status. *Blood* 55:2, 1980.

49. Epstein RB, Waxman FJ, Bennet BT, et al: *Pseudomonas* septicemia in neutropenic dogs. I. Treatment with granulocyte transfusions. *Transfusion* 14:51, 1974.

50. Higby DJ, Yates J, Henderson ES, et al: Filtration leukapheresis for granulocyte transfusion therapy. *N Engl J Med* 292:761, 1975.

51. Schiffer CA, Buchholz DH, Aisner J, et al: Clinical experience with transfusion of granulocytes obtained by continuous flow filtration leukapheresis. *Am J Med* 58:373, 1975.

52. Wiltbank TB, Nusbacher J, Higby DJ, et al: Abdominal pain in donors during filtration leukapheresis. *Transfusion* 17:159, 1977.

53. Dahlke MB, Shah SL, Sherwood WC, et al: Priapism during filtration leukapheresis. *Transfusion* 19:482, 1979.

54. Schiffer CA, Aisner AJ, Wiernik PH: Transient neutropenia induced by transfusion of blood exposed to nylon fiber filters. *Blood* 45:141, 1975.

55. Hammerschmidt DE, Craddock PR, McCullough J, et al: Complement activation and pulmonary leukostasis during nylon fiber filtration leukapheresis. *Blood* 51:721, 1978.

56. Nusbacher J, Rosenfeld SI, MacPherson JL, et al: Nylon fiber leukapheresis: Associated complement changes and granulocytopenia. *Blood* 51:359, 1978.

57. Craddock PR, Hammerschmidt DE, White JG, et al: Complement (C5a)-induced granulocyte aggregation in vitro: A possible mechanism of complement-mediated leukostasis and leukopenia. *J Clin Invest* 60:261, 1977.

58. Nusbacher J, Rosenfeld SI, Leddy JP, et al: The leukokinetic changes and complement activation associated with filtration leukapheresis. *Exp Hematol* 7(suppl 4):24, 1979.

59. French JE, Solomon JM, Fratantoni JC: Survey on the current use of leukapheresis and the collection of granulocyte concentrates. *Transfusion* 22:220, 1982.

60. McCullough J, Weiblin BJ, Deinard AR, et al: In vitro function and post-transfusion survival of granulocytes collected by continuous-flow centrifugation and by filtration leukapheresis. *Blood* 48:315, 1976.

61. Wright DG, Kauffman JC, Chusid MJ, et al: Functional abnormalities of human neutrophils collected by continuous flow filtration leukapheresis. *Blood* 46:901, 1975.

62. Applebaum FR, Norton L, Graw RG: Migration of transfused granulocytes in leukopenic dogs. *Blood* 49:483, 1977.

63. Price TH, Dale DC: Neutrophil transfusion: Effect of storage and of collection method on neutrophil blood kinetics. *Blood* 51:789, 1978.

64. Higby DJ: Granulocyte transfusions: Where now? *N Engl J Med* 305:636, 1981.

65. Strauss RG, Hester JP, Vogler WR, et al: A multicenter trial to document the efficacy and safety of a rapidly excreted analog of hydroxyethyl starch for leukapheresis with a note on steroid stimulation of granulocyte donors. *Transfusion* 26:258, 1986.

66. Lee JH, Leitman SF, Klein HG: A controlled study of the efficacy of hetastarch and pentastarch in granulocyte collections by centrifugal leukapheresis. *Blood* 86:4662, 1995.

67. Athens JW, Heab OP, Raab SO, et al: The mechanism of steroid granulocytosis. *J Clin Invest* 41:1342, 1962.

68. Mischler JM: The effects of corticosteroids on mobilization and function of neutrophils. *Exp Hematol* 5(suppl):15, 1977.

69. Higby DJ, Mishler JM, Rhomberg W, et al: The effect of a single or double dose of dexamethasone on granulocyte collection with a continuous flow centrifuge. *Vox Sang* 28:243, 1975.

70. Winton EF, Vogler WR: Development of a practical oral dexamethasone premedication schedule leading to improved granulocyte yields with the continuous-flow centrifugal blood cell separator. *Blood* 52:249, 1978.

71. Glasser L, Huestis DW, Jones JF: Functional capabilities of steroid-recruited neutrophils harvested for clinical transfusion. *N Engl J Med* 297:1037, 1977.

72. Steigbigel RT, Baum J, MacPherson JL, et al: Granulocyte bactericidal capacity and chemotaxis as affected by continuous-flow centrifugation and filtration leukapheresis, steroid administration, and storage. *Blood* 52:197, 1978.

73. Caspar CB, Segar RA, Burger J, Gmur J: Effective stimulation of donors for granulocyte transfusions with recombinant methionyl granulocyte colony-stimulating factor. *Blood* 81:2866, 1993.

74. Bensinger WI, Price TH, Dale DC: The effects of daily recombinant human granulocyte colony-stimulating factor administration on normal granulocyte donors undergoing leukapheresis. *Blood* 81:1883, 1993.

75. Adkins D, Spitzer G, Johnston M, et al: Transfusions of granulocyte-colony-stimulating factor-mobilized granulocyte components to allogeneic transplant recipients: analysis of kinetics and factors determining posttransfusion neutrophil and platelet counts. *Transfusion* 37:737, 1997

76. Jendiroba DB, Lichtiger B, Anaissie E, et al: Evaluation and comparison of three mobilization methods for the collection of granulocytes. *Transfusion* 38:722, 1998.

77. Leitman SF, Oblitas JM: Optimization of granulocytapheresis mobilization regimens using granulocyte colony stimulating factor (G-CSF) and dexamethasone (DEXA). *Transfusion* 37(suppl):67S, 1997.

78. Dale DC, Liles WC, Llewellyn C, Rodger E, Price TH: Neutrophil transfusions: kinetics and functions of neutrophils mobilized with granulocyte-colony-stimulating factor and dexamethasone. *Transfusion* 38:713, 1998.

79. Demitri GD, Griffin JD: Granulocyte colony stimulating factor and its receptor. *Blood* 78:2791, 1991.

80. Dancey JT, Deukelbeiss KA, Harker LA, Finch CA: Neutrophil kinetics in man. *J Clin Invest* 58:705, 1976.

81. Brach MA, DeVos S, Gruss HJ, Herrmann F: Prolongation of survival of human polymorphonuclear neutrophils by granulocyte-macrophage colony-stimulating factor is caused by inhibition of programmed cell death. *Blood* 80:1920 1992.

82. Bodey GP, Buckley M, Sathe YS, et al: Quantitative relationships between circulating leukocytes and infection in patients with acute leukemia. *Ann Intern Med* 64:328, 1966.

83. Raubitschek AA, Levin AS, Stites DP, et al: Normal granulocyte infusion therapy for aspergillosis in chronic granulomatous disease. *Pediatrics* 51:230, 1973.

84. Yomtovian R, Abramson J, Quie PG, McCullough J: Granulocyte transfusion therapy in chronic granulomatous disease: Report of a patient and review of the literature. *Transfusion* 21:739, 1981.

85. Elliot GR, Clay ME, Mills EL, et al: Granulocyte transfusion kinetics measured by chemiluminescence, nitroblue tetrazolium reduction, and recovery of indium-111-labeled granulocytes. *Transfusion* 26:23, 1986.

86. Ford JM, Cullen MH: Prophylactic granulocyte transfusions. *Exp Hematol* 5(suppl 1):65, 1977.

87. Schiffer CA, Aisner J, Daily PA, et al: Alloimmunization following prophylactic granulocyte transfusion. *Blood* 54:766, 1979.

88. Clift RA, Sanders JE, Thomas ED, et al: Granulocyte transfusions for the prevention of infection in patients receiving bone-marrow transplants. *N Engl J Med* 298:1052, 1978.

89. Winston DJ, Ho WG, Young LS, et al: Prophylactic granulocyte transfusions during human bone marrow transplantation. *Am J Med* 68:893, 1980.

90. Strauss RG, Connett JE, Gale RP, et al: A controlled trial of prophylactic granulocyte transfusions during initial induction chemotherapy for acute myelogenous leukemia. *N Engl J Med* 305:597, 1981.

91. Ford JM, Cullen MH, Roberts MM, et al: Prophylactic granulocyte transfusions: Results of a randomized controlled trial in patients with acute myelogenous leukemia. *Transfusion* 22:311, 1982.

92. Sutton DMC, Shumak KH, Baker MA: Prophylactic granulocyte transfusions in acute leukemia. *Plasma Ther* 3:45, 1983.

93. Higby DJ, Freeman AI, Henderson ES, et al: Granulocyte transfusions in children using filter-collected cells. *Cancer* 38:1407, 1976.

94. Ward HN: Pulmonary infiltrates associated with leukoagglutinin transfusion reaction. *Ann Intern Med* 73:689, 1970.

95. Jacob HS: Granulocyte-complement interaction. *Arch Intern Med* 138:461, 1978.

96. Wright DG, Robichaud KJ, Pizzo PA, et al: Lethal pulmonary reactions

associated with the combined use of amphotericin B and leukocyte transfusions. *N Engl J Med* 304:1185, 1981.

97. Forman SJ, Robinson GV, Wolfe JL, et al: Pulmonary reactions associated with amphotericin B and leukocyte transfusions. *N Engl J Med* 305:584, 1981.

98. DeGregorio MW, Lee WMF, Ries CA: Pulmonary reactions associated with amphotericin B and leukocyte transfusions. *N Engl J Med* 305:584, 1981.

99. Ford JM, Lucey JJ, Cullen MH, et al: Fatal graft-versus-host disease following transfusion of granulocytes from normal donors. *Lancet* 2:1167, 1976.

100. Rosen RS, Huestis DW, Corrigan JJ: Acute leukemia and granulocyte transfusion: Fatal graft-versus-host reaction following transfusion of cells obtained from normal donors. *J Pediatr* 93:268, 1978.

101. Cohen D, Weinstein H, Mihm M, et al: Nonfatal graft-versus-host disease occurring after transfusion with leukocytes and platelets obtained from normal donors. *Blood* 53:1053, 1979.

102. Graw RG, Buchner CD, Whang-Peng J, et al: Complication of bone-marrow transplantation: Graft-versus-host disease resulting from chronic-myelogenous-leukaemia leucocyte transfusions. *Lancet* 2:338, 1970.

103. Weiden PL, Zuckerman N, Hansen JA, et al: Fatal graft-versus-host disease in a patient with lymphoblastic leukemia following normal granulocytic transfusions. *Blood* 57:328, 1981.

104. Cairo MS: Granulocyte transfusions in neonates with presumed sepsis. Pediatrics 80:738, 1987.

105. McCullough J: Liquid preservation of granulocytes. *Transfusion* 20:129, 1980.

106. Lane TA: Storage of granulocyte concentrates (GC): Bacterial killing and chemotaxis. *Transfusion* 18:650, 1978.

107. McCullough J, Weiblin BJ, Quie PG: Chemotactic activity of human granulocytes preserved in various anticoagulants. *J Lab Clin Med* 84:902, 1974.

108. McCullough J, Weiblin BJ: Relationship of granulocyte ATP to chemotactic response during storage. *Transfusion* 19:764, 1979.

109. Lane TA: Granulocyte concentrate preservation: 6°C versus room temperature. *Transfusion* 18:394, 1978.

110. Lane TA: Storage of granulocyte concentrates (GC): Bacterial killing and chemotaxis. *Transfusion* 18:650, 1978.

111. McCullough J, Weiblin BJ, Peterson PK, et al: Effects of temperature on granulocyte preservation. *Blood* 52:301, 1978.

112. McCullough J: Liquid preservation of granulocytes for transfusion. *Prog Clin Biol Res* 13:185, 1977.

113. Lane TA, Lamkin GE: Hydrogen ion maintenance improves the chemotaxis of stored granulocytes. *Transfusion* 24:231, 1984.

114. Glasser L, Lane TA, McCullough J, Price TH: Neutrophil concentrates: Functional considerations, storage and quality control. *J Clin Apheresis* 1:179, 1983.

115. Lane TA, Windle BE: Granulocyte concentrate function during preservation: Effect of temperature. *Blood* 54:216, 1979.

116. Lane TA, Lamkin GE: Adherence of fresh and stored granulocytes to endothelial cells. Effect of storage temperature. *Transfusion* 28:237, 1988.

117. Lane TA, Lamkin GE: Stimulus-response coupling in fresh and stored granulocytes. *Transfusion* 28:243, 1988.

118. Babior BM, Berkman E: Granulocyte storage. *Lancet* 1:50, 1990.

119. Glasser L, Fiederlein RL, Huestis DW: Granulocyte concentrates: Glucose concentrations and glucose utilization during storage at 22°C. *Transfusion* 25:68, 1985.

120. Glasser L, Fiederlein RL: The effect of platelets and red cells on granulocytes stored at 22°C. *Transfusion* 24:310, 1984.

121. Contreras TJ, Jemionek JF, French JE, et al: Effects of plastic polymer surfaces on the liquid preservation of human granulocytes. *Transfusion* 18:650, 1978.

122. Miyamoto M, Sasakawa S: Studies on granulocyte preservation. III. Effect of agitation on granulocyte concentrates. *Transfusion* 27:165, 1987.

123. Wolber RA, Duque RE, Robinson JP, Oberman HA: Oxidative product formation in irradiated neutrophils: A cytometric analysis. *Transfusion* 27:167, 1987.

124. Buescher ES, Gallin JI: Effects of storage and radiation on human neutrophil function in vitro. *Inflammation* 11:401, 1987.

125. Lane TA: Granulocyte storage. *Transfus Med Rev* 4:23, 1990.

126. Meryman HT, Howard J: Cryopreservation of granulocytes, in The Granulocyte: Function and Clinical Utilization, edited by TJ Greenwalt, GA Jamieson, p 193, Liss, New York, 1977.

127. Hill RS, MacKinder CA: Freeze preservation of human granulocytes. *Lancet* 1:878, 1980.

128. Lionetti FJ, Hunte SM, Gore JM, et al: Cryopreservation of human granulocytes. *Cryobiology* 12:181, 1975.

129. Strauss RG: Neutrophil (granulocyte) transfusions in the new millennium. *Transfusion* 38:710, 1998.

130. Maximow A: Der Lymphozyt als gemeinsame Stammzelle der verschiedenen Blutelemente in der embryonalen Entwicklung und im postfetalen Leben der Säugetiere. *Folia Haematol* 8, 125, 1909.

131. Brecher G, Cronkite EP: Post-irradiation parabiosis and survival in rats. *Proc Soc Exp Biol Med* 77:292, 1951.

132. Levin RH, Whang J, Tjio JH, et al: Persistent mitosis of transfused homologous leukocytes in children receiving antileukemic therapy. *Science* 142:1305, 1963.

133. Goldman JM, Catovsky D, Hows J, et al: Cryopreserved peripheral blood cells functioning as autografts in patients with chronic granulocyte leukemia in transformation. *Br J Med* 13:148, 1979.

134. Korbling M, Durkin B, Ho AD, et al: Autologous transplantation of blood derived hematopoietic stem cells after myeloablative therapy in a patient with Burkitti lymphoma. *Blood* 67:529, 1986.

135. Chao NJ, Schriber JR, Grimes K, et al. Granulocyte colony stimulating factor "mobilized" peripheral blood progenitor cells accelerate granulocyte and platelet recovery after high dose chemotherapy. *Blood* 81:2031, 1993.

136. Sheridan WP, Begley CG, Juttner CA, et al: Effect of peripheral-blood progenitor cells mobilized by filgrastim (G-CSF) on platelet recovery after high-dose chemotherapy. *Lancet* 339:640, 1992.

137. Kessinger A, Armitage JO, Landmark JD, et al: Autologous peripheral hematopoietic stem cell transplantation restores hematopoietic function following marrow ablative therapy. *Blood* 71:723, 1988.

138. Reiffers J, Bernard P, David B, et al: Successful autologous transplantation with peripheral blood hematopoietic cells in a patient with acute leukemia. *Exp Hematol* 14:312, 1986.

139. Leitman SF, Read SJ. Hematopoietic progenitor cells. *Semin Hematol* 33:341, 1996.

140. Bandarenko N, Owen HG, Mair DC, et al: Apheresis: new opportunities, in Clinics in Laboratory Medicine, edited by HF Polesky, EH Perry, SJ Ilstrup, pp 907–914. Philadelphia, WB Saunders, 1996.

141. McCullough J: Quality assurance and good manufacturing practices for processing hematopoietic progenitor cells. *J Hematother* 4:493, 1995.

142. Korbling M, Przepiorka D, Huh YO, et al: Allogeneic blood stem cell transplantation for refractory leukemia and lymphoma: potential advantage of blood over marrow allografts. *Blood* 85(6):1659, 1995.

143. Bensinger W, Singer J, Appelbaum F, et al: Autologous transplantation with peripheral blood mononuclear cells collected after administration of recombinant granulocyte stimulating factor. *Blood* 81:3158, 1993.

144. To LB, Roberts MM, Haylock DN, et al: Comparison of haematologic recovery times and supportive care requirements of autologous recovery phase peripheral blood stem cell transplants, autologous bone marrow transplants, and allogeneic bone marrow transplants. *Bone Marrow Transplant* 9:277, 1992.

145. Goldberg SL, Mangan KF, Klumpp TR, et al: Complications of peripheral blood stem cell harvesting: review of 554 PBSC leukaphereses. *J Hematother* 4:85, 1995.

146. Stephens LC, Haire WD, Schmit-Pokorny K, et al: Granulocyte macrophage colony stimulating factor: high incidence of apheresis catheter thrombosis during peripheral stem cell collection. *Bone Marrow Transplant* 11:51, 1993.

147. Brecher ME, Lasky LC, Sacher RA, Issit LA (eds): Hematopoietic Progenitor Cells: Processing, Standards and Practice. American Association of Blood Banks, Bethesda, MD, 1995.

148. Bender JG, Unverzagt KL, Walker DE, et al: Identification and comparison of CD34 positive cells and their subpopulations from normal peripheral blood and bone marrow using multicolor flow cytometry. *Blood* 77:2591, 1991.

149. Lasky LC: Peripheral blood stem cell collection and use, in Cellular and Humoral Immunotherapy and Apheresis, edited by RA Sacher, DB

Brubaker, DO Kasprisin, LJ McCarthy, pp 73–85. American Association of Blood Banks, Arlington, VA 1991.

150. Richman CM, Weiner RS, Yankee RA: Increasing circulating stem cells following chemotherapy in man. *Blood* 47(6):1031, 1976.

151. To LB, Haylock DN, Kimber RJ, Juttner CA: High levels of circulating haematopoietic stem cells in the very early remission of acute non-lymphoblastic leukaemia and their collection and cryopreservation. *Br J Haematol* 58:399, 1984.

152. To LB, Roberts MM, Haylock DN, et al: The optimization of collection of peripheral blood stem cells for autotransplantation in acute myeloid leukemia. *Bone Marrow Transplant* 4:41, 1989.

153. Kosatec D, Shepherd KM, Sage RE, et al: Factors affecting blood stem cell collections following high-dose cyclophosphamide mobilization in lymphoma, myeloma, and solid tumors. *Int J Cell Cloning* (suppl 1):35, 1992.

154. To LB, Shepherd KM, Haylock DN, et al: Single high doses of cyclo-phosphamide enable the collection of high numbers of haemopoietic stem cells from the peripheral blood. *Exp Hematol* 18:442, 1990.

155. Gianni AM, Siena S, Bregni M, et al: Very rapid and complete hemato-poietic reconstitution following myeloablative treatments: the role of circulating stem cells harvested after high-dose cyclophosphamide and GM-CSF, in Bone Marrow Transplantation, 4th ed, edited by KA Kicke, G Spitzer, S Jagannath, MJ Evinger-Hodges, pp 723–731. University of Texas Press, Austin, 1989.

156. Socinski MA, Elias A, Schnipper L, et al: Granulocyte-macrophage colony stimulating factor expands the circulating haematopoietic progen-itor cell compartment in man. *Lancet* 1:1194, 1988.

157. Pettengell R, Testa NG, Swindell R, et al: Transplantation potential of hematopoietic cells released into the circulation during routine chemo-therapy for non-Hodgkins lymphoma. *Blood* 82:2239, 1993.

158. Elias AD, Ayash L, Anderson KC, et al: Mobilization of peripheral blood progenitor cells by chemotherapy and granulocyte-macrophage colony stimulating factor for hematologic support after high-dose intensi-fication for breast cancer. *Blood* 79:3036, 1992.

159. Gillespie TW, Hillyer CD: Peripheral blood progenitor cells for marrow reconstitution: mobilization and collection strategies. *Transfusion* 36:611, 1996.

160. Haas R, Hohaus S, Egerer G, et al: Recombinant human granulocyte-macrophage colony stimulating factor (rhGM-CSF) subsequent to che-motherapy improves collection of blood stem cells for autografting in patients not eligible for bone marrow harvest. *Bone Marrow Transplant* 9(6):459, 1992.

161. Lane TA: Mobilization of hematopoietic progenitor cells, in Hematopoi-etic Progenitor Cells: Processing, Standards and Practice, edited by ME Brecher, LC Lasky, RA Sacher, LA Issit, pp 59–108. American Association of Blood Banks, Bethesda, MD, 1995.

162. Lee JH, Klein HG: Collection and use of circulating hematopoietic progenitor cells in Hematology/Oncology Clinics of North America: Transfusion Medicine II, edited by PD Mintz, pp 1–22. WB Saunders, Philadelphia, 1995.

163. Siena S, Bregni M, Brando B, et al: Circulation of CD34+ hematopoietic stem cells in the peripheral blood of high-dose cyclophosphamide-treated patients: enhancement by intravenous recombinant human granulocyte-macrophage stimulating factor. *Blood* 74:1905, 1989.

164. Sutherland HJ, Eaves CJ, Lansdorp PM, et al: Kinetics of committed and primitive blood progenitor mobilization after chemotherapy and growth factor treatment and their use in autotransplants. *Blood* 83:3808, 1994.

165. Beyer J, Schwella N, Zingsem J, et al: Hematopoietic rescue after high-dose chemotherapy using autologous peripheral-blood progenitor cells or bone marrow: A randomized comparison. *J Clin Oncol* 13:1328, 1995.

166. Deeg HJ: Bone marrow and hematopoietic stem cell transplantation: Sorting the chaff from the grain, in Bone Marrow and Stem Cell Pro-cessing: A Manual of Current Techniques, edited by EM Areman, HJ Deeg, RA Sacher, pp 17–29. FA Davis, Philadelphia, 1992.

167. Dreger P, Suttorp M, Haferlach T, et al: Allogeneic granulocyte colony stimulating factor mobilized peripheral blood progenitor cells for treat-ment of engraftment failure after bone marrow transplantation. *Blood* 81:1404, 1993.

168. Russell NH, Hunter A, Rogers S, et al: Peripheral blood stem cells as an alternative of marrow for allogeneic transplantation [Letter]. *Lancet* 341:1482, 1993.

169. Weaver CH, Buckner CD, Longin K, et al: Syngeneic transplantation with peripheral blood mononuclear cells collected after the administra-tion of recombinant human granulocyte colony-stimulating factor. *Blood* 82:1981, 1993.

170. Glaspy JA, Shpall EJ, LeMaistre CF, et al: Peripheral blood progenitor cell mobilization using stem cell factor in combination with Filgrastim in breast cancer patients. *Blood* 90:2939, 1997.

171. Link H, Arseniev L, Bahre O, et al: Transplantation of allogeneic CD34+ blood cells. *Blood* 87:4903, 1996.

172. Majolino I, Corradini P, Scime R, et al: Allogeneic transplantation of unmanipulated peripheral blood stem cells in patients with multiple myeloma. *Bone Marrow Transplant* 22(5):449, 1998.

173. MacKinnon S, Papadapoulos EB, Carabasi MH, et al: Adoptive immuno-therapy evaluating doses of donor leukocytes for relapse of chronic myeloid leukemia after bone marrow transplantation: separation of graft-versus-leukemia responses from graft-versus-host disease. *Blood* 86(4):1261, 1995.

174. Majolino I, Buscemi F, Scime R, et al: Treatment of normal donors with rhG-CSF 16 micrograms/kg for mobilization of peripheral blood stem cells and their apheretic collections for allogeneic transplantation. *Haematologica* 80:219, 1995.

175. Bishop MR, Tarantolo SR, Jackson JD, et al: Allogeneic-blood stem-cell collection following mobilization with low-dose granulocyte colony-stimulating factor. *J Clin Oncol* 15:1601, 1997.

176. Schmitz N, Dreger P, Suttorp M, et al: Primary transplantation of alloge-neic peripheral blood progenitor cells mobilized by filgrastim (granulo-cyte colony-stimulating factor). *Blood* 85(6):1666, 1995.

177. Stroncek D, Clay M, Petzoldt ML, et al: Treatment of normal individuals with granulocyte-colony-stimulating factor: donor experiences and the effects on peripheral blood CD34+ cell counts and on the collection of peripheral blood stem cells. *Transfusion* 36:601, 1996.

178. Anderlini P, Pzrepiorka D, Seong D, et al: Clinical toxicity and laboratory effects of mobilization and blood stem cell apheresis from normal donors, and analysis of charges for the procedure. *Transfusion* 36:590, 1996.

179. Stroncek D, McCullough J: Policies and procedures for the establishment of an allogeneic blood stem cell programme. *Transfus Med* 7:77, 1997.

180. Bandarenko N, Brecher M, Owen H, et al: Thrombocytopenia in alloge-neic peripheral blood stem cell collections [Letter]. *Transfusion* 36:668, 1996.

181. Anderlini P, Korbling M, Dale D, et al: Allogeneic blood cell transplanta-tion: Considerations for donors [Editorial]. *Blood* 90:903, 1997.

182. Stroncek D, Clay M, Herr G, et al: Blood counts in healthy donors 1 year after the collection of granulocyte-colony-stimulating factor-mobilized progenitor cells and the results of a second mobilization and collection. *Transfusion* 37:304, 1997.

183. Reiffers J, Bernard P, Marit G, et al: Collection of blood-derived hemato-poietic stem cells and applications for autologous transplantation. *Bone Marrow Transplant* 1(suppl 1):371, 1986.

184. Gorin NC, Lopez M, Laporte JP, et al: Preparation and successful engraftment of purified CD34+ bone marrow progenitor cells in patients with non-Hodgkin's lymphoma. *Blood* 85(6):1647, 1995.

185. Hohaus S, Goldschmidt H, Ehrhardt R, Haas R: Successful autografting following myeloablative conditioning therapy with blood stem cells mobilized by chemotherapy plas rhG-CSF. *Exp Hematol* 21(4):508, 1993.

186. Jones HM, Jones SA, Watts MJ, et al: Development of a simplified single-apheresis approach for peripheral-blood progenitor cell trans-plantation in previously treated patients with lymphoma. *J Clin Oncol* 12(8):1693, 1994.

187. Urashima M, Uchiyama H, Hoshi Y, et al: Prediction of engraftment after peripheral blood stem cell transplantation by CD34+ cells in grafts. *Acta Paediatr Jpn* 35(4):325, 1993.

188. Carow CE, Hangoc G, Broxmeyer HE: Human multipotential progenitor cells (CFU-GEMM) have extensive replating capacity for secondary (CFU-GEMM): an effect enhanced by cord blood plasma. *Blood* 81:942, 1993.

189. Korbling M, Huh YO, Durett A, et al: Peripheralization and yield of donor derived primitive hematopoietic progenitor cells (CD34+ Thy-1dim) and lymphoid subsets, and possible predictors of engraftment and graft-versus-host disease. *Blood* 86:2842, 1995.

190. Bender JG, To LB, Williams S, Schwartzberg LS: Defining a therapeutic dose of peripheral blood stem cells. *J Hematother* 1:329, 1992.

191. Bensinger WI, Longin K, Appelbaum F, et al: Peripheral blood stem cells (PBSCs) collected after recombinant granulocyte colony stimulating factor (rhG-CSF): an analysis of factors correlating with the tempo to engraftment after transplantation. *Br J Haematol* 87(4):825, 1994.

192. Van der Wall E, Richel DJ, Holtkamp MJ, et al: Bone marrow reconstitution after high-dose chemotherapy and autologous peripheral progenitor cell transplantation: effect on graft size. *Ann Oncol* 5:795, 1994.

193. Kahn DG, Prilutskaya M, Cooper B, et al: The relationship between the incidence of tumor contamination and number of pheresis for stage IV breast cancer (abstr 2514). *Blood* 90(suppl 10):565a, 1997.

194. Moreb J, Cooper B, Holland K, et al: The prognostic value of immunocytochemical (ICC) analysis on bone marrow (BM) taken from patients with stage II/III breast cancer undergoing autologous transplant therapy (abstr 1703). *Blood* 90(suppl 10):383a, 1997.

195. Chen CH, Lin W, Shye S, et al: Automated enumeration of CD34+ cells in peripheral blood and bone marrow. *J Hematother* 3:3, 1994.

196. Johnsen HE: Report from a Nordic workshop on CD34+ cell analysis: technical recommendations for progenitor cell enumeration in leukapheresis from multiple myeloma patients. *J Hematother* 4:21, 1995.

197. Owens MA, Loken MR: Flow Cytometry Principles for Clinical Laboratory Practice: Quality Assurance for Quantitative Immunotyping, pp 111–127. Wiley-Liss, New York, 1995.

198. Sovalat H, Wunder E, Zimmerman R, Serke S: Multicentric determination of CD34+ cells, in Hematopoietic Stem Cells: The Mulhouse Manual, edited by E Wunder, H Sovalat, PR Henon, S Serke, p 61. AlphaMed Press, Dayton, OH, 1994.

199. Sutherland RE, Keating A, Nayar R, et al: Sensitive detection and enumeration of CD34+ cells in peripheral and cord blood by flow cytometry. *Exp Hematol* 22:1003, 1994.

200. Trischmann TM, Schepers KG, Civin CJ: Measurement of CD34+ cells in bone marrow by flow cytometry. *J Hematother* 2:305, 1993.

201. Wunder E, Sovolat H, Fritsch G, et al: Report on the European Workshop on Peripheral Blood Stem Cell Determination and Standardization—Mulhouse, France. *J Hematother* 1:131, 1992.

202. Siena S, Bregni M, Brando B, et al: Flow cytometry for clinical estimation of circulating hematopoietic progenitors for autologous transplantation in cancer patients. *Blood* 77:400, 1991.

203. Brecher ME, Sims L, Schmitz J, Shea T, Bentley SA: North American multicenter study on flow cytometric enumeration of CD34+ hematopoietic stem cells. *J Hematother* 5:227, 1996.

204. Chang A, McLachlan J, Ma DDF: Towards standardization of CD34+ cell determination: Australian Perspective (part I) [Abstract]. *J Hematother* 4:240, 1995.

205. Sutherland RE, Anderson L, Keeney M, et al: The ISHAGE guidelines for CD34+ cell determination by flow cytometry. *J Hematother* 5:213, 1996.

206. Dietz LJ, Dubrow RS, Manian BS, et al: Volumetric capillary cytometry: a new method for absolute cell enumeration. *Cytometry* 23:177, 1996.

207. Sims LC, Brecher ME, Gertis K, et al: Enumeration of CD34 positive stem cells: Evaluation and comparison of three methods. *J Hematother* 6:213, 1997.

208. Read EJ, Kunitake ST, Carter CS, et al: Enumeration of CD34+ hematopoietic progenitor cells in peripheral blood and leukapheresis products by microvolume fluorometry: a comparison with flow cytometry. *J Hematother* 6:291, 1997.

209. Hillyer CD, Lackey DA 3rd, Hart KK, et al: CD34+ progenitors and colony forming units–granulocyte macrophage are recruited during large-volume leukapheresis and concentrated by counterflow centrifugal elutriation. *Transfusion* 33(4):316, 1993.

210. Malachowski ME, Comenzo RL, Hillyer CD, et al: Large-volume leukapheresis for peripheral blood stem cell collection in patients with hematologic malignancies. *Transfusion* 32(8):732, 1992.

211. Pettengell R, Morgenstern GR, Woll PJ, et al: Peripheral blood progenitor cell transplantation in lymphoma and leukemia using a single apheresis. *Blood* 82(12):3770, 1993.

212. Bentley SA, Brecher ME, Powell E, et al: Long-term engraftment failure after marrow ablation and autologous hematopoietic reconstitution: differences between peripheral blood stem cell and bone marrow recipients. *Bone Marrow Transplant* 19:557, 1997.

213. Matsunaga T, Sakamaki S, Kohgo Y, et al: Recombinant human granulocyte-colony stimulating factor can mobilize sufficient amounts of peripheral blood stem cells in healthy volunteers for allogeneic transplantation. *Bone Marrow Transplant* 11(2):103, 1993.

214. Arseniev L, Hertenstei B, Link H, et al: Stem cell mobilization in normal donors [Letter]. *J Hematother* 7:5, 1998.

215. Gianni AM, Siena S, Bregni M, et al: Granulocyte-macrophage colony-stimulating factor to harvest haemopoietic stem cells for transplantation. *Lancet* 2:580, 1989.

216. Ho AD, Gluck S, Germond C, et al: Optimal timing for collections of blood progenitor cells following induction chemotherapy and granulocyte-macrophage colony-stimulating factor for autologous transplantation in advanced breast cancer. *Leukemia* 7:1738, 1993.

217. Bandarenko N, Sims L, Brecher M: Circulating CD34+ cell counts are predictive of CD34+ peripheral blood progenitor cell yields [Letter], *Transfusion* 37:1218, 1997.

218. Areman EM, Meehan KR, Sacher RA: Preapheresis levels of peripheral blood CD34+ cells correlate with CD34+ peripheral blood progenitor cells in autologous patients [Letter]. *Transfusion* 37:1217, 1997.

219. Elliot BC, Samson DM, Armitage S, et al: When to harvest peripheral blood stem cells after mobilization therapy: prediction of CD34+ cell yield by preceding day CD34+ concentration in peripheral blood. *J Clin Oncol* 14:970, 1996.

220. Mohle R, Murea S, Pforsich M, et al: Estimation of the progenitor cell yield in a leukapheresis product by previous measurement of CD34+ cells in the peripheral blood. *Vox Sang* 71:90, 1996.

221. Schots R, Van Riet I, Damiaens S, et al: The absolute number of circulating CD34+ cells predicts the number of hematopoietic stem cells that can be collected by apheresis. *Bone Marrow Transplant* 17:509, 1996.

222. Teshima T, Sunami K, Bessho A, et al: Circulating immature cell counts on the harvest day predict the yields of CD34+ cells collected after G-CSF plus chemotherapy-induced mobilization of peripheral blood stem cell. *Blood* 89:4660, 1997.

223. Benjamin RJ, Linsley L, Fountain D, et al: Preapheresis peripheral blood CD34+ mononuclear cell counts as predictors of progenitor cell yield. *Transfusion* 37:79, 1997.

224. Kolb HJ, Schattenberg A, Goldman JM, et al: Graft-versus-leukemia effect of donor lymphocytes marrow grafted patients. *Blood* 86(5):2041, 1995.

225. Lee JH, Klein HG: Mononuclear adoptive immunotherapy, in Hematology/Oncology Clinics of North America: Transfusion Medicine II, edited by PD Mintz, pp 1–22. WB Saunders, Philadelphia, 1995.

226. Collins RH, Piniero LA, Nemunaitis JJ, et al: Transfusion of donor buffy coat cells in the treatment of persistent or recurrent malignancy after allogeneic bone marrow transplantation. *Transfusion* 35: 1995.

227. Rosenberg SA, Lotze MT, Muul LM, et al: Observation on the systemic administration of autologous lymphokine-activated killer cells and recombinant interleukin-2 to patients with metastatic cancer. *N Engl J Med* 313:1485, 1985.

228. Rosenberg SA, Lotze MT, Muul LM, et al: A progress report on the treatment of 157 patients with advanced cancer using lymphokine-activated killer cells and interleukin-2 or high-dose interleukin-2 alone. *N Engl J Med* 316:889, 1986.

229. Klein HG, Leitman SF: Adoptive immunotherapy in the treatment of malignant disease. *Transfusion* 29:170, 1989.

230. Topalian SL, Muul LM, Solomon D, Rosenberg SA: Expansion of human tumor infiltrating lymphocytes for use in immunotherapy trials. *J Immunol Methods* 102:127, 1987.

231. Muul LM, Director EP, Hyatt C, Rosenberg SA: Large scale production of human lymphokine activated killer cells for use in adoptive immunotherapy. *J Immunol Methods* 88:265, 1986.

232. Carter CS, Leitman SF, Cullis H, et al: Use of a continuous-flow cell separator in density gradient isolation of lymphocytes. *Transfusion* 27:362, 1987.

233. Muul LM, Nason-Burchenal K, Carter CS, et al: Development of an automated closed system for generation of human lymphokine-activated killer (LAK) cells for use in adoptive immunotherapy. *J Immunol Methods* 101:171, 1987.

234. Troy AJ, Hart DNJ: Dendritic cells and cancer: Progress toward a new cellular therapy. *J Hematother* 6:523, 1997.

235. Young JW, Szabolics P, Moore MAS: Identification of dendritic cell colony-forming units among normal human CD34+ bone marrow progenitors that are expanded by c-kit ligand and yield pure dendritic cell

colonies in the presence of granulocyte/macrophage colony-stimulating factor and tumor necrosis factor-α. *J Exp Med* 182:1120, 1995.

236. Szabolics P, Moore MA, Young JW: Expansion of immunostimulatory dendritic cells among the myeloid progeny of human CD34+ bone marrow precursors cultured with *c-kit* ligand, granulocyte/macrophage colony-stimulating factor and tumor necrosis factor α. *J Immunol* 154:5841, 1995.

237. Bernhard H, Disis ML, Heimfeld S, et al: Generation of immunostimulatory dendritic cells from human CD34+ hematopoietic progenitor cells in the bone marrow and peripheral blood. *Cancer Res* 55:1099, 1995.

238. Mackensen A, Herbst B, Kohlter G, et al: Delineation of the dendritic cell lineage by generating large numbers of Birbeck granule-positive Langerhans cells from human peripheral blood progenitor cells in vitro. *Blood* 86:2699, 1995.

239. Hsu FJ, Benike C, Fagonei F, et al: Vaccination of patients with B-cell lymphoma using autologous antigen-pulsed dendritic cells. *Nat Med* 2:52, 1996.

240. Nestle FO, Alijagic S, Gilliet M, et al: Vaccination of melanoma patients with peptide- or tumor lysate-pulsed dendritic cells. *Nat Med* 4:328, 1998.

241. Tjoa BA, Simmons SJ, Bowes VA, et al: Evaluation of phase I/II clinical trials in prostate cancer with dendritic cells and PSMA peptides. *Prostate* 36:39, 1998.

242. Zhou LJ, Tedder TF: Human blood dendritic cells selectively express CD83, a member of the immunoglobulin superfamily. *J Immunol* 154:3821, 1995.

243. Hock BD, Starling GC, Daniel PB., et al: Characterization of CMRF-44, a novel monoclonal antibody to activation antigen expressed by the allostimulatory cells within peripheral blood, including dendritic cells. *Immunology* 83:573, 1974.

CHAPTER 142

PRESERVATION AND CLINICAL USE OF PLATELETS

SCOTT MURPHY

The use of platelet transfusions increased dramatically in the 1980s and peaked in 1992, following which, at least in the United States, it has remained stable. Worldwide, many methods are used for the preparation of platelets for transfusion. The "platelet-rich plasma" method and the "buffy coat method" are popular for the separation of platelets from whole blood donations in North America and in Europe, respectively. In addition, platelets separated by apheresis are gaining in popularity worldwide in order to limit donor exposure and to minimize the number of contaminating leukocytes in the preparations. Many institutions are making their platelet products universally leukoreduced at the time of their preparation. After preparation, platelets are generally stored at 20 to 24°C within plastic containers whose walls are adequately permeable to oxygen. It is optimal to agitate these preparations continuously. Storage at lower temperatures results in decreased in vivo survival after transfusion, and adequate access to oxygen and agitation are required to prevent deleterious declines in pH. Platelets stored in this fashion produce satisfactory clinical responses after storage for 5 to 7 days. Currently, storage is limited to 5 days because of concerns about overgrowth of bacteria that might have inadvertently contaminated the preparation.

The clinical response to platelet transfusion can be assessed by measuring the increment in platelet concentration achieved in the patient's blood. This generally correlates directly with the dose of platelets infused and inversely with the patient's size. Using physiologic principles, one can calculate what this response should be. Although the ideal theoretical response is occasionally achieved, on average, the response is approximately one-half of what one would predict because of immunologic and nonimmunologic clinical factors that impact negatively on the response. There is no single correct dose of platelets for all patients. On average, both the initial increment and the time to next transfusion will increase with increasing platelet dose. The appropriate dose will vary with the clinical circumstances and the patient's size and individual response to transfusion. The traditional platelet concentration that should trigger a platelet transfusion had been 20,000/μl, but studies have shown that this level can safely be reduced to 10,000/μl in stable patients. It is important to raise the transfusion trigger above this level in response to a variety of clinical circumstances that increase the likelihood of bleeding. Although most platelet transfusions are given to patients whose marrows are suppressed, occasionally platelet transfusion is indicated when the thrombocytopenia is due to massive blood loss, cardiopulmonary bypass, splenomegaly, immune-mediated thrombocytopenia, and hereditary thrombocytopenia.

The complications of platelet transfusion are almost always due to contaminating leukocytes, red cells, plasma proteins, and microorganisms. Those due to contaminating leukocytes can be reduced in frequency by prestorage leukoreduction of the platelet products. Alloimmunization to class I HLA antigens can be managed by a variety of strategies using apheresis platelet concentrates that lack the antigens to which the patient has formed antibody.

INTRODUCTION

In the 1980s and early 1990s there was a rapid increase in the use of platelet transfusion with a doubling in the United States between 1982 and 1989[1,2] (Fig. 142-1). Platelet use in the United States peaked in 1992 at 9,330,000 units with a slight decline to 7,840,000 in 1994.[3] In 1994, for the first time, platelets obtained by apheresis represented more than 50 percent of the platelets infused. The progressive increase in platelet use through the 1980s and early 1990s coincided with increasingly aggressive myelosuppressive therapy for malignancies and increased availability of platelets made possible by the development of cost-effective methods for storage of platelet concentrates.

TECHNIQUES FOR PLATELET PREPARATION

Platelet concentrates for transfusion may be obtained from routine donations of whole blood anticoagulated with citrate-based formulations or by apheresis with a variety of apheresis devices which also use citrate as the anticoagulant. Two methods of preparing platelet concentrates from whole blood are used, the platelet-rich plasma method and the buffy coat method.

In addition to appropriate platelet content, much attention is now being given to the level of contaminating leukocytes that are infused into patients. Problems produced by contaminating leukocytes will be discussed in the section on complications of platelet transfusion. In toto, these complications are sufficiently serious that many now recommend a totally leukoreduced blood supply. Blood products can be filtered during infusion at the bedside, but, for reasons to be discussed, it is probably preferable to accomplish leukoreduction at the time of preparation of the product. In the United States, an apheresis platelet concentrate or a pool of platelet-rich plasma platelet concentrates is considered leukoreduced if it contains less than 5×10^6 leukocytes. The standard in Europe is 1×10^6 leukocytes.

WHOLE-BLOOD-DERIVED PLATELET CONCENTRATES

Whole-blood-derived platelet concentrates are often termed *random-donor platelet concentrates*. This was to distinguish them from apheresis platelet concentrates derived from specific donors for specific refractory patients generally on the basis of HLA matching. Now, apheresis platelet concentrates are commonly given "randomly" to patients who do not require products from specific donors. Therefore, the term *whole-blood-derived platelet concentrates* is preferred.

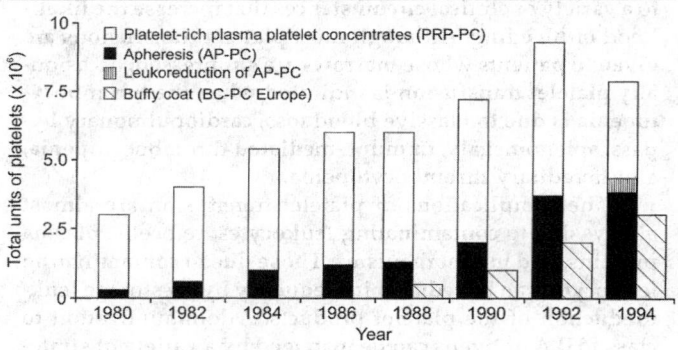

FIGURE 142-1   Trends in platelet utilization in millions of whole-blood-derived platelet concentrate equivalent units per year. The data for platelet-rich plasma platelet concentrates and apheresis platelet concentrates are from the United States as reported in references 1 to 3. In 1994, for the first time, more than half of platelet transfusions were given as apheresis platelet concentrates. Also in 1994, a small but significant fraction were leukoreduced prior to storage. Between 1988 and 1994, an increasing number of platelet concentrate transfusions were prepared by the buffy coat method in Europe, incidence estimated from reference 135.

PLATELET-RICH PLASMA PLATELET CONCENTRATES

This is the only method used in North America for whole-blood-derived platelet concentrates: 450 to 500 ml (a unit) of whole blood is held for up to 8 h at room temperature, and platelet-rich plasma is separated from red cells and buffy coat by low-speed centrifugation. After transferring the platelet-rich plasma to another bag, the plasma is centrifuged rapidly to produce a platelet pellet. Most of the plasma is removed, and then the platelet pellet is allowed to "rest" for 1 to 2 h before resuspension in approximately 50 ml of autologous citrated plasma. Without this rest period, platelets tend to clump irreversibly upon resuspension. The separated red cells are used for transfusion, while the supernatant plasma is used for transfusion or fractionation.

Over the past 20 years, technical improvements have resulted in an increase in the number of platelets in each unit from 5 to 6×10^{10} in 1975 to as much as 9 to 10×10^{10} in 1997.[4] With modern techniques an average unit should contain approximately 8×10^{10} platelets. Approximately 1 to 5×10^8 leukocytes, predominantly lymphocytes, will also be present. One unit is adequate only for the transfusion of a small child less than 30 lb in weight. To transfuse adults, 4 to 8 units need to be pooled to provide a therapeutic dose (see section on dose below).

Whole-blood-derived platelet pools of 4 to 9 units have a high level of leukocyte contamination, 0.4 to 4.0×10^9, which is three orders of magnitude higher than that of a leukoreduced transfusion. There is a system which inserts a leukocyte-reduction filter between the primary blood bag and the bag that accepts the platelet-rich plasma.[5] Thus the platelet-rich plasma is leukoreduced at the time of its preparation. This system was introduced in early 1998 for the preparation of all platelet-rich plasma platelet concentrates in Canada.

BUFFY COAT PLATELET CONCENTRATES

The buffy coat method is being used with increased frequency, particularly in Europe.[6] An initial hard centrifugation sediments all blood cells so that the plasma, buffy coat, and red cells can be collected in three separate containers. Remarkably, not only do the platelets at the top of the bag fall to the buffy coat, but also the platelets at the bottom of the bag rise to the buffy coat. Therefore, platelet yields in the buffy coat are excellent. One can prepare platelet concentrates from individual buffy coats[7] or pool 4 to 6 buffy coats, add 2 to 4 volumes

of an additive solution, centrifuge the pool at low speed to remove red cells and leukocytes, and push the supernatant through a leukoreduction filter to produce a therapeutic, leukoreduced, dose of platelets for an adult.[8,9]

The platelet-rich plasma and buffy coat methods each have their advantages and disadvantages.[6,10,11] Each produces platelets of high quality, and platelet yields are equivalent. In the buffy coat method, 20 to 25 ml of red cells are lost with the buffy coat, but an extra 70 to 80 ml of plasma can be collected. In any event, the buffy coat method is being used with increasing frequency in Europe; it is not used in North America.

APHERESIS PLATELET CONCENTRATES

One can obtain 2.5 to 10×10^{11} platelets (equivalent to 3 to 10 units of whole-blood-derived platelet concentrates) by apheresis of donors over 1 to 2 h using a variety of devices,[12–15] with an extraordinarily high level of safety for the donor.[16] The number of platelets obtained during the procedure varies according to the platelet concentration in the blood of the donor, the duration of the donation, and the efficiency of the device. The efficiency of the newest devices is such that one should expect to obtain at least 60 percent of the platelets that pass through them, and most donors begin to be quite restless if the donation time exceeds more than 90 to 120 min. Therefore, it is the wide range of the platelet concentration in the blood of normal donors, 130,000 to 500,000/μl that accounts for the wide range in platelet yields.[17] There are also devices for obtaining both apheresis platelet concentrates and a unit of red cells from the same donor at the same sitting.[18]

The goal of apheresis is to obtain a therapeutic dose of platelets for an adult from a single donor during one apheresis sitting. In a subsequent section, we will discuss current controversies concerning the appropriate dose for platelet transfusion. Current standards of the FDA in the United States state only that 75 percent of apheresis platelet products must contain more than 3.0×10^{11} platelets. While 2.5 to 3.5×10^{11} is probably a satisfactory dose for the prophylactic transfusion of a child or small adult, it is probably unsatisfactory for a large adult who is bleeding or has other clinical features that interfere with an optimal response to platelet transfusion. On the other hand, administration of high-yield platelet products to small adults and children may be wasteful. Blood centers are in the process of considering the best way to handle the manufacturing process for apheresis platelets. Consideration is being given to the preparation of products containing two or more levels of platelet content, perhaps means of 3.2×10^{11} and 6.4×10^{11} (i.e., approximately 4 and 8 whole-blood-derived units respectively). The use of the products could be tailored to the needs of individual patients.

There are two major advantages in using apheresis platelet concentrates. First, the number of donors to whom the patient is exposed is substantially reduced, thus reducing the likelihood of transmission of viral and bacterial diseases. Second, the separation technology of the various apheresis devices lends itself to the production of leukoreduced products during collection. Progressive improvements of those most recently available[12,13] has allowed the production of products with less than 1×10^6 leukocytes essentially 100 percent of the time. Figure 142-2 shows the experience of one blood center in this regard.

Prestorage leukoreduction at the blood center offers the advantage that it is carried out under standardized conditions following GMP with appropriate quality control procedures in place. Such standardization is not possible with filtration at the bedside.[19] There are reports in which bedside filtration has failed to achieve the expected beneficial results.[20]

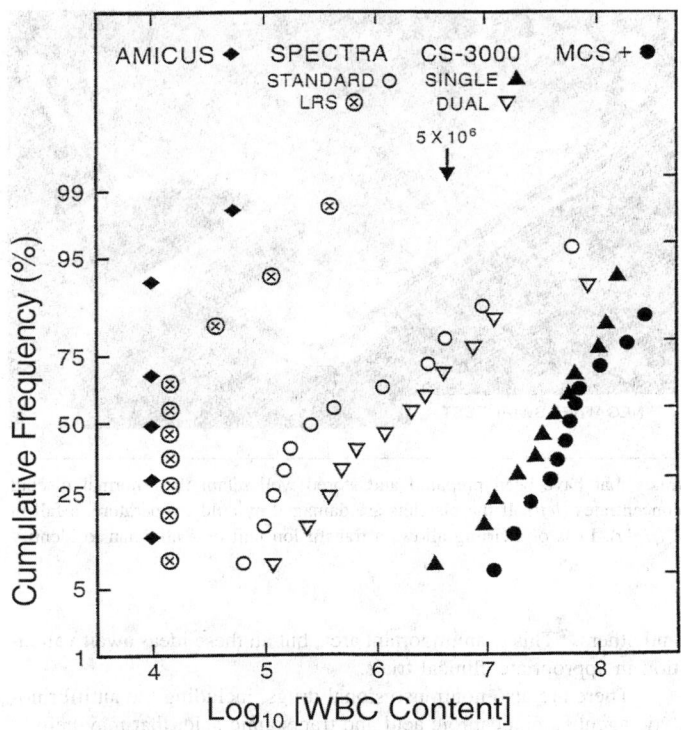

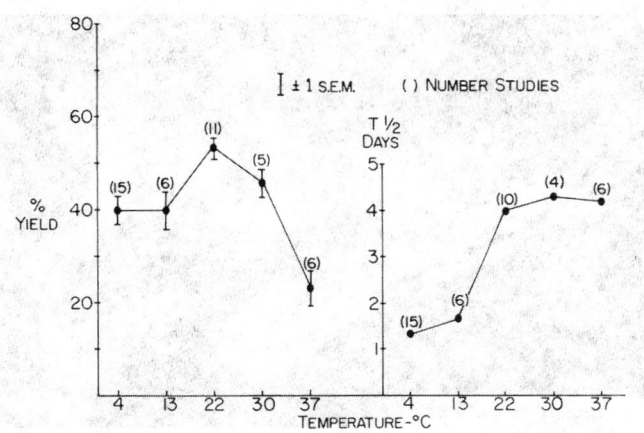

FIGURE 142-3   Relationship between storage temperature and platelet viability after transfusion. Platelet-rich plasma was obtained from normal volunteers and stored overnight at the indicated temperatures. Thereafter, the platelets were labeled with radioactive chromium and reinfused. Percent yield refers to the percent of platelets infused that circulate in the first 3 h after infusion. The 50–60% yield at 22°C (71.6°F) is a result of physiologic pooling in the spleen (see Chap. 117), not cell damage. The combination of percent yield and subsequent in vivo survival ($T_{1/2}$) is optimal at 22°C.

FIGURE 142-2   Cumulative frequency of leukocyte contents of apheresis platelet concentrates produced with six different apheresis methodologies: Fenwal Amicus, COBE Spectra (standard and leukocyte reduction system [LRS] versions), Fenwal CS-3000 (single- and dual-needle access), and Haemonetics MCS+. The newest devices, the Amicus and Spectra LRS, produce >99% products with leukocyte content less than 5×10^6, the current standard in the United States. The older procedures have a 25% (standard Spectra, dual-needle CS-3000) or 95% (single-needle CS-3000, MCS+) failure rate. Data from the American Red Cross Blood Services, Penn-Jersey Region. Reprinted from reference 136 with permission.

STORAGE OF PLATELET CONCENTRATES

LIQUID STORAGE AT 20 TO 24°C

Both whole-blood-derived and apheresis platelet concentrates may be stored for 5 days using the same principles: (1) The temperature must be 20 to 24°C.[21] (2) The storage container must be constructed of a plastic material that allows adequate diffusion of oxygen to meet the cells' metabolic needs.[22,23] (3) The platelet concentrates must be agitated during storage.[22,23]

Using radiolabeling of stored platelets (Fig. 142-3), survival after reinfusion in vivo is nearly normal if storage, even for several days, is carried out at 20 to 24°C (68.0 to 75.2°F). However, at colder temperatures, survival is dramatically shortened.[21] If oxygen influx is inadequate at 20 to 24°C (68.0 to 75.2°F), the cells will increase their production of lactic acid, leading to depletion of bicarbonate buffer and fall in pH to less than 6.2.[22,23] These acid conditions result in the platelets being rapidly cleared from the circulation after transfusion. A similar fall in pH occurs if the platelet concentrates are not agitated during storage.[23] There are data suggesting that agitation may be discontinued for up to 24 h of the 5-day storage interval.[24]

Synthetic media are also used for the storage of buffy coat platelet concentrates.[8] Definition of the optimal solution is still in progress, but it appears that it can be relatively simple, relying on acetate as an oxidative fuel for platelets.[25] The oxidation of an organic anion

such as acetate utilizes a proton from the medium, thus providing an alkalinizing effect that spares bicarbonate, the major buffer during platelet concentrate storage.[26] It is anticipated that synthetic media will soon be used for apheresis platelet concentrates as well.[27]

Some investigators have been unable to find any practical difference in clinical response between fresh and stored platelets,[28,29] but most find a reduction in recovery in vivo, with survival reduced by approximately 20 to 25 percent after 5 days of storage as judged by radiolabeling studies in normal volunteers and by the increase in platelet count in thrombocytopenic patients.[30] Furthermore, some authors have reported an even greater defect in stored platelets relative to fresh platelets in sick patients with fever, sepsis, splenomegaly, and disseminated intravascular coagulation.[31,32]

Platelet recovery and survival is as satisfactory after 7 days of storage as it is after 5 days.[33] However, when storage was extended to 7 days, bacterial overgrowth and clinical sepsis in recipients of stored platelets occurred with sufficient frequency to warrant limiting liquid storage to 5 days.[34] If methods of bacterial decontamination[35] or bacterial detection are developed,[36] it may be possible to prolong storage beyond 5 days once again.

Many platelet abnormalities have been described after ex vivo platelet storage.[37] At present, in vitro characteristics that correlate best with the capacity to circulate in vivo are retention of disc shape and good function in the hypotonic shock response.[38] With few exceptions, platelets with normal discoid morphology will circulate normally after transfusion. Platelets that are damaged by cold, acidity, or bacterial contamination generally lose their discoid morphology and become spheres. Normal discoid morphology is reflected by the "swirling" or "shimmering" appearance of well-preserved platelet concentrates during gross, visual inspection.[39] Blood bank staff and clinical personnel are urged to check platelet concentrates for this phenomenon prior to transfusion (Fig. 142-4).

The activities of coagulation factors are well maintained in the suspending plasma of platelet concentrates during storage, except for modest decreases in those of factors V and VIII.[40] Thus, a pool of 4 to 8 whole-blood-derived platelet concentrates or an apheresis platelet

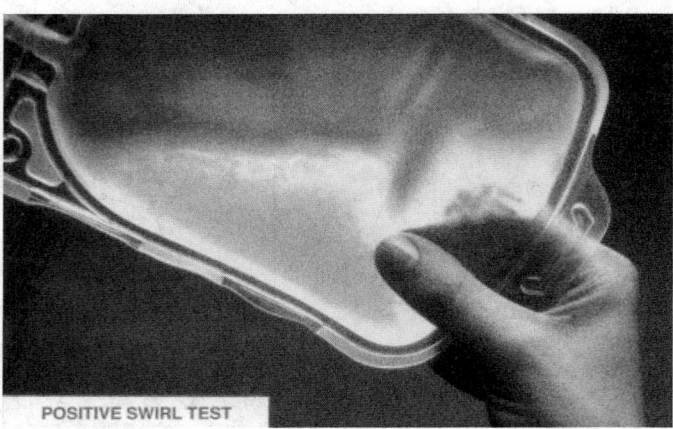
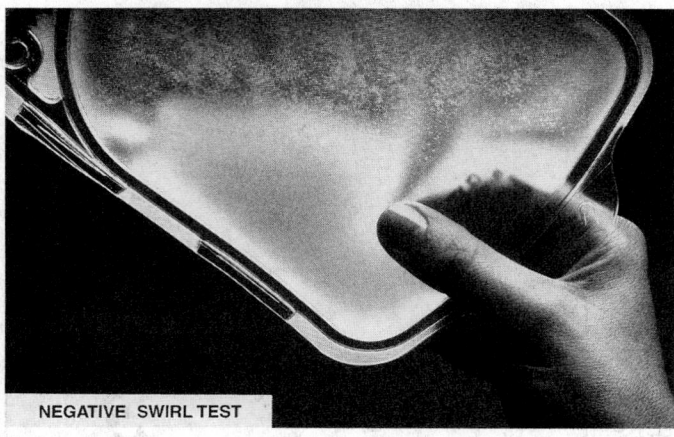

POSITIVE SWIRL TEST

NEGATIVE SWIRL TEST

FIGURE 142-4   Swirling of platelet concentrates. Platelets in platelet concentrates that have been prepared and stored well retain their normal discoid configuration, which confers a swirling or shimmering appearance to the platelet concentrates (*left*). If the platelets are damaged by cold temperature, a fall in pH, or bacterial contamination, discoid shape and the swirling appearance are lost (*right*). Loss of swirling allows a transfusion unit or a clinician to identify potentially ineffective or dangerous platelet concentrates.

concentrate provides the equivalent of 1 to 2 units of fresh-frozen plasma.

FROZEN STORAGE

The most widely used method for frozen storage employs controlled rate freezing (1°C per minute), 5% DMSO as a cryoprotective agent, rapid thawing, graded reduction of the DMSO concentration, and washing prior to infusion. In vivo viability is approximately 40 to 50 percent relative to fresh platelets.[41] Thus, this technology is both more complex and expensive and less effective than liquid storage at 20 to 24°C.[42] However, these preparations can be effective clinically[43] and may be very valuable for autologous transfusion of selected patients who may not respond well to allogeneic platelets. Platelets may be obtained before myelosuppressive therapy, then frozen and administered during subsequent periods of thrombocytopenia.[44] Newer approaches using second-messenger effectors may allow the use of lower concentrations of DMSO, which would, in turn, allow the direct infusion of platelets after thawing.[45]

FRESH WHOLE BLOOD

Children under the age of 2 who undergo complex cardiac bypass surgery have a better hemostatic response to fresh whole blood than to reconstituted blood using red cells, plasma, and platelet concentrates prepared as described above.[46] These are the only published data suggesting that the process of platelet concentrate preparation impairs platelet function. Although this conclusion has not been confirmed in a second trial, the administration of fresh whole blood is strongly endorsed by some cardiac surgeons.

LYOPHILIZED PLATELETS, PLATELET MEMBRANES, AND PLATELET SUBSTITUTES

Current methods of platelet storage are cumbersome, and the duration of storage is short. It would be ideal to have a safe and effective dried preparation with long shelf-life that one could simply rehydrate and infuse. A great deal of research is going on in this area examining platelets treated with paraformaldehyde and lyophilized platelet membrane microvesicles, fibrinogen-coated beads, albumin microspheres,

and others.[47] This is an important area, but all these ideas await validation in appropriate clinical trials.

There are also nontransfusional drugs, including the antifibrinolytic agents aminocaproic acid and tranexamic acid, that may help to stop thrombocytopenic bleeding.[48] They have been described as being effective in controlling mucosal and dental bleeding in thrombocytopenic patients without increasing the platelet concentration in the blood.

CLINICAL RESPONSE

GENERAL PRINCIPLES IN PATIENTS WITH MARROW FAILURE

Assuming that one-third of infused platelets will be pooled reversibly in a spleen of normal size (see Chap. 117) and that the recipient's blood volume is 2.5 liters/m², the infusion of 1 unit of whole-blood-derived platelet concentrate, containing 8.0×10^{10} platelets into a recipient with 1 square meter of BSA, should result in an increase in platelet count of 21,000/μl. Of course, the response to 1 unit will be inversely proportional to the patient's size, expressed as the body surface area. Thus, one can evaluate the response to a platelet transfusion by calculating the corrected count increment, or *CCI*[49]:

$$\frac{\text{Measured increase in platelet concentration} \times \text{BSA (m}^2)}{\text{Number of units infused (or number of platelets} \times 10^{11})}$$

The measurement of CCI has its critics,[50] but it is the most widely used method. Under optimal circumstances, the response should be 21,000/μl per square meter per unit infused or 26,000/μl per square meter per 10^{11} platelets infused.

In practice, in patients with thrombocytopenia secondary to marrow failure, the average CCI is approximately one-half of that expected, 10,000/μl per square meter per unit infused (Fig. 142-5).[49] Many studies have attempted to identify the factors responsible for this consistent but less than optimal response.[32,49,51–55] Alloimmunization has been incriminated, along with a variety of nonimmune factors such as platelet storage, bacterial sepsis, concomitant use of antibacterial antibiotics and amphotericin B, graft-versus-host disease, splenomegaly, disseminated intravascular coagulation, and simply having had a recent allogeneic bone marrow transplantation. It is of interest that no one factor predominates in the majority of studies, suggesting that the crucial factors vary with the populations of patients being studied.

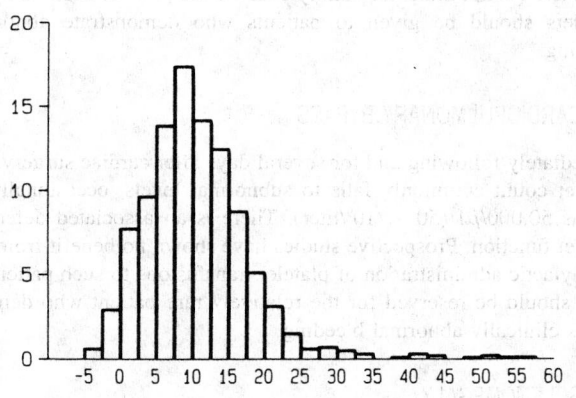

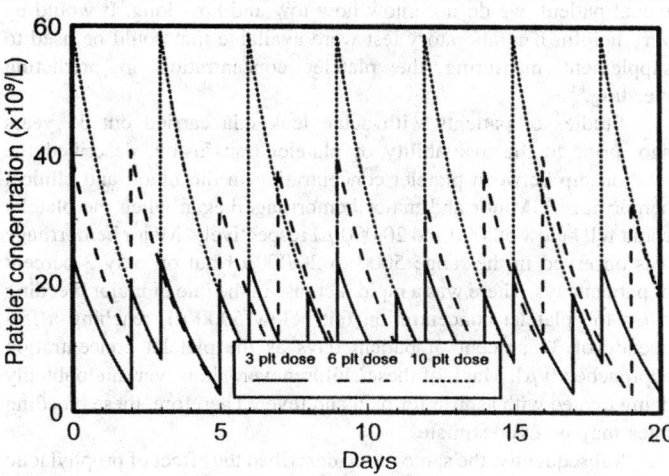

FIGURE 142-5   Rise in platelet concentration 1 h after infusion in patients with acute leukemia (redrawn from reference 49). As described in text, the increment in concentration for each unit infused has been corrected for body surface area. Without complicating factors, it should be approximately 21,000/μl (21 × 10^9/liter). The vertical axis refers to the percent of transfusions achieving the increments indicated. There is marked heterogeneity in response, with a median of approximately 10,000/μl (10 × 10^9/liter), approximately one-half of what one would predict.

FIGURE 142-6   Response to varying doses of units of whole-blood-derived platelet concentrates during repetitive transfusion of patients thrombocytopenic from marrow failure. Larger doses produce not only an initial higher increase in platelet concentration but a longer time to next transfusion. Fewer transfusion episodes are required over a 20-day transfusion period. Graph redrawn with permission from calculations in reference 58, validated by empirical data given in references 59 and 60.

The initial CCI can be measured in 10 min[56] to a few hours after the transfusion. The time until the platelet concentration returns to baseline (time to next transfusion) also varies with the immune and nonimmune factors affecting the initial CCI.[57] It also varies directly with the height of the platelet count achieved by the transfusion and, therefore, the dose of platelets administered.[58-60] This follows from the fact that platelet survival is reduced in all patients with thrombocytopenia, regardless of the cause, with progressive reduction as the platelet concentration in the blood becomes lower[61] (see Chap. 117). Therefore, everything else being equal, the larger the dose, the higher the platelet count achieved by transfusion, and the longer the time will be to the next transfusion (Fig. 142-6).

PLATELET DOSE

If the average patient has an increase in platelet concentration of 10,000/μl per square meter per unit of platelets, one can calculate the relationship between the dose administered and the platelet count achieved. Furthermore, using calculations and data from references 58 to 60, one can estimate the time to the next transfusion. For example, for the transfusion of a myelosuppressed patient of a 2-m^2 surface area and platelet count 5000/μl, these values are given in Table 142-1. The results indicate that there is no standard dose that fits all patients, regardless of size and clinical situation. For the doses given, the platelet concentrations achieved in a patient with 1-m^2 body surface would be twice those in the table. In the 1-m^2 patient, 4 units (3.2 × 10^{11}) would probably be satisfactory if the patient is not bleeding, is being transfused prophylactically, and is hospitalized so that he or she can be transfused again 24 to 48 h later, since raising the platelet concentration to 20,000 to 30,000/μl protects most thrombocytopenic patients against spontaneous, catastrophic bleeding. However, 10 units (8.0 × 10^{11}) would be a better choice if the goal was to achieve a platelet concentration over 50,000/μl because the patient was bleeding or was being prepared for an invasive procedure.[62] It is probably most critical to achieve this level of platelet concentration if the surgical field is highly vascular, as with inflammation or portal hypertension;

if there are coexisting defects in plasma coagulation; if the procedure is "blind," as in needle biopsy of the liver, when there is no opportunity to achieve hemostasis mechanically; or if the surgery is in an area where even a small hemorrhage could be disastrous, as in the central nervous system.

A higher dose might also be chosen to facilitate transfusion in the outpatient setting where a longer transfusion interval would be preferable.

However, patients vary dramatically in their responses. Therefore, the measurement of increments 1 and 24 h after transfusion is a cost-effective way to modify the dose and frequency of transfusion based on the pathophysiology of the individual patient.

PLATELET TRANSFUSION TRIGGER

Clearly, a thrombocytopenic patient who is actively bleeding requires platelet transfusion. It is more difficult to make this judgment if the platelet count is simply very low and the patient has no hemorrhagic signs or only minor ones, such as petechiae or small ecchymoses of the skin. Clinical experience suggests that if the platelet count is low enough, long enough, "spontaneous" major hemorrhage, particularly into the central nervous system, may occur. Unfortunately, in an indi-

TABLE 142-1   RELATIONSHIP BETWEEN PLATELET DOSE AND CLINICAL RESPONSE IN A PATIENT WITH A 2-M^2 BODY SURFACE WITH A PLATELET COUNT, 5000/μL, PRIOR TO TRANSFUSION

Dose		PLATELET CONCENTRATION	TRANSFUSION
× 10^{11}	UNITS*	ACHIEVED, PER μl	INTERVAL (DAYS)**
3.2	4	25,000	1.8
4.8	6	35,000	2.3
6.4	8	45,000	2.8
8.0	10	55,000	3.5

*Whole-blood-derived platelet concentrates.
**Time to return to 5000/μL.

vidual patient, we do not know how low and how long. It would be very helpful if a laboratory test were available that could be used to supplement measuring the platelet concentration in predicting bleeding.[63]

Studies of patients with acute leukemia carried out 35 years ago, prior to the availability of platelet transfusion, described the relationship between platelet concentration in the blood and clinical hemorrhage.[64] Minor and major hemorrhage began when the platelet count fell below 50,000 and 20,000/μl respectively. Major hemorrhage was observed in the range 5000 to 20,000/μl but on only 3 percent of patient days. There was a rapid increase in the rate of major bleeding when the platelet concentration fell below 5000/μl, reaching a frequency of 33 percent of patient days as the platelet concentration approached 0/μl. Many of these children were, however, undoubtedly being treated with aspirin for pain and fever. Therefore, these bleeding rates may be overestimates.

Subsequently, the same group described the effect of prophylactic platelet transfusion administered whenever the platelet count fell below 20,000/μl.[65] Although there was a striking reduction in major hemorrhage when the platelet count (measured pretransfusion) was below 5000/μl, there was no substantial change when the platelet count was in the range of 5000 to 20,000/μl. Nonetheless, for many years, this experience was used to justify prophylactic platelet transfusion whenever the platelet concentration fell below 20,000/μl, although the data actually suggested 5,000/μl as an appropriate trigger.

More recently, prospective but uncontrolled studies by one group supported the safety and efficacy of a more restrictive policy using 5000/μl as the platelet transfusion trigger.[66,67] Subsequently, three prospective studies assigned patients to one of two groups receiving prophylactic platelet transfusion at either 10,000/μl or 20,000/μl.[68-70] Uniformly, there was no increase in bleeding risk at the lower transfusion trigger, which is now being adopted by many transfusion services.[71]

However, it is just as unjustified to choose a rigid transfusion trigger as it is to choose a rigid transfusion dose. It is commonly assumed that clinical factors increase the risk of hemorrhage at any given platelet concentration. These include fever and sepsis, administration of drugs that interfere with platelet function, coexistent abnormalities of plasma coagulation factors, disseminated intravascular coagulation, and high leukocyte concentrations in the blood. Thus, it is appropriate to raise the transfusion trigger in complicated, clinically ill patients.

In addition, moderate to severe bleeding is observed in 11 to 23 percent of patients after marrow transplantation in spite of the aggressive use of prophylactic platelet transfusion and maintenance of morning platelet counts above 20,000/μl.[72,73] Gastrointestinal and urinary bleeding are most common; pulmonary and intracranial bleeding are less common. Usually, there is an identifiable anatomic cause, such as gastrointestinal ulceration, hemorrhagic cystitis, or diffuse alveolar hemorrhage. In effect, it is common in the myelosuppressed patient to be treating bleeding, not preventing it. Many centers increase the transfusion trigger to 30,000 to 50,000/μl in such cases.[72]

THROMBOCYTOPENIA DUE TO PLATELET LOSS, SEQUESTRATION, OR DESTRUCTION

MASSIVE TRANSFUSION

Dilutional thrombocytopenia will occur when massive blood loss is replaced with units of stored red cells that lack viable platelets. Following replacement of one blood volume, 35 to 40 percent of the platelets usually remain. Even when one to two blood volumes have been replaced, abnormal bleeding usually does not develop, and routine transfusion is not indicated simply because the platelet count is low.[74] Platelets should be given to patients who demonstrate abnormal bleeding.

CARDIOPULMONARY BYPASS

Immediately following and for several days after cardiac surgery, the platelet count commonly falls to subnormal levels, occasionally as low as 50,000/μl (50 $\times$ 10^9/liter). There is an associated defect in platelet function. Prospective studies have shown no benefit from the prophylactic administration of platelet transfusions to such patients.[75] They should be reserved for the relatively rare patient who demonstrates clinically abnormal bleeding.

SPLENOMEGALY

Patients with massive splenomegaly have thrombocytopenia related predominantly to excessive sequestration in a splenic pool in continuous exchange with platelets in the circulation (see Chap. 117). The platelet count rarely falls below 30,000/μl (30 $\times$ 10^9/liter) due to this mechanism alone, so that platelet transfusion is rarely considered except in anticipation of invasive procedures such as surgery and needle biopsy of the liver. Under these circumstances, depending on the degree of splenic enlargement, one may need to administer 10 to 15 units of whole-blood-derived platelet concentrates per square meter body surface area to achieve a substantial increase in platelet count. In many patients with severe splenomegaly, it may not be possible to achieve platelet count elevations even with large numbers of platelet concentrates. If such patients require elective surgery, consideration should be given to splenectomy prior to the elective procedure.

IMMUNE (IDIOPATHIC) THROMBOCYTOPENIC PURPURA (ITP)

In ITP, platelet transfusion is generally not used because the bleeding tendency is less severe than in thrombocytopenia due to diminished production, and the response to medical therapy is generally satisfactory and rapid (see Chap. 117). Furthermore, the survival of transfused platelets is relatively brief, similar to that of the patient's own platelets. Nonetheless, when there is critical bleeding or need for urgent surgery, 3 to 6 units of whole-blood-derived platelet concentrates per square meter body surface area will generally raise the platelet count for 12 to 48 h.[76] The same general principles apply to other diseases in which there is accelerated destruction of platelets, such as disseminated intravascular coagulation.

NEONATAL ALLOIMMUNE THROMBOCYTOPENIA

In this syndrome, the mother produces an alloantibody against antigens on fetal platelets that have crossed the placenta (Chap. 117). The antibody, in turn, crosses the placenta, causing in utero thrombocytopenia that may persist for weeks after delivery. Since maternal platelets are compatible, platelets harvested from the mother's blood by apheresis can produce an adequate increase in the infant's platelet count after infusion.[77] Ideally, such platelets should be concentrated in a small volume of plasma or washed, so as to avoid infusing additional antibody.

Unfortunately, it is often difficult to arrange for apheresis of the mother. Surprisingly, a randomly selected unit of platelets may raise the neonate's platelet concentration substantially.[78] If it does not, prompt serologic evaluation of the mother and father can identify the antigen to which the antibody has been formed, usually HPA-1a (Pl^{A1}). Donors lacking HPA-1a (i.e., homozygous HPA-1b) can then be recruited to support the infant.[79]

HEREDITARY THROMBOCYTOPENIA

These syndromes are rare and generally not associated with severe bleeding.[80] Since the survival of allogeneic platelets is normal, platelet transfusion is quite effective and may be used for critical bleeding and surgery.

QUALITATIVE PLATELET DISORDERS

In spite of normal platelet counts, patients with qualitative platelet disorders have a clinical bleeding tendency associated with abnormal in vitro tests of platelet function and a prolonged bleeding time in vivo. The basis may be hereditary (see Chap. 119) or acquired (see Chap. 120). Platelet transfusion is generally not indicated when the cause is extrinsic to the platelet, as in uremia, von Willebrand disease, and hyperglobulinemia, since the transfused platelets will function no better than the patient's own platelets. There are exceptions in certain types of von Willebrand's disease in which normal platelets can be used to deliver von Willebrand factor to a bleeding site (see Chap. 135). Most inherited intrinsic disorders are mild and do not require platelet transfusions even for surgery if the procedure is carried out under direct vision, so that hemostasis may be achieved mechanically. If the bleeding tendency is more severe, as in Glanzmann thrombasthenia, platelet transfusions may be necessary for more severe bleeding and surgery. The acquired defects, as in the myeloproliferative and myelodysplastic syndromes, generally do not require platelet transfusion unless there is coexistent thrombocytopenia.

POSSIBLE CONTRAINDICATIONS TO PLATELET TRANSFUSION

Concern has been voiced that platelet transfusions should not be administered to patients with forms of thrombocytopenia associated with thrombosis such as TTP and heparin-induced thrombocytopenia (see Chap. 117) since infusion of platelets might worsen the thrombotic tendency.[81,82] Unfortunately, particularly in TTP, platelet transfusion is often requested prior to invasive procedures such as the insertion of intravenous catheters for therapy with apheresis. The author's experience has been that platelet transfusions are safe in this setting. However, it seems prudent not to administer prophylactic platelet transfusions simply because the platelet concentration is low in these diseases.

COMPLICATIONS OF PLATELET TRANSFUSION

There are many complications of platelet transfusion (Table 142-2). Paradoxically, they are not due to the platelets but rather to contaminating leukocytes, red cells, plasma proteins, and microorganisms.

COMPLICATIONS DUE TO CONTAMINATING LEUKOCYTES

ALLOIMMUNIZATION TO CLASS I HLA ANTIGENS

HLA antigens are expressed on integral membrane glycoproteins. Almost all cells have Class I antigens (A, B, and C subloci), whereas only a few types of circulating leukocytes (dendritic cells, monocytes, and subsets of B cells) have Class II antigens. Primary alloimmunization to Class I HLA antigens appears to require presentation of such antigens on cells that also express Class II antigens and other costimulatory molecules.[83] There is now abundant evidence that the incidence of HLA alloimmunization can be reduced by the consistent use of leukoreduced blood products.[84,85] Transfused red cells must also be leukoreduced, since leukocytes contained in them are quite capable of inducing HLA alloimmunization.[86]

However, it remains to be seen how completely leukoreduction can eliminate alloimmunization. In one study,[87] leukoreduction had

TABLE 142-2   COMPLICATIONS OF PLATELET TRANSFUSION

Due to contaminating leukocytes
  Antibody to Class I HLA antigens
    Refractoriness to platelet transfusion
    Febrile nonhemolytic transfusion reactions (FNHTR)
  Cytokine formation
    FNHTR
  Transmission of cytomegalovirus (CMV)
  Graft-versus-host disease (GVHD)
Due to contaminating red cells
  Rh alloimmunization
  Parasites—malaria, babesiosis
Due to plasma and its contents
  Contaminating microorganisms
    Bacteria
    Viruses—HCV, HIV, HBV
    Parasites—Chagas disease
  Plasma proteins
    Urticaria
    IgA in patients with IgA deficiency
    ? FNHTR
    ABO antibodies
  Transfusion-related acute lung injury (TRALI)

almost no effect on the development of alloimmunization in patients who had been previously exposed to foreign leukocytes either through pregnancy or transfusions that had not been leukoreduced. It may be that leukoreduction will prove to be less effective in preventing secondary as opposed to primary alloimmunization. However, another trial[84] showed efficacy in such patients.

Alloimmunization to HLA should be suspected clinically if two or three consecutive platelet transfusions produce a CCI less than 3000/μl per square meter per unit.[88] It can be confirmed in the laboratory by performing a lymphocytotoxicity (LCT) assay for HLA antibody in the patient's serum. In this assay, leukocytes from 50 to 100 donors with an appropriate heterogeneity of HLA types are incubated with the patient's serum and complement. LCT is assessed microscopically. The presence of such antibody has been a good predictor of poor response to platelets from randomly selected donors[89] and improved response when platelets are matched for HLA type.[90] Many centers consider it inappropriate to issue matched platelets unless this, or a similar test, has been performed because of the belief that matching will provide little benefit if antibody is not present.[91,92]

The incidence and severity of HLA alloimmunization should be gradually decreasing as the use of leukoreduced blood products becomes increasingly popular. The following discussion is based on data accumulated before widespread leukoreduction was in use. Approximately 10 percent of patients presenting for therapy of diseases requiring platelet transfusion will already have LCT antibodies from prior transfusions and pregnancies.[93] Another 30 percent become alloimmunized during therapy, and 60 percent never do.[93] There is no known difference between those who do and do not become immunized. Among those who do, some will do so after only two to four transfusions, whereas others require dozens of transfusions.[94] The pattern and intensity of immunization varies greatly from patient to patient. An LCT assay can be characterized by the percentage of cells in the panel against which the patient's serum reacts, i.e., the percent reactive antibody (PRA). Furthermore, the pattern of reactivity can be analyzed to determine the antigens to which the patient has formed antibody. Patients may have PRA values between 4 and 100 percent (Fig. 142-7).

The majority of patients who become alloimmunized establish a level and specificity of immunization and tend to maintain that status as they continue to be transfused. However, approximately 30 percent lose their antibodies over time in spite of continuing transfusion.[95]

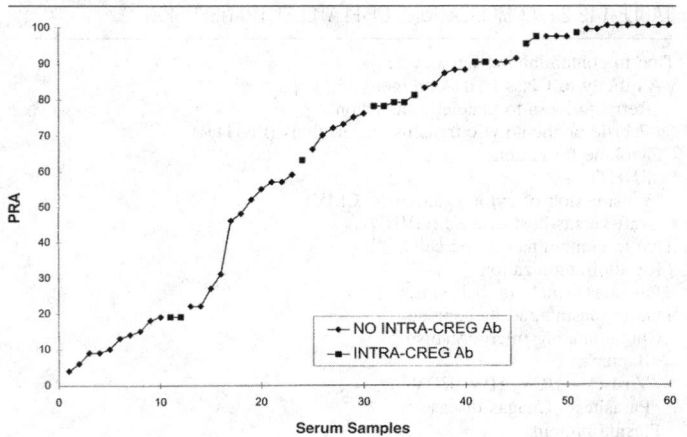

A	All 4 antigens in donor identical to those of recipient.
B1U	Only 3 antigens detected in donor; all present in recipient.
B1X	Three donor antigens identical to recipient; fourth antigen cross-reactive* with recipient.
B2U	Only 2 antigens detected in donor; both present in recipient.
B2UX	Only 3 antigens detected in donor; 2 identical with recipient, third cross-reactive.
B2X	Two donor antigens identical to recipient; third and fourth antigens cross-reactive with recipient.
C	One antigen of donor not present in recipient and not cross-reactive with recipient.
D	Two antigens of donor not present in recipient and not cross-reactive with recipient.

*Antigen in a cross-reactive group (CREG) that contains one of the patient's antigens. Revised with permission from reference 100.

FIGURE 142-7   Cumulative frequency of percent reactive antibody (PRA) by lymphocytotoxicity (LCT) assay in serum samples from 108 thrombocytopenic patients referred to a regional blood center for matched platelet support during a 6-month period. Fifty showed no reactivity, while 58 showed PRAs that varied from 4% to 100%. The squares indicate patients who had demonstrable antibody against antigens within their own cross-reactive groups, i.e., intra-CREG antibody. Data provided by Dr. Susan Hsu, American Red Cross Blood Services, Penn-Jersey Region. Reprinted from reference 136 with permission.

Thus, it is helpful to monitor antibody levels and specificity, since such patients may regain responsiveness having been previously refractory.

Cross-reactive groups (CREGs) of HLA antigens have been defined by serologic testing. Cross-reactivity among antigens in a CREG is based on the sharing of one or more public epitopes by those antigens.[96] It is common for some patients to develop antibodies to one or more public epitopes, i.e., one or more CREGs, while others develop antibodies to one or more private antigens.[97] Furthermore, some patients demonstrate intra-CREG antibodies, i.e., antibodies to antigens in the same CREG as the patient's own antigens.[98] These facts have major implications for management.

MANAGEMENT OF THE REFRACTORY PATIENT

In 1969, it was shown that refractory patients would respond to platelets from siblings who were identical for all four Class I HLA antigens.[99] In fact, this simple clinical observation remains one of the most compelling pieces of evidence supporting the role of HLA alloimmunization in platelet refractoriness. Similarly, patients could be supported by platelets from unrelated donors who were HLA-identical or closely matched. Because some patients do not make antibody to antigens within their own CREGs, it became popular to choose donors according to CREG classification, particularly BX matches, i.e., donors whose antigens are identical to or within the same CREGs as those of the patient.[100] Table 142-3 shows the categorization of such matches.

Responses were better with such matching than with random donor selection, but many BX matches failed and many C and D matches succeeded. Figure 142-7 suggests potential explanations for the relatively poor predictive capacity of this method. Some patients with relatively low PRAs have antibody to only one or two CREGs so that success with some C and D matches would be expected. On the other hand, failure of some BX matches would be expected in patients with intra-CREG antibody. Futhermore, this method generally does not provide a good match quickly. It is uncommon to find an excellent match in a blood center's inventory, and days are required to recruit and pherese one or more well-matched donors from an HLA-typed donor file.

In the late 1980s and early 1990s, practical methods for platelet cross-matching became available.[101] Many centers found that they could simply cross-match patient's serum with unselected apheresis platelet concentrates in inventory to find, within hours, a compatible product that would be successful in vivo.[51,102] However, it was recognized[102] that, in a highly immunized patient, one might cross-match with dozens of donors and not find a compatible product. For many such patients, only the identification of an A or BU match (Table 142-3) will suffice.

One other approach to these patients has been proposed.[103,104] If the PRA in the LCT assay is less than 100 percent, one should be able to identify the HLA antigens to which the patient has not formed antibody. The patient can then be supported with "antigen-negative" platelets, i.e., platelets which lack the antigens to which the patient has formed antibody. If the results of the LCT assay are known, one can often provide a product from inventory on an urgent basis using this approach.

There is no reason that one of these approaches should be chosen to the exclusion of the other two.[105] If the PRA is less than 70 percent, successful support can usually be provided by cross-matching of random products or by "antigen-negative" platelets. When the PRA is high (>80%), one can select for cross-matching the best available "antigen-negative" HLA matches and/or selectively recruit A and BU matches from an HLA-typed donor file. Some patients with common HLA types, 1,2/7,8 for example, will have dozens of A and BU matches available. Unfortunately, some patients have rare HLA types and will have no A or BU matches to recruit.

ROLE OF ABO AND PLATELET-SPECIFIC ANTIBODIES

ABO determinants are carried by both glycoproteins and glycolipids of platelets, as they are on red cells.[106] Group O patients commonly have a good response to platelets from group A or B donors, but in a subset of patients, the response can be poor[107] or very poor.[108] Thus it seems wise to observe ABO compatibility when possible.

The platelet surface carries many platelet-specific antigens (HPA, see Chap. 138) which are quite capable of eliciting a strong alloantibody response. It is surprising that there are only a few case reports of such alloantibodies accounting for refractoriness to platelet transfusion.[109–112] This area deserves further study, since it is technically difficult to identify platelet-specific antibodies when there is intense HLA alloimmunization as well. Techniques for doing so are improving.[112,113]

FEBRILE NONHEMOLYTIC TRANSFUSION REACTIONS (FNHTR)

Prior to the availability of methods for leukoreduction, approximately 20 percent of platelet transfusions were accompanied by FNHTR.[114]

Some of these reactions were undoubtedly due to antibodies in the patient directed against either leukocyte-specific or HLA antigens on leukocytes contaminating the platelet product. Leukocyte depletion by filtration during infusion reduced the frequency of these reactions, but many continued to occur.[114,115] It is now clear that contaminating leukocytes produce inflammatory cytokines such as interleukin-1, interleukin-6, interleukin-8, and tumor necrosis factor alpha during storage at 20 to 24°C and that these compounds are responsible for many FNHTR since they are not removed by bedside filtration.[116,117] These reactions provide a strong argument for routine, prestorage removal of leukocytes.

Nonetheless, FNHTR occur in approximately 2 percent of platelet transfusions even with prestorage leukoreduction.[118] The cause of these reactions is not known. They may be related to plasma proteins or products produced during storage by the platelets themselves. In these rare cases, one can wash the platelets free of plasma prior to infusion.[119]

TRANSMISSION OF CYTOMEGALOVIRUS (CMV)

In asymptomatic carriers, this virus resides in the nuclei of subsets of leukocytes with little virus free in plasma. It has been shown that the use of leukoreduced blood components is essentially equivalent to the use of components from CMV-negative donors in terms of risk of CMV transmission.[120] Since this infection is particularly dangerous for severely immunocompromised patients, such as those who have had a recent allogeneic bone marrow transplantation, some clinicians continue to use CMV-negative blood products along with leukoreduction in this select population.

GRAFT-VERSUS-HOST DISEASE (GVHD)

Immunosuppressed patients may develop GVHD from T lymphocytes present in any transfusion, including platelet transfusion. Thus, it is standard practice to treat platelet concentrates with gamma irradiation to inhibit proliferation of these T lymphocytes when the recipient had been heavily immunosuppressed.[121] Clinicians are progressively applying this practice to all patients who have received cytotoxic chemotherapy. Exposure to 5000 rad appears to have no deleterious effect on platelets. It is important to emphasize that current methods of leukoreduction do not remove enough T cells to prevent GVHD.

COMPLICATIONS OF FILTRATION OF PLATELET CONCENTRATES

Finally, there may be complications of platelet transfusion related to the removal of leukocytes by filtration of platelet concentrates at the bedside. Severe hypotension has been reported,[122] predominantly when negatively charged leukocyte reduction filters are used in patients who are receiving ACE inhibitors.[123] One proposed mechanism is that high-molecular-weight kininogen is converted to bradykinin, a potent vasodilator, by exposure to a negatively charged surface. Bradykinin is normally metabolized by ACE in a few seconds but may circulate much longer in patients receiving ACE inhibitors. Some investigators have found no clinically significant contact system activation by these filters.[124] Thus, the mechanisms behind these hypotensive reactions are still hypothetical, and more work needs to be done.

COMPLICATIONS DUE TO CONTAMINATING RED CELLS

When transfusing platelet concentrates to women of child-bearing potential who are Rh-negative, one needs to be concerned about sensitization by Rh-positive red cells contaminating infused platelets. In practice, sensitization is rather uncommon in immunosuppressed pa-

tients.[125] However, where possible, one should administer platelets from Rh-negative donors. When this is not possible, one can administer Rh immunoglobulin (RhoGAM), about 20 μg intramuscularly per unit of platelets, so that the infused red cells will be cleared prior to sensitization. A full dose of RhoGAM, 300 μg, is sufficient to suppress the immune response to 15 ml of Rh-positive red cells.

There are enough red cells contaminating platelet concentrates to transmit both malaria and babesiosis if the donor is parasitemic with these infections.

COMPLICATIONS DUE TO PLASMA AND ITS CONTENTS

CONTAMINATING MICROORGANISMS

Storage of platelet concentrates at 20 to 24°C allows proliferation to dangerous levels of bacteria that occasionally contaminate units of blood or apheresis platelet concentrates.[34] Contamination may occur because of asymptomatic bacteremia in the donor at the time of venipuncture, inadequate decontamination of the skin, or because of venipuncture through areas of the skin where bacterial colonization is deeper than can be reached by such decontamination.[126] Bacterial contamination that might not be clinically significant after 2 to 3 days of storage may become so after 5 to 7 days.[127] As previously mentioned, platelet concentrates storage is limited to 5 days for this reason.

The magnitude of this problem is commonly underestimated.[128] Estimates suggest that there may be contamination of 5 to 10 units per 10,000 whole-blood-derived platelet concentrates and 150 clinical episodes associated with severe morbidity and death in the United States per year.[129] This is 50- to 250-fold higher than the risk of mortality from transmission by transfusion of HIV or hepatitis B or C infection.

There are several potential approaches to this important problem. Because apheresis involves only one donor and one venipuncture, there may be less risk than for pooled whole-blood-derived platelet concentrates, although this has not been conclusively demonstrated. Under investigation are methods for screening platelet products for bacteria before transfusion[36] and methods of viral inactivation which also inactivate bacteria.[35] The methods of viral inactivation may inactivate T lymphocytes and prevent GVHD as well.[130]

The plasma diluent of platelet concentrates can transmit viruses such as hepatitis B and C and HIV. Recently improved methods of donor screening and testing have reduced but not eliminated this risk. As mentioned, methods for viral inactivation are being sought.[35] Transmission of the parasite, *Trypanosoma cruzi*, which is responsible for Chagas disease, has also occurred with platelet transfusion.

PLASMA PROTEINS

Many transfusion services attempt to transfuse ABO-identical platelet concentrates. However, this is not always possible. When anti-A or anti-B is transfused to a patient whose red cells carry A or B, a positive direct antiglobulin test may be observed in the laboratory, making red cell compatibility testing more difficult.[131] Actual accelerated destruction of the patient's red cells is rare.[132] However, on very rare occasions, frank acute hemolysis has been observed.[133]

As with any plasma infusion, one may encounter urticaria or anaphylactic shock in a patient with IgA deficiency and circulating anti-IgA, or transfusion-associated acute lung injury when a donor has leukocyte antibodies that can react with antigens on the leukocytes of the recipient.[134]

REFERENCES

1. Surgenor DM, Wallace EL, Hao SHS, et al: Collection and transfusion of blood in the United States, 1982–1988. *N Engl J Med* 332:1646, 1990.

2. Wallace EL, Surgenor DM, Hao HS, et al: Collection and transfusion of blood and blood components in the United States, 1989. *Transfusion* 33:139, 1993.

3. Wallace EL, Churchill WH, Surgenor DM, et al: Collection and transfusion of blood and blood components in the United States, 1994. *Transfusion* 38:625, 1998.

4. Kelley DL, Fegan RL, Ng AT, et al: High-yield platelet concentrates attainable by continuous quality improvement reduce platelet transfusion cost and donor exposure. *Transfusion* 37:482, 1997.

5. Sweeney JD, Holme S, Heaton WA, et al: White cell-reduced platelet concentrates prepared by in-line filtration of platelet-rich plasma. *Transfusion* 35:131, 1995.

6. Murphy S, Heaton WA, Rebulla P: Platelet production in the old world and the new. *Transfusion* 36:751, 1996.

7. Pietersz RN, Loos JA, Reesink HW: Platelet concentrates stored in plasma for 72 hours at 22°C prepared from buffy coats of citrate-phosphate-dextrose blood collected in a quadruple-bag saline-adenine-glucose-mannitol system. *Vox Sang* 49:81, 1985.

8. Bertolini F, Rebulla P, Riccardi D: Evaluation of platelet concentrates prepared from buffy coats and stored in a glucose-free crystalloid medium. *Transfusion* 29:605, 1989.

9. Bertolini F, Rebulla P, Marangoni F, et al: Platelet concentrates stored in synthetic medium after filtration. *Vox Sang* 62:82, 1992.

10. Heaton WAL, Rebulla P, Pappalettera M, Dzik WH: A comparative analysis of different methods for routine blood component preparation. *Transfusion* 11:116, 1997.

11. Van Delden CJ, de Wit HJC, Smit Sibinga CTH: Comparison of blood component preparation systems based on buffy coat removal: component specifications, efficiency, and process costs. *Transfusion* 38:860, 1998.

12. Adams MR, Dumont LJ, McCall M, Heaton WA: Clinical trial and local process evaluation of an apheresis system for preparation of white cell-reduced platelet components. *Transfusion* 38:966, 1998.

13. Yockey C, Murphy S, Eggers L, et al: Evaluation of the Amicus Separator in the collection of apheresis platelets. *Transfusion* 38:848, 1998.

14. Holme S, Andres M, Goermar N, Giordano GF: Improved removal of white cells with minimal platelet loss by filtration of apheresis platelets during collection. *Transfusion* 39:74, 1999.

15. Moog R, Valbonesi M, Carlier P: Collection of platelets and peripheral progenitor cells with Fresenius AS.TEC 204 blood cell separator. *J Clin Apheresis* 12:126, 1997.

16. McLeod BC, Price TH, Owen H, et al: Frequency of immediate adverse effects associated with apheresis donation. *Transfusion* 38:938, 1998.

17. Goodnough LT, Ali S, Despotis G, et al: Economic impact of donor platelet count and platelet yield in apheresis products: relevance for emerging issues in platelet transfusion therapy. *Vox Sang* 76:43, 1999.

18. Rugg N, Pitman C, Menitove JE, et al: A feasibility evaluation of an automated blood component collection system for platelets and red cells. *Transfusion* 39:460, 1999.

19. Popovsky MA: Quality of blood components filtered before storage and at the bedside: implications for transfusion practice. *Transfusion* 35:470, 1996.

20. Williamson LM, Wimperis JZ, Williamson P, et al: Bedside filtration of blood products in the prevention of HLA alloimmunization—A prospective randomized study. *Blood* 83:3028, 1994.

21. Murphy S, Gardner FH: Platelet preservation. Effect of storage temperature on maintenance of platelet viability—deleterious effect of refrigerated storage. *N Engl J Med* 280:1094, 1969.

22. Murphy S: Platelet storage for transfusion. *Semin Hematol* 22:165, 1985.

23. Murphy S, Gardner FH: Platelet storage at 22°C: role of gas transport across plastic containers in maintenance of viability. *Blood* 46:209, 1975.

24. Moroff G, George VM: The maintenance of platelet properties upon limited discontinuation of agitation during storage. *Transfusion* 30:427, 1990.

25. Murphy S: The oxidation of exogenously added organic anions by platelets facilitates maintenance of pH during their storage for transfusion at 22°C. *Blood* 85:1929, 1995.

26. Murphy S, Shimizu T, Miripol J: Platelet storage for transfusion in synthetic media: further optimization of ingredients and definition of their roles. *Blood* 86:3951, 1995.

27. Corash L, Behrman B, Rheinschmidt M, et al: Post-transfusion viability and tolerability of photochemically treated platelet concentrates (PC). *Blood* 90:267a, 1997.

28. Shanwell A, Larsson S, Aschan J, et al: A randomized trial comparing the use of fresh and stored platelets in the treatment of bone marrow transplant recipients. *Eur J Haematol* 49:77, 1992.

29. Leach MR, AuBuchon JP: Effect of storage time on clinical efficacy of single-donor platelet units. *Transfusion* 33:661, 1993.

30. Murphy S, Kahn RA, Holme S, et al: Improved storage of platelets for transfusion in a new container. *Blood* 60:194, 1982.

31. Peter-Salonen K, Bucher UE, Nydegger UE: Comparison of post-transfusion recoveries achieved with either fresh or stored platelet concentrates. *Blut* 54:207, 1987.

32. Norol F, Kuentz M, Cordonnier C, et al: Influence of clinical status on the efficiency of stored platelet transfusion. *Br J Haematol* 86:125, 1994.

33. Hogge DE, Thompson BW, Schiffer CA: Platelet storage for 7 days in second-generation blood bags. *Transfusion* 26:131, 1986.

34. Klein HG, Dodd RY, Ness PM, et al: Current status or microbial contamination of blood components: summary of a conference. *Transfusion* 37:95, 1997.

35. Lin L, Cook DN, Wiesehahn GP, et al: Photochemical inactivation of viruses and bacteria in platelet concentrates by use of a novel psoralen and long-wavelength ultraviolet light. *Transfusion* 37:423, 1997.

36. Mitchell KM, Brecher ME: Approaches to the detection of bacterial contamination in cellular blood products. *Transfusion Med Rev* 13:132, 1999.

37. Murphy S, Rebulla P, Bertolini F, et al: In vitro assessment of the quality of stored platelet concentrates. *Transfusion Med Rev* 8:29, 1994.

38. Holme S, Moroff G, Murphy S: A multi-laboratory evaluation of in vitro platelet assays: the tests for extent of shape change and response to hypotonic shock. *Transfusion* 38:31, 1998.

39. Bertolini F, Murphy S: A multicenter evaluation of reproducibility of swirling in platelet concentrates. *Transfusion* 34:796, 1994.

40. Murphy S, Martinez J, Holburn R: Stability of plasma fibrinogen during storage of platelet concentrates at 22°C. *Transfusion* 23:480, 1983.

41. Murphy S, Sayar SN, Abdou NL, et al: Platelet preservation by freezing. Use of dimethylsulfoxide as cryoprotective agent. *Transfusion* 14:139, 1975.

42. Towell BL, Levine SP, Knight WA III, et al: A comparison of frozen and fresh platelet concentrates in the support of thrombocytopenic patients. *Transfusion* 26:525, 1986.

43. Lazarus HM, Kaniecki-Green EA, Warm SE, et al: Therapeutic effectiveness of frozen platelet concentrates for transfusion. *Blood* 57:243, 1981.

44. Schiffer CA, Aisner J, Wiernik PH: Frozen autologous platelet transfusion for patients with leukemia. *N Engl J Med* 299:7, 1978.

45. Currie LM, Livesey SA, Harper JR, Connor J: Cryopreservation of single-donor platelets with a reduced dimethyl sulfoxide concentration by the addition of second-messenger effectors: enhanced retention of in vitro functional activity. *Transfusion* 38:160, 1998.

46. Manno CS, Hedbert KW, Kim HC, et al: Comparison of the hemostatic effects of fresh whole blood, stored whole blood, and components after open heart surgery in children. *Blood* 77:930, 1991.

47. Lee DH, Blajchman MA: Novel platelet products and substitutes. *Transfusion Med Rev* 12:175, 1998.

48. Mannucci PM: Hemostatic drugs. *N Engl J Med* 339:245, 1998.

49. Bishop JF, McGrath K, Wolf MM, et al: Clinical factors influencing the efficacy of pooled platelet transfusions. *Blood* 71:383, 1988.

50. Davis KB, Slichter SJ, Corash L: Corrected count increment and percent platelet recovery as measures of posttransfusion platelet response: problems and a solution. *Transfusion* 39:586, 1999.

51. Friedberg RC, Donnelly SF, Boyd JC, et al: Clinical and blood bank factors in the management of platelet refractoriness and alloimmunization. *Blood* 81:3428, 1993.

52. Klumpp TR, Herman J, Innis S, et al: Factors associated with response to platelet transfusion following hematopoietic stem cell transplantation. *Bone Marrow Transplant* 17:1035, 1996.

53. Doughty HA, Murphy MF, Metcalfe P, et al: Relative importance of immune and non-immune causes of platelet refractoriness. *Vox Sang* 66:200, 1994.

54. Alcorta I, Pereira A, Ordinas A: Clinical and laboratory factors associated with platelet transfusion refractoriness: a case-control study. *Br J Haematol* 93:220, 1996.

55. Bock M, Muggenthaler KH, Schmidt U, et al: Influence of antibiotics on posttransfusion platelet increment. *Transfusion* 36:952, 1996.

56. O'Connell B, Lee EJ, Schiffer CA: The value of 10-minute posttransfusion platelet counts. *Transfusion* 28:66, 1988.

57. Bishop JF, Matthews JP, McGrath K, et al: Factors influencing 20-hour increments after platelet transfusion. *Transfusion* 31:392, 1991.

58. Hersh JK, Hom EG, Brecher ME: Mathematical modeling of platelet survival with implications of optimal transfusion practice in the chronically platelet transfusion-dependent patient. *Transfusion* 38:637, 1998.

59. Norol F, Bierling P, Roudot-Thoraval F, et al: Platelet transfusion: a dose-response study. *Blood* 92:1448, 1998.

60. Klumpp TR, Herman JH, Gaughan JP, et al: Clinical consequences of alterations in platelet transfusion dose: a prospective, randomized, double-blind trial. *Transfusion* 39:674, 1999.

61. Hanson SR, Slichter SJ: Platelet kinetics in patients with bone marrow hypoplasia: evidence for a fixed platelet requirement. *Blood* 66:1105, 1985.

62. McVay PA, Toy PT: Lack of increased bleeding after liver biopsy in patients with mild hemostatic abnormalities. *Am J Clin Pathol* 94:747, 1990.

63. Kenet G, Lubetsky A, Shenkman B, et al: Cone and platelet analyser (CPA): a new test for the prediction of bleeding among thrombocytopenic patients. *Brit J Haematol* 101:255, 1998.

64. Gaydos LA, Freireich EJ, Mantel N: The quantitative relation between platelet count and hemorrhage in patients with acute leukemia. *N Engl J Med* 266:905, 1962.

65. Freireich EJ, Kliman A, Lawrence AG, Mantel N, Frei E: Response to repeated platelet transfusion from the same donor. *Ann Intern Med* 59:277, 1963.

66. Gmur J, Burger J, Schanz U, et al: Safety of stringent prophylactic platelet transfusion policy for patients with acute leukemia. *Lancet* 338:1223, 1991.

67. Sagmeister M, Oec L, Gmur J: A restrictive platelet transfusion policy allowing long-term support of outpatients with severe aplastic anemia. *Blood* 93:3124, 1999.

68. Heckman KD, Weiner GJ, Davis CS, et al: Randomized study of prophylactic platelet transfusion threshold during induction therapy for adult acute leukemia: 10,000/μL versus 20,000/μL. *J Clin Oncol* 15:1143, 1997.

69. Rebulla P, Finazzi G, Marangoni F, et al: The threshold for prophylactic platelet transfusions in adults with acute myeloid leukemia. *N Engl J Med* 337:1870, 1997.

70. Wandt H, Frank M, Ehninger G, et al: Safety and cost effectiveness of a 10×10^9/L trigger for prophylactic platelet transfusion compared with the traditional 20×10^9/L trigger: a prospective comparative trial in 105 patients with acute myeloid leukemia. *Blood* 91:3601, 1998.

71. Contreras M: The appropriate use of platelets: an update from the Edinburgh Consensus Conference. *Brit J Haematol* 101:10, 1998.

72. Nevo S, Swan V, Enger C, et al: Acute bleeding after bone marrow transplantation (BMT)—incidence and effect on survival. A quantitative analysis in 1,402 patients. *Blood*, 91:1469, 1998.

73. Bernstein SH, Nademanee AP, Vose JM, et al: A multicenter study of platelet recovery and utilization in patients after myeloablative therapy and hematopoietic stem cell transplantation. *Blood* 91:3509, 1998.

74. Reed RL, Ciavarella D, Heimbach DM, et al: Prophylactic platelet administration during massive transfusion. A prospective, randomized, double-blind clinical study. *Ann Surg* 203:40, 1986.

75. Simon TL, Aki Bechara, F, Murphy, W: Controlled trial of routine administration of platelet concentrates in cardiopulmonary bypass surgery. *Ann Thorac Surg* 37:359, 1984.

76. Carr JM, Kruskall MS, Kaye JA, et al: Efficacy of platelet transfusions in immune thrombocytopenia. *Am J Med* 80:1051, 1986.

77. McIntoch S, O'Brien RT, Schwartz AD, et al: Neonatal isoimmune purpura: response to platelet infusions. *J Pediatr* 82:1020, 1973.

78. Win N: Provision of random-donor platelets (HPA-1a positive) in neonatal alloimmune thrombocytopenia due to anti HPA-1a alloantibodies. *Vox Sang* 71:130, 1996.

79. Munizza M, Nance S, Keashen-Schnell MA, Sherwood W, Murphy S: Provision of HPA-1a (PLA1) negative platelets for neonatal alloimmune thrombocytopenia: screening, testing and transfusion protocol. *Immunohematology* 15:71, 1999.

80. Murphy S: Hereditary thrombocytopenia, in *Clinics in Haematology*, edited by JR O'Brien Jr, pp. 359–368. Saunders, London, 1972.

81. Bell WR, Braine HG, Ness PM, Kickler TS: Improved survival in thrombotic thrombocytopenic purpura-hemolytic uremic syndrome. *N Engl J Med* 325:398, 1991.

82. Warkentin TE, Kelton JG: Heparin and platelets *Hematol/Oncol Clin Nor Am* 4:243, 1990.

83. Kao KJ, del Rosario MLU: Role of class-II major histocompatibility complex (MHC)-antigen-positive donor leukocytes in transfusion-induced alloimmunization to donor class-I MHC antigens. *Blood* 92:690, 1998.

84. The Trial to Reduce Alloimmunization to Platelets Study Group: Leukocyte reduction and ultraviolet B irradiation of platelets to prevent alloimmunization and refractoriness to platelet transfusions. *N Engl J Med* 337:1861, 1997.

85. Vamvakas EC: Meta-analysis of randomized controlled trials of the efficacy of white cell reduction in preventing HLA-alloimmunization and refractoriness to random-donor platelet transfusions. *Transfusion Med Rev* 12:258, 1998.

86. Friedman DF, Lukas MB, Jawad A, et al: Alloimmunization to platelets in heavily transfused patients with sickle cell disease. *Blood* 88:3216, 1996.

87. Sintnicolaas K, van Marwijk Kooij M, Van Prooijen HC, et al: Leukocyte depletion of random single-donor platelet transfusions does not prevent secondary human leukocyte antigen-alloimmunization and refractoriness: a randomized prospective study. *Blood* 85:824, 1995.

88. Bishop JF, Matthews JP, Yuen K, et al: The definition of refractoriness to platelet transfusions. *Transfusion Med Rev* 2:35, 1992.

89. Hogge DE, Dutcher JP, Aisner J, et al: Lymphocytotoxic antibody is a predictor of response to random donor platelet transfusion. *Am J Hematol* 14:363, 1983.

90. McFarland JG, Anderson AJ, Slichter SJ: Factors influencing the transfusion response to HLA-selected apheresis donor platelets in patients refractory to random platelet concentrates. *Br J Haematol* 73:380, 1989.

91. Phekoo KJ, Hambley H, Schey SA, et al: Audit of practice in platelet refractoriness. *Vox Sang* 73:81, 1997.

92. Engelfriet CP, Reesink HW: Management of alloimmunized, refractory patients in need of platelet transfusions. *Vox Sang* 73:191, 1997.

93. Dutcher JP, Schiffer CA, Aisner J, et al: Long-term follow-up of patients with leukemia receiving platelet transfusions: identification of a large group of patients who do not become alloimmunized. *Blood* 58:1007, 1981.

94. Dutcher JP, Schiffer CA, Aisner J, et al: Alloimmunization following platelet transfusion: the absence of a dose-response relationship. *Blood* 57:395, 1981.

95. Lee EJ, Schiffer CA: Serial measurement of lymphocytotoxic antibody and response to nonmatched platelet transfusion in alloimmunized patients. *Blood* 70:1727, 1987.

96. Rodey GE, Neylan JF, Whelchel JD, Reves KW: Epitope specificity of HLA Class I alloantibodies I. Frequency analysis of antibodies to private versus public specificities in potential transplant recipients. *Hum Immunol* 39:272, 1994.

97. Zimmermann R, Wittmann G, Zingsem J, et al: Antibodies to private and public HLA class I epitopes in platelet recipients. *Transfusion* 39:772, 1999.

98. MacPherson BR: HLA antibody formation within the HLA-A1 cross-reactive group in multitransfused platelet recipients. *Am J Hematol* 30:228, 1989.

99. Yankee RA, Grumet FC, Rogentine GN: Platelet transfusion. The selection of compatible platelet donors for refractory patients by lymphocyte HLA typing. *N Engl J Med* 281:1208, 1969.

100. Duquesnoy RJ, Filip DJ, Rodey GE, et al: Successful transfusion of platelets "mismatched" for HLA antigens to alloimmunized thrombocytopenic patients. *Am J Hematol* 22:219, 1977.

101. Von dem Borne AEG, Ouwehand WH, Kuijpers RW: Theoretic and practical aspects of platelet crossmatching. *Transfusion Med Rev* 4:265, 1990.

102. Gelb AB, Leavitt AD: Crossmatch-compatible platelets improve corrected count increments in patients who are refractory to randomly selected platelets. *Transfusion* 37:624, 1997.

103. Bryant PC, Vayntrub TA, Schrandt HA, et al: HLA antibody enhancement by double addition of serum: use in platelet donor selection. *Transfusion* 32:839, 1992.

104. Petz LD, Garratty G, Clark BD, et al: The effectiveness of an antibody

specificity prediction (ASP) method for selecting platelets for transfusion to alloimmunized patients [Abstract]. *Blood* 86:546a, 1995.

105. Murphy S, Varma M: Selecting platelets for transfusion of the alloimmunized patient: a review. *Immunohematology* 14:117, 1998.

106. Santoso S, Kiefel V, Mueller-Eckhardt C: Blood groups A and B determinants are expressed on platelet glycoproteins IIa, IIIa, Ib. *Thromb Haemost* 65:196, 1991.

107. Lee EJ, Schiffer CA: ABO compatibility can influence the results of platelet transfusion. *Transfusion* 29:384, 1989.

108. Brand A, Sintnicolaas K, Claas FJH, et al: ABH antibodies causing platelet transfusion refractoriness. *Transfusion* 26:463, 1986.

109. Langenscheidt F, Kiefel V, Santoso S, et al: Platelet transfusion refractoriness associated with two rare platelet-specific alloantibodies (anti-Bak^a and anti-P1^{A2}) and multiple HLA antibodies. *Transfusion* 28:597, 1988.

110. Ikeda H, Mitani T, Ohnuma M, et al: A new platelet-specific antigen, Nak^a, involved in the refractoriness of HLA-matched platelet transfusion. *Vox Sang* 57:213, 1989.

111. Saji H, Maruya E, Fujii H, et al: New platelet antigen, Siba, involved in platelet transfusion refractoriness in a Japanese man. *Vox Sang* 56:283, 1989.

112. Kekomaki S, Volin L, Koistinen P, et al: Successful treatment of platelet transfusion refractoriness: the use of platelet transfusions matched for both human leucocyte antigens (HLA) and human platelet alloantigens (HPA) in alloimmunized patients with leukaemia. *Eur J Haematol* 60:112, 1998.

113. Kiefel V, Santoso S, Weisheit M, et al: Monoclonal antibody-specific immobilization of platelet antigens (MAIPA): a new tool for the identification of platelet-reactive antibodies. *Blood* 70:1722, 1987.

114. Mangano MM, Chambers LA, Kruskall MS: Limited efficacy of leukopoor platelets for prevention of febrile transfusion reactions. *Am J Clin Pathol* 95:733, 1991.

115. Goodnough LT, Riddell J, Lazarus H, et al: Prevalence of platelet transfusion reactions before and after implementation of leukocyte-depleted platelet concentrates by filtration. *Vox Sang* 65:103, 1993.

116. Heddle NM, Klama L, Singer J, et al: The role of the plasma from platelet concentrates in transfusion reactions. *N Engl J Med* 331:625, 1994.

117. Heddle NM, Klama L, Meyer R, et al: A randomized controlled trial comparing plasma removal with white cell reduction to prevent reactions to platelets. *Transfusion* 39:231, 1999.

118. Federowicz I, Barrett BB, Andersen JW, et al: Characterization of reactions after transfusion of cellular blood components that are white cell reduced before storage. *Transfusion* 36:21, 1996.

119. Buck SA, Kickler TS, McGuire M, et al: The utility of platelet washing using an automated procedure for severe platelet allergic reactions. *Transfusion* 27:391, 1987.

120. Bowden RA, Slichter SJ, Sayers M, et al: A comparison of filtered leukocyte-reduced and cytomegalovirus (CMV) seronegative blood products for the prevention of transfusion-associated CMV infection after marrow transplant. *Blood* 86:3598, 1995.

121. Leitman SF, Holland PV: Irradiation of blood products. Indications and guidelines. *Transfusion* 25:293, 1985.

122. Hume HA, Popovsky MA, Benson K, et al: Hypotensive reactions: a previously uncharacterized complication of platelet transfusion? *Transfusion* 36:904, 1996.

123. Mair B, Leparc GF: Hypotensive reactions associated with platelet transfusions and angiotensin-converting enzyme inhibitors. *Vox Sang* 74:27, 1998.

124. Scott CF, Brandwein H, Whitbread J, Colman RW: Lack of clinically significant contact system activation during platelet concentrate filtration by leukocyte removal filters. *Blood* 92:616, 1998.

125. Goldfinger D, McGinniss MH: Rh-incompatible platelet transfusion—risks and consequences of sensitizing immunosuppressed patients. *N Engl J Med* 284:942, 1971.

126. Anderson KC, Lew MA, Gorgone BC, et al: Transfusion-related sepsis after prolonged platelet storage. *Am J Med* 81:405, 1986.

127. Heal JM, Singal S, Sardisco E, et al: Bacterial proliferation in platelet concentrates. *Transfusion* 26:388, 1993.

128. AuBuchon JP, Kruskall MS: Transfusion safety: realigning efforts and risks. *Transfusion* 37:1211, 1997.

129. Svoboda R, Lipton KS: Bacterial contamination of blood components. AABB Association Bulletin #96–6, 2, 1996.

130. Grass JA, Hei DJ, Metchette K, et al: Inactivation of leukocytes in platelet concentrates by photochemical treatment with psoralen plus UVA. *Blood* 91:2180, 1998.

131. Garratty G: Problems associated with passively transfused blood group alloantibodies. *Coagulation Transfusion Med* 109:769, 1997.

132. Mair B, Benson K: Evaluation of changes in hemoglobin levels associated with ABO-incompatible plasma in apheresis platelets. *Transfusion* 38:51, 1998.

133. McManigal S, Sims KL: Intravascular hemolysis secondary to ABO incompatible platelet products. An underrecognized transfusion reaction. *Am J Clin Pathol* 111:202, 1999.

134. Ramanathan RK, Triulzi DJ, Logan TF: Transfusion-related acute lung injury following random donor platelet transfusion: a report of two cases. *Vox Sang* 73:43, 1997.

135. Hogman CF, Berseus O, Eriksson L, Gulliksson H: Buffy-coat-derived platelet concentrates: Swedish experience. *Transfusion Sci* 18:3, 1997.

136. Murphy S: Platelet transfusion therapy in *Thrombosis and Hemorrhage*, edited by J Loscalzo, AI Schafer, chap 51, 2nd ed, Williams & Wilkins, Philadelphia, 1998.

PREPARATION AND CLINICAL USE OF PLASMA AND PLASMA FRACTIONS

KENNETH D. FRIEDMAN
JAY E. MENITOVE

> Plasma collected from blood donors is provided as a blood component following minimal manipulation or as a plasma derivative after an extensive fractionation process. Plasma components include fresh-frozen plasma and the precipitate remaining after frozen plasma is thawed at 4°C (39.2°F), cryoprecipitate. Plasma components are used to replace inherited or acquired coagulation factor deficiencies, reverse the effects of warfarin when hemostasis is required urgently, and to replete plasma removed during plasma exchange therapy for thrombotic thrombocytopenic purpura. Cryoprecipitate serves as a source of fibrinogen and as a substrate for fibrin sealant. Plasma derivatives include albumin; immunoglobulin preparations; coagulation factors VIII, IX, XI, and XIII and prothrombin complex concentrates; and replacement products for antithrombin III, Cl esterase inhibitor, and α-proteinase inhibitor deficiencies.

PREPARATION AND FRACTIONATION OF PLASMA COMPONENTS AND DERIVATIVES

Plasma used for transfusion is separated from whole blood by centrifugation, tested, stored, and infused without significant modification. Plasma derivatives, including albumin, factor VIII, other hemostatic proteins, and immunoglobulins, are prepared in concentrated form following large-scale plasma fractionation procedures. This chapter addresses the preparation and clinical uses of plasma components and plasma derivatives.

PLASMA COMPONENTS

Blood banks and transfusion services provide various plasma components containing the fluid portion of donated whole blood. Plasma components are prepared from whole blood by separating the cellular

and liquid portions of blood by centrifugation or by apheresis technology in which plasma and not cellular elements are collected.

FRESH-FROZEN PLASMA

Fresh-frozen plasma (FFP) is separated within 8 h of whole-blood collection, frozen at −18°C (−0.4°F) or colder, and stored in the frozen state for up to 1 year. FFP volume varies between 180 and 300 ml. FFP contains plasma proteins and all coagulation factors. Since idealized plasma contains 1 unit of each coagulation factor, a unit of FFP contains approximately 200 units of each coagulation factor, or 7 percent of the coagulation factor activity of a 70-kg patient.[1-4]

PLASMA FROZEN WITHIN 24 H OF COLLECTION

Plasma that is frozen within 24 h of whole-blood collection contains stable coagulation factors at the same concentration as present in FFP. The levels of factors V and VIII are reduced approximately 15 percent compared to those in FFP.[4]

LIQUID PLASMA

Liquid plasma is plasma that is separated no more than 5 days after the expiration date of the whole blood. Stable coagulation factor levels are similar to those in FFP, but levels of labile factors, V and VIII, are reduced significantly.[5]

CRYO-POOR PLASMA

The supernatant plasma remaining after the removal of cryoprecipitated material is referred to as cryo-poor plasma. It is relatively deficient in fibrinogen, factor VIII, and von Willebrand factor (vWF) multimers.[4,7]

SOLVENT-DETERGENT–TREATED PLASMA

Solvent-detergent–treated (SD) plasma is a pooled plasma product that undergoes treatment with the solvent tri-(n-butyl)-phosphate (TNBP) and the detergent Triton X-100 to inactivate lipid-enveloped viruses, such as hepatitis B and C and the human immunodeficiency virus (HIV).[8-10] Plasma treated with the SD process is obtained from up to 2500 donations that are pooled together and subsequently aliquoted into 200-ml volumes. The process is not effective against nonenveloped viruses, such as hepatitis A and parvovirus, and is partially effective against emerging viruses, such as the TT virus.[11,12] The SD process does not alter or inactivate labile coagulation factors or other plasma proteins, such as fibrinogen or immunoglobulin. It lacks the largest vWF multimers.[9] SD plasma is stored in the frozen state. The cost-effectiveness of this product is unclear.[13]

DONOR RETESTED PLASMA

Donor retested plasma (DR-FFP) refers to single units of FFP prepared from repeat blood donors. DRP is prepared by making FFP from a single unit of whole blood, quarantining the plasma in the frozen state, and releasing the frozen plasma for use when the donor returns at least 112 days later and again has negative test results for hepatitis B and C and HIV. The 112-day time frame was chosen because it exceeds the ''window period'' interval during which viral transmission may occur despite negative test results for hepatitis B, C, and HIV.[14]

Acronyms and abbreviations that appear in this chapter include: aPCC, activated prothrombin complex concentrate; API, α₁-proteinase inhibitor; AT-III, antithrombin III; BU, Bethesda unit; CMV, cytomegalovirus; DDAVP, desmopressin; DEAE, diethylaminoethyl; DIC, disseminated intravascular coagulation; DR-FFP, donor retested fresh-frozen plasma; FDA, U.S. Food and Drug Administration; FFP, fresh-frozen plasma; HIV, human immunodeficiency virus; HLA, human leukocyte antigen; HTLV, human T lymphocytotropic virus; IL, interleukin; INR, international normalized ratio; ITP, immune-mediated thrombocytopenia; IVIg, intravenous immunoglobulin; MHC, major histocompatibility complex; PCC, prothrombin complex concentrate; PCR, polymerase chain reaction; PEG, polyethylene glycol; PT, prothrombin time; PTT, partial thromboplastin time; SD, solvent-detergent treated; TNBP, tri-(n-butyl)-phosphate; TNF-α, tumor necrosis factor α; TTP, thrombotic thrombocytopenic purpura; vWD, von Willebrand disease; vWF, von Willebrand factor.

CRYOPRECIPITATE

Cryoprecipitate is prepared by thawing FFP at 1 to 6°C (33.8 to 42.8°F) and recovering the precipitated material. The cold-insoluble precipitate is then refrozen and stored at -18°C (-0.4°F) or colder for up to 1 year. Cryoprecipitate contains more than 150 mg of fibrinogen, more than 80 units of factor VIII, significant amounts of vWF (including the high-molecular-weight multimers), and some fibronectin and factor XIII in less than 15-ml volume.[2,6]

CLINICAL USE OF PLASMA AND CRYOPRECIPITATE

Contemporary guidelines for the use of FFP and cryoprecipitate appeared first in 1985 in a National Institutes of Health–sponsored consensus conference.[3] Subsequently, professional associations established panels and issued reports.[1,2,4,15–17] In general, there is agreement about use of FFP for replacement of coagulation factors to treat specific coagulopathies and for use as a replacement fluid for patients with thrombotic thrombocytopenic purpura (TTP) undergoing plasma exchange therapy.

The indications for FFP, SD plasma, and donor retested plasma are similar. SD plasma is not licensed for treatment of patients with disseminated intravascular coagulation (DIC) or for use in patients with coagulation factor deficiencies related to massive blood transfusion, although it has been used successfully in these situations.[10]

INDICATIONS FOR LIQUID PLASMA AND PLASMA FROZEN WITHIN 24 H OF COLLECTION

(Table 143-1) gives the indications for the use of liquid plasma and plasma frozen within 24 h of whole-blood collection.

Congenital or Acquired Coagulation Factor Deficiencies FFP, DR-FFP, and SD plasma is indicated for the correction of known congenital or acquired coagulation factor deficiencies, such as factor II, V, VII, X, XI, and XIII deficiencies; in patients with hemorrhage; or for an anticipated surgery or invasive procedure for which specific concentrates are not available.[1–4,15–17]

Hemostasis occurs when coagulation factor concentrations are at least 20 to 30 percent of normal and when fibrinogen levels are greater than 75 mg/dl. Coagulopathy is unusual until the prothrombin time (PT) and partial thromboplastin time (PTT) exceed 1.5 to 1.8 times control values.[15,16]

Urgent Reversal of Warfarin Effect In the setting of active bleeding, pending emergency surgery, or an invasive procedure, plasma infusion is indicated if insufficient time (approximately 6 h) is available for parenteral administration of vitamin K to reverse warfarin anticoagulation [PT greater than 18 s or international normalized ratio (INR) greater than 1.6].[1–4,15–17]

Treatment of Hemorrhage in the Presence of Elevated PT or PTT[1–4,15,16] Clinical settings in which hemorrhage and elevated (greater than 1.5 times normal) PT or PTT occur include chronic liver disease, DIC, and dilutional coagulopathy.[18–23] A clear correlation between elevated PT and PTT levels and INR values has not been established. Despite this relationship, in Canada, an INR of 2.0 has

been selected as the threshold INR for recommending plasma infusion for patients with severe liver disease with active bleeding or for whom surgery or other invasive procedures are planned.[4] In general, INR should be employed as an index in patients receiving warfarin who are in steady state.

Treatment of Bleeding in the Setting of Massive Blood Transfusion When PT and PTT Are Not Obtained in a Timely Manner[20–23] In general, the use of plasma to replace coagulation factor deficiencies should be based on timely laboratory test results. If such results cannot be obtained, plasma is indicated to treat microvascular bleeding in the setting of massive transfusion (more than one blood volume) on the basis of clinical judgment alone.

Plasma Exchange for TTP FFP has been used empirically for plasma exchange therapy or as an infusion to treat patients with TTP.[24,25] Plasma therapy effectiveness may be related to the presence of autoantibodies against a metalloprotease that degrades large vWF multimers in patients with acute TTP.[26,27] Plasma removal in the exchange process removes antibody and large multimers, while replacement with normal plasma restores normal-sized multimers. In some patients with chronic, relapsing TTP, the protease is absent. Large vWF multimers serve as a platelet-aggregating cofactor in TTP. Thus, degradation of these multimers has therapeutic implications. In this regard, cyro-poor plasma has been recommended in lieu of routine plasma-exchange therapy, since cryo-poor plasma is relatively deficient in large vWF multimers.[28] The metalloprotease is present in patients with hemolytic uremic syndrome and thus may explain why plasma therapy is usually ineffective in treating patients with this syndrome.[26]

Other Uses Plasma infusions are effective in preventing acute complications of protein C deficiency and have been used in neonates with purpura fulminans. Warfarin therapy should be instituted in both disorders for therapy.[29,30] DIC and severe acquired protein C deficiency are characteristic of meningococcemia and purpura fulminans.[31] An unlicensed monoclonal antibody–purified, vapor heat–treated protein C concentrate[32] has shown remarkable promise in these patients, with control of DIC, reversal of organ dysfunction, and reduction in morbidity and mortality rates.[33,34]

Plasma is used to replace protein S during surgery or when anticoagulants cannot be given. Treatment with oral anticoagulants is effective long-term therapy.[30]

DOSE AND MONITORING FOR PLASMA TRANSFUSIONS

The volume of the infused plasma component should be sufficient to achieve at least 30 percent coagulation factor levels, 10 to 15 ml plasma per kilogram of body weight (Fig. 143-1). Urgent reversal of warfarin may require 5 to 8 ml plasma per kilogram of body weight.[2,15] Plasma is present in platelet concentrates and should be considered in calculating the plasma dose when platelets and plasma are given simultaneously. Plasma components are labeled with the ABO and Rh type of the donor; infused plasma should be ABO compatible with the recipient's red cells. Compatibility testing for plasma transfusion is not necessary.

Following infusion, subsequent dosing should be based on coagulation factor intravenous recovery half-lives, the results of repeat coagulation testing, and clinical parameters.[2]

CONTRAINDICATIONS TO PLASMA TRANSFUSIONS

Plasma components should not be used for plasma expansion, albumin supplementation, correction of hypogammaglobulinemia, treatment of hemophilia or von Willebrand disease [vWD; where desmopressin (DDAVP) or virally inactivated concentrates are available], or treatment of other congenital procoagulant or anticoagulant factor deficiencies where virally inactivated or recombinant factor concentrates are preferred.[4]

TABLE 143-1 INDICATIONS FOR PLASMA TRANSFUSIONS*

Correction of known congenital or acquired coagulation factor deficiencies (e.g., factors II, V, VII, X, XI, or XIII) in patients with hemorrhage
Urgent reversal of warfarin effect
Treatment of microvascular hemorrhage in the presence of prolonged PT, PTT, or INR
Treatment of microvascular bleeding following massive blood transfusion when timely reporting of laboratory test result is not available
Plasma exchange for TTP

*FFP, DR-FFP, and SD plasma.

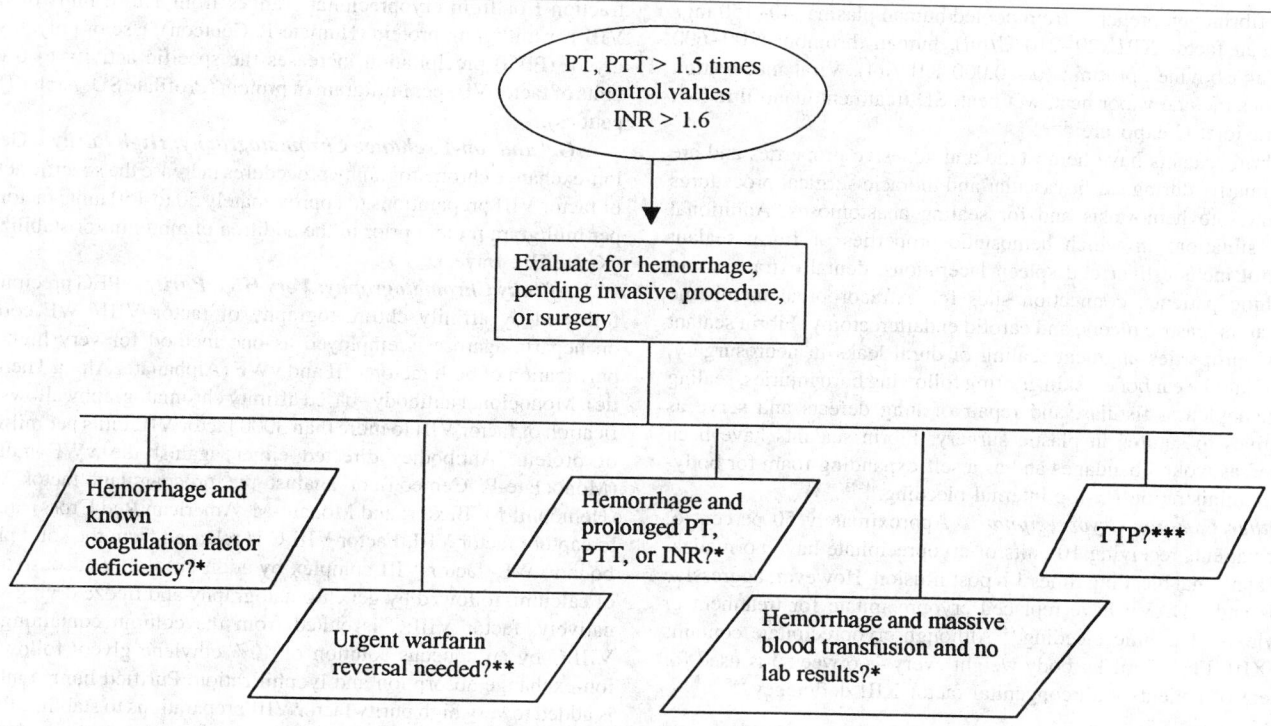

FIGURE 143-1   The decision pathway for plasma transfusions requires an evaluation of coagulation test results and clinical evidence of hemorrhage or an impending invasive procedure.
*If yes, infuse plasma, 10 to 15 ml/kg body weight. Monitor laboratory results to decide whether additional transfusions are necessary.
**If yes, infuse plasma, 5 to 8 ml/kg body weight.
***Plasma or cryo-poor plasma for exchange transfusion.

ADVERSE EVENTS ASSOCIATED WITH PLASMA TRANSFUSIONS

Plasma transfusions present the same risk as transfusion of other blood components for transmitting viral infection. The risk of viral transmission is decreased with SD-treated plasma and DR-FFP. However, hepatitis A superinfection of hepatitis C–infected patients is associated with fulminant hepatitis.[35] Intracellular viruses, such as cytomegalovirus (CMV) and HTLV-1, are not transmitted by plasma.

Allergic or anaphylactic reactions and transfusion-related acute lung injury occur infrequently. Volume overload may occur in patients with impaired cardiac reserve.[38]

Rh alloimmunization was reported following massive plasma infusion during plasma exchange therapy, presumably related to small amounts of contaminating red cells.[39] In general, plasma has a white blood cell content below that considered to cause human leukocyte antigen (HLA) alloimmunization or graft-versus-host disease, although significant numbers of leukocytes have been found in some plasma units.[40]

INDICATIONS FOR CRYOPRECIPITATE AND DOSAGE

Hypofibrinogenemia   Fibrinogen is concentrated 15- to 20-fold in cryoprecipitate compared to plasma. Commercially prepared fibrinogen concentrates are not available in the United States. Thus, cryoprecipitate is the component of choice for correction of hypofibrinogen-related bleeding or those at risk for bleeding. It is also indicated as prophylaxis in those at risk of bleeding as a result of marked hypofibrinogenemia (fibrinogen concentrations <80–100 mg/dl) facing an imminent invasive procedure or surgery.

In many instances, patients with severe hypofibrinogenemia have concomitant DIC. FFP alone may not raise the fibrinogen level to hemostatic levels (>100 mg/dl). Infusion of cryoprecipitate in doses of 1 bag per 5 kg body weight will augment fibrinogen levels by at least 75 mg/dl. Fibrinogen has a half-life of 3 to 5 days, and 50 percent of infused fibrinogen is recovered postinfusion. Additional doses should be given on the basis of laboratory measurements. For patients with inherited hypofibrinogenemia, infusions are given every other day.[1215–17]

von Willebrand Factor Replacement   Desmopressin is the preferred treatment option for patients with type I vWD. In those patients with other types of vWD or in those unresponsive to DDAVP, virally inactivated factor VIII concentrates containing adequate amounts of vWF (e.g., Humate-P) are indicated therapy. Cryoprecipitate represents an additional option for prophylactic therapy of those unresponsive to DDAVP or treatment of bleeding. About 50 percent of the vWF contained in the initial plasma is recovered in cryoprecipitate. Infusion of 1 bag of cryoprecipitate per 10 kg body weight is recommended.[215–17] Subsequent dosing should be based on an analysis of ristocetin cofactor activity, factor VIII antigen, or vWF multimer levels after transfusion. Measurement of the bleeding time to assess further dosing is not recommended.[2]

Hemophilia A   Cryoprecipitate is used infrequently for factor VIII replacement therapy in hemophilia A patients. In a 70-kg patient, factor VIII procoagulant activity levels increase approximately 2 percent for each bag of cryoprecipitate infused. Since the half-life of factor VIII is 8 to 12 h, repeat doses should be given at approximately this interval.

Fibrin Sealant   Fibrin sealants prepared by blood banks or by surgeons in operating suites, so-called homemade fibrin sealants, are prepared by mixing bovine thrombin (1000 U/ml) with an equal volume of cryoprecipitate. In May 1998, a commercial preparation was licensed by the U.S. Food and Drug Administration (FDA). This and other commercially formulated fibrin sealant preparations (Tisseel) contain fibrinogen prepared from pooled human plasma (40–150 mg/dl), human factor XIII (20–210 U/ml), human thrombin (200–600 U/ml), and bovine aprotinin (0–10,000 KIU/ml). Viral inactivation techniques include vapor heat, wet heat, SD treatment, nanofiltration, and ultraviolet C exposure.[41–43]

Fibrin sealants have hemostatic and adhesive properties and are used primarily during cardiovascular and thoracic surgical procedures as adjuncts to hemostasis and for sealing anastomoses. Additional clinical situations in which hemostatic properties of fibrin sealant are useful include liver and spleen lacerations, dental extractions in hemophilic patients, connection sites for extracorporeal membrane oxygenators, gastric ulcers, and carotid endarterectomy. Fibrin sealant adhesive properties augment sealing of dural leaks in neurosurgery, union of middle ear bones, skin grafting following burn injuries, sealing of bronchopleural fistulas, and repair of lung defects and serve as alternatives to sutures in plastic surgery. Fibrin sealants have been proposed as wound bandages and as a self-expanding foam for body-cavity administration to stop internal bleeding.[41–43]

Other Uses for Cryoprecipitate   Approximately 50 percent of uremic patients receiving 10 units of cryoprecipitate have normalization of abnormal bleeding times 1 h postinfusion. However, aggressive dialysis and DDAVP have replaced cryoprecipitate for treatment or prophylaxis of uremic bleeding.[44] Although cryoprecipitate contains factor XIII, FFP (5 ml/kg body weight every 4–6 weeks) is used for treatment of patients with congenital factor XIII deficiency.[945]

ADVERSE EVENTS ASSOCIATED WITH CRYOPRECIPITATE TRANSFUSIONS

Adverse effects associated with cryoprecipitate and fibrin sealant are similar to those associated with plasma infusion. In addition, some patients exposed to bovine thrombin develop autoantibodies to factor V that lead to hemorrhagic complications 7 to 14 days after exposure. Treatment of this complication includes infusion of FFP; possibly platelet concentrates, since platelets contain approximately 20 percent of the factor V in plasma; and immunosuppression with methylprednisolone.[46]

PLASMA DERIVATIVES

The Cohn-Oncley process is the prototype method of plasma fractionation.[47] Plasma subcomponents are separated by adding alcohol, altering the pH and temperature, and using additional chromatographic steps. The source plasma used in the fractionation process derives from volunteer and commercial donors. All donors are screened for risk factors associated with transfusion-transmitted infections, and all donations are tested for evidence of HIV and hepatitis (Fig. 143-2).[48]

FACTOR VIII CONCENTRATES (SEE TABLE 143-2)

Lyophilized factor VIII concentrates prepared from plasma pools containing as many as 20,000 donations have been distributed in the United States since the early 1970s (Table 143-2). The nomenclature for purity and the processes followed by various pharmaceutical companies to prepare various coagulation concentrates are not standardized.[49] Intermediate-purity preparations contain residual vWF, and some of these products are useful in the treatment of patients with vWD. Other contaminating proteins include fibrinogen, fibronectin, IgA, and IgG, while affinity-purified plasma-derived factor VIII preparations and recombinant products are essentially free of these contaminants.[50] Posttransfusion recovery and half-life are identical among the various preparations.[51] Major issues have been purity and viral safety.

PURIFICATION PROCEDURES[49,52,53]

Cryoprecipitation and Alcohol Precipitation: Intermediate Purity   The specific activity of factor VIII concentrates made from Cohn

fraction I or from cryoprecipitate ranges from 1 to 6 units of factor VIII per milligram protein (Humate-P, Centeon). Use of polyethylene glycol (PEG) precipitation increases the specific activity to 6 to 10 units of factor VIII per milligram of protein (Profilate SD, Alpha Therapeutics).

Gel and Ion-Exchange Chromatography: High Purity   Gel and ion-exchange chromatography procedures increase the specific activity of factor VIII preparations to approximately 50 to 150 units factor VIII per milligram protein prior to the addition of albumin for stabilization (Koate HP, Bayer).

Affinity Chromatography: Very High Purity   PEG precipitation followed by affinity chromatography of factor VIII/vWF complex on heparin-agarose is employed as one method for very high level purification of both factor VIII and vWF (Alphanate, Alpha Therapeutic). Monoclonal antibody–based affinity chromatography allows purification of factor VIII to more than 3000 factor VIII units per milligram of protein. Antibodies directed either against the vWF molecule (Monoclate-P, Centeon) or against the procoagulant factor VIII:C (Hemophil-M, Baxter; and Monarc-M, American Red Cross) are used to capture factor VIII. Factor VIII:C is released from the solid phase–bound vWF–factor VIII complex by addition of an aqueous solution of calcium, followed by gel chromatography and freeze drying. Alternatively, factor VIII:C is eluted from the column containing anti-VIII:C by an aqueous solution of 40% ethylene glycol followed by ion-exchange absorption and lyophilization. Purified human albumin is added to very high purity factor VIII preparations to stabilize the material.

Viral Inactivation   In response to transmission of hepatitis and HIV by earlier concentrates, viral inactivation methods were devised and introduced during the 1980s for pooled and/or processed plasma-derived blood products. Unfortunately, most severe hemophilic patients alive in the early 1980s had already been exposed to these infectious agents.[54] Subsequently, the efficiency of inactivation of viruses containing lipid envelopes was shown through prospective longitudinal studies of previously untransfused patients. However, transmission of nonenveloped agents, such as the hepatitis A virus, by some concentrates led to a recommendation to vaccinate patients likely to be exposed to clotting factor concentrates against hepatitis A. Hepatitis B vaccination was recommended previously.[55]

"Dry"-heated concentrates are lyophilized concentrates heated at 68°C (154.4°F) for 32 to 72 h to eliminate hepatitis risk. While partially effective against HIV,[56] "dry" heating of concentrate was not completely effective for eliminating the risk of hepatitis viruses or HIV.[495758] Prolonged dry heat (68°C for 144 h) is used in the treatment of some prothrombin complex concentrates (Proplex-T, Baxter; and Autoplex T, NABI), with dry heat at higher temperature [80°C (176°F) for 72 h] conferring viral safety for another (Konyne-80, Bayer).[59]

"Moist"-heated concentrates involve viral inactivation of lyophilized product by heating under a pressurized vapor phase (60°C for 10 h under 1190 mbar). Two prothrombin complex concentrates available in United States are so prepared (Feiba VH, Baxter; and Bebulin VH, Baxter).

Pasteurized, or "wet" heat–treated, factor concentrates include two available factor VIII concentrates (Humate-P, Centeon; and Monoclate-P, Centeon). Pasteurized concentrates do not appear to transmit HIV or hepatitis C.[49526061] However, transmission of parvovirus B19 has been reported.[62] An increase in the incidence of antibodies to factor VIII (inhibitors) found with the introduction of one pasteurized, controlled-pore, silica-adsorbed factor VIII led to a suggestion that clinicians treating hemophilia should follow serial inhibitor test results when patients change coagulation factor preparations[63]; this has not been observed with other concentrates.

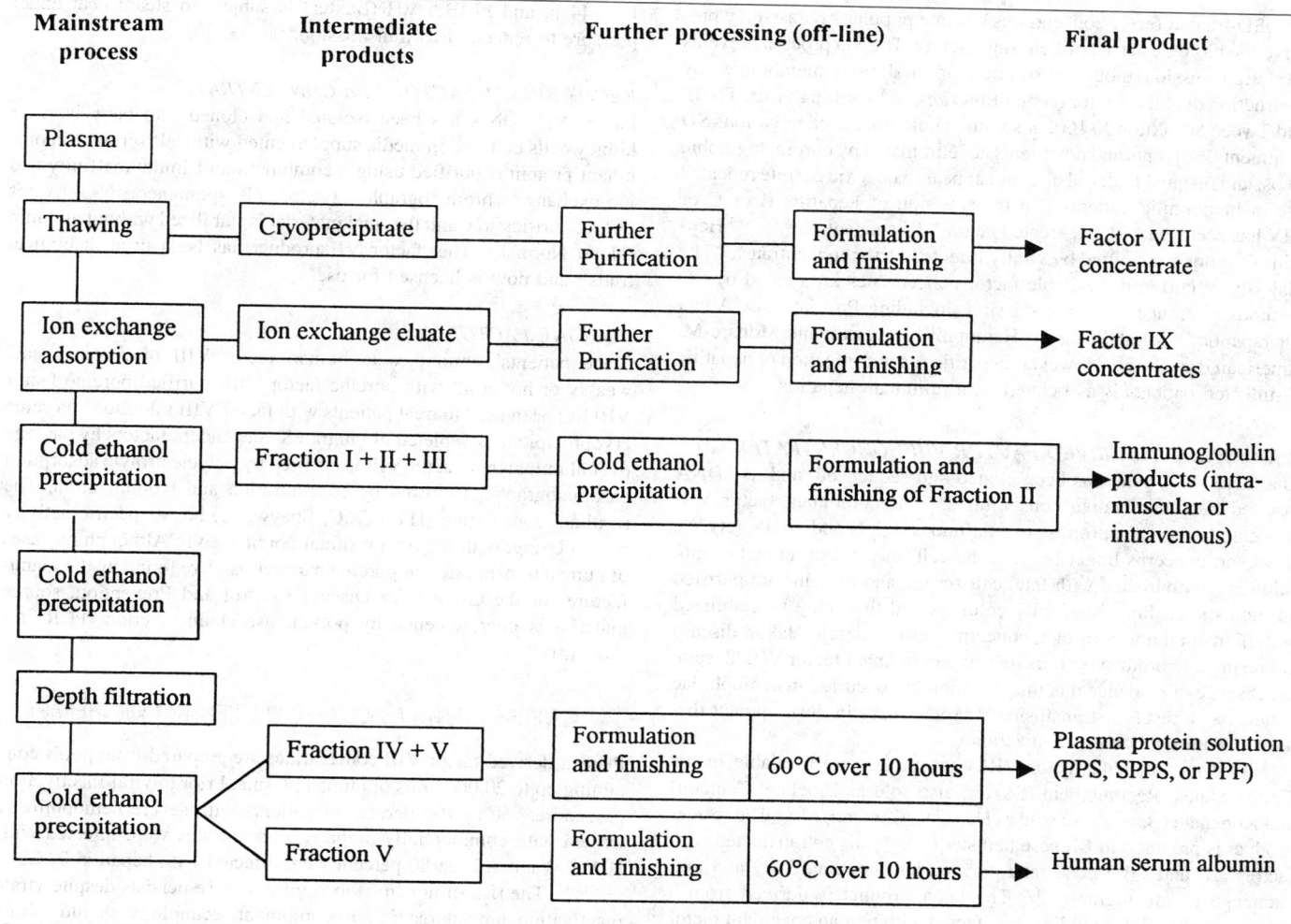

FIGURE 143-2   The cold ethanol plasma fractionation process involves multiple steps that result in various plasma derivative products. (Modified from PR Foster, B Cuthbertson: Procedures for the prevention of virus transmission by blood products, in *Blood, Blood Products and HIV*, edited by R Madhok, CD Forbes, BL Evatt, p 207, Chapman and Hall Medical, London, 1994; and DBL McClelland,[48] with permission.)

TABLE 143-2   FACTOR VIII PRODUCTS AVAILABLE IN THE UNITED STATES

Product	Manufacturer	Purity	Viral Inactivation Method
PLASMA DERIVED			
Humate-P	Centeon	Intermediate	Pasteurized 60°C 10 h
Profilate SD	Alpha	Intermediate	SD TNBP and polysorbate 80 and dry heat 60°C 36 h
Koate HP	Bayer	High	SD TNBP and polysorbate 80
HEPARIN-LIGAND OR IMMUNOAFFINITY, PLASMA DERIVED			
Alphanate	Alpha	High	SD TNBP and polysorbate 80 and dry heat 80°C 72 h
Hemophil-M	Baxter	Very high	SD TNBP and Triton X-100
Monarc-M	American Red Cross	Very high	SD TNBP and Triton X-100
Monoclate P	Centeon	Very high	Pasteurized 60°C 10 h
RECOMBINANT DNA DERIVED			
Recombinate (also Bioclate)	Baxter (also Centeon)	Ultra-high	None
Kogenate (also Helixate)	Bayer (also Centeon)	Ultra-high	None

SD-treated factor concentrates became popular because they preserve the biologic activity of clotting factors. The SD process prevents viral transmission though disruption of viral lipid membranes, by destruction of cell receptor recognition sites, or by killing virus. TNBP and Tween 80, Triton X-100, or sodium cholate are used in various SD treatments. Solvents and detergents are eliminated by chromatographic steps, and residual material does not appear to be toxic despite repeated use in hemophilic patients. No transmission of hepatitis B or C or HIV has occurred with SD-treated factor VIII concentrates.[49,57,58,64] Hepatitis G is not transmitted by virally infected factor concentrates.[65] The majority of currently available factor concentrates are treated by SD methods to reduce viral transmission (including Profilate SD, Alpha Therapeutic; Koate HP, Bayer; Hemophil-M, Baxter; and Monarc-M, American Red Cross). However, hepatitis A superinfection of hepatitis C–infected patients is associated with fulminant hepatitis.[35]

RECOMBINANT-DERIVED FACTOR VIII CONCENTRATES

The factor VIII gene has been cloned and sequenced, and its cDNA inserted into mammalian cell cultures.[66,67] Recombinant factor VIII concentrates hold the promise of continuous supply and viral safety.[68,69] However, concerns linger because the cell lines are of animal origin, cultures are nourished with fetal calf serum, and proteins are purified on monoclonal immunoaffinity columns and then may be stabilized with human albumin. In fact, concern over Creutzfeldt-Jakob disease has resulted in product withdrawals of recombinant factor VIII, despite the absence of evidence that this infection has occurred in hemophiliac patients as a result of transfusion.[70] Products are in development that do not require albumin stabilization.[71]

Two recombinant factor VIII concentrates are available in the United States: Recombinate (Baxter; also sold as Bioclate, Centeon) and Kogenate (Bayer; also sold as Helixate, Centeon).[49,72,73] The former product is prepared in Chinese hamster ovary cells cotransfected with factor VIII and vWF genes and purified by immunoaffinity and ion-exchange chromatography.[74,75] The latter product is derived from a baby hamster kidney cell line transfected with human coagulant factor VIII cDNA. The secreted protein is purified by ion-exchange chromatography and immunochromatography. Recombinant-derived factor VIII–specific activity ranges from 4000 to 7000 units of factor VIII per milligram protein prior to addition of albumin. Following infusion, the recombinant factor VIII binds to circulating vWF.[68,76] In vivo recovery and survival are similar to those for plasma-derived factor VIII.[77]

Development of factor VIII inhibitors following treatment is one of the most serious consequences of factor replacement therapy and was an early concern with the recombinant products.[68,77] Subsequent studies indicate that the cumulative incidence of inhibitors is not increased in patients treated with recombinant factor.[78,79] Although hamster and mouse proteins are present in trace amounts in the final preparations, antibodies to these proteins have not been detected.[68,72]

CONCENTRATES FOR TREATMENT OF PATIENTS WITH FACTOR VIII INHIBITORS

ACTIVATED PROTHROMBIN COMPLEX CONCENTRATES

Activated prothrombin complex concentrate (aPCC) preparations are activated spontaneously or deliberately during the manufacturing process and have been used to treat patients with inhibitors to factor VIII.[80,81] The active component or components were postulated to be either activated clotting factors (Xa or VIIa) or factor VIII complexed with phospholipid. The products are standardized by their ability to correct the clotting time of factor VIII–deficient plasma or factor VIII inhibitor plasma. Autoplex T (NABI) is dry heated at 60°C (140°F)

for 144 h, and FEIBA VH (Baxter) is subject to steam heat under pressure to reduce virus transmission.[49]

RECOMBINANT FACTOR VIIa CONCENTRATE

Factor VII cDNA has been isolated and cloned into baby hamster kidney cells cultured in media supplemented with calf serum. Recombinant protein is purified using a combination of immunoaffinity and ion-exchange chromatography. Factor VII spontaneously activates during purification, and the final material is stabilized without albumin (Novo Nordisk). This factor VII product has been used in clinical trials[82] and now is licensed for use.

PORCINE FACTOR VIII

Since patients' antibodies to human factor VIII often cross-react weakly or not at all with porcine factor VIII, purified porcine factor VIII has been used to treat patients with factor VIII inhibitor.[83] Porcine cryoprecipitate is depleted of vitamin K–dependent factors by passage over alumina; then factor VIII is purified by polyelectrolyte adsorption chromatography, followed by concentration and lyophilization. The resultant concentrate (HYATE:C, Speywood) has a specific activity of 140 U/mg, with minimal residual porcine vWF. Although no cases of human transmission of porcine parvovirus were found by the manufacturer or the Centers for Disease Control and Prevention, source material is now screened by polymerase chain reaction (PCR) for this virus.[84]

ADVERSE EVENTS ASSOCIATED WITH FACTOR VIII THERAPY

Plasma-derived factor VIII concentrates are prepared from pools containing up to 20,000 units of human plasma. Prior to viral-inactivation procedures, 60 to 100 percent of patients with severe hemophilia A treated with commercially prepared concentrates were infected with HIV,[60,135] and at least 80 percent were infected with hepatitis B, C, or G.[60,136,137] The risk of nonenveloped viral disease persists despite viral-inactivation procedures.[126,264] Recombinant technology should eliminate the risk of human transfusion-transmitted disease.

CLINICAL USE OF FACTOR VIII CONCENTRATES

SELECTION OF LEVEL FOR REPLACEMENT THERAPY

Information essential to patient management includes accurate diagnosis, the hemostatic level of factor required to achieve the therapeutic goal, the recovery of transfused factor, and the half-life of factor after transfusion. The goal of replacement therapy is to achieve hemostatic levels of the replaced factor using the lowest dose of replacement required. Guidelines for factor replacement have evolved over time; the dosage of factor VIII for various types of bleeding is discussed in Chap. 123) (also see Table 143-3 and Fig. 143-3).

BIOLOGIC HALF-LIFE AND RECOVERY

The biologic half-life of the factor replaced is used to determine the time interval for additional dosage if needed. For factor VIII, the biologic half-life is 8 to 12 h,[85] and a dose of 1 U/kg body weight will raise the circulating factor VIII level 2 percent. Factor VIII may be given twice daily. Reconstituted factor VIII concentrate loses little biologic activity at room temperature over several days[86] and does not favor bacterial growth,[86,87] allowing for continuous infusion of factor VIII. Continuous infusion avoids the unnecessarily high levels of factor VIII that occur immediately after intermittent administration and may decrease clearance of factor VIII, allowing a reduction in the total amount of factor VIII administered.[86,88] This method of administration is increasing in popularity.

TABLE 143-3   INITIAL REPLACEMENT THERAPY FOR COAGULATION FACTOR DEFICIENCY

Factor	Desired Hemostatic Level in Bleeding Surgical Patients	In Vivo Recovery, %	Biologic Half-Life	Therapeutic Dose
Fibrinogen	50–100 mg/dl	50–70	72–120 h	1 bag cryoprecipitate/5 kg body weight
Prothrombin	10–25%	50	72 h	10–20 U/kg body weight*
Factor V	25–30%	80	15–36 h	10–15 ml plasma/kg body weight* platelet transfusions may be indicated in patients with acquired V deficiency
Factor VII	10–25%	100	2–6 h	10–20 U/kg body weight*; recombinant VIIa under development
Factor VIII†		80–100	8–12 h	
Minor hemorrhage	30–40%			15–20 U/kg body weight
Major hemorrhage	80–100% for surgery			40–50 U/kg body weight
	30–50% for post-op			15–25 U/kg body weight
Invasive dental procedure	30–40%			15–20 U/kg body weight
Factor IX		40	18–24 h	
Minor hemorrhage	30–40%			30–40 U/kg body weight‡
Major hemorrhage	50–80% for surgery			50–80 U/kg body weight‡
	40% post-op			40 U/kg body weight‡
Invasive dental procedure	30–40%			30–40 U/kg body weight‡
Factor X	10–40%	50–95	24–40 h	10–20 U/kg body weight
Factor XI	20–30%	90	40–84 h	10–15 ml plasma/kg body weight; hemorrhage more likely following oral, pharyngeal, or urinary tract surgery; concentrate under development
Factor XIII	<5%	50–100	9–12 days	5 ml plasma/kg body weight every 4–6 weeks

*One unit of coagulation factor is present in each milliliter of FFP. Alternatively, PCC contains factors II and X or II, VII, and X in addition to factor IX (see Table 143-4).
†DDAVP is the treatment of choice for patients with mild or moderate hemophilia A who respond with an appropriate increase in plasma factor VIII levels.
‡Use PCC for single dose or coagulation factor IX for multiple infusions (factor IX activity is stated on the label).

CHOICE OF PRODUCT

DDAVP is the treatment of choice for patients with mild and moderate hemophilia A who respond with an appropriate rise in plasma factor VIII levels.[89] For patients with severe hemophilia A and those with mild or moderate hemophilia A who do not respond to DDAVP, factor VIII replacement is indicated. Plasma can theoretically be used to treat any factor deficiency, but the dose required to obtain a hemostatic level and the required frequency of therapy to sustain a hemostatic level would result in circulatory overload.[90] Cryoprecipitate has largely been abandoned for treatment of hemophilia A because of the lack of viral attenuation. Concentrates offer convenience and predictability in dose response. Currently available data suggest little difference regarding safety, efficacy, or convenience.[50] The choice of concentrate is problematic, since the potentially safest product, recombinant factor VIII, is both formulated with plasma-derived albumin and more expensive. Cost is a significant issue in product selection. Most physicians who treat hemophilia strongly prefer recombinant factor VIII for those patients who have never been exposed to blood products or have no evidence of transfusion-transmitted viral infections, such as hepatitis or HIV. For patients who are HIV-infected, consideration was initially given to use of highly purified factor VIII, since it caused less immunosuppression,[91,92] but other studies have shown no benefit.[93] Furthermore, these studies were all done before the advent of HIV-protease inhibitors, and other studies have shown that the progression to AIDS in hemophilia patients is similar to that in other HIV-infected individuals after age is considered.[50] For HIV-negative patients who have already been exposed to hepatitis B and C, the choice between intermediate- or high-purity factor VIII concentrate is also unclear; there is currently no evidence to suggest that exposure to the diversity of protein antigens in intermediate-purity concentrates has any negative effect on clinical course.

PRESENCE OR ABSENCE OF AN INHIBITOR

Development of an inhibitor (alloantibody) to the congenitally deficient factor is one of the most serious complications of replacement therapy. Approximately 10 to 15 percent or more of patients with hemophilia A develop an inhibitor to factor VIII, and approximately 2.5 percent of hemophilia B patients develop an antibody to factor IX.[94–97] Patients with inhibitors have severely reduced factor half-life. Patients refractory to replacement therapy require alternative means to control bleeding episodes and are candidates for induction of immune tolerance.[98,99] Most inhibitors are suspected when a patient fails to respond to replacement therapy appropriately; inhibitor titer is then quantified in vitro by the Bethesda assay.[69]

Evaluation of Acute Bleeding Episodes in Hemophilia A Patients with Inhibitors   Patients with factor VIII inhibitors are categorized as those unlikely to mount an anamnestic antibody response when exposed to allogeneic factor VIII (low responders) and those with a propensity to make such antibodies (high responders).

"Low-responder" patients usually have factor VIII inhibitors of low titer [<5–10 Bethesda units (BU)]. Hemorrhage in these patients is treated with factor VIII concentrates at a dose sufficient to overcome the effect of the anti–factor VIII antibody (20–50 U/kg plus 20 U/kg for every Bethesda unit of inhibitory activity). Following infusion, factor VIII levels should be followed to ensure that the desired effect has been attained.

"High-responder" patients have been treated with numerous approaches, and none has been entirely successful. Porcine factor VIII is used as the primary treatment modality for many "high-responder" patients if the anti–porcine antibody titer is low. Factor VIII concentrates may be effective in treating serious hemorrhage or surgical emergencies in high-responder hemophilic patients whose current inhibitor titers have decayed to less than 5 BU, but even in these patients there is the risk of anamnestic titer increases after factor VIII reexposure. When factor VIII is used, a bolus of 75 to 100 U/kg followed by continuous factor VIII infusion at 4 to 14 U/kg body weight per hour may be successful,[100] thereby taking advantage of the time dependence of inhibitor activity. Other options include prothrombin complex concentrates (PCCs), aPCC, or experimentally available recombinant factor VIIa.[101,102]

Therapeutic Options for Hemophilia A Patients with Inhibitors   Porcine factor VIII infusion may produce a persistent, measurable level of factor VIII. In general, patients with inhibitors have a lower anti–porcine factor VIII titer than anti–human factor VIII titer.[103]

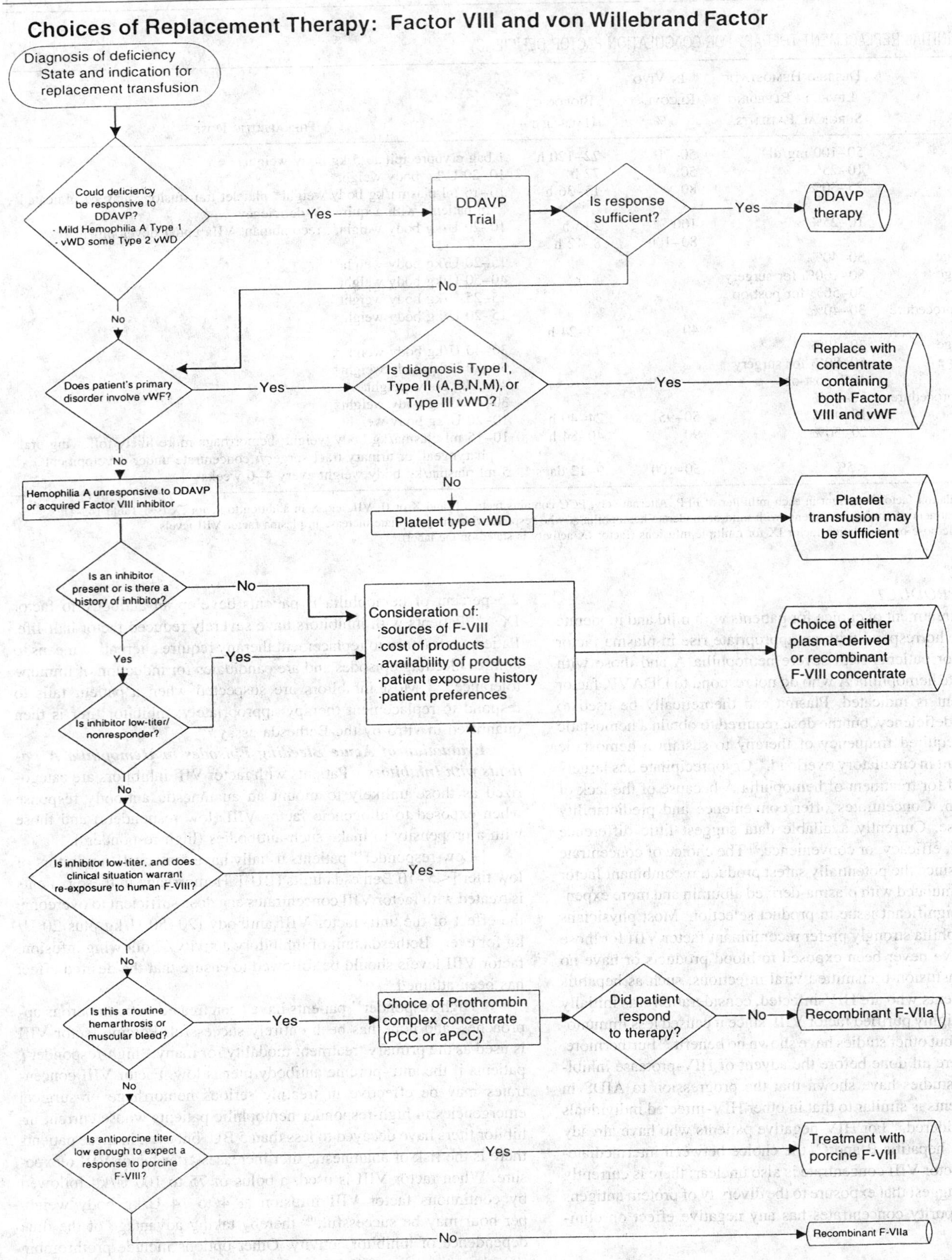

Choices of Replacement Therapy: Factor VIII and von Willebrand Factor

FIGURE 143-3   The flow diagram presents a generalized approach to the choice of replacement products for patients with factor VIII deficiency (hemophilia A) or von Willebrand disease. The algorithm may require modification based on specific patient variables and the patient's response to therapy.

An assay of the patient's inhibitor titer against porcine factor VIII and its ratio to the inhibitory effect against human factor VIII (cross-reactivity determination) should be performed and used for deciding treatment strategies. Porcine factor VIII concentrate is considered the treatment of choice for life- or limb-threatening bleeding episodes and for surgical procedures in patients with inhibitor titers less than 50 BU without antibodies to porcine factor VIII or with anti–porcine antibody levels less than 20 BU. The starting dose is 100 to 150 U/kg. Additional doses are determined by the patient's measured factor VIII response. Recovery is less and the half-life of porcine factor VIII is reduced in patients with anti–porcine inhibitor activity; measuring the 10-min posttransfusion factor VIII level rather than residual preinfusion factor VIII levels is recommended for determining efficacy in patients with low-level porcine inhibitors.[103]

Side effects include mild temperature elevation, nausea, headache, flushing, and occasional vomiting and thrombocytopenia. Patients susceptible to reactions or who have received the product previously are often treated with hydrocortisone and antihistamines intravenously. Increases of anti–porcine factor VIII titer have been reported. Porcine factor VIII is not known to transmit hepatitis or HIV.

PCCs are often used for first-line treatment of routine hemorrhages or for patients with factor VIII inhibitors that cannot be overridden (i.e., anti–human factor VIII inhibitor titer >50 BU and anti–porcine factor VIII titer >15–20 BU),[104] since prothrombin complex concentrate may bypass the deficiency in factor VIII. PCC infusions effectively control approximately 50 percent of bleeding episodes experienced by hemophilia A and B inhibitor patients,[81,105,106] but the utility of this intervention is limited by the unpredictability and short duration of some responses. Clinical parameters are followed, since there are no laboratory tests to monitor effectiveness.

The initial dose of PCC is 75 to 100 U/kg. Infusions are repeated once or twice at 8- to 12-h intervals if needed. Prolonged treatment should be avoided because of the possibility of thrombotic complications. If repeated doses are given, monitoring of the antithrombin level and for DIC is recommended; concurrent treatment with antifibrinolytic therapy should be avoided.

In one study, aPCC given as a single dose was no more effective than PCC for treatment of acute hemarthroses.[106] However, another study found that one or two doses of aPCC controlled 64 percent of mucocutaneous joint and muscle bleeding, compared to 52 percent of similar episodes in which PCC was used.[81] There are no laboratory tests to measure the effectiveness of aPCC.

Therapeutic plasma exchange has been used to transiently lower the inhibitor titer[107]; factor VIII is infused immediately following the plasmapheresis. Hemapheresis techniques, in which the patient's plasma is perfused over immunoabsorption columns containing staphylococcal protein A, have been used to reduce factor VIII and IX inhibitor levels.[98]

Recombinant factor VIIa concentrate has been used successfully in the management of acute bleeding and as perioperative prophylaxis in patients with factor VIII and XI inhibitors. The response was judged to be excellent or effective in 81 to 86 percent of surgical bleeds and 92 percent of dental extractions, with very few possible adverse events reported.[82] No markers of systemic activation of the hemostatic system were observed during the studies[82]; one patient made antibody to factor VII.[108] It is postulated that the recombinant factor VIIa interacts with tissue factor expressed at the site of vascular injury, resulting in factor X activation, thus "bypassing" the inhibited coagulation factors VIII or IX.[109] FDA approval of this product has made it a preferred treatment option.

Immune tolerance induction aimed at suppression of alloantibody production and restoration of responsiveness to factor VIII replacement therapy offers the best long-term approach for patients with inhibitors.

International registry data on 158 available patients indicate a 68 percent response rate, with best responses in patients given high-dose daily factor VIII (>100 U/kg body weight per day) and with initial inhibitor titers of less then 10 BU.[110] Tolerance was generally long lasting. Dosing schedules and adjunctive maneuvers to optimize this expensive approach to therapy are still being evaluated.[104]

Treatment of Nonhemophilic Patients with Factor VIII Inhibitors   Bleeding problems in nonhemophilic patients with inhibitors are treated with infusion of factor VIII concentrates, PCC, aPCC, or porcine factor VIII.[111–113] The antiporcine inhibitor level should be measured at presentation, and, if it is low, porcine factor VIII should be considered.[113] Since most of these patients have not previously received clotting factor concentrates, they are at risk for developing hepatitis B and should be immunized against hepatitis B. High-dose intravenous gamma globulin was reported to be effective in patients with autoantibodies, but not alloantibodies against factor VIII.[114,115] Unlike hemophilic patients with inhibitors, most nonhemophilic patients with inhibitors are responsive to prednisone or prednisone plus cytotoxic therapy.[116,117]

von WILLEBRAND DISEASE

vWD is a heterogeneous set of related bleeding conditions due to quantitative and/or qualitative abnormality of vWF. Normal vWF is required for normal plasma factor VIII levels, and decreased plasma factor VIII levels may be seen in vWD (see Chap. 135).

The most common form of vWD is type I, which accounts for approximately 80 percent of all patients with vWD.[118] The vast majority of these patients can avoid treatment with plasma-derived therapeutic products by using the drug DDAVP.[89] The optimal dose is 0.3 μg/kg DDAVP intravenously over 30 min or intranasally at a dose of 300 μg for adults or 150 μg for children. Plasma vWF and factor VIII levels are increased two- to fourfold after DDAVP, reaching a peak 30 min to 60 min after intravenous and 60 to 90 min after intranasal administration.[119] A DDAVP trial with postinfusion testing is useful, since patients' responses are variable. Doses may be repeated at intervals of 12 to 24 h, but tachyphylaxis may occur after three or four doses.[120] Patients should be counseled to avoid drinking large amounts of water for 18 h after receiving DDAVP because the residual antidiuretic activity of the drug can result in hyponatremia and seizure.[121] The risk of inducing acute thrombosis with DDAVP in patients with a predisposing factor is uncertain.[122] In patients with severe type I vWD or complete absence of vWF (type III), DDAVP will not be effective, and replacement therapy must be used.

In qualitative variants of vWD (type II vWD), DDAVP induces the release of abnormal vWF. DDAVP may be ineffective to briefly beneficial in type IIA vWD.[123] Its use is controversial in type IIB vWD, since thrombocytopenia may worsen.[124,125] In general, replacement therapy with a vWF-containing concentrate is used in these patients.

Replacement therapy with pasteurized or SD-treated factor VIII concentrates demonstrated to contain the high-molecular-weight vWF multimers is preferred over nonvirally attenuated cryoprecipitate. Data from an international retrospective study support the efficacy of this approach.[126] Filtration during the SD treatment process removes high-molecular-weight multimers of vWF, and thus cryoprecipitate made from SD-treated plasma is not recommended.[9] Monoclonal antibody–derived factor VIII concentrates and recombinant factor VIII do not contain vWF and should not be used.[127,128] The minimal hemostatic level for vWF is not as clearly established as that for factor VIII, and the role of bleeding time monitoring is unclear.[90,129] Most physicians attempt to increase the level of vWF and factor VIII to within the normal range for surgery (80–100 U/dl) and maintain it above 50 U/dl during the postoperative period. The level of correction and duration of treatment in type II variants is less clear, and often treatment must be given on an empirical basis. Factor VIII concentrates (Humate-P) are FDA licensed for this indication but are not assayed for their vWF concentration; published reports of the ratio of vWF ristocetin cofactor activity to factor VIII content help guide therapy (0.53 for Alphanate, Alpha; 2–2.7 for Humate-P, Centeon).[130,131] If the patient has had major surgery, replacement therapy must usually be given every 8 to 12 h, as in treatment of severe hemophilia. Similarly to factor VIII, infusion of 1 U/kg body weight will increase the plasma level by approximately 2 U/dl. Since the patient with vWD is fully capable of synthesizing factor VIII if normal vWF is present to stabilize the vWF/factor VIII complex, the apparent survival time of transfused factor VIII is 24 to 36 h, which is longer than the 12 h found in the hemophilic patient.[132] The transfused vWF has a normal biologic half-life in the vWD patient of 12 h.[118] A recombinant vWF product is in development.[133]

For dental extractions, a single treatment with DDAVP (for type I vWD) or replacement therapy (for type II or III vWD), together with 5 to 10 days of oral adjunctive treatment with antifibrinolytic agents (ε-aminocaproic acid or tranexamic acid) is usually adequate.

"Platelet-type" pseudo-vWD is the result of a defective vWF receptor (GPIb) on platelets and is clinically similar to type IIB vWD,[134] with loss of the plasma high-molecular-weight vWF multimers (see Chap. 135). Platelet transfusion is recommended as replacement therapy in these patients.[118]

PROTHROMBIN COMPLEX CONCENTRATES AND FACTOR IX CONCENTRATES

Table 143-4 summarizes the PCC and factor IX concentrates currently available in the United States.

PROTHROMBIN COMPLEX CONCENTRATES

PCCs were first developed in 1959, became available in the United States in 1969, and quickly became the mainstay of hemophilia B therapy. Prepared by barium sulfate precipitation followed by column chromatography on various adsorbents,[138] these intermediate-purity concentrates of vitamin K–dependent proteins had large amounts of prothrombin and thus acquired the name *PCC*. Although labeled by factor IX content, currently available PCCs contain variable amounts of factors II, VII, and X; thus, PCC may be useful for therapy of other inherited vitamin K–dependent factor deficiencies.[139] PCCs are prepared by DEAE absorption of the Cohn fraction I effluent (Konyne 80, Bayer), DEAE-Sephadex absorption, PEG precipitation (Proplex T, Baxter), or other procedures (Profilnine HT, Alpha; Bebulin VH, Baxter).[49,140]

Prolonged and repeated use of PCC is associated with adverse events, such as thrombotic complications.[141] Potential explanations included contamination with either activated coagulation factors or phospholipid.[142,143] In order to prevent these complications, second-generation factor IX concentrates contain only traces of other prothrombin complex factors.[144] Thermal stability of factor IX allowed implementation of methods to reduce the risk of virus transmission by PCC and subsequent concentrates; HIV transmission has not been associated with currently available products.[49,140]

COAGULATION FACTOR IX CONCENTRATES

AlphaNine SD (Alpha) is prepared by ion-exchange and carbohydrate ligand affinity chromatography.[145,146] Specific activity levels of 84 to 256 units of factor IX per milligram of protein have been achieved. Mononine (Centeon) is prepared by monoclonal antibody affinity chromatography. Sodium thiocyanate is used to elute factor IX from the column and also destroys HIV. Viral retention ultrafiltration, used in

---

TABLE 143-4   PROTHROMBIN COMPLEX CONCENTRATES AND FACTOR IX PRODUCTS AVAILABLE IN THE UNITED STATES

Product	Manufacturer	U/ml (Note Wide Variation)				Viral Inactivation Method
		Factor II	Factor VII	Factor IX	Factor X	
PROTHROMBIN COMPLEX CONCENTRATE						
Konyne 80 (20 or 40 ml)	Bayer	22–28	2–4	2–25	25–35	Dry heat 80°C 72 h
Profilnine, heat treated (10 or 25 ml)	Alpha	47–69	7–21	42–58	22–41	n-Heptane suspension, 60°C 20 h
Bebulin VH (20 ml)	Baxter	Similar to IX	~10% of IX	10–60; IX level indicated on label	Similar to IX	Steam heat under pressure, 60°C 10 h, 1190 mbar; 80°C 1 h, 1375 mbar
Proplex T (30 ml)	Baxter	5–6	68–91	11–22	8–10	Dry heat 60°C 144 h
COAGULATION FACTOR IX						
Mononine	Centeon	<6	<5	97	0	Sodium thiocyanate, ultrafiltration
AlphaNine SD	Alpha	6	<5	84–256	16	SD TNBP and polysorbate 80 ultra-filtration
RECOMBINANT FACTOR IX						
BeneFix	Genetics Institute	0	0	>200	0	Ultrafiltration
Activated PCC						
FEIBA VH	Baxter	—	—	—	—	Steam heat under pressure, 60°C 10 h, 1190 mbar; 80°C 1 h, 1375 mbar
Autoplex T	NABI	—	—	—	—	Dry heat 60°C 144 h

NOTE: Activated PCC used for treatment of patients with factor VIII inhibitors.
SOURCE: Compiled from Refs. 14, 15, 17, 22, and 23.

the preparation of both coagulation factor IX concentrates, confers additional viral safety.[64] The specific activity is approximately 180 units of factor IX per milligram of protein.[147] The recovery of factor IX for each of these products is at least equal to that achieved with PCC. Purified factor IX concentrates entail significantly less risk of thrombogenicity than do PCCs[148,149] and are the preferred product when more then one dose of factor is anticipated.[150] Antibody to mouse IgG or inhibitors to factor IX have not been reported to date.[147]

RECOMBINANT FACTOR IX CONCENTRATE

The challenges of producing an extensively posttranslationally modified protein such as factor IX have recently been overcome.[151] Genes for factor IX and a soluble form of a paired basic amino acid–cleaving protein (PACE-SOL) were expressed in Chinese hamster ovary cells grown in a bovine protein-free system. The expressed factor IX (BeneFix, Genetics Institute) is purified by serial nonimmunoaffinity chromatographic steps and does not require albumin stabilization, thus avoiding bovine, murine, and human protein exposure during production. Although the half-life of transfused recombinant factor IX is identical to that of plasma-derived factor, the recovery is approximately 28 percent less, requiring dose adjustment for patients switched from plasma-derived factor therapy.[152] Although minor differences in phosphorylation and sulfation of the recombinant protein have been noted, inhibitor development has not yet been a concern.

CLINICAL USE OF PROTHROMBIN COMPLEX CONCENTRATES, COAGULATION FACTOR IX CONCENTRATES, RECOMBINANT FACTOR IX, AND FACTORS XI AND XIII AND PROTEIN C CONCENTRATES

Currently, recombinant factor IX or highly purified coagulation factor IX concentrates are preferred to PCC for hemophilia B patients. Although less expensive PCCs are occasionally used when a single dose is sufficient, PCCs are inappropriate in situations where repeated replacement therapy is anticipated (e.g., perioperatively, with large-muscle hematomas, or in situations of life-threatening hemorrhage) or in individuals at increased risk of thrombotic complications, such as patients with liver dysfunction. PCCs are not advised for newborns due to hepatic immaturity; neonates should be considered for recombinant product to avoid the risks of exposure to plasma-derived products. PCC is still a good choice for patients with factor II, VII, or X deficiency when specific viral-inactivated clotting factor concentrates are not available or treatment with plasma is not feasible or ineffective. The levels of factors II, VII, and X vary with manufacturer and lot[139] (see Table 143-3).

SELECTION OF DESIRED LEVEL NEEDED FOR REPLACEMENT THERAPY

The biologic half-life of factor IX is 18 to 24 h once equilibrium is established,[153] and a dose of 1 U/kg body weight will raise the circulating factor IX level approximately 1 percent. Factor IX may be given in a single daily dose. Calculation of doses of factor IX is discussed in Chap. 123. Increasing the factor IX level to 30 to 40 percent is effective in stopping most routine hemorrhages.[146] If the bleeding is limb- or life-threatening, the factor IX level should be raised to 50 to 80 percent and maintained at 30 to 40 percent levels for 7 to 14 days with coagulation factor IX concentrates. For major surgery, the factor IX levels should be increased to 60 to 80 percent just prior to surgery and then maintained above 30 percent for 5 to 7 days and above 15 to 20 percent for 7 to 10 additional days until healing occurs. For prophylaxis against hemorrhage during times of extensive physical activity, the plasma factor IX levels should be raised to 15 to 30 percent. Levels are maintained above 1 percent for patients on primary

prophylaxis to prevent the development of joint disease, usually requiring bolus therapy every 2 to 3 days.

ADVERSE EFFECTS ASSOCIATED WITH FACTOR IX THERAPY

Prior to treatment with virally attenuated products, 45 to 57 percent of patients with severe hemophilia B had developed antibodies to HIV, and more than 80 percent were infected with hepatitis.[60,135–137,140,146] These risks have been greatly reduced by the viral attenuation procedures[49,57] and are probably eliminated through use of recombinant product.

Following administration of PCC, some patients develop transient fever, chills, headache, flushing, or tingling. PCC administration has been associated with activation of the hemostatic system, thrombosis, and sudden death from myocardial infarction.[140,141,154–156] Factor IX concentrate or recombinant factor IX use should significantly reduce this risk. PCCs are not recommended for treatment of hemostatic abnormalities occurring in patients with liver disease, since thrombotic complications have occurred following PCC infusion in some, but not all, patients. ε-Aminocaproic acid should be avoided during PCC or aPCC use.

Between 2.5 and 16 percent of hemophilia B patients develop inhibitors in response to replacement therapy,[157] which may present as failure to respond appropriately to replacement therapy or as anaphylaxis.[158] Similar to hemophilia A patients with inhibitors, those with titers less than 10 BU may respond to higher-dose therapy,[140] and those with titers over 10 BU are usually treated with PCC, aPCC, or recombinant factor VIIa. Induction of immune tolerance has been disappointing in hemophilia B, and several cases of nephrotic syndrome have developed in this setting.[159]

FACTOR XI CONCENTRATE

There is significant variability in the occurrence of bleeding episodes in patients with factor XI deficiency, which is generally a milder condition than hemophilia A or B. Hemorrhage is reported following surgical procedures in the mouth and oral pharynx or urinary tract, possibly because of the associated high levels of plasminogen activators in these areas.[207–209]

Hemorrhage is treated with plasma infusion ($\approx$10–20 ml/kg body weight) to raise factor XI activity to 20 to 30 percent. The biologic half-life of infused factor XI is 40 to 84 h, and the half-disappearance time is approximately 2 days. Factor XI concentrates are under development and have been used in Europe.[210,211] Consumptive coagulopathy and thrombotic complications have been reported with two European concentrates.[212,213]

FACTOR XIII CONCENTRATE

Factor XIII deficiency is characterized by delayed wound healing and bleeding with injuries. The very low levels required for normal function ($\approx$5%)[214] and a long half-life (288 h)[215] permit replacement therapy with plasma or cryoprecipitate.[10] Factor XIII concentrate is available in Europe.[216]

PROTEIN C CONCENTRATE

Purpura fulminans may be a presenting symptom complex of either congenital homozygous protein C deficiency[32] or acquired disorders, such as meningococcal sepsis.[33] Experience with an investigational monoclonal antibody–purified, vapor heat–treated protein C concentrate[32] has shown remarkable promise,[2,34] and studies are underway to expand this initial experience. Infusion of activated protein C into baboons was demonstrated to prevent septic shock and death in animals challenged with bacterial infusion,[12] and studies of recombinant activated protein C therapy are in clinical trial.

Choice of replacement therapy: Hemophilia B or deficiency of other Vitamin K–dependent factors

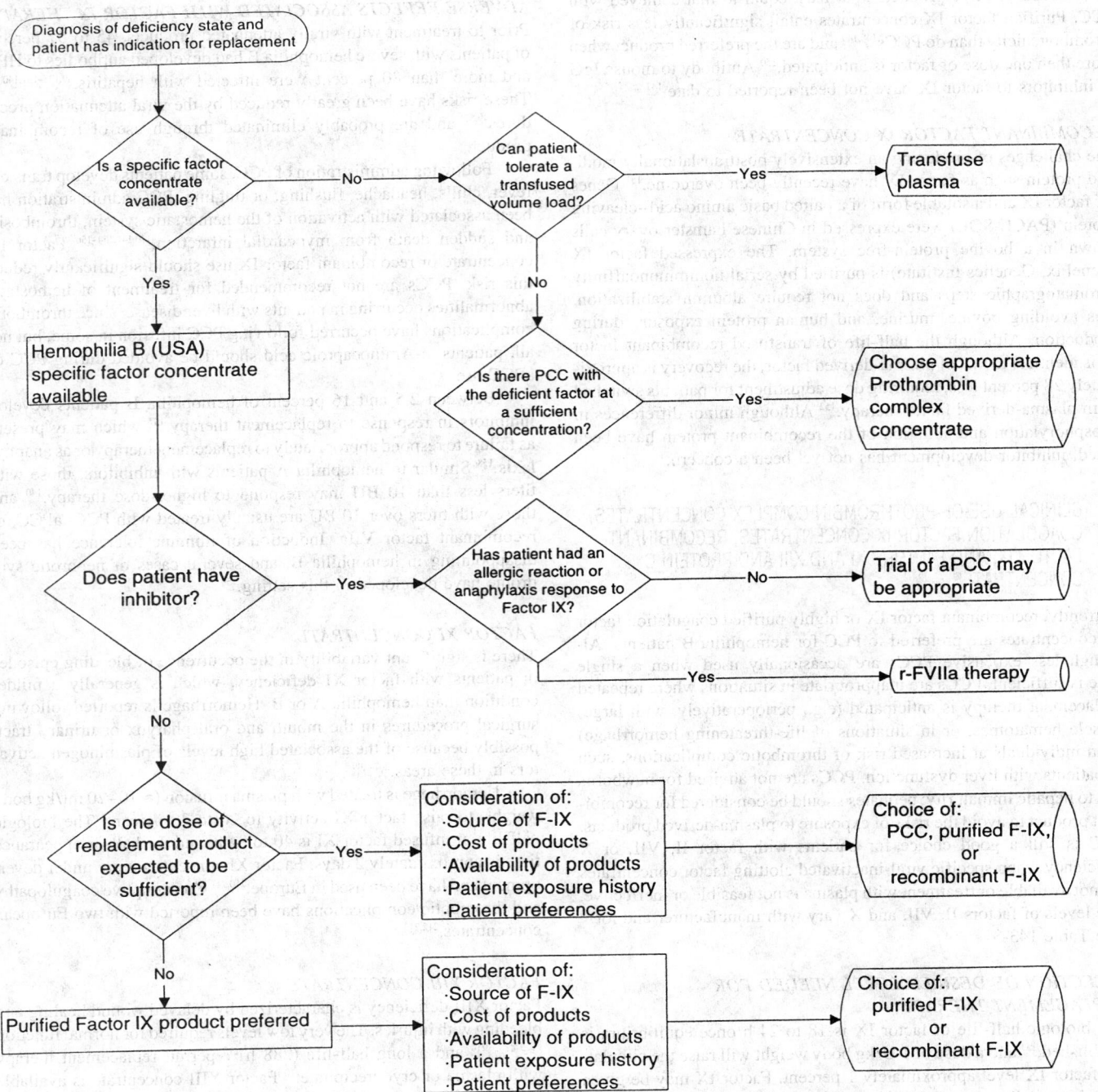

FIGURE 143-4   The flow diagram presents a generalized approach to the choice of replacement products for patients with factor IX deficiency (hemophilia B) or other vitamin K–dependent factor deficiencies. The algorithm may require modification based on the specific patient's response to therapy.

ALBUMIN AND PLASMA PROTEIN FRACTIONS

Albumin and plasma protein fractions are referred to as protein colloid solutions, in contrast to nonprotein colloid solutions, such as heta-starch, dextran, and other synthetic colloid products. Albumin and plasma protein fractions are prepared from plasma, serum, or human placentas. At least 96 percent of the total protein in albumin products

is albumin, while a minimum of 83 percent of the total protein in plasma protein fractions is albumin, with immunoglobulins constituting the remaining protein content. Albumin and plasma protein fractions are heated for 10 h or more at 60°C (140°F) to inactivate contaminating viruses. Despite concern about transmission of classic Creutzfeldt-Jakob disease by plasma derivatives, there is no evidence to indicate this has occurred.[48]

CLINICAL USE OF ALBUMIN AND PLASMA PROTEIN FRACTIONS

The purported benefits of albumin in the treatment of patients with burns or hypoalbuminia and possibly with hypovolemia were questioned in a meta-analysis of 30 randomized, controlled trials comparing recipients of albumin or plasma protein fraction with those receiving no fluid or those receiving crystalloid solution.[160] The relative risk of death after albumin administration was 1.46 for hypovolemia, 2.40 for burns, and 1.69 for hypoalbuminemia. The pooled risk of death between albumin and nonalbumin recipients was 6 percent, or 1 additional death for every 17 patients treated with albumin or plasma protein fraction.

In 26 randomized, controlled trials, there was an absolute mortality rate increase of 4 percent, or 4 extra deaths for every 100 patients resuscitated with colloids compared to crystalloids.[161]

One possible explanation for the adverse events associated with albumin administration is cardiac decompensation secondary to rapid volume replacement and edema, including pulmonary edema, because of albumin leakage from capillaries with increased permeability. In addition, colloid solutions may exert antihemostatic effects and exacerbate thrombocytopenic complications that increase blood loss. Albumin resuscitation during hypovolemic shock also impairs sodium and water excretion and thus may lead to renal insufficiency.[162]

The University Hospital Consortium guidelines for albumin usage include plasma exchange involving more than 20 ml/kg body weight and short-term usage in conjunction with diuretic therapy for patients with nephrotic syndrome and acute, severe peripheral or pulmonary edema as the only first-line indications for albumin.[163,164] These guidelines state that (1) the effectiveness of colloid solutions in the treatment of sepsis has not been demonstrated in clinical trials, (2) crystalloids are considered the initial resuscitation fluid of choice for hemorrhagic shock, (3) colloids should be used in thermal injury after the first 24 h if crystalloids fail to correct hypovolemia, (4) crystalloids are preferred to colloids to prevent complications associated with large-volume paracentesis, and (5) there is limited or inconclusive published supportive evidence for using albumin for patients with severe hypoalbuminemia.

If 25% albumin is diluted to a 5% solution, 0.9% NaCl or 5% dextrose solution should be used. Reports of hemolysis in recipients, including fatal episodes, have been associated with the use of sterile water as a diluent.[165]

IMMUNOGLOBULINS

Immunoglobulin preparations for intravenous administration are made by cold ethanol fractionation, the Cohn-Oncley process, from plasma pooled from 3000 to 10,000 donations.[166–169] The product is treated at pH 4.0 to 4.25 and stabilized with albumin, glucose, maltose, glycerin, or sucrose. The latter has been implicated in the etiology of acute renal failure resulting from osmotic injury to proximal renal tubules.[170] Intravenous immunoglobulin (IVIg) products contain more than 95 percent IgG, less than 2.5 percent IgA, and small amounts of IgM. IgG_1 varies between 55 to 70 percent, and IgG_2 from 0.7 to 2–6 percent.[166] The half-life of infused IVIg ranges from 15 to 25 days.

IVIg preparations contain antibodies against multiple infectious agents and anti-idiotype antibodies. In contrast to native IgG, 40 percent of the IgG in IVIg is present as dimers binding double-arm and single-arm $F(ab')_2$ domains. Sixty percent of the IgG is in monomeric form. IVIg also contains immunomodulating proteins, such as soluble CD4, CD8, and HLA molecules.[166]

Currently, IVIg is considered to have a minimal risk of transmitting known viruses. Donors are screened and tested for transmissible agents, and HIV and hepatitis B virus are inactivated by the fraction-ation process. Treatment with the SD process inactivates hepatitis C virus and other lipid-enveloped viruses, such as GBV-C and hepatitis G virus.[171] Prior to SD treatment and following donor testing for anti–hepatitis C virus, at least 100 cases of hepatitis C transmission occurred from one IVIg preparation, possibly because removal of donors with anti–hepatitis C antibodies resulted in a reduction of neutralizing hepatitis C antibody.[172,173] Transmission of Creutzfeldt-Jakob disease and other spongiform encephalopathy agents is theoretically possible, but the risk is considered minimal.[174] Nonetheless, batches of IVIg have been withdrawn because one or more of the donors to a large pool developed the disease subsequent to donation. This factor, production impediments related to regulatory compliance issues, and increases in usage led to shortages of IVIg products in the late 1990s.[175]

The postulated mechanisms of the immunomodulatory action of IVIg include anti-idiotypic antibody neutralization of pathologic autoantibodies; down-regulation of antibody production; suppression of cytokine activity, since IVIg contains neutralizing antibodies against IL-1a, IL-6, and TNF-α; prevention of Fc receptor–mediated phagocytosis by saturating or altering the affinity of Fc receptors; interfering with the membranolytic attack complex of complement by preventing incorporation of C3 molecules into the C5 convertase assembly; and interfering with antigen recognition by T cells through the actions of soluble CD4, CD8, and MHC-II molecules.[166]

CLINICAL USE OF INTRAVENOUS IMMUNOGLOBULINS

The FDA-approved indications for IVIg products include treatment of primary immunodeficiency, immune-mediated thrombocytopenia (ITP), Kawasaki syndrome, marrow transplantation in adults, chronic B-cell lymphocytic leukemia, and pediatric HIV-1 infection. In addition, IVIg is used for treatment of "off-label" conditions, such as posttransfusion purpura and chronic inflammatory demyelinating polyneuropathy.[166–168,175–183]

Other uses include prevention of infections in patients with stable multiple myeloma, CMV-negative recipients of CMV-positive organs, hypogammaglobulinemic neonates at risk for infection, intractable epilepsy, systemic vasculitic syndromes, warm-type autoimmune hemolytic anemia, immune-mediated neutropenia, anemia caused by parvovirus B19, neonatal alloimmune thrombocytopenia unresponsive to other treatments, dermatomyositis, polymyositis, decompensation in myasthenia gravis, and severe thrombocytopenia unresponsive to other treatments.[166–168,175,184–190]

In light of difficulties in obtaining supplies of IVIg, alternative approaches have been used to reduce IVIg usage. These include infusion of anti-D antibodies, but not monoclonal anti-D, to Rh D–positive patients with ITP and plasmapheresis for patients with autoimmune neuropathies. Intravenous anti-D has been reported to increase the platelet count by more than 50,000/μl in 46 percent of nonsplenectomized patients with ITP or HIV-related ITP.[192] Splenectomized patients with chronic ITP had minimal or no response to anti-D therapy.

ADVERSE EFFECTS OF IVIg THERAPY

Mild to moderate headaches occur in up to 10 percent of patients. Chills, myalgias, or chest discomfort may develop following the onset of therapy but respond to slowing the infusion rate. Fatigue, nausea, and fever may persist for 24 h. Anaphylactic reactions occur rarely. Aseptic meningitis has been reported with infusions ranging from 0.2 to 2 g/kg body weight. This syndrome occurs within several hours to 2 days following IVIg administration and resolves within a few days of discontinuing IVIg treatment.[193] Acute renal failure, including fatal cases, has been reported predominantly in association with higher doses of preparations containing sucrose that were used during consecutive days. This finding led to recommendations to ensure that patients are adequately hydrated, to consider the risk of sucrose-containing preparations in patients with risk factors for renal insufficiency, to limit the rate at which sucrose-containing preparations are infused, and to monitor renal function in patients receiving IVIg.[170]

SERINE PROTEASE INHIBITORS

Plasma protease inhibitors are members of the serine protease inhibitor (serpin) superfamily. They play a crucial role in regulation of the coagulation, fibrinolytic, complement, and kinin systems, as well as regulation of cellular proteases. Deficiency of certain serpins is associated with disease states; thus, several serpins have been purified from plasma and made available for therapeutic uses as concentrate.

ANTITHROMBIN

Lyophilized preparations are prepared by subfractionation using cold ethanol precipitation techniques and pasteurization. There has been no evidence of virus transmission associated with infusion of this product.[194]

Antithrombin inactivates serine proteases of the coagulation cascade through a 1:1 stoichiometric complex of the protease serine-active site and an arginine residue on antithrombin.

Antithrombin is an important regulator of factors Xa and IIa. Their deficiency is associated with increased risk for thrombosis. Standard care of patients with antithrombin deficiency and thrombosis is anticoagulation.[195] Concentrates were licensed in the United States for use limited to treatment of patients with hereditary antithrombin deficiency as prophylaxis against thrombosis following surgery or obstetric procedures and for therapeutic use when these patients had thromboembolic events.[194]

In stable patients with antithrombin deficiency, the half-life of infused antithrombin varies between 60 and 91 h, with an initial half-disappearance time of approximately 22 h. In acute DIC, antithrombin recovery is approximately one-half that achieved in stable patients; the half-life may be as short as 4 h.

Antithrombin concentrates are indicated in patients with hereditary deficiency in the peripartum period and perioperatively to minimize the risk of thrombosis and in certain acute thrombotic conditions.[196] There is debate about indications for antithrombin III (AT-III) replacement therapy in patients with acquired AT-III deficiency. Antithrombin supplementation is associated with improved heparin responsiveness in patients requiring extracorporeal circulation during surgery,[197] but the heparin resistance seen in patients incurring a thrombosis is rarely due to antithrombin deficiency.[198] Definitive clinical results have yet to be established a benefit in DIC or in liver transplantation.[196]

AT-III replacement dosage is designed to achieve an AT-III level of 120 percent following infusion. Subsequent doses ($\approx$60 percent of the loading dose) are determined empirically to maintain levels of 70 to 120 percent.[199]

C1 ESTERASE INHIBITOR

C1 esterase inhibitor regulates activation of the kinin and complement systems.[200] Hereditary deficiency results in hereditary angioedema. A concentrate available in Europe is prepared by anion-exchange chromatography, several precipitation steps, and viral inactivation by a "moist heat" treatment method.[201]

Hereditary angioedema is characterized by well-circumscribed subepithelial edema involving the extremities, face, larynx, or bowel. Complications may include acute abdominal pain or respiratory distress. Autosomal dominant C1 esterase inhibitor deficiency underlies this condition.[202] While androgens and antifibrinolytic medications may prevent attacks, replacement therapy is the only intervention

shown to shorten attacks already in progress. FFP has been used successfully during acute attacks,[203,204] but the volume of FFP required and the time required for thawing are limitations. Concentrate is available in Europe and has been shown to be effective and safe in a clinical trial.

α_1-PROTEINASE INHIBITOR

Originally called antitrypsin, α_1-proteinase inhibitor (API) is the primary physiologic inhibitor of neutrophil elastase. Autosomal recessive hereditary deficiency presents with panacinar emphysema.[205] Panacinar emphysema due to destruction of alveolar wall develops in the third to fourth decade in the patients with hereditary absence of α_1-proteinase; disease develops earlier in smokers.

A commercially prepared concentrate is made from plasma via Cohn fractionation followed by PEG anion-exchange chromatography and pasteurization (Proelastin, Bayer).

The infused material has a terminal-phase half-life of 4.4 days. After infusion, α_1-proteinase diffuses into alveolar walls, and sustained levels are found 1 week later in alveolar lavage fluid.[206] Weekly replacement therapy is indicated in individuals with hereditary α_1-proteinase deficiency and clinically evident panacinar emphysema.

REFERENCES

1. British Committee for Standards in Haematology: Working Party of the Blood Transfusion Task Force guidelines for the use of fresh frozen plasma. *Transfus Med* 2:57, 1992.
2. Practice Guidelines Development Task Force of the American College of Physicians: Practice parameter for the use of fresh-frozen plasma, cryoprecipitate, and platelets. *JAMA* 271:777, 1994.
3. Consensus Conference: Fresh frozen plasma: Indications and use. *JAMA* 235:551, 1985.
4. Expert Working Group: Guidelines for red blood cell and plasma transfusion for adults and children. *Can Med Assoc J* 156:1,1997.
5. Braunstein AH, Oberman HA: Transfusion of plasma components. *Transfusion* 24:281, 1984.
6. Howard PL, Bovill EG, Golden E: Postthaw stability of fibrinogen in cryoprecipitate stored between 1° and 6°C. *Transfusion* 31:30, 1991.
7. Leblond PF, Rock G, Herbert CA: The use of plasma as a replacement fluid in plasma exchange. *Transfusion* 38:834, 1998.
8. Horowitz B, Bonomo R, Prince AM, et al: Solvent/detergent-treated plasma: A virus-inactivated substitute for fresh frozen plasma. *Blood* 79:826, 1992.
9. Horowitz MS, Pehta JC: SD plasma in TTP and coagulation factor deficiencies for which no concentrates are available. *Vox Sang* 74:231, 1998.
10. Baudoux E, Margraff U, Coenen A, et al: Hemovigilance: Clinical tolerance of solvent-detergent treated plasma. *Vox Sang* 74:237, 1998.
11. Klein HG, Dodd RY, Dzik WH, et al: Current status of solvent/detergent-treated frozen plasma. *Transfusion* 38:102, 1998.
12. Simmonds P, Davidson F, Lycett C, et al: Detection of a novel DNA virus (TTV) in blood donors and blood products. *Lancet* 352:191, 1998.
13. AuBuchon JP, Birkmeyer JD: Safety and cost-effectiveness of solvent-detergent-treated plasma. *JAMA* 272:1210, 1994.
14. Lee HH, Allain JP: Genomic screening for blood-borne viruses in transfusion settings. *Vox Sang* 74:119, 1998.
15. Hume HA, Kronick JB, Blanchette VS: Review of the literature on allogeneic red blood cell and plasma transfusions in children, *Can Med Assoc J* 156:41, 1997.
16. Stehling LC, Doherty DC, Faust RJ, et al: Practice guidelines for component therapy. *Anesthesiology* 84:732, 1996.
17. ACOG technical bulletin: Blood component therapy. *Int J Gynecol Obstet* 48:233, 1995.
18. Ewe K: Bleeding after liver biopsy does not correlate with indices of peripheral coagulation. *Dig Dis Sci* 26:388, 1981.
19. McVay PA, Toy PTCY: Lack of increased bleeding after liver biopsy in patients with mild hemostatic abnormalities. *Am J Clin Pathol* 94:747, 1990.

20. Counts RB, Haisch C, Simon TL, et al: Hemostasis in massively transfused trauma patients. *Ann Surg* 190:91, 1979.

21. Mannucci PM, Federici AB, Sirchia G: Hemostasis testing during massive blood replacement: A study of 172 cases. *Vox Sang* 42:113, 1982.

22. Reed RL, Heimbach DM, Counts RB, et al: Prophylactic platelet administration during massive transfusion: A prospective, randomized, double-blind clinical study. *Ann Surg* 203:40, 1986.

23. Ciavarella D, Reed RL, Counts RB, et al: Clotting factor levels and the risk of diffuse microvascular bleeding in the massively transfused patient. *Br J Haematol* 67:365, 1987.

24. Rock GA, Shumak KH, Buskard NA, et al: Comparison of plasma exchange with plasma infusion in the treatment of thrombotic thrombocytopenic purpura. *N Engl J Med* 325:393, 1991.

25. Bell WR, Braine HG, Ness PM, et al: Improved survival in thrombotic thrombocytopenic purpura–hemolytic uremic syndrome: Clinical experience in 108 patients. *N Engl J Med* 325:398, 1991.

26. Furlan M, Robles R, Galbusera M: von Willebrand factor-cleaving protease in thrombotic thrombocytopenic purpura and the hemolytic-uremic syndrome. *N Engl J Med* 339:1578, 1998.

27. Tsai HM, Lian EC-Y: Antibodies to von Willebrand factor–cleaving protease in acute thrombotic thrombocytopenic purpura. *N Engl J Med* 339:1585, 1998.

28. Rock G, Shumak KH, Sutton DM, et al: Cryosupernatant as replacement fluid for plasmapheresis in thrombotic thrombocytopenic purpura. *Br J Haematol* 94:383, 1996.

29. Peters C, Casella JF, Marlar RA, et al: Homozygous protein C deficiency: Observations on the nature of the molecular abnormality and effectiveness of warfarin therapy. *Pediatrics* 81:272, 1988.

30. Greaves M, Preston FE: Clinical annotation: The hypercoagulable state in clinical practice. *Br J Haematol* 79:148, 1991.

31. Marlar RA, Endres-Brooks J, Miller C: Serial studies of protein C and its plasma inhibitor in patients with disseminated intravascular coagulation. *Blood* 66:59, 1985.

32. Dreyfus M, Magny JF, Bridey F, et al: Treatment of homozygous protein C deficiency and neonatal purpura fulminans with a purified protein C concentrate. *N Engl J Med* 325:1565, 1991.

33. Rivard GE, Michele D, Farrell C, Schwarz HP: Treatment of purpura fulminans in meningococcemia with protein C concentrate. *J Pediatr* 126:646, 1995.

34. White B, Mc Mahan C, Smith OP: Protein C replacement therapy for meningococcal induced purpura fulminans [abstr]. *Blood* 92(suppl 1):670a, 1998.

35. Vento S, Garofano T, Renzini C, et al: Fulminant hepatitis associated with hepatitis A virus superinfection in patients with chronic hepatitis C. *N Engl J Med* 338:286, 1998.

36. Sayers MH, Anderson KC, Goodnough LT, et al: Reducing the risk for transfusion-transmitted cytomegalovirus infection. *Ann Intern Med* 116:55, 1992.

37. Okuchi K, Sato H, Hinuma YA: Retrospective study on transmission of adult T cell leukemia virus by blood transfusion: Seroconversion in recipients. *Vox Sang* 46:245, 1984.

38. Case Records of the Massachusetts General Hospital. *N Engl J Med* 339:2005, 1998.

39. McBride JA, O'Hoski P, Barnes CC, et al: Rhesus alloimmunization following intensive plasma exchange. *Transfusion* 23:352, 1983.

40. Willis JI, Lown JAG, Simpson MC, Erber WN: White cells in fresh-frozen plasma: Evaluation of a new white cell-reduction filter. *Transfusion* 38:645, 1998.

41. Alving BM, Weinstein JS, Menitove JE, et al: Fibrin sealant: Summary of a conference on characteristics and clinical uses. *Transfusion* 35:783, 1995.

42. Martinowitz U, Renato S: Fibrin sealant. *Curr Opin Hematol* 3:395, 1996.

43. Radosevich M, Goubran HA, Burnouf T: Fibrin sealant: Scientific rationale, production methods, properties, and current clinical use. *Vox Sang* 72:133, 1997.

44. Weigert AL, Schafer AI: Uremic bleeding: Pathogenesis and therapy. *Am J Med Sci* 316:94, 1998.

45. Andreae MC, Amanullah A, Jamil S: Congenital factor XIII deficiency: A patient report and review of the literature. *Clin Pediatr* 36:53, 1997.

46. Christie RJ, Carrington L, Alving B: Postoperative bleeding induced by topical bovine thrombin: Report of two cases. *Surgery* 121:708, 1997.

47. Cohn EJ, Strong LE, Hughes WL Jr: Preparation and properties of serum and plasma proteins: IV. A system for the separation into fractions of the protein and lipoprotein components of biological tissues and fluids. *J Am Chem Soc* 68:459, 1946.

48. McClelland DBL: Safety of human albumin as a constituent of biologic therapeutic products. *Transfusion* 38:690, 1998.

49. Kasper CK, Lusher JM, Transfusion Practices Committee: Recent evolution of clotting factor concentrates for hemophilia A and B. *Transfusion* 33:422, 1993.

50. Berntorp E: Why prescribe highly purified factor VIII and IX concentrates? *Vox Sang* 70:61, 1996.

51. Nilsson IM, Berntorp E: Clinical efficacy of clotting factor concentrates: Survival, recovery and hemostatic capacity, in *Coagulation and Blood Transfusion*, edited by CT Smith Sibinga, PC Das, PM Mannucci, p 193. Kluwer, Dordrecht, 1991.

52. Gill JC: Therapy of factor VIII deficiency. *Semin Thromb Hemost* 19:1, 1993.

53. Gomperts ED, de Biasi R, De Vreker R, et al: The impact of clotting factor concentrates on the immune system in individuals with hemophilia. *Transfer Med Rev* 6:44, 1992.

54. Geodert JJ, Kessler CM, Aledort LM, et al: A prospective study of human immunodeficiency virus type 1 infection and the development of AIDS in subjects with hemophilia. *N Engl J Med* 321:1141, 1994.

55. Centers for Disease Control and Prevention: Hepatitis A among persons with heophilia who received clotting factor concentrate: United States, September–December 1995. *MMWR* 45:29, 1996.

56. Columbo M, Mannucci PM, Carnelli V, et al: Transmission of non-A, non-B hepatitis by heat-treated factor concentrates. *Lancet* 2:1, 1985.

57. Suomela H: Inactivation of viruses in blood and plasma products. *Transfer Med Rev* 7:42, 1993.

58. Dietrich SL, Mosley JW, Lusher JM, et al: Transmission of human immunodeficiency virus type 1 by dry-heated clotting factor concentrates. *Vox Sang* 59:129, 1990.

59. Rizza CR, Fletcher ML, Kernoff PBA: Confirmation of viral safety of dry heated factor VIII concentrate (8Y) prepared by Bio Products Laboratory (BPL): A report on behalf of U.K. Haemophilia Centre directors. *Br J Haematol* 84:269, 1993.

60. Fricke W, Augustyniak L, Lawrence D: Human immunodeficiency virus infection due to clotting factor concentrates: Results of the Seroconversion Surveillance Project. *Transfusion* 32:707, 1992.

61. Mannucci PM, Schimpf K, Brettler DB, et al: Low risk for hepatitis C in hemophiliacs given a high-purity, pasteurized factor VIII concentrate. *Ann Intern Med* 113:27, 1990.

62. Mauser-Bunschoten EP, Zaaijer HL, van Drimmelen AAJ, et al: High prevalence of parvovirus B19 IgG antibodies among Dutch hemophilia patients. *Vox Sang* 74:225, 1998.

63. Rosendaal FR, Nieuwenhuis HK, Van den Berg HM, et al: A sudden increase in factor VIII inhibitor development in multitransfused hemophilia A patients in the Netherlands. *Blood* 81:2180, 1993.

64. Soucie JM, Robertson BH, Bell BP, et al: Hepatitis A virus infections associated with clotting factor concentrate in the United States. *Transfusion* 38:573, 1998.

65. Yamada-Osaki M, Sumazaki R, Kajwara Y, et al: Natural course of HGV infection in haemophiliacs. *Br J Haematol* 102:616, 1998.

66. Gitschier J, Wood WI, Goralka TM, et al: Characterization of the human factor VIII gene. *Nature* 312:326, 1984.

67. Wood WI, Capon DJ, Simonsen CC, et al: Expression of active human factor VIII from recombinant clones. *Nature* 312:330, 1984.

68. Lusher JM, Arkin S, Abilgaard CF, et al: Recombinant factor VIII for the treatment of previously untreated patients with hemophilia A. *N Engl J Med* 328:453, 1993.

69. Bray GL, Gomperts ED, Courter S, et al: A multicenter study of recombinant factor VIII (Recombinate): Safety, efficacy, and inhibitor risk in previously untreated patients with hemophilia A. *Blood* 83:2428, 1994.

70. Evatt B, Austin H, Barnhart E, et al: Surveillance for Creutzfeldt-Jakob disease among persons with hemophilia. *Transfusion* 38:817, 1998.

71. Berntorp E: Second generation, B-domain deleted recombinant factor VIII. *Thomb Haemost* 78:256, 1997.

72. Growe GH, Poon M-C, Scarth I: International Symposium on Recombinant Factor VIII: Report of the proceedings. *Transfer Med Rev* 6:137, 1992.

73. White GC II, McMillan CW, Kingdon HS: Use of recombinant antihemo-

philic factor in the treatment of two patients with classic hemophilia. *N Engl J Med* 320:166, 1989.

74. Kaufman R: Expression and structure-function properties of recombinant factor VIII. *Transfer Med Rev* 6:235, 1992.

75. Gomperts E, Lundblad R, Adamson R: The manufacturing process of recombinant factor VIII, Recombinate. *Transfer Med Rev* 6:247, 1992.

76. Schwartz RS, Abildgaard CF, Aledort LM, et al: Human recombinant DNA-derived antihemophilic factor (factor VIII) in the treatment of hemophilia A. *N Engl J Med* 323:1800, 1990.

77. White GC, Courter S, Bray GL, et al: A multicenter study of recombinant factor VIII (Recombinate) in previously treated patients with hemophilia A: The Recombinate previously treated patient group. *Thromb Haemost* 77:660, 1997.

78. Addiego J, Kasper C, Abildgaard C, et al: Frequency of inhibitor development in haemophiliacs treated with low-purity factor VIII. *Lancet* 342:464, 1993.

79. Lusher JM: Recombinant clotting factor concentrates. *Balliere's Clin Hematol* 9:291, 1996.

80. Abildgaard CF, Penner JA, Watson-Williams EJ: Anti-inhibitor coagulant complex (autoplex) for treatment of factor VIII inhibitors in hemophilia. *Blood* 56:978, 1980.

81. Sjamsoedin LJM, Heijnen L, Mauser-Bunschoten EP, et al: The effect of activated prothrombin-complex concentrate (FEIBA) on joint and muscle bleeding in patients with hemophilia A and anti-bodies to factor VIII: A double-blind clinical trial. *N Engl J Med* 305:717, 1981.

82. Lusher J, Ingerslev J, Robert H, Hedner U: Clinical experience with recombinant factor VIIa. *Blood Coag Fibrinol* 9:119, 1998.

83. Brettler DB, Forsberg AD, Levine PH, et al: The use of porcine factor VIII concentrate (Hyate:C) in the treatment of patients with inhibitor antibodies to factor VIII. *Arch Int Med* 149:1381, 1989.

84. Vichi PJ: Hyate:C supply status letter, January 5, 1998.

85. Noe DA, Bell WR, Ness PM, et al: Plasma clearance rates of coagulation factors VIII and IX in factor-deficient individuals. *Blood* 67:969, 1986.

86. Martinowitz U, Schlman S: Continuous infusion of coagulation products. *J Pediatr Hematol Oncol* 1:471, 1994.

87. Didier ME, Fischer S, Maki DG: Reconstituted recombinant factor VIII can be safely infused continuously for at least three days: It is a poor microbial growth medium. *Blood Coag Fibrinol* 9:227, 1998.

88. Hay CR, Doughty HI, Savidge GF: Continuous infusion of factor VIII for surgery and major bleeding. *Blood Coag Fibrinol* 7(suppl 1):S15, 1996.

89. Mannucci PM: Desmopressin (DDAVP) in the treatment of bleeding disorders: The first 20 years. *Blood* 90:2515, 1997.

90. Robert HR: Highly purified factor VIII concentrates, in *Recent Advances in Hemophilia Care*, edited by CK Kasper, p 167. Alan R Liss, New York, 1990.

91. de Biasi R, Rocino A, Miraglia E, et al: The impact of a very high purity factor VIII concentrate on the immune system of human immunodeficiency virus–infected hemophiliacs: A randomized, prospective, two-year comparison with an intermediate purity concentrate. *Blood* 78:1919, 1991.

92. Mannucci PM, Gringeri A, de Biasi R, et al: Immune status of asymptomatic HIV-infected hemophiliacs: Randomized, prospective, two-year comparison of treatment with a high-purity or an intermediate-purity factor VIII concentrate. *Thromb Haemost* 67:310, 1992.

93. Hay CRM, Ludlam CA, Lowe GDO, et al: The effect of monoclonal or ion-exchange purified factor VIII concentrate on HIV disease progression: A prospective cohort camparison. *Br J Haematol* 101:632, 1998.

94. McMillan CW, Shapiro SS, Whitehurst D, et al: The natural history of factor VIII:C inhibitors in patients with hemophilia A: A national cooperative study: II. Observations on the initial development of factor VIII:C inhibitors. *Blood* 71:344, 1988.

95. Schwarzinger I, Pabinger I, Korninger C, et al: Incidence of inhibitors in patients with severe and moderate hemophilia A treated with factor VIII concentrates. *Am J Hematol* 24:241, 1987.

96. Sultan Y, French Hemophilia Study Group: Prevalence of inhibitors in a population of 3435 hemophilia patients in France. *Thromb Haemost* 67:600, 1992.

97. Ehrenforth S, Kreuz W, Scharrer I, et al: Incidence of development of factor VIII and factor IX inhibitors in haemophiliacs. *Lancet* 339:594, 1992.

98. Nilsson IM: The management of hemophilia patients with inhibitors. *Transfer Med Rev* 6:285, 1992.

99. Kasper CK: Treatment of factor VIII inhibitors. *Prog Hemost Thromb* 9:57, 1989.

100. Blatt PM, White GC II, McMillan CW, et al: Treatment of anti-factor VIII antibodies. *Thromb Haemost* 35:117, 1977.

101. Ingerslev J, Feldstedt M, Sindet-Pedersen S, et al: Control of haemostasis with recombinant factor VIIa in patients with inhibitor to factor VIII. *Lancet* 338:831, 1991.

102. Hedner U, Glazer S, Falch J: Recombinant activated factor VII in the treatment of bleeding episodes in patients with inherited and acquired bleeding disorders. *Transfer Med Rev* 7:78, 1993.

103. Fiks-Sigaud M, Bendelac L, Parquet A, et al: Comparison of anti-human and anti-porcine factor VIII inhibitor levels in 63 patients with severe haemophilia A. *Vox Sang* 64:210, 1993.

104. Hay CRM, Laurian Y, Verroust F, et al: Induction of immune tolerance in patients with hemophilia A and inhibitors treated with porcine VIIIC by home therapy. *Blood* 76:882, 1990.

105. Lusher JM, Shapiro SS, Palasczk et al: Efficacy of prothrombin-complex concentrates in hemophiliacs with antibodies to factor VIII: A multicenter therapeutic trial. *N Engl J Med* 303:421, 1980.

106. Lusher JM, Blatt PM, Penner JA, et al: Autoplex versus proplex: A controlled, double-blind study of effectiveness in acute hemarthroses in hemophiliacs with inhibitors to factor VIII. *Blood* 62:1135, 1983.

107. Slocombe GW, Newland AC, Colvin MP, et al: The role of intensive plasma exchange in the prevention and management of haemorrhage in patients with inhibitors to factor VIII. *Br J Haematol* 47:577, 1981.

108. Nicolaisen EM, Hansen LL, Poulen F, et al: Immunologic aspects of recombinant factor VII in congenital factor VII deficiency [abstr]. *Haemophilia* 2(suppl):63, 1996.

109. ten Cate H, Bauer KA, Levi M, et al: The activation of factor X and prothrombin by recombinant factor VIIa in vivo is mediated by tissue factor. *J Clin Invest* 92:1207, 1993.

110. Mariani G, Ghirardini A, Bellocco R: Immune tolerance in hempohilia: Principal results from the international registry. *Thromb Haemost* 72:155, 1994.

111. Green D, Lechner KA: Survey of 215 nonhemophilic patients with inhibitors to factor VIII. *Thromb Haemost* 45:200, 1981.

112. Lottenberg R, Kentro TB, Kitchens CS: Acquired hemophilia: A natural history study of 16 patients with factor VIII inhibitors receiving little or no therapy. *Arch Intern Med* 147:1077, 1987.

113. Morrison AE, Ludlam CA, Kessler C: Use of porcine factor VIII in the treatment of patients with acquired hemophilia. *Blood* 81:1513, 1993.

114. Sultan Y, Kazatchkine MD, Maisonneuve P, et al: Anti-idiotypic suppression of autoantibodies to factor VIII (antihaemophilic factor) by high dose intravenous gammaglobulin. *Lancet* 2:765, 1984.

115. Green D, Kwaan HC: An acquired factor VIII inhibitor responsive to high-dose gamma globulin. *Thromb Haemost* 58:1005, 1987.

116. Shaffer LG, Phillips MD: Successful treatment of acquired hemophilia with oral immunosuppressive therapy. *Ann Intern Med* 127:206, 1997.

117. Sohngen D, Specker C, Bach D, et al: Acquired factor VIII inhibitors in nonhemophilic patients. *Ann Hematol* 74:89, 1997.

118. Scott JP, Montgomery RR: Therapy of von Willebrand disease. *Semin Thromb Hemost* 19:37, 1993.

119. Lethagen S, Harris AS, Sjörin E, et al: Intranasal and intravenous administration of desmopressin: Effect on F VIII/vWF, pharmacokinetics and reproducibility. *Thromb Haemost* 58:1033, 1987.

120. Mannucci PM, Bettega D, Catteneo M: Patterns of development of tachyphylaxis in patients with hemophilia and von Willebrand disease after repeated doses of desmopressin (DDAVP). *Br J Haematol* 82:87, 1992.

121. Weinstein RE, Bona RD, Altman AJ, et al: Severe hyponatremia after repeated intravenous administration of desmopressin. *Am J Hematol* 32:258, 1989.

122. Mannucci PM: Hemostatic drugs. *N Engl J Med* 339:245, 1998.

123. Gralnick HR, Williams SB, McKeown LP, et al: DDAVP in type IIa von Willebrand's disease. *Blood* 67:465, 1986.

124. Holmberg L, Nilsson IM, Borge L, et al: Platelet aggregation induced by 1-desamino-8-D-arginine vasopressin (DDAVP) in type IIb von Willebrand's disease. *N Engl J Med* 309:816, 1983.

125. Casonato A, Sartori MT, de Marco L, et al: 1-Desamino-8-D-arginine vasopressin (DDAVP) infusion in type IIB von Willebrand's disease: Shortening of bleeding time and induction of a variable pseudothrombocytopenia. *Thromb Haemost* 64:117, 1990.

126. Keeling DM, Luddington R, Allain JP, et al: Cryoprecipitate prepared from plasma virally inactivated by the solvent detergent method. *Br J Haematol* 96:194, 1997.

127. Zimmerman TS: Purification of factor VIII by monoclonal antibody affinity chromatography. *Semin Hematol* 25(suppl 1):25, 1988.

128. Schreiber AB: The preclinical characterization of MONOCLATE factor VIII:C, antihemophilic factor (human). *Semin Hematol* 25(suppl 1):27, 1988.

129. Menache D, Aronson DL: New treatments of von Willebrand disease: Plasma-derived von Willebrand factor concentrates. *Thromb Haemost* 78:566, 1997.

130. Mannucci PM, Tenconi PM, Castaman G, et al: Comparison of four virus-inactivated plasma concentrates for treatment of severe von Willebrand disease: A cross-over randomized trial. *Blood* 79:3130, 1992.

131. Bertorp E: Plasma product treatment in various types of von Willebrand's disease. *Haemostasis* 24:289, 1994.

132. Over J, Sixma JJ, Bouma BN, et al: Survival of iodine-125-labeled factor VIII in patients with von Willebrand's disease. *J Lab Clin Med* 97:332, 1981.

133. Schwarz HP, Turecek PL, Pichler L: Recombinant factor VIII. *Thromb Haemost* 78:571, 1997.

134. Weiss HJ, Meyer D, Rabinowitz R, et al: Pseudo-von Willebrand's disease: An intrinsic platelet defect with aggregation by unmodified human factor VIII/von Willebrand factor and enhanced adsorption of its high-molecular-weight multimers. *N Engl J Med* 306:326, 1982.

135. Eyster ME, Goedert JJ, Sarngadharan MG, et al: Development and early natural history of HTLV-III antibodies in persons with hemophilia. *JAMA* 253:2219, 1985.

136. Troisi CL, Hollinger FB, Hoots WK, et al: A multicenter study of viral hepatitis in a United States hemophilic population. *Blood* 81:412, 1993.

137. Hanley JP, Jarvis LM, Hayes PC, et al: Patterns of hepatitis G viraemia and liver disease in haemophiliacs previously exposed to non-virus inactivated coagulation factor concentrates. *Thromb Haemost* 79:291, 1998.

138. Gunay U, Choi HS, Maurer HS, et al: Commercial preparations of prothrombin complex. *Am J Dis Child* 126:775, 1973.

139. Robert HR, Ebert ME: Current management of hemophilia B. *Hematol Oncol Clin North Am* 7:1269, 1993.

140. Smith KJ: Factor IX concentrates: The new products and their properties. *Transfer Med Rev* 6:124, 1992.

141. Lusher JM: Thrombogenicity associated with factor IX complex concentrates. *Semin Hematol* 28(suppl 6):3, 1991.

142. Hultin MD: Activated clotting factor in factor IX concentrates. *Blood* 54:1028, 1979.

143. Giles AR, Nesheim ME, Hoogendorn H, et al: The coagulant-active phospholipid content is a major determinant of in-vivo thrombogenicity in animal models. *Blood* 59:401, 1982.

144. Menache D, Behre HE, Orthner CL, et al: Coagulation factor IX concentrate: Method of preparation and assessment of potential in vivo thrombogenicity in animal models. *Blood* 64:1220, 1984.

145. Mannucci PM, Bauer KA, Gringeri A, et al: Thrombin generation is not increased in the blood of hemophilia B patients after the infusion of a purified factor IX concentrate. *Blood* 76:2540, 1990.

146. Goldsmith JC, Kasper CK, Blatt PM, et al: Coagulation factor IX: Successful surgical experience with a purified factor IX concentrate. *Am J Hematol* 40:210, 1992.

147. Kim HC, McMillan CW, White GC, et al: Purified factor IX using monoclonal immunoaffinity technique: Clinical trials in hemophilia B and comparison to prothrombin complex concentrates. *Blood* 79:568, 1992.

148. Menache D, Behre HE, Orthner CL, et al: Coagulation factor XI concentrate: Method of preparation and assessment of potential in vivo thrombogenicity in animal models. *Blood* 64:1220, 1984.

149. Kim HC, Matts L, Eisele J, et al: Monoclonal antibody-purified factor IX: Comparative thrombogenicity to prothrombin complex concentrate. *Semin Hematol* 28:15, 1991.

150. Kim HC, McMillan CW, White GC, et al: Clinical experience of new monoclonal antibody purified factor IX: Half-life, recovery, and safety in patients with hemophilia B. *Semin Hematol* 27:30, 1990.

151. Harrison S, Adamson S, Bonam D, et al: The manufacturing process for recombinant factor IX. *Semin Hematol* 35(suppl 2):4, 1998.

152. White GC, Beebe A, Nielsen B: Recombinant factor IX. *Thromb Haemost* 78:261, 1997.

153. Noe DA, Bell WR, Ness PM, et al: Plasma clearance rates of coagulation factors VIII and IX in factor-deficient individuals. *Blood* 67:969, 1986.

154. Hampton KK, Preston FE, Lowe GDO, et al: Reduced coagulation activation following infusion of a highly purified factor IX concentrate compared to a prothrombin complex concentrate. *Br J Haematol* 84:279, 1993.

155. Ohga S, Saito M, Matsukazi A, et al: Disseminated intravascular coagulation in a patient with haemophilia B during factor IX replacement therapy. *Br J Haematol* 84:343, 1993.

156. Fuerth JH, Mahrer P: Myocardial infarction after factor IX therapy. *JAMA* 245:1455, 1981.

157. Katz J: Prevalence of factor IX inhibitors among patients with haemophilia B: Results of a large-scale North American survey. *Haemophilia* 2:28, 1996.

158. Warrier I, Ewenstein BM, Koerper MA, et al: Factor IX inhibitors and anaphylaxis in hemophilia B. *Hematol Oncol Clin North Am* 7:1269, 1993.

159. Ewenstein BM, Takemoto C, Warrier I, et al: Nephrotic syndrome as a complication of immune tolerance in hemophilia B. *Blood* 89:1115, 1997.

160. Cochrane Injuries Group Albumin Reviewers: Human albumin administration in critically ill patients: Systematic review of randomised controlled trials. *BMJ* 317:285, 1998.

161. Schierhout G, Roberts I: Fluid resuscitation with colloid or crystalloid solutions in critically ill patients: A systematic review of randomised trials. *BMJ* 316:961, 1998.

162. Cochrane Injuries Group Albumin Reviewers. Human albumin administration in critically ill patients: systematic review of randomized clinical trials. *BMJ* 317:235, 1998.

163. Vermeulen LC, Ratko TA, Erstad BL, et al: The University Hospital Consortium guidelines for the use of albumin, nonprotein colloid, and crystalloid solutions. *Arch Intern Med* 155:373, 1995.

164. Yim JM, Vermeulen, LC, Erstad BL, et al: Albumin and nonprotein colloid solution use in US academic health centers. *Arc Intern Med* 155:2450, 1995.

165. Centers for Disease Control and Prevention: Hemolysis associated with 25% human albumin diluted with sterile water: United States, 1994–1998. *MMWR* 48:157, 1999.

166. Dalakas MC: Intravenous immune globulin therapy for neurologic diseases. *Ann Intern Med* 126:721, 1997.

167. Stiehm RE: Appropriate therapeutic use of immunoglobulin. *Transfus Med Rev* 10:203,1996.

168. NIH Consensus Conference: Intravenous immunoglobulin. *JAMA* 264:3189, 1990.

169. Buckley RH, Schiff RI: The use of intravenous immune globulin in immunodeficiency diseases. *N Engl J Med* 325:110, 1991.

170. Epstein JS, Zoon KC: Important drug warning. FDA Dear Doctor letter. Center for Biologics Evaluation and Research, Food and Drug Administration, Rockville, MD, Nov 13, 1998.

171. Nubling CM, Groner A, Lower J: GB virus C/hepatitis G virus and intravenous immunoglobulins. *Vox Sang* 75:189, 1998.

172. Yap PL: The viral safety of intravenous immune globin. *Clin Exp Immunol* 104:35, 1996.

173. Centers for Disease Control and Prevention: Outbreak of hepatitis C associated with intravenous immunoglobulin administration: United States, October 1993–June 1994. *MMWR* 43:505, 1994.

174. Brown P, Rohwer RG, Dunstan BC, et al: The distribution of infectivity in blood components and plasma derivatives in experimental models of transmissible spongiform encephalopathy. *Transfusion* 38:810, 1998.

175. Centers for Disease Control and Prevention: Availability of immune globulin intravenous for treatment of immune-deficient patients: United States, 1997–1998. *MMWR* 48:159, 1999.

176. George JN, Woolf SH, Raskob GE, et al: Idiopathic thrombocytopenic purpura: A practice guideline developed by explicit methods for the American Society of Hematology. *Blood* 88:3, 1996.

177. Newburger J, Takahashi M, Beiser AS, et al: A single intravenous infusion of gamma globulin as compared with four infusions in the treatment of acute Kawasaki syndrome. *N Engl J Med* 324:1633, 1991.

178. Sullivan KM: Immunomodulation in allogeneic marrow transplantation:

Use of intravenous immune globulin to suppress acute graft-versus-host disease. *Clin Exp Immunol* 104:43, 1996.

179. Cooperative Group for the Study of Immunoglobulin in Chronic Lymphocytic Leukemia: Intravenous immunoglobulin for the prevention of infection in chronic lymphocytic leukemia. *N Engl J Med* 319: 902, 1988.

180. Weeks JC, Tierney MR, Weinstein MC: Cost effectiveness of prophylactic intravenous immune globulin in chronic lymphocytic leukemia. *N Engl J Med* 325:81, 1991.

181. Mofenson LM, Moye J Jr, Bethel J, et al: Prophylactic intravenous immunoglobulin in HIV-infected children with CD4+ counts of 0.20 × 10^9/L or more: Effect on viral, opportunistic, and bacterial infections. *JAMA* 268:483, 1992.

182. Van der Meche FGA, Schmitz PMI, Dutch Guillain-Barré Study Group: A randomized trial comparing intravenous immune globulin and plasma exchange in Guillain-Barré syndrome. *N Engl J Med* 326:1123, 1992.

183. Mueller-Eckhardt C: Annotation: Post-transfusion purpura. *Br J Haematol* 64:419, 1986.

184. Blanchette VS, Kirby MA, Turner C, et al: Role of intravenous immunoglobulin G in autoimmune hematologic disorders. *Semin Hematol* 29(suppl 2):72, 1992.

185. Ragni MV, Bontempo FA, Myers DJ, et al: A hemorrhagic sequelae of immune thrombocytopenic purpura in human immunodeficiency virus–infected hemophiliacs. *Blood* 75:1267, 1990.

186. Lynch L, Bussel J, McFarland J, et al: Antenatal treatment of alloimmune thrombocytopenia. *Obstet Gynecol* 80:67, 1992.

187. Cullis JO, Win N, Dudley JM: Post-transfusion hyperhaemolysis in a patient with sickle cell disease: Use of steroids and intravenous immunoglobulin to prevent further red cell destruction. *Vox Sang* 69:355, 1995.

188. Charles RJ, Sabo KM, Kidd PG, Abkowitz JL: The pathophysiology of pure red cell aplasia: Implications for therapy. *Blood* 87:4831, 1996.

189. Young NS: Parvovirus infection and its treatment. *Clin Exp Immunol* 104:26, 1996.

190. Kaplan C, Murphy MF, Kroll H, et al: Feto-maternal alloimmune thrombocytopenia: Antenatal therapy with IVIgG and steroids: More questions than answers. *Br J Haematol* 100:62, 1998.

191. Hartwell EA: Use of Rh immune globulin. *Am J Clin Pathol* 110:281, 1998.

192. Scaradavou A, Woo B, Woloski S, et al: Intravenous anti-D treatment of immune thrombocytopenic purpura: Experience in 272 patients. *Blood* 89:2689, 1997.

193. Zoon KC: FDA Dear IgIV Manufacturer letter. Center for Biologics Evaluation and Review, Food and Drug Administration, Rockville, MD, Oct 3, 1994.

194. Menache D, Grossman BJ, Jackson CM: Antithrombin III: Physiology, deficiency, and replacement therapy. *Transfusion* 32:580, 1992.

195. Hathaway WE: Clinical aspects of antithrombin III deficiency. *Semin Hematol* 28:19, 1991.

196. Bucur SZ, Levy JH, Despotis GJ, et al: Uses of antithrombin III concentrate in congenital and acquired deficiency states. *Transfusion* 38:481, 1998.

197. Despotis GJ, Levine V, Joist JH, et al: Antithrombin III during cardiac surgery: Effect on response of activated clotting time to heparin and relationship to markers of hemostatic activation. *Anesth Analg* 85:498, 1997.

198. Young E, Prins M, Levine MN, Hirsh J: Heparin binding to plasma proteins: An important mechanism of heparin resistance. *Thromb Haemost* 67:639, 1992.

199. Ménaché D, O'Malley JP, Schorr JB, et al: Evaluation of the safety, recovery, half-life, and clinical efficacy of antithrombin III (human) in patients with hereditary antithrombin III deficiency. *Blood* 75:33, 1990.

200. Career FM: The C1 inhibitor deficiency: A review. *Eur J Clin Chem Clin Biochem* 30:793, 1992.

201. Kunschak M, Engl W, Maritsch F: A randomized, controlled trial to study the efficacy and safety of C1 inhibitor concentrate in treating hereditary angioedema. *Transfusion* 38:540, 1998.

202. Kunschak M, Engl W, Maritsch F, et al: A randomized, controlled trial of the study of efficacy and safety of C1 inhibitor in treating hereditary angioedema. *Transfusion* 38:540, 1998.

203. Pickering RJ, Good RA, Kelly JR, Gewurz H: Replacement therapy in hereditary angioedema: Successful treatment of two patients with fresh frozen plasma. *Lancet* 1:326, 1969.

204. Cohen G, Peterson A: Treatment of hereditary angioedema with frozen plasma. *Ann Allergy* 30:690, 1972.

205. Janus ED, Phillips NT, Carrell RW: Smoking, lung function and alpha₁ antitrypsin deficiency. *Lancet* 1:152, 1985.

206. Wewers MD, Caslaro MA, Sellers SE, et al: Replacement therapy for alpha1-antitrypsin deficiency associated with emphysema. *N Engl J Med* 316:1055, 1987.

207. Ragni MV, Sinha D, Seaman F, et al: Comparison of bleeding tendency, factor XI coagulant activity, and factor XI antigen in 25 factor XI–deficient kindreds. *Blood* 65:719, 1985.

208. Asakai R, Chung D, Davie EW, et al: Factor XI deficiency in Ashkenazi Jews in Israel. *N Engl J Med* 325:153, 1991.

209. Hancock JF, Wieland K, Pugh RE, et al: A molecular genetic study of factor XI deficiency. *Blood* 77:1942, 1991.

210. Burnouf-Radosevich M, Burnouf TA: Therapeutic, highly purified factor XI concentrate from human plasma. *Transfusion* 32:861, 1992.

211. Bolton-Maggs PHB, Wensley RT, Kernoff PBA, et al: Production and therapeutic use of a factor XI concentrate from plasma. *Thromb Haemost* 67:314, 1993.

212. Bolton-Maggs PHB, Colvin BT, Satchi G, et al: Thrombogenic potential of factor XI concentrate [letter]. *Lancet* 344:748, 1994.

213. Mannucci PM, Bauer KA, Santagostino E, et al: Activation of the coagulation cascade after infusion of a factor XI concentrate in congenitally deficient patients. *Blood* 84:1314, 1994.

214. Stirling D, Ludlam CA: Therapeutic concentrates for the treatment of congenital deficiencies of factors VII, XI, XIII. *Semin Thromb Hemost* 19:48, 1993.

215. Miloszewski K, Losowsky MS: The half-life of factor XIII in vivo. *Br J Haematol* 19:685, 1970.

216. Kitchens CS, Newcomb TF: Factor XIII. *Medicine* 58:413, 1979.

217. Gootenberg JE: Factor concentrates for treatment of factor XIII deficiency. *Curr Opin Hematol* 5:372, 1998.

218. Taylor F, Chang A, Ferrell G, et al: Protein C prevents the coagulopathic and lethal effects of *E. coli* infusion in the baboon. *J Clin Invest* 79:918, 1987.

CHAPTER 144

THERAPEUTIC HEMAPHERESIS: INDICATIONS, EFFICACY, COMPLICATIONS

BRUCE C. MCLEOD

Therapeutic hemapheresis provides a means to rapidly alter the composition of components of the blood. It can be a valuable and safe initial treatment in a number of illnesses associated with quantitative and/or qualitative abnormalities of blood cells or plasma. Cell depletions are useful in symptomatic thrombocythemia and hyperleukocytosis. Plasma exchange is useful in certain paraproteinemias, antibody-mediated disorders, and toxin-mediated diseases; it can also be used to replete a deficient plasma constituent. Red cell exchange is used primarily for severe manifestations of sickle cell disease. Selective extraction techniques are available for IgG and low-density lipoprotein, and modulation of certain immune responses is possible with photopheresis. Adverse effects with current techniques are infrequent and usually mild.

INTRODUCTION

Therapeutic hemapheresis comprises a set of related techniques in which the amount or composition of a component of the blood is manipulated for a direct therapeutic purpose, usually with a continuous-flow centrifugal blood separation instrument. Available techniques fall into the three main categories of blood cell depletion, blood component exchange, and blood component modification, as shown in Table 144-1. Excess platelets or leukocytes are the usual targets for cell depletion procedures. These procedures are currently done almost exclusively for hematologic diseases. Blood component exchanges will target plasma or red cells. Plasma exchange is beneficial in a number of antibody-mediated conditions, many of which are not usually considered hematologic diseases. Specialized techniques have been developed for on-line selective extraction of certain individual constituents such as IgG and low-density lipoproteins from plasma separated by an apheresis instrument, and for photochemical modification of separated lymphocytes (photopheresis). Donation of autologous peripheral blood stem cells with an apheresis instrument is discussed in Chapter 141.

The goal of therapeutic apheresis is usually therapeutic depletion, although infusion of normal blood constituents in quantity may also be important in some instances. Apheresis therapy depletes rapidly but does not decrease production of an abnormal blood constituent. Therefore, in most illnesses it is best used acutely to control symptoms until more definitive therapy takes effect. Chronic apheresis therapy is seldom appropriate unless more convenient treatments are ineffective or contraindicated.

Adverse effects of therapeutic apheresis with modern instruments are relatively infrequent and generally mild. Hypotension will occur in 1 to 2 percent of procedures. Hypocalcemia due to citrate infusion may also occur. Urticaria may be seen when donor plasma is infused in plasma exchange. Deaths associated with plasma exchange are rare, and most are attributable to the disease being treated rather than the apheresis therapy.[1-3]

CELL DEPLETION

PLATELETPHERESIS

With the use of hydroxyurea or anagrelide, thrombocythemia can usually be managed pharmacologically. Therapeutic plateletpheresis, however, can be valuable in patients with symptomatic thrombocythemia who require rapid reduction in their platelet count or who cannot tolerate drug therapy.[4-10] The platelet count can usually be lowered by about 50 percent with each procedure,[5] though the decrement may be less if platelets are mobilized from an enlarged spleen during apheresis. Plateletpheresis can reverse clinical manifestations of myocardial or cerebral ischemia, pulmonary embolism, and gastrointestinal bleeding. Multiple procedures at intervals of a few days are usually needed until chemotherapy takes effect. It is not known whether prophylactic plateletpheresis lowers the incidence of thrombosis or hemorrhage; however, it may prevent placental infarction and fetal death in pregnant patients with thrombocythemia.[11] Long-term plateletpheresis is logistically and financially burdensome and is seldom indicated as the sole therapy for thrombocythemia[6,12] (see Chap. 118).

LEUKAPHERESIS

The most common application of therapeutic leukapheresis is the removal of malignant leukocytes. It has been performed in both acute and chronic leukemias and in the leukemic phase of lymphoma. The usual goal is to relieve or forestall acute symptoms of hyperleukocytosis, but it has occasionally been used as a primary method of disease control.[13] Immunomodulation by removal of nonmalignant lymphocytes has also been tried[14,15] but has not become an accepted treatment for any illness.

The threshold white cell count for pulmonary and/or cerebral dysfunction (leukostasis) in patients with leukemia is not known; it may depend on rheologic variables that differ among different leukemias, and even among different patients with the same type of leukemia. Clinical manifestations of hyperleukocytosis may occur in acute myelogenous leukemia (AML) with a white cell count of $75,000/\mu l$[16,17] but are more likely when the white cell count exceeds $200,000/\mu l$.[18] Although controlled trials documenting benefit are lacking, therapeutic leukapheresis is often performed urgently in AML if the white cell count is greater than $100,000/\mu l$ because this is a risk factor for early death.[19] Patients with acute lymphocytic leukemia (ALL) are often treated similarly, even though symptoms are less frequent in this condition.[20-22] In one study of ALL patients, leukapheresis led to a lower incidence of electrolyte abnormalities.[22]

White cell removal in chronic myelogenous leukemia (CML) was one of the earliest applications of apheresis instruments in patients.[23] Repeated leukapheresis as therapy for CML also provided leukocytes for transfusion to infected neutropenic patients with acute leukemia.[24] Some CML patients had a reduction in organomegaly and amelioration of constitutional symptoms, but chronic leukapheresis did not prolong life or delay the onset of blast transformation.[25] Logistical and financial issues make this approach impractical except in unusual circumstances such as pregnancy[26] in which a delay in chemotherapy is desirable. Currently, leukapheresis therapy in CML is usually reserved for patients who have white cell counts of 300,000 to $500,000/\mu l$ and signs of leukostasis. The same may be said of chronic lymphocytic leukemia.[27,28]

In Sézary syndrome, a leukemic phase of cutaneous T cell lymphoma (CTCL), repeated leukapheresis has resulted in reduction

TABLE 144-1   THERAPEUTIC HEMAPHERESIS TECHNIQUES

Cell depletion
   Plateletpheresis
   Leukapheresis
Blood component exchange
   Plasma exchange (plasmapheresis)
   Red cell exchange
Blood component modification
   Selective extraction of a plasma constituent
   Photopheresis

---

of the number of circulating malignant (Sézary) cells and improvement or resolution of skin lesions.[29-31] More recently, photopheresis (extra-corporeal photochemotherapy) has been used to treat CTCL, especially in the erythrodermic phase.[32] In this technique, leukocytes removed by apheresis are exposed to ultraviolet A light in the presence of 8-methoxypsoralen and then returned to the patient. It is believed that photochemical damage to DNA renders the malignant cells immuno-modulatory and thereby stimulates host antitumor immunity.[33,34] Photopheresis has brought about sustained remissions in CTCL.[34]

The extent to which the white cell count should be lowered is not known with certainty for any application of therapeutic leukapheresis. Processing at least two patient blood volumes has been recommended, with reductions in white cell count of 15 to 86 percent reported in acute leukemias.[13] It is difficult to predict the outcome of a procedure because of mobilization of cells into the bloodstream, underestimation of patient blood volume by standard formulas, and patient-specific differences in the behavior of leukemic cells in a centrifugal instrument. In practice it is worthwhile to monitor the white cell count during a procedure and to continue until there is a 30 to 50 percent decline.

BLOOD COMPONENT EXCHANGES

PHYSIOLOGY

Therapeutic blood component exchange reduces the concentration of a harmful blood constituent by removal of patient material and its simultaneous replacement with a substitute lacking the unwanted constituent. In a plasma exchange, the extent of depletion of an unwanted macromolecule, X, can be estimated at any point by the formula[35]:

$$X_n = X_o e^{-n}, \text{ where}$$

n = volume exchanged, expressed in patient plasma volumes

X_o = starting concentration of X

X_n = concentration of X after exchange of n plasma volumes

e = base natural log

This formula describes an asymptotic function which predicts (assuming equilibration with extravascular substance is slow) that exchange of one plasma volume will lower the intravascular concentration of a substance by about 65 percent, while exchange of a second plasma volume will lower it by only about 23 percent more. Removal is thus more efficient in the early portion of an exchange, and for this reason many exchanges are limited to a single plasma volume. For IgG antibodies, the existence of a substantial extravascular reservoir provides a further rationale for a series of single plasma-volume exchanges separated by intervals adequate to allow reequilibration between intra- and extravascular spaces. Applied in a reciprocal manner, the formula works equally well for predicting the outcome of a red cell exchange,

although the concentration of normal red cells can be increased efficiently beyond the predicted level at the end of a procedure by infusing red cells while removing plasma.

A protein-containing replacement fluid must be given during plasma exchange. Either normal plasma or 5 percent albumin is usually chosen. The latter is preferred for most applications because it does not transmit viral infections or cause urticarial reactions and can be administered without regard to blood type. As expected, levels of IgG and IgM fall by about 63 percent after a one-plasma-volume exchange for albumin and then take several weeks to recover.[36] Coagulation factor levels also fall, with transient prolongation of the prothrombin time and partial thromboplastin time; however, clinical bleeding is not usually encountered, and all coagulant proteins except fibrinogen return to the normal range within 6 to 24 h after an exchange.[37,38] Because levels of most other plasma proteins also recover quickly between exchanges, a series of thrice-weekly exchanges of patient plasma for 5 percent albumin produces a rather selective depression in immunoglobulin levels.[39] Plasma replacement may be necessary in certain illnesses, such as thrombotic thrombocytopenic purpura (TTP), for the desired therapeutic effect. Also, plasma may be given in the final portion of an exchange to replete coagulation factors when a patient has a preexisting bleeding diathesis.

PLASMA EXCHANGE

Therapeutic plasma exchange has been used to treat several types of plasma constituent abnormalities (Table 144-2). In most instances, the goal is to remove a pathogenic immunoglobulin from the patient's blood. These cases can be subdivided depending on whether it is the antigenic specificity of the immunoglobulin or an abnormal physical property imparted to the blood by its presence (e.g., hyperviscosity) that mediates the disease process. In a few instances plasma exchange can be helpful by removing substances other than immunoglobulin (e.g., low-density lipoproteins). Finally, plasma exchange can replete a deficient factor to a higher level than plasma infusion alone.

IMMUNOGLOBULINS WITH PATHOGENIC PHYSICAL PROPERTIES

Almost all of the conditions in this category are due to monoclonal proteins. The hyperviscosity syndrome, which can be a feature of macroglobulinemia, is probably the oldest indication for therapeutic apheresis.[40-42] It is particularly amenable to plasmapheresis because IgM is distributed largely in the plasma and not in the extravascular fluid. Furthermore, since the relationship between paraprotein concentration and viscosity is nonlinear, a reduction in viscosity sufficient to relieve both hemorrhagic and ischemic symptoms can sometimes be achieved with exchange of only 500 to 1000 ml plasma by manual bag techniques. Larger automated exchanges are even more effective. Plasma exchange can also reverse clinical manifestations of cryoglobulinemia such as vasculitis, glomerulonephritis, and Raynaud phenomenon.[43-45] In both instances it is best used as a temporizing strategy until more definitive therapy directed at the protein-producing cells can take effect. However, in unusual circumstances long-term treatment can also be effective.

TABLE 144-2   INDICATION CATEGORIES FOR PLASMA EXCHANGE

Goal	Example
Immunoglobulin removal	
Abnormal physical properties	Hyperviscosity syndrome
Specific antibody	Goodpasture syndrome
Nonimmunoglobulin constituent removal	Familial hypercholesterolemia
Factor replacement	Thrombotic thrombocytopenic purpura

Plasma exchange may also be beneficial in renal failure associated with multiple myeloma.[46,47] In one prospective, randomized study of oliguric patients requiring dialysis, only patients treated with both plasma exchange and chemotherapy recovered renal function.[47]

IMMUNOGLOBULINS WITH PATHOGENIC SPECIFICITY

A number of diseases are mediated by circulating antibody specific for a host tissue antigen. Although autoreactive, some of these antibodies are probably stimulated by exposure to alloantigens (e.g., anti-HPA-1a in posttransfusion purpura). Plasma exchange therapy is useful in many such illnesses, including the examples listed in Table 144-3.

Hematologic Diseases   In posttransfusion purpura, thrombocytopenia develops abruptly about a week after a blood transfusion, in association with an alloantibody response to a platelet-specific antigen. It remains unclear how the patient's antigen-negative platelets are destroyed.[48] Plasma exchange will hasten recovery from this self-limited syndrome,[49] as will intravenous (IV) gamma globulin infusions.[50]

Plasma exchange was also reported to be beneficial in some trials in acute idiopathic thrombocytopenic purpura[51–53] but has since been superseded by IV gamma globulin.[54] In chronic idiopathic thrombocytopenic purpura associated with HIV infection or unresponsive to glucocorticoids and splenectomy, the platelet count has been reported to improve after infusions of autologous plasma that has passed through a protein A/silica affinity column.[55,56] The procedure can be done off-line on stored plasma or on-line in series with the plasma circuit of an apheresis device. The exposure to protein A is apparently immunomodulatory rather than subtractive, since the amounts of immune complexes and platelet-associated antibodies removed by the column are insufficient to account for the salutary effects.[56]

Plasma exchange is not routinely recommended in warm autoimmune hemolytic anemia[57] but may be helpful in refractory cases in combination with IV gamma globulin[58] or pulse cyclophosphamide.[59] In cold agglutinin disease, significant but transient reductions in antibody titer and in the severity of hemolysis have been reported.[60–63] Warming the extracorporeal circuit and replacement fluids in such cases is very important.

Coagulation factor inhibitors (both auto- and alloantibodies) can be removed by plasma exchange.[64–66] This alone will not control bleeding due to a high-titer inhibitor, but it may reduce the titer enough to allow replacement factor to circulate temporarily.[67,68] The replacement fluid for such exchanges should be fresh-frozen plasma. Repeated antibody removal by on-line immunoadsorption with a protein A-Sepharose affinity column, in combination with factor replacement and immunosuppression, may induce tolerance in alloimmunized hemophiliacs.[69,70]

Plasma exchange has also been tried in patients with disorders of blood cell production that can be linked to circulating antibody, including aplastic anemia,[71] pure red cell aplasia,[72,73] and lymphopenia.[74,75]

Removal of alloantibodies to red blood cells may also be accomplished by therapeutic apheresis. Both plasma exchange and isoagglutinin-specific immunoadsorption have been used to prepare patients for ABO-incompatible marrow transplants.[76–78] Alternatively, apheresis instruments can be used to remove red cells from the graft.[79] In sensitized Rh-negative women, removal of maternal IgG by plasma exchange during pregnancy to ameliorate destruction of fetal red cells[80] has been largely supplanted by intrauterine transfusion of compatible cells. Plasma exchange may still be tried, however, if therapy is needed prior to 18 to 20 weeks gestation, when intrauterine transfusion is not technically feasible.[81,82]

Neurologic Diseases   Neurologic diseases account for more plasma exchange treatments than any other category. The effectiveness of this treatment complements other evidence supporting an autoimmune etiology for several neuropathic and neuromuscular disorders.

In Guillain-Barré syndrome, early treatment with plasma exchange clearly hastens recovery[83–85] from an illness in which antibodies to myelin are frequently found,[86] possibly in response to infection with *Campylobacter jejuni* in some cases.[87–89] Antimyelin antibodies may also be found in chronic inflammatory demyelinating polyneuropathy,[90–92] and a controlled trial in this condition has shown significant improvement in patients treated with plasma exchange.[93] Chronic neuropathy in the context of a monoclonal gammopathy may also respond to plasma exchange.[94]

Myasthenia gravis and Lambert-Eaton syndrome are both mediated by autoantibodies to structures in the neuromuscular junction.[95] In the former the target is the acetylcholine receptor on the muscle cell, while antibodies in Lambert-Eaton syndrome are directed against structures in the nerve ending. Both illnesses respond to plasma exchange,[96,97] which has been most useful in severe myasthenia gravis.

Several paraneoplastic syndromes with neurologic manifestations are associated with autoantibodies; e.g., encephalomyelitis with anti-Hu, cerebellar degeneration with anti-Yo, opsoclonus-myoclonus with anti-Ri, and retinal degeneration with anti-CAR. Results from plasma exchange, however, have been disappointing.[98,99]

Renal and Rheumatic Diseases   Goodpasture syndrome of glomerulonephritis and lung hemorrhage is due to linear deposition of autoantibody to a collagen found in pulmonary and renal basement membranes.[100] Prompt intervention with plasma exchange and cyclophosphamide is the treatment of choice. By contrast, in nephritis associated with systemic lupus erythematosus, controlled trials have shown that oral cyclophosphamide plus plasma exchange is no better than oral cyclophosphamide alone.[101,102] In pauci-immune rapidly progressive glomerulonephritis, one study suggested benefit from plasma exchange in patients with dialysis-dependent renal failure[103]; however, benefit has not been seen in controlled trials in dialysis-independent patients.[103–105] Plasma exchange has been tried in patients with several categories of severe vasculitis,[106–108] but in recent studies in severe nonrenal lupus erythematosus there were excess deaths from infection when plasma exchange was added to pulse intravenous cyclophosphamide therapy.[109,110] Multiple controlled trials have shown that plasma exchange is ineffective in reversing renal transplant rejection.[111–114]

NONIMMUNOGLOBULIN CONSTITUENTS

Removal of low-density lipoproteins by plasma exchange can lower cholesterol levels and promote resorption of xanthomas and atheromas

---

TABLE 144-3   EXAMPLES OF SPECIFIC ANTIBODIES IN DISEASES TREATED WITH PLASMA EXCHANGE

Antibody Specificity	Disease
Autoantibodies	
Motor endplate acetylcholine receptor	Myasthenia gravis
Nerve ending calcium channel active zone	Lambert-Eaton myasthenic syndrome
Peripheral nerve myelin	Guillain-Barré syndrome, chronic inflammatory demyelinating polyneuropathy
Red cell I/i	Cold agglutinin disease
Factor VIII	Acquired hemophilia
a3 chain of type IV collagen	Goodpasture syndrome
Alloantibodies	
HPA-1a or other platelet antigen	Posttransfusion purpura
Anti-A, anti-B	ABO-incompatible transplant
Anti-D	Hydrops fetalis
Factor VIII	Hemophilia A inhibitor

in patients with familial hypercholesterolemia.[115,116] On-line selective extraction of lipoproteins from patient plasma can be accomplished by several chemical and immunological means,[117-119] one of which has been approved by the Food and Drug Administration for patients with severe hypercholesterolemia resistant to dietary and drug therapy.[119] Removal of phytanic acid can prevent or reverse neurologic manifestations in Refsum disease.[120] Plasma exchange can also remove excessive levels of low molecular weight drugs, toxins, and hormones that are bound to plasma proteins.[121-123]

NORMAL FACTOR REPLACEMENT

Conceptually, one could use plasma exchange (normal plasma for the patient's deficient plasma) to correct a deficiency of any plasma factor that is not available in a concentrated form. Plasma exchange can achieve higher levels (theoretically 65 percent of normal with a one-plasma-volume exchange) than simple plasma infusion, without inducing volume overload.

Thrombotic thrombocytopenic purpura responds to plasma exchange, but only if the replacement fluid is normal plasma.[124-126] Some patients will respond to simple plasma infusion, but results of treatment are better with plasma exchange,[127] suggesting that replacement of a deficient plasma factor is an important element of the therapeutic effect. The missing factor may be a specific protease, active in limiting the size of circulating von Willebrand factor multimers, which is absent from the plasma of patients.[128-130] In adult patients with idiopathic "acquired" thrombotic thrombocytopenic purpura, the deficiency may be due to an IgG inhibitor, most likely an autoantibody,[129,130] removal of which would be an additional mechanism for the beneficial effect of plasma exchange.

Repletion of coagulation factors is part of the rationale for use of plasma exchange to support patients with acute liver failure until recovery or liver transplantation.[131]

RED CELL EXCHANGE

Most red cell exchanges are done for patients with complications of sickle cell disease. Simply stated, the goal of exchanging patient cells for cells containing hemoglobin A is to create a hemoglobin mixture approximating sickle trait cells and to interrupt thereby the vicious cycle of sickling, stasis, and progressive hypoxia.[132] The proportions of hemoglobins A and S needed to accomplish this are not known with certainty, but many exchanges aim for a posttreatment hemoglobin A level above 70 percent so that a level above 50 percent will persist for several weeks. Exchange may be indicated in severe crises such as stroke,[133,134] chest syndrome,[135,136] cholestasis,[137,138] and priapism.[139,140] Exchange in the last condition is sometimes associated with neurologic events occurring up to 11 days later.[141] Although not indicated for simple pain crisis,[142] prophylactic exchange may prevent future events for patients with frequent or overlapping crises. Prophylactic red cell exchange has been recommended for pregnant patients[143,144] and prior to general anesthesia,[145] but both of these indications are currently considered controversial.[146-148]

In other applications, red cell exchange may be employed to lower parasite load in severe falciparum malaria[149,150] and babesiosis.[151,152] Exchange of red cells for a plasma substitute can be used to lower hematocrit rapidly, yet without hypovolemia, in polycythemic states[153] and to deplete iron more rapidly than simple phlebotomy in hemochromatosis.[154] Finally, exchange of plasma for red cells can rapidly raise the hematocrit without producing hypervolemia.[155]

REFERENCES

1. Sutton DMC, Nair RC, Rock G: The Canadian Apheresis Study Group. Complications of plasma exchange. *Transfusion* 29:124, 1989.

2. Strauss RG, McLeod BC: Complications of therapeutic apheresis, in *Transfusion Reactions*, edited by MA Popovsky, p 281. AABB Press, Bethesda, MD, 1996.

3. McLeod BC, Price TH, Owen H, et al: Frequency of immediate adverse effects associated with therapeutic apheresis. *Transfusion* 39:282, 1999.

4. Pineda AA, Brzica SM, Taswell HF: Continuous- and semi-continuous flow blood centrifugation systems: Therapeutic applications, with plasma-, platelet-, lympha-, and eosinapheresis. *Transfusion* 17:407, 1977.

5. Taft EG, Babcock RB, Scharfman WB, Tartaglia AP: Plateletpheresis in the management of thrombocytosis. *Blood* 50:927, 1977.

6. Panlilio AL, Reiss RF: Therapeutic plateletpheresis in thrombocythemia. *Transfusion* 19:147, 1979.

7. Greenberg BR, Watson-Williams EJ: Successful control of life-threatening thrombocytosis with a blood processor. *Transfusion* 15:620, 1975.

8. Taft EG: Apheresis in platelet disorders. *Plasma Ther* 2:181, 1982.

9. Younger J, Umlas J: Rapid reduction of platelet count in essential hemorrhagic thrombocythemia by discontinuous flow plateletpheresis. *Am J Med* 64:659, 1978.

10. Grisell DL, Mills GM: Reversible acute sensorineural loss associated with essential thrombocytosis. *Arch Intern Med* 146:1813, 1986.

11. Mercer B, Drouin J, Jolly E, d'Anjou G: Primary thrombocythemia in pregnancy: A report of two cases. *Am J Obstet Gynecol* 159:127, 1988.

12. Goldfinger D, Thompson R, Lowe C, et al: Long-term plateletpheresis in the management of primary thrombocytosis. *Transfusion* 19:336, 1979.

13. Hester J: Therapeutic cell depletion, in *Apheresis: Principles and Practice*, edited by BC McLeod, TH Price, MJ Drew, p 251. AABB Press, Bethesda, MD, 1997.

14. Klippel JH: Apheresis: Biotechnology and the rheumatic diseases. *Arthritis Rheum* 27:1081, 1984.

15. McFarland HF, Rose JW: Lymphocytapheresis in the treatment of multiple sclerosis. *Plasma Ther Transfus Technol* 3:411, 1982.

16. Fritz RD, Forkner GE, Freireich EJ, et al: The association of fatal intracranial hemorrhage and blastic "crisis" in patients with acute leukemia. *N Engl J Med* 261:59, 1959.

17. Freireich E, Thomas L, Rei E, et al: A distinctive type of intracerebral hemorrhage associated with 'blastic crisis' in patients with leukemia. *Cancer* 13:146, 1960.

18. McKee LC, Collins RD: Intravascular leukocyte thrombi and aggregates as a cause of morbidity and mortality in leukemia. *Medicine* 53:463, 1974.

19. Ventura GJ, Hester JP, Smith TL, Keating MJ: Acute myeloblastic leukemia with hyperleukocytosis: Risk factors for early mortality in induction. *Am J Hematol* 27:34, 1988.

20. Carpentieri U, Patten EV, Chamberlin PA, et al: Leukapheresis in a 3-year-old child with lymphoma in leukemic transformation. *J Pediatr* 94:919, 1979.

21. Kamen BA, Summers CP, Pearson HA: Exchange transfusion as a treatment for hyperleukocytosis, anemia, and metabolic abnormalities in a patient with leukemia. *J Pediatr* 96:1045, 1980.

22. Maurer HS, Steinharz PG, Gaynon PS, et al: The effect of initial management of hyperleukocytosis on early complications and outcome of children with acute lymphoblastic leukemia. *J Clin Oncol* 6:1425, 1988.

23. Morse EE, Carbone PP, Freireich EJ, et al: Repeated leukapheresis of patients with chronic myelocytic leukemia. *Transfusion* 6:175, 1966.

24. Morse EE, Freireich EJ, Carbone PP, et al: The transfusion of leukocytes from donors with chronic myelocytic leukemia to patients with leukopenia. *Transfusion* 6:183, 1966.

25. Hester JP, McCredie KB, Freireich EJ: Response to chronic leukapheresis procedures and survival of chronic myelogenous leukemia patients. *Transfusion* 22:305, 1982.

26. Caplan SM, Coco FV, Berkman EM: Management of chronic myelocytic leukemia in pregnancy by cell pheresis. *Transfusion* 18:120, 1978.

27. Hocker P, Pitterman E, Gobets M, Stacher A: Treatment of patients with chronic myeloid leukemia (CML) and chronic lymphocytic leukemia (CLL) by leukapheresis with a continuous flow blood cell separator, in *Leukocytes: Separation, Collection and Transfusion*, edited by JM Goldman, RM Lowenthal, p 510. Academic Press, London, 1975.

28. Goldfinger D, Capostagno V, Lowe C, : Use of long-term leukapheresis in the treatment of chronic lymphocytic leukemia. *Transfusion* 29:450, 1980.

29. Edelson R, Factor M, Andrews A, et al: Successful management of the Sézary syndrome. *N Engl J Med* 291:293, 1974.

30. Bongiovanni MB, Katz RS, Tomaszewski JE, et al: Cytapheresis in a patient with Sézary syndrome. *Transfusion* 21:332, 1981.

31. Belter SV, Knop J, Bruske K, Sorg C: Leukapheresis in the treatment of cutaneous T-cell lymphomas. *Br J Dermatol* 115:159, 1986.

32. Edelson RL, Berger C, Gasparro F, et al: Treatment of cutaneous T-cell lymphoma by extracorporeal photochemotherapy. *N Engl J Med* 316:297, 1987.

33. Marks DI, Rockman SP, Oziemski MA, Fox RM: Mechanisms of lymphocytotoxicity induced by extracorporeal photochemistry for cutaneous T cell lymphoma. *J Clin Invest* 86:2080, 1990.

34. Lim HW, Edelson RL: Photopheresis for the treatment of cutaneous T-cell lymphoma. *Hematol Oncol Clin North Am* 9:1117, 1995.

35. Chopek M, McCullough J: Protein and biochemical changes during plasma exchange, in Therapeutic Hemapheresis: A Technical Workshop, edited by EM Berkman, J Umlas, p 13. American Association of Blood Banks, Washington, DC, 1980.

36. Orlin JB, Berkman EM: Partial plasma exchange using albumin replacement: Removal and recovery of normal plasma constituents. *Blood* 56:1055, 1980.

37. Keller AJ, Chirnside A, Urbaniak SJ: Coagulation abnormalities produced by plasma exchange on the cell separator with special reference to fibrinogen and platelet levels. *Br J Haematol* 42:593, 1979.

38. Simon TL: Coagulation disorders with plasma exchange. *Plasma Ther Transfus Technol* 3:147, 1982.

39. McLeod BC, Sassetti RJ, Stefoski D, Davis FA: Partial plasma protein replacement in therapeutic plasma exchange. *J Clin Apheresis* 1:115, 1983.

40. Schwab PJ, Fahey JL: Treatment of Waldenström's macroglobulinemia by plasmapheresis. *N Engl J Med* 263:574, 1960.

41. Solomon A, Fahey JL: Plasmapheresis therapy in macroglobulinemia. *Ann Intern Med* 58:789, 1963.

42. Beck JR, Quinn BM, Meier FA, Rawnsley HM: Hyperviscosity syndrome in paraproteinemia. Managed by plasma exchange; monitored by serum tests. *Transfusion* 22:51, 1982.

43. Berkman EM, Orlin JB: Use of plasmapheresis and partial plasma exchange in the management of patients with cryoglobulinemia. *Transfusion* 20:171, 1980.

44. McLeod BC, Sassetti RJ: Plasmapheresis with return of cryoglobulin-depleted autologous plasma (cryoglobulinpheresis) in cryoglobulinemia. *Blood* 55:866, 1980.

45. Talpos G, Horrocks M, White JM, Cotton LT: Plasmapheresis in Raynaud's disease. *Lancet* 1:416, 1978.

46. Wahlin A, Lofvenberg E, Holm J: Improved survival in multiple myeloma with renal failure. *Acta Med Scand* 221:205, 1987.

47. Johnson WJ, Kyle RA, Pineda AA, et al: Treatment of renal failure associated with multiple myeloma. *Arch Intern Med* 150:863, 1990.

48. Mueller-Eckhardt C. Post-transfusion purpura: *Br J Haematol* 64:419, 1986.

49. Cimo PL, Aster RH: Post-transfusion purpura: Successful treatment by exchange transfusion. *N Engl J Med* 287:290, 1972.

50. Mueller-Eckhardt C, Kiefel V: High dose IgG for post-transfusion purpura revisited. *Blut* 57:163, 1988.

51. Branda RF, Tate DY, McCullough JJ, Jacob HS: Plasma exchange in the treatment of fulminant idiopathic (autoimmune) thrombocytopenic purpura. *Lancet* 1:688, 1978.

52. Marder VJ, Nusbacher J, Anderson FW: One-year follow-up of plasma exchange therapy in 14 patients with idiopathic thrombocytopenic purpura. *Transfusion* 21:291, 1981.

53. Blanchette VS, Hogan VA, McCombie NE, et al: Intensive plasma exchange therapy in ten patients with idiopathic thrombocytopenic purpura. *Transfusion* 24:388, 1984.

54. Bussel JB: Autoimmune thrombocytopenic purpura. *Hematol Oncol Clin North Am* 4:179, 1990.

55. Mittelman A, Bertram H, Henry DH, et al: Treatment of patients with HIV thrombocytopenia and hemolytic uremic syndrome with protein A (Prosorba column) immunoadsorption. *Semin Hematol* 26(suppl 1):15, 1989.

56. Snyder HW, Cochran SK, Balint JP, et al: Experience with Protein A-immunoadsorption in treatment resistant immune thrombocytopenic purpura. *Blood* 79:2237, 1992.

57. McLeod BC, Strauss RG, Ciavarella D, et al: Clinical applications of therapeutic hemapheresis: management of hematological disorders and cancer. *J Clin Apheresis* 8:211, 1993.

58. Hughes P, Toogood A: Plasma exchange as a necessary prerequisite for the induction of remission by human immunoglobulin in auto-immune haemolytic anemia. *Acta Haematol* 91:166, 1994.

59. Silva VA, Seder RH, Weintraub LR: Synchronization of plasma exchange and cyclophosphamide in severe and refractory autoimmune hemolytic anemia. *J Clin Apheresis* 9:120, 1994.

60. Brooks BD, Steane EA, Sheehan RG, et al: Therapeutic plasma exchange in the immune hemolytic anemias and immunologic thrombocytopenic purpura. *Prog Clin Biol Res* 106:317, 1982.

61. Silberstein LE, Berkman EM: Plasma exchange in autoimmune hemolytic anemia (AIHA). *J Clin Apheresis* 1:238, 1983.

62. Valbonesi M, Guzzini D, Zerbi D, et al: Successful plasma exchange for a patient with chronic demyelinating polyneuropathy and cold agglutinin disease due to anti-Pr$_a$. *J Clin Apheresis* 3:109, 1986.

63. Geurs F, Ritter K, Mast A, Van Maele V: Successful plasmapheresis in corticosteroid-resistant hemolysis in infectious mononucleosis: role of autoantibodies against triosephosphate isomerase. *Acta Haematol* 88:142, 1992.

64. Nilsson IM, Jonsson S, Sundqvist SB, et al: A procedure for removing high titer antibodies by extracorporeal protein-A-Sepharose adsorption in hemophilia: Substitution therapy and surgery in a patient with hemophilia B and antibodies. *Blood* 58:38, 1981.

65. Slocombe GW, Newland AC, Colvin MP, et al: The role of intensive plasma exchange in the prevention and management of haemorrhage in patients with inhibitors to factor VIII. *Br J Haematol* 47:577, 1981.

66. Zehnder JL, Keung LLK: Development of antibodies to thrombin and factor V with recurrent bleeding in a patient exposed to topical bovine thrombin. *Blood* 76:2011, 1990.

67. Lusher JM: Management of patients with factor VIII inhibitors. *Transfusion* 1:123, 1987.

68. Bona RD, Pasquale DN, Kalish RI, et al: Porcine factor VIII and plasmapheresis in the management of hemophilia patients with inhibitors. *Am J Hematol* 21:201, 1986.

69. Nilsson IM, Berntorp E, Zettervoll O: Induction of immune tolerance in patients with hemophilia and antibodies to factor VIII by combined treatment with intravenous IgG, cyclophosphamide, and factor VIII. *N Engl J Med* 318:947, 1988.

70. Uehlinger J, Button GR, McCarthy JM, et al: Immunoadsorption for coagulation factor inhibitors. *Transfusion* 31:269, 1991.

71. Austouelen R, Moe PJ, Jorstad S, Wideroe TE: Treatment of refractory aplastic anemia with plasmapheresis: Report of a case in childhood with review of the literature. *Pediatr Hematol Oncol* 7:285, 1990.

72. Means RT Jr, Dessypris EN, Krantz SB: Treatment of refractory pure red cell aplasia with cyclosporine A: disappearance of IgG inhibitor associated with clinical response. *Br J Haematol* 78:114, 1991.

73. Messner HA, Fauser AA, Curtis JE, et al: Control of antibody-mediated pure red-cell aplasia by plasmapheresis. *N Engl J Med* 304:1334, 1981.

74. Tomar RH, Kloster BE, Lamberson HV: Plasmapheresis increases T4 lymphocytes in patients with AIDS. *Am J Clin Pathol* 81:518, 1984.

75. Wenz B, Rubinstein A: Partial immunologic reconstitution of a patient with acquired agammaglobulinemia: A transient phenomenon accompanying therapeutic plasmapheresis. *Blood* 59:233, 1982.

76. Berkman EM, Caplan W, Kim GS: ABO-incompatible bone marrow transplantation: Preparation by plasma exchange and in vivo antibody absorption. *Transfusion* 18:504, 1978.

77. Bensinger WL, Baker DA, Buckner CD, et al: Immunoadsorption for removal of A and B blood group antibodies. *N Engl J Med* 304:160, 1981.

78. Bensinger WL, Baker DA, Buckner CD, et al: In vitro and in vivo removal of anti-A erythrocyte antibody by adsorption to a synthetic immunoadsorbent. *Transfusion* 21:335, 1981.

79. Braine HG, Sensenbrenner LL, Wright SK, et al: Bone marrow transplantation with major ABO incompatibility using erythrocyte depletion of marrow prior to infusion. *Blood* 60:420, 1982.

80. Rock G, Lafreniere I, Chan L, McCombie N: Plasma exchange in the treatment of hemolytic disease of the newborn. *Transfusion* 21:546, 1981.

81. Filbey D, Berseus O, Lindeberg S, Wesstrom G: A management programme for Rh alloimmunization during pregnancy. *Early Hum Dev* 15:11, 1987.

82. Watson WJ, Katz VL, Bowes WA: Plasmapheresis during pregnancy. *Obstet Gyn* 76:451, 1990.

83. The Guillain-Barré Syndrome Study Group: Plasmapheresis and acute Guillain-Barré syndrome. *Neurology* 35:1096, 1985.

84. Osterman PG, Lundemo G, Pirskanen R, et al: Beneficial effects of plasma exchange in acute inflammatory polyradiculoneuropathy. *Lancet* 2:1296, 1984.

85. French Cooperative Group on Plasma Exchange and Guillain-Barré Syndrome: Efficiency of plasma exchange in Guillain-Barré syndrome: role of replacement fluids. *Ann Neurol* 22:753, 1987.

86. Vriesendorp FJ, Mishu B, Blaser MJ, Koski CL: Serum antibodies to GM1, GD16, peripheral nerve myelin, and *Campylobacter jejuni* in patients with Guillain-Barré syndrome and controls. *Ann Neurol* 34:130, 1993.

87. Rees JH, Gregson NA, Hughes RA: Anti-ganglioside GM1 antibodies in Guillain-Barré syndrome and their relationship to *Campylobacter jejuni* infection. *Ann Neurol* 38:809, 1995.

88. Rees JH, Soudain SE, Gregson NA, Hughes RAC: *Campylobacter jejuni* infection and Guillain-Barré syndrome. *N Engl J Med* 333:1374, 1995.

89. McKhann GM, Cornblath DR, Griffen JW, et al: Acute motor axonal neuropathy: a frequent cause of flaccid paralysis in China. *Ann Neurol* 33:333, 1993.

90. Connolly AM, Pestronk A, Trotter JL, et al: High-titer selective anti-beta-tubulin antibodies in chronic demyelinating polyneuropathy. *Neurology* 43:557, 1993.

91. Simone IL, Annunziata P, Maimone D, et al: Serum and CSF anti-GM1 antibodies in patients with Guillain-Barré syndrome and chronic inflammatory demyelinating polyneuropathy. *J Neurol Sci* 114:49, 1993.

92. Khalili-Shirazi A, Atkinson P, Gregson N, Hughes RAC: Antibody response to P_0 and P_2 myelin proteins in Guillain-Barré syndrome and chronic inflammatory demyelinating polyradiculoneuropathy. *J Neuroimmunol* 46:245, 1993.

93. Dyck PJ, Daube J, O'Brien P, et al: Plasma exchange in chronic inflammatory demyelinating polyradiculoneuropathy. *N Engl J Med* 314:461, 1986.

94. Dyck PJ, Low PA, Windebank AJ, et al: Plasma exchange in polyneuropathy associated with monoclonal gammopathy of undetermined significance. *N Engl J Med* 325:1482, 1991.

95. Masselli RA: Pathophysiology of myasthenia gravis and Lambert-Eaton syndrome. *Neurol Clin* 12:285, 1994.

96. Seybold ME: Plasmapheresis in myasthenia gravis. *Ann NY Acad Sci* 505:584, 1987.

97. Lisak RP: Plasma exchange in neurologic disease. *Arch Neurol* 41:654, 1984.

98. Moll JWB, Vecht CJ: Immune diagnosis of paraneoplastic neurological disease. *Clin Neurol Neurosurg* 97:71, 1995.

99. Graus F, Rene R: Clinical and pathological advances on central nervous system paraneoplastic syndromes. *Rev Neurol (Paris)* 148:496, 1992.

100. Kalluri R, Gunwar S, Reeders ST, et al: Goodpasture syndrome: Localization of the epitope for the autoantibodies to the carboxy terminal region of the alpha 3(IV) chain of basement membrane collagen. *J Biol Chem* 266:24018, 1991.

101. Lewis EJ, Hunsicker LG, Lan S-P, et al: A controlled trial of plasmapheresis therapy in severe lupus nephritis. *N Engl J Med* 326:1373, 1992.

102. Doria A, Piccoli A, Vesco P, et al: Therapy of lupus nephritis. *Ann Med Interne* 145: 307, 1994.

103. Pusey CD, Rees AJ, Evans DJ, et al: Plasma exchange in focal necrotizing glomerulonephritis without anti-GBM antibodies. *Kidney Int* 40: 757, 1991.

104. Glöckner WM, Sieberth HG, Wichmann HE, et al: Plasma exchange and immunosuppression in rapidly progressive glomerulonephritis: a controlled, multi-center study. *Clin Nephrol* 29:1, 1988.

105. Cole E, Cattran D, Magil A, et al: A prospective randomized trial of plasma exchange as additive therapy in idiopathic crescentic glomerulonephritis. *Am J Kidney Dis* 20:261, 1992.

106. Gerraty RP, McKelvie PA, Byrne E: Aseptic meningoencephalitis in primary Sjögreni's syndrome. *Acta Neurol Scand* 88:309, 1993.

107. Jenkins HR, Jewkes F, Vujanic GM: Systemic vasculitis complicating infantile autoimmune enteropathy. *Arch Dis Child* 71:534, 1994.

108. Fauci AS, Leavitt RY: Systemic vasculitis, in *Current Therapy in Allergy, Immunology and Rheumatology*, edited by LM Liechtenstein and AS Fauci, p 149. Decker, Toronto, 1988.

109. Aringer M, Smolen J, Graninger W: Severe infections in plasmapheresis-treated systemic lupus erythematosus. *Arthritis Rheum* 41:414, 1998.

110. Schroeder JO, Schwab U, Zennet R, et al: Plasmapheresis and subsequent pulse cyclophosphamide in severe systemic lupus erythematosus. Preliminary results of the LPSG-Trial. *Arthritis Rheum* 40:S325, 1997.

111. Soulillou JP, Guyot C, Guimbretiere J, et al: Plasma exchange in early kidney graft rejection associated with anti-donor antibodies. *Nephron* 35:158, 1983.

112. Allen NH, Ayer P, Geoghegan T, et al: Plasma exchange in acute renal allograft rejection: a controlled trial. *Transplantation* 35:425, 1983.

113. Kirubakaran MG, Disney APS, Norman J, et al: A controlled trial of plasmapheresis in the treatment of renal allograft rejection. *Transplantation* 32:164, 1981.

114. Blake P, Sutton D, Cardella C: Plasma exchange in acute renal transplant rejection. *Prog Clin Biol Res* 31:698, 1990.

115. Ginsberg HN: Update on the treatment of hypercholesterolemia, with a focus on HMG-CoA reductase inhibitors and combination regimens. *Clin Cardiol* 18:307, 1995.

116. Mabuchi H, Koizumi J, Michishita I, et al: Effects on coronary atherosclerosis of long-term treatment of familial hypercholesterolemia by LDL-apheresis. *Beitr Infusionther* 23:87, 1988.

117. Lane DM, McConathy WJ, Laughlin LO, et al: Weekly treatment of diet/drug-resistant hypercholesterolemia with the heparin-induced extracorporeal low-density lipoprotein precipitation (HELP) system by selective plasma low-density lipoprotein removal. *Am J Cardiol* 71:816, 1993.

118. Knisel W, Pfohl M, Müller M, et al: Comparative long-term experience with immunoadsorption and dextran sulfate cellulose adsorption for extracorporeal elimination of low-density lipoproteins. *Clin Invest* 72:660, 1994.

119. Gordon BR, Kelsey SF, Dan P, et al: Long-term effects of low-density lipoprotein apheresis using an automated dextran sulfate cellulose adsorption system. *Am J Cardiol* 81:407, 1998.

120. Gibberd FB: Plasma exchange for Refsum's disease. *Transfus Sci* 14:23, 1993.

121. Jones JS, Dougherty J: Current status of plasmapheresis in toxicology. *Ann Emerg Med* 15:474, 1986.

122. Mercuriali F, Sirchia G: Plasma exchange for mushroom poisoning. *Transfusion* 17:644, 1977.

123. Ashkar FS, Katims RB, Smoak WM, Gilson AJ: Thyroid storm treatment with blood exchange and plasmapheresis. *JAMA* 214:1275, 1979.

124. Byrnes JJ, Moake JL, Periman P: Effectiveness of the cryosupernatant fraction of plasma in the treatment of refractory thrombotic thrombocytopenic purpura. *Am J Hematol* 34:169, 1990.

125. Welborn JL, Emrick P, Acevedo M: Rapid improvement of thrombotic thrombocytopenic purpura with vincristine and plasmapheresis. *Am J Hematol* 35:18, 1990.

126. Rock G, Shumak K, Kelton J, et al: Thrombotic thrombocytopenic purpura: Outcome in 24 patients with renal impairment treated with plasma exchange. *Transfusion* 32:710, 1992.

127. Rock GA, Shumak KH, Buskard NA, et al: Comparison of plasma exchange with plasma infusion in the treatment of thrombotic thrombocytopenic purpura. *N Engl J Med* 325:393, 1991.

128. Furlan M, Robles R, Solenthaler M, Lämmle B: Acquired deficiency of von Willebrand factor-cleaving protease in a patient with thrombotic thrombocytopenic purpura. *Blood* 91:2839, 1998.

129. Furlan M, Robles R, Galbusera M, et al: Von Willebrand factor-cleaving protease in thrombotic thrombocytopenic purpura and the hemolytic-uremic syndrome. *N Engl J Med* 339:1578, 1998.

130. Tsai H-M, Lian EC-Y: Antibodies to von Willebrand factor-cleaving protease in acute thrombotic thrombocytopenic purpura. *N Engl J Med* 339:1585, 1998.

131. Kondrup J, Almdal T, Vilstrup H, et al: High volume plasma exchange in fulminant hepatic failure. *Int J Artif Organs* 15: 669, 1992.

132. Kleinman SH, Goldfinger D: Erythrocytapheresis in sickle cell disease, in *Therapeutic Hemapheresis*, vol 2, edited by JL MacPherson, DD Kasprisin, p 129. CRC Press, Boca Raton, FL, 1985.

133. Miller ST, Jensen D, Sreedhar PR: Less intensive long-term transfusion therapy for sickle cell anemia and cerebrovascular accident. *J Pediatr* 120:54, 1992.

134. Cohen AR, Martin MB, Silber JH, et al: A modified transfusion program for prevention of stroke in sickle cell disease. *Blood* 79:1657, 1992.

135. Vichinsky EP, Syles LA, Colangelo LH, et al: Acute chest syndrome in sickle cell disease: clinical presentation and course. *Blood* 89:1787, 1997.

136. Emre U, Miller ST, Gutierez M, et al: Effect of transfusion in acute chest syndrome of sickle cell disease. *Pediatrics* 127:901, 1995.

137. Rossof AH, McLeod BC, Holmes AW, Fried W: Intrahepatic sickling crisis in hemoglobin SC disease: management by partial exchange transfusion. *Plasma Ther* 2:7, 1981.

138. Sheehy TW, Law DE, Wade BH: Exchange transfusion for sickle cell intrahepatic cholestasis. *Arch Intern Med* 140:1364, 1980.

139. Hamre MR, Harmon EP, Kirkpatrick DV, et al: Priapism as a complication of sickle cell disease. *J Urol* 145:1, 1991.

140. Chakrabarty A, Upadhyay J, Dhabuwala CB, et al: Priapism associated with sickle cell hemoglobinopathy in children: long-term effects on potency. *J Urol* 155:1419, 1996.

141. Rackoff WR, Ohene-Frempong K, Month S, et al: Neurologic events after partial exchange transfusion for priapism in sickle cell disease. *J Pediatr* 120:882, 1992.

142. Kleinman SH, Hurvitz CG, Goldfinger D: Use of erythrocytapheresis in the treatment of patients with sickle cell disease. *J Clin Apheresis* 2:170, 1984.

143. Morrison JC, Wiser WL: The use of prophylactic partial exchange transfusion in pregnancies associated with sickle cell hemoglobinopathies. *Obstet Gynecol* 48:516, 1976.

144. Cunningham FG, Pritchard JA, Mason R: Pregnancy and sickle cell hemoglobinopathies; results with and without prophylactic transfusion. *Obstet Gynecol* 62:419, 1983.

145. Esseltine DW, Baxter MRN, Bevan JC: Sickle cell states and the anaesthetist. *Can J Anaesth* 35:385, 1988.

146. Koshy M, Weiner SJ, Miller ST, et al: Surgery and anesthesia in sickle cell disease. *Blood* 86:3676, 1995.

147. Tuck SM, James CE, Brewster EM, et al: Prophylactic blood transfusions in maternal sickle cell syndromes. *Br J Obstet Gynaecol* 94:121, 1987.

148. Koshy M, Burd L, Wallace D, et al: Prophylactic red-cell transfusions in pregnant women with sickle cell disease; a randomized cooperative study. *N Engl J Med* 319:1447, 1988.

149. Yarrish RL, Janas JS, Nosanchuk JS, et al: Transfusion-acquired falciparum malaria: Treatment with exchange transfusion following delayed diagnosis. *Arch Intern Med* 142:187, 1982.

150. Kramer SL, Campbell CC, Moncreif RE: Fulminant *Plasmodium falciparum* infection treated with exchange blood transfusion. *JAMA* 249:244, 1983.

151. Cahill KM, Benach JL, Reich LM, et al: Red cell exchange: Treatment of babesiosis in a splenectomized patient. *Transfusion* 21:193, 1981.

152. Jacoby GA, Hunt JV, Kosinski KS, et al: Treatment of transfusion-transmitted babesiosis by exchange transfusion. *N Engl J Med* 303:1098, 1980.

153. Kaboth U, Rumph KW, Liersch T, et al: Advantages of isovolemic large-volume erythrocytapheresis as a rapidly effective and long-lasting treatment modality for red blood cell depletion in patients with polycythemia vera. *Ther Apheresis* 1:131, 1997.

154. Cesana M, Mandelli C, Tiribelli C, et al: Concomitant primary hemochromatosis and β-thalassemia trait: iron depletion by erythrocytapheresis and desferrioxamine. *Am J Gastroenterol* 84:150, 1989.

155. McLeod BC, Reed SR, Viernes AV, Valentino L: Rapid red cell transfusion by apheresis. *J Clin Apheresis* 9:142, 1994.

INDEX

Bold numbers indicate start of main discussion of the topic; page numbers followed by "f" or "t" indicate figures and tables respectively.